# CANCER TREATMENT

# CANCER TREATMENT

## FIFTH EDITION

## Charles M. Haskell, M.D., FACP

Professor of Medicine

UCLA School of Medicine

Director Emeritus, Wadsworth Cancer Center

VA Greater Los Angeles Healthcare System

Los Angeles, California

With 168 Contributors

## Jonathan S. Berek, M.D.

Part Editor for **Gynecologic Neoplasms**

**W.B. SAUNDERS COMPANY**

*A Harcourt Health Sciences Company*

Philadelphia   London   New York   St. Louis   Sydney   Toronto

**W.B. SAUNDERS COMPANY**
*A Harcourt Health Sciences Company*

The Curtis Center
Independence Square West
Philadelphia, Pennsylvania 19106

**Library of Congress Cataloging-in-Publication Data**

Cancer treatment/[edited by] Charles M. Haskell; with 168 contributors; Jonathan S. Berek, section editor for gynecologic neoplasms.—5th ed.

p.    cm.

Includes bibliographical references and index.

ISBN 0–7216–7833–5

1. Cancer—Treatment.    I. Haskell, Charles M.    II. Berek, Jonathan S.
   [DNLM: 1. Neoplasms—therapy.    QZ 266 C219 2001]

RC270.8.C38 2001    616.99′406—dc21                        99-089086

*Acquisitions Editor:* Marc Strauss
*Developmental Editor:* Rebecca Gruliow
*Manuscript Editor:* Jodi von Hagen
*Production Manager:* Linda Garber
*Illustration Specialist:* Walt Verbitski
*Indexer:* Dennis Dolan

CANCER TREATMENT                                ISBN 0–7216–7833–5

Printed in the United States of America.

Last digit is the print number:    9    8    7    6    5    4    3    2    1

# CONTRIBUTORS

**David S. Alberts, M.D.**
Professor of Medicine, Pharmacology and Public Health and Associate Dean for Research, University of Arizona College of Medicine; Director, Cancer Prevention and Control, Arizona Cancer Center, Tucson, Arizona
*Methods and Procedures of Cancer Chemotherapy: Intraperitoneal Chemotherapy*

**Michael Andreeff, M.D., Ph.D.**
Professor of Medicine, Department of Bone Marrow Transplantation, University of Texas M. D. Anderson Cancer Center, Houston, Texas
*Acute Myeloid Leukemia*

**James B. Atkinson, M.D.**
Professor of Surgery, UCLA School of Medicine; Attending Staff, UCLA Medical Center, Los Angeles, California
*Wilms' Tumor*

**Joseph S. Bailes, M.D.**
National Medical Director, Physician Reliance Network, Inc., Dallas, Texas
*Economic and Regulatory Issues Affecting Oncology*

**Lodovico Balducci, M.D.**
Professor of Medicine and Program Leader, Senior Adult Oncology Program, Division of Medical Oncology and Hematology, Department of Medicine, University of South Florida College of Medicine, H. Lee Moffitt Cancer Center and Research Institute, Tampa, Florida
*Cancer and Age*

**Sanford H. Barsky, M.D.**
Professor of Pathology, UCLA School of Medicine; Pathologist and Chief, Breast Pathology, UCLA Medical Center, Los Angeles, California
*Breast Cancer: Natural History and Pretreatment Assessment; In Situ Breast Cancer*

**John Barstis, M.D.**
Associate Clinical Professor of Medicine, UCLA School of Medicine, Los Angeles; Medical Director, UCLA Cancer Centers in Santa Clarita and Lancaster, California
*Gastrointestinal Problems: Stomatitis, Diarrhea, Constipation*

**Nancy L. Bartlett, M.D.**
Assistant Professor of Medicine, Washington University School of Medicine, St. Louis, Missouri
*Low-Grade Lymphoma*

**Lawrence W. Bassett, M.D.**
Iris Cantor Professor of Breast Imaging, UCLA School of Medicine, Department of Radiology, UCLA Medical Center, Los Angeles, California
*Breast Cancer: Natural History and Pretreatment Assessment*

**Ulrich Batzdorf, M.D.**
Professor of Neurosurgery, UCLA School of Medicine, Los Angeles, California
*Spinal Cord: Natural History, Diagnosis, and Staging, Surgical Treatment*

**Arie S. Belldegrun, M.D.**
Professor of Urology, Department of Urology, UCLA School of Medicine, Los Angeles, California
*Kidney*

**Robert Benjamin, M.D.**
Professor and Chairman, University of Texas M. D. Anderson Cancer Center, Houston, Texas
*Methods and Procedures of Cancer Chemotherapy: Continuous-Infusion Therapy*

**Jonathan S. Berek, M.D.**
Professor and Vice Chair; Chief, Division of Gynecologic Oncology; Director, UCLA Women's Reproductive Cancer Program, Jonsson Comprehensive Cancer Center, UCLA School of Medicine, Los Angeles, California
*Ovary and Fallopian Tubes; Vulva; Vagina*

**James R. Berenson, M.D.**
Professor of Medicine, UCLA School of Medicine; Director of Myeloma Program, Cedars-Sinai Medical Center, Los Angeles, California
*Myeloma, Macroglobulinemia, and Amyloidosis*

**Ross S. Berkowitz, M.D.**
William H. Baker Professor of Gynecology, Harvard Medical School; Co-Director, New England Trophoblastic Disease Center; Director of Gynecologic Oncology and Gynecology, Fillette Center for Women's Cancers, Brigham and Women's Hospital, Dana Farber Cancer Institute, Boston, Massachusetts
*Gestational Trophoblastic Neoplasia*

**Michael L. Berman, M.D.**
Professor, Department of Obstetrics and Gynecology, University of California, Irvine, School of Medicine and Medical Center, Irvine, California
*Cervix; Uterus*

**Sunita M. Bhuta, M.D.**
Professor of Pathology and Attending Pathologist, UCLA School of Medicine, Los Angeles, California
*Wilms' Tumor*

**Keith E. Blackwell, M.D.**
Assistant Professor, Department of Surgery, Division of Head and Neck Surgery, UCLA School of Medicine, Los Angeles, California
*Oral Cavity and Oropharynx; Nasal Cavity and Paranasal Sinuses; Nasopharynx; Salivary Glands; Larynx and Hypopharynx*

**William H. Blahd, M.D.**
Professor of Medicine, UCLA School of Medicine; Director Emeritus, Nuclear Medicine Program, VA Greater Los Angeles Healthcare System, Los Angeles, California
*Thyroid Gland*

**Jerome B. Block, M.D.**
Professor of Medicine, Harbor-UCLA Medical Center, UCLA School of Medicine, Torrance; Consultant, Kaiser-Permanente Hospital, Bellflower, California
*Paraneoplastic Syndromes*

**Clara D. Bloomfield, M.D.**
Professor of Medicine, Ohio State University; Director, Ohio State University Comprehensive Cancer Center, Columbus, Ohio
*Acute Lymphoblastic Leukemia*

**Otis W. Brawley, M.D.**
Chief, Office of Special Populations, National Cancer Institute, Bethesda, Maryland
*Principles of Cancer Screening; Cancer in Special Populations*

**John Byrd, M.D.**
Assistant Professor of Medicine, Walter Reed Army Medical Center, Washington, D.C.
*Acute Lymphoblastic Leukemia*

**Thomas C. Calcaterra, M.D.**
Professor, Department of Surgery, Division of Head and Neck Surgery, UCLA School of Medicine, Los Angeles, California
*Oral Cavity and Oropharynx; Nasal Cavity and Paranasal Sinuses; Nasopharynx; Salivary Glands; Larynx and Hypopharynx*

**Robert B. Cameron, M.D.**
Assistant Professor of Surgery and Chief, Thoracic Oncology, UCLA School of Medicine; Chief, Thoracic Surgery, West Los Angeles VA Medical Center, Los Angeles, California
*Non–Small Cell Lung Cancer*

**Dennis A. Casciato, M.D.**
Clinical Professor of Medicine, UCLA School of Medicine; Attending Physician, Hematology-Oncology Section, VA Greater Los Angeles Healthcare System, Los Angeles, California
*Metastasis of Unknown Origin; Malignant Effusions*

**Richard E. Champlin, M.D.**
Professor and Chief, Bone Marrow Transplant Section, Department of Hematology, University of Texas M. D. Anderson Cancer Center, Houston, Texas
*Blood Stem Cell and Marrow Transplantation*

**Helena R. Chang, M.D., Ph.D.**
Professor, Department of Surgery, UCLA School of Medicine; Director, Revlon/UCLA Breast Center, Los Angeles, California
*Breast Cancer: In Situ Breast Cancer, Local Treatment with Surgery*

**Linnea I. Chap, M.D.**
Assistant Professor, UCLA School of Medicine, Department of Medicine, Los Angeles, California
*Breast Cancer: Natural History and Pretreatment Assessment, Systemic Treatment for Metastases, Adjuvant Treatment, Treatment by Stage of Disease and Special Problems*

**Arvind Chaudhry, M.D., Ph.D.**
Medical Director, Holy Family Cancer Center, Spokane, Washington
*Carcinoid Tumors*

**Lee-may Chen, M.D.**
Assistant Professor, Division of Gynecologic Oncology, Department of Obstetrics and Gynecology, University of California at San Francisco School of Medicine, San Francisco, California
*Ovary and Fallopian Tubes: Ovary, Fallopian Tubes*

**Timothy Cloughesy, M.D.**
Associate Clinical Professor and Director, Neuro-Oncology Program, UCLA School of Medicine, Los Angeles, California
*Brain*

**Alistair J. Cochran, M.D., FRCP(Glasg), FRCPath**
Professor of Pathology and Surgery, UCLA School of Medicine, Los Angeles, California
*Malignant Melanoma of the Skin*

**Terry S. Coleman, J.D.**
Fox, Bennett, and Turner, Washington, D.C.
*Economic and Regulatory Issues Affecting Oncology*

**Matthew E. Conolly, M.D., FACP, FRCP**
Professor of Medicine and Anesthesiology, UCLA School of Medicine; Attending Physician, UCLA Medical Center, Los Angeles, California
*Management of Pain in the Cancer Patient*

**Anne Coscarelli, Ph.D.**
Director, Rhonda Fleming Mann Resource Center for Women with Cancer, Jonsson Comprehensive Cancer Center, Los Angeles, California
*Cancer Rehabilitation*

**E. David Crawford, M.D.**
Professor of Surgery, Division of Urology, University of Colorado Health Sciences Center, Denver, Colorado
*Prostate; Bladder, Renal Pelvis, and Ureters*

**Mary B. Daly, M.D., Ph.D.**
Adjunct Scholar, Clinical Faculty, University of Pennsylvania, Philadelphia; Director, Cancer Control Science Program, Fox Chase Cancer Center, Cheltenham, Pennsylvania
*Principles of Cancer Genetics Counseling*

**Jean B. deKernion, M.D.**
Professor of Urology and Chairman, Department of Urology, UCLA School of Medicine, Los Angeles, California
*Urethra and Penis*

**Ardie E. Delforge, B.S.N.**
Clinical Nurse Manager, Arizona Cancer Center, Tucson, Arizona
*Methods and Procedures of Cancer Chemotherapy: Intraperitoneal Chemotherapy*

**Antonio A. F. De Salles, M.D., Ph.D.**
Associate Professor, UCLA School of Medicine; Attending Surgeon, UCLA Medical Center, Los Angeles, California
*Management of Pain in the Cancer Patient*

**John F. DiPersio, M.D., Ph.D.**
Professor of Medicine, Pathology, and Pediatrics, Washington University School of Medicine, Division of Bone Marrow Transplantation and Stem Cell Biology, St. Louis, Missouri
*Clinical Use of Hematopoietic Growth Factors*

**Jeffrey J. Eckardt, M.D.**
Professor of Orthopedic Surgery and Chief, Section of Orthopedic Oncology, UCLA School of Medicine, Los Angeles, California
*Osteogenic Sarcoma; Ewing's Sarcoma*

**James E. Economou, M.D., Ph.D., FACS**
Professor of Surgery, UCLA School of Medicine, Division of Surgical Oncology, Department of Surgery, Los Angeles, California
*Gene Therapy for Cancer; Malignant Melanoma of the Skin*

**Frederick R. Eilber, M.D.**
Professor of Surgery and Chief, Division of Surgical Oncology, UCLA School of Medicine, Los Angeles, California
*Principles of Cancer Surgery; Osteogenic Sarcoma; Ewing's Sarcoma; Soft Tissue Sarcomas*

**John C. Elkas, M.D.**
Staff Physician, Department of Obstetrics and Gynecology, Walter Reed Army Medical Center, Washington, D.C.
*Vagina*

**Christos Emmanouilides, M.D., Ph.D.**
Assistant Professor of Medicine, UCLA School of Medicine; Director of Lymphoma Program, Division of Oncology, UCLA Medical Center for the Health Sciences, Los Angeles, California
*Hodgkin's Lymphoma*

**Robert E. Engstrom, Jr., M.D.**
Assistant Professor of Ophthalmology, Retina Division, UCLA School of Medicine, Los Angeles; Chief, Department of Ophthalmology, Olive View Medical Center, Sylmar, California
*Malignant Melanoma of the Eye*

**Martine Extermann, M.D.**
Associate Program Leader and Research Director, Senior Adult Oncology Program, H. Lee Moffitt Cancer Center and Research Institute, Tampa, Florida
*Cancer and Age*

**Robert Figlin, M.D.**
Professor of Medicine, UCLA School of Medicine, Division of Hematology-Oncology, Jonsson Comprehensive Cancer Center, Los Angeles, California
*Non–Small Cell Lung Cancer; Pleural Mesothelioma; Kidney*

**Richard I. Fisher, M.D.**
Dorothy W. & J. D. Stetson Coleman Professor of Oncology, Professor of Medicine, Department of Medicine, Loyola University School of Medicine; Director, Cardinal Bernardin Cancer Center; Director, Division of Hematology/Oncology, Loyola University Cancer Center, Maywood, Illinois
*Intermediate- and High-Grade Lymphomas*

**Arlene A. Forastiere, M.D.**
Professor, Department of Oncology, The Johns Hopkins University School of Medicine, Baltimore, Maryland
*Chemotherapy of Head and Neck Cancer*

**Charles A. Forscher, M.D.**
Assistant Clinical Professor, UCLA School of Medicine; Physician, Cedars-Sinai Comprehensive Cancer Center, Cedars-Sinai Medical Center, Los Angeles, California
*Osteogenic Sarcoma; Ewing's Sarcoma; Soft Tissue Sarcomas*

**Stanley R. Frankel, M.D.**
Associate Professor of Medicine, University of Maryland Medical System; Director of Clinical Studies, Greenebaum Cancer Center, University of Maryland, Baltimore, Maryland
*Acute Lymphoblastic Leukemia*

**Yao-Shi Fu, M.D.**
Professor of Pathology and Laboratory Medicine (Emeritus), UCLA School of Medicine, Los Angeles, California; Department of Pathology, Northridge Hospital, Northridge, California
*Osteogenic Sarcoma; Ewing's Sarcoma*

**James L. Gajewski, M.D.**
Associate Professor of Medicine and Deputy Chairman, Department of Blood and Marrow Transplantation, University of Texas M. D. Anderson Cancer Center, Houston, Texas
*Methods and Procedures of Cancer Chemotherapy: Vascular Access Catheters and Devices; Blood Stem Cell and Marrow Transplantation*

**Patricia A. Ganz, M.D.**
Professor, UCLA Schools of Medicine and Public Health; Director, Division of Cancer Prevention and Control Research, Jonsson Comprehensive Cancer Center, Los Angeles, California
*Cancer Rehabilitation*

**Dava J. Garcia, B.A.**
Principal Research Specialist, Arizona Cancer Center, Tucson, Arizona
*Methods and Procedures of Cancer Chemotherapy: Intraperitoneal Chemotherapy*

**Ellen R. Gaynor, M.D.**
Professor, Department of Medicine, Division of Hematology/Oncology, Loyola University Stritch School of Medicine, Maywood, Illinois
*Intermediate- and High-Grade Lymphomas*

**Francis J. Giles, M.D., MRCPI**
Associate Professor, Department of Leukemia, Division of Medicine, University of Texas M. D. Anderson Cancer Center, Houston, Texas
*Acute Myeloid Leukemia*

**Parkash Gill, M.D.**
Professor of Medicine and Pathology, University of Southern California Keck School of Medicine, Los Angeles, California
*Adult T-Cell Leukemia/Lymphoma*

**Maura L. Gillison, M.D.**
Assistant Professor, Department of Oncology, The Johns Hopkins University School of Medicine, Baltimore, Maryland
*Chemotherapy of Head and Neck Cancer*

**Tanya L. Girman, MPH, RD, CNSD**
Nutrition Support Dietitian, VA Greater Los Angeles Health-care System, Los Angeles, California
*Nutrition*

**Barbara J. Gitlitz, M.D.**
Fellow, Division of Hematology/Oncology, Department of Medicine, UCLA School of Medicine, Los Angeles, California
*Kidney*

**John A. Glaspy, M.D.**
Associate Professor of Medicine, Division of Hematology-Oncology, UCLA School of Medicine; Medical Director, Bowyer Surgical Oncology Center, Los Angeles, California
*Malignant Melanoma of the Skin*

**Matthew Bidwell Goetz, M.D.**
Professor of Clinical Medicine, UCLA School of Medicine; Chief, Infectious Diseases, VA Greater Los Angeles Health-care System, Los Angeles, California
*Infection in Cancer Patients*

**John Gohagan, Ph.D., FACE**
Chief, Early Detection Research Group, Division of Cancer Prevention, National Cancer Institute, Bethesda, Maryland
*Principles of Cancer Screening*

**David W. Golde, M.D.**
Professor of Molecular Pharmacology and Therapeutics, Cornell University Graduate School of Medical Sciences; Physician in Chief, Memorial Sloan-Kettering Cancer Center, New York, New York
*Hairy Cell Leukemia*

**Donald P. Goldstein, M.D.**
Professor of Obstetrics, Gynecology, and Reproductive Biology, Harvard Medical School; Co-Director, New England Trophoblastic Disease Center, Fillette Center for Women's Cancers, Brigham and Women's Hospital, Dana Farber Cancer Institute, Boston, Massachusetts
*Gestational Trophoblastic Neoplasia*

**Gayle B. Goldstein, Ph.D. (Psychol.)**
Director of Behavioral Health, McKenzie-Wilamette Hospital, Eugene, Oregon
*Psychosocial Care*

**H. Earl Gordon, M.D., FACS**
Professor of Surgery (Emeritus), UCLA School of Medicine; Consultant in General Surgery, VA Greater Los Angeles Healthcare System, Los Angeles, California
*Thyroid Gland*

**F. Anthony Greco, M.D.**
Medical Director, Sarah Cannon Cancer Center, Centennial Medical Center, Nashville, Tennessee
*Mediastinal Tumors; Testis*

**Peter L. Greenberg, M.D.**
Professor of Medicine, Hematology Division, Stanford University Medical Center, Stanford, California
*Myeloproliferative and Myelodysplastic Syndromes*

**Thomas M. Grogan, M.D.**
Professor of Pathology and Chief, Section of Hematopathology, University of Arizona, Tucson, Arizona
*Natural History, Diagnosis, and Staging of the Non-Hodgkin's Lymphomas*

**Steven M. Grunberg, M.D.**
Professor of Medicine, University of Vermont; Attending Physician, Fletcher Allen Healthcare, Burlington, Vermont
*Gastrointestinal Problems: Nausea and Vomiting*

**John D. Hainsworth, M.D.**
Director, Clinical Research, Sarah Cannon Cancer Center, Centennial Medical Center, Nashville, Tennessee
*Mediastinal Tumors; Testis*

**Heine H. Hansen, Ph.D., M.D.**
Professor of Oncology, University of Copenhagen; Director, The Finsen Center, National University Hospital, Copenhagen, Denmark
*Small Cell Carcinoma of the Lung*

**William J. Harrington, Jr., M.D.**
Assistant Professor of Medicine, University of Miami School of Medicine, Miami, Florida
*Adult T-Cell Leukemia/Lymphoma*

**Charles M. Haskell, M.D., FACP**
Professor of Medicine, UCLA School of Medicine; Director Emeritus, Wadsworth Cancer Center, VA Greater Los Angeles Healthcare System, Los Angeles, California
*Introduction; Principles of Cancer Chemotherapy; Antineoplastic Agents; Oncologic Emergencies: Overview of Oncologic Emergencies, Superior Vena Cava Syndrome; Nutrition; Hospice and Other End-of-Life Programs; Breast Cancer: Natural History and Pretreatment Assessment, Systemic Treatment for Metastases, Adjuvant Treatment, Treatment by Stage of Disease and Special Problems; Esophagus: Natural History and Staging of Esophageal Cancer, Chemotherapy for Esophageal Cancer, Treatment of Esophageal Cancer by Stage of Disease; Stomach: Natural History, Diagnosis, and Staging of Gastric Cancer, Radiation Therapy for Gastric Carcinoma; Chemotherapy for Gastric Cancer, Treatment of Gastric Cancer by Stage of Disease; Small Intestine; Colorectal Cancer: Natural History, Diagnosis, and Staging; Treatment by Stage of Disease; Anal Canal: Natural History, Diagnosis, and Staging, Chemotherapy, Treatment by Stage of Disease; Exocrine Pancreas: Natural History, Diagnosis, and Staging, Chemotherapy, Treatment by Stage of Disease; Liver: Natural History, Diagnosis, and Staging, Chemotherapy, Treatment by Stage of Disease; Gallbladder: Natural History, Diagnosis, and Staging, Treatment; Bile Duct Carcinomas: Natural History, Diagnosis, and Staging, Chemotherapy, Summary of Treatment; Ampulla of Vater; Adrenal Gland; Spinal Cord: Natural History, Diagnosis, and Staging, Treatment with Chemotherapy, Approach to the Patient with Suspected Spinal Cord Compression*

**Jerome M. Hershman, M.D., M.S.**
Professor of Medicine, UCLA School of Medicine; Chief, Endocrinology and Metabolism Division, VA Greater Los Angeles Healthcare System, Los Angeles, California
*Thyroid Gland*

**David M. J. Hoffman, M.D.**
Fellow, Hematology/Oncology, UCLA School of Medicine, Los Angeles, California
*Kidney*

**Christine H. Holschneider, M.D.**
Fellow, Division of Gynecologic Oncology, UCLA School of Medicine, Los Angeles, California
*Vulva*

**Richard T. Hoppe, M.D.**
Professor and Chairman, Department of Radiation Oncology; Co-Director, Cutaneous Lymphoma Clinic, Stanford University School of Medicine, Stanford, California
*Mycosis Fungoides and Other Cutaneous Lymphomas*

**Sandra J. Horning, M.D.**
Professor of Medicine, Stanford University School of Medicine, Stanford, California
*Low-Grade Lymphoma*

**William Isacoff, M.D.**
Assistant Clinical Professor of Medicine, UCLA School of Medicine, Los Angeles, California
*Exocrine Pancreas: Chemotherapy*

**Marina A. Jaramillo**
Instructor of Pathology and Hemopathology Fellow, University of Arizona, Tucson, Arizona
*Natural History, Diagnosis, and Staging of the Non-Hodgkin's Lymphomas*

**Guy J. F. Juillard, M.D.**
Professor, Department of Radiation Oncology, UCLA School of Medicine, Los Angeles, California
*Oral Cavity and Oropharynx; Nasal Cavity and Paranasal Sinuses; Nasopharynx; Larynx and Hypopharynx*

**A. Robert Kagan, M.D.**
Clinical Professor, Radiation Oncology, UCLA School of Medicine; Chief, Radiation Oncology, Southern California Kaiser Permanente Medical Group, Los Angeles, California
*Burkitt's Lymphoma; Extranodal Lymphomas*

**Carsten E. Kampe, M.D., Ph.D.**
Hematologist/Oncologist, South Austin Cancer Center, Austin, Texas
*Soft Tissue Sarcomas; Adult T-Cell Leukemia/Lymphoma*

**Michael J. Keating, M.D.**
Professor, Department of Leukemia, Division of Medicine, University of Texas M. D. Anderson Cancer Center, Houston, Texas
*Acute Myeloid Leukemia*

**Nancy Kemeny, M.D.**
Professor of Medicine, Cornell University Medical College; Attending Physician, Division of Solid Tumor Oncology, Department of Medicine, Memorial Sloan-Kettering Cancer Center, New York, New York
*Management of Liver Metastases*

**Hanna J. Khoury, M.D.**
Instructor of Medicine, Division of Bone Marrow Transplantation and Stem Cell Biology, Washington University School of Medicine, St. Louis, Missouri
*Clinical Use of Hematopoietic Growth Factors*

**Youn H. Kim, M.D.**
Associate Professor of Dermatology and Co-Director, Cutaneous Lymphoma Clinic, Stanford University School of Medicine, Stanford, California
*Mycosis Fungoides and Other Cutaneous Lymphomas*

**Nancy Klipfel, M.D.**
Pathology Resident, UCLA Medical Center, Los Angeles, California
*Wilms' Tumor*

**Kevin B. Knopf, M.D., M.P.H.**
Office of Special Populations Research, National Cancer Institute, Bethesda, Maryland
*Cancer in Special Populations*

**H. Phillip Koeffler, M.D.**
Professor of Medicine, UCLA School of Medicine; Director, Division of Hematology/Oncology, Cedars-Sinai Medical Center, Los Angeles, California
*Chronic Myelogenous Leukemia; Chronic Lymphocytic Leukemia*

**Barnett S. Kramer, M.D., M.P.H.**
Clinical Professor of Medicine, Uniformed Services University of the Health Sciences; Director, Office of Medical Applications of Research, National Institutes of Health, Bethesda, Maryland
*Principles of Cancer Screening*

**Larry K. Kvols, M.D.**
Professor of Medicine, GI Tumor Program, University of South Florida and H. Lee Moffitt Cancer Center and Research Institute, Tampa, Florida
*Carcinoid Tumors*

**Ulrik Lassen, Ph.D., M.D.**
Research Associate, The Finsen Center, National University Hospital, Copenhagen, Denmark
*Small Cell Carcinoma of the Lung*

**Sunai Leewansangtong, M.D.**
Fellow, Division of Urology, University of Colorado Health Sciences Center, Denver, Colorado
*Prostate; Bladder, Renal Pelvis, and Ureters*

**Alexandra M. Levine, M.D.**
Professor of Medicine, University of Southern California Keck School of Medicine; Chief, Division of Hematology, and Medical Director, USC/Norris Cancer Hospital, Los Angeles, California
*Acquired Immunodeficiency Syndrome–Related Lymphoma*

**Linda Liau, M.D., Ph.D.**
Assistant Professor, Division of Neurosurgery, UCLA School of Medicine, Los Angeles, California
*Brain*

**Michael C. Lill, M.B., B.S.**
Associate Professor of Medicine, UCLA School of Medicine; Director, Bone Marrow/Stem Cell Transplantation, Cedars-Sinai Medical Center, Los Angeles, California
*Hematologic Complications of Cancer and Its Treatment; Chronic Myelogenous Leukemia*

**Marcio H. Malogolowkin, M.D.**
Associate Professor of Pediatrics and Clinical Director, UCLA Medical Center, Los Angeles, California
*Retinoblastoma; Wilms' Tumor*

**Charles L. Maurer, M.D.**
Fellow in Hematology/Oncology, University of Rochester, Rochester, New York
*Adult T-Cell Leukemia/Lymphoma*

**Kenneth L. McClain, M.D., Ph.D.**
Associate Professor of Pediatrics, Baylor College of Medicine and Texas Children's Cancer Center, Houston, Texas
*Histiocytic Disorders*

**Michael T. McHale, M.D.**
Department of Obstetrics and Gynecology, Division of Gynecologic Oncology, CHAO Cancer Center, University of California, Irvine, College of Medicine, Orange, California
*Uterus*

**Frank L. Meyskens, Jr., M.D.**
Professor of Medicine and Biological Chemistry, University of California, Irvine, College of Medicine; Director, UCI Clinical Cancer Center, Orange, California
*Principles of Cancer Prevention*

**Steven A. Miles, M.D.**
Associate Professor of Medicine, Division of Hematology/ Oncology, UCLA School of Medicine, Los Angeles, California
*Kaposi's Sarcoma*

**Thomas P. Miller, M.D.**
Professor of Medicine and Chief, Section of Hematology/ Oncology, University of Arizona, Tucson, Arizona
*Natural History, Diagnosis, and Staging of the Non-Hodgkin's Lymphomas*

**Malcolm S. Mitchell, M.D.**
Professor of Medicine, Immunology, and Microbiology and Herrick Professor of Breast Cancer Immunology, Wayne State University; Program Leader of Biological Therapy, Karmanos Cancer Institute; Attending Physician, Karmanos Cancer Institute and Detroit Medical Center, Detroit, Michigan
*Principles of Biologic Therapy; Biologic Agents Approved for Use*

**Ronald T. Mitsuyasu, M.D.**
Associate Professor of Medicine, UCLA School of Medicine; Director, UCLA Center for Clinical AIDS Research and Education (CARE) Center, Los Angeles, California
*AIDS and Solid Tumors: AIDS and Cancer*

**Franco M. Muggia, M.D.**
Professor of Medicine and Anne Murnick & David H. Cogan Professor of Oncology, New York University School of Medicine; Director, Division of Medical Oncology; Program Director, Kaplan Comprehensive Cancer Center; Associate Dean, New York University Medical Center, New York, New York
*Investigational Drugs*

**Robert S. Negrin, M.D.**
Associate Professor of Medicine, Stanford University School of Medicine; Attending Physician, Stanford University Hospital, Stanford, California
*Myeloproliferative and Myelodysplastic Syndromes*

**Carol Nishikubo, M.D.**
Assistant Clinical Professor, UCLA School of Medicine; Staff Physician, VA Greater Los Angeles Medical Center, Los Angeles, California
*Oncologic Emergencies: Superior Vena Cava Syndrome; Esophagus: Natural History and Staging of Esophageal Cancer, Chemotherapy for Esophageal Cancer, Treatment by Stage of Disease; Stomach: Natural History, Diagnosis, and Staging of Gastric Cancer, Chemotherapy for Gastric Cancer, Treatment of Gastric Cancer by Stage of Disease; Management of Pulmonary Metastases*

**Dorothy J. Park, M.D.**
Assistant Professor of Medicine, UCLA School of Medicine; Program Director, Hematology/Oncology Fellowship Program, Cedars-Sinai Medical Center, Los Angeles, California
*Chronic Lymphocytic Leukemia*

**Robert G. Parker, M.D.**
Professor of Radiation Oncology, UCLA School of Medicine, Los Angeles, California
*Principles of Radiation Oncology; Breast Cancer: Radiation Therapy*

**Roman Perez-Soler, M.D.**
Professor of Medicine, New York University School of Medicine; Associate Director for Clinical Oncology and Translational Research, Kaplan Comprehensive Cancer Center, New York University Medical Center, New York, New York
*Investigational Drugs*

**Lawrence D. Petz, M.D.**
Professor of Pathology and Laboratory Medicine, UCLA School of Medicine; Co-Director, Transfusion Medicine, UCLA Medical Center, Los Angeles, California
*Transfusion Therapy for Patients with Cancer*

**Steven Piantadosi, M.D., Ph.D.**
Director of Oncology Biostatistics, The Johns Hopkins Oncology Center, The Johns Hopkins University School of Medicine, Baltimore, Maryland
*Clinical Trial Design and Interpretation of Data*

**Lawrence D. Piro, M.D.**
John Wayne Cancer Institute, 2001 Santa Monica Blvd., Suite 560, Santa Monica, California
*Hairy Cell Leukemia*

**Joseph R. Pisegna, M.D.**
Assistant Professor of Medicine, UCLA School of Medicine; Chief, Division of Gastroenterology and Hepatology, VA Greater Los Angeles Healthcare System, Los Angeles, California
*Multiple Endocrine Neoplasia; Neuroendocrine Pancreas*

**Joshua P. Prager, M.D., M.S.**
Clinical Assistant Professor, UCLA School of Medicine; Director, California Pain Medicine Centers, UCLA Medical Center, Los Angeles, California
*Management of Pain in the Cancer Patient*

**Philip C. Prorok, Ph.D.**
Acting Chief, Biometry Research Group, Division of Cancer Prevention, National Cancer Institute, Bethesda, Maryland
*Principles of Cancer Screening*

**Issam Raad, M.D.**
Professor of Medicine, Deputy Chairman of Internal Medicine Specialties, and Chief, Section of Infection Control, University of Texas M. D. Anderson Cancer Center, Houston, Texas
*Methods and Procedures of Cancer Chemotherapy: Vascular Access Catheters and Devices*

**Kenneth P. Ramming, M.D.**
Professor of Surgery (Emeritus), UCLA School of Medicine, Los Angeles; Director of Cryosurgery, Century City Cancer Center, Century City, California
*Esophagus: Surgery for Esophageal Cancer; Stomach: Surgery for Gastric Neoplasms; Small Intestine; Colorectal Cancer: Surgery; Anal Canal: Surgery; Exocrine Pancreas: Surgery; Liver: Surgery; Gallbladder: Treatment; Bile Duct Carcinomas: Surgery; Ampulla of Vater*

**Mitchell K. Rauch, M.D.**
Clinical Instructor in Urology and Fellow, Urologic Oncology, UCLA School of Medicine, Los Angeles, California
*Urethra and Penis*

**Alice Reier, M.D.**
Highland Hospital, Oakland, California
*AIDS and Solid Tumors: AIDS and Cancer, Kaposi's Sarcoma*

**Matthew Rettig, M.D.**
Assistant Professor, Department of Medicine, UCLA School of Medicine; Staff Physician, VA Greater Los Angeles Healthcare System, Los Angeles, California
*Biology of Cancer*

**C. Patrick Reynolds, M.D., Ph.D.**
Professor of Pediatrics and Pathology, University of Southern California Keck School of Medicine; Head, Developmental Therapeutics Section, Division of Hematology-Oncology, Children's Hospital of Los Angeles, Los Angeles, California
*Neuroblastoma*

**David C. Rhew, M.D.**
Assistant Professor, UCLA School of Medicine and UCLA Center for the Health Sciences; Staff Physician, VA Greater Los Angeles Healthcare System, Los Angeles, California
*Infection in Cancer Patients*

**Antoni Ribas, M.D.**
Clinical Instructor in Internal Medicine, Division of Hematology-Oncology, Department of Medicine, UCLA School of Medicine, Los Angeles, California
*Gene Therapy for Cancer*

**Gerald Rosen, M.D.**
Medical Director, St. Vincent's Comprehensive Cancer Center, New York, New York
*Osteogenic Sarcoma; Ewing's Sarcoma*

**Lee Rosen, M.D.**
Assistant Professor, Division of Hematology-Oncology, UCLA School of Medicine, Los Angeles, California
*Antineoplastic Agents*

**Peter J. Rosen, M.D.**
Professor of Clinical Medicine, UCLA School of Medicine; Director, Oncology Program, Division of Oncology, UCLA Medical Center, Los Angeles, California
*Hodgkin's Lymphoma; Noncutaneous T-Cell Lymphomas and NK Neoplasms*

**Joseph D. Rosenblatt, M.D.**
Chief, Hematology/Oncology Unit, University of Rochester, Rochester, New York
*Adult T-Cell Leukemia/Lymphoma*

**Mace L. Rothenberg, M.D.**
Associate Professor of Medicine, Vanderbilt University School of Medicine; Ingram Associate Professor of Cancer Research and Director, Phase I Drug Development, Vanderbilt-Ingram Cancer Center, Nashville, Tennessee
*Colorectal Cancer: Chemotherapy*

**Valerie W. Rusch, M.D.**
Professor of Surgery, Cornell University Medical College; Attending Surgeon, Thoracic Service, Department of Surgery, Memorial Sloan-Kettering Cancer Center, New York, New York
*Pleural Mesothelioma*

**Ahmad Sadeghi, M.D.**
Associate Professor of Radiation Oncology, UCLA School of Medicine; Chief, Radiation Therapy, VA Greater Los Angeles Healthcare System, Los Angeles, California
*Oncologic Emergencies: Superior Vena Cava Syndrome*

**Jonathan Said, M.D.**
Professor of Pathology, UCLA School of Medicine; Chief, Division of Anatomic Pathology, and Chief of Surgical Pathology, UCLA Medical Center for the Health Sciences, Los Angeles, California
*Hodgkin's Lymphoma; Noncutaneous T-Cell Lymphomas and NK Neoplasms*

**Gregory P. Sarna, M.D., FACP**
Clinical Professor of Medicine, UCLA School of Medicine; Medical Oncologist, Cedars-Sinai Comprehensive Cancer Center, Los Angeles, California
*Burkitt's Lymphoma; Extranodal Lymphomas*

**Gail Sartor, Pharm.D.**
Staff Pharmacist, Bowyer Oncology Center, University of California at Los Angeles, Los Angeles, California
*Methods and Procedures of Cancer Chemotherapy: Preparation, Administration, and Disposal of Antineoplastic Agents*

**Mark P. Sawicki, M.D.**
Associate Professor and Attending Surgeon, UCLA School of Medicine, Department of Surgery; Chief, General Surgery, VA Greater Los Angeles Healthcare System, Los Angeles, California
*Biology of Cancer; Multiple Endocrine Neoplasia; Neuroendocrine Pancreas; Adrenal Gland*

**Paul L. Schneider, M.D.**
Assistant Clinical Professor of Medicine, UCLA School of Medicine; Chair, Bioethics, VA Greater Los Angeles Healthcare System, Los Angeles, California
*Ethical Issues in Cancer Treatment*

**Robert C. Seeger, M.D.**
Professor of Pediatrics, University of Southern California Keck School of Medicine; Deputy Division Head for Research, Division of Hematology-Oncology, Children's Hospital of Los Angeles, Los Angeles, California
*Neuroblastoma*

**Michael Selch, M.D.**
Professor, Department of Radiation Oncology, UCLA School of Medicine, Los Angeles, California
*Brain; Spinal Cord: Radiation Therapy*

**William W. Shaw, M.D., FACS**
Professor and Chief, Division of Plastic and Reconstructive Surgery, UCLA School of Medicine, Los Angeles, California
*Breast Cancer: Surgical Reconstruction*

**William V. R. Shellow, M.D.**
Professor of Medicine (Dermatology), UCLA School of Medicine; Chief, Department of Dermatology, West Los Angeles VA Healthcare Center, Los Angeles, California
*Skin Cancer*

**Chia Soo, M.D.**
Resident, Department of Surgery, UCLA School of Medicine and Medical Center, Los Angeles, California
*Breast Cancer: In Situ Breast Cancer*

**Sheila Stinnett, R.N.**
Nurse Manager, UCLA Oncology Center, Los Angeles, California
*Methods and Procedures of Cancer Chemotherapy: Preparation, Administration, and Disposal of Antineoplastic Agents*

**Wendy Stock, M.D.**
Assistant Professor of Medicine, University of Illinois, Chicago, Illinois
*Acute Lymphoblastic Leukemia*

**Bradley R. Straatsma, M.D.**
Professor of Ophthalmology, Retina Division, and Director, Ophthalmic Oncology Center, Department of Ophthalmology, UCLA School of Medicine and Medical Center, Los Angeles, California
*Malignant Melanoma of the Eye*

**Hector L. Sulit, M.D.**
Assistant Clinical Professor, UCLA School of Medicine, Los Angeles; Physician, St. Mary's Medical Center, Pacific Hospital, Bellflower Medical Center, Bellflower; Gardena Medical Center, Gardena, California
*Malignant Melanoma of the Eye*

**Hassan J. Tabbarah, M.D.†**
Professor of Medicine, UCLA School of Medicine, Los Angeles; Assistant Chairman, Department of Medicine, Harbor-UCLA Medical Center, Torrance, California
*Cancer and Pregnancy*

**May Lin Tao, M.D., M.S.P.H.**
Assistant Professor of Radiation Oncology and Pediatrics, UCLA School of Medicine, Los Angeles, California
*Retinoblastoma; Wilms' Tumor*

**David M. Tishler, M.D.**
Assistant Professor of Pediatrics, University of Southern California Keck School of Medicine; Medical Director, Ambulatory Care Practice, and Medical Director, Long-Term Information Followup and Evaluation (LIFE) Program, Children's Hospital of Los Angeles and Children's Center for Cancer and Blood Diseases, Los Angeles, California
*Retinoblastoma*

**Paul R. Torrens, M.D., M.P.H.**
Professor of Health Services, UCLA School of Public Health, Los Angeles, California
*Hospice and Other End-of-Life Programs*

**Luu M. Tran, M.D.†**
Department of Radiation Oncology, VA Greater Los Angeles Healthcare System, Los Angeles, California
*Esophagus: Radiation Therapy; Stomach: Radiation Therapy for Gastric Carcinoma; Small Intestine; Colorectal Cancer: Radiation Therapy; Anal Canal: Radiation Therapy; Exocrine Pancreas: Radiation Therapy; Liver: Radiation Therapy; Gallbladder: Treatment; Bile Duct Carcinomas: Radiation Therapy; Ampulla of Vater*

**Steven J. Tucker, M.D.**
Medical Oncologist, Breast Cancer Research Program, John Wayne Cancer Institute, Santa Monica, California
*Breast Cancer: Adjuvant Treatment of Breast Cancer, Treatment by Stage of Disease and Special Problems*

**Anil Tulpule, M.D.**
Assistant Professor of Clinical Medicine, University of Southern California Keck School of Medicine and USC/Norris Cancer Hospital, Los Angeles, California
*Acquired Immunodeficiency Syndrome–Related Lymphoma*

**Andrew T. Turrisi, III, M.D.**
Professor and Chairman, Department of Radiation Oncology, Medical University of South Carolina, Charleston, South Carolina
*Non–Small Cell Lung Cancer*

**Robert A. Vescio**
Assistant Professor of Medicine, UCLA School of Medicine and Medical Center; Associate Director of Myeloma Programs, Cedars-Sinai Medical Center, Los Angeles, California
*Myeloma, Macroglobulinemia, and Amyloidosis*

**Donna L. Walker, M.D.**
Fellow in Hematology-Oncology, UCLA School of Medicine, Los Angeles, California
*Malignant Effusions*

**David K. Wellisch, Ph.D. (Psychol.)**
Professor, Department of Psychiatry and Biobehavioral Science, UCLA School of Medicine, Los Angeles, California
*Psychosocial Care*

†Deceased.

†Deceased.

**H. Rodney Withers, M.D., D.Sc.**
Professor and Chair, Department of Radiation Oncology, UCLA School of Medicine, Los Angeles, California
*Principles of Radiation Oncology*

**Diane Yamada, M.D.**
Assistant Professor, Department of Obstetrics and Gynecology, Division of Gynecologic Oncology, University of Chicago, Chicago, Illinois
*Cervix*

**Lowell S. Young, M.D.**
Clinical Professor of Medicine, University of California, San Francisco; Director, Kuzell Institute for Arthritis and Infectious Diseases, San Francisco, California
*Infection in Cancer Patients*

**Jacob Zighelboim, M.D.**
Anchor Clinic, Inc., Center for Humanistic Oncology, Beverly Hills, California
*Integrative Medicine*

# PREFACE

The goal of *Cancer Treatment* is to provide an authoritative, comprehensive, scholarly appraisal of contemporary therapy. Because of advances in molecular medicine and therapeutics, this appraisal requires a more extensive understanding of the basic science of oncology than in the past. An introduction to essential basic concepts is now included to meet this need. It is worth restating, however, that the central goal of this book is to provide the practitioner with reliable, authoritative information on contemporary treatment for the cancer patient.

This new edition is organized into 22 parts. Part I provides an overview of the principles of cancer treatment, including information on cancer biology, genetic counseling, cancer prevention and screening, and introductions to the principles of the various treatment modalities. Part II provides detailed information on drug therapy, including a series of individual drug monographs for both chemotherapeutic and biologic agents. Part III provides an overview of hematologic considerations in cancer treatment. Part IV deals with supportive care and other selected management issues. Parts V to VII deal with cancer in special populations, investigational therapy, and selected clinical practice issues. Parts VIII to XX deal with primary cancer arising in the various organ systems, Part XXI reviews selected malignant conditions associated with the acquired immunodeficiency syndrome (AIDS), and Part XXII deals with the management of metastatic cancer.

We have tried to provide useful and explicit recommendations on management, but I must stress that these recommendations are subject to change. Some of our recommendations are controversial and the subject of ongoing clinical trials. Whenever possible, we urge that patients participate in clinical trials as the best available therapy. Not only does participation advance the field, it also serves to bring the highest quality of care to the individual patient.

As in the past, I would like to dedicate this book to postgraduate physicians in training to become medical oncologists. It is worth stating that this new edition has been reorganized with the explicit requirements of the medical oncology subspecialty curriculum in mind. This curriculum requires the subspecialist to be familiar with all aspects of cancer care, including the issues that arise at the end of life. In keeping with the breadth of this curriculum and the value of the lessons that can be learned during lifelong training in this discipline, I close with the following quotation from Sherlock Holmes:

> "Education never ends, Watson. It is a series of lessons with the greatest for the last." *The Adventure of the Red Circle*
>
> Sir Arthur Conan Doyle (1859–1930)

CHARLES M. HASKELL, M.D., FACP

# ACKNOWLEDGMENTS

This new edition would not have been possible without the support of the contributing authors and their staffs. I would like to thank them collectively for their invaluable and unflagging assistance.

*Cancer Treatment* has been supported from the beginning by the highly professional and committed staff at the W.B. Saunders publishing company. For this 5th edition, I would especially like to thank Marc Strauss, Acquisitions Editor, and Rebecca Gruliow, Developmental Editor, for their support and diligence in the creation of this new edition.

I would like to thank my wife, Christine Haskell, for unstinting support in updating references from the old short form to the new complete form that is used throughout this edition. I would also like to thank Kris Langabeer, Medical Editor, for invaluable editorial assistance in preparing manuscripts for submission to the publisher.

Hassan J. Tabbarah, M.D., and Luu M. Tran, M.D., died after submission of their manuscripts for inclusion in this new edition. Both were esteemed and trusted colleagues of many years and I shall miss their wise counsel and expert advice. I join their families and close personal friends in mourning their loss.

CHARLES M. HASKELL, M.D., FACP

# CONTENTS

## NOTICE

Cancer treatment is an ever-changing field. Standard safety precautions must be followed, but as new research and clinical experience broaden our knowledge, changes in treatment and drug therapy may become necessary or appropriate. Readers are advised to check the most current product information provided by the manufacturer of each drug to be administered to verify the recommended dose, the method and duration of administration, and contraindications. It is the responsibility of the treating physician, relying on experience and knowledge of the patient, to determine dosages and the best treatment for each individual patient. Neither the publisher nor the editor assumes any liability for any injury and/or damage to persons or property arising from this publication.

THE PUBLISHER

# P A R T

# I

# PRINCIPLES OF CANCER TREATMENT

# CHAPTER 1

# INTRODUCTION

● CHARLES M. HASKELL

Heart disease (32.1%) and cancer (23.4%) are the two most common causes of death in the United States.[1] The American Cancer Society estimated that 1,221,800 new cases of cancer would develop during 1999 in the United States and that there would be 563,100 cancer deaths (>1500 Americans per day).[2] Age-specific prevalence rates are highest among the elderly, with 12% of men and 11% of women older than age 70 having been diagnosed with cancer at some point in their lives.[3]

Figure 1–1 summarizes the distribution of new cases and deaths from cancer by organ system for 1999, as estimated by the American Cancer Society. Figure 1–2 provides the

percentage of cancer deaths by tumor type and gender for the three types of cancer that caused the greatest number of deaths in the United States in 1999. Lung cancer for men and women, prostate cancer for men and breast cancer for women, and colorectal cancer for men and women account for more than half of all cancer deaths in the United States.

Clinical oncology expanded dramatically in the United States with the passage of the National Cancer Act in 1972. Special services contributing to cancer patient care are now provided by a variety of professionals: surgeons, radiation oncologists, medical oncologists, nurses, psychologists, psychiatrists, nutritionists, pharmacists, social workers, rehabili-

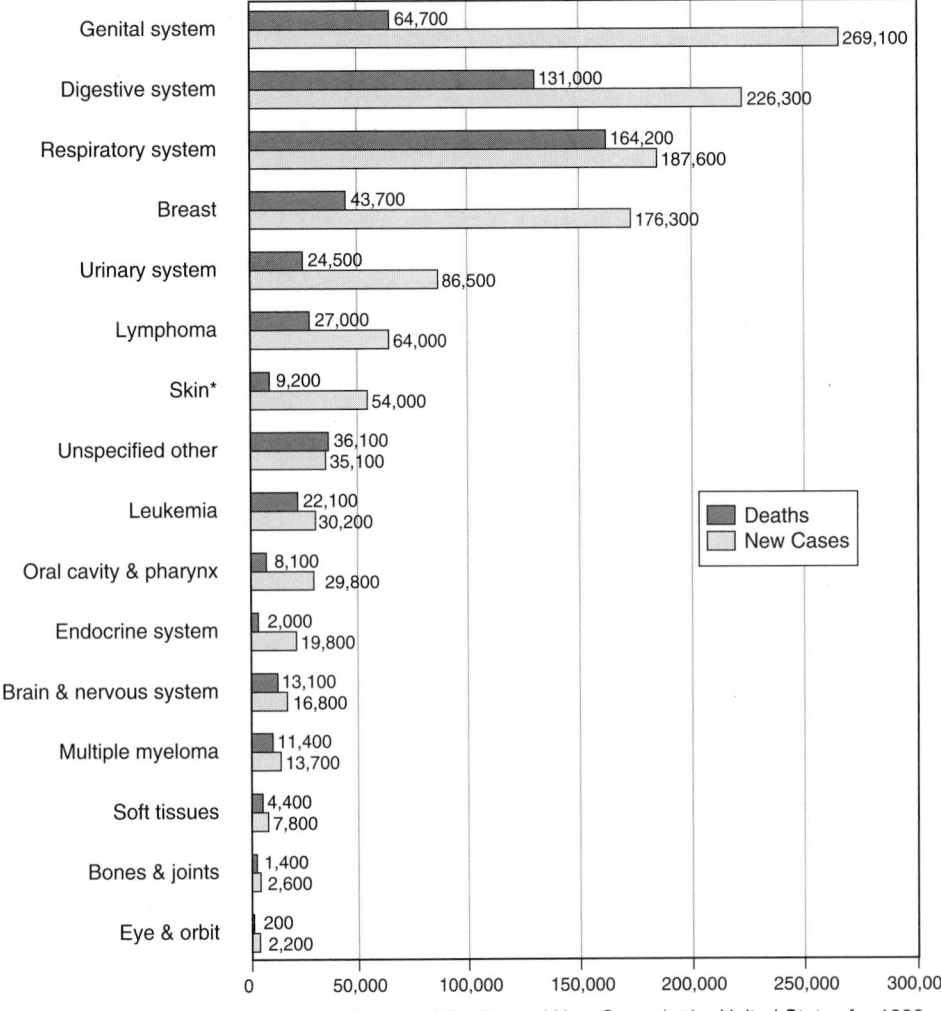

**Cancer in the United States, 1999**

**Figure 1–1.** American Cancer Society estimates of the total number of deaths from cancer and new cases of cancer by organ system in 1999 for both sexes and all ages in the United States. During this time the American Cancer Society estimates that there will be 1,221,800 new cases and 563,100 deaths from cancer overall. *Skin cancer other than squamous cell and basal cell types. (Redrawn from Landis SH, Murray T, Bolden S, Wingo PA: Cancer statistics, 1999. CA Cancer J Clin 1999;49:8–31.)

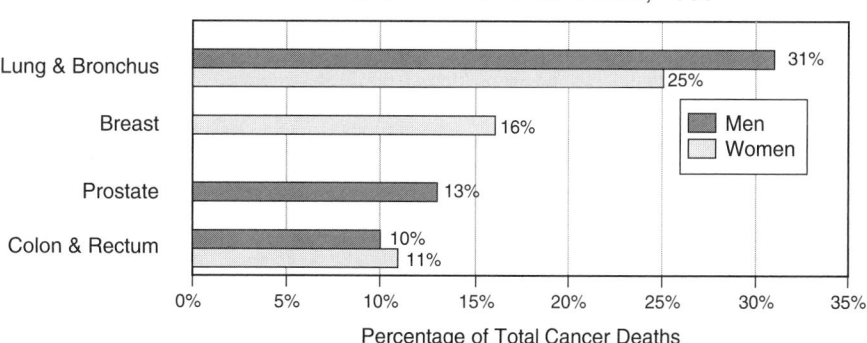

Cancer in the United States, 1999

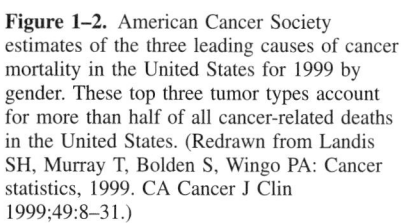

**Figure 1–2.** American Cancer Society estimates of the three leading causes of cancer mortality in the United States for 1999 by gender. These top three tumor types account for more than half of all cancer-related deaths in the United States. (Redrawn from Landis SH, Murray T, Bolden S, Wingo PA: Cancer statistics, 1999. CA Cancer J Clin 1999;49:8–31.)

tation specialists, and others. Coordination of this care remains a problem, and there is room for improvement in its delivery, as highlighted in a report sponsored by the Institute of Medicine.[4]

This expanded and diversified approach to cancer achieved some early success, especially in children. However, between 1973 and 1990, the overall incidence and mortality rates for cancer in the United States increased. Sweden also reported a rise in cancer incidence, suggesting the possibility that these populations were being exposed to increasing numbers or quantities of carcinogenic materials. This led to controversy about the true success of the "war against cancer." This controversy diminished with the release of data showing that the overall incidence and death rates from cancer have been decreasing since 1992 (Fig. 1–3).[5] This is particularly true for smoking-related cancers, which have decreased in parallel with reductions in the rate of cigarette smoking in the United States.[6]

Economic issues in cancer research and treatment are of growing concern. Several deserve explicit comment. First, continued progress is impossible without sufficient financial support for both basic and clinical research. It is important that we continue to train young clinical investigators who can help translate basic research discoveries into practical therapeutic advances.[7] A related concern is that physicians and patients must continue to support controlled clinical trials as the best way of determining the value of new

treatments. The National Cancer Institute has tried to facilitate patient entry into such studies by providing computerized access to information about clinical trials in the United States through the Physicians Data Query system.[8] The second issue relates to the reimbursement of patient care costs for clinical research. Many insurance companies refuse to cover the costs of "investigational" therapy in a formal trial but will cover the cost of one or more of the treatment arms of such trials when given as "best available therapy." This serves as an economic disincentive to clinical research. It is encouraging that one of the largest health care systems in the world—namely, the health care system of the Department of Veterans Affairs—has explicitly committed itself to the support of clinical research for Veterans Affairs cancer patients and has a sharing agreement with the National Cancer Institute to support clinical trials research.[9] Third, there is growing evidence that socioeconomic factors are critical in delivering optimal therapy.[10, 11] If individuals do not have financial access to modern cancer treatment, they will not be able to enjoy its benefits.[12]

This book represents the authors' attempts to delineate contemporary multidisciplinary cancer treatment. Part I consists of chapters summarizing basic principles of cancer biology and treatment. These chapters provide an essential perspective on the natural history of cancer, cancer prevention, early diagnosis, genetic screening, and the principles underlying each cancer treatment modality. Part II reviews

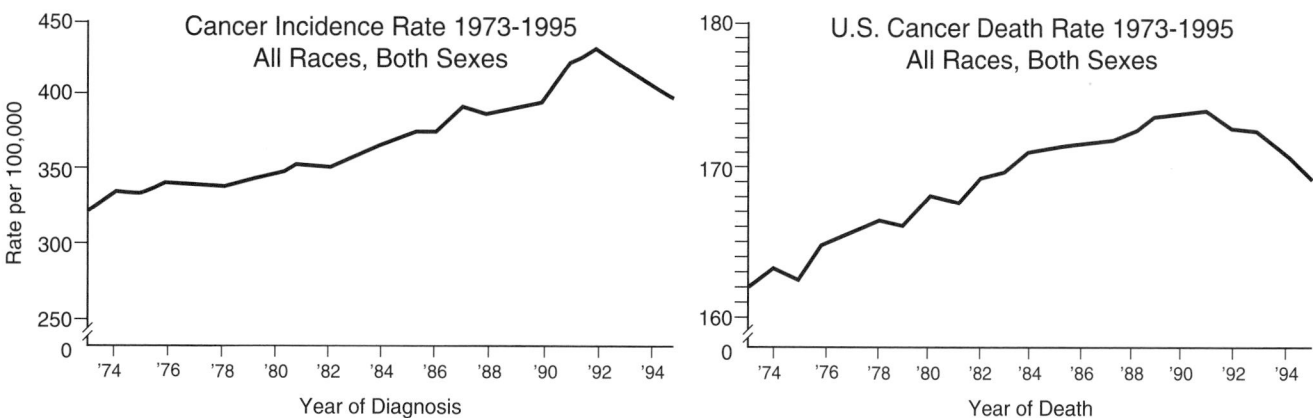

**Figure 1–3.** New cancer cases *(left)* and deaths *(right)* per 100,000 population in the United States for the years 1974 to 1994. Based on data from the National Cancer Institute and the SEER/NCHS/Census, as reported by Marshall E: The war on cancer—cancer warriors claim a victory. Science 1998;279:1842–3.)

drug therapy, including individual drug monographs on the major antineoplastic agents and the technology of drug administration. Part III reviews hematologic considerations in cancer treatment with an emphasis on hematologic supportive care. Part IV deals with the many facets of nonhematologic supportive care. Part V describes special populations afflicted with cancer. Part VI discusses investigational therapy. Part VII reviews selected clinical practice issues, including economic issues, ethics, and the use of alternative methods of cancer treatment. The remainder of the book deals with cancer involving specific sites and organ systems. Each chapter reviews the natural history of the tumor, its diagnosis and staging, and the contemporary role of the oncologic specialties in cancer treatment, with specific guidelines for management.

The remainder of this chapter provides a brief synopsis of cancer biology, an introduction to treatment planning, and some comments on selected clinical practice issues. These topics are covered in more detail in subsequent chapters.

## Natural History of Cancer

Neoplasms arise from transformed cells by a process known as *multistep carcinogenesis* (Fig. 1–4).[13] The first step in this process is called *initiation* and consists of a change in DNA that can be induced by a variety of chemical, viral, and physical agents. In most cases, the additional presence of a tumor-promoting agent is needed to complete the carcinogenic process. Individual susceptibility to malignant transformation may be influenced by genetic factors. This can relate to abnormal DNA repair mechanisms, to the variable expression of cellular oncogenes that appear to play a role in normal and abnormal cell differentiation, or to the loss of tumor suppressor genes. The immune function of the host may also be important, as illustrated by the development of Kaposi's sarcoma in patients with acquired immunodeficiency syndrome.

The number of cells in any given tissue represents the net balance of cell proliferation and programmed cell death

(apoptosis). Malignant transformation may involve an increase in proliferation or a decrease in apoptosis, or both. The importance of this balance in malignant transformation, and the competing effects of oncogenes and suppressor genes, is discussed in Chapter 2.

The subsequent growth of a transformed cell as a clone can lead to additional subclones whose acquired genetic variability results in considerable tumor cell heterogeneity within any given tumor. Tumor cells may be less genetically stable than normal cells—possibly from the activation or suppression of specific gene loci, the continued presence of carcinogens, the development of abnormal DNA repair mechanisms, or even nutritional deficiencies within the tumor. The inherent genetic instability of these cells, accompanied by variable processes of cell loss and selection, can result in advanced neoplasms with unique biologic and cytogenetic characteristics. These changes may be further accentuated by cancer treatment, as seen in the development of drug-resistant cancer cells.

Cancer may remain a locally invasive process, or it may spread to noncontiguous sites by hematogenous or lymphatic routes. Some neoplasms exhibit a relatively orderly pattern of progression. Initially, these tumors grow locally, and as they grow, tumor cells spread to and colonize the regional nodes. Finally, and only with advanced tumor size, distant metastases occur. However, it is also clear that some tumors may metastasize to distant organs prior to or coincident with their spread to regional lymph nodes. Indeed, it is not uncommon to find tumor cells in the systemic circulation in patients with patterns of disease suggesting a high risk of metastasis.

A more detailed discussion of the molecular biology of cancer is presented in Chapter 2. Genetic aspects of cancer are reviewed in Chapter 3.

Ideally, cancer should be prevented before it becomes a clinical problem. Tobacco is the largest single cause of cancer in the United States, and an estimated 400,000 individuals died in the United States in 1990 from tobacco-related diseases.[14] The importance of cancer prevention is so great that the theoretical and practical bases of this emerging

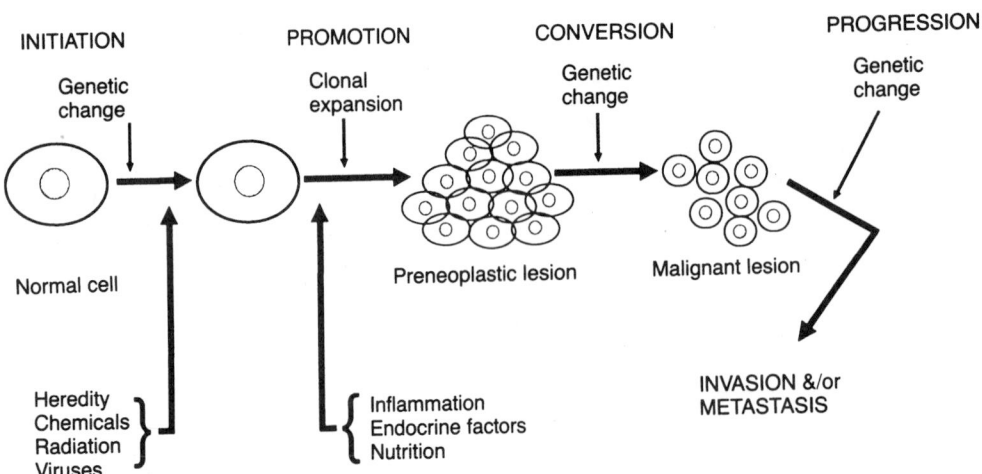

**Figure 1–4.** Schematic model of multistep carcinogenesis. *Genetic change* refers to events such as the activation of proto-oncogenes or drug-resistance genes or the inactivation of tumor suppressor genes, antimetastasis genes, or apoptosis. Genetic change may be relatively minimal, as with the translocations seen with various leukemias, or it may involve multiple sequential genetic alterations, as exemplified by the development of colon cancer.

discipline are presented in Chapter 4. Cancer screening is reviewed in Chapter 5.

## Choice of Therapy

In the past, patients in the United States rarely questioned the therapy recommended by their physicians. Physicians were guided by the golden rule of the Judeo-Christian tradition: "Do unto others as you would have them do unto you." Today, less authoritarian models of the physician-patient relationship are emerging in which patients retain responsibility for decisions about their own lives. Increasingly, the physician's responsibility is seen more as that of an educator, adviser, and provider of technical care. These evolving "patient autonomy" or "partnership" models in no way diminish the importance of the physician in assessing and delivering care; rather, they serve to clarify the crucial role of the patient in setting appropriate and realistic treatment goals. This revised perspective may be called the platinum rule: Do unto others as they would have you do unto them.

Establishing the goals of treatment for an individual cancer patient usually follows an assessment of three sets of factors: those related to (1) the specific tumor, (2) the available therapy, and (3) the specific patient.

### TUMOR FACTORS

The specific histologic type or subtype of a tumor and, in certain circumstances, its histologic grade are important factors in assessing prognosis and selecting therapy, as discussed subsequently in the disease-oriented chapters. The presence or absence of specific receptor molecules may influence the choice of therapy. For example, the presence or absence of hormone receptors may influence the treatment of breast cancer. The presence or absence of amplification of the HER-2/*neu* (c-*erb*B2) oncogene in breast cancer tissue helps determine whether or not it is reasonable to consider treatment with trastuzumab (Herceptin).[15]

The selection and adjustment of therapy may be affected by tumor markers in the blood, such as alpha-fetoprotein and β-human chorionic gonadotropin (β-hCG) in germ cell tumors. Additional tumor markers are being vigorously sought because of their potential value in early diagnosis and screening as well as in following the response of the patient to therapy. Examples of other tumor factors currently being investigated for clinical use include the estimation of the tumor's in vitro sensitivity to cancer chemotherapy, cytogenetic factors, and cell kinetic factors as assessed by flow cytometry. The use of laboratory tests in the management of the cancer patient is discussed in the respective disease-oriented chapters.

For most types of malignant neoplasms, the extent or stage of disease critically determines prognosis and treatment. Thus throughout this book, specific recommendations for a staging work-up are given, based on the natural history of each cancer type, and treatment recommendations for patients with various neoplasms are usually presented as a function of the tumor's stage. We have generally used the

international TNM system developed jointly by the American Joint Committee on Cancer[16] and the International Union Against Cancer.[17] The American Joint Committee on Cancer recognizes two distinct types of staging for primary, previously undiagnosed cancer as well as two additional types of staging for recurrent or fatal cancer. The two types of staging for primary cancer are (1) clinical-diagnostic staging (cTNM) for patients who have had a biopsy but are otherwise in the preoperative phase of study, and (2) postsurgical resection-pathologic staging (pTNM), which includes a complete evaluation of the surgical specimen by a pathologist. Additional types of staging include retreatment staging (rTNM) at the time of recurrent cancer and autopsy staging (aTNM) for patients who have expired.

Diagnostic imaging plays a key role in cancer staging, especially clinical staging performed before surgery. The roles of ultrasonography, standard roentgenography, computed tomography, magnetic resonance imaging, and radionuclide scanning are addressed in the individual disease-oriented chapters. Positron emission tomography scanning has added the additional dimension of function to the purely anatomic findings of more traditional imaging modalities. As such, positron emission tomographic scans are playing an increased role in cancer staging, especially in the context of possible recurrent disease and retreatment staging.

### TREATMENT FACTORS

The importance of integrating cancer treatment modalities is generally recognized. Surgery and radiation therapy are forms of local therapy that are best judged by their ability to provide local control of disease. However, local therapy cannot control systemic disease, and the proper timing of systemic treatment is important. In most tumors of childhood, such as Wilms' tumor or Ewing's sarcoma, chemotherapy is used immediately after local therapy. In adults, the value of such early systemic treatment is also well established but for a smaller number of malignancies. The theoretical basis for such adjuvant or combined modality treatment is presented in Figure 1–5.

The task of integrating cancer treatment modalities appropriately may be difficult and complex. In some hospitals, tumor boards contribute to the integration of treatment modalities. In most instances, the patient's welfare depends on the ongoing services of a flexible and sophisticated treatment team. For such patients, a team leader should be identified who can coordinate and direct the overall effort.

There is a growing body of data supporting the view that patients undergoing procedures that are technically difficult to perform do better when that care is performed at high-volume institutions. Examples of such procedures identified in a report to the Institute of Medicine include resections of all or part of the esophagus, surgery for pancreatic cancer, removal of pelvic organs, and complex chemotherapy regimens.[4] Such high-volume institutions may be found in community settings, although they are more likely to be associated with major cancer centers, such as those approved and reviewed by the National Cancer Institute.

### PATIENT FACTORS

The patient's age, sex, physical performance status, and psychological function may influence the choice of therapy

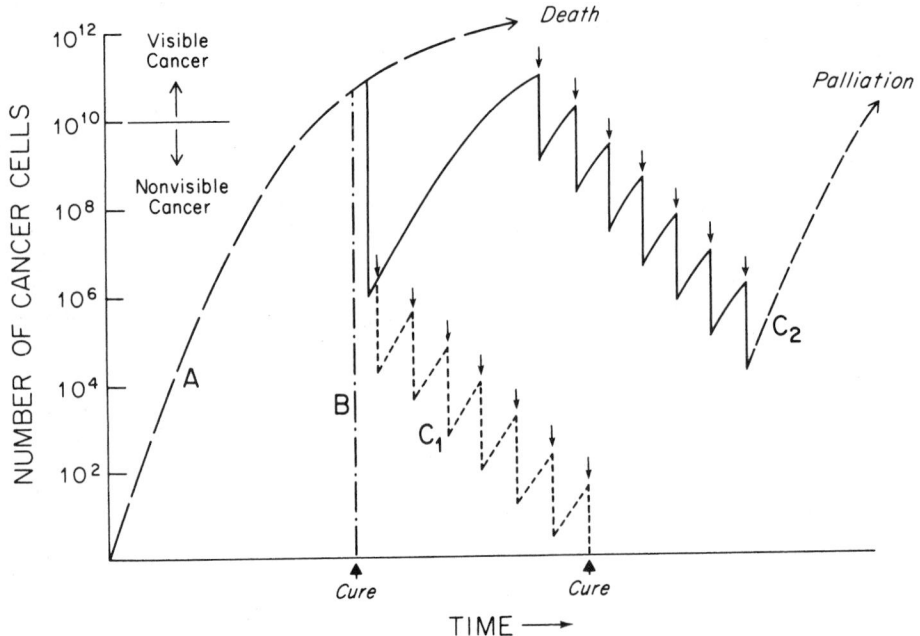

**Figure 1–5.** Schematic diagram of the natural history and treatment of a tumor. A cancer cell population of $10^{10}$ cells corresponds to 10 g of tumor, and $10^{12}$ cells corresponds to 1 kg of tumor. *Curve A* (— —) shows the growth curve for an untreated cancer. The tumor doubles about 30 times by cell division before becoming clinically evident. *Line B* (— · — · —) shows the result of successful local treatment undertaken before metastatic spread. *Lines* $C_1$ and $C_2$ illustrate two ways of adding systemic chemotherapy to local treatment, depicted as vertical arrows. In $C_2$ (—), systemic chemotherapy used for clinically evident cancer is palliative; it fails because of cancer cell resistance or patient intolerance to chemotherapy. In $C_1$ (- - - -), systemic chemotherapy is used immediately after local treatment in a patient with a high risk of recurrence from clinically occult "micrometastases." The goal of this "adjuvant" treatment is to eradicate the occult cancer before it becomes resistant to chemotherapy or the patient experiences unacceptable toxic reactions.

(this is discussed repeatedly throughout this book). For example, the presence or absence of weight loss, systemic symptoms, severe pain, complicating non-neoplastic (co-morbid) diseases, and the status of immunologic function can influence both prognosis and treatment planning. Socio-economic factors may also influence the choice of therapy, but not always in a manner beneficial to the patient. In many cases, the variety of factors that are *important to the patient* may exceed the comprehension of the physician, which further emphasizes the importance of each patient's personal values in setting treatment goals.

## TREATMENT GOALS

*Survival duration* and *quality of life* must both be considered in developing a treatment plan for individual patients. Traditionally, treatment of *curative intent* has been distinguished from that of *palliative intent*. Cure may be defined in two major ways: (1) *statistically*, based on an analysis of survival curves for *groups of patients* and (2) in a *personal* or *individual* sense, based on a retrospective analysis of what happens to the individual patient or (in some rare types of tumors) through the eradication of one or more sensitive tumor markers. In oncology, one almost always uses the word *cure* in its statistical sense, based on the analysis of survival curves.[18] Technically, cure has been accomplished when the survival curve for a group of patients with cancer is parallel to that of an age- and sex-matched control population without cancer (Fig. 1–6).[19] In other words, cure has been achieved when the forces of mortality are acting equally on the two groups of individuals.

Survival data on an appropriate control population are not always available, however, so some investigators use the appearance of a plateau or flattening of the survival curve as evidence of cure.[20, 21] In any case, cure is not simply equivalent to surviving with no evidence of disease for some arbitrary time, such as 3, 5, or even 10 years. For example, patients with primary breast cancer are at risk of recurrence for at least 15 years, and some investigators question whether this group of patients ever has a normal life expectancy. However, a large number of these patients survive longer than 10 years, and many of them ultimately die of other causes while they are free of recurrence. For the latter group, treatment is curative in a personal sense despite the fact that the potential for cure in a statistical sense for the entire group of patients may be uncertain.

Many cancer patients have tumors for which statistical cure is unlikely. Thus, much of our treatment is either palliative or directed to the prolongation of life without the likelihood of cure. It is widely held that some treatment-related morbidity and even the risk of death may be justified for patients with potentially curable tumors, especially young patients, whereas such risks are less acceptable for patients in whom the treatment goal is palliation or the modest prolongation of life.

In many cases, the most appropriate approach to the cancer patient is to consider the cancer a chronic disease that may be controlled rather than eradicated or cured. Thus, the duration and quality of survival become especially important, interdependent terms.

Discussing prognosis with the patient and family is an important part of establishing a treatment plan. Although some cultures continue to keep the diagnosis of cancer a

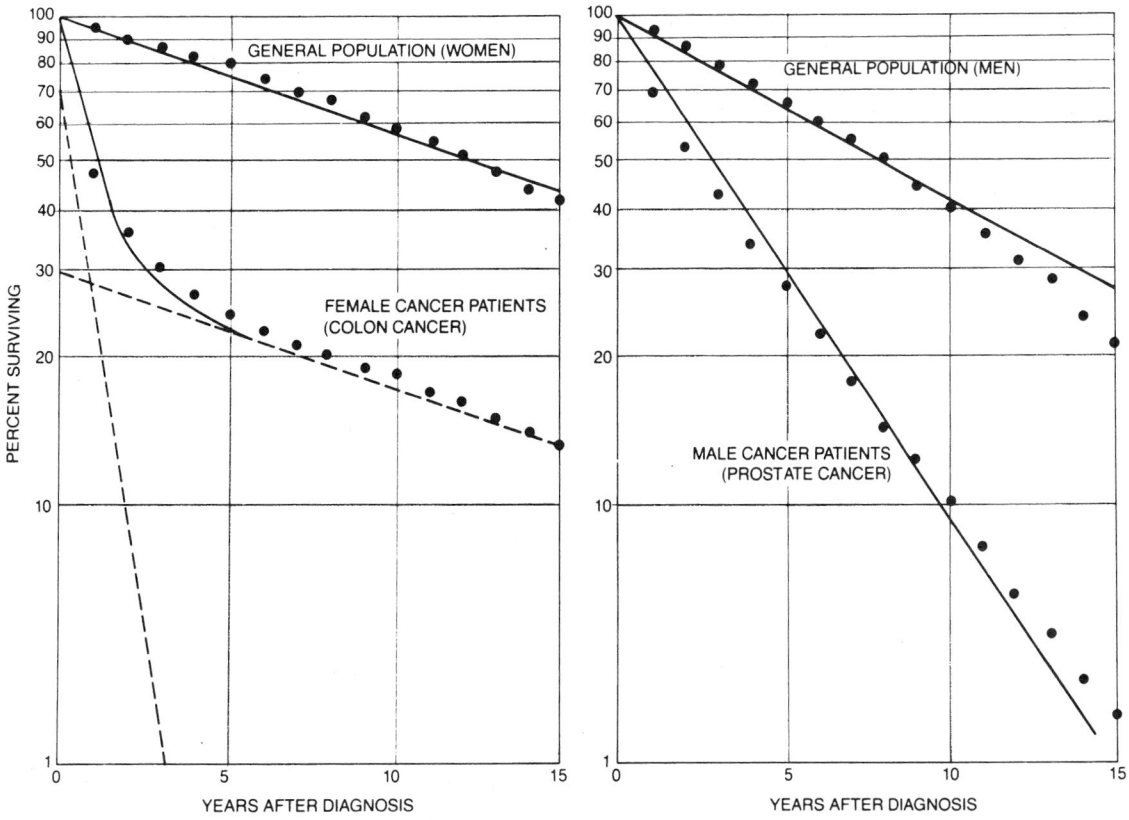

**Figure 1–6.** Cancer patients are considered cured if they die at approximately the same rate as the general population. The graph on the left compares the survival rate of Norwegian women who had colon cancer *(lower line)* to the survival rate of the general population of women who had the same age distribution *(upper line)*. The half-life of the general population was about 13 years (the time required for half of a given population to die). The survival curve for women with colon cancer is the summation of the two broken lines and shows that the women with colon cancer can be considered to fall into one of two categories: 70 percent had a half-life of 8 months, and 30 percent had a half-life of 13 years. In other words, a subgroup consisting of 30 percent of the women died at the same rate as the general population. Some cancers, in contrast, show no such subgroup and in this sense should perhaps be considered incurable by present methods. Cancer of the prostate is one example; the graph at the right compares the survival rate of Norwegian men who had prostate cancer *(lower line)* to the survival rate of similarly aged men in the general population *(upper line)*. The normal population had a half-life of 8 years, whereas the cancer patients had a half-life of 3 years. About a third of these cancer patients suffered no loss of life span as a result of their disease. (These graphs and this commentary from Cairns J: The treatment of diseases and the war against cancer. Sci Am 1985;253:53. Copyright © 1985 by Scientific American, Inc. All rights reserved.)

secret from patients, it is now established practice in the United States to be truthful with patients about their diagnoses. There are, however, many "truths" about what such a diagnosis means. One can describe prognosis and treatment in either positive or negative terms (the latter has been called *hanging crepe*). My bias is that hope should be maintained to the fullest extent possible. To that end, I have found it useful to discuss prognosis with patients in two ways. The first is from the perspective of the scientific physician, using the results of clinical trials to convey what can be expected for *groups* of patients with the same diagnosis. The other is to draw on the stories of individual patients who have done exceptionally well with the same or a similar problem. Not infrequently, it is the latter approach that a patient can hear and understand best because patients customarily think in terms of stories. Indeed, one of the rewards of becoming an experienced physician comes from personally collecting and participating in the stories that flow from the lives of individual patients.

To summarize, one must consider the quality and expected duration of life in both relative and absolute terms when establishing a treatment plan. The potential for cure should be assessed, but one should be alert to the dangers

of misusing the term in talking with individual patients. It is also important to remember that life itself is a terminal condition: It is not a question of whether an individual will die, it is a question of how and when. The patient's values thus become critical in establishing a treatment plan. To the extent that the patient fears a premature death, concern about the *duration* of survival may dominate planning. To the extent that the patient fears an altered body image or the loss of function, a concern for the *quality* of life may dominate. Most patients have a balanced view of these two concerns, but the wise physician never takes this for granted. The goals of treatment must make sense in human terms to the person with the disease—the patient.

## POST-TREATMENT FOLLOW-UP CARE

The importance of post-treatment follow-up is axiomatic. It forms one of the cornerstones of the approvals program of the American College of Surgeons, which has been a pioneer in efforts to ensure accurate follow-up of cancer patients and careful end-results reporting. However, tumor-specific guidelines for what constitutes an appropriate follow-up interval and appropriate levels of testing are not available from federal, state, or authoritative private sources for most forms of cancer. Johnson and colleagues[22] have approached this vacuum by contacting various international cancer research centers to ascertain their protocols for follow-up. Their book on this topic, *Cancer Patient Follow-up*, represents a good resource for developing an appropriate plan of follow-up care for the common forms of human cancer.

In the United States, the National Cancer Institute and the American Cancer Society have major programs aimed at reducing the risk of cancer in our society through smoking cessation, control of alcohol intake, proper dietary measures (reducing the intake of fat), and avoidance of industrial carcinogens. This effort is just as important for the cancer patient as it is for the general population. The same can be said for programs of cancer screening and early detection. A patient may be cured of one cancer only to succumb later to another form of neoplastic disease. This may occur because of chance (which is at least equal to the chance of cancer developing in the normal population), continued exposure to carcinogens (such as continued cigarette smoking), genetic predisposition (which is, fortunately, rare), or even the treatment used for the initial primary cancer (such as cancer chemotherapy or radiation therapy). It is therefore important to develop a strategy of follow-up care for the patient that includes screening for new cancer as well as surveillance for any recurrence of the original tumor. Conversely, it is also important to avoid excessive testing. Many patients assume that an early diagnosis of *metastatic* cancer is as important as an early diagnosis of the initial primary cancer. For most tumors, this is simply not true, and an excessive effort to identify early metastatic disease merely increases the cost of care and raises unrealistic expectations about the value of subsequent therapy for metastatic disease.

A related issue is the extent to which the oncologist serves as the patient's primary care physician, as opposed to serving solely as a consultant. The majority of medical oncologists prefer to work as consultants rather than as providers of primary care.[23] In many systems of capitated care, the "gatekeeper" function of the generalist or primary care physician is rigidly separated from the role of specialists, and a medical oncologist may be precluded from serving this function. In other settings, such as in the Department of Veterans Affairs, specialists may serve as primary care providers for patients with major diseases such as cancer. Either model may be chosen, as long as the patient has full access to the important contributions of both traditions: There must be attention to the particular needs of the cancer diagnosis, but one must not neglect the health maintenance and prevention needs of the patient through poor communication or organization of services.

## SUGGESTIONS FOR ADDITIONAL READING

Kiberstis P, Marx J. Frontiers in cancer research. Science 1997;278:1035–77. *Eleven articles (including an editorial and three news items) about modern cancer research and its implications for the prevention and treatment of cancer.*
Barlogie B, Foti M, Frei E III, et al (steering committee). Foundations of clinical cancer research: perspective for the 21st century. Proceedings of a Symposium to Honor Emil Freireich, M.D., on the occasion of his 70th birthday. Clin Cancer Res 1997;12:2546–2734. *Thirty-one presen-*

*tations grouped into five sessions on various aspects of clinical trials research.*
Integrating economic analysis into cancer clinical trials: the National Cancer Institute–American Cancer Society of clinical oncology economics workbook. J Natl Cancer Inst Monogr 1998;24:1–28. *An excellent introduction to planning, designing, and implementing an economic analysis of cancer clinical trials.*
Hewitt M, Simone J, eds. Ensuring quality cancer care. Report of the National Cancer Policy Board, the Institute of Medicine, and the Commission on Life Sciences, National Research Council. Washington, D.C.: National Academy Press, 1999. *The authors conclude that some individuals with cancer in the United States do not receive care known to be effective for their condition. The group makes 10 recommendations for improving this situation.*

## REFERENCES

1. NCI Fact Book, National Cancer Institute, 1997. National Institutes of Health Publication No. 98.512, May, 1998. Also available on the Internet on the Financial Management Branch home page of the NCI website: (see http://www.nci.nih.gov.)
2. Landis SH, Murray T, Bolden S, Wingo PA. Cancer statistics, 1999. CA Cancer J Clin 1999;49:8–31.
3. Feldman AR, Kessler L, Myers MH, Naughton MD: The prevalence of cancer. Estimates based on the Connecticut Tumor Registry. N Engl J Med 1986;315:1394–7.
4. Hewitt M, Simone J, eds. Ensuring quality cancer care. Report of the National Cancer Policy Board, the Institute of Medicine, and the Commission on Life Sciences, National Research Council. Washington, D.C.: National Academy Press, 1999 (233 pp).
5. Marshall E. Cancer warriors claim a victory—the war on cancer. Science 1998;279:1842–3.
6. Wingo PA, Ries LAG, Giovino GA, et al. Annual report to the nation on the status of cancer, 1973–1996, with a special section on lung cancer and tobacco smoking. J Natl Cancer Inst 1999;91:675–90.
7. Freireich EJ. The future of clinical cancer research in the next millennium. Clin Cancer Res 1997;3:2563–70.
8. Perry DJ, Sloane EM, Hubbard SM, et al. Keeping up with the cancer literature: PDQ access. J Clin Oncol 1988;6:1649–52.
9. Kizer K: National cancer strategy. Department of Veterans Affairs, VHA Directive 97-050, October 21, 1997.
10. Greenberg ER, Chute CG, Stukel T, et al. Social and economic factors in the choice of lung cancer treatment: a population-based study in two rural states. N Engl J Med 1988;318:612–7.
11. Greenwald HP. Who survives cancer? Berkeley, Calif.: University of California Press, 1992.
12. Ozonoff D, Clapp R. Cancer survival is no lottery. Lancet 1999;343:1379–80.
13. Pitot HC. The molecular biology of carcinogenesis. Cancer 1993;72: Suppl 3:962–70.
14. McGinnis JM, Foege WH. Actual causes of death in the United States. JAMA 1993;270:2207–12.
15. Pegram MD, Lipton A, Hayes DF, et al. Phase II study of receptor-enhanced chemosensitivity using recombinant humanized anti-p185HER2/neu monoclonal antibody plus cisplatin in patients with HER2/neu-overexpressing metastatic breast cancer refractory to chemotherapy treatment. J Clin Oncol 1998;16:2659–71.
16. Fleming ID, Cooper JS, Henson DE, et al, eds., American Joint Committee on Cancer Cancer Staging Manual. 5th ed. Philadelphia: Lippincott-Raven, 1997.
17. TNM Classification of Malignant Tumors. 3rd ed. Geneva: International Union Against Cancer, 1978.
18. Easson E. Possibilities for the cure of Hodgkin's disease. Cancer 1966;19:345.
19. Cairns J. The treatment of diseases and the war against cancer. Sci Am 1985;253:51–9.
20. Frei E III. Curative cancer chemotherapy. Cancer Res 1985;45:6523–37.
21. Frei E III. Re:position paper on curative cancer chemotherapy. Letter. Cancer Res 1987:3907–8.
22. Johnson FE, Virgo KS, eds. Cancer patient follow-up. St. Louis: CV Mosby, 1997 (554 pp).
23. American Society of Clinical Oncology Special Article: Status of the medical oncology workforce. J Clin Oncol 1996;14:2612–21.

# CHAPTER 2

# BIOLOGY OF CANCER

• MATTHEW RETTIG • MARK P. SAWICKI

Since the 1970s, the biology and pathogenesis of cancer have begun to be elucidated. Investigators have identified many of the molecular mechanisms that lead to the development and propagation of malignancies. Despite a protean array of molecular events that are involved in the development of any given malignancy, the common threads that link the pathogenesis of all cancers are (1) *the loss of regulation of growth* and (2) *the ability to locally invade tissues and metastasize*.

The normal physiology of growth control is complex and involves a careful balance between the death of senescent cells and the appearance of new cells. The cellular process of programmed cell death is known as *apoptosis*; new cell formation occurs as a consequence of the proliferation of mitotic cells. For the number of cells in a population to remain constant, a balance between proliferation and apoptosis must exist. When this homeostasis is perturbed, dysregulated growth results. A simple equation results:

$$\uparrow \text{Proliferation} \pm \downarrow \text{Apoptosis} \rightarrow \text{Net accumulation of cells}$$

Both benign and malignant neoplasms are characterized by increased proliferation or decreased apoptosis, or both. Malignant neoplasms generally acquire a greater number of genetic alterations in genes that regulate growth. However, dysregulated growth alone does not define a malignancy. The ability to invade local tissues and to metastasize is of equal pathophysiologic importance to the development of a malignancy. In fact, the presence of metastasis is the sine qua non for defining a neoplasm as malignant as opposed to benign. Thus, benign neoplasms have also lost some degree of growth control, but they do not by definition have the capacity to metastasize. Malignancies acquire genetic alterations that enhance local tumorigenicity and metastatic potential, and these genetic changes may overlap with those involved in loss of growth regulation, or they may be entirely different.

Tumors may arise from a variety of genetic mutations involving a variety of growth-related genes. Broadly, these genes may be categorized as gatekeepers, caretakers, and landscapers. The gatekeepers consist predominantly of oncogenes and tumor suppressor genes. Caretakers are genes involved in repairing the genome when DNA damage occurs, and the landscapers are involved in the microenvironment of the growing cell.

Ultimately, dysregulated growth and the capacity for local invasion and metastasis are the defining characteristics of a malignant neoplasm. This chapter provides an overview of the cellular and molecular physiology and pathophysiology leading to the acquisition of these characteristics. It is important to emphasize that the breadth of topics in this chapter is limited to a summary and overview, and the reader should refer to appropriate sources for more in-depth discussion of individual topics.

## The Cell Cycle, Proliferation, and Signal Transduction

According to the simple equation given earlier, the net accumulation of cells in a population occurs as a consequence of increased proliferation or decreased apoptosis (see further on). Proliferation results from a cell passing through the *cell cycle*, during which it undergoes mitosis and gives rise to two daughter cells. The cell cycle is composed of mitosis and interphase; the latter is the period between mitoses and is composed of the $G_1$, S, and $G_2$ phases (Fig. 2–1). The S phase represents the period during which DNA is synthesized, resulting in the duplication of the entire DNA content of a cell. During S phase, the DNA content of a diploid human cell goes from 2n to 4n. $G_1$ and $G_2$ are the *gap* phases during which a cell prepares for S phase and mitosis, respectively. During $G_1$ and $G_2$, protein and RNA synthesis occur, but the DNA content remains stable. Mitosis is the phase in which the nuclear and cytoplasmic material of a cell are split and divided between two daughter cells. Cells that are not passing through the cell cycle are in $G_0$ phase. $G_0$ cells are metabolically active but do not proliferate. Cells may withdraw from the cell cycle in early $G_1$ and enter $G_0$ or may be stimulated to exit $G_0$ and enter the cell cycle at $G_1$.

The cell cycle represents a complex but ordered process that is carefully regulated during the transition from one phase of the cycle to another. Generally, one phase of a cycle cannot begin until the previous phase has been successfully completed. Such careful regulation ensures that DNA is duplicated correctly and subsequently divided equally between two daughter cells. Studies involving a variety of scientific disciplines, including yeast genetics, frog biochemistry, and mammalian tissue culture, have led to our current understanding of cell cycle control.

The control of the cell cycle involves positive and negative regulatory circuits that rely on the activity of proteins known as *cyclin-dependent kinases (CDKs)*. Kinases are proteins that phosphorylate other proteins. Phosphorylation is a fundamental molecular mechanism that all eukaryotic cells employ to regulate the activity of proteins. Phosphorylation generally leads to activation of a protein, but it may also result in deactivation. Proteins that remove phosphate groups (i.e., dephosphorylation) are known as *phosphatases* and also play a crucial role in the regulation of cellular molecular circuits.

CDKs function during cell cycle *checkpoints* during all phases of the cell cycle. These checkpoints monitor the

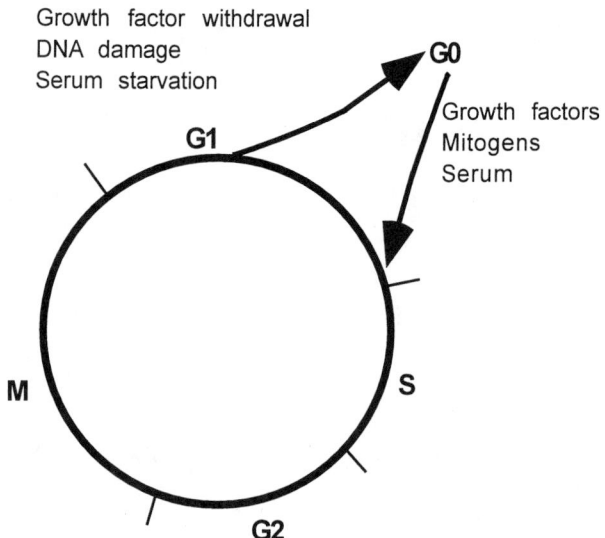

**Figure 2–1.** The cell cycle consists of four phases as illustrated. When cells proliferate, they pass through each phase of the cell cycle in a tightly regulated, ordered fashion. Nonproliferating, or resting cells, are in the $G_0$ phase. Various stimuli can induce cells to enter or exit the cell cycle primarily from the $G_1$ phase.

successful completion of a cell cycle phase before the transition to the next phase is initiated. Thus, there are checkpoints in $G_1$, S, $G_2$, and M. In higher eukaryotes, including humans, the $G_1$-S transition is perhaps the most crucial event in the cell cycle. The molecular mechanisms for the $G_1$-S transition have been well characterized and serve as a model for understanding the regulatory control of the cell cycle. Once a cell has passed the $G_1$ checkpoint, it reaches the *restriction point*, after which the cell is committed to making the transition into the S phase and beginning the duplication of its DNA. If the cell does not pass the $G_1$ checkpoint, it exits the cell cycle and enters the $G_0$ quiescent state. Alternatively, it may undergo apoptosis (see further on).

CDKs form a complex with other proteins that regulate the activity of the CDKs themselves (Fig. 2–2). Cyclins are key activating subunits,[1] whereas cyclin-dependent kinase inhibitors (CKIs) inhibit CDKs. There are many CDKs,

cyclins, and CKIs that function in the animal cell cycle. Important proteins in $G_1$-S regulation are cdk4 and cdk6, the D cyclins, and INK4 proteins (i.e., *in*hibitors of cd*k*4, which are CKIs).[2] Perhaps the most important function of the CDK complex of proteins is the regulation of the retinoblastoma protein, pRB.[3] pRB and the related proteins p130 and p107 are crucial proteins that bind to a group of transcription factors collectively known as the *E2F family of proteins*.[4] Transcription factors are proteins that enter the nucleus, bind to DNA, and regulate the transcription of genes. In its hypophosphorylated state, pRB binds to E2F proteins and prevents them from transactivating genes that are necessary for entry into S phase. When cdk4 or cdk6 performs its kinase function by phosphorylating pRB, pRB releases E2F proteins, which, in turn, increase the transcription of key proteins necessary for DNA synthesis during S phase. Among the proteins activated by the E2F proteins are dihydrofolate reductase, thymidine kinase, thymidylate synthase, and DNA polymerase-$\alpha$,[5] all of which have well-defined functions in the production of deoxyribonucleotides and the duplication of DNA.

In an adult human, three subpopulations exist with respect to the cell cycle. One subpopulation essentially remains in the cell cycle. Tissues that contain constantly cycling cells include the gastrointestinal mucosa and the epidermis. These tissues require a proliferating pool of cells to replace the senescent cells that are sloughed each day. The second subpopulation of cells remains in $G_0$ and does not have the capacity to enter the cell cycle and divide. Cells of this type are represented by neurons. In fact, humans are born with a full complement of neurons, and the number of neurons decreases every day until death, although some data in mice indicate the potential for activation of proliferation of neurons. Finally, there are cells that exist in $G_0$ but can be stimulated to enter the cell cycle. For example, when the majority of the adult liver is removed, the remaining hepatic cells enter the cell cycle, proliferate, and ultimately regenerate a liver that approximates the size and mass of the original liver. Another cell type that exists in $G_0$ but can enter the cell cycle is the hematopoietic stem cell. These cells are capable of dividing to regenerate more stem cells, or they have the capacity to differentiate into the various hematopoietic lineages in the bone marrow (leukocytes, erythrocytes,

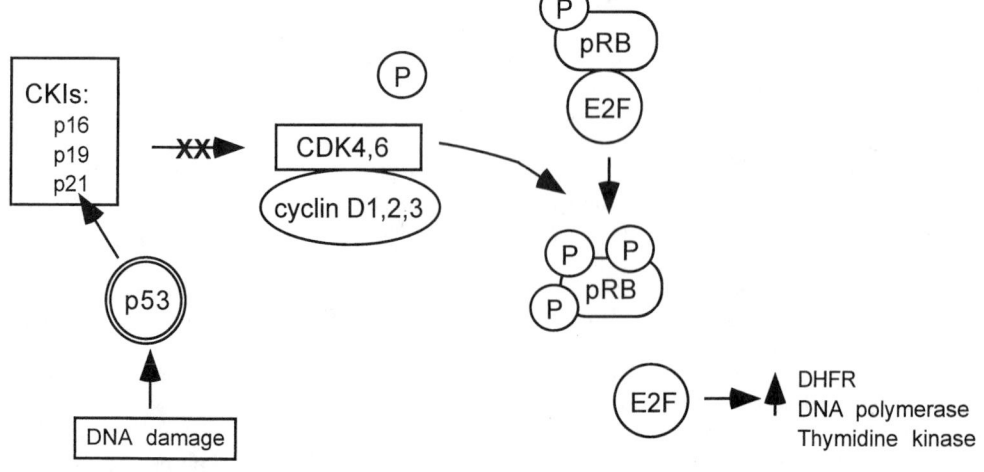

**Figure 2–2.** The principal proteins involved in the control of the $G_1$- to S-phase transition. The central protein in this transition is pRB, which in its hypophosphorylated state binds to the E2F family of transcription factors. On phosphorylation, pRB releases the E2F transcription factors, which subsequently upregulate the expression of key proteins involved in the synthesis of DNA. The phosphorylation of pRB involves an interplay of several positive and negative regulatory proteins, including cyclin-dependent kinases (CDKs), cyclins, and cyclin-dependent kinase inhibitors (CKIs).

and platelets). Because some hematopoietic stem cells exist in $G_0$, they are partially protected from the cytotoxic effects of chemotherapeutic agents, which almost all function by selectively inducing the death of cells that are in the cell cycle.

In a given population of cells, enhanced proliferation occurs when cells that are actively proliferating are maintained in the cell cycle, leading to uncontrolled proliferation; when the duration of the cell cycle is shortened; and when the percentage of cells that enter the cell cycle increases. Exogenous factors frequently stimulate cells to enter the cell cycle from $G_0$. In the preceding examples, removal of a large part of the liver or the immediate postchemotherapy state stimulates liver and hematopoietic stem cells, respectively, to exit $G_0$ and enter the cell cycle at $G_1$. In addition, there are cellular growth factors and stimulatory substances known as *mitogens* that induce the proliferation of cells by causing them to enter the cell cycle at $G_1$. Growth factors not only stimulate entry into the cell cycle from $G_0$ but also promote cells to remain in the cell cycle. This latter feat may be partially accomplished by causing the increased expression of D cyclins so that growth factor–stimulated cells can successfully phosphorylate pRB and ultimately go from $G_1$ to S phase. Activation of D cyclins may also expedite the passage of cells through $G_1$ phase.

Although we have briefly discussed some of the mutations that can affect growth factor–receptor pathways, the most common genetic alterations that affect oncogenesis involve regulators of $G_1$ progression. These oncogenic events not only facilitate entry into the cell cycle but also accelerate passage through $G_1$, generally the longest phase of the cell cycle, as well as prevent cells from exiting the cell cycle and entering $G_0$. Thus, both the number of cells that are in the cell cycle and the rapidity with which cells pass through the cell cycle are increased by genetic alterations that affect $G_1$ regulatory proteins. Indeed, most of the proteins that regulate $G_1$ progression have been affected in the molecular pathogenesis of malignancies. There are two basic types of

genetic alterations of $G_1$ regulatory proteins that can lead to enhanced proliferation. The first type results in activating mutations of genes that enhance proliferation. For example, cyclin $D_1$ is overexpressed in a variety of cancers, including B-cell lymphomas, head and neck cancers, esophageal cancer, breast cancer, and others.[6, 7] The second type of alteration leads to decreased activity of genes that retard proliferation. Inactivating mutations and deletions of CKIs including INK4a (p16) have been reported for gliomas, acute lymphoblastic leukemia, nasopharyngeal carcinoma, and many other cancers.[1, 7] The most commonly mutated gene among all human malignancies is the one that codes for p53,[8, 9] a protein that plays a key regulatory role in $G_1$ progression by activating the CKI known as *p21*.[10, 11] Inactivating mutations of p53 result in its inability to activate p21 and alter its ability to induce the apoptosis of cells that have undergone DNA damage. A more detailed description of the function of p53 is provided further on.

Although many of the genes that are mutated in human cancers are directly involved in the cell cycle, many code for proteins that function in signal transduction pathways that regulate the expression of cell cycle proteins but are not themselves directly involved in cell cycle control. Signal transduction pathways represent the biochemical mechanisms whereby a cell communicates with its extracellular environment (Fig. 2–3). Cells receive signals from this microenvironment from specific soluble proteins or proteins that make up the extracellular matrix and interact with receptors on the plasma membranes (and sometimes nuclear membrane) of cells. Alternatively, a cell may communicate with another cell by direct cell-cell contact that involves the interaction of two complementary proteins on the plasma membranes of both cells. Whether a cell receives a signal from a soluble protein or by direct cell-cell interaction, the result is activation of a signal transduction pathway. The biochemical consequence is activation of proteins, including nuclear transcription factors. These transcription factors are involved in the transactivation of the regulatory elements of

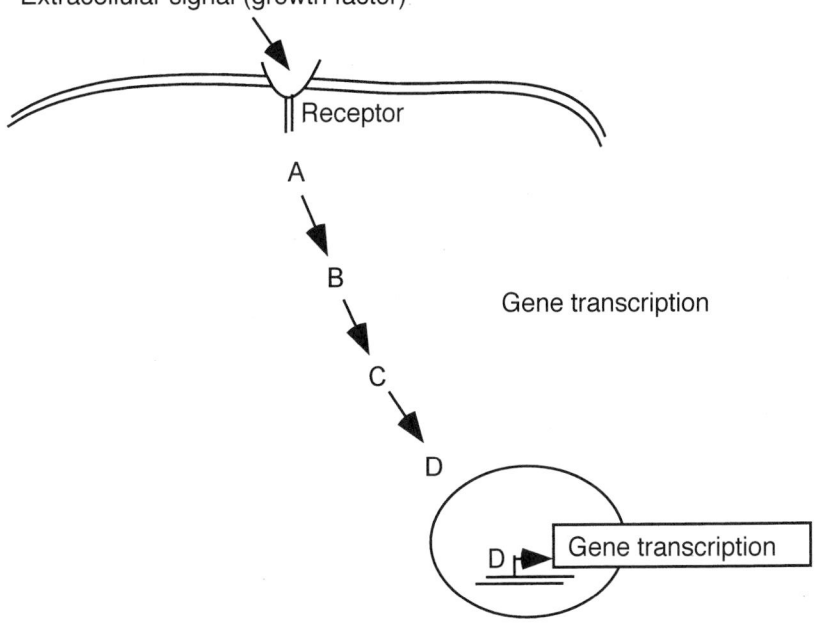

**Figure 2–3.** A schematic illustration of signal transduction. An extracellular signal, typically a growth factor or cytokine, binds to its receptor. On ligand binding, the receptor undergoes conformational changes, dimerization (or trimerization or oligomerization), or phosphorylation, or a combination, which leads to activation of other signaling proteins. These signaling proteins, or second messengers, subsequently activate other proteins so that the signal is amplified at each successive step. The typical final targets for the signal transduction pathway are transcription factors, which bind to the upstream regulatory elements of genes and result in increased gene transcription.

target genes (e.g., cyclin D) so that transcription of a target gene can be upregulated or downregulated. Increased or decreased protein synthesis occurs, and a phenotypic change (e.g., proliferation) in the cell results.

As mentioned, the interaction of an extracellular signal with a plasma membrane receptor results in the activation of a signal transduction pathway. In human cells, there are four basic types of signal transduction pathways (Fig. 2–4) that are activated on interaction of an extracellular ligand with its receptor.

- Activation of adenylate cyclase, a membrane-bound enzyme that generates cyclic adenosine monophosphate
- Activation of guanylate cyclase to generate cyclic guanine monophosphate, which is involved in retinal signals to light and mediates relaxation of smooth muscle
- Activation of phospholipase enzymes, which generates inositol 1,4,5-triphosphate, causing elevation of intracellular $Ca^{2+}$
- Activation of protein kinases—enzymes that function by phosphorylating other proteins at tyrosine residues (i.e., tyrosine kinases)—or serine or threonine (i.e., serine-threonine kinases), or both (i.e., dual specificity kinases)

These signal transduction pathways are the fundamental means by which cells communicate with their environment and are centrally involved in the regulation of proliferation and cell death. These pathways encompass innumerable different proteins at various levels of the signaling cascades. Virtually any of these proteins at any level of the signal transduction cascade can be mutated in human cells and lead to dysregulated growth. Many of the factors are outlined in a subsequent section. As an example, growth factor receptors, including the epidermal growth factor receptor (EGFR) family of proteins, are genetically altered in a variety of cancers (e.g., breast cancer). In breast cancer, HER-2/*neu* growth factor receptor is amplified (multiple copies of the gene encoding for the protein) in 30% of cases.[12] The amplification in the gene results in overexpression of HER-2-neu protein, and the degree of amplification correlates with breast cancer prognosis and proliferation in vitro.

One of the most important signal transduction pathways that is genetically altered in human malignancies is the protein kinase pathway known as the mitogen-activated protein kinase (MAPK) signal transduction pathway (Fig. 2–5). The MAPK pathway is perhaps the most well-characterized signal transduction pathway and represents a model for understanding how an extracellular signal can be transmitted to and amplified in the intracellular environment. Once a growth factor binds to its receptor, the receptor undergoes a conformational change or tyrosine phosphorylation, or both, that results in the activation of the protein known as *Grb2*, which subsequently activates an adaptor protein known as *SOS*. The Grb2/SOS complex then activates ras,[13] a monomeric G protein (i.e., guanine nucleotide-binding protein), which exchanges guanosine triphosphate (GTP) for guanosine diphosphate (GDP) and consequently is able to transmit the signal to cytoplasmic proteins as shown in Figure 2–5. The signal is amplified at each step, transcription factors are ultimately activated, and gene transcription results in the expression of proteins that regulate proliferation.[14] One of the proteins that is upregulated by the MAPK pathway is cyclin D, which facilitates both the entry into $G_1$ from $G_0$ and the transition from $G_1$ to S phase. Thus, an extracellular signal that activates a growth factor receptor may result in enhanced proliferation through increased expression of cyclin D.

Many of the genes coding for the proteins in the MAPK pathway have been shown to be mutated in human malignancies, and theoretically the mutation of any protein in the pathway could result in enhanced proliferation. Indeed, many of the MAPK pathway genes are mutated in human cancers. With respect to the pathogenesis of malignancies, the most important protein in the MAPK pathway is the ras protein, which is mutated in numerous malignancies, including 95% of pancreatic adenocarcinomas.[15] The ras protein undergoes a modification known as *farnesylation*, which results in the ability of ras to localize to the plasma membrane,[16] where it performs its signal transduction functions. Inhibitors of ras farnesylation have been developed and are currently being tested in clinical trials in a variety of cancers.

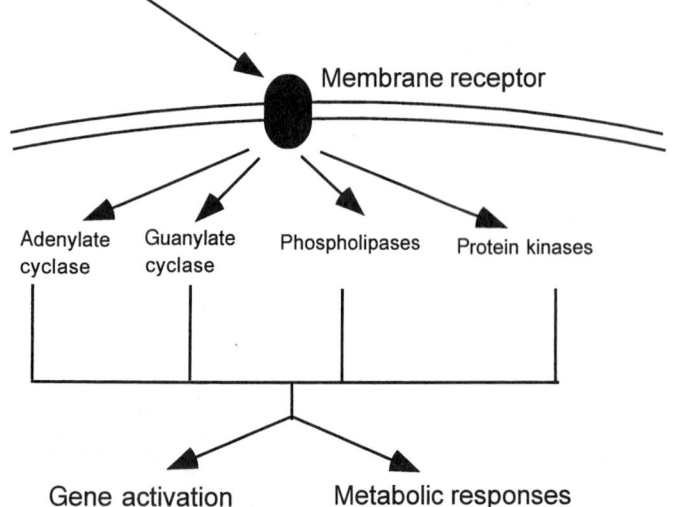

Figure 2–4. The four basic signal transduction pathways. (See text for explanation.)

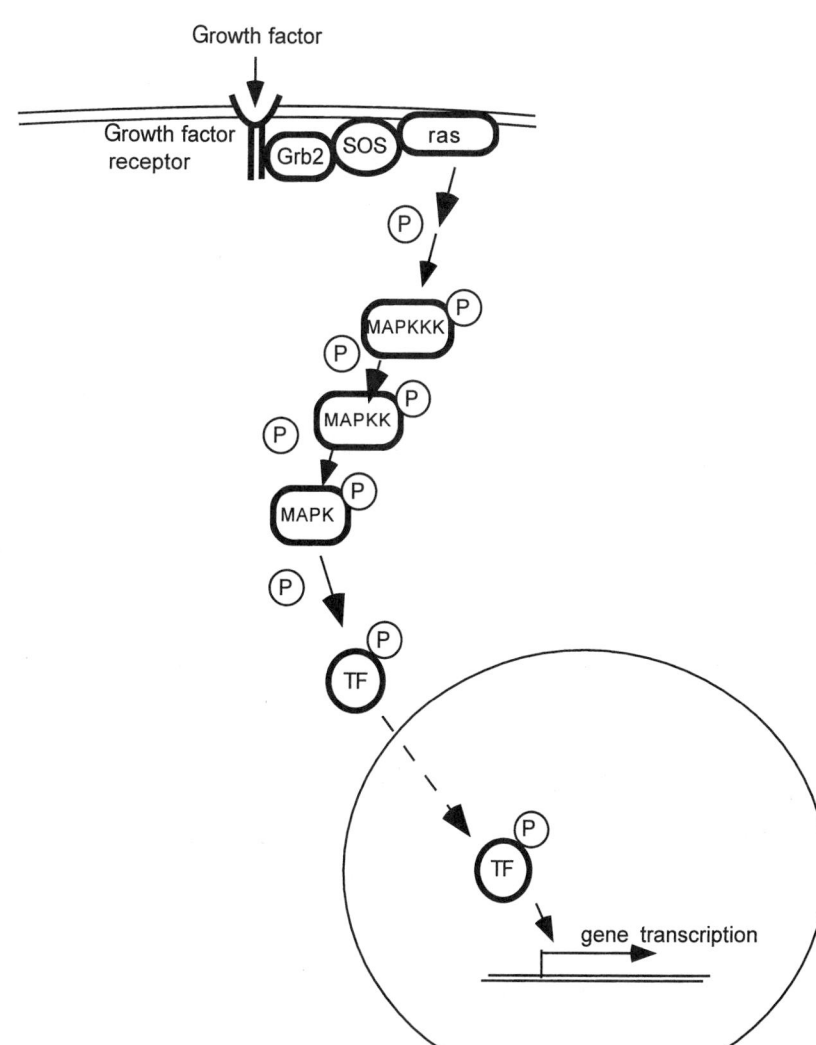

**Figure 2–5.** The mitogen-activated protein kinase (MAPK) signal transduction pathway. In this pathway, growth factors bind to plasma membrane growth factor receptors and result in tyrosine phosphorylation of the receptors. Consequently, the Grb2 associates with the receptor and recruits the adaptor protein SOS to the plasma membrane, where SOS is activated. In its activated form, SOS activates Ras, a monomeric G protein. The intermediate steps between Ras activation and downstream protein kinases have not been entirely elucidated. Nonetheless, Ras activation ultimately results in the phosphorylation of a series of serine-threonine kinases: MAPK kinase kinase (MAPKKK), MAPK kinase (MAPKK), and MAPK. MAPK may enter the nucleus, where it phosphorylates and activates nuclear transcription factors.

In summary, any component of a pathway linking an extracellular signal (i.e., growth factor) to a biochemical pathway that regulates the cell cycle may have oncogenic potential. Many of the common mutations in human cancers occur in genes that are directly involved in the cell cycle (e.g., p53, cyclin D, p21), especially at the $G_1$-S transition. Alternatively, mutations in genes involved in signal transduction pathways that indirectly regulate the cell cycle by controlling expression of cell cycle proteins also function in the pathogenesis of human malignancies.

## Apoptosis

Cell death can occur as a consequence of one of two processes: *necrosis* or *apoptosis*. Necrosis usually results from a massive tissue insult such as severe hypoxia, toxins, and conditions of energy depletion. Necrosis is an energy-independent process whereby cells that have sustained the inciting insult swell and lyse into randomly sized fragments. Inflammation results, and the cellular debris is cleared by phagocytes. Until the early 1970s, necrosis was the only identified mechanism of cell death.

In 1972, the physiologic process of apoptosis was described.[17] Since then, it has become clear that apoptosis predominates as the main physiologic process of cell death. It is clear that most if not all cells contain the genetic machinery to undergo the programmed cell death of apoptosis. Apoptosis plays an important role in embryogenesis in which it is involved in the formation of visceral organs and the shaping of limb buds, for example. In humans, apoptosis is involved in the homeostasis of many cell populations. For example, circulating granulocytes survive approximately 24 hours before they undergo apoptosis; the bone marrow represents a source of newly formed granulocytes that constantly replace those that have died by apoptosis.

When a cell undergoes apoptosis, there is a stereotypical sequence of events that is morphologically recognizable (Fig. 2–6).[18] Initially, the chromatin condenses and the nucleus fragments. Cytoplasmic blebbing occurs, followed by fragmentation of the cell into *apoptotic bodies*. Unlike necrosis, cells undergoing apoptosis do not lyse, and the plasma membrane remains intact. In addition, apoptosis does not

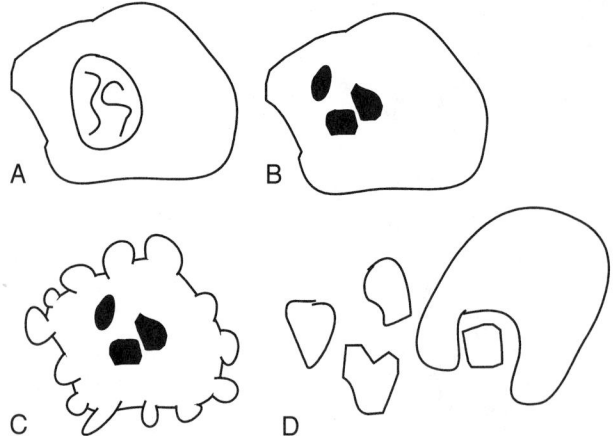

**Figure 2–6.** The morphologically recognizable steps of apoptosis. *A,* Cell before the initiation of apoptosis. The chromatin and nucleus are intact. *B,* Chromatin condenses and the nucleus begins to fragment. *C,* Cytoplasmic blebbing. *D,* Fragmentation of the cell into apoptotic bodies, which are engulfed and degraded by phagocytes.

elicit an inflammatory response, yet it does require adenosine triphosphate and is thus an energy-dependent process.

Many of the molecular pathways and molecules that are involved in apoptosis have come from studies of the nematode worm *Caenorhabditis elegans.* Study of *C. elegans* has allowed investigators to elucidate many of the molecular mechanisms of apoptosis in higher eukaryotes, including humans. Apoptosis occurs in four sequential steps: (1) commitment to programmed cell death induced by extracellular or intracellular stimuli, (2) activation of cellular proteases that are the effectors of apoptosis and functionally kill the cell, (3) engulfment of apoptotic bodies by surrounding cells, and (4) lysosomal degradation of engulfed apoptotic bodies.

The commitment to apoptosis results from a protean array of signals (Table 2–1). These signals include but are not limited to ionizing radiation (by inducing DNA damage), withdrawal of growth factors, and activation of various plasma membrane death receptors that may activate apoptotic effector proteins through signal transduction pathways. When apoptosis is induced by any of these signals, a series of proteins called *caspases* (i.e., cysteine-containing aspartate-specific proteases) are activated. Caspases are the executioners of cell death due to all known signals that induce apoptosis.[19] In humans, there are at least 10 caspases that participate in apoptosis. Caspases exist as inactive proteins that are collectively known as *zymogens.* One of the first caspases to become activated is caspase 8.[20] Once activated,

**Table 2–1.** **Factors that Induce Apoptosis**

Ionizing radiation
Cytotoxic chemotherapy
Cytokines
  Tumor necrosis factor family members
  Transforming growth factor-β
Heat
Hypoxia
Growth factor withdrawal
Glucocorticoids
Fas ligand

it cleaves other caspase zymogens by proteolysis and thereby perpetuates the caspase cascade. One of the downstream caspases is caspase 3, which is considered one of the final "executioner" caspases.[21] Caspase 3 targets several proteins, the alteration of which leads to the recognizable morphologic changes of apoptosis. Some of these target proteins include (1) an endonuclease (for chopping up DNA), (2) gesolin, a protein that binds to actin and helps cells maintain their shape, (3) p21-activated kinase-2 (PAK2), a protein that regulates the internal skeleton of cells, and (4) poly ADP-ribose polymerase (PARP), a protein that is not necessary for apoptosis but represents a good diagnostic marker for apoptosis.[22–24] Thus, the targets of the caspase system of proteins are involved in digesting DNA and maintaining the structural integrity of the cell, and alteration of these proteins leads to the morphologic changes that characterize apoptosis.

Although nuclear fragmentation is a hallmark of apoptosis, the presence of a nucleus is not necessary for apoptosis to occur, at least in some cell systems. This fact, along with studies that show that cytoplasmic extracts can result in nuclear fragmentation, indicates that apoptosis may not require new protein synthesis.[25] Thus, all the components necessary for apoptosis may exist within a cell and may be called into action by the appropriate stimulus.

Recent studies have brought to light the importance of mitochondria in apoptosis. Cytochrome c, a mitochondrial membrane protein, is released from mitochondria during apoptosis. Released cytochrome c binds to a protein called *apoptotic protease activating factor-1* (Apaf-1),[26] which, in turn, cleaves and activates caspase 9. The latter functions as an initiator of the caspase cascade, and activates caspase 3, whose "executioner" function was described earlier. That the mitochondrion plays a role in apoptosis is not surprising because many forms of cellular insult cause injury to the mitochondrial membrane and result in the release of cytochrome c.

Because the caspases represent such a potent system for executing apoptosis, cells have developed apoptotic counter-regulatory proteins called the *bcl family of proteins.* The bcl family consists of antiapoptotic and proapoptotic proteins. These proteins received their name because the first one to be described, bcl-2, was identified in a *B-c*ell *lymphoma.*[27] The bcl proteins exist in the outer mitochondrial membrane and regulate each other by forming homodimers (e.g., bcl-2:bcl-2) and heterodimers (e.g., bcl-2:bax). Their mechanisms of action are only partly understood, but it appears that they regulate release of cytochrome c and inhibit the activation of Apaf-1.[28, 29] Other proteins known as inhibitors of apoptosis can directly inhibit caspases.[30]

The final stages of apoptosis, namely, engulfment of apoptotic bodies by neighboring phagocytes and subsequent degradation, are less well understood than the first two steps of commitment to and execution of cell death. It does appear that the macromolecular components of the plasma membrane (i.e., proteins and lipids) become altered during apoptosis, which allows phagocytes to recognize and engulf apoptotic bodies. In the final stage of apoptosis, lysosomal degradation of engulfed apoptotic bodies ensues.

The role of apoptosis in the pathogenesis of malignancies has not been fully established. Apoptosis and the inhibition of apoptosis play a role in the mechanism of cytotoxicity induced by chemotherapy and radiation and resistance to these treatments, respectively. Nonetheless, inhibition of apoptosis may function in the development of malignancies. Genes that regulate apoptosis are genetically altered in a broad spectrum of cancers. The gene that codes for the bcl-2 protein represents a classic example of the way in which apoptosis plays a role in human cancers. The bcl-2 antiapoptotic protein is overexpressed in approximately 90% of human B-cell follicular lymphomas.[27] The overexpression occurs as a consequence of the translocation of the *bcl-2* gene on chromosome 18 to the immunoglobulin heavy chain (IgH) gene locus on chromosome 14. The translocation is denoted as t(14;18). The IgH locus contains constitutively active *cis* regulatory elements (i.e., promoters and enhancers) that result in high-level expression of the *bcl-2* gene, which has been juxtaposed to these regulatory elements as a consequence of the t(14;18) chromosomal translocation. The overexpression of *bcl-2* inhibits apoptosis.

Perhaps the most important gene that regulates apoptosis in human malignancies is p53. p53 and mdm2, the gene that regulates p53, are mutated in the majority of human malignancies. It is estimated that up to 70% of cancers contain a mutation of either p53 or mdm2.[8, 31, 32] p53 is mutated in 80% of colon cancers, 50% of lung cancers, and 40% of breast cancers. Germline mutations of p53 are found in the Li-Fraumeni syndrome in which patients have inherited mutations in the p53 gene and are at risk for a variety of cancers, including soft tissue sarcomas, breast cancer, brain cancer, lung cancer, leukemias, and adrenocortical tumors.

The mechanisms whereby p53 mediates apoptosis have begun to be elucidated. It functions as a transcription factor, upregulating the expression of proapoptotic genes. Some of these genes are involved in the regulation of the redox state of cells and creation of free radicals that injure mitochondrial membranes. As a consequence of mitochondrial injury, cytochrome c is released and activates the caspase cascade. The expression of bax, a proapoptotic member of the bcl family of proteins, is also upregulated by p53, and it downregulates the expression of bcl-2, an antiapoptotic protein.

If p53 plays a central role in initiating apoptosis, how is p53 itself activated? The answer is DNA damage.[33] For instance, radiation therapy and many chemotherapeutic agents kill cells by causing DNA damage, which results in p53 activation. DNA damage results in the activation of intermediary proteins, such as ATM (the gene that is mutated in ataxia telangiectasia), which, in turn, activates p53. Once p53 has been called into action, not only are proapoptotic signals induced but the cell exits the cell cycle as a consequence of the activation of p21 (a CKI) by p53, as described earlier. Thus, cells that contain mutations of p53 may be resistant to the effects of chemotherapy and radiation because p53-deficient cells may ignore the DNA injury induced by treatment. In addition, p53 mutations predispose to mutations in other genes because of the failure of cells to die in response to DNA damage. Thus, p53 plays a central role in the regulation of proliferation, apoptosis, treatment resistance, and progression of malignancies. Because p53 mutations are so common, replacement of p53 function is an ideal target for gene therapy. Indeed, gene therapy for p53 mutations is currently being studied as an approach to treating cancers that have inactivating mutations of p53, and

such therapy appears to be successful in vitro and in animal models.

In the cancerous cell, apoptosis most frequently occurs in the setting of enhanced proliferation. In fact, proliferation and apoptosis are often intimately entwined, as exemplified by the multitude of effects of p53. Thus, the specific contribution of apoptosis in the pathogenesis of malignancy is uncertain, but current research should elucidate the true role that apoptosis plays in cancer development. The focus of this chapter now turns to a more in-depth discussion of the plethora of genes that may be genetically altered in cancers, leading to enhanced proliferation and inhibition of apoptosis.

## Viral Oncogenesis

Both DNA and RNA viruses are associated with animal and human malignancies (Table 2–2). Although these viruses do not appear to play a role in the pathogenesis of the majority of human cancers, they provide a unique opportunity to study their molecular biology. DNA and RNA viruses share in common the need to integrate their genome into host DNA, and they differ in the molecular mechanisms by which they transform the host cell. DNA viruses produce proteins that inactivate the host proteins that normally act in negatively regulating the cell cycle. RNA viruses either carry altered forms of the host genes that mimic the host gene function, resulting in constitutive overactivity, or they cause insertional mutagenesis.

### RNA VIRUSES

The study of RNA tumor retroviruses such as the Rous sarcoma virus has provided great insight into genetic events leading to the development of malignancies in numerous animal models.[34] Transforming retroviruses can be broadly categorized into two groups based on their molecular mechanisms of transformation.[35] The first category of virus, called *acutely transforming retroviruses*, harbors a mutated form of their host genes.[36, 37] The v-*src* gene from the Rous sarcoma virus is the archetypal example. This gene is not necessary for the function of the virus but was accidentally pirated from the host by transduction.[38] These altered copies of host genes do not contain introns and have mutations, which often make them more active when compared with the normal host counterpart. These mutations arise because the viruses have relatively low fidelity during their replication. When these oncogenic retroviruses infect cells, they express the altered form of their captured host gene. High levels of virus-driven

*Table 2–2.* **Viruses in Human Cancer**

| Virus | Tumors |
|---|---|
| Papillomaviruses | Uterine cervix |
| Hepatitis B and C | Liver |
| Epstein-Barr virus | Bone marrow, nasopharynx |
| Human T-cell leukemia virus | Thymus, spleen |
| HHV-8 | Bone marrow |

HHV, human herpes virus.

expression of the modified host gene deregulate the host cell cycle and result in increased cell proliferation. Such virally encoded genes are called *oncogenes*.[39] Their normal host cellular counterparts are called *proto-oncogenes*. More than 100 such viral oncogenes have been described. v-*src* was the first retroviral oncogene characterized in detail, but it has not been strongly implicated in human cancers, although there is a human form of the gene SRC that is important in cell proliferation. An excellent example important in human tumors is the v-H-*ras* oncogene, which is encoded by the Harvey murine sarcoma retrovirus. Analysis of this virus quickly identified this transforming gene, which is similar to the H-*ras* gene in the host cell. When the viral form of the gene was analyzed, it was determined that there was a mutation at amino acid residue 12, which decreased the guanosine triphosphatase (GTPase) activity of the viral oncogene.[40] The GTPase component is crucial for inactivation of *ras* genes. Consequently, the viral mutation made it more active than its normal cellular counterpart. The first mutated human proto-oncogene to be identified was isolated from a bladder carcinoma cell line. This gene was highly homologous to the v-H-*ras* oncogene and was shown to be activated by a point mutation that also decreased GTPase activity.[41–44] Analysis of many different types of retroviruses has yielded similar results; that is, there are genes carried in the genome of these viruses that readily transform host cells. These genes have a variety of functions in cells and include growth factors, growth factor receptors, signal transduction proteins, and transcription factors. These genes have in common the ability to cause increased cell growth when their activity is increased. Most human tumors are not caused by oncogenic viruses but by alteration of the host native proto-oncogenes.

The second, more common category of transforming retroviruses, are called *chronic tumor viruses*. They differ from acute transforming viruses in that they do not contain oncogenes. Instead, they transform cells by insertional mutagenesis. Once inserted into the host genome, the provirus upregulates the expression of neighboring genes. Several proto-oncogenes such as c-*myc*, H-*ras*, and c-*erb*B have been targets for insertional mutagenesis in animals. For example, the avian leukemia virus induces lymphomas by integrating upstream of the c-*myc* proto-oncogenes.[45] The long terminal repeat of the provirus strongly induces the expression of the avian c-*myc* gene. The deregulated c-*myc* increases proliferation and results in tumor formation.

Other retroviruses such as HTLV-1, HTLV-2, and HIV are associated with transformation, but the mechanisms are not as well understood. Transformation by these viruses may involve virally encoded proteins that lead to transformation, but they are not pirated counterparts of human genes as in the case of the viral oncogenes. For example the HTLV-1 Tax gene is thought to induce transformation through modification of host transcription factors such as NF-kB and CREB.[46, 47]

## DNA VIRUSES

Virtually every group of DNA virus (papovaviruses, papillomaviruses, adenoviruses, herpesviruses, hepadenaviruses, poxviruses) has been shown to be associated with tumors in animals. Several DNA viruses have been implicated in human tumorigenesis. The papovaviruses, in particular simian virus 40 (SV40), have provided tremendous insight into viral oncogenesis. Although they have not been proved to cause human malignancies directly, studies have suggested that this virus is found in certain human tumors, such as osteosarcomas and mesotheliomas.[48] SV40 was initially discovered as a contaminant in the poliomyelitis vaccine prepared in rhesus monkey cells.[49] The virus was inadvertently injected into millions of individuals who received the vaccine. When injected into rodents, this virus causes brain tumors and pancreatic endocrine tumors as well as other tumors.[50]

SV40 affects cells in one of two ways. In permissive cells, the virus proceeds through a lytic cycle. Alternatively, in nonpermissive cells, the virus may integrate into the host genome and effect transformation primarily through expression of the large T antigen.[51] This protein causes transformation by binding to two key cell cycle regulatory proteins, pRB (including p 107 and p130) and p53, thereby inactivating them.[52, 53] Virtually any rodent cell overexpressing the large T antigen will become transformed. This has been extensively exploited in a variety of transgenic mouse tumor models.

Human papillomaviruses (HPV) and adenoviruses are also oncogenic. In a manner similar to SV40, these viruses cause transformation by inactivating p53 and pRB. Human adenoviruses cause upper respiratory infections in humans, but some strains are oncogenic in rodents. The transformed cells contain integrated virus and express the E1A and E1B proteins. E1A binds and inactivates pRB, whereas E1B binds p53.[54, 55]

Certain strains of HPV are oncogenic in humans. HPV 16, 18, 31, 33, and 45 are found in about 90% of human cervical cancers.[56–58] However, only a small percentage of women infected with this virus acquire cervical cancer. The transforming ability of HPV depends on the integration and expression of the E6 and E7 proteins, which bind p53 and pRB, respectively.[59, 60]

The Epstein-Barr virus is associated with nasopharyngeal carcinoma and Burkitt's lymphoma. This virus induces transformation by expression of the latent membrane protein-2 (LMP2).[61] LMP2 contains a functional antigen recognition activation motif similar to that found on T-cell and B-cell antigen receptors. This protein induces proliferation by interacting with cytoplasmic tyrosine kinases.[62]

## Oncogenes in Human Cancer

From the study of retroviruses, it became clear that the transforming gene harbored by these viruses were authentic vertebrate genes that were pirated by the virus. These seminal observations in the v-*src* gene from the Rous sarcoma virus paved the way for the discovery of other viral oncogenes and their vertebrate counterparts, proto-oncogenes. Nearly all the known retroviral oncogenes have human counterpart proto-oncogenes.

Oncogenes in general are involved in cellular growth processes and their deregulation leads to proliferation and transformation. Although there are many viral oncogenes associated with animal models of tumorigenesis, many have not been proved to be directly involved in human tumors (Table 2–3). Some of these genes are expressed at high

*Table 2–3.* Oncogene Groups

| Oncogene | Virus | Function | Activation | Human Tumors |
|---|---|---|---|---|
| *Growth Factors* | | | | |
| INT-1 | | Matrix protein | | |
| INT-2 | | Fibroblast growth factor–related protein | A | Squamous cell cancer, breast cancer, bladder cancer |
| HST | | | A | Gastric cancer, breast cancer, bladder cancer |
| SIS | | Platelet-derived growth factor | | |
| *Growth Factor Receptors* (tyrosine kinase) | | | | |
| EGFR | | Epidermal growth factor receptor | A | Squamous carcinoma, glioblastoma |
| FMS | | M-CSF receptor | P | AML |
| KIT | | Stem cell growth factor receptor | | |
| MET | | Hepatic growth factor receptor | | |
| Her-2/*neu* | None | Heregulin receptor | A | Breast cancer, prostate cancer, gastric cancer, bladder cancer |
| RET | None | Glial cell–derived neurotrophic factor receptor | P, T | Medullary thyroid cancer, papillary thyroid cancer, MEN 2 |
| TRKA | | Nerve growth factor receptor | T | Papillary thyroid cancer |
| *G Proteins* | | | | |
| H-Ras | Harvey murine sarcoma virus | Small G protein | P | Leukemia, oral cancer, thyroid cancer |
| K-Ras | Kirsten murine sarcoma virus | Small G protein | P | Pancreatic cancer, colon cancer |
| N-Ras | None | Small G protein | P | Neuroblastoma, acute leukemia |
| *Cytoplasmic Kinases* | | | | |
| BCR-ABL | Abelson murine leukemia virus | Tyrosine kinase | T | CML |
| FES/FPS | Fuginami sarcoma virus | Tyrosine kinase | | |
| FGR | | | | |
| CBL | | | | |
| HCK | None | Tyrosine kinase | | |
| LCK | None | Tyrosine kinase | | |
| PIM | | | | |
| SRC | | Tyrosine kinase | | |
| YES | | Tyrosine kinase | | |
| RAF | | Serine threonine kinase | | |
| MOS | | Serine threonine kinase | | |
| *Other Cytoplasmic Proteins* | | | | |
| CRK | Avian sarcoma virus | Adapter protein | | |
| BCL-2 | | Antiapoptosis | A | B-cell lymphoma |
| *Nuclear Proteins* | | | | |
| ERB-A | | Thyroid hormone receptor | | |
| ETS | | Transcription factor | A | AML, lymphoma |
| FOS | | Transcription factor | | |
| MYB | | Transcription factor | A | Colon cancer, AML |
| FRA | | Transcription factor | | |
| JUN | | Transcription factor | | |
| L-MYC | | Transcription factor | A | Small cell lung cancer |
| C-MYC | | Transcription factor | A | Colon cancer, breast cancer, leukemia, stomach cancer |
| N-MYC | None | Transcription factor | A | Neuroblastoma, small cell lung cancer, retinoblastoma |
| REL | | Transcription factor | A | Leukemia |
| SKI | | Transcription factor | | |
| TAL-1 | | Transcription factor | T | Leukemia |
| LYL | | Transcription factor | T | Leukemia |
| MDM2 | | | A | Sarcomas |

A, amplification of DNA; P, point mutation; AML, acute myelogenous leukemia; T, translocation; MEN 2, multiple endocrine neoplasia, type 2; CML, chronic myelogenous leukemia.

levels, for example, but there are no associated malignancies associated with this overexpression.

Viral oncogenes are overactive by virtue of mutations within key functional regions of the protein. The mechanisms of proto-oncogene activation in human tumors are more diverse (Fig. 2–7). Some genes have point mutations similar to those of the retroviral oncogenes. In other instances, chromosome translocation or DNA amplification leads to uncontrolled overexpression. Fusion genes resulting from chromosome rearrangements can lead to altered gene activity. Some genes have increased transcription for unexplained reasons.

## POINT MUTATIONS

An excellent example of mutation leading to overactivity is the *ras* family of oncogenes. The *ras* oncogenes were the first human oncogenes cloned. This group of proteins (H-*ras*, K-*ras*, and N-*ras*) is implicated in the vast majority of tumors. For example, the K-*ras* oncogene is mutated in more than 90% of pancreatic adenocarcinomas and a significant number of colon cancers.[63] *ras* proteins are part of a large family of GTPase proteins that are involved in signal transduction within the cell (see Fig. 2–5). These proteins convey signals from growth factor tyrosine kinase receptors to the nucleus, resulting in alterations in cell growth. They act through the MAPK pathway.[64] RAS functions by binding GTP and thereby becomes activated.[41] After binding GTP, RAS performs its signaling function. This function is terminated by hydrolyzing the GTP to GDP. If the GTPase activity of the *ras* protein is inhibited, the protein remains in the GTP-bound active state. This results in overactivity of the *ras* protein and excessive cell signaling without the presence of an activated receptor. When the *ras* genes are mutated, the GTPase activity is reduced and the proteins remain in the activated state for a prolonged period. The mutations resulting in increased activity are very specific. The sequenc-

ing of this gene in several types of cancer has revealed that mutations involving codons 12, 13, and 61—which are critical for the GTPase activity of the protein—result in increased *ras* activity.[65] There are several efforts afoot to develop tumor therapy based on restoring the activity of these genes.

One therapeutic target in the *ras* pathway is an enzyme important for RAS post-translational modification. In order for *ras* to become functional, it must be attached to the inner plasma membrane by a short-chain fatty acid. One of the enzymes involved in this processing, farnesyl transferase, can be effectively inhibited by several drugs that are now in clinical trials.[66] One such drug not only inhibits *ras* farnesylation but also affects other important target proteins that have not been identified. This is significant because one of the three forms of *ras* called K-*ras* can be modified by pathways independent of farnesyl transferase. Fortunately, the farnesyl inhibitors still block the growth of some tumors with K-*ras* mutations. Other drugs are being developed to target the downstream effectors of the *ras* pathway as well as the receptor tyrosine kinases (e.g., genistein).

## OVEREXPRESSION

The second major mechanism for increased activity of oncogenes is by overexpression (see Fig. 2–7). This may occur through a variety of genetic mechanisms, including chromosome translocation, DNA amplification, and enhanced gene transcription. Chromosome translocations involving the *myc* oncogene on chromosome 8 and the immunoglobin heavy chain gene on chromosome 14 result in enhanced expression of the *myc* oncogene under the immunoglobin promoter in patients with Burkitt's lymphoma and plasmacytomas.[67] Overactivity of the *myc* oncogene, which is a transcription factor, results in increased expression of genes important in promotion of the progression of the cell cycle. The *myc* gene expressed is a normal unaltered protein. Because of the

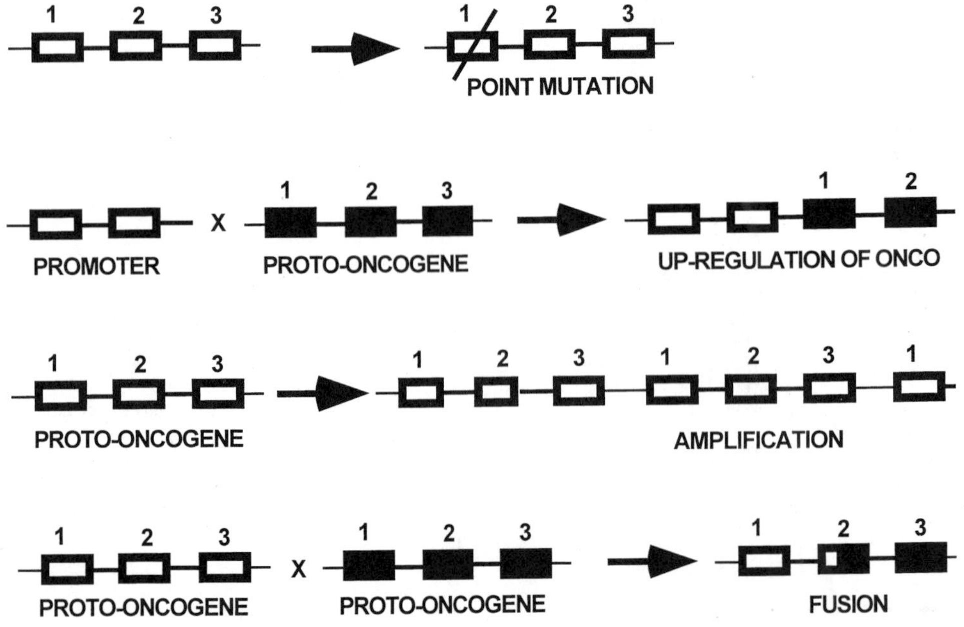

**Figure 2–7.** Mechanisms responsible for oncogene activation.

overexpression of the normal gene, the cell becomes transformed. Chromosome 8 translocations involving chromosomes 2 and 22 correspond to the kappa light chain and lambda light chain genes, respectively, and also result in dysregulated *myc* expression. Similar rearrangements lead to activation of numerous other oncogenes such as ETS-1 in acute myelogenous leukemia (AML) and small cell lymphoma and *bcl-2* in B-cell lymphomas.

DNA amplification is an important example of oncogene activation in breast cancer, in which the HER-2/*neu* oncogene is present in multiple copies within the tumor cells in more aggressive tumors.[68] This gene is a tyrosine kinase receptor, and increased expression of HER-2/*neu* results in increased mammary cell proliferation. HER-2/*neu* is highly expressed in 30% of breast cancer cases and correlates with prognosis. Its increased expression is achieved by DNA amplification, a process whereby many copies of the HER-2/*neu* oncogene are present within the tumor cells. Usually this is because there are duplications of the gene within the chromosome containing this oncogene. The excess number of copies of the gene results in higher amounts of the RNA being transcribed and consequently more protein receptor expressed on the cell surface. When the receptors are present in high numbers on the cell surface, they autophosphorylate and remain active.[69] The number of copies of the gene per cell, as well as protein expression, correlates with the aggressiveness of the tumors. This is clinically useful in planning treatment for these patients.[70, 71] One of the best examples of gene-directed therapy is the development of an antibody to the HER-2/*neu* receptor for therapy.[72] Numerous other genes are amplified in tumors such as cyclin D1 and *bcl-2* in several types of cancer, mdm2 in sarcomas, N-*myc* in neuroblastomas, and c-*myc* in breast cancer.

Some oncogenes are overexpressed either by alterations in their transcriptional machinery or mutations within their promoters. This results in overexpression of growth factors or cell signal molecules, which are important in enhancing cell growth and proliferation.

## TRANSLOCATION

The third mechanism of oncogene activation is translocation and fusion. This is the mechanism involved in chronic myelogenous leukemia and the Philadelphia chromosome that results from a reciprocal translocation between chromosomes 9q and 22q. This results in a fusion between the *abl* gene on chromosome 9 and the *bcr* gene on chromosome 22. The resultant protein has increased tyrosine kinase activity. An interesting translocation occurs between chromosomes 15 and 17 in acute promyelocytic leukemia. In this translocation, there is a fusion between the PML gene on chromosome 15 and the retinoic acid receptor α (RAR-α) on chromosome 17.[73] The fusion protein has altered DNA binding and transcriptional properties. Many of these patients respond to treatment with retinoic acid derivitives.

## Oncogenes and Mitogenic Signaling Pathways

Cell growth is a highly regulated process and to a large extent is controlled by extracellular signals. Secreted growth factors or cytokines bind to cell surface receptors that are usually tyrosine kinases with the exception of the transforming growth factor-β (TGF-β) receptor, which is a serine-threonine kinase. In the absence of serum and growth factors, cells stop proliferating and enter $G_0$. Transformed cells continue to grow independent of growth factors or at reduced requirements. How this independence is achieved is not completely understood but occurs in some tumors by activation of oncogenes that drive cell proliferation through mitogenic signaling pathways.

The best understood mitogenic pathway involves receptor tyrosine kinases such as HER-2/*neu*. Binding of the ligand to the receptor alters their conformation, which triggers the receptors to cluster and transphosphorylate each other. This phosphorylation can also be triggered in the absence of ligand if the receptors are present at high densities, as in the case of HER-2/*neu* amplification in breast cancer. Receptor phosphorylation recruits cytoplasmic proteins to the receptor, which transmit the mitogenic signal to the nucleus. Several types of cytoplasmic proteins can transmit the signal. They share a common sequence called the src homology domain-2 (SH2).[74] This protein-binding sequence was first described in the *src* oncogene and hence the name was given to the domain sequence. The SH2 domain specifically binds phosphorylated tyrosines that are present in the activated receptor. The SH2-containing cytoplasmic proteins are often enzymes whose activity is increased by phosphorylation. These include phospholipases, phosphatidylinositol 3-kinase, protein tyrosine phosphatases, and src kinases. Besides these enzymes, there are adapter proteins that do not have enzymatic activity but serve to connect to proteins that do have enzymatic activity. On binding the receptor, the SH2-containing protein is phosphorylated by tyrosine, which induces a conformational change. These changes in the SH2-containing protein facilitate binding to the next protein in the signal cascade and, if it is an enzyme, increase its activity.

One of the SH2-containing proteins attracted to the receptor is GRB2.[75] GRB2, in turn, binds to SOS, which functions as a guanine nucleotide exchange factor for RAS proteins. This activates RAS by exchanging GDP for GTP. Activated RAS may then interact with a variety of downstream targets. Activated RAS then binds to another protein, RAF, which is a serine-threonine kinase.[76] This leads to activation of the extracellular regulated kinase (ERK) pathway, which is one of the MAPK pathways.[77] *raf* activates MAPK or ERK kinase (MEK), which, in turn, activates members of the ERK family. Activated ERKs translocate to the nucleus, where they phosphorylate certain transcription factors such as *jun* and *fos*. Hence the signal that began at the outer membrane receptor tyrosine kinase has been communicated to the nucleus, where key regulatory proteins are affected. It is also apparent that constitutional activation of certain oncogenes such as *ras* by mutation in a tumor cell would lead to continuous proliferation signals. It is not clear why other members in this pathway are not commonly altered in human cancers.

## Tumor Suppressor Genes

Tumor suppressor genes, in contrast to oncogenes, normally act to slow the growth of cells. Loss of activity of such genes through mutation causes deregulation of the cell cycle, contributing to tumor formation. The initial notion that tumor suppressor genes existed was based on experiments with somatic cell hybrids and studies of retinoblastomas. Through these studies, the retinoblastoma gene became the archetypal tumor suppressor gene and elucidated the role of tumor suppressor genes in cancer. Through the study of other inherited and sporadic tumors, numerous candidate tumor suppressor genes have been identified.

Somatic cell hybrids are formed when two different somatic cells are fused together (Fig. 2–8). The resulting hybrid contains the chromosomal material from the two parent cells. Growth of the hybrid is governed by the genetic constitution of the parental cells. The ability of such hybrids to form tumors is determined by inoculating the hybrid cells into nude mice. The tumorigenicity of the hybrid is determined by comparing the growth of the hybrid cells with that of the parent cells.[78]

When human cervical carcinoma (HeLa) cells were fused with human fibroblast cells, the hybrid did not form tumors.[79, 80] This suggested that the normal parent (fibroblast) contributed genes that imposed negative growth control (a "brake" on the cell cycle) on the tumorigenic cell (HeLa). It was presumed that the negative growth control genes contributed by the normal cell were lost by the tumor cell during its transformation process. Subsequent experiments demonstrated that a small number of specific chromosomes (genes) are required to restore normal growth to a transformed cell.[81, 82] These experiments indicated that tumor formation could result from the loss of genes that normally act to suppress cell growth. Support for this hypothesis at a molecular level came from the study of retinoblastomas.

The retinoblastoma gene is the best studied example of tumor suppressor genes.[83] Retinoblastoma, a tumor of the embryonic neural retina, occurs in 1 of 20,000 children. It usually develops before 5 years of age and accounts for 1% of childhood cancer deaths. It is inherited in an autosomal

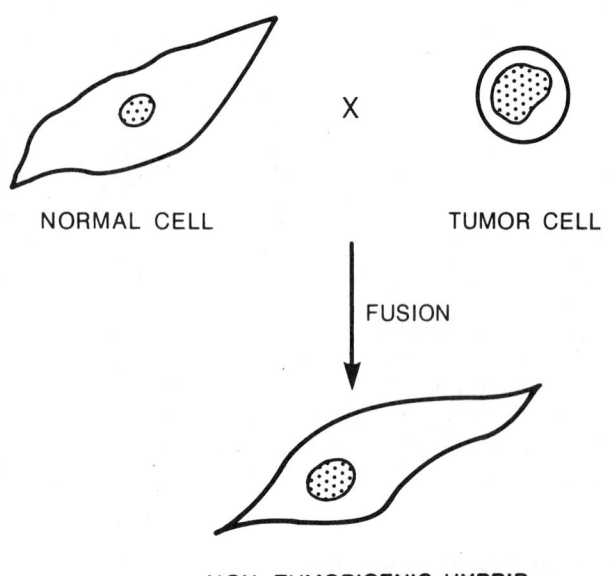

**Figure 2–8.** Somatic cell hybrid. The fusion of a normal cell with a malignant cell is shown. The resultant hybrid is nontumorigenic.

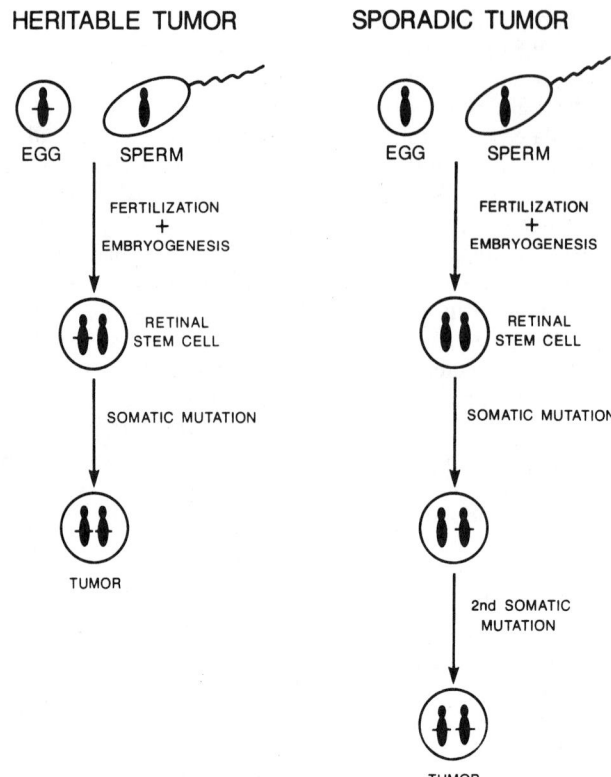

**Figure 2–9.** Knudson's two-hit hypothesis. In this model of tumor suppressor genes, both hereditary and sporadic tumors may arise from two mutations within the predisposing gene. In the hereditary form, one mutation is inherited (indicated by a slash through the chromosome symbol) and the other occurs as a random event in a somatic cell during mitosis.

dominant fashion with nearly 100% penetrance. Approximately 40% of cases are hereditary, and most of these cases represent new germline mutations. The hereditary form is usually bilateral, multifocal, and associated with an increased incidence of many other types of tumors. The sporadic form is uniformly unilateral and unifocal.

Based on epidemiologic data, Knudson postulated a genetic mechanism, the "two-hit" hypothesis, for the development of retinoblastomas (Fig. 2–9).[84] After studying patients with sporadic and hereditary retinoblastomas, he hypothesized that hereditary retinoblastomas are caused by two independent genetic mutations (or "hits") occurring within the same embryonal retinal cell. It was hypothesized that the first mutation was inherited. Inheriting one mutated gene alone was not sufficient to initiate tumor formation. Thus, although all the embryonal retinal cells have inherited the mutated gene, few go on to form tumors. Knudson argued that it required a second mutation in the embryonal retinal cell to result in a transformed retinoblastoma cell. In the familial form, one mutation would be inherited and therefore all retinal stem cells would have one mutation present at birth. The second event would occur as a somatic mutation in a random cell whose genotype (two mutations) would then favor neoplastic growth. He did not know whether these mutations occurred within the same gene or different genes.

The same two-hit hypothesis could also be applied to sporadic retinoblastomas. In the sporadic retinoblastoma, the same predisposing gene would be involved, but the origin of the mutations would be different. In contrast to hereditary tumors, sporadic tumors arise from a retinal stem cell that has two mutations occurring as independent somatic events but that result in the same tumor genotype as the familial form.

Several pieces of information led to the discovery that the mutations that Knudson described involved the retinoblastoma gene (Rb). First, cytogenetic studies of both white blood cells from children with familial retinoblastoma and tumor cells from patients with sporadic retinoblastomas showed loss of a specific portion of the long arm of chromosome 13 (13q14). Second, DNA linkage studies showed tight linkage between the esterase D locus at 13q14 and familial retinoblastoma. Third, analysis of both sporadic and familial retinoblastomas showed loss of alleles (loss of heterozygosity) for DNA markers spanning the region of 13q14.

The initial clue for the location of the retinoblastoma gene came from cytogenetic studies.[85] Karyotype analysis of the peripheral blood white blood cells of patients with familial retinoblastoma showed interstitial deletions of 13q14 in 5% of the cases. Studies in sporadic tumors showed that approximately 25% had similar interstitial deletions. Thus, deletions within 13q14 were involved in the formation of both familial and sporadic tumors.

Additional evidence that the retinoblastoma susceptibility gene was located at 13q14 came from genetic linkage studies.[86] The genetic marker esterase D mapped to 13q14 is polymorphic. By studying families who were informative for this marker (i.e., the proband is heterozygous), it was shown that the retinoblastoma susceptibility gene is linked to the esterase D gene (i.e., they are near each other on the chromosome).

The ability to show loss of alleles from DNA markers in the region spanning 13q14 in both the sporadic and familial tumors was the third clue. The impetus for this approach came from the cytogenetic studies showing a deletion involving 13q14 in a few retinoblastoma patients. This suggested that the critical event for tumor development was the

loss of genes at this band. Applying this information to Knudson's hypothesis suggested that the two mutations required to initiate tumorigenesis could inactivate both alleles of a gene at 13q14.

In patients with familial retinoblastoma, cytogenetic observations indicated that the inherited or first mutation was usually small and not easily detected; only 5% of patients had a visible change in the karyotype at 13q14. The second mutation affecting the other allele could arise through one of four possible mechanisms (Fig. 2–10).[87] First, there may be another small mutation like the first. Detecting such alterations in the retinoblastoma gene could be studied only after the gene was cloned. The other three mechanisms result in more gross changes not only involving the retinoblastoma gene but also affecting a large region surrounding the retinoblastoma gene. They include mitotic nondisjunction, both with and without duplication of the chromosome harboring the mutant allele, and mitotic recombination involving the mutant allele. These latter three mechanisms could be easily identified by analyzing the tumors with DNA markers near the retinoblastoma gene.

The genetic mechanisms involved with the second mutation could be demonstrated by showing that the tumors had allele loss for DNA markers near the retinoblastoma gene. Allele loss is identified by comparing the DNA from the patient's somatic cells (usually peripheral blood white blood cells) with that of the tumor cells. When one of the two alleles for each DNA marker is simply lost, the tumor is hemizygous for that marker. Similarly, when one allele is lost and the remaining allele is duplicated, the tumor is said to be homozygous. Collectively, these mechanisms are referred to as loss of heterozygosity (LOH). LOH could in fact be demonstrated near the putative site of the retinoblastoma gene in these tumors.

The initial approach to demonstrating LOH in tumors used the genetic marker esterase D.[88, 89] Esterase D was a convenient genetic marker because it is linked to the retinoblastoma susceptibility gene (Rb) and is polymorphic. In these experiments, patients who had both alleles in their

CONSTITUTIONAL

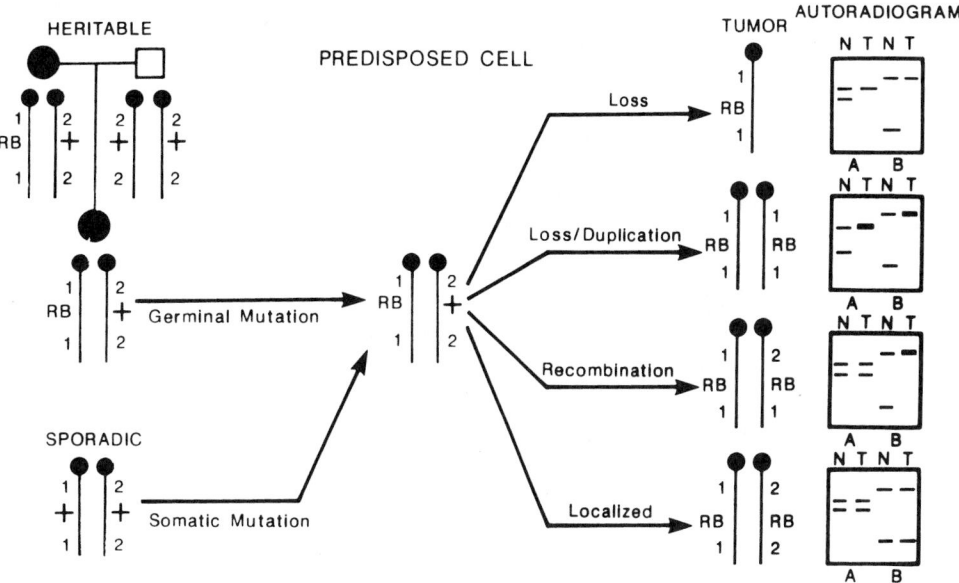

**Figure 2–10.** Mechanism of tumor suppressor gene inactivation. Illustrating the heritable form of retinoblastoma is a simple pedigree in which the son has inherited the predisposing mutated retinoblastoma allele (RB) from his mother. He also inherits a normal allele (+) from his father. One of the predisposed retinal stem cells containing one mutated allele (RB) and one normal allele (+) then undergoes one of the four hypothesized mechanisms to inactivate the normal allele. With both alleles inactivated by mutation, tumor formation ensues. Also illustrated is the sporadic case in which a random normal retinal stem cell undergoes two somatic mutations, which leads to tumor formation.

white blood cells (heterozygous) had a single esterase D allele (homozygous) in their tumors. Furthermore, in familial cases, the allele that was lost was the one inherited from the normal parent. Since the esterase D locus was homozygous in the tumor, the linked retinoblastoma gene would also be expected to be homozygous. The resultant cell would then contain only the mutant Rb allele that presumably was nonfunctional.

Further evidence of LOH in retinoblastomas was found in restriction fragment length polymorphism (RFLP) studies. DNA probes can be used to identify polymorphisms within the DNA sequence.[90] These polymorphisms result from variation in the DNA sequence that alters the restriction enzyme recognition site. This gives rise to an RFLP for that probe–restriction enzyme combination. These RFLPs are identified as distinct bands on the autoradiogram from a Southern blot. The bands on the autoradiogram represent the two parent alleles at the locus identified by the DNA marker, one from the maternally derived and one from the paternally derived chromosomal homologues. If the patient is homozygous for the DNA marker, the Southern blot will show a single allele or band. If the patient is heterozygous, the Southern blot will show two alleles or bands.

The mechanisms causing the second mutation during tumor formation can be determined by comparing the patient's somatic and tumor genotypes at each of these marker loci near the Rb locus and by examining which portion of the chromosome appears to have LOH. LOH in a tumor for a particular DNA marker is identified by comparing the autoradiographic pattern of the somatic DNA with that of the tumor. If LOH is present, one of the bands present on the autoradiogram of the somatic DNA will be absent in the tumor DNA. Such an alteration represents the loss of one of the alleles for that locus. Densitometry of the band on the autoradiogram can determine if the locus is homozygous (two copies of the allele) or hemizygous (one copy of the allele). Knowing whether the locus is hemizygous or homozygous helps determine the mechanism of the second mutation. Identifying these alterations requires that the patient be heterozygous for that DNA marker. The chance that any individual will be heterozygous for a given DNA marker varies. Therefore, for complete analysis, several markers spanning the region must be examined. Many recombinant DNA markers that identify RFLPs have been isolated that span chromosome 13 and have been used to determine somatic changes in retinoblastomas.

Southern analysis of 33 retinoblastomas showed LOH for DNA markers near the Rb locus in 24 (75%) of these tumors.[91] These mutations result from the three genetic mechanisms described earlier. In 20 of 33 cases, there was LOH at all informative loci along the entire chromosome. In 19 of these cases, densitometry of the remaining alleles suggested that each locus had become homozygous during transformation. These data are consistent with nondisjunction and duplication of the remaining abnormal homologue. In one case, the remaining alleles were hemizygous, consistent with the sole loss of chromosome 13 without reduplication. Evidence for mitotic recombination between the chromosomal homologues was found in 4 of 33 tumors. In these tumors, there was LOH for markers beginning centromeric to the Rb locus and for all distal long arm markers. Densitometry of the remaining alleles was consistent with homo-

zygosity. In 9 of 33 alleles, there was no evidence of LOH and these were presumed to involve localized events that could not be easily detected by the methods used. Other studies have substantiated these findings, with LOH at 13q14 ranging from about 10 to 60%.[92–94]

These studies suggest that the second hit is chromosomal rearrangement involving the physical loss of the wild-type allele at the retinoblastoma locus. This has been corroborated by examining cases of heritable retinoblastoma. The chromosome 13 homologue retained in the tumor was derived from the affected parent as would be predicted.[95]

The Rb gene was isolated by positional cloning techniques.[96–99] It is 180 kb and contains 27 exons that code for a 4.7-kb mRNA translated into a 105-kb nuclear phosphoprotein. The Rb gene is expressed in normal retinoblasts. Most retinoblastomas have either absent Rb mRNA or truncated or, rarely, elongated transcripts by Northern blot. The gene is mutated in 30% of cases as determined by Southern analysis, and in many cases both alleles can be found to be mutated. Southern analysis, however, provides only gross information and is insensitive to small mutations. More detailed analyses have revealed subtle changes in the gene sequence that affect the splicing of the 4.7-kb mRNA or cause premature termination of transcription. Most convincing are experiments in which the Rb gene has been reintroduced into cell lines and reversed their malignant phenotype.[100] Taken together, these data suggest that inactivation of both Rb alleles is necessary for retinoblastoma tumor formation. This is consistent with Knudson's two-hit hypothesis.[84]

One might expect that the retinoblastoma gene would show tissue-specific expression in the retina and only be mutated in retinoblastomas. It was quickly discovered, however, that the retinoblastoma gene was expressed in a variety of normal tissues. Furthermore, inactivation of the retinoblastoma gene has been implicated in the formation of several tumors, including osteosarcomas and other soft tissue sarcomas, breast cancer, small cell carcinoma of the lung, esophageal carcinoma, leukemia, and bladder cancer. It is not surprising that since the gene is ubiquitously expressed, it has been implicated in a variety of tumor types.

It is of particular interest that the retinoblastoma gene was found to be inactivated in osteosarcomas. These tumors are one of many secondary lesions found in patients with hereditary retinoblastoma. Such hereditary osteosarcomas were the first tumors, besides retinoblastomas, that were discovered to demonstrate inactivation of the retinoblastoma gene. Subsequently, it was shown that inactivation of the retinoblastoma gene is important for the development of the sporadic osteosarcomas as well as many other soft tissue sarcomas. This line of inquiry is an excellent example of how the study of a rare familial cancer syndrome has helped elucidate our understanding of the role of tumor suppressor genes in other tumors.

The retinoblastoma paradigm has provided a useful framework for the study of other tumor suppressor genes. Furthermore, it has led to the search for other possible tumor suppressor genes on other chromosomes through the use of DNA probes that systematically look for LOH in tumors.

pRB was the first tumor suppressor gene identified. The function of pRB is to regulate the progression of cells through the $G_1$ to S transition. As described earlier, when pRB is phosphorylated, it releases the E2F transcription factors that promote the synthesis of DNA synthesis–related genes. Inactivation of pRB leads to the loss of this regulatory control, and the cell continues to proliferate. Although RB is an important gatekeeper of the cell cycle, it is regulated by several other proteins that are either oncogenes or tumor suppressor genes. pRB is phosphorylated by cdk4 and cdk6 following their activation by cyclin D1, which is amplified and overexpressed in several tumors such as breast cancer and oral cancer. Overexpression of this oncogene leads to continuous phosphorylation of pRB, which effectively inactivates it as if it were deleted. An important regulator of cdk4 is p16, which inhibits the kinase function of cdk4 and functions as a tumor suppressor. Mutation inactivation of p16 has been reported in a variety of tumors.

The p53 tumor suppressor gene is a frequent target in many tumors. The primary function of p53 is to arrest cell cycle progression or initiate programmed cell death in response to cell damage. The functional role of p53 has been studied extensively in models of DNA damage. When ionizing radiation causes DNA damage, p53 is activated through a mechanism involving the ataxia-telengiectasia (ATM) protein. Activated p53 then functions as a transcription factor to induce the expression of p21, a CDK inhibitor. This delays the $G_1$ to S transition, allowing the cells time to repair the DNA damage. Alternatively, the cell may undergo apoptosis depending on the circumstances.

Other tumor suppressor genes have a variety of functions within the cell. They all share in common the theme of inactivation, which leads to increased cell growth. A group of these genes affect transcription regulation. p53 is a transcription factor, as described earlier. The Wilms' tumor gene (WT1) functions as a transcriptional repressor of some genes such as the insulin growth factor (IGF) receptor protein and an activator affecting certain genes such as the Rb-associated protein (RbAP46) important for inhibiting cell growth. The von Hippel-Lindau gene (VHL) regulates transcriptional elongation by RNA polymerase II. An important gene affected is VEGF. The multiple endocrine neoplasia type 1 gene functions as a transcription factor and represses JUN D–mediated transcription. NF2 is involved in the actin cytoskeleton organization. NF1 is a *ras*-associated GTPase-activating protein (RAS GAP). The familial polyposis coli gene, APC, is involved with β-catenin regulation.

## DNA Repair Genes

A number of genes are directly involved with DNA damage repair and function as caretakers of the genome. Inactivation of these genes leads to more frequent mutations in genes that are critical for cell growth regulation. Patients with hereditary nonpolyposis colorectal cancer (HNPCC) have a genetic predisposition to colon cancer as well as endometrial and ovarian cancer. The first clue linking this disease to DNA repair was the discovery that repeated sequences of DNA in the HNPCC tumors were not faithfully replicated during cell division. This phenomenon is called *microsatellite instability* and is so named because microsatellite sequences in DNA, for example, (CA)20, are not faithfully copied and extra base pairs are introduced into the daughter

strands during DNA replication. Drawing on knowledge of DNA repair in single-celled organisms, the human mismatch repair genes MSH-2, PMS2, and MLH-1 were found to be mutated in the germline of patients with HNPCC. Two genes that are commonly affected in patients with defects in the mismatch repair enzyme system include the gene for transforming growth factor-β and the apoptosis-inducing protein BAX. Sporadic forms of colorectal cancer also have mutations in these mismatch repair genes as well as others (GTBP, MSH3, polymerase-δ). Other genes involved in DNA repair that are also associated with the genetic predisposition to cancer include p53 (see preceding discussion), BRCA1, BRCA2, ATM, FACC, FACA, XPA, XPB, XPD, and BLM (see further on).

## Inherited Cancer Syndromes

Inherited tumor susceptibility syndromes have provided great insight into the inner workings of cancer. At least 20 known syndromes have been identified (Table 2–4). The majority of these syndromes arise through mutation of "gatekeepers" that include tumor suppressors and oncogenes. Most of these arise from mutations of tumor suppressor genes such as Rb and p53. Not surprisingly, only a few syndromes are known to arise from oncogenes (*mbt, cdk4,* and *ret*). Some inherited cancer syndromes arise from the mutation of DNA repair genes, the so-called caretakers. These include HNPCC, hereditary breast cancer, ataxia telangiectasia, xeroderma pigmentosum, and Fanconi's anemia. Although all of these are caused by mutation inactivation of DNA repair enzymes, the predisposing tumors are different in each case.

Mutations of DPC4 within the stromal cells surrounding the colon epithelia have been shown to promote colon hamartomatous polyps as well as the development of colorectal cancer in patients with familial juvenile polyposis. This is in contrast to the classic colon cancer tumor model in which the cancer grows because of a series of mutations in the epithelial stem cell. These "landscaper" defects arise because of mutations in the stromal cells that affect the microenvironment of the epithelial cells, leading to cancer formation. In this model, the epithelial cell is driven to proliferate because of changes in the microenvironment driven by defects in the surrounding stromal cells.

## Chemical Carcinogenesis

Most cancers develop as a consequence of genetic and environmental factors. Fortunately, genetics accounts for only 5% of human cancers. The balance is thought to be largely due to environmental factors (Table 2–5). There is reason for optimism as the latter effects should be largely preventable.

Chemical carcinogens vary tremendously. They share in common the ability to form covalent adducts with proteins or DNA. In some instances, they can do this directly and in others they must be activated by metabolic pathways. Once such a carcinogen binds to DNA, a DNA replication error may result during the next cell division. If this occurs within

*Table 2–4.* Inherited Cancer Syndromes

| Syndrome | Tumors | Gene | Function |
|---|---|---|---|
| Familial retinoblastoma | Retinoblastoma | Rb | Cell cycle and transcriptional regulation |
| | Osteosarcoma | | |
| Familial adenomatous polyposis | Colon and other GI tract adenomas | APC | Regulation of β-catenin |
| Li-Fraumeni syndrome | Sarcomas | p53 | Transcription factor |
| | Breast cancer | | |
| | Brain tumors | | |
| | Leukemia | | |
| Multiple endocrine neoplasia, type 1 | Parathyroid hyperplasia | MENIN | Transcription factor |
| | Pancreatic endocrine tumors | | |
| | Pituitary adenomas | | |
| Multiple endocrine neoplasia, type 2 | Medullary thyroid cancer | RET | GDNF receptor |
| | Pheochromocytoma | | |
| | Parathyroid hyperplasia | | |
| von Hippel-Lindau syndrome | Renal cancer | VHL | Regulates transcription elongation by RNA polymerase II |
| | Pheochromocytoma | | |
| | Retinal angiomas | | |
| | Hemangioblastomas | | |
| Neurofibromatosis, type I | Neurofibromas | NF1 | RAS GTPase-activating protein |
| | AML | | |
| | Brain tumors | | |
| Neurofibromatosis, type II | Acoustic neuromas | NF2 | Actin-cytoskeletal organization |
| | Meningiomas | | |
| Wilms' tumor | Wilms' tumor | WT1 | Transcription factor |
| Familial breast cancer I | Breast cancer | BRCA1 | DNA repair |
| | Ovarian cancer | | |
| Familial breast cancer II | Breast cancer | BRCA2 | DNA repair |
| | Pancreatic cancer | | |
| Hereditary nonpolyposis colorectal cancer (HNPCC) | Endometrial cancer | MSH2, | DNA mismatch repair |
| | Ovarian cancer | MLH1, | |
| | Hepatobiliary cancer | PMS1, | |
| | Urogenital cancer | PMS2 | |
| | Colorectal cancer | | |
| Cowden's disease | Breast cancer | PTEN | Phosphatase involved with P13 kinase/AKT2 signal regulation |
| | Thyroid cancer | | |
| Hereditary papillary renal cancer (HRPC) | Renal cancer | MET | Receptor for hGF |
| Familial melanoma | Melanoma and pancreatic cancer | CDKN2 (p16) | Inhibitor of cdk4 and cdk6 cyclin-dependent kinases |
| Ataxia telangiectasia (AT) | Lymphoma | ATM | DNA repair |
| Bloom's syndrome | Solid tumors | BLM | DNA helicase |
| Xeroderma pigmentosum | Skin cancer | XPB, XPA₃, XPD | DNA repair helicases |
| Fanconi's anemia | AML | FACC, FACA | DNA repair |
| Nevoid basal cell carcinoma syndrome | Basal cell skin cancer | PTCH | Receptor for hedgehog signaling molecule |
| Familial juvenile polyposis | Hamartomatous polyps | DPC4 | TGF-β signal pathway |
| | | PTEN | Phosphatase |

GI, gastrointestinal; GDNF, glial cell line–derived neurotrophic factor; hGF, human growth factor; TGF-β, transforming growth factor-β.

DNA segments that encode for proteins or within key regulatory regions, protein dysfunction may lead to altered cell growth. The metabolic pathways that cause biotransformation of these carcinogens are composed of several multigene enzyme families. Bioactivation usually leads to inactivation of toxic substances within the bloodstream. In the case of carcinogens, the "detoxification" process actually activates the offending agent.

Drug-metabolizing enzymes are broadly categorized into phase I and phase II based on their mechanism of action. Phase I enzymes include the well-known cytochrome P450 mono-oxygenase family. These are membrane-bound enzymes that oxidize carbon, nitrogen, and sulfur atoms to produce hydroxylated metabolites. Such activated metabolites, as well as the less common directly acting carcinogens,

interact with DNA by transfering an alkyl group, arylamine group, or an aralkyl group. Phase II enzymes include epoxide hydrolase, glutathione S-transferase, *N*-acetyltransferase, and sulfotransferase. These enzymes detoxify chemicals by converting them to excretable hydrophilic products.

Once a DNA strand has been modified by a carcinogen, there are several mechanisms of repair. These include direct repair by removing the adduct, mismatch repair, and base or nucleotide excision. In direct repair, the adduct is enzymatically removed from the nucleotide and the normal DNA strand remains. Several methylating agents such as *N*-methyl-*N*′-nitro-*N*-nitrosoguanidine (MNNG) can alkylate DNA to produce *O*-alkylated and *N*-alkylated products. The most biologically significant product is the *O*6-methylated derivative of guanine, which can aberrantly pair with thymine

*Table 2–5.* Human Carcinogens

| Agent | Cancer Site |
| --- | --- |
| Aflatoxin | Liver |
| Alcohol | Oral cavity, larynx, esophagus, and liver |
| Aromatic amines | Bladder |
| Alkylating agents | Leukemia |
| Estrogen | Endometrium |
| Polycyclic aromatic hydrocarbons | Skin, lung |
| Tobacco | Oral, esophagus, lung, bladder, pancreas, kidney, cervix |

instead of cytosine and result in a transition G:C to A:T during the next round of DNA replication. This alkylated product is directly repaired by *O*6-methylguanine-DNA methyltransferase (MGMT).

The mismatch repair system repairs single-base mispairs and small insertion-deletion mispairs. This system, which is operative during DNA replication, was originally described in bacteria as replication error repair. Human homologues of this system include hMSH2, hMLH1, hPMS1, hPMS2, and GTBP. This system is inefficient for repairing carcinogens because during the repair process, the mismatched base is removed instead of the offending adduct base. The nucleotide and base excision repair system is more effective and operative on bulky adducts.

Genetic susceptibility to cancer is obvious in certain inherited cancer syndromes. Less obvious, but probably more common, are genetic polymorphisms in enzymes involved in carcinogen metabolism. For example, many P450 enzymes catalyze the oxidative metabolism of chemicals, thereby making them carcinogens. Many P450 genes are polymorphic, such as CYP1A1, whose product metabolizes polycyclic aromatic hydrocarbons. Approximately 10% of the American population has a genetic polymorphism within this gene that is associated with an increased risk of lung cancer in smokers. It is hypothesized that these forms of the enzyme have higher inducibility or enhanced catalytic activity. Another enzyme, GST, is important for detoxifying reactive intermediates of polycyclic aromatic hydrocarbons and is commonly deleted from the genomes of approximately 50% of whites, with an associated increased risk of lung and bladder cancer. NAT2 deactivates carcinogens through *N*-acetylation. Many individuals are slow acetylators. Some studies suggest that these slow acetylators are at higher risk for the development of bladder cancer when exposed to certain carcinogens. Similar effects on cancer risk have been associated with polymorphisms of certain receptors, such as the aromatic hydrocarbon receptor, which results in upregulation of the P450 enzymes. These genes are an important target for chemoprevention and risk assessment. Additional studies by molecular epidemiologists will have a significant impact on the development of these strategies.

## Angiogenesis, Invasion, and Metastasis

Metastasis involves the capacity of neoplastic cells to detach from a primary tumor and disseminate to other parts of the body to form secondary tumors. It represents the major cause of death from cancers and defines a neoplasm as malignant. It requires that the neoplastic cells invade local tissues with invasion of the basement membrane. In addition, for tumors to grow beyond a minimal size, they must be able to induce angiogenesis, which is the process of the development of new blood vessels to supply necessary nutrients. Subsequently, malignant cells must detach from the primary tumor, invade into and circulate in the vasculature, and adhere to distant tissues, where tumor growth is again promoted by local invasion and angiogenesis (Fig. 2–11).

Angiogenesis plays a crucial role in the growth of both primary and metastatic tumors. In the absence of its own blood supply, a tumor is restricted in its growth by the capacity of oxygen and nutrients to diffuse; such tumors are consequently limited in size. In contrast, a tumor that is able to generate its own blood supply can theoretically grow to any size.

The process of angiogenesis is complex and involves soluble proangiogenic and antiangiogenic factors (Table 2–6) that can be produced by the tumor clone itself or by non-neoplastic cells that are present in the tumor microenvironment. Angiogenic factors act on vascular endothelial cells, resulting in their migration or proliferation, or both. Tumor necrosis factor-α stimulates migration of endothelial cells, whereas vascular endothelial growth factor (VEGF) induces endothelial cell proliferation. VEGF appears to be a relatively important factor in angiogenesis of malignancies because it is highly expressed in a variety of solid and hematologic tumors. Two VEGF receptors have been identified on endothelial cells, FLK1 and FLT1. Neutralizing antibodies to these receptors, as well as inhibition of other proangiogenic factors, have resulted in suppression of human tumors in murine models.[101] It should be noted that many of the soluble factors that are involved in angiogenesis have nonangiogenic effects, including but not limited to induction of proliferation of the tumor clone itself (e.g., epidermal growth factor and platelet derived-endothelial cell growth factor).

Antiangiogenesis factors are currently in clinical trials, including an anti-VEGF neutralizing antibody. The role of such treatment in the overall schema of cancer treatment has yet to be elucidated, but antiangiogenesis therapy is unlikely to be used alone as a mainstay of anticancer therapy. More likely, antiangiogenesis treatment will function in an ancillary role to conventional and potentially novel anticancer therapies.

The pathogenesis of invasion and metastasis involves the breakdown of basement membranes and interstitial stroma. Cancers must invade through the basement membrane, degrade the interstitial stroma, and subsequently intravasate into small blood vessels, which itself requires degradation of the endothelial basement membrane. By definition, in situ breast cancer progresses to invasive cancer when it invades through the epithelial basement membrane. After tumor cells enter the systemic circulation, and in order for a metastatic tumor to develop, tumor cells must extravasate from the blood supply, invade local stroma, and develop their own blood supply. Extravasation requires breakdown of the endothelial basement membrane, and local invasion mandates that stromal environment be degraded. This pattern of basement membrane breakdown and destruction of the interstitial stroma is mediated by a protean array of proteins. These

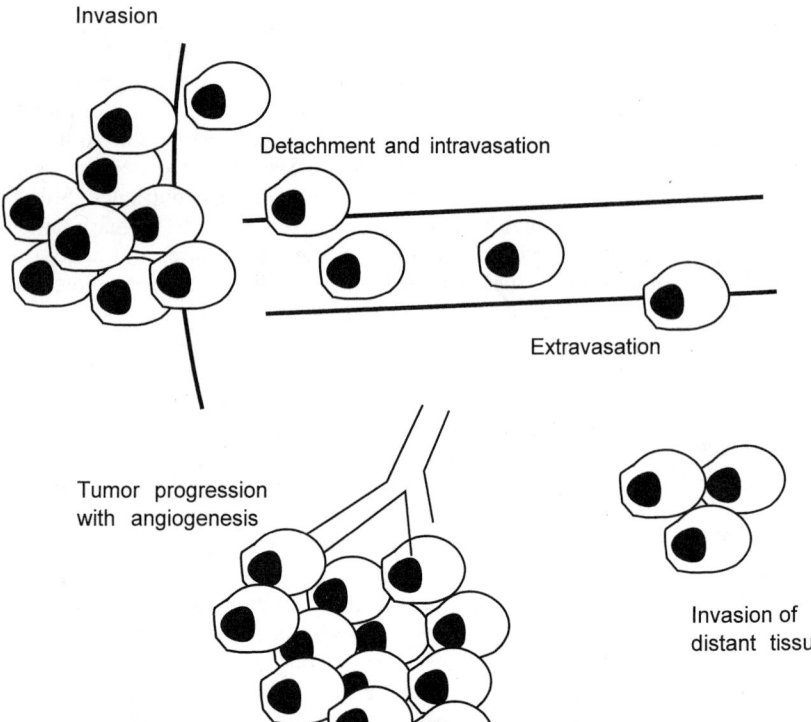

Invasion

Detachment and intravasation

Extravasation

Tumor progression with angiogenesis

Invasion of distant tissues

**Figure 2–11.** Schematic diagram of the general steps involved in metastasis.

proteins regulate invasion and metastasis through their involvement in cell-cell and cell-matrix interactions and proteolysis.

There are multiple groups of proteins involved in cell-cell and cell-matrix adhesion and interaction: integrins, CD44, the immunoglobulin superfamily, and the cadherins. Integrins are a family of transmembrane cell surface proteins that mediate cell-cell adhesion and cell adhesion to the interstitial stroma.[102, 103] The integrins consist of two subunits, the α and β subunits. There are at least 11 α subunits and 6 β subunits that form heterodimers that give rise to at least 16 different integrins. It is conceivable that both loss- or gain-of-function mutations could promote metastasis. Gain-of-function might be involved in the ability of tumor cells to adhere to distant sites of metastasis, whereas loss-of-function mutations might be involved in the capacity of tumor cells to break away from a primary tumor site.

Another protein involved in cell-cell and cell-matrix interactions is CD44. This protein may be expressed in multiple splice variants. It is physiologically involved in many cellular processes, including lymphocyte homing to lymph nodes. CD44 levels are highly expressed in numerous cancers, including colon and bladder cancer and melanoma, and CD44 levels correlate with tumor burden.[104] Introduction of CD44 into colon cancers increases their tumorigenicity in mice.

The immunoglobulin superfamily represents another group of proteins that is involved in metastasis. In particular, neural cell adhesion molecule (NCAM), or CD56, is involved in the adhesion of glioma cells to their matrix. Gliomas that lack NCAM expression are highly invasive and frequently extend several centimeters from their epicenters.

Cadherins are a group of glycoproteins that also mediate adhesion. Cadherins include B-cadherin, E-cadherin, and P-cadherin, among others, and their function is regulated by another group of proteins called *catenins* (e.g. α- and β-catenin). The tumor suppressor gene product APC binds to the catenins and may play a role in colon cancer growth and metastasis.

In addition to cell-cell and cell-matrix interactions, degradation of the interstitial stroma is a crucial process in local invasion and metastasis. A group of 18 proteins, known as *matrix metalloproteinases* (MMPs), predominantly mediate digestion of the major macromolecules in the interstitial connective tissue: collagens, fibronectin, proteoglycans, and so on. MMPs are secreted as inactive zymogens, are cleaved to form active proteases, and form an ionic bond with a central metal ion (i.e., $Zn^{2+}$) that plays a key role in the activation of MMPs. MMPs are normally secreted by the

*Table 2–6.* **Some Factors Involved in Angiogenesis**

Proangiogenic factors
    Vascular endothelial growth factor (VEGF)
    Acidic fibroblast growth factor (AFGF)
    Basic fibroblast growth factor (BFGF)
    Epidermal growth factor (EGF)
    Angiogenin
Antiangiogenic factors
    Interferons
    Tissue inhibitors of metalloproteinases (TIMPs)
    Heparinases
    Platelet factor 4
    Cartilage-derived inhibitor
    Suramin

connective tissue cells, but tumor cells may also secrete MMPs. Alternatively, MMP secretion can be stimulated by tumor products (e.g., interleukin-1β, TGF-β).

There are four groups of MMPs: collagenases, gelatinases, stromolysins, and a group of membrane-bound MMPs. When MMPs are initially secreted (except for the membrane-bound MMPs), they are activated by cleavage by plasmin. Plasmin itself is secreted as an inactive zymogen and is cleaved and activated by tissue plasminogen activator (TPA), which, in turn, is regulated by tissue plasminogen activator–inhibitor (TPAI). The timing and types of MMPs secreted likely is not a random process because for metastasis to develop, a balance between digestion of the connective tissue matrix and adhesion of cells to the matrix must exist. Thus, regulation by plasmin, TPA, and TPAI is relevant in this regard, as are a group of MMP regulator proteins known as *tissue inhibitors of metalloproteinases* (TIMPs). TIMPs form complexes with MMPs and in so doing inactivate them. TIMPs have been shown to block cell invasion in vitro and in vivo.

The balance between MMP activation and inactivation in large part determines the potential for local invasion and metastasis. Tumors that overexpress TPAI are poorly invasive, whereas low MMP expression in astrocytomas is associated with slow growth, and anaplastic astrocytomas show high MMP expression. It should be noted that the expression of proteins involved in MMP regulation does not necessarily correlate as one would predict with tumor invasiveness. Thus, high MMP expression may be associated with slowly invasive tumors. This discrepancy between MMP activation and tumor invasion and metastasis is partly explained by the fact that proteins involved in MMP regulation have other biologic effects, including regulation of proliferation and apoptosis.

Other proteins involved in degradation of the interstitial tissue matrix include cysteine and aspartic proteinases (e.g., cathepsins L, D, and B), and heparinase. Cathepsin L is overexpressed in melanoma cells, and cathepsin B is overexpressed in breast cancer. Cathepsin D overexpression increases metastasis in nude mice.

## Summary

The development of a malignant tumor requires (1) dysregulated growth and (2) the ability to invade local tissues and metastasize. Dysregulated growth results predominantly from uncontrolled proliferation, although decreased apoptosis plays a role in some cancers. Increased proliferation arises from mutations in proto-oncogenes, tumor suppressor genes, and genes that are involved in correction of spontaneous mutations. For a tumor to grow beyond a minimal size, it must also stimulate angiogenesis so that oxygen and vital nutrients can reach the growing tumor.

Once a tumor acquires the genetic changes that result in dysregulated growth, it may invade local tissue and metastasize. Invasion and metastasis require alterations in cell-cell and cell-matrix interactions and degradation of the interstitial connective tissue.

The fruits of the last several decades of research have fueled our current understanding of oncogenesis. Our understanding of the fundamental molecular mechanisms of tumor pathogenesis has already resulted in important clinical developments and will surely lead to further important advances in the understanding, diagnosis, and treatment of cancer.

## SUGGESTIONS FOR ADDITIONAL READING

Mendelsohn J, Howley PM, Israel MA, Liotta LA, eds. The molecular basis of cancer. Philadelphia: WB Saunders: 1995.

Vogelstein B, Kiuzler KW, eds. The genetic basis of human cancer. New York: McGraw-Hill, 1998.

## REFERENCES

1. Sherr CJ, Roberts JM. Inhibitors of mammalian $G_1$ cyclin-dependent kinases. Genes Dev 1995;9:1149–63.
2. Sherr CJ. $G_1$ phase progression: cycling on cue. Cell 1994;79:551–5.
3. Ewen ME, Sluss HK, Sherr CJ, et al. Functional interactions of the retinoblastoma protein with mammalian D-type cyclins. Cell 1993;73:487–97.
4. Nevins JR. E2F: a link between the Rb tumor suppressor protein and viral oncoproteins. Science 1992;258:424–9.
5. Sherr CJ. Cancer cell cycles. Science 1996;274:1672–7.
6. Hunter T, Pines J. Cyclins and cancer. II: cyclin D and CDK inhibitors come of age. Cell 1994;79:573–82.
7. Hall M, Peters G. Genetic alterations of cyclins, cyclin-dependent kinases, and Cdk inhibitors in human cancer. Adv Cancer Res 1996;68:67–108.
8. Nigro JM, Baker SJ, Preisinger AC, et al. Mutations in the p53 gene occur in diverse human tumour types. Nature 1989;342:705–8.
9. Greenblatt MS, Bennett WP, Hollstein M, Harris CC. Mutations in the p53 tumor suppressor gene: clues to cancer etiology and molecular pathogenesis. Cancer Res 1994;54:4855–78.
10. El-Deiry WS, Tokino T, Velculescu VE, et al. WAF1, a potential mediator of p53 tumor suppression. Cell 1993;75:817–25.
11. Dulic V, Kaufmann WK, Wilson SJ, et al. p53-Dependent inhibition of cyclin-dependent kinase activities in human fibroblasts during radiation-induced G1 arrest. Cell 1994;76:1013–23.
12. Slamon DJ, Clark GM, Wong SG. Human breast cancer: correlation of relapse and survival with amplification of the HER-2/*neu* oncogene. Science 1987;235:177–82.
13. Lowenstein EJ, Daly RJ, Batzer AG, et al. The SH2 and SH3-domain containing protein Grb2 links receptor tyrosine kinases to ras signaling. Cell 1992;70:431–42.
14. Nicosia RF, Bonanno E, Smith M, Yurchenco P. Modulation of angiogenesis in vitro by laminin-entactin complex. Dev Biol 1994;164:197–206.
15. Bishop JM. Molecular themes in oncogenesis. Cell 1991;64:235–48.
16. Glomset JA, Gelb MH, Farnsworth CC. Prenyl proteins in eukaryotic cells: a new type of membrane anchor. Trends Biochem Sci 1990;15:139–42.
17. Kerr JFR, Wyllie AH, Currie AR. Apoptosis: a basic biologic phenomenon with wide-ranging implications in tissue kinetics. Br J Cancer 1972;26:239–57.
18. Cotran RS, Kumar V, Robbins SL: Cellular injury and cellular death. In: Cotran RS, Kumar V, Robbins, eds. Pathologic basis of disease. 5th ed. Philadelphia: WB Saunders: 1994:1–34.
19. Williams GT, Smith CA. Molecular regulation of apoptosis: genetic controls on cell death. Cell 1993;74:777–9.
20. Muzio M, Chinnaiyan AM, Kischkel FC, et al. FLICE, a novel FADD-homologous ICE/CED-3-like protease, is recruited to the CD95 (Fas/APO-1) death-inducing signaling complex. Cell 1996;85:817–27.
21. Tewari M, Quan LT, O'Rourke K, et al. CPP32 beta, a mammalian homolog of CED-3, is a CrmA-inhibitable protease that cleaves the death substrate poly (ADP-ribose) polymerase. Cell 1995;81:801–9.
22. Enari M, Sakahira H, Yokoyama H, et al. A caspase-activated DNase that degrades DNA during apoptosis, and its inhibitor, ICAD. Nature 1998;391:43–50.
23. Kothakota S, Azuma T, Reinhard C, et al. Caspase-3-generated fragment of gelsolin: effector of morphological change in apoptosis. Science 1997;278:294–8.

24. Rudel T, Bokoch G. Membrane and morphological changes in apoptotic cells regulated by caspase-mediated activation of PAK2. Science 1997;276:1571–4.

25. Liu X, Kim CN, Yang J, et al. Induction of apoptotic program in cell-free extracts: requirements for dATP and cytochrome c. Cell 1996;86:147–57.

26. Zou H, Henzel WJ, Liu X, et al. Apaf-1, a human protein homologous to *C. elegans* CED-4, participates in cytochrome c-dependent activation of caspase-3. Cell 1997;90:405–13.

27. Tsujimoto Y, Gorham J, Cossman J, et al. The t(14;18) chromosome translocations involved in B-cell neoplasms result from mistakes in VDJ joining. Science 1985;229:1390–3.

28. Vander Heiden MG, Chandel NS, Williamson EK, et al. Bcl-x$_L$ regulates the membrane potential and volume homeostasis of mitochondria. Cell 1997;91:627–37.

29. Reed JC. Double identity for proteins of the bcl-2 family. Nature 1997;387:773–6.

30. Roy N, Deveraux QL, Takahashi R, et al. The c-IAP-1 and C-IAP-2 proteins are direct inhibtors of specific caspsases. EMBO J 1997;16:6914–25.

31. Levine AJ, Momand J, Finlay CA. The p53 tumour suppressor gene. Nature 1991;351:453–6.

32. Hollstein M, Sidransky D, Vogelstein B, Harris CC. p53 mutations in human cancers. Science 1991;253:49–53.

33. Carson DA, Lois A. Cancer progression and p53. Lancet 1995;346:1009–11.

34. Gallo RC, Wong-Staal F. Retroviruses as etiologic agents of some animal and human leukemias and lymphomas and as tools for elucidating the molecular mechanism of leukemogenesis. Blood 1982;60:545–557.

35. Varmus H. Retroviruses. Science 1988;240:1427–1435.

36. Spector DH, Smith K, Padgett T, et al. Uninfected avian cells contain RNA related to the transforming gene of avian sarcoma viruses. Cell 1978;13:371–79.

37. Stehelin D, Varmus HE, Bishop JM, Vogt PK. DNA related to the transforming gene(s) of avian sarcoma viruses is present in normal avian DNA. Nature 1976;260:170–73.

38. Swanstrom R, Parker RC, Varmus HE, Bishop JM. Transduction of a cellular oncogene: the genesis of Rous sarcoma virus. Proc Natl Acad Sci U S A 1983;80:2519–23.

39. Bishop JM. Cellular oncogenes and retroviruses. Annu Rev Biochem 1983;52:301–54.

40. Gibbs JB, Ellis RW, Scolnick EM. Autophosphorylation of v-Ha-ras p21 is modulated by amino acid residue 12. Proc Natl Acad Sci U S A 1984;81:2674–78.

41. Sweet RW, Yokoyama S, Kamata T, et al. The product of ras is a GTPase and the T24 oncogenic mutant is deficient in this activity. Nature 1984;311:273–75.

42. Reddy EP, Reynolds RK, Santos E, Barbacid M. A point mutation is responsible for the acquisition of transforming properties by the T24 human bladder carcinoma oncogene. Nature 1982;300:149–52.

43. Santos E, Tronick SR, Aaronson SA, et al. T24 human bladder carcinoma oncogene is an activated form of the normal human homologue of BALB- and Harvey-MSV transforming genes. Nature 1982;298:343–47.

44. Pulciani S, Santos E, Lauver AV, et al. Oncogenes in human tumor cell lines: molecular cloning of a transforming gene from human bladder carcinoma cells. Proc Natl Acad Sci U S A 1982;79:2845–49.

45. Hayward WS, Neel BG, Astrin SM. Activation of a cellular onc gene by promoter insertion in ALV-induced lymphoid leukosis. Nature 1981;290:475–80.

46. Hiscott J, Petropoulos L, Lacoste J. Molecular interactions between HTLV-1 Tax protein and the NF-kappa B/kappa B transcription complex. Virology 1995;214:3–11.

47. Lundblad JR, Kwok RP, Laurance ME, et al. The human T-cell leukemia virus-1 transcriptional activator Tax enhances cAMP-responsive element-binding protein (CREB) binding activity through interactions with the DNA minor groove. J Biol Chem 1998;273:19251–59.

48. Mendoza SM, Konishi T, Miller CW. Integration of SV40 in human osteosarcoma DNA. Oncogene 1998;17:2457–62.

49. Strickler HD, Rosenberg PS, Devesa SS, et al. Contamination of poliovirus vaccines with simian virus 40 (1955–1963) and subsequent cancer rates. JAMA 1998;279:292–95.

50. Uchida S, Watanabe S, Aizawa T, et al. Induction of papillary ependymomas and insulinomas in the Syrian golden hamster by BK virus, a human papovavirus. Gann 1976;67:857–65.

51. Conzen SD, Cole CN. The three transforming regions of SV40 T antigen are required for immortalization of primary mouse embryo fibroblasts. Oncogene 1995;11:2295–2302.

52. DeCaprio JA, Ludlow JW, Figge J, et al. SV40 large tumor antigen forms a specific complex with the product of the retinoblastoma susceptibility gene. Cell 1988;54:275–83.

53. Sarnow P, Ho YS, Williams J, Levine AJ. Adenovirus E1b-58kd tumor antigen and SV40 large tumor antigen are physically associated with the same 54 kd cellular protein in transformed cells. Cell 1982;28:387–94.

54. Whyte P, Buchkovich KJ, Horowitz JM, et al. Association between an oncogene and an anti-oncogene: the adenovirus E1A proteins bind to the retinoblastoma gene product. Nature 1988;334:124–29.

55. Yew PR, Berk AJ. Inhibition of p53 transactivation required for transformation by adenovirus early 1B protein. Nature 1992;357:82–5.

56. Macnab JC, Walkinshaw SA, Cordiner JW, Clements JB. Human papillomavirus in clinically and histologically normal tissue of patients with genital cancer. N Engl J Med 1986;315:1052–58.

57. McCance DJ. Human papillomavirus (HPV) infections in the aetiology of cervical cancer. Cancer Surv 1988;7:499–506.

58. Mitchell H, Drake M, Medley G. Prospective evaluation of risk of cervical cancer after cytological evidence of human papilloma virus infection. Lancet 1986;1:573–5.

59. Dyson N, Howley PM, Munger K, Harlow E. The human papilloma virus-16 E7 oncoprotein is able to bind to the retinoblastoma gene product. Science 1989;243:934–37.

60. Werness BA, Levine AJ, Howley PM. Association of human papillomavirus types 16 and 18 E6 proteins with p53. Science 1990;248:76–9.

61. Brielmeier M, Mautner J, Laux G, Hammerschmidt W. The latent membrane protein 2 gene of Epstein-Barr virus is important for efficient B cell immortalization. J Gen Virol 1996;77:2807–18.

62. Longnecker R, Druker B, Roberts TM, Kieff E. An Epstein-Barr virus protein associated with cell growth transformation interacts with a tyrosine kinase. J Virol 1991;65:3681–92.

63. Bos JL: ras oncogenes in human cancer: a review [published erratum appears in Cancer Res 1990;50:1352]. Cancer Res 1989;49:4682–89.

64. Moodie SA, Willumsen BM, Weber MJ, Wolfman A. Complexes of Ras.GTP with Raf-1 and mitogen-activated protein kinase. Science 1993;260:1658–61.

65. Manne V, Bekesi E, Kung HF. Ha-ras proteins exhibit GTPase activity: point mutations that activate Ha-ras gene products result in decreased GTPase activity. Proc Natl Acad Sci U S A 1985;82:376–80.

66. Barinaga M. From bench top to bedside. Science 1997;278:1036–9.

67. Rabbitts TH. Chromosomal translocations in human cancer. Nature 1994;372:143–9.

68. Slamon DJ, Godolphin W, Jones LA, et al. Studies of the HER-2/neu proto-oncogene in human breast and ovarian cancer. Science 1989;244:707–12.

69. Reese DM, Slamon DJ. HER-2/neu signal transduction in human breast and ovarian cancer. Stem Cells 1997;15:1–8.

70. Harbeck N, Ross JS, Yurdseven S, et al. HER-2/neu gene amplification by fluorescence in situ hybridization allows risk-group assessment in node-negative breast cancer. Int J Oncol 1999;14:663–71.

71. Press MF, Bernstein L, Thomas PA, et al. HER-2/neu gene amplification characterized by fluorescence in situ hybridization: poor prognosis in node-negative breast carcinomas. J Clin Oncol 1997;15:2894–2904.

72. Pegram MD, Lipton A, Hayes DF, et al. Phase II study of receptor-enhanced chemosensitivity using recombinant humanized anti-p185HER2/neu monoclonal antibody plus cisplatin in patients with HER2/neu-overexpressing metastatic breast cancer refractory to chemotherapy treatment. J Clin Oncol 1998;16:2659–71.

73. Fenaux P, Chomienne C, Degos L. Acute promyelocytic leukemia: biology and treatment. Semin Oncol 1997;24:92–102.

74. Pawson T, Gish GD. SH2 and SH3 domains: from structure to function. Cell 1992;71:359–62.

75. Lowenstein EJ, Daly RJ, Batzer AG, et al. The SH2 and SH3 domain-containing protein GRB2 links receptor tyrosine kinases to ras signaling. Cell 1992;70:431–42.

76. Vojtek AB, Hollenberg SM, Cooper JA. Mammalian Ras interacts directly with the serine/threonine kinase Raf. Cell 1993;74:205–14.

77. Marshall CJ. MAP kinase kinase kinase, MAP kinase kinase and MAP kinase. Curr Opin Genet Dev 1994;4:82–9.

78. Harris H. The analysis of malignancy by cell fusion: the position in 1988. Cancer Res 1988;48:3302–06.

79. Stanbridge EJ: Suppression of malignancy in human cells. Nature 1976;260:17–20.
80. Stanbridge EJ, Der C, Doerson CJ, et al. Human cell hybrids: analysis of transformation and tumorigenicity. Science 1982;215:252–59.
81. Stanbridge EJ, Flandermeyer RR, Daniels DW, Nelson-Rees A. Specific chromosome loss associated with the expression of tumorigenicity in human cell hybrids. Somat Cell Genet 1981;7:699–712.
82. Saxon PJ, Srivatson ES, Stanbridge EJ. Introduction of human chromosome 11 via microcell transfer controls tumorigenic expression of HeLa cells. EMBO J 1986;5:3461–66.
83. Marshall CJ. Tumor suppressor genes. Cell 1991;64:313–26.
84. Knudson AG Jr. Mutation and cancer: statistical study of retinoblastoma. Proc Natl Acad Sci U S A 1971;68:820–23.
85. Knudson AG Jr, Meadows AT, Nichols WW, Hill R. Chromosomal deletion and retinoblastoma. N Engl J Med 1978;295:1120–23.
86. Sparkes RS, Murphree AL, Lingua RW, et al. Gene for hereditary retinoblastoma assigned to human chromosme 13 by linkage to esterase D. Science 1983;219:971–73.
87. Dryja TP, Rapaport JM, Joyce JM, Peterson RA. Molecular detection of deletions involving band q14 of chromosome 13 in retinoblastomas. Proc Natl Acad Sci U S A 1986;83:7391–94.
88. Cavenee WK, Dryja TP, Phillips RA, et al. Expression of recessive alleles by chromosomal mechanisms in retinoblastoma. Nature 1983;305:779–84.
89. Godbout R, Dryja TP, Squire J, et al. Somatic inactivation of genes on chromosome 13 is a common event in retinoblastoma. Nature 1983;304:451–3.
90. Watkins PC. Restriction fragment length polymorphism (RFLP): applications in human chromosome mapping and genetic disease research. Biotechniques 1988;6:310–20.
91. Hansen MF, Cavenee WK. Genetics of cancer predisposition. Cancer Res 1987;47:5518–27.
92. Zhu X, Dunn JM, Phillips RA, et al. Preferential germline mutation of the paternal allele in retinoblastoma. Nature 1989;340:312–13.
93. Janson M, Kock E, Nordenskjold M. Constitutional deletions predisposing to retinoblastoma. Hum Genet 1990;85:21–4.
94. Canning S, Dryja TP. Short, direct repeats at the breakpoints of deletions of the retinoblastoma gene. Proc Natl Acad Sci U S A 1989;86:5044–48.
95. Cavenee WK, Hansen MF, Nordenskjold M, et al. Genetic origin of mutations predisposing to retinoblastoma. Science 1985;228:501–3.
96. Friend SH, Bernards R, Rogelj S, et al. A human DNA segment with properties of the gene that predisposes to retinoblastoma and osteosarcoma. Nature 1986;323:643–46.
97. Bookstein R, Lee EYH, To T, et al. Human retinoblastoma susceptibility gene: genomic organization and analysis of heterozygous intragenic deletion mutants. Proc Natl Acad Sci U S A 1988;85:2210–14.
98. Fung YKT, Murphree AL, T'Ang A, et al. Structural evidence for the authenticity of the human retinoblastoma gene. Science 1987;236:1657–61.
99. Lee WH, Bookstein R, Hong F, et al. Human retinoblastoma susceptibility gene: cloning, identification and sequence. Science 1987;235:1394–99.
100. Huang HJ, Yee JK, Shew JY, et al. Suppression of the neoplastic phenotype by replacement of the retinoblastoma gene in human cancer cells. Science 1988;242:1563–66.
101. Asano M, Yukita A, Matsumoto T, et al. Inhibition of tumor growth and metastasis by an immunoneutralizing monoclonal antibody to human vascular endothelial growth factor/vascular permeability factor 121. Cancer Res 1995;55:5296–5301.
102. Hynes RO. Integrins: versatility, modulation, and signaling in cell adhesion. Cell 1992;69:11–25.
103. Pigott R, Power C. The adhesion molecule facts book. London: Academic Press, 1993.
104. Guo Y, Kiu G, Wang X, et al. Potential use of soluble CD44 in serum as indicator of tumor burden and metastasis in patients with gastric or colon cancer. Cancer Res 1994;54:422–6.

# CHAPTER 3

# PRINCIPLES OF CANCER GENETICS COUNSELING

• MARY B. DALY

The recent cloning of genes associated with a hereditary risk of cancer has heightened public interest in personal cancer risk and has made genetic screening of some individuals with a hereditary pattern of cancer possible. The development of technology to locate and isolate cancer susceptibility genes has brought together the fields of oncology, cancer control, genetics, and genetic counseling to create a new specialty of cancer risk counseling whose goal is to communicate more accurate information about personal cancer risk profiles based on personal and family histories.[1] This new discipline provides an opportunity to educate and counsel individuals and their families about their risks for cancer, to address individual concerns about cancer, and to devise appropriate prevention and surveillance plans that are tailored to the needs of the counselee. The application of genetic risk assessment techniques to the field of cancer risk has created new clinical, social, economic, and ethical challenges and heralds a change in the medical and scientific approach to cancer prevention. This chapter places the new discipline of cancer risk counseling within the tradition of medical genetic counseling and highlights the important elements and goals of this emerging field.

## Tradition of Genetic Counseling

Advances in the field of human genetics since the 1970s have contributed substantially to our understanding of human diseases and led to improvements in prevention, early detection, and treatment. Not only have many conditions been found to follow a mendelian pattern of inheritance but subtle *acquired* genetic alterations have been identified as contributing factors in a host of additional diseases. In response to these advances, the field of genetic counseling has evolved and plays a growing role in the evaluation and risk estimation of families with known or suspected genetic conditions. Genetic counseling is practiced by a multidisciplinary team of professionals that includes medical geneticists, genetic counselors with master's degrees, primary care physicians, nurses, and social scientists who address the genetic, medical, social, psychological, and ethical concerns of their patients.

The traditional elements of genetic counseling have included (1) an accurate diagnosis of the genetic condition or predisposition; (2) an estimate of the probable cause of the disorder; (3) an estimation of the risk for future occurrences of the condition within the family based on the pattern of inheritance of the disease; (4) communication of an understanding of the genetic and medical facts of the disorder; (5) an exploration of appropriate courses of action to manage the genetic risk and to alter the risk of occurrence; and (6) ways of coping with the disorder or risk of the disorder.[2–4]

Just as important as a careful risk factor analysis and interpretation of risk to family members is attention to the psychosocial issues raised by the enhanced risk and the emotional needs of those involved.[5] Genetic counselors play an important role in providing a source of information not only about the genetic disorder, its management, and course but also about alternate social sources of information and assistance. By offering long-term follow-up and support, the counselor can help the family deal with their emotional reactions to the genetic risk and can help strengthen their coping skills and resources.[6]

Several studies have attempted to assess the effectiveness and efficacy of genetic counseling and have identified a number of common predictors of response. The use of genetic counseling services is associated with higher socioeconomic status and educational level and, in the setting of prenatal genetic conditions, with intention to have children.[7] Understanding and retention of the information received has been found to be higher among individuals who are self-referred, those with higher educational levels, and among those families at higher risk levels. Multiple counseling sessions have been shown to boost understanding and information retention.[8] Another consistent observation has been that although important, the information obtained at a genetic counseling session is not the only factor contributing to risk-related decisions. Rather, perception of risk is a concept formed over a person's lifetime and is a result of internalizing personal experiences and beliefs. Decisions made in the genetic counseling setting therefore reflect a complicated interplay of expectations, emotions, and value judgments. As a result, the genetic counselor is likely to be most successful when the information shared during genetic counseling is provided in the context of the counselee's personal orientation and belief system.

## Application of Genetic Counseling to Cancer Risk Assessment

### PURPOSE AND GOALS

Building on the practice of traditional genetic counseling, cancer risk counseling is an interactive education and communication process whose purpose is to evaluate an individual's potential risk of acquiring specific forms of cancer based on inherited susceptibilities, physiologic modulators, and lifestyle and environmental factors that contribute to cancer risk and to communicate this information in a comprehensible and sensitive way. Familial cancer risk counseling uses a broad approach to place genetic risk in the context of other related risk factors, thereby customizing it to the experiences of the individual. In addition to addressing genetic risk and its clinical management, cancer risk counseling also considers the psychosocial needs of the individual and family. Typically, the process involves the collection of perti-

nent medical, familial, and lifestyle information; documentation of cancer diagnoses; delivery of background information about cancer risks and cancer genetics; identification of specific hereditary cancer syndromes, and transmission of personalized risk estimates.[9] The ultimate goal of the education and communication process is to help the individual and other family members make informed and appropriate decisions about strategies for cancer prevention or early detection, or both.

Genetic counseling for genetic cancer risk represents a new direction in genetics and has raised some particularly interesting and difficult issues. Risk estimates for cancer may be either empirical or based on actual gene identification, but they are typically complex and sophisticated, challenging the communication skills of the counseling team. The nature of the counseling situation often requires the involvement of other family members to supply missing information or even for genetic screening, a situation that may compromise the privacy and confidentiality of the individuals seeking risk counseling or alter the dynamics within the family. The options offered by the counseling team, including genetic testing, may involve emotional and ethical dilemmas for which there are no clear answers. Despite these problematic issues, cancer risk counseling is a growing field that has tremendous potential to assist families in understanding their risk for cancer and in making informed choices for prevention.

### TARGET POPULATION

Intense media attention to the complex aspects of genetic susceptibility to disease and the recent availability of genetic tests for cancer susceptibility have produced an increased awareness of the familial contribution to cancer and have altered the way individuals perceive their risk. Individuals who seek cancer risk counseling are often highly motivated by a personal experience with cancer in their family and by concern for the risks faced by themselves and their offspring. Participants in cancer risk counseling are often self-referred, but as physicians become more aware of the importance of family history in determining an individual's risk for cancer, they are increasingly referring their patients for genetic evaluation. Although the general indication for participation in a cancer risk counseling program is a perception of increased risk for cancer based on family history or other recognized risk exposures, or both, individual participants come to the process with a wide variety of experiences, health beliefs, expectations, and needs. Therefore, an assessment of individual differences that can influence comprehension and compliance with appropriate health recommendations, is one of the primary goals of the counseling team.

### COUNSELING TEAM

Traditionally, the medical genetics counseling team has included a medical geneticist, a genetics counselor, and often the referring primary care physician, usually an obstetrician or pediatrician. Genetic counselors typically earn a masters of science degree at an accredited institution and are certified by the American Board of Genetic Counselors. Dedicated training in the field of cancer genetics has been added to the curricula of genetic counseling education programs. There is also a growing interest in genetics on the part of nurses, many of whom are beginning to seek specialized training in the field. As the field of genetic counseling has expanded to include adult diseases such as cancer, other disciplines, including oncology, molecular genetics, social work, and psychology, have joined the team to provide the multidisciplinary approach needed. Originally, cancer risk counseling programs were mainly situated in cancer centers and academic institutions, but increasingly these services are expanding to community hospitals, workplaces, and health centers, where they are often one component of a more broad-based health promotion program.

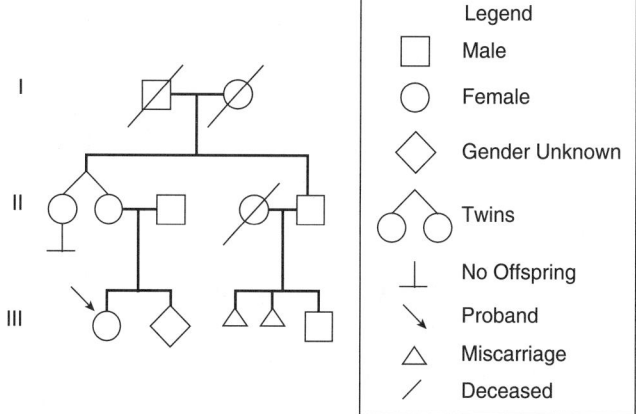

**Figure 3–1.** Family history data are graphically represented on this sample pedigree. The symbols in this pedigree follow standard recommended nomenclature to illustrate family relationships and other pedigree designations.

## COMPONENTS OF THE COUNSELING PROCESS

**Information Gathering.** The first step in evaluating an individual's risk for cancer is to assess the individual's concerns and reasons for seeking counseling to guarantee that personal needs and priorities are met in the counseling process. The next step is to collect the pertinent medical, family, and personal information to assemble a risk profile and begin to explore options for dealing with the risk (Table 3–1). A detailed family history is the cornerstone of effective genetic counseling. The counselor begins with the health of the proband and proceeds outward to include first-, second-, and third-degree relatives on both the maternal and paternal sides. In addition to cancer diagnoses by primary site, age at onset, bilaterality when appropriate, and current age or age at death are recorded. Cancer diagnoses are validated by obtaining medical records, pathology reports, or death certificates when possible. Other medical and genetic conditions that may predispose individuals to cancer risk (e.g., Crohn's disease and colon cancer, atypical ductal hyperplasia and breast cancer) should also be noted. It is important to include information about family members unaffected with cancer to appreciate overall patterns of inheritance. Information about possible consanguinity is also valuable, particularly in the consideration of recessive disorders. Ethnicity should be recorded because some inherited conditions are more common in certain ethnic groups.

Family history data are graphically represented on a pedigree, which follows standard nomenclature to illustrate family relationships and disease information[10] (Fig. 3–1). Factors that limit the informativeness of the pedigree are small

*Table 3–1.* **Basic Elements of Cancer Genetic Counseling**

Documentation of extended family medical history
Development of a family pedigree
Collection of medical records from proband and appropriate family members
Collection of information about other risk factors (biologic, environmental, lifestyle)
Careful assessment of risk
Education about cancer, genetics, and preventive options
Communication of risk estimate in clear and simple language
Development of individualized prevention and surveillance strategy
Attention to emotional and social needs and concerns of proband and family
Long-term follow-up and support

family size; early deaths in family members, precluding the possibility of them acquiring adult diseases; prophylactic surgeries that remove an organ from subsequent risk of cancer (e.g., total hysterectomy for uterine fibroids in which the ovaries are also removed); and incomplete information about the health of family members. The degree of accuracy of reporting cancer diagnoses in relatives varies by how close the relatives are to the proband, with lack of information about generation-specific cancer diagnoses in older second- or third-generation individuals, or both, being a particularly common problem encountered in pedigree generation.

The collection of a targeted medical history of the proband serves two purposes: (1) the identification of premalignant conditions associated with subsequent cancer progression and (2) the estimation of other risk factors that may interact with or modify familial cancer risk. A careful reproductive history is pertinent to a number of common cancers in women. Exogenous hormone use and other medication history is also of value. The knowledge of other medical conditions may have an impact on the management recommendations for reducing cancer risk. Caution about the use of exogenous estrogens in women with a familial predisposition of breast cancer may, for example, be tempered by a strong personal or family history of cardiovascular disease or osteoporosis.

Environmental exposures and lifestyle factors such as smoking, diet, and alcohol use and type of occupation may contribute to the overall estimation of risk, and their identification may offer opportunities for lifestyle changes to alter risk. Although occupational exposures to carcinogens such as benzene or asbestos account for a relatively small proportion of cancers, their recognition is important in elucidating patterns of cancer and in eliminating other causes among exposed individuals. Environmental exposures and lifestyles are often shared by family members and must be recognized when assessing hereditary patterns of cancer. Finally, a record of past cancer screening practices establishes a history of health promotion behavior and helps guide the counselor in making reasonable and appropriate health recommendations.

**Education About Cancer Genetics.** Genetic risk information cannot be effectively communicated in the absence of general information about cancer risk, cancer genetics, and risk estimation. Individuals faced with a familial risk of cancer must assimilate complex and often highly technical information to make informed decisions about genetic testing, cancer screening and preventive actions for themselves, and to communicate that information to other family members. An integral part of the genetic counseling process is educational preparation, provided either in a group or individual setting, to help the proband develop the understanding necessary to make informed decisions about the cancer risk. The basic educational components of cancer risk information are discussed in the following sections.

*Concepts of Cancer, Cancer risk, and Cancer Risk Factors.* The multifactorial nature of cancer is explored with an emphasis on the pathways of cancer formation and expression. Persons affected with cancer who seek counseling may be particularly interested in information about the presentation, diagnosis, and treatment of cancer. The basics of cancer epidemiology can be presented, and examples, such as the importance of hormonal regulation in breast cancer and the importance of diet in colon cancer, can be used to illustrate the role of both external factors and internal metabolism in changing normal cells to premalignant and malignant tissue.

*Role of Family History in Cancer Risk Assessment.* The interaction of shared environmental and genetic backgrounds among family members in determining risk is explored. Sample pedigrees can be used to illustrate the types of family cancer patterns (Table 3–2) and to demonstrate the concepts of vertical transmission through maternal or paternal lines, the significance of age at onset and bilaterality of disease, and penetrance issues (Fig. 3–2). With this background, the counselor can review the proband's own pedigree for the patterns expressed and the identification of pertinent risk factors.

*Role of Genes in Cancer Development.* The counselor introduces the concepts and language of chromosomes, genes, and DNA and how genetic alterations can lead to cancer. It is particularly important for the proband to under-

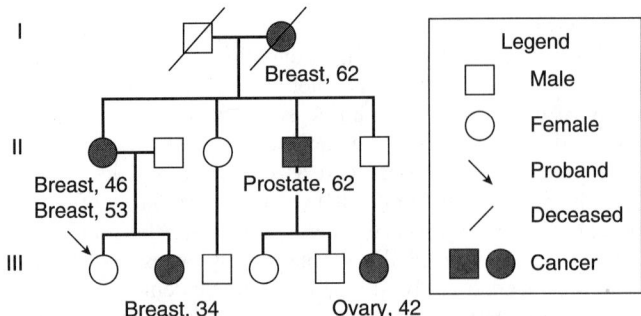

**Figure 3–2.** Sample pedigree illustrating a family history of a hereditary family cancer pattern. This pedigree demonstrates vertical (autosomal dominant) transmission of cancers, showing early ages of onset, bilaterality of disease, and increased penetrance.

stand the difference between the acquisition of genetic alterations during his or her lifetime that may affect the risk for cancer, and the inheritance of cancer-related genetic alterations from a parent, which can also be passed on to the proband's offspring. Within this context, the counselor can introduce information about cancer susceptibility genes that have been identified, such as *BRCA1, BRCA2, APC,* the hereditary nonpolyposis colorectal cancer (HNPCC) genes, and the cancer syndromes associated with each, with an emphasis on syndromes that appear to be most consistent with the proband's family history.

The educational component of cancer risk counseling is meant to be interactive, with ample opportunity for the proband to ask questions and the counselor to tailor the information to the needs of the individual.

**Personalized Assessment of Risk.** Cancer risk assessment is an attempt to quantify the probability of an individual's risk for a particular cancer using empirical models that account for a variety of personal, familial, and environmental risk factors. It is a complex process, both because it is based on imperfect and often conflicting data and because it involves probabilistic statements about the *chance* of an event occurring, concepts that are difficult to convey and to understand. The concept of risk can be presented in a variety of ways, each of which has a different interpretation. *Absolute risk* refers to the rate of cancer occurrence in the population and often serves as the background risk to which individuals compare themselves. *Relative risk* is the comparison of risk in an individual with a particular set of risk factors at a particular point in time to that of an individual without those risk factors, thus implying some magnitude of vulnerability.[11] *Cumulative risk* is the risk over a defined period calculated by accumulating relative risks over time.

Cancer risk counselors attempt to place the proband's risk of cancer within the context of population risk, both in quantitative and qualitative terms, to provide a rationale for recommended health behaviors. As a first step, the counselor refers to the family pedigree to triage families into levels of familial risk. The majority of families do not exhibit the features of hereditary cancer syndromes but rather represent the effect of a combination of multiple genetic and environmental factors that interact to increase cancer risk to a moderate degree. For these families, counselors often use empirical approaches based on epidemiologic data that provide age-specific risks of cancer in tabular formats that can

---

*Table 3–2.* **Family Cancer Patterns**

*Sporadic*

A single occurrence of a cancer occurring on one side of the family

*Familial*

A pattern of cancers on one side of the family, seen in one or more generations, that does not fit an autosomal dominant pattern of inheritance of cancer. The cancers on that side of the family do not fit a known cancer family syndrome. The pattern seen may represent a clustering of incidental cancers or may be the result of shared environmental or lifestyle factors.

*Hereditary*

A pattern of cancers on one side of the family that is seen in two or more generations in several members of the family and fits an autosomal dominant pattern of cancers. The cancers on that side of the family may fit a known cancer family syndrome.
*or*
Genetic testing performed on the proband or the proband's family member has detected a mutation in a cancer predisposition gene (e.g., *BRCA1*) and inheritance of this mutation has been established

incorporate several pertinent risk factors. For some cancers, these empirical data have actually been integrated into mathematical models that can predict cumulative risk estimates of a cancer developing over a defined period in an individual's lifetime. The *Gail model* predicts breast cancer risk from age 20 to 80 years, using a model that includes current age, age at menarche, age at first live birth, number of first-degree relatives with breast cancer, and number of breast biopsies.[12] It has been validated by the Breast Cancer Prevention Trial and is most accurate in predicting breast cancer among women screened with regular mammograms.[13] This model is now available from the National Cancer Institute on a floppy disk, the "Risk Disk," that can easily be used in the clinical setting.

The *Claus model*, based on data from the Cancer and Steroid Hormone (CASH) study, accounts for both first- and second-degree relatives with breast cancer as well as their age at onset and may be more reliable among women with limited screening.[14] As more large data sets are assembled, models for other cancer sites will also become available.

For families in whom a hereditary pattern of cancer is suspected, the cloning of rare but highly penetrant cancer susceptibility genes, such as *BRCA1* and *BRCA2*, has made available the direct assessment of mutation status, thus obviating the need for empirical risk models. Parameters, such as the Amsterdam Criteria and the Bethesda Guidelines for Hereditary Nonpolyposis Colon Cancer (HNPCC),[15, 16] have been established to identify families who are candidates for genetic testing. In addition to these sets of criteria, mathematical models are appearing that, based on features of the family history, predict the likelihood of the individual being a mutation carrier and help the counselor and clinician further refine genetic testing decisions.[17, 18] There is a growing body of literature that quantifies estimates of penetrance (actual cancer risk) among carriers of these genetic alterations, thus allowing a more precise risk estimate both for those family members who have true positive test results and for those who are not carriers.

In addition to using a variety of models developed from empirical data sets, counselors are increasingly aware that individuals seeking cancer risk counseling belong to an extended family system and often have a preconceived estimate of their cancer risk. Perceptions of risk are influenced by their own personal and familial experience of cancer and their beliefs about the causes of cancer. This risk is often perceived in absolute rather than probabilistic terms, making numerical risk estimates less cogent to their own situation.[19, 20]

**Role of Genetic Testing.** Several surveys have documented high levels of interest in tests for cancer-related genetic mutations among individuals with a family history of cancer. Common reasons cited for seeking genetic testing by individuals surveyed include concern about the risk for their children, a desire to improve their own health by more targeted screening and prevention, and the need to have an understanding of the cancer experience in the family.[21] Genetic testing for cancer, and its role, benefits, and limitations are discussed in the counseling session both in terms of the scientific merits of understanding the genetic basis of cancer and, when appropriate, as it may apply to further characterizing the cancer risk within the proband's family. The distinctions among positive, negative, inconclusive, and indeterminant test results (Table 3–3) and the technical limitations of the testing process are reviewed. The probabilistic nature of genetic test results and the potential implications for other family members must be included in the pretest counseling. A clear distinction is made between the probability of being a mutation carrier and the probability of cancer developing. Because the true frequency of genetic mutations can only be determined by large-scale population studies, which are expensive and difficult, these estimates are slow to emerge, and counselors are often faced with extrapolation of data from smaller studies performed in limited population groups. Furthermore, the prevalence of different genetic mutations may vary in different ethnic subsets of the population as a result of variations in migration patterns and the degree of genetic diversity within the group.

Estimates of penetrance of the gene—that is, the chance that a mutation will actually result in cancer in a person—are also typically derived from small studies among narrowly defined families and are difficult to apply to a particular individual unless he or she matches the characteristics of the families studied. Information on other factors that may modify gene expression is rudimentary at this point for most of the genes identified. The technologies for detecting mutations in the major cancer susceptibility genes are constantly evolving but can basically be divided into tests of gene function, such as protein truncation tests, and methods to sequence the genes directly. Protein truncation tests are misleading when the gene length is normal but its function is altered. Direct sequencing can miss certain types of mutations or large deletions, or it can detect mutations of unknown clinical significance. Many of these technical limitations will most likely be eliminated as the technology is improved and as clinical correlations are established for each mutation.

Choosing the appropriate candidates for genetic testing is based on the personal and familial characteristics that determine the prior probability of the individual being a mutation carrier. In many cases, reliable estimates of carrier status can be derived from the age and personal and family history of an individual. Examples are the Amsterdam Criteria and Bethesda Guidelines, which identify HNPCC families who are likely to be carriers of a mutation in the *MLH1* or *MSH2*

**Table 3–3. Genetic Test Results**

*True Positive*

The person is a carrier of an alteration in a known cancer-predisposing gene

*True Negative*

A person is not a carrier of a known cancer-predisposing gene that has been positively identified in another family member

*Indeterminant*

A person is not a carrier of a known cancer-predisposing gene and the carrier status of other family members is either also negative or unknown

*Inconclusive*

A person is a carrier of an alteration in a gene that currently has no known significance genes[22] (Table 3–4). When possible, it is best to consider first testing an affected family member who meets the criteria for a hereditary cancer, as that individual is the one most likely to have positive test results. When a mutation is found, additional family members can be tested with an assay that tests specifically for that particular mutation.

There are four possible interpretations of a genetic test result. If a known risk-associated mutation is found within a family, those family members who test *positive* for the mutation are considered "true positives." They are counseled that they are at increased risk for a spectrum of cancers, and options for risk management are discussed (see further on). It must be emphasized that a positive mutation result is not a positive cancer test result but rather a susceptibility estimate. A positive test result does, however, confirm a 50% chance of passing on the mutation to each biologic child of the carrier. A second outcome of a positive test result is the discovery of a variant of the gene of *unknown clinical significance*. These genes are truly altered but have not yet been clearly linked to disease risk and may represent neutral alterations in the gene structure that do not compromise its function. Over time, as more families are studied, most of these variants will most likely be separated into disease-related changes and benign changes, known as *polymorphisms*. Until then, families found to carry one of these variants must be counseled about the uncertain meaning of the result, and recommendations based on their family and personal history of disease. When a disease-related mutation has been identified in a family, subsequent family members who have negative test results for that mutation are thought to be "true negatives" whose risks for the relevant cancers are *not* increased over those of the general population. These family members may be spared the increased surveillance or

consideration of prophylactic surgery, or both, offered to carriers. They can also be reassured that they will not pass on the deleterious mutation to their offspring. Finally, when no mutation is found in any family member (which is the most common situation), the meaning of a negative test result is ambiguous. It may mean that there truly is no mutation in the family and that the family history represents a clustering of sporadic cancers; it may mean that a known disease-related mutation does exist in the family but no informative family members were available for testing; or it may mean that a mutation exists but cannot be detected by current technology. Again, counseling must emphasize the ambiguous nature of the test results. These families may still face a significantly increased risk of cancer, and management should be based on other factors.

In addition to technical limitations, genetic testing is offered with caution because of the clinical limitations in altering risk once mutation status is known as well as the potential for consequent discrimination on the part of insurers or employers, or both. The magnitude of insurance and employment risks from discrimination is currently not known but is a major concern for state and federal governmental agencies, professional societies, and the insurance industry and represents a significant barrier to genetic testing for many families. This controversial issue is being played out in the courts and in legislative efforts to protect individuals from discrimination on the basis of genetic information about that individual. In the meantime, every effort is made by the counseling team to maintain confidentiality of genetic test results. As genetic testing and counseling for adult-onset diseases becomes more widespread, the counseling approach will continue to diversify to include familial and sociocultural perspectives along with the more traditional biomedical model.

**Recommendations for Prevention.** One of the primary motivations for seeking cancer risk counseling is to identify ways to reduce or delay the risk of cancer developing, or to enhance the possibility of detecting cancer at an early, curable stage. Individuals who seek these services clearly want recommendations for the medical management of their risk from their providers. By achieving a reliable estimate of cancer risk, either by considering personal and family history or by performing genetic testing, the cancer risk counselor, working with the medical team, can help tailor primary and secondary prevention strategies to the individual. Although there are currently limited data on the long-term efficacy of prevention strategies directed at individuals with a familial or hereditary risk, clinical management decisions are being made based on the best available evidence. Recommendations fall into four general categories: (1) increased screening, (2) pharmacologic interventions (chemoprevention), (3) surgical prophylaxis, and (4) lifestyle changes.

A common recommendation for individuals with an increased risk for cancer is heightened surveillance. Because hereditary cancer syndromes are often marked by a significantly earlier age at onset, screening for early detection may be initiated at a younger age or may be repeated at more frequent intervals than is recommended for the general population, or both these methods may be used. For example, women whose family history is characterized by early-onset breast cancer or who have tested positive for a *BRCA1* or *BRCA2* mutation are advised to start annual mammography

*Table 3–4.* **Amsterdam Criteria and Bethesda Guidelines for Hereditary Nonpolyposis Colorectal Cancer (HNPCC)**

*The Amsterdam Criteria*

Histologically confirmed colorectal cancer in at least three relatives, one of whom is a first-degree relative of the other two
Occurrence of disease in at least two successive generations
Age at diagnosis <50 yr in at least one individual
Exclusion of familial adenomatous polyposis

*The Bethesda Guidelines*

Individuals with cancer in families that meet the Amsterdam Criteria
Individuals with two HNPCC-related cancers, including synchronous and metachronous colorectal cancers or associated extracolonic cancers
Individuals with colorectal cancer and a first-degree relative with colorectal cancer or HNPCC-related extracolonic cancer or a colorectal adenoma, or a combination of the preceding; one of the cancers diagnosed at age <45 yr, and the adenoma diagnosed at age <40 yr
Individuals with colorectal cancer or endometrial cancer diagnosed at age <45 yr
Individuals with right-sided colorectal cancer with an undifferentiated pattern (solid/cribriform) on histopathology diagnosed at age <45 yr
Individuals with signet-ring–cell-type colorectal cancer diagnosed at age <45 yr
Individuals with adenomas diagnosed at age <40 yr

Data from Vasen H, Mecklin J, Khan P, et al. The International Collaborative Group on Hereditary Nonpolyposis Colorectal Cancer (ICG-HNPCC). Dis Colon Rectum 1991;34:424–425 *and* Rodriguez-Bigas M, Boland C, Hamilton S, et al. A National Cancer Institute workshop on hereditary nonpolyposis colorectal cancer syndrome: meeting highlights and Bethesda guidelines. J Natl Cancer Inst 1997;89:1758–62.

between the ages of 25 and 35 years and to have clinical breast examinations every 6 to 12 months.[23] Individuals from families with a history of HNPCC are advised to begin colonoscopy at 20 to 25 years with a frequency of every 1 to 3 years, depending on findings.[24] Because of the increased risk of endometrial cancer in female carriers of an HNPCC mutation, annual transvaginal ultrasonography is also recommended starting at age 25 to 35 years. Screening recommendations are problematic for cancers like ovarian and pancreatic cancer for which no early detection method has been found to be sufficiently sensitive and specific, and for conditions like Li-Fraumeni syndrome, in which individuals are at risk for a wide spectrum of cancers during their lifetime. Conversely, members of high-risk families are ideal candidates to participate in trials of newer imaging technologies and intermediate biomarkers to improve the early detection of cancer in younger individuals.

Outcome data from chemoprevention trials is just beginning to emerge. The Breast Cancer Prevention Trial, which randomized more than 13,000 high-risk women to the antiestrogen agent tamoxifen or to placebo, found a 49% reduction in the incidence of breast cancer among women in the tamoxifen arm.[25] A second large trial comparing tamoxifen to the selective estrogen-receptor modulator raloxifene is under way. Population-based studies have established a role for aspirin and some of the nonsteroidal anti-inflammatory drugs in reducing adenoma and polyp formation in the colon.[24] Epidemiologic studies have established a role for oral contraceptives in the prevention of ovarian cancer.[26] Several phase I, II, and III trials are currently under way to study both pharmacologic agents and natural products in a preventive setting for breast, colon, prostate, lung, head and neck, cervical, and skin cancers. It is possible that an armamentarium of chemopreventive agents with well-characterized pharmacologic and toxicologic properties will eventually be available to high-risk individuals.

In certain hereditary cancer syndromes, most notably familial adenomatous polyposis and hereditary medullary cancer of the thyroid, prophylactic total colectomy and prophylactic total thyroidectomy, respectively, have been shown to be effective means of reducing cancer incidence and mortality in susceptible individuals. There is scant evidence, however, about the efficacy of prophylactic oophorectomy, mastectomy, or colectomy for other high-risk individuals. Prophylactic oophorectomy is being considered by women with a family history of ovarian cancer, particularly those who are *BRCA1/2* mutation carriers, because of the uncertainty about current screening options for early detection of ovarian cancer and the high case-fatality rate once ovarian cancer is diagnosed. Although data from the Gilda Radner Familial Ovarian Cancer Registry suggest a significant reduction in incidence among women undergoing prophylactic oophorectomy because of a strong family history of ovarian cancer,[27] the risk of subsequent peritoneal carcinomatosis is estimated to range from 1.9 to 10.7%.[28] Furthermore, premenopausal women choosing this option must consider the potential consequences of long-term hormone replacement therapy following surgically induced menopause. Similarly, prophylactic mastectomy does not completely eliminate the risk of subsequent breast cancer, although a retrospective review of 2029 women who had elected the procedure for a variety of reasons estimates a greater than 90% reduction in

risk.[29] This consideration occurs most commonly among women from high-risk families or those with known *BRCA1/2* mutations who are making treatment choices for their first primary breast cancer, given the increased rate of second cancers in the same breast as well as the contralateral breast in that setting. Another indication for the procedure among high-risk women is extremely dense breast tissue that renders both clinical breast examination and standard mammography less reliable. Studies are now under way to follow women who elect prophylactic oophorectomy or mastectomy prospectively to monitor long-term disease reduction as well as to document the variables influencing the decision to pursue prophylactic surgery and the medical and psychological consequences of the surgery.

No data exist on the impact of prophylactic colectomy for members of families with a history of HNPCC, although subtotal colectomy with iliorectal anastomosis is being recommended in HNPCC carriers with colon cancer to prevent metachronous cancers and as prophylaxis for those who present with adenomas.[24]

Finally, there is intense interest on the part of high-risk individuals about opportunities to reduce their cancer risk by changes in diet, exercise, or other lifestyle modifications that may minimize their exposure to carcinogens. Preliminary data suggest, for instance, that the use of exogenous estrogens, including oral contraceptives and estrogen replacement, may confer an increased risk for breast cancer among women with a hereditary predisposition.[30] The exact role of diet and exercise remains elusive for most cancers, although recommendations can be made on the basis of general health and ideal weight maintenance. Dietary supplementation with micronutrients and other natural products to reduce cancer risk is so far unsupported by scientific data. Long-term studies are needed to assess the role of any of these strategies in the setting of familial risk for cancer.

**Dealing with Psychosocial Issues.** An integral part of the counseling process is the attention to the psychosocial needs of the counselee. This is especially critical in the setting of counseling for cancer risk, which deals with the complexity of probabilities; it involves the entire family and may provide risk information that can become a source of discrimination. Cancer is one of the most feared diseases of modern times. Cultural beliefs about cancer, painful memories of relatives' experiences with cancer, high levels of mental stress associated with cancer-related anxiety, unresolved grief, feelings of denial, guilt, and other family dynamics all can interfere with the receipt and understanding of risk information and the formulation of strategies for risk reduction and can have a negative impact on quality of life. Both the information received during the process of genetic counseling, and the information-seeking coping style of the individual may elicit further emotional reactions, especially if the counseling involves the receipt of genetic test results. The counselor takes an active role in helping the counselee identify his or her risk status, confront fears and anxieties about the meaning of that risk, develop coping strategies to deal with both the emotional and medical components of the unique situation and coping style, and facilitate decision-making. The counselor can also assist the counselee in communicating cancer risk information to other family members, dealing with their potential reactions, and enrolling them in a counseling program. Follow-up genetic counseling sessions have been found to reinforce the information communicated in the original sessions, solidify decisions made, assess adjustment to risk status, and make referrals for specialty consultations if needed.

## CONCLUSIONS AND FUTURE DIRECTIONS

As the importance of cancer prevention and control is increasingly recognized, cancer risk counseling services are becoming a standard component of primary health care. Individuals are becoming increasingly aware of the role of their family history in their own personal cancer risk. The growing sophistication in the process of risk identification, including the use of genetic tests for cancer susceptibility genes, is stimulating research to develop risk modification and cancer prevention strategies. Several registries of high-risk families are being assembled to provide prospective data on the epidemiology and natural history of familial cancers and the effectiveness of a variety of cancer control interventions. Optimal screening protocols for members of high-risk families are being developed and evaluated. Long-term follow-up of mutation carriers will help define the spectrum of cancer risk, clinical course of hereditary cancer, and response to treatment. Central to these research efforts are ongoing studies of the short- and long-term effects of cancer risk counseling on health behaviors and quality of life. Coincidental with this are the many new educational initiatives to prepare health care professionals to become part of the cancer risk counseling team.

## SUGGESTIONS FOR ADDITIONAL READING

Statement of the American Society of Clinical Oncology. Genetic testing for cancer susceptibility. J Clin Oncol 1996;14:1730–1736.

Vogelstein B, Kinzler KW, eds. The genetic basis of human cancer. New York: McGraw-Hill, 1998 (731 pp).

## REFERENCES

1. Baty B, Venne V, McDonald J, et al. *BRCA1* testing: genetic counseling protocol development and counseling issues. J Genet Counsel 1997;6:223–44.
2. Fraser FC. Genetic counseling. Am J Hum Genet 1974;26:636–61.
3. Peters J. Familial cancer risk. I: impact on today's oncology practice. J Oncol Manag 1994;20–30.
4. Muller H. Genetic counseling and cancer. In: Weber W, Laffer U, Durig M, eds. Hereditary cancer and preventive surgery. Basel: Karger, 1990:12–18.
5. Lynch H, Harris R, Organ C, et al. Management of familial breast cancer. Arch Surg 1978;113:1061–7.
6. Kessler S. The process of communication, decision making, and coping in genetic counseling. In: Kessler S, ed. Genetic counseling: psychological dimensions. New York: Academic Press, 1979.
7. Tambor E, Bernhardt B, Chase G, et al. Offering cystic fibrosis carrier screening to an HMO population: factors associated with utilization. Am J Hum Genet 1994;55:626–37.
8. Evers-Kiebooms G, van den Berghe H. Impact of genetic counseling: a review of published follow-up studies. Clin Genet 1979;15:465–74.
9. Peters J. Familial cancer risk. II: Breast cancer risk counseling and genetic susceptibility testing. J Oncol Manag 1994;14–22.
10. Bennett R, Steinhaus K, Uhrich S, et al. Recommendations for standardized human pedigree nomenclature. Am J Hum Genet 1995;56:745–52.
11. Mahon S, Casperson D. Hereditary cancer syndrome. 1: clinical and educational issues. Oncol Nurs Forum 1995;22:763–71.
12. Gail MH, Brinton LA, Byar DP, et al. Projecting individualized probabilities of developing breast cancer for white females who are being examined annually. J Natl Cancer Inst 1989;81:1879–86.
13. Hoskins KF, Stopfer JE, Calzone KA, et al. Assessment and counseling for women with a family history of breast cancer. a guide for clinicians. JAMA 1995;273:577–85.
14. Claus E, Risch N, Thompson D. Autosomal dominant inheritance of early-onset breast cancer. Cancer 1994;73:643–51.
15. Vasen H, Mecklin J, Khan P, et al. The International Collaborative Group on Hereditary Nonpolyposis Colorectal Cancer (ICG-HNPCC). Dis Colon Rectum 1991;34:424–5.
16. Rodriguez-Bigas M, Boland C, Hamilton S, et al. A National Cancer Institute workshop on hereditary nonpolyposis colorectal cancer syndrome: meeting highlights and Bethesda guidelines. J Natl Cancer Inst 1997;89:1758–62.
17. Shattuck-Eidens D, Oliphant A, McClure M, et al. *BRCA1* sequence analysis in women at high risk for susceptibility mutations, risk factor analysis, and implications for genetic testing. JAMA 1997;278:1242–50.
18. Berry D, Parmigiani G, Sanchez J, et al. Probability of carrying a mutation of breast-ovarian cancer gene *BRCA1* based on family history. J Natl Cancer Inst 1997;89:227–38.
19. Hallowell N, Statham H, Murton F. Women's understanding of their risk of developing breast/ovarian cancer before and after genetic counseling. J Genet Counsel 1998;7:345–64.
20. Sagi M, Kaduri L, Zlotogora J, et al. The effect of genetic counseling on knowledge and perceptions regarding risks for breast cancer. J Genet Counsel 1998;7:417–34.
21. Lynch H, Lemon S, Durham C, et al. A descriptive study of *BRCA1* testing and reactions to disclosure of test results. Cancer 1997;79:2219–28.
22. Wijnen J, Khan P, Vasen H, et al. Hereditary nonpolyposis colorectal cancer families not complying with the Amsterdam criteria show extremely low frequency of mismatch-repair-gene mutations. Am J Hum Genet 1997;61:329–35.
23. Burke W, Daly M, Garber J, et al. Recommendations for follow-up care of individuals with an inherited predisposition to cancer. II: *BRCA1* and *BRCA2*. JAMA 1997;277:997–1003.
24. Burke W, Petersen G, Lynch P. Recommendations for follow-up care of individuals with an inherited predisposition to cancer. I: Hereditary nonpolyposis colon cancer. JAMA 1997;277:915–19.
25. Fisher B, Costantino J, Wickerham L, et al. Tamoxifen for prevention of breast cancer: report of the National Surgical Adjuvant Breast and Bowel Project P-1 Study. J Natl Cancer Inst 1998:90:1371–88.
26. Daly M, Obrams GI. Epidemiology and risk assessment for ovarian cancer. Semin Oncol 1998;25:255–64.
27. Piver S, Jushi M, Tsukada Y, et al. Primary peritoneal carcinoma after prophylactic oophorectomy in women with a family history of ovarian cancer. Cancer 1993;71:2751–55.
28. Eisen A, Weber B. Primary peritoneal carcinoma can have multifocal origins: implications for prophylactic oophorectomy. J Natl Cancer Inst 1998;90:797–99.
29. Hartmann L, Jenkins R, Schaid D, et al. Prophylactic mastectomy: preliminary retrospective cohort analysis. Proc Am Assoc Can Res 1997;38:1123.
30. Ursin G, Henderson B, Halle R, et al. Does oral contraceptive use increase the risk of breast cancer in women with *BRCA1/BRCA2* mutations more than in other women? Cancer Res 1997;57:3678–81.

# CHAPTER 4

# PRINCIPLES OF CANCER PREVENTION

• FRANK L. MEYSKENS, JR.

The best therapy for cancer is prevention. Advances in the identification of predisposition and testing (assessment of genetic risk), understanding the biology of early cancer formation (carcinogenesis), the development of effective screening modalities, the identification of major avoidable risk factors for cancer development, and the emerging field of chemoprevention suggest that the contribution of cancer prevention to decreasing the overall morbidity and mortality from cancer will increase rapidly in the near future. Clinical oncologists have begun to participate actively in this process, having relegated much of the development of cancer prevention in the past to epidemiologists and biologists in the research milieu and to primary care physicians and public health officials in the practical mode. Clinical oncologists need to incorporate the strategies of cancer prevention into their practices to ensure maximal health benefit and to provide continuity of care for their patients and their families.

## The Biology of Cancer Formation

An understanding of the general biologic features that underlie the formation of the cancer cell is essential to the implementation of a successful cancer prevention effort. An increasing amount of information suggests that the cancer cell develops through cumulative genetic changes[1]; many of these steps may be amenable to prescriptive intervention. The process of carcinogenesis needs to be viewed from many perspectives; an integrated approach is provided in Figure 4–1.[2] From a clinical viewpoint, the patient is normal or normal with a genetic predisposition or has an identifiable precancer or a malignancy. The designation of "normality" has become increasingly less certain and more complex as our understanding of underlying genetic risk at the cellular level has deepened. These issues are discussed in more detail in Chapters 2 and 3.

A useful way to view the issue of genetic risk may be to consider that each individual has a set point for malignant transformation of any particular cell.[3] Advances in molecular genetics have allowed a more precise identification of that risk. At one extreme are defects in key genes that inevitably result in cancer (e.g., loss of a particular gene located at chromosome 11 leads to hereditary retinoblastoma), whereas at the other extreme are situations in which multiple acquired genetic changes must occur before the fully transformed malignant cell develops (e.g., a series of mutations and deletions must occur before colon cancer develops). In either case, molecular changes in key genes occur and it is on the particular phenotypic expression that exogenous influences and factors act. The initial molecular change defines the stage of carcinogenesis known as *initiation*, whether the

alteration emanates from a hereditary genetic contribution or from acquired genetic damage from a physical, viral, or chemical carcinogen.[4] What is remarkable is that the same key molecular change occurs with high frequency for any particular cancer.[2] Furthermore, the same agent may cause a similar molecular change in a diversity of organs.[5]

Once the initial molecular damage has occurred, the cell is primed for further phenotypic change and alterations; this is the stage of carcinogenesis known as *promotion*. This step may last a long time (for decades in humans) and should be highly amenable to dietary, hormonal, or pharmacologic interventions.[6–8] Promotion is characterized by a gradual expansion of phenotypic abnormalities at the molecular and biochemical levels and eventual clinical recognition at the histologic level. A number of markers may develop during this time that can be used to predict subsequent malignant expression.[9] Some common promoters include hormones, components of cigarette smoke, ultraviolet light, and dietary substances. Many other dietary components probably serve as natural chemopreventive agents as well and put a brake on the carcinogenesis process, the most prominent example being vitamin A and its derivative β-*trans*-retinoic acid (vitamin A acid).[10] With time, the promoted cell replicates, and eventually a hyperplastic focus develops; when histologically identifiable, the lesion becomes "preneoplasia."[7, 11, 12]

The stage from histologic preneoplasia to frank malignancy may extend from months to years, is progressively accompanied by an increasing number of acquired genetic changes, should be suppressible for some time, and should be of major interest to clinical oncologists. In addition to the well-known and well-studied example of cervical dysplasia, other common precancers include leukoplakia (oropharynx), bronchial metaplasia (lung), various bladder abnormalities, colon polyps, actinic keratoses and other cutaneous changes, and dysplastic nevi (melanoma). Progression of these precancers and other premalignant lesions should be controllable in many instances with preventive intervention.[7, 13–19]

What is clear about our understanding of carcinogenesis is that the process is a continuum in which a series of discrete changes can be identified that result in a more and more autonomous cellular process. The hope is that each step may serve as a target for preventive or therapeutic intervention by which to interrupt the evolution to cancer.

## Screening as a Prevention Strategy

Classically, screening is viewed as the identification of disease in asymptomatic individuals, whereas early detection occurs in a clinically symptomatic patient. The boundary

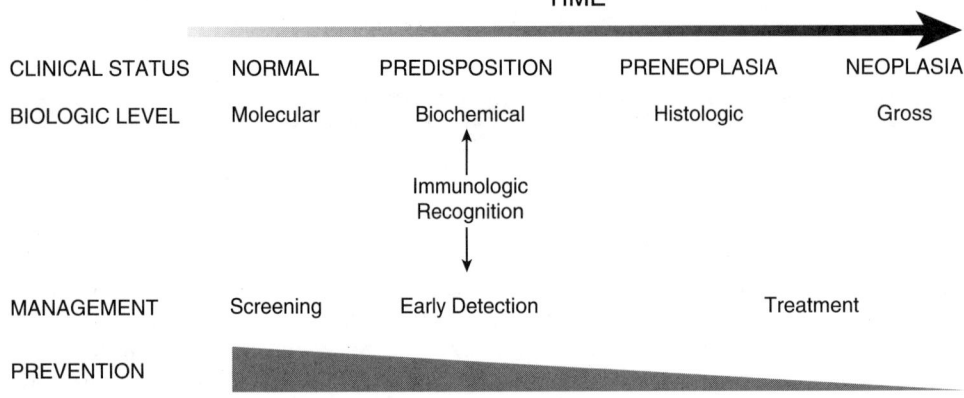

TIME

| CLINICAL STATUS | NORMAL | PREDISPOSITION | PRENEOPLASIA | NEOPLASIA |
| BIOLOGIC LEVEL | Molecular | Biochemical | Histologic | Gross |

Immunologic
Recognition

| MANAGEMENT | Screening | Early Detection | | Treatment |

PREVENTION

**Figure 4–1.** Multilevel perspective of cancer evolution and management.

between screening and early detection is becoming increasingly blurred as advances in biology allow us to identify "disease" at earlier and earlier stages.

The use of screening is an important prevention strategy. A large number of techniques have been used to screen for cancer, but the data are sufficiently impressive for only two modalities to recommend their widespread general use. These techniques include mammography in women between the ages of 50 and 69 (and probably age 40 to 49 as well) and Papanicolaou cytologic studies in sexually active women.[20, 21] Evidence for efficacy for the use of Hemoccult screening (for fecal occult blood) in colon cancer has also increased as has the use of routine flexible sigmoidoscopy in individuals older than age 50.[22, 23] The value of prostate-specific antigen (PSA) as a screening tool for identifying asymptomatic prostate cancer continues to be hotly debated, and vigorous opinions have been expressed on both sides of the issue.[24, 25] A recent randomized population-based trial suggests that screening PSA may indeed reduce mortality from prostate cancer.[26] Currently, there is no definitive information that supports the use of any technique as a screening tool for lung, bladder, stomach, or ovarian cancer, although the proponents for bronchoscopy, gastric or bladder cytologic studies, and vaginal ultrasonography are many.

The use of screening procedures in individuals at high risk for cancer because of a family or hereditary background, prior cancer, and occupational or other exposure may well be appropriate. However, the clinical indications for such screening are only now being defined, and this is a controversial and ethically challenging area of research.[27, 28] The topic of cancer screening is discussed further in Chapter 5.

## Major Avoidable Risk Factors

There are a large number of factors that can contribute to the development of human cancer. Some of the more important ones are listed in Table 4–1. It should be emphasized that cigarette smoking is the number one avoidable risk factor for morbidity and mortality from all diseases.[29] The large range of effects of cigarette smoking on organ carcinogenesis is generally not well appreciated, even by clinical oncologists.[30] In addition to its widely appreciated contribution to cancer of the lung and aerodigestive tract (larynx, oropharynx, esophagus), cigarette smoking also contributes

significantly in an etiologic fashion to the development of at least eight other cancers, including those of the bladder, kidney, cervix, pancreas, and stomach. Surprisingly, epidemiologic and biologic evidence also implicates cigarette smoking in the development of 15 to 25% of adult leukemias.[31] Overall, smoking contributes in a highly significant way to the development of more than 35% of all cancers.

The role of cigarette smoking in cancer formation extends beyond its contribution to primary carcinogenesis and tumor development. Experimental and clinical evidence shows that cigarette smoking leads to "field carcinogenesis" in target organs. This has two important implications: (1) The control of second malignancies in survivors of primary cancer is improved by discontinuation of cigarette smoking[32] and (2) suppression or inhibition of second malignancies is an important strategy in controlling cancer.[33] Clinical oncologists should be prominently involved in both areas. In well-studied carcinomas involving sites such as the aerodigestive and urologic tracts, more than 25% of the mortality in patients cured of low-stage disease results from a second malignancy in the same organ. The prevention of these malignancies has become an increasingly important strategy in the control of cancer.

Clinical oncologists need to help their patients stop smoking. What works and what does not has been well studied. In dealing with patients who smoke, following a few simple

*Table 4–1.* **Attributable Risk Factors for Cancer**

| Agent | Major Types of Cancer | Estimated Contribution to Excess Cancer Mortality (%) |
|---|---|---|
| Tobacco | Lung, oropharynx, bladder, cervix* | 30 |
| Diet | Breast, colon, prostate, aerodigestive† | 35 |
| Radiation ionizing | Lung, leukemia | 3 |
| Chemicals or occupation | Bladder, mesothelioma | 4 |

*Also evidence for pancreas, esophagus, kidney, stomach, and bone marrow (leukemia).

†Almost all cancers have shown a protective association with a vegetable-based diet.

Adapted from Doll R, Peto R. The causes of cancer: quantitative estimates of avoidable risks of cancer in the United States today. J Natl Cancer Inst 1981; 66:1191–308.

guidelines decreases the incidence of cigarette smoking, particularly in patients with a recent diagnosis of cancer[34–36]:

1. The message from the physician to stop smoking should be firm and unequivocal.

2. Cigarette smoking should be treated as a medical condition, and the patient should be given a prescription to stop smoking.

3. Specific follow-up of the status of cigarette smoking behavior and associated symptoms should be made and positive reinforcement offered by the physician and staff.

Using this simple physician-led strategy can lead to more than 50% of patients stopping smoking.

There are a large number of factors that contribute to the causation of cancer, and they are discussed in subsequent disease-related chapters. These factors include ionizing (lung, leukemia) and nonionizing (skin cancer) radiation, viruses (papilloma for the cervix and hepatitis for the liver), and chemicals (bladder, lung mesothelioma, liver). Among chemicals, aflatoxin (hepatoma), aromatic amines (bladder), asbestos (lung, mesothelioma), benzene (leukemia), and vinyl chloride (liver angiosarcoma) make a substantial contribution to the incidence of cancer.

Based on epidemiologic studies, alterations in the dietary intake of fat, fiber, and various micronutrients can increase the risk of human cancer. The magnitude of this contribution to risk in various studies varies from 10 to 70%.[37] Excess dietary fat contributes to the development of breast, colon, prostate, and endometrial cancers, and the attributable risk may be substantial. A vexing methodologic issue has been to discriminate total calories from dietary fat per se, but animal feeding studies suggest that both factors—fat and calories—contribute independently.[38] Fiber appears to demonstrate a consistently protective effect against the development of polyps and invasive cancer in the colon. In vitro and physiologic studies indicate that the mechanisms are complex and involve absorption of oxidized bile acids, decreased fecal transit time, and generation of soluble fiber products, such as butyrate, with differentiation-producing properties.[39, 40] Increased fiber in the diet may also protect against the development of breast cancer by absorbing and functionally inactivating dietary compounds that have estrogenic properties.

There are many micronutrients that have been identified as important in the development of certain cancers.[41] Most prominent among these are vitamin A, beta-carotene, ascorbic acid (vitamin C), alpha-tocopherol (vitamin E), and selenium.[38] A substantial amount of epidemiologic and laboratory data, as well as mechanistic considerations, suggest a broad role for these compounds in the natural prevention of cancer.[42]

## Chemoprevention

Chemoprevention of cancer is the prevention of cancer using dietary or chemical compounds. This modality is becoming a major new form of cancer treatment. The strategy of controlling disease by preventing its development is well established in cardiology. Examples include the use of drugs and diet to control blood pressure and cholesterol, and cardiac conditioning through exercise. Strategies for prescriptive prevention to control cancer lag about 15 years behind those of cardiology.

Since the 1970s, a body of experimental and epidemiologic evidence has accumulated supporting the notion of chemoprevention. In the 1990s, dietary compounds were targeted as possible chemoprevention agents, and myriad pharmacologic agents became available. The development of chemoprevention agents for human use is an exacting, lengthy, and demanding process.[43] The strategy parallels new drug development for therapeutic agents but differs in important ways. Some of the major issues that arise include the following:

1. Is it ethical to develop agents for use in well populations?

2. Is the maximum tolerated dose (MTD) relevant to chemoprevention? If not, what dose is?

3. Is it reasonable to perform dose de-escalation trials of drugs in which the MTD can be extrapolated from the results of therapeutic trials?

4. Since cancer usually develops after a prolonged latent period, can one identify intermediate markers of cancer risk that predict the likelihood of subsequent cancer? Would such intermediate markers be the same as other, more traditional markers of cancer risk?

The science of drug development for chemoprevention agents is in active evolution. Some of the key trials that have been completed to date are summarized in Table 4–2. Several large trials indicate that different types of vitamin A derivatives (retinoids) can reverse oral leukoplakia[44] or suppress cervical intraepithelial neoplasia.[45] Two large stud-

*Table 4–2.* **Definitive Positive Large Randomized Chemoprevention Trials**

| Target End Points | Agent | Total No. of Participants | Comment | Reference |
|---|---|---|---|---|
| Oral leukoplakia | Isotretinoin | 44 | Highly effective, toxic | Hong et al.[44] |
| Second aerodigestive cancers | Isotretinoin | 103 | Effective, toxic | Hong et al.[46] |
| Second lung cancers | Retinyl palmitate | 307 | Effective, nontoxic | Pastorino et al.[47] |
| Resected adenoma | Vitamins A, C, E | 209 | Decreased recurrent polyps, well tolerated | Roncucci et al.[69] |
| Actinic keratoses | *Trans*-retinoic acid (topical) | 455 | Effective, low toxicity | Kligman[70] |
| First skin cancer | Retinol | 2,298 | Effective, well tolerated | Moon et al.[63] |
| Stomach cancer | Multiple vitamins | 29,584 | Prevents stomach cancer, well tolerated | Blot et al.[65] |
| Cervix cancer | *Trans*-retinoic acid (topical) | 301 | Enhances regression of dysplasia, acceptable side effects | Meyskens et al.[45] |
| Breast cancer | Tamoxifen | 14,000 | Highly effective, some side effects | Fisher et al.[50] |

ies suggest that the appearance of second malignancies in the aerodigestive tract or lung can be suppressed using high doses of 13-*cis*-retinoic acid (Accutane) or retinyl palmitate (vitamin A), respectively.[46, 47] Conversely, supplementary beta-carotene produced an excess of lung cancers and mortality in two large randomized trials.[48, 49] The reduction of breast cancer incidence by 45% in women at increased risk for breast cancer who took tamoxifen has been reported and is a significant event in the field of chemoprevention.[50] However, two subsequent, smaller randomized trials have been negative,[51, 52] and coupled with the side effects of this compound, enthusiasm for tamoxifen as a chemopreventive agent has been tempered.

A major limitation of chemoprevention to date has been the side effects of the available agents. Newer studies are directed to testing lower doses of active retinoids; different, less toxic retinoids (e.g., *N*-4-hydroxyphenylretinamide); and other compounds (e.g., vitamin E, beta-carotene).[53–55]

Limited, short-term studies have been published on the chemoprevention of colon polyps and colorectal cancer. A number of agents appear to have potential efficacy, as measured by short-term changes in the frequency of polyp formation or the modulation of an appropriate intermediate biologic or biochemical end point. These compounds include vitamin C, sulindac (a nonsteroidal anti-inflammatory agent), calcium, and difluoromethylornithine (a polyamine synthesis inhibitor).[56–60] Newer, larger randomized trials will determine the efficacy of several of these agents (wheat bran fiber, sulindac, calcium, and aspirin) in the prevention of secondary polyp occurrence, and one trial is examining the role of calcium in preventing the development of secondary colon cancers.

In nonmelanoma skin cancer, beta-carotene, 13-*cis*-retinoic acid, and retinol have been found to be ineffective in preventing the development of new cutaneous cancers in patients who have had one or more skin cancers removed.[61–63] However, high doses of 13-*cis*-retinoic acid can inhibit secondary skin cancer development in patients with the genetic disease xeroderma pigmentosum.[64] In contrast, at a relatively low dose, retinol (vitamin A) inhibits the development of new skin cancers in patients with prior actinic keratoses.[63]

A large number of other trials have been reported with encouraging data that the early stages of cancer formation in the stomach (multivitamins), bladder (etretinate), and cervix (retinoic acid) may be susceptible to control by chemoprevention.[65–67]

In addition to the studies cited, there are many large chemoprevention trials in progress around the world. Large randomized trials are being conducted to determine if chemoprevention agents can prevent some major malignancies. These include the prevention of lung and head and neck cancers with lower doses of the retinoid 13-*cis*-retinoic acid and the prevention of prostate cancer with the testosterone inhibitor finasteride (Proscar), as well as studies with other compounds.[67–69] Participation by clinical oncologists in these trials is important.

Prevention of cancer will become increasingly focused as epidemiology and molecular biology converge to provide the opportunity of intervention at the earliest stages of cancer development. This will include studies in high-risk popula-

tions of individuals and, ultimately, the use of targeted agents for high-risk individuals.

Screening and early detection will become indistinguishable as reliable molecular markers are developed. Chemoprevention will serve as the therapeutic arm of this endeavor and the management of cancer will be directed toward early intervention. Clinical oncologists need to understand this new discipline, or the early care of cancer patients will default to others.

## SUGGESTIONS FOR ADDITIONAL READING

Bertram JS, Kolonel LN, Meyskens FL Jr. Rationale and strategies for chemoprevention of cancer in humans. Cancer Res 1987;47:3012–31.

Cummings S, Olopade O. Predisposition testing for inherited breast cancer. Oncology 1998;12:1227–41.

Doll R, Peto R. The cause of cancer: quantitative estimates of avoidable risks of cancer in the United States today. J Natl Cancer Inst 1981;66:1191–1308.

Henderson BE, Ross RK, Pike MC. Toward the primary prevention of cancer. Science 1991;254:1131–8.

Hong WK, Sporn MB. Recent advances in chemoprevention of cancer. Science 1997;278:1073–7.

Meyskens FL Jr. Strategies for prevention of cancer in humans. Oncology 1992;6:Suppl:16–24.

Newcombe PA, Carbone PP. The health consequences of smoking. Med Clin North Am 1992;76:305–31.

Willett WC. Diet and health: what should we eat? Science 1994;264:532–7

## REFERENCES

1. Vogelstein B, Fearon ER, Hamilton SR, et al. Genetic alterations during colorectal-tumor development. N Engl J Med 1988;319:525–32.
2. Bertram JS, Kolonel LN, Meyskens FL Jr. Rationale and strategies for chemoprevention of cancer in humans. Cancer Res 1987;47:3012–31.
3. Lippman SM, Bassford TL, Meyskens FL Jr. A quantitatively scored cancer-risk assessment tool: its development and use. J Cancer Educ 1992;7:15–36.
4. Wattenberg LW. Chemoprevention of cancer. Cancer Res 1985;45:1–8.
5. Aguilar F, Hussain SP, Cerutti P. Aflatoxin B1 induces the transversion of G→T in codon 249 of the p53 tumor suppressor gene in human hepatocytes. Proc Natl Acad Sci U S A 1993;90:8586–90.
6. Ames BN, Gold LS, Willett WC. The causes and prevention of cancer. Proc Natl Acad Sci U S A 1995;92:5258–65.
7. Lipkin M, Newmark H, Boone CW, et al. Calcium, vitamin D, and colon cancer. Cancer Res 1991;51:3069–70.
8. Henderson BE, Ross RK, Pike MC. Toward the primary prevention of cancer. Science 1991;254:1131–38.
9. Meyskens FL Jr. Biomarker intermediate endpoints and cancer prevention. J Natl Cancer Inst 1992;13:177–81.
10. Lippman SM, Kessler JF, Meyskens FL Jr. Retinoids as preventive and therapeutic anticancer agents. Part I. Cancer Treat Rep 1987;71:391–405.
11. Meyskens FL Jr. Strategies for prevention of cancer in humans. Oncology 1992;6:15–24.
12. Lippman SM, Lee JS, Lotan R, et al. Biomarkers as intermediate end points in chemoprevention trials. J Natl Cancer Inst 1990;82:555–60.
13. Lippman SM. Retinoids and aerodigestive cancers. In: DeVita VT, eds. Important advances in oncology. Philadelphia: JB Lippincott, 1992:93.
14. Sellers TA, Potter JD, Bailey-Wilson JE, et al. Lung cancer detection and prevention: evidence for an interaction between smoking and genetic predisposition. Cancer Res 1992;52:2694–7.
15. Garewal HS, Meyskens FL Jr. Retinoids and carotenoids in the prevention of oral cancer: a critical appraisal. Cancer Epidemiol Biomarkers Prev 1992;1:155–9.
16. Meyskens FL Jr. The place of chemoprevention studies in cancer prevention planning. Prog Clin Biol Res 1990;346:135–43.
17. Gensler H. Prevention of cutaneous cancers. In: Dawson M, Okamura WH, eds. Chemistry and biology of synthetic retinoids. Boca Raton, Fla.: CRC Press, 1990:467.

18. Atiba JO, Meyskens FL Jr. Chemoprevention of breast cancer. Semin Oncol 1992;19:220–9.
19. Wattenberg LW. Chemoprevention of cancer. Cancer Res 1985;45:1–8.
20. Hurley SF, Kaldor JM. The benefits and risks of mammographic screening for breast cancer. Epidemiol Rev 1992;14:101–30.
21. Cramer DW. The role of cervical cytology in the declining morbidity and mortality of cervical cancer. Cancer 1974;34:2018–27.
22. Mandel JS, Bond JH, Church TR, et al. Reducing mortality from colorectal cancer by screening for fecal occult blood. Minnesota Colon Cancer Control Study. N Engl J Med 1993;328:1365–71.
23. Shapiro S. Case-control studies of colorectal cancer mortality: is the case made for screening sigmoidoscopy? J Natl Cancer Inst 1992;84:1546–7.
24. Collins MM, Barry MJ. Controversies in prostate cancer screening. Analogies to the early lung cancer screening debate. JAMA 1996;276:1976–9.
25. Denis LJ. Prostate cancer screening and prevention: "realities and hope." Urology 1995;46:56–61.
26. Diamond GP, Belange A, Bousseau G, et al. Decrease of prostate cancer from PSA screening. Proc Am Soc Clin Oncol 1998;17:2a.
27. Cummings S, Olopade O. Predisposition testing for inherited breast cancer. Oncology 1998;12:1227–41.
28. Lerman C, Rimer BK, Engstrom PF. Cancer risk notification: phychosocial and ethical implications. J Clin Oncol 1991;9:1275–82.
29. Centers for Disease Control. Smoking attributable mortality and years of potential life lost—United States 1988. MMWR 1991;40:62.
30. Peto R, Lopez AD, Boneham J, et al. Mortality from tobacco in developed countries: indirect estimation from national vital statistics. Lancet 1992;339:1268–78.
31. Sandler DP, Shore DL, Anderson JR, et al. Cigarette smoking and risk of acute leukemia: associations with morphology and cytogenetic abnormalities in bone marrow. J Natl Cancer Inst 1993;85:1994–2003.
32. Richardson GE, Tucker MA, Venzon DJ, et al. Smoking cessation after successful treatment of small-cell lung cancer is associated with fewer smoking-related second primary cancers. Ann Intern Med 1993:119:383–90.
33. Meyskens FL Jr. Biology and intervention of the premalignant process. Cancer Bull 1991;43:475.
34. Clinical opportunities for smoking intervention: a guide for the busy physician. Washington, D.C.: National Institutes of Health Publication No. 86–2178, 1986.
35. Ockene JK: Physician-delivered interventions for smoking cessation: strategies for increased effectiveness. Prev Med 1987;16:723–37.
36. DiClemente CC, Prochaska JO, Fairhurst SK, et al. The process of smoking cessation: an analysis of precontemplation, contemplation, and preparation stages of change. J Consult Clin Psychol 1991;59:295–304.
37. Willett WC, Hunter DJ, Stampfer MJ, et al. Dietary fat and fiber in relation to risk of breast cancer. An 8-year follow-up. JAMA 1992;268:2037–44.
38. Willett WC, Stampfer MJ, Colditz GA, et al. Dietary fat and the risk of breast cancer. N Engl J Med 1987;316:22–8.
39. Light L, Lanza E, Greenwald P. Progress in diet and cancer research. Prog Clin Biol Res 1989;320:89–99
40. Reddy BS, Burill C, Rigotty J. Effects of diets high in omega-3 and omega-6 fatty acids on initiation and postinitiation stages of colon carcinogenesis. Cancer Res 1991;51:487–491.
41. Weisburger JH. Nutritional approach to cancer prevention with emphasis on vitamins, antioxidants, and carotenoids. Am J Clin Nutr 1991;53:226s–37s.
42. Meyskens FL Jr. Micronutrients. In: DeVita V, ed. Cancer principles and practice. 5th ed. New York: Lippincott-Raven, 1997:573.
43. Goodman GE. The clinical evaluation of cancer chemoprevention agents: defining and contrasting phase I, II, and III objectives. Cancer Res 1992;52:2752s–7s.
44. Hong WK, Endicott J, Itri LM, et al. 13-*cis*-retinoic acid in the treatment of oral leukoplakia. N Engl J Med 1986;315:1501–5.
45. Meyskens FL Jr, Surwit E, Moon TE, et al. Enhancement of regression of cervical intraepithelial neoplasia II (moderate dysplasia) with topically applied all-*trans*-retinoic acid: a randomized trial. J Natl Cancer Inst 1994;86:539–43.
46. Hong WK, Lipman SM, Itri LM, et al. Prevention of second primary tumors with isotretinoin in squamous-cell carcinoma of the head and neck. N Engl J Med 1990;323:795–801.
47. Pastorino U, Infante M, Maioli M, et al. Adjuvant treatment of stage I lung cancer with high-dose vitamin A. J Clin Oncol 1993;11:1216–22.
48. The Alpha-Tocopherol, Beta-Carotene Prevention Study Group: The effect of vitamin E and beta-carotene on the incidence of lung cancer and other cancers in male smokers. N Engl J Med 1994;330:1029–35.
49. Omenn GS, Goodman GE, Thornquist MD, et al. Effects of a combination of beta carotene and vitamin A on lung cancer and cardiovascular disease. N Engl J Med 1996;334:1150–5.
50. Fisher B, Costantino JP, Wickenham DL, et al. Tamoxifen for prevention of breast cancer: report of the National Surgical Adjuvant Breast and Bowel Project P-1 study. J Natl Cancer Inst 1998;90:1371–88.
51. Veronesi U, Maisonneuvre P, Costa A, et al. Prevention of breast cancer with tamoxifen: preliminary findings from the Italian randomised trial among hysterectomised women. Italian Tomoxifen Prevention Study. Lancet 1998;352:93–7.
52. Powles T, Eeles R, Ashley S, et al. Interim analysis of the incidence of breast cancer in the Royal Marsden Hospital tamoxifen randomised chemoprevention trial. Lancet 1998;352:98–101.
53. Lippman SM, Batsakis JG, Toth BB, et al. Comparison of low-dose isotretinoin with beta carotene to prevent oral carcinogenesis. N Engl J Med 1993;328:15–20.
54. Garewal HS, Meyskens FL Jr, Killen D, et al. Response of oral leukoplakia to beta-carotene. J Clin Oncol 1990;8:1715–20.
55. Chiesa F, Tradata N, Marazza M, et al. Prevention of local relapses and new localisations of oral leukoplakias with the synthetic retinoid fenretinide (4-HPR). Preliminary results. Eur J Cancer B Oral Oncol 1992;28:97–102.
56. Bussey HJ, DeCosse JJ, Deschner EE, et al. A randomized trial of ascorbic acid in polyposis coli. Cancer 1982;50:1434–9.
57. Giardiello FM, Hamilton SR, Krush AJ, et al. Treatment of colonic and rectal adenomas with sulindac in familial adenomatous polyposis. N Engl J Med 1993;328:1313–6.
58. Lipkin M, Newmark H. Effect of added dietary calcium on colonic epithelial-cell proliferation in subjects at high risk for familial colonic cancer. N Engl J Med 1985;313:1381–4.
59. Rigau J, Piquae JM, Rubio E, et al. Effects of long-term sulindac therapy on colonic polyposis. Ann Intern Med 1991;115:952–4.
60. Meyskens FL Jr, Gerner EW, Emerson S, et al. Effect of alpha-difluoromethylornithine on rectal mucosal levels of polyamines in a randomized, double-blinded trial for colon cancer prevention. J Natl Cancer Inst 1998;90:1212–18.
61. Greenberg ER, Baron JA, Stukel TA, et al. A clinical trial of beta carotene to prevent basal-cell and squamous-cell cancers of the skin. The Skin Cancer Prevention Study Group. N Engl J Med 1990;323:789–95.
62. Tangrea JA, Edwards BK, Taylor PR, et al. Long-term therapy with low-dose isotretinoin for prevention of basal cell carcinoma: a multicenter clinical trial. Isotretinoin-Basal Cell Carcinoma Study Group. J Natl Cancer Inst 1992;84:328–32.
63. Moon TE, Levine N, Cartmel B, et al. Effect of retinol in preventing squamous cell skin cancer in moderate-risk subjects: a randomized, double-blind, controlled trial. Southwest Skin Cancer Prevention Study Group. Cancer Epidemiol Biomarkers Prev 1997;6:949–56.
64. Kraemer KH, DiGiovanna JJ, Moshell AN, et al. Prevention of skin cancer in xeroderma pigmentosum with the use of oral isotretinoin. N Engl J Med 1988;318:1633–7.
65. Blot WJ, Li JY, Taylor PR, et al. Nutrition intervention trials in Linxian, China: supplementation with specific vitamin/mineral combinations, cancer incidence, and disease-specific mortality in the general population. J Natl Cancer Inst 1993;85:1483–92.
66. Alfthan O, Tarkkanen J, Greohn P, et al. Tigason (etretinate) in prevention of recurrence of superficial bladder tumors. A double-blind clinical trial. Eur Urol 1983;9:6–9.
67. Fisher B. The evolution of paradigms for the management of breast cancer: a personal perspective. Cancer Res 1992;52:2371–83.
68. Donodeo F. Prevention trial for prostate cancer piques public interest. J Natl Cancer Inst 1993;85:1801–2.
69. Roncucci L, Di Donato P, Carati L, et al. Antioxidant vitamins or lactulose for the prevention of the recurrence of colorectal adenomas. Colorectal Cancer Study Group of the University of Modena and the Health Care District 16. Dis Colon Rectum 1993;36:227–34.
70. Kligman AM. In: Marks R, ed. Retinoids in cutaneous malignancy. Cambridge: Blackwell Scientific, 1991:66.

# CHAPTER 5

# PRINCIPLES OF CANCER SCREENING*

• OTIS W. BRAWLEY • PHILIP C. PROROK •
• JOHN GOHAGAN • BARNETT S. KRAMER •

Screening is an important element in any cancer control program. It is a means of detecting disease early in asymptomatic populations. The goal of cancer screening is not simply to diagnose cancer in an early preclinical stage in asymptomatic individuals. The true goal of screening is to decrease the morbidity and mortality of cancer through early detection. Although advances in technology are making it easier to diagnose disease, it is imperative to understand that early detection does not guarantee benefit.[1] For screening to be useful, the test or procedure must detect cancer earlier, and there must be evidence that treatment at this earlier, preclinical stage of disease results in an improved outcome compared with treatment at later stages of disease.

Screening interventions are performed on asymptomatic, presumably healthy individuals. The examinations, tests, and procedures are not necessarily diagnostic. They are performed to assess suspicion and to indicate whether or not a diagnostic work-up is in order. Screening is most likely to benefit a population when the targeted neoplasms are common.

For widespread use, a screening test or procedure must be safe, convenient, acceptable to the public, and relatively inexpensive. It must also be accurate and reliable. Accuracy reflects the intervention's ability to discriminate disease. The four indices of accuracy are sensitivity, specificity, positive predictive value, and negative predictive value (Table 5–1). *Sensitivity* is the proportion designated positive by the screening test among all individuals who have the disease, whereas *specificity* is the proportion designated negative by the test among all those who do not have the disease. The *positive predictive value* is the proportion of individuals testing positive who have the disease and, similarly, *negative predictive value* is the proportion of individuals with a negative test result who do not have the disease.

The prevalence of disease has tremendous influence on the positive predictive value of a test (Table 5–2). Screening is usually most efficient and economic when performed in populations with a high prevalence of the targeted disease. Reasonably high specificity is required for screening examinations, whereas sensitivity need not be extremely high. High sensitivity is necessary for diagnostic testing, but high specificity is not as critical.

## Biases of Screening

Screening is subject to a number of biases that can suggest benefit when there is none.

*Lead-time bias* occurs when a screening test does not have an impact on the natural history of the disease but merely prolongs the time the subject is aware of the disease (Fig. 5–1). The magnitude of lead-time bias is a function of the test's sensitivity, the testing interval, and the duration of the disease's preclinical phase. It is important to note that increased survival from diagnosis by itself is not a legitimate measure of the effectiveness of screening because the treatment may not affect the natural history of the disease. The survival may simply be artificially lengthened by the amount of the lead time.

*Length bias* is seen when slowly growing, less aggressive cancers are detected during screening. Cases diagnosed between scheduled screening tests, because of the onset of symptoms, are more aggressive, on average, and are associated with worse survival. The inherent properties of the tumors found during screening, and not an improvement in those properties due to screening, are responsible for the screened population enjoying better survival. Overdiagnosis is a type of length bias.

*Selection bias* results when a population screened differs from the general population with which it is compared. Individuals volunteering to be screened may be more health conscious than the general population, and this may affect results (the "healthy volunteer effect"), or they may be motivated to participate because of a risk factor not found in the general population.

The reservoir of some undetected malignancies is large. Improved technology, together with the increased use of such technology in screening, has the potential to amplify the documented prevalence and incidence of these cancers without beneficial effect. Some lesions that fulfill the criteria of malignancy by histologic standards may be of no clinical significance. Identification of these lesions involves a special type of length bias known as *overdiagnosis*. Screening can increase the number of cases of a specific cancer and even create the false impression of an epidemic. It can also give the appearance of a stage shift and increased survival duration without necessarily reducing mortality rates.

The value of a screening intervention is best determined by submitting it to the scientific method. This means testing it in a well-designed, randomized, controlled trial that takes into account the biases inherent with screening. In a randomized, controlled screening trial, two like populations are established by random assignment. One population receives the medical standard of care (which may be no screening at all), and the other receives the research intervention. Over time, the two populations are compared to determine if the intervention group benefits when compared with the control group, using cause-specific population mortality as the primary end point. When the screened population has a better

*All material in this chapter is in the public domain, with the exception of any borrowed figures or tables.

*Table 5–1.* Definition of Terms

| Term | Definition |
|------|------------|
| Sensitivity | The proportion of persons with the conditions who test positive: $a/(a + c)$ |
| Specificity | The proportion of persons without the condition who test negative: $d/(b + d)$ |
| Positive predictive value | The proportion of persons with a positive test who have the condition: $a/(a + b)$ |
| Negative predictive value | The proportion of persons with a negative test who do not have the condition: $d/(c + d)$ |

| | | CONDITION PRESENT | CONDITION ABSENT |
|---|---|---|---|
| a = True positive | Positive test | a | b |
| b = False positive | | | |
| c = false negative | Negative test | c | d |
| d = True negative | | | |

cause-specific mortality rate, it implies that screening and treatment lead to increased survival. A randomized, controlled screening trial generally involves thousands of persons and lasts for years.

Other, less definitive study designs are also employed in estimating the effectiveness of screening practices. The relative value of different kinds of evidence of screening benefit can be ranked as follows, from strongest to weakest:

- The results of randomized clinical trials
- The findings of controlled trials without randomization (e.g., subject assignment by birth date or date of clinic appointment)
- The findings of cohort or case-control analytic studies
- The results of multiple time series studies, with or without the intervention
- The opinions of respected authorities based on clinical experience, descriptive studies, or reports of experts

For interpreting screening studies, the best measure of benefit is when a screening procedure leads to decreased cause-specific mortality in a randomized trial. Studies demonstrating a reduction in the incidence of advanced-stage disease, an increase in survival, and a shift in stage are generally considered weaker evidence of benefit. Early detection of cancer can be of apparent benefit to the individual without a true advantage, and there can even be a net harm. Indeed, even if the test has high sensitivity, the intervention may not be of benefit to the patient. The person screened is at risk for the following:

- Unnecessary morbidity due to the screening intervention itself
- Morbidity associated with the work-up of positive test results (both true-positive and false-positive results)
- Excess morbidity and costs from treatment of true-positive test results, even if life is extended by treatment
- The emotional and social repercussions of false-positive results
- The potential overtreatment of indolent lesions of no threat (overdiagnosis)
- The false reassurance of a false-negative test

The psychosocial impact of cancer screening, no matter what the result of the test, should not be underestimated.[2] Screening and the unnecessary treatment that results from it can also be of substantial financial burden to society.

*Table 5–2.* **Positive Predictive Value as a Function of Sensitivity, Specificity, and Disease Prevalence\***

| Prevalence | Specificity | Sensitivity (%) | |
|------------|-------------|-----|------|
| | | 0.8 | 0.95 |
| 5/1000 | 0.95 | 7 | 9 |
| | 0.999 | 80 | 83 |
| 1/10,000 | 0.95 | 0.2 | 0.2 |
| | 0.999 | 7 | 9 |

\*Positive predictive value (PPV) as determined by the following formula:

$$PPV = \frac{(Prevalence)(Sensitivity)}{(Prevalence)(Sensitivity) + (1 - Prevalence)(1 - Specificity)}$$

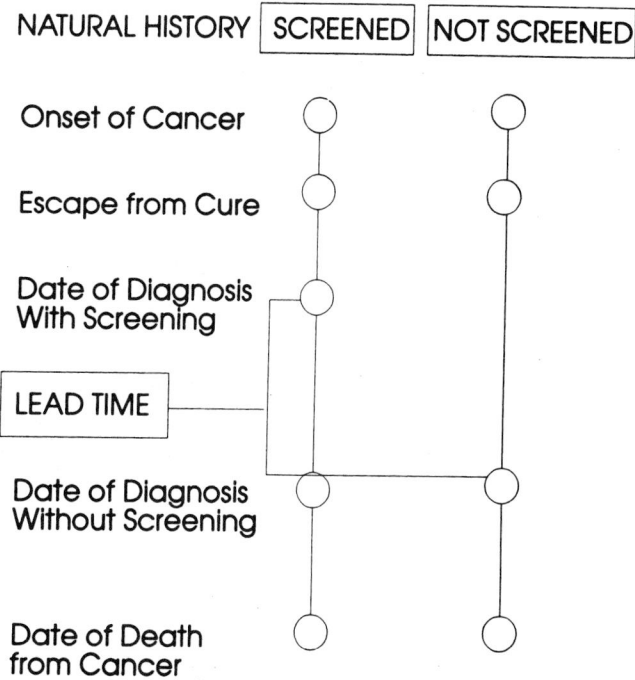

**Figure 5–1.** Lead-time bias.

## Screening for Specific Cancers

Table 5–3 summarizes the screening recommendations of the U.S. Preventive Services Task Force (USPSTF),[1] the Canadian Task Force on Preventive Health Care,[2, 3] the American College of Physicians,[4–6] and the American Cancer Society.[7–9] The National Cancer Institute has developed a series of separate state-of-the-art statements summarizing the literature and attaching levels of evidence to screening studies. Cancer treatment and screening information is available from the National Cancer Institute's Cancer Information Service (1-800-4-CANCER) and the Physicians Data Query (PDQ) system (fax number 1-301-402-5874) or http://cancer-net.nci.nih.gov/.

To date, only generalized breast, colon, and cervical cancer screening has been shown to be beneficial through scientific studies. Special surveillance of those with a high risk or personal history of a specific cancer may be prudent; however, few studies have been conducted to assess the value of this practice. Genetic screening capable of identifying large numbers of individuals at increased risk of specific neoplasms is becoming available.[10, 11] It must be carefully evaluated.

### BREAST CANCER

The fact that lives are saved by screening women older than age 50 with mammography alone or mammography with breast examination has been demonstrated in a number of

*Table 5–3.* Screening Recommendations for Asymptomatic, Normal-Risk Subjects

| Test or Procedure | American Cancer Society | U.S. Preventive Services Task Force | Canadian Task Force on Preventive Health Care | American College of Physicians |
|---|---|---|---|---|
| Sigmoidoscopy | Age 50 and older every 5 yr | Older than age 50 no recommendation Younger than age 50 not recommended | No recommendation | Older than age 50 every 3–5 yr or barium enema every 5 yr |
| Fecal occult blood testing | Age 50 and older every yr | No recommendation | Age 18–39 recommendation against Age older than 40 no recommendation | Older than age 50 every yr |
| Digital rectal examination | Age 50 and older every yr | No recommendation | No recommendation | Not considered |
| Prostate-specific antigen | Offer to men age 50 and older every yr with information | Recommendation against | Recommendation against | No recommendation |
| Papanicolaou test | Women beginning at age 18 yearly × 3 and then every 1–3 yr at physician's discretion | Females at onset of sexual activity to age 65 every 1–3 yr | Women at age 18–69 annually once sexually active or at age 18 then every 3 yr after two normal test results | Women at age 20–65 every 3 yr |
| Pelvic examination | Women age 18–40 every 1–3 yr with Papanicolaou test Older than age 40 every yr | Not recommended, advise adnexal palpation during examination for other reasons | Not recommended, advise adnexal palpation during examination for other reasons | Not considered |
| Endometrial tissue sampling | At menopause if at risk because of obesity or unopposed estrogen use and at physician's discretion | Not considered | Recommendation against | Not considered |
| Breast self-examination | Age 20 and older monthly | No recommendation | No recommendation | Not considered |
| Breast clinical examination | Women age 20–40 every 3 yr Women older than age 40 every yr | Women age 40 and older every yr | Women age 50 and older every yr | Women age 40 and older every yr |
| Mammography | Women age 40–49 every 1–2 yr Women age 50 and older every yr | Women age 50–75 every 1–2 yr | Women older than age 50 every yr | Women older than age 50 every yr |
| Complete skin examination | Age 20–39 every 3 yr | Not recommended | Poor evidence to include or exclude persons of normal risk | Not considered |

This table is a summary of the screening procedures recommended for the general population by the American Cancer Society, the U.S. Preventive Services Task Force, the Canadian Task Force on Preventive Health Care, and the American College of Physicians. "Normal-risk subjects" refers to asymptomatic persons who have no risk factors, other than age or gender, for the targeted condition.

well-designed trials. These studies indicate that screening for breast cancer can decrease the breast cancer mortality rate by approximately 30%. There is insufficient scientific evidence to make an informed decision regarding the screening of women younger than age 50 who are at normal risk. Analysis of eight large randomized trials showed a 17% reduction in breast cancer death for women entering the trials when they were age 40 to 49. This reduction occurred 15 years after the start of screening. Little or no reduction was evident during the first 10 years after screening started, meaning that some of the 17% reduction observed may be due to cancers detected after age 50.

Recommendations on when mammography should begin and how frequently it should be performed vary and are a matter of considerable controversy.[12] Breast self-examination has not been proved to decrease mortality, even though it is recommended as prudent by many organizations.[13, 14]

## COLORECTAL CANCER

A randomized study in Minnesota indicates that annual fecal occult blood testing using hydrated specimens decreases mortality from colorectal cancer by approximately one third after 13 years of follow-up.[15] Two European trials have found a 15% and an 18% reduction, respectively, in mortality with biennial screening for fecal occult blood.[16, 17] A subset of the Minnesota trial screened for fecal occult blood biennially was found to have a 21% reduction in mortality when compared with control after 18 years of follow-up.[15]

From 1 to 5% of persons tested are found to have positive fecal occult blood tests, and approximately 10% of these positive test results are from invasive cancer and 20 to 30% from adenomas.[10] There may be increased sensitivity for fecal occult blood when specimens are rehydrated before testing, at a cost of lower specificity.[18]

Digital rectal examination for rectal cancer has been assessed in a case-control study. It was not associated with a statistically significant reduction in mortality.[19]

Two case-control studies provide suggestive evidence that regular screening of individuals older than age 50 with sigmoidoscopy can decrease mortality.[19, 20] It is estimated that 25 to 35% of polyps can be discovered with the rigid sigmoidoscope, 50 to 55% with the 35-cm flexible scope, and 65 to 75% with the 60-cm scope. Diagnosis of polyposis by sigmoidoscopy should lead to evaluation of the entire colon with colonoscopy or barium enema, or both. The optimal interval for screening sigmoidoscopy has not been established.

## CERVICAL CANCER

Population cohort and quasiexperimental studies have demonstrated the value of Papanicolaou smears in decreasing cervical cancer mortality.[21, 22] These results have been corroborated in case-control studies. Most guidelines and recommendations advise regular Papanicolaou testing for all women who are or have been sexually active or have reached age 18. These recommendations further state that Papanicolaou smears should be repeated every 1 to 3 years at the physician's discretion. A substantial public health problem is the failure of older women to get cervical cancer screening. More than 25% of those diagnosed with cervical cancer are past age 65.[23]

The use of vaginal smears for women who have had a hysterectomy with removal of the cervix for a benign condition suggests little or no benefit.[24]

## SKIN CANCER

Visual examination of all skin surfaces by the individual or by a medical provider has been used in screening for basal and squamous cell cancers and melanoma. Well-designed trials have not been performed to evaluate whether mortality rates will decrease from such screening. Epidemiologic studies imply a decrease in melanoma mortality with aggressive screening. Scotland and Australia have among the highest incidence rates of melanoma in the world. Aggressive screening and public health education campaigns in Scotland and Australia may have had a positive impact in this disease.[25, 26] In Scotland, the proportion of patients diagnosed with thin, good-prognosis melanoma has risen from 38 to 62%, whereas that of those with thick, poor-prognosis tumors has fallen from 34 to 15%. Australia has stabilized its population-based mortality rates.

## LUNG CANCER

Lung cancer is the leading cause of cancer death in men and women in the United States. Screening modalities that have been evaluated in large series include screening chest radiography and sputum cytologic examination. When compared with the control group, those screened did show that lung cancer screening detects cancer at an earlier stage, and survival from diagnosis to death is increased. The latter is likely a lead-time bias, as there was no significant reduction in lung cancer mortality. All the controlled trials to date have had low statistical power.[27, 28]

## PROSTATE CANCER

Prostate cancer has become the most common non–skin cancer diagnosis in men. Much of this increase is due to an emphasis on screening with the prostate-specific antigen (PSA) test. This is true even though there is significant debate among experts as to whether prostate cancer screening is effective, with some authorities being concerned that there may be a net harm.[29–31] The biologic behavior of prostate cancer makes screening prone to length and lead-time bias (especially overdiagnosis).

A population-based study in Sweden compared prostate cancer rates in the early 1960s to rates in the early 1980s. Survival rates increased dramatically as methods of diagnosis changed. The investigators estimated that at least one third of cancers diagnosed in 1980 to 1984 were of the nonlethal type and all cancers diagnosed from 1960 to 1964 were of the lethal type. Similar observations have been made by comparing the incidence and mortality patterns of American white men to that of British white men. American men have had a substantially higher age-adjusted incidence since the 1980s, with nearly identical age-adjusted mortality rates.[32]

The most common prostate cancer screening modalities are the digital rectal examination (DRE)[21] and the serum PSA.[22] Both DRE and PSA clearly detect many asymptomatic cancers, but there is a high prevalence of indolent, clinically insignificant prostate cancer in the male population older than age 50. The use of free to complexed PSA is gaining increased use in an attempt to differentiate a PSA elevation due to benign prostatic hyperplasia from that due to prostate cancer.[33] Its use is still controversial. Transrectal ultrasonography is not widely used as a screening tool but is commonly used in the diagnostic work-up of an abnormal DRE or PSA test.

Most organizations have never advocated prostate cancer screening and those that have advocated it have moved toward some type of informed consent or education before performing the test. Most would agree that if a patient is to be screened, he should be given a choice and informed that no well-designed prospective, randomized trial has been conducted to test the true benefit of prostate cancer screening. Available tests are good at diagnosing prostate cancer, but our technology cannot reliably distinguish tumors that are lethal, but still curable, from those that are of little or no threat to health.[29, 34, 35]

## OVARIAN CANCER

Ovarian cancer screening is, in general, not recommended.[36] Palpation of the adnexa is insensitive and nonspecific when used in screening for ovarian cancer. Transvaginal ultrasonography has not proved beneficial, nor has cancer antigen-125 (CA-125) screening. CA-125 screening is an excellent example of the harm that screening can cause. In one clinical study, 0.6% of 900 women had a serum CA-125 level greater than 35 U/ml. This implies that if 100,000 women were tested, 600 would be identified as having an abnormal value. The prevalence of ovarian cancer in the female adult population is approximately 20 per 100,000. This means that the test would identify 600 women who would undergo further evaluation to identify 20 cases of ovarian cancer. This evaluation may be only an ultrasound examination, but some patients will ultimately undergo an exploratory laparotomy. It should be noted that many of the 20 women identified as having ovarian cancer will still have incurable advanced disease.

## Conclusions

Technical innovations are leading to increasing numbers of screening interventions, and the public's increasing awareness of the cancer problem is leading to an increased demand for screening. Tests that are more sensitive can be mistakenly accepted as better because they detect a broader spectrum of disease that includes a subgroup whose natural history and response to intervention are unknown. Likewise, the lead-time and length biases of early detection can cause therapies to be mistakenly interpreted as effective.

Screening interventions and their appropriate application must be carefully evaluated before their use is widely encouraged in screening programs. When health care practitioners offer a screening test to apparently healthy subjects, there is the implicit promise of benefit. Careful assessment of screening tests and procedures requires patience and is best performed through application of the scientific method and the use of controlled clinical trials.

## SUGGESTIONS FOR ADDITIONAL READING

Black CB, Welch HG. Advances in diagnostic imaging and overestimations of disease prevalence and the benefits of therapy. N Engl J Med 1993;328:1237–43. *A discussion of scientific advances in diagnostic imaging and how this has led to diagnosis of disease that in the past would never have been diagnosed and treated. It is difficult to assess the benefits of technical advances because of the biases associated with improved imaging.*

Guide to Clinical Preventive Services: Report of the U. S. Preventive Services Task Force. Philadelphia: Lippincott-Raven, 1996. *The USPSTF is a panel of experts convened by the Assistant Secretary for Health of the Department of Health and Human Services. Their recommendations summarize the findings of an extremely rigorous literature review looking for evidence of efficacy.*

Hayward RSA, Steinberg EP, Ford DE. Preventive care guidelines: 1991. Ann Intern Med 1991;114:758–83. *An overview of preventive interventions and guidelines recommended for clinical practice by a number of organizations.*

The Canadian Guide to Clinical Preventive Health Care. Ottawa: Health Canada, 1994.

Fletcher SW, Black W, Harris R, et al. Report of the International Workshop on Screening for Breast Cancer. J Natl Cancer Inst 1993;85:1644–56. *An overview of the results of the major breast cancer screening trials.*

Kramer BS, Brown ML, Prorok PC. Prostate cancer screening: what we know and what we need to know. Ann Intern Med 1993;119:914–23. *An overview of the issues in prostate cancer screening with serum prostate-specific antigen.*

## REFERENCES

1. U.S. Preventive Services Task Force. Guide to Clinical Preventive Services: Report of the U.S. Preventive Services Task Force. Philadelphia: Lippincott-Raven, 1996.
2. Canadian Task Force on the Periodic Health Examination. Canadian guide to clinical preventive health care. Ottawa: Health Canada, 1994.
3. Doherty VR, MacKie RM. Reasons for poor prognosis in British patients with cutaneous malignant melanoma. Br Med J 1986;292:987–9.
4. Hayward RS, Steinberg EP, Ford DE, et al. Preventive care guidelines: 1991. American College of Physicians. Canadian Task Force on the periodic health examination. United States Preventive Services Task Force. Ann Intern Med 1991;114:758–83.
5. Ransohoff DF, Lang CA. Screening for colorectal cancer with the fecal occult blood test: a background paper. American College of Physicians. Ann Intern Med 1997;126:811–22.
6. Anonymous. Screening for prostate cancer. American College of Physicians. Ann Intern Med 1997;126:480–4.
7. Mettlin C, Smart CR. Breast cancer detection guidelines for women aged 40 to 49 years: rationale for the American Cancer Society reaffirmation of recommendations. American Cancer Society. CA Cancer J Clin 1994;44:248–55.
8. Mettlin C, Jones G, Averette H, et al. Defining and updating the American Cancer Society guidelines for the cancer-related checkup: prostate and endometrial cancers. CA Cancer J Clin 1993;43:42–6.
9. Anonymous. Update January 1992: the American Cancer Society guidelines for the cancer-related checkup. CA Cancer J Clin 1992;42:44–5.
10. Biesecker BB, Boehnke M, Calzone K, et al. Genetic counseling for families with inherited susceptibility to breast and ovarian cancer. JAMA 1993;269:1970–4.
11. Hughes C, Gomez-Caminero A, Benkendorf J, et al. Ethnic differences

in knowledge and attitudes about BRCA1 testing in women at increased risk. Patient Educ Couns 1997;32:51–62.

12. Anonymous. National Institutes of Health Consensus Development Conference Statement: breast cancer screening for women ages 40–49, January 21–23, 1997. National Institutes of Health Consensus Development Panel. J Natl Cancer Inst 1997;89:1015–26.

13. Fletcher SW, Black W, Harris R, et al. Screening for breast cancer. J Natl Cancer Inst 1994;86:558–61.

14. Fletcher SW. Breast cancer screening among women in their forties: an overview of the issues. J Natl Cancer Inst Monogr 1997;5–9.

15. Mandel JS, Bond JH, Church TR, et al. Reducing mortality from colorectal cancer by screening for fecal occult blood. Minnesota Colon Cancer Control Study. N Engl J Med 1993;328:1365–71.

16. Hardcastle JD, Thomas WM, Chamberlain J, et al. Randomised, controlled trial of faecal occult blood screening for colorectal cancer. Results for first 107,349 subjects. Lancet 1989;1:1160–64.

17. Kronborg O, Fenger C, Olsen J, et al. Randomised study of screening for colorectal cancer with faecal occult-blood test. Lancet 1996;348:1467–71.

18. Ahlquist DA, Wieand HS, Moertel CG, et al. Accuracy of fecal occult blood screening for colorectal neoplasia. a prospective study using Hemoccult and HemoQuant tests. JAMA 1993;269:1262–67.

19. Herrinton LJ, Selby JV, Friedman GD, et al. Case-control study of digital-rectal screening in relation to mortality from cancer of the distal rectum. Am J Epidemiol 1995;142:961–4.

20. Newcomb PA, Norfleet RG, Storer BE, et al. Screening sigmoidoscopy and colorectal cancer mortality. J Natl Cancer Inst 1992;84:1572–75.

21. Benedet JL, Anderson GH, Matisic JP. A comprehensive program for cervical cancer detection and management. Am J Obstet Gynecol 1992;166:1254–59.

22. Makuc DM, Freid VM, Kleinman JC. National trends in the use of preventive health care by women. Am J Public Health 1989;79:21–6.

23. Mandelblatt JS, Phillips RN. Cervical cancer: how often—and why—to screen older women. Geriatrics 1996;51:45–8.

24. Pearce N, Bethwaite P. Social class and male cancer mortality in New Zealand, 1984–7. N Z Med J 1997;110:200–2.

25. Holman CD, James IR, Gattey PH, Armstrong BK. An analysis of trends in mortality from malignant melanoma of the skin in Australia. Int J Cancer 1980;26:703–9.

26. Doherty VR, MacKie RM. Reasons for poor prognosis in British patients with cutaneous malignant melanoma. Br Med J 1986;292:987–9.

27. Melamed MR, Flehinger BJ, Zaman MB, et al. Screening for early lung cancer. Results of the Memorial Sloan-Kettering study in New York. Chest 1984;86:44–53.

28. Eddy DM. Screening for lung cancer. Ann Intern Med 1989;111:232–7.

29. Lu-Yao GL, Potosky AL, Albertsen PC, et al. Follow-up prostate cancer treatments after radical prostatectomy: a population-based study. J Natl Cancer Inst 1996;88:166–73.

30. Coley CM, Barry MJ, Fleming C, et al. Early detection of prostate cancer. II: Estimating the risks, benefits, and costs. American College of Physicians. Ann Intern Med 1997;126:468–79.

31. Coley CM, Barry MJ, Fleming C, Mulley AG. Early detection of prostate cancer. I: Prior probability and effectiveness of tests. The American College of Physicians. Ann Intern Med 1977;126:394–406.

32. Shibata A, Ma J, Whittemore AS. Prostate cancer incidence and mortality in the United States and the United Kingdom. J Natl Cancer Inst 1998;90:1230–1.

33. Recker F, Kwiatkowski MK, Piironen T, et al. Free-to-total prostate-specific antigen (PSA) ratio improves the specificity for detecting prostate cancer in patients with prostatism and intermediate PSA levels. Br J Urol 1998;81:532–8.

34. Shibata A, Ma J, Whittemore AS. Prostate cancer and mortality in the United States and the United Kingdom. J Natl Cancer Inst 1998;90:1230–1.

35. Brawley OW. Prostate carcinoma incidence and patient mortality: the effects of screening and early detection. Cancer 1997;80:1857–63.

36. Anonymous. Screening for ovarian cancer: recommendations and rationale. American College of Physicians. Ann Intern Med 1994;121:141–2.

# CHAPTER 6

# PRINCIPLES OF CANCER SURGERY

• FREDERICK R. EILBER

Surgical excision is the oldest and most tested therapeutic modality for the treatment of cancer. Early surgical attempts, however, often resulted in the death of the patient or rapid local recurrence of the malignant neoplasm. Outcomes such as these were largely due to operative and immediate postoperative problems, such as excessive blood loss, difficult anesthesia, and respiratory insufficiency, all of which required a hurried, suboptimal operation. With advances such as blood transfusions, the use of antibiotics, tracheostomy to prevent airway obstruction, and nasogastric decompression of the stomach, the surgical treatment of cancer became safe and effective. Operative deaths were greatly reduced, and therapeutic results improved.

Despite these major advances in the surgical preoperative and postoperative care of patients, it soon became clear that surgical treatment of malignant neoplasms was a "limited" type of cancer therapy. We now realize that surgical techniques are effective only in the area of the primary tumor or regional lymphatics and do nothing for the neoplasm outside the operative field. There have been numerous attempts to extend the operative procedure to encompass additional contiguous anatomic structures, for example, the supraradical operations for carcinoma of the stomach and breast. These attempts, by and large, have not proved efficacious. The surgical excision is not at fault because tumor spread is usually already well beyond the confines of the operative field.

To understand the principles of cancer surgery, it is helpful to divide its application into four basic topics: (1) the diagnostic biopsy, (2) the surgical treatment of the primary tumor, (3) the treatment of regional lymphatics and metastases, and (4) the combinations of various modes of therapy. A discussion of these principles is followed by guidelines for integrating surgery into a treatment plan for the individual patient.

## Diagnostic Biopsy

Since different types of neoplasms have their own responses to the various modalities of therapy, a histologic diagnosis is imperative in planning the appropriate management of malignant disease. For example, cancer of the parotid gland is not a single disease because there are at least 10 different histologic types of cancer that affect this gland, each with a different response and cure rate. An accurate histopathologic diagnosis may therefore be critical in tailoring the surgical procedure to the needs of the patient.

Biopsy is a crucial procedure in the diagnosis of malignant disease in that it provides the pathologist with adequate samples of tumor. Adequate, in this instance, means a fragment of tissue that is representative of the tumor and is neither crushed nor contaminated. Careful handling of the tissues is mandatory. Noncrushing techniques to preserve nodal architecture, electron microscopy for sarcomas, and immediate touch preparations for lymphomas may be needed for histopathologic diagnosis.

Several biopsy techniques are available to the practicing physician, including exfoliative cytology, punch biopsy, incisional biopsy, excisional biopsy, shave biopsy, and needle aspiration biopsy.

In planning the type of biopsy to be used and the site to be sampled, it is important to consider the eventual methods of treatment. If surgery is contemplated, the biopsy should be performed by an individual familiar with the various surgical procedures. Tumors have a propensity for seeding and contaminating biopsy incisions; therefore, when en bloc surgical procedures are performed, it is essential to include the biopsy site or incision in the subsequent operation. A biopsy site that is far removed from the potential operative incision can severely jeopardize later attempts for surgical control of the tumor and will result in a compromised operation or severe wound healing problems.

Since the core of many neoplasms is necrotic and sometimes infected, it is usually preferable to perform the biopsy at the periphery of the tumor, specifically at the interface of the advancing tumor margin. In addition to providing less necrotic tissue, a biopsy at the tumor margin affords the pathologist an opportunity to evaluate the invasion of normal tissue. Many tumors have a low mitotic rate (e.g., tumors of the parathyroid gland) and therefore their cytologic features are insufficient for determining malignancy; thus, their invasive characteristics may be the only clue to tumor type.

In addition to the biopsy, an immediate frozen section is valuable. It affords the surgeon the knowledge that adequate tissue for final diagnosis has been obtained, obviating the need for rebiopsy for another tissue sample. For example, an immediate frozen section should be taken whenever a breast mass is excised because if the tissue contains malignant cells, the remainder of the specimen can be submitted for special studies such as a biochemical estrogen receptor analysis or special stains for lymphoma. It is impossible to perform many of these studies after the specimen is placed in formaldehyde for permanent section.

Lymph node biopsy deserves further comment. Before this technique is employed in the head and neck area, the primary tumor needs to be identified. Examination should include palpation and direct or indirect visualization of the oral cavity, oropharynx, hypopharynx, and larynx.[1] If the primary tumor site is found, it should be biopsied. Such a biopsy may be more meaningful, and it may spare a scar on the neck, which itself could make subsequent evaluation and surgical procedures more difficult.

Needle biopsy has several advantages over incisional or excisional biopsies. It is easier to perform, has fewer complications, and causes little tissue reaction. The primary prerequisite for this method is the pathologist's familiarity with the interpretation of needle biopsy specimens. Second, an adequate quantity and quality of tissue must be obtained. The major drawback of needle biopsy is a false-negative result if the malignant tumor is missed by the needle.

In summary, biopsy for histologic diagnosis is a crucial technique in the management of the cancer patient. All too often, the biopsy procedure has been performed by an inexperienced surgeon who does not appreciate the importance of the procedure and its role in subsequent treatment. Inappropriate biopsy by the wrong person often results in a pathology report stating "tissue inadequate for diagnosis; suggest rebiopsy." *Biopsy should be performed only by a trained surgeon who is prepared to undertake definitive surgical treatment.*

## Treatment

### PRIMARY TUMOR

The primary goal of cancer surgery is the complete eradication of local and regional tumor. The biology and natural history of each neoplasm must be taken into consideration before any surgical procedure is undertaken. Knowledge of the most common avenues of spread for the various histologic types of neoplasm is essential for ultimate success in primary tumor therapy. This involves obtaining adequate margins of normal tissue surrounding the neoplasm.

The techniques of cancer surgery are nearly identical to those of general surgery except for the following:

1. A bloodless surgical field is necessary during a cancer operation because the appearance of the tissue is important in terms of gross visualization of tumor spread.

2. To achieve a wide surgical margin of normal uninvolved tissue, the line of incision should not contain visible or palpable tumor. This differs from other types of general surgery in that liberal frozen sections of the operating margins are a necessity. These margins must include any suspicious areas, the limits of the surgical excision in depth and length, and the margins of the adjacent nerves in neoplasms that have the potential for perineural spread. If the tumor is visualized, the wide normal tissue margin required has not been achieved.

3. Finally, and most important, to accomplish adequate removal of the neoplasm, the cancer surgeon must employ a three-dimensional approach to the tumor, including its length, width, and depth. This should be carefully planned before the operation so that the margins of the procedure will be adequate and ensure normal tissue planes.

Table 6–1 gives examples of the most common neoplasms encountered and the essential adequate tissue margin required for complete surgical therapy. The rationale for an "adequate" tissue margin is based on the fact that surgical excisions that do not include a given amount of normal tissue result in a high recurrence rate, even though the tumors appear to be grossly excised ("cleared"). Obviously,

*Table 6–1.* **Adequate Normal Tissue Margins for Primary Malignancy Treated by Surgery Alone**

| Histology | Normal Tissue Margin |
|---|---|
| Melanoma | 2 cm |
| Sarcoma | Origin to insertion of involved muscles and fascia or one joint above for bone |
| Breast | Entire breast |
| Colon | 5 cm |
| Squamous cell carcinoma of head and neck | 2 cm minimum |

this reasoning must take into account the biology of the particular neoplasm in terms of its ability to spread through the organ, whether mucosally or submucosally, along fascial planes, or along nerves.

A problem that is not uncommon for the cancer surgeon is to find that the final report from the pathologist shows a less than adequate margin. At this juncture, his or her options are to operate further, do nothing but careful follow-up, or employ adjuvant chemotherapy or radiotherapy. In this setting, the word "adjuvant" is often used to cover an inadequate surgical procedure. The surgeon should assess the potential morbidity and mortality of reoperation, which must encompass not only the positive margin but also the entire operative field.

The final area of consideration concerns reconstruction of the primary tumor site. The goals of surgical treatment for cancer patients should include eradication of the cancer in association with satisfactory physiologic function and acceptable cosmetic results. All too often, the large, extensive surgical procedures are time-consuming, and important decisions or procedures for subsequent functional or cosmetic results may occur at the end of the procedure when the surgeon is fatigued. Many authors suggest that the primary excision be followed by a tumor-free period before any reconstructive procedures are initiated. This principle, although sound, imposes multiple operations and severe cosmetic deformities on many patients. An alternative approach to this problem is the surgical team method, in which one member of the team is responsible for ablating the tumor without concern for preservation of adjacent tissues for reconstruction, and the second member performs the reconstruction without concern for the tumor excision. This team approach enables the first surgeon to be somewhat more aggressive than if he or she had to be concerned with reconstruction.

## LOCAL WOUND SEEDING

Although the most efficacious method for preventing local recurrence is wide excision, several additional principles are worthy of discussion. A key consideration is to include liberally any biopsy incision or needle track into the en bloc excision.

Numerous techniques have been attempted to prevent seeding of tumors into the operative field or transplanting tumor cells from the primary tumor to another site. These methods include irrigation of the wound with tumoricidal solutions (such as 0.5% formaldehyde or sterile water) to lyse any residual cells that may be present or the use of various "no-touch" techniques, including minimal palpation of the tumor and early ligation of the blood supply to prevent any dislodgment of the tumor cells into the venous circulation during the time of the operation.[2] In some cases, these techniques have been extended to the application of a tourniquet to the extremities prior to performing the biopsy to prevent dissemination of the tumor.

Early ligation of the blood supply, wide normal tissue margins, and no visualization of the tumor necessitate a much more radical surgical procedure to achieve wound healing than does a lesser excision. Although these various techniques to reduce local recurrence are controversial, their theoretical value has led to their widespread acceptance.

If a second area of the body requires operation at the time of tumor excision, all gloves and instruments must be changed. This principle further prevents any wound seeding or transplantation of tumor cells from the primary tumor to a distant site. These precautions should be employed routinely when a skin graft is required to cover defects because there have been numerous instances of seeding various solid neoplasms to the distant skin graft donor site. Thus, the same principles that prevail for operating on infectious processes must be employed to prevent seeding to a distant wound.

## REGIONAL LYMPHATICS

In addition to contiguous spread, most solid tumors have a propensity for dissemination via local lymphatics to the regional lymph nodes. Therefore, careful surgical consideration must be given to the regional lymphatics and the possibility of regional node dissection.

Random sampling of one regional lymph node to determine nodal spread has not been of value because examination of a single random node does not ensure the absence of occult metastases in adjacent nonexcised nodes. Furthermore, in patients with palpable disease in the neck, it has been found that once the size of a lymph node exceeds 3 cm, the tumor is extranodal and involves the perinodal fat and the lymphatic channels. Local excision of the area is inadequate for treatment of the perinodal spread. Therefore, surgical techniques for en bloc excision of regional lymph nodes have been devised for the neck, axillae, and pelvic and inguinal areas.

If a regional lymphadenectomy is contemplated for the treatment of clinically evident regional metastases or as a means of histologic determination of the stage of disease, the appropriate regional lymph nodes must be dissected. An example of this problem is the parotid group of lymph nodes. Squamous cell carcinomas, basal cell carcinomas, and melanomas of the forehead, cheek, and scalp region drain primarily to this area.[3] Since these lymph nodes are within the capsule of the parotid gland, it is obvious that a superficial parotidectomy is required to remove them. Failure to perform such a procedure leaves potentially malignant nodes in the intervening parotid lymphatics.

In some circumstances, such as for selected patients with breast cancer, it may be possible to limit the extent of a node dissection by identifying the sentinel lymph node.[4] This involves injecting the primary tumor with a blue dye or radioactive substance that can be used to identify the first lymph node draining that area of the tumor. Many clinicians consider a negative sentinel lymph node examination performed by a surgeon who has mastered the technique to be adequate evidence of negative nodes, thus saving the patient from the morbidity of a more complete lymphatic dissection. The procedure is not useful, however, when performed by surgeons without adequate experience and technical expertise in the procedure. This topic is further discussed in Chapter 35 in the section on surgical treatment of breast cancer.

## DISTANT METASTASES

It is often assumed that the patient with disseminated disease is not a candidate for surgical procedures. It must be emphasized, however, that there is a certain percentage of these patients, albeit a small one, with truly isolated metastases that are amenable to complete surgical excision. Such metastatic sites include the solitary cerebral or hepatic metastasis, pulmonary metastases, an isolated metastasis that appears after a long disease-free interval or metastases that are multiple but have a prolonged doubling time associated with a controlled primary tumor, multiple subcutaneous metastases that present cosmetic problems, and bowel metastases that cause life-threatening obstruction or bleeding. Surgical treatment for these metastatic lesions may result in long-term tumor control or even cure, and palliation may be achieved in many of these patients.[5] To deny such patients the potential benefit of surgical treatment is inappropriate.

Additional surgical treatment for patients with distant metastases may include the placement of intrahepatic catheters for infusion chemotherapy. Attempts at dearterialization of the liver and hepatic artery ligation, combined with infusion, have been numerous and are, by and large, experimental. However, the results obtained from placement of an intra-arterial catheter for 5-fluorouracil (5-FU) infusion for inoperable hepatoma have shown significant long-term palliation. Although catheters can be placed percutaneously via the brachial or femoral route, their placement directly into the hepatic artery at laparotomy provides relatively problem-free, long-term function and less impairment of normal activity.

## RADIATION THERAPY

Much has been written about the combination of surgery and radiation therapy for the management of cancer. In general, two settings for combining these modalities can be identified: (1) preplanned combined-modality treatment, as discussed in many chapters in this book, and (2) radiation therapy employed as a "rescue" technique when the surgical procedure has proved incomplete or inadequate. In the latter setting, high-dose radiation may be required for control, the major difficulty being local complications, including difficult wound healing. This should be anticipated if possible, and techniques should be employed that will minimize this problem. Specifically, single incisions, as opposed to multibranched ones, should be used, and every effort should be made to cover major blood vessels. This is especially important in the groin and neck, where carotid and femoral ruptures are often fatal. In these areas, covering an exposed artery with skin or muscle flaps has proved to be of great value. As a final concern, preoperative radiation therapy in some areas may predispose the patient to the formation of a fistula. In some cases, a controlled fistula may be preferred, such as one formed by the use of a pharyngoscope to prevent leakage of saliva into an irradiated field.[6]

## CHEMOTHERAPY

Surgical procedures for patients who are receiving chemotherapy require little, if any, alteration. In most instances, local tissue healing has not been a significant problem. The major difficulties involve hemostasis in patients who are pancytopenic or thrombocytopenic. In these instances, platelet transfusions may be necessary. Because of the necessary normal fibroblastic repair process that must take place for surgical healing, one must consider the duration of fibroblast suppression by the various chemotherapeutic drugs. There are few quantitative data regarding this issue, but certain guidelines appear reasonable. For methotrexate (MTX) and the alkylating agents, the maximal effect is usually about a week and, if possible, the surgical procedure should be delayed until after this period. Doxorubicin (Adriamycin), dacarbazine (DTIC), and the nitrosoureas affect fibroblasts for 10 to 16 days, and operative procedures should therefore be postponed longer if possible. Obviously, in emergency situations, operations can and have been performed under less than ideal circumstances, and wound healing has not been significantly delayed. Stay sutures in abdominal incisions for patients receiving large doses of chemotherapy have been useful.

Because many patients require long-term chemotherapy, there may be a problem with collapse of the accessible venous system after prolonged drug infusion. This may be severe enough to warrant the creation of an artificial route for vascular access, as discussed in Chapter 12, Vascular Access.

Some investigators advocate "debulking" surgery as an adjunct to chemotherapy. This involves the removal of the major part of the tumor but not all of it.[7] Rationale for this came from observations that the bulk of the tumor, in terms of the total number of cells in the leukemias and lymphomas, was reduced by sequential courses of chemotherapy. This result can be achieved with radiation therapy to some extent in that the percentage of cells killed correlates with increased doses of radiation. Those who would transfer this concept to surgical procedures suggest that one can remove a portion of the tumor and then return to remove another portion of the tumor or that one can remove 80% of the tumor and rely on radiation and chemotherapy to destroy the residual. In practice, however, incomplete excision of a tumor often results in excessive blood loss and carries a high risk. Furthermore, such a procedure can seed tumor cells into areas that would otherwise not be at risk. Finally, as after any surgical procedure, the blood supply to the area is compromised, making radiation or chemotherapy more difficult. Therefore, unless the primary tumor can be removed in toto, it is usually prudent to perform a biopsy of the site, visualize the extent of the tumor, and cease the operation to reconsider treatment options.

## TIMING OF DEFINITIVE SURGERY

Once a diagnosis of operable cancer is established, most patients want immediate surgery. However, this is not always possible or appropriate. The immediate surgical excision of a primary tumor is based on the premise that the tumor is excised before dissemination of tumor cells, yet we know that any clinically evident tumor has been present in the patient for a prolonged period. Furthermore, the exact time that it takes for a tumor to metastasize is unclear because it is obvious that some tumors metastasize early in the preclinical stage, whereas others achieve enormous proportions before any metastases are evident. Clearly, some immediate surgical procedures, such as amputation for osteogenic sarcoma or immediate resection for Wilms' tumor, have not provided increased cures or a reduction of disease recurrence.

Because the time interval for metastasis is unknown in almost all tumors, it becomes apparent that accurate diagnosis by histologic means and a thorough search by various diagnostic procedures to determine the stage of the tumor should be performed as expeditiously as possible. The advantages of the knowledge gained by this delay far outweigh the disadvantages of inappropriate treatment. To proceed with treatment with inadequate knowledge of the tumor is more harmful for the patient than the 1- or 2-week delay required for adequate preoperative evaluation.

## NUTRITION

A significant advance in the surgical therapy of patients with malignant disease has been a better understanding of nutritional support. The use of intravenous hyperalimentation and the administration of various high-calorie materials via the alimentary tract have proved extremely useful in the surgical management of patients. The result is clear in patients with cachexia from carcinoma of the esophagus or those with severe disability following radiation therapy. Nasogastric feeding of high-calorie solutions and intravenous hyperalimentation prior to operation have markedly reduced the mortality and morbidity rates of the surgical procedures for carcinomas of the esophagus and for patients who have undergone radiation therapy. Earlier fears that alimentation or calories, or both, would cause rapid tumor growth have not been borne out by experience. Therefore, a period of alimentation before the surgical procedure is essential for the patient who is undernourished. Further discussion of this aspect of treatment is given in Chapter 21.

## Guidelines for Integrating Surgery into a Treatment Plan

When considering surgery for the cancer patient, the physician must be concerned with four major topics: (1) tumor factors, (2) patient factors, (3) the treatment team, and (4) the treatment goals.

## TUMOR FACTORS

The anatomic location constitutes an important tumor factor. Some tumors, such as those located in the nasopharynx, cannot be treated by surgical resection because an adequate margin of normal tissue cannot be achieved. Those that intimately involve major blood vessels (e.g., cancer of the lung involving the aorta) or bilaterally involve an essential organ, such as the liver, clearly do not benefit from surgical treatment.

Certain histologic types of tumor are not treated by surgical resection. For example, lymphomas, leukemias, and small cell carcinoma of the lung are not treated by surgical resection because these tumors are disseminated at the outset, and local control is not the major consideration.

Another major tumor factor is stage. Clearly, if a patient has widespread metastatic disease, long-term local control is not as important as it is in patients who have localized disease. When examination reveals fixed regional lymph nodes, nodes that are greater than 3 cm in diameter, or multiple palpable lymph nodes, surgical resection alone usually results in a probability of local recurrence that is greater than 50%. A patient with such findings may therefore require more treatment than simple surgical excision.

A most important tumor factor concerns the size of the primary tumor. In general, larger tumors respond more favorably to surgical therapy than to other modalities of treatment. Chemotherapy and radiation therapy require an excellent blood and oxygen supply to cause destruction, whereas surgical resection does not. Thus, large localized tumors that tend to have necrotic centers and poor blood supplies are best treated with surgical resection.

## PATIENT FACTORS

Age and general health are important patient factors. Older patients frequently tolerate surgical procedures better than radiation therapy or chemotherapy. Although this seems somewhat paradoxical, the physiologic insult from surgical resection is relatively brief (4 to 5 days), whereas that from radiation therapy or chemotherapy tends to be much more prolonged. Certainly, important consideration must be given to the patient's medical history because those who have had recent cerebrovascular accidents or cardiovascular catastrophes or those who have uncontrolled diabetes tend to be poor surgical candidates because of the high postoperative mortality rate. The social history of the patient must be taken into account and any concurrent diseases evaluated. Finally, and probably most important, the patient's desire for treatment must be assessed. Surgical resection in a patient who does not want an operation, even though it may be the most effective means for tumor control, is not appropriate.

## TREATMENT TEAM

The experience and expertise of the treatment team must be closely matched to each patient's needs. In many cases, the sophisticated resources of a cancer center or major medical center are not required for optimal treatment of the individual patient. However, for some tumors, treatment in a community setting may seriously jeopardize the patient's welfare. In making such an assessment, the primary physician should carefully consider the adequacy of local resources for the patient in surgery, radiation therapy, and chemotherapy. For example, a patient with a primary bone tumor may require the close cooperation of specialists in orthopedic surgery, head and neck surgery, plastic surgery, radiation therapy, and chemotherapy. Such a combination of talents may be difficult to assemble away from a cancer center.

## TREATMENT GOALS

Just as the considerations for surgical resection are important, so too are those of the goals of treatment. Different surgical procedures are performed to achieve specific treatment goals, for example, palliation versus complete tumor eradication. Certainly, total eradication of all viable tumor cells requires a much more extensive surgical procedure than does a palliative resection; either may be justified, depending on the situation.

## CONCLUSIONS

A dogmatic statement of when surgical resection, radiation therapy, or chemotherapy should be applied is not possible because each or all may have a place in the treatment of a cancer patient. The judicious integration of each of these modalities is currently being tested, with some exciting results. These studies are designed to search for a realistic appreciation of each type of therapy, examining its advantages, limitations, and complications to achieve the optimal effect and to provide the best chance for long-term survival of the patient with cancer.

Tumor factors, patient factors, treatment team availability, and treatment goals must be considered prior to any therapy. Evaluation of the primary tumor and the regional lymphatics and the possibility of distant metastases is especially important for assessing the possibility of effective tumor control. However, from a social and emotional point of view, patients need to have one physician who directs the treatment course, even though multiple treatment modalities may be required.

## SUGGESTIONS FOR ADDITIONAL READING

Caputo GM, Gross RJ. Medical consultation on surgical services: an annotated bibliography. Ann Intern Med 1993;118:290–7. *An excellent listing of key articles relevant to preoperative consultations and assessments for patients scheduled for surgical procedures.*

Eisenberg BL. Introduction: surgical management of recurrent cancer. Semin Oncol 1993;20:399–551. *An excellent series of reviews on the role of surgery in the management of locally recurrent and metastatic cancer.*

Reynolds C, Mick R, Donohue JH, et al. Sentinel lymph node biopsy with metastasis: can axillary dissection be avoided in some patients with breast cancer? J Clin Oncol 1999;17:1720–6. *The authors conclude that selected patients with small breast cancers may be adequately staged by the sentinel lymph node procedure.*

## REFERENCES

1. Jesse RH, Perez CA, Fletcher GH. Cervical lymph node metastasis: unknown primary cancer. Cancer 1973;31:854–9.
2. Turnbull RB Jr, Kyle K, Watson FR, Spratt J. Cancer of the colon: the influence of the no-touch isolation technic on survival rates. Ann Surg 1967;166:420–7.
3. Storm FK, Eilber FR, Sparks FC, Morton DL. A prospective study of parotid metastases from head and neck cancer. Am J Surg 1977;134:115–9.
4. Giuliano AE. Mapping a pathway for axillary staging: a personal perspective on the current status of sentinel lymph node dissection for breast cancer. Arch Surg 1999;134:195–9.
5. Holmes EC, Morton DL. Pulmonary resection for sarcoma metastases. Orthop Clin North Am 1977;8:805–10.
6. Ballantyne AJ. In: Neoplasia of the Head and Neck. Chicago; Year Book Medical, 1974:85.
7. Silberman AW. Surgical debulking of tumors. Surg Gynecol Obstet 1982;155:577–85.

# CHAPTER 7

# PRINCIPLES OF RADIATION ONCOLOGY

• ROBERT G. PARKER • H. RODNEY WITHERS

Radiation oncology is a clinical medical specialty in which ionizing radiations are used to treat patients with cancers or, occasionally, selected benign diseases. The radiation oncologist is supported by medical physicists, who ensure accuracy of the dose administered, and radiation therapists, who operate the large machines that deliver the treatment.

The most common objective of radiation treatment of cancer is eradication of the tumor with preservation of the structure and function of normal tissues. For radiation therapy, as for surgery, this means local-regional control of tumor cells in patients without evidence of metastases, which implies a careful pretreatment evaluation as well as long-term post-treatment observation. Another common indication is the palliation of symptoms from either the primary tumor or metastases to improve the quality of life.

Radiation therapy is effective in controlling a variety of malignant tumors and is a component in the management of about half of all patients with cancer.[1, 2] Therefore, about 15% of the population will at some time receive radiation therapy.[3] The effectiveness of radiation therapy, like surgery, must be judged by the frequency of local-regional tumor control in relation to the incidence and severity of treatment-induced morbidity.

The characteristic of the types of radiations used in radiation oncology is that they are sufficiently energetic to cause ionization of atoms in tissue. This results in the formation of highly reactive radicals in a well-defined, restricted volume. Such controlled radiochemical changes are a form of localized cytotoxicity that is different from chemotherapy because of its straightforward, simple, and direct pharmacokinetics. Radiation therapy does not require absorption at a distant site, transportation via blood vessels, or diffusion from vessels into the tissues. Therefore, the unique characteristic of radiation therapy is that it is relatively free of systemic toxicity, which limits chemotherapy. Also, it is free of the anatomic restraints that often limit surgery. Such freedom from systemic toxicity and anatomic restrictions permits the destruction of sizable masses of tumor cells, with the preservation of structure, function, and cosmesis of normal tissues. In practice, radiation therapy is most effective when the number of tumor cells is limited, therefore requiring only modest doses for their elimination, and when the tumor has not destroyed adjacent normal tissue, thus allowing its preservation.

Thus, the best results are obtained in early-stage tumors or when the surgeon can remove the main bulk of the tumor without the need for a radical operation. Another advantage of radiation therapy, compared with surgery, is the lesser influence of a patient's concurrent medical problems, such as cardiac or pulmonary disease, on the application of treatment. Patients receiving radiation therapy infrequently require general anesthesia, hospitalization, or intensive or emergency care related to the treatment itself. A disadvantage is that it requires several weeks of daily administration. Although the overall treatment time may be a disadvantage for some patients, the short daily treatment (approximately 10 to 20 minutes) can usually be given on an outpatient basis, permitting continuation of normal activities. In addition, the frequent contact with members of the medical team (radiation oncologists, physicists, therapists, nurses, social workers) can provide a strong patient support system.

Central to the radiation treatment of the patient with cancer is the radiation oncologist, a physician trained in human cancer biology and the medical use of ionizing radiation. As noted many years ago by Buschke,[4] such a physician has full and exclusive responsibility for the patient under his or her care, just as the surgeon does for the surgical treatment of the patient with cancer. This responsibility includes independence of opinion (including disagreement) about diagnosis and management; control of the actual treatment, including medications; an obligation to respond at any time; and the necessity of close cooperation with other involved physicians.

## Biophysical Basis of Radiation Therapy

Ionizing radiations are characterized by the mechanism of energy dissipation—namely, ionization (and excitation) of atoms and molecules in the absorption material (i.e., tissue). These radiations may be electromagnetic (x-rays, gamma rays) or corpuscular (electrons, protons, heavy ions, neutrons, alpha particles). Regardless of their origin (e.g., x-rays or electrons from linear accelerators, gamma rays from $^{60}$Co or $^{137}$Cs, neutrons from a cyclotron), the basic biophysical mechanisms of action of all types of ionizing radiations are similar.

In mammalian cells and tissues, the physical absorption of energy from ionizing radiations is followed by radiochemical events that may occur within $10^{-10}$ seconds.[5] Interactions with water result in products such as hydrogen free radicals, hydroxyl free radicals, hydroxyl ions, hydrogen, and hydrogen peroxide. Inasmuch as these free radicals have a short lifetime ($10^{-5}$ to $10^{-10}$ seconds), their range of action is limited by the restricted time available for diffusion. The presence of oxygen can prolong the lifetime of ionized molecules and thereby increase (by up to a factor of 3) the radiosensitivity of a cell. Conversely, sulfhydryl-containing compounds (e.g., amifostine) can scavenge free radicals and thereby protect the cell. These effects of oxygen and sulfhydryls require their presence at the time of irradiation. Other agents, particularly the halogenated pyrimidines 5-bromodeoxyuridine and iododeoxyuridine, can increase the susceptibility of DNA to radiation injury. However, to achieve a radiosensitizing effect they must already be incorporated into the DNA, requiring administration before irradiation.

## DOSIMETRY: PHYSICAL AND BIOLOGIC

**Physical Dosimetry.** The dose of ionizing radiation can be measured more accurately than can any other medication. This provides the opportunity and responsibility for precise and careful clinical use. For decades, radiation doses in patients were extrapolated from exposure doses measured in air (i.e., the roentgen). Current clinical use requires the measurement of the absorbed dose at the anatomic point of interest. On the basis of the 1980 recommendations of the International Commission on Radiation Units and Measurements (ICRU),[6] doses are now quantified in units of gray (Gy). One gray equals 1 joule per kilogram of absorber, equivalent to 100 rad in the old terminology. Alternatively, 1 cGy equals 1 rad. In some situations, the dose can be measured directly in the patient through the use of small-volume receptors (e.g., thermoluminescent capsules, diodes). In clinical practice, it is unusual to measure the dose directly because accurate dosimetry at any specific anatomic site can be predicted by the use of computerized dosimetry data obtained from measurement in phantoms constructed to have tissue absorption and inhomogeneities similar to those present in the human. The total doses required to achieve high rates of tumor control vary from as low as 25 to 30 Gy for seminomas to about 70 Gy for squamous carcinomas and adenocarcinomas, all doses being given in daily fractions of about 2 Gy.

**Biologic Dosimetry.** The effectiveness per unit of radiation dose can vary. For example, per unit of dose, neutrons are more effective than x-rays, whereas x-rays vary in their effectiveness, depending on the size of a daily dose or the dose rate. Thus, 1 Gy of neutrons is more lethal to cells than 1 Gy of x-rays, and 1 Gy of x-rays given at a high dose rate is more lethal than 1 Gy of x-rays given at a low dose rate. However, the total doses can be adjusted to allow for these differences. Because these adjustments of total doses to achieve a constant effect may vary between tumors and normal tissues, it is possible to increase (or decrease) the therapeutic index merely by changing the dose per sitting or the dose rate.

For proper clinical use, it is the biologically effective

dose that is of concern: the biologic effectiveness of an accurately measured total physical dose is modified by dose rate, dose increment size when the total dose is given as a series of dose fractions, overall time and temporal pattern of application, anatomic part and tissue volume irradiated, and to some extent host factors that can influence radiosensitivity. The quantitative aspects of determining isoeffective doses with change in fraction size or overall time, or both, have received a great deal of attention. Formulas exist for such calculations.[7] No single formula can be applied to all tissues because there are substantial variations in the radiosensitivity within the shoulder region of cell-survival curves and because repopulation kinetics are highly variable from tissue to tissue and among tumors.[8, 9]

## DELIVERY SYSTEMS FOR RADIATION THERAPY

**External Beams.** Modern radiation therapy has been made possible by the development of equipment capable of generating and precisely delivering very high energy radiations. These energies are expressed as kVp (peak kilovoltage on the x-ray tube) or MV, (million electron volts potential). Radiations with peak energies greater than 1 to 2 MV (usually >4 MV) are arbitrarily labeled supervoltage or megavoltage and are used almost exclusively for external-beam therapy. Widespread use of megavoltage therapy began with the introduction of $^{60}$Co teletherapy units, but the most common source is now the linear accelerator (LINAC). Current conventional clinical use of radiations is limited mainly to high-energy x-rays or high-energy electrons from linear accelerator units, with some use of gamma rays from a cobalt machine or beta rays from radioisotopes. Other types of ionizing radiations, such as protons, neutrons, and heavy ions, have limited and special applications.

The penetration of a treatment beam increases in direct proportion to the energy of the photons. This facilitates delivery of high doses to deep-seated tumors, but there are also other important clinically exploitable characteristics of megavoltage beams: skin sparing, reduced absorption in bone, high dose rates, and reduced lateral scattering into adjacent tissues. These additional characteristics are especially advantageous for avoiding skin reactions and when short treatment times (e.g., in children or uncomfortable patients) and precise normal tissue sparing (e.g., the lens in the treatment of retinoblastoma) are particularly important.

Another advantage of megavoltage accelerators is that they can generate electrons. These high-energy particles are useful in certain treatment situations because they have a finite range in tissue, with a sharp drop in dose over a few millimeters with lower energy electrons or more than a few centimeters with high energies. This permits irradiation of superficial tumors with a rapid fall-off in dose to underlying structures.

**Interstitial or Intracavitary Sources.** Interest in the use of radiation sources introduced into tissues (interstitial) or body cavities (intracavitary) has been revived in part by the generation of radioactive isotopes in atomic reactors or cyclotrons (e.g., $^{60}$Co, $^{137}$Cs, iridium 192, and iodine 125) and can be used in highly adaptable, flexible, custom-made applicators, replacing inflexible radium needles. These radioactive sources are usually "afterloaded" under remote con-

trol into preimplanted applicators. This has several advantages: the exact position of the applicators can be checked radiographically to ensure they are well positioned before they are loaded, the sources are introduced and removed under remote control without exposure to medical personnel, and during prolonged treatments lasting hours or days, the sources can be withdrawn temporarily to a special safe storage during nursing and other activities. Also, the dose distribution from such remote afterloaded radioisotopes can be "tailored" to the shape of the tumor by varying the duration for which each of a multiplicity of sources remains within its applicator. A variation of this concept is to move one source in a computer-controlled stepwise manner continually throughout an array of applicator tubes, varying the duration of "residence" at each step to deliver the dose in a predetermined distribution in and around the tumor volume.

The application of radioactive sources within or adjacent to the tumor is called *brachytherapy*. It usually requires an operative procedure and delivers concentrated radiation doses into tumor-bearing tissues. These doses are relatively high when compared with the doses received by the surrounding normal tissues.

**Targeted Therapy.** A technique that can bring a radioisotope into close contact with the tumor is exemplified by the systemic administration of iodine 131 to a patient in whom thyroid cancer metastases demonstrate uptake of a tracer dose of the isotope. This principle of targeting a radioisotope to deposits of tumor is now being applied in other ways, most notably by attaching radioisotopes to one or more monoclonal antibodies that seek out tumor antigens.

**Large-Field Radiation Therapy.** Interest in total-body irradiation (TBI) from an external source has been revived both as a systemic treatment of lymphomas and leukemias and as a method of immunosuppression and eradication of bone marrow prior to the transplantation of donor bone marrow. It has also been combined with intensive chemotherapy for elective treatment of patients who are predicted to be at high risk for the later appearance of overt systemic metastases (e.g., patients with breast cancer and a large number of positive axillary lymph nodes).

## Biologic Basis of Radiation Therapy

Although the basic physical and chemical changes incited by ionizing radiation occur almost instantaneously (within $10^{-12}$ seconds), the observed wide spectrum of biologic effects may be recognized over a broad range of time, from within seconds (signs of central nervous system damage from pulsed high doses) to hours (nausea, vomiting) to days (skin erythema) to weeks (hematopoietic suppression, desquamation) to years (myelitis, fibrosis) to decades (carcinogenesis) to generations (mutagenic changes). The variation in the time course of the development of sequelae reflects different mechanisms of induction of the various effects. The most relevant effect for radiation therapy of cancer is the death of cells. In some tissues, a proportion of the cells die quickly from induction of apoptosis. However, most cell killing results from misrepair or failure of repair of double-strand breaks in DNA, an injury that translates into death of the cell only when its capacity to reproduce itself is tested by mitotic division. Thus, the rate of expression of cell killing in various tissues depends on the rate at which its component cells turn over. In bone marrow and various squamous and mucosal surfaces, where cell turnover is relatively fast, effects may become evident in days or weeks, whereas in other tissues with low proliferative activity, such as fibrovasculature, muscles, nerve tracts, renal tubules, and bones, the manifestation of cell sterilization may not be evident for months or years.

## CELLULAR RESPONSES

Modern radiobiology of mammalian cells dates to the introduction of cell culture methods by Puck and Marcus.[10] They made possible the quantitative correlation of reproductive cell death with the dose of radiations. Mammalian cell-survival curves are constructed by determining the reduction in the number of surviving cells as a function of increasing radiation dose. For a specific dose increment, a constant proportion, not an absolute number, of cells is killed. This proportional, or exponential, relationship is most easily displayed on semilogarithmic paper. The steeper the slope—that is, the smaller the dose required for a specific amount of cell killing—the greater the radiosensitivity.

X-ray survival curves for most mammalian cells exhibit an initial "shoulder" region, with a downward slope becoming steeper with increase in dose. This is most easily understood in terms of "single-hit" and accumulative injury to DNA. Although other mechanisms for cell killing exist, the usual one is considered to be the induction of double-strand breaks in DNA. These may arise by a single hit of dense ionization or may result from the spatial and temporal proximity of two or more separately induced single-strand breaks, which then effectively become a double-strand break. Single-strand breaks are much more frequent than double-strand breaks but are repaired efficiently and are rarely lethal. Double-strand breaks are mostly repaired as well but are more prone to misrepair, which disrupts the genome. The most common form of cell death involves an ultimate loss of its reproductive integrity. Interphase death by apoptosis is increasingly recognized as another mode of radiation cytotoxicity. The relative contributions of apoptotic and mitotic death may vary with a number of factors, for example, proliferative activity and gene mutations.

The shoulder shape of the dose-survival curve reflects a linear dose response from single-hit nonrepairable injury, to which is added interacting multihit injury, which becomes increasingly more effective the more numerous the pre-existing single-strand breaks, that is, with an increase in dose. This second (accumulative) type of injury causes a progressive downward curvature in the survival curve as dose is increased. In effect, the dose-survival curve is a direct (linear) logarithmic reduction from single-hit injury, described by $e^{-\alpha d}$, where $\alpha$ is a coefficient for single-hit killing specific for the cell and the type of radiation, to which is added a logarithmic reduction proportional to the dose squared, that is, $(e^{-\beta d2})$, where $\beta$ is the coefficient for multihit killing. The combined survival response is therefore described by

$$\text{Surviving fraction of cells} = e - (\alpha d + \beta d^2)$$

Obviously, the relative contributions of single-hit ($\alpha$ type) and multihit ($\beta$ type) injury will determine how quickly the survival curve bends downward (i.e., the higher the $\alpha/\beta$ ratio, the more slowly the curve bends downward). "Sublethal" injury in the cell, which results from the accumulative $\beta$-type injury, is repaired over a few hours,[11] allowing cells without lethal injury to shed their sublethal lesions and return to their preradiation status. Thus, the higher the ratio of $\beta$- to $\alpha$-type injury, the greater the reduction in lethality that results from dividing the total dose into multiple smaller fractions, that is, the lower the $\alpha/\beta$ ratio, the more the rate of cell killing will change with change in dose.[7] It is of practical importance to the radiation oncologist that because of the nonlinearity of the x-ray dose-survival curve, the effectiveness of treatment is not a direct function of total dose but rather is determined by the size of the dose per fraction as well as the total dose. Although there are no qualitative differences in the form of dose-survival curves for normal and malignant cells, important quantitative differences exist, especially at doses on the order of 2 Gy. This is a commonly used daily dose fraction, for which most cell survival is still traced by the shoulder region of the survival curve. Subtle differences in survival from each daily dose fraction can be exploited to increase the therapeutic index because a difference in relative survival increases exponentially in proportion to the number of fractions into which the total dose is divided. Thus, if the ratio of cell survival in normal and malignant cells following exposure to 2 Gy were 6/5 (60% survival vs. 50% survival), the ratio after 35 fractions of 2 Gy would be $(6/5)^{35} = 590$, other factors being equal.

## RADIOSENSITIVITY, RADIORESISTANCE, AND RADIOCURABILITY

Radiosensitivity is a measure of the susceptibility to cellular injury by ionizing radiations. The injury may be lethal through interruption of the cell's capacity to reproduce indefinitely (reproductive death) or, less commonly, through structural degeneration independent of the reproductive cycle (interphase death), commonly by apoptosis.

Often the terms *radiosensitive* and *radioresistant* are misused clinically to describe roughly the rate of reduction in the size of a tumor. Actually, the gross response of a tumor depends not only on tumor cell killing but also on the rate at which tumor cells die and are cleared. Since most lethally irradiated cells die as a result of DNA injury and disruption of their reproductive integrity, the rate at which they die reflects their division cycle activity: rapidly proliferating normal tissues show an early response, slowly proliferating tissues may not manifest injury for months or years. Tumors show a wide range of response rates, although mostly they regress over several weeks. Nevertheless, some tumors in which cells have long replication cycles may not fully express lethal damage for months or even years, and a biopsy should not be performed if they are still regressing. Also, some tumors contain a large component of inert intercellular matrix and may regress only slowly and incompletely (e.g., nodular sclerosing Hodgkin's disease, some sarcomas and teratocarcinomas, craniopharyngiomas, and meningiomas), whereas some may show no significant regression despite being permanently controlled (e.g., chondrosarcomas, glomus tumors).

Clinically, radiocurability is the important concept. Assuming that the tumor has not disseminated to distant organs, local radiocurability is much more dependent on the size and location of a tumor and, to some extent, its histologic characteristics than on its rate of regression during treatment, even though rapid regression is commonly a favorable prognostic sign.

The number of clonogenic cells (i.e., those capable of infinite reproduction) in a tumor is a major determinant of radiocurability: the more cells, the higher the dose required to cure the tumor. The threshold sigmoid curve for tumor control (Fig. 7–1) illustrates that below a certain (threshold) dose there is no control of tumors, but once the number of surviving clonogenic cells is reduced to close to 1, further dose is increasingly likely to eliminate the last survivors, leading to a rapid increase in the proportion of tumors sterilized. Thus, in practice, to have a finite chance of cure of a primary tumor by radiation therapy alone requires administration of doses above a threshold, and the more the dose exceeds that threshold, the greater the chances of cure. Conversely, it is pointless to give doses below the threshold except for palliation.

The dose response for elective irradiation of presumed subclinical spread of tumor is different from that for macroscopic (primary or metastatic) disease. Because there is a broad range of metastatic cell burdens within a series of patients, some are cured even without elective irradiation (i.e., they have zero metastatic cell burden), others with small numbers are controlled by low doses, whereas those with a large burden may require 50 Gy or more for a high probability of cure. There are two important consequences of this wide distribution of metastatic cell burden among patients harboring subclinical disease:

1. Adjuvant therapy (chemotherapy or radiation) should be given promptly so that small metastatic burdens, which grow much faster than do large deposits, will not become large and "escape" from cure.

2. Given promptly, there will be a proportion of patients in whom even relatively low doses of x-irradiation will be effective in reducing the incidence of local-regional recurrence. This contrasts with the threshold in the dose response for clinically detectable disease.

Other factors that are important in limiting local control of a primary tumor may be variations in intrinsic radiosensitivity, persistent hypoxia, and accelerated regrowth by clonogenic tumor cells during protracted treatment regimens. In practice, some tumors are easily cured with low doses (e.g., seminomas), but most of the common radiocurable tumors require high doses. A few (e.g., glial tumors) are rarely cured even with very high doses.

## BIOLOGIC BASIS FOR DOSE FRACTIONATION

Often, radiation therapy is aimed at cure and is conventionally delivered in five doses per week for durations of 3 to 8 weeks. A common daily dose fraction is 2 Gy (200 cGy, with total doses in 2-Gy fractions ranging from less than 30 Gy (for seminoma) to about 40 Gy for Hodgkin's disease, to 50 Gy for areas of presumed subclinical metastatic deposits in lymph nodes, to about 66 to 70 Gy, or even more, for primary squamous or adenocarcinomas. Other dose fractionation schemes exist, both as standard practice and as experimental protocols. Palliative treatment is commonly given more quickly to lower total doses in larger dose fractions (e.g., 30 Gy in 10 fractions of 3 Gy). However, with our increasing understanding of the biology of dose fractionation, a greater diversity of treatment options has developed.

Dose fractionation enhances the therapeutic ratio.[7, 12, 13] Four biologic phenomena contribute to this differential between the responses of tumors and normal tissues: repair of cellular injury, repopulation by surviving cells, redistribution of surviving cells within the division cycle, and reoxygenation of tumor cells (the 4 Rs).

**Repair of Cellular Injury.** When a tissue is exposed to low doses (e.g., 2 Gy), most of the cell killing results from single-hit injury. If higher doses are given, the contribution from interactions between sublethal lesions (β-type injury) increases, a mechanism more effective in killing the target cells in slowly responding normal tissues such as the fibrovasculature, muscle, or nervous system than in killing the malignant clonogens in tumors.[14] Since sublethal β-type injury can be repaired,[11] the use of small dose fractions minimizes injury to slowly responding normal tissues, with little impact on the tumor response. For example, a total dose of 24 Gy in 6-Gy fractions is equivalent to about 48 Gy in 2-Gy fractions for slowly responding normal tissue such as spinal cord, whereas for killing clonogenic cells in squamous carcinoma, 24 Gy in six fractions is probably equivalent to less than 32 Gy in 2-Gy fractions.[15] Clearly, the increasing "tolerance" of the slowly responding normal tissues that can be obtained with reduction in dose per fraction permits administration of higher, more effective doses to the tumor.

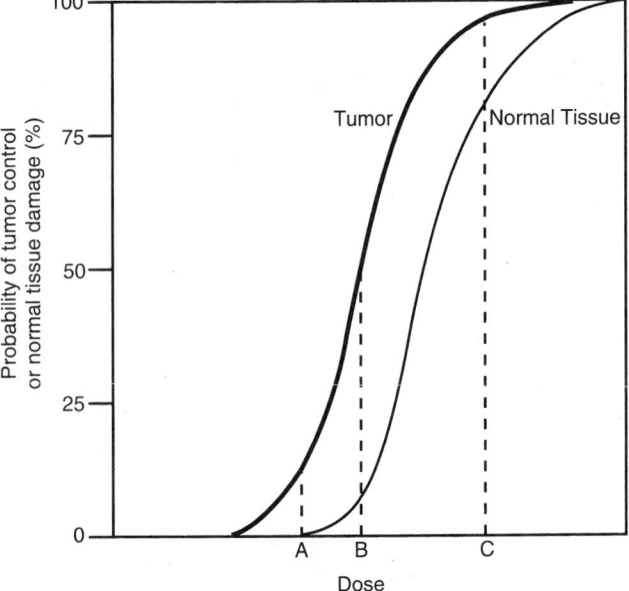

**Figure 7–1.** The relation between x-ray dose and outcome of radiotherapy. At any given dose—for example, A, B, or C—there is a balance between tumor control and complications. The dose prescribed depends on factors relating to the tumor, normal tissues, and the whole patient. (From Withers H. Biological basis of radiation therapy for cancer. Lancet 1992;339:157, © by The Lancet Ltd.)

**Redistribution of Surviving Cells Within the Division Cycle.** Mammalian cells vary in their radiosensitivity as they progress through the mitotic division cycle.[16] In general, $G_0$ and late S-phase cells are the most resistant, and late $G_2$ and mitotic (M) cells are the most sensitive. Each daily 2-Gy dose fraction in a standard course of x-ray therapy preferentially kills cells in the sensitive phases of the cycle. During the intervals between successive dose fractions, the relatively more resistant, and therefore surviving, subpopulations redistribute through the division cycle. This redistribution out of resistant phases leads to a net radiosensitizing effect by the time a proliferative cell population is exposed to another dose (e.g., 24 hours later). This occurs to a lesser extent, or not at all, in nonproliferating or slowly proliferating target cells in slowly responding normal tissues. Thus, small dose fractions are relatively more damaging to a proliferating tumor than to slowly cycling, late-responding normal tissue. (This radiobiologic phenomenon can be extrapolated to support the use of continuous infusion, rather than bolus injection of chemotherapeutic agents.)

**Reoxygenation.** Tumors commonly outstrip the growth of their new vasculature and become hypoxic, with or without overt evidence of necrosis. Hypoxic cells are significantly (2.5 to 3 times) more radioresistant than are euoxic cells, even when the level of hypoxia is still compatible with viability.[17] With large dose fractions, even a small proportion of hypoxic cells could limit radiocurability because the euoxic cells are sterilized early in the exposure, leaving a relatively radioresistant cohort against which the latter part of the dose is increasingly less effective. If during the course of multiple exposures to low doses (e.g., 2 Gy) a fraction of the tumor cell population remained hypoxic, they would soon dominate among the survivors because of their greater radioresistance. Thus, after several days of treatment, the tumor would be 2.5 to 3 times more resistant than at the beginning, with no such change in the continuously euoxic tissues. However, with repeated small doses, the lethally injured euoxic cells die, permitting better access to oxygen for previously hypoxic cells. Provided that this process of "reoxygenation"[18] continues efficiently enough to ensure that the percentage of hypoxic cells remains low (e.g., less than 10%), the hypoxic cells will exert only a minor influence on the overall response to repeated exposure to doses on the order of 2 Gy.

**Repopulation.** Repopulation of surviving cells within rapidly proliferating, acutely responding normal tissues—such as the mucosa of the aerodigestive tract, bone marrow, and skin—is essential to their tolerating high doses and is an important phenomenon leading to an increase in the therapeutic index from protracted, fractionated radiation therapy.[9] A limit to the magnitude of therapeutic gain from this phenomenon is imposed by the lack of a similar regenerative response in the slowly responding normal tissues such as the fibrovasculature, bones, muscles, nerves, and kidneys. Furthermore, there is now extensive evidence for an accelerated repopulation response in most tumor types.[9] In head and neck cancer, the median doubling time shortens from 45 to 60 days before treatment begins to 3 to 4 days late in a standard 6- to 8-week treatment regimen. On average, this tumor regrowth is less efficient than regeneration in normal tissues in terms of both a longer lag period before it begins and a slower rate after it begins.

Since no gain from repopulation is realized by late-responding normal tissues, the optimal design of a fractionated treatment regimen is to deliver the "tolerance" dose for late sequelae (in small doses to maximize the favorable differential effects of repair of sublethal injury) in as short an overall time as tolerated by acutely responding normal tissues (to limit the extent of repopulation in the tumor).

## BIOLOGIC EFFECT OF CHANGES IN DOSE RATE

Cell killing can be modified by altering the radiation dose rate.[19] As the dose rate decreases, cell killing per unit dose decreases because cells repair sublethal injury during the exposure. Biologically, low dose rates are analogous to an infinite number of small dose increments, with a shallower dose-survival curve characteristic of the initial shoulder region of the cell-survival curve.

The same biologic advantages as result from using small dose fractions are gained from the low dose rates used in brachytherapy. The biggest rate of change in effectiveness occurs over the range of 0.01 to 0.1 Gy/min, the very range used in most TBI preceding bone marrow transplantation. This is reflected in the divergent incidences of sequelae reported from different centers administering TBI.

## MODIFIED FRACTIONATION PATTERNS

As discussed, cellular and tissue responses to ionizing radiations can be modified by the pattern of radiation application, that is, by the size of each dose fraction and overall duration of treatment.

**Hyperfractionation.** As the size of dose increments increases, the severity of late responses increases relative to that of early responses.[7, 14, 15] Therefore, treatment patterns of a few large fractions (hypofractionation) disproportionately increase the late sequelae in normal tissues compared with the acute reactions and tumor responses and should be avoided except for short-term palliation. Conversely, a therapeutic differential between late-responding normal tissues and acutely responding tumor cells, derived from differences in repair capacities and division cycle redistribution kinetics, may be exploited clinically by using a larger number of smaller dose fractions. Such "hyperfractionation" involving two or more dose increments daily requires intervals of more than 6 hours to allow complete repair of sublethal injury in normal cells. If a daily dose of 2 Gy is changed to a twice per day regimen, given in the same overall time, the total doses can be increased by about 15% because of an increased tolerance of late-responding normal tissues. A 30% reduction in local recurrence rates in oropharyngeal carcinomas has been achieved by hyperfractionation in a European Organization for Research in Cancer Therapy (EORTC) randomized trial.[20]

**Accelerated Treatment.** If the overall time of treatment is prolonged without an increase in total dose, the frequency of tumor control decreases because tumor cells, like cells in acutely responding normal tissues, accelerate their growth rate, although only after an initial lag period following the start of treatment.[9, 14] Therefore, the overall treatment time should be as short as is compatible with acceptable acute toxicity in normal tissues. The shortening of overall treatment time using the same total dose (accelerated treatment) should be useful not only for rapidly growing tumors but also in the presumably much larger group that manifest early acceleration despite a fairly slow pretreatment growth rate.

Acceleration should not involve large dose fractions; instead, the overall time should be shortened by increasing the frequency of administration of small dose fractions. In practice, this has been achieved in the following ways:

- By delivering "boost" doses to the main tumor mass during, rather than at the end of, treatment of the initial field (which is larger to include subclinical extensions of tumor)[20]
- By delivering the treatment regimen in two parts (roughly halves), each given as multiple fractions per day in 7 to 12 days, separated by an interval of 10 to 14 days to permit the brisk acute reactions to subside and yet shorten the total duration of treatment[21]
- By treating with one or more doses per day 6 or 7 days per week, sometimes a lower total dose is tolerated than is tolerated with "standard" therapy[22]
- Interstitial and intracavitary brachytherapy is also a form of accelerated treatment because the total dose can be delivered to a small volume in a few days.

## DRUG-RADIATION INTERACTIONS

An advantage from using a combination of radiation and drugs may be realized if the drug selectively radiosensitizes tumor cells or if the two agents act additively and selectively against tumor cells without a similar additive effect in toxicity. Some drugs are known to radiosensitize hypoxic tumor cells selectively—for example, the nitroimidazoles—whereas others are selectively toxic to hypoxic cells.[23] A problem in proving these agents to be useful adjuvants is that not all tumors contain hypoxic cells in sufficient quantity to limit radiocurability, and hence it becomes necessary to identify patients with severely hypoxic or poorly reoxygenating tumors.

Most chemotherapeutic agents are useful when combined with radiation therapy because of their additive tumor cytotoxicity as well as their independent toxicity for normal tissues; alternatively they may provide a greater recovery potential for normal tissue in the interval between administration of the two modalities.

## Clinical Principles

Although the importance of technologic developments should not be minimized, the critically important component of clinical radiation therapy remains the optimal use of such sophisticated technology. The optimal use of excellent facilities requires a cooperative effort by highly trained radiation oncologists, physicists, dosimetrists, and the radiation therapists who actually operate the treatment machines.

## PRETREATMENT EVALUATION OF THE PATIENT

Like other therapeutic methods, radiation therapy has definite indications and contraindications for clinical application. The use of this powerful modality, which often eradicates cancer but can also create morbidity, involves careful evaluation of many factors.

It is essential that the diagnosis be firmly established prior to the institution of treatment. Initial diagnostic proof should be based on the study of a specimen obtained by biopsy. Exceptions (when therapy can be licensed without documented histologic findings) are rare and are related to unreasonable threats posed by the biopsy itself, such as in patients with tumors of the midbrain, brain stem, or optic tract. In the case of recurrence, or in the treatment of metastases, histologic documentation of the tumor is also desirable but is less essential, and evidence obtained by other means, such as clinical findings, roentgenograms, isotope scans, or sometimes serum titers of biologic markers (e.g., alpha-fetoprotein, prostate-specific antigen) is often adequate. For example, although an initial pulmonary lesion requires biopsy identification, post-treatment regrowth or the identification of a second lesion on chest roentgenogram may be adequate evidence for treatment.

Histologic identification of tumor type, an assessment of tumor cell activity within a particular tumor type (grading), and assessment of gene expression are useful pretherapeutic predictors of biologic behavior. However, such evidence is a poor predictor of radioresponsiveness or radiocurability. Epidermoid carcinoma and adenocarcinoma are comparably radioresponsive, yet the advisability of treatment and outcome are related to other factors, such as tumor site and extent. For example, the advisability of radiation therapy for epidermoid carcinoma arising in the floor of the mouth is related not to histologic differentiation but to other factors, including preservation of function. The anatomic site of origin and the extent of a cancer are often more important than tumor type when deciding whether or not irradiation is appropriate. Thus, an epidermoid carcinoma that is limited to a freely movable vocal cord should be irradiated, whereas one that is large and has destroyed laryngeal function could make surgery preferable because the rate of cure with retained function is low. In contrast, a pulmonary epidermoid carcinoma without spread to the mediastinum usually should be resected, but extension of such a tumor to the mediastinum causing superior vena cava compression makes regional irradiation preferable. Alternatives to irradiation of a potentially responsive cancer also may be preferred because of an adjacent bone growth center in a young person. Identification of extensive intracranial metastases might make any treatment of the primary lesion or regional spread unnecessary. Commonly, treatment alternatives are best discussed in a multispecialty tumor board.

## TREATMENT GOALS

After evaluation of the patient, the objective of radiation therapy must be defined. If the cancer is potentially radiocurable, a high dose should be prescribed, with less attention to other factors such as patient inconvenience or cost. If treatment is to be palliative, avoidance of sequelae that are acceptable in curative treatment assumes more importance, as do patient convenience and cost.

In the actual treatment planning, not only identifiable gross tumor but also sites of high risk of spread must be delineated. Irradiation of clinically nondetectable (subclinical) tumor, such as in the abdominal para-aortic nodes in patients with seminoma of the testis or the cervical nodes in patients with epidermoid carcinoma of the oral tongue, can be effective in eliminating subclinical metastases using modest doses that are unlikely to cause morbidity.[24, 25]

Depending on factors such as the size and histologic characteristics of the primary tumor and its characteristic patterns of spread, doses to different sites in the same patient may vary, and actual delivery may require an integration of different types of radiations from several radiation sources, the aim being to deliver a dose that is sufficient to eliminate the tumor burden from each anatomic site. Thus, in cancers of the prostate gland, uterine cervix, or oral cavity, the primary site with the largest tumor volume may have a course of external-beam therapy supplemented by the insertion of radioactive materials (brachytherapy) to deliver a very high dose to the volume bearing the main mass of tumor cells. In contrast, regional structures containing subclinical metastases, such as lymph nodes in the pelvis or neck, require a smaller dose for control of the relatively small tumor burden and may be homogeneously irradiated to a lower dose from an external source (teletherapy). The "tailoring" of the dose distribution to maximize the therapeutic differential requires a carefully constructed treatment plan.

As is the case with any medication, the total dose of ionizing radiations must be related to the pattern and overall time of application. For example, a total dose of 6000 cGy delivered in five equal increments per week for 6 consecutive weeks is not biologically equal to the same total dose delivered in six larger increments given at weekly intervals, nor is a course split into two parts the same as a continuous course. As a general rule, a course of cancer therapy should involve small dose increments (to minimize late toxicity), given in as short an overall time as is consistent with acute toxicity (to minimize the risk of "escape" of the tumor through accelerated growth). Regardless of the detailed design of a course of radiation therapy, the underlying concept is to eliminate every clonogenic cancer cell in the local tumor and regional metastatic sites. This requires doses that vary depending on the number of tumor cells (mass vs. micrometastases) and the histologic characteristics of the tumor; these factors also account for the tolerance of the incidentally irradiated normal tissues.

## TECHNICAL CONSIDERATIONS

Several procedures precede the initiation of radiation therapy. The target volume, including the tumor, is accurately defined in three dimensions on the basis of physical examination, visual aids (i.e., radiographs, computed tomographic scans, magnetic resonance imaging), and a knowledge of both tumor biology and anatomy. The best method for selectively irradiating the tumor is chosen from several alternatives in which beam energy, direction of delivery, and field size are ultimately optimized with the help of a simulator and a treatment planning computer system. The simulator is a machine that mimics the characteristics of the treatment machine except that it operates at the low energies needed for diagnostic radiography (and fluoroscopic) capabilities. Also, it is common to use a computed tomography–based

imaging system. The computer software permits rapid generation of dose distributions throughout the irradiated tissues. Two-dimensional dose-calculation algorithms are standard, but three-dimensional algorithms are increasingly available to provide better visualization of possible dose distributions within the presumed tumor volume and incidentally irradiated normal tissues.

Based on the requirements for the individual patient, immobilization devices and other treatment aids—such as custom blocks to shape the radiation portals and wedges or beam compensators, or both, to alter the patterns of absorption of the radiation beams—are designed and assembled. A common new alternative is to program the movements of built-in beam collimators (jaws) to vary the shape of the beam before or during treatment, or both. Doses at selected sites are calculated (or sometimes measured). Finally, the accuracy of the treatment application is checked on the actual device (linear accelerator, $^{60}$Co unit) by means of radiographs obtained before the start of treatment and at intervals (e.g., weekly) during the course of "fractionated" doses. Modern accelerators include treatment monitoring computers, which prevent the machine from operating except at the prescribed settings; in addition, "real-time" imaging devices are becoming available for monitoring beam alignment at all times during treatment.

It is increasingly common to "conform" all or part of the prescribed tumor dose to the tumor by the use of "beam's-eye" viewing of dose distribution around the whole three-dimensional image of the tumor during treatment planning. In this way, it is possible to "wrap" the dose around the target volume using multiple planar or noncoplanar beams or by continually varying the intensity of a beam of radiation focused on the tumor as the machine rotates (arcs) around the body.

## SIDE EFFECTS

Every effective therapeutic procedure can cause complications. In radiation oncology, the incidence of undesirable treatment sequelae has been reduced by the introduction of megavoltage equipment; better standardization of dosimetry; more careful, computer-assisted treatment planning; advances in the understanding of radiation biology; and more stringent mechanisms of quality control.

The art of radiation oncology lies both in determining the appropriate risk-benefit ratio for each individual patient and in planning treatment to achieve that goal.

In curative therapy (which composes at least 70% of the clinical practice of most radiation oncologists), it is clear that both tumor control and complications increase with dose and that in good practice there must be some incidence of complications (Table 7–1; see also Fig. 7–1). Many factors affect the best compromise in a given patient, such as the probability of achieving cure; the probability of distant metastases and, related to these factors, the goal of treatment; the nature, severity, and consequences of possible complications; and the wishes of the patient with respect to risk and benefit.

The side effects of radiation therapy are usually localized to the body site irradiated, there being few of the systemic side effects common with chemotherapy. For example, alo-

*Table 7–1.* Radiation Complications

|  | Organ | Injury | CD$_{5/5}$* (cGy) | CD$_{5/50}$† (cGy) | Portion of Organ |
|---|---|---|---|---|---|
| Potentially severe or fatal radiation injury | Bone marrow | Pancytopenia, aplasia | 250 | 450 | Whole |
|  |  |  | 3000 | 4000 | Segmental |
|  | Liver | Hepatitis | 2500 | 4000 | Whole |
|  | Stomach | Ulcer, hemorrhage | 4500 | 5500 | 100 cm$^2$ |
|  | Intestine | Ulcer, perforation | 4500 | 5500 | 400 cm$^2$ |
|  | Rectum | Stricture, ulcer | 6000 | 8000 | 100 cm$^2$ |
|  | Brain | Infarct, necrosis | 6000 | 7000 | Whole |
|  |  |  | 7000 | 8000 | 25% |
|  | Spinal cord | Infarct, myelitis, necrosis | 4500 | 5500 | 10 cm |
|  | Heart | Pericarditis | 4500 | 5500 | 60% |
|  | Lung | Acute and chronic pneumonitis | 3000 | 3500 | 100 cm$^2$ |
|  | Kidney | Acute and chronic nephrosclerosis | 1500 | 2500 | Whole |
|  | Fetus | Death | 200 | 400 | Whole |
| Potentially mild or moderately severe radiation injury | Bladder | Contracture | 6000 | 8000 | Whole |
|  | Testes | Sterilization | 100 | 200 | Whole |
|  | Ovary | Sterilization | 200–300 | 625–1200 | Whole |
|  | Lens | Cataract | 500 | 1200 | Whole or part |
|  | Vagina | Ulcer, fistula | 9000 | 10,000 | Whole or part |
|  | Breast (child) | No development | 1000 | 2500 | Whole |
|  | Breast (adult) | Atrophy, necrosis | >5000 | >10,000 | Whole |

*CD$_{5/5}$, dose to which a given population of patients is exposed at standard time-dose fractionation resulting in a 5% complication rate within 5 yr after treatment.

†CD$_{5/50}$, dose to which a given population of patients is exposed at standard time-dose fractionation resulting in a 50% complication rate within 5 yr after treatment.

Data from Moosa AR, et al. Comprehensive textbook of oncology. Baltimore: Williams & Wilkins, 1985:267. Copyright, Williams & Wilkins, 1985. Modified from Rubin P. Clinical Oncology. Rochester: American Cancer Society, 1978.

pecia occurs only in the treatment field, and nausea and vomiting usually occur only after irradiation of the upper abdomen.

The clinically important late sequelae of radiation therapy, which become manifested months or even years after treatment, should occur in less than 5 to 10% of patients and need to be viewed in the perspective of the probability of tumor control and the impact of the complication on the quality of life. A colostomy that is made necessary by bowel stenosis, which is produced infrequently in curing a patient with stage III cancer of the cervix, is described as a complication, whereas it is a necessary sequela of a planned abdominal perineal resection for cancer of the colon. Balancing the impact of sequelae in normal tissues against the chances of cure is the crux of clinical practice and must take into account the patient's attitude and preferences.

## COMBINATION THERAPY

As is discussed throughout this book, radiation therapy is being increasingly combined with surgery, chemotherapy, therapy with biologic agents, or any combination thereof. The objective of such combined modalities must be improvement of local and regional control of tumor and, hopefully, some decrease in the incidence of metastatic growth, commonly with a concomitant reduction in morbidity. This aim is best achieved by an initial multidisciplinary plan tailored to the particular patient's circumstances rather than by ad hoc attempts to rescue the failures of one modality by the other. Both surgery and radiation therapy may be directed to the same anatomic site (with either modality being performed first), with the intent of improving local tumor control, such as in patients with malignant tumors of the hypopharynx or paranasal sinuses, breast, rectum, or soft tissues. Alternatively, the modalities may be directed to adjacent but

different anatomic sites in an attempt to supplement local tumor control by improved regional control, such as in patients with cancers arising in the tongue or testis.

Whether radiation therapy precedes or follows surgery depends on the different objectives of treatment and the preferences of the involved physicians. The interval between the application of each treatment method should be planned to minimize additive complications without dissipating any advantage in tumor control that might result from the growth of residual tumor or regional micrometastases. With preoperative irradiation, this time interval until surgery should be long enough to permit resolution of the early radiation response of the fibrovasculature and other relevant tissues and, in some cases, to permit sufficient tumor regression to facilitate surgery. Depending on the dose and purpose of preoperative irradiation, this interval may be as short as 1 day to as long as 6 weeks. With postoperative irradiation, it is necessary to permit some healing of the wound but avoid significant regrowth of subclinical deposits in the tumor bed or lymphatics. Irradiation has its most adverse effect on the early stages of wound healing but should normally not interfere with wound strength if delayed for 7 to 20 days postoperatively. The growth rate of microscopic cancer may be faster than suggested by the growth rate of the detectable primary tumor, with doubling times being as short as 3 to 4 days. For these reasons, postoperative adjuvant radiation therapy should not be delayed unnecessarily (e.g., beyond 2 to 3 weeks) and may be started before wound healing is complete without prejudicing ultimate wound strength.

Combinations of radiation therapy and chemotherapy increased strikingly in the late 1990s. Usually the objectives of each are complementary. Radiation therapy is usually directed at primary tumor masses and regional nodes, whereas systemic treatment is aimed at widespread metastases, either documented or predicted while still imperceptible. Chemotherapeutic agents may modify the response of tumor and normal tissues to irradiation, usually as an additive effect.

Most drugs used for chemotherapy appear to kill cells independently of, and therefore additively to, irradiation. Some cytotoxic drugs (e.g., platinum compounds) may produce some radiosensitization, but none has been shown to sensitize tumor cells selectively. Cells are usually more radioresistant in the S-phase than in other phases of the mitotic cycle, whereas cytotoxic drugs are commonly more effective in killing S-phase cells. Achievement of a therapeutic gain from these potentially complementary phase-specific sensitivities requires a selectively greater effect on the tumor than on irradiated normal tissues, which will depend on closer coordination in the timing of administration of the two modalities than has been characteristic of most clinical trials.

An unusual effect of dactinomycin and doxorubicin is their ability to induce a "recall" reaction in tissues that have been previously irradiated; the mechanism is unknown.

Because a proportion of solid tumors contain hypoxic but viable cells, drugs that are selectively toxic to hypoxic cells hold promise. Drugs that selectively radiosensitize hypoxic cells have been identified and subjected to clinical trials. Although a meta-analysis has suggested improved local tumor control rates with hypoxic cell radiosensitizers,[26] dramatic improvements require better identification of that subset of tumors whose response to a course of fractionated radiation therapy is limited by hypoxic cells.

Whether cytotoxic agents act independently or by synergism, providing an additive effect or antagonism, it must be remembered that the clinical objective is to improve the ratio of tumor cell killing to normal tissue damage (therapeutic ratio). Interaction, of itself, is not sufficient.

The necessity of correlating the therapeutic capacity of radiation oncology, cancer biology, radiobiology of cancers and normal tissues, and physics, as well as continuous performance evaluation and analysis of long-term results, should make it evident that the selection of patients for radiation therapy should involve consultation with the radiation oncologist, preferably in a multidisciplinary clinic setting, and should not be the unilateral decision of the referring physician, regardless of competence in his or her chosen medical specialty. Thus, the selection of patients for radiation therapy must ultimately be made by the radiation oncologist, just as the selection for surgery or chemotherapy must be the decision of the surgeon or medical oncologist.

## Conclusions

The clinical use of ionizing radiations dates to the discovery of x-rays in 1895 and the recognition of natural radioactivity in 1896. However, the physical foundations of their therapeutic application, the development and distribution of megavoltage generators, the training of substantial numbers of physicians and support personnel, and even an elementary knowledge of radiobiology are far more recent developments.

The prospects for better therapeutic use of ionizing radiations in the future are good owing to both research developments and education. Research objectives include a better understanding of cancer biology, favorable modifications of the radiosensitivity of both tumors and normal tissues, better prediction of possible limiting factors in radiocurability in individual patients (e.g., tumor hypoxia or regrowth potential), better definition of targets, better dose delivery systems

through the use of new imaging devices, computer-assisted treatment planning and delivery, refined use of adjuvants, and more effective strategies for multidisciplinary treatment.

However, a great improvement in the multimodality therapy for cancer could be achieved immediately if all patients received what is currently acknowledged as the best available treatment. This requires that individual physicians appreciate the potential of available treatment modalities, especially the advantage of multidisciplinary consultation at the time of initial diagnosis and treatment and development of a treatment strategy.

## SUGGESTIONS FOR ADDITIONAL READING

Vokes EE (chairman). Concomitant chemoradiotherapy for solid tumors: rationale and clinical experience. Semin Oncol 1992;19(Suppl 11):1–108. *Fifteen reports on this subject presented at a conference in 1991.*

Hill RP, Tannock IF, eds. The Basic Science of Oncology. 3rd ed. New York: McGraw-Hill, 1998.

Perez CA, Brady LW, eds. Principles and practice of radiation oncology. 3rd ed. Philadelphia: JB Lippincott, 1998.

## REFERENCES

1. Buschke FJ, Parker RG. Radiation therapy in cancer management. New York: Grune & Stratton, 1972.
2. Kramer S, Herring DF. The patterns of care study: a nationwide evaluation of the practice of radiation therapy in cancer management. Int J Radiat Oncol Biol Phys 1976;1:1231–6.
3. Withers HR. Biological basis of radiation therapy for cancer. Lancet 1992;339:156–9.
4. Buschke FJ. What is a radiotherapist? Radiology 1962;79:319–21.
5. Boag JW. The time scale in radiobiology. In: Nygaard OF, Adler HI, Sinclair WK, eds. Radiation research: biomedical, chemical, and physical perspectives. Proceedings of the fifth International Congress of Radiation Research. Seattle, Wash., July 14–20, 1974. New York: Academic Press, 1975:9–29.
6. International Commission on Radiation Units and Measurements (ICRU). Report No. 33, 1980, 1–25.
7. Thames HD, ed. Fractionation in radiotherapy. New York: Taylor & Francis, 1987.
8. Steel GG, ed. Growth kinetics of tumors. New York: Oxford University Press, 1977.
9. Tepper JL, ed. Seminars in radiation oncology. Vol. 3. Philadelphia: WB Saunders, 1993.
10. Puck TT, Marcus PI. Action of x-rays on mammalian cells. J Exp Med 1956;103:653.
11. Elkind MM, Sutton H. X-ray damage and recovery in mammalian cells in culture. Nature 1959;184:1293.
12. Coutard H: Sur les delais d'apparition et d'evolution des reactions des la peau et der muqueses de la bouche et du pharynx provoquées par ler rayons x. CR Soc Biol (Paris) 1922;86:1140.
13. Regaud C, Blanc J. Action des rayons x sur les diverses générations de la lignée spermatique. Extreme sensibilité des spermatogomes á ces rayons. CR Soc Biol (Paris) 1906;41:163.
14. Thames HD, Peters LJ, Withers HR, Fletcher GH. Accelerated fractionation vs hyperfractionation: rationales for several treatments per day. Int J Radiat Oncol Biol Phys 1983;9:127–38.
15. Withers H. Biologic basis of radiation therapy. In: Perez CA, Brady LW, eds. Principles and Practice of Radiation Oncology. Philadelphia: JB Lippincott, 1987:67–98.
16. Sinclair WK, Morton RA. X-ray sensitivity during the cell generation cycle of cultured Chinese hamster cells. Radiat Res 1966;29:450–74.
17. Gray LH, Conger AD, Ebert M, et al. The concentration of oxygen dissolved in tissues at the time of irradiation as a factor in radiotherapy. Br J Radiol 1953;26:638.
18. Kallman RF. The phenomenon of reoxygenation and its implications for fractionated radiotherapy. Radiology 1972;105:135–42.
19. Hall EJ. Radiation dose-rate: a factor of importance in radiobiology and radiotherapy. Br J Radiol 1972;45:81–97.

20. Horiot JC, Le Fur R, N'Guyen T, et al. Hyperfractionation versus conventional fractionation in oropharyngeal carcinoma: final analysis of a randomized trial of the EORTC cooperative group of radiotherapy. Radiother Oncol 1992;25:231–41.
21. Peters LJ, Ang KK, Thames HD, et al. In: Perez CA, Brady LW, eds. Principles and practice of radiation oncology. 2nd ed. Philadelphia: Lippincott-Raven, 1992.
22. Maciejewski B, Skladowski K, Pilecki B, et al. Randomized clinical trial on accelerated 7 days per week fractionation in radiotherapy for head and neck cancer. Preliminary report on acute toxicity. Radiother Oncol 1996;40:137–45.

23. Brown JM, Yu NY, Brown DM, Lee, WW. SR-2508: a 2-nitroimidazole amide which should be superior to misonidazole as a radiosensitizer for clinical use. Int J Radiat Oncol Biol Phys 1981;7:695–703.
24. Fletcher GH. Elective irradiation of subclinical disease in cancers of the head and neck. Cancer 1972;29:1450–4.
25. Withers HR, Peters LJ, Taylor JM. Dose-response relationship for radiation therapy of subclinical disease. Int J Radiat Oncol Biol Phys 1995;31:353–9.
26. Overgaard J. Clinical evaluation of nitroimidazoles as modifiers of hypoxia in solid tumors. Oncol Res 1994;6:509–18.

# CHAPTER 8

# PRINCIPLES OF CANCER CHEMOTHERAPY

● CHARLES M. HASKELL

It is axiomatic that systemic (metastatic) cancer should be treated systemically. Lissauer demonstrated the anticancer effect of potassium arsenite (Fowler's solution) in 1865, but the modern age of systemic therapy more properly dates from the early 1940s, when Huggins and Hodges showed that patients with prostate cancer benefited from the administration of estrogen. By 1950, the rate of introduction of useful new agents began to accelerate (Table 8–1), and subsequent research in tumor cell biology, pharmacology, and immunology has led to more rational drug therapy.

There are two major types of systemic therapy: cancer chemotherapy and biologic therapy. Cancer chemotherapy involves the use of cytotoxic drugs and hormones, whereas immunotherapy involves the use of biologic molecules known collectively as *biologic response modifiers* (BRMs). There is considerable overlap between these two types of therapy, and they are increasingly employed together in various combinations, either as separate agents or as investigational immunoconjugates. Both are complex, but certain principles and unifying concepts aid in their selection and rational use. This chapter summarizes these concepts for cancer chemotherapy. The principles and use of biologic therapy are covered in Chapter 9, and the use of hematopoietic growth factors is discussed in Chapter 15. Individual antineoplastic agents are discussed in more detail in Chapter 10, where they are listed in alphabetical order by generic name.

## Selective Toxicity

The clinically useful antineoplastic agents are more toxic to sensitive malignant cells than to normal cells of the tumor-bearing host. They are said to exhibit selective toxicity. Cancer chemotherapy inhibits cancer through several potential mechanisms. It may induce cell death through specific and nonspecific means (cytotoxicity), it may suppress cancer cells for variable periods without inducing cell death (cytostatic effects) and, rarely, it may induce cell differentiation.[1]

Biologic therapy, or *immunotherapy* as it is sometimes known, is more likely to alter the balance of biologic factors that control the growth and dormancy of cells or their differentiation, or both. Biologic therapy can, however, be cytotoxic to cancer cells and induce cell death. It may also be extremely toxic, as exemplified by cardiovascular collapse from interleukin-2 (IL-2)[2] and the retinoic acid syndrome seen with the use of all-*trans*-retinoic acid.[3]

Malignant tissues are largely composed of dividing cells that synthesize DNA at some point in their life cycle. Cancer cells use large amounts of glucose as a source of energy to permit the exaggerated use of amino acids and nucleosides in the synthesis of DNA. This pattern of metabolism is nonspecific because it is also seen in fetal or regenerating tissue. What appears to be unique with neoplastic tissues, however, is an altered pattern of gene expression, especially a failure of the cancer cell to control or cease gene expression and to control the rate of cell division.

Selective toxicity of chemotherapeutic agents is possible because of quantitative differences between malignant and normal cells (i.e., there are differences in the amounts of certain chemicals or in the rates of various chemical reactions). The fact that these differences are quantitative rather than qualitative results in at least some degree of injury to normal tissues during treatment. It is important to emphasize that the differences between normal and malignant tissues may be slight. Many regenerating normal tissues have a high proliferative capacity rivaling, and in some instances exceeding, that of malignant tissues. Such normal tissues, including bone marrow elements, gastrointestinal epithelium, and hair follicles, bear the brunt of the toxic effects of certain anticancer drugs. The rapidly proliferating normal cells and cancer cells are not always equally vulnerable. It is apparent, however, that the margin of safety is often narrow, and the success of chemotherapy is not simply a matter of excessive toxicity for rapidly proliferating neoplasms.[4]

The most useful chemotherapeutic agents interact with important enzymes or substrates that are acted on by enzyme systems, or both. For most agents, the target is an enzyme

*Table 8–1.* Development of Chemotherapeutic Agents

| Approximate Date | Agent | Diseases Treated | Approximate Date | Agent | Diseases Treated |
|---|---|---|---|---|---|
| 1865 | Potassium arsenite | Leukemias, various malignancies | 1970–1980 | Doxorubicin | Sarcomas and a wide spectrum of other tumors |
| 1893 | Coley's toxins | Various malignancies | | Bleomycin | Lymphomas, head and neck cancer |
| 1941 | Estrogens | Prostate and breast carcinomas | 1980–1990 | Tamoxifen | Breast cancer |
| | Androgens | Breast cancer | | Leuprolide | Prostate cancer |
| 1945 | Nitrogen mustard | Lymphomas, solid tumors | | Flutamide | Prostate cancer |
| 1948–1950 | Adrenocorticosteroids | Leukemias, lymphomas, multiple myeloma | | Etoposide | Germ cell tumors, small cell lung cancer |
| | Methotrexate | Acute leukemia, choriocarcinoma | | Streptozocin | Islet cell carcinoma |
| 1950–1955 | Busulfan | Chronic granulocytic leukemia | | Interferons | Hairy cell leukemia, Kaposi's sarcoma |
| | 6-Mercaptopurine | Acute leukemia | | Mitoxantrone | Acute leukemia, some solid tumors |
| | Actinomycin D | Wilms' tumor, testicular tumors, choriocarcinoma | | Octreotide acetate | Carcinoid and islet cell carcinomas |
| 1955–1960 | 5-Fluorouracil | Carcinomas of breast and gastrointestinal tract | | Ifosfamide | Refractory germ cell tumors |
| | Progestins | Endometrial carcinoma | | Carboplatin | Refractory ovarian carcinoma |
| | Cyclophosphamide | Lymphomas, solid tumors | 1990 + | Fludarabine | Chronic lymphocytic leukemia |
| | Mitotane | Adrenal carcinoma | | | |
| | Vinca alkaloids | Lymphomas, acute leukemia, miscellaneous tumors | | Pentostatin | Hairy cell leukemia |
| | | | | Cladribine | Hairy cell leukemia |
| | Mitomycin C | Gastrointestinal tumors | | Paclitaxel | Refractory ovarian carcinoma, breast cancer |
| 1960–1965 | Hydroxyurea | Chronic granulocytic leukemia | | Docetaxel (Taxotere) | Breast and ovarian cancer |
| | Procarbazine | Hodgkin's disease | | Vinorelbine | Breast cancer |
| | Cytarabine | Acute leukemia | | Gemcitabine | Pancreatic cancer |
| | Mithramycin | Testicular tumors | | Capecitabine | Colorectal cancer |
| | Nitrosoureas | Lymphomas, brain tumors, solid tumors | | Topotecan | Ovarian cancer |
| | Daunorubicin | Acute leukemia | | | |
| 1965–1970 | L-Asparaginase | Acute leukemia | | | |
| | Dacarbazine | Melanoma | | | |
| | Cisplatin | Testicular and ovarian tumors | | | |

or substrate that is related to DNA synthesis or function and, consequently, these drugs appear to exert their major toxic and antitumor effects by inhibiting cells that undergo DNA synthesis at some time in their life cycle. These effects can result in nonspecific cell death leading to necrosis, or they may initiate a carefully modulated and controlled series of events known as *programmed cell death*, or *apoptosis* (Fig. 8–1).[5] Apoptosis is important in embryogenesis, cell differentiation, immune system remodeling, and the ultimate cytotoxicity of many (if not most) cancer chemotherapeutic agents. It involves packaging damaged cell material into lipid bilayer particles, which can then be internalized by adjacent cells.

Myriad factors contribute to selective toxicity. The cancer cell is a complex entity that may have lost important genetic controls through gene deletion or amplification, as discussed in Chapter 2. Normal genes flanking those lost could be a target for cancer chemotherapy.[6] Altered receptors may also occur from specific translocations, such as the t(15;17) chromosomal translocation seen with acute promyelocytic leukemia. In this case, there is fusion of part of a retinoid receptor gene on chromosome 17 with a gene termed *PML* on chromosome 15.[7] Consequently, the cell is sensitive to all-*trans*-retinoic acid.

In most cases, there is no clear-cut qualitative difference between any given neoplasm and its related normal cellular counterpart. Such neoplasms nevertheless may contain a variety of potentially sensitive receptor molecules. This diversity, or heterogeneity, may relate to subclonal evolution of the cells or to peculiarities in the life cycles of the various cells in the tumor. Drug resistance may differ accordingly. Ultimately, drug action depends on a direct interaction of the drug or its active metabolite or metabolites with a specific target molecule. The ability of a given drug or drug combination to reach cellular receptors is a function of its pharmacokinetic properties. Successful chemotherapy depends on multiple pharmacologic and biologic factors. For any given antineoplastic drug, the net effect on the host is often referred to as the drug's therapeutic index (i.e., a ratio of the doses at which therapeutic effect and toxicity occur).

Cancer chemotherapeutic agents are usually discussed in groups that reflect either the origin of the drug or their predominant mechanism of action. The major classes of agents include the alkylating agents, antitumor antibiotics, plant derivatives, antimetabolites, hormonal agonists and antagonists, and a variety of miscellaneous agents. Each of these groups is discussed briefly here, and a schematic diagram of their biochemical target molecules is given in Figure 8–2. A more detailed discussion of selected, important drugs appears in Chapter 10.

Normal Cell

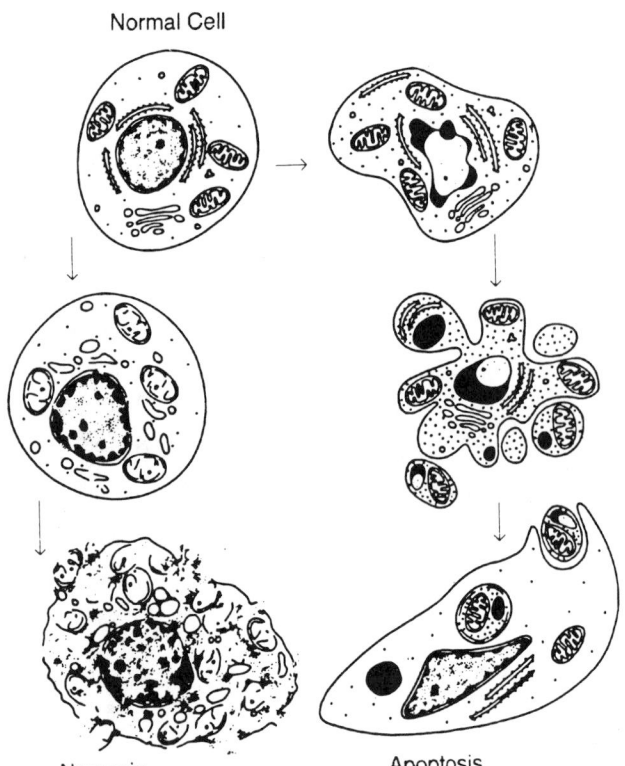

Necrosis                    Apoptosis

**Figure 8–1.** Programmed cell death (apoptosis). (From Kerr JFR, Harmon BV. Curr Comm Cell Mol Biol 1991;3:5–29.)

## Classes of Agents

### ALKYLATING AGENTS AND RELATED COMPOUNDS

The classic alkylating agents are highly reactive compounds that have the ability to substitute alkyl groups (e.g., $R\text{-}CH_2\text{-}CH_2^+$) for the hydrogen atoms of certain organic compounds. In most instances, this substitution involves the formation of an ethylenimmonium ion intermediate (Fig. 8–3). Although many cellular substances can be alkylated in this way, the alkylation of nucleic acids, primarily DNA, is the critical cytotoxic action for most of these compounds. Alkylation may produce breaks in the DNA molecule, cross-linking of its twin strands (interstrand cross-linking), cross-linking within the same strand of DNA (intrastrand cross-linking), or various combinations of these effects, interfering with DNA replication and the transcription of RNA. Similar breaks in the DNA molecule are produced by certain kinds of ionizing radiations so that the classic alkylating agents are said to be radiomimetic. The effects of alkylators, similar to the corresponding ones of irradiation, are often visible microscopically as abnormalities of chromosome structure, and both are mutagenic, teratogenic, and potentially carcinogenic. The classic alkylating agents, which are discussed more fully in Chapter 10, include the following: mechlorethamine (nitrogen mustard), chlorambucil, melphalan, cyclophosphamide, ifosfamide, thiotepa, and busulfan.

A number of nonclassic alkylating agents also damage DNA and proteins, but through diverse and complex mechanisms, such as methylation or chloroethylation, that differ from those of the classic alkylators. The nonclassic alkylating agents, discussed in Chapter 10, include the following: dacarbazine (DTIC), carmustine (BCNU), lomustine (CCNU), cisplatin, carboplatin, procarbazine, and altretamine.

## ANTIBIOTICS

The clinically useful antitumor antibiotics are natural products of various strains of the soil fungus *Streptomyces*. They produce their tumoricidal effects by one or more mechanisms. All the antibiotics are capable of binding to DNA, usually by interposition between base pairs (a process called *intercalation*), with subsequent uncoiling of the DNA helix. This distortion impairs the ability of DNA to serve as a template for DNA synthesis or RNA synthesis, or both. These drugs may also damage DNA by the formation of free radicals (compounds that possess an unpaired electron) and the chelation of important metal ions. They may also act as inhibitors of topoisomerase II, a critical enzyme in cell division. Drugs of this class, discussed in Chapter 10, include the following: doxorubicin (Adriamycin), daunorubicin, idarubicin, mitoxantrone, bleomycin, dactinomycin, mitomycin C, plicamycin (mithramycin), and streptozocin.

## PLANT DERIVATIVES

Through folklore, random screening, and chance observation, plants have provided some of the most useful antineoplastic agents. Four groups of agents from this class are reviewed in Chapter 10: the vinca alkaloids (vincristine and vinblastine), the epipodophyllotoxins (etoposide and teniposide), the taxanes (paclitaxel and docetaxel [Taxotere]), and the camptothecins (topotecan and irinotecan).

The vinca alkaloids are extracted from the common periwinkle plant (*Vinca rosea* Lin, more properly known as *Catharanthus roseus*). This plant was originally screened for bioactive alkaloids by pharmaceutical chemists because of the use of these plants as hypoglycemic agents by natives in several parts of the world. The hypoglycemic properties of the extracts were not impressive; however, their marrow-suppressive and other cytotoxic effects were readily apparent, and vincristine and vinblastine have well-established roles in the treatment of cancer. These agents bind to microtubular proteins found in dividing cells and the nervous system. This binding alters the dynamics of tubulin addition and loss at the ends of mitotic spindle microtubules, rather than by depolymerizing the microtubules themselves. Because these microtubules are essential contractile proteins of the mitotic spindle of dividing cells, this binding leads to mitotic arrest. Similar proteins make up an important part of nervous tissue so that these agents are neurotoxic.

Podophyllin is an extract of the roots of the plant *Podophyllum peltatum*, commonly known as the May apple or mandrake. It was described as an excellent emetic in 1731, and in 1862 its topical use for cancerous growths was described. It has been a common component of various folk remedies (e.g., Carter's Little Liver Pills), including remedies for cancer. In 1947, it was shown that podophyllin induced metaphase arrest, so it was tested more extensively

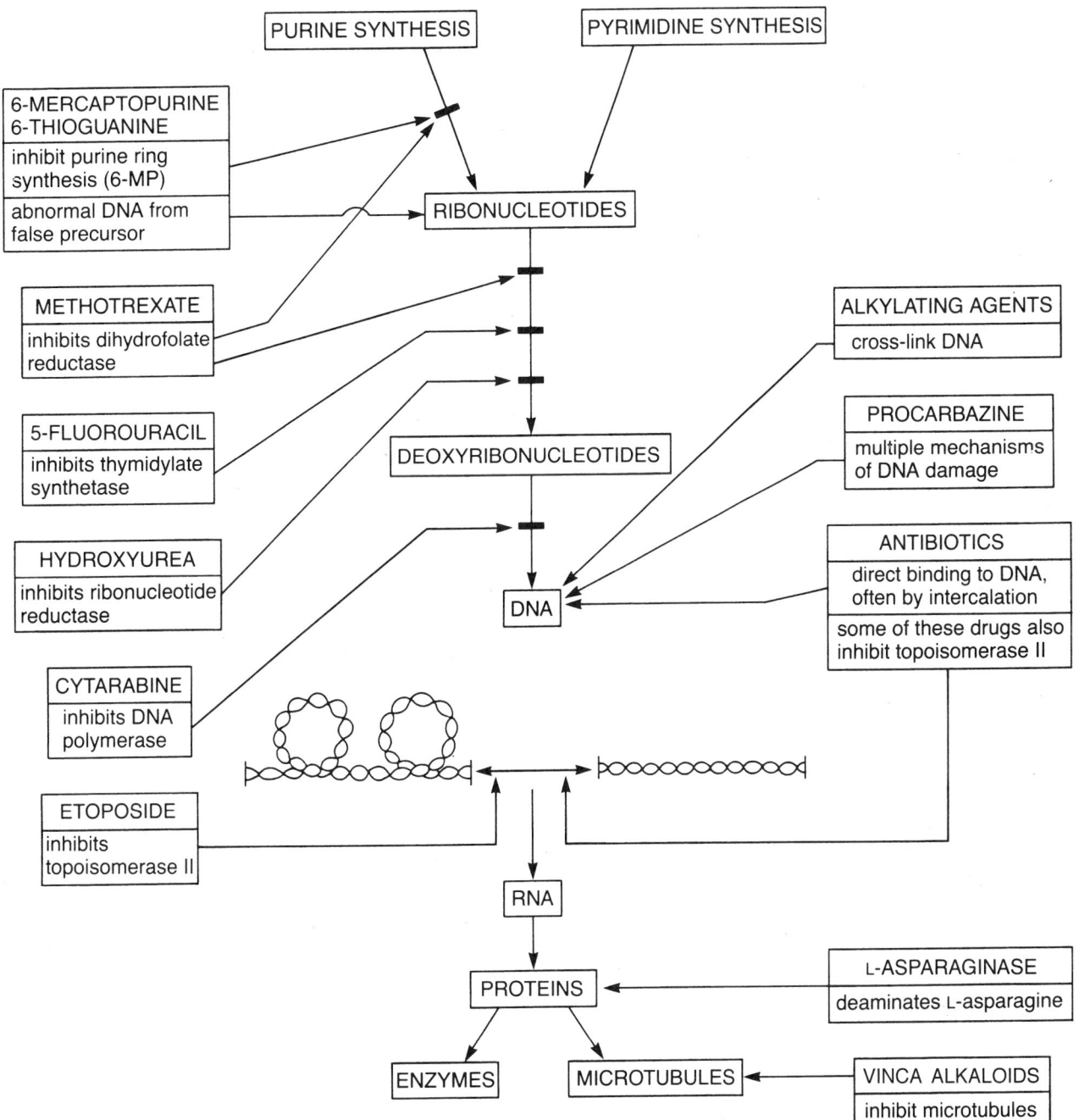

**Figure 8–2.** Summary of the mechanisms and sites of action of selected drugs used in cancer chemotherapy. (Isomeric forms of DNA redrawn from Glisson BS, Ross WE. DNA topoisomerase II: a primer on the enzyme and its unique role as a multidrug target in cancer chemotherapy. Pharmacol Ther 1987;32:89.)

as an antineoplastic agent. It proved to be highly toxic and ineffective. In 1963, Sandoz started a semisynthetic podophyllin derivative program that resulted in two derivatives known as VP-16 (etoposide [VePesid], NSC-141540) and VM-26 (teniposide [Vumon]).

The epipodophyllin derivatives of podophyllin that were tested did not interfere with microtubules; rather, they inhibited an important cellular enzyme called *topoisomerase II*. Because many clinicians are unfamiliar with the role of topoisomerase II in cell biology, and because of the emerging importance of this enzyme as a target of cancer chemother-

apy, a few comments about this enzyme are in order. Every mammalian chromosome contains about 5 cm of helical DNA that has to be packaged into a nucleus with an approximate diameter of 5 to 10 μm. This packaging involves forming numerous loops and kinks around various structures, which requires unraveling the DNA double helix. This unraveling process involves two sets of nuclear enzymes that are able to catalyze the interconversion of topologic isomers of DNA, hence the name topoisomerases. Two types of these enzymes are recognized. Type I causes temporary breaking and rejoining of single-strand DNA, allowing the DNA helix

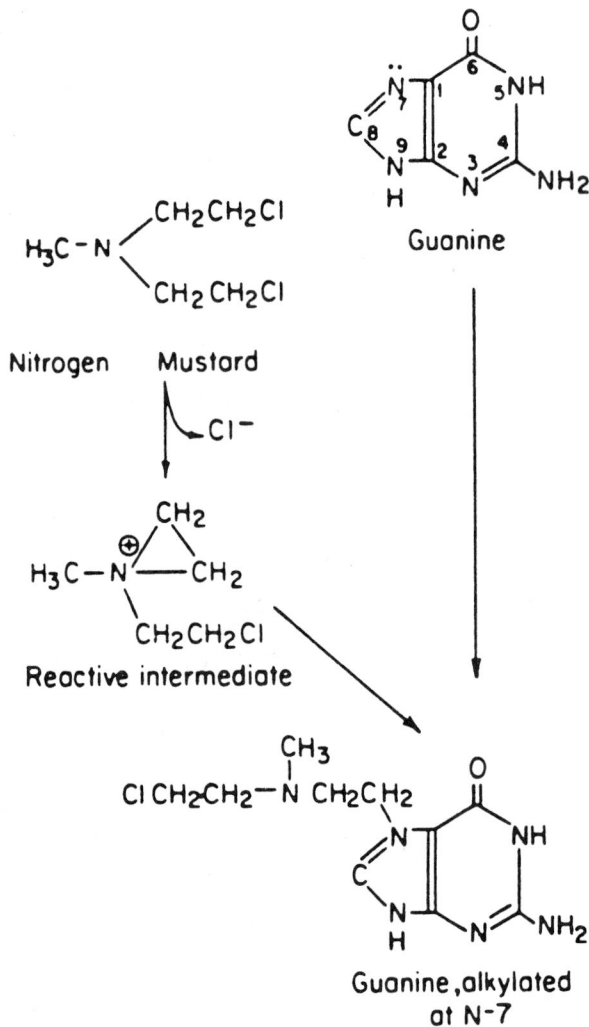

**Figure 8–3.** Mechanism of action of classic alkylating agents. Reactions leading to alkylation at the N-7 position of guanine by mechlorethamine (nitrogen mustard). (From Erlichman C. The pharmacology of anticancer drugs. In: Tannock IF, Hill RP, eds. The basic science of oncology. New York: Pergamon Press, 1987:297.)

to change its twist. Type II temporarily cleaves both strands of the DNA helix, which is followed by transient relaxation of DNA twist and a process called *strand passage*. Topoisomerase II participates in this reaction by forming a transient enzyme-DNA complex. Etoposide binds to the transient enzyme-DNA complex, causing it to become stabilized. Given the importance of topoisomerase II to DNA replication, recombination, transcription, and repair, this binding can have profound implications for cell function.

Paclitaxel (Taxol) is a derivative of the bark of the yew tree from the Pacific Northwest of the United States. Docetaxel is a derivative of needles of the European yew tree. They are unique and interesting drugs with complex effects on microtubules that differ from those of the other plant derivatives, as described in Chapter 10.

The camptothecins are alkaloidal extracts from an Asian tree, *Camptothecin acuminata*. There are two clinically available forms of camptothecin available—topotecan and irinotecan. They are unique in being specific inhibitors of topoisomerase I, resulting in stabilization of the cleavable

complex formed between single-stranded DNA and the enzyme. Topotecan is commercially available for the treatment of metastatic ovarian cancer refractory to other agents. Irinotecan is used in the treatment of colorectal cancer.

## ANTIMETABOLITES

The antimetabolites are structural analogues of normal metabolites that are required for cell function and replication. As such, they work by interacting with cellular enzymes. There are three ways in which antimetabolites or their biotransformed active products may interact with enzymes and damage cells: (1) by substituting for a metabolite that is normally incorporated into a key molecule, making the key molecule function abnormally; (2) by competing successfully with a normal metabolite for the occupation of the catalytic site of a key enzyme; and (3) by competing with a normal metabolite that acts at an enzyme regulatory site (the allosteric or noncatalytic site) to alter the catalytic rate of a key enzyme.

Of the many antimetabolites that have been developed and tested, 12 are discussed in Chapter 10: methotrexate, 5-fluorouracil (5-FU), floxuridine (FUDR), capecitabine, gemcitabine, cytarabine, 6-mercaptopurine (6-MP), 6-thioguanine, deoxycoformycin, fludarabine, 2-chloro-2′-deoxyadenosine, and hydroxyurea.

## HORMONAL AGENTS

Endocrine manipulation is an effective therapy for several forms of neoplastic disease. The empirical use of various hormonal agents preceded by many years any rational understanding of how endocrine manipulation might work, but advances in endocrinology and molecular biology promise to revolutionize the understanding and potential use of such treatment. This revolution relates to the dramatic expansion of knowledge about a variety of newly defined growth factors and growth factor inhibitors in cell biology.

Hormones appear to function by interacting with and binding to specific receptors. These receptors may be located on the cellular membrane, within the cytoplasm, or within the nucleus of the target cell. Steroid hormones, such as estrogen, bind mainly to specific nuclear or cytoplasmic receptor proteins that are characteristic of the target cell (Fig. 8–4). After binding, the hormone-receptor complex undergoes a three-dimensional structural rearrangement (called *receptor transformation* or *activation*), followed by binding to DNA. The subsequent biochemical events are incompletely understood but include the synthesis of messenger RNA (transcription), followed by the translation of this information into new protein synthesis through the action of transfer RNA and the polysomes. In some cases, the new protein is a receptor for yet another hormone ($H_2$ and pathway A in Fig. 8–4). In other situations, a single hormone may be sufficient to achieve the final biologic effect through the production of one or more specific growth factors (pathway B in Fig. 8–4). There may be additional factors modulating this model of steroid hormone action, such as biotransformation of one hormone to another by intracellular enzymes or cross-reactivity between one hormone or its

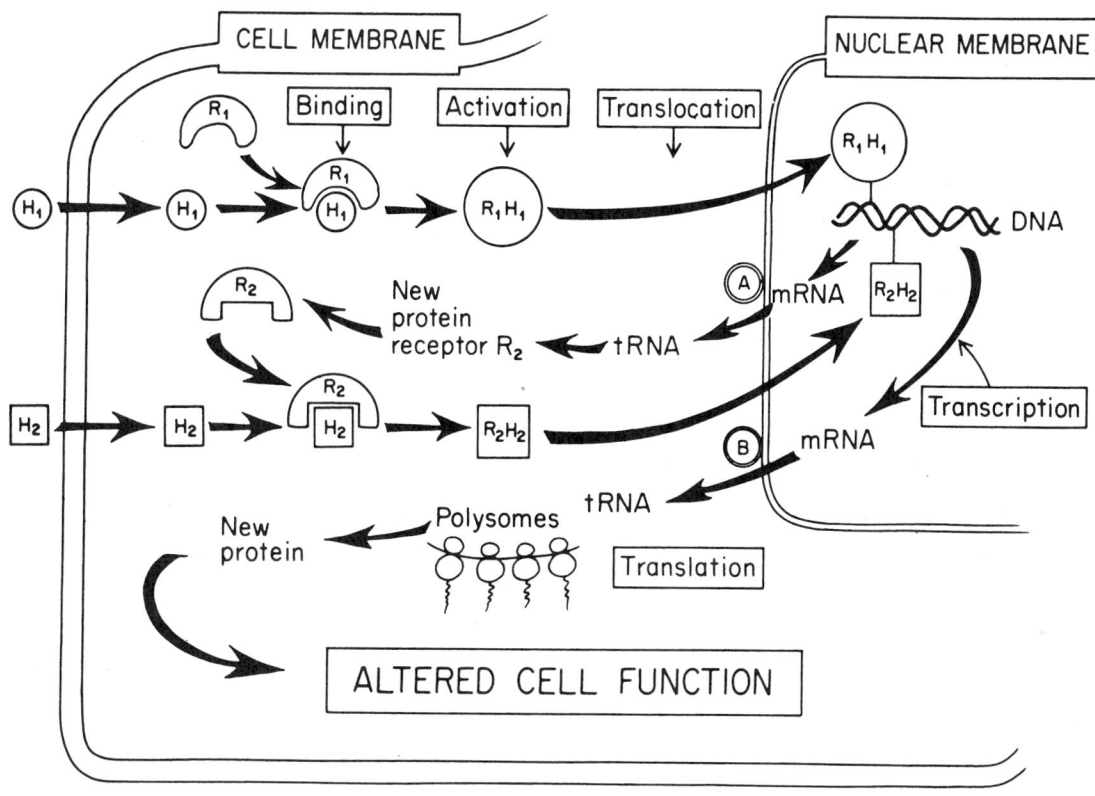

**Figure 8–4.** Mechanism of steroid hormone action.

metabolites and another class of receptors. As discussed in Chapter 35, in the sections on natural history and systemic therapy, hormone receptors are an important consideration in choosing therapy for some tumors, such as breast cancer.

Three patterns of hormone secretion, distribution, and action are recognized: (1) the endocrine pattern, in which a hormone is released in one area of the body and acts on a receptor elsewhere; (2) the paracrine pattern, in which the hormone is released by one cell and the receptor for the hormone is found on an adjacent cell in the same tissue; and (3) the autocrine pattern, in which a cell produces and releases a hormone that then acts directly on one of its own receptors (Fig. 8–5). Each of these patterns is discussed briefly.

In the past, endocrinology has been largely concerned with interactions of various endocrine hormones released by the hypothalamus and acting on the pituitary, thyroid, parathyroid, and adrenal glands as well as on the testes, ovaries, and pancreas. These vital interactions are described in standard textbooks of endocrinology and internal medicine and are not repeated here.

Paracrine mechanisms of hormone action appear to be especially important in the function of a wide variety of newly described growth factors. Some of these, such as the interleukins and interferons, are discussed further in Chapter 9. Others, such as human granulocyte colony–stimulating factor (G-CSF) and granulocyte-macrophage colony-stimulating factor (GM-CSF), are discussed in Chapter 15.

Autocrine mechanisms of hormone action may explain why some cancer cells are autonomous. In this model, the cancer cell is capable of producing its own growth factors, freeing the cell from dependence on a paracrine or endocrine source of a necessary growth-promoting material. Two examples of this mechanism of autologous growth stimulation are bombesin in small cell lung cancer and several autocrine and paracrine cytokines in acquired immunodeficiency syndrome–related Kaposi's sarcoma.

A wide variety of hormones and hormone antagonists have been developed for potential use in oncology. Some are widely used, such as tamoxifen and corticosteroids, whereas others are rarely used. A complete discussion of all of the available hormonal agents is beyond the scope of this book. Only the following selected hormonal agents are reviewed in Chapter 10: diethylstilbestrol, tamoxifen, megestrol acetate,

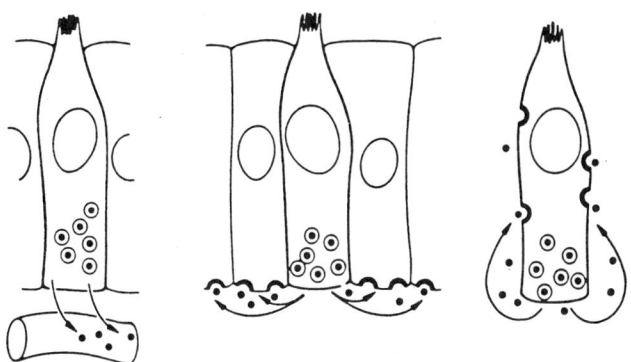

**Figure 8–5.** Diagrammatic representation of autocrine *(right)*, paracrine *(center)*, and endocrine *(left)* secretion. Regulatory chemical messengers are shown in latent form within the cell. The thickened, semicircular regions of the cell membrane represent receptor sites. (From Todaro G. Tumor growth factors. In: Fortner JG, Rhoads JE, eds. Accomplishments in cancer research 1986. Philadelphia: JB Lippincott, Co, 1987:150.)

dexamethasone, prednisone, aminoglutethimide, leuprolide, goserelin, flutamide, and octreotide acetate.

## MISCELLANEOUS AGENTS

A variety of other mechanisms exist, which are difficult to classify, for a small group of agents discussed in Chapter 10. These agents include L-asparaginase, mitotane (*o,p'*-DDD), estramustine, and levamisole.

# Pharmacokinetic Factors

Pharmacokinetic factors that alter the concentration over time of a critical drug or its active metabolites at the primary site of action must be considered in the use of cancer chemotherapeutic drugs. The most important factor is drug dosage, but the route of drug administration and absorption, transport and biodistribution, biotransformation (metabolism), excretion, and interactions among drugs are also important. These are discussed briefly in this section. More detailed information related to specific drugs is found in Chapter 10.

## DOSE INTENSITY

Most antineoplastic agents have a steep dose-response curve so that choosing the dose of chemotherapy is a serious concern. The most appropriate guide to choosing dosage is the function of the dose-limiting target organ or organs. In most cases, this target is the bone marrow, but occasionally it may be the kidneys or some other organ. In general, dosage is dictated by guidelines derived from prior empirical studies in groups of patients rather than from measurements of drug concentrations in the body fluids of the individual patient. An exception to this is methotrexate given in high dosage, in which measurements of the concentration of the drug in blood may be a vital consideration in safe administration.

Drug dosage is generally determined as a function of body surface area rather than body weight. This convention was adopted because of pioneering research by Freireich and colleagues[8] relating the maximal tolerated doses of chemotherapy in multiple species to body weight and body surface area. It became apparent that interspecies comparisons of dose were far more accurate using body surface area than weight; however, the pertinence of this convention has been questioned. Because the bone marrow is the dose-limiting organ for most drugs used in chemotherapy, and the amount of normal marrow in a person correlates much more closely to weight than to body surface area, some investigators consider weight to be the best guide to drug dosage for agents that suppress the bone marrow.[9]

There has been increasing concern that cancer patients may be receiving inadequate doses of chemotherapy because of inappropriate dose reductions by physicians who are excessively worried about drug toxicity. Improper dose reductions should be avoided, and chemotherapy should not be used as a placebo. Debate on this issue has raised the question of whether or not the standard dose regimens are sufficiently intense. One way of studying the importance of drug dosage in clinical trials is to determine the dose intensity used in the study. As used by Hryniuk and associates,[10] *dose intensity* is defined as the amount of each drug given per unit time (expressed as milligrams per square meter per week), regardless of the schedule used. This definition assumes that the schedule of drug administration is not critical and that the maximal tolerated dose of chemotherapy is the best dose. Both of these assumptions can be questioned (see subsequent discussion); there is uncertainty about the most appropriate definition of dose intensity.[11] Nevertheless, the concept of dose intensity continues to play a key role in clinical trial development.

The debate about dose intensity has been broadened to include several related concepts. Alternative ways of expressing the relationship between dose and response include the concepts of *peak dose*, *cumulative dose*, *dose rate*, *dose density*, and *sequential dose*. The relative importance of these concepts in comparison to standard dose intensity is under investigation.

## ROUTE OF ADMINISTRATION AND ABSORPTION

Diverse routes of drug administration may be used in oncology to optimize drug availability at the tumor target site (Fig. 8–6). For example, one may administer drugs orally, intravenously, intramuscularly, or intra-arterially. In many cases, the use of intravenous or intra-arterial chemotherapy

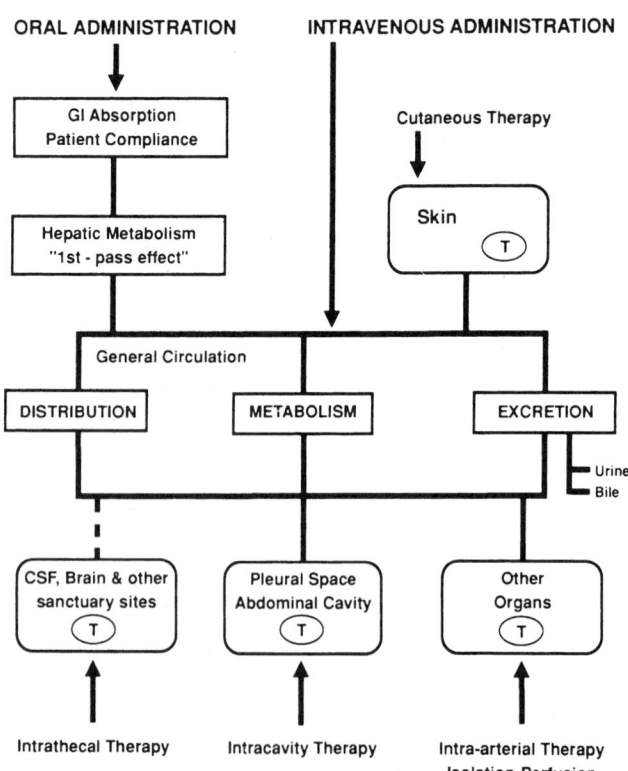

**Figure 8–6.** Factors influencing the pharmacokinetics of cancer chemotherapeutic agents following administration by a variety of routes. CSF, cerebrospinal fluid; GI, gastrointestinal; T, target molecule.

may be facilitated by the use of vascular access catheters, as discussed in Chapter 12. One may also choose to use a drug locally, such as on the skin or by instillation into the pleural space, bladder, abdominal cavity, or cerebrospinal fluid.

Careful selection of the route of administration may improve the antitumor effect of a given drug by allowing it to reach high concentrations in the area of greatest clinical need, but some routes of administration pose special problems. Two examples are given to illustrate this concern. First, it makes intuitive sense to use chemotherapy by regional arterial infusion, but the pharmacokinetic theory of such treatment has yet to be fully validated. Specifically, few studies have taken into account drug streaming from the site of infusion or the importance of regional blood flow differences between normal tissue and the regional tumor. In most cases, it has been difficult to prove a survival benefit of the use of such regional therapy compared with more traditional systemic routes of administration. Second, one must be wary of unusual forms of toxicity when drugs are used by some routes of administration. For example, vincristine and daunorubicin are both well-tolerated drugs when given intravenously, but both have caused lethal neurotoxicity when injected by error directly into the cerebrospinal fluid.

One specialized route of administration involves isolation perfusion of an extremity with large doses of alkylating agents for regional melanoma. Other specialized routes of administration include the use of totally implanted pumps for the continuous intravenous or intra-arterial administration of drugs,[12] the chemoembolization of tumors by the intra-arterial administration of cytotoxic drugs contained within ethylcellulose microcapsules,[13] the use of tourniquets after the administration of drugs to extremities as a way of postponing systemic transport,[14] the use of an intraperitoneal catheter to deliver high doses of drug to the peritoneal cavity,[15] the submucosal injection of drugs into the anal region for pelvic malignancies,[16] and the use of drug aerosols to increase the concentration of drugs in the bronchi.[17]

## DISTRIBUTION AND TRANSPORT

The distribution and transport of drugs may influence drug therapy (see Fig. 8–6). After a drug is absorbed, it may be bound to serum albumin or other blood components. It may then enter or pass through various body compartments, including vascular spaces and extracellular spaces, and into cells. In some cases, drugs may accumulate in certain areas as a result of binding, active transport, or high solubility in fat. The converse of this is that some drugs may be excluded from certain areas because of factors influencing distribution, including the blood supply of the tumor. If tumor cells are in an area of the body that is inaccessible to anticancer drugs, the drug concentration over time for those drugs is negligible, and the cancer cells survive. This phenomenon is sometimes referred to as the *sanctuary effect*. An example of such a sanctuary is the cerebrospinal fluid, where tumor cells appear to be relatively inaccessible to most anticancer drugs by virtue of the blood-brain barrier. Factors influencing the ability of a drug to cross the blood-brain barrier include its relative ionization at physiologic pH values, its molecular size, and its lipid solubility.

Because most anticancer drugs exert their effects by interacting with intracellular target molecules, the ability of a particular drug or its active metabolites to get into the cancer cell is a vital concern. For some drugs, entry into the cell is an active process. For example, some alkylating agents depend on a membrane-carrier transport system for cell entry (e.g., cisplatin, nitrogen mustard), whereas others do not (e.g., mitomycin C, nitrosoureas). For some macromolecules, there may also be important intracellular transport processes needed to achieve the ultimate biologic effect.

Attempts to improve treatment by increasing the delivery of toxic agents to areas of tumor include hyperthermia; or a variety of delivery vehicles such as phospholipid vesicles (liposomes), magnetic albumin microspheres, erythrocytes, DNA or nonspecific proteins; and monoclonal antibodies.

## BIOTRANSFORMATION

The metabolism of a given drug may be an important consideration. Some drugs are inactive before administration, requiring biotransformation to achieve an active form. One example of this is cyclophosphamide, which is metabolized in the liver from an inactive to an active form. The importance of biotransformation can be illustrated with a simple example. Patients with malignant pleural effusions are frequently treated by the instillation of drugs into the pleural space, and success usually depends on a direct local drug effect. Consequently, cyclophosphamide, which requires hepatic biotransformation, should not be used for such local therapy.

## EXCRETION

The liver and kidneys are the most common routes of excretion for chemotherapeutic drugs. Their function may be critical to the success of therapy, and great care is often needed in the use of drugs when either of these organs is functioning abnormally. Examples of drugs that require dosage reductions in the face of liver dysfunction include doxorubicin and vincristine. Examples of drugs that require reasonably normal renal function for safe use include high-dose methotrexate, cisplatin, and streptozocin. Table 8–2 lists specific guidelines for dosage adjustments of chemotherapeutic agents according to renal function.[18] More detailed guidelines for adjusting drug doses in the face of liver or renal problems are also given for each drug in Chapter 10.

Excretory organs may also be damaged by cancer treatment, as a direct result of a given drug or as a result of successful therapy. For example, acute leukemia is sensitive to chemotherapy, and successful treatment results in the elaboration of large amounts of uric acid from the breakdown of the nucleic acids of destroyed cancer cells. Uric acid is relatively insoluble in urine, resulting in a loss of renal function called *uric acid nephropathy*.

## DRUG INTERACTIONS

A variety of drug interactions may occur in clinical medicine. Because a hospitalized patient commonly receives nine

*Table 8–2.* Dosage Adjustments for Renal Insufficiency

| Chemotherapeutic Agents | Urinary Excretion (%) | Percent Total Dose Creatinine Clearance (ml/min) | | |
|---|---|---|---|---|
| | | >50 | 10–50 | <10 |
| *Alkylating Agents* | | | | |
| Busulfan | 0 | 100 | 100 | 100 |
| Cisplatin | 45 | 100 | 0 | 0 |
| Chlorambucil | 0 | 100 | 100 | 100 |
| Cyclophosphamide* | 50 | 100 | 75 | 50 |
| Ifosfamide | 60–80 | 100 | 75 | 50 |
| Mechlorethamine | 0 | 100 | 100 | 100 |
| *Antimetabolites* | | | | |
| Azacitidine | 90 | 100 | 50 | 20 |
| Azathioprine*,†,‡ | 0 | 100 | 75 | 50 |
| Cytosine arabinoside | 5–8 | 100 | 100 | 90 |
| 5-Fluorouracil* | 4–11 | 100 | 100 | 100 |
| Hydroxyurea | 80 | 100 | 50 | 20 |
| Methotrexate (low dose) | 25–40 | 100 | 75 | 50 |
| Methotrexate (high dose) | 25–40 | 100 | 0 | 0 |
| 6-Mercaptopurine | 30–50 | 100 | 75 | 50 |
| 6-Thioguanine | 30 | 100 | 50 | 20 |
| *Antibiotics* | | | | |
| Actinomycin D | 10 | 100 | 100 | 80 |
| Bleomycin | 60–70 | 100 | 75 | 50 |
| Daunorubicin | 15 | 100 | 100 | 75 |
| Doxorubicin | 5–10 | 100 | 100 | 80 |
| Mithramycin (low dose) | 25–40 | 100 | 75 | 50 |
| Mithramycin (high dose) | 25–40 | 100 | 0 | 0 |
| Mitomycin C | 15–20 | 100 | 100 | 75 |
| *Plant Derivatives* | | | | |
| Etoposide | 45 | 100 | 75 | 50 |
| Teniposide | 45 | 100 | 75 | 50 |
| Vinblastine | 5–10 | 100 | 100 | 80 |
| Vincristine | 5–10 | 100 | 100 | 80 |
| *Nitrosoureas§* | | | | |
| BCNU | 50–75 | 100 | 75 | 50 |
| CCNU | 50–75 | 100 | 75 | 50 |
| Streptozocin | 50–60 | 100 | 0 | 0 |
| *Miscellaneous Agents* | | | | |
| L-Asparaginase | 0 | 100 | 100 | 100 |
| Dacarbazine | 20–50 | 100 | 75 | 50 |
| Procarbazine | 70–80 | 100 | 50 | 25 |

*Hemodialyzable.

†Metabolites, including 6-mercaptopurine, are primarily excreted in the urine: No parent compound is detectable.

‡75% dose reduction is recommended with the concomitant use of xanthine oxidase inhibitors.

§Nitrosoureas are excreted mainly as urinary metabolites. Little of the parent nitrosourea is excreted in the urine.

Adapted from Raymond JR. Nephrotoxicities of antineoplastic and immunosuppressive agents. Curr Probl Cancer 1984;8:4–5, by permission of the author and Year Book Medical Publishers.

1. Direct chemical or physical interaction
2. Interaction during intestinal absorption
3. Interaction at plasma or blood transport sites
4. Interaction at the cellular receptor site
5. Interaction by accelerated or inhibited metabolism
6. Altered acid-base balance, leading to changes in drug distribution and renal clearance
7. Alterations of renal or liver function that influence rates of excretion
8. Alterations in membrane or intracellular transport mechanisms
9. Alterations in cellular biochemical pathways and drug resistance

Specific examples of drug interactions as they relate to cancer chemotherapy may be cited (see the individual drugs in Chapter 10 for a detailed discussion and references). Nitrogen mustard and many of its derivatives are highly reactive compounds. Direct chemical inactivation in physical mixtures of drugs in infusion solutions is a likely problem. Oral absorption of methotrexate may be altered by concomitant use of antibiotics that suppress gastrointestinal microbial flora. Methotrexate is bound and transported on serum albumin, and aspirin and sulfonamides are known to displace this drug, increasing free drug levels and drug toxicity. Cellular transport of specific drugs may be altered by other drugs. One example of this alteration appears to be inhibition of methotrexate transport across cell membranes by L-asparaginase.

Interactions may occur by accelerated or inhibited metabolism, such as suppression of pseudocholinesterase by some alkylating agents, potentially leading to prolonged apnea if succinylcholine is used during general anesthesia. It is important to emphasize the possibility that allopurinol, a potent xanthine oxidase inhibitor, may profoundly affect the metabolism of 6-MP, a purine analogue. Clinically, this effect may result in markedly augmented toxicity when the two drugs are used in combination, so one should decrease the dose of 6-MP when it is used with allopurinol. This drug interaction occurs because of first-pass metabolism of 6-MP by the liver when the drug is given orally; this drug interaction does not appear to occur with intravenous 6-MP, as discussed in Chapter 10. Cancer chemotherapy may also reduce the plasma levels of important drugs. An important example of this is the reduced plasma level of phenytoin that can occur with a variety of chemotherapeutic drugs and drug combinations, leading to a potential increase in seizure activity.[19] Patients receiving phenytoin and other anticonvulsants should have blood levels of these agents monitored during chemotherapy. Examples of drug interactions involving changes in liver or renal function are discussed in a subsequent section.

Drug interactions that may reduce acquired drug resistance to cancer chemotherapy are of particular interest and an area of active investigation. A number of drugs are currently being studied for possible use in overcoming such drug resistance.[20]

Drug interactions are important because they may antagonize a desired antitumor effect, they may increase drug toxicity, or they may reverse (rescue) normal cells from undesirable toxic reactions. These interactions are discussed

or more drugs at the same time, and because there are many opportunities for the development of clinically important drug interactions in the care of the cancer patient, this subject warrants a brief review. Drug interactions may occur by a variety of mechanisms, some of which are as follows:

subsequently in this chapter under the principles of combination chemotherapy and in Chapter 10.

## Drug Toxicity

The usefulness of cancer chemotherapy is often limited by toxic reactions. One must be thoroughly familiar with the spectrum of toxicity seen with antineoplastic drugs. In the sections that follow, the major classes of drug toxicity are given with selected comments on management. References for toxicity relating to specific drugs appear in Chapter 10. Appendix B provides guidelines for grading acute and subacute toxicity, as recommended by the National Cancer Institute. Some forms of drug toxicity are discussed further in specific chapters in Parts III and IV of this book.

### HEMATOLOGIC TOXICITY

Hematologic toxicity is the most dangerous form of toxicity for many of the antineoplastic drugs used in clinical practice. Its most common form is neutropenia, with an attendant high risk of infection, although thrombocytopenia and bleeding may also occur and can be life-threatening. Chemotherapy can also induce qualitative defects in the function of polymorphonuclear leukocytes and platelets, further aggravating the clinical impact of bone marrow suppression. Because of the critical importance of this problem in cancer chemotherapy, a classification of drugs according to their myelosuppressive potential and the time course of recovery from granulocytopenia is given in Table 8–3. Several schemes for grading the severity of myelosuppression exist. As a point of reference, Table 8–4 gives the system for grading myelosuppression that is used by the National Cancer Institute (see also Appendix B).

Patients who develop grade 4 toxicity from chemotherapy may require hospitalization for observation and, frequently, treatment for infection or bleeding. Courses of chemotherapy are generally postponed until myelosuppression abates. Patients who develop grade 3 or grade 4 toxicity are usually given reduced doses of myelosuppressive agents (25 to 50%) once myelosuppression has resolved, or they may receive subsequent courses of chemotherapy with G-CSF (see Chapter 15). When G-CSF is used with chemotherapy, it is important to confirm that the neutrophil count has exceeded 10,000/$\mu$L while the patient is on the G-CSF and that the neutrophil count 24 or more hours later remains adequate to allow the reinstitution of chemotherapy.

Some drugs cause cumulative myelosuppression, which may rarely lead to prolonged, severe pancytopenia. This situation is particularly true of certain alkylating agents, including the nitrosoureas and mitomycin C. Great care must attend their use, including careful attention to the platelet count. Mitomycin C has also been associated with the activation of clotting factors and microangiopathic hemolytic anemia. This and other rare hematologic complications of cancer and its treatment are reviewed in Chapter 13.

Marrow stem cells do not develop resistance to chemotherapy; rather, if anything, they may suffer irreversible damage with treatment. This situation has led to great inter-

**Table 8–3.** Timing of Drug-Induced Myelosuppression*

| Category† | Drug | Nadir of Granulocytes (Days) | Recovery (Days) |
|---|---|---|---|
| I | Mechlorethamine | 7–15 | 28 |
| | Melphalan | 10–12 | — |
| | Busulfan | 11–30 | 24–54 |
| | Carmustine | 26–30 | 35–49 |
| | Lomustine | 40–50 | 60 |
| | Semustine‡ | 28–63 | 82–89 |
| | Cytarabine | 12–14 | 22–24 |
| | Vinblastine | 5–9 | 14–21 |
| | Etoposide | 10–14 | 16–21 |
| II | Cyclophosphamide | 8–14 | 18–25 |
| | 5-Fluorouracil | 7–14 | 20–30 |
| | 6-Mercaptopurine | 7 | 14–21 |
| | Methotrexate | 7–14 | 14–21 |
| | Actinomycin D | 15 | 22–25 |
| | Procarbazine | 25–36+ | 35–50+ |
| | Doxorubicin | 6–13 | 21–24 |
| | Dacarbazine | 21–28 | 28–35 |
| | Mitomycin C | 28–42 | 42–56 |
| III | Vincristine | 4–5 | 7 |
| | Bleomycin | — | — |
| | L-Asparaginase | — | — |
| | Cisplatin | — | — |
| | Hormones | — | — |

*These are approximate intervals. The precise time course of myelosuppression may vary with the dose, route, and schedule of drug administration as well as with the patient's hematopoietic reserve.

†Categories: I, primarily myelosuppressive toxicity; II, myelosuppressive but other toxicities equally important; III, rarely cause granulocytopenia.

‡Experimental drug.

Modified from Henderson ES. In: Dimitrov NV, Nodine JH, eds. Drugs and hematologic reactions. New York: Grune & Stratton, 1974; and Creaven PJ, Mihich E. Semin Oncol 1977;4:147.

est in the development of experimental programs of autologous bone marrow transplantation or peripheral blood stem cell support, or both, as a way of overcoming the dose-limiting importance of the bone marrow in cancer chemotherapy, as discussed in Chapter 16.

### GASTROINTESTINAL TOXICITY

**Nausea and Vomiting.** Anorexia, nausea, and vomiting are among the most common and distressing acute reactions to a wide variety of cancer chemotherapeutic agents. From

**Table 8–4.** Grades of Myelosuppression*

| Toxicity Grade | Cell Count (1000 Cells/$\mu$L) | | |
| | WHITE BLOOD CELLS | GRANULOCYTES† | PLATELETS |
|---|---|---|---|
| 0 | 4.0 | 2.0 | 100 |
| 1 | 3.0–3.9 | 1.5–1.9 | 75–99 |
| 2 | 2.0–2.9 | 1.0–1.4 | 50–74 |
| 3 | 1.0–1.9 | 0.5–0.9 | 25–49 |
| 4 | <1.0 | <0.5 | <25 |

*As recommended for international use by Miller AB, Hoogstraaten B, Staquet M, Winkler A. Reporting results of cancer treatment. Cancer 1981;47:207.

†Granulocytes include segmented and juvenile neutrophils.

the point of view of most patients, nausea and vomiting are the most important side effects of cancer chemotherapy. The physical consequences of this problem may include tearing of the esophagus (Mallory-Weiss syndrome), weight loss, generalized malaise, dehydration, and electrolyte imbalances. The psychological consequences of vomiting include the development of anticipatory nausea (35% of cases) or anticipatory vomiting (16%); either of these may influence the patient to reject subsequent chemotherapy.

The frequency of emesis from chemotherapy varies markedly from agent to agent. Table 8–5 provides a classification of the emetogenic potential of chemotherapeutic agents. The subchapter on nausea and vomiting in Chapter 19 provides an expanded discussion of the pathophysiology and treatment of this important complication.

**Mucositis.** Stomatitis, odynophagia (painful swallowing), esophagitis, and peptic ulcer disease may complicate the use of cancer chemotherapy. These conditions are usually self-limited, but they may cause considerable discomfort. It is important to consider possible causes other than chemotherapy in these patients because this may influence therapy. Specifically, one should rule out possible infection (such as with *Candida*, herpesvirus, or *Clostridium difficile*), local infiltration of tissues by tumor, or damage from acid reflux or other physical factors. Whenever possible, good oral hygiene should be maintained to prevent this complication. In some cases, mucositis can be at least partially prevented by the use of ice chips in the mouth for 30 minutes during chemotherapy.[21] These problems are discussed further in Chapter 19 in the subchapter Stomatitis.

**Diarrhea.** Diarrhea is usually self-limited and mild; however, in some patients, it may be severe. For patients receiving 5-FU or FUDR, there may be profound diarrhea, especially when the antimetabolite is given in combination with leucovorin. When diarrhea is severe, patients require hospitalization and intravenous fluids. Octreotide acetate should also be used if possible because it markedly shortens the duration of severe symptoms and hospitalization.[22] As with mucositis, one should rule out possible infection (such as with *Candida*, herpesvirus, or *C. difficile*) as a contributing

factor to diarrhea in cancer patients. This important complication is discussed further in Chapter 19 under Diarrhea.

**Constipation.** Autonomic neuropathy from the vinca alkaloids can cause severe constipation and even rare instances of bowel obstruction. Preventive therapy with stool softeners and laxatives should be used when patients are treated with these agents. This complication is discussed further in Chapter 19 under Constipation.

## IMMUNOSUPPRESSION

Most of the commonly used antineoplastic agents are capable of suppressing cellular and humoral immunity.[23] Immunosuppression varies tremendously, however, depending on the precise dose and schedule of drug administration and whether the drug is used alone or as part of a multidrug combination. In view of evidence implicating host immunologic factors in the control of certain tumors (see Chapter 9), the potential effect of cancer chemotherapeutic drugs on the immune system becomes increasingly important. The clinical importance of immunosuppression is complex and unclear. Immunosuppression is generally considered an undesirable side effect of cancer chemotherapy because it predisposes patients to various infectious complications, as discussed in Chapter 20. The impact of immunosuppression on the natural history of cancer is unpredictable, however; it may be a necessary part of the antineoplastic efficacy of some drugs.[24]

The normal immune response involves an extremely complex interaction between cellular and humoral factors. A simplified version of the immune system as it relates to cancer is shown in Figure 8–7, which distinguishes between events involving humoral immunity and those involving cellular immunity. Figure 8–7 does not distinguish between the primary and the secondary responses to an antigen, and it does not attempt to portray the multitude of humoral factors that participate in intercellular communication. The initial stages of antigen recognition and processing involve macrophages, thymus-dependent lymphocytes (T cells), or bursa- or bone marrow–dependent lymphocytes (B cells). Interactions between these cell lines are also possible, and subsequent amplification mechanisms follow. Amplification of the immune system may arise by clonal expansion, in which lymphocyte blastogenesis occurs with a proliferation of selected cell populations. Recruitment and activation of other cell lines may also ensue through the elaboration of various cytokines. The final stage of immune effect involves a complex interaction of one or more of these elements. Table 8–6 gives selected examples of how various cancer chemotherapeutic agents interact with the stages of the immune response shown in Figure 8–7.

The acute immunosuppressive effects of most drugs used in cancer chemotherapy do not extend for prolonged periods beyond the time of active drug administration. Hersh[25] has studied this problem in patients receiving 5-day courses of intensive combination chemotherapy. The immunologic factor studies included macrophage entry into experimental inflammatory sites (the skin window), response to primary antigenic stimulation, and lymphocyte blastogenic response to phytohemagglutinin (Fig. 8–8). There is a marked decrease in all these host defenses during treatment; however,

*Table 8–5.* **Emetogenic Potential of Cancer Chemotherapy**

| Emetogenic Potential | Agent |
| --- | --- |
| High | Cisplatin |
| | Mechlorethamine |
| | Streptozocin |
| | Dacarbazine |
| | Carmustine |
| | Dactinomycin |
| Moderate | Cyclophosphamide |
| | Doxorubicin |
| | Carboplatin |
| | Mitomycin |
| | L-Asparaginase |
| Low | Fluorouracil |
| | Methotrexate |
| | Etoposide |
| | Vincristine |
| | Bleomycin |

Adapted from Strum SB, McDermed JE, Pileggi J, et al. Intravenous metoclopramide: prevention of chemotherapy-induced nausea and vomiting: a preliminary evaluation. CANCER, Vol. 53, 1984, 1432. Copyright © 1984 American Cancer Society. Adapted by permission of Wiley-Liss, Inc., a subsidiary of John Wiley & Sons, Inc.

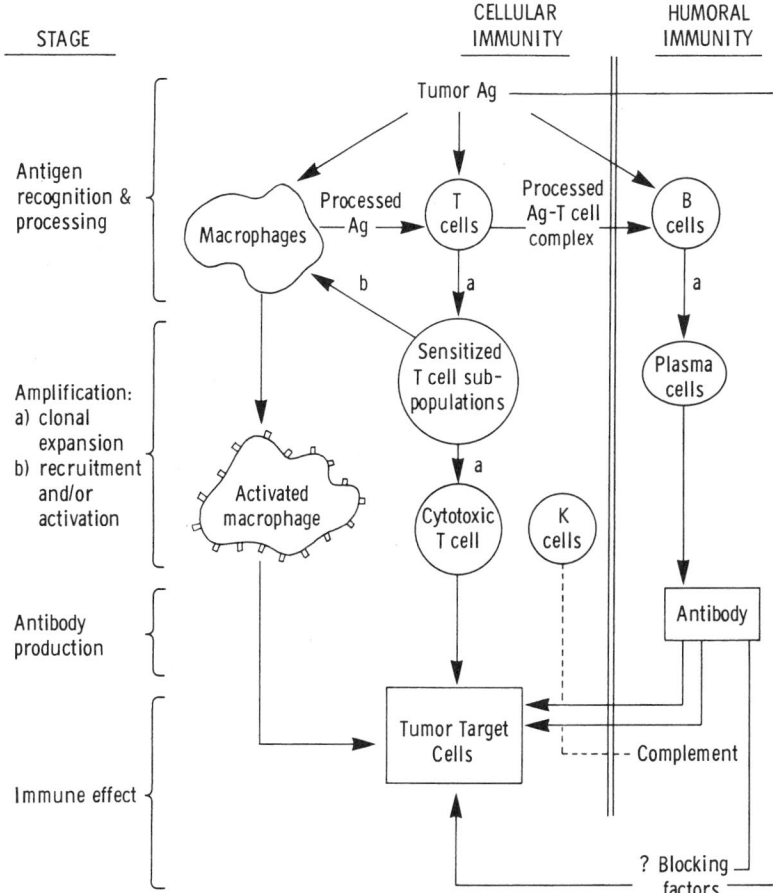

**Figure 8–7.** Diagrammatic representation of the immune response to a tumor antigen (Ag). The successive stages of the immune response are depicted on the left side of the diagram. T cell, thymus-dependent lymphocyte; B cell, bursa- or bone marrow–derived lymphocyte; K cell, natural killer cells bearing neither T-cell nor B-cell markers. (Reproduced, with permission, from the Annual Review of Pharmacology and Toxicology, Vol 17, copyright 1977 by Annual Reviews Inc., from Haskell CM. Annu Rev Pharmacol Toxicol 1977;17:179.)

within 2 or 3 days, there is complete or nearly complete recovery of immune function. In some patients, an *immunologic overshoot* may occur during the recovery period. When such 5-day courses of combination chemotherapy are given every 2 to 4 weeks, the patient's immunologic function is normal most of the time.

Cancer chemotherapy may also result in chronic, delayed immunosuppression.[26] The importance of this finding is uncertain; nevertheless, it deserves consideration in assessing the long-term risks of chemotherapy.

Immunologic theories of cancer cause and pathogenesis are in ferment, and time and research are needed to resolve many conflicts. In terms of cancer chemotherapy, the practical result of almost all contemporary thought on the immune system is that clinicians should strive for programs of cancer treatment that are minimally immunosuppressive whenever possible. Even if one believes that the immune system does not play an important role in the pathogenesis of cancer, it is clearly an important host defense mechanism for many of the complications that occur during treatment. Specifically, infections commonly lead to the death of patients with advanced cancer, and impaired immunity may contribute to such deaths.

## DERMATOLOGIC REACTIONS

The most important skin reactions seen with chemotherapy include local necrosis from drug extravasation, alopecia,

*Table 8–6.* **Stages of the Immune Response Inhibited by Drugs and Irradiation**

| Antigen Recognition, Processing, or Both | Amplification | Antibody Production | Immune Effect |
|---|---|---|---|
| Cyclophosphamide | Cyclophosphamide | Cyclophosphamide | Corticosteroids |
| Irradiation | Actinomycin D | | Antilymphocyte serum |
| Actinomycin D | 5-Fluorouracil | | |
| Corticosteroids | 6-Mercaptopurine | | |
| Antilymphocyte serum | Cytarabine | | |
| | L-Asparaginase | | |
| | Vinca alkaloids | | |

Reprinted, with permission, from the Annual Review of Pharmacology and Toxicology. Vol. 17, copyright 1977 by Annual Reviews Inc., from Haskell CM. Immunologic aspects of cancer chemotherapy. Annu Rev Pharmacol Toxicol 1977;17:179.

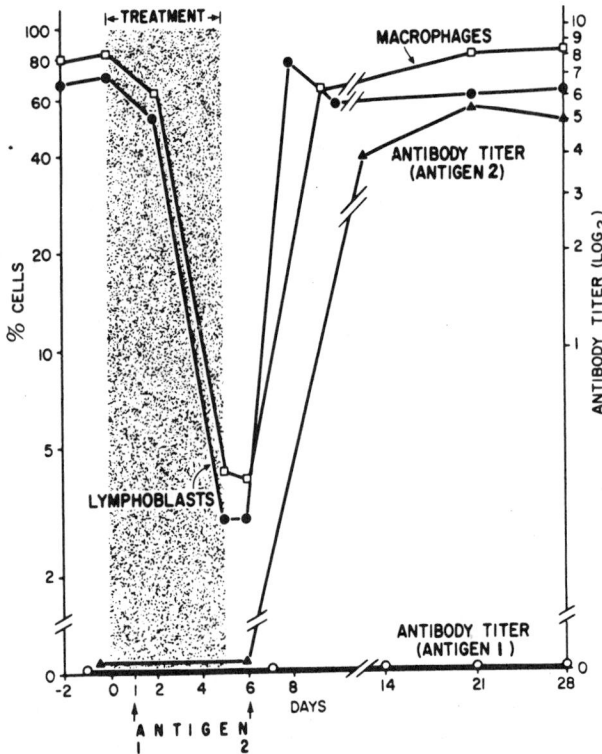

**Figure 8–8.** Effects of intensive intermittent chemotherapy on host defense mechanisms. (From Hersh EM. Modification of host defense mechanisms. In: Holland JF, Frei E III, eds. Cancer medicine. Philadelphia: Lea & Febiger, 1973:681.)

and allergic or hypersensitivity reactions.[27] Less serious skin reactions include changes in skin pigmentation, photosensitivity reactions, nail problems (transverse banding or, rarely, nail loss), folliculitis (with dactinomycin), and radiation recall reactions. Experimental data show an inhibitory effect of chemotherapy on wound healing, although this has rarely been reported as a clinical problem. Nevertheless, it is probably prudent to postpone intensive chemotherapy after major operations at least until the early phases of wound repair have been completed (i.e., at 7 to 10 days).[28, 29]

**Drug Extravasation.** Skin necrosis may result from the extravasation of certain vesicant drugs during intravenous therapy. Agents associated with modest to severe soft tissue injury on extravasation are listed in Table 8–7. The severity of reaction is a function of the drug doses extravasated, and it varies from local erythema to extensive tissue necrosis. Rarely, extravasation may occur at a site of recent venipuncture, far from the site of drug injection.[30] Even with meticulous attention to the details of drug administration, the incidence of serious extravasation is about 1 in 1000 venipunctures.

The management of drug extravasation is controversial, although all authorities advise informing the patient carefully about this problem in advance of treatment and promptly discontinuing the intravenous injection if the patient experiences any pain. If extravasation is suspected, the intravenous needle should be removed immediately without the local injection of any drug or diluent. If the vesicant is an antitumor antibiotic, the patient should be advised to apply ice packs to tolerance and elevate the extremity for 24 hours.

If the patient received an anthracycline antibiotic, such as doxorubicin or daunorubicin, the area should be examined by fluorescence microscopy.[31] If the area of suspected extravasation shows no evidence of fluorescence, necrosis is highly unlikely. If fluorescence is found, the entire area should be resected, with placement of a skin graft for larger defects. If the vesicant is a vinca alkaloid, the manufacturer advises the use of warm compresses rather than ice packs.

**Alopecia.** Alopecia is the most common cutaneous side effect of chemotherapy, and it may have severe emotional impact on some patients. It is extremely common in patients treated with doxorubicin or cyclophosphamide, but with high dosage it is also likely after mechlorethamine, paclitaxel, methotrexate (except when followed by leucovorin rescue), 5-FU, vincristine, bleomycin, and hydroxyurea. A number of other drugs may exacerbate alopecia, especially when these drugs are used in various combinations.

Alopecia is almost always reversible, but there may be a delay of several weeks after treatment before regrowth begins. It is possible to prevent or minimize alopecia in many patients through the use of an ice turban—crushed ice in plastic bags applied to the scalp for 10 minutes before and for 30 minutes after drug administration.[32] This technique is variably effective as a function of the drug or drugs being used and their single dose, total dose, route, and schedule of administration. It is not for use in patients with leukemia, lymphoma, or mycosis fungoides or when tumor cells may be present in the scalp.[33] It should also be used with caution in patients with vasculitis, prior cranial irradiation, or cryoglobulinemia.

**Photosensitivity.** Photosensitivity generally takes the form of phototoxicity or chemical injury to the skin, resulting in a sunburn reaction with erythema, edema, blisters, hyperpigmentation, and desquamation or peeling. Rarely, photoallergy, resembling contact dermatitis with immediate wheal-and-flare reactions or delayed reactions, may occur. Dacarbazine is the only agent that is a common cause of

*Table 8–7.* **Cancer Chemotherapeutic Agents Associated with Moderate-to-Severe Soft Tissue Injury from Extravasation**

| Commercially Available Drugs | Investigational Agents |
| --- | --- |
| Dactinomycin | Aclarubicin |
| Daunorubicin (Cerubidine) | Amonafide (Nafidimide) |
| Doxorubicin (Adriamycin) | Adozelesin |
| Idarubicin (Idamycin) | Carubicin (carminomycin) |
| Mechlorethamine | Chromomycin A3 |
| Melphalan | Detorubicin |
| Mitomycin | Didemnin B |
| Paclitaxel (Taxol) | Doxorubicin–DNA complex |
| Streptozocin | Elsamicin |
| Vinblastine | Epirubicin |
| Vincristine | FK-973 |
| | Galactitol |
| | Maytansine |
| | Menogaril |
| | Mitoguazone (methyl-GAG) |
| | Pirarubicin (THP-Adriamycin) |
| | Vindesine (DAVA) |
| | Zorubicin (Rubidazone) |

Adapted from Ajani JA, Dodd LG, Daugherty K, et al. Taxol-induced soft-tissue injury secondary to extravasation: characterization by histopathology and clinical course. J Natl Cancer Inst 1994;86:51.

photosensitivity, whereas less common offenders include 5-FU, methotrexate, procarbazine, and vinblastine.

## VASCULAR AND HYPERSENSITIVITY REACTIONS

The most serious form of hypersensitivity seen with chemotherapy is anaphylaxis.[34] Anaphylaxis is most commonly seen with L-asparaginase, but it may rarely occur with a wide variety of other antineoplastic agents, such as cyclophosphamide, doxorubicin, cisplatin, intravenous melphalan, and high-dose methotrexate.[35] Lesser degrees of hypersensitivity have been reported with procarbazine and etoposide (VP-16) and with topical mechlorethamine. Paclitaxel also commonly causes a vascular hypersensitivity reaction (see discussion of paclitaxel in Chapter 10). Docetaxel can cause severe anasarca, which is presumed to occur on the basis of hypersensitivity.

Bleomycin can cause a unique hyperpyrexic reaction, with clinical findings similar to anaphylaxis, as well as Raynaud's phenomenon and a scleroderma-like reaction. These problems appear to be even greater when bleomycin is used in combination with other drugs. For example, severe, life-threatening vascular disease may result from the use of vinblastine, bleomycin, and cisplatin chemotherapy in patients with germ cell tumors.[36]

Acral erythema with vasculitis, probably resulting from immune complex deposition, has been reported with induction chemotherapy followed by granulocyte transfusions. Cytarabine may rarely cause a distinctive syndrome of fever, conjunctival suffusion, and maculopapular rash that can be prevented by corticosteroids.[37]

Vascular and hypersensitivity reactions are rare, but, depending on the mechanism and severity of the reaction, they may require cessation of treatment and the use of adjunctive measures. This problem has been reviewed elsewhere.[38, 39] The larger problem of drug fever from all causes has also been reviewed.[40]

## HEPATIC TOXICITY

Hepatic toxicity is an uncommon problem in cancer chemotherapy, but when it occurs, it may be serious. The range of toxicity includes transient elevations of transaminase enzymes with cytarabine and the nitrosoureas (including streptozocin), fibrosis and cirrhosis with methotrexate, cholestasis and possible hepatic necrosis with 6-MP or mithramycin, fatty metamorphosis with L-asparaginase, and cholecystitis or cholangitis, or both, from the infusion of 5-FU or FUDR into the hepatic artery. Fatal hepatic necrosis has been reported as a consequence of high-dose chemotherapy following haloalkane anesthesia, especially with the use of high-dose methotrexate.

Hepatic veno-occlusive disease, which presents with hepatomegaly and ascites similar clinically to that of the Budd-Chiari syndrome, can result from chemotherapy. This disease is a rare complication of treatment with conventional doses of dacarbazine, 6-MP, 6-thioguanine, azathioprine, cytarabene, and radiation, but it is not rare in patients receiving high-dose treatment (usually with bone marrow transplantation) with cyclophosphamide, carmustine, lomustine, busul-

fan, and mitomycin C.[41] The importance of this complication is emphasized by data from the Johns Hopkins Oncology Center.[42] In 235 patients undergoing bone marrow transplantation, 22% developed veno-occlusive disease, which was fatal in 47%. Overall, veno-occlusive disease was the third most common cause of death in the entire series of patients. Similar results have been reported from Seattle, where 54% of transplanted patients developed veno-occlusive disease, which was frequently complicated by renal and cardiopulmonary failure as well.[43] Guidelines for the management of hepatic toxicity vary with each drug, as discussed in Chapter 10.

## PANCREATIC TOXICITY

Acute pancreatitis is a rare complication of cancer chemotherapy, but it has been described with L-asparaginase, corticosteroids, and cytarabine and rarely in patients receiving combination chemotherapy. It has also been described as part of the tumor lysis syndrome in patients with lymphoma.

## PULMONARY TOXICITY

A variety of drugs may cause profound pulmonary disturbances, especially in patients who have received prior pulmonary irradiation. Methotrexate, cytarabine, mitomycin C, procarbazine, and most alkylating agents can cause pulmonary dysfunction in occasional patients. The most common form of pulmonary toxicity, however, is pulmonary fibrosis from the use of a nitrosourea or bleomycin. In rare cases, the severity of fibrosis is sufficiently severe to justify single-lung transplantation.[44]

Bleomycin is the most important cause of pulmonary toxicity because it is a common constituent of curative regimens of chemotherapy. Although the fibrosis caused by bleomycin is somewhat dose related, occurring most frequently at doses greater than 400 units, the range of doses associated with this complication is wide. The incidence also appears increased after bleomycin is used in combination with other drugs and when it is given to patients with reduced renal function. For more information on the pulmonary complications of chemotherapy, see the discussion of specific drugs in Chapter 10.

## CARDIAC TOXICITY

Doxorubicin, daunorubicin, and high doses of cyclophosphamide may all cause cardiac damage. This damage represents the major dose-limiting toxicity of doxorubicin and daunorubicin, as discussed in Chapter 10. 5-FU has also been reported to cause cardiac problems, but only on a sporadic basis. These problems include angina, left ventricular dysfunction, and a variety of other less typical cardiac abnormalities.[45]

## GENITOURINARY TOXICITY

Hemorrhagic cystitis occurs in about 10% of patients treated with cyclophosphamide, but it rarely occurs with other agents except for ifosfamide. The free radical scavenger mesna given with cyclophosphamide or ifosfamide can reduce, if not eliminate, this complication for both agents. The kidney can be damaged by a variety of drugs but most prominently by high doses of methotrexate or 6-MP and by standard doses of mithramycin, streptozocin, mitomycin C, L-asparaginase, and cisplatin. Uric acid nephropathy may also be a problem for some patients, although this can generally be prevented by the use of allopurinol and hydration. Drug-induced renal dysfunction may alter the pharmacokinetics of other drugs, leading to increased toxicity. For example, cisplatin may change the renal clearance of bleomycin, with a marked change in bleomycin toxicity. The problem of dose adjustment for cancer chemotherapy in the face of renal dysfunction is addressed in Table 8–2. Other aspects of genitourinary toxicity from chemotherapy are reviewed by Rieselbach.[46]

## NEUROTOXICITY

Many, if not most, patients with cancer develop neurologic problems from either the cancer or its treatment at some point in the natural history of their disease. Differential diagnosis may be the key to effective management, so a thorough understanding of the neurologic consequences of cancer chemotherapy is important. The major forms of neurologic toxicity are the following[47]: (1) arachnoiditis, myelopathy, or encephalomyelopathy from the use of intrathecal drugs (methotrexate, cytarabine, or thiotepa); (2) chronic encephalopathies and the somnolence syndrome (from cranial irradiation and methotrexate or cytarabine, usually given by the intrathecal route); (3) acute encephalopathies (as with 1 and 2, plus L-asparaginase, high-dose methotrexate, 5-FU, procarbazine, hexamethylmelamine, azacitidine, high-dose cytarabine, and other experimental agents, or intracarotid drug use); (4) peripheral neuropathies (from vinca alkaloids, taxanes, cisplatin, altretamine, procarbazine, cytarabine, azacitidine, or etoposide (VP-16); (5) acute cerebellar syndromes or ataxia (with 5-FU, procarbazine, altretamine); and (6) miscellaneous forms of neurotoxicity.

The miscellaneous forms of neurotoxicity are extremely varied. Examples include cranial nerve paresis (from vinca alkaloids, cisplatin, or 5-FU), ototoxicity (from cisplatin), autonomic dysfunction (from vinca alkaloids and procarbazine), and the syndrome of inappropriate antidiuretic hormone (from vinca alkaloids, cyclophosphamide, and cisplatin). There may be subtle changes in cognition seen with a variety of antineoplastic agents, as reviewed by Silberfarb.[48] Many patients may experience clinic-associated odors and tastes when away from the clinic. These experiences have been called *pseudohallucinations*, and they are closely associated with pretreatment nausea and extensive chemotherapy. There may also be true alterations of taste and smell with chemotherapy, especially with doxorubicin, carmustine, and vincristine. Epileptic seizures have been induced by a variety of drugs, including cisplatin and chlorambucil. Neurotoxicity is discussed further in Chapter 10 in the context of the individual drugs.

## OCULAR TOXICITY

Vision may be affected by drugs. Most notably, high-dose cyclophosphamide has been reported to cause transient blurred vision in children, several alkylating agents may cause cataracts, tamoxifen may damage the retina, and cisplatin can cause optic nerve damage. Conjunctivitis is a common, rapidly reversible problem with multiple agents.

## SEXUALITY AND GONADAL FUNCTION

A variety of drugs, but most prominently the alkylating agents and procarbazine, can cause azoospermia and amenorrhea.[49] Post-therapy gynecomastia and impotence may also result from Leydig cell dysfunction. Variable degrees of gonadal and sexual dysfunction may result from cancer itself, as seen most prominently in male patients with Hodgkin's disease or testicular tumors. Sperm storage before the initiation of chemotherapy may be of social and psychological value, but it is not unusual to find that sperm storage is unrealistic before treatment because of poor testicular function. Oocyte and embryo cryopreservation (for future in vitro fertilization) can also be offered to women. The reversibility of gonadal dysfunction varies with the age of the patient and the type of chemotherapy. For most adults, the return of fertility is highly variable. Children appear to be more tolerant of chemotherapy. In a large retrospective study of 2283 long-term survivors of childhood or adolescent cancer, the relative fertility was 85% of normal.[50] Endocrine studies and psychological counseling about sexual function may be helpful in the management of patients scheduled to receive chemotherapy, as reviewed by Chapman.[51] Patients should be counseled against conceiving children during active chemotherapy because congenital malformations may result, especially when cytarabine, methotrexate, or an alkylating agent is given during the first trimester of pregnancy.[52, 53] The available data suggest, however, that most patients who receive chemotherapy during the second or third trimester have normal offspring.[54, 55] Chapter 27 and an excellent review[56] provide further discussion of the topic of cancer and cancer treatment during pregnancy.

## SECOND MALIGNANCIES

Many of the commonly employed antineoplastic drugs are mutagenic as well as teratogenic. Some, including procarbazine and the alkylating agents, are clearly carcinogenic.[57–59] This carcinogenic potential is primarily seen as delayed acute leukemia in patients treated with polyfunctional alkylating agents and inhibitors of topoisomerase II, such as etoposide and the anthracycline antibiotics. The pattern of leukemogenesis with these two groups of drugs differs as follows: (1) Polyfunctional alkylating agents tend to cause myelodysplasia with a latency of 4 to 5 years that evolves into acute myelogenous leukemia associated with deletions of chromosomes 5 and 7; (2) topoisomerase II inhibitors tend to cause acute myelogenous leukemia with a latency of less than 3 years associated with 11q23 translocations and the M4/M5 FAB subtypes. Both types of leukemogenesis appear to be increased in patients receiving dose-intensive therapy, as opposed to standard-dose treatment, and the highest risk appears to occur in patients receiving high doses of both an alkylating agent and a topoisomerase II inhibitor. Chemotherapy has also been associated with cases of delayed non-Hodgkin's lymphoma and solid tumors, especially after the use of the MOPP (mechlorethamine, vincristine [Oncovin], procarbazine, prednisone) regimen for advanced Hodgkin's disease. Delayed carcinogenesis is becoming one of the most important concerns in evaluating the curative potential and therapeutic index of combination chemotherapy. Because of the importance of this problem, the available evidence on the carcinogenic potential of chemotherapy, as reviewed by the International Agency for Research on Cancer, is summarized in Table 8–8.

The carcinogenic potential of many chemotherapeutic agents poses safety problems for health care professionals as well as patients. In the past, these drugs were commonly prepared by physicians or nurses without special precautions. This approach is no longer acceptable, largely because of evidence that unprotected individuals preparing such drugs appear to have higher than normal levels of mutagens in their urine,[60, 61] and those who become pregnant appear to have a higher rate of fetal loss.[62] Now it is accepted practice for cancer chemotherapeutic agents to be prepared solely by

*Table 8–8.* Anticancer Drugs Causing Cancer

| Category | Drug |
| --- | --- |
| Human carcinogen (group 1) | Azathioprine |
| | Busulfan |
| | Certain combination chemotherapy regimens (including MOPP)* |
| | Chlorambucil |
| | Conjugated estrogens† |
| | Cyclophosphamide |
| | Diethylstilbestrol |
| | Melphalan |
| Probable human carcinogen (group 2A) | Combined oral contraceptives† |
| | Nitrogen mustard |
| | Oxymetholone |
| | Procarbazine |
| Probable human carcinogen (group 2B) | Actinomycin D |
| | Doxorubicin (Adriamycin) |
| | Carmustine (BCNU)‡ |
| | Lomustine (CCNU)‡ |
| | Cisplatin |
| | Dacarbazine |
| | Ethinyl estradiol |
| | Norethisterone |
| | Estradiol-17 |
| | Estrone |
| | Progesterone |
| | Sequential oral contraceptives† |
| | Thiotepa |
| Unclassifiable (not a carcinogen or data inadequate) | Bleomycin |
| | 5-Fluorouracil |
| | 6-Mercaptopurine |
| | Methotrexate |
| | Megestrol acetate |
| | Prednisone |
| | Vinblastine |
| | Vincristine |

*Mechlorethamine, vincristine (Oncovin), procarbazine, prednisone (MOPP); other combinations associated with delayed leukemia include the combinations of cisplatin, vinblastine, plus bleomycin (Cancer 1986;57:984) and cisplatin plus etoposide (Blood 1987;70:1414).

†The compounds responsible for carcinogenesis have not been identified.

‡A related investigational nitrosourea, methyl-CCNU (semustine), clearly causes leukemia (N Engl J Med 1983;309:1079).

From the International Agency for Research on Cancer of the World Health Organization. IARC monographs on the evaluation of the carcinogenic risk of chemicals to humans. Suppl. 4 to Vols. 1–29, Lyon, France, 1982.

trained people (usually pharmacists) inside a biohazard safety hood while wearing protective clothing and disposable gloves made from either latex or polyvinyl chloride. The subsequent administration of the drug to the patient is performed with care taken not to cause aerosols or gross spills, and the empty syringe and tubing are disposed of as toxic waste. Special spill kits should be readily available in case of accidental contamination of the environment around the patient. Further details of this important subject have been published.[63, 64]

## MISCELLANEOUS COMPLICATIONS

A wide variety of other complications may occur.[65] About 5% of patients treated with cyclophosphamide, methotrexate, and 5-FU adjuvant chemotherapy for breast cancer experience myalgias and arthralgias after the completion of treatment.[66] This syndrome of postchemotherapy rheumatism appears to be a benign and self-limited process, which can rarely occur after chemotherapy directed against other neoplasms as well.[67] Electrolyte problems, abnormal glucose metabolism, pituitary insufficiency, hypercholesterolemia, adrenal insufficiency, fever, aseptic necrosis of the femoral heads, pathologic fractures, hemolytic anemia, nasal cartilage necrosis, and suppression of growth are other examples of rare complications seen with some drugs, as detailed in Chapter 10. The prudent physician should be aware of the known complications of cancer chemotherapy and be alert to the possible emergence of new and currently unknown side effects.

## DELAYED TOXICITY

As more cancer patients are cured with chemotherapy, delayed complications will become more apparent and important. It has been estimated that 40% of the more than 7800 children cured of cancer each year will develop a late adverse effect of combined-modality therapy.[68] The most serious delayed effect in most studies is the development of second neoplasms, but delayed cardiac problems, learning disabilities, and fertility disorders are also common. Examples of studies of the long-term effects of chemotherapy include reports on testicular cancer, paratesticular rhabdomyosarcomas in children, and acute lymphoblastic leukemia. The Late Effects Study Group is a consortium of 12 pediatric oncology centers in North America and Western Europe that is systematically studying this problem in children. It is hoped that more detailed studies of this problem will permit better guidelines for prevention, early diagnosis, and treatment.

## Biologic Factors

The cancer cell is a variable and fluctuating target, and its sensitivity to various drugs differs from one form of cancer to another. Several aspects of this biologic variability warrant specific comment, including the role of the cell cycle of individual cells in drug sensitivity, the importance of tumor cell population growth kinetics, the kinetics of tumor cell killing by drugs (the *log cell kill hypothesis*), and tumor cell drug resistance.

## CELL CYCLE

The life cycle of normal and neoplastic cells starts with mitosis, or cell division (Fig. 8–9), as discussed in detail in Chapter 2. After the cell has completed its division, it enters the $G_1$ phase, or the first gap phase, which for a long time was considered a quiescent phase by cell biologists. When cells stop proliferating and come to rest, they usually do so in the $G_1$ phase. Occasionally, cells rest for prolonged periods; this phenomenon is usually referred to as $G_0$; alternatively the cell can be described as dormant. On emerging from $G_1$, the cell begins a phase of active DNA synthesis, which has been termed the *S phase*. In this phase, the cellular content of DNA is doubled. Once the S phase begins, several things happen in rapid succession. The enzymes necessary for DNA synthesis, including those involved in purine and pyrimidine biosynthesis, and the enzymes necessary for the formation of macromolecular nucleic acids increase in specific activity. After the DNA content of the cell has doubled, the phase of DNA synthesis is complete, and the cell enters the $G_2$ phase. This phase was also once thought to be a quiescent period, but it is now clear that RNA synthesis and protein synthesis are required before the cell can construct a mitotic apparatus and begin division.

The cellular and molecular events that control and regulate the cell cycle are the subject of intense research, particularly the signaling events that control the process, as discussed in Chapter 2. Abnormalities in cell signaling, as influenced by a variety of oncogenes, appear to be involved in carcinogenesis as well as having implications for the efficacy of cancer chemotherapy. It is likely that the methods of molecular biology will clarify the relationship among cell cycle–regulated genes, oncogenes, growth factors, receptors for growth factors, and cell-signaling chemicals.

These considerations appear to be critical to the action of some chemotherapeutic agents. Agents that are effective only during a particular phase of the cell cycle, such as the S phase of cellular DNA synthesis, are called *phase-specific*. Agents whose action is prolonged and independent of any specific cell cycle phase are called *phase-nonspecific*. This distinction between specific and nonspecific agents is relative rather than absolute. Some experts in cell kinetics make additional distinctions, separating the phase-nonspecific drugs into those that demonstrate increased killing of proliferating tissues as opposed to nonproliferating tissue (cycle-specific drugs) versus those that show no such specificity (cycle-nonspecific drugs).[69, 70] Another distinction that is sometimes made is that of *self-limited cell killing*.[71] Drugs of this type (e.g., methotrexate), which kill cells in DNA synthesis, simultaneously inhibit other cells from starting DNA synthesis and prevent these cells from entering the sensitive phase of the cycle.

The concept of differential drug efficacy during specific phases of the life cycle of proliferating malignant cells has important theoretical and practical implications for cancer therapy.[72] Agents that are most effective during the S phase may be ineffective inhibitors of cell populations with a slow turnover and high percentage of dormant cells. S phase–specific drugs also require frequent administration or administration by continuous infusion so that the drug is present when tumor cells enter this critical time in their life cycle. Conversely, alkylating agents and other drugs that interact primarily with macromolecular DNA (e.g., doxorubicin) seem to be largely independent of the cell replication cycle and are effective against tumors with relatively low proliferative activity. Such non–phase-specific drugs may generally be given on a variety of schedules of drug administration.

## GROWTH OF CELL POPULATIONS

Although all cells pass through the same sequence of phases, differences exist between populations of normal cells and populations of cancer cells in their number and distribution in the replication cycle. Normal and neoplastic cells may be influenced by growth factors, and populations of both appear to contain more dividing cells when the population size is small and fewer dividing cells when it is large: The young fetus grows rapidly, and the postnatal child grows more slowly. This relationship between size and growth rate may be expressed quantitatively in two ways:

1. As a function of population doubling times (time for any given number of cells to double in number)
2. As a function of the growth fraction (the fraction of cells undergoing division at any one time)

Figure 8–10 presents a logarithmic plot of human fetal and childhood growth versus time[73] and includes specific data on the cell population doubling times during growth. Early growth is clearly exponential, with a high growth fraction and short doubling times. As time passes, the doubling time increases, and the growth fraction decreases. This change probably relates to population pressures that reduce the growth rate; this may also relate to the development of dormant populations of cells. The specific equation describing a decreased growth rate over time was originally derived by the 19th century mathematician Gompertz, and biologic growth that conforms to this pattern is referred to as *gom-*

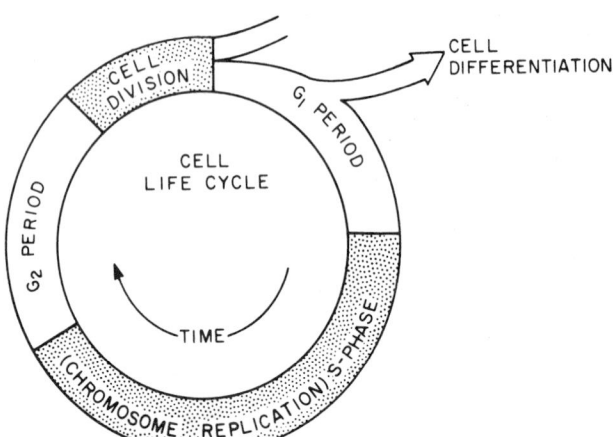

**Figure 8–9.** The cell cycle: D, cell division; $G_1$, the phase preceding active DNA synthesis; S, the phase of DNA synthesis; $G_2$, the premitotic resting phase.

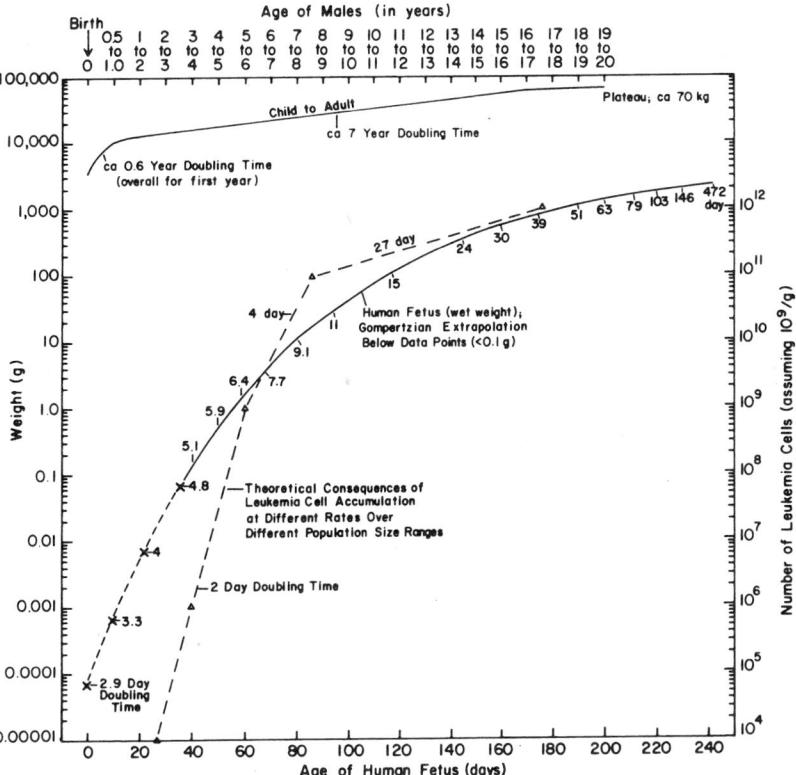

**Figure 8–10.** Human fetal and childhood growth as a gompertzian process and the theoretical consequences of accumulation of leukemic cells at different rates over varying population ranges. (From Skipper HE, Perry S. Kinetics of normal and leukemic leukocyte populations and relevance to chemotherapy. Cancer Res 1970;30:1883.)

*pertzian* growth. The growth rates of normal and neoplastic tissues may be complex. Either may demonstrate exponential growth or gompertzian growth for short periods,[74] and both may at times demonstrate dormancy.

## LOG CELL KILL HYPOTHESIS

At any given exposure, antineoplastic drugs kill a variable fraction of cells, from a few to a maximum of about 99.99%. Because of the consistency of this fractional cell killing in experimental animal tumor systems, it has been proposed that tumor cell killing is fractional in humans as well. This concept has been termed the *log cell kill hypothesis*, in part because the kinetics of killing approximate a first-order geometric process. As a result of this hypothesis, the fractional cell kill observed in experimental studies with chemotherapy is often expressed in logarithmic terms. Because the body burden of tumor cells in humans with advanced malignancies may be greater than $10^{12}$ cells (1 kg), and because the best one can hope for with a single maximal exposure of tumor cells to a drug appears to be somewhere between 2 and 5 logs of cell kill, treatment must be repeated many times to achieve control (see Fig. 1–5).

Theoretically, this hypothesis suggests that chemotherapeutic drugs may not be capable of eradicating any given population of tumor cells. Numerous studies with experimental animal tumors have proved the curative potential of cancer chemotherapy, however. There is evidence that immunologic approaches to therapy may be more effective than chemotherapy when the tumor cell mass is small; however, it may be ineffective against large tumor cell masses. The

order of magnitude for this latter effect is approximately 0.1 mg of tumor in most model systems, or about $10^5$ cells.[75]

## DRUG RESISTANCE AND TUMOR CELL HETEROGENEITY

The clinical usefulness of a chemotherapeutic agent may be severely limited by the emergence of a line of malignant cells resistant to that drug. It is common clinical experience to find that the first trial of a given drug administered to a cancer patient is successful and that subsequent trials are progressively less successful, until no apparent beneficial effect is achieved.

A number of cellular mechanisms are probably involved in drug resistance (e.g., altered metabolism of the drugs [decreased activation or increased deactivation], impermeability of the cell to the active compound or accelerated drug elimination from the cell, altered specificity of an inhibited enzyme, increased production of a target molecule, increased repair of cytotoxic lesions, or the bypassing of an inhibited reaction by alternative biochemical pathways). In some cases, resistance to one drug may confer resistance to other, biochemically distinct drugs. There are three groups of drug resistance mechanisms that deserve particular comment: (1) classic multiple drug resistance (mdr-1), (2) atypical multiple drug resistance, and (3) resistance related to DNA repair and molecular detoxification.

**Classic Multiple Drug Resistance.** The multiple drug resistance gene (*mdr-1*) produces a transmembrane glycoprotein known as P glycoprotein (Pgp).[76] In the presence of intracellular adenosine triphosphate (ATP), this glycoprotein pumps toxic chemicals from the inside of the cell to the extracellular environment. This pump results in the efflux of a variety of antineoplastic agents, most prominently the vinca alkaloids, anthracycline antibiotics, and dactinomycin. The hallmark of this mechanism is the simultaneous acquisition of resistance to all of these agents after exposure to only one member of the group and the lack of cross-resistance with other drugs (e.g., an antimetabolite, alkylating agent, or bleomycin). This is called *pleiotropic drug resistance*. The efflux of these agents caused by Pgp can be inhibited by a variety of agents, including calcium channel antagonists, cyclosporine, calmodulin inhibitors (such as phenothiazines), and other agents. Inhibitors of Pgp are being studied for potential clinical use in the hope of reversing this form of resistance in patients.

**Atypical Multiple Drug Resistance.** Other mechanisms of multiple drug resistance are also being studied. These may be grouped into three subgroups: (1) changes in drug efflux unrelated to Pgp, (2) changes in drug uptake, and (3) changes in drug metabolism.[77] Multiple drug resistance may also occur through quantitative and qualitative changes in topoisomerase II. This critical enzyme is the target of a number of drugs, and resistance to one may confer resistance to another such drug.

**DNA Repair and Molecular Detoxification**

*Glutathione and Glutathione S-Transferase Isoenzymes.* Glutathione is an intracellular thiol that is essential in the synthesis of DNA precursors. Enzymatic reactions involving glutathione are also involved in detoxifying toxic chemicals, repairing DNA damage, and acting as free radical scavengers. Glutathione and glutathione S-transferase are probably involved in resistance to classic and nonclassic alkylating agents by drug inactivation, increased metabolism and detoxification, DNA repair, or combinations of these effects. This common mechanism probably explains resistance to a variety of chemically related antineoplastic agents.

*06-Alkylguanine DNA Alkyltransferase.* This enzyme is important in resistance to nonclassic alkylating agents that are toxic to cells through methylation (dacarbazine, procarbazine) or chloroethylation (carmustine, lomustine), as discussed in Chapter 10. Investigational agents aimed at reversing this form of resistance are under development.

**Tumor Cell Heterogeneity and the Goldie-Coldman Hypothesis.** There is an analogy between the development of resistance to drugs in cancer therapy and the appearance of antibiotic-resistant strains of bacteria during the course of an infection. Both may be approached by changing drugs or, less often, by using larger doses of the same drug. The use of drug combinations is also a way of attempting to avert or overcome drug resistance. Drawing an analogy between the drug treatment of cancer and infections has gained increasing acceptance from work based on the somatic mutation theory. It is likely that resistant mutants arise spontaneously early in the natural history of cancer. The likelihood of a resistant line developing appears to be closely related to cell number, such that one or more resistant lines are likely to be present before most human malignancies become evident clinically (Goldie-Coldman hypothesis).[78] This hypothesis probably contributes to the inverse relationship between tumor cell mass and curability by drugs, and it provides a rationale for using high-dose chemotherapy as soon as possible after the diagnosis of malignancy in patients at high risk of relapse.[79]

**In Vitro Predictive Tests.** An important tool for the experimental study of drug resistance, called the *clonogenic assay*, was introduced by Salmon and coworkers in 1978.[80] This assay involved testing the drug sensitivity of human tumor explants grown in vitro. The clonogenic assay has been widely studied for potential use as a predictive test in choosing chemotherapy for individual patients and as a screening test for potentially useful new drugs. The clonogenic assay and several other related assays, such as the ATP bioluminescence assay and the fluorescent cytoprint assay, appear to be fairly good at predicting drug resistance, but they are rarely used in the routine clinical management of individual cases. These assays appear to be powerful tools for studies of tumor cell biology, and they are used for drug screening. The technology of in vitro sensitivity testing for new drugs is sufficiently advanced that the National Cancer Institute no longer uses animal tumor systems in screening for new antineoplastic agents.

## Combination Chemotherapy

Most of the successful programs of cancer chemotherapy involve the use of multiple antineoplastic agents employed together, sometimes following complex schedules of drug administration. This approach is commonly referred to as combination chemotherapy. The major rationale for the use of such combinations is tumor cell drug resistance, resulting from biochemical or cytokinetic factors. Most of the successful programs of combination chemotherapy were developed by empirical trial and error but share certain common features. These features are summarized as follows:

1. Only drugs that are active against the tumor in question are included in the combination, with the exception of certain drugs that are inactive against tumors but that minimize dangerous toxicity to normal tissues. Such drugs are often called *rescue* agents.

2. Drugs that are included have different mechanisms of action to minimize the possibility of drug resistance.

3. Drugs that are chosen generally have different toxic side effects, allowing the administration of full or nearly full doses of each of the active agents.

Contemporary efforts to develop improved programs of combination chemotherapy generally involve three different approaches: (1) biochemical modulation, (2) cytokinetic approaches, and (3) optimal sequencing of different agents.

### BIOCHEMICAL MODULATION

The therapeutic index of some drugs, notably the antimetabolites, may be increased or decreased by the presence of other drugs or normal metabolites, or both.[81] This has been termed *biochemical modulation* and is best illustrated by contemporary studies of 5-FU. At least six chemicals have been used to modulate the antitumor effects of 5-FU, as discussed in Chapters 10 and 43. At present, leucovorin is the only member of the following group of compounds that has been firmly established to achieve true biochemical modulation of 5-FU with beneficial effects for the patient:

1. Methotrexate
2. Thymidine

3. PALA [*N*-(phosphonacetyl)-L-aspartate]
4. Allopurinol
5. Uridine
6. L-Leucovorin (citrovorum factor)

Only one of these chemicals is clearly cytotoxic when used alone—methotrexate. Both thymidine and PALA have some minimal antineoplastic activity, but the key here is that all these approaches are presumed to involve important modulations of 5-FU cytotoxicity. These agents serve as exceptions to the first principle of combination chemotherapy given—that combinations should include only drugs active against cancer. It is likely that further studies of biologic response modifiers and drugs that reduce drug resistance, which may themselves lack antitumor cytotoxicity, will provide additional examples of biochemical modulation by inactive agents. In regard to 5-FU, at least two biomodulatory agents are known (interferon and levamisole), as discussed in Chapter 43 under Chemotherapy of Colorectal Cancer.

## CYTOKINETIC APPROACHES

Most antineoplastic agents are ineffective against nonproliferating cells ($G_0$). This population of tumor cells probably limits the potential curability of cancer by chemotherapy, so there has been interest in trying to recruit these cells into cell division so that they can be killed by drugs. One means has been through reduction of tumor cell mass by surgery (debulking). Other approaches include the synchronization of cells by giving one agent that kills or temporarily arrests cells in one phase (e.g., mitotic arrest by vincristine), followed by the use of S phase–specific chemotherapeutic agents (such as cytarabine) sometime later. Elaborate combinations based on cytokinetic principles have been developed, but their superiority over other combinations remains uncertain.

Another potentially important aspect of cytokinetics has been addressed by Norton and Simon.[82] These investigators were perplexed by the fact that complete remissions could be achieved with chemotherapy used against a wide variety of neoplasms but that these remissions were not durable. For some tumors, the patients relapsed with histologically identical tumors that retained biochemical drug sensitivity to the same drugs (e.g., Hodgkin's disease). They reasoned that some factor in addition to biochemical drug resistance was involved—cytokinetic resistance. They presumed that this factor related to the gompertzian growth of tumors, such that the rate of tumor regrowth increases as the tumor shrinks. They reasoned that the level of therapy adequate to initiate a regression may not be sufficient to sustain the regression and produce cure. Norton and Simon proposed two ways in which this problem might be overcome. The first, which they termed *intensification*, involves the use of a certain combination of agents as induction therapy, followed by an increased dose level of the whole combination or its individual components. The second method, which they termed *crossover intensification*, was to abandon the original agents once remission was obtained and to use new agents, perhaps in combination but always with an aggressive dose schedule. The concept of intensification, with or without crossover, has been labeled the *Norton-Simon hypothesis*. It is an intriguing concept but one that remains unproven.

## SEQUENCING AND SCHEDULING CHEMOTHERAPEUTIC AGENTS

Most investigators prefer to use intermittent courses of intensive combination chemotherapy rather than continuous programs of drug administration. This approach tends to maximize tumor cell killing, is usually better tolerated by patients, and appears to minimize immunosuppression. There is concern, however, that intermittent therapy may occasionally be suboptimal, especially for patients with tumors that regrow more rapidly than the bone marrow can recover from any given cycle of treatment. Particularly for the non-Hodgkin's lymphomas, nearly continuous programs of therapy are being studied. In addition, because of concern about the reduced dose intensity that can result from combination chemotherapy, some trials are exploring sequential single-agent therapy in high dosage as an alternative to traditional combination chemotherapy.[83] Choosing the most appropriate sequence of agents can be complicated and controversial, as reviewed by Day.[84]

A relatively unexplored question in cancer treatment is that of choosing the optimal time of day for drug administration. Practical considerations have made it difficult to study the importance of circadian rhythms to chemotherapy, but some investigators are exploring the possibility that chemotherapy could be given more safely and more effectively by using it at specific times of the day or night.[85] If such scheduling proves to be more effective than standard treatment, improvements in the technology of drug delivery through automated pumps and other delivery devices could make this approach to treatment clinically practical.

## Combined-Modality Therapy

The need to combine the available treatment modalities optimally was emphasized in Chapter 1, and this remains a dominant theme throughout this book. Animal tumor systems have provided imperfect guides to this important subject. At present, the question of how to combine therapy optimally has centered on how and when to use various forms of adjuvant therapy. The dominant model of adjuvant therapy has been the use of systemic chemotherapy shortly after the completion of local treatment with surgery or radiation therapy. A variation on this theme has been the use of various biologic response modifiers after local treatment, alone or combined with chemotherapy. In either case, the usual goal of adjuvant systemic therapy is to convert a palliative form of treatment to a curative form of therapy. The theoretical basis for this goal rests with the fact that systemic therapy for advanced disease eventually fails because of tumor cell drug resistance or host intolerance. By giving the systemic therapy at a time when metastatic disease is only micrometastatic, the hope is that the tumor will be more sensitive to chemotherapy for biochemical and cytokinetic reasons. As a consequence, the fractional cell kill accomplished at that time may be sufficient to eradicate all remaining tumor, whereas the same fractional kill would be only palliative in patients with larger tumor cell numbers. This situation is diagrammatically depicted in Figure 1–5.

An alternative model for combining local and systemic

therapy is commonly referred to as *neoadjuvant therapy*.[86] This term refers to the immediate use of chemotherapy before local therapy with the intent of (1) increasing the potential for local control by surgery or radiation therapy, or both, and (2) giving chemotherapy at the earliest possible time in the hope that any micrometastatic disease present may still be sensitive to chemotherapy. As for improving local control, this relates to at least two concerns. First is the possibility that effective chemotherapy may reduce the size of a lesion, making it easier to eradicate. Second, because chemotherapy primarily inhibits the growing outer margin of a tumor, it is theoretically possible that cells shed from this margin would be less able to implant and grow after chemotherapy. This concern may be particularly important for large sarcomas, in which accidental wound contamination occurs commonly.

In large measure, adjuvant therapy and neoadjuvant therapy remain the subjects of numerous clinical trials. The principles underlying these two approaches appear to be well established for several groups of tumors.

## Guidelines for the Use of Chemotherapy

It is critically important to establish and observe certain basic tenets for the use of cancer chemotherapeutic agents in a clinical setting. In general, the following guidelines have proved useful:

1. Use chemotherapeutic agents only when a diagnosis of malignancy has been established histologically.
2. Determine whether the malignancy is known to respond to the treatment in a reasonable percentage of cases in a manner that is beneficial to the patient or whether the treatment is a useful adjunct to surgery or radiation therapy in the management or cure of malignancy.
3. For patients with metastatic disease, follow objective tumor markers if possible to determine the response of the tumor to chemotherapy.
4. Do not use chemotherapeutic agents unless proper supportive facilities are available and the patient is capable of cooperation.

These points are worthy of elaboration. The difficulties in treating a patient blindly (i.e., without a tissue diagnosis) may be so great that one experience is enough to drive the lesson home that anticancer drugs are never given without a diagnosis of malignancy. An example of a situation when one might be tempted to initiate a blind therapeutic trial is that of the patient who is suspected of having lymphoma because of fever, weight loss, constitutional symptoms, and a downhill course. When such patients are subsequently proved to have tuberculosis, occult fungal infection, or a carcinoma, the prior use of chemotherapeutic agents is often an embarrassment to the physician and a disservice to the patient. An extension of this basic tenet of chemotherapy is that these agents are rarely, if ever, used in a diagnostic trial to determine the extent or type of malignancy.

The most important criterion for the clinical use of chemotherapy is that of anticipated benefit. In some patients, chemotherapy is given with curative intent, even when there is extensive disease. In others, chemotherapy may play a role in achieving cure but only when combined with other treatment modalities. For a much larger group of patients, the role of chemotherapy is primarily palliative, although it may provide some prolongation of life as well as control

**Table 8–9.** Role of Chemotherapy in the Treatment of Cancer*

*Used Alone with Curative Intent*

Gestational trophoblastic neoplasia
Testicular cancer
Hodgkin's lymphoma
Diffuse large cell lymphoma
Burkitt's lymphoma
Acute lymphoblastic leukemia
Acute myelogenous leukemia

*Used with Curative Intent as Part of Combined-Modality Therapy*

Wilms' tumor
Ewing's sarcoma
Osteosarcoma
Breast cancer
Ovarian cancer
Chronic myelogenous leukemia (BMT)
Epidermoid carcinoma of anus
Epidermoid carcinoma of larynx
Colorectal carcinoma (adjuvant)
Cervical cancer

*Used to Prolong Life or to Palliate Symptoms, or Both*

Small cell lung cancer
Lymphocytic lymphoma, nodular
Extragonadal germ cell tumors
Chronic lymphocytic leukemia
Prostatic carcinoma
Metastatic carcinoma (nonvisceral) of unknown primary origin
Kaposi's sarcoma
Endometrial carcinoma
Adrenal carcinoma
Islet cell carcinoma
Bladder cancer
Neuroblastoma
Multiple myeloma
Soft tissue sarcomas
Mycosis fungoides
Hairy cell leukemia
Carcinoid tumors
Malignant melanoma
Esophageal carcinoma
Non–small cell cancer
Gastric cancer (adjuvant chemoradiotherapy)
Colorectal carcinoma (metastatic disease)

*Of Minimal Value in Prolonging Life or Palliating Symptoms in Patients with Advanced or Metastatic Disease*

Epidermoid carcinomas of
  Cervix
  Head and neck
  Unknown primary origin
Adenocarcinomas of
  Stomach
  Pancreas
  Liver
  Bile ducts
  Unknown primary origin
Thyroid carcinoma
Renal carcinoma
Brain tumors

*For the purposes of this table, chemotherapy includes hormonal therapy and interferon.
BMT, bone marrow transplant.

of symptoms. Finally, for another large group of patients, chemotherapy is of little value; when given, it is with the hope of benefit for the individual patient but without supportive data for the use of chemotherapy from clinical trials in groups of patients. For the latter group, it is often preferable to consider chemotherapy an investigational modality. The groups of tumors that correspond to these four types of benefit are listed in Table 8–9. The reader is referred to Chapter 1 for further comments on developing treatment goals for the individual patient as well as to the respective disease-oriented chapters for specific drug regimens.

Because chemotherapeutic agents are potentially toxic, one should strive to follow objective markers of response in patients with metastatic disease. For example, objective markers may include a decrease in the size of the tumor, disappearance of hypercalcemia, disappearance of paraprotein in the serum, return of an infiltrated bone marrow to normal, or disappearance of a tumor marker such as alphafetoprotein, β-human chorionic gonadotropin, prostate-specific antigen, or carcinoembryonic antigen. The most important guideline to response is the size of measurable tumor masses. Standardized response criteria for cancer chemotherapy, based on objective measurements of tumor size, are given in Table 8–10. A newer approach to assessing response measuring only a single dimension has been proposed by a consortium of experts from the United States and Europe, but the role of this new measurement in clinical trials is uncertain at the time of this writing.[87]

Even objective measurements of tumor size are prone to observer errors, so response rates to chemotherapy that are derived from such measurements are best considered approximations. An extensive bibliography on observer variability in medicine has been compiled by Feinstein,[88] whereas two groups of oncologists have explicitly studied the interobserver variability of measuring tumor size.[89, 90] On the basis of these studies, it is prudent to estimate the false-positive rate of a partial response to be 5 to 10%, based solely on measuring errors. Such errors are even larger for measurements in some locations, such as masses in the abdomen or liver.

Subjective improvement, such as a decrease in pain, is a less satisfactory indication of drug action, although an objective assessment of performance status may provide important information about a patient's overall condition and quality of life. The Karnofsky Performance Status scale is the best guide to quantifying the functional status of the patient.[91] An alternative scale is that recommended by the American Joint Committee on Cancer.[92] Both of these scales (Table 8–11) are based on an assessment of functional status by a physician or another member of the health care team. Alternatively, these scales can be adapted for self-administration by patients for clinical research purposes.[93]

Quality of life has emerged as an active research discipline with its own distinct basic science.[94] Osoba[95] has reviewed this topic and identified six lessons about the measurement of quality of life that are especially pertinent in oncology: (1) Health-related quality of life (HQL) is a multidimensional matter and should be measured with multidimensional instruments; (2) observers are poor judges of how patients feel about their HQL; (3) it is possible to achieve high rates of compliance in the collection of self-reported HQL data; (4) HQL can be improved by aggressive chemotherapy; (5) symptoms are associated with disruptions in HQL that are quantifiable; and (6) pretreatment HQL appears to predict on-treatment HQL and survival.

Because of their narrow margins of safety, chemotherapeutic agents should not be used unless the physician is prepared to monitor potential toxicities to normal tissues, as previously detailed in this chapter. This means close and frequent follow-up visits, including history taking for symptoms of toxicity (e.g., nausea, vomiting, and dysuria), a physical examination with particular attention to the skin and mucous membranes, a white blood cell count, and a platelet count. It is also mandatory that the patient be truly informed about the potential risks and benefits of therapy and be prepared to cooperate with the physician in the use of this toxic modality.

The choice of a specific dose of chemotherapy warrants particular attention. Age, nutritional status, prior chemotherapy or radiation therapy, blood count, bone marrow reserve, renal and hepatic function, and condition of the patient must all be considered. Frequently, reduced doses of drugs are required for patients at high risk of toxicity, as defined by such factors. For many programs of combination chemother-

*Table 8–10.* **Response Criteria Used in Cancer Chemotherapy**

| Response | Biodimensional* | Unidimensional† |
|---|---|---|
| *Complete Response (CR)* | Complete disappearance of all signs and symptoms of cancer, lasting at least 1 mo | Complete disappearance of all signs and symptoms of cancer, lasting at least 1 mo |
| *Partial Response (PR)* | A ≥50% reduction in sum of products of greater and lesser diameters of all measured lesions lasting at least 1 mo and an absence of any new lesions during treatment | A ≥30% decrease in the sum of maximal diameters of individual tumors |
| *Progressive Disease (PD)* | A ≥25% increase in sum of products of greater and lesser diameters of all measured lesions or development of new lesions | A ≥30% increase in the sum of maximal diameters of individual tumors |

*World Health Criteria.
†From James K, Eisenhauer E, Christian M, et al. Measuring response in solid tumors: unidimensional versus bidimensional measurements. Natl Cancer Inst 1999;91:523–8.

*Table 8–11.* **Karnofsky and American Joint Committee on Cancer (AJCC) Performance Status Scales**

| Description | Karnofsky Scale (%) | AJCC Scale | Description |
|---|---|---|---|
| Normal; no complaints; no evidence of disease | 100 | H0 | Normal activity |
| Able to carry on normal activity; minor signs or symptoms of disease | 90 | | |
| Normal activity with effort; some signs or symptoms of disease | 80 | H1 | Symptomatic and ambulatory; cares for self |
| Cares for self; unable to carry on normal activity or to do active work | 70 | | |
| Requires occasional assistance but is able to care for most of own needs | 60 | H2 | Ambulatory >50% of time; occasionally needs assistance |
| Requires considerable assistance and frequent medical care | 50 | | |
| Disabled; requires special care and assistance | 40 | H3 | Ambulatory ≤50% or less of time; nursing care needed |
| Severely disabled; hospitalization indicated, although death not imminent | 30 | | |
| Very sick; hospitalization necessary; active supportive treatment necessary | 20 | H4 | Bedridden; may need hospitalization |
| Moribund, fatal processes progressing rapidly | 10 | | |
| Dead | 0 | | |

Data from Karnofsky DA. In: MacLeod CM, ed. Evaluation of chemotherapeutic agents. New York: Columbia University Press, 1949:191, and Beahrs OH, ed. American Joint Committee on Cancer: manual for staging of cancer. 4th ed. Philadelphia: JB Lippincott, 1992.

apy, dose adjustment guidelines have been developed, as given in the disease-oriented chapters of this book. One must avoid dose reduction for trivial reasons, however. DeVita has proposed that the most "toxic" chemotherapy is that which is ineffective.[96] In this case, the patient may die of undertreated cancer. Clinicians must seek an optimal dose of chemotherapy for patients—one that avoids the errors of either undertreatment or overtreatment.

## Clinical Trials

The experimental use of chemotherapeutic agents falls within the province of the clinical investigator, as discussed

*Table 8–12.* **Types of Clinical Trials**

| Phase | Goal | Comment |
|---|---|---|
| I | Determine MTD for a given schedule of a drug in humans | Mechanism of action, likely toxicities, and probable useful schedule are generally available from preclinical animal studies. Patients do not have to have measurable disease for study entry. |
| II | Determine whether or not the drug is active against specific neoplasms | MTD of a drug is used in patients with different kinds of measurable cancer. Response rate is determined, and rare side effects are looked for. |
| III | Compare ≥2 drugs, drug schedules, or drug doses to define clinical value of a new therapy more precisely | This is usually conducted as a randomized clinical trial, with control group receiving standard treatment. In some cases, this may include use of a placebo or use of supportive care without chemotherapy. |

MTD, maximum tolerated dose.

at length in Chapter 29. The decision to use an experimental therapy instead of older, more established treatments requires a careful assessment of the relative risks and benefits of the new and old treatments plus the informed consent of the patient. It also requires an awareness of economic factors in patient care because some forms of health insurance do not cover the costs of investigational therapy.[97] This situation has posed a serious impediment to the continuation of many trials, despite the fact that for many neoplastic diseases a clinical trial is the treatment of choice.[98] The importance of clinical trials to improving the treatment for patients with cancer cannot be overemphasized. For many of the diseases discussed in this book, the most appropriate therapy involves participation in a clinical trial.

Investigational drugs that are administered to a single patient almost never yield useful information and may do harm. Consequently, these drugs are nearly always evaluated by a series of clinical trials, as summarized in Table 8–12. Selected investigational drugs are reviewed briefly in Chapter 31. Clinical trial design is discussed in Chapter 29.

### SUGGESTIONS FOR ADDITIONAL READING

Perry MC, ed. The chemotherapy source book. 2nd ed. Baltimore: Williams & Wilkins, 1996. *This is an encyclopedic review of chemotherapy.*

Chabner BA, Longo D, eds. Cancer chemotherapy: principles and practice. 2nd ed. Philadelphia: JB Lippincott, 1995. *This book is a comprehensive review of chemotherapy.*

Canal P, Chatelut E, Guichard S. Practical treatment guide for dose individualization in cancer chemotherapy. Drugs 1998;56:1019–38. *This article is an excellent review of alternative methods for individualizing the starting dose of chemotherapy.*

### REFERENCES

1. Beere HM, Hickman JA. Differentiation: a suitable strategy for cancer chemotherapy? Anticancer Drug Des 1993;8:299–322.

2. Atkins MB, Sparano J, Fisher RI, et al. Randomized phase II trial of high-dose interleukin-2 either alone or in combination with interferon alfa-2b in advanced renal cell carcinoma. J Clin Oncol 1993;11:661–70.

3. Frankel SR, Eardley A, Lauwers G, et al. The "retinoic acid syndrome" in acute promyelocytic leukemia. Ann Intern Med 1992;117:292–6.

4. Armitage JO. Tumor proliferative rate and response to chemotherapy. Ann Intern Med 1992;116:771–3. editorial.

5. Kerr JFR. In: Tomei LD, ed. Apoptosis: the molecular basis of cell death. New York: Cold Spring Harbor Laboratory Press, 1991:5.

6. Frei E III. Gene deletion: a new target for cancer chemotherapy. Lancet 1993;322:662–4.

7. Warrell RP Jr, de The H, Wang ZY, Degos L. Acute promyelocytic leukemia. N Engl J Med 1993;329:177–89.

8. Freireich EJ, Gehan EA, Rall DP, et al. Quantitative comparison of toxicity of anticancer agents in mouse, rat, hamster, dog, monkey, and man. Cancer Chemother Rep 1966;50:219.

9. Vriesendorp HM, Vriesendorp R, Vriesendorp FJ. Prediction of normal tissue damage induced by cancer chemotherapy. Cancer Chemother Pharmacol 1987;19:273–6.

10. Hryniuk WM, Figueredo A, Goodyear M. Applications of dose intensity to problems in chemotherapy of breast and colorectal cancer. Semin Oncol 1987;14:Suppl 4:3–11.

11. Longo DL, Duffey PL, DeVita VT Jr, et al. The calculation of actual or received dose intensity: a comparison of published methods. J Clin Oncol 1991;9:2042–51.

12. Vogelzang NJ, Ruane M, Ratain MJ, et al. A programmable and implantable pumping system for systemic chemotherapy: a performance analysis in 52 patients. J Clin Oncol 1987;5:1968–76.

13. Willmott N. Chemoembolization in regional cancer chemotherapy: a rationale. Cancer Treat Rev 1987;14:143–56.

14. Karakousis CP. Tourniquet infusion versus hyperthermic perfusion. Cancer 1982;49:850–8.

15. Myers CE. The clinical setting and pharmacology of intraperitoneal chemotherapy: an overview. Semin Oncol 1985;12:Suppl 4:12–6.

16. Shafik A, Haddad S, Elwan F, et al. Anal submucosal injection: a new route for drug administration in pelvic malignancies. II: Methotrexate anal injection in the treatment of advanced bladder cancer. Preliminary study. J Urol 1988;140:501–5.

17. Tatsumura T, Koyama S, Tsujimoto M, et al. Further study of nebulisation chemotherapy, a new chemotherapeutic method in the treatment of lung carcinomas: fundamental and clinical. Br J Cancer 1993; 68:1146–9.

18. Raymond JR. Nephrotoxicities of antineoplastic and immunosuppressive agents. Curr Probl Cancer 1984;8:1–32.

19. Fischer DS, Knobf MT, Durivage HJ. The cancer chemotherapy handbook. 4th ed. St. Louis: CV Mosby, 1993:10–19.

20. Raderer M, Scheithauer W. Clinical trials of agents that reverse multidrug resistance: a literature review. Cancer 1993;72:3553–63.

21. Rocke LK, Loprinzi CL, Lee JK, et al. A randomized clinical trial of two different durations of oral cryotherapy for prevention of 5-fluorouracil-related stomatitis. Cancer 1993;72:2234–8.

22. Cascinu S, Fedeli A, Fedeli SL, Catalano G. Control of chemotherapy-induced diarrhea with octreotide: a randomized trial with placebo in patients receiving cisplatin. Oncology 1994;51:70–3.

23. Harris JE. The immunology of malignant disease. 2nd ed. St. Louis: CV Mosby, 1976:370.

24. Spreafico F. On the immunopharmacology of cancer chemotherapeutics. Behring Inst Mitt 1984;74:230–8.

25. Hersh EM. Modification of host defense mechanisms. In: Holland JF, Frei E III, eds. Cancer medicine. Philadelphia: Lea & Febiger, 1973:681.

26. Layween L, Levinsky RJ, Butler M. Long-term abnormalities in T and B lymphocyte function in children following treatment for acute lymphoblastic leukaemia. Br J Haematol 1981;49:251–8.

27. Dunagin WG. Clinical toxicity of chemotherapeutic agents: dermatologic toxicity. Semin Oncol 1982;9:14–22.

28. Ferguson MK. The effect of antineoplastic agents on wound healing. Surg Gynecol 1982;154:421–9.

29. Falcone RE, Nappi JF. Chemotherapy and wound healing. Surg Clin North Am 1984;64:779–94.

30. Johnston-Early A, Cohen MH. Mitomycin C–induced skin ulceration remote from infusion site. Cancer Treat Rep 1981;65:529.

31. Andersson AP, Dahlstrom KK. Clinical results after doxorubicin extravasation treated with excision guided by fluorescence microscopy. Eur J Cancer 1993;29A:1712–4.

32. Dean JC, Griffith KS, Cetas TC, et al. Scalp hypothermia: a comparison of ice packs and the Kold Kap in the prevention of doxorubicin-induced alopecia. J Clin Oncol 1983;1:33–7.

33. Witman G, Cadman E, Chen M. Misuse of scalp hypothermia. Cancer Treat Rep 1981;65:507–8.

34. Bochner BS, Lichtenstein LM. Anaphylaxis. N Engl J Med 1991; 324:1785–90.

35. Weiss RB, Baker JR Jr. Hypersensitivity reactions from antineoplastic agents. Cancer Metastasis Rev 1987;6:413–32.

36. Doll DC, List AF, Greco FA, et al. Acute vascular ischemic events after cisplatin-based combination chemotherapy for germ-cell tumors of the testis. Ann Intern Med 1986;105:48–51.

37. Shah SS, Rybak ME, Griffin TW. The cytarabine syndrome in an adult. Cancer Treat Rep 1983;67:405–6.

38. Weiss RB, Bruno S. Hypersensitivity reactions to cancer chemotherapeutic agents. Ann Intern Med 1981;94:66–72.

39. Doll DC, Ringenberg QS, Yarbro JW. Vascular toxicity associated with antineoplastic agents. J Clin Oncol 1986;4:1405–17.

40. Mackowiak PA, LeMaistre CF. Drug fever: a critical appraisal of conventional concepts: an analysis of 51 episodes in two Dallas hospitals and 97 episodes reported in the English literature. Ann Intern Med 1987;106:728–33.

41. Carreras E, Granena A, Rozman C. Hepatic veno-occlusive disease after bone marrow transplant. Blood Rev 1993;7:43–51.

42. Jones RJ, Lee KS, Beschorner WE, et al. Venoocclusive disease of the liver following bone marrow transplantation. Transplantation 1987;44:778–83.

43. McDonald GB, Hinds MS, Fisher LD, et al. Veno-occlusive disease of the liver and multiorgan failure after bone marrow transplantation: a cohort study of 355 patients. Ann Intern Med 1993;118:255–67.

44. Santamauro JT, Stover DE, Jules-Elysee K, Maurer JR. Lung transplantation for chemotherapy-induced pulmonary fibrosis. Chest 1994;105:310–2.

45. Robben NC, Pippas SW, Moore JO. The syndrome of 5-fluorouracil cardiotoxicity: an elusive cardiopathy. Cancer 1993;71:493–509.

46. Rieselbach RE, ed. Cancer and the kidney. Philadelphia: Lea & Febiger, 1982.

47. Kaplan RS, Wiernik PH. Neurotoxicity of antineoplastic drugs. Semin Oncol 1982;9:103–30.

48. Silberfarb PM. Chemotherapy and cognitive defects in cancer patients. Annu Rev Med 1983;34:35–46.

49. Barton C, Waxman J. Effects of chemotherapy on fertility. Blood Rev 1990;4:187–95.

50. Byrne J, Mulvihill JJ, Myers MH, et al. Effects of treatment on fertility in long-term survivors of childhood or adolescent cancer. N Engl J Med 1987;317:1315–21.

51. Chapman RM. Effect of cytotoxic therapy on sexuality and gonadal function. Semin Oncol 1982;9:84–94.

52. Sieber SM, Adamson RH. Toxicity of antineoplastic agents in man, chromosomal aberrations, antifertility effects, congenital malformations, and carcinogenic potential. Adv Cancer Res 1975;22:57–155.

53. Schafer AI. Teratogenic effects of antileukemia chemotherapy. Arch Intern Med 1981;14:514–5.

54. Blatt J, Mulvihill JJ, Ziegler JL, et al. Pregnancy outcome following cancer chemotherapy. Am J Med 1980;69:828–32.

55. Van Thiel DH, Ross GT, Lipsett MB. Pregnancies after chemotherapy of trophoblastic neoplasms. Science 1970;169:1326–7.

56. Doll DC, Ringenberg QS, Yarbro JW. Management of cancer during pregnancy. Arch Intern Med 1988;148:2058–64.

57. Dorr FA, Coltman CA Jr. Second cancers following antineoplastic therapy. Curr Probl Cancer 1985; 9:1–43.

58. Levine EG, Bloomfield CD. Leukemias and myelodysplastic syndromes secondary to drug, radiation, and environmental exposure. Semin Oncol 1992;19:47–84.

59. Smith A, Rubinstein L, Ungerleider RS. Therapy-related acute myeloid leukemia following treatment with epipodophyllotoxins: estimating the risks. Med Pediatr Oncol 1994;23:86–98.

60. Falck K, Grohn P, Sorsa M, et al. Mutagenicity in urine of nurses handling cytostatic drugs. Lancet 1979;1:1250–1.

61. Caudell KA, Vredevoe DL, Dietrich MF, et al. Quantification of urinary mutagens in nurses during potential antineoplastic agent exposure: a pilot study with concurrent environmental and dietary control. Cancer Nurs 1988;11:41–50.

62. Selevan SG, Lindbohm ML, Hornung RW, Hemminik K. A study of occupational exposure to antineoplastic drugs and fetal loss in nurses. N Engl J Med 1985;313:1173–8.

63. McEvoy GK, ed. American Hospital Formulary Service: drug information 94. Bethesda, Md.: American Society of Hospital Pharmacists, 1994.
64. Arrington DM, McDiarmid MA. Comprehensive program for handling hazardous drugs. Am J Hosp Pharm 1993;50:1170–4.
65. Cadman E. Toxicity of chemotherapeutic agents. In: Becker FF, ed. Cancer, A comprehensive treatise. Vol. 5. New York: Plenum Publishing, 1977:59–111.
66. Loprinzi CL, Duffy J, Ingle JN. Postchemotherapy rheumatism. J Clin Oncol 1993;11:768–70.
67. Michl I, Zielinski CC. More postchemotherapy rheumatism. J Clin Oncol 1993;11:2051–2.
68. Mahaney FX Jr. Late effects of childhood cancer treatment can be life threatening. J Natl Cancer Inst 1992;84:293–5.
69. Bruce WR. The action of chemotherapeutic agents at the cellular level and the effects of these agents on hematopoietic and lymphomatous tissue. Can Cancer Conf 1967;7:53–64.
70. Valeriote F, van Putten L. Proliferation-dependent cytotoxicity of anticancer agents: a review. Cancer Res 1975;35:2619–30.
71. Wheeler GP, Bowdon BJ, Adamson DJ, Vail MH. Comparison of the effects of several inhibitors of the synthesis of nucleic acids upon the viability and progression through the cell cycle of cultured H. Ep. no. 2 cells. Cancer Res 1972;32:2661–9.
72. Perry S. Cell kinetics and cancer therapy: history, present status, and challenges. Cancer Treat Rep 1976;60:1699–704.
73. Skipper HE, Perry S. Kinetics of normal and leukemic leukocyte populations and relevance to chemotherapy. Cancer Res 1970;30:1883–97.
74. Retsky MW, Swartzendruber DE, Wardell RH, Bame PD. Is gompertzian or exponential kinetics a valid description of individual human cancer growth? Med Hypotheses 1990;33:95–106.
75. Perez CA, Stewart CC, Wagner B. Experimental observations on the significance of cell burden in tumor control. Cancer 1974;34:113–21.
76. Beck WT. The cell biology of multiple drug resistance. Biochem Pharmacol 1987;36:2879–87.
77. Moscow JA, Cowan KH. Multidrug resistance. J Natl Cancer Inst 1988;80:14–20.
78. Goldie JH, Coldman AJ. A mathematic model for relating the drug sensitivity of tumors to their spontaneous mutation rate. Cancer Treat Rep 1979;63:1727–33.
79. DeVita VT Jr. The James Ewing lecture. The relationship between tumor mass and resistance to chemotherapy: implications for surgical adjuvant treatment of cancer. Cancer 1983;51:1209–20.
80. Salmon SE, Hamburger AW, Soehnlen B, et al. Quantitation of differential sensitivity of human-tumor stem cells to anticancer drugs. N Engl J Med 1978;298:1321–7.
81. Damon LE, Cadman EC. The metabolic basis for combination chemotherapy. Pharmacol Ther 1988;38:73–127.
82. Norton L, Simon R. The Norton-Simon hypothesis revisited. Cancer Treat Rep 1986;70:163–9.
83. Haskell CM. SWOG-9313. Curr Clin Trials Oncol 1994;1:P–646.
84. Day RS. Treatment sequencing, asymmetry, and uncertainty: protocol strategies for combination chemotherapy. Cancer Res 1986;46:3876–85.
85. Hrushesky JM, Bjarnason GA. Circadian cancer therapy. J Clin Oncol 1993;11:1403–17.
86. Frei E III. What's in a name—neoadjuvant. J Natl Cancer Inst 1988;80:1088–9.
87. James K, Eisenhauer E, Christian M, et al. Measuring response in solid tumors: unidimensional versus bidimensional measurements. J Natl Cancer Inst 1999;91:523–8.
88. Feinstein AR. A bibliography of publications on observer variability. J Chron Dis 1985;38:619–32.
89. Moertel CG, Hanley JA. The effect of measuring error on the results of therapeutic trials in advanced cancer. Cancer 1976;38:388–94.
90. Warr D, McKinney S, Tannock I. Influence of measurement error on assessment of response to anticancer chemotherapy: proposal for new criteria of tumor response. J Clin Oncol 1984;2:1040–6.
91. Schag CC, Heinrich RL, Ganz PA. Karnofsky performance status revisited: reliability, validity, and guidelines. J Clin Oncol 1984;2:187–93.
92. Fleming ID, Cooper JS, Henson DE, et al, eds. AJCC cancer staging manual. 5th ed. Philadelphia, JB Lippincott, 1997.
93. Loprinzi CL, Laurie JA, Wieand HS, et al. Prospective evaluation of prognostic variables from patient-completed questionnaires. North Central Cancer Treatment Group. J Clin Oncol 1994;12:601–7.
94. Guyatt GH, Feeny DH, Patrick DL. Measuring health-related quality of life. Ann Intern Med 1993;118:622–9.
95. Osoba D. Lessons learned from measuring health-related quality of life in oncology. J Clin Oncol 1994;12:608–16.
96. DeVita VT. Dose-response is alive and well. J Clin Oncol 1986;4:1157–9. editorial.
97. Antman K, Schnipper LE, Frei E III. The crisis in clinical cancer research: third-party insurance and investigational therapy. N Engl J Med 1988;319:46–8.
98. Gelber RD, Goldhirsch A. Can a clinical trial be the treatment of choice for patients with cancer? J Natl Cancer Inst 1988;80:886–7.

# CHAPTER 9

# PRINCIPLES OF BIOLOGIC THERAPY

• MALCOLM S. MITCHELL

## Overview

The treatment of cancer through biologic approaches, which has variously been called *biologic therapy, biotherapy,* or *biomodulation,* refers to any therapeutic alteration of the host-tumor relationship (except direct killing of the tumor) that improves the ability of a tumor-bearing host to reject the tumor.[1] Biologic therapy therefore encompasses the use of substances that assist the bone marrow in recovering from cytotoxic treatments, antagonize carcinogenesis, or inhibit metastasis, as well as approaches usually grouped into the category of "immunotherapy." The need for more effective systemic therapy for metastatic cancer than now exists has led oncologists to an ever-increasing interest in biologic approaches. Theoretically at least, these approaches offer a less toxic, more physiologic, and more selective way of overcoming a tumor than do frontal assaults aimed at destroying it. The demonstration that several types of biologic therapy are effective in animal models and human clinical trials has lent credence to this approach.

Although biologic therapy is broader than immunotherapy, the majority of biomodulators (biologic response modifiers) in current use are immunotherapeutic materials. Therefore, the main emphasis of this chapter is on forms of immunotherapy. A background of immunologic principles is provided to permit an understanding of the subsequent discussion of specific agents. The basic types of biomodulators and the tentative conclusions permitted by the results of clinical trials are also discussed. Particular attention is paid to active specific immunotherapy with vaccines and adoptive immunotherapy with lymphocytes, including cytotoxic T lymphocytes (CTLs). I also present some general principles that may be emerging about biologic therapy, which differ from those concerning chemotherapy, especially regarding the relationship of remission to survival. Although biomodulation has been studied most extensively in melanoma and breast cancer—from which most examples are drawn—principles derived from trials in those diseases have implications for the application of biologic therapy to many other malignancies.

## OBSERVATIONS SUPPORTING HOST-TUMOR IMMUNE INTERACTIONS

A number of clinical observations in the past suggested a possible role for immunologic reactivity against human cancers, including (1) documented spontaneous regressions; (2) regression of distant metastases following surgical removal of the primary tumor, as in the shrinkage or disappearance of lung metastases after nephrectomy in renal cell carcinoma; (3) an increased incidence of certain tumors in immunosuppressed patients; (4) a higher incidence of cancer in the elderly (who have a less intact immune system); and (5) dormancy of metastatic disease for many years after successful local therapy of the primary lesion. Even the log cell kill hypothesis (that cytotoxic agents kill a fixed percentage rather than a fixed number of cancer cells with each cycle) at least indirectly supports the necessity for a host response to effect complete remissions. Complete responses would probably be impossible were it not for the ability of host-related factors, or more specifically the immune response to the tumor, to eliminate the residual tumor burden.

## ANTIGENICITY VERSUS IMMUNOGENICITY OF TUMORS

After more than three decades of work in animals and humans, there is no doubt that tumors have at least the potential for eliciting an immune response in the tumor-bearing host. The controversies about this point have been resolved as we have learned how the immune system perceives tumor antigens. An important distinction, which helps explain discrepancies in early experiments, is that a tumor may be *antigenic*—that is, it may have peptides or saccharides, or both, that distinguish it from normal tissue counterparts—but may not be *immunogenic,* that is, it may be unable to evoke an immune response. The antigens may so closely resemble normal cellular components that they are weakly immunogenic or nonimmunogenic. Antigens may also be shed as soluble materials in small amounts into the bloodstream (a poor route of immunization), which is another possible reason for the weak immunogenicity of autologous tumors in situ. In addition, the major histocompatibility complex (MHC) antigens that present portions of the tumor antigens (antigenic determinants, or *epitopes*) to the immune system, which we discuss further on, may be down-regulated (absent), which leads to failure of the immune system to recognize the tumor.

## OVERVIEW OF THE IMMUNE RESPONSE

The immune response to tumors may be broadly subclassified into an antibody-mediated (humoral) response and a cell-mediated response. The weight of evidence supports a more important role for cell-mediated immunity in the destruction of malignant cells. Dendritic cells (DCs), which process and present antigens, thymus-derived small lymphocytes (T cells), and macrophages are pivotal cells in that process.

**Dendritic Cells.** DCs have become recognized as the most important of the antigen-processing and -presenting cells in the body. They are highly mobile cells of myeloid lineage closely related to monocytes, which are found in the skin and lymphoid tissues. These important cells convey antigens from the skin to the lymph nodes, degrade protein antigens to their constituent peptides, and present the immunogenic peptides (epitopes) to T-helper and T-cytotoxic cells. DCs are the only cells that can prime naive T cells to a new antigen and can also present antigens the body has already seen to memory T cells. When tumor vaccines are administered (discussed later), it is likely that DCs play a large role in the processing and presentation of those antigens. Some newer vaccination strategies involve using the patient's own DCs to prepackage the tumor antigens and then injecting the DCs intradermally.

**T Cells.** T lymphocytes are derived from bone marrow precursors that migrate during embryonic development to the thymus. There they undergo differentiation and maturation prior to their subsequent migration to all lymphatic organs and lymph node regions. From these locations, they circulate through the peripheral blood to target areas, such as sites of tumor, in response to tumor antigens and consequent release of soluble mediators from cells called *cytokines.* The recirculation of T cells from the bloodstream to the lymph enables lymphatic organs throughout the body to respond to a tumor that is present in only one site and drained by only one group of lymph nodes.

T lymphocytes may be further subdivided into T helper cells, cytotoxic T lymphocytes (CTLs), and suppressor T cells. The T helper (*Cluster Determinant 4; CD4$^+$*) cell has a specific receptor that is genetically programmed to recognize an antigenic peptide (epitope) presented by MHC class II molecules on antigen-presenting cells, such as DCs and macrophages. After receiving a second signal from the antigen-presenting cell through another molecule-molecule interaction, the T helper cell is activated and produces a variety of small peptides called *lymphokines.* The interaction of accessory molecules B7-1 and B7-2 (CD80 and CD86, respectively) with CD28 on the T helper cell is critical for production of the second signal for activation. Lymphokines stimulate other T helper cells, macrophages, and CTLs. Thus, the T helper cells function as a command center, directing the function of a variety of other cells within the immune system. It is important to note that without the second signal provided by the accessory molecule on the antigen-presenting cell, the interaction of the epitope with the T-cell receptor would lead to anergy rather than immunologic stimulation.

T helper cells that produce interferon (INF)-γ, interleukin (IL)-2, and tumor necrosis factor-α (TNF-α) are classified as T helper 1 (TH1) cells, whereas those that make IL-4, IL-5, IL-6, and IL-10 are called T helper 2 (TH2) cells. TH1 cells assist in cell-mediated immunity, whereas TH2 cells interact with B lymphocytes in antibody production. Because it is primarily the cellular immune response that participates in the rejection of tumors, TH1 cells are considered more desirable than TH2 cells to assist in that process. In humans, T helper 0 (TH0) cells producing both types of cytokines have also been identified with some frequency.

CTLs are for the most part CD8$^+$ cells that are able to lyse tumor cells in vitro. Under certain conditions in vitro, CD4$^+$ T cells are also capable of lysing tumors. Whether CTLs function extensively as cytotoxic cells directly destroying cancer cells in vivo has not been conclusively established. CTLs also produce a number of lymphokines, which may be important in vivo, especially if CD4 cells are lacking. In fact, the effectiveness of CTLs in vivo has been more closely related to their production of lymphokines than their cytotoxicity in vitro. Production of cytokines by CTLs follows the same general pattern as with T helper cells, with CTL1 and CTL2 subcategories. In vivo, it is possible that the production of cytokines, and elicitation of other cells such as macrophages, is more important than direct cytolysis judging from the immunohistologic characteristics of tumor nodules being rejected after specific immunotherapy.

The third type of T cell, the suppressor T cell, may not be a distinct subclass identified by a CD phenotype. Suppressor lymphokines, such as transforming growth factor-$\beta$ (TGF-$\beta$) and IL-10, released from CD4$^+$ and CD8$^+$ cells may be more important than a specific subclass of T cell in causing suppression. T suppressor cells normally function as an "off switch" for an immune system previously activated by an antigen. However, tumors are capable of activating suppressor influences and inappropriately downregulating the immune response as a mechanism of their survival. Among the important lymphokines released by T cells are INF-$\gamma$, TNF-$\alpha$ and TNF-$\beta$ (both of which are also produced by macrophages), IL-2, IL-4, IL-6, and IL-10. Of these, IL-2 has been the most thoroughly investigated in humans. IL-2 is a powerful stimulatory lymphokine, which binds to T cells via both a 55-kd chain (Tac receptor) and a 75-kd chain. Together, the two chains form a high-affinity receptor through which a stimulatory signal is transduced into the lymphocyte.

CTLs, like T helper cells, are genetically programmed to recognize certain epitopes. It is likely that CTLs interact with tumor epitopes presented by MHC class I molecules on DCs and tumor cells, and in the presence of lymphokines they proliferate and become activated. The CTLs can then kill the tumor cells specifically through the secretion of substances that destroy the integrity of the tumor cell membrane.

**Macrophages.** Macrophages are derived from common myeloid progenitor cells and circulate through the peripheral blood (where they are known as *monocytes*) to their final tissue destinations, including spleen, liver, and lung, where they mature into tissue macrophages. Although both C3 and Fc receptors are present on the surface of macrophages, MHC class II molecules are the most vital surface markers of the macrophage for an antitumor immune response. It is in the context of the class II molecule that macrophage-derived DCs perform their critical function as antigen-presenting cells, together with specialized cells (such as astrocytes of the brain) in certain tissues.

Macrophages subserve a number of other important functions as well. Tumoricidal macrophages have been demonstrated in vitro, usually with assays of 16 hours or more. These cells require close contact with the tumor cell but do not phagocytize their targets. Instead, these killer macrophages exert their antitumor killing effects through the release of nitric oxide, superoxide radicals, hydrogen peroxide, serine proteases, and possibly TNF-$\alpha$.

Macrophages have the dual role of presenting tumor antigens to T helper cells, especially memory T cells, and participating in nonspecific killing after being activated by lymphokines such as INF-$\gamma$ released by T cells. Macrophages also release their own soluble mediators (such as TNF-$\alpha$ and IL-1), which further augment the immune response by activating other macrophages and T cells. They may also produce inhibitory substances, such as prostaglandin E2 (PGE$_2$), that downregulate immunity by inhibiting T cell and natural killer (NK) cell proliferation. An excess of these suppressor macrophages, which are normally present in bone marrow (as shown in the mouse), is responsible for the poor delayed hypersensitivity responses found in head and neck and lung squamous carcinomas.

Biopsy specimens of human tumors undergoing immunologically mediated regression show that an overwhelming majority of the effector cells present consist of macrophages and T cells.[2–4] This suggests that these two cell types are paramount in tumor rejection.

**Natural Killer Cells and Lymphokine-Activated Killer Cells.** NK cells are large granular lymphocytes that compose approximately 10 to 15% of peripheral blood lymphocytes. They display the surface antigens CD16, which binds to the Fc portion of antibody, and CD56. They lack the ubiquitous CD3 receptor found on T lymphocytes as well as surface immunoglobulin that is present on B lymphocytes.[5]

NK cells appear to function as a nonspecific primitive tumor surveillance mechanism. Nude mice, which are T-cell–deficient but have functional NK cells, do not display an increased incidence of spontaneous tumor development. This is in contrast to mice with low or absent NK cell activity, which have a high incidence of spontaneous tumors and in which tumors are more easily induced.[6] In humans, low NK cell activity, as seen in X-linked immunodeficiency disorders and Chédiak-Higashi syndrome, is associated with an increased incidence of lymphoreticular malignancies despite normal T- and B-cell function.[7]

NK cells can lyse several human tumor cell lines, predominantly leukemia and lymphoma cells, without requiring prior tumor antigen exposure. Their method of binding to tumor cells is through adhesion molecules such as intercellular adhesion molecule-1 (ICAM-1) and through a variant of MHC class I molecules. The mechanism by which they cause cytolysis has not been completely delineated, although adenosine triphosphate, perforins, esterases, and TNF-$\alpha$ have all been suggested as mediators. Although CTLs require the presentation of tumor peptides by classic MHC class I molecules on the cell surface, the presence of MHC class I makes the tumor cell *resistant* to NK cells. Tumors that have downregulated their MHC class I molecules, and have thereby become resistant to conventional CTLs, simultaneously acquire sensitivity to NK cells. Unfortunately, it does not appear that this new sensitivity facilitates their rejection in vivo.

IL-2 binds to NK cells via its 75-kd portion, inducing them to proliferate and activating them to kill a wider range of tumor targets. These hyperactivated NK cells are more commonly referred to as *lymphokine-activated killer* (LAK) *cells.*[8] LAK cells, like NK cells, attach to tumor cells via nonspecific adhesion molecules rather than specific receptors, do not require prior sensitization for their activity, and also possess lysosomal granules. LAK cells are able to kill a variety of NK-cell–resistant tumor cell lines and may require a lower effector cell/tumor ratio than do NK cells to kill a certain tumor burden.

Although LAK cells have a certain selectivity for tumor cells, they are not entirely specific for these tumor targets, displaying a low level of killing against non-neoplastic cells such as endothelial cells, fibroblasts, and lymphocytes. LAK-like activity can also be displayed by T cells stimulated by high levels of IL-2 in the absence of specific antigens.[9] Thus, the high doses of IL-2 given in numerous therapeutic trials induce LAK activity in a morphologically heterogeneous group of lymphocytes, including both NK and T cells.

**Antibody-Mediated Immunity.** Antibody-mediated (humoral) immunity probably plays a lesser role than do cell-mediated processes in immune reactivity to human tumors. In general, antibodies can bind to tumor cells via antigen-combining sites while also binding complement, thereby bringing the tumor cell and complement in close proximity and possibly leading to the disruption of tumor cell membranes. In addition, and perhaps more important, antibodies can bind to Fc receptors on macrophages, neutrophils, NK cells, and LAK cells or to antigens on the tumor cells. By either or both of these mechanisms, the effector cells may be bound more tightly to their tumor targets. The effector cells can then lyse the tumor cells, a process called *antibody-dependent cell-mediated cytotoxicity.* This action of humoral and cell-mediated immunity in concert may be used therapeutically with combination strategies of administering IL-2 and monoclonal antibody (mAb).[10]

# The Nature of Tumor Antigens

Most tumor antigens that have been studied are proteins, especially glycoproteins. The increased understanding of the presentation of peptides by MHC molecules (which contain specific anchor points for the peptides) to CTLs has made it clear that most, if not all, antigens that stimulate CTLs are proteins. These need not be surface or structural proteins of the cell because peptides from cytoplasmic proteins can be processed in the endoplasmic reticulum, where the MHC molecules are assembled, and become associated with the MHC molecules there. The MHC molecules are then transported to the surface of the cell with the tumor-associated peptides already attached to them. Peptides that evoke an immune response are known as *epitopes,* a term from Jerne's idiotype network hypothesis of immunologic regulation.[11] Proteosomes in the cytoplasm degrade proteins into constituent peptides, which are then transported into the endoplasmic reticulum by the transporter associated with antigen processing (TAP). When tumors downregulate their immunogenicity as a means of evading immunologic detection, it is often the MHC molecule or the TAP that is lacking, leading to lack of expression of the epitope. Upregulation of epitopes by INFs, especially INF-α and INF-γ, can be accomplished through their effects on MHC molecules, ex-

pression of genes for the TAP, and proteosomal processing of proteins.

Although no convincing evidence exists that sugars can be recognized by T-cell receptors, gangliosides and saccharides can elicit humoral responses[12, 13] and can protect mice against tumors bearing those molecules. CTLs may recognize a portion of the saccharide structure surrounding a core peptide such as those present on mucins of adenocarcinomas.[14]

Among the protein antigens thus far described are (1) tyrosinase—an enzyme involved in melanin formation found in nearly all melanomas, (2) the MAGE (*me*lanoma *a*nti*ge*n) group—found in melanomas and 20% of breast cancers,[15] (3) MART-1 (*m*elanoma *a*ntigen *r*ecognized by *T* cells), or Melan-A,[16] and (4) oncogene proteins such as HER-2/*neu,* mutated p21*ras,* and mutated p53. All these materials can generate both antibodies and T-cell responses and are of at least potential use in cancer vaccines. HER-2/*neu* is found in 20 to 30% of women with breast cancer and in ovarian cancer, in which it portends a poor prognosis. Yet paradoxically, HER-2/*neu* encodes a 185-kd extracellular domain protein that has a number of immunogenic regions, which can serve as stimulants and targets of immunity.

In adenocarcinomas such as breast, ovarian, lung, or pancreatic cancers, the ubiquitous surface mucin MUC1 is another useful immunogen. MUC1 is an approximately 400-kd glycoprotein extending from the cell membrane, composed of a core protein—a series of 60 to 100 tandem repeats of a 20 amino acid sequence—to which oligosaccharide side chains are attached. MUC1 is more highly expressed in carcinomas than in normal tissues, in which it is usually cryptic on the basolateral surface, and is different from normal mucins in its composition. Glycosylation of the mucin in breast cancer cells is impaired, which results in truncated oligosaccharides rather than luxuriant polysaccharide side chains. Unlike most proteins (which have a heterogeneous amino acid composition in their various regions), because of its repetitive nature, fragments of MUC1 that are of approximately 20 amino acids contain at least one epitope, and larger fragments represent the totality of the epitopes. The most immunogenic portion of the molecule, the (A)PDTRPAP [(alanine)-proline-aspartic acid-threonine-arginine-proline-alanine-proline] region, is recognized by mouse antibodies and T cells and by human CTLs. Peptides of 16 to 100 amino acids have been used in various vaccines, usually conjugated to the large protein keyhole limpet hemocyanin (KLH), mixed with a potent adjuvant. CTLs recognizing specific HLA-A2–restricted epitopes have been identified in immunized patients.[17] Synthetic oligosaccharides of the side chains, such as sialyl-Tn, are also immunogenic in humans, eliciting IgG and IgM antibody responses.[18]

Carcinoembryonic antigen (CEA), the first "tumor-specific" antigen described, can elicit immune responses in humans and may also prove to be a useful immunogen for cancer vaccines against colon carcinoma and other tumors that express that substance.[19] Although CEA is secreted extracellularly, it is also expressed in the cancer cell of origin and thus may serve as a target for antibodies and T cells.

In lymphomas and multiple myeloma, a monoclonal immunoglobulin molecule is expressed on the surface of the tumor cell. The antigen-combining region of that molecule, which confers uniqueness on the immunoglobulin, is called the *idiotype*.[11] For lymphomas and myelomas, the idiotype is their tumor-associated antigen. The idiotype can thus be used as a target for mAbs (anti-idiotype antibodies) or as an immunogen in a therapeutic vaccine to stimulate humoral or perhaps cell-mediated immunity to those hematologic malignancies.

Solid tumors have no idiotype expressed on them, but anti-idiotype antibodies can nonetheless be used to immunize against solid tumor epitopes. If one makes a mAb (called *Ab 1*) against solid tumor cells bearing tumor antigens and then secondarily makes antibodies against that antibody (*Ab 2*), a proportion of the antiantibodies will be directed against the idiotype, which is the most variable portion of the immunoglobulin molecule. Some of those anti-idiotype antibodies will resemble the original tumor antigens, either in structure or, more likely, through their effect on the immune system.[11] Thus, anti-idiotype antibodies can be used to generate humoral or cell-mediated immunity directed against the original tumor antigens of the solid tumor, even without knowing their exact chemical nature.

## Cytokines

*Cytokines* is the term used to denote low-molecular-weight peptide mediators secreted by cells such as leukocytes and fibroblasts. *Lymphokines* are cytokines made by T cells, whereas *monokines* are monocyte-macrophage–made mediators. Thus, IL-2 is a lymphokine, whereas granulocyte-macrophage colony-stimulating factor (GM-CSF) is a cytokine (a monokine) but not a lymphokine. *Chemokines* are a class of related substances—chemical attractants of cells secreted by other cells. Cytokines are growth factors and stimulators of the same and other types of cells. They can have "positive" or "negative" effects, either activating or suppressing their activity on the other cells, especially at different doses. For example, IL-2 stimulates T helper cells, CTLs, and NK cells, and at high levels causes T cells and NK cells to kill tumor cells nonspecifically. An important new cytokine is IL-12, made by T cells and DCs, which activates T cells and NK cells. IL-12 channels T helper cells into the TH1 pathway, acting collaboratively with costimulatory molecules such as CD80 and CD86 to activate the TH1 cells.[20] IL-6 and IL-7 are also T-cell stimulators, which act in concert with IL-2.

Although the generalization is not entirely true—particularly for IL-4, which has many positive effects on T cells—the lymphokines made by TH2 cells and by some tumor cells may divert T cells into the TH2 pathway. That would lead to a less effective rejection response to the tumor. Among these TH2 lymphokines are IL-4, IL-5, and IL-10. These lymphokines may be considered "suppressive" in the sense of selecting against TH1 cells. TGF-β and PGE2 are more consistently suppressive of T-cell immunity and may be elicited by the tumor from infiltrating leukocytes to subvert immunity. PGE2 from "suppressor" macrophages is also responsible for the general anergy in delayed hypersensitivity responses found in patients with squamous cell tumors of the head and neck or lung. Inhibition of the proliferation of T cells is the major mechanism of action of PGE2.

Peroxide and superoxide molecules from phagocytic cells also play a role in downregulating T-cell and NK-cell activity. Histamine receptors on the phagocytic cells can be stimulated by the histamine molecule itself, which abrogates the suppressive activity and permits the activated T cells and NK cells to continue as killer cells. This strategy is being used in an ongoing trial in melanoma.

## Types of Immunotherapy

An understanding of the immune response to tumor cells immediately suggests therapeutic approaches based on that process. For example, one might try to stimulate the patient with tumor antigens, or perhaps the epitopes themselves, to use the entire pathway of immunization. Lymphokines released normally in the process might be synthesized and given in large amounts to stimulate effector cells. The effector cells themselves might be used to short-circuit the process of immunization, in conjunction with lymphokines to sustain them in vivo. To prepare the tumor-bearing host for immunization, an attempt to replete deficient immunologic subpopulations might be made. Finally, one might consider upregulating the patient's own tumor in vivo to permit the activated immune system to recognize the epitopes on the tumor cells optimally. All these approaches have been explored, singly or together, under the heading of *immunotherapy* in the treatment of human cancers.

I have categorized immunotherapy into the following five subtypes[1, 21]:
1. Active: stimulation of the intrinsic immune system of the host. This may be further divided into:
   a. Nonspecific: the use of microbial or synthetic agents known as adjuvants to activate nonspecific effector cells (macrophages, NK cells, LAK cells, or neutrophils). Examples of adjuvants are gram-negative bacterial endotoxins, usually "detoxified" by removal of a phorphoryl group; mycobacterial cell walls; and whole mycobacteria such as bacille Calmette-Guérin (BCG). QS-21, from the *Saponaria* tree, and the growth factor GM-CSF are other examples. Complex adjuvants combining several elements, such as endotoxin and mycobacterial cell walls, such as Detox, are also available.
   b. Specific: the use of tumor-associated antigens in the form of irradiated whole tumor cells, extracts, lysates, whole proteins, DNA, RNA, synthetic peptides, or saccharides. These antigens permit the activation of specific T cells as helper cells, memory cells, and effector cells. Therapeutic vaccines require specific antigens and usually combine them with nonspecific adjuvant materials (active nonspecific immunotherapy) for improved potency.
2. Passive: the transfer of rapidly cleared antitumor factors. Included in this group are mAbs, given either alone or conjugated to toxins such as ricin, chemotherapeutic agents, or radionuclides such as iodine 131. Therapy with cytokines is also appropriate to this category, but we will address them in the section Adoptive Immunotherapy because they have usually been administered in conjunction with lymphoid cells.
3. Adoptive: the transfer of effector cells to the host. These

cells were transferred from one animal to a syngeneic recipient in mouse models (hence "adoptive"), but in humans this term more usually refers to the reinfusion of ex vivo activated cells, especially T cells.

4. Restorative: the repletion of a depressed immune response. This is usually attempted through the inhibition of suppressor macrophages with prostaglandin inhibitors or of T suppressor lymphocytes with low-dose cyclophosphamide. Stimulation of thymic precursors into mature thymocytes by levamisole is another approach in this category.

5. Cytomodulatory: the upregulation of tumor-associated antigens and MHC antigens on the cell surface of tumor cells, thereby making them more easily identifiable by effector cells, particularly CTLs. INF-$\gamma$, INF-$\alpha$, and TNF-$\alpha$ are among the cytokines with this capacity.

## Suggestions from Mouse Models

Although they do not apply in every detail to human cancers, data from mouse models may have some relevance as general guidelines. The most successful mouse experiments were in immunoprophylaxis, where the tumor cells were inoculated after or together with the immunotherapy. True immunotherapy, involving tumors that had been allowed to grow before treatment (sometimes to a size of $\geq 4$ mm), usually required debulking by treatment with a chemotherapeutic agent to which the tumor was partially sensitive, such as cyclophosphamide. Although cytoreductive therapies may prove to be helpful before immunotherapy is applied, it is not necessary in either mice or humans to use them to produce a discernible shrinkage of the tumor by the immunotherapy. Nevertheless, treatment when the tumor burden is small (minimal residual disease) puts the immune system at an advantage, compared with the treatment of many billions of tumor cells in macroscopic metastases.

Highly immunogenic tumors, such as those induced by viruses or carcinogens, are not entirely relevant models for human tumors, which are often weakly immunogenic. Spontaneous tumors are best to study but are difficult to work with because close surveillance of mice for long periods is required to obtain them. Sublines of passaged tumors with low immunogenicity, such as the B16 melanoma, are good alternatives. The principle that has emerged in this case is that upregulation of the tumor cells is essential for them to be able to elicit a rejection reaction in vivo and, by extension, for the production of therapeutic vaccines. Insertion of genes for substances such as INF-$\gamma$ has proved useful, as has simply incubating the tumor cells for 1 to 2 days with the cytokine. If the tumor cells in the vaccine lack costimulatory molecules, rendering them nonimmunogenic, insertion of the genes for those molecules, particularly CD80 and CD86, has conferred immunogenicity on the tumor cells. Even with immunogenic tumors, additional costimulation has improved their stimulation of T cells, as measured by proliferation in vitro. Insertion of cytokine genes, which enables the tumor to attract and activate immune cells, has also been exploited, with GM-CSF, IL-2, and IL-4 emerging as important cytokines for this process.[22, 23] GM-CSF itself can be given

together with tumor cell vaccines as an adjuvant rather than transducing its gene into the tumor cell.

## Active Nonspecific Immunotherapy

Active nonspecific immunotherapy—which was explored extensively in the 1970s—used a variety of substances, but mainly those derived from microbes. They included BCG and its derivatives, including methanol-extract residue and muramyl dipeptide, the minimal component of mycobacterial cell wall that is capable of evoking an immune response; *Salmonella* endotoxin (especially detoxified endotoxin, as in the combination adjuvant DETOX); *Corynebacterium parvum* (now called *Propionibacterium acnes*); and poly I:C. The mechanism of action of these nonspecific therapies is principally through the stimulation of DCs and macrophages. Macrophages can lyse tumor cells directly after such activation, and both macrophages and DCs release T-cell–stimulatory mediators such as TNF-$\alpha$ and IL-1. The activation of T cells may, in turn, further activate the macrophages through INF-$\gamma$ in an amplifying circuit.

The two uses for BCG that have exploited its most reproducible activity include intravesical administration in bladder cancer[24] and intralesional use for intradermal melanoma nodules. These may simply be examples of nonspecific inflammatory effects locally, without a true immunostimulatory activity. Although there were some positive reports regarding BCG's effects on tumor responses or prolongation of response duration following BCG administration after initial chemotherapy, many trials produced negative reports. The reason for the lack of consistent systemic activity was not clear. However, the nonspecific activation of macrophages may include both tumoricidal and suppressor subtypes, which may directly oppose one another.[25, 26] Most of all, the lack of a specific component, that is, tumor antigens, may well be the factor that was consistently lacking in the early use of nonspecific active immunotherapy.

## Active Specific Immunotherapy

Active specific immunotherapy is epitomized by the use of therapeutic vaccines (sometimes called *theraccines* to distinguish them from true prophylactic vaccines). Vaccines have most typically comprised either autologous materials (from the same tumor-bearing individual) or allogeneic materials (from cell lines derived from a second party but carrying antigens common to the type of tumor). They may be composed of killed whole tumor cells or tumor fragments, either of which must contain antigens that can be recognized by the immune system. Because most tumors are at best weakly immunogenic, the point behind the use of therapeutic vaccines is to re-present tumor antigens in a way that forces the host's immune system to recognize them and then to attack the host's own tumor through common antigens. The use of potent adjuvants, such as those described in the section Active Nonspecific Immunotherapy, is essential to boost the stimulation by the relatively weak tumor antigens.

Tumor vaccines have an intrinsic theoretical advantage

over other forms of immunotherapy in that memory T cells specific for that disease may be generated. Therefore, unlike cytokines, whose effect is lost shortly after the completion of administration, vaccination may elicit antitumor immunity some time after immunization is completed and also have long-term effects resulting from immunologic memory. It is clear that the antitumor response seen in humans is a T-cell–mediated effect, as biopsies taken from responding sites show perivascular infiltration by T cells and a predominance of macrophages and T cells (of both CD4 and CD8 lineage) at the tumor site.

Active specific immunotherapy has been most widely and successfully used against melanoma. A wide variety of preparations, from whole cells to surface gangliosides, has been used. Only a brief representative sampling is presented here. The reader is referred to a volume of the *Annals of the New York Academy of Sciences*[27] and a review[28] devoted entirely to this subject for a more complete description.

## AUTOLOGOUS AND ANTI-IDIOTYPE VACCINES

Although the re-presentation of tumor antigens found on a host's tumor theoretically should best be achieved when an autologous tumor is used as the source of immunogens, in practice the responses to autologous vaccines have generally been disappointing. For example, although Laucius and colleagues observed two complete responses (CRs) and two partial responses (PRs) in 18 patients treated with autologous tumor cells and BCG,[29] these effects were transient (2 to 4 months) and occurred in nodal and subcutaneous sites. Berd and associates observed four CRs and one PR (median duration of response = 10 months) in 40 patients (12.5%) treated with vaccine derived from autologous tumor cells and BCG.[30] Responding sites included skin, subcutaneous tissue, nodes, lung, and possibly liver. The use of hapten-modified tumor cells has improved the delayed hypersensitivity response to those cells and may have increased the relapse-free interval in a phase II trial.[31]

The observation that selected viruses could enhance the immunogenicity of tumor cells ultimately led to clinical trials of therapeutic vaccines composed of such virally transformed tumor cells. Although most studies using this approach have been conducted in the adjunctive (surgical adjuvant) setting, evidence of tumor shrinkage in skin nodules and lymph nodes was found in 7 of 13 patients treated with Newcastle disease virus–induced melanoma cell lysates.[32]

Vaccines composed of anti-idiotype mAbs may mimic those comprising tumor antigens (see earlier section on the nature of tumor antigens). An anti-idiotype mimicking a high-molecular-weight melanoma antigen elicited one CR (in lymph nodes) and six minor responses in 35 patients.[33] With a closely related anti-idiotype, Melimmune (IDEC Pharmaceuticals) and the adjuvant muramyl dipeptide, we induced a CR of liver and lung metastases that has now lasted more than 6 years and tumor shrinkage or stable disease in another 5 of 24 melanoma patients.[34] Unfortunately, other trials with Melimmune were less successful and did not support its further development.

## IDIOTYPE VACCINES IN LYMPHOMA

Lymphomas each have a monoclonal immunoglobulin idiotype on their surface, characteristic of the clone of B cells that gave rise to them. This idiotype can serve as a tumor-specific antigen for targeting and immunization. Idiotype vaccination has been used by Hsu and colleagues for several years, most recently in the form of autologous antigen-pulsed DCs.[35] This form of therapy was highly successful in a small pilot study and will be pursued further. The immunogenicity of the monoclonal tumor idiotype appears to be considerably stronger than that of the tumor-associated antigens of solid tumors. Thus, one would hope that vaccines will be of particular usefulness for this class of tumor.

## ALLOGENEIC VACCINES

I have reviewed this subject, both from a broad perspective[36] and more narrowly focused on experience with a single vaccine.[37] The interested reader is encouraged to consult those and other reviews for a more detailed treatment of this subject.

Bystryn elicited one PR and one case of long-term stability in 13 patients treated with a melanoma vaccine composed of antigens shed by cultured melanoma cell lines.[38] The author has obtained an improved survival in patients given this preparation after removal of the primary tumor provided that the patients experienced a delayed-type hypersensitivity reaction to the material.

In 1988 and 1990, we first described the results of phase I and phase II trials with a vaccine composed of allogeneic melanoma lysates and the adjuvant DETOX.[39, 40] A low dose of cyclophosphamide (350 mg/m$^2$) preceded the course of vaccine in half of the patients. An increase in precursors of CTLs was noted in the blood of 50% of the patients between 2 and 6 weeks after beginning immunization. More important, CRs and PRs were noted, with regressions often beginning after the first injection. Our experience (now extending over a period of more than 14 years) shows a response rate of approximately 15%, with 5% CRs and 10% PRs in 109 patients treated with lysate vaccines made in our laboratory. Responses were elicited in sites such as the lung, lymph nodes, subcutaneous tissue, breast, liver, and small intestine.[4] The median duration of these responses on the vaccine treatment was 21 months. Although many of these patients went on to other treatments, such as INF-α, IL-2, or chemotherapy after vaccine, their survival dating from their initial dose of vaccine under these varied circumstances was striking. The median duration of survival in a cohort of 13 patients with major objective responses was 46 months. Four patients have now survived long term: two patients for more than 10 years, one patient for more than 12 years, and one patient for more than 13 years. In contrast, the expected median survival for patients with metastatic melanoma is only 7 to 8 months. Morton and colleagues[41] have also observed similar improvements in survival of their cohort of 68 patients with metastatic melanoma given irradiated whole melanoma cells and BCG in a phase II trial. They reported a median duration of survival of 23.1 months, with a 5-year survival rate of 26%.

It was not necessary to achieve complete remissions to elicit improved survival. Many of our patients have lived with stable or very slowly growing identifiable tumor nodules on computed tomographic scans but without the development of new metastatic masses, particularly at dire sites such as the liver. This is in direct contrast to chemotherapy, in which complete remissions are usually necessary to effect improved survival.

## VACCINES IN MINIMAL RESIDUAL DISEASE

As strongly suggested by animal models, the use of vaccines in the surgical adjuvant setting (minimal residual disease) to prevent or delay recurrence has yielded some of the most promising results. Several investigators have reported uncontrolled trials wherein improved disease-free survival and overall survival relative to historical controls have been observed.[31–33] These results warrant prospective randomized trials using those or similar vaccines. In melanoma, there are several randomized, controlled trials with vaccines in progress in stage II and stage III disease, but they have not yet been analyzed. A Southwest Oncology Group (SWOG) trial of Melacine versus observation in patients with resected stage II melanoma (1.5 to 4 mm depth) was analyzed in March 2000. Fewer relapses were seen in the vaccine-treated group ($P = 0.04$) based on intent-to-treat analysis.

An improvement in disease-free interval and survival was also noted by Hanna and Hoover in colon cancer in a randomized comparison of autologous immunization plus BCG adjuvant versus observation.[42] Although differences between the groups narrowed over a span of 7 years, there appeared to be at least an initial advantage in the immunized group.

## DEFINED VACCINES

Livingston has used the melanoma-associated gangliosides GM2 and GD2 with the adjuvant BCG to try to immunize melanoma patients with minimal residual disease.[12] The author successfully generated IgM antibodies in those patients, indicative of a primary response, and also IgG antibodies, signifying a secondary response. However, cell-mediated immunity (CTLs or T helper cells) has not yet been demonstrated. Although no statistically significant improvement in survival or disease-free interval was obtained, newer constructs of GM2 attached to an immunogenic carrier molecule, and combined with a more potent adjuvant, offer the potential of a better clinical effect.

In mouse models, immunization with saccharides of the ubiquitous mucin expressed on the surface of adenocarcinomas has protected against those tumors, as well as treated them, in conjunction with cyclophosphamide.[43] These encouraging results have stimulated those investigators to treat human adenocarcinomas, such as those of the colon, lung, pancreas, breast, and ovary. Clinical responses, principally measured as prolonged survival, appear to be present in patients with breast cancer treated with a saccharide (sialyl-Tn) vaccine including DETOX.[44, 45] Those with the highest level of antibody response have had the longest survival.

A vaccine with p185 (the extracellular domain protein encoded by the HER-2/*neu* oncogene) as the antigen has been tested in rhesus monkeys, where it elicited cytostatic antibodies and both T helper and CTLs against the human protein and its peptides.[46] HER-2/*neu* is immunogenic in humans too, making a whole cell or peptide vaccine likely in the near future. Since approximately 20 to 30% of women with breast cancer overexpress HER-2/*neu* protein and ap-

pear to have a poorer prognosis than do others with breast cancer, a trial of a vaccine approach in that situation may be appropriate. At present, the only immunotherapy that has been tried is with trastuzumab (Herceptin, Genentech), a monoclonal antibody (mAb) against the p185 extracellular domain protein. Single peptide vaccines have also been used in melanoma and breast cancer, with limited success. Among these are MAGE-1, MART-1, and MUC1. It appears that the peptides are capable of stimulating some degree of immunity in humans, but profound objective clinical remissions have not yet been obtained.

Some generalizations may be drawn from experience thus far with tumor vaccines. Most notably, unlike systemic chemotherapy, the beneficial effects of cancer vaccines have been elicited without significant systemic toxicity. Except for minimal fever, the toxicity of vaccines is local, at the sites of injection, and is easily remedied by discontinuing the adjuvant. Anaphylactic reactions were absent, as were serious autoimmune phenomena, although patchy vitiligo was occasionally noted in patients responding to melanoma vaccines. Vaccines are probably of most use in the adjunctive ("adjuvant") setting in patients with minimal residual disease. Randomized, controlled trials are in progress to test that assertion conclusively. Nevertheless, responses in metastatic sites have also been noted in approximately 10 to 20% of patients, often for years. Survival of patients with metastatic disease (specifically melanoma) who respond to vaccines has been improved in comparison with historical controls and with the survival of the group as a whole. The potential exists for the further development of this easily tolerated and clearly efficacious therapy of both residual and metastatic disease, preferably combined with cytokines and adoptive cellular therapy.

Peptide vaccines may be scientifically more desirable because of their purity and known composition, but individual peptides recognized by CTLs or helper T cells (9 or 15 amino acids, respectively) have caused few objective responses. Polyvalent peptide vaccines and whole protein or DNA-based vaccines, all simulating the whole cell vaccines or lysates in their content, can now be constructed. Several investigators have used newer versions of "crude" vaccines, fusing whole cancer cells with DCs[47] or inserting lysates into DCs and then injecting the DCs as the vaccine vehicle.[48] Packaging of multiple peptides or genes encoding them within DCs and administration of the DCs with a potent adjuvant is a method of immunization that will receive increasing attention in the next several years.

## REGULATORY STATUS OF VACCINES

Only one vaccine has yet been approved for clinical use in cancer. Melacine (Mitchell/Corixa) was approved in Canada in 1999 and may soon be examined by the U.S. Food and Drug Administration (FDA). Cancer VAX (being studied by Morton) is undergoing international clinical trial under FDA auspices, and extracts of melanoma cells (being studied by Bystryn), hapten-modified autologous melanoma vaccines (being studied by Berd), and GM2 ganglioside conjugated to KLH (GMK) (being studied by Livingston) are all undergoing national evaluative trials. MUC1 and sialyl-Tn (Theratope) breast cancer vaccines (provided by Biomira) are also in international phase II and III trials. An autologous colon carcinoma vaccine (being studied by Hanna) has been extensively tested by the Eastern Cooperative Oncology Group but has not yet been given FDA approval.

## Passive Immunotherapy

Köhler and Milstein developed a method of generating mAbs: a clonally derived population of antibodies highly specific for a particular antigenic determinant (epitope) from hybridomas.[49] Each hybridoma was derived from the fusion of a myeloma cell (which provided immortality to the fusion product) with an immunoglobulin-secreting B lymphocyte, thereby producing a constant source of antibody.[50] The enthusiasm and hope behind the application of this technology to human malignancies as a "magic bullet" specific for cancer cells have been tempered by clinical experience, but mAb therapy remains an area of intense research interest.

The rationale behind mAb administration is that the mAb will act as a bridge to bring either complement or an immune effector cell into close proximity with the tumor cell, thereby promoting tumor cell lysis. The mAb can also be used to bring other materials with cytotoxic activity into contact with the tumor cell. Presumably no normal counterparts will be targeted if the mAb is sufficiently tumor-specific. As with all other forms of immunotherapy, the in vivo mechanism of action of mAbs is uncertain, despite the rationale. It is possible that mAb is cytostatic in the absence of complement or that it influences the metabolism of the cell completely apart from immunologically based effects.

In their application to clinical practice, a number of limitations of mAbs have been identified. These include (1) cross-reactivity with normal tissues; (2) uptake in lymphoid organs, including spleen and lymph nodes; (3) binding to circulating antigen instead of the tumor cell; (4) "antigenic modulation" (loss of surface antigen) of the tumor; (5) development of human antimouse antibodies, which prevent chronic administration of mAb; (6) sanctuary sites, such as the central nervous system, that are not easily penetrated; and (7) antigenic heterogeneity of tumor cell populations.[51]

An early trial of mAb generated against the idiotype region of surface immunoglobulin on low-grade non-Hodgkin's lymphoma showed clinical activity, eliciting several complete remissions.[52] However, the mAb eventually selected for an antigen-negative variant subpopulation of lymphoma cells, "antigenic modulation" became ineffective. INF-α has been combined with mAb treatment in lymphomas and appears to enhance antitumor activity, perhaps by its cytomodulatory actions.[53]

A chimeric mAb—genetically engineered to be mostly human on a mouse background—generated against CD20, which is a marker characteristic of B cells present on more than 90% of B lymphoma cells, has shown considerable activity against non-Hodgkin's lymphomas. This mAb, rituximab (Rituxan, IDEC Pharmaceuticals), caused remissions in 48% of patients with relapsed low-grade or follicular lymphoma in a multicenter trial, with a 13-month projected median duration of response.[54] For patients with chemotherapy-resistant disease, or as first-line therapy, this mAb may be of considerable usefulness with little toxicity.

mAb infusions have also been studied in melanoma. Included among these are R-24 (a mAb generated against the GD3 ganglioside) and 3F8 (specific for the GD2 ganglioside), which have produced response rates of approximately 17 to 22%. Responses were seen mainly in subcutaneous sites and lymph nodes, although occasional responses were noted in other sites. mAb trials in other solid tumor types have produced less activity.

An important addition to the treatment of HER-2/*neu*–positive breast cancer is trastuzumab, a chimeric (humanized) mouse antibody that does not elicit human antimouse antibodies that might neutralize its activity. Trastuzumab reacts against a 185-kd extracellular domain protein, causing a variety of effects on the cancer cell, including cytostasis in the absence of complement in vitro. As with other mAbs, a variety of other mechanisms of action in vivo are possible but not yet definitively determined. Clinical remissions, mainly partial, have been noted in 14 to 25% of patients, with a suggestion that higher response rates may be elicited when the mAb is combined with anthracycline chemotherapy. Cardiac dysfunction with the combination compromises its usefulness, and FDA approval is limited to the mAb used alone.

Studies have been performed with mAbs conjugated with cytotoxic chemotherapeutic agents,[55] radioisotopes such as [131]I, yttrium 90[56], or potent toxins such as ricin A chain.[57] Occasional responses have been obtained with each of these approaches, which have not yet reached their full potential therapeutically. Some difficulties in the use of immunoconjugates include (1) unstable attachment of the toxic material to the mAb, (2) toxicity, (3) inability to generate sufficient amounts of the immunoconjugate, and (4) inability of the conjugate to be internalized by the tumor target. Nevertheless, the success of unconjugated mAbs such as trastuzumab and rituximab suggests that immunoconjugates may yet be a strong addition to the biologic armamentarium.

## Adoptive Immunotherapy

The transfer of T helper or T effector cells is a direct way to attack an immunogenic tumor in vivo. Many precedents for this form of treatment exist in animal models, the most relevant of which may be those of the University of Washington group.[58] In their work, CD4 cells were more effective than CD8 cells in transferring immunity to a syngeneic mouse. However, in mice with little or no immunity (severe combined immunodeficiency [SCID] mice), CD8 cells have direct effects on transplanted human tumors.

### HIGH-DOSE INTERLEUKIN-2 AND LYMPHOKINE-ACTIVATED KILLER CELLS

In humans, the first extensive studies of adoptive immunotherapy were performed by Rosenberg and colleagues. That group used a combination of thrice-daily bolus infusions of IL-2 and ex vivo–cultivated LAK cells.[59] Subsequent trials conducted by these authors and others have confirmed activity, especially in renal cancer and melanoma, with response rates of approximately 15 to 25%.[60–62]

The most severe toxicity of high-dose bolus IL-2 consists

of a "capillary-leak syndrome," with peripheral edema and sometimes pulmonary edema, hypotension, respiratory insufficiency, and azotemia. Mental depression and suicidal impulses have also occurred. Intensive care unit monitoring proved essential in early trials, and only patients with an excellent performance status should be considered for this type of treatment.

Since IL-2 has a short serum half-life, several investigators have attempted to use continuous infusions, both to improve effectiveness and to perhaps diminish toxicity by maintaining lower peak levels.[63] Although clinical regressions in melanoma, renal carcinoma, and occasionally other tumors have been noted, the response rates and the toxicity are not very different from those with bolus infusions (unpublished data).[64, 66] In addition, as experience with constant infusions of IL-2 has grown, the consensus is that it is more toxic than the equivalent bolus dose.[65]

Although mouse models indicated that ex vivo–cultured LAK cells improved the response to IL-2, it is now clear in humans that IL-2 alone is sufficient and perhaps desirable. There does not appear to be a significant relationship between tumor response and number of LAK cells infused,[66] nor has increased LAK activity in the blood consistently been associated with response.[67] Studies attempting to emulate the original National Cancer Institute experience have failed to show a significant difference in response rates, response duration, or median survival of IL-2 alone compared with IL-2 plus LAK cells.[60] A 1993 prospective, randomized trial comparing bolus IL-2 with bolus IL-2 plus LAK cells showed no significant difference in response rates or survival, with only a trend toward increased survival in the combination arm for patients with melanoma.[62]

Some have suggested that the only consistent effect of the addition of LAK cells to IL-2 is an increase in toxicity. LAK cells are not specific for tumor targets and do not home selectively to the tumor after intravenous infusion. Cytotoxicity of LAK cells against nonmalignant cells such as vascular endothelial cells occurs, accounting for the increased toxicity of the IL-2 plus LAK cell regimen.[68] Albertini and colleagues found a higher incidence of fever, hypotension, and decline in Karnofsky performance status in patients treated with LAK cells plus IL-2 than in those given IL-2 alone.[69] It has been asserted, but not proved, that in vitro selection of a specific subpopulation of LAK cells through their adherence to plastic (adherent LAK cells, or A-LAK cells) will improve the therapeutic index of this therapy.[70]

## ADOPTIVE IMMUNOTHERAPY WITH TUMOR-INFILTRATING LYMPHOCYTES

If LAK cells have little therapeutic effect as adoptive immunotherapy, what of more specific effector cells? A good deal of attention has been given to tumor-infiltrating lymphocytes (TILs).[71] T cells isolated from tumor biopsy specimens and cultured with autologous tumor cells to expand the number of specific antitumor CTL cells were then reinfused into the autologous host with metastatic disease. Unlike LAK cells, radiolabeled TILs traveled to metastatic sites. Response rates as high as 38% in metastatic melanoma have been reported with IL-2 and TILs.[72] Large-scale confirmatory trials are

difficult to perform, and only relatively few studies have looked at tumor types other than melanoma.[73–75]

Considerable attention has been paid to using TILs as a vehicle for transporting genes for the expression of lymphokines such as INF-α or TNF-α to the tumor site.[71] It is hoped that the lymphocytes will be self-activating in vivo, without requiring (toxic) systemic administration of lymphokines. This approach is only in its infancy, and its therapeutic advantages have not yet been demonstrated.

Among the practical problems with TIL generation are (1) the requirement for an accessible tumor mass, (2) the need to culture TILs for several months before sufficient specific T cells are generated, (3) difficulty in generating an adequate number of TILs for therapy, and (4) variations in the composition of the TIL (CD4+ vs. CD8+) from patient to patient. These factors have limited cooperative group trials of this therapeutic option, which could provide more substantial evidence that TIL adds benefit to IL-2 alone.

## ADOPTIVE IMMUNOTHERAPY WITH PEPTIDE-SPECIFIC CYTOTOXIC T LYMPHOCYTES

It is now feasible to produce immunized peptide-specific CTLs in vitro. Both antigen-presenting cells and CD8+ CTL precursors are present in the peripheral blood, and large numbers of each may be obtained from leukapheresis specimens. The process usually requires only 3 to 4 weeks, yielding nearly a billion CTLs routinely from $1 \times 10^{10}$ peripheral blood mononuclear cells. The leukapheresis may be performed in cancer patients or normal HLA-matched donors. Antigen-presenting cells such as autologous DCs may be used in this process. *Drosophila melanogaster* (fruit fly) cells transduced with HLA-A2.1, ICAM-1, and CD80 were also used in our clinical trial (Mitchell MS, et al, unpublished data, 2000). The cell membrane of *Drosophila* is essentially a "blank slate" without human self-peptides onto which tumor epitopes can be inserted for presentation to T cells. *Drosophila* cells disintegrate at 37° C and are not transferred into patients. In a phase I trial, we tested CTLs immunized against a tyrosinase monomer epitope as a prototype for this approach. Eleven patients were given a total of $5 \times 10^8$ CTLs in three to five daily infusions, without additional IL-2, and experienced no toxicity. One partial remission (mediastinal and iliac lymph nodes) lasting more than 3 months was noted. In the future, the administration of IL-2 and perhaps other T-cell growth factors will be desirable to improve the in vivo survival of the infused T cells. As with in vivo vaccination, many epitopes, rather than one, should be used as immunogens in vitro.

## OUTPATIENT SCHEDULES OF INTERLEUKIN-2 ALONE

A practical approach that would permit medical oncologists who practice apart from large medical centers to administer IL-2 would involve lower-dose IL-2 schedules. Lower dose schedules would avert some of the toxicity and thus the need for hospitalization. Single daily bolus infusions and subcutaneous administration of IL-2 have given results comparable to higher dose regimens, at least in melanomas and renal cell carcinomas, and with less toxicity. These regimens have permitted the outpatient administration of IL-2, with only a rare need for hospitalization and relatively few patients having to discontinue treatment because of overwhelming toxicity.

Our group used single daily intravenous boluses of IL-2 (usually 21.6 million IU/m$^2$/day) for 5 consecutive days on 2 consecutive weeks, preceded by 350 mg/m$^2$ of cyclophosphamide, to treat metastatic melanoma.[74, 75] This cycle was repeated twice more, with the course covering a 2-month period. The response rate (PRs and CRs) in 39 patients was 26%. It was 28% including a "minor" responder whose tumor shrank 44% and then remained stable for more than 4 years. Evidence emerged from that study, from a vantage point of 5 years, that the cohort of responders (but not the group as a whole) may have had improved survival. The median survival for the responders was 18 months, with 27% of the patients living more than a year and 10% living more than 2 years. The longest responder lived 50 months. Other investigators have subsequently shown that subcutaneous self-administered low-dose IL-2 had significant clinical activity alone or when combined with INF-α in melanomas and renal carcinoma, with relatively little toxicity.[76, 77]

## ADOPTIVE IMMUNOTHERAPY FOR OTHER TUMORS

Although adoptive immunotherapy has been most commonly investigated in melanoma and renal cancer, antitumor responses have also been reported in non-Hodgkin's lymphoma and breast, lung, ovarian, and colon cancers.[78–81] This suggests that this therapy may be combined with other modalities, including cytotoxic chemotherapy, in these other tumor types. Adoptive immunotherapy may find an important niche in states of "minimal residual disease" following dose-intensive chemotherapy. This includes patients who undergo bone marrow transplantation in which bone marrow and peripheral blood are available for in vitro immunologic stimulation with tumor antigens as well as patients who received high-dose chemotherapy and are being supported by peripheral stem cells and colony-stimulating factors.

Several trials using the adoptive transfer of "killer" macrophages have been initiated in the past, but the filtering action of the reticuloendothelial system theoretically limits this therapy. Regional (e.g., intraperitoneal) administration may be one way to circumvent this potential problem.

## CONCLUSIONS AND PERSPECTIVE ON ADOPTIVE IMMUNOTHERAPY

Although high doses of bolus intravenous IL-2 (equivalent to 22 million IU/m$^2$ every 8 hours) were originally thought to be more effective than lower doses, particularly in renal cell carcinoma, a dose-response relationship has not been well established in any tumor. Certainly, lower doses appear to cause clinical responses, although the precise definition of "low dose" has not been established. In any case, there seems to be at least a plateau after a certain dose level, unlike in chemotherapy, where more is generally better.

Adoptive immunotherapy with T lymphocytes (CTLs) is potentially highly selective for tumor cells, whereas LAK cell therapy adds little to IL-2 alone. Selectivity depends on the differences between a tumor and its normal tissue counterpart. Cytotoxicity of normal cells accounts for some of the toxicity of adoptive immunotherapy.

Cytokines have a number of toxicities, which may be considerable in degree at higher doses, but the toxicity is different from that of chemotherapy. Fatigue, depression (sometimes leading to suicidal impulses), flu-like signs and symptoms (especially high fever), capillary-leak syndrome, and damage to myocardium are some of the effects found with IL-2, which is the most extensively studied of the cytokines. Many or most of these toxic effects can be controlled by careful attention to dose and supporting medications, such as indomethacin and antidepressants.

Tumor types such as melanoma and renal cancer, for which chemotherapy does not generally improve survival and often elicits a poor objective response, may be treated with resulting long-term survival in some patients. Standard definitions of objective response based solely on degree of regression[82] are not entirely applicable. Many investigators have seen evidence of long-term stable disease, minor response, or partial remissions following adoptive immunotherapy, sometimes without maintenance treatment. Nevertheless, the duration of response is generally longest in patients with CRs,[83] and the 10% of patients who live 10 years or more are drawn from that group.

The future use of adoptive immunotherapy will probably involve defined populations of CD8$^+$ and CD4$^+$ T cells in combination, each specifically immunized against the relevant epitopes in vitro. Since these cells can be obtained from the peripheral blood and are at least as effective as those drawn from more difficult to obtain sources, the technology involved will be more generally available to oncologists.

## Restorative Immunotherapy

Deficient subpopulations of T cells can be repleted by the administration of thymic hormones and levamisole, which may have a similar activity. In some conditions, such as oat cell lung carcinoma, deficient T cells have been identified, but clinical studies looking for low CD4/CD8 T-cell ratios, for example, have been rare. This has prevented a more directed approach to repletion as a clinical strategy before attempts to increase antitumor immune responses by other means.

Often the problem is not an absolute decrease in the number of T cells but in suppressor influences exerted on them—influences secreted or elicited by the tumor. Both suppressor macrophages and suppressor T-cell influences have been identified. Suppressor macrophages appear to inhibit cellular immunity at least in part through a PGE$_2$-mediated mechanism. Nonsteroidal anti-inflammatory drugs, including indomethacin, have shown some ability to depress the function of suppressor macrophages.

Histamine antagonists, including cimetidine, ranitidine, and famotidine, have shown biomodulatory effects such as inhibiting T suppressor cells, increasing endogenous serum levels of IL-2, and enhancing CTL and NK-cell activity. Occasional cases of partial responses in various tumor types have been described. Although sporadic reports of clinical responses have been published, most studies of agents such as cimetidine as a single agent in melanoma and renal cancer have shown little or no activity.[84]

Several chemotherapeutic agents administered in less than the usual therapeutic dose have enhanced cell-mediated immunity.[85, 86] Chemotherapeutic agents such as cyclophosphamide can reduce immunosuppressive soluble mediators (such as C-reactive protein) and diminish the absolute number or function of T suppressor lymphocytes. Although immunomodulatory doses of chemotherapy may not be active against malignancies as single agents, they may have potential in combination with other biomodulators, as in the case of cyclophosphamide with IL-2. Other potential effects could include reduction of interferon-induced resistance to NK cells; increasing NK cell activity; damaging tumor cell membranes, thereby making tumor cells more susceptible to effector cells; and stimulating the production of cytokines such as IL-2.[87]

As more knowledge is gained about the importance of cytokines such as IL-10 and TGF-β in downmodulating immune responses as well as the degree to which tumors evoke those cytokines, new strategies will be devised that specifically address "suppressor" cells from that perspective. Blocking IL-10 and TGF-β by specific mAbs or antisense RNA is a potential option that has not yet been fully exploited.

## Cytomodulatory Immunotherapy

Tumor cells may potentially evade immune recognition and destruction through loss or reduced expression of their MHC molecules or downregulation of TAP expression, or both. This leads to poor expression of tumor epitopes and camouflage from detection by T cells. Several agents, such as TNF-α and the INFs, appear to be useful in alleviating this problem.

INFs are low-molecular-weight proteins produced by leukocytes or fibroblasts (INF-α and INF-β) and T lymphocytes (INF-γ), which were originally discovered through their antiviral properties. INFs have a remarkably wide range of other biologic functions: they increase NK cell activity, have a direct antiproliferative effect on tumor cells, induce tumor cell differentiation, and exhibit antiangiogenic activity. The toxicity of INFs comprises flu-like symptoms (fever, malaise, fatigue); central and peripheral nervous system problems, especially depression and peripheral neuropathies; hepatic dysfunction (exacerbated significantly by alcohol consumption); and decreased leukocytes and platelets.

INF-γ increases the expression of MHC class I and II molecules and tumor epitopes on tumor cells. INF-α is similar, although it lacks a major effect on MHC class II. Interferons also increase expression of adhesion molecules such as ICAM-1 on tumor cells, which are involved in their interaction with the reciprocal molecules (specifically LFA-1 for ICAM-1) on T and LAK cells. Interferons can increase the expression of antigens such as CEA, TAG-72, and CA-125 on some tumor lines. These actions support the use of INFs to upregulate antigens on the patient's tumor in combination with therapies that increase the immune response against that tumor.

The major effects of INF-α, thus far the only interferon released for general oncologic use, have been on hematologic malignancies. Hairy cell leukemia, low-grade lymphomas, chronic myelogenous leukemia, and multiple myeloma are all susceptible to treatment. Solid tumors have been more resistant, with response rates of 20% or less.[88–90] The major exception to the usefulness of INF-α may be in melanoma, in which a high-dose regimen was shown to extend the median survival of patients by 1 year, relative to untreated controls.[91] The optimal dose of INF-α has not been established, but it is clear that not only high-dose regimens are effective. Tolerable regimens less than 10 million units/m²/day, subcutaneously three times per week, have caused responses in metastatic melanoma patients, particularly after administration of active specific immunotherapy.[92]

Perhaps the most potentially useful effect of INF-α is its cytomodulatory activity, which would make it an important component of a combination with other biomodulators. We noted responses in 8 of 18 melanoma patients who received INF-α after failing to respond to Melacine.[93] Five of the 8 patients had site-specific CRs, and one patient died of another cause in 1 year, still with a clinical CR. The median duration of survival of responders to INF-α was 36 months; for the entire group it was 10 months. Those patients who had a clinical response at 4 months, when we could be certain whether response or progression had occurred, had a 75% likelihood of living more than 1 year, whereas those who had not responded to interferon had a 13% likelihood.

The 18 patients were immunized, with increased precursors of CTLs in the blood, but failed to have a clinical response after receiving Melacine. It is possible that the CTLs generated by the vaccination were unable to attack tumor targets that had downregulated their tumor epitopes or MHC molecules, or both. INF-α treatment may have upregulated those antigens, enabling the CTLs to destroy the tumor. A similar approach seeking to use immunomodulatory effects of interferon has combined it with IL-2. Several investigators have seen objective tumor responses primarily in melanoma and renal cancer, although it is unclear whether the combination produces increased antitumor activity compared with each agent alone.[77]

The high toxicity and lack of clinical activity of systemically administered TNF-α have been disappointing.[94] Similarly, INF-γ has, in general, not been shown to be active as a single agent in malignancy.[95] Nonetheless, both agents have proven cytomodulatory activity and may achieve their maximal effectiveness in combination with other biomodulators. TNF-α may also be useful in combination with chemotherapy for the treatment of in-transit melanoma metastases on the extremities.

## Combination Immunotherapy

A logical next step in immunotherapy is the combination of biomodulators from different categories. Possible theoretical advantages of this approach include (1) additive or synergistic effects with agents that act by different mechanisms, (2) the ability to use lower doses of each agent in a combination, and (3) concurrent or sequential administration to create the optimal milieu for tumor cell killing through upregulation of tumor epitopes or recruitment of several populations of effector cells into the tumor site. Although chemotherapy is often immunosuppressive, certain agents might be used in this combination for their immunostimulatory effects. For example, low doses of cisplatin, mitomycin C, and doxorubicin augment rather than suppress an immune response.[96, 97]

Based on animal studies showing synergism between IL-2 and INF-α, intravenous INF-α was combined with bolus intravenous IL-2 in patients with melanoma. A response rate of 39%, including three CRs and 10 PRs, was seen.[98] Other studies using IL-2, LAK cells, INF, and immunomodulatory doses of cyclophosphamide and doxorubicin have been reported.[102]

It is too early to assess definitively whether combinations of biomodulators are superior to each component of the combination alone. However, there is some indirect support for this approach. The original studies with leukocyte-extracted INF-α prior to the advent of recombinant material showed response rates of approximately 20 to 35% in patients with breast cancer with a preparation containing less than 1% interferon.[100] This is in contrast to recombinant INF-α studies, which have shown virtually no antitumor activity against this cancer.[101, 102] One implication is that a combination of cytokines might be efficacious. Similarly, antitumor effects have been seen with low-dose cyclophosphamide and IL-2 in previously treated breast cancer. Because of the complexity of the immune system, it is unlikely that even large quantities of only a single soluble mediator would suffice to stimulate an optimal antitumor immune response.

## Combining Immunotherapy with Cytotoxic Chemotherapy

A clear theoretical rationale exists for the combination of cytotoxic agents and immunotherapy. Cytotoxic chemotherapy may reduce the absolute number of tumor targets that effector cells would need to kill. Resistance of a tumor to chemotherapeutic agents does not alter its susceptibility to lysis by immunologic means, that is, there is no cross-resistance. Another postulated function of cytoreductive therapy is that it clears the bone marrow and lymphoid organs for subsequent repopulation by cytokine-induced effector cells.[103] This phenomenon may actually be due to a compensatory release of endogenous cytokines from other lymphoid organs, thereby enhancing the growth of infused T cells. The lack of myelosuppression seen with biomodulators could allow better tolerability of combination regimens. Damage of tumor cell membranes may make target cells more susceptible to immune-mediated lysis. Finally, standard-dose and even dose-intensive chemotherapy regimens that do not damage stem cells do not interfere with the induction of TILs with IL-2. It would therefore seem reasonable to treat patients sequentially with chemotherapy followed by immunotherapy, or perhaps with an alternating regimen.

Several chemoimmunotherapy regimens have shown response rates greater than 50% in metastatic melanoma.[104, 105] These regimens consisting of three- or four-drug chemother-

apy plus INF-α and IL-2 are for the most part highly toxic, having the combined toxicity of chemotherapy and the cytokines. Durable responses are approximately 10%, which are conceivably attributable to the biologic therapy, judging from results with IL-2 alone. It is debatable whether the increase in short-term remissions justifies the toxicity endured by the majority of patients, who do not achieve durable responses. In addition, once this combination therapy has failed, further treatment options are extremely limited. On at least theoretical grounds, one must be extremely careful to use immunotherapy after the immunosuppressive effects of chemotherapy have dissipated to avoid nullifying the immunostimulatory activity.[91] The time at which immunosuppression caused by powerful chemicals such as the alkylating agents (e.g., bis-chloroethyl-nitrosourea [BCNU]) has ceased should be restudied with modern methods because studies in an earlier era necessarily lacked the sophistication in assays that is now possible.

## Colony-Stimulating Factors

Granulocyte colony-stimulating factor (G-CSF) and GM-CSF are discussed in Chapter 9. In vitro data indicate that they may mediate tumor cell lysis through the generation of tumoricidal macrophages and neutrophils. Early clinical trials involving GM-CSF to evaluate its potential to activate tumoricidal macrophages have been reported[106] and one PR was seen in a patient with sarcoma.[107] Although significant activity in neoplastic disease with G-CSF has not been seen in these relatively small studies to date, the potential of these biomodulators in the generation of antitumor effector cells requires further evaluation.

A theoretical caveat should be noted, however. GM-CSF has the potential to affect the tumor-host relationship adversely. Some breast cancer cell lines produce GM-CSF constitutively, which acts as a growth factor. In addition, the secreted GM-CSF can elicit suppressor macrophages, which downregulate proliferation of T cells.[108] Thus, by these two mechanisms, GM-CSF might conceivably enhance the growth of the breast cancer in vivo and should be used systemically with caution when this is likely to be a problem.

As we noted in an earlier section, the insertion of a gene for GM-CSF amplifies the immunogenicity of some tumors in mice by attracting antigen-processing and -presenting cells such as DCs and macrophages and stimulating their production of cytokines.[22] The importance of that observation is the pinpointing of a specific cytokine that has adjuvant properties. It is likely from animal models that GM-CSF can act as a potent adjuvant in humans when mixed with a tumor vaccine, but that issue remains to be studied in detail.

## Antiangiogenesis

Blood vessel blocking (antiangiogenic) agents are important new biologic materials in the fight against cancer. A primary tumor cannot be nourished by diffusion from capillaries if it exceeds a distance of six to eight cell layers, or approximately 100 μm. Thus, a tumor that does not generate its own new blood supply from the arteries supplying the tissue where the tumor is located will remain small.[112] If the immune response that we have been discussing is active, the tumor will presumably be eradicated by it at that size. Similarly, a tumor must generate neovasculature to metastasize. Vasculature induced by tumor cells must migrate into the tumor tissue as a second important step in nourishing a primary tumor, allowing tumor cells to spread to distant sites and then permitting the metastatic cells themselves to vascularize. Furthermore, metastatic tumor sites must continually revascularize, unlike normal organs. Thus, antiangiogenesis may be crucial in preventing primary tumors from flourishing, in preventing metastasis, and in causing regression of established metastases. Since normal organs do not continually revascularize, antiangiogenic materials do not have deleterious effects on them, although wound healing is adversely affected.

Cytokines made by the tumor, particularly basic fibroblast growth factor (bFGF), vascular endothelial growth factor (VEGF), and TNF-$\alpha$, stimulate vascular endothelial cells as one early step in this invasive process. Regulatory elements on the tumor cell and the tumor vasculature include the integrins, a family of substances that interact with the substratum. An important integrin is $\alpha v\beta 3$, which attaches to the arginine-glycine-aspartic acid (R-G-D) motif on various molecules, such as fibronectin, vitronectin, laminin, and collagen, and $\alpha 5\beta 1$, which is far more specific, binding to fibronectin. Both serve to control the process of invasion of the stroma and attachment to vascular endothelium.[111] Matrix metalloproteinases from the tumor that stimulate vascular endothelium is another means by which a tumor's invasion of the vasculature is accomplished.

One group of antiangiogenic materials consists of antibodies to an integrin such as $\alpha v\beta 3$ or $\alpha 5\beta 1$, which block the interaction of the integrin with its ligand. Antagonists of the various growth factors that stimulate the vascular endothelium constitute another potential class of antiangiogenic agents. In addition, matrix metalloproteinase inhibitors, such as the experimental agent marimastat (British Biotech), are also capable of antiangiogenesis. An antibody against $\alpha v\beta 3$ integrin that blocks the vascularization and growth of human breast cancer in an animal model[111] is in phase I trials, whereas marimastat is in phase II clinical trials for the treatment of a variety of chemotherapy-resistant cancers, such as those of the lung and pancreas. Thalidomide, originally introduced as an anxiolytic and sedative agent, has been approved for use as an antiangiogenic material. Indeed, many of its effects on the limbs of the developing fetus were probably due to that property. Clinical trials of angiostatin and endostatin are imminent, and indeed many of the largest pharmaceutical houses plan trials of antiangiogenic materials within the next few years. This area of research, which has moved slowly since Folkman's original hypotheses of the late 1960s and early 1970s, has, like other areas of biologic research, received a strong impetus from discoveries in molecular science about the mediators and receptors involved in the process.

## General Conclusions About Biologic Therapy

Although data from randomized trials are only now emerging, one of the most important features of biologic therapy already appears to be its ability to increase the life span of patients who respond. Cohorts of responding patients given vaccines (usually for melanoma) in early or metastatic disease or IL-2 or INF-$\alpha$ have had survivals far exceeding the life expectancy of similar patients given chemotherapy or no treatment. Survival for years rather than months has become more frequent, even though metastatic disease has not always been completely eradicated. The prevention of further metastases, to additional organs and to additional sites within affected organs, has been more important in the prolongation of survival than shrinkage of existing lesions. This stands in direct contrast with chemotherapy, in which only complete remissions have translated into improved survivals. In our clinical trials of biologic therapies, we have continued treatment until progression of disease occurs, accepting stability of disease as perhaps indicative of a response in the first 2 to 3 months. Long-term stability ($>6$ months) is also considered tantamount to a response because increased survivals have been noted in this group of patients as well as in those with shrinkage of index lesions.

The quality of life of patients on biologic treatments is often nearly normal, particularly with vaccines, although some forms of treatment, such as IL-2, are accompanied by a variety of nontrivial side effects that are quite different from those of chemotherapy. An improvement in the quality of life would be consistent with the rationale that spurred the use of biologic approaches to cancer treatment: that they are innately nondestructive, more physiologic, and more efficient in detecting microscopic residua of cancer cells.

Biologic therapy differs from chemotherapy and should not be judged entirely by the same criteria. Biomodulators generally fail to adhere to conventional "dose-response" standards. The optimal biologic dose is usually significantly less than the maximum tolerated dose, which is different from most types of chemotherapy. Indeed, dose intensity considerations are paramount in that form of treatment.[112] Since there is no cross-resistance of tumors, that is, resistance to both chemotherapy and biologic therapy, clinical responses are possible in generally chemotherapy-resistant tumors (such as melanoma and renal cancer) as well as in more chemotherapy-sensitive tumors (such as breast cancer) that have become resistant. Also, biologic therapy takes some time to achieve its effects, in some cases 6 months or more for interferon. That means that rampant disease must first be halted by chemotherapy. A judgment about whether the biologic therapy has been effective should be delayed until clear evidence of progression of disease is found.

It is always necessary to use new anticancer agents singly to test their toxicity and efficacy before venturing to treat with combinations. We are now at the point where many phase I and phase II studies of single biomodulators have been completed. Rational combinations are now feasible with the information gained from studying the immunologic effects of single agents. These extend beyond combinations of cytokines to include cancer vaccines with adoptive T-cell immunotherapy and the addition of cytokines such as the INFs to upregulate the display of tumor antigens in situ. That strategy would enhance the ability of specific immunotherapeutic approaches to find their intended target in vivo. Biologic approaches to cancer are near or at the point of joining cytotoxic therapies in an equal partnership—alone or in carefully planned sequential combinations.

# REFERENCES

1. Mitchell MS. Biomodulation: a classification and overview. In: Reif AE, Mitchell MS, eds. Immunity to cancer. Orlando: Academic Press, 1985:401–11.

2. Hersey P, Murray E, Grace J, McCarthy WH. Current research on immunopathology of melanoma: analysis of lymphocyte populations in relation to antigen expression and histological features of melanoma. Pathology 1985;17:385–91.

3. Rubin JT, Elwood LJ, Rosenberg SA, Lotze MT. Immunohistochemical correlates of response to recombinant interleukin-2–based immunotherapy in humans. Cancer Res 1989;49:7086–92.

4. Mitchell MS. Active specific immunotherapy of cancer: therapeutic vaccines ("theraccines") for the treatment of disseminated malignancies. In: Mitchell MS, ed. Biological approaches to cancer treatment: biomodulation. New York: McGraw-Hill, 1992:326–51.

5. Robertson MJ, Ritz J. Biology and clinical relevance of human natural killer cells. Blood 1990;76:2421–38.

6. Herberman RB, Ortaldo JR. Natural killer cells: their roles in defenses against disease. Science 1981;214:24–30.

7. Roder JC, Haliotis T, Klein M, et al. A new immunodeficiency disorder in humans involving NK cells. Nature 1980;284:553–55.

8. Grimm EA, Mazumder A, Zhang HZ, Rosenberg SA. Lymphokine-activated killer cell phenomenon. Lysis of natural killer-resistant fresh solid tumor cells by interleukin 2–activated autologous peripheral blood lymphocytes. J Exp Med 1982; 155:1823–41.

9. Lanier LL, Phillips JH. Human thymic and peripheral blood non–MHC-restricted cytotoxic lymphocytes. Med Oncol Tumor Pharmacother 1986;3:247–54.

10. Harel W, Shau H, Hadley CG, et al. Increased lysis of melanoma by in vivo-elicited human lymphokine-activated killer cells after addition of antiganglioside antibodies in vitro. Cancer Res 1990;50:6311–15.

11. Jerne NK. Towards a network theory of the immune response. Ann Immunol (Paris) 1974;125C:373–89.

12. Livingston PO. Approaches to augmenting the IgG antibody response to melanoma ganglioside vaccines. Ann N Y Acad Sci 1993;690:204–13.

13. Longenecker BM, Reddish M, Koganty R, MacLean GD. Immune responses of mice and human breast cancer patients following immunization with synthetic sialyl-Tn conjugated to KLH plus Detox adjuvant. Ann NY Acad Sci 1993;690:276–91.

14. Magarian-Blander J, Domenech N, Finn OJ. Specific and effective T-cell recognition of cells transfected with a truncated human mucin cDNA. Ann NY Acad Sci 1993;690:231–43.

15. Van der Bruggen P, Traversari C, et al. A gene encoding an antigen recognized by cytolytic T lymphocytes on a human melanoma. Science 1991;254:1643–47.

16. Kawakami Y, Robbins PF, Rosenberg SA. Human melanoma antigens recognized by T lymphocytes. Keio J Med 1996; 45:100–8.

17. Reddish MA, MacLean GD, Koganty RR, et al. Anti-MUC1 class I restricted CTLs in metastatic breast cancer patients immunized with a synthetic MUC1 peptide. Int J Cancer 1998; 76:817–23.

18. Longenecker BM, MacLean GD. Prospects for mucin epitopes in cancer vaccines. Immunologist 1993;1:89–93.

19. Tsang KY, Zaremba S, Nieroda CA, et al. Generation of human cytotoxic T-cells specific for human carcinoembryonic antigen (CEA) epitopes from patients immunized with recombinant vaccinia-CEA (rV-CEA) vaccine. J Natl Cancer Inst 1995;87:

20. Tahara H, Lotze MT. Antitumor effects of interleukin-12 (IL-12): applications for the immunotherapy and gene therapy of cancer. Gene Ther 1995;2:96–106.

21. Mitchell MS. Biological approaches to cancer treatment: biomodulation. New York: McGraw-Hill, 1992.

22. Pardoll DM, Golumbek P, Levitsky H, Jaffee E. Molecular engineering of the antitumor immune response. Bone Marrow Transplant 1992;9:Suppl 1:182–6.

23. Dranoff G, Jaffee E, Lazenby A, et al. Vaccination with irradiated tumor cells engineered to secrete murine granulocyte-macrophage colony-stimulating factor stimulates potent, specific and long-lasting anti-tumor immunity. Proc Natl Acad Sci USA 1993;90:3539–43.

24. Sarosdy MF, Lamm DL. Long-term results of intravesical bacillus Calmette-Guerin therapy for superficial bladder cancer. J Urol 1989;142:719–22.

25. Klimpel GR, Henney CS. BCG-induced suppressor cells. J Immunol 1978;120:563–69.

26. Bennett JA, Rao VS, Mitchell MS. Systemic bacillus Calmette-Guérin activates natural suppressor cells. Proc Natl Acad Sci USA 1978;75:5142–44.

27. Bystryn J-C, Ferrone S, Livingston P (eds). Specific immunotherapy of cancer with vaccines. Ann NY Acad Sci 1993;690:1–411.

28. Mitchell MS. Active specific immunotherapy of melanoma. Br Med Bull 1995;51:631–46.

29. Laucius JF, Bodurtha AJ, Mastrangelo MJ, Bellet RE. A phase II study of autologous irradiated tumor cells plus BCG in patients with metastatic malignant melanoma. Cancer 1977;40:2091–93.

30. Berd D, Maguire HJ, McCue P, Mastrangelo MJ. Treatment of metastatic melanoma with an autologous tumor-cell vaccine: clinical and immunologic results in 64 patients. J Clin Oncol 1990;8:1858–67.

31. Berd DA, Maguire HC Jr, Schuchter LM, et al. Autologous hapten-modified melanoma vaccine as postsurgical adjuvant treatment after resection of nodal metastases. J Clin Oncol 1997;15:2359–70.

32. Murray DR, Cassel WA, Torbin AH, et al. Viral oncolysate in the management of malignant melanoma. II: Clinical studies. Cancer 1977;40:680–86.

33. Mittelman A, Chen ZJ, Kageshita T, et al. Active specific immunotherapy in patients with melanoma. A clinical trial with mouse antiidiotypic monoclonal antibodies elicited with syngeneic anti-high-molecular-weight-melanoma–associated antigen monoclonal antibodies [published erratum appears in J Clin Invest 1991;87:757]. J Clin Invest 1990;86:2136–44.

34. Quan WDY Jr, Dean GE, Spears L, et al. Active specific immunotherapy of metastatic melanoma with an anti-idiotype vaccine: a phase I/II trial of I-Mel-2 plus SAF-m. J Clin Oncol 1997;15:2103–10.

35. Hsu FJ, Benike C, Fagnoni F, et al. Vaccination of patients with B-cell lymphoma using autologous antigen-pulsed dendritic cells. Nat Med 1996;2:52–7.

36. Mitchell MS. A personal (biased) perspective on cancer "vaccines." Oncol Res 1997;9:459–65.

37. Mitchell MS. Perspective on the use of allogeneic vaccines for melanoma. Semin Oncol 1998;25:623–35.

38. Bystryn JC. Immunogenicity and clinical activity of a polyvalent melanoma antigen vaccine prepared from shed antigens. Ann NY Acad Sci 1993;690:190–203.

39. Mitchell MS, Kan-Mitchell J, Kempf RA, et al. Active specific immunotherapy of melanoma. Phase I trial of allogeneic melanoma lysates and a novel adjuvant. Cancer Res 1988;48:5883–93.

40. Mitchell MS, Harel W, Kempf RA, et al. Active-specific immunotherapy for melanoma. J Clin Oncol 1990;8:856–69.

41. Morton DL, Foshag LJ, Hoon DS, et al. Prolongation of survival in metastatic melanoma after active specific immunotherapy with a new polyvalent melanoma vaccine [published erratum appears in Ann Surg 1993;217:309]. Ann Surg 1992;216:463–82.

42. Hanna MG Jr, Hoover HC Jr. Active specific immunotherapy as an adjunct to the treatment of metastatic solid tumors. In: Reif AE, Mitchell MS, ed. Immunity to cancer. New York: Academic Press, 1985:429–42.

43. MacLean GD, Reddish M, Koganty RR, et al. Immunization of breast cancer patients using a synthetic sialyl-Tn glycoconjugate plus Detox adjuvant. Cancer Immunol Immunother 1993;36:215–22.

44. MacLean GD, Bowen-Yacyshyn MB, Samuel J, et al. Active immunization of human ovarian cancer patients against a common carcinoma (Thomsen-Friedenreich) determinant using a synthetic carbohydrate antigen. J Immunother 1992;11:292–305.

45. MacLean GD, Reddish M, Koganty RR, Longenecker BM. Immunization of breast cancer patients using a synthetic sialyl-Tn glycoconjugate plus Detox adjuvant. Cancer Immunol Immunother 1993;36:215–22.

46. Fendly B, Kotts C, Wong WLT, et al. Successful immunization of rhesus monkeys with the extracellular domain of p185 HER-2. A potential approach to human breast cancer. Vaccine Res 1993;2:129–39.

47. Gong J, Chen D, Kashiwaba M, Kufe D. Induction of antitumor activity by immunization with fusions of dendritic and carcinoma cells. Nat Med 1997;3:558–61.

48. Nestle FO, Alijagic S, Gilliet M, et al. Vaccination of melanoma patients with peptide- or tumor lysate–pulsed dendritic cells. Nat Med 1998;4:328–32.

49. Köhler G, Milstein C. Continuous cultures of fused cells secreting antibody of predefined specificity. Nature 1975; 256:495–97.

50. Köhler G, Milstein C. Derivation of specific antibody-producing tissue culture and tumor lines by cell fusion. Eur J Immunol 1976;6:511–19.

51. Biddle WC, Foon KA. Monoclonal antibodies in therapy: alone or conjugated with drugs. In: Mitchell MS, ed. Biological approaches to cancer treatment: biomodulation. New York: McGraw-Hill, 1992:209–51.

52. Meeker TC, Lowder J, Maloney DG, et al. A clinical trial of anti-idiotype therapy for B cell malignancy. Blood 1985;65:1349–63.

53. Brown SL, Miller RA, Horning SJ, et al. Treatment of B-cell lymphomas with anti-idiotype antibodies alone and in combination with alpha interferon. Blood 1989;73:651–61.

54. McLaughlin P, Grillo-Lopez AJ, Link BKLR, et al. Rituximab chimeric anti-CD20 monoclonal antibody therapy for relapsed indolent lymphoma: half of patients respond to a four-dose treatment program. J Clin Oncol 1998;16:2825–33.

55. Oldham RK. Custom-tailored drug immunoconjugates in cancer therapy. Mol Biother 1991;3:148–62.

56. Larson SM, Carrasquillo JA, McGuffin RW, et al. Use of I-131 labeled, murine Fab against a high molecular weight antigen of human melanoma: preliminary experience. Radiology 1985;155:487–92.

57. Spitler LE, del Rio M, Khentigan A, et al. Therapy of patients with malignant melanoma using a monoclonal antimelanoma antibody–ricin A chain immunotoxin. Cancer Res 1987;47:1717–23.

58. Greenberg PD, Klarnet JP, Kern DE, et al. Specific adoptive immunotherapy. In: Mitchell MS, ed. Immunity to cancer. II. New York: Academic Press, 1989:349–62.

59. Rosenberg SA, Lotze MT, Muul LM, et al. Observations on the systemic administration of autologous lymphokine-activated killer cells and recombinant interleukin-2 to patients with metastatic cancer. N Engl J Med 1985;313:1485–92.

60. Fisher RI, Coltman CA Jr, Doroshow JH, et al. Metastatic renal cancer treated with interleukin-2 and lymphokine-activated killer cells: a phase II clinical trial. Ann Intern Med 1988;108:518–23.

61. Margolin KA, Rayner AA, Hawkins MJ, et al. Interleukin-2 and lymphokine-activated killer cell therapy of solid tumors: analysis of toxicity and management guidelines. J Clin Oncol 1989;7:486–98.

62. Rosenberg SA, Lotze MT, Yang JC, et al. Prospective randomized trial of high-dose interleukin-2 alone or in conjunction with lymphokine-activated killer cells for the treatment of patients with advanced cancer [published erratum appears in J Natl Cancer Inst 1993;85:1091]. J Natl Cancer Inst 1993;85:622–32.

63. West WH, Tauer KW, Yanelli JR, et al. Constant-infusion recombinant interleukin-2 in adoptive immunotherapy of advanced cancer. N Engl J Med 1987;316:898–905.

64. Dillman RO, Oldham RK, Tauer KW, et al. Continuous interleukin-2 and lymphokine-activated killer cells for advanced cancer: a National Biotherapy Study Group trial. J Clin Oncol 1991;9:1233–40.

65. Cetus Consensus Conference on Interleukin-2, Scottsdale, Arizona, 1993.

66. Dutcher JP, Gaynor ER, Boldt DH, et al. A phase II study of high-dose continuous infusion interleukin-2 with lymphokine-activated killer cells in patients with metastatic melanoma. J Clin Oncol 1991;9:641–48.

67. Dutcher JP. Lymphokine-activated killer cells/tumor-infiltrating lymphocytes therapy: efficacy, toxicity, controversies. J Clin Apheresis 1990;5:80–2.

68. Lotze MT, Carrasquillo JA, Weinstein JN, et al. Monoclonal antibody imaging of human melanoma. Radioimmunodetection by subcutaneous or systemic injection. Ann Surg 1986;204:223–35.

69. Albertini MR, Sosman JA, Hank JA, et al. The influence of autologous lymphokine-activated killer cell infusions on the toxicity and antitumor effect of repetitive cycles of interleukin-2. Cancer 1990;66:2457–64.

70. Melder RJ, Whiteside TL, Vujanovic NL, et al. A new approach to generating antitumor effectors for adoptive immunotherapy using human adherent lymphokine-activated killer cells. Cancer Res 1988;48:3461–69.

71. Rosenberg SA. Karnofsky Memorial Lecture. The immunotherapy and gene therapy of cancer. J Clin Oncol 1992;10:180–99.

72. Dillman RO, Oldham RK, Barth NM, et al. Continuous interleukin-2 and tumor-infiltrating lymphocytes as treatment of advanced melanoma. A national biotherapy study group trial. Cancer 1991;68:1–8.

73. Topalian SL, Solomon D, Avis FP, et al. Immunotherapy of patients with advanced cancer using tumor-infiltrating lymphocytes and recombinant interleukin-2: a pilot study. J Clin Oncol 1988;6:839–53.

74. Kradin RL, Kurnick JT, Lazarus DS, et al. Tumour-infiltrating lymphocytes and interleukin-2 in treatment of advanced cancer. Lancet 1989;1:577–80.

75. Oldham RK, Dillman RO, Yannelli JR, et al. Continuous infusion interleukin-2 and tumor-derived activated cells as treatment of advanced solid tumors: a National Biotherapy Study Group trial. Mol Biother 1991;3:68–73.

76. Mitchell MS, Kempf RA, Harel W, et al. Effectiveness and tolerability of low-dose cyclophosphamide and low-dose intravenous interleukin-2 in disseminated melanoma. J Clin Oncol 1988;6:409–24.

77. Mitchell MS. Chemotherapy in combination with biomodulation: a 5-year experience with cyclophosphamide and interleukin-2. Semin Oncol 1992;19:80–7.

78. Atzpodien J, Körfer A, Franks CR, et al. Home therapy with recombinant interleukin-2 and interferon-alpha 2b in advanced human malignancies. Lancet 1990;335:1509–12.

79. Atzpodien J, Kirchner H. The out-patient use of recombinant human interleukin-2 and interferon alfa-2b in advanced malignancies. Eur J Cancer 1991;27:Suppl 4:S88–91

80. Weber JS, Yang JC, Topalian SL, et al. The use of interleukin-2 and lymphokine-activated killer cells for the treatment of patients with non-Hodgkin's lymphoma. [see comments] J Clin Oncol 1992;10:33–40.

81. Spicer DV, Kelley A, Herman R, et al. Low-dose recombinant interleukin-2 and low-dose cyclophosphamide in metastatic breast cancer. Cancer Immunol Immunother 1992;34:424–6.

82. Eberlein TJ, Schoof DD, Jung SE, et al. A new regimen of interleukin 2 and lymphokine-activated killer cells. Efficacy without significant toxicity. Arch Intern Med 1988;148:2571–76.

83. Bernstein ZP, Goldrosen MH, Vaickus L, et al. Interleukin-2 with ex vivo activated killer cells: therapy of advanced non–small-cell lung cancer. J Immunother 1991;10:383–7.

84. Oken MM, Creech RH, Tormey DC, et al. Toxicity and response criteria of the Eastern Cooperative Oncology Group. Am J Clin Oncol 1982;5:649–55.

85. Rosenberg SA, Lotze MT, Yang JC, et al. Experience with the use of high-dose interleukin-2 in the treatment of 652 cancer patients. Ann Surg 1989;210:474–84.

86. Armitage JO, Sidner RD. Antitumour effect of cimetidine. [letter] Lancet 1979;1:882–3.

87. Ehrke MJ, Mihich E, Berd D, Mastrangelo MJ. Effects of anticancer drugs on the immune system in humans. Semin Oncol 1989;16:230–53.

88. Berd D, Maguire HJ, Mastrangelo MJ. Potentiation of human cell-mediated and humoral immunity by low-dose cyclophosphamide. Cancer Res 1984;44:5439–43.

89. Mitchell MS. Combining chemotherapy with biological response modifiers in the treatment of cancer. J Natl Cancer Inst 1988;80:1445–50.

90. Creagan ET, Schaid DJ, Ahmann DL, Frytak S. Disseminated malignant melanoma and recombinant interferon: analysis of seven consecutive phase II investigations. J Invest Dermatol 1990;95:188S–92S.

91. VanderMolen LA, Steis RG, Duffey PL, et al. Low- versus high-dose interferon alfa-2a in relapsed indolent non-Hodgkin's lymphoma. J Natl Cancer Inst 1990;82:235–8.

92. Ratain MJ, Vardiman JW, Golomb HM. The role of interferon in the treatment of hairy cell leukemia. Semin Oncol 1986;13:21–8.

93. Kirkwood JM, Strawderman MH, Ernstoff MS, et al. Interferon alfa-2b adjuvant therapy of high-risk resected cutaneous melanoma: the Eastern Cooperative Group Trial EST 1684. J Clin Oncol 1996;14:7–17.

94. Mitchell MS, Jakowatz J, Harel W, et al. Increased effectiveness of interferon-alfa 2b following active specific immunotherapy for melanoma. J Clin Oncol 1994;12:402–11.

95. Jakubowski AA, Casper ES, Gabrilove JL, et al. Phase I trial of intramuscularly administered tumor necrosis factor in patients with advanced cancer. J Clin Oncol 1989;7:298–303.

96. Ernstoff MS, Trautman T, Davis CA, et al. A randomized phase I/II study of continuous versus intermittent intravenous interferon gamma in patients with metastatic melanoma. J Clin Oncol 1987;5:1804–10.

97. Kempf RA, Mitchell MS. Effects of chemotherapeutic agents on the immune response. I. Cancer Invest 1984;2:459–66.

98. Kempf RA, Mitchell MS. Effects of chemotherapeutic agents on the immune response. II. Cancer Invest 1985;3:23–33.

99. Rosenberg SA, Lotze MT, Yang JC, et al. Combination therapy with interleukin-2 and alpha-interferon for the treatment of patients with advanced cancer. J Clin Oncol 1989;7:1863–74.

100. Sznol M, Clark JW, Smith JW, et al. Pilot study of interleukin-2 and lymphokine-activated killer cells combined with immunomodulatory

doses of chemotherapy and sequenced with interferon alfa-2a in patients with metastatic melanoma and renal cell carcinoma. J Natl Cancer Inst 1992;84:929–37.

101. Borden EC, Holland JF, Dao TL, et al. Leukocyte-derived interferon (alpha) in human breast carcinoma. The American Cancer Society phase II trial. Ann Intern Med 1982;97:1–6.

102. Sherwin SA, Mayer D, Ochs JJ, et al. Recombinant leukocyte A interferon in advanced breast cancer. Results of a phase II efficacy trial. Ann Intern Med 1983;98:598–602.

103. Laszlo J, Hood L, Cox E, Goodwin B. A randomized trial of low doses of alpha interferon in patients with breast cancer. J Biol Response Mod 1986;5:206–10.

104. Rosenberg SA, Lotze MT, eds. The immunotherapy of cancer: from laboratory to bedside. New York: Wiley-Liss, 1990:383.

105. Richards JM. Sequential chemoimmunotherapy for metastatic melanoma. Semin Oncol 1991;18:91–5.

106. Legha SS, Ring S, Eton O, et al. Development of a biochemotherapy regimen with concurrent administration of cisplatin, vinblastine, dacarbazine, interferon alfa, and interleukin-2 for patients with metastatic melanoma. J Clin Oncol 1998;16:1752–59.

107. Bukowski RM, Murthy S, McLain D, et al. Phase I trial of recombinant granulocyte-macrophage colony-stimulating factor in patients with lung cancer: clinical and immunologic effects. J Immunother 1993;13:267–74.

108. Steward WP, Scarffe JH, Austin R, et al. Recombinant human granulocyte macrophage colony stimulating factor (rhGM-CSF) given as daily short infusions—a phase I dose-toxicity study. Br J Cancer 1989;59:142–5.

109. Fu YX, Watson GA, Kasahara M, Lopez DM. The role of tumor-derived cytokines on the immune system of mice bearing a mammary adenocarcinoma. I: Induction of regulatory macrophages in normal mice by the in vivo administration of rGM-CSF. J Immunol 1991;146:783–9.

110. Folkman J. Tumor angiogenesis: therapeutic implications. Nw Engl J Med 1971;285:1182–6.

111. Varner JA, Cheresh DA. Tumor angiogenesis and the role of vascular cell integrin αvβ3. Important Adv Oncol 1996;69–87.

112. Brooks PC, Stromblad S, Klemke R, et al. Anti-integrin αvβ3 blocks human breast cancer growth and angiogenesis in human skin. J Clin Invest 1995;96:1815–22.

113. Levin L, Hryniuk WM. Dose intensity analysis of chemotherapy regimens in ovarian carcinoma. J Clin Oncol 1987;5:756–67.

## ACKNOWLEDGMENT

It is a pleasure to acknowledge the invaluable contribution of Dr. Walter Quan, Jr. to the preparation of the version of this chapter that appeared in the Fourth Edition of this book.

# P A R T

# II

# DRUG THERAPY

# CHAPTER 10

# ANTINEOPLASTIC AGENTS

• CHARLES M. HASKELL • LEE ROSEN

This chapter reviews selected commercially available drugs used in cancer chemotherapy. Investigational agents are discussed in Chapter 31, and biologic agents, such as interferon and interleukin-2 (IL-2), are discussed in Chapters 9 and 11. The drugs are discussed by generic name in alphabetic order as listed in Table 10–1. A glossary of terms is given in Table 10–2.

The efficacy, pharmacology, toxicity, and administration of each drug are briefly reviewed, followed by selected references. Drugs that are especially important in the curative therapy of cancer are discussed more completely than drugs of more peripheral interest. The spectrum of toxicity is summarized by organ system, with an emphasis on those organ systems that are of greatest importance in assessing the safety of each drug.

The reader who wants more detailed information about each drug should consult the package insert or any of the following annually updated volumes: *Drug Information*, published by the American Society of Health Systems Pharmacists,[1] and *USP DI,* published by the U.S. Pharmacopeia.[2] Drug information in lay language also is published by the U.S. Pharmacopeia.[3] This publication is an excellent resource for writing consent forms in lay language and for patient education. Scholarly reviews of the drugs, with extensive references, can be found in several additional books.[4, 5]

Chapter 8 reviews the principles of cancer chemotherapy and provides additional guidelines for the use of these agents, including the management of toxic side effects. Several points are pertinent to nearly all of the drugs discussed in this chapter, and they are listed here for emphasis.

1. With the exception of the corticosteroids, luteinizing hormone–releasing hormone (LHRH) and gonadotropin-releasing hormone (GnRH) agonists, levamisole, octreotide, and perhaps asparaginase and the Vinca alkaloids, the drugs in this chapter should be considered potential carcinogens. Ideally, the preparation of these agents for parenteral administration should be performed by a pharmacist or other

*Table 10–1.* **Drugs Reviewed in This Chapter**

| Generic Name | U.S. Trade Name(s)* | Generic Name | U.S. Trade Name(s)* |
|---|---|---|---|
| Altretamine | Hexalen | Idarubicin | Idamycin |
| Amifostine | Ethyol | Ifosfamide | Ifex |
| Aminoglutethimide | Cytadren | Irinotecan | Camptosar |
| Asparaginase and pegaspargase | Elspar and Oncaspar | Leuprolide | Lupron |
| Bleomycin | Blenoxane | Levamisole | Ergamisol |
| Busulfan | Myleran | Lomustine | CeeNu |
| Capecitabine | Xeloda | Mechlorethamine | Mustargen |
| Carboplatin | Paraplatin | Megestrol | Megace |
| Carmustine | BiCNU | Melphalan | Alkeran |
| Chlorambucil | Leukeran | Mercaptopurine | Purinethol |
| Cisplatin | Platinol | Methotrexate | Methotrexate, Methotrexate LPF Sodium |
| Cladribine | Leustatin | Mitomycin | Mutamycin |
| Cyclophosphamide | Cytoxan, Neosar | Mitotane | Lysodren |
| Cytarabine | Cytosar-U | Mitoxantrone | Novantrone |
| Dacarbazine | DTIC-Dome | Octreotide | Sandostatin |
| Dactinomycin | Cosmegen | Paclitaxel | Taxol |
| Daunorubicin | Cerubidine | Pentostatin | Nipent |
| Dexamethasone | Decadron, Hexadrol | Plicamycin | Mithracin |
| Diethylstilbestrol | | Prednisone | Deltasone, Sterapred, Prednicen-M |
| Docetaxel | Taxotere | Procarbazine | Matulane |
| Doxorubicin | Adriamycin PFS or RDF, Rubex | Streptozocin | Zanosar |
| Estramustine | Emcyt | Tamoxifen | Nolvadex |
| Etoposide | VePesid | Teniposide | Vumon |
| Floxuridine | FUDR | Thioguanine | Tabloid brand Thioguanine |
| Fludarabine | Fludara | Thiotepa | Thioplex |
| Fluorouracil | Fluorouracil, Efudex | Topotecan | Hycamtin |
| Flutamide | Eulexin | Vinblastine | Velban |
| Gemcitabine | Gemzar | Vincristine | Oncovin |
| Goserelin | Zoladex | Vinorelbine | Navelbine |
| Hydroxyurea | Hydrea | | |

*U.S. trade names as listed in the Physicians' Desk Reference. 53rd ed. (PDR 1999). Montvale, N.J.: Medical Economics Data Production Co, 1994. This publication provides convenient access to the detailed information available in the package insert for each drug discussed in this chapter.

*Table 10–2.* Glossary

| Term(s) | Definition* |
|---|---|
| Acute | Toxicity developing within 24 hr of drug administration |
| Delayed | Toxicity developing after 24 hr but within 6 to 8 wk of drug administration |
| Short-term | Acute and delayed reactions combined |
| Late or long-term | Toxicity developing months to many years after drug administration, or persisting or unresolved short-term toxicity |
| Expected | Reaction that develops in >75% of patients |
| Common | Reaction that develops in 25 to 75% of patients |
| Uncommon or occasional | Reaction in <25% of patients |
| Rare | Reaction in 5% of patients |
| Very rare | Reaction in <1% of patients |
| Mild to moderate | NCI toxicity grades 1 or 2 |
| Severe | NCI toxicity grades 3 or 4 |
| FDA pregnancy category A | Adequate and well-controlled studies have failed to demonstrate a risk to the fetus in the first trimester of pregnancy, and there is no evidence of risk in later trimesters |
| FDA pregnancy category B | Adverse effects have not been demonstrated in animal reproduction studies, but there are no adequate and well-controlled studies of pregnant women |
| FDA pregnancy category C | Adverse effects on the fetus have been demonstrated in animal reproduction studies. There are no adequate and well-controlled studies of humans, but potential benefits may warrant use of the drug in pregnant women despite potential risks |
| FDA pregnancy category D | Adverse effects on pregnancy are established through adverse reaction data from investigational or marketing experience or other studies in humans, but potential benefits may warrant the use of the drug by pregnant women despite these potential risks |
| FDA pregnancy category X | Studies of animals or humans have demonstrated fetal abnormalities and/or there is positive evidence of human fetal risk. The risks involved in the use of the drug in pregnant women clearly outweigh potential benefits |

*NCI (National Cancer Institute) toxicity grades are listed in Appendix B. The frequency and severity of various toxic side effects may be strongly influenced by the dose and schedule of drug administration, the performance status of the patient, prior treatment, age, concurrent treatment, and other factors. The frequency of side effects in different studies may vary accordingly.

FDA, Food and Drug Administration.

trained professional working in a controlled environment, as discussed in Chapter 12. Residual drug and contaminated waste should be disposed of as toxic waste.

2. The Food and Drug Administration (FDA) classifies the embryotoxic and teratogenic effects of drugs into five categories (see Table 10–2). With the exception of octreotide, which is FDA category B, all of the drugs discussed in this chapter have been or could be classified as C, D, or X. Furthermore, the presence or absence of these drugs in breast milk is usually unknown. Consequently, antineoplastic agents are generally contraindicated during pregnancy and breast-feeding. Chapter 27 discusses this concern further.

3. Patients with highly responsive malignancies and large tumor burdens are susceptible to uric acid nephropathy and the tumor lysis syndrome (see Chapters 8 and 18). These patients should be considered for concurrent therapy with allopurinol and hydration.

4. Patients with an active viral infection and patients considered for live virus vaccination are at risk of disseminated viral complications with most of the drugs used in oncology. It is usually prudent to avoid the use of chemotherapy during episodes of active infection.

5. Extravasation of some of the drugs used in oncology causes severe tissue damage. Such drugs are best administered through a central venous catheter or through the tubing of a smoothly running intravenous infusion line with close observation by a health professional (extravasation precautions). The management of drug extravasation is discussed in Chapter 8.

6. The influence of the patient's age on the pharmacology and use of these drugs is frequently uncertain. Pediatric doses of chemotherapeutic agents are often different from those in adults, and appropriate ways to modify drug doses for patients in the geriatric age group are usually poorly defined. Given these facts, we wish to point out that these brief drug reviews are strongly oriented toward adults. Physicians interested in chemotherapy for the extremes of the human life span should consult the manufacturer's literature on each drug for guidance.

7. The efficacy section for each drug focuses on the use of the drug to treat cancer with curative or major palliative intent. Off-label and investigational uses are discussed in the respective disease-oriented chapters. Reimbursement for such off-label therapy in the United States can be a difficult issue for both physicians and patients. The Association of Community Cancer Centers publishes a quarterly bulletin dealing with the costs of drugs and reimbursement issues.[6] Information about specific drug regimens for specific diseases can be found in the disease-oriented chapters.

8. We have tried to ensure that dosage recommendations are in agreement with the standards of practice at the time of this writing. These recommendations can change, however; thus, we urge the reader to check the manufacturer's recommended dosage and schedule of administration to be certain that changes have not been made in the recommended dose or in the contraindications and precautions for administration. This is especially important for those drugs that are new or unfamiliar to the reader. Conversely, it must be emphasized that in many serious conditions drug therapy should be individualized, and expert judgment may lead to the use of a higher dose or a different schedule or route of administration than is included in the manufacturer's recommendations.

## REFERENCES

1. McEvoy GK, ed. AHFS drug information 2000. Bethesda, Md: American Society of Health Systems Pharmacists, 2000:xviii.
2. American Medical Association, Division of Drugs and Toxicology. Chicago: American Medical Association, 1995.
3. USP DI. Oncology drug information (1999–2000) 3rd ed. Rockville, Md: US Pharmacopeial Convention, 1998.

4. USP DI. Advice for the patient: drug information in lay language. Vol. II. Rockville, Md: U.S. Pharmacopeia.
5. Perry MC, ed. The chemotherapy source book. 2nd ed. Baltimore: Williams & Wilkins, 1996 (1518 pp).
6. Jewler D (pub dir). Association of community cancer centers compendia-based drug bulletin. 11600 Nebel St., Suite 201, Rockville, Md. 20852 (Telephone: 301-984-9496).

## Altretamine

Altretamine was originally synthesized as a derivative of melamine, a plastic widely used in the manufacture of dishes, automobile parts, and other items of daily use.[1] It is a synthetic s-triazine derivative that functions as a nonclassic alkylating agent. It is also known as hexamethylmelamine, HMM, HXM, Hexalen, and NSC-13875.

### EFFICACY

Altretamine has a wide spectrum of antitumor activity in humans.[1] It is marketed as a single agent for the palliative treatment of recurrent or persistent ovarian cancer following first-line therapy with alkylating agents.[2]

### PHARMACOLOGY

**Mechanism of Action.** Altretamine is structurally related to the alkylating agent triethylenemelamine, but it lacks cross-resistance to alkylating agents and does not cause alkylation in vitro.[3] N-demethylation appears to be the major metabolic pathway for hexamethylmelamine, and there is a correlation between demethylation and antitumor activity. The mechanism of action of this drug remains unclear, although some form of alkylation is suspected. The drug is considered cell cycle phase nonspecific.

**Resistance.** The mechanisms of resistance are poorly defined but are presumed to be similar to those of the alkylating agents.

**Pharmacokinetics.** Altretamine is easily absorbed by the oral route, but it undergoes extensive and rapid first-pass demethylation in the liver to pentamethylmelamine and tetramethylmelamine.[4] Altretamine and its metabolites are variably bound to plasma proteins, and the plasma levels of altretamine itself are unpredictable. The metabolites are cleared by the kidneys (90% by 72 hours), but less than 1% of the unmetabolized parent drug appears in urine. The methylated metabolites appear to accumulate in the central nervous system (CNS). The elimination half-life appears to be about 4 to 13 hours.

**Drug Interactions.** Induction of demethylation in animals by the administration of phenobarbital markedly reduces the efficacy of altretamine.[5] Cimetidine slows the metabolism of altretamine, potentially increasing its toxicity.[6] Concurrent treatment with altretamine and antidepressants of the monoamine oxidase (MAO) inhibitor class can cause severe hypotension. Pyridoxine may decrease the toxicity and efficacy of altretamine.[7] The drug may exacerbate the symptoms of porphyria, based on its in vitro effects on porphyrin metabolism.[8]

### TOXICITY

**Overview.** Common forms of short-term toxicity include mild to moderate myelosuppression, nausea and vomiting, and neurotoxicity. Any of these may prove dose limiting and can be severe in rare cases. Long-term toxicity is poorly defined but is presumed to include delayed carcinogenesis.

**Hematologic.** Mild to moderate neutropenia occurs in about 5% of patients, mild to moderate thrombocytopenia in about 10%, and anemia in about a third of patients. The nadir counts usually occur 3 or 4 weeks after starting treatment and resolve within 2 or 3 weeks.

**Digestive System.** Mild to moderate nausea, with or without emesis, occurs in about a third of patients. Anorexia, abdominal cramps, and diarrhea occasionally occur. Hepatic toxicity is very rare.

**Neurologic.** Peripheral neuropathy and CNS reactions occur in about a third of patients. These effects can include paresthesia, hyperesthesia, hyperreflexia, decreased sensation, decreased position sense, ataxia, dizziness, vertigo, agitation, hallucinations, confusion, lethargy, depression, and coma. The neurotoxicity occurs with prolonged therapy and is readily reversed by discontinuing treatment.

**Other/Rare**

*Immunologic.* Altretamine can cause hypersensitivity reactions.

*Mucocutaneous.* Skin rashes, hyperpigmentation, pruritus, and alopecia can occur.

*Cardiovascular.* Hypotension can occur when the drug is given with MAO inhibitors.

*Ocular.* Reversible ocular disturbances occur as part of neurologic toxicity.

*Genitourinary.* Cystitis and azotemia can occur.

*Reproductive.* Toxicity data place altretamine in FDA pregnancy category D.

*Endocrine-Metabolic.* Weight loss can occur.

*Carcinogenicity.* The drug is considered potentially carcinogenic. Leukemia has been reported as a second neoplasm.

### DOSAGE AND ADMINISTRATION

Altretamine is available as 50-mg capsules. The recommended dosage is 260 mg/m²/day in four divided oral doses after meals and at bedtime. This dose is given as intermittent courses lasting either 14 or 21 consecutive days in a 28-day cycle. The manufacturer recommends regular neurologic examinations and at least a monthly complete blood count (CBC) during therapy. Altretamine should be discontinued temporarily (for 14 days or longer) for any of the following:

1. Gastrointestinal intolerance unresponsive to symptomatic treatment
2. Leukopenia (white cell count [WCC] <2000/μL) or neutropenia (absolute neutrophil count [ANC] <1000/μL)
3. Thrombocytopenia (platelets <75,000/μL)
4. Progressive neurotoxicity

If symptoms resolve or stabilize, the drug can be restarted at 200 mg/m²/day. If neurologic symptoms continue to progress on the reduced dosage schedule, altretamine should be discontinued.

## REFERENCES

1. Foster BJ, Harding BJ, Leyland-Jones B, Hoth D. Hexamethylmelamine: a critical review of an active drug. Cancer Treat Rev 1986;13:197–217.
2. Manetta A, Tewari K, Podczaski ES. Hexamethylmelamine as a single second-line agent in ovarian cancer: follow-up report and review of the literature. Gynecol Oncol 1997;66:20–6.
3. Lee CR, Faulds D. Altretamine: a review of its pharmacodynamic and pharmacokinetic properties, and therapeutic potential in cancer chemotherapy. Drugs 1995;49:932–53.
4. Damia G, D'Incalci M. Clinical pharmacokinetics of altretamine. Clin Pharmacokinet 1995;28:439–48.
5. Paolini A, D'Incalci M. Effect of phenobarbital pretreatment on the metabolism and antitumor activity of hexamethylmelamine. Cancer Treat Rep 1986;70:513–6.
6. Hande K, Combs G, Swingle R, et al. Effect of cimetidine and ranitidine on the metabolism and toxicity of hexamethylmelamine. Cancer Treat Rep 1986;70:1443–5.
7. Wiernik PH, Yeap B, Vogl SE, et al. Hexamethylmelamine and low or moderate dose cisplatin with or without pyridoxine for treatment of advanced ovarian carcinoma: a study of the Eastern Cooperative Oncology Group. Cancer Invest 1992;10:1–9.
8. Cochâon AC, Aldonatti C, San Martâin de Viale LC, Wainstok de Calmanovici R. Evaluation of the porphyrinogenic risk of antineoplastics. J Appl Toxicol 1997;17:171–7.

## Amifostine

Amifostine is an aminothiol compound originally developed as a radiation protective agent.[1] It is also known as Ethyol, gammaphos, S-2-3 (3-aminopropylamino) ethyl-phosphorothionic acid, and WR 2721.

## EFFICACY

Amifostine is available for the reduction of cisplatin-induced cumulative nephrotoxicity in patients with advanced ovarian cancer, non–small cell lung cancer, or advanced solid tumors of non–germ cell origin. The drug is also being studied for possible use in protecting patients from the neurologic toxicity of cisplatin[2] and the oral toxicity of radiation therapy.[3] Several studies suggest that the treatment is cost effective as well as clinically effective.[4]

The drug is not recommended for patients with neoplasms that can potentially be cured with cisplatin because of concern raised by animal studies that amifostine may interfere with the antitumor efficacy of cisplatin. Concern has also been raised about the methods used in evaluating the efficacy of this class of drugs. For example, Phillips and Tannock have concluded that this class of agents has biologic activity but that efficacy has not been completely established because of methodologic flaws in the available studies.[5]

## PHARMACOLOGY

Amifostine is metabolized by alkaline phosphatase to an active thiol metabolite that acts as a free radical scavenger.[6] It is freely soluble in water and is quickly distributed to tissues after intravenous administration. The elimination half-life is about 8 minutes, with the predominant route of elimination being through rapid metabolism and uptake into tissues.

The concomitant use of antihypertensive or other hypotension-inducing agents should be avoided because of the potential for adverse drug interactions with amifostine.

## TOXICITY

The major dose-limiting toxicity for amifostine is hypotension, which usually occurs about 14 minutes after starting the infusion and lasts 5 to 15 minutes. This is usually asymptomatic, but it can result in dizziness or fainting. Nausea and vomiting can also occur and may be severe. Hypocalcemia may occur, resulting in paresthesias or muscle cramps.

Allergic reactions have been reported, including rare chills, skin rash, or sneezing. Somnolence has been reported and may be severe. Infrequent, usually minor side effects include a feeling of being unusually warm or cold, flushing or redness of the face or neck, and singultus.

## DOSAGE AND ADMINISTRATION

Amifostine is provided as a 500-mg single-dose vial that must be reconstituted in normal saline and then further diluted for administration. The usual dosage for nephrotoxicity prophylaxis with cisplatin is 910 mg/m² of body surface area over a 15-minute period once a day, beginning 30 minutes before cisplatin.[7] The infusion should be temporarily discontinued if the systolic blood pressure decreases significantly from baseline. It may be resumed if the blood pressure returns to normal within 5 minutes and the patient is asymptomatic. If this does not occur, subsequent courses of amifostine should be given at a lower dose (740 mg/m² of body surface area).

## REFERENCES

1. Klingermann MM, Shaw MT, Slavik M, Yuhas JM. Phase I clinical studies with WR-2721. Cancer Clin Trials 1980;3:217–21.
2. DiPaola RS, Schuchter L. Neurologic protection by amifostine. Semin Oncol 1999;26:2 Suppl 7:82–8.
3. Bohuslavizki KH, Klutmann S, Brenner W, et al. Salivary gland protection by amifostine in high-dose radioiodine treatment: results of a double-blind placebo-controlled study. J Clin Oncol 1998;16:3542–9.
4. Calhoun EA, Bennett CL. Pharmacoeconomics of amifostine in ovarian cancer. Semin Oncol 1999;26:2 Suppl 7:102–7.
5. Phillips KA, Tannock IF. Design and interpretation of clinical trials that evaluate agents that may offer protection from the toxic effects of cancer chemotherapy. J Clin Oncol 1998;16:3179–90.
6. Links M, Lewis C. Chemoprotectants: a review of their clinical pharmacology and therapeutic efficacy. Drugs 1999;57:293–308.
7. Dorr RT, Holmes BC. Dosing considerations with amifostine: a review of the literature and clinical experience. Semin Oncol 1999;26:2 Suppl 7:108–19.

## Aminoglutethimide

Aminoglutethimide is an analogue of the commercially available hypnotic glutethimide (Doriden).[1] The drug was introduced as an anticonvulsant in 1958, but it was withdrawn by the FDA in 1966 because prolonged use caused unexpected adrenal suppression. Aminoglutethimide is also known as Cytadren.

## EFFICACY

Aminoglutethimide has been approved by the FDA in the United States for the treatment of Cushing's syndrome.[2] The drug is also used as an alternative to adrenalectomy in the treatment of breast cancer. There is investigational interest in the use of aminoglutethimide in combination with flutamide withdrawal for patients with advanced prostate cancer.[3]

## PHARMACOLOGY

**Mechanisms of Action and Resistance.** Aminoglutethimide blocks adrenal steroidogenesis by inhibiting the enzymatic conversion of cholesterol to pregnenolone. In normal individuals, but not in patients with adrenocorticotropic hormone (ACTH)-independent carcinomas, aminoglutethimide therapy is accompanied by a markedly increased level of ACTH (up to sevenfold), which can produce adrenocortical hypertrophy and a resumption of steroid synthesis. Thus, in patients with breast cancer, a glucocorticosteroid must also be given to suppress the reflex increase in ACTH output. This is usually done with hydrocortisone.[4] An additional important mechanism of action derives from aminoglutethimide's ability to block the peripheral conversion (aromatization) of androgenic precursors to estrogens. Aminoglutethimide also appears to stimulate its own metabolism when given in high doses for prolonged periods.[5] More detailed discussions of the mechanisms of action and resistance of aminoglutethimide are available.[6, 7]

**Pharmacokinetics.** Aminoglutethimide is well absorbed by the oral route. About 20 to 25% of the drug is bound to blood cells or protein, and it is cleared from plasma with a half-life of about 12 hours. Renal clearance of unchanged drug accounts for 35 to 43% of an administered dose within 48 hours. The drug easily crosses the blood-brain barrier in animals.

**Drug Interactions.** Aminoglutethimide can alter the metabolism of estrogen and other drugs by inducing microsomal enzymes.[8, 9] Larger doses of coumarin anticoagulants are needed when given with aminoglutethimide,[10] and it stimulates the metabolism of dexamethasone (making dexamethasone an inappropriate choice for concomitant therapy). Alcohol can augment the toxic side effects of aminoglutethimide.

## TOXICITY

**Overview.** Adrenal suppression is expected in all patients when full doses of aminoglutethimide are used. Common short-term toxic side effects include a febrile maculopapular skin rash, hypotension, mild nausea, and neurologic changes such as lethargy and somnolence. Myelosuppression is rare but can be life threatening.

**Digestive.** Mild nausea, vomiting, and anorexia are occasional (about 12%). Hepatotoxicity is rare, but it can include cholestatic jaundice as part of a syndrome that mimics systemic lupus erythematosus.[11]

**Mucocutaneous.** A pruritic macular rash, which is sometimes associated with fever, occurs in about 15% of patients during the first 2 to 3 weeks of treatment. It generally disappears in 4 to 7 days despite continuation of treatment. If the rash continues or worsens, aminoglutethimide is discontinued. The reaction is presumed to be a hypersensitivity reaction, but this has not been proved. Rare effects include pustular psoriasis, desquamation, and oral ulceration.

**Cardiovascular.** Orthostatic dizziness occurs in 5% of patients; tachycardia occurs in 2.5%.

**Neurologic.** Lethargy (40%), somnolence (33%), ataxia (10%), and headache can occur. These reactions generally abate by lowering the dose of aminoglutethimide; the dose often can later be gradually increased again to a full dose without severe toxicity.

**Endocrine-Metabolic.** Adrenal suppression, including suppression of aldosterone production, is an expected consequence of therapy. This may result in hyponatremia, hypochloremia, and hyperkalemia. Hypercholesterolemia can occur.[12] Masculinization, hypothyroidism,[13] weight gain, hypoglycemia, and facial fullness may rarely occur.

**Other and Rare Reactions**

*Immunologic.* Immunologic reactions include urticaria and a peculiar skin rash that is presumed to be due to hypersensitivity (see Mucocutaneous section). Hypersensitivity reactions associated with cholestatic jaundice have been reported.

*Hematologic.* Myelosuppression occurs in less than 1% of patients. Extremely rare fatalities due to agranulocytosis have occurred, however, and it is unknown whether it is safe to rechallenge the patient with aminoglutethimide if neutropenia has been severe or prolonged.

*Pulmonary.* Alveolar damage with hemorrhage has occurred.[14] Pulmonary eosinophilia has been reported.[15]

*Ocular.* Nystagmus can occur.

*Musculoskeletal.* Myalgia and leg cramps may occur.

*Genitourinary.* Severe hyponatremia can develop when the drug is given simultaneously with diuretics.[16]

*Reproductive.* Aminoglutethimide is classified in FDA pregnancy category D. Normal pregnancies have occurred while taking the drug, but it can cause fetal harm, including pseudohermaphroditism.

*Carcinogenicity.* The carcinogenicity of aminoglutethimide is uncertain.

## DOSAGE AND ADMINISTRATION

Aminoglutethimide is available as 250-mg tablets. The usual oral maintenance dosage is 250 mg four times daily. Lower doses may be used initially for several weeks to induce the metabolism of the drug and minimize CNS side effects. Hydrocortisone (but not dexamethasone) is given three times daily in a dose that is sufficient to suppress the blood level of dehydroepiandrosterone sulfate to less than 25% of the control level. This initially involves a total dosage of 100 mg daily (divided into three doses of 20, 20, and 60 mg) for 2 weeks; the subsequent maintenance dose is 20 to 30 mg of hydrocortisone orally in the morning or in divided doses during the day. Mineralocorticoid replacement (such as fludrocortisone) may also be necessary. In Europe, low-dose aminoglutethimide (250 mg twice a day) without hydrocortisone has been used as first-line endocrine treatment for advanced breast cancer.[17]

Patients receiving aminoglutethimide should be monitored for hypotension at regular intervals and should be assessed and treated for adrenal suppression as needed, especially at times of added stress. They should be advised of possible drowsiness from treatment, and the manufacturer advises patients not to drive or operate dangerous machinery while taking the drug.

## REFERENCES

1. Dao TL. Estrogen synthesis in human breast tumor and its inhibition by testololactone and bromoandrostenedione. Cancer Res 1982; 42:Suppl:3338S–41.
2. Comi RJ, Gorden P. Long-term medical treatment of ectopic ACTH syndrome. South Med J 1998;91:1014–8.
3. Sartor O, Cooper M, Weinberger M. Surprising activity of flutamide withdrawal, when combined with aminoglutethimide, in treatment of "hormone-refractory" prostate cancer [published erratum appears in J Natl Cancer Inst 1994;86:463]. J Natl Cancer Inst 1994;86:222–7.
4. Santen RJ, Wells SA, Runic S, et al. Adrenal suppression with aminoglutethimide. I: Differential effects of aminoglutethimide on glucocorticoid metabolism as a rationale for use of hydrocortisone. J Clin Endocrinol Metab 1977;45:469–79.
5. Lønning PE, Kvinnsland S, Thorsen T, Ueland PM. Alterations in the metabolism of oestrogens during treatment with aminoglutethimide in breast cancer patients. Preliminary findings. Clin Pharmacokinet 1987;13:393–406.
6. Lønning PE, Kvinnsland S. Mechanisms of action of aminoglutethimide as endocrine therapy of breast cancer. Drugs 1988;35:685–710.
7. Yue W, Brodie AM. Mechanisms of the actions of aromatase inhibitors 4-hydroxyandrostenedione, fadrozole, and aminoglutethimide on aromatase in JEG-3 cell culture. J Steroid Biochem Mol Biol 1997;63:317–28.
8. Kvinnsland S, Lønning PE, Ueland PM. Aminoglutethimide as an inducer of microsomal enzymes. Part 1: Pharmacological aspects. Breast Cancer Res Treat 1986;7:Suppl:S73–6.
9. Lønning PE. Aminoglutethimide enzyme induction: pharmacological and endocrinological implications. Cancer Chemother Pharmacol 1990;26:241–4.
10. Cropp JS, Bussey HI. A review of enzyme induction of warfarin metabolism with recommendations for patient management. Pharmacotherapy 1997;17:917–28.
11. Perrault DJ, Domovitch E. Aminoglutethimide and cholestasis. Ann Intern Med 1984;100:160.
12. Bonneterre J, Nguyen M, Hecquet B, Cappelaere P. Aminoglutethimide-induced hypercholesterolaemia. Lancet 1984;1:912–3.
13. Figg WD, Thibault A, Sartor AO, et al. Hypothyroidism associated with aminoglutethimide in patients with prostate cancer. Arch Intern Med 1994;154:1023–5.
14. Rodman DM, Hanley M, Parsons P. Aminoglutethimide, alveolar damage, and hemorrhage. Ann Intern Med 1986;105:633.
15. Bell SC, Anderson EG. Pulmonary eosinophilia associated with aminoglutethimide. Aust N Z J Med 1998;28:670–1.
16. Bork E, Hansen M. Severe hyponatremia following simultaneous administration of aminoglutethimide and diuretics. Cancer Treat Rep 1986;70:689–90.
17. Cocconi G, Bisagni G, Ceci G, et al. Low-dose aminoglutethimide with and without hydrocortisone replacement as a first-line endocrine treatment in advanced breast cancer: a prospective randomized trial of the Italian Oncology Group for Clinical Research. J Clin Oncol 1992;10:984–9.

## Asparaginase and Pegaspargase

In 1953, Kidd[1] discovered that guinea pig serum inhibited several rodent neoplasms. The antitumor component of guinea pig serum was later shown to be the enzyme L-asparaginase,[2] and related enzymes with antitumor activity were subsequently extracted from various bacteria. Asparaginase is a high-molecular-weight bacterial enzyme of known amino acid sequence,[3] but its tertiary chemical structure is unknown. Two forms of asparaginase are available in the United States and are derived from *Escherichia coli* (type EC-2). The first is known as Elspar, L-asparaginase, colaspase, and NSC-109229. The second is known as pegaspargase, Oncaspar, polyethylene glycol–modified L-asparaginase, and PEG-L-asparaginase. Asparaginase derived from *Erwinia carotovora* is known as *Erwinia* L-asparaginase and NSC-106977.

### EFFICACY

Asparaginase is used in the treatment of acute lymphoblastic leukemia (ALL), either in relapse or at initial diagnosis.[4] It is not useful in maintaining remission in this disease, and it should not generally be used as a single agent. It is also used in the treatment of lymphoblastic lymphoma. Pegaspargase is indicated for patients who are candidates for asparaginase therapy despite a prior hypersensitivity reaction to the agent.

### PHARMACOLOGY

**Mechanism of Action.** Asparaginase is unique among antineoplastic agents in causing all of its known cytotoxicity through an extracellular mechanism. After parenteral administration, it acts by deaminating extracellular L-asparagine, an amino acid that is generally considered nonessential. However, L-asparagine appears to be an essential amino acid for protein synthesis by some cells because they lack an adequate level of another enzyme, asparagine synthetase. The intracellular deficiency of asparagine synthetase renders the cell susceptible to extracellular depletion of the amino acid L-asparagine. This ultimately results in apoptosis.[5]

Because most L-asparaginase preparations also contain some L-glutaminase activity, it is possible that some of their cytotoxicity is related to depletion of L-glutamine as well.[6] The postmitotic $G_1$ phase of the cell cycle is especially sensitive to L-asparaginase.

**Resistance.** Resistance is a result of derepression or induction of the enzyme asparagine synthetase.[7]

**Pharmacokinetics.** After parenteral administration, unaltered *E. coli* L-asparaginase distributes into a body space that is only 20 to 30% greater than the plasma volume. In humans, plasma levels after intramuscular injection are about half those after intravenous injection, although both routes are effective in reducing the plasma level of L-asparagine. The drug is slowly cleared from plasma, with biexponential half-lives of 0.5 and 2.5 days. Little L-asparaginase reaches the cerebrospinal fluid (CSF) or urine, but appreciable concentrations appear in pleural effusions and lymph. Nevertheless, the intravenous route is as effective as the intrathecal route for depleting L-asparagine from the CSF.[8] Clearance from the body appears to be accomplished primarily by the reticuloendothelial system.

Pharmacokinetic studies of pegaspargase have demonstrated an apparent volume of distribution equal to plasma volume and no urinary excretion.[9] A comparative study of the plasma half-lives of three preparations of L-asparaginase found the following half-life values: pegaspargase, 5.73 ± 3.24 days; *E. coli* L-asparaginase, 1.24 ± 0.17 days; and *Erwinia* L-asparaginase, 0.65 ± 0.13 days.[10]

**Drug Interactions.** Pretreatment with L-asparaginase antagonizes the effects of methotrexate (MTX) by reducing the production of MTX polyglutamates.[11] The hepatic toxicity of asparaginase can increase the toxicity of drugs that are metabolized by the liver. Some authorities recommend giving asparaginase after prednisone and vincristine when these drugs are used together because of drug interactions predicted by in vitro studies. The clinical importance of these interactions has not been established in humans.

Patients with pre-existing coagulation disorders are at a greater risk than normal of developing thrombotic complications from the drug.[12]

## TOXICITY

**Overview.** Asparaginase has a unique spectrum of toxicity, including relatively frequent hypersensitivity reactions (3 to 73%) that can include anaphylaxis (>1%), prominent inhibition of protein synthesis by the liver with protean effects on metabolism, pancreatitis (1%), hyperglycemia requiring insulin (4%), and thrombosis (4%).

**Hematologic.** Myelosuppression is rare, but results of laboratory studies of coagulation are nearly always abnormal (all treated patients have reduced levels of clotting factors II, V, VII, VIII, IX, X, fibrinogen, and antithrombin III, of both the functional and antigenic types).[13] It has been curious that such profound clotting factor abnormalities should be so rarely associated with clinically important thrombosis or bleeding. This may relate to the frequent observation that both clotting factors and antithrombin III are depressed,[14] although this has not been the case in all studies.[15] Other factors may therefore be important, such as the observation that some patients developing thrombosis during asparaginase therapy develop an altered von Willebrand's factor molecule.[16] In another study, protein C and protein S did not appear to play a role in asparaginase-induced thrombosis.[17] Although rare, fatal intracranial bleeding or thrombosis may occur. Nevertheless, aggressive clotting factor replacement is indicated for patients with this complication because it is potentially reversible and compatible with good quality survival.[18]

**Immunologic.** The most dangerous reaction is anaphylaxis, which reportedly occurs in 3 to 73% of patients. Patients who develop allergic reactions after responding to L-asparaginase from *E. coli* may be treated relatively safely with another antigenic source of the enzyme (such as pegaspargase or L-asparaginase from *E. carotovora*). The incidence of dose-limiting hypersensitivity reactions reported with pegaspargase in previously sensitive and nonsensitive patients is stated to be 23% and 5% respectively. The overall incidence of life-threatening anaphylaxis is about 1%. The drug is minimally immunosuppressive.

**Digestive System.** Nausea and vomiting are common but rarely severe. Hepatic toxicity is common but reversible (depressed lipoprotein synthesis, decreased serum albumin level, elevated serum cholesterol level, fatty liver).[19] Severe

pancreatitis can occur and may rarely prove fulminant and lethal. Successful treatment of pancreatitis in this setting has been reported with somatostatin[20] and a synthetic protease inhibitor.[21]

**Neurologic.** A syndrome of somnolence and lethargy that mimics hepatic encephalopathy is a common reaction. The problem is readily reversible in most patients by stopping treatment. Rarely, a Parkinson-like condition develops and is rapidly reversed by discontinuing the drug.

**Endocrine-Metabolic.** Abnormal laboratory values are common, including hyperlipidemia, depressed serum cholesterol, and depressed serum lipoprotein lipase. These and many of the other toxic effects of L-asparaginase can be explained by its ability to inhibit protein synthesis.[22] However, these forms of toxicity are complex, and other explanations have been suggested. For example, it has been proposed that some of the toxicity may in fact be due to the glutaminase activity rather than the asparaginase activity of the available enzyme preparation.[6, 23] Disordered glucose metabolism can occur rarely (either with or without pancreatitis).

**Other and Rare Reactions.** Chills and drug fever can occur and may progress to fatal hyperthermia. The drug is a potent contact irritant to the skin, lungs, and mucous membranes (especially the eyes). Care must be taken to correlate the results of laboratory tests with the actual clinical status of the patient. Many laboratory test abnormalities that may result are relatively trivial but, if misinterpreted, may lead to inappropriate cessation of asparaginase therapy. An example is hyperamylasemia, suggesting pancreatitis. The clinician should be aware that hyperamylasemia of salivary origin may occur and requires no change in therapy.[24]

*Mucocutaneous.* Pruritus, alopecia, nail whiteness and ridging, erythema simplex, and aphthous stomatitis can occur.

*Cardiovascular.* Chest pain, hypertension, severe hypotension, and tachycardia (with anaphylaxis) can occur.

*Pulmonary.* These effects include cough, epistaxis, severe bronchospasm, and upper respiratory tract infections.

*Musculoskeletal.* Musculoskeletal reactions include diffuse and local pain, arthralgias, joint stiffness, and cramps.

*Genitourinary.* Azotemia (usually prerenal), hemorrhagic cystitis, and proteinuria can occur.

*Reproductive.* Asparaginase is classified in FDA pregnancy category C.

*Carcinogenicity.* The drug is not mutagenic in the Ames test. Testing for carcinogenesis in animals is incomplete, but the available data suggest that the drug is not carcinogenic.

## DOSAGE AND ADMINISTRATION

*E. coli* L-asparaginase is available in vials containing 10,000 IU. The recommended dosage of L-asparaginase is 6000 IU/m² intramuscularly given three times weekly for a total of nine doses.[25] Generally, it is used as one of many drugs for the induction of remission in patients with ALL.

Pegaspargase (polyethylene glycol–modified *E. coli* L-asparaginase) is available in single-dose vials containing 3750 IU/5 ml of solution. Because of its longer half-life, the usual dosage is 2500 IU/m² intramuscularly or intravenously every 14 days in children with a body surface area of greater than or equal to 0.6 m². The maximal volume of injection is 2 ml in any one site. If the drug is given intravenously, it should be given over 1 to 2 hours. The manufacturer cautions that freezing destroys the activity of pegaspargase and that frozen samples of the drug should be discarded.

L-asparaginase is contraindicated in patients with pancreatitis or a history of pancreatitis. It is also contraindicated in patients with significant hemorrhagic toxicity and severe anaphylaxis from prior asparaginase therapy.

Because of the high frequency and risk of anaphylaxis with L-asparaginase therapy, it is essential that emergency supplies (including epinephrine, diphenhydramine, and hydrocortisone) and a physician who is experienced in resuscitation be available each time a patient is given the drug. The patient should be observed for anaphylaxis at least an hour after drug administration. The manufacturer of *E. coli* L-asparaginase recommends performing a skin test (2 units intradermally with an hour of observation time) before administering the first dose of asparaginase and again before re-treatment if more than a week has elapsed since the last dose of the drug.

## REFERENCES

1. Kidd JG. Regression of transplanted lymphomas induced in vivo by means of normal guinea pig serum. J Exp Med 1953;98:583–606.
2. Broome JD. Evidence that the L-asparaginase activity of guinea pig serum is responsible for its antilymphoma effects. Nature 1961;191:1114–5.
3. Maita T, Matsuda G. The primary structure of L-asparaginase from *Escherichia coli*. Hoppe Seylers Z Physiol Chem 1980;361:105–17.
4. Mèuller HJ, Boos J. Use of L-asparaginase in childhood ALL. Crit Rev Oncol Hematol 1998;28:97–113.
5. Story MD, Voehringer DW, Stephens LC, Meyn RE. L-Asparaginase kills lymphoma cells by apoptosis. Cancer Chemother Pharmacol 1993;32:129–33.
6. Ollenschläger G, Roth E, Linkesch W, et al. Asparaginase-induced derangements of glutamine metabolism: the pathogenetic basis for some drug-related side-effects. Eur J Clin Invest 1988;18:512–6.
7. Haskell CM, Canellos GP. L-Asparaginase resistance in human leukemia—asparagine synthetase. Biochem Pharmacol 1969;18:2578–80.
8. Woo MH, Hak LJ, Storm MC, et al. Cerebrospinal fluid asparagine concentrations after *Escherichia coli* asparaginase in children with acute lymphoblastic leukemia. J Clin Oncol 1999;17:1568–73.
9. Ho DH, Brown NS, Yen A, et al. Clinical pharmacology of polyethylene glycol-L-asparaginase. Drug Metab Dispos 1986;14:349–52.
10. Asselin BL, Whitin JC, Coppola DJ, et al. Comparative pharmacokinetic studies of three asparaginase preparations. J Clin Oncol 1993;11:1780–6.
11. Keating M, Holmes R, Lerner S, Ho D. L-Asparaginase and PEG asparaginase—past, present, and future. Leuk Lymphoma 1993;10:153–7.
12. Nowak-Gèottle U, Wermes C, Junker R, et al. Prospective evaluation of the thrombotic risk in children with acute lymphoblastic leukemia carrying the MTHFR TT 677 genotype, the prothrombin G20210A variant, and further prothrombotic risk factors. Blood 1999;93:1595–9.
13. Liebman HA, Wada JK, Patch MJ, McGehee W. Depression of functional and antigenic plasma antithrombin III (AT-III) due to therapy with L-asparaginase. Cancer 1982;50:451–6.
14. Homans AC, Rybak ME, Baglini RL, et al. Effect of L-asparaginase administration on coagulation and platelet function in children with leukemia. J Clin Oncol 1987;5:811–7.
15. O'Meara A, Daly M, Hallinan FH. Increased antithrombin III concentration in children with acute lymphatic leukaemia receiving L-asparaginase therapy. Med Pediatr Oncol 1988;16:169–74.
16. Pui CH, Chesney CM, Weed J, Jackson CW. Altered von Willebrand factor molecule in children with thrombosis following asparaginase-

prednisone-vincristine therapy for leukemia. J Clin Oncol 1985;3:1266–72.
17. Pui CH, Chesney CM, Bergum PW, et al. Lack of pathogenetic role of proteins C and S in thrombosis associated with asparaginase-prednisone-vincristine therapy for leukaemia. Br J Haematol 1986;64:283–90.
18. Alberts SR, Bretscher M, Wiltsie JC, et al. Thrombosis related to the use of L-asparaginase in adults with acute lymphoblastic leukemia: a need to consider coagulation monitoring and clotting factor replacement. Leuk Lymphoma 1999;32:489–96.
19. Haskell CM, Canellos GP, Leventhal BG, et al. L-Asparaginase: therapeutic and toxic effects in patients with neoplastic disease. N Engl J Med 1969;281:1028–34.
20. Cheung YF, Lee CW, Chan CF, et al. Somatostatin therapy in L-asparaginase–induced pancreatitis. Med Pediatr Oncol 1994;22:421–4.
21. Murakawa M, Okamura T, Shibuya T, et al. Use of a synthetic protease inhibitor for the treatment of L-asparaginase–induced acute pancreatitis complicated by disseminated intravascular coagulation. Ann Hematol 1992;64:249–52.
22. Haskell CM: L-Asparaginase: human toxicology and single agent activity in nonleukemic neoplasms. Cancer Treat Rep 1981;65:suppl:4:57–9.
23. Durden DL, Salazar AM, Distasio JA. Kinetic analysis of hepatotoxicity associated with antineoplastic asparaginases. Cancer Res 1983;43:1602–5.
24. Adams LJ, Antonow DR, Ash R, McClain CJ. Salivary hyperamylasemia after L-asparaginase therapy. Cancer Treat Rep 1985;69:1437–8.
25. Ortega JA, Nesbit ME Jr, Donaldson MH, et al. L-Asparaginase, vincristine, and prednisone for induction of first remission in acute lymphocytic leukemia. Cancer Res 1977;37:535–40.

# Bleomycin

Bleomycin is an antibiotic complex that was isolated in 1962 from a strain of *Streptomyces verticillus* that was obtained from soil from a Japanese coal mine. It can be separated into at least 13 fractions designated as A1 to A6, AN2, and B1 to B6. Although fraction A2 is probably the most active, the proportion of the various fractions has varied slightly from batch to batch without any apparent impact on the potency of the clinically used mixture. Only rarely has biologic or analytic inequivalence of commercial formulations of bleomycin been reported.[1] Other names and abbreviations for the drug include Blenoxane, BLM, Bleo, and NSC-125066.

## EFFICACY

Bleomycin plays a critical role in the curative treatment of testicular cancer using combination chemotherapy.[2] It is also widely used in the management of lymphomas. It is rarely used as a single agent, although it has modest activity against a variety of tumors, including squamous cell carcinomas arising in a number of sites (head and neck, cervix, penis, skin, vulva).

## PHARMACOLOGY

**Mechanism of Action.** Bleomycin is a bifunctional compound consisting of a DNA binding site and an active redox site. The redox site binds the ferrous form of iron, resulting in an intermediate complex [bleomycin-Fe(II)-$O_2$]. DNA is subsequently cleaved when the ferrous ion donates an electron to oxygen. The DNA fragmentation that results from this reaction includes single- and double-strand breaks in DNA.[3] Diverse evidence supports the importance of iron and oxygen in the fragmentation of DNA by bleomycin.[4] For example, the cytotoxicity of bleomycin is markedly increased by exposure of cells to high concentrations of oxygen in the presence of iron, but it is rendered nontoxic in vitro when iron is removed from the system, and bleomycin does not cleave DNA under anaerobic conditions. Furthermore, bleomycin toxicity in vivo is reduced by agents that chelate iron, counteract the formation of superoxide, or change the state of oxygenation in the cell.[3]

The amount of bleomycin-induced DNA fragmentation varies tremendously from cell to cell.[5] This is in marked contrast to the effects of gamma irradiation, which has a more homogeneous effect on DNA. Bleomycin exerts complex and variable effects on the cell cycles of different cell lines.[6] For example, it is more damaging to nonproliferating cells than to most proliferating cells, but in some cell culture systems it has $G_2$ specificity and it is capable of partially synchronizing the population of cells. Overall, the effects are sufficiently diverse and unpredictable from cell line to cell line for bleomycin to be classified as phase nonspecific.

Bleomycin is uniquely toxic to the lungs and skin. Although this may be explained in part by patterns of drug metabolism, other possible explanations are being studied. For example, bleomycin stimulates fibroblast proliferation in vitro.[7] It also increases superoxide production in some subpopulations of alveolar macrophages,[8] and in cigarette smokers it causes alveolar macrophages to release hydrogen peroxide.[9] This reaction may also have an immunologic component, as suggested by the release of cytokines after intratracheal instillation of the drug in rats,[10] the modulation of pulmonary fibrosis in the BALB/c mouse by cyclophosphamide-sensitive T cells,[11] and evidence that neutralization of the CXC chemokine (macrophage inflammatory protein–2) attenuates bleomycin-induced pulmonary fibrosis.[12] Also, as could be predicted from the mechanism of action of the drug, experimental pulmonary damage can be decreased by deferoxamine[13] and increased by hyperoxia.[14] In hamsters, niacin therapy seems to attenuate lung fibrosis through increasing the intracellular levels of nicotinamide-adenine dinucleotide (NAD) and adenosine triphosphate (ATP).[15]

**Resistance.** The degradative enzyme bleomycin hydrolase plays a key role in the resistance of normal tissues to bleomycin therapy.[16, 17] Genetically engineered mice without this enzyme have no other mechanism for bleomycin deamination, and most of these mice fail to survive the neonatal period, suggesting an important general role for the enzyme in epidermal integrity. Bleomycin hydrolase is found in tumor cells, liver, and kidney,[18] but it is lacking or markedly deficient in pulmonary and epidermal tissues. In mice, bleomycin-induced pulmonary fibrosis can be prevented by adenovirus-mediated transfer of the bacterial bleomycin resistance gene.[19] In cell culture, bleomycin resistance has been associated with changes in cellular uptake of the drug, reduced ability to damage DNA, and increased rates of DNA repair.[20, 21] Some of these effects may involve bleomycin hydrolase, but others are currently unexplained.

**Pharmacokinetics.** After intravenous injection, bleomycin is rapidly cleared from plasma, with a half-life of about 2 hours. The drug is metabolized to active and inactive compounds, although its detailed metabolic fate in humans has not been determined. In one study, intracellular internalization of bleomycin involved a receptor-mediated endocytosis mechanism.[22] Unchanged bleomycin reaches high concentrations in the skin, lungs, kidneys, peritoneum, and lymphatics, but the concentration is low in the bone marrow.[23] Bleomycin is cleared primarily by the kidneys, and clearance is markedly reduced in patients with a creatinine clearance less than 35 ml/min. The dose of bleomycin should be reduced as much as 50% in patients with severe renal failure (creatinine clearance <10 ml/min).[24]

**Drug Interactions.** Various drugs may increase the cytotoxicity of bleomycin. Examples include anesthetic agents, the radioprotective aminothiol WR-1065,[25] other antineoplastic agents (especially drugs that act by intercalation and nucleoside antimetabolites[26]), bromodeoxyuridine, and inhibitors of calmodulin from some but not all anatomic locations.[27] Cisplatin can decrease the renal elimination of bleomycin, resulting in increased bleomycin pulmonary toxicity.[28, 29] The drug is more toxic in patients with a strong history of cigarette smoking.[30] One study has suggested an increased risk of pulmonary toxicity in patients treated with granulocyte colony-stimulating factor (G-CSF),[31] but other randomized studies do not support this conclusion.[32] In animals, vitamin A pretreatment reduces the frequency and severity of lung damage.[33] In animals, amifostine has been reported to decrease the risk of bleomycin-induced lung injury.[34]

## TOXICITY

**Overview.** The predominant side effects are pulmonary fibrosis, mucocutaneous ulceration and erythema, digestive complaints, and rare vascular and hypersensitivity reactions.

**Immunologic.** Bleomycin can cause a rare, fulminant reaction that is characterized by high fever, hypotension, cardiorespiratory collapse, and death.[35] Although this reaction is assumed to be a form of anaphylaxis, its cause is not clear. It usually occurs in patients who have lymphoma and are receiving large single doses of the drug, but it can occur with small initial doses and after prior full-dose therapy. A test dose of bleomycin is usually used to avert this complication, especially in patients with lymphoma. The drug is not clinically immunosuppressive.

**Digestive System.** Anorexia, nausea, vomiting, and weight loss are common. Anorexia and weight loss may be prolonged despite cessation of treatment.

**Mucocutaneous.** Mucocutaneous toxicity occurs in about 50% of patients. This may include severe skin reactions (erythema, hyperpigmentation, hyperkeratosis, systemic sclerosis, loss of fingernails, ulceration) as well as lesser degrees of mucositis and alopecia. Nearly all these mucocutaneous lesions are dose related and reversible, although Raynaud's phenomenon may rarely progress to gangrene. Raynaud's phenomenon has been reported in about 40% of patients receiving combination chemotherapy for testicular cancer.[36] As with idiopathic Raynaud's phenomenon, the severity of this reaction can be reduced by nifedipine.[37] Iloprost, a prostacyclin analogue with both vasodilatory and platelet inhibitory effects, may also be useful.[38] Extravasation injury is not a problem with bleomycin, but thrombophlebitis can occur at the injection site. A single case of neutrophilic eccrine hidradenitis has been reported after the use of bleomycin.[39]

**Pulmonary.** Pulmonary toxicity is dose limiting and occurs in about 10% of patients. Histologic examination of the lung shows interstitial edema, intra-alveolar hyaline membrane formation, hyperplasia of type II alveolar macrophages, and, in advanced stages, collagen deposition.[40] Rarely, cavitating pulmonary granulomas may occur. Very rarely, pulmonary toxicity may mimic metastatic nodules.[41] Lethal pulmonary fibrosis occurs in about 1 to 2% of patients.[42] Rarely, pulmonary dysfunction is a result of a hypersensitivity reaction that is responsive to corticosteroids, in which case the patient usually has fever, diffuse pulmonary infiltrates, and eosinophilia.[43] In some cases, severe pneumonitis may require long-term corticosteroid therapy over many months. However, when bleomycin pneumonitis progresses to pulmonary fibrosis, there is no effective therapy. The usual cause of death in patients with pulmonary fibrosis is respiratory failure, although rarely death is caused by spontaneous pneumothorax.

Factors associated with a higher risk of pulmonary fibrosis include prior or concomitant radiation therapy, pre-existing pulmonary disease, high-dose oxygen during anesthesia, age greater than 70 years, the use of single doses greater than 26 units/m² or cumulative total doses greater than 400 units, and the use of bleomycin in combination chemotherapy programs.[42]

Early diagnosis of pulmonary dysfunction is important, because the outcome depends on the severity of the toxicity at diagnosis and whether or not bleomycin is continued in the presence of minimal toxicity. The role of serial pulmonary function tests in making an early diagnosis is controversial. Ginsberg and Comis[42] advise serial determinations of the diffusion capacity of carbon monoxide ($D_{LCO}$), with discontinuation of bleomycin for values less than or equal to 40% of the pretreatment value. Other authorities recommend the use of serial pulmonary function tests, especially total lung capacity.[44] The manufacturer has recommended obtaining a chest radiograph every 1 to 2 weeks during treatment to aid in early diagnosis; however, radiographic changes usually occur later than the development of symptomatic dyspnea and rales. We have relied primarily on clinical findings to monitor patients on bleomycin. Specifically, patients should be carefully questioned for symptoms of minimal dyspnea and examined for the presence of fine crackling rales before every dose of the drug. Chest radiography is best used as an adjunct to exclude other causes of pulmonary dysfunction, such as infection, radiation pneumonitis, drug reaction, or progressive tumor. Rarely, problematic cases may require open lung biopsy to establish the diagnosis. Very rarely, bleomycin pulmonary toxicity may mimic metastatic nodules.

### Other and Rare Reactions

**Hematologic.** Myelosuppression is rare and of minor importance.

**Cardiovascular.** An acute chest pain syndrome has been reported in about 3% of patients, but this does not require discontinuation of the drug.[45] Bleomycin can cause severe thrombotic microangiopathy[46] and other acute vascular ischemic events,[47] including pulmonary veno-occlusive disease.[48]

**Ocular.** Cataracts occur in rats, but this has not been a clinical problem in humans.

**Neurologic.** Disorientation and aggressive behavior can occur.

**Musculoskeletal.** These effects include soft tissue calcifications.

**Genitourinary.** Hematuria and cystitis can occur.

**Reproductive.** Toxicity data fit with FDA pregnancy category D.

**Carcinogenicity.** Bleomycin is mutagenic, but its carcinogenic potential is uncertain.

## DOSAGE AND ADMINISTRATION

Bleomycin is available as 15-unit vials for reconstitution and injection. The regular dosage schedule is 10 to 20 units/m² given intravenously, intramuscularly, or subcutaneously weekly or twice weekly, with close observation of the patient for signs of pulmonary toxicity (see Toxicity).

For reasons discussed previously, patients with malignant lymphoma should be treated initially with 2 units or less of bleomycin for the first two doses. If there is no reaction to these test doses, the regular dosage schedule may be used. In lymphoma patients who respond, reduced maintenance doses of 1 unit daily or 5 units weekly may be given. Bleomycin has also been used by the intracavitary route in a dose of 60 to 120 units for the management of malignant effusions (see Chapter 103). Continuous intra-arterial, intravenous, and subcutaneous infusions of bleomycin have been tried, but these routes of administration are not widely used.

Although dosage limitation is an imperfect way of avoiding pulmonary toxicity, it is prudent to limit the total lifetime dose of bleomycin to a maximum of 400 units. The use of bleomycin in combination with other cytotoxic drugs, with radiation therapy, or with hyperthermia may intensify the mucocutaneous, vascular, and pulmonary toxicity of the drug. Care should be used in the administration of anesthesia to patients who have been treated with bleomycin because fatal pulmonary edema may result. This problem can be minimized by using the lowest possible concentrations of oxygen and only modest fluid replacement during anesthesia.

## REFERENCES

1. Dorr RT, Meyers R, Snead K, Liddil JD. Analytical and biological inequivalence of two commercial formulations of the antitumor agent bleomycin. Cancer Chemother Pharmacol 1998;42:149–54.
2. Levi JA, Raghavan D, Harvey V, et al. The importance of bleomycin in combination chemotherapy for good-prognosis germ cell carcinoma. Australasian Germ Cell Trial Group. J Clin Oncol 1993;11:1300–5.
3. Sebti SM, Lazo JS. Metabolic inactivation of bleomycin analogs by bleomycin hydrolase. Pharmacol Ther 1988;38:321–9.
4. Teicher BA, Holden SA, Cathcart KN, Herman TS. Effect of various oxygenation conditions and fluosol-DA on cytotoxicity and antitumor activity of bleomycin in mice. J Natl Cancer Inst 1988;80:599–603.
5. Ostling O, Johanson KJ. Bleomycin, in contrast to gamma irradiation, induces extreme variation of DNA strand breakage from cell to cell. Int J Radiat Biol 1987;52:683–91.
6. Twentyman PR. Bleomycin—mode of action with particular reference to the cell cycle. Pharmacol Ther 1983;23:417–41.
7. Moseley PL, Hemken C, Hunninghake GW. Augmentation of fibroblast proliferation by bleomycin. J Clin Invest 1986;78:1150–4.
8. Zeidler RB, Yarbro JW, Conley NS. Bleomycin increases superoxide

production in the most active alveolar macrophage subpopulation. Int J Immunopharmacol 1987;9:691–6.

9. Lower EE, Strohofer S, Baughman RP. Bleomycin causes alveolar macrophages from cigarette smokers to release hydrogen peroxide. Am J Med Sci 1988;295:193–7.

10. Jordana M, Richards C, Irving LB, Gauldie J. Spontaneous in vitro release of alveolar-macrophage cytokines after the intratracheal instillation of bleomycin in rats: characterization and kinetic studies. Am Rev Respir Dis 1988;137:1135–40.

11. Schrier DJ, Phan SH. Modulation of bleomycin-induced pulmonary fibrosis in the BALB/c mouse by cyclophosphamide-sensitive T cells. Am J Pathol 1984;116:270–8.

12. Keane MP, Belperio JA, Moore TA, et al. Neutralization of the CXC chemokine, macrophage inflammatory protein-2, attenuates bleomycin-induced pulmonary fibrosis. J Immunol 1999;162:5511–8.

13. Chandler DB, Butler TW, Briggs DD III, et al. Modulation of the development of bleomycin-induced fibrosis by deferoxamine. Toxicol Appl Pharmacol 1988;92:358–67.

14. Goad ME, Tryka AF, Witschi HP. Acute respiratory failure induced by bleomycin and hyperoxia: pulmonary edema, cell kinetics and morphology. Toxicol Appl Pharmacol 1987;90:10–22.

15. O'Neill CA, Giri SN. Biochemical mechanisms for the attenuation of bleomycin-induced lung fibrosis by treatment with niacin in hamsters: the role of NAD and ATP. Exp Lung Res 1994;20:41–56.

16. Schwartz DR, Homanics GE, Hoyt DG, et al. The neutral cysteine protease bleomycin hydrolase is essential for epidermal integrity and bleomycin resistance. Proc Natl Acad Sci U S A 1999;96:4680–5.

17. Zheng W, Johnston SA. The nucleic acid binding activity of bleomycin hydrolase is involved in bleomycin detoxification. Mol Cell Biol 1998;18:3580–5.

18. Sebti SM, Jani JP, Mistry JS, et al. Metabolic inactivation: a mechanism of human tumor resistance to bleomycin. Cancer Res 1991;51:227–32.

19. Tran PL, Weinbach J, Opolon P, et al. Prevention of bleomycin-induced pulmonary fibrosis after adenovirus-mediated transfer of the bacterial bleomycin resistance gene. J Clin Invest 1997;99:608–17.

20. Lazo JS, Braun ID, Labaree DC. Characteristics of bleomycin-resistant phenotypes of human cell sublines and circumvention of bleomycin resistance by liblomycin. Cancer Res 1989;49:185–90.

21. Urade M, Ogura T, Mima T, Matsuya T. Establishment of human squamous carcinoma cell lines highly and minimally sensitive to bleomycin and analysis of factors involved in the sensitivity. Cancer 1992;69:2589–97.

22. Pron G, Mahrour N, Orlowski S, et al. Internalisation of the bleomycin molecules responsible for bleomycin toxicity: a receptor-mediated endocytosis mechanism. Biochem Pharmacol 1999;57:45–56.

23. Onuma T, Holland JF, Masuda H, et al. Microbiological assay of bleomycin: inactivation, tissue distribution, and clearance. Cancer 1974;33:1230–8.

24. Bennett WM, Singer I, Golper T, et al. Guidelines for drug therapy in renal failure. Ann Intern Med 1977;86:754–83.

25. Hoffmann GR, Sayer AM, Littlefield LG. Potentiation of bleomycin by the aminothiol WR-1065 in assays for chromosomal damage in GO human lymphocytes. Mutat Res 1994;307:273–83.

26. Begleiter A, Peniuk H, Israels LG, Johnston JB. Inhibition of repair of bleomycin-induced DNA strand breaks by 2'-deoxycoformycin and its effect on antitumor activity in L5178Y lymphoblasts. Biochem Pharmacol 1992;44:2229–33.

27. Hait WN, Byrne TN, Piepmeier J. The effect of calmodulin inhibitors with bleomycin on the treatment of patients with high grade gliomas. Cancer Res 1990;50:6636–40.

28. Sleijfer S, van der Mark TW, Schraffordt Koops H, Mulder NH. Enhanced effects of bleomycin on pulmonary function disturbances in patients with decreased renal function due to cisplatin. Eur J Cancer 1996;32A:550–2.

29. Bennett WM, Pastore L, Houghton DC. Fatal pulmonary bleomycin toxicity in cisplatin-induced acute renal failure. Cancer Treat Rep 1980;64:921–4.

30. Senan S, Paul J, Thomson N, Kaye SB. Cigarette smoking is a risk factor for bleomycin-induced pulmonary toxicity. Eur J Cancer 1992;28A:2084.

31. Matthews JH. Pulmonary toxicity of ABVD chemotherapy and G-CSF in Hodgkin's disease: possible synergy. Lancet 1993;342:988.

32. Bastion Y, Reyes F, Bosley A, et al. Possible toxicity with the association of G-CSF and bleomycin. Lancet 1994;343:1221–2.

33. Habib MP, Lackey DL, Lantz RC, et al. Vitamin A pretreatment and bleomycin induced rat lung injury. Res Commun Chem Pathol Pharmacol 1993;81:199–208.

34. Nici L, Calabresi P. Amifostine modulation of bleomycin-induced lung injury in rodents. Semin Oncol 1999;26:2 Suppl 7:28–33.

35. Carter JJ, McLaughlin ML, Bern MM. Bleomycin-induced fatal hyperpyrexia. Am J Med 1983;74:523–5.

36. Vogelzang NJ, Bosl GJ, Johnson K, Kennedy BJ. Raynaud's phenomenon: a common toxicity after combination chemotherapy for testicular cancer. Ann Intern Med 1981;95:288–92.

37. Hantel A, Rowinsky EK, Donehower RC. Nifedipine and oncologic Raynaud phenomenon. Ann Intern Med 1988;108:767. letter.

38. Wigley FM, Wise RA, Seibold JR, et al. Intravenous iloprost infusion in patients with Raynaud phenomenon secondary to systemic sclerosis. A multicenter, placebo-controlled, double-blind study. Ann Intern Med 1994;120:199–206.

39. Scallan PJ, Kettler AH, Levy ML, Tschen JA. Neutrophilic eccrine hidradenitis: evidence implicating bleomycin as a causative agent. Cancer 1988;62:2532–6.

40. Bedrossian CWM, Luna MA, Mackay B, Lichtiger B. Ultrastructure of pulmonary bleomycin toxicity. Cancer 1973;32:44–51.

41. Ben Arush MW, Roguin A, Zamir E, et al. Bleomycin and cyclophosphamide toxicity simulating metastatic nodules to the lungs in childhood cancer. Pediatr Hematol Oncol 1997;14:381–6.

42. Ginsberg SJ, Comis RL. The pulmonary toxicity of antineoplastic agents. Semin Oncol 1982;9:34–51.

43. Holoye PY, Iuna MA, Mackay B, Bedrossian CW. Bleomycin hypersensitivity pneumonitis. Ann Intern Med 1978;88:47–9.

44. Wolkowicz J, Sturgeon J, Rawji M, Chan CK. Bleomycin-induced pulmonary function abnormalities. Chest 1992;101:97–101.

45. White DA, Schwartzberg LS, Kris MG, Bosl GJ. Acute chest pain syndrome during bleomycin infusions. Cancer 1987;59:1582–5.

46. Jackson AM, Rose BD, Graff LG, et al. Thrombotic microangiopathy and renal failure associated with antineoplastic chemotherapy. Ann Intern Med 1984;101:41–4.

47. Doll DC, List AF, Greco FA, et al. Acute vascular ischemic events after cisplatin-based combination chemotherapy for germ-cell tumors of the testis. Ann Intern Med 1986;105:48–51.

48. Rose AG. Pulmonary veno-occlusive disease after chemotherapy with bleomycin. Hum Pathol 1984;15:199.

# Busulfan

This bifunctional alkylating agent was developed by D.A.G. Galton of the United Kingdom in 1953. It is an alkyl sulfonate and is unrelated chemically to mechlorethamine. Other names include Myleran, BSF, and NSC-750.

## EFFICACY

Busulfan is used to treat chronic myelocytic leukemia. It is occasionally used to treat patients with polycythemia and other myeloproliferative disorders, and the drug is used in some preparative regimens for bone marrow transplantation (BMT).

## PHARMACOLOGY

**Mechanisms of Action and Resistance.** Busulfan is considered a classic bifunctional alkylating agent that has phase-nonspecific effects on the cell cycle. DNA cross-linking appears to be primarily of the intrastrand type. Resistance is probably a result of mechanisms similar to those described for other agents of this class, but detailed studies are not available.

**Pharmacokinetics.** Busulfan is effective by the oral

route. Its pharmacokinetic characteristics are as follows. Oral absorption is rapid, and the subsequent blood levels are linearly related to dose. The drug is rapidly and extensively metabolized by glutathione *S*-transferase enzymes found in liver and intestine,[1] resulting in rapid clearance from the plasma (half-life about 2.5 hours) and only minimal excretion of unchanged drug in the urine (about 1% at 24 hours). There is no apparent accumulation of the drug when doses are administered once every 24 hours, although busulfan is irreversibly and extensively bound to proteins in vivo (32% to plasma proteins and 47% to blood cells). On the basis of high-dose studies with BMT, it appears that the drug readily enters the CSF, resulting in concentrations comparable to those achieved in plasma. The pharmacokinetics of high-dose busulfan are different in children from those in adults, with lower drug levels in blood after standard high-dose administration.[2] Some authors advise close pharmacokinetic monitoring of the drug when given in high doses because of interindividual differences in blood levels.[3]

**Drug Interactions.** Concomitant busulfan and thioguanine therapy can cause esophageal varices and hepatic toxicity (4%). Phenytoin alters busulfan pharmacokinetics at high doses and may inhibit its effectiveness.[4]

## TOXICITY

**Overview.** Dose-limiting myelosuppression is the predominant form of toxicity at usual doses. This can develop suddenly, and it may result in prolonged but usually reversible pancytopenia. Additional forms of toxicity may be seen with high-dose therapy in preparation for BMT.

**Hematologic.** The major dose-limiting toxicity of busulfan is bone marrow suppression. This relates to multiple effects on the bone marrow, including changes in hematopoietic stem cells and cortical bone and marrow stromal cells. With long-term oral administration, the drug occasionally produces abrupt reductions in the WCC and the platelet count, which may be irreversible.

**Digestive System.** Oral busulfan occasionally causes gastrointestinal distress (nausea, vomiting, diarrhea, anorexia, and weight loss). Patients receiving BMT can also develop moderate to severe mucositis that is usually associated with diarrhea. Reversible cholestatic jaundice occasionally occurs with standard dose therapy. BMT recipients may develop fatal veno-occlusive disease (about 20% in adults, 0 to 5% in children).[5]

**Mucocutaneous.** Fragility and anhidrosis of the skin may occur, as well as cheilosis and a dry mouth. With prolonged administration, hyperpigmentation (melanoderma) that resembles Addison's disease or porphyria cutanea tarda (about 10%) can develop, as can alopecia and a variety of skin rashes (resembling those seen with allopurinol, as well as erythema nodosum, erythema multiforme, and bullous eruptions). BMT recipients are very susceptible to radiation-recall skin reactions.[6]

**Other and Rare Reactions**

*Immunologic.* Urticaria can occur.

*Cardiovascular.* Hypotension can occur, as can endocardial fibrosis at high doses.

*Pulmonary.* Intra-alveolar pulmonary fibrosis (busulfan lung) and endocardial fibrosis are well-established, rare complications. A single case report describes pulmonary alveolar proteinosis complicating busulfan therapy.[7]

*Ocular.* Cataracts may occur at standard doses; blurred vision can occur with high doses for BMT.

*Neurologic.* Asthenia is common; myasthenia gravis occurs rarely with standard doses. BMT recipients may develop dizziness, confusion, and seizures.[8, 9]

*Genitourinary.* Hemorrhagic cystitis may occur.

*Reproductive.* Toxicity data place busulfan in FDA pregnancy category D. Sterility is likely (azoospermia, ovarian failure).

*Endocrine-Metabolic.* Gynecomastia and adrenal insufficiency can occur.

*Carcinogenicity.* The drug is carcinogenic, with well-documented cases of leukemia and other tumors in humans. Cytologic dysplasia of almost any organ may occur.

## DOSAGE AND ADMINISTRATION

Busulfan is available as 2-mg scored tablets. An intravenous preparation for use in the transplant setting is under development but not widely available.[10] Induction therapy for adult patients with chronic myelocytic leukemia usually involves the daily oral intake of 1.8 mg/m$^2$ or 60 μg/kg of body weight of the drug until the WCC (which is measured at least once weekly) falls to within the range of 10,000 to 15,000/μL. The drug is discontinued at that time and resumed when a monthly WCC exceeds 50,000/μL. Some clinicians also use maintenance therapy in selected patients, especially those with short periods of remission from induction therapy (<3 months). The maintenance dose is usually 1 to 3 mg/day (see Chapter 86). Dosages before BMT vary from 8 to 16 mg/kg in divided doses over 4 days.[11, 12]

## REFERENCES

1. Gibbs JP, Yang JS, Slattery JT. Comparison of human liver and small intestinal glutathione *S*-transferase-catalyzed busulfan conjugation in vitro. Drug Metab Dispos 1998;26:52–5.
2. Grochow LB, Krivit W, Whitley CB, Blazar B. Busulfan disposition in children. Blood 1990;75:1723–7.
3. Masson E, Zamboni WC. Pharmacokinetic optimisation of cancer chemotherapy: effect on outcomes. Clin Pharmacokinet 1997;32:324–43.
4. Hassan M, Oberg G, Bjorkholm M, et al. Influence of prophylactic anticonvulsant therapy on high-dose busulphan kinetics. Cancer Chemother Pharmacol 1993;33:181–6.
5. Vassal G, Hartmann O, Benhamou E. Busulfan and veno-occlusive disease of the liver. Ann Intern Med 1990;112:881. letter.
6. Vassal G, Hartmann O, Habrand JL, et al. Enhanced cutaneous radiation effects following high-dose busulfan therapy. Cancer Chemother Pharmacol 1989;23:117–8.
7. Aymard J-P, Gyger M, Lavallee R, et al. A case of pulmonary alveolar proteinosis complicating chronic myelogenous leukemia: a peculiar pathologic aspect of busulfan lung? Cancer 1984;53:954–6.
8. Vassal G, Deroussent A, Hartmann O, et al. Dose-dependent neurotoxicity of high-dose busulfan in children: a clinical and pharmacological study. Cancer Res 1990;50:6203–7.
9. Vasta S, Scime R, Indovina A, Majolino I. CNS toxicity and high-dose busulphan in three patients undergoing bone marrow transplantation. Haematologica 1992;77:189.
10. Schuler US, Ehrsam M, Schneider A, et al. Pharmacokinetics of intravenous busulfan and evaluation of the bioavailability of the oral formulation in conditioning for haematopoietic stem cell transplantation. Bone Marrow Transplant 1998;22:241–4.
11. Peters WP, Henner WD, Grochow LB, et al. Clinical and pharmacologic

effects of high dose single agent busulfan with autologous bone marrow support in the treatment of solid tumors. Cancer Res 1987;47:6402–6.
12. Vassal G, Deroussent A, Challine D, et al. Is 600 mg/m² the appropriate dosage of busulfan in children undergoing bone marrow transplantation? Blood 1992;79:2475–9.

# Capecitabine

Capecitabine, 5'-deoxy-5-fluoro-*N*-[(pentyloxy)carbonyl]-cytidine, is a promising new drug in the treatment of advanced breast and colorectal cancers. Marketed as Xeloda, the drug is delivered orally and has an activity profile similar to that of infusional 5-fluorouracil.

## EFFICACY

In the United States, capecitabine is currently approved for use in advanced breast cancer that is resistant to both paclitaxel and an anthracycline-containing regimen. It is also for patients who cannot receive additional (or any) anthracycline therapy. A multicenter single-agent open label trial was conducted in the United States and Canada in patients who had advanced breast cancer and who had been treated previously with paclitaxel and anthracycline therapy or could not receive anthracycline therapy.[1] Of 162 patients, 77% were paclitaxel resistant, 41% were anthracycline resistant, and 31% were resistant to both. Of the 43 patients resistant to both, 25.6% had a partial response to capecitabine; no complete responses were seen. Median duration of response was 154 days (range, 63 to 233 days).

Because of its similar mechanism of action to infusional 5-fluorouracil (5-FU), capecitabine is active in colorectal cancer as well.[2, 3] No definitive studies have yet been published to document the drug's activity. Large trials are currently under way.

## PHARMACOLOGY

**Mechanism of Action.** Once absorbed from the gastrointestinal tract, capecitabine is hydrolyzed in the liver via carboxylesterases into 5'-deoxy-5-fluorocytidine (5'-DFCR). Then an enzyme known as cytidine deaminase converts 5'-DFCR to 5'-deoxy-5-fluorouridine (5'-DFUR). Finally, thymidine phosphorylase hydrolyzes 5'-DFUR to the active drug 5-FU. The section on 5-FU provides a detailed discussion of that drug's mechanisms of action and resistance.

**Pharmacokinetics.** Once converted to 5-FU, the pharmacokinetics of capecitabine and 5-FU are similar.[4] Capecitabine itself exhibits fairly linear pharmacokinetics, with peak blood levels in 1.5 hours and peak 5-FU levels achieved around 30 minutes later. Food reduces the rate and amount of drug absorption. There is also a high degree of interpatient variability. The area under the curve (AUC) of 5-FU was about 34% higher on day 14 than on day 1 of therapy. Capecitabine is primarily bound to human albumin. Most of the administered capecitabine is excreted in the urine.

**Drug-Drug Interactions.** There are no known interactions between capecitabine and other drugs with the exception of Maalox, a commercial brand of antacid.[5] Patients taking Maalox immediately after capecitabine had a mild increase in $C_{max}$ (16%) and AUC (35%).

## TOXICITIES

**Overview.** Capecitabine is relatively well tolerated and has a side effect profile similar to that of infusional 5-FU. The toxicities discussed hereafter are taken from the package insert.

**Gastrointestinal.** The most common side effects of capecitabine are gastrointestinal. Nausea and vomiting (severe in 4%), diarrhea (severe in 11%), stomatitis (severe in 4%), and abdominal pain (severe in 4%) were reported most often. Patients can also develop constipation, dyspepsia and, less commonly, bowel obstruction, rectal bleeding, esophagitis, and gastritis.

**Hepatobiliary.** Fourteen percent of patients treated in the pivotal trials with capecitabine developed a grade 3 or higher hyperbilirubinemia (bilirubin >1.5 times the upper limit of normal). The manufacturer recommends that treatment with capecitabine be stopped if the bilirubin value rises to greater than 1.5 times normal and be resumed only when the bilirubin levels fall below this. Subsequent doses may be modified accordingly.

**Dermatologic.** Similar to infusional 5-FU, capecitabine induces a hand-foot syndrome that was labeled severe in 13% of treated patients. Fewer patients described dermatitis and nail changes.

**Hematologic.** Capecitabine can cause myelosuppression. Neutropenia ($<900/\mu L$) occurred in 3% of patients, anemia (hemoglobin $<7.9$ g/dl) in 2%, and thrombocytopenia (platelets $<50,000/\mu L$) in 1%. Rarely did treatment cease because of hematologic toxicity.

**Other.** Other side effects reported in the pivotal trials included fatigue, fever, paresthesias, headache, dizziness, insomnia, anorexia, dehydration, myalgia, and edema. All were reported rarely.

*Reproductive.* Toxicity data place capecitabine in FDA pregnancy category D.

*Carcinogenicity.* Long-term studies in animals have not been carried out. The carcinogenic potential of this drug is low to nonexistent.

## DOSAGE AND ADMINISTRATION

Capecitabine is manufactured as tablets of 150 mg (light peach color) and 500 mg (peach color) each. Tablets may be kept at room temperature. The approved dosage is 2500 mg/m²/day in two divided doses (1250 mg/m² each). The drug should be taken twice daily for 2 weeks, followed by 1 week of rest. The manufacturer recommends taking the drug with food at the end of a meal. If toxicity occurs, doses may be modified according to a table provided in the package insert. To summarize that table, the drug should be discontinued for any grade 2 or greater toxicity and held until the side effect resolves to grade 1 or less. In the event of a second occurrence of a grade 2 toxicity or the first occurrence of a grade 3 or 4 toxicity when the drug is resumed, doses should be reduced by at least 25% (and greater for more frequent or more severe side effects). Dosing in patients with hepatic or renal dysfunction has not been formally studied.

## REFERENCES

1. Blum JL, Jones SE, Buzdar AU, et al. Multicenter phase II study of capecitabine in paclitaxel-refractory metastatic breast cancer. J Clin Oncol 1999;17:485–93.
2. Cassidy J, Dirix L, Bissett D, et al. A phase I study of capecitabine in combination with oral leucovorin in patients with intractable solid tumors. Clin Cancer Res 1998;4:2755–61.
3. Meropol NJ. Oral fluoropyrimidines in the treatment of colorectal cancer. Eur J Cancer 1998;34:1509–13.
4. Mackean M, Planting A, Twelves C, et al. Phase I and pharmacologic study of intermittent twice-daily oral therapy with capecitabine in patients with advanced and/or metastatic cancer. J Clin Oncol 1998;16:2977–85.
5. Reigner B, Clive S, Cassidy J, et al. Influence of the antacid Maalox on the pharmacokinetics of capecitabine in cancer patients. Cancer Chemother Pharmacol 1999;43:309–15.

# Carboplatin

There is great interest in the development of cisplatin analogues that might retain efficacy while having reduced toxicity.[1] Carboplatin (CBDCA, JM-8, Paraplatin) was developed at Michigan State University for this purpose.

## EFFICACY

Carboplatin appears to have the same spectrum of antitumor activity as cisplatin but with a very different spectrum of drug toxicity. The choice of platinum analogue is usually based on the type of tumor, the intent of treatment, and the pharmacologic characteristics of other drugs used in the treatment regimen.[2]

## PHARMACOLOGY

**Mechanism of Action.** Carboplatin and cisplatin are considered to share the same mechanisms of cytotoxicity. Binding to DNA occurs with both drugs, following a similar aquation reaction. This process is much slower for carboplatin than for cisplatin, however, leading to marked differences in clinical pharmacology and toxicity.[3, 4] Both drugs are cell cycle phase nonspecific. Cell death from carboplatin results from either apoptosis or necrosis, depending on the cell line.[5]

**Resistance.** The mechanisms of resistance are thought to be the same as for cisplatin.

**Pharmacokinetics.** Carboplatin is rapidly removed from blood, with a half-life of about 2.5 hours. However, the reduced aquation reaction of carboplatin results in a greater percentage of the active moiety in blood than with cisplatin. In one study, 4 hours after injecting each drug, the level of ultrafilterable, non–protein-bound platinum in plasma was 76% for carboplatin and 10% for cisplatin.[6] More than 60% of carboplatin is excreted in the urine as unchanged drug, compared with 25 to 40% of cisplatin. Both cisplatin and

carboplatin undergo tubular reabsorption following glomerular filtration,[7] but renal retention of carboplatin is less than that of cisplatin.[8] Interindividual differences in pharmacokinetics for carboplatin may explain the poor predictability of toxicity after doses determined by using a single dose level based on body weight or body surface area.[9] Alternative methods for choosing a starting dose of the drug are described subsequently.

**Drug Interactions.** Biomodulation of carboplatin action has been reported by pretreatment of patients with cyclophosphamide,[10] the use of diethyldithiocarbamate chemoprotection,[11, 12] and concurrent treatment with taxanes.[13] IL-1 reportedly speeds recovery from thrombocytopenia.[14] Hyperthermia may increase the therapeutic index of carboplatin.[15] Ototoxicity may be increased by concurrent use of ototoxic drugs,[16] and renal toxicity can be increased by the use of aminoglycoside antibiotics. Nonsteroidal anti-inflammatory drugs (NSAIDs) reportedly enhance the cytotoxicity of carboplatin.[17] Other drug interactions are likely, as discussed for cisplatin. Both cisplatin and carboplatin can serve as potentiators of radiation therapy.[18] Aluminum causes precipitation of the drug in solution and reduces the potency of carboplatin. Chemoprotectants, such as amifostine, may reduce the toxicity of carboplatin; the extent to which tumor cells are also protected is uncertain.[19]

## TOXICITY

**Overview.** Dose-related, cumulative myelosuppression is the predominant dose-limiting toxicity. Vomiting is expected but is usually minimal in severity. Anaphylaxis occurs in about 2% of patients and can be life threatening. Other toxic side effects are similar to those of cisplatin but are generally much less severe. In a high-dose setting, carboplatin may rarely cause a life-threatening syndrome of multiorgan failure including acute renal failure, mental obtundation, cardiac decompensation, and, in some cases, acute myopathy.[20]

**Hematologic.** The dose-limiting adverse effect of carboplatin is myelotoxicity. Thrombocytopenia occurs about 3 weeks after treatment, followed a few days later by leukopenia. Recovery usually occurs by 4 weeks, but as many as one half of patients require as long as 5 to 6 weeks for full recovery. Consequently, a 21-day re-treatment cycle is unrealistic for this agent. The severity of thrombocytopenia is sometimes used as a guide to subsequent dosage adjustments. Anemia may be cumulative and require transfusions or erythropoietin. Hemolytic anemia can occur rarely.

**Immunologic.** Although rare (about 2% of patients), hypersensitivity reactions, including anaphylaxis, can occur, either with or without prior cisplatin exposure.[21] Some authors recommend pretreatment skin testing to help identify high-risk patients.[22]

**Digestive System.** Gastrointestinal toxicity is seen with carboplatin, but the severity of this reaction is far less than with cisplatin. Specifically, about 75% of patients have emesis, but this is almost always minimal. An elevated alkaline phosphatase level occurs in about one third of patients; transaminase elevations occur less frequently. True hepatic damage is only rarely seen with standard doses of carboplatin, but it can be life threatening with high-dose therapy. Other effects include abdominal pain (17%), diarrhea (6%), and constipation (6%).

**Neurologic.** Peripheral neuropathy is rare with carboplatin (about 4 to 6%), as is clinical ototoxicity (1%). These reactions are more frequent and severe in patients pretreated with cisplatin and in those older than 65 years. When carboplatin is used at high dose in preparation for BMT, severe ototoxicity is much more likely than with standard doses.[23] In one pediatric series, significant ototoxicity occurred in 82% of the patients.[24]

**Genitourinary.** Nephrotoxicity occurs in fewer than 25% of patients, and it is far less severe than with cisplatin. Carboplatin treatment does not require the administration of large fluid loads or mannitol. Electrolyte abnormalities are common, with hypomagnesemia occurring in about one third of patients, but electrolyte changes are rarely serious or difficult to manage. Rarely, carboplatin has been associated with hemorrhagic cystitis, presumably due to toxicity to transitional epithelium of the collecting system and bladder.[25]

**Other and Rare Reactions.** A flu-like asthenia syndrome occurs in about 1% of patients.

*Mucocutaneous.* Alopecia occurs in 3% of patients; pain occurs at the site of injection in 1%; and mucositis is rare.

*Cardiovascular.* Cardiac failure and vascular events have been reported, but their relationship to carboplatin is uncertain.

*Pulmonary.* Pulmonary embolism has been reported, but its relationship to carboplatin is uncertain.

*Ocular.* Optic neuritis is a very rare complication with standard doses; high-dose therapy increases the risk of blindness.[26]

*Reproductive.* Toxicity data place carboplatin in FDA pregnancy category D.

*Carcinogenicity.* The drug is mutagenic and potentially carcinogenic. Cases of secondary myelodysplasia and acute leukemia have been reported after its use.[27]

## DOSAGE AND ADMINISTRATION

Carboplatin is supplied in 50-, 150-, and 450-mg vials for reconstitution and intravenous administration, usually in 5% dextrose solution. Aluminum needles should not be used because of incompatibility with carboplatin. Although the drug has been given by the intra-arterial and intraperitoneal routes and by continuous intravenous infusions, it is usually administered as intermittent intravenous injections over 15 minutes or longer every 4 weeks. Commonly used intravenous doses range from 300 to 360 mg/m². As a single agent in patients refractory to other chemotherapy, the usual starting dose is 360 mg/m². Patients with renal dysfunction require lower doses (such as 250 mg/m² for a creatinine clearance of 41 to 59 ml/min or 200 mg/m² for a creatinine clearance of 16 to 40 ml/min). Aggressive hydration and electrolyte support are not required as they are for cisplatin. Much higher doses have been used as preparation for autologous BMT.[28]

Dosage adjustments can be made using either of two methods listed in Table 10–3. In the first, a CBC is measured several times during therapy, and subsequent doses of carboplatin are modified as a function of the severity of myelosuppression. An alternative high-dose schedule may be used,

*Table 10–3.* Dose Adjustments for Carboplatin

**Dose Adjustments Based on Nadir Blood Counts***

| NADIR ANC | NADIR PLATELETS | DOSE (AS A % OF PRIOR DOSE) |
|---|---|---|
| >2000 | >100,000 | 125 |
| 500–2000 | 50,000–100,000 | 100 |
| <500 | <50,000 | 75 |

**Dose Adjustments Based on Pharmacokinetic Data (AUC)†**

Dose for previously untreated patients:
  Dose (mg) = target AUC (6–8 mg/ml/min) − (CrCl + 25)
Dose for previously treated patients:
  Dose (mg) = target AUC (4–6 mg/ml/min) − (CrCl + 25)

*From Egorin MJ, Van Echo DA, Olman EA, et al. Prospective validation of a pharmacologically based dosing scheme for the *cis*-diamminedichloroplatinum (II) analogue diamminecyclobutanedicarboxylatoplatinum. Cancer Res 1985;45:6502. The nadir represents the lowest absolute neutrophil count (ANC) or platelet count in cells per microliter (fl); only one dose escalation should be made.

†From Calvert AH, Newell DR, Gumbrell LA, et al: Carboplatin dosage: Prospective evaluation of a simple formula based on renal function. J Clin Oncol 1989;7:1748. AUC, area under the curve from pharmacokinetic measurements. CrCl, creatinine clearance.

especially in patients treated with curative intent. The regimen is based on the creatinine clearance and desired AUC for carboplatin.[29] Additional dose reductions may be appropriate for geriatric patients, but these should be based on physiologic age rather than mere chronologic age.[30] A pediatric dosing formula based on glomerular filtration rate is also under investigation.[31]

## REFERENCES

1. Lebwohl D, Canetta R. Clinical development of platinum complexes in cancer therapy: an historical perspective and an update. Eur J Cancer 1998;34:1522–34.
2. Lokich J, Anderson N. Carboplatin versus cisplatin in solid tumors: an analysis of the literature [erratum published in Ann Oncol 1998;9:341]. Ann Oncol 1998;9:13–21.
3. Knox RJ, Friedlos F, Lydall DA, Roberts JJ. Mechanism of cytotoxicity of anticancer platinum drugs: evidence that *cis*-diamminedichloroplatinum(II) and *cis*-diammine-(1,1-cyclobutanedicarboxylato)platinum(II) differ only in the kinetics of their interaction with DNA. Cancer Res 1986;46:1972–9.
4. Terheggen PM, Dijkman R, Begg AC, et al. Monitoring of interaction products of *cis*-diamminedichloroplatinum(II) and *cis*-diammine(1,1-cyclobutanedicarboxylato)platinum(II) with DNA in cells from platinum-treated cancer patients. Cancer Res 1988;48:5597–603.
5. Yee S, Kamradt JM, Nielsen LC, et al. Carboplatin-induced cell death in model prostate cancer systems. Anticancer Res 1998;18:4475–82.
6. Harland SJ, Newell DR, Siddik ZH, et al. Pharmacokinetics of cis-diammine-1,1-cyclobutane dicarboxylate platinum (II) in patients with normal and impaired renal function. Cancer Res 1984;44:1693–7.
7. Sorensen BT, Stromgren A, Jakobsen P, et al. Renal handling of carboplatin. Cancer Chemother Pharmacol 1992;30:317–20.
8. Ewen C, Perera A, Hendry JH, et al. An autoradiographic study of the intrarenal localisation and retention of cisplatin, iproplatin and paraplatin. Cancer Chemother Pharmacol 1988;22:241–5.
9. Duffull SB, Robinson BA. Clinical pharmacokinetics and dose optimisation of carboplatin. Clin Pharmacokinet 1997;33:161–83.
10. Gore ME, Hills CA, Siddik ZH, et al. Priming reduces the bone marrow toxicity of carboplatin. Eur J Cancer Clin Oncol 1987;23:75–80.
11. Rothenberg ML, Ostchega Y, Steinberg SM, Young RC. High-dose carboplatin with diethyldithiocarbamate chemoprotection in treatment of women with relapsed ovarian cancer. J Natl Cancer Inst 1988;80:1488–92.
12. Qazi R, Chang AY, Borch RF, et al. Phase I clinical and pharmacokinetic study of diethyldithiocarbamate as a chemoprotector from toxic

effects of cisplatin [erratum published in J Natl Cancer Inst 1989;81:461]. J Natl Cancer Inst 1988;80:1486–8.

13. Obasaju CK, Johnson SW, Rogatko A, et al. Evaluation of carboplatin pharmacokinetics in the absence and presence of paclitaxel. Clin Cancer Res 1996;2:549–52.

14. Smith JW II, Longo DL, Alvord WG, et al. The effects of treatment with interleukin-1 alpha on platelet recovery after high-dose carboplatin. N Engl J Med 1993;328:756–61.

15. Robins HI, Cohen JD, Schmitt CL. Phase I clinical trial of carboplatin and 41.8 degrees C whole-body hyperthermia in cancer patients. J Clin Oncol 1993;11:1787–94.

16. Kennedy IC, Fitzharris BM, Colls BM, Atkinson CH. Carboplatin is ototoxic. Cancer Chemother Pharmacol 1990;26:232–4.

17. Duffy CP, Elliott CJ, O'Connor RA, et al. Enhancement of chemotherapeutic drug toxicity to human tumour cells in vitro by a subset of nonsteroidal anti-inflammatory drugs (NSAIDs). Eur J Cancer 1998; 34:1250–9.

18. Douple EV, Richmond RC, O'Hara JA, Coughlin CT. Carboplatin as a potentiator of radiation therapy. Cancer Treat Rev 1985;12:Suppl A:111–24.

19. Links M, Lewis C. Chemoprotectants: a review of their clinical pharmacology and therapeutic efficacy. Drugs 1999;57:293–308.

20. Grigg A, Szer J, Skov K, Barnett M. Multi-organ dysfunction associated with high-dose carboplatin therapy prior to autologous transplantation. Bone Marrow Transplant 1996;17:67–74.

21. Tonkin KS, Rubin P, Levin L. Carboplatin hypersensitivity: case reports and review of the literature. Eur J Cancer 1993;29A:1356–7.

22. Weidmann B, Mulleneisen N, Bojko P, Niederle N. Hypersensitivity reactions to carboplatin: report of two patients, review of the literature and discussion of diagnostic procedures and management. Cancer 1994;73:2218–22.

23. Cavaletti G, Bogliun G, Zincone A, et al. Neuro- and ototoxicity of high-dose carboplatin treatment in poor prognosis ovarian cancer patients. Anticancer Res 1998;18:3797–802.

24. Parsons SK, Neault MW, LaVita L, et al. Proc Am Soc Clin Oncol 1994;13:417.

25. Agraharkar M, Nerenstone S, Palmisano J, Kaplan AA. Carboplatin-related hematuria and acute renal failure. Am J Kidney Dis 1998;32:E5.

26. O'Brien ME, Tonge K, Blake P, et al. Blindness associated with high-dose carboplatin. Lancet 1992;339:558.

27. Colon-Otero G, Malkasian GD, Edmonson JH. Secondary myelodysplasia and acute leukemia following carboplatin-containing combination chemotherapy for ovarian cancer. J Natl Cancer Inst 1993;85:1858–60.

28. Elias AD, Ayash LJ, Eder JP, et al. Escalating doses of carboplatin with high-dose ifosfamide using autologous bone marrow as support: a phase I study. J Cancer Res Clin Oncol 1991;117:Suppl 4:s208–13.

29. Calvert AH, Newell DR, Gumbrell LA. Carboplatin dosage: prospective evaluation of a simple formula based on renal function. J Clin Oncol 1989;7:1748–56.

30. Cornelison TL, Reed E. Dose intensity analysis of high-dose carboplatin in refractory ovarian carcinoma relative to age. Cancer 1993;71:Suppl 2:650–5.

31. Newell DR, Pearson AD, Balmanno K. Carboplatin pharmacokinetics in children: the development of a pediatric dosing formula. The United Kingdom Children's Cancer Study Group. J Clin Oncol 1993;11:2314–23.

# Carmustine

In the mid-1960s, scientists at the Southern Research Institute developed a group of lipophilic alkylating agents known as nitrosoureas. Carmustine was the first of two such agents to become commercially available in the United States. The drug is also known as BCNU, BiCNU, bis-chloroethyl-nitrosourea, and NSC-409962.

## EFFICACY

Carmustine is FDA approved for the treatment of brain tumors, Hodgkin's disease, myeloma, and the non-Hodgkin's lymphomas. The drug is also used in combination with other agents against a variety of neoplasms.

## PHARMACOLOGY

**Mechanism of Action.** The nitrosoureas undergo extensive biotransformation in vivo, leading to a variety of biologic effects.[1] The primary mechanism of action of the nitrosoureas involves hydrolysis to a chloroethyldiazonium ion, which can chloroethylate DNA and undergo a subsequent reaction to form cross-links, and to a substituted isocyanate that can carbamoylate intracellular molecules. Chloroethylation is analogous to alkylation yet different. Chloroethylation involves the formation of a chloroethyl adduct at the $O^6$ position on guanine. Subsequently, this forms an internal cyclic $N^1O^6$-ethanoguanine intermediate that rearranges to an interstrand cross-link between guanine and cytosine. This cross-linking is extremely cytotoxic. The drug is usually classified as cell cycle phase nonspecific.

Emerging data on the genetic specificity of carmustine-induced DNA damage suggest that the Jun kinase signal transduction pathway may be especially sensitive to the drug and that tumor necrosis factor (TNF) may be an important mediator of carmustine-induced cytotoxicity.[2]

**Resistance.** There is at least partial cross-resistance between carmustine and other alkylating agents, suggesting shared mechanisms of resistance. A specific DNA repair protein known as $O^6$-alkylguanine DNA alkyltransferase is responsible for repair of both monofunctional and cyclic $N^1O^6$-ethanoalkylations at the $O^6$ position on guanine.[3] A secondary role is played by the excision repair pathway. The use of $O^6$-benzylguanine and other specific inhibitors of $O^6$-alkyltransferase is under investigation as a way to improve the efficacy of this class of drugs.[4]

**Pharmacokinetics.** Carmustine undergoes extensive oxidation by hepatic *N*-demethylation enzymes to active and inactive products. The parent drug is not significantly bound to serum proteins, but the metabolites are extensively bound. The drug and its metabolites are very lipid soluble and cross the blood-brain barrier with ease. These are widely distributed in the body, including breast milk. Excretion occurs primarily via the kidneys (80%). The plasma clearance of carmustine is rapid, with an approximate half-life of 15 to 20 minutes. The drug is not hemodialyzable. The pharmacokinetics of high-dose carmustine appear to be the same as for the standard dose.

Relatively little is known about the pharmacokinetics of drug access and accumulation of cancer chemotherapeutic agents by tumor tissue. One study of the pharmacokinetics of positron-labeled carmustine in patients with brain tumors found a markedly longer clearance time of carmustine from the tumor than from surrounding normal brain tissue.[5]

**Drug Interactions.** Several studies suggest that the cytotoxicity of nitrosoureas may be increased in the presence of several different drugs, including the radiation sensitizer misonidazole, amphotericin B, acetohydroxamic acid analogues of 3-nitropyrazole, 2-nitroimidazoles,[6] and α-difluoromethylornithine.[7] The antineoplastic activity of carmustine may also be increased by TNF.[8] Cimetidine slows the metabolism of carmustine, potentially leading to increased myelosuppression.[9]

## TOXICITY

**Overview.** Delayed and cumulative myelosuppression, local pain at the injection site, nausea, and pulmonary toxicity are the predominant toxic side effects of carmustine. Rare toxic reactions with standard doses of the nitrosoureas may become more common or fatal when high doses are used and are followed by autologous BMT.

**Hematologic.** The major dose-limiting side effect of carmustine is delayed bone marrow depression, commonly occurring about 4 weeks after a given dose of drug and resolving by about 6 weeks. Cumulative myelosuppression can occur.

**Digestive System.** Nausea and vomiting can be severe and usually start 3 to 6 hours after carmustine is given. The duration is short, usually lasting less than 1 day of each cycle. Hepatic dysfunction can occur rarely with standard doses (cholestasis with predominant damage to the epithelial cells of large bile ducts) but is more common with higher doses (up to 26% of patients). At high doses, veno-occlusive disease of the liver can also occur.

**Mucocutaneous.** Carmustine can cause severe local pain at the injection site and conjunctival suffusion. These may be difficult to control despite alterations in the rate of drug administration or the concentration of the solution being injected. Rarely, stomatitis and alopecia can occur. The nitrosoureas are occasionally used topically for the treatment of mycosis fungoides. Topical therapy can be complicated by the development of contact dermatitis, hyperpigmentation, telangiectasis, pruritus, and a Nikolsky-like epidermal separation in uninvolved, inflamed skin.

**Pulmonary.** Patients who receive prolonged therapy with nitrosoureas have a high risk of pulmonary fibrosis. The approximate frequency of this complication by 3 years is about 20 to 30% with a mortality rate of about 50%.[10] This risk is especially great after a cumulative dose of 1400 mg/m$^2$. Delayed pulmonary fibrosis can also occur in patients who are apparently asymptomatic for periods of 7 to 12 years. In one study of children with brain tumors treated with carmustine, the risk of delayed pulmonary fibrosis was an additional 24% and all the patients studied demonstrated some degree of pulmonary dysfunction.[11] The mechanism of this toxicity is unknown, but concomitant radiation therapy, pre-existing lung disease, and smoking all appear to increase the frequency and severity of the complication.[12] Pulmonary toxicity occurs in about 30 to 40% of patients after high-dose therapy in the transplantation setting. In one study, prophylactic prednisone was effective in preventing the development of symptomatic pulmonary dysfunction in high-risk patients identified by DLco pulmonary function testing.[13]

### Other and Rare Reactions

*Immunologic.* Hypersensitivity reactions and minimal immunosuppression may occur.

*Cardiovascular.* Myocardial ischemia has been reported, but usually only in the setting of high doses for BMT.[14]

*Ocular.* Optic neuritis, rarely with blindness, can occur. This is more common with investigational administration by the intracarotid route and in high doses with autologous BMT.

*Neurologic.* Disorientation, lethargy, ataxia, and dysarthria can occur. Encephalomyelopathy may occur with transplant doses.

*Genitourinary.* Delayed renal dysfunction with decreased kidney size, progressive azotemia, and in some cases renal failure have been reported with standard doses given for prolonged periods. The hemolytic-uremic syndrome can occur with very high doses.

*Reproductive.* Toxicity data place carmustine in FDA pregnancy category D.

*Endocrine-Metabolic.* Gynecomastia can occur.

*Carcinogenicity.* The drug is carcinogenic. Leukemia is of particular concern, and lesser forms of myelodysplasia may also develop.

## DOSAGE AND ADMINISTRATION

Carmustine is marketed in a package containing a 100-mg vial of the drug and a 3-ml vial of absolute alcohol. Each vial is reconstituted with alcohol and then diluted further with 27 ml of sterile water for injection. This is again diluted into 100 ml or more of normal saline or 5% dextrose in water and administered as a 1- to 2-hour infusion. The usual dose of carmustine is 150 to 200 mg/m$^2$ as a single intravenous injection every 6 weeks. Patients with pre-existing bone marrow depression or extensive prior bone marrow-suppressive therapy require lower doses, and prolonged treatment may necessitate further dose reductions. When carmustine is used as preparation for BMT, the dose is usually 600 mg/m$^2$.

## REFERENCES

1. McCormick JE, McElhinney RS. Nitrosoureas from chemist to physician: classification and recent approaches to drug design. Eur J Cancer 1990;26:207–21.
2. Rhee CH, Ruan S, Chen S, et al. Characterization of cellular pathways involved in glioblastoma response to the chemotherapeutic agent 1,3-bis(2-chloroethyl)-1-nitrosourea (BCNU) by gene expression profiling. Oncol Rep 1999;6:393–401.
3. Gonzaga PE, Brent TP. Affinity purification and characterization of human O6-alkylguanine-DNA alkyltransferase complexed with BCNU-treated, synthetic oligonucleotide. Nucleic Acids Res 1989;17:6581–90.
4. Gerson SL, Zborowska E, Norton K, et al. Synergistic efficacy of O6-benzylguanine and 1,3-bis(2-chloroethyl)-1-nitrosourea (BCNU) in a human colon cancer xenograft completely resistant to BCNU alone. Biochem Pharmacol 1993;45:483–91.
5. Diksic M, Sako K, Feindel W. Pharmacokinetics of positron-labeled 1,3-bis(2-chloroethyl)nitrosourea in human brain tumors using positron emission tomography. Cancer Res 1984;44:3120–4.
6. Wong K-H, Wallen CA, Wheeler KT. Chemosensitization of the nitrosoureas by 2-nitroimidazoles in the subcutaneous 9L tumor model: pharmacokinetic and structure-activity considerations. Int J Radiat Oncol Biol Phys 1990;18:1043–50.
7. Hunter KJ, Deen DF, Pellarin M, Marton LJ. Effect of alpha-difluoromethylornithine on 1,3-bis(2-chloroethyl)-1-nitrosourea and cis-diamminedichloroplatinum(II) cytotoxicity, DNA interstrand cross-linking, and growth in human brain tumor cell lines in vitro. Cancer Res 1990;50:2769–72.
8. Jones AL, Millar JL, Millar BC, et al. Enhanced anti-tumor activity of carmustine (BCNU) with tumor necrosis factor in vitro and in vivo. Br J Cancer 1990;62:776–80.
9. Volkin RL, Shadduck RK, Winkelstein A, et al. Potentiation of carmustine–cranial irradiation–induced myelosuppression by cimetidine. Arch Intern Med 1982;142:243–5.
10. Weiss RB, Poster DS, Penta JS. The nitrosoureas and pulmonary toxicity. Cancer Treat Rev 1981;8:111–25.
11. O'Driscoll BR, Hasleton PS, Taylor PM, et al. Active lung fibrosis up to 17 years after chemotherapy with carmustine (BCNU) in childhood. N Engl J Med 1990;323:378–82.

12. Limper AH, McDonald JA. Delayed pulmonary fibrosis after nitrosourea therapy. N Engl J Med 1990;323:407–9.
13. Kalaycioglu M, Kavuru M, Tuason L, Bolwell B. Empiric prednisone therapy for pulmonary toxic reaction after high-dose chemotherapy containing carmustine (BCNU). Chest 1995;107:482–7.
14. Kanj SS, Sharara AI, Shpall EJ, et al. Myocardial ischemia associated with high-dose carmustine infusion. Cancer 1991;68:1910–2.

# Chlorambucil

Chlorambucil, an aromatic derivative of mechlorethamine, was developed at the Chester Beatty Research Institute in England. It is the slowest acting and generally least toxic of the alkylating agents in common use. Other names include Leukeran, Chl, and NSC-3088.

## EFFICACY

Chlorambucil is used almost exclusively in the management of chronic lymphocytic leukemia (CLL). It does, however, have antitumor activity against a wide range of neoplasms, including malignant lymphomas, multiple myeloma, Waldenström's macroglobulinemia, polycythemia rubra vera, ovarian neoplasms, trophoblastic neoplasms, testicular tumors, some solid tumors, and a variety of non-neoplastic conditions.

## PHARMACOLOGY

**Mechanisms of Action and Resistance.** The mechanisms of action and resistance for chlorambucil are probably similar, if not the same, as those for mechlorethamine.[1] In vitro studies suggest that DNA repair enzymes are important in resisting the effects of chlorambucil.[2] In another study, both glutathione *S*-transferase and multidrug-resistance protein 1 (MRP 1), which is responsible for a drug efflux pump, were important mechanisms of resistance to chlorambucil-induced cytotoxicity.[3]

**Pharmacokinetics.** Chlorambucil is easily absorbed after oral administration, leading to peak plasma levels after 2 to 4 hours. Gastrointestinal absorption is by passive diffusion, and food can interfere with this process. Chlorambucil is metabolized in the liver to an alkylating metabolite, phenylacetic acid mustard, which is further degraded before being excreted by the kidneys. The terminal plasma half-life of chlorambucil is 1.5 hours, whereas it is 2.4 hours for phenylacetic acid mustard. Chlorambucil and its metabolites are only minimally excreted by the kidneys (about 1%), and they are extensively bound to plasma proteins (about 99%). It is unknown whether the drug crosses the blood-brain barrier. The process of cellular influx and efflux of chlorambucil and phenylacetic acid mustard for CLL cells appears to be by passive diffusion rather than by an energy-dependent process.

**Drug Interactions.** No significant drug interactions are known.

## TOXICITY

**Overview.** As with other classic alkylating agents, the predominant toxic side effect of chlorambucil is myelosup-

pression. The manufacturer recommends advising patients of the following additional toxic side effects: hypersensitivity reactions, drug fever, hepatotoxicity, infertility, seizures, gastrointestinal toxicity, and second malignancies.

**Hematologic.** Bone marrow suppression is the major and dose-limiting side effect of chlorambucil. This usually occurs gradually and is fully reversible; however, with prolonged therapy or excessive doses, it may be irreversible and lead to pancytopenia.

**Digestive System.** Nausea, vomiting, anorexia, and diarrhea can occur, but they are not common or severe in most cases. Hepatotoxicity can occur (mild and transient increases in transaminase enzymes).

**Other and Rare Reactions.** Drug fever and a peculiar wasting syndrome can occur.

*Immunologic.* Hypersensitivity reactions involving the skin are rare but potentially serious (discussed later). Immunosuppression occurs but is rarely severe. Herpes zoster can occur during treatment, and it can be exacerbated by chlorambucil therapy.

*Mucocutaneous.* Dermatitis and alopecia can occur; mucositis is rare. There are rare reports of skin rash progressing to erythema multiforme, toxic epidermal necrolysis, and Stevens-Johnson syndrome.

*Pulmonary.* Pulmonary fibrosis, especially with high doses or prolonged therapy, can occur. Interstitial pneumonitis (T-lymphocytic alveolitis) can occur.[4]

*Ocular.* Unspecified ocular damage has been reported very rarely.

*Neurologic.* Peripheral neuropathy, tremors, confusion, ataxia, flaccid paresis, and hallucinations can occur. In children, seizures have been reported. Reversible neurotoxicity is not uncommon after very high dose treatment with autologous BMT.

*Musculoskeletal.* Muscular twitching can occur.

*Genitourinary.* Sterile cystitis may occur.

*Reproductive.* Toxicity data place chlorambucil in FDA pregnancy category D.

*Endocrine-Metabolic.* Both reversible and permanent sterility have occurred in men and women.

*Carcinogenicity.* The drug is mutagenic and carcinogenic; it has been associated with acute leukemia in patients given the drug after renal transplantation.[5]

## DOSAGE AND ADMINISTRATION

Chlorambucil is available as 2-mg tablets for oral administration. The initial dose is usually 0.1 to 0.2 mg/kg/day given as a single dose on an empty stomach. Once the desired effect is achieved, usually in 3 to 6 weeks, maintenance therapy with 2 to 4 mg/day may be considered. It is important for the maintenance dosage not to exceed these levels and for a CBC to be obtained weekly. An alternative program of treatment in CLL involves the administration of chlorambucil every 2 to 4 weeks in a single dose of 0.4 mg/kg. Responses are excellent with this schedule, and toxicity is minimal.[6] Patients with lymphoma may be treated with 16 mg/m²/day for 5 days every 4 weeks.[7]

## REFERENCES

1. Begleiter A, Goldenberg GJ, Anhalt CD, et al. Mechanisms of resistance to chlorambucil in chronic lymphocytic leukemia. Leuk Res 1991;15:1019–27.

2. Mèuller MR, Buschfort C, Thomale J, et al. DNA repair and cellular resistance to alkylating agents in chronic lymphocytic leukemia. Clin Cancer Res 1997;3:2055–61.
3. Morrow CS, Smitherman PK, Diah SK, et al. Coordinated action of glutathione *S*-transferase (GSTs) and multidrug resistance protein 1 (MRP1) in antineoplastic drug detoxification: mechanism of GST A1-1- and MRP-associated resistance to chlorambucil in MCF7 breast carcinoma cells. J Biol Chem 1998;273:20114–20.
4. Crestani B, Jaccard A, Israel-Biet D, et al. Chlorambucil-associated pneumonitis. Chest 1994;105:634–6.
5. Ho WKW, Robertson MR, Macdonald GJ, et al. Association of acute leukaemia with chlorambucil after renal transplantation. Lancet 1994;343:1298–9.
6. Knospe WH, Loeb V Jr, Huguley CM Jr. Proceedings: bi-weekly chlorambucil treatment of chronic lymphocytic leukemia. Cancer 1974;33:555–62.
7. Portlock CS, Fischer DS, Cadman E. High-dose pulse chlorambucil in advanced, low-grade non-Hodgkin's lymphoma. Cancer Treat Rep 1987;71:1029–31.

# Cisplatin

In 1965, Rosenberg and coworkers discovered that replication of *E. coli* could be inhibited by passing an electric current between platinum electrodes in nutrient broth containing ammonium and chloride ions.[1] It was soon learned that this inhibition was caused by the release of platinum complexes, and a wide variety of platinum compounds are now known to inhibit animal and human tumors. The first and most important member of this new class of agents is *cis*-diamminedichloroplatinum(II) (cisplatin; DDP; Platinol).

## EFFICACY

Cisplatin is one of the most widely used drugs in oncology. It is used with curative intent in combination with other drugs in the treatment of tumors of the ovary and testis, and it is widely used in the palliative treatment of cancers of the bladder, head, neck, cervix, and lung and for osteosarcoma, neuroblastoma, and others.

## PHARMACOLOGY

**Mechanism of Action.** Cisplatin is an inorganic complex formed by an atom of platinum(II) surrounded by chlorine and ammonia atoms in the *cis* position of the horizontal plane. Both neutrality of charge and the *cis* position are required for the platinum complex to exert its antitumor effects. In plasma, which is a high-chloride environment, the cisplatin complex is thought to be un-ionized, thus allowing passage of the drug into cells. Inside the cell, where the chloride concentration is low, water displaces the chloride ligands of the complex, forming positively charged platinum complexes that are highly reactive. These complexes inhibit DNA synthesis to a much greater extent than RNA synthesis or protein synthesis. The most important form of binding appears to be with adjacent N7 nitrogens of guanine residues in DNA, leading to intrastrand cross-linking, but numerous other forms of binding may also occur, including interstrand cross-linking of DNA (which can be highly sequence specific[2]), DNA-protein cross-links, and binding to messenger RNA. The major biochemical consequence of this binding to DNA is inhibition of DNA as a template for cell replication. This results in apoptosis at higher doses of cisplatin in some systems, whereas at lower doses it results in failure to overcome a block in $G_2$.[3] Increasingly, cisplatin-induced changes in the regulation and deregulation of $G_2$ checkpoint proteins appear to be important in determining the cytotoxicity of the drug, at least in some cell systems.[4] An emerging area of potential importance to oncology is the role of telomeres in aging and carcinogenesis. In one study, cisplatin caused telomere loss as an additional form of cytotoxicity.[5] The significance of this finding remains to be explained.

**Resistance.** Cellular resistance to cisplatin is highly complex and potentially influenced by a host of drugs, including other cytotoxic agents. Some of the mechanisms found in resistant cell lines are as follows: (1) decreased cellular accumulation of cisplatin,[6] (2) increased glutathione synthesis,[7] (3) increased DNA–drug adduct repair,[8] (4) increased tolerance for unrepaired DNA lesions,[9] and (5) increased extracellular transport of a glutathione-platinum complex through an ATP-dependent glutathione S-conjugate export pump (GS-X pump).[10] Many of these mechanisms are also seen with a variety of other alkylating agents and irradiation,[11] but cisplatin does not generally demonstrate cross-resistance with other alkylating agents. Rather, there is often cross-resistance with various antimetabolites, such as 5-FU and MTX.[12] Of uncertain importance, but of interest because of the burgeoning oncogene literature, is the finding of increased resistance to cisplatin in NIH 3T3 cells transformed by *ras* oncogenes.[13] In other studies, activation of *src* was more important to drug resistance than activation of *ras* oncogenes.[14]

**Pharmacokinetics.** There are considerable interindividual differences in the pharmacokinetics of cisplatin, and the drug may be given in a wide variety of doses, schedules, and routes of administration. After standard intravenous administration, cisplatin is widely distributed in the body, although it does not enter brain tissue or the CSF to any appreciable extent. Plasma clearance of total platinum is biphasic, with an initial half-life of 25 to 49 minutes and a terminal half-life of 58 to 73 hours. Cisplatin is nonenzymatically transformed to one or more inactive metabolites, and these are extensively bound to plasma proteins (90%). These metabolites also reach high concentrations in the kidneys, liver, and intestines, and they may persist in these tissues for months after drug administration. The unbound, untransformed, cytotoxic form of cisplatin has different pharmacokinetics. It is cleared more rapidly from plasma after intravenous administration, with an initial half-life of 8 to 30 minutes and a terminal half-life of 40 to 48 minutes. Cisplatin is metabolized in the liver, and there is evidence for enterohepatic recirculation of the drug. Cisplatin appears to cross the placenta, especially late in pregnancy. It does not appear to be excreted into human milk. The principal route of excretion is the kidneys, and renal function is the key determinant of safe use. Free cisplatin is cleared both by glomerular filtration and by renal tubular secretion. Renal toxicity can be reduced by induction of high urine flow rates with either mannitol or furosemide, by drug administration at the time of maximal urine flow as determined by circadian rhythms, and by giving cisplatin in combination with verapamil and cimetidine. None of these maneuvers appears to interfere with the antitumor effectiveness of cisplatin. Some other approaches to reducing renal toxicity, such as infusing cisplatin in hypertonic saline or using intravenous thiosulfate as an antidote, may reduce the efficacy of cisplatin, based on studies in animals.

The pharmacology of cisplatin appears to be similar in children, adolescents, and adults. The pharmacokinetic properties of cisplatin have been studied in patients receiving 5-day continuous infusions of the drug,[15] injection into the peritoneal cavity,[16] into CSF by way of an Ommaya's reservoir,[17] and into various arteries,[18, 19] as well as during isolation perfusion.[20]

**Drug Interactions.** The cytotoxicity of cisplatin can be decreased by thio compounds, such as the commercially available drug amifostine, even if these are administered a short time after the platinum complex.[21] The cytotoxicity of cisplatin can be increased by concurrent use of all-*trans*-retinoic acid[22] or gemcitabine.[23]

Acquired and intrinsic drug resistance to cisplatin can be modified by a host of drugs. These include calcium channel blockers, calmodulin inhibitors, dipyridamole, cyclosporine, methylxanthines, antifungal agents, agents that deplete glutathione (buthionine sulfoximine), drugs that inhibit energy metabolism (lonidamine), drugs that inhibit DNA repair (novobiocin, ganciclovir, and others), signal transduction modulators (phorbol esters), hormonal agents (tamoxifen), nicotinamide, caffeine,[24] and antioxidants[25] (such as *N*-acetylcysteine).

The toxicity of cisplatin is increased by drugs that influence renal function, such as the aminoglycoside antibiotics. Ototoxicity may be increased by the concurrent use of cisplatin with the following: (1) high-dose cytarabine[26] and (2) other ototoxic drugs, especially in the presence of renal dysfunction. Phenytoin levels may be decreased by cisplatin, so phenytoin levels should be closely monitored during cisplatin therapy. Cisplatin may potentiate the effects of radiation therapy. Allergic reactions to cisplatin appear to be more common when the drug is given with IL-2.[27] The clinical importance of these interactions is yet to be determined.[28]

## TOXICITY

**Overview.** Vomiting, renal dysfunction, and mild to moderate peripheral neuropathy are the predominant forms of toxicity at standard doses. The pattern of dose-limiting toxicity changes to myelosuppression and severe neuropathy for patients receiving very high doses of cisplatin. A case of massive cisplatin overdose caused by accidental substitution for carboplatin has been documented.[29]

**Hematologic.** Unlike other alkylating agents, cisplatin is associated with bone marrow suppression that is usually mild to moderate at standard doses. When it does occur, the nadir WCC and platelet count are at 18 to 23 days, and recovery is usually complete by day 39 (with a range reported by the manufacturer of 13 to 62 days). In some patients, cisplatin-induced anemia is related to erythropoietin deficiency caused by the renal toxicity of cisplatin.[30] This can be treated by the administration of erythropoietin. Other hematologic effects are rare, including hemolytic anemia (which may be increased by re-treatment), increased levels

of plasma iron, abnormal porphyrin metabolism, and mobilization of lead from bone or fat deposits within the body.

**Digestive System.** Severe nausea and vomiting occur in nearly all patients. They can be immediate or may be delayed for 1 or more days. The severity of this reaction can result in the Mallory-Weiss syndrome. Diarrhea, liver toxicity, and pancreatitis occur rarely.

**Neurologic.** Tinnitus or high-frequency hearing loss occurs in about 30% of patients, and significant neuropathy occurs in about 50%.[31] Nearly all patients develop paresthesia with treatment, and it is persistent in about 40% of cases. Other forms of neurotoxicity may also occur, including loss of taste, vestibular dysfunction, Lhermitte's sign, and seizures. Neuropathy is morphologically correlated with tissue accumulation of cisplatin.[32] High-dose therapy can result in severe ototoxicity.

**Genitourinary.** Renal dysfunction occurs in about 25% of patients and is usually dose limiting. There may be a permanent reduction of renal glomerular filtration rate, but renal tubular function usually returns to normal after completion of therapy. The severity and frequency of renal dysfunction led many physicians to abandon the use of cisplatin when it was first studied, until it was demonstrated that the kidneys could be protected by mannitol diuresis. It appears that the renal toxicity of cisplatin is due to the inactive metabolites of the drug and not to cisplatin itself. The clinical consequences of renal damage may include tubular dysfunction with severe hypocalcemia, hypokalemia, and hypomagnesemia; renal salt wasting with severe hyponatremia and hypovolemia (about 10% of cases); hyperuricemia; and, very rarely, the syndrome of inappropriate secretion of antidiuretic hormone (SIADH). Very rare cases of the hemolytic-uremic syndrome may also occur. Renal damage may be increased by the use of aminoglycoside antibiotics and possibly by the concomitant use of antihypertensive medications. Indeed, hypertension itself has been reported after the intra-arterial use of cisplatin. The electrolyte abnormalities can be life threatening, so prophylaxis with magnesium sulfate is important. Cumulative or delayed nephrotoxicity does not appear to be a problem in patients receiving moderate doses of cisplatin with adequate hydration. Prior renal transplantation is not a contraindication to the use of cisplatin.[33]

**Other and Rare Reactions.** Singultus, drug fever, and a gingival platinum line all are rare.

*Immunologic.* Effects include anaphylactic reactions with wheezing, tachycardia, hypotension, and facial edema. Cisplatin has variable effects on the immune system in animals, ranging from immunosuppression to immunostimulation.

*Mucocutaneous.* Alopecia and Raynaud's phenomenon may occur. Local pain can occur at the injection site. Skin necrosis, cellulitis, or fibrosis can result from drug extravasation.

*Cardiovascular.* Cardiotoxicity has been reported, including bradycardia, left bundle branch block, and ST-T wave changes with congestive heart failure. There is a possible association with acute vascular ischemic events when cisplatin is combined with other drugs in the treatment of testicular cancer. A single case of toxic shock syndrome following cisplatin use has been reported.[34]

*Pulmonary.* Effects include nonspecific respiratory complaints (of uncertain relationship to the drug).

*Ocular.* Decreased peripheral vision can occur with standard doses, and more severe retinal damage with high-dose therapy.

**Musculoskeletal.** Muscle cramps and myalgia can occur.

**Reproductive.** Toxicity data place cisplatin in FDA pregnancy category D. Reduced fertility is common (about a third of male patients with testicular cancer remain capable of insemination).

**Endocrine-Metabolic.** Gynecomastia can occur; one study found a selective induction of follicle-stimulating hormone (FSH) during cisplatin therapy.[35]

**Carcinogenicity.** Cisplatin may cause second malignancies (primarily acute leukemia as a very rare event, with some authors ascribing the neoplasm to other concurrent chemotherapeutic agents).[36]

## DOSAGE AND ADMINISTRATION

Cisplatin is available in the form of a white powder in vials containing 10 mg. It is much more stable when reconstituted with sterile saline than with sterile water, and it is moderately sensitive to light. It should not be allowed to come in contact with aluminum needles or infusion tubing, because a brown precipitate forms. A variety of schedules and doses of intravenous cisplatin have been used, such as weekly bolus injections or intermittent courses repeated every 3 to 4 weeks consisting of either five daily injections (20 mg/m²/day) or continuous infusions of 2 to 120 hours' duration. The most widely used infusion schedules consist of either high-dose (100 to 120 mg/m²) cisplatin given over 2 to 6 hours in the hospital or lower doses (50 mg/m²) infused over 2 hours either in the hospital or in an outpatient clinic.

All these regimens must be given with large volumes of fluid, but the details of the infusion protocol vary with the dose used. Vogl and associates[37] have recommended a 2-hour schedule for outpatients receiving 50 mg/m² every 3 to 4 weeks. This involves giving 2 L of 0.45% saline–5% dextrose over 2 hours to ensure hydration, plus 40 mg furosemide at the start of the infusion and 12.5 g mannitol along with the cisplatin to ensure diuresis. When higher doses are used, we have generally hydrated the patient in the hospital with 1 L of 5% dextrose in 0.45% normal saline (D5/0.45NS) containing 10 mEq potassium chloride over 2 to 2.5 hours, followed by cisplatin dissolved in 1 L of D/5/0.45NS with 25 g mannitol given over 2 to 2.5 hours, followed by postdrug hydration over 2.5 to 3 hours with 1250 ml D5/0.45NS with 10 mEq potassium chloride/L. Serum magnesium levels should be monitored, with intramuscular or intravenous magnesium sulfate supplementation as needed.

On the basis of pharmacokinetic studies showing similar AUC results for free cisplatin after bolus, 3-hour, and 24-hour infusions, plus the clinical impression that the antitumor effectiveness of these schedules is equivalent, the choice among these regimens can be individualized according to the disease being treated and the preferences of the patient and physician.

Whatever program or schedule is used, a pretreatment audiogram, serum creatinine level, and creatinine clearance value should be obtained. Patients with pre-existing ototoxicity (decreased hearing in the 1000- to 4000-cycles/sec range) or creatinine clearance of less than 50 ml/min should probably be excluded from cisplatin treatment. Anephric patients or those on chronic dialysis may nevertheless be treated because they have already lost the use of their kidneys.

## REFERENCES

1. Rosenberg B, Van Camp L, Krigas T. Inhibition of cell division in *Escherichia coli* by electrolysis products from a platinum electrode. Nature 1965;205:698–9.
2. Zou Y, Van Houten B, Farrell N. Sequence specificity of DNA-DNA interstrand cross-link formation by cisplatin and dinuclear platinum complexes. Biochemistry 1994;33:5404–10.
3. Ormerod MG, Orr RM, Peacock JH. The role of apoptosis in cell killing by cisplatin: a flow cytometric study. Br J Cancer 1994;69:93–100.
4. Links M, Ribeiro J, Jackson P, et al. Regulation and deregulation of G2 checkpoint proteins with cisplatin. Anticancer Res 1998;18:4057–66.
5. Ishibashi T, Lippard SJ. Telomere loss in cells treated with cisplatin. Proc Natl Acad Sci U S A 1998;95:4219–23.
6. Schmidt W, Chaney SG. Role of carrier ligand in platinum resistance of human carcinoma cell lines. Cancer Res 1993;53:799–805.
7. Godwin AK, Meister A, O'Dwyer PJ, et al. High resistance to cisplatin in human ovarian cancer cell lines is associated with marked increase of glutathione synthesis. Proc Natl Acad Sci U S A 1992;89:3070–4.
8. Oldenburg J, Begg AC, van Vugt MJ. Characterization of resistance mechanisms to *cis*-diamminedichloroplatinum(II) in three sublines of the CC531 colon adenocarcinoma cell line in vitro. Cancer Res 1994;54:487–93.
9. de Graeff A, Slebos RJ, Rodenhuis S. Resistance to cisplatin and analogues: mechanisms and potential clinical implications. Cancer Chemother Pharmacol 1988;22:325–32.
10. Ishikawa T, Ali-Osman F. Glutathione-associated *cis*-diamminedichloroplatinum(II) metabolism and ATP-dependent efflux from leukemia cells: molecular characterization of glutathione-platinum complex and its biological significance. J Biol Chem 1993;268:20116–25.
11. Ozols RF, Masuda H, Hamilton TC. Mechanisms of cross-resistance between radiation and antineoplastic drugs. NCI Monogr 1988;6:159–65.
12. Scanlon KJ, Kashani-Sabet M, Miyachi H, et al. Molecular basis of cisplatin resistance in human carcinomas: model systems and patients. Anticancer Res 1989;9:1301–12.
13. Sklar MD. Increased resistance to *cis*-diamminedichloroplatinum(II) in NIH 3T3 cells transformed by *ras* oncogenes [published erratum appears in Cancer Res 1988;48:3889]. Cancer Res 1988;48:793–7.
14. Masumoto N, Nakano S, Fujishima H, et al. v-*src* induces cisplatin resistance by increasing the repair of cisplatin-DNA interstrand cross-links in human gallbladder adenocarcinoma cells. Int J Cancer 1999;80:731–7.
15. Bues-Charbit M, Gentet JC, Bernard JL, et al. Continuous infusion of high-dose cisplatin in children: pharmacokinetics of free and total platinum. Eur J Cancer Clin Oncol 1987;23:1649–52.
16. Casper ES, Kelsen DP, Alcock NW, Lewis JL Jr. Ip cisplatin in patients with malignant ascites: pharmacokinetic evaluation and comparison with the IV route. Cancer Treat Rep 1983;67:235–8.
17. Gormley PE, Gangji D, Wood JH, Poplack DG. Pharmacokinetic study of cerebrospinal fluid penetration of *cis*-diamminedichloroplatinum(II). Cancer Chemother Pharmacol 1981;5:257–60.
18. Kelsen DP, Hoffman J, Alcock N, et al. Pharmacokinetics of cisplatin regional hepatic infusions. Am J Clin Oncol 1982;5:173–8.
19. Ginos JZ, Cooper AJ, Dhawan V: [13N]cisplatin PET to assess pharmacokinetics of intra-arterial versus intravenous chemotherapy for malignant brain tumors. J Nucl Med 1987;28:1844–52.
20. Wile AG, Kar R, Cohen RA, Jakowatz JG. The pharmacokinetics of cisplatin in experimental regional chemotherapy. Cancer 1987;59:695–700.
21. Hausheer FH, Kanter P, Cao S, et al. Modulation of platinum-induced toxicities and therapeutic index: mechanistic insights and first- and second-generation protecting agents. Semin Oncol 1998;25:584–99.
22. Aebi S, Krèoning R, Cenni B, et al. All-*trans*-retinoic acid enhances cisplatin-induced apoptosis in human ovarian adenocarcinoma and in squamous head and neck cancer cells. Clin Cancer Res 1997;3:2033–8.
23. Peters GJ, Bergman AM, Ruiz van Haperen VW, et al. Interaction

between cisplatin and gemcitabine in vitro and in vivo. Semin Oncol 1995;22:4 Suppl 11:72–9.

24. Takahashi M, Yamamoto Y, Hatori S, et al. Enhancement of CDDP cytotoxicity by caffeine is characterized by apoptotic cell death. Oncol Rep 1998;5:53–6.

25. Roller A, Weller M. Antioxidants specifically inhibit cisplatin cytotoxicity of human malignant glioma cells. Anticancer Res 1998;18:4493–7.

26. Atkins JN, Muss HB, Capizzi RL, et al. Phase I study of high-dose cytarabine and cisplatin in patients with advanced malignancy. Cancer Treat Rep 1985;69:897–9.

27. Heywood GR, Rosenberg SA, Weber JS. Hypersensitivity reactions to chemotherapy agents in patients receiving chemoimmunotherapy with high-dose interleukin 2. J Natl Cancer Inst 1995;87:915–22.

28. Timmer-Bosscha H, Mulder NH, de Vries EG. Modulation of *cis*-diamminedichloroplatinum(II) resistance: a review. Br J Cancer 1992;66:227–38.

29. Chu G, Mantin R, Shen YM, et al. Massive cisplatin overdose by accidental substitution for carboplatin. Toxicity and management. Cancer 1993;72:3707–14.

30. Wood PA, Hrushesky WJ. Cisplatin-associated anemia: an erythropoietin deficiency syndrome. J Clin Invest 1995;95:1650–9.

31. Cersosimo RJ. Cisplatin neurotoxicity. Cancer Treat Rev 1989;16:195–211.

32. Gregg RW, Molepo JM, Monpetit VJ, et al. Cisplatin neurotoxicity: the relationship between dosage, time, and platinum concentration in neurologic tissues, and morphologic evidence of toxicity. J Clin Oncol 1992;10:795–803.

33. Lindley CM, Gordon TR, Tremont SJ. Cisplatin-based chemotherapy in a renal transplant recipient [see comments in Cancer 1992;69:3015–6]. Cancer 1991;68:1113–7.

34. Berman AC, Boly LR. Cisplatin therapy–associated recurrent toxic shock syndrome. West J Med 1991;155:415–6.

35. LeBlanc GA, Kantoff PW, Ng SF, et al. Hormonal perturbations in patients with testicular cancer treated with cisplatin. Cancer 1992;69:2306–10.

36. Greene MH. Is cisplatin a human carcinogen? J Natl Cancer Inst 1992;84:306–12.

37. Vogl SE, Zaravinos T, Kaplan BH, Wollner D. Safe and effective two-hour outpatient regimen of hydration and diuresis for the administration of *cis*-diamminedichloroplatinum(II). Eur J Cancer Clin Oncol 1981;17:345–50.

# Cladribine

The lymphocytes of infants with severe combined immunodeficiency disease lack the enzyme adenosine deaminase, resulting in cell death from toxic levels of intracellular purine nucleosides. Cladribine, a nucleoside analogue of deoxyadenosine, was synthesized by Carson and colleagues as a new kind of purine antimetabolite on the basis of these facts.[1] It was specifically designed to be active in lymphoid cells lacking adenosine deaminase, as reviewed by Beutler[2] and by Saven and Piro.[3] The drug is also known as 2-chloro-2-deoxyadenosine, 2-CdA, CdA, Leustatin, and NSC-105014.

## EFFICACY

Cladribine is FDA approved as an orphan drug for the treatment of hairy cell leukemia.[4] The drug also has activity against mycosis fungoides, low-grade malignant lymphomas,[5, 6] acute leukemia,[7] and CLL.[8]

## PHARMACOLOGY

**Mechanism of Action.** Cladribine is one of a new group of purine antimetabolites that depend on the relative activities of three enzymes: deoxycytidine kinase, deoxynucleotidase, and adenosine deaminase. Cells with a high ratio of deoxycytidine kinase to deoxynucleotidase allow the passive intracellular accumulation of cladribine, where it is phosphorylated by deoxycytidine kinase. The product of phosphorylation is relatively resistant to deamination by adenosine deaminase, leading to further accumulation and further activation to the toxic metabolite, 2-chloro-2'-deoxy-D-adenosine triphosphate (2-CdATP). The active metabolites of cladribine interfere with the repair of single-strand DNA breaks, and the broken pieces of DNA activate the enzyme poly(ADP-ribose) polymerase. This results in the depletion of NAD and ATP and the disruption of cellular metabolism. 2-CdATP may also be incorporated into DNA, resulting in a defective DNA molecule.[9] Interestingly, deoxycytidine kinase may be activated during inhibition of DNA synthesis by cladribine, thus resulting in a form of post-translational drug activation.[10] Ultimately, apoptosis occurs.[11] Cladribine is cell cycle phase nonspecific because of its combined inhibition of DNA synthesis and repair. It is effective against both dividing and nondividing cells.

**Resistance.** Cells with a low ratio of deoxycytidine kinase to deoxynucleotidase are resistant to cladribine. One report of four patients noted no apparent cross-resistance with fludarabine in patients with CLL.[12] However, another study of 28 patients found strong cross-resistance between the two drugs.[13] In patients with hairy cell leukemia, no cross-resistance was observed between pentostatin and cladribine.[14]

**Pharmacokinetics.** The drug is given by continuous infusion.[15] It is widely distributed in the body, including the CSF. In adults, the initial half-life is short (36 minutes) but its terminal half-life is long (approximately 7 hours). Plasma protein binding is about 20%. Animal studies suggest that the primary route of excretion is renal, with only minimal hepatic excretion. In a large study of children, the plasma clearance was slower than reported for adults, with a terminal half-life of about 20 hours.[16] With repeated daily dosing, the ratio of drug in CSF to that in plasma was about 23%. Renal clearance was highly variable but averaged 51% of total systemic clearance (range, 11 to 85%).

**Drug Interactions.** Cladribine may increase the level of uric acid, which raises the potential of adverse interactions with other drugs that affect uric acid metabolism. The clinical importance of this observation is uncertain.

## TOXICITY

**Overview.** Myelosuppression is the predominant toxicity (reported by the manufacturer as severe in 70% of patients), but other, less serious reactions are common, as follows: fatigue (45%), nausea (28%), rash (27%), headache (22%), and injection-site reactions (19%). Nonhematologic toxicity is usually mild to moderate in severity.

**Hematologic.** Myelosuppression is dose related and dose limiting. Prolonged bone marrow hypocellularity has been reported in about a third of patients, and some studies have shown myelosuppression to be cumulative. Other effects include purpura (10%), petechiae (8%), and epistaxis (5%).

**Immunologic.** Prolonged suppression of CD4 lymphocyte counts is expected in virtually all patients, leading to significant immunosuppression. Because of the severity of immunosuppression, transfusion-associated graft-versus-host disease can occur in patients recently treated with cladribine.[17]

**Digestive System.** Nausea is common, but it is usually mild and easily controlled. Other effects include anorexia (17%), vomiting (13%), diarrhea (10%), constipation (9%), abdominal pain (6%), and rare pancreatitis.

**Mucocutaneous.** Skin rashes are frequent (27%), with less frequent reactions as follows: injection-site reactions (19%), pruritus (6%), local pain (6%), and erythema (6%).

**Neurologic.** These reactions include headache (22%), dizziness (9%), and insomnia (7%). Very rare reactions include motor weakness, paresthesia, paraparesis, or quadriparesis (irreversible but seen primarily with high-dose therapy).

**Other/Rare.** The following reactions also occur: fever (69%, usually associated with infection), fatigue (45%), chills (9%), asthenia (9%), diaphoresis (9%), malaise (7%), and trunk pain (6%).

***Cardiovascular.*** Edema occurs in 6% of patients, and tachycardia in 6%.

***Pulmonary.*** Abnormal breath sounds occur in 11%, cough in 10%, and shortness of breath in 7% of patients.

***Musculoskeletal.*** Myalgia occurs in 7% of patients and arthralgia in 5%.

***Genitourinary.*** Renal toxicity is rare at normal doses, but it is life threatening and common (45%) with high-dose therapy. Rare cases of the tumor lysis syndrome have been reported in patients with CLL.[18, 19]

***Reproductive.*** Toxicity studies place cladribine in FDA pregnancy category D. Cladribine impairs fertility in monkeys, but its effect on human fertility is unknown.

***Carcinogenicity.*** The drug causes DNA damage and should be presumed to be potentially carcinogenic, although carcinogenicity in animals and humans has not been established with certainty.

## DOSAGE AND ADMINISTRATION

Cladribine is available in 20-ml vials containing drug in a concentration of 1 mg/ml. The planned dose of cladribine should be passed through a Millex filter provided with the drug before further dilution. It is then diluted in bacteriostatic normal saline for outpatient use or normal saline alone for inpatient use. Dextrose solution causes degradation of cladribine and should not be used. The drug is stable for at least 7 days at room temperature when prepared for outpatient infusion. The dosage for patients with hairy cell leukemia is 0.1 mg/kg/day as a single continuous infusion for 7 days. The infusion can be given as outpatient therapy with the full 7-day dosage in 50 to 100 ml of bacteriostatic normal saline, or to inpatients as a daily dosage in 500 ml of normal saline. Higher doses, using five daily intravenous infusions, are under investigation.[20] The drug should be used with caution or not at all in patients with pre-existing bone marrow suppression or renal insufficiency.

## REFERENCES

1. Carson DA, Kaye J, Seegmiller JE. Lymphospecific toxicity in adenosine deaminase deficiency and purine nucleoside phosphorylase deficiency: possible role of nucleoside kinase(s). Proc Natl Acad Sci U S A 1977;74:5677–81.
2. Beutler E. Cladribine (2-chlorodeoxyadenosine). Lancet 1992; 340:952–6.
3. Saven A, Piro LD. 2-Chlorodeoxyadenosine: a newer purine analog active in the treatment of indolent lymphoid malignancies. Ann Intern Med 1994;120:784–91.
4. Piro LD, Carrera CJ, Carson DA, Beutler E. Lasting remissions in hairy-cell leukemia induced by a single infusion of 2-chlorodeoxyadenosine. N Engl J Med 1990;322:1117–21.
5. Kay AC, Saven A, Carrera CJ, et al. 2-Chlorodeoxyadenosine treatment of low-grade lymphomas. J Clin Oncol 1992;10:371–7.
6. Hoffman M, Tallman MS, Hakimian D, et al. 2-Chlorodeoxyadenosine is an active salvage therapy in advanced indolent non-Hodgkin's lymphoma. J Clin Oncol 1994;12:788–92.
7. Santana VM, Mirro J Jr, Kearns C, et al. 2-Chlorodeoxyadenosine produces a high rate of complete hematologic remission in relapsed acute myeloid leukemia. J Clin Oncol 1992;10:364–70.
8. Piro LD, Carrera CJ, Beutler E, Carson DA. 2-Chlorodeoxyadenosine: an effective new agent for the treatment of chronic lymphocytic leukemia. Blood 1998;72:1069–73.
9. Yuh SH, Tibudan M, Hentosh P. Analysis of 2-chloro-2'-deoxyadenosine incorporation into cellular DNA by quantitative polymerase chain reaction. Anal Biochem 1998;262:1–8.
10. Sasvâari-Szâekely M, Spasokoukotskaja T, Szâoke M, et al. Activation of deoxycytidine kinase during inhibition of DNA synthesis by 2-chloro-2'-deoxyadenosine (cladribine) in human lymphocytes. Biochem Pharmacol 1998;56:1175–9.
11. Leoni LM, Chao Q, Cottam HB, et al. Induction of an apoptotic program in cell-free extracts by 2-chloro-2'-deoxyadenosine 5'-triphosphate and cytochrome c. Proc Natl Acad Sci U S A 1998;95:9567–71.
12. Juliusson G, Elmhorn-Rosenborg A, Liliemark J. Response to 2-chlorodeoxyadenosine in patients with B-cell chronic lymphocytic leukemia resistant to fludarabine. N Engl J Med 1992;327:1056–61.
13. O'Brien S, Kantarjian H, Estey E, et al. Lack of effect of 2-chlorodeoxyadenosine therapy in patients with chronic lymphocytic leukemia refractory to fludarabine therapy. N Engl J Med 1994;330:319–22.
14. Saven A, Piro LD. Complete remissions in hairy cell leukemia with 2-chlorodeoxyadenosine after failure with 2'-deoxycoformycin. Ann Intern Med 1993;119:278–83.
15. Santana VM, Mirro J Jr, Harwood FC, et al. A phase I clinical trial of 2-chlorodeoxyadenosine in pediatric patients with acute leukemia. J Clin Oncol 1991;9:416–22.
16. Kearns CM, Blakley RL, Santana VM. Pharmacokinetics of cladribine (2-chlorodeoxyadenosine) in children with acute leukemia. Cancer Res 1994;54:1235–9.
17. Zulian G, Roux R, Tiercy J-M, et al. Transfusion-associated graft-versus-host disease (TGVHD) in a patient treated with cladribine (2-CDA, 2-chlorodeoxyadenosine) demonstrated by PCR amplification of DNA minisatellites and HLA-DR oligotyping. Proc Am Soc Clin Oncol 1994;13:113.
18. Dann EJ, Gillis S, Polliack A, et al. Brief report: tumor lysis syndrome following treatment with 2-chlorodeoxyadenosine for refractory chronic lymphocytic leukemia. N Engl J Med 1993;329:1547–8.
19. Trendle MC, Tefferi A. Tumor lysis syndrome after treatment of chronic lymphocytic leukemia with cladribine. N Engl J Med 1994;330:1090.
20. Larson RA, Mick R, Spielberger RT, et al. Dose-escalation trial of cladribine using five daily intravenous infusions in patients with advanced hematologic malignancies. J Clin Oncol 1996;14:188–95.

## Cyclophosphamide

Cyclophosphamide is a chemical derivative of mechlorethamine synthesized in Germany in 1958. It was developed as a potential inert alkylating agent that could be activated preferentially by tumor-associated intracellular enzymes. Cyclophosphamide is widely used around the world and is known by a multitude of different names, including Cytoxan, CTX, CPM, CYC, Neosar, Endoxan, and NSC-26271. Its fascinating history has been reviewed by Brock.[1]

## EFFICACY

Cyclophosphamide may be used as a single agent in the treatment of Burkitt's lymphoma, but its greatest use in oncology is in combination chemotherapy. Examples of tumors treated with such combinations include a variety of malignant lymphomas, breast cancer, ovarian carcinomas, small cell lung cancer, neuroblastoma, multiple myeloma, mycosis fungoides, retinoblastoma, soft tissue sarcomas, Ewing's sarcoma, and some forms of leukemia. It is also used as an immunosuppressive agent in the treatment of some nonmalignant diseases.

## PHARMACOLOGY

**Mechanism of Action.** Cyclophosphamide acts as a classic alkylating agent resulting in apoptosis[2, 3] but with some unique features.[4] It was initially synthesized as a potential inert transport form of mechlorethamine, with the expectation that cancer cells would preferentially activate the drug. This early premise has proved overly simplistic. Cyclophosphamide is extensively metabolized in vivo to active and inactive metabolites (see an extensive review by Sladek[5]). Initially, the drug is biotransformed in the liver by specific cytochrome P450 mixed-function oxidase enzymes to 4-hydroxycyclophosphamide and aldophosphamide.[6] These are noncytotoxic transport forms of the drug that exist in equilibrium as tautomers. These tautomers of cyclophosphamide readily enter cells, where they are spontaneously and enzymatically degraded to inactive metabolites by aldehyde dehydrogenase (aldehyde oxygenase) or undergo spontaneous conversion to the cytotoxic metabolites phosphoramide mustard and acrolein. Activation may also occur by a process known as *co-oxidation,* which forms oxygen radicals and acrolein via prostaglandin H synthase.[7] These toxic metabolites can be generated in situ by some tissues other than liver, including the lung.[8] Phosphoramide mustard and acrolein are responsible for very different forms of cytotoxicity. Most studies suggest that phosphoramide mustard is responsible for all or nearly all of the antineoplastic activity of cyclophosphamide. This occurs as shown previously for other alkylating agents of the bis-chloroethyl amine type. Conversely, acrolein accounts for the urothelial toxicity and perhaps the pulmonary toxicity of the drug. In animals, acrolein-induced hemorrhagic cystitis can be prevented by the free radical scavenger *N*-acetylcysteine without abrogating the antineoplastic efficacy of cyclophosphamide. Another free radical scavenger, mesna, prevents cyclophosphamide-induced hemorrhagic cystitis in humans.

Although the qualitative pattern of cyclophosphamide metabolism is well known, relatively little is known about interindividual differences in the quantitative production of the various metabolites. Nevertheless, several important points can be made. First, it appears that the rate of the initial biotransformation of cyclophosphamide to its two transport forms is relatively unimportant to its ultimate cytotoxicity. Thus, drugs that modify the activity of the hepatic microsomal enzymes rarely cause clinically important drug interactions. This also explains the relatively wide range of values for the plasma clearance of cyclophosphamide in different studies. Second, it appears that most of the produc-tion of phosphoramide mustard and acrolein occurs in two places: within cells and within the collecting system of the genitourinary tract. This makes it highly unlikely that the use of a free radical scavenger, such as mesna, would inactivate the antineoplastic activity of cyclophosphamide, even when the two are given concurrently. Third, the intracellular concentrations of aldehyde dehydrogenase in many tumor cells appear to be much lower than those in the liver and most other normal cells. Thus, such tumor cells have a reduced capacity to inactivate the transport forms of cyclophosphamide before they become cytotoxic. This may explain, at least in part, the relative selective toxicity of cyclophosphamide compared with that of other alkylating agents. Like other alkylating agents, cyclophosphamide is considered cell cycle phase nonspecific.

**Resistance.** Drug resistance is thought to be mediated primarily by DNA repair enzymes, such as $O^6$-methylguanine-DNA methyltransferase.[9] Another form of resistance involves glutathione metabolism, which is important in protecting cells from oxidative damage. Acquired resistance to the drug in animals, for example, has been associated with increased activity of the glutathione *S*-transferase group of enzymes,[10] and glutathione depletion has been found to be a determinant of sensitivity of human leukemia cells in vitro to cyclophosphamide and its metabolites.[11]

**Pharmacogenetics.** Pharmacogenetic differences in the metabolism of cyclophosphamide have been described, and they have potentially important clinical consequences. The best example of this appears to be a polymorphism for the enzyme aldehyde dehydrogenase.[12] Patients with a deficiency of this enzyme produce much less carboxyphosphamide and more phosphoramide mustard than usual.[13]

**Pharmacokinetics.** Cyclophosphamide is equally effective by the oral and intravenous routes of administration.[14] It is not directly effective by intracavitary administration because it requires activation in the liver prior to exerting its systemic effect. Cyclophosphamide itself is not bound to albumin, whereas its metabolites are (about 50%). Owing to moderate lipid and water solubility, the drug and its metabolites are widely distributed to the extracellular water spaces of the body, and a small amount may reach the CSF, breast milk, sweat, saliva, and synovial fluid. The disappearance of injected cyclophosphamide from plasma is biexponential, with an average longer half-life of 4 to 6.5 hours; however, the half-life of the drug may be shortened after the use of repeated large daily doses. This is especially so when the drug is used in very high doses with BMT. Excretion takes place primarily via the kidneys, where unchanged drug constitutes almost 30% of the total. Because of the potential for altered pharmacokinetics at higher dose rates, some authorities recommend therapeutic drug monitoring in this setting.[15]

**Drug Interactions.** Cyclophosphamide can inhibit pseudocholinesterase, leading to an increased risk of apnea during anesthesia that includes the use of succinylcholine.[16] Cyclophosphamide can inhibit cholinesterase, leading to the potential for increased toxicity from cocaine. The risk of cardiomyopathy is increased in patients treated with cyclophosphamide in combination with high-dose cytarabine or anthracycline antibiotics (doxorubicin). One report describes liver necrosis in four patients who were also receiving azathioprine.[17] Cimetidine, but not ranitidine, enhances the hematologic toxicity of cyclophosphamide.[18, 19]

Mesna and *N*-acetylcysteine decrease the urotoxicity of cyclophosphamide. Fluconazole reduces the metabolic conversion of cyclophosphamide to its active metabolites in children.[20] The clinical impact of this inhibition is currently unclear.

Preliminary data suggest that the apoptosis induced by 4-hydroperoxycyclophosphamide, a metabolite of cyclophosphamide, may be amplified by co-treatment with IL-3 and IL-6.[21] Herceptin, a new antibody directed against HER-2/*neu*, synergistically increases cyclophosphamide cytotoxicity in vitro.[22] Topoisomerase I inhibitors interact in a synergistic fashion with cyclophosphamide in human brain tumor cell lines.[23]

## TOXICITY

**Overview.** Myelosuppression and hemorrhagic cystitis are the usual forms of dose-limiting toxicity with standard doses. High-dose therapy for BMT can cause a wide variety of other important multisystem reactions.

**Hematologic.** Bone marrow suppression is the major dose-limiting toxicity for cyclophosphamide, with a nadir of leukopenia after pulse intravenous therapy at about 8 to 14 days, with recovery 1 or 2 weeks later. Neutropenia is usually more severe than thrombocytopenia. In patients with CLL, hemolytic anemia may rarely be induced by cyclophosphamide. Moderate to severe immunosuppression may also occur, as well as immune augmentation. With very high dose therapy, a temporary reduction in plasma fibrinolytic activity occurs and can be prevented by granulocyte-macrophage colony-stimulating factor (GM-CSF) therapy.[24]

**Digestive System.** Nausea and vomiting are common with high-dose therapy, and diarrhea and hemorrhagic colitis may occasionally occur. Mild hepatic toxicity is rare.

**Mucocutaneous.** Alopecia is a frequent side effect; it is advisable to warn patients of this complication beforehand so that they may prepare for the possibility by obtaining a wig if desired. Alternatively, the use of scalp hypothermia may be considered in selected patients, as discussed in Chapter 8. Pigmented fingernails or skin, or both, may occur, as well as dermatitis. Mucositis and stomatitis develop only rarely.

**Cardiovascular.** Cardiac damage has been associated with very high doses (180 mg/kg or more over 4 or fewer days or >1.55 g/m$^2$/day times four) and, rarely, electrocardiologic abnormalities may occur with standard doses. In one study, exercise-induced changes in diastolic function were found in all patients following transplantation doses of cyclophosphamide, whereas resting diastolic function was normal.[25] This was interpreted as evidence for low-grade, delayed cardiotoxicity after transplantation doses of cyclophosphamide. Cardiotoxicity has been correlated with pharmacokinetics,[26] and it appears less likely when the drug is given on a twice-daily schedule than with a single daily dose in the transplant setting.[27]

**Genitourinary.** About 15% of patients develop hemorrhagic cystitis. The severity of this syndrome varies from microscopic hematuria alone to massive hematuria with obstructive uropathy due to clots. The problem is probably more likely in patients who have also received radiation therapy to the bladder, and it may be a more serious problem when it occurs in children. Stillwell and Benson[28] have reported a series of 100 patients with hemorrhagic cystitis induced by cyclophosphamide. Major symptoms were gross hematuria (78%) and irritative voiding symptoms (45%). Cystectomy was required in nine patients, and bladder cancer developed in five. Dehydration probably increases the risk of hemorrhagic cystitis. Rarely, hemorrhagic cystitis may prove lethal, and its treatment may require such maneuvers as instillation of formalin into the bladder or urinary diversion.[29] Even in the absence of hemorrhagic cystitis, the drug can cause urinary bladder fibrosis[30] and bladder cancer.[31] Mesna appears to be effective in suppressing hemorrhagic cystitis in the setting of BMT, when very high doses of cyclophosphamide may be used.[32] Mesna is not more effective than hyperhydration[33] or continuous bladder irrigation,[34] but it is probably better tolerated by patients.

**Other and Rare Reactions.** Fever, diaphoresis, facial flushing, nasal congestion, and a metallic taste in the mouth can occur.

*Immunologic.* Anaphylaxis rarely occurs after intravenous doses. The drug is a potent immunosuppressive agent; it may be especially toxic for suppressor-inducer T cells.[35] Immunosuppression is rarely a clinical problem, however, in patients with cancer.

*Pulmonary.* Pulmonary fibrosis can occur.

*Ocular.* These effects include transient myopia[36] and cataracts.

*Neurologic.* Headache and dizziness can occur.

*Reproductive.* Toxicity data place cyclophosphamide in FDA pregnancy category D. Reduced fertility, including sterility, is common.

*Endocrine-Metabolic.* Water intoxication has been reported when the drug is given in high doses (50 mg/kg or greater) with large fluid loads, especially in children. This results from a direct antidiuretic effect of cyclophosphamide and its metabolites on renal tubules, and it can be prevented by the concomitant use of intravenous furosemide. If diuretics are used with cyclophosphamide, it is important to avoid alkalization of the urine because this may exacerbate the bladder toxicity of the drug. Hypothyroidism can occur.

*Carcinogenicity.* Cyclophosphamide is carcinogenic, especially for the bladder and bone marrow.[37]

## DOSAGE AND ADMINISTRATION

Cyclophosphamide is available in the United States as oral tablets (25- and 50-mg strengths) and as a lyophilized or nonlyophilized powder for intravenous administration (vials of 100, 200, and 500 mg and 1 and 2 g). The usual oral dosage for continuous therapy with single-agent cyclophosphamide is 1 to 2.5 mg/kg/day in divided doses. The best guides to regulating the oral dosage are the response of the disease and the WCC, which should be maintained at approximately 3500 to 4000/μL. For rare clinical situations in which single-agent, intermittent high-dose treatment is preferred, cyclophosphamide may be given intravenously in a dose of 40 to 50 mg/kg divided over a period of 2 to 5 days. Doses in this range should be given with concomitant intravenous hydration (500 to 1000 ml of normal saline).

Because of the important role of renal excretion, patients with severe renal failure requiring an intravenous alkylating agent should probably be considered for another drug, such as mechlorethamine or thiotepa. Patients with renal failure receiving low-dose oral cyclophosphamide should have the interval between doses doubled.[38] Guidelines for reducing the dose of cyclophosphamide in patients with lesser degrees of renal dysfunction are given in Chapter 8. Other dosages and schedules of drug administration for cyclophosphamide when combined with other drugs are given in the disease-oriented chapters.

## REFERENCES

1. Brock N. Oxazaphosphorine cytostatics: past-present-future. Seventh Cain Memorial Award lecture. Cancer Res 1989;49:1–7.
2. Naruse I, Keino H, Kawarada Y. Antibody against single-stranded DNA detects both programmed cell death and drug-induced apoptosis. Histochemistry 1994;101:73–8.
3. Meyn RE, Stephens LC, Hunter NR, Milas L. Induction of apoptosis in murine tumors by cyclophosphamide. Cancer Chemother Pharmacol 1994;33:410–4.
4. Wang JY, Prorok G, Vaughan WP. Cytotoxicity, DNA cross-linking, and DNA single-strand breaks induced by cyclophosphamide in a rat leukemia in vivo. Cancer Chemother Pharmacol 1993;31:381–6.
5. Sladek NE. Metabolism of oxazaphosphorines. Pharmacol Ther 1988;37:301–55.
6. Chang TKH, Weber GF, Crespi CL, Waxman DJ. Differential activation of cyclophosphamide and infosphamide by cytochromes P-450 2B and 3A in human liver microsomes. Cancer Res 1993;53:5629–37.
7. Kanekal S, Kehrer JP. Evidence for peroxidase-mediated metabolism of cyclophosphamide. Drug Metab Dispos 1993;21:37–42.
8. Patel JM. Metabolism and pulmonary toxicity of cyclophosphamide. Pharmacol Ther 1990;47:137–46.
9. Mattern J, Eichhorn U, Kaina B, Volm M. O6-Methylguanine-DNA methyltransferase activity and sensitivity to cyclophosphamide and cisplatin in human lung tumor xenografts. Int J Cancer 1998;77:919–22.
10. McGown AT, Fox BW. A proposed mechanism of resistance to cyclophosphamide and phosphoramide mustard in a Yoshida cell line in vitro. Cancer Chemother Pharmacol 1986;17:223–6.
11. Crook TR, Souhami RL, Whyman GD, McLean AE. Glutathione depletion as a determinant of sensitivity of human leukemia cells to cyclophosphamide. Cancer Res 1986;46:5035–8.
12. Boddy AV, Furtun Y, Sardas S, et al. Individual variation in the activation and inactivation of metabolic pathways of cyclophosphamide. J Natl Cancer Inst 1992;84:1744–8.
13. Hadidi A-HFA, Coulter CE, Idle JR. Phenotypically deficient urinary elimination of carboxyphosphamide after cyclophosphamide administration to cancer patients. Cancer Res 1988;48:5167–71.
14. Fleming RA. An overview of cyclophosphamide and ifosfamide pharmacology. Pharmacotherapy 1997;17:5 Part 2:146S–54S.
15. Petros WP, Colvin OM. Metabolic jeopardy with high-dose cyclophosphamide? Not so fast. Clin Cancer Res 1999;5:723–4.
16. Dillman JB. Safe use of succinylcholine during repeated anesthetics in a patient treated with cyclophosphamide. Anesth Analg 1987;66:351–3.
17. Shaunak S, Munro JM, Weinbren K, et al. Cyclophosphamide-induced liver necrosis: a possible interaction with azathioprine. QJM 1988;67:309–17.
18. Anthony LB, Long QC, Struck RF, Hande KR. The effect of cimetidine on cyclophosphamide metabolism in rabbits. Cancer Chemother Pharmacol 1990;27:125–30.
19. Alberts DS, Mason-Liddil N, Plezia PM, et al. Lack of ranitidine effects on cyclophosphamide bone marrow toxicity or metabolism: a placebo-controlled clinical trial. J Natl Cancer Inst 1991;83:1739–42.
20. Yule SM, Walker D, Cole M, et al. The effect of fluconazole on cyclophosphamide metabolism in children. Drug Metab Dispos 1999;27:417–21.
21. Bullock G, Tang C, Tourkina E, et al. Effect of combined treatment with interleukin-3 and interleukin-6 on 4-hydroperoxycyclophosphamide-induced programmed cell death or apoptosis in human myeloid leukemia cells. Exp Hematol 1993;21:1640–7.
22. Pegram M, Hsu S, Lewis G, et al. Inhibitory effects of combinations of HER-2/neu antibody and chemotherapeutic agents used for the treatment of human breast cancers. Oncogene 1999;18:2241–51.
23. Janss AJ, Cnaan A, Zhao H, et al. Synergistic cytotoxicity of topoisomerase I inhibitors with alkylating agents and etoposide in human brain tumor cell lines. Anticancer Drugs 1998;9:641–52.
24. Bazzan M, Pannocchia A, Tarella C, et al. Reduction of plasma fibrinolytic activity following high-dose cyclophosphamide is neutralized in vivo by GM-CSF administration. Haematologica 1993;78:105–10.
25. Lele SS, Durrant ST, Atherton JJ, et al. Demonstration of late cardiotoxicity following bone marrow transplantation by assessment of exercise diastolic filling characteristics. Bone Marrow Transplant 1996; 17:1113–8.
26. Ayash LJ, Wright JE, Tretyakov O, et al. Cyclophosphamide pharmacokinetics: correlation with cardiac toxicity and tumor response. J Clin Oncol 1992;10:995–1000.
27. Braverman AD, Antin JH, Plappert MT, et al. Cyclophosphamide cardiotoxicity in bone marrow transplantation: a prospective evaluation of new dosing regimens. J Clin Oncol 1991;9:1215–23.
28. Stillwell TJ, Benson RC Jr. Cyclophosphamide-induced hemorrhagic cystitis: a review of 100 patients. Cancer 1988;61:451–7.
29. Johnson WW, Meadows DC. Urinary-bladder fibrosis and telangiectasia associated with long-term cyclophosphamide therapy. N Engl J Med 1971;284:290–4.
30. Brock N, Pohl J, Stekar J. Studies on the urotoxicity of oxazaphosphorine cytostatics and its prevention. 2: Comparative study on the uroprotective efficacy of thiols and other sulfur compounds. Eur J Cancer Clin Oncol 1981;17:1155–63.
31. Pedersen-Bjergaard J, Ersboll J, Hansen VL, et al. Carcinoma of the urinary bladder after treatment with cyclophosphamide for non-Hodgkin's lymphoma. N Engl J Med 1988;318:1028–32.
32. Hows JM, Mehta A, Ward L, et al. Comparison of mesna with forced diuresis to prevent cyclophosphamide-induced haemorrhagic cystitis in marrow transplantation: a prospective randomised study. Br J Cancer 1984;50:753–6.
33. Shepherd JD, Pringle LE, Barnett MJ, et al. Mesna versus hyperhydration for the prevention of cyclophosphamide-induced hemorrhagic cystitis in bone marrow transplantation. J Clin Oncol 1991;9:2016–20.
34. Vose JM, Reed EC, Pippert GC, et al. Mesna compared with continuous bladder irrigation as uroprotection during high-dose chemotherapy and transplantation: a randomized trial. J Clin Oncol 1993;11:1306–10.
35. Kuroi K, Sato Y, Yamaguchi Y, Toge T. Modulation of suppressor cell activities by cyclophosphamide in breast cancer patients. J Clin Lab Anal 1994;8:123–7.
36. Arranz JA, Jimenez R, Alvarez-Mon M. Cyclophosphamide-induced myopia. Ann Intern Med 1992;116:92–3.
37. Levine E, Bloomfield CD. Leukemias and myelodysplastic syndromes secondary to drug, radiation, and environmental exposure. Semin Oncol 1992;19:47–8.
38. Bennett WM, Singer I, Golper T, et al. Guidelines for drug therapy in renal failure. Ann Intern Med 1977;86:754–83.

# Cytarabine

A wide variety of nucleoside analogues have been tested for both antineoplastic and antiviral properties. These analogues are readily transported into rapidly dividing cells and require only a single metabolic step (phosphorylation to a nucleotide) to enter the de novo pathway of nucleotide triphosphate synthesis. Adenine nucleoside analogues are of great interest for their potential antiviral properties; analogues of cytosine have not been useful as antiviral compounds, but cytarabine, an analogue of deoxycytidine in which the sugar moiety is altered, is useful in cancer chemotherapy. Cytarabine is also known as cytosine arabinoside, ara-C, Cytosar-U, arabinosyl cytosine, 1-arabinofuranosylcytosine, Tarabine PFS, and NSC-63878.

## EFFICACY

Cytarabine is almost always used with other drugs in the treatment of acute myelogenous leukemia (AML).

## PHARMACOLOGY

**Mechanism of Action.** Cytarabine cytotoxicity depends on three interrelated factors.[1] First, cytarabine must be converted to its lethal triphosphate derivative, ara-CTP. The process involves multiple factors, including the levels of nucleoside transport, phosphorylation, deamination, and the levels of competing metabolites, particularly deoxy-CTP. Second, the antiproliferative effects of cytarabine relate to the ability of ara-CTP to interfere with one or more DNA polymerases and the degree to which it is incorporated into elongating DNA strands. These effects lead to DNA fragmentation and chain termination. Third, the ultimate fate of the cell is determined by the extent to which a threshold level of cytarabine-mediated DNA damage is exceeded, thereby inducing apoptosis. The induction of apoptosis is influenced by components of the signal transduction pathways (such as protein kinase C) and the expression of various oncogenes (especially *bcl*-2 and c-*Jun*).

Cytarabine cytotoxicity is highly specific for the S phase of the cell cycle, and its effective use is highly schedule dependent. This has important implications for the clinical use of the drug.

**Resistance.** Resistance to cytarabine is multifactorial. At low doses, the rate of accumulation in cells is determined primarily by the rate of transport across the cell membrane; at high doses, the rate of phosphorylation to ara-CTP appears to be the critical determinant of toxicity.[2] The crucial activation of cytarabine to ara-CTP is mediated by a series of nucleoside and nucleotide kinases, the first of which is deoxycytidine kinase. This is balanced by at least one and possibly other degradative enzymes that are present in plasma and in some cells (cytidine and deoxycytidylate deaminases). Other mechanisms of resistance have been postulated, including an altered affinity of DNA polymerase for ara-CTP or changes in the pool size of the competitive natural substrate deoxy-CTP. Resistance in a hamster model has also been related to the level of CTP synthetase, but this has not been demonstrated in cells from patients with leukemia.[3] Resistance may also relate to alterations in the factors that control apoptosis, such as the levels of oncogenes and the function of signal transduction.[4, 5]

**Pharmacokinetics.** The pharmacokinetics of cytarabine are largely determined by cytidine deaminase, which is found in high concentrations in the gastrointestinal mucosa, liver, and granulocytes. The terminal half-life of cytarabine disappearance from plasma is 2 to 2.5 hours irrespective of drug dose, and most of the drug is excreted in the urine as the inactive metabolite uracil arabinoside. Only moderate concentrations of cytarabine cross the blood-brain barrier with standard treatment, but the drug is reasonably well tolerated by the intrathecal route. When so given, it disappears more slowly from the CSF, with a half-life of 2 to 11 hours, which relates to the paucity of cytidine deaminase in the CSF. This makes intrathecal cytarabine an alternative to MTX for treatment of meningeal leukemia; unfortunately, such treatment may also be associated with neurotoxicity, and it is probably less effective than MTX.

Cytarabine cytotoxicity is a function of both drug concentration and duration of exposure. Because cytarabine is an S-phase–specific drug, the duration of cell exposure to the drug during this vulnerable phase of the cell cycle is critical, as discussed in Chapter 8. In humans, bolus doses of cytarabine as large as 4.2 g/m$^2$ are well tolerated because of the rapid inactivation of the parent drug and the brief period of cell exposure. On the other hand, a constant infusion of cytarabine for 48 hours with a total dose of 1 g/m$^2$ yields severe myelosuppression. Because of the S-phase specificity and short plasma half-life of cytarabine, great effort has been expended to develop prolonged schedules of drug administration.

A more detailed discussion of the pharmacokinetics of cytarabine at low doses, standard doses, high doses, and by intrathecal administration is beyond the scope of this chapter. Potential differences between the pharmacokinetics of cytarabine in adults and children have been reviewed.[6] Because the drug is schedule dependent, there is great interest in the use of the drug by continuous infusion. Preliminary data suggest that the optimal use of this high-dose schedule is to start treatment with a bolus injection and to follow this with a continuous infusion of the drug.[7]

**Drug Interactions.** The elimination of cytosine arabinoside triphosphate, a neurotoxic metabolite, may be decreased by nephrotoxic drugs. This can result in neurotoxic reactions such as confusion, lethargy, and ataxia.[8] The absorption of oral digoxin (but not digitoxin) can be reduced by chemotherapy. Limited data suggest that cytarabine may antagonize the antibiotic effectiveness of gentamicin and flucytosine. Limited data suggest that numerous drugs may enhance the antitumor cytotoxicity of cytarabine. These include thymidine, tetrahydrouridine (to inhibit degradation of cytarabine), uracil arabinoside, IL-3, hydroxyurea (through inhibition of ribonucleotide reductase[9]), GM-CSF (through altered intracellular metabolism of cytarabine[10]), dipyridamole (through intracellular cytarabine trapping[11]), and possibly other drugs as well.[12] Pretreatment with etoposide and teniposide inhibits the in vitro formation of cytarabine toxic metabolites, so it has been suggested that these two drugs should not precede cytarabine in clinical trials of combination chemotherapy.[13] However, the high protein binding of etoposide in plasma (96%) abrogates this effect in vivo, resulting in no impairment of ara-CTP formation in leukemic cells in treated patients.[14]

## TOXICITY

**Overview.** Myelosuppression is dose limiting, and it represents the most important major toxic side effect at standard doses. At high doses, the cytarabine syndrome occurs, including central and peripheral neuropathy, hemorrhagic conjunctivitis, keratitis, severe gastrointestinal ulceration, severe pulmonary distress, and hepatic toxicity.

**Hematologic.** Depression of normal leukopoiesis and thrombopoiesis appears after about a week of treatment. The nadir of granulocytopenia usually occurs 12 to 14 days after starting therapy, and recovery is usually complete by 3 weeks. However, intensive supportive therapy may be needed during that interval. Cytarabine can induce striking megaloblastic changes in bone marrow cells, sometimes leading to difficulties in morphologic interpretation. This may be accompanied by multiple chromosome breaks found on cytogenetic analysis.[15]

**Immunologic.** Cytarabine is a potent inhibitor of the

primary immune response, but it has minimal effects against established immunity. It is of interest that immunosuppression may vary markedly with the dose of the drug. Specifically, low doses in animal systems may preferentially suppress humoral immunity, whereas much larger doses of cytarabine are required to suppress cell-mediated immunity. Nevertheless, cytarabine can itself induce allergic reactions, including anaphylaxis. In children receiving high-dose cytarabine, about a third of patients develop a syndrome characterized by fever, myalgia, bone pain, and occasionally chest pain, maculopapular rash, and conjunctivitis (the cytarabine syndrome). Rarely, this syndrome may also occur in adults given low-dose cytarabine.[16] The cytarabine syndrome is presumed to be due to a hypersensitivity reaction.

**Digestive System.** Nausea, vomiting, anorexia, diarrhea, a metallic taste in the mouth, dysphagia, and abdominal pain may occur as acute forms of toxicity. Rarely, this may mimic a surgical abdomen[17] or may be associated with pseudomembranous enterocolitis due to *Clostridium difficile*.[18] Prior treatment of a patient with L-asparaginase may also predispose the patient to pancreatitis.[19] Acute pancreatitis can also occur with high-dose cytarabine without L-asparaginase therapy. Hepatic dysfunction occurs in about 7% of patients at standard doses.

**Mucocutaneous.** Stomatitis occurs in about 9% of patients with standard doses. Transient erythema can occur without exfoliation; alopecia and other rashes occur rarely. Very rarely, palmar-plantar skin changes have been noted with cytarabine use (hand-foot syndrome). Erythema and swelling of the ears may occur but usually resolve within a week.[20]

**Pulmonary.** Fatal noncardiogenic pulmonary edema has been reported as a possible complication in 24% of patients with leukemia.[21] It has been suggested that increased capillary permeability following intravenous cytarabine was the probable cause of this problem.

**Ocular.** Conjunctivitis can occur; it can be reduced with ophthalmic corticosteroids[22] or with artificial tears.[23] Blurred vision, photophobia, ocular pain, excessive tearing, and rarely keratitis can occur with high-dose cytarabine. Pseudotumor cerebri has been reported.[24]

**Neurologic.** High-dose cytarabine can cause severe neurotoxicity, especially cerebellar ataxia (16 to 40% of cases overall, severe in 7 to 18%), although this is rare with standard doses. It is more common in older patients, in men, and after shorter infusion times. In one study, the highest risk was associated with a serum creatinine level of 1.2 mg/dl, age of 40 years, and an alkaline phosphatase value three times normal.[25] It is frequently irreversible and may be fatal. Limited data suggest that cerebellar toxicity may be more common with the Quad Pharmaceuticals generic drug than with Cytosar-U, produced by Upjohn Company.[26] Other forms of neurotoxicity include aphasia, peripheral neuropathy, brachial plexus neuropathy, bilateral rectus palsy, parkinsonism, dizziness, somnolence, and, very rarely, acute demyelinating polyneuropathy with respiratory failure. Progressive ascending paralysis has also been seen with combined intrathecal and intravenous cytarabine. Severe forms of neural necrosis with death due to cytarabine may be referred to as *locked-in syndrome*.[27]

**Other and Rare Reactions.** Fever and a flu-like syndrome can occur.

*Cardiovascular.* Cardiomegaly, pericarditis, and thrombophlebitis (8% with standard doses) can occur.

*Musculoskeletal.* These effects include arthralgias and myalgias. Acute rhabdomyolysis has been reported in one patient.

*Genitourinary.* Urinary retention and hemorrhagic cystitis can occur.

*Reproductive.* Toxicity data place cytarabine in FDA pregnancy category D.

*Carcinogenicity.* The drug is mutagenic and potentially carcinogenic.

## DOSAGE AND ADMINISTRATION

Cytarabine is available for parenteral administration in vials of 100, 500, 1000, and 2000 mg. It is incompatible with a variety of drugs in solution, including nafcillin, penicillin G, oxacillin, 5-FU, carbenicillin, and heparin sodium. Lactated Ringer's solution or normal saline without preservatives should be used for reconstitution for intrathecal administration.

For the induction of remission in AML, the dosage of cytarabine when given in combination with other antineoplastic agents is 100 mg/m²/day by continuous intravenous infusion for 7 days. Alternatively, 100 mg/m² of cytarabine may be given intravenously as a bolus every 12 hours for 7 days. When cytarabine is used intrathecally, dosages ranging between 5 and 75 mg/m² given every 3 to 7 days are used. In adults, a dosage of 50 mg/m² yields peak CSF levels of 1 mM, and cytotoxic levels are maintained for about 24 hours. A commonly used intrathecal regimen is 30 mg/m² once every 4 days until the CSF findings are normal, followed by one additional dose. Other regimens may also be deployed, as discussed in the disease-oriented chapters of this book. One of the most important is high-dose cytarabine for patients with refractory lymphomas and leukemias. An example of such a regimen involves intravenous administration of cytarabine in a dosage of 2 to 3 g/m² over 1 to 3 hours every 12 hours for 2 to 6 days. This can be extremely toxic and should be used with great caution.

## REFERENCES

1. Grant S. Ara-C: cellular and molecular pharmacology. Adv Cancer Res 1998;72:197–233.
2. White JC, Rathmell JP, Capizzi RL. Membrane transport influences the rate of accumulation of cytosine arabinoside in human leukemia cells. J Clin Invest 1987;79:380–7.
3. Whelan J, Smith T, Phear G, et al. Resistance to cytosine arabinoside in acute leukemia: the significance of mutations in CTP synthetase. Leukemia 1994;8:264–5.
4. Kobayashi T, Ruan S, Jabbur JR, et al. Differential p53 phosphorylation and activation of apoptosis-promoting genes Bax and Fas/APO-1 by irradiation and ara-C treatment. Cell Death Differ 1998;5:584–91.
5. Want S, Vrana JA, Bartimole TM, et al. Agents that down-regulate or inhibit protein kinase C circumvent resistance to 1-beta-D-arabinofuranosylcytosine-induced apoptosis in human leukemia cells that overexpress Bcl-2. Mol Pharmacol 1997;52:1000–9.
6. Burke GA, Estlin EJ, Lowis SP. The role of pharmacokinetic and pharmacodynamic studies in the planning of protocols for the treatment of childhood cancer. Cancer Treat Rev 1999;25:13–27.
7. Avramis VI, Weinberg KI, Sato JK, et al. Pharmacology studies of 1-beta-D-arabinofuranosylcytosine in pediatric patients with leukemia and

lymphoma after a biochemically optimal regimen of loading bolus plus continuous infusion of the drug. Cancer Res 1989;49:241–7.

8. Damon LE, Mass R, Linker CA. The association between high-dose cytarabine neurotoxicity and renal insufficiency. J Clin Oncol 1989;7:1563–8.

9. Bhalla K, Swerdlow P, Grant S. Effects of thymidine and hydroxyurea on the metabolism and cytotoxicity of 1-β-D-arabinofuranosylcytosine in highly resistant human leukemia cells. Blood 1991;78:2937–44.

10. Reuter C, Auf der Landewehr U, Schleyer E, et al. Modulation of intracellular metabolism of cytosine arabinoside in acute myeloid leukemia by granulocyte-macrophage colony-stimulating factor. Leukemia 1994;8:217–25.

11. Yang J-L, White JC, Capizzi RL. Enhanced retention of cytosine arabinoside and its metabolites and synergistic cytotoxicity by sequential treatment with dipyridamole in L5178Y leukemia. Cancer Chemother Pharmacol 1990;26:135–8.

12. Grant S. Biochemical modulation of cytosine arabinoside. Pharmacol Ther 1990;48:29–44.

13. Ehninger G, Proksch B, Wanner T, et al. Intracellular cytosine arabinoside accumulation and cytosine arabinoside triphosphate formation in leukemic blast cells is inhibited by etoposide and teniposide. Leukemia 1992;6:582–7.

14. Liliemark J, Knochenhaur E, Gruber A, et al. On the interaction between cytosine arabinoside and etoposide in vivo and in vitro. Eur J Haematol 1993;50:22–5.

15. Karon M, Benedict WF, Rucker N. Mechanisms of 1-β-D-arabinofuranosylcytosine–induced cell lethality. Cancer Res 1972;32:2612–5.

16. Powell BL, Zekan PJ, Muss HB, et al. Ara-C syndrome during low-dose continuous infusion therapy. Med Pediatr Oncol 1986;14:310–2.

17. Johnson H, Smith TJ, Desforges J. Cytosine-arabinoside–induced colitis and peritonitis: nonoperative management. J Clin Oncol 1985;3:607–12.

18. Roda PI. *Clostridium difficile* colitis induced by cytarabine. Am J Clin Oncol 1987;10:451–2.

19. Altman AJ, Dinndorf P, Quinn JJ. Acute pancreatitis in association with cytosine arabinoside therapy. Cancer 1982;49:1384–6.

20. Krulder JWM, Vlasveld LT, Willemze R. Erythema and swelling of ears after treatment with cytarabine for leukemia. Eur J Cancer 1990;26:649–50.

21. Haupt HM, Hutchins GM, Moore GW. Ara-C lung: noncardiogenic pulmonary edema complicating cytosine arabinoside therapy of leukemia. Am J Med 1981;70:256–61.

22. Lass JH, Lazarus HM, Reed MD, Herzig RH. Topical corticosteroid therapy for corneal toxicity from systemically administered cytarabine. Am J Ophthalmol 1982;94:617–21.

23. Higa GM, Gockerman JP, Hunt AL, et al. The use of prophylactic eye drops during high-dose cytosine arabinoside therapy. Cancer 1991;68:1691–3.

24. Evers JP, Jacobson RJ, Pincus J, Zwiebel JA. Pseudotumour cerebri following high-dose cytosine arabinoside. Br J Haematol 1992;80:559–60.

25. Rubin EH, Andersen JW, Berg DT, et al. Risk factors for high-dose cytarabine neurotoxicity: an analysis of a Cancer and Leukemia Group B trial in patients with acute myeloid leukemia. J Clin Oncol 1992;10:948–53.

26. Jolson HM, Bosco L, Bufton MG, et al. Clustering of adverse drug events: analysis of risk factors for cerebellar toxicity with high-dose cytarabine. J Natl Cancer Inst 1992;84:500–5.

27. Kleinschmidt-DeMasters BK, Yeh M. "Locked-in syndrome" after intrathecal cytosine arabinoside therapy for malignant immunoblastic lymphoma. Cancer 1992;70:2504–7.

# Dacarbazine

Dacarbazine is one of several imidazole carboxamide derivatives developed in the mid-1960s under National Cancer Institute contract by scientists at the Southern Research Institute. The drug is also known as DTIC, DTIC-Dome, DIC, imidazole carboxamide, dimethyl triazeno imidazole carboxamide, and NSC-45388.

## EFFICACY

Dacarbazine is used in the treatment of malignant melanoma and lymphomas. It is less commonly used in the treatment of some endocrine tumors, sarcomas, and neuroblastoma.

## PHARMACOLOGY

**Mechanism of Action.** Although dacarbazine is a structural analogue of certain purines, its major mode of action appears to be methylation of nucleic acids. This involves the formation of $O^6$-methylguanine DNA adducts that interfere with DNA and RNA synthesis by blocking replication and transcriptional complexes.[1] These adducts are also capable of inducing mutations in the genome. Dacarbazine is cell cycle phase nonspecific, and no schedule dependence or dose-response relationship has been established.

**Resistance.** A specific DNA repair protein, $O^6$-alkylguanine-DNA alkyltransferase, is responsible for the repair of damage by methylating agents such as dacarbazine.[2] A secondary repair mechanism that is less important is the excision repair pathway.

**Pharmacokinetics.** Dacarbazine is inactive and must undergo biotransformation before exerting its cytotoxic effects. Two forms of biotransformation have been defined. The major metabolic pathway in vivo appears to be oxidative *N*-demethylation by liver microsomal enzymes. This forms alkylating metabolites that are cytotoxic for neoplastic cells; however, this process may also form products that are carcinogenic in animals. The other major pathway of biotransformation is by photodegradation to active and inactive metabolites. Dacarbazine should probably be protected from light to minimize photodegradation; however, the true importance of this is uncertain. In one animal study, photodegradation did not appear to influence the antitumor efficacy of the drug, and the investigators concluded that elaborate precautions to prevent exposure of dacarbazine to light were unnecessary.

The pharmacokinetic properties of dacarbazine include a plasma clearance half-time of about 5 hours, modest binding to plasma protein or tissues (about 20%), and excretion primarily by the kidneys. The drug has only limited access to the CNS through the blood-brain barrier.

**Drug Interactions.** Administration of dacarbazine with IL-2 leads to reduced plasma levels of dacarbazine and its metabolites[3] and a higher than expected incidence of allergic reactions.[4] The clinical significance of these effects is uncertain. Dacarbazine inhibits xanthine oxidase, so hypouricemia may be more marked when allopurinol and dacarbazine are used together.

## TOXICITY

**Overview.** Myelosuppression is the most important dose-limiting toxicity, although nausea and vomiting can also be significant problems with standard doses. Limited phase I studies suggest that dacarbazine can be given in much higher doses in the transplant setting, but this is investigational therapy.[5]

**Hematologic.** Although myelosuppression is the most common dose-limiting toxicity, it is usually only mild to moderate in severity and rarely proves to be a serious clinical problem. Eosinophilia can occasionally develop.

**Digestive System.** Acute toxicity generally includes anorexia, nausea, and moderate to severe vomiting in most patients. This often abates after two or three doses despite continued therapy, and it may be reduced by the use of antiemetics. Fatal massive hepatic necrosis with widespread thrombotic occlusion of the small hepatic veins (veno-occlusive disease) can occur rarely with standard dose therapy. The traditional view has been that this devastating complication is a rare event, with an approximate incidence of 0.01% of patients treated. However, a report from Italy suggests a higher frequency, with two cases occurring in a randomized study of 68 patients (3%).[6]

**Mucocutaneous.** Concentrated solutions of dacarbazine may be irritating to veins, and extravasation can cause severe local tissue destruction. The drug can also cause photosensitivity reactions, so patients should be advised to avoid sun exposure for several days after drug administration. Alopecia and rashes occur but are uncommon.

**Other/Rare.** A flu-like syndrome, chills, malaise, facial flushing, and a metallic taste in the mouth can occur.

**Immunologic.** Anaphylaxis can occur. In human studies, dacarbazine is minimally immunosuppressive.

**Cardiovascular.** Cardiomyopathy may occur.

**Ocular.** These effects include blurred vision.

**Neurologic.** Dizziness, paresthesia, confusion, lethargy, seizures, and peripheral neuropathy can occur.

**Musculoskeletal.** Myalgias can occur.

**Genitourinary.** Renal dysfunction is of uncertain relationship to dacarbazine.

**Reproductive.** Toxicity data place dacarbazine in FDA pregnancy category C.

**Carcinogenicity.** The drug is mutagenic and carcinogenic in animals.

## DOSAGE AND ADMINISTRATION

Dacarbazine is available in vials of 100 and 200 mg of lyophilized drug. The usual intravenous dosages range from 2.4 to 4.5 mg/kg/day for 5 to 10 days when the drug is used as a single agent. Much higher single dosages have also been used, such as 850 mg/m² of dacarbazine intravenously as a single dose every 3 to 6 weeks. However, the use of high-dose intermittent dacarbazine is probably less effective than the traditional schedule, and it has the added toxicity of hypotension and extreme nausea and vomiting. The dosage is 375 mg/m² on days 1 and 15 for Hodgkin's disease (as part of the ABVD regimen: doxorubicin [Adriamycin], bleomycin, vinblastine, dacarbazine). In selected patients with regional melanoma, dacarbazine has been used experimentally by the intra-arterial route and by isolation perfusion. It has also been used by the intrathecal route.[7] Perhaps the most widely used program of drug use is slow intravenous administration over 30 to 60 minutes in a dosage of 250 mg/m²/day for 5 days, repeated every 3 weeks. Extravasation should be avoided because dacarbazine can cause local tissue damage and severe pain.

## REFERENCES

1. Kyrtopoulos SA, Anderson LM, Chhabra SK, et al. DNA adducts and the mechanism of carcinogenesis and cytotoxicity of methylating agents of environmental and clinical significance. Cancer Detect Prevent 1997;21:391–405.
2. Souliotis VL, Valavanis C, Boussiotis VA, et al. Comparative study of the formation and repair of O6-methylguanine in humans and rodents treated with dacarbazine. Carcinogenesis 1996;17:725–32.
3. Chabot GG, Flaherty LE, Valdivieso M, Baker LH. Alteration of dacarbazine pharmacokinetics after interleukin-2 administration in melanoma patients. Cancer Chemother Pharmacol 1990;27:157–60.
4. Heywood GR, Rosenberg SA, Weber JS. Hypersensitivity reactions to chemotherapy agents in patients receiving chemoimmunotherapy with high-dose interleukin 2. J Natl Cancer Inst 1995;87:915–22.
5. Adkins DR, Irvin R, Kuhn J, et al. A phase I clinical and pharmacological profile of dacarbazine with autologous bone marrow transplantation in patients with solid tumors. Invest New Drugs 1993;11:169–79.
6. Ceci G, Bella M, Melissari M, et al. Fatal hepatic vascular toxicity of DTIC: is it really a rare event? Cancer 1988;61:1988–91.
7. Champagne MA, Silver HK. Intrathecal dacarbazine treatment of leptomeningeal malignant melanoma. J Natl Cancer Inst 1992;84:1203–4.

# Dactinomycin

The actinomycin antibiotics were discovered in 1940 and first given to patients in 1952.[1] Most have been derived from *Streptomyces parvulus,* and more than 100 analogues have been extracted or synthesized. Dactinomycin is the sole member of this group that is currently in use. The drug is also known as Cosmegen, actinomycin D, DACT, ACT-D, and NSC-3053.

## EFFICACY

Dactinomycin is primarily used in combination with surgery or radiation therapy, or both, in the treatment of Wilms' tumor, Ewing's sarcoma, and rhabdomyosarcomas. It is also used alone or in combination with other drugs in the treatment of a variety of neoplasms, especially gestational trophoblastic neoplasia, testicular seminomas, and Kaposi's sarcoma.

## PHARMACOLOGY

**Mechanism of Action.** At low concentrations in mammalian tissues, dactinomycin inhibits DNA-primed RNA synthesis by intercalating with the guanine residues of DNA. At higher concentrations, it also inhibits DNA synthesis. Additional effects may include DNA-DNA interstrand cross-links and DNA-protein cross-links.[2] The drug also inhibits topoisomerases I and II.[3] Ultimately, the drug leads to apoptosis.[4] The multiple effects of dactinomycin result in a variety of concentration-dependent changes in the life cycle of cells; the net effect, however, is best described as being phase nonspecific.

**Resistance.** Tumor resistance to dactinomycin is associated with the multiple drug resistance (mdr) phenotype and overexpression of P-glycoprotein.[5]

**Pharmacokinetics.** Dactinomycin must be administered intravenously because of its erratic oral absorption. The parent drug is extensively bound to nucleated cells and has a prolonged terminal half-life in plasma (about 36 hours). The drug undergoes only limited metabolism and is excreted unchanged by both the liver and the kidneys. Dactinomycin appears to be concentrated in bone marrow and tumor cells, but a partial blood-testis barrier exists, as well as a nearly complete blood-brain barrier. For most normal tissues, the factor that limits the ultimate concentration of dactinomycin is the blood supply to that tissue rather than the tissue's cell membrane permeability to the drug.[6]

**Drug Interactions.** No interactions have been reported.

## TOXICITY

**Overview.** At standard doses, myelosuppression and nausea are dose limiting; the drug is toxic to soft tissues, and extravasation must be avoided by taking appropriate precautions.

**Hematologic.** Dose-limiting leukopenia and thrombocytopenia occur about 1 or 2 weeks after treatment, with recovery by 3 or 4 weeks. Anemia may also occur but is rarely a problem.

**Digestive System.** Nausea and vomiting are common, usually starting about an hour after chemotherapy and lasting a few hours. Liver dysfunction, anorexia, and diarrhea can also occur rarely. Severe hepatotoxicity may be more common with high-dose intermittent schedules of administration. In a study of patients with Wilms' tumor being treated with actinomycin D plus vincristine, 3% of the patients developed this complication with standard-dose therapy, and 14% developed significant hepatic toxicity with high-dose treatment.[7] Ultrasound studies can be useful in monitoring the severity of dactinomycin-induced hepatic veno-occlusive disease and in following its response to treatment.[8]

**Mucocutaneous.** Alopecia and skin rashes can occur, including a moderately severe folliculitis[9] and various forms of brawny erythema and hyperpigmentation.[10] Glossitis, stomatitis, dysphagia, proctitis, and cheilitis occur occasionally, but these can be dose limiting in some patients. Extravasation causes severe tissue inflammation and necrosis. Delayed radiation reactions can occur (recall phenomenon).

**Other/Rare.** Fever and fatigue can occur.

**Immunologic.** Anaphylactoid reactions can occur. The drug is minimally immunosuppressive.

**Cardiovascular.** Exacerbation of doxorubicin-induced cardiomyopathy is possible.

**Musculoskeletal.** Myalgia can occur, and growth suppression can occur in children treated with radiation therapy.[11]

**Reproductive.** Toxicity data place dactinomycin in FDA pregnancy category C.

**Endocrine-Metabolic.** Hypocalcemia can occur.

**Carcinogenicity.** The drug is mutagenic and carcinogenic.

## DOSAGE AND ADMINISTRATION

Dactinomycin is available as a lyophilized powder in vials of 500 g (0.5 mg). It is incompatible with diluents containing preservatives, and it binds to some kinds of filters (cellulose ester and polytetrafluoroethylene filters). The drug is given with extravasation precautions over a period of 2 to 3 minutes, preferably through a smoothly flowing intravenous infusion line. It can also be given by intravenous infusion in 5% dextrose in water or normal saline over 20 to 30 minutes.

A number of dosage regimens have been used, and the optimal program is still unknown. A common regimen is to give 15 μg/kg intravenously (maximum single dose, 0.5 mg in children) on each of five successive days.[1] Such a course may be repeated every 3 or 4 weeks. Alternatively, a single dose of 1 mg/m[2] or greater can be given intravenously every 3 to 4 weeks.[12] Higher doses can be given as a continuous infusion over a 5-day period.[13] Lower doses may be used in treating adults with impaired bone marrow function, and extra care is needed in treating small infants. In one study comparing single-dose and divided-dose administration to patients with Wilms' tumor, the single-dose approach was superior.[14]

## REFERENCES

1. Farber S, Selman A. Waksman Conference on Actinomycins: their potential for cancer chemotherapy. Opening remarks. Cancer Chemother Rep 1974;58:Part 1:1–7.
2. Fox JMK, Byrne TD, Woods WG. Actinomycin D–associated lesions mimicking DNA-DNA interstrand crosslinks detected by alkaline elution in cultured mammalian cells. Biochem Pharmacol 1985;34:2741–7.
3. Wasserman K, Markovits J, Jaxel C, et al. Effects of morpholinyl doxorubicins, doxorubicin, and actinomycin D on mammalian DNA topoisomerases I and II. Mol Pharmacol 1990;38:38–45.
4. Cotter TG, Glynn JM, Echeverri F, Green DR. The induction of apoptosis by chemotherapeutic agents occurs in all phases of the cell cycle. Anticancer Res 1992;12:773–9.
5. Melguizo C, Prados J, Fernandez JE, et al. Actinomycin D causes multidrug resistance and differentiation in human rhabdomyosarcoma cell lines. Cell Mol Biol 1994;40:137–45.
6. Lutz RJ, Galbraith WM, Dedrick RL, et al. A model for the kinetics of distribution of actinomycin-D in the beagle dog. J Pharmacol Exp Ther 1977;200:469–78.
7. Green DM, Norkool P, Breslow NE, et al. Severe hepatic toxicity after treatment with vincristine and dactinomycin using single-dose or divided-dose schedules: a report from the National Wilms' Tumor Study. J Clin Oncol 1990;8:1525–30.
8. Schiavetti A, Matrunola M, Varrasso G, et al. Ultrasound in the management of hepatic veno-occlusive disease in three children treated with dactinomycin and vincristine. Pediatr Hematol Oncol 1996;13:521–9.
9. Epstein EH Jr, Lutzner MA. Folliculitis induced by actinomycin D. N Engl J Med 1969;181:1094–6.
10. Coppes MJ, Jorgenson K, Arlette JP. Cutaneous toxicity following the administration of dactinomycin. Med Pediatr Oncol 1997;29:226–7.
11. Wallace WHB, Shalet SM. Chemotherapy with actinomycin D influences the growth of the spine following abdominal irradiation. Med Pediatr Oncol 1992;20:177.
12. Blatt J, Trigg ME, Pizzo PA, Glaubiger D. Tolerance to single-dose dactinomycin in combination chemotherapy for solid tumors. Cancer Treat Rep 1981;65:145–7.
13. Blumenreich MS, Woodcock TM, Richman SP, et al. A phase I trial of dactinomycin intravenous infusion in patients with advanced malignancies. Cancer 1985;56:256–8.
14. Green DM, Breslow NE, Beckwith JB, et al. Comparison between single-dose and divided-dose administration of dactinomycin and doxorubicin for patients with Wilms' tumor: a report from the National Wilms' Tumor Study Group. J Clin Oncol 1998;16:237–45.

# Daunorubicin

Daunorubicin is an antitumor antibiotic developed independently in Italy and France from *Streptomyces coeruleorubidus*. It is chemically similar to doxorubicin. Other names include daunomycin, rubidomycin, Cerubidine, DNR, and NSC-82151.

## EFFICACY

Daunorubicin has a wide spectrum of activity, but its primary use is in the treatment of acute leukemia.[1]

## PHARMACOLOGY

The mechanisms of action and resistance,[2] pharmacokinetics, and drug interactions of daunorubicin are essentially the same as those of doxorubicin, with minor exceptions, such as a slightly longer elimination half-life. Of some concern is a report that ICRF-187 (dexrazoxane) may interfere with both the cardiac toxicity and the antineoplastic activity of daunorubicin.[3] It is unclear whether this is uniquely true for daunorubicin or whether this is also a problem when dexrazoxane is combined with doxorubicin.

## TOXICITY

The toxicity and precautions to be taken in the use of daunorubicin are essentially the same as for doxorubicin. Cardiac toxicity is of particular concern[4]; other major toxic side effects are myelosuppression, mucositis, and soft tissue necrosis due to extravasation. Daunorubicin is potentially carcinogenic, probably through the formation of DNA adducts by covalent binding.[5]

## DOSAGE AND ADMINISTRATION

Daunorubicin is available as a lyophilized powder in 20-mg vials. The dosage of daunorubicin in adults ranges from 30 to 60 $mg/m^2$ daily for 3 to 5 days in combination with cytarabine. A common dosage is 45 $mg/m^2$ on days 1, 2 and 3 in combination with one or more drugs, depending on the type of leukemia. The incidence of myocardial toxicity increases after a total cumulative dose of 400 to 550 $mg/m^2$ in adults and 300 $mg/m^2$ in children older than 2 years. Limiting the total lifetime dose of daunorubicin to minimize cardiotoxicity is prudent, but authorities differ on what constitutes appropriate limits. These vary from the low values just listed to a dose as high as 750 $mg/m^2$. The manufacturer recommends dose reductions for an elevated serum bilirubin or creatinine value, as follows: use three fourths the normal dose for a serum bilirubin level of 1.2 to 3 mg/dl; use one half the normal dose for a serum bilirubin level greater than 3 mg/dl or a serum creatinine level greater than 3 mg/dl.

## REFERENCES

1. Gottlieb AJ, Weinberg V, Ellison RR, et al. Efficacy of daunorubicin in the therapy of adult acute lymphocytic leukemia: a prospective randomized trial by Cancer and Leukemia Group B. Blood 1984;64:267–74.
2. Gewirtz DA. A critical evaluation of the mechanisms of action proposed for the antitumor effects of the anthracycline antibiotics Adriamycin and daunorubicin. Biochem Pharmacol 1999;57:727–41.
3. Sehested M, Jensen PB, Sorensen BS, et al. Antagonistic effect of the cardioprotector ( + )-1,2-bis(3,5-dioxopiperazinyl-1-yl)propane (ICRF-187) on DNA breaks and cytotoxicity induced by the topoisomerase II directed drugs daunorubicin and etoposide (VP-16). Biochem Pharmacol 1993;46:389–93.
4. Von Hoff DD, Rozencweig M, Layard M, et al. Daunomycin-induced cardiotoxicity in children and adults: a review of 110 cases. Am J Med 1977;62:200–8.
5. Purewal M, Liehr JG. Covalent modification of DNA by daunorubicin. Cancer Chemother Pharmacol 1993;33:239–44.

# Dexamethasone

Dexamethasone is a synthetic corticosteroid. It is also known as Decadron, Hexadrol, DXM, and DEX.

## EFFICACY

Dexamethasone is widely used in oncology for the following indications: (1) the treatment of cerebral edema due to primary or metastatic neoplasms of the nervous system, (2) as an antiemetic, (3) to prevent or suppress hypersensitivity reactions (such as with paclitaxel), and (4) as a cytotoxic hormonal component of multiagent chemotherapy regimens for a variety of tumors.

## PHARMACOLOGY

**Mechanism of Action.** Understanding of the mechanisms of action of cortisone and its synthetic derivatives is incomplete. As with other hormones, one mechanism involves binding to intracellular receptors, followed by translocation to the nucleus.[1] Other mechanisms are involved as well because some of the biochemical effects of corticosteroids occur without entry into cells and steroid insensitivity can occur irrespective of the presence of functional steroid receptors.[2] As a result of multiple interactions, corticosteroids cause a wide variety of biochemical and metabolic changes, including stimulation of hepatic protein synthesis and gluconeogenesis, inhibition of protein synthesis of peripheral tissues, and either inhibition or stimulation of lipogenesis, depending on the location of fat in the body. There may also be direct effects on steroid-sensitive enzymes, such as poly (ADP-ribose) polymerase. In many cases, the ultimate effect of corticosteroids is immunosuppression and the induction of apoptosis.[3–5]

**Resistance.** The lack of glucocorticoid receptors can result in drug resistance, as stated previously. In mice, resistance is independent of the T-cell receptor.[6] The formation of a truncated glucocorticoid receptor messenger RNA has been associated with resistance in myeloma.[7] Cortisol is transported by the multidrug-resistance gene product P-glycoprotein,[8] and overexpression of this phenotype has been associated with drug resistance in a murine thymoma cell line.[9] Overexpression of *bcl-2* is associated with resistance to dexamethasone in multiple myeloma cell lines.[10]

**Pharmacokinetics.** Dexamethasone, a potent and long-acting synthetic derivative of cortisol that is easily absorbed after oral administration, has a plasma half-life of 4 to 5 hours. The biologic half-life of dexamethasone is 1.5 to 2 times its half-life of disappearance from plasma. Dexamethasone retains a much higher proportion of its potency with time than other corticosteroids. For example, one study found that the relative potencies of hydrocortisone (cortisol), prednisone, and dexamethasone at 0, 8, and 14 hours after oral administration were as follows: hydrocortisone, 1, 1, 1; prednisone, 1.05, 3, 5.2; and dexamethasone, 17, 52, 154.[11]

**Drug Interactions.** Despite extensive information on the biochemical effects of corticosteroids used alone, very little is known about how they interact with other drugs. Of concern, however, are reports that dexamethasone may reduce the efficacy of chemotherapy directed against human malignant gliomas[12, 13] and that it may induce taxol metabolism.[14] Given the widespread use of dexamethasone as an antiemetic in cancer chemotherapy, further study of its potential interactions with antineoplastic agents is needed.

## TOXICITY

**Overview.** This potent glucocorticoid hormone has predominantly immunosuppressive and endocrine-metabolic effects, but a wide variety of other adverse reactions can also occur, including osteoporosis, aseptic necrosis of the hip, peptic ulcer disease, psychosis, and others.

**Hematologic.** Glucocorticosteroids cause neutrophilic leukocytosis, together with a reduction in circulating eosinophils, monocytes, and lymphocytes. A principal mechanism by which these steroids inhibit inflammation appears to be related to their ability to impede the access of neutrophils and monocytes to an inflammatory site. Results of granulocyte function tests remain normal with corticosteroid therapy, although monocyte-macrophage function is suppressed by such treatment.

**Immunologic.** Corticosteroids are potent immunosuppressive agents. The lymphocytopenia that is seen with corticosteroid therapy is usually transient, and it involves most lymphocyte subpopulations but most prominently suppressor T lymphocytes derived from the thymus. A primary mechanism of this action appears to be redistribution of these cells from the blood into other body compartments; however, corticosteroids may also kill lymphoid cells directly or interfere with essential lymphoid functions by inhibiting lymphoid growth factors and cytokines. These immunosuppressive changes can lead to superimposed infections of many kinds. Despite these immunosuppressive effects, dexamethasone can cause hypersensitivity reactions, including angioneurotic edema, urticaria, and anaphylactoid reactions, especially in persons who are allergic to sulfites.

**Digestive System.** Nausea, vomiting, increased appetite, anorexia, pancreatitis, and weight gain all can occur. Patients have a small (1.8%) risk of developing peptic ulcer disease while on corticosteroids.[15] Spontaneous intestinal and colonic perforations may occur in patients receiving corticosteroids and chemotherapy.[16] The key to managing this complication is early diagnosis and prompt surgical intervention. There has been one case reported of massive hepatic necrosis after chemotherapy withdrawal in a patient chronically infected with the hepatitis B virus.[17]

**Mucocutaneous.** Striae, atrophy, rash, acne, facial hair growth, ecchymoses, hirsutism, and poor wound healing can occur.

**Neurologic.** Psychosis, pseudotumor cerebri, affective changes (euphoria, depression), insomnia, headaches, muscle weakness, vertigo, dizziness, and seizures may occur. Lesser degrees of behavioral change can occur in children.[18]

**Musculoskeletal.** Myopathy, muscle wasting, osteoporosis, and aseptic necrosis of the femoral heads can occur.

**Endocrine-Metabolic.** Myriad acute and delayed reactions can occur, including sodium and water retention, potassium loss, exacerbation of diabetes mellitus, cushingoid appearance (including centripetal obesity), hyperlipidemia, hyperosmolar nonketotic coma, growth failure, amenorrhea, hirsutism, and suppression of the hypothalamic-pituitary-adrenal (HPA) axis. The effects of dexamethasone on glucose metabolism may be dose related. In one study of normal men, high-dose but not low-dose dexamethasone impaired glucose tolerance by inducing compensatory failure of pancreatic β-cells.[19]

Patients receiving corticosteroids for any prolonged period are susceptible to adrenal insufficiency at times of stress. This cannot be predicted by the duration of therapy, the dose of the corticosteroid, or the basal plasma cortisol concentration. If there is time to assess the HPA axis at the time of stress (e.g., before major surgery), the response of plasma corticotropin and cortisol either to insulin-induced hypoglycemia or to corticotropin-releasing hormone (CRH) can be measured. The CRH test is better tolerated by patients and is preferred.[20] If there is inadequate time to perform the CRH test, the patient should receive supplemental corticosteroids during the period of the emergency.[21]

**Other and Rare Reactions.** Singultus, suppression of skin test results, and exacerbation of fungal and granulomatous infections may occur.

***Cardiovascular.*** Thrombophlebitis, thromboembolism, and hypertension can occur. Myocardial rupture has been reported when dexamethasone is used after a myocardial infarction.

***Ocular.*** Glaucoma, cataracts, and exophthalmos can occur. Cataracts are especially likely when corticosteroids are combined with total-body irradiation for allogeneic BMT.[22]

***Reproductive.*** Toxicity studies place dexamethasone in FDA pregnancy category C.

***Carcinogenicity.*** No carcinogenicity is known.

## DOSAGE AND ADMINISTRATION

Dexamethasone is available in tablets of 0.25, 0.5, 0.75, 1, 1.5, 2, 4, and 6 mg. It is available as an oral solution or syrup of 0.5 mg/5 ml; as a solution for injection in strengths of 4, 10, 20, and 24 mg/ml; and in various strengths for inhalation, ophthalmic use, and intra-articular injection.

For patients with edema of the brain or spinal cord, a loading dose of 10 mg is given intravenously, followed by 4 mg intramuscularly every 6 hours until symptoms abate. For the prevention of nausea, the usual dose is 10 to 20 mg intravenously immediately before the administration of the emetogenic chemotherapy.

Dexamethasone is not an appropriate drug for programs of alternate-day steroid administration. The recommended dose and schedule of administration for corticosteroids vary with each of the diseases just mentioned; therefore, details are provided elsewhere in this book.

Suppression of the HPA axis is variable, but with prolonged daily treatment it may be severe and prolonged.[23] As a consequence, patients with malignant diseases are usually treated with very large doses for the minimal period necessary to achieve the desired clinical response. If corticosteroid treatment has been given for 2 weeks or less, it can be discontinued abruptly. Patients treated for longer periods should generally have steroid administration slowly withdrawn. If prolonged maintenance treatment is required, it is usually preferable to administer the corticosteroids on alternate days or, if that fails, as a single dose of a short-acting compound each morning. Patients who have been on corticosteroids for long periods may subsequently suffer unusual withdrawal symptoms. Dixon and Christy[24] have reviewed this problem and have provided guidelines for withdrawal in such patients.

There is some controversy about the importance of countermeasures directed against some of the other potential complications of corticosteroid treatment. For example, the value of using $H_2$-blocking agents for the prevention of peptic ulcer disease is uncertain. Likewise, the use of prophylactic potassium administration should be decided on an individual basis because the net potassium balance varies from patient to patient.

## REFERENCES

1. Boumpas DT, Chrousos GP, Wilder RL, et al. Glucocorticoid therapy for immune-mediated diseases: basic and clinical correlates. Ann Intern Med 1993;119:1198–208.
2. Darbre PD, King RJ. Progression to steroid insensitivity can occur irrespective of the presence of functional steroid receptors. Cell 1987;51:521–8.
3. Montani MS, Tuosto L, Giliberti R, et al. Dexamethasone induces apoptosis in human T cell clones expressing low levels of Bcl-2. Cell Death Differ 1999;6:79–86.
4. Wood AC, Waters CM, Garner A, Hickman JA. Changes in c-*myc* expression and the kinetics of dexamethasone-induced programmed cell death (apoptosis) in human lymphoid leukaemia cells. Br J Cancer 1994;69:663–9.
5. Adebodun F, Post JF. $^{31}P$ NMR characterization of cellular metabolism during dexamethasone-induced apoptosis in human leukemic cell lines. J Cell Physiol 1994;158:180–6.
6. Sierra-Honigmann MR, Murphy PA. T cell receptor–independent immunosuppression induced by dexamethasone in murine T helper cells. J Clin Invest 1992;89:556–60.
7. Moalli PA, Pillay S, Weiner D, et al. A mechanism of resistance to glucocorticoids in multiple myeloma: transient expression of a truncated glucocorticoid receptor mRNA. Blood 1992;79:213–22.
8. van Kalken CK, Broxterman HJ, Pinedo HM, et al. Cortisol is transported by the multidrug resistance gene product P-glycoprotein. Br J Cancer 1993;67:284–9.
9. Bougeois S, Gruol DJ, Newby RF, Rajah FM. Expression of an mdr gene is associated with a new form of resistance to dexamethasone-induced apoptosis. Mol Endocrinol 1993;7:840–51.
10. Gazitt Y, Fey V, Thomas C, Alvarez R. Bcl-2 overexpression is associated with resistance to dexamethasone, but not melphalan, in multiple myeloma cells. Int J Oncol 1998;13:397–405.
11. Meikle AW, Tyler FH. Potency and duration of action of glucocorticoids. Effects of hydrocortisone, prednisone and dexamethasone on human pituitary-adrenal function. Am J Med 1977;63:200–7.
12. Weller M, Schmidt C, Roth W, Dichgans J. Chemotherapy of human malignant glioma: prevention of efficacy by dexamethasone? Neurology 1997;48:1704–9.
13. Wolff JE, Denecke J, Jèurgens H. Dexamethasone induces partial resistance to cisplatinum in C6 glioma cells. Anticancer Res 1996;16:805–9.
14. Anderson CD, Wang J, Kumar GN, et al. Dexamethasone induction of taxol metabolism in the rat. Drug Metab Dispos 1995;23:1286–90.
15. Messer J, Reitman D, Sacks HS, et al: Association of adrenocorticosteroid therapy and peptic-ulcer disease. N Engl J Med 1983;309:21–4.
16. Torosian MH, Turnbull AD. Emergency laparotomy for spontaneous intestinal and colonic perforations in cancer patients receiving corticosteroids and chemotherapy. J Clin Oncol 1988;6:291–6.
17. Thung SN, Gerber MA, Klion F, Gilbert H. Massive hepatic necrosis after chemotherapy withdrawal in a hepatitis B virus carrier. Arch Intern Med 1985;145:1313–4.
18. Drigan R, Spirito A, Gelber RD. Behavioral effects of corticosteroids in children with acute lymphoblastic leukemia. Med Pediatr Oncol 1992;20:13–21.
19. Matsumoto K, Yamasaki H, Akazawa S, et al. High-dose but not low-dose dexamethasone impairs glucose tolerance by inducing compensatory failure of pancreatic beta-cells in normal men. J Clin Endocrinol Metab 1996;81:2621–6.
20. Schlaghecke R, Kornely E, Santen RT, Ridderskamp P. The effect of long-term glucocorticoid therapy on pituitary-adrenal responses to exogenous corticotropin-releasing hormone. N Engl J Med 1992;326:226–30.
21. Christy NP. Pituitary-adrenal function during corticosteroid therapy: learning to live with uncertainty. N Engl J Med 1992;326:266–7.
22. Tichelli A, Gratwohl A, Egger T, et al. Cataract formation after bone marrow transplantation. Ann Intern Med 1993;119:1175–80.
23. Byyny RL. Withdrawal from glucocorticoid therapy. N Engl J Med 1976;295:30–2.
24. Dixon RB, Christy NP. On the various forms of corticosteroid withdrawal syndrome. Am J Med 1980;68:224–30.

## Diethylstilbestrol

The pioneering work of Huggins and Hodges and of Haddow and colleagues in the 1940s established the usefulness of estrogen therapy. Many estrogen analogues have been synthesized, but the prototypic estrogenic compound in oncology is diethylstilbestrol (DES). It is a nonsteroidal estrogen that is potent, inexpensive, effective by oral administration, and relatively long lasting in its effect, as compared with natural estrogens. DES diphosphate is a closely related compound that is commercially known as Stilphostrol.

### EFFICACY

Although largely replaced by less toxic alternatives, DES has a time-honored historical place in the management of men with metastatic prostate cancer and postmenopausal women with metastatic breast cancer.

### PHARMACOLOGY

**Mechanism of Action.** Estrogen is thought to inhibit prostate cancer indirectly through inhibition of androgen production, resulting in a form of androgen suppression therapy. An alternative mechanism has been described in hormone-insensitive prostate cancer cell lines. In one study, DES directly induced apoptosis in the absence of receptors for DES, suggesting a possible role for DES against androgen-insensitive prostate neoplasms.[1] In breast cancer, the effects of estrogen appear to be dependent on interactions with specific receptors for estrogen, as discussed in Chapter 8. At low physiologic doses, estrogen may stimulate the growth of breast cancer, whereas at higher pharmacologic doses, estrogen may suppress the tumor's growth.

**Resistance.** This is poorly understood but probably relates to changes in the level or function of intracellular estrogen receptors.

**Pharmacokinetics.** In addition to its rapid and complete oral absorption, DES may be absorbed through the skin. After absorption, the drug is metabolized by the liver; however, the rate of inactivation is relatively slow, with an elimination half-life of about 24 hours. Some of the metabolites of DES are biologically active. For example, one study demonstrated irreversible modification of histone nuclear proteins by reactive metabolites of DES.[2] In another study, an oxidative metabolite of DES was responsible for estrogen-dependent gene regulation.[3]

**Drug Interactions.** The combined effects of DES and cancer chemotherapy are complex and poorly studied (see Chapter 8). In some cases, such combinations are antagonistic, whereas in others there may be an additive or even synergistic effect. Two examples of a potentially beneficial effect of estrogen on cancer chemotherapy can be cited. In one study, estrogen potentiated the DNA damage and cytotoxicity seen with drugs that act against topoisomerase II in human breast cancer cells.[4] In another study, estradiol enhanced the uptake and cytotoxicity of doxorubicin in human breast cancer cells in vitro.[5]

## TOXICITY

**Overview.** This nonsteroidal estrogen can cause thromboembolic problems in both sexes. In men, it causes androgen suppression that can result in gynecomastia. The main problems in women are dose-related nausea and vomiting, urinary stress incontinence, and the rare development of uterine adenocarcinomas.

**Digestive System.** Dose-related nausea and vomiting can occur, as do rare abdominal bloating and cramps. Cholestatic jaundice is a rare complication that is largely confined to patients receiving high-dose therapy. The risk of gallbladder disease is increased two- to threefold by postmenopausal estrogen replacement therapy.

**Cardiovascular.** DES therapy poses a very low risk of thrombophlebitis, embolism, and hypertension. The most important long-term risk in men appears to be the development of coronary artery disease. In one case-control study, 25% of the men receiving DES for prostate cancer developed cardiovascular problems, compared with no such complications in men undergoing orchiectomy.[6]

**Genitourinary.** Rare endometriosis and uterine fibroids may occur. Urinary stress incontinence occurs commonly in women.

**Endocrine-Metabolic.** Salt and water retention in patients with cardiac, liver, or renal disease may occur. Hypercalcemia in women can occur with breast cancer. Aggravation of chronic cystic mastitis may occur. In men, gynecomastia may develop, but this is relatively easy to prevent with a single 900-cGy dose of radiation therapy to each breast before estrogen administration or with 1200 to 1500 cGy divided into three fractions.[7] Gynecomastia is much more difficult to treat once it becomes symptomatic. If radiation therapy is used in this setting, dosages vary from 2000 cGy in five fractions to 4000 cGy in 20 fractions.[8] Breakthrough uterine bleeding, spotting, changes in menstrual flow, and amenorrhea all can occur in women taking estrogens before menopause. Increased triglycerides and hirsutism may occur. Induction of glucose intolerance is rare.

**Other/Rare.** Chloasma and melasma may occur; activation of porphyria is rare.

**Immunologic.** Both short-term[9] and delayed immunosuppression can occur.[10] Hypersensitivity reactions are theoretically possible but are extremely rare.

**Mucocutaneous.** Rash and pruritus may occur; erythema nodosum or erythema multiforme is rare.

**Ocular.** Intolerance of contact lenses, optic neuritis, and retinal thrombosis may occur.

**Neurologic.** Migraine exacerbations can occur, as well as headache, dizziness, depression, and stroke.

**Musculoskeletal.** Increased bone pain from flare reactions can occur.

**Reproductive.** DES can cause changes in libido in women and impotence in men. Toxicity data place DES in FDA pregnancy category X because of the induction of congenital anomalies when taken by women during pregnancy.

**Carcinogenicity.** DES is a potential carcinogen, although the quantitative importance of this is uncertain. When an estrogen is combined with a progestin as an oral contraceptive, the combination has a protective effect against endometrial and ovarian carcinomas.[11] However, the risk of breast cancer is increased when estrogens and progestational agents are combined in the treatment of normal-weight postmenopausal women.[12] Other tumors have also been reported, including hepatic adenomas and uterine carcinomas, but only rarely.

Estrogen has achieved some notoriety because of the development of vaginal adenomas in daughters of estrogen-treated pregnant patients (lifetime risk of 1/1000 to 1/10,000). DES exposure in utero has been linked to reproductive tract abnormalities in both male and female offspring, but a potential role in testicular carcinogenesis remains controversial. Currently, there is no evidence of transgenerational effects beyond those seen in the immediate offspring of DES-exposed mothers.[13]

## DOSAGE AND ADMINISTRATION

Tablets of DES are available in Canada (Stilbestrol) in doses ranging from 0.1 to 1.0 mg. The optimal dose of DES in carcinoma of the prostate is controversial but ranges from 1 to 3 mg. Although higher doses have been used, these have been associated with an increased risk of death due to cardiovascular disease. The dosage of DES in postmenopausal women with metastatic breast cancer is usually 5 mg thrice daily. In a randomized comparative study of 523 postmenopausal patients with breast cancer, dosages of 1.5, 15, 150, or 1500 mg/day were given.[14] In general, this study demonstrated the superiority of higher dose treatment over very low dose treatment.

## REFERENCES

1. Robertson CN, Roberson KM, Padilla GM, et al. Induction of apoptosis by diethylstilbestrol in hormone-insensitive prostate cancer cells. J Natl Cancer Inst 1996;88:908–17.
2. Roy D, Pathak DN. Histone nuclear proteins are irreversibly modified by reactive metabolites of diethylstilbestrol. J Toxicol Environ Health 1995;44:449–59.
3. Chae K, Lindzey J, McLachlan JA, Korach KS. Estrogen-dependent

gene regulation by an oxidative metabolite of diethylstilbestrol, diethylstilbestrol-4'4''-quinone. Steroids 1998;63:149–57.

4. Epstein RJ, Smith PJ. Estrogen-induced potentiation of DNA damage and cytotoxicity in human breast cancer cells treated with topoisomerase II-interactive antitumor drugs. Cancer Res 1988;48:297–303.

5. Bontenbal M, Sonneveld P, Foekens JA, Klijn JG. Oestradiol enhances doxorubicin uptake and cytotoxicity in human breast cancer cells (MCF-7). Eur J Cancer Clin Oncol 1988;24:1409–14.

6. Henriksson P, Johansson SE. Prediction of cardiovascular complications in patients with prostatic cancer treated with estrogen. Am J Epidemiol 1987;125:970–8.

7. Fass D, Steinfeld A, Brown J, Tessler A. Radiotherapeutic prophylaxis of estrogen-induced gynecomastia: a study of late sequelae. Int J Radiat Oncol Biol Phys 1986;12:407–8.

8. Chou JL, Easley JD, Feldmeier JJ, et al. Effective radiotherapy in palliating mammalgia associated with gynecomastia after DES therapy. Int J Radiat Oncol Biol Phys 1988;15:749–51.

9. Kalland T, Campbell T. Effects of diethylstilbestrol on human natural killer cells in vitro. Immunopharmacology 1984;8:19–25.

10. Wingard DL, Turiel J. Long-term effects of exposure to diethylstilbestrol. West J Med 1988;149:551–4.

11. Anonymous. Cancer risks of oral contraception. Lancet 1989;1:21–2.

12. Schairer C, Lubin J, Troisi R, et al. Menopausal estrogen and estrogen-progestin replacement therapy and breast cancer risk. JAMA 2000;283:485–91.

13. Giusti RM, Iwamoto K, Hatch EE. Diethylstilbestrol revisited: a review of the long-term health effects. Ann Intern Med 1995;122:778–88.

14. Wittes JT, Kaufman RJ. Diethylstilbestrol in breast cancer: dose-response analysis. JAMA 1977;238:1362–3.

# Docetaxel

Docetaxel is a relatively new semi-synthetic taxane, another in this class of microtubule spindle inhibitors. It is derived from the needles of the European yew tree, *Taxus baccata,* and has a broad spectrum of antitumor activity. Also called Taxotere and RP56976, docetaxel is currently approved for treating locally advanced or metastatic breast cancer.

## EFFICACY

Early preclinical and clinical studies demonstrated activity in several tumor types. The drug has been approved by the FDA for use in locally advanced and metastatic breast cancer, for which it was shown to be effective in patients who had previously progressed through alkylator-based or anthracycline-based chemotherapy.[1, 2] In addition, the drug has been tested across the spectrum of patients with breast cancer. Another trial confirmed efficacy in metastatic disease already resistant to paclitaxel, particularly in patients who had only brief exposures to that agent.[3] Other studies of breast cancer reveal docetaxel to be active as a single agent in first-line therapy for metastatic disease[4] and as part of combination adjuvant therapy.[5]

Docetaxel is also extremely active in non–small cell lung cancers. At least two trials have reported activity in combination with either gemcitabine or cisplatin in patients with advanced disease not previously treated.[6, 7] Finally, several smaller clinical trials have demonstrated efficacy alone or in combination with other agents in cancers of the prostate, head and neck, ovary, pancreas, and urothelial system.[8–11]

## PHARMACOLOGY

The mechanisms of action and resistance are essentially the same as for the prototype taxane, paclitaxel. Two identified differences have emerged from laboratory testing. The first is that docetaxel generates tubulin polymers that differ structurally from those generated by paclitaxel, and unlike paclitaxel, docetaxel does not alter the number of protofilaments in the bound microtubules.[12]

**Pharmacokinetics.** The pharmacokinetics of docetaxel have been examined in several of the early clinical trials with the agent.[13] The drug behaves according to a three-compartment model, with a rapid $\alpha$-half-life and delayed terminal phase clearance. There appears to be no difference in metabolism across gender, age groups, or ethnicities. Dexamethasone premedication does not alter clearance either. Fecal elimination was the principal route of excretion, and involvement of the hepatic cytochrome P450 system in the drug's metabolism is postulated. Patients with liver damage had decreased clearance of the drug, as would be predicted.

**Drug Interactions.** No adverse drug interactions with docetaxel are known.

## TOXICITY

**Overview.** Dose-limiting toxicities include myelosuppression and hypersensitivity reactions, although the latter are of a different nature than those caused by paclitaxel. All patients should be premedicated with corticosteroids to reduce the severity of hypersensitivity reactions and the fluid retention that is described later. The following information is obtained from the package insert and the pivotal trials in patients with metastatic breast cancer.

**Hematologic.** Neutropenia, whose median nadir occurs 8 days after drug administration, is the major dose-limiting side effect of docetaxel. It is not cumulative and is reversible. Absolute neutrophil counts less than $500/\mu L$ occurred in 76% of patients but lasted more than 7 days in only 4.3% of cycles. Anemia was observed in 89.5% of patients, although rarely was it severe. Thrombocytopenia is much less common. Patients with hepatic dysfunction experience more myelosuppression, as can be predicted from the drug's routes of excretion. Routine growth factor use is not recommended.

**Hypersensitivity Reactions.** Mild to severe (life-threatening) hypersensitivity reactions occasionally occur, usually during the first two cycles of docetaxel therapy. Most of these are minor reactions (mild flushing, drug fever, chest tightness, dyspnea, or chills) that resolve when therapy is temporarily interrupted and appropriate medications given. More severe hypersensitivity reactions are rare and include angioedema, hypotension, bronchospasm, or skin rash; they require the immediate cessation of the docetaxel infusion and aggressive supportive care. Hypersensitivity reactions are more common in patients with hepatic dysfunction, and their frequency and severity are decreased when the patient is pretreated for 1 to 3 days with corticosteroids.

**Fluid Retention.** This was a common side effect observed in early trials with docetaxel. A syndrome consisting of edema, weight gain, and occasionally pleural or pericardial effusions with or without ascites was commonly observed and was reduced in frequency with corticosteroid premedication. Even with such premedication, moderate fluid retention was seen in 17.4% of patients, the condition was severe in approximately 6%, and interruptions in therapy were required in 1.7% of cases. The symptoms resolve following completion of therapy and are more common as therapy continues.

**Cutaneous.** Docetaxel can cause skin eruptions, usually an erythema of the extremities, which can be followed by desquamation. Dose reductions can be effective in mitigating the side effects. Alopecia occurs in 80% of patients, but it almost always resolves after the completion of chemotherapy.

**Neurologic.** Seven percent of the patients with anthracycline-resistant breast cancer experienced symptoms of peripheral neuropathy. This can become severe following cumulative doses of 600 mg/m². The symptoms resolve when therapy is discontinued. Fatigue was seen in patients treated in docetaxel clinical trials. As always, it is difficult to determine what role advanced disease had in the etiology of patients' fatigue.

**Gastrointestinal.** Nausea, vomiting, and diarrhea were rare events, severe in only 8.2% of patients. Stomatitis, however was observed in 42.3% of treated patients (5.3% severe).

**Cardiovascular.** Cardiovascular abnormalities (arrhythmias, hypotension, and others) were observed only rarely, not nearly equaling the incidence of those with paclitaxel.

## DOSAGE AND ADMINISTRATION

Docetaxel comes in 20- and 80-mg vials, each with an accompanying sterile diluent vial. Final premix concentration is 10 mg/ml when the two are combined. Care should be taken to allow the polysorbate 80 foam to dissipate prior to further mixing. The premix solution should be further diluted in 250 ml using normal saline or 5% dextrose solutions in concentrations not to exceed 0.9 mg/ml. The drug should be administered intravenously over an hour in non-PVC, non-DEHP equipment. Diluted solution should be stored in glass containers or plastic bags (polypropylene, polyolefin) (see Paclitaxel).

Recommended dosages for the treatment of anthracycline-resistant metastatic breast cancer are 60 to 100 mg/m² every 3 weeks. Proper dose reductions are required for patients experiencing severe hematologic toxicity. The manufacturer suggests reducing the dose to 75 mg/m² for patients who have febrile neutropenia, neutrophil counts less than 500/μL for longer than 7 days, severe cutaneous eruptions, or severe peripheral neuropathies.

Corticosteroids should be coadministered with docetaxel in regimens such as dexamethasone 8 mg twice daily beginning the day before and continuing through the day after docetaxel therapy. This can reduce both hypersensitivity reactions and the side effects of fluid retention. No specific dose reductions are required for the elderly. Safety in children is currently unknown.

## REFERENCES

1. Ravdin PM, Burris HA III, Cook G, et al. Phase II trial of docetaxel in advanced anthracycline-resistant or anthracenedione-resistant breast cancer. J Clin Oncol 1995;13:2879–85.
2. Valero V, Holmes FA, Walters RS, et al. Phase II trial of docetaxel: a new, highly effective antineoplastic agent in the management of patients with anthracycline-resistant metastatic breast cancer. J Clin Oncol 1995;13:2886–94.
3. Valero V, Jones SE, Von Hoff DD, et al. A phase II study of docetaxel in patients with paclitaxel-resistant metastatic breast cancer. J Clin Oncol 1998;16:3362–8.
4. Fumoleau P, Chevallier B, Kerbrat P, et al. A multicentre phase II study of the efficacy and safety of docetaxel as first-line treatment of advanced breast cancer: report of the Clinical Screening Group of the EORTC. Ann Oncol 1996;7:165–71.
5. Nabholtz JM, Tonkin K, Smylie M, et al. Review of docetaxel and doxorubicin-based combinations in the management of breast cancer: from metastatic to adjuvant setting. Semin Oncol 1999;26:Suppl 3:10–6.
6. Georgoulias V, Kouroussis C, Androulakis N, et al. Front-line treatment of advanced non–small-cell lung cancer with docetaxel and gemcitabine: a multicenter phase II trial. J Clin Oncol 1999;17:914–20.
7. Zalcberg J, Millward M, Bishop J, et al. Phase II study of docetaxel and cisplatin in advanced non–small-cell lung cancer. J Clin Oncol 1998;16:1948–53.
8. Petrylak DP, Macarthur RB, O'Connor J, et al. Phase I trial of docetaxel with estramustine in androgen-independent prostate cancer. J Clin Oncol 1999;17:958–67.
9. Schoffski P, Weihkopf T, Ganser A. Advanced head and neck cancer and clinical experience of an effective new agent: docetaxel. Anticancer Res 1998;18:4751–6.
10. Kavanagh JJ, Kudelka AP, de Leon CG, et al. Phase II study of docetaxel in patients with epithelial ovarian carcinoma refractory to platinum. Clin Cancer Res 1996;2:837–42.
11. de Wit R, Kruit WH, Stoter G, et al. Docetaxel (Taxotere): an active agent in metastatic urothelial cancer, results of a phase II study in non–chemotherapy-pretreated patients. Br J Cancer 1998;78:1342–5.
12. Pronk LC, Stoter G, Verweij J: Docetaxel (Taxotere): single agent activity, development of combination treatment and reducing side-effects. Cancer Treat Rev 1995;21:463–78.
13. Bruno R, Hille D, Riva A, et al. Population pharmacokinetics/pharmacodynamics of docetaxel in phase II studies in patients with cancer. J Clin Oncol 1998;16:187–96.

# Doxorubicin

Doxorubicin, an anthracycline antibiotic discovered in Italy, is a derivative of *Streptomyces peucetius* var. *caesius*. It differs from daunorubicin by only a single hydroxyl group on carbon 14. As a consequence, doxorubicin is sometimes referred to as hydroxydaunorubicin. Other names include Adriamycin RDF, Adriamycin PFS, Rubex, DOX, ADR, and NSC-123127.

Intensely potent doxorubicin analogues are under development, based on structure-activity relationships. These have been reviewed by Farquhar and colleagues.[1]

## EFFICACY

Doxorubicin has one of the widest spectrums of antitumor activity ever observed, being effective against lymphomas, leukemias, soft tissue sarcomas, and a wide variety of carcinomas. It is one of the most important drugs used in oncology.

## PHARMACOLOGY

**Mechanism of Action.** Doxorubicin is cytotoxic through a host of mechanisms. It can be directly cytotoxic to the cell membrane without entry into tumor cells. Once inside the cell, it can intercalate with DNA and alkylate DNA through covalent binding, resulting in DNA cross-linking and the inhibition of DNA synthesis. Doxorubicin can inhibit topoisomerases I and II, it can interfere with DNA strand separation and helicase activity, and it can lead to enzyme-catalyzed iron-mediated free radical formation and lipid peroxidation.[2, 3] Ultimately, these effects result in the induction of apoptosis.[4, 5] The relative importance of these various mechanisms, including their interactions with the oncogene and signal transduction pathways involved with apoptosis, remains to be determined.

Doxorubicin can cause severe cardiac toxicity. A variety of mechanisms for cardiac toxicity have been proposed, including (1) cardiac lipid oxidation by free radicals in the presence of iron, (2) enzyme inhibition, (3) mitochondrial effects, (4) changes in cardiac calcium transport, (5) release of vasoactive substances, (6) increased phospholipase activity within the heart, and (7) direct changes in vascular perfusion induced by the drug. These changes may result either from doxorubicin itself or from its major metabolite, doxorubicinol. The leading hypothesis for anthracycline-induced cardiotoxicity involves the oxidation of cardiac tissue by free radicals in the presence of iron.[6] However, direct evidence for this in patients with cancer is lacking. Indeed, there is evidence that patients with cancer may have increased baseline levels of cardiac lipid peroxidation and that doxorubicin administration markedly inhibits this process.[7]

**Cancer Cell Resistance.** There are two major groups of mechanisms for doxorubicin resistance: classic mdr related to expression of P-glycoprotein (discussed in Chapter 8) and a variety of P-glycoprotein–independent mechanisms. Inhibition of mdr by calcium channel antagonists,[8] antisense cDNA for protein kinase C,[9] tamoxifen,[10] and cyclosporine[11] is a subject of intense investigation. P-glycoprotein–independent mechanisms are less clearly understood but include such things as decreased formation of DNA single- and double-strand breaks, increased glutathione transferase activity, increased DNA repair through the induction of DNA mismatch repair proteins,[12] and altered doxorubicin-topoisomerase interactions. As for topoisomerase II interactions, there may be different modes of anthracycline interaction relative to DNA cleavage and for overcoming drug resistance.[13] Intracellular drug sequestration,[14] increased intracellular alkalization of the pH,[15] and reduced levels of NAD phosphate (NADPH)[16] may also have a role in resistance. In human breast cancer cells in vitro, inhibition of apoptosis was considered the cause of doxorubicin resistance.[17] It is hoped that some of these mechanisms of drug resistance may be amenable to reversal by specific drug therapy, such as that reported for the in vitro use of oxalyl bis(N-phenyl)-hydroxamic acid.[18]

**Cardiac Resistance.** A variety of cardioprotective drugs has been studied. Examples include the use of the bispiperazinedione dexrazoxane; the use of liposome encapsulation of doxorubicin; the administration of a wide variety of putative antidotes, including free radical scavengers such as vitamin E or N-acetylcysteine, monohydroxyethylrutoside, ICRF-159, coenzyme Q10, carnitine, adenosine, and Damvar; and the use of inhibitors of vasoactive substances (cimetidine, diphenhydramine, phentolamine, and propranolol). The most useful of these approaches involves dexrazoxane.[19] Dexrazoxane and its metabolites may reduce cardiac toxicity by displacing iron from anthracycline-iron complexes.[20] In one study of patients with advanced breast cancer treated with doxorubicin, cardiotoxicity was reduced from 47% to 6% with dexrazoxane without any loss of antitumor responses.[21] In another study using dose-intense doxorubicin and paclitaxel, dexrazoxane reduced cardiotoxicity without reducing the frequency of antitumor responses.[22] Confirmation of reduced cardiotoxicity without reduced cancer cell cytotoxicity during doxorubicin therapy is eagerly awaited. Meanwhile, the use of dexrazoxane is limited to situations where doxorubicin is administered with palliative intent in the setting of advanced disease and prolonged drug use.

**Pharmacokinetics.** After bolus intravenous injection, doxorubicin undergoes extensive biotransformation in the liver to active and inactive metabolites. The drug is extensively bound to plasma proteins and tissues (about 70%), is excreted primarily in the bile (40 to 50%), and persists in plasma for prolonged periods. Doxorubicin and its major metabolites are cleared slowly from plasma, with terminal half-lives of 18 to 32 hours. Doxorubicin is widely distributed in the body and in breast milk. Limited data suggest that doxorubicin can cross the placenta into fetal tissue, although fetal damage occurs only rarely. The drug does not cross the blood-brain barrier to any appreciable extent. Limited data in patients undergoing hemodialysis suggest that the AUC for plasma levels of doxorubicin and its major metabolite are higher in patients requiring hemodialysis than in patients with normal renal function.[23] Hyperthermia markedly augments the intracellular accumulation of doxorubicin[24]; the importance of this to clinical practice is uncertain.

When doxorubicin is given by slow continuous infusion, the peak plasma level is less than with bolus injection and less of the drug is found in cardiac tissue.[25] However, for comparable doses, the AUC drug levels are similar.

**Drug Interactions.** Doxorubicin is a potent radiosensitizing agent, and radiation-recall reactions can be potentially serious. Radiation therapy may also increase the risk of delayed cardiac toxicity from doxorubicin.

Increased toxicity from doxorubicin may occur when it is combined with other cytotoxic agents. For example, when doxorubicin is given with continuous infusions of cytarabine, as in the treatment of acute leukemia, a fatal necrotizing colitis may occur.[26] Interferon may augment the effectiveness of doxorubicin in patients with advanced follicular lymphoma.[27] Streptozocin may prolong the elimination half-life of doxorubicin, so dose reduction is advised when the drugs are used together. Cyclosporine increases the delayed toxicity of doxorubicin in mice and rats, presumably by inhibiting P-glycoprotein and altering the normal pharmacokinetics of the drug.[28] 1,25-Dihydroxyvitamin $D_3$ enhances the susceptibility of breast cancer cells to doxorubicin-induced oxidative damage.[29] Herceptin enhances the antitumor activity of doxorubicin against HER-2/*neu*–overexpressing human breast cancer xenografts.[30] Paclitaxel modifies the pharmacokinetics of doxorubicin, so care must be taken in using paclitaxel and doxorubicin in novel combinations that have not been proved safe and effective in clinical trials.[31]

Novobiocin[32] and the cardiac glycoside ouabain[33] reduce the inhibition of topoisomerase II by doxorubicin, resulting in reduced cytotoxicity. These effects are not mediated by changes in doxorubicin influx or efflux.

Interactions of doxorubicin with other cytotoxic agents may be highly schedule dependent, as demonstrated by Zoli and colleagues.[34] For example, sequential doxorubicin followed by paclitaxel is synergistic in vitro. If gemcitabine is given either immediately before or 24 hours after the doxorubicin-paclitaxel sequential therapy, the effect is antagonistic. However, if gemcitabine is given 48 hours after the doxorubicin-paclitaxel combination, the effect is synergistic.

## TOXICITY

**Overview.** The major short-term, dose-limiting toxic side effects are myelosuppression and mucositis; cardiac toxicity is the major long-term dose-limiting toxicity. Local tissue necrosis can be severe if extravasation occurs, and nearly all patients develop alopecia.

**Hematologic.** Myelosuppression is the most common short-term dose-limiting toxicity of doxorubicin. The nadir is usually at 10 to 14 days, with recovery by day 21.

**Digestive System.** Relatively severe nausea and vomiting are common, but these can usually be prevented with aggressive antiemetic therapy. Anorexia and diarrhea also occur, but these are much less common (about 10% of patients). Very rarely, necrotizing colitis can occur.

**Mucocutaneous.** Stomatitis occurs in about 10% of patients. Total or near-total alopecia occurs in nearly every patient but is completely reversible at the conclusion of therapy. Necrosis of tissues occurs if doxorubicin is allowed to extravasate at the site of injection. The hand should be avoided as a site for injection because extravasation in this area is especially dangerous. The extent of infiltration may be difficult to determine visually, but rhodamine-filtered fluorescence microscopy can accurately delineate the extent of injury and serve as a guide to debridement and possible skin grafting.[35] Patients with obvious extravasation should be promptly treated with ice packs to tolerance[36, 37] and considered for possible skin grafting by a plastic surgeon. Unfortunately, no effective antidote currently exists for the treatment of doxorubicin extravasation. Other cutaneous reactions are also possible, including hyperpigmentation, skin rashes, plantar callus formation, onycholysis with epidermolysis, reduced wound healing after surgery, and subcutaneous ulceration in patients receiving the drug by the intra-arterial route.

**Cardiovascular.** The most important delayed dose-limiting toxicity of doxorubicin is cardiac damage. Two major forms of cardiac damage occur. First, acute changes may occur at any time and after any dosage. These usually take the form of an arrhythmia, which is nearly always a minor problem. In one study of patients monitored with a Holter monitor, minor arrhythmias occurred in 3% in the first hour after an infusion and in 24% in 1 to 24 hours.[38] Rarely, an acute syndrome of myopericarditis may also occur and is often fatal.[39] The second major form of cardiac damage is delayed congestive heart failure, which may develop many years after the cessation of therapy. This is associated with characteristic histologic changes, including fragmentation and dropout of myofibrils, mitochondrial swelling, and intracellular inclusions. These histologic changes are initially focal, but with continued treatment the changes become diffuse.[40] Despite these histologic changes, vigorous therapy

of congestive heart failure is indicated because patients may survive even severe episodes of left ventricular dysfunction.[41]

There is no totally safe dose of doxorubicin or daunorubicin below which cardiotoxicity is lacking; however, symptomatic cardiotoxicity is rare at lifetime total doses of less than 400 mg/m². Subclinical cardiac damage is extremely common. In one study of 115 children with ALL treated with doxorubicin-based chemotherapy and followed a median of 6.4 years (range of 1 to 15 years), 57% had abnormal cardiac function.[42]

Numerous attempts to predict preclinical cardiac toxicity have been reported. These include the use of serial myocardial biopsies, serial electrocardiograms, serial cardiac enzyme determinations, measurement of the systolic time interval, QRS-Korotkoff's measurements, echocardiography, and radionuclide cineangiography. Measuring atrial natriuretic peptide as a marker for cardiotoxicity has also been reported.[43] Some of these procedures have proved to be sensitive indicators of myocardial damage, but their ability to predict patients who will develop clinical congestive heart failure is uncertain, and their regular use adds substantially to the cost of care.

**Other and Rare Reactions.** Facial flushing, fever, and chills are very rare. Doxorubicin may sensitize tissue to radiation therapy; therefore, great care must be exercised in combining these two modalities. Enhanced radiation toxicity has been manifested clinically as increased immediate toxicity (e.g., esophagitis from radiation therapy at lower doses than usual) or as a recall phenomenon when doxorubicin is given after previous radiation therapy. Although it is difficult to predict these reactions quantitatively, it has been suggested that one guideline to combining these treatments is to equate a full course of doxorubicin to approximately 1000 cGy of radiation.[44]

*Immunologic.* Anaphylaxis occurs very rarely. Cross-sensitivity with lincomycin has been reported. The anthracyclines are minimally immunosuppressive.

*Ocular.* Conjunctivitis and increased lacrimation are very rare.

*Musculoskeletal.* One case of generalized muscle weakness has been reported.

*Genitourinary.* Renal failure is very rare.[45] Patients should be informed that their urine may turn red after treatment because doxorubicin is red, and that this is harmless.

*Reproductive.* Doxorubicin is mutagenic and teratogenic (FDA pregnancy category D).

*Carcinogenicity.* The drug is mutagenic and carcinogenic in animals and should be considered a potentially carcinogenic drug.

## DOSAGE AND ADMINISTRATION

Doxorubicin is available in vials of 10, 20, 50, 100, and 150 mg. The larger vials are intended for multiple-dose use, and one must be careful to avoid inadvertent overdoses.[46] Doxorubicin is physically incompatible in solutions with numerous drugs used in supportive care, including heparin, aminophylline, cephalothin, dexamethasone, sodium phosphate, diazepam, hydrocortisone, and furosemide. It is also incompatible with some antineoplastic agents, including fluorouracil and MTX.

Doxorubicin is usually given as a single intravenous dose of 60 to 75 mg/m$^2$ infused slowly over about 4 to 5 minutes, observing precautions to avoid extravasation. Alternatively, the drug can be given in the same dose as a continuous infusion over 2 to 4 days through a central venous access line (see Chapter 12, Vascular Access), or it can be divided into two or three daily bolus injections. Doses are repeated every 3 weeks with all of these schedules.

If cardiac disease is suspected prior to the initiation of doxorubicin therapy, it is prudent to obtain a baseline resting radionuclide angiocardiogram with measurement of the left ventricular ejection fraction (LVEF). Patients with a baseline LVEF of 30% should not be given doxorubicin.[47] In patients with LVEF values of greater than 30% but less than 50%, sequential studies should be performed and doxorubicin should be discontinued if the LVEF decreases 10% or reaches an LVEF value of 30%.

The standard way of trying to avoid cardiotoxicity has been to limit the total dose of anthracycline given to a patient. On the basis of early clinical experience, the commonly used guideline has been 550 mg/m$^2$ lifetime total dose. For patients with previous mediastinal or cardiac irradiation or during treatment with alkylating agents, the recommended maximal dose has been 450 mg/m$^2$. Other high-risk patients who should probably receive this lower maximum dose include those with previous hypertension for 5 years or more, those with pre-existing coronary, valvular, or myocardial disease, and those older than 70 years.

Reduced doses are used for patients with extensive previous chemotherapy or radiation therapy and for patients with liver dysfunction. The dose recommended by the manufacturer for patients with bilirubin levels of 1.2 to 3.0 mg/dl is 50% and for bilirubin levels greater than 3 mg/dl it is 25% of the usual dose. However, these guidelines are based on very early studies of doxorubicin use in patients with very advanced disease, and many authorities question whether or not they remain valid. Numerous controversies surround the choice of dose, route, and schedule of doxorubicin administration. For example, obesity may be important in modifying treatment. In a pharmacokinetic study, obese patients required much more time to clear doxorubicin and its major metabolite doxorubicinol than did patients of normal weight.[48] However, it is unclear how this information should be used, if at all, in modifying therapy. A wide variety of doses, schedules, and routes of doxorubicin administration have been tested. Intra-arterial administration has been used with some success,[49] but the value of this approach is limited by the high frequency of arteritis. Weekly schedules of drug administration have also been used, primarily because of reports of decreased cardiac toxicity with this schedule and studies suggesting that lower peak plasma levels of doxorubicin may be less cardiotoxic. In vitro evidence also shows that weekly therapy may be more cytotoxic to cancer cells than comparable doses of the drug given by monthly bolus schedules.[50] A commonly used dose for weekly therapy is 20 mg/m$^2$.[51]

## REFERENCES

1. Farquhar D, Cherif A, Bakina E, Nelson JA. Intensely potent doxorubicin analogues: structure-activity relationship. J Med Chem 1998;41:965–72.

2. Cummings J, Anderson L, Willmott N, Smyth JF. The molecular pharmacology of doxorubicin in vivo. Eur J Cancer 1991;27:532–5.

3. Gewirtz DA. A critical evaluation of the mechanisms of action proposed for the antitumor effects of the anthracycline antibiotics Adriamycin and daunorubicin. Biochem Pharmacol 1999;57:727–41.

4. Skladanowski A, Konopa J. Adriamycin and daunomycin induce programmed cell death (apoptosis) in tumour cells. Biochem Pharmacol 1993;46:375–82.

5. Thakkar NS, Potten CS. Abrogation of Adriamycin toxicity in vivo by cycloheximide. Biochem Pharmacol 1992;43:1683–91.

6. Speyer JL, Green MD, Kramer E, et al. Protective effect of the bispiperazinedione ICRF-187 against doxorubicin-induced cardiac toxicity in women with advanced breast cancer. N Engl J Med 1988;319:745–52.

7. Minotti G, Mancuso C, Frustaci A, et al. Paradoxical inhibition of cardiac lipid peroxidation in cancer patients treated with doxorubicin. Pharmacologic and molecular reappraisal of anthracycline cardiotoxicity. J Clin Invest 1996;98:650–61.

8. Toffoli G, Tumiotto L, Gigante M, et al. Increased chemosensitivity to doxorubicin of intrinsically multidrug-resistant human colon carcinoma cells by prolonged exposure to verapamil. Eur J Cancer 1993;29A:1776–8.

9. Ahmad S, Glazer RI. Expression of the antisense cDNA for protein kinase C alpha attenuates resistance in doxorubicin-resistant MCF-7 breast carcinoma cells. Mol Pharmacol 1993;43:858–62.

10. Chatterjee M, Harris AL. Reversal of acquired resistance to Adriamycin in CHO cells by tamoxifen and 4-hydroxy tamoxifen: role of drug interaction with alpha 1 acid glycoprotein. Br J Cancer 1990;62:712–7.

11. Bartlett NL, Lum BL, Fisher GA, et al. Phase I trial of doxorubicin with cyclosporine as a modulator of multidrug resistance. J Clin Oncol 1994;12:835–42.

12. Belloni M, Uberti D, Rizzini C, et al. Induction of two DNA mismatch repair proteins, MSH2 and MSH6, in differentiated human neuroblastoma SH-SY5Y cells exposed to doxorubicin. J Neurochem 1999;72:974–9.

13. Jensen PB, Sørensen BS, Sehested M, et al. Different modes of anthracycline interaction with topoisomerase II: separate structures critical for DNA-cleavage, and for overcoming topoisomerase II–related drug resistance. Biochem Pharmacol 1993;45:2025–35.

14. Sognier MA, Zhang Y, Eberle RL, Belli JA. Characterization of Adriamycin-resistant and radiation-sensitive Chinese hamster cell lines. Biochem Pharmacol 1992;44:1859–68.

15. Soto F, Planells-Cases R, Canaves JM, et al. Possible coexistence of two independent mechanisms contributing to anthracycline resistance in leukaemia P388 cells. Eur J Cancer 1993;29A:2144–50.

16. Gao JP, Friedman S, Lanks KW. The role of reduced nicotinamide adenine dinucleotide phosphate in glucose- and temperature-dependent doxorubicin cytotoxicity. Cancer Chemother Pharmacol 1993;33:191–6.

17. Osmak M, Brozoviâc A, Ambrioviâc-Ristove A, et al. Inhibition of apoptosis is the cause of resistance to doxorubicin in human breast adenocarcinoma cells. Neoplasma 1998;45:223–30.

18. Choudhuri SK, Chatterjee A. Reversal of resistance against doxorubicin by a newly developed compound, oxalyl bis(N-phenyl)hydroxamic acid in vitro. Anticancer Drugs 1998;9:825–32.

19. Green MD, Alderton P, Gross J, et al. Evidence of the selective alteration of anthracycline activity due to modulation of ICRF-187 (ADR-529). Pharmacol Ther 1990;48:61–9.

20. Buss JL, Hasinoff BB. The one-ring open hydrolysis product intermediates of the cardioprotective agent ICRF-187 (dexrazoxane) displace iron from iron-anthracycline complexes. Agents Actions 1993;40:86–95.

21. Speyer JL, Green MD, Zeleniuch-Jacquotte A, et al. ICRF-187 permits longer treatment with doxorubicin in women with breast cancer [erratum published in J Clin Oncol 1992;10:867]. J Clin Oncol 1992;10:117–27.

22. Sparano JA, Speyer J, Gradishar WJ, et al. Phase I trial of escalating doses of paclitaxel plus doxorubicin and dexrazoxane in patients with advanced breast cancer. J Clin Oncol 1999;17:880–6.

23. Yoshida H, Goto M, Honda A, et al. Pharmacokinetics of doxorubicin and its active metabolite in patients with normal renal function and in patients on hemodialysis. Cancer Chemother Pharmacol 1994;33:450–4.

24. Sakaguchi Y, Maehara Y, Inutsuka S, et al. Laser flow cytometric studies on the intracellular accumulation of anthracyclines when combined with heat. Cancer Chemother Pharmacol 1994;33:371–7.

25. Cusack BJ, Young SP, Driskell J, Olson RD. Doxorubicin and doxorubicinol pharmacokinetics and tissue concentrations following bolus injection and continuous infusion of doxorubicin in the rabbit. Cancer Chemother Pharmacol 1993;32:53–8.

26. Yates J, Glidewell O, Wiernik P, et al. Cytosine arabinoside with daunorubicin or Adriamycin for therapy of acute myelocytic leukemia: a CALGB study. Blood 1982;60:454–62.
27. Solal-Celigny P, Lepage E, Brousse N, et al. Recombinant interferon alfa-2b combined with a regimen containing doxorubicin in patients with advanced follicular lymphoma. Groupe d'Etude des Lymphomes de l'Adulte. N Engl J Med 1993;329:1608–14.
28. Colombo T, Zucchetti M, D'Incalci M. Cyclosporin A markedly changes the distribution of doxorubicin in mice and rats. J Pharmacol Exp Ther 1994;269:22–7.
29. Ravid A, Rocker D, Machlenkin A, et al. 1,25-Dihydroxyvitamin $D_3$ enhances the susceptibility of breast cancer cells to doxorubicin-induced oxidative damage. Cancer Res 1999;59:862–7.
30. Baselga J, Norton L, Albanell J, et al. Recombinant humanized anti-HER2 antibody (Herceptin) enhances the antitumor activity of paclitaxel and doxorubicin against HER2/*neu* overexpressing human breast cancer xenografts. Cancer Res 1998;82:2343–9.
31. Gianni L, Viganáo L, Locatelli A, et al. Human pharmacokinetic characterization and in vitro study of the interaction between doxorubicin and paclitaxel in patients with breast cancer. J Clin Oncol 1997;15:1906–15.
32. Smith PJ, Bell SM. A DNA topoisomerase II–independent route for novobiocin-mediated resistance to DNA binding agents. Cancer Chemother Pharmacol 1990;26:257–62.
33. Lawrence TS, Davis MA. The influence of $Na^+,K(^+)$-pump blockade on doxorubicin-mediated cytotoxicity and DNA strand breakage in human tumor cells. Cancer Chemother Pharmacol 1990;26:163–7.
34. Zoli W, Ricotti L, Barzanti F, et al. Schedule-dependent interaction of doxorubicin, paclitaxel and gemcitabine in human breast cancer cell lines. Int J Cancer 1999;80:413–6.
35. Duray PH, Cuono CB, Madri JA. Demonstration of cutaneous doxorubicin extravasation by rhodamine-filtered fluorescence microscopy. J Surg Oncol 1986;31:21–5.
36. Dorr RT, Alberts DA, Stone A. Cold protection and heat enhancement of doxorubicin skin toxicity in the mouse. Cancer Treat Rep 1985;69:431–7.
37. Harwood KVS. Treatment of anthracycline extravasation—recommendations for practice. J Clin Oncol 1987;5:1705.
38. Steinberg JS, Cohen AJ, Wasserman AG, et al. Acute arrhythmogenicity of doxorubicin administration. Cancer 1987;60:1213–8.
39. Bristow MR, Thompson PD, Martin RP, et al. Early anthracycline cardiotoxicity. Am J Med 1978;65:823–32.
40. Bristow MR. Drug-induced heart disease. Amsterdam, Elsevier/North-Holland Biomed Press, 1980:191.
41. Moreb JS, Oblon DJ. Outcome of clinical congestive heart failure induced by anthracycline chemotherapy. Cancer 1992;70:2637–41.
42. Lipshultz SE, Colan SD, Gelber RD, et al. Late cardiac effects of doxorubicin therapy for acute lymphoblastic leukemia in childhood. N Engl J Med 1991;324:808–15.
43. Bauch M, Ester A, Kimura B, et al. Atrial natriuretic peptide as a marker for doxorubicin-induced cardiotoxic effects. Cancer 1992;69:1492–7.
44. Mayer EG, Poulter CA, Aristizabal SA. Complications of irradiation related to apparent drug potentiation by Adriamycin. Int J Radiat Oncol Biol Phys 1976;1:1179–88.
45. Burke JF Jr, Laucius JF, Brodovsky HS, Soriano RZ. Doxorubicin hydrochloride-associated renal failure. Arch Intern Med 1977;137:385–8.
46. Curran CF. Acute doxorubicin overdoses. Ann Intern Med 1991;115:913–4.
47. Schwartz RG, McKenzie WB, Alexander J, et al. Congestive heart failure and left ventricular dysfunction complicating doxorubicin therapy: seven-year experience using serial radionuclide angiocardiography. Am J Med 1987;82:1109–18.
48. Rodvold KA, Rushing DA, Tewksbury DA. Doxorubicin clearance in the obese. J Clin Oncol 1988;6:1321–7.
49. Haskell CM, Silverstein MJ, Rangel DM, et al. Multimodality cancer therapy in man: a pilot study of Adriamycin by arterial infusion. Cancer 1974;33:1485–90.
50. Milano G, Cassuto-Viguier E, Fischel JL. Doxorubicin weekly low dose administration: in vitro cytotoxicity generated by the typical pharmacokinetic profile. Eur J Cancer 1992;28A:1881–5.
51. Torti FM, Bristow MR, Howes AE, et al. Reduced cardiotoxicity of doxorubicin delivered on a weekly schedule: assessment by endomyocardial biopsy. Ann Intern Med 1983;99:745–9.

# Estramustine

Estramustine phosphate is a molecule combining estradiol and nornitrogen mustard. It was developed in the hope that the estrogen moiety would allow specific targeting of hormonally responsive tissues. It is also known as Emcyt, estramustine phosphate, and NSC-89199.

## EFFICACY

The drug is marketed for the palliative therapy of advanced prostate cancer refractory to hormonal therapy.[1]

## PHARMACOLOGY

**Mechanism of Action.** The available evidence suggests that the drug has a unique mechanism of action unrelated to the original premise that estramustine phosphate would act as a carrier form of an alkylating agent. Unlike other alkylating agents, estramustine phosphate does not directly damage DNA. Rather, after dephosphorylation in vivo to estramustine, the drug binds hydrophobically to the structural proteins of the nucleus, the nuclear matrix,[2] and microtubular proteins.[3, 4] In addition, estramustine binds to a putative estramustine-binding protein (EMBP) in the rat prostate,[5] and it appears to block the secretion of collagenase during in vitro tumor cell invasion studies.[6] Estramustine also interacts with the P-glycoprotein efflux pump in some cell lines, potentially altering the intracellular concentrations of other cytotoxic agents.[7] It may also act directly as an androgen antagonist.[8] Ultimately, these effects result in apoptosis.[9]

**Resistance.** Estramustine resistance has been associated with modified patterns of tubulin expression,[10] with reduced levels of intracellular EMBP, reduced levels of tau expression in human prostatic carcinoma cells,[11] and modifications of estramustine efflux.[12] Further studies are needed to clarify the relative importance of these various mechanisms.

**Pharmacokinetics.** After oral administration, estramustine phosphate undergoes extensive presystemic dephosphorylation starting in the gastrointestinal tract. In one study of five patients with prostate cancer, the relative bioavailability of the drug was 44% as a result of incomplete absorption.[13] Estramustine itself is very stable and is resistant to enzymatic hydrolysis.[14] Consequently, the terminal half-life of the drug is relatively long (10 to 20 hours). Prolonged treatment with estramustine phosphate produces elevated total plasma concentrations of estradiol that are similar to those in patients with prostate cancer treated with estradiol.

**Drug Interactions.** The absorption of the drug can be inhibited by milk, milk products, and calcium-rich foods or drugs. Estramustine increases the radiation sensitivity of glioblastoma cells.[15, 16] Potential interactions exist with other cytotoxic agents because of estramustine's ability to inhibit P-glycoprotein.[7] Clodronate increases the oral bioavailability of estramustine.[17]

Several studies suggest that estramustine may be a rational drug to combine with chemotherapeutic agents that act against microtubular proteins. Preliminary results suggest that estramustine may augment the effects of vinblastine, paclitaxel, or etoposide against metastatic, hormone-resistant prostate cancer.[18]

## TOXICITY

**Overview.** The adverse effects from estramustine are similar to those of DES. Nausea and vomiting are the major dose-limiting side effects, but fluid retention and thrombotic events are also of concern. The drug should be used with caution in patients with diabetes mellitus, hypertension, liver or renal dysfunction, and a history of coronary artery disease or cerebrovascular disease. It is contraindicated in patients with a history of hypersensitivity to nitrogen mustard or estrogen and in patients with active thrombophlebitis or thromboembolic disorders.

**Digestive System.** Nausea and vomiting are common and may be severe enough to require cessation of treatment. These usually decrease with continued therapy. Anorexia and diarrhea occur rarely. Liver damage can occur (rare elevations of bilirubin, transaminase enzymes, or both). Elevated amylase levels, lipase levels, or both are rare.

**Endocrine-Metabolic.** The following can occur: fluid retention (common), hypercalcemia (rare), hypophosphatemia (rare), decreased glucose tolerance (rare), painful breasts or gynecomastia (common), and decreased libido and impotence.

**Other and Rare Reactions.** Any side effect of DES is a potential side effect of estramustine.

*Hematologic.* Myelosuppression is uncommon and rarely dose limiting.

*Immunologic.* Hypersensitivity reactions are rare; there is definite cross-reactivity with estrogens and mechlorethamine.

*Mucocutaneous.* Skin rash and alopecia may occur.

*Cardiovascular.* Thrombophlebitis, myocardial infarction, hypertension, and congestive heart failure can occur.

*Genitourinary.* A single case of the hemolytic-uremia syndrome has been reported after the use of estramustine.[19]

*Pulmonary.* Pulmonary emboli, dyspnea, pulmonary infiltrates, and fibrosis.

*Ocular.* Lacrimation may be increased.

*Neurologic.* Stroke can occur.

*Reproductive.* Toxicity data place estramustine in FDA pregnancy category C (contraception recommended).

*Carcinogenicity.* Estramustine is potentially carcinogenic.

## DOSAGE AND ADMINISTRATION

Estramustine is available as 140-mg capsules. The drug is used orally in a daily dose of 14 mg/kg divided into three or four doses. Because absorption may be impaired by milk, the drug is taken at least 1 hour before or 2 hours after meals.

## REFERENCES

1. Benson R, Hartley-Asp B. Mechanisms of action and clinical uses of estramustine. Cancer Invest 1990;8:375–80.
2. Tew KD, Erickson LC, White G, et al. Cytotoxicity of estramustine, a steroid-nitrogen mustard derivative, through non-DNA targets. Mol Pharmacol 1983;24:324–8.
3. Mareel MM, Storme GA, Dragonetti CH, et al. Antiinvasive activity of estramustine on malignant MO4 mouse cells and on DU-145 human prostate carcinoma cells in vitro. Cancer Res 1988;48:1842–9.
4. Laing N, Dahllèof B, Hartley-Asp B, et al. Interaction of estramustine with tubulin isotypes. Biochemistry 1997;36:871–8.
5. Pousette Å, Bjork P, Forsgren B, Carlström K. Mouse monoclonal antibodies against rat estramustine binding protein. J Steroid Biochem 1987;26:509–12.
6. Wang M, Stearns ME. Blocking of collagenase secretion by estramustine during in vitro tumor cell invasion. Cancer Res 1988;48:6262–71.
7. Speicher LA, Barone LR, Chapman AE, et al. P-glycoprotein binding and modulation of the multidrug-resistant phenotype by estramustine. J Natl Cancer Inst 1994;86:688–94.
8. Want LG, Liu XM, Kreis W, Budman DR. Androgen antagonistic effect of estramustine phosphate (EMP) metabolites on wild-type and mutated androgen receptor. Biochem Pharmacol 1998;55:1427–33.
9. Vallbo C, Bergenheim AT, Bergstrèom P, et al. Apoptotic tumor cell death induced by estramustine in patients with malignant glioma. Clin Cancer Res 1998;4:87–91.
10. Sangrajrang S, Denoulet P, Laing NM, et al. Association of estramustine resistance in human prostatic carcinoma cells with modified patterns of tubulin expression. Biochem Pharmacol 1998;55:325–31.
11. Sangrajrang S, Denoulet P, Millot G, et al. Estramustine resistance correlates with tau over-expression in human prostatic carcinoma cells. Int J Cancer 1998;77:626–31.
12. Laing NM, Belinsky MG, Kruh GD, et al. Amplification of the ATP-binding cassette 2 transporter gene is functionally linked with enhanced efflux of estramustine in ovarian carcinoma cells. Cancer Res 1998;58:1332–7.
13. Gunnarsson PO, Andersson SB, Johansson SA, et al. Pharmacokinetics of estramustine phosphate (Estracyt) in prostatic cancer patients. Eur J Clin Pharmacol 1984;26:113–9.
14. Punzi JS, Duax WL, Strong P, et al. Molecular conformation of estramustine and two analogues. Mol Pharmacol 1992;41:569–76.
15. Yoshida D, Piepmeier J, Weinstein M. Estramustine sensitizes human glioblastoma cells to irradiation. Cancer Res 1994;54:1415–7.
16. Bergenheim AT, Zackrisson B, Elfverson J, et al. Radiosensitizing effect of estramustine in malignant glioma in vitro and in vivo. J Neurooncol 1995;23:191–200.
17. Kylmèalèa T, Castrâen-Kortekangas P, Seppèanen J, et al. Effect of concomitant administration of clodronate and estramustine phosphate on their bioavailability in patients with metastasized prostate cancer. Pharmacol Toxicol 1996;79:157–60.
18. Hudes G. Estramustine-based chemotherapy. Semin Urol Oncol 1997;15:13–9.
19. Tassinari D, Sartori S, Panzini I, et al. Hemolytic-uremic syndrome during therapy with estramustine phosphate for advanced prostatic cancer. Oncology 1999;56:112–3.

# Etoposide

Etoposide is one of two semisynthetic epipodophyllotoxins developed by pharmaceutical chemists at Sandoz.[1,2] These drugs are derived from the root of the plant *Podophyllum peltatum,* which is commonly known as the May apple or mandrake plant. Etoposide is also known as VP-16, VePesid, VP-16-213, EPEG, epipodophyllotoxin, and NSC-141540.

## EFFICACY

Etoposide is used in the curative treatment of testicular cancer and extragonadal germ cell tumors and as palliative therapy for a wide variety of other malignancies, including lung cancer, leukemias and lymphomas, Kaposi's sarcoma, gynecologic neoplasms, and selected tumors of unknown primary origin and others.

## PHARMACOLOGY

**Mechanism of Action.** Unlike the parent compound podophyllin, etoposide does not bind to tubulin and does not interfere with the formation of the spindle apparatus in dividing cells. It is known to cause single-strand breaks in DNA as well as other forms of DNA damage. It appears that at least two mechanisms of DNA damage result from use of etoposide.[3] The first involves interference with the scission-reunion reaction of mammalian topoisomerase II by stabilizing a cleavable complex. The second involves metabolic activation of oxidation-reduction reactions to produce derivatives that can bind directly to cellular DNA. This process leads to a series of early events (formation of DNA-protein cross-links, DNA single-strand breaks, and DNA double-strand breaks) and later events (secondary DNA fragmentation, or cell death).[4] Morphologically, cell death occurs by apoptosis.[5, 6] Identification of the genes involved in etoposide-induced apoptosis and their relationship to oncogenes and signal transduction pathways are under investigation.[7]

Because of the inhibition of topoisomerase II, etoposide is highly schedule dependent, with a predominant effect on late S phase and $G_2$. It appears that etoposide acts synergistically when combined with some other drugs, especially cytarabine, cisplatin, and hydroxyurea.[8] The basis for this synergy is being explored.

**Resistance.** Resistance to etoposide appears to be multifactorial.[9, 10] Several mechanisms are well established. Resistance can be due to changes in the amount or specificity of DNA topoisomerase II enzymes.[11] For example, the phosphorylation state of the enzyme influences drug resistance,[12] and the activity of topoisomerase II may be markedly diminished in resistant lines, in some cases in association with overexpression of the mdr phenotype.[13] In some systems, reduced drug uptake is associated with resistance, whereas in others DNA repair appears to play a role.[14] ATP depletion abrogates the ability of etoposide to inhibit topoisomerase II.[15] Resistance to etoposide-induced apoptosis has also been related to failure to activate upstream effectors of caspase activity.[16]

**Pharmacokinetics.** Etoposide is a highly schedule-dependent drug that is available for both oral and intravenous administration. Consequently, pharmacologic aspects of etoposide therapy are especially important.[17] The drug is poorly water soluble, and its oral absorption has been considered erratic.[18] About 50% of an oral dose is absorbed, but this varies among patients, and increasing the oral dose of etoposide does not result in a linear increase in plasma level.[19] Preliminary data suggest that measuring unbound etoposide pharmacokinetics after oral administration may be useful in individualizing therapy.[20] The bioavailability of oral etoposide does not appear to be influenced by food, so fasting is unnecessary prior to taking the drug.[21]

Published studies of drug clearance after intravenous administration have shown highly variable results, with terminal plasma clearance half-life values of 3 to 11 hours.[18] There is no suggestion that dose adjustments based on age, sex, relative body weight, or creatinine clearance can eliminate this variability.[22] The rate of drug clearance appears to be faster in children than adults. The drug is protein bound and undergoes hepatic metabolism to a variable extent. The primary metabolite appears to be an etoposide glucuronide.[23]

The major metabolite of etoposide appears to distribute widely in the body, with a volume of distribution roughly equal to total body water. Nevertheless, little of the drug crosses the blood-brain barrier. The major excretory route is by renal clearance (about 35%).[18] The available data suggest that etoposide doses should be reduced for patients with renal dysfunction. No dosage adjustments appear to be necessary for patients with hepatic dysfunction, provided they have normal renal function.[24]

**Drug Interactions.** Radiosensitization can occur, including radiation-recall reactions.[25, 26] Several drugs appear to increase the cytotoxic effects of etoposide, either directly or through reducing drug resistance. These include low-dose MTX,[27] trimetrexate,[28] dipyridamole,[29] cyclosporine,[30, 31] topoisomerase I inhibitors, and alkylating agents.[32] The drug interaction with MTX appears to relate to an etoposide-induced partial recirculation of extracellular-intracellular MTX into the blood after etoposide administration.[33] The effect of cyclosporine appears to be primarily one of altering etoposide pharmacokinetics, leading to higher levels of drug exposure and greater leukopenia for a given dose.[34] The sequence of drug use in combination chemotherapy regimens may be important. In one study of small cell lung cancer, the optimal sequence was cisplatin followed by etoposide.[35] In another study, etoposide followed by paclitaxel was more effective than the concurrent administration of the two drugs together.[36] Some evidence suggests that hypersensitivity reactions may be more common in patients treated with etoposide and other antineoplastic agents.[37] Warfarin anticoagulation may be enhanced in patients receiving etoposide-based chemotherapy; thus, the International Normalized Ratio should be carefully monitored during concurrent warfarin and etoposide treatment.[38]

## TOXICITY

**Overview.** The major dose-limiting toxicity is myelosuppression, but potentially lethal hypersensitivity reactions have been reported in 1 to 2% of patients treated. The drug is contraindicated in patients who are hypersensitive to etoposide or any of its components.

**Hematologic.** The usual dose-limiting toxicity of etoposide is myelosuppression, with 60 to 91% of patients experiencing mild leukopenia (WCC $<4000/\mu L$) and 3 to 17% severe leukopenia (WCC $<1000/\mu L$). The time to the nadir of the WCC is 10 to 14 days, with recovery by day 16 to 21. Previous chemotherapy or radiation therapy increases myelosuppression and may be cause for the initial use of a lower dose. In the high-dose setting of BMT, etoposide has been shown to disrupt bone marrow stromal cell function, as well as normal hematopoiesis.[39]

**Immunologic.** Anaphylactoid reactions occur in 1 to 2% of patients. These are characterized by chills, fever, tachycardia, bronchospasm, dyspnea, and frequently hypotension. These reactions usually respond to prompt cessation of drug infusion and the administration of pressor agents, corticosteroids, antihistamines, or volume expanders, as needed. Very rarely this reaction can be fatal. There is some evidence that these reactions may be more common when etoposide is combined with paclitaxel.[40] They may also be increased in patients with leukemia or lymphoma treated with combination chemotherapy. For example, 51% of patients with Hodgkin's disease treated with vinblastine, etoposide, prednisone, and doxorubicin developed hypersensitivity reactions in one study.[40]

**Digestive System.** Digestive complaints are relatively common, especially with oral therapy, but these are rarely severe or dose limiting. The reactions reported and their relative frequencies are as follows: nausea and vomiting (31 to 43%), anorexia (10 to 13%), and diarrhea (1 to 13%). Very rare reactions include constipation, dysphagia, abdominal cramps, parotitis, and a peculiar aftertaste in the mouth. Mild hepatic dysfunction occurs rarely, principally as hyperbilirubinemia and increased transaminase levels. Acute transient parotitis has been reported after high-dose etoposide.[41]

**Mucocutaneous.** Alopecia (8 to 66%) is usually mild but can be severe in rare patients. Stomatitis is rarely a problem (1 to 6%). Very rarely, patients develop pruritus, radiation-recall skin reactions, phlebitis, hyperpigmentation, and local pain at the site of injection. The hand-foot syndrome has been reported with chronic administration of etoposide.[42] With very high dose therapy, a generalized pruritic erythematous maculopapular rash has been reported and was consistent with perivasculitis.

**Cardiovascular.** Rapid administration of the drug can cause transient hypotension in 1 to 2% of patients, but this reaction does not appear to occur with slower infusion rates. Congestive heart failure can ensue when the drug is given with large amounts of normal saline. Hypertension can occur rarely as part of hypersensitivity reactions. Vasospastic angina[43] and acute myocardial infarction[44] have been reported in patients with no known cardiac risk factors.

**Other and Rare Reactions.** Fever and a metallic taste in the mouth can occur.

**Pulmonary.** Bronchospasm, dyspnea, and even apnea can rarely occur as part of hypersensitivity reactions. A fatal case of pulmonary toxicity associated with oral etoposide has been reported.[45]

**Ocular.** Transient cortical blindness and optic neuritis are rare. Severe ocular and orbital toxicity have been reported after intracarotid administration of etoposide and carboplatin.[46]

**Neurologic.** The following neurologic effects can occur: peripheral neuropathy (1 to 2%) and somnolence and fatigue (3%). Moderate self-limited neuropathy is more common after high-dose therapy and autologous BMT (4%).[47]

**Musculoskeletal.** Muscle cramps can occur.

**Reproductive.** Toxicity data place etoposide in FDA pregnancy category D. The drug is embryotoxic in mice.[48] About 50% of women older than 40 years develop premature anovulation after etoposide therapy.[49]

**Endocrine-Metabolic.** Metabolic acidosis can occur.

**Carcinogenicity.** Etoposide is mutagenic[50] and carcinogenic; it clearly causes myelodysplasia and AML in humans.[51, 52] The AML seen after the use of topoisomerase inhibitors is usually different from the AML seen with alkylating agents. The disease occurs relatively quickly after treatment and is associated with different chromosomal abnormalities.

## DOSAGE AND ADMINISTRATION

Etoposide is provided as a 50-mg capsule for oral use. Two formulations are available for parenteral administration: (1)

etoposide (20 mg/ml) dissolved in alcohol and polyethylene glycol for slow infusions and (2) etoposide phosphate (100-mg base) for direct administration after reconstitution in saline or dextrose solutions. They are equally effective, but etoposide phosphate is more convenient to use because it is water soluble and does not have to be diluted in larger volumes of fluid and administered by slow infusion.[53] Etoposide is incompatible with idarubicin in solution. The planned dose of etoposide is usually diluted with normal saline or 5% dextrose to a final concentration of 0.4 mg/ml. Higher concentrations of drug are less stable and may precipitate.

Etoposide is given orally and by slow intravenous infusion over 30 to 60 minutes. The drug should not be given by rapid intravenous injection because this can cause serious hypotension. Etoposide phosphate can be given quickly because it is water soluble and does not require the use of toxic diluents. Usual intravenous dosages are 50 to 100 mg/m$^2$/day for 3 to 5 days with repeat doses every 3 to 4 weeks. The oral dose is double that of the intravenous dose. An alternative oral regimen calls for prolonged low-dose treatment with the drug. For example, in a study of women with ovarian cancer, a fixed dose of 100 mg orally per day was given for 14 days every 3 weeks.[54] In another study involving patients with small cell lung cancer, the oral dosage used was 50 mg/m$^2$/day for 21 consecutive days.[55] Further study is needed to clarify the optimal way to use oral etoposide.[56]

The dose of etoposide is reduced for renal failure but not for liver dysfunction. Creatinine clearance values of 10 to 50 ml/min call for a dose reduction of 25%, whereas a creatinine clearance value less than 10 ml/min calls for a 50% reduction.

## REFERENCES

1. Stähelin HF, von Wartburg A. The chemical and biological route from podophyllotoxin glucoside to etoposide: ninth Cain Memorial Award lecture. Cancer Res 1991;51:5–15.
2. Hande KR. Etoposide: four decades of development of a topoisomerase II inhibitor. Eur J Cancer 1998;34:1514–21.
3. van Maanen JMS, Retel J, de Vries J, Pinedo HM. Mechanism of action of antitumor drug etoposide: a review. J Natl Cancer Inst 1988;80:1526–33.
4. Kamesaki S, Kamesaki H, Jorgensen TJ, et al. bcl-2 protein inhibits etoposide-induced apoptosis through its effects on events subsequent to topoisomerase II–induced DNA strand breaks and their repair [erratum published in Cancer Res 1994;54:3074]. Cancer Res 1993;53:4251–6.
5. Okamoto-Kubo S, Nishio K, Heike Y, et al. Apoptosis induced by etoposide in small-cell lung cancer cell lines. Cancer Chemother Pharmacol 1994;33:385–90.
6. Sun XM, Snowden RT, Dinsdale D, et al. Changes in nuclear chromatin precede internucleosomal DNA cleavage in the induction of apoptosis by etoposide. Biochem Pharmacol 1994;47:187–95.
7. Wang Y, Rea T, Bian J, et al. Identification of the genes responsive to etoposide-induced apoptosis: application of DNA chip technology. FEBs Lett 1999;445:269–73.
8. Ratain MJ, Schilsky RL, Wojack BR, et al. Hydroxyurea and etoposide: in vitro synergy and phase I clinical trial. J Natl Cancer Inst 1988;80:1412–6.
9. Sinha BK, Haim N, Dusre L, et al. DNA strand breaks produced by etoposide (VP-16,213) in sensitive and resistant human breast tumor cells: implications for the mechanism of action. Cancer Res 1988;48:5096–100.
10. Ferguson PJ, Fisher MH, Stephenson J, et al. Combined modalities of resistance in etoposide-resistant human KB cell lines. Cancer Res 1988;48:5956–64.
11. Giaccone G, Gazdar AF, Beck H, et al. Multidrug sensitivity phenotype

of human lung cancer cells associated with topoisomerase II expression. Cancer Res 1992;52:1666–74.

12. Devore RF, Corbett AH, Osheroff N. Phosphorylation of topoisomerase II by casein kinase II and protein kinase C: effects on enyzme-mediated DNA cleavage/religation and sensitivity to the antineoplastic drugs etoposide and 4'(9-acridinylamino)methane-sulfon-m-anisidide. Cancer Res 1992;52:2156–61.

13. Takigawa N, Ohnoshi T, Ueoka H, et al. Establishment and characterization of an etoposide-resistant human small cell lung cancer cell line. Acta Med Okayama 1992;46:203–12.

14. Chiron M, Demur C, Pierson V, et al. Sensitivity of fresh acute myeloid leukemia cells to etoposide: relationship with cell growth characteristics and DNA single-strand breaks. Blood 1992;80:1307–15.

15. Sorensen M, Sehested M, Jensen PB. Effect of cellular ATP depletion on topoisomerase II poisons: abrogation of cleavable-complex formation by etoposide but not by amsacrine. Mol Pharmacol 1999;55:424–31.

16. Zhao EG, Song Q, Cross S, et al. Resistance to etoposide-induced apoptosis in a Burkitt's lymphoma cell line. Int J Cancer 1998;77:755–62.

17. Clark PI, Slevin ML. The clinical pharmacology of etoposide and teniposide. Clin Pharmacokinet 1987;12:223–52.

18. Creaven PJ. The clinical pharmacology of VM26 and VP16-213: a brief overview. Cancer Chemother Pharmacol 1982;7:133-40.

19. Harvey VJ, Slevin ML, Joel SP, et al. The effect of dose on the bioavailability of oral etoposide. Cancer Chemother Pharmacol 1986;16:178–81.

20. Perdaems N, Bachaud JM, Rouzaud P, et al. Relation between unbound plasma concentrations and toxicity in a prolonged oral etoposide schedule. Eur J Clin Pharmacol 1998;54:677–83.

21. Harvey VJ, Slevin ML, Joel SP, et al. The effect of food and concurrent chemotherapy on the bioavailability of oral etoposide. Br J Cancer 1985;52:363–7.

22. Miya T, Goya T, Yanagida O, et al. The influence of relative body weight on toxicity of combination chemotherapy with cisplatin and etoposide. Cancer Chemother Pharmacol 1998;42:386–90.

23. Hande K, Anthony L, Hamilton R, et al. Identification of etoposide glucuronide as a major metabolite of etoposide in the rat and rabbit. Cancer Res 1988;48:1829–34.

24. Hande KR, Wolff SN, Greco FA, et al. Etoposide kinetics in patients with obstructive jaundice. J Clin Oncol 1990;8:1101–7.

25. Giocanti N, Hennequin C, Balosso J, et al. DNA repair and cell cycle interactions in radiation sensitization by the topoisomerase II poison etoposide. Cancer Res 1993;53:2105–11.

26. Etoposide enhances the lethal effect of radiation on breast cancer cells with less damage to mammary gland cells. Cancer Chemother Pharmacol 1999;43:284–6.

27. Erba E, Sen S, Lorico A, D'Incalci M. Potentiation of etoposide cytotoxicity against a human ovarian cancer cell line by pretreatment with non-toxic concentrations of methotrexate or aphidicolin. Eur J Cancer 1992;28:66–71.

28. Fry DW. Cytotoxic synergism between trimetrexate and etoposide: evidence that trimetrexate potentiates etoposide-induced protein-associated DNA strand breaks in L1210 leukemia cells through alterations in intracellular ATP concentrations. Biochem Pharmacol 1990;40:1981–8.

29. Isonishi S, Kirmani S, Kim S, et al. Phase I and pharmacokinetic trial of intraperitoneal etoposide in combination with the multidrug-resistance-modulating agent dipyridamole. J Natl Cancer Inst 1991;83:621-6.

30. Slater LM, Cho J, Wetzel M. Cyclosporin A potentiation of VP-16: production of long-term survival in murine acute lymphatic leukemia. Cancer Chemother Pharmacol 1992;31:53–6.

31. Yahanda AM, Alder KM, Fisher GA, et al. Phase I trial of etoposide with cyclosporine as a modulator of multidrug resistance. J Clin Oncol 1992;10:1624–34.

32. Janss AJ, Cnaan A, Zhao H, et al. Synergistic cytotoxicity of topoisomerase I inhibitors with alkylating agents and etoposide in human brain tumor cell lines. Anticancer Drugs 1998;9:641–52.

33. Paâl K, Horvâath J, Csâaki C, et al. Effect of etoposide on the pharmacokinetics of methotrexate in vivo. Anticancer Drugs 1998;9:765–72.

34. Lum BL, Kaubisch S, Yahanda AM, et al. Alteration of etoposide pharmacokinetics and pharmacodynamics by cyclosporine in a phase I trial to modulate multidrug resistance. J Clin Oncol 1992;10:1635–42.

35. Maksymiuk AW, Jett JR, Earle JD, et al. Sequencing and schedule effects of cisplatin plus etoposide in small-cell lung cancer: results of a North Central Cancer Treatment Group randomized clinical trial. J Clin Oncol 1994;12:70–6.

36. Felip E, Massuti B, Camps C, et al. Superiority of sequential versus concurrent administration of paclitaxel with etoposide in advanced non-small cell lung cancer: comparison of two phase II trials. Clin Cancer Res 1998;4:2723–8.

37. Hudson MM, Weinstein HJ, Donaldson SS, et al. Acute hypersensitivity reactions to etoposide in a VEPA regimen for Hodgkin's disease. J Clin Oncol 1993;11:1080–4.

38. Le AT, Hasson NK, Lum BL. Enhancement of warfarin response in a patient receiving etoposide and carboplatin chemotherapy. Ann Pharmacother 1997;31:1006–8.

39. Gibson LF, Fortney J, Landreth KS, et al. Disruption of bone marrow stromal cell function by etoposide. Biol Blood Marrow Transplant 1997;3:122–32.

40. Friedland D, Gorman G, Treat J. Hypersensitivity reactions from taxol and etoposide. J Natl Cancer Inst 1993;85:2036.

41. Crump M, Brandwein JM, Scott JG, et al. Acute transient parotitis after high dose etoposide and autologous bone marrow transplantation. Bone Marrow Transplant 1990;6:259–61.

42. Schey SA, Cooper J, Summerhayes M. The "hand-foot syndrome" occurring with chronic administration of etoposide. Eur J Haematol 1992;48:118–9.

43. Yano S, Shimada K. Vasospastic angina after chemotherapy with carboplatin and etoposide in a patient with lung cancer. Jpn Circ J 1996;60:185–8.

44. Airey CL, Dodwell DJ, Joffe JK, Jones WG. Etoposide-related myocardial infarction. Clin Oncol (R C Radiol) 1995;7:135.

45. Dajczman E, Srolovitz H, Kreisman H, Frank H. Fatal pulmonary toxicity following oral etoposide therapy. Lung Cancer 1995;12:81–6.

46. Lauer AK, Wobig JL, Shults WT, et al. Severe ocular and orbital toxicity after intracarotid etoposide phosphate and carboplatin therapy. Am J Ophthalmol 1999;127:230–3.

47. Imrie KR, Couture F, Turner CC, et al. Peripheral neuropathy following high-dose etoposide and autologous bone marrow transplantation. Bone Marrow Transplant 1994;13:77–9.

48. Agarwal K, Mukherjee A, Sen S. Etoposide (VP-16): cytogenetic studies in mice. Environ Mol Mutagen 1994;23:190–3.

49. Matsui H, Seki K, Sekiya S, Takamizawa H. Reproductive status in GTD treated with etoposide. J Reprod Med 1997;42:104–10.

50. Maraschin J, Dutrillaux B, Aurias A. Chromosome aberrations induced by etoposide (VP-16) are not random. Int J Cancer 1990;46:808–12.

51. Stine KC, Saylors RL, Sawyer JR, Becton DL. Secondary acute myelogenous leukemia following safe exposure to etoposide. J Clin Oncol 1997;15:1583–6.

52. Kollmansberger C, Beyer J, Droz JP, et al. Secondary leukemia following high cumulative doses of etoposide in patients treated for advanced germ cell tumors. J Clin Oncol 1998;16:3386–91.

53. Schacter L. Etoposide phosphate: what, why, where, and how? Semin Oncol 1996;23:6 Suppl 13:1–7.

54. Hoskins PJ, Swenerton KD. Oral etoposide is active against platinum-resistant epithelial ovarian cancer. J Clin Oncol 1994;12:60–3.

55. Johnson DH, Greco FA, Strupp J, et al. Prolonged administration of oral etoposide in patients with relapsed or refractory small-cell lung cancer: a phase II trial. J Clin Oncol 1990;8:1613–7.

56. Greco FA. Etoposide: seeking the best dose and schedule. Semin Oncol 1992;19:6Suppl 14:59–63.

# Floxuridine

Floxuridine is one of a number of fluorinated pyrimidines developed for the treatment of gastrointestinal neoplasms. It is also known as 5-fluoro-2$N$-deoxyuridine, FUDR, 5-FUDR, and NSC-27640.

## EFFICACY

FUDR is used in the treatment of primary and metastatic neoplasms of the liver.

## PHARMACOLOGY

**Mechanisms of Action and Resistance.** These are discussed with the more widely used fluoropyrimidine 5-FU.

**Pharmacokinetics.** FUDR is erratically absorbed by the oral route. When single bolus doses of FUDR are administered intravenously, most of the drug is rapidly catabolized to 5-FU. However, when it is infused slowly, most of the drug is anabolized to an active metabolite (5-fluoro-2'-deoxyuridine-5'-phosphate). This metabolite is a potent inhibitor of thymidylate synthetase. When FUDR is given by hepatic arterial infusion, more than 95% of the drug undergoes first-pass clearance by normal liver.

**Drug and Radiation Interactions.** When FUDR is administered to the liver by the intra-arterial route, concomitant dexamethasone therapy may reduce FUDR-induced hepatic toxicity.[1] Also see the discussion of 5-FU.

## TOXICITY

FUDR causes toxic side effects that are similar to those of 5-FU, although their frequency is different. Because FUDR is nearly completely extracted from a single pass of blood in the hepatic artery, it is no surprise that the most important toxic side effect is cholangitis and liver dysfunction. This takes the form of sclerosis of the intrahepatic bile ducts or the extrahepatic bile ducts, or both; cirrhosis is also possible. Gastric mucosal injury can also occur with arterial infusion chemotherapy.[2] Further discussions of the problems of hepatic arterial infusion appear in Chapters 46 and 104. The complications of vascular access devices are discussed in Chapter 12, Vascular Access.

## DOSAGE AND ADMINISTRATION

FUDR is available in vials of 500 mg for injection. FUDR is marketed solely for use as a continuous intra-arterial infusion, usually via the hepatic artery for patients with primary or metastatic tumor in the liver. When FUDR is used for this purpose, the dosage varies from 0.1 to 0.6 mg/kg daily, usually for 14 to 21 days, with a rest period of 2 weeks between courses. When toxicity supervenes, the hepatic arterial line is maintained with an infusion of sterile saline until the toxicity subsides. An alternative mode of administration is with an Infusaid pump. This device is recharged every 2 weeks because of drug stability concerns, although studies in Europe suggest that FUDR is stable for at least 30 days.[3] In one study, treatment interruptions and complications were lower using an implanted pump compared with the use of external infusion devices.[4]

## REFERENCES

1. Kemeny N, Seiter K, Niedzwiecki D, et al. A randomized trial of intrahepatic infusion of fluorodeoxyuridine with dexamethasone versus fluorodeoxyuridine alone in the treatment of metastatic colorectal cancer. Cancer 1992;69:327–34.
2. Doria MI Jr, Doria LK, Faintuch J, Levin B. Gastric mucosal injury after hepatic arterial infusion chemotherapy with floxuridine: a clinical and pathologic study. Cancer 1994;73:2042–7.
3. Sadjak A, Wintersteiger R. Compatibility of morphine, baclofen, floxuridine and fluorouracil in an implantable medication pump. Arzneimittelforschung 1995;45:93–8.
4. Fordy C, Burke D, Earlam S, et al. Treatment interruptions and complications with two continuous hepatic artery floxuridine infusion systems in colorectal liver metastases. Br J Cancer 1995;72:1023–5.

# Fludarabine

Fludarabine phosphate is one of several new purine nucleoside analogues developed for the management of chronic lymphoproliferative diseases.[1, 2] The drug is also known as Fludara, fludarabine phosphate, 2-fluoroadenine arabinoside-5-phosphate, 2-fluoro-ara-AMP, FAMP, 2-Fl-AMP, and NSC-312887.

## EFFICACY

Fludarabine is FDA approved for the management of B-cell CLL after failure of standard alkylating agent therapy.[3, 4] The drug is being actively studied for potential use in other low-grade hematologic malignancies.[5]

## PHARMACOLOGY

**Mechanism of Action.** Fludarabine phosphate is dephosphorylated to fludarabine in serum and transported into cells by a carrier-mediated process.[6] Inside the cell, the drug is converted by deoxycytidine kinase to its cytotoxic nucleotide fludarabine triphosphate (2-fluoro-ara-ATP). This active metabolite has multiple intracellular toxic effects, but most prominently it inhibits DNA polymerase, ribonucleotide reductase, and DNA primase, resulting in the inhibition of DNA synthesis. At high concentrations, other effects on RNA and protein synthesis may also occur. Ultimately, fludarabine causes apoptosis.[7, 8]

**Resistance.** The amount of cross-resistance between cladribine, fludarabine, and pentostatin is variable and incomplete.[9] Resistance to fludarabine is probably related most closely to low levels of its activating enzyme, deoxycytidine kinase, but other factors may also be important.

**Pharmacokinetics.** Dephosphorylation occurs within minutes after intravenous administration. Limited data suggest that the drug is subsequently distributed widely in the body, especially to the liver, kidneys, and spleen. It is likely, but not proved, that the drug distributes to the CSF and CNS. Elimination of the drug is either biphasic or triphasic at standard doses. Using a biphasic model, the initial and delayed half-lives were reportedly 36 minutes and more than 9 hours, respectively. Renal elimination plays a role in excretion, with about 24% of the drug excreted within 24 hours in one study. At higher doses, urinary excretion was higher (41 to 60%).

Preliminary pharmacokinetic studies of oral fludarabine suggest that the plasma AUC after oral dosing is similar to that with intravenous administration.[10]

**Drug Interactions.** Concomitant use with pentostatin can cause severe and even fatal pulmonary toxicity. This occurred in four of six patients in one study, so this combination should not be used. Fludarabine potentiates the conversion of intracellular cytarabine to its active metabolite (ara-CTP), potentially augmenting the antileukemic effect of cytarabine.[11]

## TOXICITY

**Overview.** Myelosuppression is the most important and dose-limiting toxicity. Other important adverse effects include fever, chills, infection, nausea, vomiting, malaise, fatigue, anorexia, weakness, and, in patients with CLL, severe hemolytic anemia. Neurotoxicity is also common but is usually reversible at standard doses. At high doses, severe neurotoxicity occurs, including blindness and death in some patients. Concomitant use of fludarabine with pentostatin is contraindicated because the combination causes fatal pulmonary toxicity.

**Hematologic.** Dose-related, dose-limiting, usually reversible myelosuppression occurs in up to 75% of patients. This can be severe, with pancytopenia, and anemia may require transfusions. Rarely, this may progress to fatal myelofibrosis.[12] Two of 11 patients in one trial developed marked eosinophilia.[13] Hemolytic anemia has been reported in patients with CLL. Treatment with corticosteroids and discontinuation of fludarabine is effective in most cases, but the complication can be severe, is frequently life threatening, and can be fatal. Rechallenge with fludarabine after one episode of fludarabine-associated hemolytic anemia should not be attempted. Rechallenge was associated with an 88% incidence of recurrent hemolysis in one series.[14] Autoimmune thrombocytopenia has also been reported.[15]

**Immunologic.** Anaphylaxis has been reported, but it is extremely rare. Pulmonary hypersensitivity reactions occur in up to 6% of patients (possibly as an exacerbation of prior lung damage from chlorambucil). Fludarabine is profoundly cytotoxic to CD4 lymphocytes, resulting in marked immunosuppression.

**Digestive System.** Nausea and vomiting, usually mild to moderate in severity, occur in up to 36% of patients. Other adverse effects include anorexia (up to 34%), diarrhea (up to 15%), gastrointestinal bleeding (up to 13%), and other effects in up to 5 to 6% of patients (esophagitis, constipation, dysphagia, altered taste perception, abnormal liver function test results, cholelithiasis, liver failure, and pancreatitis).

**Mucocutaneous.** Fludarabine use has been associated with the following: stomatitis (up to 9%), maculopapular rash (up to 15%), pruritus and seborrhea (up to 5%), and very rare alopecia. In one patient, a maculopapular rash after one cycle of treatment progressed to nearly fatal epidermal necrolysis (pemphigus) following a second cycle of treatment.[16] Re-treatment of patients who develop a rash on therapy should be avoided.

**Cardiovascular.** Adverse effects are seen in 12 to 38% of patients treated for CLL. These include edema (up to 19%), angina (up to 6%), and a variety of other effects of uncertain relationship to fludarabine in up to 5% of patients (congestive heart failure, arrhythmias, chest pain, myocardial infarction, deep vein thrombosis, phlebitis, transient ischemic attacks, aneurysm, and pericardial effusion).

**Pulmonary.** Adverse pulmonary effects occur in 14 to 69% of patients treated for CLL. Pneumonia has been reported in 9 to 22%, as has cough (up to 44%), dyspnea (up to 22%), upper respiratory tract infection (up to 16%), pharyngitis (up to 9%), and allergic pneumonitis or hemoptysis (up to 6%). The pulmonary hypersensitivity reaction is a delayed effect, with an onset of 3 to 28 days after drug administration during the third or later course of treatment. Because all of these patients had been previously treated with chlorambucil, it is possible that this reaction represents delayed alkylating agent pulmonary damage induced or exacerbated by fludarabine.

**Neurologic.** During early high-dose trials, delayed, potentially irreversible, or fatal neurologic toxicity occurred in up to 36% of patients. This appeared 21 to 60 days after drug administration and included mental status changes, generalized seizures, flaccid or spastic paralysis with or without quadriparesis, blurred vision, blindness, and, in some cases, coma. Severe neurotoxicity is rare at standard doses and is more likely to be reversible.[17] Mild to moderate neurotoxicity occurs in 21 to 69% of patients receiving standard doses. These include weakness (up to 65%), pain (up to 44%), malaise (up to 22%), fatigue (up to 38%), paresthesia (up to 12%), visual disturbances (up to 15%), hearing abnormalities (up to 6%), and sleep disorders or headache (up to 3%). Very rarely, other diverse effects have been reported, including agitation, confusion, peripheral neuropathy, wrist drop, depression, cerebellar syndrome, equilibrium disturbances, somnolence, and coma.

**Musculoskeletal.** Myalgia occurs in up to 16% of patients, and osteoporosis and arthralgia occur in up to 6%.

**Other/Rare.** Fever occurs in up to 69% of patients, infection in up to 44%, and diaphoresis in up to 13%.

*Ocular.* Cortical blindness occurs with high-dose fludarabine therapy.

*Genitourinary.* Adverse effects are uncommon (12 to 22% of patients). Reported problems include urinary tract infection (up to 15%) and a variety of rare adverse effects (<5% each), including dysuria, urinary hesitancy, hematuria, abnormal renal function test results, proteinuria, and renal failure. Hemorrhagic cystitis is a rare complication. The tumor lysis syndrome with renal insufficiency occurs rarely. The National Cancer Institute has estimated the risk of clinically significant tumor lysis syndrome at 0.33% (26 of 6137 patients treated).[18]

*Reproductive.* Toxicity data place fludarabine in FDA pregnancy category D. Animal studies suggest that the drug can impair male fertility.

*Endocrine-Metabolic.* Fludarabine can cause the tumor lysis syndrome, with all its complex metabolic problems. Hyperglycemia has been reported in up to 6% of patients.

*Carcinogenicity.* The drug is mutagenic in some systems. Although no instances of human cancer caused by fludarabine are known, it should be considered a potential carcinogen.

## DOSAGE AND ADMINISTRATION

Fludarabine is available as a lyophilized powder in vials of 50 mg for injection. It is reconstituted in normal saline or 5% dextrose solution. The usual dosage is 25 mg/m²/day given as an intravenous infusion over about 30 minutes daily for 5 days, repeated every 4 weeks. The dose may be decreased or delayed for toxicity, and the drug should probably be discontinued in patients who develop neurotoxicity. Because fludarabine is cleared primarily by the kidneys, it should be used cautiously in patients with renal dysfunction. Guidelines for dose adjustments in patients with renal failure are not available.

## REFERENCES

1. Ross SR, McTavish D, Faulds D. Fludarabine: a review of its pharmacological properties and therapeutic potential in malignancy. Drugs 1993;45:737–59.
2. Cheson BD. The purine analogs—a therapeutic beauty contest. J Clin Oncol 1992;10:352–5.
3. Sorensen JM, Vena DA, Fallavollita A, et al. Treatment of refractory chronic lymphocytic leukemia with fludarabine phosphate via the group C protocol mechanism of the National Cancer Institute: five-year follow-up report. J Clin Oncol 1997;15:458–65.
4. O'Brien S, Kantarjian H, Beran M, et al. Results of fludarabine and prednisone therapy in 264 patients with chronic lymphocytic leukemia with multivariate analysis–derived prognostic model for response to treatment. Blood 1993;82:1695–700.
5. Adkins JC, Peters DH, Markham A. Fludarabine: an update of its pharmacology and use in the treatment of haematological malignancies. Drugs 1997;53:1005–37.
6. Plunkett W, Gandhi V, Huang P, et al. Fludarabine: pharmacokinetics, mechanisms of action, and rationales for combination therapies. Semin Oncol 1993;20:5 Suppl 7:2–12.
7. Zinzani PL, Buzzi M, Farabegoli P, et al. Apoptosis induction with fludarabine on freshly isolated chronic myeloid leukemia cells. Haematologica 1994;79:127–31.
8. Zinzani PL, Buzzi M, Farabegoli P, et al. Induction of "in vitro" apoptosis by fludarabine in freshly isolated B–chronic lymphocytic leukemia cells. Leuk Lymphoma 1994;13:95–7.
9. Kraut EH. Cross-resistance to purine analogs in hairy cell leukemia. Ann Intern Med 1994;120:247–8.
10. Foran JM, Oscier D, Orchard J, et al. Pharmacokinetic study of single doses of oral fludarabine phosphate in patients with "low-grade" non-Hodgkin's lymphoma and B-cell chronic lymphocytic leukemia. J Clin Oncol 1999;17:1574–9.
11. Gandhi V, Robertson LE, Keating MJ, Plunkett W. Combination of fludarabine and arabinosylcytosine for treatment of chronic lymphocytic leukemia: clinical efficacy and modulation of arabinosylcytosine pharmacology. Cancer Chemother Pharmacol 1994;34:30–6.
12. Palomera L, Azaceta G, Varo MJ, et al. Fatal myelofibrosis following fludarabine administration in a patient with indolent lymphoma. Haematologica 1998;83:1045–6.
13. Lèarfars G, Udâen-Blohmâe AM, Samuelsson J. Fludarabine, as well as 2-chlorodeoxyadenosine, can induce eosinophilia during treatment of lymphoid malignancies. Br J Haematol 1996;94:709–12.
14. Weiss RB, Freiman J, Kweeder SL, et al. Hemolytic anemia after fludarabine therapy for chronic lymphocytic leukemia. J Clin Oncol 1998;16:1885–9.
15. Bay JO, Fouassier M, Bâeal D, et al. Autoimmune thrombocytopenia after six cycles of fludarabine phosphate in a patient with chronic lymphocytic leukemia. Hematol Cell Ther 1997;39:209–12.
16. Braess J, Reich K, Willert S, et al. Mucocutaneous autoimmune syndrome following fludarabine therapy for low-grade non-Hodgkin's lymphoma of B-cell type. Ann Hematol 1997;75:227–30.
17. Cohen RB, Abdallah JM, Gray JR, Foss F. Reversible neurologic toxicity in patients treated with standard-dose fludarabine phosphate for mycosis fungoides and chronic lymphocytic leukemia. Ann Intern Med 1993;118:114–6.
18. Cheson BD, Frame JN, Vena D, et al. Tumor lysis syndrome: an uncommon complication of fludarabine therapy of chronic lymphocytic leukemia. J Clin Oncol 1998;16:2313–20.

# Fluorouracil

Fluorouracil is an antimetabolite developed by Heidelberger and Ansfield in 1957 as a structural analogue of the important DNA precursor thymine. The drug is also known as 5-fluorouracil, 5-FU, Efudex, and NSC-19893.

## EFFICACY

5-FU is useful in the treatment of carcinomas of the breast and gastrointestinal tract. It may also be useful in the treatment of a variety of other neoplasms and topically in the treatment of some malignant and premalignant skin diseases.[1]

## PHARMACOLOGY

**Mechanism of Action.** 5-FU is a prodrug that enters cells by a carrier-mediated process, followed by intracellular phosphorylation to a series of metabolites.[2] These metabolites produce the equivalent of two separate drugs because they are formed in different amounts depending on the schedule of drug administration. The most important metabolite and mechanism of action is 5-fluorodeoxyuridylate (5-FdUMP), which joins with $N5,N10$-methylenetetrahydrofolate (MTHF) to form a covalent ternary complex with the enzyme thymidylate synthetase. The level of MTHF is a critical determinant of the effectiveness of 5-FU and FUDR by this mechanism because only in the presence of adequate levels of MTHF does covalent binding occur. At low levels of MTHF, the inhibition is incomplete and transient. 5-FdUMP may also be incorporated into DNA, with subsequent effects on DNA repair and the induction of strand breaks resulting in a defective DNA molecule.

The other important metabolite is fluorouridine triphosphate (FUTP), which inhibits RNA metabolism. This relates primarily to the incorporation of FUTP into RNA, leading to inhibition of nuclear RNA. Other, biochemical effects include the formation of 5-FU nucleotide sugars and the inhibition of the use of preformed uracil in RNA synthesis by blocking uracil phosphatase.[3,4] An additional novel mechanism involves binding of 5-FU itself to uracil DNA glycosylase, an important base excision repair enzyme.[5] This effect occurs in nonproliferating human cell populations.

A complete understanding of the mechanism of action of the fluoropyrimidine analogues requires a detailed assessment of their metabolic interconversions in both normal and tumor tissues. Clearly, the intracellular activation of 5-FU and FUDR by several enzymes (most importantly thymidine kinase, uridine kinase, and phosphoribosyltransferase) is an obligatory step for the cytotoxicity of these drugs. In addition, the degradation of these drugs and metabolites by the liver and some other tissues is also important.

The impact of 5-FU on the cell cycles of normal and malignant cells is complex, with significant differences being seen between various cells and cell lines. Salient features include the following: (1) 5-FU has profound effects on the progression of cells through the cell cycle, most noticeably the $G_1$ and S phases; (2) 5-FU kills cells in both S and non–S phases of the cell cycle; (3) 5-FU is a proliferation-dependent agent; and (4) increasing the period of exposure of cells to 5-FU dramatically increases cytotoxicity, such that cells that appear resistant during a short period of exposure may become sensitive if the interval of treatment is prolonged.

**Resistance.** Resistance to the biochemical effects of the fluoropyrimidines is complex. In most cases, resistance is due to changes in the metabolism of 5-FU or to altered effects of the metabolites of 5-FU. For example, resistance to 5-FU may be due to a deficiency of 5-FU anabolism, a deficiency of 5-FU transport, a depletion of essential cosubstrates, enhanced catabolism of 5-FU, enhanced intracellular uridine concentrations, and alterations in the intracellular levels of deoxythymidine triphosphate. Another mechanism of resistance is mediated through changes in the major target enzyme thymidylate synthetase.[6] Yet another involves alterations in deoxyuridine triphosphatase, which is a component of the uracil misincorporation-misrepair pathway.[7] Many other alterations are also possible, including altered enzyme kinetics, enhanced accumulation of the substrate deoxyuridine monophosphate (dUMP), decreased retention of 5-FdUMP, rapid recovery of new enzyme synthesis, gene amplification, decreased stability of the ternary complex, depletion of folate cofactors, and decreased polyglutamation of folates. In the past, the levels of degradative enzymes found in various tissues have been considered a possible explanation for the differential cytotoxicity of 5-FU in colon cancer and in adjoining normal colon tissue. However, attempts to exploit such differences have been largely unsuccessful, so the clinical relevance of these differences appears minimal. A possible exception is the observation that patients with dihydropyrimidine dehydrogenase deficiency, a key enzyme in 5-FU catabolism, are susceptible to life-threatening toxicity.[8, 9]

There appears to be a lack of cross-resistance between short-term bolus therapy with 5-FU and continuous exposure therapy with 5-FU.[2, 10] This phenomenon is thought to be a result of differences in the relative inhibition of DNA and RNA synthesis by these distinctly different schedules of drug administration.

**Pharmacokinetics.** 5-FU is erratically absorbed by the oral route, so it is generally given parenterally. After rapid intravenous injection, 5-FU rapidly diffuses into all body compartments, including the nervous system and malignant effusions.[4] It is quickly cleared from plasma, with a half-life of 10 to 20 minutes after a rapid intravenous injection of 15 mg/kg. Maximum plasma levels with this dose reach $10^{-4}$ to $10^{-3}$ M, but by 3 hours 5-FU is not measurable in plasma ($<10^{-8}$ M). In contrast to its rapid clearance from plasma, 5-FU and its metabolites may persist for prolonged periods in some tissues, including some tumors. The extent of such trapping can be assessed by nuclear magnetic resonance spectroscopy.[11, 12] Preliminary studies suggest that such trapping may increase the likelihood of a clinical response to 5-FU in patients with colorectal cancer.[13] In mice, the active metabolite of 5-FU has been shown to persist in bone marrow and tumor cells for 7 days after a single intravenous injection. This may explain the prolonged effect of intermittent single doses of 5-FU in humans. It should be noted that 5-FU demonstrates nonlinear pharmacokinetics with repeated administration and that there is a good correlation between the plasma AUC versus time ($C \times T$) and clinical toxicity.[14] Stated in another way, total-body clearance of the drug decreases with increasing 5-FU doses, probably because the sites of degradation become saturated. The drug is pri-

marily degraded by the liver (about 80%), but renal and pulmonary excretion also occur.

When given by hepatic arterial infusion, more than 50% of 5-FU undergoes first-pass clearance by a normal liver.[15] The extent of hepatic extraction is markedly affected, however, by the dose and duration of infusion. For example, the hepatic extraction of 5-FU given by hepatic arterial infusion was 20 to 60% at a dose of 1000 mg/m²/day, whereas it was 90% when the dose was reduced to 780 mg/m²/day.

The clinical pharmacology of 5-FU is complex, and its study is highly dependent on technologic advances. Different individuals metabolize 5-FU in different ways, leading to interest in determining the fluorouracil phenotype of patients as a guide to drug administration.[16] Because of the presence of fluorine in the drug, 5-FU can be studied in vivo using nuclear magnetic resonance spectroscopy and positron emission tomography.[17] The details of 5-FU metabolism in humans require further definition, especially when 5-FU is combined with leucovorin or other drugs.

**Drug and Radiation Interactions.** The cytotoxicity of the fluoropyrimidines may be altered by coadministration of other drugs or metabolites, such as MTX,[18] leucovorin,[19] dipyridamole,[20] thymidine, uridine, interferon,[21] cimetidine,[22] sparfosate (PALA),[23] and allopurinol.[24] Levamisole is commonly given with 5-FU for adjuvant therapy of colorectal cancer; the use of these drugs together may result in an increased frequency of some rare forms of toxicity, specifically cerebral demyelinating disease[25] and hepatic dysfunction that may mimic metastatic disease.[26]

The most important drug interaction of 5-FU is with leucovorin. This involves the covalent binding of 5-FdUMP to thymidylate synthetase with the formation of a ternary complex with the reduced folate cofactor MTHF. Administration of leucovorin increases this binding and thereby increases 5-FU cytotoxicity. MTX therapy depletes the availability of this cofactor and may thereby inhibit 5-FU toxicity. However, prolonged use of MTX leads to the intracellular formation of MTX polyglutamates, and these promote tighter binding of thymidylate synthetase by 5-FdUMP, thereby increasing 5-FU cytotoxicity. In a meta-analysis of clinical trials combining 5-FU and MTX, the response rate was doubled and survival improved in patients with colon cancer.[27] Double modulation may also be accomplished by the combined use of leucovorin and interferon.[28, 29] 5-FU is considered a radiosensitizing agent,[30, 31] although this effect is less intense than with many other antineoplastic agents.

## TOXICITY

**Overview.** The toxicity of 5-FU is strongly influenced by the dosage used and the route and duration of drug administration. When 5-FU is given by weekly bolus injection, bone marrow suppression is the main form of toxicity. When the drug is given by continuous intravenous infusions or when it is given with leucovorin, oral mucositis and diarrhea become the predominant forms of toxicity. Patients with dihydropyrimidine dehydrogenase deficiency are more susceptible to the toxic effects of 5-FU.[8, 9]

**Hematologic.** In the early days of 5-FU use, severe bone marrow suppression was a major problem with the schedules of drug administration used. Megaloblastic changes in the peripheral blood smear could be seen as an early event, and some patients developed complete marrow aplasia. However, the schedules currently used only rarely cause this degree of marrow suppression. Nevertheless, severe, life-threatening depression of the bone marrow can still occur, and 5-FU should not be given without extremely close supervision of the patient and his or her hematologic status. This is particularly true in patients with limited bone marrow reserve, either from previous therapy or from involvement of the marrow by tumor. Very rarely, 5-FU has been associated with acute immune hemolytic anemia.[32] 5-FU causes a dose-dependent, reversible echinocytosis that temporarily increases blood viscosity and the transit time of red blood cells (RBCs) through small pores.[33] This appears to be caused by intercalation of 5-FU in the outer hemileaflet of the RBC membrane.

**Digestive System.** Anorexia, nausea, vomiting, and diarrhea can occur with any of the schedules of drug administration currently in use, but these are especially common when the drug is given by continuous infusion or with leucovorin. Diarrhea, when it occurs, is an indication for withholding 5-FU therapy. When 5-FU is given with leucovorin, diarrhea due to enterocolitis can assume life-threatening proportions. This severe diarrhea usually responds to therapy with octreotide acetate.[34] Other gastrointestinal problems that require cessation of treatment include cholecystitis and common duct stricture associated with hepatic artery infusion of 5-FU or FUDR. When 5-FU is given with levamisole, mild to moderate reversible hepatic dysfunction occurs in about 40% of patients.[26] The most common change is an increase in the serum alkaline phosphatase level, but total bilirubin and transaminase enzyme levels may also increase. In some cases, these changes are associated with an increase in the serum carcinoembryonic antigen level and the appearance of a fatty liver on computed tomographic scan or liver biopsy specimens. These changes may simulate hepatic metastasis.

**Mucocutaneous.** Ulceration of the buccal mucosa is common. The usual sequence of events visible to the physician includes erythema of the buccal mucosa, followed by a patchy white membrane and ulceration. Ice chips in the mouth for a 30-minute period during bolus injection therapy are effective in preventing oral stomatitis in the majority of patients.[35] When seen, stomatitis is an indication for withholding 5-FU therapy. Other common reactions include reversible alopecia, maculopapular rash, photosensitivity, hyperpigmentation (especially over sites of intravenous injections), skin atrophy, nail changes, and the palmar-plantar erythrodysesthesia syndrome (commonly known as the hand-foot syndrome).[36] Although the hand-foot syndrome is nearly always associated with continuous infusion therapy, it has also been reported in patients receiving weekly bolus therapy.[37] In one case report, a nicotine patch (7.0 mg) was effective prophylaxis for moderately severe desquamative dermatitis due to 5-FU.[38] Pyridoxine therapy (150 mg daily) may also be useful.[39]

**Other and Rare Reactions.** A single case report of nasal cartilage necrosis following high-dose 5-FU has been published.[40] Fever and epistaxis are rare complications.

*Immunologic.* Allergic reactions to 5-FU have been reported, including rare cases of anaphylaxis. The drug is immunosuppressive in humans.

*Cardiovascular.* There are numerous reports of cardiac ischemia associated with 5-FU, especially when the drug is given by continuous infusion in patients with pre-existing cardiac disease. The incidence of this reaction was 0.55% in a series of 910 patients receiving standard doses; the pathophysiology in each case was consistent with coronary artery vasospasm.[41] With high-dose continuous infusion therapy, the incidence was 7.6%. The most likely explanation for this side effect is the transient echinocytosis that occurs with drug administration (see Hematologic Toxicity). Thrombophlebitis may also occur with therapy.[42]

*Ocular.* Conjunctivitis, nasal discharge, photophobia, and excessive lacrimation (due to tear duct stenosis) can occur occasionally. Acute toxic optic neuropathy is a rare complication.[43]

*Neurologic.* Reversible somnolence, disorientation, confusion, euphoria, cerebellar ataxia, nystagmus, headache, and pyramidal tract signs may develop in as many as 2% of patients. Rare cases of severe cerebral demyelinating disease have been reported from the combination of 5-FU plus levamisole.[25]

*Endocrine-Metabolic.* 5-FU therapy reduces total plasma cholesterol levels.[44]

*Reproductive.* Toxicity studies place 5-FU in pregnancy category D; the drug is presumed to inhibit gametogenesis, but this has not been proved in humans.

*Carcinogenicity.* 5-FU is mutagenic in some systems but not all; the risk of carcinogenesis is uncertain.

**Topical 5-FU.** This is generally considered to be free of systemic toxicity, although a variety of local skin reactions may occur, including pain, burning, pruritus, and hyperpigmentation. Less frequent reactions include localized telangiectasia, reactivation of herpes simplex infections, chronic scaling and suppuration, and the very rare development of bullous pemphigoid.

## DOSAGE AND ADMINISTRATION

5-FU is available in vials or ampules of 500 mg. It is stable at room temperature for prolonged periods if protected from light, but it is incompatible with the following drugs in solution: cisplatin, cytarabine, daunorubicin, diazepam, doxorubicin, and idarubicin.

The optimal dose, route of administration, and schedule for 5-FU have yet to be determined. Although it is used by some physicians as arterial infusion therapy in the treatment of carcinomas involving the liver, the value of this approach is controversial. 5-FU has also been given orally, but erratic absorption and variable plasma concentrations have led to general abandonment of this route.[45] Therefore, the drug is most commonly given by intravenous injection. Fortunately, the dual role of the liver and kidneys in removing 5-FU from the body is so efficient that one need not modify the dose of 5-FU in patients with liver or kidney dysfunction.[4] Some of the more common ways of using 5-FU are as follows.

**Continuous Intravenous Infusions.** Intermittent continuous intravenous therapy is given in a dosage of about 1000 mg/m$^2$/day for 5 days (range, 650 to 1300 mg/m$^2$/day), with repeat courses every 28 days. Protracted venous infusion schedules are also used, especially in combination with radiation therapy in adjuvant therapy for rectal cancer. The dosage in this setting is 225 mg/m²/day throughout the period of radiation therapy.[46] It should be noted that there can be considerable fluctuation in drug plasma concentrations using portable pumps for continuous infusion therapy. This problem can be minimized by using daily changes of 100-ml drug cartridges containing diluted 5-FU.[47]

**Intravenous Bolus Injections.** The package insert describes an intensive loading regimen of daily bolus injections. Because of the serious toxicity of this schedule, many clinicians prefer to use one or the other of two modifications of this standard loading course. The first is a minor modification in which bolus 5-FU is given for 5 days in a daily dose of 12 mg/kg, provided the patient maintains a normal WCC and has no mucositis or diarrhea. Such 5-day cycles of treatment are then repeated at 4- to 5-week intervals, depending on the response of the patient. Another alternative is to give 5-FU on a weekly basis. This involves weekly administration of 5-FU by rapid intravenous injection without a loading dose. Doses are titrated to avoid major toxicity and drug-related deaths, and patients can be treated on an ambulatory basis. The dosage for the first 4 weeks is 15 mg/kg/wk; if possible, this is increased to 20 mg/kg/wk thereafter (maximum dose, 1 g). An adequate course is considered to be one that produces either an objective antitumor response or mild toxicity. If toxicity supervenes, 5-FU is discontinued until the symptoms have subsided, and it is then resumed at a dose that is lower by 5 mg/kg. Weekly 5-FU has been associated with much less drug toxicity than is encountered with intermittent weekly courses of the drug, but the response rates for some tumors may also be less. It is not clear, however, that the lower response rates have biologic significance because overall survival results with the two approaches to treatment are equivalent.

**5-FU with Leucovorin.** The many variations of this combination are beyond the scope of this discussion. The value of combined 5-FU and leucovorin has been confirmed by a meta-analysis of studies in patients with colorectal cancer.[48] A commonly used regimen involves giving monthly 5-day cycles of intravenous bolus 5-FU in a dosage of 425 mg/m²/day following a bolus intravenous injection of leucovorin in a dosage of 20 mg/m²/day a month apart to start, with repeat courses thereafter every 5 weeks.[49] An alternative, more toxic regimen involves weekly administration of leucovorin as a 2-hour infusion in a dosage of 500 mg/m² with a midinfusion bolus injection of 5-FU in a dosage of 500 mg/m². In one randomized study comparing these regimens, the weekly regimen caused more diarrhea and more hospitalizations and was more expensive than the 5-day regimen.[50]

## REFERENCES

1. Pinedo HM, Peters GF. Fluorouracil: biochemistry and pharmacology. J Clin Oncol 1988;6:1653–64.
2. Sobrero AF, Aschele C, Bertino JR. Fluorouracil in colorectal cancer—a tale of two drugs: implications for biochemical modulation. J Clin Oncol 1997;15:368–81.
3. Ardalan B, Glazer R. An update on the biochemistry of 5-fluorouracil. Cancer Treat Rev 1981;8:157–67.
4. Myers CE, Diasio R, Eliot HM, Chabner BA. Pharmacokinetics of the fluoropyrimidines: implications for their clinical use. Cancer Treat Rev 1976;3:175–83.
5. Wurzer JC, Tallarida RJ, Sirover MA. New mechanism of action of the cancer chemotherapeutic agent 5-fluorouracil in human cells. J Pharmacol Exp Ther 1994;269:39–43.
6. Spears CP, Gustavsson BG, Berne M, et al. Mechanisms of innate resistance to thymidylate synthase inhibition after 5-fluorouracil. Cancer Res 1988;48:5894–900.
7. Canman CE, Radany EH, Parsels LA, et al. Induction of resistance to fluorodeoxyuridine cytotoxicity and DNA damage in human tumor cells by expression of *Escherichia coli* deoxyuridine triphosphatase. Cancer Res 1994;54:2296–8.
8. Harris BE, Carpenter JT, Diasio RB. Severe 5-fluorouracil toxicity to dihydropyrimidine dehydrogenase deficiency: a potentially more common pharmacogenetic syndrome. Cancer 1991;68:499–501.
9. Houyau P, Gay C, Chatelut E, et al. Severe fluorouracil toxicity in a patient with dihydropyrimidine dehydrogenase deficiency. J Natl Cancer Inst 1993;85:1602–3.
10. Sobrero AF, Aschele C, Guglielmi AP, et al. Synergism and lack of cross-resistance between short-term and continuous exposure to fluorouracil in human colon adenocarcinoma cells. J Natl Cancer Inst 1993;85:1937–44.
11. Presant CA, Wolf W, Albright MJ, et al. Human tumor fluorouracil trapping: clinical correlations of in vivo 19F nuclear magnetic resonance spectroscopy pharmacokinetics. J Clin Oncol 1990;8:1868–73.
12. Peters GJ, Lankelma J, Kok RM, et al. Prolonged retention of high concentrations of 5-fluorouracil in human and murine tumors as compared with plasma. Cancer Chemother Pharmacol 1993;31:269–76.
13. Presant CA, Wolf W, Waluch V, et al. Association of intratumoral pharmacokinetics of fluorouracil with clinical response. Lancet 1994;343:1184–7.
14. Von Groeningen CJ, Pinedo HM, Heddes J, et al. Pharmacokinetics of 5-fluorouracil assessed with a sensitive mass spectrometric method in patients on a dose escalation schedule. Cancer Res 1988;48:6956–61.
15. Ensminger WD, Rosowsky A, Raso V, et al. A clinical-pharmacological evaluation of hepatic arterial infusions of 5-fluoro-2′-deoxyuridine and 5-fluorouracil. Cancer Res 1978;38:3784–92.
16. Schilsky RL. Biochemical and clinical pharmacology of 5-fluorouracil. Oncology 1998;12:10 Suppl 7:13–8.
17. Hull WE, Port RE, Herrmann R, et al. Metabolites of 5-fluorouracil in plasma and urine, as monitored by 19F nuclear magnetic resonance spectroscopy, for patients receiving chemotherapy with or without methotrexate pretreatment. Cancer Res 1988;48:1680–8.
18. Marsh JC, Bertino JR, Katz KH, et al. The influence of drug interval on the effect of methotrexate and fluorouracil in the treatment of advanced colorectal cancer. J Clin Oncol 1991;9:371–80.
19. Grogan L, Sotos FA, Allegra CJ. Leucovorin modulation of fluorouracil. Oncology 1993;7:63–72.
20. Trump DL, Egorin MJ, Forrest A, et al. Pharmacokinetic and pharmacodynamic analysis of fluorouracil during 72-hour continuous infusion with and without dipyridamole. J Clin Oncol 1991;9:2027–35.
21. Sparano JA, Wadler S, Diasio RB, et al. Phase I trial of low-dose, prolonged continuous infusion fluorouracil plus interferon-alfa: evidence for enhanced fluorouracil toxicity without pharmacokinetic perturbation. J Clin Oncol 1993;11:1609–17.
22. Harvey VJ, Slevin ML, Dilloway MR, et al. The influence of cimetidine on the pharmacokinetics of 5-fluorouracil. Br J Clin Pharmacol 1984;18:421–30.
23. Martin DS, Kemeny NE. Modulation of fluorouracil by N-(phosphonacetyl)-L-asparate: a review. Semin Oncol 1992;19:Suppl 3:49–55.
24. Howell SB, Wung WE, Taetle R, et al. Modulation of 5-fluorouracil toxicity by allopurinol in man. Cancer 1981;48:1281–9.
25. Kimmel DW, Schutt AJ. Multifocal leukoencephalopathy: occurrence during 5-fluorouracil and levamisole therapy and resolution after discontinuation of chemotherapy. Mayo Clinic Proc 1993;68:363–5.
26. Moertel CG, Fleming TR, Macdonald JS, et al. Hepatic toxicity associated with fluorouracil plus levamisole adjuvant therapy. J Clin Oncol 1993;11:2386–90.
27. Meta-analysis of randomized trials testing the biochemical modulation of fluorouracil by methotrexate in metastatic colorectal cancer: advanced Colorectal Cancer Meta-Analysis Project. J Clin Oncol 1994;12:960–9.
28. Steger GG, Mader RM, Djavanmard MP, et al. Double modulation of 5-fluorouracil by high-dose leucovorin and interferon alpha 2b in advanced colorectal cancer: a phase I and a phase II study of weekly administration. J Cancer Res Clin Oncol 1994;120:314–8.
29. Sinnige HAM, Timmer-Bosscha H, Peters GF, et al. Combined modulation by leucovorin and alpha-2a interferon of fluoropyrimidine mediated growth inhibition. Anticancer Res 1993;13:1335–40.

30. Bruso CE, Shewach DS, Lawrence TS. Fluorodeoxyuridine-induced radiosensitization and inhibition of DNA double strand break repair in human colon cancer cells. Int J Radiat Oncol Biol Phys 1990;19:1411–7.
31. Miller EM, Kinsella TJ. Radiosensitization by fluorodeoxyuridine: effects of thymidylate synthase inhibition and cell synchronization. Cancer Res 1992;52:1687–94.
32. Sandvei P, Nordhagen R, Michaelsen TE, Walthuis K. Fluorouracil (5-FU) induced acute immune haemolytic anaemia. Br J Haematol 1987;65:357–9.
33. Baerlocher GM, Beer JH, Owen GR, et al. The antineoplastic drug 5-fluorouracil produces echinocytosis and affects blood rheology. Br J Haematol 1997;99:426–32.
34. Cascinu S, Fedeli A, Fedeli SL, Catalano G. Octreotide versus loperamide in the treatment of fluorouracil-induced diarrhea: a randomized trial. J Clin Oncol 1993;11:148–51.
35. Rocke LK, Loprinzi CL, Lee JK, et al. A randomized clinical trial of two different durations of oral cryotherapy for prevention of 5-fluorouracil-related stomatitis. Cancer 1993;72:2234–8.
36. Lokich JD, Moore C. Chemotherapy-associated palmar-plantar erythrodysesthesia syndrome. Ann Intern Med 1984;101:798–9.
37. Atkins JN. Fluorouracil and the palmar-plantar erythrodysesthesia syndrome. Ann Intern Med 1985;102:419.
38. Kingsley EC. 5-Fluorouracil dermatitis prophylaxis with a nicotine patch. Ann Intern Med 1994;120:813.
39. Mortimer JE, Anderson I. Weekly fluorouracil and high-dose leucovorin: efficacy and treatment of cutaneous toxicity. Cancer Chemother Pharmacol 1990;26:449–52.
40. Ashford RFU, Mughal T, Goold MA, et al. Nasal cartilage necrosis following high-dose 5-FU: a case report. Cancer Treat Rep 1982;66:1884.
41. Keefe DL, Roistacher N, Pierri MK. Clinical cardiotoxicity of 5-fluorouracil. J Clin Pharmacol 1993;33:1060–70.
42. Gradishar W, Vokes E, Schilsky R, et al. Vascular events in patients receiving high-dose infusional 5-fluorouracil-based chemotherapy: the University of Chicago experience. Med Pediatr Oncol 1991;9:8–15.
43. Adams JW, Bofenkamp TM, Kobrin J, et al. Recurrent acute toxic optic neuropathy secondary to 5-FU. Cancer Treat Rep 1984;68:565–6.
44. Stathopoulos GP, Stergiou GS, Perrea-Kostarelis DN, et al. Influence of 5-fluorouracil on serum lipids. Acta Oncol 1995;34:253–6.
45. Cohen JL, Irwin LE, Marshall GJ, et al. Clinical pharmacology of oral and intravenous 5-fluorouracil (NSC-19893). Cancer Chemother Rep 1974;58:Part 1:723–31.
46. O'Connell MJ, Martenson JA, Wieand HS, et al. Improving adjuvant therapy for rectal cancer by combining protracted-infusion fluorouracil with radiation therapy after curative surgery. N Engl J Med 1994;331:502–7.
47. Etienne MC, Milano G, Lagrange JL, et al. Marked fluctuations in drug plasma concentrations caused by use of portable pumps for fluorouracil continuous infusion. J Natl Cancer Inst 1993;85:1005–7.
48. Modulation of fluorouracil by leucovorin in patients with advanced colorectal cancer: evidence in terms of response rate. Advanced Colorectal Cancer Meta-Analysis Project. J Clin Oncol 1992;10:896–903.
49. O'Connell MJ. A phase III trial of 5-fluorouracil and leucovorin in the treatment of advanced colorectal cancer: a Mayo Clinic/North Central Cancer Treatment Group study. Cancer 1989;63:1026–30.
50. Buroker TR, O'Connell MJ, Wieand HS, et al. Randomized comparison of two schedules of fluorouracil and leucovorin in the treatment of advanced colorectal cancer. J Clin Oncol 1994;12:14–20.

# Flutamide

Flutamide is a nonsteroidal antiandrogen. It is also known as Eulexin.

## EFFICACY

Flutamide is used for the treatment of prostate cancer. The best established indication for its use is in combination with an LHRH agonist, such as leuprolide, for the palliative treatment of advanced prostate cancer.[1] Flutamide is used in this context to prevent the androgen flare reaction that sometimes results from the use of an LHRH agonist. Long-term flutamide use, as part of total androgen blockade, is more controversial.[2] Flutamide withdrawal, either alone[3] or in combination with aminoglutethimide,[4] may also be useful in the treatment of prostate cancer.

## PHARMACOLOGY

**Mechanism of Action.** Flutamide has demonstrated potent antiandrogenic effects in animal studies.[5] This is thought to occur by inhibition of androgen uptake or nuclear binding of androgen in target tissues, or both. It does not appear to relate to any direct effect on the production of androgens by the adrenal glands.[6] The fact that flutamide withdrawal can result in a secondary response in patients with advanced prostate cancer raises the possibility that flutamide may also act as an agonist in vivo. This phenomenon has been reported for antiandrogens in vitro, and it deserves further study.[3, 7]

**Resistance.** Mechanisms of resistance are incompletely defined.

**Pharmacokinetics.** The drug is rapidly and completely absorbed after oral administration.[8] It is rapidly metabolized to active and inactive metabolites, with the putative active hydroxylated product reaching a maximum plasma level by 2 hours. The active metabolite approaches steady-state levels after the fourth dose, at which time it is 94 to 96% bound to plasma proteins. The plasma clearance of this metabolite is 6 to 10 hours. The vast majority of the drug is excreted by the kidneys, with about half of this as unchanged drug.

**Drug and Radiation Interactions.** Flutamide can increase the prothrombin time in patients on long-term warfarin therapy. Close monitoring of prothrombin times is recommended when warfarin and flutamide are used together.

## TOXICITY

**Overview.** The principal effect of flutamide is to induce an androgen deficiency state in men. This can cause hot flashes (61%), loss of libido (36%), impotence (33%), and gynecomastia (9%). Other important effects include diarrhea (12%), which is usually mild, and hepatic dysfunction (1 to 9%), which can be severe and life threatening.

**Digestive System.** Nausea, vomiting, and diarrhea occur in 11 to 12% of patients. These tend to be mild, although diarrhea is severe in about 5% of patients. Anorexia develops in about 4% of patients Hepatic dysfunction may occur and can be life threatening. In one study, less than 1% of patients developed hepatic dysfunction, ranging from elevated levels of transaminase enzymes alone to clinically apparent hepatitis.[9] In a prospective study undertaken to estimate the frequency of hepatic dysfunction, 2 of 22 carefully monitored patients (9%) developed hepatic dysfunction.[10] One patient in this series developed hepatic necrosis and died. Others have reported fatal hepatic necrosis and hepatic encephalopathy as well.[11] It is prudent to monitor liver function in patients treated with this drug and to withdraw therapy promptly if elevated liver enzyme values are found.

**Endocrine-Metabolic.** The most frequent side effects of flutamide therapy are those associated with low serum androgen levels. These include hot flashes (61%), loss of libido (36%), impotence (about 33%), and gynecomastia (9%). In a sense, these are not side effects because the goal of therapy in patients with prostate cancer is to induce medical castration. Galactorrhea and tender gynecomastia can also occur.

**Other and Rare Reactions.** Edema affects 4% of patients.

*Hematologic.* Mild myelosuppression can occur, with rare leukopenia (3%) and thrombocytopenia (1%). Anemia is thought to occur about 6% of the time, although one trial of 19 men demonstrated mild anemia in all of the patients.[12] Hemolytic anemia, macrocytic anemia, and methemoglobinemia may also occur but only very rarely. One case report describes cyanosis unresponsive to methylene blue.[13]

*Immunologic.* Hypersensitivity reactions are rare.

*Mucocutaneous.* Rash occurs in 3% of patients; very rarely, photosensitivity occurs (erythema, bullous reactions, ulceration, epidermal necrolysis).[14]

*Cardiovascular.* Hypertension occurs in 1%.

*Pulmonary.* Nonspecific changes occur in 1%.

*Neurologic.* CNS reactions occur in 1% (drowsiness, confusion, depression, anxiety, nervousness).

*Musculoskeletal.* Myalgia and other minor complaints occur in 2%.

*Genitourinary.* Miscellaneous minor changes occur in a geriatric population (2%). The urine can change to amber or yellow-green, presumably from a drug metabolite.

*Reproductive.* Toxicity data place flutamide in FDA pregnancy category D.

*Carcinogenicity.* The drug is not mutagenic in the Ames test, but it causes testicular interstitial cell adenomas at all doses in rats. The carcinogenic potential of the drug is incompletely defined.

## DOSAGE AND ADMINISTRATION

The drug is available as a 125-mg capsule. The usual dosage is 250 mg three times daily at 8-hour intervals, for a total daily dose of 750 mg. An LHRH agonist or orchiectomy is used as concurrent therapy. Because of potential liver toxicity, periodic liver function tests should be performed.

## REFERENCES

1. Crawford ED, Eisenberger MA, McLeod DG, et al. A controlled trial of leuprolide with and without flutamide in prostatic carcinoma [erratum published in N Engl J Med 1989;321:1420]. N Engl J Med 1989;321:419–24.
2. Denis L, Murphy GP. Overview of phase III trials on combined androgen treatment in patients with metastatic prostate cancer. Cancer 1993;72:12 Suppl:3888–95.
3. Scher HI, Kelly WK. Flutamide withdrawal syndrome: its impact on clinical trials in hormone-refractory prostate cancer. J Clin Oncol 1993;11:1566–72.
4. Sartor O, Cooper M, Weinberger M, et al. Surprising activity of flutamide withdrawal, when combined with aminoglutethimide, in treatment of "hormone-refractory" prostate cancer [erratum published in J Natl Cancer Inst 1994;86:463]. J Natl Cancer Inst 1994;86:222–7.
5. Labrie F. Mechanism of action and pure antiandrogenic properties of flutamide. Cancer 1993;72:12 Suppl:3816–27.
6. Carlström K, Pousette A, Stege R. Flutamide has no effect on adrenal androgen response to acute ACTH stimulation in patients with prostatic cancer. Prostate 1990;17:219–25.
7. Brandes LJ, Queen GM, LaBella FS. Salutary clinical response of prostate cancer to antiandrogen withdrawal: assessment of flutamide in an in vitro paradigm predictive of tumor growth enhancement. Clin Cancer Res 1997;3:1357–61.
8. Brogden RN, Clissold SP. Flutamide: a preliminary review of its pharmacodynamic and pharmacokinetic properties, and therapeutic efficacy in advanced prostatic cancer. Drugs 1989;38:185–203.
9. Gomez JL, Dupont A, Cusan L, et al. Incidence of liver toxicity associated with the use of flutamide in prostate cancer patients. Am J Med 1992;92:465–70.
10. Cetin M, Demirci D, Unal A, et al. Frequency of flutamide induced hepatotoxicity in patients with prostate carcinoma. Hum Exp Toxicol 1999;18:137–40.
11. Wysowski DK, Freiman JP, Tourtelot JB, Horton ML III. Fatal and nonfatal hepatotoxicity associated with flutamide. Ann Intern Med 1993;118:860–4.
12. Ornstein DK, Beiser JA, Andriole GL. Anaemia in men receiving combined finasteride and flutamide therapy for advanced prostate cancer. BJU Int 1999;83:43–6.
13. Kouides PA, Abboud CN, Fairbanks VF. Flutamide-induced cyanosis refractory to methylene blue therapy. Br J Haematol 1996;94:73–5.
14. Yokote R, Tokura Y, Igarashi N, et al. Photosensitive drug eruption induced by flutamide. Eur J Dermatol 1998;8:427–9.

# Gemcitabine

Gemcitabine, 2′,2′-difluorodeoxycytidine, received wide attention when its initial approval in the United States was based not only on its antitumor efficacy but also on its ability to improve patients' quality of life. A synthetic nucleoside analogue, the drug is structurally similar to cytarabine but has a different spectrum of activity. It is currently marketed as Gemzar.

## EFFICACY

At present, gemcitabine is approved for use in pancreatic and non–small cell lung cancers. In phase III clinical trials, gemcitabine significantly improved patients' symptoms in locally advanced or metastatic pancreatic cancer. In one trial, untreated patients randomly assigned to treatment with gemcitabine had an improved clinical benefit response and a modest survival advantage compared with those treated with 5-FU.[1] In a similar trial, those who had been previously treated with 5-FU similarly received benefit.[2] Gemcitabine has also been studied extensively in advanced non–small cell lung cancer. In combination with cisplatin, the drug is effective as first-line therapy in advanced disease.[3] As a single agent, it is an effective second-line treatment as well.[4] In phase II trials published to date, the drug has demonstrated at least modest activity, alone and in combination, in cancers of the head and neck, kidneys, ovaries, breasts, bile ducts, testicles, and bladder.[5–11]

## PHARMACOLOGY

**Mechanism of Action.** Similar to other antimetabolites, gemcitabine exerts its effect by prohibiting DNA chain elongation. The drug requires intracellular phosphorylation using deoxycytidine kinase (dCk) in order for it to affect DNA synthesis through inhibition of DNA polymerases.[12] Gemcitabine is a more potent inhibitor of DNA synthesis than cytarabine (perhaps accounting for its broader spectrum of antitumor activity) owing to its ability to create a positive feedback loop for its own intracellular activation. Blocking ribonucleotide reductase, the agent can prevent de novo nucleoside production, which ultimately leads to more available enzyme for gemcitabine's own in vivo activity. This drug appears to exert its maximal effect on cells undergoing DNA synthesis (S phase) and on cells at the boundary between the first growth phase ($G_1$) and the S phase.[13]

**Resistance.** As can be inferred, cells lacking in dCk are resistant to the effects of drugs such as gemcitabine and cytarabine. More recent experiments describe functional nucleoside transporters presumably required for gemcitabine influx into cancer cells. Cells lacking these transporters would be resistant to the drug's effects (and toxicities).[14]

**Pharmacokinetics.** Pharmacokinetic studies reveal gemcitabine to be metabolized almost exclusively in the kidneys. When the drug is given as approved (30-minute infusions), it has a short half-life (range, 32 to 94 minutes) and a high clearance according to a two-compartment model.[15] Longer infusions have been studied, with, as expected, longer half-lives. Clearance can be reduced in the elderly and in women of all age groups. No specific information is known about dose reductions for those with renal or hepatic impairment.

**Drug Interactions.** There are no known drug-drug interactions.

## TOXICITY

**Overview.** Myelosuppression is this agent's dose-limiting toxicity. Generally speaking, gemcitabine can be administered with ease to a majority of patients. The following description of the incidence of drug side effects is taken from the package insert and the pivotal trials in patients with pancreatic cancer.

**Hematologic.** Although this is the drug's dose-limiting toxicity, less than 1% of patients discontinued therapy for hematologic abnormalities. Nearly 20% of studied patients required RBC transfusions; less than 1% required platelet transfusions. In the pancreatic cancer pivotal trials, only 7% experienced neutrophil counts below 500/$\mu$L, although 62% had some sort of neutropenia during treatment. Doses should of course be modified for those patients experiencing severe neutropenia or thrombocytopenia.

**Gastrointestinal.** Nausea and vomiting occur (up to 69%) but are usually quite mild. Antiemetic prophylaxis can generally be accomplished with agents such as the phenothiazines. Rarely, stronger premedication is required. Although diarrhea has been reported (19%), it is also often mild, as are the rare side effects of mucositis and liver function abnormalities.

**Dermatologic.** The original phase I trials of gemcitabine reported a 20% incidence of a generalized pruritic maculopapular rash, which required interruption of treatment. In the subsequent pivotal trials in pancreatic cancer, the rash was observed in nearly 30%, although of only mild to moderate severity. It now requires discontinuing the drug only rarely.

**Fever.** Fever was the most common nonhematologic side effect in early gemcitabine studies. In subsequent trials, it occurred in 41% of patients, considerably out of proportion to the incidence of infection. The drug-induced fever can be accompanied by flu-like symptoms, which resolve spontaneously after discontinuing the drug. The syndrome is easily managed with supportive care.

**Edema.** Gemcitabine can cause peripheral edema (20%), with less than 1% of patients needing to stop therapy.

**Other.** Other reported side effects included alopecia (15%), mild peripheral neuropathies (10%), and an extremely rare drug-induced pneumonitis.

## DOSAGE AND ADMINISTRATION

Gemcitabine is available for parenteral administration in vials of 200 mg and 1 g, which should be reconstituted with normal saline to a maximum concentration of 40 mg/ml. Care should be taken to avoid infusing solutions that appear to contain particulate matter or discoloration.

Adult dosing of gemcitabine is 1000 mg/m$^2$ intravenously weekly over 30 minutes. The drug should be given sequentially for 7 weeks (or until toxicity) before it is discontinued for a week. Subsequent cycles should include 3 weeks of therapy followed by a week of rest. Prior to each week of treatment, patients should be monitored with CBCs. For neutrophil counts between 500 and 999/$\mu$L or platelet counts between 50,000 and 99,000/$\mu$L, the dose should be reduced by 25%. For lower neutrophil or platelet counts, the drug should be withheld until the toxicity resolves. For patients who complete an entire first 7-week cycle without myelosuppression (neutrophil counts always >1500/$\mu$L and platelet counts >100,000/$\mu$L), gemcitabine dose may be escalated by 25%.

Finally, patients' renal and hepatic function should be monitored carefully, and those who are elderly should be observed more often because clearance can be impaired by age and hepatorenal function.

## REFERENCES

1. Burris HA III, Moore MJ, Andersen J, et al. Improvements in survival and clinical benefit with gemcitabine as first-line therapy for patients with advanced pancreas cancer: a randomized trial. J Clin Oncol 1997;15:2403–13.
2. Rothenberg ML, Moore MJ, Cripps MC, et al. A phase II trial of gemcitabine in patients with 5-FU–refractory pancreas cancer. Ann Oncol 1996;7:347–53.
3. Crino L, Scagliotti G, Marangolo M, et al. Cisplatin-gemcitabine combination in advanced non–small-cell lung cancer: a phase II study. J Clin Oncol 1997;15:297–303.
4. Crino L, Mosconi AM, Scagliotti GV, et al. Gemcitabine as second-line treatment for relapsing or refractory advanced non–small cell lung cancer: a phase II trial. Semin Oncol 1998;25:Suppl 9:23–6.
5. Fountzilas G, Athanassiades A, Kalogera-Fountzila A, et al. Paclitaxel in combination with carboplatin or gemcitabine for the treatment of advanced head and neck cancer. Semin Oncol 1997;24:Suppl 19:S19-28–32.
6. Rohde D, Thiemann D, Wildberger J, et al. Treatment of renal cancer patients with gemcitabine (2′,2′-difluorodeoxycytidine) and interferons: antitumor activity and toxicity. Oncol Rep 1998;5:1555–60.
7. Friedlander M, Millward MJ, Bell D, et al. A phase II study of gemcitabine in platinum pre-treated patients with advanced epithelial ovarian cancer. Ann Oncol 1998;9:1343–5.
8. Possinger K, Kaufmann M, Coleman R, et al. Phase II study of

gemcitabine as first-line chemotherapy in patients with advanced or metastatic breast cancer. Anticancer Drugs 1999;10:155–62.

9. Raderer M, Hejna MH, Valencak JB. Two consecutive phase II studies of 5-fluorouracil/leucovorin/mitomycin C and of gemcitabine in patients with advanced biliary cancer. Oncology 1999;56:177–80.

10. Bokemeyer C, Gerl A, Schoffski P, et al. Gemcitabine in patients with relapsed or cisplatin-refractory testicular cancer. J Clin Oncol 1999;17:512–6.

11. Lorusso V, Pollera CF, Antimi M, et al: A phase II study of gemcitabine in patients with transitional cell carcinoma of the urinary tract previously treated with platinum. Italian Co-operative Group on Bladder Cancer. Eur J Cancer 1998;34:1208–12.

12. Guchelaar H-J, Richel DJ, van Knapen A. Clinical, toxicological and pharmacological aspects of gemcitabine. Cancer Treat Rev 1996;22:15–31.

13. Huang P, Plunkett W. Fludarabine- and gemcitabine-induced apoptosis: incorporation of analogs into DNA is a critical event. Cancer Chemother Pharmacol 1995;36:181–8.

14. Mackey JR, Mani RS, Selner M, et al. Functional nucleoside transporters are required for gemcitabine influx and manifestation of toxicity in cancer cell lines. Cancer Res 1998;58:4349–57.

15. Storniolo AM, Allerheiligen SR, Pearce HL. Preclinical, pharmacologic, and phase I studies of gemcitabine. Semin Oncol 1997;24:Suppl 7:S7-2–7.

# Goserelin

Goserelin acetate is a potent analogue of LHRH, also known as a GnRH agonist analogue.[1] The drug is also known as Zoladex, ICI 118630, and NSC-606864.

## EFFICACY

Goserelin has been approved by the FDA for the palliative treatment of advanced prostate cancer as an alternative to orchiectomy. It is also used for the palliative treatment of breast cancer in premenopausal and perimenopausal women.[2] It is being studied for possible therapeutic use for a variety of benign gynecologic conditions.[3] Goserelin has the same spectrum of antitumor efficacy as leuprolide, but it is less expensive.

## PHARMACOLOGY

**Mechanisms of Action and Resistance.** See the discussion of leuprolide, which has an identical mechanism of action.

**Pharmacokinetics.** Goserelin is supplied as a small continuous-release pellet for subcutaneous administration. Two preparations are available, a 3.6-mg implant for use monthly and a 10.8-mg implant for use every 3 months.

After subcutaneous insertion of the 3.6-mg implant, peak drug concentrations in serum are achieved by 12 to 15 days. Absorption is slow after initial insertion, but after 8 days absorption is rapid and continuous for the remainder of the 28-day dosing period. With such 28-day dosing, the serum testosterone level is kept at levels seen in surgically castrated men. As with leuprolide, when goserelin is used for the first time there is a temporary surge of luteinizing hormone (LH), FSH, and sex hormones (testosterone in men and estrogen in women).

The pharmacodynamic effects of the 10.8-mg preparation are similar to those of the 3.6-mg pellet, except for less reliable suppression of estrogen in female patients. The peak plasma level is reached more quickly than with the 3.6-mg preparation.

Elimination of goserelin is primarily renal (>90%), with the liver providing a smaller component of elimination (<10%).

**Drug and Radiation Interactions.** None is known.

## TOXICITY

**Overview.** Goserelin induces medical orchiectomy in men and medical oophorectomy in women, with all of the symptoms of hypogonadism. The most prominent changes are hot flashes, decreased libido, reduced bone mass, and, in men, decreased erections. Goserelin can initially induce a surge of testosterone in men that can exacerbate bone pain, cause ureteral obstruction due to prostate enlargement, and precipitate cord compression in patients with epidural metastases.

**Reproductive.** Toxicity data place goserelin in FDA pregnancy category X. The drug is contraindicated in nursing and pregnant women.

**Endocrine-Metabolic.** The following effects can occur: hot flashes (6%); sexual dysfunction (21%); decreased erections (18%); gynecomastia (1 to 5%); and gout, hyperglycemia, and weight gain (1 to 5%).

**Other and Rare Reactions.** The following effects can occur: lethargy (8%), edema (7%), sweating (6%), and chills and fever (1 to 5%).

*Hematologic.* Anemia occurs in 1 to 5% of patients.

*Immunologic.* LHRH agonist analogues are known to cause hypersensitivity reactions, antibody production, and very rare anaphylaxis.[4, 5]

*Digestive System.* The following effects can occur: anorexia (5%); nausea (5%); and constipation, diarrhea, ulcer, and emesis (1 to 5%).

*Mucocutaneous.* Rash is observed in 6% of patients.

*Cardiovascular.* Congestive heart failure occurs in 5% of patients; arrhythmias, cerebrovascular accident, hypertension, myocardial infarction, peripheral vascular disorders, and chest pain occur in 1 to 5%.

*Pulmonary.* Upper respiratory tract infections are intercurrent in 7% of patients; exacerbation of chronic obstructive pulmonary disease occurs in 5%.

*Ocular.* Unspecified abnormalities, such as blurred vision, occur in less than 1% of patients.

*Neurologic.* The following effects can occur: dizziness (5%); insomnia (5%); and anxiety, depression, and headache (1 to 5%).

*Musculoskeletal.* Transient increases in bone pain can occur in patients with bone metastases (flare reaction). Prolonged use of goserelin is associated with bone loss equivalent to that seen in postmenopausal women. Relapsing polychondritis with cutaneous manifestations has been reported in a single patient.[6]

*Genitourinary.* Lower urinary tract disorders occur in 13% of patients; renal insufficiency, urinary obstruction, and urinary tract infection occur in 1 to 5%.

*Carcinogenicity.* Goserelin is not mutagenic in vitro, and it has not been associated with delayed second malignancies in humans. In rats given massive doses of the drug, an increased incidence of benign pituitary macroadenomas was found. Massive doses in mice have been associated with histiocytic sarcomas of the bone marrow. The relevance of these animal neoplasms to human carcinogenesis is unknown.

## DOSAGE AND ADMINISTRATION

Goserelin is provided as a sterile, totally biodegradable pellet containing the equivalent of 3.6 mg of goserelin acetate in a disposable syringe device. The pellet is inserted under the skin of the upper abdominal wall through a 16-gauge needle after preparing the skin, usually with an alcohol swab and a local anesthetic. A single pellet is administered subcutaneously every 28 days. In the event that the pellet must be removed, it can be localized by ultrasonography. This preparation may be used in both women with breast cancer and men with prostate cancer.

The 10.8-mg pellet is used in a similar fashion every 3 weeks for men with prostate cancer but not for women with breast cancer.

Goserelin is contraindicated during pregnancy, in women who are breast-feeding, and in patients with known hypersensitivity to the drug or its constituents.

## REFERENCES

1. Conn PM, Crowley WF Jr. Gonadotropin-releasing hormone and its analogs. Annu Rev Med 1994;45:391-405.
2. Taylor CW, Green S, Dalton WS, et al. Multicenter randomized clinical trial of goserelin versus surgical ovariectomy in premenopausal patients with receptor-positive metastatic breast cancer: an intergroup study. J Clin Oncol 1998;16:994-9.
3. Perry CM, Brogden RN. Goserelin: a review of its pharmacodynamic and pharmacokinetic properties, and therapeutic use in benign gynaecological disorders. Drugs 1996;51:319-46.
4. MacLeod TL, Eisen A, Sussman GL. Anaphylactic reaction to synthetic luteinizing hormone-releasing hormone. Fertil Steril 1987;48:500-2.
5. Raj SG, Karadsheh AJ, Guillot RJ, et al. Case report: systemic hypersensitivity reaction to goserelin acetate. Am J Med Sci 1996;312:187-90.
6. Labarthe MP, Bayle-Lebey P, Bazex J. Cutaneous manifestations of relapsing polychondritis in a patient receiving goserelin for carcinoma of the prostate. Dermatology 1997;195:391-4.

# Hydroxyurea

Although it was synthesized in 1869 and found to be bone marrow suppressive in 1928, hydroxyurea was not used as a treatment for cancer until the early 1960s. Hydroxyurea is a small, relatively simple antimetabolite. It is also known as Hydrea, hydroxycarbamide, OH-urea, and NSC-32065.

## EFFICACY

Hydroxyurea is used in the treatment of chronic granulocytic leukemia and to a lesser extent in the management of polycythemia vera and other myeloproliferative syndromes. It may be of occasional use in carcinomas of the prostate, ovary,

lung, kidney, and head and neck. Hydroxyurea appears to be useful in the management of sickle cell anemia.[1] Investigational high-dose therapy is being studied for possible use in BMT[2] and as an agent for the modification of multiple drug resistance.[3] It is being studied as a potential inhibitor of the human immunodeficiency virus (HIV).[4]

## PHARMACOLOGY

**Mechanism of Action.** Hydroxyurea inhibits ribonucleotide reductase—an enzyme that is essential to DNA synthesis—by quenching the tyrosyl free radical at the active site of the M2 protein subunit of the enzyme.[5] This leads to selective inhibition of DNA synthesis through the depletion of essential DNA precursors (deoxyribonucleoside triphosphates). Cell death then occurs in the S phase, with a resultant synchronization of surviving cells.[6] Cell death itself occurs through apoptosis.[7] The cytotoxicity of the drug is limited to dividing cells and does not appear to include any important inhibition of RNA or protein synthesis. It does, however, have several other interesting effects. First, it increases the production of fetal hemoglobin, which has an inhibitory effect on polymerization of sickle cell hemoglobin.[8] These effects form the basis for hydroxyurea therapy of sickle cell disease. Second, it may cause direct chemical damage of DNA. Free radical scavengers have been reported to protect against this damage.[9] The drug has been reported to inhibit DNA repair,[5] and it accelerates the loss of extrachromosomally amplified genes from tumor cells, including amplified drug resistance genes.[10]

**Resistance.** Resistance to hydroxyurea is complex, with most studies pointing to the key role of ribonucleotide reductase in drug resistance. This may be due to changes in the enzyme itself or to gene amplification resulting in increased intracellular levels of the enzyme.[11, 12] Resistance may also be associated with coamplification of genes for ornithine decarboxylase and ribonucleotide reductase.[13]

**Pharmacokinetics.** Hydroxyurea is readily absorbed from the gastrointestinal tract and reaches a maximal plasma level by 2 hours after a single oral dose. It is metabolized to a free radical nitroxide and transported widely. The plasma clearance varies from 2 to 5 hours, leading to essentially zero plasma levels by 24 hours. Hydroxyurea readily crosses the blood-brain barrier, and it is excreted into breast milk. About a third to a half of an administered dose is excreted unchanged in the urine; the other half is metabolized by the liver and excreted as respiratory carbon dioxide and urea. Limited studies of long-term intravenous infusions of hydroxyurea suggest that this approach to treatment is feasible in future investigational trials.[14]

**Drug and Radiation Interactions.** Hydroxyurea appears to enhance the DNA breakage and cytotoxic effects of radiation therapy and several chemotherapeutic drugs, such as the intercalating antibiotics and cytarabine.[15] It may also modulate the activity of purine antimetabolites and inhibitors of topoisomerase II.[16] The clinical importance of these interactions is under investigation.

## TOXICITY

**Overview.** Myelosuppression is the predominant toxic side effect of the drug. Other, usually minor effects include stomatitis, nausea, reversible dermatologic reactions, and rare neurologic changes.

**Hematologic.** The most important adverse reaction from hydroxyurea is bone marrow depression, involving leukopenia, megaloblastic anemia, and, rarely, thrombocytopenia. If myelosuppression develops, recovery may be delayed by previous bone marrow–suppressive therapy or radiation therapy.

**Immunologic.** Rare hypersensitivity reactions occur, including cross-sensitivity to tartrazine dye.

**Digestive System.** Nausea and vomiting are uncommon, and when they occur they are generally only mild to moderate in severity. Constipation, diarrhea, and anorexia are rare. Hepatic dysfunction (elevated levels of transaminase enzymes and very rare jaundice) can occur.

**Mucocutaneous.** Mucositis is rare. Occasional alopecia, hyperpigmentation, scaling, atrophy, nail changes, radiation-recall reactions, maculopapular rash, pruritus, and erythema of the hands, feet, or face can occur. Leg ulceration appears to be more common with long-term therapy and may require skin grafts for management.[17]

**Other and Rare Reactions.** Flu-like reactions, malaise, and drug fever[18] can occur.

**Pulmonary.** Pulmonary dysfunction due to edema,[19] acute alveolitis,[20] or interstitial pneumonitis[21] occurs rarely.

**Neurologic.** Very rarely, headache, dizziness, drowsiness, disorientation, hallucinations, and seizures can occur.

**Genitourinary.** Azotemia, proteinuria, and dysuria all are rare.

**Reproductive.** Toxicity data place hydroxyurea in FDA pregnancy category D. The drug is teratogenic in animals, so its use in pregnant women should be avoided. A case of pregnancy during hydroxyurea therapy for sickle cell disease has been reported.[22] The infant was normal, but the pregnancy was complicated by vaso-occlusive crises.

**Carcinogenicity.** The drug is mutagenic; its carcinogenic potential is uncertain. Multiple skin tumors have been reported with long-term use of the drug,[23, 24] and it probably increases the risk of acute leukemia in patients with polycythemia rubra vera.[25, 26]

## DOSAGE AND ADMINISTRATION

Hydroxyurea is available as 500-mg capsules. The drug is usually given as a single daily oral dose of 20 to 30 mg/kg to patients with chronic granulocytic leukemia. If the patient is unable to swallow capsules, the contents of the capsule can be emptied into a glass of water and immediately taken. Hydroxyurea is used in the treatment of various solid tumors. When it is combined with radiation therapy, an intermittent dose of 80 mg/kg is generally administered every 3 days. Hydroxyurea should not be given to patients with pre-existing marked bone marrow suppression (WCC <2500/μL or platelets <100,000/μL). It should be used with caution in elderly patients and in patients with renal dysfunction.

## REFERENCES

1. Maier-Redelsperger M, Labie D, Elion J. Long-term hydroxyurea treatment in young sickle cell patients. Curr Opin Hematol 1999;6:115–20.
2. Vaughan WP, Bierman PJ, Reed EC, et al. High-dose hydroxyurea in autologous bone marrow transplantation: a promising "new" agent. Semin Oncol 1992;19:Suppl 9:110–5.
3. Christen RD, Shalinsky DR, Howell SB. Enhancement of the loss of multiple drug resistance by hydroxyurea. Semin Oncol 1992;19:Suppl 9:94–100.
4. Romanelli F, Pomeroy C, Smith KM. Hydroxyurea to inhibit human immunodeficiency virus-1 replication. Pharmacotherapy 1999;19:196–204.
5. Yarbro JW. Mechanism of action of hydroxyurea. Semin Oncol 1992;19 Suppl 9:1–10.
6. Skog S, Tribukait B, Wallstrom B, Eriksson S. Hydroxyurea-induced cell death as related to cell cycle in mouse and human T-lymphoma cells. Cancer Res 1987;47:Part 1:6490–3.
7. Gui CY, Jiang C, Xie HY, Qian RL. The apoptosis of HEL cells induced by hydroxyurea. Cell Res 1997;7:91–7.
8. Charache S. Mechanism of action of hydroxyurea in the management of sickle cell anemia in adults. Semin Hematol 1997;34:3:Suppl 3:15–21.
9. Przybyszewski WM, Malec J. Hydroxyurea, methotrexate and adriblastine can mediate non-enzymatic reduction of nitroblue tetrazolium with NADH which is inhibited by superoxide dismutase. Biochem Pharmacol 1987;36:3312–4.
10. Von Hoff DD, Waddelow T, Forseth B, et al. Hydroxyurea accelerates loss of extrachromosomally amplified genes from tumor cells. Cancer Res 1991;51:6273–9.
11. Carter GL, Cory JG. Cross-resistance patterns in hydroxyurea-resistant leukemia L 1210 cells. Cancer Res 1988;48:5796–9.
12. Choy BK, McClarty GA, Chan AK, et al. Molecular mechanisms of drug resistance involving ribonucleotide reductase: hydroxyurea resistance in a series of clonally related mouse cell lines selected in the presence of increasing drug concentrations. Cancer Res 1988;48:2029–35.
13. Ask A, Persson L, Rehnholm A, et al. Development of resistance to hydroxyurea during treatment of human myelogenous leukemia K562 cells with alpha-difluoromethylornithine as a result of coamplification of genes for ornithine decarboxylase and ribonucleotide reductase R2 subunit. Cancer Res 1993;53:5262–8.
14. Blumenreich MS, Kellihan MJ, Joseph UG, et al. Long-term intravenous hydroxyurea infusions in patients with advanced cancer. Cancer 1993;71:2828–32.
15. Minford J, Kerrigan D, Nichols M, et al. Enhancement of the DNA breakage and cytotoxic effects of intercalating agents by treatment with sublethal doses of 1-beta-D-arabinofuranosylcytosine or hydroxyurea in L1210 cells. Cancer Res 1984;44:5583–93.
16. Schilsky RL, Ratain MJ, Vokes EE, et al. Laboratory and clinical studies of biochemical modulation by hydroxyurea. Semin Oncol 1992;19 Suppl 9:84–9.
17. Kato N, Kimura K, Yasukawa K, Yoshida K. Hydroxyurea-related leg ulcers in a patient with chronic myelogenous leukemia: a case report and review of the literature. J Dermatol 1999;26:56–62.
18. Cheung AY, Browne B, Capen C. Hydroxyurea-induced fever in cervical carcinoma: case report and review of the literature. Cancer Invest 1999;17:245–8.
19. Bauman JL, Shulruff S, Hasegawa GR, et al. Fever caused by hydroxyurea. Arch Intern Med 1981;141:260–1.
20. Jackson GH, Wallis J, Ledingham J, et al. Hydroxyurea induced acute alveolitis in a patient with chronic myeloid leukaemia. Cancer Chemother Pharmacol 1990;27:168–9.
21. Quintâas-Cardama A, Pâerez-Encinas M, Gonzalez S, et al. Hydroxyurea-induced acute interstitial pneumonitis in a patient with essential thrombocythemia. Ann Hematol 1999;78:187–8.
22. Diav-Citrin O, Hunnisett L, Sher GD, Koren G. Hydroxyurea use during pregnancy: a case report in sickle cell disease and review of the literature. Am J Hematol 1999;60:148–50.
23. Stasi R, Cantonetti M, Abruzzese E. Multiple skin tumors in long-term treatment with hydroxyurea. Eur J Haematol 1992;48:121–2.
24. Best PJ, Petitt RM. Multiple skin cancers associated with hydroxyurea therapy. Mayo Clin Proc 1998;73:961–3.
25. Weinfeld A, Swolin B, Westin J. Acute leukaemia after hydroxyurea therapy in polycythaemia vera and allied disorders: prospective study of efficacy and leukaemogenicity with therapeutic implications. Eur J Haematol 1994;52:134–9.
26. Sterkers Y, Preudhomme C, Laèl JL, et al. Acute myeloid leukemia and myelodysplastic syndromes following essential thrombocythemia treated with hydroxyurea: high proportion of cases with 17p deletion. Blood 1998;91:616–22.

# Idarubicin

Idarubicin was developed as a structural analogue of dauno-rubicin by deleting the methoxy group from position 4 of the chromophore ring. Other names for this agent include Idamycin, 4-demethoxydaunorubicin, and NSC-256439.

## EFFICACY

The drug is marketed for the treatment of AML (see Chapter 84). Preliminary data suggest that it may be superior to daunorubicin for this purpose.[1] Idarubicin is being studied for possible use in the treatment of myelodysplastic syndromes[2] and ALL[3] and as a part of preparative regimens before allogeneic BMT.[4]

## PHARMACOLOGY

**Mechanisms of Action and Resistance.** The fundamental mechanisms of action and resistance are probably the same as those for doxorubicin and daunorubicin, although minor differences have been reported in the quantitative spectrum of molecular effects. Idarubicin is more lipid soluble than daunorubicin, leading to more rapid cellular uptake and enhanced DNA damage. The drug is considered cell cycle nonspecific, although the S phase is probably more sensitive than the other phases. It may be more effective than other anthracyclines in cells expressing the mdr phenotype.[5, 6] Idarubicin is less affected by topoisomerase II–related multidrug resistance than is daunorubicin.[7]

**Pharmacokinetics.** Idarubicin is poorly absorbed orally. After intravenous administration, the drug is metabolized in the liver to several metabolites, including idarubicinol. It is predominantly excreted in bile (about 25%), with only minimal urinary excretion (2 to 3%). The average elimination half-life of idarubicinol is about 22 hours, whereas the half-life for idarubicin is about 55 hours. Both idarubicin and idarubicinol cross the blood-brain barrier into the CSF (20% and 10% respectively).[8]

**Drug and Radiation Interactions.** These are presumed to mirror those reported for doxorubicin and daunorubicin.

## TOXICITY

The spectrum of toxicity and precautions for use are essentially identical to those for doxorubicin and daunorubicin.

## DOSAGE AND ADMINISTRATION

Idarubicin is available as a lyophilized powder for intravenous injection in vials of 5 and 10 mg. Incompatibilities are similar to those described for doxorubicin.

The usual dosage is 12 mg/m² by slow infusion over 10 to 15 minutes daily for 3 days, combined with cytarabine. Precautions are identical to those described for doxorubicin, including the use of extravasation precautions, although the maximal cumulative dose for avoiding cardiotoxicity has not been established.

## REFERENCES

1. AML Collaborative Group. A systematic collaborative overview of randomized trials comparing idarubicin with daunorubicin (or other anthracyclines) as induction therapy of acute myeloid leukaemia. Br J Haematol 1998;103:100–9.
2. Estey EH, Kantarjian H, Keating M. Idarubicin plus continuous-infusion high-dose cytarabine as treatment for patients with acute myelogenous leukemia or myelodysplastic syndrome. Semin Oncol 1993;20:Suppl 8:1–5.
3. Bassan R, Battista R, Viero P, et al. Intensive therapy for adult acute lymphoblastic leukemia: preliminary results of the idarubicin/vincristine/L-asparaginase/prednisolone regimen. Semin Oncol 1993;20:Suppl 8:39–46.
4. Muus P, Donnelly P, Schattenberg A. Idarubicin-related side effects in recipients of T-cell depleted allogeneic bone marrow transplants are schedule dependent. Semin Oncol 1993;20:Suppl 8:47–52.
5. Berman E, McBride M. Comparative cellular pharmacology of daunorubicin and idarubicin in human multidrug-resistant leukemia cells. Blood 1992;79:3267–73.
6. Petrini M, Mattii L, Valentini P, et al. Idarubicin is active on MDR cells: evaluation of DNA synthesis inhibition on P388 cell lines. Ann Hematol 1993;67:227–30.
7. Fukushima T, Inoue H, Takemura H, et al. Idarubicin and idarubicinol are less affected by topoisomerase II-related multidrug resistance than is daunorubicin. Leukemia Res 1998;22:625–9.
8. Ganzina F, Pacciarini MA, Di Pietro N. Idarubicin (4-demethoxydaunorubicin). A preliminary overview of preclinical and clinical studies. Invest New Drugs 1986;4:85–105.

# Ifosfamide with Mesna

Infosfamide was synthesized in the mid-1960s in West Germany as an isomer of cyclophosphamide in which one chloroethyl group is present on each of the nitrogen atoms. Initial preclinical studies of the drug demonstrated severe dose-limiting urothelial toxicity. However, the use of ifosfamide with the free radical scavenger mesna has led to a renaissance of interest in the drug.[1] Other names for ifosfamide include isophosphamide, Ifex, IFOS, and NSC-109724. Other names for mesna include mesnum, Mesnex, sodium-2-mercaptoethanesulfonate, uromitexan, and NSC-113891.

## EFFICACY

Ifosfamide has a broad spectrum of activity against both animal and human tumors. This spectrum is very similar to that of cyclophosphamide, although there are clearly some differences. Specifically, ifosfamide appears to be more active than cyclophosphamide against testicular cancer and sarcomas.

## PHARMACOLOGY

**Mechanism of Action.** The mechanism of action of ifosfamide is presumed to be identical to that of cyclophosphamide, although subtle differences in the molecular pharmacology of the two drugs are possible because of the different locations of the two chloroethyl chains. Namely, both chloroethyl groups are on a single nitrogen for cyclophosphamide, whereas they are on different nitrogen molecules separated by a phosphorus for ifosfamide. Despite this difference in chemical structure, most authorities ascribe the differences in cytotoxicity to subtle differences in their metabolism. Specifically, ifosfamide undergoes a slower rate of initial hydroxylation in the liver, and it undergoes a high order of dechloroethylation of the alkylating side chain. This results in a marked loss of alkylating activity. Mesna does not inhibit the antitumor activity of ifosfamide.[2] As with cyclophosphamide, ifosfamide is considered cell cycle phase nonspecific.

**Resistance.** Ifosfamide appears to be cross-resistant with cyclophosphamide in L1210 leukemia in mice, but some investigators consider cyclophosphamide and ifosfamide to be non–cross-resistant when used against certain animal and human tumors, especially lymphomas. Nevertheless, mechanisms of resistance are probably the same for the two drugs.

### Pharmacokinetics

*Ifosfamide.* The metabolic transformations of ifosfamide are identical to those of cyclophosphamide; however, the alterations in structure affect the relative rates of these metabolic changes, leading to different pharmacokinetics for the two isomers. Compared with cyclophosphamide, much more of the drug is excreted into the urine as unchanged drug (about 50% of ifosfamide compared with <10% for cyclophosphamide). There is also greater conversion of ifosfamide to inactive metabolites through the mechanism of dechloroethylation.

The plasma clearance of ifosfamide is schedule dependent. With large single doses (3.8 to 5.0 g/m$^2$), the terminal half-life is about 16 hours. When divided daily doses of ifosfamide are given (1.6 to 2.4 g/m$^2$), the terminal half-life is about 7 hours. There is only modest penetration of the drug past the blood-brain barrier into the CSF.

Ifosfamide may be unique among the alkylating agents in being schedule dependent. Five-day courses of the drug are considered better than single-day bolus therapy. This is thought to relate to autoinduction of its own metabolism.[3]

*Mesna.* After intravenous injection, mesna is rapidly oxidized to its only known metabolite, dimesna. This disulfide is physiologically inert and rapidly constitutes more than 75% of the dose injected. The vast majority of the injected mesna and its metabolite remain within the vascular system until undergoing rapid glomerular filtration. The plasma half-life in humans is about 1.5 hours.

**Drug Interactions.** Acetylcysteine and mesna decrease the urotoxicity of ifosfamide. Prior or concurrent use of cisplatin may increase the neurotoxicity[4] and nephrotoxicity[5] of the drug. Sedatives, such as lorazepam and opiates, may potentiate the neurotoxicity of ifosfamide. Methylene blue may be an antidote for cerebral toxicity due to ifosfamide.[6]

## TOXICITY

**Overview.** Preclinical studies have shown mesna to be relatively nontoxic. No teratogenic or mutagenic effects have been identified with the drug. Only with high doses of mesna has any toxicity in humans been seen, and that appears to be limited to gastrointestinal toxicity. For all practical purposes, the adverse effects of ifosfamide and mesna therapy should be ascribed to ifosfamide. The predominant toxic side effects of ifosfamide are myelosuppression and urotoxicity, but alopecia, nausea, vomiting, and CNS effects can also occur.

**Hematologic.** Myelosuppression is dose related and dose limiting, following the same pattern as with cyclophosphamide. Very rarely, patients develop coagulation problems. Ifosfamide can cause stomatocytosis, and mesna can cause echinocytosis.[7] These RBC changes are associated with increased whole blood viscosity and are reversible.

**Digestive System.** Nausea and vomiting of a moderate to severe degree occur in up to 58% of patients. Anorexia, diarrhea, and constipation occur rarely. Transient elevations in liver function tests have been reported. Acute pancreatitis has been reported in two patients.[8]

**Mucocutaneous.** Alopecia is common (83 to 100%). Rare effects include urticaria, phlebitis, and stomatitis. Dermatitis is very rare. Hyperpigmentation has also been reported.[9] Stomatitis is dose limiting when ifosfamide is given in high doses. Propantheline reportedly protects the oral mucosa in such patients.[10]

**Neurologic.** CNS toxicity has been reported in numerous clinical trails of ifosfamide, with an incidence varying between 0 and 50% (average incidence, 12%). This usually takes the form of a reduced level of arousal, but this can progress through somnolence to coma and even death. Other CNS findings include confusion, hallucinations, forgetfulness, cerebellar signs, weakness, incontinence, and seizures. The signs of CNS toxicity usually start within 2 hours of a bolus dose and abate spontaneously within 1 to 3 days of cessation of ifosfamide. There has been no specific treatment for this condition in the past other than discontinuing ifosfamide therapy and avoiding drugs with known CNS effects. However, prophylaxis and reversal of ifosfamide encephalopathy have been reported with methylene blue (50 mg methylene blue in a 2% aqueous solution given as a slow intravenous injection).[6] There is some indication that CNS toxicity is dose related; pharmacogenetic differences may also be noted in the rate of dichloroethylation involved in the syndrome.[11] Peripheral neuropathy is also a rare complication of the drug.

**Genitourinary.** Hemorrhagic cystitis was such a prominent finding in the early clinical trials of ifosfamide that the full spectrum of toxicity could not be appreciated. It is now clear that hemorrhagic cystitis can be almost completely prevented by the use of mesna, and the drug is therefore marketed as a kit that includes this agent.

High-dose ifosfamide by continuous infusion has caused renal failure despite the use of mesna, and standard doses have caused subclinical nephrotoxicity. In one study of 120 pediatric patients, 66% developed proximal tubular wasting of amino acids and 38% had phosphate loss.[5] Prior nephrectomy and cisplatin administration were associated with a higher frequency of renal dysfunction. In another pediatric study, 22% of patients had significant renal dysfunction 1 year after ifosfamide administration. Five percent of the entire group developed severe nephrotoxicity (Fanconi's syndrome).[12] In another study, 41% of patients developed tubular dysfunction and 6% developed glomerular dysfunction. Nine percent developed severe nephrotoxicity, which was associated with cumulative ifosfamide doses of 45 g/m$^2$ and age younger than 3 years.[13] Rickets can be a late complication of this form of nephrotoxicity,[14] even in children without apparent acute nephrotoxicity.[15] It is apparent that ifosfamide can cause both tubular and glomerular damage, even with mesna, and these may develop after treatment is completed and may be progressive in some patients.[16] Patients receiving ifosfamide may require electrolyte repletion, including bicarbonate and potassium.

**Other and Rare Reactions.** Fever, fatigue, malaise, and increased salivation all occur in 1% of patients.

*Immunologic.* The drug is immunosuppressive, and it causes very rare hypersensitivity reactions.

*Cardiovascular.* Cardiac toxicity can occur at very high doses[17] but is extremely rare with standard doses. Hypertension (<1%) and hypotension (<1%) may also occur.

*Pulmonary.* Rare unspecified toxicity may occur.

*Ocular.* Blurred vision may occur.

*Reproductive.* Toxicity data place ifosfamide in FDA pregnancy category D. The drug is teratogenic and can induce sterility.

*Endocrine-Metabolic.* Electrolyte abnormalities (especially asymptomatic metabolic acidosis) and SIADH may occur (see also Genitourinary section).

*Carcinogenicity.* The drug is considered a potential carcinogen.

## DOSAGE AND ADMINISTRATION

Ifosfamide is available in 1- and 3-g vials packaged with 200- and 400-mg ampules of mesna, respectively. The usual dosage schedule of ifosamide for germ cell tumors is 1.2 g/m$^2$ given as a slow intravenous infusion over at least 30 minutes daily for 5 consecutive days, with repeat cycles every 3 weeks provided there has been hematologic recovery. Ifosfamide is given with 2 L of intravenous hydration per day plus mesna. Intravenous mesna is given with ifosfamide at 20% of the ifosfamide dose prior to and at 4 and 8 hours after each dose of ifosfamide, for a total dose that is 60% of the ifosfamide dose. Mesna is incompatible with cisplatin, so they cannot be administered concurrently through the same tubing. The optimal schedule, dose, and route of ifosfamide and mesna administration are still under study. Many authorities prefer to use ifosfamide by continuous infusion. Ifosfamide and mesna are stable for 9 days at temperatures up to 27° C.[18] This makes the drug a reasonable candidate for studies of continuous ambulatory infusion using an ambulatory pump.[19]

When continuous infusion therapy is chosen, mesna is given at the same dose at the same time continuously following a loading dose of mesna equal to 6 to 10% of the total ifosfamide dose. Overall, the mesna dose for continuous infusion is 100% of the ifosfamide dose.

## REFERENCES

1. Zalupski M, Baker LH. Ifosfamide. J Natl Cancer Inst 1988;80:556–66.
2. Bokemeyer C, Schmoll HJ, Ludwig E, et al. The antitumor activity of ifosfamide on heterotransplanted testicular cancer cell lines remains unaltered by the uroprotector mesna. Br J Cancer 1994;69:863–7.
3. Lind MJ, Roberts HL, Thatcher N, Idle JR. The effect of route of administration and fractionation of dose on the metabolism of ifosfamide. Cancer Chemother Pharmacol 1990;26:105–11.
4. Pratt CB, Goren MP, Meyer WH, et al. Ifosfamide neurotoxicity is related to previous cisplatin treatment for pediatric solid tumors. J Clin Oncol 1990;8:1399–401.
5. Rossi R, Godde A, Kleinebrand A, et al. Unilateral nephrectomy and

6. Küpfer A, Aeschlimann C, Wermuth B, Cerny T. Prophylaxis and reversal of ifosfamide encephalopathy with methylene-blue. Lancet 1994;343:763–4.
7. Reinhart WH, Baerlocher GM, Cerny T, et al. Ifosfamide-induced stomatocytosis and mesna-induced echinocytosis: influence on biorheological properties of blood. Eur J Haematol 1999;62:223–30.
8. Gerson R, Serrano A, Villalobos A, et al. Acute pancreatitis secondary to ifosfamide. J Emerg Med 1997;15:645–7.
9. Teresi ME, Murry DJ, Cornelius AS. Ifosfamide-induced hyperpigmentation. Cancer 1993;71:2873–5.
10. Oblon DJ, Paul SR, Oblon MB, Malik S. Propantheline protects the oral mucosa after high-dose ifosfamide, carboplatin, etoposide and autologous stem cell transplantation. Bone Marrow Transplant 1997;20:961–3.
11. Wainer IW, Ducharme J, Franvil CP, et al. Ifosfamide stereoselective dichloroethylation and neurotoxicity. Lancet 1994;343:982–3.
12. Suarez A, McDowell H, Niaudet P, et al. Long-term follow-up of ifosfamide renal toxicity in children treated for malignant mesenchymal tumors: an International Society of Pediatric Oncology report. J Clin Oncol 1991;9:2177–82.
13. Loebstein R, Atanackovic G, Bishai R, et al. Risk factors for long-term outcome of ifosfamide-induced nephrotoxicity in children. J Clin Pharmacol 1999;39:454–61.
14. Pratt CB, Meyer WH, Jenkins JJ, et al. Ifosfamide, Fanconi's syndrome, and rickets. J Clin Oncol 1991;9:1495–9.
15. Beckwith C, Flaharty KK, et al. Fanconi's syndrome due to ifosfamide. Bone Marrow Transplant 1993;11:71–3.
16. Prasad VK, Lewis IJ, Aparicio SR, et al. Progressive glomerular toxicity of ifosfamide in children. Med Pediatr Oncol 1996;27:149–55.
17. Quezado ZMN, Wilson WH, Cunnion RE, et al. High-dose ifosfamide is associated with severe, reversible cardiac dysfunction. Ann Intern Med 1993;118:31–6.
18. Radford JA, Margison JM, Swindell R, et al. The stability of ifosfamide in aqueous solution and its suitability for continuous 7-day infusion by ambulatory pump. Cancer Chemother Pharmacol 1990;26:144–6.
19. Loeffler TM, Weber FW, Hausamen TU. Ambulatory high-dose 5-day continuous-infusion ifosfamide combination chemotherapy in advanced solid tumors: a feasibility study. J Cancer Res Clin Oncol 1991;117:Suppl 4:S125–8.

## Irinotecan

Irinotecan, an agent with broad clinical activity, represents one of the first new drugs in a long time to be approved for use in advanced colorectal cancer. A semisynthetic derivative created from the *Camptotheca acuminata* tree, irinotecan acts by inhibiting the enzyme topoisomerase I. It is also known as CPT11 and Camptosar.

## EFFICACY

At present, irinotecan is approved in the United States for use in 5-FU–resistant advanced metastatic colorectal cancer. It was given fast-track approval for this indication because of the efficacy observed in three multicenter, open label phase II trials.[1, 2]

In these phase II trials, patients with advanced colorectal cancer that had progressed through only one prior 5-FU–based regimen were treated on the current U.S. schedule with 125 mg/m$^2$ weekly for 4 weeks, followed by a 2-week break. Prior adjuvant therapy was allowed if it occurred at least 6 to 12 months before the 5-FU regimen for advanced disease. In one group, patients were treated at 150 mg/m$^2$/wk, but this dosage was abandoned because of a perceived high rate of neutropenic fevers. Similarly, some patients were treated with 100 mg/m²/wk, but this too was abandoned because of perceived inferiority to the currently approved dose. Among the patients treated at the approved dosage of 125 mg/m²/wk, the overall response rate was 15% (95% confidence interval [CI] 10 to 20.1%). A larger group was found to have stable disease. Survival in these three different trials ranged from 8.1 to 10.7 months. Statistics for other clinical trials conducted in Europe (response, survival, and so on) appeared similar when irinotecan was given at 350 mg/m² every 3 weeks.[3] Since irinotecan was initially approved, other studies that explore the drug's efficacy have been completed. Two large phase III trials were conducted in Europe. The first compared the 350 mg/m² dose versus best supportive care in 5-FU–refractory patients.[4] Here, overall survival with irinotecan was statistically significantly longer at 6 months (73% vs. 54%), 9 months (53% vs. 29%) and 1 year (36% vs. 14%, $p = 0.0001$). Quality of life, as measured by the EORTC QLQ-C30 questionnaire, was also improved. A second study compared the 350 mg/m² dosage versus the best estimated infusional 5-FU dosage (de Gramont, Lokich, or German AIO regimens) in patients who previously had progressed through a first 5-FU–based regimen for advanced disease.[5] Here again, survival was improved with irinotecan therapy (45% vs. 32%, $p = 0.035$). Comparable quality of life measurements were seen between the two arms. No statistical differences were seen in medical care consumption or in side effects of diarrhea, nausea and vomiting, fatigue, or pain. With these two phase III trials, irinotecan's role in second-line therapy was secured.

A multicenter U.S. trial in untreated advanced colorectal cancer demonstrated a potential role for irinotecan as first-line therapy.[6] In this trial, 683 patients were randomly assigned to irinotecan alone, 5-FU/leucovorin alone on the Mayo Clinic schedule, or the combination irinotecan/5-FU/leucovorin. Patients treated with the three-drug combination had a significantly higher response rate (40% vs. 22% for 5-FU/leucovorin, $p = 0.001$) and a longer median time-to-treatment failure (54 months vs. 3.9 months for 5-FU/leucovorin, $p = 0.005$). A statistically significant improvement in overall survival was not observed. A second study, conducted in Europe in 385 patients, found a similar advantage to combination irinotecan/5-FU/leucovorin therapy when compared with 5-FU/leucovorin alone as first-line therapy.[7] The investigators reported improved response (41% vs. 23%, $p < 0.001$) and 1-year survival (69% vs. 59%, $p = 0.03$) for the three-drug combination.

Further ongoing studies are examining the role of irinotecan in adjuvant therapy for colorectal cancer, and an oral formulation is being developed. The drug has broad activity in other cancers as well. Studies using single agents and drug combinations have shown efficacy in small cell and non–small cell lung cancers and in cancers of the cervix, ovary, esophagus, stomach, breast, and brain, as well as in leukemias and lymphomas.[8–11]

## PHARMACOLOGY

Irinotecan is a camptothecin analogue. The camptothecins were discovered as part of a government program to screen biologic products for clinical use.[12] In preclinical studies, the camptothecins were active against a broad range of tumor types. In the earliest human trials, however, they were extremely toxic. It was not until the 1980s, when it was discovered how the camptothecins work specifically and how to modify the chemical structure to make the drugs more tolerable, that more rapid development of this class proceeded.

**Mechanism of Action.** The camptothecins are inhibitors of topoisomerase I, an enzyme that occurs naturally in all cells, in all phases of the cell cycle.[13] During cell replication, topoisomerase I attaches to the tightly wound double-strand DNA and allows a break in one of the strands. The DNA can then unwind, the broken strand is repaired, topoisomerase I declines, and the replication fork proceeds. Irinotecan, like other drugs in its class, binds to topoisomerase I, preventing the strand break from being repaired and preventing topoisomerase I from detaching. As the replication fork proceeds, it encounters the strand breakage and the cell cannot divide. In this way, the camptothecins transform the naturally occurring and essential topoisomerase I into a cell poison.

Irinotecan is a prodrug, cleaved via carboxylesterases to its active compound SN-38. SN-38 is one of the most potent camptothecins synthesized to date and itself is from 2 to 2000 times stronger than irinotecan itself. The converting enzyme activity may influence how well irinotecan works in a particular patient.[14]

**Resistance.** Little is know about the mechanisms of resistance to irinotecan. Investigators have postulated inherent or induced changes in topoisomerase I itself or decreased expression of the enzyme.[15] P-glycoprotein–associated multidrug resistance has been demonstrated in selected cell lines.[16]

**Pharmacokinetics.** The pharmacokinetics for irinotecan are well described in the literature.[17, 18] After intravenous drug administration, plasma levels of irinotecan decrease rapidly, with a mean terminal half-life of about 6 hours. The terminal half-life of SN-38, however, is around 10 hours. Most of the irinotecan is excreted via the urine, whereas hepatic glucuronidation and biliary excretion are the principal metabolic routes for SN-38. Because of this, patients with hepatic dysfunction (e.g., bilirubin level >2.0 g/dl) should not be given this drug or should be given reduced doses. No reductions in dose are required for patients with liver metastases and normal liver function.

**Drug-Drug Interactions.** Irinotecan has no known drug-drug interactions. In early clinical trials, prochlorperazine-induced akathisia was found to be more common in irinotecan-treated patients. The package insert recommends avoiding prochlorperazine for 24 hours after irinotecan administration.

## TOXICITY

**Overview.** Leukopenia and diarrhea are the two principal side effects of irinotecan. The following information is obtained from the package insert and the pivotal trials conducted in colorectal cancer:

**Hematologic.** Leukopenia, neutropenia, and lymphocytopenia all were commonly seen in the pivotal trials with irinotecan. Fifty-four percent of patients had some sort of neutropenia; only 11.5% had neutrophil counts less than 500/μL. Those who had previously received pelvic irradiation were more likely to experience grade 3 or 4 neutropenia (48% vs. 24%). Patients with elevated serum bilirubin levels, as expected, had a greater chance of developing neutropenia. Severe anemia and thrombocytopenia were rare.

**Gastrointestinal.** Two common types of gastrointestinal toxicity are seen with irinotecan therapy. The first, occurring within 24 hours of drug administration, is a result of a cholinergic reaction.[19] Symptoms can include abdominal cramping, nausea, vomiting, sweating or flushing, and diarrhea. In one study, these cholinergic symptoms occurred in 79% of patients receiving the drug (250 mg/m² every 2 weeks), were mild to moderate in nature, and lasted 2 to 390 minutes (median ~16 minutes) after treatment.[20] These early cholinergic symptoms are easily relieved with 0.25 to 1 mg of atropine given intravenously. Prophylactic atropine is not required or helpful because the symptoms do not occur regularly in the same patient. Slowing the infusion or using a regimen with lower doses can also alleviate the cholinergic reaction.

More common is what is referred to as late diarrhea. Nearly 88% of all patients treated with irinotecan experience some diarrhea, at a median of 11 days following drug administration. With prompt recognition and use of high-dose loperamide (see Dose and Administration, later), the incidence of severe grade IV diarrhea was only 4%. The diarrhea does require careful dose adjustments but does not appear to be cumulative. The diarrhea is thought to be secretory, but the precise mechanism is yet undefined.[21]

Other gastrointestinal side effects included nausea and vomiting, occurring in 86% and 66% of patients, respectively (severe in 16% and 12%). Patients also complained of anorexia, stomatitis, constipation, and dyspepsia rarely.

**Dermatologic.** Alopecia can be expected in about 50% of patients.

**Pulmonary.** In the U.S. pivotal trials, pulmonary events were rare. In early testing of irinotecan in Japan, however, a few cases of probable drug-induced pneumonitis were seen. With extensive testing now in several different disease types, these effects have not been seen again, making the issue puzzling.

**Other and Rare Reactions**

*Reproductive.* Toxicity data place irinotecan in FDA pregnancy category D.

*Carcinogenicity.* Long-term carcinogenicity studies have not been performed with irinotecan. Topoisomerase I inhibitors have been associated with leukemia, so it is presumed that the drug poses at least some risk of carcinogenesis.

## DOSAGE AND ADMINISTRATION

Irinotecan is available in vials containing 40 and 100 mg of active drug. The drug should be diluted in normal saline or 5% dextrose solutions (preferred) to a concentration of 0.12 to 1.1 mg/ml. Solutions in 5% dextrose, stored at 2° C to 8° C and protected from light, are stable for 48 hours. Storage of solutions prepared with normal saline is not safe because of a tendency for visible particulates to form. Solutions kept at room temperature should be used within 6 hours.

The schedule currently approved in the United States is 125 mg/m² of irinotecan weekly for 4 weeks, followed by a 2-week hiatus. The drug is infused intravenously over 90 minutes. Premedication with dexamethasone and occasionally an additional antiemetic is recommended. Doses should be adjusted weekly based on the neutrophil counts and the amount of diarrhea (if any) experienced by the patient. In Europe, irinotecan is given as 350 mg/m² intravenously over 30 minutes every 3 weeks. With the higher doses, one sees more neutropenia, fairly similar diarrhea, and a higher incidence of the cholinergic reaction. The two regimens are currently being compared head to head in a multicenter clinical trial to determine if there are any differences in response or toxicity.

For patients experiencing the cholinergic reaction during or soon after irinotecan infusion, atropine, 0.25 to 1.0 mg, should be given intravenously. Prophylactic atropine is not recommended. Cholinergic symptoms include nausea, vomiting, facial flushing, sweating, abdominal cramping, and diarrhea.

At the first sign of loose stools or an increase of two bowel movements above baseline, patients should begin taking loperamide.[22] We recommend 4 mg of loperamide followed by 2 mg every 2 hours until the patient is free of diarrhea for 12 hours. Even in the middle of the night, patients are urged to set alarms to wake up every 4 hours to take 4 mg of loperamide. Proper education about how to recognize the diarrhea early and adherence to the loperamide regimen are key to making this a safe drug. Indeed, in the pivotal colorectal cancer trials, once patients were taking loperamide correctly, the incidence of severe (grade IV) diarrhea fell from 14 to 4%.

## REFERENCES

1. Rothenberg ML, Cox JV, DeVore RF, et al. A multicenter, phase II trial of weekly irinotecan (CPT-11) in patients with previously treated colorectal carcinoma. Cancer 1999;85:786–95.
2. Rothenberg ML, Eckardt JR, Kuhn JG, et al. Phase II trial of irinotecan in patients with progressive or rapidly recurrent colorectal cancer. J Clin Oncol 1996;14:1128–35.
3. Rougier P, Bugat R, Douillard JY, et al. Phase II study of irinotecan in the treatment of advanced colorectal cancer in chemotherapy-naive patients and patients pretreated with fluorouracil-based chemotherapy. J Clin Oncol 1997;15:251–60.
4. Cunningham D, Pyrhonen S, James RD, et al. Randomised trial of irinotecan plus supportive care versus supportive care alone after fluorouracil failure for patients with metastatic colorectal cancer. Lancet 1998;352:1413–8.
5. Rougier P, Van Cutsem E, Bajetta E, et al. Randomised trial of irinotecan versus fluorouracil by continuous infusion after fluorouracil failure in patients with metastatic colorectal cancer. Lancet 1998;352:1407–12 and 1634.
6. Saltz LB, Locker PK, Pirotta N, et al. Weekly irinotecan (CPT-11), leucovorin (LV), and fluorouracil (FU) is superior to daily × 5 LV/FU in patients (PTS) with previously untreated metastatic colorectal cancer (CRC). Proc Am Soc Clin Oncol 1999;18:233a. abstract 898.
7. Douillard JY, Cunningham D, Roth AD, et al. A randomized phase III trial comparing irinotecan (IRI) + 5FU/Folinic acid (FA) to the same schedule of 5FU/FA in patients (PTS) with metastatic colorectal cancer (MCRC) as front line chemotherapy (CT). Proc Am Soc Clin Oncol 1999;18:233a. abstract 899.
8. Verschraegen CF, Levy T, Kudelka AP, et al. Phase II study of irinotecan in prior chemotherapy-treated squamous cell carcinoma of the cervix. J Clin Oncol 1997;15:625–31.
9. Rosen LS. Irinotecan in lymphoma, leukemia, and breast, pancreatic, ovarian, and small-cell lung cancers. Oncology 1998;12:Suppl 6:103–9.
10. Friedman HS, Petros WP, Friedman AH, et al. Irinotecan therapy in adults with recurrent or progressive malignant glioma. J Clin Oncol 1999;17:1516–25.

11. Ilson D, Enzinger P, Saltz L, et al. Phase II trial of weekly irinotecan + cisplatin in advanced gastric cancer. Proc Am Soc Clin Oncol 1999;18:259a. abstract 994.

12. Wall ME, Wani MC. Camptothecin discovery to clinic. In: Pantazis P, Giovanella BC, Rothenberg ML, eds. The camptothecins from discovery to the patient. New York: New York Academy of Sciences, 1996;803:1–12.

13. Liu LF, Duann PU, Lin Ching-Tai, et al. Mechanism of action of camptothecin. In: Pantazis P, Giovanella BC, Rothenberg ML, eds. The camptothecins from discovery to the patient. New York: New York Academy of Sciences, 1996;803:44–9.

14. Chen SF, Rothenberg ML, Clark G, et al. Human tumor carboxylesterase activity correlates with CPT-11 cytotoxicity in vitro. Proc Am Assoc Cancer Res 1994;35:365.

15. Takimoto CH, Arbuck SG. The camptothecins. In: Chabner BA, Longo DL, eds. Cancer chemotherapy and biotherapy principles and practice. 2nd ed. Philadelphia: Lippincott-Raven, 1996:463–84.

16. Chu XY, Suzuki H, Ueda K, et al. Active efflux of CPT-11 and its metabolites in human KB-derived cell lines. J Pharmacol Exp Ther 1999;288:735–41.

17. Sparreboom A, de Jonge MJ, de Bruijn P, et al. Irinotecan (CPT-11) metabolism and disposition in cancer patients. Clin Cancer Res 1998;4:2747–54.

18. Chabot GG. Clinical pharmacokinetics of irinotecan. Clin Pharmacokinet 1997;33:245–59.

19. Gandia D, Abigerges D, Armand JP, et al. CPT-11–induced cholinergic effects in cancer patients. J Clin Oncol 1993;11:196–7.

20. Petit RG, Rothenberg ML, Mitchell EP, et al. Cholinergic symptoms following CPT-11 infusion in a phase II multicenter trial of 250 mg/m² irinotecan (CPT-11) given every two weeks. Proc Am Soc Clin Oncol 1997;17:268a. abstract 953.

21. Saliba F, Hagipantelli R, Misset JL, et al. Pathophysiology and therapy of irinotecan-induced delayed-onset diarrhea in patients with advanced colorectal cancer: a prospective assessment. J Clin Oncol 1998; 16:2745–51.

22. Armand JP, Terret C, Couteau C, Rixe O. CPT-11: the European experience. Ann N Y Acad Sci 1996;803:282–91.

# Leuprolide

Leuprolide acetate is a synthetic analogue of GnRH. It is also known as Lupron and Lupron Depot.

## EFFICACY

The major indication for leuprolide is the palliative management of advanced prostate cancer.[1] Leuprolide is usually started in combination with flutamide, as discussed in Chapter 50. Leuprolide also has activity against breast cancer.[2]

## PHARMACOLOGY

**Mechanism of Action.** Naturally occurring GnRH is a decapeptide that is synthesized in the hypothalamus. On arrival in the anterior pituitary gland, it selectively stimulates the release of LH and FSH. The physiology of this process has been definitively reviewed.[3] Because of chemical modifications of the naturally occurring hormone, leuprolide is a more potent agonist than GnRH during short-term therapy, whereas its principal effect during long-term administration is inhibition of gonadotropin secretion. This results in suppression of ovarian and testicular steroid hormone synthesis. The precise mechanism of action is undefined, but it is apparent that continuous treatment with leuprolide desensi-

tizes endocrine organs by decreasing both the number of pituitary GnRH receptors and the number of testicular LH receptors. Leuprolide may also have complex effects involving the inhibition or induction of enzymes controlling steroid hormone synthesis, the aberrant secretion of LH, and possibly the secretion of an LH molecule with altered biologic activity. This inhibitory effect is independent of the presence or absence of estrogen receptors in the tumors. In males, the net effect of leuprolide administration is a reduction of testosterone to castration levels within 2 to 4 weeks. In females, both ovarian estrogen and androgen synthesis are inhibited. These effects may persist for years with continuous therapy, although a slow rise in FSH concentrations may be noted in males despite continuous therapy.

**Resistance.** Mechanisms of resistance are unclear.

**Pharmacokinetics.** Because leuprolide is a polypeptide, it is degraded in the gastrointestinal tract and must therefore be given parenterally. It is rapidly and nearly completely absorbed after subcutaneous injection. Its distribution and metabolism are largely unknown in humans, although it has been reported to be about 7 to 15% bound to serum proteins in vitro. Its elimination half-life appears to be about 3 hours after intravenous administration. The depot preparation gives plasma levels of about 0.8 ng/ml. This slowly declines over a period of several weeks, with undetectable levels by 8 to 12 weeks.

**Drug Interactions.** No interactions have been reported.

## TOXICITY

**Overview.** The predominant forms of toxicity are hot flashes in men and amenorrhea with menopausal symptoms in women. In men with prostate cancer, transient increases in bone pain, exacerbation of cord compression, and ureteral obstruction can occur, as well as impotence and testicular atrophy.

**Cardiovascular.** A wide spectrum of cardiovascular toxicity occasionally occurs. The most common effects are electrocardiographic changes suggestive of ischemia (<20%), peripheral edema (<15%), hypertension (<10%), and a long list of rare adverse effects. These include angina, myocardial infarction, cardiac arrhythmias, transient ischemic attacks, pulmonary embolus, and phlebitis.

**Musculoskeletal.** Osteoporosis can potentially result from hypoestrogenism in women. Bone pain with flare reactions occurs in less than 10% of patients. Rare effects include myalgia, asthenia, arthralgia, and ankylosing spondylitis.

**Endocrine-Metabolic.** The most frequent side effect is hot flashes (40 to 77%), which rarely require cessation of treatment. Decreased libido, testicular atrophy, and impotence are common results of therapy in men being treated for prostate cancer. Gynecomastia is a relatively rare event. In women receiving leuprolide for breast cancer, amenorrhea and vaginal bleeding occasionally occur. Other rare effects include diabetes mellitus, hypercalcemia, hyperuricemia, thyromegaly, a peculiar body odor, and weight gain. Mean total cholesterol and triglyceride levels were increased modestly in one study (11% and 27%, respectively), but the authors considered the impact of leuprolide on cardiovascular risk factors to be questionable.[4]

**Other and Rare Reactions.** The most important side

effect of leuprolide is temporary exacerbation of signs or symptoms of the tumor being treated. Thus, men with partial obstruction of the urinary tract due to metastatic prostate cancer may develop complete obstruction. Similarly, a man with metastatic prostate cancer involving a spinal vertebra may develop increasing back pain or even spinal cord compression with treatment. Transiently increased bone pain can also occur in women with breast cancer. Very rare miscellaneous effects include lymphadenopathy, fever, infection, and hypoproteinemia.

*Hematologic.* Rarely, leukopenia and anemia may occur.

*Immunologic.* The multiple-dose vial of leuprolide contains benzyl alcohol. This solvent can cause local hypersensitivity reactions in rare patients. Anaphylaxis has been reported in one patient treated with leuprolide.[5]

*Digestive System.* Minor nausea, anorexia, and constipation are occasional side effects. Transient minor elevations of transaminase enzymes can occur. Rarely, dysphagia, diarrhea, peptic ulcer disease, and gastrointestinal bleeding may occur.

*Mucocutaneous.* Hair growth or loss, dry mouth, pruritus, hyperpigmentation, local skin reactions at sites of injection, and dermatitis occur rarely and are usually of minor importance.

*Pulmonary.* Pulmonary emboli, dyspnea, and infiltrates all are rare.

*Ocular.* Rarely, blurred vision may occur.

*Neurologic.* Uncommon changes similar to those seen in menopause can occur (insomnia, dizziness, headaches, depression). Rarely, a variety of other effects are seen, including anxiety, taste changes, lethargy, paresthesia, memory problems, mood swings, nervousness, numbness, hearing problems, and syncope. In a study of 10 men, stage 4 sleep was frequently disrupted as part of the hypogonadal state.[6]

*Genitourinary.* Rarely, dysuria, hematuria, bladder spasms, testicular pain, penile pain, and incontinence may occur.

*Reproductive.* Toxicity data place leuprolide in FDA pregnancy category X. Although normal pregnancies have occurred despite the use of leuprolide,[7] the drug is contraindicated during pregnancy.

*Carcinogenicity.* The drug is not considered mutagenic or carcinogenic.

## DOSAGE AND ADMINISTRATION

Leuprolide is available in kits of various doses for administration daily, monthly, every 3 months, or every 4 months. The daily dose is given subcutaneously, and the depot preparations are given intramuscularly. Because patients with prostate cancer may experience exacerbations shortly after initiation of therapy, it is recommended that patients at risk of bone pain, cord compression, or urinary obstruction start with daily doses of leuprolide for about 2 weeks before switching to one of the depot preparations. Many authorities also advise the use of an antiandrogen during the initiation phase of therapy as a way of preventing the androgen flare reaction.

The usual dose of leuprolide for patients with prostate cancer is 1 mg daily by subcutaneous injection, 7.5 mg of the depot suspension intramuscularly once a month, 22.5 mg

once every 3 months, or 30 mg every 4 months. The drug is available as a kit that includes the requisite needles, syringes, and drug for convenient daily self-administration by the patient. The manufacturer recommends periodic monitoring of patients with determinations of blood testosterone and prostate-specific antigen levels.

## REFERENCES

1. Sharifi R, Soloway M. Clinical study of leuprolide depot formulation in the treatment of advanced prostate cancer. The Leuprolide Study Group. J Urol 1990;143:68–71.
2. The Leuprolide Study Group. Leuprolide versus diethylstilbestrol for metastatic prostate cancer. N Engl J Med 1984;311:1281–6.
3. Conn PM, Crowley WF Jr. Gonadotropin-releasing hormone and its analogues. N Engl J Med 1991;324:93–103.
4. Eri LM, Urdal P, Bechensteen AG. Effects of the luteinizing hormone–releasing hormone agonist leuprolide on lipoproteins, fibrinogen and plasminogen activator inhibitor in patients with benign prostatic hyperplasia. J Urol 1995;154:100–4.
5. MacLeod TL, Eisen A, Sussman GL. Anaphylactic reaction to synthetic luteinizing hormone–releasing hormone. Fertil Steril 1987;48:500–2.
6. Leibenluft E, Schmidt PJ, Turner EH, et al. Effects of leuprolide-induced hypogonadism and testosterone replacement on sleep, melatonin, and prolactin secretion in men. J Clin Endocrinol Metab 1997;82:3203–7.
7. Chang SY, Soong YK. Unexpected pregnancies exposed to leuprolide acetate administered after the mid-luteal phase for ovarian stimulation. Hum Reprod 1995;10:204–6.

# Levamisole

Levamisole is a low-molecular-weight synthetic anthelmintic drug used widely in veterinary medicine. It has been studied for many years as a potential form of immunotherapy in patients with cancer, usually as an adjunct to chemotherapy.[1] It is also known as Ergamisol.

## EFFICACY

Levamisole is FDA approved as an adjunct to 5-FU in the adjuvant therapy of high-risk colorectal carcinoma (see Chapter 43). Other uses for the drug are investigational. Levamisole has highly variable effects as an immune stimulant in experimental animal tumor systems.[1] No firm conclusions about the drug have been possible, except that levamisole does not increase resistance to tumor inoculations in immunologically normal animals.[2–4] Levamisole has been extensively studied in humans as a possible immune stimulant, and initial results suggest benefit.[5, 6] Several randomized clinical trials found that levamisole therapy was associated with longer remissions in some patients. However, levamisole alone is not capable of inducing remissions. The only use for the drug appears to be that of an adjuvant with other drugs.[7] The results have been decidedly mixed, however. Some clinical trials have shown an adverse effect from the use of levamisole. The Veterans Administration Lung Cancer Group study showed that when levamisole was added to doxorubicin chemotherapy for advanced lung cancer, the levamisole-treated patients experienced increased toxicity and diminished survival.[8] In another study, levamisole appeared to have an adverse effect on the outcome in breast cancer.[9] In yet another study, levamisole was associated with an increased late death rate in patients with colorectal cancer.[10] It does not improve the results of 5-FU therapy in patients with metastatic colorectal cancer.[11]

## PHARMACOLOGY

**Mechanism of Action.** The mechanism of levamisole-induced augmentation of 5-FU chemotherapy is unknown. One study suggests it may be due to inhibition of tyrosine phosphatases by levamisole,[12] but this requires confirmation. Other putative mechanisms involve complex and varied effects of levamisole on the immune system. For example, one study demonstrated downregulation of CD59 (protectin) expression on human colorectal adenocarcinoma cell lines by levamisole, which may have rendered the colorectal cells more susceptible to complement lysis.[13] Most of the studies of the immunopharmacology of levamisole predate current concepts of cytokine interactions in the immune system and are thus incomplete. These older studies do demonstrate that levamisole stimulates immune responses in immunodepressed hosts. For example, mice have displayed enhanced resistance to *Brucella abortus* infection after being given levamisole.[14] In humans, antibody responses to influenza were increased after levamisole treatment.[15] Delayed cutaneous hypersensitivity responses have been augmented or restored by levamisole administration in patients with cancer.[16] Studies of patients with cancer have demonstrated increased levels of neopterin and decreased levels of soluble IL-2 receptors in patients given levamisole.[17] One of these studies also showed increased expression of CD64 and class I and class II major histocompatibility antigens on monocytes.[18] The addition of interferon caused no augmentation of the effects noted with levamisole. In another study, levamisole reduced the expression of major histocompatibility complex class I expression in colorectal and breast carcinoma cell lines.[18] Further studies are needed to clarify the mechanisms of action of this agent.

**Resistance.** Mechanisms of resistance are unclear.

**Pharmacokinetics.** The drug is readily absorbed after oral administration. Extensive metabolism of levamisole occurs in the liver, with only about 5% of the drug excreted unchanged into urine. The elimination half-life is 3 to 4 hours.

**Drug Interactions.** Levamisole can increase the levels of phenytoin. Levamisole also increases the levels of warfarin, leading to prolongation of the prothrombin time during concurrent therapy with both drugs.[19] Levamisole can cause a disulfiram (Antabuse)-like effect when given with alcohol. Adverse effects are more common when levamisole is administered with 5-FU. Whether this is due to simple additive toxicity or some other form of drug interaction is unknown. Preliminary in vitro studies suggest that levamisole potentiates the cytotoxicity of radiation therapy.[20]

## TOXICITY

**Overview.** Most patients tolerate levamisole despite minor toxicity, but nausea, neurologic reactions, hepatic dysfunction, neutropenia, and a variety of rare reactions are dose limiting in some patients.

**Hematologic.** Myelosuppression is unusual when levamisole is used alone, but rarely it can be life threatening. When levamisole is combined with 5-FU, myelosuppression is more severe than when either of the drugs is used alone.[21] Some cases of agranulocytosis have occurred with doses higher than those used in adjuvant therapy in patients treated for rheumatoid arthritis, probably on the basis of autoimmune neutrophil destruction.[22] Agranulocytosis is usually accompanied by a flu-like illness, and patients should be cautioned to report any such occurrence. Reversible thrombocytopenia has been reported.[23]

**Digestive System.** Nausea is common, but emesis is unusual. Anorexia, diarrhea, constipation, and a bitter taste in the mouth can occur. When 5-FU is given with levamisole, mild to moderate, reversible hepatic dysfunction occurs in about 40% of patients.[24] The most common change is an increase in the serum alkaline phosphatase level, but total bilirubin and transaminase enzyme levels may also increase. In some cases, these changes are associated with an increase in the serum carcinoembryonic antigen level and the appearance of a fatty liver on computed tomographic scan or liver biopsy specimens. These changes may simulate hepatic metastasis.

**Neurologic.** Although rare, the following have been reported: insomnia, headache, anxiety, dizziness, agitation, depression, tardive dyskinesia, parkinsonian reactions, confusion, nightmares, hallucinations, paranoia, somnolence, coma, paresthesia, tremor, ataxia, spasms, jitters, sensory stimulation, and very rarely seizures. When levamisole is combined with 5-FU, a severe encephalopathy-like syndrome associated with demyelination occurs rarely.[25, 26]

**Other and Rare Reactions.** Chills and a metallic taste are uncommon.

*Immunologic.* Immune augmentation is the presumed mechanism of action for levamisole, but hypersensitivity reactions are rare. In one study, levamisole augmented antibody responses without modulation of cellular cytotoxicity.[27]

*Mucocutaneous.* Stomatitis occurs occasionally. Alopecia is rare, as are rashes, pruritus, periorbital edema, and exfoliative dermatitis. A case of bilateral ear lobe necrosis due to levamisole-induced occlusive vasculitis has been reported in a child.[28]

*Cardiovascular.* Hypertension, hypotension, and chest pain all are rare.

*Ocular.* Conjunctivitis and blurred vision are rare.

*Musculoskeletal.* Fatigue, flu-like syndrome (myalgia, arthralgia, fever), proximal muscle weakness, and arthritis all are rare.

*Genitourinary.* Proteinuria and renal dysfunction are rare.

*Reproductive.* Toxicity studies place levamisole in FDA pregnancy category C.

*Endocrine-Metabolic.* Edema, fluid retention, hyperlipidemia, and vaginal bleeding all are rare. A single case of levamisole-induced SIADH has been reported.[29]

*Carcinogenicity.* Adequate animal studies of carcinogenesis have not been performed. The available data suggest that levamisole probably is not carcinogenic.

## DOSAGE AND ADMINISTRATION

The drug is available as 50-mg tablets in blister packages of 36 tablets. The usual dosage (in combination with 5-FU) is

50 mg every 8 hours for 3 consecutive days, with repeat courses every 2 weeks for 1 year (a total of 26 treatments).

## REFERENCES

1. Stevenson HC, Green I, Hamilton JM, et al. Levamisole: known effects on the immune system, clinical results, and future applications to the treatment of cancer. J Clin Oncol 1991;9:2052–66.
2. Potter CW, Carr I, Jennings R, et al. Levamisole inactive in treatment of four animal tumours. Nature 1974;249:567–9.
3. Johnson RK, Houchens DP, Gaston MR, Goldin A. Effects of levamisole (NSC-177023) and tetramisole (NSC-102063) in experimental tumor systems. Cancer Chemother Rep 1975;59:697–705.
4. Hopper DG, Pimm MV, Baldwin RW. Levamisole treatment of local and metastatic growth of transplanted rat tumours. Br J Cancer 1975;32:345–51.
5. Rojas AF, Feierstein NJ, Mickiewicz E, et al. Levamisole in advanced human breast cancer. Lancet 1976;1:211–5.
6. Anonymous. Immunopotentiation with levamisole in resectable bronchogenic carcinoma: a double-blind controlled trial; Study Group for Bronchogenic Carcinoma. Br Med J 1975;3:461–4.
7. Spreafico F. Use of levamisole in cancer patients. Drugs 1980;20:105–16.
8. Davis S, Mietlowski W, Rohwedder JJ, et al. Levamisole as adjuvant to chemotherapy in extensive bronchogenic carcinoma: a Veterans Administration Lung Cancer Group Study. Cancer 1982;50:646–51.
9. Executive Committee of the Danish Breast Cancer Cooperative Group. Increased breast-cancer recurrence rate after adjuvant therapy with levamisole: a preliminary report. Lancet 1980;2:824–7.
10. Chlebowski RT, Lillington L, Nystrom JS, Sayre J. Late mortality and levamisole adjuvant therapy in colorectal cancer. Br J Cancer 1994;69:1094–7.
11. Bandealy MT, Gonin R, Loehrer PJ, et al. Prospective randomized trial of 5-fluorouracil versus 5-fluorouracil plus levamisole in the treatment of metastatic colorectal cancer: a Hoosier Oncology Group trial. Clin Cancer Res 1998;4:935–9.
12. Kovach JS, Svingen PA, Schaid DJ. Levamisole potentiation of fluorouracil antiproliferative activity mimicked by orthovanadate, an inhibitor of tyrosine phosphatase. J Natl Cancer Inst 1992;84:515–9.
13. Bjørge L, Matre R. Down-regulation of CD59 (protectin) expression on human colorectal adenocarcinoma cell lines by levamisole. Scand J Immunol 1995;42:512–6.
14. Renoux G, Renoux M. Stimulation of anti-*Brucella* vaccination in mice by tetramisole, a phenyl-imidothiazole salt. Infect Immun 1973;8:544–8.
15. Brugmans J, Schuermans V, De Cock W, et al. Restoration of host defense mechanisms in man by levamisole. Life Sci 1973;13:1499–504.
16. Tripodi D, Parks LC, Brugmans J. Drug-induced restoration of cutaneous delayed hypersensitivity in anergic patients with cancer. N Engl J Med 1973;289:354–7.
17. Janik J, Kopp WC, Smith JW II, et al. Dose-related immunologic effects of levamisole in patients with cancer. J Clin Oncol 1993;11:125–35.
18. Goodrich KH, Alvarez X, Holcombe RF. Effect of levamisole on major histocompatibility complex class I expression in colorectal and breast carcinoma cell lines. Cancer 1993;72:225–30.
19. Wehbe TW, Warth JA. A case of bleeding requiring hospitalization that was likely caused by an interaction between warfarin and levamisole. Clin Pharmacol Ther 1996;59:360–2.
20. Hayostek CJ, Koval TM. Radiosensitization of human tumor cells with levamisole. Cancer Res 1992;52:3228–30.
21. Longrâee L, Focan C, Bury J, et al. Levamisole adds granulocyte toxicity to 5-FU–based chemotherapies in adjuvant treatment of Dukes B-C colorectal cancer: a preliminary report. Anticancer Res 1995;15:1561–4.
22. Ruuskanen O, Remes M, Makela AL, et al. Levamisole and agranulocytosis. Lancet 1976;2:958–9.
23. Winquist EW, Lassam NJ. Reversible thrombocytopenia with levamisole. Med Pediatr Oncol 1995;24:262–4.
24. Moertel CG, Fleming TR, Macdonald JS, et al. Hepatic toxicity associated with fluorouracil plus levamisole adjuvant therapy. J Clin Oncol 1993;11:2386–90.
25. Kimmel DW, Schutt AJ. Multifocal leukoencephalopathy: occurrence during 5-fluorouracil and levamisole therapy and resolution after discontinuation of chemotherapy. Mayo Clin Proc 1993;68:363–5.
26. Luppi G, Zoboli A, Barbieri F, et al. Multifocal leukoencephalopathy associated with 5-fluorouracil and levamisole adjuvant therapy for colon cancer: a report of two cases and review of the literature. Ann Oncol 1996;7:412–5.
27. Tempero MA, Haga Y, Sivinski C, et al. Immunologic effects of levamisole in mice and humans: evidence for augmented antibody response without modulation of cellular cytotoxicity. J Immunother Emphasis Tumor Immunol 1995;17:47–57.
28. Menni S, Pistritto G, Gianotti R, et al. Ear lobe bilateral necrosis by levamisole-induced occlusive vasculitis in a pediatric patient. Pediatr Dermatol 1997;14:477–9.
29. Tweedy CR, Silverberg DA, Scott L. Levamisole-induced syndrome of inappropriate antidiuretic hormone. N Engl J Med 1992;326:1164.

## Lomustine

Lomustine is the second of two nitrosoureas commercially available in the United States.[1] It is closely related chemically to carmustine. Lomustine is also known as 1-(2-chloroethyl)-3-cyclohexyl-1-nitrosourea, CCNU, CeeNU, and NSC-79037.

### EFFICACY

Lomustine is FDA approved for the treatment of brain tumors and Hodgkin's disease. It is also used in various drug combinations against other tumors.

### PHARMACOLOGY

The pharmacology of lomustine is similar to that of carmustine, with the following exceptions. Oral absorption is excellent, so lomustine is given orally rather than by the intravenous route. Lomustine is rapidly and completely biotransformed to active metabolites within minutes of absorption. The peak plasma levels for the metabolites occur by about 3 hours, and the elimination half-life is about 72 hours. Preliminary studies suggest that weekly therapy with lomustine may have an acceptable toxicity profile for further study.[2]

### TOXICITY

The spectrum of systemic toxicity and the precautions for the use of lomustine are essentially the same as for carmustine. The major difference between the two drugs is the absence of local pain with lomustine. Overdosage has been reported, resulting in multiorgan failure.[3]

### DOSAGE AND ADMINISTRATION

Lomustine is available as 10-, 40-, and 100-mg capsules for oral administration. The usual dosage is 100 to 130 mg/m² every 6 weeks. A patient with pre-existing bone marrow depression or extensive prior bone marrow–suppressive therapy requires lower doses, and prolonged treatment commonly requires further dose reductions or delays based on an assessment of nadir blood counts. Patients with renal dysfunction should receive reduced doses (see Chapter 8 for guidelines), and all patients need aggressive antiemetic therapy.

## REFERENCES

1. Hoogstraten B, Gottlieb JA, Caoili E, et al. CCNU (1-(2-chloroethyl)-3-cyclohexyl-1-nitrosourea, NSC-79037) in the treatment of cancer: phase II study. Cancer 1973;32:38–43.
2. Koller CA, Gorski CC, Benjamin RS, et al. A phase I trial of weekly lomustine in patients with advanced cancer. Cancer 1994;73:236–9.
3. Trent KC, Myers L, Moreb J. Multiorgan failure associated with lomustine overdose. Ann Pharmacother 1995;29:384–6.

# Mechlorethamine

During World War I, it was noted that mustard gas poisoning caused bone marrow aplasia, dissolution of lymphoid tissue, and gastrointestinal ulceration. During World War II, chemical warfare experimentation showed that nitrogen mustard could shrink some tumors, thus launching the field of cancer chemotherapy. Mechlorethamine, the parent compound for thousands of derivatives, is also known as Mustargen, HN2, nitrogen mustard, and NSC-762.

## EFFICACY

Mechlorethamine has a time-honored place in the treatment of disseminated Hodgkin's disease and other lymphomas, including mycosis fungoides. It is also used in the treatment of malignant effusions. Although mechlorethamine has activity against a variety of other neoplasms, it is rarely used for other tumors.

## PHARMACOLOGY

**Mechanism of Action.** After the formation of an ethylenimmonium ion intermediate, mechlorethamine alkylates a wide variety of biologic molecules. The major target of alkylation is DNA, which can be damaged by inter- and intrastrand cross-linking, depurination, and ring cleavage. These reactions all tend to involve binding to the N7 nitrogen of guanine. In addition, in some cell lines, altered expression and transcription of the topoisomerase II gene may occur.[1] In cell culture, mechlorethamine cytotoxicity leads to apoptosis.[2]

**Resistance.** Resistance to mechlorethamine is complex and involves many possible biochemical alterations, including altered cellular uptake, increased production of nucleophilic substances that may compete with mechlorethamine for binding to DNA, and increased DNA repair mechanisms.

**Pharmacokinetics.** Mechlorethamine is so highly reactive that it rapidly interacts with water during its reconstitution, and its cellular damage occurs within minutes of administration. The elimination half-life is about 15 minutes. Because it is altered so rapidly by all tissues, less than

0.01% of administered mechlorethamine can be recovered in the urine. It can be used without dose modification in patients with renal or hepatic dysfunction.

**Drug and Radiation Interactions.** The cytotoxicity of mechlorethamine is antagonized by thiosulfate. The drug causes radiosensitization.

## TOXICITY

**Overview.** This prototypical alkylating agent causes dose-limiting myelosuppression and emesis as its main side effects.

**Hematologic.** Myelosuppression is the main dose-limiting toxicity of mechlorethamine. The infection and bleeding associated with bone marrow depression are the most dangerous toxic side effects of the drug. The nadir of the decline in the WCC and platelet count usually occurs within 7 to 15 days of injection. The reduction may be greater in a patient whose bone marrow has been damaged by previous chemotherapy, radiation therapy, or malignant infiltration. The WCC and platelet count usually return to normal by the fourth week following drug administration. Patients with CLL are susceptible to mechlorethamine-induced hemolytic anemia.

**Digestive System.** Nausea and vomiting occur in up to 90% of patients. They usually start 1 to 3 hours after therapy and are usually severe. Aggressive antiemetic therapy is needed. Other gastrointestinal toxicity is rare but can include diarrhea, jaundice, anorexia, and peptic ulcer disease.

**Mucocutaneous.** Herpes zoster may be precipitated by therapy, and the acute phase should pass before treatment is resumed. Skin breakdown can occur in areas of drug extravasation, and intravenous therapy can cause vein irritation with hyperpigmentation, thrombosis, or thrombophlebitis. Alopecia, mucositis, and a poorly understood maculopapular skin rash can occur rarely. Erythema multiforme develops very rarely. Topical use frequently causes a delayed cutaneous hypersensitivity reaction that may require desensitization.[3]

**Other and Rare Reactions.** Drug fever can occur but is rare. When the drug is given by intracavitary administration, it may cause severe local irritation with pain and cardiac arrhythmias, depending on the site of administration. The manufacturer states that the drug should not be used in patients with foci of acute or chronic suppurative inflammation because mechlorethamine may contribute to the rapid development of extensive amyloidosis.

*Immunologic.* Systemic hypersensitivity reactions such as angioedema and anaphylaxis can occur but are very rare. The drug is only minimally immunosuppressive.

*Cardiovascular.* High-dose therapy can cause cardiac damage.[4]

*Pulmonary.* Most alkylating agents can cause pulmonary infiltrates in rare patients, although this is not specifically reported with mechlorethamine.

*Neurologic.* Some patients experience tinnitus, decreased hearing (rare), and a metallic taste in the mouth. Toxic encephalopathies may rarely occur with standard doses of mechlorethamine, but experimental use of high-dose therapy frequently causes this problem. The spectrum of changes can include weakness, headache, drowsiness, lightheadedness, vertigo, convulsions, progressive paralysis, paresthesia, cerebral degeneration, coma, and death.

*Genitourinary.* Uric acid nephropathy is rare.

*Reproductive.* Toxicity studies place mechlorethamine in FDA pregnancy category D. The drug is teratogenic and can cause amenorrhea, azoospermia, and sterility.

*Endocrine-Metabolic.* High-dose therapy may cause hypocalcemia.[4]

*Carcinogenicity.* The drug is carcinogenic.

## DOSAGE AND ADMINISTRATION

Mechlorethamine is supplied as 10-mg vials for injection. It is usually used as one of a combination of drugs (see Chapter 87). On those rare occasions when mechlorethamine is used alone, the usual dose is 0.4 mg/kg by intravenous bolus injection. For intracavitary administration, the dose is 0.2 to 0.4 mg/kg. It is commonly injected directly into intravenous tubing through which physiologic saline solution is running. Because mechlorethamine is a vesicant, gloves are worn during its preparation and care is taken to avoid infiltration into the soft tissues or splashing on the exposed skin or conjunctivas of the patient or physician. If such skin exposure does occur, sodium thiosulfate can be used locally as an antidote.[5] Guidelines for local administration of mechlorethamine ointment are given in Chapter 93.

## REFERENCES

1. Tan KB, Mattern MR, Boyce RA, Schein PS. Unique sensitivity of nitrogen mustard–resistant human Burkitt lymphoma cells to novobiocin. Biochem Pharmacol 1988;37:4411–3.
2. O'Connor PM, Wassermann K, Sarang M, et al. Relationship between DNA cross-links, cell cycle, and apoptosis in Burkitt's lymphoma cell lines differing in sensitivity to nitrogen mustard. Cancer Res 1991;51:6550–7.
3. Waldorf DS, Haynes HA, Van Scott EJ. Cutaneous hypersensitivity and desensitization to mechlorethamine in patients with mycosis fungoides lymphoma. Ann Intern Med 1967;67:282–90.
4. Hartmann DW, Robinson WA, Mangalik A, et al. Unanticipated side effects from treatment with high-dose mechlorethamine in patients with malignant melanoma. Cancer Treat Rep 1981;65:327–8.
5. Dorr RT, Soble M, Alberts DS. Efficacy of sodium thiosulfate as a local antidote to mechlorethamine skin toxicity in the mouse. Cancer Chemother Pharmacol 1988;22:299–302.

# Megestrol Acetate

Many progestins with primarily progestational activity and minimal androgenic and fluid-retaining effects are available. One of the progestins most widely used in oncology is megestrol acetate, also known as Megace.

## EFFICACY

Megestrol acetate is used primarily in the palliative management of carcinomas of the breast or endometrium. It has also been approved by the FDA for the treatment of anorexia and cachexia in patients with acquired immunodeficiency syndrome (AIDS). The drug may also be useful in ameliorating two groups of symptoms that occur in patients with cancer, as follows: (1) cancer cachexia,[1, 2] and (2) at low dosages (20 mg twice daily), palliative management of hot flashes in men and women after gonadal ablation therapy for prostate cancer and breast cancer. The latter use, however, may abrogate the effects of hormonal therapy for prostate cancer.[3] Megestrol acetate does not appear to be useful in the treatment of prostate cancer.[4]

## PHARMACOLOGY

**Mechanism of Action.** Megestrol acetate is a progestin with antiestrogenic activity. In postmenopausal women with breast cancer, it causes profound suppression of plasma estrogen levels.[5] It also inhibits the release of LH, stimulates the growth of the endometrium, and produces typical progestational changes in the acinar cells of the breast. Its mechanism of action is unclear but is presumed to involve interaction with intracellular hormone receptors. In one study, the closely related drug medroxyprogesterone acetate was shown to bind to receptors for estrogen, progesterone, and androgens.[6] Androgen receptor binding appeared to be especially crucial to the cytotoxicity of the drug. Megestrol acetate appears to influence the differentiation of adipocytes in vitro.[7]

Some evidence suggests that megestrol acetate improves clinical symptoms of the cancer anorexia-cachexia syndrome by downregulation of cytokine production by peripheral blood mononuclear cells.[8]

**Resistance.** Mechanisms of resistance are complex and multifactorial. In one study, resistance involved both increased growth factor expression and decreased progesterone receptor levels.[9]

**Pharmacokinetics.** The drug is well absorbed, followed by metabolism in the liver and excretion in the urine as steroid metabolites and inactive compounds. It has a long elimination half-life (about 15 to 20 hours).

**Drug Interactions.** Megestrol acetate given concurrently with chemotherapy in vitro induces cell cycle arrest in hematopoietic precursors.[10] It has been shown to reverse, at least partially, multidrug resistance to doxorubicin, vincristine, or both in cancer cell lines.[11] Medroxyprogesterone acetate appears to be a radiation-sensitizing agent.[12] Interferons enhance progesterone receptor levels in endometrial cancer cells in vitro[13]; it is unclear whether this effect can be exploited for therapy. Megestrol acetate has been reported to antagonize cisplatin cytotoxicity in vitro, probably by upregulating cellular metallothionein and glutathione levels.[14]

## TOXICITY

**Overview.** Hormonal therapy with megestrol acetate comes as close to being nontoxic as any cytotoxic agent used in oncology. The predominant adverse effect is weight gain, but thromboembolic events and gastrointestinal distress may also occur in rare patients.

**Digestive System.** At high doses, diarrhea and constipation have been seen. At normal doses, the drug is very well tolerated save for rare nausea, vomiting, diarrhea, flatulence, abdominal cramps, constipation, dyspepsia, dry mouth, and increased salivation. Oral candidiasis has been reported during treatment in immunosuppressed patients with AIDS.

**Cardiovascular.** Hypertension, congestive heart failure, chest pain or pressure, palpitations, peripheral edema, thrombophlebitis, and thromboembolism all are rare or unusual and generally mild and fully reversible.

**Reproductive.** Toxicity studies place megestrol acetate in FDA pregnancy category D; the manufacturer states in addition that the drug is contraindicated during the first 4 months of pregnancy. Vaginal bleeding, menstrual irregularity, hot flashes, decreased libido, and amenorrhea are common.

**Endocrine-Metabolic.** Hypercalcemia is a rare side effect of high-dose therapy. Insulin resistance causing diabetes mellitus can occur rarely.[15] Fluid retention and edema may occur, and weight gain is nearly always seen. Gynecomastia can occur in men. The pituitary-adrenal axis can be suppressed by the drug, leading to reduced levels of cortisol.[16] Severe hyperglycemia due to megestrol acetate has been reported rarely.[17] This appears to be due to insulin resistance rather than insulinopenia.[18]

**Other and Rare Reactions.** Tumor flare (with or without hypercalcemia) can occur rarely. A single case of increased bone pain followed by an excellent clinical response has been reported following the use of megestrol acetate.[19] A case of transient, reversible superior vena cava syndrome related to megestrol acetate administration has been reported.[20] The drug is porphyrogenic in animals and should be used with caution in patients with known porphyria.

**Hematologic.** Hematologic effects are insignificant in women with cancer. Anemia and leukopenia have been reported in patients with AIDS-related cachexia.

**Mucocutaneous.** Alopecia, pruritus, sweating, and rash are rare.

**Pulmonary.** Hyperpnea and dyspnea are rare. A patient treated with radiation therapy and medroxyprogesterone acetate developed fatal pulmonary toxicity.[12] This was considered the result of radiation sensitization.

**Ocular.** Amblyopia is very rare.

**Neurologic.** Headache, insomnia, asthenia, paresthesia, confusion, seizure, depression, neuropathy, hypesthesia, and abnormal thinking all are rare and generally limited to patients with AIDS.

**Musculoskeletal.** Carpal tunnel syndrome is rare.

**Genitourinary.** Urinary frequency, urinary incontinence, and urinary tract infection all are rare.

**Carcinogenicity.** The drug is not a known carcinogen in humans, but it causes breast cancer in dogs, and a patient with AIDS-related cachexia developed a sarcoma.

## DOSAGE AND ADMINISTRATION

Megestrol acetate is available as 20- and 40-mg tablets and as an oral suspension of 200 mg/5 ml. It has been used in a variety of doses, ranging from 40 to 1600 mg orally per day. For breast cancer, the optimal dosage is 160 mg/day[21] (usually given as 40 mg four times a day, but some physicians use either 80 mg twice daily or even 160 mg once daily).[22] For endometrial cancer, the dose is 40 to 320 mg/day in divided doses. When used for the treatment of anorexia and

cachexia in patients with AIDS, the recommended adult initial dose is 800 mg/day (20 ml/day of the oral suspension) for 1 month, followed by 400 to 800 mg/day for 3 more months. For patients with advanced cancer and the cancer anorexia/cachexia syndrome, doses ranging from 160 mg/day to 480 mg/day appear to be optimal.[23] The dose recommended by the manufacturer for the treatment of cancer cachexia is 400 to 800 mg/day.

## REFERENCES

1. Aisner J, Tchekmedyian NS, Tait N, et al. Studies of high-dose megestrol acetate: potential applications in cachexia. Semin Oncol 1988;15:Suppl 1:68–75.
2. Tchekmedyian NS, Tait N, Moody M, Aisner J. High-dose megestrol acetate: a possible treatment for cachexia. JAMA 1987;257:1195–8.
3. Sartor O, Eastham JA. Progressive prostate cancer associated with use of megestrol acetate administered for control of hot flashes. South Med J 1999;92:415–6.
4. Osborn JL, Smith DC, Trump DL. Megestrol acetate in the treatment of hormone refractory prostate cancer. Am J Clin Oncol 1997;20:308–10.
5. Lundgren S, Helle SI, Lonning PE. Profound suppression of plasma estrogens by megestrol acetate in postmenopausal breast cancer patients. Clin Cancer Res 1996;2:1515–21.
6. Hackenberg R, Hawighorst T, Filmer A, et al. Medroxyprogesterone acetate inhibits the proliferation of estrogen- and progesterone-receptor negative MFM-223 human mammary cancer cells via the androgen receptor. Breast Cancer Res Treat 1993;25:217–24.
7. Hamburger AW, Parnes H, Gordon GB, et al. Megestrol acetate–induced differentiation of 3T3-L1 adipocytes in vitro. Semin Oncol 1988;15:Suppl 1:76–8.
8. Mantovani G, Macciáo A, Lai P, et al. Cytokine involvement in cancer anorexia/cachexia: role of megestrol acetate and medroxyprogesterone acetate on cytokine downregulation and improvement of clinical symptoms. Crit Rev Oncog 1998;9:99–106.
9. Murphy LC, Dotzlaw H, Wong MS, et al. Mechanisms involved in the evolution of progestin resistance in human breast cancer cells. Cancer Res 1991;51:2051–7.
10. Quesada AR, Jimeno JM, Marquez G, Aracil M. Cell cycle arrest of human hematopoietic progenitors induced by medroxyprogesterone acetate. Exp Hematol 1993;21:1413–8.
11. Chang AY. Megestrol acetate as a biomodulator. Semin Oncol 1998;25:2 Suppl 6:58–61.
12. De Greve J, Warson F, Deleu D, Storme G. Fatal pulmonary toxicity by the association of radiotherapy and medroxyprogesterone acetate. Cancer 1985;56:2434–6.
13. Angioli R, Untch M, Sevin BU, et al. Enhancement of progesterone receptor levels by interferons in AE-7 endometrial cancer cells. Cancer 1993;71:2776–81.
14. Pu YS, Cheng AL, Chen J, et al. Megestrol acetate antagonizes cisplatin cytotoxicity. Anticancer Drugs 1998;9:733–8.
15. Henry K, Rathgaber S, Sullivan C, McCabe K. Diabetes mellitus induced by megestrol acetate in a patient with AIDS and cachexia. Ann Intern Med 1992;116:53–4.
16. Loprinzi CL, Jensen MD, Jiang NS, Schaid DJ. Effect of megestrol acetate on the human pituitary-adrenal axis. Mayo Clin Proc 1992;67:1160–2.
17. Rose PG. Hyperglycemia secondary to megestrol acetate for endometrial neoplasia. Gynecol Oncol 1996;61:139–41.
18. Jain P, Girardi LS, Sherman L, et al. Insulin resistance and development of diabetes mellitus associated with megestrol acetate therapy. Postgrad Med J 1996;72:365–7.
19. Greenwald ES. Megestrol acetate flare. Cancer Treat Rep 1983;67:405.
20. Abulafia O, Sherer DM. Recurrent transient superior vena cava-like syndrome possibly associated with megestrol acetate. Obstet Gynecol 1995;85:899–901.
21. Kornblith AB, Hollis DR, Zuckerman E, et al. Effect of megestrol acetate on quality of life in a dose-response trial in women with advanced breast cancer. The Cancer and Leukemia Group B. J Clin Oncol 1993;11:2081–9.
22. Carpenter JT Jr, Peterson L. Use of megestrol acetate in advanced

breast cancer on a single-daily-dose schedule. Semin Oncol 1985;12:Suppl 1:40–2.

23. Gebbia V, Testa A, Gebbia N. Prospective randomised trial of two dose levels of megestrol acetate in the management of anorexia-cachexia syndrome in patients with metastatic cancer. Br J Cancer 1996;73:1576–80.

# Melphalan

Melphalan, a phenylalanine derivative of mechlorethamine, was synthesized by Bergel and Stock in 1953. It is commercially available in the United States for oral or intravenous administration and is known by several names (Alkeran, phenylalanine mustard, L-PAM, L-sarcolysin).

## EFFICACY

Melphalan is used primarily in the treatment of multiple myeloma. In the past it was also used against breast cancer and ovarian cancer. High-dose parenteral melphalan has been used in the treatment of regional melanoma by the isolation-perfusion technique.[1] High-dose melphalan with stem cell rescue is used in the treatment of advanced multiple myeloma.[2]

## PHARMACOLOGY

**Mechanisms of Action and Resistance.** These are thought to be similar to those of mechlorethamine and chlorambucil. The predominant effect is interstrand cross-linking of DNA by alkylation of the N7 position of guanine. Glutathione plays an important role in drug resistance with this and other alkylating agents, and its modulation is being studied for possible therapeutic use.[3, 4] The cellular influx and efflux process of melphalan appears to be active, probably by means of the large neutral amino acid carrier system. This is probably responsible for at least one form of melphalan resistance.[5] Poly (ADP-ribose) polymerase may also be involved in melphalan resistance.[6]

**Pharmacokinetics.** Oral absorption of melphalan is erratic, with bioavailability varying from 32 to 100% (72% mean). The time to peak plasma level is about 6 hours, but this also varies greatly. After absorption, the drug undergoes spontaneous degradation to one of two hydrolysis products. The drug is not metabolized in the liver. Melphalan is extensively bound by serum albumin (40 to 75%, depending on the dose of melphalan and individual variability). Its plasma half-life appears to be about 1.5 hours. Although the average patient excretes only a small proportion of the drug via the kidneys (about 20 to 35%), there is enormous individual variability of renal excretion, even after intravenous administration (3 to 93%). The drug is capable of crossing the blood-brain barrier via the neutral amino acid transporter.[7]

**Drug Interactions**

*Increased Toxicity.* Severe renal failure has been reported in patients receiving cyclosporine after intravenous melphalan. Intravenous melphalan may reduce the threshold for carmustine-induced pulmonary toxicity. Cisplatin-induced renal dysfunction may alter the pharmacokinetics of melphalan and cause increased toxicity. Nalidixic acid and intravenous melphalan given together may increase the incidence of severe hemorrhagic necrotic enterocolitis in pediatric patients.

*Decreased Effectiveness.* Food and cimetidine can reduce oral absorption of the drug, leading to inadequate treatment. Interferon increases plasma elimination of melphalan in patients with cisplatin-induced renal dysfunction, potentially reducing the effectiveness of melphalan in this setting. Melphalan is incompatible in solution with amphotericin B and with chlorpromazine hydrochloride.[8]

## TOXICITY

**Overview.** The predominant and dose-limiting toxicity is myelosuppression. This is more common and severe with intravenous than with oral therapy. A variety of other effects are occasionally seen, especially with high-dose treatment, including hypersensitivity reactions in about 2% of patients.

**Hematologic.** As with other classic alkylating agents, the major dose-limiting toxicity of melphalan is reversible myelosuppression. Irreversible myelosuppression can also occur as a very rare event. Very rarely, melphalan has been reported to cause hemolytic anemia.[9]

**Digestive System.** High-dose melphalan frequently causes nausea and vomiting, but this problem is rare with standard oral dosage regimens. Diarrhea is rare. Veno-occlusive disease of the liver is rare and occurs only with high-dose intravenous therapy.

**Other and Rare Reactions**

*Immunologic.* Hypersensitivity reactions range from skin rashes to anaphylaxis, with an approximate frequency of 2% with the intravenous preparation.[10] Immunosuppression occurs, but not to a clinically important severity.

*Mucocutaneous.* Mucositis, alopecia, and skin ulceration in areas of intravenous drug extravasation all are rare.

*Cardiovascular.* Vasculitis is rare. Paroxysmal atrial fibrillation has been reported after high-dose melphalan with stem cell support.[11]

*Pulmonary.* Pulmonary fibrosis and interstitial fibrosis are rare.

*Genitourinary.* Melphalan is generally considered to be free of serious genitourinary toxicity, although hyperuricemia may result from tumor lysis. Patients with multiple myeloma frequently have renal dysfunction, making assessment of drug toxicity difficult. High-dose melphalan with stem cell support has been reported to improve renal function for such patients and is not a contraindication to treatment.[12]

*Ocular.* Cataracts are rare.

*Reproductive.* Toxicity studies place melphalan in FDA pregnancy category D. Infertility and menstrual irregularity are common.

*Endocrine-Metabolic.* SIADH has been reported with intravenous high-dose melphalan.[10]

*Carcinogenicity.* Melphalan is mutagenic and is a definite leukemogen in humans. It is probably more carcinogenic than cyclophosphamide.[13] It is known to cause pulmonary dysplasia after prolonged use.

## DOSAGE AND ADMINISTRATION

Melphalan is available for oral use as 2-mg tablets and for injection as 50-mg vials. When melphalan is given on a daily oral basis, severe and somewhat unpredictable myelosuppression may occur. Because the time of onset and the severity of myelosuppression are more predictable with intermittent schedules, it is generally preferable to use the drug as an intermittent pulse of treatment, as described by Alexanian and coworkers.[14] This intermittent program uses a dosage of 0.25 mg/kg/day for 4 to 5 days, with courses repeated at 4- to 6-week intervals. Because of the effect of food on its oral bioavailability, melphalan should be taken several hours before eating. The dose of oral melphalan should be reduced modestly in the presence of renal failure. More specific guidelines for this are given in Chapter 8.

The standard intravenous dosage of melphalan is 16 mg/$m^2$ infused over 15 to 20 minutes every 2 weeks for four doses, followed by 4-week intervals as tolerated. This dose should be reduced by up to 50% for patients with renal insufficiency (blood urea nitrogen, 30 mg/dl). Preliminary results from investigational high-dose therapy (140 mg/$m^2$), even without autologous bone marrow rescue, are encouraging.[15] The maximal dose of melphalan combined with stem cell support appears to be 200 mg/$m^2$ during a 90-minute period given on two separate occasions.[16]

## REFERENCES

1. Van der Zee J, Kroon BB, Nieweg OE, et al. Rationale for different approaches to combined melphalan and hyperthermia in regional isolated perfusion. Eur J Cancer 1997;33:1546–50.
2. Samuels BL, Bitran JD. High-dose intravenous melphalan: a review. J Clin Oncol 1995;13:1786–99.
3. Bailey HH, Mulcahy RT, Tutsch KD, et al. Phase I clinical trial of intravenous L-buthionine and sulfoximine and melphalan: an attempt at modulation of glutathione. J Clin Oncol 1994;12:194–205.
4. Chen G, Waxman DJ. Role of cellular glutathione and glutathione S-transferase in the expression of alkylating agent cytotoxicity in human breast cancer cells. Biochem Pharmacol 1994;47:1079–87.
5. Moscow JA, Swanson CA, Cowan KH. Decreased melphalan accumulation in a human breast cancer cell line selected for resistance to melphalan. Br J Cancer 1993;68:732–7.
6. Bramson J, Prevost J, Malapetsa A, et al. Poly (ADP-ribose) polymerase can bind melphalan damaged DNA. Cancer Res 1993;53:5370–3.
7. Cornford EM, Young D, Paxton JW, et al. Melphalan penetration of the blood-brain barrier via the neutral amino acid transporter in tumor-bearing brain. Cancer Res 1992;52:138–43.
8. Trissel LA, Martinez JF. Physical compatibility of melphalan with selected drugs during simulated Y-site administration. Am J Hosp Pharm 1993;50:2359–63.
9. Eyster ME. Melphalan (Alkeran) erythrocyte agglutinin and hemolytic anemia. Ann Intern Med 1967;66:573–7.
10. Sarosy G, Leyland-Jones B, Soochan P, Cheson BD. The systemic administration of intravenous melphalan. J Clin Oncol 1988;6:1768–82.
11. Olivieri A, Corvatta L, Montanari M, et al. Paroxysmal atrial fibrillation after high-dose melphalan in five patients autotransplanted with blood progenitor cells. Bone Marrow Transplant 1998;21:1049–53.
12. Reiter E, Kalhs P, Keil F, et al. Effect of high-dose melphalan and peripheral blood stem cell transplantation on renal function in patients with multiple myeloma and renal insufficiency: a case report and review of the literature. Ann Hematol 1999;78:189–91.
13. Greene MH, Harris EL, Gershenson DM, et al. Melphalan may be a more potent leukemogen than cyclophosphamide. Ann Intern Med 1986;105:360–7.
14. Alexanian R, Haut A, Khan AU, et al. Treatment for multiple myeloma: combination chemotherapy with different melphalan dose regimens. JAMA 1969;208:1680–5.
15. Cunningham D, Paz-Ares L, Gore ME, et al. High-dose melphalan for multiple myeloma: long-term follow-up data. J Clin Oncol 1994;12:764–8.
16. Weaver CH, Zhen B, Schwartzberg LS, et al. Phase I-II evaluation of

rapid sequence tandem high-dose melphalan with peripheral blood stem cell support in patients with multiple myeloma. Bone Marrow Transplant 1998;22:245–51.

# Mercaptopurine

Mammalian cells use preformed purines or those made de novo within the cell as essential components of RNA, DNA, and coenzymes. Therefore, purine analogues were of early interest in the historic development of cancer chemotherapy. Hitchings and Elion were awarded the Nobel Prize for Medicine and Physiology in 1988 for developing four such agents.[1] One of these antimetabolites is mercaptopurine. Mercaptopurine is also known as 6-mercaptopurine, 6-MP, Purinethol, and NSC-755.

## EFFICACY

6-MP is primarily used in the treatment of ALL, especially in children. Oral therapy is standard, but intravenous therapy has many advantages that are being studied in clinical trials.[2, 3]

## PHARMACOLOGY

**Mechanism of Action.** 6-MP must be activated by the enzyme thiopurine methyltransferase (TPMT) as a minimal requirement for cytotoxicity.[4] 6-MP is converted to 6-thioguanine (6-TG) ribotide or one of its products, and in this form it is incorporated into DNA.[5, 6] 6-MP also inhibits de novo purine synthesis directly.[7] Inhibition of purine synthesis involves several interrelated metabolic steps, including direct inhibition of the conversion of amino-imidazole carboxamide ribonucleotide (AICR) to inosine and indirect inhibition of AICR synthesis after conversion to a methylated form (6-methylmercaptopurine riboside [6-MMPR]). The latter occurs by a novel mechanism: The 6-MMPR acts as a pseudoregulatory inhibitor of the allosteric, or controlling, site of the enzyme that catalyzes the formation of AICR. Thus, 6-MP inhibits cells by three different mechanisms: (1) incorporation into DNA, leading to an abnormal DNA molecule; (2) inhibition of the active site of an important enzymatic step in purine synthesis; and (3) inhibition of the allosteric site of an important enzyme in purine synthesis.

In murine leukemic cell lines exposed to thiopurines, survival curves display a phenomenon termed *paradoxic cytotoxicity*, defined as a decrease in cytotoxicity with increasing drug concentration. This has been attributed to perturbations of the cell cycle with higher doses, but an alternative explanation involves the relative concentrations of thiol- and non–thiol-containing metabolites at different doses.[8] Specifically, the thionucleotide that is incorporated into DNA is more toxic to cell growth and does not increase with higher drug concentrations, whereas desulfurated metabolites that interfere with DNA incorporation of thionucleotides increase in a linear fashion with dose. These results have been interpreted as showing a unique mechanism of detoxification in which higher drug doses result in the production of a comparatively potent "self-rescue" agent.

6-MP influences cell cycle progression in highly complex ways.[7] To summarize these effects, 6-MP is considered to be cell cycle phase specific but self-limited. Data relevant to possible schedule dependence in humans are scant.

**Resistance.** The 6-thiopurines are not cross-resistant to other chemotherapeutic drugs used in clinical practice, but 6-MP and 6-TG are cross-resistant to each other. There are myriad types of resistance to 6-MP treatment involving alterations of intracellular drug metabolism.[9]

**Pharmacokinetics.** 6-MP is efficiently absorbed after oral administration, but extensive first-pass metabolism by xanthine oxidase occurs in the liver.[10] Only about 10 to 20% of an oral dose reaches the bloodstream under normal circumstances, although this increases to about 60% in the presence of the xanthine oxidase inhibitor allopurinol. About 10 to 40% of a 6-MP dose is excreted in the urine as unchanged drug. The elimination half-life is about 6 to 8 hours. Only negligible levels of 6-MP cross the blood-brain barrier. Because of first-pass metabolism, the bioavailability of oral 6-MP is variable and somewhat unpredictable.[11]

Preclinical pharmacology, phase I and II trials, and pharmacokinetic studies of intrathecal 6-MP suggest that this route of administration may be useful.[12] This investigational route of administration deserves further study.

**Pharmacogenetics.** The critical enzyme in 6-MP metabolism is TPMT. This enzyme varies in the population: About 85% of whites have high levels of the enzyme, about 14% have intermediate levels, and about 1 patient in 300 has very low values.[13, 14] Patients with high levels of TPMT are very tolerant of standard dose 6-MP and are at risk of undertreatment with standard protocols. Patients with very low levels of TPMT are at risk of severe, life-threatening toxicity with very low doses of 6-MP. There is increasing interest in identifying these patients before they are treated with 6-MP in order to optimize therapy, preferably by determining the pharmacokinetics of 6-MP after a test dose[15] or by monitoring RBC levels of TPMT during therapy.[16]

**Drug Interactions**

*Increased Toxicity.* Xanthine oxidase is essential to the degradation of 6-MP. Allopurinol, which inhibits xanthine oxidase, markedly inhibits the first-pass metabolism of oral 6-MP by the liver. As a consequence, the oral dose of 6-MP must be reduced to 25 to 33% of the usual dose in patients receiving concurrent allopurinol. The intravenous dose of investigational 6-MP and oral doses of thioguanine do not have to be changed because they are unaffected by first-pass metabolism. The concurrent use of doxorubicin or the use of hepatotoxic drugs may increase the incidence of 6-MP–associated hepatotoxicity. Olsalazine has been reported to increase the toxicity of 6-MP, probably because of olsalazine-induced noncompetitive inhibition of TPMT.[17] Sulfasalazine and its metabolite 5-aminosalicylic acid are also noncompetitive inhibitors of TPMT; thus, they should also be considered candidates for the same adverse drug-drug interaction.[18]

*Drug Antagonism.* Nondepolarizing muscle relaxants, such as tubocurarine and pancuronium, are antagonized by 6-MP. These neuromuscular relaxants must be given in two to four times the usual dose when combined with 6-MP.[19]

The dose of the anticoagulant coumarin must also be increased when given with 6-MP.[20]

*Therapeutic Interactions.* The antineoplastic effect of 6-MP combined with cytarabine is markedly increased by subsequent use of asparaginase.[21] This synergy is due to the increased apoptosis noted with this sequence of drug administration.

## TOXICITY

**Overview.** Myelosuppression and hepatic toxicity are the major dose-limiting adverse effects of 6-MP.

**Hematologic.** Myelosuppression is expected and is dose limiting. The neutrophil nadir occurs at about 7 days, and recovery is complete by 14 to 21 days.

**Immunologic.** Mild to moderate immunosuppression is expected and may contribute to infectious complications during treatment. A single case of serum sickness due to 6-MP has been reported.[22]

**Digestive System.** The drug is usually well tolerated, but occasional nausea, emesis, anorexia, diarrhea, intestinal ulceration, malabsorption, and abdominal cramps may occur. Moderate to severe cholestatic jaundice that can progress in rare cases to hepatic necrosis, fibrosis, and very rarely death can occur.[23] This problem may be exacerbated by the concomitant use of hepatotoxic drugs or drugs that undergo extensive hepatic metabolism (such as doxorubicin). Two patients with inflammatory bowel disease developed pancreatitis while taking 6-MP.[24]

**Mucocutaneous.** Stomatitis can occur, resembling thrush, but frank ulceration is very rare. Hyperpigmentation can rarely occur, as well as a papular skin rash that can develop after withdrawal of oral 6-MP.[25]

**Other and Rare Reactions**

*Systemic.* Fever can occur.

*Neurologic.* Headaches can occur.

*Genitourinary.* Hematuria and crystalluria can occur after very large doses.[26]

*Reproductive.* Toxicity studies place 6-MP in FDA pregnancy category D.

*Endocrine-Metabolic.* Suppression of thyroid function[27] and hyperuricemia due to tumor lysis can occur.

*Carcinogenicity.* 6-MP is mutagenic, but the carcinogenic potential of the drug appears to be minimal.

## DOSAGE AND ADMINISTRATION

6-MP is available as 50-mg tablets. Commonly used oral maintenance doses of 6-MP range from 50 to 100 mg/m²/day. Unlike 6-TG, the dose of oral 6-MP should be reduced to 25 to 33% of the usual dose in patients receiving concurrent allopurinol therapy. The manufacturer recommends careful monitoring of both hematologic and liver function in patients treated with 6-MP. Treatment should be discontinued for myelosuppression with or without infection. Immediate cessation of therapy is also needed if the patient develops anorexia, clinical jaundice, right upper quadrant tenderness, hepatomegaly, or any evidence of liver enzyme deterioration.

Pharmacokinetic considerations and several clinical trials suggest that the daily dose of 6-MP should be given in the evening, not in the morning.[28] Several studies have demonstrated therapeutic failure because of poor compliance by patients.[29] Strategies for dealing with this problem include confirmation of drug effect by periodic measurements of 6-MP metabolites in blood and by electronic monitoring of the actual doses of chemotherapy taken by the patient.[30]

## REFERENCES

 1. Hitchings GH, Elion GB. The chemistry and biochemistry of purine analogs. Ann N Y Acad Sci 1954;60:195.
 2. Pinkel D. Intravenous mercaptopurine: life begins at 40. J Clin Oncol 1993;11:1826–31.
 3. Lockhart S, Plunkett W, Jeha S, et al. High-dose mercaptopurine followed by intermediate-dose cytarabine in relapsed acute leukemia. J Clin Oncol 1994;12:587–95.
 4. Krynetski EY, Krynetskaia NF, Yanishevski Y, Evans WE. Methylation of mercaptopurine, thioguanine, and their nucleotide metabolites by heterologously expressed human thiopurine S-methyltransferase. Mol Pharmacol 1995;47:1141–7.
 5. Tidd DM, Paterson AR. A biochemical mechanism for the delayed cytotoxic reaction of 6-mercaptopurine. Cancer Res 1974;34:738–46.
 6. Nelson JA, Carpenter JW, Rose LM, Adamson DJ. Mechanisms of action of 6-thioguanine, 6-mercaptopurine, and 8-azaguanine. Cancer Res 1975;35:2872–8.
 7. Bokkerink JPM, Stet EH, De Abreu RA, et al. 6-Mercaptopurine: cytotoxicity and biochemical pharmacology in human malignant T-lymphoblasts. Biochem Pharmacol 1993;45:1455–63.
 8. Adamson PC, Balis FM, Hawkins ME, et al. Desulfuration of 6-mercaptopurine: the basis for the paradoxical cytotoxicity of thiopurines in cultured human leukemic cells. Biochem Pharmacol 1993;46:1627–36.
 9. van Scoik KG, Johnson CA, Porter WR. The pharmacology and metabolism of the thiopurine drugs 6-mercaptopurine and azathioprine. Drug Metab Rev 1985;16:157–74.
10. Zimm S, Collins JM, Riccardi R, et al. Variable bioavailability of oral mercaptopurine: is maintenance chemotherapy in acute lymphoblastic leukemia being optimally delivered? N Engl J Med 1983;308:1005–9.
11. Koren G, Ferrazini G, Sulh H, et al. Systemic exposure to mercaptopurine as a prognostic factor in acute lymphocytic leukemia in children. N Engl J Med 1990;323:17–21.
12. Adamson PC, Balis FM, Arndt CA, et al. Intrathecal 6-mercaptopurine: preclinical pharmacology, phase I/II trial, and pharmacokinetic study. Cancer Res 1991;51:6079–83.
13. Escousse A, Guedon F, Mounie J, et al. 6-Mercaptopurine pharmacokinetics after use of azathioprine in renal transplant recipients with intermediate or high thiopurine methyl transferase activity phenotype. J Pharm Pharmacol 1998;50:1261–6.
14. Lennard L, Lilleyman JS. Individualizing therapy with 6-mercaptopurine and 6-thioguanine related to the thiopurine methyltransferase genetic polymorphism. Ther Drug Monit 1996;18:328–34.
15. Mawatari H, Kato Y, Nishimura S, et al. Reversed-phase high-performance liquid chromatographic assay method for quantitating 6-mercaptopurine and its methylated and non-methylated metabolites in a single sample. J Chromatogr B Biomed Sci Appl 1998;716:392–6.
16. Giverhaug T, Bergan S, Loennechen T, et al. Analysis of methylated 6-mercaptopurine metabolites in human red blood cells: comparison of two methods. Ther Drug Monit 1997;19:663–8.
17. Lewis LD, Benin A, Szumlanski CL, et al. Olsalazine and 6-mercaptopurine-related bone marrow suppression: a possible drug-drug interaction. Clin Pharmacol Ther 1997;62:464–75.
18. Szumlanski CL, Weinshilboum RM. Sulphasalazine inhibition of thiopurine methyltransferase: possible mechanism for interaction with 6-mercaptopurine and azathioprine. Br J Clin Pharmacol 1995;39:456–9.
19. Chapple DJ, Clark JS, Hughes R. Interaction between atracurium and drugs used in anaesthesia. Br J Anaesth 1983;55:Suppl 1:17S–22S.
20. Spiers ASD, Mibashan RS. Increased warfarin requirement during mercaptopurine therapy: a new drug interaction. Lancet 1974;2:221–2. letter.
21. Nandy P, Periclou AP, Avramis VI. The synergism of 6-mercaptopurine plus cytosine arabinoside followed by PEG-asparaginase in human leukemia cell lines is due to increased cellular apoptosis. Anticancer Res 1998;18:727–37.
22. Andersen JM, Tiede JJ. Serum sickness associated with 6-mercaptopurine in a patient with Crohn's disease. Pharmacotherapy 1997;17:173–6.
23. Krawitt EL, Stein JH, Kirkendall WM, Clifteon JA. Mercaptopurine hepatotoxicity in a patient with chronic active hepatitis. Arch Intern Med 1967;120:729–34.
24. Bank L, Wright JP. 6-Mercaptopurine-related pancreatitis in 2 patients with inflammatory bowel disease. Dig Dis Sci 1984;29:357–9.
25. Kirk JA, Rogers M, Menser MA, et al. Unusual skin rash following withdrawal of oral 6-mercaptopurine in children with leukemia. Med Pediatr Oncol 1987;15:281–4.
26. Duttera MJ, Carolla RS, Gallelli JF, et al. Hematuria and crystalluria after high-dose 6-mercaptopurine administration. N Engl J Med 1972;287:292–4.
27. Jubiz W, Nolan G. The effects of 6-mercaptopurine (6-MP) on the thyroid gland. Endocrinology 1974;94:1583–6.
28. Schmiegelow K, Glomstein A, Kristinsson J, et al. Impact of morning versus evening schedule for oral methotrexate and 6-mercaptopurine on relapse risk for children with acute lymphoblastic leukemia. J Pediatr Hematol Oncol 1997;19:102–9.
29. Schmiegelow K, Schrøder H, Gustafsson G, et al. Risk of relapse in childhood acute lymphoblastic leukemia is related to RBC methotrexate and mercaptopurine metabolites during maintenance chemotherapy. J Clin Oncol 1995;13:345–51.
30. Lau RC, Matsui D, Greenberg M, Koren G. Electronic measurement of compliance with mercaptopurine in pediatric patients with acute lymphoblastic leukemia. Med Pediatr Oncol 1998;30:85–90.

# Methotrexate

The introduction of folic acid antagonists by Farber and colleagues in 1948 marked the beginning of an important new phase in the history of cancer chemotherapy. Many folic acid analogues have been developed and used clinically, but an early compound, MTX, is the one currently used. The drug is also known as methotrexate sodium, Methotrexate LPF, Rheumatrex, amethopterin, and NSC-740.

## EFFICACY

MTX is used in three main ways: (1) in standard doses given by either the oral or the parenteral routes, (2) by intrathecal administration, and (3) in very high doses followed by leucovorin (high-dose MTX with rescue).

**Standard-Dose Therapy.** Systemic MTX in standard doses is an important drug in the treatment of acute leukemia, gestational trophoblastic neoplasia, mycosis fungoides, and carcinomas of the head and neck and the breast. Conventional doses of MTX are also used in a variety of nonmalignant conditions, especially severe psoriasis (possibly through induction of keratinocyte differentiation[1]) and debilitating rheumatoid arthritis.[2]

**Intrathecal Therapy.** Intrathecal MTX is a standard part of the treatment of some forms of acute leukemia, either as prophylaxis or as treatment of active leptomeningeal leukemia. Intrathecal MTX is also used in the treatment of meningeal carcinomatosis.

**High-Dose MTX with Leucovorin Rescue.** This is used primarily in the adjuvant therapy of osteosarcoma. Less frequently it is used in the treatment of childhood acute leukemia and in several aggressive regimens of combination chemotherapy for advanced non-Hodgkin's lymphoma.

## PHARMACOLOGY

**Mechanism of Action.** MTX and its polyglutamate metabolites compete avidly for the folate binding site of the enzyme dihydrofolate reductase (DHFR).[3, 4] Tight but reversible binding to DHFR leads to blockage of tetrahydrofolate synthesis and depletion of reduced folate cofactors in the cell, resulting primarily in decreased synthesis of thymidine and purine nucleotides. The polyglutamate form of MTX also inhibits other enzymes within the cell, especially AICR, transformylase, and thymidylate synthase.[5] Ultimately, these effects result in apoptosis.[6]

MTX is relatively cell cycle phase specific, although this effect is self-limited. Consequently, clinical use of MTX exhibits schedule dependence, as discussed in Chapter 8.

**Resistance.** Biochemical resistance to MTX is multifactorial and may involve any one or more of the following steps. First, uptake of MTX into the cell is an active process involving a single carrier system shared with folic acid and L-leucovorin,[7, 8] whereas MTX efflux occurs by a different mechanism with at least three components that have different sensitivities to specific inhibitors.[9] Resistance can therefore occur by reduced influx or increased efflux of MTX. Second, intracellular MTX can act directly or be converted to noneffluxing long-chain MTX polyglutamate species.[10] Although both forms of MTX are cytotoxic, the polyglutamate form can remain within the cell for prolonged periods and cause substantial cytotoxicity. Thus, reduced conversion of MTX to the polyglutamate form can be a mechanism of resistance, and enhanced conversion of MTX to polyglutamates by some tumor cell lines can result in enhanced killing of tumor compared with normal cells.[5, 10, 11] In one study, this form of increased sensitivity was associated with hyperdiploid ALL cells (>50 chromosomes).[12] A third mechanism of resistance involves the target molecule DHFR. Resistance to MTX has been related to altered amounts of the enzyme, primarily through gene amplification,[13] to changes in the affinity of DHFR for MTX,[14] and through a mutation involving a residue 9 to 12 nm away from the enzyme active site.[15] Additional mechanisms of possible resistance include a decrease in the level of thymidylate synthase activity in resistant cells,[16] decreased cell growth itself (presumably because of a proliferation-dependent reduction in the formation of polyglutamate forms of MTX[17]), and perhaps other unknown mechanisms.

It is well known that the cytotoxicity of MTX can be reversed by leucovorin (citrovorum factor, L-leucovorin calcium). Leucovorin is readily converted to other forms of reduced folate within the cell, including a polyglutamate form, which can then act as methyl donors for a variety of biochemical reactions. At low doses of MTX, leucovorin efficiently bypasses the block of DHFR; however, at high MTX levels, relatively higher doses of leucovorin are needed because both MTX and leucovorin compete for intracellular transport. The use of leucovorin to overcome the cytotoxic effect of MTX is commonly referred to as *leucovorin rescue*.[14] Other forms of rescue have also been studied, including the use of thymidine[18] and the enzyme carboxypeptidase.[19, 20] Pretreatment of patients with 5-FU also allows higher than normal doses of MTX to be delivered, even without leucovorin rescue.[21]

**Pharmacokinetics.** After intravenous administration, MTX is bound to serum albumin and widely distributed in body water, except for the nervous system. MTX is retained in the kidneys for several weeks and is retained in the liver for months. Clearance from plasma is triphasic: It is very

rapid initially, but the half-life of the critical phase (which starts 12 to 36 hours after the intravenous dose) is 8 to 12 hours. The precise rate of clearance may be variable from patient to patient, depending on the dose and the route of drug administration, the adequacy of renal function, and the presence or absence of so-called third-space depots (e.g., an effusion in the chest or abdomen).

Most aspects of the clinical use and toxicity of MTX can be understood as a function of the duration of time tissues are exposed to critical threshold MTX concentrations. Complete suppression of DNA synthesis by MTX commonly requires an extracellular MTX concentration of $10^{-8}$ M or more, with the resultant presence of unbound MTX or MTX polyglutamates within the cell. The duration of a cell's exposure to free intracellular MTX or MTX polyglutamates is also critical. Indeed, for toxicity to occur, both the concentration threshold and the time threshold for the tissue must be exceeded, and the severity of the toxicity is particularly determined by the extent to which the time threshold is exceeded. For bone marrow and gut epithelium, the plasma concentration threshold and the time threshold appear to be $2 \times 10^{-8}$ M and about 42 hours, respectively. Estimated concentration thresholds for toxicity in various tissues are $10^{-3}$ M for the kidneys with alkaline urine, $10^{-4}$ M for the kidneys with acid urine, and $10^{-9}$ to $10^{-7}$ M for the lungs and liver.[22] Unfortunately, the time threshold for many of these tissues is uncertain.

**Drug Interactions.** Numerous potential and well-demonstrated drug interactions exist for MTX. For example, the delivery of MTX to tissues may be influenced by a variety of factors. MTX is 50 to 70% bound by intravascular serum albumin, and hypoalbuminemia or drugs may displace MTX from albumin. The use of gut-sterilizing antibiotics may cause increased MTX toxicity by eliminating the gut bacteria, which, in part, degrade the MTX that is given orally or that enters into the enterohepatic circulation phase of its distribution.[23, 24] Similarly, gastrointestinal obstruction may lead to sustained serum MTX concentrations.[25] A variety of drugs may affect the ability of MTX to enter or leave cells. For example, cephalothin and hydrocortisone inhibit MTX accumulation by human leukemia cells, whereas high concentrations of vincristine enhance MTX accumulation, apparently by inhibiting MTX efflux from the cell. Estrogens can induce MTX resistance in vitro, but the mechanism is uncertain.[26]

As a practical matter, the pharmacokinetic alterations and drug interactions just described are rarely a clinical problem. However, one pharmacokinetic consideration is of vital importance—that of renal clearance. MTX is very insoluble in acidic solutions, so alkalization of the urine leads to augmented renal clearance. Anything that reduces renal function can increase MTX toxicity, including such commonly used drugs as the aminoglycoside antibiotics and cisplatin-based chemotherapy. Moreover, because the drug is secreted in part by the kidneys (and the liver via the bile), drugs that inhibit the secretion of MTX may increase toxicity. Some of these potential drug interactions are sufficiently well demonstrated to discuss individually.

*Aspirin.* Aspirin competes with MTX for renal elimination, and it can displace MTX from its binding site on albumin. Concurrent use of salicylates thus can increase MTX toxicity.[27, 28]

*Sulfonamides.* Sulfonamides can displace MTX from albumin, leading to increased MTX toxicity.[29]

*Nonsteroidal Anti-inflammatory Drugs.* Numerous studies suggest that concurrent use of MTX with NSAIDs leads to increased toxicity.[30] The mechanism is uncertain but probably involves changes in renal blood flow or MTX clearance by the kidneys in the presence of NSAIDs. One study suggests possible differences among various NSAIDs. Pharmacokinetic changes were prominent with ibuprofen, whereas ketoprofen, flurbiprofen, and piroxicam caused no significant change in MTX pharmacokinetics.[31]

*Probenecid.* This drug reduces the renal tubular secretion of MTX, and it can thus increase MTX toxicity when used concurrently. For example, in a patient with rheumatoid arthritis, this drug interaction resulted in life-threatening pancytopenia.[32] Trimethoprim can also falsely elevate MTX blood level measurements.

*Trimethoprim.* This antibiotic is an inhibitor of DHFR; concurrent use with MTX can lead to enhanced MTX toxicity,[33] including pancytopenia.[34]

*Other.* Macrolide antibiotics can prolong plasma clearance of MTX, leading to potentially serious increased toxicity.[35] The index case received ketoprofen, which is chemically related to erythromycin.

## TOXICITY

**Overview.** The major dose-limiting toxicity of MTX is myelosuppression, but other forms of toxicity are important, including mucositis, nausea, abdominal distress, malaise, undue fatigue, chills and fever, and decreased resistance to infection. The pattern of toxicity differs by the dose and route of administration. Because the most common use of MTX is standard dose therapy, the spectrum of toxicity with this mode of use is summarized first. Subsequently, toxicities unique to intrathecal and high-dose therapy with leucovorin rescue are separately described.

**Hematologic.** Neutropenia is dose related, with a nadir of granulocytopenia at 7 to 14 days and recovery by day 14 to 21. Thrombocytopenia tends to parallel the level of neutropenia; anemia is less of a problem. Myelosuppression is a strong indication for postponing therapy, especially in patients receiving MTX for one of several nonmalignant conditions. Even low-dose therapy is capable of inducing prolonged pancytopenia. Immune hemolytic anemia occurs rarely.

**Digestive System.** Nausea and vomiting are unusual with standard doses, as are anorexia, hematemesis, and melena. Diarrhea can occur and is an indication for discontinuing MTX therapy. The drug should be used with extreme caution or not at all in patients with ulcerative colitis or peptic ulcer disease. Liver dysfunction may occur, primarily in patients receiving long-term low-dose therapy. This can take the form of acutely elevated transaminase enzyme levels, which usually return to normal after discontinuing therapy. However, chronic hepatotoxicity with liver fibrosis and cirrhosis can also occur. Chronic toxicity tends to occur after long-term therapy, and it can be fatal. MTX should be used with caution or not at all in patients taking other hepatotoxic drugs or in patients with pre-existing liver disease. Chronic

hepatic damage has been considered sufficiently serious to warrant yearly liver biopsy in patients receiving MTX for psoriasis or rheumatoid arthritis.

**Mucocutaneous.** Proliferating epithelial cells are a major target of toxicity. The buccal mucosa is particularly vulnerable, and stomatitis is a strong indication for interrupting MTX treatment. Mucositis is common and occurs with dose-related frequency and severity. This can include conjunctivitis and excessive lacrimation. Other skin reactions are unusual but can include erythema or rash, pruritus, urticaria, alopecia, photosensitivity, depigmentation or hyperpigmentation, acneiform rash, furunculosis, exfoliative dermatitis, distal erythema with desquamation, formation of bullas, folliculitis, ecchymosis, and telangiectases. MTX has been reported to reactivate thermal burns.[36]

**Pulmonary.** A dry, nonproductive cough or nonspecific pneumonitis occasionally develops during treatment at any dose level.[37] MTX should be discontinued immediately because this can progress to a severe form of lung disease characterized by dyspnea, hypoxia, and an increasing infiltrate on chest radiographs. This interstitial pneumonitis can progress to chronic interstitial obstructive pulmonary disease or even death.

**Genitourinary.** The following can occur: renal toxicity with hematuria due to large doses; rare renal tubular necrosis and renal failure, especially with high-dose treatment; and proteinuria due to suboptimal hydration with high-dose MTX.[38]

**Other and Rare Reactions**

*Systemic.* Fever, chills, and malaise can occur. The manufacturer recommends that MTX be used with extra caution in patients with debility.

*Immunologic.* Anaphylaxis is very rare; immunosuppression is usually mild to moderate, but it may become severe in patients with pre-existing immunosuppression.

*Cardiovascular.* Vasculitis can occur.

*Ocular.* Conjunctivitis, excessive lacrimation, cataracts, photophobia, and blurred vision all are rare. Cortical blindness is very rare with high doses.

*Neurologic.* Leukoencephalopathy can occur following intravenous MTX as well as after high-dose MTX with rescue in patients treated previously with cranial or cranial-spinal irradiation. The leukoencephalopathy may persist despite cessation of drug therapy. Transient neurologic dysfunction can also occur in patients receiving high-dose MTX with leucovorin rescue. This syndrome can include behavioral changes, focal sensorimotor changes, and abnormal reflexes. CNS changes listed by the manufacturer also include headache, drowsiness, aphasia, hemiparesis, and convulsions.

*Musculoskeletal.* Osteoporotic fracture, arthralgia, and myalgia can occur.

*Reproductive.* Toxicity studies place MTX in FDA pregnancy category X. Reversible oligospermia, impaired fertility, menstrual dysfunction, and vaginal discharge can occur; congenital malformations have been reported but are rare.[39]

*Endocrine-Metabolic.* The following effects are possible: loss of libido and impotence, diabetes mellitus, and hyperuricemia with tumor lysis.

*Carcinogenicity.* Animal and human evidence for and against carcinogenicity is not conclusive. Three cases of bladder cancer in patients on low-dose MTX and cortico-steroids have been reported,[40] and further surveillance for second neoplasms is thus needed.

**Intrathecal Methotrexate.** This route of MTX administration may be associated with acute, subacute, and delayed forms of neurotoxicity.[41] Acutely, symptomatic chemical arachnoiditis occurs in 5 to 40% of patients within 12 hours of drug administration. The signs and symptoms of this problem mimic those of other forms of meningitis. This is usually a self-limited process, but in one case, this was lethal in a patient receiving intraventricular MTX.[42] Subacute toxicity usually takes the form of a myelopathy or encephalopathy developing days to weeks after starting intrathecal MTX. This reaction is most common in patients who have received 5 to 11 treatments, for a total MTX dose of 90 to 192 mg.[41] The major manifestation of this form of subacute toxicity is motor dysfunction of brain or spinal cord origin, which can rarely progress to paraplegia. This myelopathy or encephalopathy may be permanent, but most cases resolve by reducing the dose of MTX or discontinuing its use. Seizures may also represent a form of subacute toxicity. Delayed neurotoxicity is extremely rare in patients receiving intrathecal MTX alone but increases in importance when cranial irradiation or other intrathecal drugs are used as well. In such patients, the delayed toxicity can take the form of cerebral atrophy with concomitant abnormalities of psychological and intellectual function.

Several possible mechanisms of neurotoxicity have been postulated, including toxic inhibition of neurotransmitter synthesis, possible pharmacologic differences in drug clearance from the CSF, and the presence of benzyl alcohol as a preservative in the standard preparation of MTX. The latter problem has been corrected by the commercial availability of preservative-free MTX, which should always be used when intrathecal therapy or high-dose therapy is planned.

**High-Dose Methotrexate with Rescue.** Although most patients have minimal side effects, any of the problems described for conventional MTX therapy can occur with high-dose treatment. Furthermore, several forms of toxicity are of great concern. Renal failure may result from high-dose MTX, probably because of the direct deposition of MTX within the kidneys.[43] Dialysis for the removal of MTX in these patients is ineffective, but charcoal hemoperfusion, either alone[44] or combined with hemodialysis,[45, 46] has proved useful. Unfortunately, leucovorin is incapable of rescuing patients from established tissue damage; the need to anticipate its potential use in high-risk patients is thus emphasized. Other potential (but rare) side effects of high-dose MTX include chemical pleuritis, erythema and desquamation, ocular irritation, transient (benign) hepatotoxicity, anaphylaxis, and a transient encephalopathy that does not preclude further treatment. Transient testicular failure has been reported in one half of men receiving high-dose MTX, but MTX has no apparent effect on ovarian function.[47] Very rarely, optic nerve damage can result in blindness.

Despite the generally mild nature of the side effects of high-dose MTX in most patients, it must be emphasized that treatment with high-dose MTX is potentially very dangerous and even lethal. MTX blood levels should be readily avail-able, and the staff should be carefully trained to follow the many details of safe administration described next.

## DOSAGE AND ADMINISTRATION

MTX is available in the following forms: as a lyophilized powder for injection in vials of 20, 50, 100, 250, and 1000 mg; as a 25 mg/ml preservative-free isotonic solution for injection in vials of 50, 100, 200, and 250 mg; as a 2.5 mg/ml preservative-free isotonic solution for injection in a 5-mg vial; as a 25 mg/ml preservative-free isotonic solution for injection in vials of 50 and 250 mg; and as 2.5-mg tablets. It is considered vital that a preservative-free form be used both for intrathecal and for high-dose treatment with leucovorin rescue. The drug is reconstituted with water or other solutions, and it is often diluted further in normal saline or 5% dextrose in water. It is incompatible in solution with numerous drugs, including bleomycin, doxorubicin, idarubicin, prednisolone, droperidol, metoclopramide, and ranitidine.

**Conventional Systemic Treatment.** MTX is usually given in single doses of 25 to 75 mg/m² intravenously, intramuscularly, or orally once or twice weekly, depending on the disease being treated. Doses of this magnitude cause peak plasma concentrations of $1 \times 10^{-6}$ M to $1 \times 10^{-5}$ M. Clearance is reasonably complete by 1 to 2 days, and in the absence of previous marrow dysfunction or renal disease, leucovorin is not required. This dose may be titrated up or down, depending on the patient's tolerance.[48] In this regard, it should be noted that plasma levels of MTX are comparable after low oral or low intravenous doses of MTX, but they are predictable at higher doses only when the intravenous route of administration is used.

Patients should be closely monitored with frequent blood counts, urinalysis, renal and liver function tests, and chest radiographs. Patients with renal impairment, pleural effusion, or other third-space accumulation of fluid are at especially high risk of toxicity. These patients should be considered for MTX treatment only if absolutely necessary. Fluid should be removed before therapy if possible. Such patients may require blood level measurements of MTX and should probably receive leucovorin, as per published guidelines for high-dose MTX with rescue.

**Intrathecal Methotrexate.** The usual dose of MTX for injection into the lumbar subarachnoid space in adults is 6 to 12 mg/m², up to a maximum of 15 mg. Preservative-free MTX (Methotrexate LPF Sodium) is dissolved in 10 ml of saline or artificial CSF. This dose is given twice weekly until evidence of leukemic involvement disappears. It is then administered monthly. In the case of prophylactic treatment, a total of five doses is given in league with whole-brain radiation therapy. The normal half-life for clearance from the CSF is approximately 12 hours. This is associated with a slow rise in the plasma MTX concentration, with cytotoxic levels being maintained for as long as 48 hours. This curve contrasts with the more rapid disappearance of MTX from plasma after intravenous administration. For patients whose lives would be jeopardized by myelosuppression, several low doses of leucovorin (3 to 6 mg every 6 hours) should be started 24 hours after intrathecal MTX is given. This

*Table 10–4.* **Guidelines for the Use of High-Dose Methotrexate and Rescue**

Administration of MTX should be delayed until recovery if:
    White blood cell count is <1500/μL
    Neutrophil count is <200/μL
    Platelet count is <75,000/μL
    Serum bilirubin level is >1.2 mg/dl
    Serum glutamic-pyruvic transaminase level is >450 units
    Mucositis is present, until there is evidence of healing
    Persistent pleural effusion is present; this should be drained dry before infusion
Adequate renal function must be documented.
    Serum creatinine level must be normal, and creatinine clearance must be >60 ml/min, before initiation of therapy.
    Serum creatinine level must be measured before each subsequent course of therapy. If serum creatinine level has increased
        by 50% compared with a prior value, creatinine clearance must be measured and documented to be >60 ml/min (even if
        serum creatinine level is still within normal range).
Patients must be well hydrated and must be treated with sodium bicarbonate for urinary alkalization.
    Administer 1000 ml/m² of intravenous fluid over 6 hr before initiation of MTX infusion. Continue hydration at 125 ml/m²/hr
        (3 L/m²/day) during MTX infusion, and for 2 days after infusion has been completed.
    Alkalize urine to maintain pH above 7.0 during MTX infusion and leucovorin calcium therapy. This can be accomplished by
        administration of sodium bicarbonate orally or by incorporation into separate intravenous solution.
Repeat serum creatinine and serum MTX 24 hr after starting MTX and at least once daily until MTX level is below $5 \times 10^{-8}$
    mol/L (0.05 μmol/L).
Table 10–5 provides guidelines for leucovorin calcium dosage based on serum MTX levels. Patients who experience delayed
    early MTX elimination are likely to develop nonreversible oliguric renal failure. In addition to appropriate leucovorin
    therapy, these patients require continuing hydration and urinary alkalization and close monitoring of fluid and electrolyte
    status until serum MTX level has fallen to below 0.05 μmol/L and renal failure has resolved.
Some patients will have abnormalities in MTX elimination or abnormalities in renal function after MTX administration. These
    are significant but less severe than abnormalities described in Table 10–5. These abnormalities may or may not be associated
    with significant clinical toxicity. If significant clinical toxicity is observed, leucovorin rescue should be extended for an
    additional 24 hr (total, 14 doses over 84 hr) in subsequent courses of therapy. The possibility that a patient is taking other
    medications that interact with MTX should be considered (see earlier discussion).

MTX, methotrexate.
From the Immunex product brochure on methotrexate, revised November 1997.

delay is necessary because a metabolite of leucovorin readily crosses the blood-brain barrier, and its premature use would abrogate the effect of MTX against the CSF leukemia cells.

When intrathecal MTX is given as part of induction therapy for patients without leptomeningeal involvement by ALL, there is evidence that the intrathecal therapy adds to the systemic effect of the induction chemotherapy regimen.[49]

**High-Dose Methotrexate with Rescue.** Many variations of this approach to treatment have been described. Variations of these high-dose regimens are included in many programs of combination chemotherapy, as discussed in the disease-oriented chapters. However, the primary use of high-dose MTX with leucovorin rescue at this time is in the adjuvant therapy of osteosarcoma, as discussed in Chapter 81. The starting dose for MTX in the usual regimens is 12 g/m². This is followed by leucovorin in a dosage of 15 mg orally every 6 hours for 10 doses starting at 24 hours after the start of the MTX infusion. Repeat courses may be given as frequently as once weekly, depending on the precise regimen used. If 12 g/m² does not result in a peak serum MTX concentration of 1000 mol/L ($10^{-3}$ mol/L) at the end of the MTX infusion, the dose may be escalated to 15 g/m² in subsequent courses. If the patient is vomiting or is unable to tolerate oral medication, leucovorin is given intravenously or intramuscularly at the same dose and schedule. Tables 10–4 and 10–5 summarize the precautions and safety guidelines recommended by the manufacturer when doses of this magnitude are used.

*Table 10–5.* **Leucovorin Rescue Schedules Following Treatment with Higher Doses of Methotrexate**

| Clinical Situation | Laboratory Findings | Leucovorin Dosage and Duration |
|---|---|---|
| Normal MTX elimination | Serum MTX level approximately 10 μmol/L at 24 hr after administration, 1 μmol/L at 48 hr, and <0.2 μmol/L at 72 hr | 15 mg PO, IM, or IV q 6 hr for 60 hr (10 doses starting at 24 hr after start of MTX infusion) |
| Delayed late MTX elimination | Serum MTX level remaining >0.2 μmol/L at 72 hr, and >0.05 μmol/L at 96 hr after administration | Continue 15 mg PO, IM, or IV q 6 hr until MTX level is <0.05 μmol/L |
| Delayed early MTX elimination and/or evidence of acute renal injury | Serum MTX level of 50 μmol/L at 24 hr, or 5 μmol/L at 48 hr after administration; *or* a 100% increase in serum creatinine level at 24 hr after MTX administration (e.g., increase from 0.5 mg/dl to level of 1.0 mg/dl) | 150 mg IV q 3 hr until MTX level is <1 μmol/L, then 15 mg IV q 3 hr until MTX level is <0.05 μmol/L |

From the Immunex product brochure on methotrexate revised November 1997.
MTX, methotrexate; PO, orally; IM, intramuscularly; IV, intravenously.

# REFERENCES

1. Schwartz PM, Barnett SK, Atillasoy ES, Milstone LM. Methotrexate induces differentiation of human keratinocytes. Proc Natl Acad Sci U S A 1992;89:594–8.
2. Bannwarth B, Labat L, Moride Y, Schaeverbeke T. Methotrexate in rheumatoid arthritis: an update. Drugs 1994;47:25–50.
3. Waltham MC, Holland JW, Robinson SC, et al. Direct experimental evidence for competitive inhibition of dihydrofolate reductase by methotrexate. Biochem Pharmacol 1988;37:535–9.
4. Bertino JR. Karnofsky Memorial Lecture. Ode to methotrexate. J Clin Oncol 1993;11:5–14.
5. Baram J, Allegra CJ, Fine RL, Chabner BA. Effect of methotrexate on intracellular folate pools in purified myeloid precursor cells from normal bone marrow. J Clin Invest 1987;79:692–7.
6. Genestier L, Paillot R, Fournel S, et al. Immunosuppressive properties of methotrexate: apoptosis and clonal deletion of activated peripheral T cells. J Clin Inves 1998;102:322–8.
7. Henderson GB, Tsuji JM, Kumar HP. Transport of folate compounds by leukemic cells: evidence for a single influx carrier for methotrexate, 5-methyltetrahydrofolate, and folate in CCRF-CEM human lymphoblasts. Biochem Pharmacol 1987;36:3007–14.
8. Gifford AJ, Kavallaris M, Madafiglio J, et al. P-glycoprotein–mediated methotrexate resistance in CCRF-CEM sublines deficient in methotrexate accumulation due to a point mutation in the reduced folate carrier gene. Int J Cancer 1998;78:176–81.
9. Henderson GB, Tsuji JM. Identification of the bromosulfophthalein-sensitive efflux route for methotrexate as the site of action of vincristine in the vincristine-dependent enhancement of methotrexate uptake in L1210 cells. Cancer Res 1988;48:5995–6001.
10. Pizzorno G, Mini E, Coronnello M, et al. Impaired polyglutamylation of methotrexate as a cause of resistance in CCRF-CEM cells after short-term, high-dose treatment with this drug. Cancer Res 1988;48:2149–55.
11. Chabner BA, Allegra CJ, Curt GA, et al. Polyglutamation of methotrexate: is methotrexate a prodrug? J Clin Invest 1985;76:907–12.
12. Whitehead VM, Vuchich MJ, Lauer SJ, et al. Accumulation of high levels of methotrexate polyglutamates in lymphoblasts from children with hyperdiploid (greater than 50 chromosomes) B-lineage acute lymphoblastic leukemia: a Pediatric Oncology Group study. Blood 1992;80:1316–23.
13. Schimke RT. Methotrexate resistance and gene amplification. Mechanisms and implications. Cancer 1986;57:1912–7.
14. Bertino JR. Clinical pharmacology of methotrexate. Med Pediatr Oncol 1982;10:401–11.
15. Dicker AP, Waltham MC, Volkenandt M, et al. Methotrexate resistance in an in vivo mouse tumor due to a non-active-site dihydrofolate reductase mutation. Proc Natl Acad Sci U S A 1993;90:11797–801.
16. Curt GA, Jolivet J, Carney DN, et al. Determinants of the sensitivity of human small-cell lung cancer cell lines to methotrexate. J Clin Invest 1985;76:1323–9.
17. Fernandes DJ, Sur P, Kute TE, Capizzi RL. Proliferation-dependent cytotoxicity of methotrexate in murine L5178Y leukemia. Cancer Res 1988;48:5638–44.
18. Grem JL, King SA, Sorensen JM, Christian MC. Clinical use of thymidine as a rescue agent from methotrexate toxicity. Invest New Drugs 1991;9:281–90.
19. Adamson PC, Balis FM, McCully CL, et al. Methotrexate pharmacokinetics following administration of recombinant carboxypeptidase-G2 in rhesus monkeys. J Clin Oncol 1992;10:1359–64.
20. DeAngelis LM, Tong WP, Lin S, et al. Carboxypeptidase G2 rescue after high-dose methotrexate. J Clin Oncol 1996;14:2145–9.
21. White RM. 5-Fluorouracil modulates the toxicity of high dose methotrexate. J Clin Pharmacol 1995;34:1156–65.
22. Bleyer WA. Methotrexate: clinical pharmacology, current status and therapeutic guidelines. Cancer Treat Rev 1977;4:87–101.
23. Zaharko DS, Bruckner H, Oliverio VT. Antibiotics alter methotrexate metabolism and excretion. Science 1969;166:887–8.
24. Cohen MH, Creaven PJ, Fossieck BE, et al. Effect of oral prophylactic broad spectrum nonabsorbable antibiotics on the gastrointestinal absorption of nutrients and methotrexate in small cell bronchogenic carcinoma patients. Cancer 1976;38:1556–9.
25. Evans WE, Tsiatis A, Crom WR, et al. Pharmacokinetics of sustained serum methotrexate concentrations secondary to gastrointestinal obstruction. J Pharm Sci 1981;70:1194–8.
26. Thibodeau PA, Bissonnette N, Bâedard SK, et al. Induction by estro-

gens of methotrexate resistance in MCF-7 breast cancer cells. Carcinogenesis 1998;19:1545–52.
27. Mandel MA. The synergistic effect of salicylates on methotrexate. Plast Reconstr Surg 1976;57:733–7.
28. Paxton JW. Protein binding of methotrexate in sera from normal beings: effect of drug concentration, pH, temperature, and storage. J Pharmacol Methods 1981;5:203–13.
29. Taylor JR, Halprin KM. Effect of sodium salicylate and indomethacin on methotrexate–serum albumin binding. Arch Dermatol 1977; 113:588–91.
30. Thyss A, Milano G, Kubar J, et al. Clinical and pharmacokinetic evidence of a life-threatening interaction between methotrexate and ketoprofen. Lancet 1986;1:256–8.
31. Tracy TS, Worster T, Bradley JD, et al. Methotrexate disposition following concomitant administration of ketoprofen, piroxicam and flurbiprofen in patients with rheumatoid arthritis. Br J Clin Pharmacol 1994;37:453–6.
32. Basin KS, Escalante A, Beardmore TD. Severe pancytopenia in a patient taking low dose methotrexate and probenecid. J Rheumatol 1991;18:609–10.
33. Jeurissen ME, Boerbooms AM, van de Putte LB. Pancytopenia and methotrexate with trimethoprim-sulfamethoxazole. Ann Intern Med 1989;111:261.
34. Govert JA, Patton S, Fine RL. Pancytopenia from using trimethoprim and methotrexate. Ann Intern Med 1992;117:877–8.
35. Thyss A, Milano G, Renee N, et al. Severe interaction between methotrexate and a macrolide-like antibiotic. J Natl Cancer Inst 1993;85:582–3.
36. Sotos GA, Liebmann JE, Kohler DR, Longo DL. Reactivation of thermal burn by methotrexate. J Natl Cancer Inst 1992;84:1936–8.
37. Schoenfeld A, Mashiach R, Vardy M, Ovadia J. Methotrexate pneumonitis in nonsurgical treatment of ectopic pregnancy. Obstet Gynecol 1992;80:520–1.
38. Kovacs GT, Paal C, Somlo P, et al. Proteinuria due to suboptimal hydration with high-dose methotrexate therapy. Cancer Chemother Pharmacol 1993;33:262–3.
39. Kozlowski RD, Steinbrunner JV, MacKenzie AH, et al. Outcome of first-trimester exposure to low-dose methotrexate in eight patients with rheumatic disease. Am J Med 1990;88:589–92.
40. Millard RJ, McCredie S. Bladder cancer in patients on low-dose methotrexate and corticosteroids. Lancet 1994;343:1223–3.
41. Bleyer WA, Byrne TN. Leptomeningeal cancer in leukemia and solid tumors. Curr Probl Cancer 1988;12:181–238.
42. ten Hoeve RF, Twijnstra A. A lethal neurotoxic reaction after intraventricular methotrexate administration. Cancer 1988;62:2111–3.
43. Abelson HT, Fosburg MT, Beardsley GP, et al. Methotrexate-induced renal impairment: clinical studies and rescue from systemic toxicity with high-dose leucovorin and thymidine. J Clin Oncol 1983;1:208–16.
44. Bouffet E, Frappaz D, Laville M, et al. Charcoal haemoperfusion and methotrexate toxicity. Lancet 1986;1:1497.
45. Molina R, Fabian C, Cowley B Jr: Use of charcoal hemoperfusion with sequential hemodialysis to reduce serum methotrexate levels in a patient with acute renal insufficiency. Am J Med 1987;82:350–2.
46. Relling MV, Stapleton FB, Ochs J, et al. Removal of methotrexate, leucovorin, and their metabolites by combined hemodialysis and hemoperfusion. Cancer 1988;62:884–8.
47. Shamberger RC, Rosenberg SA, Seipp CA, Sherins RJ. Effects of high-dose methotrexate and vincristine on ovarian and testicular functions in patients undergoing postoperative adjuvant treatment of osteosarcoma. Cancer Treat Rep 1981;65:739–46.
48. Evans WE, Pratt CB. Effect of pleural effusion on high-dose methotrexate. Clin Pharmacol Ther 1978;23:68–72.
49. Thyss A, Suciu S, Bertrand Y, et al, for the EORTC Cancer Children's Leukemia Cooperative Group. Systemic effect of intrathecal methotrexate during the initial phase of treatment of childhood acute lymphoblastic leukemia. J Clin Oncol 1997;15:1824–30.

# Mitomycin

Mitomycin is an antitumor antibiotic that was initially isolated from *Streptomyces caespitosus* in 1958.[1] The drug is also known as Mutamycin, mitomycin C, MMC, and NSC-26980.

## EFFICACY

Mitomycin is mainly used as a single agent in intravesical treatment of superficial bladder carcinoma.[2] The drug has modest activity against a wide variety of tumors, and it is used in several drug combinations. However, the severe adverse effects of the drug limit its use. Mitomycin is not indicated for primary management of any human malignancy.

## PHARMACOLOGY

**Mechanism of Action.** Unlike most antitumor antibiotics, mitomycin is activated in vivo to a bifunctional or trifunctional alkylating agent.[3] After activation, it binds preferentially to the guanine and cytosine moieties of DNA, leading to cross-linking of DNA and inhibition of DNA synthesis and function.[4] Mitomycin is toxic to both hypoxic and aerobic cells, probably by activation through separate hypoxic and aerobic enzyme systems.[5] The increased toxicity seen in hypoxic human cells makes mitomycin an attractive candidate for combined-modality therapy with radiation therapy.[6] Mitomycin is cell cycle phase nonspecific.

**Resistance.** Resistance is complex and involves multiple mechanisms. In one highly resistant cell line, resistance was associated with P-glycoprotein (the mdr phenotype), elevated levels of glutathione *S*-transferase expression, and reduced levels of topoisomerase II.[7] In another system, resistance was correlated with the level of the enzyme NADPH:cytochrome P450.[8] There is usually cross-resistance between mitomycin and other alkylating agents.

**Pharmacokinetics.** Intravenous mitomycin is rapidly cleared from plasma (terminal half-life, 48 minutes), primarily by metabolism in the liver and rapid distribution into intracellular compartments.[9] Metabolism in the liver does not appear to be changed by drugs that induce microsomal drug metabolism.[10] In animals, the highest concentrations of mitomycin occur in the kidneys. Renal clearance also occurs, although this is a minor route of excretion (8 to 10%).[9] The drug does not appear to cross the blood-brain barrier. When mitomycin is given by the intravesical route, only minimal amounts are absorbed, as discussed in a detailed pharmacokinetic study.[11]

**Drug Interactions.** Vinblastine appears to increase the risk of mitomycin-induced pulmonary toxicity. Mitomycin may potentiate the cardiomyopathy associated with doxorubicin and other anthracycline antibiotics.

## TOXICITY

**Overview.** Myelosuppression occurs in a dose-related, cumulative fashion that is somewhat delayed compared with most other antineoplastic agents. Genitourinary toxicity (hemolytic-uremic syndrome) and pulmonary toxicity are rare but potentially dose limiting and fatal. The drug is contraindicated in patients who develop hypersensitivity reactions

with its use, and it should not be used in patients with bleeding or coagulation disorders, thrombocytopenia, or a creatinine value greater than 1.7 mg/dl.

**Hematologic.** The major toxicity of intravenous mitomycin is myelosuppression (about two thirds of patients). This reaction is usually delayed, cumulative, and occasionally fatal. Patients who have had extensive prior chemotherapy or radiation therapy may be especially susceptible to this problem, and patients who respond to mitomycin but who experience severe bone marrow suppression require reduced doses of the drug. Significant myelosuppression is rare with intravesical use of mitomycin.

**Digestive System.** Nausea and vomiting occasionally occur with intravenous mitomycin but generally not after intravesical therapy. The vomiting typically occurs 1 to 2 hours after drug administration. Nausea is usually mild, but it can persist for several days. Anorexia, diarrhea, hematemesis, and abdominal pain may also occur on rare occasion. Severe hepatic damage can occur occasionally.[12] This may take the form of veno-occlusive disease, especially when high-dose therapy is used.[13]

**Mucocutaneous.** Local pain, thrombophlebitis, and severe tissue damage may occur in areas of drug administration, even without obvious drug extravasation. These reactions are usually immediate, but they may be delayed for weeks or months and develop in sites some distance from the original injection. Skin grafting may be required for this problem when it is severe. Alopecia (4%), stomatitis, photosensitivity, desquamation, and pruritus are rare complications.

**Pulmonary.** Interstitial pneumonitis (often with hemoptysis) can be severe, but it occurs in fewer than 10% of patients.[14] Treatment of this form of pulmonary toxicity consists of high-dose corticosteroids and immediate cessation of mitomycin therapy.[15] About 40% of these patients develop progressive pulmonary insufficiency despite high doses of corticosteroids.[16] Rarely, bronchospasm and pulmonary fibrosis may occur. Acute, severe bronchospasm can occur a few minutes to several hours after the administration of vincristine or vinblastine in some patients who have received prior mitomycin treatment. Pulmonary edema can also occur as part of the hemolytic-uremic syndrome (65%). Unfortunately, serial pulmonary function tests are not predictive of pulmonary toxicity.[17]

**Neurologic.** Fatigue, lethargy, weakness, headache, paresthesia, confusion, drowsiness, and syncope all are rare. Neurologic abnormalities can also occur as part of the hemolytic-uremic syndrome (16%).

**Genitourinary.** Patients treated with mitomycin by bladder instillation may develop asymptomatic ulcers at biopsy sites in the bladder. A biopsy of these should be performed to rule out persistent cancer, but they usually represent areas of delayed healing. One patient developed bladder calcification after bladder instillation therapy. Delayed renal dysfunction occurs in about 2% of patients treated with systemic mitomycin as a dose-related sclerotic reaction of the glomerulus that causes a rising serum creatinine level. This may be associated with microangiopathic hemolytic anemia and thrombocytopenia and may thus resemble the hemolytic-uremic syndrome.[18] This syndrome may be exacerbated by the administration of blood products, and it is rarely seen with doses of mitomycin less than 60 mg. The mortality rate of the syndrome is about 50%. The cause is unknown. Optimal treatment of this complication has not been established, but some authorities advise plasmapheresis, either with or without plasma exchange and corticosteroids.

#### Other and Rare Complications

*Systemic.* Fever is rare.

*Immunologic.* Mitomycin is minimally immunosuppressive.

*Cardiovascular.* Some evidence suggests that the use of mitomycin with doxorubicin may lead to a higher incidence of cardiomyopathy than otherwise expected. Hypertension can occur as part of the hemolytic-uremic syndrome. Edema and thrombophlebitis can occur rarely.

*Ocular.* Blurred vision can occur.

*Reproductive.* Toxicity studies place mitomycin in FDA pregnancy category D. The drug is mutagenic and teratogenic.

*Carcinogenicity.* Mitomycin is carcinogenic in animals and presumably in humans.

## DOSAGE AND ADMINISTRATION

Mitomycin is available in vials containing 5, 20, and 40 mg of lyophilized drug. It is reconstituted in water and injected intravenously through a freely flowing intravenous line over 2 to 5 minutes, or it is administered as an intravesical instillation. When used as a single agent, the usual intravenous dosage of mitomycin is 10 to 20 mg/m$^2$ every 6 to 8 weeks. Some authorities recommend a maximal total cumulative dose of 50 mg/m$^2$ to avoid excessive toxicity to the lungs, liver, and kidneys. For bladder instillation, the dosage is 20 to 40 mg mixed with 20 to 40 ml of water or saline, with repeat instillations every 1 to 2 weeks.

The manufacturer recommends an initial dose of 20 mg/m$^2$ for patients who have completely recovered from prior chemotherapy, with subsequent dose adjustments after 6 to 8 weeks based on nadir blood counts. The same dose can be repeated for patients with a normal CBC and a nadir WCC of 3000 and platelet count of 75,000 μL. Patients with a nadir WCC of 2000 to 2999 μL or platelet count of 25,000 to 74,999 μL receive a 70% dose of mitomycin when their CBC recovers. Patients with a WCC less than 2000 μL or a platelet count less than 25,000 μL receive 50% of the prior mitomycin dose when their CBC recovers.

## REFERENCES

1. Crooke ST, Bradner WT. Mitomycin C: a review. Cancer Treat Rev 1976;3:121–39.
2. Doll DC, Weiss RB, Issell BF. Mitomycin: ten years after approval for marketing. J Clin Oncol 1985;3:276–86.
3. Tomasz M, Palom Y. The mitomycin bioreductive antitumor agents: cross-linking and alkylation of DNA as the molecular basis of their activity. Pharmacol Ther 1997;76:73–87.
4. Tomasz M, Lipman R, Chowdary D, et al. Isolation and structure of a covalent cross-link adduct between mitomycin C and DNA. Science 1987;235:1204–8.
5. Belcourt MF, Hodnick WF, Rockwell S, Sartorelli AC. Exploring the mechanistic aspects of mitomycin antibiotic bioactivation in Chinese hamster ovary cells overexpressing NADPH:cytochrome C (P-450) reductase and DT-diaphorase. Adv Enzyme Regul 1998;38:111–33.
6. Sartorelli AC. Therapeutic attack of hypoxic cells of solid tumors: presidential address. Cancer Res 1988;48:775–8.
7. Hoban PR, Robson CN, Davies SM. Reduced topoisomerase II and elevated alpha class glutathione S-transferase expression in a multidrug resistant CHO cell line highly cross-resistant to mitomycin C. Biochem Pharmacol 1992;43:685–93.
8. Bligh HF, Bartoszek A, Robson CN. Activation of mitomycin C by NADPH:cytochrome P-450 reductase. Cancer Res 1990;50:7789–92.
9. Dorr RT. New findings in the pharmacokinetic, metabolic, and drug-resistance aspects of mitomycin C. Semin Oncol 1988;15:Suppl 4:32–41.
10. Kerpel-Fronius S, Verwey J, Stuurman M, et al. Pharmacokinetics and toxicity of mitomycin C in rodents, given alone, in combination, or after induction of microsomal drug metabolism. Cancer Chemother Pharmacol 1988;22:104–8.
11. Dalton JT, Wientjes MG, Badalament RA, et al. Pharmacokinetics of intravesical mitomycin C in superficial bladder cancer patients. Cancer Res 1991;51:5144–52.
12. Perry MC. Hepatotoxicity of chemotherapeutic agents. Semin Oncol 1982;9:65–74.
13. Lazarus HM, Gottfried MR, Herzig RH. Veno-occlusive disease of the liver after high-dose mitomycin C therapy and autologous bone marrow transplantation. Cancer 1982;49:1789–95.
14. Verweij J, van Zanten T, Souren T, et al. Prospective study on the dose relationship of mitomycin C–induced interstitial pneumonitis. Cancer 1987;60:756–61.
15. Chang AY, Kuebler JP, Pandya KJ, et al. Pulmonary toxicity induced by mitomycin C is highly responsive to glucocorticoids. Cancer 1986;57:2285–90.
16. Okuno SH, Frytak S. Mitomycin lung toxicity: acute and chronic phases. Am J Clin Oncol 1997;20:282–4.
17. Castro M, Veeder MH, Mailliard JA, et al. A prospective study of pulmonary function in patients receiving mitomycin. Chest 1996;109:939–44.
18. Cantrell JE Jr, Phillips TM, Schein PS. Carcinoma-associated hemolytic-uremic syndrome: a complication of mitomycin C chemotherapy. J Clin Oncol 1985;3:723–34.

## Mitotane

Mitotane, a derivative of the insecticide DDT, causes necrosis and atrophy of the adrenal cortex. It is also known as *o,p'*-DDD, Lysodren, and NSC-38721.

## EFFICACY

Mitotane is used in the treatment of inoperable adrenocortical carcinoma, both the functional and the nonfunctional types, and as treatment for selected patients with Cushing's syndrome.[1-3] An objective response to mitotane has also been reported in a single case of malignant Leydig's cell tumor of the testis.[4] Clinical benefit has been reported in about 50% of cases of adrenocortical carcinoma treated with mitotane, and in rare cases with residual tumor after operation, mitotane appears to have been curative.[2,5]

## PHARMACOLOGY

**Mechanism of Action.** Mitotane is tightly and rapidly bound to the mitochondria of the adrenal cortex, and this action leads to marked inhibition of the conversion of cholesterol to ACTH-induced steroids.[6] Mitotane covalently binds to adrenal proteins, resulting in direct destruction of adrenal cortical tissues[7] and peripheral extra-adrenal stimulation of cortisol metabolism.[8] It may also modify peripheral androgen metabolism.[9] Mitotane does not inhibit aldosterone synthesis, but spironolactone appears to abrogate the adrenal suppression seen with the drug.[10] Because of this, the two should not be used together.

**Resistance.** Resistance is unknown.

**Pharmacokinetics.** Approximately 40% of an oral dose is absorbed, with subsequent distribution to all tissues and storage in fat. Mitotane is metabolized to a water-soluble metabolite by the liver and kidneys and eliminated slowly, with a terminal half-life of 18 to 159 days. The metabolite distributes minimally across the blood-brain barrier. Oral absorption can be enhanced experimentally by the administration of the drug in fatty vehicles, such as milk or oil emulsions.[11] Daily doses of 5 to 15 g lead to plasma concentrations of 10 to 90 μg/ml of unchanged drug and 30 to 50 μg/ml of a metabolite. The optimal plasma concentrations of mitotane are probably in the range of 10 to 20 μg/ml, although one study considered levels less than 14 μg/ml to be insufficient.[12] Antitumor responses were rare in patients with blood levels less than 10 μg/ml, and neurotoxicity was excessive with blood levels more than 10 μg/ml. Its extensive deposition in fat results in measurable levels of mitotane in blood many months after its withdrawal.[13, 14] About 25% of an oral dose ultimately appears in the urine as a water-soluble metabolite. Because of irregular absorption and the apparent importance of optimal blood levels, it has been suggested that plasma concentrations of the drug should be monitored regularly.[13] In most centers in the United States, this is not feasible, and no studies confirm this recommendation.

**Drug Interactions.** A variety of drug interactions are possible because mitotane induces hepatic microsomal enzymes in animals. This could theoretically influence the use of drugs such as barbiturates, coumarin anticoagulants, and phenytoin, but confirmatory studies of clinically significant interactions are lacking. Mitotane is uricosuric, and it may lead to a variety of laboratory test abnormalities of questionable significance, including hypouricemia, hypercholesterolemia, and decreased serum protein-bound iodine. The effects of mitotane can be blocked by spironolactone, so use of the latter should be avoided.[10] Mitotane can cause CNS depression, and its administration with other CNS depressants can result in additive neurotoxicity.

The potential of mitotane to modify the cytotoxicity of other antineoplastic agents against human adrenocortical carcinoma cells in vitro has been studied.[15] Mitotane increased the activity of anthracyclines and cisplatin, but no potentiation was seen with etoposide.

## TOXICITY

**Overview.** The most common reactions are nausea, vomiting, diarrhea, neurologic changes, and dermatitis. These reactions can usually be managed by the use of a lower dose of mitotane.

**Digestive System.** About 80% of patients develop gastrointestinal disturbances, usually anorexia, nausea, vomiting, or some combination of these. Diarrhea is less common (about 20%). Levels of transaminase enzymes, alkaline phosphatase, and bilirubin may be mildly elevated. Severe toxicity is very rare.

**Mucocutaneous.** About 15% of patients develop a maculopapular rash. The rash tends to be transient and does not appear to be dose related. In some patients, the rash abates despite continued treatment at the same dose. Less common side effects include chloasma, alopecia, urticaria, hyperpigmentation, erythema multiforme, periorbital or facial swelling, and scaling of the paranasal area.

**Neurologic.** About 40% of patients develop CNS effects. Lethargy and somnolence are the most common adverse effects, and they can be severe initially. Less commonly, patients complain of dizziness or frank vertigo. Other possible reactions include mental depression, headache, irritability, confusion, tremors, weakness, and fatigue. Rare adverse reactions include difficulties with speech, decreased hearing, memory impairment, neuropathy, ataxia, myelopathy, hallucinations, psychosis, and frank encephalopathy. Prolonged administration of mitotane can result in permanent brain damage and functional impairment. While taking mitotane, the patient must be warned to avoid tasks requiring mental alertness, and he or she should be carefully monitored for the development of behavioral or neurologic problems.

**Endocrine-Metabolic.** Adrenal insufficiency develops in most patients. Exogenous steroids should be administered and mitotane discontinued if the patient sustains severe trauma or shock. Hypouricemia and hypercholesterolemia frequently occur; gynecomastia is rare.

**Other/Rare**

*Systemic.* Flushing and fever can occur.

*Hematologic.* Leukopenia and thrombocytopenia may occur. In a series of six patients, mitotane caused a clinically relevant defect of platelet function with a prolonged bleeding time.[16] Nevertheless, clinical bleeding is rarely a problem.

*Immunologic.* Hypersensitivity reactions are very rare.

*Cardiovascular.* Hypertension and orthostatic hypotension can occur.

*Pulmonary.* Wheezing and dyspnea may occur.

*Ocular.* The following effects can occur: blurred vision, diplopia, papilledema, cataracts, optic neuritis, retinal hemorrhages, and toxic retinopathy.

*Musculoskeletal.* Arthralgia, myalgia, and generalized aching can occur.

*Genitourinary.* Proteinuria, hematuria, and hemorrhagic cystitis may occur.

*Reproductive.* Toxicity studies place mitotane in FDA pregnancy category C.

*Carcinogenicity.* There are no animal or human data available on which to base an assessment of risk.

## DOSAGE AND ADMINISTRATION

Mitotane is available as 500-mg tablets. The usual initial dosage is 2 to 6 g/day in three to four divided doses. The dose is gradually increased until a mildly toxic level is identified and the dose is then reduced and continued as long as clinical benefits are observed. The stable dose is usually in the range of 9 to 10 g daily, but tolerance varies widely between 2 and 16 g daily. Responses can occur as late as 3 months after starting treatment, so it is important not to discontinue drug administration too soon. Patients who respond to treatment are generally continued on therapy indefinitely. Plasma cortisol levels should be measured periodically to assess the effectiveness of treatment in reducing elevated levels of cortisol due to tumor and to ensure adequate residual adrenal function. Measurements of urinary 17-hydroxycorticosteroids or 17-ketosteroids are not useful owing to the extra-adrenal effects of the drug.[8, 9]

The manufacturer recommends initiating mitotane therapy in the hospital. An alternative approach is to initiate therapy with concomitant corticosteroid replacement therapy on an outpatient basis with frequent physician visits. At times of stress, such as with trauma or infection, corticosteroid doses should be increased. Patients should be warned that mitotane may impede their ability to drive a car or operate machinery. They should be monitored closely for neurologic function, especially after prolonged therapy (>2 years). Some clinicians recommend that patients have periodic liver function tests during treatment.

## REFERENCES

1. Hutter AM Jr, Kayhoe DE. Adrenal cortical carcinoma: results of treatment with *o,p*′DDD in 138 patients. Am J Med 1966;41:581–92.
2. Becker D, Schumacher OP. *O,p*′DDD therapy in invasive adrenocortical carcinoma. Ann Intern Med 1975;82:677–9.
3. Temple TE Jr, Jones DJ Jr, Liddle GW, Dexter RN. Treatment of Cushing disease: correction of hypercortisolism by *o,p*′DDD without induction of aldosterone deficiency. N Engl J Med 1969;281:801–5.
4. Azer PC, Braunstein GD. Malignant Leydig cell tumor: objective tumor response to *o,p*′-DDD. Cancer 1981;47:1251–5.
5. Dickstein G, Schechner C, Arad E, et al. Is there a role for low doses of mitotane (*o,p*′-DDD) as adjuvant therapy in adrenocortical carcinoma? J Clin Endocrinol Metabol 1998;83:3100–3.
6. Martz F, Straw JA. Treatment with *o,p*′-DDD (mitotane) decreased cytochrome P-450, heme, and microsomal protein content in the dog adrenal cortex in vivo. Res Commun Chem Pathol Pharmacol 1976;13:83–92.
7. Cai W, Counsell RE, Schteingart DE, et al. Adrenal proteins bound by a reactive intermediate of mitotane. Cancer Chemother Pharmacol 1997;39:537–40.
8. Hart MM, Reagan RL, Adamson RH. The effect of isomers of DDD on the ACTH-induced steroid output, histology and ultrastructure of the dog adrenal cortex. Toxicol Appl Pharmacol 1973;24:101–13.
9. Hellman L, Badlow HL, Zumoff B. Decreased conversion of androgens to normal 17-ketosteroid metabolites as a result of treatment with *o,p*′-DDD. J Clin Endocrinol Metab 1973;36:801–3.
10. Wortsman J, Soler NG. Mitotane: Spironolactone antagonism in Cushing's syndrome. JAMA 1977;238:2527.
11. Moolenaar AJ, van Slooten H, van Seters AP, Smeenk D. Blood levels of *o,p*′-DDD following administration in various vehicles after a single dose and during long-term treatment. Cancer Chemother Pharmacol 1981;7:51–4.
12. Haak HR, Hermans J, van de Velde CJ, et al. Optimal treatment of adrenocortical carcinoma with mitotane. Br J Cancer 1994;69:947–51.
13. von Slooten H, van Seters AP, Smeenk D, Moolenaar AJ. *O,p*′-DDD (mitotane) levels in plasma and tissues during chemotherapy and at autopsy. Cancer Chemother Pharmacol 1982;9:85–8.
14. Leutenegger M, Caron J, Couchot J, et al. [Plasma determination of *o,p*′-DDD. Clinical value.] Nouv Presse Med 1977;6:566.
15. Villa R, Orlandi L, Berruti A, et al. Modulation of cytotoxic drug activity by mitotane and lonidamine in human adrenocortical carcinoma cells. Int J Oncol 1999;14:133–8.
16. Haak HR, Caekebeke-Peerlinck KM, van Seters AP, Briet E. Prolonged bleeding time due to mitotane therapy. Eur J Cancer 1991;27:638–41.

## Mitoxantrone

Mitoxantrone was developed by American Cyanamid Company and the Midwest Research Institute in the hope that a synthetic aminoanthraquinone might retain the antitumor spectrum of an anthracycline without causing cardiotoxicity.[1, 2] The drug is also known as Novantrone, dihydroxyanthracenedione, DHAD, DHAQ, and NSC-301739.

## EFFICACY

Mitoxantrone is marketed in the United States for the treatment of acute nonlymphocytic leukemia.[3] It is active against a variety of other tumors, including breast cancer, prostate cancer, ovarian cancer, and lymphomas.

## PHARMACOLOGY

**Mechanism of Action.** Mitoxantrone accumulates in cells as monomers, aggregates, a naphthoquinoxaline metabolite, and drug-target complexes.[4] Mitoxantrone intercalates into DNA and causes interstrand and intrastrand cross-linking. It binds electrostatically to the phosphate backbone of DNA, causes DNA strand breaks, and causes trapping of DNA-topoisomerase II complexes on cellular DNA. Some evidence shows that the sequence of DNA binding is specific to sites prior to pyrimidine (3′–5′) purine sequences, a finding that is consistent with the fact that the mitoxantrone side chains lie in the major groove.[5] Consequently, the drug is a potent inhibitor of both DNA and RNA synthesis and causes nuclear aberrations and chromosomal scattering.[6] Ultimately, cell death occurs by apoptosis.[7–9] The drug is cell cycle phase nonspecific, although it does induce a $G_2$ block in the cell cycle with an increase in cellular RNA and polyploidy. The drug causes only minimal free radical formation and lipid peroxidation (compared with doxorubicin).

**Resistance.** Multiple mechanisms contribute to mitoxantrone resistance. Low-level mitoxantrone resistance is due to the presence of a novel, energy-dependent drug efflux pump similar to P-glycoprotein and the multidrug resistance–associated protein.[10] Resistance also involves the mechanisms described for doxorubicin, namely overexpression of P-glycoprotein (mdr), alterations of topoisomerase II, and overexpression of glutathione *S*-transferase.[11, 12] The cardiac toxicity of mitoxantrone in animal models is reduced by dexrazoxane,[13] but not to the extent as with doxorubicin.[14] Dexrazoxane reduces the cardiac toxicity of mitoxantrone in patients with leukemia.[15]

**Pharmacokinetics.** Following intravenous administration, the drug disappears rapidly from plasma and is widely distributed and bound to tissues. The drug is excreted as unchanged drug and as two major metabolites. Both renal excretion (6 to 11% over 5 days) and hepatobiliary elimination (25% over 5 days) are limited, whereas overall elimination of the drug is slow (mean half-life, 24 to 37 hours). Saturation of mitoxantrone elimination does not occur, even with the very high doses used in the setting of BMT.[16] No adjustment of dose is recommended for either renal or hepatic dysfunction. The drug is not eliminated by hemodialysis.[17]

**Drug Interactions.** Mitoxantrone increases the cytotoxicity seen with both radiation therapy and hyperthermia,[18] and it may cause synergistic cytotoxicity in combination with cytarabine.[19] Synergistic cytotoxicity is also seen with TNF.[20]

## TOXICITY

**Overview.** Although developed and marketed as a less cardiotoxic alternative to doxorubicin, mitoxantrone has a similar spectrum of toxicity as anthracycline antibiotics. Myelosuppression is the major short-term toxic side effect of mitoxantrone, whereas cardiac toxicity is the major limiting factor for long-term treatment. Other common effects include nausea, vomiting, mucositis, and alopecia.

**Hematologic.** Dose-limiting neutropenia is expected 10 to 14 days after treatment, with recovery by day 21. Recovery time can be shortened by GM-CSF, potentially allowing more dose-intense therapy.[21] Thrombocytopenia and anemia may also occur, but these tend to be less severe than neutropenia. Myelosuppression is likely to be more severe in patients with pre-existing marrow dysfunction.

**Digestive System.** The drug is moderately emetogenic, but this can usually be prevented with aggressive use of antiemetics. Diarrhea and abdominal pain may rarely occur. Minor and transient elevations of levels of transaminase enzymes occasionally occur, as may hyperbilirubinemia.

**Mucocutaneous.** Alopecia, mucositis, phlebitis, and soft tissue damage due to drug extravasation are less severe than with doxorubicin; nevertheless, severe local reactions, including ulceration and cellulitis, have been reported. Severe alopecia is very rare (about 1% of patients). The scleras may temporarily turn blue or blue-green, and delayed bluish discoloration of the nails may occur. Conjunctivitis is an occasional side effect, and onycholysis a very rare event.[22]

**Cardiovascular.** Although mitoxantrone was originally developed with the hope of retaining the antineoplastic activity of the anthracyclines while reducing the risk of cardiotoxicity, it is clear that mitoxantrone can induce both acute and chronic congestive heart failure.[23] As with the anthracyclines, this is related to the total lifetime dose of drug received. When mitoxantrone is used for nonleukemic neoplasms, the manufacturer reports a 2.6% risk of congestive heart failure for cumulative doses of 140 mg/m$^2$, but it rises to 13% when the dose exceeds this level. Prior exposure to doxorubicin or daunorubicin probably increases the risk of congestive heart failure due to mitoxantrone.

**Genitourinary.** Patients should be warned that their urine may turn blue-green. Renal failure, hyperuricemia, and the tumor lysis syndrome all are rare.

**Other and Rare Reactions**

*Systemic.* Fever may occur.

*Immunologic.* Allergic reactions, such as hypotension, dyspnea, and urticaria and other rashes, occur rarely. The drug is immunosuppressive in animals, but little is known about the importance of this in humans.

*Pulmonary.* Cough can occur.

*Neurologic.* Headache and seizures can occur.

*Reproductive.* Toxicity studies place mitoxantrone in FDA pregnancy category D. Amenorrhea may occur.

*Carcinogenicity.* The drug is mutagenic in animals and bacteria. Human and animal carcinogenesis data are incomplete, but the drug is probably carcinogenic.

## DOSAGE AND ADMINISTRATION

Mitoxantrone is available as a concentrated solution of 2 mg/ml in vials of 20, 25, and 30 mg. It is incompatible in solution with heparin or hydrocortisone sodium phosphate. The drug is diluted in at least 50 ml of normal saline or dextrose in water and infused intravenously with extravasation precautions over a period of not less than 3 minutes and preferably 15 to 30 minutes. The usual dosage of mitoxantrone for induction therapy of acute nonlymphocytic leukemia in combination with cytarabine is 12 mg/m$^2$ daily on days 1 to 3, given as a slow intravenous infusion over 15 to 30 minutes. A common dosage for single-agent use against other neoplasms is 12 mg/m$^2$ every 3 or 4 weeks. The same administration precautions used for doxorubicin and daunorubicin are used for mitoxantrone.

There have been anecdotal reports of responses of leptomeningeal leukemia and lymphoma to mitoxantrone administered by the intrathecal route,[24] but this has also been associated with paraplegia and other neurologic dysfunction.[25] The manufacturer discourages the use of this route, even as an investigational therapy. High-dose therapy with mitoxantrone is under investigation.[26]

## REFERENCES

1. White RJ, Durr FE. Development of mitoxantrone. Invest New Drugs 1985;3:85–93.
2. Shenkenberg TD, Von Hoff DD. Mitoxantrone: a new anticancer drug with significant clinical activity. Ann Intern Med 1986;105:67–81.
3. Dunn CJ, Goa KL. Mitoxantrone: a review of its pharmacological properties and use in acute nonlymphoblastic leukaemia. Drugs Aging 1996;9:122–7.
4. Feofanov A, Sharonov S, Fleury F, et al. Quantitative confocal spectral imaging analysis of mitoxantrone within living K562 cells: intracellular accumulation and distribution of monomers, aggregates, naphthoquinoxaline metabolite, and drug-target complexes. Biophys J 1997; 73:3328–36.
5. Panousis C, Phillips DR. DNA sequence specificity of mitoxantrone. Nucleic Acid Res 1994;22:1342–5.
6. Faulds D, Balfour JA, Chrisp P, et al. Mitoxantrone: a review of its pharmacodynamic and pharmacokinetic properties, and therapeutic potential in the chemotherapy of cancer. Drugs 1991;41:400–49.
7. Bhalla K, Ibrado AM, Tourkina E, et al. High-dose mitoxantrone induces programmed cell death or apoptosis in human myeloid leukemia cells. Blood 1993;82:3133–40.
8. Bellosillo B, Colomer D, Pons G, Gil J. Mitoxantrone, a topoisomerase II inhibitor, induces apoptosis of B-chronic lymphocytic leukaemia cells. Br J Haematol 1998;100:142–6.
9. Bettaieb A, Plo I, Mansat-De Mas V, et al. Daunorubicin- and mitoxantrone-triggered phosphatidylcholine hydrolysis: implication in drug-induced ceramide generation and apoptosis. Mol Pharmacol 1999;55:118–25.
10. Hazzlehurst LA, Foley NE, Gleason-Guzman MC, et al. Multiple mechanisms confer drug resistance to mitoxantrone in the human 8226 myeloma cell line. Cancer Res 1999;59:1021–8.
11. Kamath N, Grabowski D, Ford J, et al. Overexpression of P-glycoprotein and alterations in topoisomerase II in P388 mouse leukemia cells selected in vivo for resistance to mitoxantrone. Biochem Pharmacol 1992;44:937–45.
12. Peters WHM, Roelofs HM. Biochemical characterization of resistance to mitoxantrone and Adriamycin in Caco-2 human colon adenocarcinoma cells: a possible role for glutathione S-transferases. Cancer Res 1992;52:1886–90.
13. Shipp NG, Dorr RT, Alberts DS, et al. Characterization of experimental mitoxantrone cardiotoxicity and its partial inhibition by ICRF-187 in cultured neonatal rat heart cells. Cancer Res 1993;53:550–6.
14. Alderton PM, Gross J, Green MD. Comparative study of doxorubicin, mitoxantrone, and epirubicin in combination with ICRF-187 (ADR-529) in a chronic cardiotoxicity animal model. Cancer Res 1992;52:194–201.
15. Lemez P, Maresova J. Efficacy of dexrazoxane as a cardioprotective agent in patients receiving mitoxantrone- and daunorubicin-based chemotherapy. Semin Oncol 1998;25:4 Suppl 10:61–5.

16. Richard B, Launay-Iliadis MC, Iliadis A, et al. Pharmacokinetics of mitoxantrone in cancer patients treated by high-dose chemotherapy and autologous bone marrow transplantation. Br J Cancer 1992;65:399–404.
17. Boros L, Cacek T, Pine RB, Battaglia AC. Distribution characteristics of mitoxantrone in a patient undergoing hemodialysis. Cancer Chemother Pharmacol 1992;31:57–60.
18. Mitoxantrone. Med Lett Drugs Ther 1988;30:67–8.
19. Heinemann V, Murray D, Walters R, et al. Mitoxantrone-induced DNA damage in leukemia cells is enhanced by treatment with high-dose arabinosylcytosine. Cancer Chemother Pharmacol 1988;22:205–10.
20. Valenti M, Cimoli G, Mariani GL, et al. Potentiation of TNF-mediated cell killing by mitoxantrone: relationship to DNA single-strand break formation. Biochem Pharmacol 1993;46:1199–206.
21. Schiller JH, Storer B, Arzoomanian R, et al. Phase I trial of mitoxantrone and granulocyte-macrophage colony-stimulating factor (GM-CSF) in patients with advanced solid malignancies. Invest New Drugs 1993;11:291–300.
22. Mitchell PLR, Harvey VJ. Mitozantrone-induced onycholysis. Eur J Cancer 1992;28:243–4.
23. Cassidy J, Merrick MV, Smyth JF, Leonard RC. Cardiotoxicity of mitozantrone assessed by stress and resting nuclear ventriculography. Eur J Cancer Clin Oncol 1988;24:935–8.
24. Laporte JP, Godefroy W, Verny A, et al. Intrathecal mitozantrone. Lancet 1985;2:160.
25. Lakhani AK, Zuiable AG, Pollard CM, et al. Paraplegia after intrathecal mitozantrone. Lancet 1986;2:1393.
26. Mollgard L, Tidefelt U, Sundman-Engberg B, et al. High single dose of mitoxantrone and cytarabine in acute non-lymphocytic leukemia: a pharmacokinetic and clinical study. Ther Drug Monit 1998;20:640–5.

# Octreotide Acetate

Somatostatin, a naturally occurring cyclic tetradecapeptide hormone, appears to be an endogenous growth inhibitor. It is found in high concentrations in the hypothalamus, stomach, pancreas, and intestine. The clinical potential of somatostatin was appreciated for many years, but its short duration of action (half-life in the circulation of about 3 minutes) made its systemic use impractical. Octreotide acetate, a long-acting analogue of somatostatin, was synthesized in 1982 by a Sandoz research team in Basel, Switzerland.[1, 2] It was approved by the FDA in 1988. The drug is also known as Sandostatin and SMS 201-995.

## EFFICACY

Octreotide has been approved by the FDA specifically for the treatment of symptoms in patients with metastatic carcinoid and vasoactive intestinal peptide–secreting tumors (VIPomas). Elevated levels of tumor markers in these patients may decrease, but objective tumor regressions generally do not occur. The drug may also be useful in the symptomatic treatment of nonmalignant neuroendocrine tumors,[3] in reducing diarrhea due to 5-FU toxicity[4] and AIDS,[5] as treatment for ectopic ACTH syndrome[6] (see Chapter 18), and in reducing emesis in patients with bowel obstruction.[7] It is being studied for a wide variety of other indications as well.[8]

## PHARMACOLOGY

**Mechanism of Action.** Among the major effects of somatostatin are the inhibition of the release of pituitary growth hormone and, under certain conditions, prolactin. Somatostatin also suppresses the secretion of serotonin and the secretions of the endocrine pancreas, stomach, and intestine (including gastrin, vasoactive intestinal peptide, insulin, glucagon, secretin, motilin, and pancreatic polypeptide). Somatostatin has indirect antiproliferative effects of uncertain cause and a direct antiproliferative action that is mediated by intratumor somatostatin receptors.[9]

Many of these effects have been demonstrated for octreotide acetate as well, although the precise mechanism of action against any given tumor type may differ. Among other things, inhibition of these gut hormones acts to slow gastrointestinal transit time and to regulate water and electrolyte transport across the gut.[10, 11] The symptomatic benefit of octreotide acetate in patients with carcinoid syndrome or VIPomas is probably explained by such effects. However, direct antiproliferative effects in vitro have been demonstrated for octreotide. For example, octreotide inhibits the growth of IL-6–dependent and IL-6–independent human multiple myeloma cell lines.[12] In this system, octreotide activates somatostatin receptor signaling, leading to apoptosis.

**Resistance.** Resistance is unknown.

**Pharmacokinetics.** Octreotide acetate requires parenteral administration because of its peptide chemical structure. After subcutaneous injection, it is absorbed rapidly and completely, with peak concentrations being reached 0.4 hour after administration. The drug distributes into an apparent volume of 13.6 L and has an apparent elimination half-life from plasma of about 1.5 hours. Nevertheless, the biologic duration of effect may be as long as 12 hours, depending on the tumor being treated. The distribution of the drug into RBCs is negligible, but 65% is bound to plasma proteins. About 32% of a given dose of the drug is excreted unchanged in the urine, and patients with renal failure requiring dialysis have about half the clearance of normal subjects.

The impact of cirrhosis on the pharmacokinetics of octreotide has been studied.[13] The average clearance of octreotide was about two-thirds normal in both compensated and decompensated cirrhotic patients, with a corresponding increase in the maximum serum concentration in the cirrhotic patients. The serum half-life was prolonged in cirrhosis, and equilibration between plasma and ascitic fluid in decompensated cirrhotic patients was delayed. The authors concluded that cirrhosis markedly alters the pharmacokinetics of octreotide.

**Drug Interactions.** Octreotide may decrease absorption of nutrients and some drugs. One case of transplant rejection was presumed to result from octreotide-induced malabsorption of cyclosporine. Octreotide can cause glucose intolerance, so blood glucose levels should be monitored carefully in patients receiving concurrent therapy with sulfonylureas, insulin, diazoxide, corticosteroids, and dextrose. Because of shifts in fluid balance and electrolytes, the manufacturer also advises extra care in the concurrent use of octreotide with thiazide diuretics and β-blockers.

## TOXICITY

**Overview.** Octreotide is well tolerated by most individuals, but 15 to 20% of patients develop cholelithiasis. Other gastrointestinal complaints are uncommon during the early weeks of therapy, and they tend to abate with time.

**Digestive System.** As with natural somatostatin, octreotide can cause cholelithiasis (15 to 20% of patients), which may require acute surgical intervention. This is probably related to prolongation of large bowel transit time by octreotide, which increases the proportion of deoxycholic acid in fasting serum (and, by implication, in bile).[14] Patients should be monitored periodically for gallbladder disease by ultrasound examination of the gallbladder and bile ducts. Uncommon effects include nausea (10%), diarrhea (7%), abdominal pain or discomfort (7%), loose stools (4%), vomiting (4%), and steatorrhea (1 to 2%). Very rare reactions include constipation, flatulence, hepatitis, jaundice, a slight increase in levels of liver enzymes, rectal spasm, gastrointestinal bleeding, dyspepsia, a fluttering sensation in the abdomen, and abnormal-appearing stools.

**Mucocutaneous.** Transient minor pain at the injection site occurs in about 8% of patients. Other reactions are rare but may include flushing (1.4%), edema (1%), flaking of the skin, bruising, bleeding from superficial wounds, rash, and pruritus. Thinning of the hair and hair loss are said to be rare but appear to be common in patients with prior scalp radiation therapy.[15]

**Endocrine-Metabolic.** Less than 3% of patients develop hypoglycemia, hyperglycemia, and urine hyperosmolarity. Less than 1% develop hypothyroidism, decreased libido, and galactorrhea. Octreotide has long-term effects on markers of bone metabolism, most notably prolonged elevation of parathormone levels.[16] The significance of these changes is uncertain.

**Other and Rare Reactions.** The manufacturer lists a wide variety of largely trivial toxic side effects occurring in less than 1% of patients. These include rhinorrhea, dry mouth, hyperhidrosis, hyperdipsia, chills, fever, throat discomfort, increased blood level of creatine phosphokinase, and arm pain.

*Hematologic.* No hematologic side effects are known.

*Immunologic.* The preparation does not appear to be particularly immunogenic.

*Cardiovascular.* Less than 1% of patients develop hypertension, dyspnea, thrombophlebitis, cardiac ischemia, congestive heart failure, palpitations, chest pain, or orthostatic hypotension. It has also been associated rarely with bradycardia.[17]

*Ocular.* Very rarely, a burning sensation can occur.

*Neurologic.* About 2% of patients develop headache. Other, very rare reactions include dizziness, weakness, fatigue, anxiety, depression, convulsions, anorexia, drowsiness, vertigo, hyperesthesia, pounding in the head, irritability, insomnia, forgetfulness, malaise, nervousness, shakiness, syncope, tremor, and Bell's palsy.

*Musculoskeletal.* Very rarely, backache, muscle pain, muscle cramps, arthralgia, shoulder and leg pain, and chest wall pain can occur.

*Genitourinary.* Oliguria, pollakiuria, prostatitis, and urine hyperosmolarity each occur in less than 1% of patients.

*Reproductive.* Toxicity studies place octreotide in FDA pregnancy category B (not an animal teratogen; not studied adequately in pregnant women).

*Carcinogenicity.* Octreotide is not mutagenic in animals. Animal and human carcinogenicity testing is incomplete, but it is unlikely that octreotide is carcinogenic.

## DOSAGE AND ADMINISTRATION

Octreotide is available in two ampule sizes: (1) 1-ml ampules containing 50 $\mu g$/ml, 100 $\mu g$/ml, and 500 $\mu g$/ml and (2) 5-ml multidose vials of 200 $\mu g$/ml and 1000 $\mu g$/ml. Octreotide acetate is incompatible with 10% fat emulsion. The initial dosage is 50 $\mu g$ administered subcutaneously once or twice daily. Subsequently, the number of injections and dosage may be gradually increased on the basis of a patient's tolerance and response. For patients with carcinoid tumors, the daily dosage of octreotide acetate during the first 2 weeks of treatment varies from 100 to 600 $\mu g$ in two to four divided doses (mean, 300 $\mu g$/day). In clinical trials, the usual maintenance dosage was 150 $\mu g$ three times daily, but it ranged from 50 to 1500 $\mu g$/day (with the usual maximum being 750 $\mu g$/day). For patients with VIPomas, the daily dosage is 200 to 300 $\mu g$ in two to four divided doses during the first 2 weeks of therapy (range, 150 to 750 $\mu g$/day). Doses higher than 450 $\mu g$/day are almost never required for these patients. The maintenance dose for VIPomas and carcinoid tumors may vary and should be adjusted for each patient, depending on the clinical response. The dosage of octreotide for 5-FU–induced diarrhea is 100 $\mu g$ twice daily for 3 days.[4]

The manufacturer recommends that the drug be inspected visually for particulate matter and discoloration prior to administration. If present, the drug should be discarded. This point is important to emphasize because the long-term nature of this treatment mandates self-administration by most patients, just as with the use of insulin by diabetic patients. Furthermore, patients should be cautioned to rotate the sites of injection and to avoid multiple injections in the same location.

The drug may also be used intravenously in an emergency, such as for patients developing severe episodes of carcinoid syndrome during an operative procedure. The dosage is the same as that used subcutaneously. In healthy volunteers, intravenous bolus injections of 1000 $\mu g$ have been given without serious complication.

A long-acting form of somatostatin became available in 1999 for use in patients who have benefited from the use of the immediate dose preparation. It is available as a suspension for intragluteal injection in vials of 10, 20, and 30 mg. The maintenance dose for patients with gastrointestinal tumors is 30 mg every 4 weeks.[18, 19] It offers the potential convenience of once-monthly administration for patients who benefit from the standard regimen.

## REFERENCES

1. Schally AV. Oncological applications of somatostatin analogues. Cancer Res 1988;48:6977–85.
2. Gorden P, Comi RJ, Maton PN, Go VL. NIH conference: somatostatin and somatostatin analogue (SMS 201-995) in treatment of hormone-secreting tumors of the pituitary and gastrointestinal tract and non-neoplastic diseases of the gut. Ann Intern Med 1989;110:35–50.
3. Battershill PE, Clissold SP. Octreotide: a review of its pharmacodynamic and pharmacokinetic properties, and therapeutic potential in

conditions associated with excessive peptide secretion. Drugs 1989;38:658–702.

4. Cascinu S, Fedeli A, Fedeli SL, Catalano G. Octreotide versus loperamide in the treatment of fluorouracil-induced diarrhea: a randomized trial. J Clin Oncol 1993;11:148–51.
5. Cello JP, Grendell JH, Basuk P, et al. Effect of octreotide on refractory AIDS-associated diarrhea: a prospective, multicenter clinical trial. Ann Intern Med 1991;115:705–10.
6. Woodhouse NJY, Dagogo-Jack S, Ahmed M, Judzewitsch R. Acute and long-term effects of octreotide in patients with ACTH-dependent Cushing's syndrome. Am J Med 1993;95:305–8.
7. Khoo D, Hall E, Motson R, et al. Palliation of malignant intestinal obstruction using octreotide. Eur J Cancer 1994;30A:28–30.
8. Mosdell KW, Visconti JA. Emerging indications for octreotide therapy. Am J Hosp Pharm 1994;51:1184–92.
9. Weckbecker G, Raulf F, Bodmer D, Bruns C. Indirect antiproliferative effect of the somatostatin analog octreotide on MIA PaCa-2 human pancreatic carcinoma in nude mice. Yale J Biol Med 1997;70:549–54.
10. Dueno MI, Bai JC, Santangelo WC, Krejs GJ. Effect of somatostatin analog on water and electrolyte transport and transit time in human small bowel. Dig Dis Sci 1987;32:1092–6.
11. Vinik AI, Tsai ST, Moattari AR, et al. Somatostatin analogue (SMS 201-995) in the management of gastroenteropancreatic tumors and diarrhea syndrome. Am J Med 1986;81:Suppl 6B:23–40.
12. Georgii-Hemming P, Stromberg T, Janson ET, et al. The somatostatin analog octreotide inhibits growth of interleukin-6 (IL-6)–dependent and IL-6–independent human multiple myeloma cell lines. Blood 1999;93:1724–31.
13. Ottesen LH, Flyvbjerg A, Jakobsen P, Bendtsen F. The pharmacokinetics of octreotide in cirrhosis and in healthy man. J Hepatol 1997;26:1018–25.
14. Veysey MJ, Thomas LA, Mallet AI, et al. Prolonged large bowel transit increases serum deoxycholic acid: a risk factor for octreotide induced gallstones. Gut 1999;44:675–81.
15. Jönsson A, Manhem P. Octreotide and loss of scalp hair. Ann Intern Med 1991;115:913.
16. Legovini P, De Menis E, Breda F, et al. Long-term effects of octreotide on markers of bone metabolism in acromegaly: evidence of increased serum parathormone concentrations. J Endocrinol Invest 1997;20:434–8.
17. Herrington AM, George KW, Moulds CC. Octreotide-induced bradycardia. Pharmacotherapy 1998;18:413–6.
18. Gillis JC, Noble S, Goa KL. Octreotide long-acting release (LAR): a review of its pharmacological properties and therapeutic use in the management of acromegaly. Drugs 1997;53:681–99.
19. Rubin J, Ajani J, Schirmer W, et al. Octreotide acetate long-acting formulation versus open-label subcutaneous octreotide acetate in malignant carcinoid syndrome. J Clin Oncol 1999;17:600–6.

# Paclitaxel

Paclitaxel is a complex plant alkaloid derived from the bark of the Pacific yew tree, *Taxus brevifolia*. It was discovered in the late 1960s as part of a National Cancer Institute screening program involving 35,000 natural materials. The drug is highly lipophilic and insoluble in water. Because of this, it is provided in solution with polyoxyethylated castor oil (Cremophor EL). The drug is the first of a novel new class of agents—the taxanes.[1] Paclitaxel is also known as Taxol and NSC-125973.

## EFFICACY

The drug is FDA approved for the palliative treatment of carcinomas of the ovary, breast, and lung, and as second-line therapy for patients with Kaposi's sarcoma.[2] Other indications are less certain. The full spectrum of efficacy has not been defined.

## PHARMACOLOGY

**Mechanism of Action.** Paclitaxel is a novel microtubule inhibitor that works by stabilizing intracellular microtubules in susceptible cells.[3–5] The drug promotes the assembly of microtubules from tubulin dimers and prevents depolymerization by binding to the β subunit of tubulin.[6] This stabilization inhibits the normal dynamic reorganization of the microtubule network that is required at interphase. The morphologic result of microtubule stabilization is the induction of abnormal bundles of microtubules throughout the cell cycle and multiple "asters" of microtubules during mitosis. The stabilization of microtubules leads ultimately to apoptosis.[7]

Paclitaxel and bacterial lipopolysaccharides activate murine macrophages to express TNF-α and to downregulate their TNF-α receptors.[8] These changes are accompanied by induction of five additional genes in characteristic patterns. The role of these effects on the toxicity and efficacy of paclitaxel remains to be defined.

Cremophor EL is used as a solvent for paclitaxel. Preliminary data suggest that Cremophor EL itself may have cytotoxic effects.[9, 10] It induces a cell cycle block distinct from that seen with paclitaxel, and it inhibits multiple drug resistance. Further study is needed to define the clinical importance of these observations.

**Resistance.** Two mechanisms are known: (1) Resistant cells can evolve with abnormal microtubules that require the presence of taxol for normal function[11] and (2) resistance can be mediated by P-glycoprotein and the mdr gene.[12] Cremophor EL, the vehicle for paclitaxel, is itself an inhibitor of P-glycoprotein at dose levels achieved during clinical therapy.[13] The importance of this effect in clinical practice is uncertain.

**Pharmacokinetics.** After parenteral administration, paclitaxel is metabolized in the liver by cytochrome P450 isozymes.[14] It is avidly bound by proteins (89 to 98%), and 1 to 13% is excreted in the urine as unchanged drug, indicating extensive nonrenal clearance. It is widely distributed in the body, including to ascitic fluid (40%), and has biphasic plasma clearance, with a terminal elimination half-life that varies from 5 to 17 hours following 1-hour and 6-hour infusions in doses ranging from 15 to 275 mg/m².

Hepatic metabolism is extensive in animals and humans, with high concentrations of the drug in bile. However, the effects of hepatic and renal function on drug metabolism and clearance have not been studied extensively. Preliminary results in one patient with renal failure confirm that the drug can be given safely in that setting,[15] and reduced doses appear reasonable in patients with hepatic dysfunction, based on results in 81 patients.[16]

Pharmacokinetic studies in children receiving very high doses show that both distribution and elimination of paclitaxel are saturable.[17] In this study, estimates of paclitaxel systemic exposure correlated with toxicity better than dose. In another pharmacokinetic study in adults, the measurement of the duration of plasma concentrations above the threshold of 0.1 μmol/L was the best predictor of myelosuppression.[18] If these results are confirmed, measurements of drug levels may prove useful in future studies of more dose-intense therapy.

**Drug and Radiation Interactions.** Paclitaxel contains a

polyoxyethylated castor oil vehicle (Cremophor EL). Patients sensitive to this form of castor oil may also be sensitive to paclitaxel. The drug is metabolized by P450 enzymes in the liver that are inducible by barbiturates and benzodiazepine.[14, 19] Therefore, it is likely that a variety of drug interactions will be identified in the future. When the drug is combined with cisplatin, paclitaxel should be administered first because of excessive toxicity with the opposite sequence.[20] In vitro data suggest that ketoconazole can inhibit the metabolism of paclitaxel. Limited studies combining paclitaxel and vinorelbine (Navelbine) suggest an increased rate and severity of neurotoxicity and antitumor cross-resistance with the combination, presumably secondary to their sharing microtubules as their target molecule.[21] In vitro cytotoxicity studies suggest that paclitaxel may antagonize the antitumor efficacy of etoposide and doxorubicin.[22] A single case report implicates possible cross-sensitivity between paclitaxel and etoposide.[23] Paclitaxel is a moderate radiosensitizing agent for some, but not all, human cell lines.[24] This process appears to require the production of a $G_2/M$ cell cycle block. Preliminary data suggest that paclitaxel is especially effective against tumors that overexpress HER-2/*neu*.[25] Some authorities consider combined doxorubicin and paclitaxel therapy more cardiotoxic than either drug used alone, but this view is controversial.[26]

## TOXICITY

**Overview.** Dose-limiting toxicities include myelosuppression, hypersensitivity reactions, arrhythmias, and neuropathy. The frequency of these reactions varies, depending on the schedule of drug administration. The hypersensitivity reaction requires pretreatment prophylaxis with corticosteroids, diphenhydramine, and a histamine $H_2$-receptor antagonist.

**Hematologic.** Neutropenia (>90%) can be severe and is dose limiting, with a nadir at 8 to 11 days and recovery by day 21. Anemia and thrombocytopenia are less common and less severe problems. Myelosuppression is more likely in heavily pretreated patients, especially those receiving cisplatin. The manufacturer recommends that paclitaxel not be given to patients with a baseline ANC of less than 1500/μL.

**Immunologic.** Approximately 40% of patients develop histamine-related hypersensitivity reactions that may include cutaneous flushing, hypotension, bronchospasm, and bradycardia. Angioedema, diaphoresis, urticaria, and abdominal and extremity pain may also occur. About half of these reactions occur within 2 or 3 minutes of the first dose of therapy. Severe life-threatening hypersensitivity reactions occur in about 2% of patients. Anaphylaxis has been reported but occurs only rarely.[27] Reactions are more common with short infusion times, but the rate of hypersensitivity reactions is about the same with infusions, ranging from 3 to 24 hours. Premedication of patients with a corticosteroid, antihistamine, and $H_2$ blocker is highly recommended. Paclitaxel is contraindicated in patients with a prior history of hypersensitivity reactions to drugs using Cremophor EL as a solvent (e.g., cyclosporine and teniposide). In vitro, Cremophor EL has been shown to activate human complement, providing a possible mechanism for treatment-related hypersensitivity reactions.[28] Successful re-treatment with paclitaxel after ma-

jor hypersensitivity reactions has been reported,[29, 30] but the safety of this procedure has been questioned.[31]

**Digestive System.** Patients may develop mild to moderate nausea and vomiting (59%), diarrhea (43%), anorexia, and changes in taste. Rarely, paralytic ileus can occur. Eighteen cases of gastrointestinal necrosis have been reported; this should be suspected in patients who are receiving paclitaxel and who present with neutropenic fever and abdominal pain.[32] Four patients have developed unexplained bowel perforation.[33] Minor hepatic function abnormalities can occur, including an increase in serum bilirubin level (8%), alkaline phosphatase (23%), aspartate aminotransferase (serum glutamic-oxaloacetic transaminase, 16%), and alanine aminotransferase (serum glutamic-pyruvic transaminase, 33%). *C. difficile*–associated diarrhea occurs in about 2% of patients treated with standard doses of paclitaxel, and the risk of *C. difficile* infection increases to 20% in patients treated with high-dose regimens.[34]

**Mucocutaneous.** Many patients develop mild to moderate mucositis (39%), usually by 3 to 7 days and lasting about a week. It is characterized by diffuse ulceration of the lips, oral cavity, and pharynx, and it can extend to the esophagus. Severe alopecia is the rule, occurring 14 to 21 days after starting therapy and often affecting all areas of the body, including the eyebrows and pubic area. This process is reversible, and regrowth may occur after five to seven cycles in patients receiving ongoing therapy. Extravasation can cause phlebitis, cellulitis, and frank ulceration, so extravasation precautions are necessary.[35, 36] Paclitaxel is a radiosensitizing agent, and severe radiation-recall dermatitis can occur.[37, 38] Acral erythema due to paclitaxel has been reported.[39]

**Cardiovascular.** Bradycardia (10%) and hypotension (23%) can occur as part of a hypersensitivity reaction. Electrocardiographic changes occur frequently (33%), but severe changes are rare (about 1%). Ventricular tachycardia and atypical chest pain occur infrequently, and myocardial infarction is a very rare complication.[40–42] In one case of death due to congestive heart failure, electron microscopy demonstrated peculiar subsarcolemmic concentric lamellar bodies that may be uniquely associated with paclitaxel.[43] Sudden death can occur; one such event occurred 7 days after paclitaxel treatment.[44] Overall, 5% of patients at one center experienced serious cardiac toxicity.[20] Some centers routinely use cardiac monitoring for the first course of therapy, but this is not a universally applied precaution. The manufacturer recommends frequent vital sign monitoring during treatment, especially during the first hour of treatment. Rare cases of thrombosis have been reported.[45]

**Neurologic.** Peripheral neuropathy occurs in more than 60% of patients early in the course of treatment. It is mostly sensory and begins after the first or second dose.[46] Neuropathy is usually mild and only rarely dose limiting. When peripheral neuropathy is severe, a dose reduction of 20% for all subsequent courses of paclitaxel is recommended. Peripheral neuropathy is more common with long infusion times, with higher doses, and in patients with conditions predisposing to neuropathy, such as diabetes mellitus or prior abuse of alcohol. Rarely, generalized weakness, headaches, and seizures may occur. Transient encephalopathy has been reported in two patients.[47] Despite the high frequency of neuropathy, pre-existing neuropathy is not considered a contraindication to the use of paclitaxel. Ototoxicity does not appear to be a problem with paclitaxel.

**Musculoskeletal.** Myalgia and arthralgia (55% overall, 4% severe) can begin within 2 or 3 days of starting therapy, but they resolve within 2 to 4 days and are diminished by NSAIDs. These symptoms are dose related and may be intensified by filgrastim (G-CSF). Low-dose prednisone (10 mg BID starting 24 hours after the completion of chemotherapy and continuing for a total of 5 days) has been reported to relieve myalgias and arthralgias significantly in 85% of cases not adequately controlled by NSAIDs.[48]

**Other and Rare Reactions**

*Systemic.* Fatigue may occur.

*Pulmonary.* Interstitial pneumonitis due to delayed-type hypersensitivity has been reported in less than 1% of cases.[49, 50] It usually responds well to parenteral corticosteroids. Lung fibrosis has been reported in a patient treated with combined paclitaxel and carboplatin.[51] Pulmonary lipid embolism was fatal in one case.[52]

*Genitourinary.* Minor azotemia can occur.

*Reproductive.* Toxicity studies place paclitaxel in FDA pregnancy category D. The drug reduces the fertility of rats and is embryo-fetal toxic in rabbits. It is unknown whether paclitaxel is distributed into breast milk.

*Endocrine-Metabolic.* Elevation of serum triglycerides can occur.

*Carcinogenicity.* The drug is mutagenic in vitro and in vivo, but its potential for carcinogenicity is uncertain.

## DOSAGE AND ADMINISTRATION

Paclitaxel is available as a concentrated solution in vials of 30 mg. It is diluted in normal saline or in 5% dextrose solution to a final concentration of 0.3 to 1.2 mg/ml. Paclitaxel is stable for 27 hours at room temperature. The solution may appear hazy, but it should not contain particulate matter. The drug is incompatible with polyvinyl chloride (PVC) bags and infusion sets owing to leaching of a plasticizing agent by the concentrated drug solution. The diluted drug should be stored in bottles (glass, polypropylene) or plastic bags (polypropylene, polyolefin), and administration should be through polyethylene-lined administration sets. Plasticized PVC containers and administration sets are not recommended. Paclitaxel should be administered through intravenous tubing with an in-line filter with a microporous membrane not greater than 0.22 μm. Filter devices with short-inlet and short-outlet PVC coating (such as the IVEX-2 filters from Abbott Laboratories) can be used if necessary for diluted drug but not for the concentrated form of paclitaxel. Sets can be configured for administration using portable infusion pumps.[53] The detailed pharmaceutical properties of paclitaxel have been reviewed.[54]

The optimal dose, duration of infusion, and use of paclitaxel with colony-stimulating factors have yet to be determined.[55] Commonly used regimens follow.[2] For breast cancer, the dose is 175 mg/m² over 3 or 24 hours with repeat cycles every 21 days. For ovarian cancer, the dose is 135 mg/m² or 175 mg/m² over 3 or 24 hours every 21 days. For Kaposi's sarcoma, the dose is 135 mg/m² over 3 or 24 hours every 21 days. And, for non–small cell lung cancer, cisplatin in a dose of 75 mg/m² is given first, followed by paclitaxel

in a dose of 135 mg/m² administered over 24 hours, with repeat cycles every 21 days for the duration of therapy. None of these regimens requires coadministration of a colony-stimulating factor. Higher doses of paclitaxel can be given when a patient is also treated with G-CSF.[56, 57] However, there may be a plateau on the dose-response curve for paclitaxel, so it is unclear that dose-intense therapy is superior to standard doses.[55]

Prior to the administration of paclitaxel, the patient is premedicated to avoid hypersensitivity reactions. One program of premedication calls for the oral or intravenous administration of dexamethasone in a dosage of 20 mg for solid tumors and 10 mg for patients with Kaposi's sarcoma approximately 12 and 6 hours before paclitaxel administration, followed by the following intravenous medications 30 to 60 minutes before paclitaxel: diphenhydramine (50 mg intravenously) and ranitidine (50 mg intravenously) or famotidine (20 mg intravenously). More intensive regimens may also be considered, especially for patients who are retreated after prior hypersensitivity reactions.[29]

Minor symptoms of hypersensitivity during an infusion (such as flushing, minor dyspnea, hypotension, or tachycardia) do not require cessation of therapy. However, severe hypersensitivity reactions (such as hypotension requiring vasopressors, bronchospasm requiring bronchodilators, angioedema, or generalized urticaria) require immediate cessation of treatment. The manufacturer states that patients who develop severe hypersensitivity reactions should not be rechallenged with paclitaxel.

The manufacturer recommends withholding subsequent courses of treatment until the ANC has increased to greater than 1500/μL and the platelet count exceeds 100,000/μL. The dose should be reduced 20% for patients who develop severe neutropenia or neuropathy. Recommendations for dose adjustments for liver or renal dysfunction are not available, but the manufacturer recommends caution in using paclitaxel in patients with liver dysfunction because the drug is metabolized by the liver. Limited data suggest that dose reduction solely for advanced age is not necessary.[58]

## REFERENCES

1. Rowinsky EK. The development and clinical utility of the taxane class of microtubule chemotherapy agents. Ann Rev Med 1997;48:353–74.
2. Paclitaxel. USP DI 2000. Oncology drug information, 3rd ed. Englewood, Co.: Micromedix; 1999–2000:339–45.
3. Rowinsky EK, Cazenave LA, Donehower RC. Taxol: a novel investigational antimicrotubule agent. J Natl Cancer Inst 1990;82:1247–59.
4. Matsuoka H, Furusawa M, Tomoda H, Seo Y. Difference in cytotoxicity of paclitaxel against neoplastic and normal cells. Anticancer Res 1994;14:163–7.
5. Amos LA, Lowe J. How Taxol stabilises microtubule structure. Chem Biol 1999;6:R65–9.
6. Rao S, Horwitz SB, Ringel I. Direct photoaffinity labeling of tubulin with taxol. J Natl Cancer Inst 1992;84:785–8.
7. Bhalla K, Ibrado AM, Tourkina E, et al. Taxol induces internucleosomal DNA fragmentation associated with programmed cell death in human myeloid leukemia cells. Leukemia 1993;7:563–8.
8. Manthey CL, Brandes ME, Perera PY, Vogel SN. Taxol increases steady-state levels of lipopolysaccharide-inducible genes and protein-tyrosine phosphorylation in murine macrophages. J Immunol 1992;149:2459–65.
9. Fjällskog M-L, Frii L, Bergh J. Is Cremophor EL, solvent for paclitaxel, cytotoxic? Lancet 1993;342:873.
10. Liebmann J, Cook JA, Lipschultz C, et al. The influence of Cremophor

EL on the cell cycle effects of paclitaxel (Taxol) in human tumor cell lines. Cancer Chemother Pharmacol 1994;33:331–9.

11. Cabral FR. Isolation of Chinese hamster ovary cell mutants requiring the continuous presence of Taxol for cell division. J Cell Biol 1983;97:22–9.

12. Jachez B, Nordmann R, Loor F. Restoration of Taxol sensitivity of multidrug-resistant cells by the cyclosporine SDZ PSC 833 and the cyclopeptolide SDZ 280-446. J Natl Cancer Inst 1993;85:478–83.

13. Webster L, Linsenmeyer M, Millward M, et al. Measurement of Cremophor EL following Taxol: plasma levels sufficient to reverse drug exclusion mediated by the multidrug-resistant phenotype. J Natl Cancer Inst 1993;85:1685–90.

14. Cresteil T, Monsarrat B, Alvinerie P, et al. Taxol metabolism by human liver microsomes: identification of cytochrome P450 isozymes involved in its biotransformation. Cancer Res 1994;54:386–92.

15. Schilder LE, Egorin MJ, Zuhowski EG, Rossof AH. The pharmacokinetics of taxol in a dialysis patient. Proc Am Soc Clin Oncol 1994;13:136.

16. Venook AP, Egorin M, Rosner GL, et al. Phase I and pharmacokinetic trial of paclitaxel in patients with hepatic dysfunction: CALGB 9264. J Clin Oncol 1998;16:1811–9.

17. Sonnichsen DS, Hurwitz CA, Pratt CB, et al. Saturable pharmacokinetics and paclitaxel pharmacodynamics in children with solid tumors. J Clin Oncol 1994;12:532–8.

18. Huizing MT, Keung AC, Rosing H, et al. Pharmacokinetics of paclitaxel and metabolites in a randomized comparative study in platinum-pretreated ovarian cancer patients. J Clin Oncol 1993;11:2127–35.

19. Monsarrat B, Royer I, Wright M, Cresteil T. Biotransformation of taxoids by human cytochromes P450: structure-activity relationships. Bull Cancer (Paris) 1997;84:125–33.

20. Rowinsky EK, Gilbert MR, McGuire WP, et al. Sequences of taxol and cisplatin: a phase I and pharmacologic study. J Clin Oncol 1991;9:1692–703.

21. Fazeny B, Zifko U, Meryn S, et al. Vinorelbine-induced neurotoxicity in patients with advanced breast cancer pretreated with paclitaxel—a phase II study. Cancer Chemother Pharmacol 1996;39:150–6.

22. Viallet J, Tsao MS, Gallant G. Etoposide and doxorubicin antagonize the in vitro activity of paclitaxel in human non–small cell lung cancer cell lines. Lung Cancer 1996;15:93–101.

23. Friedland D, Gorman G, Treat J. Hypersensitivity reactions from taxol and etoposide. J Natl Cancer Inst 1993;85:2036.

24. Liebmann J, Cook JA, Fisher J, et al. In vitro studies of Taxol as a radiation sensitizer in human tumor cells. J Natl Cancer Inst 1994;86:441–6.

25. Baselga J, Seidman AD, Rosen PP, Norton L. HER2 overexpression and paclitaxel sensitivity in breast cancer: therapeutic implications. Oncology 1997;11:3 Suppl 2:43–8.

26. Martin M, Lluch A, Ojeda B, et al. Paclitaxel plus doxorubicin in metastatic breast cancer: preliminary analysis of cardiotoxicity. Semin Oncol 1997;24:5 Suppl 17:S17-26–30.

27. Ciesielski-Carlucci C, Leong P, Jacobs C. Case report of anaphylaxis from cisplatin/paclitaxel and a review of their hypersensitivity profiles. Am J Clin Oncol 1997;20:373–5.

28. Szebeni J, Muggia FM, Alving CR. Complement activation by Cremophor EL as a possible contributor to hypersensitivity to paclitaxel: an in vitro study. J Natl Cancer Inst 1998;90:300–6.

29. Peereboom DM, Donehower RC, Eisenhauer EA, et al. Successful retreatment with taxol after major hypersensitivity reactions. J Clin Oncol 1993;11:885–90.

30. Olson JK, Sood AK, Sorosky JI, et al. Taxol hypersensitivity: rapid retreatment is safe and cost effective. Gynecol Oncol 1998;68:25–8.

31. Laskin MS, Lucchesi KJ, Morgan M. Paclitaxel rechallenge failure after a major hypersensitivity reaction. J Clin Oncol 1993;11:2456–7.

32. Seewaldt VL, Cain JM, Goff BA, et al. A retrospective review of paclitaxel-associated gastrointestinal necrosis in patients with epithelial ovarian cancer. Gynecol Oncol 1997;67:137–40.

33. Seewaldt V, Cain JM, Greer BE, et al. Bowel complications with taxol therapy. J Clin Oncol 1993;11:1198.

34. Husain A, Aptaker L, Spriggs DR, Barakat RR. Gastrointestinal toxicity and *Clostridium difficile* diarrhea in patients treated with paclitaxel-containing chemotherapy regimens. Gynecol Oncol 1998;71:104–7.

35. Ajani JA, Dodd LG, Daugherty K, et al. Taxol-induced soft-tissue injury secondary to extravasation: characterization by histopathology and clinical course. J Natl Cancer Inst 1994;86:51–3.

36. Herrington JD, Figueroa JA. Severe necrosis due to paclitaxel extravasation. Pharmacotherapy 1997;17:163–5.

37. Raghavan VT, Bloomer WD, Merkel DE. Taxol and radiation recall dermatitis. Lancet 1993;341:1354.

38. McCarty MJ, Peake MF, Lillis P, Vukelja SJ. Paclitaxel-induced radiation recall dermatitis. Med Pediatr Oncol 1996;27:185–6.

39. De Argila D, Dominguez JD, Iglesias L. Taxol-induced acral erythema. Dermatology 1996;192:377–8.

40. Rowinsky EK, McGuire WP, Guarnieri T, et al. Cardiac disturbances during the administration of taxol. J Clin Oncol 1991;9:1704–12.

41. Laher S, Karp SJ. Acute myocardial infarction following paclitaxel administration for ovarian carcinoma. Clin Oncol (R Coll Radiol) 1997;9:124–6.

42. Hekmat E. Fatal myocardial infarction potentially induced by paclitaxel. Ann Pharmacother 1996;30:1110–2.

43. Jekunen A, Heikkila P, Maiche A, Pyrhonen S. Paclitaxel-induced myocardial damage detected by electron microscopy. Lancet 1994;343:727–8.

44. Alagaratnam TT. Sudden death 7 days after paclitaxel infusion for breast cancer. Lancet 1993;342:1232–3.

45. Sevelda P, Mayerhofer K, Obermair A, et al. Thrombosis with paclitaxel. Lancet 1994;343:727.

46. Forsyth PA, Balmaced C, Peterson K, et al. Prospective study of paclitaxel-induced peripheral neuropathy with quantitative sensory testing. J Neurooncol 1997;35:47–53.

47. Perry JR, Warner E. Transient encephalopathy after paclitaxel infusion. Neurology 1996;46:1596–9.

48. Markman M, Kennedy A, Webster K, et al. Use of low-dose oral prednisone to prevent paclitaxel-induced arthralgias and myalgias. Gynecol Oncol 1999;72:100–1.

49. Fujimori K, Yokoyama A, Kurita Y, et al. Paclitaxel-induced cell-mediated hypersensitivity pneumonitis: diagnosis using leukocyte migration test, bronchoalveolar lavage and transbronchial lung biopsy. Oncology 1998;55:340–4.

50. Khan A, McNally D, Tutschka PJ, Bilgrami S. Paclitaxel-induced acute bilateral pneumonitis. Ann Pharmacother 1997;31:1471–4.

51. Sotiriou C, van Houtte P, Klastersky J. Lung fibrosis induced by paclitaxel. Support Care Cancer 1998;6:68–71.

52. Brandwein MS, Rosen M, Harpaz N, et al. Fatal pulmonary lipid embolism associated with taxol therapy. Mt Sinai J Med 1988;55:187–9.

53. Goldspiel BR, Kohler DR, Koustenis AG, et al. Paclitaxel administration using portable infusion pumps. J Clin Oncol 1993;11:2287–8.

54. Trissel LA. Pharmaceutical properties of paclitaxel and their effects on preparation and administration. Pharmacotherapy 1997;17:5 Pt 2:133S–9S.

55. Rowinsky EK. The taxanes: dosing and scheduling considerations. Oncology 1997;11:3 Suppl 2:7–19.

56. Kohn EC, Sarosy G, Bicher A, et al. Dose-intense taxol: high response rate in patients with platinum-resistant recurrent ovarian cancer. J Natl Cancer Inst 1994;86:18–24.

57. Link CJ Jr, Bicher A, Kohn EC, et al. Flexible granulocyte colony-stimulating factor dosing in ovarian cancer patients who receive dose-intense taxol therapy. Blood 1994;83:1188–92.

58. Lichtman SM, Zaheer W, Gal D, et al. No increased risk of Taxol toxicity in older patients. J Am Geriatr Soc 1996;44:472–4.

# Pentostatin

Pentostatin is an antitumor antibiotic derived from *Streptomyces antibioticus*.[1, 2] It is also known as 2N-deoxycoformycin, DCF, Nipent, and NSC-218321.

## EFFICACY

Pentostatin has been used alone[1, 3] as well as in combination with cytarabine[4] in the treatment of a wide variety of lymphoid malignancies. It is especially effective against hairy cell leukemia, inducing complete remissions in 84% of patients in one large trial.[5] It also appears to be useful in other indolent lymphoid malignancies, such as CLL, prolymphocytic leukemia, and mycosis fungoides.[2, 6, 7] The drug is too toxic for use against most acute leukemias, with the possible exception of adult T-cell leukemia and lymphoma[2] and prolymphocytic leukemias.[8] The immunosuppressive effects of the drug are being studied as possible treatments for graft-versus-host disease, graft rejection, and some autoimmune diseases (such as multiple sclerosis).[9]

## PHARMACOLOGY

**Mechanism of Action.** Pentostatin is a potent inhibitor of adenosine deaminase, an important enzyme found in high concentration in lymphoid tissue.[2] This leads to elevated levels of adenine deoxynucleotides (e.g., deoxyadenosine 5'-triphosphate), which in the presence of deoxyadenosine leads to cell death. This is associated with depletion of ATP levels, with a concomitant reduction in cell energy and reduced cyclic adenosine monophosphate formation. Additional effects include the incorporation of the triphosphate form of pentostatin into DNA and formation of DNA strand breaks.[2] Deficient adenosine deaminase activity can cause immunosuppression, and the enzyme plays a role in the metabolism of some anticancer drugs, especially cytarabine.

**Resistance.** Resistance is not yet defined.

**Pharmacokinetics.** The drug is used solely by parenteral routes of administration. Plasma clearance is biexponential, with the alpha phase ranging between 30 and 85 minutes and the beta phase between 5 and 15 hours. At 24 hours, urinary recovery of the drug ranges from 32 to 48%.[2] Nevertheless, inhibition of adenosine deaminase persists for more than 1 week after a single dose of pentostatin. This suggests that substantial intracellular accumulation of the drug may occur, although this does not appear to involve extensive binding to tissues. There is ample evidence that the total-body clearance of pentostatin varies with creatinine clearance. For example, the elimination half-life may exceed 18 hours for patients with a creatinine clearance of less than 50 ml/min. Dose modifications based on abnormal renal function are therefore necessary.

**Drug Interactions.** Concurrent treatment with pentostatin and fludarabine is contraindicated because of a high rate of fatal pulmonary toxicity. Fatal cardiac toxicity has been reported with the combination of pentostatin and cyclophosphamide.[10] Allopurinol may increase the frequency of liver and renal dysfunction in patients treated with pentostatin. Pentostatin inhibits the degradation of vidarabine and increases its cytotoxicity.

## TOXICITY

**Overview.** Toxicity is clearly a function of drug dose and underlying disease.[2] In patients with solid tumors and indolent lymphoid malignancies treated with standard doses, lymphopenia is seen with little other toxicity. Patients with renal dysfunction or a poor performance status tolerate the drug poorly. Higher doses cause myelosuppression as well as renal, liver, pulmonary, and CNS toxicity. Concurrent therapy with fludarabine is contraindicated because of a high probability of lethal pulmonary toxicity.

**Hematologic.** Neutropenia and lymphopenia are common

(60%), but they are usually quantitatively minor. About a third of patients develop anemia and thrombocytopenia, and 3 to 10% develop hemorrhage. Rarely, myelodysplastic syndromes may develop after the use of pentostatin.[11, 12] Patients treated with pentostatin are extremely susceptible to overwhelming infections, even when they have normal granulocyte counts. In some cases, infections are fatal; therefore, these patients should be aggressively treated with the same antibiotic regimens used for neutropenic fever, even when the neutrophil count appears to be adequate.[13]

**Immunologic.** Hypersensitivity reactions occur in 11% of patients,[14] including hypersensitivity vasculitis, which is very rare.[15] The fact that pentostatin inhibits the formation of interferon in vitro raises the theoretical possibility of reduced resistance to viral infections.[16]

**Digestive System.** Easily controlled nausea and vomiting occur in 53% of patients, elevated liver enzymes in 19%, diarrhea in 15%, anorexia in 16%, and abdominal pain, constipation, and flatulence in less than 10%; altered taste and reversible hepatitis are rare.

**Mucocutaneous.** Stomatitis may occur; rash occurs in 26% of patients and dry skin in 17%.

**Cardiovascular.** Chest pain, arrhythmias, abnormal electrocardiographic findings, and thrombophlebitis all occur in less than 10% of patients.

**Pulmonary.** Cough occurs in 17% of patients and bronchitis, dyspnea, pneumonia, and edema in less than 10%. Fatal pulmonary failure can occur when pentostatin is given with fludarabine.

**Neurologic.** The following effects can occur: fatigue (29%); pain (20%); lassitude, confusion, headache (13%); and sleep disorders, slurred speech, depression, hallucinations, abnormal thinking, agitation, anxiety, confusion, dizziness, nervousness, and somnolence (all <10%). Cerebral edema, seizures, and coma all are very rare. These CNS reactions are usually minor, but they can be severe and life threatening.

**Musculoskeletal.** Myalgia occurs in 11% of patients, and back pain and arthralgia in less than 10%.

**Other and Rare Reactions.** The following reactions can occur: fever (42%); chills (11%); flu-like syndrome (<10%); malaise (<10%); ear pain (<10%); and pharyngitis, rhinitis, and sinusitis (<10%).

**Ocular.** Abnormal vision and eye pain occur in less than 10% of patients; keratoconjunctivitis is rare.

**Genitourinary.** Hematuria and dysuria occur in less than 10% of patients; increased blood urea nitrogen or creatinine level occurs in less than 10%. Acute tubular necrosis with renal failure is rare.

**Reproductive.** Toxicity studies place pentostatin in FDA pregnancy category D. Studies of dogs demonstrated mild seminiferous tubule degeneration. Formal fertility tests have not been completed.

**Endocrine-Metabolic.** Weight loss and peripheral edema occur in less than 10% of patients.

**Carcinogenicity.** Animal carcinogenesis studies have not been performed. The drug can induce chromosomal abnormalities in animals and should be considered carcinogenic until proved otherwise.

## DOSAGE AND ADMINISTRATION

Pentostatin is available as a lyophilized powder in vials of 10 mg. It is reconstituted with sterile water or normal saline.

Patients with hairy cell leukemia who have failed to respond to interferon treatment and have a good performance status, good renal function (creatinine clearance >60 ml/min), and good hepatic function are treated with 4 mg/m$^2$ of pentostatin intravenously every 2 weeks. The dose is administered by intravenous bolus or diluted and given over 20 minutes or longer. An additional 500 to 1000 ml of hydration is given before and after each treatment. Patients with a poor performance status (Eastern Cooperative Oncology Group 3) receive 2 mg/m$^2$ of the drug. The manufacturer recommends continued treatment until complete remission is achieved, at which time two additional courses are given and the drug is discontinued. Patients with a partial response should continue treatment for as long as a year. If no response is seen by 6 months, the drug should be discontinued. The manufacturer recommends withholding or discontinuing pentostatin if severe reactions develop. The following are listed as indications for discontinuing or withholding treatment: severe rash (discontinue), nervous system toxicity, hypersensitivity reactions, active infection, and renal dysfunction (discontinue or decrease dose to 2 mg/m$^2$).

## REFERENCES

1. Dillman RO. A new chemotherapeutic agent: deoxycoformycin (pentostatin). Semin Hematol 1994;31:16–27.
2. O'Dwyer PJ, Wagner B, Leyland-Jones B, et al. 2'-Deoxycoformycin (pentostatin) for lymphoid malignancies: rational development of an active new drug. Ann Intern Med 1988;108:733–43.
3. Major PP, Agarwal RP, Kufe DW. Clinical pharmacology of deoxycoformycin. Blood 1981;58:91–6.
4. Gray DP, Grever MR, Siaw MF, et al. 2'Deoxycoformycin (DCF) and 9-beta-D-arabinofuranosyladenine (Ara-A) in the treatment of refractory acute myelocytic leukemia. Cancer Treat Rep 1982;66:253–7.
5. Cassileth PA, Cheuvart B, Spiers AS, et al. Pentostatin induces durable remissions in hairy cell leukemia. J Clin Oncol 1991;9:243–6.
6. Ho AD, Ganeshaguru K, Knauf WU, et al. Clinical response to deoxycoformycin in chronic lymphoid neoplasms and biochemical changes in circulating malignant cells in vivo. Blood 1988;72:1884–90.
7. Ho AD, Thaler J, Willemze R, et al. Pentostatin (2'deoxycoformycin) for the treatment of lymphoid neoplasms. Bone Marrow Transplant 1989;4:Suppl 1:60–2.
8. Dohner H, Ho AD, Thaler J, et al. Pentostatin in prolymphocytic leukemia: phase II trial of the European Organization for Research and Treatment of Cancer Leukemia Cooperative Study Group. J Natl Cancer Inst 1993;85:658–62.
9. Dighiero G. Adverse and beneficial immunological effects of purine nucleoside analogues. Hematol Cell Ther 1996,38:Suppl 2:S75–81.
10. Gryn J, Gordon R, Bapat A, et al. Pentostatin increases the acute toxicity of high dose cyclophosphamide. Bone Marrow Transplant 1993;12:217–20.
11. Psiachou-Leonard E, Bain BJ. Persistent bone marrow failure with dysplastic features following pentostatin therapy for hairy cell leukaemia. Clin Lab Haematol 1998;20:195–7.
12. Orchard JA, Bolam S, Oscier DG. Association of myelodysplastic changes with purine analogues. Br J Haematol 1998;100:677–9.
13. O'Dwyer PJ, Spiers AS, Marsoni S. Association of severe and fatal infections and treatment with pentostatin. Cancer Treat Rep 1986;70:1117–20.
14. O'Dwyer PJ, King SA, Eisenhauer E, et al. Hypersensitivity reactions to deoxycoformycin. Cancer Chemother Pharmacol 1989;23:173–5.
15. Steinmetz JC, DeConti R, Ginsburg R. Hypersensitivity vasculitis associated with 2-deoxycoformycin and allopurinol therapy. Am J Med 1989;86:498–9.
16. Slomiany DJ, Woldehawariat G, Petryshyn RA. Chemotherapeutic purine analogs alter the level of interferon-beta mRNA induced by poly I-poly C in cultured osteosarcoma cells. J Interferon Cytokine Res 1997;17:245–54.

# Plicamycin

Plicamycin is an antibiotic derived as a natural product of *Streptomyces plicatus*. The drug is also known as mithramycin, Mithracin, and NSC-24559.

## EFFICACY

The primary use of plicamycin is in the treatment of hypercalcemia (see Chapter 18), although the drug is used less frequently for this purpose since the advent of bisphosphonate therapy. In the past, the drug was also used in the palliative treatment of embryonal cell carcinoma of the testis, but this use has been almost completely replaced by combination chemotherapy regimens that are given with curative intent. A single case of Paget's disease of bone that appears to have been cured by plicamycin has been reported.[1]

## PHARMACOLOGY

**Mechanism of Action.** Plicamycin binds to the GC and AT regions of DNA and inhibits DNA, RNA, and protein synthesis. The drug is known to block the hypercalcemic effect of pharmacologic doses of vitamin D, and it can inhibit the effect of parathormone on osteoclasts. However, it is unclear whether or not these latter effects explain the hypocalcemic effect of the drug. Other interesting effects of plicamycin are under investigation. For example, it avidly binds the c-Ki-*ras* promoter region of DNA, resulting in complete abrogation of its function.[2] In another study, plicamycin was a powerful inducer of erythroid differentiation of human K562 cells in vitro, raising the possibility that the drug may be useful in treating hematologic diseases characterized by abnormal expression of β-globin genes.[3]

Plicamycin is cell cycle phase nonspecific, but late $G_1$ and $G_2$ phases may be somewhat more sensitive.

**Resistance.** Mechanisms of resistance are not clearly defined. They are probably similar to those of other antitumor antibiotics, such as dactinomycin.

**Pharmacokinetics.** Plicamycin preferentially distributes to Kupffer's cells in the liver, renal tubular cells, and areas of active bone resorption. The drug also crosses the blood-brain barrier.[4] A single dose reaches its peak effect by 72 hours, and the duration of effect from a single dose is 7 to 10 days. The drug is eliminated by the renal route.

**Drug Interactions.** Plicamycin-induced hypoprothrombinemia may increase the activity of warfarin anticoagulation. Caution should be exercised when combining plicamycin with any drug known to reduce platelets or clotting factors because of the known impact of plicamycin on coagulation.[4]

## TOXICITY

**Overview.** Myelosuppression and a hemorrhagic diathesis are the main dose-limiting toxicities, but a variety of other problems that can occur can be severe, unpredictable, and life threatening. Plicamycin is contraindicated in patients with thrombocytopenia, thrombocytopathy, coagulation disorders, other forms of bleeding diathesis, and pre-existing bone marrow functional impairment.

**Hematologic.** Plicamycin causes only minor and temporary myelosuppression at commonly used doses. Prolonged daily administration of high-dose therapy can cause life-threatening myelosuppression and a severe bleeding diathesis. However, death due to hemorrhage, presumably as a result of disseminated intravascular coagulation, has occurred with as little as one dose of the drug given for the treatment of hypercalcemia.[5]

**Digestive System.** Anorexia, nausea, vomiting, and diarrhea can occur, but they are rarely a serious problem. About 16% of patients develop mild, reversible hepatic dysfunction with low-dose therapy.[6]

**Mucocutaneous.** Stomatitis and skin eruptions (acneiform rash, hyperpigmentation, toxic epidermal necrolysis) can occur but only rarely. Severe tissue damage occurs with extravasation.

**Other/Rare.** Malaise, fever, and facial flushing can occur.

*Immunologic.* Minimal, if any, immunosuppression can occur.

*Neurologic.* Headache, apprehension, depression, nervousness, and lethargy may occur.

*Genitourinary.* Renal dysfunction can occur. It is usually minor but may be severe.

*Reproductive.* Toxicity data place plicamycin in FDA pregnancy category X (the drug is contraindicated during pregnancy). The drug inhibits spermatogenesis in rats.

*Endocrine-Metabolic.* Hypocalcemia, hypomagnesemia, hypophosphatemia, and hypokalemia can occur.

*Carcinogenicity.* Formal testing has not been completed. The drug should be considered carcinogenic until proved otherwise.

## DOSAGE AND ADMINISTRATION

Plicamycin is available as a lyophilized powder in 2.5-mg vials. It is reconstituted in sterile water and then further diluted in saline or dextrose in water for intravenous infusion. The drug is incompatible with trace element solutions, iron, and cellulose ester filters.

When plicamycin is used in the treatment of hypercalcemia due to bone destruction by metastatic malignancy, a dosage of 25 µg/kg may be given intravenously every 2 or 3 days until an acceptable calcium level is achieved. The manufacturer recommends that this be given over a 4- to 6-hour period because rapid injections may cause more severe gastrointestinal side effects. Care must be taken to prevent extravasation because the drug can be locally irritating. Because of this risk, the dose of plicamycin may also be given by intravenous push over 20 to 30 minutes. If the initial course of treatment is successful, intermittent doses one to three times weekly may serve to maintain the response.

## REFERENCES

1. Ryan WG, Fordham EW. Mithramycin and Paget's disease revisited. Ann Intern Med 1984;100:771.
2. Vigneswaran N, Mayfield CA, Rodu B, et al. Influence of GC and AT specific DNA minor groove binding drugs on intermolecular triplex formation in the human c-Ki-*ras* promoter. Biochemistry 1996;35:1106–14.
3. Bianchi N, Osti F, Rutigliano C, et al. The DNA-binding drugs mithramycin and chromomycin are powerful inducers of erythroid differentiation of human K562 cells. Br J Haematol 1999;104:258–65.
4. Yarbro JW, Bailes JS, Baker LH, et al. Plicamycin. In:USP DI oncology drug information. Rockville, Md.: U.S. Pharmacopeia, 1998:350–353.
5. Brumpt I, Baglin A, Alterescu R, Goguel A. [Fatal complications of a single infusion of mithramycin.] Nouv Presse Med 1981;10:3853–4.
6. Green L, Donehower RC. Hepatic toxicity of low doses of mithramycin in hypercalcemia. Cancer Treat Rep 1984;68:1379–81.

# Prednisone

Prednisone is a synthetic corticosteroid with wide use in oncology. It is also known as Deltasone, Sterapred, Prednicen-M, PRED, and others.

## EFFICACY

Prednisone is an important constituent of many drug combinations used in the treatment of malignant hematopoietic tumors. It also has a place in the palliative treatment of many solid tumors, such as carcinomas of the breast and prostate, and in the treatment of several complications of cancer, including thrombocytopenia, hemolytic anemia, and hypercalcemia. It is widely used in the treatment of immune-mediated diseases.[1]

## PHARMACOLOGY

**Mechanisms of Action and Resistance.** See Dexamethasone.

**Pharmacokinetics.** One can separate the commonly used corticosteroids into those with a relatively short duration of action and low potency and those with a prolonged duration of action and great relative potency. Hydrocortisone (cortisol) and prednisone are relatively weak corticosteroids with a short duration of action. After oral administration, their respective plasma half-lives are approximately 1.5 and 3.5 hours. The biologic half-life of these two corticosteroids is 1.5 to 2 times the half-time of disappearance from plasma. Prednisone retains much less of its potency with time compared with dexamethasone. For example, one study found that the relative potencies of hydrocortisone (cortisol), prednisone, and dexamethasone at 0, 8, and 14 hours after oral administration were as follows: hydrocortisone, 1, 1, 1; prednisone, 1.05, 3, 5.2; and dexamethasone, 17, 52, 154.[2]

**Drug Interactions.** Relatively little is known about drug interactions involving prednisone. In one tissue culture study, the antitumor effects of 6-MP and cytarabine were inhibited by prednisolone, whereas prednisolone had no inhibitory effect on daunorubicin or MTX.[3] However, in a subsequent study,[4] these investigators showed a synergistic effect with cytarabine and a glucocorticoid with a different schedule of drug use. The clinical importance of these preliminary results is uncertain, but they do suggest the need for more detailed assessment of this issue.

## TOXICITY

The spectrum of toxic side effects and precautions for the use of prednisone are similar to those of dexamethasone.

## DOSAGE AND ADMINISTRATION

Prednisone is available as tablets of 1, 2.5, 5, 10, 20, 25, and 50 mg. Oral solutions of 1 mg/ml and 5 mg/ml are also available. Various doses are used, depending on the precise regimen of treatment. Commonly used dosages in oncology include 40 mg/m²/day for 14 days every 28 days and 100 mg/m²/day for 5 days repeated every 3 or 4 weeks. For some chronic conditions, alternate-day prednisone treatment may be used to maintain a beneficial response.[5] Precautions and guidelines for withdrawal of corticosteroid therapy are discussed in the section on dexamethasone.

## REFERENCES

1. Boumpas DT, Chrouros GP, Wilder RL, et al. Glucocorticoid therapy for immune-mediated diseases: basic and clinical correlates. Ann Intern Med 1993;119:1198–208.
2. Meikle AW, Tyler FH. Potency and duration of action of glucocorticoids: effects of hydrocortisone, prednisone and dexamethasone on human pituitary-adrenal function. Am J Med 1977;63:200–7.
3. Gledhill RM, Norman MR. Antagonism of drugs used in leukaemia therapy to the killing of human lymphoblastoid cells by steroid. Br J Cancer 1981;44:467–71.
4. Gledhill RM, Edwards AJ, Norman MR. Synergistic killing of human leukaemic lymphoblasts by glucocorticoids and cytosine arabinoside. Br J Cancer 1983;47:649–57.
5. MacGregor RR, Sheagren JN, Lipsett MB, Wolff SM. Alternate-day prednisone therapy: evaluation of delayed hypersensitivity responses, control of disease and steroid side effects. N Engl J Med 1969;280:1427–31.

# Procarbazine

Procarbazine is a unique antineoplastic agent that was initially synthesized as a potential MAO inhibitor.[1] The drug is also known as Matulane, Ibenzmethyzin, Natulan, *N*-methylhydrazine, and NSC-77213.

## EFFICACY

Procarbazine is used primarily in the treatment of advanced Hodgkin's disease. As a single agent, it yields a response rate of about 50%; however, these responses rarely last longer than 2 or 3 months, and it is therefore nearly always used in combination with other drugs. The most commonly used regimen is MOPP, described by DeVita and colleagues,[2] in which mechlorethamine, vincristine (Oncovin), procarbazine, and prednisone are combined (see Chapter 87). Procarbazine is less useful in the treatment of other kinds of lymphoma, and it is of marginal value as a single agent in the treatment of bronchogenic carcinoma and brain tumors. It is being studied as a component of multiagent regimens for the treatment of advanced brain tumors.[3]

## PHARMACOLOGY

**Mechanism of Action.** Procarbazine has multiple sites of action, so it is difficult to classify its mechanism of cytotoxicity precisely.[4] It inhibits incorporation of many small precursors into DNA, and it can inhibit RNA and protein synthesis by a process known as methylation.[5] This involves the formation of $O^6$-methylguanine DNA adducts that interfere with DNA and RNA synthesis by blocking replication and transcriptional complexes.[6] Damaging DNA involves the biotransformation of procarbazine to one or more azoxy metabolites.[7] The *N*-oxidation that is required for this biotransformation involves certain forms of cytochrome P450 in the liver and is therefore susceptible to drug interactions involving this enzyme system. The most important metabolite appears to be azoxy 2-procarbazine, which causes single-strand breaks in DNA through direct strand scission and spontaneous depurination of methylated DNA.[7] In addition, procarbazine inhibits the transmethylation of methyl groups of methionine into transfer RNA, and the drug can release hydrogen peroxide during the process of auto-oxidation, which may attack protein sulfhydryl groups bound to DNA. The drug is cell cycle phase nonspecific.

It has been proposed that the inhibition of spermatogenesis by procarbazine may involve a different metabolic pathway than that proposed for its major antineoplastic effects.[8] Hormonal pretreatment suppresses sperm production and appears to provide some protection against procarbazine-induced testicular damage.[9] The mechanism of this effect is uncertain, although it is associated with suppression of intratesticular testosterone levels.[10]

**Resistance.** A specific DNA repair protein, $O^6$-alkylguanine DNA alkyltransferase, is responsible for the repair of damage by methylating agents such as procarbazine. A secondary repair mechanism that is less important is the excision repair pathway. Another mechanism may be mismatch repair deficiency.[11] Preliminary studies suggest that the level of $O^6$-alkylguanine DNA alkyltransferase may be reduced in tumors with p53 mutations, thus causing increased sensitivity to methylating agents such as procarbazine.[12] Resistance develops rapidly in most tumors when procarbazine is used as a single antineoplastic agent. Procarbazine is not cross-resistant to other alkylating agents or to other commonly used antineoplastic drugs.

**Pharmacokinetics.** Procarbazine is well absorbed from the gastrointestinal tract. It is metabolized by RBCs and by microsomal enzymes in the liver to azoprocarbazine. It is widely distributed in the body, including the CSF. Its overall elimination half-life is about 1 hour. The major route of excretion is the kidneys, although less than 5% of the drug is excreted unchanged by this route.[1]

**Drug Interactions.** A wide variety of drugs and foods may potentiate the toxic side effects of procarbazine, especially neurologic reactions.

*Drugs.* The following drugs may potentiate toxic side effects of procarbazine: MAO inhibitors (such as pargyline); tricyclic antidepressants (such as imipramine, nortriptyline, amitriptyline, desipramine); antihypertensives; sympathomimetic agents (such as ephedrine, pseudoephedrine, isoproterenol, epinephrine); phenothiazines; narcotic analgesics (such as meperidine); antihistamines; and barbiturates. With alcohol, a peculiar flushing syndrome may occur, not unlike that seen with disulfiram (Antabuse). Concomitant exposure to anticonvulsant drugs during procarbazine therapy appears to increase the risk of procarbazine-induced hypersensitivity reactions.[13]

*Foods.* Tyramine-rich foods (such as ripe cheese, imported beer, some wines), chocolate, and fava beans may potentiate toxic side effects of procarbazine.

## TOXICITY

**Overview.** Myelosuppression is the major dose-limiting toxicity. Other important side effects include nausea and vomiting, hepatic dysfunction, and neurologic effects. A disulfiram-like reaction can occur when the drug is taken while drinking alcohol.

**Hematologic.** Mild to moderate bone marrow suppression commonly occurs and is the dose-limiting toxicity. This may be delayed in some patients. As with other hydrazine derivatives, procarbazine rarely causes hemolytic anemia, with hemoglobin denaturation and the formation of Heinz bodies in RBCs.

**Digestive System.** Anorexia, nausea, and vomiting occur frequently, but these tend to subside with continued treatment. Diarrhea and constipation are rare complaints. Liver function test results are occasionally abnormal. Rare reported side effects include clinical jaundice, ascites, hematemesis, melena, dysphagia, anorexia, and abdominal pain.

**Mucocutaneous.** Allergic skin rashes can occur, as can photosensitivity and urticaria.[14] On the basis of a study in patients with brain tumors, a skin rash should be used as an indication to discontinue the drug.[15] Stomatitis and xerostomia occur infrequently, as well as pruritus, alopecia, hyperpigmentation, and flushing.

**Neurologic.** Mild to moderate neurotoxicity commonly occurs. As many as one third of patients treated with procarbazine develop disorders of consciousness (somnolence, depression, nightmares, apprehension, nervousness, confusion, slurred speech, agitation, psychosis), and peripheral neuropathies have been reported in 17% of these patients. Ataxia occasionally occurs. The neurotoxic effects of procarbazine are rarely dose limiting and probably arise from a combination of its weak MAO inhibitory properties and decreased pyridoxal 5-phosphate levels. This gives rise to numerous potential drug interactions, the most important being with tricyclic antidepressants and a disulfiram-like reaction with alcohol ingestion (discussed earlier).

**Other and Rare Reactions.** These include intercurrent infections, hearing loss, fever, diaphoresis, lethargy, weakness, fatigue, edema, chills, and hoarseness.

**Immunologic.** Immunosuppression is not a major problem. Generalized allergic reactions have been reported rarely.

*Cardiovascular.* Orthostatic hypotension, tachycardia, and syncope can occur. Hypertensive reactions can occur through drug interactions with sympathomimetic agents and tricyclic antidepressants resulting from MAO inhibition.

*Pulmonary.* Pleuropulmonary reactions with fever, cough, pneumonitis, and pleural effusions can occur.[16] These can be delayed and life threatening.[17]

*Ocular.* The following reactions may occur: photophobia, diplopia, papilledema, and retinal hemorrhages.

*Musculoskeletal.* Myalgia and arthralgia can occur.

*Genitourinary.* Patients may develop urinary frequency, hematuria, and nocturia.

*Reproductive.* Toxicity studies place procarbazine in FDA pregnancy category D. The drug is mutagenic and teratogenic. Procarbazine commonly causes severe azoospermia. The possibility that this may be due to a different metabolic pathway than the antitumor effects of the drug raises the possibility of preventing this complication.[8] Although several approaches have been studied, including the use of steroid contraceptives[18] and the use of thiol-containing antioxidants, none can be recommended.

*Endocrine-Metabolic.* Gynecomastia may occur in prepubertal boys and boys in early puberty; menstrual irregularities can occur.

*Carcinogenicity.* Procarbazine is one of the most potent carcinogens used in oncology; many cases of leukemia and myelodysplasia have been reported.[1, 19, 20]

## DOSAGE AND ADMINISTRATION

Procarbazine is available as 50-mg capsules. The drug is almost always used as part of the MOPP or C-MOPP (C-M = cyclophosphamide) combination regimen for the treatment of Hodgkin's lymphoma (see Chapter 87) in a dosage of 100 mg/m$^2$ on days 1 to 14 of each course. When used alone, procarbazine is generally given in a dosage of 2 to 4 mg/kg body weight daily by mouth for the first week. If this dosage is tolerated, the daily dose is increased to 4 to 6 mg/kg/day. Procarbazine is discontinued when grade 1 leukopenia or thrombocytopenia arises and is reinstituted at a lower dosage (50 to 100 mg/day) when hematologic recovery occurs.

The dose of procarbazine should be reduced in patients with impaired renal, liver, or bone marrow function. Careful attention to the many potential drug interactions is a crucial part of drug administration. The manufacturer recommends prompt cessation of therapy for any of the following: (1) CNS signs or symptoms (e.g., paresthesia, neuropathy, confusion), (2) WCC less than 4000/μL, (3) platelet count less than 100,000/μL, (4) hypersensitivity reactions, (5) stomatitis of any degree, (6) diarrhea, and (7) hemorrhage or bleeding tendency.

## REFERENCES

1. Spivack SD. Drugs 5 years later: procarbazine. Ann Intern Med 1974;81:795–800.
2. DeVita VT Jr, Serpick AA, Carbone PP. Combination chemotherapy in the treatment of advanced Hodgkin's disease. Ann Intern Med 1970;73:881–95.
3. Kim L, Hochberg FH, Thornton AF, et al. Procarbazine, lomustine, and vincristine (PCV) chemotherapy for grade III and grade IV oligoastrocytomas. J Neurosurg 1996;85:602–7.
4. Pletsa V, Valavanis C, van Delft JH, et al. DNA damage and mutagenesis induced by procarbazine in lambda lacZ transgenic mice: evidence that bone marrow mutations do not arise primarily through miscoding by O6-methylguanine. Carcinogenesis 1997;18:2191–6.
5. Schold SC Jr, Brent TP, von Hofe E, et al. O6-alkylguanine-DNA alkyltransferase and sensitivity to procarbazine in human brain-tumor xenografts. J Neurosurg 1989;70:573–7.
6. Souliotis VL, Kaila S, Boussiotis VA, et al. Accumulation of O6-methylguanine in human blood leukocyte DNA during exposure to

procarbazine and its relationships with dose and repair. Cancer Res 1990;50:2759–64.

7. Erikson JM, Tweedie DJ, Ducore JM, Prough RA. Cytotoxicity and DNA damage caused by the azoxy metabolites of procarbazine in L1210 tumor cells. Cancer Res 1989;49:127–33.

8. Horstman MG, Meadows GG, Yost GS. Separate mechanisms for procarbazine spermatotoxicity and anticancer activity. Cancer Res 1987;47:1547–50.

9. Meistrich ML, Wilson G, Zhang Y, et al. Protection from procarbazine-induced testicular damage by hormonal pretreatment does not involve arrest of spermatogonial proliferation. Cancer Res 1997;57:1091–7.

10. Meistrich ML, Wilson G, Ye WS, et al. Relationship among hormonal treatments, suppression of spermatogenesis, and testicular protection from chemotherapy-induced damage. Endocrinology 1996;137:3823–31.

11. Duke researchers link brain tumor drug resistance to mismatch repair deficiency. Compr Ther 1997;23:622–3.

12. Russell S, Ye YW, Waber PG, et al. p53 mutations, *O6*-alkylguanine DNA alkyltransferase activity, and sensitivity to procarbazine in human brain tumors. Cancer 1995;75:1339–42.

13. Lehmann DF, Hurteau TE, Newman N, Coyle TE. Anticonvulsant usage is associated with an increased risk of procarbazine hypersensitivity reactions in patients with brain tumors. Clin Pharmacol Ther 1997;62:225–9.

14. Giguere JK, Dougas DM, Lupton GP, et al. Procarbazine hypersensitivity manifested as a fixed drug eruption. Med Pediatr Oncol 1988;16:378–80.

15. Coyle T, Bushunow P, Winfield J, et al. Hypersensitivity reactions to procarbazine with mechlorethamine, vincristine, and procarbazine chemotherapy in the treatment of glioma. Cancer 1992;69:2532–40.

16. Garbes ID, Henderson ES, Gomez GA, et al. Procarbazine-induced interstitial pneumonitis with a normal chest x-ray: a case report. Med Pediatr Oncol 1986;14:238–41.

17. Brooks BJ Jr, Hendler NB, Alvarez S, et al. Delayed life-threatening pneumonitis secondary to procarbazine. Am J Clin Oncol 1990;13:244–6.

18. de la Calle JFV, Jegou B. Protection by steroid contraceptives against procarbazine-induced sterility and genotoxicity in male rats. Cancer Res 1990;50:1308–15.

19. Sieber SM, Adamson RH. Toxicity of antineoplastic agents in man, chromosomal aberrations, antifertility effects, congenital malformations, and carcinogenic potential. Adv Cancer Res 1975;22:57.

20. Arseneau JC, Canellos GP, Johnson R, DeVita VT Jr. Risk of new cancers in patients with Hodgkin's disease. Cancer 1977;40:4 Suppl:1912–6.

# Streptozocin

Streptozocin is a synthetic antibiotic originally derived from *Streptomyces achromogenes*. Its structure consists of a nitrosourea moiety interposed between a methyl group and a glucosamine.[1] The drug is also known as Zanosar, streptozotocin, and NSC-85998.

## EFFICACY

Streptozocin is mainly used in the treatment of endocrine tumors of the pancreas, especially islet cell carcinomas. Carcinoid tumors and lymphomas may also be treated with this agent.

## PHARMACOLOGY

**Mechanism of Action.** Streptozocin has multiple effects on cells, and its complete mechanism of action is uncertain. The predominant mechanism appears to involve methylation of guanine residues in DNA, which is analogous to but different from alkylation of DNA by classic alkylating agents.[2] Methylation involves the formation of $O^6$-methylguanine DNA adducts that interfere with DNA and RNA synthesis by blocking replication and transcriptional complexes. These adducts are also capable of inducing genomic mutations. The drug is known to inhibit DNA synthesis and to interfere with the biochemical reactions of NAD, reduced NAD (NADH), and some key enzymes involved in gluconeogenesis.[3] These effects ultimately result in apoptosis.[4, 5] However, the high degree of β-cell selectivity remains unexplained.[6] As with the other nitrosoureas, streptozocin is cell cycle phase nonspecific.

**Resistance.** Despite structural similarities, streptozocin is not cross-resistant with the other nitrosoureas. A specific DNA repair protein, $O^6$-methylguanine DNA methyltransferase, is responsible for the repair of damage by methylating agents such as streptozocin. The excision pathway is a secondary repair mechanism. However, studies in human brain tumor cell lines suggest that other undefined mechanisms of resistance may also be important for this drug.[7] Mechanisms of resistance for pancreatic islet cells are also under investigation. In one study, metabolic activation of islet cells improved resistance to streptozocin.[8]

**Pharmacokinetics.** Streptozocin is administered parenterally, and it is rapidly distributed into extracellular spaces. Its biologic half-life in the body is about 40 minutes, and its half-time of plasma clearance is approximately 13 minutes. It is metabolized by the liver and excreted by the kidneys. When streptozocin is given by the hepatic arterial route, hepatic extraction is about 5%.

**Drug Interactions.** Hepatic dysfunction due to streptozocin may cause problems when the drug is combined with drugs that are metabolized by the liver. An example of such an adverse interaction has been reported for doxorubicin.[9] Because of potential additive renal toxicity, streptozocin should not be used with other nephrotoxic drugs. Limited data suggest that phenytoin may decrease the effectiveness of streptozocin. The use of streptozocin with other nitrosoureas (lomustine, carmustine) may be associated with especially severe myelosuppression.

## TOXICITY

**Overview.** Renal dysfunction is the dose-limiting toxicity, but the drug can induce diabetes mellitus. Nausea and vomiting can be severe, whereas myelosuppression tends to be modest in severity. Liver dysfunction, diarrhea, and myelosuppression are occasional problems.

**Hematologic.** Mild hematologic toxicity occurs in about 20% of treated patients. Cumulative toxicity in the form of anemia may occur in patients treated with multiple courses of drug. Patients may develop eosinophilia. On very rare occasions, myelosuppression has been severe and fatal.

**Digestive System.** Streptozocin frequently causes moderate or severe nausea and vomiting that should be aggressively pretreated. Anorexia, abdominal cramps, and diarrhea occur less frequently. About 25% of patients develop mild hepatic dysfunction.

**Mucocutaneous.** The drug is locally irritating to tissues, and severe necrosis can occur after drug extravasation.

**Genitourinary.** The most important adverse effect of streptozocin is renal toxicity, which occurs in 25 to 75% of patients. It is dose related, cumulative, and potentially severe or fatal. Renal toxicity usually starts as proteinuria with or without azotemia, and this can progress to renal tubular acidosis and renal failure. In one early series, 5 of 52 patients died of renal failure.[3] With newer dose schedules and alert attention to renal function, this high mortality rate should be avoidable. Close monitoring of renal function with urinalysis, blood urea nitrogen measurement, and weekly creatine clearance determination is recommended. The appearance of proteinuria or deterioration of renal function is an indication for interrupting therapy. Despite these precautions, delayed chronic renal failure may occur.[10] Several cases of nephrogenic diabetes insipidus have been reported.

**Other and Rare Reactions.** Fever may occur.

**Immunologic.** Rarely, dramatic febrile hypersensitivity reactions may occur.[11, 12]

**Neurologic.** Patients receiving streptozocin by continuous infusion may experience mild confusion, lethargy, and depression.

**Reproductive.** Toxicity studies place streptozocin in FDA pregnancy category C. Sterility can occur.

**Endocrine-Metabolic.** Variable hyperglycemia occurs with the drug, and severe hypoglycemia can be a rare complication of treatment in patients with insulinoma.

**Carcinogenicity.** The drug is mutagenic and potentially carcinogenic.[13]

## DOSAGE AND ADMINISTRATION

Streptozocin is available as a lyophilized powder in vials containing 1 g of drug. It is reconstituted with dextrose in water or normal saline. There are no important incompatibilities of the drug with other drugs or infusion equipment. Streptozocin may be given with extravasation precautions as a weekly regimen or as an intermittent 5-day regimen. The first involves a weekly intravenous dosage of 1 g/m² given over 30 to 60 minutes for two doses, with possible escalation to 1.5 g/m²/wk for another two doses if there is no response.[1, 3] The consecutive-day regimen calls for 500 mg/m² by intravenous bolus daily for 5 days, with repeat courses every 6 weeks until optimal benefit is achieved.

## REFERENCES

1. Iwasaki M, Ueno M, Ninomiya K, et al. Alkyl streptozotocin analogues with improved biological activities. J Med Chem 1976;19:918–23.
2. Pegg AE. Mammalian O6-alkylguanine-DNA alkyltransferase: regulation and importance in response to alkylating carcinogenic and therapeutic agents. Cancer Res 1990;50:6119–29.
3. Broder LE, Carter SK. Pancreatic islet cell carcinoma. II: Results of therapy with streptozotocin in 52 patients. Ann Intern Med 1973;79:108–18.
4. Murata M, Takahashi A, Saito I, Kawanishi S. Site-specific DNA methylation and apoptosis: induction by diabetogenic streptozotocin. Biochem Pharmacol 1999;57:881–7.
5. Saini KS, Thompson C, Winterford CM, et al. Streptozotocin at low doses induces apoptosis and at high doses causes necrosis in a murine pancreatic beta cell line, INS-1. Biochem Mol Biol Int 1996;39:1229–36.
6. Eizirik DL, Sandler S, Ahnstrom G, Welsh M. Exposure of pancreatic islets to different alkylating agents decreases mitochondrial DNA content but only streptozotocin induced long-lasting functional impairment of B-cells. Biochem Pharmacol 1991;42:2275–82.
7. Bobola MS, Tseng SH, Blank A, et al. Role of O6-methylguanine-DNA methyltransferase in resistance of human brain tumor cell lines to the clinically relevant methylating agents temozolomide and streptozotocin. Clin Cancer Res 1996;2:735–41.
8. Burkart V, Brenner HH, Hartmann B, Kolb H. Metabolic activation of islet cells improves resistance against oxygen radicals or streptozocin, but not nitric oxide. J Clin Endocrinol Metab 1996;81:3966–71.
9. Chang P, Riggs CE Jr, Scheerer MT, et al. Combination chemotherapy with Adriamycin and streptozotocin. II: Clinicopharmacologic correlation of augmented Adriamycin toxicity caused by streptozotocin. Clin Pharmacol Ther 1976;20:611–6.
10. Perry DJ, Weiss RB. Nephrotoxicity of streptozocin. Ann Intern Med 1982;96:122.
11. Shah KA, Greenwald E, Levin J, et al. Streptozocin-induced eosinophilia and fever: a case report. Cancer Treat Rep 1982;66:1449–51.
12. Garnick MB, Ernst T, Martinez F. Acute febrile reaction to streptozocin. N Engl J Med 1984;311:798.
13. Mauer SM, Lee CS, Najarian JS, Brown DM. Induction of malignant kidney tumors in rats with streptozotocin. Cancer Res 1974;34:158–60.

# Tamoxifen

Tamoxifen was synthesized in 1966 by Harper and Walpole in Great Britain as an antifertility drug.[1] However, its antiestrogenic properties led to its evaluation in the treatment of breast cancer in 1970, and it is now widely used for the treatment of this disease. It is also known as Nolvadex, tamoxifen citrate, TAM, Tam, and NSC-180973.

## EFFICACY

Tamoxifen is FDA approved for the treatment of breast cancer in the following settings: (1) as adjuvant therapy for women with negative axillary lymph nodes; (2) as adjuvant therapy for postmenopausal women with positive axillary lymph nodes; and (3) as treatment of advanced disease in both men and women, especially for tumors that are positive for estrogen receptors (see Chapter 35, Adjuvant Treatment, for further discussion). It is also FDA approved for "reduction of the risk of breast cancer" in high-risk women without breast cancer (see Chapter 35, Natural History and Pretreatment Assessment, for discussion).[2–5]

In addition to its anticancer effects, tamoxifen appears to have beneficial effects on cardiovascular risk factors[6–9] and bone density in postmenopausal women.[10–13] In the meta-analysis of tamoxifen in the adjuvant treatment of breast cancer, the drug was associated with a 25% reduction in deaths due to cardiovascular disease.[14] The effects on bone and cardiovascular risk factors appear to be limited to the period when tamoxifen is actually taken.[15]

Tamoxifen has been reported to benefit patients with psoriasis,[16] malignant melanoma,[17] and brain tumors.[18] It is being studied as a potential agent to reverse pleiotropic drug resistance.[19] Further study of these potential indications is needed before tamoxifen can be recommended for patients with these conditions.

## PHARMACOLOGY

**Mechanism of Action.** The precise mechanism of action for tamoxifen is uncertain, although many biologic effects have been documented with its use.[20] Tamoxifen appears to be a weakly estrogenic compound that is capable of tight competitive binding to cytoplasmic estrogen receptors. The antiestrogen-receptor complex itself appears to suppress the genome of the breast cancer cell,[21] and this receptor binding probably represents the first step in the complex sequence of events that inhibits tumors.[22] There may also be substantial binding to other intracellular structures (type II sites) that are not classic high-affinity estrogen receptors.[23] Receptor binding ultimately leads to endocrine and nonendocrine effects within the cell. Some of these are summarized here briefly.

**Endocrine Effects.** Endocrinologic effects of tamoxifen differ in premenopausal and postmenopausal women. In postmenopausal women, serum estrogen levels remain low and the normally elevated gonadotropin levels decrease with tamoxifen therapy. Nevertheless, tamoxifen causes mild estrogenic effects in postmenopausal patients, such as uterine bleeding and vaginal cornification. In many premenopausal women, however, serum estrogen levels are strikingly elevated and gonadotropin levels are either unchanged or slightly increased.[24]

**Nonendocrine Effects.** Tamoxifen has been associated with numerous biochemical changes, at least some of which appear to be independent of binding to estrogen receptors. At present, these observed changes do not provide a complete pathophysiologic explanation of tamoxifen's mechanism of action. They are listed here as an introduction to the complexity of the topic. Tamoxifen and its metabolites interact specifically with protein kinase C, a key enzyme in cellular growth regulation.[25, 26] Tamoxifen appears to be a calcium channel antagonist,[27] and it may bind to other receptor complexes, such as those for muscarinic cholinergic drugs.[28] There have been a variety of effects on transforming growth factor-$\alpha$ and -$\beta$ (TGF-$\alpha$ and TGF-$\beta$) that inhibit the growth of breast cancer cells in vitro. Specifically, tamoxifen downregulates secretion of TGF-$\alpha$, an epidermal cell growth stimulator,[29, 30] and increases secretion of TGF-$\beta$, an inhibitor of breast cancer cell growth.[31] The drug seems to stimulate human natural killer cells[32, 33] and modulate human mononuclear cells.[34] Tamoxifen can be activated by microsomal liver enzymes to form DNA adducts.[35] The active metabolite of tamoxifen, hydroxytamoxifen, can directly induce structural changes in membranes,[36] and tamoxifen itself can act as an antioxidant to protect membranes, such as cardiac microsomes.[37] Tamoxifen can inhibit angiogenesis,[38] upregulate estrogen receptors,[39] and stimulate the expression of some oncogenes (c-*fos*).[40] Finally, the growth of some estrogen receptor–negative cells can be markedly inhibited by tamoxifen by unknown mechanisms.[41]

**Resistance.** Resistance is multifactorial and may differ between individual patients and cell types. About half of the cases of tamoxifen resistance relate to a lack of estrogen receptor within the resistant cell.[42] Additional mechanisms of resistance could include alterations in estrogen receptor structure and function, alterations in postreceptor interactions, changes in paracrine interactions, and pharmacologic alterations.[43] Many of these mechanisms have been demonstrated, at least in some patients, but others have not.[44] For example, rare cases of resistance have been related to structural mutations in estrogen receptor.[45] Other studies have shown a change in receptor function, such that the receptor

interprets tamoxifen as an estrogen while a pure antiestrogen continues to be suppressive.[46] In one study, this transformation occurred after 2 to 5 years of tamoxifen therapy, which was interpreted as a potential explanation for the time-limited value of adjuvant tamoxifen in women with breast cancer.[47] Another mechanism involves the development of altered patterns of tamoxifen metabolism, leading to metabolites that act as estrogens rather than as antiestrogens.[48] Finally, one study associated acquired resistance to tamoxifen with reduced intratumoral accumulation of the drug in resistant cells.[49] This acquired resistance is common and has an interesting correlate. It appears to be associated with an increased frequency of P-glycoprotein expression in tamoxifen-resistant cell lines.[50] This may be an important factor in resistance to chemotherapy after tamoxifen therapy in patients with advanced disease.

**Pharmacokinetics.** Tamoxifen is readily absorbed after oral administration. The drug undergoes extensive hepatic metabolism with multiple metabolic products, the most important of which appears to be *N*-desmethyltamoxifen. The pattern of metabolism may be important in the development of drug resistance, as previously stated. The distribution of tamoxifen and its metabolites in the body is incompletely defined, but limited data suggest that high levels are present in bile and endometrial tissues. The drug does not appear to cross the blood-brain barrier in appreciable amounts,[51] but it can cause neurotoxicity. Tamoxifen has a long biologic half-life, presumably because of the high level of plasma protein binding and enterohepatic recirculation. The distribution half-life of tamoxifen is about 7 to 14 hours, and its elimination half-life is greater than 7 days. The predominant route of excretion appears to be the feces, mainly as various conjugates, with only a small amount of excretion in urine.

**Drug Interactions.** Tamoxifen increases the anticoagulant effect of warfarin. Great care should be exercised when the two drugs are administered together.[52] Patients receiving concurrent tamoxifen and bromocriptine have increased serum levels of tamoxifen and *N*-desmethyltamoxifen. Tamoxifen inhibits P-glycoprotein and is being studied for possible clinical use for this purpose.[53–55] It may also inhibit drug resistance to cisplatin, but the mechanism of this interaction is uncertain.[56] The antineoplastic effects of tamoxifen appear to be enhanced by somatostatin analogues, such as octreotide.[57]

**Interference with Laboratory Tests**

*Thyroid Function Tests.* Increased thyroglobulin levels can result in apparently elevated serum thyroxine levels without evidence of clinical hyperthyroidism.

*Estrogen Receptor Measurements.* False-negative estrogen receptor measurements can occur if tests are performed during or shortly after tamoxifen use. It is recommended that these determinations be delayed until 4 to 6 weeks after discontinuing tamoxifen.

## TOXICITY

**Overview.** The majority of patients have no adverse effects from tamoxifen. The most common side effects are hot flashes, nausea, and vomiting, which occur in up to 25% of patients. These are rarely severe enough to require cessation of therapy. The most serious toxicity is delayed second neoplasms, especially endometrial carcinoma. The increasing use of tamoxifen for prolonged periods in the adjuvant setting is a relatively recent development. A full appreciation of the possible long-term consequences of tamoxifen use requires more time.

**Hematologic.** Temporary thrombocytopenia and leukopenia occur occasionally (<20%), but these are self-limited and generally minor in severity. Anemia is only rarely a problem. Venous thrombosis may occur,[58] and one study found that long-term tamoxifen use (>2 years) tended to reduce levels of both antithrombin III and protein C.[59] A randomized study of tamoxifen versus a placebo in normal women, however, found no increase in the incidence of thromboembolic events on tamoxifen.[60] Hemorrhagic episodes have been reported as very rare events. A single case of fatal hepatocellular damage and agranulocytosis has been reported.[61]

**Digestive System.** About 10% of patients have nausea, which may be severe and associated with vomiting and the need to discontinue treatment. Rare effects include anorexia, a distaste for food, diarrhea, constipation, abdominal cramps, and very rarely the development of benign liver cysts.[62] Abnormal hepatic enzyme changes can occur, and, more rarely, severe hepatic abnormalities have developed, including fatty changes, cholestasis, hepatitis, hepatic necrosis, and death.

**Endocrine-Metabolic.** Hot flashes occur in about 25% of patients. Weight gain is common, even when the drug is accompanied by dietary intervention.[63] Clonidine by patch delivery system is sometimes helpful for hot flashes, but the benefit is modest at best.[64] An increase in bone pain or hypercalcemia, or both, can occur in patients with breast cancer metastatic to bone.[65, 66] In one series, these occurred in 2.3% of cases, with a median time of onset of 7 days (range 4 to 11 days).[66] This flare reaction is rarely fatal, and it does not necessarily preclude subsequent successful treatment with tamoxifen. Indeed, many of these patients will later enjoy an excellent response to tamoxifen treatment. Treatment for the tamoxifen flare reaction includes supportive care, temporary interruption of tamoxifen administration, and subsequent reinstitution of tamoxifen starting at a lower dose. The physiologic basis of this reaction is uncertain, although tamoxifen can stimulate the release of bone-resorbing activity by cultured human breast cancer cells.[67] Very rarely, tamoxifen has been associated with the tumor lysis syndrome after a tamoxifen flare.[68] Tamoxifen raises the serum level of thyroxine-binding globulin, but this is not associated with physiologically important changes in thyroid function.[69] Preliminary studies suggest that long-term use of tamoxifen can provide some protection against postmenopausal loss of bone minerals, so it may help prevent osteoporosis (see Efficacy). Limited studies suggest that tamoxifen acts as an estrogen agonist on the liver, resulting in a salutary effect on the composition of blood lipids (see Efficacy), including a reduction of total cholesterol and low-density lipoprotein cholesterol.[70, 71] However, an improved lipid profile has not been established with certainty because at least one patient developed severe lipemia from tamoxifen use.[72]

**Carcinogenicity.** Tamoxifen is a potent carcinogen in rats, causing hepatocellular carcinomas at all dose levels.[73] This is probably because of the formation of carcinogenic tamoxifen DNA adducts in rat liver.[74] Tamoxifen adducts are not formed in human liver, and hepatocellular carcinoma is not a risk of tamoxifen therapy. Thus, the carcinogenic potential of tamoxifen is considered highly species specific.

In women, endometrial hyperplasia, polyps, endometrial cancer, and very rare ovarian neoplasms have been reported during the use of tamoxifen. Seven cases of müllerian adenosarcomas of the uterus have been reported.[75] Two case-control studies in Europe strongly support an association between tamoxifen and endometrial cancer.[76, 77] In addition, two prospectively randomized trials demonstrate an increased risk of endometrial cancer. The first of these is a large Swedish randomized study summarized in the package insert for tamoxifen. In this study, tamoxifen was given for 2 to 5 years at 40 mg/day. Twenty-three of 1372 patients randomized to receive tamoxifen versus 4 of 1357 patients randomized to observation alone developed uterine cancers (relative risk 5.6, $p < 0.001$). The second prospective randomized trial is NSABP trial B-14, which involved patients with node-negative, estrogen receptor–positive, invasive breast cancer.[78] This study included 2843 patients assigned to placebo or tamoxifen and 1220 tamoxifen-treated patients who were registered but not randomized. After 8 years of follow-up for the randomized patients, the annual hazard rate for endometrial cancer was 0.2 per 1000 in the placebo group and 1.6 per 1000 in the tamoxifen-treated group. This represents a 7.5-fold increase in the relative risk of developing endometrial cancer by taking tamoxifen. Most of these uterine carcinomas were diagnosed at an early stage, but aggressive disease was not uncommon and four of the patients died of endometrial cancer. It is fair to conclude that tamoxifen is capable of inducing endometrial cancer in a small proportion of women. A reasonable estimate of this risk for 5 years of treatment is 1.3 cases per 1000 women treated per year (for a total of 6.3 cases per 1000 women treated).[79]

The manufacturer recommends immediate reporting of any abnormal vaginal bleeding and routine gynecologic care for all women receiving tamoxifen. Specifically, an annual pelvic examination is indicated for patients receiving tamoxifen therapy. There is evidence that transvaginal ultrasonography is useful in diagnosing endometrial cancer, but there is no evidence that ultrasonography should be part of the routine follow-up or pretreatment screening of these patients. Ultrasound examination yields a high frequency of false-positive findings, and results are difficult to interpret.[80, 81] The National Cancer Institute has been working with the American College of Obstetricians and Gynecologists and the Society of Gynecologic Oncologists to develop consensus recommendations for management of this problem.[82]

**Other and Rare Reactions**

*Ocular.* Dose-related, reversible ocular toxicity is occasionally seen. With standard doses, the incidence of retinopathy or keratopathy, or both, was 6.3% in one prospective study of 63 patients[83] and 0.9% in another study of 274 patients.[84] Ocular findings consist of crystalline retinal deposits, macular edema, and corneal changes.[85] Extensive retinal lesions and macular edema with visual impairment are rare and are primarily reported in patients receiving high-dose tamoxifen. Less extensive retinal changes may be seen after long-term low-dose therapy, and isolated retinal crystals without visual symptoms may occur. After tamoxifen withdrawal, almost all ocular abnormalities resolve, with the exception of retinal opacities. Special screening for ocular toxicity is probably not warranted, given its low incidence and favorable prognosis.

*Immunologic.* Hypersensitivity reactions are extremely rare.

*Mucocutaneous.* Skin rash, erythema, and mild hair loss can occur; radiation-recall reactions are very rare.[86]

*Cardiovascular.* The following reactions can occur: occasional peripheral edema, very rare purpuric vasculitis,[87] occasional thrombophlebitis, and an improved lipid profile for cardiovascular disease (see Efficacy).

*Pulmonary.* Pulmonary emboli are very rare; one case of tamoxifen-induced asthma has been reported.[88]

*Neurologic.* Rarely, depression, dizziness, lightheadedness, headache, confusion, fatigue, lassitude, and other forms of reversible CNS dysfunction occur.[89] One patient developed an organic delusional syndrome that resolved within 2 to 4 weeks of discontinuing therapy.[90] Neurotoxicity is more common and can be dose limiting with investigational megadose therapy (400 mg/m$^2$ followed by 150 mg/m$^2$ twice daily).

*Musculoskeletal.* A case of dermatomyositis has been reported.[91] Occasional leg cramps are possible. Bone pain can occur (see Endocrine section). A possible effect is suppression of postmenopausal osteoporotic changes (see Efficacy).

*Genitourinary.* Vaginal bleeding, vaginal discharge, menstrual irregularities, pruritus vulvae, endometriosis, and, rarely, the development of uterine carcinomas (see Carcinogenicity) can occur. Priapism occurred in one patient; ovarian cysts are rare.

*Reproductive.* The drug is teratogenic in animals and genotoxic in rats.[92] The package insert states that the drug is FDA pregnancy category D, but it also states that pregnancy is contraindicated during tamoxifen therapy. In women, dyspareunia and decreased orgasm can occur with intercourse.[93] In men, decreased libido (29%) and impotence can occur, leading to a high attrition rate in men (21%).[94]

## DOSAGE AND ADMINISTRATION

Tamoxifen is available as 10-mg and 20-mg tablets. It has been given in varying dosages of 10 to 80 mg/day in divided doses, but the usual dose is 20 mg daily. Because the bioavailability of tamoxifen is equivalent for once-daily and twice-daily administration,[95] we prefer the once-daily schedule.

The manufacturer recommends that tamoxifen be used with caution in patients with leukopenia and thrombocytopenia, and periodic blood counts are advised. Patients with pre-existing hyperlipoproteinemia should have periodic monitoring of serum triglyceride and cholesterol levels. Women should be advised to report any vaginal bleeding, and it should be investigated promptly. The National Cancer Institute has advised that all women taking tamoxifen as part of a sponsored clinical trial should sign a consent form acknowledging awareness of the risk of potentially lethal uterine cancer and that they should have an annual pelvic examination during therapy. Some authorities also advise periodic uterine ultrasound evaluations for cancer screening. Tamoxifen is contraindicated in patients with known hypersensitivity to the drug.

## REFERENCES

1. Harper MJK, Walpole AL. Contrasting endocrine activities of *cis* and *trans* isomers in a series of substituted triphenylethylenes. Nature 1966;212:87.
2. Fisher B, Costantino JP, Wickerham DL, et al. Tamoxifen for prevention of breast cancer: report of the National Surgical Adjuvant Breast and Bowel Project P-1 Study. J Natl Cancer Inst 1998;90:1371–88.
3. Fisher B. National Surgical Adjuvant Breast and Bowel Project breast cancer prevention trial: a reflective commentary. J Clin Oncol 1999;17:1632–9.
4. Chlebowski RT, Collyar DE, Somerfield MR, Pfister DG. American Society of Clinical Oncology technology assessment on breast cancer risk reduction strategies: tamoxifen and raloxifene. J Clin Oncol 1999;17:1939–55.
5. Day R, Ganz PA, Costantino JP, et al: Health-related quality of life and tamoxifen in breast cancer prevention: a report from the National Surgical Adjuvant Breast and Bowel Project P-1 Study. J Clin Oncol 1999;17:2659–69.
6. Love RR, Wiebe DA, Newcomb PA, et al. Effects of tamoxifen on cardiovascular risk factors in postmenopausal women. Ann Intern Med 1991;115:860–4.
7. Rutqvist LE, Mattsson A. Cardiac and thromboembolic morbidity among postmenopausal women with early-stage breast cancer in a randomized trial of adjuvant tamoxifen: the Stockholm Breast Cancer Study Group. J Natl Cancer Inst 1993;85:1398–406.
8. Thangaraju M, Kumar K, Gandhirajan R, Sachdanandam P. Effect of tamoxifen on plasma lipids and lipoproteins in postmenopausal women with breast cancer. Cancer 1994;73:659–63.
9. Dziewulska-Bokiniec A, Wojtacki J, Skokowski J, Kortas B. The effect of tamoxifen treatment on serum cholesterol fractions in breast cancer women. Neoplasma 1994;41:13–6.
10. Fentiman IS, Saad Z, Caleffi M, et al. Tamoxifen protects against steroid-induced bone loss. Eur J Cancer 1992;28:684–5.
11. Love RR, Mazess RB, Barden HS, et al. Effects of tamoxifen on bone mineral density in postmenopausal women with breast cancer. N Engl J Med 1992;326:852–6.
12. Ward RL, Morgan G, Dalley D, Kelly PJ. Tamoxifen reduces bone turnover and prevents lumbar spine and proximal femoral bone loss in early postmenopausal women. Bone Miner 1993;22:87–94.
13. Kristensen B, Ejlertsen B, Dalgaard P, et al. Tamoxifen and bone metabolism in postmenopausal low-risk breast cancer patients: a randomized study. J Clin Oncol 1994;12:992–7.
14. Early Breast Cancer Trialists' Collaborative Group. Systemic treatment of early breast cancer by hormonal, cytotoxic, or immune therapy: 133 randomised trials involving 31,000 recurrences and 24,000 deaths among 75,000 women. Lancet 1992;339:71–85.
15. Cuzick J, Allen D, Baum M, et al. Long term effects of tamoxifen: biological effects of Tamoxifen Working Party. Eur J Cancer 1992;29A:15–21.
16. Boyd AS, King LE Jr. Tamoxifen-induced remission of psoriasis. J Am Acad Dermatol 1999;41:5 Part 2:887–9.
17. Rusthoven JJ. The evidence for tamoxifen and chemotherapy as treatment for metastatic melanoma. Eur J Cancer 1998;34:Suppl 3:S31–6.
18. Mastronardi L, Puzzilli F, Ruggeri A. Tamoxifen as a potential treatment of glioma. Anticancer Drugs 1998;9:581–6.
19. Leonessa F, Jacobson M, Boyle B, et al. Effect of tamoxifen on the multidrug-resistant phenotype in human breast cancer cells: isobologram, drug accumulation, and Mdr) 170,000 glycoprotein (gp 170) binding studies. Cancer Res 1994;54:441–7.
20. Wakeling AE, Bowler J. Biology and mode of action of pure antioestrogens. J Steroid Biochem 1988;30:141–7.
21. Coezy E, Borgna JL, Rochefort H. Tamoxifen and metabolites in MCF7 cells: correlation between binding to estrogen receptor and inhibition of cell growth. Cancer Res 1982;42:317–23.
22. Borgna JL. The elucidation of the antiestrogen and antitumoral mechanisms of tamoxifen. Bull Cancer 1994;81:29–37.
23. Leo G, Cappiello G, Poltronieri P, et al. Tamoxifen binding sites heterogeneity in breast cancer: a comparative study with steroid hormone receptors. Eur J Cancer 1991;27:452–6.
24. Sunderland MC, Osborne CK. Tamoxifen in premenopausal patients with metastatic breast cancer: a review. J Clin Oncol 1991;9:1283–97.
25. O'Brian CA, Ward NE, Anderson BW. Role of specific interactions between protein kinase C and triphenylethylenes in inhibition of the enzyme. J Natl Cancer Inst 1988;80:1628–33.

26. Fujimoto N, Katzenellenbogen BS. Alteration in the agonist/antagonist balance of antiestrogens by activation of protein kinase A signaling pathways in breast cancer cells: antiestrogen selectivity and promoter dependence. Mol Endocrinol 1994;8:296–304.

27. Greenberg DA, Carpenter CL, Messing RO. Calcium channel antagonist properties of the antineoplastic antiestrogen tamoxifen in the PC12 neurosecretory cell line. Cancer Res 1987;47:70–4.

28. Batra S. Interaction of antiestrogens with binding sites for muscarinic cholinergic drugs and calcium channel blockers in cell membranes. Cancer Chemother Pharmacol 1990;26:310–2.

29. Koga M, Sutherland RL. Epidermal growth factor partially reverses the inhibitory effects of antiestrogens on T 47D human breast cancer cell growth. Biochem Biophys Res Commun 1987;146:739–45.

30. Noguchi S, Motomura K, Inaji H, et al. Down-regulation of transforming growth factor-alpha by tamoxifen in human breast cancer, Cancer 1993;72:131–6.

31. Knabbe C, Zugmaier G, Schmahl M, et al. Induction of transforming growth factor beta by the antiestrogens droloxifene, tamoxifen, and toremifene in MCF-7 cells. Am J Clin Oncol 1991;14:Suppl 2:S15–20.

32. Mandeville R, Ghali SS, Chausseau JP. In vitro stimulation of human NK activity by an estrogen antagonist (tamoxifen). Eur J Cancer Clin Oncol 1984;20:983–5.

33. Robinson E, Rubin D, Mekori T, et al. In vivo modulation of natural killer cell activity by tamoxifen in patients with bilateral primary breast cancer. Cancer Immunol Immunother 1993;37:209–12.

34. Teodorczyk-Injeyan J, Cembrzynska-Nowak M, Lalani S, Kellen JA. Modulation of biological responses of normal human mononuclear cells by antiestrogens. Anticancer Res 1993;13:279–83.

35. Pathak DN, Bodell WJ. DNA adduct formation by tamoxifen with rat and human liver microsomal activation systems. Carcinogenesis 1994;15:529–32.

36. Custodio JBA, Almeida LM, Madeira VM. The active metabolite hydroxytamoxifen of the anticancer drug tamoxifen induces structural changes in membranes. Biochim Biophys Acta 1993;1153:308–14.

37. Wiseman H, Cannon M, Arnstein HR, Halliwell B. Tamoxifen inhibits lipid peroxidation in cardiac microsomes: comparison with liver microsomes and potential relevance to the cardiovascular benefits associated with cancer prevention and treatment by tamoxifen. Biochem Pharmacol 1993;45:1851–5.

38. Gagliardi A, Collins DC. Inhibition of angiogenesis by antiestrogens. Cancer Res 1993;53:533–5.

39. Noguchi S, Motomura K, Inaji H, et al. Up-regulation of estrogen receptor by tamoxifen in human breast cancer. Cancer 1993;71:1266–72.

40. Kirkland JL, Murthy L, Stancel GM. Tamoxifen stimulates expression of the c-*fos* proto-oncogene in rodent uterus. Mol Pharmacol 1993;43:709–14.

41. Croxtall JD, Emmas C, White JO, et al. Tamoxifen inhibits growth of oestrogen receptor-negative A549 cells. Biochem Pharmacol 1994;47:197–202.

42. Johnston SRD, Dowsett M, Smith IE. Towards a molecular basis for tamoxifen resistance in breast cancer. Ann Oncol 1992;3:503–11.

43. Katzenellenbogen BS. Antiestrogen resistance: mechanisms by which breast cancer cells undermine the effectiveness of endocrine therapy. J Natl Cancer Inst 1991;83:1434–5.

44. Johnston SR. Acquired tamoxifen resistance in human breast cancer—potential mechanisms and clinical implications. Anticancer Drugs 1997;8:911–30.

45. Karnik PS, Kulkarni S, Liu XP, et al. Estrogen receptor mutations in tamoxifen-resistant breast cancer. Cancer Res 1994;54:349–53.

46. Wakeling AE. Are breast tumors resistant to tamoxifen also resistant to pure antiestrogens? J Steroid Biochem Mol Biol 1993;47:107–14.

47. Norris JD, Paige LA, Christensen DJ, et al. Peptide antagonists of the human estrogen receptor. Science 1999;285:744–6.

48. Osborne CK. Mechanisms for tamoxifen resistance in breast cancer: possible role of tamoxifen metabolism. J Steroid Biochem Mol Biol 1993;47:83–9.

49. Johnston SRD, Haynes BP, Smith IE. Acquired tamoxifen resistance in human breast cancer and reduced intra-tumoral drug concentration. Lancet 1993;342:1521–2.

50. Keen JC, Miller EP, Bellamy C, et al. P-glycoprotein and resistance to tamoxifen. Lancet 1994;343:1047–8.

51. Noguchi S, Miyauchi K, Imaoka S, Koyama H. Inability of tamoxifen to penetrate into cerebrospinal fluid. Breast Cancer Res Treat 1988;12:317–8.

52. Tenni P, Lalich DL, Byrne MJ. Life threatening interaction between tamoxifen and warfarin. Br Med J 1989;298:93.

53. Kirk J, Houlbrook S, Stuart NS, et al. Selective reversal of vinblastine resistance to multidrug-resistant cell lines by tamoxifen, toremifene and their metabolites. Eur J Cancer 1993;29A:1152–7.

54. Millward MJ, Lien EA, Robinson A, Cantwell BM. High-dose (480 mg/day) tamoxifen with etoposide: a study of a potential multi-drug resistance modulator. Oncology 1994;51:79–83.

55. Trump DL, Smith DC, Ellis PG, et al. High-dose oral tamoxifen, a potential multidrug-resistance-reversal agent: phase I trial in combination with vinblastine. J Natl Cancer Inst 1992;84:1811–6.

56. McClay EF, Albright KD, Jones JA, et al. Tamoxifen modulation of cisplatin cytotoxicity in human malignancies. Int J Cancer 1993;55:1018–22.

57. Pollak M. Enhancement of the anti-neoplastic effects of tamoxifen by somatostatin analogues. Digestion 1996;57:Suppl 1:29–33.

58. Auger MJ, Mackie MJ. Effects of tamoxifen on blood coagulation. Cancer 1988;61:1316–9.

59. Pemberton KD, Melissari E, Kakkar VV. The influence of tamoxifen in vivo on the main natural anticoagulants and fibrinolysis. Blood Coagul Fibrinolysis 1993;4:935–42.

60. Jones AL, Powles TJ, Treleaven JG, et al. Haemostatic changes and thromboembolic risk during tamoxifen therapy in normal women. Br J Cancer 1992;66:744–7.

61. Ching CK, Smith PG, Long RG. Tamoxifen-associated hepatocellular damage and agranulocytosis. Lancet 1992;339:940.

62. Nand S, Gordon LI, Brestan E, et al. Benign hepatic cyst in a patient on antiestrogen therapy for metastatic breast cancer. Cancer 1982;50:1882–3.

63. Rose DP, Connolly JM, Chlebowski RT, et al. The effects of low-fat dietary intervention and tamoxifen adjuvant therapy on the serum estrogen and sex hormone–binding globulin concentrations of postmenopausal breast cancer patients. Breast Cancer Res Treat 1993;27:253–62.

64. Goldberg RM, Loprinzi CL, O'Fallon JR, et al. Transdermal clonidine for ameliorating tamoxifen-induced hot flashes. J Clin Oncol 1994;12:155–8.

65. O'Connell TX. Hypercalcemia induced by tamoxifen. Am J Surg 1981;141:277–8.

66. Legha SS, Powell K, Buzdar AU, Blumenschein GR. Tamoxifen-induced hypercalcemia in breast cancer. Cancer 1981;47:2803–6.

67. Valentin-Opran A, Eilon G, Saez S, Mundy GR. Estrogens and antiestrogens stimulate release of bone resorbing activity by cultured human breast cancer cells. J Clin Invest 1985;75:726–31.

68. Cech P, Block JB, Cone LA, Stone R. Tumor lysis syndrome after tamoxifen flare. N Engl J Med 1986;315:263–4.

69. Gordon D, Beastall GH, McArdle CS, Thomson JA. The effect of tamoxifen therapy on thyroid function tests. Cancer 1986;58:1422–5.

70. Bagdade JD, Wolter J, Subbaiah PV, Ryan WG. Effects of tamoxifen treatment on plasma lipids and lipoprotein lipid composition. J Clin Endocrinol Metab 1990;70:1132–5.

71. Bruning PF, Bonfrer JM, Hart AA, et al. Tamoxifen, serum lipoproteins and cardiovascular risk. Br J Cancer 1988;58:497–9.

72. Brun LD, Gagne C, Rousseau C, et al. Severe lipemia induced by tamoxifen. Cancer 1986;57:2123–6.

73. Williams GM, Iatropoulos MJ, Djordjevic MV, Kaltenberg OP. The triphenylethylene drug tamoxifen is a strong liver carcinogen in the rat. Carcinogenesis 1993;14:315–7.

74. Busch H. Adducts and tamoxifen. Semin Oncol 1997;24:1 Suppl 1:S1-98–104.

75. Clement PB, Oliva E, Young RH. Müllerian adenosarcoma of the uterine corpus associated with tamoxifen therapy: a report of six cases and a review of tamoxifen-associated endometrial lesions. Int J Gynecol Pathol 1996;15:222–9.

76. Fornander T, Hellstrom AC, Moberger B. Descriptive clinicopathologic study of 17 patients with endometrial cancer during or after adjuvant tamoxifen in early breast cancer. J Natl Cancer Inst 1993;85:1850–5.

77. van Leeuwen FE, Benraadt J, Coebergh JW, et al. Risk of endometrial cancer after tamoxifen treatment of breast cancer. Lancet 1994;343:448–52.

78. Fisher B, Costantino JP, Redmond CK, et al. Endometrial cancer in tamoxifen-treated breast cancer patients: findings from the National Surgical Adjuvant Breast and Bowel Project (NSABP) B-14. J Natl Cancer Inst 1994;86:527–37.

79. Loret de Mola JR. Endometrial changes with chronic tamoxifen use. Curr Opin Obstet Gynecol 1997;9:160–4.

80. Goldstein SR. Unusual ultrasonographic appearance of the uterus in patients receiving tamoxifen. Am J Obstet Gynecol 1994;170:447–51.
81. Hulka CA, Hall DA. Endometrial abnormalities associated with tamoxifen therapy for breast cancer: sonographic and pathologic correlation. Am J Roentgenol 1993;160:809–12.
82. Friedman MA, Trimble EL, Abrams JS. Tamoxifen: trials, tribulations, and trade-offs. J Natl Cancer Inst 1994;86:478–9.
83. Pavlidis NA, Petris C, Briassoulis E, et al. Clear evidence that long-term, low-dose tamoxifen treatment can induce ocular toxicity: a prospective study of 63 patients. Cancer 1992;69:2961–4.
84. Tang T, Shields J, Schiffman J, et al. Retinal changes associated with tamoxifen treatment for breast cancer. Eye 1997;11:Part 3:295–7.
85. Nayfield SG, Gorin MB. Tamoxifen-associated eye disease: a review. J Clin Oncol 1996;14:1018–26.
86. Parry BR. Radiation recall induced by tamoxifen. Lancet 1992;340:49.
87. Drago F, Arditi M, Rebora A. Tamoxifen and purpuric vasculitis. Ann Intern Med 1990;112:965–6.
88. Smith RP, Dewar JA, Winter JH. Tamoxifen-induced asthma. Lancet 1993;341:772.
89. Pluss JL, DiBella NJ. Reversible central nervous system dysfunction due to tamoxifen in a patient with breast cancer. Ann Intern Med 1984;101:652.
90. Ron IG, Inbar MJ, Barak Y, et al. Organic delusional syndrome associated with tamoxifen treatment. Cancer 1992;69:1415–17.
91. Harris AL, Smith IE, Snaith M. Tamoxifen-induced tumour regression associated with dermatomyositis. Br Med J 1982;284:1674–5.
92. White IN, de Matteis F, Davies A, et al. Genotoxic potential of tamoxifen and analogues in female Fischer F344/n rats, DBA/2 and C57BL/6 mice and in human MCL-5 cells. Carcinogenesis 1992;13:2197–203.
93. Mortimer JE, Boucher L, Baty J, et al. Effects of tamoxifen on sexual function in patients with breast cancer. J Clin Oncol 1999;17:1488–92.
94. Anelli TF, Anelli A, Tran K, et al. Tamoxifen administration is associated with a high rate of treatment-limiting symptoms in male breast cancer patients. Cancer 1994;74:74–7.
95. Buzdar AU, Hortobagyi GN, Frye D, et al. Bioequivalence of 20-mg once-daily tamoxifen relative to 10-mg twice-daily tamoxifen regimens for breast cancer. J Clin Oncol 1994;12:50–4.

# Teniposide

Teniposide is an epipodophyllotoxin derivative that is closely related to etoposide. It is also known as VM-26, Vumon, thenylidene-lignan-P, PTG, and NSC-122819.

## EFFICACY

The spectrum of efficacy for teniposide is very similar to that of etoposide, but its main use has been in children with ALL.

## PHARMACOLOGY

**Mechanism of Action.** Teniposide, like etoposide, causes dose-dependent DNA strand breakage, most likely as a result of the ability of the two drugs to stimulate the formation of a cleavable complex between DNA-topoisomerase II and DNA.[1, 2] Studies suggest that this cleavable complex may act as a replication fork barrier at a specific genomic site in the c-*myc* gene in mammalian cells.[3] This leads to irreversible DNA damage and cytotoxicity in proliferating cells, including the inhibition of cell cycle progression prior to mitosis during the late S or early $G_2$ phases. As a consequence, the efficacy of teniposide is highly dependent on the schedule of drug administration. Other effects of teniposide include the formation of free radicals and orthoquinone species via biologic oxidation of the drug and degradation of nuclear DNA.[4]

**Resistance** (see Etoposide).

**Pharmacokinetics.** Teniposide is administered intravenously in a solution that contains Cremophor EL as a solvent. The drug is extensively (99%) bound to plasma albumin, and there is extensive metabolic conversion to inactive metabolites in the liver.[1] Only about 10% of the drug is excreted unchanged in the urine. Plasma levels decline biexponentially, with a terminal half-life of 5 hours. The drug gains only limited access to the CSF in normal patients, but higher levels are achieved in patients with brain tumors.

The plasma levels achieved with various schedules and doses of teniposide, as well as the pharmacokinetics of the drug, differ widely among individuals. The pharmacokinetics of the drug may also be different in patients with newly diagnosed ALL compared with treated patients with recurrent ALL.[5] Using a prolonged intravenous infusion and monitoring of plasma drug levels, investigators noted a clear correlation between the mean clearance of drug, the steady-state concentration of teniposide in plasma, and antitumor response. In one study, 10 of 10 patients responded to teniposide when the mean plasma concentration was greater than 12 mg/L, whereas only 5 of 13 patients with values less than this level responded ($p<0.01$).[6] Because of these variations, individual dosage adjustments for toxicity are common.

Compared with etoposide, teniposide demonstrates much more protein binding, has greater cellular uptake, and has a longer half-life, and less of the drug is excreted in urine.

**Drug Interactions.** Anticonvulsant medications, such as phenobarbital, phenytoin, and carbamazepine, significantly increase the clearance of teniposide.[7] Sedative antiemetics in children may cause unexpected somnolence and hypotension. Tolbutamide, sodium salicylate, and sulfamethizole displace teniposide from sites of protein binding. These drugs could therefore increase the toxicity of teniposide if used together. MTX does not influence the pharmacokinetic profile of teniposide; however, teniposide slightly prolongs the clearance of MTX, and the level of intracellular MTX in vitro is increased by teniposide. The clinical significance of these interactions is uncertain.

## TOXICITY

**Overview.** Myelosuppression is dose limiting, but serious hypersensitivity reactions may also limit therapy. Rapid infusions of the drug must be avoided because they can cause acute life-threatening hypotension. The toxicity of teniposide may be especially severe in elderly patients and in those with a poor performance status.[8]

**Hematologic.** The drug is nearly always used with other drugs in the treatment of ALL. In this setting, virtually all patients develop myelosuppression by 10 to 14 days, and recovery may be protracted. Neutropenia predominates, but severe anemia and thrombocytopenia should also be expected.

**Immunologic.** Anaphylaxis is rare, but other forms of hypersensitivity occur in 2 to 11% of patients, depending on the type of clinical trial.[9] These can include chills, fever, hypotension or hypertension, bronchospasm, tachycardia, facial flushing, urticaria, diaphoresis, fever, and periorbital edema. The cause of this reaction is uncertain, but it may be related to the Cremophor EL (polyoxyethylated castor oil) component of the vehicle or teniposide itself. Hypersensitivity reactions appear to be especially common among patients with brain tumors and neuroblastoma. There is no cross-sensitivity between etoposide and teniposide.

**Digestive System.** Nausea and vomiting (29%) and diarrhea (33%) are common but tend to be mild and easily managed. Anorexia is an infrequent effect. Rarely, mild hepatic damage occurs (increased levels of bilirubin and transaminase enzymes in <1% of patients).

**Mucocutaneous.** Alopecia (9%) is uncommon but can progress to total baldness. Stomatitis is common (76%) but it is usually mild to moderate in severity and easily managed. Phlebitis at sites of intravenous injection can occur, but severe extravasation injury is unlikely. At high doses, teniposide can cause a severe skin rash (3%).

**Other and Rare Reactions.** Fever occurs in 3% of patients; occlusion of vascular access devices from precipitated drug during prolonged infusions is rare.

*Pulmonary.* Bronchospasm and dyspnea with hypersensitivity reactions can occur; a single case of fulminant pulmonary hyaline membrane disease has been reported.[10]

*Neurologic.* Fatigue, peripheral neuropathy (paresthesia), and seizures can rarely occur (<1%). At high doses and with various antiemetic regimens, acute CNS depression with somnolence and hypotension have been observed, probably in part because of increased blood alcohol levels from the teniposide preparation and interactions with depressive antiemetic drugs.[11]

*Cardiovascular.* Hypotension can occur with rapid infusions and as part of hypersensitivity reactions. No other cardiovascular or electrocardiographic problems have been noted.

*Genitourinary.* Mild renal dysfunction can occur (elevated blood urea nitrogen and serum creatinine levels in rare patients).

*Reproductive.* Teniposide is classified as FDA pregnancy category D.

*Carcinogenicity.* Teniposide is mutagenic and carcinogenic. AML has been reported to occur after its use.

## DOSAGE AND ADMINISTRATION

Teniposide is provided in 50-mg vials. It is more stable in glass containers than plastic containers, but it can be stored in plastic containers for up to 8 hours if the diluent is normal saline. It is administered by slow intravenous infusion using extravasation precautions over a period of at least 30 to 60 minutes. The patient must be observed closely for hypotension and other signs of hypersensitivity during the infusion and for at least an additional hour after the infusion is completed. If hypersensitivity occurs, it should be treated vigorously with antihistamines, corticosteroids, epinephrine, intravenous fluids, and other supportive measures, as clinically indicated.

A representative dose of teniposide for the induction of remission in combination with cytarabine in patients with ALL is 165 mg/m² twice weekly for eight or nine doses.

Teniposide is contraindicated in patients with a history of severe hypersensitivity to Cremophor EL or teniposide itself.

## REFERENCES

1. Cragg G, Suffness M. Metabolism of plant-derived anticancer agents. Pharmacol Ther 1988;37:425–61.
2. Grem JL, Hoth DF, Leyland-Jones B, et al. Teniposide in the treatment of leukemia: a case study of conflicting priorities in the development of drugs for fatal diseases. J Clin Oncol 1988;6:351–79.
3. Catapano CV, Carbone GM, Pisani F, et al. Arrest of replication fork progression at sites of topoisomerase II-mediated DNA cleavage in human leukemia CEM cells incubated with VM-26. Biochemistry 1997;36:5739–48.
4. Tepper CG, Studzinski GP. Teniposide induces nuclear but not mitochondrial DNA degradation. Cancer Res 1992;52:3384–90.
5. Evans WE, Rodman JH, Relling MV, et al. Differences in teniposide disposition and pharmacodynamics in patients with newly diagnosed and relapsed acute lymphocytic leukemia. J Pharmacol Exp Ther 1992;260:71–7.
6. Rodman JH, Abromowitch M, Sinkule JA, et al. Clinical pharmacodynamics of continuous infusion teniposide: systemic exposure as a determinant of response in a phase I trial. J Clin Oncol 1987;5:1007–14.
7. Baker DK, Relling MV, Pui CH, et al. Increased teniposide clearance with concomitant anticonvulsant therapy. J Clin Oncol 1992;10:311–5.
8. Cerny T, Pedrazzini A, Joss RA, Brunner KW. Unexpected high toxicity in a phase II study of teniposide (VM-26) in elderly patients with untreated small cell lung cancer (SCLC). Eur J Cancer Clin Oncol 1988;24:1791–4.
9. O'Dwyer PJ, King SA, Fortner CL, Leyland-Jones B. Hypersensitivity reactions to teniposide (VM-26): an analysis. J Clin Oncol 1986;4:1262–9.
10. Commers JR, Foley JF. Pulmonary hyaline membrane disease occurring in the course of VM-26 therapy. Cancer Treat Rep 1979;63:2093–5.
11. Mcleod HL, Baker DK Jr, Pui CH, Rodman JH. Somnolence, hypotension, and metabolic acidosis following high-dose teniposide treatment in children with leukemia. Cancer Chemother Pharmacol 1991;29:150–4.

# Thioguanine

6-TG is a purine antimetabolite developed by Hitchings and Elion in the early 1950s. It is also known as 6-thioguanine, Tabloid brand Thioguanine, aminopurine-6-thiol-hemihydrate, and NSC-752. The pharmacology of 6-TG is very similar to that of 6-MP, save for the role of xanthine oxidase in metabolism, but 6-MP is far more widely used than 6-TG.

## EFFICACY

6-TG is used solely for the treatment of leukemia, although it is only rarely included in contemporary regimens. 6-TG may be a reasonable alternative to 6-MP for patients who have ALL and low levels of the enzyme TPMT.[1] 6-TG and 6-MP are being directly compared for efficacy in childhood lymphoblastic leukemia in a European clinical trial.[2]

## PHARMACOLOGY

**Mechanism of Action.** Unlike 6-MP, 6-TG is not metabolized by TPMT. It is therefore not subject to the pharmacokinetic uncertainties that are so important with 6-MP therapy (see discussion of 6-MP). 6-TG does have to be activated to its ribonucleotide as a minimal requirement for cytotoxicity. The drug is then incorporated into DNA as a false purine base. This appears to be its major mechanism of action,[3] although an additional cytotoxic effect is related to its incorporation into RNA.[4] 6-TG is considered to be cell cycle S-phase specific, but data relevant to possible schedule dependence in humans are scant.

**Resistance.** Mechanisms of resistance are probably similar to those to 6-MP. There is evidence that 6-TG cytotoxicity may require an intact mismatch repair mechanism; cells that are deficient in mismatch repair of DNA are resistant to 6-TG.[5] The 6-thiopurines are not cross-resistant to other chemotherapeutic drugs used in clinical practice, but 6-MP and 6-TG are cross-resistant to each other.

**Pharmacokinetics.** The drug is erratically absorbed by mouth and reaches maximum plasma concentrations about 8 hours after drug administration. Extensive metabolism to several metabolites occurs in the liver, but this process is not dependent on xanthine oxidase. The incorporation of 6-TG into the DNA of bone marrow is usually very small after a single oral dose, but after five daily doses, the guanine of DNA is largely replaced by 6-TG. Urinary excretion of unchanged drug is negligible. The elimination half-life is about 11 hours.

An intravenous preparation is under investigation as continuous infusion therapy[6] and as bolus therapy.[7]

**Drug Interactions.** There is no drug interaction with allopurinol because 6-TG is not metabolized by xanthine oxidase. 6-TG has been associated with a high frequency of nodular regenerative hyperplasia of the liver with esophageal varices when given for prolonged periods with busulfan. 6-TG has been reported to increase the radiation sensitivity of two murine fibrosarcomas.[8] Its potential for clinical radiosensitization in humans is uncertain.

## TOXICITY

**Overview.** Myelosuppression is the most important toxicity and is dose limiting, but hepatotoxicity and gastrointestinal distress can also occur.

**Hematologic.** Myelosuppression is expected and dose limiting.

**Digestive System.** Nausea, vomiting, and anorexia may occur, but they tend to be mild and easily managed. Cholestatic jaundice may occur, but it is generally reversible. Rarely, hepatic veno-occlusive disease may occur.[9, 10] Diarrhea is common and can be severe. Very rarely, intestinal necrosis and perforation have been reported in patients receiving combination chemotherapy regimens that include 6-TG. Esophageal varices have been reported with thioguanine and busulfan (see Drug Interactions).

**Mucocutaneous.** Stomatitis, rash, and dermatitis can occur.

**Other and Rare Reactions**

*Immunologic.* Immunosuppression occurs, but it is generally not a clinical problem. Hypersensitivity reactions are extremely rare.

*Neurologic.* Peripheral neuropathy is rare.

*Genitourinary.* Uric acid nephropathy due to tumor lysis may occur.

*Reproductive.* Toxicity studies place 6-TG in FDA pregnancy category D.

*Endocrine-Metabolic.* Hyperuricemia due to the tumor lysis syndrome is very rare with preventive measures.

*Carcinogenicity.* 6-TG is mutagenic and should be considered potentially carcinogenic in humans until proved otherwise.

## DOSAGE AND ADMINISTRATION

6-TG is available as 40-mg tablets. When used alone, the dosage of 6-TG is 2 mg/kg/day; if no leukocyte depression is noted by 4 weeks, one may cautiously increase the dosage to 3 mg/kg/day. The drug should be discontinued immediately if any evidence of hepatitis or cholestasis is observed by clinical or laboratory examination.

## REFERENCES

 1. Lennard L, Lilleyman JS. Individualizing therapy with 6-mercaptopurine and 6-thioguanine related to the thiopurine methyltransferase genetic polymorphism. Ther Drug Monit 1996;13:328–34.
 2. Lancaster DL, Lennard L, Rowland K, et al. Thioguanine versus mercaptopurine for therapy of childhood lymphoblastic leukaemia: a comparison of haematological toxicity and drug metabolite concentrations. Br J Haematol 1998;102:439–43.
 3. Ling YH, Chan JY, Beattie KL, Nelson JA. Consequences of 6-thioguanine incorporation into DNA on polymerase, ligase, and endonuclease reactions. Mol Pharmacol 1992;42:802–7.
 4. Carrico CK, Sartorelli AC. Effects of 6-thioguanine on RNA biosynthesis in regenerating rat liver. Cancer Res 1977;37:1876–82.
 5. Glaab WE, Risinger JI, Umar A, et al. Resistance to 6-thioguanine in mismatch repair-deficient human cancer cell lines correlates with an increase in induced mutations at the HPRT locus. Carcinogenesis 1998;19:1931–7.
 6. Kitchen BJ, Balis FM, Poplack DG, et al. A pediatric phase I trial and pharmacokinetic study of thioguanine administered by continuous I.V. infusion. Clin Cancer Res 1997;3:713–7.
 7. Ingle JN, Twito DI, Suman VJ, et al. Evaluation of intravenous 6-thioguanine as first-line chemotherapy in women with metastatic breast cancer. Am J Clin Oncol 1997;20:69–72.
 8. Kim JH, Alfieri AA, Kim SH, Hong SS. Radiosensitization of two murine fibrosarcomas with 6-thioguanine. Int J Radiat Oncol Biol Phys 1990;18:583–6.
 9. Gill RA, Onstad GR, Cardamone JM, et al. Hepatic veno-occlusive disease caused by 6-thioguanine. Ann Intern Med 1982;96:58–60.
10. Krivoy N, Raz R, Carter A, Alroy G. Reversible hepatic veno-occlusive disease and 6-thioguanine. Ann Intern Med 1982;96:Part 1:788.

# Thiotepa

The initial chemical reaction that mechlorethamine undergoes before alkylation involves the formation of an ethylenimmonium ion. Compounds with this structure were therefore screened for antitumor activity, and several were found to be active. Thiotepa, a relatively stable sulfur-containing compound, has remained available since its clinical introduction in 1953. Other names for this drug include Thioplex, triethylenethiophosphoramide, TESPA, TSPA, and NSC-6396.

## EFFICACY

The spectrum of tumors sensitive to thiotepa is nearly identical to that of mechlorethamine. The major use of the drug currently is in the treatment of metastatic breast cancer as part of a drug combination known as VATH (vinblastine, doxorubicin, thiotepa, fluoxymesterone) or as a replacement for cyclophosphamide in patients who develop hemorrhagic cystitis. Thiotepa is also used by intracavitary administration in selected patients with malignant pleural or pericardial effusions, as intravesical therapy for bladder cancer, and, rarely, for the treatment of leptomeningeal carcinomatosis. There is interest in the experimental use of high-dose thiotepa with autologous BMT.

## PHARMACOLOGY

**Mechanisms of Action.** Thiotepa undergoes glutathione-dependent biotransformation to its metabolite monoglutathionylthiotepa.[1] The drug then acts as a trifunctional alkylating agent, as discussed previously for the bifunctional agent mechlorethamine. It is cell cycle phase nonspecific.

**Resistance.** The manufacturer notes that the drug has not demonstrated cross-resistance with cyclophosphamide in one animal tumor system and has shown impressive cytotoxicity in vitro relative to other alkylating agents. Unfortunately, others have found a poor correlation between the in vitro and in vivo activity of this agent. On balance, it would appear that the mechanisms of resistance are probably identical to those discussed for mechlorethamine.

**Pharmacokinetics.** Unlike mechlorethamine, thiotepa is not a vesicant and is reasonably stable in solution after it has been prepared for parenteral administration. It is erratically absorbed from the gastrointestinal tract and from serosal surfaces. After intravenous administration, the drug rapidly undergoes extensive metabolism. The plasma half-life is therefore short (about 1.5 hours). About 60% of an intravenous dose is excreted in the urine within 24 to 72 hours, but only about 1% of this is unchanged drug. When thiotepa has been used in very high dosage followed by BMT, the pharmacokinetic results have been similar to those with standard dose therapy, suggesting that metabolic clearance mechanisms for the drug require extremely high doses before saturation occurs.

**Drug Interactions.** Increased neuromuscular blockade with prolonged respiratory depression occurred in one patient treated with intraperitoneal thiotepa 90 minutes after pancuronium.[2]

## TOXICITY

**Overview.** In standard doses, this polyfunctional alkylating agent has a spectrum of toxicity that is nearly identical to that of mechlorethamine, except that it is not a vesicant and seldom causes vomiting. When the drug is combined in high doses with GM-CSF, thrombocytopenia is dose limiting.[3] When thiotepa is used as intravesical therapy, it may also cause lower abdominal pain, hematuria, bladder irritability, and, rarely, hemorrhagic cystitis. In the transplant setting, neuromuscular complications are common, and stupor and coma are dose limiting.[4] Dermatologic complications are also common with high-dose therapy.

**Hematologic.** Myelosuppression is dose related and dose limiting. After intravenous thiotepa administration, the leukocyte nadir occurs at 10 to 14 days, with subsequent rapid recovery in most patients, depending on the dose used. After intracavitary or intravesical administration, myelosuppression is unpredictable. At least one death due to myelosuppression has occurred after intravesical treatment.

**Digestive System.** Mild nausea and vomiting can occur. Lower abdominal pain has been reported after intravesical therapy.

**Other and Rare Reactions.** Fever and tightness in the throat are rare effects.

*Immunologic.* Immunosuppression (modest) can occur; hypersensitivity reactions are extremely rare.

*Mucocutaneous.* Local pain can occur at the injection site. Alopecia, hives, rash, and pruritus may occur.

*Pulmonary.* Prolonged apnea can occur when thiotepa is given with succinylcholine (see Drug Interactions).

*Ocular.* Periorbital depigmentation can occur after ocular administration (not an approved route of administration).

*Neurologic.* Headache, dizziness, lower extremity weakness, pain, and paresthesia can occur. Spinal cord demyelination may occur after intrathecal administration (not an approved route of administration).

*Genitourinary.* Hemorrhagic cystitis can result from intravesical therapy.

*Reproductive.* Toxicity studies place thiotepa in FDA pregnancy category D. Decreased spermatogenesis, menstrual irregularity, and sterility may occur.

*Carcinogenicity.* Thiotepa is mutagenic and carcinogenic.

## DOSAGE AND ADMINISTRATION

Thiotepa is available in 15-mg vials for intravenous administration. The usual intravenous dosage of thiotepa when used alone is 0.3 to 0.4 mg/kg, repeated at 1- to 4-week intervals, depending on the response and tolerance of the patient. In the transplant setting, doses up to 900 mg/m² have been used.[5] The intrapleural dosage of thiotepa is generally double that of mechlorethamine when used in a comparable situation—namely, 0.6 to 0.8 mg/kg. However, it is more stable than mechlorethamine and need not be prepared at the bedside. The usual dosage for intravesical administration for patients with superficial bladder tumors is 30 to 60 mg in 30 to 60 ml of distilled water. It is probably better to use 30 ml than 60 ml of diluent because this results in a higher dosage rate of thiotepa to the tumor, but it does not increase systemic toxicity.[6]

Thiotepa is contraindicated in patients with known hypersensitivity to the drug. The manufacturer advises against its use in patients with pre-existing hepatic, renal, or bone marrow damage.

## REFERENCES

1. Cnubben NH, Rommens AJ, Oudshoorn MJ, Van Bladeren PHJ. Glutathione-dependent biotransformation of the alkylating drug thiotepa and transport of its metabolite monoglutathionylthiotepa. Cancer Res 1998;58:4616–23.
2. Bennett EJ, Schmidt GB, Patel KP, Grundy EM. Muscle relaxants, myasthenia, and mustards? Anesthesiology 1977;46:220–1.
3. O'Dwyer PJ, LaCreta FP, Schilder R, et al. Phase I trial of thiotepa in combination with recombinant granulocyte-macrophage colony-stimulating factor. J Clin Oncol 1992;10:1352–8.

4. Fischer DS. The cancer chemotherapy handbook. 4th ed. St. Louis: CV Mosby, 1993:194.
5. Bowers C, Adkins D, Dunphy F, et al. Dose escalation of mitoxantrone given with thiotepa and autologous bone marrow transplantation for metastatic breast cancer. Bone Marrow Transplant 1993;12:525–30.
6. Masters JR, McDermott BJ, Harland S, et al. ThioTEPA pharmacokinetics during intravesical chemotherapy: the influence of dose and volume of instillate on systemic uptake and dose rate to the tumor. Cancer Chemother Pharmacol 1996;38:59–64.

# Topotecan

Topotecan is a semisynthetic derivative of the *Camptotheca acuminata* tree, one of two agents in this class new to the market. It acts as a topoisomerase I inhibitor and is active against a few different tumor types. The drug is generally well tolerated. Topotecan is also known as Hycamtin.

## EFFICACY

In the United States, topotecan is approved for use in advanced ovarian cancer and refractory small cell lung cancer. It is interesting that the drug has an apparently different spectrum of activity from other drugs in its class.

Early studies revealed topotecan to be active as a single agent as second-line therapy for metastatic ovarian cancers. In patients whose cancer progressed during or after one platinum-containing regimen and who were randomly assigned to topotecan or paclitaxel, those treated with topotecan had a higher response rate and a longer time to tumor progression.[1] In a second study of women whose disease had progressed through one or two prior regimens, usually platinum or paclitaxel, or both, topotecan was also effective.[2] Future studies will define the role of the drug as up-front therapy in this disease. A small phase I trial has shown the safety of intraperitoneal administration, perhaps to be used eventually if proved efficacious for those with diffuse carcinomatosis.[3]

Two other studies led to approval of topotecan use in small cell lung cancer. One study described its effectiveness in refractory disease[4]; another found the agent to be at least as effective as combination therapy with cyclophosphamide, doxorubicin, and vincristine therapy in refractory disease.[5] Toxicity and survival were quite similar between the two groups.

In other smaller studies, topotecan has been found effective against a broad range of pediatric tumors, head and neck cancer, and various hematologic malignancies including AML, myelodysplastic syndromes, chronic myelomonocytic leukemia, and multiple myeloma.[6–10]

## PHARMACOLOGY

**Mechanisms of Action and Resistance.** As with irinotecan, topotecan is a camptothecin analogue (see Irinotecan for a more complete discussion of the mechanism of action). As such, it exerts its effect by binding to topoisomerase I and preventing DNA replication. Little is known about mechanisms of resistance to topotecan or why one member of the camptothecin class can have such a different spectrum of activity from another. One study suggests that in human leukemia cell lines, resistance is the result of diminished topoisomerase I–DNA adducts that render the drug less effective.[11]

**Pharmacokinetics.** Topotecan usually behaves according to a two-compartment model, with linear pharmacokinetics in the dose range of 0.5 to 3.5 mg/m$^2$.[12] It has a plasma half-life of 2 to 3 hours, with approximately 30% of the drug excreted in the urine. In patients with hepatic impairment, plasma drug clearance decreases by about one third, but patients surprisingly were able to tolerate full doses of topotecan. The parent compound, with a preserved active lactone ring, undergoes a reversible hydrolysis reaction in which the opened-ring form predominates at physiologic pH.

**Drug Interactions.** Administration of topotecan and G-CSF the same day resulted in prolonged neutropenia. Similarly, combinations of topotecan and cisplatin resulted in severe myelotoxicity. No other information is known about drug-drug interactions.

## TOXICITY

**Overview.** Topotecan's main dose-limiting side effect is myelosuppression. The following information was taken from the package insert and from the pivotal trials carried out in patients with ovarian cancer.

**Hematologic.** At recommended doses, 60% of patients had severe neutropenia (granulocytes <500/μL) during the first course of therapy. The severe neutropenia occurred in 40% of all courses of the drug. The median nadir was at 11 days and had a median duration of 7 days. Febrile neutropenia occurred in just over one fourth of patients, and prophylactic G-CSF was given in 27% of second courses with topotecan. Platelet values declined below 25,000/μL (grade 4) in 26% of patients, with 13% of patients requiring transfusions. Severe anemia, defined as hemoglobin less than 8 g/dl, occurred in 40% of patients, with 56% requiring RBC transfusions.

**Gastrointestinal.** Severe nausea and vomiting were rare (10% and 9%, respectively), although milder symptoms occurred quite commonly (77% and 58%). Routine antiemetic prophylaxis was not used. Nearly half the patients described some sort of diarrhea, although it was severe in only 5%. Constipation was reported in 39% (3% severe) of patients.

**Neurologic.** Mild headaches (21%) and mild paresthesias (9%) were reported in these clinical trials.

**Other Reactions.** Allergic reactions were extremely rare.

*Reproductive.* Toxicity studies place topotecan in FDA pregnancy category D.

*Carcinogenicity.* There is some evidence linking topoisomerase I inhibitors with human leukemia, but long-term animal studies of carcinogenicity have not been carried out. The drug is genotoxic and should be presumed to be potentially carcinogenic.

## DOSAGE AND ADMINISTRATION

Topotecan is available in 4-mg single-dose vials. Each vial should be reconstituted with 4 ml of sterile water and then diluted in either normal saline or 5% dextrose solutions. The drug is given intravenously over 30 minutes.

Recommended dosages in ovarian cancer or small cell lung cancer are 1.5 mg/m² daily for 5 days, repeated every 21 days. The manufacturer recommends a minimum of four courses because median time to response in the pivotal ovarian studies was 9 to 12 weeks. Prior to therapy, patients should have neutrophil counts higher than 1500/μL and platelet counts greater than 100,000/μL. If severe neutropenia develops during therapy, the dose can be reduced by 0.25 mg/m² daily or G-CSF can be used prophylactically the day after the fifth daily dose. No dose adjustment appears necessary for a serum bilirubin value up to 10 mg/dl. For patients with creatinine clearance between 20 and 39 ml/min, the topotecan dose should be 0.75 mg/m². No information about more severe renal impairment exists.

## REFERENCES

1. ten Bokkel Huinink W, Gore M, Carmichael J, et al. Topotecan versus paclitaxel for the treatment of recurrent epithelial ovarian cancer. J Clin Oncol 1997;15:2183–93.
2. Bookman MA, Malmstrom H, Bolis G, et al. Topotecan for the treatment of advanced epithelial ovarian cancer: an open-label phase II study in patients treated after prior chemotherapy that contained cisplatin or carboplatin and paclitaxel. J Clin Oncol 1998;16:3345–52.
3. Plaxe SC, Christen RD, O'Quigley J, et al. Phase I and pharmacokinetic study of intraperitoneal topotecan. Invest New Drugs 1998;16:147–53.
4. Ardizzoni A, Hansen H, Dombernowsky P, et al. Topotecan, a new active drug in the second-line treatment of small-cell lung cancer: a phase II study in patients with refractory and sensitive disease. The European Organization for Research and Treatment of Cancer Early Clinical Studies Group and New Drug Development Office, and the Lung Cancer Cooperative Group. J Clin Oncol 1997;15:2090–6.
5. von Pawel J, Schiller JH, Shepherd FA, et al. Topotecan versus cyclophosphamide, doxorubicin, and vincristine for the treatment of recurrent small-cell lung cancer. J Clin Oncol 1999;17:658–67.
6. Nitschke R, Parkhurst J, Sullivan J, et al. Topotecan in pediatric patients with recurrent and progressive solid tumors: a Pediatric Oncology Group phase II study. J Pediatr Hematol Oncol 1998;20:315–8.
7. Robert F, Soong SJ, Wheeler RH. A phase II study of topotecan in patients with recurrent head and neck cancer: identification of an active new agent. Am J Clin Oncol 1997;20:298–302.
8. Crump M, Lipton J, Hedley D, et al. Phase I trial of sequential topotecan followed by etoposide in adults with myeloid leukemia: a National Cancer Institute of Canada Clinical Trials Group Study. Leukemia 1999;13:343–7.
9. Beran M, Estey E, O'Brien SM, et al. Results of topotecan single-agent therapy in patients with myelodysplastic syndromes and chronic myelomonocytic leukemia. Leuk Lymphoma 1998;31:521–31.
10. Kraut EH, Crowley JJ, Wade JL, et al. Evaluation of topotecan in resistant and relapsing multiple myeloma: a Southwest Oncology Group study. J Clin Oncol 1998;16:589–92.
11. Kaufmann SH, Svingen PA, Gore SD, et al. Altered formation of topotecan-stabilized topoisomerase I–DNA adducts in human leukemia cells. Blood 1997;89:2098–104.
12. Dennis MJ, Beijnen JH, Grochow LB, van Warmerdam LJ. An overview of the clinical pharmacology of topotecan. Semin Oncol 1997;24:Suppl 5:S5-12–18.

## Vinblastine

Vinblastine is a very large plant alkaloid derived from *Cantharanthus roseus,* the common periwinkle plant. Vinblastine and vincristine, two closely related plant alkaloids that have been used since the late 1950s, are referred to as vinca alkaloids. Vinblastine is also known as Velban, vinblastine sulfate, vincaleukoblastine, VLB, VBL, and NSC-49842.

## EFFICACY

Vinblastine is used primarily in combination with other drugs, especially in the curative treatment of Hodgkin's disease. It is also used in the treatment of testicular cancer, non-Hodgkin's lymphomas, Kaposi's sarcoma, histiocytic disorders, drug-resistant choriocarcinoma, and breast cancer. Occasional benefit may attend its use for lung cancer, renal carcinoma, and carcinomas of the head and neck. It has sometimes been used in pregnant patients with Hodgkin's disease as a palliative therapy pending delivery of the infant. Continuous infusion of low-dose vinblastine has been used successfully as immunosuppressive treatment for autoimmune hemolytic anemia and idiopathic thrombocytopenic purpura, although a randomized trial found that bolus treatment is just as effective.[1]

## PHARMACOLOGY

**Mechanism of Action.** Vinblastine avidly binds to critical microtubular proteins within cells.[2] This binding alters the dynamics of tubulin addition and loss at the ends of mitotic spindle microtubules, ultimately blocking microtubule assembly.[3] Because these microtubules are essential contractile proteins of the mitotic spindle of dividing cells, this binding leads to mitotic arrest. Similar proteins make up an important part of nervous tissue. In addition, at high concentrations, vinblastine can kill nonproliferating cells and exert complex effects on RNA and protein synthesis. Vinblastine has also been reported to block the cellular utilization of glutamic acid, thus inhibiting purine synthesis, the citric acid cycle, and urea formation. Vinblastine arrests cells in the $G_2/M$ phase of the cell cycle and subsequently induces apoptosis.[4]

**Resistance.** Vinblastine resistance is primarily related to P-glycoprotein and the mdr phenotype caused by the mdr gene.[5] Other mechanisms are under investigation, including alternative drug efflux and uptake mechanisms, as discussed in separate references related to specific drug interactions discussed subsequently.

**Pharmacokinetics.** Vinblastine is light sensitive. The drug is marketed solely for use by the intravenous route. After intravenous administration, plasma clearance is triphasic and prolonged, with respective half-lives of 3.7 hours, 1.6 hours, and 24.8 hours. The kinetics of drug clearance from plasma are nonlinear and primarily influenced by changes in liver function. Vinblastine binds extensively to blood and other cellular elements, with the tissue affinities being in the order of plasma→platelets→RBCs→leukocytes. The drug is metabolized in part in the liver to another active compound, deacetylvinblastine. It is excreted primarily in bile as biodegraded products, and very little is excreted in the urine as unchanged drug. The pharmacology of vinblastine, with its primary excretion via the liver, explains the added toxicity that occurs when the drug is given to patients with liver disease. The drug does not cross the blood-brain barrier in appreciable amounts.

**Drug Interactions.** Vinblastine toxicity is increased by liver disease. Vinblastine resistance can be reduced or reversed experimentally by a variety of agents, including tamoxifen and toremifene,[6] phenytoin,[7] cyclosporine analogues,[8, 9] forskolin derivatives,[10] paclitaxel,[11] inhibitors of calmodulin,[12] chlorpromazine,[13] an anti-BP–glycoprotein monoclonal antibody (HUB-241),[14] and components of grapefruit juice.[15] The clinical importance of these interactions is unclear. Hypersensitivity reactions with pulmonary insufficiency may be more common when vinblastine is given in combination with mitomycin, especially in patients with pre-existing pulmonary symptoms. Simultaneous treatment with phenytoin can reduce blood levels of the anticonvulsant and increase seizure activity.

## TOXICITY

**Overview.** Myelosuppression is the major dose-limiting toxicity, but neuropathy can rarely be dose limiting as well. Patients should be informed of possible constipation, jaw pain, pain in organs containing tumor, alopecia, nausea, and vomiting. Because of hepatic clearance, the toxicity of vinblastine may be more severe in patients with liver dysfunction.

**Hematologic.** Bone marrow suppression, manifested most commonly as dose-related granulocytopenia, is the most frequent and dangerous toxicity. The nadir of granulocytopenia occurs 5 to 10 days after a given dose, with resolution by another 7 to 14 days. Myelosuppression is more common in patients with pre-existing bone marrow suppression, generalized debility, or ulcerated areas of skin.

**Digestive System.** Constipation is the most common and troublesome gastrointestinal complaint. Anorexia, nausea, vomiting, abdominal pain, ileus, diarrhea, anorexia, and abdominal cramps can occur, but these symptoms tend to be mild and self-limited. Rectal bleeding from ulceration of the duodenum or rectum occurs very rarely.

**Mucocutaneous.** Alopecia is common but is reversible and usually incomplete. Stomatitis and pharyngitis are occasional complications of vinblastine use. The drug is a severe local irritant, so thrombophlebitis and local tissue necrosis may be seen, especially following drug extravasation. Photosensitivity reactions and skin vesiculation are very rare complications. A single case of a radiation-recall reaction has been reported in a patient with Kaposi's sarcoma and AIDS.[16] Raynaud's phenomenon and digital gangrene have been associated with sequential vinblastine-bleomycin therapy in five patients with Kaposi's sarcoma.[17] The authors concluded that the reaction was directly related to the total dose of vinblastine given and that it was not solely due to bleomycin.

**Neurologic.** Malaise, weakness, and, rarely, neurologic problems can occur with vinblastine use. These include a wide variety of forms of peripheral neuropathy (such as paresthesia, paralysis, loss of deep tendon reflexes), autonomic neuropathy (constipation, paralytic ileus, orthostatic hypotension, urinary retention), and other changes, such as vocal cord paralysis, severe pain in the jaw or other locations, Raynaud's phenomenon, depression, dizziness, headache, and seizures. Neurologic effects are dose related and relatively rare with standard doses, but they can be permanent and disabling.

**Other and Rare Reactions.** Pain in tumor-containing tissue with drug administration, malaise, and fever all are rare.

**Immunologic.** Minimal immunosuppression can occur; hypersensitivity reactions, including dyspnea and severe bronchospasm, are very rare.

**Cardiovascular.** Hypertension, myocardial ischemia,[18] and Raynaud's phenomenon can occur (usually when vinblastine is given with bleomycin).

**Pulmonary.** Vinblastine is not considered toxic to the lungs, but pulmonary toxicity with severe dyspnea and bronchospasm secondary to vinblastine use has been reported in two patients who also received mitomycin.[19]

**Ocular.** Severe irritation with inadvertent direct exposure to the drug may occur.

**Musculoskeletal.** Myalgia (usually with associated neuropathy) and bone pain can occur.

**Reproductive.** Mutagenesis and teratogenesis have been reported in animals.[20] Aspermia can occur in men. Toxicity studies place vinblastine in FDA pregnancy category D.

**Endocrine-Metabolic.** SIADH has been reported in three patients with breast cancer.[21] Tumor lysis syndrome can occur.

**Carcinogenicity.** Although second neoplasms have occurred after combination chemotherapy with regimens including vinblastine, there is no compelling evidence in humans or animals that vinblastine is carcinogenic.

## DOSAGE AND ADMINISTRATION

Vinblastine is available as a lyophilized powder in 10-mg vials and as a 1 mg/ml solution. The drug is incompatible with furosemide, heparin, and Infusaid pumps. It is usually reconstituted with normal saline for intravenous injection. When vinblastine is dispensed, the manufacturer states that the container or syringe holding the drug must be enclosed in an overwrap bearing the statement "Do not remove covering until moment of injection. Fatal if given intrathecally. For IV use only." Management of patients mistakenly given intrathecal vinblastine is considered a medical emergency; treatment guidelines are provided in the package insert.

Vinblastine is administered intravenously, with extreme care being taken to avoid extravasation because of its ability to cause local tissue damage. The usual intravenous starting dosage when used alone is 0.1 mg/kg, given once weekly until the desired effect is achieved or until bone marrow depression precludes further treatment. This dosage may be titrated upward to as high as 0.3 mg/kg/wk in some patients. When used as maintenance therapy, vinblastine is generally given every 1 or 2 weeks, as tolerated. Continuous low-dose infusions of vinblastine have been used in the treatment of advanced cancer,[22] but this approach is of controversial value and the manufacturer advises against the use of daily low-dose therapy with vinblastine because severe, unexpected toxicity has developed with such schedules in the past.

Patients with liver disease should receive reduced doses of vinblastine. One guideline for this is to use a 50% reduction in dose for patients with total serum bilirubin levels greater than 3.0 mg/dl. No change in dose is required for patients with renal dysfunction.

## REFERENCES

1. Facon T, Caulier MT, Wattel E, et al. A randomized trial comparing vinblastine in slow infusion and by bolus I.V. injection in idiopathic thrombocytopenic purpura: a report on 42 patients. Br J Haematol 1994;86:678–80.
2. Tucker RW, Owellen RJ, Harris SB. Correlation of cytotoxicity and mitotic spindle dissolution by vinblastine in mammalian cells. Cancer Res 1977;37:4346–51.
3. Jordan MA, Thrower D, Wilson L. Mechanism of inhibition of cell proliferation by Vinca alkaloids. Cancer Res 1991;51:2212–22.
4. Tashiro E, Simizu S, Takada M, et al. Caspase-3 activation is not responsible for vinblastine-induced Bcl-2 phosphorylation and G$_2$/M arrest in human small cell lung carcinoma Ms-1 cells. Jpn J Cancer Res 1998;89:940–6.
5. Horio M, Gottesman MM, Pastan I. ATP-dependent transport of vinblastine in vesicles from human multidrug-resistant cells. Proc Natl Acad Sci U S A 1988;85:3580–4.
6. Kirk J, Houlbrook S, Stuart NS, et al. Selective reversal of vinblastine resistance in multidrug-resistant cell lines by tamoxifen, toremifene and their metabolites. Eur J Cancer 1993;29A:1152–7.
7. Kawamura KI, Grabowski D, Weizer K, et al. Modulation of vinblastine cytotoxicity by dilantin (phenytoin) or the protein phosphatase inhibitor okadaic acid involves the potentiation of anti-mitotic effects and induction of apoptosis in human tumour cells. Br J Cancer 1996;73:183–8.
8. Cabot MC, Giuliano AE, Han TY, Liu YY. SDZ PSC 833, the cyclosporine A analogue and multidrug resistance modulator, activates ceramide synthesis and increases vinblastine sensitivity in drug-sensitive and drug-resistant cancer cells. Cancer Res 1999;59:880–5.
9. Kusunoki N, Takara K, Tanigawara Y, et al. Inhibitory effects of a cyclosporin derivative, SDZ PSC 833, on transport of doxorubicin and vinblastine via human P-glycoprotein. Jpn J Cancer Res 1998;89:1220–8.
10. Hunter J, Hirst BH, Simmons NL. Transepithelial vinblastine secretion mediated by P-glycoprotein is inhibited by forskolin derivatives. Biochem Biophys Res Commun 1991;181:671–6.
11. Syed SK, Christopherson RI, Roufogalis BD. Vinblastine transport by membrane vesicles from human multidrug-resistant CCRF-CEM leukaemia cells: inhibition by taxol and membrane permeabilising agents. Biochem Mol Biol Int 1993;30:743–53.
12. Ido M, Lagace L, Chafouleas JG. Increased sensitivity to vinca alkaloids in cells overexpressing calmodulin by gene transfection. Cancer Res 1990;50:6554–8.
13. Syed SK, Christopherson RI, Roufogalis BD. Reversal of vinblastine transport by chlorpromazine in membrane vesicles from multidrug-resistant human CCRF-CEM leukaemia cells. Br J Cancer 1998;78:321–7.
14. Rittmann-Grauer LS, Yong MA, Sanders V, Mackensen DG. Reversal of vinca alkaloid resistance by anti-P-glycoprotein monoclonal antibody HYB-241 in a human tumor xenograft. Cancer Res 1992;52:1810–6.
15. Takanaga H, Ohnishi A, Matsuo H, Sawada Y. Inhibition of vinblastine efflux mediated by P-glycoprotein by grapefruit juice components in caco-2 cells. Biol Pharm Bull 1998;21:1062–6.
16. Nemechek PM, Corder MC. Radiation recall associated with vinblastine in a patient treated for Kaposi sarcoma related to acquired immune deficiency syndrome. Cancer 1992;70:1605–6.
17. Hladunewich M, Sawka C, Fam A, Franssen E. Raynaud's phenomenon and digital gangrene as a consequence of treatment for Kaposi's sarcoma. J Rheumatol 1997;24:2371–5.
18. Subar M, Muggia FM. Apparent myocardial ischemia associated with vinblastine administration. Cancer Treat Rep 1986;70:690–1.
19. Konits PH, Aisner J, Sutherland JC, Wiernik PH. Possible pulmonary toxicity secondary to vinblastine. Cancer 1982;50:2771–4.
20. Sieber SM, Adamson RH. Toxicity of antineoplastic agents in man, chromosomal aberrations, antifertility effects, congenital malformations, and carcinogenic potential. Adv Cancer Res 1975;22:57–155.
21. Fraschini G, Recchia F, Holmes FA. Syndrome of inappropriate antidiuretic hormone secretion associated with hepatic arterial infusion of vinblastine in three patients with breast cancer. Tumori 1987;73:513–6.
22. Ratain MJ, Vogelzang NJ. Phase I and pharmacological study of vinblastine by prolonged continuous infusion. Cancer Res 1986;46:4827–30.

# Vincristine

Vincristine is a large plant alkaloid that is closely related chemically to vinblastine. The drug is also known as Oncovin, vincristine sulfate, VCR, Vcr, leurocristine, and NSC-67574.

## EFFICACY

Vincristine, in combination with other drugs, is FDA approved and listed by the manufacturer as indicated for the treatment of ALL, Hodgkin's disease, the non-Hodgkin's lymphomas, neuroblastoma, Wilms' tumor, and rhabdomyosarcomas.

Vincristine has also been used in the treatment of breast cancer, some brain tumors, soft tissue sarcomas other than rhabdomyosarcomas, Kaposi's sarcoma, cervical carcinoma, and small cell carcinoma of the lung, although these are not specifically listed by the manufacturer as indications. It is occasionally used to treat some nonmalignant conditions, most notably immunogenic thrombocytopenia.[1]

## PHARMACOLOGY

**Mechanisms of Action and Resistance.** As with vinblastine, the primary mechanism of action for vincristine is inhibition of microtubule assembly, and resistance is primarily mediated by P-glycoprotein. One study suggests that myeloperoxidase may mediate another form of vincristine resistance.[2] This may explain the relatively low efficacy of vincristine in AML (which contains large amounts of myeloperoxidase) compared with ALL (which lacks myeloperoxidase). Other studies implicate both P-glycoprotein and glutathione in vincristine resistance.[3–5] Another mechanism of resistance may involve nitric oxide.[6] Vincristine arrests cells in the G$_2$/M phase of the cell cycle and causes at least partial synchronization of cells in vitro.[7]

**Pharmacokinetics.** With a single exception, the pharmacology of vincristine is very similar to that of vinblastine. It is clear that both of the vinca alkaloids are extensively bound to tissues (primarily tubulin) and slowly eliminated from the body; are metabolized in the liver and excreted primarily in bile to the stool and minimally by way of the kidneys; are bound to serum proteins and the formed elements of the blood; and cross the blood-brain barrier poorly. However, although slow, the serum clearance rates are strikingly different, with vinblastine being cleared nearly sevenfold more rapidly.[8] This may explain the different patterns of toxicity of the two agents.

**Drug Interactions.** These are probably the same as for vinblastine, although megestrol acetate has been reported to augment vincristine toxicity in vitro without augmenting vinblastine toxicity.[9] Another drug that enhances the in vitro cytotoxicity of vincristine is indomethacin.[10] In vivo, several drugs without known neurotoxic effects have been reported to increase vincristine-related neurotoxicity. Itraconazole caused this drug-drug interaction in two patients in one report,[11] and severe atypical neuropathy has been reported with the combined use of vincristine and hematopoietic colony-stimulating factors.[12] Because of the greater neurotoxicity of vincristine compared with vinblastine, neuroactive drugs should be used with caution during vincristine treatment, especially in elderly patients.

## TOXICITY

**Overview.** Neurologic toxicity is dose limiting; alopecia is common; myelosuppression is negligible. Most side effects are dose related and reversible, but neurotoxicity can persist for months after the discontinuation of therapy in some patients, and it may be disabling in very rare patients. *Of note are continued reports of inadvertent, lethal intrathecal and intraventricular administration of vincristine. Precautions must be taken to prevent this tragic and avoidable complication.*

**Digestive System.** Constipation due to autonomic neuropathy is common (see Neurologic section). Other gastrointestinal effects are rare, including nausea, vomiting, paralytic ileus, anorexia, diarrhea, intestinal necrosis or perforation, abdominal cramps, and pancreatitis.

**Mucocutaneous.** Alopecia (20 to 70% of patients), rare stomatitis, a rare rash, and localized phlebitis or necrosis with drug extravasation can occur. Extravasation precautions are mandatory.

**Neurologic.** The most important toxic reaction due to vincristine is a mixed motor-sensory and autonomic neuropathy due to extensive binding with tubulin within the nervous system. Its earliest manifestation is depression of the Achilles tendon reflex, followed by paresthesia of the fingers and toes. If the drug is continued, weakness, muscle pain, and sensory impairment may develop. Further treatment may produce severe, generalized motor weakness and, rarely, quadriparesis. Very rarely, convulsions may occur.[13] Autonomic neuropathy is manifested by constipation, ileus, or, rarely, bowel obstruction. Bowel and bladder atony mimicking spinal cord compression may also occur.[14] Vincristine use has been linked to severe pain in the jaw, pharynx, bones, back, or extremities. Decreased singing ability has been reported,[15] and at high doses, auditory dysfunction has been reported.[16] Recovery from most of these changes is possible by withdrawing the drug, but motor weakness may be irreversible. Vincristine-induced ileus, however, may respond to treatment with metoclopramide.[17]

Although neuropathy is bothersome to patients, mild to moderate dysfunction appears to be necessary for an antitumor effect by this drug. However, patients must be closely monitored to avoid severe neurotoxicity. One guide to therapy is to discontinue vincristine use if patients develop paresthesia proximal to the distal interphalangeal joints of the hands or if any motor weakness occurs. This may easily be tested by having patients attempt to walk on their heels. The bowel problems due to vincristine can usually be avoided by the use of stool softeners and cathartics. If these are insufficient, vigorous cleansing enemas and discontinuation of vincristine may be necessary.

Lethal myeloencephalopathy has been reported on numerous occasions after inadvertent administration of vincristine by the intrathecal or intraventricular routes.[18–21] It is crucial to take steps to prevent this human error. Serious neurotoxicity has been reported with experimental use of five consecutive daily doses of the drug.[22] Several drugs have been reported to increase vincristine toxicity, including itraconazole[11] and hematopoietic colony-stimulating factors.[12]

Pre-existing neurologic disorders may predispose to more severe forms of neurotoxicity. This may be true for patients without obvious neurologic problems but with a family history of a neurologic disease. A good example of this is Charcot-Marie-Tooth disease. Two studies have demonstrated that a family history of this problem can contribute to markedly augmented vincristine neuropathy in apparently normal persons.[23, 24]

**Other and Rare Reactions.** Weight loss is rare, drug fever in children is rare,[25] and headache is rare.

*Hematologic.* Unlike vinblastine, only minimal acute myelosuppression follows the use of vincristine in standard doses. Occasional patients may develop delayed anemia, leukopenia, or thrombocytopenia that is mild and generally not dose related.

*Immunologic.* Very rare cases of hypersensitivity with edema, rash, and anaphylaxis have occurred.[26]

*Cardiovascular.* Hypertension and hypotension can occur. Myocardial infarction may occur.[27] Myocardial infarction may be more likely in patients who have undergone prior mediastinal irradiation.[28]

*Pulmonary.* Acute dyspnea and bronchospasm can occur when the drug is given in combination with mitomycin.

*Ocular.* Diplopia, ptosis, photophobia, optic atrophy, and a variety of other rare neuropathic ocular changes have been reported. Cortical blindness is a particularly catastrophic potential side effect.[29]

*Musculoskeletal.* Myalgia, jaw pain, and bone pain can occur (see Neurologic section).

*Genitourinary.* Polyuria, dysuria, and urinary retention due to bladder atony can occur.

*Reproductive.* Azoospermia may occur, especially in children and adolescents.[30] The drug is teratogenic. Toxicity studies place vincristine in FDA pregnancy category D.

*Endocrine-Metabolic.* SIADH may occur, as may tumor lysis syndrome with hyperuricemia.

*Carcinogenicity.* Vincristine is not a known mutagen or carcinogen.

## DOSAGE AND ADMINISTRATION

Vincristine is provided as a solution in vials of 1, 2, and 5 mg. It is incompatible with furosemide, idarubicin, polysiloxane containers used in portable delivery devices, and some infusion-line filters.

Vincristine is administered intravenously because of erratic oral absorption. As with vinblastine, this must be performed carefully owing to the severe local tissue destruction that results from extravasation. It is usually administered by rapid intravenous bolus injection in weekly dosages of 1.4 mg/m² for adults and 1.5 to 2.0 mg/m² for children. Some authorities recommend a maximum total single dose in adults of 2.0 mg. This maximum dose is controversial,[31] however, and for some programs of chemotherapy this limit on the dose is not applied (see discussion of Hodgkin's lymphoma in Chapter 87). A 50% dose reduction is recommended for patients with hepatic dysfunction and a direct bilirubin value great than 3 mg/dl.

There is no specific antidote for vincristine overdosage, but plasmapheresis may be useful in attenuating neuropathy.[32] The manufacturer provides the following warning: "The intrathecal administration of Oncovin usually results in death. Syringes containing this product should be labeled 'WARNING—FOR IV USE ONLY.' " A protocol for immediate management of inadvertent intrathecal vincristine is provided in the package insert.

## REFERENCES

1. Ries CA. Vincristine for treatment of refractory autoimmune thrombocytopenia. N Engl J Med 1976;295:1136.
2. Schlaifer D, Cooper MR, Attal M, et al. Potential strategies for circumventing myeloperoxidase-catalyzed degradation of vinca alkaloids. Leukemia 1994;8:668–71.
3. Whelan RDH, Waring CJ, Wolf CR, et al. Over-expression of P-glycoprotein and glutathione S-transferase pi in MCF-7 cells selected for vincristine resistance in vitro. Int J Cancer 1992;52:241–6.
4. Loe DW, Almquist KC, Deeley RG, Cole SP. Multidrug resistance protein (MRP)-mediated transport of leukotriene C4 and chemotherapeutic agents in membrane vesicles: demonstration of glutathione-dependent vincristine transport. J Biol Chem 1996;271:9675–82.
5. Loe DW, Deeley RG, Cole SP. Characterization of vincristine transport by the M(r) 190,000 multidrug resistance protein (MRP): evidence for cotransport with reduced glutathione. Cancer Res 1998;58:5130–6.
6. Ogura T, DeGeorge G, Tatemichi M, Esumi H. Suppression of antimicrotubule agent-induced apoptosis by nitric oxide: possible mechanism of a new drug resistance. Jpn J Cancer Res 1998;89:199–205.
7. Klein HO, Adler D, Doering M, et al. Investigations on pharmacologic induction of partial synchronization of tumor cell proliferation: its relevance for cytostatic therapy. Cancer Treat Rep 1976;60:1959–79.
8. Balis FM, Holcenberg JS, Bleyer WA. Clinical pharmacokinetics of commonly used anticancer drugs. Clin Pharmacokinet 1983;8:202–32.
9. Tansan S, Koc Y, Aydin H, et al. Augmentation of vincristine cytotoxicity by megestrol acetate. Cancer Chemother Pharmacol 1997;39:333–40.
10. Kobayashi S, Okada S, Yoshida H, Fujimura S. Indomethacin enhances the cytotoxicity of VCR and ADR in human pulmonary adenocarcinoma cells. Tohoku J Exp Med 1997;181:361–70.
11. Gillies J, Hung KA, Fitzsimons E, Soutar R. Severe vincristine toxicity in combination with itraconazole. Clin Lab Haematol 1998;20:123–4.
12. Weintraub M, Adde MA, Venzon DJ, et al. Severe atypical neuropathy associated with administration of hematopoietic colony-stimulating factors and vincristine. J Clin Oncol 1996;14:935–40.
13. Hurwitz RL, Mahoney DH Jr, Armstrong DL, Browder TM. Reversible encephalopathy and seizures as a result of conventional vincristine administration. Med Pediatr Oncol 1988;16:216–9.
14. Raphaelson MI, Stevens JC, Newman RP. Vincristine neuropathy with bowel and bladder atony, mimicking spinal cord compression. Cancer Treat Rep 1983;67:604–5.
15. Rezvani K, Bain BJ, Coulter CA. Loss of singing ability caused by vincristine. Clin Lab Haematol 1988;20:47–8.
16. Lugassy G, Shapira A. A prospective cohort study of the effect of vincristine on audition. Anticancer Drugs 1996;7:525–6.
17. Garewal HS, Dalton WS. Metoclopramide in vincristine-induced ileus. Cancer Treat Rep 1985;69:1309–11.
18. Al Ferayan A, Russell NA, Al Wohaibi M, et al. Cerebrospinal fluid lavage in the treatment of inadvertent intrathecal vincristine injection. Childs Nerv Syst 1999;15:87–9.
19. Meggs WJ, Hoffman RS. Fatality resulting from intraventricular vincristine administration. J Toxicol Clin Toxicol 1998;36:243–6.
20. Michelagnoli MP, Bailey CC, Wilson I, et al. Potential salvage therapy for inadvertent intrathecal administration of vincristine. Br J Haematol 1997;99:364–7 and 1998;101:398.
21. Lau G. Accidental intraventricular vincristine administration: an avoidable iatrogenic death. Med Sci Law 1996;36:263–5.
22. Jochimsen PR. Subacute vincristine toxicity following five consecutive daily doses. Am J Clin Oncol 1982;5:437–41.
23. Graf WD, Chance PF, Lensch MW, et al. Severe vincristine neuropathy in Charcot-Marie-Tooth disease type 1A. Cancer 1996;77:1356–62.
24. Neumann Y, Toren A, Rechavi G, et al. Vincristine treatment triggering the expression of asymptomatic Charcot-Marie-Tooth disease. Med Pediatr Oncol 1996;26:280–3.
25. Ishii E, Hara T, Mizuno Y, Ueda K. Vincristine-induced fever in children with leukemia and lymphoma. Cancer 1988;61:660–2.
26. Gassel WD, Gropp C, Havemann K. Acute allergic reaction due to vincristine sulfate: a case report. Oncology 1984;41:403–5.
27. Federman DG, Henry G. Chemotherapy-induced myocardial necrosis in a patient with chronic lymphocytic leukemia. Respir Med 1997;91:565–7.
28. von Hoff DD, Rozencweig M, Piccart M. The cardiotoxicity of anticancer agents. Semin Oncol 1982;9:23–33.
29. Merimsky O, Loewenstein A, Chaitchik S. Cortical blindness—a catastrophic side effect of vincristine. Anticancer Drugs 1992;3:371–3.
30. Rautonen J, Koskimies AI, Siimes MA. Vincristine is associated with the risk of azoospermia in adult male survivors of childhood malignancies. Eur J Cancer 1992;28A:1837–41.
31. Sulkes A, Collins JM. Reappraisal of some dosage adjustment guidelines. Cancer Treat Rep 1987;71:229–33.
32. Pierga JY, Beuzeboc P, Dorval T, et al. Favourable outcome after plasmapheresis for vincristine overdose. Lancet 1992;340:185.

## Vinorelbine

Vinorelbine is the newest of the vinca alkaloid drugs. It is a semisynthetic derivative, 5'-nor-anhydrovinblastine, first identified in the 1970s. This too is broadly active against many tumor types and is also known as Navelbine. Its advantage over other agents in its class is thought to be an improved toxicity profile.

### EFFICACY

Vinorelbine's approved indication in the United States is in the treatment of advanced non–small cell lung cancer, either alone or in combination with cisplatin.[1] For patients with stage III lung cancers, the drug is given together with cisplatin. The pivotal trial designs were interesting in that a North American study of stage IV cases randomly assigned untreated subjects to Navelbine or 5-FU, a regimen not commonly used for the disease. Those treated with vinorelbine had a survival advantage. Further studies of lung cancer have shown superiority of the combination vinorelbine plus cisplatin to cisplatin alone.[2] Newer lung cancer studies are examining the role of triplet combinations and trying to determine whether one of several doublets is better than another in first-line therapy.

Early clinical testing found the drug active in advanced breast cancer, a finding later confirmed by a host of clinical trials. Vinorelbine is an effective single agent as first- or second-line therapy in anthracycline-resistant metastatic breast cancer.[3] It is also safely and effectively given as part of combination regimens that do not contain anthracyclines.[4] Further investigation will define the agent's role as adjuvant therapy or in various other combinations for more advanced disease.

Other trials demonstrate activity of vinorelbine in cancers of the cervix, ovary, head and neck, and esophagus, as well as in lymphoma (Hodgkin's and non-Hodgkin's).[5–10] Even more studies in various stages of completion are examining the role of vinorelbine alone and in combinations for many different disease indications.

## PHARMACOLOGY

**Mechanism of Action.** As with the other vinca alkaloids, vinorelbine exerts its antitumor effects via inhibition of the mitotic spindle apparatus. Interestingly, when vincristine also caused depolymerization of axonal microtubules (leading clinically to neuropathies), equivalent doses of vinorelbine did not. This may explain why the neurotoxicity is thought to be less for this agent than for others in its class.[11] Vinorelbine was also observed to have a selective production of mitotic tubulin paracrystallization, which might account for improved clinical efficacy compared with other vinca alkaloids.[12]

**Mechanisms of Resistance.** Unfortunately, vinorelbine is similarly affected by the P-glycoprotein, multidrug-resistance system.[13]

**Pharmacokinetics.** Vinorelbine has a large volume of distribution and behaves according to a three-compartment model.[14] It has a rapid initial decay but a prolonged terminal phase, probably because of delayed efflux from peripheral compartments. The terminal phase half-life is as great as 40 hours. It is mainly metabolized in the liver, with small amounts also appearing in the urine after dosing. Although no specific information is known about dose adjustments in patients with renal or hepatic impairment, it follows from experience with other vinca alkaloids that care should be taken when dosing these groups of patients.

In early studies, vinorelbine demonstrated high binding also to platelets and lymphocytes, perhaps accounting for the drug's activity in hematologic malignancies. Pharmacokinetics are not known to be influenced by coadministration of other agents.

**Drug Interactions.** There are no known adverse drug interactions with vinorelbine. However, this is likely to change, given the number of drug interactions identified for other vinca alkaloids.

## TOXICITY

**Overview.** Vinorelbine is extremely well tolerated. Its major dose-limiting side effect is myelosuppression, predominantly leukopenia. The following information is obtained from the package insert and the pivotal trials performed using patients with lung cancer.

**Hematologic.** As stated earlier, vinorelbine's principal toxicity is leukopenia, occurring in more than 90% of patients at some point in their clinical course. Severe neutropenia ($<500/\mu L$) was found in just greater than 30% of patients. Nadirs occurred within 7 to 10 days of drug administration and usually resolved within 7 to 14 days. Only 9% of patients were admitted to the hospital as a result of complications of the neutropenia; the toxicity does not appear to be cumulative over time. Severe anemia and thrombocytopenia were rare. Routine growth factor administration is not recommended.

**Neurologic.** Although the incidence of peripheral neuropathies was much less than that with other vinca alkaloids, nearly a quarter of patients experienced some sensorimotor symptoms. In only 1% of patients was the neuropathy labeled severe.

**Gastrointestinal.** Mild to moderate nausea and vomiting were indeed observed with administration of vinorelbine but did not require routine prophylactic administration of antiemetics. Other frequent complaints included constipation, diarrhea, anorexia, and stomatitis; these were almost always mild in nature.

**Dermatologic.** Alopecia occurred in 12% of patients and was often mild. The drug is a vesicant, as are the other drugs in its class. Injection site reactions were mild.

**Other Reactions**

*Reproductive.* Toxicity studies place vinorelbine in FDA pregnancy category D.

*Carcinogenicity.* Long-term carcinogenicity studies in animals have not been carried out.

## DOSAGE AND ADMINISTRATION

Vinorelbine is supplied in 10-mg and 50-mg vials, each diluted in sterile water for injection at a concentration of 10 mg/ml. The drug may either be diluted in a syringe (with normal saline or 5% dextrose solutions to a concentration between 1.5 and 3.0 mg/ml) or into an intravenous bag containing normal saline, 5% dextrose, 0.45% normal saline, 0.45% normal saline with 5% dextrose, lactated Ringer's solution, or Ringer's solution (at concentrations between 0.5 and 2.0 mg/ml). In either case, the drug should be given through a freely flowing intravenous line over 6 to 10 minutes, followed by at least 75 to 125 ml of fluid to flush the line.

The recommended dosage in non–small cell lung cancer is 30 mg/m$^2$ weekly until toxicity or disease progression. Doses should be halved for neutrophil counts between 1000 and 1499/$\mu$L or a total bilirubin level between 2.1 and 3.0 mg/dl. For neutrophil counts less than 1000/$\mu$L, the drug should be held until toxicity resolves. For patients with a bilirubin level greater than 3.0 mg/dl, the weekly dosage of vinorelbine should be 7.5 mg/m$^2$.

## REFERENCES

1. Bunn PA Jr, Vokes EE, Langer CJ, Schiller JH. An update on North American randomized studies in non–small cell lung cancer. Semin Oncol 1998;25:Suppl 9:2–10.
2. Wozniak AJ, Crowley JJ, Balcerzak SP, et al. Randomized trial comparing cisplatin with cisplatin plus vinorelbine in the treatment of advanced non–small-cell lung cancer: a Southwest Oncology Group study. J Clin Oncol 1998;16:2459–65.
3. Weber BL, Vogel C, Jones S, et al. Intravenous vinorelbine as first-line and second-line therapy in advanced breast cancer. J Clin Oncol 1995;13:2722–30.
4. Turpin F, Lluch A, Closon MH, et al. Treatment with a nonanthracycline regimen in advanced breast cancer: vinorelbine, cyclophosphamide, and 5-fluorouracil with folinic acid. Am J Clin Oncol 1999;22:196–8.
5. Pignata S, Silvestro G, Ferrari E, et al. Phase II study of cisplatin and vinorelbine as first-line chemotherapy in patients with carcinoma of the uterine cervix. J Clin Oncol 1999;17:756–60.
6. Burger RA, DiSaia PJ, Roberts JA, et al. Phase II trial of vinorelbine

in recurrent and progressive epithelial ovarian cancer. Gynecol Oncol 1999;72:148–53.
7. Degardin M, Oliveira J, Geoffrois L, et al. An EORTC-ECSG phase II study of vinorelbine in patients with recurrent and/or metastatic squamous cell carcinoma of the head and neck. Ann Oncol 1998; 9:1103–7.
8. Conroy T, Etienne PL, Adenis A, et al. Phase II trial of vinorelbine in metastatic squamous cell esophageal carcinoma: European Organization for Research and Treatment of Cancer Gastrointestinal Treat Cancer Cooperative Group. J Clin Oncol 1996;14:164–70.
9. Devizzi L, Santoro A, Bonfante V, et al. Vinorelbine: a new promising drug in Hodgkin's disease. Leuk Lymphoma 1996;22:409–14.
10. Balzarotti M, Santoro A, Tondini C, et al. Activity of single agent vinorelbine in pretreated non-Hodgkin's lymphoma. Ann Oncol 1996;7:970–2.
11. Fellous A, Ohayon R, Vacassin T, et al. Biochemical effects of Navelbine on tubulin and associated proteins. Semin Oncol 1989;16:Suppl 4:9–14.
12. Johnson SA, Harper P, Hortobagyi GN, Pouillart P. Vinorelbine: an overview. Cancer Treat Rev 1996;22:127–142.
13. Adams DJ, Knick VC. P-glycoprotein–mediated resistance to 5'-nor-anhydrovinblastine (Navelbine). Invest New Drugs 1995;13:13–21.
14. Wargin WA, Lucas VS. The clinical pharmacokinetics of vinorelbine (Navelbine). Semin Oncol 1994;21:Suppl 10:21–7.

# CHAPTER 11

# BIOLOGIC AGENTS APPROVED FOR USE

• MALCOLM S. MITCHELL

The biologic agents that are approved for clinical use and described in the following sections are listed in Table 11–1.

## Interleukin-2

### EFFICACY

Interleukin-2 (IL-2) is effective in, and approved by the Food and Drug Administration (FDA) for the treatment of, metastatic renal cell carcinoma and metastatic melanoma. IL-2 has been used principally to treat renal cell carcinoma, melanoma, and lymphomas. It has some activity, but has been less widely tested, in the treatment of breast cancer. Although high-dose bolus and intravenous regimens were first applied, more recent studies indicate effectiveness at much lower doses as well.

Rosenberg and colleagues[1, 2] introduced high-dose IL-2 therapy for melanoma and renal cell carcinoma, in which bolus intravenous (IV) doses of the lymphokine were injected every 8 hours. These trials usually included adoptive cellular immunotherapy, with lymphokine-activated killer (LAK) cells or tumor-infiltrating lymphocytes. This treatment resulted in 19% objective response rates and long-term survival in 10% of patients. Patients with complete responses were those who had the long responses (40 ± 54+ months median), whereas partial responses lasted 6 months (melanoma) or 20 months (renal cell cancer).

### PHARMACOLOGY

Of all the lymphokines produced by T helper cells, IL-2 has been the most thoroughly investigated in humans. IL-2 is a powerful stimulatory lymphokine of approximately 15 kd that binds to T cells via both a 55 kd chain (Tac receptor) and a 75 kd chain. Together, the two chains form a high-affinity receptor through which a stimulatory signal is transduced into the lymphocyte. IL-2 is produced by recombinant DNA technology by inserting a human gene for IL-2 into *Escherichia coli*. The recombinant IL-2 differs from the native human IL-2 in several ways: (1) it lacks the N-terminal alanine, (2) it is not glycosylated (*E. coli* do not glycosylate proteins), (3) a serine was purposely substituted for a cysteine at amino acid 125, and (4) the aggregation state is likely to be different from the native IL-2. Nevertheless, the in vitro immunologic activities of recombinant IL-2 are the same as those of the native molecule.

IL-2 stimulates mitogenesis of T lymphocytes, stimulates long-term growth of IL-2–dependent T-cell lines, enhances lymphocyte-mediated cytotoxicity, induces interferon-γ (INF-γ), and induces natural killer and LAK cell production from lymphocytes.

IL-2 has a serum half-life of approximately 7 minutes after IV administration, which suggested to some the use of continuous IV administration. Particularly when given subcutaneously (SC) or intramuscularly (IM), bolus IL-2 treatments nevertheless appear to be as effective as continuous IV administration and have less toxicity.

### TOXICITY

The toxicity of IL-2 includes capillary leak syndrome, with peripheral and pulmonary edema, wheezing (an early form

**Table 11–1.** Biologic Agents Approved for Clinical Use

| Generic Name | Other Names |
|---|---|
| Aldesleukin | Interleukin-2 |
| | IL-2 |
| | Proleukin |
| Interferon alfa | Interferon alfa-2a, recombinant |
| | Interferon alfa-2b, recombinant |
| | Interferon alfa-n3 |
| | Alferon N |
| | Intron A |
| | Roferon-A |
| | Wellferon |
| Trastuzumab | Herceptin |
| Rituximab | Rituxan |
| | Anti-CD20 monoclonal antibody |

of capillary leak syndrome), hives, fatigue, depression (sometimes with suicidal ideation), arthralgias, myalgias, nausea, vomiting, diarrhea, dehydration (due to lack of desire for fluids, fluid loss, and poor fluid intake), and eosinophilia. Changes in mental status are often significant, sometimes leading to suicidal ideation and actual suicide, and are potentiated by combination of IL-2 with INF-α. Hospitalization is often required for the high-dose regimen, including treatment in an intensive care treatment unit or equivalent for an average of 10 days. A mortality rate of 2% was found in the early, high-dose trials but is now less than 1%.

## DOSAGE AND ADMINISTRATION

IL-2 is supplied as a white to off-white lyophilized cake in single-use vials. IL-2 may be given intravenously or SC. When reconstituted with 1.2 ml of sterile water for injection, each ml contains 18 million IU, or 1.1 mg protein. Mannitol, sodium dodecyl sulfate (as a solubilizing agent), and sodium phosphate (as a buffer) are also present, all at a pH of 7.5. IL-2 should be stored in a refrigerator before and after reconstitution and should be used within 48 hours of reconstitution. Note that the amount of IL-2 supplied per vial has not changed since it was first formulated and remains 21.6 million IU/vial. Many of the early studies were performed after using 1.0 ml of water to remove the IL-2, which led to a concentration of 21.6 million IU/ml. Reconstitution with 1.2 ml permits all the material to be removed more efficiently but changes the concentration per milliliter to 18 million IU/ml.

The recommended dosage schedule, which derives directly from the early work of Rosenberg and colleagues,[1, 2] is 600,000 IU/kg every 8 hours for a maximum of 14 doses over 5 days. This is given by a 15-minute IV infusion. The treatment may be repeated after 9 days of rest for a maximum of 28 doses per course. Most patients cannot receive all the projected days of treatment because of toxicity, which must be monitored closely with this level of treatment. The course should not be repeated more often than every 7 to 8 weeks, and effectiveness and toxicity should be evaluated in the interim.

Alternative routes and schedules of IL-2 have also been described, especially at lower doses and by the SC route. Although FDA approval and package insert recommendations are for high-dose IV treatment only, it is clear that lower doses are also effective at approximately the same level of response and are less toxic, permitting more frequent administration, self-administration, and home therapy.

Several lower dose regimens of IL-2 in the outpatient setting have been used with some success.[3–5] In melanoma, three "cycles" of IL-2 at 21.6 million IU/m² preceded by cyclophosphamide, 350 mg/m² on day −3 have yielded response rates (approximately 25%) similar to those of higher dose regimens. Others have used even lower dose regimens with equal success in melanoma and renal cell carcinoma.[6] These outpatient regimens can be used at home because IL-2 can be self-administered SC. A "cycle" of "low-dose" IL-2 treatment in our hands has consisted of a pretreatment dose of cyclophosphamide on day −3, followed by IL-2, 21.6 million IU/m² SC (originally given IV) on days 1 to 5 and 8 to 12. The cycle is repeated twice

more with a 7-day respite between the last day of IL-2 administration and the next pretreatment dose of cyclophosphamide. Maintenance treatment, consisting of a 2-week cycle of cyclophosphamide plus IL-2 given once every 6 to 8 weeks, is given after one or two complete courses if there is no progression of disease. This maintenance treatment can be continued indefinitely. Patients with metastatic melanoma have tolerated this treatment for 4 to 5 years. It is uncertain how long treatment must be continued in long-term responders.

IL-2 combined with INF-α reportedly produced response rates somewhat higher than IL-2 alone.[7] Toxicity of the two agents has been considerable particularly at high-dose levels. In particular, the neurologic and mental side effects have been disturbing, with suicidal impulses in several patients with no prior history of psychological problems. The combination has been most useful for renal cell carcinomas in our experience. We use a "flat" dose of INF-α of 1 million units three times per week SC, together with a low-dose cyclophosphamide plus IL-2 regimen on days 1 to 5 and 8 to 12. Note that the IL-2 here is at a dose of 7.5 million IU/m²/day, *not* 21.6 million IU/m²/day. Maintenance IL-2 administration follows the same guidelines as that with IL-2 alone. This regimen is well tolerated even by elderly individuals, and we have used it in several such patients to maintain a clinical response for more than 2 years.

## REFERENCES

1. Rosenberg SA, Lotze MT, Yang JC, et al. Experience with the use of high-dose interleukin-2 in the treatment of 652 cancer patients. Ann Surg 1989;210:474–84.
2. Rosenberg SA, Lotze MT, Yang JC, et al. Prospective randomized trial of high-dose interleukin-2 alone or in conjunction with lymphokine-activated killer cells for the treatment of patients with advanced cancer [published erratum appears in J Natl Cancer Inst 1993;85:1091]. J Natl Cancer Inst 1993;85:622–32.
3. Mitchell MS, Kempf RA, Harel W, et al. Effectiveness and tolerability of low-dose cyclophosphamide and low-dose intravenous interleukin-2 in disseminated melanoma. J Clin Oncol 1988;6:409–24.
4. Mitchell MS. Chemotherapy in combination with biomodulation: a 5-year experience with cyclophosphamide and interleukin-2. Semin Oncol 1992;19:80–7.
5. Sleijfer DT, Janssen RA, Buter J, et al. Phase II study of subcutaneous interleukin-2 in unselected patients with advanced renal cell cancer on an outpatient basis. J Clin Oncol 1992;10:1119–23.
6. Atzpodien J, Kirchner H. The outpatient use of recombinant human interleukin-2 and interferon alfa-2b in advanced malignancies. Eur J Cancer 1991;27:Suppl 4:S88–91.
7. Rosenberg SA, Lotze MT, Yang JC, et al. Combination therapy with interleukin-2 and alpha-interferon for the treatment of patients with advanced cancer. J Clin Oncol 1989;7:1863–74.

## Interferon-α

### EFFICACY

Two pharmaceutical companies produce interferon-alfa (INF-α); the products differ from each other by one amino acid but appear to be identical in their activity. Intron A (interferon alfa-2b) is manufactured by Schering-Plough, whereas Hoffmann-LaRoche produces Roferon-A (interferon alfa-2a). Interferon alfa is officially approved for use by the FDA in patients 18 years of age or older. It is useful in the treatment of hairy cell leukemia,[1] which is the indication for which the FDA originally approved it. Only 2 million IU/m² SC or IM three times per week is required for this highly sensitive tumor. Interferon alfa is also useful for the treatment of low-grade lymphomas, chronic myelogenous leukemia, and multiple myeloma. In general, interferon alfa is of relatively greater value for the treatment of hematologic malignancies, even though the absolute number of such malignancies is small.[2-4]

In solid tumors, INF-α also has activity, although perhaps less than in hematologic malignancies.[2] High-dose INF-α, that is, 20 million IU/m² intravenously for 1 week, followed by 10 million IU/m² SC three times per week for the remainder of a year, has been approved for use in preventing recurrence of melanoma following resection of stage III (lymph node–positive) disease. Although evidence on extension of survival is still conflicting, with one study showing improvement and another none, improvement in relapse-free survival was established in two studies. A national trial in progress comparing the combination of "low-dose" interferon alfa in combination with Melacine melanoma vaccine with high-dose INF-α seeks to determine whether only the high-dose regimen is effective in this stage of melanoma.* INF-α is also used in acquired immunodeficiency syndrome (AIDS)–related Kaposi's sarcoma at 30 million IU/m² three times per week SC or IM. INF-α is also part of a successful regimen for the treatment of renal cell carcinoma.

Chronic hepatitis B, which is a precursor to hepatoma, particularly in Asia, is also treatable with interferon alfa at a dose of 30 to 35 million IU/week.

## PHARMACOLOGY

The interferons are a family of molecules with pleiotropic activity on viral replication and tumor cells. Interferon alfa is produced by recombinant DNA technology, with a human leukocyte IFN-α gene inserted into *E. coli*. It has a molecular weight of 19,271 d and is water soluble. After subcutaneous or intramuscular injection, peak concentrations are reached in 3 to 12 hours. INF-α has an elimination half-life of 3 hours. After IV administration, peak concentrations are reached at the end of the infusion, with an elimination half-life of 2 hours. INF-α was undetectable 4 hours after IV administration but persisted until 16 hours after subcutaneous or intramuscular administration.

Although the exact mechanisms of action leading to beneficial activity on the course of cancer are unknown, effects such as inhibition of tumor cell replication, stimulation of macrophages and natural killer cells, upregulation of tumor antigens and major histocompatibility complex molecules on tumor cells, and direct augmentation of specific lymphocyte-mediated cytotoxicity against tumor cells may all contribute to its efficacy.

## TOXICITY

Toxic effects include fever, headache, fatigue, myalgia, mental depression, anorexia, nausea, hypotension, leukopenia,

thrombocytopenia, abnormal liver function test results (chemical hepatitis), and paresthesias.[5] These effects are generally dose-related and may range from severe to minimal. Paresthesias have occasionally forced discontinuation of treatment when they proved unrelated to dose. Mental depression bordering on suicidal ideation has been related to high-dose therapy, and patients with a history of depression should probably be excluded from that form of treatment.

## DOSAGE AND ADMINISTRATION

INF-α is supplied as a powder in several dosage strengths, with accompanying water for injection. For example, interferon alfa-2b is supplied as 3 million, 5 million, 10 million, 18 million, 25 million, and 50 million IU/vial. Most forms of interferon alfa must be reconstituted and injected by syringe, but "pens" are now available that contain the material in a form suitable for injection at various dosages that are chosen by turning a dial on the barrel.

The dosage schedules used in various diseases have already been discussed. Many schedules of INF-α were used to treat solid tumors, but some attempt was made later to study dose-response relationships. It is interesting that high doses of interferon alfa suppress immunologic functions, whereas lower doses are immunostimulatory to macrophage and natural killer cell activity. Hairy cell leukemia is the most sensitive of the tumors, requiring very small doses, but the treatment of metastatic melanoma and renal cell carcinoma does not require very large doses either. The schedule used in the successful adjunctive trial against melanoma was derived from a South African study that used very high dose therapy, but it is uncertain whether such high doses are absolutely required.

## REFERENCES

1. Ratain MJ, Vardiman JW, Golomb HM. The role of interferon in the treatment of hairy cell leukemia. Semin Oncol 1986;13:21–8.
2. Kirkwood JM, Ernstoff ME. Potential applications of the interferons in oncology. Semin Oncol 1986;13:48–56.
3. Brown SL, Miller RA, Horning SJ, et al. Treatment of B-cell lymphomas with anti-idiotype antibodies alone and in combination with alpha interferon. Blood 1989;73:651–61.
4. VanderMolen LA, Steis RG, Duffey PL, et al. Low- versus high-dose interferon alfa-2a in relapsed indolent non-Hodgkin's lymphoma. J Natl Cancer Inst 1990;82:235–8.
5. Quesada JR, Talpaz M, Rios A, et al. Clinical toxicity of interferons in cancer patients: a review. J Clin Oncol 1986;4:234–43.

## Trastuzumab (Herceptin)

### EFFICACY

Trastuzumab (Herceptin, Genentech) is a genetically engineered, humanized (chimeric) mouse monoclonal antibody to c-*erb*B2/*neu* (HER-2/*neu*) extracellular domain protein. It has caused clinical responses in approximately 15% of patients with breast cancer. A complete response rate of 2% has been observed, with the remainder partial responses. In combination with paclitaxel, cisplatin, or doxorubicin,

---

*Melacine melanoma vaccine, discussed in Chapter 9, was approved for use in Canada in November 1999 too late for inclusion in this chapter.

response rates approaching 25% have been observed, but no formal randomized comparison has been made with trastuzumab alone to confirm an additive effect of chemotherapy. Since approximately 20 to 30% of women with breast cancer have the HER-2/*neu* oncogene, and approximately 20% of them respond to trastuzumab, 4% of all women with breast cancer benefit from the monoclonal antibody. However, from a different perspective, patients with the oncogene—which usually confers a poorer prognosis—who have exhausted cytotoxic therapies and are still viable now have an alternative treatment of potential benefit.

## PHARMACOLOGY

Trastuzumab binds to the HER-2/*neu* p185 extracellular domain protein with considerable affinity and specificity. It is an IgG1κ antibody containing human framework regions with the mouse variable regions that bind to the target protein. It is produced in Chinese hamster ovary cells and has a serum half-life of 5.8 days at therapeutic doses. No change in this half-life was found in patients with diminished renal function or advanced age. Trastuzumab inhibits proliferation of human tumor cells that overexpress HER-2/*neu,* and can mediate antibody-dependent cellular cytotoxicity.

## TOXICITY

Anaphylactic reactions have not been observed because the antibody is essentially a human immunoglobulin despite its origin as a mouse antibody. In fact, side effects are generally mild, including chills, fever, pain, asthenia, nausea, vomiting, diarrhea, increased cough, headache, dyspnea, infection, rhinitis, and insomnia.[1] However, in a study with cisplatin and trastuzumab in combination, the toxicity was no different and no greater than that of cisplatin alone.[2] In combination with anthracyclines, it has been reported that cardiotoxicity, relatively uncommon with trastuzumab alone, is increased. Class III to class IV cardiac dysfunction was found in 19% of patients who received anthracyclines and cyclophosphamide with trastuzumab. It is best to exert extreme caution when using the antibody in this setting with combination chemotherapy or with anthracyclines alone. Leukopenia, anemia, diarrhea, and abdominal pain were also increased in combination with chemotherapy. Approval was granted by the FDA for the use of trastuzumab alone in breast cancer patients previously treated with chemotherapy. Approval for use of trastuzumab with paclitaxel was granted for breast cancer patients who had not received chemotherapy.

## DOSAGE AND ADMINISTRATION

Trastuzumab is supplied as a lyophilized sterile powder containing 440 mg trastuzumab per vial under vacuum. Included in the same carton is 30 ml of bacteriostatic water for injection containing 1.1% benzyl alcohol. The standard schedule consists of a loading dose of 4 mg/kg IV followed by weekly IV doses of 2 mg/kg. Variations on this schedule include a loading dose of 250 mg IV and weekly doses of 100 mg IV when the mAb is combined with chemotherapy.[2] Doses larger than 500 mg have not been given.

## REFERENCES

1. Goldenberg MM. Trastuzumab, a recombinant DNA-derived humanized monoclonal antibody, a novel agent for the treatment of metastatic breast cancer. Clin Ther 1999;309–18.
2. Pegram MD, Lipton A, Hayes DF, et al. Phase II study of receptor-enhanced chemosensitivity using recombinant humanized anti-p185HER2/neu monoclonal antibody plus cisplatin in patients with HER2/neu overexpressing metastatic breast cancer refractory to chemotherapy treatment. J Clin Oncol 1999;16:2659–71.

# Rituximab (Rituxan; Anti-CD20 Monoclonal Antibody)

## EFFICACY

Rituximab targets the CD20 marker on B lymphomas. More than 90% of B-cell lymphomas and chronic lymphocytic leukemias express CD20, as do 50% of pre–B-cell acute lymphoblastic leukemias. CD20 is absent from pre-B cells, hematopoietic stem cells, normal plasma cells, and other normal tissues. CD20 is not normally shed from the cell surface and so presents a stable marker of the B-cell lineage. Responses have been obtained in 48% of patients with relapsed indolent low-grade or follicular lymphomas. Six percent of responses were complete responses, and the remainder were partial responses.[1] In this pivotal multicenter study, the time to onset of response was 50 days, and the median duration of response was projected to be 10 to 12 months. The mechanisms of action of the antibody are probably several, including antibody-dependent cell-mediated cytotoxicity and direct apoptotic effects on the tumor cells, and perhaps complement-mediated cytotoxicity, all of which have been shown in vitro.

## PHARMACOLOGY

Rituximab is a humanized (chimeric), genetically engineered mouse monoclonal antibody to the CD20 marker on B cells, which is also present on B-cell lymphomas. It is produced in Chinese hamster ovary cells and purified by affinity and ion-exchange column chromatography. Rituximab is an IgGκ monoclonal antibody, with mouse light and heavy chain variable region sequences but human constant region sequences. Its approximate molecular weight is 145,000 d. Since rituximab is largely a human antibody, it does not generate human antimouse antibodies (<1% of patients) and would be expected to be cleared at approximately the same rate as native human Ig, with a half-life of 7 days. In patients with lymphomas, however, the clearance of a first infusion is much more rapid, approximately 60 hours, because of attachment to tumor tissues and normal B cells. After the fourth infusion, a half-life of 174 hours, or approximately 7 days, was observed. There is a great variability in serum half-life in all patients because of variability of tumor burden. Normal B cells in circulation and in lymph nodes are rapidly depleted after IV administration of rituximab. This depletion is sustained for 6 to 9 months after treatment in the great majority of patients. Recovery of B-cell levels usually occurs by 12 months. IgG and IgM serum levels were reduced in approximately 14% of patients 5 to 11 months after treatment; the remainder showed no reductions.

## TOXICITY

Fever, chills, and rigors were found in most patients (80%) during the first infusion of rituximab. Nausea, urticaria, pruritus, bronchospasm, fatigue, headache, dyspnea, and a feeling of swelling of the throat or tongue were also frequent. These effects occurred within 30 to 120 minutes of the beginning of the infusion and resolved with slowing or interruption of the infusion. Supportive care with IV saline, diphenhydramine (Benadryl), and acetaminophen was also helpful. During subsequent infusions, the incidence of infusion-related toxicity decreased to 40%. Anaphylactic reac-

tions such as angioedema and bronchospasm were found in a minority of patients (8 to 14%) and were treated with epinephrine. Serious anaphylaxis (angioedema) was found in only one patient.

## DOSAGE AND ADMINISTRATION

Rituximab is supplied in sterile, preservative-free, single-use vials of 100 mg and 500 mg to be stored at 2° to 8° C. The recommended dose is 375 mg/m² given as an IV infusion, once weekly for four doses on days 1, 8, 15, and 22. IV push or boluses should not be given.

## REFERENCE

1. McLaughlin P, Grillo-Lopez AJ, Link BK, et al. Rituximab chimeric anti-CD20 monoclonal antibody therapy for relapsed indolent lymphoma: half of patients respond to a four-dose treatment program. J Clin Oncol 1998;16:2825–33.

# CHAPTER 12

# METHODS AND PROCEDURES OF CANCER CHEMOTHERAPY

## PREPARATION, ADMINISTRATION, AND DISPOSAL OF ANTINEOPLASTIC AGENTS

• Gail Sartor • Sheila Stinnett

Since the initiation of chemotherapy, side effects involving patients receiving chemotherapeutic agents have been well documented in the literature. Only years later, however, did it become apparent there was risk to health care workers as well. In the late 1970s and early 1980s, medical journals began publishing letters to the editor indicating the rising concerns of health care workers.[1–3] Studies of nurses administering chemotherapy and pharmacists preparing these agents began appearing in the literature.[4–6] These studies suggested mutagenicity in urine and chromosome changes, raising questions about the risk of handling these agents. Some studies supported the causal relationship between handling chemotherapeutic agents and exposure to them, whereas others did not.[7, 8] It became increasingly evident that exposure to antineoplastic agents was potentially hazardous to personnel and caregivers, and studies now show that many chemotherapeutic agents may cause irritation to those preparing these drugs for administration.[9, 10]

## Areas Affected by Specific Agents

### SKIN

Mechlorethamine (nitrogen mustard) is a strong irritant and blistering agent.[11] Precautions must be taken to avoid spills

to the skin because chemical burns may occur. Inhalation of aerosol may cause irritation to mucous and bronchial membranes. Other agents may irritate the skin, including bis-chloroethyl-nitrosourea (BCNU)[12, 13] and fluorouracil.[14]

### EYES

Most incidents of eye irritation have been reported following accidental splashing of chemicals into the eye. It was reported that methotrexate caused tearing and conjunctival irritation in three nurses after they handled this drug.[10] Other agents that have been documented as causing ocular irritation are vinblastine,[15, 16] etoposide, and carmustine.[17] All instances of ocular irritation followed accidental exposure to the eye by splashing, either when mixing or administering these drugs.

### SYSTEMIC REACTIONS

Many of the reports of systemic side effects were reported in the late 1970s and early 1980s. In 1976, Gundersen[18] reported respiratory symptoms and urticaria in two nurses who prepared and administered methotrexate and cyclophosphamide. One nurse experienced relief of symptoms by using a mask and ventilation. In another report, pharmacists reported lightheadedness, dizziness, and facial flushing while preparing dacarbazine and cisplatin.[19] Use of a horizontal laminar flow hood decreased these symptoms.

## ALLERGIC REACTION

Repeated exposure has been indicated in sensitized factory workers who worked in the production of melphalan.[20] Symptoms included asthma, dermatitis, rhinitis, and sinusitis. One nurse reported urticaria, rash, and difficulty in breathing when handling an investigational substance; her symptoms increased with subsequent exposure (personal communication, 1999).

## Methods of Exposure

An increasing number of chemotherapy exposures and a decreased use of protective measures have been positively correlated with the number of reported acute symptoms.[21] As documented later in the section on safe handling of cytotoxic drugs, inhalation of chemotherapy agents can occur during preparation, initial administration, and cessation of therapy as well as during disposal of equipment at any time. Inhalation may also occur during a spill or when transporting these chemicals. Handling excreta poses another risk for inhalation and direct contact exposure.

Exposure during preparation and administration can occur at any time during the process. Examples of the opportunities for risk include the following: when removing medication from vials; when opening ampules; when transferring drugs from syringes to bags; while connecting bags, bottles, or tubing to the patient; from tubing that is broken or leaking; and by overfilling syringes.[21] Disposal of syringes, bags, and tubing creates additional exposure to staff, as does disposing of linen soaked in body fluids of people who have recently received chemotherapy. Ingestion may occur by inadvertently splashing medication into the face or mouth and through contact with contaminated food, food containers, or smoking materials. Absorption can occur through direct exposure to the skin, by needle stick, or by direct contact with the eye.

## Protection for Personnel

Compliance with protective standards is clearly warranted because studies reveal that 40% of nurses do not routinely wear protective gear when working with antineoplastics.[22, 23] To decrease the risk to medical personnel preparing, administering, and disposing of cytotoxic agents, worker protection guidelines were published in 1983 by the U.S. Public Health Service.[24] Since then, guidelines reflecting the current knowledge have been published and revised by an organization of hospital pharmacists and the Oncology Nursing Society (ONS).

## Safe Handling, Preparation, Administration, and Disposal of Cytotoxic Agents

The safe handling of antineoplastic agents includes certain practices in all settings (Table 12–1). Any personnel involved with administering and disposing of cytotoxic agents must wear protective clothing whenever they come in contact with these agents. Appropriate protective gear consists of gowns, gloves, and masks suitable to the task. The ONS Guidelines, published in 1996,[25] reflect the accumulated knowledge assembled at this time and offer general recommendations for safe practice.

### GOWNS

Gowns should be disposable, nonpermeable, and lint-free. They should have a closed front with the opening down the back, long sleeves, and cuffs that fit snugly around the wrists. Laboratory coats or other absorbent gowns used for patient care do not meet these criteria.[26]

### GLOVES

Suggested gloves are the latex, powder-free ones that are recommended by the manufacturer for this purpose. Gloves should be changed every 30 to 60 minutes or when torn or contaminated by cytotoxic agents. Any person with a latex allergy should use a glove made of nitrile or a double glove consisting of a polyvinyl chloride (PVC) glove under a latex glove.[27] Hands should be washed before and after wearing gloves. Care should be taken not to snap the glove when removing.

### MASKS

Cytotoxic agents should be prepared under a class II or III vertical airflow biologic safety cabinet.[28] Eye protection and face wear should be worn if splashes are anticipated or if sprays or aerosols are to be used.

### PERSONNEL ADMINISTERING CYTOTOXIC AGENTS

Only persons who have been trained in the administration of cytotoxic agents should administer these agents.[29–31] Personnel should wear appropriate gown, gloves, and facemask as necessary.[29] When administering cytotoxic agents, the Occupational Safety and Health Administration (OSHA), American Society of Hospital Pharmacists, and ONS suggest the following procedure: The necessary equipment (absorbent pad, alcohol swabs, medication, and gauze pads) is assembled in a resealable plastic bag, which is used afterward for the disposal of the used equipment. Also the appropriate gown, gloves, and mask are prepared.

Hands should be washed before and after wearing gloves. Gloves and gown should be changed immediately if they become torn or contaminated. To administer cytotoxic

*Table 12–1.* **Guidelines for Safe Handling and Disposal of Antineoplastic Agents**

*Drug Preparation*

1. All antineoplastic drugs should be prepared by specially trained individuals in a centralized area to minimize interruptions and risk of contamination
2. Drugs are prepared in a class II biologic safety cabinet (vertical laminar airflow hood) with vents to the outside, if possible. The blower is left on 24 hours a day, 7 days per week. The hood is serviced regularly according to the manufacturer's recommendations
3. Eating, drinking, smoking, and applying cosmetics in the drug preparation area are prohibited
4. The work surface is covered with a plastic absorbent pad to minimize contamination. This pad is changed immediately in the event of contamination and at the completion of drug preparation each day or shift
5. The prescribed drug is prepared using aseptic technique according to the physician's orders, other pharmaceutical resources, or both
6. Disposable surgical latex unpowdered gloves are used when handling the drugs. Gloves should be changed hourly, or immediately if torn or punctured
7. A disposable long-sleeved gown made of lint-free fabric with knitted cuffs and closed front is worn during drug preparation
8. A thermoplastic (Plexiglas) face shield or goggles and a powered air-purifying respirator should be used if a biologic safety cabinet is not available
9. Priming of all IV tubing is carried out under the protection of the hood because exposure can result when connecting and disconnecting IV tubing; when injecting the drug into the IV line; when removing air from the syringe or infusion line; and when leakage occurs at the tubing, syringe, or stopcock connection
10. Other measures to guard against drug leakage during drug preparation include venting the vial and using large-bore needles, Luer-lok fittings, and sterile gauze or sponge around the neck of the vial during needle withdrawal. Aerosolization may also be minimized by attaching an aerosol protection device (Cytoguard, Bristol-Myers Squibb, Princeton, NJ 08543) to the vial of drug before adding the diluent
11. Once reconstituted, the drug is labeled according to institutional policies and procedures; the label should include the drug's vesicant properties and antineoplastic drug warning
12. Antineoplastic drugs are transported in an impervious packing material and are marked with a distinctive warning label
13. Personnel responsible for drug transport are knowledgeable of procedures to be followed in the event of drug spillage

*Drug Administration*

1. Chemotherapeutic agents are administered by registered professional nurses who have been specially trained and designated as qualified, according to specific institutional policies and procedures
2. Before administering the drugs, the nurse ensures that informed consent has been given and clarifies any misconceptions the patient might have regarding the drugs and their side effects
3. Appropriate laboratory results are evaluated and found to be within acceptable levels
4. Measures to minimize side effects of the drugs are carried out before drug administration (hydration, antiemetics, antianxiety agents, and patient comfort)
5. An appropriate route for drug administration is ensured according to the physician's order
6. Personal protective equipment is worn, including disposable latex surgical gloves and a disposable gown made of a lint-free, low-permeability fabric with a closed front, long sleeves, and elastic or knit closed cuffs
7. The work surface is protected with a disposable absorbent pad
8. Drugs are administered according to established institutional policies and procedures
9. Documentation of drug administration, including adverse reactions, is made in the patient's medical record
10. A mechanism for identification of the patients receiving antineoplastic agents is established for the 48-hour period after drug dispensing
11. Disposable surgical unpowdered latex gloves and a disposable gown are worn when handling body secretions, such as blood, vomitus, or excreta, from patients who received chemotherapy drugs within the previous 48 hours
12. In the event of accidental exposure, contaminated gloves and gown should be removed immediately and discarded according to official procedures
13. Wash the contaminated skin with soap and water
14. An eye that is accidentally exposed to chemotherapy should be flooded with water or isotonic eye wash for at least 5 minutes
15. After any exposure, medical evaluation must be obtained as soon as possible and the incident documented according to institutional policies and procedures

*Drug Disposal*

1. Regardless of the setting (hospital, ambulatory care, or home), all equipment and unused drugs are treated as hazardous and are disposed of according to the institution's policies and procedures
2. All contaminated equipment, including needles, are disposed of intact to prevent aerosolization, leaks, and spills
3. All contaminated materials used in drug preparation are disposed of in leakproof, punctureproof containers with a distinctive warning label and are placed in a sealable 4-mil-thickness polyethylene or 2-mil-thickness polypropylene bag with appropriate labeling
4. Linen contaminated with bodily secretions of patients who have received chemotherapy within the previous 48 hours is placed in a specially marked laundry bag, which is placed in an impervious bag that is marked with a distinctive warning label
5. In the event of a spill, personnel should don double surgical latex unpowdered gloves; eye protection; and a disposable gown made of a lint-free, low-permeability fabric with a closed front, long sleeves, and elastic or knit closed cuffs
6. Small amounts of liquids are cleaned up with gauze pads, whereas larger spills (>5 ml) are cleaned up with absorbent pads
7. Small amounts of solids or spills involving powder are cleaned up with damp cloths or absorbent gauze pads
8. The spill area is cleaned three times with a detergent followed by clean water
9. Broken glassware and disposable contaminated materials are placed in a leakproof, punctureproof container, then placed in a sealable 4-mil polyethylene or 2-mil polypropylene bag and marked with a distinctive warning label
10. Contaminated reusable items are washed by specially trained personnel wearing double surgical unpowdered latex gloves
11. The spill should be documented according to established institutional policies and procedures

From Goodman M. Delivery of cancer chemotherapy. In: Baird SB, McCorkle R, Grant M, eds. Cancer nursing: a comprehensive textbook. Philadelphia: WB Saunders, 1991:291–320.

agents, absorbent pads are placed on the work area. If using the side arm of an intravenous (IV) set, a gauze pad wrapped around the insertions site should be used to prevent possible aerosolization of the agent. All syringes should be Luer-Lok and disposed of immediately into the resealable plastic bag. If the cytotoxic agent is in an IV bag or bottle, the gauze pad should be used when spiking the container (all IV tubing should be primed in the hood and not at the bedside). All containers, syringes, and tubing should be collected in a resealable plastic bag to be disposed of in the appropriate container outside the patient's room or in a utility room. A spill kit should be readily available in the event of a spill.[25, 28, 29]

## HANDLING BODILY FLUIDS

OSHA and ASHP have accepted a standard of 48 hours as the time frame that bodily fluids may contain cytotoxic waste. The time can vary, however, depending on the agent. When handling bodily fluids, personnel or caregivers should wear gloves and gowns for the first 48 hours. If there is a possibility of a splash, face and eye protection should be worn. Gloves should be used only once, and gowns should be discarded when contaminated with bodily fluids. Bodily waste discarded into the toilet should be flushed twice, especially if there is low water pressure.

## HANDLING LINEN

OSHA and ASHP[28, 29] recommend the following when handling contaminated linen: Personnel and caregivers should wear the appropriate gloves and gown. Contaminated disposable linens should be disposed of in a puncture-proof container. Nondisposable linen should be bagged in a heavy plastic laundry bag that is appropriately labeled "chemo waste." In institutions, linen is usually handled by laundry staff wearing gloves, face protection, and heavy gowns, and the linen is laundered twice, which is sufficient for soiled laundry. In the home, linen should be washed separately twice with detergent after being collected in the manner just described.[9, 30, 32]

## Disposal Procedures

OSHA and ASHP recommend all equipment used to prepare and administer cytotoxic agents be disposed of in specifically marked puncture-proof and leakproof containers. In an institution, these containers are collected by assigned trained staff, stored in a secured area, and labeled as cytotoxic waste to be disposed of by a commercial disposal company that handles only toxic waste. The contents are either incinerated or buried. In the home, contaminated syringes and equipment used to administer cytotoxic medication should be collected in the same manner as in an institution, placed in a secured container, and transported back to the agency for disposal. Disposal of hazardous waste is controlled by local, state, and federal agencies.[29, 30]

The following procedure is recommended during an acci-

dental spill: Spill kits, either commercial or assembled, should be available in any area where cytotoxic agents are given, including the home setting. Commercially available spill kits contain the attire and equipment to clean up a spill. Spills are defined as small (<5 ml or 5 g happening outside a hood) or large (>5 ml or 5 g). Only specially trained personnel should handle a spill, to ensure the safety of personnel and patients.[31]

## Role of the Pharmacist

Most chemotherapy is prepared by pharmacists using aseptic technique in a biologic safety cabinet. Aseptic technique is a method of preparation that minimizes the chance for contamination of sterile products. Sterile products are products that, by definition, are free of living organisms; they also are void of bacterial toxins and particles that can cause fever. Special techniques and equipment are necessary to ensure that all IV medications are sterile. Aseptic technique and the use of the biologic safety cabinet are the two most important safeguards for health care workers during antineoplastic drug preparation.[33]

The basic elements of aseptic technique are designed to ensure preparation of a sterile product. Touch contamination is the most frequent cause of contamination. The operator should work at least 6 inches inside the airflow hood. A direct open path must be maintained between the filter and the area inside the hood where the work is performed. The syringe tip and plunger of the syringe should not be touched. Needle packages must be opened in the hood. Needles should never be swabbed with alcohol. Rubber stoppers on vials and the necks of ampules and the injection port of the IV bag should be cleaned with alcohol before use. The injection ports should be positioned toward the high efficiency particulate air (HEPA) filter when the admixture is prepared. The IV tubing should be attached to the IV bag while inside the biologic safety cabinet or hood.

Room air may be highly contaminated, and the biologic safety cabinet by itself cannot ensure a sterile product. Class II biologic safety cabinets are designed to protect the product, the operator, and the environment from contamination and are widely used in hospitals, laboratories, and pharmaceutical facilities. A common feature of all safety cabinets is the HEPA filter, which removes particulates and microorganisms from the environment and allows clean laminar airflow at a constant velocity over the product in the cabinet. The filter does not remove vapors or gases. A HEPA filter is able to trap 9997 to 9999 of every 10,000 particles having a diameter greater than 0.3 μ.[34]

In a typical biologic safety cabinet used for preparing chemotherapy, 30% of the air is exhausted through a HEPA filter from a common plenum, whereas the remaining 70% is recirculated through the supply HEPA filter back into the work area. HEPA-filtered air descends through the work area in a vertical laminar flow. All chemotherapy preparations should take place in a class II biologic safety cabinet or vertical laminar airflow hood that meets the standards set by the National Sanitation Foundation.[35] The biologic safety cabinet draws room air into the front intake grill, which prevents contaminants from entering the work space. The room air passes through the HEPA filter and is diffused vertically to the drug preparation area. At the work surface, the clean air splits so that half is drawn into the front intake grill and half into the rear exhaust grill. The contaminated air in the actual drug preparation area is exhausted through the front and rear grills and mixes below the work surface. The air beneath the surface is then passed through an exhaust duct and up the rear of the biologic safety cabinet until it reaches the top, where a portion of the air is recycled back into the preparation area and a portion is expelled through the exhaust HEPA filter. The vertical laminar flow hood is the only hood that should be used to prepare chemotherapeutic agents. Even if the horizontal laminar airflow hood is turned off, there can be residual cytotoxic material left behind that is blown into the operator's face once the hood is turned on again.

Compounding of cytotoxic drugs should be done on a plastic-backed paper liner that has absorptive properties. This liner allows any leaks or spills to be absorbed onto the preparation mat and keeps the chemotherapeutic drugs off the stainless steel biologic safety cabinet surface. This mat is replaced at the end of each work shift or after a spill. Preparation mats do not cover intake or exhaust grills in the biologic safety cabinet.

All doses of cytotoxic drugs should be dispensed in a clear, sealable heavy plastic bag or container to prevent accidental exposure through punctures or leaks. These doses should be delivered by hand and not through mechanical devices, such as pneumatic tubes. Any light-sensitive materials should be placed in an amber bag, then placed in the sealable plastic bag. Cytotoxic products should be clearly labeled as cytotoxic material and should include cautions for safe handling and disposal. There are inherent risks associated with the preparation and handling of cytotoxic materials. If the guidelines for safe handling and preparation are followed, however, the health care worker and the environment will be adequately protected.

## Choosing an Appropriate Dosage

### BODY SURFACE AREA

Most chemotherapy doses are calculated on the basis of body surface area (BSA), and they are expressed in milligrams per square meter. BSA is generally determined from the patient's weight and height using some type of nomogram (see Appendix A).[36] The BSA provides a method of determining a patient's dose by minimizing variations in similar-sized individuals resulting from weight; it also provides for dosage differences between adults and children.[37] Actual weights and heights should be obtained before each course of chemotherapy. Although there is no concrete agreement in the medical community, the general consensus about weight recommends that actual weight be used in the initial chemotherapy dose except when using high-dose regimens as for bone marrow transplant or in instances when dosing a person greater than 30% ideal body weight.[38]

### ALTERNATIVE METHODS FOR CHOOSING DOSAGE

In the case of specific drugs (e.g., carboplatin, methotrexate, and leucovorin), alternative methods of dosing have been evaluated to optimize dosing for the individual patient based on the pharmacokinetics of the drug. *Pharmacokinetics* is the study of drug absorption, distribution, metabolism, and excretion. *Pharmacodynamics* is the study of dose-response relationships. Each of these concepts has contributed to the understanding of therapeutic drug monitoring by helping to devise ways to individualize drug dosing in patients with cancer. The interest in these fields has led to the routine use of mathematical formulas developed by Calvert and Chatelet to determine doses for carboplatin.[39] The mathematical formulas they developed were based on pretreatment patient characteristics and desired drug effect determined by *area under the curve* (AUC).[40] AUC represents total drug exposure over time, and clearance predicts elimination of the drug from the body. Studies by Collins and colleagues[40] showed that AUC dosing is more closely correlated with drug toxicity than is a dose based on BSA.

AUC is calculated by plotting a graph of the plasma level of a drug over time and measuring the area beneath the plotted curve. This type of dosing establishes the optimal dose by showing the relationship between drug toxicity and the response rates in cancer patients, and it provides a guideline for establishing the optimal dose of carboplatin in the individual patient. Studies done by Egorin and associates[41] and Calvert and coworkers[42] showed that one could adjust carboplatin exposure based on pretreatment renal function. Calvert and coworkers[42] predicted the carboplatin AUC that would be produced by a given dose of the drug. By measuring the AUC in patients who had various levels of renal function, the investigators found that the predicted AUC equaled the actual findings later measured. The mathematical formulas they developed were based on pretreatment patient characteristics and desired drug effect determined by AUC. AUC dosing provides a reliable method to reduce the risk of carboplatin toxicity.

## Routes of Administration

The IV route is the most commonly used route for administering chemotherapy. It can be IV push, IV side arm, IV piggyback, or continuous IV infusion.[43] IV administration depends on a reliable IV route of access. Specialized techniques for obtaining intravascular access are discussed in the next section (Vascular Access Catheters and Devices). The most feared complication of IV drug administration is extravasation, which can be devastating with some drugs. The management of drug extravasation is discussed in Chapter 8.

### INTRAVENOUS PUSH

The IV push route is performed with two syringes, one with medication and the other with a flush solution, typically saline. After venipuncture, the flush syringe is attached to the needle, and a small amount of normal saline (3 to 5 ml) is injected to establish patency of the vein. The medication syringe is then attached, and the medicine is injected at the proper rate for that medicine. The flush syringe is reattached, and 5 to 10 ml of saline is pushed through to clear the line.

The push method is cost-effective because it requires a relatively small amount of time to administer.

## INTRAVENOUS SIDE ARM

The IV side arm method is preferred for vesicant administration.[44] IV tubing is attached to the vein with a free-flowing IV solution running wide open. The medication syringe is injected through the side arm (y-site), and the chemotherapy is infused. The site of administration is continually viewed by the person administering the chemotherapy in case of extravasation. The free-flowing IV solution further dilutes the chemotherapy, making it less irritating or caustic to the vein. It is important to flush the line with 20 ml of saline before administering another drug.

## INTRAVENOUS PIGGYBACK

When medications require a larger volume of dilution and longer periods of delivery, the IV piggyback method is preferred. This method is not used for vesicant medications because the person administering is not always available to observe the site. The chemotherapeutic medicine is put into a 50- to 250-ml bag of solution and administered over a specific time period. After administration is complete, the primary IV solution flushes the vein.

## CONTINUOUS INTRAVENOUS INFUSIONS

The continuous IV infusion is used for chemotherapeutic drug administration lasting more than 24 hours. The infusion period varies from 1 day to 7 days to 10 (or more) days. This method can be used for vesicant and nonvesicant medicines. Normally, vesicant medications are administered through a central line. This type of IV therapy most often employs a portable pump or implantable device that allows for patient mobility.

## REGIONAL CHEMOTHERAPY

Systemic therapy is aimed at attaining the maximum cytotoxic effect without toxicity to normal tissues, whereas regional chemotherapy is aimed at delivering chemotherapy directly to the blood vessel or cavity in which the tumor is located. Intrathecal, intra-arterial, intracavitary, and intraosseous routes are examples of this method of drug delivery. Regardless of the route of administration, specific guidelines for safe handling and disposal of chemotherapeutic agents must be followed.

## SUGGESTIONS FOR ADDITIONAL READING

American Society of Clinical Oncology. Criteria for facilities and personnel for the administration of parenteral systemic antineoplastic therapy. J Clin Oncol 1997;15:3416–7.

Carmignani SS, Raymond GG. Safe handling of cytotoxic drugs in the physician's office: a procedure manual model. Oncol Nurs Forum 1997;24:1 Suppl:41–8.

Bertelli G. Prevention and management of extravasation of cytotoxic drugs. Drug Saf 1995;12:245–5.

## REFERENCES

1. Donner AL. Possible risk of working with antineoplastic drugs in horizontal laminar flow hoods. Am J Hosp Pharm 1978;35:900.
2. Falck K, Gröhn P, Sorsa M, et al. Mutagenicity in urine of nurses handling cytostatic drugs. Lancet 1979;1:1250–1.
3. Ng LM, Jaffe N. Possible hazards of handling antineoplastic drugs. Pediatrics 1970;46:648–9.
4. Walsvik H, Klepp O, Brøgger A. Chromosome analyses of nurses handling cytostatic agents. Cancer Treat Rep 1981;65:607–0.
5. Norppa H, Sorsa M, Vainio H, et al. Increased sister chromatid exchange frequencies in lymphocytes of nurses handling cytostatic drugs. Scand J Work Environ Health 1980;6:299–301.
6. Anderson RW, Puckett WH Jr, Dana WJ, et al. Risk of handling injectable antineoplastic agents. Am J Hosp Pharm 1982;39:1881–7.
7. Staiano N, Gallelli JF, Adamson RH, Thorgeirsson SS. Lack of mutagenic activity in urine from hospital pharmacists admixing antitumour drugs. Lancet 1981;1:615–6.
8. Stiller A, Obe G, Boll I, Pribilla W. No elevation of the frequencies of chromosomal alterations as a consequence of handling cytostatic drugs: analyses with peripheral blood and urine of hospital personnel. Mutat Res 1983;121:253–9.
9. Gullo SM. Safe handling of antineoplastic drugs: translating the recommendations into practice. 1988 [classical article]. Oncol Nurs Forum 1995;22:517–5.
10. Valanis B, Shortridge L. Oncology nursing society study of antineoplastic drugs. Oncol Nurs Forum 1985;12:Suppl:1–6.
11. Thestrup-Pedersen K, Christiansen JV, Zachariae H. Precautions for personnel applying topical nitrogen mustard to patients with mycosis fungoides. Dermatologica 1982;165:108–3.
12. Frost P, DeVita VT. Pigmentation due to a new antitumor agent: effects of topical application of BCNU. Arch Dermatol 1966;94:265–8.
13. Gottlieb JA. Hazards of handling antineoplastic drugs. Pediatrics 1971;47:480.
14. Zelickson AS, Mottaz J, Weiss LW. Effects of topical fluorouracil on normal skin. Arch Dermatol 1975;111:1301–6.
15. Cordier J, Mendelsohn P. Corneal ulceration caused by an antimitotic agent. Bull Soc Ophtalmol France 1970;70:116–22.
16. McLendon BF, Bron AJ. Corneal toxicity from vinblastine solution. Br J Ophthalmol 1978;62:97–99.
17. Dorr RT. Cancer chemotherapy handbook. 2nd ed. Norwalk, CT: Appleton & Lange, 1993.
18. Gundersen S. Precautionary measures during preparation and infusion of cytostatics. Tidsskr Nor Laegeforen 1976;96:1388.
19. Ladik CF, Stoehr GP, Maurer MA. Precautionary measures in the preparation of antineoplastics. Am J Hosp Pharm 1980;37:1184–6.
20. Nava C, Briatico Vangosa G, Forni A. [Pathological manifestations in workers engaged in the production or administration of cytostatic drugs]. Boll Chim Farm 1984;123:547–1.
21. Valanis BG, Vollmer WM, Labuhn KT, Glass AG. Acute symptoms associated with antineoplastic drug handling among nurses. Cancer Nurs 1993;16:288–95.
22. Barry LK, Booher RB. Promoting the responsible handling of antineoplastic agents in the community. Oncol Nurs Forum 1985;12:41–6.
23. Valanis B, McNeil V, Driscoll K. Staff members' compliance with their facility's antineoplastic drug handling policy. Oncol Nurs Forum 1991;18:571–576.
24. U.S. Public Health Service. NIH Publication No. 83-2621. Bethesda, Md: National Institutes of Health, 1983.
25. Oncology Nursing Society. Cancer chemotherapy guidelines and recommendations for practice. Pittsburgh: Oncology Nursing Press, 1984, 1988, 1996.
26. Laidlaw JL, Connor TH, Theiss JC, et al. Permeability of four disposable protective-clothing materials to seven antineoplastic drugs. Am J Hosp Pharm 1985;42:2449–54.
27. Jackson D. Latex allergy and anaphylaxis—what to do? J IV Nurs 1995;18:33–52.
28. Occupational Safety and Health Administration. OSHA Publication No. 8-1.1. Washington, D.C.: Department of Labor, 1986.
29. ASHP technical assistance bulletin on handling cytotoxic and hazardous drugs. Am J Hosp Pharm 1990;47:1033–49.

30. Occupational Safety and Health Administration: Work practice guidelines for personnel dealing with cytotoxic (antineoplastic) drugs. Washington, D.C.: Department of Labor, 1995.

31. Welch J, Silveira J, eds. Safe handling of cytotoxic drugs: an independent study manual. 2nd ed. Pittsburgh: Oncology Nursing Press, 1997:13.

32. McNally JC. Home care. In: Groenwald SL, ed. Cancer nursing principles and practice. 3rd ed. Boston: Jones & Bartlett 1993:1403–31.

33. Wilson IP, Solimando DA. Aseptic technique as a safety precaution in the preparation of antineoplastic agents. Hosp Pharm 1981;16:575–81.

34. The Baker Company, PO Drawer E, Sanford, ME, 1990.

35. National Study Commission on Cytotoxic Exposure. Recommendations for handling cytotoxic agents. Providence, RI: National Study Commission on Cytotoxic Exposure, 1987.

36. Dubois D, Dubois EF. A formula to estimate the approximate surface area if height and weight be known. Arch Intern Med 1916;17:863–71.

37. Brown K, Hogan CM. Chemotherapy. In: Groenwald SL, Frogge MH, Goodman M, Yarbro CH, eds. Cancer nursing: principles and practice. 2nd ed. Boston: Jones & Bartlett, 1990:230–83.

38. Gelman RS, Tormey DC, Betensky R, et al. Actual versus ideal weight in the calculation of surface area: effects on dose of 11 chemotherapy agents. Cancer Treat Rep 1987;71:907–11.

39. Egorin MJ, Van Echo DA, Tipping SJ, et al. Pharmacokinetics and dosage reduction of cisdiammine (1, 1-cyclobutane di-carboxylate)–platinum in patients with impaired renal function. Cancer Res 1984;44:5432–8.

40. Collins JM, Zaharko DS, Dedrick RL, Chabner BA. Potential roles for preclinical pharmacology in phase I clinical trials. Cancer Treat Rep 1986;70:73–80.

41. Egorin MJ, Van Echo DA, Olman EA, et al. Prospective validation of a pharmacologically based dosing scheme for the cis-diamminedichloroplatinum (II) analogue diamminecyclobutanedicarboxylatoplatinum. Cancer Res 1985;45:6502–6.

42. Calvert AH, Newell DR, Gore ME. Future directions with carboplatin: can therapeutic monitoring, high-dose administration, and hematologic support with growth factors expand the spectrum compared with cisplatin? Semin Oncol 1992;19:Suppl 2:155–63.

43. Holmes BC. Administration of cancer chemotherapy agents. In: Dorr RT, Von Hoff DD, eds. Cancer chemotherapy handbook. 2nd ed. East Norwalk, CT: Appleton & Lange, 1994:61.

44. Goodman M. Delivery of cancer chemotherapy. In: Baird SB, McCorkle R, Grant M, eds. Cancer nursing: a comprehensive textbook. Philadelphia: WB Saunders, 1991:291–320.

················································

# VASCULAR ACCESS CATHETERS AND DEVICES

• James L. Gajewski  •  Issam Raad

Central venous catheters were originally introduced to provide long-term IV hyperalimentation to patients with gastrointestinal disease.[1, 2] The use of central venous catheters has become increasingly common in oncology practice because cancer patients frequently require venipuncture for diagnostic studies and for the therapeutic administration of drugs and blood products.[1] Peripheral veins rapidly collapse or undergo thrombosis, and repeated venipuncture is a source of pain, discomfort, and psychological distress. The risk of extravasation from chemotherapeutic agents may necessitate long-term central venous access with indwelling catheters.

## Catheter Selection

Early catheters were composed of polyethylene and PVC, but these stiff materials were associated with a high rate of thrombosis.[2] Polyurethane is commonly used for short-term, percutaneously placed catheters.[3] Currently, most long-term catheters are constructed of silicone elastomer (Silastic) because this soft, biocompatible material is less damaging to the intima of the vessel.[4] Venous access catheters can be grouped as follows: (1) tunneled catheters, (2) subcutaneous devices, and (3) percutaneous catheters.

### TUNNELED CATHETERS

Tunneled catheters include the Broviac, Hickman, and Groshong catheters (Bard Access Systems, Salt Lake City, UT). They are surgically introduced into a central vein and exit the body through a small stab wound in the skin some distance from the insertion site (Fig. 12–1). Groshong catheters require weekly flushing with saline, whereas Hickman

catheters need daily flushing with heparin. The choice among Broviac, Hickman, and Groshong catheters is often a matter of personal preference because the complication rates are similar.

### IMPLANTED VENOUS ACCESS PORTS

Implanted venous access ports include devices such as the Portacath, in which the catheter is connected to a subcutaneous reservoir. These reservoirs or ports are accessed with Huber needles, which are specially designed to prevent coring of the septum. Implanted venous ports have the cosmetic advantage of being entirely subcutaneous. For patients whose

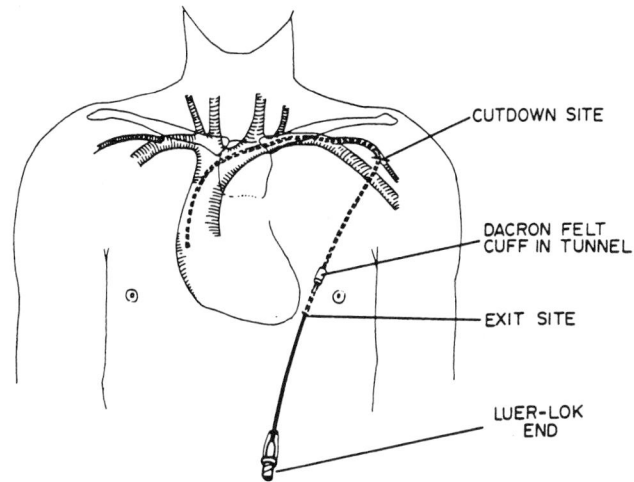

**Figure 12–1.** Proper position of Hickman, Broviac, and Groshong catheters.

central venous catheters are infrequently accessed, implanted venous ports may be preferable because of the lower infection risk.[5] Leukemia and bone marrow transplant recipients frequently require daily access to central venous catheters. Tunneled catheters spare these patients painful needle sticks and are easier to remove if the catheter becomes infected. Patients requiring daily use of access catheters are especially prone to catheter infections. Tunneled and implantable catheters are available with single and double lumens; the tunneled variety is also available with triple lumens.

## PERCUTANEOUS SILASTIC CENTRAL VENOUS CATHETERS

Percutaneous silastic central venous catheters may be placed peripherally in the basilic or cephalic vein or more centrally in the subclavian or internal jugular vein.[6–8] The costs of placing these catheters are less than those of tunneled or subcutaneous catheters. The peripherally inserted catheters can be placed by a nurse but are associated with an increased risk of local inflammation. These nontunneled, nonimplanted catheters are the easiest to remove in the event of infection or thrombus and are available with single, double, or triple lumens.

## Surgical Placement

Placement of the catheter tip in the superior vena cava at the atriocaval junction is preferred. Placement in the inferior vena cava through the saphenofemoral junction is also satisfactory but is attended by a higher infection rate. Catheters may be introduced by an open cutdown or a closed, peelaway sheath technique. The closed method using a peeled away sheath requires the introduction of a needle into either the subclavian or internal jugular veins followed by placement of a sheath through which the catheter is introduced into the vein. The sheath is then peeled away. Because this is essentially a blind technique, the complication rate for this approach has proved significantly higher in a number of series.[9, 10] The incidence of pneumothorax is approximately 6% and of subclavian vein thrombosis as high as 10%. Other documented complications include hemothorax, puncture of the subclavian artery, and injury to the brachial plexus. Rarely, deaths have been reported.

The safer and preferred method consists of cutdown of the external jugular, internal jugular, or cephalic veins. This procedure can be accomplished under local anesthesia with introduction of the catheter through a transverse venotomy. The external jugular vein, particularly the right, is the preferred vein if visible with the patient in the Trendelenburg position. In greater than 95% of attempts, a catheter can be properly positioned in the superior vena cava. Occasionally the catheter cannot be advanced past the junction of the external jugular and subclavian veins and may require a soft, floppy, vascular J wire for positioning. Suitable alternatives include the internal jugular vein, in which the catheter is introduced through a venotomy controlled by a purse-string suture. The cephalic vein is present in the deltopectoral groove but is often of insufficient caliber to accommodate double-lumen adult catheters. The cephalic vein, however, is worth considering for use with implanted ports because the reservoir can be placed over the pectoral muscle, allowing the procedure to be accomplished with one incision.

Complication rates for catheters placed by direct venous cutdown are low. There should be no incidence of pneumothorax or hemothorax, and the thrombosis rate is about 2 to 3%. After placement, a chest radiograph should be obtained to confirm placement in the superior vena cava and not the internal mammary, where there is an increased risk of hemothorax, and to rule out a pneumothorax as a result of this placement.

All tunneled catheters have a Dacron cuff, which becomes infiltrated with fibrous tissue and acts as a barrier to infection with skin organisms. Silver-impregnated cuffs have not reduced the infection risk.[11] If the Dacron cuff is positioned just beneath the skin insertion site, the catheter removal is easier. Properly maintained catheters can remain in place and function for several years.

## Care of Catheters

Tunneled and percutaneously placed catheters require meticulous care. The skin at the insertion site should be scrubbed daily with alcohol and a povidone-iodine solution and covered with a sterile dressing. Acetone should never be used because it would dissolve the catheter. The Luer-Lok connection must also be maintained with sterile technique and daily preparation with alcohol and providone-iodine solutions. Preferably the lines should be opened only once a day. The care of tunneled and implanted catheters has been well reviewed in the nursing literature.[1] All hospital, nursing, and IV services have formal policies and procedures for the care of central venous catheters. These teams play a key role in catheter care and patient education.

## Complications

### NONINFECTIOUS COMPLICATIONS

Long-term indwelling central venous catheters carry a number of potential complications. Pneumothorax and hemothorax may complicate placement and, rarely, occur long after placement. Implantable catheters have two potential sites for extravasation: (1) the needle accessing the port through the skin and (2) the connection between the implanted subcutaneous port and the catheter. Later complications include catheter migration, catheter occlusion, vein thrombosis, and catheter infection.

Catheters are placed in the operation suite under fluoroscopic guidance, so that the incidence of malposition should be low. The jet effect of rapid infusion, however, particularly in pediatric-sized catheters, can cause migration into tributaries of the superior vena cava, including the internal jugular and subclavian veins. Frequently, these malpositioned catheters may be manipulated by an intervention radiologist rather than being replaced.

A common complication is that of partial or complete

catheter occlusion. This occlusion is generally caused by fibrin sheath formation or thrombus at the tip of the catheter.[12] Generally the first indication is difficulty in aspirating blood. Such withdrawal occlusion may occur in 15% of patients. Thrombolytic agents, such as urokinase and streptokinase, are able to dissolve these fibrin clots.[13] Urokinase is preferred to streptokinase because of the lack of antigenicity and its generally high success rate. A number of catheter protocols call for the prophylactic use of fibrinolytic agents intermittently or the use of a tissue plasminogen activator.[13]

Partial or complete vein thrombosis has been associated with all types of indwelling catheters.[14] Iatrogenic superior vena cava syndrome has been reported. Predisposing risk factors for vein thrombus include infection, hypercoagulable states, and intimal damage caused by catheter insertion. The incidence of subclavian vein thrombosis is reported to range from 1 to 16% and may be heralded by arm or neck swelling. The swelling usually resolves with catheter removal. The diagnosis can be made noninvasively by nuclear venography. Some investigators have advocated prophylactic use of low-dose warfarin to reduce the incidence of thrombus formation.[15] For patients with catheter-induced subclavian vein thrombosis, the risk of pulmonary embolism may be as high as 10%.[16] Pulmonary embolisms are most common in patients with central venous catheters used for hyperalimentation. Three to 6 months of anticoagulation, following the guidelines for a deep venous thrombosis, is now recommended for patients with a catheter-induced thrombosis if the patient is not thrombocytopenic. In cancer patients, at risk for thrombocytopenia because of their disease or as a result of the therapy, the risks stemming from the use of warfarin or heparin are significant and must be balanced against a risk of a second thromboembolic event.

## INFECTIOUS COMPLICATIONS

Bloodstream infections associated with long-term central venous catheters have been reported to occur at a rate of 1 to 2 episodes per 1000 catheter days.[17–20] The infection rate in terms of frequency of infection depends on the type of catheter. Groeger and colleagues[21] reported an infection rate of 8 per 100 for subcutaneous implanted ports inserted and 43 per 100 tunneled long-term catheters. At M.D. Anderson Cancer Center, the infection rate for peripherally inserted central catheters and nontunneled subclavian central venous catheters was 1.4 per 1000 catheter days, which is comparable to what is described for Hickman catheters in the literature.[22] The cost of inserting nontunneled long-term silicone catheters is significantly lower, however, than that of Hickman tunneled catheters or implantable ports.[23] Several studies have compared the efficiency of tunneled catheters with implantable ports.[23] Several studies have compared the efficiency of tunneled catheters with implantable ports. Mueller and coworkers,[24] in a prospective randomized study, compared the complications of the two types of long-term catheters and determined no significant difference in infection rates between the two types of devices. In a prospective observational study conducted at Memorial Sloan-Kettering on 1630 long-term central venous catheters, which consisted of tunneled catheters and implantable ports, Groeger and colleagues[21] found that the incidence of infection per device per day was 12 times greater for the tunneled catheters as compared with the implantable ports.

The most frequent organisms causing catheter infections are coagulase-negative staphylococci, *Staphylococcus aureus*, and *Candida* species, particularly *Candida albicans* and *Candida parapsilosis*.[17] All three organisms produce an exopolysaccharide termed *extracellular slime*, *microbial biofilm*, or *fibrous glycocalix*. This microbial biofilm promotes the adherence of the organisms to the catheter surface. In addition, these organisms embed themselves in a biofilm and become resistant to antimicrobials, such as vancomycin. After the insertion of the central venous catheter, the reaction of the host to the foreign body is to form a fibrin sheath around the catheter. This fibrin sheath is rich in fibrin and fibronectin. Staphylococci and *Candida* bind well to fibrin and fibronectin.

Various types of infections are associated with long-term central venous catheters, including an exit site infection, port pocket abscess, tunnel infection as well as systemic infection, such as catheter-related bloodstream infections. The diagnosis of central venous catheter–related bloodstream infections before the removal of the catheter is a challenge. Catheter-related bloodstream infections have often been overdiagnosed, resulting in a wasteful removal of the central venous catheter. The clinician should check for the clinical and microbiologic data to determine whether the catheter is the source of the infection. To determine whether the catheter is the source of the bloodstream infection, the clinician should evaluate the patient for any of the following features consistent with catheter-related infection:

1. The absence of any source for the bloodstream infection caused by a likely organism, such as *Staphylococcus epidermidis*, *Staphylococcus aureus*, or *C. albicans*.
2. The presence of a catheter exit site inflammation, tunnel infection, or port pocket abscess (tenderness at the port site).
3. The presence of a differential positive quantitative blood culture whereby a quantitative blood culture drawn through the central venous catheter reveals at least fivefold the number of colonies when compared with a simultaneous quantitative blood culture drawn through a peripheral vein.[25]
4. The presence of what has been termed as the differential positivity time. Blot and colleagues[26] reported that if simultaneous qualitative blood cultures are drawn through the central venous catheter and peripheral vein, the information as to the time when the blood cultures become positive would be useful to determine whether the catheter is the source of the infection.

Usually the time at which a culture becomes positive is a function of the inoculum of organisms in that culture. If there is a time differential of 2 hours or greater between the blood culture drawn through the central venous catheter becoming positive as compared with that drawn through the peripheral vein, this is highly suggestive of a bloodstream infection.

Several interventions have been shown to be effective in preventing infections in long-term catheters. These consist of the following:

1. Maximal sterile barriers include the use of sterile gloves, a mask, a gown, and a cap, as well as using a large

drape during the insertion of the catheter. In a study at M.D. Anderson Cancer Center, maximal sterile barrier precautions decreased the risk of catheter-related bacteremia from 0.5 per 1000 catheter days to 0.02 per 1000 catheter days.[27] The use of maximal sterile barriers is now highly recommended by the Centers for Disease Control during the insertion of all types of long-term central venous catheter (including nontunneled catheters, such as peripherally inserted central catheter lines).

2. A skilled infusion therapy team has been shown to decrease the catheter-related infection rate by fivefold to eightfold.[28]

3. The use of intraluminal antibiotic lock solutions would decrease the risk of recurrent catheter-related infections if the catheter were not removed.[29] It is advisable, however, to use solutions that do not contain vancomycin, given the emerging resistance of vancomycin-resistant gram-positive organisms. A combination of minocycline and ethylenediaminetetraacetic acid (EDTA) has been used to flush catheters with prior history of infection and has been found to be highly effective in preventing recurrence.[30]

Other new innovations include a new hub antiseptic model[31] and the use of antimicrobial-impregnated catheters.[32] Catheters impregnated with antibiotics, such as minocycline and rifampin, have been shown to be highly effective in decreasing the risk of infection in polyurethane catheters used 60 days in bone marrow transplant patients. Their use in long-term silicone catheters is currently being evaluated.

The management of catheter-related infections involves decisions related to the choice of the antimicrobial agent, the duration of antimicrobial therapy, and whether to remove or retain the catheter. Infections caused by coagulase-negative staphylococci could be treated with vancomycin without the removal of the catheter.[33] The optimal duration of treatment is 7 days. For organisms such as *S. aureus*, *C. albicans*, *C. parapsilosis*, and gram-negative organisms such as *Stenotrophomonas maltophilia* or *Pseudomonas aeruginosa*, removal of the catheter should be considered.[34, 35]

Catheter removal should be considered in particular if there is a lack of early response to antimicrobial therapy. With early response to antimicrobial therapy and the use of antibiotic-antimicrobial lock solutions (such as minocycline-EDTA), however, it is possible to treat such infections without the removal of the catheter.[30] The antibiotics of choice for *S. aureus* bloodstream infection is usually nafcillin or oxacillin, unless one is dealing with a methicillin-resistant *S. aureus*. Vancomycin is the drug of choice for methicillin-resistant *S. aureus*, and the duration of therapy is at least 10 to 14 days after the removal of the catheter. For *Candida* bloodstream infections, fluconazole could be used for *C. albicans* and *C. parapsilosis* infections. Amphotericin B regimens (including lipsomal amphotericin B) are the drugs of choice for fluconazole-resistant organisms, such as *Candida krusei* or *Candida glabrata*. The duration of treatment for catheter-related candidemia is 10 to 14 days.[35]

Catheter infections complicated by a tunnel infection or port pocket abscess require removal of the catheter and treatment with appropriate antibiotics for a 10-day period. Central venous catheter–related infections that are complicated by septic thrombosis (infection of the vein associated with an infected thrombus detected by venogram or an ultrasound Doppler study) or endocarditis should be treated for 4 to 6 weeks with appropriate antimicrobial therapy.

## Summary

It has been estimated that approximately 0.5 million venous access catheters are implanted each year in the United States,[10] underscoring their indispensable role in the management of many diseases. This common use emphasizes the need for safe placement, meticulous care, and early recognition and treatment of complications.

### SUGGESTIONS FOR ADDITIONAL READING

Groeger JS, Lucas AB, Thaler HT, et al. Infectious morbidity associated with long-term use of venous access devices in patients with cancer. Ann Intern Med 1993;119:1168–74. *In 1431 consecutive patients at Memorial Sloan-Kettering Cancer Center requiring 1630 venous access devices, the rate of infection was 43% for patients with catheters and 8% for those with subcutaneous implanted ports. When analyzed by the number of infections per 1000 device days, the rate was 12-fold higher with catheters than with implanted ports. On the basis of this experience, this institution uses implanted ports whenever possible.*

Haire WD, Lieberman RP, Lund GB, et al. Obstructed central venous catheters: restoring function with a 12-hour infusion of low-dose urokinase. Cancer 1990;66:2279–85. *With a 12-hour infusion of urokinase at the rate of 40,000 units per hour, 29 of 30 catheters were salvaged. None of the patients developed bleeding or other serious complications.*

Darouiche RO, Raad II, Heard SO, et al, for the Catheter Study Group. A comparison of two antimicrobial-impregnated central venous catheters. N Engl J Med 1999;340:108.

Howell PB, Walters PE, Donowitz GR, Farr BM. Risk factors for infection of adult patients with cancer who have tunneled central venous catheters. Cancer 1995;75:1367–74.

### REFERENCES

1. Broviac JW, Cole JJ, Scribner BH. A silicone rubber atrial catheter for prolonged parenteral alimentation. Surg Gynecol Obstet 1973;136:602–6.
2. Hickman RO, Buckner CD, Clift RA, et al. A modified right atrial catheter for access to the venous system in marrow transplant recipients. Surg Gynecol Obstet 1979;148:871–5.
3. Linder LE, Curelaru I, Gustavsson B, et al. Material thrombogenicity in central venous catheterization: a comparison between soft, antebrachial catheters of silicone elastomer and polyurethane. JPEN J Parenter Enteral Nutr 1984;8:399–406.
4. Pottecher T, Forrler M, Picardat P, et al. Thrombogenicity of central venous catheters: prospective study of polyethylene, silicone and polyurethane catheters with phlebography or post-mortem examination. Eur J Anaesthesiol 1984;1:361–5.
5. Pegues D, Axelrod P, McClarren C, et al. Comparison of infections in Hickman and implanted port catheters in adult solid tumor patients. J Surg Oncol 1992;49:156–62.
6. Davidson H, Bowersox J, Lee R. Experience with Groshong versus Hickman central venous catheters. Proc ASCO 1988;7:289.
7. Raad I, Davis S, Becker M, et al. Low infection rate and long durability of nontunneled silastic catheters: a safe and cost-effective alternative for long-term venous access. Arch Intern Med 1993;153:1791–6.
8. Broadwater JR, Henderson MA, Bell JL, et al. Outpatient percutaneous central venous access in cancer patients. Am J Surg 1990;160:676–80.
9. Henriques HF 3d, Karmy-Jones R, Knoll SM, et al. Avoiding complications of long-term venous access. Am Surg 1993;59:555–8.
10. Raaf JH, Heil D. Open insertion of right atrial catheters through the jugular veins. Surg Gynecol Obstet 1993;177:295–8.
11. Groeger JS, Lucas AB, Coit D, et al. A prospective, randomized evaluation of the effect of silver impregnated subcutaneous cuffs for

preventing tunneled chronic venous access catheter infections in cancer patients. Ann Surg 1993;218:206–10.

12. Tschirhart JM, Rao MK. Mechanism and management of persistent withdrawal occlusion. Am Surg 1988;54:326–8.

13. Wachs T. Urokinase administration in pediatric patients with occluded central venous catheters. J IV Nurs 1990;13:100–2.

14. Lokich JJ, Bothe A Jr, Benotti P, Moore C. Complications and management of implanted venous access catheters. J Clin Oncol 1985;3:710–17.

15. Bern MM, Lokich JJ, Wallach SR, et al. Very low doses of warfarin can prevent thrombosis in central venous catheters: a randomized prospective trial. Ann Intern Med 1990;112:423–8.

16. Monreal M, Raventos A, Lerma R, et al: Pulmonary embolism in patients with upper extremity DVT associated to venous central lines—a prospective study. Thromb Hemost 1994;72:548–50.

17. Press OW, Ramsey PG, Larson EB, et al. Hickman catheter infections in patients with malignancies. Medicine 1984;63:189–200.

18. Decker MD, Edwards KM. Central venous catheter infections. Pediatr Clin North Am 1988;35:579–612.

19. Clarke DE, Raffin TA. Infectious complications of indwelling long-term central venous catheters. Chest 1990;97:966–72.

20. Howell PB, Walters PE, Donowitz GR, Farr BM. Risk factors for infection of adult patients with cancer who have tunneled central venous catheters. Cancer 1995;75:1367–74.

21. Groeger JS, Lucas AB, Thaler HT, et al. Infectious morbidity associated with long-term use of venous access devices in patients with cancer. Ann Intern Med 1993;119:1168–74.

22. Radd I, Davis S, Becker M, et al. Low infection rate and long durability of nontunneled silastic catheters: a safe and cost-effective alternative for long-term venous access. Arch Intern Med 1993;153:1791–6.

23. Raad II, Safar H. Long-term central venous catheters: infectious complications and cost. In: Seifert H, Jansen B, Farr BM, eds. Catheter-related infections. New York: Marcel Dekker, 1997:307–24.

24. Mueller BU, Skelton J, Callender DPE, et al. A prospective randomized trial comparing the infectious complications of the externalized catheters versus a subcutaneously implanted device in cancer patients. J Clin Oncol 1992;10:1943–8.

25. Capdevila JA, Planes AM, Palomar M, et al. Value of differential quantitative blood cultures in the diagnosis of catheter-related sepsis. Eur J Clin Microbiol Infect Dis 1992;11:403–7.

26. Blot F, Schmidt E, Nitenberg G, et al. Earlier positivity of central-venous-versus peripheral-blood cultures is highly predictive of catheter-related sepsis. J Clin Microbiol 1998;36:105–9.

27. Raad II, Hohn DC, Gilbreath BJ, et al. Prevention of central venous catheter-related infections using maximal sterile barrier precautions during insertion. Infect Control Hosp Epidemiol 1994;15:231–8.

28. Nehme AE. Nutritional support of the hospitalized patient: the team concept. JAMA 1980;243:1906–8.

29. Krzywda EA, Andris DA, Edmiston CE, Quebbeman EJ. Treatment of Hickman catheter sepsis using antibiotic lock technique. Infect Control Hosp Epidemiol 1995;16:596–8.

30. Raad I, Buzaid A, Rhyne J, et al. Minocycline and ethylenediaminetetraacetate for the prevention of recurrent vascular catheter infections. Clin Infect Dis 1997;25:149–51.

31. Segura M, Alvarez-Lerma F, Tellado JM, et al. Advances in surgical technique: a clinical trial on the prevention of catheter-related sepsis using a new hub model. Ann Surg 1996;223:363–9.

32. Darouiche RO, Raad II, Heard SO, et al, for the Catheter Study Group. A comparison of two antimicrobial-impregnated central venous catheters. N Engl J Med 1999;340:108.

33. Himenz J, Skelton J, Pizzo PA. Perspective on the management of catheter-related infections in cancer patients. Pediatr Infect Dis J 1986;5:6–11.

34. Dugdale DC, Ramsey PG. *Staphylococcus aureus* bacteremia in patients with Hickman catheters. Am J Med 1990;89:137–41.

35. Rex JH, Bennett JE, Sugar AM, et al. Intravascular catheter exchange and duration of candidemia. Clin Infect Dis 1995;21:994–6.

# CONTINUOUS-INFUSION THERAPY

• Robert Benjamin

Continuous infusions of chemotherapy, IV hydration, electrolyte replacement, parenteral nutrition, and a variety of other drugs are routinely employed in the management of patients with cancer. This section focuses primarily on administration of anticancer agents by continuous infusion but also discusses outpatient infusions of other agents used in association with, or to treat complications of, anticancer therapy. The two primary reasons to consider continuous-infusion chemotherapy are to increase antitumor efficacy or to decrease host toxicity (Table 12–2). A complete analysis of this topic is beyond the scope of this section. Interested

readers are referred to the monograph by Lokich.[1] For detailed evaluation of the recommended therapeutic regimens for any given tumor, the reader is referred to the appropriate chapter on that disease.

## Indications for Continuous-Infusion Therapy

### EFFICACY

Regarding the first reason for using continuous infusion, drugs most likely to demonstrate improved antitumor efficacy when given by continuous infusion are those that require prolonged exposure to neoplastic cells for efficacy but that have a short biologic half-life. The prime example is ara-C, which at standard doses is much more effective by continuous infusion, and common induction regimens such as *7 and 3* use an infusion schedule.[2] The most commonly used agent that shares these characteristics and is administered by continuous infusion is 5-fluorouracil (5-FU). In therapeutic regimens for squamous carcinomas, 5-day continuous-infusion 5-FU has been used in combination with short infusions of cisplatin.[3] Prolonged infusions of 5-FU have been used in primary management of patients with

*Table 12–2.* **Advantages of Continuous Infusion**

| Therapy | Benefits |
|---|---|
| Chemotherapy | |
| 5-Fluorouracil | Increased efficacy |
| Ara-C | Increased efficacy |
| Doxorubicin (Adriamycin) | Decreased cardiac toxicity |
| Bleomycin | Decreased pulmonary toxicity |
| Supportive care | |
| Mesna | Convenience |
| IV fluids | Hydration |
| Electrolytes | More efficient replacement |
| | Decreased gastrointestinal toxicity |

*Table 12–3.* **Toxicities**

*Peak-level toxicities*

Nausea
Vomiting
Acute anaphylactoid reactions
Doxorubicin (Adriamycin) cardiac toxicity
Bleomycin pulmonary toxicity
Ifosfamide neurotoxicity

*Duration-dependent toxicities*

Mucositis
Dermatitis (hand-foot syndrome)

colorectal carcinoma.[4, 5] The same approach has been used to particular advantage for radiation sensitization, as a single agent, or in combination with short infusions of cisplatin.[6] The advantage of newer oral agents, such as capecitabine and UFT (a combination of Tegafur and uracil), may modify the need for the continuous-infusion strategy with 5-FU. Drugs requiring prolonged exposure but having a long half-life can be effectively administered by repeated daily doses. Examples are the vinca alkaloids. Initial studies suggested superiority of a continuous-infusion regimen over widely interrupted therapy,[7–9] but repeated daily doses later proved to be as effective as but no more effective than continuous infusion.[10] Only logistic considerations and patient preference determine whether it is better to bring a patient back for a few minutes of treatment with such drugs every day for 5 days or to start the patient on a 5-day outpatient infusion.

## TOXICITY

The second major reason for use of continuous-infusion therapy is to avoid toxicity associated with high peak levels of chemotherapeutic agents (see Table 12–3). The most notable example is the use of continuous infusions of doxorubicin (Adriamycin) to decrease cardiac toxicity. A series of studies initiated at the M.D. Anderson Cancer Center in the late 1970s demonstrated the importance of peak levels of doxorubicin in determining cardiac toxicity.[11–14] Although 24-hour infusions decreased cardiac toxicity to a minimal extent, 48- to 96-hour infusions had a more profound effect.[15, 16] Ninety-six-hour infusions of doxorubicin permit a doubling of the safe cumulative dose from 400 mg/m² to 800 mg/m².[17] Infusions of 48 to 72 hours produce intermediate benefit. The availability of the cardioprotective agent, dexrazoxane, permits an alternative strategy for decreasing cardiac toxicity without requiring continuous infusion. Dexrazoxane adds myelosuppression, and there is a suggestion from randomized clinical trials in breast cancer that antitumor activity may possibly be minimally compromised. Such is not the case with continuous infusions of doxorubicin. Another alternative to the continuous infusion of doxorubicin is liposomal encapsulated doxorubicin (Doxil). Liposomal encapsulated doxorubicin has an extraordinarily long half-life and would be expected to decrease cardiac toxicity; however, a detailed evaluation of the cardiac toxicity of liposomal encapsulated doxorubicin is not available. Also, liposomal encapsulated doxorubicin acts similar to a long doxorubicin infusion (2 to 3 weeks in duration) with a

markedly altered toxicity spectrum (see later). Another drug with delayed peak level toxicity is bleomycin. The pulmonary fibrosis associated with cumulative bleomycin administration can be reduced by continuous infusion. Quantitative aspects of this toxicity reduction are not as well studied as those of doxorubicin cardiac toxicity.

Some drug toxicities are related to peak drug levels, and others depend on the time of exposure above a given concentration (Table 12–3). The best way to avoid peak levels is to give drugs by continuous infusion. Acute nausea and vomiting are always peak level toxicities. The nausea and vomiting of doxorubicin decrease with continuous versus rapid infusion. Similarly, the acute nausea and vomiting of cisplatin, dacarbazine, and cyclophosphamide can be reduced by continuous infusion. Modern antiemetics reduce the need to resort to infusional therapy simply to decrease nausea and vomiting, but for some patients, continuous infusions may be the only way to make chemotherapy tolerable. Facial flushing, hypotension, and pseudoanaphylactic reactions observed by overly rapid infusion of some drugs can be virtually eliminated by prolonging infusion time and reducing peak levels. In contrast, other side effects are more sensitive to the duration of exposure above a critical level than they are to peak levels. The most notable are mucositis and dermatitis (hand-foot syndrome). The longer the infusion, the more likely these toxic effects will be dose limiting. Hand-foot syndrome is seen most commonly with prolonged infusions of 5-FU or doxorubicin. A short infusion of liposomal encapsulated doxorubicin simulates a long doxorubicin infusion because of the extraordinarily long half-life of liposomal encapsulated doxorubicin and produces the same side effects. Doxorubicin-related mucositis is extremely sensitive to changes in infusion duration. For patients with dose-limiting stomatitis with 96-hour doxorubicin infusion, 48-hour infusion of the same total dose frequently ameliorates the problem to a tolerable level. For patients who cannot tolerate 48-hour doxorubicin infusions because of mucositis, rapid-infusion doxorubicin with dexrazoxane is an alternative strategy to limit mucositis and cardiac toxicity.

Myelosuppression is another side effect, which seems to have some relationship to infusion duration, although it is not as simple as mucositis (Table 12–4). For 5-FU, myelosuppression is a dose-limiting toxicity when the drug is administered by rapid infusion daily for 5 days. For a 5-day continuous infusion, there is relatively little myelosuppression, and mucositis becomes the dose-limiting toxicity. In contrast, myelosuppression from doxorubicin is the same regardless of whether the drug is given by rapid infusion on day 1 or by continuous infusion over 96 hours. If the drug is infused over 3 weeks, however, myelosuppression is reduced, and mucositis or hand-foot syndrome becomes the

*Table 12–4.* **Myelosuppression as a Function of Infusion Duration**

| Drug | Short Infusion | 3- to 5-Day Infusion | 2-Day Infusion |
|---|---|---|---|
| Ara-C | + | + + + + | NA |
| Doxorubicin (Adriamycin) | + + + + | + + + + | + |
| 5-Fluorouracil | + + + + | + | + |

NA, not available.

dose-limiting toxicity as with liposomal encapsulated doxorubicin.

A number of regimens use ifosfamide by continuous infusion to decrease acute neurologic toxicity and nephrotoxicity. A common regimen for soft tissue sarcomas, MAID, gives all three chemotherapeutic agents, doxorubicin (Adriamycin), ifosfamide, and dacarbazine, by continuous infusion simultaneously with continuous infusions of mesna, an agent designed to decrease bladder toxicity. The original data of Antman and colleagues[18] suggest decreased drug efficacy of ifosfamide when given by continuous infusion. Data from the Sarcoma Center at M.D. Anderson Cancer Center support that finding at standard[19] and high doses.[20] It is recommended that ifosfamide be given by interrupted short infusion at a rate of approximately 1 $g/m^2/hr$. Continuous infusion of mesna is employed routinely with outpatient ifosfamide therapy. This regimen allows the patient to come into the outpatient clinic and receive a relatively short infusion of ifosfamide and leave with a continuous infusion supplying mesna to protect the bladder, IV fluids to ensure adequate hydration, and electrolytes to counteract the loss of electrolytes from the renal tubular acidosis that accompanies ifosfamide administration in most cases. The IV fluids ensure adequate hydration even if the patient is nauseated and decrease the risk of further renal damage. The mesna infusion is at least as effective as repeated bolus doses of mesna and eliminates the need for patients to stay in a treatment center for 8 hours or to return at 4 and 8 hours after ifosfamide administration for the mesna doses used according to the standard schedule of drug administration. The continuous infusion of fluids and mesna requires a high-volume portable infusion pump because the mesna is usually mixed in 2 L of IV fluids, and several such pumps are now available.

Chronic electrolyte imbalance is a well-described complication of cancer chemotherapy. Cisplatin, particularly when given in high single doses, results in chronic hypomagnesemia. Although this is rarely a clinical problem, oral magnesium replacement rarely corrects hypomagnesemia, and the large doses of oral magnesium supplements required to maintain a normal magnesium level, once it has been replaced intravenously, frequently cause gastrointestinal side effects. Ifosfamide, especially at the doses required in sarcoma therapy (10 to 14 $g/m^2$), regularly results in low-grade renal tubular acidosis. Although most patients can be managed successfully with oral potassium and bicarbonate supplementation, some patients require such high doses of electrolyte replacement that it is impossible to manage them except by continuous IV infusion. Frequently, electrolytes can be concentrated in relatively small volumes and infused using a small-volume pump, but occasionally, large-volume infusions are required. I have seen one patient treated with cisplatin who also required diuretic therapy to manage doxorubicin-induced cardiomyopathy. Only with IV replacement therapy was it possible to keep up with magnesium and potassium loss, and she was maintained on continuous IV electrolyte replacement for 9 years. Another patient treated with high-dose ifosfamide required 200 to 300 mEq of potassium chloride replacement daily for more than 1 year.

## Methods and Procedures

Continuous-infusion therapy requires central venous access (covered in another section of this chapter) and an infusion pump to ensure that the drugs are given by continuous infusion. New pumps seem to appear on the market monthly, reflecting seemingly endless technologic advances. Pumps are characterized by type of drug delivery (e.g., continuous infusion, intermittent infusion), the pump mechanism, and the volume of fluid that they can deliver (Table 12–5). Although most infusion pumps used on inpatient wards deliver high volumes of fluids accurately, these pumps are usually large, heavy, and unsuited to the outpatient setting. Most ambulatory infusion pumps handle only small fluid volumes. Those designed for outpatient parenteral nutrition, however, can be used for other high-volume outpatient treatments. Because the subject of this section is continuous infusion, I shall not discuss the specialized pumps designed for intermittent infusion or patient-controlled anesthesia pumps. The reader is referred to a number of review articles for information on such specialized pumps.[21–23]

The simplest pumps from a mechanical point of view are the elastomeric reservoir pumps. Fluid is placed in the elastomeric reservoir that expands and causes pressure. The rate of deflation of the reservoir is controlled by an outlet valve, which is fixed. The only aspect of the delivery system that is variable is the viscosity of the fluid flowing through the valve. The viscosity can be influenced by the composition of the fluid as well as the temperature. Because there is no way to fine-tune the infusion rate, accuracy of these pumps is lower than for mechanical pumps but is usually within 10 to 15% of the calculated infusion rate and is satisfactory for most chemotherapy infusions. From a patient's point of view, these pumps are simplest because they require no adjustment, they are absolutely silent, and they have the lowest weight.

Another type is the syringe pump. It is the most nearly accurate ( $\pm$ 2 to 5%). Fluid delivery is regulated by mechanically advancing the plunger of a syringe, which serves as the drug reservoir. Single or multiple syringe units are available, but the volume is limited to 60 ml or less for each syringe.

Peristaltic infusion pumps are the most commonly used mechanical ambulatory pumps. They work by mechanically squeezing the administration tubing. A fluid bag, usually 65 to 250 ml, serves as the reservoir for drug administration, and special tubing is required to fit the pump. In some cases, larger infusion volumes (4 L per day on a dual-channel pump) make these pumps suitable for large-volume outpatient infusions so that they can accommodate parenteral nutrition as well as vigorous IV hydration.

Finally, cassette system pumps are used primarily for inpatient administration and large fluid volumes. The pumps work on a two-cycle mechanism: the first to fill the chamber

*Table 12–5.* **Types of Infusion Pumps**

| Type | Characteristics | Accuracy | Fluid Volume |
|---|---|---|---|
| Elastomeric reservoir pumps | Simple, light, quiet | Lowest | Small |
| Syringe pumps | Complex, heavier, noisy | Highest | Small |
| Peristaltic pumps | Complex, heavier, noisy | High | Small-large |
| Cassette pumps | Complex, very heavy, noisy | Very high | Large |

and the second to empty it and deliver the infusion to the patients. Pumps handling multiple infusion sources are used routinely for complex inpatient management of different IV solutions.

The choice of infusion pump is dictated by many factors, including the length and volume of the infusion, patient preferences, costs, reliability, and ability to instruct the patient on management of the pump when away from the hospital. The variety of pumps available today is broad enough that practically any therapy that is safe enough to be given in an ambulatory setting can now be administered without the need for hospitalization.

## REFERENCES

1. Lokich J. Cancer chemotherapy by infusion. Chicago: Precept Press, 1990:747.
2. Yates J, Glidewell O, Wiernik P, et al. Cytosine arabinoside with daunorubicin or adriamycin for therapy of acute myelocytic leukemia: a CALGB study. Blood 1982;60:454–62.
3. Kish J, Ensley J, Jacobs J, et al. A randomized trial of cisplatin (CACP) + 5-fluorouracil (5-FU) infusion and CACP + 5-FU bolus for recurrent and advanced squamous cell carcinoma of the head and neck. Cancer 1985;56:2740–4.
4. Lokich J, Ahlgren J, Cantrell J, et al. A prospective randomized comparison of protracted infusional 5-fluorouracil with or without weekly bolus cisplatin in metastatic colorectal carcinoma. A Mid-Atlantic Oncology Program study. Cancer 1991;67:14–19.
5. Seifert P, Baker L, Reed M, Vaitkevicius V. Comparison of continuously infused 5-fluorouracil with bolus injection in treatment of patients with colorectal adenocarcinoma. Cancer 1975;36:123–8.
6. Rich T, Ajani J, Morrison W, et al. Chemoradiation therapy for anal cancer: radiation plus continuous infusion of 5-fluorouracil with or without cisplatin. Radiother Oncol 1993;27:209–15.
7. Yap B, Benjamin R, Plager C, et al. A randomized study of continuous infusion vindesine versus vinblastine in adults with refractory metastatic sarcomas. Am J Clin Oncol 1983;6:235–8.
8. Yap H, Blumenschein G, Keating M, et al. Vinblastine given as a continuous 5-day infusion in the treatment of refractory advanced breast cancer. Cancer Treat Rep 1980;64:279–83.
9. Fraschini G, Yap H, Hortobagyi G, et al. Five-day continuous-infusion vinblastine in the treatment of breast cancer. Cancer 1985;56:225–9.
10. Yau J, Yap Y, Buzdar A, et al. A comparative randomized trial of vinca alkaloids in patients with metastatic breast carcinoma. Cancer 1985;55:337–40.
11. Benjamin R, Legha S, Valdivieso M, et al. Reduction of adriamycin cardiac toxicity by schedule manipulation. In: Muggia F, Young C, Carter S, eds. Anthracycline antibiotics in cancer therapy. Boston: Martinus Nijhoff, 1982:352–7.
12. Benjamin R, Ewer M, MacKay B, et al. An endomyocardial biopsy study of anthracycline-induced cardiomyopathy—detection, reversibility, and potential amelioration. Proc AACR/ASCO 1979;20:372.
13. Hortobagyi G, Frye D, Buzdar A, et al. Decreased cardiac toxicity of doxorubicin administered by continuous intravenous infusion in combination chemotherapy for metastatic breast carcinoma. Cancer 1989;63:37–45.
14. Legha S, Benjamin R, Mackay B, et al. Reduction of doxorubicin cardiotoxicity by prolonged continuous intravenous infusion. Ann Intern Med 1982;96:133–9.
15. Benjamin R, Chawla S, Ewer M, et al. Adriamycin cardiac toxicity: an assessment of approaches to cardiac monitoring and cardioprotection. In: Hacker M, Lazo J, Tritton T, eds. Organ directed toxicities of anticancer drugs. Boston: Martinus Nijhoff, 1988:41–55.
16. Benjamin R. The schedule dependency of the cardiotoxicity of adriamycin: its relevance to pharmacokinetic parameters. In: Muggia F, Green M, Speyer J, eds. Cancer treatment and the heart. Baltimore: Johns Hopkins University Press, 1992:278–85.
17. Ewer M, Benjamin R. Cardiotoxicity of chemotherapeutic drugs. In: Perry M, ed. The chemotherapy source book. Baltimore: Williams & Wilkins, 1996:649–61.
18. Antman KH, Ryan L, Elias A, et al. Response to ifosfamide and mesna: 124 previously treated patients with metastatic or unresectable sarcoma. J Clin Oncol 1989;7:126–31.
19. Benjamin RS, Legha SS, Patel SR, Nicaise C. Single-agent ifosfamide studies in sarcomas of soft tissue and bone: the M.D. Anderson Experience. Cancer Chemother Pharmacol 1993;31:Suppl 2:S174–9.
20. Patel S, Vadhan-Raj S, Papadoulos N, et al. High-dose ifosfamide in bone and soft-tissue sarcomas—results of phase II and pilot studies: dose response and schedule dependence. J Clin Oncol 1997;15:2378–84.
21. Finley R. Infusion technology: growth present choices. Highlights Antineoplastic Drugs 1995;13:13–14.
22. Finley R. Drug-delivery systems: infusion and access devices. Highlights Antineoplastic Drugs 1995;13:15–29.
23. Kwan J. High-technology I.V. infusion devices. Am J Hosp Pharm 1989;46:320–35.

······························

# INTRAPERITONEAL CHEMOTHERAPY

• David S. Alberts    • Dava J. Garcia    • Ardie E. Delforge

## Early Clinical Studies of Intraperitoneal Chemotherapy

Ovarian cancer is the leading cause of death from gynecologic cancer in the United States. In 1998, more than 25,000 women were diagnosed with ovarian cancer, and 14,500 women died of the disease.[1] Unfortunately, 70% of ovarian cancer patients are diagnosed with advanced-stage disease, and the current cure rate for these patients is less than 10%.[2] In an effort to improve long-term survival and cure rates for advanced ovarian cancer patients, intraperitoneal (IP) administration of chemotherapeutic agents is being investigated in clinical studies as a means of optimizing chemotherapy.

Because ovarian cancer typically remains confined to the peritoneal cavity for most of its natural history in most patients, it is particularly amenable to regional IP therapy. In 1978, Dedrick and colleagues[3] established a strong pharmacologic rationale for IP administration of chemotherapy. During the next decade, Howell and coworkers[4, 5] and others performed a series of phase I and pharmacokinetic trials and documented significant pharmacologic advantages (defined as the ratio of the total drug exposure of the peritoneal cavity to that of plasma) with IP administration for several important chemotherapeutic agents, including cisplatin. Phase II studies by Markman and associates[6] and others provided evidence of significant activity of IP cisplatin in the salvage setting. When IP cisplatin was administered to ovarian cancer patients with a prior response to systemic cisplatin and minimal (i.e., <1 cm) residual disease at the start of IP therapy, 15 of 36 patients (42%) achieved a pathologically documented complete response.[6]

## Phase III Studies of Intraperitoneal Cisplatin-Based Regimens as Primary Therapy of Stage III, Optimal Disease Ovarian Cancer

The promising results of phase II studies were verified by a phase III study conducted by the Southwest Oncology Group, Gynecologic Oncology Group, and Eastern Cooperative Oncology Group in patients with optimal disease (<2 cm residual disease after initial debulking laparotomy), stage III ovarian cancer.[7] Between June 1986 and July 1992, 654 patients (546 eligible patients) were randomized to receive primary chemotherapy with IP cisplatin 100 mg/m$^2$ plus intravenous (IV) cyclophosphamide 600 mg/m$^2$ or IV cisplatin 100 mg/m$^2$ plus IV cyclophosphamide 600 mg/m$^2$. Patients on the IP therapy arm survived significantly longer than patients on the IV arm (estimated median survival, 49 months vs. 41 months) and the IP/IV death hazard ratio was 0.76 (95% confidence interval, 0.61 to 0.96; $p=0.02$).

The IP therapy was well tolerated by study patients. As anticipated, grade II or greater abdominal pain was more common on the IP arm than the IV arm (2% vs. 18%; $p<0.001$); however, the pain typically resolved within 24 hours with nonopioid or mild opioid analgesics. Patients on the IP arm also experienced more pulmonary toxicity, principally transient dyspnea, as a result of base compression of the lung by the IP fluid. A lower percentage of patients on the IP arm experienced grade II or greater neutropenia, tinnitus, clinical hearing loss, and neuromuscular toxicities.

A second intergroup, phase III study of IP therapy for primary treatment of advanced, optimal disease ovarian cancer has been performed by the Gynecologic Oncology Group, Southwest Oncology Group, and Eastern Cooperative Oncology Group.[8] This study compared paclitaxel 135 mg/m$^2$ by 24-hour continuous IV infusion on day 1 followed by cisplatin 75 mg/m$^2$ IV on day 2 every 21 days for six courses with an experimental regimen of IV carboplatin AUC = 9 (as calculated by the Calvert formula) every 28 days for two courses followed by paclitaxel 135 mg/m$^2$ IV over 24 hours on day 1 plus cisplatin 100 mg/m$^2$ IP on day 2 every 21 days for six courses. When compared with the IV cisplatin-paclitaxel arm, the IP arm was associated with a significant improvement in recurrence-free survival (27.6 months vs. 22.5 months; relative risk = 0.793; $p=0.02$) and a borderline significant improvement in overall survival (median survivals of 52.9 months vs. 47.6 months; relative risk = 0.785; $p=0.056$).

The two courses of high-dose carboplatin in the experimental arm were administered in an attempt to *debulk chemically* the residual tumor and potentially optimize the IP therapy. The two cycles of IV carboplatin were associated with considerable myelosuppression, however, and hampered the administration of subsequent therapy. Of patients on the experimental arm, 19% received two or fewer courses of IP therapy. Because of the unacceptable toxicity associated with the two cycles of high-dose carboplatin, the experimental arm is not recommended. However, the results of this study strongly support the further development of IP therapy for the primary treatment of ovarian cancer.

## Patient Selection Criteria for Intraperitoneal Chemotherapy

Ovarian cancer patients with bulky residual disease (tumor nodules >2 cm in diameter) are not good candidates for IP therapy because direct diffusion of cytotoxic drugs into tumor nodules is limited to a few millimeters from the periphery.[9] A retrospective analysis of 89 ovarian cancer patients who received second-line IP cisplatin therapy at the Memorial Sloan-Kettering Cancer Center showed that the size of the largest residual tumor nodule at the initiation of salvage therapy was predictive of the likelihood of response.[6] The pathologic complete response rate at third-look surgery was 41% for patients with only microscopic disease at the start of IP therapy, versus 25% for patients with macroscopic disease less than 1 cm, versus 5% for patients with at least one tumor nodule greater than 1 cm at the start of salvage therapy.

Additionally, patients with chemoresistant tumors are not good candidates for IP therapy because they are unlikely to achieve a durable response. In a retrospective study of second-line IP cisplatin, prior response to systemically administered primary therapy was an important predictor of the likelihood of response, regardless of the size of residual tumor.[6] For example, in the group of patients with small-volume residual disease (<1 cm) at the initiation of IP therapy, the pathologic complete response rate was 42% for patients who had achieved an objective response to front-line therapy versus 7% for patients who did not achieve at least a partial response to primary chemotherapy.

IP chemotherapy has utility as primary chemotherapy for patients with optimal disease (residual disease <1 to 2 cm) following an initial exploratory laparotomy, as consolidation therapy for advanced disease patients with no pathologic evidence of disease at second-look surgery, or as salvage therapy for patients with an objective response to primary chemotherapy and minimal residual disease (<1 cm) after second-look surgery.

## Selection of Chemotherapeutic Agent for Intraperitoneal Delivery

Cytotoxic agents with slow clearance from the IP space and a rapid clearance from systemic circulation offer the greatest pharmacologic advantage with IP administration. Water-soluble agents are retained in the IP space longer than lipid-soluble drugs, and large molecules enter the systemic circulation more slowly than small molecules.

IP cisplatin has undergone extensive study and has proven efficacy in the primary and the salvage setting.[4, 6–8] Other agents that have been successfully administered by the IP route include paclitaxel,[10] floxuridine,[11] 5-FU,[12] mitoxantrone,[11] carboplatin,[13] and alfa-interferon.[13]

Although carboplatin can be administered by the IP route, cisplatin, rather than carboplatin, is the preferred platinum agent for IP administration. Los and colleagues[14] have shown in a rat tumor model that following IP administration of equimolar doses of carboplatin or cisplatin, the platinum concentration in peritoneal tumors was approximately seven fold greater in the cisplatin group than in the carboplatin group. Markman and coworkers[15] have documented a significantly higher surgically verified response rate to salvage therapy with IP cisplatin versus IP carboplatin in patients with macroscopic, small-volume residual disease ovarian cancer (71% vs. 32%; $p<0.05$).

Paclitaxel is a particularly promising agent for IP administration because it has a highly favorable pharmacokinetic profile when administered by this route. In a phase I trial conducted by the Gynecologic Oncology Group, the peritoneal drug exposure (AUC) was on average almost 1000 times greater than systemic exposure, the IP clearance rate was slow (0.42 L/m²/day), and plasma drug levels following IP administration were comparable to those achieved with 24-hour IV infusions.[10]

## Selection of Catheter for Intraperitoneal Drug Delivery

IP therapy may be administered via semipermanent or single-use catheters. Semipermanent catheters, such as the Port-A-Cath (Pharmacia, Deltec, St. Paul, MN), Tenckhoff (Quinton Instrument Co, Seattle, WA), or Groshong (Bard Access Systems, UT), are used more often than single-use catheters for IP chemotherapy administration. These catheters require surgical placement during a laparotomy or a laparoscopic procedure, and it is therefore preferable to obtain patient consent for catheter placement at the time a surgical tumor debulking is planned.

The Tenckhoff and Groshong catheters are externally accessed and require daily maintenance. In a limited retrospective study by Runowicz and associates,[16] the Tenckhoff catheter was associated with a 67% complication rate in 12 patients undergoing IP therapy (6 patients had complications that required removal of the Tenckhoff catheter). Three of the 12 patients developed bacterial peritonitis. Other complications included catheter obstruction, abdominal pain, and development of non–tumor-related masses. The authors also described their experience with single-use catheters and concluded that, in their hands, single-use catheters were superior. Waggoner and colleagues[17] have reported on their use of the Groshong catheter for IP therapy in 18 patients. There was a single case of bacterial infection at the catheter exit site in this series of patients. Other complications that occurred included one case of chemical peritonitis, one catheter obstruction related to adhesions, and leakage of fluid from the vaginal cuff in two patients. Also, two patients declined further IP therapy after developing severe nausea and vomiting and prolonged bone marrow suppression. Based on their overall experience, the authors recommended the Groshong catheter as safe and reliable for delivery of IP chemotherapy.

In contrast to the Tenckhoff or Groshong catheter, the Port-A-Cath is a totally implantable system and does not require any maintenance by the patient. Almadrones and Yerys[18] have performed a retrospective review of the use of the Port-A-Cath in 106 patients who underwent IP chemotherapy at the Memorial Sloan-Kettering Cancer Center. In this study, major complications were infrequent. Sixteen patients (15%) developed complications that required catheter removal (seven resumed IP treatment after placement of a second catheter). These complications included infection (six patients), poor distribution of IP fluid (two patients), and catheter nonfunction (eight patients). The rate of serious infections was 8.5% (nine infections in eight patients).

Some gynecologic oncologists prefer to use the IV Port-A-Cath instead of the peritoneal Port-A-Cath for IP administration of anticancer drugs. The multiple openings on the sides of the peritoneal Port-A-Cath may contribute to fibrous sheath development and a higher rate of catheter dysfunction than experienced with the IV Port-A-Cath (when implanted for IP anticancer drug administration). No prospective study has compared the complication rates associated with the use of the IV and peritoneal Port-A-Caths for IP chemotherapy administration.

Single-use systems include the Veress needle[19, 20] and percutaneous catheters.[16, 21] In a report by Menczer,[20] the Veress needle was used for 87 IP chemotherapy administrations in 32 patients, with only two cases of nonserious adverse events. The needle was inserted under local anesthesia, without aid of ultrasound, at a point midway on the line between the left anterior superior iliac spine and the umbilicus. Runowicz and coworkers[16] and Smith and associates[21] have reported the successful use of a percutaneous Drum-Cartridge catheter (Abbott Laboratories, Chicago, IL) for administration of chemotherapy and IP ³²P. In both reports, the percutaneous catheter was placed under local anesthesia (1% lidocaine [Xylocaine]) without ultrasonographic or radiologic guidance into the right or left lower quadrant. Catheter placement was generally successful during the first attempt. When multiple attempts were necessary, Smith and associates[21] reported an increased risk of complications, including bowel perforation. Once adequate flow was established, 2 L of normal saline was instilled by gravity, followed by the chemotherapeutic agents. The catheter was removed immediately after chemotherapy administration.

## Guidelines for Intraperitoneal Chemotherapy Administration

The following instructions for IP chemotherapy administration were developed for use in intergroup studies of IP chemotherapy conducted by the Southwest Oncology Group, Gynecologic Oncology Group, and Eastern Cooperative Group. They can also serve as general guidelines for IP chemotherapy administration.

1. An implantable device (typically an IV Port-A-Cath) should be surgically placed in the peritoneal cavity. If an implantable device is used, the peritoneal cavity should be accessed by a 19-gauge Huber point needle through the skin into the port following an aseptic alcohol–povidone-iodine (Betadine) preparation of the skin. At the time of catheter placement and after each chemotherapy treatment, the catheter should be flushed with saline. After the IP catheter has healed in place for 1 or 2 days, the patient can start IP chemotherapy.

2. Noninvasive imaging of IP patency and fluid distribution is not typically necessary. An imaging study should be considered, however, if installation of the dialysate is slow or the patient experiences increased pain after instillation of less than 2 L of fluid.

3. Before IP therapy administration, the peritoneal cavity should be drained as completely as possible (if ascites is present) via the peritoneal catheter.

4. Two liters of drug-containing fluid (warmed to body temperature) should be instilled into the peritoneal cavity as rapidly as possible. Instillation may require 30 to 60 minutes. If the flow rate is slow, a blood pressure cuff should be placed on the bag containing the drugs and inflated to 100 mm Hg to speed the flow. If there is difficulty instilling the full 2 L of fluid (because of patient discomfort or small size), the volume may be decreased to 1.5 L. If pain during instillation persists despite a decrease in volume and adjustment of analgesic medications, the total volume may be decreased to 1 L. Patients not able to tolerate 1 L of IP infusate should receive IV chemotherapy.

5. If IP cisplatin is being administered, concurrent with the start of the chemotherapy instillation, the patient should receive IV hydration with at least 1 L normal saline (with 3 g magnesium sulfate/L and 40 g mannitol). Patients with a history of congestive heart failure may be hydrated over an extended time period. Subsequent IV hydration is advisable for patients with inadequate oral intake.

6. Peritoneal cavity drainage is neither desirable nor indicated (no adverse consequences, other than patient discomfort, have been identified as a result of leaving the fluid in the abdomen). After completion of dialysate infusion, the catheter should be flushed with saline.

# REFERENCES

1. Landis SH, Murray T, Bolden S, Wingo PA. Cancer statistics, 1998. CA Cancer J Clin 1998;48:6–29.
2. Cannistra SA. Cancer of the ovary. N Engl J Med 1993;329:1550–9.
3. Dedrick RL, Myers CE, Bungay PM, De Vita VT Jr. Pharmacokinetic rationale for peritoneal drug administration in the treatment of ovarian cancer. Cancer Treat Rep 1978;62:1–11.
4. Howell SB, Pfeilfle CL, Wung WE, et al. Intraperitoneal cisplatin with systemic thiosulfate protection. Ann Intern Med 1982;6:845–51.
5. Howell SB. Intraperitoneal chemotherapy for ovarian cancer. J Clin Oncol 1988;6:1673–5.
6. Markman M, Reichman B, Hakes T, et al. Responses to second-line cisplatin-based intraperitoneal therapy in ovarian cancer: influence of a prior response to intravenous cisplatin. J Clin Oncol 1991;9:1801–5.
7. Alberts DS, Liu PY, Hannigan EV, et al. Intraperitoneal cisplatin plus intravenous cyclophosphamide versus intravenous cisplatin plus intravenous cyclophosphamide for stage III ovarian cancer. N Engl J Med 1996;335:1950–5.
8. Markman M, Bundy B, Benda J, et al. Randomized phase 3 study of intravenous (iv) cisplatin (cis)/paclitaxel (pac) versus moderately high dose IV carboplatin (carb) followed by iv pac and intraperitoneal (ip) cis in optimal residual ovarian cancer (oc): an intergroup trial (GOG, SWOG, ECOG). Proc ASCO 1998;17:361a.
9. Los G, Mutsaers PH, van der Vijgh WJ, et al: Direct diffusion of cis-diamminedichloroplatinum (II) in intraperitoneal rat tumors after intraperitoneal chemotherapy: a comparison with systemic chemotherapy. Cancer Res 1989;49:3380–4.
10. Markman M, Rowinsky E, Hakes T, et al. Phase I trial of intraperitoneal Taxol: a Gynecologic Oncology Group study. J Clin Oncol 1992;10:1485–91.
11. Muggia FM, Liu PY, Alberts DS, et al. Intraperitoneal mitoxantrone or floxuridine: effects on time-to-failure and survival in patients with minimal residual ovarian cancer after second-look laparotomy—a randomized phase II study by the Southwest Oncology Group. Gynecol Oncol 1996;61:395–402.
12. Walton LA, Blessing JA, Homesley HD. Adverse effects of intraperitoneal fluorouracil in patients with optimal residual ovarian cancer after second-look laparotomy: a Gynecologic Oncology Group study. J Clin Oncol 1989;7:466–70.
13. Bruzzone M, Rubagotti A, Gadducci A, et al. Intraperitoneal carboplatin with or without interferon-alpha in advanced ovarian cancer patients with minimal residual disease at second look: a prospective randomized trial of 111 patients. G.O.N.O. Gruppo Oncologic Nord Ovest Gynecol Oncol 1997;65:499–505.
14. Los G, Verdegaal EM, Mutsaers PH, McVie JG. Penetration of carboplatin and cisplatin into rat peritoneal tumor nodules after intraperitoneal chemotherapy. Cancer Chemother Pharmacol 1991;28:159–65.
15. Markman M, Reichman B, Hakes T, et al. Evidence supporting the superiority of intraperitoneal cisplatin compared to intraperitoneal carboplatin for salvage therapy of small-volume residual ovarian cancer. Gynecol Oncol 1993;50:100–4.
16. Runowicz CD, Dottino PR, Shafir MK, et al. Catheter complications associated with intraperitoneal chemotherapy. Gynecol Oncol 1986;24:41–50.
17. Waggoner SE, Johnson J, Barter J, Barnes W. Intraperitoneal therapy administered through a Groshong catheter. Gynecol Oncol 1994;53:320–5.
18. Almadrones L, Yerys C. Problems associated with the administration of intraperitoneal therapy using the Port-A-Cath system. Oncol Nurs Forum 1990;17:75–80.
19. Pfeiffer P, Asmussen L, Kvist-Poulson H, Bertelsen K. Intraperitoneal chemotherapy: introduction of a new "single-use" delivery system—a preliminary report. Gynecol Oncol 1989;35:47–9.
20. Menczer J. Use of the Veress needle for instillation of intraperitoneal chemotherapy. Gynecol Oncol 1995;59:249–50.
21. Smith HO, Gaudette DE, Goldberg GL, et al. Single-use percutaneous catheters for intraperitoneal $P^{32}$ therapy. Cancer 1994;73:2633–7.

# HEMATOLOGIC CONSIDERATIONS IN CANCER TREATMENT

# CHAPTER 13

# HEMATOLOGIC COMPLICATIONS OF CANCER AND ITS TREATMENT

● MICHAEL C. LILL

Hematologic abnormalities occur frequently in patients with neoplastic disorders. These abnormalities include increased or decreased concentrations of formed elements in the blood and changes in blood coagulation proteins. The major clinical sequelae are infection, bleeding, and thrombosis. In addition, tumor thromboembolism and veno-occlusive disease of the liver produce clinical syndromes indistinguishable from those that result from blood clotting abnormalities. Hematologic abnormalities eventually develop in almost all cancer patients. Sometimes these complications are profound and dominate the clinical picture.

In the modern era of cancer treatment, peripheral blood cytopenias resulting from chemotherapy and radiation therapy are the most frequently observed changes; these are discussed in Chapters 8 and 7, respectively. This chapter is concerned with other hematologic complications of cancer and its treatment. The reader is referred to the respective chapters for details of the treatment of infections (Chapter 20), transfusion of blood products (Chapter 14), and management of central venous catheters and their associated complications (Chapter 12, Vascular Access Catheters and Devices).

## Thrombohemorrhagic Disorders

### DISSEMINATED INTRAVASCULAR COAGULATION, VENOUS THROMBOEMBOLIC DISEASE, NONBACTERIAL THROMBOTIC ENDOCARDITIS, AND TROUSSEAU'S SYNDROME

**Disseminated Intravascular Coagulation.** There is abundant evidence that cancer cells may produce and release substances that activate procoagulant and fibrinolytic pathways; the release of such substances probably underlies the clinical development of disseminated intravascular coagulation (DIC). Procoagulant clotting factors, antithrombin III, protein C, fibrinogen, plasminogen, and platelets are consumed, and there is usually evidence of fibrinogen and fibrin degradation. The prothrombin, activated partial thromboplastin, and thrombin times become abnormal because of clotting factor depletion and the circulation of anticoagulant fibrinogen degradation products. The plasma fibrinogen level may be reduced. A positive protamine paracoagulation test indicates thrombin-mediated fibrinogen catabolism and circulating fibrin monomers. Serum fibrinogen and fibrin degradation products, fibrinopeptide A, and D-dimers are usually elevated when DIC is clinically significant. Thrombocytopenia is frequently present. When fibrin strands are formed in the microvasculature, erythrocytes may be fragmented.

None of these tests alone has sufficient sensitivity and specificity to diagnose DIC reliably, and the diagnosis is made when several test abnormalities are found in a high-risk clinical setting.

Routine laboratory tests and kinetic studies indicate that DIC is common in patients with malignancy. The mean fibrinogen turnover and platelet turnover are increased approximately threefold, although hypofibrinogenemia and thrombocytopenia may not be observed. Plasma fibrinopeptide A correlates with fibrinogen turnover and levels of fibrinogen and fibrin degradation products. The fibrinopeptide A generation rate and turnover, however, are proportionately less than the fibrinogen turnover, suggesting that thrombin-mediated fibrinogen proteolysis is only a small part of the overall enhanced fibrinogen catabolism. Heparin may normalize plasma fibrinopeptide A levels, whereas fibrinogen turnover remains accelerated. Some patients develop what appears to be primary fibrinolysis without evidence of thrombin generation.

The intensity of DIC appears to parallel the activity of the malignant disease. Of patients with metastatic cancer of various types, 95% were found to have elevated plasma fibrinopeptide A levels, compared with 20% of patients with malignancy without metastases and 10% of cancer patients with no evident disease.[1] Plasma fibrinopeptide A levels parallel disease activity in acute nonlymphocytic leukemia. Remission of DIC can accompany successful therapy of the underlying tumor. The control of the malignant disease is the most important factor in control of the coagulopathy.

In the setting of malignancy, DIC occurs in two general forms: acute and chronic. Acute DIC occurs in patients who have tumors with rapid cell division and necrosis. It may be considered a facet of the *tumor lysis syndrome*, in which tumors are rapidly lysed with effective anticancer treatment. In addition, acute DIC may accompany other serious complications of cancer or cancer treatment, including infection, hemolytic transfusion reactions, or hypotension from any cause. Acute DIC is invariably accompanied by multiple abnormal findings in coagulation tests. Chronic DIC occurs in patients whose cancers are not necessarily undergoing rapid growth or lysis; the process may be observed over weeks or months. If there are compensatory increases in clotting factor and platelet production (this is a frequent occurrence), there may be relatively few abnormalities in the coagulation tests. Plasma coagulation factor levels may even be increased, and hyperfibrinogenemia or increased levels of procoagulant factors V and VIII may be found. The activated partial thromboplastin time may be abnormally short, whereas the prothrombin time is usually prolonged, but both may be normal. The clinical complications of DIC, hemorrhage and thrombosis, do not correlate well with the extent of derangement of routine coagulation test results. Occasionally, laboratory findings suggesting fibrinolysis without DIC are found in acute and chronic leukemias and in prostate cancer. In primary fibrinolysis, as opposed to DIC, there is no evidence of thrombin generation (i.e., a negative protamine test), there is often a normal platelet count, and there is no schistocytosis; both syndromes, however, are associated with hypofibrinogenemia and high titers of fibrinogen and fibrin degradation products. Although there are no completely reliable tests to discriminate primary fibrinolysis from DIC, elevation of D-dimer levels implies lysis of cross-linked fibrin and supports a diagnosis of DIC.

Bleeding complications may occur during the course of DIC or primary fibrinolysis. Bleeding occurs from predisposed sites, such as vessel puncture sites and sites of recent surgery, biopsy, diagnostic procedures, or trauma, or there may be bruising on trivial injury. Rarely, in severe cases, spontaneous intracranial hemorrhage may occur; this complication occurs with particularly high frequency in association with acute leukemia, especially acute promyelocytic leukemia.

**Venous Thromboembolic Disease.** Venous thromboembolic disease (VTE) in cancer may be considered in two broad categories: (1) as an initial presentation of previously occult malignancy and (2) as a complication of established neoplasia or treatment of the underlying malignancy. A substantial body of evidence demonstrates that there is an increased risk of diagnosis of cancer in the years following the diagnosis of VTE. This evidence takes several forms: First, a number of series analyzed the risk of cancer in patients who were suspected of having VTE. Those who were proved to have VTE, by a variety of different techniques, had approximately a twofold increased risk of cancer relative to those shown not to have VTE.[2–7] Other investigators analyzed the development of cancer in cohorts of patients who were proved to have VTE and subdivided them into two groups: with and without known risk factors for VTE. The definition of risk factors varied from one study to another, but all of them showed the same trend, which was an increased risk of development of cancer in the idiopathic group.[8–19] A pooled analysis suggested a 4.8-fold increased risk of development of cancer in patients with idiopathic VTE relative to those with an established secondary cause.[20] Finally, two large population-based studies from Scandinavia demonstrated a 2.2-fold to 4.4-fold increased risk of diagnosis of cancer in the first 12 months following the diagnosis of VTE.[21, 22]

The most frequent malignancies detected in these studies varied with methodology; however, there were some common features. The Scandinavian studies found carcinoma of the pancreas, ovary, liver, and brain to be the most common solid tumor types associated with VTE, whereas other studies have found prostate, colorectal, lung, pancreas, and stomach to be most common.[8–11, 15, 18, 19, 21, 22] Breast cancer appears to be underrepresented.

The utility and cost-effectiveness of screening for cancer in patients with idiopathic VTE have not been formally established; however, it seems reasonable to perform at least some screening tests in this patient population. The history and physical examination should be focused on symptoms and signs of the most common cancers. Most patients with

VTE already have had a chest radiograph. Male patients greater than 50 years of age should have a prostate-specific antigen level checked. Women greater than 50 years of age who have not had a recent mammogram should have one performed. Patients older than age 50 who have not had recent sigmoidoscopy should have either colonoscopy or sigmoidoscopy. The role of abdominal and pelvic computed tomography (CT) scanning is uncertain because of its cost, potential complications, and low sensitivity and specificity.[23] The role of thoracic CT is also uncertain, although unpublished data suggest that spiral CT scans of the chest may have a role in the future in screening for lung cancer in high-risk patients.

Tumor compression of large vessels, prolonged bed rest and debility, congestive heart failure, smoking, central venous catheters, and estrogen administration contribute to the risk of development of VTE. It is generally considered, however, that patients with malignant disease have an increased risk of thrombosis even in the absence of identifiable precipitating factors.

An additional risk factor for VTE in cancer patients appears to be related to therapy. The best evidence for this is seen in breast cancer. Randomized studies of adjuvant chemotherapy have shown risks of VTE to range from 2.1 to 6% for patients receiving chemotherapy versus 0 to 0.8% for patients not receiving chemotherapy.[24–31] The risk of VTE decreased markedly once therapy was completed. The National Surgical Adjuvant Breast and Bowel Project (NSABP) randomized trial of tamoxifen as a chemopreventive agent has conclusively confirmed this association. Women older than age 50 receiving tamoxifen had approximately double the risk of VTE compared with women not receiving tamoxifen.[32] The risk of VTE seems to be higher in stage IV disease, in which 17.6% of patients receiving combination chemotherapy developed VTE.[33]

L-Asparaginase, used in the treatment of acute lymphoblastic leukemia, has also been clearly associated with increased risk of VTE, ranging from 1.1 to 14.3%.[34–36] The mechanism presumably involves inhibition of hepatic synthesis of anticoagulant proteins such as S and protein C.

Granulocyte-macrophage colony-stimulating factor (GM-CSF) has also been reported to increase the risk of thrombosis, although this is not a definite association.[37] Also, there appears to be an increased incidence of deep venous thrombosis during therapy for Hodgkin's disease. The mechanism for this increased thrombotic diathesis is unclear. Proteins C and S have been shown to fall during CMF (cyclophosphamide, methotrexate, fluorouracil) chemotherapy into the range seen with heterozygous protein C and protein S deficiencies in some patients. There is usually no significant change in antithrombin III and plasminogen levels. Protein C and antithrombin III levels can decrease during estrogen therapy for prostate cancer, and antithrombin III levels have been reported to drop in patients receiving tamoxifen for breast cancer. Plasma from patients undergoing chemotherapy for breast cancer can increase endothelial cell reactivity to platelets. In addition, thrombotic cerebrovascular accidents have been described in several patients after therapy with cisplatin, bleomycin, and vincristine for treatment of epidermoid or germ cell carcinomas. Myocardial infarctions have been reported in young patients, without risk factors for coronary disease, associated with chemotherapy with cisplatin and bleomycin. The mechanism of the acute arterial vascular events is unclear but may involve chemotherapy-induced increased vasospasm.

Venous thrombosis may involve only the deep venous system of the lower extremities. There is occasionally extensive involvement of superficial and deep veins throughout the body, however, and the inferior or superior vena cava, portal venous system, hepatic veins, veins draining the upper extremities, cerebral veins, and dural sinuses may be involved. Widespread venous thrombosis in a patient previously considered well and without risk factors for thrombosis should alert the physician to the possibility of occult malignancy. Paradoxic thromboembolism through a patent atrial septal defect has been observed.

Patients with cancer undergoing abdominal surgery have a substantially increased risk of VTE. The American Chest Physicians 1995 consensus conference reported that 40 to 80% of patients develop calf vein thrombosis and 10 to 20% develop proximal vein thrombosis.[38] The International Multicentre Trial for prevention of deep venous thrombosis demonstrated a 1.6% incidence of fatal pulmonary embolus in patients with cancer receiving no prophylaxis versus 0.5% in patients with benign conditions.[39] Prophylaxis with low-dose heparin in patients with cancer reduced the incidence of fatal pulmonary embolus to 0.4%. The presence of cancer is also an independent risk factor for death from pulmonary embolus with a hazard ratio of 2.3.[7]

All patients with malignant diseases, without contraindications to heparin therapy, undergoing major surgery should receive prophylaxis against deep venous thrombosis. A dose-response effect has been observed for dalteparin, with the incidence of deep venous thrombosis being reduced from 14.9% to 8.5% by increasing the dose from 2500 units daily to 5000 units daily.[40] Enoxaparin 30 mg daily resulted in a 14.7% incidence of deep venous thrombosis compared with heparin 5000 units three times a day, with an incidence of 18.2%.[41] These data suggest that it may be beneficial to use low-molecular-weight heparins as first-line prophylaxis. Low-molecular-weight heparins may also decrease cancer-associated mortality, but this remains to be definitively proved.[42, 43]

Patients with cancer have an increased risk of recurrence of VTE in the first 90 days after diagnosis (10% vs. 4%).[44–48] The presence of cancer is also an independent risk factor for warfarin (Coumadin)-induced bleeding.[49] Randomized studies have demonstrated that home administration of low-molecular-weight heparin is as safe as adjusted-dose heparin in the hospital.[44–46] Home administration of heparin may be preferable for many patients with cancer in whom quality of life is a major concern.

**Nonbacterial Thrombotic Endocarditis.** Nonbacterial thrombotic endocarditis (NBTE) can occur in patients with malignant disease. The overall incidence of NBTE in autopsy series has been found to be 1 to 2%. Most patients with NBTE detected at autopsy have an underlying malignancy, most frequently adenocarcinoma. The incidence of NBTE appears to be higher in certain subsets of cancer patients; it ranges from 3 to 7% at autopsy in patients with adenocarcinoma of the lung, pancreas, or prostate. NBTE can precede the diagnosis of cancer and can occur with localized disease. The aortic and mitral valves are primarily involved, with friable bland fibrinous vegetations of 1 mm

to greater than 2 cm in size; the tricuspid valve is rarely involved by itself. The diagnosis should be suspected in patients who develop one or more acute arterial events. Echocardiogram may be useful but is not highly sensitive diagnostically.

NBTE frequently results in arterial embolization; among cancer patients with arterial thromboemboli, 74% were found to have NBTE.[50] Autopsy studies of cancer patients with NBTE reveal systemic emboli in approximately 50% of cases.[51] Embolization may involve any arterial system, including cerebral, retinal, coronary, mesenteric, renal, and peripheral vasculature, and is often multiple. The cerebral and cardiac vasculatures are the most significant sites of clinical involvement. Transient neurologic symptoms can precede cerebral infarction secondary to NBTE. NBTE may also be associated with microvascular occlusion and tissue infarction secondary to DIC. DIC may cause multifocal brain infarctions in the absence of NBTE. Evidence of DIC is seen in 8 to 87% of patients with NBTE.

**Trousseau's Syndrome.** Some patients have one or more facets of a syndrome encompassing superficial or deep (or both) venous thromboembolism, NBTE, arterial thrombosis, and DIC; such associations are often referred to as *Trousseau's syndrome*. The syndrome appears in association with some types of malignancy more often than with others and can be the first manifestation of a malignancy. Table 13–1 lists the malignancies that are most commonly associated with DIC, Trousseau's syndrome, or both. Many different malignancies have been rarely associated with DIC or Trousseau's syndrome. In a review of patients who presented with clinical features of Trousseau's syndrome, adenocarcinoma of the pancreas was found in 24.2%, lung cancer in 19.8%, prostate cancer in 12.6%, gastric adenocarcinoma in 11.6%, acute leukemia in 9.3%, adenocarcinoma of the colon in 4.9%, carcinoma with unknown primary in 4.9%, ovarian cancer in 3.8%, cancer of the gallbladder in 3.3%, and miscellaneous tumors in the remaining 5.6%.[52] Most patients with pancreatic adenocarcinoma do not develop any signs of Trousseau's syndrome.

**Treatment of Disseminated Intravascular Coagulation.** It is a therapeutic dictum that the most important treatment of DIC is to alleviate identifiable precipitating factors. If malignancy per se is the cause, a successful outcome of treatment may nevertheless require time, during which the patient may be at risk of bleeding or thrombotic complications. Often the state of the art is such that eradication of

*Table 13–1.* **Common Association of Specific Types of Neoplasia with Disseminated Intravascular Coagulation or Trousseau's Syndrome or Both**

Pancreatic adenocarcinoma
Gastric adenocarcinoma
Prostatic adenocarcinoma
Ovarian adenocarcinoma
Colorectal, gallbladder adenocarcinoma
Lung cancer (all types)
Renal cell carcinoma
Hemangiosarcoma and vascular tumors
Acute promyelocytic leukemia
Acute leukemia (myeloblastic, monoblastic, lymphoblastic, undifferentiated; blast crisis of Ph1-positive chronic myelogenous leukemia)

the tumor is unlikely. Treatment of DIC in itself may become necessary. The use of blood products, such as fresh frozen plasma, cryoprecipitate, and platelet transfusion, may be of temporary value, but the benefit is short-lived if the consumptive process continues unabated.

When it is necessary to attenuate the process, especially when thrombotic complications or NBTE occurs, heparin is the treatment of choice. Heparin is superior to oral vitamin K antagonists, and prolonged therapy should be strongly considered for patients who have chronic DIC with Trousseau's syndrome. Most patients show some control with heparin anticoagulation. Patients usually require about 5 to 20 units/kg body weight/hr. Therapeutic efficacy is demonstrated by a rising platelet count and plasma fibrinogen, a negative protamine sulfate test, and decreasing titers of fibrinogen and fibrin degradation products. Once initial control is achieved, the subcutaneous route of heparin administration should be considered for convenience and outpatient feasibility. The required total daily dosage should be divided into injections at 8- or 12-hour intervals. In general, the dosage should be sufficient to optimize platelet count, fibrinogen, and serum fibrin degradation products, with a target activated partial thromboplastin time range of about 1.5 to 2 times control. Devastating clinical complications can occur when anticoagulation is discontinued; patients failing to respond to heparin rarely respond to warfarin.

**Treatment of Venous Thromboembolic Disease in Patients with Cancer.** All patients with VTE should be initially treated with heparin. This treatment may safely be carried out on an outpatient basis. All patients should receive at least 5 days of heparin treatment. Oral anticoagulation is a reasonable next step. This treatment should be continued for at least 3 months and probably for as long as the underlying malignancy is still active. Recurrent disease can be managed with low-molecular-weight heparin or insertion of a Greenfield filter.

The use of fibrinolytic inhibitors (e.g., aminocaproic acid, tranexamic acid) is seldom indicated. Treatment may be considered for patients who have bleeding from the lower urinary tract (in the absence of upper urinary tract bleeding) or for the rare patient with primary fibrinolysis. If a fibrinolytic inhibitor is given in the presence of DIC, thrombosis may result. Extreme caution is recommended in the use of fibrinolytic inhibitors. The role of fibrinolytic inhibitors in the management of DIC associated with acute promyelocytic leukemia is described subsequently.

Occasionally, acute venous thromboembolism is massive, or an extremity is threatened by an arterial embolus. In these instances, rapid clot dissolution by means of a thrombolytic agent administered systemically or locally may be considered. Currently available agents are streptokinase, urokinase, and tissue plasminogen activator. These drugs should be administered by personnel experienced in their use. A major thrombotic obstruction in the deep venous system in the thigh, pelvis, vena cava, or subclavian veins; an acute arterial embolus in a patient in whom embolectomy is impractical; and pulmonary embolism involving 30% or more of the pulmonary vascular bed (especially if accompanied by hypotension) are indications for the use of these drugs. Absolute contraindications to their use are active internal bleeding, a cerebrovascular accident within the previous 2 months, uncontrolled severe hypertension, or any known intracranial

process. In patients with cancers known to metastasize to the brain, it is wise to obtain negative results from CT scanning or magnetic resonance imaging of the brain before beginning therapy, even in the absence of neurologic findings on physical examination. Major contraindications in the cancer patient are surgery or invasive procedures (e.g., biopsies, lumbar punctures, large-gauge catheters recently placed or removed from noncompressible vessels) within the previous 10 days, a pre-existing coagulopathy, or thrombocytopenia.

Acute promyelocytic leukemia is a specific morphologic variant of acute nonlymphocytic leukemia, which is recognizable histologically by the presence of characteristic large granules and frequent Auer rods in the blast cells. It is often associated with DIC, fibrinolysis, and a severe bleeding disorder. This bleeding disorder has also developed during promyelocytic transformation of chronic myelogenous leukemia. Hypofibrinogenemia occurs more frequently in acute promyelocytic leukemia than in other morphologic variants of acute myelogenous leukemia. The pathophysiology of the bleeding disorder is complex and appears to involve a combination of procoagulant factor–associated DIC, release of plasminogen activators from endothelial and leukemic cells with concomitant activation of the fibrinolytic system, and release of proteases. Hemorrhage occurs in the skin, mucous membranes, gastrointestinal and urinary tracts, and central nervous system. Bleeding often worsens during remission induction therapy; without specific therapy, intracerebral bleeding may occur in more than half of patients. Risk factors for hemorrhage include pretreatment absolute peripheral blast and promyelocyte counts greater than 1000/$\mu$l, platelet counts less than 30,000/$\mu$l, plasma fibrinogen less than 150 mg/dl, age greater than 50, and, possibly, $\alpha_2$-antiplasmin levels less than 30% of normal. Early mortality resulting from hemorrhage may be 58% in some high-risk patients.

The treatment of acute promyelocytic leukemia has evolved dramatically over the last several years. The use of all-transretinoic acid (ATRA) substantially improves long-term, event-free survival and corrects some of the coagulation abnormalities seen in acute promyelocytic leukemia. Randomized studies have not shown any decrease in early mortality or hemorrhage in ATRA-treated patients versus chemotherapy-treated patients. Additionally, there may be an increased thrombotic risk associated with ATRA, particularly when combined with antifibrinolytic therapy.

There are no randomized studies to address the issue of optimal management of DIC in acute promyelocytic leukemia. A representative review is that of the GIMEMA group, which has reviewed their results with antihemorrhagic treatment in 268 consecutive patients with acute promyelocytic leukemia.[53] Ninety-four patients were treated with heparin, 67 with antifibrinolytic agents, and 107 with supportive care only. The incidence of early hemorrhagic death was 9.4%, with no significant difference seen between the groups. Patients who received heparin required significantly more platelet transfusions.

My current approach to management of patients with acute promyelocytic leukemia undergoing induction chemotherapy is to use intensive blood product support (i.e., fresh frozen plasma, cryoprecipitate, and platelets) and heparin during remission induction until there is a marked reduction in the number of promyelocytes and the DIC process has subsided. I usually maintain the platelet count greater than 50,000/μl and use sufficient fresh frozen plasma and cryoprecipitate to maintain the fibrinogen concentration greater than 150 mg/dl and the prothrombin time within 3 seconds of control until the coagulopathy subsides because serious bleeding has occurred at lower levels. Fatal hemorrhages (mostly intracranial) occur with an overall average of 19% (range, 10 to 25%) with the use of heparin, compared with 28% (range, 16 to 60%) in patients treated without heparin. Good results (19% total hemorrhage rate) were obtained at Harvard using only aggressive blood product support.[54] For patients who continue to bleed despite this therapy, an antifibrinolytic agent may be added to the regimen.

## CARCINOMA-ASSOCIATED THROMBOTIC MICROANGIOPATHY

Carcinoma-associated thrombotic microangiopathy is a syndrome clinically similar to thrombotic thrombocytopenic purpura and the hemolytic-uremic syndrome. Thrombocytopenia and a Coombs-negative hemolytic anemia with fragmented erythrocytes in the peripheral blood are almost invariably present. Mild renal insufficiency is common, but renal failure is unusual. Headaches, confusion, lethargy, or hemiparesis may be present. Variably severe coagulation abnormalities characteristic of DIC may be found in 50% of cases. The catabolism of radiolabeled fibrinogen has been shown to be increased in patients despite normal or near-normal plasma fibrinogen. Hyaline thrombi in the microvasculature (most frequently pulmonary) are characteristic and may contain tumor cells but not often platelets. The cause of thrombotic microangiopathy is unknown but most likely involves intravascular coagulation, tumor emboli, and endothelial damage, such as caused by immune complexes. One patient with colon carcinoma and thrombotic microangiopathy was found to have circulating immune complexes containing carcinoembryonic antigen. The syndrome has been described most frequently in patients with adenocarcinomas of the stomach (Table 13–2). It has also been described with adenocarcinomas of the breast, pancreas, ovary, prostate, and colon; with lung cancer (including extensive small cell); and with carcinoma of unknown primary. It has been described less frequently with epidermoid carcinoma, hepatoma, cholangiocarcinoma, cancer of the seminal vesicle, and hemangioendothelioma. This syndrome can occasionally be the first clinical manifestation of cancer, and its presence strongly suggests disseminated disease, although small localized gastric adenocarcinomas have been found at autopsy in some patients presenting with the syndrome. The severity of thrombocytopenia and hemolytic anemia with schistocytosis may parallel the extent of metastatic disease.

Thrombotic microangiopathy in association with malignancy is an ominous finding, and most patients do not survive 2 months. Transfusion requirements are high. Glucocorticoids and platelet-inhibitor drugs have been tried without success. Transfusions of plasma and heparinization can result in transient improvement, but heparinization should be reserved for patients who have clear laboratory evidence of DIC. In the few reported cases, heparin has not significantly altered the hemolytic process. Treatment of the malignant process (underlying disease) should be attempted whenever possible. Hematologic improvement and even remission of this syndrome have been observed with chemotherapy or hormonal therapy in responsive tumors.

## CHEMOTHERAPY-RELATED THROMBOTIC MICROANGIOPATHY

Thrombotic microangiopathy may follow the treatment of malignant disease with chemotherapeutic agents. In contrast to cancer-associated thrombotic microangiopathy, this syndrome frequently occurs with minimal or no residual disease. In addition, progressive renal insufficiency is usually a prominent feature, with approximately one third of patients requiring dialysis. This syndrome closely resembles the hemolytic-uremic syndrome. Thrombocytopenia and microangiopathic hemolytic anemia are constant findings. Coagulation abnormalities suggesting DIC may be present. Hypertension and noncardiogenic pulmonary edema frequently occur at some time during the clinical course; neurologic abnormalities are a less frequent finding. In contradistinction to cancer-associated, non–treatment-related thrombotic microangiopathy, blood products frequently exacerbate this syndrome, can precipitate pulmonary edema, and should be avoided if possible. Underlying malignancies have included adenocarcinoma of the stomach, pancreas, and colon; epidermoid cancers; carcinoma of unknown primary; hepatoma; and germ cell tumors. A surprisingly high frequency (10 to 20%) of the disease has been reported following bone marrow transplantation, with a widely varying mortality rate (0 to 80%). A few cases have been reported after treatment with cisplatin, bleomycin, and a *Vinca* alkaloid or with cyclosporin A. Most cases have occurred in association with mitomycin C chemotherapy, either alone or in combination with 5-fluorouracil or 5-fluorouracil and doxorubicin. The syndrome occurs at a median of 9.5 months after initiation of mitomycin C and is unusual in patients who have received less than 20 mg/m² of the agent. Occasionally, it can occur several months after the last dose of mitomycin C. The incidence in patients receiving mitomycin C is reported to be 4.1%.[55] Autopsy studies usually reveal microthrombi occluding the afferent renal microvasculature. There is usually minimal extrarenal involvement, primarily involving the lungs and brain. The cause is unknown but may involve mitomycin C–induced endothelial injury. In addition, immune complexes are elevated in most patients, and these complexes have been reported to induce in vitro aggregation of normal platelets.

The prognosis is grave, with a mortality rate of 70 to 80%, although the prognosis is probably better with early detection. Proteinuria and hematuria can be early signs. Most forms of therapy appear to be ineffective. Steroids, immunosuppressive agents, heparin, and platelet inhibitors have been attempted without success. Vincristine has been

*Table 13–2.* **Common Causes of Carcinoma-Associated Thrombotic Microangiopathy**

| | |
|---|---|
| Gastric adenocarcinoma | Prostate carcinoma |
| Breast adenocarcinoma | Colon carcinoma |
| Pancreatic adenocarcinoma | Lung carcinoma |
| Ovarian carcinoma | Carcinoma of unknown primary |

used successfully in two patients.[56] Plasmapheresis frequently reverses the hematologic abnormalities, but the progressive renal dysfunction is irreversible in most, although not all, patients. Staphylococcal protein A immunoperfusion has been reported to be beneficial in reversing the hematologic abnormalities and stabilizing or improving renal function in 25 of 55 patients treated.[57] Responding patients had a significantly better 1-year survival rate than nonresponding patients (61% vs. 22%). In a registry report, it was noted that treatment with staphylococcal A column immunoperfusion was associated with prolonged survival.[58] Although there are no controlled clinical trials, I recommend initial treatment with staphylococcal A column immunoperfusion. If this treatment is not available, aggressive plasmapheresis should be attempted.

## THROMBOHEMORRHAGIC COMPLICATIONS WITH L-ASPARAGINASE

L-Asparaginase is a first-line chemotherapeutic agent for lymphoblastic leukemia, although several complications are associated with its use (see Chapter 10). The drug inhibits protein synthesis, and a dose of 200 units/kg/day or 6000 units/m²/day is sufficient to reduce coagulation factor synthesis. After 4 days of treatment, serum levels of albumin, $\alpha_1$-antitrypsin, transferrin, $\alpha_2$-macroglobulin, and insulin fall, whereas gamma globulin levels rise. The prothrombin, activated partial thromboplastin, and thrombin times increase, whereas fibrinogen; factor II, V, IX, and X; antithrombin III; plasminogen; protein C; protein S; and $\alpha_2$-antiplasmin levels fall. Factor VIII and von Willebrand's factor levels are normal or increased, although qualitative abnormalities of von Willebrand's factor multimers have been demonstrated in patients with L-asparaginase–associated thrombosis. Plasma fibrinogen levels fall in virtually all treated patients, often to less than 100 mg/dl. Usually the fibrinogen level returns to normal 7 to 10 days after treatment is discontinued. Kinetic studies employing radiolabeled fibrinogen indicate that fibrinogen survival is usually unaltered during L-asparaginase therapy, suggesting that decreased fibrinogen synthesis is the cause of hypofibrinogenemia. Patients with acute lymphoblastic leukemia have increased thrombin generation at presentation. During L-asparaginase treatment, the capacity to generate thrombin in vitro is preserved, but the capacity to inhibit thrombin is decreased.

Despite major changes in coagulation studies and fibrinogen levels, bleeding complications resulting from L-asparaginase therapy appear to be rare. No bleeding complications occurred in 26 patients who had platelet counts greater than 100,000/µl. Bleeding complications may develop when treatment is associated with the development of DIC. Thrombotic complications, including stroke and venous thrombosis, have been estimated to occur in 2.1 to 4.25% of patients receiving L-asparaginase, and these may occur more frequently in older patients and in those with a prior history of a thrombotic event. Thrombotic complications can occur during or after remission induction, and they usually occur between days 16 and 29 after the institution of therapy. It is unclear but possible that reduction in antithrombin III, protein S, protein C, and plasminogen or abnormalities in the

von Willebrand factor molecule are related to the development of thrombotic complications.

For bleeding complications or severe coagulopathy during L-asparaginase therapy or for coexisting severe thrombocytopenia, treatment with fresh frozen plasma, cryoprecipitate, or platelets should be considered as appropriate. Administration of antithrombin III concentrate (2000 units every other day, or 50 units/kg daily) has been shown to prevent the usual decline in protein C, protein S, plasminogen, $\alpha_2$-antiplasmin, and factor VII, and it reduces levels of thrombin-antithrombin complexes. It is not clear whether this reduction translates into an antithrombotic activity, but in a patient at high risk, one may consider heparin prophylaxis with or without antithrombin III.

## THROMBOSIS AND HYPEREOSINOPHILIA

Eosinophilia may be associated with malignant disorders (see section on eosinophilia later in this chapter). Occasionally, eosinophil counts are extremely elevated, and complications of the hypereosinophilic syndrome may develop, including pulmonary infiltrates and Löffler's endocarditis. Hypereosinophilia may be associated with deep venous thrombosis, and Löffler's endocarditis is associated with overlying mural thrombosis and embolism.

## CONDITIONS MIMICKING THROMBOTIC DISORDERS

**Tumor Thromboembolism.** Embolic tumor masses may produce clinical syndromes that are indistinguishable from those caused by the more typical fibrin thromboemboli. Tumor emboli are found in 26% of cases at autopsy.[59] Major tumor embolism to the lungs may result in dyspnea, pleuritic pain, hemoptysis, pulmonary infarction, and pulmonary hypertension. Pulmonary tumor emboli were found in 33 of 331 autopsied patients with non–small cell lung cancer. Tumor emboli have also been described in renal cell carcinoma, testicular cancer, parotid gland tumor, thyroid cancer, hepatoma, soft tissue sarcoma, chondrosarcoma, and adrenal carcinoma. Tumor thrombi confined to the renal veins or inferior vena cava have been described in renal cell carcinoma, Wilms' tumor, and adrenal carcinoma.

Arterial tumor embolism appears to be rare. Only 12 cases were reported in a 1978 review.[60] Among patients who develop arterial tumor emboli, nearly all have primary or metastatic lung tumors. Among patients reported, the primary tumors were bronchogenic carcinoma or sarcomas in almost all cases. It has been suggested that arterial emboli are fragments of pulmonary tumor masses that have grown into pulmonary veins; rarely, arterial tumor embolism is paradoxic, occurring through a patent foramen ovale or ductus arteriosus.

**Veno-occlusive Disease of the Liver.** Veno-occlusive disease of the liver is a distinct histopathologic entity characterized clinically by tender hepatomegaly, ascites, or unexplained weight gain and by abnormal liver function tests with an elevated bilirubin level.[61] Frequently, refractoriness to platelet transfusions develops. On pathologic examination, there is nonthrombotic obliteration of the terminal hepatic venules and small sublobular veins by a reticular and collagenous intimal thickening. On clinical grounds, it is difficult to distinguish veno-occlusive disease from hepatic vein thrombosis (Budd-Chiari syndrome).

Veno-occlusive disease has been associated with hepatic radiation (usually >3000 cGy), 6-thioguanine, dacarbazine, azathioprine, and acute leukemia treated with combination chemotherapy. It is a common complication associated with allogeneic bone marrow transplantation for various disorders and was found in 53% of cases in one large series of 355 patients.[62] Because bone marrow transplant patients develop a multiplicity of clinical complications and receive numerous kinds of treatment, it has been difficult to ascertain precisely the most important predisposing factors. There is evidence that preparatory regimens, including high-dose busulfan (5 to 20 mg/kg), carmustine (450 mg/m²), or mitomycin (60 to 90 mg/m²), may have predisposed transplant patients to veno-occlusive disease. The combination of graft-versus-host disease prophylaxis with methotrexate together with conditioning with busulfan and cyclophosphamide appeared to be particularly problematic, resulting in a 70% incidence of veno-occlusive disease. Patients with pretransplant hepatitis appear to have a threefold increased incidence of veno-occlusive disease. The disease is considerably less common (4.5%) in patients undergoing autologous bone marrow transplantation.

Veno-occlusive disease is a serious and frequently lethal complication. Of 53 bone marrow transplant patients in whom it developed, the complication was considered to contribute to death in 17 (32%). Seven others had serious progressive liver disease, whereas the rest (45%) recovered at a mean of 21 days after onset.[63] The degree of elevation of bilirubin has prognostic significance. A prognostic index has been developed using elevation in bilirubin and degree of weight gain that predicts outcome from veno-occlusive disease. On occasion, however, veno-occlusive disease may remain subclinical. One prospective randomized clinical trial strongly supported a benefit for prophylactic heparin in the prevention of this disorder,[64] another suggested a benefit for prophylactic ursodiol,[65] and another suggested a benefit for prophylactic infusion of prostaglandin.[66] Case reports have suggested that some patients with severe disease may benefit from thrombolytic therapy. Currently the standard of care for this disorder is purely supportive. Spontaneous reversal of the clinical manifestations has been reported when the complication was due to 6-thioguanine or azathioprine.

## Bleeding Disorders

### COAGULOPATHIES

**Dysfibrinogenemia.** Hepatocellular carcinoma can be associated with dysfibrinogenemia. This coagulopathy is not specific for hepatoma and can be seen with other forms of serious liver injury or L-asparaginase therapy. There is usually a prolonged thrombin time, prolonged reptilase time, and disparity between the apparent fibrinogen concentration when measured by thrombin clotting assays versus heat-precipitable protein or immunologic assays. Abnormal fibrin monomer polymerization is seen. Carbohydrate analysis of the abnormal fibrinogen molecules has revealed an increased sialic acid content, the extent of which is proportional to the prolongation of thrombin time and fibrin monomer polymerization.

**Factor Deficiencies and Inhibitors.** On rare occasions, factor deficiencies can be seen with various malignancies. Circulating factor VIII inhibitors have been associated with mycosis fungoides, lymphomas, IgA myeloma, prostate carcinoma, and lung, colon, and renal carcinoma. Factor X deficiency may occur in primary amyloidosis as a result of rapid clearance by absorption onto amyloid fibrils. Improvement may result from splenectomy or melphalan and prednisone therapy. A case of severe, but remittent, factor XIII deficiency was seen in a patient with chronic myelomonocytic leukemia.[67]

**Lupus Anticoagulant.** A paraprotein with properties of a lupus anticoagulant has been described in a patient without a thrombohemorrhagic diathesis who had Waldenström's macroglobulinemia.[68] Lupus anticoagulants have also been described in multiple myeloma, monoclonal gammopathy of unknown significance, lymphoproliferative diseases, hairy cell leukemia, acute myelogenous leukemia, non-Hodgkin's lymphoma, and other malignancies. In one study, the titer of antiphospholipid antibody normalized in patients responding to treatment for acute myelogenous leukemia or non-Hodgkin's lymphoma.[69]

**von Willebrand's Syndrome.** von Willebrand's syndrome is a bleeding syndrome characterized by reduced levels of von Willebrand's factor measured by immunologic or functional (ristocetin cofactor) assays. Additional common findings are a prolonged bleeding time, prolonged activated partial thromboplastin time, and reduced factor VIII. Acquired forms of von Willebrand's syndrome have been associated with a variety of tumors predominantly hematologic in origin (Table 13–3). Included among the causes are Wilms' tumor, multiple myeloma, monoclonal gammopathy, Waldenström's macroglobulinemia, chronic lymphocytic leukemia, lymphoma, polycythemia rubra vera, and chronic myelogenous leukemia.

Both type I and type IIa von Willebrand's syndrome have been described. On the basis of in vitro studies, several mechanisms probably give rise to acquired von Willebrand's disease. None of the three cases described with Wilms' tumor had a circulating inhibitor to von Willebrand's factor, and all had improvement or cure with resection of the tumor. High serum levels of hyaluronic acid were described in one patient with Wilms' tumor, and hyaluronic acid added to normal platelet-poor plasma induces a von Willebrand–type picture. Some patients are found to have inhibitors against ristocetin cofactor, although most do not. Some patients probably have immunoglobulin binding to an inactive portion of the von Willebrand factor molecule with accelerated clearance of this complex. In one patient, improvement was noted following treatment of the lymphoma. In a case associated with Waldenström's macroglobulinemia, lymphocytes

*Table 13–3.* **Causes of Acquired von Willebrand's Disease**

| | |
|---|---|
| Wilms' tumor | Chronic lymphocytic leukemia |
| Multiple myeloma | Lymphoma |
| Monoclonal gammopathy | Polycythemia rubra vera |
| Waldenström's macroglobulinemia | Chronic myelogenous leukemia |

were able to absorb the von Willebrand factor, and there was clinical improvement following splenectomy.[70] Transient responses to desmopressin have been observed.

**Vitamin K Deficiency.** Vitamin K is obtained from the diet and from intestinal bacteria. It is fat soluble, and it requires bile salts and normal intestinal mucosa for absorption. Vitamin K is required for post-translational modification of the procoagulant factors II, VII, IX, and X and the anticoagulant factors protein C and protein S. Gamma carboxylation of these proteins is required for them to be functional, and this step requires the presence of reduced vitamin K. The reduced vitamin K is consumed in the process and is recycled via the vitamin K epoxide reductase pathway. Deficiency of reduced vitamin K may result from starvation, especially when broad-spectrum antibiotics are administered concurrently, or from biliary obstruction. The oral anticoagulants (e.g., warfarin) and aspirin in large doses (usually >3 g/day) antagonize vitamin K action by inhibiting vitamin K epoxide reductase and vitamin K reductase. Actinomycin D may antagonize vitamin K–induced correction of the prothrombin time.

The prothrombin time is the most sensitive screening laboratory test for detecting a depletion of vitamin K–dependent procoagulant factors. The activated partial thromboplastin time is less sensitive, and the thrombin time is normal. Addition of an equal volume of normal plasma to the patient's plasma corrects the prothrombin time. Correction of the prothrombin time after vitamin K administration is diagnostic.

Because malignant disease may be associated with multiple additional coagulopathies (e.g., DIC or the coagulopathy of hepatic insufficiency), it may be difficult to establish with certainty the diagnosis of vitamin K deficiency with routine laboratory tests. If the prothrombin time is prolonged, a therapeutic trial of vitamin K is usually warranted. In the adult, vitamin $K_1$, 10 mg by oral or subcutaneous routes, is sufficient when the deficiency is not related to oral anticoagulants. Parenteral administration is preferred if biliary obstruction or malabsorption is suspected. The intravenous route should be reserved for patients with active bleeding because of the risk, albeit low, of an anaphylactoid reaction. The intramuscular route of administration is not usually required and may result in the development of a significant hematoma in these patients. A dose of 50 mg may be needed to treat a serious oral anticoagulant overdose. If serious bleeding is present, the deficiency state is immediately reversible by infusion of a volume of plasma equal to 30 to 40% of the patient's estimated plasma volume (average estimated plasma volume is 45 ml/kg).

## PLATELET DISORDERS

**Thrombocytopenia.** Thrombocytopenia is a common occurrence in patients with malignant disease. It may result from extensive tumor infiltration of the bone marrow, radiation therapy, chemotherapeutic agents, other drugs, DIC or thrombotic microangiopathy, hypersplenism, infection, or post-transfusion purpura. In addition, an idiopathic thrombocytopenic purpura (ITP)–like syndrome may develop, which is characterized by selective thrombocytopenia, circulating megathrombocytes, and adequate to increased numbers of

bone marrow megakaryocytes, in the absence of other apparent causes of thrombocytopenia. This ITP-like syndrome has been reported most frequently in association with Hodgkin's disease, lymphoma, and chronic lymphocytic leukemia. It has also been infrequently seen in association with acute lymphoblastic leukemia; Waldenström's macroglobulinemia; after bone marrow transplantation; with small cell lung cancer and non–small cell lung cancer; and with colorectal, germ cell, prostate, pancreatic, epidermoid, breast, and ovarian carcinomas. The syndrome can predate the diagnosis of the tumor. On rare occasions, the ITP-like syndrome has been associated with a Coombs-positive hemolytic anemia. Cisplatin chemotherapy has also been associated with the acute development of thrombocytopenia and a Coombs-positive hemolytic anemia.

In Hodgkin's disease, the ITP-like syndrome may be the initial clinical manifestation. Although it may be the sole clinical manifestation of recurrent disease, patients considered to be in complete remission after treatment have been followed for 10 years after development of the ITP-like syndrome without recurrent disease. Hodgkin's disease, however, was found in the spleen of one patient who developed the ITP-like syndrome who was believed to have been in complete remission. Patients with Hodgkin's disease who develop the ITP-like syndrome may improve after splenectomy, although the syndrome can occur postsplenectomy. Glucocorticoids can be beneficial. Therapy of the underlying Hodgkin's disease may resolve the thrombocytopenia.

The ITP-like syndrome may precede or accompany the development of lymphoma. Prognosis is usually determined by how effectively the underlying lymphoma can be treated. In chronic lymphocytic leukemia, the syndrome may improve with glucocorticoids, alkylators, or splenectomy, although steroid failure has been reported. Glucocorticoid therapy has been reported to improve the ITP-like syndrome associated with acute lymphoblastic leukemia. A glucocorticoid, splenectomy, or vincristine may benefit patients who develop the ITP-like syndrome in association with solid tumors.

**Thrombocytosis.** Thrombocytosis is common in cancer patients, and, conversely, it can indicate an underlying malignancy. In several studies, 40% of cancer patients had platelet counts exceeding 400,000/L. Among all patients with platelet counts exceeding 500,000/L, 36% and 21% had a malignancy in two separate studies. Most cases of secondary thrombocytosis are mild or moderate in severity, with platelet counts rarely exceeding 1 million/L.

Thrombocytosis appears to be particularly common in association with all forms of lung cancer (approximate frequency 50%). This disorder has also been noted in adenocarcinomas of the gastrointestinal tract, breast, ovary, and uterus; cancer of the esophagus and liver; choriocarcinoma and retinoblastoma; Hodgkin's disease; fibrous histiocytoma; and multiple myeloma. An elevated platelet count can be seen in acute nonlymphocytic leukemia in association with rearrangement of the long arm of chromosome 3 (3q21).

Thrombocytosis may be attributed to an effect of malignancy only when other causes have been considered and excluded, including primary bone marrow disorders, iron deficiency anemia, the postsplenectomy state, infections, and other inflammatory disorders. Firm evidence that thrombocytosis secondary to a malignant disease may predispose to thrombosis is lacking. A conservative viewpoint is that thrombocytosis coupled with additional risk factors for thrombosis may contribute to a thrombotic diathesis.

Optimal therapy of secondary thrombocytosis is treatment of the underlying cause. Cytoreductive therapy for thrombocytosis per se is not generally warranted. Anticoagulation should be reserved for patients with thrombotic complications. A role for platelet-inhibitor drugs is undefined.

Essential or primary thrombocythemia is a myeloproliferative disorder that may be associated with a bleeding or a thrombotic diathesis. Patients may present with erythromelalgia, a syndrome characterized by attacks of severe burning pain, erythema, and warmth of the extremities, frequently dramatically relieved by a single aspirin. One large study of 100 consecutive patients demonstrated a low risk of significant hemorrhage (0.33%/patient year) versus a risk of thrombosis (6.6%/patient year).[71] The authors suggested that the risk of thrombosis could be reduced by decreasing the platelet count to less than 600,000/μl. This approach has not been proved in randomized, controlled clinical trials.

**Acquired Platelet Disorders.** Acquired platelet dysfunction may occur in association with lymphoma, acute and chronic leukemias, myeloproliferative disorders, hairy cell leukemia, and myelodysplastic syndromes.

## COMPLEX BLEEDING DISORDERS

**Mithramycin Therapy.** Mithramycin may be associated with the development of a bleeding disorder when doses of 25 to 50 μg/kg are given daily for 5 days or more. Ecchymosis, mucosal bleeding, hemoptysis, hematuria, and gastrointestinal bleeding may occur. Thrombocytopenia; prolongation of the bleeding time; platelet function abnormalities; reduced platelet adenosine diphosphate stores; prolongation of the prothrombin time; and reduced levels of factors II, V, and VII have been reported. Bleeding may occur without thrombocytopenia. The bleeding time usually remains prolonged for 1 to 2 weeks.

**Paraproteinemia.** Paraproteinemia may be associated with a bleeding tendency. With IgG multiple myeloma, there is a hemorrhagic diathesis in 15% of patients, and the incidence is higher with IgA multiple myeloma and Waldenström's macroglobulinemia. Paraproteins may cause prolongation of the bleeding time; platelet dysfunction; prolongation of the prothrombin, thrombin, and reptilase times; and defective fibrin monomer polymerization. Plasmapheresis may ameliorate the hemostatic defect. Bleeding is more common with high paraprotein levels. Paraproteins may function as clotting factor inhibitors and may result in or cause a hemorrhagic diathesis, as previously reviewed in this chapter.

**Antibiotic-Associated Coagulopathy.** Antibiotics are frequently required in cancer patients. Semisynthetic penicillins and some cephalosporins can induce a multifunctional hemorrhagic diathesis that can be clinically significant, especially in the presence of thrombocytopenia, renal failure, or malnutrition. Cephalosporins with a methylthiotetrazole side chain (moxalactam, cefoperazone, cefamandole, and cefotetan) can cause hypoprothrombinemia secondary to inhibition of gamma carboxylation of vitamin K–dependent clotting factors. This effect is prevented or rapidly reversed by parenteral vitamin K. In addition, semisynthetic penicillins and moxalactam induce a qualitative platelet defect characterized by decreased platelet aggregation and a prolonged bleeding time. This effect appears to be most common with carbenicillin, ticarcillin, and moxalactam; less frequent with piperacillin; and least common with mezlocillin. This platelet defect resolves within 3 to 4 days of stopping the responsible antibiotic.

**Liver Dysfunction.** Liver dysfunction may develop during the course of malignancy. The associated coagulopathy is complex. Hepatocellular failure results in decreased clotting factor synthesis and platelet dysfunction. Chronic low-grade DIC may occur and, occasionally, enhanced fibrinolysis. Factor VIII is notably unaffected, unless there is DIC. The level of plasma fibrinogen is usually preserved until liver disease is far advanced. If hypofibrinogenemia accompanies relatively mild hepatic dysfunction, DIC or primary fibrinolysis should be suspected. DIC is most likely to occur in patients with liver disease as a result of sepsis or peritoneovenous shunting. Bile salt deficiency may lead to malabsorption of vitamin K and cause vitamin K–dependent clotting factor deficiencies. Dysfibrinogenemia can occur with serious liver injuries and with hepatomas. Thrombocytopenia is common and may result from hypersplenism or shortened platelet survival. Patients with relatively mild abnormalities in coagulation tests or platelet count may have severe bleeding during a surgical operation. Thrombotic complications are unusual.

Patients with bleeding complications or those who undergo surgery usually require treatment to correct the hemostatic defects. Fresh frozen plasma, cryoprecipitate, and platelet transfusions may be employed, depending on the precise defect. Vitamin K$_1$, 10 mg parenterally, may be given. Desmopressin may result in transient improvement in the bleeding time. Heparin therapy for DIC in the liver disease setting is seldom justifiable. Fibrinolytic inhibition may be considered if attempts to control bleeding are unsuccessful, particularly if DIC is excluded.

**Renal Insufficiency.** Renal insufficiency is associated with a bleeding disorder resulting from a qualitative platelet disorder. In azotemic patients without other complications, the platelet count and prothrombin and activated partial thromboplastin times are normal. When it is necessary to correct the hemostatic defect, dialysis, infusion of cryoprecipitate, intravenous desmopressin, high-dose conjugated estrogen, or red cell transfusion or erythropoietin may be of benefit.

## Generalized Bone Marrow Disorders

Currently the most common cause of peripheral blood cytopenias in cancer patients is bone marrow hypoplasia, which results from the administration of chemotherapeutic drugs or the direct or abscopal effects of radiation therapy. The effects of chemotherapy are discussed in Chapters 8 and 10. Findings in the peripheral blood are anemia with reticulocytopenia, neutropenia, and thrombocytopenia. The bone marrow may show variable degrees of hypoplasia, megaloblastic and dysplastic changes, and redistribution of cellular maturation. Megaloblastic changes can result from chemotherapy agents

**Table 13–4.** Causes of Carcinoma-Induced Myelofibrosis

| | |
|---|---|
| Chronic myeloid leukemia | Bronchogenic carcinoma |
| Prostate cancer | Fibrosarcoma |
| Gastric adenocarcinoma | Hodgkin's disease |
| Breast carcinoma | Multiple myeloma |

and folic acid deficiency in malnourished patients and have also been due to vitamin $B_{12}$ deficiency associated with multiple myeloma in several cases. Tumor involvement of bone marrow may be associated with cytopenias or a leukoerythroblastic picture. Patients treated with alkylating agents may develop a myelodysplastic syndrome that can lead to acute leukemia.

An uncommon complication of cancer is myelofibrosis, which can mimic agnogenic myeloid metaplasia. It may be accompanied by osteosclerosis, bone marrow necrosis, or myeloid metaplasia. It is often associated with tumor involvement of the bone marrow. A wide variety of tumors have been associated with this problem (Table 13–4). Prostate cancer, gastric adenocarcinoma, breast cancer, bronchogenic carcinoma, fibrosarcoma, Hodgkin's disease, and multiple myeloma have been linked. Myelofibrosis associated with Hodgkin's disease may reverse with successful chemotherapy, and it has been reported to reverse during successful treatment of breast cancer. The myeloid fibrosis commonly associated with chronic myelogenous leukemia is completely reversible with bone marrow transplantation.

Bone marrow necrosis is a rare complication of cancer. It is accompanied by bone pain in 85% of cases, and it may be associated with a leukoerythroblastic picture, cytopenias, fat embolization, or hypercalcemia. It has been associated with myeloproliferative disorders; acute leukemias; lymphoma; and solid tumors, including gastric adenocarcinoma, cystadenocarcinoma of the ovary, and anaplastic bronchogenic carcinoma. It may accompany tumor involvement of the bone marrow with myelofibrosis. Necrotic tumor in the marrow stained with Romanowsky's dyes may stain reddish, compared with normal bluish marrow staining. Successful treatment of the underlying malignant disease led to bone marrow recovery in one case.[72]

# Erythrocyte Disorders

## ERYTHROCYTOSIS

Physiologically inappropriate erythrocytosis may accompany various neoplastic disorders and may present as the initial clinical problem. Ectopic production of erythropoietin has been demonstrated in some cases but not in others. Paraneoplastic erythropoiesis is not usually accompanied by splenomegaly and panmyelosis, which helps to discriminate it from polycythemia vera. During investigation of the course of erythrocytosis, non-neoplastic causes should be considered, including heavy smoking (carboxyhemoglobinemia), chronic lung disease, right-to-left cardiac shunts, hemoglobinopathy with aberrant oxygen binding, renal cysts, hydronephrosis, Cushing's disease, and androgen or glucocorticoid treatment. All patients with unexplained secondary erythrocytosis should undergo abdominal CT to look for renal,

adrenal, and hepatic masses or renal cysts, a careful pelvic examination to look for uterine fibroids, and a neurologic examination to look for cerebellar signs of cerebellar hemangioblastoma. An erythropoietin level may be useful in distinguishing between primary and secondary erythrocytosis.[73]

Neoplastic diseases associated with erythrocytosis are listed in Table 13–5. Among 340 patients with tumor-associated erythrocytosis, renal lesions were found in 52%, including 35% with renal cell carcinomas and 14% with benign renal lesions (cysts, hydronephrosis, and adenomas).[74] Also, 19% of the patients had hepatomas and 15% had cerebellar hemangioblastoma. Erythrocytosis occurs in 4 to 6% of patients with renal cell carcinoma; a rising hematocrit may signal tumor recurrence. After renal cell carcinoma, hepatoma is the next most frequently associated tumor. Erythrocytosis is common in patients with hepatoma, with an incidence of approximately 10%. When sought, an elevated erythrocyte mass is found more frequently. Other neoplastic causes of erythrocytosis are less common. Successful removal of the tumor or treatment of a renal cyst or hydronephrosis relieves erythrocytosis in 97% of cases.

## HYPOPROLIFERATIVE ANEMIA

Hypoproliferative anemia, which is characterized by an inappropriately low reticulocyte count, is common in cancer patients. Causative factors include the administration of chemotherapeutic drugs and radiation therapy, malnutrition, hypersplenism, iron deficiency, renal insufficiency, and other conditions mentioned previously that are generalized bone marrow disorders.

In addition, chronically ill cancer patients frequently develop the *anemia of chronic disease*, characterized by a normal reticulocyte count, a low serum iron and iron-binding capacity, normal to reduced normoblastic marrow activity, and adequate marrow iron stores with reduced numbers of sideroblasts. The cause is unknown. Iron deficiency anemia has been associated with renal cell carcinoma and is possibly caused by the diversion of iron to hemosiderin in the tumor. Erythropoietin levels are usually slightly low or appropriate for the degree of anemia. In randomized studies, treatment of anemic cancer patients with erythropoietin, 100 to 300 units/kg three times per week, resulted in significant increases in the hematocrit and significant improvement in the quality of life of the patients. About half of the patients with the hypoproliferative anemia of cancer appear to benefit from erythropoietin therapy.[75] (This topic is further discussed in Chapter 15.)

A syndrome of microcytic anemia and unbalanced globin chain synthesis, without iron deficiency or thalassemia, in a group of untreated Hodgkin's disease patients has been described.[76] The microcytic anemia and abnormal globin

**Table 13–5.** Causes of Paraneoplastic Erythrocytosis

| | |
|---|---|
| Renal neoplasia | Cerebellar hemangioblastoma |
| Hypernephroma | Adrenal tumors (including pheochromocytoma) |
| Wilms' tumor | Ovarian tumors |
| Sarcoma | Lung tumors |
| Adenoma | Uterine fibroids |
| Hepatoma | Thymoma |

*Table 13–6.* **Causes of Paraneoplastic Pure Red Cell Aplasia**

Thymoma
Lymphoma
Chronic lymphocytic leukemia
T-gamma lymphoproliferative disease
Acute lymphoblastic leukemia
Chronic myelogenous leukemia
Adenocarcinoma (breast, stomach, bile duct, unknown primary thyroid)
Bronchogenic carcinoma (including small cell type)
Azathioprine

synthesis resolved with therapy and recurred with relapse. An acquired sideroblastic anemia has been associated with chronic lymphocytic leukemia. Anemia may precede or accompany alkylator-induced leukemia.

An unusual form of hypoproliferative anemia is pure red cell aplasia (PRCA), characterized by anemia and severe reticulocytopenia, with the virtual absence of erythroid development in the bone marrow. Granulocytopoiesis and thrombopoiesis are usually preserved; they may also be affected, however, and the picture may appear to be that of pan-marrow hypoplasia.

Neoplastic disorders that have been associated with PRCA are listed in Table 13–6. The strongest association is with thymoma; about half of adults developing PRCA have a thymoma. The average age of these patients is 60 years (range, 20 to 78 years), and women are affected twice as often as men. Most thymomas are noninvasive and can be of various histologic types. Associated clinical disorders include myasthenia gravis, hypogammaglobulinemia, hypergammaglobulinemia, positive Coombs' test, pancytopenia with bone marrow hypoplasia, thrombocytopenia, and neutropenia. Thrombocytopenia or neutropenia does not usually precede PRCA, but these or aplastic anemia can develop after the onset of PRCA. Thymectomy results in improved marrow activity in only about one third of cases, suggesting that the thymoma per se is not always responsible for marrow hypofunction. PRCA may develop after thymectomy for the treatment of myasthenia gravis. Thymectomy may normalize a positive Coombs' test. PRCA secondary to thymoma may respond to alkylator therapy combined with steroids. B-cell chronic lymphocytic leukemia–associated PRCA appears to respond frequently to alkylator therapy; spontaneous remissions can also occur. Cyclosporin A caused a good response in two B-cell chronic lymphocytic leukemia PRCA patients resistant to alkylators and antithymocyte globulin.

In other neoplastic disorders, PRCA is not necessarily related to the status of the underlying tumor and can precede the diagnosis of the tumor. Improvement of PRCA has been reported following glucocorticoid or cytotoxic immunosuppressive treatment and after splenectomy.

## HEMOLYTIC ANEMIA

Hemolytic anemia is unusual in cancer patients, occurring in only 2 or 3% of cases. This form of anemia is characterized by reticulocytosis and indirect hyperbilirubinemia. When hemolysis is brisk, there may be circulating nucleated erythrocytes, and the serum lactate dehydrogenase is elevated. The peripheral blood smear should be examined, and

the direct and indirect antiglobulin (Coombs') tests should be obtained. The bone marrow shows erythroid hyperplasia when its activity has not been suppressed by chemotherapy or radiation therapy. Immediate and delayed hemolytic transfusion reactions should be considered, and acute blood loss as a cause of the anemia and reticulocytosis should also be excluded.

**Warm-Type Immune Hemolytic Anemia.** Warm-type immune hemolytic anemia is characterized by a positive Coombs' test and has been described in association with various neoplastic disorders. It may be the initial presentation. It has especially been associated with chronic lymphocytic leukemia, lymphoma, Hodgkin's disease, angioimmunoblastic lymphadenopathy with dysproteinemia, and ovarian teratomas. Additional rare associations are epidermoid carcinomas of the lung and cervix; adenocarcinomas of the stomach, ovary, breast, lung, and colon; undifferentiated carcinomas of the lung and ovary; renal cell carcinoma; small cell lung carcinoma; seminoma; Kaposi's sarcoma; multiple myeloma; thymoma; hairy cell leukemia; and T-gamma lymphoproliferative disease. Rarely an ITP-like syndrome coexists. Cisplatin has been associated with an acute, self-limited hemolysis that may be direct Coombs' positive or negative; thrombocytopenia may appear concomitantly. Methotrexate and 5-fluorouracil have also been associated with a Coombs-positive hemolytic anemia.

Warm-type immune hemolysis in Hodgkin's disease may improve with glucocorticoids or splenectomy, and spontaneous recovery has also been noted. In lymphoma, a glucocorticoid with chemotherapy or a splenectomy may be beneficial. Long-term intravenous immunoglobulin therapy may be useful in warm-type immune hemolytic anemia secondary to a lymphoproliferative disease. In solid tumors, glucocorticoids appear to be less beneficial than in idiopathic warm-type immune hemolysis. Splenectomy can benefit some, but it is frequently unsuccessful. The preferred approach is definitive tumor treatment, which can resolve the hemolytic process in most patients. Recurrent hemolysis can herald recurrent tumor.

**Cold-Type Immune Hemolytic Anemia.** Cold-type immune hemolytic anemia is often associated with abnormal serum IgM monoclonal paraproteins. Associated neoplastic disorders are B-cell lymphoproliferative disorders, including lymphoma, chronic lymphocytic leukemia, and Waldenström's macroglobulinemia. Cold agglutinin titers are frequently elevated in angioimmunoblastic lymphadenopathy with dysproteinemia.

**Microangiopathic Hemolytic Anemia.** Hemolytic anemia with fragmented erythrocytes accompanies thrombotic microangiopathy and may occur with DIC (see earlier sections).

## HEMOPHAGOCYTIC SYNDROMES

Hemophagocytic syndromes are characterized by fever, hepatosplenomegaly, cytopenias, hypertriglyceridemia, hypofibrinogenemia, and hemophagocytosis. Hemophagocytosis is usually seen in the bone marrow because this is the area from which biopsy specimens are most frequently obtained, but it can also be found in other areas of the reticuloendothelial system (e.g., lymph node biopsy specimens and liver biopsy specimens). The diagnosis may be difficult because occasionally the hemophagocytic histiocytes are rare in the bone marrow biopsy specimen. The cause is diverse, but there is a strong correlation with non-Hodgkin's lymphoma, especially peripheral T-cell lymphoma; any patient with a diagnosis of this syndrome should undergo a diagnostic work-up for non-Hodgkin's lymphoma. The prognosis of this entity is poor.

# Leukocyte Disorders

## NEUTROPHIL DISORDERS

Neutropenia may accompany any generalized bone marrow disorder. The most common causes are chemotherapy and radiation therapy. In two cases of Hodgkin's disease, neutropenia failed to respond significantly to splenectomy, then improved with chemotherapy; the cause of the neutropenia was believed to be immunologic in both cases. Reduced granulopoiesis and neutropenia are seen in T-gamma lymphocytosis, a disease also characterized frequently by anemia, thrombocytopenia, splenomegaly, polyclonal hypergammaglobulinemia, and rheumatoid arthritis. Agranulocytosis with hypogammaglobulinemia may be associated with thymoma without PRCA. Recurrent reversible agranulocytosis has been associated with *l*-mandelonitrile-β-glucuronic acid (Laetrile) treatment.

Neutrophilia regularly accompanies bacterial infection or the administration of glucocorticoids when the marrow has adequate reserve. *Left-shifted* granulocytes may enter the circulation during a leukoerythroblastic reaction. A neutrophilic leukemoid reaction occasionally accompanies malignancy. In many cases, the tumor can be demonstrated to produce a number of hematopoietic cytokines, including granulocyte colony–stimulating factor (G-CSF), GM-CSF, and macrophage colony–stimulating factor (M-CSF). The reaction may be marked by leukocyte counts exceeding 100,000/L. Mild-to-moderate leukemoid reactions (>30,000 to 50,000/L) occur in about 3% of patients with lung cancer. Neutrophilic leukemoid reactions have also been associated with angioimmunoblastic lymphadenopathy with dysproteinemia, epidermoid carcinoma of the oral cavity, adenocarcinoma of the stomach or breast, fibrous histiocytoma, splenic hemangiosarcoma, hepatoma, adrenal carcinoma, and melanoma. Neutrophilic leukemoid reactions may be distinguished from chronic myelogenous leukemia by the presence of an elevated leukocyte alkaline phosphatase score. Neutrophil dysfunction has been described in association with myelodysplastic syndromes, acute leukemias, chronic myelogenous leukemias, myelofibrosis with myeloid metaplasia, paroxysmal nocturnal hemoglobinuria, and hairy cell leukemia.

## EOSINOPHILIA

Eosinophilia may be associated with various malignant diseases. The overall incidence is about 0.5%. The disease is usually metastatic, and it has been suggested that eosinophilia is associated with tumor necrosis. Cytokines associated with eosinophilia are primarily interleukin-5 (IL-5), but also GM-CSF and IL-3. Production of GM-CSF by a lung cancer has been implicated in causation of eosinophilia in two patients.[77] Eosinophilia is usually mild, but absolute counts may occasionally exceed 25,000/μl. Clinical complications of hypereosinophilia may occur, including Löffler's endocarditis or pulmonary infiltrates.

Eosinophilia, not infrequently of an extreme degree, may accompany acute lymphoblastic leukemia and lymphomas. Eosinophilia may be present at diagnosis of the lymphoblastic disorder, may precede it, or may signal recurrence. The eosinophils may be morphologically abnormal, with hyposegmentation and hypogranularity; however, eosinophilia is considered secondary to the lymphoblastic disorder and not neoplastic per se. In a number of reported cases, the lymphoblasts have T-cell characteristics. Bone marrow eosinophilia with morphologic atypia and slight peripheral blood eosinophilia may accompany acute nonlymphocytic leukemia (M4eo) with abnormalities of the long arm of chromosome 16 (16q22). Eosinophilia is present in about 7.5 to 20% of patients with Hodgkin's disease and appears to be due to production of IL-5 by the tumor.[78] The presence of eosinophilia was a favorable prognostic factor. It is quite common in angioimmunoblastic lymphadenopathy with dysproteinemia. A syndrome in middle-aged to elderly men has been described, characterized by eosinophilia, panniculitis, polyarthralgias or polyarthritis, and pancreatic acinar cell carcinoma. Eosinophilia has been noted in association with lung cancer; adenocarcinomas of the gastrointestinal tract; hepatoma; melanoma; sarcoma; and cancer of the uterus, thyroid, cervix, penis, and adrenal glands. The use of recombinant cytokines, such as IL-2, GM-CSF, and IL-3, has also been associated with eosinophilia. IL-2 stimulates T cells to release IL-5, resulting in a secondary eosinophilia.

## MONOCYTOSIS

Monocytosis (a monocyte count >1000/μl) was noted in 21 of 100 patients with cancer in one series.[79] Most instances of monocytosis are mild, and it can occur with a wide range of neoplasms. Monocytosis is relatively common in Hodgkin's disease and has been noted in lymphoma, myeloma, and various solid tumors. Glucocorticoid treatment may cause monocytosis.

## LYMPHOCYTOPENIA

Lymphocytopenia (<100/μl) may be associated with Hodgkin's disease, angioimmunoblastic lymphadenopathy with dysproteinemia, and various solid tumors. It commonly occurs with corticosteroid therapy and postradiation therapy.

## SUGGESTIONS FOR ADDITIONAL READING

Colman RW, Hirsh J, Marder VJ, Salzman EW. Hemostasis and thrombosis: basic principles and clinical practice. 3rd ed. Philadelphia: JB Lippincott, 1994.

Levine MN, Lee AYY. Treatment of venous thromboembolism in cancer patients. Semin Thromb Hemost 1999;25:245–9.

Kakkar AK, Williamson RCN. Prevention of venous thromboembolism in cancer patients. Semin Thromb Hemost 1999;25:239–43.

Monreal M, Prandoni P. Venous thromboembolism as first manifestation of cancer. Semin Thromb Hemost 1999;25:131–6.

Büller H, Wouter ten Cate J: Primary venous thromboembolism and cancer screening (editorial). N Engl J Med 1998;338:1221–2.

Levi M, Ten Cate H. Disseminated intravascular coagulation. N Engl J Med 1999;341:586–92.

# REFERENCES

1. Peuscher FW, Cleton FJ, Armstrong L, et al. Significance of plasma fibrinopeptide A (fpA) in patients with malignancy. J Lab Clin Med 1980;96:5–14.
2. Gore JM, Appelbaum JS, Greene HL, et al. Occult cancer in patients with acute pulmonary embolism. Ann Intern Med 1982;96:556–60.
3. Goldberg RJ, Seneff M, Gore JM, et al. Occult malignant neoplasm in patients with deep venous thrombosis. Arch Intern Med 1987;147:251–3.
4. Griffin MR, Stanson AW, Brown ML, et al. Deep venous thrombosis and pulmonary embolism: risk of subsequent neoplasms. Arch Intern Med 1987;147:1907–11.
5. Nordstrom M, Lindblad B, Anderson H, et al. Deep venous thrombosis and occult malignancy: an epidemiological study. BMJ 1994;308:891–4.
6. Cornuz J, Pearson SD, Creager MA, et al. Importance of finding on the initial evaluation for cancer in patients with symptomatic idiopathic deep venous thrombosis. Ann Intern Med 1996;125:785–93.
7. Goldhaber SZ, Visani L, De Rosa M. Acute pulmonary embolism: clinical outcomes in the International Cooperative Pulmonary Embolism Registry (ICOPER). Lancet 1999;353:1386–9.
8. Aderka D, Brown A, Zelikovski A, Pinkhas J. Idiopathic deep vein thrombosis in an apparently healthy patient as a premonitory sign of occult cancer. Cancer 1986;57:1846–9.
9. Monreal M, Salvador R, Soriano V, Sabria M. Cancer and deep venous thrombosis. Arch Intern Med 1988;148:485.
10. Monreal M, Lafoz E, Casals A, et al. Occult cancer in patients with deep venous thrombosis: a systematic approach. Cancer 1991;67:541–5.
11. Prandoni P, Lensing AWA, Buller HR, et al. Deep-vein thrombosis and the incidence of subsequent symptomatic cancer. N Engl J Med 1992;327:1128–33.
12. Monreal M, Casals A, Boix J, et al. Occult cancer in patients with acute pulmonary embolism: a prospective study. Chest 1993;103:816–9.
13. Bastounis EA, Karayiannakis AJ, Makri GG, et al. The incidence of occult cancer in patients with deep venous thrombosis: a prospective study. J Intern Med 1996;239:153–6.
14. Ahmed Z, Mohyuddin Z. Deep vein thrombosis as a predictor of cancer. Angiology 1996;47:261–5.
15. Monreal M, Fernandez-Llamazares J, Perandreu J, et al. Occult cancer in patients with venous thromboembolism: which patients, which cancers. Thromb Haemost 1997;78:1316–8.
16. Hettiarachchi RJK, Lok J, Prins MH, et al. Undiagnosed malignancy in patients with deep-vein thrombosis: incidence, risk indicators, and diagnosis. Cancer 1998;83:100–5.
17. Achkar A, Laaban JP, Horellou MH, et al. Prospective screening for occult cancer in patients with venous thromboembolism. Thromb Haemost 1997;Suppl:OC-1564.abstract.
18. Rance A, Emmerich J, Guedj C, Fiessinger JN. Occult cancer in patients with bilateral deep-vein thrombosis. Lancet 1997;350:1448–9.
19. Rajan R, Levin M, Gent M, et al. The occurrence of subsequent malignancy in patients presenting with deep vein thrombosis: results from a historical cohort study. Thromb Haemost 1998;79:19–22.
20. Monreal M, Prandoni P. Venous thromboembolism as first manifestation of cancer. Thromb Haemost 1999;25:131–6.
21. Baron JA, Gridley G, Weiderpass E, et al. Venous thromboembolism and cancer. Lancet 1998;351:1077–80.
22. Sorensen HT, Mellemkjaer L, Steffensen FH, et al. The risk of a diagnosis of cancer after primary deep venous thrombosis or pulmonary embolism. N Engl J Med 1998;338:1169–73.
23. Sannella NA, O'Connor DJ, Lowell MD. "Idiopathic" deep venous thrombosis: the value of routine abdominal and pelvic computed tomographic scanning. Ann Vasc Surg 1991;5:218–22.
24. Saphner T, Tormey DC, Gray R. Venous and arterial thrombosis in patients who received adjuvant therapy for breast cancer. J Clin Oncol 1991;9:286–94.
25. Weiss RB, Tormey DC, Holland JF, Weinberg VE. Venous thrombosis during multimodal treatment of primary breast carcinoma. Cancer Treat Rep 1981;65:677–9.
26. Clahsen PE, van de Velde CJH, Julien JP, et al. Thromboembolic complications after perioperative chemotherapy in women with early breast cancer: a European Organization for Research and Treatment of Cancer Breast Cancer Cooperative Group Study. J Clin Oncol 1994;12:1266–71.
27. Levine MN, Gent M, Hirsch J, et al. The thrombogenic effect of anticancer drug therapy in women with stage II breast cancer. N Engl J Med 1988;318:404–7.
28. Fisher B, Redmond C, Legaul-Poisson S, et al. Postoperative chemotherapy and tamoxifen compared with tamoxifen alone in the treatment of positive-node breast cancer patients aged 50 years and older with tumors responsive to tamoxifen: results from the National Surgical Adjuvant Breast and Bowel Project B-16. J Clin Oncol 1990;8:1005–18.
29. Pritchard KI, Paterson AHG, Paul NA, et al. Increased thromboembolic complications with concurrent tamoxifen and chemotherapy in a randomized trial of adjuvant therapy for women with breast cancer. J Clin Oncol 1996;14:2731–7.
30. Von Tempelhoff GF, Dietich M, Hommel G, et al. Blood coagulation during adjuvant epirubicin/cyclophosphamide chemotherapy in patients with primary operable breast cancer. J Clin Oncol 1996;14:2560–8.
31. Rivkin SE, Green S, Metch B, et al. Adjuvant CMFVP and tamoxifen for post-menopausal, node-positive, and estrogen receptor-positive breast cancer patients: a Southwest Oncology Group Study. J Clin Oncol 1994;12:2078–85.
32. Fisher B, Constantino JP, Wickerham L, et al. Tamoxifen for prevention of breast cancer: report of the National Surgical Adjuvant Breast and Bowel Project P-1 Study. J Natl Cancer Inst 1998;90:1371–88.
33. Goodnough LT, Saito H, Manni A, et al. Increased incidence of thromboembolism in stage IV breast cancer patients treated with a five-drug chemotherapy regimen: a study of 159 patients. Cancer 1984;54:1264–8.
34. Gugliotta L, Mazzacconi MG, Leone G, et al. Incidence of thrombotic complications in adult patients with acute lymphoblastic leukemia receiving L-asparaginase during induction therapy: a retrospective study. Eur J Haematol 1992;49:63–6.
35. Priest JR, Ramsay NKC, Steinberz PG, et al. A syndrome of thrombosis and hemorrhage complicating L-asparaginase therapy childhood acute lymphoblastic leukemia. J Pediatr 1982;100:984–9.
36. Kucuk O, Kwaan HC, Gunnar W, Vazquez RM. Thromboembolic complications associated with L-asparaginase therapy. Cancer 1985;55:702–6.
37. Barbui T, Finazzi G, Grassi A, Marchioli R. Thrombosis in cancer patients treated with hematopoietic growth factors—a meta-analysis. Thromb Haemost 1996;75:368–71.
38. Clagett GP, Anderson FA Jr, Heit J, et al. Prevention of venous thromboembolism. Chest 1995;108:312–34.
39. International Multicentre Trial. Prevention of fatal postoperative pulmonary embolism by low doses of heparin. Lancet 1975;2:45–51.
40. Bergqvist D, Burmark US. Low-molecular-weight heparin started before surgery as prophylaxis against deep-vein thrombosis: 2500 versus 5000 anti-Xa units in 2070 patients. Br J Surg 1995;82:496–501.
41. ENOXACAN Study Group. Efficacy and safety of enoxaparin versus unfractionated heparin for prevention of deep-vein thrombosis in elective cancer surgery: a double-blind randomised multicentre trial with venographic assessment. Br J Surg 1997;84:1099–1103.
42. Green D, Hull RD, Brant R, Pineo GF. Lower mortality in cancer patients treated with low-molecular-weight versus standard heparin. Lancet 1992;339:1476.
43. Valentine K, Hull R, Pineo GF. Low-molecular-weight heparin therapy and mortality. Semin Thromb Haemost 1997;23:173–8.
44. Levine M, Gent M, Hirsch J, et al. A comparison of low-molecular-weight heparin administered primarily at home with unfractionated heparin administered in the hospital for proximal deep-vein thrombosis. N Engl J Med 1996;334:677–81.
45. Koopman MMW, Prandoni P, Piovella F, et al. Treatment of venous thrombosis with intravenous unfractionated heparin administered in the hospital as compared with subcutaneous low-molecular-weight heparin administered at home. N Engl J Med 1996;334:682–7.
46. The Columbus Investigators. Low-molecular-weight heparin in the

treatment of patients with venous thromboembolism. N Engl J Med 1997;337:657–662.

47. Prandoni P. Antithrombotic strategies in patients with cancer. Thromb Haemost 1997;78:141–4.

48. Bona RD, Sivjee KY, Hickey AD, et al. The efficacy and safety of oral anticoagulation in patients with cancer. Thromb Haemost 1995;74:1055–8.

49. Wester JPJ, deValk HW, Nieuwenhuis HK, et al. Risk factors for bleeding during treatment of acute venous thromboembolism. Thromb Haemost 1996;76:682–8.

50. Sack GH, Jr, Levin J, Bell WR. Trousseau's syndrome and other manifestations of chronic disseminated coagulopathy in patients with neoplasms: clinical, pathophysiologic, and therapeutic features. Medicine 1977;56:1–37.

51. Graus F, Rogers LR, Posner JB. Cerebrovascular complications in patients with cancer. Medicine 1985;64:16–35.

52. Bell WR, Starksen NF, Tong S, Porterfield JK. Trousseau's syndrome: devastating coagulopathy in the absence of heparin. Am J Med 1985;79:423–30.

53. Rodeghiero F, Avvisati G, Castaman G, et al. Early deaths and anti-hemorrhagic treatments in acute promyelocytic leukemia: a GIMEMA retrospective study in 268 consecutive patients. Blood 1990;75:2112–7.

54. Goldberg MA, Ginsburg D, Mayer RJ, et al. Is heparin administration necessary during induction chemotherapy for patients with acute promyelocytic leukemia? Blood 1987;69:187–91.

55. Sheldon R, Slaughter D. A syndrome of microangiopathic hemolytic anemia, renal impairment, and pulmonary edema in chemotherapy-treated patients with adenocarcinoma. Cancer 1986;58:1428–36.

56. Grem JL, Merritt JA, Carbone PP. Treatment of mitomycin-associated microangiopathic hemolytic anemia with vincristine. Arch Intern Med 1986;146:566–8.

57. Snyder HW Jr, Mittelman A, Oral A, et al. Treatment of cancer chemotherapy-associated thrombotic thrombocytopenic purpura/hemolytic uremic syndrome by protein A immunoadsorption of plasma. Cancer 1993;71:1882–92.

58. Lesesne JB, Rothschild N, Erickson B, et al. Cancer-associated hemolytic-uremic syndrome: analysis of 85 cases from a national registry. J Clin Oncol 1989;7:781–9.

59. Winterbauer RH, Elfenbein IB, Ball WC Jr. Incidence and clinical significance of tumor embolization to the lungs. Am J Med 1968;45:271–90.

60. Prioleau PG, Katzenstein AL. Major peripheral arterial occlusion due to malignant tumor embolism: histologic recognition and surgical management. Cancer 1978;42:2009–14.

61. Richardson P, Bearman SI. Prevention and treatment of hepatic venocclusive disease after high-dose cytoreductive therapy. Leuk Lymphoma 1998;31:267–77.

62. McDonald GB, Hinds MS, Fisher LD, et al. Veno-occlusive disease of the liver and multiorgan failure after bone marrow transplantation: a cohort study of 355 patients. Ann Intern Med 1993;118:255–67.

63. McDonald GB, Sharma P, Matthews DE, et al. The clinical course of 53 patients with venocclusive disease of the liver after marrow transplantation. Transplantation 1985;39:603–8.

64. Attal M, Huguet F, Rubie H, et al. Prevention of hepatic veno-occlusive disease after bone marrow transplantation by continuous infusion of low-dose heparin: a prospective, randomized trial. Blood 1992;79:2834–40.

65. Essell JH, Thompson JM, Harman GS, et al. Pilot trial of prophylactic ursodiol to decrease the incidence of veno-occlusive disease of the liver in allogeneic bone marrow transplant patients. Bone Marrow Transplant 1992;10:367–72.

66. Gluckman E, Jolivet I, Scrobohaci ML, et al. Use of prostaglandin E1 for prevention of liver veno-occlusive disease in leukaemic patients treated by allogeneic bone marrow transplantation. Br J Haematol 1990;74:277–81.

67. Petri M, Ellman L, Carey R. Acquired factor XIII deficiency with chronic myelomonocytic leukemia. Ann Intern Med 1983;99:638–9.

68. Thiagarajan P, Shapiro SS, De Marco L. Monoclonal immunoglobulin M lambda coagulation inhibitor with phospholipid specificity: mechanism of a lupus anticoagulant. J Clin Invest 1980;66:397–405.

69. Stasi R, Stipa E, Masi M, et al. Antiphospholipid antibodies: prevalence, clinical significance and correlation to cytokine levels in acute myeloid leukemia and non-Hodgkin's lymphoma. Thromb Haemost 1993;70:568–72.

70. Brody JI, Haidar ME, Rossman RE. A hemorrhagic syndrome in Waldenström's macroglobulinemia secondary to immunoadsorption of factor VIII: recovery after splenectomy. N Engl J Med 1979;300:408–10.

71. Cortelazzo S, Viero P, Finazzi G, et al. Incidence and risk factors for thrombotic complications in a historical cohort of 100 patients with essential thrombocythemia. J Clin Oncol 1990;8:556–62.

72. Carloss H, Winslow D, Kastan L, Yam LT. Bone marrow necrosis: diagnosis and assessment of extent of involvement by radioisotope studies. Arch Intern Med 1977;137:863–6.

73. Spivak JL. Serum immunoreactive erythropoietin in health and disease. Int J Cell Cloning 1990;8:Suppl 1:211–24.

74. Hammond D, Winnick S. Paraneoplastic erythrocytosis and ectopic erythropoietins. Ann N Y Acad Sci 1974;230:219–27.

75. Ludwig H, Fritz E, Leitgeb C, et al. Prediction of response to erythropoietin treatment in chronic anemia of cancer. Blood 1994;84:1056–63.

76. Fahey JL, Rahbar S, Farbstein MJ, et al. Microcytosis in Hodgkin disease associated with unbalanced globin chain synthesis. Am J Hematol 1986;23:123–9.

77. Sawyers CL, Golde DW, Quan S, Nimer SD. Production of granulocyte-macrophage colony-stimulating factor in two patients with lung cancer, leukocytosis, and eosinophilia. Cancer 1992;69:1342–6.

78. Samoszuk M, Nansen L. Detection of interleukin-5 messenger RNA in Reed-Sternberg cells of Hodgkin's disease with eosinophilia. Blood 1990;75:13–16.

79. Barrett O Jr. Monocytosis in malignant disease. Ann Intern Med 1970;73:991–2.

# CHAPTER **14**

# TRANSFUSION THERAPY FOR PATIENTS WITH CANCER

• LAWRENCE D. PETZ

Blood transfusion is essential in the supportive care of many cancer patients and makes possible a number of aggressive treatment regimens. Advances in transfusion medicine have led to a clearer delineation of appropriate indications for transfusion of red blood cells (RBCs), platelets, fresh frozen plasma (FFP), and special products such as granulocytes, irradiated cellular components, leukocyte-depleted products, and products for the prevention of transmission of cytomegalovirus (CMV) infection.

Indications for transfusion must balance the potential benefits and known risks. There has been a remarkable improvement in the safety of the blood supply in regard to transmission of infectious diseases, primarily as a result of implementing rigorous donor screening techniques and sensitive serologic tests for human immunodeficiency virus (HIV) and hepatitis C virus (Table 14–1).[1] Planned implementation of nucleic acid testing of blood products for viral disorders will significantly decrease the already low incidence of disease transmission. The risk of a fatality associated with a RBC transfusion due to ABO incompatibility resulting from a transfusion error (1/600,000 transfusions) is now about as great as the risk of acquiring HIV infection from a blood product.[2]

With the decrease in the frequency of transfusion-transmitted viral diseases, bacterial contamination of blood components, usually the result of bacteremia in an asymptomatic blood donor with subsequent bacterial proliferation during storage, is becoming relatively more common. Up to nine acute fatal reactions related to bacterial contamination are reported to the Food and Drug Administration annually in the United States.[3] There is less than a 1/million chance that a blood transfusion within the United States will be complicated by a parasitic infection such as malaria, babesiosis *(Babesia microti)*, Chagas' disease *(Trypanosoma cruzi)*, or ehrlichiosis *(Ehrlichia chaffeenis)*.[4, 5] The transmission of Creutzfeldt-Jakob disease by blood transfusion remains a theoretical concern but has never been documented in humans.[6]

## Red Blood Cell Transfusion

Administration of RBCs is indicated to promote delivery of oxygen to tissue in patients who are actively bleeding and in those who have symptomatic anemia unresponsive to specific therapy.[7, 8] Although the hemoglobin level provides incomplete information on which to base a decision as to whether transfusion is necessary, it does provide some indication of the probability of significant physiologic impairment of a patient (Table 14–2).

A point of fundamental importance is that blood volume is decreased only slightly in patients with chronic anemia because there are compensatory increases in plasma volume. Thus, transfusions in chronically anemic patients regularly cause hypervolemia, which has the potential for precipitating cardiac decompensation. Accordingly, physicians must not be too aggressive in performing transfusions in patients with severe anemia. RBCs rather than whole blood should be transfused in patients who are normovolemic, and transfusions should be carried out slowly, especially in elderly

*Table 14–1.* **The Risk of Transfusion-Transmitted Viral Infections**

| Virus | Incidence (units) |
| --- | --- |
| Human immunodeficiency virus | 1/493,000 |
| Hepatitis C virus | 1/103,000 |
| Hepatitis B virus | 1/63,000 |
| HTLV-I and HTLV-II | 1/641,000 |

HTLV, human T-cell lymphotropic virus.
Data from Schreiber GB, Busch MP, Kleinman SH, Korelitz JJ. The risk of transfusion-transmitted viral infections: the Retrovirus Epidemiology Donor Study. N Engl J Med 1996;334:1685–90.

*Table 14–2.* **Guidelines for Assessing Physiologic Impairment of the Anemic Patient and Determining Transfusion Strategy**

| Hemoglobin Level (g/dl) | Probability of Significant Impairment | Transfusion Strategy |
| --- | --- | --- |
| ≥10 | Very low | Avoid |
| 8–10 | Low | Transfusions usually can be avoided if patient is stable; they should be continued only if they produce significant improvement |
| 7–8 | Moderate | Transfusions may be indicated |
| <7 | High | Transfusions are usually indicated if other forms of therapy will not correct anemia |

patients or others with a significant risk for congestive heart failure.

Adequate oxygen-carrying capacity to maintain cardiopulmonary function can be met by a hemoglobin level of 7 g/dl (a hematocrit of approximately 21%) when the intravascular volume is adequate for perfusion.[9] Healthy patients are generally asymptomatic with hemoglobin levels greater than 8 g/dl.[9] Other studies suggest that the functional status of patients is improved by an elevation of the hemoglobin level to greater than 7 g/dl, but this improvement appears to plateau near a level of 10 g/dl. In deciding whether a specific patient should undergo transfusion, the physician should consider the patient's age, the degree of anemia, the intravascular volume, and the presence or probable existence of coexisting cardiac, pulmonary, or vascular conditions.[7–9]

Criteria for transfusion should be established by each medical staff for purposes of auditing transfusion practices. These audit criteria are not synonymous with indications for transfusion and instead are used to screen medical records for transfusions that may not have been indicated. Any health problems that influence the decision to transfuse, such as cardiac or pulmonary disease, should be documented in the medical record, especially when the transfusion is not in accord with the audit screening criteria.

Examples of proposed audit criteria for RBC transfusion are (1) active bleeding with a blood loss of 15% or more of estimated blood volume and (2) a patient who is not bleeding and has a hemoglobin level of 9 g/dl or less. The latter guideline is liberal; most published recommendations suggest a hemoglobin level of 7 or 8 g/dl. More liberal guidelines than previously recommended may be considered because of the improvements in the safety of the blood supply (see Table 14–1). The patient's hemoglobin level should be determined before transfusion, and a post-transfusion determination should be obtained to assess its effectiveness.

## Platelet Transfusion

The use of platelet transfusions has risen considerably, partly as a consequence of the increasingly intensive treatment of patients with malignancies.

## GUIDELINES FOR PLATELET TRANSFUSION[10]

1. Determine the policy for prophylactic platelet support and select the platelet count below which platelet transfusions will be used.

2. Use leukocyte-reduced RBC and platelet products to prevent HLA alloimmunization for patients who are likely to require long-term transfusion support.[11] (Leukocyte reduction of all cellular blood products other than granulocytes may become the standard of care.)

3. Perform typing of HLA-A and HLA-B antigens early in the course of therapy in patients who are likely to require long-term platelet transfusion support.

4. Use random-donor platelets for initial platelet support, either single donor (plateletpheresis) or multiple donor (pooled platelet concentrates obtained from units of whole blood).

5. Determine the post-transfusion platelet count increment after each transfusion. This may be carried out within an hour after transfusion, although it is often more practical to obtain the platelet count later during the subsequent 24 hours.

6. Determine criteria for refractoriness to platelet transfusion (see further on).

7. If refractoriness occurs, test the patient's serum for HLA antibodies and determine whether there are correctable clinical factors that may be associated with nonimmune consumption of platelets, as may be caused by sepsis, disseminated intravascular coagulation (DIC), amphotericin administration, and splenomegaly.

8. If HLA antibodies are present in a refractory patient, use HLA-matched platelets.

9. If HLA-matched platelets are not available, use cross-matched platelets or platelets chosen on the basis of compatibility with the specificity of the patient's HLA antibodies.

10. If the patient does not respond to HLA-matched, cross-matched, or antigen-compatible platelets and has thrombocytopenic bleeding, use platelets from random donors in an attempt to control bleeding and increase the dose if necessary.

## PROPHYLACTIC PLATELET TRANSFUSION

Varying opinions have been published regarding an optimal policy for prophylactic platelet transfusions.[10] Although a platelet count of 20,000/$\mu$L was frequently used in the past, evidence suggests that this number might safely be lowered (e.g., 10,000/$\mu$L) for some patients.[12, 13] However, caution is warranted if factors associated with bleeding in thrombocytopenic patients are present, such as fever (temperature >38.5° C), infection, concurrent coagulation disturbances, DIC, or hepatic failure.[10] Also, for patients with high blast counts (>100,000/$\mu$L) or those with acute progranulocytic leukemia who are receiving concomitant heparin therapy to prevent or control DIC, a count of 40,000 to 50,000/$\mu$L has been recommended.[14]

The decision to withhold platelet transfusion in severely thrombocytopenic patients should be made only by physicians with extensive experience in the management of such individuals, and platelets must be immediately available in the event of active bleeding. The major reason to withhold platelet transfusion in stable thrombocytopenic patients who are not bleeding is that each transfusion carries a risk of disease transmission. This risk must be balanced with the risk of morbidity and mortality caused by thrombocytopenia, especially intracranial hemorrhage.[15] Since the blood supply in developed countries is now remarkably safe (see Table 14–1), a policy of prophylactic transfusions would be warranted even if it prevented intracranial hemorrhage only infrequently.

## PROPHYLAXIS FOR SURGERY

Bone marrow aspiration and biopsy may be performed even in patients with severe thrombocytopenia without platelet transfusion support, provided that adequate surface pressure is applied to the site.[10]

The platelet count should be raised to greater than 50,000/$\mu$L for lumbar puncture, epidural anesthesia, insertion of indwelling lines, transbronchial biopsy, liver biopsy, laparotomy, or similar procedures.[10] A review of 167 operations in thrombocytopenic patients indicated that surgery can be performed safely if preoperative platelet transfusions are given to raise the platelet count to more than 50,000/$\mu$L.[16] For operations in critical sites, such as the brain or eyes, a platelet count of greater than 100,000/$\mu$L has been recommended.[10]

## PLATELET TRANSFUSIONS FOR PATIENTS WHO ARE BLEEDING

If a patient has a platelet count of less than 50,000/$\mu$L and has clinically significant bleeding that is thought to be due to the thrombocytopenia, a platelet transfusion to increase the platelet count to greater than 50,000/$\mu$L is indicated.

## DETERMINING THE APPROPRIATE DOSE OF PLATELETS

A number of simple methods are available to calculate the appropriate dose.

1. A dose of 1 unit/10 kg body weight can be expected to increase the platelet count by about 50,000/$\mu$L. (Each unit contains about 6 to 7 $\times$ 10$^{10}$ platelets.)

2. One plateletpheresis product contains about 3 to 4 $\times$ 10$^{11}$ platelets and is therefore equivalent to about 5 or 6 units of platelets. One plateletpheresis product should increase the platelet count of a 70-kg patient by about 50,000/$\mu$L.

3. For pediatric patients, 5 ml/kg of a random-donor platelet concentrate should increase the platelet count by 50,000/$\mu$L. A single random-donor platelet product contains about 40 ml and therefore should supply the needs of patients weighing up to about 8 kg. For patients weighing more than 8 kg, the standard dose of 1 unit/10 kg should be used.

## ASSESSING THE RESPONSE TO PLATELET TRANSFUSION

A pretransfusion platelet count should be obtained within 24 hours of ordering a platelet transfusion and as close to the time of transfusion as is practical. A post-transfusion platelet count should be obtained 10 to 60 minutes after the transfusion or at 18 to 24 hours, or both. The expected post-transfusion platelet count increment can be estimated roughly by knowing the dose of platelets and the size of the patient, as previously described. For more precise determinations, a number of formulas have been used to correct for the patient's size and the number of platelets transfused.[10] Two such formulas follow:

1. Percentage platelet recovery (R) is calculated from the platelet increment $\times$ $10^9/\mu L$ (PI), the blood volume (BV) in liters, and the platelet dose (PD) transfused ($\times$ $10^9$). The BV is calculated by multiplying the body surface area in square meters $\times$ 2.5 or weight in kilograms $\times$ 69 ml/kg in males and by 65 ml/kg in females. The formula is

$$R\ (\%) = PI \times BV \times PD^{-1} \times 100$$

2. The corrected count increment (CCI)[10] is calculated from the platelet increment (PI), the body surface area (BSA) of the patient in square meters, and the number of platelets transfused. The formula is

$$CCI = \frac{PI \times BSA}{\text{Number of platelets transfused } (\times 10^{11})}$$

The minimal standard for a successful transfusion may be considered as a percentage platelet recovery of more than 30% at 1 hour and more than 20% at 20 hours or a CCI of more than 7500 at 1 hour and more than 4500 at 20 hours.[10] CCI units are often incorrectly reported as increment per cubic millimeter, whereas they are correctly indicated as platelets per microliter per $10^{11}$ per square meter.[17]

## REFRACTORINESS TO PLATELET TRANSFUSION

A patient may be considered refractory to platelet transfusions when three consecutive platelet transfusions yield an inadequate post-transfusion increment. Poor responses may be due to alloimmunization, primarily caused by HLA antibodies, or to nonimmune causes that include fever (temperature >38.5° C), sepsis, splenomegaly,[18] DIC, bone marrow transplantation, and amphotericin therapy.[19]

Patients who are refractory to platelet transfusions from random donors and who have HLA antibodies should receive platelet transfusions from HLA-matched donors. However, platelets that are matched at HLA-A and HLA-B loci frequently are not available; in this case, one may transfuse platelets mismatched for cross-reactive HLA antigens.[20, 21] A preferable alternative is to use cross-matched platelets, which may produce adequate responses regardless of the degree of HLA matching between donor and recipient.[21–24] Another alternative is to use HLA antigen–compatible platelets, which are selected on the basis of the specificity of the patient's HLA antibodies.[10] The use of HLA-matched platelets is not indicated for refractory patients in whom HLA antibodies have not been detected.[10]

## MANAGEMENT OF PATIENTS WHO DO NOT RESPOND TO HLA-MATCHED, CROSS-MATCHED, OR HLA ANTIGEN–COMPATIBLE PLATELETS

If patients do not respond to special platelet products with an adequate post-transfusion platelet count increment, it is uncertain whether daily prophylactic transfusions will be of benefit, and some recommend that such support should be discontinued.[10] If bleeding occurs, platelet transfusions from random donors may reduce the severity of hemorrhage. Larger doses of platelets, such as the transfusion of 1 unit/10 kg, two or three times daily, may be tried empirically.

Attempts have been made to treat refractoriness in patients who are alloimmunized by using intravenous immunoglobulin[25–27] or by protein A column therapy.[28] An improvement in response to platelet transfusion has been reported in some patients, but the effects are often minimal and the therapies are expensive.

## THROMBOPOIETIN

The cloning and characterization of thrombopoietin (TPO) have profoundly changed our understanding of platelet production. TPO supports the proliferation of megakaryocytic progenitor cells and their differentiation into mature platelet-producing cells. TPO also acts in synergy with other pluripotent cytokines on the hematopoietic stem cell to augment the development of erythroid and myeloid progenitors. It is hoped that TPO may play an important role in reducing the myelosuppressive complications of naturally occurring and iatrogenic marrow failure. Clinical trials are in progress that are attempting to establish the capacity of TPO to have a favorable impact on the complications of myelosuppressive therapies and the need for platelet transfusions during iatrogenic and natural states of marrow failure.[29, 30]

## Fresh Frozen Plasma

FFP is indicated to correct deficiency of multiple clotting factors in bleeding patients or in patients who are at risk of bleeding by virtue of requiring an invasive procedure. These clotting factor deficiencies occur as a result of liver disease, vitamin K deficiency, massive bleeding, or DIC. FFP may also be used for the treatment of thrombotic thrombocytopenic purpura; for the correction of specific coagulation factor deficiencies such as antithrombin III, factors II, V, VII, IX, and XI, or protein C or S; or for the correction of warfarin therapy when reversal by vitamin K is not feasible because of time constraints.

The following are guidelines for the use of FFP.[9, 31, 32]

1. FFP can be used with active bleeding and a prolonged prothrombin time (PT) or partial thromboplastin time (PTT) (1.5 to 1.8 times the mean normal value), or both.

2. Patients with a prolonged PT or PTT at risk of bleeding because of scheduled surgery or an invasive procedure may require FFP.

3. Patients with massive bleeding who are at high risk of clotting factor deficiency may be appropriately treated with FFP while PT and PTT studies are pending.

4. There is no justification for FFP as an intravascular volume expander in patients without clotting factor deficiency, as a nutritional supplement, or as a treatment for bleeding in the absence of clotting factor deficiency.

When FFP is indicated, 10 to 15 ml/kg (about 4 to 6 units of 200 to 250 ml/unit) is often needed for initial therapy for an adult.[9, 31] Further needs should be determined by subsequent assessment of the risk of bleeding and the results of the PT and PTT.

## Granulocyte Transfusion

Interest has been renewed in granulocyte transfusions with the introduction of myeloid growth factors, for example, granulocyte colony–stimulating factor (G-CSF) in the treatment of the granulocyte donor so that extraordinary numbers of polymorphonuclear neutrophils (PMNs) can be collected for transfusion.[33, 34] One of the major reasons for the failure of some previous studies to demonstrate effectiveness was thought to be the inability to obtain adequate numbers of granulocytes for transfusion. Normal donors stimulated with recombinant human G-CSF yield markedly increased numbers of circulating granulocytes and monocytes.[34] Two- to 10-fold more cells may be harvested from these donors than from donors in whom conventional corticosteroid stimulation techniques are used, even with a single subcutaneous injection of G-CSF 12 to 16 hours before collection. Furthermore, the use of G-CSF increases the leukocyte number for several days and appears to mobilize granulocyte progenitors.

Granulocyte transfusions may be beneficial in patients with severe neutropenia ($<0.5 \times 10^9$/L PMN blood leukocytes) and progressive bacterial, yeast, and fungal infections who have failed a reasonable course (approximately 48 hours) of combination antibiotics.[34] If a decision to use granulocyte transfusions is made, the minimal dosage should be a daily infusion of 2 to $3 \times 10^{10}$ PMNs. Daily transfusions are continued either until the infection has resolved or until the blood PMN count has increased to more than $0.5 \times 10^9$.

In nonalloimmunized recipients, granulocytes from nonmatched donors can be administered safely. Patients who show evidence of alloimmunization (platelet refractoriness, antileukocyte antibodies, or repeated febrile transfusion reactions) should receive granulocyte transfusions from donors selected to be as leukocyte compatible as possible by HLA-matching or leukocyte cross-matching, or both.[34]

The use of recombinant myeloid growth factors (G-CSF and granulocyte-macrophage colony stimulating factor [GM-CSF]) in association with granulocyte transfusion for the treatment of neutropenic patients with persistent infections is under study.

## Leukocyte-Reduced Blood Components

Leukocytes, which are contained in RBC and platelet products, are the chief cause of alloimmunization to HLA antigens and leukocyte-specific antigens in transfusion recipients.[35] Leukocytes are also the vector for transfusion-associated CMV infection. Technologic advances in leukocyte reduction of cellular blood components have made it possible to reduce the number of leukocytes to fewer than $10^6$ per cellular blood product transfused. Leukocyte-reduced components minimize the incidence of febrile transfusion reac-

tions[36] and the incidence of alloimmunization and refractoriness to platelet transfusions[11, 36] and may be effective in reducing the risk of transfusion-transmitted CMV infection.[36, 37] Some data suggest that removal of leukocytes will minimize other adverse immunologic consequences of transfusion (see further on). Leukocyte reduction of all cellular blood products may become the standard of care.

## Irradiated Blood Products for Prevention of Transfusion-Associated Graft-Versus-Host Disease

Transfusion-associated graft-versus-host disease (TA-GVHD) can occur as a result of engraftment of stem cells that are present in cellular blood components, such as RBCs and platelets. This risk is not eliminated by leukocyte reduction of blood products. Patients with immunodeficiencies are at particular risk, but TA-GVHD can also occur in immunocompetent patients, particularly if the donor is homozygous for an HLA haplotype for which the patient is heterozygous.[38–41] This occurs more frequently when the donor and recipient are related than in random donor-recipient pairs.[41]

The chief clinical manifestations of TA-GVHD are fever; a scaly, maculopapular, erythematous rash; diarrhea; hepatocellular damage with marked abnormalities seen in liver function test results; and pancytopenia.[40] Skin biopsies reveal abnormalities that are characteristic but not diagnostic of GVHD. Although the diagnosis is a clinical one, strong supportive evidence can be obtained by the demonstration of circulating lymphocytes with an HLA type that is different from that of the host cells. Two characteristics of TA-GVHD that differ from the GVHD that occurs after allogeneic bone marrow transplantation are the high incidence of severe pancytopenia with hypoplastic marrow and a mortality rate of approximately 90%.[38]

Irradiation of cellular blood products with 2500 cGy is effective in preventing TA-GVHD and is the only known means of prevention. The primary indication for irradiated blood products is in immunosuppressed patients, but they are also appropriate when there is a higher than average risk of the donor being homozygous for an HLA haplotype for which the patient is heterozygous. This occurs when the donor and recipient are blood relatives or when patients receive platelet transfusions from HLA-matched donors.[41] In disorders for which there are only occasional case reports of TA-GVHD, policies regarding the use of irradiated blood components vary from institution to institution.[39] Table 14–3 lists risk groups for TA-GVHD.

## Prevention of Transfusion-Transmitted Cytomegalovirus Infection

Patients with severe immune deficiency who have never been exposed to CMV are at risk of transfusion-transmitted CMV infection. This may be associated with substantial morbidity and mortality in immunocompromised patients and can be avoided by screening blood donors to select

*Table 14–3.* **Risk Groups for Transfusion-Associated Graft-Versus-Host Disease***

*Risk Well Defined*

Bone marrow transplant recipients
Congenital immunodeficiency syndromes
Intrauterine transfusions
Transfusions from blood relatives
Premature newborns
Neonates receiving exchange transfusion
Patients receiving HLA-matched platelet transfusions
Hodgkin's disease

*Occasional Case Reports Documenting Some Risk*

Hematologic malignancies other than Hodgkin's disease
  Acute leukemia
  Non-Hodgkin's lymphoma
Solid organ transplant recipients
Solid tumors treated with chemotherapy or radiation therapy
  Neuroblastoma
  Glioblastoma
  Rhabdomyosarcoma
  Immunoblastic sarcoma

*Surprisingly, TA-GVHD has not been reported in patients with acquired immunodeficiency syndrome even though these patients have severe immunodeficiency.

those who are CMV seronegative. Published data suggest that leukocyte reduction of cellular blood products by means of modern filters reduces transmission of CMV.[37] Some institutions no longer use CMV-seronegative blood products for prevention of CMV transmission and rely on leukocyte reduction for this purpose. At other institutions, cellular blood products from CMV-seronegative donors are used, and these special products are reserved for categories of patients most likely to benefit from their use[36] (Table 14–4).

## Immunologic Consequences of Blood Transfusion

Allogeneic blood transfusion may alter host immune function in a variety of clinical settings, and there have been

*Table 14–4.* **Indications for the Use of Special Blood Products for the Prevention of Transfusion-Transmitted Cytomegalovirus Infection**

*Special Blood Products Clearly Indicated*

CMV-seronegative recipients of allogeneic bone marrow transplants from CMV-seronegative donors
CMV-seronegative patients receiving solid organ transplants from CMV-seronegative donors
CMV-seronegative patients who are candidates for allogeneic bone marrow transplantation
CMV-seronegative patients with HIV infection
CMV-seronegative pregnant women
Premature infants weighing <1200 g

*Special Blood Products Less Well Established*

CMV-seronegative autologous bone marrow transplant recipients
CMV-seronegative recipients of bone marrow or solid organ transplants from seropositive donors
CMV-seronegative patients undergoing splenectomy

*Special Blood Products Not Clearly Indicated*

CMV-seropositive recipients of bone marrow or solid organ transplants
Neonates weighing >1200 g

CMV, cytomegalovirus; HIV, human immunodeficiency virus.

some reports of detrimental effects, such as increased rates of solid tumor recurrence and an increased incidence of postoperative infections. However, meta-analyses have led to the conclusion that there is no evidence that allogeneic blood transfusion increases the risk of clinically important adverse sequelae in patients with cancer who are undergoing surgery.[42–44] Similarly, scientifically sound clinical studies unequivocally establishing the existence of an adverse effect relating perioperative transfusion to septic complications of surgery have not yet been published.[45] Randomized, controlled clinical trials need to be conducted to document the clinical significance of these potential immunologic consequences of transfusion.

## REFERENCES

1. Schreiber GB, Busch MP, Kleinman SH, Korelitz JJ. The risk of transfusion-transmitted viral infections: the Retrovirus Epidemiology Donor Study. N Engl J Med 1996;334:1685–90.
2. Linden JV, Paul B, Dressler KP. A report of 104 transfusion errors in New York state. Transfusion 1992;32:601–6.
3. Klein HG, Dodd RY, Ness PM, et al. Current status of microbial contamination of blood components: summary of a conference. Transfusion 1997;37:95–101.
4. Shulman IA. Parasitic infections and their impact on blood donor selection and testing. Arch Pathol Lab Med 1994;118:366–70.
5. Standaert SM, Dawson JE, Schaffner W, et al. Ehrlichiosis in a golf-oriented retirement community. N Engl J Med 1995;333:420–5.
6. Dealler S. A matter for debate: the risk of bovine spongiform encephalopathy to humans posed by blood transfusion in the UK. Transfus Med 1996;6:217–22.
7. Welch HG, Meehan KR, Goodnough JT. Prudent strategies for elective red blood cell transfusion. Ann Intern Med 1992;116:393–402.
8. Audet AM, Goodnough LT. Practice strategies for elective red blood cell transfusion. Ann Intern Med 1992,116:403–6.
9. Silberstein LE, Kruskall MS, Stehling LC, et al. Strategies for the review of transfusion practices [published erratum appears in JAMA 1990;263:2302]. JAMA 1989;262:1993–7.
10. Petz LD. Platelet transfusion. In: Petz LD, Swisher SN, Kleinman S, et al, eds. Clinical practice of transfusion medicine. 3 ed. New York: Churchill Livingstone, 1996:359–412.
11. Leukocyte reduction and ultraviolet B irradiation of platelets to prevent alloimmunization and refractoriness to platelet transfusions: the Trial to Reduce Alloimmunization to Platelets Study Group. N Engl J Med 1997;337:1861–9.
12. Gmur J, Burger J, Schanz U, et al. Safety of stringent prophylactic platelet transfusion policy for patients with acute leukemia. Lancet 1991;338:1223–6.
13. Aderka D, Praff G, Santo M, et al. Bleeding due to thrombocytopenia in acute leukemias and re-evaluation of the prophylactic platelet transfusion policy. Am J Med Sci 1986;291:147–51.
14. Heyman MR, Schiffer CA. Platelet transfusion therapy for the cancer patient. Semin Oncol 1990;17:198–209. review.
15. Tornebohm E, Lockner D, Paul C. A retrospective analysis of bleeding complications in 438 patients with acute leukaemia during the years 1972–1991. Eur J Haematol 1993;50:160–7.
16. Bishop JF, Schiffer CA, Aisner J, et al. Surgery in acute leukemia: a review of 167 operations in thrombocytopenic patients. Am J Hematol 1987;26:147–55.
17. Brubaker DB. Correction of the corrected count increment units. Transfusion 1993;33:358–9. letter.
18. McFarland JG, Anderson AJ, Slichter SJ. Factors influencing the transfusion response to HLA-selected apheresis donor platelets in patients refractory to random platelet concentrates. Br J Haematol 1989;73:380–6.
19. Bishop JF, McGrath K, Wolf MM, et al. Clinical factors influencing the efficacy of pooled platelet transfusions. Blood 1988;71:383–7.
20. Duquesnoy RJ, Filip DJ, Rodey GE, et al. Successful transfusion of platelets "mismatched" for HLA antigens to alloimmunized thrombocytopenic patients. Am J Hematol 1977;2:219–26.
21. Dahlke MB, Weiss KL. Platelet transfusion from donors mismatched for crossreactive HLA antigens. Transfusion 1984;24:299–302.

22. Kickler TS, Braine HG, Ness PM, et al. A radiolabeled antiglobulin test for crossmatching platelet transfusions. Blood 1983;61:238–42.
23. Moroff G, Garratty G, Heal JM, et al. Selection of platelets for refractory patients by HLA matching and prospective crossmatching. Transfusion 1992;32:633–40.
24. Petz LD. Platelet crossmatching. J Clin Pathol 1988;90:114–5. editorial.
25. Kekomeaki R, Elfenbein G, Gardner R, et al. Improved response of patients refractory to random-donor platelet transfusions by intravenous gamma globulin. Am J Med 1984;76:199–203.
26. Schiffer CA, Hogge DE, Aisner J, et al. High-dose intravenous gamma-globulin in alloimmunized platelet transfusion recipients. Blood 1984;64:937–40.
27. Kickler T, Braine HG, Piantadosi S, et al. A randomized, placebo-controlled trial of intravenous gammaglobulin in alloimmunized thrombocytopenic patients. Blood 1990;75:313–6.
28. Christie DJ, Howe RB, Lennon SS, Sauro SC. Treatment of refractoriness to platelet transfusion by protein A column therapy. Transfusion 1993;33:234–42.
29. Kaushansky K. Thrombopoietin: the primary regulator of platelet production. Blood 1995;86:419–31.
30. Kaushansky K. Thrombopoietin: understanding and manipulating platelet production. Ann Rev Med 1997;48:1–11.
31. Practice guidelines for blood component therapy: a report by the American Society of Anesthesiologists Task Force on Blood Component Therapy. Anesthesiology 1996;84:732–47.
32. Practice parameter for the use of fresh-frozen plasma, cryoprecipitate, and platelets: Fresh-Frozen Plasma, Cryoprecipitate, and Platelets Administration Practice Guidelines Development Task Force of the College of American Pathologists. JAMA 1994;271:777–81.
33. Strauss RG. Therapeutic granulocyte transfusions in 1993. Blood 1993;81:1675–8.
34. Klein HG, Strauss RG, Schiffer CA. Granulocyte transfusion therapy. Semin Hematol 1996;33:359–68.
35. Bordin JO, Heddle NM, Blajchman MA. Biologic effects of leukocytes present in transfused cellular blood products. Blood 1994;84:1703–21.
36. Engelfriet CP, Reesink HW. The use and quality control of leukocyte-depleted cell concentrates. Vox Sang 1998;75:82–92.
37. Bowden RA, Slichter SJ, Sayers M, et al. A comparison of filtered leukocyte-reduced and cytomegalovirus CMV seronegative blood products for the prevention of transfusion-associated (CMV) infection after marrow transplant. Blood 1995;86:3598–603.
38. Anderson KC, Weinstein HJ. Transfusion-associated graft-versus-host disease. N Engl J Med 1990;323:315–21.
39. Anderson KC, Goodnough LT, Sayers M, et al. Variation in blood component irradiation practice: implications for prevention of transfusion-associated graft-versus-host disease. Blood 1991;77:2096–102.
40. Greenbaum BH. Transfusion-associated graft-versus-host disease: historical perspectives, incidence, and current use of irradiated blood products. J Clin Oncol 1991;9:1889–1902.
41. Petz LD, Calhoun L, Yam P, et al. Transfusion-associated graft-versus-host disease in immunocompetent patients: report of a fatal case associated with transfusion of blood from a second-degree relative, and a survey of predisposing factors. Transfusion 1993;33:742–50.
42. McAlister FA, Clark HD, Wells PS, Laupacis A. Perioperative allogeneic blood transfusion does not cause adverse sequelae in patients with cancer: a meta-analysis of unconfounded studies. Br J Surg 1998;85:171–8.
43. Vamvakas EC. Perioperative blood transfusion and cancer recurrence: meta-analysis for explanation. Transfusion 1995;35:760–8.
44. Lapierre V, Aupaerin A, Tiberghien P. Transfusion-induced immunomodulation following cancer surgery: fact or fiction? J Natl Cancer Inst 1998;90:573–80.
45. Vamvakas EC, Moore SB. Blood transfusion and postoperative septic complications. Transfusion 1994;34:714–27.

# CHAPTER 15

# CLINICAL USE OF HEMATOPOIETIC GROWTH FACTORS

• HANNA J. KHOURY • JOHN F. DiPERSIO

The hematopoietic growth factors (HGFs) are a family of proteins that regulate the proliferation, differentiation, and viability of hematopoietic progenitor cells and mature blood elements. The recognition that circulating factors regulate red cell production dates back to the work of Carnot and Deflandre,[1] who in 1906 induced erythrocytosis in normal rabbits by infusing them with plasma from anemic animals. Sixty years later, the semisolid culture systems necessary to grow bone marrow progenitor cells in vitro were developed.[2,3] This development led to the identification of the HGFs, originally called *colony-stimulating factors* (CSFs) because they stimulated the formation of colonies of cells derived from individual bone marrow progenitors. A group of factors, termed *interleukins* (ILs), have predominant roles as regulatory proteins between leukocytes and can stimulate colony formation as well. A general term for HGF, CSF, or IL is *cytokine*. This term refers to a regulatory protein communicating between cells.[4]

This chapter focuses mainly on the emerging roles of HGFs in the supportive care of cancer patients and for the mobilization and transplantation of peripheral blood stem cells (PBSCs). Other clinical uses of HGFs are also discussed. The HGFs discussed are those already licensed for use in the United States and those currently in phase I-II clinical trials and include granulocyte CSF (G-CSF),[5] granulocyte-macrophage CSF (GM-CSF),[6] erythropoietin (EPO),[7,8] IL-11,[9,10] GM-CSF/IL-3 fusion protein (PIXY321),[11] macrophage CSF (M-CSF),[12] IL-1,[13] IL-3,[14] IL-6,[15] stem cell factor (SCF) (also called *Steel factor, c-kit ligand*, and *mast cell growth factor*),[16] thrombopoietin (TPO),[17,18] and Flk2/Flt3 ligand.

## Preclinical Considerations

### PROLIFERATIVE AND DIFFERENTIATIVE PROPERTIES

The HGFs can be classified according to the stage of hematopoietic cell differentiation affected, specifically early-stage cytokines, lineage-nonspecific cytokines, and lineage-specific cytokines. Many cytokines are capable of affecting more than one stage of differentiation, suggesting that these cytokines are highly redundant and promiscuous.

The cell at the earliest stage of differentiation has been termed the *pluripotent stem cell*. It is capable of self-renewal and differentiation.[19] Conceptually, differentiation can occur along one of three major pathways resulting in the production of (1) erythrocytes, granulocytes (neutrophils, eosinophils, and basophils), monocytes-macrophages, and megakaryocytes-platelets; (2) lymphocytes (T cells, B cells, and natural killer cells); and (3) stromal cells, endothelial cells, and fibroblasts. A presumptive scheme for lineage development is shown in Figure 15–1. Most of the HGFs can act to varying degrees alone or in synergy with other HGFs on cells at the early stages of differentiation: SCF,[20] IL-3,[14] IL-1,[21] IL-6,[22] IL-11,[23] IL-12,[23, 24] leukemia inhibitory factor (LIF),[25] Flk2/Flt3 ligand,[26] TPO,[27] GM-CSF, and G-CSF.[19] These HGFs appear to be capable of inducing self-renewal of the pluripotent stem cell. When stem cells are induced to exit the $G_0$ stage, they may self-replicate or commit to differentiate along specific pathways, or both. This decision appears to be random (also termed *stochastic*). Once the decision to differentiate is made, cell-cell interaction and the expression of cell surface receptors for the aforementioned HGFs, with subsequent binding of the HGFs, undoubtedly play a role in directing differentiation along particular pathways.[28, 29]

The HGFs that primarily affect the lineage-nonspecific stage of differentiation (i.e., after the pluripotent stem cell has exited $G_0$) are GM-CSF,[6] G-CSF,[5] IL-3,[30] and IL-4.[31] The HGFs that primarily affect the lineage-specific stages of differentiation include G-CSF,[5] EPO,[8] M-CSF,[12] IL-5,[32] and IL-11[33]-TPO[34] affecting the neutrophil, erythroid, monocyte-macrophage, eosinophil, and megakaryocyte lineages.

At present, of all the HGFs mentioned, only G-CSF, GM-CSF, EPO, and IL-11 are currently licensed for clinical use in the United States. An advisory panel at the U.S. Food and Drug Administration (FDA) has recommended that SCF be approved for the specific indication of improving stem cell mobilization in "hard-to-mobilize" patients. Many of the other HGFs (i.e., the lineage-nonspecific factors) are currently entering or are already in phase I-II clinical trials. Their applications are leading to therapy in combination or in tandem with each other or with the late-stage growth factors. The premise for combination therapy is based on the additive or synergistic effect demonstrated in various in vitro assay systems. SCF, IL-1, IL-6, and LIF do not have any significant CSF activity in vitro. All can synergize with other HGFs, however, such as GM-CSF, G-CSF, IL-3, and M-CSF, in enhancing colony growth.[28, 29, 35–40]

The timing of administration of combination therapy is probably important, as evidenced by the observation that the synergism of IL-3 with GM-CSF occurs only when IL-3 is given in tandem with GM-CSF, not simultaneously.[41] This observation can best be explained in terms of an initial expansion by IL-3 of early-stage progenitors followed by further expansion along the myeloid pathway by GM-CSF. Another approach in maximizing myelostimulation may be the use of cytokines not temporally combined but physically combined. The prototype is PIXY321, which is a genetically engineered fusion protein of GM-CSF and IL-3.[11, 42] Both IL-3 and GM-CSF have multiple biologic functions in common, further underscoring the presence of a common heterotrimeric receptor complex that can bind both molecules as well as IL-5.[32] A common-signaling subunit for the GM-CSF and IL-3 receptors may explain why IL-3 and GM-CSF share so

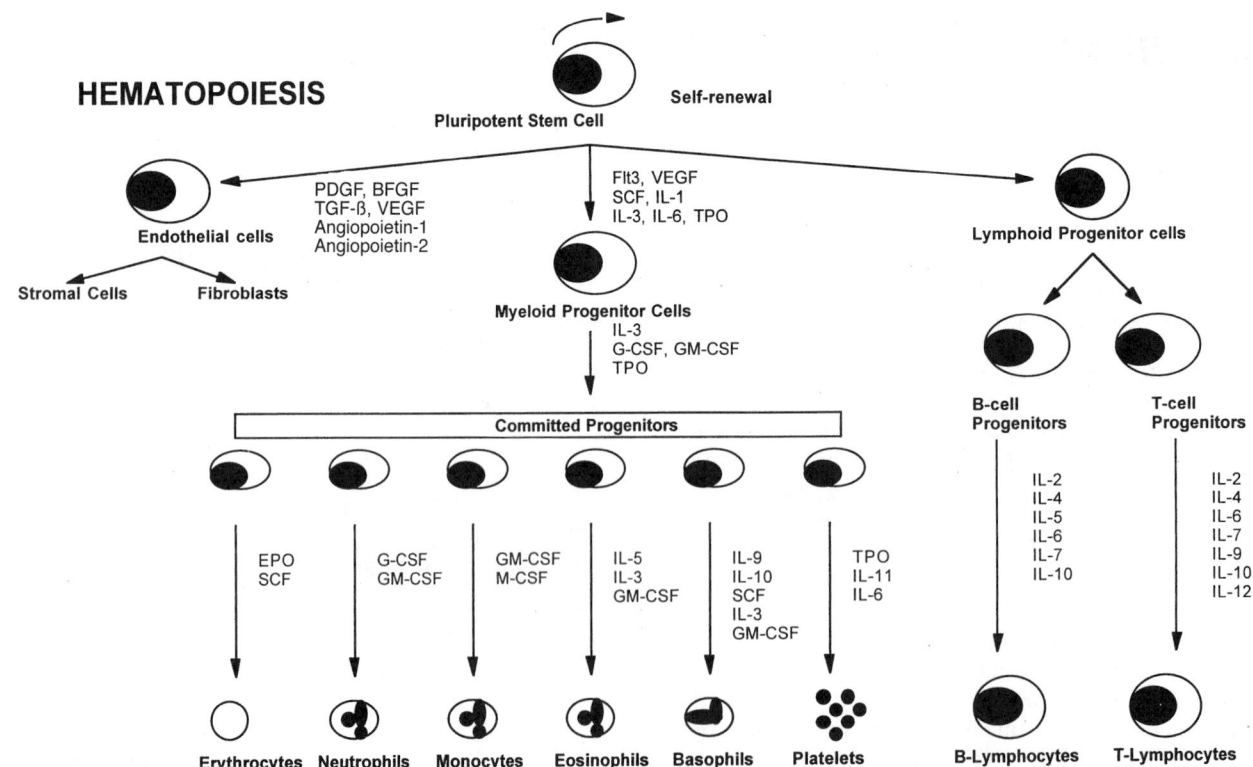

**Figure 15–1.** Schematic representation of the regulation of hematopoiesis. PDGF, platelet-derived growth factor; BFGF, basic fibroblast growth factor; TGF-β, transforming growth factor-β; VEGF, vascular epithelial growth factor; Flt3, Flt3 ligand; SCF, stem cell factor; IL, interleukin; TPO, thrombopoietin; G-CSF, granulocyte colony-stimulating factor; GM-CSF, granulocyte-macrophage colony-stimulating factor; EPO, erythropoietin; M-CSF, macrophage colony-stimulating factor.

many biologic activities. A fusion protein was constructed on the assumption that a molecule with more than one receptor-binding domain may be more active than each HGF alone.[42] Investigation of the use of chimeric molecules, which include both IL-3 agonist properties and G-CSF (*myelopoietins*), IL-3 agonist properties and TPO (*promegapoietin*), and Flt3 ligand and G-CSF (*progenipoietin*), has been completed in preclinical and phase I clinical trials.[43, 44]

New insights into cytokine biology have been possible by studying mice engineered to be homozygous deletion mutants for one or more cytokines or cytokine receptors. These *knockout* mice have provided information that challenges hypotheses of cytokine function based on tissue culture studies.[45] For example, mice deficient in GM-CSF production are not leukopenic. The only observed defect in these mice appears to be a pulmonary defect that resembles pulmonary alveolar proteinosis.[46] G-CSF,[47] EPO,[48] and TPO-deficient[49] mice are selectively neutropenic, anemic, and thrombocytopenic. G-CSF and TPO knockout mice are not absolutely neutropenic or thrombocytopenic, suggesting that other cytokines may also contribute to basal levels of neutrophils and platelets in mice and presumably in humans as well. Overall, these emerging results suggest that cytokine networks that regulate hematopoiesis are complex, with overlapping and redundant functions for some factors and unclear functions for others. To investigate these possibilities, mice deficient in multiple factors are now being studied.[50] These mice should provide further insights into the critical events of hematopoietic regulation. Data have shown complementary interactions between some neuropeptides (the tachykinins) and the cytokines in the regulation of hematopoiesis,[51] demonstrating again the multiple and complex interactions that govern hematopoiesis.

## MYELOPROTECTIVE AND RADIOPROTECTIVE PROPERTIES

Besides the positive effect on differentiation and self-renewal, some HGFs can exert an inhibitory effect.[28, 29] This inhibitory effect can be beneficial in sustaining hematopoiesis by protecting the stem cell from cytocidal therapies. This effect has been observed with several cytokines, including macrophage inflammatory protein-1α (MIP-1α),[52] IL-1,[53] IL-12,[54] transforming growth factor-β (TGF-β),[55] and SCF.[56] MIP-1α is a chemokine that appears to inhibit the movement of the stem cells from $G_1$ to S phase of the cell cycle.[13, 52] During S phase, cells are most susceptible to the cytocidal effects of cell cycle–specific (e.g., cytarabine) and non–cell cycle–specific (e.g., cyclophosphamide) agents. IL-1 protects the hematopoietic system against ionizing radiation or chemotherapeutic agents depending on the schedule of its administration. Administration of a single dose of IL-1 within 18 to 24 hours before irradiation is necessary for radioprotection, whereas administration of multiple daily doses of IL-1 is required to protect against cytotoxic chemotherapeutic agents. The radioprotective effect of IL-1 is believed to be mediated by its ability to promote the cycling and progression of progenitor cells into S phase.[57] Paradoxically, IL-1 also causes inhibition of cell cycle progression, which is protective against the apoptotic effect of chemotherapeutic drugs.[58] IL-12, through its interaction with different cytokines, has a radioprotective effect on stem cells and a sensitizing effect on gastrointestinal tissue.[59] Basic fibroblast growth factor can reverse the inhibition of hematopoiesis by TGF-β1 (a potent inhibitor of the cell cycle), leading to progenitor cell growth.[60] SCF has been shown to have radioprotective effects similar to IL-1.[13]

## STEM CELL MOBILIZATION AND EXPANSION PROPERTIES

HGFs have been shown to promote the mobilization of CD34+ human stem cells from the bone marrow to the peripheral blood when administered alone or after chemotherapy.[61] Despite intensive studies, the mechanisms that control the movement of hematopoietic progenitor cells from the bone marrow to the blood are incompletely understood. The localization of hematopoiesis to the bone marrow involves developmentally regulated adhesive interactions between primitive hematopoietic cells and the marrow stromal microenvironment.[62] This fact and the broad range of agents that can result in transient increases in blood progenitor cells led to the assumption that mobilization involves a perturbation of the adhesive interactions with stromal elements in the bone marrow.[63] The role and relative contribution of the many adhesion molecules and their ligands in the homing, lodgment, and retention of primitive hematopoietic progenitor cells within the bone marrow remain largely unknown. Studies have suggested an important contribution is made by the β-1 integrin VLA-4, whose two ligands, fibronectin and VCAM-1, are constitutively expressed by the marrow stroma.[64] Perturbation of VLA-4 function after administration of anti-VLA-4 antibody to nonhuman primates was found to induce mobilization of hematopoietic stem cells.[65] After treatment with a range of cytokines, including IL-3, GM-CSF, and SCF, CD34+ cells were shown to exhibit transient dose-dependent increases in surface VLA-4 and VLA-5 ligand binding properties followed by a return to basal activation states.[66] These data suggest that mobilization of hematopoietic progenitor cells may, at least in part, result from cytokine-induced changes in integrin function on CD34+ cells that facilitate their egress from the bone marrow. Studies have provided information on the biology and mechanism of stem cell mobilization by vastly differing cytokines, such as IL-8,[67, 68] G-CSF, and Flt-3 ligand.[69, 70] Further understanding of the mechanism of mobilization may contribute to the development of more predictable and efficacious mobilization protocols.

Ex vivo expansion of hematopoietic stem cells refers to a method of growing progenitors outside the body. Ex vivo expansion of hematopoietic stem cells can be measured using in vitro assays or in vivo human or xenogeneic transplantation models. These animal models involve the use of nonobese diabetes/SCID (NOD/SCID) mice[71, 72] or sheep fetuses.[73] The transplanted human stem cells home to and engraft in the xenogeneic bone marrow, where they proliferate and differentiate, producing large numbers of early progenitors as well as mature myeloid, erythroid, and lymphoid cells. Two assay systems have been developed to identify and quantify the stem cell population in vitro. One system generates hematopoietic progenitor colonies from culture in stroma-free liquid media, whereas the other, called the *long-*

*term culture-initiating cell system*, measures hematopoietic colonies or colony-forming cells after 5 to 6 weeks of co-culture on stromal layers. These two in vitro systems require liquid culture media that include various cytokine combinations, such as SCF, IL-1, IL-3, IL-6, G-CSF, GM-CSF, and EPO. The optimal combination offering the maximum progenitor expansion remains to be defined.[74] Cytokines that appear to have the greatest effects on expansion of early progenitors as measured in these assays include SCF, Flt-3 ligand, TPO, and IL-6.[75]

The potential advantages of the ex vivo expansion of hematopoietic stem cells include enhancement of tumor purging, progenitor cell transplantation using cord blood in adults, and ability to manipulate hematopoietic stem cells genetically.[74] The resultant *expanded* stem cell product should contain abundant mixtures of progenitors as well as pluripotent stem cells, the former preventing or ameliorating the initial phase of neutropenia and the latter sustaining long-term hematopoiesis. Preclinical studies to date suggest promise for this approach,[76–78] and reports of the clinical application of ex vivo expanded hematopoietic stem cells are emerging. Reports describe rapid and sustained hematopoietic recovery in patients receiving expanded autologous stem cells.[79, 80] The long-term engrafting capability of these ex vivo expanded CD34+ cells remains unknown, however.[81] Ex vivo expansion of CD34+ cells could be used as a source of cells for retrovirus-mediated gene transfer (e.g., insertion of the multidrug-resistance gene or other genes of interest).[82]

## ENHANCEMENT OF EFFECTOR CELL FUNCTION

HGFs not only stimulate the growth and differentiation of stem cells but also activate or enhance directly the function of mature effector cells, such as neutrophils, eosinophils, and monocytes as well as B and T lymphocytes.[83] Numerous effects on the function of these cells have been documented, including regulation of cell motility; increases in cell surface expression of various receptors, particularly those involved in adhesion and phagocytosis; augmentation of the secretion of cytokines and inflammatory mediators; and increased microbicidal activity via effects on oxidative burst and antibody-dependent cytotoxicity.[83–85] The effects can be complicated, as evidenced by the observation that brief exposure to GM-CSF primes the neutrophil for chemotaxis, whereas prolonged low doses of GM-CSF inhibit neutrophil migration (probably because of increased expression of cell surface adhesion receptors).[86] The varied effects of HGFs on the neutrophil, monocyte, and eosinophil have correlated with preclinical studies that have demonstrated enhanced antibacterial activity[84] (e.g., pretreatment with GM-CSF in immunosuppressed mice lowers *Pseudomonas*-induced or *Staphylococcus aureus*–induced mortality[87]), antifungal activity (e.g., GM-CSF, M-CSF, and IL-3 augment the fungicidal activity of human monocytes for *Candida albicans*[88]), and antiviral activity (e.g., M-CSF[89] and IL-3[90] can inhibit herpes simplex virus replication). The indication for the use of HGFs may extend from neoplastic diseases to the treatment of infectious diseases in combination with antibiotics. Despite these effects in vitro, however, thus far, no studies have demonstrated clinical benefit of HGFs in the management of patients with active infection.

HGFs are increasingly used in clinical trials to accelerate reconstitution of bone marrow function after myelosuppressive or high-dose chemotherapy in patients with solid tumors. A significant concern regarding the use of these growth factors in this setting is that while promoting repopulation of the bone marrow, they might induce growth of the underlying tumor. This concern is based on the detection of receptors of or the stimulation of cell proliferation by GM-CSF,[91] IL-3,[92] or IL-6[93] in cancer cell lines in vitro. The effects of GM-CSF, IL-3, and IL-6 were tested on tumor cells taken directly from patients with solid tumors using human tumor cloning assays.[94] Stimulation of tumor colony-forming units was observed in few instances, indicating a small likelihood that these malignant cells could be stimulated by GM-CSF, IL-3, or IL-6. There has been no clinical evidence that HGFs stimulate the growth of solid tumors in vivo.[95, 96]

Preclinical studies have demonstrated antiproliferative and antitumor effects of IL-3,[94] IL-4,[97] IL-6,[94, 98, 99] IL-7,[100] IL-12,[101] M-CSF,[25, 102] LIF,[103] and GM-CSF.[104] A report describes antitumor activity of Flt-3 ligand when administered to mice challenged with syngeneic fibrosarcoma cells.[105] Tumor growth was observed for 2.5 weeks after injection of syngeneic fibrosarcoma cells in both Flt3 ligand–treated and mouse serum albumin–treated mice. A decrease in tumor size followed by complete tumor regression was observed in 19 of 50 Flt3 ligand–treated mice as compared with only 1 of 30 mouse serum albumin–treated mice. Flt3 ligand treatment of these tumor-bearing mice appeared to induce immunologically mediated (Thy1+, CD4−, CD8+ cells) and non-immunologically mediated responses that affect tumor growth in vivo. Generation of dendritic cells may play an important role in Flt3 ligand–induced antitumor immune response. It is possible that the combination of HGFs with cytotoxic agents may potentiate antitumor activity against solid tumors.

## PREPARATIONS AND BIOLOGIC PROPERTIES

Much of what is known about the expression, structure, and function of HGFs has been made possible by the use of molecular biologic techniques permitting the isolation and molecular cloning of full-length cDNA sequences encoding these proteins. All the HGFs available for clinical use as therapeutic agents have been produced by using recombinant technology. Insertion of the cDNAs into eukaryotic, yeast, or bacterial expression systems has allowed the generation of large amounts of purified proteins necessary for adequate in vitro and in vivo studies and clinical trials. When bacterial expression systems (usually *Escherichia coli*) are used to manufacture these products, the resulting human proteins contain an additional amino acid (N terminal methionine) that is not present in the native form of the HGF. In addition, and as compared with the endogenous human HGFs, *E. coli*–derived HGFs are not glycosylated. Some manufacturers have used yeast or mammalian expression systems to generate glycosylated HGFs. The available data are not conclusive as to whether the glycosylation of HGFs has important therapeutic implications.[106]

PIXY321 is the prototype of a class of synthetic cytokines. This genetically engineered HGF was designed in an attempt to take advantage of the synergism and the enhanced multilineage stimulation of IL-3 and GM-CSF. PIXY321 consists of the active domain of recombinant human GM-CSF and recombinant human IL-3 coupled by a flexible amino-acid linker sequence.[11, 42] Although IL-3 plays a pivotal role in the stimulation of hematopoiesis, the clinical use of native IL-3 is limited by a relatively narrow therapeutic index, mainly because of the intrinsic inflammatory activity of this molecule.[107] A detailed understanding of the structure-activity relationships of IL-3 was undertaken and led to the development of several synthetic cytokines (called *synthokines*) with a high-affinity IL-3 receptor agonist activity.[108] These synthokines exhibited a significantly greater biologic activity than the recombinant human IL-3 in human hematopoietic cell proliferation and marrow colony–forming unit assays. These synthetic cytokines have been combined with other HGFs (e.g., G-CSF and TPO) to form chimeric cytokines with the hope of expanding mobilization properties and to decrease further therapy-induced myelosuppression.[42–44] It is unclear yet how much of a significant role these synthetic cytokines will play in clinical medicine. A summary of the gene location, function, and therapeutic potential of the major HGFs is presented in Table 15–1.

Histologic damage and disease is occasionally associated with increased levels of endogenous cytokines.[109, 110] This association has prompted the design of anticytokine monoclonal antibodies. For example, IL-6 is a growth factor for multiple myeloma and has constitutively been produced by some myeloma cells as an autocrine and paracrine growth factor.[111] In vitro, anti-IL-6 antibodies inhibit myeloma cell growth.[112] Studies using anti-IL-6 monoclonal antibodies demonstrated a reduction in plasma cell proliferation, serum calcium, and serum monoclonal IgG levels in myeloma patients, suggesting a clinical response.[113] The addition of anti-IL-6 monoclonal antibodies to the available therapeutic arsenal may be complementary in treating this incurable disease. Anti-IL-6 monoclonal antibodies have been used to alleviate the symptoms of a patient with Castelman's disease,[114] another IL-6–related disorder.

## PHARMACOLOGIC CONSIDERATIONS

Identification of a strict dose-response relationship for HGFs has proved difficult because there are multiple biologic end points that must be measured, and potential secondary endogenous cytokines may be produced, any of which may influence the response.[115] The response also depends on the number and type of target cells present in the bone marrow.

**Granulocyte Colony–Stimulating Factor and Granulocyte-Macrophage Colony-Stimulating Factor.** The complementary DNAs that encode G-CSF and GM-CSF have been cloned.[116–120] Both can be produced in nonglycosylated form in bacteria without any apparent compromise in biologic activities compared with native glycosylated GM-CSF and G-CSF. Glycosylation of GM-CSF appears to correlate with lower specific activity using in vitro progenitor assays.[115, 121] The highly glycosylated forms may also have

*Table 15–1.* **Characteristics of Selected Hematopoietic Growth Factors**

| Cytokine | Gene Location | Function | Potential Therapeutic Role |
|---|---|---|---|
| GM-CSF | 5q23-31 | Stimulates hematopoiesis of myeloid and macrophage lineage; activates granulocytes and macrophages | Therapy- and disease-related myelosuppression, mobilization of progenitor cells, ? antitumor agent, ? antimicrobial agent, ? gene therapy for tumors |
| G-CSF | 17q11-22 | Stimulates hematopoiesis of granulocyte lineage; activates granulocytes | Therapy- and disease-related myelosuppression, mobilization of progenitor cells |
| M-CSF | 5q23 | Stimulates monocyte growth and development; activates monocytes/macrophages | Antimicrobial agent (fungal infection), ? antitumor agent |
| EPO | 7q11-12 | Stimulates erythroid growth and development | Therapy for erythropoietin-depleted states of anemia (renal failure, malignancy-associated anemia); ? therapy for erythropoietin-replete anemic states (MDS), autologous blood donation |
| IL-1 | 2q14 | Stimulates early stages of hematopoiesis, T- and B-cell activation | Protection of marrow function during chemotherapy-radiotherapy, expansion of progenitor cells in vitro |
| IL-3 | 5q23-31 | Stimulates early stages of hematopoiesis | Mobilization of progenitor cells, therapy- and disease-related myelosuppression, expansion of progenitor cells in vitro |
| IL-6 | 7q15 | Costimulates early stages of hematopoiesis, T- and B-cell activation | Therapy-related myelosuppression, expansion of progenitor cells in vitro |
| IL-11 | 24 | Stimulates megakaryocytes | Therapy-related thrombocytopenia, reduction of therapy-related gastrointestinal toxicity |
| Thrombopoietin (TPO) | 3q26-27 | Stimulates all stages of megakaryocytosis | Mobilization of progenitor cells, ? therapy-related thrombocytopenia |
| Stem cell factor | 4q | Costimulates early stages of hematopoiesis, mast cell, and megakaryocyte growth factor | Mobiliziation of progenitor cells, ? Therapy-related myelosuppression, expansion of progenitor cells in vitro |
| Flt-3 Ligand | 19q13.319 q13.4 | Costimulates early stages of hematopoiesis, stimulates the generation of dendritic cells | Mobilization of progenitor cells, immunotherapy, gene therapy |

GM-CSF, granulocyte macrophage colony-stimulating factor; G-CSF, granulocyte colony–stimulating factor; M-CSF, macrophage colony–stimulating factor; EPO, erythropoietin; MDS, myelodysplasia.

greater immunogenicity[122] but a longer half-life.[115] The rare cases of antibody development have not been clinically significant.[115, 123, 124]

Transient leukopenia (more frequently after an intravenous bolus dose than after a subcutaneous dose) has been observed 5 to 60 minutes after the administration of GM-CSF and less frequently G-CSF.[122, 125] This effect appears to be due to rapid pulmonary sequestration of blood neutrophils.[126] The kinetic pattern of leukocytosis is somewhat different for G-CSF and GM-CSF. Daily administration of G-CSF results in a dose-dependent increase in the neutrophil count with a plateau occurring during the second week of administration. In contrast to G-CSF, daily administration of GM-CSF results in a biphasic response with an increase in neutrophils in the first 5 days, followed by a transient decrease, then a second increase that continues for another 3 to 5 days after therapy is stopped.[127] This pattern has been attributed to an initial demargination followed by increased neutrophil production. GM-CSF–stimulated neutrophils have enhanced viability in vitro and in vivo.[115, 128] Overall, there is a greater rise in the neutrophil count by G-CSF than by GM-CSF on an equimolar basis.[115] In both cases, the peripheral blood leukocytosis consists of a leftward shift in myeloid maturation (occasionally including myeloblasts), with a dose-related eosinophilia and monocytosis also noted with GM-CSF.[128]

The recommended dose of GM-CSF is 250 $\mu$g/m$^2$ or 3 to 5 $\mu$g/kg.[115, 127] The leukocytosis continues to be dose dependent beyond 3 to 5 $\mu$g/kg, but at greater than 3 $\mu$g/kg, fever and chills occur, and at greater than 20 $\mu$g/kg, side effects, such as capillary leak–type syndrome, become dose limiting.[129, 130] This capillary leak–type syndrome may be due, in part, to GM-CSF–induced release of tumor necrosis factor (TNF) and IL-1 by monocytes[131] and IL-6 by neutrophils[132] and to GM-CSF–induced tissue eosinophilia. In some cases, low doses of GM-CSF (10 $\mu$g/m$^2$) may be more myelostimulatory than standard doses.[133] The enhancement of neutrophil function in terms of adherence, phagocytosis, chemotaxis, and respiratory burst in preclinical studies mentioned previously has also been noted in clinical studies.[115, 127] The recommended dose of G-CSF is 5 $\mu$g/kg, but in contrast to GM-CSF, there does not appear to be any definite dose limit, as levels of 200,000 neutrophils have been well tolerated.[127] Bone pain often develops at doses of G-CSF exceeding 5 $\mu$g/kg.[134]

Initial clinical studies of G-CSF and GM-CSF focused on their administration via the intravenous route.[135, 136] Since then, numerous studies have shown that subcutaneous administration once or twice a day is more myelostimulatory than 2- to 4-hour intravenous infusions.[137–142] There also appears to be less GM-CSF–induced toxicity when it is given subcutaneously.[137, 139] Another mode of administration is continuous infusion. Intuitively, one would expect this to be the most myelostimulatory strategy but conceivably more toxic. This approach may be appropriate when the neutropenia is refractory to subcutaneous administration. There is as yet no evidence to support this approach, however.

GM-CSF can activate lymphocytes through unclear mechanisms because lymphocytes do not express GM-CSF receptors.[143] Long-term follow-up of lymphoma patients who have received GM-CSF after autologous bone marrow transplantation, however, did not show higher rates of relapse compared with controls in randomized studies.[144] GM-CSF, when added to IL-6, can stimulate myeloma cell growth in vitro,[145] but there has been no evidence of such an effect in clinical trials with GM-CSF in myeloma patients.[146]

**Recombinant Human Erythropoietin.** Subcutaneous administration of recombinant human EPO (rHuEPO) induces lower peak plasma EPO concentrations but a higher elimination half-life when compared with intravenous administration. Subcutaneous administration of smaller doses of rHuEPO more closely resembles the physiology of EPO production and leads to a greater efficacy than intravenous administration of larger doses.[147, 148] A variety of dosages (150 to >1000 IU/kg/wk) and administration schedules have been used outside the uremia setting. Studies using rHuEPO for the anemia of cancer employed the subcutaneous route three times per week at a dose usually at least two to five times higher than that used for renal failure.[149–151] Indicators of response are used to monitor patients treated with rHuEPO and should be interpreted in the context of its administration, especially in patients receiving transfusions, concomitant chemotherapy, or both. Increments in hemoglobin[152] ($\geq$1.0 g/dl) or in reticulocyte count[153] ($\geq$40 $\times$ 10$^9$/L) after 4 weeks have been shown to be good predictors of response to rHuEPO. Of patients treated with rHuEPO, 50% develop evidence of iron deficiency.[154] Monitoring iron status in these patients may allow prompt detection of iron deficiency and early iron supplementation therapy.

**Interleukin-11.** IL-11 is available for subcutaneous administration at a recommended dose of 50 $\mu$g/kg given once daily. In one study,[155] daily subcutaneous administration for 14 days increased the platelet counts in a dose-dependent manner. Platelet counts increased relative to the baseline 5 to 9 days after the start of dosing with IL-11. After cessation of therapy, platelet counts continued to increase for 7 days, then returned to baseline within 14 days. A therapy-related anemia, secondary to plasma volume expansion, was observed at all doses of IL-11.

### Other Hematopoietic Growth Factors

***Stem Cell Factor.*** Increases in peripheral leukocytes resulting from increases in total numbers of neutrophils, lymphocytes, monocytes, eosinophils, and basophils were observed after the infusion of SCF at a dose of 200 $\mu$g/kg/day.[156] The leukocytes and absolute number of each lineage returned to pretreatment values within 7 days of discontinuation of SCF. Platelet counts initially decreased but returned to pretreatment values by 3 weeks and thereafter. When administered with G-CSF for stem cell mobilization, the recommended dose of SCF is 20 $\mu$g/kg subcutaneously daily.

***Flt3 Ligand.*** Sustained mobilization of progenitor cells is observed with the subcutaneous administration of Flt3 ligand at a dose of 100 $\mu$g/kg/day for 14 consecutive days.[157] There is also an increase in the level of circulating dendritic cells (30-fold) and peripheral blood leukocytes (2-fold to 3-fold), partly as a result of an increase in the monocyte fraction.[158]

***Interleukin-3.*** There is a moderate, dose-dependent increase in neutrophils, platelets, and total white blood cells after continuous intravenous or subcutaneous IL-3 injection. The leukocytosis mostly consists of neutrophils, eosinophils, and lymphocytes.[159]

***Interleukin-6.*** A dose-dependent, twofold increase in the platelet count was observed in a phase I trial of recombinant human IL-6 in patients with refractory advanced malignancies.[160]

***Macrophage Colony–Stimulating Factor.*** A phase I-II trial showed a moderate, dose-dependent increase in monocytes and decrease in platelet count with the intravenous infusion of M-CSF at a daily dose of $3.0 \times 10^6$ units for 7 days.[161]

***Thrombopoietin.*** In one study,[162] a single dose of recombinant human TPO (0.3 to 2.4 µg/kg) was associated with an increase in platelet counts in a dose-related manner. This increase was observed by day 4 after the administration of TPO and peaked at a median of 12 days. Platelet response was accompanied by a dose-related increase in bone marrow megakaryocytes.

# Clinical Uses of Hematopoietic Growth Factors

Most clinical trials of HGFs have been conducted in the context of therapy of hematologic and oncologic diseases. Sufficient data from human clinical trials have accumulated to permit publication of evidence-based practice guidelines,[124, 163, 164] some of which have been updated.[165] These guidelines are a welcome initiative to inform clinicians as to the most appropriate use of these potent and expensive drugs. This section focuses primarily on the use of HGFs for supportive care of the cancer patient rendered cytopenic by chemotherapy (standard or myeloablative) and the use of HGFs for peripheral blood stem cells (PBSC) mobilization.

## CYTOPENIAS ASSOCIATED WITH CHEMOTHERAPY

Neutropenia and resultant infections can be life-threatening side effects of cancer chemotherapy. G-CSF and GM-CSF have been extensively evaluated for the prevention of myelosuppression associated with conventional chemotherapy. The efficacy of these agents was initially tested by administration immediately after chemotherapy and continuing through the anticipated period of neutropenia.[134, 166–168] These HGFs were then administered in conjunction with antibiotics for the management of febrile neutropenia.[169–174] All randomized trials have shown a modest reduction in the days of neutropenia but little or no effects on number of days of antibiotic therapy, length of hospital stay, or mortality resulting from infections. With escalating health care costs, there has been a growing interest in the assessment of economic outcomes associated with the use of HGFs.[175, 176] G-CSF and GM-CSF appear to have equal efficacy in the setting of chemotherapy-induced neutropenia, as demonstrated by a large, double-blind, randomized trial comparing these two HGFs.[177]

The American Society of Clinical Oncology (ASCO) guidelines[165] recommend that routine HGF support should be used only in patients with a greater than 40% risk of neutropenic sepsis, although these patients are often difficult to recognize. Possible factors identifying these patients include advanced age, retroviral disease, extensive marrow involvement, use of intensified regimens, poor performance status, and sepsis in a preceding course. No studies have examined the minimum dose of G-CSF or GM-CSF required in these situations.

With the introduction of myeloid growth factors, neutropenia may no longer be a dose-limiting toxicity, whereas thrombocytopenia has become a clinical problem with dose-intensive regimens. Two randomized trials evaluated the efficacy of recombinant human IL-11 in reducing the need for platelet transfusion after chemotherapy.[178, 179] In one study, 93 patients were randomized, as part of secondary prophylaxis, to receive placebo or recombinant human IL-11 at 25 µg/kg or 50 µg/kg subcutaneously once daily for 14 to 21 days beginning 1 day after chemotherapy for solid tumors or lymphoma.[178] Patients were eligible if they developed chemotherapy-induced thrombocytopenia (platelets <20,000/µL) and had received at least one platelet transfusion during the preceding cycle of chemotherapy. Approximately 30% of patients treated with recombinant human IL-11 at a dose of 50 µg/kg did not require platelet transfusions compared with 18% of patients treated with recombinant human IL-11 at a dose of 25 µg/kg and 4% of patients who received placebo ($p<0.05$). The median numbers of platelet transfusions required among the groups treated with 50 µg/kg, 25 µg/kg, and placebo were one, two, and three. The mean number of platelet transfusions required per patient was 2.2 for each of the recombinant human IL-11 groups and 3.4 for the placebo group. This difference was not statistically different. Among patients receiving recombinant human IL-11 at a dose of 50 µg/kg, the median duration of platelet counts less than 20,000/µL, 50,000/µL, and 100,000/µL was not statistically different. The incidence or severity of bleeding and the duration of hospitalization were similar for all three groups.

In another trial, women with advanced breast carcinoma were randomized to treatment with placebo or 50 µg/kg/day recombinant human IL-11 subcutaneously for 10 to 17 days after two cycles of dose-intensive cyclophosphamide (3200 mg/m²) and doxorubicin (75 mg/m²).[179] The patients were stratified by whether or not they had received prior chemotherapy. Approximately 68% of patients who received recombinant human IL-11 did not require platelet transfusions compared with 41% in the placebo group ($p=0.04$). There was no statistically significant difference in the number of platelets transfused or the duration of thrombocytopenia after the first cycle. After the second cycle of chemotherapy, the mean number of platelet transfusions required by patients who received recombinant human IL-11 was 0.8 and that for placebo-treated patients was 2.2 ($p=0.04$). The mean time to platelet recovery to greater than 100,000/µl was 15 days, 3 days earlier than the placebo-treated group.

Polyethylene glycol–conjugated recombinant human megakaryocyte growth and development factor (MGDF) is a polypeptide related to TPO that contains the receptor-binding N terminal domain of TPO. MGDF efficacy in reducing the need for platelet transfusion was also tested in patients receiving chemotherapy with carboplatin and paclitaxel for non–small cell lung cancer.[180] This randomized study showed that MGDF reduced the platelet nadir and shortened the duration of reduced platelet levels. No dose response was observed, and there was no effect on the hematocrit or the neutrophil levels. In no patient studied was the thrombocytopenia severe enough to warrant prophylactic platelet transfusion (median nadir platelet count 111,000/µL in the placebo arm vs. 188,000/µL for the MGDF group). These studies are encouraging; however, before IL-11 or MGDF achieves significant use, the criteria for their efficacy and safety should be established and made appropriate for each potential clinical application. Other cytokines, such as IL-3,[181] sequential IL-3 followed by GM-CSF,[182] PIXY321,[183] IL-6,[184] and IL-1,[185] have also undergone preliminary testing for prevention of chemotherapy-induced thrombocytopenia. The results of these studies are inconsistent, and phase III trials are warranted.

## CYTOPENIAS AFTER HIGH-DOSE CHEMOTHERAPY AND HEMATOPOIETIC CELL TRANSPLANTATION

High-dose chemotherapy and bone marrow transplantation is probably the only field in which the introduction of HGFs had a dramatic impact. HGFs are used to reduce the duration of cytopenia after high-dose therapy and stem cell transplantation and for mobilization of PBSCs.

**Autologous Bone Marrow Transplantation.** Numerous clinical trials evaluated the use of HGFs after autologous bone marrow transplantation. Randomized studies involving GM-CSF[186–189] or G-CSF[190] showed an enhanced neutrophil recovery (average reduction by 7 days in the number of days to achieve an absolute neutrophil count >500/µl, as compared with the placebo arm). Not all trials noted a statistically significant difference in the incidence of fever, frequency of infections, duration of antibiotic use, or duration of hospitalization, however.[191] No impact on relapse was noted in patients randomized to receive HGFs. HGFs had no impact on the duration of the absolute neutropenia.

Markedly increased levels of endogenous EPO are observed after autologous BMT,[192] suggesting that these patients would be unlikely to benefit from rHuEPO therapy. Randomized trials using rHuEPO did not significantly enhance recovery of erythropoiesis in this setting.[193, 194]

**Allogeneic Bone Marrow Transplantation.** The initial trials of HGFs were carried out in patients undergoing autologous rather than allogeneic bone marrow transplantation because of concerns that HGFs might interact with immunocompetent cells to promote graft-versus-host disease or graft failure.[195] The few available randomized studies of GM-CSF[196–198] or G-CSF[199] demonstrated an accelerated neutrophil recovery (by an average of 5 days) after allogeneic bone marrow transplantation between matched siblings, without promoting graft-versus-host disease or graft failure. The neutrophil recovery may not be as rapid as that seen in the autologous setting.[196, 197] Based on the encouraging results with the use of HGFs in matched sibling transplants, trials using GM-CSF in patients receiving transplants from unrelated donors were undertaken. No clinical benefit, however, was demonstrated with the use of GM-CSF in this setting.[200, 201]

Endogenous EPO production is frequently inadequate in response to the degree of anemia in recipients of allogeneic bone marrow transplantation.[202] The reasons for this less-than-optimal response, which has not been noted in patients undergoing autologous transplantation, are not clear, but infection, cyclosporine, and graft-versus-host disease could all play a role. Three randomized studies have shown that rHuEPO in high doses (200 to 300 IU/kg three times per week) reduces transfusion requirements during the first 2 months after allogeneic bone marrow transplantation, whereas lower doses were less effective.[203–205]

Although complete sustained engraftment is usually seen after allogeneic transplantation, 10% fail to engraft or, after engraftment, experience a period of poor graft function. These patients have a dismal survival, largely as a result of a high incidence of fatal infections. In a phase II trial, patients with graft failure treated with GM-CSF were observed to have a decreased 100-day mortality compared with historical controls.[206] In one randomized trial, the use of GM-CSF alone led to a higher survival rate at 100 days as compared with the sequential use of GM-CSF plus G-CSF.[207]

***Peripheral Blood Stem Cell Transplantation.*** The benefit of HGFs after infusion of PBSCs has been demonstrated. In two randomized trials, time to neutrophil engraftment was significantly reduced (by an average of 5 days) in patients receiving G-CSF alone[208] or in combination with GM-CSF[209] after autologous PBSC transplantation. The impact of HGFs on the incidence of fever, frequency of infections, duration of antibiotic use, and duration of hospitalization remains to be defined but is, at best, minimal.

Theoretically, until an adequate number of mature neutrophil precursors have been generated by the stem cell product, there might not be any benefit for using HGFs, especially for terminally acting growth factors. The optimal timing for the use of HGFs has been evaluated in the bone marrow[210, 211] and in the PBSC[212] transplant setting. The results of these studies suggest that delaying HGF administration for 8 days after transplantation (rather than starting 1 day after transplantation) is not associated with any significant delay in neutrophil recovery.

Current data suggest a more rapid myeloid recovery in patients who receive myeloid HGFs (specifically G-CSF and GM-CSF) after stem cell transplantation. The required duration and starting point for initiation of these growth factors is less well defined. Sequential IL-3 and GM-CSF,[213] PIXY321,[183] and IL-6 with GM-CSF[214] have been tested in clinical trials, but the results have been inconclusive.

## PERIPHERAL BLOOD PROGENITOR MOBILIZATION

Peripheral blood has gradually replaced bone marrow as the major source of hematopoietic progenitor cell support for patients undergoing transplantation for hematologic and nonhematologic malignancies. PBSC transplantation has several advantages when compared with bone marrow transplantation: The procurement of stem cells does not require hospitalization or exposure to anesthesia, and the duration of cytopenia after myeloablative therapy is shortened. Mobilization of PBSCs can be accomplished with chemotherapy plus HGFs or with HGFs alone.

**Mobilization with Chemotherapy Plus Hematopoietic Growth Factors**

Although chemotherapy alone can produce increases in the concentration of progenitors in the peripheral blood,[215] numerous phase II studies demonstrated additional stem cell mobilization when HGFs were added after chemotherapy. HGFs reduced chemotherapy-induced myelotoxicity and allowed the collection of more progenitors with less leukapheresis.[216–218] Many different myelosuppressive chemotherapy protocols have been used in conjunction with cytokines for mobilization. GM-CSF was the first cytokine shown to enhance blood progenitor cell mobilization when given after chemotherapy[219] but is less commonly used than G-CSF. The dose of G-CSF used is 3 to 6 μg/kg/day,[218] usually started on the day after chemotherapy and continued until the completion of leukapheresis. This daily dose is lower than the 10 to 24 μg/kg/day dose given when G-CSF is used alone for mobilization, but there seems to be no cost saving because the duration required is longer (8 to 12 days compared with 4 to 6 days when G-CSF is given without chemotherapy). In addition, 20 to 30% of patients receiving chemotherapy and HGFs for PBSC mobilization require admission for fever and neutropenia. Sequential administration of IL-3 and GM-CSF after chemotherapy was shown to enhance mobilization as compared with GM-CSF alone.[220] A report from a randomized trial investigating the efficacy of PBSC mobilization using SCF after chemotherapy showed a beneficial effect of the combination of G-CSF and SCF compared with G-CSF alone (fivefold increases in the median CD34+ cells).[221] Preliminary data suggest that PIXY321 given after cyclophosphamide mobilizes a similar number of stem cells when compared with GM-CSF.[222]

### Mobilization with Hematopoietic Growth Factors Alone

*Granulocyte Colony–Stimulating Factor.* G-CSF increases the level of PBSCs in a dose-dependent manner.[223] The minimal dose of G-CSF is yet to be defined. Data suggest that dose escalation beyond 10 μg/kg/day appears to enhance mobilization only minimally.[224] After 4 to 5 days of treatment, the level of PBSCs increases 40-fold to 80-fold and returns to baseline values within 6 days after cessation of G-CSF.[225] The rate of neutrophil and platelet recovery is higher after G-CSF–mobilized PBSCs over steady-state PBSCs and bone marrow.[226–228]

*Granulocyte-Macrophage Colony-Stimulating Factor.* Although GM-CSF has been approved for mobilization in the United States, G-CSF is used more frequently. Initial reports described an 18-fold increase in peripheral blood colony-forming unit–granulocyte-macrophage (CFU-GM) after 3 to 7 days of GM-CSF administered at 4 to 64 μg/kg/day as a continuous intravenous infusion.[229] Later reports described a more modest fourfold to ninefold increase in peripheral blood CFU-GM.[230–232] The kinetics of mobilization of GM-CSF appears to be similar to that of G-CSF, with peak levels of CD34+ cells observed after four to six doses of G-CSF or GM-CSF.

*Other Agents.* SCF has only modest effects on hematopoietic progenitor cell proliferation in vitro, and its mobilization effect in humans when given alone is also negligible. The combination of SCF and G-CSF was synergistic, demonstrating a fourfold higher CD34+ mobilization yield as compared with G-CSF alone.[15]

Although *IL-3* has a proliferative effect on primitive hematopoietic cells in vitro, its mobilization activity when given alone is minimal.[233]

*Flt3 ligand* stimulates the proliferation of primitive progenitors cells in vitro, with only modest proliferation properties as a single agent. Data demonstrated synergism between Flt3 ligand and G-CSF for mobilization of PBSCs in mice.[234] Preliminary results from clinical studies in humans have been reported. Flt3 ligand was safe and well tolerated when

administered to a dose of 100 μg/kg/day for 14 consecutive days to normal healthy volunteers.[157] Sustained mobilization of progenitor cells was observed with elevated circulating levels of CD34+ cells persisting for 1 week after the last dose of Flt3 ligand. Circulating dendritic cells were also increased 30-fold after Flt3 ligand administration.[158] The effects of combining Flt3 ligand with GM-CSF or G-CSF were examined in a randomized double-blind study of 72 healthy volunteers.[235] Subjects received daily subcutaneous injections of Flt3 ligand plus GM-CSF, Flt3 ligand plus G-CSF, or G-CSF (10 μg/kg) alone. Peak levels of circulating CD34+ cells were increased twofold after the use of Flt3 ligand combined with either G-CSF or GM-CSF compared with G-CSF alone. In contrast to mobilization with G-CSF alone, mobilization of CD34+ cells by the Flt3 ligand combinations was sustained for 10 days. Flt3 ligand combined with G-CSF or GM-CSF greatly increased dendritic cells in peripheral blood to levels equivalent to those seen with Flt3 ligand alone.

The mobilization potential of *TPO* has been reported.[236] In a phase I trial, 12 cancer patients with normal hematopoiesis received a single dose of recombinant human TPO before chemotherapy. Recombinant human TPO at doses of 1.2 to 2.4 μg/kg increased peripheral blood concentrations of CD34+ cells (mean 3.6-fold to 5.5-fold). The effects of combining recombinant human TPO with G-CSF were examined in a randomized phase II trial of patients with breast cancer.[237] Patients received a single intravenous injection of recombinant human TPO at 0.6 μg/kg, 1.2 μg/kg, or 2.4 μg/kg or three doses of intravenous recombinant human TPO at 0.3 μg/kg or 0.6 μg/kg followed by G-CSF 5 μg/kg subcutaneously twice daily until $3 \times 10^6$ or more CD34+ cells/kg were collected. The highest CD34+ yield was achieved when patients were mobilized with the combination of G-CSF and the three 0.6 μg/kg doses of recombinant human TPO. No toxicity was reported with this combination.

The updated ASCO guidelines[165] suggest that HGFs can be routinely used as adjuncts to allogeneic and autologous progenitor cell transplantation, for mobilization of PBSCs, and to speed hematopoietic reconstitution after bone marrow or PBSC transplantation. Administration of HGFs in cases of engraftment failure is also warranted.

## USE OF CYTOKINES IN LEUKEMIA PATIENTS

The use of HGFs in patients undergoing treatment for leukemia has been studied in the supportive care setting to abrogate therapy-induced cytopenias or as potential agents for recruitment of myeloblasts into S phase before exposure to cell cycle–specific chemotherapeutic agents. Because of the potential to stimulate leukemic cells through cytokine exposure, there was initial reluctance to explore the use of these agents in diseases such as acute leukemia. Neutrophil recovery can be accelerated with GM-CSF[238] or G-CSF,[166] but a positive effect on secondary end points, such as duration of antibiotic use and length of hospital stay, is uncertain. Most cases of acute myeloid leukemia (AML) occur in patients older than age 60, a group of patients in whom intensive chemotherapy is associated with a high risk of treatment-related toxicity and mortality. A number of double-blind, randomized, controlled trials using GM-CSF[239–241] and G-

CSF[242, 243] to promote myeloid recovery after induction chemotherapy in AML were designed to address specifically the benefit of these HGFs in elderly patients. These studies demonstrated a somewhat shorter period of neutropenia in patients receiving HGFs, but serious infections were not reduced. In some studies, the use of HGFs was associated with a higher remission rate,[242] but neither short-term nor overall survival was improved. There was no risk of stimulating leukemic cells in any of these studies. Similar results were reported with the use of G-CSF in patients with acute lymphoblastic leukemia.[166, 244–246] From these data, it appears that the use of HGFs to shorten the duration of neutropenia in patients with acute leukemia may be, at most, modest. The routine use of GM-CSF or G-CSF after acute leukemia induction therapy cannot be recommended. Perhaps different strategies using HGFs other than G-CSF or GM-CSF, applied in other ways, may contribute to improved outcome of acute leukemia patients undergoing standard induction chemotherapy.

GM-CSF can recruit leukemic cells into S phase in vivo.[247] Attempts to recruit cells into S phase before the administration of cell cycle–specific therapy may increase therapeutic benefit of ara-C. A few trials have evaluated this approach in AML patients.[247–249] Although initial results of pretreatment with GM-CSF were disappointing,[247] a more recent study suggested that this strategy may be appropriate in AML.[249] In this trial, the complete remission rates, mortality rate from resistant disease, and incidence of infectious events were similar in the GM-CSF and placebo groups, but a longer disease-free survival was observed in the GM-CSF group (48% vs. 21% in the placebo group; $p = 0.003$). This benefit was observed mainly in the cohort of younger patients (aged 55 to 64) and was only marginal in patients 65 years old and older. Further evaluations of optimal conditions for the use of myeloid growth factors in AML are needed.

The updated ASCO guidelines[165] suggest that primary administration of HGFs can be used after completion of induction chemotherapy in patients 55 years old and older. HGFs administered before or concurrently with chemotherapy for priming effects was not recommended outside clinical trials.

## DISEASE-RELATED CYTOPENIAS

**Myelodysplasia.** Given the relatively poor risk-benefit ratio of intensive chemotherapy for most myelodysplastic patients (i.e., those >60 years), many physicians adopt a "watch and wait" approach, intervening with administration of HGFs singly, in combination, or together with low-dose chemotherapy at the time of progressive cytopenia. The use of GM-CSF or G-CSF for the treatment of neutropenia associated with MDS resulted in an increase in neutrophil counts in a modest number of patients.[250, 251] For some patients with multilineage abnormalities, treatment with multiple or broader-acting HGFs,[252] such as IL-3[253] or PIXY321,[254] was associated with an increase in neutrophil and platelet count. A concern in patients treated with myeloid-enhancing cytokines for MDS has been the possibility of increasing the percentage of myeloblasts and the transformation to AML. Randomized trials with GM-CSF[255] or G-CSF,[256] reported in

abstract form only, suggest that these HGFs may not influence the rate of progression to AML. There have been no direct comparative studies or published randomized, placebo-controlled, double-blind studies of GM-CSF or G-CSF versus supportive care in patients with MDS, however.[257] Such studies are needed to determine their impact on the incidence of infections, leukemic progression, and overall survival.

Anemia and the requirement of blood transfusion is a significant problem in the management of most MDS patients. Because the basic defect resides within the stem cell, the serum level of endogenous EPO is often not diminished in the anemia of MDS.[258] Pharmacologic doses of rHuEPO were administered to patients with MDS with the hope to overcome the block in maturation of red cell precursors.[259] Overall, 15 to 20% of patients respond to rHuEPO treatment, but most responders are not transfusion dependent, and the doses required to achieve response are greater than 450 IU/kg/wk.[259–261] Factors predicting response to rHuEPO therapy include serum EPO less than 100 mU/ml, refractory anemia FAB-subtype, female gender, and normal karyotype.[262, 263] The response rate to rHuEPO increases to approximately 40% when rHuEPO and G-CSF are used in combination in MDS patients.[264] Approximately 50% of responding patients, however, require both G-CSF and rHuEPO to maintain an effective response.[265] This observation suggests that synergy between G-CSF and rHuEPO exists in vivo for the production of red cells in MDS.[257, 266] The updated ASCO guidelines[165] suggest that intermittent administration of HGFs may be considered in a subset of MDS patients with severe neutropenia and recurrent infections.

**Human Immunodeficiency Virus Infections.** Cytopenia in human immunodeficiency virus (HIV) infection is multifactorial, with immune factors, drugs, infection, bone marrow infiltration, and HIV infection per se all playing a part. Treatment-related myelosuppression is a major limiting factor in therapy of HIV and its complications. A significant number of patients have been shown to respond to rHuEPO with a decreased transfusion requirement and improved quality of life.[267] Greater responses were observed in patients with low endogenous EPO levels (<500 IU/ml). G-CSF and GM-CSF have been used with variable dosing intervals to maintain absolute neutrophil count greater than $1.5 \times 10^9$/L, enabling continuation of combination drug therapy for the treatment of HIV infection, prophylaxis, treatment of infectious complications, or chemotherapy.[268]

**Agranulocytosis and Neutropenia.** HGFs have been used with encouraging results for the treatment of drug-induced[269] and congenital agranulocytosis.[270] Children with Kostmann's syndrome show a remarkable response to G-CSF, although evidence suggests that mutation of the G-CSF receptor may confer an increased risk of transformation to myelodysplasia and acute leukemia.[271] G-CSF has been shown to have a beneficial effect on neutropenia and the resulting symptoms from infectious complications in patients with cyclic neutropenia.[272]

**Anemia Associated with Malignancy.** The cause of anemia in cancer patients is often multifactorial. Red cell production can be affected by a variety of pathophysiologic mechanisms, including chemotherapy and radiotherapy, bleeding, bone marrow infiltration, and immune factors. When the erythroid lineage is not a part of the malignant clone, the anemia is often characterized by an inappropriately low EPO level for the degree of anemia. Occasionally the anemia responds to therapy with rHuEPO, resulting in a reduction in transfusion requirements and improved quality of life.[149, 150] The associated anemia seen in patients with myeloma responds better than anemias associated with solid tumors.[149] Given that only about 50% of cancer patients are significant responders to rHuEPO, that only relatively small increments in hemoglobin are seen in these patients, and that the risk of transfusions remains relatively low,[273] it is difficult to recommend rHuEPO as a cost-effective alternative to conventional transfusion therapy in cancer patients without the benefit of formal economic analyses.

## OTHER USES OF HEMATOPOIETIC GROWTH FACTORS

**Antimicrobial Agents.** In a phase I trial, recombinant human M-CSF was administered in combination with standard antifungal treatment for refractory fungal infections after bone marrow transplantation[274]; 6 of 24 patients showed resolution of infection. A continued long-term follow-up of these patients showed a greater survival rate for the patients who received M-CSF as compared with historical controls treated with standard antifungal medications alone.[275] Clinical resolution of severe drug-resistant chronic mucocutaneous candidiasis after the administration of GM-CSF has been described.[276] Ongoing multicenter randomized, controlled trials in allogeneic marrow recipients treated with high doses of steroids for graft-versus-host disease should elucidate the role of GM-CSF in the prevention of invasive fungal infections.

**Myeloprotection and Radioprotection.** In a phase I clinical study, BB-10010, a variant of MIP-1α, was well tolerated, and no maximum tolerated dose was defined, with 300 μg/kg administered subcutaneously and 100 μg/kg intravenously.[277] A randomized phase II trial evaluated the potential myeloprotective effect of a 7-day regimen of BB-10010 administered at two dose levels (30 and 100 μg/kg) in combination with standard doses of 5-fluorouracil, doxorubicin (Adriamycin), and cyclophosphamide (FAC) chemotherapy for women with breast cancer.[278] The myeloprotection was assessed in terms of neutrophil recovery rate in each 21-day cycle of FAC treatment, mobilization of PBSCs, and quality of the progenitor cells in the bone marrow before and after six cycles of FAC. No difference in neutrophil nadir or incidence of febrile neutropenia was noted between the treated and nontreated groups. There was, however, a trend for an improved neutrophil recovery beyond three cycles of FAC in the BB-10010 group. Mobilization of granulocyte-macrophage colony-forming cells (GM-CFCs) was enhanced by BB-10010 with a 25-fold increase over pretreatment values.

Published studies indicating the use of HGFs after radiation therapy are not yet available. Myeloprotective HGFs, such as IL-1 and SCF, may prove effective in minimizing radiotherapy-induced myelosuppression.[58, 123, 279]

**Antitumor Agents.** A phase I trial of M-CSF demonstrated moderate antitumor activity in 2 of 14 patients with solid tumors.[280] None of 11 patients in a phase I trial of IL-

6 showed a response. There was evidence of lymphocyte activation, however.[160]

**Recombinant Human Erythropoietin and Autologous Blood Donation.** Autologous blood donation is becoming increasingly popular,[281] and the feasibility of this is much enhanced by rHuEPO therapy. Patients who would benefit most from rHuEPO therapy are those whose initial hematocrit is 33 to 39% and whose surgical blood losses are anticipated to be 1000 to 3000 ml. The most cost-effective regimen may be four weekly subcutaneous doses of rHuEPO, starting at 100 units/kg, with increases to 600 units/kg, if necessary, to produce evidence of reticulocyte response.[282]

**Granulocyte Colony–Stimulating Factor and Granulocyte Transfusions.** Even with the use of HGFs after transplant or HGF-mobilized PBSCs, there is still a period of absolute neutropenia in the post-transplant period, during which patients are at risk for developing life-threatening infections. Administration of G-CSF to normal marrow donors is well tolerated and allowed for the collection of 5-fold to 10-fold more neutrophils than collected without G-CSF.[283] When these cells are administered to neutropenic patients, they exhibit a prolonged intravascular survival.[283, 284] These observations, the progress in modern apheresis techniques,[285] and red cell depletion of granulocyte components[286] have revived the research interest in therapeutic[287, 288] and prophylactic[289–291] granulocyte transfusions.

**Thrombopoietin and Volunteer Platelet Donations.** With modern techniques of platelet apheresis, relatively small increases in peripheral blood platelet counts result in large increases in the number of platelets that can be recovered. A randomized, placebo-controlled, blinded, crossover, sequential dose-escalation study was designed to test the safety and efficacy of MGDF (a pegylated truncated Mpl ligand) in healthy platelet donors.[292] The resulting apheresis products were transfused into cancer patients with chemotherapy-induced grade IV thrombocytopenia. MGDF given to normal subjects in a single dose of 3 μg/kg increased the yield of platelets by a factor of nearly four and was associated with a quadrupling of platelet counts in the recipients of the apheresed platelets. The safety profile of TPO in healthy donors remains to be proved, however, and must remain excellent before the drug can be used to improve the efficacy of platelet-transfusion therapy.

## Hematopoietic Growth Factor–Associated Toxicities

### GRANULOCYTE COLONY–STIMULATING FACTOR

G-CSF is usually well tolerated. Medullary bone pain is the most frequent side effect observed in patients receiving G-CSF, with 15 to 39% of recipients complaining of this symptom.[124] Other adverse effects include headaches, generalized musculoskeletal pain, and exacerbation of underlying inflammatory skin disease, such as eczema[293] or psoriasis.[294] Cutaneous eruption histologically resembling Sweet's syndrome (neutrophilic dermatoses)[295] with occasional dermal eosinophilia[296] and injection site reactions have been rarely noted with G-CSF. Increased serum levels of alkaline phosphatase and lactate dehydrogenase are common and are thought to reflect the release of enzymes from high numbers of leukocytes rather than liver or muscle toxicity.[297] To date, the development of anti-G-CSF antibodies has not been reported. Two reports describe an anaphylactic-like reaction that was associated with G-CSF administration.[298, 299] One case of de novo leukocytoclastic vasculitis has been reported.[300] A case of spontaneous splenic rupture after G-CSF administration in an allogeneic donor of PBSCs has been reported.[301]

## GRANULOCYTE-MACROPHAGE COLONY-STIMULATING FACTOR

GM-CSF is generally well tolerated. Adverse effects observed in patients receiving GM-CSF include low-grade fever, bone pain, flu-like symptoms with myalgias, and localized eruption at the site of the subcutaneous injection.[296, 302, 303] Route of administration may be an important variable in the incidence of side effects, with intravenous dosing more frequently accompanied by generalized rash and *first dose reaction* (transient flushing, dyspnea, transient hypoxemia, tachycardia, and hypotension), whereas subcutaneous administration has been associated with local reaction at the injection site.[304] Antibodies to GM-CSF have been identified in approximately 4% of those tested,[124] but the clinical significance of such antibodies is uncertain. Exacerbation by GM-CSF of underlying autoimmune disease, such as leukocytoclastic vasculitis,[305] thyroiditis,[306] rheumatoid arthritis,[307] and idiopathic thrombocytopenic purpura,[308] has been noted. Anaphylaxis is extremely rare with GM-CSF.[309] One report describes splenic enlargement and rupture that was associated with GM-CSF administration.[310]

## RECOMBINANT HUMAN ERYTHROPOIETIN

rHuEPO is remarkably well tolerated. Adverse reactions have been described mostly in chronic renal failure patients, with development of hypertension and seizures.[7] Outside of the renal failure setting, there are no reports of significant side effects. Aggravation of splenomegaly has been occasionally observed in patients with myeloproliferative disorders.[311] Only a few cases of antibodies against EPO have been demonstrated in patients treated with rHuEPO, which can cause resistance to rHuEPO therapy.[147]

## INTERLEUKIN-11

The most common adverse effects observed in patients receiving IL-11 include peripheral edema, dyspnea, pleural effusions, and conjunctival injection.[179] Transient atrial arrhythmias and dilutional anemia were also reported.[155]

## OTHER HEMATOPOIETIC GROWTH FACTORS

Virtually all patients who have been given *SCF* developed a pruritic wheal and flare response at the injection site approximately 120 minutes after subcutaneous injection.[312]

Moderate to severe anaphylactic-like reactions, believed to be mast cell mediated and dose related, were observed in 23% of patients in a phase I-II trial.[313] With standard prophylactic medication regimens including both H$_1$ and H$_2$ antihistamines and inhaled albuterol, SCF-induced adverse events have been less frequently observed in phase II and III trials.[314]

*Flt3 ligand* is well tolerated. Localized injection site reactions similar to those observed with SCF and IL-3 have been reported.[235] Flt3 ligand does not activate mast cells and is not associated with systemic anaphylactoid reactions.

Flu-like symptoms are common with the administration of *IL-3*,[315, 316] and headache appears to be dose limiting.[163]

Side effects of *IL-3* plus *GM-CSF* are similar to those with GM-CSF alone.[181, 317]

Fever and a dose-dependent normocytic anemia develop in most patients treated with *IL-6*[318]; hepatotoxicity and cardiac arrhythmias are dose-limiting factors.[160]

The most significant side effect associated with the use of recombinant human *M-CSF* is a dose-related, transient thrombocytopenia.[12, 319] In contrast, the human urinary M-CSF is better tolerated, with no significant adverse effect on platelet counts.[320] Ophthalmologic side effects (iritis, conjunctivitis) are other significant clinical toxicities observed with high-dose recombinant human M-CSF.[12] A case of mobilization of leukemic blasts has been reported during treatment with M-CSF.[321]

Recombinant human *TPO*[162] and *MGDF*[180] are well tolerated, and no significant side effects have been reported so far. The major concern with repeated subcutaneous injections of MGDF, TPO, or related compounds is the generation of neutralizing antibodies that cross-react with endogenous TPO, resulting in prolonged and life-threatening thrombocytopenia. At least three such cases have been observed after the repeated subcutaneous administration of MGDF to patients receiving sequential cycles of dose-intensive chemotherapy and to at least one normal platelet donor after multiple exposures to MGDF. Native TPO and its recombinant variants appear to be significantly immunogenic, especially when given repetitively via the subcutaneous route.

## Future Perspectives

Several novel indications for the use of HGFs are currently being investigated. Intradermal injection of myeloid HGFs was shown to improve wound healing in patients with leprosy,[322] chronic leg ulcers, diabetic foot ulcers,[323] or cutaneous Kaposi's sarcoma lesions.[324] GM-CSF was shown to enhance keratinocyte growth and Langerhans' cell recruitment, contributing to faster wound healing.[325] G-CSF[326] and GM-CSF applied locally[324, 326] or subcutaneously[327] may prove to be beneficial in preventing oral mucositis after myeloablative chemotherapy or radiotherapy. Several preclinical studies have reported the effectiveness of GM-CSF[328] and M-CSF[329] in antitumor immunity and tumor vaccination. It has been speculated that this effect may be due to the ability of GM-CSF to promote T-cell activation[330] and differentiation of dendritic cells[331] and the ability of M-CSF to stimulate tumoricidal activity of monocytes-macrophages through antibody-independent[332] and antibody-dependent[333] cytotoxicity. Ex vivo expansion of progenitor cells for gene therapy is another area of active cytokine research.

The availability of pharmacologic quantities of HGFs has broadened the horizon for studies in basic science and clinical investigation. It has been clearly demonstrated that HGFs shorten the duration of myelosuppression after chemotherapy, particularly high-dose chemotherapy and stem cell rescue. Administration of HGFs has been instrumental in facilitating autologous and allogeneic PBSC mobilization. Clinically significant disease stimulation and recurrence has not been demonstrated in studies to date. Although HGFs do not appear to affect survival, their effect on quality of life may be significant. Some randomized studies have demonstrated the effectiveness of myeloid HGFs in facilitating early discharge from the hospital. Cost-effectiveness remains a key element in the era of managed care. Future phase III studies evaluating the clinical benefits of newer cytokines need to include pharmacoeconomic analyses of the adjusted costs associated with the addition of those HGFs.

## REFERENCES

1. Carnot P, Deflandre C. Sur l'activite hemopoietique des differents organes au cours de la regeneration du sang. Cr Hebd Acad Sci 1906;143:432–5.
2. Pluznik DH, Sachs L. The cloning of normal "mast" cells in tissue culture. J Cell Comp Physiol 1965;66:319–24.
3. Bradley TR, Metcalf D. The growth of mouse bone marrow cells in vitro. Aust J Exp Biol Med Sci 1966;44:287–99.
4. Crosier PS, Clark SC. Basic biology of the hematopoietic growth factors. Semin Oncol 1992;19:349.
5. Tabbara IA. Granulocyte colony-stimulating factor. South Med J 1993;86:350.
6. Shadduck RK. Granulocyte-macrophage colony-stimulating factor: present use and future directions. Semin Hematol 1992;29:Suppl 3:38.
7. Spivak JL. Recombinant erythropoietin. Annu Rev Med 1993;44:243.
8. Tabbara IA. Erythropoietin: biology and clinical applications. Arch Intern Med 1993;153:298.
9. Telper I, Elias L, Smith JW, et al. A randomized placebo-controlled trial of recombinant human interleukin-11 in cancer patients with severe thrombocytopenia due to chemotherapy. Blood 1996;87:3607–14.
10. Issacs C, Robert NJ, Bailey FA, et al. Randomized placebo-controlled study of recombinant human interleukin-11 to prevent chemotherapy-induced thrombocytopenia in patients with breast cancer receiving dose-intensive cyclophosphamide and doxorubicin. J Clin Oncol 1997;15:3368–77.
11. Williams DE, Park LS. Hematopoietic effects of a granulocyte-macrophage colony-stimulating factor/interleukin-3 fusion protein. Cancer 1991;67:2705.
12. Munn DH, Cheung NK. Preclinical and clinical studies of macrophage colony-stimulating factor. Semin Oncol 1992;19:395.
13. Bernstein SH, Kufe DW. Future of basic/clinical hematopoiesis research in the era of hematopoietic growth factor availability. Semin Oncol 1992;19:441.
14. Ganser A. Clinical results with recombinant human interleukin-3. Cancer Invest 1993;11:212.
15. Glaspy J, LeMaistre CF, Lill M, et al. Dose-response of 7 day administration of recombinant methionyl human SCF in combination with G-CSF for progenitor cell mobilization in patients with stage II–IV breast cancer. Blood 1995;86:463a.
16. McNiece IK, Zsebo KM. The role of stem cell factor in the hematopoietic system. Cancer Invest 1993;11:724–9.
17. Vadhan-Raj S, Murray LJ, Bueso-Ramos C, et al. Stimulation of megakaryocyte and platelet production by a single dose of recombinant human thrombopoietin in patients with cancer. Ann Intern Med 1997;26:731–3.
18. Fanucchi M, Glaspy J, Crawford J, et al. Effects of polyethylene glycol-conjugated recombinant human megakaryocyte growth and development factor on platelet counts after chemotherapy for lung cancer. N Engl J Med 1997;336:404–9.
19. Ogawa M. Differentiation and proliferation of hematopoietic stem cells. Blood 1993;81:2844.
20. Broxmeyer HE, Cooper S, Lu L, et al. Effect of murine mast cell growth factor (c-kit proto-oncogene ligand) on colony formation by human marrow hematopoietic progenitor cells. Blood 1991;77:2142.
21. Mochizuki DY, Eisenman JR, Conlon PJ, et al. Interleukin 1 regulates hematopoietic activity, a role previously ascribed to hemopoietin 1. Proc Natl Acad Sci U S A 1987;84:5267.
22. Otuska T, Thacker JD, Hogge DE. The effects of interleukin 6 and interleukin 3 on early hematopoietic events in long-term cultures of human marrow. Exp Hematol 1991;19:1042.
23. Quesniaux VF. Interleukins 9, 10, 11 and 12 and kit ligand: a brief overview. Res Immunol 1992;143:385.
24. Hirayama F, Katayama N, Neben S, et al. Synergistic interaction between IL-12 and steel factor in support of proliferation of murine lymphohematopoietic progenitors in culture. Blood 1994;83:92–8.
25. Estrov Z, Talpaz M, Wetzler M, et al. The modulatory hematopoietic activities of leukemia inhibitory factor. Leuk Lymphoma 1992;8:1–7.
26. Namikawa R, Muench MO, et al. Regulatory roles of ligand for Flk2/Flk3 tyrosine kinase receptor on human hematopoiesis. Stem Cells 1996;14:388–95.
27. Katayama N, Itoh R, Sugawara T, et al. Role of C-MPL and its ligand thrombopoietin in early hematopoiesis. Leuk Lymphoma 1997;28:51–6.
28. Metcalf D. Lineage commitment of hemopoietic progenitor cells in developing blast cell colonies: influence of colony-stimulating factors. Proc Natl Acad Sci U S A 1991;88:11310–4.
29. Moore MA. Clinical implications of positive and negative hematopoietic stem cell regulators. Blood 1991;78:1.
30. Lopez AF, To LB, Yang YC, et al. Stimulation of proliferation, differentiation, and function of human cells by primate interleukin 3. Proc Natl Acad Sci USA 1987;84:2761.
31. Kishi K, Ihle JN, Urdal DL, et al. Murine B-cell stimulatory factor-1 (BSF-1)/interleukin-4 (IL-4) is a multilineage colony-stimulating factor that acts directly on primitive hemopoietic progenitors. J Cell Physiol 1989;139:463.
32. Sanderson CJ. Interleukin-5, eosinophils, and disease. Blood 1992;79:3101.
33. Bree A, Schlerman F, Timony G, et al. Pharmacokinetics and thrombopoietic effects of recombinant human IL-11 in nonhuman primates and rodents. Blood 1991;78:132a.
34. de Sauvage FJ, Hass PE, Spencer SD, et al. Stimulation of megakaryocytopoiesis by the c-Mpl ligand. Nature 1994;369:569:533–8.
35. Carrington PA, Hill RJ, Stenberg PE, et al. Multiple in vivo effects of interleukin-3 and interleukin-6 on murine megakaryocytopoiesis. Blood 1991;77:34.
36. Neben TY, Loebelenz J, Hayes L, et al. Recombinant human interleukin-11 stimulates megakaryocytopoiesis and increases peripheral platelets in normal and splenectomized mice. Blood 1993;81:901.
37. Monroy RL, Davis TA, Donahue RE, et al. In vivo stimulation of platelet production in a primate model using IL-1 and IL-3. Exp Hematol 1991;19:629.
38. Briddell RA, Brandt JE, Leemhuis TB, et al. Role of cytokines in sustaining long-term human megakaryocytopoiesis in vitro. Blood 1992;79:332.
39. Ikebuchi K, Wong GG, Clark SC, et al. Interleukin 6 enhancement of interleukin 3-dependent proliferation of multipotential hemopoietic progenitors. Proc Natl Acad Sci U S A 1987;84:9035.
40. McNiece IK, Langley KE, Zsebo KM. Recombinant human stem cell factor synergises with GM-CSF, G-CSF, IL-3 and I EPO to stimulate human progenitor cells of the myeloid and erythroid lineages. Exp Hematol 1991;19:226.
41. Donahue RE, Seehra J, Metzger M, et al. Human IL-3 and GM-CSF act synergistically in stimulating hematopoiesis in primates. Science 1988;241:1820.
42. Larsen A, Davis T, Curtis BM, et al. Expression cloning of a human granulocyte colony-stimulating factor receptor: a structural mosaic of hematopoietin receptor, immunoglobulin, and fibronectin domains. J Exp Med 1990;172:1559.
43. DiPersio JF, Abboud CN, Winter JN, et al. Phase I/II study of mobilization of PBSC by SC-68420 in patients with breast cancer or lymphoma. Blood 1997;90:97a.
44. Abboud CN, DiPersio JF, Frenette G, et al. Phase I/II study to

determine the safety and tolerability of SC-70935 in patients with relapsed lymphoma receiving ESHAP. Blood 1997;90:173a.

45. Metcalf D. The granulocyte-macrophage regulators: reappraisal by gene activation. review. Exp Hematol 1995;23:569.

46. Dranoff G, Crawford AD, Sadelain M, et al. Involvement of granulocyte-macrophage colony-stimulating factor in pulmonary homeostasis. Science 1994;264:713.

47. Lieschke GJ, Grail D, Hodgson G, et al. Mice lacking granulocyte colony-stimulating factor have chronic neutropenia, granulocyte, and macrophage progenitor cell deficiency, and impaired neutrophil mobilization. Blood 1994;84:1737.

48. Wu H, Liu X, Lodish HF. Generation of committed erythroid BFU-E and CFU-E progenitors does not require erythropoietin or the erythropoietin receptor. Cell 1995;83:59.

49. de Sauvage FJ, Shiuh-Ming L, et al. Deficiencies in early and late stages of megakaryocytopoiesis in TPO-KO mice. Blood 1995;86:1007a.

50. Lieschke GJ, Stanley E, Grail D, et al. Mice lacking both macrophage and granulocyte-macrophage colony-stimulating factor have macrophages and coexistent osteopetrosis and severe lung disease. Blood 1994;84:27.

51. Rameshwar P, Gascon P, et al. Hematopoietic modulation by the tachykinins. Acta Haematol 1997;98:59–64.

52. Graham GJ, Wright EG, Hewick R, et al. Identification and characterization of an inhibitor of haemopoietic stem cell proliferation. Nature 1990;344:442.

53. Neta R, Vogel SN, Plocinski JM, et al. In vivo modulation with anti-interleukin-1 (IL-1) receptor (p80) antibody 35F5 of the response to IL-1: the relationship of radioprotection, colony-stimulating factor, and IL-6. Blood 1990;76:57.

54. Neta R, Oppenheim JJ, Wang JM, et al. Synergy of IL-1 and c-kit ligand (KL) in radioprotection of mice correlates with IL-1 upregulation of mRNA and protein expression for c-kit on bone marrow cells. J Immunol 1994;153:1536.

55. Keller JR, Mantel C, Sing GK, et al. Transforming growth factor beta 1 selectively regulates early murine hematopoietic progenitors and inhibits the growth of IL-3-dependent myeloid leukemia cell lines. J Exp Med 1988;168:737.

56. Zsebo KM, Smith KA, Hartley CA, et al. Radioprotection of mice by recombinant rat stem cell factor. Proc Natl Acad Sci U S A 1992;89:9464.

57. Neta R, Sztein MB, Oppenheim JJ, et al. Bone marrow cells are induced to cycle following administration of IL-1. J Immunol 1987;139:1861.

58. Neta R, Keller JK, Ali N, et al. Contrasting mechanisms of myeloprotective effects of IL-1 against ionizing radiation and cytoablative 5-fluorouracil (5-FU). Radiat Res 1996;145:624.

59. Neta R. Modulation of radiation damage by cytokines. Stem Cells 1997;15:87.

60. Gabrilove JL, Wong G, Bollenbacher E, et al. Basic fibroblast growth factor counteracts the suppressive effects of transforming growth factor-beta 1 on human myeloid progenitor cells. Blood 1993;81:909.

61. To LB, Haylock DN, Simmons PJ, Juttner CA. The biology and clinical uses of blood stem cells. Blood 1997;89:2233–58.

62. Long MW. Blood cell cytoadhesion molecules. Exp Hematol 1992;20:288.

63. Turner ML. Regulation of hematopoietic progenitor cell migration, mobilization and homing. Stem Cells 1994;12:227.

64. Williams DA, Rios M, et al. Fibronectin and VLA-4 in haematopoietic stem cell-microenvironment. Nature 1991;352:438–41.

65. Papayannopoulou T, Nakamoto B. Peripheralization of hemopoietic progenitors in primates treated with anti-VLA-4 integrin. Proc Natl Acad Sci Usa 1993;90:9374.

66. Levesque JP, Haylock DN, Simmons PJ. Cytokine regulation of proliferation and cell adhesion are correlated events in human CD34+ hematopoietic progenitors. Blood 1996;88:1168.

67. Laterveer L, Lindley IJ, Heemeskerk DP, et al. Rapid mobilization of hematopoietic progenitor cells in rhesus monkeys by a single intravenous injection of interleukin-8. Blood 1996;87:781–8.

68. Liu F, Poursine-Laurent J, Link DC. The G-CSF receptor is required for the mobilization of murine hematopoietic progenitors into peripheral blood by cyclophosphamide or IL-8 but not Flt-3 ligand. Blood 1997;90:2522–8.

69. Brasel K, McKenna HJ, Charrier K, et al. Synergistic effects in vivo of Flt-3 ligand with GM-CSF or G-CSF in mobilization of colony forming cells in mice. Blood 1997;90:3781–8.

70. Lyman SD, Jacobsen SE. c-kit ligand and Flt-3 ligand: stem/progenitor cell factors with overlapping yet distinct activities. Blood 1998;41:1101–34.

71. Bhatia M, Bonnet D, Kapp U, et al. Quantitative analysis reveals expansion of human hematopoietic repopulating cells after short-term ex vivo culture. J Exp Med 1997;186:619.

72. Conneally E, Cashman J, Petzer A, et al. Expansion in vitro of transplantable human cord blood stem cells demonstrated using a quantitative assay of their lympho-myeloid repopulating activity in nonobese diabetic-scid/scid mice. Proc Natl Acad Sci U S A 1997;94:9836.

73. Zanjani ED, Almeida-Porada G, Flake AW. The human/sheep xenograft model: a large animal model of human hematopoiesis. Int J Hematol 1996;63:179.

74. Lange W, Henschler R, Mertelsmann R. Biological and clinical advances in stem cell expansion. Leukemia 1996;10:943–5.

75. Piacibello W, Sanavio F, Garetto L, et al. Differential growth factor requirement of primitive cord blood hematopoietic stem cell for self-renewal and amplification vs. proliferation and differentiation. Leukemia 1998;12:718–27.

76. Migliaccio G, Migliaccio AR, Druzin ML, et al. Long-term generation of colony-forming cells in liquid culture of CD34+ cord blood cells in the presence of recombinant human stem cell factor. Blood 1992;79:2620.

77. Haylock DN, To LB, Dowse TL, et al. Ex vivo expansion and maturation of peripheral blood CD34+ cells into the myeloid lineage. Blood 1992;80:1405.

78. Brugger W, Mocklin W, Heimfeld S, et al. Ex vivo expansion of enriched peripheral blood CD34+ progenitor cells by stem cell factor, interleukin-1 beta (IL-1 beta), IL-6, IL-3, interferon-gamma, and erythropoietin. Blood 1993;81:2579.

79. Brugger W, Heimfeld S, Berenson R, et al. Reconstitution of hematopoiesis after high-dose chemotherapy by autologous progenitor cells generated ex vivo. N Engl J Med 1995;333:283.

80. Williams SF, Lee WJ, Bender JG, et al. Selection and expansion of peripheral blood CD34+ cells in autologous stem cell transplantation for breast cancer. Blood 1996;87:1687.

81. Shimizu Y, Kabayashi M, Zanjani ED. Engraftment of cultured human hematopoietic cells in sheep. Blood 1998;91:3688–92.

82. Bregni M, Magni M, Siena S, et al. Human peripheral blood hematopoietic progenitors are optimal targets of retroviral-mediated gene transfer. Blood 1992;80:1418.

83. Coffey RG, ed. Granulocyte responses to cytokines. New York: Marcel Dekker, 1992.

84. Rose RM. The role of colony-stimulating factors in infectious disease: current status, future challenges. Semin Oncol 1992;19:415–21.

85. Rapaport AP, Abboud CN, DiPersio JF, et al. Granulocyte-macrophage colony-stimulating factor (GM-CSF) and granulocyte colony-stimulating factor (G-CSF): receptor biology, signal transduction, and neutrophil activation. Blood Rev 1992;6:43.

86. Weisbart RH, Kwan L, Golde DW, et al. Human GM-CSF primes neutrophils for enhanced oxidative metabolism in response to the major physiological chemoattractants. Blood 1987;69:18.

87. Mayer P, Schutze E, Lam C, et al. Recombinant murine granulocyte-macrophage colony-stimulating factor augments neutrophil recovery and enhances resistance to infections in myelosuppressed mice. J Infect Dis 1991;163:584.

88. Wang M, Friedman H, Djeu JY. Enhancement of human monocyte function against *Candida albicans* by the colony-stimulating factors (CSF): IL-3, granulocyte-macrophage-CSF, and macrophage-CSF. J Immunol 1989;143:671.

89. Ho RJ, Chong KT, Merigan TC. Antiviral activity and dose optimum of recombinant macrophage colony-stimulating factor on herpes simplex genitalis in guinea pigs. J Immunol 1991;146:3578.

90. Chan WL, Ziltener HJ, Liew FY. Interleukin-3 protects mice from acute herpes simplex virus infection. Immunology 1990;71:358.

91. Baldwin GC, Golde DW, Widhopf GF, et al. Identification and characterization of a low-affinity GM-CSF receptor on primary and cultured human melanoma cells. Blood 1991;78:609–15.

92. Pedrazzoli P, Bacciocchi G, Bergamaschi G, et al. Effects of granulocyte-macrophage colony-stimulating factor and interleukin-3 on small cell lung cancer cells. Cancer Invest 1994;12:283.

93. Miki S, Iwano M, Yamamot M. IL-6 functions and in vitro autocrine growth factor in renal cell carcinomas. FEBS Lett 1989;250:607–10.

94. Izquierdo MA, Degen D, Meyers L, et al. Effects of the hematopoietic

growth factors GM-CSF, IL-3 and IL-6 on human tumor colony-forming units taken directly from patients. Ann Oncol 1995;6:927–32.

95. Ohsaka A, Kitagawa S, Ikeda K, et al. Enhanced neutrophil functions in a patient with colony-stimulating activity-producing lung cancer. J Intern Med 1991;230:459.

96. Satoh H, Abe Y, Katoh Y, et al. Bladder carcinoma producing granulocyte colony-stimulating factor: a case report. J Urol 1993;149:843.

97. Toi M, Bicknel R, Harris AL. Inhibition of colon and breast carcinoma cell growth by IL-4. Cancer Res 1992;52:275.

98. Givon T, Slavin S, Haran-Ghera N, et al. Antitumor effects of human recombinant interleukin-6 on acute myeloid leukemia in mice and in cell cultures. Blood 1992;79:2392.

99. Eisenthal A, Kashtan H, Rabau M, et al. Antitumor effects of recombinant interleukin-6 expressed in eukaryotic cells. Cancer Immunol Immunother 1993;36:101.

100. Alderson MR, Tough TW, Ziegler SF, et al. IL-7 induces cytokine secretion and tumourocidal activity by human peripheral blood monocytes. J Exp Med 1991;173:923–30.

101. Gateley MK, Wolitzky AG, Quinn PM, et al. Regulation of human cytolytic lymphocyte response by IL-12. Cell Immunol 1992;143:127–42.

102. Suzu S, Yokota H, Yamada M, et al. Enhancing effect of human monocytic colony-stimulating factor on monocyte tumoricidal activity. Cancer Res 1989;49:5913.

103. Verfaille C, McGlave P. Leukemia inhibitory factor/human interleukin for DA cells: a growth factor that stimulates the in vitro development of multipotential human hematopoietic progenitors. Blood 1991; 77:263–70.

104. Yamashita Y, Nara N, Aoki N. Antiproliferative and differentiative effect of granulocyte-macrophage colony-stimulating factor on a variant human small cell lung cancer cell line. Cancer Res 1989;49:5334.

105. Lynch DH, Andreasen A, Maraskovsky E, et al. Flt3 ligand induces tumor regression and antitumor immune responses in vivo. Nat Med 1997;3:625–31.

106. Costa JJ. The therapeutic use of hematopoietic growth factors. Allergy Clin Immunol 1998;101:1–6.

107. Dezlinger C, Walther J, Wilmanns W, et al. Interleukin-3 enhances the endogenous leukotriene production. letter. Blood 1993;81:2466.

108. Thomas JW, Baum CM. Potent IL-3 receptor agonist with selectively enhanced hematopoietic activity relative to recombinant human IL-3. Proc Natl Acad Sci U S A 1995;92:3779.

109. Metcalf D. The consequences of excess levels of haemopoietic growth factors. Br J Haematol 1990;75:1.

110. Thorpe R, Wadhwa M, Bird CR, et al. Detection and measurement of cytokines. Blood Rev 1992;6:133.

111. Kawano M, Hirano T, Matsuda T, et al. Autocrine generation and requirement of BSF-2/IL-6 for human multiple myelomas. Nature 1988;332:83.

112. Klein B, Zhang XG, Jourdan M, et al. Interleukin-6 is a major myeloma cell growth factor in vitro and in vivo especially in patients with terminal disease. Curr Top Microbiol Immunol 1990;166:23.

113. Suzuki H, Yasukawa K, Saito T, et al. Anti-human interleukin-6 receptor antibody inhibits human myeloma growth in vivo. Eur J Immunol 1992;22:1989.

114. Beck JT, Hsu SM, Wijdenes J, et al. Brief report: alleviation of systemic manifestations of Castleman's disease by monoclonal anti-interleukin-6 antibody. N Engl J Med 1994;330:602.

115. Lieschke GJ, Burgess AW. Granulocyte colony-stimulating factor and granulocyte-macrophage colony-stimulating factor. N Engl J Med 1992;327:28.

116. Wong GG, Wick JS, Temple PA, et al. Human GM-CSF: molecular cloning of the complementary DNA and purification of the natural and recombinant proteins. Science 1985;228:810.

117. Cantrell MA, Anderson D, Cerretti DP, et al. Cloning, sequence, and expression of a human granulocyte/macrophage colony-stimulating factor. Proc Natl Acad Sci U S A 1985;82:6250.

118. Souza LM, Boone TC, Gabrilove J, et al. Recombinant human granulocyte colony-stimulating factor: effects on normal and leukemic myeloid cells. Science 1986;232:61.

119. Nagata S, Tsuchiya M, Asano S, et al. Molecular cloning and expression of cDNA for human granulocyte colony-stimulating factor. Nature 1986;319:415.

120. Zsebo KM, Cohen AM, Murdock DC, et al. Recombinant human granulocyte colony stimulating factor: molecular and biological characterization. Immunobiology 1986;172:175.

121. Mayer P, Lam C, Obenaus H, et al. Recombinant human GM-CSF induces leukocytosis and activates peripheral blood polymorphonuclear neutrophils in nonhuman primates. Blood 1987;70:206.

122. Moonen P, Mermod JJ, Ernst JF, et al. Increased biological activity of deglycosylated recombinant human granulocyte/macrophage colony-stimulating factor produced by yeast or animal cells. Proc Natl Acad Sci U S A 1987;84:4428.

123. Williams DE, Park LS. Hematopoietic effects of a granulocyte-macrophage colony-stimulating factor/interleukin-3 fusion protein. Cancer 1991;67:2705.

124. American Society of Clinical Oncology. American Society of Clinical Oncology recommendations for the use of hematopoietic colony-stimulating factors: evidence-based, clinical practice guidelines. J Clin Oncol 1994;12:2471–508.

125. Devereaux S, Linch DC, Costa D, et al. Transient leucopenia induced by granulocyte-macrophage colony-stimulating factor. Lancet 1987; 2:1523.

126. Morstyn G, Campbell L, Lieschke G, et al. Treatment of chemotherapy-induced neutropenia by subcutaneously administered granulocyte colony-stimulating factor with optimization of dose and duration of therapy. J Clin Oncol 1989;7:1554.

127. Fleischman RA. Clinical use of hematopoietic growth factors. Am J Med Sci 1993;305:248.

128. Lord BI, Gurney H, Chang J, et al. Haemopoietic cell kinetics in humans treated with rGM-CSF. Int J Cancer 1992;50:26.

129. Steward WP, Scarffe JH, Austin R, et al. Recombinant human granulocyte macrophage colony stimulating factor (rhGM-CSF) given as daily short infusions phase I dose-toxicity study. Br J Cancer 1989;59:142.

130. Lieschke GL, Maher D, O'Connor M, et al. Phase I study of intravenously administered bacterially synthesized granulocyte-macrophage colony-stimulating factor and comparison with subcutaneous administration. Cancer Res 1990;50:606.

131. Peters WP, Shogan J, Shpall EJ, et al. Recombinant human granulocyte-macrophage colony-stimulating factor produces fever. Lancet 1988;1:950.

132. Cicco NA, Lindemann A, Content J, et al. Inducible production of interleukin-6 by human polymorphonuclear neutrophils: role of granulocyte-macrophage colony-stimulating factor and tumor necrosis factor-alpha. Blood 1990;75:2049.

133. Kurzrock R, Talpaz M, Gomez JA, et al. Differential dose-related haematological effects of GM-CSF in pancytopenia: evidence supporting the advantage of low- over high-dose administration in selected patients. Br J Haematol 1991;78:352.

134. Crawford J, Ozer H, Stoller R, et al. Reduction by granulocyte colony-stimulating factor of fever and neutropenia induced by chemotherapy in patents with small-cell lung cancer. N Engl J Med 1991;325:164.

135. Socinski MA, Cannistar SA, Elias A, et al. Granulocyte-macrophage colony-stimulating factor expands the circulating haematopoietic progenitor cell compartment in man. Lancet 1988;1:1194.

136. Gabrilove J, Jakubowski A, Scher H, et al. Effect of granulocyte colony-stimulating factor on neutropenia and associated morbidity due to chemotherapy for transitional cell carcinoma of the urothelium. N Engl J Med 1988;318:1414–22.

137. Cebon JS, Bury RW, Lieschke GJ, et al. The effects of dose and route of administration on the pharmacokinetics of granulocyte-macrophage colony-stimulating factor. Eur J Cancer 1990;26:1064.

138. Herrmann F, Ganser A, Lindemann A, et al. Stimulation of granulopoiesis in patients with malignancy by recombinant human granulocyte-macrophage colony-stimulating factor: assessment of two routes of administration. J Biol Resp Mod 1990;9:475.

139. Rosenfeld CS, Sulecki M, Evans C, et al. Comparison of intravenous versus subcutaneous recombinant human granulocyte-macrophage colony-stimulating factor in patients with primary myelodysplasia. Exp Hematol 1991;19:273.

140. Cebon J, Lieschke GJ, Bury RW, et al. The dissociation of GM-CSF efficacy from toxicity according to route of administration: a pharmacodynamic study. Br J Haematol 1992;80:144.

141. Edmonson JH, Hartmann LC, Long HJ, et al. Granulocyte-macrophage colony-stimulating factor: preliminary observations on the influences of dose, schedule, and route of administration in patients receiving cyclophosphamide and carboplatin. Cancer 1992;70:2529.

142. Hovgaard DI, Mortensin BT, Schifter S, et al. Clinical pharmacokinetic studies of a human haemopoietic growth factor, GM-CSF. Eur J Clin Invest 1991;22:45.

143. Kimura H, Ishibashi T, Shikama Y, et al. Interleukin-1 beta (IL-1

beta) induces thrombocytosis in mice: possible implication of IL-6. Blood 1990;76:2493.

144. Rabinowe SN, Neuberg D, Bierman PJ, et al. Long-term follow-up of a phase III study of recombinant human granulocyte-macrophage colony-stimulating factor after autologous bone marrow transplantation for lymphoid malignancies. Blood 1993;81:1903.

145. Zhang X-G, Bataille R, Jourdan M, et al. Granulocyte-macrophage colony-stimulating factor synergizes with interleukin-6 in supporting the proliferation of human myeloma cells. Blood 1990;76:2599.

146. Barlogie B, Jagannath S, Dixon DO, et al. High-dose melphalan and granulocyte-macrophage colony-stimulating factor for refractory multiple myeloma. Blood 1990;76:677.

147. Cazzola M, Mercuriali F, Brugnara C. Use of recombinant human erythropoietin outside the setting of uremia. Blood 1997;89:4248–67.

148. Kaufman JS, Reda DJ, Fye CL, et al. Subcutaneous compared with intravenous epoietin in patients receiving hemodialysis. N Engl J Med 1998;339:578–83.

149. Ludwig H, Fritz E, Kotzmann H, et al. Erythropoietin treatment of anemia associated with multiple myeloma. N Engl J Med 1990;322:1639.

150. Platanias LC, Miller CB, Mick R, et al. Treatment of chemotherapy-induced anemia with recombinant human erythropoietin in cancer patients. J Clin Oncol 1991;9:2021.

151. Cascinu S, Fedeli A, Fedeli SL, et al. Cisplatin-associated anaemia treated with subcutaneous erythropoietin. Br J Cancer 1993;67:156.

152. Najman A, Silingardi V, Spriano M, et al. Recombinant human erythropoietin in the anemia associated with multiple myeloma or non-Hodgkin lymphoma: dose finding and identification of predictors of response. Blood 1995;86:4446.

153. Cazzola M, Ponchi L, Pedrotti C, et al. Prediction of response to recombinant human erythropoietin in anemia of malignancy. Haematologica 1996;81:434.

154. Eschbach J, Egrie J, Downing M, et al. Correction of the anemia of end-stage renal disease with recombinant human erythropoietin. N Engl J Med 1987;316:73–8.

155. Gordon M, McCaskill-Stevens W, Battiato L, et al. A phase I trial of recombinant human IL-11 in women with breast cancer receiving chemotherapy. Blood 1996;87:3615.

156. Andrews RG, Knitter GH, Bartelemez SH, et al. Recombinant human stem cell factor, a c-kit ligand, stimulates hematopoiesis in primates. Blood 1991;78:1975–80.

157. Lebsack ME, McKenna HJ, Hoek JA, et al. Safety of FLT3 ligand in healthy volunteers. Blood 1997;90:170a.

158. Maraskovsky E, Roux E, Teepe M, et al. FLT3 ligand increases peripheral blood dendritic cells in healthy volunteers. Blood 1997;90:581a.

159. Lindemann A, Ganser A, Herrmann F, et al. Biologic effects of recombinant human interleukin-3 in vivo. J Clin Oncol 1991;9:2120.

160. Weber J, Yang JC, Topalian SL, et al. Phase I trial of subcutaneous interleukin-6 in patients with advanced malignancies. J Clin Oncol 1993;11:499.

161. Motoyoshi K, Takaku F, Kusumoto K, et al. Phase I and early phase II studies on human urinary macrophage colony-stimulating factor. Jpn J Med 1982;21:187–91.

162. Vadhan-Raj S, Murray LJ, Bueso-Ramos C, et al. Stimulation of megakaryocyte and platelet production by a single dose of recombinant human thrombopoietin in patients with cancer. Ann Intern Med 1997;26:731–3.

163. Rowe JM, Ciobanu N, Ascencao J, et al. Recommended guidelines for the management of autologous and allogeneic bone marrow transplantation. Ann Intern Med 1994;120:143–57.

164. Byrne JL, Haynes AP, Russel NH. Use of hematopoietic growth factors: commentary on the ASCO/ECOG guidelines. Blood Rev 1997;11:16–27.

165. American Society of Clinical Oncology. Update of recommendations for the use of hematopoietic growth factors: evidence-based clinical practice guidelines. J Clin Oncol 1996;14:1957–60.

166. Ohno R, Tomonaga M, Kobayashi T, et al. Effect of G-CSF after intensive induction therapy in relapsed or refractory acute leukemia. N Engl J Med 1990;323:871–7.

167. Gerhatz HH, Engelhaed M, Meusers P, et al. A randomized, double-blind placebo controlled phase III study of rhGM-CSF as adjunct to induction treatment of high-grade NHL. Blood 1993;82:2329–39.

168. Pettengel R, Gurney H, Radford GA, et al. G-CSF to prevent dose limiting neutropenia in NHL: a randomized controlled trial. Blood 1992;80:1430–6.

169. Maher DW, Lieschke GJ, Green M, et al. Filgrastim in patients with chemotherapy-induced febrile neutropenia: a randomized controlled trial. Ann Intern Med 1994;121:492–501.

170. Riikonen P, Saarinen UM, Makipernaa A, et al. Recombinant human granulocyte-macrophage colony-stimulating factor in the treatment of febrile neutropenia: a double-blind placebo controlled study in children. Pediatr Infect Dis J 1994;13:197–202.

171. Mayordomo JI, Riviera F, Diaz-Puente MT, et al. Improvement of chemotherapy-induced neutropenic fevers by administration of colony-stimulating factors. J Natl Cancer Inst 1995;87:803–8.

172. Anaissie E, Vartivarian S, Bodey GP, et al. Randomized comparison between antibiotics alone and antibiotics plus granulocyte-macrophage colony-stimulating factor in cancer patients with fever and neutropenia. Am J Med 1996;100:17–23.

173. Bierma B, deVries EG, Willemse PH, et al. Efficacy and tolerability of recombinant human granulocyte-macrophage colony-stimulating factor in patients with chemotherapy-related leukopenia and fever. Eur J Cancer 1990;26:932–6.

174. Hartmann LC, Tschetter LK, Habermann TM, et al. Granulocyte colony-stimulating factor in severe chemotherapy-induced afebrile neutropenia. N Engl J Med 1997;336:1776–80.

175. Glaspy JA. Economic outcomes associated with the use of hematopoietic growth factors. Oncology 1995;9:93–105.

176. Chouaid C, Bassinet L, Fuhrman C, et al. Routine use of G-CSF is not cost-effective and does not increase patient comfort in the treatment of small cell lung cancer: an analysis using a Markov model. J Clin Oncol 1998;16:2700–7.

177. Beveridge RA, Miller JA, Kales AN, et al. Randomized trial comparing the tolerability of rhGM-CSF and rhG-CSF in cancer patients receiving myelosuppressive chemotherapy. Support Care Cancer 1997;5:289–98.

178. Telper I, Elias L, Smith JW, et al. A randomized placebo-controlled trial of recombinant human interleukin-11 in cancer patients with severe thrombocytopenia due to chemotherapy. Blood 1996;87:3607–14.

179. Issacs C, Robert NJ, Bailey FA, et al. Randomized placebo-controlled study of recombinant human interleukin-11 to prevent chemotherapy-induced throbocytopenia in patients with breast cancer receiving dose-intensive cyclophosphamide and doxorubicin. J Clin Oncol 1997;15:3368–77.

180. Fanucchi M, Glaspy J, Crawford J, et al. Effects of polyethylene glycol-conjugated recombinant human megakaryocyte growth and development factor on platelet counts after chemotherapy for lung cancer. N Engl J Med 1997;336:404–9.

181. D'Hondt V, Weynants P, Humblet Y, et al. Dose dependent IL-3 stimulation of thrombopoiesis and neutropoiesis in patients with small-cell lung cancer before and following chemotherapy. J Clin Oncol 1993;11:2063–71.

182. Steward WP, Verweji J, Somers R, et al. Granulocyte-macrophage colony-stimulating factor allows safe escalation of dose-intensity of chemotherapy in metastatic adult soft tissue sarcomas: a study of the European Organization for Research and Treatment of Cancer Soft Tissue and Bone Sarcoma Group. J Clin Oncol 1993;11:15.

183. Vose JM, Pandite AN, Beveridge RA, et al. Granulocyte-macrophage colony-stimulating factor/interleukin-3 fusion protein versus granulocyte-macrophage colony-stimulating factor after autologous bone marrow transplantation for non-Hodgkin's lymphoma: results of a randomized double-blind trial. J Clin Oncol 1997;15:1617–23.

184. Crawford J, Figlin R, Chang A, et al. Phase I/II trial of recombinant human IL-6 and G-CSF following ICE chemotherapy in patients with advanced non-small cell lung cancer. Blood 1993;82:1452a.

185. Brugger W, Frisch J, Schulz G, et al. Sequential administration of IL-3 and GM-CSF following standard-dose combination chemotherapy with etoposide, ifosfamide, and cisplatin. J Clin Oncol 1992;10:1452–9.

186. Nemunaitis J, Rabinowe SN, Singer JW, et al. Recombinant granulocyte-macrophage colony-stimulating factor after autologous bone marrow transplantation for lymphoid cancer. N Engl J Med 1991;324:1773.

187. Gorin N, Coiffier B, Hayat M, et al. Recombinant human granulocyte-macrophage colony-stimulating factor after high-dose chemotherapy and autologous bone marrow transplantation with unpurged and purged marrow in non-Hodgkin's lymphoma: a double-blind placebo-controlled trial. Blood 1992;80:1149.

188. Khwaja A, Yong K, Jones HM, et al. The effect of macrophage

colony-stimulating factor on haemopoietic recovery after autologous bone marrow transplantation. Br J Haematol 1992;81:288.

189. Brandt SJ, Peters WP, Atwater SK, et al. Effects of recombinant human granulocyte-macrophage colony-stimulating factor on hematopoietic reconstitution after high-dose chemotherapy and autologous bone marrow transplantation. N Engl J Med 1988;318:869–76.

190. Stahel RA, Jost LM, Cerny T, et al. Randomized study of recombinant human granulocyte colony-stimulating factor after high-dose chemotherapy and autologous bone marrow transplantation for high-risk lymphoid malignancies. J Clin Oncol 1994;12:1931–8.

191. Gulati SC, Bennett CL. Granulocyte-macrophage colony-stimulating factor (GM-CSF) as adjunct therapy in relapsed Hodgkin disease. Ann Intern Med 1991;116:177.

192. Lazurus HM, Goodnough LT, Goldwasser E, et al. Serum erythropoietin levels and blood component therapy after autologous bone marrow transplantation: implications for erythropoietin therapy in this setting. Bone Marrow Transplant 1992;10:71.

193. Locatelli F, Zecca M, Pedrazzoli P, et al. Use of recombinant human erythropoietin after bone marrow transplantation in pediatric patients with acute leukemia: effect of erythroid repopulation in autologous versus allogeneic transplants. Bone Marrow Transplant 1994;13:403.

194. Chao NJ, Scriber JR, Long GD, et al. A randomized study of erythropoietin and granulocyte colony-stimulating factor versus placebo and G-CSF for patients with Hodgkin's and non-Hodgkin's lymphoma undergoing autologous marrow transplantation. Blood 1994; 83:2823–8.

195. Appelbaum FR. Allogeneic marrow transplantation and the use of hematopoietic growth factors. Stem Cells 1995;13:344–50.

196. Powles R, Smith C, Milan S, et al. Human recombinant GM-CSF in allogeneic bone-marrow transplantation for leukaemia: double-blind, placebo-controlled trial. Lancet 1990;336:1417.

197. De Witte T, Gratwohl A, van der Lely N, et al. Recombinant human granulocyte-macrophage colony-stimulating factor accelerates neutrophil and monocyte recovery after allogeneic T-cell-depleted bone marrow transplantation. Blood 1992;79:1359.

198. Nemunaitis J, Rosenfeld C, Ash R, et al. Phase III double-blind trial of recombinant human granulocyte-macrophage colony-stimulating factor following after allogeneic bone marrow transplantation. Bone Marrow Transplant 1995;15:949–54.

199. Masoaka T, Takaku F, Kato S, et al. Recombinant human granulocyte colony-stimulating in allogeneic bone marrow transplantation. Exp Hematol 1989;17:1047–50.

200. Nemunaitis J, Anasetti C, Storb R, et al. Phase II trial of recombinant human granulocyte-macrophage colony-stimulating factor in patients undergoing allogeneic bone marrow transplantation from unrelated donors. Blood 1992;79:2572–7.

201. Anasetti C, Anderson G, Appelbaum FR, et al. Phase III study of rhGM-CSF in allogeneic marrow transplantation from unrelated donors. Blood 1993;82:454a.

202. Beguin Y, Clemons GK, Oris R, et al. Circulating erythropoietin after bone marrow transplantation: inappropriate response to anemia in allogeneic transplants. Blood 1991;77:868.

203. Klaesson S, Ringden O, Ljungman P, et al. Reduced blood transfusion requirements after allogeneic bone marrow transplantation: results of a randomized, double-blind study with high-dose erythropoietin. Bone Marrow Transplant 1994;13:397.

204. Link H, Boogaerts MA, Fauser AA, et al. A controlled trial of recombinant human erythropoietin after bone marrow transplantation. Blood 1994;84:3327.

205. Biggs JC, Atkinson KA, Booker V, et al. Prospective randomized, double-blind trial of the in vivo use of recombinant human erythropoietin in bone marrow transplantation from HLA-identical sibling donors. The Australian Bone Marrow Transplant Study Group. Bone Marrow Transplant 1995;15:129.

206. Nemunaitis J, Singer JW, Buckner CD, et al. The use of recombinant human granulocyte-macrophage colony-stimulating factor in graft failure after bone marrow transplantation. Blood 1990;76:245–53.

207. Weisdorf DJ, Verfaillie CM, Davies SM, et al. Hematopoietic growth factors for graft failure after bone marrow transplantation: a randomized trial of granulocyte-macrophage colony-stimulating factor versus sequential granulocyte-macrophage colony-stimulating factor plus granulocyte colony-stimulating factor. Blood 1995;85:3452–6.

208. Klumpp TR, Mangan KF, Goldberg SL, et al. Granulocyte colony-stimulating factor accelerates neutrophil engraftment following peripheral blood stem cell transplantation: a prospective randomized trial. J Clin Oncol 1995:13;1323–7.

209. Spitzer G, Adkins DR, Spencer V, et al. Randomized study of growth factors post peripheral blood stem cell transplant: neutrophil recovery is improved with modest clinical benefit. J Clin Oncol 1994;12:661–70.

210. Vey N, Molnar S, Faucher C, et al. Delayed administration of granulocyte colony-stimulating factor after autologous bone marrow transplantation: Effect on granulocyte recovery. Bone Marrow Transplant 1994;14:779–82.

211. Khwaja A, Mills W, Leveridge K, et al. Efficacy of delayed granulocyte colony-stimulating factor after autologous bone marrow transplantation. Bone Marrow Transplant 1993;11:479–82.

212. Schwartzberg L, Birch R, Weaver C, et al. The effect of varying duration of G-CSF on neutrophil engraftment and supportive care following peripheral blood progenitor cell infusion. Blood 1994;84:91a.

213. Fay JW, Lazarus HM, Herzig R, et al. Sequential administration of IL-3 and GM-CSF after autologous bone marrow transplantation for malignant lymphoma: a phase I/II multicenter trial. Blood 1994;84:2151–7.

214. Fay JW, Collins R, Pineiro L, et al. Concomitant administration of IL-6 and GM-CSF following autologous bone marrow transplantation: a phase I trial. Blood 1993;82:1707a.

215. Richman CM, Weiner RS, Yankee RA. Increase in circulating stem cells following chemotherapy in man. Blood 1976;47:1031.

216. Elias AD, Ayash L, Anderson KC, et al. Mobilization of peripheral blood progenitor cells by chemotherapy and granulocyte-macrophage colony-stimulating factor for hematologic support after high dose intensification for breast cancer. Blood 1992;79:3036.

217. Haas R, Mohle R, Fruhauf S, et al. Patients characteristics associated with successful mobilizing and autografting of peripheral blood progenitor cells in malignant lymphoma. Blood 1994;83:3787.

218. Scwartzberg LS, Birch R, Hazelton B, et al. Peripheral blood stem cell mobilization by chemotherapy with and without recombinant human granulocyte colony-stimulating factor. J Hematother 1992;1:317.

219. Gianni AM, Bregni M, Siena S, et al. Recombinant human granulocyte-macrophage colony-stimulating factor reduces hematologic toxicity and widens clinical applicability of high-dose cyclophosphamide treatment in breast cancer and non-Hodgkin's lymphoma. J Clin Oncol 1990;8:768.

220. Brugger W, Bross K, Frisch L, et al. Mobilization of peripheral blood progenitor cells by sequential administration of interleukin-3 and granulocyte-macrophage colony-stimulating factor following polychemotherapy with etoposide, ifosfamide and cisplatin. Blood 1992;70:1193.

221. Weaver A, Chang J, Wrigley E, et al. Randomized comparison of progenitor-cell mobilization using chemotherapy, SCF, and G-CSF or chemotherapy plus G-CSF alone in patients with ovarian cancer. J Clin Oncol 1998;16:2601–12.

222. Winter GN, Lazarus HM, Rademaker AF, et al. Comparison of PIXY321 and GM-CSF for mobilization of peripheral blood progenitor cells in advanced breast cancer. Blood 1995;86:578a.

223. Duhrsen U, Villeval JL, Boyd D. Effects of recombinant human granulocyte colony-stimulating factor on hematopoietic progenitor cells in cancer patients. Blood 1988;72:2074.

224. Weaver CH, Birch R, Greco FA, et al. Mobilization and harvesting of peripheral blood stem cells: randomized evaluations of different doses of filgrastim. Br J Haematol 1998;100:338–47.

225. Sheridan WP, Begley CG, Juttner CA, et al. Effect of peripheral blood progenitor cells mobilized by G-CSF on platelet recovery after high doses chemotherapy. Lancet 1992;339:640.

226. Huan SD, Hester J, Spitzer G, et al. Influence of mobilized peripheral blood cells on the hematopoietic recovery by autologous marrow and recombinant human granulocyte-macrophage colony-stimulating factor after high-dose cyclophosphamide, etoposide, and cisplatin. Blood 1992;79:3388.

227. Chao NJ, Schriber JR, Grimes K, et al. Granulocyte colony-stimulating factor "mobilized" peripheral blood progenitor cells accelerate granulocyte and platelet recovery after high-dose chemotherapy. Blood 1993;81:2031.

228. Peters WP, Rosner G, Ross M, et al. Comparative effects of granulocyte-macrophage colony-stimulating factor (GM-CSF) and granulocyte colony-stimulating factor (G-CSF) on priming peripheral blood progenitor cells for use with autologous bone marrow after high-dose chemotherapy. Blood 1993;81:1709.

229. Socinski MA, Cannistar SA, Elias A, et al. Granulocyte-macrophage

colony-stimulating factor expands the circulating haematopoietic progenitor cell compartment in man. Lancet 1988;1:1194.

230. Haas R, Ho AD, Bredthauer U, et al. Successful autologous transplantation of blood stem cells mobilized with recombinant human granulocyte-macrophage colony-stimulating factor. Exp Hematol 1990;18:94.

231. Aglietta M, Piacibello W, Sanavio F, et al. Kinetics of human hemopoietic cells after in vivo administration of granulocyte-macrophage colony-stimulating factor. J Clin Invest 1995;83:551.

232. Villeval JL, Duhrsen U, Morstyn G, et al. Effects of recombinant human granulocyte-macrophage colony-stimulating factor on progenitor cells in patients with advanced malignancies. Br J Haematol 1990;74:36.

233. Vose JM, Kessinger A, Bierman PJ, et al. The use of recombinant human IL-3 for mobilization of peripheral blood stem cells in previously treated patients with lymphoid malignancies. Int J Cell Cloning 1992;10:62.

234. Molineux G, Mccrea C, Yan XO, et al. Flt3 ligand synergizes with granulocyte colony-stimulating factor to increase neutrophil numbers and to mobilize peripheral blood stem cells with long-term repopulating potential. Blood 1997;89:3998–4004.

235. Lebsack ME, McKenna HJ, Hoek J, et al. FLT3 ligand administered in combination with GM-CSF or G-CSF to healthy volunteers. Proc ASCO 1998;18:78a.

236. Murray LJ, Luens KM, Estrada MF, et al. Thrombopoietin mobilizes CD34+ cell subsets into peripheral blood and expands multilineage progenitors in bone marrow of cancer patients with normal hematopoiesis. Exp Hematol 1998;26:207–16.

237. Somlo G, Sniecinski I, Brent J, et al. Recombinant human thrombopoietin in combination with G-CSF is safe and effective as peripheral blood progenitor cell mobilizer. Blood 1997;90:565a.

238. Buchner T, Hiddemann W, Koenigsmann M, et al. Recombinant human granulocyte-macrophage colony-stimulating factor after chemotherapy in patients with acute myeloid leukemia at higher age or after relapse. Blood 1991;78:1190.

239. Stone RM, Berg DT, George SL, et al. Granulocyte-macrophage stimulating factor after initial chemotherapy for elderly patients with primary acute myeloid leukemia. N Engl J Med 1995;332:1671–7.

240. Rowe JM, Andersen JW, Mazza JJ, et al. A randomized placebo-controlled Phase III study of granulocyte-macrophage colony-stimulating factor in adult patients (>55 to 70 years of age) with acute myeloid leukemia: a study of the Eastern Cooperative Oncology Group. Blood 1995;86:457.

241. Lowenberg B, Suciu S, Archimbaud E, et al. Use of recombinant human granulocyte-macrophage colony-stimulating factor during and after remission induction chemotherapy in patients aged 61 years and older with AML: final report of AML-11, a phase III randomized study of the Leukemia Cooperative Group of European Organization for the Research and Treatment of Cancer Cooperative Group. Blood 1997;90:2952.

242. Dombret H, Chastang C, Fenaux P, et al. A controlled study of recombinant human granulocyte colony-stimulating factor in elderly patients after treatment for acute myeloid leukemia. N Engl J Med 1995;332:1678–83.

243. Godwin JE, Kopecky KJ, Head DR, et al. A double-blind placebo-controlled trial of granulocyte colony-stimulating factor in elderly patients with previously untreated acute myeloid leukemia: a Southwest Oncology Group study. Blood 1998;91:3607–15.

244. Ottmann OG, Hoelzer D, Gracien E, et al. Concomitant granulocyte colony-stimulating factor and induction chemoradiotherapy in adult acute lymphoblastic leukemia: a randomized phase III trial. Blood 1995;86:444–50.

245. Pui CH, Boyett JM, Hughes WT, et al. Human granulocyte colony-stimulating factor after induction chemotherapy in children with acute lymphoblastic leukemia. N Engl J Med 1997;336:1781–7.

246. Larson RA, Dodge RK, Linker CA, et al. A randomized controlled trial of filgrastim during remission induction and consolidation chemotherapy for adults with acute lymphoblastic leukemia: CALGB study 9111. Blood 1998;92:1556–64.

247. Estey EH, Thall PF, Kantarjian H, et al. Treatment of newly diagnosed acute myelogenous leukemia with granulocyte-macrophage colony-stimulating factor (GM-CSF) before and during continuous-infusion high-dose ara-C + daunorubicin: comparison to patients treated without GM-CSF. Blood 1992;79:2246.

248. Bettelheim P, Valent P, Andreeff M, et al. Recombinant human granu-locyte-macrophage colony-stimulating factor in combination with standard induction chemotherapy in de novo acute myeloid leukemia. Blood 1991;77:700.

249. Witz F, Sadoun A, Perrin MC, et al. A placebo-controlled study of recombinant human granulocyte-macrophage colony-stimulating factor administered during and after induction treatment for de novo acute myeloid leukemia in elderly patients. Blood 1998;91:2722–30.

250. Vadhan-Raj S, Keating M, LeMaistre A, et al. Effects of recombinant human granulocyte-macrophage colony-stimulating factor in patients with myelodysplastic syndrome. N Engl J Med 1987;317:1545–52.

251. Negrin RS, Haeuber DH, Nahler A, et al. Maintenance treatment of patients with myelodysplastic syndromes using recombinant human granulocyte colony-stimulating factor. Blood 1990;76:36–43.

252. Ganser A, Seipelt G, Lindemann A, et al. Effects of recombinant human interleukin-3 in patients with myelodysplastic syndromes. Blood 1990;76:455.

253. Kurzrock R, Talpaz M, Estrov Z, et al. Phase I study of recombinant human interleukin-3 in patients with bone marrow failure. J Clin Oncol 1991;9:1241–50.

254. Vadhan-Raj S, Jeha S, Broxmeyer HE, et al. Stimulation of hematopoiesis by PIXY321 in patients with bone marrow failure. Blood 1993;82:1449a.

255. Schuster MW, Larson RA, Thompson JA, et al. GM-CSF for MDS: Results of a multicenter randomized controlled trial. Blood 1990;76:318a.

256. Greenberg P, Taylor K, Larson RA, et al. Phase III randomized multicentric of G-CSF vs. observation for myelodysplastic syndromes. Blood 1993;82:196a.

257. Ganser A, Hoelzer D. Treatment of myelodysplastic syndromes with hematopoietic growth factors. Hematol Oncol North Am 1992;6:633.

258. Aul C, Arning M, Runde V, et al. Serum erythropoietin concentrations in patients with myelodysplastic syndromes. Leuk Res 1991;15:571.

259. Stein RS, Abels RI, Krantz SB, et al. Pharmacologic doses of recombinant human erythropoietin in the treatment of myelodysplastic syndromes. Blood 1991;78:1658–63.

260. Goy A, Belanger C, Casadevail N, et al. High doses of intravenous recombinant erythropoietin for the treatment of anaemia in myelodysplastic syndrome. Br J Haematol 1993;84:232.

261. Hellstrom-Lindberg E. Efficacy of erythropoietin in the myelodysplastic syndromes: a meta-analysis of 205 patients from 17 studies. Br J Haematol 1995;89:67–71.

262. Stenke L, Wallvik J, Celsing F, et al. Prediction of response to treatment with rhEPO in myelodysplastic syndromes. Leukemia 1993;7:1324–7.

263. Rose EH, Abels RI, Nelson RA, et al. The use of rHuEpo in the treatment of anemia related to myelodysplasia. Br J Haematol 1995;89:831–7.

264. Negrin RS, Stein R, Vardiman J, et al. Treatment of anemia of myelodysplasic syndromes using recombinant human G-CSF in combination with erythropoietin. Blood 1993;82:737–43.

265. Hellstrom-Lindberg E, Ahlgren T, Beguin Y, et al. Treatment of anemia in myelodysplastic syndromes with granulocyte colony-stimulating factor plus erythropoietin: results from a randomized phase II study and long-term follow-up of 71 patients. Blood 1998;92:68–75.

266. Negrin RS, Stein R, Doheerty K, et al. Maintenance treatment of the anemia of myelodysplasic syndromes with recombinant human G-CSF and erythropoietin: evidence of in vivo synergy. Blood 1996;87:4076–81.

267. Fisch M, Galpin JE, Levine JD, et al. Recombinant human erythropoietin for patients with AIDS treated with zidovudine. N Engl J Med 1990;322:1488–93.

268. Scadden DT. Cytokine use in the management of HIV disease. J Acquir Immune Defic Syndr Hum Retrovirol 1997;16:S23–9.

269. Sprikkelman A, deWolf JT, Vellenga E, et al. The application of hematopoietic growth factors in drug-induced agranulocytosis: a review of 70 cases. Leukemia 1994;8:2031–8.

270. Bonilla MA, Gillio AP, Ruggeiro M, et al. Effects of recombinant human granulocyte colony-stimulating factor on neutropenia in patients with congenital agranulocytosis. N Engl J Med 1989;320:1574–80.

271. Dong F, Brynes RK, Tidow N, et al. Mutations in the gene for granulocyte colony-stimulating factor receptor in patients with acute myeloid leukemia preceded by severe congenital neutropenia. N Engl J Med 1995;333:487–93.

272. Hammond WP, Price TH, Souza LM, et al. Treatment of cyclic

neutropenia with granulocyte colony-stimulating factor. N Engl J Med 1989;320:1306–11.

273. Schreiber GB, Busch MP, Kleinman SH, et al. The risk of transfusion-transmitted viral infections. N Engl J Med 1996;334:1685–90.

274. Nemunaitis J, Meyers JD, Buckner CD, et al. Phase I trial of recombinant human macrophage colony-stimulating factor in patents with invasive fungal infections. Blood 1991;78:907.

275. Nemunaitis J, Shannon-Dorcy K, Appelbaum F, et al. Long-term follow-up of patients with invasive fungal disease who received adjunctive therapy with recombinant human M-CSF. Blood 1993;82:1422–7.

276. Shabar E, Kriboy N, Pollack S. White cell enhancement in the treatment of severe candidosis. Lancet 1995;86:974–5.

277. Marshall E, Powles R, Millar A, et al. Clinical effects of human MIP-1α administration to humans: a phase I study in cancer patients and normal healthy volunteers with the genetically engineered variant, BB-10010. Eur J Cancer 1998;34:1023–9.

278. Clemmons MJ, Marshall E, Durig J, et al. A randomized phase-II study of BB-10010 in patients with advanced breast cancer receiving 5-fluorouracil, Adriamycin, and cyclophosphamide chemotherapy. Blood 1998;92:1532–40.

279. Zachariah B. Case report: role of granulocyte colony stimulating factor in radiotherapy. Am J Med Sci 1992;304:252.

280. Redman BG, Flaherty L, Chou TH, et al. Phase I trial of recombinant M-CSF by rapid intravenous infusion in patients with cancer. J Immunother 1992;12:50–4.

281. Wallace EL, Churchill WH, Surgenor DM, et al. Collection and transfusion of blood and blood components in the United States, 1992. Transfusion 1995;35:802–12.

282. Goodnough LT, Monk TG, Andriole GL. Erythropoietin therapy. N Engl J Med 1997;336:933–8.

283. Bensinger WI, Price TH, Dale DC, et al. The effects of daily recombinant human granulocyte colony-stimulating factor administration on normal granulocyte donors undergoing leukapheresis. Blood 1993;81:1883–8.

284. Caspar CB, Seger RA, Burger G, et al. Effective stimulation of donors for granulocyte transfusions with recombinant methionyl G-CSF. Blood 1993;81:2866–71.

285. Adkins D, Ali S, Despotis G, et al. Granulocyte collection efficiency and yield are enhanced by the use of higher interface offset during apheresis of donors given granulocyte colony-stimulating factor. Transfusion 1998;38:557–64.

286. Adkins D, Johnston M, Walsh J, et al. Hydroxyethylstarch sedimentation by gravity ex-vivo for red cell reduction of granulocyte apheresis components. J Clin Apheresis 1998;13:56–61.

287. Swerdlow B, Deresinski S. Development of *Aspergillus* sinusitis in a patient receiving amphotericin B: treatment with granulocyte transfusions. Am J Med 1984;76:162–6.

288. Spielberger RT, Falleroni MJ, Coene AJ, et al. Concomitant amphotericin B therapy, granulocyte transfusions, and GM-CSF administration for disseminated infection with fusarium in a granulocytic patient. Clin Infect Dis 1993;16:528–0.

289. Adkins D, Spitzer G, Johnston M, et al. Transfusions of G-CSF mobilized granulocyte components to allogeneic transplant recipients: analysis of kinetics and factors determining post-transfusion neutrophil and platelet counts. Transfusion 1997;37:737–48.

290. Brown RA, Adkins D, Goodnough L, et al. Infusion of granulocytes collected from HLA-identical sibling donors reduces the duration of neutropenia following allogeneic PBSC transplant. Blood 1996; 88:261b.

291. Adkins D, Goodnough L, Brown RA, et al. G-CSF mobilized granulocyte components transfused into autologous transplant recipients results in significant and sustained absolute neutrophil count increments. Blood 1997;90:126b.

292. Kuter D, McCullough J, DiPersio JF, et al. Treatment of platelet donors with pegylated recombinant human growth and development factor increases circulating platelet counts and platelet apheresis yields and increases platelet increments in recipients of platelets transfusions. Blood 1997;90:579a.

293. Ross HG, Moy LA, Kaplan R, et al. Bullous pyoderma gangrenosum after granulocyte colony-stimulating factor treatment. Cancer 1991;68:441.

294. Negrin RS, Haeuber DH, Nagler A, et al. Treatment of myelodysplastic syndromes with recombinant human granulocyte colony-stimulating factor: a phase I–II trial. Ann Intern Med 1989;110:976.

295. Mehregan DR, Fransway AF, Edmonson JH, et al. Cutaneous reactions to granulocyte-monocyte colony-stimulating factor. Arch Dermatol 1992;128:1055.

296. Park JW, Mehrotra B, Barnett BO, et al. The Sweet syndrome during therapy with granulocyte colony-stimulating factor. Ann Intern Med 1992;116:996.

297. Anderlini P, Przepiorka D, Seong D, et al. Clinical toxicity and laboratory effects of granulocyte-colony-stimulating factor mobilization and blood cell apheresis from normal donors, and analysis of charges for the procedure. Transfusion 1996;36:590–5.

298. Jayesimi I, Giralt SS, Wood J. Subcutaneous granulocyte colony-stimulating factor and acute anaphylaxis. N Engl J Med 1991;325:587.

299. Adkins D. Anaphylactoid reaction in a normal donor given granulocyte colony-stimulating factor. J Clin Oncol 1998;16:812–3.

300. Schliesser G, Pratte H, Lohmeyer J. Leukocytoclastic vasculitis complicating granulocyte colony-stimulating factor (G-CSF) induced neutrophil recovery in T gamma-lymphocytosis with severe neutropenia. Ann Hematol 1992;65:151.

301. Becker PS, Wagle M, Matous S, et al. Spontaneous splenic rupture following administration of G-CSF: occurrence in an allogeneic donor of peripheral blood stem cells. Biol Blood Marrow Transplant 1997;3:108.

302. Biesma Bvellenga E, Willemse PH, et al. Effects of hematopoietic growth factors on chemotherapy-induced myelosuppression. Crit Rev Oncol Hematol 1992;13:107–34.

303. Steger GC, Locker G, Rainer H, et al. Cutaneous reactions to GM-CSF in inflammatory breast cancer. N Engl J Med 1992;327:286.

304. Lieschke GJ, Maher D, O'Connor M, et al. Phase I study of intravenously administered bacterially synthesized granulocyte-macrophage colony-stimulating factor and comparison with subcutaneous administration. Cancer Res 1990;50:606–14.

305. Dreicer R, Schiller JH, Carbone PP. Granulocyte-macrophage colony-stimulating factor and vasculitis. Ann Intern Med 1989;111:91.

306. Hoekman K, VonBlomberg-van der Flier BM, Wagstaff J, et al. Reversible thyroid dysfunction during treatment with GM-CSF. Lancet 1991;338:541.

307. De Vries EG, Willemse PH, Biesma B, et al. Flare-up of rheumatoid arthritis during GM-CSF treatment after chemotherapy. Lancet 1991;338:517.

308. Lieschke GJ, Maher D, O'Connor M, et al. Phase I study of intravenously administered bacterially synthesized granulocyte-macrophage colony-stimulating factor and comparison with subcutaneous administration. Ann Intern Med 1989;110:357.

309. Bokemeyer C, Schmoll HJ, Harstrick A, et al. A phase I/II study of a stepwise dose-escalated regimen of cisplatin, etoposide and ifosfamide plus granulocyte-macrophage colony-stimulating factor (GM-CSF) in patients with advanced germ cell tumors. Eur J Cancer 1993;29A:924.

310. Zimmer BM, Berdel WE, Ludwig WD, et al. Fatal spleen rupture during induction chemotherapy with rhGM-CSF priming for acute monocytic leukemia: clinical case report and in vitro studies. Leuk Res 1993;17:277.

311. Cazzola M, Ponchio L, Beguin Y, et al. Subcutaneous erythropoietin for treatment of refractory anemia in hematologic disorders: results of a phase I/II clinical trial. Blood 1992;79:29.

312. Costa JJ, Demetri GD, Harrist TJ, et al. Recombinant human stem cell factor (kit ligand) promotes human mast cell and melanocyte hyperplasia and functional activation in vivo. J Exp Med 1996;183:2681–6.

313. Moskowitz CH, Stiff P, Gordon MS, et al. Recombinant methionyl human stem cell factor and filgrastim for peripheral blood progenitor cell mobilization and transplantation in non-Hodgkin's lymphoma patients—results of a phase I/II trial. Blood 1997;89:3136–47.

314. Glaspy J, Davis MW, Parker WR, et al. Biology and clinical potential of stem cell factor. Cancer Chemother Pharmacol 1996;38:S53–7.

315. Ganser A, Lindemann A, Seipelt G, et al. Effects of recombinant human interleukin-3 in patients with normal hematopoiesis and in patients with bone marrow failure. Blood 1990;76:666.

316. Biesma B, Willemse PH, Mulder NH, et al. Effects of interleukin-3 after chemotherapy for advanced ovarian cancer. Blood 1992;80:1141.

317. Ganser A, Lindemann A, Ottmann OG, et al. Sequential in vivo treatment with two recombinant human hematopoietic growth factors (interleukin-3 and granulocyte-macrophage colony-stimulating factor) as a new therapeutic modality to stimulate hematopoiesis; results of a phase I study. Blood 1992;79:2583.

318. Van Gameren MM, Willemse PH, Mulder NH, et al. Effects of recombinant human IL-6 in cancer patients: a phase I/II study. Blood 1994;84:1434–41.
319. Cole DJ, Sanda MG, Yang JC, et al. Phase I trial of recombinant human M-CSF administered by continuous intravenous infusion in patients with metastatic cancer. J Natl Cancer Inst 1994;86:39–45.
320. Masaoka T, Shibata H, Ohno R, et al. Double blind test of human urinary M-CSF for allogeneic and syngeneic bone marrow transplantation: effectiveness of treatment and 2-year follow-up for relapse of leukemia. Br J Haematol 1990;76:501–5.
321. Yasuda N, Ohmori S, Usui T. Mobilization of myeloblasts with 5q– abnormality during treatment with macrophage colony-stimulating factor. Am J Hematol 1995;48:60.
322. Kaplan G, Walsh G, Guido LS, et al. Novel responses of human skin to intradermal recombinant GM-CSF: Langerhans cell recruitment, keratinocyte growth and enhanced wound healing. J Exp Med 1992;175:1717–28.
323. Gough A, Clapperton M, Rolando N, et al. Randomized placebo-controlled trial of G-CSF in diabetic foot infection. Lancet 1997;350:855–9.
324. Ketley NJ, Newland AC. Haematopoietic growth factors. Postgrad Med J 1997;73:213–21.
325. Jyung RW, Wu L, Pierce GF, et al. Granulocyte-macrophage colony-stimulating factor and granulocyte colony-stimulating factor: differential action on incisional wound healing. Surgery 1994;115:325–34.
326. Karthaus M, Rosenthal C, Huebner G, et al. Effects of topical oral G-CSF on oral mucositis: a randomized placebo-controlled trial. Bone Marrow Transplant 1998;22:781–5.
327. Dunphy F, Kim H, Dunleavy T, et al. GM-CSF ameliorates radiation mucositis. Blood 1997;90:184b.
328. Dunussi-Joannopoulos K, Dranoff G, Weinstein HJ, et al. Gene immunotherapy in murine acute myeloid leukemia: granulocyte-macrophage colony-stimulating factor tumor cell vaccines elicit more potent antitumor immunity compared with B7 family and other cytokine vaccines. Blood 1998;91:222–30.
329. Morita T, Ikeda K, Douzono M, et al. Tumor vaccination with macrophage colony-stimulating factor tumor-producing lewis lung carcinoma in mice. Blood 1996;88:955–61.
330. Westermann J, Aicher A, Kopp J, et al. GM-CSF modulates cellular immune response: upregulation of costimulatory molecules, increased cytotoxicity and enhancement of T cell activation in cancer patients. Blood 1997;90:174a.
331. Dranoff G, Mulligan RC. Gene transfer as cancer therapy. Adv Immunol 1995;58:417.
332. Suzu S, Yakota H, Yamanda M, et al. Enhancing effect of human monocytic colony-stimulating factor on monocyte tumoricidal activity. Cancer Res 1989;49:5913.
333. Sanda MG, Bolton E, Mulle JJ, et al. In vivo administration of recombinant macrophage colony-stimulating factor induces macrophage-mediated antibody-dependent cytotoxicity of tumor cells. J Immunother 1992;12:132.

# CHAPTER 16

# BLOOD STEM CELL AND MARROW TRANSPLANTATION

• JAMES L. GAJEWSKI • RICHARD E. CHAMPLIN

Blood stem cell and bone marrow transplantation is a therapeutic modality enabling the administration of dose-intensive chemotherapy or radiation therapy, or both, for treatment of hematologic malignancies, lymphopoietic malignancies, and select solid tumors by infusing hematopoietic progenitors to prevent prolonged pancytopenia. The dose of antineoplastic agents that can be administered clinically is limited by toxicity to normal tissues. For most agents, bone marrow suppression and pancytopenia is the dose-limiting toxicity. The doses of irradiation and many drugs can be substantially escalated to more effective levels if followed by transplantation of hematopoietic progenitors to rescue the patient from severe, prolonged myelosuppression. For dose-intensive therapy to be successful, the neoplasm must exhibit a dose-dependent response to chemotherapy or irradiation so that one (or possibly several) courses of intensive combined-modality treatment and bone marrow transplantation can eradicate the malignant cells. The treatment of cancer with blood stem cell and marrow transplantation and dose-intensive therapy is an increasingly effective treatment for a wide range of malignant diseases (Table 16–1).

Although blood and marrow transplantation has been viewed as hematopoietic support, it is increasingly designed to be a vehicle for administering cellular therapy for treatment of malignancy. The marrow produces the formed elements of the blood, including granulocytes, macrophages, erythrocytes, and platelets as well as T and B lymphocytes. These mature cells of the peripheral blood are derived from a complex hierarchy of hematopoietic stem cells that reside in the bone marrow. Hematopoietic stem cells have a dual capacity for self-renewal and differentiation. The most primitive cells, pluripotent stem cells, give rise to committed stem cells, which are restricted to a single line of differentiation. Transplantation of a relatively small number of pluripotent stem cells can reconstitute hematopoiesis and immunity in appropriately prepared recipients. Immunopoiesis after blood and marrow transplantation provides additional therapeutic benefit in reducing relapse risk for some types of cancer.

Sources of bone marrow include (1) *syngeneic* transplants involving a genetically identical twin donor, (2) *allogeneic* transplants from one person to another, and (3) *autologous* transplants using a patient's own hematopoietic cells. Autologous and syngeneic transplants are associated with less risk

*Table 16–1.* **Malignancies Effectively Treated by Bone Marrow Transplantation**

| *Allogeneic and Syngeneic Transplants* | *Autologous Transplants* |
| --- | --- |
| Acute myelogenous leukemia | Acute myelogenous leukemia |
| Acute lymphoblastic leukemia | Acute lymphoblastic leukemia |
| Chronic myelogenous leukemia | Chronic lymphocytic leukemia |
| Chronic lymphocytic leukemia | Chronic myelogenous leukemia |
| Lymphoma and Hodgkin's disease | Lymphoma |
| Myeloma | Hodgkin's disease |
| Neuroblastoma | Neuroblastoma |
| | Breast carcinoma |
| | Germ cell carcinoma of testes |

because the cells are not rejected and do not mediate graft-versus-host disease (GVHD). Allogeneic transplants have a greater rate of complications because of these potential immunologic problems but can be applied to patients with marrow involvement by their malignancy and can confer greater immune-mediated graft-versus-malignancy effect.

Historically the commonest source of allogeneic bone marrow transplantation has been from a human leukocyte antigen HLA-identical sibling donor. Increasingly, partially HLA-matched family donors, closely matched unrelated donors, and related and unrelated chord blood donors have been used. Essential to identifying a prospective donor and understanding the risks and benefits of allogeneic blood and marrow transplantation is the HLA system, the major histocompatibility complex in humans. The HLA system is encoded by genes present in several closely linked loci on the short arm of chromosome 6. Class I loci include HLA-A, HLA-B, and HLA-C. Class II loci include HLA-DR, HLA-DRW, HLA-DQ, and HLA-DP. These loci were originally defined serologically using antisera obtained from multiparous women. Molecular technology employing allele-specific or sequence-specific oligonucleotide typing is being increasingly used to define specific antigen with far greater resolution than serotyping. Matching with higher-resolution molecular typing is reducing the risks of immunologic complications with allogeneic transplantation.[1] The HLA system is not the only mediator of immunologic complications in allogeneic transplantation. HLA genotypically identical siblings develop immunologic complications with blood and marrow transplantation because of mismatching in poorly defined minor histocompatibility antigens. The only easily identified minor histocompatibility antigen is the HY antigen. The likelihood of mismatching for these minor antigens increases as the disparity in HLA increases between donor and recipient. It has been impossible in mismatch HLA transplants to assign relative risk of immunologic complications to either HLA mismatching or minor antigen mismatching.

Immunosuppressive conditioning treatment is required to allow sustained engraftment after allogeneic bone marrow transplants. More intensive pretransplant immunosuppression is required for marrow transplantation than is necessary to prevent rejection of solid organ allografts, such as the kidney, liver, or heart. A typical scheme for blood stem cell and bone marrow transplantation is shown in Figure 16–1. The immunosuppressive preparative treatment administered before transplantation should virtually ablate the recipient's immunity, including T-lymphocyte and natural killer cell function. In addition, the preparative therapy probably needs to provide space in the bone marrow microenvironment to allow engraftment of hematopoietic stem cells. The intensity of immunosuppressive therapy required varies depending on the immunocompetence of the recipient, the composition of the transplanted cells, the HLA disparity between donor and recipient, and whether the goal of therapy is complete donor chimera. Most preparative regimens for malignancies were maximally dose intensive, which resulted in myeloablation and totally impaired recipient immunity. As evidence has emerged that allogeneic immunopoiesis is tumor suppressive and potentially tumoricidal, newer, less toxic preparative regimens have been developed. These new regimens are not myeloablative but remain immunosuppressive to permit allogeneic hematopoietic and immunopoietic engraftment.[2] Donor-derived allogeneic cellular immunity is used to treat the malignancy.

The preparative regimen generally involves chemotherapy alone or in combination with irradiation. After the conditioning therapy is completed, the blood or marrow cells are infused intravenously. The cells circulate transiently, and sufficient numbers of stem cells home to the bone marrow to restore hematopoiesis and immunopoiesis. Allogeneic transplants require approximately 1 to 5 $\times$ 10$^8$ nucleated bone marrow cells per kilogram of recipient body weight to achieve engraftment.[1] The peripheral blood progenitor cell regimen requires harvesting 3 to 4 $\times$ 10$^6$ CD34$^+$ cells/kg of recipient body weight to achieve engraftment. Approximately 1 to 5 $\times$ 10$^7$ marrow cells/kg are sufficient for syngeneic or autologous transplants.[2] For autologous engraftment, 1 to 2 $\times$ 10$^6$ CD34$^+$ cells/kg are needed. Bone marrow dosing criteria were developed before identifying CD34 as a surrogate marker for the pluripotent hematopoietic stem cell. Peripheral blood counts are profoundly suppressed because of the effects of the conditioning treatment but generally recover within 10 to 30 days.

Engraftment of donor cells can be documented by acquisition of donor-type cell surface antigens, isoenzymes, chromosome markers, or DNA restriction fragment-length polymorphisms or by polymerase chain reactions of micro-

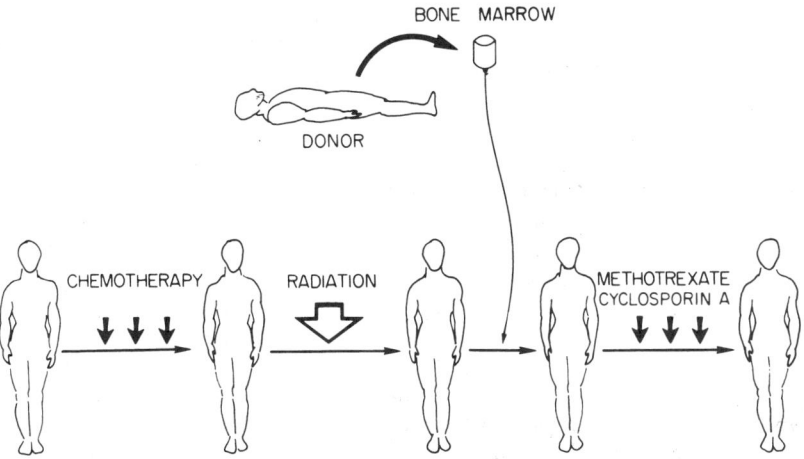

**Figure 16–1.** Scheme of bone marrow transplantation from an allogeneic donor. The transplant recipient receives chemotherapy or radiation, or both, as immunosuppressive conditioning treatment followed by intravenous infusion of bone marrow cells from a normal donor. After transplantation, further immunosuppressive treatment with cyclosporine or methotrexate, or both, is administered to prevent graft-versus-host disease.

satellite regions. After successful transplantation, cells of the hematologic and immunologic systems are primarily derived from the blood or marrow donor, although in some cases mixed chimerism occurs in which both donor-derived and recipient-derived cells are present. Parenchymal cells of visceral organs and most mesenchymal cells remain host in origin. Endothelial cells within the muscular system may be of donor origin.

Only a few patients have an HLA-identical sibling donor. As family size decreases, the odds of a family match also decrease. Related donor-recipient pairs that are mismatched for only one A, B, or D HLA locus or HLA phenotypically identical pairs have had a higher incidence of acute GVHD, but survival rates are similar to those of transplants between HLA-identical siblings for advanced-stage hematologic malignancies.[3] Historically, recipients mismatched for two or more loci have poorer results, with a high risk of graft rejection, GVHD, and other complications. With use of peripheral blood progenitor cells that have been aggressively T-cell depleted (4 to 5 log reduction), results with haploidentical transplants are dramatically improving.

Unrelated donor transplants continue to increase. Because of the tremendous polymorphism of the HLA loci, it is unlikely that a patient would be HLA identical with an unrelated individual. With worldwide registries including more than 3.8 million individuals, 30 to 40% of patients have an HLA-A, HLA-B, and HLA-DR identical donor by low resolution.[3] HLA gene frequencies vary considerably between racial groups, and linkage dysequilibrium occurs such that some haplotypes occur commonly, but approximately 50% of people have rare haplotypes. Unrelated donor transplants are increasingly successful, although the incidence and severity of GVHD are increased compared with transplants from HLA genotypically identical siblings. This increase is presumably related to greater genetic disparity with unrelated donors; these pairs are more likely to be mismatched for HLA variants and minor histocompatibility loci than related donors. Use of related and unrelated umbilical cord blood donation is increasing. Umbilical cord blood is harvested by drawing it at time of delivery. Banks of unrelated cryopreserved cord blood have been established. Umbilical cord blood has less risk of GVHD than cells obtained from pediatric or adult donors. The cell numbers collected are low, and use of cord blood donors is associated with a 20% graft failure risk in adults.[4]

The optimal choice of donor for a given recipient needing an allogeneic progenitor cell transplant still depends on clinical circumstances. Unless a syngeneic or HLA genotypically identical sibling has an underlying risk of a genetic defect or viral infection and is in poor health, it is rare to choose an unrelated donor over a family donor. For chronic myelogenous leukemia (CML), it may be preferable to consider an HLA genotypically identical sibling donor over a syngeneic donor for the superior outcome with a graft-versus-tumor effect. The choice between a partially matched family donor, unrelated donor, or cord blood is more problematic. The first issue in the decision tree analysis is how good is the matching and what type of cell processing support is available. When a related donor mismatched for two or more HLA-A, HLA-B, or HLA-DR antigens is being considered, these types of allogeneic transplants have reasonable success rates only with aggressive T-cell depletion of the stem cells by

the cell-processing laboratory. The advantage of related donors is that the donors are usually readily available. Unrelated donors require a 2- to 6-month search process and are usually not immediately available. If an unrelated donor is matched to the recipient by high-resolution molecular techniques for HLA-A, HLA-B, HLA-C, HLA-DR, and HLA-DQ loci, one report shows survival may be equivalent for an unrelated donor transplant to an HLA genotypically identical sibling transplant. Identifying such an optimally matched donor is difficult, and any mismatched loci compromise outcome. Umbilical cord blood can be obtained quickly, but it may be hard to obtain. Mixing cord blood from different donors should not be employed except in a research study. Cord blood should be considered only if a cell dose is greater than 1.5 to $3 \times 10^7$/kg with documented viability. Given the small number of cells in a unit of cord blood, it is not possible to do immunophenotyping of cord blood to establish a CD34$^+$ cell/kg standard.

For autologous transplantation, the patient must first undergo collection, cryopreservation, and storage of bone marrow or peripheral blood progenitor cells (Fig. 16–2). Both marrow collection and peripheral blood progenitor cell collection should occur at a time when the bone marrow is normally cellular and preferably does not contain malignant cells. At a later time, the patient can receive intensive marrow-ablative chemotherapy, irradiation, or both followed by reinfusion of the cryopreserved marrow to restore hematopoiesis. With current techniques, marrow cryopreservation can be reliably performed, and the stored cells can remain viable for more than 5 years.

Progenitors capable of reconstituting hematopoiesis can be collected from the peripheral blood by repeated leukapheresis. Circulating progenitors are rare but can be mobilized with hematopoietic growth factors, with or without cytoreductive chemotherapy after cytoreduction and with granulocyte colony–stimulating factor (G-CSF) or granulocyte-macrophage colony-stimulating factor (GM-CSF) stimulation. Peripheral blood progenitors were initially an alternative source of hematopoietic cells for transplantation but are now largely replacing bone marrow. Peripheral blood progenitors were initially also a potential source for patients with bone marrow involvement by malignant cells, although it remains to be determined if the level of contaminating malignant cells is less in the peripheral blood. Peripheral blood cells are relatively enriched for differentiated progenitors, and transplantation of large numbers of peripheral blood cells results in more rapid recovery of granulocytes and platelets than does marrow transplantation. A major area of research involves development of systems for ex vivo expansion of hematopoietic progenitors from blood or bone marrow. To date, this expansion has been impossible to achieve without having differentiation of the pluripotent stem cell.

One potential limitation of autologous transplantation is the possibility that the marrow or blood progenitors may be contaminated by malignant cells at the time of collection. A number of investigators are evaluating techniques to detect submicroscopic involvement by tumor and approaches to deplete occult malignant cells selectively from the normal bone marrow cells before cryopreservation by ex vivo treatment with antitumor monoclonal antibodies, antibody-toxin conjugates, chemotherapy, or physical techniques. An alter-

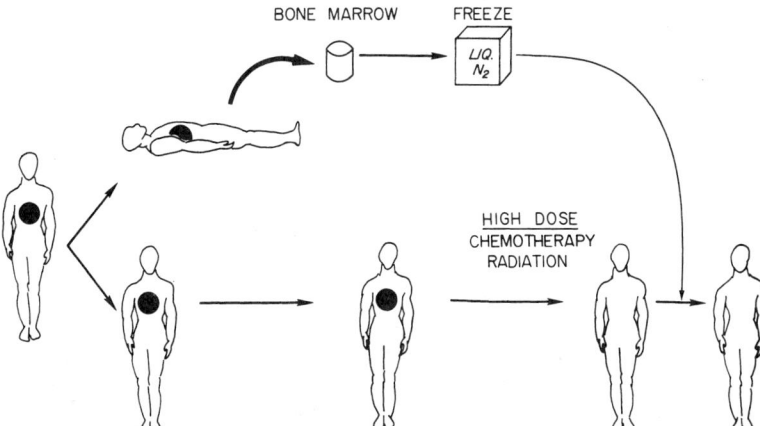

**Figure 16–2.** Scheme of autologous bone marrow transplantation.

native method is to select positively hematopoietic stem cells. CD34$^+$ cells represent less than 1% of the bone marrow but encompass progenitors capable of reconstituting hematopoiesis. Highly enriched CD34$^+$ selected cells have been used for autologous bone marrow or blood stem cell transplants, resulting in rapid hematologic recovery. The best purging comes with combining positive selection of CD34$^+$ cells with negative depletion of tumor cells.

## Potential Complications of Dose-Intensive Therapy with Bone Marrow Transplantation

Intensive chemoradiotherapy and bone marrow transplantation may be associated with a number of serious complications (Table 16–2), including toxicity from the pretransplant conditioning regimen; infections resulting from granulocytopenia or post-transplant immunodeficiency; graft failure; and, in the case of allogeneic transplants, transplant rejection and GVHD. In all, fatal complications generally occur in 5 to 15% of autologous transplant recipients and 20 to 40% of patients receiving allogeneic transplants for malignancy.

### HEMATOLOGIC TOXICITY

Patients receiving dose-intensive therapy and bone marrow transplantation develop profound pancytopenia lasting approximately 2 to 4 weeks until the transplanted cells restore hematopoiesis and immunopoiesis. During the period of granulocytopenia, life-threatening infectious complications may occur. GM-CSF and G-CSF have been shown to accelerate hematopoietic recovery after autologous marrow trans-

*Table 16–2.* **Potential Complications of Allogeneic Bone Marrow Transplantation**

Toxicity of high-dose chemotherapy and irradiation
Graft rejection
Acute and chronic graft-versus-host disease
Post-transplant immunodeficiency and infections
Interstitial pneumonitis
Secondary malignancy

plantation or to improve hematopoiesis in patients with graft failure. Neither G-CSF nor GM-CSF prevents the nadir of granulocytes, but the granulocytopenic period is shortened by approximately 1 week. Neither factor affects erythrocyte or platelet recovery. Use of these growth factors reduces the number of febrile days and shortens the period of hospitalization. Transplants of peripheral blood progenitor cells have been shown to produce more rapid recovery of platelets than bone marrow transplants. Thrombopoietic growth factors have only marginally improved platelet recovery.

### ORGAN TOXICITY

Pretransplant cytotoxic preparative regimens approach the limit of tolerance for several tissues. Severe toxicity may occur involving the lung, heart, liver, nervous system, and, rarely, other tissues. Organs affected vary depending on the drugs and radiotherapy regimens involved. Fatal hepatic veno-occlusive disease occurs in approximately 5% of patients undergoing transplantation for leukemia.[4–6] This disease is more common in older patients; patients with pre-existing liver function abnormalities, active hepatitis B or C infections; and patients who have received extensive previous chemotherapy. Pneumonitis ascribed to toxicity of the conditioning regimen occurs in 5 to 10% of patients[7]; this is particularly common with bis-chloroethyl-nitrosourea (BCNU) or alkylating agent–based regimens or in patients undergoing transplantation after mediastinal radiotherapy.[8, 9] This situation is often difficult to distinguish from pneumonitis related to cytomegalovirus (CMV) or other viral infections. Unexplained dypsnea and hypoxemia observed 1 to 9 months after transplantation are the presenting symptoms of pneumonitis. This diagnosis must be considered. The use of bronchoscopy to rule out an infectious cause, particularly a viral infection, must be done quickly. Early administration of steroids is necessary to avoid a fatal outcome. Cardiac toxicity is common with high-dose cyclophosphamide regimens, particularly when combined with BCNU or other alkylating agents. Central nervous system complications are relatively uncommon, but dementia or leukoencephalopathy may occur. Endocrine complications may develop but are generally not life-threatening. Hypothyroidism commonly occurs as a delayed complication 6 months to 2 years after transplantation.

Intensive combined-modality therapy typically results in sterility for men and women, although gonadal endocrine function and ejaculation are usually intact. Cataracts are a common delayed complication of total-body irradiation. Bladder toxicity resulting from high-dose cyclophosphamide chemotherapy also is a common problem. This problem is probably mediated by acrolein, a metabolite of 4-hydroxy-cyclophosphamide that is toxic to transitional epithelium. Hemorrhagic cystitis may develop acutely or as a delayed complication weeks to months later. Mesna, a uroprotective agent that binds to acrolein, has been reported to reduce the risk of urinary toxicity of cyclophosphamide in bone marrow transplant patients without inhibiting its therapeutic effects. Hemorrhagic cystitis has been observed with other agents and may be due to viral infection. Initial treatment is always bladder irrigation. If that fails, carboprost, a prostaglandin $E_2$ inhibitor, which causes local vasoconstriction, has had some success. The other option is surgery to do cauterization or fulguration with formalin. On rare occasions, a cystectomy needs to be performed.

## GRAFT REJECTION AND GRAFT-VERSUS-HOST DISEASE

For patients receiving allogeneic transplants, graft rejection may occur, mediated by host T lymphocytes or natural killer cells. Preparative regimens involving total-body irradiation or the combination of busulfan and cyclophosphamide are sufficiently immunosuppressive so that graft rejection from an HLA-identical donor is rare. Patients receiving transplants from HLA-nonidentical donors and recipients of T lymphocyte–depleted transplants have a greater risk of rejection.

A more frequent problem is GVHD. Two forms of GVHD have been identified: acute and chronic. Acute GVHD results from engraftment of immunocompetent cells from the donor bone marrow that react against recipient tissues. The pathophysiology of acute GVHD is incompletely defined but is initially mediated by T lymphocytes reacting against disparate host antigens. The incidence and clinical manifestations of GVHD are affected by several factors, including the degree of genetic disparity between the donor and recipient, patient age, the toxicity of the conditioning regimen, and the nature and quantity of the transplanted cells. Besides HLA compatibility issues, donor factors include age, parity if female, number of transfusion exposures, and donor sex. Primary target organs include skin, liver, lymphoid tissues, and gastrointestinal tract. Moderate to severe acute GVHD occurs in 30 to 60% of HLA-identical transplants, typically develops within 30 to 100 days, and is fatal in approximately half of affected patients.[10, 11] In HLA genotypically identical sibling transplant recipients, preliminary reports indicate that the use of peripheral blood progenitor cells as the source of hematopoietic support may result in less acute GVHD because of faster engraftment and less organ toxicity. Chronic GVHD may be increased in recipients of HLA-identical peripheral blood progenitor cell transplants, particularly if the number of $CD34^+$ cells/kg recipient body weight exceeds $8 \times 10^6$ cells/kg.[5] GVHD occurs more frequently after HLA-mismatched transplants, and the incidence increases with recipient age. For syngeneic and autologous transplants, GVHD should not occur, although a syndrome resembling acute GVHD suggests that abnormal regulation of immunity may participate in the pathogenesis of this disorder. This syndrome may be imitated by giving immunosuppression to syngeneic or autologous graft recipients and abruptly withdrawing it.

Several approaches have been proposed to prevent or treat acute GVHD. Most patients have received prophylactic post-transplant immunosuppressive treatment with cyclosporine or tacrolimus, usually combined with methotrexate or corticosteroids for 3 to 6 months.[12] Results with tacrolimus may be slightly improved compared with cyclosporine, but the principal benefit of tacrolimus is that the drug level is predictive of toxicity. Patients who develop acute GVHD are generally treated with high-dose corticosteroids, such as methylprednisolone at 2 mg/kg.[13] Patients with steroid-resistant GVHD have a poor prognosis, although some respond to additional immunosuppressive therapy, such as antithymocyte globulin. There is considerable interest in the role of cytokines in the pathophysiology of GVHD. Interleukin (IL)-1 and tumor necrosis factor have been implicated, and anticytokine therapy may be useful for prophylaxis or treatment. Potential agents include soluble IL-1 or tumor necrosis factor receptor, IL-1 receptor antagonist, or IL-10. These agents are under study.

Depletion of T lymphocytes from the donor bone marrow or peripheral blood progenitor cells before transplantation is an alternate approach to prevent GVHD. The most common techniques include agglutination with lectins and E rosette depletion or treatment with anti–T cell monoclonal antibodies. These techniques are effective in reducing the incidence and severity of GVHD. Immunologic recovery does not appear to be compromised, but the risk of graft failure because of rejection is increased. The mechanism by which T lymphocytes facilitate engraftment is unclear; one possibility is a graft-versus-host effect abrogating residual host immunocompetent cells, but T lymphocytes facilitate engraftment in $F_1$ offspring to parent transplants in mice, a combination in which rejection occurs, but GVHD is absent.[14] Growth factors or cytokines released by T lymphocytes may be involved, or a subset of T lymphocytes may actively facilitate engraftment by direct cellular interaction. Patients receiving T lymphocyte–depleted transplants have also had a greater risk of leukemia relapse, indicating that marrow T lymphocytes may contribute to the beneficial graft-versus-leukemia (GVL) effect. The increased risk of relapse in T-cell–depleted transplants is less if the donor is HLA mismatched with the recipient. T-lymphocyte depletion may ultimately be clinically useful if more effective immunosuppressive and antileukemic preparative regimens can be developed.

Chronic GVHD is a distinct clinical syndrome affecting approximately 25% of transplant recipients who survive more than 6 months.[15, 16] Two thirds of affected patients have preceding acute GVHD, but it develops de novo in one third of patients. The incidence of chronic GVHD increases with recipient age. Chronic GVHD may be increased in recipients of allogeneic peripheral blood progenitor grafts. Peripheral blood progenitor cells have 1 to 2 logs more T lymphocytes than bone marrow graft. Chronic GVHD has protean clinical manifestations similar to those seen in several rheumatologic and autoimmune disorders, such as progressive systemic sclerosis, systemic lupus erythematosus, Sjögren's syndrome, and primary biliary cirrhosis. Chronic GVHD is a disease of disordered immunity; patients have a spectrum of immune-related abnormalities, including profound immunodeficiency, autoantibodies, and excessive nonspecific suppressor T-cell activity. Affected patients often die of infections, and most centers recommend the long-term use of prophylactic antibiotics, such as penicillin or trimethoprim-sulfamethoxazole, for these patients.

Chronic GVHD may develop in two forms: a limited form involving localized areas of the skin and an extensive form with generalized skin and multisystem involvement. The limited form does not require therapy. The systemic form of chronic GVHD is more serious and responds poorly to treatment. Corticosteroids, antithymocyte globulin, and other immunosuppressive or cytotoxic agents are usually ineffective in advanced disease. Prednisone alone or the combination of prednisone with azathioprine or cyclosporine is beneficial in patients with early chronic GVHD. Thalidomide has been effective in some patients. Photopheresis and psoralens plus ultraviolet A therapy has been effective for patients with skin-only chronic GVHD.

Some patients develop obliterative bronchiolitis, a delayed form of respiratory failure caused by obstructive terminal airway disease 6 months to 2 years after transplantation.[17, 18] This illness often results in recurrent pneumothorax and progressive respiratory insufficiency, which is often fatal. Its pathogenesis is poorly defined but typically occurs in patients with chronic GVHD and is usually not associated with a documented infection. No effective therapy has been reported.

## IMMUNODEFICIENCY

Allogeneic transplant recipients have a severe immunodeficiency involving T and B cells. The most profound abnormalities occur within the first 4 to 6 months, followed by slow recovery over the next year.[19, 20] Patients with chronic GVHD continue to have a profound immunodeficiency for prolonged periods. They have an opsonization defect and are prone to infection from encapsulated organisms, such as pneumococcus. Antibiotic prophylaxis is often recommended for these patients. Intensive preparative regimens virtually ablate the host immune system. T and B lymphocytes as well as macrophages, monocytes, and other myeloid cells are subsequently produced from precursor cells present in the donor bone marrow. The number of circulating T and B cells returns to normal levels within 6 weeks, but functional studies of these cells are abnormal for at least 1 year. There is a marked decrease in CD4 T-helper and inducer and CD8 T-suppressor and cytotoxic subsets during the immediate post-transplant period but more rapid recovery of CD8$^+$ cells, resulting in a reversal of the CD4/CD8 ratio. This abnormality does not appear to be related to GVHD. Nevertheless, patients with GVHD may exhibit delayed normalization of T-cell subsets, and the ratio may remain abnormal for prolonged periods in those with chronic GVHD. Bone marrow transplant recipients also show increased numbers of immature or activated T cells. Immune reconstitution after the less intensive preparative regimens remains to be studied. Recipients of syngeneic or autologous transplants also have a period of immunodeficiency, but their recovery

may be more rapid, and post-transplant infections are less severe than in allogeneic transplant recipients.

## INFECTIONS

Allogeneic and autologous marrow transplant recipients are predisposed to develop a number of infectious complications. During the immediate post-transplant period, patients have granulocytopenia and a high incidence of bacterial and fungal infections. Mucosal herpes simplex infections are also common during this period but seldom disseminate; prophylactic treatment with acyclovir may decrease their incidence. Viral gastroenteritis may also occur and may be confused with manifestations of GVHD.

Allogeneic marrow transplant patients are at risk for opportunistic infections, particularly from viral and parasitic agents. Most centers require patients to remain locally until 100 days after transplantation for close monitoring and antibiotic prophylaxis. Herpes zoster is common within the first year of transplantation. It is generally confined to a single dermatome, but fatal dissemination may occur. Abdominal zoster may present severe subxyphoid abdominal pain. Treatment with high-dose acyclovir is beneficial in patients with disseminated disease, multiple dermatome zoster, and ocular zoster and may prevent dissemination in immunocompromised patients with localized involvement. Valacyclovir and fanciclovir may be alternatives for patients with single dermatome herpes zoster.

Interstitial pneumonitis is one of the major complications of allogeneic marrow transplantation, occurring in approximately 10 to 25% of patients, usually within the first 4 months.[7] More than half of these cases are associated with CMV infections.[21] Exogenous CMV infections can be acquired via blood product transfusions. CMV-seropositive recipients are at high risk for CMV disease from reactivation of latent endogenous infection. Recipients of HLA-mismatched transplants are at a higher risk for CMV disease. In general, CMV disease is less of a problem now than in the early 1990s because of better molecular diagnostics and treatment of antigenemia or PCR-positive seroconversion prior to active disease. *Pneumocystis carinii*, adenovirus, echovirus, respiratory syncytial virus, and herpes varicella-zoster are involved in some cases. Factors important in the development of interstitial pneumonitis include age, GVHD, post-transplant immunodeficiency, and drug-related or radiation-related lung injury. The severity of GVHD is a major risk factor. Heavily pretreated patients have a higher incidence, particularly patients who have received thoracic or mediastinal radiation therapy. Patients receiving total-body irradiation at a low-dose rate and those receiving cyclosporine rather than methotrexate after transplantation have a lower incidence of interstitial pneumonitis.

Several approaches to the prevention or treatment of interstitial pneumonitis have been evaluated. Prophylactic treatment with trimethoprim-sulfamethoxazole is effective in preventing *P. carinii* infections. For CMV-seronegative recipients, acquisition of CMV can be prevented by selecting blood products from CMV-seronegative donors. Several trials have indicated that passive immunization with immune globulin containing a high titer of antibodies to CMV can modify or prevent serious CMV infections and reduce the incidence of interstitial pneumonitis. CMV-seropositive patients have latent virus present and are at high risk for reactivation pneumonitis after transplantation. Prophylaxis with acyclovir has been reported to reduce modestly the rate of CMV pneumonitis. Ganciclovir has greater in vitro activity against CMV. The combination of ganciclovir and intravenous immune globulin has been effective for patients with early CMV infections but is generally ineffective for patients with symptomatic pneumonitis. Ganciclovir has been studied as prophylactic treatment to prevent CMV infection in seropositive recipients. Ganciclovir reduces the incidence of CMV infection, but it frequently produces granulocytopenia, and its use has not been shown to improve survival. Rather than relying on growing CMV tissue cultures, patients are now being screened with antigen testing or by molecular techniques using polymerase chain reaction. Treatment before sufficent viral load can grow in culture has been beneficial in a randomized trial.

Autologous transplant patients recover immunity more quickly than patients with allogeneic transplants and have a much lower risk of infection after recovery of peripheral blood counts. A small fraction of autograft recipients develop late infections. *P. carinii* infection most frequently occurs in patients with lymphoid malignancies, and prophylactic sulfamethoxazole-trimethoprim is indicated. CMV infection may occur in heavily immunocompromised patients and should be considered in any patient with interstitial infiltrates or unexplained hypoxic dypsnea. For autograft recipients who received BCNU, it is important to differentiate CMV interstitial pneumonitis from late allergic BCNU pneumonitis. BCNU-related pneumonitis responds quickly to corticosteroids, whereas corticosteroids can exacerbate CMV pneumonitis.

## SECOND MALIGNANCIES

The high-dose chemotherapy and radiation treatment regimens for bone marrow transplantation are potentially carcinogenic and may predispose to the development of secondary malignancies. Second malignancies rarely occur after marrow transplantation. Cytogenetic abnormalities observed before cryopreserving autologous progenitor cells can clonally expand and cause acute myelogenous leukemia (AML) or myelodysplasia after transplantation. Solid tumors, particularly sarcomas and thyroid cancer, are increased in allogeneic transplants receiving total-body irradiation, but the risk is only approximately 1 in 250 long-term survivors. Lymphoproliferative disorders in donor-derived B lymphocytes related to Epstein-Barr infection may occur, particularly in heavily immunosuppressed patients with intravenous antithymocyte globulin or anti–T cell antibody therapy or HLA-mismatched or T cell–depleted transplants. These B-lymphocyte malignancies frequently respond to an allogeneic T-lymphocyte infusion from the donor of $1 \times 10^5$ CD3$^+$ cells/kg.

## Results of Bone Marrow Transplantation for Treatment of Malignancy

### LEUKEMIA

Marrow transplantation has been most extensively evaluated for treatment of leukemias. Autologous and allogeneic trans-

plants attempt to take advantage of the cytotoxic effects of the high-dose preparative regimen. Allogeneic marrow recipients potentially also benefit from an immune-mediated GVL effect from the transplanted donor cells. The mechanism and cell populations involved with GVL are incompletely understood. T-cell clones reactive with human leukemia cells have been described, and T cell–depleted allogeneic transplants have had a higher relapse rate. Lymphokine-activated killer and natural killer cells may also contribute. Leukemia-specific antigens have not been described for human acute leukemias and CML, and the recognition mechanism for GVL is unknown. The potential mechanism need not require recognition of leukemia-specific antigens; reactivity may be directed at host hematopoietic tissue in general, preventing repopulation by normal and leukemic host–derived hematopoietic cells.

Clinical data indicate a critical role for GVL in preventing the recurrence of leukemia after allogeneic bone marrow transplantation. Occasionally, patients with leukemia achieve remission only after the development of acute GVHD. Recipients who develop GVHD have a lower incidence of leukemia relapse than patients without GVHD. This antileukemic effect correlates best with the presence of chronic GVHD. The impact of acute GVHD is uncertain, but the lowest rate of relapse occurs in patients with acute and chronic GVHD. Patients with AML or CML receiving transplants from identical-twin donors have a significantly higher risk of relapse than allogeneic bone marrow transplant recipients. In CML patients relapsing after transplantation, infusion of peripheral blood leukocytes from the transplant donor has effectively reinduced remission. The newer, less intensive nonmyeloablative preparative regimen can be safely administered without hematopoietic cellular support. With allogeneic cellular support, these regimens have induced remission, whereas giving the regimen without allogeneic cellular support has not induced a remission. HLA mismatched and unrelated donor transplants have been associated with lower relapse rates.

Immunosuppressive treatments designed to prevent GVHD also affect the rate of leukemia relapse. Cyclosporine can reduce the GVL effect in animal models, and patients with acute lymphoblastic leukemia (ALL) receiving posttransplant cyclosporine have a higher relapse rate than patients receiving methotrexate. There is a significantly lower rate of acute GVHD with cyclosporine and methotrexate treatment compared with cyclosporine alone after transplantation, but the combination results in a higher rate of leukemia relapse in patients with AML, abrogating any improvement in disease-free survival. The impact of tacrolimus is still being studied. Use of allogeneic peripheral blood progenitors may have a lower relapse rate. This is speculated to be secondary to the extra log of T-lymphocyte infusion with the graft.

T-cell depletion of donor bone marrow is the most effective means of preventing acute and chronic GVHD, but this approach is associated with a substantial increase in the risk of recurrent leukemia; the net effect is either no change or worsening of disease-free survival in all forms of leukemia. In HLA mismatched or unrelated transplants, T-cell depletion has not been associated as strongly with an increased risk of relapse and, for some patients, may improve survival.

It is important to understand the mechanisms of leukemic

*Table 16–3.* **Approximate Percentage Survival at 5 Years or Longer in Acute Myelogenous Leukemia with Bone Marrow Transplantation or Conventional Chemotherapy**

|  | BMT (%) | Chemotherapy (%) |
| --- | --- | --- |
| First remission | 40–65 | 10–50 |
| Second remission | 30–50 | 10 |
| Partial remission/early relapse | 30 | 0 |
| Relapse | 10–20 | 0 |

BMT, bone marrow transplantation.

recurrence after bone marrow transplantation. In most patients who relapse, the leukemic cells are of recipient (host) origin, indicating failure of the treatment regimen to eradicate completely all leukemic cells. Improvement in the treatment outcome for these patients requires the development of a more effective antileukemic therapy. There have been several cases reported, however, in which the leukemia appears to have recurred in donor cells, indicating that under some circumstances the leukemia may be reinduced. There are alternative explanations of this phenomenon that must be considered, including microenvironmental or regulatory abnormalities or somatic cell hybridization with transfer of oncogenic DNA between a recipient leukemia cell and normal donor hematopoietic cells.

## ACUTE MYELOGENOUS LEUKEMIA

Marrow transplantation has been extensively used for the treatment of patients with AML. The objective is to administer high-dose chemoradiotherapy to eradicate the malignant cells followed by transplantation of normal marrow to rescue the patient from severe myelosuppression. Results primarily

depend on the stage of the leukemia, the leukemia cytogenetics, the age of the recipient, and the HLA matching between the donor and recipient at the time of transplantation.

Allogeneic marrow transplantation has been extensively evaluated in patients with AML. Results are summarized in Table 16–3. Most patients have received high-dose cyclophosphamide and 9 to 15 Gy total-body irradiation with or without other chemotherapy or the combination of busulfan and cyclophosphamide. Most patients achieve complete remission. Approximately 25% of patients with refractory leukemia receiving syngeneic marrow transplants have achieved prolonged disease-free survival, the major cause of treatment failure being relapse of leukemia.[22] For recipients of allogeneic marrow transplants with induction failure or leukemia in relapse, actuarial 5- to 10-year survival is approximately 20%.[23, 24] The major causes of treatment failure are GVHD, interstitial pneumonitis, and recurrent leukemia. Approximately 70% of patients experience recurrence of leukemia within 2 years. More intensive regimens designed to have greater antileukemic activity have been associated with a high rate of complications resulting from toxicity, and overall survival has improved. Intensive chemoradiotherapy and bone marrow transplantation can be curative in a small proportion of patients with otherwise end-stage AML.

Data indicate that results are improved by employing bone marrow transplantation as the initial treatment of leukemic relapse rather than attempting reinduction of remission with chemotherapy and performing bone marrow transplantation in a second remission (Fig. 16–3). The best results of allogeneic marrow transplantation are achieved in patients in first remission. The rationale for this approach includes treatment of the patients with a relatively low burden of malignant cells before the development of resistant leukemia. In addition, patients in remission are generally in better medical condition than patients with advanced leukemia and

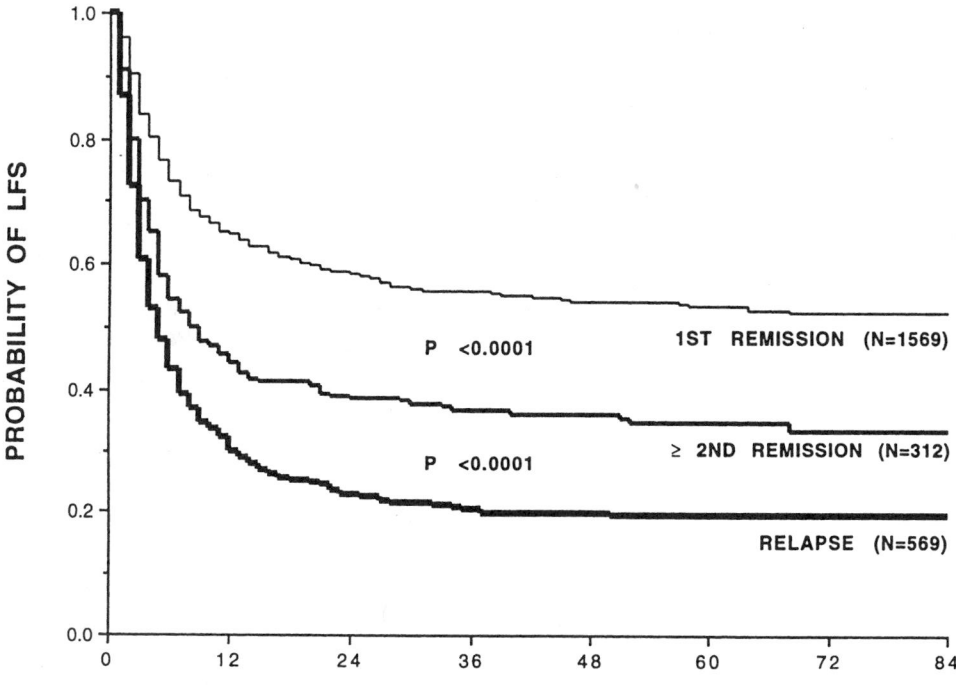

**Figure 16–3.** Leukemia-free survival (LFS) after allogeneic bone marrow transplantation for patients with acute myelogenous leukemia (AML). (Data from the International Bone Marrow Transplant Registry.)

can tolerate better the intensive preparative regimen. Most centers have limited transplantation to patients younger than 55 years of age who have an HLA-identical sibling donor. The nonmyeloblative regimen has opened the option of allogeneic transplantation to patients up to 75 years. Most studies report a low risk of leukemic relapse, generally 20 to 30%, and actuarial survival is 40 to 65% at 3 to 5 years. The major causes of treatment failure were GVHD, interstitial pneumonitis, and leukemic relapse. Patient age appears to be an important prognostic factor, and the best results have been reported in patients younger than age 20 (Fig. 16–4).

One setting in which bone marrow transplantation may be particularly useful is the treatment of patients with preleukemia or therapy-related AML. Conventional therapy is often unsuccessful in these patients because of the failure of normal hematopoietic cells to recover after induction chemotherapy. Intensive marrow-ablative chemoradiotherapy with bone marrow transplantation has been successful in preliminary studies, producing complete remissions and restoring normal hematopoiesis in selected patients.

The results of bone marrow transplantation for patients with AML in first remission must be compared with data reported with standard-dose chemotherapy using regimens involving intensive consolidation, maintenance programs, or both. There is a wide range of reported results for standard chemotherapy among centers, with actuarial disease-free survival reported to be 10 to 50% at 3 to 5 years. A number of prognostic factors have been reported that predict for prolonged duration of remission, such as initial white blood cell count, histologic subtype, cytogenetic data, presence of an antecedent preleukemic syndrome, and response to initial induction chemotherapy.

Several controlled trials comparing allogeneic bone marrow transplantation with combination chemotherapy have been reported in patients with AML in first remission. Each

study has shown a significantly lower relapse rate in patients receiving bone marrow transplantation. Marrow transplantation, however, is more likely to be associated with fatal treatment-related complications than is chemotherapy. Two trials reported an advantage in disease-free survival with marrow transplantation. Allogeneic transplantation with a HLA-matched sibling has generally improved survival compared with standard-dose chemotherapy, especially among patients with standard-risk or high-risk cytogenetics. Autologous transplantation results have generally been equivalent to chemotherapy. A Southwest Oncology Group (SWOG) trial did not show an advantage to transplantation over chemotherapy. The Medical Research Council (MRC) 10th trial, which stratified patients by cytogenetic risk groups, showed superior outcomes with autologous transplantation in high, intermediate, and poor prognostic groups. With an intention-to-treat analysis, better results with allogeneic transplantation compared with chemotherapy were observed only in the intermediate prognostic group. The good prognostic group did well with all treatments. The poor prognostic group did poorly, in part, because four cycles of chemotherapy were given before patients being transplanted. Most patients relapsed during the 4 to 6 months of receiving postremission consolidation therapy and were transplanted after relapse.

Based on the age-dependent results of bone marrow transplantation, most data suggest that allogeneic bone marrow transplants from an HLA-identical sibling or one antigen HLA-AB, HLA-DR–mismatched related donor are indicated in children and young adults with AML in first remission. It is uncertain whether adults should be treated with allogeneic bone marrow transplantation in first remission or receive postremission chemotherapy with marrow transplantation at the time of relapse. For recipients with only an unrelated donor or family mismatched donor or a family mismatched donor for two or more HLA-A, HLA-B, HLA-DR antigens

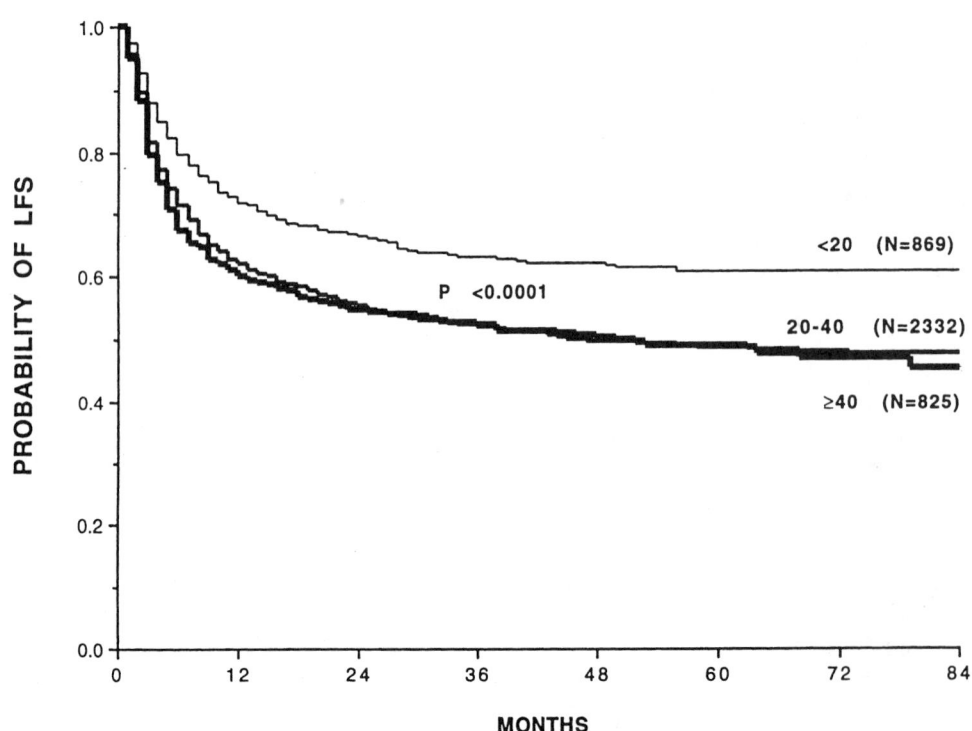

**Figure 16–4.** Effect of age on LFS for good-risk patients receiving allogeneic marrow transplantation from an HLA-identical sibling for early leukemia. (Data from the International Bone Marrow Transplant Registry.)

should be transplanted only after relapse, unless there are poor-risk cytogenetics or an antecedent hematologic disorder. Further studies are required to identify prognostic factors that allow selection of patients who would be best treated with either chemotherapy or bone marrow transplantation. Alternatively, assays to detect minimal numbers of leukemia cells may allow selection of patients at high risk to relapse and may guide selection of therapy.

Autologous bone marrow transplantation has been evaluated as an approach to AML patients who lack an HLA-identical donor. Patients undergo procurement and cryopreservation of bone marrow cells while in remission. They may then receive similar marrow ablative chemoradiotherapy followed by reinfusion of the cryopreserved hematopoietic cells to restore hematopoiesis. The major limitation is the high likelihood that the *remission* bone marrow may be contaminated by small numbers of leukemic cells, which would be cryopreserved and reinfused with the autologous marrow. For patients with a cytogenetic marker, cytogenetics should be run immediately before cryopreservation of hematopoietic cells. The autologous marrow would not be likely to mediate the favorable GVL effect as described for allogeneic transplantation, making eradication of the systemic leukemia in the patient more difficult.

For patients receiving autologous marrow transplants while in relapse,[25, 26] the major problem has been rapid relapse of leukemia; the median duration of remission has been 3 to 5 months, and less than 10% of patients survived 1 year. Better results have occurred with autologous marrow transplantation in patients in first or second remission. Relapse of leukemia remains a major problem, but approximately 20 to 40% of patients transplanted in second remission have achieved greater than 2-year disease-free survival. These data indicate that this approach can be successful and that relapse of leukemia may not invariably occur.

A number of techniques have been explored to deplete occult leukemic cells from the harvested bone marrow in vitro before cryopreservation. Immunologic approaches using anti-AML monoclonal antibodies or pharmacologic agents, such as 4-hydroperoxycyclophosphamide or mafosfamide, have been studied. Although some of the best results are reported in series using purged marrow, no controlled studies have been done, and the efficacy of purging remains to be determined. After autotransplantation, patients may relapse from leukemia cells that survive the systemic high-dose chemotherapy or from leukemia cells present in the transplanted marrow. Studies in which the autologous marrow was marked in vitro using a retrovirus showed the presence of the marker within leukemia cells after relapse, demonstrating that malignant cells present in the autologous marrow infusion can contribute to relapse. Development of effective purging techniques is probably necessary.

Novel agents under evaluation potentially to improve antileukemic efficacy include the use of etoposide in the preparative regimen. The use of radionuclide-conjugated antimyeloid monoclonal antibodies or bone-seeking radioconjugates can target the malignant cells or marrow with little systemic toxicity.

For relapsed AML patients lacking a sibling or syngeneic donor, whether to pursue an unrelated donor transplant, haploidentical transplant, or autologous transplant depends on circumstances. Autologous transplant should be considered only in patients who are in a well-established remission and in whom the autologous progenitor cells were harvested during remission documented by cytogenetics and molecular assays. Because it often takes 2 to 6 months to identify an unrelated donor and procure marrow, the patient's disease status must allow this lead time. Unrelated cord blood can be obtained more quickly but is not an optimal option for adults because of the high graft failure rate. Aggressively T cell–depleted haploidentical bone marrow transplantation can salvage 20 to 30% of relapsed AML patients. To achieve this success rate with haploidentical bone marrow transplantation, the cell-processing laboratory needs to have technology available to reduce T cells by 4 to 5 logs, while still infusing greater than 6 million CD34$^+$ cells/kg.

## ACUTE LYMPHOBLASTIC LEUKEMIA

Bone marrow transplantation is an effective treatment for ALL. Recipients have usually received preparative regimens of high-dose cyclophosphamide with or without other chemotherapy and total-body irradiation (7.5 to 10 Gy) in a single dose or 15 Gy in fractionated schedules. Results are summarized in Table 16–4.

Because most newly diagnosed children and many adults with ALL achieve prolonged remission with conventional chemotherapy, transplantation has generally been reserved for patients after relapse. The prognosis with standard-dose chemotherapy for patients with bone marrow relapse depends on the duration of first remission. Longer initial remissions are associated with a higher probability of achieving a second remission and longer second remissions. The GVL effect is less in ALL than in AML and CML. The rarity of allogeneic donor lymphocyte infusion restoring donor chimera after ALL relapses supports this premise. Patients with active leptomeningeal leukemia should have the disease treated before transplant.

Studies in children with ALL in second remission report a 5-year disease-free survival of 40 to 64%.[27, 28] Prognostic factors at diagnosis and the length of initial remission correlate with the risk of relapse after a transplant in second remission in most but not all studies. The International Bone Marrow Transplant Registry compared results of chemotherapy and bone marrow transplantation in children with ALL treated while in second remission. Transplants were superior to chemotherapy in children relapsing within 18 months of achieving the first remission. Persons relapsing at 18 to 36 months showed a slight but insignificant advantage with bone marrow transplantation. Children relapsing more than

*Table 16–4.* **Approximate Percentage Survival at 5 Years or Longer in Acute Lymphoblastic Leukemia with Bone Marrow Transplantation or Conventional Chemotherapy**

|  | BMT (%) | Chemotherapy (%) |
| --- | --- | --- |
| First remission | 40–60 | 20–60 |
| Second remission | 30–50 | <10 |
| Third remission | 25 | 0 |
| Relapse | 10–20 | 0 |

BMT, bone marrow transplantation.

36 months after achieving remission or after completing maintenance chemotherapy had similar results with both therapies. Adults with recurrent ALL have a poor prognosis with chemotherapy and should probably receive a transplant in second remission if a suitable donor is available[29]; their anticipated long-term survival is 20 to 30%.

An important clinical question is which patients, if any, should receive bone marrow transplants while in first remission. Children with standard-risk ALL have a good prognosis with chemotherapy alone and should not be considered. The aforementioned advances in chemotherapy for high-risk children with ALL result in extended survival in about 70%. Consequently, it is reasonable to postpone transplantation in these patients until after relapse. Possible exceptions are children younger than 6 months old or those with deleterious cytogenetic abnormalities of t(9:22) or t(4:11); these patients have an extremely poor prognosis.

Several centers have initiated trials of marrow transplantation in high-risk adult patients in first remission. Preliminary results indicate relapse rates of 20 to 30% and disease-free survival of approximately 33 to 75% at 3 years. Patient age, initial white blood cell count, lactate dehydrogenase concentration, B-cell or T-cell surface phenotype, and cytogenetic data have been used as prognostic factors. Improved results have been reported, with intensive induction and maintenance chemotherapy regimens producing a 5-year disease-free survival of 30 to 50% of adults or children with poor prognostic features, with the exception of patients with t(9:22) or t(4:11).[30–32] Survival data from the International Bone Marrow Transplant Registry are summarized in Figure 16–5. Because of the considerable variability in the results of both chemotherapy and bone marrow transplantation in high-risk ALL, it is not possible to analyze critically their relative efficacy. Controlled clinical trials are required with patients carefully stratified for known prognostic factors.

Adults with the Philadelphia chromosome are best treated in first remission with allogeneic transplantation, with results ranging from 33 to 60% disease-free survival.[33, 34]

Recurrent leukemia is a major problem in patients with ALL after bone marrow transplantation. Approaches to overcoming this problem include the use of high-dose fractionated radiation, high-dose cytarabine, etoposide, or other chemotherapeutic agents and the use of post-transplant treatment. Intentional induction of limited GVHD has also been attempted to provide an additional antileukemia effect. None of these approaches has been convincingly shown to reduce the relapse rate or to improve survival in controlled trials.

Autologous bone marrow transplantation has also been evaluated in patients with ALL. In contrast to the situation in AML, a number of monoclonal antibodies to leukemia-associated antigens are available in ALL that are nonreactive with normal hematopoietic progenitors. These include antibodies to the common ALL antigen (CALLA) or a number of T-cell or B-cell antigens. Many patients have received autologous transplants using bone marrow that was treated ex vivo with one or more of these antibodies and complement. Although each of these antigens is expressed on subpopulations of normal lymphoid cells, they are not present on hematopoietic progenitors, and engraftment and immunologic recovery have consistently occurred. Limitations to this technique include probable antigenic heterogeneity among neoplastic cells, and it is unclear if leukemic stem cells express these cell surface antigens. Although selected patients with ALL in second remission have achieved prolonged remissions after receiving intensive chemotherapy, total-body irradiation, and autologous marrow transplantation using anti-CALLA antibody and complement-treated marrow, most autologous transplants have results with long-term survival of 20% or less.[35, 36] These data are difficult to

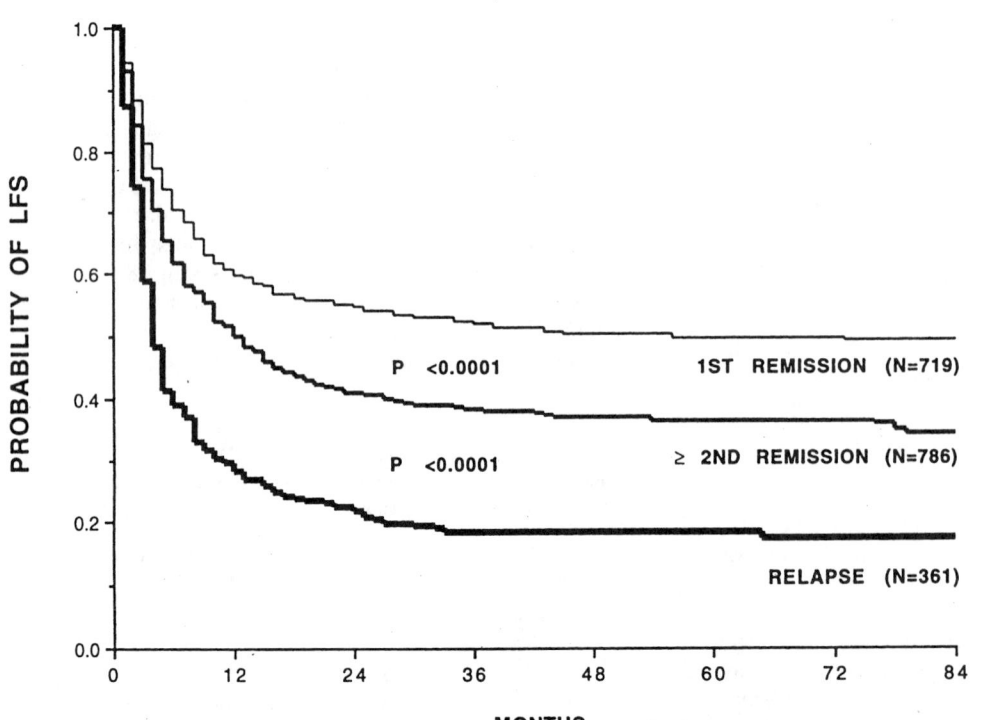

**Figure 16–5.** LFS after allogeneic bone marrow transplantation for patients with acute lymphoblastic leukemia (ALL). (Data from the International Bone Marrow Transplant Registry.)

interpret because many of the successful cases involved patients with a relatively good prognosis with conventional treatment, such as patients who relapse after a long first remission and in whom maintenance therapy has been discontinued. Results in patients with average or poor prognostic features have been much less encouraging.

## CHRONIC MYELOGENOUS LEUKEMIA

CML is a hematologic malignancy characterized by excessive clonal proliferation of myeloid cells and their progenitors. In greater than 90% of cases, the Philadelphia chromosome (t(9:22)) is a marker of the malignant clone. The disease can be divided into two phases, an initial *chronic phase*, in which cell maturation is normal, followed by transformation to an *acute phase* (blast crisis), characterized by maturation arrest at the level of the myeloblast or lymphoblast. Some patients develop a transient *accelerated phase* before the development of overt blast crisis.

Allogeneic or syngeneic bone marrow transplantation is an effective treatment for CML, capable of producing long-term disease-free survival. Approximately 20% of syngeneic recipients transplanted in blast crisis have survived free of disease greater than 5 years, demonstrating that the intensive marrow-ablative therapy can eradicate even far-advanced disease in some patients.[37] Better results have been reported for patients receiving allogeneic or syngeneic bone marrow transplantation while in the chronic phase, with an actuarial survival of 65% at more than 5 years. If the transplant is performed within 1 to 2 years of diagnosis from an allogeneic HLA genotypically identical sibling donor, survival is 80 to 90%.[38, 39]

More than 4000 patients with CML have received allogeneic marrow transplantation from an HLA-identical sibling donor. Survival data are summarized in Figure 16-6. Most patients have received high-dose cyclophosphamide and total-body irradiation as the antileukemic preparative regimen before bone marrow transplantation. The combination of busulfan and cyclophosphamide without radiotherapy appears equally effective. In a phase III trial, patients with CML in the chronic phase up to age 55 with an HLA-identical sibling were randomized to receive a preparative regimen of either cyclophosphamide and 12-Gy fractionated total-body irradiation or busulfan and cyclophosphamide. With a median follow-up of 2 years, approximately 80% of patients in both arms were alive, with a relapse rate of approximately 10%.[40] The new intravenous busulfan has far less toxicity with the lack of erratic oral absorption and is preferable to oral busulfan. Intravenous busulfan has not been compared with total-body irradiation plus cyclophosphamide. It has not been possible to improve the antileukemic efficacy of the preparative regimen with additional systemic chemotherapy or radiation without a concomitant increase in toxicity.

Although most patients achieve a complete hematologic and cytogenetic remission from the marrow-ablative preparatory regimen, overall results depend on the stage of the disease at the time of transplantation. For patients undergoing bone marrow transplantation during blast crisis, approximately 10 to 20% become long-term survivors and remain in continuous complete remission. Patients who are in the accelerated phase have approximately a 35% chance of 5-year disease-free survival, whereas patients undergoing transplantation in the chronic phase have a 50 to 85% chance of long-term disease-free survival. The major cause of treatment failure for patients with advanced CML is leukemia relapse. Patients transplanted in blast crisis have a 60% relapse rate, compared with 20% for patients in the chronic phase.

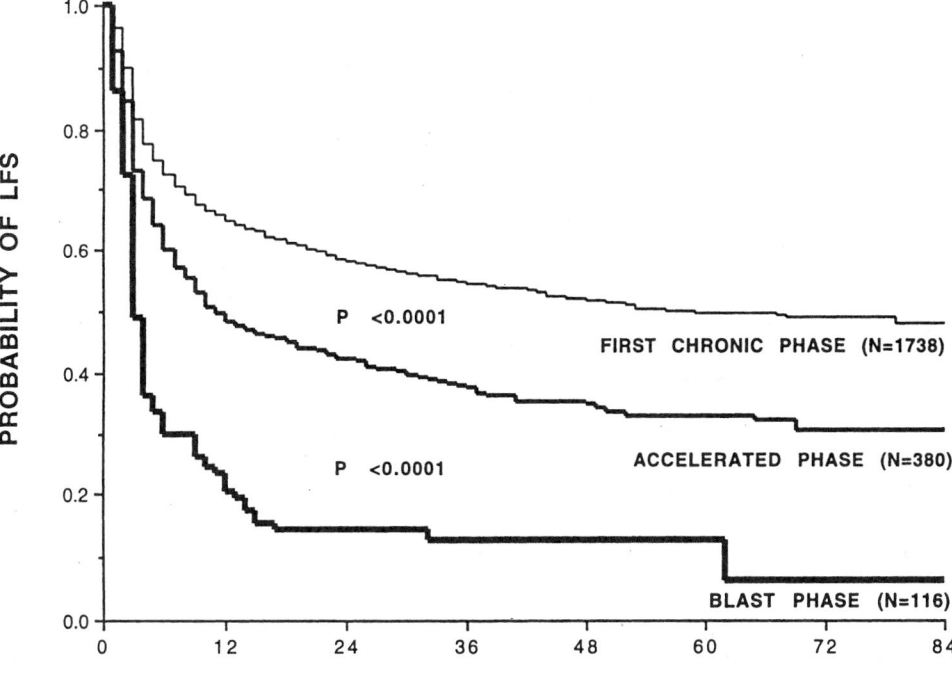

**Figure 16-6.** LFS after allogeneic bone marrow transplantation for patients with chronic myelogenous leukemia (CML). (Data from the International Bone Marrow Transplant Registry.)

The major limitation of allogeneic bone marrow transplantation is the risk of transplant-related complications. The high-dose chemotherapy and radiation preparative regimens are sufficiently immunosuppressive that graft rejection is rare with transplantation of unmodified HLA-matched marrow. Acute GVHD is a major problem, however, occurring in 20 to 35% of patients receiving combination post-transplant immunosuppressive therapy. Life-threatening, regimen-related toxicity and infectious complications may occur. Of patients, 20 to 30% have died from treatment-related complications within 6 months of the procedure.

Clonal evolution, the development of additional chromosome abnormalities in patients with chronic-phase CML, often precedes clinical features of transformation. The presence of an additional Philadelphia chromosome, or trisomy 8, or deletion of a fragment of 17q in bone marrow transplantation recipients has been associated with a worse prognosis with nontransplant therapies and an increased risk of relapse after transplantation. In other studies, clonal evolution as an isolated finding has not had prognostic implications for bone marrow transplantation.

Splenomegaly is a characteristic feature in CML and a major site of disease involvement. The presence of marked splenomegaly at diagnosis is reported to be an adverse prognostic factor after bone marrow transplantation, and some investigators have recommended pretransplant splenectomy or splenic radiation to eliminate a potential site of residual disease. The presence of splenomegaly at the time of bone marrow transplantation, however, has not been associated with a greater risk of relapse. Marked splenomegaly at the time of transplantation can impair the response to platelet transfusions and delay the time to hematologic recovery. Prior splenectomy is associated with a shorter interval to engraftment but possibly a higher risk of GVHD. Routine use of splenectomy is recommended only for patients with marked splenomegaly or hypersplenism.

Myelofibrosis is a poor prognostic feature associated with accelerated CML. This myelofibrosis can be reversed by allogeneic bone marrow transplantation. The presence of myelofibrosis prolongs the interval to hematologic recovery and increases the risk of graft failure.

The major prognostic factors predicting transplant outcome are stage of the disease, age, interval from diagnosis to transplant, and HLA compatibility between donor and recipient. Patients transplanted in the first two decades of life have superior survival than older recipients. Allogeneic bone marrow transplantation offers the only potential for long-term control of the disease and makes this a reasonable treatment option even for patients in their 40s. This effect of interval from diagnosis to bone marrow transplantation was due to a lower risk of treatment-related mortality and a lower relapse rate. Prior therapy with busulfan was also associated with a greater risk of transplant-related mortality than the use of hydroxyurea.

The best results of allogeneic bone marrow transplantation have been achieved in patients during the early chronic phase. If a transplant is to be performed, delaying the procedure in a clinically stable patient can only increase the risk of treatment failure. The risks and potential benefits of early bone marrow transplantation must be balanced against the risk of delaying the treatment, that is, transformation to blast crisis. Given the risk of transplant-related complications, some patients have opted to delay transplantation. There are, however, no reliable tests to detect imminent transformation of the leukemia, and results are clearly inferior if transplantation is performed after the development of the accelerated phase or a blast crisis.

The alternatives to transplantation remain alfa-interferon–based approaches. Approximately 30% of newly diagnosed patients achieve a complete hematologic and cytogenetic remission if alfa-interferon is given in conjunction with cytarabine; median duration of survival exceeds 8 years among respondents.[41] A randomized French trial demonstrated improved survival with the combination.[42] These data using alfa-interferon in patients with early chronic-phase CML have prompted some centers to delay the use of bone marrow transplantation in older adults for approximately 6 months to 1 year to allow for a trial of alfa-interferon. Patients failing to have hematologic control and patients without a complete cytogenetic remission within this interval could then be referred for allogeneic bone marrow transplantation. This approach delays incurring the risks associated with bone marrow transplantation, and a small fraction of patients achieve remissions exceeding 5 years with alfa-interferon alone. The concern with this approach is progression of the CML while receiving alfa-interferon therapy, which would compromise the success of subsequent bone marrow transplantation. Because the interval from diagnosis to bone marrow transplantation is an important prognostic factor, this approach may potentially have an adverse effect on the rate of long-term survival. In a preliminary analysis at the M.D. Anderson Cancer Center, prior alfa-interferon therapy did not lead to a greater risk of graft failure, GVHD, or other transplant complications in HLA-identical sibling transplants.[43] This situation may be different in recipients of unrelated or mismatched related donor transplants because some preliminary data implicate alfa-interferon with increasing HLA expression on selected organ tissues. The Seattle program showed best results in unrelated transplant recipients, younger than age 32 with an HLA-A, HLA-B, HLA-C, HLA-DR, HLA-DQ molecularly matched donor. In that group of patients, survival with unrelated donor transplant was 85% if done within 1 year of diagnosis with less than 6 months of alfa-interferon. If greater than 6 months of alfa-interferon was given, survival dropped to 55%. For older patients or patients with a less well-matched donor, survival was poorer. Another series showed improved results in patients who received alfa-interferon for greater than 6 months. For patients younger than age 32 for whom a completely molecularly matched unrelated donor can be identified, it is reasonable to pursue a transplant or alfa-interferon shortly after diagnosis. Older CML chronic-phase patients or those for whom only a mismatched donor can be identified should receive a trial of alfa-interferon and cytarabine.

Considerable data indicate that the high-dose preparative regimen does not completely eliminate all malignant cells in patients with CML and that an important GVL effect is necessary to prevent relapse. Most patients have small numbers of Philadelphia chromosome–positive cells identified by cytogenetics or by polymerase chain reaction analysis for bcr gene rearrangement. Many patients receiving unmodified transplants have remained in hematologic remission, and the Philadelphia chromosome–positive cells may spontaneously disappear in later analyses. In recipients of T cell–depleted marrow, however, greater than 90% of patients with cytogenetic relapse progress to an overt clinical relapse.[44, 45] These data support the concept that the GVL effect is largely mediated by alloreactive T cells present in donor marrow. Infusion of donor T lymphocytes can ultimately salvage 90% of CML patients relapsing in a chronic phase. Typically, these cells are collected in one to two leukophereses. The optimal dose in HLA-identical siblings is $1 \times 10^7$ CD3$^+$ cells/kg. The response for conversion of patients to donor hematopoiesis takes about 3 to 12 months. Patients typically become cytopenic 4 to 6 weeks after infusion of the donor lymphocytes. The long duration before a response is seen is probably why this approach works best in indolent disease, such as CML in chronic phase, myeloma, and chronic lymphocytic leukemia (CLL), and less well in AML and is rarely effective in ALL. GVHD can occur with donor lymphocyte infusions and is a major risk if the donor is more of a mismatch from the patient than an HLA-identical sibling.

Autologous transplants for CML involve collection and cryopreservation of bone marrow or peripheral blood stem cells during the chronic phase of the disease. Patients later receive intensive chemotherapy alone or combined with total-body irradiation, followed by reinfusion of cryopreserved autologous cells. The objective of this approach is to restore the early chronic phase and, if possible, diploid hematopoiesis. Because Philadelphia chromosome–positive cells are reinfused, cure is not possible. Some patients have transiently recovered apparently normal hematopoiesis without the Philadelphia chromosome. The Philadelphia chromosome–positive leukemia cells, however, almost always become dominant again within a short interval, and the disease recurs. A major limitation of autotransplantation for advanced CML is resistance of the acute-phase cells to intensive chemoradiotherapy. Another approach has been to attempt to collect autologous marrow or blood progenitor cells when they contain predominantly diploid cells. Marrow is harvested from patients in a partial or complete cytogenetic remission after alfa-interferon or intensive chemotherapy. The cells may be treated in vitro to separate normal from leukemic cells by a variety of developmental approaches, including separation on the basis of HLA-DR expression or with treatment in long-term culture. Gene-marking studies have shown that CML cells collected and cryopreserved as part of a harvest can contribute to relapse. Although most patients transplanted with autografts in the accelerated phase or blast crisis achieve a brief second chronic phase, the median duration is only 4 months, and less than 30% survive 1 year. This therapy must be considered of marginal benefit and cannot be routinely recommended. There have been some attempts to prolong the duration of the chronic phase by performing autotransplants in patients still in the chronic phase using bone marrow collected in cytogenetic remission or the early chronic phase. Results have not been encouraging.

## CHRONIC LYMPHOCYTIC LEUKEMIA

CLL is the most prevalent form of leukemia. It is a clonal disorder with proliferation and accumulation of small lymphocytes, usually of B-cell lineage. The disease has an indolent natural history but is incurable with available treatments. Historically, few marrow transplants have been performed in this disease because CLL primarily affects the elderly, and the marrow is heavily involved with malignant cells, precluding autologous transplantation. CLL is generally sensitive to alkylating agents and radiation; their use is limited by myelosuppression. High-dose cyclophosphamide, total-body irradiation, and allogeneic bone marrow transplantation have been effective in producing prolonged disease-free survival in selected younger patients with this disease. This disease has been sensitive to less intensive nonablative regimens using fludarabine and cyclophosphamide followed by allogeneic hematopoietic progenitor cells. CLL is also responsive to donor lymphocytes for treatment of relapse after allogeneic bone marrow transplantation.

A number of developments have allowed the evaluation of bone marrow transplantation in patients with CLL. Fludarabine (9-β-D-arabinofuranosyl-2-fluoroadenine monophosphate) has been established as an effective agent for the management of CLL. About 35% of patients treated with fludarabine achieve a complete or nodular complete remission, allowing autologous bone marrow harvest and transplantation. Responding patients have a time to progression of 21 months, and all ultimately relapse.

The technology for depletion of malignant leukemia cells (i.e., purging) has become available to deplete small numbers of residual leukemia cells present in the autologous marrow. Autologous bone marrow transplantation using monoclonal antibody–purged autologous marrow has been evaluated, producing complete remissions in patients with advanced disease. The responses here have been far less durable than the allogeneic transplant. If an allogeneic donor, related or unrelated, can be identified, this is the preferable treatment option.

## LYMPHOMA

Syngeneic, allogeneic, and autologous marrow transplants have been studied in patients with non-Hodgkin's lymphoma. Autologous bone marrow transplantation has been extensively studied in patients with relapsed or resistant large cell lymphoma and immunoblastic lymphoma. Patients have received intensive chemotherapy alone, such as BEAC (BCNU, etoposide, ara-C, cyclophosphamide), or cyclophosphamide plus total-body irradiation–based regimens. Results have been highly variable. Most patients achieve complete remission with this treatment, and approximately 20 to 60% of patients have survived in remission for several years. The Parma study was a randomized trial comparing standard salvage chemotherapy in first-relapse large cell lymphoma with standard chemotherapy plus autologous bone marrow transplantation. Only after 7 years of follow-up, the bone marrow transplantation–treated patients showed significantly better survival rates than those treated with standard chemotherapy. The best results have been noted in patients treated in a second remission or with a relapse that is still responsive to chemotherapy. Encouraging results have been reported in patients receiving autologous transplants in partial remission after initial induction therapy for large cell lymphoma. Toxicity has been a major problem, particularly in heavily pretreated and debilitated patients, and severe hepatic, cardiac, and pulmonary toxicity may occur. Allogeneic bone marrow transplantation was less preferred for large cell and immunoblastic lymphoma. For patients with marrow involvement or for those whose disease is refractory to standard chemotherapy, allogeneic bone marrow transplantation can still salvage 33% of patients. For patients with chemotherapy-responsive disease or in an advanced remission, allogeneic transplants result in a 60% survival rate. Whether an allogeneic-matched sibling transplant is preferable over an autologous transplant remains debatable. Lymphoblastic lymphoma has not been well studied in the bone marrow transplantation literature. Most have been transplanted after recurrence as ALL. For this population, allogeneic bone marrow transplantation is preferable to autologous bone marrow transplantation. For lymphoblastic lymphoma not relapsing as ALL, there are insufficient data to recommend autologous or allogeneic transplant. Burkitt's lymphoma and leukemia have not been responsive to an allogeneic GVL effect. Autologous bone marrow transplantation has been successful but only in remission. For Burkitt's lymphoma, preparative regimens should preferably contain cyclophosphamide. Mantle cell lymphoma, an aggressive lymphoma, has proved to be resistant to standard chemotherapy. Allogeneic bone marrow transplantation has shown a 90% survival rate in patients transplanted after their first remission and 30% for patients transplanted during relapse. Autologous bone marrow transplantation has been successful in first remission with a 75% long-term remission. Beyond first remission, autologous bone marrow transplantation has been less successful for mantle cell lymphoma.

Autologous transplantation has been evaluated for patients with low-grade lymphoma. Low-grade lymphomas are generally sensitive to alkylating agents and radiation. Effective use of these agents in conventional therapy is limited by myelosuppression. One concern in applying autologous bone marrow transplantation to patients with low-grade lymphoid malignancies is the propensity of these diseases to involve the bone marrow as part of their natural history. Techniques have been developed for selectively purging malignant lymphoid cells from normal bone marrow cells using ex vivo treatment with monoclonal antibodies against lymphoid cell surface antigens that do not cross-react with normal hematopoietic progenitors. Normal bone marrow cells can be separated from malignant B cells using monoclonal antibody and complement treatment or immunomagnetic beads. Many centers employ ex vivo treatment of the harvested autologous marrow to deplete malignant cells. For clinical bone marrow harvests, purging techniques generally achieve approximately a 2- to 3-log reduction of malignant cells, and these systems cannot effectively deplete cells from patients with clinically involved marrow. Gribben and colleagues[46] reported significantly better disease-free survival in patients receiving autologous transplants that were successfully purged free of evidence of residual lymphoma by *bcl-2* gene rearrangement by the polymerase chain reaction. Similar to CLL, low-grade lymphomas have proven sensitive to allogeneic transplants. Results have shown a 60% 5-year disease survival, even in refractory patients. The indolent nature of this disease allows donor lymphocyte infusions to be a treatment after relapse following allogeneic bone marrow transplantation. Allogeneic transplant is now the preferred option for low-grade lymphoma given the difficulty in purging lymphoma cells from the marrow or peripheral blood.

## HODGKIN'S LYMPHOMA

Despite combination chemotherapy and radiation treatment, many patients with Hodgkin's lymphoma fail to achieve a durable complete remission. Patients with recurrent disease may respond to additional standard-dose chemotherapy, but most ultimately die of the disease. High-dose chemotherapy and autologous bone marrow transplantation is an effective treatment capable of producing sustained remissions in selected high-risk patients with Hodgkin's lymphoma and is widely considered as the treatment of choice for patients who fail to respond durably to systemic chemotherapy.

Patients with systemic relapse after combination chemotherapy, such as MOPP (mechlorethamine, vincristine [Oncovin], procarbazine, prednisone), with a first remission duration greater than 12 months can be retreated with MOPP with a complete response rate greater than 90%,[47] although most of these patients ultimately relapse.[48] The prognosis is worse for those relapsing within 1 year; salvage chemotherapy with MOPP, ABVD (doxorubicin [Adriamycin], bleomycin, vinblastine, dacarbazine), or comparable regimens produces only a 29 to 50% complete response rate, and less than 20% remain disease-free at 5 years.[49, 50] In addition to a long disease-free interval, favorable prognostic features include good performance status, involvement of a limited number of nodal sites, absence of visceral disease, and absence of B symptoms. For patients in a second systemic relapse, long-term disease-free survival with conventional chemotherapy is rare.

For patients with recurrent Hodgkin's lymphoma, treatment with high-dose chemotherapy or chemotherapy and total-body irradiation with autologous bone marrow transplantation results in a complete remission rate of greater than 50 to 80% and a 20 to 60% disease-free survival at 3 to 5 years.[51–55] Although no controlled trials have been reported, results in patients with initial remissions of less than 1 year appear superior to those reported with standard-dose salvage chemotherapy. Controversy remains regarding the selection of patients for autologous bone marrow transplantation as well as defining the most effective preparative regimen.

Initial studies used cyclophosphamide in combination with total-body irradiation. Total-body irradiation is not an ideal treatment for Hodgkin's lymphoma; it is not possible to administer whole-body doses greater than 15 Gy in humans, and radiation doses exceeding 40 Gy are necessary to control active sites of disease when treated with local radiation therapy. Patients with Hodgkin's lymphoma frequently receive mediastinal radiation as part of their initial therapy; these patients have a high rate of radiation pneumonitis if they are later treated with total-body irradiation. High-dose chemotherapy regimens have been better tolerated. The most commonly used regimens involve a nitrosourea, alkylating agents, and etoposide. The CBV regimen (cyclophosphamide, BCNU, and etoposide [VP-16]) has been the most frequently used. The doses employed have varied widely from center to center: cyclophosphamide, 4.5 to 6.0 g/m$^2$; BCNU, 300 to 600 mg/m$^2$; and etoposide, 1200 to 2400 mg/m$^2$. With increasing dose, there is an increased rate of extramedullary toxicity, and treatment-related mortality has varied from 5 to greater than 20%. It is unclear if the higher dose regimens result in superior long-term disease-free survival. Other regimens have been studied, but there is no evidence that any are superior to CBV.

Prognostic factors for response and survival after autologous bone marrow transplantation include age, performance status, disease stage at transplantation, number of extranodal sites, number of prior treatment regimens, and response to prior chemotherapy and radiation treatment. These factors are similar to prognostic factors for patients receiving salvage chemotherapy. Patients with all favorable prognostic features have greater than 70% disease-free survival at 4 years compared with approximately 20% for patients with adverse prognostic factors.[54] These patient-related and disease-related factors have such a major impact on response and survival that it is difficult to compare treatment regimens between centers or in different subsets of patients in which prognostic features vary or are not well defined. It is also difficult to compare autologous marrow transplantation with salvage chemotherapy because of differences in eligibility, patient selection, time censoring, and prognostic factors.

The optimal roles and interaction of salvage chemotherapy and autologous bone marrow transplantation are uncertain. Some centers have performed autologous transplantation as the first treatment of relapse. Others have instituted several courses of a salvage chemotherapy program, such as DHAP (dexamethasone, high-dose ara-C, cisplatin [Platinol]), with collection of the autologous marrow between courses and institution of the dose-intensive therapy with autologous bone marrow transplantation after achieving maximal cytoreduction with the salvage regimen. This latter approach has the appeal of providing treatment immediately after relapse, collecting the marrow between courses, and employing the high-dose regimen at the time of minimal tumor burden.

Allogeneic bone marrow transplantation has the potential advantage that the donor bone marrow is unambiguously free of malignant cells, and the donor-derived lymphoid cells may have an immunotherapeutic effect, analogous to GVL. Allogeneic bone marrow transplantation is, however, associated with a greater risk of morbidity and mortality because of the immunologic complications of the procedure, graft rejection, GVHD, post-transplant immunodeficiency, and infections resulting in treatment-related mortality in approximately 40% of patients. Relatively few allogeneic transplants have been performed in patients with Hodgkin's lymphoma. Studies in patients with advanced disease probably not suitable for autologous transplantation have a 15 to 20% salvage rate with HLA-matched sibling bone marrow transplantation. It is difficult to draw firm conclusions because of patient selection and differences in prognostic features, but most centers prefer to use autologous transplants because of the lower risk of treatment-related mortality.

## MULTIPLE MYELOMA

Autologous bone marrow transplantation is increasingly used to treat myeloma. A randomized trial showed an advantage of autologous bone marrow transplantation over standard chemotherapy. The preparative regimen studied was high-dose melphalan. Another randomized trial demonstrated better survival with two cycles than with one cycle of high-dose melphalan with peripheral blood progenitor cells. Autologous transplants have been associated with prolonged survival, but they rarely show prolonged progression-free survival. Autologous transplants have been studied for patients up to age 65 years. The patients most likely to benefit from autologous transplant are those treated for primary resistant disease or responding disease with low $\beta_2$-microglobulin and lactate dehydrogenase levels who are treated within 1 year of diagnosis.

Because myeloma is typically a disease of the elderly, only a small fraction can be considered for allogeneic bone marrow transplantation. Allogeneic bone marrow transplantation has been studied in selected young patients with multiple myeloma who have relapsed or progressed during standard chemotherapy. Patients have generally received high-dose melphalan and total-body irradiation or busulfan and cyclophosphamide–based preparative regimens. Most have achieved clinical remission with marked reduction or disappearance of the paraprotein, and approximately one third have survived 1 to 3 years free of relapse. Allogeneic transplants have been shown to rescue patients after relapse following autologous bone marrow transplantation. Patients with poor prognostic features, such as any abnormality of chromosome 13, should be considered for allogeneic bone marrow transplantation early in their treatment plan.

## PEDIATRIC SOLID TUMORS

Autologous bone marrow transplantation has been studied in the treatment of a range of pediatric solid tumors using cryopreserved bone marrow or peripheral blood hematopoietic stem cells. Marrow transplantation may be particularly useful in the treatment of several pediatric tumors, such as neuroblastoma and Ewing's sarcoma, which are highly sensitive to a number of chemotherapeutic agents and radiation yet have a poor prognosis in patients with advanced disease.

Patients with far advanced or recurrent neuroblastoma have a dismal prognosis with standard treatment. Several studies are currently in progress using high-dose, combined-modality therapy and allogeneic marrow transplantation or autologous marrow transplantation in these patients.[56–59] Neuroblastoma frequently involves the bone marrow. Monoclonal antibodies to neuroblastoma-related antigens can be used to detect microscopic bone marrow involvement and to purge metastatic neuroblastoma cells from the marrow before cryopreservation. Peripheral blood progenitor transplants have also been used, although tumor cells may contaminate blood. Gene-marking studies of autologous marrow demonstrate that malignant cells infused in the autotransplant can contribute to relapse. The most encouraging results have been reported with treatment of patients at an earlier point in their disease and with the use of more intensive pretransplant conditioning regimens involving combination chemotherapy and total-body irradiation and either allogeneic or autologous marrow transplantation.

Ewing's sarcoma is another potential candidate tumor for autologous bone marrow transplantation. It is responsive to chemotherapy and irradiation and rarely involves the bone marrow. High-dose melphalan or cyclophosphamide and total-body irradiation with autologous bone marrow transplantation can produce complete remissions in patients with relapsed Ewing's sarcoma, but these responses are usually brief. Intensive chemoradiotherapy with autologous bone marrow transplantation may be more effective in consolidation treatment as part of first-line therapy.

## BREAST CANCER

**Background.** Breast cancer has been the most common and most controversial disease treated by autologous transplantation. Most chemotherapeutic agents active against breast cancer exhibit a dose-dependent antitumor response; increasing dose results in increased cytotoxicity. The dose response of antimetabolites plateaus at the point of maximal inhibition of the targeted metabolic pathway, but DNA-damaging agents, such as alkylating agents and platinum derivatives, have increasing antitumor effects across a broad dosage range. The maximal dose of most agents is limited by myelosuppression. Dose escalation is possible, however, if followed by intravenous infusion of bone marrow or peripheral blood progenitors to regenerate hematopoiesis. The high-dose chemotherapy regimens used with autologous marrow or blood stem cell transplantation include combinations of alkylating agents and related drugs, such as cyclophosphamide, melphalan, thiotepa, carmustine, cisplatin, or carboplatin. Taxanes are now being studied in bone marrow transplantation preparative regimens. The doses of these agents can be typically increased threefold over standard doses when followed by autologous bone marrow or blood stem cell transplantation. In hematologic malignancies, dose-intensive therapy has been most effective in patients with a minimal burden of chemotherapy-sensitive tumor cells. This finding provides a theoretical rationale for the use of high-dose chemotherapy with hematopoietic support for the adjuvant therapy of breast cancer.

**Adjuvant Therapy.** The best results in nonrandomized trials of autologous transplants for patients with breast cancer have been as adjuvant therapy in patients with locoregional disease at high risk of relapse. High-dose chemotherapy combined with autologous bone marrow transplantation has been evaluated as an adjuvant therapy for patients with high-risk stage II and III disease. High-risk disease has generally been defined as stage II disease with 10 or more positive axillary nodes; stage III disease, particularly failures of neoadjuvant therapy; and inflammatory breast cancer. Five-year disease-free survival with standard adjuvant therapy ranges from 25 to 57% for these patients. In phase II studies of autologous transplant, approximately 50 to 85% of these high-risk patients survive free of relapse at 5 years.[60]

Three randomized studies in the adjuvant setting had preliminary data presented at a national meeting in 1999. One of these studies was subsequently discredited because of data falsification.[61] Two studies comparing transplant with standard chemotherapy regimens given for a prolonged course, beyond that which is currently used, did not show a survival advantage compared with transplant.[62, 63] One of these studies demonstrated a reduction in relapse rate that may translate into a future survival advantage.

One of the concerns of high-dose therapy is that it may increase the risk of therapy-related leukemia and myelodysplasia. The aforementioned studies demonstrated that this problem was more severe in patients receiving prolonged chemotherapy than in patients receiving a shorter duration of dose-intensive therapy, such as that used in transplantation. Follow-up of these studies has been short (2 to 3 years), however. Longer follow-up is clearly needed, possibly as long as 10 years.

**Transplantation for Metastatic Disease.** Studies in patients with chemotherapy-responsive metastatic breast cancer have documented that autologous transplantation significantly increases the complete response rate to greater than 50%. For patients with metastatic disease transplanted in complete remission, 20 to 40% have progression-free survival at 4 years, which is the best rate reported for patients with metastatic breast cancer. Favorable prognostic factors in these patients include responsiveness to standard-dose chemotherapy, limited tumor bulk and number of disease sites, absence of liver involvement, and good performance status. Another approach to transplantation for patients with advanced metastatic disease is allogeneic transplantation, which has the theoretical advantage over autologous transplantation of the graft-versus-tumor effect. Preliminary studies of this approach from the M.D. Anderson Hospital have demonstrated long-term responses in 20% of patients.[64] Despite these suggestive findings, the only randomized trial reported to date of high-dose chemotherapy followed by hematopoietic support versus standard chemotherapy has shown no significant difference in survival.[65]

## OTHER SOLID TUMORS

A similar approach with autologous bone marrow transplantation has been used for the treatment of other chemotherapy-responsive solid tumors in adults, including testicular and germ cell carcinomas, ovarian cancer, and small cell carcinoma of the lung. Testicular carcinoma is a chemotherapy-responsive malignancy that is frequently cured using standard-dose, cisplatin-based chemotherapy. Patients failing first-line and second-line chemotherapy regimens have received high-dose chemotherapy and autologous marrow transplants. Response rates are high, and a few have achieved long-term remissions; responses in most patients are usually of short duration. Patients have been generally heavily pretreated and debilitated and tolerate high-dose therapy poorly. Given the efficacy of standard chemotherapy in this disease, only a small fraction of patients is eligible for trials of autologous transplantation.

Dose-intensive chemotherapy is being increasingly used for treating ovarian cancer. Similar to breast cancer, this tumor is sensitive to alkylating agents, platinum-based chemotherapy agents and taxanes, and topoisomerase I inhibitors. Transplants have not been used commonly in the adjuvant setting but have a role for patients with low-bulk disease after a second-look laporatory and for patients with chemotherapy-sensitive low-bulk relapsed disease.

Autologous transplants have been extensively studied in small cell lung cancer using preparative regimens of chemotherapy alone or cyclophosphamide and total-body irradiation. Patients with extensive disease or relapsed carcinoma have generally had only brief responses and modest clinical benefit. In some studies, better results have been obtained as consolidation therapy for patients with limited small cell lung cancer with prolongation of remission duration. Few patients are long-term survivors, and the efficacy of this approach remains to be established. A number of malignancies that are poorly responsive to conventional treatment have been treated with high-dose chemotherapy and autologous marrow transplantation, including melanoma, colon and other gastrointestinal carcinomas, and non–small cell lung cancer. These patients have generally received escalated doses of single agents, such as melphalan or carmustine, or combinations of alkylating agents. This high-dose treatment has increased response rates, but these responses are usually brief, and it is unclear if overall survival is improved. Controlled clinical trials are required to assess the efficacy of this treatment approach versus conventional management of these patients.

Allogeneic transplantation is under investigation for patients with renal cell carcinoma and malignant melanoma. Successful treatment of a patient with metastatic renal cell carcinoma with a nonmyeloablative allogeneic peripheral blood progenitor-cell transplant was considered to be evidence for probable graft-versus-tumor effect.[66] Further study is needed before such a graft-versus-tumor effect can be considered an established benefit of allogeneic transplantation for patients with solid tumors.

## Future Directions

Important questions remain regarding the optimal use and the role of hematopoietic transplantation. The use of autologous bone marrow and blood stem cell transplantation should be restricted to cancer research centers, and all patients should be entered into ongoing clinical trials. Participation by all bone marrow transplantation patients in clinical trials is essential because this is a rapidly evolving technology. Blood and marrow transplantation is moving into a new regulatory environment. The U.S. Food and Drug Administration (FDA) has several regulatory measures under consideration. Health insurance payors are credentialing blood and marrow transplant physicians and facilities. Although there is no specific board in blood and marrow transplantation, physicians are generally boarded in hematology, oncology, immunology, or pediatric hematology-oncology. The community of marrow transplanters has set up the Foundation for the Accreditation of Hematopoietic and Cellular Transplant Centers (FAHCT) to inspect and accredit blood and marrow transplant centers. The FAHCT accreditation process credentials the physician, facility, and cell-processing laboratory as an integrated program providing this service. The American Association of Blood Banks is willing to inspect and credential just the cell-processing laboratory. The FAHCT and AABB hope their standards will meet or exceed all pending FDA regulations.

The cost of high-dose chemotherapy and bone marrow or peripheral blood stem cell transplantation is primarily related to the length of hospitalization for supportive care, blood product transfusions, and antibiotic treatment for granulocytopenic infections. The typical length of hospitalization is 3 to 5 weeks. There has been an effort to transfer a major portion of care to the outpatient clinic. Well-organized outpatient infusion centers can administer dose-intensive treatment to stable patients, and with rapid hematologic recovery induced by growth factors and peripheral blood progenitor cells, patients may not routinely require admission. Typically, bone marrow transplants are paid by case rate or a fixed payment. Although occasional transplants are denied as experimental, this is increasingly uncommon. The case rate payment has forced provider institutions to confront costs of complications. There is a movement to use less mucositis-producing chemotherapy agents because these often have prolonged inpatient hospitalization. With new antibiotics and hematopoietic growth factors, toxicities and costs are decreasing. Transplants are being done to cure cancer. Society does not want providers to forego using a drug that improves response and survival rate by 5 to 10% simply because it adds 2 to 3 days of hospitalization because of mucositis.

Improvement in the results of autologous bone marrow transplantation for solid tumors requires the development of more effective treatment regimens that are not excessively toxic to normal tissues. A number of chemotherapeutic agents can be escalated to two to five times their standard dosage in the setting of autologous marrow transplantation, including cyclophosphamide, melphalan, busulfan, carmustine, lomustine, mitomycin C, etoposide, and amsacrine. Further phase I and II clinical studies are required to determine the efficacy and nonhematopoietic toxicity of other chemotherapeutic agents in high doses. Candidate drugs should have documented efficacy in standard dosage, have toxicity limited primarily to the bone marrow, and lack substantial nonmarrow toxicity. Novel classes of drugs, including anthrapyrazoles, topoisomerase I inhibitors, and taxanes, have activity against many cancers and may be important components of future high-dose, combination-chemotherapy regimens. Targeted radiation therapy, such as monoclonal antibody–radionuclide immunoconjugates and bone-seeking isotopes such as holmium, are under active evaluation as a means to target radiotherapy to the tumor; this approach has little systemic toxicity other than myelosuppression, which can be ameliorated by autologous marrow or blood stem cell transplantation.

Dose intensity is important to achieve the maximal cytoreduction with available chemotherapeutic agents. It may be possible to improve results further using strategies to overcome drug resistance mechanisms, such as administration of inhibitors to P-glycoprotein or chemoprotectant agents.

Kinetic resistance and the presence of poorly vascularized tumor masses are factors that limit the effectiveness of a single course of high-dose chemotherapy. Greater overall dose intensity may be achieved by repeated courses of therapy. The ability to collect large numbers of marrow and peripheral blood hematopoietic cells allows the administration of two to four courses of treatment. Nonhematopoietic toxicity may be cumulative, and some dose reduction is necessary for multiple-course regimens to achieve optimal cytoreduction with acceptable toxicity.

The collection of bone marrow or peripheral blood hematopoietic cells offers the potential for ex vivo genetic therapy to improve treatment results. Transfection of genes for drug resistance, such as the multiple drug resistance gene (*mdr-1*), into normal marrow cells may allow better tolerance to subsequent chemotherapy with agents such as doxorubicin, vinca alkaloids, and paclitaxel (Taxol). Alternative strategies include transfecting cytokine genes into hematopoietic cells or directly into the malignant cells to enhance immune reactivity against the tumor. Animal models used to test tumor vaccines have shown better immune stimulators when administering a vaccine after high-dose therapy. No one has been able to explain this phenomenon, but it probably relates to the re-education of the system that occurs during what has been described as the recapitulation of immunologic ontogeny. Given these data as well as the well-described graft-versus-leukemia-lymphoma effect, several studies are underway with allogeneic transplants for solid tumors. Results are preliminary, but responses have been reported for breast cancer, renal cell carcinoma, and melanoma. Other efforts are underway to mimic an allogeneic transplant by doing immune stimulation in autologous transplant. Most often, this stimulation is done by incubating the hematopoietic progenitors with IL-2 and administering IL-2 after transplantation. Fundamentally, blood and marrow transplant is cellular therapy. In the allogeneic transplant setting, laboratory research efforts are underway to create and infuse antigen-specific immune cells that attack tumors and pathogens but spare the normal donor organs and tissues. Much research is under way to understand the cellular interaction observed in autologous and allogeneic bone marrow transplantation but, in particular, the graft-versus-tumor effect and effectors of GVHD. Future trials using gene therapy or immune modulation will manipulate these processes to try to improve the efficacy of transplantation to treat cancer.

## SUGGESTIONS FOR ADDITIONAL READING

Shea TC. Introduction: current issues in high-dose chemotherapy and stem cell support. Bone Marrow Transplant 1999;23:Suppl 2:S1–5.

Champlin R, Khouri I, Kornblau S, et al. Reinventing bone marrow transplantation: reducing toxicity using nonmyeloablative, preparative regimens and induction of graft-versus-malignancy. Curr Opin Oncol 1999;11:87–95.

Shpall EJ. The utilization of cytokines in stem cell mobilization strategies. Bone Marrow Transplant 1999;23:Suppl 20:S13–9.

Porter DL, Antin JH. The graft-versus-leukemia effects of allogeneic cell therapy. Annu Rev Med 1999;50:369–86.

Marks DI, Otton S, Williamson E, Bird JM. Unrelated donor bone marrow transplantation in adults: some current controversies. Leuk Lymphoma 1999;32:459–66.

Glaspy JA. Economic considerations in the use of peripheral blood progenitor cells to support high-dose chemotherapy. Bone Marrow Transplant 1999;23:Suppl 2:S21–7.

Gammie JS, Pham SM. Simultaneous donor bone marrow and cardiac transplantation: can tolerance be induced with the development of chimerism? Curr Opin Cardiol 1999;14:126–32.

## REFERENCES

1. Thomas E, Storb R, Clift RA, et al. Bone-marrow transplantation (first of two parts). N Engl J Med 1975;292:832–43.
2. Appelbaum FR, Herzig GP, Graw RG, et al. Study of cell dose and storage time on engraftment of cryopreserved autologous bone marrow in a canine model. Transplantation 1978;26:245–48.
3. Beatty PG, Dahlberg S, Mickelson EM, et al. Probability of finding HLA-matched unrelated marrow donors. Transplantation 1988; 45:714–8.
4. McDonald GB, Sharma P, Matthews DE, et al. The clinical course of 53 patients with venocclusive disease of the liver after marrow transplantation. Transplantation 1985;39:603–8.
5. Shulman HM, Hinterberger W. Hepatic veno-occlusive disease—liver toxicity syndrome after bone marrow transplantation. Bone Marrow Transplant 1992;10:197–214.
6. McDonald GB, Hinds MS, Fisher LD, et al. Veno-occlusive disease of the liver and multiorgan failure after bone marrow transplantation: a cohort study of 355 patients. Ann Intern Med 1993;118:255–67.
7. Weiner RS, Bortin MM, Gale RP, et al. Interstitial pneumonitis after bone marrow transplantation: assessment of risk factors. Ann Intern Med 1986;104:168–75.
8. Jochelson M, Tarbell NJ, Freedman AS, et al. Acute and chronic pulmonary complications following autologous bone marrow transplantation in non-Hodgkin's lymphoma. Bone Marrow Transplant 1990;6:329–31.
9. Jones RB, Matthes S, Shpall EJ, et al. Acute lung injury following treatment with high-dose cyclophosphamide, cisplatin, and carmustine: pharmacodynamic evaluation of carmustine. J Natl Cancer Inst 1993;85:640–7.
10. Nash RA, Pepe MS, Storb R, et al. Acute graft-versus-host disease: analysis of risk factors after allogeneic marrow transplantation and prophylaxis with cyclosporine and methotrexate. Blood 1992;80:1838–45.
11. Gale RP, Bortin MM, van Bekkum DW, et al. Risk factors for acute graft-versus-host disease. Br J Haematol 1987;67:397–406.
12. Storb R, Deeg, HJ, Whitehead J, et al. Methotrexate and cyclosporine compared with cyclosporine alone for prophylaxis of acute graft versus host disease after marrow transplantation for leukemia. N Engl J Med 1986;314:729–35.
13. Martin PJ, Schoch G, Fisher L, et al. A retrospective analysis of therapy for acute graft-versus-host disease: initial treatment. Blood 1990;76:1464–72.
14. Lapidot T, Lubin I, Terenzi A, et al. Enhancement of bone marrow allografts from nude mice into mismatched recipients by T cells void of graft-versus-host activity. Proc Natl Acad Sci U S A 1990;87:4595–9.
15. Shulman HM, Sullivan KM, Weiden PL, et al. Chronic graft-versus-host syndrome in man: a long-term clinicopathologic study of 20 Seattle patients. Am J Med 1980;69:204–17.
16. Sullivan KM, Agura E, Anasetti C, et al. Chronic graft-versus-host disease and other late complications of bone marrow transplantation. Semin Hematol 1991;28:250–9.
17. Ralph DD, Springmeyer SC, Sullivan KM, et al. Rapidly progressive air-flow obstruction in marrow transplant recipients: possible association between obliterative bronchiolitis and chronic graft-versus-host disease. Am Rev Respir Dis 1984;129:641–4.
18. Schwarer AP, Hughes JM, Trotman-Dickenson B, et al. A chronic pulmonary syndrome associated with graft-versus-host disease after allogeneic marrow transplantation. Transplantation 1992;54:1002–8.
19. Lum LG. The kinetics of immune reconstitution after human marrow transplantation. Blood 1987;69:369–80.
20. Keever CA, Small TN, Flomenberg N, et al. Immune reconstitution following bone marrow transplantation: comparison of recipients of T-cell depleted marrow with recipients of conventional marrow grafts. Blood 1989;73:1340–50.
21. Meyers JD. Prevention and treatment of cytomegalovirus infection after marrow transplantation. Bone Marrow Transplant 1988;3:95–104.
22. Fefer A, Cheever MA, Thomas ED, et al. Bone marrow transplantation for refractory acute leukemia in 34 patients with identical twins. Blood 1981;57:421–30.
23. Forman SJ, Schmidt GM, Nademanee AP, et al. Allogeneic bone marrow transplantation as therapy for primary induction failure for patients with acute leukemia. J Clin Oncol 1991;9:1570–4.
24. Biggs JC, Horowitz MM, Gale RP, et al. Bone marrow transplants may cure patients with acute leukemia never achieving remission with chemotherapy. Blood 1992;80:1090–3.
25. Dicke KA, Spitzer G. Evaluation of the use of high-dose cytoreduction with autologous marrow rescue in various malignancies. Transplantation 1986;41:4–20.
26. Gorin NC, David R, Stachowiak J, et al. High dose chemotherapy and autologous bone marrow transplantation in acute leukemias, malignant lymphomas and solid tumors: a study of 23 patients. Eur J Cancer 1981;17:557–68.

27. Sanders JE, Thomas ED, Buckner CD, Doney K. Marrow transplantation for children with acute lymphoblastic leukemia in second remission. Blood 1987;70:324–6.

28. Brochstein JA, Kernan NA, Groshen S, et al. Allogeneic bone marrow transplantation after hyperfractionated total-body irradiation and cyclophosphamide in children with acute leukemia. N Engl J Med 1987;317:1618–24.

29. Herzig RH, Bortin MM, Barrett AJ, et al. Bone-marrow transplantation in high-risk acute lymphoblastic leukaemia in first and second remission. Lancet 1987;1:786–9.

30. Gaynor J, Chapman D, Little C, et al. A cause-specific hazard rate analysis of prognostic factors among 199 adults with acute lymphoblastic leukemia: the Memorial Hospital experience since 1969 [published erratum appears in J Clin Oncol 1988;6:1522]. J Clin Oncol 1988;6:1014–30.

31. Hoelzer D, Thiel E, Löffler H, et al. Prognostic factors in a multicenter study for treatment of acute lymphoblastic leukemia in adults. Blood 1988;71:123–31.

32. Linker CA, Levitt LJ, O'Donnell M, et al. Improved results of treatment of adult acute lymphoblastic leukemia. Blood 1987;69:1242–8.

33. Forman SJ, O'Donnell MR, Nademanee AP, et al. Bone marrow transplantation for patients with Philadelphia chromosome-positive acute lymphoblastic leukemia. Blood 1987;70:587–8.

34. Barrett AJ, Horowitz MM, Ash RC, et al. Bone marrow transplantation for Philadelphia chromosome-positive acute lymphoblastic leukemia. Blood 1992;79:3067–70.

35. Kersey JH. The role of marrow transplantation in acute lymphoblastic leukemia. J Clin Oncol 1989;7:1589–90.

36. Billett AL, Kornmehl E, Tarbell NJ, et al. Autologous bone marrow transplantation after a long first remission for children with recurrent acute lymphoblastic leukemia. Blood 1993;81:1651–7.

37. Fefer A, Cheever MA, Greenberg PD, et al. Treatment of chronic granulocytic leukemia with chemoradiotherapy and transplantation of marrow from identical twins. N Engl J Med 1982;306:63–68.

38. Thomas ED, Clift RA, Fefer A, et al. Marrow transplantation for the treatment of chronic myelogenous leukemia. Ann Intern Med 1986;104:155–63.

39. Goldman JM. Bone marrow transplantation for chronic myelogenous leukemia. Curr Opin Oncol 1992;4:259–63.

40. Clift RA, Buckner CD, Thomas ED, et al. Marrow transplantation for patients in accelerated phase of chronic myeloid leukemia. Blood 1994;84:4368–73.

41. Talpaz M, Kantarjian H, Kurzrock R, et al. Interferon-alpha produces sustained cytogenetic responses in chronic myelogenous leukemia: Philadelphia chromosome-positive patients. Ann Intern Med 1991;114:532–8.

42. Guilhot F, Chastang C, Michallet M, et al. Interferon alfa-2b combined with cytarabine versus interferon alone in chronic myelogenous leukemia. French Chronic Myeloid Leukemia Study Group. N Engl J Med 1997;337:223–9.

43. Giralt SA, Kantarjian HM, Talpaz M, et al. Effect of prior interferon alfa therapy on the outcome of allogeneic bone marrow transplantation for chronic myelogenous leukemia. J Clin Oncol 1993;11:1055–61.

44. Arthur CK, Apperley JF, Guo AP, et al. Cytogenetic events after bone marrow transplantation for chronic myeloid leukemia in chronic phase. Blood 1988;71:1179–86.

45. Offit K, Burns JP, Cunningham I, et al. Cytogenetic analysis of chimerism and leukemia relapse in chronic myelogenous leukemia patients after T cell-depleted bone marrow transplantation. Blood 1990;75:1346–55.

46. Gribben JG, Freedman AS, Neuberg D, et al. Immunologic purging of marrow assessed by PCR before autologous bone marrow transplantation for B-cell lymphoma. N Engl J Med 1991;325:1525–33.

47. Rizzoli V, Mangoni L, Carlo-Stella C. Autologous bone marrow transplantation in acute myelogenous leukemia. Leukemia 1992;6:1101–6.

48. Longo DL, Duffey PL, Young RC, et al. Conventional-dose salvage combination chemotherapy in patients relapsing with Hodgkin's disease after combination chemotherapy: the low probability for cure. J Clin Oncol 1992;10:210–8.

49. Bergsagel DE. Salvage treatment for Hodgkin's disease in relapse. J Clin Oncol 1987;5:525–6.

50. Tannir N, Hagemeister F, Velasquez W, Cabanillas F. Long-term follow-up with ABDIC salvage chemotherapy of MOPP-resistant Hodgkin's disease. J Clin Oncol 1983;1:432–9.

51. Carella AM, Carlier P, Congiu A, et al. Nine years' experience with ABMT in 128 patients with Hodgkin's disease: an Italian study group report. Leukemia 1991;5:Suppl 1:68–71.

52. Phillips GL, Reece DE. Clinical studies of autologous bone marrow transplantation in Hodgkin's disease. Clin Haematol 1986;15:151–66.

53. Chopra R, Linch DC, McMillan AK, et al. Mini-BEAM followed by BEAM and ABMT for very poor risk Hodgkin's disease. Br J Haematol 1992;81:197–202.

54. Jagannath S, Armitage JO, Dicke KA, et al. Prognostic factors for response and survival after high-dose cyclophosphamide, carmustine, and etoposide with autologous bone marrow transplantation for relapsed Hodgkin's disease. J Clin Oncol 1989;7:179–85.

55. Vose JM, Armitage JO. Bone marrow transplantation for Hodgkin's disease and lymphoma. Annu Rev Med 1993;44:255–63.

56. August CS, Serota FT, Koch PA, et al. Treatment of advanced neuroblastoma with supralethal chemotherapy, radiation, and allogeneic or autologous marrow reconstitution. J Clin Oncol 1984;2:609–16.

57. Hartmann O, Valteau-Couanet D, Vassal G, et al. Prognostic factors in metastatic neuroblastoma in patients over 1 year of age treated with high-dose chemotherapy and stem cell transplantation: a multivariate analysis in 218 patients treated in a single institution. Bone Marrow Transplant 1999;23:789–95.

58. Ladenstein R, Philip T, Lasset C, et al. Multivariate analysis of risk factors in stage 4 neuroblastoma patients over the age of one year treated with megatherapy and stem-cell transplantation: a report from the European Bone Marrow Transplantation Solid Tumor Registry. J Clin Oncol 1998;16:953–65.

59. Seeger RC, Villablanca JG, Matthay KK, et al. Intensive chemoradiotherapy and autologous bone marrow transplantation for poor prognosis neuroblastoma. Prog Clin Biol Res 1991;366:527–33.

60. Peters WP, Ross M, Vredenburgh JJ, et al. High-dose chemotherapy and autologous bone marrow support as consolidation after standard-dose adjuvant therapy for high-risk primary breast cancer. J Clin Oncol 1993;11:1132–43.

61. Bezwoda WR. Randomized, controlled trial of high dose chemotherapy (HD-CNVp) versus standard dose (CAF) chemotherapy for high risk, surgically treated, primary breast cancer. Proc Am Soc Clin Oncol 1999;18:2a. study discredited because of data falsification. New York Times, February 5, 2000, p. A7.

62. The Scandinavian Breast Cancer Study Group 9401. Results from a randomized adjuvant breast cancer study with high dose chemotherapy with CTCb supported by autologous bone marrow stem cells versus dose escalated and tailored FEC therapy. Proc Am Soc Clin Oncol 1999;18:2a. abstract.

63. Peters W, Rosner G, Vredenburgh J, et al. A prospective, randomized comparison of two doses of combination alkylating agents (AA) as consolidation after CAF in high-risk primary breast cancer involving ten or more axillary lymph nodes (LN): preliminary results of CALGB 9082/SWOG 9114/NCIC MA-13. Proc Am Soc Clin Oncol 1999;18:1a. abstract.

64. Ueno N, Rondon G, Mirza N, et al. Allogeneic peripheral blood progenitor cell transplantation for poor-risk patients with metastatic breast cancer. J Clin Oncol 1998;16:986–93.

65. Stadtmauer EA, O'Neill A, Goldstein LJ, et al. Conventional-dose chemotherapy compared with high-dose chemotherapy plus autologous hematopoietic stem-cell transplantation for metastatic breast cancer. Philadelphia Bone Marrow Transplant Group. N Engl J Med 2000;342:1069–76.

66. Childs RW, Clave E, Tisdale J, et al. Successful treatment of metastatic renal cell carcinoma with a nonmyeloablative allogeneic peripheral-blood progenitor-cell transplant: evidence for a graft-versus-tumor effect. J Clin Oncol 1999;17:2044–9.

# SUPPORTIVE CARE AND SELECTED MANAGEMENT ISSUES

# CHAPTER 17

# ONCOLOGIC EMERGENCIES

...................................

## OVERVIEW OF ONCOLOGIC EMERGENCIES

• Charles M. Haskell

Oncologic emergencies may be defined as complications of cancer or its treatment that are life threatening or capable of inducing irreversible disability if not managed promptly.[1] They may occur at the time of the initial diagnosis of cancer, during the course of active cancer treatment (usually as a complication of therapy), or later in the natural history of the cancer as a result of progressive disease or delayed toxic side effects of chemotherapy. Table 17–1 provides a general overview of the varied forms of oncologic emergencies, with cross-references to appropriate chapters elsewhere in the book and to other sources of detailed information on the subject. The only problem listed in Table 17–1 that is discussed in detail in this chapter is the superior vena cava (SVC) syndrome. It is only rarely an emergency, but it is widely categorized as such, and its importance justifies a separate discussion. Emergencies that may occur in any patient, with or without a diagnosis of cancer, are not reviewed here because their management is a standard part of general medicine and surgery.

*Table 17–1.* **Overview of Oncologic Emergencies**

| Organ System | Specific Emergency | Suggested Reading |
|---|---|---|
| Cardiovascular | SVC syndrome | Chapters 17 and 103 |
| | Cardiac tamponade | Chapter 103 |
| Respiratory | Acute large airway obstruction | Chapters 36–39 |
| | | Hanowell and Waldron[2] |
| | Pulmonary hemorrhage | Benumof[3] |
| | Respiratory failure | |
| Renal and metabolic | Obstructive uropathy | Chapters 18, 50–53 |
| | Urate nephropathy and tumor lysis | Hirshberg and Greenberg[4] |
| | | Long[5] |
| | Hypercalcemia | |
| Gastrointestinal | Obstruction | Chapters 40–49 |
| | Perforation | Forrest et al[6] |
| | Hemorrhage | Arregui[7] |
| | | Langhorne et al[8] |
| | | Tai and Chia[9] |
| Hematologic | Leukostasis | Chapter 13 |
| | Hyperviscosity | Chapter 99 |
| | DIC | Chapter 13 |
| | Thrombocytopenia | Chapter 13 |
| | Neutropenia | Chapter 13 |
| | Neutropenic fever | Chapters 13 and 20 |
| Neurologic | Spinal cord compression | Chapter 73 |
| | Raised intracranial pressure | Chapter 72 |
| | Seizures | Chapter 72 |
| Miscellaneous | Orbital and intraocular metastases | De Potter[10] |
| | Bone pain | Chapter 22 |
| | Gynecologic hemorrhage | Chapter 57 |

SVC, superior vena cava; DIC, disseminated intravascular coagulation.

## REFERENCES

1. Price CGA, Price P. Acute emergencies in oncology: general overview. In: Peckham M, Pinedo HM, Veronesi U, eds. Oxford textbook of oncology. Oxford: Oxford University Press, 1995:2193–201.
2. Hanowell LH, Waldron RJ, eds. Airway management. Philadelphia: Lippincott-Raven, 1996.
3. Benumof JL, ed. Airway management: principles and practice. St. Louis: CV Mosby, 1996.
4. Hirshberg SJ, Greenberg RE. Urologic issues of palliative care. In: Berger AM, Portenoy RK, Weissman DE, eds. Principles and practices of supportive oncology. Philadelphia: Lippincott-Raven, 1998:371–83.
5. Long WS. Primary renal failure. In: Berger AM, Portenoy RK, Weissman DE, eds. Principles and practices of supportive oncology. Philadelphia: Lippincott-Raven, 1998:385–98.
6. Forrest APM, Carter DC, Macleod IB, eds. Principles and practice of surgery. 3rd ed. Edinburgh: Churchill Livingstone, 1995.
7. Arregui ME, ed. Principles of laparoscopic surgery: basic and advanced techniques. New York: Springer-Verlag, 1995.
8. Langhorne NB, Asch MR, Jaffer N. Palliation of gastrointestinal obstruction with expendable metallic stents: 3 case reports. Can Assoc Radiol J 1997;48:327–32.
9. Tai LS, Chia YW. Endoscopic Nd:YAG laser treatment of inoperable lower gastrointestinal cancer. Ann Acad Med Singapore 1996;25:712–6.
10. De Potter P: Ocular manifestations of cancer. Curr Opin Ophthalmol 1998;9:100–4.

# SUPERIOR VENA CAVA SYNDROME

• Carol Nishikubo • Ahmed Sadeghi • Charles M. Haskell

The SVC syndrome was first described by Hunter in 1757. The initial case was the result of a luetic aortic aneurysm, and a host of other nonmalignant causes of the syndrome were later described. With the rise of successful treatment for conditions such as thyroid goiter, syphilis, and tuberculosis, malignant tumors have become the most common cause of the SVC syndrome. The differential diagnosis of this problem, however, must still include a wide variety of nonmalignant problems, which vary in frequency in different clinical settings. For example, the frequency of benign causes of the SVC syndrome in patients in general hospitals ranges from 10 to 25%, whereas it is 0 to 3% in patients seen in cancer clinics.[1] Because the benign and malignant causes of the SVC syndrome are treated differently, every reasonable effort to make a diagnosis should precede therapy for this condition.

## Natural History, Diagnosis, and Prognosis

### PATHOPHYSIOLOGY AND CLASSIFICATION

The SVC is particularly vulnerable to obstruction by primary bronchial and lymphoid tumors or metastatic mediastinal nodes because it is a thin-walled vessel with a low venous pressure surrounded by lymph nodes that drain areas that are commonly involved by cancer. It is situated to the right of the midline anterior to the trachea and right mainstem bronchus and posterior to the sternum. The lymph nodes that surround the SVC drain the structures in the right and the lower parts of the left thoracic cavity.

The location of the SVC makes it apparent why the most common tumor associated with the SVC syndrome is bronchogenic carcinoma (75% of all cases) and why the syndrome is more common with right-sided lesions (4:1). Lymphomas account for 15% of cases, with metastatic malignancies making up approximately 7%. Of patients with lung cancer, 3 to 12% develop SVC syndrome,[2, 3] and approximately 8% of patients with lymphoma have symptoms of SVC syndrome in the course of their disease. A wide variety of malignancies can cause the SVC syndrome, including such unlikely primary tumors as prostate cancer, acute myelogenous leukemia, cervical cancer, and primary mediastinal germ cell tumors. Benign causes of SVC syndrome include substernal goiter, mediastinal granulomatous diseases (histoplasmosis, tuberculosis), other mediastinal infections (pyogenic, actinomycosis), pericarditis, idiopathic fibrosing mediastinitis, benign mediastinal neoplasms such as bronchogenic cysts, and central venous catheters.

Obstruction of the SVC can be due to extrinsic compression, intraluminal obstruction, or infiltration of the vessel wall. Malignant neoplasms characteristically cause extrinsic compression, although this situation may be complicated by intrinsic obstruction from complicating thrombosis.

## CLINICAL FEATURES AND DIAGNOSIS

The SVC syndrome is characterized by edema and suffusion of the neck, face, upper extremities, and, on occasion, upper torso as well as by dilatation of collateral veins on the chest and abdomen and progressive dyspnea, cough, and orthopnea. As the cerebral venous pressure rises, headaches, vertigo, drowsiness, stupor, and unconsciousness can become manifested.

The speed with which the syndrome develops depends on the nature of the obstruction and its rate of change. For example, fast-growing tumors do not allow sufficient time for collateral circulation to develop, and the SVC syndrome may develop rapidly. A kinked vascular catheter may cause a rapidly progressive, acute form of the SVC syndrome. Lesions above the azygos vein are generally better tolerated because this important link between the upper torso and the SVC allows compensatory collateral circulation. When the SVC syndrome is caused by a vascular catheter, the frequency of this complication appears to be related to the location of the device. For example, in a study from France, 8 of 28 (29%) patients with malpositioned catheters in the upper left part of the vena cava developed the SVC syndrome.[4] Subsequent insistence on replacement of malpositioned catheters reduced the frequency of the SVC syndrome to 1%.

After making a clinical diagnosis of the SVC syndrome, the clinician must establish an anatomic and histopathologic diagnosis if possible. In the past, invasive diagnostic procedures were avoided in these patients, and early radiation therapy was recommended to prevent irreversible nervous system injury and to avoid pulmonary complications. Contemporary studies, however, suggest that most of these patients can undergo invasive diagnostic procedures with reasonable safety, including bronchoscopy with endobronchial biopsy, thoracentesis, pleural biopsy, percutaneous fine-needle aspiration cytology under computed tomography (CT) guidance, surgical lymph node biopsies, and mediastinoscopy or thoracotomy.

The SVC syndrome is only rarely an emergency, and optimal therapy cannot be planned without anatomic localization of the lesion or lesions and an accurate histologic diagnosis. Anatomic localization is usually performed by thoracic CT. In one series, CT identification of collateral vessels predicted the presence of the SVC syndrome with a sensitivity of 96% and a specificity of 92%.[5] If there is any doubt about the anatomic nature of the problem, magnetic resonance imaging (MRI) clearly shows vascular pathologic features and provides etiologic suggestions based on the intensity of T1-weighted and T2-weighted signals.[6] If one is forced to treat without a histologic diagnosis, however, there is at least some evidence in the literature that treatment directed at the most likely clinicopathologic entity is reasonable and associated with some patients living for prolonged periods.[7]

Few studies have dealt with thrombus versus tumor as the basis for the SVC syndrome. Patients may show an excellent antitumor response from radiation therapy, only to have no improvement in symptoms. This situation most certainly relates to the continued presence of thrombosis rather than persistent tumor.

## PROGNOSIS

The prognosis of a patient with SVC syndrome relates mainly to the histologic type of the primary tumor. The median survival for bronchogenic carcinoma presenting with the syndrome is 3 to 5 months with treatment. Other nonthoracic primary tumors that metastasize to the mediastinum have similar prognoses. The prognoses of malignant lymphomas that produce this syndrome relate to the stage of the disease as well as to the histologic type of lymphoma. For many of these patients, the prognosis is good.

## Treatment

### SURGICAL THERAPY

First-line therapy for patients presenting with SVC syndrome resulting from malignancy in most cases involves radiation, chemotherapy, or both, as is discussed subsequently. There are cases, however, that are resistant to these procedures or that recur after initial treatment that may benefit from surgical intervention. Surgical approaches to the SVC syndrome include bypass grafts, radical excision with vein grafting, and stenting with expandable metallic stents. Outcomes in patients treated with stents as first-line therapy or in patients who have previously failed or recurred following initial radiation therapy have resulted in high rates of resolution of clinical symptoms (68 to 100%).[8, 9] Results have been somewhat better with treating SVC syndrome caused by extrinsic compression as opposed to cases caused by intraluminal disease.[10] The complication rates in most series have been fairly low, consisting of recurrent obstruction, thrombosis and, rarely, bleeding, pulmonary edema, and stent migration.[9, 10] The comparable overall response rates achieved over a shorter time than observed with radiation have led some authors to suggest that stenting may be considered as first-line therapy in some patients.[11]

### RADIATION THERAPY

Radiation therapy is extremely useful in the treatment of SVC syndrome. The total dose of radiation therapy depends on the primary tumor and the stage of disease. For epithelial tumors that are limited to local or regional areas, doses in the range of 5000 to 6600 cGy given over 5 to 7 weeks are needed for treatment with curative intent. If there is distant disease, lower doses over shorter periods of time are warranted for treatment of palliative intent. Lymphomas are more sensitive than epithelial tumors to radiation therapy, requiring 3500 to 4500 cGy given in 180- to 200-cGy fractions over 4 to 5 weeks.

In the past, the initial daily doses of radiation therapy have been controversial because of concern about the risk of radiation edema. Rubin and coworkers[12] found that faster and longer relief of symptoms was obtained by using large initial fractions of radiation rather than beginning with small fractions and slowly increasing the daily dose. They noted that morbidity did not increase in patients receiving this high-dose therapy (400 cGy times three doses). The fear of producing additional compromise of the SVC by radiation therapy from edema after large fractions of irradiation appears to be unfounded. For patients with small cell lung cancer, however, the necessity of delivering these initial high doses of radiation was brought into question. Chan and colleagues[13] observed no differences in response rates or survival over a range of initial doses delivered to their patients. For this subset of patients, with tumors that are traditionally sensitive to radiation therapy, the high-dose therapy may not be required.

The portal of irradiation is designed to encompass the primary tumor and mediastinal, hilar, and any adjacent pulmonary parenchymal lesions. If there is an upper lobe lung lesion or superior mediastinal adenopathy, the supraclavicular nodes are usually included in the radiation portal. For lymphoma, the field is generally extended to include adjacent node-bearing areas, including the cervical, mediastinal, and axillary areas. The response rates from irradiation are 75 to 95%, with relief usually noted within 1 week and lasting 20 to 23 weeks. In a series by Davenport and colleagues,[14] 33 of 35 patients with SVC syndrome responded to high initial fraction (4 Gy times three doses) and high total dose (30 to 50 Gy) radiation. The two patients who failed to respond had large thrombi occluding the SVC at autopsy. There were no instances of exacerbation of symptoms or severe complications.

### CHEMOTHERAPY

Chemotherapy is a rational form of treatment for the SVC syndrome resulting from cancers that are generally sensitive to chemotherapy, such as small cell lung cancer and malignant lymphoma. For example, in a series of 26 patients with the SVC syndrome caused by small cell carcinoma of the lung, 22 had chemotherapy alone. The SVC syndrome was resolved in all 22 cases by 7 days.[15] A European study similarly concludes that intensive chemotherapy is the first line of therapy for small cell lung cancer.[16] Chemotherapy is as good as radiation therapy for the emergency treatment of these patients, and the high incidence of concurrent systemic metastases in small cell carcinoma favors the earliest possible use of chemotherapy. Chemotherapy is especially useful when the location and size of the neoplasm are such that a large volume of lung would have to be irradiated to encompass the tumor bulk fully. If the tumor responds to chemotherapy, any subsequent radiation therapy can be given to a smaller port, sparing substantial portions of normal lung. Similar considerations hold for the management of malignant lymphoma.

### SUPPORTIVE CARE

Steroids have been advocated for severe cases of the SVC syndrome associated with respiratory compromise. Rarely, successful chemotherapy for small cell lung cancer may lead to a temporary exacerbation of the SVC syndrome because of edema. Corticosteroid treatment is useful if this unusual complication occurs.[17] Diuretics can be quite effective in providing immediate decompression, but the response is short lived unless specific antitumor therapy is given.

Anticoagulation has been used with radiation therapy to prevent or treat thrombosis, although its value has not been established. In one study of thromboembolic events in patients with malignant SVC syndrome, two fatal thromboembolic events occurred in 10 patients receiving no anticoagulation, whereas there were two fatal episodes of cranial hemorrhage in 20 patients who did receive anticoagulation. The authors concluded that a randomized trial is required to resolve the relative merits of using or not using anticoagulation in these patients.[18] Thrombolytic therapy, with streptokinase, urokinase, or a recombinant plasminogen activator, has also been tried with some success in preliminary reports. Further work is needed, however, to define the optimal use of these agents.[19]

## Summary of Treatment

The SVC syndrome is only rarely an oncologic emergency. It is nearly always possible to obtain anatomic localization and a specific pathophysiologic diagnosis (including tissue) using modern diagnostic techniques and to plan treatment according to the specific cause of the syndrome. The most common malignancy causing the SVC syndrome is small cell carcinoma of the lung, which should generally be treated first with chemotherapy. Radiation therapy may or may not be required subsequently, depending on the response of the patient and the specific guidelines for treatment of the disease used by the treating physician. Similarly, lymphomas may be treated initially with chemotherapy or radiation therapy, or both, depending on the specific histologic type and stage of lymphoma. Unresolved issues in the management of the SVC syndrome include the extent of vascular imaging needed before the initiation of therapy and the roles, if any, of stenting, anticoagulation, and thrombolytic therapy.

### SUGGESTIONS FOR ADDITIONAL READING

Schindler N, Vogelzang RL. Superior vena cava syndrome: experience with endovascular stents and surgical therapy. Surg Clin North Am 1999;79:683–94.

## REFERENCES

1. Schraufnagel DE, Hill R, Leech JA, Pare JA. Superior vena caval obstruction: is it a medical emergency? Am J Med 1981;70:1169–74.
2. Falk S, Fallon M. ABC of palliative care: emergencies. Br Med J 1997;315:1525–8.
3. Stewart IE. Superior vena cava syndrome: an oncologic complication. Semin Oncol Nurs 1996;12:312–7.
4. Puel V, Caudry M, LeMetayer P, et al. Superior vena cava thrombosis related to catheter malposition in cancer chemotherapy given through implanted ports. Cancer 1993;72:2248–52.
5. Kim HJ, Kim HS, Chung SH. CT diagnosis of superior vena cava syndrome: importance of collateral vessels. AJR Am J Roentgenol 1993;161:539–42.
6. Giron J, Durand G, Benezet O, Senac JP. Contribution of magnetic resonance imaging to the exploration of the mediastinum. Rev Pneumol Clin 1993;49:129–36.
7. Loeffler JS, Leopold KA, Recht A, et al. Emergency prebiopsy radiation for mediastinal masses: impact on subsequent pathologic diagnosis and outcome. J Clin Oncol 1986;4:716–21.
8. Tanigawa N, Sawada S, Mishima K, et al. Clinical outcome of stenting in superior vena cava syndrome associated with malignant tumors: comparison with conventional treatment. Acta Radiol 1998;39:669–74.
9. Hochrein J, Bashore TM, O'Laughlin MP, Harrison JK. Percutaneous stenting of superior vena cava syndrome: a case report and review of the literature. Am J Med 1998;104:78–84.
10. Entwisle KG, Watkinson AF, Reidy J. Case report: migration and shortening of a self-expanding metallic stent complicating the treatment of malignant superior vena cava stenosis. Clin Radiol 1996;51:593–5.
11. Nicholson AA, Ettles DF, Arnold A, et al. Treatment of malignant superior vena cava obstruction: metal stents or radiation therapy. J Vasc Interv Radiol 1997;8:781–8.
12. Rubin P, Green J, Holzwasser G, et al. Superior vena cava syndrome. Radiology 1963;81:388–401.
13. Chan RH, Dar AR, Yu E, et al. Superior vena cava obstruction in small-cell lung cancer. Int J Radiat Oncol Biol Phys 1997;38:513–20.
14. Davenport D, Ferree C, Blake D, Raben M. Radiation therapy in the treatment of superior vena caval obstruction. Cancer 1978;42:2600–3.
15. Dombernowsky P, Hansen HH. Combination chemotherapy in the management of superior vena caval obstruction in small-cell anaplastic carcinoma of the lung. Acta Med Scand 1978;204:513–6.
16. Urban T, Lebeau B, Chastang C, et al. Superior vena cava syndrome in small-cell lung cancer. Arch Intern Med 1993;153:384–7.
17. Sand JJ, Rosenthal CJ. Obstruction of the superior vena cava after chemotherapy. Arch Intern Med 1985;145:364–5.
18. Adelstein DJ, Hines JD, Carter SG, Sacco D. Thromboembolic events in patients with malignant superior vena cava syndrome and the role of anticoagulation. Cancer 1988;62:2258–62.
19. Escalante CP. Causes and management of superior vena cava syndrome. Oncology 1993;7:61–8.

# CHAPTER 18

# PARANEOPLASTIC SYNDROMES

• JEROME B. BLOCK

Paraneoplastic syndromes are a group of disorders associated with *specific* neoplasms that have signs and symptoms that cannot be ascribed to local tumor invasion. These syndromes are the result of a wide variety of tumor-derived biologic mediators. In most cases, the primary tumor is clinically evident before the onset of a paraneoplastic syndrome, but in rare cases the tumor is occult.

Historically, clubbing of the nails is the oldest known paraneoplastic syndrome. Signs typical of clubbing were discovered in 2500-year-old archaeologic excavations from Mesoamerica in the Western Hemisphere.[1] The condition was described by Hippocrates (460–375 BC) and later named *pachydermatoperiostosis* by Friedreich in 1868. The term *paraneoplastic syndrome* is more recent, with the first citations appearing under this term in the *Index Medicus* in 1974.

The molecular mechanisms of paraneoplastic syndromes are varied and have yet to be fully unraveled. In an early review of the subject, Nathanson and Hall[2] proposed that the pathogenesis of these syndromes was due to (1) embryonic derepression of tumor cells leading to production of atypical (for the tissue site of primary tumor) amounts of biologically active hormones or (2) tumor-initiated antigen-antibody interactions resulting in a variety of neurologic or neurovascular disorders.

Initially, many of the endocrine-metabolic syndromes were considered to be due to *ectopic* hormone production by tumors derived from non–hormone-producing tissues. An example of this is Cushing's syndrome resulting from adrenocorticotropic hormone (ACTH) production by lung cancer.[3, 4] The work of Odell and associates,[5] however, showed that the term *ectopic* was a misnomer because normal tissues as well as many tumors can synthesize immunoreactive ACTH. This immunoreactive ACTH is precursor ACTH or pro-opiomelanocortin (POMC) and largely biologically inactive.[6] Tumors associated with Cushing's syndrome have considerably more POMC than normal tissues and metabolize it sufficiently to produce an excess of biologically active ACTH.

Odell proposed that paraneoplastic syndromes are due to one or more of the following: (1) protein hormone or hormone precursor production by a tumor; (2) stimulation by the tumor of an antibody that demonstrates cross-reactivity with tumor and with normal cellular antigens (i.e., the nervous system); (3) other syndromes characterized by the production of paracrine or autocrine substances; and (4) rarely, tumor metabolism of steroid or other hormone precursors. An unequivocal diagnosis of a paraneoplastic endocrine-metabolic hormone syndrome broadly requires three features: (1) There must be a temporal correlation between changes in tumor size and serum levels of the biologic mediator. (2) There should be an increase in the pulmonary venous-arterial concentration gradient for the mediator

across the tumor bed and an increased concentration of the mediator in the tumor. (3) There should be evidence that the tumor cells are synthesizing and secreting the biologic mediator or its precursor.

The time between onset of a paraneoplastic syndrome and tumor diagnosis may be remarkably long or difficult to establish. Many syndromes persist for years before diagnosis, as may be the case for small cell or carcinoid tumors causing neurologic syndromes or, in another example, dermatoses heralding lymphomas or gastrointestinal cancers. Early tumor identification may prevent further irreversible tissue damage caused by the paraneoplastic process and increase the likelihood, with appropriate treatment, of remission or reversal of the syndrome.

Recognition of paraneoplastic syndromes is important in the management of cancer. Their recognition may lead to an earlier diagnosis of malignancy than would otherwise be the case. The clinical severity of the syndrome can be used as a guide to the response of the neoplasm to therapy. Also, the quality of the patient's life can sometimes be improved by effective palliative therapy of the syndrome. In the future, a better understanding of these syndromes may also result in new therapies.

This chapter discusses common endocrine-metabolic, neuromuscular, and dermatologic paraneoplastic syndromes, with an emphasis on the clinical setting of the syndromes, their diagnosis, and management. Excellent reviews are available for the reader interested in more details.[7, 8] Some paraneoplastic syndromes are not addressed, for example, the common syndrome of cachexia of malignancy (see Chapter 21),[9] and virtually every known hormone (with the possible exception of thyroid and steroid hormones), or hormone-releasing factor, has been shown to be produced by a tumor. These are all potential candidates for causing a paraneoplastic syndrome. Because of such heterogeneous hormone production, several paraneoplastic syndromes may occur in the same patient, particularly with small cell lung cancer and amine precursor uptake and decarboxylation (APUD)–derived tumors (see Chapter 67).[10–13] Table 18–1 lists some common paraneoplastic syndromes associated with specific tumor histologic features.

## Endocrine-Metabolic Syndromes

### SYNDROME OF INAPPROPRIATE SECRETION OF ANTIDIURETIC HORMONE

**Background.** Antidiuretic hormone (ADH), or arginine vasopressin (AVP), is a 9-amino acid peptide that is secreted by the hypothalamus to maintain the constancy of plasma

*Table 18–1.* **Paraneoplastic Syndromes More Commonly Associated with Certain Tumor Histology**

| Tumor Cell Type | Paraneoplastic Syndrome |
| --- | --- |
| Squamous cell carcinoma, all sites (e.g., lung, cervix) | Humoral hypercalcemia<br>Acanthosis nigricans |
| Small cell carcinoma, pulmonary and genitourinary type | SIADH<br>ANF secretion<br>Lambert-Eaton syndrome<br>Ectopic ACTH production (Cushing's syndrome)<br>Central nervous system degenerative disorders<br>Peripheral neuronopathy<br>Autonomic neuronopathy<br>Retinopathy |
| Carcinoid and neuroectodermal tumors | Ectopic ACTH production (Cushing's syndrome)<br>Humoral hypercalcemia |
| Lymphomas | Pemphigus<br>Humoral hypercalcemia<br>Nephrotic syndrome<br>Dermatomyositis/polymyositis |
| Plasma cell dyscrasias | Peripheral neuropathy<br>POEMS variants |
| Melanoma | Acanthosis nigricans variants<br>Retinopathy<br>Humoral hypercalcemia |
| Adenocarcinoma of ovary, fallopian tubes | Retinopathy |
| All grade I tumors | Trousseau's syndrome<br>Acanthosis nigricans variants<br>Multiple eruptive seborrheic keratoses |
| Breast | Humoral hypercalcemia<br>Retinopathy<br>Cerebellar degenerative diseases |
| Lung, often adenocarcinoma | Hypertrophic pulmonary osteoarthropathy |
| Thymic tumors | Myasthenic syndrome<br>Ectopic ACTH production (Cushing's syndrome)<br>Red cell aplasia |
| Mesenchymal tumors (benign and sarcomatous) | Osteomalacia<br>Humoral hypoglycemia |

SIADH, syndrome of inappropriate secretion of antidiuretic hormone; ANF, atrial natriuretic factor; ACTH, adrenocorticotropic hormone; POEMS, polyneuropathy, organomegaly, endocrinopathy, M protein myeloma, skin changes.

osmolarity.[14, 15] In healthy individuals, plasma osmolarity is maintained between 286 and 294 mOsm/kg of body weight. Vascular osmoreceptors are sensitive to changes of greater than or equal to 1% in plasma osmolarity, resulting in changes in AVP release. The AVP prohormone, preprovasopressin-neurophysin (propressophysin), a 164-amino acid peptide, is found in the magnocellular neurons of the supraoptic and paraventricular nuclei of the hypothalamus. Its products, AVP and neurophysin, are released into the circulation. Receptors for AVP are found in the kidney, blood vessels, and pituitary. AVP regulates free water clearance through its effects on renal tubules.

Hyponatremia is the primary biochemical indicator of clinically inappropriate secretion of ADH. Hyponatremia associated with lung cancer was first described in 1938. The syndrome of inappropriate secretion of ADH (SIADH) was described in 1957 and associated with ADH production by tumors in 1963. The most common cause of SIADH is small cell lung cancer.[16] Other common causes of SIADH are other forms of lung cancer (1 to 5%), carcinoid tumors, and, rarely, other tumors.

The serum ADH level is increased in 32 to 46% of patients with small cell lung cancer, and abnormal tolerance to a water load is seen in 53 to 68% of patients with this tumor.[17, 18] The full-blown clinical syndrome, however, is present in only 9 to 14% of cases. The extent of elevation of serum AVP or other AVP prohormone products is directly related to the extent of disease. Because of this relationship, it has been suggested that AVP might serve as a tumor marker for the assessment of treatment.

Eighty-eight percent of patients with small cell lung cancer have at least one of the four degradation products of the neurophysin portion of AVP prohormone in their serum, and 65% have elevated serum neurophysin.[19] The syndrome is also seen with other lung cancers, lymphoma, Ewing's sarcoma, thymoma, and pancreatic and duodenal cancer. SIADH has been reported with squamous cell head and neck cancer alone[20] and after induction chemotherapy and with radical neck dissection in head and neck cancer.[21] Although AVP production by these tumors has often been demonstrated, their location in the neck and their spread to the mediastinum raise the contributing issue of physiologic secretion of atrial natriuretic factor (ANF) secondary to the spread of these tumors.

SIADH is rare in the absence of measurable increases in AVP. The exclusive role of AVP in such syndromes has been questioned, however, because of increased understanding of the influence of the 28-amino acid peptide ANF in causing states of hyponatremia.[22, 23] AVP and ANF have been shown to be produced by tumors, together or separately, in hyponatremic SIADH-like states. ANF receptors are found in endothelium, the adrenal cortex, and the kidneys. Physiologic release of ANF is affected by changes in baroreceptors located in the arterial system (carotid sinus, aortic arch, afferent glomerular arterioles). ANF release may occur by indirect tumor involvement, as in lung cancer with mediastinal spread, or by a reduction in intravascular volume produced by metastatic disease to the pericardium with tamponade. Compounding the complexity of the syndrome is the observation that a reduction of effective arterial volume produces a baroreceptor-mediated, non–osmotic-dependent, physiologic release of AVP, perhaps operating through AVP vascular receptors. The compounds AVP, ANF, angiotensin II, endothelin-1, brain natriuretic peptide (which shares 70% amino acid homology with ANF),[24] and C-type natriuretic peptide all play a role in vascular tone and may influence intravascular volume, osmotic pressure, ADH secretion, and salt excretion. Although these other peptides have not been proven to cause paraneoplastic syndromes, they could potentially do so. Some authorities prefer the term *syndrome of inappropriate antidiuresis* in place of SIADH to emphasize that ADH is not the only possible cause of this hyponatremic syndrome.[25]

**Diagnosis.** The differential diagnosis of hyponatremia in patients with cancer includes the following:

1. Laboratory hyponatremia generally results from other molecules in the plasma giving a falsely low laboratory measurement for serum sodium. When the measured se-

rum osmolality is normal but the calculated osmolality ($2[Na^+]$ + glucose/18 + blood urea nitrogen/2.8) is low, large amounts of blood lipids or macromolecular proteins are often found.

2. Hyponatremia associated with volume depletion and urinary sodium less than 20 mEq/L may be seen with vomiting, fluid sequestration, diarrhea, and excessive sweating. A urinary sodium value greater than 20 mEq/L with volume depletion is noted with diuretic use, nephrogenic salt loss, mineralocorticoid deficiency, osmotic diuresis, metabolic alkalosis, and renal tubular acidosis.

3. Hyponatremia associated with volume expansion and a urinary sodium less than 20 mEq/L can be seen in congestive heart failure, cirrhosis, and the nephrotic syndrome. A urinary sodium greater than 20 mEq/L is commonly associated with acute or chronic renal failure. Euvolemic states with hyponatremia include SIADH, glucocorticoid deficiency, hypothyroidism, psychogenic polydipsia, physical and emotional stress states, and a variety of pharmacologic agents, including phenothiazine and tricyclic antidepressants (Table 18–2). Cisplatin can cause salt-losing nephritis, which can result in hypovolemia, and possibly cause the liberation of intracellular AVP or ANF occurring with chemotherapy-induced tumor necrosis.

4. SIADH in cancer is often a diagnosis of exclusion, but most euvolemic cancer patients with hyponatremia have SIADH. In such patients, the criteria for making a diagnosis of SIADH are as follows:
   a. Serum sodium less than 135 mEq/L, with
   b. Plasma osmolality less than 280 mOsm/kg, and
   c. Urine osmolality greater than 100 mOsm/kg, with
   d. Absence of decreased urinary sodium (i.e., sodium >20 mEq/L).

A small percentage of patients with small cell lung cancer and SIADH have no increase in the blood level of AVP. These cases may be due to a postulated *reset* of osmoreceptors[26] in cancer patients or to the secretion of ANF. These *reset osmostat* patients usually have mild hyponatremia in the range of 125 to 130 mEq/L and have no defect in urine dilution so that hyponatremia usually does not worsen or become clinically symptomatic.[27]

**Treatment.** The treatment of hyponatremia resulting from SIADH is influenced by the degree of depression in serum sodium and the duration of the hyponatremic state. More rapidly developing and more profound hyponatremia is clinically dangerous in terms of mortality and irreversible neurologic morbidity. Caution is required in reversing the hyponatremic state. Generally, for the more gradually acquired

hyponatremic states when serum sodium is in excess of 120 mEq/L, fluid restriction to less than 1 L/day represents adequate corrective therapy. For more severe and symptomatic hyponatremia, infusion of 3% saline at a rate of 0.1 ml/kg/min for 24 hours, or about 1 mmol/hr, should increase serum sodium by 10 mmol/L after 24 hours of therapy. Careful repetitive monitoring of serum sodium is required so that the serum sodium does not rise more than 25 mmol/L for the first 48 hours of therapy.[28] A rapid and inappropriate correction of serum sodium has been associated with central pontine myelinolysis and other neurologic damage,[29] particularly when hyponatremia is of short duration. Regulating the rise of serum sodium to approximately 10% per day of therapy is said to decrease significantly the risk of this neurologic complication. The addition of furosemide to hypertonic saline infusions has also been highly successful in the treatment of hyponatremia. Demeclocycline (1 g/day over 1 to 2 weeks), fluorocortisone (0.1 to 0.3 mg twice daily), and lithium carbonate are useful in the long-term treatment of the asymptomatic hyponatremia states.

Chemotherapy directed against the tumor associated with the SIADH syndrome has been reported to cause sudden shock and death. In one report,[30] tumor tissue contained significant amounts of ANF, and shock developed without congestive heart failure after chemotherapy. The pathogenesis of this reaction was thought to involve chemotherapy-induced tumor lysis with the acute release of ANF.

## CUSHING'S SYNDROME RESULTING FROM ECTOPIC ADRENOCORTICOTROPIC HORMONE–PRODUCING TUMORS

**Background.** Classic, fully expressed Cushing's syndrome is characterized by hypertension, plethora, central nervous system abnormalities including psychosis, cutaneous hyperpigmentation, edema, glucose intolerance, abnormal fat distribution, and hypokalemic alkalosis.[31] The cardinal features of the syndrome are those of protein catabolism (i.e., striae, ecchymoses, and proximal muscle weakness). The syndrome may be either pituitary dependent, such as with an ACTH-producing pituitary adenoma, hyperplasia, or Nelson's syndrome (pituitary ACTH-producing adenomas after adrenalectomy), or pituitary independent, as in ectopic tumor production of ACTH or primary adrenal adenoma, carcinoma, or hyperplasia.[32, 33] The association of nonadrenal carcinoma with Cushing's syndrome has been recognized since 1928. Most Cushing's syndrome patients have pituitary adenomas, whereas an estimated 2 to 10% of Cushing's syndrome cases have ectopic causes.[3]

Cushing's syndrome from non–pituitary-dependent, ectopic ACTH-producing tumors has been reported with all malignancies other than sarcomas. The most frequent causes are as follows: small cell lung cancer (50%); thymic tumors (10%); carcinoids (10%); pheochromocytoma (5%); medullary carcinoma of the thyroid (5%); and bronchial adenocarcinoma (5%). The syndrome is relatively rare, even in patients with these tumors. Delisle and colleagues[34] reviewed 840 patients with small cell lung cancer and noted an incidence of 1.6% of clinical ectopic ACTH-producing syndrome; Kohler and Trump[35] found evidence of only 2.4% for Cushing's syndrome in similar cancer patients. On rare

*Table 18–2.* **Drugs Associated with Hyponatremia-like Pattern in Cancer Patients**

| | |
|---|---|
| Tricyclic antidepressants | Chlorpropamide |
| *Vinca* alkaloids | Nonsteroidal anti-inflammatory agents |
| Cyclophosphamide | Diuretics |
| Cisplatin | Oral hypoglycemic agents |
| Clofibrate | Anticonvulsants |
| Levamisole | Acetaminophen |
| Carbamazepine | Butyrophenone |
| Monoamine oxidase inhibitors | |

occasions, the syndrome has also been described with histologically benign diseases, including Whipple's disease,[36] certain inflammatory masses, and mammary hyperplasia.[37] Pituitary-driven, ACTH-dependent Cushing's syndrome is considerably commoner in women, whereas ectopic ACTH syndromes are approximately equally distributed between men and women, perhaps because of the predominant cause of small cell lung cancer.[38]

Studies of the biology of ACTH and its precursor proteins have led to a better understanding of ACTH production by tumors and new approaches to the differential diagnosis of clinical Cushing's syndrome, formerly characterized mainly by ACTH serum levels measured by older radioimmunoassay techniques. These latter techniques have demonstrated that almost all normal tissues have small but demonstrable amounts of immunoreactive ACTH that also contain β-melanocyte–stimulating hormone (β-MSH) immunoreactivity. This material has a high molecular weight of approximately 31,000 without ACTH-like biologic activity. It is apparent that many carcinomas and the serum of many patients with lung cancer have large amounts of this high-molecular-weight, immunoreactive ACTH substance and that there is less biologically active ACTH in these tissues. The development of newer sandwich immunoradiometric assays (IRMA) has permitted the specific and ready identification of biologically active ACTH, as distinct from those nonactive, high-molecular-weight ACTH molecules that are now thought to represent enzymatic degradation products of POMC, the ACTH precursor molecule.[39] Almost all cancers produce increased quantities of POMC. For example, 50% of patients with lung cancer have increased circulating POMC products, perhaps reflecting tumors that have more effective translation of messenger RNA for the immunoreactive POMC or that have lost mechanisms to prevent continual expression of the POMC gene. Clinical Cushing's syndrome is seen only in tumors, usually of defined histology, that are able to convert POMC enzymatically to biologically active ACTH. Small cell lung cancer and carcinoid and thymic tumors constitute more than half of the cancers clinically presenting with Cushing's syndrome. Melanoma, gastrinoma, and any of the APUD neuroectodermal tumors can also produce the syndrome. In ectopic production of ACTH, more than 75% of the tumors are found in the chest.[40] These latter tumors may be clinically occult because of their small size.

Typically, small bronchial carcinoids present diagnostic problems in the lung, in that they are often less than 1 cm in diameter; in contrast, thymic carcinoids are usually greater than 2 cm.[38] The most dramatic observations on tumor size and ectopic ACTH is that of clinically occult, tiny, pulmonary neuroendocrine *tumorlets*, which may produce Cushing's syndrome secondary to corticotropin secretion for more than a decade before a diagnosis is made.[41] The differences between these tumorlets and the customary bronchial carcinoid are that bronchial carcinoids are solitary, centrally located, do metastasize, and have a long median survival after diagnosis; tumorlets are multiple (often hundreds), are peripherally located, rarely metastasize, and have a short survival after diagnosis.

Because enzymatic conversion of POMC by cancers yields various peptide products, these too may aid in the differential diagnosis of Cushing's syndrome.[42] Ectopic ACTH-producing tumors seem to secrete preferentially greater amounts of POMC peptides produced by endopeptidases as well as apparently distinct POMC products that are not found circulating either in true Cushing's disease or in primary adrenal causes of Cushing's syndrome.[43] Table 18–3 presents the known POMC peptides found in Cushing's disease or in the ectopic ACTH syndrome. Endopeptidases PC1 and PC2 found in small cell lung and bronchial carcinoid are responsible for processing POMC to pro-ACTH and further POMC fragments. Assays for POMC may not be as sensitive as those for pro-ACTH.[44, 45] Assays for these peptides may greatly facilitate distinguishing pituitary-dependent from primary adrenal causes of hypercortisolism. The presence of the POMC fragments has been recognized since the early work of Yalow and Berson[46] in 1971 using older radioimmunoassay techniques. It is now recognized that only small amounts of complete ACTH appear in the circulation with ectopic ACTH tumors, but these small amounts are of sufficient biologic activity to produce the syndrome.

The observation that small cell lung cancer and carcinoid and other neuroendocrine tumors associated with ectopic ACTH production frequently have somatostatin receptors[47] on tumor cells has represented a new direction in diagnosis and treatment of Cushing's syndrome.[48] Normal pituitary glands and pituitary adenomas usually do not express somatostatin receptors and do not, accordingly, respond to administered somatostatin analogues with an attendant fall in serum ACTH or cortisol. In contrast, the neuroendocrine tumors producing ACTH (and other hormones) usually have decreased ACTH production after administration of somatostatin analogues when receptors for somatostatin are present.[49, 50] There are at least five somatostatin receptors identified with varying binding affinities for the analogues[51]; their demonstration signals a new phase in diagnosis and treatment of non–pituitary-dependent, nonadrenal causes of Cushing's syndrome.

**Diagnosis.** Paraneoplastic Cushing's syndrome is a heterogeneous disorder, and the differential diagnosis of the syndrome is complex, as summarized in Table 18–4. The most important distinction is between pituitary-dependent and non–pituitary-dependent, nonadrenal causes of Cushing's syndrome. This distinction is made biochemically, with supplemental radiographs as needed to define the presence of adenomas or other tumors. Some of the advantages and disadvantages of specific tests for different forms of the syndrome are discussed in the following paragraphs.

*Table 18–3.* **Metabolism of the ACTH Precursor Peptide Pro-opiomelanocortin (POMC)**

| |
|---|
| POMC peptide fragments in cancer and associated with normal ACTH production |
|     N terminal fragment |
|     Joining peptide |
|     ACTH |
|     β-Lipotropic hormone |
|     β-Endorphin |
|     γ-Lipotropic hormone |
| Other ectopic ACTH-producing, cancer-associated peptides |
|     γ-Melanocyte-stimulating hormone |
|     β-Melanocyte-stimulating hormone |
|     Corticotropin-like intermediate lobe polypeptide |

ACTH, adrenocorticotropic hormone.

*Table 18–4.* **Metabolic Diagnosis of ACTH-Producing Tumor**

| | Pituitary Dependent | Non–Pituitary Dependent, Nonadrenal Ectopic |
|---|---|---|
| Basal serum cortisol | Moderately or slightly elevated | Slightly to markedly elevated |
| Serum ACTH levels | Slightly elevated or normal | Slightly to markedly elevated |
| Metyrapone response | High response | Little or no response |
| Response to high-dose dexamethasone (8 mg × 2 days) | Most cases show a 50% reduction in urinary 17-hydroxysteroids* | Usually no reduction in steroid excretion or serum ACTH† |
| Sensitivity to HP axis | Present | Lost |
| Response to ovine CRH infusion (10 μg IV) | Supraresponse of 20–50% above baseline normal increase | |
| Cortisol levels | | |
| ACTH levels | Supraresponse of 20–50% above baseline normal increase | Little change or slight increase‡ |
| Response to DDAVP (10–15 μg IV) | >50% increase above baseline for serum cortisol | No increase in serum cortisol |
| Response to octreotide (200 μg SC q 4 hr) | No change in ACTH or cortisol | Suppression of serum ACTH and cortisol |

*15–30% of cases of Cushing's disease do not suppress.

†In approximately 50% of carcinoid tumors producing ACTH and Cushing's syndrome, the metabolic response to dexamethasone is similar to that of pituitary-dependent Cushing's disease.

‡Ectopic ACTH-producing tumors with concomitant production of CRH and ectopic CRH-producing tumors respond similarly to pituitary-dependent Cushing's syndrome.
ACTH, adrenocorticotropic hormone; HP, hypothalamic-pituitary; CRH, corticotropin-releasing hormone; DDAVP, 1-deamino-(8-D-arginine)-vasopressin.

Immunoreactive ACTH is found in the serum of more than 70% of patients with lung cancer. Odell and colleagues[5] found that the mean ACTH radioimmunoreactive serum level was 53.5 pg/ml in control patients, 69.2 pg/ml in patients with pulmonary obstructive disease, and 131.8 pg/ml in 75 patients with lung cancer, all without clinical Cushing's syndrome. Only a few of these had appreciable circulating biologically active ACTH.

The clinical features of Cushing's syndrome are rarely fully developed in ectopic tumor production of ACTH resulting from small cell lung cancer, perhaps because the rapidity of tumor growth limits the time available for the development of the full clinical syndrome. In states of ectopic ACTH production, the predominant clinical features are those of profound muscle wasting, hypokalemia, glucose intolerance, alkalosis, and edema. Although few patients develop full Cushing's syndrome, all have at least one of its clinical features. Hypokalemia and alkalosis, which may be profound, occur in 90% of patients with ectopic ACTH syndromes, reflecting an excess of mineralocorticoids. In contrast, hypokalemia in Cushing's disease is uncommon, usually occurring in less than 10% of patients.[52] Although features of typical cushingoid fat distribution and hyperpigmentation are uncommon in the ectopic ACTH syndromes, syndromes associated with the slow-growing neuroendocrine tumors, such as carcinoid tumors, bronchial adenomas, gastrinomas, pheochromocytomas, and medullary thyroid cancer, may permit the more complete expression of a *Cushing's disease* clinical picture. In these tumors, biochemical differentiation from Cushing's disease may not be possible using classic challenge or suppression clinical tests (see Table 18–4).

The metabolic and laboratory abnormalities characteristic of ectopic ACTH syndromes are usually more extreme than pituitary-dependent causes of Cushing's syndrome. In contrast to Cushing's disease and adrenal causes of hypercortisolism, most small cell lung cancer ectopic syndromes are characterized by ACTH secretion, which is insensitive to circulating glucocorticoid levels, yielding high serum levels.

The reasons for insensitivity to circulating cortisol excess as manifested by continued ACTH production in ectopic ACTH syndromes is not fully understood. One demonstrated reason is the production of an aberrant glucocorticoid receptor transcription in the presence of a normal receptor gene.[53] Other causes for glucocorticoid resistance may be defective flucorticoid receptor function, receptor signaling defects, or abnormalities in the POMC gene itself. Ectopic ACTH syndromes resulting from bronchial carcinoid may not demonstrate glucocorticoid resistance in the high-dose dexamethasone test. Although clinical Cushing's syndrome is rare in small cell lung cancer (1.5 to 5%), 50% of small cell lung cancer patients have hypercortisolism. High urinary levels of cortisol and a serum ACTH level greater than 200 pg/ml usually signify an ectopic syndrome (see Table 18–4). Clinically covert ectopic ACTH syndromes are common, however, and may give patterns of cortisol production and ACTH plasma levels quite similar to those of Cushing's disease, particularly when the ectopic tumor is a carcinoid tumor. The classic features of ACTH responsiveness testing and the integrity of the pituitary hypothalamic axis have been (1) dexamethasone suppression,[54] (2) corticotropin-releasing hormone (CRH) administration,[55] and (3) metyrapone stimulation.[56] Features of the ectopic ACTH syndrome include loss of the hypothalamic-pituitary-adrenal axis sensitivity to hormonal changes and serum hypercortisolism. This loss yields a loss of diurnal variation in cortisol production and extremely high levels of serum ACTH in the face of concomitant and extreme hypercortisolism. Cases resulting from ectopic CRH production by tumors may mimic pituitary-dependent syndromes with regard to biochemical challenge testing (see Table 18–4) relating to serum ACTH levels.

The noted excess of mineralocorticoids in ectopic ACTH syndromes is mirrored by high serum cortisol/corticosterone ratios (>80), which may be contrasted to ratios of 10 in Cushing's disease and healthy people.[57] A defect in 11β-dehydrogenase activity for steroid conversion has been related to high ACTH and high cortisol levels in the ectopic

ACTH syndromes. Affected patients have elevated serum cortisol, corticosteroids, and 11-deoxycorticosteroids.

In the diagnosis of Cushing's syndrome, rare cases may require catheterization of the petrosal veins with ACTH measurement across the pituitary bed, often with CRH infusion to differentiate pituitary-dependent Cushing's syndrome from ectopic production of ACTH.[58] When no mass is seen in the pituitary on computed tomography (CT) scan or magnetic resonance imaging (MRI),[59] however, and it remains important to make the noted distinction in diagnosis, catheterization is recommended to detect a peripheral vein–petrosal vein ACTH gradient. In Cushing's disease, 20 to 30% of patients may have a negative CT scan or MRI of the pituitary, yet a microadenoma may be found by surgical exploration. For catheterization procedures, simultaneous catheterization of the right and left petrosal veins is recommended. The specificity of petrosal sinus catheterization in Cushing's disease or other pituitary-dependent, ACTH-producing syndromes is 100% except for the rare ectopic CRH-producing or CRH/ACTH–producing tumor.[60]

The invasive radiologic techniques to differentiate pituitary-dependent versus non–pituitary-dependent causes of Cushing's syndrome are the subject of some discussion.[61, 62] Bilateral inferior petrosal sinus catheterization requires skill and the need for CRH injection to minimize false-negative rates. The risk of serious morbidity for the procedure is about 1 per 1000 studies. Bilateral catheterization of the jugular venous bulb may rule out pituitary-dependent Cushing's syndrome with a high degree of specificity, but a negative examination necessitates higher level catheterization,[63–65] in either the inferior petrosal sinuses or the cavernous sinus, the latter requiring no CRH administration.[64, 66, 67] The arena of radiologic diagnosis is, however, a controversial one[65] because of the potential for venous dilutional error, improper catheter tip placement, pulsatile excretion and ACTH, and the loss of specificity when dynamic MRI is used in place of stand CT scans of the sella. *Incidentalomas* of the pituitary are found in 27% of autopsies[68] and 61% of MRI studies; the false-negative rate for MRI of the sella varies between 8 and 25%.[65]

ACTH secretion and an increase in serum cortisol 20 to 50% greater than basal levels are typical of pituitary-dependent causes of Cushing's syndrome on infusion of ovine CRH and administration of metyrapone. The test is less useful and specific, however, in patients with ectopic CRH-producing tumors and in some patients with carcinoid tumors. These changes, however, are specific for approximately 90% of Cushing's syndrome and may approach 100% when combined with a positive high-dose dexamethasone suppression test.[69]

The vasopressin analogue desmopressin (1-deamino-8-D-arginine-vasopressin [DDAVP]), a nontoxic, less expensive (than CRH) compound without appreciable clinical vasopressor activity at usual doses, is being evaluated in the differential diagnosis of Cushing's disease. Early studies with 5- to 10-μg injections of desmopressin have shown a rise in serum ACTH and cortisol of greater than 50% above baseline in pituitary-dependent Cushing's syndrome. DDAVP evoked no ACTH rise in these studies, either in patients with adrenal causes of Cushing's syndrome or in the few patients studied with ectopic ACTH-producing tumors. Because of its low cost and the greater induced changes in ACTH and cortisol

from baseline than are seen with CRH infusion, DDAVP may prove useful in diagnosing difficult cases of Cushing's syndrome.[70]

Given such biochemical and metabolic overlap in determining the cause of Cushing's syndrome, the use of IRMA measurements of ACTH and the peptide products of POMC enzymatic degradation by tumors seems to offer new hope for ready and specific laboratory diagnosis of the ectopic ACTH syndromes. Because adrenal causes of Cushing's syndrome are not associated with elevated plasma ACTH, and non–pituitary-dependent tumors predominantly excrete POMC peptides relative to the biologically active ACTH, measurements of β-MSH and γ-lipotropic hormone (γ-LPH) seem to be quite useful diagnostically. A high ratio of β-MSH/γ-LPH (see Table 18–3) is a feature of the ectopic tumor production syndromes. White and coworkers[71] measured ACTH precursors in pituitary-dependent and pituitary-independent syndromes, noting precursor serum levels to average 37 pmol/L and 3697 pmol/L. The ratio of precursor to biologically active ACTH was 5 for pituitary-dependent syndromes and 58 for pituitary-independent (ectopic) ACTH syndromes.

The presence of somatostatin receptors on neuroendocrine tumors, such as carcinoid tumors and small cell lung cancer, has led to the use of somatostatin analogues to inhibit ACTH production and to aid further in differential diagnosis of hypercortisolism states.[47, 48, 72] Octreotide in doses of 300 to 1500 μg/day quickly returns serum ACTH and cortisol levels toward normal in patients with ectopic syndromes. Other diagnostic studies using radiolabeled somatostatin analogues have proved useful in identifying most clinical sites of ectopic ACTH production.[48, 72] In instances in which the tumor has been shown in vitro to have appropriate somatostatin receptors, all ectopic production sites are identifiable. Because of high background uptake, tomographic scintigraphy with high isotope doses is recommended. For abdominal studies, high doses of indium 111–labeled analogues, such as indium 111–DPTA octreotide, indium 111 pentatreotide, and indium 111 Tyr3-octreotide, have been used. The pentatreotide analogue is excreted predominantly by the kidneys, offering added use in abdominal scans for tumors. Isotope doses of 100 to 200 MBq have been used for scanning. The isotopic studies are particularly relevant to the diagnosis of bronchial adenomas because these are characteristically small (0.3 to 1.5 cm) and may escape detection by CT scan. A report using radiolabled somatostatin analogue identified a 7-mm bronchial adenoma causing an ectopic ACTH-producing syndrome. Radiolabeled somatostatin analogues used in the differential diagnosis of Cushing's syndrome are enhanced by the observation that pituitary adenomas and adrenal cancers do not take up the isotopes. Although localization of ectopic ACTH production by carcinoid and related neuroendocrine tumors has been quite useful, experience with small cell lung cancers with ectopic ACTH production has been more limited. When somatostatin analogues are selected for treatment of ectopic syndromes, it is believed that useful therapeutic responses are more likely when tumor receptors are identified by tissue analysis or by isotope scanning. Of further interest is the observation that treatment with the progestin antagonist-agonist RU 486 (mifepristone) may enhance expression of somatostatin receptors. This agent may improve the diagnostic utility of the analogue approach, and it may prove useful in therapy as well.[71]

**Treatment.** Treatment of ectopic ACTH syndromes is concerned with management of the malignancy and management of the metabolic abnormalities, which are often the dominant causes of clinical morbidity. In small cell lung carcinoma with Cushing's syndrome resulting from ectopic ACTH production, prognosis is grave. One study[73] showed that 82% of affected patients died within 54 days of initiating chemotherapy, whereas 25% died in that period when small cell lung cancer presented without clinical Cushing's syndrome. Patients with Cushing's syndrome usually die from infection. In a study[34] of small cell lung carcinoma with ectopic ACTH syndrome, patients had a median survival of 5.5 months, although 5 of the 14 patients presented with limited disease. For carcinoid tumors with ectopic ACTH production, prognosis is not as poor; thymic carcinoid tumors with Cushing's syndrome have a 10-year survival of 35% and a median survival of 5 years.[74]

These observations have led to the view that optimal management of small cell lung carcinoma with Cushing's syndrome requires initial control of the metabolic abnormalities over a 1- to 2-week period before initiating myelotoxic antitumor chemotherapy or surgery. Because control of hypercortisolism and its effects may be critical to survival, it is fortunate that a variety of agents are available and useful in most instances of Cushing's syndrome. Table 18–5 lists current medical approaches available to control the glucocorticoid excess in patients with ectopic ACTH-producing tumors.

Bilateral adrenalectomy or removal of the tumor source of ACTH remains the best and most rapid approach to hormonal control, although this may not always be feasible because of concurrent illness or the debilitating effects of hypercortisolism. Most physicians favor initial reduction of glucocorticoid production by the use of mitotane (1,1-dichlorodiphenyldi-chloroethane ortho-p'-DDD), ketoconazole,[75] aminoglutethimide, or RU 486.[76] Bromocriptine has also been reported to reverse ectopic ACTH secretion and the symptoms of glucocorticoid excess.[77] Other than with bromocriptine and RU 486, there is appreciable clinical toxicity in about 50% of patients.

The somatostatin analogue octreotide may be useful in treatment, especially for patients with carcinoid tumors producing ACTH. The efficacy of octreotide has been challenged,[78] but it appears quite efficacious and is associated with tolerable toxicity.[48, 78, 79] In one review of results that were not correlated with tumor somatostatin receptors, octreotide's use in carcinoid and related tumors resulted in five of nine patients having a reduced serum cortisol level, of which four returned to normal.[69] ACTH levels also were reduced in seven of these nine patients and returned to normal in four. The authors observed that gastrinomas responded better to octreotide than carcinoid tumors of the lung.

The glucocorticoid receptor antagonist-agonist RU 486, although still an investigational agent, may have special value in reversing the hypokalemic alkalosis of the ectopic ACTH syndromes as well as the psychoses seen frequently.[80] In contrast to the other therapeutic agents for Cushing's syndrome, RU 486 produces clinical improvement without significant changes in serum cortisol or urinary corticosteroid excretion. The agent is also being evaluated as potentially inducing tumor somatostatin receptor expression in the ectopic ACTH syndromes, offering added potential for somatostatin analogues used in diagnosis and therapy.

Because of the danger of induced adrenal insufficiency with agents such as aminoglutethimide, mitotane, and RU 486, 24-hour urinary free cortisol measurements while receiving therapy have been recommended to anticipate the desired antiadrenal effects of such drugs and to guide the initiation of adrenal replacement therapy.

Although the ACTH-producing tumors present important diagnostic and therapeutic challenges with respect to glucocorticoid metabolism, small cell carcinoma and carcinoid tumors frequently and concomitantly produce a variety of other hormones. These peptide hormones as well as other paracrine and autocrine factors may have important effects on survival, response to therapy, and prognosis. More than one paraneoplastic syndrome may appear in the same patient.[81, 82]

## HYPERCALCEMIA

**Background.** Hypercalcemia in malignancy has received increasing attention since its early description in the 1930s by Gutman. The prevalence of hypercalcemia in newly diagnosed lung cancer, the most common antecedent tumor causing hypercalcemia, was 0.52% of 9006 new patients referred to a comprehensive cancer center.[83] The frequencies of hypercalcemia developing during the clinical course of nonhematologic malignancies in one series were as follows: epidermoid lung cancer (25%); breast cancer (20%); squamous carcinoma of the head and neck, the esophagus, and the cervix (19%); and renal cell carcinoma (8%).[84] In other broad surveys, the common cancers associated with hypercalcemia were breast and lung cancer, which together constituted approximately one half of incident cases, whereas uterine, cervical, esophageal, and head and neck cancer; lymphoma; multiple myeloma; and renal cell cancer equally contributed to the remaining number of cases.[85, 86]

The cause of hypercalcemia in cancer patients was initially considered to be secondary to bony metastatic disease causing bone resorption and liberation of calcium into the serum, as typified by breast cancer and osteolytic multiple myeloma. Of breast cancer patients, however, 85% develop bony metastatic disease, and only 15% of these have hyper-

*Table 18–5.* **Medical Treatment of Cushing's Syndrome Resulting from Ectopic ACTH Production**

| Drug | Dosage | Site of Action |
|------|--------|----------------|
| Metyrapone | 250–6000 mg/day PO | Adrenal gland |
| Ketoconazole* | 400–800 mg/day PO | Adrenal gland |
| Aminoglutethimide* | 1000–1500 mg/day PO | Adrenal gland |
| RU 486* | 10–20 mg/kg/day IM or PO | Glucocorticoid tissue receptors |
| Octreotide | 100–300 µg SC q 8 hr daily | Tumor somatostatin receptors |
| Bromocriptine | 20–30 mg/day PO | Dopamine receptors |
| Ortho-p'DDD* | 10 g/day PO | Adrenal gland |

*May require glucocorticoid replacement (i.e., dexamethasone 1.0 mg PO daily).

calcemia.[87] Twenty-five percent of hypercalcemic breast cancer patients have no bone metastases.[88] Small cell lung cancer patients frequently have bony metastatic disease, but hypercalcemia is rare, whereas epidermoid lung cancer is responsible for almost all lung cancer–associated hypercalcemia, and rarely is there concomitant bony metastatic disease. In one report,[89] 66% of small cell lung cancer patients had bony metastases, but none had hypercalcemia, whereas 27% of the squamous cell lung cancer patients had hypercalcemia, but none had bony metastases.

These observations have led to the concept that hypercalcemia in cancer, when not caused by the rare complicating parathyroid adenoma or hyperplasia, is most frequently due to humoral factors liberated directly or indirectly by the tumor and is not due to simple bony erosion by expanding erosive metastatic cancer.[90, 91] As such, humoral hypercalcemia may then be considered a typical and common paraneoplastic syndrome.

Understanding the humoral hypercalcemia of malignancy was dramatically aided by discovery of the parathyroid hormone–related protein (PTHrP) in patients with hypercalcemia.[92–96] Such a protein was suggested by Albright in 1941. PTHrP, whose gene is located on chromosome 12, exists as three peptide isomers of 139, 141 the most dominant PTHrP gene product, or 173 amino acids and shares homology with native parathyroid hormone (PTH) in 8 of the first 13 amino acids at the amino terminal portion of the molecule (1–34). This is the site of biologic activity for bone resorption and renal effects on phosphate resorption, calciuria, and α-hydroxylase activity. PTHrP circulates in the serum predominantly in the 1–74 and 109–138 amino acid fragments; in renal failure, the 109–138 amino acid terminal fragment is retained and may increase 10-fold above levels of the 1–74 fragment. In tumor tissue, 22- to 23-kd PTHrP amino acid fragments are found, whereas there is accumulation of a 10-kd fragment in pleural effusions.[97] New IRMA techniques now permit measurement of PTH and PTHrP at two sites within these molecules so that there is no immunologic cross-reactivity with the 84-amino acid PTH molecule. Current assay techniques are much improved over those used in the past.[98] Clinically, PTHrP hypercalcemia is more rapid in onset than that of primary hyperparathyroidism and causes symptoms to occur at a lower than expected level of serum calcium; it is unlikely to find clinical keratopathy, renal calculi, pruritus, or the osteopenia characteristic of primary hyperparathyroidism, with its more chronic course of persistent hypercalcemia.

Table 18–6 lists the clinical and biologic characteristics of hypercalcemia accompanying elevated PTH and PTHrP, which share clinical effects and affinity for bone and renal PTH receptors. In PTHrP-related hypercalcemia, there is usually an absence of induced renal α-hydroxylase activity so that serum 1,25-dihydroxyvitamin $D_3$ is usually, but not invariably, low.[99] In contrast, there are increased hydroxylase and serum vitamin D levels with primary hyperparathyroidism.[100, 101] Because renal receptors for PTHrP (at the amino *terminal end* of the molecule) are present, it is of interest that the PTHrP 1–141 amino acid moiety has less resorptive capacity in bone assay systems than either the PTH 1–34 or the 1–74 PTHrP fragment. Fukumoto and colleagues[102] postulated a circulating inhibitor in hypercalcemic cancer patients accounting for reduced renal α-hydroxylase expres-

*Table 18–6.* **Clinical and Laboratory Findings in Hypercalcemia Resulting from Primary Hyperparathyroidism (PHP) or Parathyroid Hormone–Related Protein (PTHrP)**

|  | PTHr | PHP |
|---|---|---|
| CNS symptoms at lower levels of hypercalcemia | Yes* | No |
| Normal or reduced serum 1,25-dihydroxyvitamin $D_3$ | Yes | No |
| Acidosis | Yes | No |
| Decreased renal reabsorption of phosphorus | Yes | No |
| Pruritus | No | Yes |
| Alkalosis | No | Yes |
| Renal calculi | No | Yes |
| Band keratopathy | No | Yes |
| Osteomalacia and bone remodeling | No | Yes |
| Activates renal α-hydroxylase | No | Yes |
| Osteopenia | No | Yes |
| Increased urinary cAMP | Yes | Yes |
| Hypercalciuria | Yes | Yes |
| Elevated osteocalcin (bone GLA protein) | No | No |

*Yes, Common; no, uncommon.
CNS, central nervous system; cAMP, cyclic adenosine monophosphate.

sion.[103] A PTHrP fragment cleaved near the carboxyl terminal of the mentioned 1–141 amino acid fragment has been shown to possess inhibitory action on osteoclastic bone-resorbing activity.[104] The amount of this putatively inhibitory carboxyl fragment 107–111 (termed *osteostatin*), relative to the amounts of PTHrP 1–74 circulating fragments, may influence levels of induced hypercalcemia as well as inhibit renal α-hydroxylase induction. Circulating cytokines (interleukin-6 [IL-6] and tumor necrosis factor [TNF]) may inhibit the expression of renal α-hydroxylase as well.[105]

Although PTHrP was first detected in the blood of patients with cancer and is rarely detected in the serum of healthy individuals, or only at very low levels, it is found in a variety of fetal and normal adult tissues, in breast milk, and in other body fluids.[106] The normal biologic function of PTHrP is not fully understood. It (1) is involved in the transplacental transfer of calcium; (2) is a smooth muscle relaxant; (3) regulates cell proliferation, differentiation, and apoptosis; and (4) is probably a developmental factor because disruption of its gene or its receptor is lethal in fetal or postpartum life.[107] Placental transfer of calcium and fetal calcium homeostasis may be localized in the 75–84 amino acid fragment of the molecule as well as in the 35–94 fragment; fragments 1–34 and 1–36 have been shown to have growth-regulating and hypercalcemic action; the 109–141 fragment inhibits osteoclast function; and the 63–78 and the 1–74 fragments are characteristic of humoral hypercalcemia of malignancy.[98] Elevations of serum PTHrP are found with many epithelial and hematologic malignancies in association with hypercalcemia, especially with tumors of squamous cell histology. Among patients with solid tumors and hypercalcemia, 71% have an elevated (>2 pmol/ml) serum PTHrP; 85% of those without bony metastases have elevated PTHrP.[108] PTHrP is usually not present in the serum or is found at only low levels in solid tumor patients without hypercalcemia; serum levels are low or undetectable in normal subjects.

The quantitative level of serum PTHrP does not predict the severity of clinical hypercalcemia.[109] This poor correlation probably relates to complex interactions of the various circulating PTHrP fragments and other factors that are active

*Table 18–7.* **Identified Clinical Tumor Products Influencing Hypercalcemia of Malignancy**

| Promoting Net Bone Resorption and Increased Serum Calcium | Inhibiting Net Bone Resorption and Decreased Serum Calcium |
|---|---|
| Parathyroid hormone | Calcitonin |
| Parathyroid hormone–related protein | α interferon |
| Colony-stimulating factors | Transforming growth factor β |
| Tumor necrosis factor α and β | Osteocalcin (bone GLA protein) |
| Interleukin-1, 2- and -6 | Osteostatin |
| Prostaglandin $E_2$ | |
| Transforming growth factor α | |
| Corticosteroids | |
| 1,25-Dihydroxyvitamin $D_3$ | |
| 1,24(R)Dihydroxyvitamin $D_3$ | |
| Tumor-derived procathepsin D | |

at the bone, renal, or gut level in regulating serum calcium levels. Such interactions, however, are not yet fully understood. Tumor-induced or tumor-secreted circulating factors, lymphokines, and cytokines that influence osteoclast function include 1,25-dihydroxyvitamin $D_3$, PTH, PTHrP, IL-1 and IL-6, TNF-α and TNF-β, and colony-stimulating factors.[110, 111] The blood ionized calcium level is affected by the following components of calcium metabolism: (1) local bone resorption and remodeling, (2) renal calcium absorption and excretion, (3) gastrointestinal calcium absorption, and (4) renal and other tissue sites for the synthesis of 1,25-dihydroxyvitamin $D_3$. General and tumor-related factors that may influence these components of calcium metabolism are summarized in Tables 18–7 and 18–8.

Using older and then standard radioimmunoassays for PTH, elevations of PTHrP associated with hypercalcemia usually demonstrated normal or slightly low PTH serum levels. This apparent lack of normal responsiveness of PTH to an elevated serum calcium level has been clarified through use of the new double-site IRMA technology. With these current assays, PTH is usually low or undetectable in the humoral hypercalcemia of malignancy associated with elevated PTHrP[97]; if serum PTH is found to be increased in that setting, concomitant primary hyperparathyroidism or the ectopic production of PTH should be expected as occurring either in the same tumor-producing PTHrP or in another producing only PTH.[97, 112, 113]

Certain clinical tumors are unique in relation to their association with humoral hypercalcemia. Table 18–8 summarizes the factors resulting in humoral hypercalcemia in the various clinical cancers. Although lung cancer is commonly associated with serum calcium elevation, this relationship is largely with squamous cell cancers; small cell (oat) lung cancer is much less commonly associated with hypercalcemia, as noted previously. In contrast, ovarian small cell carcinoma, which may be histologically difficult to distinguish from ovarian gonadoblastoma, dysgerminoma, or clear cell carcinoma, is characteristically associated with humoral hypercalcemia.[114] In another review of 75 patients with ovarian cancer of this type, 67% had hypercalcemia.[115] Hypercalcemia is now recognized as the most common paraneoplastic syndrome in ovarian cancer, and patient prognosis seems quite poor in all stages other than stage IA. Ovarian oat cell cancer hypercalcemia may be due to PTHrP secretion,[115, 116] although early published reports did not always include such levels. Elevated serum calcitriol is also reported with ovarian small cell cancer along with elevated PTHrP.[117] In one report, however, the ectopic production of PTH by an ovarian tumor was noted.[118]

Although elevated serum PTHrP has been found in most solid tumors presenting with elevated serum calcium, it is low or undetectable in greater than 92% of patients with primary hyperparathyroidism and elevated in only about one third of hematologic malignancies with hypercalcemia.[119] These elevations of PTHrP are not common in patients with myeloma but are characteristic in patients with adult T-cell lymphoma.

The hematologic malignancies present a complex and often mixed picture with regard to observed hypercalcemic mechanisms. Of interest is the predominant role of PTHrP in most patients with hypercalcemia and adult human T-cell lymphotropic virus (HTLV-1) lymphoma.[120] In this disease, hypercalcemia may be due to induction of the PTHrP gene on chromosome 12 by HTLV-1, which also may activate the *tax* gene, which stimulates production by these lymphoma cells of IL-2 and the IL-2 receptor, furthering net bone resorption (see Table 18–7). Although elevated calcitriol is seen in some of these adult T-cell lymphomas,[121] increased synthesis of 1,25-dihydroxyvitamin $D_3$, which results in hypercalcemia, is characteristic of acquired immunodeficiency syndrome (AIDS)-related lymphoma[122] and has been suggested to be the predominant cause of hypercalcemia in Hodgkin's and non-Hodgkin's lymphoma.[123] Dysregulated vitamin D metabolism in these lymphomas results in elevated calcitriol levels and increased osteoclastic effects.

*Table 18–8.* **Defined Causes of Hypercalcemia in Cancer**

| Tumor | Major Cause | Minor Cause |
|---|---|---|
| Squamous cell carcinoma (any site), most other solid tumors | PTHrP | Leukokines and osteokines (breast cancer) |
| Small cell ovarian cancer, B-cell lymphoma, myeloma | ? PTHrP, leukokines, osteokines | Ectopic PTH secretion, PTHrP, synthesis of 1,25-dihydroxyvitamin $D_3$ |
| Adult T-cell lymphoma | PTHrP, leukokines | Increased synthesis of 1,25-dihydroxyvitamin $D_3$, prostaglandins |
| AIDS-associated lymphoma, non-Hodgkin's lymphoma | Increased synthesis of 1,25-dihydroxyvitamin $D_3$, prostaglandins | PTHrP, leukokines |
| Small cell cancer (rarely) of lung and ovary | PTHrP | PTH, 1,24(R)dihydroxyvitamin $D_3$ |

PTHrP, parathyroid hormone–related protein; PTH, parathyroid hormone; AIDS, acquired immunodeficiency syndrome.

Calcitriol may act with IL-1 and TNF as well in lymphomas. Hypercalcemia is more characteristic of the aggressive high-grade and intermediate-grade non-Hodgkin's lymphomas, in which 30% of cases occur. There is a 1.4% frequency of hypercalcemia among all lymphomas, and published reports show an underrepresentation in Hodgkin's disease with nodular sclerosis histology. Lymphomas with a *starry-sky* histology as a result of macrophages appear to be more associated with hypercalcemia. Hypercalcemia in low-grade B-cell malignancies is, in general, uncommon.[124] Such tumors, other than myeloma, are featured by micro-osteoclastic bone resorption when bone metastases occur, causing bone remodeling that does not release calcium into the circulation. In myeloma, micro-osteoclastic activity is not elevated. There is no increased micro-osteoclastic activity in the absence of bone marrow involvement by these B-cell lymphomas.[125]

Perhaps the best evidence for the primary role of humoral factors in hypercalcemia of malignancy is the series of experimental studies in nude mouse tumor models. In these studies, human tumors associated with hypercalcemia and the specific production of PTHrP, IL-6, or IL-1 were transplanted and grew in the mouse model. Resultant hypercalcemia was prevented or effectively reduced by treatment with specific antihuman PTHrP, IL-6, or IL-1 antibodies and not by the relevant antimouse antibodies.[126, 127]

Other causes of hypercalcemia in cancer include the approximate 7% of patients with primary hyperparathyroidism or ectopic production of PTH.[118] There is one report of a small cell lung cancer producing 1,24(R)-dihydroxyvitamin $D_3$,[128] which has biologic activity equal to that of 1,25-dihydroxyvitamin $D_3$.

Myeloma bone resorption and hypercalcemia, although occasionally influenced by PTHrP, seem to occur almost exclusively in the clinical setting of osteolytic bone lesions or diffuse osteopenia. The hypercalcemia is caused predominantly by cytokines,[129] mainly IL-1 and prostaglandins made by the surrounding stromal cells, perhaps under stimulation by PTHrP, IL-6, IL-1, and TNF. Myeloma cells themselves may also make PTHrP as well as these cytokines, inhibiting bone osteoblastic activity. In about 15% of patients with myeloma, there are no lytic bone lesions at the time of diagnosis, and in some other myeloma patients, bone lesions are sclerotic.[130] These patients often have increased bone GLA protein (osteocalcin), which stimulates osteoblastic activity. Such myeloma patients are usually found to have an M protein lambda light chain dysproteinemia caused by IgG or IgA and more rarely by IgM.[131, 132]

In this *sclerotic myeloma* and in other plasma cell disorders associated with sclerotic bone lesions, there is often an associated peripheral motor or sensory neuronopathy along with components of the POEMS syndrome (polyneuropathy, organomegaly, endocrinopathy, M protein myeloma, and skin changes [e.g., hyperpigmentation, hypertrichosis, or thickening])[133] and Castleman's syndrome (angiofollicular lymph node hyperplasia, characterized by blood vessel proliferation and sheaths of monoclonal plasma cells between the lymph node follicles).[134] In a large review of plasma cell dyscrasias with sclerotic bone lesions at the Mayo Clinic, 84% of the 38 patients with accompanying polyneuropathy had osteosclerotic bone lesions, and 86% of the time these patients also had the multiorgan involvement seen in POEMS; 5 of the 38 patients reviewed fulfilled all POEMS criteria.[135] In this

patient group, 87% had an abnormal M protein in the serum that was usually an IgA lambda, and 94% of the patients had a lambda light chain protein, IgG, IgA, or IgM. The characteristic diffuse plasmacytic infiltration of the bone marrow (>10% plasma cells) with painful osteolytic bone lesions typical for classic myeloma may be contrasted with osteosclerotic, neuronopathic myeloma, in which marrow plasma cell infiltration is less than 5% and plasmacytomatous sclerotic lesions are more typical.[136] Because Castleman's syndrome also has been reported with features of POEMS and M protein–associated polyneuropathy, current opinion supports a general plasma cell dyscrasia syndrome that encompasses sclerotic myeloma, POEMS, and Castleman's syndrome.

The Crow-Fukase and Takatsuki syndromes (no longer described only in Japanese men) are prominently associated with coronary and general vascular insufficiency related to an increased concentration of IgG or IgA M component lambda light chains.[133, 137] These syndromes also have POEMS features and perhaps should also be considered as part of the sclerotic myeloma spectrum.[138] Hypercalcemia is rare in these patient groups, but if it occurs in these or in any patient with elevated serum proteins as a result of excessive amounts of IgG or IgM immunoglobulin production, serum ionized calcium is normal, and symptoms caused by hypercalcemia are absent. Each mole of IgG myeloma protein binds 4 mol of serum calcium at the lambda light chain Fab fragment.[139] The role of IL-6 has been explored in these diseases and may be more reflective of disease status in myeloma and Castleman's syndrome than in the POEMS syndrome.[140, 141] IL-6 has been viewed as being responsible for *uncoupling* of bone in vivo, that is, blocking the formation of new bone (osteoblastic activity) in the face of excessive absorption of bone by osteoclasts, mediated by PTHrP and other cytokines.[142] In tumor-bearing mice, antibodies to IL-6 block such uncoupling and permit remodeling of bone in the face of continued PTHrP tumor secretion.

One of the newer directions resulting from the understanding of the biologic mediators of hypercalcemia is to assess their relevance to clinical metastatic pattern and prognosis. This thinking may have been stimulated by observations on the customarily *limited* disease presentation of small cell lung cancer when accompanied by the paraneoplastic endocrine syndrome of ectopic ACTH production and certain neurologic syndromes (see later). Recognizing the association of PTHrP with breast cancer, several authors[143, 144] noted that in 92% of patients with breast cancer, bony metastases, and hypercalcemia, there was elevated serum PTHrP, whereas only 36% of patients without hypercalcemia but with bony metastases had an elevated serum PTHrP, and only 9% of normocalcemic breast cancer patients without bony metastases had elevated serum PTHrP. Approximately 60% of primary breast cancer specimens were immunohistochemically positive for PTHrP. Staining correlated with the presence of progesterone receptors but not for lymph node status, tumor size, tumor grade, or the presence of estrogen receptors, and 92% of breast cancer metastases to bone were immunohistochemically positive for PTHrP. Analysis of other organ metastases showed PTHrP positive only 17% of the time. These studies suggest that an assay for an elevated PTHrP in the primary tumor may predict a future bony metastatic pattern, possibly assisting in decisions for prevention of skeletal metastases with the bisphosphonates.[145] In early controlled studies from Leiden in 170 patients with breast cancer treated with or without pamidronate, the treated group had less bony complications than the control group. In a clodronate study, the treated group had less hypercalcemia (25 vs. 52 control), fewer vertebral fractures (84 vs. 124 control), and fewer overall skeletal complications (219 vs. 305 control).[146] In contrast, 100% of prostate cancers stain for PTHrP, but hypercalcemia is rare even with extensive bone metastases. Bisphosphonate effects on bone healing in patients with prostate cancer have been modest.[147] Animal data in vivo demonstrate that the presence of PTHrP in tumors favors skeletal metastasis growth.[142, 148, 149]

**Diagnosis.** Measurement of an elevated serum calcium value (8.5 to 10.5 mg/dl) in the presence of such symptoms as somnolence, coma, confusion, nausea and vomiting, polyuria, or a shortened QT interval on electrocardiogram usually leads to the appropriate diagnosis. Bone pain may also be a symptom. In symptomatic patients with normal or borderline elevated serum calcium and hypoalbuminemia, measured calcium levels may be approximately corrected by adding 0.8 mg/dl or 0.2 mmol for each 10 g of albumin per liter of serum concentration less than a normal value of 40 g/L. The differential diagnosis should include various granulomatous diseases, such as sarcoid, which may occasionally accompany lymphoma, and hypervitaminosis D. An unusual cause of symptomatic hypercalcemia occurring during cancer therapy and that may be life-threatening is the *tumor flare* reaction associated with hormonal management of breast cancer when extensive bony metastases are present. The incidence is about 3 to 7% of treated patients, usually occurring within 2 to 14 days of initiating any hormonal therapy other than surgical ablation. Patients present with classic findings of acute hypercalcemia, along with bone pain, and increased serum alkaline phosphatase. Such episodes are said to portend a favorable response to therapy and are readily managed. Conventional combination cytotoxic chemotherapy for 1 to 2 weeks during hormone initiation may prove as useful and, when given concomitantly with hormones, may prevent flare reactions. The relative effectiveness of concomitant treatment with a bisphosphonate has not been fully evaluated but will probably prove useful as well.

**Treatment.** Table 18–9 lists the agents available for the treatment of humoral hypercalcemia in cancer. Agents are grouped on the basis of their general use for all the hypercalcemic states and in relation to the specific causes of hypercalcemia. For many tumors, the cause of hypercalcemia is multifactorial, so that the response of the patient to therapy should be carefully followed.

There are several excellent reviews of therapy for hypercalcemia in malignancy.[147, 150, 151] Infused saline is the cornerstone of therapy, and many patients with mild or somewhat moderate hypercalcemia have normalized serum calcium after adequate hydration. Saline is primarily for volume repletion and expansion because polyuria, hypovolemia, and resulting impaired renal calcium excretion are frequently associated with an elevated serum calcium. In addition, presentation of a saline load to the renal distal loop facilitates calciuresis, which may be enhanced further by addition of a loop diuretic, such as furosemide. Thiazide diuretics should not be used and have been associated with facilitating hypercalcemia by inducing renal calcium absorption in exchange with sodium.

When moderate or high serum calcium levels are present and the use of bisphosphonates is planned, measurements of serum PTHrP and urinary cyclic adenosine monophosphate (cAMP) should be considered to confirm that the cause of the hypercalcemia is one that would be amenable to treat-

**Table 18–9.** Agents for Clinical Treatment Related to the Pathogenesis of Hypercalcemia

| | Dosage | Toxicity |
|---|---|---|
| *General Use* | | |
| Normal saline | 2–3 L/ml/day IV | Volume overload |
| Furosemide | 20–60 mg/day IV | Hypomagnesemia |
| Neutral phosphate | 100 mmol/IV over 24 hr/day | Metastatic calcinosis |
| WR-2721 (amifostine) | Experimental agent | |
| *PTHrP Elevations* | | |
| Calcitonin | 2–8 U/kg SC or IM | None |
| Plicamycin (mithramycin) | 15–24 µg/kg IV over 4–24 hr | Disorders of protein metabolism Hemorrhagic effects |
| Etidronate (Didronel) | 7.5 mg/kg IV daily × 5–7 in saline | Increased serum PO$_4$ |
| Gallium nitrate (Ganite) | 200 mg/m$^2$ IV daily over 5 days | Renal toxicity |
| Pamidronate (Aredia) | 60–90 mg IV over 8 hr | Fever, PO$_4$ depletion |
| Clodronate (not in U.S.) | 500 mg in saline IV over 4 hr; 300 mg IV over 4 hr daily × 5 | Osteolysis |
| Octreotide | 150 µg SC TID | Little |
| *Elevated Synthesis of 1,25-Dihydroxyvitamin D$_3$* | | |
| Prednisone | 40–60 mg/day PO | Little with short duration of use |
| *Increased Prostaglandin Synthesis* | | |
| Indomethacin | 50–150 mg/day PO | Little with short duration of use |

PTHrP, parathyroid hormone–related protein.

ment with osteoclast inhibitors. Measurement of urinary hydroxyproline excretion has been used as an indirect measure of inhibition of osteoclast function by the bisphosphonates,[152] although excretion in malignancy may be an unreliable measure of bone formation. More recent approaches to assessment of adequacy of bisphosphonate osteoclast inhibition have relied on the urinary excretion of pyridinolene and deoxypyridinolene.[153] Calcitonin's effect is mediated through binding of osteoclast receptors; its onset of action is the most prompt among agents used to treat hypercalcemia. The effectiveness of bisphosphonates has made the role of calcitonin an archaic one in contemporary hypercalcemia management. Repeated use often results in tachyphylaxis, but it is unclear whether concomitant use of corticosteroids would reverse this observed resistance to calcitonin. The predominant role of corticosteroids is in the management of hypercalcemia in which calcitriol effects are prominent. Plicamycin (mithramycin) inhibits the effects on bone osteoclasts of vitamin D and PTHrP. Gallium nitrate (Ganite) inhibits osteoclasts. The bisphosphonates etidronate, pamidronate, and clodronate inhibit the brush border of osteoclasts, resulting in structural changes and inhibited function in these cells.

Currently, it is believed that pamidronate, alone or in combination with calcitonin, offers the most rapid and effective treatment for hypercalcemia when the predominant cause is tumor production of PTHrP. In emergent clinical situations, calcitonin (300 international units intramuscularly every 6 hours) and pamidronate (90 mg intravenously over 3 hours) have proved effective.[154] The dose of pamidronate chosen relates to the severity of the hypercalcemia and to whether a high dose is necessary to overcome low-dose bisphosphonate resistance.[155] Single doses of pamidronate are as effective as divided multiple doses; normocalcemic levels are usually reached 3 to 7 days after therapy is initiated, with a median of 4 days. Total doses of pamidronate of 80 mg give a 90 to 95% success rate for normocalcemia when osteolysis is the predominant disorder.[155] Orally active bisphosphonates may be useful in the subsequent outpatient management of hypercalcemia.

Bisphosphonate toxicity is largely renal and is believed to be related to calcium-phosphonate crystallization in the blood and rapidity of infusion. Because pamidronate is given in smaller doses owing to its greatly enhanced effects on bone resorption, toxicity is minimal and readily prevented by prolonging infusion. Correction of hypercalcemia usually results in recovery from all symptoms, usually within 24 to 48 hours of return to normal of the serum calcium. A fall in serum PTHrP does not occur with serum calcium fall after bisphosphonate therapy, although serum PTH levels may rise to normal after therapy of humoral hypercalcemia of malignancy.[156] In some reports using bisphosphonates, bone pain may not resolve as readily; calcitonin, because of its apparent analgesic effect in cancer, may aid in the control of this hypercalcemic symptom. Prednisone's effects are predominantly related to inhibition of macrophage α-hydroxylase activity and absorption of intestinal calcium; lowering of the serum calcium may occur without tumor shrinkage.

Octreotide therapy (150 μg subcutaneously every 8 hours) has been effective after failure of conventional therapy with fluids and calcitonin.[157] It is not clear whether this somatostatin analogue's mechanism of action is mediated through inhibition of PTHrP tumor cell secretion, in a manner similar to the agent's effects in the ectopic ACTH syndromes, or through effects on calcitriol production. Both mechanisms have been suggested as related to hypercalcemia, but appropriate correlative clinical measurements are largely lacking.

Certain chemotherapeutic agents, such as cisplatin, are associated with calciuresis and may have a role in managing hypercalcemic states or tumors associated commonly with hypercalcemia. Because hypercalcemia can be anticipated in most cancers, prevention should be considered to be of clinical importance. Maintenance of adequate hydration and intravascular volume and avoidance of diuretic therapy for hypertension are helpful. Oral neutral phosphates (250 to 400 mg daily) and phytic acid are less commonly used since the advent of bisphosphonate therapy.

Patient survival in hypercalcemia is often short, usually less than 90 days even when the hypercalcemia is corrected, perhaps signaling ineffective tumor therapy. Failure to correct hypercalcemia in the face of adequate treatment with conventional and correctly selected agents and recurrent hypercalcemia imply rapid tumor growth and short survival. Recurrent hypercalcemia in head and neck cancer after a period of cancer therapy had a more ominous prognosis than initial hypercalcemia on presentation before any therapy of the tumor in one study.[158] Hypercalcemia occurring in association with small cell cancer of the ovary is notoriously difficult to treat with conventional agents, perhaps resulting in that tumor's poor prognosis.

For children, therapy of hypercalcemia of malignancy must be carefully monitored for development of hypocalcemia, hypomagnesemia, and hypophosphatemia.[159] For mild hypercalcemia, a dose of 0.5 to 1.0 mg/kg of pamidronate intravenously is useful, whereas 2 mg/kg is recommended for severe hypercalcemia or for patients with severe bone involvement. In patients with AIDS or Kaposi's sarcoma, the agent foscarnet has produced hypercalcemia, usually transient,[160] as well as other disturbances in mineral metabolism. The retinoids 9-cis-retinoic acid (Panretin), isotretinoin, and etretinate have all been reported to cause elevated serum calcium. All-*trans*-retinoic acid, used to treat acute promyelocytic leukemia, also produces bone pain and hypercalcemia.[161]

## HYPOCALCEMIA

Symptomatic hypocalcemia in malignancy is clinically uncommon, although laboratory measurements demonstrating a low serum calcium (<2.25 to 2.65 mmol/L) are not unusual.[162] In a review of patients with bony metastatic disease, hypocalcemia was commoner (16%) than hypercalcemia (9%), whereas among 7610 cancer patients evaluated over a 1-year period, hypocalcemia was observed in 1.6% of patients. Hypocalcemia is usually seen in the setting of osteoblastic metastatic disease to bone, typically in prostate cancer but less commonly in breast and lung cancer. In most patients with cancer and hypocalcemia, hypoalbuminemia is present owing to a variety of causes, such as malnutrition, sepsis, hypomagnesemia, and chemotherapy. When this occurs, ionized serum calcium is rarely low, and the patient is not symptomatic. In the occasional cancer patient in whom

*Table 18–10.*  **Clinical Findings in Hypocalcemia**

Central nervous system irritability
Tetanus
Seizures
Cardiac arrhythmia
Heart failure
Hypotension
Calcifications in brain
Papilledema
Cataracts
Skin and mental changes
Prolonged ST interval on electrocardiogram

there is rapid healing of bone metastases, acute pancreatitis, or rapid osteoblastic proliferation, hypocalcemic symptoms may become evident. Table 18–10 lists the broad clinical symptoms associated with hypocalcemia; concurrent hypomagnesemia is frequently present and may compound symptoms.

The most profound, clinically important reductions in serum calcium accompany acute, massive tumor lysis as seen after treatment of leukemias and lymphomas that are exquisitely sensitive to chemotherapy.[163] For example, in Burkitt's lymphoma, adult T-cell leukemia, and various high-grade B-cell malignancies, the pattern of acute hyperkalemia, azotemia, acidosis, lactic acidemia, hyperphosphatemia, hyperuricemia, and hypocalcemia with occasional death as a result of cardiac arrhythmia is called the *tumor lysis syndrome*. Symptomatic tumor lysis is rare, occurring in only about 6% of patients; however, characteristic biochemical changes for the syndrome are quite common. Table 18–11 summarizes the laboratory aspects of the tumor lysis syndrome.

Therapy of the syndrome consists predominantly of intravenous fluids, with administration of dextrose and saline at 4 to 6 L/day and allopurinol, 600 mg/day by mouth initially for 2 days, then 300 mg/day for 7 days. The role of alkalinization has been questioned because of the concern for further induced hypocalcemia caused by alkalosis-fostered precipitation of calcium phosphate salts in the tissues.

Tumor-associated osteomalacia is a rare but recognized paraneoplastic syndrome.[164, 165] Most reported cases occur in younger patients with mesenchymal soft tissue neoplasms. Tumors may be benign or malignant. Ninety percent of the cases involve the head and neck, and 50% are in the bone. In adults, myeloma, neurofibromatosis, and prostate cancer are seen with osteomalacia syndromes. Symptoms and bone

*Table 18–11.*  **Laboratory Characteristics of the Tumor Lysis Syndrome**

| | Hande et al (100 patients)* (%) | Cohen et al (46 patients)† (%) |
|---|---|---|
| Hyperuricemia | 25 | 3.9 |
| Hyperphosphatemia | 32 | 52 |
| Hyperkalemia | 11 | 9 |
| Hypocalcemia | 9 | 57 |
| Azotemia | 25 | 30 |

*Data from Hande KR: Am J Med 1993; 94:133.
†Data from Cohen AF: Am J Med 1980; 68:486.

loss may precede localization of the tumor by several years because the tumor may be quite small. Circulating tumor osteolytic factors are presumed responsible for the syndrome, which usually features hypophosphatemia, asymptomatic hypocalcemia, low or normal levels of 1,25-dihydroxyvitamin $D_3$, and no abnormalities in serum PTH levels. Surgical resection cures greater than 90% of patients, and approximately 57% improve with partial resection. Medical therapy consists of oral phosphate and vitamin D.

## HYPOGLYCEMIA

Non–insulinoma-associated hypoglycemia, or non–islet cell tumor hypoglycemia (NICTH), also called the *Doege-Potter syndrome*,[166] has been noted in malignancy since 1930. Usually occurring in patients with tumors of mesenchymal origin, in 85% of cases, the tumors are greater than 1 kg in weight and have been reported as large as 20 kg. In 40% of patients, the tumors are retroperitoneal or intrathoracic (30%) and less commonly are intraperitoneal (29%) or peripheral. The tumor is usually a spindle cell sarcoma; other tumors include hepatoma. These tumors are thought to secrete insulin-like growth factor II[167] (IGF-II), and the normal plasma ratio of IGF-II to IGF-I is uniquely raised, resulting in hypoglycemia.[168] The normal ratio of IGF-I to IGF-II is less than 0.2. There is characteristic low or unmeasurable plasma insulin, plasma C peptide, proinsulin, and a blood glucose value less than 3.0 mmol/L.

Most tumors associated with NICTH overexpress IGF-11 and secrete increased amounts of a 10- to 15-kd protein known as *big* IGF-II. In normals, 80% of IGF activity is carried in a 150-kd ternary complex (IGF-I, IGF–binding protein [IGF-BP-3], and a 85-kd glycoprotein, which is the acid labile subunit). The remainder of IGF activity is carried in a 50-kd binary complex of IGFs bound to IGF-BP-1, IGF-BP-2, and IGF-BP-4. Limited proteolysis of IGF-BP-3 shifts the distribution by the secretion of *big* IGF-II; the ternary complex formation is inhibited, resulting in a shift to the 50-kd component, which can leave the vascular compartment readily and cause hypoglycemia.[169–173] Symptoms of hypoglycemia, other than hypoglycemia-related mental changes and coma, are due to the release of the counterregulatory hormones epinephrine and glucagon, producing tremulousness, sweating, pallor, and hypotension. Treatment is palliative and surgical; however, there is some evidence that growth hormone may be useful as well as diazoxide, steroids, somatostatin, and glucagon infusions.[171] For hepatoma-associated hypoglycemia, ethanol injections into the tumor bed have proved useful[172] as well as growth hormone.[173]

## Paraneoplastic Neurologic Syndromes

### BACKGROUND

Neurologic disorders associated with cancer have been noted since the early 20th century. Denny-Brown in 1948 described a primary sensory neuropathy with lung carcinoma. Subsequently the cause of these syndromes was related to antibodies cross-reacting to shared normal nerve tissue and tumor

*Table 18–12.* Neurologic Paraneoplastic Syndromes and Associated Cancers

| Neurologic Syndrome | Cancer |
|---|---|
| Subacute sensory neuropathy | Small cell lung cancer |
| Subacute motor neuropathy | Hodgkin's disease, lymphoma |
| Peripheral motor polyneuropathy | Myeloma |
| Amyloid polyneuropathy | Myeloma |
| Autonomic motor myenteric neuropathy | Small cell lung cancer |
| Brachial plexus neuropathy | Hodgkin's disease |
| Myasthenia gravis | Thymoma |
| Lambert-Eaton syndrome | Small cell lung cancer |
| Symmetric sensorimotor neuropathy | Carcinoma, lymphoma, myeloma |
| Amyotrophic lateral sclerosis | Non–small cell lung cancer, renal cancer |
| Encephalomyelitis | Small cell lung cancer |
| Cerebellar degeneration (Purkinje cell loss) | Breast, ovary, small cell lung cancer |
| Opsoclonus/myoclonus | Ovary, breast, fallopian tube, neuroblastoma, small cell lung cancer |
| Necrotizing myelopathy | Small cell lung cancer, lymphoma |
| Retinopathy and uveopathy | Breast cancer, small cell cancer of cervix and genital tract, melanoma, uterine cancer, and, rarely, non–small cell lung cancer |
| Neuromyeloencephalitis | Small cell lung cancer |
| Intestinal and gastrointestinal myenteric plexopathy | Small cell lung cancer |

carcinoma of the lung, whereas HuC and Hel-1 are noted only in the cerebral cortex.[178, 179] In some paraneoplastic neurosensory neuropathies, however, tissue localization of the shared antigen may not be identified; in those instances, CD8$^+$ T-cell infiltration of sensory neurons, sympathetic ganglia, and hippocampal regions causes symptoms suggesting other antigenic stimuli.[180] Table 18–12 lists most of these defined syndromes and the predominantly associated cancer, and Table 18–13 describes the predominant antineuronal antibodies and their frequently associated syndromes. Syndromes frequently overlap clinically but differ in their associated antibody, tumor, and response to therapy; although antibodies may cross-react with immunohistochemical techniques, they may be separated by Western blot analysis. The frequency of the paraneoplastic sensory and motor peripheral neuropathies is ascribed perhaps to more ready penetration of antineuronal autoantibodies into peripheral nerves and dorsal root ganglia because of an ineffective blood–nerve root–ganglion barrier, as contrasted with the more efficient blood-brain barrier.[181, 182]

Neurologic symptoms in the cancer patient are usually not due to a paraneoplastic syndrome. Among 5124 neurologic consultations in a cancer referral center, the causes of the complaints were usually direct tumor effects and were as follows: mental status change owing to metabolic causes, intracranial metastases, and headache without a found cause. Back or neck pain complaints were caused by bone metastases in 30% of patients, paravertebral mass in 9%, epidural metastases in 33%, meningeal tumor in 4%, and plexopathy in 8%.[183]

## CEREBELLAR DEGENERATION

Syndromes associated with cerebellar degeneration as a result of Purkinje cell loss are varied and are estimated to occur in approximately 2 patients in every 1000 cases of cancer. Visual loss, vertigo, and truncal ataxia characterize the syndrome. In women, paraneoplastic cerebellar degeneration is most typically associated with breast adenocarcinoma, with a seemingly special additional relationship with endometrial and fallopian tube cancers that are small cell in type.[184-186] The anti-Yo antibody (see Table 18–13) is directed against Purkinje cells and breast tumor cells with their shared antigen; it is not found in normal subjects or in other patients without the syndrome, and the antigen is found only in patients with breast cancer and the cerebellar degeneration

cell antigens, provoking a nonspecific cellular immune inflammatory response involving the nervous tissue and perivascular spaces.[174] Antibody synthesis is demonstrable in the brain.[175] The resulting clinical sensory and motor neuronitis and encephalomyelitis are the most common of the paraneoplastic neurologic syndromes[176] and are often caused by multiple circulating specific antibodies.

Paraneoplastic syndromes are now defined by location of induced neurologic deficit, the associated tumors, and the molecular characteristics of the tissue antigen and circulating antibody. These cross-reacting antibodies have been shown to localize in the brain in the areas responsible for clinical abnormalities.[177]

For example, the major tissue antigens in these syndromes are the HU antigens HuD, HuC, and Hel-1. HuD messenger RNA is found in the cerebral cortex and in small cell

*Table 18–13.* Antibody-Mediated Neurologic Paraneoplastic Syndrome

| Antibody | Antigen Molecular Weight (kd) | Syndrome |
|---|---|---|
| Anti-Yo | 62 | Purkinje cell degeneration |
| | 34 | |
| Anti-Hu (ANNA-type I) | 35–40 | Varieties of neuronal encephalopathies, intestinal pseudo-obstruction |
| Anti-Ri (ANNA-type II) | 55 | Opsoclonus/myoclonus usually in adult with breast cancer |
| | 80 | |
| Antiretinal Ab | 26; also 20–24, 65, 145 | Cancer-associated retinopathy |
| Anti-VGCC, synaptotagmin | 58 | Lambert-Eaton syndrome |
| Anti-AChR | | Myasthenia gravis |
| Antimyenteric plexus | Polyclonal IgG | Intestinal pseudo-obstruction |

syndrome. The DNA binding antibody circulates in the serum, at a titer greater than 500, and is less common in the cerebrospinal fluid with titers greater than 100. Anti-Yo has immunoreactivity distinct from anti-Hu, the antineuronal antibody characteristic of small cell lung cancer,[187] which can cause a similar cerebellar clinical picture. Although anti-Yo antibodies may react immunologically with anti-Hu sera, they can be distinguished further from anti-Hu on Western blot analysis.[188] Tumors in the anti-Yo Purkinje cell destructive syndrome express polyclonal immunoglobulins, including CDR (cerebellar degeneration gene) 62- and 34-kd proteins, which are not seen in patients without the associated syndrome. These proteins are termed *class II antigens* and are similar to normal tissue antigens, such as carcinoembryonic antigen (CEA). The characteristic anti-Yo antibodies are present in the serum or cerebrospinal fluid in approximately 50% of cases.

Patients with paraneoplastic cerebellar degeneration have been found to have anti-Yo (PCA-1) antibodies as well as antibodies to P/Q specific voltage-gated neuronal calcium channels.[189] Most occurred in women with ovarian, breast, and other gynecologic cancers and may be associated with encephalopathy and neuropathy. In a study of 172 patients with positive PCA-1 antibodies and cerebellar degeneration with ovarian cancer, 37% had antibodies to P/Q or N type calcium channels, 7% had both; in patients with ovarian cancer but no cerebellar degeneration, 1% had circulating PCA-1 antibodies, and none were found in healthy women. Among these women with circulating antibodies, 83 had ovarian cancer, 28 had breast cancer, and the remainder had other gynecologic cancers. Among those with cerebellar degeneration, 15% had ovarian cancer and antibodies to P/Q-type calcium channels. Fifteen others had extrapyramidal signs, seizures, neuropathy, trigeminal signs, and mixed sensorimotor neuropathy. Nine patients had more than one primary tumor. Current recommendations for women with risk from breast and gynecologic malignancy are that they be screened with immunofluorescent techniques for anti-Yo, anti-HU, and amphiphysin antibodies as well as immunoprecipitation tests for P/Q-type and N-type calcium channel antibodies so that early aggressive therapy can be instituted. The authors point out that PCA-1 antibodies, rather than being only markers for cerebellar degeneration, are also markers for the presence of breast or gynecologic malignancy,[189] whereas others believe that Western blot methodology is needed to distinguish antibodies and the clinical syndromes.[190] Some paraneoplastic cerebellar degeneration cases with components of encephalitis and sensory neuropathy are associated with anti-Hu antibody[191]; Lambert-Eaton syndrome also has been observed with a separate cerebellar degeneration syndrome resulting from anti-Hu antibodies.[12, 13, 192]

Rarely, paraneoplastic cerebellar degeneration occurs with optic neuritis and prominent visual symptoms. This syndrome may be distinguished from cancer-associated retinopathy clinically and is associated with antibodies to CV2 and oligodendrocytic antigen found in the optic chiasm, spinal cord, cerebellum, and brain stem. In such patients, antibodies against Hu, Yo, and Ri by immunohistochemical and Western blot techniques are negative.[193]

Uncommonly, small cell lung cancer is associated with the cerebellar degeneration syndrome, but in these cases, signs of encephalitis or peripheral neuronopathies are frequently found also.[181, 194] Antibodies against Purkinje cells are found in 40% of small cell lung cancer tumor cells with or without the paraneoplastic cerebellar degeneration syndrome. When tumors give rise to anti-Hu antibodies, the clinical syndrome is associated with high titers of anti-Hu antibody in the serum or cerebrospinal fluid.[192] These anti-Hu antibodies, which are found in other neurologic paraneoplastic syndromes (see later), have considerable homology with the amino acid hexapeptide sequence Phe-Leu-Glu-Asp-Val-Asp, which is in $\alpha_2$-macroglobulin and in $\alpha_1$-trypsin inhibitors.[181] Because these compounds may play a promoting role in tumor growth and metastasis, their postulated inhibition by anti-Hu antibodies suggests an antitumor role for the antibodies.[195] Patients with paraneoplastic neurologic syndromes characteristically present with more limited stage of disease.

The response to therapy (steroids, plasmapheresis) is usually poor; however, atypical reports noted complete responses to intravenous high-dose gamma globulin and to chemotherapy.[192] The cerebellar degenerative syndrome typically antedates cancer detection. In one report, 70% of patients had cerebellar disease that antedated cancer detection by 2 to 41 months.[187, 192] Reversibility may relate to duration of symptoms and attendant neurologic damage before the correct diagnosis.

## NEURONAL ENCEPHALOPATHIES

Neuronal encephalopathies include paraneoplastic sensory neuropathy and encephalomyelitis. This syndrome complex is associated with the anti-Hu antibody and is limited to patients with small cell lung cancer.[195] The clinical picture can be cerebellar or cerebral in focus or give the appearance of panencephalitis (or both), and it is found in approximately 3 in 1000 cancer patients. Sensory symptoms occur in 59% of cases, mental changes and seizures in 21%, motor signs in 14%, cerebellar signs in 13%, and brain stem signs in 11% at presentation; autonomic dysfunction is found in 16% of patients.[196] Patients with high anti-Hu titers usually have a paraneoplastic syndrome, and the presence of these antibodies is 92% specific for the presence of small cell lung cancer; other patients may have low titers without the syndrome. In the studies cited previously, 11% of 71 patients with the syndrome clinically had anti-Hu antibodies (low titer) without discernible tumor.

Almost all patients with small cell lung cancer express the Hu antigen in tumor, although serum antibodies are rare. Because the Hu D gene in these tumors has not been shown to have mutated,[197] some mechanism for antibody development other than simple ectopic antigen expression of Hu appears necessary to break immune tolerance in these patients. Paraneoplastic sensory neuronopathy is often associated with anti-Hu antibodies. These antibodies were found in 40 of 126 patients with suggestive clinical features of the syndrome. In this setting, the antibody test demonstrates 99% sensitivity and 82% specificity for the condition. In some cases, the neuropathy was due to antibodies directed against amphiphysin, a 66-kd protein related to axon electrical guidance, and to another 106-kd protein.[198] Other paraneoplastic sensory neuropathies have been related to an antiganglioside antibody in hepatoma, associated with cryo-globulinemia.[199]

Although response to therapy is rare, the syndrome has remitted with chemotherapy and has been associated with at least one case of apparent spontaneous tumor regression.[200] Small cell carcinoma, when associated with clinical anti-Hu neurologic syndromes, has been reported to present more commonly as limited-stage tumors[194] in most of the patients with neurologic deficit, in contrast to patients without the syndrome, who present with advanced disease 85% of the time. The more benign stage of anti-Hu–positive small cell lung cancer is not related to survival because most patients die of infection or respiratory failure[195]; only one third of patients die as a result of progressive tumor growth. The paraneoplastic neurologic syndrome may be commoner in females, which is thought typical for autoimmune disorders, although there is a study showing a male preponderance.[192]

## OPSOCLONUS-MYOCLONUS

The syndrome of opsoclonus-myoclonus is seen with neuroblastoma and osteoblastoma in the child; in the adult, breast cancer and fallopian tube cancer predominate.[201, 202] It is characterized by anti-Ri antibodies, which share immunohistochemical characteristics with anti-Hu antibodies but may be distinguished by Western blot analysis. The adult disease is usually responsive to prednisone. Anti-Ri antibodies are found more commonly in the spinal fluid rather than the serum. When the syndrome is associated with small cell cancer of the lung or genital tract, anti-Hu antibodies are present. Patients with breast, ovary, or uterine carcinoma who have elements of the neuronal encephalopathies usually have anti-Hu antibodies, whereas others with prostate cancer, neuroblastoma, and chondrosarcoma may not have the antibody.

On rare occasions, some adult patients with the syndrome also show a multifocal pattern of defects, including encephalitis and dementia. In such cases, RNA-binding antibodies to Nova-1 (distributed in the brain stem, spinal cord, and subcortical central nervous system) or to Nova-2 (distributed in the neocortex and hippocampus) may be demonstrated and can lead to highly variable signs and symptoms that can progress to stupor or coma.[203, 204]

## CANCER-ASSOCIATED RETINOPATHY

Cancer-associated retinopathy[205–208] is seen most commonly with breast adenocarcinoma and with small cell carcinoma of the cervix, endometrium, and upper respiratory tract. The associated autoantibodies are characteristically directed against a 23-kd retinal antigen, recoverin, that reacts with tumor cell antigens and with retinal and choroidal tissues, leading to destruction of photoreceptors. A syndrome of (1) ring scotoma, (2) photosensitivity, and (3) attenuated retinal vessels along with (4) visual acuity loss is called *cancer-associated retinopathy*. There is an occasional response to prednisone. Other syndromes have been reported with autoantibodies to müllerian cells in the retina and ophthalmic nerve but without cross-reaction to the 23-kd protein.[209] Differentiation from various causes of night blindness is

important because the syndrome may be the earliest indicator of an occult carcinoma.

The rare glucagonoma syndrome may also give central scotomata but is also associated with dementia, ataxia, nystagmus, and optic atrophy. In addition, there are angular stomatitis, diarrhea, lower limb weakness, necrotizing migrating erythema, and diabetes mellitus. Low serum levels of amino acids may accompany the syndrome. Response to somatostatin analogues or to chemotherapy has been reported.[210]

## LAMBERT-EATON SYNDROME

The Lambert-Eaton syndrome is due to defective cholinergic electrical impulse transmission along peripheral motor nerves and presents clinically as weakness, decreased reflexes, and autonomic dysfunction.[211] Although patients may not have malignancy (i.e., 25% of women with the syndrome are free of tumor), all patients have IgG antibodies directed against neural presynaptic, potassium-mediated, voltage-gated calcium channels that interfere with acetylcholine release. Symptoms include muscle weakness, loss of tendon reflexes, and autonomic dysfunction. Sixty percent of patients with the syndrome have small cell lung cancer,[212] but others with non–small cell lung cancer may also have the syndrome.[213] Although estimates of incidence of Lambert-Eaton syndrome in small cell lung cancer have been as high as 14%, contemporary clinical studies suggest that a 3% incidence is more appropriate. The synaptic vesicle protein synaptotagmin is a 58-kd protein associated with N-type calcium channels[214] in nerves and neuronal granular secreting cells as well as in small cell lung cancer tumor lines and is believed to give rise to autoantibodies that may cause the Lambert-Eaton syndrome.[215] These antibodies have produced the syndrome in the rat.[216]

There are now numerous recognized types of voltage-gated calcium channels (P/Q, N, L, P, T)[217–219] in differing tissues and cell lines. L-type channels are found in the cardiovascular system and are sensitive to dihydropyridines; N-type, P-type, and Q-type channels have been found in amphibian nerve terminals; P/Q-type channels are characteristically mammalian.[220] In some patients, IgG antibodies react with voltage-gated L-type channels; other patients with Lambert-Eaton syndrome have antibodies that react with neither N-type nor L-type channels but are believed to react with P-type channels. These studies suggest a heterogeneity to the antibody-mediated causes of Lambert-Eaton syndrome. The 58-kd IgG has considerable homology with other Lambert-Eaton syndrome antibodies targeting to w-conotoxin, a protein closely associated with voltage-gated calcium channels in various tissues and cell lines.[213, 221, 222] This antibody is found in the sera of patients with systemic lupus erythematosus or in sera positive for rheumatoid factor, but tests for the antibodies may serve as a screening tool for the Lambert-Eaton syndrome.

The differential diagnosis of the Lambert-Eaton syndrome includes myasthenia gravis.[223] The latter disease is usually associated with thymic hyperplasia, and a thymic tumor (thymoma) is present only 15 to 20% of the time. The associated findings in myasthenia gravis of cytopenias, decreased gamma globulin, polymyositis, and susceptibility to nonbacterial opportunistic infections are not characteristic of the Lambert-Eaton syndrome; in thymomas, pemphigus skin lesions are common.[224] The pathogenesis of myasthenia gravis is believed to involve circulating acetylcholine receptor–specific T cells. These T cells are thought to be generated by autoimmune reactivity involving antigens in thymus myoid cells and skeletal muscle, which share the acetylcholine receptor antigen. Table 18–14 presents some clinical differences between the myasthenic syndromes.

Because circulating acetylcholine receptor antibodies often rise after thymectomy, other aspects of autoimmunity are being explored. For example, antibodies to interferon alfa and to IL-2 are common in late-onset myasthenia gravis.[225] Further myasthenic crises have been observed after bone marrow transplantation with and without concurrent graft-versus-host disease[226, 227] and in an AIDS-like syndrome with *Pneumocystis carinii* pneumonia.[228, 229]

Patients with Lambert-Eaton syndrome may present with more complex neurologic deficits, including those typical for cerebellar degeneration. In this regard, the IgG antisynaptotagmin antibodies have been shown to produce in vitro toxicity in small cell tumor cell lines and in Purkinje cells.[213, 215] Other patients with cerebellar symptoms have been reported with serum anti-w-conotoxin and anti-Hu antibodies. Treatment with plasmapheresis and high-dose gamma globulin has been reported to improve the clinical picture of the Lambert-Eaton syndrome.[230] In another patient, successful treatment of small cell lung cancer cleared the neurologic symptoms.

Therapy of the Lambert-Eaton syndrome is often rewarding. Plasma exchanges every 6 to 8 weeks or treatment with azathioprine (2.5 mg/kg/day) is useful in producing remission. 3,4-Diaminopyridine is the drug of choice for short-term acute therapy of the disease; doses of 10 to 100 mg/day are recommended.[231] Intravenous immunoglobulin (400 mg/kg/day for 5 days or 1 g/kg/day for 2 days) often produces complete clinical neurologic remissions. Neurologic improvement with effective antitumor therapy is vari-

able.[232] Use of high-dose intravenous immunoglobulin has been associated with transient hyperviscosity[233] and complications such as stroke and thrombosis. Caution with the agent's use in the elderly and in those with arterial disease has been recommended. As was noted for anti-Hu-related syndromes in small cell lung cancer, patients with the Lambert-Eaton syndrome present with more limited tumor stage, but, in contrast to small cell lung cancer with anti-Hu syndromes, survival is better with the associated Lambert-Eaton paraneoplastic syndrome. Myasthenia gravis treatment includes neostigmine, pyridostigmine, surgery, and immunosuppression. High-dose intravenous gamma globulin (0.4 g/kg/day for 5 days) has also proved useful. Response to therapy is related to early diagnosis and minimal presenting symptoms.

## GASTROINTESTINAL MYENTERIC PLEXOPATHIES (OGILVIE'S SYNDROME)

Symptoms of stomach and bowel obstruction, esophageal achalasia, and biliary dilation with obstruction have been observed in cancer without demonstrable physical obstruction by, for example, tumor or stricture.[234–236] In many instances, these symptoms are associated with cancer, usually small cell lung cancer. Pathologic evaluation demonstrates neuronal damage and infiltration by CD8 and T lymphocytes resulting from enteric IgG polyclonal antibodies in the myenteric and submucosal plexus of the stomach or bowel. In other cases of jaundice, a similar cause may be present in T-cell lymphoma,[237] hypernephroma,[238] and Hodgkin's disease.[239] In some of these patients, there may be overlap with clinical features of anti-Hu-associated paraneoplastic syndromes. Therapy with octreotide and intravenous high-dose gamma globulin has been useful in relieving pseudo-obstructive symptoms when diagnosed early.

Severe intestinal pseudo-obstruction can be a life-threatening[240] complication, with a high risk of perforation. Although emergency colostomy is at times indicated, other therapeutic measures include the use of water-soluble contrast enemas[241] and neostigmine treatment with a dose of 2.5 mg in 100 ml saline over 60 minutes with electrocardiogram monitoring of heart rate and conduction[241]; neostigmine is contraindicated in patients receiving β-blockers, in patients with acidosis, and in patients with a recent myocardial infarction.

## MISCELLANEOUS PARANEOPLASTIC NEUROLOGIC DISORDERS

Several other paraneoplastic neurologic disorders have been described. The stiff-man syndrome[242–245] is seen in breast cancer. It is characterized by muscular rigidity and is associated with antibodies against amphiphysin, a 128 kd synaptic protein.[244, 246] These patients may be distinguished from others without cancer and others with renal cell cancer, small cell lung cancer, and prostate cancer who have antibodies against glutamic acid decarboxylase, which is enzymatically important for neural transmission and generation of the neural inhibitor gamma amino butyric acid.[247, 247a, 247b] Rarely, these patients may present with gastrointestinal dysmotility

*Table 18–14.* **Comparison of Lambert-Eaton Syndrome and Myasthenia Gravis**

| | Lambert-Eaton Syndrome | Myasthenia Gravis |
|---|---|---|
| Associated tumor | Small cell carcinoma of the lung in 60–70% | Thymoma in 15–20% |
| Response to tetanic muscle stimulation | Progressively stronger | Progressively weaker |
| Response to pyridostigmine | Poor | Good |
| Location of defect in acetylcholine release | Presynaptic | Usually postsynaptic |
| Associated antibody | Usually anti-Hu | Anti–acetylcholine receptor |
| Ocular and bulbar muscle weakness | Absent | Present |
| Associated myenteric plexopathy | Present | Absent |
| Response to high-dose IV gamma globulin | Good | Useful |

and seizures. Other paraneoplastic disorders are characterized by clinical symptoms paralleling localizing lesions in the brain, such as limbic encephalitis[243, 246] or temporal lobe epilepsy.[248] Disorders of neural transmission due to gamma amino butyric acid inhibition are often helped by therapy with diazepam; steroids, plasmapheresis, and intravenous gammaglobulin may also be useful for the reversal of autoimmunity.

## Paraneoplastic Dermatologic Diseases

### BACKGROUND

A broad spectrum of dermatologic disorders have been related to cancer.[212] Because both dermatoses and malignancy are clinically common, it became important to define paraneoplastic dermatologic disorders as occurring other than coincidentally. Such definitions include (1) the dermatosis

occurring in cancer patients more frequently than chance with a close temporal relationship for both disorders, (2) the cancer and the dermatosis having parallel courses of clinical activity, and (3) the dermatologic disorder being associated with distinctive and uniform tumor types. Table 18–15 is a compilation of the more commonly recognized paraneoplastic dermatologic diseases grouped by clinical presentation. Their clinical expression usually results from autoimmune polyclonal antibodies being deposited in the epidermis and epidermal-dermal interface of the skin or in blood vessels, causing rashes, erosion, or bullae in the skin or vascular abnormalities. Epidermal growth factors appear to be related to the proliferative and hyperkeratotic dermatologic signs in the paraneoplastic disorders.

### PEMPHIGUS-LIKE DISORDERS

One of the common and better characterized paraneoplastic disorders of the skin is paraneoplastic pemphigus.[249–251] It is

*Table 18–15.* **Sporadic, Noninherited Cutaneous Paraneoplastic Syndromes**

| Clinical Dermatosis | Syndromes | Associated Cancer | Frequency |
|---|---|---|---|
| ***Pigmentation Disorders*** | | | |
| Depigmentation in elderly | Vitiligo | GI, gallbladder | 7% |
| Zebra skin | Erythema | Lung, uterus | 100% |
| Brown-black warty lesions | Acanthosis nigricans | Carcinoma in abdomen (lung cancer) | 86% (4–10%) |
| ***Hyperkeratotic Lesions*** | | | |
| Hypertrichosis, red tongue papillae | Lanuginosa acquisita | Lung, GI, urinary tract, bladder, breast | 100% |
| Dry, thick skin | Ichthyosis | Hodgkin's disease | Often |
| Eruptive seborrheic keratoses | Leser-Trélat sign | GI | 43% |
| Gray thick skin and increased psoriasiform rash on fingers, toes, ears, nose | Paraneoplastic acrokeratosis (Bazex's syndrome) | Upper aerodigestive tract, vulva, prostate (larynx) | 100% (50%) |
| Eruptive verrucous lesions | Florid cutaneous papillomatosis | GI | 100% |
| | Tripe palms | Lung cancer | 94% |
| ***Erythemas, Ulcers, and Bullae*** | | | |
| Acantholytic bullae | Pemphigus vulgaris | Lymphoma, thymoma | Infrequent |
| Erosion of buccal mucosa and periumbilical area | Lichen planus pemphigoid | Pararenal, paravertebral, intraperitoneal tumors | Occasional |
| Bullae of face | Porphyria liver and arms | Liver, cutanea tarda | Frequent |
| Erythematous, crusted perioral lesions | Glucagonoma syndrome | Pancreas | 100% |
| Lilac color to face with erythema | Dermatomyositis, genital | GI, lung (female) | 10–15% |
| ***Nodules and Papules*** | | | |
| Acute neutrophilic dermatitis | Sweet's syndrome, atypical pyoderma gangrenosum | Leukemia, myeloma | Infrequent |
| Blue-red nodules | Sarcoidosis | Lymphoma | Increased association |
| Panniculitis, fever | Nodules, fat necrosis | Pancreas | Rare |
| Yellow-brown or red papules | Multicentric reticulosis | Pancreas GI, lung, ovary, sarcoma | Occasional |
| ***Miscellaneous*** | | | |
| Digital ischemia | Atypical Raynaud's phenomenon | Kidney, GI, ovary, stomach, pancreas | 100% |
| Migrating thrombophlebitis with low-grade DIC, emboli, nonbacterial endocarditis | Trousseau's syndrome | Stomach, colon | 40% |
| Vasculitis | | Lymphoma and leukemia (epithelial cancers) | Infrequent (rare) |

GI, gastrointestinal; DIC, disseminated intravascular coagulation.

characterized by mucosal erosion, polymorphous skin eruptions, and blistering over the trunk and extremities; commonly, there is also blistering of palms and soles, giving the appearance of lichen planus or erythema multiforme. Histologically, there is epidermal vacuolization at the epidermal-dermal interface, acantholysis, keratinocyte necrosis, and intraepidermal cell detachment. Direct immunofluorescence histochemical studies demonstrate polyclonal IgG and complement deposition on epithelial intercellular surfaces and in the epidermal basement membrane zone; IgA and IgM deposition has also been seen. Paraneoplastic pemphigus is associated with lymphomas, thymoma, chronic lymphatic leukemia, spindle cell sarcomas, and, rarely, benign tumors. Pathogenesis is believed to be related to the development of autoantibodies to the desmosomal proteins desmoplakin I (250 kd) and desmoplakin II (210 kd). These desmosomal antigens are not expressed by the tumor cells of the associated lymphomas but are expressed commonly by squamous and basal cell keratinocytes; however, the syndrome is not seen with basal and squamous cell skin cancers. The antibody reaction to these characteristic desmoplakins aids in the differential diagnosis of other blistering pemphigus-like lesions. Pemphigus vulgaris and pemphigus foliaceus have antibody reactivity to a complex of desmosomal-adherence junctional pro-mins termed *plakoglobin*. Pemphigus vulgaris is associated with a 130-kd antigen, and pemphigus foliaceus has an antibody to a 160-kd protein. Bullous pemphigoid is characterized by an autoantibody to a 230-kd antigen that shares some homology with the 250-kd and 210-kd desmoplakin antigens of paraneoplastic pemphigus; diagnostic overlap may occur, but diagnosis can usually be clarified by indirect immunofluorescent studies using various epithelial models for antibody targeting (Table 18–16).

There has been a long association of malignancy with pemphigus lesions, particularly pemphigus vulgarus (e.g., about one third of patients with pemphigus lesions and tumor have a thymoma).[224, 252] Molecular characterization of these skin disorders may delineate associations more firmly and clarify these syndromes. Clinical and laboratory diagnostic criteria for blistering lesions are not always clear-cut. Overlap may occur in a variety of benign and malignant disorders that are not sufficiently common to meet the criteria of paraneoplastic association.[253] Treatment with steroids may be of benefit; however, the disease parallels growth patterns of the underlying malignancy. Rarely, there is epithelial autoimmune disease involving the lung and gastrointestinal tract in paraneoplastic pemphigus[254] as well as the conjunctiva.[255]

## BAZEX SYNDROME

Bazex syndrome, a paraneoplastic cutaneous syndrome, also termed *paraneoplastic acrokeratosis*, is usually associated, in men, with squamous cell cancers of the upper aerodigestive tract and less commonly, in women, with vulvar, esophageal, and uterine tumors. Clinically, there is a psoriasiform rash with acral distribution affecting the nails, ears, nose, fingers, toes, and, to a limited extent, elbows and knees.[256, 257]

## ACANTHOSIS NIGRICANS, TRIPE PALMS, AND LESER-TRÉLAT SIGN

Acanthosis nigricans is a thickened, hyperpigmented lesion that often involves the axillae, neck, or submammary skin and is associated with cancer. The association with lung cancer is 5%, but the association with gastrointestinal malignancy is 37%. Of interest is the frequent association of acanthosis nigricans with other paraneoplastic syndromes, such as *tripe palms*, a thickening of the skin of the palms of the hands (exophytic dermatoglyphics), which then resembles pig stomach mucosa. When tripe palms occurs with acanthosis nigricans, there is an associated gastric carcinoma in 55% of cases. Tripe palms alone is commonly seen with squamous cell carcinomas of the tongue and to a lesser extent with gastric and lung carcinoma. One patient with melanoma had tripe palms, acanthosis nigricans, and paraneoplastic pemphigus.[258]

Eruptive seborrheic keratosis, termed the *Leser-Trélat sign*,[259] is associated with gastrointestinal cancer in 43% of cases but may also be seen in association with multiple skin tags (acrochordons, which have an association with colon cancer and colonic polyps) and acanthosis nigricans. A possible common role for transforming growth factor-α in stimulating these clinically varied hyperplastic cutaneous paraneoplastic signs has been suggested.[260] The rare polycystic ovarian syndrome[261] of excess growth hormone (gigantism and acromegaly), insulin resistance, diabetes mellitus, and hyperandrogenism has been associated with acanthosis nigricans, further supporting a role for growth factors causing this dermatologic abnormality.

## Miscellaneous Syndromes of Uncertain Pathogenesis

A variety of other paraneoplastic associations have been suggested, including paraneoplastic nephrogenous diabetes

*Table 18–16.* **Diagnostic Characteristics of Pemphigus Lesions**

| Skin Disorder | Antigens | Epithelial Indirect Immunohistochemical Antibody Reactivity | | |
|---|---|---|---|---|
| | | HUMAN STRATIFIED SQUAMOUS | RAT TRANSITIONAL BLADDER | MONKEY ESOPHAGEAL |
| Paraneoplastic pemphigus | Desmoplakin I (250 kd), desmoplakin II (210 kd) | Present | Present | Present |
| Pemphigus vulgaris | 130 kd | Present | Absent | Present |
| Pemphigus foliaceus | 160 kd | Present | Absent | Present |
| Bullous pemphigoid | 230 kd | Present | Absent | Present |

insipidus,[262, 263] heart disease,[264] glomerulonephropathies,[265–267] polymyositis,[268] rheumatologic diseases,[269–272] Raynaud's phenomenon,[273] vasculitis,[274] and hypercoagulability.[275, 276] There is lack of agreement on the extent of some of these associations with cancer and the likely mechanism involved. The subject is well discussed by Bunn.[277] Hematologic syndromes are discussed in Chapter 13.

## Summary

The identification and study of paraneoplastic syndromes have led to broad understanding of the cause of a variety of tissue injuries and clinical symptoms associated with cancer. The use of appropriate animal models has confirmed and elucidated these associations and led to important new directions in cancer treatment. Molecular studies of ectopic ACTH or POMC and PTHrP fragments secreted or found in tumors have shown these compounds to be structurally and often functionally unique[278] and readily separable from hormones produced by nonmalignant, normal tissues. In this sense, ectopic hormones made by tumors are *ectopic* only in their being compounds that share biologic activity with other compounds made at traditional sites in nonmalignant tissues. Study of paraneoplastic syndromes now offers increasing opportunities for early diagnosis of cancer and new directions in predicting a tumor's clinical biology and sensitivity to therapy and may provide new target molecules for therapeutic intervention in the future.

## SUGGESTIONS FOR ADDITIONAL READING

Cohen PR, Kurzrock R. Mucocutaneous paraneoplastic syndromes. Semin Oncol 1997;24:334–59.

Hall TC. Paraneoplastic syndromes: mechanisms. Semin Oncol 1997; 24:269–76.

Maesaka JK, Mittal SK, Fishbane S. Paraneoplastic syndromes of the kidney. Semin Oncol 1997;24:373–81.

Odell WD. Endocrine/metabolic syndromes of cancer. Semin Oncol 1997;24:299–317.

Posner JB, Dalmau JO. Paraneoplastic syndromes affecting the central nervous system. Ann Rev Med 1997;48:157–66.

Sanders DB. Lambert-Eaton myasthenic syndrome: clinical diagnosis, immune-mediated mechanisms, and update on therapies. Ann Neurol 1995;37:Suppl 1:S63–73.

Staszewski H. Hematological paraneoplastic syndromes. Semin Oncol 1997;24:329–33.

## REFERENCES

1. Martínez-Lavín M, Mansilla J, Pineda C, et al. Evidence of hypertrophic osteoarthropathy in human skeletal remains from pre-Hispanic Mesoamerica. Ann Intern Med 1994;120:238–41.
2. Nathanson L, Hall TC. A spectrum of tumors that produce paraneoplastic syndromes: lung tumors: how they produce their syndromes. Ann N Y Acad Sci 1974;230:367–77.
3. Imura H. Ectopic hormone syndromes. Clin Endocrinol Metab 1980;9:235–260.
4. Odell W. Ectopic ACTH secretion: a misnomer. Endocrinol Metab Clin North Am 1991;20:371–9.
5. Odell W, Wolfsen A, Yoshimoto Y, et al. Ectopic peptide synthesis: a universal concomitant of neoplasia. Trans Assoc Am Phys 1977;90:204–25.
6. Odell WD. Ectopic ACTH secretion: a misnomer. Endocrinol Metab Clin North Am 1991;20:371–9.
7. Schiller JH, Jones JC. Paraneoplastic syndromes associated with lung cancer. Curr Opin Oncol 1993;5:335–42.
8. Abeloff MD. Paraneoplastic syndromes: a window on the biology of cancer. N Engl J Med 1987;317:1598–1600.
9. Nelson KA, Walsh D, Sheehan FA. The cancer anorexia-cachexia syndrome. J Clin Oncol 1994;12:213–25.
10. Richardson GE, Johnson BE. Paraneoplastic syndromes in lung cancer. Curr Opin Oncol 1992;4:323–33.
11. Richardson GE, Johnson BE. The biology of lung cancer. Semin Oncol 1993;20:105–127.
12. Blumenfeld AM, Recht LD, Chad DA, et al. Coexistence of Lambert-Eaton myasthenic syndrome and subacute cerebellar degeneration: differential effects of treatment. Neurology 1991;41:1682–5.
13. Fueyo J, Gomez-Manzano C, Pascual J, Pou A. Paraneoplastic syndromes. Neurology 1993;43:236.
14. Kovacs L, Robertson GL. Syndrome of inappropriate antidiuresis. Endocrinol Metab Clin North Am 1992;21:859–75.
15. Moses AM, Scheinman SJ. Ectopic secretion of neurohypophyseal peptides in patients with malignancy. Endocrinol Metab Clin North Am 1991;20:489–506.
16. Zerbe R, Stropes L, Robertson G. Vasopressin function in the syndrome of inappropriate antidiuresis. Annu Rev Med 1980;31:315–27.
17. Comis RL, Miller M, Ginsberg SJ. Abnormalities in water homeostasis in small cell anaplastic lung cancer. Cancer 1980;45:2414–21.
18. Comis RL, Miller M, Ginsberg SJ. Abnormalities in water homeostasis in small cell anaplastic lung cancer. Cancer 1980;45:2414–21.
19. Maurer LH, O'Donnell JF, Kennedy S, et al. Human neurophysins in carcinoma of the lung: relation to histology, disease stage, response rate, survival, and syndrome of inappropriate antidiuretic hormone secretion. Cancer Treat Rep 1983;67:971–6.
20. Kavanagh BD, Halperin EC, Rosenbau LC, et al. Syndrome of inappropriate secretion of antidiuretic hormone in a patient with carcinoma of the nasopharynx. Cancer 1992;69:1315–9.
21. Wenig BL, Heller KS. The syndrome of inappropriate secretion of antidiuretic hormone (SIADH) following neck dissection. Laryngoscope 1987;97:467–70.
22. Cogan E, Debieve MF, Pepersack T, Abramow M. Natriuresis and atrial natriuretic factor secretion during inappropriate antidiuresis. Am J Med 1988;84:Pt 1:409–18.
23. Kamoi K, Ebe T, Hasegawa A, et al. Hyponatremia in small cell lung cancer: mechanisms not involving inappropriate ADH secretion. Cancer 1987;60:1089–93.
24. Rubin SA, Levin ER. Clinical review 53: the endocrinology of vasoactive peptides: synthesis to function. J Clin Endocrinol Metab 1994;78:6–10.
25. Robertson GL. Syndrome of inappropriate antidiuresis. N Engl J Med 1989;321:538–9.
26. Wall BM, Crofton JT, Share L, Cooke CR. Chronic hyponatremia due to resetting of the osmostat in a patient with gastric carcinoma. Am J Med 1992;93:223–8.
27. Wall BM, Crofton JT, Share L, Cooke CR. Chronic hyponatremia due to resetting of the osmostat in a patient with gastric carcinoma. Am J Med 1992;93:223–8.
28. Ayus JC, Krothapalli RK, Arieff AI. Treatment of symptomatic hyponatremia and its relation to brain damage: a prospective study. N Engl J Med 1987;317:1190–5.
29. McDonald GA, Dubose TD Jr: Hyponatremia in the cancer patient. Oncology 1993;7:55–64.
30. Shimizu K, Nakano S, Nakano Y, et al. Ectopic atrial natriuretic peptide production in small cell lung cancer with the syndrome of inappropriate antidiuretic hormone secretion. Cancer 1991;68:2284–8.
31. Jex RK, van Heerden JA, Carpenter PC, Grant CS. Ectopic ACTH syndrome: diagnostic and therapeutic aspects. Am J Surg 1985;149:276–82.
32. Howlett TA, Drury PL, Perry L, et al. Diagnosis and management of ACTH-dependent Cushing's syndrome: comparison of the features in ectopic and pituitary ACTH production. Clin Endocrinol 1986;24:699–713.
33. Trainer PJ, Grossman A: The diagnosis and differential diagnosis of Cushing's syndrome. Clin Endocrinol 1991;34:317–30.
34. Delisle L, Boyer MJ, Warr D, et al: Ectopic corticotropin syndrome and small-cell carcinoma of the lung: clinical features, outcome, and complications. Arch Intern Med 1993;153:746–52.

35. Kohler PC, Trump DL. Ectopic hormone syndromes. Cancer Invest 1986;4:543–554.
36. Fernandez JF, Ordoñez NG, Schultz PN, Samaan NA. Paraneoplastic hypercalcemia in thymic hyperplasia. Am J Clin Oncol 1992; 15:453–6.
37. Khosla S, van Heerden JA, Gharib H, et al. Parathyroid hormone-related protein and hypercalcemia secondary to massive mammary hyperplasia. N Engl J Med 1990;332:1157.
38. Newell-Price J, Trainer P, Besser M, Grossman A. The diagnosis and differential diagnosis of Cushing's syndrome and pseudo-Cushing's states. Endocr Rev 1998;19:647–72.
39. Schteingart DE. Ectopic secretion of peptides of the proopiomelanocortin family. Endocrinol Metab Clin North Am 1991;20:453–71.
40. Vincent JM, Trainer PJ, Reznek RH, et al. The radiological investigation of occult ectopic ACTH-dependent Cushing's syndrome. Clin Radiol 1993;48:11–17.
41. Arioglu E, Doppman J, Gomes M, et al. Cushing's syndrome caused by corticotropin secretion by pulmonary tumorlets. N Engl J Med 1998;339:883–6.
42. Clark AJL, Newell-Price J. Ectopic hormone production. In: Grossman A, ed. Clinical endocrinology. Oxford: Blackwell Scientific, 1993:917.
43. Thomas L, Leduc R, Thorne BA, et al. Kex2-like endoproteases PC2 and PC3 accurately cleave a model prohormone in mammalian cells: evidence for a common core of neuroendocrine processing enzymes. Proc Natl Acad Sci USA 1991;88:5297–301.
44. White A, Gibson S. ACTH precursors: biological significance and clinical relevance. Clin Endocrinol 1998;48:251–5.
45. Stewart PM, Gibson S, Crosby SR, et al. ACTH precursors characterize the ectopic ACTH syndrome. Clin Endocrinol 1994;40:199–204.
46. Yalow RS, Berson SA. Size heterogeneity of immunoreactive human ACTH in plasma and in extracts of pituitary glands and ACTH-producing thymoma. Biochem Biophys Res Commun 1971;44:439–45.
47. Lamberts SW, de Herder WW, Krenning EP, Reubi JC. A role of (labeled) somatostatin analogs in the differential diagnosis and treatment of Cushing's syndrome. J Clin Endocrinol Metab 1994;78:17–19.
48. Phlipponneau M, Nocaudie M, Epelbaum J, et al. Somatostatin analogs for the localization and preoperative treatment of an adrenocorticotropin-secreting bronchial carcinoid tumor. J Clin Endocrinol Metab 1994;78:20–4.
49. Reubi JC, Kvols LK, Waser B, et al. Detection of somatostatin receptors in surgical and percutaneous needle biopsy samples of carcinoids and islet cell carcinomas. Cancer Res 1990;50:5969–77.
50. Reubi JC, Krenning E, Lamberts SW, Kvols L. In vitro detection of somatostatin receptors in human tumors. Metabolism 1992;41:Suppl 2:104–10.
51. Reubi JC, Kvols L, Krenning E, Lamberts SW. Distribution of somatostatin receptors in normal and tumor tissue. Metabolism 1990;39:Suppl 2:78–81.
52. White A, Clark AJ, Stewart MF. The synthesis of ACTH and related peptides by tumours. Baillieres Clin Endocrinol Metab 1990;4:1–27.
53. Parks LL, Turney MK, Detera-Wadleigh S, Kovacs WJ. An ACTH-producing small cell lung cancer expresses aberrant glucocorticoid receptor transcripts from a normal gene. Mol Cell Endocrinol 1998;142:175–81.
54. Dichek HL, Nieman LK, Oldfield EH, et al. A comparison of the standard high dose dexamethasone suppression test and the overnight 8-mg dexamethasone suppression test for the differential diagnosis of adrenocorticotropin-dependent Cushing's syndrome. J Clin Endocrinol Metab 1994;78:418–22.
55. Nieman LK, Oldfield EH, Wesley R, et al. A simplified morning ovine corticotropin-releasing hormone stimulation test for the differential diagnosis of adrenocorticotropin-dependent Cushing's syndrome. J Clin Endocrinol Metabol 1993;77:1308–12.
56. Avgerinos PC, Nieman LK, Oldfield EH, Cutler GB Jr. A comparison of the overnight and the standard metyrapone test for the differential diagnosis of adrenocorticotrophin-dependent Cushing's syndrome. Clin Endocrinol 1996;45:483–91.
57. Walker BR, Campbell JC, Fraser R, et al. Mineralocorticoid excess and inhibition of 11 beta-hydroxysteroid dehydrogenase in patients with ectopic ACTH syndrome. Clin Endocrinol 1992;37:483–92.
58. Oldfield EH, Doppman JL, Nieman LK, et al. Petrosal sinus sampling with and without corticotropin-releasing hormone for the differential diagnosis of Cushing's syndrome. N Engl J Med 1991;325:897–905 [published erratum N Engl J Med 1992;326:1172].
59. Hermus AR. In: Casanueva F, ed. Recent advances in basic and clinical neuroendocrinology. New York: Elsevier, 1989:351.
60. Grossman AB, Howlett TA, Perry L, et al. CRF in the differential diagnosis of Cushing's syndrome: a comparison with the dexamethasone suppression test. Clin Endocrinol 1988;29:167–78.
61. Doppman JL, Oldfield EH, Nieman LK. Bilateral sampling of the internal jugular vein to distinguish between mechanisms of adrenocorticotropic hormone-dependent Cushing syndrome. Ann Intern Med 1998;128:33–6.
62. Mamelak AN, Dowd CF, Tyrrell JB, et al. Venous angiography is needed to interpret inferior petrosal sinus and cavernous sinus sampling data for lateralizing adrenocorticotropin-secreting adenomas. J Clin Endocrinol Metabol 1996;81:475–81.
63. Oldfield EH, Doppman JL. Petrosal versus cavernous sinus sampling. J Neurosurg 1998;89:890–3.
64. Trainer PJ. Too much of a good thing. Clin Endocrinol 1998;49:285–286.
65. Miller DL, Doppman JL, Peterman SB, et al. Neurologic complications of petrosal sinus sampling. Radiology 1992;185:143–7.
66. Teramoto A. Petrosal versus cavernous sinus sampling response. J Neurosurg 1998;89:892–3.
67. Teramoto A, Yoshida Y, Sanno N, Nemoto S. Cavernous sinus sampling in patients with adrenocorticotrophic hormone-dependent Cushing's syndrome with emphasis on inter- and intracavernous adrenocorticotropic hormone gradients. J Neurosurg 1998;89:762–8.
68. Tabarin A, Laurent F, Catargi B, et al. Comparative evaluation of conventional and dynamic magnetic resonance imaging of the pituitary gland for the diagnosis of Cushing's disease. Clin Endocrinol 1998;49:293–300.
69. Grossman A. New uses for an old peptide: desmopressin and Cushing's syndrome. Clin Endocrinol 1993;38:461–2.
70. Malerbi DA, Mendonca BB, Liberman B, et al. The desmopressin stimulation test in the differential diagnosis of Cushing's syndrome. Clin Endocrinol 1993;38:463–72.
71. White A, Stewart S, Gibson SR, et al. ACTH precursors characterize the ectopic ACTH syndrome. J Endocrinol 1992;132:Suppl:155. abstract.
72. Lamberts SW, Krenning EP, Reubi JC. The role of somatostatin and its analogs in the diagnosis and treatment of tumors. Endocr Rev 1991;12:450–82.
73. Dimopoulos MA, Fernandez JF, Samaan NA, et al. Paraneoplastic Cushing's syndrome as an adverse prognostic factor in patients who die early with small cell lung cancer. Cancer 1992;69:66–71.
74. Wick MR, Scott RE, Li CY, Carney JA. Carcinoid tumor of the thymus: a clinicopathologic report of seven cases with a review of the literature. Mayo Clin Proc 1980;55:246–54.
75. Farwell AP, Devlin JT, Stewart JA. Total suppression of cortisol excretion by ketoconazole in the therapy of the ectopic adrenocorticotropic hormone syndrome. Am J Med 1988;84:1063–6.
76. Laue L, Gallucci W, Loriaux DL, et al. The antiglucocorticoid and antiprogestin steroid RU 486: its glucocorticoid agonist effect is inadequate to prevent adrenal insufficiency in primates. J Clin Endocrinol Metab 1988;67:602–6.
77. Lamberts SW, Klijn JG, de Quijada M, et al. The mechanism of the suppressive action of bromocriptine on adrenocorticotropin secretion in patients with Cushing's disease and Nelson's syndrome. J Clin Endocrinol Metabol 1980;51:307–11.
78. Cheung NW, Boyages SC. Failure of somatostatin analogue to control Cushing's syndrome in two cases of ACTH-producing carcinoid tumours. Clin Endocrinol 1992;36:361–7.
79. Bertagna X, Favrod-Coune C, Escourolle H. Suppression of ectopic adrenocorticotropin secretion by the long-acting somatostatin analog octreotide. J Clin Endocrinol Metab 1989;68:988–91.
80. van der Lely AJ, Foeken K, van der Mast RC, Lamberts SW. Rapid reversal of acute psychosis in the Cushing syndrome with the cortisol-receptor antagonist mifepristone (RU 486). Ann Intern Med 1991;114:143–4.
81. Murakami O, Takahashi K, Sone M, et al. An ACTH-secreting bronchial carcinoid: presence corticotropin-releasing hormone, neuropeptide Y and endothelin-1 in the tumor tissue. Acta Endocrinol 1993;128:192–6.
82. O'Brien T, Young WF Jr, Davila DG, et al. Cushing's syndrome associated with ectopic production of corticotrophin-releasing hormone, corticotrophin and vasopressin by a phaeochromocytoma. Clin Endocrinol 1992;37:460–7.

83. Vassilopoulou-Sellin R, Newman BM, Taylor SH, Guinee VF. Incidence of hypercalcemia in patients with malignancy referred to a comprehensive cancer center. Cancer 1993;71:1309–12.
84. Strewler GJ, Nissenson RA. Peptide mediators of hypercalcemia in malignancy. Annu Rev Med 1990;41:35–44.
85. Strewler GJ, Nissenson RA. Hypercalcemia in malignancy. West J Med 1990;153:635–40.
86. Rosol TJ, Capen CC. Mechanisms of cancer-induced hypercalcemia. Lab Invest 1992;67:680–702.
87. Ralston SH, Gallacher SJ, Patel U, et al. Comparison of three intravenous bisphosphonates in cancer-associated hypercalcaemia. Lancet 1989;2:1180–1182.
88. Coleman RE, Rubens RD. The clinical course of bone metastases from breast cancer. Br J Cancer 1987;55:61–6.
89. Bender RA, Hansen H. Hypercalcemia in bronchogenic carcinoma: a prospective study of 200 patients. Ann Intern Med 1974;80:205–8.
90. Mundy GR. Ectopic production of calciotropic peptides. Endocrinol Metab Clin North Am 1991;20:473–87.
91. Mundy GR. Pathophysiology of cancer-associated hypercalcemia. Semin Oncol 1990;17:Suppl 5:10–15.
92. Broadus AE. Identification of the parathyroid-related peptide. In: Halloran BP, ed. Parathyroid hormone-related protein: normal physiology and its role in cancer. Boca Raton, FL: CRC Press, 1992:1–23.
93. Stewart AF, Broadus AE. Clinical review 16: parathyroid hormone-related proteins: coming of age in the 1990s. J Clin Endocrinol Metab 1990;71:1410–4.
94. Bilezikian JP. Parathyroid hormone-related peptide in sickness and in health. N Engl J Med 1990;322:1151–3.
95. Martin TJ. Properties of parathyroid hormone-related protein and its role in malignant hypercalcemia. Q J M 1990;76:771–86.
96. Stewart AF, Horst R, Deftos LJ, et al. Biochemical evaluation of patients with cancer-associated hypercalcemia: evidence for humoral and nonhumoral groups. N Engl J Med 1980;303:1377–83.
97. Ratcliffe WA, Hutchesson AC, Bundred NJ, Ratcliffe JG. Role of assays for parathyroid-hormone-related protein in investigation of hypercalcaemia. Lancet 1992;339:164–7.
98. Bucht E, Rong H, Pernow Y, et al. Parathyroid hormone-related protein in patients with primary breast cancer and eucalcemia. Cancer Res 1998;58:4113–6.
99. Schilling T, Pecherstorfer M, et al. Parathyroid hormone-related protein (PTHrP) does not regulate 1,25-dihydroxyvitamin D serum levels in hypercalcemia of malignancy. J Clin Endocrinol Metab 1993;76:801–3.
100. Broadus AE, Horst RL, Lang R, et al. The importance of circulating 1,25-dihydroxyvitamin D in the pathogenesis of hypercalciuria and renal-stone formation in primary hyperparathyroidism. N Engl J Med 1980;302:421–6.
101. Ralston SH, Cowan RA, Robertson AG, et al. Circulating vitamin D metabolites and hypercalcaemia of malignancy. Acta Endocrinol 1984;106:556–63.
102. Fukumoto S, Matsumoto T, Yamoto H, et al. Suppression of serum 1,25-dihydroxyvitamin D in humoral hypercalcemia of malignancy is caused by elaboration of a factor that inhibits renal 1,25-dihydroxyvitamin D3 production. Endocrinology 1989;124:2057–62.
103. Burtis WJ, Brady TG, Orloff JJ, et al. Immunochemical characterization of circulating parathyroid hormone-related protein in patients with humoral hypercalcemia of cancer. N Engl J Med 1990;322:1106–12.
104. Fenton AJ, Kemp BE, Hammonds RG Jr, et al. A potent inhibitor of osteoclastic bone resorption within a highly conserved pentapeptide region of parathyroid hormone-related protein; PTHrP[107–111]. Endocrinology 1991;129:3424–26.
105. Scher HI, Yagoda A. Bone metastases: pathogenesis, treatment, and rationale for use of resorption inhibitors. Am J Med 1987;82:6–28.
106. Ratcliffe WA, Norbury S, Heath DA, Ratcliffe JG. Development and validation of an immunoradiometric assay of parathyrin-related protein in unextracted plasma. Clin Chem 1991;37:678–85.
107. Wysolmerski JJ, Stewart AF. The physiology of parathyroid hormone-related protein: an emerging role as a developmental factor. Annu Rev Physiol 1998;60:431–60.
108. Bundred NJ, Ratcliffe WA, Walker RA, et al. Parathyroid hormone related protein and hypercalcaemia in breast cancer. BMJ (Clin Res Ed) 1991;303:1506–9.
109. Mallette LE. The hypercalcemias. Semin Nephrol 1992;12:159–90.
110. Seyberth HW, Segre GV, Morgan JL, et al. Prostaglandins as mediators of hypercalcemia associated with certain types of cancer. N Engl J Med 1975;293:1278–83.
111. Komiya I, Yamaguchi K, Miyake Y, et al. Retroperitoneal neurilemoma presenting with humoral hypercalcemia associated with markedly elevated plasma prostaglandin levels. Cancer 1991;68:1086–91.
112. Strewler GJ, Budayr AA, Clark OH, Nissenson RA. Production of parathyroid hormone by a malignant nonparathyroid tumor in a hypercalcemic patient. J Clin Endocrinol Metab 1993;76:1373–5.
113. Yoshimoto K, Yamasaki R, Sakai H, et al. Ectopic production of parathyroid hormone by small cell lung cancer in a patient with hypercalcemia. J Clin Endocrinol Metab 1989;68:976–81.
114. Dickersin GR, Kline IW, Scully RE. Small cell carcinoma of the ovary with hypercalcemia: a report of eleven cases. Cancer 1982;49:188–97.
115. Benrubi GI, Pitel P, Lammert N. Small cell carcinoma of the ovary with hypercalcemia responsive to sequencing chemotherapy. South Med J 1993;86:247–8.
116. Bakri YN, Akhtar M. Gonadal dysgerminoma-seminoma associated with severe hypercalcemia. Acta Obstet Gynaecol Scand 1993;72:57–9.
117. Hoekman K, Tjandra YI, Papapoulos SE. The role of 1,25-dihydroxyvitamin D in the maintenance of hypercalcemia in a patient with an ovarian carcinoma producing parathyroid hormone-related protein. Cancer 1991;68:642–7.
118. Nussbaum SR, Gaz RD, Arnold A. Hypercalcemia and ectopic secretion of parathyroid hormone by an ovarian carcinoma with rearrangement of the gene for parathyroid hormone. N Engl J Med 1990;323:1324–8.
119. Senba M, Kawai K, Chiyoda S, Takahara O. Metastatic liver calcification in adult T-cell leukemia-lymphoma associated with hypercalcemia. Am J Gastroenterol 1990;85:1202–3.
120. Dazai Y, Katoh I, Hara Y, et al. Two cases of adult T-cell leukemia associated with acute pancreatitis due to hypercalcemia. Am J Med 1991;90:251–4.
121. Fukumoto S, Matsumoto T, Ikeda K, et al. Clinical evaluation of calcium metabolism in adult T-cell leukemia/lymphoma. Arch Intern Med 1988;148:921–5.
122. Adams JS, Fernandez M, Gacad MA, et al. Vitamin D metabolite-mediated hypercalcemia and hypercalciuria patients with AIDS- and non-AIDS-associated lymphoma. Blood 1989;73:235–9.
123. Seymour JF, Gagel RF. Calcitriol: the major humoral mediator of hypercalcemia in Hodgkin's disease and non-Hodgkin's lymphomas. Blood 1993;82:1383–94.
124. Davies SV, Vora J, Wardrop CA. Parathyroid hormone related protein (PTHrP) in hypercalcaemia of lymphoproliferative disease. J Clin Pathol 1993;46:188.
125. Rossi JF, Chappard D, Marcelli C, et al. Micro-osteoclast resorption as a characteristic feature of B-cell malignancies other than multiple myeloma. Br J Haematol 1990;76:469–75.
126. Yoneda T, Alsina MA, Chavez JB, et al. Evidence that tumor necrosis factor plays a pathogenetic role in the paraneoplastic syndromes of cachexia, hypercalcemia, and leukocytosis in a human tumor in nude mice. J Clin Invest 1991;87:977–85.
127. Kukreja SC, Shevrin DH, Wimbiscus SA, et al. Antibodies to parathyroid hormone-related protein lower serum calcium in athymic mouse models of malignancy-associated hypercalcemia due to human tumors. J Clin Invest 1988;82:1798–1802.
128. Shigeno C, Yamamoto I, Dokoh S, et al. Identification of 1,24(R)-dihydroxyvitamin D3-like bone-resorbing lipid in a patient with cancer-associated hypercalcemia. J Clin Endocrinol Metab 1985;61:761–68.
129. Evely RS, Bonomo A, Schneider HG, et al. Structural requirements for the action of parathyroid hormone-related protein (PTHrP) on bone resorption by isolated osteoclasts. J Bone Miner Res 1991;6:85–93.
130. Driedger H, Pruzanski W. Plasma cell neoplasia with osteosclerotic lesions: a study of five cases and a review of the literature. Arch Intern Med 1979;139:892–6.
131. Bataille R, Chappard D, Marcelli C, et al. Osteoblast stimulation in multiple myeloma lacking lytic bone lesions. Br J Haematol 1990;76:484–7.
132. Bataille R, Delmas PD, Chappard D, Sany J. Abnormal serum bone GLA protein levels in multiple myeloma: crucial role of bone formation and prognostic implications. Cancer 1990;66:167–72.
133. Bardwick PA, Zvaifler NJ, Gill GN, et al. Plasma cell dyscrasia with polyneuropathy, organomegaly, endocrinopathy, M protein, and skin changes: the POEMS syndrome: report on two cases and a review of the literature. Medicine 1980;59:311–22.
134. Feigert JM, Sweet DL, Coleman M, et al. Multicentric angiofollicular

lymph node hyperplasia with peripheral neuropathy, pseudotumor cerebri, IgA dysproteinemia, and thrombocytosis in women: a distinct syndrome. Ann Intern Med 1990;113:362–7.

135. Miralles GD, O'Fallon JR, Talley NJ. Plasma-cell dyscrasia with polyneuropathy: the spectrum of POEMS syndrome. N Engl J Med 1992;327:1919–23.

136. Paredes JM, Mitchell BS. Multiple myeloma: current concepts in diagnosis and management. Med Clin North Am 1980;64:729–42.

137. Kato T, Kaneko E, Numano F, et al. Vasospastic angina in Crow-Fukase Syndrome. Am Heart J 1992;124:505–7.

138. Chan WC, Hargreaves H, Keller J. Giant lymph node hyperplasia with unusual clinicopathologic features. Cancer 1984;53:2135–9.

139. Merlini G, Fitzpatrick LA, Siris ES, et al. A human myeloma immunoglobulin G binding four moles of calcium associated with asymptomatic hypercalcemia. J Clin Immunol 1984;4:185–96.

140. Yoshizaki K, Matsuda T, Nishimoto N, et al. Pathogenic significance of interleukin-6 (IL-6/BSF-2) in Castleman's disease. Blood 1989; 74:1360–7.

141. Mandler RN, Kerrigan DP, Smart J, et al. Castleman's disease in POEMS syndrome with elevated interleukin-6. Cancer 1992;69:2697–703.

142. Nagai Y, Yamato H, Akaogi K, et al. Role of interleukin-6 in uncoupling of bone in vivo in a human squamous carcinoma coproducing parathyroid hormone-related peptide and interleukin-6. J Bone Miner Res 1998;13:664–72.

143. Powell GJ, Southby J, Danks JA, et al. Localization of parathyroid hormone-related protein in breast cancer metastases: increased incidence in bone compared with other sites. Cancer Res 1991;51:3059–61.

144. Southby J, Kissin MW, Danks JA, et al. Immunohistochemical localization of parathyroid hormone-related protein in human breast cancer. Cancer Res 1990;50:7710–6.

145. van Holten-Verzantvoort AT, Bijvoet OL, et al. Reduced morbidity from skeletal metastases in breast cancer patients during long-term bisphosphonate (APD) treatment. Lancet 1987;2:983–5.

146. Paterson AH, Powles TJ, Kanis JA, et al. Double-blind controlled trial of oral clodronate in patients with bone metastases from breast cancer. J Clin Oncol 1993;11:59–65.

147. Clarke NW, Holbrook IB, McClure J, George NJ. Osteoclast inhibition by pamidronate in metastatic prostate cancer: a preliminary study. Br J Cancer 1991;63:420–3.

148. Guise TA, Yin JJ, Taylor SD, et al. Evidence for a causal role of parathyroid hormone-related protein in the pathogenesis of human breast cancer-mediated osteolysis. J Clin Invest 1996;98:1544–9.

149. Yaghoobian J, Morieux C, Denne MA, et al. Pamidronate corrects the down-regulation of the renal parathyroid hormone (PTH)/PTH-related peptide (PTHrP) receptor mRNA in rats bearing Walker tumors. Horm Metab Res 1998;30:249–55.

150. Gallacher SJ, Ralston SH, Fraser WD, et al. A comparison of low versus high dose pamidronate in cancer-associated hypercalcaemia. Bone Miner 1991;15:249–56.

151. Gucalp R, Ritch P, Wiernik PH, et al. Comparative study of pamidronate disodium and etidronate disodium in the treatment of cancer-related hypercalcemia. J Clin Oncol 1992;10:134–42.

152. Uebelhart D, Gineyts E, Chapuy MC, Delmas PD. Urinary excretion of pyridinium crosslinks: a new marker of bone resorption in metabolic bone disease. Bone Miner 1990;8:87–96.

153. Dodwell DJ, et al. The management of skeletal metastases and hypercalcemia of osteoclast inhibition. In: Rubens RD, ed. Management of bone metastases and hypercalcemia by osteoclast inhibition. Toronto: Hogrefe & Huber, 1990:76–80.

154. Coleman RE, Purohit OP. Osteoclast inhibition for the treatment of bone metastases. Cancer Treat Rev 1993;19:79–103.

155. Pecherstorfer M, Thiébaud D. Treatment of resistant tumor-induced hypercalcemia with escalating doses of pamidronate (APD). Ann Oncol 1992;3:661–3.

156. Blind E, Raue F, Meinel T, et al. Levels of parathyroid hormone-related protein (PTHrP) in hypercalcemia of malignancy are not lowered by treatment with the bisphosphonate BM 21.0955. Horm Metab Res 1993;25:40–4.

157. Anstey A, Gowers L, Vass A, Robson AO. Ovarian dysgerminoma presenting with hypercalcaemia: case report and review of the literature. Br J Obstet Gynaecol 1990;97:641–4.

158. Sridhar KS, Hussein AM. Hypercalcemia in head and neck squamous-cell carcinoma. Am J Clin Oncol 1990;13:388–93.

159. Kutluk T, Akyüz C, Yalcin B, et al. Use of pamidronate in the management of acute cancer-related hypercalcemia in children. Med Pediatr Oncol 1998;31:39.

160. Aboulafia DM, Bundow D, Weaver C, Yokum RC. Retinoid-induced hypercalcemia in a patient with Kaposi sarcoma associated with acquired immunodeficiency syndrome. Am J Clin Oncol 1998;21:513–7.

161. Barba R, Gómez-Rodrigo J, Marco J, et al. Transient foscarnet-induced hypercalcaemia. AIDS 1998;12:1930–1.

162. Abramson EC, Gajardo H, Kukreja SC. Hypocalcemia in cancer. Bone Miner 1990;10:161–9.

163. Hall TC, Griffiths CT, Petranek JR. Hypocalcemia—an unusual metabolic complication of breast cancer. N Engl J Med 1966;275:1474–7.

164. Weidner N, Bar RS, Weiss D, Strottmann MP. Neoplastic pathology of oncogenic osteomalacia/rickets. Cancer 1985;55:1691–705.

165. Ryan EA, Reiss E. Oncogenous osteomalacia: review of the world literature of 42 cases and report of two new cases. Am J Med 1984;77:501–12.

166. Chandalia HB, Boshell BR. Hypoglycemia associated with extrapancreatic tumors: report of two cases with studies on its pathogenesis. Arch Intern Med 1972;129:447–56.

167. Marks V. Recognition and differential diagnosis of spontaneous hypoglycaemia. Clin Endocrinol 1992;37:309–16.

168. Fukuda I, Hizuka N, Takano K, et al. Characterization of insulin-like growth factor II (IGF-II) and IGF binding proteins in patients with non-islet-cell tumor hypoglycemia. Endocr J 1993;40:111–9.

169. Sharma N, Jain S, Kumari S, Varma S. Hypercalcaemia with radiographic abnormalities in chronic myeloid leukaemia. Postgrad Med J 1998;74:301–303.

170. Jones JI, Clemmons DR. Insulin-like growth factors and their binding proteins: biological actions. Endocr Rev 1995;16:3–34.

171. Hoff AO, Vassilopoulou-Sellin R. The role of glucagon administration in the diagnosis and treatment of patients with tumor hypoglycemia. Cancer 1998;82:1585–92.

172. Saigal S, Nandeesh HP, Malhotra V, Sarin SK. A case of hepatocellular carcinoma associated with troublesome hypoglycemia: Management by cytoreduction using percutaneous ethanol injection. Am J Gastroenterol 1998;93:1380–1.

173. Hunter SJ, Daughaday WH, Callender ME, et al. A case of hepatoma associated with hypoglycaemia and overproduction of IGF-II (E-21): beneficial effects of treatment with growth hormone and intrahepatic adriamycin. Clin Endocrinol 1994;41:397–401.

174. Henson PA, Hoffman HL, Urich H. Encephalomyelitis with carcinoma. Brain 1985;88:449–64.

175. Furneaux HF, Reich L, Posner JB. Autoantibody synthesis in the central nervous system of patients with paraneoplastic syndromes. Neurology 1990;40:1085–91.

176. Chad DA, Recht LD. Neuromuscular complications of systemic cancer. Neurol Clin 1991;9:901–18.

177. Anderson NE, Rosenblum MK, Graus F, et al. Autoantibodies in paraneoplastic syndromes associated with small-cell lung cancer. Neurology 1988;38:1391–8.

178. Manley GT, Smitt PS, Dalmau J, Posner JB. Hu antigens: reactivity with Hu antibodies, tumor expression, and major immunogenic sites. Ann Neurol 1995;38:102–10.

179. Hainfellner JA, Kristoferitsch W, Lassmann H, et al. T-cell-mediated ganglionitis associated with acute sensory neuronopathy. Ann Neurol 1996;39:543–7.

180. Ichimura M, Yamamoto M, Kobayashi Y, et al. Tissue distribution of pathological lesions and Hu antigen expression in paraneoplastic sensory neuronopathy. Acta Neuropathol 1998;95:641–8.

181. Posner JB, Furneaux HM. Paraneoplastic syndromes. In: Waksman BH, ed. Immunologic mechanisms in neurologic and psychiatric disease. New York: Raven Press, 1990:187–219.

182. Panegyres PK, Reading MC, Esiri MM. The inflammatory reaction of paraneoplastic ganglionitis and encephalitis: an immunohistochemical study. J Neurol 1993;240:93–7.

183. Clouston PD, DeAngelis LM, Posner JB. The spectrum of neurological disease in patients with systemic cancer. Ann Neurol 1992;31:268–73.

184. Waterhouse DM, Natale RB, Cody RL. Breast cancer and paraneoplastic cerebellar degeneration. Cancer 1991;68:1835–41.

185. Furneaux HM, Rosenblum MK, Dalmau J, et al. Selective expression of Purkinje-cell antigens in tumor tissue from patients with paraneoplastic cerebellar degeneration. N Engl J Med 1990;322:1844–1851.

186. Graus F, René R. Clinical and pathological advances on central ner-

vous system paraneoplastic syndromes. Rev Neurol 1992;148:496–501.

187. Moll JW, Henzen-Logmans SC, Splinter TA, et al. Diagnostic value of anti-neuronal antibodies for paraneoplastic disorders of the nervous system. J Neurol Neurosurg Psychiatry 1990;53:940–3.

188. Moll JW, Henzen-Logmans SC, Van der Meché FG, Vecht CH. Early diagnosis and intravenous immune globulin therapy in paraneoplastic cerebellar degeneration. J Neurol Neurosurg Psychiatry 1993;56:112.

189. Lennon VA, Kryzer TJ. Neuronal calcium channel autoantibodies coexisting with type 1 Purkinje cell cytoplasmic autoantibodies (PCA-1 or "anti-Yo"). Neurology 1998;51:327–9.

190. Tanaka K, Motomura M, Nakao Y, et al. Absence of anti-P/Q calcium channel antibody in the sera of patients with anti-Yo antibody-positive paraneoplastic cerebellar degeneration. Neurology 1997;49:895–6.

191. Kiers L, Altermatt HJ, Lennon VA. Paraneoplastic anti-neuronal nuclear IgG autoantibodies (type I) localize antigen in small cell lung carcinoma. Mayo Clin Proc 1991;66:1209–16.

192. Dalmau J, Furneaux HM, Rosenblum MK, et al. Detection of the anti-Hu antibody in specific regions of the nervous system and tumor from patients with paraneoplastic encephalomyelitis/sensory neuronopathy. Neurology 1991;41:1757–64.

193. de la Sayette V, Bertran F, Honnorat J, et al. Paraneoplastic cerebellar syndrome and optic neuritis with anti-CV2 antibodies: clinical response to excision of the primary tumor. Arch Neurol 1998;55:405–8.

194. Dalmau J, Furneaux HM, Gralla RJ, et al. Detection of the anti-Hu antibody in the serum of patients with small cell lung cancer—a quantitative Western blot analysis. Ann Neurol 1990;27:544–52.

195. Batson OA, Fantle DM, Stewart JA. Paraneoplastic encephalomyelitis: dramatic response to chemotherapy alone. Cancer 1992;69:1291–3.

196. Dalmau J, Graus F, Rosenblum MK, Posner JB. Anti-Hu–associated paraneoplastic encephalomyelitis/sensory neuronopathy: a clinical study of 71 patients. Medicine 1992;71:59–72.

197. Carpentier AF, Voltz R, DesChamps T, et al. Absence of HuD gene mutations in paraneoplastic small cell lung cancer tissue. Neurology 1998;50:1919.

198. Molinuevo JL, Graus F, Serrano C, et al. Utility of anti-Hu antibodies in the diagnosis of paraneoplastic sensory neuropathy. Ann Neurol 1998;44:976–80.

199. Hatzis GS, Delladetsima I, Koufos C. Hepatocellular carcinoma presenting with paraneoplastic neurologic syndrome in a hepatitis B surface antigen-positive patient. J Clin Gastroenterol 1998;26:144–7.

200. Darnell RB, DeAngelis LM. Regression of small-cell lung carcinoma in patients with paraneoplastic neuronal antibodies. Lancet 1993; 341:21–2.

201. Luque FA, Furneaux HM, Ferziger R, et al. Anti-Ri: an antibody associated with paraneoplastic opsoclonus and breast cancer. Ann Neurol 1991;29:241–51.

202. Dropcho EJ, Kline LB, Riser J. Antineuronal (anti-Ri) antibodies in a patient with steroid-responsive opsoclonus-myoclonus. Neurology 1993;43:207–11.

203. Yang YY, Yin GL, Darnell RB. The neuronal RNA-binding protein Nova-2 is implicated as the autoantigen targeted in POMA patients with dementia. Proc Natl Acad Sci USA 1998;95:13254–9.

204. Darnell RB. Onconeural antigens and the paraneoplastic neurologic disorders: at the intersection of cancer, immunity, and the brain. Proc Natl Acad Sci USA 1996;93:4529–36.

205. Kornguth SE. Neuronal proteins and paraneoplastic syndromes. N Engl J Med 1989;321:1607–8.

206. Thirkill CE, FitzGerald P, Sergott RC, et al. Cancer-associated retinopathy (CAR syndrome) with antibodies reacting with retinal, optic-nerve, and cancer cells. N Engl J Med 1989;321:1589–94.

207. Jacobson DM, Thirkill CE, Tipping SJ. A clinical triad to diagnose paraneoplastic retinopathy. Ann Neurol 1990;28:162–7.

208. Rizzo JF 3d, Gittinger JW Jr. Selective immunohistochemical staining in the paraneoplastic retinopathy syndrome. Ophthalmology 1992; 99:1286–9.

209. Rush JA. Paraneoplastic retinopathy in malignant melanoma. Am J Ophthalmol 1993;115:390–1.

210. Holmes A, Kilpatrick C, Proietto J, Green MD. Reversal of a neurologic paraneoplastic syndrome with octreotide (Sandostatin) in a patient with glucagonoma. Am J Med 1991;91:434–6.

211. Elrington GM, Murray NM, Spiro SG, Newsom-Davis J. Neurological paraneoplastic syndromes in patients with small cell lung cancer: a prospective survey of 150 patients. J Neurol Neurosurg Psychiatry 1991;54:764–7.

212. Bady B, Vial C, Chauplannaz G. [Lambert-Eaton syndrome: clinical and electrophysiological study of 18 cases associated with lung cancer]. Rev Neurol 1992;148:513–9.

213. O'Neill JH, Murray NM, Newsom-Davis J. The Lambert-Eaton myasthenic syndrome: a review of 50 cases. Brain 1988;111:Pt 3:577–96.

214. Lennon VA, Lambert EH. Autoantibodies bind solubilized calcium channel-omega-conotoxin complexes from small cell lung carcinoma: a diagnostic aid for Lambert-Eaton myasthenic syndrome. Mayo Clin Proc 1989;64:1498–504.

215. Leveque C, Hoshino T, David P, et al. The synaptic vesicle protein synaptotagmin associates with calcium channels and is a putative Lambert-Eaton myasthenic syndrome antigen. Proc Natl Acad Sci USA 1992;89:3625–9.

216. Rosenfeld MR, Wong E, Dalmau J, et al. Cloning and characterization of a Lambert-Eaton myasthenic syndrome antigen. Ann Neurol 1993;33:113–20.

217. Takamori M, Hamada T, Komai K, et al. Synaptotagmin can cause an immune-mediated model of Lambert-Eaton myasthenic syndrome in rats. Ann Neurol 1994;35:74–80.

218. Cruz LJ, Olivera BM. Calcium channel antagonists: omega-conotoxin defines a new high affinity site. J Biol Chem 1986;261:6230–3.

219. Perin MS, Brose N, Jahn R, Südhof TC. Domain structure of synaptotagmin (p65). J Biol Chem 1991;266:623–9.

220. Lang B, Waterman S, Pinto A, et al. The role of autoantibodies in Lambert-Eaton myasthenic syndrome. Ann N Y Acad Sci 1998;841:596–605.

221. Kim YI, Neher E. IgG from patients with Lambert-Eaton syndrome blocks voltage-dependent calcium channels. Science 1988;239:405–8.

222. Leys K, Lang B, Johnston I, Newsom-Davis J. Calcium channel autoantibodies in the Lambert-Eaton myasthenic syndrome. Ann Neurol 1991;29:307–14.

223. Greenberg DA. Calcium channels and neuromuscular disease. Ann Neurol 1994;35:131–2.

224. Drachman DB, de Silva S, Ramsay D, Pestronk A. Humoral pathogenesis of myasthenia gravis. Ann N Y Acad Sci 1987;505:90–105.

225. Beeson D, Bond AP, Corlett L, et al. Thymus, thymoma, and specific T cells in myasthenia gravis. Ann N Y Acad Sci 1998;841:371–87.

226. Koski SL, Mackey JR, Mackey DS. Myasthenia gravis post allogeneic bone marrow transplantation revisited. Bone Marrow Transplant 1998;22:403–4.

227. Mackey JR, Desai S, Larratt L, et al. Myasthenia gravis in association with allogeneic bone marrow transplantation: clinical observations, therapeutic implications and review of literature. Bone Marrow Transplant 1997;19:939–42.

228. Lefvert AK, Björkholm M. Antibodies against the acetylcholine receptor in hematologic disorders: implications for the development of myasthenia gravis after bone marrow grafting. N Engl J Med 1987;317:170.

229. Asherson GL, Webster DM. Thymus and immune deficiency. In: Asherson GL, Webster ABD, eds. Diagnosis and treatment of immunodeficiency diseases. Oxford: Blackwell Scientific Publications, 1980:78–98.

230. Díez-Tejedor E, Tejada J, Ramos MJ, et al. Response to combined therapy with plasmapheresis and high doses of immunoglobulin in Lambert-Eaton syndrome. Neurologia 1994;9:76–7.

231. McEvoy KM, Windebank AJ, Daube JR, Low PA. 3,4-Diaminopyridine in the treatment of Lambert-Eaton myasthenic syndrome. N Engl J Med 1989;321:1567–71.

232. Bird SJ. Clinical and electrophysiologic improvement in Lambert-Eaton syndrome with intravenous immunoglobulin therapy. Neurology 1992;42:1422–3.

233. Dalakas MC. High-dose intravenous immunoglobulin and serum viscosity: risk of precipitating thromboembolic events. Neurology 1994;44:223–6.

234. Lennon VA, Sas DF, Busk MF, et al. Enteric neuronal autoantibodies in pseudoobstruction with small-cell lung carcinoma. Gastroenterology 1991;100:137–42.

235. Schuffler MD, Baird HW, Fleming CR, et al. Intestinal pseudo-obstruction as the presenting manifestation of small-cell carcinoma of the lung: a paraneoplastic neuropathy of the gastrointestinal tract. Ann Intern Med 1983;98:129–34.

236. Yapp RG, Siegel JH. Unexplained biliary tract dilatation in lung cancer patients. Endoscopy 1992;24:593–5.

237. Watterson J, Priest JR. Jaundice as a paraneoplastic phenomenon in a T-cell lymphoma. Gastroenterology 1989;97:1319–22.

238. Walsh PN, Kissane JM. Nonmetastatic hypernephroma with reversible hepatic dysfunction. Arch Intern Med 1968;122:214–22.

239. Vickers SM, Niederhuber JE. Hodgkin's disease associated with neurologic paraneoplastic syndrome. South Med J 1997;90:839–44.

240. Dorudi S, Berry AR, Kettlewell MG. Acute colonic pseudo-obstruction. Br J Surg 1992;79:99–103.

241. Turégano-Fuentes F, Muñoz-Jiménez F, Del Valle-Hernández E, et al. Early resolution of Ogilvie's syndrome with intravenous neostigmine: a simple, effective treatment. Dis Col Rectum 1997;40:1353–7.

242. Posner JB. Paraneoplastic syndromes. Curr Opin Neurol 1997;10:471–476.

243. Dropcho EJ. Neurologic paraneoplastic syndromes. J Neurol Sci 1998;153:264–78.

244. Dropcho EJ. Antiamphiphysin antibodies with small-cell lung carcinoma and paraneoplastic encephalomyelitis. Ann Neurol 1996;39:659–67.

245. Folli F, Solimena M, Cofiell R, et al. Autoantibodies to a 128-kd synaptic protein in three women with the stiff-man syndrome and breast cancer. N Engl J Med 1993;328:546–51.

246. David C, Solimena M, De Camilli P. Autoimmunity in stiff-man syndrome with breast cancer is targeted to the C-terminal region of human amphiphysin, a protein similar to the yeast proteins, Rvs167 and Rvs161. FEBS Lett 1994;351:73–9.

247. Rosen L, DeCamilli P, Butler M, et al. Stiff-man syndrome in a woman with breast cancer: an uncommon central nervous system paraneoplastic syndrome. Neurology 1998;50:94–8.

247a. Levy LM, Dalakis MC, Floeter MK. The stiff-person syndrome: an autoimmune disorder affecting neurotransmission of gamma-aminobutyric acid. Ann Intern Med 1999;131:522–30.

247b. Vincent A, Grimaldi LM, Martino G, et al. Antibodies of [125]I-glutamic acid decarboxylase in patients with stiff man syndrome. J Neurol Neurosurg Psychiatry 1997;62:395–7.

248. Petit T, Janser JC, Achour NR, et al. Paraneoplastic temporal lobe epilepsy and anti-Yo autoantibody. Ann Oncol 1997;8:919.

249. Anhalt GJ, Kim SC, Stanley JR, et al. Paraneoplastic pemphigus: an autoimmune mucocutaneous disease associated with neoplasia. N Engl J Med 1990;323:1729–35.

250. Berg WA, Fishman EK, Anhalt GJ. Retroperitoneal reticulum cell sarcoma: a cause of paraneoplastic pemphigus. South Med J 1993;86:215–7.

251. Burtis WJ, Brady TG, Orloff JJ. Immunochemical characterization of circulating parathyroid hormone-related protein in patients with humoral hypercalcemia of cancer. N Engl J Med 1990;322:1106–2.

252. Cohen PR, Kurzrock R. Malignancy-associated tripe palms. J Am Acad Dermatol 1992;27:Pt 1:271–2.

253. Helm TN, Camisa C, Valenzuela R, Allen CM. Paraneoplastic pemphigus: A distinct autoimmune vesiculobullous disorder associated with neoplasia. Oral Surg Oral Med Oral Pathol 1993;75:209–13.

254. Mutasim DF, Pelc NJ, Anhalt GJ. Paraneoplastic pemphigus. Dermatol Clin 1993;11:473–81.

255. Lam S, Stone MS, Goeken JA, et al. Paraneoplastic pemphigus, cicatricial conjunctivitis, and acanthosis nigricans with pachydermatoglyphy in a patient with bronchogenic squamous cell carcinoma. Ophthalmology 1992;99:108–13.

256. Handfield-Jones SE, Matthews CN, Ellis JP, et al. Acrokeratosis paraneoplastica of Bazex. J R Soc Med 1992;85:548–50.

257. Bolognia JL, Brewer YP, Cooper DL. Bazex syndrome (acrokeratosis paraneoplastica): an analytic review. Medicine 1991;70:269–80.

258. Ellis DL, Kafka SP, Chow JC, et al. Melanoma, growth factors, acanthosis nigricans, the sign of Leser-Trélat, and multiple acrochordons: a possible role for alpha-transforming growth factor in cutaneous paraneoplastic syndromes. N Engl J Med 1987;317:1582–7.

259. Cohn MS, Classen RF. The sign of Leser-Trélat associated with adenocarcinoma of the rectum. Cutis 1993;51:255–7.

260. Wilgenbus K, Lentner A, Kuckelkorn R, et al. Further evidence that acanthosis nigricans maligna is linked to enhanced secretion by the tumour of transforming growth factor alpha. Arch Dermatol Res 1992;284:266–70.

261. Unal A, Sahin Y, Kelestimur F. Acromegaly with polycystic ovaries, hyperandrogenism, hirsutism, insulin resistance and acanthosis nigricans: a case report. Endocr J 1993;40:207–11.

262. Nobels F, Colemont L, Goethals M, Abs R. Nephrogenic diabetes insipidus: an unusual presentation of recurrent rectal cancer. Cancer 1991;68:2056–2059.

263. Feibusch J, Barbosa-Saldivar JL, Bernstein RS, Robertson GL. Tumor-associated nephrogenic diabetes insipidus. Ann Intern Med 1980;92:797–8.

264. Naschitz JE, Yeshurun D, Abrahamson J, et al. Ischemic heart disease precipitated by occult cancer. Cancer 1992;69:2712–20.

265. Norris SH. Paraneoplastic glomerulopathies. Semin Nephrol 1993;13:258–72.

266. Zech P, Colon S, Pointet P, et al. The nephrotic syndrome in adults aged over 60: etiology, evolution and treatment of 76 cases. Clin Nephrol 1982;17:232–6.

267. Kaplan BS, Klassen J, Gault MH. Glomerular injury in patients with neoplasia. Annu Rev Med 1976;27:117–25.

268. Manchul LA, Jin A, Pritchard KI, et al. The frequency of malignant neoplasms in patients with polymyositis-dermatomyositis: a controlled study. Arch Intern Med 1985;145:1835–9.

269. McCarty GA. Autoantibodies and their relation to rheumatic diseases. Med Clin North Am 1986;70:237–61.

270. Marcus RM, Grayzel AI. A lupus antibody syndrome associated with hypernephroma. Arthritis Rheum 1979;22:1396–8.

271. Salem NB. Lupus antibody syndrome with intestinal lymphoma. Arthritis Rheum 1980;23:613–4.

272. Johnson JJ, Leonard-Segal A, Nashel DJ. Jaccoud's-type arthropathy: an association with malignancy. J Rheumatol 1989;16:1278–80.

273. DeCross AJ, Sahasrabudhe DM. Paraneoplastic Raynaud's phenomenon. Am J Med 1992;92:571–2.

274. Sánchez-Guerrero J, Gutiérrez-Ureña S, Vidaller A, et al. Vasculitis as a paraneoplastic syndrome: report of 11 cases and review of the literature. J Rheumatol 1990;17:1458–62.

275. Sack GH Jr, Levin J, Bell WR. Trousseau's syndrome and other manifestations of chronic disseminated coagulopathy in patients with neoplasms: clinical, pathophysiologic, and therapeutic features. Medicine 1977;56:1–37.

276. Nachman RL, Silverstein R. Hypercoagulable states. Ann Intern Med 1993;119:819–27.

277. Bunn PA Jr, Ridgway EC. Paraneoplastic syndromes. In: DeVita VT, ed. Cancer: principles and practice of oncology. 4th ed. Philadelphia: JB Lippincott, 1993:2026–71.

278. White A, Clark AJ. The cellular and molecular basis of the ectopic ACTH syndrome. Clin Endocrinol 1993;39:131–41.

# CHAPTER 19

---

# GASTROINTESTINAL PROBLEMS

........................................

## NAUSEA AND VOMITING

• Steven M. Grunberg

---

Nausea and vomiting are not the toxicities of chemotherapy most feared by medical professionals. Other toxicities, such as neutropenic fever following the administration of severely myelosuppressive agents or renal failure after nephrotoxic agents, may constitute true oncologic emergencies and be immediately life-threatening. Although dehydration, electrolyte imbalance, and Mallory-Weiss tears of the esophagus may result from vomiting, the more common sequelae for patients experiencing nausea and vomiting caused by insufficient antiemetic protection are emotional distress and decreased quality of life. Toxicities such as neutropenia or renal insufficiency may develop and resolve without symptomatic manifestations. Nausea and vomiting are immediately apparent. It is therefore not surprising that nausea and vomiting have been identified as the toxicities of chemotherapy most feared by the patient.[1]

## Mechanisms of Emesis

To understand chemotherapy-induced nausea and vomiting, it is necessary to understand the vomiting process. It is not a pathologic process but rather a physiologic process in which the body attempts to rid itself of toxic substances. This reaction is controlled by a reflex arc with multiple afferent limbs, a coordinating area (vomiting center), and multiple efferent pathways that activate and coordinate the muscle groups necessary for a successful vomiting response. The afferent limbs include (1) the chemoreceptor trigger zone (CTZ) pathway, in which substances released into the cerebrospinal fluid activate the CTZ; (2) the peripheral pathway, initiated by relevant neurotransmitter receptors found in the gut wall that send messages to the vomiting center by way of the vagus nerve; (3) the cerebrocortical pathway, which is activated by learned associations; and (4) the vestibular pathway, in which changes in position (motion sickness) lead to activation of the vomiting center. The various components of this reflex arc communicate by way of neurotransmitters and neurotransmitter receptors; the goal of antiemetic therapy has therefore been to identify the relevant neurotransmitter receptors in the emetic pathway and to attempt to disrupt their function.

The major determinant of the emetic potential of a chemotherapeutic regimen is the intrinsic emetogenicity of the chemotherapeutic agents themselves (Table 19-1). These agents may be classified as those that will virtually always cause vomiting if given without antiemetics (e.g., high-dose cisplatin) to those with virtually no intrinsic emetogenicity (e.g., vincristine, bleomycin).[3] Emetogenicity can be further increased through the use of combination chemotherapy, which requires estimation of the additive or synergistic effects of multiple agents.[3] However, emetic potential can then be modified by numerous additional factors (Table 19-2). Regarding the chemotherapeutic agents themselves, emetogenicity is affected by dose and schedule. In terms of patient characteristics, a high-risk profile for chemotherapy-induced emesis can be developed that includes age (younger), gender (female), and lack of a history of heavy alcohol use. Preconceptions of the incidence and severity of chemotherapy-induced emesis (based largely on reports of the experience of patients before modern antiemetics were developed) may also have an adverse effect and should be proactively combated with careful patient education prior to the initiation of chemotherapy.

## History of Antiemetic Development

Modern antiemetic practice began with randomized trials in the early 1960s that demonstrated that standard-dose phenothiazines were effective antiemetics for the prevention of chemotherapy-induced nausea and vomiting.[4] However, these trials were performed with 5-fluorouracil (5-FU), a mildly emetogenic chemotherapeutic agent, as the challenge agent. As moderately emetogenic agents (anthracyclines) and severely emetogenic agents (cisplatin) were developed, standard-dose phenothiazines proved inadequate. The substituted benzamide metoclopramide had the theoretical advantage of being both a dopamine ($D_2$) receptor antagonist like the phenothiazines and a prokinetic agent. Early antiemetic trials of metoclopramide were unsuccessful. However, escalation of the metoclopramide dose to a total of 10 mg/kg resulted in significant antiemetic protection, even against high-dose cisplatin.[5] This antiemetic protection could be further improved through the simultaneous administration of a corticosteroid such as dexamethasone.[6] However, high-dose metoclopramide could produce significant antidopaminergic toxicity as well,[7] and concomitant use of an antihistamine and a benzodiazepine to counteract this toxicity was often necessary. It was soon appreciated that high-dose metoclopramide functioned both as a $D_2$-receptor antagonist and as a serotonin (5-hydroxytryptamine-3 [5-HT$_3$]) receptor antagonist[8] and that much of the antiemetic effect resided in the 5-HT$_3$ antagonist properties. Thus it became possible to

*Table 19–1.* **Emetogenic Potential of Single Chemotherapeutic Agents**

| Level 1 | Level 2 | Level 3 | Level 4 | Level 5 |
|---|---|---|---|---|
| FREQUENCY OF EMESIS <10% | FREQUENCY OF EMESIS 10–30% | FREQUENCY OF EMESIS 30–60% | FREQUENCY OF EMESIS 60–90% | FREQUENCY OF EMESIS >90% |
| Bleomycin | Docetaxel | Cyclophosphamide $\leq$750 mg/m$^2$ | Carboplatin | Carmustine >250 mg/m$^2$ |
| Busulfan | Etoposide | Cyclophosphamide (oral) | Carmustine $\leq$250 mg/m$^2$ | Cisplatin $\geq$59 mg/m$^2$ |
| Chlorambucil (oral) | 5-Fluorouracil <1000 mg/m$^2$ | Doxorubicin 20–60 mg/m$^2$ | Cisplatin <50 mg/m$^2$ | Cyclophosphamide >1500 mg/m$^2$ |
| 2-Chlorodeoxyadenosine | Gemcitabine | Epirubicin $\leq$90 mg/m$^2$ | Cyclophosphamide | Dacarbazine |
| Fludarabine | Methotrexate | Hexamethylmelamine (oral) | >750 mg/m$^2$ $\leq$1500 mg/m$^2$ | Mechlorethamine |
| Hydroxyurea | >50 mg/m$^2$ <250 mg/m$^2$ | Idarubicin | Cytarabine >1 g/m$^2$ | Streptozocin |
| Methotrexate $\leq$50 mg/m$^2$ | Mitomycin | Ifosfamide | Doxorubicin >60 mg/m$^2$ | |
| L-Phenylalanine mustard (oral) | Paclitaxel | Methotrexate | Methotrexate >1000 mg/m$^2$ | |
| Thioguanine (oral) | | 250–1000 mg/m$^2$ | Procarbazine (oral) | |
| Vinblastine | | Mitoxantrone <15 mg/m$^2$ | | |
| Vincristine | | | | |
| Vinorelbine | | | | |

Adapted from Hesketh PJ, Kris MG, Grunberg SM, et al. Proposal for classifying the acute emetogenicity of chemotherapy. J Clin Oncol 1997;15:103–9.

*Table 19–2.* **Factors Affecting Emetogenicity of Chemotherapeutic Agents**

| Factor | Increased Emetogenicity |
| --- | --- |
| Dose of drug | Higher |
| Duration of infusion | Shorter |
| Age | Younger |
| Gender | Female |
| Heavy alcohol use | None |

separate antiemetic efficacy from antidopaminergic toxicity through the development of specific 5-HT$_3$ antagonists. The present generation of 5-HT$_3$ antagonists that are commercially available in the United States (ondansetron, granisetron, and dolasetron) is the result of this effort, and these agents provide excellent antiemetic protection without antidopaminergic toxicity.[9–11] This antiemetic protection is further enhanced through the concomitant use of corticosteroids.[12]

At present, the "gold standard" for acute antiemetic protection against highly or moderately emetogenic chemotherapeutic agents is a combination of a 5-HT$_3$ antagonist and a corticosteroid.[12, 13] A 5-HT$_3$ antagonist, a corticosteroid, or an antidopaminergic agent (such as a phenothiazine) may be sufficient for mildly emetogenic chemotherapeutic agents. Although the 5-HT$_3$ antagonists differ in potency and in serum half-life, schedule of administration does not appear to be an important consideration. A single adequate dose of one of these agents administered prior to chemotherapy provides maximal antiemetic protection equivalent to that obtained by divided doses[14] or by a 24-hour infusion.[15] Route of administration is also not a key issue because oral (tablet or syrup) and intravenous preparations at full dose appear to have equivalent efficacy.[16, 17] The important consideration is administration of a full dose of appropriate antiemetics prior to the emetogenic challenge.

There has been controversy concerning the determination of "full dose" for intravenous 5-HT$_3$ antagonists and for dexamethasone. Approved doses in Europe and in the United States for ondansetron range from 8 mg to 32 mg, whereas doses for granisetron range from 10 µg/kg to 3 mg. These discrepancies may be explained by the relatively flat dose-response curve[18] and excellent toxicity profile of 5-HT$_3$ antagonists once a threshold dose has been surpassed. Although any dose greater than the threshold will be effective, the optimal dose would be the minimal dose in this range. An international consensus conference[19] recommended the following intravenous doses: ondansetron, 8 mg; granisetron, 10 µg/kg; or dolasetron, 1.8 mg/kg. Recommended oral doses are approximately twice as high. The recommended intravenous dose for dexamethasone is 20 mg.[20]

## Families of Antiemetics

Antiemetic agents may be classified by their site of action and by their chemical family.[21] The anticholinergic agents (e.g., scopolamine) can cause sedation and dry mouth. These agents are of little use against chemotherapy-induced emesis but are effective against motion sickness. The antidopamin-

ergic agents include the phenothiazines (prochlorperazine, chlorpromazine, thiethylperazine, perphenazine, and promethazine), the butyrophenones (droperidol, haloperidol, and domperidone), and the substituted benzamides (metoclopramide, trimethobenzamide, alizapride, and cisapride). Potential toxicities of these agents include extrapyramidal reactions, sedation, hypotension, anxiety, and depression. Standard-dose phenothiazines can be effective antiemetics against mildly or moderately emetogenic chemotherapeutic agents. Butyrophenones have a cost-benefit ratio somewhat lower than the phenothiazines and therefore have little practical role in this area. All these agents have increased efficacy with dose escalation.[5, 22, 23] The best studied of these agents at high dose is metoclopramide, which has antiserotonergic as well as antidopaminergic activity and can have excellent antiemetic efficacy. The antiserotonergic (5-HT$_3$) agents (ondansetron, granisetron, dolasetron) maintain antiemetic efficacy better than high-dose metoclopramide without severe toxicity.[24] The toxicities of the antiserotonergic agents include mild headache, lightheadedness, diarrhea, and occasional elevation of transaminase levels.[9]

Other families of antiemetic agents include the benzodiazepines, corticosteroids, and cannabinoids. The benzodiazepines (lorazepam, alprazolam, diazepam) are sedatives and anxiolytic agents that have little intrinsic antiemetic effect but may be valuable in decreasing the anxiety associated with the chemotherapy experience and in blunting the learned response of anticipatory vomiting.[25] The mechanism of action of the corticosteroids is unknown. Corticosteroids may aggravate diabetes and exacerbate underlying psychiatric conditions, but the side effects in most patients are mild.[26] Corticosteroids (dexamethasone, methylprednisolone) are moderately effective single-agent antiemetics and potentiate the antiemetic activity of virtually all other classes of antiemetic agents. Cannabinoids (dronabinol, nabilone) are also moderately effective antiemetics but have a relatively severe toxicity profile that includes dysphoria, hallucinations, sedation, dizziness, and disorientation.[27] The dysphoria of cannabinoids can be blocked through the administration of a low-dose phenothiazine.[28] Because of the poor cost-benefit ratio and the regulatory burden of prescription, however, cannabinoids are usually used only if other standard agents have failed to achieve antiemetic control.

## Delayed and Anticipatory Emesis

The preceding discussion concentrated on the management of acute vomiting—the vomiting seen within 24 hours of the administration of chemotherapy. Although this is historically the most intense period of nausea and vomiting in the patient who does not receive adequate antiemetic therapy, emesis both before chemotherapy (anticipatory vomiting) and extending for several days after chemotherapy (delayed vomiting) can also be disruptive and require additional medical care. These forms of vomiting have different mechanisms of action and require different remedies. Anticipatory vomiting can best be described as a learned response conditioned by a previous experience of vomiting with chemotherapy.[29] Anticipatory vomiting could thus appear at any time in the treatment cycle if the appropriate stimulus appears. Classic anticipatory vomiting appears before the administration of chemotherapy on a second or later treatment cycle and thus cannot be confused with a direct effect of the chemotherapy itself. Both anxiolytics[30] and behavioral modification techniques[31] have been used with some success against anticipatory vomiting. However, the best method of prevention is avoidance of the initial uncontrolled stimulus. Thus the best prevention for anticipatory vomiting is effective and aggressive use of antiemetics from the initiation of chemotherapy. Delayed vomiting is a physical result of chemotherapy and appears 2 days or more after the administration of cisplatin or some moderately emetogenic agents (such as cyclophosphamide or the anthracyclines).[32] However, the mechanism of delayed vomiting is different from that of acute vomiting, as evidenced by the relative lack of control gained with standard antiemetics. Corticosteroids appear to be the most effective single agents for delayed vomiting and may provide protection for about 20% of patients. Although single-agent metoclopramide has only a minor effect, a combined 4-day regimen of metoclopramide and corticosteroid was more effective for the prevention of delayed vomiting than corticosteroid alone.[33] Oral ondansetron has been found to be equivalent in efficacy to oral metoclopramide in this setting.[34] An exciting area of current research is the use of NK-1 receptor antagonists (for which the natural ligand is substance P).[35] These agents have only a minor effect on acute vomiting but appear to be more effective in preventing delayed vomiting than any other agents described to date.[36, 37] Large-scale randomized trials will be necessary to confirm these promising results.

## Future Challenges

The history of rational antiemetic therapy has been based on the sequential discovery of significant neurotransmitters and neurotransmitter receptors. The recent description of the NK-1 receptor antagonists emphasizes that this process is not yet complete. However, additional areas of antiemetic theory and practice still need to be explored. Cancer anorexia is similar in presentation to chemotherapy-induced nausea and may provide fertile ground for comparison of effective remedies and the development of a common theoretical base. It should also be noted that several of the receptors that are important in chemotherapy-induced emesis have a significant role in pathways of pain and analgesia, suggesting a unified model for several areas of supportive care. Investigation of this overlap may provide improved understanding and more effective agents for both antiemesis and analgesia. Major strides have been made in the control of chemotherapy-induced emesis, but the results are not yet perfect. More accurate models and more effective agents for control of emesis can only improve the quality of life of our patients and make chemotherapy more tolerable.

## REFERENCES

1. Coates A, Abraham S, Kaye SB, et al. On the receiving end—patient perception of the side effects of cancer chemotherapy. Eur J Cancer Clin Oncol 1983;19:203–8.
2. Seigel LJ, Longo DL. The control of chemotherapy-induced emesis. Ann Intern Med 1981;95:352–9.
3. Hesketh PJ, Kris MG, Grunberg SM, et al. Proposal for classifying the acute emetogenicity of cancer chemotherapy. J Clin Oncol 1997;15:103–9.
4. Moertel CG, Reitemeier RJ, Gage RP. A controlled clinical evaluation of antiemetic drugs. JAMA 1963;186:116–8.
5. Gralla RJ, Itri LM, Pisko SE, et al. Antiemetic efficacy of high-dose metoclopramide: randomized trials with placebo and prochlorperazine in patients with chemotherapy-induced nausea and vomiting. N Engl J Med 1981;305:905–9.
6. Allan SG, Cornbleet MA, Warrington PS, et al. Dexamethasone and high-dose metoclopramide: efficacy in controlling cisplatin induced nausea and vomiting. Br Med J 1984;289:878–9.
7. Tortorice PV, O'Connell MB. Management of chemotherapy-induced nausea and vomiting. Pharmacotherapy 1990;10:129–45.
8. Fozard JR, Mobarok Ali AT. Blockage of neuronal tryptamine receptors by metoclopramide. Eur J Pharmacol 1978;49:109–12.
9. Grunberg SM, Stevenson LL, Russell CA, McDermed JE. Dose-ranging phase I study of the serotonin antagonist GR 38032F for prevention of cisplatin-induced nausea and vomiting. J Clin Oncol 1989;7:1137–41.
10. Navari RM, Kaplan HG, Gralla RJ, et al. Efficacy and safety of granisetron, a selective 5-hydroxytryptamine-3 receptor antagonist, in the prevention of nausea and vomiting induced by high-dose cisplatin. J Clin Oncol 1994;12:2204–10.
11. Kris MG, Grunberg SM, Gralla RJ, et al. Dose-ranging evaluation of the serotonin antagonist dolasetron mesylate in patients receiving high-dose cisplatin. J Clin Oncol 1994;12:1045–9.
12. Roila F, Tonato M, Cognetti F, et al. Prevention of cisplatin-induced emesis: a double-blind multicenter randomized crossover study comparing ondansetron and ondansetron plus dexamethasone. J Clin Oncol 1991;9:675–8.
13. Italian Group for Antiemetic Research. Dexamethasone, granisetron, or both for the prevention of nausea and vomiting during chemotherapy for cancer. N Engl J Med 1995;332:1–5.
14. Beck TM, Hesketh PJ, Madajewicz S, et al. Stratified, randomized, double-blind comparison of intravenous ondansetron administered as a multiple-dose regimen versus two single-dose regimens in the prevention of cisplatin-induced nausea and vomiting. J Clin Oncol 1991;10:1969–75.
15. Marty M, d'Allens H, Groupe Multicentrique Français. Etude randomisée en double-insu comparant l'efficacité de l'ondansetron selon deux modes d'administration: injection unique et perfusion continue. Cah Cancer 1990;2:541–6
16. Perez EA, Hesketh P, Sandbach J, et al. Comparison of single-dose oral granisetron versus intravenous ondansetron in the prevention of nausea and vomiting induced by moderately emetogenic chemotherapy: a multicenter, double-blind, randomized parallel study. J Clin Oncol 1998;16:754–60.
17. White L, McKenna CJ, Zhestkova N, et al. A comparison of oral ondansetron syrup and intravenous ondansetron regimens given in combination with oral dexamethasone for the prevention of emesis and nausea in paediatric patients receiving moderately/highly emetogenic chemotherapy. Proc Am Soc Clin Oncol 1998;17:50a. abstract.
18. Grunberg SM. Antiemetic drugs: essential pharmacology. In: Tonato M, ed. Antiemetics in the supportive care of cancer patients. Berlin: Springer, 1996:25–33.
19. Gandara DR, Roila F, Warr D, et al. Consensus proposal for 5HT₃ antagonists in the prevention of acute emesis related to highly emetogenic chemotherapy: dose, schedule, and route of administration. Support Care Cancer 1998;6:237–43.
20. Italian Group for Antiemetic Research. Double-blind, dose-finding study of four intravenous doses of dexamethasone in the prevention of cisplatin-induced acute emesis. J Clin Oncol 1998;16:2937–42.
21. Grunberg SM, Hesketh PJ. Control of chemotherapy-induced emesis. N Engl J Med 1993;329:1790–6.
22. Carr BI, Blayney DW, Goldberg DA, et al. High doses of prochlorperazine for cisplatin-induced emesis: a prospective, random, dose-response study. Cancer 1987;60:2165–9.
23. Grunberg SM, Gala KV, Lampenfield M, et al. Comparison of the antiemetic effect of high-dose intravenous metoclopramide and high-dose intravenous haloperidol in a randomized double-blind crossover study. J Clin Oncol 1984;2:782–7.
24. Hesketh PJ. Comparative trials of ondansetron versus metoclopramide

in the prevention of acute cisplatin-induced emesis. Semin Oncol 1992;19(4 Suppl 10):33–40.

25. Greenberg DB, Surman OS, Clarke J, Baer L. Alprazolam for phobic nausea and vomiting related to cancer chemotherapy. Cancer Treat Rep 1987;71:549–60.
26. Herrstedt J, Aapro MS, Smyth JF, Del Favero A. Corticosteroids, dopamine antagonists, and other drugs. Support Care Cancer 1998;6:204–14.
27. Tyson LB, Gralla RJ, Clark RA, et al. Phase I trial of levonantradol in chemotherapy-induced emesis. Am J Clin Oncol 1985;8:528–32.
28. Cunningham D, Forrest GJ, Soukop M, et al. Nabilone and prochlorperazine: a useful combination for emesis induced by cytotoxic drugs. Br Med J 1985;291:864–5.
29. Morrow GR, Rosco JA, Kirshner JJ, et al. Anticipatory nausea and vomiting in the era of 5-HT$_3$ antiemetics. Support Care Cancer 1998;6:244–7.
30. Razavi D, Delvaux N, Farvacques C, et al. Prevention of adjustment disorders and anticipatory nausea secondary to adjuvant chemotherapy: a double-blind, placebo-controlled study assessing the usefulness of alprazolam. J Clin Oncol 1993;11:1384–90.
31. Morrow GR, Morrell C. Behavioral treatment for the anticipatory

nausea and vomiting induced by cancer chemotherapy. N Engl J Med 1982;307:1476–80.
32. Kris MG, Gralla RJ, Clark RA, et al. Incidence, course, and severity of delayed nausea and vomiting following the administration of high-dose cisplatin. J Clin Oncol 1985;3:1379–84.
33. Kris MG, Gralla RJ, Tyson LB, et al. Controlling delayed vomiting: double-blind randomized trial comparing placebo, dexamethasone alone, and metoclopramide plus dexamethasone in patients receiving cisplatin. J Clin Oncol 1989;7:108–14.
34. Italian Group for Antiemetic Research. Ondansetron versus metoclopramide, both combined with dexamethasone, in the prevention of cisplatin-induced delayed emesis. J Clin Oncol 1997;15:124–30.
35. Rudd JA, Jordan CC, Naylor RJ. The action of the tachykinin 1 receptor antagonist, CP 99,994, in antagonizing the acute and delayed emesis induced by cisplatin in the ferret. Br J Pharmacol 1996;119:931–6.
36. Navari R, Reinhardt RR, Gralla RJ, et al. Reduction of cisplatin-induced emesis by a selective neurokinin-1-receptor antagonist. L-754,030 Antiemetic Trials Group. N Engl J Med 1999;340:190–5.
37. Hesketh PJ, Gralla RJ, Webb RT, et al. Randomized phase II study of the neurokinin-1 antagonist CJ-11,974 in the control of cisplatin-induced emesis. J Clin Oncol 1999;17:338–43.

# STOMATITIS

• John Barstis

No complication of cancer treatment is more acutely distressing than stomatitis. The oral cavity, normally a delicately balanced and exquisitely sensitive portal, can become a site of extreme discomfort. Stomatitis, or oral mucositis, is defined as the inflammation of the oral mucous membranes. Such inflammation affects one's sense of taste and smell, as well as nutrition and hydration, and may well reduce the ability to take oral medications. When severe, stomatitis may necessitate parenteral care. Furthermore, the compromised mucosa can act as a portal for the systemic entry of infectious pathogens. The monetary costs are illustrated by an M.D. Anderson Cancer Center study of this problem. Patients with mucositis stayed in hospital 3 to 6 days longer and experienced fever 2 to 4 days longer than did patients without mucositis.[1]

## Pathophysiology

The mucosal layer serves multiple functions, providing a physical and chemical barrier for the epithelium below it. In symbiosis with normal flora, it acts to limit and remove potential pathogens. Normal oral mucosa turns over approximately every 5 to 16 days.[2]

Chemotherapy and radiation therapy can damage the mucosal layer and dramatically slow its return to normal function. Pre-existing oral pathologic conditions then become important. The American Dental Association estimates that 70% of Americans have some form of gum disease by age 18. Caries, periodontal disease, and occlusal pathologic conditions are the most frequent sources of oral pathogens.[3] Loss of the intact mucosal layer leads to exposure of underlying connective tissue stroma and its nervous innervation, causing pain. In a patient who otherwise has normal immune function, stomatotoxicity from chemotherapy or radiation

therapy can form lesions 5 to 7 days after the start of treatment that heal fully in 2 to 3 weeks. The first finding is asymptomatic erythema. Raised, discrete, slightly painful white patches appear next, followed by larger, often confluent ulcers with pseudomembranes. The ulcers are acutely painful; when present in the posterior pharynx, they cause dysphagia, which, in turn, compromises nutrition and further delays regeneration of the healthy mucosal layer.[4, 5]

Stomatitis can occur after most types of chemotherapy but is a frequent side effect with certain agents and creates a dose-limiting toxicity with a few agents. It has been estimated that mucositis occurs in 30 to 40% of patients receiving standard chemotherapy and in up to 90% of patients receiving high-dose chemotherapy or bone marrow transplantation.[6]

The most frequently used chemotherapy protocol that produces dose-limiting stomatitis is 5-FU with leucovorin. In some series, this occurs in as many as 75% of patients. In a report using patient diaries from patients receiving bolus treatment, oral symptoms started by day 4, reached a maximum on days 7 to 11, and began resolving on day 12.[7] It has been reported that women receiving 5-FU–based chemotherapy developed more severe mucositis than did men.[8, 9] Other classes of agents that commonly cause stomatitis include antimetabolites (especially methotrexate), alkylating agents, and anthracyclines (especially doxorubicin).

## Assessment

Many different approaches have tried to characterize stomatitis objectively.[10–12] The National Cancer Institute's common toxicity grading scale is shown in Table 19–3. Individual assessment of patients with oral symptoms should include

*Table 19–3.* **National Cancer Institute Grading of Mucositis***

| Grade | Criteria |
|-------|----------|
| 1 | Painless ulcers, erythema, or mild soreness in the absence of lesions |
| 2 | Painful erythema, edema, or ulcers present, but patient can eat or swallow |
| 3 | Painful erythema, edema or ulcers requiring intravenous hydration |
| 4 | Severe ulceration or patient requires parenteral or enteral nutritional support or prophylactic intubation |

*The criteria for grading mucositis from bone marrow transplantation differ slightly.

grading of the process and looking for thrush, herpes-like lesions, and dental problems.

## Prevention and Treatment

Prior to treatment, a careful dental examination is recommended in chemotherapy patients and is mandatory in head and neck radiotherapy settings. In the latter, attention to oral pathologic conditions by an experienced dental oncologist is the standard of care. Attention to oral hygiene from the beginning of any chemotherapy regimen is important.[4, 13] Surveillance cultures for bacterial and fungal pathogens have not generally proved of value.[14]

The optimal approach to prevention and treatment of stomatitis has not been established. Extensive research exists, but the results are conflicting and inadequate for consensus development. Many studies are not randomized, and those that are generally involve small numbers of patients. Meaningful cross-study comparisons can be almost impossible because of vastly different cancers and cancer treatments, such as 5-FU versus bone marrow transplantation. Different studies of the same agent for stomatitis vary widely in terms of time of initiation, dose, schedule, and combination with other treatments. The nosocomial profile of the study site can also affect findings of infectious aspects of stomatitis. Nonetheless, some useful approaches have been devised.

Most institutions have individualized prevention and treatment approaches that are empirically derived. Goals of intervention include elimination of pathogens, gentle removal of adherent mucous and pseudomembranes, protective coating of sensitive tissues, and elimination of pain. Rinses with saline, ice, dilute hydrogen peroxide, sodium bicarbonate, and chlorhexidine have frequently been employed for disinfecting and debriding. Over-the-counter antacids (e.g., Maalox, Mylanta), sucralfate, or diphenhydramine are the most commonly used coating agents.[15] Viscous lidocaine is the most widely used topical anesthetic. Its use before meals can allow better intake when severe dysphagia is present.[5] Because it will deaden sensation of the tongue on contact, swabbing or focused application is preferable to many patients. Mixtures or "cocktails" of these agents can provide significant subjective benefit to patients, although there are no data to confirm any approach as uniformly superior. The optimal method may be to start with a protocol but be sensitive to patient preference and substitute empirically.

Studies to assess the value of elimination of oral microbes have most often used chlorhexidine, a potent disinfectant formulated for oral use. Although it can measurably decrease oral bacterial counts and has demonstrated an ability to remove some bacterial pathogens, most investigators have found no decrease in mucositis.[16, 17] In some cases, chlorhexidine has caused an increase in oral discomfort.[18, 19] Some trials using antibiotic mouthwashes or lozenges for this purpose have shown clinical benefit. As with disinfectants, the use of oral antibiotics, while diminishing bacterial counts, does not reliably decrease mucositis.[20, 21] Evidence exists that prophylactic use of nystatin is not effective[5, 17] and is locally irritating in some patients. The widely accepted effectiveness of fluconazole for systemic prophylaxis has provided an alternative in prolonged neutropenia. In less immunocompromised settings, a high degree of suspicion and early therapeutic intervention can be the best strategy. The use of acyclovir for prevention of herpes morbidity is accepted in the highest risk persons, those with a clinical history of the infection, or those undergoing very aggressive therapy.[22] Such therapy is discussed further on.

Cryotherapy (oral cooling with ice) has been reported to be beneficial for patients receiving 5-FU–containing regimens, especially 5-FU and leucovorin.[23, 24] Such an approach has been routinely used at the Mayo Clinic; patients who received a bolus dose of 5-FU and leucovorin removed their dentures, if present, placed ice chips in their mouths 5 minutes before treatment, and replenished them continuously for 30 minutes. No significant benefit was derived with a longer duration of cooling.[25] Cryotherapy has not been widely reported with other chemotherapy agents and is clearly not feasible with infusion therapy.

As discussed, bonding or coating agents have been widely employed for their subjective benefit. They have received extensive study for objective effectiveness as well. Sucralfate is the most widely investigated. It is designed to aid the healing of peptic ulcers and appears to work primarily by forming an ionic bond with local proteins, thus creating a barrier to harmful substances. Studies have used sucralfate prophylactically with radiotherapy or chemotherapy. Results are at best conflicting regarding its ability to decrease the incidence or severity of stomatitis.[26-28] They do, however, often confirm its ability to reduce the pain from this condition.[29]

The relationship of neutropenia to stomatitis has received much attention. Researchers have shown that oral tissue neutrophils repopulate sooner than do circulatory neutrophils and that growth factors enhance both.[30] The literature includes reports about the prophylactic or therapeutic use of colony-stimulating factors, either in the form of granulocyte colony-stimulating factor (G-CSF) or granulocyte-macrophage colony-stimulating factor (GM-CSF). Both grade and duration of mucositis have been diminished in some, but not all, studies. Many small pilot trials have used these agents subcutaneously, and others have used a dilute G-CSF mouthwash.[31-34] Interventions with other biologic and immune substances have been reported, but the size of the studies was too small to allow conclusions. These interventions included subcutaneous and oral administration of immunoglobulin[35] and transforming growth factor-$\beta_3$.[36, 37]

Other miscellaneous agents have been studied. Allopurinol has been tested as a mouthwash in patients receiving 5-

FU regimens. Results have been conflicting, including a negative outcome in a randomized trial by the North Central Treatment Group. All patients treated by this group received cryotherapy; those in other studies did not.[38, 39] The rationale for using allopurinol is that by inhibiting the enzyme orotidylate decarboxylase and decreasing the metabolites fluorodeoxyuridylate and fluorouridine, local toxicity will be diminished. Decreased pain and healing time have been reported in preliminary studies of dinoprostone or prostaglandin $E_2$; however, the mechanism is not understood.[40] Capsaicin, the active ingredient in chili peppers, has been studied and found effective in nonmalignant pain syndromes. Another study has reported decreased oral pain of stomatitis in cancer patients.[41] Existing studies on the use of vitamins and antioxidants in this setting are limited and generally fail to show benefit, although in one randomized study with 18 patients, vitamin E provided benefit.[42]

Special attention to mucositis is a standard part of the regimen in any type of bone marrow transplant or high-dose chemotherapy setting. Prolonged neutropenia increases the risk of oral infections, which may be difficult to distinguish visually from purely inflammatory processes. This risk is modified to a variable degree by various prophylactic measures for systemic infection, including attempted oral and gut sterilization and systemic antibiotics. The most frequent viral infections are herpes simplex, varicella zoster, and cytomegalovirus.[43–45] Routine prophylaxis for herpes simplex is used in seropositive patients. In a study by Schubert and colleagues, herpes simplex virus infection occurred in 37% of 627 allogeneic bone marrow transplant recipients. Of the 233 patients with infection, 231 were seropositive before transplantation.[45] A novel approach in high-dose treatment with etoposide is the use of the anticholinergic propantheline to induce xerostomia because etoposide is extensively secreted into the saliva. Local concentrations of chemotherapeutic agents and toxicity are then minimized.[46] However, large trials have not yet been performed.

---

*Table 19–4.* **Management of Stomatitis**

*Expectant Management in High-Risk Settings*

Pretreatment dental evaluation and treatment of oral pathologic conditions
Dilute hydrogen peroxide gargle; disinfectants optional (unproven benefits)
Consider cryotherapy with ice for bolus 5-FU therapy (see text)
Prophylaxis with acyclovir for patients who are seropositive for herpes simplex virus
Prophylaxis with fluconazole for *Candida* species in severe or prolonged cases

*Treatment Options for Symptomatic Process*

Mixtures to be used empirically, then guided by patient preference:
   Coating agents: sucralfate, antacids, sodium bicarbonate
   Disinfectants: dilute hydrogen peroxide, chlorhexidine
   Anesthetics agents: viscous lidocaine, diphenhydramine
Trial of capsaicin for topical analgesic effect
Neutrophil growth factors if severe neutropenia persists
Systemic treatment for infectious components
   Acyclovir for herpes simplex virus
   Fluconazole, clotrimazole (Mycelex) troches, or nystatin for *Candida* species

5-FU, 5-fluorouracil.

---

## Summary of Treatment

This section has outlined a variety of measures that can be used for the anticipation, prevention, assessment, and management of stomatitis. Table 19–3 provides the National Cancer Institute system for grading mucositis. Table 19–4 provides a summary of measures to consider in the expectant management of stomatitis in high-risk settings as well as treatment options for established, symptomatic stomatitis.

### SUGGESTIONS FOR ADDITIONAL READING

Berger AM, Kilroy TJ. Oral complications of cancer therapy. In: Berger AM, Portenoy AK, Weissman DE, eds. Principles and practice of supportive oncology. Philadelphia: Lippincott-Raven, 1998:223–36.
Peterson DE, Schubert MM. Oral toxicity. In: Perry MC, ed. The chemotherapy source book. Baltimore: Williams & Wilkins, 1997:571–94.

### REFERENCES

1. Manzullo E, Chambers M, Tooth B, et al. Outcomes and resource utilization in cancer patients with oral and gastrointestinal complications of chemotherapy. Proc Am Soc Clin Oncol 1998;17:416a. abstract.
2. Peterson DE, Schubert MM: Oral toxicity. In: Perry MC, ed. The chemotherapy source book. 2nd ed. Baltimore: Williams & Wilkins; 1997:571.
3. Poland J. Prevention and treatment of oral complications in the cancer patient. Oncology 1991;5:45–50.
4. Berger AM, Kilroy TJ. Oral complications of cancer therapy. In: Berger AM, Portenoy RK, Weissman DE, eds. Principles and practice of oncology. Philadelphia: Lippincott-Raven, 1998:223–30.
5. Sonis ST, Haley JD. Pharmacologic attenuation of chemotherapy-induced oral mucositis. Exp Opin Invest Drugs 1996;5:1155–62.
6. Dodd MJ, Facione NC, Dibble SL, et al. Comparison of methods to determine the prevalence and nature of oral mucositis. Cancer Pract 1996;4:312–8.
7. Meropol GH, Clamon JR, Lu ZJ, et al. Measuring the impact of mucositis on quality of life. Proc Am Soc Clin Oncol 1997;16:77a.
8. Zalcberg J, Cunningham D, Rath U, et al. Modulated 5FU: female gender and increasing age are associated with significantly more grade 3 or 4 leukopenia and mucositis. Proc Am Soc Clin Oncol 1996;15:201.
9. Weinerman B, Rayner H, Venne A, et al. Increased incidence and severity of stomatitis in women treated with 5-fluorouracil and leucovorin. Proc Am Soc Clin Oncol 1998;17:305a.
10. Sonis ST, Costello KA: A database for mucositis induced by cancer chemotherapy. Eur J Cancer B Oral Oncol 1995;31B:258–60.
11. Tardieu C, Cowen D, Thirion X, et al. Quantitative scale of oral mucositis associated with bone marrow transplantation. Eur J Cancer B 1996;32B:381–7.
12. Schubert MM, Williams BE, Lliod ME, et al. Clinical assessment scale for the rating of oral mucosal changes associated with bone marrow transplantation: development of an oral mucosal index. Cancer 1992;69:2469–77.
13. Consensus Conference. Oral complications of cancer therapies: diagnosis, prevention and treatment. Conn Med 1989;53:595.
14. Feld R. The role of surveillance cultures in patients likely to develop chemotherapy-induced mucositis. Support Care Cancer 1997;5:371–5.
15. Berger AM, Kilroy TJ: Oral complications. In: DeVita VT, Hellman S, Rosenberg SH, eds. Cancer: principles and practice of oncology. Philadelphia: Lippincott-Raven, 1997:2714–25.
16. Epstein JB, Vickars L, Spinelli J, et al. Efficacy of chlorhexidine and nystatin rinses in prevention of oral complications in leukemia and bone marrow transplantation. Oral Surg Oral Med Oral Pathol 1992;73:682–9.
17. Ferretti GA, Raybould TP, Brown AT, et al. Chlorhexidine prophylaxis for chemotherapy- and radiotherapy-induced stomatitis: a randomized double-blind trial. Oral Surg Oral Med Oral Pathol 1990;69:331–8.
18. Foote RL, Loprinzi CL, Frank AR, et al. Randomized trial of a chlorhexidine mouthwash for alleviation of radiation-induced mucositis. J Clin Oncol 1994;12:2630–3.

19. Wahlin YB. Effects of chlorhexidine mouth rinse on oral health in patients with acute leukemia. Oral Surg Oral Med Oral Pathol 1989;68:279–87.

20. Symonds RP, McIlroy P, Khorrami J, et al. The reduction of radiation mucositis by selective decontamination antibiotic pastilles: a placebo-controlled double-blind trial. Br J Cancer 1996;74:312–7.

21. Bondi E, Baroni C, Prete A, et al. Local antimicrobial therapy of oral mucositis in paediatric patients undergoing bone marrow transplantation. Oral Oncol 1997;33:322–6.

22. Ahmed T, Engelking C, Szalyga J, et al. Propantheline prevention of mucositis from etoposide. Bone Marrow Transplant 1993;12:131–2.

23. Mahood DJ, Dose AM, Loprinzi AL, et al. Inhibition of fluorouracil-induced stomatitis by oral cryotherapy. J Clin Oncol 1991;9:449–52.

24. Stefano C, Fedeli A, Fedeli LF, et al. Oral cooling (cryotherapy): an effective treatment for the prevention of 5-fluorouracil–induced stomatitis. Oral Oncol Eur J Cancer B 1994;30B:234–6.

25. Rocke LK, Loprinzi CL, Lee JK, et al. A randomized clinical trial of two different durations of oral cryotherapy for prevention of 5-fluorouracil–related stomatitis. Cancer 1993;72:2234–8.

26. Loprinzi CL, Ghosh C, Camoriano J, et al. Phase III–controlled evaluation of sucralfate to alleviate stomatitis in patients receiving fluorouracil-based chemotherapy. J Clin Oncol 1997;15:1235–8.

27. Makkonen TA, Bostrom P, Vilja P, et al. Sucralfate mouth washing in the prevention of radiation-induced mucositis: a placebo-controlled double-blind randomized study. Int J Radiat Oncol 1994;30:177–82.

28. Allison R. Salagen, carafate elixir, and diflucan elixir minimizes mucositis. Proc Am Soc Clin Oncol 1998;17:52a.

29. Epstein JB, Wong FLW. The efficacy of sucralfate suspension in the prevention of oral mucositis due to radiation therapy. Int J Rad Oncol Biol Phys 1994;28:693–8.

30. Graham JL, Ramenghi U, O'Connor MP, at al: Studies of oral neutrophil levels in patients receiving G-CSF after autologous marrow transplantation. Br J Haematol 1992;82:589–95.

31. Chi KH, Chen CH, Chan WK, et al. Effect of granulcyte-macrophage colony-stimulating factor on oral mucositis in head and neck cancer patients after cisplatin, fluorouracil, and leucovorin chemotherapy. J Clin Oncol 1995;13:2620–8.

32. Iwase M, Yoshiwa M, Kakuta S, et al. Clinical trial of recombinant colony-stimulating factor for chemotherapy-induced neutropenia patients with oral cancer. J Oral Maxillofac Surg 1997;58:836–40.

33. Karthaus M, Rosenthal C, Paul H, et al. Effect of topical oral G-CSF application on oral mucositis in high-grade lymphoma patients treated with HD-methotrexate—results of a randomized placebo-controlled trial. Proc Am Soc Clin Oncol 1998;17:61a.

34. Ibrahim EM, al-Muhim FA. Effect of granulocyte-macrophage colony-stimulating factor on chemotherapy-induced oral mucositis in non-neutropenic cancer patients. Med Oncol 1997;14:47–51.

35. Mose S, Adamietz IA, Saran F, et al. Can prophylactic application of immunoglobulin decrease radiotherapy-induced oral mucositis? Am J Clin Oncol 1997;20:407–11.

36. Sonis ST, Van Vugt AG, Brien JP, et al. Transforming growth factor-beta$_3$–mediated modulation of cell cycling and attenuation of 5-fluorouracil–induced oral mucositis. Oral Oncol 1997;33:47–54.

37. Wymenga ANM, van der Graaf WT, Hofstra LF, et al. Phase I study of CGP-46614 (TGF-β$_3$) mouthwash as prevention for chemotherapy-induced mucositis. Proc Am Soc Clin Oncol 1998;17:72a.

38. Porta C, Moroni M, Nastasi G: Allopurinol mouthwashes in the treatment of 5-fluorouracil–induced stomatitis. Am J Clin Oncol 1994;17:246–7.

39. Loprinzi CL, Cianflone SG, Dose AM, et al. A controlled evaluation of an allopurinol mouthwash as prophylaxis against 5-fluorouracil–induced stomatitis. Cancer 1990;65:1879–82.

40. Labar B, Mrsic M, Pavletic Z, et al. Prostaglandin E$_2$ for prophylaxis of oral mucositis following BMT. Bone Marrow Transplant 1993;11:379–82.

41. Berger A, Henderson M, Nadoolman W, et al. Oral capsaicin provides temporary relief for mucositis pain secondary to chemotherapy/radiation therapy. J Pain Symptom Manage 1995;10:243–8.

42. Wadleigh RG, Redman RS, Graham ML, et al. Vitamin E in the treatment of chemotherapy-induced mucositis. Am J Med 1992;92:481–4.

43. Schubert MM. Oral manifestations of viral infections in immunocompromised patients. Curr Opin Dentistry 1991;1:384–97.

44. Eisen D, Essell J, Broun ER. Oral cavity complications of bone marrow transplantation. Semin Cutan Med Surg 1997;16:265–72.

45. Schubet MM, Peterson DE, Flournoy N, et al. Oral and pharyngeal herpes simplex infection after allogeneic bone marrow transplantation: analysis of factors associated with infection. Oral Surg Oral Med Oral Pathol 1990;70:286–93.

46. Oblon DJ, Paul SR, Oblon MB, et al. Propantheline protects the oral mucosa after high-dose ifosfamide, carboplatin etoposide, and autologous stem cell transplantation. Bone Marrow Transplant 1997;20:961–3.

......................................

# DIARRHEA

• John Barstis

---

Although there is no universally accepted clinical definition of diarrhea, it can generally be said to exist when bowel movements are excessive in both frequency and liquid content. The quantitative definition of diarrhea most frequently used is stool weight of more than 200 g/day.[1] A patient usually requires no precise criteria to know if he or she has diarrhea. It is a frequent problem in cancer patients and has the potential to cause great morbidity. Consequences include dehydration; nutritional, electrolyte, and albumin losses; and deleterious effects on a patient's psychological, immune, and functional status.

## Pathophysiology

It has been estimated that 9 L of fluid enters a normal gastrointestinal tract in 1 day: 2 L by ingestion, 1.5 L as saliva, 2.5 L as gastric juices, and 3 L as biliary, pancreatic, and small intestine secretions. The small intestine absorbs 8 L of fluid, whereas 800 ml is absorbed in the colon, leaving an average of 200 ml/day liquid in the feces.[2] Absorption is achieved by multiple active and passive transport mechanisms for electrolytes, bile salts, and nutrients in the small intestine, and Na$^+$ in the colon. Perhaps the most important of these mechanisms is the Na$^+$-glucose cotransport mechanism in the small intestine. The secretory function in both the large and small intestines is carried out by active Cl$^-$ transport, with Na$^+$ and water following passively.[3] Absorptive and secretory mechanisms are independent, with the former often less affected in diarrhea. Consequently, the ingestion of glucose-electrolyte solutions usually remains beneficial in severe secretory diarrhea.[4] Of special concern in cancer patients is the effect that bowel surgeries, chemotherapy, and radiotherapy may have on bowel neurologic function and mucosal integrity, which, in turn, adversely affect motility and absorptive capacity. Treatment-related diarrhea in cancer patients frequently involves combinations in varying proportions of secretory, absorptive, and transit time disorders.[5] The normal gastric mucosa replaces itself every 2 to 3 days; the intestinal mucosa regenerates itself about once every 7 days.[6, 7] The time necessary for this layer to recover is highly variable, depending on the type and extent of damage. For example, in transient radiation injury, gut epithelium can completely regenerate in less than 14 days, but with more severe injury growth is markedly slowed.[8]

## Causes of Diarrhea

A comprehensive review of the causes of diarrhea is beyond the scope of this chapter, but there are many causes of importance to cancer patients. Although a rigid classification is artificial, causes can be grouped according to their predominant mechanism (Table 19–5).

In surgical patients, deranged motility may result from postgastrectomy dumping syndromes,[9] ileocecal valve resection,[10] or short-bowel syndromes. A study by Papa and colleagues found that diarrhea was much less frequent if less than 10 cm of terminal ileum was resected and more than 10 cm of colon was left above the peritoneal reflection.[11]

Osmotic diarrhea occurs in the presence of any nonabsorbable solute, most commonly laxatives. Endocrine tumors can cause secretory diarrhea by producing secretagogue transmitters, for example, carcinoid tumors produce catecholamines, histamine, kinins, prostaglandin, and serotonin; Zollinger-Ellison syndrome resulting from a gastrinoma produces gastrin; pheochromocytoma produces catecholamines; medullary thyroid cancer produces calcitonin; and non–β-cell pancreatic adenomas produce a variety of peptides. Tumors that predominantly make one such peptide—vasoactive polypeptide—are termed *vipomas*. These tumors may produce a watery diarrhea and hypokalemia-hypochlorhydria syndrome. Studies have shown markedly decreased colonic transit time in some of these patients.[12]

Bacterial endotoxins, chemotherapy, radiation therapy, and graft-versus-host disease all cause an inflammatory response by damaging intestinal epithelium and thus causing diarrhea through the release of prostaglandins and their potent secretagogue effect, which interferes with both normal motility and absorption.[13] *Clostridium difficile* pseudomembranous enterocolitis that occurs after administration of broad-spectrum antibiotics is the predominant cause of infectious diarrhea in oncology patients.[14, 15] It is of special importance to note that this type of enterocolitis can also be observed in chemotherapy patients who have not received antibiotics.[16, 17]

*Table 19–5.* **Causes of Diarrhea**

> Osmotic diarrhea
>     Laxatives
>     Tube feedings
> Surgery
>     Postgastrectomy dumping syndrome
>     Short-bowel syndrome
>     Terminal ileum-ileocecal valve resection
> Secretory diarrheas
>     Carcinoid tumors
>     Gastrinomas and Zollinger-Ellison syndrome
>     Medullary thyroid cancer
>     Non–beta-cell pancreatic adenomas
>     Pheochromocytomas
>     Vipomas
> Inflammatory damage
>     Graft-versus-host disease
>     Radiation therapy
>     Infectious diarrhea
>         *Clostridium difficile* from antibiotic use
>         *C. difficile* from chemotherapy
>         Methicillin-resistant *Staphylococcus aureus*
> Chemotherapy or biologic therapy induced
>     5-FU–based regimens
>     Cisplatin
>     Topoisomerase I inhibitors
>         Irinotecan (CPT-11)
>         Oral topotecan
>     Cytarabine
>     Methotrexate
>     Interleukin-2
> Medications
>     Broad-spectrum antibiotics
>     Diuretics (thiazides, furosemide)
>     Cardiac medications
> Paraneoplastic syndromes
>     Autonomic neuropathy
>     Ectopic hormone secretion from nonendocrine tumors

## Assessment

Diarrhea can be encountered in cancer patients in two very different settings. In the first, diarrhea may be therapy related or have an obvious cause. In these cases, there is evidence that extensive initial work-ups are not of benefit.[15, 18] Consequently, the approach is empirical and interventional. The patient's chemotherapy flow chart and radiation history may provide the best information to predict the course and duration of this process.

In the second setting, an unknown cause poses a great risk to a cancer patient already compromised in multiple ways. An adequate history should then be taken regarding the frequency and consistency of stools and their color as well as if blood is present. Fever, abdominal pain, and tenesmus are pertinent conditions. A complete knowledge of the patient's drug history, including alternative agents, is critical. Abdominal and rectal examinations should be performed to exclude the presence of a partial bowel obstruction that allows only liquids to pass.[19]

If the cause is not obvious at this point, a *C. difficile* stool assay should be performed, because of its prevalence in oncology settings. Gram stains and stool cultures for pathogens may reveal *Staphylococcus, Campylobacter,* or *Candida.* Guaiac testing may help reveal tumors or severe mucosal damage.

In all cases, the process should be documented in an objective manner. The National Cancer Institute's common toxicity scale is presented in Table 19–6. The recommendations of a consensus conference about the assessment, grading, and treatment of chemotherapy-induced diarrhea have been published.[40]

*Table 19–6.* **National Cancer Institute Toxicity Scale for Diarrhea**

| Grade | Criteria |
|-------|----------|
| 1 | Increase of <4 stools/day over pretreatment |
| 2 | Increase of 4–6 stools/day or nocturnal stools |
| 3 | Increase of >7 stools/day or incontinence; need for parenteral support for dehydration |
| 4 | Physiologic consequences requiring intensive care; hemodynamic collapse |

## Approach to Treatment

A summary of the management of diarrhea is provided in Table 19–7. For mild diarrhea, a conservative approach may suffice, especially if the cause is understood. Withdrawal of any exacerbating or causative factors is important, such as milk products, caffeine, alcohol, and foods high in fat or fiber. In patients who are being fed by tube, adding fiber and avoiding concurrent antibiotics have decreased liquid stools in some, but not all, studies.[20, 21] Oral intake of glucose-electrolyte solutions is more effective than water or electrolyte solutions alone because of cotransport mechanisms.[4]

There are a number of medications that may be helpful in specific situations. *C. difficile* colitis requires appropriate antibiotics. Bismuth subsalicylate (Pepto-Bismol) helps symptomatically in infectious diarrhea.[12] Simethicone, in pills or formulated with antacid, may reduce gas-related intestinal distention caused by fermentation. In some prostaglandin-mediated secretory disorders, prostaglandin E inhibitors such as salicylate and indomethacin have been reported to be effective.[22] Other agents reported to be somewhat effective in reducing secretory processes include calcium channel blockers, phenothiazines, and clonidine.[12] Kaolin-pectin binds osmotically active substances and can thicken stools but has little documented therapeutic benefit.[19] Trials of cholestyramine have shown benefit in radiation-induced cases of diarrhea.[23]

*Table 19–7.* **Summary of Treatment for Diarrhea**

*Identify and eliminate underlying cause*
Discontinue chemotherapy
Discontinue suspected medications
Obtain stool assay for *Clostridium difficile;* start appropriate
  antibiotics
*Begin supportive therapy*
Intensive oral rehydration with water-glucose-electrolyte solutions
Appropriate dietary management
  Avoid high-fat, high-fiber foods and dairy products
  Frequent small meals high in complex carbohydrates and protein
*12–24 hours later if inadequate response*
Add loperamide, 2 mg every 4 hr, continue 12 hr after resolution
Give 2 mg every 2 hr if preceding dosage fails or if patient treated
  with irinotecan
*12–24 hours later if inadequate response*
Begin octreotide, 150 μg subcutaneously TID
If no response in 12–24 hours, increase to a maximum of 500 μg
  TID
Consider entry into clinical trial for maximal doses of octreotide,
  if available
*12–24 hours later or immediately if National Cancer Institute
  Grade 3 or 4*
Begin intravenous fluids
Admit to hospital

For more serious cases of diarrhea, opioid congeners are the most frequently used agents. Opioids slow transit time markedly, allowing increased absorption of water from the intestine. They also increase ileocecal tone, inhibit the defecation reflex, and inhibit anorectal sphincter relaxation.[24, 25] Agents used for analgesia have antidiarrheal activity but also have other undesirable side effects. Loperamide usually is the initial choice in this group because it has few side effects as well as the highest antidiarrheal/analgesic ratio among opioid agents. It does not cross the blood-brain barrier. The recommended dose is 2 mg every 4 hours as needed. In trials with the chemotherapy agent irinotecan (CPT-11), a dose of 2 mg every 2 hours regularly has been found to be well tolerated and more effective than the standard dose. This dose exceeds the manufacturer's recommendations. Diphenoxylate, although similar chemically to meperidine, clinically has a favorable therapeutic profile for diarrhea. At the usual maximal dose of 20 mg/day, analgesia and sedation are uncommon. As in the general medical population, these agents may be contraindicated when inflammatory bowel disease, infectious diarrhea, or partial bowel obstruction is present.[23]

The most effective agent in current use for severe diarrhea is octreotide. It is a long-acting, eight–amino acid analogue of the cyclic tetradecapeptide somatostatin. Somatostatin is a potent inhibitor of endocrine and exocrine secretion. Inhibition is achieved by binding to specific cell surface receptors.[26] Octreotide was first demonstrated to be effective in treating the aggressive secretory processes caused by endocrine tumors.[27] It has also been shown to be well tolerated and effective when used for diarrhea resulting from chemotherapy. Randomized trials comparing it to loperamide have shown it to be superior after 5-FU and other types of chemotherapy.[28, 29] In a study by Kalofonos and colleagues, complete resolution of 5-FU–induced diarrhea was achieved in 59% of patients at a dose of 0.1 mg TID, and 95% of patients at a dose of 0.5 mg TID.[30] No side effects were noted in either group. Currently an Intergroup trial, E1295, is under way to answer questions about the optimal octreotide dose and the amount of benefit it has over loperamide. Patients are randomized to one of three arms: octreotide, 150 μg TID; octreotide, 1500 μg TID; or loperamide, 6 mg followed by 2 mg after each bowel movement to a maximum of 16 mg/day. All groups are treated for 5 days and are then assessed. Octreotide at a dose of 0.15 mg BID was ineffective at preventing 5-FU–associated diarrhea in 11 patients in a study at Roswell Park Institute.[31] It has been demonstrated to be successful in high-dose chemotherapy, bone marrow transplantation, and patients with acute graft-versus-host disease.[32, 33]

Diarrhea from topoisomerase I inhibitors requires special consideration. Irinotecan is the one most associated with this toxicity, but oral topotecan has also been reported to cause this clinical picture.[34] An immediate cholinergic syndrome can occur that may include diarrhea, but it is effectively treated with 0.25 to 1 mg of atropine. Delayed diarrhea of grade 3 or 4 severity occurs in more than one third of patients, beginning from 8 hours to 1 week after administration. Treatment at present consists of institution of loperamide, 2 mg every 2 hours for up to 3 days.[35, 36] The enkephalinase inhibitor acetorphan is under study to potentiate or possibly replace loperamide.[37, 38] A similar agent has been reported beneficial in decreasing cisplatin-induced diarrhea.[39]

## SUGGESTIONS FOR ADDITIONAL READING

Wadler S, Benson AB, Engleking C, et al. Recommended guidelines for the treatment of chemotherapy-induced diarrhea. J Clin Oncol 1998;16:3169–78.

Brunton LL. Agents affecting gastrointestinal water flux and motility. In: Hardman JG, Limbard LL, eds. Goodman & Gilman's the pharmacological basis of therapeutics. 9th ed. New York: McGraw-Hill, 1996:917–28.

## REFERENCES

1. Friedman LS, Isselbacher KJ. Diarrhea and constipation. In: Fauci AS, Braunwald E, Isselbacher KJ, eds. Harrison's principles of internal medicine. 14th ed. New York: McGraw-Hill, 1998:237.
2. Kaunitz JD, Barrett KE, McRoberts JA. Electrolyte secretion and absorption: small intestine and colon. In: Yamada T, Alpers DH, Owyang DH, et al, eds. Textbook of gastroenterology. 2nd ed. Philadelphia: JB Lippincott, 1995:327.
3. Field M, Rao MC, Chang EB. Intestinal electrolyte transport and diarrheal disease. N Engl J Med 1989;321:800–6.
4. Friedman LS, Isselbacher KJ. Diarrhea and constipation. In: Fauci AS, Braunwald E, Isselbacher KJ, eds. Harrison's principles of internal medicine. 14th ed. New York: McGraw-Hill, 1998:236.
5. Mercadante S. Diarrhea, malabsorption and constipation. In: Berger AM, Portenoy AK, Weissman DE, eds. Principles and practice of supportive oncology. Philadelphia: Lippincott-Raven, 1998:191–7.
6. Madara J. Epithelial responses to disease and injury. In: Yamada T, Alpers DH, Owyang DH, et al, eds. Textbook of gastroenterology. 2nd ed. Philadelphia: JB Lippincott, 1995:152.
7. Podolsky DK, Babyatsky MW. Growth and differentiation of the gastrointestinal tract. In: Yamada T, Alpers DH, Owyang DH, et al, eds. Textbook of gastroenterology. 2nd ed. Philadelphia: JB Lippincott, 1995:561.
8. Nostrant TT, Robertson JM, Lawrence TS. Radiation injury. In: Yamada T, Alpers DH, Owyang DH, et al, eds. Textbook of gastroenterology. 2nd ed. Philadelphia: JB Lippincott, 1995:2538.
9. Sawyers JL. Management of postgastrectomy syndromes. Am J Surg 1990;159:8–14.
10. Ben-Chaim J, Shenfield O, Goldwasser B, et al. Does the use of the ileocecal region in reconstructive surgery cause persistent diarrhea? Eur Urol 1995;27:315–8.
11. Papa MZ, Karni T, Koller M, et al. Avoiding diarrhea after subtotal colectomy with primary anastomosis in the treatment of colon cancer. J Am Coll Surg 1997;184:269–72.
12. Powell DW. Approach to the patient with diarrhea. In: Yamada T, Alpers DH, Owyang DH, et al, eds. Textbook of gastroenterology. 2nd ed. Philadelphia: JB Lippincott, 1995:813–40.
13. Friedman LS, Isselbacher KJ. Diarrhea and constipation. In: Fauci AS, Braunwald E, Isselbacher KJ, eds. Harrison's principles of internal medicine. 14th ed. New York: McGraw-Hill, 1998:239–41.
14. Nielsen H, Daugaard G, Tvede M, et al. High prevalence of *Clostridium difficile* diarrhea during intensive therapy for disseminated germ cell cancer. Br J Cancer 1992;66:666–7.
15. Cirisano FD, Greenspoon JS, Stenson R, et al. The etiology and management of diarrhea in the gynecologic oncology patient. Gynecol Oncol 1993;50:45–8.
16. Anand A, Glatt AE. *Clostridium difficile* infection associated with antineoplastic chemotherapy: a review. Clin Infect Dis 1993;17:109–13.
17. Kamthan AG, Bruckner HW, Hirschman SZ, et al. *Clostridium difficile* diarrhea induced by cancer chemotherapy. Arch Intern Med 1992;152:1715–7.
18. Cascinu S, Catalano G. Have enteric infections a role in 5-fluorouracil–associated diarrhea? Support Care Cancer 1995; 3:322–3.
19. Mercadante S. Diarrhea in terminally ill patients: pathophysiology and treatment. J Pain Symptom Manage 1995; 10:298–309.
20. Reese JL, Means ME, Hanrahan K, et al. Diarrhea associated with tube feedings. Oncol Nurs Forum 1996;23:59–66.
21. Pesola GR, Hogg JE, Elissa N, et al. Hypertonic nasogastric tube feedings: do they cause diarrhea? Crit Care Med 1990; 18:1378–82.
22. Nostrant TT, Robertson JM, Lawrence TS. Radiation injury. In: Yamada T, Alpers DH, Owyang DH, et al, eds. Textbook of gastroenterology. 2nd ed. Philadelphia: JB Lippincott, 1995:2524–32.
23. Danielsson A, Nyhlin H, Persson H, et al. Chronic diarrhoea after radiotherapy for gynecologic cancer: occurence and aetiology. Gut 1991;32:1180–7.
24. Bouvier M, Grimaud JC, Naudy B, et al. Effects of morphine on electrical activity of the rectum in man. J Physiol 1987; 388:153–61.
25. DeLuca A, Coupar IM. Insights into opioid action in the intestinal tract. Pharmacol Ther 1996;69:103–15.
26. Weckbecker G, Raulf F, Stolz B, et al. Somatostatin analogs for diagnosis and treatment of cancer. Pharmacol Ther 1993; 60:245–64.
27. Harris AG. Octreotide in the treatment of disorders of the gastrointestinal system. Drug Invest 1992;499(Suppl):1–54.
28. Cascinu S, Fedeli A, Fedeli SL, et al. Octreotide versus loperamide in the treatment of fluorouracil-induced diarrhea: a randomized trial. J Clin Oncol 1993;11:148–51.
29. Gebbia V, Carreca I, Testa A, et al. Subcutaneous octreotide versus oral loperamamide in the treatment of diarrhea following chemotherapy. Anti-Cancer Drugs 1993; 4:443–5.
30. Kalofonos HP, Naxakis S, Christopoulou A, et al. Octreotide acetate in the treatment of fluorouracil-induced diarrhea. Proc Am Soc Clin Oncol 1997;16:71a. abstract.
31. Meropol NJ, Blumenson LE, Creaven PJ. Octreotide does not prevent diarrhea in patients treated with weekly 5-fluorouracil plus high-dose leucovorin. Am J Clin Oncol 1998;21:135–8.
32. Wasserman E, Hornedo J, Hidalgo M, et al. Octreotide (SMS-201-995) in the treatment of severe diarrhea secondary to high-dose chemotherapy. Proc Am Soc Clin Oncol 1996;15:549. abstract.
33. Ipoliti C, Champlin R, Bugazia N, et al. Use of octreotide in the symptomatic management of diarrhea induced by graft-versus-host disease in patients with hematologic malignancies. J Clin Oncol 1997;15:3350–4.
34. Creemers GJ, Gerrits CJ, Eckhardt JH, et al. Phase I and pharmacologic study of oral topotecan administered twice daily fo 21 days to adult patients with solid tumors. J Clin Oncol 1997;15:1087–93.
35. Pitot HC, Wender DB, O'Connell MJ, et al. Phase II trial of irinotecan on patients with metastatic colorectal carcinoma. J Clin Oncol 1997;15:2910–9.
36. Merrouche Y, Extra JM, Abigerges D, et al. High dose–intensity of irinotecan administered every 3 weeks in advanced cancer patients: a feasibility study. J Clin Oncol 1997;15:1080–6.
37. Merrouche Y, Bugat R, Brunet R, et al. High-dose acetorphan versus acetorphan plus loperamide in the treatment of CPT-11–induced diarrhea: preliminary report of a randomized phase II study in patients with advanced colorectal cancer. Proc Am Soc Clin Oncol 1996;15:211.
38. Goncalves E, da Costa L, Abigerges D, et al. A new enkephalinase inhibitor as an alternative to loperamide in the prevention of diarrhea induced by CPT-11. J Clin Oncol 1996;14:2144–6. letter.
39. Kris MG, Gralla RJ, Clark RA, et al. Control of chemotherapy-induced diarrhea with the synthetic enkephalin BW942C: a randomized trial with placebo in patients receiving cisplatin. J Clin Oncol 1988;6:663–8.
40. Wadler S, Benson AB, Engelking C, et al. Recommended guidelines for the treatment of chemotherapy-induced diarrhea. J Clin Oncol 1998;16:3169–78.

...........................................

# CONSTIPATION

• John Barstis

As with diarrhea, there is no consistently accepted definition of constipation. The most easily quantified measure is a decrease in stool frequency to less than three times a week. Although subjective, authorities also refer to difficulties with defecation, such as straining, pain, or sense of incomplete evacuation, as another defining characteristic.[1] Stool weight quantification and consistency, although relevant, are not diagnostic criteria. There is no disagreement, however, about the cost to individuals and society from constipation, including harm to a patient's nutrition, functional status, and psychological well-being. One must then add the distress to family and caregivers and the cost of hospital emergency room visits and admissions to have an adequate appreciation of the problem.

## Etiology and Pathophysiology

Normal intestinal physiology is briefly reviewed in the section Stomatitis. Any factor that causes a decrease in motility or secretion or an increase in absorption can lead to constipation. In abnormal as well as normal function, these three mechanisms are all closely interrelated. In addition, the local functions of the anorectal region that are required for normal defecation are of major importance. They include rectal tone, capacity and sensation, and anal sphincter reflexes.[2]

In a palliative care setting, frail patients may be immobile, resulting in supine positioning, bedpan use, lack of access to bathroom facilities, loss of privacy, and diminished oral intake and stool bulk. This, in turn, leads to progressive loss of normal tone and sensation in the anorectal region and resultant constipation. Neurologic and mechanical changes from surgery or the presence of a mass may also produce constipation of anorectal origin.[3]

Many medications can cause constipation. Opioids are the primary agents; the attributes that are so therapeutic for diarrhea become pathogenic in this setting. The list of effects of this class of agents on the bowel is long and growing. They include inhibition of both contraction of longitudinal smooth muscle and secretion of intestinal secretagogues. They increase colonic circular muscle tone and decrease overall intestinal transit time. There is subsequent increased intestinal absorption of fluid and electrolytes. Further, opioids cause impairment of normal anorectal tone and sensation, leading to profound bowel dysfunction.[4]

There are many other drugs commonly encountered in an oncology setting that may contribute to constipation. These include tricyclic antidepressants, anticonvulsants, diuretics, and calcium and aluminum compound antacids. The $5HT_3$ inhibitor antiemetics also tend to cause constipation in some patients.[5]

Certain chemotherapeutic agents can be associated with serious constipation. Vinca alkaloids can cause acute or, more rarely, late autonomic neuropathy. Clinical sequelae range from acute constipation to an ileus that mimics obstruction.[5]

## Prevention Strategies

An approach to the prevention and treatment of constipation is given in Table 19–8. The initial assessment of the patient must include a rectal examination by a member of the medical team. Information obtained will include the presence or absence of a mass, quantity and consistency of stool in the rectal vault, and rectal tone. Some palliative care experts include a routine abdominal radiograph when feasible and score the amount of stool present.[6]

The initial interventions must be holistic. One of the basic commandments of palliative care is to keep a patient ambulatory for as long as possible and to maximize remaining mobility after that. Physical therapy and a bed trapeze may prove of value. There should be careful education of patient and caregivers and optimization of medical equipment and the immediate environment. Upright posture and exercise appropriate for the setting stimulate peristalsis and bowel awareness and thus bowel movements.[7] A second supportive care tenet is that a bowel regimen must always accompany the use of opioids because constipation with their use is a near certainty.

Altering fiber intake in the diet has been studied. Most researchers have found that attempting to increase fiber is ineffective in preventing or treating constipation in the setting of advanced cancer.[8, 9] Hydration is accepted as at least somewhat beneficial both preventively and therapeutically, but it is often difficult to achieve orally.[10]

*Table 19–8.* **Sequence of Treatment for Constipation**

*Maintenance of Adequate Bowel Function*

Encourage movement and ambulation
Ensure adequate hydration
Maintain bowel awareness
Administer stool softener–senna combination on a regular schedule
Add and titrate regular lactulose, starting at 30 ml/day as needed

*Lack of Bowel Movement for 3 Days or Patient Uncomfortable*

Assess consistency of stool and need for disimpaction
Intervention from below first to avoid abdominal pain
  Biscadoyl suppositories if stool is soft
  Fleet-type enemas, glycerin suppositories if stool is hard

*Constipation Unrelieved by Preceding Interventions*

Continue lactulose, increasing dose up to 30 ml QID as needed
Use magnesium citrate or polyethylene glycol-electrolyte solution
  (GoLytely) only when preceding procedure is ineffective after
  48 hr

## Treatment

Often if hard stool is present, the initial intervention must be disimpaction. Glycerine suppositories are useful with hard stools because they soften and lubricate rectal contents, promoting less painful defecation. Bisacodyl suppositories are stimulants and are an appropriate first measure if stool is adequately soft. Small-volume phosphate enemas may be effective, but if large-volume or high-colonic enemas are needed, one must use isotonic saline. Large-volume phosphate enemas, as well as water or soap and water enemas, are potentially dangerous.[10, 11] If impaction is present, rectal approaches may be the best initial therapy because oral agents that stimulate peristalsis may cause abdominal pain.

Laxatives are categorized as softening agents or as stimulants of peristalsis, but no agent works purely by either mechanism. The first agents tried are usually stool softeners, which work by lowering the surface tension of stool, promoting penetration of hard stool by water and fats. Stool softeners usually are best given with a mild stimulant of peristalsis, especially when counteracting opioid effects. Senna is the most widely used.[12, 13]

Two of the most potent laxatives acceptable for long-term use are the nonabsorbable sugars lactulose and sorbitol. Lactulose is a synthetic disaccharide that is poorly absorbed from the digestive tract. There is no enzymatic degradation in the small intestine, so it reaches the colon intact, where it is metabolized to lactic acid and causes an increase in oncotic pressure, softening the stool. Although this colon-specific action makes it an ideal long-term laxative, the initial effect is usually delayed for 24 to 48 hours. It should be titrated to the desired results. The usual dose range is from 15 ml/day to 30 ml BID, and occasionally higher. Large doses can cause bloating; some patients are bothered by flatulence or an overly sweet taste. Lactulose is more expensive than first-line laxatives listed previously, and for this reason sorbitol has been recommended as an alternative. A randomized study by Lederle and colleagues in elderly patients comparing lactulose to sorbitol found the two equally effective and well tolerated.[14]

## SUGGESTIONS FOR ADDITIONAL READING

Mercadante S. Diarrhea, malabsorption, and constipation. In: Berger AM, Portenoy AK, Weissman DE, eds. Principles and practice of supportive oncology. Philadelphia: Lippincott-Raven, 1998:191–205.

Brunton LL. Agents affecting gastrointestinal water flux and motility. In: Hardman JG, Limbard LL, eds. Goodman & Gilman's the pharmacological basis of therapeutics. 9th ed. New York: McGraw-Hill, 1996:917–28.

## REFERENCES

1. Friedman LS, Isselbacher KJ. Diarrhea and constipation. In: Fauci AS, Braunwald E, Isselbacher KJ, eds. Harrison's principles of internal medicine. 14th ed. New York: McGraw-Hill, 1998:242.
2. Wald A. Approach to the patient with constipation. In: Yamada T, Alpers DH, Owyang DH, et al, eds. Textbook of gastroenterology. 2nd ed. Philadelphia: JB Lippincott, 1995:864–9.
3. Richter I. Choice of laxative in treatment of constipation. Home Healthcare Consultant 1997;4:28–41.
4. Bouvier M, Grimaud JC, Naudy B, et al. Effects of morphine on electrical activity of the rectum in man. J Physiol 1987;388:153–61.
5. DeLuca A, Coupar IM. Insights into opioid action in the intestinal tract. Pharmacol Ther 1996;69:103–15.
6. Glare P, Lickiss NP. Unrecognized constipation in patients with advanced cancer: a recipe for disaster. J Pain Symptom Manage 1992;7:369–71.
7. Seynaeve C, deMulder PH, Lane-Allman E, et al. The 5-HT$_3$ antagonist ondansetron re-establishes control in refractory emesis induced by non-cisplatin chemotherapy. Clin Oncol 1991;3:199–203.
8. Rowinski EK, Donehower RC. Microtubule targeting drugs. In: Perry MC, ed. The chemotherapy source book. 2nd ed. Baltimore: Williams & Wilkins, 1997:387–414.
9. Bruera E, Suarez-Almazor M, Velasco A, et al. The assessment of constipation in terminal cancer patients admitted to a palliative care unit: a retrospective review. J Pain Symptom Manage 1994;9:515–9.
10. Mercadante S. Diarrhea, malabsorption, and constipation. In: Berger AM, Portenoy AK, Weissman DE, eds. Principles and practice of supportive oncology. Philadelphia: Lippincott-Raven, 1998:200–204.
11. Pike BF, Phillippi PJ, Lawson EH. Soap colitis. N Engl J Med 1971;285:217–8.
12. Sykes NP. Current approaches to the management of constipation. Cancer Surv 1994;21:137-46.
13. Tadesco FJ. Laxative use in constipation. Am J Gastroenterol 1985;80:303–9.
14. Lederle FA, Busch DL, Mattox KM, et al. Cost-effective treatment of constipation in the elderly: a randomized double-blind comparison of sorbitol and lactulose. Am J Med 1990;89:597–601.

# CHAPTER 20

# INFECTION IN CANCER PATIENTS

• DAVID C. RHEW • LOWELL S. YOUNG • MATTHEW BIDWELL GOETZ

It has often been stated that the major problems regarding the clinical management of patients with neoplastic diseases are those that involve the diagnosis, treatment, and prevention of infection. This is probably an overstatement because problems with infection pertain primarily to individuals who have malignancies of the hematopoietic system. What is clear, however, is that since the 1960s, the complications of bleeding and organ failure have been largely controlled by measures such as platelet and blood component transfusions, and there now exist a variety of supportive therapies for circulatory collapse, respiratory failure, and renal failure.

The treatment of certain neoplasms, particularly that of lymphomas and leukemias, is particularly aggressive with the use of protocols aimed at destroying malignant cells. The risk of infection remains high with these disorders. Much of the progress that has been made in the treatment of the acute leukemias and the lymphomas has coincided with the availability of potent new antimicrobial agents that hold microbial pathogens at bay, while permitting antineoplastic agents to affect the underlying disease favorably. In most patients with solid tumors, the problem of infection is not nearly as omnipresent as in individuals with hematologic malignancies. As increasingly aggressive new chemotherapeutic protocols (including autologous bone marrow transplantation) are introduced to treat solid tumors, however, infections similar to those frequently encountered in leukemia patients should be anticipated. Patients with solid malignancies usually have a more rapid recovery of bone marrow function and shorter periods of neutropenia. Nonetheless, the clinician must be alerted to the possibility of serious infection whenever antineoplastic and immunosuppressive agents are used.

Although most oncologists are cognizant of the challenge of infection, there are many unresolved controversies about diagnostic, therapeutic, and prophylactic approaches. Many of the practices that are commonly in use are based on strongly held beliefs or longstanding convictions rather than on rigorously executed clinical trials. Definitive clinical trials to establish the worth of certain approaches are expensive, difficult to undertake, and often difficult to analyze. There is increasing pressure on clinicians with a subspecialty in infectious diseases in the oncologic setting to question seriously measures that are not cost-effective.

## Host Defects That Predispose to Infection

Table 20–1 summarizes what may be considered the conventional wisdom regarding the immunologic impairments associated with certain neoplastic disorders. For example, in acute leukemia, normal circulating neutrophils and monocytes are largely replaced by blast cells, which do not function well in the phagocytizing and killing of bacterial and fungal agents.

Hodgkin's disease has long been considered the premier example of a naturally occurring disorder of cell-mediated immunity. A more typical example in the present hospital setting of a patient with a disorder of cell-mediated immunity is the individual diagnosed with acquired immunodeficiency syndrome (AIDS). Before the advent of antimicrobial chemotherapy, patients with Hodgkin's disease developed tuberculosis and cryptococcal meningitis even if they had not received antineoplastic therapy.[1] This fact provides evidence that a defect in cell-mediated immunity predisposes a patient to infection caused by granuloma-inciting organisms. In con-

trast, with multiple myeloma, there is aberrant production of monoclonal antibodies, such that levels of antibody against the pyrogenic microorganisms, such as pneumococci, are significantly depressed. Patients with myeloma are prone to infection caused by a variety of encapsulated microorganisms (e.g., *Streptococcus pneumoniae*, *Haemophilus influenzae*, and *Neisseria meningitidis*).

In the modern chemotherapeutic era, use of cytotoxic drugs, immunosuppressive agents, and irradiation may exacerbate or potentiate an underlying immunologic defect. The use of corticosteroids in patients with Hodgkin's disease may further impair cell-mediated immunity. The use of corticosteroids, alkylating agents, and antimetabolites may reduce functional antibody levels in multiple myeloma. Corticosteroids given to patients with acute leukemia may impair granulocyte and mononuclear cell mobilization. Also in these cases, alkylating agents, antimetabolites, and radiation therapy may suppress leukopoiesis, exacerbating a functional defect in circulating neutrophils.

In clinical practice, the use of multiple anticancer agents, often in a rotating fashion with or without radiation therapy, causes the association between the various underlying diseases and specific infectious complications to become blurred. For example, infections from *Nocardia* and *Listeria* have been more typically associated with Hodgkin's disease and impaired cell-mediated immunity. When one corrects for the fact that Hodgkin's disease is relatively more common than acute leukemia, however, the overall incidence of these specific infections in the latter disorder is not that rare.[2] Similarly, although the major underlying disorder in chronic lymphocytic leukemia is hypogammaglobulinemia, which increases the risk for infection with encapsulated microorganisms and enteric bacteria, when fludarabine, a purine analogue, is included in the treatment regimen, opportunistic infections by *Pneumocystis carinii*, *Mycobacterium tuberculosis*, *Listeria*, and other pathogens normally controlled by cell-mediated immunity occur with increased frequency.[3]

## Epidemiologic Considerations

An epidemiologic approach to the nature of infection in the cancer patient is important because of the implications relating to its prevention and control. Broadly speaking, patterns of infection can be divided into two major categories that have been recognized since the 19th century. *Exogenous infections* are those due to microbes that are not part of the normal host flora and are transmitted from person to person or from the environment to the susceptible individual. *En-*

*Table 20–1.* **Immune Defects Present in Neoplastic Diseases**

| Host Defect | Neoplastic Disease | Therapy Causing Similar Defect |
|---|---|---|
| Impaired phagocytic function | Acute leukemia | Corticosteroids |
| Phagocyte mobilization | | Alkylating agents |
| Neutropenia | | Antimetabolites |
| Impaired cell-mediated immunity | Hodgkin's disease | Corticosteroids |
| | Hairy cell leukemia | Antilymphocyte globulin |
| Decreased antibody levels | Multiple myeloma | Alkylating agents |
| | Chronic lymphocytic leukemia | Antimetabolites |

*dogenous infections* are those caused by the host's native microbial flora.

## EXOGENOUS INFECTIONS

Classic methods developed to create physical barriers between patients and hospital personnel and the use of *protective isolation*, with accordant rituals of masking and gowning procedures, have all been directed toward limiting exogenous infection. In the hospital setting, infection with *Pseudomonas aeruginosa*, *Serratia marcescens*, and *Klebsiella* spp. may be transmitted by exposure to contaminated inhalation therapy equipment or pressure-monitoring devices or even through the administration of contaminated intravenous fluids. Transmission of staphylococci and enterococci to high-risk patients has been linked to human carriers. Contaminated aerosols may also lead to acquisition of infection by *Aspergillus*, varicella-zoster virus, respiratory syncytial virus, adenovirus, and influenza.

Acquisition of hospital-associated pathogens is of special concern because of the increased prevalence of antimicrobial resistance in such microbes. The development of antimicrobial resistance is promoted by the inappropriate use of antimicrobial agents, especially those with a broad spectrum of activity. Resistance of *Staphylococcus aureus* to methicillin (methicillin-resistant *S. aureus* [MRSA]) and of *Enterococcus* spp. to vancomycin (vancomycin-resistant *Enterococcus* [VRE]) represent major problems in many hospital and cancer center settings. Similarly, hospital-acquired infections by highly resistant gram-negative bacilli and organisms with plasmid-mediated β-lactamases (e.g., extended-spectrum β-lactamases) pose challenging problems for treatment.[4] Concerns regarding the spread of these organisms and for the future development and spread of vancomycin-intermediate and vancomycin-resistant strains of *S. aureus* have prompted the development and implementation of strict environmental and antimicrobial control measures.[5–7]

## ENDOGENOUS INFECTIONS

Most normal individuals harbor tremendous numbers of aerobic and anaerobic gram-negative rods, and half the population may be carriers of staphylococci. There has been a great temptation to assume that the organisms that cause gram-negative rod bacteremia, one of the most common causes of life-threatening infection in the cancer patient, are endogenous. This concept is only partially correct. *Escherichia coli*, which is part of the normal flora of the human gastrointestinal tract, is usually the most common organism isolated from bacteremic infections in cancer patients. Septicemias caused by *Klebsiella* and *Pseudomonas* spp. usually have a different mode of transmission, and recognition of this is important. These species are not part of the normal gastrointestinal flora, and attempts to colonize normal, healthy individuals with *P. aeruginosa* via the oral route have been largely unsuccessful. Nonetheless, when a patient has a neoplasm or some other serious underlying disease, these organisms are able to colonize the upper respiratory passageways and the gastrointestinal tract successfully. In the cancer patient, such colonization may precede septicemia by days if not weeks.[2] Organisms not normally found in the gastrointestinal tract that are resistant to multiple antibiotics may colonize mucosal surfaces of an immunosuppressed host, particularly when antimicrobial agents have been administered. Bacteremic infection or serious localized infections may ensue following small breaks or ulceration in the gastrointestinal mucosa secondary to chemotherapy or neutropenia, or both. Food, ornamental plants, medicines, and contaminated fluids and drinking water have been identified as sources of bacterial colonization. Prudent epidemiologic control measures in the hospital setting have been implemented in an attempt to minimize these sources of infection.[8]

Organisms that infect via an indwelling vascular catheter are usually those normally found on the skin, and such infections are properly classified as being of endogenous origin. Although attention has focused on the proper management of indwelling plastic devices such as the Foley urinary catheter in the control of nosocomial infection, a common practice in the oncology setting has been the tendency to use long-term indwelling vascular catheters of the Hickman or Broviac type or completely indwelling catheters (Portacath). The rationale for using these devices is clear and appealing. They are threaded into the superior vena cava, allowing for the easy delivery of large volumes of needed fluid and blood components. Some of these devices have a second tubing, making it possible to draw blood from the patient. Although skillful insertion of such catheters under rigorous conditions in the operating room can be associated with a low risk of serious infection, some, including endocarditis, can still result.[9]

*S. aureus*, coagulase-negative staphylococci, *Candida*, *Corynebacterium*, and gram-negative rods are the most common catheter-associated pathogens. Coagulase-negative staphylococci and corynebacteria are usually considered relatively avirulent, yet they can cause severe and occasionally fatal bacteremia, especially in immunocompromised patients. This fact further emphasizes that virulence of microbial pathogens can be defined only in terms of the status of the host. Even carefully inserted vascular devices in the high-risk patient may provide the opportunity for nonpathogenic organisms to gain footholds. These infections are often accompanied by minimal signs of inflammation because of the impaired host response. Persistent fever in patients with catheters should be a clear warning to consider these devices a source of infection and to obtain blood cultures through each vascular channel.

In addition, reactivation of endogenous pathogens acquired from previous environmental exposure can occur in cancer patients during and after immunosuppressive chemotherapy. Important examples include reactivation of latent infection by tuberculosis, endemic mycoses (e.g., *Histoplasma capsulatum* and *Coccidioides immitis*), herpesviruses (herpes simplex, cytomegalovirus, and varicella-zoster virus), and parasites (e.g., *Toxoplasma gondii* and *Strongyloides stercoralis*). Serologic evidence also suggests that *P. carinii* may commonly establish latency during childhood.[10] Each of these latent infectious processes may become reactivated if a previously infected individual subsequently develops a neoplasm that is treated with immunosuppressive or cytotoxic therapy, or both.

# Clinical Syndromes of Infection

Many reviews of infection in the cancer patient include extensive lists of the types of microorganisms isolated from patients with fever, septicemia, or evidence of specific organ infection. These reviews can be helpful in estimating the statistical probability of specific infectious processes. For instance, a major category of microbial pathogens that needs consideration is the one including aerobic bacteria: *S. aureus* is the most important among the gram-positive bacteria, and *E. coli*, *K. pneumoniae*, and *P. aeruginosa* are important among the gram-negative rods. These organisms can cause rapidly progressive serious infections in virtually every organ system.

Rigorous diagnostic studies fail to disclose the cause of fever in 50 to 80% of febrile cancer patients.[1] There has been intense speculation as to the causes of such febrile illnesses. Underlying disease could be one of the confounding variables as well as drug reactions or hypersensitivity reactions that are still poorly understood. Another plausible suggestion is that high fevers in neutropenic patients who nonetheless have negative blood cultures result from localized aerobic and anaerobic infection around the gastrointestinal tract that has not yet spread into the bloodstream. Regardless of what may be the cause of fever, it is a widespread clinical practice to give patients who have total granulocyte counts of less than 500/mm[3] an empirical course of antimicrobial therapy. Most febrile neutropenic patients without confirmed bacterial infection improve after systemic antimicrobial agents are given,[1] and in these cases, empirical therapy may be adequately treating as-yet-unidentified infectious agents.

The clinician usually does not know the nature of the causative organism at the time of the first clinical presentation or symptom complex. Table 20–2 summarizes the types of agents that might be encountered in certain clinical syndromes and provides a useful initial guide to the differential diagnosis of septicemia, disseminated skin infections, infections of the central nervous system (CNS), lung infections, pain on swallowing, and diarrhea. The possibilities that are enumerated should give the physician the proper clinical focus for the initiation of diagnostic procedures as well as the selection of empirical antimicrobial therapy.

## SEPTICEMIA

Septicemia in the cancer patient may signal invasive infection from various anatomic sites. Bloodstream infections with *S. aureus*, coagulase-negative staphylococci, *Corynebacterium jeikeium* (JK), and *Candida* spp. are frequently secondary to infected intravascular devices, although contamination must be considered when single blood cultures reveal coagulase-negative staphylococci. Other bacteremias may provide the first clinical evidence of an underlying malignancy. For example, bacteremia resulting from *Streptococcus bovis* often occurs in association with a gastrointestinal malignancy, particularly colon cancer.[11] Similarly, 70% of bacteremias resulting from *Clostridium septicum* are associated with either colon cancer or leukemia.[12]

Although the incidence of bacteremia is generally increased in cancer patients, this risk is profoundly influenced by the degree of granulocytopenia. When mucositis is present, the risk of sepsis increases substantially when the granulocyte count falls to less than 500 cells/$\mu$l and becomes formidable when there are less than 100 cells/$\mu$l. Such patients are at special risk for bloodstream infection by *K. pneumoniae*, *E. coli*, *P. aeruginosa*, and other aerobic gram-negative bacilli (e.g., *Proteus* spp., *Serratia* spp., *Enterobacter* spp., *Acinetobacter* spp., *Stenotrophomonas maltophilia*, *Burkholderia cepacia*) as well as by fungi (primarily by *Candida* spp., although *Trichospora* spp. and *Fusarium* spp. may also be isolated).

## HIGH FEVER WITH EVIDENCE OF CUTANEOUS DISSEMINATION

Classically, the organisms that result in cutaneous lesions are *Staphylococcus aureus* and *P. aeruginosa*. Although staphylococcal disease was once a common infection in leukemia patients, it was on the wane until the introduction of long-term indwelling vascular catheters. The lesions associated with *S. aureus* are usually purulent and metastatic and, on aspiration and gram staining, show abundant gram-positive cocci in grape-like clusters. In the neutropenic patient, however, purulent inflammation is often absent.

*P. aeruginosa* is the prototypical gram-negative organism that causes cutaneous lesions.[13] This organism has a tendency to produce a vasculitis and round or oval bull's-eye lesions that develop a colorful vesicular or necrotic center (ecthyma gangrenosum). Most patients with *Pseudomonas* sepsis do not have ecthyma gangrenosum, however, and the factors that lead to this particular clinical manifestation are poorly understood. The appearance of these lesions is not diagnostic of *Pseudomonas* infection. Other aerobic gram-negative rods, such as *Aeromonas hydrophila*, *Stenotrophomonas maltophilia*, nonhalophilic *Vibrio* spp. such as *V. vulnificus*, members of the family Enterobacteriaceae, and rarely streptococci, may also produce such lesions.[14, 15]

Systemic fungal infections may also present with high fever and cutaneous lesions. Of these, *Candida* spp., particularly *C. tropicalis*, stand out as a common cause of nummular or coin-like lesions. *Aspergillus* spp., fungi belonging to the order Mucorales (the agents of mucormycosis), *Pseudallescheria boydii*, and dermatophytes, however, can cause cutaneous lesions secondary to embolization, direct extension, and thrombosis. *Aspergillus* and Mucorales isolates are well-known causes of necrotizing vasculitis in the lung and in the CNS. These processes may also involve the skin. Lesions on the gums, mouth, and palate as well as on the skin may be seen with histoplasmosis and paracoccidioidomycosis. Skin lesions are commonly reported in patients with disseminated coccidioidomycosis, cryptococcosis, and blastomycosis.

Viral diseases can present with cutaneous lesions that are usually easily recognized. Varicella-zoster and herpes simplex viruses cause vesicular lesions on an erythematous base, and it is difficult to distinguish between the two on the basis of appearance. At times, the clinical presentation of herpes zoster can be aberrant in immunocompromised patients.[16] Cytomegalovirus infections can occasionally present with an erythematous rash.

*Table 20–2.* Infectious Disease Syndromes and Causative Agents in the Cancer Patient

| Pattern of Involvement | Bacteria | Fungi | Viruses | Parasites |
|---|---|---|---|---|
| Disseminated disease with skin lesions (vasculitis or abscesses, or both) | *Staphylococcus aureus*<br>*Pseudomonas aeruginosa*<br>*Aeromonas hydrophila*<br>Other gram-negative bacteria<br>*Nocardia*<br>Noncholera *Vibrios*<br>*Mycobacterium* | *Candida*<br>*Aspergillus*<br>*Histoplasma*<br>*Zygomycetes*<br>*Sporothrix schenckii*<br>*Pseudallescheria*<br>*Trichosporon* | Herpes simplex<br>Varicella-zoster | |
| Diffuse interstitial pneumonia* | Any gram-negative or gram-positive bacteria, including *Nocardia* and *Mycobacterium*<br>*Chlamydia* | *Aspergillus*<br>*Candida*<br>*Mucor*<br>*Pneumocystis carinii* | Herpes simplex<br>Varicella-zoster<br>Cytomegalovirus<br>Influenza<br>Respiratory syncytial virus<br>Adenovirus | *Toxoplasma gondii*<br>*Strongyloides stercoralis* |
| Central nervous system infection, meningoencephalitis, possibly brain abscess | *Listeria monocytogenes*<br>*Nocardia*<br>*S. aureus*<br>*P. aeruginosa*<br>*Mycobacterium tuberculosis* | *Cryptococcus neoformans*<br>*Aspergillus fumigatus*<br>*Zygomycetes*<br>*Candida* | Varicella-zoster<br>Herpes simplex | |
| Oroesophageal syndromes | Anaerobes<br>Aerobes: streptococci and gram-negative rods, particularly *P. aeruginosa* | *Candida*<br>*Aspergillus* | Herpes simplex<br>Cytomegalovirus | |
| Diarrhea | *Clostridium difficile*<br>*Salmonella*<br>*Shigella*<br>*Campylobacter* | | *Adenovirus*<br>*Coxsackievirus*<br>*Rotavirus* | *Giardia lamblia*<br>*Cryptosporidium*<br>*Isospora belli* |

*Consider also underlying disease, radiation, and drug reactions.

## DIFFUSE PNEUMONIA

Diffuse pneumonias attract urgent clinical attention owing to the frequency of rapidly progressing respiratory symptoms. The cancer patient is also prone to lobar pneumococcal pneumonia, gram-negative pneumonia that presents as a bacteremic or embolic complication from another site, aspiration pneumonia resulting from impaired consciousness, and obstructive pneumonia resulting from partial obstruction of the bronchus by tumor.

Cancer patients who present with diffuse interstitial pneumonia must be urgently evaluated, particularly when the illness is accompanied by evidence of arterial hypoxemia. There is no question but that the rapid administration of appropriate antimicrobial and other supportive therapy is essential if the best clinical results are to be obtained. Virtually every type of gram-positive and gram-negative organism may cause severe pneumonia in cancer patients. Some of the organisms responsible for diffuse interstitial pneumonia are listed in Table 20–2.

**Fungal Infections.** The agent *P. carinii* was previously classified as a protozoan but is now recognized as a fungus. *P. carinii* pneumonia often presents as a diffuse, bilateral patchy or interstitial infiltrate associated with arterial hyposaturation and represents an important cause of pneumonia in the cancer patient with T-cell dysfunction. Acute lymphoblastic leukemia, Hodgkin's lymphoma, rhabdosarcoma, and use of corticosteroids have been implicated as risk factors for acquiring *P. carinii* pneumonia in the cancer patient.[17] In the neutropenic patient, *Aspergillus* spp. are a common cause of pulmonary infection that often presents as a cavitating, pleural-based pulmonary infiltrate in association with pleu-

ritic chest pain. Infection caused by members of the order Mucorales (the agents of mucormycosis) may present in a similar manner. *Cryptococcus neoformans* is a less common cause of pulmonary infection but should be suspected in settings of disseminated cryptococcosis. Despite the fact that *Candida* spp. are frequently recovered from respiratory secretions, *Candida* pneumonia is rare in the absence of disseminated candidiasis. Pneumonia caused by the agents of endemic mycoses should be suspected in patients who possess appropriate regional demographics. Confusion may ensue when patients who have previously resided in endemic areas for histoplasmosis (the Mississippi and Ohio River Valleys and Central America) or coccidioidomycosis (the San Joaquin Valley of California and other desert areas in the southwest United States) develop reactivation disease after moving to another part of the United States and becoming immunocompromised. Blastomycosis (found primarily in the southeastern and south central United States) and paracoccidioidomycosis (found in South America) reactivate less often.

**Parasitic Infections.** The parasitic infections have received much attention in immunosuppressed cancer patients. Toxoplasmosis can occasionally involve the lung, although it is more common for *T. gondii* to invade the brain and cause mass lesions. *Strongyloides stercoralis* is a common intestinal pathogen that can invade systemically and cause lung infiltrates in immunocompromised patients. Diagnosis of this condition is suggested by the recovery of the parasite in the stool, but on direct sampling of lung secretions, an abundant number of organisms may also be detected.

**Viral Infections.** The herpesviruses are an important

cause of respiratory infection. The most important agent in the group causing progressive lung infiltrates in multiple transfused patients and recipients of marrow transplants is cytomegalovirus. This agent can cause a lethal progressive pneumonia. Herpes simplex viruses can cause necrotizing as well as diffuse pneumonias. Their occurrence, however, has been relatively less common than that of cytomegalovirus. Additionally, influenza virus, respiratory syncytial virus, parainfluenza virus, and adenovirus may cause pneumonia.

**Other Pathogens.** There appears to be a higher incidence of *Legionella pneumophila* infections in patients receiving immunosuppressive therapy relative to other nonimmunosuppressed individuals subjected to equivalent environmental exposure.[18] Additionally, adults with altered host defenses have been reported to have lung infections resulting from *Chlamydia* spp.[19]

## CENTRAL NERVOUS SYSTEM INFECTIONS

It is useful to categorize infections of the CNS by the site of involvement. Some patients develop meningitis, others have a brain abscess, and a third group has encephalomyelitis.

**Meningitis.** In contrast to the normal population in which *Streptococcus pneumoniae*, *H. influenzae*, and *N. meningitidis* constitute 70% of the bacterial meningitides, approximately one third of CNS infections in cancer patients are fungal, with *C. neoformans* being the most commonly isolated pathogen. Also noteworthy is that *L. monocytogenes*, responsible for 1% of the bacterial meningitides occurring in the general population, is the most common bacterium producing meningitis in the immunocompromised host.[20]

**Brain Abscess.** Opportunistic pathogens are the offending agents in almost three quarters of cancer patients who develop a brain abscess. *Nocardia* and *Aspergillus* are particularly frequent offenders in this regard. This situation contrasts with the normal population, in whom the most common causes are gram-positive cocci, such as *S. aureus*, streptococci, and anaerobes.

**Encephalomyelitis.** Encephalomyelitis, manifested by diffuse parenchymal invasion of the CNS, most commonly results from infection with herpesviruses and *T. gondii*. The latter agent frequently presents as a CNS mass lesion in patients with compromised host defenses.[21]

**Diagnosis.** For the clinician, there is often little difference among the clinical presentations of meningitis, brain abscess, and encephalomyelitis. Fever, headache, and impaired consciousness should trigger immediate diagnostic studies to rule out the presence and nature of a CNS infection. Mild confusion and agitation, with or without fever, should trigger clinical suspicion. The development of neurologic symptoms, even in individuals likely to have CNS metastases, can be a valuable clue to the early diagnosis of an infectious problem. Clinicians should be aware that peripheral neutropenia can result in a low CNS inflammatory response. The classic signs and symptoms of neurologic impairment, such as dizziness, vertigo, and nuchal rigidity, may be absent, but extensor plantar responses are common findings in patients with mass lesions.

## OROESOPHAGEAL INFECTION

Infections involving the oropharynx and the esophagus are common in patients with neoplastic diseases. These infections are highly symptomatic and may lead to markedly reduced or impaired nutrition, compromising the host's ability to deal with infection.

Upper gastrointestinal colonization with organisms such as *Candida* spp. has usually been ascribed to alterations in normal flora via the use of antibiotics. In addition, the use of anticancer agents further compromises host defenses and increases the risk of mucosal candidiasis. Ulcerations caused by cancer chemotherapy can become the nidus of invasive gram-positive, gram-negative, and anaerobic infections. Although anaerobic organisms are quite abundant in the mouth and esophagus and can cause serious infections of the head and neck region, infections in that area are more often due to mixed aerobic and anaerobic processes.

Difficulty in swallowing and substernal burning have always been considered to be synonymous with *Candida* esophagitis. Nonetheless, there is abundant evidence that *Aspergillus* spp., cytomegalovirus, and herpesviruses can cause lesions in the esophagus that are clinically and symptomatically identical to those secondary to *Candida*. Esophageal infection with *Candida* or herpes may occur in the absence of simultaneous oropharyngeal involvement. The barium swallow examination does not allow differentiation among various causes. Only endoscopy with biopsy or culture, or both, can establish the diagnosis with certainty. Complications of esophageal infection include dissemination, perforation, and bleeding.

## DIARRHEAL SYNDROMES

The onset of diarrhea, which is frequently ignored, should be viewed with concern. *Salmonella*, *Shigella*, and *Campylobacter* are common bacterial pathogens of the gut, and they may appear in patients with cellular immune deficiencies or in recipients of corticosteroid therapy. The isolation of these organisms may reflect a nosocomial infection hazard. Diarrhea caused by *Clostridium difficile* is a common complication of antibiotic therapy. *C. difficile* should be suspected in patients with fever and diarrhea who have received an antibacterial agent or chemotherapy within 3 weeks before the onset of the diarrhea.[22] *C. difficile* not only may cause severe colitis but also may be a risk factor for VRE bacteremia in patients with acute leukemia who have VRE colonization.[23] Giardiasis should be considered if patients are hypogammaglobulinemic. Recipients of bone marrow transplants may be at risk for diarrhea caused by adenovirus, rotavirus, and coxsackievirus.[24] In the setting of severe neutropenia, diarrhea may be a manifestation of necrotizing enterocolitis (typhlitis). This process may be due to infection by *C. septicum*, *C. tertium*, or *C. perfringens* or to infection by mixed bowel flora and must be differentiated from disease caused by *C. difficile*.[25–28]

## Clinical Approach to the Patient

Careful observation and willingness to institute prompt diagnostic studies and therapeutic intervention provide the cornerstone for management of the oncology patient who is prone to develop infection. Fever should be compulsively evaluated despite the fact that high-risk patients are likely to have multiple episodes of fever, some of which may be related to drugs or to transfusion. Each episode necessitates thorough investigation because the status of a patient may be rapidly altered by chemotherapy. The urgency of the clinical response should be determined by a careful consideration of the underlying host defect, including the white blood cell count, the nature and effect of antineoplastic therapy, and prior use of antibiotic therapy. The individual who should be most urgently investigated is the one whose host defenses are most severely compromised and in whom fever is accompanied by an increased respiratory rate, a change in mental status, the presence of agitation or apprehensiveness, and any hemodynamic instability.

At the first sign of infection, multiple blood cultures should be obtained as should cultures of local sites, such as urine, stool, and sputum (if good specimens can be obtained). Routine blood tests should consist of a complete blood count with differential and transaminase, sodium, potassium, creatinine, and blood urea nitrogen levels.[29] A chest radiograph should be obtained to rule out pneumonia. The chest film is especially important in the elderly patient, who may not manifest typical signs or symptoms of pneumonia, such as fever and cough.[30] One of the most challenging clinical situations is the rapid development of diffuse lung infiltrates. These are probably most expeditiously diagnosed by transbronchial biopsy; open lung biopsy is a more definitive procedure but entails greater risks.[31] In the severely neutropenic thrombocytopenic patient, bronchoalveolar lavage may be the preferred noninvasive diagnostic procedure.[32]

The presence of new cutaneous lesions offers an excellent opportunity for aspiration, biopsy, and culture.[33] A cutaneous lesion may provide even more valuable information than blood cultures because bacteremia may be a transient event. Our advice on observation of such lesions, even in the thrombocytopenic patient, is to carry out a diagnostic aspiration after careful cleansing of the skin.

Evaluation of patients for suspected CNS infection should include careful examination of the cerebrospinal fluid. If there is any hint of elevated intracranial pressure, however, urgent computed tomography or magnetic resonance imaging of the brain should be carried out before lumbar puncture. Bacterial infection of the meninges with gram-negative rods is usually the result of an embolic-septicemic phenomenon. Radionuclide scanning and electroencephalography are less important diagnostic tools.

Serologic tests can be ordered. Some time may elapse before the results of these tests are available, however, and few clinical decisions regarding starting or stopping antimicrobial therapy are based on serologic results. In certain situations, the best example of which is the cryptococcal antigen test in spinal fluid, the diagnosis of a specific infectious process can be made with great certainty. Such technology has not been extended to other infectious disease processes, and there is great debate about the value of other assays to detect antibodies, antigens, and metabolic products related to *Candida* spp.[34–36] Our own position at this time is that most of the serodiagnostic tests yield limited information.

The decision to administer antibiotic therapy is based on clinical judgment, and one should be quick to alter treatment depending on the results of cultures or the availability of new information after the patient has been started on empirical therapy. Empirical antimicrobial therapy is warranted for all episodes of fever (defined as a single oral temperature of >38.3° C [101° F] or >38.0° C [100.4° F] over at least 1 hour) in patients with neutropenia (defined as neutrophil count <500/μL or <1000/μL with a predicted decline to <500/μL).[29]

## ANTIMICROBIAL THERAPY

Specific therapeutic recommendations for all the major infectious complications that occur in the cancer patient are beyond the scope of this chapter, but they may be found in many sources[1, 29] as well as in annually updated reviews of antimicrobial therapy, such as the *Medical Letter on Drugs and Therapeutics*. Treatment algorithms for febrile patients with neutropenia have been developed by the Infectious Diseases Society of America.[29] These recommendations represent a combination of evidence-based information and consensus-obtained expert opinion and are summarized in Table 20–3.[37] If a specific pathogen is isolated from blood, body fluid, or a tissue, antimicrobial therapy may be more specifically tailored based on identification of the species and in vitro susceptibility testing. Every hospital microbiology laboratory should issue updated reports on the incidence of isolation of major bacterial pathogens as well as profiles of their in vitro antimicrobial susceptibility. A practicing physician should be alerted to any institutional problems of infection or any noteworthy patterns of drug resistance, which could affect the decision-making process regarding antibiotic therapy. There are major differences from institution to institution with respect to the incidence of *Pseudomonas* and *Aspergillus* infections. Some hospitals have experienced epidemics or large clusters of cases, whereas others have infrequently reported or documented these problems. The same can be said regarding the risk of *Pneumocystis* infection in leukemic children; different institutions using identical chemotherapeutic protocols have noted a vast variation in the incidence of this complication. There should be close ties between the microbiology laboratory, infection control personnel, and those directly responsible for management of patients with altered immunity.

Empirical antimicrobial regimens should cover the spectrum of the most likely causes of systemic and rapidly progressing infection (see Table 20–3). Realistically, such therapy must begin before results of cultures and susceptibility tests are available (which still usually takes a minimum of 2 days). In the cancer patient, the most likely pathogens include gram-positive organisms, such as staphylococci, pneumococci, and streptococci, and gram-negative organisms, such as Enterobacteriaceae and *Pseudomonas*. Coverage of more unusual pathogens, such as *L. monocytogenes*, should be included in high-risk situations, such as patients receiving large doses of corticosteroids or those with Hodgkin's disease. Attention must be paid to identifying a specific site of infection, evaluation of which may suggest or prove the presence of a particular pathogen. The presence of underlying medical illnesses and the likelihood of a specific micro-

*Table 20–3.* **Guidelines for Use of Antimicrobial Agents in Patients With Fever (>38.3° C) and Neutropenia (<500/μL)**

Initial antimicrobial choices
    Monotherapy with ceftazidime, imipenem, cefepime, or meropenem. All with or without vancomycin (as per listed indications)
    Combination therapy (aminoglycoside + either antipseudomonal β-lactam or antipseudomonal carbapenem*). Preferred for high-risk patients.† All
       with or without vancomycin (as per listed indications)
    Indications for adjunctive, initial empirical use of vancomycin
       Severe mucositis
       Quinolone prophylaxis
       Known colonization with methicillin-resistant *Staphylococcus aureus* or penicillin-resistant or cephalosporin-resistant *Streptococcus pneumoniae*
       Obvious catheter-related infection
       Hypotension
Reassessment after 3 days
    Management of patients who become afebrile within the first 3 days of antimicrobial treatment
       No cause identified
          Low-risk‡ patient: consider changing antibiotic to oral antibiotic (cefixime or quinolone) and discharge
          Other patients: continue current antibiotic regimen
       Cause identified: adjust to appropriate treatment for the specific pathogen
    Management of patients who have persistent fever despite 3 days of antimicrobial treatment
       Re-evaluate patient for source of fever
       If a source of fever becomes apparent, adjust to appropriate treatment for the specific pathogen or for pathogens likely to be found at site of
        infection (e.g., addition of metronidazole for intra-abdominal or perirectal infection or vancomycin for catheter-related infection)
       If no cause remains apparent
          If patient unchanged and clinically stable, consider stopping vancomycin if this antibiotic has been empirically started
          If progressive disease, add vancomycin and initiate dual gram-negative bacillary coverage if this has not previously been administered
          If patient remains febrile despite 5–7 days of antimicrobial therapy, and resolution of neutropenia is not imminent, add amphotericin B with or
            without concomitant change of other antimicrobials
Duration of antimicrobial therapy
    Afebrile by day 3
       If neutrophil count is ≥500/μL by day 7, stop antimicrobial therapy after 7 days
       If neutrophil count is <500/μL at day 7
          Low-risk‡ patient: stop antimicrobials when afebrile for 5–7 days
          Other patients: continue antibiotics
    Persistent fever of uncertain origin despite recommended antimicrobial therapy
       If neutrophil count is ≥500/μL after 4–5 days: reassess
       If neutrophil count is <500/μL: continue antimicrobial therapy for 2 weeks, reassess, and stop if no substantiation of infection
       Consider empirical use of amphotericin B
Empirical use of antivirals: not recommended for routine use
Use of colony-stimulating factors: not routine; consider in certain cases with predicted worsening of course

   *Antipseudomonal β-lactams and carbapenems include ticarcillin, ticarcillin-clavulanate, piperacillin, piperacillin-tazobactam, mezlocillin, ceftazidime, cefepime, imipenem, and meropenem. Limited data suggest that amikacin plus ceftriaxone may also be sufficient in selected patient populations.[37]
   †High-risk patients are those with a neutrophil count of <100/μL, with severe mucositis, or who are clinically unstable.
   ‡Low-risk patients are defined as having a neutrophil count of more than 100/μL, being medically and oncologically stable, and having community-acquired infections.
   Adapted from Hughes WT, Armstrong D, Bodey GP, et al: 1997 guidelines for the use of antimicrobial agents in neutropenia patients with unexplained fever. Clin Infect Dis 1997;25:551–73.

biologic cause appropriately alter the choice of empirical antimicrobial therapy (see Table 20–3).

**Non-neutropenic Patients.** A cephalosporin, such as cephalothin, cefazolin, or cefoxitin, has been used with an aminoglycoside as an alternative to antipseudomonal penicillin for community-acquired infections in cancer patients who are not neutropenic. This regimen gives dual-agent coverage for *K. pneumoniae* and methicillin-susceptible *S. aureus*. In centers in which community-acquired *Pseudomonas aeruginosa*, *Serratia marcescens*, *Enterobacter* spp., and indole-positive *Proteus* spp. are known to be infrequent pathogens, such an approach has considerable merit in patients with intact neutrophil responses.

**Combination Regimens.** The basic regimen that we have employed since the 1970s in the treatment of febrile neutropenic patients has been the combination of an aminoglycoside, such as gentamicin or amikacin, and an antipseudomonal penicillin (ticarcillin, ticarcillin-clavulanate, mezlocillin, piperacillin, or piperacillin-tazobactam), cephalosporin (ceftazidime or cefepime), or carbapenem (imipenem or meropenem). The rationale for this approach, which has its weaknesses, is that such combinations give broad coverage of the likely gram-negative and gram-positive pathogens, including

at least one drug for all of the agents present. Such a combination approach offers dual-agent coverage of *P. aeruginosa*, the organism associated with the highest mortality rate from gram-negative bacteremia in cancer patients.[38] It has been repeatedly demonstrated that combination therapy is often synergistic and that in vitro synergism correlates with improved clinical results.[39] The selection of a specific regimen should be based on knowledge of the profile of antimicrobial resistance and the frequency with which various microorganisms are isolated locally.

With the availability of several different broad-spectrum β-lactam agents, one could consider using two agents, such as ceftazidime and piperacillin, instead of an aminoglycoside combined with a β-lactam agent. Although the experience with such a double β-lactam agent combination has been acceptable, there have been few patients treated who have had serious systemic *Pseudomonas* infection.[40] Such a regimen of piperacillin and ceftazidime might be more appropriate for patients who are older (>50 years of age) or have pre-existing renal disease or eighth cranial nerve dysfunction, but their advantage over other regimens, including monotherapy, has not been conclusively demonstrated.[41, 42]

**Monotherapy Regimens.** The increasing availability of

new antimicrobial agents of greater potency and broader spectrum has brought new hopes to the field of antimicrobial therapy. Studies in neutropenic patients have shown that administration of ceftazidime, cefepime, meropenem, or imipenem as monotherapy provides comparable results to combination therapy regimens that usually contain a β-lactam compound plus an aminoglycoside.[43–48] These regimens offer the advantage of decreased nephrotoxicity and ototoxicity for patients who are at substantial risk for such toxicity as a consequence of their chemotherapeutic regimen. Reservations must be expressed, however, that use of these clinical studies often results in frequent modifications of treatment and that the clinical studies have enrolled relatively few patients with the more challenging gram-negative infections, such as bacteremias caused by *P. aeruginosa* and *Enterobacter* spp. Because of concerns regarding inducible resistance, some authors recommend avoidance of third-generation cephalosporins (e.g., ceftazidime) in the treatment of serious *Enterobacter* infections and instead recommend the use of a broad-spectrum agent, such as cefepime or a carbapenem, or combination therapy with an aminoglycoside.[4, 49] Similarly, in the treatment of serious *P. aeruginosa* infections, acquisition of resistance during the course of monotherapy is common and can result in clinical failure.[4] For cancer patients with profound and persistent neutropenia (as defined by neutrophil counts <100/μL), it still seems prudent to prescribe combinations that include antipseudomonal β-lactam agents plus an aminoglycoside as initial empirical therapy. Monotherapy with quinolones is not recommended.[29]

**Use of Vancomycin.** With the current resurgence in gram-positive infection, many clinicians advocate the concurrent addition of vancomycin for empirical therapy to provide improved coverage of MSRA and methicillin-resistant, coagulase-negative staphylococci. The so-called front loading of vancomycin does not appear to have a significant impact in reducing overall morbidity and mortality in adult patients.[43, 50] Instead, vancomycin is most appropriately initiated when staphylococcal or α-hemolytic organisms are recovered from blood cultures. Concerns about the inappropriate use of vancomycin stem not only from the cost and toxicity of this agent but also from the emergence of VRE. In response, clinical guidelines for the appropriate use of vancomycin have been published.[51] These guidelines do not recommend the empirical use of vancomycin for febrile neutropenic patients, unless there is clinically obvious evidence of an infection caused by staphylococci (such as inflammation around the exit site of a vascular catheter) or a positive blood culture for gram-positive bacteria pending final identification and sensitivity of the organism. Although the early use of vancomycin does not improve the outcome of patients with staphylococcal bacteremia, it does benefit patients who prove to have bacteremia caused by α-hemolytic (viridans) streptococci.[39, 43, 50] Early empirical use of vancomycin may be considered in circumstances in which a high proportion of febrile illnesses are due to α-hemolytic streptococcal bacteremia, as occurs in profoundly neutropenic patients with severe mucositis who have received quinolone prophylaxis.[52, 53] Similarly, early empirical use of vancomycin may be appropriate in patients who are known to be colonized by MSRA or penicillin-resistant *S. pneumoniae*. Use of vancomycin may be indicated if fevers and other evidence of infection persist or progress despite empirical treatment with

a non–vancomycin-containing regimen (see Table 20–3).[29] Vancomycin may be discontinued after day 3 if culture results do not demonstrate an indication for vancomycin, even if the patient is not improved.

**Outpatient Therapy.** The risk of infection and the response to antibiotic therapy in cancer patients are largely determined by the magnitude and the duration of neutropenia. The risk of infection begins to increase as the neutrophil count drops to less than 1000/μl and is greatest at counts less than 100/μl.[54–56] Bacteremia accompanies 20% of infections occurring in the setting of such profound neutropenia. In this context, validated criteria have been developed that define febrile neutropenic patients who are at low risk for significant complications.[55, 57] These patients are defined by being medically and oncologically stable and having community-acquired infections. Pilot studies suggest that in carefully selected patients, treatment with brief periods of hospitalization followed by outpatient therapy with oral or intravenous antimicrobials is reasonably safe and effective.[58–60] Even in controlled studies, many patients treated in this fashion may develop complications such as hypotension, require admission for persistent fever, or require alteration of their antimicrobial regimen.[59] These studies, although they provide encouragement that outpatient treatment may be possible in carefully selected, low-risk, febrile, neutropenic patients, warrant further validation, and their current application requires careful patient selection.[61]

**Antimicrobial Selection.** Antimicrobial treatment should include first-line therapy against identified and suspected pathogens. For example, ampicillin or penicillin is the agent of choice for *Listeria* infection. In vitro studies have demonstrated synergy against *L. monocytogenes* when combining either ampicillin or penicillin with an aminoglycoside. None of the cephalosporins are significantly active against *L. monocytogenes*. Coagulase-negative staphylococci and *Corynebacterium* frequently infect indwelling vascular catheters. Although there has been general satisfaction with the use of such catheters that minimize the need for frequent venipunctures, there are significant hazards for infection with organisms such as *Corynebacterium*, coagulase-negative staphylococci, gram-negative rods, and *Candida* spp. Vancomycin is the most effective agent for infections with coagulase-negative staphylococci, which, when found in association with vascular catheter infection or hospitalization, are nearly uniformly methicillin resistant. Trimethoprim-sulfamethoxazole (TMP-SMZ) is the agent of choice for the initial therapy of the patient with *P. carinii* pneumonia. Additionally, TMP-SMZ is a broad-spectrum antibacterial agent with significant activity against other important pathogens, including *L. monocytogenes*, *Nocardia asteroides*, and *Stenotrophomonas maltophilia*. The response of an interstitial pneumonia to TMP-SMZ is not diagnostic of *Pneumocystis* infection because of the broad antibacterial spectrum of the drug combination. Combinations of antipseudomonal fluoroquinolones (e.g., ciprofloxacin) given parenterally with an antipseudomonal β-lactam may represent an alternative to aminoglycoside-containing regimens. Azithromycin and levofloxacin are now recommended as preferred agents for patients with legionnaires' disease.[62, 63] Although it should never be used alone, the addition of rifampin is advised for the treatment of legionnaires' disease in severely ill or immunocompromised patients, especially if the primary therapy is not with azithromycin or a fluoroquinolone.[63]

In the seriously ill patient with infection, no clinician should assume that a standard recommended dosage of antimicrobial agents can be relied on to achieve therapeutic levels. This is particularly true with the aminoglycosides, in which there is a narrow range between therapeutic and toxic levels. In our experience, many patients receive doses of aminoglycosides that are too low, and this situation has been associated with therapeutic failure. With the ready availability of assay techniques, aminoglycoside blood levels should be measured at frequent intervals (such as two to three times per week initially) in critically ill patients with septicemia resulting from gram-negative rods.

There has been considerable interest in the use of once-daily dosing of aminoglycosides. Several meta-analyses have shown that such therapy is equally effective and no more toxic than the traditional every-8-hour dosing of these antimicrobials.[64] This dosing scheme offers the potential advantage of ensuring that all patients achieve a therapeutic aminoglycoside serum concentration with the first administered dose. Although concerns have been raised regarding the efficacy of once-daily aminoglycoside therapy for neutropenic patients, several analyses have found no diminution of the effectiveness of such therapy in this setting.[65, 66]

Another issue that is widely discussed is the advisability of changing antibiotic therapy once a specific pathogen has been isolated. For instance, if a highly susceptible *E. coli* is isolated from blood cultures, there is the question of whether or not therapy with expensive agents, such as piperacillin or imipenem, should be replaced by ampicillin, with or without an aminoglycoside. Our experience has been that in patients who are not markedly neutropenic, the use of one effective agent gives results that are similar to the use of two or more antimicrobials.[67] In the high-risk neutropenic patient, however, we would continue dual-drug coverage of a serious bacteremic infection resulting from gram-negative rods if the total neutrophil count remained less than 500/μL.

**Antifungal Therapy.** Perhaps the most challenging therapeutic area related to infections in cancer patients is antifungal chemotherapy. This challenge is compounded by the fact that the diagnosis of systemic fungal disease in the cancer patient is often difficult to establish. Organisms such as *Candida* spp., which are the most common opportunistic fungal pathogens, readily colonize mucosal surfaces. It is difficult, if not impossible, on clinical grounds to distinguish colonization from systemic disease. *Candida* esophagitis refractory to topical nystatin or orally administered azoles (e.g., fluconazole, itraconazole, ketoconazole) may require systemic doses of amphotericin B. Similarly, in patients from whom yeasts are repeatedly cultured from multiple sites, such as from the oropharynx and the stool, or in patients who do not have a urinary catheter but have repeated isolations of yeast from the urine, the diagnosis of systemic candidiasis should be strongly suspected. Although robust data support the treatment of *C. albicans* bloodstream infections with either fluconazole or amphotericin B,[68] there are insufficient data on which to recommend the use of fluconazole for treatment of presumed or proven *Candida* infections in neutropenic patients.[69, 70] Amphotericin B should be considered the first-line antifungal agent when infection by azole-resis-

tant *Candida* spp. (e.g., *C. krusei*) is identified or strongly suspected.[71]

Other fungal infections that occur sufficiently often for comment include mucormycosis, aspergillosis, and reactivated mycotic infections, such as histoplasmosis and coccidioidomycosis. Aspergillosis is initially a lung infection that can spread systemically (particularly to the brain); it is characterized by necrotizing vasculitis and a proclivity to lung infarction and cavitation. The development of cavitary pulmonary infiltrates in patients receiving broad-spectrum antibacterial agents is strongly suggestive of aspergillosis or mucormycosis.[72, 73] Such situations justify the initiation of amphotericin B therapy, even without confirmatory cultures.

A major dilemma is the management of the patient who is neutropenic and receiving immunosuppressive anticancer therapy but in whom there are no clues (e.g., positive blood cultures) to the cause of persistent fever. Two randomized studies support the concept that patients who do not respond to an initial broad-spectrum antibacterial regimen should receive empirical amphotericin B. In these studies, patients who received broad-spectrum antibiotics as well as amphotericin B seemed to defervesce more rapidly and develop significantly fewer opportunistic fungal infections than did those who continued to receive broad-spectrum antibiotics alone.[74, 75] Of note, patients randomized to discontinue systemic antibiotics developed a high incidence of shock or rebound bacterial infections.[74]

Although the results are consistent with our own experience, there are problems with using a rigid formula for starting empirical antifungal therapy in patients who do not respond to antibacterial agents. Our policy has been to observe a patient taking systemic antibacterial treatment for 5 to 7 days. This is approximately the median time required for defervescence in clinical trials of antimicrobial therapy for neutropenic fever.[29] If the patient defervesces, we generally (1) treat for a conventional period if a causative organism is identified or (2) stop systemic antimicrobials in 3 to 7 days following defervescence and resolution of clinical signs of infection, even if no pathogen is isolated. More prolonged therapy should be considered for patients who have prolonged, severe neutropenia; extensive mucositis; or skin ulceration. Before the initiation of treatment with amphotericin B, it is essential that the patient be critically reassessed to rule out the presence of nonfungal infection. This reappraisal should include a review of all previous culture results; a review of the adequacy of serum concentrations of antibiotics, especially aminoglycosides; a careful physical examination; evaluation of all vascular catheters and other invasive devices; reculture of blood and specific sites of infection; chest radiographs; and careful diagnostic imaging of any anatomic region, such as the abdomen or sinus, suspected of harboring infection. Additional studies may be performed to identify relatively infrequent causes of fever, such as infection with *T. gondii*, herpesviruses, enteric protozoa, mycobacteria, and *Chlamydia* spp., as suggested by the clinical setting.

If the patient is febrile and persistently neutropenic, we consider the initiation of empirical amphotericin B after 7 febrile days. The interval before the initiation of amphotericin B might be prolonged, however, if there is a good reason to suspect other causes of persistent fevers, if the patient's neutrophil count exceeds 500/μL, or if the white blood cell count is slowly rising. Conversely, the 7-day period might be shortened or empirical amphotericin B initiated more rapidly if there are strong clues to an underlying systemic fungal infection, such as (1) the isolation of *Candida* spp. from urine in a patient without a Foley catheter, (2) the documentation of lung infiltrates increasing or progressing in the face of broad-spectrum antibacterial coverage, or (3) the appearance of eye lesions consistent with *Candida* endophthalmitis, which is an unusual occurrence in the markedly neutropenic patient. More detailed discussions regarding the timing of empirical antifungal therapy and the duration of antimicrobial therapy in general have been published elsewhere[29] and are summarized in Table 20–3.

The availability of the new azole antifungal agents has provided important new therapeutic options. Although fluconazole and itraconazole inhibit medically important yeasts, such as *Candida* spp., *Cryptococcus* spp., and *Coccidioides immitis*, only itraconazole has clinically important activity against *Histoplasma capsulatum*, *Blastomyces dermatitidis* and, to a lesser extent, *Aspergillus*. These agents also have the advantage of oral administration. Although studies primarily performed in AIDS patients demonstrate the efficacy of fluconazole in treating esophageal candidiasis (100 mg/day) and in the therapy of cryptococcal meningitis (400 mg/day), amphotericin B, with or without concomitant flucytosine, remains the preferred treatment for most patients with cryptococcal meningitis.[76] There may be an advantage to combining an agent such as fluconazole with flucytosine, providing rapid antiyeast therapy with two oral agents. Some centers where fluconazole has been used extensively have observed the emergence of infection by fluconazole-resistant isolates of *Candida* (primarily *C. krusei*, although resistant *C. glabrata* and *C. albicans* have also been reported).[71, 77, 78]

Renal failure is a worrisome aspect of conventional amphotericin B therapy. Fluconazole therapy is a less nephrotoxic alternative to amphotericin B, but, as noted, its use is often limited in the presence of azole-resistant molds and fluconazole-resistant yeasts. Studies have demonstrated the usefulness of new formulations of amphotericin (e.g., amphotericin B lipid complex [ABLC, Abelcet], amphotericin B colloidal dispersion [ABCD, Amphotec], and liposomal amphotericin [AmBisome]) in treating invasive fungal infections (e.g., aspergillosis, candidiasis, cryptococcal meningitis, mucormycosis, fusariosis), owing to the lower rate of associated nephrotoxicity, febrile reactions, and cardiorespiratory complications compared with conventional amphotericin B formulated in deoxycholate.[79, 80] To date, however, none of these formulations has demonstrated superiority over conventional amphotericin B in treating documented fungal infections, and until further studies become available, the use of the new formulations of amphotericin (which are substantially more expensive than traditional amphotericin) should be restricted for patients who are intolerant or refractory to conventional amphotericin B.[79]

**Antiviral Therapy.** Progress has been made in the chemotherapy of viral infections.[81, 82] Acyclovir, famciclovir, and valacyclovir are clinically effective in the treatment of herpes simplex and varicella-zoster infections and have largely replaced the use of adenine arabinoside.[83] Famciclovir and valacyclovir offer the advantage of being somewhat better absorbed by the gastrointestinal tract than is acyclovir. Ganciclovir, foscarnet, and cidofovir are active against cytomegalovirus. The latter two agents, in contrast to ganciclovir, which is active only against acyclovir-susceptible herpes simplex virus and varicella-zoster virus isolates, are also active against acyclovir-resistant isolates. All these agents have significant toxicity: The toxicity of ganciclovir is primarily suppression of myelopoiesis, whereas foscarnet and cidofovir can cause profound electrolyte abnormalities and renal failure. The combination of antiviral chemotherapy plus high-titered cytomegalovirus immune globulin may improve survival in selected patients with cytomegalovirus pneumonia.[84]

Infection resulting from respiratory syncytial virus may be treated with ribavirin. Also, rimantadine and amantidine are efficacious against influenza A infections when administered within the first few days of infection.

## PREVENTIVE MEASURES

**Laminar Airflow Units.** Susceptibility to infection varies widely among patients who are receiving chemotherapy, but the group at highest risk consists of individuals with hematologic malignancies who are rendered neutropenic by additional chemotherapy or radiation, or both. Many efforts have been directed at minimizing the exposure of high-risk patients to important pathogens. Over the years, these efforts have taken several forms, but that which has received the greatest attention (and correspondingly has represented the greatest investment in hospital facilities) has been the so-called protective environment with laminar airflow or high-efficiency particulate air filtration. The basic unit is designed to isolate a single patient from all direct contact and consistently provide a unidirectional flow of sterile, filtered air. The air is essentially *germ free*, but the problem of infection from other routes persists.

Although a number of studies have attested to the effectiveness of the laminar airflow unit in reducing infection, some issues obscure the evaluation of their ultimate efficacy.[85] They are expensive to build and maintain, and a strong argument has been raised that they are not cost-effective. The reason why patients managed in protected environments have fewer infections is still debatable. Most patients who have been managed in laminar airflow rooms have also received prophylactic oral antimicrobials that (1) suppress the endogenous fecal flora or (2) kill or inhibit organisms that may be acquired and colonize the gastrointestinal tract. The excellent filtering capacity of most laminar airflow systems appears to account for the absence of *Aspergillus* infection in patients managed for the duration of chemotherapy in such units. The use of laminar airflow per se would be expected to have little impact on gram-negative infections originating from the gastrointestinal tract. As demonstrated by Schimpff and collaborators,[85] administration of oral nonabsorbable antibiotics with antipseudomonal activity to neutropenic patients in a nonisolation setting has been associated with almost as much reduction of infection and comparable leukemia remission rates as observed in patients managed in laminar airflow units who also were given oral nonabsorbable antibiotics.

**Antibiotic Regimens.** Prevention of infection by administering prophylactic antibiotics may be useful for selected cancer patients. TMP-SMZ is the most effective agent for preventing *P. carinii* pneumonia and should be considered for patients at high risk for *P. carinii* pneumonia (e.g., prolonged use of high doses of corticosteroids, acute lymphocytic leukemia, AIDS). Although TMP-SMZ also has antimicrobial activity against several gram-positive and gram-negative bacteria, no study has demonstrated improved survival with prophylactic use of TMP-SMZ.[29] Rapid emergence of resistance has been observed in some settings, and the overall reduction of infection shown in two studies was partially offset by the number of resistant infections in patients who received TMP-SMZ prophylaxis.[86, 87]

Toxicity from TMP-SMZ and emergence of resistant organisms remain a concern and have prompted the study of alternative prophylactic agents, particularly those that might have better antipseudomonal activity. Norfloxacin, ciprofloxacin, and ofloxacin have been used with success in controlled studies of bacterial infection in neutropenic patients and have demonstrated delays in the appearance of fever and in some studies significant reductions in gram-negative bacillary infections. Studies comparing the prophylactic use of quinolones (ofloxacin or ciprofloxacin) versus TMP-SMZ have demonstrated that quinolone prophylaxis is more effective in decreasing the incidence of gram-negative bacillary infections in afebrile neutropenic patients. The overall use of systemic antibiotics in cancer patients, however, does not appear to be obviated by prophylactic quinolones; there has been little evidence to show that these agents decrease the duration of hospitalization, decrease systemic antimicrobial use, permit use of larger doses of anticancer agents, or improve survival, and in contrast to TMP-SMZ, quinolones cannot be used for prophylaxis against *Pneumocystis* infection. Quinolone prophylaxis has resulted in the development of quinolone-resistant gram-negative bacilli. For these reasons, routine use of quinolone prophylaxis is controversial.[29, 52, 53] Because many of the quinolones lack activity against gram-positive pathogens, several trials have evaluated the utility of adding agents with activity against these microorganisms to the prophylactic regimen. Even in these circumstances, meta-analyses have failed to demonstrate convincing clinical benefit.[52]

Regarding antifungal prophylaxis, although oral fluconazole appears to reduce the incidence of invasive and noninvasive fungal disease in bone marrow transplant patients, only superficial infections are prevented in patients with leukemia per se.[88–90] Routine use of fluconazole has also been associated with increased colonization of fluconazole-resistant organisms, including *C. krusei* and some strains of *C. glabrata*. Fluconazole has no activity against molds, in contrast to itraconazole, which has demonstrated activity against *Aspergillus* spp. Prophylaxis with itraconazole has not demonstrated a decrease in *Aspergillus* infections.[91] Routine prophylaxis with antifungal agents is not recommended for cancer patients.[29] Prophylaxis with low doses of intraluminal vancomycin has demonstrated benefit in preventing gram-positive catheter infections. Because of the concern for increasing microbial resistance against vancomycin, however, routine use of vancomycin prophylaxis is not recommended.[29, 51]

Although consideration of antimicrobial prophylaxis is warranted in certain situations, the final decision requires careful consideration of the proven benefits of the prophylactic regimen, the issues relating to side effects and drug interactions, and the potential development of antimicrobial resistance. One exception, in which antimicrobial prophylaxis is effective, regards the prophylaxis of tuberculosis. Purified protein derivative skin testing is warranted before initiation of immunosuppressive therapy for patients with epidemiologic risk factors for exposure to tuberculosis. Patients with positive tuberculin skin tests should receive isoniazid (INH) prophylaxis.[92]

**Immunization.** The response to vaccines is diminished in cancer patients. Nevertheless, the Advisory Committee on Immunization Practices has recommended that patients who require immunosuppressive chemotherapy (including corticosteroids), organ or bone marrow transplant patients, and patients with leukemia, lymphoma (e.g., Hodgkin's), multiple myeloma, or metastatic cancer receive the pneumococcal and the influenza vaccine.[93, 94] Vaccination should be administered before chemotherapy. Cancer patients who undergo scheduled splenectomy should receive the pneumococcal vaccine before removal of the spleen. Tetanus-diphtheria (Td) vaccination is also recommended for patients with or without cancer. This vaccine should be routinely given every 10 years. Immunization with live viruses, as a general rule, should not be administered during chemotherapy. Use of gamma globulin to bolster humoral antibody levels has not been successful, and active immunization with pneumococcal and pseudomonal antigens has proved disappointing.

**Granulocyte Transfusions.** An approach to reducing the risk of bacterial infection is to augment host defenses through the use of granulocyte transfusions. For many years, an argument for granulocyte transfusions was the belief that any increment in the functional leukocyte pool might be beneficial to the host. The early belief that patients who were neutropenic did not recover unless they received granulocytes, however, was not supported by studies of aggressive antimicrobial therapy in neutropenic patients.[95] Even in studies claiming a benefit from transfused granulocytes, there was no difference in survival rates between the transfused and the control groups when analyzed 3 to 4 weeks after entry into the study.[96, 97] Although investigators were initially enthusiastic about this approach, the use of prophylactic transfusions on a daily basis is not only exceedingly expensive, but also carries serious additional risks and fails to affect survival. No one seriously questions the role of granulocytes in human host defenses, but the quantity of therapeutic granulocytes delivered via transfusions cannot possibly approach that which the normal host can make for himself or herself in the presence of a serious infection.[98] Our present policy is to reserve therapeutic granulocyte transfusions for patients with documented infection who do not respond to appropriate antibacterial therapy and colony-stimulating factors.[29, 99]

**Colony-Stimulating Factors.** The use of granulocyte colony–stimulating factor and granulocyte-macrophage colony-stimulating factor has largely supplanted therapeutic granulocyte transfusions for patients with persistent fever and refractory documented bacterial infections. There is little question that the use of these factors significantly raises the circulating neutrophil count, but there have been some questions about the quality of cells stimulated in this manner. Some clinical studies have shown the definite benefit in terms of decreased duration of neutropenia, decreased episodes of fever, decreased use of systemic antibiotics, and decreased hospitalization.[100] Convincing and consistent evidence that the use of these colony-stimulating factors improves survival or overall results in the treatment of cancer (i.e., improved remission rates, improved overall response rates, or decreased infectious mortality in patients with established infections) is still lacking, however.[29, 101]

Recommendations from the American Society of Clinical Oncology stipulate that colony-stimulating factors should not be routinely used for the primary (before chemotherapy) or secondary (after chemotherapy) prophylaxis of neutropenia-associated episodes of fever or infection.[102] These guidelines also do not call for the routine use of colony-stimulating factors as adjuncts to treatment for the febrile neutropenic patient. The guidelines, however, acknowledge certain situations in which use of colony-stimulating factors may be of benefit, although meager evidence currently exists to support these indications, such as administering colony-stimulating factors together with antibiotics for patients with features predictive of clinical deterioration (e.g., sepsis, fungal infection, severe pneumonia).

## MANAGEMENT OF VASCULAR CATHETERS

Another subject that is frequently debated relates to the usage of long-term indwelling vascular catheters for hyperalimentation and intravenous therapy. Serious infections related to such indwelling catheters are now a common experience, including cases of bacterial and fungal endocarditis.

It cannot be assumed that bacteremia in a patient with an indwelling vascular catheter arises from the catheter or that the catheter becomes a source of secondary infection. Other peripheral blood cultures should be drawn to confirm the bacteremia as well as samples of blood drawn through the catheter. Appropriate systemic antibiotic therapy should be started, and in most cases empirical therapy should be administered if the patient develops high fever.

If the organism isolated from a suspected catheter infection is a coagulase-negative *Staphylococcus* (e.g., *S. epidermidis*) or *Corynebacterium*, our policy is to attempt to suppress the infection with the best available antimicrobial therapy. This therapy usually includes the addition of vancomycin and possibly concomitant therapy with rifampin if supported by in vitro studies. Care must be taken to infuse antibiotic through the various channels of the indwelling vascular catheter. Even with initially successful therapy, 20% of these infections may recur.[103] As a rule, simple exit site infections can be managed without removal of the catheter, whereas tunnel infections invariably require removal, especially if *Pseudomonas aeruginosa* is recovered. Port pocket infections as seen with completely implanted catheters are usually due to *S. aureus* and require removal of the device.[104]

As well as being determined by the presence of local complications of infection (e.g., tunnel infection, septic thrombophlebitis), the urgency of removal of an infected long-term central catheter is determined by the identity of the infecting microorganism. For locally uncomplicated infections with low virulence microorganisms, a patient might continue to receive cancer treatment while the catheter-associated infection is suppressed. If fever and bacteremia persist in the face of suppressive therapy, the only choice is to remove the catheter. Treatment of catheter-related bacter-

emias resulting from *S. aureus* or fungi is often unsuccessful, however, without removal of the indwelling device. A prospective interventional study has demonstrated that failure to remove *S. aureus*–infected intravascular devices substantially increases the risk of relapse or death.[105] Observational studies have demonstrated that retaining an infected catheter in the setting of fungemia is associated with a poorer outcome.[106, 107] As a general rule, in catheter-related bacteremias resulting from highly virulent pathogens, such as *S. aureus* or fungi, the best course is to remove the catheter as soon as feasible. Although catheter-related bacteremias resulting from gram-negative rods are similarly difficult to treat without catheter removal, most gram-negative bacteremias do not involve the catheter.[108, 109] Finally, although catheter-related bacteremia resulting from atypical mycobacteria is rare, such infections require removal of the catheter.

## SUGGESTIONS FOR ADDITIONAL READING

Rubin RH, Young LS. Clinical approach to infections in the compromised host. 3rd ed. New York: Plenum, 1994. *This is the largest published book that deals specifically with management of immunocompromised hosts.*

Pizzo PA. Drug therapy: management of fever in patients with cancer and treatment-induced neutropenia. N Engl J Med 1993;328:1323–32. *This is an excellent review from the viewpoint of a pediatric oncologist.*

Hughes WT, Armstrong D, Bodey GP, et al. 1997 guidelines for the use of antimicrobial agents in neutropenic patients with unexplained fever. Infectious Diseases Society of America. Clin Infect Dis 1997;25:551–73. *This is a comprehensive literature review of prophylactic and empirical antimicrobial therapy with specific algorithms for clinical situations. Some guidelines are provided for the choice of antimicrobial agents and for the organization and analysis of clinical studies of antimicrobial agents in the febrile neutropenic patient.*

Brown AE, White MH. Controversies in the management of infections in immunocompromised patients. Clin Infect Dis 1993;17:Suppl 2:S317–551. *This Memorial Sloan-Kettering Cancer Center symposium issue addresses virtually all the controversies that surround the infectious disease management of immunosuppressed patients.*

## REFERENCES

1. Rubin RH, Young LS. Clinical approach to infection in the compromised host. 3rd ed. New York: Plenum, 1994.
2. Young LS. Nosocomial infections in the immunocompromised adult. Am J Med 1981;70:398–404.
3. Morrison VA. The infectious complications of chronic lymphocytic leukemia. Semin Oncol 1998;25:98–106.
4. Pitout JDD, Sanders CC, Sanders WE Jr. Antimicrobial resistance with focus on β-lactam resistance in gram-negative bacilli. Am J Med 1997;103:51–9.
5. CDC. Interim guidelines for prevention and control of staphylococcal infection associated with reduced susceptibility to vancomycin. MMWR Morb Mortal Wkly Rep 1997;46:626–30.
6. Smith TL, Pearson ML, Wilcox KR, et al. Emergence of vancomycin resistance in *Staphylococcus aureus*. N Engl J Med 1999;340:493–501.
7. Sieradzki K, Roberts RB, Haber SW, Tomasz A. The development of vancomycin resistance in a patient with methicillin-resistant *Staphylococcus aureus* infection. N Engl J Med 1999;340:517–23.
8. Rhame FS. The inanimate environment. In: Bennett JV, Brachman PS, eds. Hospital infections. 4th ed. Philadelphia: Lippincott-Raven, 1998:299–324.
9. Greene JN. Catheter-related complications of cancer therapy. Infect Dis Clin North Am 1996;10:255–95.
10. Meuwissen JH, Tauber I, Leeuwenberg AD, et al. Parasitologic and serologic observations of infection with *Pneumocystis* in humans. J Infect Dis 1977;136:43–9.

11. Klein RS, Catalano MT, Edberg SC, et al. *Streptococcus bovis* septicemia and carcinoma of the colon. Ann Intern Med 1979;560–2.
12. Koransky JR, Stargel MD, Dowell VRJ. *Clostridium septicum* bacteremia: its clinical significance. Am J Med 1979;66:63–6.
13. Whitecar JP Jr, Luna M, Bodey GP. *Pseudomonas* bacteremia in patients with malignant diseases. Am J Med Sci 1970;260:216–23.
14. Vartivarian SE, Papadakis KA, Palacios JA, et al. Mucocutaneous and soft tissue infections caused by *Xanthomonas maltophilia*: a new spectrum. Ann Intern Med 1994;121:969–73.
15. Shapiro RL, Altekruse S, Hutwagner L, et al. The role of Gulf Coast oysters harvested in warmer months in *Vibrio vulnificus* infections in the United States, 1988–1996. J Infect Dis 1998;178:752–9.
16. Gallagher JG, Merigan TC. Prolonged herpes-zoster infection associated with immunosuppressive therapy. Ann Intern Med 1979; 91:842–6.
17. Sepkowitz KA, Brown AE, Armstrong D. *Pneumocystis carinii* pneumonia without acquired immunodeficiency syndrome: more patients, same risk. Arch Intern Med 1995;155:1125–8.
18. Stout JE, Yu VL. Legionellosis. N Engl J Med 1997;337:682–7.
19. Meyers JD, Hackman RC, Stamm WE. *Chlamydia trachomatis* infection as a cause of pneumonia after human marrow transplantation. Transplantation 1983;36:130–4.
20. Chernik NL, Armstrong D, Posner JB. Central nervous system infections in patients with cancer. Medicine (Baltimore) 1973;52:563–81.
21. Israelski D, Remington J. Toxoplasmosis in the non-AIDS immunocompromised host. In: Remington J, Schwartz M, eds. Current clinical topics in infectious diseases. Vol. 13. Boston, Mass.: Blackwell Scientific Publications, 1993:322–56.
22. DeMaio J, Bartlett JG. Update on diagnosis of *Clostridium difficile*–associated diarrhea. Curr Clin Top Infect Dis 1995;15:97–114.
23. Roghmann MC, McCarter RJJ, Brewrink J, et al. *Clostridium difficile* infection is a risk factor for bacteremia due to vancomycin-resistant enterococci (VRE) in VRE-colonized patients with acute leukemia. Clin Infect Dis 1997;1056–99.
24. Yolken RH, Bishop CA, Townsend TR, et al. Infectious gastroenteritis in bone-marrow-transplant recipients. N Engl J Med 1982;306:1010–2.
25. Alpern RJ, Dowell VRJ. *Clostridium septicum* infections and malignancy. JAMA 1969;209:385–8.
26. Wade DS, Nava HR, Douglass HOJ. Neutropenic enterocolitis: clinical diagnosis and treatment. Cancer 1992;69:17–23.
27. Song HK, Kreisel D, Canter R, et al. Changing presentation and management of neutropenic enterocolitis. Arch Surg 1998;133:979–82.
28. Gomez L, Martino R, Rolston KV. Neutropenic enterocolitis: spectrum of the disease and comparison of definite and possible cases. Clin Infect Dis 1998;27:695–9.
29. Hughes WT, Armstrong D, Bodey GP, et al. 1997 guidelines for the use of antimicrobial agents in neutropenic patients with unexplained fever. Clin Infect Dis 1997;25:551–73.
30. Venkatesan P, Gladman J, Macfarlane JT, et al. A hospital study of community acquired pneumonia in the elderly. Thorax 1990;45:254–8.
31. Shelhamer JH, Toews GB, Masur H, et al. Respiratory disease in the immunosuppressed patient. Ann Intern Med 1992;117:415–31.
32. Kahn FW, Jones JM. Analysis of bronchoalveolar lavage specimens from immunocompromised patients with a protocol applicable in the microbiology laboratory. J Clin Microbiol 1988;26:1150–1.
33. Wolfson JS, Sober AJ, Rubin RH. Dermatologic manifestations of infection in the compromised host. Ann Rev Med 1983;34:205–17.
34. Walsh TJ, Merz WG, Lee JW, et al. Diagnosis and therapeutic monitoring of invasive candidiasis by rapid enzymatic detection of serum D-arabinitol. Am J Med 1995;99:164–72.
35. Christensson B, Wiebe T, Pehrson C, Larsson L. Diagnosis of invasive candidiasis in neutropenic children with cancer by determination of D-arabinitol/L-arabinitol ratios in urine. J Clin Microbiol 1997;35:636–40.
36. Reiss E, Morrison CJ. Nonculture methods for diagnosis of disseminated candidiasis. Clin Microbiol Rev 1993;6:311–23.
37. The International Antimicrobial Therapy Cooperative Group of the European Organization for Research and Treatment of Cancer. Efficacy and toxicity of single daily doses of amikacin and ceftriaxone versus multiple daily doses of amikacin and ceftazidime for infection in patients with cancer and granulocytopenia. Ann Intern Med 1993;119:584–93.
38. Young LS, Meyer-Dudnik PV, Hindler J, Martin WJ. Aminoglycosides in the treatment of bacteraemic infections in the immuno-compromised host. J Antimicrob Chemother 1981;8:Suppl A:121–32.

39. Shenep JL, Hughes WT, Roberson PK, et al. Vancomycin, ticarcillin, and amikacin compared with ticarcillin-clavulanate and amikacin in the empirical treatment of febrile, neutropenic children with cancer. N Engl J Med 1988;319:1053–8.
40. Young LS. Double beta-lactam therapy in the immunocompromised host. J Antimicrob Chemother 1985;16:4–6.
41. De Jongh CA, Joshi JH, Thompson BW, et al. A double beta-lactam combination versus an aminoglycoside-containing regimen as empiric antibiotic therapy for febrile granulocytopenic cancer patients. Am J Med 1986;80:101–11.
42. Winston DJ, Ho WG, Bruckner DA, Champlin RE. Beta-lactam antibiotic therapy in febrile granulocytopenic patients: a randomized trial comparing cefoperazone plus piperacillin, ceftazidime plus piperacillin, and imipenem alone. Ann Intern Med 1991;115:849–59.
43. Elting LS, Rubenstein EB, Rolston KV, Bodey GP. Outcomes of bacteremia in patients with cancer and neutropenia: observations from two decades of epidemiological and clinical trials. Clin Infect Dis 1997;25:247–59.
44. Rolston KV, Berkey P, Bodey GP, et al. A comparison of imipenem to ceftazidime with or without amikacin as empiric therapy in febrile neutropenic patients. Arch Intern Med 1992;152:283–91.
45. Pizzo PA, Hathorn JW, Hiemenz J, et al. A randomized trial comparing ceftazidime alone with combination antibiotic therapy in cancer patients with fever and neutropenia. N Engl J Med 1986;315:552–8.
46. De Pauw BE, Deresinski SC, Feld R, et al. The Intercontinental Antimicrobial Study Group. Ceftazidime compared with piperacillin and tobramycin for the empiric treatment of fever in neutropenic patients with cancer: a multicenter randomized trial. Ann Intern Med 1994;120:834–44.
47. Biron P, Fuhrmann C, Cure H, et al. Cefepime versus imipenem-cilastatin as empirical monotherapy in 400 febrile patients with short duration neutropenia. J Antimicrob Chemother 1998;42:511–8.
48. Cometta A, Calandra T, Gaya H, et al. Monotherapy with meropenem versus combination therapy with ceftazidime plus amikacin as empiric therapy for fever in granulocytopenic patients with cancer. Antimicrob Agents Chemother 1996;40:1108–15.
49. Chow JW, Fine MJ, Shlaes DM, et al. *Enterobacter* bacteremia: clinical features and emergence of resistance during therapy. Ann Intern Med 1991;115:585–90.
50. EORTC International Antimicrobial Therapy Cooperative Group and the National Cancer Institute of Canada—Clinic Trials Group. Vancomycin added to empirical combination antibiotic therapy for fever in granulocytopenic cancer patients. J Infect Dis 1991;163:951–8.
51. Hospital Infection Control Practices Advisory Committee (HICPAC). Recommendations for preventing the spread of vancomycin resistance. Infect Control Hosp Epidemiol 1995;16:105–13.
52. Cruciani M, Rampazzo R, Malena M, et al. Prophylaxis with fluoroquinolones for bacterial infections in neutropenic patients: a meta-analysis. Clin Infect Dis 1996;23:795–805.
53. Engels EA, Lau J, Barza M. Efficacy of quinolone prophylaxis in neutropenic cancer patients: a meta-analysis. J Clin Oncol 1998;16:1179–87.
54. Schimpff SC. Empiric antibiotic therapy for granulocytopenic cancer patients. Am J Med 1986;80:Suppl 5C:13–20.
55. Talcott JA, Finberg R, Mayer RJ, Goldman L. The medical course of cancer patients with fever and neutropenia: clinical identification of a low-risk subgroup at presentation. Arch Intern Med 1988;148:2561–8.
56. Rubin M, Hathorn JW, Pizzo PA. Controversies in the management of febrile neutropenic cancer patients. Cancer Invest 1988;6:167–84.
57. Talcott JA, Siegel RD, Finberg R, Goldman L. Risk assessment in cancer patients with fever and neutropenia: a prospective, two-center validation of a prediction rule. J Clin Oncol 1992;10:316–22.
58. Rubenstein EB, Rolston K, Benjamin RS, et al. Outpatient treatment of febrile episodes in low-risk neutropenic patients with cancer. Cancer. 1993;71:3640–6.
59. Talcott JA, Whalen A, Clark J, et al. Home antibiotic therapy for low-risk cancer patients with fever and neutropenia: a pilot study of 30 patients based on a validated prediction rule. J Clin Oncol 1994;12:107–14.
60. Malik IA, Khan WA, Karim M, et al. Feasibility of outpatient management of fever in cancer patients with low-risk neutropenia: results of a prospective randomized trial. Am J Med 1995;98:224–31.
61. Rolston KV, Rubenstein EB, Freifeld A. Early empiric antibiotic therapy for febrile neutropenia patients at low risk. Infect Dis Clin North Am 1996;10:223–37.

62. Edelstein PH. Antimicrobial chemotherapy for Legionnaires' disease: a review. Clin Infect Dis 1995;21:S265–76.

63. Edelstein PH. Antimicrobial chemotherapy for Legionnaires disease: time for a change. Ann Intern Med 1998;129:328–30.

64. Ali MZ, Goetz MB. A meta-analysis of the relative efficacy and toxicity of single daily dosing versus multiple daily dosing of aminoglycosides. Clin Infect Dis 1997;24:796–809.

65. Barza M, Ioannidis JP, Cappelleri JC, Lau J. Single or multiple daily doses of aminoglycosides: a meta-analysis. Br Med J 1996;312:338–45.

66. Hatala R, Dinh TT, Cook DJ. Single daily dosing of aminoglycosides in immunocompromised adults: a systematic review. Clin Infect Dis 1997;24:810–5.

67. Anderson ET, Young LS, Hewitt WL. Antimicrobial synergism in the therapy of gram-negative rod bacteremia. Chemotherapy 1978;24:45–54.

68. Rex JH, Bennett JE, Sugar AM, et al. A randomized trial comparing fluconazole with amphotericin B for the treatment of candidemia in patients without neutropenia. N Engl J Med 1994;331:1325–30.

69. Anaissie EJ, Vartivarian SE, Abi-Said D, et al. Fluconazole versus amphotericin B in the treatment of hematogenous candidiasis: a matched cohort study. Am J Med 1996;101:170–6.

70. Viscoli C, Castagnola E, Van Lint MT, et al. Fluconazole versus amphotericin B as empirical antifungal therapy of unexplained fever in granulocytopenic cancer patients: a pragmatic, multicentre, prospective and randomised clinical trial. Eur J Cancer 1996;32A:814–20.

71. Wingard JR, Merz WG, Rinaldi MG, et al. Increase in *Candida krusei* infection among patients with bone marrow transplantation and neutropenia treated prophylactically with fluconazole. N Engl J Med 1991;325:1274–7.

72. Meyer RD, Young LS, Armstrong D, Yu B. Aspergillosis complicating neoplastic disease. Am J Med 1973;54:6–15.

73. Meyer RD, Rosen P, Armstrong D. Phycomycosis complicating leukemia and lymphoma. Ann Intern Med 1972;77:871–9.

74. Pizzo PA, Robichaud KJ, Gill FA, Witebsky FG. Empiric antibiotic and antifungal therapy for cancer patients with prolonged fever and granulocytopenia. Am J Med 1982;72:101–11.

75. EORTC International Antimicrobial Therapy Cooperative Group. Empiric antifungal therapy in febrile granulocytopenic patients. Am J Med 1989;86:668–72.

76. van der Horst CM, Saag MS, Cloud GA, et al. Treatment of cryptococcal meningitis associated with the acquired immunodeficiency syndrome. N Engl J Med 1997;337:15–21.

77. Boschman CR, Bodnar UR, Tornatore MA, et al. Thirteen-year evolution of azole resistance in yeast isolates and prevalence of resistant strains carried by cancer patients at a large medical center. Antimicrob Agents Chemother 1998;42:734–8.

78. Pfaller MA, Jones RN, Messer SA, et al. National surveillance of nosocomial blood stream infection due to *Candida albicans*: frequency of occurrence and antifungal susceptibility in the SCOPE Program. Diagn Microbiol Infect Dis 1998;31:327–32.

79. Wong-Beringer A, Jacobs RA, Guglielmo BJ. Lipid formulations of amphotericin B: clinical efficacy and toxicities. Clin Infect Dis 1998;27:603–18.

80. Walsh TJ, Finberg RW, Arndt C, et al. Liposomal amphotericin B for empirical therapy in patients with persistent fever and neutropenia. N Engl J Med 1999;340:764–71.

81. Hirsch MS, Schooley RT. Drug therapy: treatment of herpesvirus infections. N Engl J Med 1983;309:963–70.

82. Whitley RJ. Viral encephalitis. N Engl J Med 1990;323:242–50.

83. Whitley RJ, Lakeman F. Herpes simplex virus infections of the central nervous system: therapeutic and diagnostic considerations. Clin Infect Dis 1995;20:414–20.

84. Snydman DR. Cytomegalovirus immunoglobulins in the prevention and treatment of cytomegalovirus disease. Rev Infect Dis 1990;12:Suppl 7:S839–48.

85. Schimpff SC, Greene WH, Young VM, et al. Infection prevention in acute nonlymphocytic leukemia: laminar air flow room reverse isolation with oral, nonabsorbable antibiotic prophylaxis. Ann Intern Med 1975;82:351–8.

86. Dekker AW, Rozenberg-Arska M, Sixma JJ, Verhoef J. Prevention of infection by trimethoprim-sulfamethoxazole plus amphotericin B in patients with acute nonlymphocytic leukaemia. Ann Intern Med 1981;95:555–9.

87. Gualtieri RJ, Donowitz GR, Kaiser DL, et al. Double-blind randomized study of prophylactic trimethoprim/sulfamethoxazole in granulocytopenic patients with hematologic malignancies. Am J Med 1983;74:934–40.

88. Goodman JL, Winston DJ, Greenfield RA, et al. A controlled trial of fluconazole to prevent fungal infections in patients undergoing bone marrow transplantation. N Engl J Med 1992;326:845–51.

89. Winston DJ, Chandrasekar PH, Lazarus HM, et al. Fluconazole prophylaxis of fungal infections in patients with acute leukemia: results of a randomized placebo-controlled, double-blind, multicenter trial. Ann Intern Med 1993;118:495–503.

90. Menichetti F, Del Favero A, Martino P, et al. Preventing fungal infection in neutropenic patients with acute leukemia: fluconazole compared with oral amphotericin B. Ann Intern Med 1994;120:913–8.

91. Bohme A, Just-Nubling G, Bergmann L, et al. Itraconazole for prophylaxis of systemic mycoses in neutropenic patients with haematological malignancies. J Antimicrob Chemother 1996;38:953–61.

92. American Thoracic Society. Treatment of tuberculosis and tuberculosis infection in adults and children. Am J Respir Crit Care Med 1994;149:1359–74.

93. Anonymous. Prevention and control of influenza: recommendations of the Advisory Committee on Immunization Practices (ACIP). MMWR Morb Mortal Wkly Rep 1997;46:RR-9:1–25.

94. Anonymous. Prevention of pneumococcal disease: recommendations of the Advisory Committee on Immunization Practices (ACIP). MMWR Morb Mortal Wkly Rep 1997;46:RR-8:1–24.

95. Love LJ, Schimpff SC, Schiffer CA, Wiernik PH. Improved prognosis for granulocytopenic patients with gram-negative bacteremia. Am J Med 1980;68:643–8.

96. Vogler WR, Winton EF. A controlled study of the efficacy of granulocyte transfusions in patients with neutropenia. Am J Med 1977;63:548–55.

97. Alavi JB, Root RK, Djerassi I, et al. A randomized clinical trial of granulocyte transfusions for infection in acute leukemia. N Engl J Med 1977;296:706–11.

98. Boggs DR. Transfusion of neutrophils as prevention or treatment of infection in patients with neutropenia. N Engl J Med 1974;290:1055–62.

99. Bhatia S, McCullough J, Perry EH, et al. Granulocyte transfusions: efficacy in treating fungal infections in neutropenic patients following bone marrow transplantation. Transfusion 1994;34:226–32.

100. Crawford J, Ozer H, Stoller R, et al. Reduction by granulocyte colony-stimulating factor of fever and neutropenia induced by chemotherapy in patients with small-cell lung cancer. N Engl J Med 1991;325:164–70.

101. Hoelzer D. Hematopoietic growth factors—not whether, but when and where. N Engl J Med 1997;336:1822–4.

102. American Society of Clinical Oncology. Update of recommendations for the use of hematopoietic colony-stimulating factors: evidence-based clinical practice guidelines. J Clin Oncol 1996;14:1957–60.

103. Raad II, Davis S, Khan A, et al. Catheter removal affects recurrence of catheter-related coagulase-negative staphylococci bacteremia. Infect Control Hosp Epidemiol 1992;13:215–21.

104. Groeger JS, Lucas AB, Thaler HT, et al. Infectious morbidity associated with long-term use of venous access devices in patients with cancer. Ann Intern Med 1993;119:1168–74.

105. Fowler VG, Sanders LL, Sexton DJ, et al. Outcome of *Staphylococcus aureus* bacteremia according to compliance with recommendations of infectious diseases specialists: experience with 244 patients. Clin Infect Dis 1998;27:478–86.

106. Nguyen MH, Peacock JEJ, Tanner DC, et al. Therapeutic approaches in patients with candidemia: evaluation in a multicenter, prospective, observational study. Arch Intern Med 1995;155:2429–35.

107. Nucci M, Silveira MI, Spector N, et al. Risk factors for death among cancer patients with fungemia. Clin Infect Dis 1998;27:107–11.

108. Press OW, Ramsey PG, Larson EB, et al. Hickman catheter infections in patients with malignancies. Medicine (Baltimore) 1984;63:189–200.

109. Elting LS, Bodey GP. Septicemia due to *Xanthomonas* species and non-aeruginosa *Pseudomonas* species: increasing incidence of catheter-related infections. Medicine (Baltimore) 1990;69:296–306.

# CHAPTER 21

# NUTRITION

• CHARLES M. HASKELL • TANYA L. GIRMAN

The importance of good nutrition to health is widely appreciated by physicians and patients alike. There is enormous interest in the potential prevention of cancer through nutritional approaches, as discussed in Chapter 4 and in many books written for the general public. Many patients as well as some physicians believe that nutritional management may have direct cytotoxic effects against cancer and that this should constitute another form of systemic therapy. Credence for this view comes from a growing appreciation of retinoic acid and related compounds in the treatment of cancer. The best example is the use of retinoids in the treatment of acute promyelocytic leukemia, as discussed in Chapter 84. Despite the popular appeal of special diets, however, dietary treatment of cancer is in its infancy, and there is no scientific evidence that dietary manipulation is an effective primary therapy for established cancer.[1] For now, everyone should be advised to follow a prudent diet, such as that recommended by the American Cancer Society (Table 21–1) and the U.S. Department of Agriculture and U.S. Department of Health and Human Services (Fig. 21–1).

The nutritional status of the patient can have an important impact on the efficacy of cancer treatment. For example, malnourished patients are at risk of infections because of immunosuppression, they may have impaired wound healing after surgery,[2] and malnutrition may exacerbate the side effects of chemotherapy and radiation therapy. This chapter discusses the role of nutrition in the supportive care of the cancer patient.

## Incidence

Weight loss and malnutrition frequently accompany advanced cancer. Although some patients with resectable cancer have normal nutritional status, malnutrition has been reported to occur in 50% of patients treated for advanced solid tumors.[3] The frequency of moderate to severe malnutrition, which is commonly referred to as *cancer cachexia*, varies from 15 to 40% at the initial presentation of cancer and occurs in 80% of patients with advanced disease.[4] Early satiety occurs in 40 to 60% of patients.[5, 6] The anorexia-cachexia syndrome is considered by some authorities to be the most common cause of death in patients with cancer.[7]

## Pathogenesis

A variety of factors can modify the nutritional status of the cancer patient. These can be broadly grouped into nonmeta-

bolic and metabolic causes of malnutrition. In some patients, these categories overlap, especially for patients with the cancer anorexia-cachexia syndrome.

## NONMETABOLIC CAUSES OF MALNUTRITION

Myriad nonmetabolic problems may cause malnutrition in the cancer patient. Common examples of nonmetabolic causes include the following: decreased appetite, resulting from altered taste and smell as a result of cancer or its treatment; odynophagia and dysphagia, resulting from cancer of the aerodigestive tract; mechanical obstruction of the gastrointestinal tract at any level; hepatic insufficiency; blind loop syndromes in patients previously treated with surgery for gastric cancer or peptic ulcer disease; and psychological factors that may result in anorexia, diarrhea, early satiety, malabsorption, or nausea and vomiting. Diarrhea, nausea, vomiting, and stomatitis from cancer chemotherapy can lead to malnutrition, as discussed in Chapter 19. Treatment with opioids for cancer-related pain can result in anorexia and weight loss. Radiation therapy can cause anorexia through multiple mechanisms.

## METABOLIC CAUSES OF MALNUTRITION

The principal metabolic cause of malnutrition in the cancer patient is the cancer anorexia-cachexia syndrome. The syndrome is characterized by loss of appetite and food intake that is inadequate for the patient's metabolic needs. The syndrome may be complicated by pain; psychological effects, such as aversion to specific foods; and altered gastrointestinal function, such as abnormalities of taste, problems with digestion and absorption, early satiety, gastric stasis, constipation, xerostomia, and nausea. Cancer cachexia also may affect the patient's quality of life. Fatigue and weakness may decrease the patient's ability to shop, prepare meals, and eat. A negative body self-image and decreased physical functioning may lead to depression and a reduction in social contacts.

*Table 21–1.* **American Cancer Society Guidelines on Diet, Nutrition, and Cancer**

Choose most of the foods you eat from plant sources
Limit intake of high-fat foods, particularly from animal sources
Be physically active
Achieve and maintain a healthy weight
Limit consumption of alcoholic beverages, if you drink at all

From American Cancer Society's Cancer Facts & Figures 1999. Atlanta, GA, American Cancer Society, 1999:29, reprinted with permission.

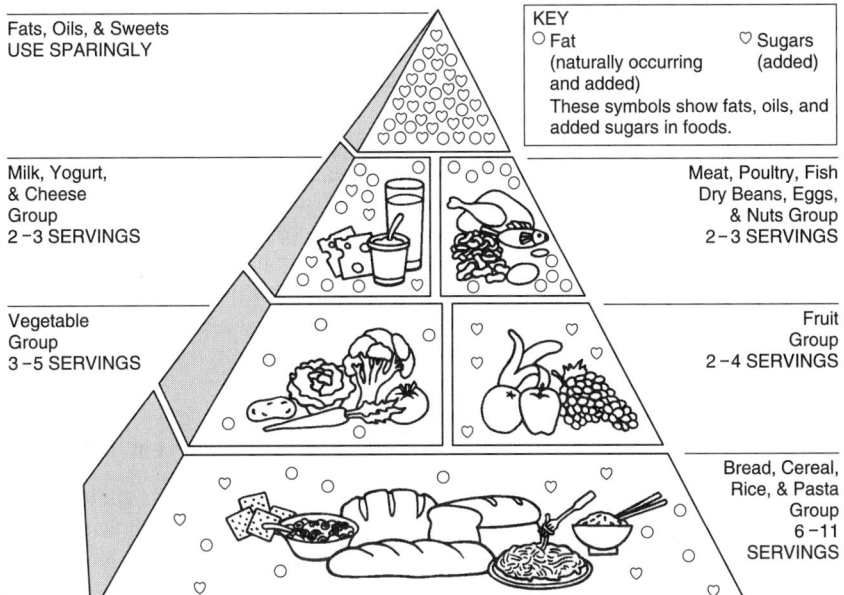

KEY
○ Fat
(naturally occurring
and added)
♡ Sugars
(added)
These symbols show fats, oils, and
added sugars in foods.

Fats, Oils, & Sweets
USE SPARINGLY

Milk, Yogurt,
& Cheese
Group
2–3 SERVINGS

Meat, Poultry, Fish
Dry Beans, Eggs,
& Nuts Group
2–3 SERVINGS

Vegetable
Group
3–5 SERVINGS

Fruit
Group
2–4 SERVINGS

Bread, Cereal,
Rice, & Pasta
Group
6–11
SERVINGS

**Figure 21–1.** Food guide pyramid: a guide to daily food choices. (From the U.S. Department of Agriculture and U.S. Department of Health and Human Services.)

Cancer cachexia includes metabolic, hormonal, and cytokine-related abnormalities that result in progressive wasting.[8] Cancer patients do not have downregulated gluconeogenesis, the usual adaptive response of starvation. Instead, protein catabolism and lipolysis occur at rapid rates to maintain high rates of hepatic glucose synthesis. Relative insulin resistance may occur such that glucose uptake and use is decreased, particularly in the muscles, subsequently causing proteolysis and glycogenic amino acid production. Lipolysis related to the insulin resistance is characterized by excess fatty acid oxidation, regardless of fat and calorie intake. Decreased intake and absorption leads to increased rates of glycerol and free fatty acid turnover in the cancer patient. As a result, cancer patients develop hypertriglyceridemia and decreased lipoprotein lipase levels, leading to decreased adipocyte triglyceride synthesis, while also depleting fat stores for further gluconeogenesis.

The biochemical basis of this syndrome has been reviewed by Nelson and colleagues.[7] Some of the features that serve to distinguish cancer cachexia and starvation cachexia are summarized in Table 21–2.

*Table 21–2.* **Characteristics of Starvation Versus Cancer Cachexia**

| Starvation | Cancer |
|---|---|
| Preferential mobilization of fat, sparing skeletal muscle | Equal mobilization of fat and skeletal muscle |
| Decreased basal metabolic rate | Normal or increased basal metabolic rate |
| Liver atrophy | Increased liver size and metabolic activity |
| Normal lipoprotein lipase | Reduced lipoprotein lipase; acute-phase protein reaction; increased Cori cycle activity |
| Reduced glucose turnover | Normal or increased glucose turnover |
| Decreased protein breakdown | Increased protein breakdown |

From Nelson KA, Walsh D, Sheehan FA. The cancer anorexia-cachexia syndrome. J Clin Oncol 1994;12:213–25.

## Evaluation of Nutrition Status in the Cancer Patient

The cornerstone of nutritional assessment is a detailed history and physical examination by an experienced clinician. Early identification of patients at risk for malnutrition, combined with appropriate multidisciplinary intervention, better supports a patient's body composition, functional status, and quality of life than delayed interventions during the terminal stages of cancer. The usual symptoms of cancer-related malnutrition are anorexia, early satiety, fatigue, and malaise. Accompanying signs on physical examination may include visible evidence of muscle atrophy or myopathy, loss of fat deposits, and generalized edema. Laboratory studies associated with cancer cachexia include anemia; decreased lymphocytes; decreased serum carrier proteins, such as albumin, transferrin, prealbumin, and retinol-binding protein;[9] glucose intolerance; evidence of deficient trace metal and vitamin levels, if measured; and abnormal delayed cutaneous hypersensitivity tests.

### BASIC SCREENING TESTS

Three tests are particularly useful for the initial screening for cancer cachexia and the need for supplementary nutrition. These include the body mass index (BMI), the determination of the rate of weight loss, and the serum albumin. Numerous other assessment tools are also available[10–15] and may be used in making a more detailed nutritional assessment. For example, modified versions of the Subjective Global Assessment of Nutritional Status have been developed for use with oncology patients specifically.[16, 17]

**Body Mass Index.** The BMI may be determined from widely available tables giving the BMI as a function of height and weight, or it may be calculated as follows:

$$BMI = weight\ (kg)/height\ (m^2)$$

BMI values between 18.5 and 24.9 are considered normal.[18] Values greater than 25 constitute being overweight, whereas values greater than 30 constitute obesity. Although 18.5 is the lower limit of normal, some authorities consider values less than 22 to be indicative of possible protein-calorie malnutrition, especially in cancer patients.[19]

**Weight Loss.** Weight loss is usually determined by obtaining a careful history from the patient. Frequently, weight loss is the symptom that prompts a patient to seek a medical evaluation. The severity of weight loss is a function of the amount of weight lost compared with usual body weight and the time over which the loss occurred. The percent weight change is calculated as follows:

$$\text{Percent weight change} = \frac{[\text{usual weight} - \text{actual weight}] \times 100}{\text{usual weight}}$$

Weight loss can be characterized as *significant* as follows:[5]

- 1 to 2% change over 1 week
- 5% change over 1 month
- 7.5% change over 3 months
- 10% change over 6 months

Weight change in excess of these limits may be characterized as severe. The maximal lean body mass wasting an individual can withstand is approximately 40% before death ensues.[20] The presence of edema should be considered when interpreting any weight changes.

**Serum Albumin.** Albumin is synthesized in the liver and has a half-life of about 20 days. The normal serum concentration is greater than 3.5 g/dl. In hospitalized patients, hypoalbuminemia is associated with anergy and an increased risk of infections. It is also associated with increased morbidity and mortality from numerous causes and is considered a marker of poor prognosis. It is not a definitive marker of nutritional status, however, because it also can be influenced by other factors, such as liver disease, nephrotic syndrome, malabsorption, injury, infection, or surgery, and it may be affected by shifts in fluid balance.

## OTHER MEASURES

Numerous other tools and tests are available for a more precise assessment of nutritional status in the cancer patient, including additional blood tests (transferrin, total lymphocyte counts, and prealbumin levels), urine studies (nitrogen balance, creatine height index), immune function studies (delayed hypersensitivity skin tests), anthropometric studies (measurements of triceps skinfold or arm muscle circumference), or combinations of these. A full discussion of these techniques and the prognostic indices based on these measurements is beyond the scope of this chapter.

A qualified nutrition professional, such as a registered dietitian, should be part of the multidisciplinary cancer treatment team. This is especially true for patients scheduled for highly invasive or aggressive forms of therapy, or the treatment may result in longer hospital stays, increased health care costs, and increased morbidity and mortality. The reader interested in a detailed review of these additional nutritional assessment techniques is referred to an excellent review of this topic by Apovian and colleagues.[19] In addition to the initial screening and nutritional assessment, serial reassessments should be scheduled to monitor impact and tolerance of recommended nutritional interventions.

## Treatment of Malnutrition in the Cancer Patient

Nutritional support may take the form of oral supplements, enteral therapy via tubes placed at various levels of the gastrointestinal tract (orogastric, nasoenteric, gastrostomy, jejunostomy) or by parenteral nutrition. For most patients, nutrition should be given orally or enterally; total parenteral nutrition (TPN) is only rarely indicated in adults with cancer. Figure 21–2 provides one approach to determining the most appropriate route of nutritional supplementation for malnourished cancer patients.

### ENTERAL NUTRITION

In addition to preventing weight loss and other nutritional deficits, the focus of nutrition counseling and education should include a discussion of the cancer therapy planned and its potential side effects that may impair eating. This process requires individualization of the meal plan and prepares the patient to make diet adjustments should intake problems occur when the cancer treatment is initiated. When the patient is not consuming enough calories or when fatigue is preventing meal preparation and intake, oral supplements may be initiated. Oral supplements may be commercially available products or fortified foods that the patient or caregiver prepares. Supplements may include high-protein shakes made with powdered milk in whole milk and mixed with various flavoring agents. Registered dietitians may provide suggestions for other methods of creating additional nutrient-dense foods to optimize the patient's oral intake

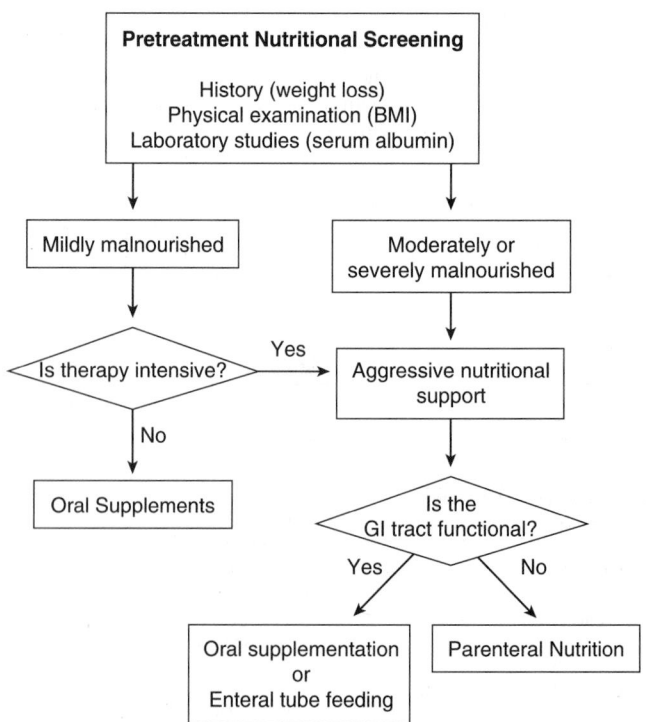

**Figure 21–2.** An approach to nutrition for malnourished cancer patients being considered for treatment of major palliative or curative intent. BMI, body mass index; GI; gastrointestinal.

before more aggressive nutritional intervention is pursued. Specific suggestions for diet modifications to prevent nutritional deficits are provided in a detailed review by Kelly.[21] If the patient is not able to meet nutritional needs with augmentation of oral intake, enteral tube feedings should be considered, if the gastrointestinal tract is functional.

**Indications for Enteral Nutrition.** Enteral feeding provides several advantages over parenteral nutrition, including enhanced immune function, improved nitrogen balance, increased safety of administration compared with central venous catheters, and reduced cost of administration. Enteral feedings require access to an adequately functioning gastrointestinal tract.

**Complications of Enteral Nutrition.** With appropriate monitoring, the complications associated with enteral feedings may be minimized or prevented. Standardized feeding protocols may be available in the institution to provide a specific monitoring schedule and plan of feeding administration. Enteral feeding complications can be categorized as mechanical, gastrointestinal, infectious, or metabolic in nature.

*Mechanical Complications.* Mechanical complications may be related to the enteral tube composition or positioning as well as the size of the feeding tube. Adequate flushing of the tube with water is necessary to maintain tube patency and prevent lumen occlusion. The use of soft, small-bore feeding tubes promotes patient comfort. Ideally, tubes made of biocompatible materials, such as silicone or polyurethane, rather than rubber-based or vinyl-based tubes, should be used. Tubes made of biocompatible materials decrease skin irritation, sinusitis, and otitis media.

*Gastrointestinal Complications.* The most prevalent gastrointestinal complications include diarrhea, nausea, and vomiting. Concurrent drug therapy, the enteral formula being administered, or both may affect the patient's usual bowel habits. Predisposing conditions, such as diabetes, malabsorption syndromes (such as short bowel syndrome, pancreatitis, and radiation enteritis), hypoalbuminemic malnutrition, or gastrointestinal infections (e.g., *Clostridium difficile* or blind loop syndromes), may also result in diarrhea of seemingly sudden onset, especially after a prolonged period of time with inadequate or no enteral intake. Patients with a prolonged hospital stay and broad-spectrum antibiotic use may acquire *C. difficile*, which results in a secretory diarrhea. Other conditions related to the malignancy (carcinoid, vipomas, pancreatic cancer with exocrine insufficiency) may also result in a secretory diarrhea, which is suspected when diarrhea persists for more than 24 hours after discontinuing enteral feedings. Medications frequently associated with diarrhea onset include antacids containing magnesium, phosphorus supplements, and sorbitol-containing medications, such as elixirs. If a new medication has been added or the dose increased in the patient's treatment regimen, diarrhea may ensue.

*Infectious Complications.* The main serious infectious risk is aspiration. Strict adherence to proper formula preparation, storage, handling, and administration may prevent contamination of the enteral formula and reduce infectious complications.

*Metabolic Complications.* Fluid balance, electrolyte balance, and nutrient metabolism alterations may be minimized and prevented with appropriate monitoring and formula ad-

justments. Potential drug-nutrient interactions may be avoided with careful monitoring.

## PARENTERAL NUTRITION

If parenteral nutrition is chosen after following the algorithm in Figure 21–2, one must choose between total parenteral nutrition (TPN) or peripheral parenteral nutrition. If central venous access is difficult to obtain, the duration of parenteral nutrition is expected to be less than 2 weeks, and the patient can tolerate a large fluid load, peripheral parenteral nutrition is a reasonable alternative. Otherwise, TPN is preferred using a central venous line. Peripherally inserted central catheters are an increasingly common route of obtaining central access, but they must be inserted by a certified clinician.

**Indications for Parenteral Nutrition.** In the past, there was intense interest in the use of parenteral nutrition in the support of the cancer patient, either as preoperative therapy or as prolonged therapy in patients receiving chemotherapy. After numerous studies[22, 23] and a position paper from the American College of Physicians,[24] parenteral nutrition has largely been abandoned in contemporary management for most patients with cancer. An exception to this conclusion may be the use of TPN in the setting of bone marrow transplantation,[25, 26] but this conclusion is not supported by all studies.[27] Severely malnourished patients with esophageal cancer may also benefit from parenteral nutrition before esophagectomy, chemoradiotherapy, or a combination of the two. Another broad group of patients for whom parenteral nutrition may be indicated are those with severe malnutrition and self-limited, treatment-associated toxicities that preclude the use of enteral nutrition for 7 to 10 days or longer.[28] The American Society for Parenteral and Enteral Nutrition published a revised set of guidelines for the use of nutritional support in adult and pediatric patients in 1993.[29] It defines the subset of oncologic patients that may benefit from adjunctive TPN:

1. Enteral and parenteral nutrition supplementation may benefit severely malnourished cancer patients in whom treatment toxicity is expected to preclude oral intake for more than 1 week. Patients in this subset should receive nutritional support at the onset of cancer therapy.
2. Specialized nutrition support is not routinely indicated for well-nourished or mildly malnourished patients undergoing surgery, chemotherapy, or radiation therapy, and in whom adequate oral intake is anticipated.
3. TPN is unlikely to benefit patients with advanced cancer whose malignancy is documented as unresponsive to chemotherapy or radiation therapy.

**Complications of Parenteral Nutrition.** If parenteral nutrition is used, it must be monitored carefully, and the patient must be informed of the numerous complications that may occur. Complications can be grouped as mechanical, metabolic, infectious, or gastrointestinal in origin.

*Mechanical Complications.* Mechanical complications may include pneumothorax, subclavian artery injury, embolism (air or catheter), venous thrombosis, or catheter malposition.

*Metabolic Complications.* The most important metabolic

complication is hyperglycemia, which may be complicated by hyperosmolar nonketotic coma. Other complications include hypoglycemia, hyperkalemia (especially in the presence of renal dysfunction), carbon dioxide retention, hyperchloremic metabolic acidosis, azotemia, essential fatty acid deficiency, hypertriglyceridemia, hypophosphatemia, hypocalcemia, hypomagnesemia, hypokalemia, and bleeding from vitamin K deficiency. Patients with prolonged inadequate feeding combined with the sudden, rapid infusion of parenteral nutrition may also be at risk for refeeding syndrome. Refeeding syndrome may be a metabolic consequence of aggressive nutritional support in patients who have had chronic inadequate nutrient intake, resulting in a marasmic type of malnutrition. Severe hypophosphatemia has traditionally been the hallmark of this syndrome, but a broader definition includes other electrolyte abnormalities, such as severe hypokalemia, hypomagnesemia, or both as well as fluid or glucose intolerance.[30] Patients particularly at risk of refeeding syndrome are those who have been experiencing anorexia and may have resulting decreased functional reserve of the organ systems.[31] In a prospective study of 106 cancer patients, the incidence of refeeding syndrome was 24.5%.[32] Cardiac, pulmonary, and renal systems may be overwhelmed by sudden intake of high levels of nutrients, leading to congestive heart failure. The body adapts to the refeeding by shifting potassium, phosphorus, and magnesium intracellularly, with resulting low serum levels of these electrolytes. The patient may experience heart dysrhythmias. Low magnesium may cause hypocalcemia that is resistant to correction until serum magnesium levels are normal. Carbohydrate administration stimulates insulin secretion, which, in turn, limits sodium and water excretion.[33] Recommendations to prevent refeeding syndrome are to initiate calorie goals at 20 kcal/kg/day and protein at 1 to 1.2 g/kg/day and to increase slowly to full nutritional goal over 1 to 2 weeks. Long-term adverse consequences of parenteral nutrition administration include osteomalacic bone disease and possible trace element deficiencies for chromium and selenium.[30]

*Infections.* Catheter sepsis and infection at the skin site of the TPN catheter occurs commonly. In a prospective study of 827 patients, the rate of infection overall was 1 infection per 1000 days of parenteral nutrition.[34] A dedicated port of access for parenteral nutrition alone may minimize the risk of infection. Nonfemoral lines are also associated with less risk of infection.[35] Management of vascular access lines is described in Chapter 12, Vascular Access.

*Gastrointestinal Complications.* Fatty liver, cholestasis, cholelithiasis, and gastrointestinal atrophy may occur, particularly after long-term use of TPN.

## Treatment of Cancer Cachexia

The only curative treatment for cancer cachexia is eradication of the underlying malignancy. All other efforts are palliative and must be applied in an individualized fashion based on the needs of the patient. Treatment with enteral or parenteral nutrition is of unproven value, as is treatment with a variety of unproven drugs (cyproheptadine,[36] hydrazine sulfate,[37, 38] anabolic steroids,[6] pentoxifylline[39]). General sup-

portive care should be provided as needed. General supportive care includes the control of pain (Chapter 22), mucositis, xerostomia (Chapter 19, Stomatitis), nausea and vomiting (Chapter 19, Nausea and Vomiting), constipation (Chapter 19, Constipation), and depression (Chapter 24). Nutritional consultation is important, and the following drugs may be considered for further stimulation of the appetite.

*Metoclopramide* is effective in the treatment of delayed gastric emptying and gastroparesis in the cancer patient occurring after opioid or tricyclic antidepressant therapy.[4] In one study, 17 of 20 patients with advanced cancer had decreased anorexia with the use of this drug.[40] It may also be helpful in patients with refractory nausea unassociated with specific chemotherapeutic agents. A reasonable dose is 10 mg orally before meals and at bedtime. Side effects include dystonic reactions, especially in young women. The drug is contraindicated in patients with a history of dyskinesis. Hyperactivity is a common side effect that generally responds to a reduction in dosage.

*Megestrol acetate* in high dosage is approved by the U.S. Food and Drug Administration for the treatment of anorexia and cachexia in patients with acquired immunodeficiency syndrome (AIDS). Beneficial effects on appetite vary with dosage, from 30% at standard doses of 160 mg/day to 96% with doses 10 times higher.[41, 42] The major clinical problem with this drug is edema. Another problem is its high cost. For cancer patients, treatment is usually initiated at 160 mg/day rather than at the higher doses approved for patients with AIDS. Further discussion of this drug is given in Chapter 10. An alternative to megestrol acetate is medroxyprogesterone acetate.

*Dexamethasone* has been shown to improve appetite without side effects in several studies.[43–45] Nelson and colleagues[7] provide the following guidelines for the use of dexamethasone to stimulate the appetite and improve well-being. Initially the patient is given 4 mg of dexamethasone every morning after food. The dose can be increased to 4 mg twice daily if necessary, with the second dose at noon. Dexamethasone is not given later in the day because it may cause insomnia. A histamine $H_2$ blocker, such as ranitidine, is used to prevent gastric irritation. Dexamethasone should be avoided in diabetic patients, and it should be discontinued immediately if the patient develops any evidence of proximal myopathy. Nelson and colleagues[7] consider dexamethasone to be particularly useful in patients with asthenia and in those needing an anti-inflammatory coanalgesic for pain management. Treatment is recommended for short-term use only, however, because controlled studies in the cancer patient have not shown a prolonged benefit, and these drugs may have many unacceptable side effects,[46] including edema, muscle weakness, dysphoria, hypocalcemia, hyperglycemia, and immune suppression.

*THC*, or delta-9-tetrahydrocannabinol (dronabinol, Marinol), has several potential beneficial effects in patients with cancer. In addition to serving as an antiemetic, it stimulates appetite and promotes weight gain.[47, 48] These effects are modest, however, and they are accompanied by significant side effects. For example, in a study of 15 mg/day orally of THC, side effects included dizziness, fluid retention, somnolence, and feelings of dissociation (especially in elderly patients).[49] Nelson and colleagues[7] have found a lower dose more acceptable. In a study of 2.5 mg orally three times daily 1 hour after meals, varying degrees of appetite stimulation, weight gain, increased calorie count, and improved sense of well-being were noted. The timing of the dose was important, and elderly patients were given THC initially after breakfast and lunch only. The authors consider THC to be particularly useful in patients with mild depression because it causes mood elevation, but it should be avoided in patients who require other psychotropic medications. Nausea can occur with the use of THC, and it may require cessation of therapy.

The choice of drug is determined by cost, side effects, and convenience. In general, lacking contraindications, Nelson and colleagues[7] rank the effective drugs in the order discussed here—metoclopramide ⟹ megestrol acetate ⟹ dexamethasone ⟹ THC. It is hoped that further studies will identify better drugs than those currently available.

## SUGGESTIONS FOR ADDITIONAL READING

American College of Physicians. Parenteral nutrition in patients receiving cancer chemotherapy (position statement). Ann Intern Med 1989; 110:734–6.

Nelson KA, Walsh D, Sheehan FA. The cancer anorexia-cachexia syndrome (review). J Clin Oncol 1994;12:213–25.

Weitzman S. Alternative nutritional cancer therapies. Int J Cancer 1998;11:Suppl:69–72.

Apovian CM, Still CD, Blackburn GL. Nutrition support. In: Berger A, et al eds. Principles and practice of supportive oncology. Philadelphia: Lippincott-Raven, 1998:571.

## REFERENCES

1. Weitzman S. Alternative nutritional cancer therapies. Int J Cancer 1998;11:Suppl:69–72.
2. Haydock DA, Hill GL. Impaired wound healing in surgical patients with varying degrees of malnutrition. JPEN J Parenter Enteral Nutr 1986;10:550–4.
3. De Wys WD, Begg D, Lavin PT, et al. Prognostic effect of weight loss prior to chemotherapy in cancer patients. Am J Med 1980;69:491–7.
4. Willox JC, Corr J, Shaw J, et al. Prednisolone as an appetite stimulant in patients with cancer. Br Med J 1984;288:27.
5. Curtis EB, Krech R, Walsh TD. Common symptoms in patients with advanced cancer. J Palliat Care 1991;7:25–9.
6. Armes PJ, Plant HJ, Allbright A, et al. A study to investigate the incidence of early satiety in patients with advanced cancer. Br J Cancer 1992;65:481–4.
7. Nelson KA, Walsh D, Sheehan FA. The cancer anorexia-cachexia syndrome. J Clin Oncol 1994;12:213–25.
8. Puccio M, Nathanson L. The cancer cachexia syndrome. Semin Oncol 1997;24:277–87.
9. Bourry J, Milano G, Caldan C, Schneider M. Assessment of nutritional proteins during the parenteral nutrition of cancer patients. Ann Clin Lab Sci 1982;12:158–62.
10. Buzby GP, Mullen JL, Matthews DC, et al. Prognostic nutritional index in gastrointestinal surgery. Am J Surg 1980;139:160–7.
11. Hickman DM, Miller RA, Rombeau JL, et al. Serum albumin and body weight as predictors of postoperative course in colorectal cancer. JPEN J Parenter Enteral Nutr 1980;4:314–6.
12. Klidjian AM, Archer TJ, Foster KJ, et al. Detection of dangerous malnutrition. JPEN J Parenter Enteral Nutr 1982;6:119–21.
13. Seltzer MH, Bastidas JA, Cooper DM, et al. Instant nutritional assessment. J Parenter Enteral Nutr 1979; 3:157–9.
14. Seltzer MH, Slocum BA, Cataldi-Betcher EL, et al. Instant nutritional assessment: absolute weight loss and surgical mortality. JPEN J Parenter Enteral Nutr 1982;6:218–21.
15. Nutrition Screening Initiative. Nutrition interventions manual for pro-

fessionals caring for older Americans. Washington, D.C.: Nutrition Screening Initiative, 1992.
16. Ottery FD. Modification of Subjective Global Assessment (SGA) of Nutritional Status (NS) for oncology patients. 19th Clinical Congress, American Society for Parenteral and Enteral Nutrition, Miami, Fla., January 15–18, 1995. abstract 119.
17. Ottery FD. Rethinking nutrition support of the cancer patient: the new field of nutritional oncology. Semin Oncol 1994;21:770–8.
18. National Heart, Lung, and Blood Institute Expert Panel on the Identification, Evaluation, and Treatment of Overweight and Obesity in Adults. Executive summary of the clinical guidelines on the identification, evaluation, and treatment of overweight and obesity in adults. J Am Diet Assoc 1998;98:1178–91.
19. Apovian CM, Still CD, Blackburn GL. Nutrition support. In: Berger A, et al, eds. Principles and practice of supportive oncology. Philadelphia: Lippincott-Raven, 1998:571.
20. Mora RJ. Malnutrition: organic and functional consequences. World J Surg 1999;23:530–5.
21. Kelly K. An overview of how to nourish the cancer patient by mouth. Cancer 1986;58:1897–1901.
22. Detsky AS, Baker JP, O'Rourke K, Goel V. Perioperative parenteral nutrition: a meta-analysis. Ann Intern Med 1987;107:195–203.
23. Veterans Affairs Total Parenteral Nutrition Cooperative Study Group. Perioperative total parenteral nutrition in surgical patients. N Engl J Med 1991;325:525–32.
24. American College of Physicians. Parenteral nutrition in patients receiving cancer chemotherapy (position paper). Ann Intern Med 1989;110:734–6.
25. Uderzo C, Rovelli A, Bonomi M, et al. Total parenteral nutrition and nutritional assessment and leukaemic children undergoing bone marrow transplantation. Eur J Cancer 1991;27:758–62.
26. Weisdorf SA, Lysne J, Wind D, et al. Positive effect of prophylactic total parenteral nutrition on long-term outcome of bone marrow transplantation. Transplant 1987;43:833–8.
27. Szeluga DJ, Stuart RK, Brookmeyer R, et al. Nutritional support of bone marrow transplant recipients: a prospective, randomized clinical trial comparing total parenteral nutrition to an enteral feeding program. Cancer Res 1987;47:3309–16.
28. Souba WW. Nutritional support. In: De Vita V, Hellman S, Rosenberg SA, eds. Principles and practice of oncology. 5th ed. Philadelphia: Lippincott-Raven, 1997:2841.
29. American Society for Parenteral and Enteral Nutrition. Guidelines for the use of parenteral and enteral nutrition in adult and pediatric patients. JPEN J Parenter Enteral Nutr 1993;17:4Suppl:1SA–52SA.
30. Solomon SM, Kirby DF. The refeeding syndrome: a review. JPEN J Parenter Enteral Nutr 1990;14:90–7.
31. Torun B, Chew F. Protein-energy malnutrition. In: Shills ME, Olson JA, Shike M, eds. Modern nutrition in health and disease. Philadelphia: Lea & Febiger, 1994.
32. Gonzalez AG, Fajardo RA, Gonzalez FE. The incidence of the refeeding syndrome in cancer patients who receive artificial nutritional treatment. Nutr Hosp 1996;11:98–101.
33. Matz R. Parallels between treated and uncontrolled diabetes and the refeeding syndrome with emphasis on fluid and electrolyte abnormalities. Diabetes Care 1994;17:1209–13.
34. Tokars JI, Cookson ST, McArthur MA, et al. Prospective evaluation of risk factors for bloodstream infection in patients receiving home infusion therapy. Ann Intern Med 1999;131:340–7.
35. Harden JL, Kemp L, Mirtallo J. Femoral catheters increase risk of infection in total parenteral nutrition patients. Nutr Clin Pract 1995;10:60–6.
36. Kardinal CG, Loprinzi CL, Schaid DJ, et al. A controlled trial of cyproheptadine in cancer patients with anorexia and/or cachexia. Cancer 1990;65:2657–62.
37. Loprinzi CL, Kuross SA, O'Fallon JR, et al. Randomized placebo-controlled evaluation of hydrazine sulfate in patients with advanced colorectal cancer. J Clin Oncol 1994;12:1121–5.
38. Kosty MP, Fleishman SB, Herndon JE 2nd, et al. Cisplatin, vinblastine, and hydrazine sulfate in advanced, non-small-cell lung cancer: a randomized placebo-controlled, double-blind phase III study of the Cancer and Leukemia Group B. J Clin Oncol 1994;12:1113–20.
39. Ottery FD. Supportive nutrition to prevent cachexia and improve quality of life. Semin Oncol 1995;22:98–111.
40. Nelson KA, Walsh TD. Metoclopramide in anorexia caused by cancer-associated dyspepsia syndrome (CADS). J Palliat Care 1993;9:14–8.

41. Tchekmedyian NS, Tait N, Moody M, Aisner J. High-dose megestrol acetate: a possible treatment for cachexia. JAMA 1987;257:1195–8.
42. Loprinzi CL, Michalak JC, Schaid DJ, et al. Phase III evaluation of four doses of megestrol acetate as therapy for patients with cancer anorexia and/or cachexia. J Clin Oncol 1993;11:762–7.
43. Moertel CG, Schutt AJ, Reitemeier RJ, Hahn RG. Corticosteroid therapy of preterminal gastrointestinal cancer. Cancer 1974;33:1607–9.
44. Bruera E, Roca E, Cedaro L, et al. Action of oral methylprednisolone in terminal cancer patients: a prospective randomized double-blind study. Cancer Treat Rep 1985;69:751–4.
45. Loprinzi CL, Kugler JW, Sloan JA, et al. Randomized comparison of megestrol acetate versus dexamethasone versus fluoxymesterone for

the treatment of cancer anorexia/cachexia. J Clin Oncol 1999; 17:3299–306.
46. Tchekmedyian NS, Heber D. Cancer and AIDS cachexia: mechanisms and approaches to therapy. Oncology 1993; 7:55–9.
47. Ekert H, Waters KD, Jurk IH, et al. Amelioration of cancer chemotherapy-induced nausea and vomiting by delta-9-tetrahydrocannabinol. Med J Aust 1979;2:657–9.
48. Benowitz NL, Jones RT. Cardiovascular and metabolic considerations in prolonged cannabinoid administration in man. J Clin Pharmacol 1981;21:Suppl:214S–23S.
49. Curtis EB, Walsh TD. Prescribing practices of a palliative care service. J Pain Symptom Manage 1993;8:312–6.

# CHAPTER 22

# MANAGEMENT OF PAIN IN THE CANCER PATIENT

• MATTHEW E. CONOLLY • JOSHUA P. PRAGER •
• ANTONIO A. F. DE SALLES •

*"Pain is a more terrible lord of mankind than even death itself."*

Albert Schweitzer

## Impact of Pain

When presented with the diagnosis of incurable malignancy, the patient is plunged into an existential crisis. As the initial shock recedes, the prospect of dying in unrelieved pain then becomes a dominant concern. Frequently, that fear becomes a reality because many physicians, exhibiting a deep-rooted and irrational phobia of opiates, offer inadequate responses to the patient's pain. Many physicians seem more comfortable closing their eyes to the suffering over which they preside. Even physicians willing to use analgesic drugs in an appropriate manner often ignore the fact that pain is a complex issue with mental, social, and spiritual as well as physical components. If we ignore the former aspects, no matter what we do about the merely physical pain, the patient's suffering will not be relieved.

Palliative care, as it is best understood, has been too long in coming, largely because of the destructive economic pressures of managed care. Home hospice care has been offered as a cost-effective alternative, but often the caregiver on whom the burden of heavy nursing falls is elderly and infirm or untrained in the necessary skills. To avoid spending money, patients are left to spend their remaining days in misery. For good reason, at least one state has legalized physician-assisted suicide, and others are expected to follow suit.

### PREVALENCE OF PAIN

Bonica[1] estimates that 51% of all cancer patients experience pain and that pain occurs in 74% of those with advanced disease. Consequently, more than 1 million Americans expe-

rience cancer-related pain each year; worldwide the figure is measured in the tens of millions. This problem is exacerbated in some countries by extraordinarily restrictive laws concerning the availability of opiates. Bonica determined that among the 74% of patients with pain from advanced disease, roughly 50% could be categorized as having moderate to severe pain, and 25 to 30% had excruciating pain. That patients should suffer in the United States is a matter of great professional shame because it is not that physicians lack the means of alleviating suffering, but that, as individuals, they lack either the knowledge or the courage to exploit the tools available.[2]

### SOURCES OF PAIN

For a rational approach to the management of pain, the physician must understand where the pain is coming from. It has been pointed out[3] that the physical pain encountered by cancer patients is commonly due to not one but two, three, or even more processes going on simultaneously. Not all pain is necessarily related directly to the malignancy. It is important for the treating physician not only to obtain a clear diagnostic view of the sources of pain at the outset, but also *frequently* to reanalyze the situation because the sources of pain may alter radically as the disease progresses.

A. Pain may be directly related to the tumor as a result of
   Bony metastases
   Soft tissue infiltration
   Nerve compression
B. Pain may be indirectly related to the malignancy because of
   Infection (e.g., cellulitis, deep abscess formation)
   Intestinal obstruction
   Massive edema or ascites
   Immobility of a paralyzed limb
C. Pain may be a result of therapeutic interventions:
   Acute postoperative pain (largely inexcusable)

Chronic postsurgical pain (e.g., from neuroma formation, phantom-limb pain)

Radiation therapy (e.g., acutely, as mastalgia caused by postlumpectomy radiation, or chronically, as a result of postradiation fibrosis entrapping nerve trunks)

Painful peripheral neuropathy (e.g., from vinca alkaloids, platinum-based chemotherapy)

Peptic ulceration (paradoxically this *may* be painless)

Opiate-induced constipation (almost always avoidable)

## IMMUNOLOGIC CONSEQUENCES OF UNRELIEVED PAIN

Important studies have revealed that, in addition to being a major component of suffering, pain may exert other directly harmful effects. It has been shown that the activity of natural killer cells, an essential component of the body's defense system, is depressed by unrelieved pain.[4] Page and colleagues[5] have raised serious questions about the impact of pain on prognosis. Rats were subjected to laparotomy, in the course of which tumor cells were implanted in the abdominal cavity. The animals were then subdivided into two groups, one of which was given adequate postoperative analgesia, whereas the other received none. In the animals with unrelieved postoperative pain, the tumor spread faster and grew more aggressively. Although such data may not be directly extrapolated to humans, they raise extremely provocative questions about the importance of pain control in general and about postoperative pain control in particular. One has to ask whether 5-year survival figures may not be distorted in situations in which there has been failure to provide adequate postoperative analgesia.

## REASONS FOR FAILURE TO CONTROL PAIN

Bonica[6] defines where the root of failure to control pain lies. It is most commonly in ignorance of the following:

- Duration of action of the drugs used
- Dose equivalence (e.g., between one opiate and another)
- Bioavailability of medications when given orally
- The most appropriate way to schedule doses
- Mythical nature of addiction and respiratory depression
- Fear of legal prosecution for prescribing large doses of narcotics
- Interindividual susceptibility to pain
- The consequences of unrelieved pain

**Duration of Action.** Duration of action is directly related to the half-life of the drug in question. For the most part, the half-lives of commonly used opiates are 2 to 4 hours (see Table 22–8). If pain is to be controlled at all times, narcotics need to be given with a frequency corresponding to the rate at which the drug in question is removed from the body. In practical terms, in patients with normal renal and hepatic function, this means that (except for methadone and levorphanol) opiates need to be given on a *strictly 4-hourly basis*, unless a sustained-release preparation is being used. In the case of morphine, there is a metabolite, morphine-6-glucuronide, that (most unusually for a metabolite) is a more potent narcotic agonist than the parent compound.

It accumulates in the face of renal failure; it is not readily dialyzed and may result in long-lasting opiate effects. For other agents, such as nonsteroidal anti-inflammatory drugs (NSAIDs), the half-lives may be considerably longer (see later), and a less frequent dosing schedule suffices.

**Dose Equivalence.** Frequently the need arises to change a patient from one opiate to another, perhaps because of an unfavorable side-effect profile. Suggested conversion factors are included in Table 22–6. Physicians commonly discharge a patient from the hospital substituting a small dose of an oral agent, such as Percocet, for the infusion of morphine on which the patient had been stabilized. As night follows day, the resurgence of often quite intolerable pain is entirely predictable.

**Bioavailability.** Most opiates are poorly absorbed from the gastrointestinal tract. Only about one third of an oral dose of morphine is absorbed. In the case of hydromorphone, the absorption is even lower (20%). This situation presents no problem as long as the physician makes suitable allowance when changing from parenteral to oral dosage forms. For example, a patient receiving morphine intravenously at a rate of 10 mg/hr requires $10 \times 3 \times 4$ mg every 4 hours (i.e., 120 mg every 4 hours by mouth). NSAIDs have a much higher bioavailability, and, in changing from parenteral to oral ketorolac, for example, no such correction would be needed.

**Time-Contingent Administration.** Analgesics for the cancer patient should *never* be given "p.r.n. pain" (on an as-needed basis for pain), even though this approach is widely practiced. It has been well established[7] that once pain is allowed to break through, more analgesics are required to regain control, and drug toxicity becomes more probable. The constant recurrence of pain (the condition necessary to trigger another dose) serves only to escalate the patient's level of anxiety and creates a climate of conflict between the patient and the caregivers.

**Myth of Addiction.** Common sense should dictate that, in patients with irrecoverable disease, addiction should be the last thing on anyone's mind. Such is the societal fear of drug-related problems, however, that this is not the case.[8] There is moreover a widespread inability to distinguish between true addiction (the overwhelming psychological craving for a drug to experience its euphorigenic effects) and physical dependence. The latter is a state in which abrupt cessation of administration of an agonist leads to withdrawal symptoms, as may occur not only with opiates, but also with quite dissimilar agents, such as clonidine.[9] The popular, but shockingly erroneous, belief is that once a patient receives opiates, addiction becomes likely, if not inevitable. This notion has its origins in the surveys carried out 40 or more years ago, in which established addicts were asked about the source of their addiction and commonly placed the blame on a physician's prescription of, for example, postoperative analgesics.[10, 11] In more appropriate studies, in which *normal* subjects requiring opiates have been examined before and after exposure to these drugs, an entirely different picture emerges. In one study, by Perry and Heidrich,[12] the records of 10,000 patients with significant burn injuries were studied. After drawn-out and painful courses, requiring prolonged treatment with opiates, only 22 of 10,000 patients were considered to have a drug problem, and they had the problem before the injury occurred. In a briefly reported study of

11,882 patients receiving opiates of unspecified type, for varied durations, Porter and Jick[13] found only 4 patients who were thought to have developed any kind of drug problem, and in only 1 (of 11,882) was it considered serious.

The clinician should be aware of so-called pseudoaddiction, in which the patient *appears* to be exhibiting drug-seeking behavior but which, in reality, is a desperate quest for adequate analgesic therapy, provoked by poor clinical management of the pain. As Wall[14] has pointed out, it has been "a disgraceful episode in the history of medicine that doctors and scientists allowed themselves to join a mass hysteria which confused the tremendous benefits of narcotics for the patient in pain with the social abuse of the same compounds."

*Respiratory depression* is an acknowledged side effect of opiate overdose.[15] It has been shown, however, that pain, which is a powerful stimulant to respiration,[16] is capable of counteracting the effect of opiates on respiratory drive. It is always safe to give opiates in increasing doses, as long as the dose is titrated against pain levels and is increased only to the point at which the pain is obliterated.[17, 18] In a patient thus stabilized on opiates, should an invasive procedure, such as a cordotomy, be carried out to provide relief of pain, the previously tolerated dose of opiates would become an overdose, and, under those special conditions, respiratory depression could ensue if the dose were not reduced in anticipation.[19, 20]

*Legal barriers* have played a major role in preventing many patients from obtaining the opiates they need to control their pain. These barriers usually take the form of fear, on the part of the physician, of prosecution from overzealous governmental agencies.[21, 22] These fears are undoubtedly heightened by the veiled threat of ongoing governmental surveillance contained in the triplicate prescription programs adopted by several states[23] and are fostered by the ignorance and insane witch-hunt mentality pervading some states' medical board members, as has been seen in Florida. Changes in the laws of California and Texas have provided some relief. The statement, "Quantity and chronicity of prescribing will be judged on the basis of the diagnosis and treatment of the targeted symptoms, and *neither of these factors are prima facie evidence of inappropriate or excessive prescribing,*"[24] is refreshing. More changes are needed. Internationally, several countries still have laws that savagely restrict the availability of opiates to all their citizens. Despite all the international discussions over the past decade that have led to an increase in the legitimate consumption of morphine in most developed countries, 11 countries report a *decline* in its use in the last few years. The fact that one particular country with a population of 800 million can record its total annual use of morphine as 83 kg indicates that virtually no effective pain control exists there. Numerous countries continue to use meperidine in preference to morphine, despite its drawbacks. Despite the rapid increase in the medical use of morphine in the United States, the diversion of legitimate morphine toward unlawful consumption is small, being no greater than it was several years ago.[25]

*Interindividual susceptibility to pain* is a poorly studied phenomenon. From the work of Woolf[26] and others, it appeared that tissue injury may lead to changes in neuronal function within the spinal cord, heightening the intensity of pain and widening the area in which it is perceived (the

*wind-up* phenomenon). Failure to recognize this phenomenon as a possible factor in the intensity of the patient's pain has caused many physicians to dismiss patient complaints as drug seeking for its own sake.

From mouse studies, it also appears that, in some animals, there is an inherited susceptibility to pain, traceable to a deficiency in opiate receptors.[27] In such animals, a larger dose of opiates is needed to achieve the same effect as in *normal* subjects. It is not unreasonable to expect that the same heterogeneity may occur in humans, although this is not known. With such factors as these in mind, it is to be expected that there would be widely differing reports on the part of patients as to how much opiate they require to control their pain, and the temptation to label complainers as *drug seeking* should be subject to critical scrutiny.

The *consequences of inadequately relieved pain* are rarely considered. The immunologic considerations alluded to previously, however, to say nothing of quality-of-life issues, must spur every caregiver who becomes aware of them on to achieve better pain control.

## Options for Treating Pain

### DIRECT INTERVENTIONS FOR THE RELIEF OF CANCER PAIN

Wherever possible, the pain should be attacked at the source. This attack may take the form of surgical intervention, be it draining an abscess, reduction and fixation of a pathologic fracture, or relief of intestinal obstruction. At other times, a more appropriate intervention might be radiation therapy. As discussed elsewhere in this book, radiation may be an extremely effective way of reducing pain from bony metastases or from the perineal pain of recurrent rectosigmoid carcinoma. Strontium 89 is for many patients with bony metastases an effective form of localized radiotherapy. Being selectively taken up at sites of osteoblastic activity, this beta-emitting isotope is uniquely effective in concentrating radiation at the sites of bony metastases. It is specifically indicated in situations in which the metastases are too numerous and widespread to permit conventional irradiation (e.g., multiple sites on both sides of the diaphragm). In a study of 118 patients with painful skeletal metastases (mostly from prostate, breast, and lung cancer), 47.5% reported substantial or complete remission of symptoms. A further 40.7% reported mild improvement, whereas fewer than 5% claimed no benefit at all. Benefit seems less likely in bony metastases from cancers other than prostate, breast, and lung. Pain relief lasted approximately 3 months in the first instance. For metastases associated with prostate, breast, and lung cancer, strontium 89 could be given repeatedly, with similar periods of relief (in the case of breast cancer, the duration of symptomatic relief extended from 3 to 5.3 months after the fifth dose of strontium 89).[28] In a review of three other studies confined to prostate cancer, it was found that each treatment lasted about 3 months and could be repeated, with symptomatic relief. Overall survival time was not increased. Myelosuppression was observed, but it was not of significant magnitude. It is not an adequate substitute for conventional radiotherapy in situations in which impending spinal cord compression exists.[29]

Pharmacology may sometimes provide a form of direct intervention. In the treatment of the pain of skeletal metastases, calcitonin, in doses of 100 to 200 units one to four times per day for periods of up to 17 months, seems to have been helpful in several (but not all) studies.[30–33]

A direct attack on osteoclasts, which are involved in bone destruction by metastases, may also give substantial relief of bone pain. For this purpose, the bisphosphonates, which are widely used in treating osteoporosis, have been prescribed. A study involving clodronate[34] and several others using pamidronate[35] have yielded encouraging results, especially (but not exclusively) in the case of breast cancer and multiple myeloma. Olpadronate has produced comparable responses in metastatic prostate cancer.[36] Some data suggest that these agents may not only inhibit osteoclasts, but also may exert a direct antitumor effect.[37]

Muscle spasm is a common source of considerable pain, and this too can be treated with specific pharmacology, rather than being blocked out by analgesics. Baclofen, given orally or by means of intrathecal infusion (see later) may give dramatic relief.[38]

Even in situations in which surgical correction or radiation is not appropriate, other interventions may be considered, including nerve blocks or neurosurgical procedures, as discussed in subsequent sections of this chapter. Much can be achieved by means of analgesic therapy, however, without the discomfort and risk of invasive procedures.

## PHARMACOLOGIC CONTROL OF CANCER PAIN

Eventually, in most patients with incurable malignancy, it becomes necessary for the physician to draw on the extensive pharmacologic resources available for the control of pain. Analgesic drugs available fall into three categories: (1) nonopiate analgesics, (2) opiate analgesics, and (3) *adjuvant* analgesics (Table 22–1).

Frequent reference is made to the *analgesic ladder*,[39, 40] which describes a sequential deployment of all the above-listed analgesics, in a sequence supposed to represent increasing potency to control the pain. Although this approach may have some usefulness, analogous to the now outmoded *stepped care* approach to hypertension, it does not take into account the complexity of pain and the multitude of sources that may be active. Instead, it regards *pain* as a single symptom to be obliterated. A more thoughtful approach, based on careful repeated clinical assessments of the sources of the pain, as described previously, in full knowledge of the differing modes of action of the available drugs, is more likely to produce the desired result.

*Table 22–1.* **Categories of Analgesic Drugs**

| Nonopiate Analgesics | Opiates | Adjuvant Agents |
|---|---|---|
| Acetaminophen | Weak opiates | Heterocyclic antidepressants |
| Nonsteroidal anti-inflammatory drugs | Potent opiates Full agonists Partial agonists Agonist-antagonists | Anticonvulsants Psychotropic agents |

## Nonopiate Analgesics

### ACETAMINOPHEN

Acetaminophen is a widely used analgesic, of moderate potency. In conventional doses, it is safe and is often used for prolonged periods.[41] In high single doses (10 to 15 g), it may be acutely hepatotoxic. Such toxicity is not seen in normal practice, but it is important to remember that not only is acetaminophen a common over-the-counter agent available in unlimited amounts, but also it is a component of many prescription-only analgesics, such as Anexsia, Darvocet-N, DHC Plus, Esgic, Lorcet, Lortab, Percocet, Phenaphen, Roxicet, Talacen, Tylox, Vicodin, Vicodin ES, Wygesic, and Zydone. Some of these preparations may contain 750 mg of acetaminophen per capsule or tablet, so the potential for the unwitting consumption of a larger than intended dose of acetaminophen does exist. If this should occur in the context of debilitating illness, with malnutrition and disease-related hepatic damage, additional hepatotoxicity might arise,[42] although pertinent data are sparse. A total daily dose no greater than 4.0 g is generally accepted as safe to use over a prolonged period.

### NONSTEROIDAL ANTI-INFLAMMATORY DRUGS

NSAIDs comprise a large and heterogeneous group of agents. They are derived from several dissimilar parent compounds (Table 22–2), and individual patients react differently to the various groups of NSAIDs. If the response to one NSAID is not satisfactory, before abandoning this valuable class of drugs, the physician should try to use an NSAID from another chemical group.

NSAIDs may be extremely effective in providing pain relief, especially in the context of bony metastases. Among skilled hospice physicians, it is often found that, in managing bone pain, the appropriate use of NSAIDs may permit the use of opiates to be sharply curtailed or even, for a while, suspended (West T, personal communication, 1986). Although NSAIDs are normally administered by mouth and occasionally by suppository, ketorolac has been approved for intramuscular injection. Although valuable for acute pain relief, especially postoperatively, in the extended treatment of cancer pain, repeated intramuscular injections are not useful. A report of success with prolonged intravenous infusions of ketorolac in controlling the bone pain of a patient with disseminated prostatic cancer,[43] however, suggests a way in which parenteral NSAIDs might be more useful in treating cancer pain.

Numerous side effects are associated with the use of NSAIDs. The most common is gastrointestinal irritation or ulceration with attendant bleeding that can be massive. This side effect occurs regardless of the route of administration because of the impact of NSAIDs in the systemic circulation on prostaglandin formation. It may be lessened by the administration of antacids or by one of the antisecretory agents now available to reduce gastric acidity ($H_2$ blockers, such as ranitidine; ion-pump inhibitors, such as omeprazole; or the prostaglandin analogue misoprostol). This side effect is more common with ketorolac and less prominent with naproxen, but it can occur with any NSAID and may occur without premonitory symptoms.

*Table 22–2.* **Nonsteroidal Anti-Inflammatory Drugs***

| Salicylates | Carboxylic Acid Derivatives | | | Oxicams |
| | PROPIONIC ACID DERIVATIVES | ACETIC ACID DERIVATIVES | ANTHRANILIC ACID DERIVATIVES | |
| --- | --- | --- | --- | --- |
| Aspirin | Ibuprofen | Indomethacin | Mefenamic acid | Piroxicam |
| Salsalate | Naproxen | Ketorolac | Floctafenine† | |
| Diflunisal | Fenoprofen | Diclofenac | Meclofenamate | |
| | Flurbiprofen | Nabumetone | | |
| Choline magnesium trisalicylate | Ketoprofen | Etodolac | | |
| | Fenbufen† | Sulindac | | |
| | | Tolmetin | | |
| Sodium salicylate | | | | |

*The two currently available COX-2 selective inhibitors do not fit into this scheme. Celecoxib (Celebrex) is a sulfonamide derivative. Rofecoxib (Vioxx) is a furinone.
†Currently not available in the United States.

Platelet function is compromised by many NSAIDs. Aspirin is the most troublesome in this regard because once the platelet cyclooxygenase is acetylated, its activity is permanently abolished, and restoration of platelet function requires the synthesis of a totally new population of platelets. With many of the other NSAIDs, cyclooxygenase is *reversibly* inhibited. As the plasma level of NSAID declines, platelet activity returns to normal. This difference is perhaps of little practical importance while the patient is receiving continuous therapy, but at least a fairly rapid reversal is ensured if therapy needs to be discontinued because of bleeding. Of greater practical importance is the *lack* of significant antiplatelet effect in ketorolac, the little known nonacetylated salicylates, such as salsalate[44] and choline magnesium trisalicylate,[45] as well as the new COX-2 selective inhibitors.

Renal function may sometimes become severely compromised by NSAID-induced papillary necrosis. None of the available agents is devoid of this potential, although it has been reported that sulindac (Clinoril) is less likely to cause such problems; this is because it has to undergo metabolic transformation (reduction) to its active (sulfide) form in the liver and is deactivated by other enzymes in the kidneys. As a practical issue, in the management of cancer pain, NSAID-induced renal damage is rarely a matter of great concern.

Diuretic action may be inhibited, and fluid retention with dependent edema can occur. The renal excretion of certain important drugs, such as digoxin, methotrexate, cyclosporine, and lithium, may be compromised by the coadministration of NSAIDs. Hepatotoxicity is possible but rare with agents other than acetaminophen.

A few patients develop life-threatening bronchospasm when exposed to small doses of NSAIDs. Although often referred to as an allergic reaction, bronchospasm is now thought to be due to the diversion of arachidonic acid into leukotriene production as a result of cyclooxygenase inhibition. True allergies can also develop to NSAIDs and can be fatal. Cross-reactivity between NSAIDs may occur. NSAIDs may interfere with the metabolism of warfarin and potentiate its anticoagulant effect. Pharmacologic profiles of the commonly used NSAIDs follow.

**Salicylates.** *Aspirin* is the original NSAID. It irreversibly inhibits platelet cyclooxygenase. Gastric irritation and ulceration are fairly common. Ulceration can cause severe bleeding without necessarily causing pain. It is rapidly absorbed from the gut and has an effective half-life of 2 to 3 hours. It should be used with care in patients with pre-existing renal disease. In overdose, it can produce severe metabolic derangements, which may be difficult to treat, especially in children. Aspirin potentiates the action of oral anticoagulants and methotrexate. The usual dose is 0.5 to 1.0 g every 4 to 6 hours, with a daily maximum of 6000 mg.

*Diflunisal* (Dolobid) is a new derivative. It has a long half-life and so may be given on a twice-daily schedule. Side effects are similar to those of aspirin. The usual dose is 250 to 500 mg every 12 hours. At the lower dose, antiplatelet effects are minimal. The maximal recommended dose is 1500 mg/day.

*Salsalate* (Disalcid) is hydrolyzed to two molecules of salicylic acid in the gut or, following absorption, in the plasma. Its initial half-life is 3 to 4 hours but, similar to aspirin, its metabolism quickly comes to obey zero order kinetics, as the process of hydrolysis becomes saturated at conventional doses. This leads to a slowing of elimination so that a twice-daily dosing schedule is appropriate. It has less gastrointestinal toxicity than aspirin and no antiplatelet effect. The maximum recommended daily dose is 3000 mg.

*Choline magnesium trisalicylate* (Trilisate) has the advantage of water solubility so that a liquid dosage form exists. Gastric irritation is less than with aspirin, and it does not interfere with platelet function. It has a long duration of action and need only be given once or twice a day. A typical dose is 500 mg, with a recommended daily maximum of 3000 mg.

*Sodium salicylate* is rarely used. It is available in oral form and, in some countries, as an injectable preparation. Oral absorption is erratic.

**Propionic Acid Derivatives.** *Ibuprofen* (Motrin, Nuprin, Brufen) is rapidly absorbed from the gut. It causes less gastrointestinal irritation than aspirin. The half-life is approximately 2 hours. The usual dose is 200 to 400 mg every 4 hours. The maximum daily dose should not exceed 3200 mg.

*Naproxen* (Naprosyn, Anaprox, Laraflex) has a long half-life (12 hours) and need be given only two to three times a day. Gastrointestinal side effects are less common than with aspirin or ibuprofen. The usual starting dose is 250 mg three times a day, and the total daily dose should not exceed 1250 mg/day.

*Fenoprofen* (Nalfon, Fenopron) has a half-life of 3 hours

and needs to be given correspondingly frequently. Equipotent doses of fenoprofen cause fewer gastrointestinal side effects than aspirin. In general, it is well tolerated compared with other NSAIDs. The usual dose is 200 mg every 4 hours. Beyond that level, the dose-response curve is flat, and little benefit is gained by increasing the dose further. The daily total should not exceed 3200 mg.

*Flurbiprofen* (Ansaid, Froben) is well absorbed from the gut and has a half-life of 4 to 6 hours. The recommended dose is 25 to 50 mg every 4 to 6 hours. The dose-response curve is linear to a dose of 150 mg. The recommended total daily dose is 200 to 300 mg.

*Ketoprofen* (Orudis, Oruvail) has a half-life of 2 to 4 hours. It differs from the other NSAIDs in that it inhibits the synthesis not only of prostaglandins, but also the other product of the arachidonic acid cascade, the leukotrienes. In theory, this should make its effects more steroid-like because steroids also inhibit the production of leukotrienes and prostaglandins (albeit by inhibiting phospholipase-mediated release of the precursor, arachidonic acid). Doses of 50 mg are said to be better than 650 mg of aspirin and as effective as 90 mg of codeine. Beyond that point, the dose-response curve is flat so that no advantage follows any further dose increase. It is rapidly absorbed from the gut. The oral dose should not exceed 300 mg/day.

**Acetic Acid Derivatives.** *Indomethacin* (Indocin, Indocid) is rapidly and completely absorbed from the gut. It has a half-life of 4 to 12 hours. Side effects are common, especially gastric irritation and bilateral frontal headaches. It may interfere with the adaptation necessary for night vision. Particularly in the elderly, indomethacin may cause confusion. Inhibition of the action of furosemide is quite marked. A dose of 50 mg of indomethacin is thought to be equivalent to 650 mg of aspirin. It may be taken by mouth or in suppository form. Few patients can tolerate more than 200 mg/day.

*Ketorolac* (Toradol) is unique in the United States in being available for injection as well as for enteral administration. It is quite potent, 30 mg by injection being as effective as 10 to 12 mg morphine. Thereafter, as with all the other NSAIDs, there is little further increase in effect. Its use as a continuous intravenous infusion (not a U.S. Food and Drug Administration [FDA]-approved use) was described previously. Gastrointestinal absorption is rapid and complete. The half-life is about 5 to 6 hours. Gastric irritation is prominent, and the oral product was removed from the German market for a while because of this. For this reason also, the manufacturers encourage short-term administration only, which limits its usefulness in treating cancer pain. The maximum oral dose should not exceed 90 mg/day.

*Diclofenac* (Voltaren, Voltarol) is an enteric-coated, controlled-release preparation. An immediate-release form, diclofenac potassium (Cataflam) has been marketed in the United States. Diclofenac is well absorbed from the gut but subject to extensive first-pass metabolism. The half-life is about 2 hours. Gastric lesions are less common than with indomethacin or naproxen but remain a potential hazard. Influence on bleeding and clotting times appears to be minimal. Only the oral preparation is available in the United States, but an injectable form exists in the United Kingdom. The maximum oral dose should not exceed 200 mg/day.

*Nabumetone* (Relafen) is well absorbed from the gut.

It is converted in vivo to its active form, 6-methoxy-2-naphthylacetic acid, which has a half-life of about 24 hours. Gastric erosions seem less common than with naproxen or aspirin. It may be given once or twice daily, in a total dose of 1000 to 2000 mg.

*Etodolac* (Lodine) is well absorbed from the gut but is extensively and variably metabolized in the liver so that some dose titration may be needed. The half-life is about 7 hours. Doses range from 200 to 400 mg every 6 to 8 hours; a daily maximum of 1200 mg is recommended.

*Sulindac* (Clinoril), similar to nabumetone, is a well-absorbed prodrug, being reduced in vivo from its sulfoxide form to a sulfide, which has a half-life of about 16 hours. Adverse effects on the gastrointestinal and renal systems appear to be less common than with many other NSAIDs. The recommended dose is 200 mg twice a day.

*Tolmetin* (Tolectin) is comparable to other agents in this group. Animal studies have raised the possibility of ocular toxicity. Its adverse effects are typical of the other NSAIDs. The half-life is about 5 hours. It should be administered on an every-6-hour basis. The maximum recommended daily dose is 1800 mg.

**Anthranilic Acid Derivatives.** *Mefenamic acid* (Ponstel) not only inhibits prostaglandin production but also acts as a prostaglandin antagonist at the receptor level. It causes the gastrointestinal side effects usually associated with NSAIDs and may cause a troublesome diarrhea. The manufacturers do not advocate its use for more than 1 week at a time, so it does not seem to be useful in cancer-related pain.

*Meclofenamate* (Meclomen), like mefenamic acid, not only inhibits prostaglandin production, but also acts as a prostaglandin antagonist at the receptor level. The half-life is reported to be 1 to 2 hours. There is an active metabolite, 3-hydroxymethyl meclofenamic acid, which is only about one fifth as active as the parent compound, but it has a half-life of about 15 hours so that plasma levels do not reach a plateau for about 4 days. Meclofenamate appears to have less potential for causing gastric bleeding than does aspirin, and it has a negligible effect on platelet function. It does, however, cause diarrhea. The dose should not exceed 100 mg every 6 hours.

*Floctafenine* (Idarac) is not available in the United States. It is mainly intended for short-term use and is unsuited to use in treating cancer-related pain.

**Oxicams.** *Piroxicam* (Feldene) has a long duration of effect, the half-life being 30 to 86 hours. It is usually given in a single daily dose of 20 mg. It has a profile of effects and side effects common to the NSAIDs as a whole. It is expensive.

## CYCLOOXYGENASE-2 INHIBITORS

A novel development has grown out of the recognition that cyclooxygenase, the enzyme responsible for the formation of prostaglandins from arachidonic acid, is not uniform throughout the body. The enzyme responsible for the formation of gastroprotective prostaglandins (cyclooxygenase type 1 [COX-1]) is different from that involved in prostaglandin production in inflammatory processes (COX-2). Recognition of this difference spurred the development of compounds tailored specifically to block the catalytic site of the COX-2

*Table 22–3.* Side Effects of Heterocyclic Antidepressants Used in Pain Management

| Drug | Typical Dose Range (mg/day) | Orthostatic Hypotension | Sedation | Anticholinergic Effects |
|---|---|---|---|---|
| *First generation* | | | | |
| Amitriptyline | 10–150 | + + | + + + | + + + |
| Nortriptyline | 25–150 | + | + | + + |
| Imipramine | 20–150 | + + + | + | + + + |
| Desipramine | 25–200 | + + | 0 | + |
| Doxepin | 30–300 | + + | + + + | + + |
| Trimipramine | 75–250 | + + | + + + | + + |
| Clomipramine | 20–200 | + + | + + | + + |
| *Second generation* | | | | |
| Maprotiline | 75–200 | + | + + | + |
| Trazodone | 50–300 | + + | + + + | + / − |
| *Third generation* | | | | |
| Fluoxetine | 20–80 | + / − | + | + |
| Paroxetine | 10–40 | + / − | + + | + |
| Sertraline | 50–200 | + / − | + / − | + / − |

Adjust doses slowly. Use lower doses in the elderly.

enzyme. Exactly what the value of this approach will be remains to be determined. In particular, the role of COX-2 inhibitors in treating cancer pain has yet to be explored. The coadministration of any nonselective NSAID will immediately vitiate the sophisticated pharmacology that these new compounds represent.

## Adjuvant Agents

A heterogeneous group of agents has been found effective in reducing certain pain, particularly that associated with nerve damage, which is fortunate because such pain may respond poorly to conventional analgesics, although some dispute this notion.[46] This collection of drugs includes heterocyclic antidepressants; anticonvulsants; and, although less commonly used because of concern about tardive dyskinesia, the neuroleptics. Although sometimes effective when used singly, it may be necessary to give two or even all three types of adjuvant drugs in combination to gain the desired relief.

For the purposes of pain management in the cancer patient, the monoamine oxidase inhibitors are not considered because they have numerous side effects and can cause other problems by inhibiting the metabolism of many of the other drugs that may be given, such as the opiates.[47]

**Heterocyclic Antidepressants.** Heterocyclic antidepressants are usually the preferred agents because they have less toxicity than the other two groups, even though side effects are sometimes pronounced, especially in the older patient. They are said to be particularly effective against the burning component of neuropathic pain. The literature is conflicting as to whether the older agents are superior to the newer, more serotonin-selective agents, such as fluoxetine. Many of these drugs are subject to variable metabolism, the same dose producing a plasma level that may vary 20-fold in any given group of patients.[48] Unless the plasma levels are measured, a full-dose titration should be undertaken before these drugs are abandoned as ineffective. The most common side effects are listed in Table 22–3. There is no doubt that the most problematic side effects, especially in older patients, are sedation, orthostatic hypotension, and anticholinergic effects, which manifest themselves as dry mouth, urinary retention, and severe constipation.

**Anticonvulsants.** Anticonvulsants may be the best agents to use for the shooting, lancinating, or hyperesthetic pain that often accompanies neuronal damage. Carbamazepine, phenytoin, valproic acid, and clonazepam have been the

*Table 22–4.* Anticonvulsants Used as Adjunctive Analgesics

| Medication | Dose Range (mg/day) | Common Side Effects and Toxicity |
|---|---|---|
| Carbamazepine | 200–1600 | Sedation, ataxia, nausea and vomiting. Serious marrow depression is rare. Serious hepatotoxicity is even less common, but both can be fatal |
| Clonazepam | 2–8 | Sedation |
| Phenytoin | 200–400 | Hyperplasia of gums. Skin changes (acne, hirsutism). Enzyme induction may increase metabolism of other drugs. Saturable (zero order) kinetics may result in unexpectedly large increase in plasma level after small dose change, causing ataxia and other CNS effects. Monitor blood levels |
| Valproic acid | 1500–3000 | Nausea and vomiting. Hepatotoxicity (most common when taking numerous other drugs); pancreatitis |
| Gabapentin | 900–3600 | Fatigue, somnolence, dizziness, ataxia, diplopia |

CNS, central nervous system.

most widely used drugs in this situation.[49] More recently, gabapentin and lamotrigine have been introduced. Gabapentin especially has gained widespread acceptance. Toxicity, especially the leukopenia and hepatotoxicity seen with carbamazepine, is commonly regarded as a major concern, although, in fact, such toxicity is rare. Dose titration is important, especially with carbamazepine, which should be used in doses to 1200 mg/day (if tolerated) before concluding that the drug is ineffective. Dose ranges and side effects are listed in Table 22–4.

**Local Anesthetics.** Local anesthetics may be an important and underused resource, especially in treating neurogenic pain. The anticonvulsant drugs and the polycyclic antidepressants, often used to treat such pain, also share local anesthetic properties. Brose and Cousins[50] reported the efficacy of subcutaneous infusions of lidocaine sufficient to maintain a plasma level of 2 to 5 $\mu$g/ml in three patients whose pain was refractory to all other interventions, including epidural and intrathecal opiates. Good pain relief without significant toxicity was maintained for 6 months by this means.

# Opiates

Opiates have been in use for more than 5000 years, mention being made of them in ancient Sumerian writings. The Greeks, Romans, Hebrews, and Arabs were all familiar with the analgesic properties of the juice of the poppy plant. As chemistry has allowed, numerous derivatives of the original alkaloids have been developed. Although opiate receptors have long been recognized, the discovery of the natural agonists that exogenous opioids mimic was comparatively recent, beginning with the discovery of enkephalins[51] in Kosterlitz' laboratory. The synthesis of selective agonists has enabled us to discern the heterogeneity of opiate receptors. Thus far, $\mu_1$, $\mu_2$, $\delta$, and $\kappa$ receptors have been identified, although this knowledge has not yet been exploited clinically. Clinically available opiate agonists also exhibit heterogeneity (Table 22–5). In broad terms, opiates may be classified as weak or strong and according to whether they have a purely stimulatory effect on the opiate receptors (full agonists) or whether they stimulate at low doses but block

the receptors at higher concentrations (agonist-antagonist type). Of this latter group, all except for buprenorphine have a ceiling on their analgesic effect below that of the full agonists and are also termed *partial agonists*. The full agonists differ among themselves in terms of potency (Table 22–6), but the maximal achievable pain relief is the same for all of them. Higher potency merely means that the agonist in question produces maximal pain relief with fewer milligrams than would an agonist of lesser potency. Bioavailability is another important source of variability between opiates when the oral route is being used (Table 22–7).

Despite important individual differences described subsequently, there are certain features common to all opiates:

1. All can cause nausea, which may be severe, so that it is not uncommon to have to coadminister an antiemetic. Transdermal scopolamine is often adequate, and the convenience of a patch that needs to be replaced only once every 3 days is important. At other times, the nausea can be intractable, and even new potent antiemetics, such as ondansetron, may not overcome it. One agent, insufficiently recognized in the United States, is methotrimeprazine. It is orally active, although no oral preparation is marketed in the United States. It can be given by intramuscular injection or by intravenous infusion. In the United Kingdom, it is not

*Table 22–6.* **Potency of Major Opiates Relative to Morphine (Morphine = 1)**

| | | |
|---|---|---|
| *Weak Agonists* | Codeine | 1:$\frac{1}{12}$ |
| | Propoxyphene | 1:$\frac{1}{24}$ |
| *Moderate Potency* | Dihydrocodeine | Not established |
| | Hydrocodone | Not established |
| *Strong Agonists* | Diamorphine | 1:2 |
| | Fentanyl | 1:100 |
| | Levorphanol | 1:5 |
| | Hydromorphone | 1:5 |
| | Meperidine | 1:$\frac{1}{8}$ |
| | Methadone | 1:1 rising to 1:3* |
| | Oxycodone | 1:2† |
| | Oxymorphone | 1:5 |

*Methadone *appears* to be more potent than morphine because its longer half-life allows higher plateau concentrations to develop with prolonged dosing.

†Oxycodone (available only in oral form) appears twice as potent because of greater bioavailability.

*Table 22–5.* **Opiate Agonists**

| | Full Agonists | Agonist-Antagonists |
|---|---|---|
| *Weak Agonists* | Codeine | |
| | Propoxyphene | |
| *Moderate Potency* | Dihydrocodeine | Pentazocine |
| | Hydrocodone | |
| *Strong Agonists* | Diamorphine* | Nalbuphine |
| | Fentanyl | Buprenorphine |
| | Levorphanol | Butorphanol |
| | Hydromorphone | |
| | Meperidine | |
| | Methadone | |
| | Morphine | |
| | Oxycodone | |
| | Oxymorphone | |

*Available in Canada and the United Kingdom, but not in the United States.

*Table 22–7.* **Bioavailability**

| | Full Agonists | Oral to Parenteral Dose Ratios (Parenteral = 1) |
|---|---|---|
| *Weak Agonists* | Codeine | 1:1.5 |
| | Propoxyphene | Not injected |
| *Moderate Potency* | Dihydrocodeine | 1:1 |
| | Hydrocodone | Not injected |
| *Strong Agonists* | Diamorphine | 1:1.5 |
| | Fentanyl | Not established |
| | Levorphanol | 1:2 |
| | Hydromorphone | 1:5 |
| | Meperidine | 1:4 |
| | Methadone | 1:2 |
| | Morphine | 1:3 |
| | Oxycodone | 1:1.5 |
| | Oxymorphone | Not taken orally |

uncommonly mixed in the same syringe as the opiate and given by subcutaneous infusion by means of a portable patient-controlled analgesia infusion device.[52] It confers the added benefit of a considerable analgesic effect.[53, 54] The main disadvantages are that it is sedating, and it has some potential for causing orthostatic hypotension.

2. Constipation is an almost entirely avoidable side effect but often becomes a major problem because of inappropriate use of laxatives. Stool softeners should be used in adequate amounts, which means the equivalent of eight 100-mg capsules of docusate (Colace) per day. If this is insufficient, docusate can be supplemented with bowel stimulants, such as bisacodyl (Dulcolax) or senna (Senokot), eight tablets per day. A bowel stimulant should not be given if the gut has not been prepared with a stool softener because this may merely provoke regional bowel spasm, making a bad situation worse. A number of reports describe the use of oral naloxone as a means of overcoming opiate-induced constipation. Given by mouth, it gains access to the myenteric plexus, but because of low absorption, little enters the systemic circulation so that full-scale opiate antagonism does not occur.[55, 56] To avoid such an undesirable effect, it is suggested that the dose of naloxone be limited to 20% of the prevailing 24-hr morphine dose, up to 12 mg every 6 hours. One practical difficulty in this approach in a managed care environment is that insurance carriers are quick to label this as *experimental* even now, and refuse to pay for it.

3. Tolerance may develop to a surprising degree, although it is never absolute (i.e., morphine never totally loses its effect through prior use). There is not always complete cross-tolerance between all opiates so that efficacy at low dose may be regained by changing to another opiate. Tolerance is the inevitable result of receptor downregulation, which itself is the inevitable effect of the prolonged administration of an agonist. It is the basis of physical dependency and the well-known withdrawal reactions but is not to be confused with the entirely different phenomenon of addiction (see the introductory section of this chapter).

4. Allergy may develop to the opiates. Commonly the problem may be avoided by changing to another opiate. Frequently, patients may erroneously report allergy, when what they had experienced was flushing of the skin caused by histamine release.

5. Pruritus, especially in the facial area and particularly after spinal administration of the opiate, is believed to be a central effect.

6. Other central side effects include sedation, confusion, hallucinations, coma, and, in extremely high doses, myoclonic jerks and grand mal seizures.

7. There appears to be considerable interindividual variability in the response of any given patient to each individual opiate. No one opiate is inherently superior in all patients because patients who fail to obtain adequate pain relief from one opiate given at the maximum tolerable dose may do so from another.[57]

## SIGNIFICANT FEATURES OF INDIVIDUAL OPIATES

**Codeine.** Codeine is a widely used opioid, despite its low potency as an analgesic. For convenience, it is commonly given in combination with acetaminophen because this is classified as a Schedule III drug, whereas, given singly, it is Schedule II. The disadvantage of such combinations is that the amount of narcotic that can be given without risk of acetaminophen-induced hepatotoxicity is limited. The availability of codeine is overly restricted in the United States. In Britain, for example, acetaminophen with codeine is an over-the-counter preparation, and it causes no problems. In the cancer patient, once significant pain has developed, codeine is too weak an analgesic to be of much use, but, like all opiates, it can cause nausea and constipation.

**Propoxyphene.** Propoxyphene, a congener of methadone, is less potent than codeine and more expensive. It is supplied as a single agent (Darvon) and with acetaminophen (Darvocet-N 50, Darvocet-N 100, and Wygesic). The potential benefit of the active metabolite (norpropoxyphene), which has a local anesthetic effect, has not been adequately evaluated. Side effects are similar to those seen with codeine. It is a Schedule IV drug.

**Dihydrocodeine.** Although available in Europe for more than 30 years, only in the 1990s has dihydrocodeine been approved for oral use in the United States. It is available only in combination with acetaminophen and caffeine (DHC Plus) or with aspirin and caffeine (Synalgos DC). It may be twice as potent as codeine,[58] although this is open to question.[59] It is classified as a Schedule III drug. It has been largely eclipsed by hydrocodone-containing preparations.

**Hydrocodone.** Hydrocodone appears to be more powerful than dihydrocodeine, although exact potency ratios are unknown. It is most widely used in combination with acetaminophen (Anexsia, Lorcet, Lortab, Vicodin, Vicodin ES, and Zydone) or with aspirin (Damason-P and Lortab ASA). The drawback of having to give unwanted acetaminophen or aspirin may be overcome by using Hycodan. This is a combination of hydrocodone and homatropine, intended as a cough suppressant. The prescriber must ensure that the patient will not be harmed by the homatropine included in the mixture by excluding those with, for example, narrow-angle glaucoma, asthma, and prostatism. All hydrocodone-containing preparations are classified as Schedule III agents. It is not well known that hydrocodone can be obtained as a stand-alone product, and many compounding pharmacists are willing to prepare capsules of pure hydrocodone, but this is then classified as a Schedule II drug, requiring a triplicate-type prescription in those states that use them.

**Diamorphine (Heroin).** The most controversial and maligned of all the major narcotics, heroin is not available as a legal therapeutic agent in the United States. It is endowed with no spectacular analgesic properties because once it enters the body, it is rapidly transformed into morphine. Nevertheless, heroin does have certain advantages:

- It is more soluble than morphine, and more analgesic effect can be gained with smaller injections (of importance chiefly for intramuscular administration).
- Its oral absorption is significantly better than that of morphine so that fewer mistakes would be made in conversions from parenteral to oral dose forms.
- It is more lipid soluble than morphine so that when used subcutaneously, absorption is probably more reliable. When given intrathecally or epidurally, there can be greater certainty that the drug will be absorbed into the spinal cord at the level at which it was inserted. There is less

likelihood that it will remain in the cerebrospinal fluid and cause respiratory depression or other central side effects as it drifts rostrally. When the issue of legalizing heroin was discussed in Washington years ago, there were no really *clean* data for review, so the measure was not passed. Although cancer patients probably would be better off with heroin than without it, the time and energy it would take to change the political climate are probably not justified, given the other options available to treat cancer pain. In the United Kingdom, where heroin is available, it continues to be widely used.

**Fentanyl.** Long used in anesthesiology, fentanyl (Duragesic) has become available as a medication for the ambulatory patient, in the form of a transdermal patch. This development was possible (as with any drug given by transdermal patches) because of its low molecular weight and extremely high potency (see Table 22–6), which means that an effective dose is in the microgram range. Being a lipophilic drug, central side effects seem to be more common than with morphine or hydromorphone (Conolly ME, unpublished observations, 1990). For the transdermal patch to be effective, it must remain securely stuck to the skin. Many patients do not press around the edge of the patch firmly enough or long enough for the contact adhesive to form an adequate bond. The pharmacokinetics of this dosage form differ from other forms of opiate administration. It takes 17 hours for the plasma level to reach steady state (and correspondingly long for the level to decline once the patch is removed). Drug delivery is, to a large extent, regulated by the membrane within the patch, but skin blood flow and the prevailing room temperature must influence the rate of removal from the skin. Patients who are vasoconstricted, hypovolemic, or, for other reasons, exhibit impaired cardiovascular function will probably not absorb transdermally administered fentanyl as well as anticipated. There is no means of altering the dose at short notice to alleviate breakthrough pain with the patch alone. A buccal form of fentanyl (Actiq), however, has been introduced to deal with the issue of breakthrough pain.[60] The relatively high cost of the patch may limit its general acceptance, but for a selected subset of patients unable to take opiates by mouth and unwilling to use a patient-controlled analgesia pump, transdermal fentanyl is a useful addition. It is conventional for the patches to be changed every 72 hours, but it is common for patients to find that the patches require replacement every 48 hours (Conolly ME, unpublished observations, 1993). There is one report of the successful use of the fentanyl analogue, sufentanyl, administered sublingually to control breakthrough pain in a patient unwilling to accept a patient-controlled analgesia device.[61]

**Levorphanol.** Levorphanol (Levo-Dromoran) is about five times as potent as morphine, but its pharmacodynamic profile is essentially the same. It has a significantly longer half-life (Table 22–8) so that repeated dosing may result in a significantly higher body load than would occur with morphine. When given orally, it is slightly better absorbed than morphine is (see Table 22–7).

**Hydromorphone.** Hydromorphone (Dilaudid) is an opiate of major importance. It has a higher potency than morphine (see Table 22–6), but this is of less importance than its relative lipid insolubility. This property often makes it

**Table 22–8.** Half-Lives of Commonly Used Opiates

| | Full Agonists | Half-Life (hr) |
|---|---|---|
| *Weak Agonists* | Codeine | 3 |
| | Propoxyphene* | 6–12 |
| *Moderate Potency* | Dihydrocodeine | 3–5 |
| | Hydrocodone | 3–4 |
| *Strong Agonists* | Diamorphine | 3 |
| | Fentanyl | 3–4 |
| | Levorphanol | 12–16 |
| | Hydromorphone | 2–3 |
| | Meperidine | 2–4 |
| | Methadone | 24–96 |
| | Morphine | 2–4 |
| | Oxycodone | 2–5 |
| | Oxymorphone | Unknown |

*Propoxyphene has an active metabolite, norpropoxyphene, which has local anesthetic properties comparable to lidocaine, which may be important in treating neurogenic pain. Its half-life is 30 to 36 hours.

possible to maintain good pain control without undesirable side effects, such as sedation and hallucinations. It has a lower bioavailability and a slightly shorter half-life than morphine (see Tables 22–7 and 22–8), differences that are easily accommodated. Like morphine, hydromorphone is extensively metabolized, and some of the metabolites may accumulate, especially in renal failure, and cause neurotoxicity.[62] There is currently no clinically available controlled-release formulation of this drug, but such a preparation is currently undergoing clinical trials in Canada,[63, 64] and will shortly be introduced in the United States. The only tablet sizes available until more recently (2 mg and 4 mg) are inappropriately small, given the high doses sometimes needed in treating severe pain. The introduction of an 8-mg tablet is an improvement. A significant disadvantage of hydromorphone is that although the oral form is about the same price as morphine, the powder needed to make the drug up for infusion is five times as expensive.

**Meperidine.** Meperidine (Demerol) is not a good drug for the control of pain in the cancer patient. It has a relatively low analgesic potency. Oral absorption is less than for morphine, whereas intramuscular injections are painful, produce extensive tissue damage, and result in erratic absorption. Intravenous administration sometimes causes an unexpectedly large increase in heart rate. Meperidine is sometimes selected in the belief that it causes less spasm in the sphincter of Oddi than do other opiates, but measurements of biliary pressure through biliary T-tubes indicate that the effects of meperidine and morphine are almost the same. Fentanyl increases biliary pressure considerably more and pentazocine considerably less.[65] A serious problem associated with the use of meperidine in large doses or for prolonged periods of time is that normeperidine, one of its metabolites, with a long half-life (15 to 35 hours), may accumulate.[66] This accumulation is especially likely in the context of renal or hepatic dysfunction but may occur in healthy individuals if the daily dose exceeds 1500 mg. Normeperidine has diminished analgesic properties but is a cerebral irritant, which can cause agitation, confusion, and grand mal seizures. These are not reversed by naloxone[67] and respond poorly to conventional anticonvulsants, presumably because of the persistence of the cerebral irritant that provoked the seizure in the first place. The coadministration of meperidine with monoamine oxidase inhibitors produces a severe reaction characterized by excitation, delirium, hyperpyrexia, and convulsions or severe respiratory depression.[68]

**Methadone.** Methadone (Dolophine) is a difficult drug to use because of its pharmacokinetic characteristics. In acute single-dose studies, it is equipotent with morphine. It is somewhat better absorbed from the intestine, most authoritative texts suggesting a bioavailability of 50%.[69, 70] Estimates of half-life vary widely. When first administered, the half-life is generally reported as being between 24 and 35 hours, but with prolonged administration it may rise to about 50 hours.[71] Having a long half-life, methadone exhibits a more prolonged effect than morphine and, as would be expected, takes a correspondingly long time to reach steady-state levels when given on a regular schedule. This situation may create a trap for the unwary, for if a patient achieves rapid pain control on a given dose and is then discharged from the hospital, within 10 to 14 days, the patient may develop symptoms of opiate overdose. This risk may be reduced by prolonging the interval between doses once the patient is sent home and by introducing the drug at a dose some 30% less than what the ultimate dose is expected to be. Methadone is extensively metabolized in the liver. Rifampin and phenytoin may accelerate its metabolism, producing an acute withdrawal state,[72] whereas cimetidine may reduce the rate of metabolism and cause toxicity.[73] Although some patients seem to do better on methadone than other opiates, most find that the prolonged half-life makes rapid dose adjustment difficult. Being more lipid-soluble than morphine, central side effects are more common.

**Morphine.** Morphine remains the gold standard by which all other opiates should be judged. Inexpensive and available in a wide variety of dosage forms, it is without question one of the most valuable drugs available for the control of severe pain. Primarily, it should be considered as an oral agent. Bioavailability is low (30%) but consistent. Although in former times it was given as a component of a pain *cocktail*, such as the Brompton Mixture (named after the Brompton Hospital in London), it is now usual to give it alone, to begin with as an elixir or as an immediate-release tablet. Once the dose required to achieve pain control has been established, it can then be given in the form of a controlled-release tablet. Two such tablets are on the market in the United States, MS Contin (known as MST Continus in the United Kingdom) and Oramorph SR. Both of these are available in a range of dose sizes, which is important, given the extremely wide dosage requirements seen among patients. MS Contin is available in 15-, 30-, 60-, 100-, and 200-mg tablets. Oramorph SR is available in 30-, 60-, and 100-mg sizes. Both are effective products, but the few comparative studies that have been published indicate that morphine absorption is somewhat greater from MS Contin than from Oramorph SR.[74] Absorption from MS Contin is not influenced by the presence of food in the gut,[75] whereas in the case of Oramorph SR, there are modest but significant differences.[76] A comparison in terms of pain relief between the 90-mg MS Contin and the (now obsolete) 90-mg Oramorph SR showed a clear advantage in favor of MS Contin.[77] No comparison between the 100-mg Oramorph and the 90-mg MS Contin is available. Both these preparations are designed to make possible a twice-daily (every 12 hours) dosing schedule, which substantially reduces the burden of constant medication.[78, 79] In opting to use controlled-release morphine tablets, some caveats need to be kept in mind:

1. It is inappropriate to begin therapy with a controlled-release preparation. Initial dose titration requires an immediate-release form of the medication.

2. Controlled-release tablets cannot be crushed to facilitate swallowing or administration through a feeding tube because this disrupts the tablet matrix on which the controlled release depends.

3. Gastrointestinal motility should not be impaired. When it is, absorption may be impaired, and should further doses be taken and motility abruptly improve (as, for example, in the postoperative situation), unexpectedly large amounts of morphine may be rapidly absorbed. A fatality has been reported from this cause.[80, 81]

4. Any preparation that releases its contents over a 12-hour period necessarily requires a functionally normal distal bowel. If a patient with an ileostomy is changed from an immediate-release to a controlled-release dosage form, the result may be disastrous, if the tablet falls into the ileostomy bag with much of its contents undischarged (Conolly ME, unpublished observation, 1989).

One unorthodox use of MS Contin (not advocated by the manufacturers because it does not conform with FDA labeling but described in the hospice literature) has been as a suppository. Embedded in cold-hardened butter, these small tablets can be easily inserted into the rectum and exhibit a bioavailability comparable to that seen after oral dosing. This technique has principally been of use in situations in which oral dosing was no longer possible and parenteral administration could not be initiated promptly.

To a limited extent, morphine has been given as sublingual pellets. Despite the small surface area of the oral cavity, sufficient drug may be absorbed to exert a worthwhile analgesic effect.

The metabolic fate of morphine has attracted interest as it has become apparent that morphine, like meperidine, has active metabolites, which may accumulate in renal failure. In contrast to meperidine, however, one active metabolite, morphine-6-glucuronide, mimics the parent compound in that it is an analgesic. Most extraordinarily for a metabolite, it is 10 to 40 times more active than morphine itself, and it appears to contribute materially to the analgesic effect of morphine[82, 83] as well as to toxicity in patients with renal failure.[84, 85]

It has been claimed that the preponderant metabolite, morphine-3-glucuronide, may exert an *antagonistic* effect at the opiate receptors. This effect could contribute to tolerance,[86] and it has been suggested that some cases of intractable or paradoxic pain (which seems to increase as the dose of morphine is advanced) may be due to excessive amounts of morphine-3-glucuronide relative to the levels of morphine-6-glucuronide.[87, 88] Concentrations of these metabolites relative to the concentration of morphine are greater after oral than after intravenous administration,[89] indicating that significant first-pass metabolism occurs in the intestinal mucosa, as has been shown for other drugs.[90]

Morphine, more than the other opiates, has been used in a variety of patient-controlled analgesia devices (such as the Pharmacia CADD-PCA pump, Pharmacia Deltec, St. Paul, MN) designed to deliver a constant basal infusion, together with the option of self-administered extra doses of predetermined size at a predetermined frequency, for breakthrough pain. Once programmed, the pump can be electronically locked to prevent deliberate or accidental maladministration. Venous access is not required for such infusions; absorption from the subcutaneous tissues is quite adequate, provided that no more that 2 to 3 ml is infused per hour. To keep the volume of infusate within that limit, concentrations of 50 mg morphine/ml may be needed. Such high concentrations may produce local irritation and subcutaneous plaque formation. To prevent this, it is the practice at this center to add dexamethasone, 0.04 to 0.06 mg/ml, to the infusate. If more than 100 mg/hr is required, it becomes necessary to use a secure venous access (peripherally inserted central catheter [PICC] line or Hickman catheter) or to change to hydromorphone, with its high potency and greater solubility. Fentanyl in general is not used in this way because of its higher cost and the fact that it is available only as a single-strength solution (50 μg/ml). This is one situation in which heroin would be advantageous. It has been our experience with morphine that the infusion site needs to be changed every 3 days to prevent local irritation, subcutaneous plaque formation with impaired absorption, and infection. With hydromorphone, the infusion site may be changed less often.[91] Given that modest level of care, we have been able to maintain patients at home for periods ranging from a few weeks to 4 years, without difficulty. Although these pumps are expensive (costing $450/month to rent), they are extremely reliable and allow many patients to retain dignity, mobility, and a high degree of comfort far into the course of their disease.

Even with the most aggressive dose titration, in a small number of patients, adequate pain relief cannot be obtained with systemically administered opiates. For such patients, a technique has been developed in the form of intrathecal opiate infusions (see later). Only morphine is approved by the FDA for this purpose at present.

**Oxycodone.** Oxycodone (Roxicodone) is an underused, little-known opiate, at least as a stand-alone medication. Most practitioners know it in the form of Percocet and Percodan. It is generally regarded as a weak opiate, but only because these fixed-dose combinations contain just 5 mg of oxycodone per tablet. If used as a medication in its own right, oxycodone has about the same potency as morphine. It has some advantage, in that, being less lipid soluble, it tends to cause fewer central side effects.[92] It is substantially better absorbed from the gut than is morphine, with estimates of its bioavailability ranging from 70 to 87%.[93, 94] Its chief disadvantage is that the immediate-release tablet size (5 mg) is far too small. Parenteral oxycodone is not available in the United States. A sustained-release form of oxycodone (OxyContin) has proved to be an invaluable addition for many patients.[95-98] Like MS Contin, it is designed to be given every 12 hours,[99, 100] although persuading tradition-bound physicians to use it in this way is no small task.

**Oxymorphone.** Oxymorphone (Numorphan) is available in parenteral and suppository form in the United States. It is approximately 5 to 10 times more potent than morphine, but its pharmacologic profile is otherwise similar.

## TECHNIQUE FOR RAPID PAIN CONTROL USING OPIATE INFUSIONS

It is not an uncommon experience for a patient to be admitted as an emergency for the control of pain that has escalated beyond the level of endurance. If an infusion were simply to be initiated, it would take approximately five half-lives of the drug employed to achieve steady-state concentrations. For morphine or hydromorphone, it would be approximately 15 hours before the adequacy (or otherwise) of the chosen dose would be known. If too low a dose had been selected, a further 15 hours would have to elapse before the effect of the dose change would be known. A far more effective way to establish the dose rapidly is as follows:

An initial dose is chosen on the basis of whatever history is available (such as the effect of an injection in the emergency department), and the response is observed. In the absence of any such history, a prudent dose, for example, 5 mg of morphine, is injected. If no pain relief is secured within 20 minutes, the dose is increased by 25%, and this cycle is repeated until such time as pain is controlled. The patient is then observed until the pain begins to return. At this stage, knowing the total amount of drug administered to begin with ($D_o$ mg), the quantity still in the body ($D_t$ mg) can be calculated from the formula:

$$D_t = D_o \times e^{-kt}$$

where $k$, the rate constant of elimination, $= 0.693$/half-life ($t_{1/2}$), and $t$ is the time (in hours) that it took for pain to return.

The required information, the rate at which the opiate must be infused ($\frac{D}{T}$) to maintain the body load at or slightly above $D_t$, is calculated by rearranging the standard formula for describing the relationship between the infusion rate and steady-state concentration ($C_{ss}$):

$$C_{ss} = \frac{D}{T} \times \frac{t_{1/2} \cdot 1.44}{\text{Volume of distribution}}$$

Because this approach deals with opiates in terms of body load and not plasma concentration, which bears an uncertain relationship to central effect, the value $D_t$ is substituted for $C_{ss}$, and the term *volume of distribution* is removed from the equation, which then simplifies and rearranges to

$$\frac{D}{T} = \frac{C_{ss}}{t_{1/2} \times 1.44}$$

It has been our experience in this center (Conolly ME, unpublished observations, 1992) that, usually within 3 to 6 hours, using this simple approach, satisfactory pain control can be secured. Some midcourse correction may be needed in the ensuing day or two to allow for tolerance, alteration of metabolite levels (see earlier), and progression of the disease.

## NARCOTICS FOR THE DYING PATIENT PROTOCOL

It is generally accepted (in theory) that dying patients should be given whatever opiates they require to control their pain. It is also acknowledged that the popular notion that adequate pain control shortens life is a misconception. In practice, however, we have found that many physicians, especially among the ranks of the resident staff, have some difficulty in incorporating these two facts into their care of the terminally ill. Once or twice a year, a dying patient is *revived* with naloxone, given in response to a slowed respiration rate. The results are predictably distressing for all concerned. To ease the minds of physicians caught up in this situation and to emphasize that the patient is dying of the disease, *regardless of the medication that is prescribed*, we place such patients on the hospital-approved *Narcotics for the Dying Patient* protocol,[101] which explicitly states that dying patients are entitled to the greatest degree of comfort that can be secured and that they are not to be denied narcotics because of changes in their vital signs.

## BARBITURATES FOR THE DYING PATIENT PROTOCOL

Rarely, especially so given the availability of spinal blocks, do we encounter patients who are not adequately relieved by opiates, even when pushed to the level of significant toxicity. In those few cases, we have, for several years, employed a barbiturate infusion, similar to that described by Truog and colleagues.[102] In essence, this approach requires giving patients a general anesthetic and maintaining them in a state of coma until death supervenes naturally. Owing to the long half-life of barbiturates, progressive accumulation would occur in the face of a continuous infusion, for as long as 10 days, which itself might bring about the patient's death. To avoid this situation (for euthanasia is unlawful and morally unacceptable), care should be taken to give only as much barbiturate as is needed to maintain comfortable sleep.

## ANESTHESIOLOGY TECHNIQUES FOR CONTROL OF CANCER PAIN

Nerve blocks with local anesthetics can serve diagnostic and therapeutic purposes in the management of cancer pain. When local anesthetics cannot provide long-term control of the pain, neurolysis may be indicated. Opioids, administered neuraxially (epidurally or intrathecally), may control pain when all other forms of treatment have failed.

## DIAGNOSTIC BLOCKS

Local anesthetics interfere with the neural transmission of noxious stimuli and can often provide immediate relief of pain.[103] This approach does not usually provide a long-term solution but may aid in localizing the origin of the pain. It may also provide further useful information to guide treatment. Diagnostic blocks should not be performed in isolation but should be regarded as one component of a comprehensive physical and psychological evaluation.

**Anatomic Localization of Sources of Pain.** Anatomic localization of sources of pain can be achieved in various ways. A definitive diagnosis is established when alleviation of pain is produced by the injection of low concentrations of local anesthetics directly into superficial areas of exquisite sensitivity.[104] Blocking specific somatic nerves can rule out or confirm the suspected source of pure nociceptive pain.

**Sympathetically Mediated Pain in Nonvisceral Structures.** Sympathetically mediated pain in nonvisceral struc-

tures can be demonstrated by means of diagnostic nerve blocks. These blocks should be performed at anatomic sites where sympathetic and somatic fibers are anatomically separated. Such sites include the following:

Lumbar sympathetic chain
Celiac plexus
Splanchnic nerves
Cervicothoracic sympathetic chain (stellate ganglion)

In the extremities, intravenous sympathetic blockade (e.g., with guanethidine) can also help to diagnose sympathetically mediated pain.

An alternative method for achieving sympathetic blockade is by using differential concentrations of local anesthetics epidurally or intrathecally.[105] In addition to pain relief, there are usually changes in blood flow and skin temperature to the affected area after all forms of sympathetic blocks.

**Somatic and Visceral Pain.** Somatic and visceral pain can be distinguished using local anesthetic blocks. Diagnostic confusion can occur when the body wall is overlooked as the source of the pain in favor of visceral structures. Examples include trunk pain involving the abdomen, chest, and pelvis. Often, somatic pain can be dramatically relieved by injections into rib cartilages or soft tissues. Intercostal blocks improve pain emanating from the chest wall. Conversely the visceral origins of epigastric or poorly defined lower chest pain can be identified using celiac plexus or splanchnic blocks. Similarly, stellate ganglion (sympathetic block) can confirm a diagnosis of chest pain of visceral origin. When attempting to distinguish somatic from visceral pain, it is often useful to compare efficacy of analgesia of somatic and visceral blocks.

**Prognostic Local Anesthetic Blocks.** Prognostic local anesthetic blocks are often beneficial in predicting the effects of procedures intended to be permanently destructive of neural structures. Such destructive procedures include injecting absolute alcohol or phenol or neurosurgical procedures such as cordotomy or rhizotomy. The purpose of the prognostic block, performed before these destructive procedures, is to allow the patients temporarily to feel the sensations that they will experience after the more permanent procedure is performed.[106] This procedure provides the patient and the physician valuable additional information with which to decide whether or not to carry out the procedure. The prognostic block may mimic the numbness, dysesthesias, and other effects on sensory and motor function as well as the pain relief likely to be produced by the destructive procedure. Prognostic nerve blocks are useful but not fully predictive, in part, because the plasticity of the nervous system confounds the ability to make long-term predictions. For instance, when a spinal rhizotomy is performed, an alternate pain pathway may develop with time, eventually leaving the patient without permanent complete pain relief.[107]

## SYMPATHETIC BLOCKS FOR THE TREATMENT OF PAIN

Visceral pain not amenable to other therapies may respond to sympathetic blockade. The nociceptive pathways from the abdominal and thoracic viscera accompany the efferent sympathetic nerves. Stimulation of these nerves gives rise to segmental reflexes, which may cause skeletal muscle spasm or sympathetic hyperactivity. Once activated, this state may be exacerbated by stimulation of hypothalamic autonomic centers that cause catecholamine release and generally increase sympathetic tone. Systemic narcotic agonists have limited usefulness in treating the resultant pain because they are not directed against its pathogenesis. The three most commonly used sympathetic blocks are the stellate ganglion (cervicothoracic), celiac plexus, and lumbar sympathetic blocks. Other blocks that are less commonly used in the management of cancer pain include superior hypogastric plexus block and block of the ganglion of Walther.[108]

**Stellate Ganglion Blocks.** Stellate ganglion blocks interrupt sympathetic outflow to the head, neck, and arm as well as to the viscera of the thorax. The ganglion is formed by the fusion of the inferior cervical and first thoracic paravertebral sympathetic ganglia. It lies at the base of the neck, anterior to the junction of the transverse process of the first thoracic vertebra and the first rib. Frequently, it extends superiorly to the level of the seventh cervical transverse process.

The technique of blocking the stellate ganglion involves injecting at the level of C6. By performing the block at this level, the risk of pneumothorax is reduced. When the medication is injected in the proper fascial plane, it spreads freely within the craniocaudal axis. Volumes injected vary between 5 and 20 ml, and spread varies from C6–T2 to C3–T5.

Success of the block is usually indicated by the development of an ipsilateral Horner's syndrome (ptosis, miosis, anhydrosis) as well as increases in ipsilateral arm temperature greater than 1° C. Also commonly encountered are nasal congestion, hoarseness, and facial warmth.

It is *imperative* to draw back on the syringe before injection to avoid intravascular injection or introduction of local anesthetic directly into the cerebrospinal fluid. Potential complications include vertebral or carotid artery injection resulting in seizures, high spinal block producing respiratory arrest or bradycardia, pneumothorax, vocal cord paralysis, vasovagal syncope, and orthostatic hypotension. Because of the proximity of numerous significant structures, the advisability of a neurolytic block of the stellate ganglion is controversial.

Problems responsive to stellate ganglion block include pain in the head, pain from a Pancoast tumor, or pain from vascular insufficiency (such as Raynaud's disease) in the upper extremity. Neuropathic pain caused by tumor involvement, postherpetic neuralgia, radiation therapy, and chemotherapy may also benefit from this procedure.

**Celiac Plexus Block.** Celiac plexus block is one of the most commonly used and effective nerve blocks in the management of cancer pain.[109] This plexus is the largest of the great sympathetic plexuses. It innervates the abdominal viscera. It lies at the level of the upper portion of the vertebral body of L1, in the retroperitoneal space, anterior to the spine and crura of the diaphragm and behind the stomach and bursa of the omentum. The plexus is periaortic in location and is actually a diffuse complex of interconnected neural fibers embedded in fatty tissue. Various structures come together to form the plexus. Specifically, these include the greater splanchnic nerves (T5–9), the lesser splanchnic nerves (T10–11,) and the least splanchnic nerve (T12) as well as the actual celiac ganglia, fibers of both

vagus nerves, and the superior and inferior mesenteric ganglia. This conglomeration represents preganglionic thoracic branches and white rami from adjacent sympathetic nerves.

Afferent sensory nerve fibers that travel with the sympathetic and parasympathetic fibers transmit visceral nociceptive signals. The plexus can transmit pain from the colon, small intestine, abdominal aorta, mesentery, adrenal glands, pancreas, spleen, liver, stomach, and diaphragm. Blocking the plexus may interrupt pain impulses from all these organs.

There are numerous approaches to blocking the celiac plexus. Posterior techniques include the retrocrural, transcrural, and transaortic approaches. Various anterior approaches are also used. Preprocedure preparation includes establishment of intravenous access and prehydration. Most blocks are performed under radiologic guidance (either computed tomography [CT] or fluoroscopy). For a prognostic block, 5 to 20 ml of local anesthetic is injected on each side.

A common side effect is orthostatic hypotension. Complications include aortic or vena caval puncture resulting in retroperitoneal hematoma. Pneumothorax and puncture of the liver, spleen, pancreas, ureter, and kidney have been reported. Complications of neurolysis are discussed subsequently.

The most common indication for performing a celiac plexus block is treatment of upper abdominal and referred back pain caused by pancreatic carcinoma. It is also useful for other cancer pain involving the upper and mid-abdomen as well as acute and chronic visceral disease. Pain associated with hepatic embolization for therapy of carcinoma is also amenable to celiac plexus block.

**Lumbar Sympathetic Block.** Lumbar sympathetic block is most useful for diagnosis and treatment of sympathetically maintained pain unrelated to cancer. This includes reflex sympathetic dystrophy and inoperable ischemic pain. Lower extremity pain of neoplastic origin is predominantly somatically mediated. Often, however, sympathetic mediation must be ruled out. In patients with rectal or cervical carcinoma, tumor involvement of the lumbar sympathetic nerves can give rise to painful distal syndromes. Radiation fibrosis of the lumbar plexus can produce neuropathic pain that mimics sympathetically maintained pain and may be treated successfully with lumbar sympathetic block.[110]

The lumbar sympathetic ganglia are found in a fascial plane anterolateral to the vertebral bodies of L2 and L3. The approach for the block is posterior. For the prognostic block, 20 ml of local anesthetic is employed. Block at L2 alone usually provides a sympathectomy to the entire leg. Common complications and side effects include orthostatic hypotension, spinal or epidural injection resulting in somatic block, injury to the kidney or ureter, and genitofemoral block.

## NEUROLYSIS

Local anesthetic blocks have only a transient effect on cancer pain. More permanent results may be obtained by destroying the sympathetic and somatic nerves with neurolytic agents. Proper patient selection is essential. Understanding of the agents and their side effects and complications is important.

**Patient Selection.** Optimal patient selection is the key to success with neurolysis. Prognostic blocks should have demonstrated significant pain relief. Aggressive conventional pharmacologic management should have failed because of lack of efficacy or intolerable side effects. The block should not exacerbate the underlying medical condition or accelerate its course. Bodily functions important to the patient, such as bowel or bladder control and ambulation, should not be compromised. Contraindications to needle introduction, such as coagulopathy or sepsis, should be ruled out. Nondestructive procedures, such as neuraxial narcotics, should be deemed inappropriate. In the case of somatic blocks, the pain should be limited to as small a number of dermatomes as possible.

Patients should understand the risks and benefits of neurolysis. Realistic expectations should be fostered. These expectations should be partially based on the outcome of the prognostic block and should include the understanding that successful pain control does not treat the underlying problem.

**Neurolytic Agents.** These include absolute ethyl alcohol, phenol, ammonium sulfate, silver nitrate, and chlorocresol. Alcohol and phenol are the most commonly used and are discussed here.

Absolute ethyl alcohol is extremely irritating to local tissues and causes considerable temporary pain on injection. For this reason, local anesthetics are sometimes injected before the alcohol to blunt the burning sensation. The mechanism of action of alcohol in neurolysis is believed to involve dehydration of neural tissue, extracting cholesterol, phospholipid, and cerebrosides. Mucoprotein and lipoprotein precipitate from the myelin sheath. Alcohol is commonly used for neurolysis of peripheral nerves, cranial nerves, lumbar sympathetics, and the celiac plexus. Typically the effect of alcohol-induced neurolysis lasts 1 year.

Commonly occurring problems after alcohol neurolysis include persistent pain at the site of injection, paresthesia, hyperesthesia, and postinjection neuritis.[111] Systemic hypotension is expected and may be attenuated by prehydration and the use of vasopressors. Care must be taken to avoid inadvertent injection into unintended motor or sensory nerves. Needles should be flushed before being removed to avoid leaving alcohol along their tracks. Because the volume required to produce the blocks is small (20 ml per side), alcohol intoxication is extremely rare.

Phenol is the only agent used more commonly than alcohol for neurolysis to treat intractable cancer pain. Phenol injection is considerably less painful than alcohol injection. The initial effect produced is thought to be similar to a reversible local anesthetic.

The effect of phenol on nerve fibers is related to its concentration, which ranges from 5 to 8%. At low concentrations, unmyelinated C fibers are selectively blocked. Sympathetic transmission is also differentially blocked at lower concentrations. As the concentration increases, there is more effect on the myelinated fibers.[112] As with alcohol, extravasation of phenol into the tissues can produce sloughing, and needles need to be flushed free of phenol before removal to avoid creating a track. The effect of phenol is usually less profound and of shorter duration than that of alcohol.

Alcohol and phenol can also be used to perform intrathecal neurolysis. Subarachnoid neurolysis produces good pain relief with either agent. This technique is mentioned here for completeness. Details of this procedure are described elsewhere.[113, 114]

## NEURAXIAL NARCOTICS

Patients who do not derive adequate pain relief from systemic narcotics (usually because of dose-limiting side effects) have a further therapeutic option in the form of narcotics delivered into the epidural space or directly into the cerebrospinal fluid (intrathecal). This technique is a valuable alternative to the irreversible neuroablative procedures, which may be associated with risks of loss of function and independence. In contrast to specifically targeted nerve blocks, neuraxial narcotics may be used to treat multiple foci of pain, which are typically present in metastatic disease. This approach can provide dramatic improvement in cancer pain control when other approaches have failed.

The *locus of action* explains why minute doses of medications can achieve such profound effects. The largest concentration of opioid receptors are found in laminas II and III (substantia gelatinosa) of the dorsal horn of the spinal cord.[115] The dorsal horn is the principal site of action of nociceptive modulation and suppression. Here, opioid agonists act at $\mu$ and $\delta$ receptors, changing neuronal membrane hyperexcitability, making the neurons more refractory to further excitation.[116] Consequently, neurotransmitter release is inhibited, and an inhibition of nociceptive transmission develops.

Neuraxial narcotics can be injected intermittently or can be delivered continuously by epidural or intrathecal infusion. Narcotics administered epidurally cross the meninges, dissolve in the cerebrospinal fluid, and act in the same fashion as intrathecally administered narcotics. Because only a small portion of epidurally administered medication reaches the cerebrospinal fluid, however, approximately 10 times as much medication must be given epidurally as intrathecally to achieve equivalent analgesia.

Spinal drug delivery methods range from simple to highly sophisticated systems. The simplest technique involves the percutaneous placement of an exteriorized epidural[117] or intrathecal catheter, which is taped in place. This catheter allows intermittent or continuous spinal administration of the opiate. A greater length of the exteriorized catheter may be buried subcutaneously if it is placed through a paraspinous incision than if it is introduced percutaneously. It is possible to bury such catheters entirely beneath the skin, attaching the distal end to a subcutaneous injection port. The most sophisticated system by which intraspinal narcotics can be administered is to use a totally implanted intrathecal catheter, which delivers medications from an implanted, externally programmable, variable-rate pump.[118] Pumps for this purpose have been perfected and are commercially available (Medtronics, Inc, Minneapolis, MN). These pumps can deliver a constant infusion or may be set up to follow a complex sequence of steps, in which different infusion rates are automatically delivered at set times of the day. Before such an elaborate and expensive system is implanted, it is essential that the patient have a trial injection of neuraxial narcotics to confirm efficacy and a lack of unacceptable side effects. Also, a psychological determination that the patient could adjust to living with such a permanent device is essential before implantation.

Typically, at roughly monthly intervals, the patient must attend the clinic where high-concentration, preservative-free morphine is used to refill the pump, by percutaneous injection, and adjustments are made to the infusion rate as necessary. Preservative-free morphine has been the drug of choice for continuous intrathecal infusion and is currently the only narcotic preparation that is approved by the FDA.

Complications related to intrathecal infusion are few but important. Because the opioid is injected almost directly into the receptor site, the dose necessary for pain control is several orders of magnitude smaller than the dose injected systemically. Mild side effects, such as nausea, vomiting, and pruritus, may occur. Pruritus is a common complaint, although it usually subsides in a few days. The most important side effect is respiratory depression. To avoid this side effect, trials of morphine infusion must be performed in an environment prepared to treat this complication. It is advisable to have a complete respiratory function evaluation before placement of a continuous intrathecal infusion device. Respiratory depression can be reversed by intravenous naloxone.

In the initial phase of enthusiasm for this technique, it was thought that tolerance would not develop when opioids were infused intrathecally. After several years of experience, however, tolerance has been recognized as a limitation of the efficacy of intrathecal opioid infusion.[119] Other opioids, such as fentanyl, may be used intermittently in place of morphine to lessen the development of tolerance, although none is FDA approved for this purpose as yet. Overall the reported efficacy of intrathecal infusion varies from 70 to 90% during a median follow-up time of 6 months.[120–122]

Baclofen (a derivative of the inhibitory neurotransmitter γ-aminobutyric acid) has been approved for intrathecal use to treat chronic spasticity.[123]

Both epidural and intrathecal narcotics have assumed a prominent role in the management of cancer pain. Epidural narcotics may be delivered from external pumps and can be mixed with dilute concentrations of a local anesthetic. Such external delivery systems offer certain advantages, such as easy changing of medication and easy refilling, coupled with sophisticated patient-controlled analgesia. Major disadvantages are the need for a spinal catheter to be connected to an external device, with the inevitably increased risks of infection and the limitations on activity necessary for protection of the catheter and its entry site. Although they have lower initial costs, in the long run, they have higher monthly maintenance costs than internal systems.

Internal systems, which use implantable pumps, built to extremely high specifications, are expensive. Currently, to place such a pump costs about $20,000. One has to consider, however, the level of comfort that it alone may provide (coupled with the need to impose fewer restrictions on the patient's activity) as well as the rather considerable costs of providing a steady supply of medication cassettes for the external devices described previously. Overall maintenance costs for the implanted devices may ultimately be lower than those of external pumps.[124]

# Neurosurgical Aspects of Cancer Pain Control

Roughly one third of patients with cancer pain gain inadequate benefit from medical treatment. Severe side effects and poor pain control greatly impair the quality of life for these patients. Many physicians tend to refer such patients to a neurosurgeon late in the course of their disease, when they are already severely debilitated and have become poor surgical candidates. The likelihood that they could then benefit from the neurosurgical procedure is small because by then most have become bedridden.

Alternative approaches to pain management should always be considered as soon as it becomes clear that other, less invasive treatments are failing to maintain the patient pain free and functional. Nerve blocks performed by the anesthesiologist (see earlier) often prove helpful and frequently serve as a diagnostic strategy for future neurosurgical intervention. The chief aim of any neurosurgical procedure is to provide the patient with a pain-free terminal phase, without the need for high doses of analgesic drugs that often impair cognition.

Neurosurgical procedures can be directed toward

- Alleviation of pressure on neuronal structures caused by encroachment on nerves by tumor
- Delivery of drugs directly to the central nervous system
- Augmentation of pain-controlling pathways by electric stimulation
- Interruption of pain pathways

These surgical options are discussed subsequently (Table 22–9).

## NEURONAL DECOMPRESSION

The best approach for the treatment of pain is always removal of the causative factor. Tumor encroachment on neuronal structures, particularly of peripheral nerves and spinal cord, can cause excruciating pain that often responds poorly

*Table 22–9.* **Common Neurosurgical Procedures Used to Control Cancer Pain**

Relief of neural compression by tumor
  Spinal nerves
  Cranial nerves
  Brachial plexus
  Lumbar plexus
  Sacral plexus
  Spinal cord
Delivery of drugs directly to the CNS
  Epidural—spinal canal
  Intrathecal—spinal canal, intraventricular
Augmentation of pain-controlling pathways by electric stimulation
  Deep brain stimulation
  Cortical stimulation
  Dorsal column stimulation
  Peripheral nerve stimulation
Interruption of pain pathways in the peripheral nervous system or CNS
  Rhizotomy
  Ganglionectomy
  Cordotomy
  Dorsal root entry zone lesion
  Commissural myelotomy
  Thalamotomy
  Cingulotomy
  Mesencephalotomy
  Chemical hypophysectomy

CNS, central nervous system.

to medical management. Decompression of these structures should be the first goal of the neurosurgeon.[125] Detailed work-up with imaging studies, such as magnetic resonance imaging (MRI) and CT scans, must be performed before any surgical plan is developed. For example, intracranial metastatic lesions involving the trigeminal nerve can cause severe facial pain. Detailed imaging studies of the base of the skull may provide essential details of the anatomic relationship of the tumor to the gasserian ganglion or trigeminal trunk. A craniotomy for removal of the tumor compressing the trigeminal nerve should be considered along with the use of radiotherapy or radiosurgery. Depending on what is achieved during surgery, section of branches of the trigeminal nerve may also be necessary. Such procedures are discussed in the section on neuroablative procedures.

Spinal involvement by metastatic disease can cause pain at any level of the spine. Intractable occipital and neck pain may be secondary to invasion and destruction of the atlanto-occipital joint. Likewise, atlantoaxial tumor invasion may cause odontoid fracture and instability. This diagnosis is obtained by dynamic plain radiographs, MRI, and CT scans. Surgery for decompression and stabilization of these structures may completely alleviate pain and instability.[126] Invasion of a vertebral body can cause vertebral collapse and instability at any level of the spine. In the thoracic region, instability is less common because of the rib cage. The pain generated usually follows a dermatomal distribution. Radiation therapy to the region frequently controls pain. When steroids and radiation therapy fail to control pain, resection of the vertebral body, spinal nerve decompression, and reconstruction with methyl methacrylate may be indicated.

Involvement of the thoracolumbar junction and lumbar spine is often a more difficult diagnostic problem. The pain takes on a more diffuse quality, frequently described as sacroiliac pain. Dynamic plain radiographs, MRI, CT scans, and, if necessary, a myelogram may disclose tumor invasion of the spinal canal, root compression, vertebral collapse, or subluxation. Surgical decompression followed by spine stabilization by instrumentation may be the treatment of choice for such pain.[127] Every available spinal procedure for tumor resection and vertebral stabilization is indicated when the general medical condition of the patient permits and life expectancy is reasonable.[128] This decision must be made by the team taking care of the patient, including the medical oncologist, the pain management group, the anesthesiologist, and the neurosurgeon.

Pain involving limbs, shoulder, or sacral region secondary to brachial, lumbar, or sacral plexus infiltration is hard to treat. Techniques to expose these plexuses to permit resection of tumor tissue have been developed but have yielded uncertain results.[129] Radiation therapy remains the best initial approach, although its results diminish with time. Other neurosurgical approaches, as discussed subsequently, might be required.

## DELIVERY OF DRUGS DIRECTLY TO THE CENTRAL NERVOUS SYSTEM

The least invasive procedures are obviously the most desirable for control of pain in patients in poor condition and with short life expectancy. Direct infusion of opioids intrathecally or epidurally (as described earlier) has gained popularity since its conception in the early 1980s. Poletti and associates[130] devised a method to permit continuous infusion of morphine into the subarachnoid space of the spine to control cancer pain. The surgery is simple. The intrathecal catheter is placed transcutaneously and is connected to a continuous delivery system, which is buried in the abdominal subcutaneous tissue. The operation is performed under light sedation and local anesthesia at our institution. Patients return every 2 to 4 weeks to allow the reservoir in the pump to be refilled. Complications with this procedure are rare. The surgically related complications are infection, pump migration, seroma formation around the pump, and catheter disconnection.

Patients with upper neck and facial pain have been treated with intraventricular infusion of opioids.[131, 132] Placement of an intraventricular catheter connected to an infusion system located in the subcutaneous tissue in the anterior chest wall is a relatively simple neurosurgical procedure. This approach has been rewarding, with a low complication rate.[133] Intracranial hemorrhage related to catheter placement is extremely rare. Infection, pump malfunction, and catheter disconnection are possible complications. As in the case of intrathecal infusion at the spinal level, these problems should be suspected when analgesia fails. Plain radiographs usually show catheter disconnection, and MRI or CT scan may disclose any intracranial mishap.

## AUGMENTATION OF PAIN-CONTROLLING PATHWAYS BY ELECTRIC STIMULATION

The idea of applying deep brain stimulation to control pain arose from the experimental work of Olds and Milner in 1954.[134] They described a positive analgesic effect of deep brain stimulation in laboratory animals. In 1969, Raynolds[135] showed that stimulation of the periaqueductal region of rats prevented the typical responses to nociceptive stimulation. This finding led to increased research into pain pathways as well as to the study of the release of endogenous opioids by stimulation of specific areas of the brain.[136]

Knowledge accumulated in the laboratory was quickly applied to the treatment of persistent pain in humans. The first trial in humans was performed by Heath and Mickle in 1960,[137] who implanted electrodes in the septal area. Success with this technique has been reported to range from 22 to 94%.[138–146] This approach, although controversial, confers the benefit of avoiding permanent interruption of central nervous system pathways or destruction of nuclei, which must occur with ablative procedures. Because the results obtained by this approach have been inconsistent, however, only a few centers throughout the world use these techniques.

Stimulation of three main areas in the brain have been found to be effective for pain control: the periaqueductal gray, the periventricular gray, and the ventroposterolateral and ventroposteromedial nuclei of the thalamus. Periaqueductal gray and periventricular gray stimulation is applied for diffuse pain, whereas ventroposteromedial and ventroposterolateral stimulation is applied for localized neurogenic pain.[146]

Stimulation of somatosensory pathways to control pain is

based on the gate theory of Melzack and Wall.[147] This theory provides a mechanism not only for the effect of ventroposteromedial and ventroposterolateral stimulation, but also for pain control achieved by transcutaneous peripheral nerve[148, 149] and dorsal column stimulation.[150] These procedures are apparently more successful for treatment of chronic pain of nonmalignant origin than cancer pain.[151] The use of electric stimulation for cancer-related pain has been advocated for phantom-limb pain, nerve injury pain, sympathetic dystrophies, and postherpetic neuralgia.[129] Stimulation of the motor cortex for control of severe intractable pain has been reported.[152]

The variability of the results may be merely the effect of the lack of a dependable commercially available electrode or to selection of different targets on the part of the authors.[141] The data of Young and Brechner[146] are encouraging. This technique may represent the solution for several cases of severe, diffuse cancer pain that responds poorly to systemic or intrathecal opioids[146] and certainly deserves further study.

## INTERRUPTION OF PAIN PATHWAYS IN THE PERIPHERAL OR CENTRAL NERVOUS SYSTEM

Destructive procedures have been progressively abandoned over the years. The idea of impairing function, even when it represents abolition of pain, is not well accepted by the patient. This idea also induces in the surgeon a feeling of failure because he or she is, in fact, destroying the nervous system. Nevertheless, neurosurgical interruption of pain pathways or the limbic system can provide pronounced relief of pain. Destructive surgery should be considered only when all other options for pain control have failed.

**Rhizotomy and Ganglionectomy.** Rhizotomy and ganglionectomy represent peripheral interruption of pain pathways. The major disadvantage of these procedures is the complete loss of sensory function in the corresponding dermatome.

The surgeon shares with the anesthesiologist percutaneous techniques of rhizotomy or ganglionectomy, such as alcohol, phenol, and glycerol injection.[153, 154] Radiofrequency rhizotomy is usually performed by neurosurgeons. These procedures are performed under local anesthesia and with fluoroscopic guidance. The patient cooperates with the surgeon in identifying the roots that, when severed, lead to pain relief.[155] When percutaneous procedures fail, surgical section under general anesthesia is undertaken. Rhizotomy can also cause loss of motor function if the particular nerve root carries motor fibers. Section of the posterior rootlets in the spinal canal or removal of the sensory ganglion (ganglionectomy) avoids any motor compromise. When several roots or ganglia are involved at the upper or lower extremities level, motor function can become severely compromised by the concomitant loss of proprioception. Rhizotomies and ganglionectomies are reserved for malignant pain related to sensory cranial nerves, thoracic wall pain, and somatic pain. The main drawback of rhizotomies and ganglionectomies is the short duration of pain relief, usually measured in months, and the possible later onset of severe deafferentation pain in the denervated area.

**Cordotomy and Myelotomy.** Cordotomy is the most common destructive procedure performed for cancer pain. Pain relief after a cordotomy, with few exceptions, lasts 18 months. The life expectancy of the patient is an important factor in the decision to perform a cordotomy. The best candidates for cordotomies are patients with unilateral pain below the T12 dermatome. Bilateral pain relief, however, and analgesia up to the C5 dermatome can be obtained.[156] The surgical technique was described by Spiller and Martin in 1912.[157] Since then, improvements in the surgical procedure and development of a technique for percutaneous cordotomy at the C2 level have made this procedure safe, and it can provide excellent control of cancer pain in 90% of patients.[158–160] The complication rate increases dramatically when bilateral cordotomy is performed. Complications are urinary incontinence, hemiparesis, and paraparesis. Death from respiratory arrest in cases of bilateral cordotomy performed above the C4 level may occur because of diaphragmatic paralysis. Complications related to open surgery, such as infection and cerebrospinal fluid leakage, can also occur.

Pain and temperature pathways are separated from those of touch and proprioception in the spinal cord. The spinothalamic tract (pain and temperature) is located in the contralateral anterior quadrant of the spinal cord, whereas the gracile and cuneatus tracts (proprioception and touch) are located in the ipsilateral posterior column.[161] This unique anatomic distribution allows for obliteration of pain and temperature sensation in the site of the pain, with preservation of touch and proprioception, which are indispensable for motor function. After a cordotomy, patients must be warned to be careful with the extremity deprived of pain and temperature perception to avoid injuries.

The unique crossing of the pain fibers in the commissure of the spinal cord allows for another operation to control pain. This operation is called *commissural myelotomy* and consists of longitudinal midline section of the spinal cord at the dermatome level of the pain.[162] The complication rate with this operation is higher than that of cordotomy, and it is rarely performed.[163]

**Intracranial Ablative Procedures.** Bilateral disconnection of the limbic system usually affords control of cancer pain without somatic sensory loss,[164] and a remarkable decrease in opioid intake may be observed after such disconnection.[165] The affective (*suffering*) component of the patient's distress is abolished, and, although still present, the pain no longer bothers the patient.[166] The site of choice for limbic system disconnection is the cingulate gyrus. MRI provides excellent visualization of the cingulate gyrus for stereotactic lesion placement. Ablation of the cingulate gyrus can be performed by radiofrequency thermocoagulation or by radiosurgery.[167]

Several other targets that might improve the control of cancer pain have been described. Stereotactic guidance, supplemented by electric stimulation to confirm the accurate localization of the desired target, makes the procedures anatomically reliable. Although effective, however, pain relief by these central procedures is short lasting.[168]

1. Mesencephalotomy has been advocated for control of intractable facial, arm, and entire body contralateral pain.[169] Side effects of mesencephalotomy are formidable, consisting of ocular motor palsies, dysesthesias, and anesthesia dolorosa. This procedure has largely been abandoned.[170]

2. Thalamotomy directed to the spinothalamic tract relay nuclei, ventroposteromedian and lateral, provides control of pain in the opposite side of the body with accompanying contralateral hypoesthesia.[171]

3. Destruction of less specific sensory thalamic nuclei, such as the intralaminar, centrum medianum, parafascicularis, and pulvinar nuclei also provide variable control of pain.[168]

## Conclusion

Physicians can do vastly more for patients than is often done. Fear of unrelieved pain should not stalk patients in the way that it does. Physicians have an obligation to exploit to the full the many drugs and procedures now available to ensure that patients do not endure unnecessary pain. In addition to all that we have at our disposal now, the future holds out the prospect of a better understanding of the drugs available and of other agents to come.

The issue of tolerance is one that commonly arises in the context of prolonged opiate usage. It has become clear that this is not just a matter of receptor downregulation, but the involvement of separate cellular pathways. The proposed mechanisms are extremely complex and are beyond the scope of this chapter. Much attention, however, has focused on the role of pathways involving excitatory amino acids, such as N-methyl-D-aspartate (NMDA). To this end, agents known to have NMDA receptor antagonist properties and agents that selectively block L-type calcium channels have been explored. These agents include dextromethorphan, amantadine, and nimodipine. In our hands, these agents have been disappointing (Conolly ME, unpublished observations, 1997), but a morphine-dextromethorphan combination (Morphidex) may be marketed in the near future.

From the skin of a poisonous Ecuadoran tree frog, a chemical, epibatidine, has been isolated that in animal tests proved to be 200 times more potent an analgesic than morphine. It could not be reversed by naloxone,[172] and subsequent research confirmed that this compound exerted its effects through nicotinic cholinergic receptors. Epibatidine itself was too toxic for use in humans, but a derivative of it (ABT 294) is being studied by Abbott Laboratories (North Chicago, IL). Another toxin, in this case one produced by the Conus sea snail with which it paralyzes passing fish, has been modified to produce a highly selective calcium channel–blocking agent (Ziconotide), which is being studied as an intrathecal medication with a profound ability to block pain pathways.

Death is immutable, but, in the conquest of pain, there is always hope.

## REFERENCES

1. Bonica JJ, ed. The management of pain. Philadelphia: Lea & Febiger, 1990:402.
2. Von Roenn JH, Cleeland CS, Gonin R, et al. Physician attitudes and practice in cancer pain management. Ann Intern Med 1993;119:121–6.
3. Twycross RG, Fairfield S. Pain in far advanced cancer. Pain 1982;14:303–10.
4. Liebeskind J. Pain can kill. Pain 1991;44:3–4.
5. Page GG, Ben-Eliyahu S, Yirmiya R, et al. Morphine attenuates surgery-induced enhancement of metastatic colonization in rats. Pain 1993;54:21–8.
6. Bonica JJ, ed. The management of pain. Philadelphia: Lea & Febiger, 1990:12.
7. Twycross RG. Relief of pain. In: Saunders CM, ed. The management of terminal malignant disease. London: Edward Arnold, 1984:64.
8. Clark HW, Sees KL. Opioids, chronic pain and the law. J Pain Symptom Manage 1983;8:297–305.
9. Conolly ME, Briant RH, George CF, et al. A cross-over comparison of clonidine and methyldopa in hypertension. Eur J Clin Pharmacol 1972;4:222–7.
10. Friedman DP. Perspectives on the medical use of drugs of abuse. J Pain Symptom Manage 1990;5:Suppl 1:S2–5.
11. Portenoy RK. Chronic opioid therapy in nonmalignant pain. J Pain Symptom Manage 1990;5:Suppl 1:S46–62.
12. Perry S, Heidrich G. Management of pain during debridement: a survey of U.S. burn units. Pain 1982;13:267–80.
13. Porter J, Jick H. Addiction rare in patients treated with narcotics. N Engl J Med 1980;302:123.
14. Wall PD. Neuropathic pain. Pain 1990;43:267–8.
15. Jaffe JH, Martin WR. Opioid analgesics and antagonists In: Goodman AG, Gilman LS, eds. The pharmacological basis of therapeutics. New York: Macmillan, 1985:500.
16. Glynn CJ, Lloyd JW, Folkhard S. Ventilatory response to intractable pain. Pain 1981;11:201–11.
17. Hanks GW, Twycross RG. Pain, the physiological antagonist of opioid analgesics. Lancet 1984;1:1477–8.
18. Walsh TD, Baster R, Bownman K, et al. High dose morphine and respiratory function in chronic cancer pain. Pain 1981;Suppl 1:S39.
19. Jaffe JH, Martin WR. Opioid analgesics and antagonists. In: Goodman AG, Gilman LS, eds. The pharmacological basis of therapeutics. New York: Macmillan, 1985:507.
20. Wells CJ, Lipton S, Lahverta J. Respiratory depression after percutaneous cervical antero-lateral cordotomy in patients on slow-release oral morphine. Lancet 1984;1:739.
21. Stanley R. Legal questions over pain relief worrying medical community. Austin American Statesman, October 31, 1992.
22. Pulley M. Doctors thrust, consumers parry enforcement issue. Business Journal, February, 1993.
23. Jorenson DE. Federal and state regulation of opioids. J Pain Symptom Manage 1990;5:Suppl 1:S12.
24. Stasney CR, Stratton Hill C. Pain control and the Texas State Board of Medical Examiners. Texas State Board of Medical Examiners Newsletter 1993;15:1.
25. Joranson DE. Availability of opioids for cancer pain: recent trends, assessment of system barriers, new World Health Organization guidelines, and the risk of diversion. J Pain Symptom Manage 1993;8:353–60.
26. Woolf CJ. Functional plasticity of the flexor withdrawal reflex in the rat following peripheral tissue injury. Adv Pain Res Ther 1985;9:193–201.
27. Mogil JS, Marek P, O'Toole LA, et al. Mu-opiate receptor binding is up-regulated in mice selectively bred for high stress-induced analgesia. Unpublished observations.
28. Kasalicky J, Krajska V. The effect of repeated strontium-89 chloride therapy on bone pain palliation in patients with skeletal cancer metastases. Eur J Nucl Med 1998;25:1362–7.
29. Brundage MD, Crook JM, Lukka H. Use of strontium-89 in endocrine-refractory prostate cancer metastatic to bone. Cancer Prev Control 1998;2:79–87.
30. Hindley AC, Hill EB, Leyland MJ, et al. A double-blind controlled trial of salmon calcitonin in pain due to malignancy. Cancer Chemother Pharmacol 1982;9:71–4.
31. Szanto J, Jozsef J, Rado J, et al. Pain killing with calcitonin in patients with malignant tumors. Oncology 1986;43:69–72.
32. Roth A, Kolaric K. Analgesic activity of calcitonin in patients with painful osteolytic metastases. Breast Cancer Oncol 1986;43:283–7.
33. Bloomqvist C, Elomaa I, Porkka L, et al. Evaluation of salmon calcitonin treatment in bone metastases from breast cancer—a controlled trial. Bone 1988;9:45–51.
34. Ernst DS, MacDonald RN, Paterson AHG, et al. A double-blind, crossover trial of intravenous clodronate in metastatic bone pain. J Pain Symptom Manage 1992;7:4–11.
35. Ripamonti C, Fulfaro F, Ticozzi C, et al. Role of pamidronate diso-

dium in the treatment of metastatic bone disease. Tumori 1998;84:442–55.

36. Pelger RCM, Hamdy NAT, Zwinderman AH, et al. Effects of the bisphosphonate olpadronate in patients with carcinoma of the prostate to the skeleton. Bone 1998;22:403–8.

37. Mundy GR, Yoneda T. Bisphosphonates as anticancer drugs. N Engl J Med 1998;339:398–400.

38. Fodstad H, Ljunggren BCA. Baclofen and carbamazepine in supraspinal spasticity. J R Soc Med 1991;84:747–8.

39. World Health Organization. Cancer pain relief. Geneva: World Health Organization, 1986.

40. World Health Organization. Cancer pain relief and palliative care. Geneva: World Health Organization Technical Report Series 804, 1990.

41. Bradley JD, Brandt KD, Katz BP, et al. Comparison of an anti-inflammatory dose of ibuprofen, an analgesic dose of ibuprofen and acetaminophen in the treatment of patients with osteoarthritis of the knee. N Engl J Med 1991;325:87–91.

42. Whitcomb DC. Low dose acetaminophen hepatotoxicity is more closely associated with diminished food intake than chronic ethanol use. Gastroenterology 1992;102:A909.

43. Klein DS, Edwards LW. Continuous intravenous ketorolac infusion for the treatment of cancer pain. Am J Pain Manage 1993;3:179–80.

44. Estes D, Kaplan K. Lack of platelet effect with the aspirin analog, salsalate. Arthritis Rheum 1980;23:1303–7.

45. Zucker MB, Rothwell KG. Differential influences of salicylate compounds on platelet aggregation and serotonin release. Curr Ther Res 1978;23:194–9.

46. Portenoy RK, Foley KM, Inturrisi CE. The nature of opioid responsiveness and its implications for neuropathic pain: new hypotheses derived from studies of opioid infusions. Pain 1993;43:273–86.

47. Monks R, Merskey H. Psychotropic drugs. In: Wall PD, Melzack R, eds. Textbook of pain. Edinburgh: Churchill Livingstone, 1989;711.

48. Sjoqvist F, Borga O, Orme ML. Fundamentals of clinical pharmacology. In: Avery GS, ed. Drug treatment. Sydney: Adis Press, 1980:32.

49. Swerdlow M: The use of anticonvulsants in the management of cancer pain. In: Erdmann W, Oyamma T, Pernack MJ, eds. The pain clinic. Utrecht, The Netherlands: VNU Scientific Press, 1985:9.

50. Brose WG, Cousins MJ. Subcutaneous lidocaine for treatment of neuropathic cancer pain. Pain 1991;45:145–8.

51. Hughes J. Isolation of an endogenous compound from the brain with pharmacological properties similar to morphine. Brain Res 1975;88:295–308.

52. Baines MJ. Control of other symptoms. In: Saunders CM, ed. The management of terminal malignant disease. London: Edward Arnold, 1984:109.

53. Bloomfield S, Simard-Savoie S, Bernier J, et al. Comparative analgesic activity of levopromazine and morphine in patients with chronic pain. Can Med Assoc 1964;90:1156–9.

54. Beaver WT, Wallenstein SL, Houde RW, et al. Comparison of the analgesic effects of methotrimeprazine and morphine in patients with cancer. Clin Pharmacol Ther 1966;4:436–46.

55. Culpepper-Morgan JA, Inturrisi CE, Portenoy RK, et al. Treatment of opioid-induced constipation with oral naloxone: a pilot study. Clin Pharmacol Ther 1992;52:90–5.

56. Sykes NP. An investigation of the ability of oral naloxone to correct opioid-related constipation in patients with advanced cancer. Palliat Med 1996;10:135–44.

57. Galer BS, Coyle N, Pasternak GW, et al. Individual variability in the response to different opioids. Pain 1992;49:87–91.

58. Swerdlow M. General analgesics used in pain relief: pharmacology. Br J Anaesth 1967;39:699–712.

59. Seed JC, Wallenstein SL, Houde RW, et al. A comparison of the analgesic and respiratory effects of dihydrocodeine and morphine in man. Arch Int Pharmacodynam 1958;116:293–339.

60. Christie JM, Simmons M, Patt R, et al. Dose-titration, multicenter study of oral transmucosal fentanyl citrate for the treatment of breakthrough pain in cancer patients using transdermal fentanyl for persistent pain. J Clin Oncol 1998;16:3238–45.

61. Kunz KM, Thiesen JA, Schroeder ME. Severe episodic pain: management with sublingual sufentanyl. J Pain Symptom Manage 1993;8:189–90.

62. Babul N, Darke AC. Putative role of hydromorphone metabolites in myoclonus. Pain 1992;51:260–1.

63. Hays H, Hagen N, Thirlwell M, et al. Comparative clinical efficacy

and safety of immediate release and controlled release hydromorphone for chronic severe cancer pain. Cancer 1994;15:1808–16.

64. Hagen NA, Babul N. Comparative clinical efficacy and safety of a novel controlled-release oxycodone formulation and controlled-release hydromorphone in the treatment of cancer pain. Cancer 1997;79:1428–37.

65. Radnay PA, Brodman E, Mankikar D, et al. The effect of equianalgesic doses of fentanyl, morphine, meperidine and pentazocine on common bile duct pressure. Anaesthesist 1980;29:26–9.

66. Szeto HH, Inturrisi CE, Houde R, et al. Accumulation of normeperidine, an active metabolite of meperidine, in patients with renal failure or cancer. Ann Intern Med 1977;86:738–41.

67. Martin WR. Pharmacology of opioids. Pharmacol Rev 1983;35:283–323.

68. Jaffe JH, Martin WR. Opioid analgesics and antagonists. In: Goodman AG, Gilman LS, eds. The pharmacological basis of therapeutics. New York: Macmillan, 1985:516.

69. Jaffe JH, Martin WR. Opioid analgesics and antagonists. In: Goodman AG, Gilman LS, eds. The pharmacological basis of therapeutics. New York: Macmillan, 1985:519.

70. US Pharmacopeia Dispensing Information. 12th ed. Vol 1B:2089.

71. Anggard E, Nilsson M-I, Holmstrand J, et al. Pharmacokinetics of methadone during maintenance therapy: pulse labeling with deuterated methadone in the steady state. Eur J Clin Pharmacol 1979;16:53–7.

72. Jaffe JH, Martin WR. Opioid analgesics and antagonists. In: Goodman AG, Gilman LS, eds. The pharmacological basis of therapeutics. New York: Macmillan, 1985:518.

73. Twycross RG. Relief of pain. In: Saunders CM, ed. The management of terminal malignant disease. London: Edward Arnold, 1984:64–90.

74. Hunt TL, Kaiko RF. Comparison of the pharmacokinetic profiles of two oral controlled-release morphine formulations in healthy young adults. Clin Ther 1991;13:482–8.

75. Kaiko RF, Lazarus H, Cronin C, et al. Controlled-release morphine bioavailability (MS Contin tablets) in the presence and absence of food. Hospice J 1990;6:17–30.

76. Kaiko R, Grandy R, Thomas G, et al. A single-dose study of the effect of food ingestion and timing of dose administration on the pharmacokinetic profile of 30 mg sustained-release morphine sulfate tablets. Curr Ther Res 1990;47:869–78.

77. Bloomfield SS, Cissell GB, Mitchell J, et al. Analgesic efficacy and potency of two oral controlled-release morphine preparations. Clin Pharmacol Ther 1993;53:469–78.

78. Mignault GG, Latreille J, Viguié F, et al. Control of cancer-related pain with MS Contin: a comparison between 12-hourly and 8-hourly administration (see comments). J Pain Symptom Manage 1995;10:416–22.

79. Warfield CA. Controlled-release morphine tablets in patients with chronic cancer pain: a narrative review of controlled clinical trials. Cancer 1998;15:2299–306.

80. Brahams D. Death of patient participating in trial of oral morphine for relief of postoperative pain. Lancet 1984;1:1083–4.

81. Vere D. Death from sustained release morphine sulphate. Lancet 1984;1:1477.letter.

82. Portenoy RK, Thaler HT, Inturrisi CE, et al. The metabolite morphine-6-glucuronide contributes to the analgesia produced by morphine infusion in patients with pain and normal renal function. Clin Pharmacol Ther 1992;51:422–31.

83. Faura CC, Moore A, Horga JF, et al. Morphine and morphine-6-glucuronide plasma concentrations and effect in cancer pain. J Pain Symptom Manage 1996;11:95–102.

84. Osborne RJ, Joel SP, Slevin ML. Morphine intoxication in renal failure: the role of morphine-6-glucuronide. Br Med J 1986;292:1548–9.

85. Sear JW, Hand CW, Moore RA, McQuay HJ. Studies on morphine disposition: influence of renal failure on the kinetics of morphine and its metabolites. Br J Anaesth 1989;62:28–32.

86. Smith MT, Watt JA, Cramond T. Morphine-3-glucuronide—a potent antagonist of morphine analgesia. Life Sci 1990;47:579–85.

87. Bowsher D. Paradoxical pain. Br Med J 1993;306:473–4.

88. Janicki PK. Pharmacology of morphine metabolites. Curr Rev Pain 1997;1:264–70.

89. Osbourne R, Joel S, Trew D, et al. Morphine and metabolite behavior after different routes of administration: demonstration of the importance of the active metabolite morphine-6-glucuronide. Clin Pharmacol Ther 1990;47:12–9.

90. Conolly ME, Davies DS, Dollery CT, et al. Metabolism of isoprenaline in dog and man. Br J Pharmacol 1972;46:458–72.
91. Bruera E, MacEachern T, Macmillan K, et al. Local tolerance to subcutaneous infusions of high concentrations of hydromorphone: a prospective study. J Pain Symptom Manage 1993;8:201–4.
92. Poyhia R, Vainio A, Kalso E. A review of oxycodone's clinical pharmacokinetics and pharmacodynamics. J Pain Symptom Manage 1993;8:63–7.
93. Kalso E, Vainio A. Morphine and oxycodone hydrochloride in the management of cancer pain. Clin Pharmacol Ther 1990;47:639–46.
94. Leow KP, Smith MT, Williams B, et al. Single-dose and steady-state pharmacokinetics and pharmacodynamics of oxycodone in patients with cancer. Clin Pharmacol Ther 1992;52:487–95.
95. Reder RF, Oshlack B, Miotto JB, et al. Steady-state bioavailability of controlled-release oxycodone in normal subjects. Clin Ther 1996;18:95–105.
96. Benziger DP, Kaiko RF, Miotto JB, et al. Differential effects of food on the bioavailability of controlled-release oxycodone tablets and immediate-release oxycodone solution. J Pharm Sci 1996;85:407–10.
97. Heiskanen T, Kalso E. Controlled-release oxycodone and morphine in cancer related pain. Pain 1997;73:37–45.
98. Bruera E, Belzile M, Pituskin E, et al. Randomized, double-blind, cross-over trial comparing safety and efficacy of oral controlled-release oxycodone with controlled-release morphine in patients with cancer pain. J Clin Oncol 1998;16:3222–9.
99. Parris WC, Johnson BW, Croghan MK, et al. The use of controlled-release oxycodone for the treatment of chronic cancer pain: a randomized, double-blind study. J Pain Symptom Manage 1998;16:205–11.
100. Kaplan R, Parris WC, Citron ML, et al. Comparison of controlled-release and immediate-release oxycodone tablets in patients with cancer pain. J Clin Oncol 1998;16:3230–7.
101. McCarty K, Rosemark R, Katz RL. Narcotic policy for terminally ill patients. Semin Anesth 1991;10:175–9.
102. Truog RD, Berde CB, Mitchell C, et al. Barbiturates in the care of the terminally ill. N Engl J Med 1992;327:1678–82.
103. Boas RA, Cousins MJ. Chronic pain and local anesthetic neural blockade, diagnostic neural blockade. In: Cousins MJ, Bridenbaugh PO, eds. Neural blockade. Philadelphia: JB Lippincott, 1986:885–98.
104. Porges P. Local anesthetics and the treatment of cancer pain. Recent Results Cancer Res 1984;89:127–36.
105. Raj P. Local anesthetic blockade. In: Patt RB, ed. Cancer pain. Philadelphia: JB Lippincott, 1993:329–41.
106. Bonica JJ, ed. The management of pain. Philadelphia: Lea & Febiger, 1990:438, 1886.
107. Loeser JD. Dorsal rhizotomy for the relief of chronic pain. J Neurosurg 1972;36:745–50.
108. Plancarter VR, Patt RB: Neurolytic blocks of the sympathetic axis. In: Patt RB, ed. Cancer pain. Philadelphia: JB Lippincott, 1993:377–423.
109. Thompson GE, Moore DC, Bridenbaugh PO, et al. Abdominal pain and alcohol celiac plexus nerve block. Anesth Analg 1977;56:1–5.
110. Evans RJ, Watson CPN. Lumbosacral plexopathy in cancer patients. Neurology 1985;35:1392–3.
111. Jain S. Nerve blocks. In: Warfield CA, ed. Principles and practice of pain management, New York: McGraw-Hill, 1993:379.
112. Wood KA. The use of phenol as a neurolytic agent: a review. Pain 1978;5:205–29.
113. Cousins MJ, ed. Chronic pain and neurolytic neural blockade. Philadelphia: JB Lippincott, 1988:1053.
114. Warfield CA, ed. Principles and practice of pain management. New York: McGraw-Hill, 1993:531.
115. Cousins MJ, Mather LE. Intrathecal and epidural administration of opioids. Anesthesiology 1984;61:276–310.
116. Zieglgansberger W: Opiate actions on mammalian spinal neurons. Int Rev Neurobiol 1984;25:243–67.
117. DuPen SL, Peterson DG, Bogosian AC, et al. A new permanent exteriorized epidural catheter for narcotic self-administration to control cancer pain. Cancer 1987;59:986–993.
118. Waldman SD, Coombs DW. Selection of implantable narcotics delivery systems. Anesth Analg 1989;68:377–84.
119. Yaksh TL, Onofrio BM. Retrospective consideration of doses of morphine given intrathecally by chronic infusion in 163 patients by 19 physicians. Pain 1987;31:211–23.
120. Coombs DW, Maurer LH, Saunders RL, Gaylor M. Outcomes and complications of continuous intra-spinal narcotic analgesia for cancer pain control. J Clin Oncol 1984;2:1414–20.
121. Penn RD, Paice JA. Chronic intrathecal morphine for intractable pain. J Neurosurg 1987;67:182–6.
122. Yaksh TL, Onofrio BM. Retrospective consideration of doses of morphine given intrathecally by chronic infusion in 163 patients by 19 physicians. Pain 1987;31:211–23.
123. Cedarbaum JM, Schleifer LS. Drugs for treatment of Parkinson's, spasticity and acute muscle spasm. In: Goodman LS, Gilman AG, eds. Pharmacological basis of therapeutics. New York: Macmillan, 1990:479.
124. Bedder M, Burchiel K, Larson A. Cost analysis of two implantable narcotic delivery systems. J Pain Symptom Manage 1991;6:368–73.
125. Boraas MC: Palliative surgery. Semin Oncol 1985;12:368–74.
126. Sundaresan N, Galicich JH, Lane JM, et al. Treatment of odontoid fractures in cancer patients. J Neurosurg 1981;52:187–92.
127. Sundaresan N, Galicich JH, Lane JM, et al. Treatment of epidural cord compression by vertebral body resection and stabilization. J Neurosurg 1985;63:676–84.
128. Sundaresan N, DiGiancinto GV, Hughes JEO. Surgical treatment of spinal metastases. Clin Neurosurg 1986;33:503–22.
129. Sundaresan N, DiGiancinto GV, Hughes JEO. Neurosurgery in the treatment of cancer pain. Cancer 1989;63:2365–77.
130. Poletti CE, Cohen AM, Todd DP, et al. Cancer pain relieved by long-term epidural morphine with permanent indwelling systems for self-administration. J Neurosurg 1981;55:581–4.
131. Leavens ME, Hill CS, Cech DA, et al. Intrathecal and intraventricular morphine for pain in cancer patients: initial study. J Neurosurg 1982;56:41–5.
132. Lobato RD, Madrid JL, Lorenza MD, et al. Intraventricular morphine for the control of pain in terminal cancer patients. J Neurosurg 1983;59:627–33.
133. Obbens EA, Hill SC, Leavens ME, et al. Intraventricular morphine administration for control of chronic cancer pain. Pain 1987;28:61–8.
134. Olds J, Milner B. Positive reinforcement produced by electrical stimulation of the septal area and other regions of the rat brain. J Comp Physiol Psychol 1954;47:419–27.
135. Raynolds DV. Surgery in the rat during electrical analgesia induced by focal brain stimulation. Science 1969;164:444–5.
136. Hammond DL. Control systems for nociceptive afferent processing: the descending inhibitory pathways. In: Yaksh TL, ed. Spinal afferent processing. New York: Plenum Press, 1986:363.
137. Heath RG, Mickle WA. Evaluation of seven years experience with depth electrode studies in human patients. In: Ramey ER, O'Doherty DS, eds. Electrical studies on the unanesthetized brain. New York: Hoeber, 1960:214.
138. Richardson DE, Akil H. Long term results of periventricular gray self-stimulation. Neurosurgery 1977;1:199–202.
139. Hosobuchi Y, Admans JE, Linchitz R. Pain relief by electrical stimulation of the central gray matter in humans and its reversal by naloxone. Science 1977;197:183–5.
140. Mazars G, Merienne L, Ciolocca C. Comparative study of electrical stimulation of posterior thalamic nuclei, periaqueducatal gray, and other midline mesencephalic structures in man. Adv Pain Res Ther 1979;3:541–6.
141. Boivie J, Meyerson BA. A correlative anatomical and clinical study of pain suppression by deep brain stimulation. Pain 1982;13:113–26.
142. Lazorthes Y, Siegfried J, Gouarderes C, et al. Periventricular gray matter stimulation versus chronic intrathecal morphine in cancer pain. Adv Pain Res Ther 1983;5:467–75.
143. Meyerson BA. Electrical stimulation procedures: effects, presumed rationale, and possible mechanisms. Adv Pain Res Ther 1983;5:495–534.
144. De Salles AAF, Katayama Y, Becker DP, Hayes R. Pain suppression induced by electrical stimulation of the pontine parabrachial region. J Neurosurg 1985;62:397–407.
145. Baskin DS, Mehler WR, Hosobuchi Y, et al. Autopsy analysis of the safety, efficacy and cartography of electrical stimulation of the central gray in humans. Brain Res 1986;371:231–6.
146. Young RF, Brechner T. Electrical stimulation of the brain for relief of intractable pain due to cancer. Cancer 1986;57:1266–72.
147. Melzack R, Wall PD. Pain mechanisms: a new theory. Science 1964;150:971–8.
148. Barolat G. Percutaneous retroperitoneal stimulation of the sacral plexus. Stereotact Funct Neurosurg 1991;56:250–7.
149. Nashold BS, Goldner JL. Electrical stimulation of peripheral nerves for relief of intractable chronic pain. Med Instrum 1975;9:224–5.

150. Holsheimer J, Struijk JJ, Rijkhoff NJM. Contact combinations in epidural spinal cord stimulation: a comparison by computed modeling. Stereotact Funct Neurosurg 1991;56:220–33.
151. Long DM. Surgical therapy of chronic pain. Neurosurgery 1980;6:317–28.
152. Tsubokawa T, Katayama Y, Yamamoto T, et al. Chronic motor cortex stimulation in patients with thalamic pain. J Neurosurg 1993;78:393–401.
153. Singler RC. Alcohol neurolysis of sciatic and femoral nerves. Anesth Analg 1981;60:532–3.
154. Sahni KS, Pieper DR, Anderson R, et al. Relation of hypesthesia to the outcome of glycerol rhizolysis for trigeminal neuralgia. J Neurosurg 1990;72:55–8.
155. Tobler WD, Tew JM, Cosman E, et al. Improved outcome in the treatment of trigeminal neuralgia by percutaneous stereotactic rhizotomy with a new, curved tip electrode. Neurosurgery 1983;12:313–7.
156. Batzdorf U, Weingarten SM. Percutaneous cordotomy: a simplified approach to management of intractable pain. West J Med 1970;112:21–6.
157. Spiller WG, Martin E. The treatment of persistent pain of organic origin in the lower part of the body by division of the anterolateral column of the spinal cord. JAMA 1912;58:1489–90.
158. Mullen S. Percutaneous cordotomy. J Neurosurg 1971;35:360–6.
159. Levin AB, Cosman ER. Thermocouple-monitored cordotomy electrode. J Neurosurg 1980;53:266–8.
160. Batzdorf U, Bentson JR. Use of metrizamide for percutaneous cordotomy. J Neurosurg 1983;59:545–7.
161. Kahle W. Nervous system and sensory organs. New York: Georg Thieme Verlag, 1986:298.
162. Sopurek K. Commissural myelotomy. J Neurosurg 1969;31:524–7.
163. Cook AW, Kawakami Y. Commissural myelotomy. J Neurosurg 1977;47:1–6.
164. Folz EL, White LE Jr. Pain relief by frontal cingulumotomy. J Neurosurg 1962;19:89–100.
165. Hassenbush SJ, Pillay PK, Barnett GH. Radiofrequency cingulotomy for intractable cancer pain using stereotaxis guided by magnetic resonance imaging. Neurosurgery 1990;27:220–3.
166. Hurt RW, Ballantine HT. Stereotactic anterior cingulate lesions for persistent pain: a report on 68 cases. Clin Neurosurg 1974;21:334–51.
167. De Salles AAF, Hariz M. Functional radiosurgery. In: De Salles AAF, Goetsch SJ, eds. Stereotactic surgery and radiosurgery. Madison, Wisc.: Medical Physics Publishing, 1993:390.
168. Laitinen LV. Functional stereotactic surgery for movement disorder, pain and behavioral disorder. In: De Salles AAF, Goetsch SJ, eds. Stereotactic surgery and radiosurgery. Madison, Wisc.: Medical Physics Publishing, 1993:95.
169. Frank F, Tognetti F, Gaist G, et al. Stereotaxic rostral mesencephalotomy in treatment of malignant faciothoracobrachial pain syndromes. J Neurosurg 1982;56:807–11.
170. Laitinen LV. Mesencephalotomy and thalamotomy for chronic pain. In: Lunsford LD, ed. Modern stereotactic neurosurgery. Boston: Martinus Nijhoff, 1988:269.
171. Richardson DE. Thalamotomy for control of chronic pain. Acta Neurochir 1974;21:Suppl:77–88.
172. Spande TF, Garraffo HM, Edwards MW, et al. Epibatidine: a novel (chloropyridyl) azabicycloheptane with potent analgesic activity from an Ecuadoran poison frog. J Am Chem Soc 1992;114:3475–78.

# CHAPTER 23

# CANCER REHABILITATION

• PATRICIA A. GANZ • ANNE COSCARELLI

*I couldn't sleep at the time I was told I had cancer because of the fear of what was happening. After the surgery I could talk with the doctor, read some books, and know more about it, how treatable it is, and I haven't felt the fear for the longest time. I'm beginning to look at cancer as a chronic disease, something that I have, that I have to take care of, take medicine, maybe have regular checkups to keep an eye on it. The idea that I'm going to die tomorrow doesn't happen anymore. I feel much better.*

From an interview with a 37-year-old woman
1 month after surgery for breast cancer.

## General Considerations

Advances in treatment have led to prolonged survival for many individuals diagnosed with cancer, and it is estimated that nearly half of all newly diagnosed cancer patients will survive for more than 5 years.[1] Many patients are disease free but experience sequelae from cancer treatments that impair function in several spheres. Others live with active cancer for many years, with symptomatic problems controlled by surgery, hormones, chemotherapy, or radiation therapy—for these individuals, cancer is truly a chronic disease. Many patients have advanced cancer at the time of diagnosis and suffer considerable functional impairment as a direct result of the disease. Rehabilitation interventions are appropriate for all of these individuals who are living with cancer.

Early work in cancer rehabilitation focused on the problems of acutely hospitalized patients who frequently underwent physically disabling surgical procedures.[2] Current perspectives on cancer rehabilitation see it as a field concerned with many broad areas of human function, including physical, psychological, social, and vocational activities. As suggested by Cullen,[3] the major goal of contemporary cancer rehabilitation is to help each patient achieve maximum function in all of these areas within the limitations imposed by the disease or its treatment. Mellette[4] has suggested that "cancer rehabilitation is the process aimed at *prevention* of the physical and psychosocial dysfunction which may result from the disease or its treatment." As part of this process, physicians must anticipate sequelae and initiate preventive interventions.

The treatment of cancer has increased in complexity, leading to new kinds of rehabilitation problems. Surgical procedures are often less extensive than in preceding decades (e.g., radical mastectomy vs. modified radical mastectomy vs. segmental mastectomy with radiation; limb salvage therapy in the treatment of sarcomas); however, to limit the extent of surgery, the patient receives adjunctive chemotherapy or radiation therapy, which increases the length and the toxicities of treatment. Multimodal therapy, combining two or three treatment approaches, is now standard for many curable cancers. The rehabilitation and recovery process is prolonged for these intensively treated patients compared with previous times when surgery was the sole form of treatment. Primary treatment frequently extends from 6 months to 1 year, and the combined side effects of multimodal therapy can affect all areas of function (physical, psychosocial, vocational, and economic).[5] Rehabilitation programs for cancer patients must address all of these potential problem areas.

Functional status and quality of life have been fundamental concerns of oncologic practice since 1949, when Karnofsky and Burchenal[6] developed a clinical scale to quantify the functional performance of cancer patients (see Table 8–11).[7] In the 1990s, there has been increasing interest in the systematic assessment of health-related quality of life in cancer patients using standardized, self-administered measures.[8] Health-related quality of life is a multidimensional construct that includes the subjective appraisal of the patient's physical, mental, and social well-being.[9, 10] Although quality of life assessments are more commonly used in clinical trials and in research settings,[11, 12] more user-friendly approaches with computerized or scannable scoring systems have been developed.[13, 14] Quality of life outcomes are also key goals of contemporary cancer rehabilitation. Rehabilitation interventions can help maximize the functional status of individuals with cancer and reduce the morbidity associated with the disease and its treatments. They can also address the psychosocial and vocational problems associated with cancer and lead to improvements in well-being. Quality of life measures are well suited for assessing rehabilitation outcomes.[13]

## Identification and Assessment of Rehabilitation Needs

Effective intervention can be provided only when the physician and health care team identify the rehabilitation needs of the patient. A systematic rehabilitation needs assessment should be performed at the time of diagnosis, with periodic reassessment of needs as the treatment and disease progress. The literature documents, however, that physicians do not regularly or effectively identify cancer rehabilitation problems or recommend appropriate management interventions.[15–17] These needs often escape detection unless they are severe or the patient or family brings them to someone's attention. Some physical problems, such as pain, may be more regularly assessed, but most rehabilitation problems are not (e.g., psychosocial, vocational, and economic)[16] because most physicians have not been trained to address these concerns. Also, an accepted method of comprehensive assessment has not been readily available for clinicians.

In the 1990s, greater attention has been given to the assessment of rehabilitation problems as part of research protocols. Out of these studies have come several assessment methodologies, including functional assessment scales from the Medical College of Virginia,[18] a comprehensive interview,[19] and a self-report survey instrument called the *Cancer*

*Rehabilitation Evaluation System* (CARES) (formerly called the *Cancer Inventory of Problem Situations*).[13, 20, 21] These instruments were developed as research tools; however, CARES has been used as a clinical tool in a randomized trial evaluating rehabilitation needs and interventions.[22–25] CARES has considerable potential for facilitating the rapid identification of rehabilitation problems that need further follow-up, evaluation, and intervention. More widespread clinical and research use of this assessment tool should determine its efficacy in conjunction with specific rehabilitation interventions.

Certain kinds of rehabilitation needs are *treatment-phase specific*. For example, patients with *newly diagnosed cancer* receiving curative treatment frequently face an array of physical and constitutional problems that are the immediate consequences of major surgical procedures or combined-modality therapy. Psychological distress commonly occurs from the knowledge that one has a potentially fatal illness. For individuals who require amputations or disfiguring surgical procedures, restoration of physical defects is a major part of the rehabilitation process. Increasingly, chemotherapy and radiation are playing a larger role in the primary treatment of cancer. Patients experience short-term and long-term physical side effects from these treatment modalities, and sometimes temporary or permanent interruption of employment occurs.

With *recurrent cancer*, patients face many of the same rehabilitation problems that occur at diagnosis. Depending on the site of recurrence, pain and physical dysfunction can be prominent problems. Psychological distress often peaks at the time of recurrence because this usually signals the beginning of palliative rather than curative treatment approaches. Side effects from treatments can contribute to physical symptoms. Nutrition and weight maintenance are serious problems for some patients. Depending on the individual's type of employment and occupation (self-employed, blue collar, or white collar), vocational and economic problems may develop at this time.[26–30]

Patients with *advanced metastatic cancer* share many of the same problems that other patients face; however, they have some unique problems that are specific to this phase of the illness. They often face progressive deterioration in physical function and increasing dependence on others. Although pain is not a universal concomitant of advanced cancer, it is frequent in this setting. Uncontrolled pain leads to further decline in physical abilities. Psychosocial concerns related to death and dying occupy the patient and the family support network at this time. Financial, legal, and insurance problems present additional burdens for many families. Rehabilitation efforts should include regular reassessment as patients make the transition into a new phase of illness.

## Approach to Common Rehabilitation Problems

### PHYSICAL PROBLEMS

Physical problems are among the most frequent rehabilitation problems facing patients.[15] To a large extent, the physical impact of cancer and its treatment depend on the degree of physical dysfunction the patient experiences at the time of diagnosis and the extent to which the cancer is treatable or has manifestations that are reversible. The intensity of the physical rehabilitation intervention relates to the type of cancer, its treatment, and the Karnofsky Performance Status of the patient. For example, a patient undergoing curative surgery for breast cancer sometimes requires short-term physical therapy to restore arm mobility, whereas a patient with advanced metastatic breast cancer with a pathologic hip fracture needs intensive physical therapy to restore mobility. The patient with the hip fracture benefits from working with an occupational therapist to assist her in activities of daily living (grooming, bathing, eating, toileting).

Ideally, all patients suffering from physical problems related to their cancer should be evaluated for physical therapy intervention. Physicians do not always recognize these physical problems until they become severe.[15] An early consultation with a physiatrist (a physician with training in rehabilitation medicine) or a physical therapist can facilitate prompt intervention. Established physical therapy interventions for dealing with various surgical treatments (thoracotomy, mastectomy or axillary node dissection, amputation of limbs, radical neck dissection) exist and should be offered to patients undergoing such treatment. In centers with well-developed cancer rehabilitation programs, patients are seen by the rehabilitation service preoperatively in preparation for the postoperative physical limitations and the specific interventions that will be employed.[31, 32]

For patients with advanced cancer, physical therapy interventions are used to maintain mobility, to improve stamina, and to retain activities of daily living. Assistive devices can be used by these patients to improve physical function and quality of life. Patients with neurologic deficits (brain metastases, spinal cord compression syndrome, peripheral neuropathies) often benefit from a physical rehabilitation intervention. Consultation with the hospital rehabilitation service before the patient's discharge from the hospital is invaluable and maximizes the patient's chance of maintaining physical function and independence while at home.

Physical rehabilitation is important for patients living with cancer as a chronic illness. This importance is readily demonstrated by data from a survey we completed of 500 patients with colorectal, lung, and prostate cancer who on average had been living with the disease for more than 3 years. Figure 23–1 shows the wide range of physical and constitutional problems these patients experience. We found that more than 80% of this sample reported problems with ambulation, and for more than 50% of the sample, this problem was severe. These patients also reported difficulty with activities of daily living (colorectal, 41%; lung, 69%; prostate, 40%). These physical problems occurred in this relatively functional sample whose average Karnofsky Performance Status scores were greater than 80% and with more than 40% of each group having no evidence of active disease. Physicians should not hesitate to obtain the advice and consultation of a physical therapist when the patient has difficulties with walking and activities of daily living. Physical therapy assessment and intervention can be provided in the home if the patient is unable to visit an outpatient treatment center.

## PSYCHOSOCIAL PROBLEMS

Psychosocial problems, such as anxiety, depression, worry, marital or partner difficulties, sexual problems, and interper-

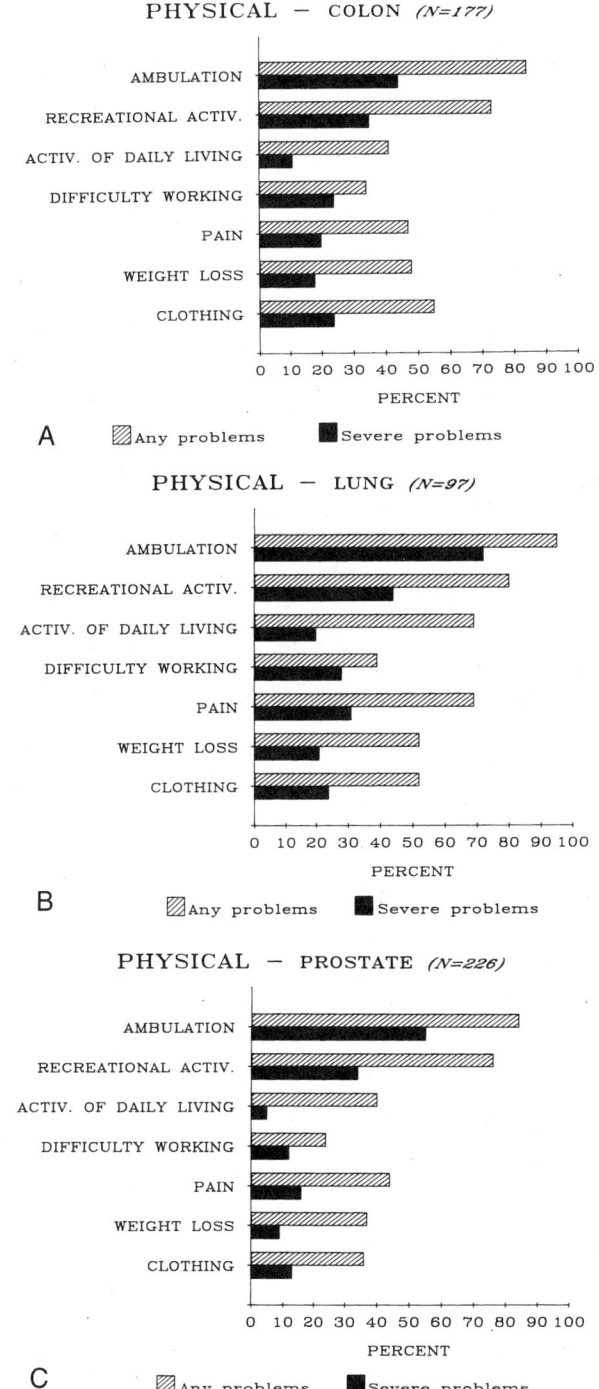

**Figure 23–1.** Constitutional and physical problems in colon (*A*), lung (*B*), and prostate (*C*) cancer patients living with cancer for more than a year since diagnosis.

sonal communication problems, occur with considerable frequency in cancer patients. These problems are less obvious than physical difficulties and are less likely to be acknowledged by the patient or recognized by the physician. Patients tend to emphasize their physical problems and may not want to burden the physician with their psychosocial concerns. Psychosocial problems tend to fluctuate with the clinical course of the illness. Patients generally experience the most difficulty at the time of diagnosis, at recurrence, or with approaching death. Needs assessment should occur at these times as well as during more stable periods. Frequently, psychosocial distress is aggravated by declining physical abilities[33]; maintenance of physical function is important. In our sample of colorectal, lung, and prostate cancer patients living for more than 1 year after their cancer diagnosis, we found a wide range of psychosocial problems (Fig. 23–2). We also found that individuals with more advanced disease or more disfiguring surgery appeared to have the most difficulties (Schag CC, Heinrich RL, Ganz PA, unpublished data, 1988).

Most cancer patients cope successfully with psychological difficulties; however, some need and benefit from professional interventions.[34] Psychological distress should be managed with appropriate psychotropic medications (antidepressants, anxiolytics)[35] and referral to mental health professionals who have experience working with cancer patients or medically ill persons. Short-term professional counseling should be encouraged to address psychological problems before they become severe. Often patients and physicians have negative stereotypes about mental health interventions. A physician treating patients with cancer can benefit from developing a working relationship with a mental health professional. This relationship can aid the physician in reassur-ing the patient that psychological assistance is an appropriate component of patient care rather than an indication of mental illness. Patients often need substantial reassurance and education about the help that they can receive. Support groups often prove useful for cancer patients, and local units of the American Cancer Society are an excellent resource for obtaining information about ongoing groups in the community. Support groups vary considerably in their structure and format (time limited vs. ongoing; disease specific vs. heterogeneous; family vs. patient only); however, they may have less associated stigma and are a good first referral for some patients. The individual patient's needs and attitudes have to be considered. Psychosocial issues are discussed in greater detail in Chapter 24.

## SEXUAL PROBLEMS

Sexual problems are relatively common in the general population of healthy individuals, and the cancer experience can exacerbate old problems and create new ones.[36, 37] Fatigue from treatment (surgery, radiation, or chemotherapy) or from progressive cancer usually leads to a decline in sexual desire and a loss of interest in sexual activity. Body image is

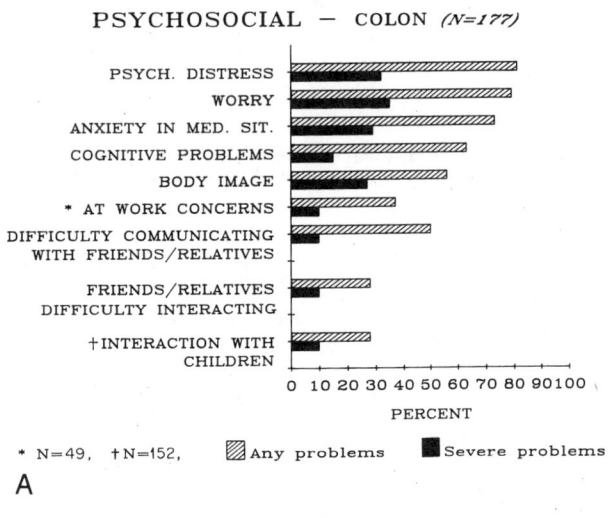

A

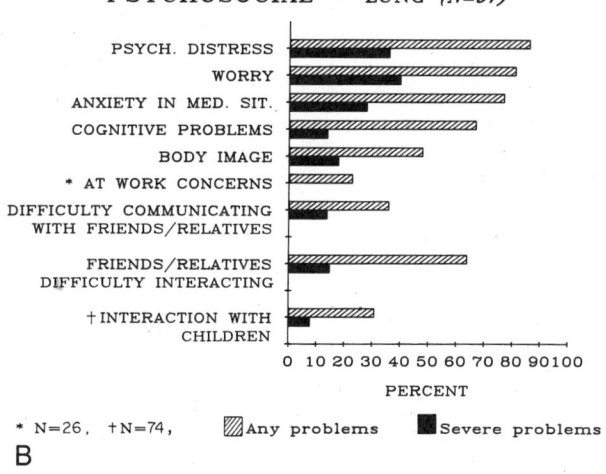

B

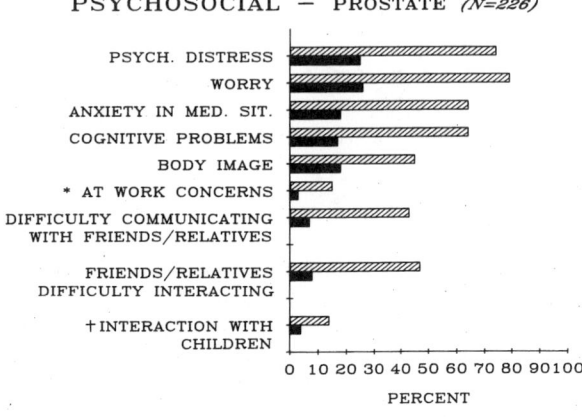

C

**Figure 23–2.** Psychosocial problems in colon (*A*), lung (*B*), and prostate (*C*) cancer patients living with cancer for more than a year since diagnosis. Psych. distress, anxiety, depression, feeling overwhelmed by emotions about the cancer; worry, concerns about not being able to care for self, worry about how family will manage if patient dies, worry about recurrence or whether treatments are working; anxiety in med. sit., nervous when having diagnostic tests, blood drawing, waiting to see the doctor, going to the hospital, seeing other patients receive treatment; at work concerns, concerns about being fired, communication with boss and coworkers, concerns about job performance.

distorted through weight loss, hair loss, and physical scars, leading to a loss of feeling sexually attractive. After abdominal and pelvic surgical procedures (prostatectomy, abdominoperineal resection, retroperitoneal lymph node dissection), innervation to pelvic organs may be damaged, causing impotence or physical problems that lead to sexual dysfunction. Other surgical procedures (vaginectomy, penectomy, radical vulvectomy) remove tissues that are important for sexual activity, with resultant functional impairment. For women with breast cancer or endometrial cancer, early menopause and estrogen deficiency may precipitate sexual dysfunction (e.g., decreased libido, vaginal dryness).[38] Currently, there is considerable interest in management of these symptoms with nonestrogen alternatives as well as in the evaluation of the safety of hormone replacement therapy.

Despite the importance of sexual function for the patient and his or her partner, most physicians do not systematically address the impact of cancer and its treatment on sexual function before therapy. As with many other rehabilitation problems, sexual problems are usually overlooked, unless the patient is assertive or presents in a crisis situation. As a first step, physicians should at least review the patient's present level of sexual activity and discuss the potential impact of therapy. Awareness of these potential problems helps the patient adapt to post-treatment difficulties. Pretreatment discussion of sexuality and intimacy provides a baseline for comparison during subsequent re-evaluation of the patient after treatment. Once specific problems are identified, physicians and other members of the health care team can successfully implement several simple interventions that do not require extensive training in sex therapy. Although it is beyond the scope of this chapter to detail the specific interventions, there are a number of excellent reviews of this topic.[39–43]

## DIET AND NUTRITION

Diet and nutrition are important components in the patient's rehabilitation program, especially for patients receiving radiation and chemotherapy. In extreme states of malnutrition, intravenous hyperalimentation may be an important intervention.[44] More often, however, less intensive nutritional therapies are appropriate, such as the use of commercially available dietary supplements. A consultation with the hospital dietitian can identify current dietary patterns and help plan ways to supplement the diet. Family members should be included in these meetings and discussions because of their involvement in the planning and preparation of meals. Dietitians can educate patients about how to increase caloric intake while still providing meals that are palatable. Cancer patients undergoing treatment often have changes in taste for food, and their eating habits may change. Making family members aware of these common problems can prevent battles related to food and eating and can help the family in planning meals that maintain the patient's weight. Studies have demonstrated substantial benefit from megestrol acetate as an appetite stimulant and an aid to preventing cachexia.[45]

Patients sometimes modify their diets in an attempt to eliminate putative carcinogens or to follow fad diets that are reported to treat cancer. This activity should be discouraged if there is a risk of significant weight loss or nutrient depletion. If the diet has no negative health impact on the patient,

however, it may provide some sense of control over a situation that is out of personal control. The physician should be alert to the patient's adoption of unusual diets and fads because these may signal other unmet psychological concerns.

## FAMILY AND SOCIAL PROBLEMS

The cancer diagnosis adds considerable stress to otherwise supportive and stable social networks. Family and social problems that predate the diagnosis of cancer can contribute to rehabilitation difficulties. The physician should assess the characteristics and quality of the patient's support network early on because members of the patient's family are often crucial to accomplishing the treatment goals. With the patient's permission, it is useful to share information with the family about the patient's disease and the treatment plan. Conflicts within the family and lack of social support need to be identified early because these problems can have a negative impact on the patient's care. As the patient's functional status declines, additional assistance might be required at home. Knowledge of the patient's available support determines when referral to a home care agency might be helpful. A wide variety of services are available to patients and their families to help them deal with the impact of the cancer diagnosis and treatment. Services range from specific information about cancer and its treatment; to individual, family, or group psychological counseling; to provision of concrete services such as transportation, assistance with meals, household chores, and nursing care. A social worker is usually the most appropriate person to evaluate the patient's supportive care needs and to determine what resources are most appropriate.

## VOCATIONAL AND ECONOMIC PROBLEMS

Vocational and economic problems are common among cancer patients. The impact of the cancer diagnosis is often most serious for those in blue-collar occupations,[27, 29, 30] with more flexibility in work schedules being available for individuals with higher levels of education and employment status. Until major reform occurs in the U.S. health care system, health insurance benefits will be linked to employment. Currently, loss of employment leads to the discontinuation of health insurance benefits. In addition, cancer is usually considered an excluded pre-existing condition that often makes it difficult to obtain new health insurance coverage. To maintain health insurance, many cancer patients are reluctant to change jobs, and they experience "job lock" as a result. Although many patients successfully negotiate modifications in their work schedules to accommodate their cancer treatment schedules, some patients may feel threatened by the employer or by the fear of losing their job. The physician can play an important role as an advocate for the patient under these circumstances and can intervene by educating the employer about the patient's abilities and prognosis. This intervention can be accomplished by early contact with the employer to describe the length of time the patient is likely to be disabled or what accommodations could be made at work to allow the patient to continue working while receiving chemotherapy or radiation treatments.[46] The Rehabilitation Act of 1973 provides some protection for cancer patients,[47] and a number of states have legislation that protects the employment rights of cancer patients, especially in relation to hiring discrimination and reasonable accommodation during treatment. The Americans with Disabilities Act of 1991 now gives federal protection to cancer patients. Vocational counseling should be considered for individuals who lose their jobs or who are unable to continue in their previous type of employment secondary to the effects of cancer or its treatment.

Cancer treatment is expensive and has a major impact on the patient's financial resources.[29, 48, 49] In our sample of colon, lung, and prostate cancer patients, 29 to 43% reported some economic problems. A number of studies have examined the nonreimbursable out-of-pocket expenses associated with cancer treatment, and they are considerable.[50, 51] To deal with this problem, the physician should make a brief assessment of the patient's financial status and promptly refer the patient (when appropriate) for social service evaluation to determine whether other sources of income are available. It may be appropriate for some patients with advanced cancer to file for Social Security disability benefits early because this may take many months to process.

## Patients with Unique Rehabilitation Problems

### HEAD AND NECK CANCER

Head and neck cancer patients share a common set of problems despite a wide variety of specific cancer sites within this anatomic region. Surgery and radiotherapy are the mainstay of treatment; however, chemotherapy is being used more frequently in the neoadjuvant setting.[52–54] Most head and neck cancers are associated with tobacco and alcohol abuse by the patient. These habits are associated with a variety of complex psychosocial problems related to addiction and lack of social support, and these factors may complicate treatment and rehabilitation.

Pretreatment dental evaluation is critical in patients receiving radiotherapy because post-treatment xerostomia can accelerate the development or progression of dental caries. Osteoradionecrosis is a serious late complication of radiation treatment. Trauma to the irradiated bone hastens this process. All dental extractions should be completed before the initiation of radiation treatment, and careful oral hygiene should be maintained during and after treatment. Compliance with oral hygiene regimens must be emphasized as a preventive strategy in this group of patients.

Maintenance of adequate nutrition is a problem for patients with cancers of the head and neck because deglutition may be directly affected by the primary tumor or as a consequence of treatment. Liquid nutritional supplements play an important role in the rehabilitation of these patients, and nasogastric feedings may be required if oral intake is inadequate. Consultation with a dietitian is frequently helpful.

Many patients require a radical neck dissection as part of definitive surgical treatment. The accessory nerve is usually severed as part of this procedure, leading to denervation of the trapezius muscle. This denervation results in serious shoulder dysfunction, which is physical and cosmetic. The trapezius muscle is responsible for upward rotation of the shoulder during abduction and flexion and is the major stabilizer of the scapula. The loss of this muscle leads to shoulder malalignment and motor dysfunction, resulting in an inability to push, lift, or carry heavy objects. Shoulder range of motion is usually limited and painful. Physical therapy interventions are available to address these problems and should be an integral part of the rehabilitation of these patients.[31] If motor dysfunction results from the radical neck dissection, range of motion exercises directed by a physical therapist can facilitate the recovery process.

Cosmetic restoration of physical defects resulting from surgery to parts of the face or oropharynx (nose, orbit, maxilla, or mandible) is an important problem for patients with head and neck cancer. Maxillofacial prosthodontists are subspecialists who design individualized prosthetic devices for these patients. These prostheses are used to restore function and cosmesis. Without cosmetic rehabilitation, there may be continued and worsening psychological distress in these patients. Preparation of the maxillofacial prosthesis is a multistep process, with pretreatment evaluation of the patient and several evaluations in the post-treatment period. Final prosthesis preparation does not occur until complete healing of the involved tissues many months after diagnosis, surgery, and radiation treatment. In the interim, a temporary prosthesis is used. Patients are in considerable need of psychological support during the period of adaptation to their physical loss, especially before completion of surgical reconstruction or prosthetic restoration.

Restoration of speech is an additional area of particular concern for head and neck cancer patients. Tumors of the nose, mouth, pharynx, and larynx cause a variety of speech deficits. At the extreme is the patient with a total laryngectomy, who needs training in esophageal speech or in using one of several prosthetic devices that permit transmission of sounds generated in the neck to the oral cavity to produce audible speech. Patients who undergo partial or total glossectomy are also candidates for speech therapy intervention and may require prosthetic devices to assist in the speech rehabilitation process. The psychological consequences of the loss of speech are legion and must be dealt with preoperatively as well as postoperatively. Laryngectomee support groups can be found in many communities and can serve as an invaluable resource to patients and their families.

### BREAST CANCER

Breast cancer patients are another special population with unique rehabilitation needs. As the most common cancer occurring in women, breast cancer has had extensive evaluation in the rehabilitation and the psychosocial literature.[5, 55–59] The primary treatment of breast cancer is associated with a high frequency of physical and psychological problems.[25, 60] The radical mastectomy (extensive surgery that includes removal of the pectoral muscles) has largely been replaced by the modified radical mastectomy and breast conservation surgery. Although axillary node dissection is still performed with contemporary surgery, arm and shoulder dysfunction is much less frequent than occurred historically with more radical surgery. Nevertheless, patients still experi-

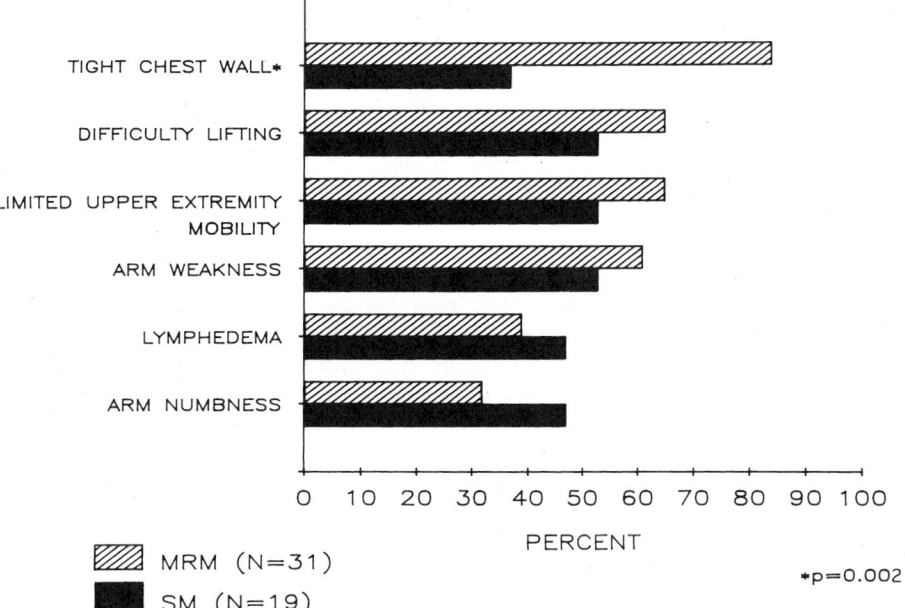

**Figure 23–3.** Most frequent physical problems related to primary surgical treatment in newly diagnosed breast cancer patients interviewed 1 month after surgery. MRM, modified radical mastectomy; SM, segmental mastectomy with axillary dissection. (From Ganz PA, Schag CC, Polinsky ML, et al. Rehabilitation needs and breast cancer: the first month after primary therapy. Breast Cancer Res Treat 1987;10:243.)

ence psychosocial and cosmetic rehabilitation problems secondary to loss of the breast.

Patients who undergo breast conservation surgery usually have a wide excision of the breast tumor and an axillary dissection. Subsequently the patient receives primary radiation therapy to the remaining breast tissue, usually over the course of 5 to 6 weeks. In our experience, these patients have upper extremity mobility problems that are identical to those seen in patients undergoing the modified radical mastectomy[60] and, in general, have the same range of physical problems as those reported by patients receiving a mastectomy (Figs. 23–3 and 23–4). Frequent problems include fatigue, limited upper extremity mobility, difficulty lifting, arm weakness, difficulty doing household chores, and arm

numbness. In another publication,[24] we demonstrated that during the year after breast cancer surgery, there were no significant differences in quality of life, psychosocial adjustment, or performance status in patients receiving mastectomy or breast conservation surgery. The patients who received conservation surgery, however, experienced significantly fewer problems with clothing and body image. These findings have been noted by others.[61]

With either type of breast cancer surgery, the axillary dissection increases the potential risk of lymphedema. All breast cancer patients should be cautious in avoiding trauma or infection involving the extremity with the axillary dissection. Once lymphedema is established, it is difficult to combat. Conservative management for mild edema includes ele-

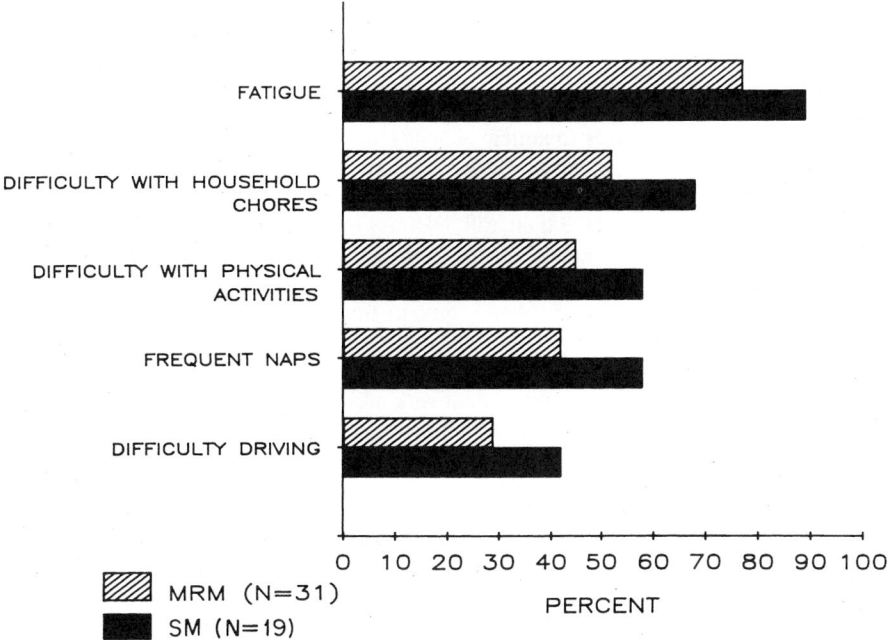

**Figure 23–4.** Most frequent constitutional and physical problems after primary surgical treatment in newly diagnosed breast cancer patients interviewed 1 month after surgery. Difficulty with physical activities refers to sports and recreational activities. MRM, modified radical mastectomy; SM, segmental mastectomy with axillary dissection. (From Ganz PA, Schag CC, Polinsky ML, et al. Rehabilitation needs and breast cancer: the first month after primary therapy. Breast Cancer Res Treat 1987;10:243.)

vation of the extremity, salt restriction, diuretics, and an exercise program. For more severe cases, intermittent pneumatic compression or manual lymphatic drainage is useful for redistribution of fluid from the extremity. This fluid redistribution can be maintained by use of a supportive garment or sleeve. For massive lymphedema that is refractory or whose onset is several years after the primary surgery, recurrence of the tumor in the axillary area should be ruled out by use of radiographic studies with computed tomography or magnetic resonance imaging.

Restoration of physical appearance is important for the woman who has had a mastectomy. The chest wall is usually tender in the immediate postoperative period, and purchase of a permanent breast prosthesis should be deferred for several weeks. A temporary prosthesis made from soft, lightweight material (cotton, lamb's wool, nylon stockings) can be pinned into the brassiere before a permanent prosthesis is purchased. An American Cancer Society Reach-to-Recovery volunteer provides a temporary prosthesis when she visits the patient. In addition, the volunteer often provides a list of stores in the local community that provide fitting and selection of a permanent prosthesis. These permanent breast prostheses come in a wide variety of sizes, weights, and materials at a range of costs. Patients should be encouraged to examine a number of brands before purchasing one. Many specialty shops also provide a range of special garments for use by mastectomees (e.g., bathing suits, night gowns).

Surgical reconstruction of the breast should be offered to all women who choose or require a total mastectomy. The specific reconstructive procedure depends on the type of primary surgery performed and the condition of the remaining tissue. The development of tissue expanders has aided in the reconstruction of women whose overlying chest wall skin is relatively taut. Immediate reconstruction can be done at the time of the initial mastectomy using a tissue expander, an implant, or a transrectus abdominis muscle (TRAM) flap. Breast reconstruction often requires a number of surgical procedures, including reduction mammoplasty for the remaining breast, and not all women choose to have additional surgery. Nevertheless, the option of reconstruction should be discussed with patients as part of the rehabilitation program.

The psychosocial impact of breast cancer surgery has been extensively studied and is not explored in detail here.[24, 55–57] Currently, breast cancer treatment extends over many months beyond surgery owing to primary radiation treatment or adjuvant chemotherapy. Multimodal therapy has many associated side effects that take their toll. Women today are frequently burdened with detailed information about prognostic factors and survival statistics. They are also asked to participate in the choice of surgical or adjuvant treatments, which may contribute to increased anxiety or concerns about recurrence. A number of interventions are available to deal with the side effects of chemotherapy treatment, and support groups or individual psychotherapy is helpful to many patients.

Problems with sexuality and body image are frequently reported after breast cancer surgery.[25, 58, 62] It is important for the patient's partner to view the mastectomy scar early in the postoperative period, especially at the time the patient herself first sees the scar. In this way, the couple can share in the loss and deal with the recovery together. Several reports suggest that patients undergoing breast conservation have less disruption of body image than those undergoing mastectomy.[24, 61, 63–65] Radiation and chemotherapy treatments frequently lead to a decrease in sexual desire and impaired vaginal lubrication, with a resultant decline in the frequency of sexual intercourse. Premature menopause can exacerbate this situation[38] because estrogen replacement therapy is generally contraindicated. Sexual therapy with a qualified psychotherapist may be useful for couples in whom a preillness sexual pattern has not been re-established after the cessation of primary cancer treatment.

## OSTOMY CARE

Patients who require an ostomy as part of cancer treatment have special rehabilitation needs.[66] These include patients with rectal or sigmoid colon cancers and patients with a variety of pelvic tumors (bladder, cervix, uterus) for whom a urinary diversion is required. An enterostomal therapist should see the patient before surgery to provide information and reassurance about the ostomy, its function, and its care. The therapist can aid the surgeon in identifying the best location for the stoma to ensure that it can be easily managed by the patient and that it will be adequately supported and be away from the belt line or body folds.

In the immediate postoperative period, the enterostomal therapist begins direct teaching with the patient on the care of the stoma and the use of appliances. If the patient has difficulty adjusting to the stoma, the emotional response can impair the teaching process. The patient must be encouraged to view the stoma site as well as touch it to develop independence and self-confidence regarding self-care. Periodic home care visits by an enterostomal therapist after the patient's discharge from the hospital facilitates the recovery process and engenders patient confidence in independent self-care. Meticulous skin care should be emphasized and monitored.

During the early postoperative period, the patient and family members can benefit from peer support, such as that available through the United Ostomy Association. A volunteer visitor with an ostomy can provide reassurance as a living example of an individual who has successfully adapted to life with a stoma. Many local chapters of the organization have regular support groups and periodicals that are helpful. During the months following surgery, the patient should be encouraged to resume usual activities and work, including sexual activity. Sexual rehabilitation of the ostomate must address the physical loss of pelvic organs as well as the presence of the stoma or appliance and the psychological impact of the changes in personal bodily function related to elimination. Preoperative discussion of the sexual impact of treatment (see earlier) is extremely important in this population of patients.

## AMPUTATION

Amputations for bone and soft tissue cancers lead to a wide range of physical and psychological rehabilitation problems for patients receiving this treatment. The functional impairment relates to the location and extent of the primary tumor. In contrast to amputations done for benign conditions, amputations for cancer may be radical and include such procedures as a hemipelvectomy or forequarter amputation. A preoperative assessment should be performed to prepare the prostheses and to orient patients to the postoperative rehabilitation program. Crutch walking can be introduced postoperatively when balance is better and there is no pain. Rigid dressings are recommended in the postoperative period to decrease pain and the potential for phantom limb sensation. A physical therapy program should be encouraged in the postoperative period to maintain strength and prevent contractures. The prosthesis cannot be used until the stump shrinkage is complete, and at that time the patient needs gait training and assistance in ambulation.

Bone and soft tissue cancers are primarily tumors of children, adolescents, and young adults. Patients at these life stages can be especially vulnerable to psychological problems. School is usually interrupted, particularly if the patient requires adjuvant chemotherapy. Recreational and social activities have to be modified. Counseling should be offered to the patient and family to deal with the disruption caused by the cancer treatment as well as to deal with long-term problems of physical and vocational rehabilitation.

## Rehabilitation Problems of Long-Term Survivors

There is a growing population of long-term survivors of cancer treatment, ranging from survivors of pediatric cancers, to young adults with Hodgkin's disease or testicular cancer, to adults with breast or colorectal cancer.[67, 68] These gains in survivorship have been accomplished through increasingly complex primary treatments, usually combining surgery, chemotherapy, and radiation. There are possible long-term sequelae from each of these treatments, and there can be potentiation of toxicities when treatments are combined.[69, 70]

### DELAYED EFFECTS

Delayed effects from primary curative therapy may not become manifest until many years after primary treatment. For example, radiation injury to normal tissues can be relatively mild during acute treatment but may demonstrate more chronic injury over the ensuing years. The lungs, heart, bladder, intestines, and other soft tissue organs are most likely to manifest these changes. The effects of radiation are potentiated by several chemotherapeutic agents that are radiosensitizers or that by themselves may cause damage to these organs (e.g., bleomycin, doxorubicin). Radiation therapy and chemotherapy are also potentially carcinogenic, so that delayed second neoplasms can be a problem. Radiation injury to the brain and central nervous system has been described in children receiving central nervous system prophylaxis for acute leukemia. Although eradication of leukemia from the meninges has greatly lengthened survival, it has been at the cost of serious cognitive disability and learning disorders in many children. Some children have suffered growth retardation from radiation injury to long bones and the spine. For some pediatric tumors, chemother-

apy has taken on a more strategic role because of this complication. Newer treatment protocols are studying innovative approaches that modify toxicity without the sacrifice of cure. Increasingly, rehabilitation efforts must begin to examine these long-term problems and devise preventive interventions to deal with them.

### INFERTILITY

Infertility as a consequence of cancer therapy is an important problem as more and more cancer patients are expected to survive and be cured. Relatively little information is available about gonadal dysfunction and how it might be prevented. Several chemotherapy drugs (primarily alkylating agents) and radiation therapy are directly toxic to normal gonadal tissue, and often little can be done to eliminate the use of these treatments if cure is the goal of therapy. Potential infertility should be discussed with the patient before the initiation of treatment. In a survey of 121 men who had undergone curative treatment for nonseminomatous testicular cancer, Schover and Von Eschenbach[71] found that 56.9% of the sample reported that they produced no semen and that more than 20% of the sample had frequent anxiety related to infertility and lack of semen. Infertility is also a concern for survivors of Hodgkin's disease. Fobair and colleagues[72] found that 19% of 165 patients who wanted to have children after cure of Hodgkin's disease were infertile.

Treatment planning for individuals likely to be cured of cancer must begin to take these findings into account. For men, it is possible to make use of sperm banking, although many men with newly diagnosed cancer may have azoospermia secondary to the acute illness. Oophoropexy is recommended to decrease the dose of radiation to the ovaries for women receiving radiation treatment for Hodgkin's disease. A report from Santoro and associates[73] suggests that ABVD (doxorubicin [Adriamycin], bleomycin, vinblastine, dacarbazine) has less gonadal toxicity for both sexes than MOPP (mechlorethamine, vincristine [Oncovin], procarbazine, prednisone); the initial treatment plan for a patient with Hodgkin's disease might take this into consideration.

### EMPLOYMENT PROBLEMS

Employment discrimination can be a serious problem for the cancer survivor, as noted earlier. This is often a more serious problem for the young cancer survivor without a prior work history. Even the military once discriminated against individuals with a cancer history.[74] Fobair and colleagues[72] reported that 42% of their sample of 403 long-term survivors of Hodgkin's disease had difficulties at work related to the cancer experience. The passage of the Americans with Disabilities Act may help decrease discrimination based solely on a cancer history. Employment has value beyond the income it provides, including a sense of pride and self-worth. The cancer survivor who experiences overt or subtle discrimination is deprived of this opportunity.

### INSURANCE PROBLEMS

Health and life insurance may be difficult or impossible for the cancer survivor to obtain, even after a lengthy disease-free interval.[75] Large group health insurance policies are often the best solution because they rarely exclude pre-existing illnesses. Life insurance policies may be impossible to obtain or can have such high premiums that they are unaffordable. Both of these areas have to be addressed with the increasing numbers of long-term survivors who are denied access to insurance coverage.

## Rehabilitation Resources

Only a few centers in the United States have established programs in cancer rehabilitation, and these are generally in large cancer hospitals or in centers where there has been an individual with an interest in this field as a specialty.[31, 32] More often, the rehabilitation problems of cancer patients are addressed through the hospital's general rehabilitation department. The cancer patient's physician plays an important role in identifying rehabilitation problems and coordinating the patient's care in the community. Because the physician's time is limited, cost-efficient and time-efficient methods of evaluation and referral must be developed. The physician must also provide the emotional support necessary to ensure that the patient follows through on the recommendations and referrals that are made. Effective combinations of skilled interviewing techniques (exploratory questions such as, "Is this a problem for you?" or "Have you experienced the following?") and the use of problem inventories (e.g., CARES [discussed earlier]) can facilitate identification of critical problems. Once the physician reviews the problem list for a specific patient, recommendations and specific referrals can be made. The physician can refer patients to the hospital rehabilitation department or to community agencies that deal with rehabilitation of the cancer patient. Home care agencies are excellent sources for rehabilitation services for homebound patients.

### REHABILITATION TEAM

Members of the rehabilitation team include the physiatrist, physical therapist, occupational therapist, enterostomal therapist, vocational counselor, social worker, psychologist, prosthetist-orthotist, rehabilitation nurse, speech pathologist, and maxillofacial prosthodontist. Other members might include a psychiatrist, dietitian, sex therapist, dentist, and dental hygienist. Ideally a team approach should be used to determine the rehabilitation plan for each cancer patient; in some centers, site-specific rehabilitation teams have been organized to plan and deliver rehabilitation services most effectively.[18] Team members should evaluate the patient before primary treatment in preparation for the anticipated functional limitations and to provide education about the required post-treatment rehabilitation interventions. Post-treatment morbidity can be reduced by taking a preventive approach rather than by waiting until problems become severe and more difficult to manage.

### COMMUNITY RESOURCES

Community resources are invaluable to staff and patients. Resources range from concrete services (durable medical equipment, assistive devices, nursing, and other home care services), to information and psychological support services (American Cancer Society, United Ostomy Association, Lost Chord Society), to assistance with financial and insurance problems (state department of social services, Department of Veterans Affairs, Social Security, Medicare, Medicaid, office of vocational rehabilitation–state education department, Legal Aid Society). Depending on the community, more specialized resources may be available, with many cancer-specific services being associated with hospitals and cancer centers.

## Summary and Conclusions

With advances in treatment that have occurred during the 1990s, cancer has become a chronic disease for many patients. The price of increased longevity has sometimes been the persistence of mild to severe functional impairment as a result of the disease or its treatment. Rehabilitation of the cancer patient should focus on preventive interventions to decrease functional impairment and to maximize the quality of the individual patient's life. The physician can begin this process by carefully evaluating the several components of function (physical, psychosocial, vocational, economic) in each patient before treatment and by recommending interventions that minimize the subsequent negative effects.

### SUGGESTIONS FOR ADDITIONAL READING

Schover LR. Sexuality and fertility after cancer. New York: John Wiley & Sons, 1997.

Ganz PA, Hirji K, Sim M-S, et al. Predicting psychosocial risk in patients with breast cancer: a potentially cost-effective approach. Med Care 1993;31:419–31.

Ganz PA, Schag CAC, Lee JJ, Sim M-S. The CARES: a generic measure of health-related quality of life for cancer patients. Qual Life Res 1992;1:19–29.

Ganz PA, Rowland JH, Desmond K, et al. Life after breast cancer: understanding women's health-related quality of life and sexual functioning. J Clin Oncol 1998;16:501–14.

Hoffman B, ed. A cancer survivor's almanac: charting your journey. Minneapolis, Minn.: Chronimed Publishing, 1996.

Osoba D. Lessons learned from measuring health-related quality of life in oncology. J Clin Oncol 1994;12:608–16.

### REFERENCES

1. DeVita VT. Testimony to the Committee on Appropriations, United States House of Representatives, March 7, 1984.
2. University of Texas, M.D. Anderson Hospital and Tumor Institute. Rehabilitation of the cancer patient. Proceedings of the Annual Clinical Conferences on Cancer, 1970. Chicago: Year Book Medical Publishers, 1972.
3. Cullen JR. Cancer rehabilitation in the 1980s. In: Cancer rehabilitation. Proceedings of the Western States Conference on Cancer Rehabilitation. Palo Alto, Calif.: Bull Publishing, 1982.
4. Mellette S. Workshop presentation, National Cancer Institute, Bethesda, Md. September 11, 1987.
5. Meyerowitz BE, Sparks FC, Spears IK. Adjuvant chemotherapy for breast carcinoma: psychosocial implications. Cancer 1979;43:1613.
6. Karnofsky DA, Burchenal JH. In: Macleod CM, ed. Evaluation of chemotherapeutic agents. New York: Columbia University Press, 1949.

7. Schag CAC, Heinrich RL, Ganz PA. Karnofsky performance status revisited: reliability, validity, and guidelines. J Clin Oncol 1984;2:187.

8. Strain JJ. The evolution of quality of life evaluations in cancer therapy. Oncology 1990;4:Suppl:22.

9. Aaronson NK. Quality of life: what is it? How should it be measured? Oncology 1988;2:69.

10. Cella DF, Cherin EA. Quality of life during and after cancer treatment. Compr Ther 1988;14:69.

11. Cella DF, Tulsky DS. Measuring quality of life today: methodological aspects. Oncology 1990;4:Suppl:29.

12. Moinpour CM, Feigl P, Metch B, et al. Quality of life end points in cancer clinical trials: review and recommendations. J Natl Cancer Inst 1989;81:485.

13. Schag CAC, Heinrich RL. Development of a comprehensive quality of life measurement tool: CARES. Oncology 1990;4:135.

14. Cella DF, Bonomi AE, Leslie WT, et al. Quality of life and nutritional well-being: measurement and relationship. Oncology 1993;7:Suppl:105.

15. Lehmann J, DeLisa J, Warren G, et al. Cancer rehabilitation: assessment of need, development and evaluation of a model of care. Arch Phys Med Rehab 1978;59:410.

16. Habeck RV, Blandford KK, Sacks R, et al. WCCC Cancer Rehabilitation and Continuing Care Needs Assessment Study Report. Madison, Wisc.: Wisconsin Clinical Cancer Center, Cancer Control Program, Grant No. NCI-CA-16405, 1981.

17. Houts PS, Yasko JM, Kahn SB, et al. Unmet psychological, social, and economic needs of persons with cancer in Pennsylvania. Cancer 1986;58:2355.

18. Mellette SJ. Development and utilization of rehabilitation and continuing care resources and services for cancer patients. Final report NCI Contract N01-CN-65287. Richmond, Va.: Medical College of Virginia/Virginia Commonwealth University Cancer Center, 1977.

19. Gordon W, Friedenbergs I, Diller L, et al. Efficacy of psychosocial intervention with cancer patients. J Consult Clin Psychol 1980;48:743.

20. Schag CC, Heinrich RL, Ganz PA. Cancer Inventory of Problem Situations: An instrument for assessing cancer patients' rehabilitation needs. J Psychosoc Oncol 1983;1:11.

21. Schag CAC, Heinrich RL, Aadland RL, Ganz PA. Assessing problems of cancer patients: psychometric properties of the Cancer Inventory of Problem Situations. Health Psychol 1990;9:83.

22. Ganz PA, Rofessart J, Polinsky ML, et al. A comprehensive approach to the assessment of cancer patients' rehabilitation needs: The Cancer Inventory of Problem Situations and a companion interview. J Psychosoc Oncol 1986;4:27.

23. Ganz PA, Schag CC, Cheng H. Assessing the quality of life—a study in newly-diagnosed breast cancer patients. J Clin Epidemiol 1990;43:75.

24. Ganz PA, Schag CAC, Lee JJ, et al. Breast conservation versus mastectomy: is there a difference in psychological adjustment or quality of life in the year after surgery? Cancer 1992;69:1729.

25. Schag CAC, Ganz PA, Polinsky ML, et al. Characteristics of women at risk for psychosocial distress in the year after breast cancer. J Clin Oncol 1993;11:783.

26. Feldman FL. Work and cancer health histories: a study of the experience of recovered patients. San Francisco, Calif.: American Cancer Society (California Division), 1976.

27. Feldman FL. Work and cancer health histories: a study of the experiences of recovered blue-collar workers. Oakland, Calif.: American Cancer Society (California Division), 1978.

28. Feldman FL. Work and cancer health histories: work expectations and experiences of youth with cancer histories. Oakland, Calif.: American Cancer Society (California Division), 1980.

29. Greenleigh Associates, Inc. Report on the social, economic and psychological needs of cancer patients in California. Oakland, Calif.: American Cancer Society (California Division), 1979.

30. Barofsky I. Job discrimination: a measure of the social death of the cancer patient. In: Cancer rehabilitation. Proceedings of the Western States Conference on Cancer Rehabilitation. Palo Alto, Calif.: Bull Publishing, 1982.

31. Dietz JH Jr. Rehabilitation oncology. Somerset, N.J.: John Wiley & Sons, 1981.

32. Gunn AE. Cancer rehabilitation. New York: Raven Press, 1984.

33. Cassileth BR, Lusk EJ, Brown LL, et al. Psychosocial status of cancer patients and next of kin: normative data from the Profile of Mood States. J Psychosoc Oncol 1985;3:99.

34. Derogatis LR, Morrow GR, Fetting J, et al. The prevalence of psychiatric disorders among cancer patients. JAMA 1983;249:751.

35. Derogatis LR, Feldstein M, Morrow G, et al. A survey of psychotropic drug prescriptions in an oncology population. Cancer 1979;44:1919.

36. Andersen BL. Sexual functioning morbidity among cancer survivors. Cancer 1985;55:1835.

37. Schover LR. Sexuality and fertility in urologic cancer patients. Cancer 1987;60:553.

38. Schover LR. The impact of breast cancer on sexuality, body image, and intimate relationships. CA Cancer J Clin 1991;41:112.

39. Schover LR, Fife M. Sexual counseling of patients undergoing radical surgery for pelvic or genital cancer. J Psychosoc Oncol 1985;3:21.

40. Schover LR, Evans RB, Von Eschenbach AC. Sexual rehabilitation in a cancer center: diagnosis and outcome in 384 consultations. Arch Sex Behav 1987;16:445.

41. Wasow M. Sexuality assessment as a tool for sexual rehabilitation in cancer patients. Sex Disabil 1982;5:28.

42. Von Eschenbach AC, Schover LR. Sexual rehabilitation of cancer patients. In: Gunn AE, ed. Cancer rehabilitation. New York: Raven Press, 1984.

43. Andersen BL. How cancer affects sexual functioning. Oncology 1990;4:81.

44. Ota DM, Cox LC, Copeland EM. Nutritional support of the cancer patient. In: Gunn AE, ed. Cancer rehabilitation. New York: Raven Press, 1984.

45. Loprinzi CL. Pharmacologic management of cancer anorexia/cachexia. Oncology 1993;7:Suppl:101.

46. ASCO Committee on Patient Advocacy. The physician as the patient's advocate. J Clin Oncol 1993;11:1011.

47. Sigel CJ. Legal recourse for the cancer patient-returnee: the Rehabilitation Act of 1973. Am J Law Med 1984;10:309.

48. Houts PS, Harvey HA, Simmonds MA, et al. Characteristics of patients at risk for financial burden of cancer and its treatment. J Psychosoc Oncol 1985;3:15.

49. Lansky S, Black J, Cairns N. Childhood cancer: medical costs. Cancer 1983;52:762.

50. Lansky S, Cairns N, Clark G, et al. Childhood cancer: nonmedical costs of the illness. Cancer 1979;43:403.

51. Houts P, Lipton A, Harvey H, et al. Nonmedical costs to patients and their families associated with outpatient chemotherapy. Cancer 1984;53:2388.

52. Jacobs C, Goffinet D, Goffinet L, et al. Chemotherapy as a substitute for surgery in the treatment of advanced resectable head and neck cancer: a report from the Northern California Oncology Group. Cancer 1987;60:1178.

53. Dimery IW, Hong WK. Overview of combined modality therapies for head and neck cancer. J Natl Cancer Inst 1993;85:95.

54. Department of Veterans Affairs Laryngeal Cancer Study Group. Induction chemotherapy plus radiation compared with surgery plus radiation in patients with advanced laryngeal cancer. N Engl J Med 1991;324:1685.

55. Meyerowitz BE. Psychosocial correlates of breast cancer and its treatment. Psychol Bull 1980;8:108.

56. Lewis FM, Bloom JR. Psychosocial adjustment to breast cancer: a review of selected literature. Int J Psychiatry Med 1978–79;9:1.

57. Holland JC, Jacobs E. Psychiatric sequelae following surgical treatment of breast cancer. Adv Psychosom Med 1986;15:109.

58. Schain W, Edwards BK, Gorrell CR, et al. Psychosocial and physical outcomes of primary breast cancer therapy: mastectomy vs. excisional biopsy and irradiation. Breast Cancer Res Treat 1983;3:377.

59. Burdick D. Rehabilitation of the breast cancer patient. Cancer 1975;36:645.

60. Ganz PA, Schag CC, Polinsky ML, et al. Rehabilitation needs and breast cancer: the first month after primary therapy. Breast Cancer Res Treat 1987;10:243.

61. Kiebert GM, deHaes JCJM, van de Velde CJH. The impact of breast-conserving treatment and mastectomy on the quality of life of early-stage breast cancer patients: a review. J Clin Oncol 1991;9:1059.

62. Wolberg WH, Romsaas EP, Tanner MA, et al. Psychosexual adaptation to breast cancer surgery. Cancer 1989;63:1645.

63. Sanger CK, Reznikoff M. A comparison of the psychological effects of breast-saving procedures with the modified radical mastectomy. Cancer 1981;48:2341.

64. Taylor SE, Lichtman RR, Wood JV, et al. Illness-related and treatment-related factors in psychological adjustment to breast cancer. Cancer 1985;55:2506.
65. Findlay PA, Lippman ME, Danforth D Jr, et al. Mastectomy versus radiotherapy as treatment for stage I-II breast cancer: a prospective randomized trial at the National Cancer Institute. World J Surg 1985;9:671–5.
66. Hurny C, Holland J. Psychosocial sequelae of ostomies in cancer patients. CA Cancer J Clin 1985;35:170.
67. Mullan F. Seasons of survival: reflections of a physician with cancer. N Engl J Med 1985;312:270.
68. Koocher GP, O'Malley JE. The Damocles syndrome: psychosocial consequences of surviving childhood cancer. New York: McGraw-Hill, 1981.
69. Loescher LJ, Welch-McCaffrey D, Leigh SA, et al. Surviving adult cancers. Part 1: physiologic effects. Ann Intern Med 1989;111:411.
70. Welch-McCaffrey D, Hoffman B, Leigh SA, et al. Surviving adult cancer. Part 2: psychosocial implications. Ann Intern Med 1989;111:517.
71. Schover LR, Von Eschenbach AC. Sexual and marital relationships after treatment for nonseminomatous testicular cancer. J Urol 1985;25:251.
72. Fobair P, Hoppe RT, Bloom J, et al. Psychosocial problems among survivors of Hodgkin's disease. J Clin Oncol 1986;4:805.
73. Santoro A, Bonadonna G, Valagussa P, et al. Long-term results of combined chemotherapy-radiotherapy approach in Hodgkin's disease: superiority of ABVD plus radiotherapy versus MOPP plus radiotherapy. J Clin Oncol 1987;5:27.
74. Feldman FL. In: Cancer rehabilitation. Palo Alto, Calif.: Bull Publishing, 1982.
75. Holmes GE, Baker A, Hassanein RS, et al. The availability of insurance to long-time survivors of childhood cancer. Cancer 1986;57:190.

# CHAPTER 24

# PSYCHOSOCIAL CARE

• DAVID K. WELLISCH • GAYLE B. SURDAM

A diagnosis of cancer is widely feared[1–3] and can result in serious social, personal, and economic costs. As survival rates improve with modern therapy, there is increasing focus on issues relating to the quality of life and the psychosocial aspects of cancer care. This chapter reviews the psychosocial consequences of the diagnosis and the treatment of cancer, and it presents guidelines for determining patients' levels of psychosocial adjustment and suggested interventions linked to each level. Also considered are the special issues of home care of cancer patients, alternative treatments, management of cancer pain, and the role of stress and emotions in medical illness.

## Adaptation to Cancer

Cancer is a stressful life event that can cause numerous adverse physical and psychological changes. A report by Cohen[4] included the following description:

> Developing symptoms of illness and undergoing medical treatment can be highly stressful events. Many people take for granted their health and abilities to carry out daily activities and to fulfill social roles. Since this view of oneself as being healthy, able, and having normal physique is central to most people's image and evaluation, becoming ill can be a shock to a person's sense of security and to his or her self-image. Not only does it threaten the customary view of oneself, but it further underscores that one is indeed vulnerable . . . that life is uncertain, that one may have little control over events, and that one's life may be changed in major respects.

Facing the possibility of disabling illness, death, mutilation, pain, altered future goals and plans, loss of important body parts, separation from family, alienation from friends, and loss of or change in physical functioning is a challenge to an individual's self-concept.

## SELF-CONCEPT

Becoming a *cancer patient* may result in three types of change in self-concept: changes in appearance and physical functioning, reduction in the sense of personal control, and acknowledging one's own mortality.

**Physical Function.** Changes in physical functioning can be associated with tumor growth, metastases, surgical treatment, chemotherapy, and radiation therapy. Although changes in appearance obviously have an impact on body image, changes in physical function may cut deeper because a person's sense of self-worth may be deeply influenced by a reduced physical competence. For example, hysterectomy may raise issues concerning a woman's attractiveness and the feminine role, but for a younger patient, the greatest loss may be fertility. Emotional distress and a reduction of self-esteem have been observed after mastectomy, particularly for women whose self-worth was predicated on their body image or attractiveness.[5–8] For other women, survival itself is a greater concern.[9]

Debilitation associated with chemotherapy,[10, 11] advancing disease, or pain[12, 13] may affect a person's perception of his or her ability to meet role demands and personal expectations. The patient confronts loss of (or reduction in) status, self-sufficiency, employability, and feelings of independence and mastery. Given these changes, the patient must readjust his or her goals and expectations or, at various points, experience hopelessness, feelings of worthlessness, and depression. An example of how this may happen is illustrated in the following case.

### CASE 1

A 54-year-old man who was a cigarette smoker and now has lung cancer presented for pain management with post-thoracotomy pain. He was a bachelor and had no children or relatives. He reported that he had few friends. His major interest was his work as an accountant. He reported that up to this point he had led a satisfying life with few problems. He had no history of psychiatric difficulties or substance abuse (except for cigarette addiction). When he was evaluated for his pain, he was found to be moderately to severely depressed. This depression was attributed to the fact that his respiratory difficulties, weakness, and pain precluded employment. It was evident that this individual gained feelings of satisfaction, mastery, status, and autonomy through employment, and when he became unable to pursue this avenue, his life lacked purpose, and depression followed. Psychosocial recommendations included helping him to develop other interests, such as drawing and assisting nursing home residents.

Each patient faced with changes in physical appearance or function, or both, must be aided in evaluating his or her situation on the basis of individual expectations, needs, and standards of performance and functioning.

**Personal Control.** A threatening, unexpected event such as cancer can undermine a person's sense of control over his or her body and life, and this may cause depression.[14, 15] Lack of control, loss of autonomy, and uncertainty are experiences common to the cancer patient. Submission to multiple tests and treatment procedures, coupled with uncertainty about the course of the disease, may contribute to feelings of dependence, helplessness, anxiety, and depression in degrees varying with the person's feelings about dependence and independence.[3] Enhancement of the sense of control can be achieved, to some degree, by helping the patient understand as much as possible about the disease and its treatment[16] and by encouraging the patient to be an active and informed participant in decisions regarding treatment. The helplessness and dependency associated with hospitalization and treatment can be reduced by encouraging self-care as much as possible.[17, 18]

**Mortality.** Issues of mortality often cannot be avoided when a person is diagnosed as having cancer. With recurrence, severe pain, or continuing disability, fear surrounding death and uncertainty about outcome become paramount. Coping with death means facing the unknown, considering the meaning of death and life, experiencing the pain of the losses that occur at death, making practical arrangements, communicating with loved ones, living in as satisfying a way as possible, and resolving the conflict between wanting to grasp life and letting go.[19]

## COPING WITH CANCER

Although sadness, dysphoria, anger, guilt, and fear are typical concomitants of the experience of having cancer, only a few patients suffer significant long-term emotional impairment.[20] The task of the person with a diagnosis of cancer is to cope with these new social, physical, and emotional demands. *Coping* is defined as a process of mastering harmful, threatening, or challenging conditions that tax or exceed adaptive capacities or for which previous learned responses are inappropriate.[21–23]

One factor in evaluating coping is the unit of time. Are long-term or short-term consequences of more interest? A coping strategy that is effective on a short-term basis may prove to be ineffective and perhaps destructive in the long run. For example, if a patient minimizes the threat of a suspicious lump, it may immediately reduce overwhelming

anxiety but interfere with seeking treatment. Minimization may be an appropriate strategy in situations in which there is no beneficial action to take, such as waiting for a laboratory result.

A person's developmental stage, cultural background, and personal needs, motivations, and standards determine the effectiveness of coping. For staff members who treat the cancer patient, understanding the phenomenology and developmental stage of the patient can often be of greater importance than having absolute standards of adequate coping.

**Phenomenology.** An understanding of the meaning of the disease to the patient makes his or her emotional and behavioral responses comprehensible. Cancer holds a special significance for each individual. Illness may be viewed as a challenge, a punishment, an enemy, a weakness, a relief, a strategy, an irreparable loss, damage, an attention getter, or a value.[23] The meaning of the disease and the meanings attributed to each aspect of treatment determine the patient's emotional reactions, coping strategies, and treatment decisions. For example, individuals hold different attitudes toward chemotherapy. Various patients have described chemotherapy as follows: "Chemotherapy is insurance against cancer recurrence." "Chemotherapy is a last resort; I must be dying." "Chemotherapy is horrible; I certainly don't want to lose my hair or feel nauseated all the time." "I went into a deep depression when my doctor told me I'd need chemotherapy for only 6 months rather than a year; I thought he gave up on me." These attitudes toward chemotherapy may determine whether or not the patient will receive chemotherapy, how the patient will approach the treatment, the feelings the patient will experience during treatment, the patient's reactions to side effects, and the patient's attitudes toward recurrence or absence of recurrence. Confusing or even seemingly irrational reactions can often be interpreted by understanding the patient's beliefs and priorities.

**Stage of Development.** Developmental stage is an important determinant of patient attitudes toward the disease and treatment. Each stage of development is associated with particular concerns that dictate attitudes toward one's body, interpersonal relationships, feelings of independence, and investment in work. For example, adolescents maintain a high level of investment in physical appearance; hair loss may have a more profound emotional effect for this age group than for older individuals. Adolescents are also involved with a struggle for independence from parental control; the lack of control and dependency associated with hospitalization may be more disturbing for them. Issues of fertility are of greater concern to a younger adult than to an older person, and issues concerning completion of professional tasks are generally of most concern to a middle-aged adult.[19]

**Coping Strategies.** Coping strategies vary from patient to patient and even in the same patient during the course of the disease. Three strategies commonly used by cancer patients are denial, search for meaning, and problem solving.

*Denial.* Denial is one of the most frequently discussed strategies in the literature. Contrary to psychoanalytic theories of psychopathology that define denial as a primitive and maladaptive defense, there is empirical and clinical evidence to support the notion that denial can be an adaptive mechanism for a person faced with a stress as threatening as cancer.[24]

The full implications of having cancer are so overwhelming that they must be adjusted to gradually. Denial encompasses a diverse set of processes,[25] ranging from the delusional denial of illness to selective misinterpretation of fact to reduce threatening aspects.[23] The goal of denial is "to reduce a threatening portion of reality in order to allow the person to function under less psychic stress."[26] Cancer patients commonly engage in denial.[27–29] Use of denial as a coping strategy has been associated with lower levels of anxiety and fear[30, 31]; lower corticosteroid levels, indicating lower stress[31, 32]; higher levels of functioning[31, 33]; and higher probability of recurrence-free survival.[34]

Denial-like coping processes involve costs as well as benefits.[25] Denial can clearly interfere at points during the disease when problem-focused, action-oriented coping strategies are appropriate, such as seeking consultation or treatment.

*Search for Meaning.* Search for meaning is the act of understanding why an event has occurred, its impact, and its significance.[16] Although it is difficult for anyone to be certain about the cause of his or her cancer (except in cases of lung cancer in smokers), most cancer patients demonstrate a need to discover meaning in the cancer experience by attributing causality.[16, 35] Evidence suggests that patients attribute their cancers to stress, carcinogens (drugs and environmental), hereditary factors, diet, and accidents.[16]

Search for meaning also involves a life reappraisal process prompted by the cancer. The individual attempts to reframe or restructure his or her life meaningfully according to the significance the cancer holds. For example, one patient with breast cancer reported that she reordered priorities in her life after her disease was diagnosed; she now "knows what is important and what is not." Other patients find that they are more appreciative of "the simple things" in life. Still others change their lifestyles (e.g., spend more time with their families, change their diets, exercise, slow down the pace of their lives, or change careers).

*Problem Solving.* Problem-solving modes of coping involve attempting to gain a sense of mastery over the cancer by engaging in actions and behaviors aimed at combating the disease and its ill effects.[4] This behavior may involve attempting to change one's lifestyle to lessen the probability of recurrence, seeking information about the disease and treatment, engaging in appropriate treatment, and fighting the side effects of treatment. It is obvious how adaptive this coping strategy is, although under certain circumstances, such as when there are no further appropriate steps to take, it can prove to be damaging or exhausting. The patient who continues to have advancing disease, yet frantically travels the globe searching for "the cure," may lose the support of family and friends, suffer financial hardship, and avoid dealing with inevitabilities.

## Problems in Adaptation

In general, most cancer patients ultimately adapt to their disease. There are, however, many who, at some time or another over the course of the disease, demonstrate significant behavioral or emotional difficulties requiring consultation. Senescu[3] has developed a useful guide to help identify difficulties in adaptation in cancer patients. The following events are indicative of short-term or long-term breakdown in coping abilities and suggest the need for psychological or psychiatric consultation:

1. Emotional responses of the patient endanger his or her welfare by interfering with the ability to seek appropriate treatment or to cooperate with necessary procedures. Evaluation should be undertaken in patients who interfere with their own welfare by avoiding treatment or making treatment decisions that demonstrate impaired judgment or who display inappropriate paranoia regarding procedures or extreme anger at staff. Impaired judgment may result from depression, organicity, psychosis, or personality disturbance.

2. Emotional responses of the patient cause greater pain and distress than the disease itself. Increase in disease-related impairment may appear excessive given the realities of the disease and treatment. Inability to carry out daily activities, hypochondriasis, somatization of feelings (e.g., spastic colon), extreme reactions to the side effects of treatment, inappropriate overreliance on medications, and anxiety or generalized distress that increase disability and pain are indicative of emotional reactions that compound the patient's difficulties.

3. Emotional responses of the patient interfere with daily functions, such as work and relationships, or cause the patient to curtail (or give up) his or her usual sources of gratification. This refers to a situation in which personal factors, not disease or treatment factors, interfere with functions that the patient is physically capable of carrying out. Such interfering factors may be depression, social withdrawal, or lack of interest or pleasure in typical activities.

4. Emotional responses of the patient result in personality or behavioral disorganization associated with conventional psychiatric symptoms, such as severe or vegetative depression, psychosis, self-destructiveness, suicidal ideation, extreme inappropriate anger and hostility, and general misinterpretation and distortion of environmental events.

## PSYCHOSOCIAL LEVELS OF ADJUSTMENT

Individuals vary in their ability to cope with a life-threatening illness and in their appropriateness for various forms of psychosocial intervention. Before proceeding with medical treatment, it is helpful to assess briefly the patient's level of psychosocial adjustment to anticipate difficulties and, it is hoped, prevent emotional crises. We have identified three levels of psychosocial adjustment based on characteristics of the patient, his or her family, and previous life experiences (Table 24–1). Most of this information can be obtained during an initial interview with a patient and a review of previous records.

The level 1 patient demonstrates appropriate affect, including anger, fear, and sadness, in response to detection, diagnosis, and treatment of cancer. This patient usually has a solid support system and a previous history of effectively coping with different problems of living. Such a patient responds well to a cooperative relationship with staff and requires minimal, if any, psychological intervention.

The level 2 patient often reports a history of moderate depression, anxiety, or significant traumatization in the past.

*Table 24–1.* Level of Psychosocial Adjustment

| Psychosocial Characteristics | Level 1 | Level 2 | Level 3 |
|---|---|---|---|
| Prior psychiatric history | None | Some history of depression, anxiety, or trauma | Significant history; may involve: chemical dependency, major depression, multiple significant losses, serious personality disorder |
| Prior coping history | Good–excellent | Good–fair | Fair–poor |
| Quality of family support | Good–excellent | Good–fair; separation difficulties, conflict | Dysfunctional |
| Quality of affect | Appropriate fears, some anxiety, appropriate sadness | Extreme fears, moderate anxiety, moderate depression | Generalized anxiety, moderate–severe depression, extreme fears, extreme anger |
| Coping with disease and treatment | Resolution of feelings about diagnosis; considers treatment options with a realistic balance of hope and concern for the future | Denial, lack of clarity, ambivalence over treatment choice | Extreme denial, confusion over disease course, severe ambivalence about treatment |
| Proneness to anticipatory problems | Not prone to anticipatory problems | Moderate–high | Severe anticipatory anxiety, nausea, vomiting |

On diagnosis, the level 2 patient may demonstrate moderate to high levels of agitation, dysphoria, and anxiety. There is usually an unwillingness to accept the diagnosis, and the patient may refuse to consider treatment options or future-oriented decisions. Family members range from being overly involved (e.g., speaking for the patient, demonstrating difficulties in separation) to expressing their anger and resentment in overtly destructive ways. As discussed later, psychosocial interventions serve a critical role in the management of these patients and their families.

A significant prior psychiatric history, which often involves chemical dependency, major depression, disorganizing anxiety, and serious personality disturbance, characterizes the level 3 patient. These patients are often visibly depressed, with suicidal ideation, difficulty concentrating, and extreme agitation. During treatment, there are often angry outbursts toward caretakers and hostile or passive-dependent encounters with staff. Most efficacious psychosocial interventions are aimed at helping staff and family members deal with their own feelings related to such patients and to facilitating productive interaction by setting limits and addressing emotional needs.

## Psychosocial Intervention

Although interventions used with a particular patient depend on the presenting problems, there are general goals involved in psychosocial intervention with the cancer patient. These goals include (1) enabling the patient to function, physically, socially, and emotionally, at the highest level possible within the constraints of the disease and treatment; (2) enabling the patient to make adaptive decisions regarding treatment; (3) mobilizing and potentiating the patient's support system; (4) helping the patient maintain his or her sense of personal control and integrity; (5) helping the patient realistically plan for the future; (6) helping the patient mourn for losses, such as the loss of former self, dreams, plans, and goals; the potential loss of relationships; and the loss of certain physi-

cal capabilities, body functions, and body parts; and (7) helping the patient resolve issues surrounding terminality and mortality, if appropriate. Working within this framework, the mental health professional uses a variety of skills and methods appropriate for problems experienced by the patient with cancer.

Table 24–2 outlines the various psychosocial intervention strategies recommended for patients at each level of adjustment. The following case examples illustrate how psychosocial interventions are implemented with patients and staff according to a patient's level of psychosocial adjustment. These intervention strategies are discussed later in more depth.

### CASE 2 (LEVEL 1)

A 36-year-old man with chronic myelogenous leukemia was admitted for bone marrow transplantation. He had several close friends and was currently involved in a significant relationship. His girlfriend was open, supportive, and willing to visit him on a regular basis. He had no previous history of significant psychological problems or difficulties. His parents were appropriately concerned but not overly involved.

Psychosocial interventions were minimal and involved brief, infrequent visits oriented toward (1) helping the patient find activities to help deal with the boredom of prolonged hospitalization and isolation and (2) providing supportive counseling to help deal with his anger over diagnosis and fears of death and dying. The patient's friends and family members obtained support and received needed information from the group sessions held on the unit.

### CASE 3 (LEVEL 2)

A 30-year-old married man with Hodgkin's disease and preleukemia was admitted for a bone marrow transplant. He had demonstrated moderate levels of anxiety and depression on admission and was perceived by staff as demanding and angry. According to the patient, he and his wife had been having marital problems, including poor communication and sexual difficulties, for the past 2 years. They had a 4-year-old child who was demonstrating behavioral problems. Although the patient had achieved financial success, he was dissatisfied with his

*Table 24–2.* **Appropriate Psychosocial Intervention for Each Level of Adjustment**

| Interventions | Level 1 | Level 2 | Level 3 |
|---|---|---|---|
| Individual therapy | Brief, once a week, supportive | Two times a week; relationship oriented, grief resolution | Frequent and extended daily visits, ventilation, clarifying, limit setting, little or no dynamic/interpreting work |
| Behavioral approaches | Progressive muscle relaxation, can use audiotape, self-hypnosis | Relaxation training/hypnosis; improving coping strategies, reframing of negative experiences | Relaxation procedures and hypnosis only with therapist present |
| Family therapy | Optional support group; information and education | Support group plus occasional family therapy | Family therapy with patient and without, sessions directive and aimed at limit setting |
| Psychopharmacologic | Rarely | Often necessary as requested; usually tricyclic antidepressants | Usually necessary; benzodiazepines, antidepressants, and occasionally phenothiazines |
| Staff issues | Usually not necessary | Staff often have difficulty dealing with family members of patient and in helping patient cope with anxiety and depression | Additional psychological consultation usually necessary; provide ventilation and support for staff members and behavioral planning and resolve staff splitting |

accomplishments and viewed his achievements as meaningless and unimportant.

Intervention consisted of helping this man cope with his anxiety and existential crisis through individual therapy sessions. He learned hypnosis and relaxation on audiotapes by listening several times a day. He was also given permission and opportunity to express his feelings of anger and sadness in individual sessions. Marital sessions focused on increasing communication between husband and wife and providing tools for dealing with the son's behavioral problems. Special arrangements were made to place their child in day-care facilities to allow increased peer involvement and nurturance during the crisis situation. Consultation with staff emphasized the importance of setting realistic limits with the patient and not attending to negative attention-getting behaviors (e.g., spilling urine), while reinforcing positive coping behaviors (e.g., walking around and eating).

### CASE 4 (LEVEL 3)

A 34-year-old woman with acute myelogenous leukemia was referred for a psychological consultation. The patient had a long history of alcohol and polydrug abuse starting at age 15. This patient had been treated in the past for chronic pain and numerous other medical problems. Notes in her medical chart indicated the presence of behavioral and compliance issues. Her family history revealed a dysfunctional family unit with role confusion, including unresolved anger and grief. The patient's father and uncles had died of complications related to alcohol abuse. The patient's mother was unable to leave her daughter's side and was overly involved with treatment decisions to the exclusion of the patient's husband. During treatment, the patient was extremely demanding and uncooperative when her mother was present. Family members often abused privileges around the unit in terms of following hospital rules and policies.

The most important intervention was in helping nursing and medical staff to ventilate their frustration and anger in an appropriate manner. Also, the liaison psychologist educated staff on behavioral management issues and limit setting. Critical medical decisions (e.g., "do not resuscitate") were discussed with the psychologist present to facilitate communication and minimize splitting between staff members. The patient's mother was given permission and encouraged to leave her daughter's room every day for a specified hour. To minimize additional

conflict, the patient was given choices regarding treatment options and a reasonable amount of control over scheduling of medication and procedures.

The next section discusses specific psychological approaches that are used by mental health professionals to facilitate adaptive coping in patients with cancer.

## BEHAVIORAL APPROACHES

Behavioral approaches involve replacing maladaptive behaviors with adaptive ones. In contrast to individual psychotherapies, which focus on underlying conflicts and verbal exploration of feelings, needs, and motivations, behavioral treatment focuses on the reduction of dysfunctional symptoms and the strengthening of problem solving and coping capabilities. These approaches are most appropriate for specific symptoms, such as pain, nausea, and anxiety.

**Hypnosis, Relaxation, and Guided Imagery.** These techniques are discussed together because the use of one usually implies the use of at least one of the other two. In addition to treating pain (which is discussed in another section of this chapter as well as in Chapter 22), hypnosis and relaxation have been used successfully in relieving anxiety, preparing for difficult medical procedures, and treating insomnia.[36] Hypnosis is also useful in helping a person regain a sense of control over his or her bodily responses,[37] circumventing feelings of helplessness and depression.[38]

Relaxation training and hypnosis have been effective in the treatment of anticipatory and post-treatment nausea and vomiting associated with chemotherapy.[39, 40] Evidence suggests that these techniques reduce anxiety and physiologic arousal (reducing gastrointestinal upset), distract the patient from triggering stimuli, and increase feelings of control.[41, 42] Various combinations of hypnosis, relaxation, meditation, and guided imagery have been suggested and used in an attempt to influence the immune response.[43, 44] Simonton[45] reported greater than expected frequency of tumor remission and regression in a population in which conventional treatment was supplemented by meditation and guided imagery.

The technique involves deep-breathing exercises with meditation, visualization of the immune system destroying the tumor, and instillation of positive attitudes about the body's ability to defend itself.

## PSYCHOTHERAPEUTIC APPROACHES

**Family Therapy.** Family therapy involves meeting with the whole or parts of the patient's family unit. This therapy can involve the patient and spouse or partner, the patient's children and spouse, the children alone, or even the spouse alone. Key issues in family-oriented counseling of the cancer patient are (1) improving communication about the illness and its impact on family relationships and (2) developing more favorable family-based support, not only for the patient but also for the other family members. Often a small number of such meetings can lead to dramatic changes in the emotional environment of the cancer patient's family. When a family is given permission to communicate about the illness and a model is provided of how to do so, much of the family-based tension is reduced.

**Individual Therapy.** Individual therapy, which involves meeting with the cancer patient alone, allows the patient to ventilate feelings that otherwise might not be expressed. The purposes of individual therapy are to strengthen psychological defenses, to enhance emotional coping, and to reduce the sense of fearful isolation. Individual therapy with the cancer patient differs from that undertaken with noncancer patients in at least two important areas. First, the therapist does not attempt to interpret or reduce the cancer patient's psychological defenses to reach deeper to more unconscious issues, as would be done in conventional therapy. The cancer patient's psychological defenses are left intact and untouched; they protect the patient from deep and profound fears associated with serious illness and mortality. Second, the use of formal psychoanalytic techniques (e.g., therapist as an infrequent verbalizer) is counterproductive and inappropriate with the cancer patient. The therapist is not silent or reflective but rather is active, supportive, and often self-revealing.

Individual sessions can be as few as one or last for several years, depending on the premorbid personality of the patient, the type of cancer, the programs available, and family availability.

**Group Therapy.** Group therapy with cancer patients may include patients only or patients plus family members. The group's discussion may focus on emotional or coping issues alone or may focus partly on lecture material and partly on emotional aspects. Groups may include patients with a mixture of organ sites and diagnoses or may be homogeneous as to diagnosis or organ site. Group therapy can provide a valuable means to help cancer patients feel less alone, to feel less like "the only one with cancer," and to understand better what they are experiencing.

In our clinical experience, groups function best with a leader who is a trained mental health professional. Group anxiety may be reduced by use of a mixed lecture-discussion format. For two reasons, we recommend that treating physicians not attend the group. First, patients sometimes need to ventilate about the physician and would be hesitant to do so in the physician's presence. Second, with the treating physicians present, the focus usually becomes a medical question-and-answer session rather than one that allows exploration of emotional concerns and support among members.

**Sex Therapy.** A vital area of any marital relationship involves sexual function. Cancer and its treatments often result in altered sexual function, although not necessarily an obliteration of sexual function as many couples believe. With cancer patients, the need for education and support in the sexual area can be profound. Cancer patients and their partners may be prone to sexual dysfunction based on either physical or psychological problems. These may be biologic, psychological, or interpersonal, or a mixture of these factors, in response to the disease and its treatment. Sex therapy is generally short term (5 to 10 sessions) and may include a combination of education, support, and behavioral techniques directed toward reducing conflicts that inhibit sexual functioning and toward enhancing sexual activity within the limits of capability for both partners.

## Home Care

Most cancer patients live with a family member in a home setting.[46] They also spend considerably more time at home than in the hospital during their illnesses. The literature on the psychosocial problems of cancer patients and their families has focused primarily on the settings of the hospital or the clinic, with far less attention given to the home situation.

In an article on the feasibility of home care for cancer patients, an oncologist stated[47]:

> Home care is not for everyone; the feasibility must be individually determined by assessing the needs of the patient and the ability of the family to meet these needs. Even when the physical facilities are adequate, the emotional adjustments that must be made should not be minimized.

Home care of the cancer patient presents stresses and benefits. In regard to the stresses, studies have found sleep disorders in 77% of family members engaged in home care[46]; physical and mental exhaustion, especially in the primary caretaker[47]; and significantly more anxiety, depression, and irritability in patients at home than in those in an inpatient hospital setting.[48] In terms of the benefits, home care patients have been shown to reflect greater independence and to have lower (self-rated) pain scores.[49] Home care is considerably cheaper. For example, there was a 300% decrease in costs in the last month of life for home-managed adult patients compared with a matched hospitalized group of adult patients,[49] and hospital care was eight times more expensive for hospitalized pediatric cancer patients with terminal or advanced disease than for a matched group of home care patients.

In attempting to assess how able a family may be to deal with home care for a terminal family member with cancer, several criteria have been suggested.[50] These include the following:

1. *Who constitutes the family unit?* Who are the significant figures in this family? Do the family members whom the health care team expect to assume major responsibility actually live outside the patient's home? Will all of the responsibility fall on one family member who really has no backup?

2. *What are the family boundaries?* Are the family boundaries blurred so that younger children will be given expectations for the emotional or physical care of the patient and for the patient's spouse far beyond their abilities? Are the boundaries rigid so that the family will have greater difficulties in allowing visiting health care professionals to enter the family physically or emotionally?

3. *Where is the family in the developmental life cycle?* In our research, we have found that the older couple facing home care for one spouse almost always needs extensive homemaking interventions and visiting health professional visits but rarely needs psychotherapeutic help for their relationship. The younger couple facing home care for one spouse needs less extensive homemaking or visiting health professional services but often needs psychotherapeutic help for their relationship.[51]

4. *What are the communication patterns in the family?* The family that has never been easily able to communicate and that during the patient's illness is engaged in a conspiracy of silence is probably at a high risk for problems in managing the homebound cancer patient.

5. *How has the family coped with crisis in the past?* The family's response to the present illness should be viewed as an example, albeit extreme, of their previous history of coping with crises. The assessment of this history is vital to evaluate their current capacities.

6. *What is the family's capability to care for the patient?* Family members may, out of a deep sense of obligation, guilt, or other emotional drives, wish to care for the patient at home and frequently want to do so without outside intervention. The family's actual physical, emotional, situational, and fiscal resources must be carefully evaluated to assess the feasibility of such an undertaking. For example, the elderly spouse with disabling arthritis or the younger spouse with full-time work and no other source of income, however well meaning, is not a suitable candidate for this task. The following case examples serve to reflect some, but by no means all, of the problems faced by families caring for a dying member at home.

### CASE 5

A 50-year-old unmarried man was dying at home of lung cancer that had metastasized widely, producing pain, paralysis, and depression. He had been divorced many years before and was being cared for in his final months by his sister, age 46, who had come to live with him. The sister had no problems with the management of her brother's medications or other aspects of his physical care. Occasional visits by a visiting nurse and phone calls from the patient's oncologist were sufficient. The major problem was her brother's all-encompassing, stifling dependency on her. This dependency was an extension of his lifelong pattern of imposing impossible demands on significant others. Now, he was using fear and guilt to keep the sister at home by his side. The sister was becoming increasingly resentful, angry, and depressed by her brother's relentless dependency needs. The psychological consultant needed to make three major interventions. They involved (1) helping the sister set definitive limits and separate when needed, (2) increasing psychotherapy with the patient to attempt to halt the regression that was leading the patient to feel like an infant abandoned by his mother, and (3) helping the patient and his sister to widen their base of support so that the patient could be somewhat more comfortable staying with others when his sister took time off.

This case reflects the stresses of middle-aged siblings dealing with cancer. The major problem here was not physical exhaustion but rather the enormous stresses of the increased dependency needs of the ill patient and the loss of independence in the well partner. Although these issues are not novel for the older couple, they are unique and frightening for the younger couple, such as this sister and brother.

### CASE 6

A family was caring for the terminally ill daughter, a young woman in her 20s dying of leukemia. The patient's family consisted of her mother and father, both in their late 40s, and a teenage younger brother. The family all knew that the patient had left the hospital for the last time and that this was the final stage of her illness at home. The family felt panic about what to do when their daughter actually was dying and died. In reality, they did well and were with her, in the absence of any health professionals, when she died early in the morning. Her last hours were relatively peaceful. Several issues that had concerned the family in the time leading up to her death remained important in the postdeath bereavement period, however. The family felt a sense of estrangement from the patient's primary physician before her death. The physician had not communicated extensively with the home care–visiting nurse agency. The agency, apparently waiting for directions from the physician, was not in extensive communication with the family about what to do at the end. The family, not knowing protocol, waited. In psychotherapy during the bereavement period, one key emotional theme expressed by the family was feeling abandoned by the home care team and primary physician. Another key theme was, "In the absence of the team, did we do the right things?"

This case elucidates the absolute necessity of effective systemwide communication and coordination by physicians, nurses, and mental health personnel in home care work. Even though the family did well, their fearful sense of "flying by the seat of the pants" in this situation demands better links between the team and the family.

## Patient Involvement in Unorthodox Cancer Treatments

One of the most psychologically complicated aspects of the cancer experience is that of the patient's attraction to and involvement in unorthodox treatments. This situation presents myriad issues for the patient, the family, and especially the health care team.

**Who Seeks Such Treatments?** A well-conducted study on the subject of unorthodox treatments presented some surprising conclusions.[52] In this study, 660 patients were interviewed, of whom 282 participated in conventional therapy alone, 325 participated in conventional and unorthodox therapies, and 53 participated in unorthodox therapy alone. The results showed that patients began unorthodox treatment almost as often when their disease was local as when it was distant (and terminal). Patients who sought and participated in unconventional treatments were better educated than those who used conventional therapy alone.

**Why Do Patients Seek Such Treatments?** Patients choose unconventional treatments because of beliefs about causes of cancer, feelings about treatments, and reactions to the physician-patient relationship. In regard to cause, unorthodox practitioners offer simple explanations of cancer as having to do with underlying systemic disorders of the body (eating, elimination, or emotional or spiritual stress). These appeal to the patient's desperate search for manageable answers to the all-encompassing question, "Why me?" Unorthodox treatments can be pleasant, free of side effects, and given in nonhospital settings. Orthodox and conventional cancer treatments are viewed as weakening the body unnecessarily and as not treating the *true* systemic disorder, while inducing severe side effects.

In the previously cited study, the quality of the physician-patient relationship was related to seeking unorthodox treatment.[52] Patients receiving only conventional therapy were more likely to report positive relationships with physicians than were patients receiving conventional plus unorthodox treatment. Least-positive perceptions of the physician-patient relationship were reported by patients receiving unconventional therapies alone. The training backgrounds of the practitioners offering unorthodox treatment in this study were investigated. Of the practitioner sample, 60% had M.D. degrees, and 81% of the physicians were trained in the United States.[52] These figures parallel a study in England, in which 60% of unorthodox practitioners were also found to be physicians.[53] Several common features are noted in regard to unorthodox practitioners, which include the following[54]:

1. They are isolated from established scientific facilities and associates.
2. They do not use regular channels of communication (current, reputable scientific journals).
3. They claim that prejudice of conventional medicine hinders their efforts.
4. Their method of treatment is often secret and available only from them, or the mode of administration depends on special judgment that can be learned only from them.
5. They may use proven drugs or other methods of (established) treatment as adjuvants to the unproven therapy, and, if a favorable effect on cancer is shown, claim that it is the result of their unproven remedy.

The following case reflects some of the complicated psychodynamics involved in the area of unorthodox cancer treatment.

## CASE 7

An attractive single woman in her early 30s was self-referred for a *psychological crisis* following a biopsy for breast cancer that had proved positive 2 months earlier. She related that she had spent much of the 2 months since the positive diagnosis attempting to obtain disconfirmation of it. When no conventional practitioners provided disconfirmation, she began seeing a series of unorthodox practitioners who offered her a bewildering array of explanations and interventions for the problem. She kept unearthing more information on unorthodox approaches that led her in a seemingly endless quest for the *right* approach. Rather than calming her, this quest brought an increasing sense of anxiety verging on panic. In the evaluation, it became clear that she was heavily invested in her body image, that she feared her bodybuilder boyfriend would abandon her if she had breast surgery and hence a less than perfect body, and that she believed that no man would ever be interested in her if he learned she had undergone breast surgery. Several interventions were performed to help her deal more effectively with her problem:

1. Contacting and linking the patient with a surgical oncologist, who arranged for her to be educated about factors such as conservative breast surgery and breast reconstruction. This was initially done by a nurse oncologist from the surgeon's office. This link served as a bonding and as a desensitization step toward working with the surgeon.
2. Arranging for the patient to be given low-dose anxiolytic medication temporarily so that she could calm down enough to hear the information to be presented.
3. Seeing the patient's boyfriend alone to see if he could be supportive. He was most cooperative, saying, "I never said I would reject her; she said I would."
4. Arranging conjoint sessions with the couple in which his support of her was clarified and the fact that she was projecting her own feelings of negativity and fears of abandonment onto him was demonstrated. The patient was able to proceed with conventional treatment.

This case reflects several issues. First is the vital importance of the formation of a relationship with a competent physician who can convey appropriate information about treatment to the patient. This patient was too anxious initially to hear the information and was so phobic about surgical oncologists that their presence precipitated anxiety attacks. Second, the deconditioning of this anxiety and the formation of a working physician-patient emotional alliance was necessary as a prerequisite to actual treatment of any sort. The patient's experience of the "merry-go-round" of unorthodox cancer treatments was common. Once a patient is in this network, the sense of compulsion to go from one practitioner, clinic, or method to the next is almost too much to withstand. This compulsion may well come to involve visits to Mexico, the Bahamas, Asia, or Europe. With this patient, the effect of this mass of contradictory information was to escalate her sense of panic and obsessional thinking. Third, the necessity arose to help the patient deal with her own distressed feelings, which she was projecting onto others. She saw her boyfriend as rejecting, whereas actually she was rejecting her own image of an altered body. She saw the surgical oncologists as cold and unempathetic, but she had not been able to give any one of them a chance to form a relationship with her.

## Pain

It is estimated that approximately one third of intermediate-stage cancer patients and 60 to 80% of those with advanced disease experience moderate to severe pain.[55] The differential diagnosis of pain and its management by physical or pharmacologic means are discussed in Chapter 22. This section emphasizes the management of pain from a psychological perspective.

For the cancer patient, pain is more than an aversive sensory experience; it has particular meaning and significance.[13] Cancer pain may signal advancing disease, approach of death, increasing physical disability, reduction in autonomous functioning, dependence on family and health care providers, interpersonal problems, reduced social functioning, reduced sense of personal control, and lowered self-esteem. These changes may result in anxiety about the course of the disease, frustration and anger at perceived therapeutic failure, and depression associated with debilitation, dependency, helplessness, and hopelessness. It follows that patients with pain frequently report difficulties in sleeping, reduced appetite, weight loss, nausea and vomiting associated with medication,[55] difficulties in concentration, and reduced abilities to carry out daily functions. These symptoms compound their distress.

Assessment of pain is a difficult task because (1) it may not have a simple one-to-one relationship with tissue damage or body lesions[56, 57] and (2) it consists of the perception of sensation and the patient's psychological reaction to it,[58, 59] neither of which can be seen or felt by others. Pain is generally evaluated psychologically through subjective report and behavioral observation. Because most people describe pain in a nonarbitrary manner,[60] an objective questionnaire, such as the McGill Pain Questionnaire,[61] may also be useful in difficult cases by providing accurate information regarding the patient's sensory, affective, and evaluative pain experience.

An adequate assessment of pain from a psychological point of view must go beyond the usual questions of pain severity, duration, and quality (e.g., sharp, dull, burning). One must also evaluate the patient's affect. For example, is the patient stoic, tearful, angry, hopeless, or bland while describing the pain? The patient's behavior must also be noted. For example, how is the patient's behavior toward pain influenced by those around him or her? Does he or she become distressed about the pain when others are around? Do others undertake things for the patient when pain occurs? Does the patient avoid complaining about the pain when family members are around?

## GENERAL TREATMENT CONSIDERATIONS

Cancer pain may be improperly managed because of outdated guidelines in this area.[55] Patients with moderate to severe pain may be given inadequate doses of narcotics because of misconceptions about the risk of addiction to these drugs.[55, 62, 63] A smaller number of patients are inappropriately overtreated with narcotics and *snowed under*.[55, 62] The quality of remaining life may be compromised for both these groups of patients. Effective treatment of cancer patients with pain requires the following to be considered:

1. An attempt should be made to understand the patient's attitudes toward and beliefs about specific treatments. These attitudes are indicative of patient compliance with and responsiveness to therapy. For example, a patient who believes that taking medications represents weakness may attempt to delay treatment until the pain becomes unbearable and suffer needlessly. In many circumstances, attitudes can be explored, misconceptions corrected, or treatment agreements made.

2. An effort should be made to pinpoint expectations regarding treatment procedures. Unrealistically high expectations of a nerve block, for instance, can result in disappointments or frustration even when some pain relief is obtained. Some cancer patients with pain deny all problems other than their pain or experience their pain as the focus for all their distress.[55] In these cases, pain relief is usually unsatisfactory. Finally, inadequate understanding of the side effects of treat-

ment and lack of perceived choice in decisions regarding treatment may influence response.

3. For refractory chronic cancer pain, the patient should be referred to a multidisciplinary cancer pain clinic or to a cancer pain specialist. The patient should be referred before too many unsuccessful remedies have accumulated to minimize patient hopelessness and resistance.

4. When there is a high level of functional overlay (i.e., the pain is exacerbated by psychological factors, such as anxiety or depression), psychotropic medications, psychological support, and behavioral techniques may be helpful in pain reduction.

5. It is more effective to schedule regularly timed doses of pain medication than to prescribe on an as-needed basis.[62] When taking medications on an as-needed basis, some patients wait until the pain becomes severe before taking the prescribed dosages, creating greater difficulty in pain control. As-needed prescriptions reinforce complaints of pain because medications are contingent on pain behavior.[64] Giving regularly scheduled dosages whether or not pain is present may help reduce the patient's attention to pain and allow one to stay ahead of the pain.[65]

## BEHAVIORAL INTERVENTION

Behavioral intervention entails the substitution of pain behaviors with more adaptive, pain-reducing behaviors. It also involves the modification of affective, cognitive, and environmental mediators of pain and pain behavior. This approach is based on the assumption that emotional arousal, beliefs about pain, and environmental responses (e.g., family attention) influence the experience and expression of pain.

Behavioral treatment is highly diverse and individualized. Relaxation, hypnosis, and biofeedback techniques are used to enable the patient to replace dysfunctional responses that exacerbate pain, such as anxiety, pain focusing, and helplessness, with more adaptive responses, such as deep relaxation and feelings of comfort and control. Cognitive-behavioral techniques involve helping the patient to replace self-defeating attitudes toward pain with more adaptive coping-oriented responses.[66] For example, appropriate candidates for this strategy are those who panic when pain is present, think that the pain is definitely indicative of a recurrence, automatically associate the pain with death, or believe that there is no way to control the pain. These patients could learn to (1) slow down and relax and (2) problem solve appropriately (e.g., visit the physician to have a work-up for recurrence and employ appropriate methods of pain control). Such approaches reduce anxiety, enable the patient to solve problems rationally, and increase feelings of competency and control.

Other behavioral management techniques involve evaluating the particular aspects in the environment that exacerbate pain or reinforce pain behavior. These techniques are unique to each patient and his or her situation. For instance, a patient who receives support and attention only when he or she is in pain is being reinforced for that experience. Appropriate intervention might entail (1) having family members give the patient attention at times other than when he or she is in pain; (2) exploring and modifying patient behaviors and family relationships that lead to a situation in which the patient gets attention and support only for pain; and (3) teaching the patient strategies for independent coping with pain, such as relaxation or self-hypnosis, to dissociate family relationships from pain events. Patients who escape responsibilities may also be reinforced for having pain.

## HYPNOSIS AND RELAXATION

Relaxation is the state of lowered physiologic, emotional, and cognitive arousal. Hypnosis, which has been used successfully in reducing cancer pain, is believed to be a state of relaxation accompanied by heightened suggestibility.[67–70] Intensity, quality, and duration of pain experience have been successfully altered under hypnosis.[70, 71] Kroger[37] reports that 20% of his patients can control their discomfort and another 40% can drastically reduce narcotic ingestion. The mechanism by which hypnosis is effective in reducing pain is unclear; it may reduce pain by blocking perception,[37] reducing anxiety,[36, 65] separating sensation from distress,[72] providing suggestions of comfort,[71] instilling amnesiac processes,[72] and increasing an individual's sense of well-being and personal control.[36]

### CASE 8

A 46-year-old man with lung cancer and metastatic disease to the kidney and femur had been complaining of groin and sacral pain for 2 years. On presentation, this patient reported severe pain at the base of the spine (an 8.5 on a 1-to-10 scale, with 10 being the most pain imaginable). The pain was of a constant, stabbing, sharp nature. He could not lie on his back, and his activities were extremely limited. He had been taking hydromorphone (Dilaudid) (8 mg every 4 hours), methadone (10 mg every 12 hours), and oxazepam (Serax) (as needed up to 120 mg/day). The patient was also drinking large amounts of alcohol to help with sleep. He was severely depressed, his memory and concentration were significantly impaired, and he was unable to sustain attention for more than a few minutes. He had lost 15 pounds in the last few weeks. Treatment consisted of gradually tapering the oxazepam over 2 weeks and eventually eliminating it. The hydromorphone was also stopped. An antidepressant (imipramine) was added at bedtime, starting at 25 mg and increasing to 150 mg. Also, methadone was administered in a dose of 5 mg every 6 hours initially, but as the disease progressed, the patient received 20 mg every 6 hours. A series of epidural and caudal nerve blocks was also administered.

The patient was taught relaxation exercises and self-hypnosis. His friends and family were educated about his disease and given an opportunity to discuss their feelings concerning the patient's illness and their own caretaking responsibilities. The patient was provided with supportive psychotherapy once a week. After 6 weeks, the patient's pain level was a 2 on a scale of 1 to 10. He was much more active and able to sit normally and to drive himself to medical appointments. He was gaining weight and sleeping more regularly.

A great deal of attention has been focused on the role of emotions in physical health and illness. The following section discusses the empirical investigations of the relationship between stress, emotions, and physical illness.

## Stress, Emotions, and Cancer

Although particular studies investigating the relationship between stress and disease are open to methodologic or theoret-ical criticism, most reviewers[73–76] agree that the bulk of the empirical evidence indicates that individuals who have been exposed to a high degree of recent life stress have greater degeneration of overall health, more disease of the upper respiratory tract, more allergies, greater incidence of hypertension, and greater risk of sudden cardiac death and coronary disease than do individuals who have been exposed to much lower degrees of life stress. Several reviews of research on lower animals[77–80] suggest that psychosocial factors, particularly psychological stress, affect immunologic functioning.

Most of the evidence with humans suggests that stress is associated with an increased incidence of diseases against which the immune system defends and is associated with diminished immunocompetence as determined in a variety of in vitro assays. Stress has been related to tumor growth and to changes in neurochemical, hormonal, and immunologic functioning.[81, 82] Acute stress has been associated with depletion of catecholamines, increases in corticosteroids, immunosuppression, and accelerated tumor growth.[81, 83] Chronic stress has not been definitely proven to influence neurochemical, hormonal, and immunologic systems or tumor growth.[84]

Psychological factors or personality characteristics have been associated with the development, growth, and spread of tumors. Premorbid psychosocial variables that have been associated with the development of cancer are as follows: a significant loss suffered by individuals predisposed to depression, despair, and helplessness[85]; hopelessness[86]; emotional constriction[87]; lack of warm parental relationship[88]; excessive use of denial and repression[89, 90]; and inability to express hostility.[91, 92] Pettingale and associates[93] studied the relationship between immunosuppressive serum alpha globulin (IgA), which may play a role in the development of breast cancer, and anger suppression in a sample of patients with either benign breast disease or breast cancer. Their finding of a significant association between IgA and anger suppression suggests, but does not demonstrate, a plausible biologic pathway linking emotion and biologic risk status. A baseline initial study[94] and a 10-year follow-up assessment of a subsample[95] of breast cancer patients found a relationship between hydrocortisone metabolic excretion and adequacy of psychological defenses, assessed by interview-based ratings.

Temoshok[96] showed, as a first step, that a tumor variable—higher mitotic rate (indicating faster cell division)—and a host response finding—less lymphocyte infiltration at tumor base—significantly differentiated subjects who had disease progression from those with no evidence of disease at follow-up. They then showed that these two biologic factors were significantly related to ratings of emotional expression in a videotaped structured interview (i.e., more emotional expression was positively related to the favorable prognostic indicators of more lymphocyte infiltration and lower mitotic rate of the tumor).

Research in this area is problematic because many studies are retrospective and lack appropriate control groups.[97] A multitude of factors probably contribute to carcinogenesis, of which personality and coping style may account for only a fraction of the variance. An example of the problems raised by lack of information on these questions is the belief that the personality of an individual contributed to the development of cancer. This belief may lead to derogation of the patient by others and self-blame and guilt on the part of the patient, which would serve only to increase the problems of the cancer patient. A more productive approach is to provide cancer patients with opportunities for open expression of feelings and for learning adaptive coping strategies.

Grossarth-Mahcek[98] demonstrated significantly longer survival rates of patients undergoing therapy specially designed to help with expression of previously inhibited needs and feelings. Investigators have demonstrated a significant positive relationship between enhanced relaxation—using biofeedback,[99] imagery,[98] and hypnosis—and immune response.[99]

## Psychosocial Issues of the Medical and Nursing Staff

One of the paradoxes of behavioral science efforts in cancer is that little attention has been focused on the emotional experience of the physician or nurse in cancer medicine. The extensive focus on the experience of the patient and family appears to embody the assumption that the health care deliverers are untouched by the emotional turmoils generated by cancer. Perhaps it is assumed by behavioral scientists and by health care deliverers alike that cancer treatment personnel, through the processes of clinical work and experience, become *objective* and somehow distance themselves from these conflicts. Such assumptions are fallacious; the high turnover rates of oncology nurses in inpatient settings testify to the existence of such stresses.

The physician or nurse dealing with cancer must learn to strike an emotional balance between aloofness and overinvolvement. To be too aloof is to avoid vital contact with the patient; to become too involved ensures ultimate emotional devastation, making it impossible to help any patient. This is not to say, however, that experiences of personnel do not register at an unconscious level and begin to take a toll in ways that are covert and yet negative. These experiences may become manifested through depression, disinterest in work, irritability, withdrawal, or emotional unavailability to colleagues and family members alike. The physician and nurse must be taught to identify within themselves the signs of escalating depression, which might include (1) sleep disorders, especially waking in the early hours of the morning with severe anxieties; (2) irritability, such that colleagues, staff, and family members distance themselves and reduce feedback; (3) highly disturbing, symbolic dreams latently expressing patient-related feelings; and (4) a sense of feeling overwhelmed, such that each task seems intimidating.

Mental health professionals who deal with severely disturbed or disturbing individuals—such as those who are chronically suicidal—know that the shortest route to professional incompetence and personal despair is (1) to feel solely responsible for all aspects of the patient's treatment and (2) to keep one's feelings about the situation completely internalized. The need to widen the base of communication and responsibility is vital for one's emotional survival. The oncologist who chooses to practice in isolation exacerbates personal pressure, but even in this situation, communication with one's staff about patients and families and the feelings

they generate can make the difference between professional emotional survival and nonsurvival. One must accept the need to use mental health professionals in patient management as critical to the emotional maintenance of the cancer physician or nurse. When certain patients overtax the staff resources, it should be realized that referral of these patients does not signify failure on the part of the health care providers.

Maintenance of mental health for the physician and nurse demands more than communication about patients and open interaction with colleagues. It is vital for the physician and nurse to organize a lifestyle that allows complete emotional disconnection from cancer and cancer patients when not in the clinical setting. If the professional allows cancer to dominate his or her life to the point of allowing no time for other, unrelated activities, with the expectation that all emotional gratifications and rewards will come from this area, problems will certainly follow. It is only when the physician or nurse dealing with cancer considers his or her emotional maintenance to be as important as that of the patient that high-quality care can be assured.

## SUGGESTIONS FOR ADDITIONAL READING

Cassileth BR, Lusk GJ, Strouse TB, et al. Psychosocial status in chronic illness groups: a comparative analysis of six diagnostic groups. N Engl J Med 1984;311:506–11.

Bloom JR. Psychological response to mastectomy. Cancer 1987;59:189–96.

Fawzy FI, Kemeny MD, Fawzy NW, et al. A structured psychiatric intervention for cancer patients. Arch Gen Psychiatry 1990;47:729–35.

Ganz PA, Schag CC, Polinsky ML, et al. Rehabilitation needs and breast cancer: the first month after primary therapy. Breast Cancer Res Treat 1987;10:243–53.

Derogatis LR, Morrow GR, Fetting J, et al. The prevalence of psychiatric disorders among cancer patients. JAMA 1983;249:751–7.

Holland JC, Morrow GR, Schmale A, et al. A randomized clinical trial of alprazolam versus progressive muscle relaxation in cancer patients with anxiety and depressive symptoms. J Clin Oncol 1991;9:1004–11.

Massie MJ, Holland JC. The cancer patient with pain: psychiatric complications and their management. Med Clin North Am 1987;71:243–58.

Northhouse L. The impact of cancer on the family: an overview. Int J Psychiatry Med 1984;14:215–42.

Spiegel D. Psychosocial intervention in cancer. J Natl Cancer Inst 1993;85:1198–205. *This article provides a concise summary of a mini-symposium on this topic presented to the National Cancer Advisory Board in 1992.*

Whippen DA, Canellos GP. Burnout syndrome in the practice of oncology: results of a random survey of 1,000 oncologists. J Clin Oncol 1991;9:1916–21. *Burnout was reported by 56% of those responding to the survey.*

## REFERENCES

1. Clark RL. Psychological reactions of patients and health care professionals to cancer. In: Cullen JW, ed. Cancer: the behavioral dimensions. New York: Raven Press, 1976:xv–xxvi.
2. Stehlin JS Jr, Beach KH. Psychological aspects of cancer therapy: a surgeon's viewpoint. JAMA 1966;197:100–4.
3. Senescu RA. The development of emotional complications in the patient with cancer. J Chronic Dis 1963;16:813.
4. Cohen F. Coping with the stresses of illness. In: Stone GC, ed. Health psychology. San Francisco: Jossey-Bass, 1979:217.
5. Bard M., Sutherland AM. Psychological impact of cancer and its treatment. IV: Adaptation to radical mastectomy. Cancer 1955;8:656–72.
6. Polivy J. Psychological effects of mastectomy on a woman's feminine self-concept. J Nerv Ment Dis 1977;164:77–87.

7. Renneker R. Psychological problems of adjustment to cancer of the breast. JAMA 1952;148:833.

8. Schain W, Edwards BK, Gorrell CR, et al. Psychosocial and physical outcomes of primary breast cancer therapy: mastectomy vs excisional biopsy and irradiation. Breast Cancer Res Treat 1983;3:377–82.

9. Worden JW, Weisman AD. The fallacy in postmastectomy depression. Am J Med Sci 1977;273:169–75.

10. McArdle CS, Calman KC, Cooper AF, et al. The social, emotional and financial implications of adjuvant chemotherapy in breast cancer. Br J Surg 1981;68:261–4.

11. Meyerowitz BE, Sparks FC, Spears IK. Adjuvant chemotherapy for breast carcinoma: psychosocial implications. Cancer 1979;43:1613–8.

12. Bond MR. Psychologic and emotional aspects of cancer pain. In: Bonica JJ, ed. Advances in pain research and therapy. Vol 2. New York: Raven Press, 1979:81–8.

13. Chapman CR. Psychologic and behavioral aspects of cancer pain. In: Bonica JJ, ed. Advances in pain research and therapy. Vol 2. New York: Raven Press, 1979:45–58.

14. Seligman MEP. Helplessness. San Francisco: WH Freeman & Co, 1975.

15. Abramson LY, Seligman ME, Teasdale JD. Learned helplessness in humans: critique and reformulation. J Abnorm Psychol 1978;87:49–74.

16. Taylor SE. Adjustment to threatening events: a theory of cognitive adaptation. 10th Katz-Newcomb Lecture presented at the University of Michigan, April 1982.

17. Klagsbrun SC. Cancer, emotions, and nurses. Am J Psychiatry 1970;126:1237–44.

18. Miller CL, Denner PR, Richardson VE. Assisting the psychosocial problems of cancer patients: a review of current research. Int J Nurs Stud 1976;13:161–6.

19. Kalish RA. Coping with death. In: Ahmed P, ed. Living and dying with cancer. New York: Elsevier, 1981:37–49.

20. Rainey LC. Toward a more positive perspective. In: Ahmed P, ed. Living and dying with cancer. New York: Elsevier, 1981:223–39.

21. Roskies E. Considerations in developing a treatment program for the coronary prone (type A) behavior pattern. In: Davidson PO, ed. Behavioral medicine: changing health lifestyles. New York: Brunner/Mazel, 1980:299–331.

22. Lazarus RS. Stress-related transactions between person and environment. In: Pervin LA, ed. Perspectives in interactional psychology. New York: Plenum Publishing, 1978:287–327.

23. Lipowski ZJ. Psychosomatic medicine in the seventies: an overview. Am J Psychiatry 1977;134:233–44.

24. Hamburg DA. Coping behavior in life-threatening circumstances. Psychother Psychosom 1974;23:13–25.

25. Lazarus RS. The costs and benefits of denial. In: Breznitz S, ed. The denial of stress. New York: International Universities Press, 1983:1.

26. Hackett TP, Cassem NH. Development of a quantitative rating scale to assess denial. J Psychosom Res 1974;18:93–100.

27. Shands HC. Psychological mechanisms in patients with cancer. Cancer 1951;4:1159.

28. Cobb B. Patient-responsible delay of treatment of cancer. Cancer 1954;7:920.

29. Peck A. Emotional reactions to having cancer. Am J Roentgenol Rad Ther Nucl Med 1972;114:591–9.

30. Moses R, Cividali N. Differential levels of awareness of illness: their relation to some salient features in cancer patients. Ann N Y Acad Sci 1966;125:984–94.

31. Katz JL, Weiner H, Gallagher TF, Hellman L. Stress, distress, and ego defenses: psychoendocrine response to impending breast tumor biopsy. Arch Gen Psychiatry 1970;23:131–42.

32. Wolff CT. Relationship between psychological defenses and mean urinary 17-hydroxycorticosteroid excretion rates. Psychosom Med 1964;26:576.

33. Sanders JB, Kardinal CG. Adaptive coping mechanisms in adult acute leukemia patients in remission. JAMA 1977;238:952–4.

34. Greer S, Morris T, Pettingale KW. Psychological response to breast cancer: effect on outcome. Lancet 1979;2:785–7.

35. Abrams RD. Guilt reactions in patients with cancer. Cancer 1953;6:474.

36. Hilgard ER. Hypnosis in the relief of pain. Los Altos, Calif.: William Kaufmann, 1975.

37. Kroger WS. Clinical and experimental hypnosis. 2nd ed. Philadelphia: JB Lippincott, 1977.

38. Steggles S, Stam HJ, Fehr R, Aucoin P. Hypnosis and cancer: an annotated bibliography 1960–1985. Am J Clin Hypn 1987;29:281–90.

39. Lyles JN, Burish TG, Krozely MG, Oldham RK. Efficacy of relaxation training and guided imagery in reducing the aversiveness of cancer chemotherapy. J Consult Clin Psychol 1982;50:509–24.

40. Redd WH, Andresen GV, Minagawa RY. Hypnotic control of anticipatory emesis in patients receiving cancer chemotherapy. J Consult Clin Psychol 1982;50:14–9.

41. Burish TG. Variables in behavioral oncology: overview and assessment of current issues. In: Fox BH, ed. Impact of psychoendocrine systems in cancer and immunity. Toronto: Hogrefe, 1984.

42. Burish TG. Conditioned nausea and vomiting in cancer chemotherapy: treatment approaches. In: Burish TG, ed. Cancer, nutrition, and eating behavior: a biobehavioral perspective. Hillsdale, N.J.: Erlbaum, 1985:205–24.

43. Bowers KS, Kelly P. Stress, disease, psychotherapy, and hypnosis. J Abnorm Psychol 1979;88:490–505.

44. Simonton OC, Matthews-Simonton S, Sparks TF. Psychological intervention in the treatment of cancer. Psychosomatics 1980;21:226–7, 231–3.

45. Simonton OC. Getting well again. Los Angeles: JP Tarcher, 1978.

46. Rose MA. Problems families face in home care. Am J Nurs 1976;76:416–8.

47. Rosenbaum EH, Rosenbaum IR. Principles of home care for the patient with advanced cancer. JAMA 1980;244:1484–7.

48. Hinton J. Comparison of places and policies for terminal care. Lancet 1979;1:29–32.

49. Yates J. A comparative study of home nursing care of patients with advanced cancer. In: Proceedings of the Third National Conference on Human Values and Cancer. New York: American Cancer Society, 1981:207–18.

50. Gordon A, Roney A. Hospice and the family: a systems approach to assessment. Am J Hospice Care 1984;1:31–3.

51. Wellisch DK. Evaluation of psychosocial problems of the homebound cancer patient. II: The relationship of disease and patient sociodemographic variables to family problems. J Psychosoc Oncol 1983;1:3:1–17.

52. Cassileth BR, Lusk EJ, Strouse TB, Bodenheimer BJ. Contemporary unorthodox treatments in cancer medicine: a study of patients, treatments, and practitioners. Ann Intern Med 1984;101:105–12.

53. Lister J. Current controversy on alternative medicine. N Engl J Med 1983;309:1524–7.

54. American Cancer Society: Unproven methods of cancer management. New York: American Cancer Society, 1982.

55. Bonica JJ. Importance of the problem. In: Bonica JJ, ed. Advances in pain research and therapy. Vol 2. New York: Raven Press, 1979:1–12.

56. Foley KM. In: Bonica JJ, ed. Advances in pain research and therapy. Vol 2. New York: Raven Press, 1979.

57. Mersky H. In: Smith WL, ed. Pain: meaning and management. New York: Spectrum Publications, 1980:71.

58. Twycross RG. The assessment of pain in advanced cancer. J Med Ethics 1978;4:112–6.

59. Fordyce WE. Learning processes in pain. In: Sternbach RA, ed. The psychology of pain. New York: Raven Press, 1978:49–72.

60. Kremer EF, Atkinson JH Jr, Ignelzi RJ. Pain measurement: the affective dimensional measure of the McGill pain questionnaire with a cancer pain population. Pain 1982;12:153–63.

61. Melzack R. The McGill Pain Questionnaire: major properties and scoring methods. Pain 1975;1:277–99.

62. Lewis BJ. Pharmacologic approaches. In: DeVita VT, ed. Cancer: principles and practice of oncology. Philadelphia: JB Lippincott, 1982.

63. Marks RM, Sachar EJ. Undertreatment of medical inpatients with narcotic analgesics. Ann Intern Med 1973;78:173–81.

64. Fordyce WE. Chronic pain. In: Pomerleu OF, ed. Behavioral medicine: theory and practice. Baltimore: Williams & Wilkins, 1979:125.

65. Kroger WS. Hypnosis and behavior modification: imagery conditioning. Philadelphia: JB Lippincott, 1976.

66. Turk D. Cognitive behavioral techniques in the management of pain. In: Foreyt J, ed. Cognitive behavior therapy: research and application. New York: Plenum Publishing, 1978.

67. Caracappa JM. Hypnosis in terminal cancer. Am J Clin Hypn 1963;5:205.

68. Crasilneck HB, Hall JA. Clinical hypnosis in problems of pain. Am J Clin Hypn 1973;15:153–61.

69. Sacerdote P. Theory and practice of pain control in malignancy and other protracted or recurring painful illnesses. Int J Clin Exp Hypn 1970;18:160–80.

70. Sacerdote P. Erickson's approaches to hypnosis and psychotherapy. In:

Zeig JK, ed. Ericksonian approaches to hypnosis and psychotherapy. New York: Brunner/Mazel, 1982:336.

71. Erickson MH. Hypnotherapy: an exploratory casebook. New York: Irvington Publishers (John Wiley & Sons), 1979.

72. Hilgard ER. The alleviation of pain by hypnosis. Pain 1975;1:213–31.

73. Dohrenwend BS, ed. Stressful life events: their nature and effects. New York: John Wiley & Sons, 1974.

74. Jenkins CD. Recent evidence supporting psychologic and social risk factors for coronary disease. N Engl J Med 1976;294:1033–8.

75. Rabkin JG, Struening EL. Life events, stress, and illness. Science 1976;194:1013–20.

76. Minter RE, Kimball CP. Life events and illness onset: a review. Psychosomatics 1978;19:334–9.

77. Borysenko M, Borysenko J. Stress, behavior, and immunity: animal models and mediating mechanisms. Gen Hosp Psychiatry 1982;4:59–67.

78. Monjan AA. In: Psychosocial factors, stress, and immune processes. Ader R, ed. Psychoneuroimmunology. New York: Academic Press, 1981:185–228.

79. Riley V. Psychoneuroendocrine influences on immunocompetence and neoplasia. Science 1981;212:1100–9.

80. Rogers MP, Dubey D, Reich P. The influence of the psyche and the brain on immunity and disease susceptibility: a critical review. Psychosom Med 1979;41:147–64.

81. Borysenko JZ. Behavioral-physiological factors in the development and management of cancer. Gen Hosp Psychiatry 1982;4:69–74.

82. Sklar LS, Anisman H. Stress and cancer. Psychol Bull 1981;89:369–406.

83. Stein M, Schiavi RC, Camerino M. Influence of brain and behavior on the immune system. Science 1976;191:435–40.

84. Schmale A, Iker H. The psychological setting of uterine cervical cancer. Ann N Y Acad Sci 1966;125:807–13.

85. LeShan LL. In: Kissen DM, LeShann LL. International conference on the psychosomatic aspects of neoplastic disease. Cambridge: JB Lippincott, 1964.

86. Visintainer MA, Volpicelli JR, Seligman ME. Tumor rejection in rats after inescapable or escapable shock. Science 1982;216:437–9.

87. Kissen DM. Personality characteristics in males conducive to lung cancer. Br J Med Psychol 1963;36:27.

88. Thomas CB, Duszynski KR. Closeness to parents and the family constellation in a prospective study of five disease states: suicide, mental illness, malignant tumor; hypertension and coronary heart disease. Johns Hopkins Med J 1974;134:251–70.

89. Bahnson CB. Psychophysiological complementarity in malignancies: past work and future vistas. Ann NY Acad Sci 1969;164:319–34.

90. Dattore PJ, Shontz FC, Coyne L. Premorbid personality differentiation of cancer and noncancer groups: a test of the hypothesis of cancer proneness. J Consult Clin Psychol 1980;48:388–94.

91. Bacon CL. A psychosomatic survey of cancer of the breast. Psychosom Med 1952;14:453.

92. LeShan LL. Some recurrent life history patterns observed in patients with malignant disease. J Nerv Ment Dis 1956;124:460.

93. Pettingale KW, Greer S, Tee DE. Serum IgA and emotional expression in breast cancer patients. J Psychosom Res 1977;2:395–9.

94. Katz JL, Ackman P, Rothwax Y, et al. Psychoendocrine aspects of cancer of the breast. Psychosom Med 1970;32:1–18.

95. Gorzynski JG, Holland J, Katz JL, et al. Stability of ego defenses and endocrine responses in women prior to breast biopsy and ten years later. Psychosom Med 1980;42:323–8.

96. Temoshok L. Biopsychosocial studies on cutaneous malignant melanoma: psychosocial factors associated with prognostic indicators, progression, psychophysiology and tumor-host response. Soc Sci Med 1985;20:833–40.

97. Fox BH. Premorbid psychological factors as related to cancer incidence. J Behav Med 1978;1:45–133.

98. Grossarth-Mahcek R. Psychotherapy research in oncology. In: Steptoe A, ed. Health care and human behavior. London: Academic Press, 1984:325.

99. Rossi EL. The psychobiology of mind-body healing. Ontario: WW Newport, 1986.

# CHAPTER 25

# HOSPICE AND OTHER END-OF-LIFE PROGRAMS

• PAUL R. TORRENS • CHARLES M. HASKELL

One of the most interesting developments in cancer care has been the emergence of end-of-life programs for the care of terminally ill patients. This includes the development of hospice programs around the world as well as the emergence of palliative medicine as a distinct specialty. Although much has been written about hospice care and palliative medicine, it is not widely recognized that these concepts are continuing to evolve as new modalities for cancer treatment and palliation appear. The exact role of an individual hospice or palliative care program in the continuum of cancer care in a community may vary, depending on the availability of other types of supportive services in that community. It is imperative that every health care professional who works with cancer patients understand the principles of end-of-life care as practiced by hospices and palliative medicine specialists so that their benefits and strengths can be integrated more appropriately into a comprehensive program of care for patients.

## Background

### HOSPICE MOVEMENT

Much of the current interest in hospice care originated with the landmark work of Saunders at St. Christopher's Hospice in London. Although this facility was not the first to concentrate solely on the care of the dying, Saunders' purposeful and vigorous writing and teaching made it a leading institution for innovation in hospice care.[1–5] St. Christopher's was also the first hospice program to recognize the need for improved professional education and training in the care of the dying, and it provided international leadership in the development of other hospice programs all around the world.

After the opening of St. Christopher's in 1967, similar programs soon began to appear in various parts of England and Scotland. Many of these programs shared the same model of organization as St. Christopher's in that they were separate, freestanding units that were developed solely to provide inpatient care for dying patients.

By the early 1970s, news of the work at St. Christopher's began to spread across the United States and Canada, and by the mid-1970s, four important programs of different types were established in Montreal, New Haven, Marin County (California), and New York City. In 1974, a new program for the care of the dying was established at the Royal Victoria Hospital in Montreal; in contrast to the separate freestanding hospices that had been developed in Great Britain, this hospice program was located on a nursing unit directly within the hospital itself and was closely integrated into all hospital functions. At the same time, in New Haven, Connecticut, a group of health care professionals associated with Yale University organized a hospice program that initially did not have an inpatient unit of its own but concentrated on providing professional care to the dying in their own homes. In more recent years, the program has added a freestanding inpatient unit, but its major emphasis remains on care of patients at home. In 1976 in Marin County, California, just north of San Francisco, a group of community leaders came together to form a community-based, volunteer-staffed hospice program whose purpose was to support and extend the already existing medical, nursing, and support services in the community. In the beginning, this program did not provide inpatient services or home care services of a traditional nature, but instead concentrated on providing a new array of services, such as bereavement counseling, that were not already available in the community. Finally, in the mid-1970s at St. Luke's Hospital in Manhattan, an in-hospital support team was formed to provide technical assistance and coordination of care to health care professionals and programs that were already providing care to cancer patients at the hospital. The philosophy here was not to provide an entirely new service for the care of the dying but rather to build on and integrate better what was already being done.

At the time these early hospice programs were developing, there was relatively little experience in important areas such as pain control, bereavement counseling, psychosocial support for cancer patients and their families, and provision of nursing and treatment services at home. As a result, hospice programs often became widely involved in aspects of cancer care that were much broader than just the care of terminally ill patients, either because these other programs did not exist or because the experience and range of the hospice programs were broader and more advanced. Over the years, as other forms of supportive care for cancer patients have developed, hospice programs have been able to concentrate more specifically on the care of terminally ill patients for whom there is no hope of cure.

After the early development of the pilot programs in the 1970s, the growth of hospice programs in the United States was explosive. In the 10-year period from 1977 to 1987, the number of U.S. hospice programs increased from approximately 50 in 1977 to approximately 1900 in 1987, of which about half operated from a hospital base and half from a community base.[6] A survey by the Joint Commission on Accreditation of Hospitals in 1986 revealed that the primary diagnosis in their patients was almost exclusively cancer (92%).[7]

The most significant development in hospice care in the

United States came in 1982 when a hospice benefit was added to the Medicare program on a 3-year trial basis and was then made permanent in 1986. The Congressional legislation was passed in overwhelming fashion, drawing support from those who altruistically wanted to improve the care of the dying and from those who were more interested in the hospice's impact on the rising costs of hospital care for dying patients. These twin themes of improved quality of patient care and reduced hospital costs continue to predominate in hospice activities today, often supporting one another and also often in conflict.

To take advantage of the Medicare hospice benefit, a Medicare-eligible patient must be terminally ill, with a survival prognosis of 6 months or less, and must elect the hospice benefit. In doing so, such a patient relinquishes other Medicare benefits and agrees that the hospice program will provide for all his or her needs except for the services of the patient's attending physician. The benefits in the Medicare hospice package include nursing care; medical social services; consulting physician services; counseling services; home health aide and homemaker services; physical, occupational, and speech therapy services; volunteer and bereavement services; medical supplies and durable medical equipment; and medication for symptom control. Short-term inpatient care, along with short-term respite and home nursing care, is also covered. The patient's eligibility for these services must be periodically evaluated and recertified at 90, 180, and 210 days. Under the terms of the Medicare hospice benefit, it is the program's responsibility to develop a coordinated plan of care, which the program must then supervise and carry out, either with its own services or with services that are obtained from other providers. In return, the hospice program is reimbursed on a per diem basis for one of four levels of care:

1. Routine home care, in which the patient is at home and receiving care; this should account for 80% of all hospice days.
2. Continuous home care, in which the patient is at home and receiving continuous and primarily nursing care during a period of more severe difficulties that involve a need for greater services.
3. General inpatient care, in which inpatient services are required for acute pain or symptom control.
4. Inpatient respite care, in which the patient is receiving inpatient care to relieve the primary caregiver at home for up to 5 days.

To participate in the Medicare hospice benefit, a program must meet certain specific requirements demanded by Medicare and must be formally certified. In states in which hospice licensing laws exist,[8] the programs must be licensed to be eligible for Medicare reimbursement.

The importance of the Congressional hospice Medicare legislation and the subsequent inclusion of hospice care as a permanent Medicare benefit cannot be emphasized enough. The legislation represented an acceptance of hospice care as a legitimate health care service and a valued addition to the system of health care in the United States. It mandated a certain form of organization and provision of services that a hospice program must offer to be certified by Medicare, indirectly bringing a standardization of programs and services that was quite constructive.[8] The inclusion of the hospice benefit under Medicare provided a steady, predictable stream of financial support for hospice programs that has allowed them to broaden their range of services and strengthen their organizational structures. The long-term success of the hospice movement in the United States has depended, in large part, on the availability of Medicare funding for approved programs. It is also clear that the Medicare benefit has broadened the access to hospice programs for the elderly far beyond what it otherwise might have been.

In addition to the growth and expansion of hospice programs since the introduction of the Medicare hospice benefit in 1986, there has been growth and expansion of a wide variety of individual services that are needed by cancer patients but are not necessarily offered through recognized hospice programs. These include home intravenous line services, total parenteral nutrition programs, special transportation programs, psychological support services, and others. Many of these services are used individually by physicians and others to augment and strengthen their cancer care of patients; many of these same services may be brought together with other individual services to create a formal hospice program. Whether they are considered separately or together, there has been an extraordinary expansion in the availability of individual cancer support services that benefit individual cancer patients and provide potential building blocks for more formal hospice programs.

**Palliative Medicine.** As the hospice movement gained momentum, it became clear that physicians with special knowledge and skills in the delivery of hospice care were needed. In some cases, these physicians were part of the hospice movement itself, whereas in others, palliative medicine developed as an alternative to the hospice approach. This alternative development was especially true in settings where the available hospice programs were perceived as being outside the mainstream of medicine.

The term *palliative medicine* has been defined by Doyle[9] as "the study and management of patients with active, progressive, far-advanced disease for whom the prognosis is limited and the focus of care is quality of life." The discipline is recognized as a specific subspecialty by the American Board of Hospice and Palliative Medicine, with its first examination for special qualifications in palliative medicine being given in 1996.[10]

## ROLE OF MEDICAL ONCOLOGY IN PALLIATIVE CARE

Many medical oncologists consider palliative care to be an essential part of the subspecialty.[11] The importance of palliative medicine to the practice of medical oncology has been recognized formally by the American Society of Clinical Oncology (ASCO), which devoted considerable attention to the topic at its annual meeting in 1998. Subsequently the ASCO Board of Directors published the following principles, which they considered essential to providing a humane system of cancer care during the last phase of life.[12]

- Cancer care is centered around the longstanding, continuous relationship between the primary oncologist or other physician with training and interest in end-of-life care and the patient.

- Cancer care is responsive to the patient's wishes and to the parents' wishes if the patient is a child.
- Cancer care is based on truthful, sensitive, empathic communication with the patient; care is family centered as well as child focused.
- Cancer care optimizes quality of life throughout the course of an illness through meticulous attention to the myriad physical, spiritual, and psychosocial needs of the patient and family.

## Principles of Hospice Care and Designation as a Hospice Program

As mentioned previously, the early years of the hospice movement in the United States saw many different types of hospice programs develop, each providing some slight variant of the basic ideas and principles of hospice care developed originally at St. Christopher's in London. These different programs grew up in different types of organizations ranging from already existing health care programs, such as hospitals and home health agencies, to more informal, community-based volunteer groups. Over the years, the variety of sponsoring organizations has been maintained, but a much greater clarification and standardization of hospice *program* or *package* has emerged.[13] This clarification and standardization has had two parts: first, a more legal and formalistic development, involving licensing or certification,[14] and second, an agreement to an overall set of guiding principles.

From a funding perspective, it is critical for a hospice program to have formal designation by Medicare as an approved provider of the Medicare hospice benefit package. To obtain this designation, a hospice program must show that it can either provide or obtain under contract a specific set of services and must make formal application to Medicare to become an approved provider. In states in which there is formal licensing, the program must also be licensed by the state. The formal designation of a hospice program as an approved provider of the hospice Medicare benefit is important to physicians and their patients because it means that the services provided are paid for by Medicare; patients who obtain hospice services from non–Medicare-certified programs have to pay for those services from their own funds.[15]

There are many hospice programs that are neither licensed (because they operate in states that do not require licensure) nor certified by Medicare (because they have chosen not to seek that certification). These programs may be equal in quality and range of services to programs that are licensed or certified, and they probably adhere to the same set of general principles of hospice care that characterize the licensed Medicare-certified hospice programs.[16] Any physician or patient seeking hospice care should determine whether the hospice program in question does adhere to these general principles and whether it is organized according to them.[17]

The basic principles of hospice care as developed by Saunders and her colleagues in London have been reaffirmed by the leaders of the National Hospice Association in the 1970s. These are as follows:

1. Hospice programs are organized to provide care for terminally ill patients and their families. The unit of care for a hospice is the patient and the family together; the definition of *family* is determined by the patient and may include nonrelatives.

2. Care is provided by an interdisciplinary team that may include physicians, nurses, social workers, psychologists, spiritual ministers, volunteers, and others.

3. Care is provided under the terms of a specific written plan that is developed by the interdisciplinary team and is coordinated by the hospice program.

4. Care is provided on a 24-hour-a-day, 7-day-a-week basis. Services should be readily available, and communication between patient and family and the interdisciplinary team should be direct and easy.

5. Significant attention and preventive action should be directed toward control of pain and toward alleviation of physical symptoms, such as constipation, oral infections, and bedsores, before they become a major concern; this is particularly true with regard to control of pain by the use of anticipatory doses of pain-control medication. There is also recognition that pain not only is physical but is also made up of emotional, psychological, and spiritual components.

6. Active treatment of patients' problems should be carried out as needed and as appropriate to ease their distress; hospice care does not mean nontreatment of a medical condition, but rather selective treatment as appropriate to ease pain and suffering. The concentration of care is on improvement of the quality of life and not necessarily on extending it; the focus is on palliative care, not curative treatment.

7. Bereavement services and counseling should be available to family members for an extended period after the patient's death; these services may include one-on-one counseling, support groups, and telephone encouragement and support. For family members with obvious and continuing serious problems, referral to appropriate therapy or support services is carried out.

8. Hospice programs provide for a continuum of inpatient and home care services through an integrated administrative structure that links the individual services to the written treatment plan. These services may be either directly provided by the hospice program itself or provided under contract by other organizations or individuals.

## Major Issues in Hospice Care

There are certain major issues related to hospice care of which oncologists involved in the care of dying patients should be aware and which are most likely to predominate in any further development of hospice programs.

### ARE HOSPICE PROGRAMS NECESSARY ANY LONGER?

Hospice programs were developed initially because suitable programs for the care of the dying were not available. The standard treatment sites, particularly those for cancer patients, did not provide an appropriate range of counseling, patient and family support, home care services, and other supportive services that were needed to provide compassionate care for patients and their families. The existing treatment sites and personnel were focused on the challenges of active treatment and cure but were not as knowledgeable about or interested in the relief and palliation of suffering in patients for whom active treatment was no longer a realistic option.

Hospice programs, in England and the United States, began somewhat in protest over the lack of these supportive services. They assumed a *fugitive* posture outside the organized health care system, as much in rebuke of the system as for any other reason; they were also started outside the established system because few individuals within it were interested or ready to support these new efforts. Early hospice advocates willingly assumed this outsider role, and in some cases that role became a way of life.

Now, by contrast, most of the ideas, principles, and programs that the early hospice leaders advocated have been accepted as valuable additions to the cancer treatment continuum. There is no longer any reasonable argument that hospice programs are anything other than a well-needed extension of good patient care—in this case, to the patient's family and home. Hospice programs have shown the way, documented the results, and generally rewritten the textbooks on what *comprehensive care* for cancer patients should be.

In the process, a variety of individual new services have appeared in traditional cancer care programs that were once available only in hospice programs or other *outsider* programs.[18] Psychological services for patients and their families, home infusion services, respite care, and advanced pain-control techniques have all now become part of any comprehensive cancer program that claims to be excellent in the range and quality of its services.[19] The questions then arise: With the expansion of support and ancillary services to cancer patients within the comprehensive cancer program, is there any further need for hospice programs? Cannot the work be done by a combination of already existing support services without the creation of an entirely new organization structure or vehicle called a *hospice*?

The answer to the first question, from hospice workers and health care professionals involved in cancer care in general, seems to be strongly positive, for two primary reasons. The first reason why hospice programs are still needed is that they provide a focused, well-coordinated program for a wide variety of services that might otherwise be scattered, poorly linked, and without any overall plan for coordination and delivery. The organizers of hospice programs have learned how to bring together an array of diverse services and professionals, focusing them specifically on the needs of individual patients and their families and doing it in ways that save money. The quality of care improves; the cost of care is held down; and, most important, the patient and family have a sense of support, communication, compassion, and completion that might otherwise be lacking. Hospice programs provide an organizational way of doing well and efficiently what otherwise might not be done.

The second major reason why hospice programs are still needed is that they remind health care professionals and leaders about the special needs of the dying and their families. Hospice programs serve as a means of providing for the needs of the dying, of training personnel to serve the dying, and of learning about better ways to serve the dying. Without hospice programs, this constant reminder of the fact that dying patients require our particular interest and compassion might be slowly eroded.

All hospice programs need not be totally freestanding, separate from comprehensive cancer programs, and providing all the individual services themselves. Although hospice programs are certainly necessary and appropriate, they may be developed by the use of existing individual services drawn together to provide a coordinated package of services. In the same fashion, they do not necessarily need to be completely separate from larger programs of comprehensive cancer care; instead, they can (and should) easily be integrated into these cancer programs as a logical extension of their services. Hospice programs are an integral part of the continuum of cancer care and as such are more important than ever, not less. This importance is increasingly recognized by the presence of palliative medicine as a formal part of the medical school curriculum.[20]

## DISCOURAGEMENT OF MEDICAL TREATMENT AND EUTHANASIA AND ASSISTED DEATH

In the past, when hospice programs were first beginning, questions were regularly posed to individuals working in them: "Don't hospice programs refuse medical treatment to their patients? Aren't hospices places to which individuals are admitted and where no active medical care is provided?" The implication of medical nihilism was widespread and difficult to refute fully.

Over the years, however, the practical experience of hospice care has made it clear that hospices do provide active care for patients' medical problems, and such care is appropriate for the individual patient. The difference is that the care is supplied to ease pain and suffering, to control distress, and to handle temporary or nonessential conditions; it is not provided as a possible long-term cure, and it is not automatically given just to extend life. Medical treatment is provided within the general framework of palliation, not cure.

Questions have also begun to be raised in some circles about the appropriateness of some form of medically assisted death, if that is what the particular patient wishes. The argument here is that patients should have the right to obtain assistance in actively dying if that is their choice. Supporters of this view say that patients should not be forced to accept passively a slow, painful, obvious, and inevitable death if they do not wish to. Because hospice programs deal specifically and only with dying patients, suggestions have been made that perhaps hospice programs should be studying more carefully the entire question of medically assisted death for their patients.[21, 22]

Many hospice workers are appalled by any suggestion that their program should be involved in any type of active assistance in the dying process because this would be in direct contradiction to many of the basic contentions about hospice programs. In the fall of 1992, when Proposition 161 (Death with Dignity Act) was being proposed for the general ballot through the initiative process in California, the California State Hospice Association formally opposed the Act and explained its position by saying, "We believe that legalizing physician-assisted suicide is not in the best interests of the dying, their families, and society . . . Hospice has a long

tradition of acting as an advocate of the rights and dignity of dying persons and their families . . . We believe the Death with Dignity Initiative, however well intended, may open the door for abuses of the rights and dignity of dying people."[23] Earlier, in 1990, the National Hospice Organization (NHO) issued a statement on euthanasia that, although affirming "a patient's right to refuse unwanted medical intervention including the provision of artificially supplied hydration and nutrition . . . rejects the practice of voluntary euthanasia and assisted suicide in the care of the terminally ill."[24] The NHO went on to argue that "hospice care is an alternative to voluntary euthanasia and assisted suicide . . . hospice care neither hastens nor postpones death." These early views on the role of euthanasia in hospice programs have been sustained over time.[24]

Individual hospice workers may support the general idea of medically assisted suicide, but the hospice movement in general and hospice programs in particular have been careful to avoid any suggestion that they will become involved in medically assisted death as part of the program. They generally believe that medically assisted suicide contradicts the overall purposes and principles of hospice care; their support of such practices might confuse these purposes in the eyes of the public and undermine the confidence that the public has developed in hospice programs in general.

## HOSPICE AS A MEANS OF REDUCING HEALTH CARE COSTS

One of the predominant motives for congressional approval of hospice care as a Medicare benefit was the belief that it would help control health care costs and would reduce Medicare expenditures for care of the dying.[25] Much of the initial enthusiasm for hospice programs had been based on the assumption that they would be a major force in the reduction of health care costs in general.

The evidence has not shown that hospice programs necessarily reduce the total expenditures for dying patients throughout the United States, although they do seem to reduce the hospital costs of individual patients.[26-36] These seemingly contrasting findings are based on the fact that the passage of the Medicare hospice benefit expanded the availability of hospice programs, increased the use of these services, and expanded the number of total persons being served. Although the cost per case for dying Medicare recipients who previously would have been hospitalized for the final dying period has been reduced by hospice programs, the total expenditures for the entire class of Medicare beneficiaries have increased.[37, 38] Probably the major long-term benefit from the expanded Medicare hospice benefit has not been a savings in expenditures but rather an improvement in quality, access to care, and use of services.[39, 40]

## HIGH-TECHNOLOGY SERVICES AND PALLIATIVE CARE

The summer 1993 issue of *California Hospice Report*, the regular publication of the California State Hospice Association, discussed a topic that is giving rise to serious concerns among hospice leaders across the United States: the changing mix of patients in hospice programs and the changing (higher technology) array of services being expected and requested by hospice patients and their families.[41] The impact of high-technology services in health care is being felt by hospice programs, and many questions need to be answered.

One impact of high-technology services in health care is that patients are being kept under active treatment for a much longer time and are referred to hospice programs when they are nearer and nearer to death. (Some hospice programs report that one third of their patients are referred to them only 2 weeks before death.) The shorter time frame results from much more active treatment and a reluctance to let go of the hope for a cure. The result is that patients come into hospice programs in a seriously debilitated state, requiring a high level of service, and with a short period to provide any real stabilizing, compassionate impact. The persistence of high-technology treatment for a longer period before referral to hospice programs results in a similarly high level of services and care for a much shorter time once the patient is referred.

An equally serious technology-related problem for hospice programs is the demand for high-technology palliative care services, services that require more expensive instrumentation or professional staff involvement, with resultant higher overall costs. Examples such as the increased demand for and use of total parenteral nutrition regimens, patient-controlled anesthesia, subcutaneous pumps, skin patches, and other new drug administration systems are easily identified. The state of the art in palliative, not curative, care is becoming characterized by increasingly higher technology and increasing expense. An approach to patient care that began with a determinedly antitechnology attitude is now in danger of making use of increasingly higher technology itself.

Because hospice programs receive fixed, per diem reimbursements for their services from Medicare, their primary source of revenue, and must exist within carefully fixed budgets, the arrival of high-technology palliative care makes all the previous financial projections inadequate for the Medicare program that must find the money to pay for the increasingly expensive services. With increasing frequency, hospice programs are being forced to decide whether to provide palliative services on the basis of the cost of those services because of increasing technology, not on the basis of effectiveness. Although the rest of the health care field has had to make these difficult decisions for some time, it is a new experience for most hospice programs and one that is making hospice workers uneasy.[42]

## CHALLENGE OF ACQUIRED IMMUNODEFICIENCY SYNDROME TO HOSPICE PROGRAMS

Hospice programs are facing important new challenges as a result of the acquired immunodeficiency syndrome (AIDS) epidemic. As many experienced hospice workers discovered, just when it was thought that hospice programs knew much of what there was to learn about the care of the dying, the AIDS epidemic came along and posed entirely new sets of challenges.[43, 44]

First, patients with AIDS who need hospice care are different from the population currently seen in most hospice programs, from the point of view of age, social status, and psychological characteristics. The present hospice population is generally older, is middle-class, and has family available to assist in their care; for the most part, they have minimal or average previous psychological difficulties, aside from those raised by the prospect of death. Dying AIDS patients are more likely to be younger, not regularly employed, and not middle class in values or in possessions. They may be estranged from their families and friends because of homosexuality or intravenous drug use, and they often carry a heavy burden of previous psychological problems related to drug use, homosexuality, or hemophilia. If the death of the present typical hospice patient with cancer can be seen as complex, the death of a minority-group, intravenous drug–using AIDS patient is obviously much more difficult and complex for all concerned.

A second challenge presented by the dying AIDS population is the financial one: How will the necessary terminal care for AIDS patients be financed, when many of these patients are completely uninsured or have insurance benefits that do not cover the range of services needed? With the number of human immunodeficiency virus (HIV)–positive cases increasing each year, the costs of caring for AIDS cases are soaring.[45]

The third challenge presented by dying AIDS patients arises from the uniquely infectious nature of AIDS and the potential for transmission of the disease to caregivers. Although many health care professionals and hospice volunteers are willing to work with the present dying population in hospice programs, it is not clear that they would be as willing to care for potentially infectious AIDS patients. Although the potential risk to hospice professionals and volunteers of acquiring AIDS by caring for AIDS patients is small, the psychological barrier to full and enthusiastic care for AIDS patients is real and must be taken into consideration. One positive development has been the development of a number of special AIDS hospice programs, such as the London Lighthouse and the Midway Mission Hospice in London; the Casey House in Toronto; and others in New York, San Francisco, and Los Angeles. It may be that future hospice care of dying AIDS patients will be provided by special AIDS hospice programs, although this would be a sad and fragmenting development for the hospice movement.

## SUGGESTIONS TO PHYSICIANS CONSIDERING HOSPICE PROGRAMS FOR PATIENTS

Most physicians in general medicine or surgical practice at some time have patients who may be appropriate candidates for a hospice program.[46] All oncologists regularly encounter such patients. What are the factors that physicians should review when considering hospice programs for their patients?[47, 48] If a palliative medicine specialist is to be consulted, what would be the elements of such a consultation?[49]

As a first consideration, physicians must review their own views about death and dying, their views about their role in such cases, and in particular their own values and standards. Questions they need to answer include the following: Do they believe that active treatment should be continued vigorously, even when it seems unlikely that positive results will follow? Do they believe that only a limited amount of pain medication should be used and only in response to actual pain, or do they believe that pain medication should be given at higher doses in a preventive fashion to block even the possibility of pain? How much do they believe that patients and families should enter into the decisions to continue previous treatment regimens or begin new ones? Are referring physicians comfortable turning over the complete care of the patient to another physician in the hospice program, or do they expect to remain completely involved and in charge of the patient's care until the patient's death? Physicians should examine these and related questions and should review their own values and beliefs about death and dying well in advance of the need to put them into effect because it makes involvement with the dying patient easier and more effective.

For the individual physician interested in finding an appropriate hospice program for a patient, the process is now comparatively simple. An inquiry to the hospital's social work department or home care program is one way to begin, as are inquiries to the local visiting nurse service or the local chapter of the American Cancer Society. In more difficult cases, inquiries might be directed to the central office of the NHO in Arlington, Virginia, which keeps an updated directory of hospice programs in existence throughout the United States. In states in which hospice licensure is required, a telephone call to the state health department or state licensing agency should result in a list of licensed programs in the physician's locality.

Once the names of appropriate hospice programs have been obtained, the physician should call the various programs and inquire about the range of services offered, the charge to the patient for these services, and the conditions (if any) attached to the possible acceptance of patients. These conditions may be related to whether or not all curative treatment must be stopped before a patient can be accepted, how close to death the patient must be, and whether the patient is at home or still hospitalized. It is important to know whether the hospice has a medical staff of its own that takes on the responsibility for total patient care or whether it expects the referring physician to continue to be actively responsible for decisions regarding the patient.

The physician may request the names of other physicians who have used the hospice program in the past for their patients and may want to request the names of families that have been served by the hospice program in the past, to obtain an idea of patient satisfaction with the program. Because each hospice program probably has a medical director or a coordinator of patient care services, the physician may wish to talk to that person to get a better idea of how the specific hospice program functions. If a physician believes that the patient needs only certain selected services provided by the hospice program, it is in order to question whether it is possible to obtain only those specific services and not the whole hospice program. In general, most good hospice programs are pleased to be asked these questions because it allows them to interact more directly with the physician and eventually provide better care for the patient.

Before using any hospice program, the referring physician must review the individual case to determine whether the program can fulfill the patient's needs and whether it is, in fact, an improvement over the present pattern of care.[50] If the patient's pain is well controlled, if the patient's physical condition is well served by adequate nursing care, and if the patient and family are handling the emotional stresses in satisfactory fashion, there may be no need for referral to a hospice program. Close review of the situation may reveal significant areas of unmet needs for the patient, the family, or both, and referral to a hospice may be appropriate. It is vitally important that the referring physician discuss entry into a hospice program with the patient and the family in an open and complete fashion. It is essential that all involved understand the implications and agree to the referral before it is made. In many cases, patients have already considered such a referral and are relieved and grateful when it is made.

As a final consideration, all concerned physicians must carefully review the services that are available at their hospital or in their community for improved care of the dying. One of the most important reasons for encouraging active physician participation in the daily care of dying patients is to enable them to understand better and appreciate the range of problems that afflict dying patients and their families and the array of services needed to alleviate these problems. It is only when physicians know in detail what it takes to ease the pain and suffering of dying patients that they can review the services offered by their hospitals and determine whether they are adequate. If the services are not adequate, it may be an important role for the concerned physician to arrange that additional services be developed. Whether this development is formalized into an organization called a *hospice* or whether it merely consists of upgrading and improving services that already exist is not important. What is important is that all physicians, all hospitals, and all dying patients have available to them the range of services that are currently thought to be necessary to deliver high-quality, compassionate, and effective terminal care.

## SUGGESTIONS FOR ADDITIONAL READING

Caring for the dying: identification and promotion of physician competency. Reprint of educational resource documents and personal narratives. Philadelphia: American Board of Internal Medicine, 1998. (See *http://www.abim.org*.)

Doyle D, Hanks GWC, MacDonald N, eds. Oxford textbook of palliative medicine. New York: Oxford University Press, 1993.

Berger AM, Portenoy RK, Weissman DE, eds. Principles and practice of supportive oncology. Philadelphia: Lippincott-Raven, 1998.

## REFERENCES

1. Saunders C. A therapeutic community: St. Christopher's Hospice. In: Schoenberg B, ed. Psychosocial aspects of terminal care. New York: Columbia University Press, 1972.
2. Saunders C. The challenge of terminal care. In: Symington T, ed. Scientific foundations of oncology. London: Heinemann, 1976.
3. Saunders C. Hospice care. Am J Med 1978;65:726–8.
4. Saunders C. The management of terminal illness. London: Arnold Publishers, 1978.
5. Saunders C. Hospice: the living idea. Philadelphia: WB Saunders, 1981.
6. McCann BA. Hospice care in the United States: the struggle for definition and survival. J Palliat Care 1988;4:16–8.
7. Longo D. The nature, process, and modes of hospice care delivery: final analytic report. Contract No. 500-85-0022. Chicago: Joint Commission on Accreditation of Hospitals, 1987.

8. Health Care Financing Administration. Medicare hospice manual (HCFA Publication No. 21). Washington, D.C.: Government Printing Office, 1983.
9. Doyle D. Palliative medicine: a time for definition? Palliat Med 1993;7:253–5.
10. Holman GH, Smith DC. Board certification in palliative care for U.S. physicians. Officers and Trustees of the American Board of Hospice and Palliative Medicine. J Pain Symptom Manage 1999;17:309–10.
11. Cherny NI, Catane R. Palliative medicine and the medical oncologist: Defining the purview of care. Hematol Oncol Clin North Am 1996;10:1–20.
12. American Society of Clinical Oncology. Cancer care during the last phase of life. J Clin Oncol 1998;16:1986–96.
13. Joint Commission on Accreditation of Hospitals. Hospice Standards Manual. Chicago: Joint Commission on Accreditation of Hospitals, 1983.
14. Olson SL. The Michigan model: a year review of hospice licensure. Mich Med 1986;85:632–4.
15. Tehan C. Has success spoiled hospice? Hastings Center Report 1985;15:10–3.
16. Greer D, Mor V. How Medicare is altering the hospice movement. Hastings Cent Rep 1985;15:5–9.
17. Mor V, Schwartz R, Laliberte L, Hiris J. An examination of the effect of reimbursement and organizational structure on the allocation of hospital staff time. Home Health Care Serv Q 1985;6:101–18.
18. Abel EK. The hospice movement: institutionalizing innovation. Int J Health Serv 1986;16:71–85.
19. Benjamin H. From victim to victor: the Wellness Community Guide to fighting for recovery for cancer patients and their families. Los Angeles: Tarcher/St. Martin's Press, 1987.
20. Barnard D, Quill T, Hafferty FW, et al. Preparing the ground: contributions of the preclinical years to medical education for care near the end of life. Working Group on the Pre-clinical Years of the National Consensus Conference on Medical Education for Care Near the End of Life. Acad Med 1999;74:499–505.
21. Byock IR. The hospice clinician's response to euthanasia/physician assisted suicide. Hospice J 1994;9:1–8.
22. Miller RJ. Hospice and the do-not-resuscitate order. Hospice J 1991;7:67–77.
23. Beresford L. Calif Hospice Rep 1992;10:1. editorial.
24. Begley AM. Response to the National Council for Hospice and Specialist Palliative Care Services—voluntary euthanasia: the council's view. Nurs Ethics 1999;6:157–61.
25. Emanuel EJ, Emanuel LL. The economics of dying: the illusion of cost savings at the end of life. see comments. N Engl J Med 1994;330:540–4.
26. Wales J, Kane R, Robbins S, et al. UCLA hospice evaluation study: methodology and instrumentation. Med Care 1983;21:734–44.
27. Kane RL, Wales J, Bernstein L, et al. A randomised controlled trial of hospice care. Lancet 1984;1:890–4.
28. Kane RL, Berstein L, Wales J, Rothenberg R. Hospice effectiveness in controlling pain. JAMA 1985;253:2683–6.
29. Kane RL, Klein SJ, Bernstein L, et al. Hospice role in alleviating the emotional stress of terminal patients and their families. Med Care 1985;23:189–97.
30. Greer DS, Mor V, Sherwood S, et al. National hospice study analysis plan. J Chronic Dis 1983;36:737–80.
31. Mor V. Overview of the National Hospice Study design. In: Green D, ed. Final report of the National Hospice Study. Providence, R.I.: Brown University Program in Medicine and Center for Health Care Research, 1984.
32. Birnbaum HG, Kidder D. What does hospice cost? Am J Public Health 1984;74:689–97.
33. Mor V, Kidder D. Cost savings in hospice: final results of the National Hospice Study. Health Serv Res 1985;20:407–22.
34. Greer DS, Mor V, Morris JN, et al. An alternative in terminal care: results of the National Hospice Study. J Chronic Dis 1986;39:9–26.
35. Morris JN, Suissa S, Sherwood S, et al. Last days: a study of the quality of life of terminally ill cancer patients. J Chronic Dis 1986;39:47–62.
36. Raftery JP, Addington-Hall JM, MacDonald LD, et al. A randomized controlled trial of the cost-effectiveness of a district co-ordinating service for terminally ill cancer patients. Palliat Med 1996;10:151–61.
37. Davis FA. Medicare hospice benefit: early program experiences. Health Care Financing Rev 1988;9:99–111.
38. Kidder D. The effects of hospice coverage on Medicare expenditures. Health Serv Res 1992;27:195–217.
39. Wallston KA, Burger C, Smith RA, Baugher RJ. Comparing the quality of death for hospice and non-hospice cancer patients. Med Care 1988;26:177–82.
40. Hughes SL, Cummings J, Weaver F, et al. A randomized trial of the cost effectiveness of VA hospital-based home care for the terminally ill. Health Serv Res 1992;26:801–17.
41. Beresford L. Calif Hospice Rep 1993;11:1. editorial.
42. Government Accounting Office: Medicare program provisions and payments discourage hospice participation. Washington, D.C., 1989.
43. Amenta M. AIDS and the hospice community. Binghamton, N.Y.: Hayworth Press, 1992.
44. O'Neill JF, Alexander CS. Palliative medicine and HIV/AIDS. Prim Care 1997;24:607–15.
45. Jonsen A. The social impact of AIDS in the United States. Washington, D.C.: National Academy of Science Press, 1993.
46. Moinpour CM, Polissar L. Factors affecting place of death of hospice and non-hospice cancer patients. Am J Public Health 1989;79:1549–51.
47. Hyman RB, Bulkin W. Physician reported incentives and disincentives for referring patients to hospice. Hospice J 1990;6:39–64.
48. Schonwetter RS, Teasdale TA, Storey P, Luchi RJ. Estimation of survival time in terminal cancer patients: an impedance to hospice admissions? Hospice J 1990;6:65–79.
49. Weissman DE. Consultation in palliative medicine. Arch Intern Med 1997;157:733–7.
50. Rhymes J. Hospice care in America. JAMA 1990;264:369–72.

# PART

# V

# CANCER IN SPECIAL POPULATIONS

# CHAPTER 26

# CANCER IN SPECIAL POPULATIONS

• OTIS W. BRAWLEY • KEVIN B. KNOPF

Population studies of cancer demonstrate tremendous disparities in cancer incidence, mortality, and survival among populations. Narrowing and eliminating disparities among populations is a significant challenge in cancer prevention and control. The term *special populations* refers to groups that have disparate cancer incidence or mortality rates or have decreased access to adequate cancer screening and treatment. Some also refer to these populations as *vulnerable* or *at risk* populations.[1, 2] Special populations have been defined by race, ethnicity, nationality, and socioeconomic status.

Studying the variation in cancer rates among populations provides clues to the causes, risk factors, and forces that influence the development and progression of cancer. Some American populations have rates higher than the majority white population and some populations have rates lower than that of the majority white population. A mistake commonly made in interpretation of epidemiologic data is to confuse correlation with high incidence or high mortality in a population with causation.[3] A statistical correlation does not necessarily imply causation. Demographic data showing a higher cancer rate in a specific group versus another are merely a comparison. They can be used to form scientific hypotheses about causes of the differences but should not be considered as definitive evidence of cause.[4]

## Cancer Rates in Special Populations

Annually, the National Cancer Institute Surveillance Epidemiology and End Results Program and the National Center for Health Statistics publish cancer incidence and mortality rates for the United States.[5] Rates for selected cancers are shown in Tables 26–1 to 26–4. Race and ethnicity in the numerator are based on information abstracted from medical records or death certificates. The U.S. Bureau of the Census provides population counts used in the denominator of the calculated rates. Incidence and mortality rates for some racial or ethnic groups must be interpreted cautiously. These rates are less precise for Hispanics, Asian-Pacific Islanders, and Native Americans than are rates for larger populations such as blacks and whites because of smaller population size. Rates are averaged over 5 years to provide more reliable data.

Overall, cancer incidence and mortality rates are higher in men than in women. Among Americans, black men have the highest overall cancer rates and non-Hispanic white men have the second highest. The major causes of cancer death among American men are cancers of the lung, prostate, colon, and rectum. Cancers of the liver and stomach are leading causes of death among Asian-Pacific Islander, His-

panic, and Native American populations. Among women, racial and ethnic differences are not as extreme. Cancers of the lung, breast, colon, and rectum are major causes of cancer death in American women. Native American women have a significant risk of cancer of the gallbladder.

The varying rates of some cancers have been linked to biologic, environmental, and lifestyle factors, which can vary with race, ethnicity, socioeconomic, and other factors.

## BREAST CANCER

The known risk factors for breast cancer are early age at onset of menarche, late age at onset of menopause, first full-term pregnancy after age 30, and history of premenopausal breast cancer in a relative.[6, 7] In addition, obesity, nulliparity, and urban residence have been linked to increased risk of breast cancer.[8] Obesity has also been linked to increased stage at diagnosis.[9] Cultural differences among the races and ethnicities likely have a great influence on the differences in breast cancer risk. Early-onset menarche is more common among some populations and has been linked to dietary variance, which is of course influenced by culture and socioeconomics. Culture and socioeconomic status also influence childbirth patterns and risk of obesity.[10]

## PROSTATE CANCER

The recorded incidence of prostate cancer increased dramatically in the United States in the early 1990s because of the availability of the serum prostate-specific antigen screening test.[11] Black and white Americans have mortality rates far higher than do other American populations. The reasons are largely unknown. It may be due to a shared genetic influence or shared environmental influences (which include diet). Men with a family history of the disease are at higher risk.[12, 13] Certain genetic polymorphisms (minor changes in DNA sequences) that are thought to increase the risk of prostate cancer have been found to predominate in some racial or ethnic groups. Variation in polymorphic alleles of genes associated with modest fluctuations in risk could explain a large proportion of the difference in population risk for prostate cancer.[12]

There is also the suggestion that the Asian diet, which is high in soy content and low in animal fat, may prevent prostate cancer and that the American diet, which is high in animal fat, may encourage prostate carcinogenesis.[14] Asians migrating to the United States are at higher risk than those who remain in their native countries. Second- and third-generation Asian Americans who acculturate into the white

*Table 26–1.* **Selected Cancers, Females: Incidence Rates and Ratios, 1990–1995**

| | Breast | | Lung and Bronchus | | Colon | | Stomach | | Liver | | Cervix | |
|---|---|---|---|---|---|---|---|---|---|---|---|---|
| | RATE PER 100,000 | RATIO | RATE PER 100,000 | RATIO | RATE PER 100,000 | RATIO | RATE PER 100,000 | RATIO | RATE PER 100,000 | RATIO | RATE PER 100,000 | RATIO |
| White | 113.2 | 1.0 | 43.4 | 1.0 | 37.2 | 1.0 | 4.2 | 1.0 | 1.7 | 1.0 | 8.5 | 1.0 |
| White Hispanic | 73.2 | 0.6 | 20.7 | 0.5 | 25.6 | 0.7 | 8.1 | 1.9 | 3.2 | 1.9 | 17.0 | 2.0 |
| White non-Hispanic | 117.7 | 1.0 | 45.8 | 1.1 | 38.2 | 1.0 | 3.8 | 0.9 | 1.6 | 0.9 | 7.2 | 0.8 |
| Black | 99.0 | 0.9 | 46.4 | 1.1 | 45.5 | 1.2 | 7.6 | 1.8 | 2.6 | 1.5 | 12.1 | 1.4 |
| Native American | 31.9 | 0.3 | 14.1 | 0.3 | n/c | n/c | n/c | n/c | n/c | n/c | n/c | n/c |
| Asian-Pacific Islander | 71.4 | 0.6 | 22.4 | 0.5 | 31.2 | 0.8 | 11.1 | 2.6 | 6.1 | 3.6 | 10.2 | 1.2 |
| Hispanic | 69.3 | 0.6 | 19.8 | 0.5 | 24.3 | 0.7 | 7.7 | 1.8 | 3.0 | 1.8 | 16.0 | 1.9 |

Based on SEER data: Incidence and mortality rates, age-adjusted, rate per 100,000.
n/c, not calculated (too few cases to calculate).
From Ries LAG, Kosary CL, Hankey BF, et al. SEER cancer statistics review, 1973–1995. Bethesda, Md: National Cancer Institute, 1998.

*Table 26–2.* **Selected Cancers, Females: Mortality Rates and Ratios, 1990–1995**

| | Breast | | Lung and Bronchus | | Colon | | Stomach | | Liver | | Cervix | |
|---|---|---|---|---|---|---|---|---|---|---|---|---|
| | RATE PER 100,000 | RATIO | RATE PER 100,000 | RATIO | RATE PER 100,000 | RATIO | RATE PER 100,000 | RATIO | RATE PER 100,000 | RATIO | RATE PER 100,000 | RATIO |
| White | 26.0 | 1.0 | 33.6 | 1.0 | 14.6 | 1.0 | 2.6 | 1.0 | 1.9 | 1.0 | 2.5 | 1.0 |
| White Hispanic | 16.1 | 0.6 | 11.5 | 0.3 | 8.9 | 0.6 | 4.6 | 1.8 | 3.2 | 1.7 | 3.7 | 1.5 |
| White non-Hispanic | 26.6 | 1.0 | 34.9 | 1.0 | 14.9 | 1.0 | 2.5 | 1.0 | 1.9 | 1.0 | 2.4 | 1.0 |
| Black | 31.5 | 1.2 | 32.7 | 1.0 | 20.1 | 1.4 | 5.6 | 2.2 | 2.9 | 1.5 | 6.2 | 2.5 |
| Native American | 11.7 | 0.5 | 19.6 | 0.6 | 8.7 | 0.6 | 3.1 | 1.2 | 2.6 | 1.4 | 3.8 | 1.5 |
| Asian-Pacific Islander | 11.6 | 0.4 | 15.0 | 0.4 | 9.0 | 0.6 | 6.4 | 2.5 | 5.1 | 2.7 | 2.8 | 1.1 |
| Hispanic | 15.3 | 0.6 | 11.0 | 0.3 | 8.5 | 0.6 | 4.4 | 1.7 | 3.1 | 1.6 | 3.5 | 1.4 |

Based on SEER data: Incidence and mortality rates, age-adjusted, rate per 100,000.
From Ries LAG, Kosary CL, Hankey BF, et al. SEER cancer statistics review, 1973–1995. Bethesda, Md: National Cancer Institute, 1998.

Table 26–3. Selected Cancers, Males: Incidence Rates and Ratios, 1990–1995

| | Prostate | | Lung and Bronchus | | Colon | | Stomach | | Liver | | Oral Cavity and Pharynx | |
|---|---|---|---|---|---|---|---|---|---|---|---|---|
| | RATE PER 100,000 | RATIO | RATE PER 100,000 | RATIO | RATE PER 100,000 | RATIO | RATE PER 100,000 | RATIO | RATE PER 100,000 | RATIO | RATE PER 100,000 | RATIO |
| White | 150.3 | 1.0 | 74.3 | 1.0 | 53.8 | 1.0 | 9.8 | 1.0 | 4.6 | 1.0 | 15.0 | 1.0 |
| White Hispanic | 109.1 | 0.7 | 42.1 | 0.6 | 37.4 | 0.7 | 15.8 | 1.6 | 8.9 | 1.9 | 9.7 | 0.6 |
| White non-Hispanic | 153.8 | 1.0 | 77.6 | 1.0 | 55.2 | 1.0 | 9.2 | 0.9 | 4.1 | 0.9 | 15.7 | 1.0 |
| Black | 224.3 | 1.5 | 114.4 | 1.5 | 59.4 | 1.1 | 17.2 | 1.8 | 7.8 | 1.7 | 21.0 | 1.4 |
| Native American | 46.4 | 0.3 | 25.1 | 0.3 | 21.9 | 0.4 | n/c | n/c | n/c | n/c | n/c | n/c |
| Asian-Pacific Islander | 82.2 | 0.5 | 52.4 | 0.7 | 47.2 | 0.9 | 20.5 | 2.1 | 16.3 | 3.5 | 11.3 | 0.8 |
| Hispanic | 104.4 | 0.7 | 40.0 | 0.5 | 35.6 | 0.7 | 15.0 | 1.5 | 8.4 | 1.8 | 9.2 | 0.6 |

Based on SEER data: Incidence and mortality rates, age-adjusted, rate per 100,000.
n/c, not calculated (too few cases to calculate).
From Ries LAG, Kosary CL, Hankey BF, et al. SEER cancer statistics review, 1973–1995. Bethesda, Md: National Cancer Institute, 1998.

Table 26–4. Selected Cancers, Males: Mortality Rates and Ratios, 1990–1995

| | Prostate | | Lung and Bronchus | | Colon | | Stomach | | Liver | | Oral Cavity and Pharynx | |
|---|---|---|---|---|---|---|---|---|---|---|---|---|
| | RATE PER 100,000 | RATIO | RATE PER 100,000 | RATIO | RATE PER 100,000 | RATIO | RATE PER 100,000 | RATIO | RATE PER 100,000 | RATIO | RATE PER 100,000 | RATIO |
| White | 24.1 | 1.0 | 70.7 | 1.0 | 21.8 | 1.0 | 5.7 | 1.0 | 4.2 | 1.0 | 3.9 | 1.0 |
| White Hispanic | 17.4 | 0.7 | 33.9 | 0.5 | 13.9 | 0.6 | 8.6 | 1.5 | 7.2 | 1.7 | 3.2 | 0.8 |
| White non-Hispanic | 24.4 | 1.0 | 72.5 | 1.0 | 22.2 | 1.0 | 5.6 | 1.0 | 4.0 | 1.0 | 3.9 | 1.0 |
| Black | 55.0 | 2.3 | 102.0 | 1.4 | 28.0 | 1.3 | 12.7 | 2.2 | 7.0 | 1.7 | 8.8 | 2.3 |
| Native American | 14.2 | 0.6 | 40.0 | 0.6 | 10.5 | 0.5 | 6.1 | 1.1 | 5.1 | 1.2 | 3.7 | 0.9 |
| Asian-Pacific Islander | 10.9 | 0.5 | 35.1 | 0.5 | 13.6 | 0.6 | 11.2 | 2.0 | 13.4 | 3.2 | 3.0 | 0.8 |
| Hispanic | 16.8 | 0.7 | 32.4 | 0.5 | 13.2 | 0.6 | 8.2 | 1.4 | 6.8 | 1.6 | 3.0 | 0.8 |

Based on SEER data: Incidence and mortality rates, age-adjusted, rate per 100,000.
n/c, not calculated (too few cases to calculate).
From Ries LAG, Kosary CL, Hankey BF, et al. SEER cancer statistics review, 1973–1995. Bethesda, Md: National Cancer Institute, 1998.

American culture have rates of prostate cancer approaching white Americans.

## LUNG CANCER

Lung cancer is the second most common nonskin cancer and the leading cause of cancer death among Americans. Incidence and mortality rates vary by race and ethnicity, primarily because there are cultural differences in smoking.[15, 16] Compared with white Americans, black Americans smoke more menthol cigarettes. The anesthetic quality of menthol cigarettes allows deeper and longer inhalation. Poorer populations have also been shown to smoke cigarettes more completely. Certain polymorphisms in genes coding for enzymes such as those of the cytochrome P450 system have been associated with an increased risk of lung cancer. These genetic polymorphisms do vary among populations, but their effect on cancer rates is unknown.[17–20]

## COLORECTAL CANCER

Colorectal cancer is the second most common cause of cancer death among Americans as a whole. Studies of migrants from areas of low risk to areas of high risk have shown that risk is modifiable.[21] Rates of Japanese and Chinese immigrants to the United States are higher than those of Japanese and Chinese individuals who remain in their native countries. Colorectal cancer appears to increase with certain dietary changes. Second- and third-generation Asian Americans who acculturate to the mainstream American culture have rates of colorectal cancer that approach those of white Americans.[21, 22]

## HEPATIC CANCER

Hepatoma or primary cancer of the liver accounts for only 1.5% of all cancers in the United States. It is the second leading cause of cancer death among Chinese American men. Nearly 70% of hepatocellular cancers are associated with hepatitis B or hepatitis C (so-called viral hepatitis).[23] Viral hepatitis is endemic in certain areas of Asia. In Africa and Asia, certain types of mold and aflatoxins in stored food are an added risk factor.[24]

## GASTRIC CANCER

Gastric cancer is one of the five leading causes of cancer death among many Asian and Hispanic American populations.[25] Rates have apparently dropped because of the declining use of salted, smoked, and pickled meats and the increased use of refrigeration. These are all influences that are mediated by culture and socioeconomic status. *Helicobacter pylori* infection of the stomach has been linked to gastric ulcer and gastric cancer.

## CERVICAL CANCER

Cervical cancer was once the leading cause of cancer death in American women. Screening has had a significant impact on the early detection and reduction in mortality of this disease. The primary cause of cervical cancer is the human papillomavirus (HPV).[26] Exposure to HPV is in some ways influenced by socioeconomic status because HPV is sexually transmitted.[27] Some populations may have higher rates of cervical dysplasia and cervical cancer because they are infected with more aggressive strains of HPV.[28–30] Cervical cancer rates are currently very high among Vietnamese American women. This is likely because of a lack of screening over a prolonged period. Cervical cancer rates are also higher in black and Hispanic Americans. There are significant barriers to screening, early detection, and adequate treatment of cervical cancer in many special populations.[27]

## CANCERS OF THE HEAD AND NECK

Head and neck cancers include those of the nasopharynx, mouth, and larynx. These cancers affect men disproportionately. Cancer of the nasopharynx occurs with high frequency in Asians. Americans who have immigrated from China, Vietnam, Laos, Cambodia, and the Philippine Islands have higher rates of nasopharyngeal cancer when compared with white Americans. The cause is thought to be related to consumption of fermented foods and salted fish. Exposure to the Epstein-Barr virus and certain dust and smoke particles may also increase risk.[31, 32] Squamous cell carcinomas of the mouth and throat are also heavily linked to smoking and drinking, which may vary by socioeconomic and class status.

# Population Categories

Populations are frequently described by race, ethnicity, or socioeconomic status. These terms are not well understood and are frequently misused. For example, race is often used as a surrogate for socioeconomic status, and this can occasionally lead to the inappropriate inference that race is a cancer risk factor. The categories in Tables 26–1 through 26–4 are racial and ethnic categories as defined by the U.S. Office of Management and Budget (OMB) Directive 15.[33] The U.S. National Cancer Institute has published beyond the OMB classifications, often using nationality of origin, especially among America's diverse Asian population.[5, 34, 35] This effort is limited because the National Cancer Institute has published data dependent on data collected from other federal agencies that use only the OMB definitions.

## RACE

Race, as used in the OMB categorization, has no scientific or biologic basis.[36] The directive has been updated several times, the last time being in 1998. The categories are not based on taxonomic efforts of physicians, anthropologists, or biologists. The categories are social constructs reflecting the history and current status of race relations in the United States. It is a classification scheme that is of value for social science research; however, inferences about the causes of cancer and racial genetics require extreme caution. Although race should not be used as a scientific category, it may be viewed as a surrogate to identify social and cultural subgroups whose environmental exposures may be similar.

Racial categorization originated in the 18th century.[36] The traditional racial categories are Asian or mongoloid, negroid or African, and Caucasian. Biologically distinct races do not exist and likely never did. Racial groups are overlapping statistical groups based on combinations of visible anatomic traits. These traits are superficial and are not transmitted by genetic clusters. The genetic basis of race is the subject of political controversy; indeed, science has found no genetic basis for race and racial classification. Over the past 400 years, there has been much miscegenation between European and black African populations in the United States. Indeed, by some estimates, more than three quarters of Americans who identify themselves as black or African American have a blood relative who identifies himself or herself as white or Caucasian.[37] The "one-drop" rule in which a person with just one African ancestor is considered black is still practiced in the United States. This is the ultimate example of how unscientific racial classification is.

## ETHNICITY

The OMB directive recognizes Hispanic as an ethnicity. These are individuals from the Spanish-speaking cultures of North, South, and Central America. In the newest OMB directive, Hispanics can also classify themselves as black, white, or Native American. The anthropologic and medical sociologic literature use a different definition of ethnicity. In this definition, many ethnicities exist, and ethnicity involves how one sees oneself and how one is "seen by others as part of a group on the basis of presumed ancestry and sharing a common destiny with others on the basis of this background."[38] Common threads that may tie one to an ethnic group include skin color, religion, language, customs, ancestry, and occupational or regional features. In addition, persons belonging to the same ethnic group share a unique history different from that of other ethnic groups.[35, 38–40]

The "boundaries" of ethnic identity are unclear. Ethnic identities are circumstantial.[38] Some may identify themselves as belonging to a particular group in one context and to another group in a different context. Ethnicity is flexible, fluid, and perceived. It is not rigid or fixed. This has been made more complex by the increased number of mixedethnicity families in the United States, where individuals may claim two or more ethnicities or give different ethnic identifications at different times or for different purposes.

It is useful in medical and epidemiologic research to distinguish ethnic groups from one another provided that researchers are clear on the nature and source of human variation (e.g., cultural, behavioral patterns, lifestyle, and other environmental influences) and their relationship to health. Membership in an ethnic group may be associated with behavioral, environmental, and other extrinsic factors that may increase or decrease the likelihood of an illness. Thus, the availability of pertinent information for a diversity of ethnic groups would assist both those involved in health research and the population as a whole by indicating if any ethnic differences need to be explored further. Such research, however, can be accomplished only by clearly identifying population groups and understanding that human identity is not static or mutually exclusive.

## SOCIOECONOMIC STATUS

Health status is highly correlated to those with higher socioeconomic status enjoying greater health. Indeed, many problems have been linked to low socioeconomic status, such as crime, poor education, ill health and poor health habits, and inadequate access to health care.[41, 42] A substantial body of literature suggests that cancer incidence and mortality are higher among persons in the lower socioeconomic strata.[43, 44] Socioeconomic indicators include education, income, and occupation.[45] There is controversy over which indexes have appropriately or inappropriately assessed socioeconomic status to characterize social determinants of health. The European literature uses the term *deprivation,* taking into account numerous markers of wealth and education. Variables of increased deprivation have been correlated with increased cancer mortality.[15, 46, 47] Health care disparities among socioeconomic strata have been found to persist in an equalaccess health care system.[48]

# Cancer Etiology

The causes of cancer are genetic (intrinsic) or environmental (extrinsic), or both.[49] Most cancer causes involve some geneenvironment interaction. The relationships among race, ethnicity, socioeconomic status, and environment often are not appreciated. Some have made the mistake of attributing the health disparities among groups to intrinsic racial or ethnic differences. Race, ethnicity, and socioeconomics can be correlated with unnamed and at times unidentified environmental influences that cause cancer, cause a delay in diagnosis of cancer, or cause less than optimal treatment of cancer. Access to and convenience of care play a large role in this arena. In the United States, 17% of the population is without any health insurance, and a disproportionate number of these individuals are members of special populations.

## GENETICS AND CANCER

Although biologic and especially phenotypic differences clearly exist among the racial groups as commonly defined in the United States, these differences usually track poorly with skin color. The prevalence of a specific gene can be higher in a specific population, but that population is unlikely to monopolize that gene.[50] Most genetic differences that have been correlated or associated with race should be considered familial and not racial. A specific gene or series of genes can be conserved among families. A closed society will conserve genetic traits within that society. Segregation on basis of race, ethnicity, economics, or other factors can lead to increased prevalence of a specific gene or series of genes in the segregated population. This has been demonstrated in other diseases with a well-defined genetic basis, such as Tay-Sachs disease, cystic fibrosis, and sickle cell disease.[50] Each of these diseases has a higher prevalence in, but is not exclusive to, a specific racial or ethnic group. As America becomes more interracial, these genetic differences will lessen.

There is no reason to believe that there is a natural selection for cancer in any racial or ethnic group. The genetic mutations associated with cancer have been found in persons of all races and ethnicities in which they have been sought.[51–53] Mutations of the BRCA-1 and BRCA-2 genes have been isolated in families in which women are at high risk for the development of breast and ovarian cancer. Although mutations of BRCA-1 and BRCA-2 have been found in women of all races, three specific mutations are common, but not exclusive, to individuals who identify themselves as Ashkenazi Jews.[51, 54, 55] These mutations are likely common among Jewish families because of ethnic segregation among families.

Just as there are genetic differences that predispose to cancer, there are genetic differences in how some individuals metabolize drugs (pharmacogenetics).[56] For example, the action of *N*-acetyltransferase, which is involved in the metabolism of many drugs, varies by racial and ethnic groups. Approximately 50% of American whites and American blacks have "slow"-acetylating enzymes, whereas 90% of Asians have fast-acetylating enzymes.[57]

The same pathways through which drugs are metabolized are often involved in the detoxification of environmental toxins and carcinogens, and thus variations in detoxification enzymes may lead to variations in cancer risk. Detoxifying enzymes, such as those of the cytochrome P450 system and the glutathiones, have polymorphisms.[58, 59] Some polymorphisms are more efficient enzymes than others. The prevalence of certain phenotypes is higher in certain groups or populations than in others.

One cytochrome P450 enzyme, CYP1A1, has had four major polymorphisms identified to date, with frequencies that vary among racial and ethnic groups.[19] Certain polymorphisms of CYP1A1 may confer increased susceptibility to lung cancer.[60, 61] The varying frequency may explain some racial and ethnic differences in cancer rates among populations.[62] The hydroxylation of the drug debrisoquine by another P450 CYP2D6 enzyme varies several hundred–fold.[63] "Extensive" metabolizers of the antihypertensive agent debrisoquine have a greater risk for lung cancer than do "poor" or "intermediate" metabolizers. Extensive metabolizers apparently hydroxylate large amounts of the tobacco-specific *N*-nitrosamine, forming a more carcinogenic compound. There are also population differences in polymorphisms of alcohol dehydrogenase, glucose-6-phospodiesterase, and a number of other enzymes.[64, 65]

Although a specific gene or series of genes can be conserved within a relatively closed population such as an extended family, genetic variation within a race is significant.[36, 66] Indeed, genetic variation within a race is greater than among races. Genetic variation in a population can be assessed by estimating the level of DNA heterozygosity or polymorphism. These variations include differences in blood group antigens and DNA sequence variations in enzymes and nuclear restriction fragment-linked polymorphisms. Also, variation can be found in the sequences of mitochondrial DNA, which is transmitted maternally and in base pair sequences (microsatellites) that occur all across the genome.

## ENVIRONMENT AND CANCER

There are certain biologic factors that track with certain racial or ethnic groups and may predispose to the development of cancer. Some of these differences are familial or inherited; others are heavily influenced by nutritional, social, cultural, behavioral, and other environmental factors.[67] Important knowledge about the environmental influences on the etiology of cancers has been gained through studies of similar populations in different environments.

Culture and ethnicity may influence cancer risk through dietary habits. Several studies have shown that migration from areas of low risk to areas of high risk increases the risk of the disease.[68–70] This presumably occurs through the adoption of habits in the area of high incidence or loss of protective factors found in the area of low risk. Prentice and Sheppard [71] found that the incidence of breast cancer in 21 countries showed a 5.5-fold increase in countries with the highest fat intake (45% of daily caloric intake) compared with those with the lowest fat intake (15% of daily caloric intake). Margetts and colleagues correlated dietary fat intake with risk of cancer of the prostate and breast.[72] When Italian immigrants to Australia were studied, it was found that the age-adjusted breast cancer mortality rate doubled over a nearly 20-year period in those who adopted the regional high-fat diet, nearly equaling the Australian rates. The dietary pattern followed in certain parts of the Mediterranean is thought to reduce the risk of cancer.[40] In addition, there is a growing body of evidence that moderate consumption of wine may lead to a decreased risk of cancer.

In migration studies performed before the prostate-specific antigen screening era, Japanese migrants to the United States were shown to have a marked increase in prostate cancer compared with men in their native lands,[73] although the rates of prostate cancer in Japanese Americans are still less than those of whites.[34] Prostate cancer incidence rates are very low in eastern Europe and Russia. Polish immigrants to the United States acquire significantly higher rates on migration. Men of African heritage in Brazil, Jamaica, and the United States have a higher prostate cancer incidence; this suggests that there may be a genetic component to prostate cancer.[74–76]

The use of alcohol and tobacco products has been linked to a number of cancers. Patterns in alcohol and tobacco use vary by economic status, social situation, and culture. The prevalence and manner of smoking vary considerably by race and ethnicity.[19, 77–79] They are also correlated with social condition and socioeconomic status. These cultural differences can manifest as biologic differences in addiction and possibly even different lung cancer rates.

Some cancer differences among populations are associated with environmental factors unique to a particular geographic region. Indeed, some cancers that were once speculated to be due to a genetic predisposition of the population were later found to be due to environmental exposure. For example, inhabitants of Linxian, a county in the Henan province of north central China, have one of the highest rates of esophageal squamous cell carcinoma in the world. Most squamous cell cancer in low-risk groups is due to alcohol and tobacco consumption. This was ruled out as the cause of esophageal cancer in Linxian, and genetic susceptibility was suspected. The causative agent in this high-risk population is now thought to be high-level exposure to polycyclic aromatic hydrocarbons in the food chain of the region.[80] Similarly, the African form of Burkitt's lymphoma was once thought to be due to a genetic predisposition among Africans, but it has been related to infection with the Epstein-Barr virus and has increased in prevalence in areas where malaria is endemic.[81]

Melanoma is a disease that is caused by an environmental stimulus (sun exposure). It affects individuals with light complexions disproportionately. Persons of African and Asian heritage are known to get melanoma but have a much lower risk than whites. It is perhaps the only cancer in which race is a definite risk factor, but even melanoma risk is mediated by skin pigmentation and not race or ethnicity. For melanoma, particularly, a higher incidence and mortality have been found in persons of high socioeconomic status.[16, 47, 82, 83] This is postulated to be due to a greater amount of leisure time, which could correlate with sun exposure, a known risk factor for melanoma.[84]

## Special Populations and Cancer Outcomes

It is well appreciated that black Americans have poorer cancer outcomes when compared with whites.[85] Unfortunately, there are few data on Hispanics, Asians, and Native Americans to determine whether their outcomes are better or worse than those of whites. Race has become intimately entwined in medical perceptions about the biologic behavior of tumors. Racial disparities in breast cancer are better studied than those in any other cancer. Correlations among race, socioeconomic status, and outcomes in breast cancer are discussed here, but lessons in breast cancer are likely applicable to other diseases.

When compared with white Americans, black Americans have a lower incidence of breast cancer but greater mortality from it. It is accepted that, as a group, a larger proportion of black women present with higher stage tumors and with more aggressive pathologic conditions when compared with whites.[86, 87] These are poor prognostic factors, suggesting differences in biology. Many use these facts to argue that there are racial differences in the biology of breast cancer. Some assume there are differences in the genetics predisposing to the tumors that black women develop versus the tumors that white women get. Indeed, when the genetics of black and white women with breast cancer were carefully studied, HER-2/*neu* overexpression was similar in blacks and whites, as were aberrations in p53 status.[88–90]

The assumption of inherent racial differences in genetics fails to take into account a great deal of evidence that there are numerous extrinsic influences causing differences in breast cancer. Black women had a lower mortality rate from

breast cancer when compared with white women prior to 1981. The disparity in mortality has increased every year since. Race is far less important when stage and socioeconomic factors are considered.[91, 92] Socioeconomic status likely even has some effect on grade of tumor at diagnosis. A case-control study that adjusted for age and stage at diagnosis[93] found black-white differences but also found that the pathologic features of tumors in white women of high socioeconomic status were more favorable than those in white women of lower socioeconomic status. This is highly suggestive of an extrinsic influence associated with socioeconomic status that is responsible for the increasing disparity.

The increased proportions of blacks presenting with advanced disease may in part be explained by delays in reporting symptoms. In a case-control study comparing black and white women with breast cancer, Coates and colleagues[94] demonstrated that the median time from recognition of symptoms to medical consultation was longer for black women than for white women. The authors were unable to relate the delay in seeking treatment directly to increased mortality, but it is a likely contributor. Other studies suggest that delay in reporting symptoms was a significant factor in stage of disease at diagnosis and survival.[95, 96]

Data suggest that both black and white cancer patients living in census tracts with lower median education and incomes are diagnosed in later disease stages than are patients in census tracts with higher median education and incomes.[97] Blacks as a group are disproportionately poorer. Despite the consistent and strong association of social class with health status, the extent to which racial and ethnic disparities in cancer screening reflect social class is rarely addressed.[98] Poverty is associated with lower mammographic screening rates and less access to adequate medical care. This can result in delays in presentation even after symptoms are noticed.

Considerable effort has been put into encouraging women to obtain breast cancer screening. A substantial scientific literature has been developed concerning methods to increase minority participation in screening programs in special populations.[99] Much of the work focuses on tailoring messages so that they are culturally acceptable and educating the health educator and health care giver to be culturally sensitive.[100] Trends in breast cancer screening rates showed an increase in use during the final years of the 1990s for women from most racial ethnic groups. Data from the National Health Interview[35, 40] indicate that in 1992, 48% of black women, 51.6% of white women, and 47% of Hispanic women older than age 50 reported having had a mammogram in the previous 2 years. By 1994, 56% of black women, 56% of white women, and 50% of Hispanic women older than age 50 reported having had a clinical breast examination and a mammogram.[100]

Dietary history and nutritional status are significant extrinsic influences on breast cancer etiology. In a study of blacks and whites in Connecticut, Jones and colleagues[9] found evidence that the higher prevalence of severe obesity among black women may also help explain their relative disadvantage of being diagnosed at a later stage of breast cancer. It has been suggested that racial differences in survival may be partly explained by differences in nutritional status.[101] Black women are disproportionately overweight when compared with whites, and obesity in black women has been linked to poverty and other social issues. The National Cancer Institute black-white Cancer Study[102] assessed a cohort of 1960 women diagnosed with breast cancer from 1975 to 1979. After adjusting the data for stage of disease, socioeconomic status, and other prognostic factors, McWhorter and Mayer determined that black women had poorer survival rates than whites. Within each stage, lower levels of serum albumin and hemoglobin and higher relative body weight were more common among blacks and were independently associated with poorer survival. Adjustment for these variables substantially reduced the excess mortality rate among blacks.

Numerous case series have reported black-white differences in outcome. Many of these studies have not normalized for treatment disparities.[103] In a retrospective review of Department of Defense (DOD) medical beneficiaries with breast cancer, black women were found to have a decrease in survival when compared with whites. The 5-year mortality rate for black women was 24.8% compared with 18.1% for white women.[104] In the United States Surveillance Epidemiology and End Results (SEER) registry, the 5-year mortality rate was 34.2% for black women and 18.4% for white women. These observations suggest that ready access to medical facilities and the full complement of treatment options that are standard for all DOD patients improves survival rates for black women. However, a significant unexplained difference in survival still exists between black and white military beneficiaries. The improved prognosis among women treated in the military system, while not an equalization of risk, is still clear, solid evidence of the positive impact of equal access to health care. The authors did not adjust for differences in body mass index or treatment received. These types of adjustments, as well as an assessment of cultural differences, might have equalized risk.

Analysis of racial subsets in clinical trials is difficult and should be carried out cautiously.[105] When assessing outcomes in breast cancer clinical trials, equal treatment yields equal outcomes regardless of race.[106, 107] After adjustment for other prognostic factors, race appears to have no independent prognostic significance in survival. These results suggest that early detection and appropriate therapy among black patients could result in a reduction in the current disparity in breast carcinoma mortality between blacks and whites.

In an analysis of two clinical trials, conducted by the National Surgical Adjuvant Breast and Bowel Project in women with lymph node–negative breast carcinoma, Dignam and colleagues[106] found comparable responses for black women and their white peers. Among patients with estrogen receptor–negative tumors, the overall 5-year survival rate for blacks was 83%, compared with 85% for white Americans. The black patients also had a 5-year, disease-free survival rate of 71%, compared with 74% for whites. In patients with estrogen receptor–positive tumors, the overall 5-year survival rate was 93% for blacks and 92% for whites. The 5-year, disease-free survival rate was 81% for blacks and 80% for whites. Therefore, black and white patients with localized breast carcinoma benefit equally from systemic therapy.

Roach and colleagues[107] assessed black-white outcomes in a Cancer and Leukemia Group B study of 1572 patients, (12% black, 84% white) to determine the effect of high-dose, standard-dose, and low-dose CAF (cyclophosphamide,

doxorubicin, fluorouracil) in women with node-positive breast cancer. The trial demonstrated that adjuvant chemotherapy, when given appropriately, has a positive impact on mortality. After adjustment for other well-known prognostic factors, race had no independent prognostic significance for survival in this study.

Several case series and case-control trials have demonstrated that equal treatment yields equal outcome among breast cancer patients. Gordon[108] examined the outcome in 1392 patients (253 blacks, 1132 whites, and 7 individuals of other races) treated in multi-institutional prospective trials from 1974 to 1985. A multivariate analysis, using Cox proportional hazards model, indicated that socioeconomic status was a significant indicator of disease-free survival and overall survival, but race was not.

Franzini and colleageus[43] looked at 163 black, 205 Hispanic, and 964 white American women with breast cancer treated at M.D. Anderson Cancer Center from 1987 to 1991. The patient outcomes in this case-control study were adjusted for age, stage, histologic characteristics, and type of treatment. The results of a univariate and multivariate analysis again showed that race was not a significant predictor of survival after adjusting for socioeconomic status and disease characteristics. Socioeconomic status was a significant predictor after all adjustments were made.

Nomura and colleagues[109] conducted a case-control study of 182 Japanese and 161 white breast cancer patients diagnosed and treated in Hawaii during 1975 to 1980. Obesity was linked to increased mortality. By the end of 1987, obese Japanese women had a relative risk of death of 3.5 (95% confidence interval [CI], 1.3 to 10.0) compared with nonobese subjects. Among whites, those with a high-fat diet were found to have a relative risk of death of 3.2 (95% CI, 1.2 to 8.6). When Japanese and white patients were compared with each other, there was no significant difference in survival.

Heimann and colleagues[110] compared the outcome of 1037 white and 481 black breast cancer patients treated at the University of Chicago from 1946 to 1987. The 20-year, disease-free survival rate did not differ by race among women with the same stage of cancer. Race was not an independent factor influencing outcome.

Perkins and colleagues[91] conducted an investigation into the survival rates of black and white breast cancer patients treated at M.D. Anderson from 1958 to 1987. In univariate analysis, survival was quite different among the races. After controlling for socioeconomic status, stage, and treatment, the relative risk (RR) of death at 5 years was not statistically significantly different (RR = 1.12; 95% CI, 1.0 to 1.25). Socioeconomic status, stage, and type of treatment were significant factors influencing outcome. Race was not a significant factor.

Although case series and data from clinical trials overwhelmingly support the concept that equal treatment yields equal outcomes regardless of race, patterns of cancer care studies show that care received often differs among populations categorized by race or ethnicity. For example, it has been demonstrated that black women with breast cancer are less likely to receive aggressive or stage-appropriate therapy when compared with whites.[111] In a study of SEER data using more than 36,900 breast cancer cases, blacks were found to be treated nonsurgically more often than were whites, (odds ratio, 1.4; 95% CI, 1.2 to 1.7) or were found to have no cancer-directed therapy (odds ratio, 1.7; 95% CI, 1.3 to 2.3). Even after adjusting by logistic regression for differences in age, stage, and histologic features, these variables still strongly influenced 5-year survival. More recent assessment of SEER data shows that the trend in disparate treatment continues. Blacks with breast cancer are less likely to receive radiation therapy after lumpectomy or adjuvant chemotherapy.[111, 112] The reasons for this and other disparities in breast cancer care are an active area of research. Some studies have suggested that cultural differences in the acceptance of having a disease and in acceptance of treatment are important.[96] In other cases, treatment differences may be due to disparities in co-morbid diseases, making aggressive therapy inappropriate. Blacks, Hispanics, and other special populations do have a disproportionate amount of hypertension and cardiovascular and other co-morbid diseases.[113] Socioeconomic barriers, such as lack of insurance and lack of access to treatment as well as racial and socioeconomic discrimination, are also likely factors in such disparities.[42, 114]

Although the preceding discussion focused on breast cancer, there are studies showing that equal treatment yields equal outcome in prostate,[115] colon,[116] and lung cancer.[117, 118] Race should not be a factor in medical care. There are also studies that show clearly defined differences by race in patterns of care for cancers of the colon,[119, 120] prostate,[121–123] lung,[124] endometrium,[125] and cervix.[126] Blacks disproportionately receive less aggressive cancer care or less appropriate therapies when compared with whites. The full effect of these disparities in treatment on mortality is unknown. It should be noted that these disparities have been shown to exist in the treatment of other diseases such as cardiac disease,[127] and few studies of cancer treatment practice patterns have been performed in populations other than black and white.

Evidence shows that many of these disparities are often due to socioeconomic barriers that are prevalent among many populations, including a substantial portion of white Americans.[114] Socioeconomic barriers to care go beyond just affording care and include difficulty accessing care. Obtaining transportation to physician visits can be a significant barrier to optimal therapy. Other barriers to optimal care cannot be as easily generalized. Some patients refuse therapy because of fear of disease or fear of the medical system. In some cultures, fatalism (the feeling of having no control) is a significant influence on behavior.[96] Fear of the medical system is common in a number of populations because of bad personal experiences in accessing medical care or knowledge of some terrible tragedies in which medical personnel have taken advantage of vulnerable individuals.[128] Unfortunately, some treatment disparities are likely due to some forms of discrimination, both conscious and subconscious.[129, 130]

## Conclusion

There is no question that the risk of many cancers varies substantially by categories such as race, ethnic group, and socioeconomic status. Important clues to cancer etiology may come from investigating the differences in risk across subgroups of the population, but this requires tremendous caution. Race has been legitimized by its use in medical literature and practice, but it is a label that is unnecessary for proper diagnosis and treatment of disease in humans. Assumptions about disease that are made because a race has been assigned can result in negative consequences for individual patients and inaccurate genetic inferences for populations. The effect of ethnicity, which includes culture, diet, language, religion, and other social factors, can have significant impact on cancer etiology and treatment. The effect of socioeconomic status on cancer is also significant.

Much can be learned through the study of cancer rates of various populations. This knowledge benefits all who are at risk for the disease. Racial and ethnic groups as used in data published by the U.S. government are defined by sociopolitical, not scientific, criteria. Cancer incidence and mortality rates are influenced by numerous extrinsic factors. Extrinsic or environmental factors include diet, socioeconomic status, and cultural factors that often correlate with race and ethnicity. The prevalence of a gene or genetic mutation is often higher in a particular population when compared with another. Although a specific gene or series of genes can be conserved within a relatively closed population, genetic variation within a given population or race is significant.[36] Although there has been interest in how the pharmacology of drugs differs among populations, the most pressing issue in the control of cancer in special populations is making quality care available to all. Evidence shows that in numerous cancers equal treatment yields equal outcome regardless of race. There is also evidence that a significant proportion of the population does not receive optimal cancer therapies.

## SUGGESTIONS FOR ADDITIONAL READING

Krieger N, Quesenberry C Jr, Peng T, et al. Social class, race/ethnicity, and incidence of breast, cervix, colon, lung, and prostate cancer among Asian, black, Hispanic, and white residents of the San Francisco Bay Area, 1988–92 (United States). Cancer Causes Control 1999;10:525–37. *This study demonstrates the importance of considering socioeconomic factors in assessing the epidemiology of cancer in special populations.*

Yood MU, Johnson CC, Blount A, et al. Race and differences in breast cancer survival in a managed care population. J Natl Cancer Inst 1999;91:1487–91.

Freeman HP. The meaning of race in science—considerations for cancer research: concerns of special populations in the National Cancer Program. Cancer 1998;82:219–25.

## REFERENCES

1. Aday LA. At risk in America: the health and health care needs of vulnerable populations in the United States. New York: Jossey-Bass, 1993.
2. Guidry JJ, Aday LA, Zhang D, Winn RJ. Cost considerations as potential barriers to cancer treatment. Cancer Pract 1998;6:182–7.
3. Rimer BK. Correlation is not causation. Am J Public Health 1998;88:832–3.
4. Kaufman JS, Cooper RS, McGee DL. Socioeconomic status and health in blacks and whites: the problem of residual confounding and the resiliency of race. see comments. Epidemiology 1997;8:621–8.
5. Ries LAG, Kosary CL, Hankey BF, et al. SEER Cancer Statistics Review, 1973–1995. Bethesda, Md: National Cancer Institute, 1998.
6. Gail MH, Brinton LA, Byar DP, et al. Projecting individualized probabilities of developing breast cancer for white females who are being examined annually. J Natl Cancer Inst 1989;81:1879–86.

7. Benichou J, Gail MH, Mulvihill JJ. Graphs to estimate an individualized risk of breast cancer. J Clin Oncol 1996;14:103–10.

8. Ziegler RG, Hoover RN, Nomura AM, et al. Relative weight, weight change, height, and breast cancer risk in Asian-American women. J Natl Cancer Inst 1996;88:650–60.

9. Jones BA, Kasi SV, Curnen MG, et al. Severe obesity as an explanatory factor for the black/white difference in stage at diagnosis of breast cancer. Am J Epidemiol 1997;146:394–404.

10. Gordon NH, Crowe JP, Brumberg DJ, Berger NA. Socioeconomic factors and race in breast cancer recurrence and survival. Am J Epidemiol 1992;135:609–18.

11. Potosky AL, Kessler L, Gridley G, et al. Rise in prostatic cancer incidence associated with increased use of transurethral resection. see comments. J Natl Cancer Inst 1990;82:1624–8.

12. Shibata A, Whittemore AS. Genetic predisposition to prostate cancer: possible explanations for ethnic differences in risk. Prostate 1997;32:65–72.

13. Whittemore AS, Wu AH, Kolonel LN, et al. Family history and prostate cancer risk in black, white, and Asian men in the United States and Canada. Am J Epidemiol 1995;141:732–40.

14. Kolonel LN, Nomura AM, Cooney RV. Dietary fat and prostate cancer: current status. J Natl Cancer Inst 1999;91:414–28.

15. Law MR, Morris JK. Why is mortality higher in poorer areas and in more northern areas of England and Wales? J Epidemiol Community Health 1998;52:344–52.

16. Pearce N, Bethwaite P. Social class and male cancer mortality in New Zealand, 1984–7. NZ Med J 1997;110:200–2.

17. Ishibe N, Wiencke JK, Zuo ZF, et al. Susceptibility to lung cancer in light smokers associated with CYP1A1 polymorphisms in Mexican- and African-Americans. Cancer Epidemiol Biomarkers Prev 1997;6:1075–80.

18. London SJ, Daly AK, Leathart JB, et al. Genetic polymorphism of CYP2D6 and lung cancer risk in African-Americans and Caucasians in Los Angeles County. see comments. Carcinogenesis 1997;18:1203–14.

19. Garte S. The role of ethnicity in cancer susceptibility gene polymorphisms: the example of CYP1A1. Carcinogenesis 1998;19:1329–32.

20. Taioli E, Ford J, Trachman J, et al. Lung cancer risk and CYP1A1 genotype in African Americans. Carcinogenesis 1998;19:813–7.

21. Le Marchand L, Wilkens LR, Kolonel LN, et al. Associations of sedentary lifestyle, obesity, smoking, alcohol use, and diabetes with the risk of colorectal cancer. Cancer Res 1997;57:4787–94.

22. Shimizu H, Mack TM, Ross RK, Henderson BE. Cancer of the gastrointestinal tract among Japanese and white immigrants in Los Angeles County. J Natl Cancer Inst 1987;78:223–8.

23. El-Serag HB, Mason AC. Rising incidence of hepatocellular carcinoma in the United States. N Engl J Med 1999;340:745–50.

24. Evans AA, O'Connell AP, Pugh JC, et al. Geographic variation in viral load among hepatitis B carriers with differing risks of hepatocellular carcinoma. Cancer Epidemiol Biomarkers Prev 1998;7:559–65.

25. El-Serag HB, Sonnenberg A. Ethnic variations in the occurrence of gastroesophageal cancers. J Clin Gastroenterol 1999;28:135–9.

26. Kjellberg L, Wang Z, Wiklund F, et al. Sexual behaviour and papillomavirus exposure in cervical intraepithelial neoplasia: a population-based case-control study. J Gen Virol 1999;80:391–8.

27. Liu L, Deapen D, Bernstein L. Socioeconomic status and cancers of the female breast and reproductive organs: a comparison across racial/ethnic populations in Los Angeles County, California (United States). Cancer Causes Control 1998;9:369–80.

28. Nindl I, Rindfleisch K, Teller K, et al. Cervical cancer, HPV 16 E6, variant genotypes, and serology. letter. Lancet 1999;353:152.

29. Hildesheim A. Human papillomavirus variants: implications for natural history studies and vaccine development efforts. editorial; comment. J Natl Cancer Inst 1997;89:752–3.

30. Burger RA, Monk BJ, Kurosaki T, et al. Human papillomavirus type 18: association with poor prognosis in early stage cervical cancer. see comments. J Natl Cancer Inst 1996;88:1361–8.

31. Sung NS, Edwards RH, Seillier-Moiseiwitsch F, et al. Epstein-Barr virus strain variation in nasopharyngeal carcinoma from the endemic and non-endemic regions of China. Int J Cancer 1998;76:207–15.

32. Atula S, Auvinen E, Grenman R, Syrjanen S. Human papillomavirus and Epstein-Barr virus in epithelial carcinomas of the head and neck region. Anticancer Res 1997;17:4427–33.

33. Anonymous. Recommendations from the Interagency Committee for the Review of the Racial and Ethnic Standards to the Office of Management and Budget concerning changes to the Standards for the Classification of Federal Data on Race and Ethnicity (directive 15). Washington, D.C., General Printing Office, 97 A.D.; 62(131), 36873–36946.

34. Anonymous. Racial/ethnic patterns of cancer in the United States 1988–1992. Bethesda, Md: National Cancer Institute, 1996.

35. National Center for Health Statistics. Health, United States, 1995. 1996; Hyattsville, Md: U.S. Public Health Service.

36. Witzig R. The medicalization of race: scientific legitimization of a flawed social construct. Ann Intern Med 1996;125:675–9.

37. Freeman HP. The meaning of race in cancer of the breast. comment. Cancer J Sci Am 1997;3:76–7.

38. Zenner W. Encyclopedia of cultural anthropology. New York: Henry Holt, 1996:393–5.

39. American Anthropological Association. AAA response to OMB directive 15: Race and Ethnic Standards for Federal Statistics and Administrative Reporting. Arlington, Va: American Anthropological Association, 1997.

40. de Lorgeril M, Salen P, Martin JL, et al. Mediterranean dietary pattern in a randomized trial: prolonged survival and possible reduced cancer rate. Arch Intern Med 1998;158:1181–7.

41. Levine A, Nidiffer J. Beating the odds: how the poor get to college. San Francisco: Jossey-Bass, 1996.

42. Andrulis DP. Access to care is the centerpiece in the elimination of socioeconomic disparities in health. see comments. Ann Intern Med 1998;129:412–6.

43. Franzini L, Williams AF, Franklin J, et al. Effects of race and socioeconomic status on survival of 1,332 black, Hispanic, and white women with breast cancer. Ann Surg Oncol 1997;4:111–8.

44. Freeman H. Race, poverty, and cancer. J Natl Cancer Inst 1991;83:526–7.

45. Adler NE, Boyce T, Chesney MA, et al. Socioeconomic status and health: the challenge of the gradient. Am Psychol 1994;49:15–24.

46. Brewster DH, Black RJ. Breast, lung, and colorectal cancer incidence and survival in South Thames region, 1987–1992: the effect of social deprivation. letter; comment. J Public Health Med 1998;20:236–8.

47. Smith D, Taylor R, Coates M. Socioeconomic differentials in cancer incidence and mortality in urban New South Wales, 1987–1991. Aust NZ J Public Health 1996;20:129–37.

48. Andrulis DP. Access to care is the centerpiece in the elimination of socioeconomic disparities in health. Ann Intern Med 1998;129:412–6.

49. Doll R, Peto R. The causes of cancer: quantitative estimates of avoidable risks of cancer in the United States today. J Natl Cancer Inst 1981;66:1191–308.

50. Liu ET. The uncoupling of race and cancer genetics. Cancer 1998;83:1765–9.

51. Neuhausen S, Gilewski T, Norton L, et al. Recurrent BRCA2 6174delT mutations in Ashkenazi Jewish women affected by breast cancer. Nat Genet 1996;13:126–8.

52. Fitzgerald MG, MacDonald DJ, Krainer M, et al. Germ-line BRCA1 mutations in Jewish and non-Jewish women with early-onset breast cancer. see comments. N Engl J Med 1996;334:143–9.

53. Keoun B. Ashkenazim not alone: other ethnic groups have breast cancer gene mutations, too. news. J Natl Cancer Inst 1997;89:8–9.

54. Offit K, Gilewski T, McGuire P, et al. Germline BRCA1 185delAG mutations in Jewish women with breast cancer. Lancet 1996;347:1643–5.

55. Phillips KA, Nichol K, Ozcelik H, et al. Frequency of p53 mutations in breast carcinomas from Ashkenazi Jewish carriers of BRCA1 mutations. J Natl Cancer Inst 1999;91:469–73.

56. Flaws JA, Bush TL. Racial differences in drug metabolism: an explanation for higher breast cancer mortality in blacks? Med Hypotheses 1998;50:327–9.

57. Bouchardy C, Mitrunen K, Wikman H, et al. N-acetyltransferase NAT1 and NAT2 genotypes and lung cancer risk. Pharmacogenetics 1998;8:291–8.

58. Ishibe N, Wiencke JK, Zuo ZF, et al. Susceptibility to lung cancer in light smokers associated with CYP1A1 polymorphisms in Mexican- and African-Americans. Cancer Epidemiol Biomarkers Prev 1997;6:1075–80.

59. Nyberg F, Hou SM, Hemminki K, et al. Glutathione S-transferase mu1 and N-acetyltransferase 2 genetic polymorphisms and exposure to tobacco smoke in nonsmoking and smoking lung cancer patients and population controls. Cancer Epidemiol Biomarkers Prev 1998;7:875–83.

60. Taioli E, Ford J, Trachman J, et al. Lung cancer risk and CYP1A1 genotype in African Americans. Carcinogenesis 1998;19:813–7.

61. Wu X, Amos CI, Kemp BL, et al. Cytochrome P450 2E1 DraI polymorphisms in lung cancer in minority populations. Cancer Epidemiol Biomarkers Prev 1998;7:13–8.

62. Kim JA, Kuban DA, el-Mahdi AM, Schellhammer PF. Carcinoma of the prostate: race as a prognostic indicator in definitive radiation therapy. Radiology 1995;194:545–9.

63. Armstrong M, Fairbrother K, Idle JR, Daly AK. The cytochrome P450 CYP2D6 allelic variant CYP2D6J and related polymorphisms in a European population. Pharmacogenetics 1994;4:73–81.

64. Maezawa Y, Yamauchi M, Toda G, et al. Alcohol-metabolizing enzyme polymorphisms and alcoholism in Japan. Alcohol Clin Exp Res 1995;19:951–4.

65. Hanke JZ. Genetic susceptibility to toxic substances and its relationship to carcinogenesis. IARC Sci Publ 1984;59:99–106.

66. Freeman HP. The meaning of race in science—considerations for cancer research: concerns of special populations in the National Cancer Program. Cancer 1998;82:219–25.

67. Doll R, Peto R. The causes of cancer: quantitative estimates of avoidable risks of cancer in the United States today. J Natl Cancer Inst 1981;66:1191–308.

68. Le Marchand L, Wilkens LR, Kolonel LN, et al. Associations of sedentary lifestyle, obesity, smoking, alcohol use, and diabetes with the risk of colorectal cancer. Cancer Res 1997;57:4787–94.

69. Le Marchand L, Kolonel LN. Cancer in Japanese migrants to Hawaii: interaction between genes and environment. Rev Epidemiol Sante Publique 1992;40:425–30.

70. Shimizu H, Mack TM, Ross RK, Henderson BE. Cancer of the gastrointestinal tract among Japanese and white immigrants in Los Angeles County. J Natl Cancer Inst 1987;78:223–8.

71. Prentice RL, Sheppard L. Validity of international, time trend, and migrant studies of dietary factors and disease risk. Prev Med 1989;18:167–79.

72. Margetts BM, Hopkins SM, Binns CW. Nutrient intakes in Italian migrants and Australians in Perth. Food Nutrition 1981;38:7–10.

73. Haenszel W, Kurihara M. Studies of Japanese migrants. I: Mortality from cancer and other diseases among Japanese in the United States. J Natl Cancer Inst 1968;40:43–68.

74. Glover FEJ, Coffey DS, Douglas LL, et al. The epidemiology of prostate cancer in Jamaica. J Urol 1998;159:1984–6.

75. Bouchardy C, Mirra AP, Khlat M, et al. Ethnicity and cancer risk in Sao Paulo, Brazil. Cancer Epidemiol Biomarkers Prev 1991;1:21–7.

76. Brawley OW. Prostate cancer and black men. Semin Urol Oncol 1998;16:184–6.

77. Flint AJ, Yamada EG, Novotny TE. Black-white differences in cigarette smoking uptake: progression from adolescent experimentation to regular use. Prev Med 1998;27:358–64.

78. Griesler PC, Kandel DB. Ethnic differences in correlates of adolescent cigarette smoking. J Adolesc Health 1998;23:167–80.

79. Faulkner DL, Merritt RK. Race and cigarette smoking among United States adolescents: the role of lifestyle behaviors and demographic factors. Pediatrics 1998;101:E4

80. Roth MJ, Strickland KL, Wang GQ, et al. High levels of carcinogenic polycyclic aromatic hydrocarbons present within food from Linxian, China, may contribute to that region's high incidence of oesophageal cancer. letter. Eur J Cancer 1998;34:757–8.

81. Araujo I, Foss HD, Bittencourt A, et al. Expression of Epstein-Barr virus-gene products in Burkitt's lymphoma in Northeast Brazil. Blood 1996;87:5279–86.

82. Faggiano F, Partanen T, Kogevinas M, Boffetta P. Socioeconomic differences in cancer incidence and mortality. IARC Sci Publ 1997;138:65–176.

83. Rimpela AH, Pukkala EI. Cancers of affluence: positive social class gradient and rising incidence trend in some cancer forms. Soc Sci Med 1987;24:601–6.

84. Aase A, Bentham G. Gender, geography and socio-economic status in the diffusion of malignant melanoma risk. Soc Sci Med 1996;42:1621–37.

85. Grady KE, Lemkau JP, McVay JM, Reisine ST. The importance of physician encouragement in breast cancer screening of older women. Prev Med 1992;21:766–80.

86. Edwards MJ, Gamel JW, Vaughan WP, Wrightson WR. Infiltrating ductal carcinoma of the breast: the survival impact of race. J Clin Oncol 1998;16:2693–9.

87. Lyman GH, Kuderer NM, Lyman SL, et al. Importance of race on breast cancer survival. Ann Surg Oncol 1997;4:80–7.

88. Elledge RM, Clark GM, Chamness GC, Osborne CK. Tumor biologic factors and breast cancer prognosis among white, Hispanic, and black women in the United States. J Natl Cancer Inst 1994;86:705–12.

89. Krieger N, Van Den Eeden SK, Zava D, Okamoto A. Race/ethnicity, social class, and prevalence of breast cancer prognostic biomarkers: a study of white, black, and Asian women in the San Francisco bay area. Ethn Dis 1997;7:137–149.

90. Weiss SE, Tartter PI, Ahmed S, et al. Ethnic differences in risk and prognostic factors for breast cancer. Cancer 1995;76:268–74.

91. Perkins P, Cooksley CD, Cox JD. Breast cancer. Is ethnicity an independent prognostic factor for survival? Cancer 1996; 78:1241–7.

92. Eley JW, Hill HA, Chen VW, et al. Racial differences in survival from breast cancer. Results of the National Cancer Institute black/white Cancer Survival Study. JAMA 1994;272:947–54.

93. Chen VW, Correa P, Kurman RJ, et al. Histological characteristics of breast carcinoma in blacks and whites. Cancer Epidemiol Biomarkers Prev 1994;3:127–35.

94. Coates RJ, Bransfield DD, Wesley M, et al. Differences between black and white women with breast cancer in time from symptom recognition to medical consultation. black/white Cancer Survival Study Group. J Natl Cancer Inst 1992;84:938–50.

95. Howard DL, Penchansky R, Brown MB. Disaggregating the effects of race on breast cancer survival. Fam Med 1998;30:228–35.

96. Lannin DR, Mathews HF, Mitchell J, et al. Influence of socioeconomic and cultural factors on racial differences in late-stage presentation of breast cancer. JAMA 1998;279:1801–7.

97. Wells BL, Horm JW. Stage at diagnosis in breast cancer: race and socioeconomic factors. Am J Public Health 1992;82:1383–5.

98. Hoffman-Goetz L, Breen NL, Meissner H. The impact of social class on the use of cancer screening within three racial/ethnic groups in the United States. Ethn Dis 1998;8:43–51.

99. Rimer BK. Interventions to enhance cancer screening. Cancer 1998;83:1770–4.

100. Rimer BK, Glassman B. Tailoring communications for primary care settings. Methods Inf Med 1998;37:171–7.

101. Coates RJ, Clark WS, Eley JW, et al. Race, nutritional status, and survival from breast cancer. J Natl Cancer Inst 1990;82:1684–92.

102. McWhorter WP, Mayer WJ. black/white differences in type of initial breast cancer treatment and implications for survival. Am J Public Health 1987;77:1515–7.

103. Roach M, Alexander M. The prognostic significance of race and survival from breast cancer: a model for assessing the reliability of reported survival differences. J Natl Med Assoc 1995;87:214–9.

104. Wojcik BE, Spinks MK, Optenberg SA. Breast carcinoma survival analysis for African American and white women in an equal-access health care system. Cancer 1998;82:1310–8.

105. Freedman LS, Simon R, Foulkes MA, et al. Inclusion of women and minorities in clinical trials and the NIH Revitalization Act of 1993—the perspective of NIH clinical trialists. Control Clin Trials 1995;16:277–85.

106. Dignam JJ, Redmond CK, Fisher B, et al. Prognosis among African-American women and white women with lymph node negative breast carcinoma: findings from two randomized clinical trials of the National Surgical Adjuvant Breast and Bowel Project (NSABP). Cancer 1997;80:80–90.

107. Roach M, Cirrincione C, Budman D, et al. Race and survival from breast cancer: based on Cancer and Leukemia Group B Trial 8541. Cancer J Sci Am 1997;3:107–12.

108. Gordon NH. Association of education and income with estrogen receptor status in primary breast cancer. Am J Epidemiol 1995;142:796–803.

109. Nomura AM, Marchand LL, Kolonel LN, Hankin JH. The effect of dietary fat on breast cancer survival among Caucasian and Japanese women in Hawaii. Breast Cancer Res Treat 1991;18 (Suppl 1):S135–41.

110. Heimann R, Ferguson D, Powers C, et al. Race and clinical outcome in breast cancer in a series with long-term follow-up evaluation. J Clin Oncol 1997;15:2329–37.

111. Diehr P, Yergan J, Chu J, et al. Treatment modality and quality differences for black and white breast-cancer patients treated in community hospitals. Med Care 1989;27:942–58.

112. Breen N, Wesley MN, Merril RM, Johnson K. The relationship of socio-economic status and access to minimum expected therapy among female breast cancer patients in the National Cancer Institute black-white Cancer Survival Study. Ethn Dis 1999;9:111-25.

113. McGee D, Cooper R, Liao Y, Durazo-Arvizu R. Patterns of comorbidity and mortality risk in blacks and whites. Ann Epidemiol 1996;6:381–5.
114. Thomson GE. Discrimination in health care. editorial; comment. Ann Intern Med 1997;126:910–2.
115. Optenberg SA, Thompson IM, Friedrichs P, et al. Race, treatment, and long-term survival from prostate cancer in an equal-access medical care delivery system. JAMA 1995;274:1599–1605.
116. Akerley WL, Moritz TE, Ryan LS, et al. Racial comparison of outcomes of male Department of Veterans Affairs patients with lung and colon cancer. Arch Intern Med 1993;153:1681–8.
117. Graham MV, Geitz LM, Byhardt R, et al. Comparison of prognostic factors and survival among black patients and white patients treated with irradiation for non–small-cell lung cancer. J Natl Cancer Inst 1992;84:1731–5.
118. Greenwald HP, Polissar NL, Borgatta EF, et al. Social factors, treatment, and survival in early-stage non–small-cell lung cancer. Am J Public Health 1998;88:1681–4.
119. Cooper GS, Yuan Z, Rimm AA. Racial disparity in the incidence and case-fatality of colorectal cancer: analysis of 329 United States counties. Cancer Epidemiol Biomarkers Prev 1997;6:283–5.
120. Cooper GS, Yuan Z, Landefeld CS, Rimm AA. Surgery for colorectal cancer: race-related differences in rates and survival among Medicare beneficiaries. Am J Public Health 1996;86:582–6.
121. Harlan L, Brawley O, Pommerenke F, et al. Geographic, age, and racial variation in the treatment of local/regional carcinoma of the prostate. J Clin Oncol 1995;13:93–100.
122. Klabunde CN, Potosky AL, Harlan LC, Kramer BS. Trends and black/white differences in treatment for nonmetastatic prostate cancer. Med Care 1998;36:1337–48.
123. Mettlin C, Murphy GP, Menck H. Trends in treatment of localized prostate cancer by radical prostatectomy: observations from the Commission on Cancer National Cancer Database, 1985–1990. Urology 1994;43:488–92.
124. Greenwald HP, Polissar NL, Borgatta EF, et al. Social factors, treatment, and survival in early-stage non–small cell lung cancer. Am J Public Health 1998;88:1681–4.
125. Hicks ML, Phillips JL, Parham G, et al. The National Cancer Data Base report on endometrial carcinoma in African-American women. Cancer 1998;83:2629–37.
126. Russell AH, Shingleton HM, Jones WB, et al. Diagnostic assessments in patients with invasive cancer of the cervix: a national patterns of care study of the American College of Surgeons. Gynecol Oncol 1996;63:159–65.
127. Schulman KA, Berlin JA, Harless W, et al. The effect of race and sex on physicians' recommendations for cardiac catheterization. N Engl J Med 1999;340:618–26.
128 Gamble VN. Under the shadow of Tuskegee: African Americans and health care. Am J Public Health 1997;87:1773–8.
129. Thomson GE. Discrimination in health care. Ann Intern Med 1997;126:910–2.
130. Anonymous. Social inequalities and cancer. IARC Sci Publ 1997;138:1–15.

# CHAPTER 27

# CANCER AND PREGNANCY

• HASSAN J. TABBARAH

## Background

### INCIDENCE

The incidence of cancer in pregnancy is not well determined. It is reported to be neither frequent nor rare. A review of medical records in two hospitals in Washington, D.C., placed the incidence at 1 cancer in 1003 pregnancies.[1] One may expect at least 3472 cases of cancer during pregnancy each year in the United States by estimating that 3.5 million live births occur annually. This represents 0.8% of the 422,000 women who develop cancer (excluding carcinoma in situ and nonmelanotic skin cancer) and 2.2% of women between the ages of 15 and 44.[2] Information from the Third National Cancer Survey indicates that approximately 13% of all cancers in women occur during the reproductive period.[3] The cancers most likely to occur during this period, in decreasing order of frequency, are thyroid cancer, cancer of the uterine cervix, melanoma, neoplasms of the bones and joints, lymphomas, and central nervous system (CNS) neoplasms.[3] Almost 50% of thyroid cancers and more than one third of uterine cervical cancers occur in women between the ages of 15 and 44. The cancers most likely to be seen in pregnant women, in decreasing order of frequency, are cancer of the breast, cancer of the uterine cervix, cancer of the thyroid,

cancer of the ovary, lymphomas, and colon cancer. The National Cancer Registry of the German Republic reported 355 cases of cancer in women between the ages of 15 and 44 from 1970 to 1979. In the same period, there were approximately 2 million live births. Uterine cervical cancer was the most frequent malignancy, followed by breast cancer, ovarian cancer, lymphoma, melanoma, and leukemia.[4]

### PREDISPOSING RISKS OF CANCER IN PREGNANT WOMEN

The factors that increase the risk of cancer in the female population may also increase that risk during pregnancy. Pregnancy and breast-feeding may decrease the risk of epithelial ovarian cancer. The estimated relative risks of epithelial ovarian cancer are approximately 0.6 for women who have ever been pregnant and 0.6 for women who have ever breast-fed.[5] The risks of gestational trophoblastic disease are increased in women who become pregnant after the age of 40. Pregnancy appears to have no effect on the development or the natural history of uterine cervical malignancy.[6] The incidence of human papillomavirus infection is five times higher in pregnant Western women than in Chinese women, yet the incidence of uterine cervical cancer is higher in Chinese women than in American women.[7] It has been reported that the immunologic status of pregnant women is permissive to viral infections and that spontaneous regression of cervical lesions caused by the cytopathic effects of papillomavirus and herpes simplex virus, type 2 occurs after delivery.[8] Pregnancy may immunize against breast cancer, as evidenced by case studies that demonstrated the presence of a tumor-specific antigen, MUC1, on both fetal and cancer tissue.[9]

## INTERACTION OF PREGNANCY WITH MALIGNANCY

An important reason for the belief that pregnancy adversely affects the clinical course of cancer is seen in the immunologic behavior that characterizes both conditions. The immunologic changes in pregnancy include depression of cellular immunity; the presence of circulating blocking factors that permit the tolerance of antigenic tissues (probably immunoglobulin); the immunosuppressive effects of various hormones such as estrogen, progesterone, and human chorionic gonadotropin; the presence of suppressor T cells; the presence of leukocyte migration enhancement factor; and decreased red blood cell immune adherence.[10, 11] Available pertinent information and relevant issues about the interaction of pregnancy with malignancy in the most common specific cancer sites are addressed in the following sections.

**Breast Cancer.** There is epidemiologic evidence that breast-feeding protects against breast cancer, especially in the years immediately following pregnancy.[12] Case-control studies in a total of 12,666 Swedish patients with breast cancer were compared with 62,121 age-matched control subjects. This study showed that pregnancy has a dual effect on the risk of breast cancer: It transiently increases the risk after childbirth but reduces the risk in later years. A plausible explanation is that pregnancy increases the short-term risk of breast cancer by stimulating the growth of cells that have undergone the early stages of malignant transformation and that it confers long-term protection by inducing the differentiation of normal mammary stem cells that have the potential for neoplastic change.[13] Whether pregnancy adversely affects or exacerbates cancer of the breast remains controversial. Some centers report that breast cancer during pregnancy is a highly aggressive disease with an attendant poor prognosis. Others suggest that the prognosis for gestational breast cancer is no different from that for age- and stage-matched nonpregnant controls. At the University of California, Los Angeles (UCLA), the occurrence of breast cancer during pregnancy was analyzed over a period of 15 years with special reference to overall survival, prognosis, and correlation with estrogen-receptor status and HER-2/*neu* oncogene expression.[14] The UCLA experience supported the opinion that breast cancer during pregnancy carries a poor prognosis and is usually hormone receptor–negative. No increased expression of HER-2/*neu* oncogene was detected to explain the poorer prognosis.[14] Similarly, a study from the Princess Margaret Hospital covering a period of 54 years between 1931 and 1985[12] found that coincidental pregnancy, and to a lesser degree coincidental lactation, in women with breast cancer was detrimental to survival, whereas subsequent preg-

nancy had no effect on survival.[15] In a report describing 5652 women with primary breast cancer aged 45 years or younger, a diagnosis of breast cancer sooner than 2 years after childbirth was associated with poor survival.[16] Another study of 5725 women with breast cancer showed no increase in the risk of miscarriage or induced abortion after breast cancer treatment.[17] In contrast, a 35-year multi-institutional study from the University of South Carolina and New York Medical College found that gestational breast cancer—when diagnosed, accurately staged, and treated aggressively—shows a potentially favorable outcome, with survival statistics comparable to those of a nonpregnant cohort.[18] A report from the European Association for Cancer Research suggested that for equal stages, the prognosis of patients with breast cancer associated with pregnancy is similar to that of patients with breast cancer who are not pregnant.[19] Disease-free survival was almost identical in both groups (37 and 38% at 8 years, respectively), but the nonpregnant control group had a longer survival (42% vs. 50% for the control at 8 years, $p = 0.049$). The control group had a higher chance of having stage I disease (23% vs. 9%) than did the breast cancer patients with associated pregnancy. When matched for age and stage, the survival was identical in both groups (42% at 8 years).[19] An analysis showed that the survival of women with breast carcinoma is not decreased by subsequent pregnancy in any of the published series. Nevertheless, several biases may be present, making the results less than conclusive because no prospective studies are available.[20]

**Malignant Lymphomas in Pregnancy.** The immunologic alterations associated with pregnancy have limited, if any, relevance to the etiology of non-Hodgkin's lymphoma or chronic lymphocytic leukemia. Changing reproductive pattern is an unlikely contributor to the marked increase in incidence in non-Hodgkin's lymphoma seen in many populations.[21] Studies show that pregnancy does not exacerbate Hodgkin's disease or adversely affect the mean duration of survival. Conversely, Hodgkin's disease has no effect on the course of gestation or delivery or on the incidence of spontaneous abortion or prematurity. Abortion does not influence the course of patients with Hodgkin's disease.

Offspring of either men or women with previous Hodgkin's disease have a slight but negligible increased risk of developing Hodgkin's disease.[22, 23] One study showed no effect of parity within marriage on the incidence of Hodgkin's disease in women age 40 to 80. With respect to prognosis, parity was found to have a beneficial influence in 15- to 56-year-old women. Excess mortality in mothers who have two children and Hodgkin's disease compared with otherwise equal mothers with two children and without Hodgkin's disease was significantly lower than the corresponding excess mortality among childless women. By contrast, there were strong indications of an increase in excess mortality from Hodgkin's disease across marital parity for women age 40 to 80.[24]

Non-Hodgkin's lymphoma during pregnancy is usually, but not always, associated with an aggressive histologic appearance. However, there are reports suggesting that pregnancy may stabilize non-Hodgkin's lymphoma because the disease was seen to progress after delivery.[25] Burkitt's lymphoma may take a progressive course during pregnancy and often involves the breast and ovaries. During pregnancy, intermediate- and high-grade lymphomas result in a high mortality rate if untreated. The first successful pregnancy associated with advanced intermediate-grade non-Hodgkin's lymphoma was reported in 1977 and attributed to aggressive combination chemotherapy.[26] Another report documented that through varied therapeutic programs, the management of non-Hodgkin's lymphoma in pregnant women can result in long-term survival and a satisfactory outcome for mother and fetus.[27]

**Melanoma.** Melanoma in women occurs during the reproductive years, there being a peak incidence in the third and fourth decades of life. Endocrine changes during pregnancy have been suspected of influencing the clinical behavior of melanoma. For example, there is increased pigmentation during pregnancy owing to increased stimulation of melanocytes, and estrogen-receptor protein has been demonstrated in malignant melanoma.[28] Reports describing the regression of melanoma during pregnancy and its recurrence after delivery have been conflicting. Melanoma during pregnancy usually carries a poor prognosis, but once the disease is diagnosed, the course is not worse than expected, considering the stage of the disease and the primary site.[29, 30]

A retrospective Canadian study comparing the survival rates of pregnant women with melanoma and those of melanoma patients who were never pregnant showed no significant difference between the two groups.[31] It was reported that during pregnancy, a 34-year-old housewife noticed ulceration, bleeding, and a rapid increase in the size of a congenital mole on the right forearm.[32] Immediately after a spontaneous abortion (third month), coincidentally or as a result of the abortion, the mole stopped growing, no further bleeding occurred, and the local irritation disappeared. Subsequent excision proved the mole to be a Clark's level V malignant melanoma.[32]

In one study, women who had previously been pregnant and had current melanoma had better prognoses, stage for stage, than did women with current melanoma who had never been pregnant.[33] Most authors, however, seem to agree that there is no significant difference in melanoma survival between pregnant and nonpregnant women and that the endocrine condition of pregnancy or therapeutic abortion, or both, has no influence on the course of the disease.[34] The same authors[26] reported a higher frequency of trunk lesions and more frequent nodal metastases in pregnant patients and in patients with mole activation related to pregnancy. One study found that melanomas associated with pregnancy were of more advanced stage at the time of treatment than were those found in women who were not pregnant. Nevertheless, the 10-year survival rates were the same.[28] In the absence of nodal metastases, the 5-year disease-free survival rates for melanomas or for mole activation related to pregnancy are the same as those in nonpregnant patients.[34]

**Cancer of the Uterine Cervix.** Carcinoma of the uterine cervix is the most common malignancy associated with pregnancy. It typically occurs in the reproductive years of life and is diagnosed in 1 of every 2200 deliveries. Approximately 3% of all carcinomas of the cervix are diagnosed in pregnant women.[35–37] In a study in Norway that investigated pregnancy outcome after laser surgery for cervical intraepithelial neoplasia, a strong relationship between conization and low birth weight was found, but no difference in birth weight was observed after vaporization.[38]

**Endometrial Cancer.** In a prospective study of 765,756 Norwegian women, a decrease in the risk of endometrial carcinoma with an increasing number of full-term pregnancies was observed ($p<0.001$). The reduction in risk associated with the first pregnancy was more pronounced than that observed for any subsequent pregnancy. The risk of endometrial carcinoma increased with increasing time since the last birth. The reduction in risk among parous women compared with nulliparous women diminished with increasing time since the last birth. For endometrial carcinoma, the decrease in risk with increasing age at first and last birth disappeared after adjustment for time since the last birth. For sarcomas, however, the relationship of age at childbirth and the time since the last birth seemed to be of minor importance as an independent risk factor.[39]

**Thyroid Cancer.** Thyroid cancer occurs most often in young women. It is relatively rare, and its relationship to pregnancy is not well documented in the literature. The general impression is that pregnancy does not stimulate the growth of thyroid cancer. Its presence is not a significant cause for the prevention of pregnancy or an indication for therapeutic abortion.[40, 41] Most thyroid cancers are papillary in histologic appearance.

**Ovarian Cancer.** The incidence of ovarian cancer is 1 per 9000 to 25,000 deliveries.[42] Some authors suggest that pregnancy may actually protect against the development of ovarian cancer. Only 5% of ovarian tumors found during pregnancy are malignant, compared with 15 to 20% of the ovarian tumors found in nonpregnant women.[43] Miller and colleagues described a successful term pregnancy following conservative debulking surgery for a stage IIIA serous tumor of the ovary with low malignant potential; normal ovarian function was preserved.[44]

**Gastrointestinal Cancer.** Cancer of the gastrointestinal tract has an estimated incidence of 1 in 100,000 pregnancies. Most such cancers are of the colorectum.[45] There appears to be a high ratio of rectal to colon cancer, which is the reverse of that seen in the general population. This is probably due to a selection bias caused by the obstetric attention given to the pelvis during pregnancy.[46] It is suggested that pregnancy does not influence the growth of cancer and that the cancer poses no threat to the fetus. However, it is reported that the prognosis for pregnant women with colon cancer is dismal, with no 5-year survivors. In contrast, the 5-year survival rate for rectal cancer in pregnant women is 62.5%, which is comparable to the survival rate in nonpregnant women with rectal cancer.[46]

**Tumors of the Central Nervous System.** The CNS tumors affected adversely by pregnancy include pituitary adenomas, craniopharyngiomas, and meningiomas. The pituitary tumors may or may not be hormonally active. Pregnancy is usually associated with an enlarged pituitary gland as a result of hyperplasia of the acidophilic prolactin-secreting cells.[47] During pregnancy, all pituitary tumors increase in size, and craniopharyngiomas may enlarge rapidly.[48] Approximately 40% of patients develop symptoms about 10 to 14 weeks after the beginning of pregnancy, and all these patients receive treatment with surgery or radiation therapy.

**Pregnancy After Bone Marrow Transplantation.** Multiple case reports and a few studies showed more than 250 births from bone marrow transplant recipients. Bone marrow transplant patients receive high-dose chemotherapy and often radiation as well. These agents are associated with gonadal dysfunction, and the fertility of patients after bone marrow transplant is of concern because these patients are often young persons who wish to resume a normal quality of life, which for many patients involves the desire to have children. The issue of counseling bone marrow transplant patients about fertility, pregnancy complications, and potential birth defects is becoming increasingly complex and warrants further investigation.[49]

**Metastasis to the Fetus.** The placenta and fetus are at little risk from maternal cancer, particularly when it is not disseminated. The infrequency of fetal involvement suggests that protective mechanisms may exist for the placenta and fetus. Reports of the mother's cancer being transmitted to the fetus are scanty. Metastases from the maternal tumor to the fetus are reported to occur in malignant melanoma (the most common), followed by breast cancer and malignant lymphomas. Such metastases are so rare that, except perhaps for malignant melanoma, they are not a significant consideration in the discussion of cancer in pregnancy. The propensity for melanoma to involve the placenta and fetus remains difficult to explain. The mother invariably has disseminated disease. Thirty-five cases in which metastasis to the placenta or fetus occurred have been described in the literature.[50] In 26 of the 35 cases, the placenta was involved, and in 11 cases the fetus showed evidence of metastasis. In only two instances were the placenta and the fetus involved at the same time.

A report of five cases of primary fetal cancer (three neuroblastomas, one melanoma, and one leukemia) without dissemination to the mother supports the theory of a placental barrier to neoplastic transmission.[1] Careful examination of the placenta of women who have or have had cancer, as well as careful observation of the infant if the mother has or has had melanoma or lymphoma, is recommended. A 1-month-old infant was reported to have died from intracerebral hemorrhage due to metastatic choriocarcinoma to the brain that presumably originated in the placenta.[51]

# Diagnostic and Therapeutic Concerns in the Pregnant Patient

Clinicians who care for pregnant women with cancer face serious medical and social problems that affect the maternal and fetal outcome. Planning therapy is complicated by information that is limited and sometimes contradictory and by complex emotional, religious, and ethical considerations. Ideally, the physician's objectives are to cure the patient of her cancer and deliver a healthy, viable infant; however, both these goals may not always be achievable.

## DIAGNOSTIC INTERVENTIONS

The diagnosis of cancer during pregnancy poses a challenging dilemma. Once the cancer is suspected, an expedient histologic diagnosis should be obtained. Delay in diagnosis may jeopardize the chances of survival. When the diagnosis is established, treatment should be similar to that for the nonpregnant patient.

The diagnostic difficulties posed by pregnant women with cancer are not different from those faced in nonpregnant patients except in a few primary cancer sites. These difficulties are caused mostly by the normal physiologic changes of pregnancy. These specific changes are addressed separately as they influence specific neoplasms.

**Breast Cancer.** During pregnancy, there is an increase in firmness and nodularity with hypertrophy of breast tissue. These physiologic changes obscure subtle masses, causing them to blend in and feel like the rest of the breast tissue. A mammogram during pregnancy is not easy to read because of the increased water content of the breast tissue and the loss of contrasting fatty tissue that usually defines a mass. Ultrasonography is a safe and accurate way to differentiate between solid and cystic lesions. Aspiration of a breast lesion is useful because a cyst or galactocele disappears and solid masses such as fibroadenoma, papilloma, and lipoma persist. In a series of 105 benign biopsies in pregnant women, only 70% of patients had conditions that were also present in nonpregnant women, and 29% had changes peculiar to gestation such as galactocele, lobular hyperplasia, and lactational mastitis.[52]

Surgeons are usually reluctant to perform a breast biopsy during pregnancy. In a Memorial Sloan-Kettering series, less than 20% of cancers were diagnosed and treated during pregnancy, and almost 50% were diagnosed and treated within 12 weeks after delivery. As a result of such reluctance, the median size of breast tumors at the time of postpartum diagnosis was 3.5 cm.[53]

The problems that face the surgeon while performing a breast biopsy are secondary to the physiologic changes that occur during pregnancy or lactation. The increased vascularity requires special attention to hemostasis. Milk is an excellent culture medium that promotes infection. Milk fistulas may develop after a breast biopsy but may be prevented by having the patient cease lactation before the biopsy is performed. Helpful measures include the use of firm breast binders, application of ice packs, and administration of bromocriptine to lower the level of prolactin and dry up breast milk. To reduce infection, prophylactic antibiotics are given before biopsy. A breast pump should be used to express and discard the milk containing antibiotics given to the mother. Biopsy of a central lesion has a higher chance of inducing a milk fistula than does biopsy of a peripheral lesion. There is no contraindication to core needle biopsy (Tru-Cut) or to needle aspiration of the breast. An experienced cytologist is needed who can differentiate between the macronuclei seen in benign breast tissue during pregnancy and the macronuclei of malignancy.[54] Incisional biopsy is an excellent alternative to excisional biopsy. Local anesthesia is safe and preferable, although general anesthesia is acceptable.

**Cancer of the Uterine Cervix.** Diagnosis of cancer of the uterine cervix is similar in pregnant and nonpregnant women because there are no pathophysiologic alterations of the cervical epithelium during pregnancy that can be confused with malignancy. Vaginal bleeding as a sign of cervical cancer is infrequent in pregnant women. If a Papanicolaou's (Pap) smear is abnormal, definitive diagnosis should be pursued with the same determination as in a nonpregnant woman. Colposcopic study and directed biopsy must be performed when indicated.[35–37]

**Malignant Melanoma.** Melanoma has a peak incidence

in women between 30 and 40 years of age, which is considered to be a reproductive period in the Western world. As a principle, any suspicious change in a pigmented cutaneous lesion during pregnancy warrants an immediate biopsy and appropriate treatment with the same determination required for a nonpregnant patient. Biopsy can be performed easily with local anesthesia.

**Malignant Lymphomas.** The occurrence of Hodgkin's disease in pregnancy is not unusual, considering that the mean age for such a diagnosis is 32 to 35 years. The incidence of Hodgkin's disease in pregnancy is reported to be 1 in 1000 to 1 in 6000 deliveries.[22, 23] Conversely, non-Hodgkin's lymphoma is a disease that is diagnosed at a mean age of 42 years, thus knowledge of and experience in its management during pregnancy is limited. Again, as a matter of principle, any suspicious lymph node should be biopsied as expediently in pregnant women as in nonpregnant women.

## STAGING PROCEDURES AND THE DILEMMA OF IONIZING RADIATION

Malignancy in pregnant patients should be clinically staged by complete physical examination, complete blood count, and serum biochemical tests as used for staging cancer in nonpregnant women. The only studies that should be avoided, if possible, are those that expose the fetus to ionizing radiation.

Pregnancy is divided into three periods. The first and earliest is known as the preimplantation period, which extends from the time of conception to days 10 to 14. During this period, radiation will result in the death of the embryo.[55] The second period is that of organogenesis and lasts from days 10 to 14 through the eighth week of gestation. The organogenesis period is the most sensitive to ionizing radiation. Mice who are exposed to as low a dose as 0.18 Gy have a 20% incidence of severe malformations, mostly in the CNS, and a 100% incidence of CNS malformations when exposed to 2 Gy.[55] Pregnant women exposed to an air dose of 0.01 to 0.09 Gy delivered babies with an 11% incidence of microcephaly and mental retardation, compared with 4% in a nonirradiated control group.[56] The third and final period is the fetal period, which extends from the eighth week of gestation to term. Radiation exposure during the fetal period of gestation is much less likely to produce congenital abnormalities than exposure during the organogenesis period. Dose for dose, microcephaly is four to five times less common if radiation exposure occurs during the fetal period than if it occurs during the organogenesis period.[56] After about 30 weeks of gestation, radiation-induced congenital defects are extremely rare.[57] Interruption of pregnancy is not routinely recommended by the American Academy of Pediatrics and the American College of Radiology if the fetus has been exposed to less than 0.05 Gy. If the fetus was exposed to more than 0.1 Gy, therapeutic abortion is recommended.[58] The risk of radiation-induced leukemia in the offspring at 10 years is reported to be 1 in 2000 versus 1 in 3000 in the unexposed control for a 0.02-Gy exposure.[59]

If a decision for therapeutic termination of pregnancy is made, all necessary studies can be obtained without any need for concern.

## STAGING STUDIES

**Ultrasonography.** Ultrasonography of the abdomen and pelvis may be ordered when indicated without much concern about significant adverse effects to the mother or fetus. The current recommended fetal exposure limit for ultrasonography is 94 mW/cm$^2$ spatial peak temporal average intensity.[60]

### Radiographic Studies

*Biologic Effects of Radiation.*[61] All ionizing radiation is harmful, and no data are available to indicate whether there is a threshold below which no harmful effects will occur. Radiation levels should be kept at the lowest practical level, and the maximal permissible dose should never be thought of as perfectly safe.

The roentgen (R) is a unit of radiation exposure. In the SI system, exposure is expressed in terms of "coulombs per kilogram of air." This definition is relatively meaningless to physicians in the United States. In familiar terms, a roentgen is the approximate exposure to the body surface of an anteroposterior film of the abdomen in a patient of average thickness. As a measure of exposure, the roentgen is independent of area or field size. The rad is the unit of absorbed dose measured in energy of radiation deposited per gram of irradiated material (1 rad = 100 erg/g). The gray (Gy) is the SI unit for the absorbed dose. The relation between the gray and the rad is as follows: 1 Gy = 100 rad and 1 rad = 1 cGy (centigray). Thus, 1 cGy is the same as 1 rad, and 1 Gy is equivalent to 100 rad. The rem is the unit of absorbed dose equivalent. It is used only in radiation protection and is a measure of the biologic effectiveness of radiation. The SI unit of absorbed dose equivalent is the sievert (Sv), and 1 Sv = 100 rem. The absorbed dose equivalent is equal to the absorbed dose multiplied by a quality factor (QF). Because the QF for x-rays is 1, the rad and rem are equal. In fact, at diagnostic energy levels, the roentgen, rad, and rem may all be considered equal. Therefore, 1 R = 1 rad = 1 rem = 1 cGy. The mGy is one tenth of a cGy. The mrad is one thousandth of a rad.

*Plain X-Ray Films.* Table 27–1 lists the radiation exposures for specific plain x-ray examinations as projected in the Federal Register (Veterans Affairs medical centers)[62] or as determined by the Nationwide Evaluation of X-Ray Trends.[63] Fetal shielding is advisable when plain x-ray examinations are performed. Fetal shielding in the later months of pregnancy obscures the lower lung fields.

A lymphangiogram may be obtained when indicated in patients with Hodgkin's disease. A plain x-ray film of the abdomen is taken after the injection of contrast material and results in a fetal exposure of about 0.01 Gy.

*Computed Tomography.* The dose values in computed tomography (CT) depend primarily on four different factors: single scan image quality, radiation detection and efficiency, details of scan motion, and multiple scan geometry. The patient dosage usually increases with increased transverse resolution and increased contrast resolution. The maximal surface dose ranges from 2 to 10 mGy per study if five or more slices are taken, although internal doses are 25 to 35% less. The surface dose per study values may be in excess of 200 mGy, depending on the type of scanner (rotary translate or pure rotary motion).[64] CT of the head with abdominal shielding provides negligible x-ray exposure to the fetus.[65] Consequently, prudent use of clinically indicated CT may be

*Table 27–1.* **Radiation Exposures**

| Examination | Mean ESE (mrad)* | |
|---|---|---|
| | NATIONWIDE EVALUATION OF X-RAY TRENDS | VETERANS AFFAIRS MEDICAL CENTERS |
| Chest (PA) | 22 | 30 |
| Skull (lateral) | 240 | 300 |
| Abdomen (AP) | 640 | 750 |
| Cervical spine (AP) | 240 | 250 |
| Thoracic spine (AP) | 720 | 900 |
| Full spine (AP) | 320 | 300 |
| Lumbosacral spine (AP) | 800 | 1000 |
| Retrograde pyelogram (AP) | 720 | 900 |
| Feet (DP) | 200 | 270 |
| Dental (bitewing, periapical) | | 700 |

*ESE, entrance skin exposure determined by the Nationwide Evaluation of X-Ray Trends program for a patient having the following body part thicknesses: head, 15 cm; neck, 13 cm; thorax, 23 cm; abdomen, 23 cm; and foot, 8 cm.

PA, posteroanterior; AP, anteroposterior; DP, dorsal plantar.

Data from Radiation protection guidance to federal agencies for diagnostic x-rays. Part V: federal register for VA medical centers, Feb. 1, 1978, and Nationwide evaluation of x-ray trends, HEW Publication, FDA 78-8056.

considered during pregnancy because the fetal dose can be calculated before ordering the scan. As a principle, however, CT of the chest and abdomen should be avoided during pregnancy, and CT of the pelvis should not be performed. In a typical scanning sequence over the pelvic region of a pregnant woman, the fetal dose may range from about 30 to 100 mGy.[64] In a report from Germany, the radiation exposure to the fetus exceeded 20 mGy in 50% of the pregnant patients undergoing CT of the pelvis.[66]

*Mammography.* The exposure from mammography for one film-screen is estimated to be 320 mrad for skin dose and 60 to 75 mrad for glandular dose (4 cm–thick breast). Mammographic examination may require one to three film-screens.[67] Exposure may vary from one x-ray machine to another.

**Embryo Uterine Exposure for Selected X-Ray Projection.**[68] Table 27–2 lists breast, ovary, and embryo uterine exposure levels for selected x-ray projections in millirads.

**Internal Radiation Doses in Diagnostic Nuclear Medicine.** Table 27–3 depicts the internal radiation doses received from diagnostic nuclear medicine procedures.[69] Table 27–4 shows the dose for the embryo in centigray per millicurie administered.[70] The Nuclear Regulatory Commission sets limits on the amount of activity that can be used. Iodine 131 is not used in diagnostic studies in pregnant patients because of its strong radiation effects.

Bone scans may be ordered when indicated. The radiation dose from a bone scan to the fetus during pregnancy is approximately 6.6 mrad/mCi. This would result in 99 mrad, assuming a conventional 15-mCi dose of technetium 99m when methylene diphosphate is used.

It is prudent to exclude a bone scan from the initial evaluation of a patient, even when indicated, until the termination of organogenesis or until a decision concerning the fetus has been made. Baker described a modified bone scan with lower exposure to be used in pregnant women.[71]

The dose to the developing fetus from a liver scan is 7 mrad/mCi administered. This results in 14 to 21 mrad to the fetus from a conventional 2- to 3-mCi dose of technetium 99m sulfur colloid.

In general, with nuclear medicine, it is advisable to hydrate pregnant patients well and have them void frequently after a study is completed to empty any isotope concentrated in the bladder via renal excretion.

*Table 27–2.* **Organ Doses for Common Radiographic Examinations (Adult Females)**

| Examination | No. of Examinations Per Year (millions) | Organ Dose (mrad) | | |
|---|---|---|---|---|
| | | BREASTS | OVARIES | UTERUS/EMBRYO |
| Chest | 21.8 | 14 | 0.06 | 0.06 |
| Skull | 1.4 | — | <0.01 | <0.01 |
| Cervical spine | 1.5 | — | <0.01 | <0.01 |
| Ribs | 0.53 | 411 | 0.4 | 0.5 |
| Shoulder (one) | 1.0 | 77 | <0.01 | <0.01 |
| Thoracic spine | 0.77 | 276 | 0.6 | 0.6 |
| Cholecystogram | 2.3 | — | 6.0 | 5.0 |
| Lumbar spine | 1.4 | — | 405 | 408 |
| Upper gastrointestinal tract | 2.9 | 53 | 45 | 48 |
| KUB | 1.4 | — | 212 | 263 |
| Barium enema | 1.9 | — | 787 | 822 |
| Lumbosacral spine | 0.8 | — | 640 | 639 |
| Intravenous pyelogram | 1.7 | — | 636 | 814 |
| Pelvis | 1.2 | — | 148 | 194 |
| Hip (one) | 1.0 | — | 78 | 128 |
| Full spine (chiropractic) | 0.11 | 234 | 100 | |
| Mammography (xeroradiography) | 2.0 | 766 | | Negligible |
| Mammography (film-screen) | | 212 | | Negligible |

KUB, kidney, ureter, and bladder.
From Kereias JG, ed. Handbook of radiation doses in nuclear medicine and diagnostic x-ray. Boca Raton: CRC Press, 1988:211.

*Table 27–3.* Internal Radiation Dose in Diagnostic Nuclear Medicine

| Organ | Administered Activity (mCi) | Agent | Critical Organ | Approximate Total Dose (rad) |
|---|---|---|---|---|
| Thyroid | 1.0 | $^{99m}$TcO$_4$ | Thyroid | 0.34 |
| | 0.2 | $^{123}$I | Thyroid | 4 |
| Bone | 20 | $^{99m}$Tc-phos | Skeleton | 0.8 |
| Liver | 3.0 | $^{99m}$Tc-sc | Liver | 1.02 |
| Tumor | 3 | $^{67}$Ga-citrate | Colon | 2.7 |
| Kidneys | 2 | $^{99m}$Tc-gluco | Kidneys | 0.6 |
| | 0.03 | $^{131}$I-hippurate | Kidneys | 0.003 |
| | | | Bladder wall | 0.36 |
| Lungs | 3 | $^{99m}$Tc-microsph | Lung | 0.63 |
| Heart | 2 | $^{201}$Tl | Kidneys | 0.8 |
| | 20 | $^{99m}$Tc-RBC | Blood | 1 |
| Gallbladder | 1–8 | $^{99m}$Tc-disofenin | Gallbladder wall | 0.39–3.12 |

From Harbert JC: Absorbed dose estimates from radionuclides. Clin Nucl Med 1984;9:210.

**Magnetic Resonance Imaging.** In general, magnetic resonance imaging (MRI) is not believed to be hazardous to the fetus. However, a variety of mechanisms can potentially produce harmful interaction between electromagnetic fields and a fetus. The Food and Drug Administration requires labeling of MRI systems to indicate that "safety of MRI when used to image the fetus and infants has not been established." Thus, it is inadvisable to use MRI routinely in pregnant women unless it is absolutely indicated and the clinician feels it is necessary in order to avoid ionizing radiation.[72]

## THERAPEUTIC ABORTION

As discussed earlier, pregnancy per se does not make the prognosis worse for the newly diagnosed cancer patient receiving standard treatment. Therefore, a therapeutic abortion cannot be recommended solely on the grounds that it is necessary for prolonging the life of the mother. In most cases, therapeutic abortion provides no survival benefits in addition to those provided by standard therapy. Conversely, it may be strongly recommended when fetal damage might or would occur from the planned radiation therapy (fetal dose >0.1 Gy) or chemotherapy. Diagnosis and treatment may be greatly simplified by performing a therapeutic abortion, but in the end it is the parents' responsibility to make an informed decision.

*Table 27–4.* Dose Estimates for the Embryo

| Radiopharmaceutical | Centigray/Millicurie Administered |
|---|---|
| $^{90m}$Tc-sulfur colloid (normal) | 0.007 |
| $^{90m}$Tc-sodium pertechnetate | |
| Resting population | 0.037 |
| Nonresting population | 0.039 |
| $^{123}$I-sodium iodide (15%) | 0.032–0.10 |
| $^{123}$I-sodium rose bengal | 0.13–0.68 |

From Smith EM, Warner GG. Estimates of radiation dose to the embryo from nuclear medicine procedures. J Nucl Med 1976;17:836–9.

## Problems and Indications for Delaying Treatment

A significant delay in treatment of a patient with cancer is likely to be detrimental. When referred to a physician, a pregnant woman with a suspicious lesion deserves an expedient histologic diagnosis so that her chances of survival are not compromised. Once the diagnosis is established, she should be treated in the same way as a nonpregnant woman. Fears of fetal exposure to radiation should not deter the physician from ordering the appropriate diagnostic tests to stage the cancer provided that precautions are taken to protect the fetus. Surgery can be performed when indicated with the patient under local or general anesthesia, with no significantly increased risk.[53] Treatment may be delayed in the circumstances described in the following sections.

### EARLY PREGNANCY: FIRST 20 WEEKS

**Lymphoma.** Patients with indolent or low-grade non-Hodgkin's lymphoma or Hodgkin's disease that does not need to be treated immediately may be observed and treatment delayed until after the first trimester if possible, unless significant progression is noted.[73]

**Breast Cancer.** Adjuvant chemotherapy, when indicated for breast cancer, should be delayed until after the first trimester.[74, 75]

**Cervical Cancer.** Conization of the uterine cervix should be delayed until the end of the first trimester in both carcinoma in situ and invasive carcinoma.[76] This decreases the incidence of spontaneous abortion.

### LATE PREGNANCY: LAST 20 WEEKS OR LESS

**Lymphoma.** The treatment of indolent or low-grade non-Hodgkin's lymphoma or Hodgkin's disease may be delayed until the postpartum period, and strong consideration should be given to an early delivery.

**Cancer of the Uterine Cervix.** Uterine cervical cancer treatment by radiation therapy or surgery may be delayed until the postpartum period, with strong consideration of cesarean section when the fetus is viable. Vaginal delivery does not seem to affect prognosis in uterine cervical cancer, and survival is the same whether the delivery is vaginal or by cesarean section.

## Principles of Treatment

The decisions that must be made for pregnant women with cancer are difficult for both physicians and patients. The data regarding the outcome for the mother and fetus are scanty, involving only small numbers of patients with conflicting findings. Fortunately, however, the incidence of cancer in pregnant women is relatively low. The results and side effects of the available forms of treatment—that is, surgery, chemotherapy, and radiation therapy—as reported in the medical literature, are summarized in the following sections.

### SURGERY

Surgery can be performed using local or general anesthesia with no ill effects during the entire three trimesters of pregnancy.

**General Anesthesia.** General anesthesia is necessary for major surgical procedures, such as mastectomy, with or without axillary dissection; wide or deep local excision of melanoma, with or without lymph node dissection; colon resection; and hysterectomy. General anesthesia is difficult in pregnant women because of increased blood volume, increased heart rate, increased cardiac output, increased stroke volume, decreased blood pressure, decreased peripheral vascular resistance, increased glomerular filtration rate, decreased blood urea nitrogen levels, decreased creatinine levels, increased platelet count, increased fibrinogen level, supine positional hypotension, prolonged gastric emptying, elevated diaphragm, decreased pulmonary functional capacity, hypervascularity of the respiratory tract mucosa, and albumin levels decreased by almost 20% in the second trimester.[77]

The risks of teratogenesis from general anesthetic drugs are nonexistent.[78] Nitrous oxide and halothane interfere in vitro with nucleic acid synthesis, but no deleterious effects have been detected in humans.[79, 80] These agents have the theoretical advantage of relaxing the uterine musculature, and they reduce the incidence of premature labor. The occurrence of premature labor depends more on the surgical site, being more common with lower abdominal or pelvic operations, and drugs are available for its reversal. It is rare in breast and thoracic surgery. Postoperative monitoring for uterine contractions should be continued until the effects of anesthesia abate. Obstetric and maternal-fetal health consultations should be obtained. Fetal monitoring should be used so that patterns of fetal distress may be detected and treated by a fine adjustment in the amount of anesthetic drugs used. In one report,[52] only one fetal death occurred among 134 patients receiving general anesthesia during pregnancy.

### CHEMOTHERAPY

The availability of effective adjuvant chemotherapy has created a difficult management problem. For example, surgery alone is inadequate for any woman with stage II or III breast cancer and would constitute undertreatment for approximately 30% of women with stage I disease. Chemotherapy is not advisable in early pregnancy (first trimester). It may be given when absolutely indicated, but it carries a significantly increased risk for the fetus. Chemotherapy given during the second trimester of pregnancy is less hazardous but is also associated with adverse effects, although less frequently. Chemotherapy during the last trimester is least hazardous. In a report from the Princess Margaret Hospital,[74, 75] 21 pregnant women who received chemotherapy during a 30-year period were evaluated retrospectively for cancer involving all sites and histologic types. There were five women with breast cancer, four with Hodgkin's disease, four with leukemia, four with melanoma, two with non-Hodgkin's lymphoma, one with ovarian cancer, and one with rhabdomyosarcoma. Among 13 women treated during the first trimester, five carried the fetus to term, four had spontaneous abortions, and four had elective abortions. Two of the five women who carried to term had children with major malformations: one child born to a mother who had received MOPP (mechlorethamine, vincristine, procarbazine, prednisone) for stage IVB Hodgkin's disease died of hydrocephalus. Another infant whose mother had received bacille Calmette-Guérin for stage I Clark's level III melanoma had cardiac abnormalities. Four women were treated during the second trimester, resulting in one stillbirth, one therapeutic abortion, and two live births. The stillbirth occurred 9 days after the mother was treated for acute myelogenous leukemia. At birth, the fetus appeared normal except for areas of bruising and petechiae. All four women who received chemotherapy during the third trimester had normal live births. Among the live births, the mean birth weight of infants exposed to chemotherapy in utero was significantly lower than that of infants born to matched controls. The gestational ages of this group were also significantly less because of a higher proportion of preterm deliveries, as labor was induced to permit more aggressive treatment of the mother.

A report from the M.D. Anderson Cancer Center[81] described 11 women in whom breast cancer was diagnosed during pregnancy and noted that chemotherapy was not begun until after the first trimester and consisted of 5-fluorouracil, 1000 mg/m$^2$; doxorubicin, 50 mg/m$^2$; and cyclophosphamide, 500 mg/m$^2$, every 28 days. There were ten normal infants (three delivered by cesarean section); one was neutropenic and experienced respiratory distress. All infants survived, and at 24 months of follow-up all had reached normal developmental milestones.[80] In contrast, another report described eight pregnant women with Hodgkin's disease treated with combination chemotherapy during the first trimester, resulting in no apparent malformations in the infants born to these women.[25] Regimens reported to be safe for use in pregnant women with non-Hodgkin's lymphoma include COP-BLEO (cyclophosphamide, Oncovin [vincristine], prednisone, bleomycin), CHOP (cyclophosphamide, hydroxydaunomycin, Oncovin, prednisone), and MACOP-B (methotrexate, Adriamycin [doxorubicin], cyclophosphamide, Oncovin, prednisone, bleomycin).[82, 83]

In general, the drug effect on the fetus is related to dosage, gestational age, synergism with other drugs, and the teratogenicity of the individual drugs. Vinblastine can be used with minimal risk to the fetus. Antimetabolites are to be avoided because they accumulate in the amniotic fluid and intrauterine growth retardation has been observed with their use. The placenta is readily traversed by all cytotoxic drugs. In 1989, Garber[84] reviewed the teratogenic effects of approximately 20 cytotoxic drugs as described in 300 reports. In 71 patients who received chemotherapy during the first trimester of pregnancy, the fetal malformation rate was 12.7%.

## RADIATION THERAPY

Because of the potential teratogenicity of radiation therapy at any point in pregnancy, radiation therapy for a woman who wants to maintain her pregnancy should be limited to radiation fields above the diaphragm. Analysis of fetal exposure to supradiaphragmatic radiation confirms that the dosage from internal scatter increases during pregnancy as the uterus rises toward the xiphoid, and the benefits of abdominal shielding are limited.[85, 86] An expected fetal exposure exceeding 0.1 Gy has been suggested as the threshold for recommending therapeutic abortion.

Radiation therapy to the breast as an alternative to mastectomy requires a standard breast radiation therapy course of about 50 Gy. This exposes the fetus to 0.1 Gy early in pregnancy and up to 2 Gy or more in late pregnancy. A large amount of radiation reaches the fetus from internal scatter in the mother, and this cannot be reduced by external shielding. The quantity of such radiation depends on the distance of the fetus from the field center, the field size, and the energy source. Thus, if the fetus is less than 12 weeks' gestation, 50 Gy will result in an exposure to the fetus of 0.1 to 0.15 Gy, and toward the end of pregnancy the fetal structure is a distance of 10 cm from the field center and will receive 2 Gy for the same treatment course.[59]

Therefore, radiation therapy is contraindicated in the first trimester of pregnancy and should be avoided in late pregnancy because of increased internal radiation scatter. An exception to this recommendation may be the patient with non-bulky Hodgkin's stage IA cervical or axillary disease. Such a patient could be treated with modified fields and modified dose irradiation and further therapy deferred until after delivery. A report from M.D. Anderson concluded that radiation therapy is an appropriate initial treatment for stages IA and IIA supradiaphragmatic Hodgkin's disease in pregnant women during the second and third trimesters provided that special attention is paid to treatment and shielding techniques.[87] The outcome has not been shown to be adversely affected by pregnancy, and after the first 8 weeks of gestation, the risk to the fetus appears minimal. Four to five half-value layers of lead were used to shield the uterus during radiation therapy. The estimated total dose to the midterm fetus ranged from 0.014 to 0.055 Gy for treatment with 6 MeV and from 0.1 to 0.136 Gy for treatment with cobalt 60. Of the 25 pregnant women with Hodgkin's disease, 7 were in the first, 10 were in the second, and 8 were in the third trimester. Before treatment, 6 patients in the first trimester had an abortion and 3 patients in the third trimester had normal deliveries. All the remaining 16 patients subsequently delivered normal infants and underwent further staging and treatment as needed.

## Conclusions

There are no absolute guidelines or definitive recommendations for treating pregnant women with cancer. In addition, general guidelines can never substitute for clinical judgment, and the oncologist should be prepared to alter the original plan when necessary. Most of the available information is derived from case studies, retrospective analysis of findings from a small number of patients observed or treated in a particular setting, or selected groups of patients treated by physicians using different treatment modalities. Therefore, the treatment of pregnant women with cancer should be individualized to suit their specific needs.

As a reasonable principle, oncologists usually counsel therapeutic abortion for afflicted women who are in the first half of pregnancy. In the second half of pregnancy, most patients can be followed carefully and therapy postponed until induction of delivery at 32 to 36 weeks. Chemotherapy and radiation therapy should not be used during the first trimester because they would inflict the most harm to the fetus during this intricate developmental period. Chemotherapy may be given during the last trimester without significant adverse effects to the fetus. Radiation therapy should be avoided during late pregnancy if possible and preferably should be delayed until after delivery to protect the fetus from internal radiation scatter.

## SUGGESTIONS FOR ADDITIONAL READING

Blatt J. Pregnancy outcome in long-term survivors of childhood cancer. Med Pediatr Oncol 1999;33:29–33. *Long-term follow-up suggests that these survivors are at risk of having spontaneous abortions, but their offspring do not appear to have an increased risk of congenital anomalies or cancer.*

Berry DL, Theriault RL, Holmes FA, et al. Management of breast cancer during pregnancy using a standardized protocol. J Clin Oncol 1999;17:855–61. *The authors considered chemotherapy a reasonable option during the second and third trimesters of pregnancy.*

Hensley ML, Reichman BS. Fertility and pregnancy after adjuvant chemotherapy for breast cancer. Crit Rev Oncol Hematol 1998;28:121–8.

Sorosky JI, ed. Cancer complicating pregnancy. Obstet Gynecol Clin North Am 1998;25:273–450.

## REFERENCES

1. Potter JF, Schoeneman M. Metastasis of maternal cancer to the placenta and fetus. Cancer 1970;25:380–8.
2. Vital Statistics Report. Annual summary for the United States, 1979. U.S. Department of Health and Human Services. Vol. 28. 1980:1–29.
3. Third National Cancer Survey. Incidence Data. Natl Cancer Inst Monogr 1975;41:108–11.
4. Haas JF. Pregnancy in association with a newly diagnosed cancer: a population-based epidemiologic assessment. Int J Cancer 1984;34:229–35.
5. Gwinn ML, Lee NC, Rhodes PH, et al. Pregnancy, breast feeding, and oral contraceptives and the risk of epithelial ovarian cancer. J Clin Epidemiol 1990;43:559–68.
6. Smith EB, Creasman WT. Preinvasive and invasive cervical neoplasia in pregnancy. In: Gleicher N, ed. Principles of medical therapy in pregnancy. New York: Plenum, 1985:1112–7.
7. Collins RJ, Ngan HY, Hsu C, et al. Human papillomavirus infection in the cervix of pregnant females in Hong Kong. Cytopathology 1990;1:147–52.
8. Dalbert D, Mural J, Bartt O, et al. Colposcopic, histologic, and virologic study on the epithelial pathology of the uterine cervix in pregnancy. Cervix Lower Female Genital Tract 1987;5:31–8.

9. Botelho F, Clark DA. How might pregnancy immunize against breast cancer? Am J Reprod Immunol 1998;39:279–83.

10. Gleicher N, Siegel I. Common denominators of pregnancy and malignancy. In: Gleicher N, ed. Reproductive immunology. New York: Alan R. Liss, 1981:339–53.

11. Gleicher N, Deppe G, Cohen CJ. Common aspects of immunologic tolerance in pregnancy and malignancy. Obstet Gynecol 1979;54:335–42.

12. Enger SM, Ross RK, Henderson B, Bernstein L. Breastfeeding history, pregnancy experience, and risk of breast cancer. Br J Cancer 1997;76:118–23.

13. Lambe M, Hsieh C, Trichopoulos D, et al. Transient increase in the risk of breast cancer after giving birth. N Engl J Med 1994;331:5–9.

14. Wolin M, Giuliano A, Glaspy J. Breast cancer in pregnancy: The UCLA experience. meeting abstract. Proc Annu Meet Am Soc Clin Oncol 1990;9:A171.

15. Clark RM. Breast cancer and pregnancy. meeting abstract. Presented at the seventh annual meeting of the European Society of Therapeutic Radiation Oncologists, The Hague, The Netherlands, September 5–8, 1988, p 35.

16. Kroman N, Wohlfahrt J, Andersen KW, et al. Time since childbirth and prognosis in primary breast cancer: population-based study. Br J Med 1997;315:851–5.

17. Kroman N, Jensen MB, Melbye M, et al. Should women be advised against pregnancy after breast-cancer treatment? Lancet 1997;350:319–22.

18. Greene FL, Leis HP. Management of breast cancer in pregnancy. meeting abstract. Proc Proc Annu Meet Am Soc Clin Oncol 1989;8:94.

19. Schlanger H, Ben Yosef R, Baras M, Catane R. The effect of pregnancy at diagnosis on the prognosis in breast cancer. meeting abstract. Presented at the 10th biennial meeting of the European Association of Cancer Research, Galway, Ireland, September 10–13, 1989, p 80.

20. Surbone A, Petrek JA. Childbearing issues in breast carcinoma survivors. Cancer 1997;79:1271–8.

21. Adami HO, Tsaih S, Lambe M, et al. Pregnancy and risk of non-Hodgkin's lymphoma: a prospective study. Int J Cancer 1997;70:155–8.

22. Thomas PRM, Peckham MJ: The investigation and management of Hodgkin's disease in the pregnant patient. Cancer 1976;38:1443–51.

23. Redman JR, Bajorunas DR, Lacher MJ. Hodgkin's disease: pregnancy and progenity. In: Lacher MJ, Redman JR, eds. Hodgkin's disease. Philadelphia: Lea & Febiger, 1990:244–66.

24. Kravdal O, Hansen S. The importance of childbearing for Hodgkin's disease: new evidence from incidence and mortality models. Int J Epidemiol 1996;25:737–43.

25. Aviles A, Diaz-Maqueo JC, Torras V, et al. Non-Hodgkin's lymphomas and pregnancy: presentation of 16 cases. Gynecol Oncol 1990;37:335–7.

26. Ortega J. Multiple agent chemotherapy including bleomycin of non-Hodgkin's lymphoma during pregnancy. Cancer 1977;40:2829–35.

27. Habermann Tjohansen K, Colgan J, Witzig T, et al. The synchronous presentation of non-Hodgkin's lymphoma and pregnancy. meeting abstract. Proc ASCO 1990;9:1026.

28. George PA, Fortner JG, Pack GT. Melanoma with pregnancy. Cancer 1960;13:854–9.

29. McCulloch PB, Dent PB. Melanoma. In: Allen HH, Nisker JA, eds. Cancer in pregnancy: therapeutic guidelines. Mount Kisco, New York: Futura, 1986:205–24.

30. Cascinelli N, MacKie R, Bufalino R, et al. Melanoma and pregnancy. Advances in the biology and clinical management of melanoma. meeting abstract. Thirty-fifth annual clinical conference and 24th annual special pathology program, Houston, Texas, November 20–23, 1991, pp 26–27.

31. Elwood JM, Coldman AJ. Previous pregnancy and melanoma prognosis. Lancet 1978;2:1000–1.

32. Riberti Cmarola G, Bertani A. Malignant melanoma: the adverse effect of pregnancy. Br J Plast Surg 1981;34:338–9.

33. Hersey P, Morgan G, Stone DE, et al. Previous pregnancy as a protective factor against death from melanoma. Lancet 1977;1:451–2.

34. Shiu MG, Schottenfeld D, MacLean B, et al. Adverse effect of pregnancy on melanoma: a reappraisal. Cancer 1976;37:181–7.

35. Gilotra PM, Lee FY, Krupp PJ, et al. Carcinoma in situ of the cervix uteri in pregnancy. Surg Gynecol Obstet 1976;142:396–8.

36. Jolles CJ. Gynecologic cancer associated with pregnancy. Semin Oncol 1989;16:417–24.

37. Bianco V, Gilardi EM, Lomonico S. Cervical screening programs as

they appear through pregnant women. Cervix Low Female Genital Tract 1987;5:251–6.

38. Forsmo S, Hansen MH, Jacobsen BK, Oian P. Pregnancy outcome after laser surgery for cervical intraepithelial neoplasia. Acta Obstet Gynecol Scand 1996;75:139–43.

39. Albrektsen G, Heuch I, Tretli S, Kvale G. Is the risk of cancer of the corpus uteri reduced by a recent pregnancy: a prospective study of 765,756 Norwegian women. Int J Cancer 1995;6:485–90.

40. Rosvoll RV, Winship T. Thyroid carcinoma and pregnancy. Surg Gynecol Obstet 1965;121:1039–42.

41. Hill CS Jr, Clark RL, Wolf M. The effect of subsequent pregnancy on patients with thyroid carcinoma. Surg Gynecol Obstet 1966;122:1219.

42. Karlen JR, Akbari A, Cook WA. Dysgerminoma associated with pregnancy. Obstet Gynecol 1979;53:330–5.

43. Novak ER, Lambrou CD, Woodruff JD. Ovarian tumors in pregnancy. Obstet Gynecol 1975;46:401–6.

44. Miller DM, Ehlen TG, Saleh EA. Successful term pregnancy following conservative debulking surgery for a stage IIIA serous low-malignant-potential tumor of the ovary: a case report. Gynecol Oncol 1997;66:535–8.

45. Girard RM, Lamarch J, Baillot R. Carcinoma of the colon associated with pregnancy. Dis Colon Rectum 1981;24:473–5.

46. O'Leary JA, Pratt JH, Symmonds RE. Rectal carcinoma and pregnancy. Obstet Gynecol 1967;30:862–8.

47. Magyar DM, Marshall JR. Pituitary tumors and pregnancy. Am J Obstet Gynecol 1978;132:739–51.

48. Sachs BP, Smith SK, Cassar J, et al. Rapid enlargement of a craniopharyngioma in pregnancy. Br J Obstet Gynecol 1978;5:557–8.

49. Gulati SC, Van Poznak C. Pregnancy after bone marrow transplantation. J Clin Oncol 1998;16:1978–85.

50. Rothman LA, Cohen CJ, Astarloa J. Placental and fetal involvement by maternal malignancy. Am J Obstet Gynecol 1973;116:1023–34.

51. Chandra SA, Gilbert EF, Vaseskul C, et al. Neonatal intracranial choriocarcinoma. Arch Pathol Lab Med 1990;114:1079–82.

52. Byrd BF, Bayer DS, Robertson JC, et al. Treatment of breast tumors associated with pregnancy and lactation. Ann Surg 1962;155:940–7.

53. Petrek JA, Dukoff R, Rogatko A. Prognosis of pregnancy-associated breast cancer. Cancer 1991;67:869–72.

54. Bottles K, Taylor RN. Diagnosis of breast masses in pregnant and lactating women by aspiration cytology. Obstet Gynecol 1985;66:765–85.

55. Hall EJ. Effects of radiation on the developing embryo. In: Hall EJ, ed. Radiobiology for the radiologist. New York: Harper & Row, 1973:231–9.

56. Miller R, Mulvihill S. Small head size after atomic radiation. Teratology 1976;14:355–7.

57. Orr JW, Shingleton HM. Cancer in pregnancy. Curr Probl Cancer 1983;8:1–50.

58. Wallack MK, Wolff JA Jr, Bedwinek J, et al. Gestational carcinoma of the female breast. Curr Probl Cancer 1983;7:1–58.

59. Brent RL. The effect of embryonic and fetal exposure to x-ray, microwaves, and ultrasound: counseling the pregnant and nonpregnant patient about these risks. Semin Oncol 1989;16:347–68.

60. Kremkau FW. Biologic effects and safety. In: Rumack CM, ed. Diagnostic ultrasound. St. Louis: Mosby-Year Book, 1991:19–29.

61. Curry TS III, Dowdey JE, Murry RC Jr, eds. Christensen's Physics of Diagnostic Radiology. 4th ed. Philadelphia, Lea & Febiger, 1990:372–375.

62. Radiation Protection Guidance to Federal Agencies for Diagnostic X-rays. Part V: Federal Register for VA Medical Centers, Feb. 1, 1978.

63. NEXT (Nationwide Evaluation of X-ray Trends). HEW Publication, FDA 78–8056. 1978.

64. Rothenberg LN, Pentlow KS. Radiation dose in CT. Radiographics 1992;12:1225–43.

65. Felmlee JP, Gray JE, Leetzow ML, Price JC. Estimated fetal radiation dose from multislice CT studies. AJR 1990;154:185–90.

66. Panzer W, Zankl M. A method for estimating embryo doses resulting from computed tomographic examinations. Br J Radiol 1989;62:936–9.

67. Kopans DB. Breast imaging. Philadelphia: JB Lippincott, 1989:38.

68. Kereias JG, ed. Handbook of Radiation Doses in Nuclear Medicine and Diagnostic X-ray. Boca Raton, Florida: CRC Press, 1988:211.

69. Harbert JC, Pollina R. Absorbed dose estimates from radionuclides. Clin Nucl Med 1984;9:210–21.

70. Smith EM, Warner GG. Estimates of radiation dose to the embryo from nuclear medicine procedures. J Nucl Med 1976;17:836–9.

71. Baker J, Ali A, Groch MW, et al. Bone scanning in pregnant patients with breast carcinoma. Clin Nucl Med 1987;12:519–24.
72. NIH Consensus Conference. Magnetic resonance imaging. JAMA 1988;259:2132–8.
73. Doll DC, Ringenberg S, Yarbro JW. Management of cancer during pregnancy. Arch Intern Med 1988;148:2058–64.
74. Zemlickis D, Lishner M, Degendorfer P, et al. Maternal and fetal outcome after breast cancer in pregnancy. Am J Obstet Gynecol 1992;166:781–7.
75. Zemlickis D, Lishner M, Degendorfer P, et al. Fetal outcome after in utero exposure to cancer chemotherapy. Arch Intern Med 1992;152:573–6.
76. Allen HH, Nisker JA. Cancer in pregnancy. In: Allen HH, eds. Cancer in pregnancy. Mount Kisco, New York: Futura, 1986:3–8.
77. Baron WM. The pregnant surgical patient. Ann Intern Med 1984;101:683.
78. Melmed AP. Anesthesia principles and technique in pregnancy. In: Cherry SH, eds. Medical, surgical and gynecologic complications of pregnancy. Baltimore: Williams & Wilkins, 1985:664–87.
79. Pedersen H, Finster M. Anesthetic risks in the pregnant surgical patient. Anesthesiology 1979;51:439–51.
80. Nunn FJ. Faulty cell replication, abortion, congenital abnormalities. Int Anesthesiol Clin 1981;19:82–3.
81. Theriault R, Walters R, Holms F, et al. Management of breast cancer during pregnancy. Proc ASCO 1992;11:86.
82. Ward F, Weiss RB. Lymphoma and pregnancy. Semin Oncol 1989;16:397–409.
83. Nantel S, Parboosingh J, Poon M. Treatment of an aggressive non-Hodgkin's lymphoma during pregnancy with MACOP-B chemotherapy. Med Pediatr Oncol 1990;18:143–5.
84. Garber JE. Long-term follow-up of children exposed in utero to antineoplastic agents. Semin Oncol 1989;16:437–44.
85. Zucali R, Marchesini R, DePalo G. Abdominal dosimetry for supradiaphragmatic irradiation of Hodgkin's disease in pregnancy. Tumori 1981;67:203–8.
86. Wong PS, Rosemark PJ, Wexler MC, et al. Doses to organs at risk from mantle field radiation therapy using 10 MV x-rays. Mt Sinai Med J 1985;52:216–20.
87. Woo SY, Fuller LM, Cundiff JS, et al. Radiotherapy during pregnancy for clinical stages IA–IIA Hodgkin's disease. Radiat Oncol Biol Phys 1992;23:407–12.

# CHAPTER 28

# CANCER AND AGE

• LODOVICO BALDUCCI • MARTINE EXTERMANN

In the Western world, the population older than age 65 has been progressively expanding since the 1950s.[1] The causes of this unprecedented epidemiologic phenomenon include prolonged life expectancy and a reduced natality rate. At the turn of the 20th century, the age profile of the US population looked like a pyramid, with a wide base of individuals younger than 20 years and a small top of older individuals; today the profile looks more like a square because the young base has shrunk and the older top has enlarged.[2] In geriatric circles, this shift in age profile is referred to as "squaring of the pyramid." In some European countries, such as Italy, the population older than 65 years has already exceeded the population younger than 20 years. In the United States, this event is expected to occur around the year 2010 if the current trends in population growth persist.[3]

The aging of the population has important social as well as medical implications. When compared with the 1950s, the medical panorama today includes a higher prevalence of chronic diseases associated with a higher prevalence of comorbidity and polypharmacy and a spiraling use and cost of medical services.[4, 5] In dealing with a population with limited life expectancy and affected by multiple chronic conditions, the goals of treatment have shifted from cure to preservation of function and quality of life (Fig. 28–1).[6] After age 50, the incidence of chronic diseases increases, and disease and disability may precede death by several years. This gap may become as wide as 20 years for older individuals. The main goal of geriatric medicine is to close this gap of dependence and discomfort (compression of morbidity). In addition, numerous novel problems have emerged that are specific to the older population. As functional reserve and life expectancy become progressively more restricted, the therapeutic index of many forms of

treatment is reduced because the benefits are lessened and the risks enhanced.[4] The biology of many diseases may change with the age of the patient; new diseases, such as dementia and osteoporosis, become more common; and the influence of social support on the effectiveness of treatment becomes more prominent.

Cancer is a major problem for the older population: The increase in cancer incidence has paralleled the aging of the population, and cancer is second only to cardiovascular disease as a cause of death for persons older than age 65 (Fig. 28–2).[7] In addition, cancer is a major cause of morbidity and disability. Cancer control is essential to compression of morbidity. Paradoxically, most information related to cancer management was obtained from a younger population[8, 9]:

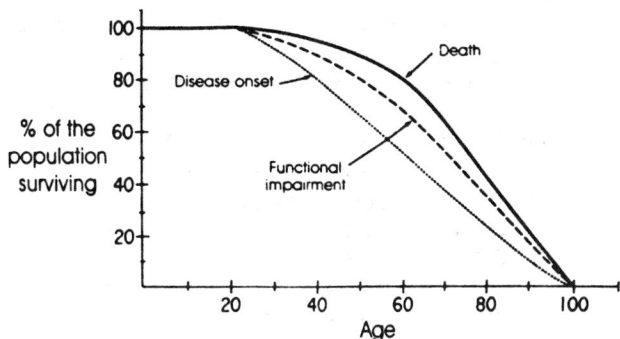

**Figure 28–1.** The incidence of disease precedes death for approximately 30 years, and the incidence of disability for approximately 20 years. The goal of geriatric medicine is to delay the occurrence of disease and disability (compression of morbidity). (From Manton KG, Soldo BJ. Dynamics of health changes in the oldest old. Milbank Q 1985;63:210–9.)

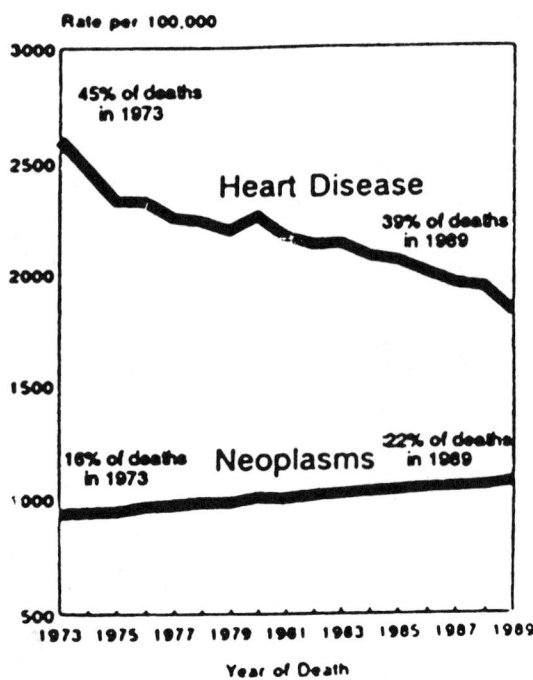

**Figure 28–2.** Causes of death in the population older than 65 years. As cardiovascular diseases decline, cancer progressively becomes a more common cause of death. (From Berlin NI. The conquest of cancer. Cancer Invest 1995;13:540–50.)

only recently have a number of publications addressed the specific problems of cancer in the elderly.[10–19]

This chapter explores the biologic interactions of cancer and age and the principles of cancer control in the older person and proposes a research agenda for approaching unsolved issues.

## Extent of the Problem

The incidence of most malignancies increases with age (Fig. 28–3).[1, 2] Currently, 50% of all neoplasms occur in the 12% of persons older than age 65: It is expected that as many as 60% of all neoplasms will affect older persons by the year 2010.

What are the clinical implications of the high concentration of malignancies among the elderly? Do older persons die of their cancer or with their cancer? The answer to this basic clinical question involves two parts. First, cancer-related mortality has declined for individuals younger than 65 years but has increased for older persons.[7] Cancer is indeed relevant to the survival and health of older individuals. This increment reflects several factors, including increased incidence of cancer, ineffective antineoplastic treatment for older persons, suboptimal use of preventive measures, restricted access to timely diagnosis and treatment of cancer, and poor tolerance of treatment.[20–23] These factors are partly reversible and represent a major target of ongoing research to improve cancer control in the older person. Second, cancer is particularly relevant in persons aged 65 to 85. After age 85, the incidence of many malignancies de-

clines and so does the incidence of cancer-related deaths, partly because of a rise in competitive causes of death.[24–28]

The association of cancer and aging may be accounted for by two nonmutually exclusive explanations. First, carcinogenesis is a time-consuming process, whose end product—cancer—becomes manifested several years from its initiation. According to this hypothesis, cancer is one of the prices one pays for getting old. The variation in incidence of different neoplasms is partly accounted for by this hypothesis (see Fig. 28–3). Although the incidence of lung cancer increases up to age 70 and drops thereafter, the incidence of colorectal or prostate cancer keeps rising after age 85. Seemingly, the duration of carcinogenesis is longer for neoplasms whose peak incidence occurs later in life. Second, older individuals may be more susceptible to the effects of late-stage carcinogens (promoters). Several lines of evidence support this possibility (Table 28–1). Experiments in rodents showed that older animals were more prone to the development of tumors than were younger animals after exposure to late-stage carcinogens, including 7, 12-dimethyl benz [*a*] anthracene and methylnitrosourea.[29] When the tissues of older animals were transplanted into younger animals, the application of the carcinogen induced more tumors in the transplanted tissue than it did in the adjacent tissues of the younger animals. This experiment indicated that increased susceptibility to carcinogenesis was a function of the age of the tissue, rather than of the animal, and presumably was independent from the systemic effects of aging, such as immune senescence.[29] Also, this effect appeared to be tissue specific: It was more marked for the cutaneous, hepatic, and lymphatic tissues and was not apparent in the nervous or mesenchymal tissues.[29] Several molecular changes occur in

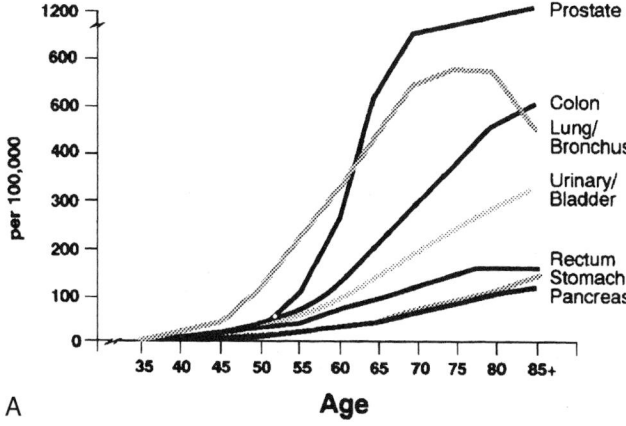

A

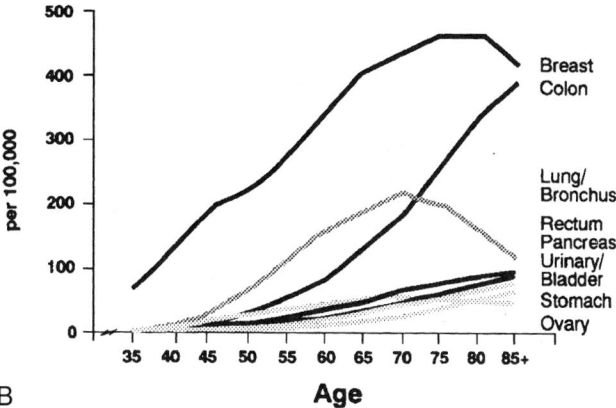

B

**Figure 28–3.** Age-related incidence of cancer in men *(A)* and women *(B).* (From Yancik RM, Ries LA. Cancer in the older person: magnitude of the problem. How do we apply what we know? In: Balducci L, Lyman GH, Ershler WB. Comprehensive geriatric oncology. London: Harwood Academic, 1998:95–104, copyright 1998; Overseas Publishers Association N.V.)

aging cells, including formation of DNA adducts and DNA hypomethylation.[29–32] These changes may lead to activation of proto-oncogenes and inhibition of antioncogenes and mimic the initial stages of carcinogenesis. Thus, the older person may have a higher concentration of "initiated" cells, which are susceptible to the action of late-stage carcinogens (Fig. 28–4). This finding may have important clinical consequences because the effects of late-stage carcinogens are offset by chemoprevention.[33] Campisi has raised the possibility that proliferative senescence might predispose to cancer.[34] Proliferative senescence is the loss of proliferative capacity

*Table 28–1.* **Age and Susceptibility to Late-Stage Carcinogens (Promoters)**

Experimental studies
    Increased susceptibility of older rodents and older tissues to late-stage carcinogens
Proliferative senescence and cancer
Molecular changes of aging
Epidemiologic findings
    Logarithmic increase in the incidence of some cancers (skin, prostate) with aging

by aging phenotypic cells and is associated with genomic changes, release of cellular substances that may stimulate carcinogenesis in neighboring tissues, and resistance to apoptosis.

Epidemiologic findings include the geometric increase in the incidence of skin cancer and prostate cancer with age, which suggests enhanced susceptibility of these tissues to carcinogenesis in the aged, and the emergence of new cancer epidemics among older individuals.[35, 36] The incidence of some malignancies has increased dramatically in the older population since 1950. The incidence of non-Hodgkin's lymphomas (NHLs) has increased 80% in persons older than 60 years,[17, 37, 38] that of malignant brain tumors has increased almost sevenfold[39–41] in individuals past 70 years, and that of squamous cell carcinoma of the skin has also increased severalfold.[35, 36] More prolonged exposure to the sun may account for the increment in skin cancer. In the case of other tumors, a cause is not clearly evident. Improved detection rates from more accurate diagnostic techniques seem to play at most a marginal role in the increased incidence of brain tumors.[39] Older persons may be more susceptible than younger persons to environmental carcinogens and may represent a natural monitor system for new carcinogens in the environment. Barbone and colleagues reported that the risk of lung cancer secondary to an airborne carcinogen in Trieste, Italy, increased with the age of the subject at the time of exposure to the carcinogen.[42]

Although aging and cancer may follow similar molecular pathways, it would be inappropriate to consider cancer a normal consequence of aging because important molecular differences exist between these two processes. For example, the cellular concentration of telomerases declines during normal aging but persists unchanged in many neoplastic systems. This enzyme is essential to the support of the proliferative ability of the cells because it prevents shortening of DNA telomeres.[43, 44] Also, the expression of the p16 gene is enhanced during normal aging and is lacking in most cancer cells. p16 encodes the cyclin-dependent kinase 4 (cdk4) that activates an inhibitor of cell proliferation.[45, 46]

In conclusion, age is definitely a risk factor for cancer. Age may be associated with an increased susceptibility of some tissues to environmental carcinogens, and this susceptibility may explain the epidemics of NHL and brain tumors in older persons. This increased susceptibility to environmental carcinogens may make older individuals ideal candidates for chemoprevention. Although aging and carcinogenesis may follow, to some extent, the same molecular pathways, they diverge for a number of molecular characteristics, and under no circumstances can cancer be considered a consequence of normal aging.

## Biology of Cancer and Age

The prognosis of some common neoplasms varies with the age of the patient (Table 28–2). In exploring these variations, it may be useful to consider cancer growth as a function of the "seed" (the inherent aggressiveness of the tumor cell) and of the "soil" (the ability of the tumor host to support cancer growth).[47]

It is reasonable to expect a concentration of more indolent

**AGE 20**                                                    **AGE 80**

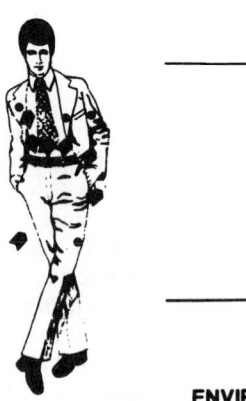
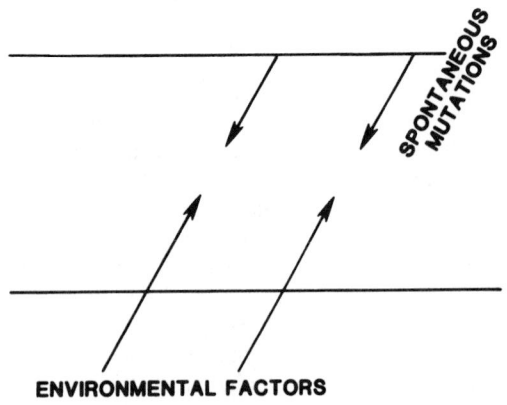
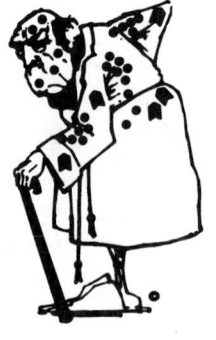

**Figure 28–4.** A number of age-related molecular changes mimic the early stages of carcinogenesis. As a consequence, older individuals have a much higher concentration of cells that are susceptible to late-stage carcinogens than do younger individuals.

ENVIRONMENTAL FACTORS

- CELLS IN LATE CARCINOGENIC STAGES
- LATE STAGE CARCINOGENS

tumors in older individuals (Fig. 28–5). By a process of natural selection, the bearers of aggressive neoplasms are eliminated by their disease at an earlier age, whereas the bearers of more indolent neoplasms survive to an older age. The influence of the age of the tumor host on tumor growth was well documented by Ershler.[47] This author found that the same load of transplantable tumors, such as Lewis' lung carcinoma and B16 melanoma, caused more metastasis and shorter survival in younger mice than in older mice. The mechanisms through which the organisms modulate tumor growth are largely unknown. Aging involves declining production of the sex hormones that stimulate the growth of breast, prostate, and endometrial cancer.[48] Aging is generally associated with immune senescence, which may modulate tumor growth in different ways. In the case of highly immu-

nogenic tumors, the loss of T-cell function may result in enhanced tumor growth; in the case of other cancers, such as breast cancer, immune senescence may delay tumor growth.[47–49] Several authors found that the growth of breast cancer was stimulated by a cytokine produced by the mononuclear cells infiltrating the tumor, and the concentration of these mononuclear cells decreased with the age of the patient.[50, 51] Aging is associated with a decline in the production of some growth factors, such as insulin-like growth factor I, and with increased serum concentrations of interleukin-6 (IL-6) which stimulate proliferation of lymphoid tissue.[52–54]

Table 28–2 offers some explanations of the different behavior of common neoplasms in younger and older individuals. In the case of acute myelogenous leukemia (AML),

*Table 28–2.* **Examples of Neoplasms Whose Prognosis Varies with Age**

| Cancer | Age-Related Changes | Mechanisms |
|---|---|---|
| Acute myelogenous leukemia (AML) | Decreased remission rate<br>Increased mortality in induction | Higher prevalence of myeloblasts expressing MDR-1<br>Higher prevalence of unfavorable chromosomal patterns<br>Neoplastic involvement of the pluripotent hemopoietic precursor |
| Large-cell non-Hodgkin's lymphoma (NHL) | Decreased duration of complete remission<br>Higher recurrence rate | Possibly increased plasma concentration of interleukin-6 (IL-6) |
| Celomic ovarian cancer | Decreased response to chemotherapy<br>Decreased duration of response | Unknown |
| Breast cancer | More indolent disease with higher prevalence of bone and soft tissue metastases and lower prevalence of visceral metastases | Higher prevalence of hormone receptor–rich, well-differentiated tumors<br>Decreased cellular proliferation<br>Decreased mononuclear cell infiltration of the tumor<br>Possibly decreased production of growth factors such as transforming growth factor-β and insulin-like growth factor-I |
| Non-small cell cancer of the lung (NSCLC) | Clinical presentation at an earlier stage | Unknown |

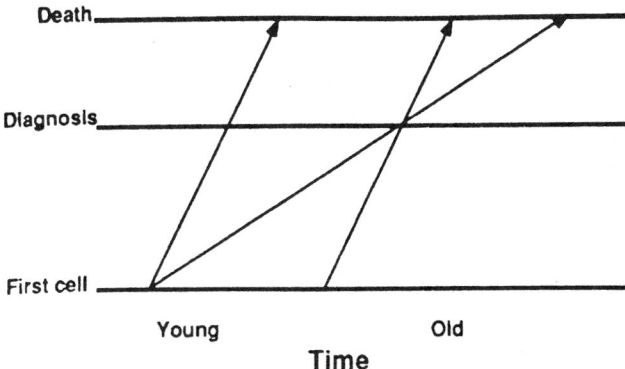

**Figure 28–5.** Theoretical explanation of the concentration of more indolent tumors in older individuals. Individuals with very aggressive tumors are killed when young, and a higher concentration of more indolent tumors is found in the older population from a process of natural selection.

the nature of the seed clearly changes with the age of the patient. Willman demonstrated that the prevalence of multidrug resistance was 57% among patients older than 60 years with acute leukemia and 21% among younger patients.[55] The prevalence of unfavorable chromosomal changes also increased with the age of the patient.[55] Another unfavorable feature of AML in the elderly is neoplastic involvement of pluripotent hemopoietic precursors, which may critically reduce the reserve of hemopoietic stem cells available for regeneration of the bone marrow after induction chemotherapy.[56, 57] In breast cancer, both the seed and the soil may influence the growth of the tumor. A number of studies showed that the prevalence of well-differentiated, hormone receptor–rich tumor increases with age, whereas the tumor proliferation rate decreases.[19, 51, 58–59] The prevalence of metastases to the bones and soft tissues is higher among older women, whereas the prevalence of visceral, life-threatening metastases is lower in this population.[19, 60, 61] The mononuclear cell reaction to the primary tumor also declines with the age of the patient.[50, 51] The end result is a more indolent tumor.[62–64] Veronesi and colleagues[64] provided a convincing demonstration that the behavior of breast cancer changes with age (Fig. 28–6). After breast quadrantectomy and in the absence of postoperative irradiation, 17% of women younger than 55 years experienced a recurrence of their disease at 3 years, but only 3% of older women did.[64] Increased circulating concentrations of IL-6 may be responsible for the worse prognosis of large-cell NHL in the elderly.[53, 54]

Age-related changes in tumor biology should not determine the management of cancer in the individual patient. Age itself is a poor predictor of individual outcome. Although the prognosis of NHL worsens with age, at least 30% of patients with this disease are curable after age 60; thus, a remission of lymphoma should be aggressively pursued with the most active chemotherapy.[17, 37, 38, 65] Breast cancer–related mortality is higher in older women than in younger women, although the disease becomes more indolent with age.[66] These findings are not surprising: Given the increasing prevalence of breast cancer with age, the absolute number of older women with aggressive breast cancer is higher than that for younger women, although the percentage

of women with aggressive cancer declines with age. The treatment of individual patients should be based on the characteristics of the tumor and on the ability of the patient to withstand treatment, not on the patient's chronologic age.

## Cancer Prevention in the Older Patient

Cancer prevention is subdivided into primary and secondary prevention.[37, 67–69] Primary prevention is directed toward reversing carcinogenesis and involves elimination of environmental carcinogens and chemoprevention.[37, 67–69] Secondary prevention involves early detection of cancer by screening asymptomatic persons at risk.[68, 69]

Contrary to a common prejudice, older persons are good candidates for primary prevention of cancer owing to an increased susceptibility to late-stage carcinogens. A person is never too old to adopt a healthy diet and daily exercise and to cease smoking. Chemoprevention of cancer is becoming more and more popular, and older persons are ideal candidates for this technique.[70] Retrospective randomized controlled studies showed that both estrogen antagonists[70–72] and selective modulators of estrogen receptors[73] effectively prevent breast cancer in women at risk, that is, women older than 60 years and women with a personal or family history of breast cancer. Randomized studies also showed that retinoids prevent smoking-related neoplasms in the head and neck areas,[74] whereas retrospective analyses suggest that estrogens prevent colorectal and ovarian cancer[75, 76] and nonsteroidal anti-inflammatory drugs (NSAIDs) may prevent colorectal cancer.[77] Despite these encouraging results, chemoprevention still belongs more to the realm of clinical research than to that of clinical practice. A number of issues

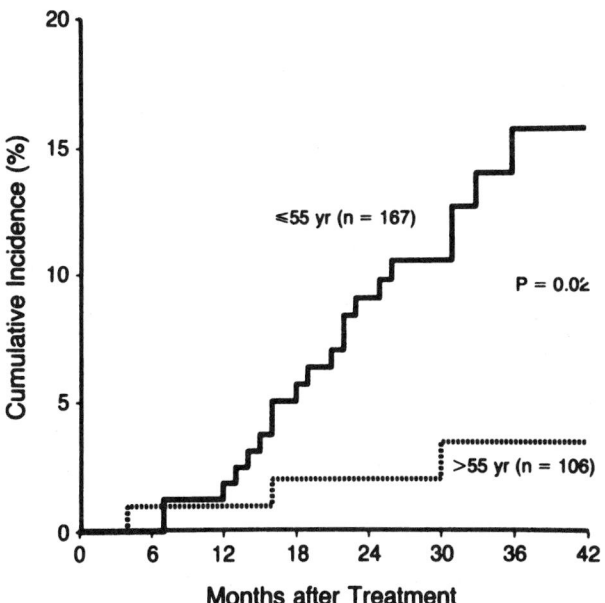

**Figure 28–6.** The incidence of local breast cancer recurrence at 3 years from mastectomy was 17% in women younger than age 55 and 3% among older women. (From Veronesi U, Luini A, Del Vecchio M, et al. Radiotherapy after breast-conserving surgery in women with localized cancer of the breast. N Engl J Med 1993;328:1587–1591.)

remain to be addressed, including the duration and long-term side effects of treatment.

Secondary prevention is currently the best established form of cancer prevention: Forms of cancer screening that have reduced cancer-related mortality include serial mammography for breast cancer,[19, 78] annual fecal occult blood testing for cancer of the large bowel,[79] serial cervical Papanicolaou's (Pap) smears for cervical cancer–related mortality for women younger than 40 years,[80] and possibly serial determinations of prostate-specific antigen (PSA) levels for prostate cancer[81, 82] and serial determinations of alpha-fetoprotein and liver ultrasonography for hepatocellular carcinoma in carriers of hepatitis B and hepatitis C.[83] Serial determination of serum calcitonin in persons with a family history of multiple endocrine neoplasia, type I syndrome also may reduce the mortality related to medullary carcinoma of the thyroid.[84] The value of secondary prevention of cancer in the older person is not well established. For example, only three of seven controlled studies of mammography included women up to age 70, and of these only two included women up to age 75[85] (Table 28–3). All three studies failed to show clearly that mammography reduced mortality for women past 65 years. Only a historically controlled study, done in Holland, showed some benefit for women aged 65 to 75, and the results of this study are far from conclusive.[86]

Several factors may influence the effectiveness of screening asymptomatic older persons with cancer.[67–69] The positive predictive value of some screening tests, such as mammography, may increase because the prevalence of breast cancer increases with the age of the population. At the same time, the detection of new cancers may decrease because most neoplasms were detected by previous examinations. Also, the death-preventing potential of screening may disappear in a population with limited life expectancy.

A number of barriers impede the access that older persons have to cancer screening. They include transportation, limited mobility, economic restrictions, dementia, and lack of information.[87] Since the 1980s, cancer screening has become more acceptable to the older population, mainly because of

*Table 28–3.* **Screening Mammography Trials**

| Study | Age-Range (Yr) | Relative Risk of Breast Cancer Death (Screened/Controls) |
|---|---|---|
| *Prospectively Controlled Studies of Screening Mammography* | | |
| Hip | 40–64 | .65 (.46–.92) |
| Malmo | 45–39 | .81 (.62–1.07) |
| Edinburgh | 45–64 | .84 (.63–1.12) |
| Kopparbergh | 40–74 | .64 (.45–.90) |
| Ostergotland | 40–74 | .74 (.55–.99) |
| Canadian2 | 50–59 | .97 (.62–1.52) |
| Stockholm | 40–64 | .8 (.53–1.22) |
| Gothenburg | 40–59 | .86 (.54–1.37) |
| *Historically Controlled Trials of Screening Mammography* | | |
| BCDDP | 59–74 | — |
| Dom | 50–64 | .52 (.32–.83) |
| Florence | 40–70 | .53 (.33–.85) |
| Nijmegen | 35–65 | .51 (.26–.99) |
| UK | 45–64 | .76 (.54–1.08) |

*Table 28–4.* **Guidelines for Screening Older Persons for Cancer***

| Cancer | Who to Screen | How to Screen |
|---|---|---|
| Breast | Life expectance ≥3 yr | Biennial mammography Physical examination of the breast at each physician visit |
| Colorectum | Life expectancy ≥3 yr | Annual fecal occult blood examination Possible endoscopy every 5 yr |
| Prostate | Men age 50–70 | Serial PSA determinations Serial rectal examination |
| Cervix | Women older than 60 yr who did not undergo previous screening | Pelvic examination and Pap smear at least every 5 yr |

*These guidelines apply to persons at average risk of cancer, that is, persons without a previous history of cancer in that particular organ.
PSA, prostate-specific antigen; Pap, Papanicolaou's.

the support of primary care providers[88, 89] who have encouraged screening.

In the absence of more conclusive evidence, the screening of older individuals for cancer should be directed by common sense. We follow the guidelines described in Table 28–4. We believe it is important not to put an upper age limit for screening patients for breast and colorectal cancer because the diagnosis of either cancer may be beneficial even when early treatment is not clearly associated with survival benefits. Partial and even total mastectomy are simple procedures that do not require more than 1 day of hospitalization and may be performed with local anesthesia in patients with poor cardiopulmonary reserve. Timely mastectomy may prevent the local complications of breast cancer such as pain, infection, bleeding, and unsightly fungating masses. In cancer of the large bowel, an elective colectomy is preferable to emergency colostomy because emergency surgery is particularly risky for older individuals.[90] Also, a number of local procedures, such as laser surgery, Bicap, and the use of rectal prostheses, may prevent large bowel obstruction in patients who are unfit for surgery.[91] Since the initial benefits of screening were seen 3 years after the institution of the screening program, a life expectancy of at least 3 years appears to be a reasonable condition for screening older individuals. In all studies of breast cancer, annual and biennial mammography appeared comparable.[78] Biennial mammography greatly reduces the cost and inconvenience for older individuals. Seemingly, the value of physical examination of the breast by physician or nurse may increase in the older population, because the breast atrophies, the subcutaneous fat becomes less prominent, and new nodules become easier to appreciate. The physical examination of the breast may be performed in a short time, in any medical office, and with minimal cost and inconvenience.

Only annual determination of fecal occult blood proved beneficial in a randomized controlled study for colorectal cancer screening.[79] Several authorities believe that some form of endoscopy every 5 years may also be beneficial.[79]

In a randomized Canadian study, serial determination of serum PSA produced a decline in prostate cancer–related mortality.[82] These results are controversial because only a small proportion of the target population underwent screening; however, the conclusions are supported by uncontrolled American studies that showed that the incidence of advanced prostate cancer in the United States decreased since PSA screening was instituted.[81] The best interval between consecutive PSA determinations is unknown at present. We recommend that screening stop after age 70 because there is no evidence that any treatment of early prostate cancer is beneficial after this age.[92]

A study by Celentano and Klassen showed that the incidence of invasive cervical cancer increased among women age 60 and older in recent years.[93] The same study showed that serial pelvic examinations reduced the death rate from cervical cancer among these women. The women most at risk were those who had never had screening prior to age 60 and those who had not undergone screening in the prior 10 years.

# Cancer Treatment in the Older Person

The management of cancer in the older person hinges on two questions: "Is the patient able to tolerate life-prolonging treatment? Is the treatment going to improve the survival and the symptoms of the patient?" We address the issue of treatment tolerance in this section and the issue of patient selection in the next.

## SURGERY

The mortality related to general surgery[90] or thoracic surgery[94] does not appear to rise with the age of the patient (up to age 80) for elective procedures. However, the incidence of postsurgical complications and the length of hospital stay do increase with age.[95–97] Older patients are particularly at risk of dying from emergency surgery because of a high incidence of gram-negative sepsis.[90, 98] This high mortality rate reflects the limited functional reserve of the older patient and underlines the importance of early detection of digestive cancer in these patients. Early detection may allow elective procedures in most patients. Also, elderly patients are more likely to present with co-morbid conditions that may worsen surgical outcome.[5, 27, 99–104] A number of surgical advances have reduced the extent of the resection and the need for general anesthesia and are particularly beneficial for the elderly. They include partial mastectomy,[105] transanal resection for rectal cancer,[106] intraluminal tumor ablation in the digestive and respiratory tracts,[91] and stereotactic surgery in the central nervous system.[107] Anesthesia has become much safer for older individuals, including those older than age 100.[108]

## RADIATION THERAPY

Radiation therapy is particularly well tolerated by older individuals: two large European series of several thousand patients[109, 110] showed that the incidence of grade III and grade IV toxicity in patients past age 70 who were receiving curative therapy was less than 5%. Zachariah and colleagues reported similar figures for patients age 80 and older.[111] New forms of radiation therapy that promise to be particularly beneficial to the elderly include brachytherapy for prostate cancer and radiosurgery for brain tumors.[112] Hyperfractionated radiation therapy appears to be more effective than standard radiation therapy for tumors of the lung, esophagus, and upper airways, but it is also more toxic. The experience with this technique in older individuals is limited at present. The experience with chemoradiation therapy[113] is also limited.

## CYTOTOXIC CHEMOTHERAPY

The pharmacologic behavior of antineoplastic agents used in cytotoxic chemotherapy may undergo a number of age-related changes (Table 28–5). Probably, the most consistent age-related physiologic change is a progressive decline in glomerular filtration rate (GFR), which leads to a decline in the elimination of drugs such as methotrexate, bleomycin, carboplatin, and fludarabine, that are excreted through the kidneys.[12–15, 48] Careful dosing of these drugs may decrease the risk of complications in elderly patients.[12, 13, 114, 115] In treating patients with reduced GFR, a couple of considerations are also important. First, a number of drugs, such as the anthracyclines, give origin to active metabolites that are excreted renally, although the parent compound is eliminated through the bile. For example, 80% of the activity of idarubicin is due to the alcohol idarubicinol. In the presence of renal insufficiency, the excretion of idarubicinol is reduced and the toxicity of idarubicin enhanced.[116] The same occurs with cytarabine in high doses. The neurotoxic metabolite ara-uridine accumulates in the circulation of patients with renal insufficiency and causes cerebellar symptoms.[117] Second, a number of compensatory mechanisms make it difficult to predict the pharmacokinetics of different agents in individual patients. Burkowski and associates reported that the renal clearance of dichloromethotrexate but not the total clearance of the drug, declined with the age of the patient, suggesting that excretion by different mechanisms may occur.[118] Alternative mechanisms of excretion may explain the

*Table 28–5.* **Age-Related Changes in the Pharmacology of Antineoplastic Agents**

Pharmacokinetics
  Decreased elimination of drugs excreted through the kidney
  Variable activation and elimination of drugs metabolized in the liver
  Decreased volume of distribution of water-soluble drugs
    Decreased total water content
    Decreased cellular mass
    Decreased concentration of circulating albumins
    Anemia
Pharmacodynamics
  Increased prevalence of multidrug resistance
    MDR-1
    Impaired apoptosis
    Tumor anoxia
    Reduce tumor growth fraction
Enhanced toxicity to normal tissues
  Myelotoxicity
  Mucositis
  Cardiotoxicity
  Peripheral and central neurotoxicity

many different areas under the curve (AUC) experienced by different patients receiving the same doses of chemotherapy.[119]

The decline in volume of distribution of water-soluble agents is associated with an increased concentration of these drugs in the circulation and enhanced toxicity. Although the measurement of the total body water is available only in research settings, the measurement of the cellular mass may help direct the doses of hydrosoluble agents. The ratio of circulating cysteine/cystine provides a reliable measurement of the cellular mass.[120] The influence of anemia on drug toxicity is of particular interest because anemia may be reversible with erythropoietin. Several compounds, including the anthracyclines, the anthracendiones, the natural and synthetic alkaloids, the epipodophyllotoxins, and the taxanes, are heavily bound to red blood cells.[13] In the presence of anemia, the concentration of free drugs in the circulation is increased and the risk of complications enhanced.[121]

Pharmacodynamic changes may lessen the effectiveness of chemotherapy. Several forms of multidrug resistance have been described in neoplasms of the elderly. As already mentioned, the prevalence of myeloblasts expressing MDR-1 increases with age in patients with AML.[55] The incidence of neoplasms expressing the Bcl-2 gene, whose product prevents apoptosis, also increases with age.[122, 123] As the growth of some tumors becomes slower because of restriction of the tumor growth fraction, the target of cycle-active chemotherapy is also reduced. Anoxic tumor cells are resistant to megavoltage radiation therapy and alkylating agents. A higher concentration of anoxic tumor cells from reduced angiogenesis has been described in aged mice, and the same is likely in older individuals.[124] Other potential mechanisms of drug resistance include an increased concentration of glutathione reductase; an abnormal structure of enzymes that are targets of chemotherapy, such as dihydrofolate reductase and topoisomerase I and II; and abnormal intracellular drug transport and metabolism.[12, 13] Pharmacodynamic changes may also lead to enhanced drug toxicity. For example, Rudd and colleagues reported that the clearance of cisplatin-induced DNA adducts was delayed in the monocytes of older individuals.[125]

Age is associated with a decline in the functional reserve of many organ systems. The vulnerability of these organs to chemotherapy may thus be enhanced. In at least three studies, the myelotoxicity of chemotherapy did not appear to increase with the age of the patients. Newcomb and Carbone reviewed the experience accumulated by the Eastern Cooperative Oncology Group (ECOG) over 20 years.[9] Christman and coworkers reviewed the experience of women with metastatic breast cancer treated according to the protocols of the Piedmont Oncology Group.[126] Ibrahim and colleagues reviewed cases of metastatic breast cancer treated at M.D. Anderson Cancer Center over 20 years.[127] A number of considerations temper the generalization of these studies, however. First, patients older than age 70 represented a minority of all patients (12% in the study of Newcomb and Carbone, 8% in the study of Christman). Second, only a small minority of these patients were older than 75 years. Third, the doses of drugs were generally lower than those used in current studies. Seemingly, these patients embodied a small, healthy fringe of older patients—hardly representative of the older population at large.

A number of studies showed that the severity and duration of myelodepression increase after age 70.[128–130] Gomez and colleagues studied patients age 60 to 85 with large-cell NHL treated with CHOP (cyclophosphamide, hydroxydaunomycin [doxorubicin], Oncovin [vincristine], prednisone) and showed that the incidence of febrile neutropenia was 7% among those age 60 to 69, and 43% among the oldest, despite the use of granulocyte-macrophage colony-stimulating factor (GM-CSF).[130] The incidence of thrombocytopenia was 12% among the younger patients and 70% among the older patients.

The incidence of mucositis also increases with age and is particularly serious with the use of fluorinated pyrimidines.[131] Both a decreased reserve in mucosal stem cells and a decreased metabolism of the drug may contribute to mucositis.[132] The tissue concentration of dihydropyrimidine dehydrogenase (DPD) declines progressively with the age of the patient. Mucositis has resulted in a number of deaths among persons age 65 and older from volume depletion and shock.[133]

The incidence of cardiomyopathy, a complication of anthracyclines, anthracendiones, mitomycin C, and cyclophosphamide in high doses, shows a clear relation to patient age.[134] Peripheral neurotoxicity is a complication of several plant derivatives—including taxanes, vinca alkaloids, and epipodophyllotoxins—and of cisplatin.[135] Cerebellar toxicity may result from high doses of cytarabine,[117] and acute and chronic mental status changes may result from the simultaneous administration of radiation to the brain and cytotoxic chemotherapy.[136] Some agents, including ifosfamide, may cause subtle cognitive changes, such as loss of short-term memory and delirium. Seemingly these changes may precipitate dementia in patients with early cognitive decline.[136]

A number of provisions may reduce the risks of chemotherapy in older individuals (Table 28–6). The formula of Kintzel and Dorr[115] allows dose adjustment of compounds that are excreted or whose active and toxic metabolites are excreted through the kidney:

$$\text{Adjusted Dose} = (\text{standard dose}) \times f[Kf - 1] + 1$$

where $Kf$ = patient's creatinine clearance/120/min and f = fraction of the compound or active metabolite excreted through the kidney.

The most accurate clinical estimate of the GFR is provided by the formula of Cockroft and Gault.[137] Especially for a GFR of 50 ml/min or more, this formula reflected the clearance of radioactive hippurate better than did the calculation of the creatinine clearance based on 24-hour urine collection.[137] A reasonable approach is to adjust the first dose of the drug to renal function and to escalate the following doses according to the nadir blood counts.

The continuous intravenous infusion of doxorubicin may enhance the risk of mucositis.[138] Daily or weekly small doses of the drug may avoid cardiomyopathy without the emergence of other side effects.[139]

In about 60% of patients, hemoglobin levels may be maintained at 10 g/dl or greater with erythropoietin.[140] This approach has two advantages: It may lessen the risk of drug-related complications and it may improve the general well-being of the patient by relieving fatigue. According to most studies, an 8-week trial of erythropoietin at 10,000 units three times per week or 40,000 units weekly is necessary to

**Table 28–6. Prevention of Chemotherapy-Related Risks in Older Individuals**

Pharmacologic provisions
  Dose adjustment of renally excretable agents to the patient's
    glomerular filtration rate
  Administration of anthracyclines by continuous intravenous
    infusion or small daily doses
  Maintenance of hemoglobin levels ≥11 g/dl
Use of antidotes to drug toxicity
  Myelodepression
    G-CSF, GM-CSF
    Interleukin-11
  Cardiomyopathy
    Dexrazoxane
    Digoxin
  Nephrotoxicity
    Amifostine
  Peripheral neurotoxicity
    Glutamic acid
    Pyridoxine
Prophylactic treatment of complications
  Sulfamethoxazole/trimethoprim in patients with prolonged
    neutropenia
  Fluid resuscitation of patients with diarrhea and mucositis
Use of alternative drugs
  Gemcitabine
  Vinorelbine
  Taxanes in low weekly doses

G-CSF, granulocyte colony–stimulating factor; GM-CSF, granulocyte-macrophage colony-stimulating factor.

obtain the best effect. If after 2 months of treatment hemoglobin levels do not increase 1 g/dl or more, and there is no reduction in the need for transfusion, 2 months of an additional trial at double dose may be indicated. The use of red blood cell transfusions to maintain levels of hemoglobin at 11 g/dl or greater is not indicated because of the risk of transfusion-related disease and refractoriness to more transfusions.

Of the antidotes to drug toxicity, granulocyte colony–stimulating factor (G-CSF) and GM-CSF appear indicated in persons age 70 and older who are receiving moderately toxic chemotherapy such as CHOP for lymphoma or cyclophosphamide-doxorubicin for breast cancer.[140-142] In these patients, the risk of neutropenic fever is higher than the threshold generally recommended for these compounds to be cost-effective. Also, neutropenic infections may be associated with increased mortality in older individuals.[143] IL-11 may prevent life-threatening thrombocytopenia, but it is not clear if it can be recommended for routine prophylactic use in older individuals.[144] Dexrazoxane is definitely indicated when doses of doxorubicin 300 or greater mg/m² or greater are planned and when doxorubicin is used in persons with borderline cardiac function.[145] As dexrazoxane may enhance chemotherapy-related myelodepression,[145] its routine use in patients receiving lower doxorubicin doses does not appear indicated. Although digoxin is not approved in the United States for the prevention of doxorubicin cardiomyopathy, this compound proved effective in an old Israeli study.[146] The substitution of dexrazoxane with digoxin may result in substantial savings. Amifostine, a thiol derivative, is approved in the United States for the prevention of nephrotoxicity from high doses of cisplatin.[147] This compound may also prevent cisplatin-related neuropathy, anthracycline-

related cardiomyopathy, and myelodepression from alkylating agents.[147] High cost and severe side effects, including hypotension and emesis, have prevented further study of this compound in the elderly.

Although the use of glutamic acid decreased the risk of vincristine-related neuropathy in an older study,[148] this compound did not encounter wide favor and currently is not available. Pyridoxine is routinely used for this purpose, but the effectiveness of this compound has been documented only in the treatment of fluorouracil-related neuropathy.[149, 150]

The early intervention of aggressive fluid resuscitation may be life-saving in older individuals, whose limited functional reserve makes them particularly vulnerable to volume depletion.[133]

A number of new drugs allow the safe treatment of debilitated patients because of a favorable toxicity profile.[151] Gemcitabine has a wide spectrum of action that includes pancreatic neoplasms, non–small cell lung cancer, cancer of the breast, and transitional-cell carcinoma.[152-155] Vinorelbine (Navelbine)[156] and low weekly doses of taxanes[157] are effective in breast and non–small cell lung cancer.

Other drugs may substitute for doxorubicin with a reduced risk of cardiotoxicity. They include the anthracendiones mitoxantrone and losoxantrone[151] and the liposomal anthracyclines.[158] An advantage of the anthracendiones is their high level of tolerability, with a minimal incidence of alopecia and fatigue. More studies are needed, however, to establish whether the activity of these agents is comparable to that of doxorubicin. In two randomized, controlled studies of NHL, mitoxantrone appeared less active than doxorubicin.[159, 160] From the previous discussion, a number of clinical guidelines may be derived for the management of patients age 70 or older with chemotherapy (Table 28–7). These guidelines are in a state of continuous evolution. Interventions that may be added in the near future include the prophylactic use of erythropoietin in patients who are not anemic[161] and the prophylactic use of IL-11.[144]

## BIOLOGIC THERAPY FOR CANCER

Biologic therapy for cancer is of special interest to older individuals for two reasons. First, reversal of immune senes-

**Table 28–7. General Recommendations for Cytotoxic Chemotherapy in Persons Age 70 and Older**

1. Adjust first doses of renally excretable drugs to the patient's GFR
2. Escalate successive doses according to nadir counts
3. Try to maintain hemoglobin levels ≥11 mg/dl
4. Routinely use G-CSF or GM-CSF for chemotherapy with moderate myelodepression (CHOP, CA, CAF)
5. Use IL-11 after an episode of thrombocytopenia requiring platelet transfusions
6. Consider low daily doses of doxorubicin
7. Consider substitution of doxorubicin with mitoxantrone in the management of breast cancer or with liposomal anthracyclines
8. Use dexrazoxane when planning total doses of doxorubicin ≥300 mg/m²
9. Institute fluid resuscitation in patients with mucositis or diarrhea, or both, following chemotherapy

GFR, glomerular filtration rate; G-CSF, granulocyte colony–stimulating factor; GM-CSF, granulocyte-macrophage colony-stimulating factor; CHOP, cyclophosphamide, hydroxydaunomycin, Oncovin, prednisone; CA, cyclophosphamide, Adriamycin; CAF, cyclophosphamide, Adriamycin, fluorouracil; IL-11, interleukin-11.

cence may offset the growth of some tumors in the elderly. Second, biologic treatment is generally not associated with myelodepression and mucositis, which are particularly burdensome for the older patient. Current methods of biologic therapy include recombinant interferon alfa, IL-2, and monoclonal antibodies such as rituximab and trastuzumab.

Interferon at low doses, as used in the management of hairy cell leukemia, chronic myelogenous leukemia and other myeloproliferative disorders, and lymphomas, appears to be well tolerated in patients of all ages.[12] However, high doses of interferon, as used in the adjuvant treatment of melanoma, are associated with catatonic delirium in approximately 40% of patients age 70 and older.[162] Ongoing studies are evaluating methylphenidate (Ritalin) for the prevention of this major complication. The experience with IL-2 is limited in older individuals. At low subcutaneous doses, this agent appears to be tolerated by most patients of any age. However, the effectiveness of this treatment is questionable.

Rituximab induces a durable response in at least 40% of follicular lymphomas, the prevalence of which is highest among older individuals.[163] The only serious complication of this agent is a rare form of capillary leak, which is preventable by slow infusion of the drug. Trastuzumab, a monoclonal antibody targeted to the epidermal growth factor receptor, promises to improve the control of breast cancer with overexpression of the Her-2/*neu* oncogene.[164] The experience in older individuals is limited. The only concern results from a report that trastuzumab may potentiate the cardiotoxicity produced by anthracyclines.

### ORGAN PRESERVATION IN THE TREATMENT OF PRIMARY TUMORS

Organ preservation in lieu of radical surgery is achievable for cancer of the anus, the larynx, the esophagus, the bladder, and the rectum with the combination of chemotherapy and radiation therapy.[113] Organ preservation avoids the stress and the difficulty of prolonged rehabilitation in older individuals.

### PALLIATIVE TREATMENT

Palliative treatment of older individuals also presents special problems.[165, 166] For example, NSAIDs are associated with gastritis and renal insufficiency in older individuals, whereas narcotics may cause constipation, nausea and vomiting, and delirium. Also, the pharmacology of narcotics is unpredictable. The half-life of active morphine metabolites, such as morphine 3 sulfate and morphine-6-glucuronide, is more prolonged with a decline in the GFR. Also the balance of $\mu$ and $\delta$ narcotic receptors in the central nervous system may shift with age. As a result, the benefits of narcotics may be reduced and the complications enhanced. A special problem is the assessment of pain in older patients.[167] The roots of this problem include stoicism, an inability to use the pain scales, poor communication, and fear of the complications of narcotics.

Antineoplastic treatment, which has improved the survival and quality of life in patients with cancer, may be both effective and safe in older individuals. In addition to the precautions already described, patient selection is critical to the success of treatment in older individuals. The following section addresses the individualized management of the older cancer patient.

## The Older Person with Cancer

The distinctive characteristic of the older population, especially persons past the age of 70, is diversity (Table 28–8). The assessment of this diversity enables the practitioner to make individualized decisions in older cancer patients based on life expectancy and tolerance of treatment. Life expectancy is influenced by function, co-morbidity, and cognition.[168–170] The functional status of the older person is commonly assessed as activities of daily living (ADL)[171] and Instrumental Activities of Daily Living (IADL).[172] ADLs reflect the ability of a person to provide self-care and include feeding, transferring, grooming, toileting, dressing, and continence. IADLs reflect the person's ability to live independently and include cooking; using the phone, check book, and transportation; doing the laundry, housekeeping, and shopping; and taking medications. Siu and colleagues found that the 2-year mortality rate of persons age 70 and older correlated with the degree of dependence and rose from 8% for those who were totally independent to 42% for those who were institutionalized.[169] A number of direct tests of function have been proposed, including chair stand, walking speed, 360-degree turn, grip strength, reaching down and hand grasp. The advantage of these tests is their simplicity and time-effectiveness. However, the reproducibility of some tests is questionable, and their relation to outcome is unestablished.[173] At the same time, self-reporting of function by elderly patients is not always reliable.[173]

*Table 28–8.* **Elements of Diversity**

Function
    Performance status (PS)
    Activities of Daily Living (ADL)
    Instrumental Activities of Daily Living (IADL)
Co-morbidity
    Number of co-morbid conditions
    Co-morbidity index
Cognition
    Folstein's Mini-mental Status (MMS)
    Dementia Rating Scale (DRS)
Nutrition
    Mininutrition Assessment (MNA)
Social conditions
    Income
    Marital status
    Caregiver
    Living conditions
Depression
Polypharmacy
Geriatric syndromes
    Dementia
    Delirium
    Depression (new, with accentuated anhedonia)
    Falls ($\geq$3 unexplained falls yearly)
    Incontinence (continuous and irreversible)
    Osteoporosis
    Failure to thrive
    Neglect and abuse

The number of co-morbid conditions increases the risk for competitive causes of deaths. For women age 65 and older with breast cancer and no other co-morbidity, Satariano and Regland found the risk of dying of breast cancer to be 12-fold higher than that among women with three or more co-morbid conditions.[99] In addition to the number of co-morbid conditions, it is important to assess the seriousness of each condition. Several co-morbidity scales have been proposed to derive a co-morbidity index.[174] Of these, Charlson's scale[175] and the Cumulative Index of Related Symptoms—Geriatrics (CIRS-G)[176] have widespread use. Charlson's scale is brief and simple but of poor sensitivity; the CIRS-G is lengthy and cumbersome but highly sensitive. Of the patients enrolled in the Senior Adult Oncology Program at the H. Lee Moffitt Cancer Center in Tampa, Florida, 34% according to Charlson's scale and 94% according to the CIRS-G presented with significant co-morbidity.[177] In the same study, Extermann and colleagues tried to establish whether a single index could reflect function and co-morbidity but found poor correlation among co-morbidity, ADL, IADL, and ECOG performance status.[177]

Patient survival is inversely related to the severity of dementia.[178] Folstein's mini-mental status (MMS), which is easy and quick to administer and highly reproducible, scores mental status between 30 (normal) and 0 (lowest).[178] With the MMS one can distinguish mild, moderate, and severe dementia with scores of 25 to 30, 18 to 25, and less than 18, respectively. The Dementia Rating Scale (DRS) requires special training to administer but is very sensitive to early cognitive dysfunctions, unlike the MMS.[179] Early cognitive dysfunction is important for two reasons. First, progression of dementia may be halted with medications,[180] and second, patients with early dysfunction may be vulnerable to the cognitive complications of cancer chemotherapy.[136] In addition, the DRS is designed to discriminate among different types of dementia.

Tolerance of treatment has been predicted by the patient's performance status.[181] The classic performance status scales, such as the Karnofski and ECOG scales, may be inadequate for the older person because they are not age weighted. A moderate correlation between performance status and IADL was found by Fratino and colleagues[182] and by our group ($p = 0.61$).[177] Monfardini and colleagues determined that IADL dependence compromised the administration of chemotherapy to older cancer patients.[183] Seemingly, co-morbid conditions may reveal the vulnerability of specific organs to chemotherapy.

Other conditions are also relevant to the management of older individuals. Prevention of malnutrition may improve the patient's sense of general well-being and ameliorate the side effects of chemotherapy, in addition to avoiding the complications specific to malnutrition. Good nutritional status reduces the risk of surgical complications, and patients with cancer of the upper airways and upper digestive tract are particularly vulnerable to malnutrition.[184] Older patients at risk of malnutrition are identified with the mini–nutritional assessment (MNA), which has been validated in the older population of the Western world.[185] Risk factors include involuntary weight loss of 5% or more of the original body weight, body weight greater than 10% lower than ideal body weight, cancer of the upper airways and digestive tract, history of malabsorption, and erratic eating habits (fewer than two full meals a day). These patients require a more detailed assessment of nutritional history and status to identify a specific deficiency. Effective interventions include nutritional counseling, patency of the digestive tract, and provision of regular meals.

The prevalence of depression increases with age, is often associated with changes in living conditions (e.g., disability, a move to an assisted-living facility, death of a spouse), and may be precipitated by the diagnosis of cancer. In older persons, depression is often difficult to detect and is manifested mainly as anhedonia and withdrawal. A useful screening tool for depression is the Geriatric Depression Scale.[186] Without screening, depression often goes undiagnosed.

Identification of the caregiver is critical.[187] Most older patients undergoing cancer treatment depend on the assistance of another person for a number of issues, including transportation, business, feeding, and support. Generally the caregiver is an elderly spouse, also with limited functional reserve, or an adult child with a family of his or her own. The caregiver is subject to three types of pressure: to provide the best care to the patient, to allay tensions within the family, and to fulfill pre-existing obligations. Exhaustion in the caregiver is a common and devastating occurrence that usually compromises the treatment of the patient. This may be prevented by setting realistic goals and expectations, illustrating likely difficulties and possible solutions, explaining common family dynamics, and indicating sources of support and respite.

The use of multiple medications increases with the age of the population.[188] Common problems include duplication of medications, drug interactions, and unnecessary and potentially harmful medications. Alternative forms of cancer treatment are becoming increasingly common, even among older patients. These problems are generated and compounded by the absence of a primary care provider, the increasing availability of over-the-counter medications, and the common practice of exchanging prescription medications among members of the same family or the same retirement community. The interview with a pharmacist may correct many of these problems and institute a more organized drug program.

The geriatric syndromes represent a number of disorders that are characteristic of aging (see Table 28–7).[189] The presence of one or more geriatric syndromes qualifies a person not only as old but also as a frail elderly person (see further on). These syndromes need qualifications that distinguish them from similar disorders occurring in younger individuals. Delirium is an acute change in mental status. In older individuals, delirium may be the first manifestation of a mild respiratory or urinary tract infection, even in the absence of fever, and may also complicate other conditions that do not affect the central nervous system, such as acute myocardial infarction or pulmonary embolism. Falls should be frequent (at least three in a year), and without identifiable cause. Fecal or urinary incontinence should be repeated and irreversible. Osteoporosis should involve a spontaneous fracture or a decrement in bone mineral density of at least two standard deviations from the age-adjusted norms. Failure to thrive is the inability of some older individuals to gain weight and to improve their function despite adequate care, including adequate food and fluid intake.

Frailty is a landmark of aging.[190] The frail person is the

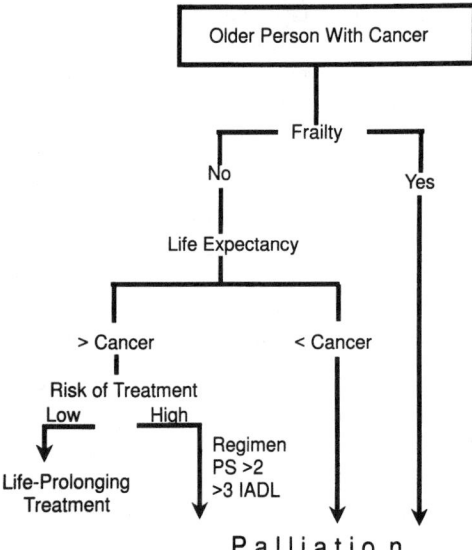

**Figure 28–7.** Guidelines for the treatment of older individuals with cancer based on life expectancy and Comprehensive Geriatric Assessment.

person without functional reserve. Frail elderly use the whole functional reserve for basic living activities. Any stress, no matter how minimal, may cause failure of these living activities and death. The definition of frailty includes one or more geriatric syndromes or age 85 and older, or three or more co-morbid conditions, or dependence in one or more ADLs, or a combination of these factors.

The estimate of life expectancy and treatment tolerance, and the definition of frailty, allow the design of an algorithm for the management of older individuals (Fig. 28–7). Obviously, this algorithm is susceptible to evolution with ongoing development in the field.

## Perspectives

The issues related to cancer and aging may be both general and tumor specific (Table 28–9). In the previous discussion we referred to patients age 70 and greater as older patients. This is a legitimate classification because prevalence of diversity in various realms increases steeply after age 70.[191]

*Table 28–9.* **Issues of Cancer and Aging**

General issues
    Molecular markers of aging
    Molecular markers of tumor-host interactions
    Pharmacologic studies
    Chemotherapy in frail patients
    Assessment of palliative response
    Rehabilitation
    Quality of life
Specific issues: breast cancer
    Necessity of radiation therapy after partial mastectomy
    Value of lymph node dissection
    Medical treatment of primary breast cancer
    Adjuvant hormonal therapy of the oldest old
    Adjuvant chemotherapy of women older than age 70

We also adopted the common geriatric distinction of young old (age 70 to 80), old old (age 80 to 84), and oldest old (age 85 and older). A reliable marker of aging that is more objective than chronologic age is highly desirable but still unattained. Circulating levels of IL-6 are increased in some geriatric syndromes, but no good correlation exists between levels of IL-6 and life expectancy or functional reserve. A promising marker is the ratio of cystine to thiolic groups (s/d) in the circulation, which reflects the total cellular mass. The ratio increases predictably with age and with cancer progression.[120] Future studies may explore the relation of s/d to survival, treatment tolerance, volume of distribution of water-soluble agents, nutritional therapy, and failure to thrive. This ratio may also allow confirmation of a common suspicion—that cancer and age are synergistic in their catabolic effects.

A better understanding of tumor-host interactions may provide important prognostic information, but no markers of this interaction are available for clinical use. Circulating levels of IL-6 predict a poor prognosis for large-cell lymphoma[52–54] but not for multiple myeloma.[192] Markers of special interest include the mononuclear cell infiltration and the angiogenesis of primary breast cancer.[50, 51]

The pharmacologic changes in older individuals are largely hypothetical.[12–14, 193, 194] Few studies have assessed the actual pharmacology of antineoplastic agents in the elderly. Parameters of immediate clinical applications include the relationship between GFR and drug elimination and the influence of hemoglobin concentration and cellular mass on drug toxicity.[120, 121] A proactive measure that may provide substantial information on the pharmacology of aging is the inclusion of patients age 70 and older in phase I studies.

New drugs, including vinorelbine and gemcitabine, may provide the palliation of choice for frail patients with cancer because of their favorable toxicity profile.[151] A number of new agents, such as angiogenesis inhibitors and monoclonal antibodies, may also be found suitable for this use and may blur the boundaries between life-prolonging treatment and pure palliation in frail individuals.

The assessment of pain, fatigue,[195] and quality of life[196, 197] is essential for the evaluation of the treatment outcome. In older patients, symptom scales are often not practical because of cognitive, visual, and auditory limitations. Also, quality of life scales have not been calibrated to age. Overcash and coworkers validated the Functional Assessment Cancer Treatment (the instrument of the ECOG) in individuals age 65 and older.[198] Qualitative research, which employs open-ended questions, text analysis, and story telling, may represent a valid alternative for the study of quality of life in the elderly.[199]

Breast cancer represents an excellent example of treatment-related issues that are age specific.[19] The need for postoperative irradiation after partial mastectomy has been questioned. A number of retrospective studies showed that the incidence of local recurrences declined with age, and in a prospective study, Veronesi and colleagues showed that the recurrence rate at 3 years was 17% for women younger than age 65 and 3% for those older than 65 years (see Fig. 28–6).[64] Although well tolerated,[200] radiation therapy to the breast is costly and time-consuming. An ongoing intergroup study explores this issue by comparing partial mastectomy and tamoxifen with and without postoperative radiation therapy in women age 70 and older.

The need for axillary dissection also has been questioned. The diffusion of lymph node mapping and sentinel lymph node biopsy may void this controversy, since only women with a positive sentinel lymph node undergo further dissection.[201]

The British Breast Cancer Campaign Trial showed that treatment of primary breast cancer with tamoxifen results in survival rates comparable to those of surgery plus tamoxifen in women age 70 and older.[202] However, the local progression rate was much higher for patients treated medically. A study by the European Organization for Research and Treatment of Cancer (EORTC) showed that surgery might improve survival after 5 years.[203] Considering the negligible morbidity of mastectomy, we question the benefit of a pure medical approach to primary breast cancer.

According to the most recent Oxford meta-analysis, adjuvant treatment with estrogen antagonists decreased the breast cancer–related mortality of women of all ages by approximately 30%,[72] although the data for women past 80 years are scarce. The benefit of adjuvant chemotherapy declined with the age of the patients, however.[204] This contrast is of special interest. Had this decline been due to competitive causes of deaths, it should also be observed with hormonal treatment. One must invoke either decreased efficacy of chemotherapy or increased risk of treatment-related mortality. This area definitely deserves randomized, controlled trials.

Other neoplasms involving age-specific questions include the acute leukemias; the NHLs; cancer of the large bowel, prostate, lung, cervix, and ovaries; and malignant melanoma.

## Conclusions

Increasingly, the practitioner has to face questions related to the prevention and treatment of cancer in older individuals, for example: "Are the interventions that are beneficial in younger individuals also beneficial for the elderly?" This chapter outlines the present status of knowledge and areas of potential research. We conclude the following:

- Cancer is a major clinical problem for persons age 65 to 85.
- Older persons may be at increased risk for late-stage carcinogens, and primary prevention of cancer is reasonable for older persons.
- The biology of some tumors changes with age, because of changes in the tumor cell itself or in the ability of the patient to support tumor growth.
- There are no conclusive studies demonstrating the benefits of cancer screening in persons older than age 70, but some form of screening appears reasonable for persons with a life expectancy of 3 years or more.
- The mortality from elective cancer surgery does not increase significantly up to age 80, but the mortality from emergency surgery increases progressively after age 60.
- Radiation therapy is well tolerated by person of all ages.
- A number of provisions may ameliorate the risk of cytotoxic chemotherapy in the elderly, including dose adjust-

ment of drugs that undergo renal excretion, correction of anemia, and the use of antidotes to drug toxicity.
- Individualized treatment must be based on a comprehensive geriatric assessment, including function, co-morbidity, cognition, identity of caregiver, nutrition, emotions, pharmacy, and presence of geriatric syndromes.
- Frail elderly individuals have no functional reserve and may benefit from palliative treatment only.

Areas of future research include the following:

- Interactions in the prevention of cancer and age
- Molecular markers of aging
- Markers of tumor-host interaction
- Pharmacologic studies of cancer chemotherapy in the elderly, exploring excretion mechanisms that do not include renal excretion, relationship of the AUC of drugs to anemia and cellular mass
- Palliative use of cytotoxic and biologic agents in older individuals
- Assessment of pain and quality of life in the older person

## REFERENCES

1. LaVecchia C, Levi F, Lucchini F, Negri E: International perspective of cancer and aging. In: Balducci L, Lyman GH, Ershler WB. Comprehensive geriatric oncology. London: Harwood Academic, 1998:19–94.
2. Yancik RM, Ries LA. Cancer in the older person: magnitude of the problem. How do we apply what we know? In: Balducci L, Lyman GH, Ershler WB. Comprehensive geriatric oncology. London: Harwood Academic, 1998:95–104.
3. Taeuber CM. Sixty five plus in America. revised edition. Current population reports special studies, P23–178RV. Washington DC: U.S. Government Printing Office, 1993.
4. Balducci L, Lyman GH. Cancer in the elderly: epidemiologic and clinical implications. Clin Geriatr Med 1997;13:1–14.
5. Fried LP, Storer DJ, King DE, et al. Diagnosis of illness presentation in the elderly. J Am Geriatr Soc 1991;39:117–23.
6. Manton KG, Soldo BJ. Dynamics of health changes in the oldest old. Milbank Q 1985;63:210–9.
7. Berlin NI. The conquest of cancer. Cancer Invest 1995;13:540–50.
8. Begg CB, Cohen JL, Ellerton J. Are the elderly predisposed to toxicity from cancer chemotherapy? An investigation using data from the Eastern Cooperative Oncology Group. Cancer Clin Trials 1980;3:369–74.
9. Newcomb PA, Carbone PP. Cancer treatment and age: patient perspectives. J Natl Cancer Inst 1993;85:1580–84.
10. Monfardini S, Yancik RM. Cancer in the elderly: meeting the challenge of an aging population. J Natl Cancer Inst 1993;85:532–8.
11. Ershler WB, Longo DL. Aging and cancer: issues of basic and clinical sciences. J Natl Cancer Inst 1997;89:1489–97.
12. Cova D, Beretta G, Balducci L. Chemotherapy of the older person with cancer. In: Balducci L, Lyman GH, Ershler WB. Comprehensive geriatric oncology. London: Harwood Academic, 1998:429–42.
13. Balducci L, Extermann M. Cancer chemotherapy in the older patient: what the medical oncologist needs to know. Cancer 1997;80:1317–22.
14. Kimmick G, Fleming R, Muss H, Balducci L. Cancer chemotherapy in older adults: a tolerability perspective. Drugs Aging 1997;10:134–49.
15. Baker SD, Grochow L. Pharmacology of cancer chemotherapy in the older person. Clin Geriatr Med 1997;13:169–83.
16. Lowemberg B, Aittoun R, Kerkhofs H, et al. On the value of intensive remission-induction chemotherapy in elderly patients of 65+ years with acute myeloid leukemia: a randomized phase III study of European Organization for Research and Treatment of Cancer Leukemia group. J Clin Oncol 1989;7:1268–74.
17. O'Reilly SE, Connors JM, Macpherson N, et al. Malignant lymphomas in the elderly. Clin Geriatr Med 1997;13:251–64.
18. Monfardini S, Carbone A. Non-Hodgkin's lymphomas. In: Balducci L, Lyman GH, Ershler WB. Comprehensive geriatric oncology. London: Harwood Academic, 1998:577–94.

19. Balducci L, Silliman RA, Baekey P. Breast cancer: an oncologic perspective. In: Balducci L, Lyman GH, Ershler WB. Comprehensive geriatric oncology. London: Harwood Academic, 1998:629–60.

20. Guadagnoli E, Shapiro C, Gurwitz JH, et al. Age-related patterns of care: evidence against ageism in the treatment of early-stage breast cancer. J Clin Oncol 1997;15:2338–44.

21. Greenfield S, Blanco DM, Elashoff RM, et al. Patterns of care related to age of breast cancer patients. JAMA 1987;257:2766–70.

22. Goodwin JS. Factors affecting the diagnosis and the treatment of older persons with cancer. In: Balducci L, Lyman GH, Ershler WB. Comprehensive geriatric oncology. London: Harwood Academic, 1998:115–22.

23. Mor V, Masterson-Allen S, Goldberg RJ, et al. Relationship between age at diagnosis and treatment received by cancer patients. J Am Geriatr Soc 1985;33:585–9.

24. Saltzstein SL, Behling CA, Baergen RN. Features of cancer in nonagenarians and centenarians. J Am Geriatr Soc 1998;46:994–8.

25. Flaker JM, Kiely DK. A practical approach to identifying mortality-related factors in established long-term care residents. J Am Geriatr Soc 1998;46:1012–15.

26. Bain MRS, Harvey JC, Muir CS. Epidemiology research in aging: perspectives and limitations. In: Balducci L, Lyman GH, Ershler WB. Comprehensive geriatric oncology. London: Harwood Academic, 1998;105–14.

27. Stanta G, Campagner L, Cavallieri F, Giarelli L. Cancer in the oldest old: what we learned from autopsy studies. Clin Geriatr Med 1997;13:55–68.

28. Caranasos GJ. Prevalence of cancer in older persons living at home and in institutions. Clin Geriatr Med 1997;13:15–31.

29. Anisimov I. Age as a risk factor in multistage carcinogenesis. In: Balducci L, Lyman GH, Ershler WB. Comprehensive geriatric oncology. London: Harwood Academic, 1998:157–78.

30. Fernandez Pol JA. Growth factors, oncogenes and aging. In: Balducci L, Lyman GH, Ershler WB. Comprehensive geriatric oncology. London: Harwood Academic, 1998:179–96.

31. Lee SW, Wei JY. Molecular interactions of aging and cancer. Clin Geriatr Med 1997;13:69–78.

32. Kim S, Jiang JC, Kirchman PA, et al. Cellular and molecular aging. In: Balducci L, Lyman GH, Ershler WB. Comprehensive geriatric oncology. London: Harwood Academic, 1998.

33. Minton S, Shaw G. Chemoprevention of cancer in the older person. In: Balducci L, Lyman GH, Ershler WB. Comprehensive geriatric oncology. London: Harwood Academic, 1998:307–24.

34. Campisi J. Aging and cancer: the double edged sword of proliferative senescence. J Am Geriatr Soc 1997;45:482–90.

35. Glass AG, Hoover RH. The emerging epidemic of melanoma and squamous cell cancer. JAMA 1989;262:2097–100.

36. Laszlo Keller K, Fenske NA, Glass LF. Cancer of the skin in the older patient. Clin Geriatr Med 1997;13:339–62.

37. Balducci L, Ballester O. Non-Hodgkin's lymphoma in the elderly. Cancer Control JHLMCC 1996;3:Suppl:5–14.

38. Ballester O, Moscinski L, Spiers A, Balducci L. Non-Hodgkin's lymphomas in the older person: a review. J Am Geriatr Soc 1992;20:277–84.

39. Greig NH, Ries LG, Yancik R, et al. Increasing annual incidence of primary brain tumors in the elderly. J Natl Cancer Inst 1990; 82:1621–4.

40. Flowers A. Brain tumors. In: Balducci L, Lyman GH, Ershler WB. Comprehensive geriatric oncology. London: Harwood Academic, 1998:703–20.

41. Fernandez PM, Brem S. Malignant brain tumors in the elderly. Clin Geriatr Med 1998;13:327–38.

42. Barbone F, Bovenzi M, Cavallieri F, et al. Air pollution and lung cancer in Trieste, Italy. Am J Epidemiol 1995;141:1161–9.

43. Shay JW. Molecular pathogenesis of aging and cancer: are telomeres and telomerase the connection? J Clin Pathol 1997;50:799–800.

44. DeLange T. Telomeres and senescence: ending the debate. Science 1998;279:334–5.

45. Vogt M. Independent induction of senescence by p16INK4a and p21CIP1 in spontaneously immortalized human fibroblasts. Cell Growth Differ 1998;9:139–46.

46. Yeager TR. Overcoming cellular senescence in human cancer pathogenesis. Genes Dev 1998;12:163–74.

47. Ershler WB. Tumor-host interactions, aging, and tumor growth. In: Balducci L, Lyman GH, Ershler WB. Comprehensive geriatric oncology. London: Harwood Academic, 1998:201–12.

48. Duthie EH. Physiology of aging: relevance to symptoms, perceptions, and treatment tolerance. In: Balducci L, Lyman GH, Ershler WB. Comprehensive geriatric oncology. London: Harwood Academic, 1998:247–62.

49. Burns EA, Goodwin JS. Immunological changes of aging. In: Balducci L, Lyman GH, Ershler WB. Comprehensive geriatric oncology. London: Harwood Academic, 1998:213–22.

50. Kurz HM, Jacquemier J, Amalric R, et al. Why are local recurrences after breast-conserving surgery more frequent in older patients? J Clin Oncol 1990;10:141–52.

51. Nixon AJ, Neuberg D, Hayes DF. Relationship of patient's age to pathologic features of the tumor and prognosis for patients with stage I and II breast cancer. J Clin Oncol 1994;12:888–94.

52. Ershler WB. Interleukin 6: a cytokine for gerontologists. J Am Geriatr Soc 1993;41:176–81.

53. Seymour JF, Talpaz M, Cabanillas F, et al. Serum interleukin 6 levels correlate with prognosis in diffuse large cell lymphoma. J Clin Oncol 1995;13:575–82.

54. Preti HA, Cabanillas F, Talpaz M, et al. Prognostic value of serum interleukin 6 in diffuse large cell lymphoma. Ann Intern Med 1997;127:186–94.

55. Willman CL. The prognostic significance of the expression and function of multidrug resistance transporter proteins in acute myeloid leukemia: studies of the Southwest Oncology Group Leukemia research program. Semin Hematol 1997;34:Suppl 5:25–33.

56. Extermann M. Acute leukemia in the elderly. Clin Geriatr Med 1997;13:227–44.

57. Buchner T. Treatment of acute myeloid leukemia in the older patient. In: Balducci L, Lyman GH, Ershler WB. Comprehensive geriatric oncology. London: Harwood Academic, 1998:545–50.

58. Daidone MG, Luisi A, Silvestrini R, et al. Biologic characteristics of primary breast cancer in the elderly. In: Balducci L, Lyman GH, Ershler WB. Comprehensive geriatric oncology. London: Harwood Academic, 1998:197–200.

59. Valentinis B, Silvestrini R, Daidone MG, et al. 3H-thymidine labeling index, hormone receptors, and ploidy in breast cancer in elderly patients. Breast Cancer Res Treat 1991;20:19–24.

60. Heimann R, Hellman S. Aging, progression and phenotype in breast cancer. J Clin Oncol 1998;16:2686–92.

61. Holmes FF. Clinical evidence for changes in tumor aggressiveness with age. In: Balducci L, Lyman GH, Ershler WB. Comprehensive geriatric oncology. London: Harwood Academic, 1998:223–8.

62. Galante E, Cerrotta AM, Crippa A. Outpatient treatment of clinically node-negative breast cancer in elderly women. Cancer Control JHLMCC 1994;1:344–9.

63. Wazer DE, Erban JK, Robert NJ, et al. Breast conservation in elderly women for clinically negative axillary lymph nodes without axillary dissection. Cancer 1994;74:878–83.

64. Veronesi U, Luini A, Del Vecchio M, et al. Radiotherapy after breast-conserving surgery in women with localized cancer of the breast. N Engl J Med 1993;328:1587–91.

65. Greil R. Prognosis and management strategies of lymphatic neoplasias in the elderly. Oncology 1998;55:189–217.

66. Host H, Lund E. Age as a prognostic factor in breast cancer. Cancer 1986;57:2217–21.

67. Balducci L, Barry P. A practical approach to the screening of asymptomatic older person with cancer. In: Balducci L, Lyman GH, Ershler WB. Comprehensive geriatric oncology. London: Harwood Academic, 1998:325–32.

68. Robinson B, Beghe C. Cancer screening in the elderly. Clin Geriatr Med 1997;13:97–118.

69. Edmiston K, Costanza M. Cancer screening in the older person. In: Balducci L, Lyman GH, Ershler WB. Comprehensive geriatric oncology. London: Harwood Academic, 1998:333–50.

70. Ragaz J, Coldman A. Survival impact of adjuvant tamoxifen on competing causes of mortality in breast cancer survivors, with analysis of mortality from contralateral breast cancer, cardiovascular events, endometrial cancer, and thromboembolic episodes. J Clin Oncol 1998;16:2018–24.

71. Veronesi U, Maisonneuve P, Costa A, et al. Prevention of breast cancer with tamoxifen: preliminary findings from the Italian Randomised Trial among hysterectomised women. Lancet 1998;352:93–7.

72. Early Breast Cancer Trialist Collaborative Study: Tamoxifen for early breast cancer: an overview of randomised trials. Lancet 1998;1451–67.

73. Cummings SR, Norton L, Eckert S, et al. Raloxifene reduces the risk

of breast cancer and may decrease the risk of endometrial cancer in postmenopausal women. Two year finding from the Multiple Outcomes of Raloxifene Evaluation Trial. Proc Am Soc Clin Oncol 1998;16:2a.

74. Hong WK, Sporn MB. Recent advances in chemoprevention of cancer. Science 1997;278:1073–7.

75. Fernandez E, LaVecchia C, Braga C, et al. Hormone replacement therapy and risk of colon and rectal cancer. Cancer Epidemiol Biomark Prev 1998;7:329–34.

76. Narod SA, Risch H, Moslehi R, et al. Oral contraceptives and the risk of hereditary ovarian cancer. N Engl J Med 1998;339:424–8.

77. Smalley W, DuBois RN. Colorectal cancer and non-steroidal anti-inflammatory drugs. Adv Pharmacol 1997;39:1–20.

78. Kerlikowske K, Grady D, Rubin SM, et al. Efficacy of screening mammography: a meta-analysis. JAMA 1995;273:149–54.

79. Toribara NW, Sleisinger MH. Screening for colorectal cancer. N Engl J Med 1995;332:861–7.

80. Goldberg TH, Chavin SI. Preventive medicine and screening in older adults. J Am Geriatr Soc 1997;45:344–54.

81. Balducci L, Pow-Sang J, Friedland J, Diaz J. Prostate cancer. Clin Geriatr Med 1997;13:307–26.

82. Labrie F, Dupont A, Candas B, et al. Decrease of prostate cancer death by screening: first data from the Quebec Prospective and Randomized Study. Proc Am Soc Clin Oncol 1998;16:2a.

83. McMahon BJ, London T. Workshop on screening for hepatocellular carcinoma. J Natl Cancer Inst 1991;83:916–21.

84. Melvin KEW, Miller HH, Tashjian AH. Early diagnosis of medullary carcinoma of the thyroid by means of calcitonin assay. N Engl J Med 1971;285:1115–9.

85. Nystrom L, Rutqvist LE, Wall S, et al. Breast cancer screening with mammography: overview of Swedish randomized trials. Lancet 1993;341:973–8.

86. vanDijck JAAM, Holland R, Verbeeck ALM, et al. Efficacy of mammographic screening in the elderly: a case-referent study in the Nijmegen program in the Netherlands. J Natl Cancer Inst 1994;86:934–8.

87. Fox SA, Roetzheim RG, Kington RS. Barriers to cancer prevention in the older person. In: Balducci L, Lyman GH, Ershler WB. Comprehensive geriatric oncology. London: Harwood Academic, 1998:351–62.

88. Coleman EA, Feuer EJ. Breast cancer screening among women from 65 to 74 years of age in 1987–1988 and in 1991. Ann Intern Med 1992;117:991–6.

89. Blustein J, Weiss LJ. The use of mammography by women aged 75 and older: factors related to health, functioning and age. J Am Geriatr Soc 1998;48:941–6.

90. Berger DH, Roslyn JJ. Cancer surgery in the elderly. Clin Geriatr Med 1997;13:119–42.

91. Pinkas H, Pencev D, Brady PG. The role of endoscopy in the management of gastrointestinal cancer. In: Balducci L, Lyman GH, Ershler WB. Comprehensive geriatric oncology. London: Harwood Academic, 1998:501–24.

92. Chodak GW, Thisted RA, Gerber GS, et al. Results of conservative management of clinically localized prostate cancer. N Engl J Med 1994;330:242–8.

93. Celentano DD, Klassen AC. The impact of aging on screening for cervical cancer. In: Balducci L, Lyman GH, Ershler WB. Geriatric oncology. Philadelphia: JB Lippincott, 1992:105–17.

94. Antonia SJ, Robinson LA, Ruckdeschel JC, Wagner H. Lung cancer. In: Balducci L, Lyman GH, Ershler WB. Comprehensive geriatric oncology. London: Harwood Academic, 1998:610–28.

95. Khuri SF, Daley J, Henderson W, et al. The national Veterans Administration Surgical Risk Study: risk adjustment for the comparative assessment of quality of surgical care. J Am Coll Surg 1995;180:519–53.

96. Karl RC, Smith SK, Fabri PJ. Validity of major cancer operations in elderly patients. Ann Surg Oncol 1995;2:107–13.

97. Fong Y, Blumgart LH, Fortner JG, et al. Pancreatic and liver resection for malignancy is safe and effective for the elderly. Ann Surg 1995;222:426–37.

98. Donegan WL. Operative treatment of cancer in older patients by general surgeon. In: Balducci L, Lyman GH, Ershler WB. Geriatric oncology. Philadelphia: JB Lippincott, 1992:151–9.

99. Satariano WA, Ragland DR. The effect of comorbidity on 3-year survival of women with primary breast cancer. Ann Intern Med 1994;120:104–10.

100. Coebergh JWW, Janssen-Heijnen MLG, Razenberg PPA. Prevalence of co-morbidity in newly diagnosed patients with cancer: a population-based study. Crit Rev Oncol Hematol 1998;27:97–100.

101. Piccirillo JF, Feinstein AR. Clinical symptoms and comorbidity: significance for the prognostic classification of cancer. Cancer 1996;77:834–42.

102. Goodwin JS, Samet JM, Hunt WC. Determinants of survival in older cancer patients. J Natl Cancer Inst 1996;88:1031–8.

103. Flacker JM, Kiely DK. A practical approach to identifying mortality-related factors in established long-term care residents. J Am Geriatr Soc 1998;46:1012–5.

104. Bennahum DA, Forman WB, Vellas B, et al. Life-expectancy, comorbidity, and quality of life: a framework of reference for medical decisions. Clin Geriatr Med 1997;13:33–54.

105. Fisher B, Anderson S, Friedman MH. Reanalysis and results after 12 years of follow-up in a randomized clinical trial comparing total mastectomy with lumpectomy with and without irradiation in the treatment of breast cancer. N Engl J Med 1995;333:1456–61.

106. Rounaet P, Saint Aubert B, Fabre JM, et al. Conservative treatment for low rectal carcinoma by local excision with or without radiotherapy. Br J Surg 1993;80:1452–6.

107. Barnett GH, Kormos DW, Steiner CP, et al. Use of a frameless, armless stereotactic wand for brain tumor localization with two-dimensional and three-dimensional neuroimaging. Neurosurgery 1993;33:4–18.

108. Warner MA, Saletel RA, Schroeder DR, et al. Outcomes of anesthesia and surgery in people 100 years of age and older. J Am Geriatr Soc 1998;46:988–93.

109. Olmi P, Ausili-Cefaro GP, Balzi M, et al. Radiotherapy in the aged. Clin Geriatr Med 1997;13:143–68.

110. Scalliet P, Pignon T. Radiotherapy in the elderly. In: Balducci L, Lyman GH, Ershler WB. Comprehensive geriatric oncology. London: Harwood Academic, 1998:421–8.

111. Zachariah B, Casey L, Balducci L. Radiation therapy of the oldest old cancer patient: a study of effectiveness and toxicity. J Am Geriatr Soc 1995;43:1–3.

112. Brada M, Laing R. Radiotherapy/stereotactical external beam radiotherapy for malignant brain tumors: the Royal Marsden Hospital experience. Recent Results Cancer Res 1994;135:91–104.

113. Balducci L, Trotti A. Organ preservation: an effective and safe form of cancer treatment. Clin Geriatr Med 1997;13:185–202.

114. Gelman RS, Taylor SG. Cyclophosphamide, methotrexate and 5-fluorouracil chemotherapy in women more than 65 years old with advanced breast cancer. The elimination off age-trend in toxicity by using doses based on creatinine clearance. J Clin Oncol 1984;2:1406–14.

115. Kintzel PE, Dorr RT. Anticancer drug renal toxicity and elimination: dosing guidelines for altered renal function. Cancer Treat Rev 1995;21:33–64.

116. Doroshow JH. Anthracyclines and anthracendiones. In: Chabner BA, Longo DL, eds. Cancer chemotherapy and biotherapy. Philadelphia: Lippincott-Raven, 1996:409–34.

117. Rubin EH, Andersen JW, Berg DT, et al. Risk factors for high-dose cytarabine neurotoxicity: an analysis of a cancer and leukemia group B trial in patients with acute myeloid leukemia. J Clin Oncol 1992;10:948–53.

118. Burkowski JM, Duerr M, Donehower RC, et al. Relation between age and clearance rate of nine investigational anticancer drugs from phase I pharmacokinetic data. Cancer Chem Pharmacol 1994;33:493–6.

119. Gurney H. Dose calculation of anticancer drugs: a review of current practices and introduction of an alternative. J Clin Oncol 1996;14:2590–611.

120. Hack V, Breitkreutz R, Kinscherf R, et al. The redox state as a correlate of senescence and wasting and as target for therapeutic interventions. Blood 1998;92:59–67.

121. Balducci L, Hardy CH. Anemia of aging: a model of erythropoiesis in cancer patients. Cancer Control JHLMCC 1998;5:Suppl 1:17–21.

122. Hannun YA. Apoptosis and the dilemma of cancer chemotherapy. Blood 1997;89:1845–53.

123. Fischer DE. Apoptosis, chemotherapy, and aging. In: Balducci L, Lyman GH, Ershler WB. Comprehensive geriatric oncology. London: Harwood Academic, 1998:237–45.

124. Rockwell O, Hughes CS, Kennedy KA. Effects of host age on microenvironmental heterogeneity and efficacy of combined modality treatment in solid tumors. Int J Rad Oncol Biol Phys 1991;20:259–63.

125. Rudd GN, Hartley GA, Souhani RL. Persistence of cisplatin-induced interstrand crosslinking in peripheral blood mononuclear cells from elderly and younger individuals. Cancer Chemother Pharmacol 1995;35:323–6.

126. Christman K, Muss HB, Case D, et al. Chemotherapy of metastatic breast cancer in the elderly. JAMA 1992;268:57–62.

127. Ibrahim N, Buzdar A, Frye D, et al. Should age be a determinant factor in treating breast cancer patients with combination chemotherapy? Proc Am Soc Clin Oncol 1993;12:68.

128. Rowe J, Andersen JW, Mazza JJ, et al. A randomized placebo-controlled phase III study of granulocyte-macrophage colony–stimulating factor in adult patients (>55 to 70 years of age) with acute myelogenous leukemia: a study of the Eastern Cooperative Oncology Group. Blood 1995;86:457–62.

129. Bastion Y, Blay J-Y, Divine M, et al. Elderly patients with aggressive Non-Hodgkin's lymphoma: disease presentation, response to treatment, and survival. J Clin Oncol 1997;15:2945–53.

130. Gomez H, Mas L, Casanova L. Elderly patients with aggressive Non-Hodgkin's lymphoma Treated with CHOP chemotherapy plus granulocyte-macrophage colony stimulating factor: identification of two age subgroups with differing hematological toxicity. J Clin Oncol 1998;16:2352–8.

131. Stein BN, Petrelli NJ, Douglass HO, et al. Age and sex are independent predictors of 5-fluorouracil toxicity. Cancer 1995;75:11–17.

132. Balducci L, Phillips DM, Davis KM, et al. Systemic treatment of advanced cancer in the elderly. Arch Gerontol Ger 1988;7:119–50.

133. Petrelli N, Douglass HO, Herrera L, et al. The modulation of fluorouracil with leucovorin in metastatic colorectal carcinoma: a prospective randomized phase III trial. J Clin Oncol 1989;7:1419–26.

134. Allen A. The cardiotoxicity of chemotherapeutic drugs. Semin Oncol 1992;19:529–42.

135. Tuxen MK, Hansen SW. Neurotoxicity secondary to antineoplastic drugs. Cancer Treat Rev 1994;20:191–214.

136. McDonald DR. Neurotoxicity of chemotherapeutic agents. In: Perry MC. The chemotherapy source book. Baltimore: Williams & Wilkins, 1997:745–66.

137. Waller DC, Fleming JS, Ramsay B, et al. The accuracy of creatinine clearance with and without urine collection as a measure of glomerular filtration rate. Postgrad Med J 1991;67:42–6.

138. Legha SS, Benjamin RS, Mackay B, et al. Reduction of doxorubicin cardiotoxicity by prolonged continuous intravenous infusion. Ann Intern Med 1982;96:133–9.

139. Basser RL, Green MD. Strategies for prevention of anthracycline cardiotoxicity. Cancer Treat Rev 1993;19:57–77.

140. Glaspy J, Bukowski R, Steinberg D, et al. Impact of therapy with epoetin alfa on clinical outcomes in patients with non-myeloid malignancies during cancer chemotherapy in community oncology practices. J Clin Oncol 1997;15:1218–31.

141. Lyman GH, Lyman CG, Sanderson RA, Balducci L. Decision analysis of hematopoietic growth factor use in patients receiving cancer chemotherapy. J Natl Cancer Inst 1993;85:488–93.

142. Zagonel V, Pinto A, Monfardini S. Strategies to prevent chemotherapy-related toxicity in the older person. In: Balducci L, Lyman GH, Ershler WB. Comprehensive geriatric oncology. London: Harwood Academic, 1998:481–500.

143. Greene JN. Management of infectious complications. In: Balducci L, Lyman GH, Ershler WB. Comprehensive geriatric oncology. London: Harwood Academic, 1998:733–42.

144. Isaacs C, Robert NJ, Bailey FA, et al. Randomized placebo-controlled study of recombinant human interleukin 11 to prevent chemotherapy-induced thrombocytopenia in patients with breast cancer receiving dose-intensive cyclophosphamide and doxorubicin. J Clin Oncol 1997;15:3368–77.

145. Swain SM, Whaley FS, Gerber MC, et al. Cardioprotection with dexrazoxane for doxorubicin-containing therapy in advanced breast cancer. J Clin Oncol 1997;15:1318–32.

146. Guthrie D, Gibson AL. Doxorubicin cardiotoxicity: possible role of digoxin in its prevention. Br Med J 1997;2:1447–9.

147. Kemp G, Rose P, Lurain J, et al. Amifostine pretreatment for protection against cyclophosphamide-induced and cisplatin-induced toxicities: results of a randomized control trial in patients with advanced ovarian cancer. J Clin Oncol 1996;14:2101–12.

148. Jackson DV, Wells HB, Atkins JN, et al. Amelioration of vincristine neurotoxicity by glutamic acid. Am J Med 1988;84:1016–22.

149. Vukelja SJ. Pyridoxine for the palmar-plantar erythrodysthesis syndrome. Ann Intern Med 1989;111:688–9.

150. Fabian CJ. Pyridoxine therapy for palmar-plantar erythrodysesthesia associated with continuous 5-fluorouracil infusion. Invest New Drugs 1990;8:57–63.

151. Eckardt JR, Von Hoff DD. New antineoplastic agents of interest for the older patient. In: Balducci L, Lyman GH, Ershler WB. Comprehensive geriatric oncology. London: Harwood Academic, 1998:443–70.

152. Burris HA, Moore MJ, Andersen J, et al. Improvement in survival and clinical benefits with gemcitabine as front-line therapy for patients with advanced pancreatic cancer: a randomized trial. J Clin Oncol 1997;15:2403–13.

153. Anderson H, Lund B, Bach F, et al. Single-agent activity of weekly gemcitabine in advanced non-small cell lung cancer: a phase II study. J Clin Oncol 1994;12:1821–6.

154. Blackstein M, Vogel CL, Ambinder R, et al. Phase II study of gemcitabine in patients with metastatic breast cancer. Proc Am Soc Clin Oncol 1996;15:A135.

155. DeLena M, Gridelli C, Lorusso V, et al. Gemcitabine activity in resistant stage IV bladder cancer. Proc Am Soc Clin Oncol 1996;15:A-622.

156. Goa KL, Faulds D. Vinorelbine. A review of its pharmacological properties and clinical use in cancer chemotherapy. Drugs Aging 1994;5:200–7.

157. Klaasen U, Harstrick A, Schleucher N, et al. Activity- and schedule-dependent interactions of paclitaxel, etoposide and hydroperoxy-ifosfamide in cisplatin-sensitive and refractory human ovarian carcinoma. Br J Cancer 1996;74:224–8.

158. Gill PS, Espina BM, Muggia F, et al. Phase I/II clinical and pharmacokinetic evaluation of liposomal daunorubicin. J Clin Oncol 1995;13:996–1003.

159. Sommerveld P, de Ridder M, van de Lelie H, et al. Comparison of doxorubicin and mitoxantrone in the treatment of elderly patients with advanced diffuse non-Hodgkin's lymphoma using CHOP vs. CNOP chemotherapy. J Clin Oncol 1995;13:2530–39.

160. Tirelli U, Errante D, Van Glabbeke M, et al. CHOP is the standard regimen in patients ≥70 years of age with intermediate-grade or high-grade non-Hodgkin's lymphoma: results of a randomized study of the European Organization for Research and Treatment of Cancer Lymphoma Cooperative Study Group. J Clin Oncol 1998;16:27–34.

161. Del Mastro L, Venturini M, Lionetto R, et al. Randomized phase III trial evaluating the role of erythropoietin in the prevention of chemotherapy-induced anemia. J Clin Oncol 1997;15:2715–21.

162. Nozaki O, Takagi C, Takaoka K, et al. Psychiatric manifestations accompanying interferon therapy for patients with chronic hepatitis C: an overview of cases in Japan. Psychiatry Clin Neurosci 1997;51:175–80.

163. Coiffier B, Ketterer N, Haioun C, et al. A randomized phase II study of rituximab at two dosages in patients with relapsed or refractory intermediate or high-grade lymphoma or in elderly patients in first line therapy. Proc Am Soc Hematol 1997;2271.

164. Cobleigh M, Vogel CL, Tripathy D, et al. Efficacy and safety of herceptin (humanized anti-HER-2 antibody) as a single agent in women with HER2 overexpression who relapsed following chemotherapy for metastatic breast cancer. Proc Am Soc Clin Oncol 1998;17:97a.

165. Shehaan DC, Forman WB. Symptomatic management of the older person with cancer. Clin Geriatr Med 1997;13:203–20.

166. Cleary JF. Cancer pain in the elderly. In: Balducci L, Lyman GH, Ershler WB. Comprehensive geriatric oncology. London: Harwood Academic, 1998:753–64.

167. Bernabei R, Gambassi G, Lapane K, et al. Management of pain in elderly patients with cancer. JAMA 1998;279:1877–82.

168. Beghe C, Balducci L. Geriatric oncology: perspectives from decision analysis. Arch Gerontol Geriatr 1990;10:141–62.

169. Siu AL, Moshita L, Blaustein J. Comprehensive geriatric assessment in a day hospital. J Am Geriatr Soc 1994;42:1094–9.

170. Inouye SK, Peduzzi PN, Robison JT, et al. Importance of functional measures in predicting mortality among older hospitalized patients. JAMA 1988;279:1187–93.

171. Katz S, Ford AB, Moskowitz RW, et al. Studies of illness in the aged: the index of ADL, a standardized measure of biological and psychosocial function. JAMA 1963;185:914–9.

172. Lawton MP, Brady EM. Assessment of older people: self-maintaining instrumental activities of daily living. Gerontologist 1969;9:179–86.

173. Tager IB, Swanson A, Satariano WA. Reliability of physical performance and self-reported functional measures in an older population. J Gerontol Med Sci 1998;53A:M295–M300.

174. Exterman M, Balducci L. Practical proposals for clinical protocols in elderly patients with cancer. In: Balducci L, Lyman GH, Ershler WB. Comprehensive geriatric oncology. London: Harwood Academic, 1998:263–70.

175. Charlson M, Szatrowski TP, Peterson J, et al. Validation of a combined comorbidity index. J Clin Epidemiol 1994;47:1245–51.

176. Conwell Y, Forbes NT, Cox C, et al. Validation of a measure of physical illness burden at autopsy: the cumulative illness rating scale. J Am Geriatr Soc 1993;41:38–41.

177. Extermann M, Overcash J, Lyman GH, et al. Comorbidity and functional status are independent in older cancer patients. J Clin Oncol 1998;16:1582–87.

178. Folstein MF, Folstein SE, McHugh PR. The Folstein mini-mental state examination: a practical method for grading the cognitive state of patients for the clinician. J Psychiatr Res 1975;12:189–98.

179. Salmon DP, Thal LJ, Buttes N, et al. Longitudinal evaluation of dementia of the Alzheimer type. Neurology 1990;40:1225–30.

180. Sunderland T. Cholinergic therapy and beyond. Am J Geriatr Psychiatry 1998;6:s56–s63.

181. Finkelstein DM, Ettinger DS, Ruckdeschel JC. Long-term survivors in metastatic non–small cell lung cancer: an Eastern Cooperative Oncology Group study. J Clin Oncol 1986;4:702–9.

182. Fratino L, Serraino D, LaConca G, et al. Is the Comprehensive Geriatric Assessment (CGA) more useful than performance status (PS) to evaluate the treatment choice in the elderly patients (EP) with haematological malignancies (HM)? XV Riunione Nazionale di Oncologia Sperimentale e Clinica. Cagliari, 4–7 Ottobre 1997. Tumori 1997;83:Suppl 1:244–87.

183. Monfardini S, Aapro M, Ferrucci L, et al. Cancer in the elderly. Eur J Cancer 1993;29A, 16, 2325–30.

184. Tchkmedyian NS, Heber D. Nutritional therapy. In: Balducci L, Lyman GH, Ershler WB. Comprehensive geriatric oncology. London: Harwood Academic, 1998;765–80.

185. Guigoz Y, Vellas B, Garry PJ. Mini-nutritional assessment: a practical assessment tool, for grading the nutritional status of elderly patients. In: Facts, Research and Interventions in Geriatrics 1997, New York: Springer, 1997:15–60.

186. Koenig HG, Ford SM, Sibert TE. Screening for depression in elderly patients. In: Vellas BJ, Albarede L, Garry PJ. Facts and research in gerontology journal, 1995. New York: Springer, 1995:119–30.

187. Haley WE, Ehrbar LA, Schonwetter RS. Family caregiving issues. In: Balducci L, Lyman GH, Ershler WB. Comprehensive geriatric oncology. London: Harwood Academic, 1998:805–12.

188. Corcoran ME. Polypharmacy in the older patient. In: Balducci L, Lyman GH, Ershler WB. Comprehensive geriatric oncology. London: Harwood Academic, 1998:525–32.

189. Vinograd CH, Gerety MB, Chung M, et al. Screening for frailty: criteria and predictors of outcome. J Am Geriatr Soc 1991;39:778–84.

190. Strawbridge WJ, Shema SJ, Balfour JL, et al. Antecedents of frailty over three decades in an older cohort. J Gerontol Social Sci 1998;53B:s9–s16.

191. Balducci L, Schonwetter R, Grey J, et al. Individualized treatment of the older cancer patient. Proc Am Geriatr Soc 1990;58.

192. Ballester O, Vesole D, Corrado C. Multiple myeloma. In: Balducci L, Lyman GH, Ershler WB. Comprehensive geriatric oncology. London: Harwood Academic, 1998:595–609.

193. Sotaniemi EA, Arranto AJ, Pelkonen O, et al. Age and cytochrome P450-linked drug metabolism in humans: an analysis of 226 subjects with equal histopathologic conditions. Clin Pharm Ther 1997;61:331–9.

194. Bonetti A, Franceschi T, Apostoli G, et al. Cisplatin pharmacokinetics in elderly patients. Ther Drug Monit 1994;16:477–82.

195. Broeckel J, Jacobsen P, Horton J, et al. Characteristics and correlates of fatigue after adjuvant chemotherapy for breast cancer. J Clin Oncol 1998;16:1689–96.

196. Cella D. Quality of life in advanced non-small cell lung cancer: results from the Eastern Cooperative Oncology Group Study E5592. Proc Am Soc Clin Oncol 1997;16:2a.

197. Balducci L. Quality of life of the older person with cancer. Drugs Aging 1994;4:313–24.

198. Overcash J, Extermann M, Parr J, Balducci L. Validation of the FACT-G in the older cancer patient. Proceedings of the 4th Conference on Cancer in the Elderly, Rome, Italy, 1998.

199. Maly RC. Qualitative research for the study of cancer and aging. Hematol Oncol Clin 2000;14:79–88.

200. Wyckoff JJ, Greenberg H, Sanderson R, et al. Breast irradiation in the older woman: a toxicity study. J Am Geriatr Soc 1994;42:150–2.

201. Albertini JJ, Lyman GH, Cox C, et al. Lymphatic mapping and sentinel node biopsy in the patient with breast cancer. JAMA 1996;276:1818–22.

202. Bates T, Riley DL, Houghton J, et al. Breast cancer in elderly women: a Cancer Research Campaign trial comparing treatment with tamoxifen and optimal surgery with tamoxifen alone. The Elderly Breast Cancer Working Party. Br J Surg 1991;78:591–4.

203. Mustacchi G, Lattaier J, Milani S, et al. Tamoxifen versus surgery plus tamoxifen as primary treatment for elderly patients with breast cancer: combined data from the "GRETA" and the "CRC" trial. Proc Am Soc Clin Oncol 1998;17:99a.

204. Early Breast Cancer Trialist Collaborative Group. Systemic treatment of early breast cancer by hormonal, cytotoxic or immune therapy: 133 randomised trials involving 31,000 recurrences and 24,000 deaths among 75,000 women. Lancet 1992;339:1–15 and 71–85.

## ACKNOWLEDGMENT

The authors wish to thank Anita Klamo for her most valuable editorial assistance.

# PART

# VI

# INVESTIGATIONAL THERAPY

# CHAPTER 29

# CLINICAL TRIAL DESIGN AND INTERPRETATION OF DATA

• STEVEN PIANTADOSI

In this chapter, I review concepts that are helpful in designing and interpreting clinical trials. The subject of clinical trials is a broad one, and I discuss only a portion of it. However, excellent materials are available that cover other important topics, including history and policy,[1, 2] general discussions,[3–12] cancer trials specifically,[13–21] ethics,[22–26] prognostic factor analyses,[27, 28] and reporting.[29–44]

The premise of this chapter is that clinicians are best served by understanding and emphasizing the design and interpretation of trials instead of their analysis. Clinicians usually do not have sufficient statistical background to analyze clinical trials reliably on their own. This matter is best left to the trial methodologists. However, a well-designed and well-executed trial usually provides clinically useful evidence with a simple analysis, the understanding of which is essential for the clinician.

In oncology, clinical trials are usually classified as phase I (pharmacologic), phase II (developmental), or phase III (comparative). These different types of trials have important design differences and substantially different roles in the development of new cancer therapies. I attempt to present a common perspective on all types of trials and emphasize statistical ways of thinking that can improve the design and interpretation of each of these studies. Because of their size, complexity, and importance in assessing relative efficacy, phase III studies receive more attention in this chapter.

The chapter begins by outlining some of the sources of uncertainty in inferences from clinical trials. Phase I and phase II trials are then discussed briefly. Next, I outline points in the design and conduct of phase III studies. Finally, both the analysis and the reporting of results are discussed.

## Bias and Variability

A clinical trial is a true experimental design. This means that the investigator specifies and controls the entry of subjects into the study, the assignment of treatments, the ascertainment of end points, and the analysis. Other types of investigations, some of which are also valuable to medical science, do not control all these components of a study. These control points illustrate the potential sources of uncertainty that affect medical investigations. The most convincing clinical trials use methods to control and minimize sources of uncertainty in each of these control points.

Two qualitatively different types of uncertainty or error can result when making inferences about clinical trials. They are bias (systematic error) and variability (random error). Both types of error can be controlled by using proper design, but neither error can be reliably controlled by analysis alone.

## BIAS

Although many sources and types of bias have been described,[44, 45] they all produce systematically high or low mistaken estimates of the true treatment effect. In any medical study, it is important to understand the relative magnitudes of bias and random error. In oncology, treatment effects that are about the same magnitude as potential biases are often clinically important. Furthermore, we seldom know the relative magnitude or direction of bias. For these reasons, control of systematic errors is especially important.

Most sources of bias can be controlled by appropriate use of (1) eligibility criteria, (2) quantitative end points, (3) impartial treatment assignment (in comparative trials), (4) treatment masking, (5) active end point ascertainment, (6) analysis of all study participants in accord with the trial design, and (7) adhering to a priori clinical hypotheses when reporting results.

Patients who agree to participate in a clinical trial are usually not representative of the population with the disease (selection bias). Although this can affect the external validity of the study, it may have little effect on the estimates of treatment differences. When the comparison group is subject to the same selection effect, as in randomized studies, relative treatment effects are estimated without bias and may well generalize to patients who do not meet the eligibility criteria. More damaging biases arise from exclusion of patients after study entry, loss of data for reasons associated with outcome or prognosis, differential assessment of end points in treatment groups, and retrospective definitions or analyses. For example, it often seems clinically appropriate to exclude patients because of "nonevaluability" or "noncompliance" with the study. However, compliance is both an outcome and a predictor. One cannot employ statistical methods assuming that compliance is only a predictor (e.g., make exclusions based on outcomes) without the potential for bias.

In some circumstances, data are missing for reasons associated with outcome. This can occur, for example, in time-to-event studies when a recurrence or death event is not observed because the patient has not returned to clinic for follow-up visits. Commonly used life-table methods assume that such study subjects are alive or, at best, censored at the time of last follow-up. This might result in an underreporting of events and can be corrected only by actively ascertaining the status of all patients periodically.

## RANDOM ERROR

The two types of random error that can result from a formal hypothesis test are shown in Table 29–1. The type I error is

*Table 29–1.* **Type I and Type II Random Errors Arising from Statistical Hypothesis Tests**

| Result of Hypothesis Test | True State of Nature | |
|---|---|---|
| | H₀ TRUE | H₀ FALSE |
| Reject H₀ | Type I error | No error |
| Do Not Reject H₀ | No error | Type II error |

a "false-positive" error and occurs if there is no treatment effect or difference, but the investigators wrongly conclude that there is. The chance of making a type I error is usually under the control of the investigator, even during the *analysis*, because the type I error is controlled by the level of significance chosen for statistical tests.

There are circumstances in which the type I error must be carefully considered when designing a clinical trial. When investigators examine accumulating data and repeatedly perform statistical tests, as is done in sequential or group sequential monitoring of clinical trials, failure to account for the effect of such repeated hypothesis tests increases the type I error rate. This is discussed in more detail further on.

The type II error is a "missed effect," which occurs when investigators fail to detect a treatment difference that is actually present. The *power* of a clinical trial is the chance of not making a type II error, that is, declaring a treatment effect of a specified size to be statistically significant. The type II error can be controlled only by proper design (i.e., a sufficiently large sample size) and not by any procedures used in the analysis of the study. The type II error depends on the hypothesized treatment difference: Declaring small differences to be statistically significant requires large samples, whereas even small trials have high power to detect large differences.

A common error is to design clinical trials whose power to detect clinically important treatment effects is low. For example, a small study may yield a high power to detect a large treatment difference. However, clinicians may be genuinely interested in modest or small treatment effects. A small study will usually have low power to reliably detect such differences. There is little sense in undertaking a trial when the chance of missing a clinically important effect is larger than the chance of finding it.

## Noncomparative Trials

### PHASE I TRIALS

Oncology clinical trials that focus on the dosing, toxicity, and side effects of new drugs are usually termed *phase I trials*. Their purpose is to study drug distribution, metabolism, excretion, and toxicity and, in the case of cytotoxic drugs, to determine the dose associated with tolerable and reversible side effects. Until recently, statistical thinking did not contribute extensively to the design of these studies. Instead, they were conducted using designs that evolved mostly in response to ethical and practical concerns. In oncology, these studies were often carried out in patients who had been treated previously with standard therapies.

The design concepts commonly used in phase I trials include (1) selection, in advance, of a small set of drug doses to be tried; (2) treatment of a small number of patients (e.g., three individuals) at each dose with toxicity monitoring; (3) decision rules for stopping the trial if toxicities in excess of a prespecified frequency are seen; and (4) escalation to the next higher dose if the stopping criteria are not met. When the stopping criteria are met, the dose chosen for subsequent trials is usually the one preceding the terminating dose. Often, between three and six additional patients are studied at that dose, with the total number of patients treated usually being fewer than 25 to 30.

This type of design alleviates certain practical and ethical problems in administering agents with unknown properties to humans. For example, it tends to minimize the number of patients treated at toxic doses of the drug. However, these same properties also tend to select conservative doses. Improved phase I designs have been suggested that correct this problem.[46, 47] In these designs, doses are not prespecified but are determined from the current results and a parametric form of the dose-toxicity curve. Also, the final sample size of the trial is not fixed in advance but depends on the toxicities seen. These designs have great promise, but it remains to be seen if they will be widely adopted.

### PHASE II TRIALS

After determining the pharmacologic properties of a new drug and a clinically useful dose, developmental trials focus on obtaining evidence of treatment feasibility and efficacy. These are usually termed *phase II trials*. For this discussion, I consider trials that use tumor response as an end point for evidence of efficacy. Two types of designs are commonly used: fixed sample size and staged. In fixed sample size trials, the number of study subjects is chosen in advance—for example, to yield a specified precision in the estimated response rate. Staged designs employ a treatment evaluation after groups of subjects have been entered, permitting early termination of accrual if high or low response rates are observed. Excellent working designs can be obtained from only two stages.[48]

Numerous other statistical issues arise in the design and evaluation of phase II trials, including patient selection, how to quantitatively evaluate response, patient exclusions, and the role of randomization. Space does not permit the discussion of these issues here. Reviews can be found in an article by Buyse and colleagues.[7]

**Sample Size for Phase II Trials.** Consider a phase II trial in which patients with ovarian cancer are treated with chemotherapy prior to surgical resection. A complete response, defined as *the absence of macroscopic and microscopic tumor at the time of surgery,* is expected to occur 55% of the time. We would like the 95% confidence interval of our estimate to be +15%. Approximate 95% confidence intervals for a proportion, *p,* are

$$p \pm 1.96 \times \sqrt{\frac{p(1-p)}{n}}$$

where *n* is the number of patients tested and 1.96 is the quantile from the normal distribution corresponding to a two-sided probability of 5%. Using this formula,[1] we have

$0.15 = 1.96 \times \sqrt{0.55(1 - 0.55)/n}$. Thus, $n = 42$ patients needed to meet the requirements for precision. Because 55% is just an estimate of the proportion and some patients may not complete the study, the actual sample size used would be increased to allow for dropouts. Accrual rates on previous similar studies may be used to estimate the expected duration of this study.

This example can be simplified slightly to yield a useful, but rough, rule of thumb for estimating sample sizes needed for proportions. Because $p(1 - p)$ is maximal for $p = 0.5$, an approximate and conservative relationship between $n$, the sample size, and $w$, the width of the 95% confidence interval, is $n = 1/w^2$. To achieve a precision of $+10\%$ (0.10), 100 patients are needed and a precision of $+20\%$ (0.20) requires 25 patients. This inverse-square relationship demands large sample sizes for high precision. This approximation is not valid for proportions that deviate greatly from 0.5. For example, for proportions less than about 0.2 or greater than about 0.8, exact binomial or other methods should be used to estimate precision and sample size.

For staged designs, more sophisticated methods are needed for sample-size estimation. [48]

## Comparative Trials

### DESIGNING PHASE III TRIALS

Designing phase III trials involves detailed discussions with investigators to resolve questions such as the following:

1. What is the best population to study?
2. Are the treatment methods unambiguously defined?
3. How will patients be allocated to treatment groups?
4. How will outcomes be measured, and what can be done to ensure that measurements will be obtained on all patients in all treatment groups?
5. What design features will minimize loss to follow-up and promote compliance to the treatment protocol?

Some points of good design for comparative trials are listed in Table 29–2. Most of these concerns must be addressed simultaneously.

**Quantifying Objectives.** Converting clinical objectives into quantitative measurements is a necessary but sometimes difficult task. Suppose we are interested in knowing whether

*Table 29–2.* **Helpful Concepts for Phase III Trial Design**

1. Select quantitative study objectives to meet clinical goals.
2. Define study population using eligibility and exclusion criteria. External validity may be enhanced by using broad criteria.
3. Realistically assess accrual resources using similar trials or surveys.
4. Specify treatments, treatment modifications, and methods of assigning patients to treatment.
5. Define study end points. Define methods and time of end-point assessment.
6. Calculate quantitative properties of design (power against meaningful alternatives, sample size, trial duration).
7. Establish procedures for collecting, editing, and quality-controlling data.

Adapted from Piantadosi S. Biostatistics for clinical trials. In: Abeloff M, Armitage J, Lichter A, Niederhuber J, eds. Clinical oncology. New York: Churchill Livingstone, 1995:339–54.

a certain therapy is associated with "lower toxicity." The measurement of toxicity is not automatically well defined and involves at least three aspects. The first is a window of time during which adverse events are likely to be the result of therapy. The second is a list of specific toxicities to be included. The third is a list of diagnostic criteria required to establish each diagnosis definitively.

Outcomes such as recurrence and death are often used in clinical trials because they can be treated quantitatively and are less subject to bias than are subjective measurements. Also, they usually correspond to definitive clinical questions. However, even quantitative outcomes can be weakened by passive ascertainment or postentry selection effects that affect one treatment group more than another.

**Study Population.** Differences in study populations resulting from different eligibility criteria probably explain many of the differences from seemingly identical clinical trials. Even when several institutions use identical protocols, interpretation of eligibility criteria and type of patients enrolled contribute to differences in results. Thus, trials from different institutions or within different periods, or both, may not be comparable even if the eligibility criteria are the same. This is one reason that randomized concurrent controls are so important for comparative trials.

It is well known that adverse outcomes such as drug toxicity and operative morbidity can be reduced by the careful selection of patients. Age restrictions can reduce the number and severity of many chemotherapy toxicities, although such restrictions are seldom made explicit. Eligibility criteria can be used to define a homogeneous study population, reducing variability in outcomes. However, if those excluded have the same response as those included, the trial would be needlessly prolonged. Some end points may be evaluated more easily if complicating factors are prevented by patient exclusion. For example, if patients with recent malignancies are excluded from a breast cancer trial, evaluation of recurrence and second primary lesions might be simpler.

**Estimate Accrual.** Low accrual is a preventable cause of early study termination. Investigators should be aware of the accrual rate required to complete a study in a certain fixed period of time, that is, a "best case" projection. Most researchers would like to see comparative treatment trials completed within 5 years and pilot or feasibility studies finished within 1 or 2 years. Disease prevention trials may take longer. In any case, the accrual rate required to complete a study within the time targeted can be determined easily from the total sample size required.

*Realistic* estimates of accrual rates are essential. The number of patients with a specific diagnosis can often be determined easily from hospital or clinic records but is an overestimate of potential study accrual. It must be reduced by the proportion of subjects likely to meet the eligibility criteria, and again by the proportion of those willing to participate in the trial (e.g., consenting to randomization). This latter proportion is usually less than half. Study duration can then be projected based on this potential accrual rate, which might be one fourth to one half of the patient population.

Investigators can project trial duration based on a "worst case" accrual. The study may still be feasible under such plans. Accrual estimates from outside institutions may be suspect. Is the study feasible as a single-institution trial? A formal survey of potential participants can be accomplished easily. Eligibility forms for patients seen prior to initiating the study can be filled out and sent to the coordinating center. These will provide a useful estimate of accrual.

**Treatment Specification.** Control of treatments and their allocation is a defining characteristic of true experimental designs. In practical situations, explicit plans are needed for modifications in the treatment of individual patients. To satisfy scientific objectives, essential components of the therapy should be guided by the protocol, but modifications that are unlikely to affect the outcome should be left to the treating physician.

Physicians participating in trials are always obligated to replace protocol treatments with others when they feel that it is in the best interest of the patient. However, sufficient flexibility in the treatment specification—especially concerning complications, toxicity, or side effects—may permit most patients to continue following the protocol. This could contribute more information to the trial results and enhance the credibility of the study report.

**Defining End Points and Methods of Assessment.** Three types of end points are frequently used in oncology trials: (1) continuously varying measurements, (2) dichotomous outcomes, and (3) event times. Each of these is discussed briefly.

Examples of measurements that can vary continuously over some range include many laboratory values, blood or serum levels of drugs or metabolites, functional measures, and physical dimensions. In the study population, these measurements have a probability distribution that can often be characterized by a mean and variance. This type of outcome is most useful when the primary effect of a treatment is to raise or lower the average measure in a population. Typical statistical tests that can detect differences such as these include the *t*-test (or a nonparametric analogue) and analyses of variance (for more than two groups). To control the effect of more than one factor simultaneously on outcome, linear regression models might be used.

Some outcomes have only two possible values. For example, a lesion might be present or absent. Other examples include some imprecise measurements such as tumor size, which might be described only as responding or not, and outcomes such as infection, which either is present or is not. Outcomes such as these are often summarized as a proportion. Comparing proportions might be performed using statistical tests such as the chi-squared test. Another useful summary is the odds ratio. The effect of prognostic factors or confounders on odds ratios can often be modeled using regression methods.

Event times, such as survival and recurrence times, are common and useful outcome measurements in clinical trials. Other intervals might be of clinical importance, such as time to hospital discharge or time spent on a ventilator. A complicating aspect of event-time outcomes is the possibility of censoring. This means that some subjects under observation may not experience the event by the end of the study. Using the information in the censored observation time correctly requires some special statistical procedures that lead to estimating event-time or "survival" distributions (e.g., life tables). Median times or proportions at fixed times are sometimes used to summarize these outcomes. The most

useful summary of event-time data is the hazard or failure rate.

There has been much discussion among clinical trialists concerning the use of "intermediate end points," which become known early after treatment but are reliably associated with definitive outcomes. Examples include premalignant lesions in cancer prevention and CD4 lymphocyte counts in acquired immunodeficiency syndrome. Intermediate end points are probably not as relevant to cancer treatment studies as to these other areas of study. One exception in oncology is the use of prostate-specific antigen to monitor prostate cancer recurrence.

**Treatment Allocation: Randomization.** Randomization is one of the most effective means for reducing bias because it guarantees that treatment assignment will not be confounded with patient prognostic factors. Randomization provides control over prognostic factors even if they are unknown to the investigators, and it also provides a basis for the validity of statistical tests.

One argument against randomization is that it is unnecessary because confounders can be controlled in the analysis by using statistical adjustment procedures. The extent to which this can be done relies on two additional assumptions: (1) the investigators have measured the confounders in the experimental subjects and (2) the assumptions of the statistical models or other adjustment procedures are known to be correct. Randomization is a more reliable method than adjustment because it controls bias without these assumptions.

**Quantitative Properties of the Design (Precision, Power, Duration).** It is not possible to specify a universally valid approach to answering questions about sample size and power in phase III trials; here I provide some basic ideas and examples. For a statistically oriented review, see Donner.[49] Computer software is available to perform many power and sample-size calculations,[50] but most programs are written for a statistician.

Comparative clinical trials are often designed to yield statistical hypothesis tests with desirable properties, such as a high power to detect important clinical differences. In trials with event time as the primary end point, the power of the study depends on the number of events (e.g., recurrences or deaths) observed. Under fairly flexible assumptions, one method of calculating power and sample size[51] requires that the size of such a study should satisfy

$$d = \frac{4(Z_\alpha + Z_\beta)^2}{(\log(\Delta))^2}$$

where $d$ is the total number of events needed on the study, $\Delta$ is the ratio of hazards in the two treatment groups, and $Z_\alpha$ and $Z_\beta$ are the normal quantiles for the type I and II error rates.

For example, to detect a hazard rate of 2 as being statistically significantly different from 1 using a two-sided 0.05 $\alpha$-level test with 90% power requires

$$\frac{4(1.96 + 1.282)^2}{(\log(2))^2} = 88 \; events.$$

Additional values for $\Delta$ and $d$ are shown in Table 29–3. Note that $d$ is not the final sample size. A sufficient number of patients must be enrolled in the study so as to yield 88 events in an interval of time appropriate for the trial. For

*Table 29–3.* **Total Events Required to Detect Hazard Ratios as Being Significantly Different from 1.0***

| Δ | Events |
|---|--------|
| 1.25 | 844 |
| 1.50 | 256 |
| 1.75 | 134 |
| 2.00 | 88 |
| 2.25 | 64 |
| 2.50 | 50 |

*All trials assume a two-sided 0.05 α-level test and 90% power.

example, if 50% of patients remain event free (censored) at the end of the trial, 176 subjects are required. In general, the sample size, *n,* is

$$n = \frac{d}{1 - p},$$

where *p* is the proportion censored.

## Trial Conduct

### MANAGING DATA

Processing information from patients in a clinical trial involves at least five components: (1) eligibility check and registration-randomization; (2) data acquisition from the source (clinical record); (3) editing, error checking, and quality control; (4) monitoring and interim reporting; and (5) analysis. When these components are properly performed, they reduce the frequency and severity of data errors. Space does not permit a thorough discussion of this subject; the first four components are summarized in the following section, and the fifth is discussed subsequently.

Eligibility check and registration constitute a simple but important quality control point. The knowledge that eligibility will be impartially checked causes many investigators to take entry criteria more seriously.

Data acquisition from the clinical record must be performed by an individual with sufficient clinical, protocol, and medical record knowledge. In some cases this requires the investigator's expertise, whereas in other circumstances a research nurse or data specialist can succeed. It is not necessary to record all the information needed for the care of the patient in the study database. Only items that correspond to the outcomes and objectives of the study are needed. Ideally, one would not collect any items that do not need analysis. Increasingly, it is necessary to audit significant portions of the clinical data collected to guarantee reliability.

Numerous quality control checks and edits are necessary to be certain that the database produced from paper records accurately represents the clinical record. For example, audits may compare the database with the chart. Within a single patient's record, computerized checks of bounds and internal consistency can be performed. When reviewed by a knowledgeable person, lists and summaries of the data can trap many errors.

Monitoring ongoing trials serves several purposes. It provides an opportunity for the investigators to review accumulating data related to administrative aspects of the study such as accrual rates and delinquent observations. Complication and toxicity rates can be reviewed to be certain that the type, frequency, and severity of such events are reasonable. Also, efficacy end points can be reviewed, following appropriate statistical guidelines, to satisfy ethical concerns.

Plans for monitoring and early stopping of accrual are another element of good trial design that can greatly alleviate problems in conducting studies. Researchers have an ethical obligation to learn about treatment differences as quickly as possible and to minimize the number of patients who are given a convincingly inferior treatment. By planning for early termination of accrual when unexpectedly large differences are observed, investigators can make a clinical trial more acceptable to other researchers and trial participants. A full discussion of sequential and group sequential methods for use in this context is beyond the scope of this chapter. These methods are now commonly used with well-described techniques.[52–61] Investigators can ensure that monitoring methods are effectively implemented by having the accumulating data reviewed formally at intervals by a monitoring committee.

Repeatedly performing statistical significance tests on accumulating data increases the overall type I error. If 10 interim analyses were conducted with the conventional significance level of 0.05, the resulting overall type I error could be as high as 15%. This inflation of the type I error can be even higher if many interim observations of the data are performed. To control the overall type I error, investigators must prospectively plan the analysis points and the significance levels to use, each of which will be smaller than the overall significance level.

For example, in a clinical trial comparing response rates and testing for significance after each third of the patients are accrued, a frequently used group sequential method[55] requires that the analyses be conducted with significance levels of 0.00052, 0.0142, and 0.046 to control the overall type I error at the conventional 5%. Note that the final analysis is conducted employing a significance level near, but less than, the usual 5%. Early in the trial, achieving statistical significance is more difficult.

A second reason for terminating a trial early is when interim analyses demonstrate the near equivalence of the treatments and continuing the trial would be unlikely to demonstrate clinically significant differences. In this circumstance, early discontinuance has been based on "conditional power" calculations.[61] Using this technique reduces the size and length of trials that show no effect or treatment difference but still yields clinically useful information.

## Analysis and Interpretation

The exact procedures necessary for analyzing a clinical trial depend on the design and purposes of the study. To meet their objectives, pharmacologic studies require modeling and estimation of physiologic parameters in each patient, whereas comparative trials usually require population summaries of relative or absolute treatment effects and confidence intervals. Analyses for these differing types of studies seem to have little in common. However, when we consider that all trials should inform us about the population being studied, the need for unbiased statistical estimation of clinical effects, and the need to summarize data in the most clinically useful form, much common ground is evident.

The approach that I recommend for analysis and interpretation emphasizes estimation rather than hypothesis testing.[35–41] Measuring and reporting clinical effects and associated estimates of variability (or confidence intervals) are more informative than reporting only formal tests of statistical hypotheses and *p* values.

In this spirit, I discuss the following basic concepts in the analysis and interpretation of clinical trials (Table 29–4). These steps are conceptual and do not necessarily occur in the order listed. Also, some steps are relevant only to randomized or comparative trials.

## INTENTION TO TREAT

Many factors contribute to patients failing to complete the assigned therapy on a trial, including severe side effects, disease progression, strong preference for a different treatment, and a change of mind. Thus, adherence to treatment is both an outcome and a predictor. Although there are often clinical perspectives that suggest it is mostly a predictor, this is not the case in general. Bias will likely result if adherence is assumed to be only a predictor.

To be certain that the trial results closely reflect the effect of the treatment, the eligibility criteria should exclude patients with characteristics that might prevent them from completing the therapy. For example, if the therapy is lengthy, perhaps only patients with good performance status should be eligible. If the treatment is highly toxic, only patients with normal function in major organ systems will be likely to complete the therapy.

*Table 29–4.* **Helpful Concepts for Trial Analysis and Interpretation**

1. Approach trial with a plan to analyze all patients entered in treatment group to which they were assigned. This is "intent to treat" principle. Plan to analyze all patients who met eligibility criteria.
2. Examine data and correct errors.
3. Qualitatively and quantitatively describe population on study. For comparative trials, verify comparability of treatment groups.
4. Estimate effect of treatment and other prognostic factors individually on major outcome. Estimate confidence intervals for these effects.
5. Use standard statistical methods or models to estimate treatment effect while adjusting for
   a. Statistically significantly imbalanced prognostic factors.
   b. Strong or influential prognostic factors, whether imbalanced or not.
   c. Any prognostic factor for which it is important to demonstrate convincing control.
6. Address secondary clinical questions. Any analyses not protected by randomization should correspond to clinical hypotheses stated as study objectives. Use methods to control prognostic factors for these analyses.
7. Consider repeating steps 1–6 after excluding ineligible patients, i.e., patients who are ineligible based on entry criteria.
8. Cautiously conduct exploratory or hypothesis-generating analyses:
   a. Any comparison suggested by data and not by hypothesis.
   b. Any comparison that excludes patients based on postentry criteria.
   c. Subset analyses.
      These should never be the "primary" analysis.

Adapted from Piantadosi S. Biostatistics for clinical trials. In: Abeloff M, Armitage J, Lichter A, Niederhuber J, eds. Clinical oncology. New York: Churchill Livingstone, 1995:339–54.

Following these considerations, the most important analysis in a randomized trial includes all patients entered in the trial, regardless of postentry events. Patients are analyzed with respect to the assigned treatment. This analysis is referred to as the "intention to treat" analysis. It is possible to exclude patients who were retrospectively found not to meet the eligibility criteria—that is, those who were mistakenly entered in the study—without creating bias. Only eligibility or pre-entry criteria should be used to make such exclusions. If patients are excluded based on "evaluability" or other postentry criteria, the possibility of bias increases.

## EXAMINING THE DATA

Knowledgeable investigators can prevent many problems in analyzing clinical trials by correcting errors that become apparent after inspecting the data. With the widespread use of computers to manage clinical information, it is possible to produce results from clinical studies without carefully examining the data. This is unfortunate because even a cursory examination of raw data by a technically knowledgeable person can detect many errors of importance to the analysis.

Some of the errors that can be detected by inspection include (1) missing data, (2) incorrect decimal points, (3) failure to convert numeric codes for special values, (4) out of range or impermissible values, (5) mislabeled variables, (6) coding and recoding errors, and (7) corrections attributable to investigator memory (especially in small studies).

## DESCRIBING THE STUDY POPULATION

Clinical trials are studies of well-defined and often relatively small cohorts. Although the eligibility criteria define a target population of particular interest, the patients actually accrued in a trial may differ because of either chance or institutional characteristics. Investigators should describe the cohort actually accrued, particularly with regard to important prognostic factors. Simple population measures and summary statistics usually suffice for this purpose. This process is also both a byproduct of, and valuable in, error checking.

Often in randomized studies, the first table presented in the report is intended to show the comparability of treatment groups. Statistically nonsignificant differences between the treatment groups do not guarantee the absence of influential imbalances but only demonstrate the effectiveness of randomization. Even so, demonstrating balance increases confidence in the validity of the findings. Although statistically significant differences between groups are a concern, nonsignificant imbalances in strong prognostic factors can also influence treatment comparisons. This is discussed more completely in the paragraphs on deciding when to adjust (see further on). Conversely, statistically significant imbalances are not necessarily influential because the imbalance may occur in a weak prognostic factor.

## TREATMENT AND PROGNOSTIC EFFECTS

Odds ratios are useful summaries of data when describing the effects of dichotomous variables, for example, differ-

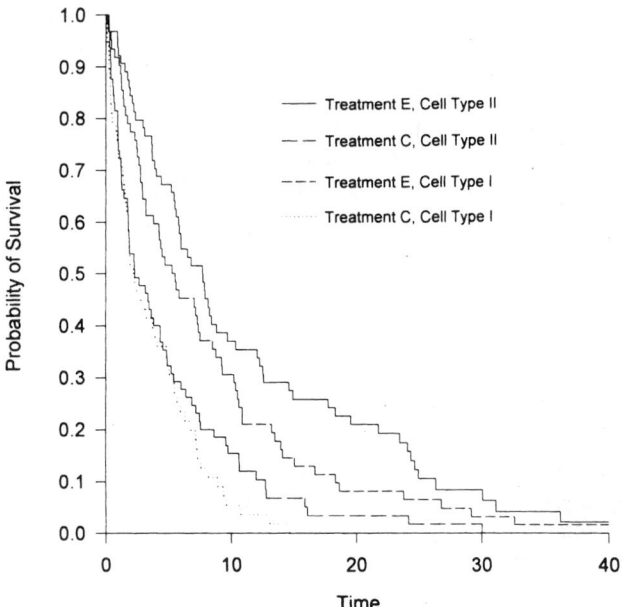

**Figure 29–1.** Survival by treatment group and cell type in a hypothetical clinical trial.

ences in the probability of response. Similarly, hazard ratios are useful for describing differences in risk of failure (survival) over time.

To illustrate these and other aspects of the estimation of clinical effects, data from a simulated randomized trial comparing two treatments (C and E) for treatment of central nervous system tumors are considered. The advantage to using simulated data, aside from convenience, is that the "true" treatment and covariate effects are known. In this case, the true treatment effects were a twofold odds of response and a 1.5-fold risk of death in favor of treatment E. For pathologic type, the odds of response was threefold and the risk of death was twofold, both in favor of cell type I. Response and survival were independent of one another. In what follows, the estimated effects differ from these values because of random variation.

Simple randomization was employed in this study, with 120 patients receiving treatment C and 130 patients receiving treatment E. Study end points were response and survival. Differences in response and survival attributable to pathologic type are also thought to be important. Nonparametric estimates of survival for subgroups defined by treatment–pathologic type combinations are shown in Figure 29–1.

**Odds and Hazard Ratios.** Response data for the two treatment groups are shown in Table 29–5. The estimated

**Table 29–5. Responses to Treatments for Central Nervous System Tumors**

| Treatment | Outcome | |
|---|---|---|
| | RESPONSE | NO RESPONSE |
| Group C | 26 | 94 |
| Group E | 36 | 94 |

**Table 29–6. Example of Odds Summary Data**

| Group | Cell Type | Patients | Responses | Response Odds |
|---|---|---|---|---|
| C | I | 9 | 49 | 0.183 |
| | II | 17 | 45 | 0.377 |
| | Overall | 26 | 94 | 0.277 |
| E | I | 8 | 57 | 0.140 |
| | II | 28 | 37 | 0.757 |
| | Overall | 36 | 94 | 0.383 |

response probability for treatment C was 0.217, compared with 0.277 for treatment E. The odds of response for treatment C is

$$odds_C = \frac{p}{1 - p} = \frac{0.217}{0.783} = 0.277.$$

A more useful quantity for judging the relative effect of treatment on response is the odds ratio. The estimate of the overall odds ratio for group E versus group C, $OR_{EC}$, is

$$\widehat{OR_{EC}} = \frac{94 \times 36}{94 \times 26} = 1.38$$

Because the odds of response for treatment E is higher than that for treatment C, this might be a clinically important difference regardless of the *p* value. The decision to use the odds ratio of E versus C or vice versa is purely a matter of convenience.

The results relating pathologic type and response are shown in Table 29–6. In treatment group C, the odds ratio for cell type II versus cell type I is 0.377/0.183 = 2.06. In treatment group E, the corresponding ratio is 5.39. Thus, it appears that cell type II is more likely to respond than cell type I, and this is explored further later in the analysis.

For event-time end points, the quantities of interest are the number of events in the groups and the total follow-up or exposure time (in years) (Table 29–7). The total exposure time is obtained by summing all follow-up times without regard to censoring. This represents the aggregate time at risk for the group. Thus, the estimated overall hazard of death in group C, $\hat{\lambda}_c$, is

$$\hat{\lambda}_C = \frac{119}{734} = 0.162 \; per \; person\text{-}year,$$

and for group E is

**Table 29–7. Example of Hazard Summary Data**

| Group | Cell Type | Patients | Exposure Time | Deaths | Hazard |
|---|---|---|---|---|---|
| C | I | 58 | 213 | 57 | 0.268 |
| | II | 62 | 522 | 62 | 0.119 |
| | Overall | 120 | 734 | 119 | 0.162 |
| E | I | 65 | 316 | 64 | 0.203 |
| | II | 65 | 694 | 61 | 0.088 |
| | Overall | 130 | 1010 | 125 | 0.124 |

$$\hat{\lambda}_E = \frac{125}{1010} = 0.124 \; per \; person\text{-}year.$$

The hazard ratio, $\Delta$, is

$$\Delta = \frac{\hat{\lambda}_C}{\hat{\lambda}_E} = \frac{0.162}{0.124} = 1.31.$$

From these data, we would conclude that the risk of death following treatment C is higher and that this difference might be of clinical importance. Here also, pathologic type appears to influence the risk of death. The estimated hazard ratios for cell type II versus cell type I are 0.443 and 0.433 for treatments C and E. The effect of pathologic type is explored later in more detail.

**Confidence Intervals.** A confidence interval is a region in which we believe that a true parameter lies. More rigorously, confidence intervals are probability statements about an estimate and not about the true parameter value. A 95% confidence interval indicates the region that would contain the true parameter value 95% of the time if we repeated the experiment. The value of confidence intervals is that they convey both the magnitude of the estimated clinical effect and a sense of its precision.

Continuing with the example of the randomized clinical trial, we first consider confidence intervals for the probability of response. Using the methods outlined for sample size in phase II trials, an approximate 95% confidence interval for the probability of response for treatment C is

$$0.217 \pm 1.96 \times \sqrt{\frac{0.217(1 - 0.217)}{120}} = 0.217 \pm 0.073 - [0.143, 0.290]$$

Similarly, an approximate 95% confidence interval for response for treatment E is $0.277 \pm 0.076 = [0.200, 0.354]$. Because of the large sample size and the intermediate size of the probabilities, these intervals are close to those that would be obtained using the binomial distributions, which are [0.147, 0.301] and [0.202, 0.362] for groups C and E, respectively.

Calculating approximate confidence intervals for odds and hazard ratios is easier on a log scale than on the "natural" scale. Converting from these to confidence intervals on the "natural" scale is simple. An approximate confidence interval for the log odds ratio for C versus E is

$$\log \{1.31\} \pm Z_\alpha \times \sqrt{\frac{1}{94} + \frac{1}{26} + \frac{1}{94} + \frac{1}{36}},$$

where $Z_\alpha$ is the point on normal distribution exceeded with probability $\alpha/2$ (e.g., for $\alpha = 0.05$, $Z_\alpha = 1.96$). This yields a confidence interval of [0.309, 0.850] for the log odds ratio or [0.73, 2.34] for the odds ratio. Because the 95% confidence interval for *dOREC* includes 1, the difference is not "statistically significant." In fact, the statistical test of the null hypothesis *H0: dOREC = 1* has significance level $p = 0.27$.

A similar method can be used for the hazard ratio. An approximate confidence interval for the log hazard ratio is

$$\log \{1.38\} \pm Z_\alpha \times \sqrt{\frac{1}{119} + \frac{1}{125}}.$$

This yields a confidence interval of [0.071, 0.573] for the log hazard ratio or [1.07, 1.77] for the hazard ratio. This 95% confidence interval excludes 1.0, indicating a "statistically significant" difference in the death rates between the groups.

**Why *p* Values Do Not Summarize Data.** The *p* value is helpful for characterizing the error from hypothesis tests but has properties that make it a poor summary of clinical effects. In particular, the size of a *p* value is a consequence of two things: the magnitude of the estimated effect and its variability (which is itself a consequence of sample size). Thus, the *p* value partially reflects the size of the experiment, which has no real biologic importance. The *p* value also obscures the magnitude of the treatment difference, which does have major biologic importance.

One often hears "the effect might be statistically significant in a larger sample." However, any effect other than zero is statistically significant in a large enough sample. Investigators should focus on the magnitude and clinical significance of an estimated treatment effect rather than on its *p* value.

## ADJUSTMENTS

Clinical trial statisticians disagree on the need for performing any adjusted analyses in randomized clinical trials. However, information gathered by adjusting for covariates can often help explain observed effects; that is, the difference in estimated treatment effects before and after adjustment often conveys useful knowledge. Furthermore, nonrandomized studies, such as cohort studies, are invariably analyzed with adjustment for confounders or prognostic factors. Errors due to confounding can arise in randomized clinical trials because of chance imbalances. This seems to provide a good rationale for examining the results of adjusted analyses.

Using statistical models and regression, investigators can estimate the treatment effect while adjusting for prognostic factors. One should consider adjusting for variables that meet any of the following three criteria: (1) prognostic factors that are statistically significantly imbalanced between the treatment groups; (2) strong or influential prognostic factors, whether imbalanced or not; or (3) to prove that a particular prognostic factor does not artificially create the treatment effect.

**Accounting for Multiple Effects.** The essential idea in adjustment is to relate the outcome to one or more predictor variables using a statistical model. The model consists of a structural equation, an error term, parameters (biologic constants), and empirical components (the observed data). If the model is approximately correct, it should predict the observed data "well" provided that we choose appropriate parameter values. Conversely, we can choose those parameter values that make the predictions and data "close" in some well-defined way. This latter sense is the way in which most statistical models are used. Trustworthy fitting methods exist (e.g., maximal likelihood) to estimate the best parameter values. Models also provide a means for obtaining confidence intervals, testing hypotheses, and even revising the model itself.

We return to the hypothetical randomized clinical trial of the previous section in which pathologic type appeared to influence response rate and survival. For response, an appro-

*Table 29–8.* **Logistic Regression Models Illustrating Adjusted Treatment Effects**

| Model | Variable | Odds Ratio | 95% Confidence Limits | *p* Value |
|---|---|---|---|---|
| 1 | E vs. C | 1.39 | 0.78–2.47 | 0.27 |
| 2 | Cell type I vs. II | 3.42 | 1.83–6.41 | <0.001 |
| 3 | E vs. C | 1.45 | 0.79–2.63 | 0.23 |
|   | Cell type I vs. II | 3.47 | 1.85–6.52 | <0.001 |

priate statistical model is the logistic regression model, the results of which are shown in Table 29–8. Models 1 and 2 show the overall odds ratios, confidence limits, and *p* values for treatment and pathologic type considered individually. Model 3 shows the joint effects of pathologic type and treatment group on response. When the effect of treatment is taken into account, cell type I is seen to have a higher response odds. Because the estimated odds ratios do not change much after adjustment, this suggests that pathologic type and treatment have nearly independent effects on response.

For the survival end point, the results of proportional hazards regression models, a widely used method, are shown in Table 29–9. The estimated hazard ratios are quantitatively similar to those determined in the previous section and show a higher risk for cell type II. Differences are due to different methods of calculation. The effect of treatment controlling for pathologic type is significant. The adjusted hazard ratios (model 3) also suggest independent effects for pathologic type and treatment on survival time. Note that the significance test for the treatment group hazard ratio differs slightly from the approximate calculation presented earlier but that the estimated hazard ratio is nearly identical. This difference highlights the point made previously about viewing *p* values cautiously.

## REPEATING ANALYSES

There are circumstances in which one would like to know if the exclusion of some patients from the analysis on the basis of clinical criteria affects the results. One such situation is the exclusion of ineligible patients in a randomized trial. Exclusions based on eligibility criteria do not violate the intention to treat principle because patients are still analyzed according to the treatment group to which they were assigned. In other circumstances, investigators may feel the

need to exclude eligible patients because of compelling clinical reasons. One can consider repeating the first six steps of analysis (see Table 29–4) after doing so. Provided that the fraction of patients excluded is small, say 5%, and affects both treatment groups equally (if the trial is comparative), it is likely that the results will agree with the "all patients randomized" analysis. This is as much an argument not to exclude patients as it is to allow exclusions.

## DATA EXPLORATION

Clinicians are generally agreeable (appropriately so) to conducting exploratory analyses of their data because many of these analyses are "explanatory" in nature. They offer the possibility of revealing more biologic structure than the rigorous analyses suggested by the experimental design. In other words, exploratory analyses are those that do not follow directly from the design of the experiment. Unfortunately, the results from these types of analyses can be unreliable. Therefore, the best role for exploratory analyses is to generate hypotheses to be tested more rigorously in the future.

Exploratory analyses may be unreliable for the following reasons:

1. A comparison suggested by the data and not by prior hypothesis is likely to have a type I error larger than the level of the test. This occurs because investigators find interesting, and test, only those differences that are large, most of which are probably due to chance.

2. Most poststudy classifications are based on variables that are both responses and predictors. Simple analyses that assume that such a variable is purely a predictor will likely be biased.

3. Subset analyses can easily be influenced by uncontrolled prognostic factors.

4. Testing differences between large numbers of subsets can lead to "significant" differences purely by chance (i.e., inflated type I error).

For these reasons, exploratory analyses should never be the primary analysis of a clinical trial.

## Publication of Trial Results

In this section, I outline basic reporting guidelines (Table 29–10) that follow the approach of estimation and confidence intervals. These guidelines should be helpful for reporting many types of clinical trials. They might also be useful for reviewing and interpreting published reports of trials or prognostic factor analyses. Published reports of clinical trial results are subject to constraints that analyses are not. For example, reports require a consensus among investigators and must undergo an imperfect editorial process prior to publication, whereas analyses can, and should, be more exploratory. The best chance of reaching a consensus among study investigators is to conduct analyses that draw strength from the design of the trial (as opposed to those that are speculative). These will likely have a certain minimal content and structure.

*Table 29–9.* **Proportional Hazards Regression Models Illustrating Adjusted Treatment Effects**

| Model | Variable | Hazard Ratio | 95% Confidence Limits | *p* Value |
|---|---|---|---|---|
| 1 | E vs. C | 1.25 | 0.97–1.61 | 0.08 |
| 2 | Cell type I vs. II | 2.12 | 1.63–2.76 | <0.001 |
| 3 | E vs. C | 1.30 | 1.01–1.68 | 0.04 |
|   | Cell type I vs. II | 2.16 | 1.65–2.81 | <0.001 |

*Table 29–10.* **Helpful Concepts for Reporting and Reviewing Results of Clinical Trials**

1. Report all clinically relevant descriptions of trial population, possibly including patients who met eligibility criteria but chose not to participate.
2. Describe those patients who were retrospectively found to have failed eligibility criteria and those patients who failed to complete assigned treatment.
3. Report all statistical methods and assumptions made.
4. Report estimated treatment effects (log odds ratios or hazard ratios), confidence intervals, and significance levels of tests of no treatment effect (*p* values). Absolute treatment effects may be as clinically relevant as relative treatment effects.
5. When appropriate, report adjusted estimates of treatment effects, confidence intervals, and *p* values.
6. Report any differences between "intention to treat" analyses and "eligible patient" analyses, if performed. If "treatment received" analyses are clinically compelling, report these and how they differ from "intention to treat" results.
7. Results with strong biologic or clinical justification and *p* values near 0.05 could be called "statistically significant."
8. Results without biologic or clinical back-up or those that seem contradictory should be reported but interpreted with caution.
9. Represent exploratory or hypothesis-generating analyses accurately and cautiously.

Adapted from Piantadosi S. Biostatistics for clinical trials. In: Abeloff M, Armitage J, Lichter A, Niederhuber J. Clinical oncology. New York: Churchill Livingstone, 1995:339–54.

## DESCRIBING THE STUDY POPULATION

Clinically relevant descriptions of both the study and the target population should be reported. It may also be important to describe patients who met the eligibility criteria but chose not to participate in the trial, when this information is available. The need for this might arise when patients from a large group are asked to participate but many refuse. As pointed out earlier, it may be difficult to generalize from these situations. For nonrandomized designs, even detailed descriptions of the study group may not provide a convincing basis on which to make comparisons with other studies. Thus, comparison is not the motivation, but thoroughness is.

## TREATMENT AND ELIGIBILITY FAILURES

As mentioned, it is acceptable to perform statistical analyses on only the subset of eligible patients, even when eligibility is corrected in retrospect. This does not create bias in the estimate of relative effects within the trial. Investigators should report patients who were retrospectively found to have failed the eligibility criteria as well as patients who failed to complete the assigned treatment.

There are situations in which a large fraction of patients complete the assigned therapy but may receive additional therapy not specified by the protocol or design of the trial. For example, patients with esophageal cancer may undergo resection and chemotherapy and have a variety of second-line treatments if signs of disease progression or recurrence are observed. If some of these latter treatments are active, the results of an initial treatment comparison based on recurrence or survival may be skewed. In fact, in general it is difficult or impossible to use the statistical information in studies that permit "crossovers" either to new treatments or to the other treatment arm. One cannot exclude these patients but can use only the information up to the time that the assigned treatment is stopped.

## STATISTICAL METHODS AND ASSUMPTIONS

Readers should be made aware of any assumptions made in both the design and the analysis of a clinical trial. The assumptions and limitations of many common statistical procedures are well understood by clinicians. However, the readers of clinical trial reports should be convinced that the data analyst has verified all important assumptions and reported the methods in detail for less well-known statistical procedures. Examples of assumptions that are often made in analysis, often violated by the data, and also likely to be consequential are distributional assumptions underlying the *t*-test or other statistical hypothesis tests, error distributions in linear regression analyses, and proportionality of hazards in life-table regressions.

For example, the *t*-test assumes that the distributions being compared are normal with equal variances. It can yield incorrect results when either of these assumptions is false, particularly if distributions are not symmetric. Proportional hazards regression models most often assume that the effect of predictors is to multiply a baseline risk and that the multiplicative factor is constant over time. Although the model is robust to departures from this assumption (i.e., it will often yield the correct estimates of relative risk and significance levels anyway), it is helpful to validate the assumptions.

## UNIVARIATE ANALYSES

It is likely that the data analyst will test the effect of all potentially important prognostic variables on the major outcomes. For these univariate analyses, investigators should report estimated treatment effects (odds ratios or hazard ratios), confidence intervals, and significance levels of tests of no treatment effect (*p* values). This does not preclude presenting other displays of univariate analyses (e.g., survival curves or 2 × 2 tables) if these analyses are especially relevant. However, the investigators should keep in mind that univariate analyses, particularly in uncontrolled studies, are subject to confounding. Consequently, these analyses should probably not be emphasized or presented in excessive detail.

## ADJUSTED ANALYSES

In a randomized trial, the univariate comparison of treatment groups is a simple and valid summary. However, many investigators attempt to show that the treatment effect is not due to any measured confounders by using adjusted analyses. The best style of reporting multivariate analyses is the same or similar to that for univariate effects. However, the adjusted analyses reported are usually selected from a larger set of less informative or preliminary results. As an example, consider a life-table regression model attempting to predict time to cancer recurrence. The "best" (most predictive but parsimonious) model might be built using a step-down procedure from a large set of potential prognostic factors. Each step in the analysis need not be reported, but the final model is a major objective of the analysis.

For multiple regression analyses, investigators usually report adjusted estimates of treatment effects, confidence intervals, and *p* values. Not all prognostic factors retained in multiple regression models must be "statistically significant." It is often useful to keep nonsignificant effects in a multiple regression model to demonstrate convincingly that the treatment effect persists in their presence.

## NEGATIVE FINDINGS

When no statistically significant treatment effect or difference is found, the power of the study is sometimes called into question. However, the absence of a significant difference is not the same as evidence of no effect. Because clinical effects are measured by risk ratios rather than *p* values, guidelines given previously emphasizing estimated treatment differences rather than hypothesis tests are important. Helpful advice regarding negative clinical trials is provided by Detsky and Sackett.[42] Power calculations performed after the study is completed are rarely, if ever, helpful.

## EFFECT OF PATIENT EXCLUSIONS

Although I have emphasized the value of the intent to treat principle and related analyses, in practice many exploratory analyses are performed. Investigators should report any differences between "intention to treat" analyses and "eligible patient" analyses. If subset analyses are performed, discrepancies between these and the major analyses of the clinical trial should be reported.

## WHAT IS SIGNIFICANT?

The *p* value should not be the only criterion for "significance." Results with strong biologic or clinical justification and *p* values near 0.05 are "statistically significant." When biologic justification is strong, effect estimates are large, and confidence intervals or *p* values indicate significance near conventional levels, it seems appropriate to label these results as "statistically significant." Conversely, results with no biologic or clinical justification or those that seem paradoxical should be reported and interpreted with caution, even when *p* values are smaller than 0.05. There is no way to separate type I errors from truly significant results except to rely on additional evidence and biologic rationale. It is wise to report cautiously results that seem not to make sense.

## EXPLORATORY ANALYSES

Exploratory or hypothesis-generating analyses should only be informally reported. They should not be emphasized as the primary findings of a clinical trial unless supported by the design and a priori hypothesis.

## Summary and Conclusions

In developing new cancer treatments, investigators are often interested in treatment effects and differences that are about the same size as the variability or the bias that is a part of all clinical studies. The only solution for making valid inferences in the face of these potential errors is to properly design, conduct, and analyze clinical trials. There are a small number of important design considerations to help control bias and random errors, including the use of randomization, blinding, stratification, adequate sample size, planned interim monitoring, and minimizing postentry exclusions.

Clinical trials have limitations, partly because of the rigor required to implement them. Investigators contemplating the use of these important scientific tools should focus most efforts on the design aspects of the study and concern themselves little with analysis. This is because most of the serious errors that can be made when performing clinical trials can be prevented or minimized by correct design. In this regard, consultation with an experienced clinical trial methodologist early in the design stage of an investigation will be of enormous benefit.

When analyzing and reporting the results of clinical trials, investigators should follow a simple approach. The purpose of a trial is to estimate an effect or treatment difference, which, if present, would have clinical utility when treating new patients. Procedures or methods that do not facilitate estimating and reporting the treatment effect with precision and without bias are likely to mislead investigators. Often in clinical trials, investigators are interested in estimates of odds or hazard ratios between treatment groups.

These ideas suggest that the most useful results from clinical trials are estimated risk ratios and their confidence limits. Especially in oncology studies, in which disease progression, recurrence, and death are of interest, estimates of risk difference are very relevant. Hypothesis tests and associated *p* values, although often (or exclusively) reported, are of lesser utility because they do not fully summarize the data. These recommendations are similar to those in many journals.

Despite some technical disagreement among statisticians regarding the need for adjusted analyses for imbalanced prognostic factors, I believe that it is wise to see if treatment effects change after accounting for imbalances. When this occurs, it seems likely that it will be of clinical interest. Although I discourage analyses that exclude any patients who meet the eligibility criteria, some circumstances will require that this be done (e.g., when a patient refuses to participate after randomization). Investigators should report, and emphasize as primary, those analyses that include all eligible patients.

## SUGGESTIONS FOR ADDITIONAL READING

Piantadosi S. Clinical trials: a methodologic perspective. New York: John Wiley & Sons, 1997:590 pp and 1 computer disk (3 1/2 inch). System requirements: IBM-compatible PC.

International Committee of Medical Journal Editors: Uniform requirements for manuscripts submitted to biomedical journals. Ann Intern Med 1988;108:258–65. *This is a useful reference for putting into perspective problems associated with reporting study results.*

# REFERENCES

1. Bull JP: The historical development of clinical therapeutic trials. J Chronic Dis 1959;10:218–48.
2. Office of Technology Assessment, U.S. Congress. The impact of randomized clinical trials on health policy and medical practice: background paper. Washington, D.C.: U.S. Government Printing Office, OTA-BP-H-22, 1983.
3. Meinert CL. Clinical trials. Oxford: Oxford University Press, 1986.
4. Silverman WA. Human experimentation: a guided step into the unknown. Oxford: Oxford University Press, 1985.
5. Shapiro SH. Clinical trials: issues and approaches. New York: Marcel Dekker, 1983.
6. Pocock SJ. Clinical trials: a practical approach. New York: John Wiley & Sons, 1983.
7. Buyse ME, Staquet MJ, Sylvester RJ, eds. Cancer clinical trials: methods and practice. Oxford: Oxford University Press, 1984.
8. Leventhal BG. Research methods in clinical oncology. New York: Raven Press, 1988.
9. Freidman LM. Fundamentals of clinical trials. Boston: John Wright, 1981.
10. Armitage P. The design of clinical trials. Aust J Stat 1979;21:266–281.
11. Louis TA, Mosteller F, McPeek B. Timely topics in statistical methods for clinical trials. Annu Rev Biophys Bioeng 1982;11:81–104.
12. Lewis JA. Clinical trials: statistical developments of practical benefit to the pharmaceutical industry (with discussion). J R Stat Soc A 1983;146:362–393.
13. Leventhal BG. An overview of clinical trials in oncology. Semin Oncol 1988;15:414–22.
14. Piantadosi S. Principles of clinical trial design. Semin Oncol 1988;15:423–33.
15. Peto R, Pike MC, Armitage P, et al. Design and analysis of randomized clinical trials requiring prolonged observation of each patient. I: Introduction and design. Br J Cancer 1976;34:585–612.
16. Peto R, Pike MC, Armitage P, et al. Design and analysis of randomized clinical trials requiring prolonged observation of each patient. II: analysis and examples. Br J Cancer 1977;35:1–39.
17. Byar DP, Simon RM, Friedewald WT, et al. Randomized clinical trials: perspectives on some recent ideas. N Engl J Med 1976;295:74–80.
18. Piantadosi S, Saijo N, Tamura T. Basic design considerations for clinical trials in oncology. Jpn J Cancer Res 1992;83:547–58.
19. Armitage P. Statistical methods in medical research. Oxford: Blackwell Scientific, 1987:172–175.
20. Simon RM. Design and conduct of clinical trials. In: DeVita VT, Jr, Rosenberg SA, Hellman S, eds. Cancer: principles and practice of oncology. 4th ed. Philadelphia: JB Lippincott: 1993:418.
21. Green SB. Randomized clinical trials: design and analysis. Semin Oncol 1981;8:417–23.
22. Taves DR. Minimization: a new method of assigning patients to treatment and control groups. Clin Pharmacol Ther 1974;15:443–53.
23. Schafer A. The ethics of the randomized clinical trial. N Engl J Med 1977;307:719–24.
24. Burkhardt R, Kienle G. Basic problems in controlled trials. J Med Ethics 1983;9:80–4.
25. Vere DW. Problems in controlled trials—a critical response. J Med Ethics 1983;9:85–9.
26. Royall R. Ethics and statistics in randomized clinical trials. Stat Sci 1991; 6:52–88.
27. Byar DP. Identification of prognostic factors. In: Buyse ME, Staquet MF, Sylvester RJ, eds. Cancer clinical trials: methods and practice. Oxford: Oxford University Press, 1984:210.
28. George SL. Identification and assessment of prognostic factors. Semin Oncol 1988;15:462–71.
29. International Committee of Medical Journal Editors. Uniform requirements for manuscripts submitted to biomedical journals. Ann Intern Med 1988;108:258–65.
30. Bailar JC III, Mosteller F. Guidelines for statistical reporting in articles for medical journals: amplifications and explanations. Ann Intern Med 1988;108:266–73.
31. Altman DG, Gore SM, Gardner MJ, Pocock SJ. Statistical guidelines for contributors to medical journals. Br Med J 1983;286:1489–93.
32. Mosteller F, Gilbert JP, McPeek B. Reporting standards and research strategies for controlled trials—agenda for the editors. Control Clin Trials 1980;1:37–58.
33. Berry G. Statistical guidelines and statistical guidance. Med J Aust 1987;146:408–9.
34. DerSimonian R, Charette LJ, McPeek B, Mosteller F. Reporting on methods in clinical trials. N Engl J Med 1982;306:1332–7.
35. Berry G. Statistical significance and confidence intervals. Med J Aust 1986;144:618–9.
36. Simon R. Confidence intervals for reporting results of clinical trials. Ann Intern Med 1986;105:429–35.
37. Gardner MJ, Altman DG. Confidence intervals rather than *p* values: estimation rather than hypothesis testing. Br Med J 1986;292:746–50.
38. Braitman LE. Confidence intervals extract clinically useful information from data. Ann Intern Med 1988;108:296–8.
39. Berger J. Are p-values reasonable measures of accuracy? In: Manley BFJ, Lam FC, eds. Pacific Statistical Congress. New York: Elsevier-North Holland, 1986.
40. Berger J, Selke T. Testing a point null hypothesis: the irreconcilability of p-values and evidence. J Am Stat Assoc 1987;82:112–139.
41. Rothman K. Significance questing. Ann Intern Med 1986;105:445–7.
42. Detsky AS, Sackett DL. When was a "negative" clinical trial big enough? How many patients you needed depends on what you found. Arch Intern Med 1985;145:709–12.
43. Freiman JA, Chalmers TC, Smith H Jr, Kuebler RR. The importance of beta, the type II error, and sample size in the design and interpretation of the randomized control trial: Survey of 71 "negative" trials. N Engl J Med 1978;299:690–4.
44. Sackett DL. Bias in analytic research. J Chronic Dis 1979;32:51–63.
45. Chalmers TC. The control of bias in clinical trials. In: Shapiro SH, Louis TA, eds. Clinical trials: issues and approaches. New York: Marcel Dekker, 1983:115.
46. O'Quigley J, Chevret S. Methods for dose-finding studies in cancer clinical trials: a review and results of a Monte Carlo study. Stat Med 1991;10:1647–64.
47. Goodman SN, Zahurak ML, Piantadosi S. Some practical improvements in the continual reassessment method for phase I studies. Stat Med 1995;14:1149–61.
48. Simon R. Optimal two-stage designs for phase II clinical trials. Control Clin Trials 1989;10:1–10.
49. Donner A. Approaches to sample size estimation in the design of clinical trials—a review. Stat Med 1984;3:199–214.
50. Piantadosi S. Clinical trials design program. Cambridge: BIOSOFT, 1990.
51. George SL, Desu MM. Planning the size and duration of a clinical trial studying the time to some critical event. J Chronic Dis 1974;27:15–24.
52. Anscombe FJ. Sequential medical trials. J Am Stat Assoc 1963;58:365–383.
53. Armitage P, McPherson CK, Rowe BC. Repeated significance tests on accumulating data. J R Stat Soc A 1969;132:235–244.
54. Pocock SJ. Group sequential methods in the design and analysis of clinical trials. Biometrika 1977;64:191–9.
55. O'Brien PC, Fleming TR. A multiple testing procedure for clinical trials. Biometrics 1979;35:549–56.
56. Hughes MD, Pocock SJ. Stopping rules and estimation problems in clinical trials. Stat Med 1988;7:1231–42.
57. Berry DA. Interim analyses in clinical trials: classical versus Bayesian approaches. Stat Med 1985;4:521–6.
58. Gail MH. Monitoring and stopping clinical trials. In: Mike V, Stanley K, eds. Statistics in medical research. New York: John Wiley & Sons, 1982.
59. O'Fallon JR. Policies for interim analysis and interim reporting of results. Cancer Treat Rep 1985;69:1101–6.
60. DeMets DL. Practical aspects in data monitoring: a brief review. Stat Med 1987;6:753–60.
61. Lan KKG, Simon R, Halperin M. Stochastically curtailed tests in long-term clinical trials. Comm Stat 1982;C1:207–219.

# CHAPTER 30

# GENE THERAPY FOR CANCER

• ANTONI RIBAS • JAMES E. ECONOMOU

Gene transfer techniques are powerful tools for cancer treatment. Both viral vectors and physical methods enable the introduction of foreign genetic material into target cells, thereby generating cells that did not exist before in nature. How we use these techniques will guide the benefit our patients will receive. So far, with more than 300 clinical protocols approved and more than 3000 patients treated in gene medicine protocols worldwide, the majority in cancer, the biggest contribution of gene therapy has been increased knowledge about the biology of cancer.[1] Gene marking studies in human patients were the first type of gene medicine protocols approved and have established the biology of tumor infiltrating lymphocytes[2] as well as the contribution of contaminating cancer cells to tumor relapses after autologous bone marrow transplants.[3] Clinical trials using gene transfer techniques to treat cancer patients have yielded some provocative responses, but more usually they have highlighted the complexity of cancer biology and the need for increased understanding and continued research to develop effective new treatments.

Gene therapy is limited by the availability of vector systems to introduce foreign genes in vitro and in vivo. Several systems, including viral and physical methods, are available and are used in different situations according to their characteristics. Genes used for experimental cancer therapies include prodrug enzymes, replacement of tumor suppressor genes, disruption of dominant oncogene expression, genes that confer protection to chemotherapy, and genes intended to stimulate the immune system to recognize and reject the autologous cancer cells. The continuously increasing list of cloned genes allows them to be tested as therapeutic approaches for cancer.

## Methods of DNA Transfer into Cells

### VIRAL VECTORS

Viruses have the ability to transfer genetic material (DNA or RNA) from cell to cell. Their life cycle consists of an infection phase, in which they attach to host cells through specific binding of a virus-attachment protein to a cellular receptor, which enables the virus to penetrate the cell. During the next phase, they replicate and express the virus genome in the host cell. Once inside the cytoplasm or nucleus, the virus is uncoated and uses the host cell's replication machinery to its advantage. This enables the virus to synthesize its own proteins and genetic material to generate multiple progeny viruses. During the final phase of viral infection, the mature virions eventually overwhelm the host cell and lead to the burst of infective virions. Understanding the viral

cycle allowed the engineering of viral particles that take advantage of the ability of viruses to penetrate cells and express their genomic information, but these particles do not go on to the later phases of progeny virion assembly and burst. By deleting critical genes from the viral backbone (*gag, pol,* and *env* genes in retroviruses, early region [E1] in adenoviruses), viruses are rendered replication deficient, but they maintain the ability to infect cells and express some genes. The critical replication genes that are taken out of the viral backbone are introduced into cell lines (called *packaging cell lines),* which will then enable the assembly of the defective viral particles that have the ability to infect a single target cell. The gene used for gene transfer *(transgene)* is introduced in the place left by the deleted viral genes, and its expression is guided by a promoter that has the ability to be "turned on" permanently in the host cells.

Several modified viral vectors (retrovirus, adenovirus, adeno-associated virus, lentivirus, pox virus, and herpes virus) have been used for gene transfer. Each vector system has different characteristics that can be an advantage or disadvantage for gene therapy approaches.

**Retrovirus.** Retroviruses were the earliest gene vector systems and the ones used in the majority of clinical trials to date.[4] They have an RNA genome that is reverse transcribed into DNA and then integrated into the genome of the infected cell, leading to a long duration of expression. Other advantages include the accommodation of a relatively large insert (up to 10 kb) and low immunogenicity. Their main disadvantages are a low transduction efficiency, the potential oncogenicity due to random genome insertion, their susceptibility to complement-mediated lysis, and the requirement of replicating target cells for transduction. These characteristics make them suitable for in vitro transduction of tissue culture cancer cell lines as used in many tumor vaccine clinical trials but gives them limited in vivo applications. In one approach, however, the ability to transduce only replicating cells was used to selectively target glioblastoma cancer cells.[5] In the central nervous system (CNS), the only replicating cells would be the cancer cells because neurons do not cycle during adult life. Since retroviruses infect cycling cells only, glioblastoma cells can be targeted selectively to express the genes coded by the retroviral vector. Future developments with these vectors will include engineering their receptors to target specific receptors in cancer cells as well as the production of complement-resistant vectors[4].

**Lentivirus.** Three of the favorable characteristics of retroviruses—integration, duration of expression, and low immunogenicity—are maintained in lentiviruses.[6] These members of the retrovirus family, of which the human immunodeficiency virus is a member, have an additional characteristic that gives them considerable potential in gene medicine, that is, the ability to infect both dividing and nondividing cells. Their main disadvantage is safety concerns.

**Adenovirus.** Adenoviruses have also been used extensively in gene transfer protocols, mainly because of the practical need to transduce both dividing and resting cells.[7] Their main advantages are the low toxicity profile of the wild-type viruses in humans, a very high transduction efficiency, the ability to obtain high concentrations of viral particles, and a wide range of susceptible targets, which include dividing and quiescent cells. Other characteristics include no integration of the transgene in the host genome (the virus remains episomal) and a short duration of expression. Although these characteristics may be a disadvantage for some applications (e.g., they are unsuited to correct gene abnormalities), they are an advantage for other applications when a transient high level of expression is needed in a tumor or tissue. Disadvantages include a smaller insert size compared with retroviruses (up to 5 kb); their high immunogenicity, which precludes repeated in vivo administration; and a short duration of in vivo transgene expression. Future developments with these vectors will include the generation of vectors with higher insert capacity and lower immunogenicity that are devoid of most adenoviral genes (called "gutless" vectors)[8] and the production of receptor-targeted vectors.

A new field of adenovirus use in cancer treatment is the engineering of replication-competent viruses. The idea would be to engineer viruses that generate a replicative cycle in cancer cells, leading to cytotoxic death from the burst of viral progeny, but that are unable to replicate in normal human tissues. The first virus used according to this hypothesis is an E1B-deleted adenoviral vector that would have a replication advantage in p53-negative cells (most cancer cells), whereas the presence of wild-type p53 in normal cells would not sustain viral replication.[9] Other selective replication-competent adenovirus strategies involve the generation of defective adenoviruses in which the E1A gene is expressed from a tumor-specific promoter. If the alpha-fetoprotein (AFP) promoter is used, the E1A gene will be expressed only in AFP-positive hepatocellular carcinoma cells, and virus progeny will be produced only in these cells. Another strategy is the cotransfection of tumor cells with an E1 replication–defective adenovirus together with a plasmid expressing the E1 gene, or to take advantage of the E1-substituting activity of interleukin-6 (IL-6) produced by some tumor cells to generate replication-competent environments in tumors.[10]

**Adeno-Associated Virus.** Adeno-associated viruses (AAVs) are small single-stranded DNA viruses that require the presence of a helper adenovirus to initiate a productive viral infection. In the absence of a helper virus, wild-type AAVs produce no progeny virus in the infected host cells and instead integrate selectively in the short arm of chromosome 19. This life cycle enables the engineering of AAV vectors for gene therapy: they can be produced in vitro using helper adenoviruses and will not produce infective particles after targeting cells in vitro or in vivo in the absence of helper viruses.[11] Their advantages are low immunogenicity because they have limited structural genes plus the ability to infect nonreplicating cells and to achieve sustained gene expression. However, recombinant AAV vectors without the *rep* gene lose the specificity for chromosome 19 integration,

which removes one of their advantages, making it possible to integrate the transgene in an oncogene region, which is a concern for carcinogenic transformation of the host cells. Their main disadvantages are a small insert ($<5$ kb), the current inefficient production process that leads to low viral titers, and the possible contamination with helper virus.

**Herpes Simplex Virus.** The use of herpes simplex virus as a gene therapy vector has been proposed mainly because of its ability to establish a latent infection in the brain. The main advantages are that it can accommodate a very large gene insert and infect resting cells.[12] However, the biology of its large genome (150 kb), containing more than 80 genes, has not been fully characterized and its potential for development into useful gene therapy vectors awaits further study. The high viral toxicity and immunogenicity further limit its current use.

**Other Viruses.** Other viral vectors include vaccinia virus, which can accommodate large inserts but is cytotoxic for the host cell; fowlpox and canarypox, which are unable to replicate in mammalian cells; baculovirus; SV40; Epstein-Barr virus; and the recent description of the use of live Sabin poliovirus vaccine as a gene therapy vector.[13, 14] Finally, hybrid systems have been reported in which a retroviral vector is packaged into an adenoviral capsule, enabling the transduction of cells that are usually inaccessible to retroviral transduction while maintaining the ability of retrovirus to integrate into the host genome.

## NONVIRAL VECTORS

Several physical methods have been used to transfect cells in vitro, including calcium-phosphate precipitation, liposome encapsulation, electroporation, or gene gun. Since plasmid DNA is relatively simple to produce and store and is safer than viral vectors, the possibility to use plasmid DNA for in vivo approaches has been actively investigated. The use of naked DNA in the form of a eukaryotic expression vector has considerable promise as a method for genetic immunization. Naked plasmid DNA expressing a foreign protein under control of a suitable promoter may be propelled into the skin using a gene gun or injected into a skeletal muscle.[15, 16] DNA is taken up by cells (myocytes, fibroblasts) in which it remains as an episome (not integrated into the genome) and is transcribed and translated with expression of the vector-encoded protein. The gene products are taken up by host antigen-presenting cells, and antigenic fragments are presented in the context of major histocompatibility class I (MHC) antigens. This causes activation of host immune cells, which results in generation of cytolytic T cells (CTLs) and antibody-producing B cells.[17, 18] This vaccination strategy provides exceptionally long-lasting immunity, which is an attractive feature for DNA-based vaccines, particularly with respect to the generation of T-cell responses to defined tumor antigens.

Liposomes are positively charged lipid membranes that can form complexes with DNA. These liposome-DNA complexes can fuse with cell membranes, permitting the transfer of DNA into cells. The efficiency of liposome-mediated gene transfer is considerably higher than with naked DNA for single-cell transfection in vitro, as well as intratumoral gene transfer of plasmid DNA in vivo.

# Strategies for Cancer Gene Therapy

Various strategies have been developed for gene therapy in cancer. They include using prodrug-converting enzymes, drug resistance genes, tumor suppressor or oncogene therapy, anti-angiogenic approaches, cytokine-based therapies, and genetic immunotherapy. Table 30–1 summarizes the gene medicine clinical trials approved by the U.S. Food and Drug Administration up until 1999 and describes the therapeutic strategy, the transgene used, and the targeted cancer sites.

## ENZYME-PRODRUG GENE THERAPY

Genes encoding for prodrug-converting enzymes, also known as "suicide" genes, convert a nontoxic precursor drug into a toxic metabolite. The prototype enzyme is the herpes simplex virus thymidine kinase (HSVtk) gene. HSVtk adds a phosphate group to ganciclovir, which is then converted to its triphosphate form by cellular enzymes. This leads to inhibition of DNA replication and cell death. Human thymidine kinase has a much lower affinity for ganciclovir, and therefore no toxic triphosphate compounds are produced in untransfected human cells. This enzyme has been used in a number of vector backbones (retroviral, adenoviral, AAV) to direct conversion of ganciclovir into toxic metabolites within solid tumors in vivo. Direct intratumoral vector injection or placement of vector-producing packaging cell lines in the tumor bed leads to in vivo transduction of tumor cells. Subsequent systemic administration of ganciclovir results in pronounced tumor inhibition in a variety of experimental tumors. An interesting feature of HSVtk-based gene therapy is that not all cells within the tumor need to be transduced to achieve tumor regression, a phenomenon known as the *bystander effect*. In vitro, this effect has been demonstrated to be mediated by the cell-to-cell transfer of toxic compounds through gap junctions and by the transfer of phosphorylated ganciclovir from dying transduced cells to naive neighboring cancer cells. There is also a systemic bystander effect in vivo, leading to antitumor responses in tumor sites distant from the ones treated with the HSVtk gene. This systemic effect is immune-mediated because it is not noted in nude mice.[19] Phase I and II clinical trials using this approach have been started for the treatment of tumors of the CNS, ovarian and breast carcinomas, mesothelioma, and melanoma, with some responses in cancer patients with very advanced disease.[20, 21] A phase III clinical trial has been initiated following the promising results of phase I and II trials using this system. In this trial, which is open to more than 40 centers in North America and Europe, patients with brain tumors have a retroviral packaging cell line implanted into the tumor bed after surgical resection. The packaging cell line will produce vectors containing HSVtk that will transduce dividing tumor cells, and ganciclovir is administered 7 days later. A variation of this approach is the use of the suicide gene to selectively target graft hematopoietic cells used in allogeneic bone marrow transplants,[22] as is the case of the appearance of life-threatening graft-versus-host reactions.

Cytosine deaminase (CD) from *Escherichia coli* catalyzes the conversion of the prodrug 5-fluorocytosine to the toxic 5-fluorouracil (5-FU) and has also been used as a suicide gene. Expression of the CD gene allows a high local concentration of the chemotherapeutic agent 5-FU in the tumor.[23] This prodrug-converting enzyme has been used in experimental models of gastrointestinal malignancies and in a clinical trial in colon cancer. The combination of cytochrome P450 and cyclophosphamide or ifosfamide has also been tested in brain and pancreatic tumors.

Although earlier approaches with prodrug-converting enzyme employed vectors in which the suicide gene was expressed constitutively by a strong viral promoter, second-generation vectors have been tested using tumor-specific promoters.[24] The carcinoembryonic antigen (CEA) promoter has been used to drive the CD gene expression in CEA-positive adenocarcinomas.[25, 26] Therefore, the toxic products of the suicide gene are produced only in the cancer cells.

## CHEMOPROTECTION GENE THERAPY

Repeated administration of chemotherapy agents is more effective than a single administration. However, repeated cycles of high-dose chemotherapy and hematopoietic stem cell transplantation are not feasible because of the limiting capacity of hematopoietic progenitors to survive several cycles of supralethal doses of chemotherapy. However, if the hematopoietic progenitors used for the first transplantation were modified in vitro to become chemotherapy resistant, repeated high-dose cycles would be feasible. Toward this goal, the multiple drug resistance gene (MDR1) has been introduced into bone marrow or peripheral blood-derived hematopoietic stem cells. The MDR1 gene produces a P-glycoprotein that functions as a cellular efflux pump responsible for the resistance to various cytotoxic drugs. MDR-transduced hematopoietic stem cells are then resistant to systemically administered chemotherapeutic agents. This allows the administration of repeated cycles of high-dose chemotherapy with little marrow toxicity.[27] Other potential drug resistance genes include dihydrofolate reductase, topoisomerase II, and methylguanine methyltransferases. Caveats of this approach include the dose-limiting toxicity to nonhematopoietic organs and the fear that the transduction of a small population of contaminating tumor cells in the graft may produce drug-resistant tumors.

## TUMOR SUPPRESSOR GENE AND ANTISENSE ONCOGENE THERAPY

Mutations in p53 are found in a large percentage of human cancers. Restoration of wild-type p53 expression in cells with deleted or defective p53 is sufficient to cause apoptosis or growth arrest. This has been accomplished using retroviral, adenoviral, and nonviral gene delivery vectors expressing wild-type p53, with impressive results in vitro and in animal models. Additionally, wild-type p53 transfection into nonmutated p53 tumor cells also induces apoptotic tumor cell death. p53 gene therapy has also been proposed as chemotherapy-sensitizing treatment. DNA cross-linking agents such as cisplatin would damage the tumor DNA, and the addition of high levels of wild-type p53 would recognize the DNA damage and lead the cell to apoptotic death.[28]

p53-based clinical trials are being conducted for a number

*Table 30–1.* **Human Clinical Trials Approved by the U.S. Food and Drug Administration**

| Therapeutic Approach | Gene Transferred | Cancer Site |
|---|---|---|
| Gene marking<br>In vitro transduction | Neo resistance gene | Advanced cancers–TILs<br>Melanoma-TILs<br>Kidney-TILs<br>Ovarian-TILs<br>AML, CML, CLL-BMT<br>NHL-BMT<br>Myeloma-BMT<br>Breast-BMT<br>Leukemia-CTLs<br>Hodgkin-CTLs |
| Prodrug<br>In vivo transduction | HSVtk | Ovarian<br>Brain<br>Mesothelioma<br>Prostate<br>Head and neck<br>Leptomeningeal carcinomatosis<br>Hepatic metastases |
| Prodrug<br>In vitro transduction | HSVtk | Myeloma–donor leukocytes<br>Leukemia–donor leukocytes |
| Prodrug<br>In vivo transduction | Cytosine deaminase | Colon |
| Drug resistance<br>In vitro transduction | MDR | Ovarian<br>Breast<br>Testicular |
| Tumor suppressor gene<br>In vivo transduction | p53 | NSCLC<br>Head and neck<br>Hepatic metastases |
| Tumor suppressor gene<br>In vivo transduction | Rb | Bladder |
| Tumor suppressor gene<br>In vivo transduction | BRCA-1 | Ovarian |
| Oncogene<br>In vivo transduction | c-*fos* antisense | Breast |
| Oncogene<br>In vivo transduction | c-*myc* antisense | Prostate |
| Oncogene<br>In vivo transduction | Anti-*erb*B2 single-chain antibody gene | Ovarian |
| Oncogene<br>In vivo transduction | BCR/ABL antisense | CML |
| Oncogene<br>In vivo transduction | E1A | Breast<br>Ovarian |
| Immunotherapy<br>In vitro transduction | IL-2 | Advanced cancers<br>Neuroblastoma<br>Melanoma<br>Kidney<br>Small cell lung cancer<br>Colon<br>Glioblastoma<br>Breast<br>NHL<br>Prostate<br>Ovarian |
| Immunotherapy<br>In vivo transduction | IL-2 | Advanced cancers<br>Prostate |
| Immunotherapy<br>In vitro transduction | IL-4 | Kidney<br>Brain |
| Immunotherapy<br>In vitro transduction | IL-7 | Melanoma |
| Immunotherapy<br>In vitro transduction | IL-12 | Melanoma<br>NHL<br>Breast<br>Head and neck |
| Immunotherapy<br>In vitro transduction | GM-CSF | Kidney<br>Prostate |
| Immunotherapy<br>In vivo transduction | GM-CSF | Melanoma<br>Sarcoma |
| Immunotherapy<br>In vitro transduction | IFN-γ | Melanoma<br>Neuroblastoma<br>Prostate |

*Table continued on opposite page*

*Table 30–1.* Human Clinical Trials Approved by the U.S. Food and Drug Administration (Continued)

| Therapeutic Approach | Gene Transferred | Cancer Site |
|---|---|---|
| Immunotherapy In vitro transduction | TNF-α | Melanoma-TIL |
| Immunotherapy In vitro transduction | B7 (CD80) | Ovarian Breast Small cell lung cancer |
| Immunotherapy In vitro transduction | Insulin-like growth factor antisense Factor antisense | Brain |
| Immunotherapy In vitro transduction | TGF-β antisense | Brain |
| Immunotherapy In vivo transduction | HLA-B7 | Advanced cancers Melanoma Colon Kidney Breast Head and neck NHL |
| Genetic immunization In vivo transduction | CEA | Advanced cancers Colon Breast Lung |
| Genetic immunization In vivo transduction | PSA | Prostate |
| Genetic immunization In vivo transduction | MART-1 | Melanoma |
| Genetic immunization In vivo transduction | gp 100 | Melanoma |

TILs, tumor-infiltrating lymphocytes; BMT, bone marrow transplantation; CTLs, cytotoxic T lymphocytes; AML, acute myelocytic leukemia; CML, chronic myelocytic leukemia; CLL, chronic lymphocytic leukemia; NHL, non-Hodgkin's lymphoma; NSCLC, non–small cell lung cancer.

of malignancies in which treatment has proved feasible and effective. Treatment of head and neck cancers with adenoviral p53 is being carried out in an outpatient setting with minimal toxicity. Reported clinical trial results in lung cancer, head and neck cancers, and hepatocellular carcinoma are more encouraging than expected.[29–31] It was believed that to be totally successful the tumor suppressor gene had to be targeted to every single cancer cell in the host, a situation that is unrealistic using the currently available vectors. The encouraging results in early-phase clinical studies may be influenced by other factors, such as a local and immune-based bystander effect similar to the one seen in suicide gene therapy strategies.

Another novel strategy to exploit the p53 status of tumors is the use of adenoviruses deleted in the E1B region, which has already been commented on.[9] The adenoviral E1B 55-kd gene product is capable of binding to, and inactivating, the p53 gene product, thereby enabling the virus to overcome restrictions imposed on viral replication by the host cell cycle. In hosts with tumors carrying p53 mutations, a wild-type adenovirus will have difficulty replicating in p53 wild-type normal cells (due to p53 block) but will have a replication advantage in the p53-mutated tumor cells. If the adenovirus is modified to lack expression of the E1B 55-kd protein, it will have further difficulty replicating in p53 wild-type normal cells (the effect of p53 will not be blocked by the adenoviral E1B gene product), while maintaining replication ability in p53-null tumor cells. However, the p53 selective effect of the E1B-deleted vector *dl*1520 has been questioned in several reports. These selective replication-competent viruses are currently in clinical trials for head and neck, pancreatic, and hepatocellular cancers.

Only a single mutant allele of an oncogene is required to confer a malignant phenotype to a cell. To inhibit oncogene expression, antisense constructs have been employed to inhibit translation of the oncogene messenger RNA. They will bind to the message and inhibit the translation of the gene product because they have the mirror image of base pair sequences contained in the oncogene messenger RNA. This strategy has been applied with some success to the *ras* family of oncogenes in pancreatic cancers, c-*fos* in breast cancer, and c-*myc* in leukemias and prostate cancer.[32]

## INHIBITION OF ANGIOGENESIS

Antiangiogenesis strategies are an appealing approach for cancer treatment. To inhibit blood vessel formation or selectively target neoformed endothelial cells in tumors, several strategies have been proposed. They include the transfection of endothelial cells with mutated, signaling-defective vascular endothelial growth factor (VEGF) receptor gene, treatment with VEGF antisense constructs, or engineered adenoviral vectors carrying cytokine or suicide genes under an endothelial-specific promoter.

## CYTOKINE-BASED TUMOR VACCINES

Gene therapy approaches have been used in an attempt to generate or increase antitumor immune responses. This strategy is based on the existence of tumor antigens and the ability of the immune system to recognize them. The progressive description of several genes and peptide epitopes specifically recognized by T cells on cancer cells has established the existence of tumor antigens. Direct evidence of powerful, clinically relevant, antitumor cellular immune responses comes from responses in melanoma and renal carcinoma following systemic cytokine treatment[33] and the clinical responses observed after donor leukocyte infusions in leukemia patients relapsing after allogeneic bone marrow transplants.[34] The major advantage of this approach is that it is suitable for the treatment of metastatic tumors, since the transgene does not have to be targeted to every single cancer cell.

Although tumor cells have tumor antigens, they are presented poorly to the immune system. Induction of tumor antigen–specific T-cell immunity has several requirements. The tumor antigen must be correctly processed and presented in the context of MHC molecules together with costimulatory molecules such as B7 to deliver additional signals to the T lymphocytes. Proinflammatory cytokines provide a favorable environment for the clonal activation and proliferation of antigen-reactive T lymphocytes. Tumor cells are poor antigen presenters because they frequently downregulate MHC expression, do not express costimulatory ligands and, instead of producing stimulatory cytokines, they produce immunosuppressive substances such as transforming growth factor β (TGF-β), prostaglandins, and IL-10.

Tumor cell vaccines genetically engineered to secrete proinflammatory cytokines were developed to increase the efficiency of antigen presentation and immune stimulation by tumor cells. This strategy exploits the paracrine nature of cytokine production, in which regional expression of the cytokine at the site of tumor cell antigens would be more effective in generating immune responses. To achieve similar levels of cytokine expression at the tumor site, cytokines would have to be given systemically at doses that are too toxic. Virtually all tested cytokines reduce the tumorigenicity of genetically engineered tumor cells in animal models. Cytokines tested include IL-1, IL-2, IL-3, IL-4, IL-6, IL-7, IL-12, interferon-α and interferon-γ, tumor necrosis factor (TNF)-α and TNF-β, macrophage colony–stimulating factor, granulocyte colony–stimulating factor, and granulocyte-macrophage colony-stimulating factor (GM-CSF).[35–43] Reduced tumorigenicity in vivo is caused by the influx of host effector cells such as natural killer cells, macrophages, granulocytes, host antigen-presenting cells, and T lymphocytes. The nonspecific inflammatory response will recruit enough specific T-cell effectors to render these animals immune to a rechallenge of the parental untransduced tumor. Among the most effective cytokines in generating antitumor protection is GM-CSF, a cytokine with no immunostimulatory effects on T lymphocytes. The mechanism by which GM-CSF–based tumor vaccines work is by attracting and activating host antigen-presenting cells, such as dendritic cells, which migrate to the injection site, take up antigens from the transduced tumor cells, and process and present them to the immune system.[44] These experimental findings have spawned clinical trials using autologous tumor cell vaccine–transduced cytokine vectors that include IL-2, IL-4, IL-7, IL-12, GM-CSF, and interferon-γ.

Costimulatory molecules provide an important second signal for T-cell activation. Transducing costimulatory molecule genes like B7.1 (CD80) and B7.2 (CD86) into tumor cells would allow them to provide the first signal (antigen) and the second signal (costimulation), thereby acting as surrogate antigen-presenting cells.[44–46] An alternative explanation of why B7 transduction works is its ability to inhibit Fas ligand–mediated T cell–receptor–induced apoptosis, a mechanism used by tumor cells to protect themselves against the attack of cytotoxic T lymphocytes. These efforts have met with success in experimental models and are in clinical trials. Another approach aimed at making tumor cells better antigen presenters is the transfection of MHC class II molecules to tumor cells. Tumors usually express varying levels of MHC class I molecules but, except for some melanomas and leukemias, usually do not express class II molecules. Physiologically, only professional antigen-presenting cells express MHC class II molecules. Immune responses are initiated by the initial activation of CD4 cells that recognize antigenic epitopes expressed by class II molecules, a situation that normally occurs only if professional antigen-presenting cells process antigens taken up from dying tumor cells. Expressing MHC class II molecules in tumor cells bypasses the requirement of antigen-presenting cell processing, thereby making the tumor cells the initiators of an immune response against their own antigens. A variation of these strategies is fusing tumor cells with professional antigen-presenting cells such as B cells or dendritic cells.[47–49]

Tumor cells produce immunosuppressive factors, including TGF-β, IL-6, IL-10, prostaglandins, and insulin-like growth factor. A strategy known as *inhibiting the inhibitors* has been proposed to introduce an antisense construct of these tumor-produced immune inhibitors to downregulate their expression. When the modified cells are injected into the patient as a vaccine, the lack of immune inhibitors may allow the generation of an immune response to antigens presented by the tumor cells that before were not recognized as antigenic because of the presence of the inhibitor.[50]

The ex vivo manipulation and transduction of autologous tumor cells, however, is labor intensive, and recent efforts have been directed toward in vivo transduction of tumor with either cytokine genes or costimulatory molecules, or both. Such an approach requires vectors that generate high transduction efficiencies and levels of cytokine expression. Recombinant adenovirus, AAVs, and poxvirus vectors are suitable for these strategies. In vivo gene delivery carries the risk of systemic leak of the viral vector. Even if carefully injected into the tumor, this phenomenon has been documented in animal models and accounts for much of the toxicity of these tumor-directed transduction strategies.[43, 51] It is for this reason that transcriptionally specific, second-generation vectors have been developed. As described earlier, these vectors involve replacing the constitutive (always "turned on") viral promoters used to drive these genes with the regulatory sequences that are specific for certain tumor histologies. Promoters for the CEA antigen, AFP, and tyrosinase genes will direct synthesis of their gene products only in tumor cells producing these tumor markers or enzymes (adenocarcinomas, hepatocellular carcinomas, and melanomas, respectively).[25, 51, 52] This genetic manipulation should add an important degree of biologic safety and increased therapeutic ratio to these in vivo approaches.

Nonviral vectors have also been used to transfect tumor cells in vivo to attract immune effector cells to the site of tumor vaccines. One approach is the transduction of tumor cells with a lipid complex containing the HLA-B7 gene

(Allovectin-7) in HLA-B7–negative patients. This would generate a nonspecific immune response against the allo-MHC molecule that would also attract sufficient specific effectors to generate a protective response against the tumor antigens, thereby resulting in an immune attack on nontransduced cancer cells.[53, 54] Another strategy is the in vivo administration of cationic vectors expressing the IL-2 gene (Leuvectin).

## GENETIC IMMUNIZATION

The concept of genetic immunization involves the use of tumor antigen genes to vaccinate against cancers expressing these same antigens. Peptides derived from antigen genes are presented by MHC molecules on the surface of cells. Tumors usually express only class I molecules. To initiate an effective immune response, their antigens have to be taken up and processed by professional antigen-presenting cells. This allows the tumor-derived antigenic epitopes, which are 10 to 35 amino acids long, to be presented by MHC class II restriction. Peptide–MHC class II complexes are recognized by CD4 cells, which will activate the antigen-presenting cell through the CD40-ligand–CD-receptor system. Activated antigen-presenting cells will increase MHC class I and class II complex expression, costimulatory molecules, adhesion molecules, and activating cytokine expression (IL-12), which will enhance their ability to stimulate CD8 effector cells. CD8 cells will become antigen-specific killers when recognizing 8- to 10–amino acid–long peptides derived from the same antigen presented by MHC class I molecules on the surface of the activated antigen-presenting cells, and will then traffic the body searching for and killing other cells presenting the same epitope–MHC class I molecule.

This increased knowledge of how antigen-specific cellular immune responses are generated and regulated and the identification and cloning of tumor antigen genes make genetic immunization feasible. In melanoma, antigens include MART1, gp100, tyrosinase, p15, TRP-1, and β-catenin.[55, 56] Surprisingly, all these tumor-rejection antigens were found to be normal, nonmutated differentiation antigens that are present in normal melanocytes and melanomas. Despite the exposure of the immune system to these melanocyte lineage "self"-antigens, immunologic tolerance was not generated. These findings in melanoma have generated considerable interest in the use of other self-antigens expressed by other human cancers as suitable targets for immunotherapy, for example, CEA antigen, prostate-specific antigen, Her-2/*neu*, mutated *ras*, wild-type and mutant p53, and others.

With the identification and cloning of potential tumor-rejection antigens, various strategies to immunize hosts genetically to these defined antigens are now being tested. GM-CSF–transduced tumor cell vaccines, in which host antigen-presenting cells are attracted to the vaccine site to stimulate immunity, are one form of genetic immunotherapy to undefined tumor antigens. Another genetic immunization strategy involves the intramuscular injection or the biolistic delivery of naked DNA encoding tumor-antigen genes.

Among professional antigen-presenting cells, dendritic cells are the most potent described. Dendritic cells are bone marrow derived and characterized by dendritic morphologic features; high mobility; expression of high levels of MHC class I and class II molecules, costimulatory molecules such as B7.1 and B7.2, and adhesion molecules; and the ability to present antigen to naive T cells in an MHC-restricted fashion. It is possible to generate large numbers of dendritic cells from hematopoietic precursors. Both bone marrow and peripheral blood progenitors may be cultured in cytokines such as stem cell factor, GM-CSF, TNF-α, and IL-4 to yield highly enriched, potent, differentiated dendritic cells.[57–60] In animal models and in clinical trials, synthetic tumor-antigen peptides, which are known to bind specific MHC class I alleles, can be loaded onto dendritic cells, which are then used to immunize the host. This peptide-based dendritic cell strategy is capable of inducing protective CTL responses.[61–64] Even when the tumor antigens have not been defined, putative tumor antigen can be eluted from the dissected tumor and loaded onto dendritic cells, or tumor lysates containing tumor antigen proteins can be macropinocytosed by DC and processed and presented on the surface together with MHC molecules.[65, 66] Finally, an exciting strategy is the possibility of genetically engineered dendritic cells to express defined tumor antigens. A tumor antigen gene therapy vector, such as an adenoviral vector, may be used to transduce dendritic cells in vitro. The dendritic cells will properly process the tumor antigen, and different antigenic peptides derived from that gene will be displayed on the cell surface in an MHC-restricted fashion. These dendritic cells are then administered to the patient to generate tumor antigen–specific responses. This approach has several potential advantages, including the continuous expression of antigenic peptides, the potential for both MHC class I and class II presentation, and the simultaneous presentation of multiple antigenic peptide determinants derived from the tumor-antigen polypeptide.[67–70] A variation of this approach is the transfection of DC with tumor-derived or antigen-derived RNA, a strategy that has also been shown to generate antigen-specific protection.[71] These strategies are currently in clinical trials and should provide important insight into what is in fact an autoimmune response to a self-protein.

## Concluding Remarks

The number of clinical cancer gene therapy trials being initiated each year increases exponentially, and early results have promise. Continued investigation will generate better vector systems, vectors capable of specifically recognizing tumor cells, increased knowledge about the benefits and pitfalls of current strategies, and tailored therapies based on the mechanisms involved in malignant transformation and tumor growth.

## SUGGESTED ADDITIONAL READING

Anderson WF. The best of times, the worst of times. Science 2000; 288:627–9. *This commentary briefly summarizes the successes, caveats and challenges of current gene therapy strategies.*

Regulatory Issues: Department of Health and Human Services National Institutes of Health Recombinant DNA Advisory Committee minutes of meeting June 12–13, 1997. Hum Gene Ther 1998;9:391–445. *This article contains a detailed list of human gene therapy protocols that have been approved to date by this committee.*

Roth JA, Cristiano RJ. Gene therapy for cancer: what have we done and where are we going? J Natl Cancer Inst 1997;89:21–39. *This article provides a detailed description of treatment strategies and delivery systems for cancer gene therapy.*

Gómez-Navarro J, Curiel DT, Douglas JT. Gene therapy for cancer. Eur J Cancer 1999;35:867–85.

Jenks S. Gene therapy death—"everyone has to share in the guilt" [news]. J Natl Cancer Inst 2000;92:98–100. *Despite the promise of gene therapy, the modality is not without risk. This commentary relates to the death of a patient treated with a non–cancer-related gene that was inserted using an adenovirus vector.*

Cavazzana-Calvo M, Hacein-Bey S, de Saint Basile G, et al. Gene therapy of human severe combined immunodeficiency (SCID)-X1 disease. Science 2000;288:669–72. *This report from Paris describes successful gene therapy lasting at least 10 months in two infants. These data strongly suggest that SCID-X1 can be treated successfully by this technique.*

# REFERENCES

1. Rosenberg SA, Blaese RM, Brenner MK, et al. Human gene marker/therapy clinical protocols. Hum Gene Ther 1997;8:2301–38.
2. Rosenberg SA, Aebersold P, Cornetta K, et al. Gene transfer into humans—immunotherapy of patients with advanced melanoma, using tumor-infiltrating lymphocytes modified by retroviral gene transduction. N Engl J Med 1990;323:570–8.
3. Brenner MK, Rill DR, Holladay MS, et al. Gene marking to determine whether autologous marrow infusion restores long-term haemopoiesis in cancer patients. Lancet 1993;342:1134–7.
4. Anderson WF. Human gene therapy. Nature 1998;392:25–30.
5. Culver KW, Ram Z, Wallbridge S, et al. In vivo gene transfer with retroviral vector-producer cells for treatment of experimental brain tumors. see comments. Science 1992;256:1550–2.
6. Poeschla EM, Wong-Staal F, Looney DJ. Efficient transduction of nondividing human cells by feline immunodeficiency virus lentiviral vectors. Nat Med 1998;4:354–7.
7. Bett AJ, Prevec L, Graham FL. Packaging capacity and stability of human adenovirus type 5 vectors. J Virol 1993;7:5911–21.
8. Mitani K, Graham FL, Caskey CT, Kochanek S. Rescue, propagation, and partial purification of a helper virus-dependent adenovirus vector. Proc Natl Acad Sci U S A 1995;92:3854–8.
9. Bischoff JR, Kirn DH, Williams A, et al. An adenovirus mutant that replicates selectively in p53-deficient human tumor cells. Science 1996;274:373–6.
10. Douglas JT, Rogers BE, Rosenfeld ME, et al. Targeted gene delivery by tropism-modified adenoviral vectors. Nat Biotechnol 1996;14:1574–8.
11. Kotin RM. Prospects for the use of adeno-associated virus as a vector for human gene therapy. Hum Gene Ther 1994;5:793–801.
12. Glorioso J, Bender MA, Fink D, DeLuca N. Herpes simplex virus vectors. Mol Cell Biol Hum Dis Ser 1995;5:33–63.
13. Mandl S, Sigal LJ, Rock KL, Andino R. Poliovirus vaccine vectors elicit antigen-specific cytotoxic T cells and protect mice against lethal challenge with malignant melanoma cells expressing a model antigen. Proc Natl Acad Sci U S A 1998;95:8216–21.
14. Levitsky HI. Canarypox virus vectors for gene transfer in cancer immunotherapy. editorial; comment. J Natl Cancer Inst 1997;89:408–9.
15. Wolff JA, Malone RW, Williams P, et al. Direct gene transfer into mouse muscle in vivo. Science 1990;247:1465–8.
16. Conry RM, LoBuglio AF, Curiel DT. Polynucleotide-mediated immunization therapy of cancer. Semin Oncol 1996;23:135–47.
17. Corr M, Lee DJ, Carson DA, Tighe H. Gene vaccination with naked plasmid DNA: mechanism of CTL priming. J Exp Med 1996;184:1555–60.
18. Doe B, Selby M, Barnett S, et al. Induction of cytotoxic T lymphocytes by intramuscular immunization with plasmid DNA is facilitated by bone marrow–derived cells. Proc Natl Acad Sci U S A 1996;93:8578–83.
19. Freeman SM, Ramesh R, Marrogi AJ. Immune system in suicide gene therapy. Lancet 1997;349:2–3.
20. Alvarez RD, Curiel DT. A phase I study of recombinant adenovirus vector-mediated intraperitoneal delivery of herpes simplex virus thymidine kinase (HSV-TK) gene and intravenous ganciclovir for previously treated ovarian and extraovarian cancer patients. Hum Gene Ther 1997;8:597–613.
21. Sterman DH, Treat J, Litzky LA, et al. Adenovirus-mediated herpes simplex virus thymidine kinase/ganciclovir gene therapy in patients with localized malignancy: results of a phase I clinical trial in malignant mesothelioma. Hum Gene Ther 1998;9:1083–92.
22. Garcia-Sanchez F, Pizzorno G, Fu SQ, et al. Cytosine deaminase adenoviral vector and 5-fluorocytosine selectively reduce breast cancer cells 1 million-fold when they contaminate hematopoietic cells: a potential purging method for autologous transplantation. Blood 1998;92:672–82.
23. Mullen CA, Coale MM, Lowe R, Blaese RM. Tumors expressing the cytosine deaminase suicide gene can be eliminated in vivo with 5-fluorocytosine and induce protective immunity to wild type tumor. Cancer Res 1994;54:1503–6.
24. Dachs GU, Patterson AV, Firth JD, et al. Targeting gene expression to hypoxic tumor cells. Nat Med 1997;3:515–20.
25. Osaki T, Tanio Y, Tachibana I, et al. Gene therapy for carcinoembryonic antigen–producing human lung cancer cells by cell type–specific expression of herpes simplex virus thymidine kinase gene. Cancer Res 1994;54:5258–61.
26. Tanaka T, Kanai F, Okabe S, et al. Adenovirus-mediated prodrug gene therapy for carcinoembryonic antigen–producing human gastric carcinoma cells in vitro. Cancer Res 1996;56:1341–5.
27. Deisseroth AB, Pizzorno G. The use of chemotherapy resistance in cancer treatment. Cancer J Sci Am 1997;3:60–9.
28. Fujiwara T, Grimm EA, Mukhopadhyay T, et al. Induction of chemosensitivity in human lung cancer cells in vivo by adenovirus-mediated transfer of the wild-type p53 gene. Cancer Res 1994;54:2287–91.
29. Clayman GL, el-Naggar AK, Lippman SM, et al. Adenovirus-mediated p53 gene transfer in patients with advanced recurrent head and neck squamous cell carcinoma. J Clin Oncol 1998;16:2221–32.
30. Roth JA, Swisher SG, Merritt JA, et al. Gene therapy for non–small cell lung cancer: a preliminary report of a phase I trial of adenoviral p53 gene replacement. Semin Oncol 1998;25:33–7.
31. Swisher SG, Roth JA. Gene therapy for human lung cancers. Surg Oncol Clin North Am 1998;7:603–16.
32. Narayanan R, Akhtar S. Antisense therapy. Curr Opin Oncol 1996;8:509–15.
33. Rosenberg SA. Karnofsky Memorial Lecture: the immunotherapy and gene therapy of cancer. J Clin Oncol 1992;10:180–99.
34. Giralt SA, Kolb HJ. Donor lymphocyte infusions. Curr Opin Oncol 1996;8:96–102.
35. Pardoll DM. Cancer vaccines. Immunol Today 1993;14:310–6.
36. Golumbek PT, Lazenby AJ, Levitsky HI, et al. Treatment of established renal cancer by tumor cells engineered to secrete interleukin-4. Science 1991;254:713–6.
37. Fearon ER, Pardoll DM, Itaya T, et al. Interleukin-2 production by tumor cells bypasses T-helper function in the generation of an antitumor response. Cell 1990;60:397–403.
38. Gansbacher B, Zier K, Daniels B, et al. Interleukin-2 gene transfer into tumor cells abrogates tumorigenicity and induces protective immunity. J Exp Med 1990;172:1217–24.
39. Gansbacher B, Bannerji R, Daniels B, et al. Retroviral vector-mediated gamma-interferon gene transfer into tumor cells generates potent and long-lasting antitumor immunity. Cancer Res 1990;50:7820–5.
40. McBride WH, Thacker JD, Comora S, et al. Genetic modification of a murine fibrosarcoma to produce interleukin-7 stimulates host cell infiltration and tumor immunity. Cancer Res 1992;52:3931–7.
41. McBride WH, Dougherty GD, Wallis AE, et al. Interleukin-3 in gene therapy of cancer. Folia Biol (Praha) 1994;40:62–73.
42. Dranoff G, Jaffee E, Lazenby A, et al. Vaccination with irradiated tumor cells engineered to secrete murine granulocyte-macrophage colony-stimulating factor stimulates potent, specific, and long-lasting anti-tumor immunity. Proc Natl Acad Sci U S A 1993;90:3539–43.
43. Toloza EM, Hunt K, Swisher S, et al. In vivo cancer gene therapy with a recombinant interleukin-2 adenovirus vector. Cancer Gene Ther 1996;3:11–7.
44. Huang AY, Golumbek P, Ahmadzadeh M, et al. Role of bone marrow–derived cells in presenting MHC class I–restricted tumor antigens. Science 1994;264:961–5.
45. Huang AY, Bruce AT, Pardoll DM, Levitsky HI. Does B7-1 expression confer antigen-presenting cell capacity to tumors in vivo? J Exp Med 1996;183:769–76.
46. Wu TC, Huang AY, Jaffee EM, et al. A reassessment of the role of B7-1 expression in tumor rejection. J Exp Med 1995;182:1415–21.
47. Guo Y, Wu M, Chen H, et al. Effective tumor vaccine generated by fusion of hepatoma cells with activated B cells. Science 1994;263:518–20.

48. Gong J, Chen D, Kashiwaba M, Kufe D. Induction of antitumor activity by immunization with fusions of dendritic and carcinoma cells. Nat Med 1997;3:558–61.

49. Gong J, Chen D, Kashiwaba M, et al. Reversal of tolerance to human MUC1 antigen in MUC1 transgenic mice immunized with fusions of dendritic and carcinoma cells. Proc Natl Acad Sci U S A 1998;95:6279–83.

50. Fakhrai H, Dorigo O, Shawler DL, et al. Eradication of established intracranial rat gliomas by transforming growth factor beta antisense gene therapy. Proc Natl Acad Sci U S A 1996;93:2909–14.

51. Bui LA, Butterfield LH, Kim JY, et al. In vivo therapy of hepatocellular carcinoma with a tumor-specific adenoviral vector expressing interleukin-2. Hum Gene Ther 1997;8:2173–82.

52. DiMaio JM, Clary BM, Via DF, et al. Directed enzyme prodrug gene therapy for pancreatic cancer in vivo. Surgery 1994;116:205–13.

53. Rubin J, Galanis E, Pitot HC, et al. Phase I study of immunotherapy of hepatic metastases of colorectal carcinoma by direct gene transfer of an allogeneic histocompatibility antigen, HLA-B7. Gene Ther 1997;4:419–25.

54. Stopeck AT, Hersh EM, Akporiaye ET, et al. Phase I study of direct gene transfer of an allogeneic histocompatibility antigen, HLA-B7, in patients with metastatic melanoma. J Clin Oncol 1997;15:341–9.

55. Rosenberg SA. The immunotherapy of solid cancers based on cloning the genes encoding tumor-rejection antigens. Annu Rev Med 1996;47:481–91.

56. Boon T, Coulie P, Van den Eynde B. Tumor antigens recognized by T cells. Immunol Today 1997;18:267–8.

57. Inaba K, Inaba M, Romani N, et al. Generation of large numbers of dendritic cells from mouse bone marrow cultures supplemented with granulocyte/macrophage colony-stimulating factor. J Exp Med 1992;176:1693–702.

58. Romani N, Gruner S, Brang D, et al. Proliferating dendritic cell progenitors in human blood. J Exp Med 1994;180:83–93.

59. Steinman RM, Pack M, Inaba K. Dendritic cell development and maturation. Adv Exp Med Biol 1997;417:1–6.

60. Young JW, Szabolcs P, Moore MA. Identification of dendritic cell colony-forming units among normal human CD34$^+$ bone marrow progenitors that are expanded by c-kit-ligand and yield pure dendritic cell colonies in the presence of granulocyte/macrophage colony-stimulating factor and tumor necrosis factor alpha. J Exp Med 1995;182:1111–9.

61. Mayordomo JI, Zorina T, Storkus WJ, et al. Bone marrow–derived dendritic cells pulsed with synthetic tumour peptides elicit protective and therapeutic antitumour immunity. Nat Med 1995;1:1297–302.

62. Mayordomo JI, Loftus DJ, Sakamoto H, et al. Therapy of murine tumors with p53 wild-type and mutant sequence peptide-based vaccines. J Exp Med 1996;183:1357–65.

63. Porgador A, Snyder D, Gilboa E. Induction of antitumor immunity using bone marrow-generated dendritic cells. J Immunol 1996;156:2918–26.

64. Celluzzi CM, Mayordomo JI, Storkus WJ, et al. Peptide-pulsed dendritic cells induce antigen-specific CTL-mediated protective tumor immunity. J Exp Med 1996;183:283–7.

65. Zitvogel L, Mayordomo JI, Tjandrawan T, et al. Therapy of murine tumors with tumor peptide-pulsed dendritic cells: dependence on T cells, B7 costimulation, and T helper cell 1–associated cytokines. J Exp Med 1996;183:87–97.

66. Nestle FO, Alijagic S, Gilliet M, et al. Vaccination of melanoma patients with peptide- or tumor lysate–pulsed dendritic cells. Nat Med 1998;4:328–32.

67. Ribas A, Butterfield LH, McBride WH, et al. Genetic immunization for the melanoma antigen MART-1/melan-A using recombinant adenovirus-transduced murine dendritic cells. Cancer Res 1997;57:2865–9.

68. Brossart P, Goldrath AW, Butz EA, et al. Virus-mediated delivery of antigenic epitopes into dendritic cells as a means to induce CTL. J Immunol 1997;158:3270–6.

69. Specht JM, Wang G, Do MT, et al. Dendritic cells retrovirally transduced with a model antigen gene are therapeutically effective against established pulmonary metastases. J Exp Med 1997;186:1213–21.

70. Song W, Kong HL, Carpenter H, et al. Dendritic cells genetically modified with an adenovirus vector encoding the cDNA for a model antigen induce protective and therapeutic antitumor immunity. J Exp Med 1997;186:1247–56.

71. Boczkowski D, Nair SK, Snyder D, Gilboa E. Dendritic cells pulsed with RNA are potent antigen-presenting cells in vitro and in vivo. J Exp Med 1996;184:465–72.

# CHAPTER 31

# INVESTIGATIONAL DRUGS

● ROMAN PEREZ-SOLER ● FRANCO M. MUGGIA

Anticancer drug development is a dynamic and rapidly changing field, with many agents entering clinical trials at a given point and many others being abandoned because of intolerable or unexpected toxicities or, more often, lack of efficacy. Less than 10% of new anticancer agents that enter phase I evaluation are eventually approved. This high failure rate is due to the inability of currently available animal tumor models to predict for clinical antitumor activity. The term *investigational cancer drugs* covers a large and heterogeneous group of compounds at different stages of development and regulatory approval process. This chapter concerns itself with small-molecule anticancer drugs that are not yet commercially available in the United States but that are actively studied in the clinic based on a new mechanism of action, promising preclinical profile, or preliminary evidence of encouraging antitumor activity and tolerability in early clinical trials. Excluded from this review are biologic agents (proteins, oligopeptides, genes, and so on) and vaccines.

We cover at least six different types of investigational agents:

1. *Agents that have been approved in foreign countries but not in the United States and for which efforts are under way seeking such approval.* The oral 5-fluorouracil formulation UFT (to be marketed as Orzel), the thymidylate synthase (TS) inhibitor raltitrexed (Tomudex), and the platinum compound oxaliplatin approved in Japan and Europe, respectively, are good examples of this group of agents. The Food and Drug Administration (FDA) has recognized the desirability of formalizing procedures allowing "expanded access" to drugs that are available elsewhere but have not attained approved indications in the United States.[1] An analysis of 46 drugs included in such expanded access available since March 1996 reveals 21 chemotherapeutic agents, 11 hormones, 5 immunomodulators, and a small miscellaneous group of radiation sensitizers, herbal medicines, and supportive care preparations. Some of these drugs have since gained approval in the United States, and others have been dropped by the foreign sponsor.

2. *Agents that have been approved in the United States for a particular indication and that continue to be studied*

*in the clinic for other indications.* A major emerging trend in the United States is to approve drugs for certain narrow indications, and any other uses are considered "investigational" until such time that trials addressing a specific new use gain additional FDA-approved indications. Although the FDA has never regulated commercially available drugs used "off label" (only limiting the distribution of information by the manufacturer), the restriction of coverage by third-party carriers for the increasingly more expensive drug market to approved indications only constitutes the major barrier to such off-label prescribing. As a result, off-label use of drugs is becoming increasingly difficult out of the context of a clinical trial, thus blurring the distinction between investigational and off-label use of commercially available drugs. This has encouraged submissions of Supplementary New Drug Applications by industry.

3. *New formulations of approved drugs.* An important emerging trend has been the focus on developing oral formulations of the major classic chemotherapeutic drugs, an approach previously ignored because of concerns about the reproducibility of the absorption pattern for most existing chemotherapeutic agents. There are currently at least five different oral fluoropyrimidine agents in clinical development, one of them already approved in the United States, and two oral formulations of camptothecin drugs (topotecan and 9-nitrocaptothecin). Also, many years of efforts in the area of drug delivery systems have resulted in the approval of a variety of liposome and polyethylene glycol formulations of different agents (e.g., L-asparaginase), and this approach continues to be explored for other agents requiring daily administration such as granulocyte colony–stimulating factor for different indications.

4. *Analogues of existing agents designed and selected for clinical development because of an improved toxicity profile or a broader spectrum of antitumor activity.* The best example of this approach is the significant efforts placed on identifying analogues that are not subject to the classic mechanisms of acquired drug resistance, namely, transmembrane transporters and DNA repair. Examples of agents in this category are many of the new anthracyclines and the diaminocyclohexane platinum compounds.

5. *New chemical entities that exert their therapeutic effects on newly identified cellular and molecular targets; in many cases these chemicals are claimed to be specific for tumor cells.* In the late 1990s, advances in our understanding of cancer biology and genetics led to intensive efforts to rationally design or identify from large combinatorial chemistry libraries agents that exert their antitumor activity by interfering with pathways involved in dysregulated tumor cell growth, angiogenesis, the cell cycle, apoptosis, telomerase, and tumor invasion. Many compounds targeting these pathways are now actively being developed in the clinic. Because many of these agents are not classic cytotoxic compounds and are probably more tumor specific than the classic chemotherapeutic agents, there is extensive discussion about whether the end point of phase I trials with these agents should be the determination of the optimal biologic dose (dose that effectively inhibits the targeted enzyme) rather than the maximal tolerated dose.

6. *Modulators of antitumor activity and toxicity.* In addition to the previous five groups of investigational agents, a number of drugs are under investigation for their resistance-reversal potential in combination with conventional cytotoxic agents. Conversely, following the successful introduction of dexrazoxane and amifostine, a number of other normal tissue cytoprotective agents that may block the toxicities of anthracyclines and cisplatin are under active investigation.

## Established Antitumor Drug Classes

### TOPOISOMERASE II INHIBITORS

**Anthracyclines.** Doxorubicin, daunorubicin, and idarubicin continue to be the standard agents in the topoisomerase II family. Efforts in the anthracycline area have been focused on enhancing their therapeutic index through liposome delivery and on developing analogues that are mechanistically different or offer the potential of a reduced cellular efflux. Two liposomal formulations of doxorubicin and daunorubicin are approved for clinical indications against human immunodeficiency virus–related Kaposi's sarcoma (Caelyx or Doxil,[2] and DaunoXome[3]). These formulations consist of small (about 100 nm in diameter), nonleaky liposomes that have a prolonged plasma circulation time because they contain phospholipids with a high transition temperature (DaunoXome, Gilead) and pegylated phospholipids (Doxil or Caelyx, Alza). As a result, with time these liposomes tend to localize in tissues with leaky vessels. Both formulations are now being studied in a variety of solid tumors. In particular, Caelyx has shown promising antitumor activity in patients with recurrent ovarian carcinoma.[4] Another liposomal-doxorubicin formulation (TLC D-99, The Liposome Co.) is under investigation for metastatic breast cancer because of expectations of reduced cardiac and other toxicities.[5] This formulation consists of small (about 100 nm in diameter) liposomes that release the drug quickly after intravenous administration and that result in reduced cardiac drug levels compared with free doxorubicin.

Several anthracycline analogues are under active investigation. Annamycin (Aronex) is a highly lipophilic analogue that incorporates the 4-demethoxy modification of idarubicin and the 4'epi hydroxyl group of epirubicin. It is ideally suited for liposome delivery and is not a substrate for P-glycoprotein. It is being tested in a liposome formulation in patients with acute leukemia and metastatic breast cancer that is refractory to anthracyclines and has significant activity by the oral route.[6] AD-32 (Anthra) is another lipophilic, non–cross-resistant anthracycline that has undergone wide phase III testing for local-regional administration, either intravesically or intraperitoneally, because of its favorable depot characteristics and enhanced tissue penetration properties.[7] The morpholino derivatives MX2[8] and methoxymorpholino doxorubicin[9] (Pharmacia) offer the potential advantage of greatly enhanced potency, and they are also poor substrates for the P-glycoprotein and other drug efflux mechanisms. Although annamycin and AD-32 are topoisomerase II poisons, the morpholino compounds are alkylating agents and therefore mechanistically distinct from the parent compound. Hepatotoxicity was observed in the phase I study of methoxymorpholino doxorubicin. Some of the morpholino compounds are also potentially active by the oral route.

**Anthrapyrazoles.** These compounds were synthesized as DNA-binding drugs sharing the three-ring structure of the anthracenediones (e.g., mitoxantrone), but with a reduced potential for cardiotoxicity by substituting an imine for a carbonyl in the B ring, thus reducing the degree of free radical generation. As with amsacrine, anthracyclines, and anthracenediones, these compounds bind to DNA, inhibiting its synthesis and causing topoisomerase II–induced DNA strand breaks. Conversely, the potential for anthrapyrazoles to induce activated oxygen species is several times less than it is for doxorubicin. The initial phase II trial of losoxantrone (DuP 941) in patients with advanced breast cancer at the Royal Marsden Hospital reported 2 complete and 17 partial responses among 30 patients evaluated. Untreated patients accounted mostly for this high response rate, but 4 of 6 responses were documented in patients who had been treated previously with CMF (cyclophosphamide, methotrexate, 5-fluorouracil).[10] Randomized studies have been performed in previously untreated metastatic breast cancer, demonstrating that losoxantrone improves the response rate and progression-free survival when given with paclitaxel over that achieved by paclitaxel alone.[11]

**Other Topoisomerase II Inhibitors.** Other compounds that act as topoisomerase II poisons are being developed. Elinafide (LU 79553, Knoll) is a bisnaphtalamide with DNA intercalating and topoisomerase II poisoning action, which has shown activity in multidrug-resistant cell lines. Its dose-limiting toxicities are neutropenia and a reversible neuromuscular syndrome.[12] Olivacine (S 16020, Servier) is a topoisomerase II inhibitor that also has activity in multidrug-resistant cell lines and is currently in phase I studies.[13] NSC 655649 is a rebeccamycin analogue with DNA intercalating and topoisomerase II inhibitory activity. Its dose-limiting toxicity is myelosuppression.[14] TOP-53 (Taiho Pharmaceutical) is an etoposide analogue with enhanced water solubility. Limiting toxicities observed in a recently completed phase I trial include myelosuppression and liver and lung toxicity.[15] Two other interesting compounds under development have both topoisomerase I and topoisomerase II poisoning activity. TAS-103 is a quinoline developed by Taiho Pharmaceutical, which tends to accumulate in the lung and has shown enhanced antitumor activity in different models of lung tumors. It is currently in phase I studies in the United States and its limiting toxicity is neutropenia.[16] The other, intoplicine (RPR 60475),[17] has liver toxicity and myelosuppression as dose-limiting toxicities. This dual mechanism of action is of interest because combinations of topoisomerase I and topoisomerase II poisons appear to be antagonistic when administered together and synergistic when given sequentially.

## ANTIFOLATES

Several compounds have been introduced that target enzymes other than dihydrofolate reductase. Folate antagonists, such as lometrexol, that are excellent substrates of folylpolyglutamyl synthetase (FPGS) and inhibit glycinamide ribonucleotide formyltransferase (GARFT) were among the first to be introduced into trial but were associated with cumulative hematologic toxicity. Other derivatives targeting this enzyme are undergoing phase I investigation because of their promising activity in xenograft models and higher potency compared with lometrexol; they are AG2034, developed by protein structure–based drug design,[18] and LY309887.[19]

Structure-activity relationships identified powerful thymidylate synthase (TS) inhibitors among this class of agents, which resulted in the successful clinical development of raltitrexed (Tomudex)—an agent that has been approved in Europe as a drug equivalent to 5-fluorouracil (5-FU) for advanced colorectal cancer.[20] Combining 5-FU or irinotecan with raltitrexed has yielded encouraging leads,[21] and its potential as a radiosensitizer is also being explored. ZD 9331, a TS inhibitor that does not require FPGS for activation and therefore may have a different spectrum of activity, is undergoing phase I evaluation.[22] A multitargeted antifolate (MTA, LY 231514, Lilly) that inhibits TS, dihydrofolate reductase, and GARFT has advanced beyond phase I study,[23] has shown antitumor activity in non–small cell lung cancer and malignant mesothelioma, and is also being tested in combination with 5-FU. Its limiting toxicity is myelosuppression.

## FLUOROPYRIMIDINES AND OTHER NONFOLATE THYMIDYLATE SYNTHASE INHIBITORS

5-FU continues to occupy center stage in the treatment of colorectal cancer, and its therapeutic index is likely improved by prolonged exposure and by the administration of reduced folates. Orally administered prodrugs have been under active investigation, initially in Japan and more recently throughout the world. Capecitabine (Xeloda, Roche) is a fluoropyrimidine carbamate, which was rationally designed as an orally available antitumor agent. It crosses the intestinal tract intact, is transformed into 5′-DFUR in the liver and into 5-FU primarily in tumor tissues under the action of pyrimidine nucleoside phosphorylase. It has become available for the treatment of anthracycline- and taxane-refractory breast cancer.[24] Other prodrugs under development include UFT (tegafur and uracil at a 1:4 molar ratio, Bristol Myers–Squibb),[25] S1 (tegafur, 5-chloro-2,4-didroxypyridine m-CDHP, and potassium oxonate)[26] and BOF-A2 (emitefur and 3-cyano-2,6-dihydropyrimidine)[27]; they have been mostly targeted against colorectal cancer. They all combine a 5-FU prodrug with an inhibitor of its catalysis and, in the case of S1, also with an inhibitor of nucleotide formation in the gastrointestinal tract (potassium oxonate) that results in decreased gastrointestinal toxicity. Evidence that inhibition of dihydropyrimidine dehydrogenase improves the antitumor activity of 5-FU and markedly enhances its bioavailability has also spurred the development of a suicide inhibitor of the enzyme (eniluracil) and small daily doses of oral 5-FU. Phase III comparative studies of this strategy for colorectal cancer, as well as combination studies with radiation for head and neck cancer, are maturing.[28]

A nonfolate inhibitor of TS, nolatrexed (Thymitaq, AG-337), represents drug development by rational design based on the structure of TS and its active site. It has proceeded beyond phase I to a number of phase II studies consisting of a daily schedule for 5 consecutive days of infusion therapy (daily × 5). On this schedule, only hematologic toxicity has been observed, and transient elevations in plasma deoxyuridine levels provide evidence for its biochemical effects.[29]

Classic fluoropyrimidines continue to be explored widely in combination with leucovorin as biochemical modulation based on presumably selective enhanced TS inhibition. Another strategy under investigation is selective rescue of bone marrow and other normal tissues by uridine, inhibiting the incorporation of fluorouridinetriphosphate into RNA. PN401 is an oral prodrug of uridine that is under study; it permits substantially higher doses of 5-FU to be administered[30] and has also been used as a rescue agent after inadvertent overdosing of 5-FU. In addition, S1 (see previously) contains oxonic acid that selectively protects against gastrointestinal toxicity.

## NUCLEOSIDES

Azacytidine and deoxyazacytidine are derivatives with long-term clinical experience that are receiving renewed attention for their demethylating properties. They are being investigated in solid tumors in which inactivation of certain genes by methylation is thought to play an important role in their pathogenesis.[31] Gemcitabine's success has attracted attention to cytosine nucleoside analogues, and some of these agents are proceeding to clinical trials. BCH-4556 is a novel nucleoside with an L configuration. It is incorporated into DNA but lacks the critical hydroxyl moiety required for chain elongation, which results in complete DNA chain termination. It is undergoing phase I clinical trials in Canada.[32]

## TOPOISOMERASE I INHIBITORS

Different camptothecin analogues, in addition to topotecan and CPT-11, are in clinical development using a variety of schedules of administration. 9-Amino camptothecin (IDEC Pharmaceuticals, Inc) was one of the most active agents in preclinical models when a twice-weekly depot schedule of administration was used but had little activity by intravenous administration. Its development has been hampered by its lack of water solubility. It is currently being studied in a colloidal dispersion using a daily × 5 short infusion schedule. Its limiting toxicity is myelosuppression.[33, 34] 9-Nitro camptothecin (RFS 2000, SuperGen, Inc) is being developed in an oral formulation. This agent is a prodrug of 9-amino camptothecin. Its main limiting toxicity is myelosuppression. Mild to moderate chemical cystitis has been observed in about 20% of patients. A few responses have been observed in patients with pancreatic cancer. Combination studies with gemcitabine and radiotherapy are being planned. GI 147211 (Glaxo), a somewhat more potent version of topotecan, is currently being developed in a liposome formulation in collaboration with Nexstar.[35] Liposomes with a long circulation time are a rational delivery system for camptothecins because they may provide a slow drug release system, accumulate passively in tumors, and protect the drug from inactivation (opening of lactone ring) by plasma components. DX-8951f (Daichi), a fluorinated compound, is being developed because of its increased potency and broader spectrum of antitumor activity.[36] Several phase I studies exploring different schedules are in progress in the United States and Europe. The dose-limiting toxicity appears to be myelosuppression and the spectrum of toxicities similar to that of topotecan. In addition to 9-nitro camptothecin, topotecan is also being developed in an oral formulation. Its absorption in the gastrointestinal tract is reproducible and on the order of 30%. It is currently being studied in a daily × 5 schedule. Using this schedule, doses that result in an area under the curve equivalent to that obtained with intravenous administration have been shown to result in equivalent antitumor activity in ovarian carcinoma patients and small cell lung cancer patients but to produce significantly less neutropenia, thus suggesting that myelosuppression but not antitumor activity may be related to plasma peak levels. Diarrhea has been observed in a small proportion of patients. More prolonged schedules of administration are planned, and they may be ideally suited to combination with radiation therapy.

## ANTITUBULIN AGENTS

RPR 109881A is a new taxoid selected for its ability to circumvent P-glycoprotein–mediated resistance.[37] It has shown activity both in vitro and in vivo in models that are resistant to paclitaxel and, as is the case in many analogues that are not substrates for P-glycoprotein, it has also shown an ability to cross the blood-brain barrier. Different phase I studies using different schedules of administration are in progress. Myelosuppression is the dose-limiting toxicity. Responses in patients with non–small cell lung cancer and head and neck cancer have been observed. LU 103793 (Knoll) is an analogue of dolastatin 15, which inhibits microtubule assembly and tubulin polymerization by binding to tubulin at sites distinct from the vinca alkaloids and taxanes. In a completed phase I study, the limiting toxicity was neutropenia.[38] CI-980 is a novel mitotic spindle inhibitor that binds at the colchicine site and has shown activity against multidrug-resistant cell lines in preclinical systems. It is currently being evaluated in different phase II trials using a 3-day continuous infusion schedule.[39]

## PLATINUM ANALOGUES

After years of intensive search for more effective platinum analogues, the compound oxaliplatin (Sanofi) is emerging as a promising new antitumor agent. Oxaliplatin belongs to the family of the diaminocyclohexane (DACH) analogues, which have a cyclohexane group attached to the two amino groups. It has been known for a long time that this modification confers a lack of cross-resistance. The mechanism of the lack of cross-resistance is unknown but most likely is related to the inability of cisplatin-resistant cells to repair DACH-Pt-DNA adducts as effectively as $(NH_3)_2$-Pt-DNA adducts. Several DACH compounds have been evaluated in the clinic since 1985 without success for a variety of reasons. Tetraplatin (ormaplatin) turned out to cause significantly more neurotoxicity than did oxaliplatin, and its development was abandoned. This is thought to be secondary to the fastest and more predominant transformation of tetraplatin into DACH-Pt-Cl2, whereas oxaliplatin tends to remain in its aquated species for a more prolonged period.[40] The dose-limiting toxicity of oxaliplatin is a sensory neuropathy that appears to be easily reversible. The incidence of grade 2 to grade 3 neuropathy is about 10% after six cycles. Ototoxicity is not a side effect of oxaliplatin. Myelosuppression is uncommon and not severe when oxaliplatin is used as a single agent.[41] Oxaliplatin has shown modest single-agent antitumor activity against a variety of solid tumors, mainly colorectal and non–small cell lung cancer. Remarkable synergism with 5-FU was observed in vitro,[42] and this combination has been reported to produce a remarkable response rate in patients with colorectal carcinoma whose disease had progressed after treatment with 5-FU. Oxaliplatin has already been approved for this indication in France. Studies leading to its approval in the United States are in progress. Other potential indications include lung cancer, head and neck cancer, and ovarian carcinoma.

L-NDDP (M.D. Anderson Cancer Center) is a lipophilic DACH-Pt compound designed for liposome delivery. It is formulated in large multilamellar liposomes that measure 1 to 3 μm in diameter. Initial phase I trials by intravenous administration indicated that its dose-limiting toxicity is myelosuppression. Because of its depot characteristics, it is currently being explored for the treatment of malignant mesothelioma and ovarian carcinoma by the intracavitary route. Clinical trials by intravenous administration in patients with colorectal carcinoma, renal cell carcinoma, and non–small cell lung cancer are also in progress.

JM-216 (Bristol Myers–Squibb) is a *cis*-diammine compound with toxicologic efficacy properties similar to those of carboplatin; it is being developed for oral administration.[43] Remarkable activity in small cell lung cancer has already been reported. The oral formulation will ensure exploration of new daily schedules that may be advantageous in combination with radiation. Platinum drugs are also being tested in combination with protective drugs such as amifostine, and with modulators such as tirapazamine (see further on).

SPI-77 is a liposomal formulation of cisplatin developed by Sequus. Stealth liposomes similar to those developed for Caelyx are used. Phase I clinical trials are in progress. The maximal tolerated dose has not been reached at 300 mg/m². No myelosuppression or renal toxicity has been seen at this dose level. Neurotoxicity has been observed and may be the limiting toxicity of this formulation.

A depot cisplatin formulation using a polymeric gel is also being developed by Matrix Pharmaceuticals for intratumoral administration. Studies in head and neck cancer and melanoma are in progress.[44]

## Miscellaneous Antitumor Drugs

Temozolomide (Schering-Plough) is a DTIC (dimethyl triazeno imidazole carboxamide [dacarbazine]) analogue that is stable at acid pH, thus allowing for 100% oral bioavailability, and with excellent penetration into the central nervous system. In vivo studies demonstrated excellent activity against central nervous system tumors that are resistant to the nitrosoureas. Using a daily × 5 schedule, activity was observed in patients with malignant gliomas and melanomas, as well as other solid tumors. Combination studies in patients with brain tumors and melanomas are in progress.

Carzelesin (Pharmacia-Upjohn) is a novel DNA minor groove–binding, sequence-specific alkylating agent. It is an analogue of the potent antibiotic CC-1065–like adozelesin and bizelesin. Broad phase II evaluation has shown that the drug is well tolerated but with only limited antitumor activity against a variety of solid tumors. Cumulative myelosuppression has been of concern with this group of drugs.[45]

## Toxicity Protectors and Antitumor-Action Enhancers (Modulators)

Amifostine is the first FDA-approved chemoprotective agent. Amifostine selectively protects the normal organs, including bone marrow, kidney, and peripheral nervous system, from chemotherapy- and radiotherapy-induced damage. Amifostine is an organic thiophosphate that is diphosphorylated by alkaline phosphatase to an activated thiol form. The basis for its lack of protection in tumor tissues is their decreased alkaline phosphatase activity. Numerous ongoing phase II and phase III studies are exploring the use of amifostine as a cytoprotective agent in patients with a variety of solid tumors treated with radiation or drug combinations containing platinum compounds, antitubulin agents, and taxanes.[46, 47]

Tirapazamine (Sanofi) is a novel bioreductive agent with selective cytotoxicity against hypoxic tumor cells; it is being explored as a radiosensitizer and a potentiator of cisplatin antitumor activity. Several studies in which it was used in combination with cisplatin in patients with non–small cell lung cancer, cervical cancer, and head and neck cancer have shown encouraging results. In patients with non–small cell lung cancer, a response rate of 25% and a median survival of 39 weeks have been observed. Toxicities have included muscle cramps, gastrointestinal symptoms, vomiting, and hearing loss in 13% of patients, which was reversible. No increased myelosuppression was observed.

PSC-833 (Novartis) is an analogue of cyclosporine that has shown a remarkable ability to reverse P-glycoprotein–mediated resistance both in vitro and in vivo. It is being evaluated in combination with different chemotherapeutic agents in acute leukemia and different solid tumors in which classic multidrug resistance may be involved. Responses have in general been disappointing, thus suggesting that classic multidrug resistance is just one of multiple concomitant mechanisms of resistance in most human cancers.[48]

## Antitumor Agents Directed Toward New Molecular Targets

### SIGNAL TRANSDUCTION PATHWAYS

Tyrosine kinase activation is the initial step in a variety of signal transduction pathways involved in dysregulated neoplastic growth. Specific inhibitors of the various tyrosine kinases involved in these pathways have been identified and are rapidly entering clinical evaluation.

The epidermal growth factor receptor (EGFR) pathway is involved in the pathogenesis of a number of solid tumors, including head and neck cancer, non–small cell lung cancer, renal cell carcinoma, and cervical cancer, among others.[49] The monoclonal antibody C225 (Imclone Systems) blocks EGFR, inhibits its tyrosine kinase function, and exerts a cytostatic effect in most tumor cells with high EGFR expression.[50] In addition, and similar to the anti *erb*-B2 antibody trastuzumab (Herceptin) (Genentech),[51] it has shown marked synergism in vivo with different chemotherapeutic agents, including cisplatin, paclitaxel, and doxorubicin. A variety of small molecules that are selective inhibitors of EGFR tyrosine kinase have been identified from large combinatorial chemistry libraries. Two of these compounds have reached clinical evaluation (ZD 1839, Zeneca; CP 358774, Pfizer).[52, 53] In preclinical studies, these compounds showed a cytostatic effect in tumors expressing EGFR. In contrast with studies with C225 and trastuzumab, combinations with different chemotherapeutic agents showed an additive effect but no synergism. In completed phase I studies, the limiting toxicity appears to be some type of folliculitis. Studies in combination with chemotherapy are in progress. A similar compound developed by Warner-Lambert has not yet entered clinical trials.

Platelet-derived growth factor (PDGF) signaling has been implicated in the aberrant growth of many cancers. SU101 (Sugen) is an inhibitor of PDGF–tyrosine kinase.[54] In preclinical studies, SU101 was found to inhibit the growth of PDGF-dependent tumor cell growth and cause cell cycle arrest. To date, several phase I and phase II trials have been completed. The dose-limiting toxicity of SU101 was altered mental status due to cerebral edema, and responses were seen in patients with brain tumors, non–small cell lung cancer, and prostate cancer.

Other specific tyrosine kinase inhibitors include SU5416 (Sugen),[55] which is a specific inhibitor for the vascular endothelial growth factor (VEGF) receptor Flt-1 tyrosine kinase and is being developed as an antiangiogenic agent (see further on) and CEP 2563 (TAP Holdings),[56] an inhibitor of the neurotropin family of growth factor receptor–linked tyrosine kinases. Both compounds are currently being evaluated in phase I clinical trials.

Three protein kinase inhibitors are currently in clinical development: Bryostatin, a natural marine compound (Bristol Myers–Squibb),[57] CGP 41251 (Novartis),[58] and UCN-01 (National Cancer Institute).[59] Bryostatin is a macrocytic lactone isolated from a marine animal. Its antitumor activity appears to stem from the modulation of protein kinase C (PKC). Several schedules have been explored in phase I studies. The limiting toxicities were myalgias and phlebitis at the site of injection. CGP 41251, *N*-benzoyl staurosporine, has just completed phase I clinical evaluation. The drug is well tolerated, with side effects limited to nausea and vomiting at doses that cause PKC inhibition in vivo. UCN-01, 7 hydroxy-staurosporine, is a potent PKC inhibitor, which has shown potent direct inhibition of cell cycle–dependent kinases and selective antiproliferative effects in p53-mutated cell lines. A phase I clinical study has been completed. The limiting toxicities include hyperglycemia, myalgias, and hypophosphatemia. The development of these agents is being pursued in combination with chemotherapeutic agents.

## RAS FARNESYL TRANSFERASE INHIBITORS

Farnesylation of ras proteins has been identified as a promising target in tumor therapy because of the occurrence of mutated *ras* in a wide variety of human cancers. Inhibition of the farnesylation of ras proteins reverses the transformation caused by mutated *ras*.[60] Several small chemical entities that inhibit ras farnesylation have been developed during the last few years by Schering-Plough (SCH 66336), Merck (L-744832), Janssen (R115777), and Bristol Myers–Squibb, and have entered clinical trials in the United States. Interestingly, these compounds have shown striking antitumor activity in both *ras*-mutated and nonmutated preclinical tumor models. In addition to these specific inhibitors, perillyl alcohol, a monoterpene that inhibits *ras* function, is also being evaluated.

## METALLOPROTEINASE INHIBITORS

Metalloproteinases comprise a multigene family of enzymes that degrade a wide range of matrix protein substrates, including collagens, laminin, fibronectin, and elastin. High expression of these enzymes occurs in cancer and is related to the ability of the tumors to metastasize as well as to one of the pathways by which angiogenesis occurs. Inhibiting the deregulation of proteolysis and mobility required for invasion, metastasis, and angiogenesis offers a novel strategy for cancer treatment. The following specific inhibitors of metalloproteinases have entered clinical trials: BAY12-9566 (Bayer), Marimastat (British Biotechnology), AG3340 (Agouron), and D2163 (Chiron). These compounds differ in their specificity for the different metalloproteinases. Marimastat and BAY12-9566 are in phase II and phase III trials as single agents and in combination with cytotoxic agents.[61]

## ANTIANGIOGENIC AGENTS

The widespread interest stimulated by Folkman's pioneering work and the publicity over the dramatic effects of angiostatin and endostatin on achieving regression of transplanted murine tumors have resulted in a growing list of drugs introduced in clinical trials for their effects in inhibiting tumor angiogenesis.

Antiangiogenic agents currently in clinical trials include some of the conventional chemotherapeutic drugs such as paclitaxel and topoisomerase I inhibitors,[62] inhibitors of matrix metalloproteinases, thalidomide, the fumigillin analogue TNP-470 (TAP Holdings),[63] CAI (National Cancer Institute), the polysaccharide CM-101 (CarboMed),[64] specific inhibitors of the VEGF-linked tyrosine kinase (SU5416, Sugen),[55] and monoclonal antibodies to VEGF (Genentech), the VEGF receptor, and the integrins associated with neovascularization.

In the early 2000s, a variety of new anticancer compounds, many of them directed toward new molecular targets, are expected to reach clinical trials. As we make progress toward understanding how tumor cells are able to escape normal cell growth regulatory pathways, as the cell cycle machinery of tumor cells is elucidated and tumor-specific alterations in the function of the different cyclin-dependent kinases identified, and as differences in the apoptotic pathways between normal and tumor cells are unveiled, it is expected that many new targets and strategies for therapeutic intervention will be recognized. This body of knowledge should result in the introduction of many new potentially effective antitumor agents. Changes in clinical trial design, including redefinition of eligibility criteria and end points, will have to be implemented as we move progressively from testing cytotoxic, non–tumor-specific agents to tumor-specific agents with well-defined biochemical targets. A major challenge will be our ability to test expeditiously all the new compounds. As the number of new agents reaching clinical evaluation grows exponentially, the availability of patients for clinical trials may become a real limiting step in our drug development efforts. Hopefully, our improved knowledge of cancer biology should also result in the development of more predictable antitumor activity screening systems, thus preventing the introduction into clinical trials of compounds with a low probability of improved clinical efficacy over existing agents.

## SUGGESTIONS FOR ADDITIONAL READING

Gelmon KA, Eisenhauer EA, Harris AL, et al. Anticancer agents targeting signaling molecules and cancer cell environment: challenges for drug development? J Natl Cancer Inst 1999;91:1281–7.

Cragg GM, Newman DJ. Discovery and development of antineoplastic agents from natural sources. Cancer Invest 1999;17:153–63.

Phillips KA, Tannock IF. Design and interpretation of clinical trials that evaluate agents that may offer protection from the toxic effects of cancer chemotherapy. J Clin Oncol 1998;16:3179–90.

Mayer LD. Future developments in the selectivity of anticancer agents: drug delivery and molecular target strategies. Cancer Metastasis Rev 1998;17:211–8.

Frei E 3rd. Clinical trials of antitumor agents: experimental design and timeline considerations. editorial. Cancer J Sci Am 1997;3:127–36.

## REFERENCES

1. Kobayashi K, Vaccari L, Cutler E, et al. Expanded access to investigational cancer (CA) therapies (Rx) in the U.S. that have been approved in other countries: 1998 update. Tenth NCI-EORTC symposium on new drugs in cancer therapy. Amsterdam, June 16–19, 1998. Ann Oncol 1998;9 Suppl 2:177. abstract.

2. Gabizon AA. Clinical trials of liposomes as carriers of chemotherapeutic agents: synopsis and perspective. In: Lasic DD, Papahadjopoulos D, eds. Medical applications of liposomes. The Netherlands: Elsevier Science B.V., 1998:625–34.

3. Gill PS, Wernz J, Scadden DT, et al. Randomized phase III trial of liposomal daunorubicin versus doxorubicin, bleomycin, and vincristine in AIDS-related Kaposi's sarcoma. J Clin Oncol 1996;2353–64.

4. Muggia FM, Hainsworth JD, Jeffers S, et al. Phase II study of liposomal doxorubicin in refractory ovarian cancer: antitumor activity and toxicity modification by liposomal encapsulation. J Clin Oncol 1997;15:987–93.

5. Harris L, Winer E, Batist G, et al. Phase III study of TLC D-99 (liposome encapsulated doxorubicin) vs. free doxorubicin (DOX) in patients with metastatic breast carcinoma (MBC). Proc Am Soc Clin Oncol 1998;17:124a.

6. Zou Y, Ling YH, Van NT, et al. Antitumor activity of the lipophilic and partially non–cross resistant anthracycline annamycin entrapped in liposomes. Cancer Res 1994;54:1479–84.

7. Greenberg R, Bahnson RR, Wood D, et al. Initial report on intravesical administration of N-trifluoroacetyladriamycin-14-valerate (AD 32) to patients with refractory superficial transitional cell carcinoma of the urinary bladder. Urology 1997;49:471–5.

8. Underhill C, Clarke K, Green M, et al. MX2 (KRN8602), an active new agent with low toxicity in high-grade malignant glioma. Tenth NCI-EORTC symposium on new drugs in cancer therapy. Amsterdam, June 16–19, 1998. Ann Oncol 1998;9 Suppl 2:170. abstract.

9. Bakker M, Droz JP, Hanauske AR, et al. Updated report on a feasibility and pharmacokinetic study of FCE 23762 every 4 weeks in solid tumor patients. Ninth NCI-EORTC symposium on new drugs in cancer

therapy. Amsterdam, March 12–15, 1996. Ann Oncol 1996;7 Suppl 1:97. abstract.

10. Talbot DC, Smith IE, Mansi JL, et al. Anthrapyrazole CI941: a highly active new agent in the treatment of advanced breast cancer. J Clin Oncol 1991;9:2141–7.

11. Kaufman PA, Harris R, Skillings J, et al. Losoxantrone + paclitaxel versus paclitaxel alone as first-line chemotherapy for metastatic breast cancer (MBC): final results of a phase III randomized trial. Proc Am Soc Clin Oncol 1998;17:124a.

12. Martin M, Casado A, Benavides A, et al. Phase I study of Elinafide in solid tumors. Tenth NCI-EORTC symposium on new drugs in cancer therapy. Amsterdam, June 16–19, 1998. Ann Oncol 1998;9 Suppl 2:63. abstract.

13. Awada A, Eftekhari P, Piccart MJ, et al. Phase I clinical and pharmacokinetic study of S16020 (Olivacine). Tenth NCI-EORTC symposium on new drugs in cancer therapy. Amsterdam, June 16–19, 1998. Ann Oncol 1998;9 Suppl 2:64. abstract.

14. Rizzo J, Renouf J, Eckhardt SG, et al. Cytochrome P-450 metabolism of the rebeccamycin analog NSC655649. Tenth NCI-EORTC symposium on new drugs in cancer therapy. Amsterdam, June 16–19, 1998. Ann Oncol 1998;9 Suppl 2:61. abstract.

15. Sasaki Y, Ohashi Y, Minami H, et al. A phase I trial of TOP-53 by hybrid dose escalation strategy based on PGDE and CRM. Tenth NCI-EORTC symposium on new drugs in cancer therapy. Amsterdam, June 16–19, 1998. Ann Oncol 1998;9 Suppl 2:64. abstract.

16. Iyer L, Mortell MA, Azuma R, et al. Glucuronidation of TAS-103 by uridine diphosphate glucuronosyltransferase (UGT) isoforms 1a1 and 2: Possible implication of TAS-103 toxicity in Gilbert's syndrome. Tenth NCI-EORTC symposium on new drugs in cancer therapy. Amsterdam, June 16–19, 1998. Ann Oncol 1998;9 Suppl 2:61. abstract.

17. van Gijn R, ten Bokkel Huinink WW, Rodenhuis S, et al. Phase I and pharmacologic study with the novel topoisomerase I/II inhibitor intoplicine administered as a 24-hour infusion. Tenth NCI-EORTC symposium on new drugs in cancer therapy. Amsterdam, June 16–19, 1998. Ann Oncol 1998;9 Suppl 2:66. abstract.

18. Jansen G, Peters GJ, Kathmann I, et al. Membrane transport and biological activity of stereoisomers AG2032 and AG2034; novel inhibitors of glycinamide ribonucleotide formyltransferase. Tenth NCI-EORTC symposium on new drugs in cancer therapy. Amsterdam, June 16–19, 1998. Ann Oncol 1998;9 Suppl 2:154. abstract.

19. Aylesworth C, Baker SD, Stephenson J, et al. Phase I and pharmacokinetic (PK) study of the glycinamide ribonucleotide formyltransferase inhibitor LY309887 as a bolus every 3 weeks with folic acid. Tenth NCI-EORTC symposium on new drugs in cancer therapy. Amsterdam, June 16–19, 1998. Ann Oncol 1998;9 Suppl 2:159. abstract.

20. Touroutoglou N, Pazdur R. Thymidylate synthase inhibitors. Clin Cancer Res 1996;2:227–43.

21. Schwartz GK, Kemeny N, Bertino J, et al. Interim results of phase I trial suggest that "Tomudex™" (raltitrexed) may act synergistically with 5-fluorouracil (5-FU) in patients with advanced colorectal cancer. Tenth NCI-EORTC symposium on new drugs in cancer therapy. Amsterdam, June 16–19, 1998. Ann Oncol 1998;9 Suppl 2:159. abstract.

22. Aylesworth C, Baker SD, Stephenson J, et al. Phase I and pharmacokinetic (PK) study of the glycinamide ribonucleotide formyltransferase inhibitor LY309887 as a bolus every 3 weeks with folic acid. Tenth NCI-EORTC symposium on new drugs in cancer therapy. Amsterdam, June 16–19, 1998. Ann Oncol 1998;9 Suppl 2:159. abstract.

23. Rinaldi DA, Burris HA, Dorr FA, et al. Initial phase I evaluation of the novel thymidylate synthase inhibitor, LY231514, using the modified continual reassessment method for dose escalation. J Clin Oncol 1995;13:2842–50.

24. O'Shaughnessy J, Moiseyenko V, Bell D, et al. A randomized phase II study of Xeloda™ (capecitabine) vs. CMF as first-line chemotherapy of breast cancer in women aged ≥55 years. Proc Am Soc Clin Oncol 1998;17:103a.

25. Ota K, Taguchi T, Kimura K. Report on nationwide pooled data and cohort investigation in UFT Phase II study. In: DeVita VT Jr, Hellman S, Rosenberg SA, eds. Cancer: principles and practice of oncology. 5th ed. Vol. 1. Philadelphia: Lippincott-Raven, 1997:450.

26. Taguchi T, Ohtsu A, Sakata Y, et al. Late phase II study of S-1 in patients with advanced colorectal cancer in Japan. Tenth NCI-EORTC symposium on new drugs in cancer therapy. Amsterdam, June 16–19, 1998. Ann Oncol 1998;9 Suppl 2:164.

27. Geyer C, Nemunaitis J, Hoff P, et al. Phase I trial of BOF-A2 (emitefur): a novel oral fluorinated pyrimidine. Tenth NCI-EORTC sympo-

sium on new drugs in cancer therapy. Amsterdam, June 16–19, 1998. Ann Oncol 1998;9 Suppl 2:167. abstract.

28. Vokes EE, Humerickhouse R, Dolan E, et al. Phase I study of the dihydropyrimidine dehydrogenase (DPD) inhibitor eniluracil (GW776C85) and oral 5-FU with concomitant radiotherapy (XRT) for recurrent or advanced head and neck cancer (HNC). Tenth NCI-EORTC symposium on new drugs in cancer therapy. Amsterdam, June 16–19, 1998. Ann Oncol 1998;9 Suppl 2:156. abstract.

29. Taylor GA, Estlin EJ, Pinkerton CR, et al. Deoxyuridine plasma levels during the phase I study of nolatrexed in children with advanced cancer. Tenth NCI-EORTC symposium on new drugs in cancer therapy. Amsterdam, June 16–19, 1998. Ann Oncol 1998;9 Suppl 2:161. abstract.

30. Hidalgo M, Villalona-Calero MA, Britten C, et al. A phase I and pharmacokinetic (PK) study of PN401 as a rescue agent for escalating doses of 5 fluorouracil (5-FU) in patients with cancer. Tenth NCI-EORTC symposium on new drugs in cancer therapy. Amsterdam, June 16–19, 1998. Ann Oncol 1998;9 Suppl 2:163. abstract.

31. Gabbara S, Bhagwat AS. The mechanism of inhibition of DNA (cytosine-5)-methyltransferases by 5-azacytosine is likely to involve methyl transfer to the inhibitor. In: DeVita VT Jr, Hellman S, Rosenberg SA, eds. Cancer: principles and practice of oncology. 5th ed. Vol. 1. Philadelphia: Lippincott-Raven, 1997:451.

32. Stephenson J Jr, Baker SD, Aylesworth C, et al. A phase I safety and pharmacokinetic (PK) study of BCH-4556, a novel L-nucleoside antimetabolite, on a daily × 5 day every 21-day schedule in patients with solid neoplasms. Tenth NCI-EORTC symposium on new drugs in cancer therapy. Amsterdam, June 16–19, 1998. Ann Oncol 1998;9 Suppl 2:156. abstract.

33. Punt CJA, de Jonge MJA, Sarreboom A, et al. Phase I and pharmacologic study on the topoisomerase I inhibitor [PEG 1000] 9-aminocamptothecin (9-AC) given orally to patients (PTS) with solid tumors. Proc Am Soc Clin Oncol 1998;17:197a.

34. Robert F, Zhang R, Dallaire B, Shuey S. A phase I trial of a daily × 5 intravenous bolus schedule of 9-aminocamptothecin in patients with solid tumors. In: New York University Post-Graduate Medical School, Kaplan Comprehensive Cancer Center, eds. The Ninth Conference on DNA Topoisomerases in Therapy. New York: NYU School of Medicine, 1998:13.

35. Wanders J, Dombernowsky P, Nielsen D, et al. A phase II study with GI147211 (GW211) in small cell lung cancer (SCLC). Proc Am Soc Clin Oncol 1998;17:474a.

36. Rowinsky EK. Future development of topoisomerase I inhibitors. Tenth NCI-EORTC symposium on new drugs in cancer therapy. Amsterdam, June 16–19, 1998. Ann Oncol 1998;9 Suppl 2:14. abstract.

37. Slaughter M, Dumas P, Hoff PM, et al. Clinical and pharmacokinetic study of RPR 109881A (RPR): a phase I trial of a novel taxoid derivative administered as a 24-hour continuous infusion. Tenth NCI-EORTC symposium on new drugs in cancer therapy. Amsterdam, June 16–19, 1998. Ann Oncol 1998;9 Suppl 2:100. abstract.

38. Gallagher M, Allen SL, Stevenson J, et al. Phase I trial of the dolastatin-15 analogue LU-103793 (cemadotin) every other day for three doses. Tenth NCI-EORTC symposium on new drugs in cancer therapy. Amsterdam, June 16–19, 1998. Ann Oncol 1998;9 Suppl 2:101. abstract.

39. Vokes EE, Arrieta R, Lad T, et al. A phase II trial of CI-980 in advanced non–small cell lung cancer. Tenth NCI-EORTC symposium on new drugs in cancer therapy. Amsterdam, June 16–19, 1998. Ann Oncol 1998;9 Suppl 2:100. abstract.

40. Luo FR, Stanko J, Chaney SG. Pharmacokinetical and neurotoxicological comparison of oxaliplatin, ormaplatin, and their biotransformation products. Proc Am Assoc Cancer Res 1998;39:596–7.

41. O'Dwyer PJ, Johnson SW, Hamilton TC. Cisplatin and its analogues. In: DeVita VT Jr, Hellman S, Rosenberg SA, eds. Cancer: principles and practice of oncology. 5th ed. Vol. 1. Philadelphia: Lippincott-Raven, 1997:418–32.

42. Maindrault-Goebel F, de Gramont A, Louvet C, et al. Bi-monthly oxaliplatin with leucovorin (LV) and 5-fluorouracil (5FU) in pretreated metastatic colorectal cancer (FOLFOX6). Proc Am Soc Clin Oncol 1998;17:273a.

43. Groen HJM, Smit EF, Bauer J, et al. A phase II study of oral platinum JM-216 as first-line treatment in small cell lung cancer (SCLC). Proc Am Soc Clin Oncol 1996;15:378.

44. Newlands ES, Stevens MFG, Wedge SR, et al. Temozolomide: a review of its discovery, chemical properties, pre-clinical development and clinical trials. Cancer Treat Rev 1997;23:35–61.

45. van Tellingen O, Schaaf LJ, Punt CJA, et al. In vitro and in vivo bone marrow toxicity assays in the clinical development of new drugs: carzelesin as an example. Tenth NCI-EORTC symposium on new drugs in cancer therapy. Amsterdam, June 16–19, 1998. Ann Oncol 1998;9 Suppl 2:54. abstract.

46. Alberts D, Bleyer WA. Future development of amifostine in cancer treatment. Semin Oncol 1996;23:90–9.

47. von Pawel J, von Roemeling R. Survival benefit from Tirazone™ (tirapazamine) and cisplatin in advanced non–small cell lung cancer (NSCLC) patients: final results from the international phase III Catapult I trial. Proc Am Soc Clin Oncol 1998;17:454a.

48. Advani R, Lum BL, Fisher GA, et al. A phase I trial of doxorubicin, paclitaxel, and PSC 833 (PSC) as a modulator of multidrug resistance (MDR) in refractory solid tumors. Proc Am Soc Clin Oncol 1998;17:199a.

49. Perez-Soler R, Mendelsohn J. Growth factor receptors as a target for therapy. In: Roth JA, Cox JD, Hong WK, eds. Lung cancer. Cambridge, MA: Blackwell Science, 1998:309–41.

50. Perez-Soler R, Shin DM, Donato N, et al. Tumor studies in patients with head and neck cancer treated with humanized anti-epidermal growth factor (EGFR) monoclonal antibody C225 in combination with cisplatin. Proc Am Soc Clin Oncol 1998;17:393a.

51. Slamon D, Leyland-Jones B, Shak S, et al. Addition of Herceptin™ (humanized anti-Her2 antibody) to first-line chemotherapy for HER2 overexpressing metastatic breast cancer (HER2 ± MBC) markedly increases anticancer activity: a randomized, multinational controlled phase III trial. Proc Am Soc Clin Oncol 1998;17:98a.

52. Woodburn JR, Barker AJ, Gibson KH, et al. ZD1839, an epidermal growth factor tyrosine kinase inhibitor selected for clinical development. Proc Am Assoc Cancer Res 1997;38:633.

53. Pollack VA, Savage DM, Baer DA, et al. Therapy of human carcinomas in athymic mice by inhibition of EGF receptor-mediated signal transduction with CP-358774: dynamics of receptor inhibition and antitumor effects. Proc Am Assoc Cancer Res 1997;38:633.

54. Williamson RA, Yea CM, Robson PA, et al. Dihydro-orotate dehydrogenase is a high affinity binding protein for A771726 and mediator of a range of biological effects of the immunomodulatory compound. J Biol Chem 1995;270:22467–72.

55. Rosen LS, Kabbinavar F, Rosen P, et al. Phase I trial of SU5416, a novel angiogenesis inhibitor in patients with advanced malignancies. Proc Am Soc Clin Oncol 1998;17:218a.

56. Bhargava P, Marshall J, Dahut W, et al. Phase I study of CEP-2563 dihydrochloride in patients with advanced cancer. Tenth NCI-EORTC symposium on new drugs in cancer therapy. Amsterdam, June 16–19, 1998. Ann Oncol 1998;9 Suppl 2:111. abstract.

57. Prendivilli J, Crowther D, Thatcher N, et al. A phase I study of intravenous bryostatin 1 in patients with advanced cancer. Br J Cancer 1993;68:418–24.

58. Propper D, McDonald A, Thavasu P, et al. Phase I study of the protein kinase C inhibitor CGP 41251: tolerability and effects on signal transduction ex-vivo. Tenth NCI-EORTC symposium on new drugs in cancer therapy. Amsterdam, June 16–19, 1998. Ann Oncol 1998;9 Suppl 2:112. abstract.

59. Akinaga S, Gomi K, Morimoto M, et al. Antitumor activity of UCN-01, a selective inhibitor of protein kinase C, in murine and human tumor models. Cancer Res 1991;51:4888–92.

60. Sepp-Lorenzino L, Zhenping M, Rands E, et al. A peptidomimetic inhibitor of farnesyl: protein transferase blocks the anchorage-dependent and -independent growth of human tumor cell lines. Cancer Res 1995;55:5302–9.

61. Grochow LB. Preclinical and clinical pharmacology of matrix metalloproteinase inhibitors (MMPIs). Tenth NCI-EORTC symposium on new drugs in cancer therapy. Amsterdam, June 16–19, 1998. Ann Oncol 1998;9 Suppl 2:11. abstract.

62. Clendeninn NJ, Johnston A. Phase II trials of Thymitaq™ (AG337) in six solid tumor diseases. Ninth NCI-EORTC symposium on new drugs in cancer therapy. Amsterdam, The Netherlands. Ann Oncol 1996;7 Suppl 1:86.

63. Stadler WM, Shapiro CL, Sosmann J, et al. A multi-institutional study of the angiogenesis inhibitor TNP-470 in metastatic renal cell carcinoma (RCC). Proc Am Soc Clin Oncol 1998;17:310a.

64. Hellerqvist CG, Wamil BD, Yakes M, et al. CM101 treatment overrides tumor-induced immunosuppression and induces apoptosis in adenocarcinoma metastasis. Proc Am Soc Clin Oncol 1998;17:449a.

# VII

# CLINICAL PRACTICE ISSUES

# CHAPTER 32

# ECONOMIC AND REGULATORY ISSUES AFFECTING ONCOLOGY

• JOSEPH S. BAILES • TERRY S. COLEMAN

The late 1990s saw a number of important economic and regulatory issues affecting medicine in general and oncology in particular. The issues affecting oncology have largely, although not universally, been resolved favorably, but the favorable resolution has not always come easily. The high costs of health care will continue to induce the government and private insurers to seek payment reductions and other restrictions that will adversely affect oncology.

In terms of the overall health care system, the emphasis within the fee-for-service sector has been on developing fee schedules and fixed-payment methods that bundle together various services and pay for them at a predetermined price. The more significant long-term development is the increased importance of managed care, particularly the use of capitated and similar systems in which health care providers are placed at financial risk with respect to the services they furnish to their patients. The development of managed care not only is affecting the nature of the payment systems but also is bringing about a reorganization of the medical delivery system as various players reposition themselves for a managed care regime.

This chapter provides an overview of the economic and regulatory issues facing oncology, with particular emphasis on the effects of these broad developments and also touching on some of the more specific concerns.

## Insurance Coverage

As is well understood, there are numerous gaps in insurance coverage under the health care system in the United States. A large number of Americans are uninsured at any given time, and many of those who are insured have limited coverage.

Cancer patients historically have had particular problems as a result of "medical underwriting" and exclusions under insurance policies for pre-existing conditions. Such practices and exclusions are designed by insurance companies to protect themselves from adverse selection by sick individuals, but they have had severe effects in the case of patients with chronic diseases like cancer. If a cancer patient attempted to change insurance carriers because of a new job, a spouse's new job, or for other, often unavoidable reasons, an exclusion for pre-existing conditions denied coverage for a time for treatment related to the cancer. Medical underwriting may exclude the patient from coverage altogether.

Federal legislation was enacted in 1996 to prevent medical underwriting for group health insurance and in certain limited situations for individual insurance. The result should be increased coverage of the population, including cancer patients.

## Specific Coverage Issues

In addition to the general problem of uninsured individuals, there are specific coverage issues that arise with respect to cancer patients who are eligible for benefits under public or private health plans. These coverage limitations can be the source of much difficulty.

### DRUG COVERAGE

Since chemotherapy is such an important aspect of cancer treatment, insurance coverage of drugs is a major issue. A significant problem confronting many cancer patients is a limited drug benefit under their insurance plans. Although drugs administered to inpatients and outpatients are generally covered under insurance plans, oral and other self-administered drugs frequently are not, except when the expense is so large that it triggers a major medical benefit. There are also frequently gaps in coverage even when a drug benefit exists, especially for indications not reflected in a drug's approved labeling or when an investigational drug is used as part of a chemotherapy regimen.

**Off-Label Uses of Drugs.** The Food and Drug Administration (FDA) approves drugs based on the proposed labeling submitted by the manufacturer, and the indications for use included in the FDA-approved labeling are those that the manufacturer has demonstrated are safe and effective to the FDA's satisfaction. Once a drug has been approved by the FDA, however, physicians are legally permitted to prescribe the drug for any purpose without limitation to the indications set forth in the approved labeling.

In the case of anticancer drugs, the indications for use in the FDA-approved labeling are ordinarily specific to the particular malignancies for which the drug was first tested successfully. After a drug is marketed, researchers may use the drug to treat other types of malignancies or under different conditions of use (e.g., different dosages) than appear in the FDA-approved labeling. Indeed, it has been estimated that more than half the uses of anticancer drugs are for purposes that are not included in the approved labeling.

The policies of third-party payers on covering such "off-label" uses differ somewhat, but in general insurers look to the major drug use compendia and the peer-reviewed literature and will pay for uses that are supported by those sources.

*Medicare.* For a number of years, Medicare's policy has been that it allows its carriers to reimburse for off-label uses of approved drugs "taking into consideration the generally accepted medical practice in the community."[1] Under this longstanding policy, Medicare covered many cancer chemotherapy drugs, but coverage lacked uniformity across the United States because it depended on local assessments of generally accepted medical practice.

To remedy this lack of uniformity, Congress enacted legislation effective in 1994 for drugs "used in an anticancer chemotherapeutic regimen."[2] Under this law, Medicare is required to cover any off-label use that is listed in any one of the major drug-use compendia (the *United States Pharmacopoeia–Drug Information* and the *American Hospital Formulary Service*) or that is supported by articles in certain peer-reviewed journals. The list of approved journals includes the major cancer-related journals as well as the important general medicine publications.

There is a potential difference in the standards for Medicare coverage between an off-label use that is listed in a compendium and one that is merely supported by the literature. In the case of a compendium listing, Medicare is automatically required to cover the listed use. In the case of a literature-supported use, each carrier remains free to evaluate the literature and determine whether the published articles in fact support the use. Since there is a lag between the time that articles are published and the time that the compendia are revised to take them into account, it is likely that there will continue to be some lack of uniform coverage during that period. There is also inconsistency in the standards that carriers apply in assessing the literature, with some demanding reports of phase III trials, whereas others are willing to confer coverage based on less elaborate studies.

*Medicaid.* Medicaid's policy on coverage of off-label uses is more complicated. Generally, state Medicaid programs are required by federal law to cover all off-label uses that are listed in one of the drug-use compendia identified earlier. A state may, however, establish a formulary and exclude from the formulary any drug, or use of a drug, that does not have a "significant, clinically meaningful therapeutic advantage in terms of safety, effectiveness, or clinical outcome" compared with other drugs that are included in the formulary.[3] Any excluded drug must nevertheless be available to patients on a case-by-case basis if authorized by the state prior to use.

*Private Insurance.* Coverage of off-label drug uses by private insurers varies but typically resembles Medicare's policy in its reliance on the major compendia and published literature. A number of states have enacted statutes that require private insurers to cover the recognized off-label uses of cancer drugs and, in a few cases, drugs for other conditions. These laws apply only to insurance, however, and not to self-insured employers because of a federal law that prohibits state regulation of employee benefits.

**Medicare Drug Coverage.** Medicare does not include a benefit for most self-administered drugs. Many of the new injectable biologic drugs, such as the hematopoietic growth factors, can be self-administered subcutaneously but are also administered by health care professionals. This results in a potential issue of coverage under Medicare, which excludes coverage of drugs that "cannot" be self-administered. Medicare policy, however, is that it covers drugs that are not "usually" self-administered.[4] Under this policy, Medicare is paying for growth factors except when the drugs are in fact self-administered.

Although Medicare does not have a drug benefit as such, there are a few circumstances in which the program covers drugs. First, drugs, including oral drugs, are covered as part of the benefits for inpatient hospital services, nursing facility services, and hospice services, and therefore drugs provided to patients of these facilities are covered. (As discussed further on, however, when there is a fixed payment for all services furnished to a hospital inpatient or hospice patient, there is no extra payment to cover drugs.)

Second, drugs that cannot be self-administered are covered by Medicare when they are furnished incident to a physician's professional service and are included in the physician's bill. Chemotherapy and other injectable drugs furnished in the office are covered under this provision. For this coverage to apply, Medicare requires that the physician be present in the office suite and immediately available to provide assistance and direction, although a nurse or other assistant may actually administer the drug. In addition, if a nonphysician administers the drug, that person must be employed by the physician, rather than be the employee of a hospital or other entity.[5] Under legislation, a physician assistant or nurse practitioner can substitute for the physician in supervising chemotherapy administered to Medicare patients if such a role is within the individual's permitted scope of practice under state law and if Medicare is billed in the name of the nonphysician.

Third, drugs are covered as part of the durable medical equipment benefit when they are administered through pumps that are reimbursed as durable medical equipment.[6] This coverage applies to both ambulatory infusion pumps and stationary equipment used in the patient's home, but it does not extend to disposable pumps, which are not considered durable medical equipment.

In addition to these injectable drugs, Medicare covers a small number of oral drugs, including several anticancer chemotherapy agents. Coverage of chemotherapy agents is limited to oral drugs that have an injectable counterpart used for the same indication. Currently, four drugs qualify under this provision—cyclophosphamide, etoposide, melphalan, and methotrexate. Oral antiemetics given in conjunction with chemotherapy are also covered provided that they are administered within 48 hours of the chemotherapy and are a full replacement for intravenous antiemetics.

## NEW TECHNOLOGIES

A persistent issue, under both public and private health plans, relates to the coverage of new procedures and technologies. Since all health plans exclude coverage of items and services that are considered *experimental* or *investigational* (or some similar term), any innovation faces an obstacle until it is regarded as standard practice. These provisions have proved troublesome in oncology because so many patients undergo nonstandard treatment.

Coverage in such situations can vary considerably among insurers. Some insurers will deny coverage of the patient care costs for any service designated as investigational and may take the use of an informed consent form as evidence that the service was investigational.

Obstacles to coverage may be especially formidable in the case of expensive technologies. Even though cost generally is not explicitly a factor in determining whether insurance coverage exists, a high-cost procedure will be carefully scrutinized with respect to its investigational status, whereas a new low-cost procedure may draw little attention.

**Applicable Criteria.** A number of formal programs have been established to evaluate new technologies to determine whether they should be covered by insurance. Among private insurers, the most active may be the Blue Cross and Blue Shield Association's Technical Evaluation Program. This program, which provides nonbinding advisory opinions to local Blue Cross and Blue Shield plans, does not rely on community practice standards or consensus but only on scientific evidence.

The Technical Evaluation Program uses the following criteria, which are similar to factors of other evaluators, to determine whether to cover a particular technology:

- The technology must have final approval from the appropriate government regulatory bodies.
- The scientific evidence must permit conclusions concerning the effect of the technology on health outcomes.
- The technology must improve the net health outcome.
- The technology must be as beneficial as any established alternatives.
- The technology must be attainable outside investigational settings.[7]

Medicare uses somewhat analogous criteria in deciding whether particular services should be covered:

- The service must be safe and effective. Medicare will rely on either general acceptance by the medical community or on authoritative evidence.
- The service must not be experimental or investigational. A service furnished for research purposes in accordance with predetermined rules is considered experimental or investigational.
- The service must be appropriate under the circumstances. This requirement means that the service is commensurate with the patient's medical needs and is furnished by qualified personnel.[8]

These criteria are ordinarily interpreted and applied by individual Medicare carriers, although carrier medical directors also discuss coverage of particular drugs among themselves. Medicare is in the process of revising its process for making coverage decisions, which it intends to make more public.

In the case of all insurers, the best route to obtaining a determination that a procedure is no longer experimental is usually the publication of articles in peer-reviewed journals that support the safety and effectiveness of the procedure. Oncologists who are developing new procedures and new uses of drugs should be mindful of the importance of literature to insurance coverage and should seek to publish studies involving new procedures as quickly as possible.

**Clinical Trials.** The most disadvantageous situation for insurance coverage is a clinical trial because the very existence of the trial is often viewed as conclusive evidence that the procedure being furnished is experimental. Although it may be justifiable under the limiting language of insurance plans to deny coverage of the aspects of the trial that are truly experimental, when coverage is denied it often extends to all aspects of the patient's care, including patient care costs that would have been incurred even if the patient had undergone standard therapy.

Various legislative efforts have been initiated to require Medicare and other insurers to cover the patient care costs associated with clinical trials, but none has been successful so far. In reality, many patient care costs associated with clinical trials are in fact covered by insurance because insurers are not aware that the services were furnished as part of trials. The continuing threat of coverage denial and its occasional manifestation, however, are important barriers to clinical trials and must be eliminated to maximize the development of new cancer therapies.

## Fee-for-Service Payment Issues

Third-party payers are increasingly concerned with imposing cost controls in the fee-for-service sector. Many of these controls take the form of fee schedules or fixed-amount payment methods.

### HOSPITAL INPATIENT SERVICES

In 1983, Medicare began implementing a prospective payment system for inpatient hospital services in which the payment rates are fixed in advance and, except in rare cases, do not vary in accordance with the costs incurred in treating a particular patient. The amount of the payment is determined by the diagnosis-related group (DRG) into which each patient is classified. This system has been adopted by a number of Medicaid programs and some other payers and may be used even more widely in the future.

In a nonsurgical patient, the DRG classification is largely determined by the patient's principal diagnosis at the time of admission. In a patient who has had one or more operating room procedures, the DRG is also based on the most resource-intensive procedure furnished to the patient during the admission.

Payment amounts are determined by multiplying an assigned "weight" for each DRG by a conversion factor, known as the *standardized amount*. The weights are intended to reflect relative resource use and are determined by estimating the average costs that hospitals incur for treating patients classified into each DRG. Each year, the Medicare program examines hospital cost data and adjusts DRG weights that appear to be out of line. The standardized amount was initially set at a level based on aggregate Medicare expenditures under the previous reimbursement system and has subsequently been subject to annual adjustments that are influenced by factors such as the federal government's budget deficit.

Like other fixed-price payment mechanisms, the theory underlying the DRG-based payment system is that a fixed payment will induce hospitals to operate more efficiently to avoid losses or to create profits. Since hospitals are required to report their costs to Medicare each year, the government can monitor hospital efficiency and know the extent to which it needs to adjust payment rates. Thus, Medicare can capture the benefits of the induced efficiencies by lowering payment rates or raising them less than would otherwise have been the case.

A fixed-price payment mechanism can be expected to have effects on the use of new technologies and procedures. If a new technology would lower the cost of treating a patient while the Medicare payment remains unchanged, the system creates a strong incentive to adopt the new technology. Conversely, if a new procedure costs more but is used because it promises better outcomes or other improvements, hospitals may be reluctant to adopt the new technology because they could incur losses.

Medicare does not assess the value of particular new technologies in determining whether to increase DRG weights (and hence payment amounts). Instead, the Health Care Financing Administration (HCFA) adjusts the DRG weights based on whatever costs hospitals incurred in the prior period under review. Thus, if hospitals are willing to incur increased costs to adopt a new technology, eventually the DRG weight will be increased to reflect those new costs, or a new DRG will be created solely for the new technology based on the higher costs incurred.

For example, bone marrow transplants were initially reimbursed at an amount that was only a fraction of their actual costs because they were classified into a DRG that consisted largely of much simpler procedures. Only after sufficient Medicare data had been accumulated on actual bone marrow transplants was a new DRG established (at a much higher payment rate) exclusively for such transplants.

Fixed-price payment methods will undoubtedly continue to be a problem in the future, as cancer therapy appears to be moving in the direction of highly sophisticated and expensive procedures. HCFA will not allow the use of cost data from clinical trials and other non-Medicare sources to set the hospital payment rate, and thus adequate payment for new cancer treatments will often require that hospitals furnish a new treatment at a financial loss while at least a year's worth of Medicare cost data are accumulated and then analyzed by HCFA. Additional protections may have to be adopted by the U.S. Congress to ensure that payment restrictions do not unduly interfere with the dissemination of new technologies.

## HOSPITAL OUTPATIENT SERVICES

The federal government is developing a fixed-price payment system for hospital outpatient department services for use by Medicare. This development has potentially broader significance than may be apparent. As in the case of the DRG system, it is likely that the fee schedule for Medicare outpatient services—at least its structure, if not the actual payment rates—will be adopted by other payers as well. Moreover, since Medicare wants to have reimbursement policies that create a "level playing field" and do not favor a particular site of service, eventually the same fee schedule will probably apply to both physician offices and outpatient departments.

Historically, Medicare reimbursed hospitals for the costs

they incurred in providing outpatient department services. More recently, however, the U.S. Congress reduced Medicare payments for outpatient departments to 94.2% of operating costs and 90% of capital costs to help reduce the federal budget deficit.

In the case of outpatient department ambulatory surgery and radiology services (including therapeutic radiology), the payment methods are more complex. In the late 1990s, the U.S. Congress observed that Medicare paid significantly more for procedures performed in the outpatient department than for the same procedures furnished in physicians' offices or ambulatory surgery centers. As a result, hospital payments were reduced partially toward the lower amounts that are paid in the other settings. Hospitals are paid the lesser of their costs or a blended rate, 42% of which is based on each hospital's own costs and 58% of which is based on the ambulatory surgery center or the physician's office payment rate.

The outpatient department remains a major area in the Medicare program for which payment is not based on fee schedules or fixed payments. At the same time, growth of outpatient department services has been rapid as more procedures are transferred from inpatient status. Consequently, there has been substantial effort to develop a fixed-price system.

Initial research on developing an outpatient payment method focused on a diagnosis-related system like that used for inpatients. It was determined, however, that diagnosis is a poor predictor of resources used in an outpatient department visit.

Development efforts therefore switched to the use of "ambulatory patient groups," which have become known as *ambulatory patient classifications* (APCs). In patients undergoing procedures, APCs would not be based on diagnosis but on a core procedure. The fee schedule payment amount for the APC would constitute payment for that core procedure as well as for associated costs. HCFA has not yet disclosed what other services would be considered covered by the payment amount, but the amount could cover associated laboratory and minor radiologic services, drugs, and supplies. For medical visits, the APC would apparently be based on the patient's diagnosis and other factors. Unlike the inpatient system, in which a single DRG covers each admission, it would be permissible to have multiple APCs that were applicable to the same outpatient department encounter. The U.S. Congress passed legislation requiring HCFA to implement an outpatient hospital fee schedule in 1999, although HCFA may seek to delay implementation.

The principal issue for oncology raised by the impending outpatient department fee schedule relates to the treatment of chemotherapy administration and the related drugs. The APC system will have far fewer categories of services than exist in the fee schedule for physician services. Consequently, there may be only one or two fees for chemotherapy administration, each of which would encompass a variety of administration methods and treatment lengths. In addition, HCFA may seek to pay for the chemotherapy agents themselves by grouping drugs into a small number of categories and paying the same amount for each category, regardless of the specific drugs and amounts used. Such a system could result in substantial financial losses when certain drugs are used and would therefore create new and potentially undesirable incentives for hospitals with respect to chemotherapy.

Another issue related to the outpatient department is the level of hospital charges. As for other services, Medicare beneficiaries are responsible for 20% of the payment amount that Medicare allows. In cost-based reimbursement used for the outpatient department, the 20% is not based on a hospital's costs, because they cannot be calculated at the time of service; instead, beneficiaries are obligated to pay 20% of the hospital's charges.

Although at one time hospital charges were approximately equal to their costs, charges have increased much more rapidly than costs. As a consequence, Medicare beneficiaries currently pay about half of total payments for outpatient department services (instead of the 20% assumed), and the percentage is expected to rise to 68% by the end of the 1990s.[9] In cancer patients receiving chemotherapy, this 20% coinsurance can be a substantial burden. As part of the move to the outpatient department fee schedule, however, the U.S. Congress is requiring HCFA to phase out the large patient payments by increasing the fee schedule amounts. After the phase-in period, patients will be responsible only for 20% of the fee schedule amount, which will be a substantial reduction from their current responsibility in many circumstances.

## PAYMENT FOR PHYSICIAN SERVICES

Historically, private insurance paid for physician services based on physician charges, subject to a limitation that payment does not exceed the physician's usual charge or the customary and reasonable charge in the community. For many years, Medicare had a similar policy, in which payments were limited by the lower of the physician's customary charge and the local prevailing charge. In addition, beginning in 1974, the prevailing charge used in this limitation was allowed to increase each year only by the amount of inflation in the estimated cost of operating a physician's office. In 1992, however, Medicare introduced a radically different payment method based on relative values. The system is being adopted by other payers and may eventually become universal.

**Resource-Based Relative Value Scale.** The Medicare fee schedule for physician services is established on a resource-based relative value scale (RBRVS). A "resource-based" system is intended to pay for physician services according to the resources used in providing each service (including the time and intensity of the physician's personal effort) but not to consider factors such as the value of the service to the patient or, directly, the physician's training and experience.

A primary motivation for adopting the RBRVS was the belief that procedures were overcompensated under the prior system compared with cognitive physician work. Thus, the fee schedule redistributed substantial Medicare payments from surgical procedures to evaluation and management services.

In addition, the RBRVS includes geographic adjustment factors to reflect local variations in office expenses and wages. The effect of these adjustments is to narrow greatly the range of differences in payment amounts around the United States compared with the range that existed before implementation of the fee schedule, since variations are now based solely on objective differences in costs. The RBRVS generally redistributed payments from physicians in large cities to those in smaller cities and rural areas.

*Relative Values.* Despite its name, the Medicare RBRVS is in reality not yet fully resource based. The relative value for each physician service has three components: relative value units for physician work, practice expenses, and malpractice insurance. The physician work component was resource based from inception of the fee schedule in 1992, but the component for practice expenses does not become resource based until a phase-in period begins in 1999. Conversion of the malpractice insurance component to being resource based is still further in the future.

The relative value of the physician work component was determined by "magnitude estimation" according to a method developed by Hsiao and colleagues.[10, 11] Using this method, physicians subjectively compared the time and intensity of various procedures to a reference procedure, which is assigned a value of 100. This process was carried out by groups of specialists for procedures within their specialties. The resulting relative value scales for each specialty were then aligned on a common scale through the values of procedures that were either common to more than one specialty or were viewed as being similar. Finally, all the relative values were proportionately adjusted so that the value of an intermediate office visit would equal exactly 1.

The appropriate method for making the practice expense component resource based is much more controversial. The first method advanced by HCFA involved estimating the staff time, supplies, and equipment used in providing key reference services. This method would have reallocated substantial Medicare funds from certain specialties, particularly surgeons, to other specialties, including medical and radiation oncology. To reduce the impact on the disadvantaged specialties, HCFA subsequently proposed a different approach based on each specialty's current overall expenses. As the proposal currently stands, this latter approach would not particularly assist medical oncology and would disadvantage radiation oncology.

The outcome of this debate has not been resolved as of this writing and, whatever general approach is adopted by HCFA, there will be numerous refinements over the next few years. Many oncologists believe that Medicare payments for office-based chemotherapy administration are inadequate, and they look forward to a resource-based fee schedule to correct that shortfall. It is not yet clear, however, whether the ostensible resource-based method to be adopted by HCFA will actually recognize the costs involved in office-based chemotherapy administration.

*Conversion Factor.* Under the Medicare fee schedule, the relative value for a particular service is multiplied by a conversion factor (denominated in dollars) to determine the payment amount. Initially, in 1992, the conversion factor was set at a budget-neutral amount intended to pay out the same aggregate amount under the fee schedule as would have been paid out under the prior system. Subsequently, the conversion factor has been increased based on the combined effect of an inflation adjustment and a reward (or penalty) for compliance (or noncompliance) with a target amount.

The target amount was initially called the *volume perfor-*

*mance standard rate of increase* and is now known as the *sustainable growth rate.* Both attempt to control the growth in the aggregate volume and intensity of physician services provided to Medicare patients. If aggregate services are less than the standard, the conversion factor is increased faster than the rate of inflation, and the reverse is true if aggregate services exceed the standard. The sustainable growth rate is rather restrictive, and some experts believe it will cause the conversion factor actually to decline in the relatively near future.

**Chemotherapy Administration.** There are a surprisingly large number of issues surrounding payment for chemotherapy administration. Most involve the issue of whether there should be separate payment for particular items or services, or whether payment for those items or services is already covered by the payment for another service. These issues exemplify the growing trend toward bundling items and services together and making a single payment for the group regardless of the particular services furnished.

An example is the payment for chemotherapy administration by push (CPT 96408) and infusion (CPT 96410) on the same day. The CPT manual directs that the physician should report separate codes for each parenteral method of administration. Nevertheless, since insurers are not governed by the CPT, some will not pay separately for a push administration on the same day as they pay for an infusion. Medicare also had that policy during 1992 but subsequently decided to pay for both CPT 96408 and CPT 96410 on the same day. Medicare, however, will pay for only one push service per day, regardless of how many drugs are administered.

Another issue is whether there is a separate payment for placement of the needle or for port access. Although Medicare does not recognize such a payment (considering it part of the chemotherapy administration service), some other insurers do make a separate payment.

Finally, there is the issue of separate payments for supplies. Medicare's policy is that it generally considers the costs of supplies to be included in the payment for the related service, and the payment amounts for the services were computed on that basis. Separate payments for supplies are made only in unusual circumstances in which the lack of a separate payment for a relatively expensive supply (e.g., a surgical tray) could cause the procedure to be performed in the hospital outpatient department, and this policy will be in effect only until the practice expense component fee schedule is revised to become resource based.

**Chemotherapy Management.** An issue of controversy is the proper method of reporting and billing the physician's management services related to chemotherapy. At present, Medicare takes the position that all physician evaluation and management services are included in the visit codes and that the chemotherapy administration codes cover only the technical aspects of the procedure. As a result, if chemotherapy is administered to inpatients or in the hospital outpatient department (where the physician does not bill for the technical aspects of the chemotherapy administration), there is no Medicare payment for the physician's services apart from the visit services.

Some private insurers do not follow Medicare's lead on this point. They view the chemotherapy administration codes as composed of both a technical and a professional component. Thus, in the hospital setting, a physician may bill a chemotherapy administration code with modifier "-26" to indicate the professional component of chemotherapy administration, in addition to the visit code.

It is possible that Medicare will change its policy in the future and make a separate payment for chemotherapy management. If it does, the payment amount may be determined by setting a relative value based on the amount of work involved in chemotherapy management that exceeds the work covered by a visit unrelated to chemotherapy.

**Limitations on Physician Charges.** Physicians who are Medicare-participating physicians or otherwise take Medicare claims on assignment are limited to the Medicare allowed amount (which is paid 80% by Medicare and 20% by the patient). In unassigned claims, physicians are limited to charging 115% of the Medicare-allowed amount. Since the allowed amount for nonparticipating physicians is 95% of the normal amount, charges are limited to 109.25% of the fee schedule amount (i.e., 115% of 95%).

These limitations have led to questions about whether particular practices would violate the limitation or another rule. Approaches that some physicians have considered include billing patients for the entire cost of supplies for which Medicare no longer pays separately or billing patients for telephone consultations (for which Medicare makes no payment). In the case of supplies, billing the patient would clearly be prohibited because Medicare considers the supplies to be paid for by the payment for the related visit or procedure. Billing for a telephone call may be less clearly prohibited, but Medicare would generally take the position that telephone calls are included in the payment for the associated visit and therefore cannot be billed separately to the patient.

Some physicians have suggested that they should be able to contract with Medicare patients for services at any charge level if the patient agrees to pay the entire charge and not seek reimbursement from Medicare. In 1997, Congress enacted provisions allowing physicians to opt out of Medicare and set their charges as they wish, but the restrictions on such action are so severe that only a small number of physicians have elected this course.

**Payment for Drugs Administered by Physicians.** Third-party payer policies on paying for physician-administered drugs evidence a remarkable divergence in approach. Private insurers sometimes pay full charges for drugs without applying any kind of "usual, customary, and reasonable" or similar limitation. By contrast, Medicare's policy is, in essence, to reimburse physicians only for the cost of the drugs themselves, with overhead and administration costs considered covered by payments for office visits or for drug administration. Other private insurers take a middle course, paying more than Medicare but less than the physician's charges.

Medicare's allowable amount for a drug is the lower of the physician's charge or 95% of the published average wholesale price (AWP). AWP is, in theory, the average price at which pharmacists and physicians can purchase a drug from a wholesaler. There are commercial services that publish AWPs, which they determine based on, to varying extent, information from drug manufacturers and surveys of wholesalers.

The use of published AWP as the benchmark for third-party reimbursement is a source of continuing controversy because drugs are frequently available for purchase at prices less than the AWP, sometimes substantially less. The issue was settled for Medicare at least temporarily in 1997 when the U.S. Congress lowered the basis for Medicare reimbursement from the AWP to 95% of the AWP. Despite this action, there have been new proposals to substitute actual acquisition cost for the AWP method as a basis for reimbursement.

A complicating factor in drug reimbursement methods is the variability in prices paid. This variation is both a function of the purchaser (large-volume purchasers frequently pay much less) and time (discounts come and go). The variability makes any system that is designed to pay for drugs on a cost pass-through, or estimated acquisition cost, basis difficult to administer fairly.

Since the current Medicare payment for chemotherapy administration services is generally viewed as being less than the costs incurred by physicians, the current payment level for drugs is important to maintaining the viability of oncologists' practices. Accordingly, further reductions in drug payments would probably need to be accompanied by increased payments for chemotherapy administration. Drug payment policy continues to be a contentious issue that is likely to be revisited by the U.S. Congress.

# Managed Care

The accelerating growth of managed care has many economic and policy implications for oncology and the rest of medicine. Some of these are reviewed in the following sections.

## USE OF SPECIALISTS AND SPECIALIZED FACILITIES

One concern relates to the use of specialists. Managed care organizations typically prefer to have patients handled by primary care physicians to the extent possible. Indeed, referrals to specialists may be discouraged by financial incentives applicable to the primary care physicians who act as gatekeepers. The failure of managed care organizations to use pediatric oncologists is frequently identified in oncology as a particular shortcoming.

Based on the use of specialists in existing prepaid group practice health maintenance organizations, it has been estimated that there would be a large surplus of specialists if all medicine in the United States was delivered through such systems. The degree of projected surplus varies among specialties, with hematology-oncology estimated to have a 50% surplus—a relatively small percentage compared with the estimates for some other specialties.[12] One of the major issues confronting oncologists in the coming years as managed care becomes more pervasive is whether such a surplus will in fact materialize and, if it does, how physicians will adapt to it.

A related issue is the extent to which managed care organizations will use specialized facilities such as the comprehensive cancer centers or other sophisticated treatment centers. This issue not only has a bearing on the quality of care available to cancer patients enrolled in managed care organizations but also relates to the availability of patients for enrollment in the clinical trials conducted at these institutions. If cancer patients are treated almost entirely in community hospitals, the national program for clinical trials would have to be redesigned or trials could not be undertaken.

There are two possible general approaches to these issues. Under one approach, there could be regulatory controls on managed care organizations, requiring them to use specialists and specialized facilities under certain circumstances to ensure patients access to high-quality care. An alternative approach would rely on measurement of, and publicity regarding, health outcomes and patient satisfaction in each managed care organization so that consumers could make more informed choices among managed care plans. It remains to be seen whether either of these approaches will be adopted.

## RESTRUCTURING OF DELIVERY AND PAYMENT SYSTEMS

In preparation for the anticipated growth in managed care, there is currently substantial activity among physician practices, hospitals, and other entities aimed at forming larger networks and integrated delivery systems. It is thought that these larger organizations will be better able to compete in the managed care arena. For example, insurers operating managed care programs that want to establish a network of participating providers may find it easier to contract with large preformed groups than to assemble a network composed of many small practices.

The desire of managed care organizations to use capitation and case-rate payment methods may also give an advantage to large delivery systems, since large organizations may be in a better position to contract on such terms. Small groups of physicians may lack both the data necessary to estimate the costs of treating patients accurately and a patient population large enough to spread the risk involved.

The ultimate outcome of this restructuring is far from clear, but it seems likely that there will be many more large providers than exist today. It is possible that in any given geographic area, a handful of large networks or integrated delivery systems will dominate. It is unclear whether specialists such as oncologists can continue to operate independently in such a regime or whether they must become part of large multispecialty networks or integrated systems. These issues will, however, plainly dominate the economic aspects of medical practice in the early 2000s.

# Self-Referral Prohibitions and Related Issues

An issue of importance is legal restrictions on "self-referral." Based on a few studies indicating that physicians who own diagnostic equipment are more likely to order tests than those who do not, the federal government and some state governments have enacted restrictions on physicians and providers referring patients to facilities in which they have an interest or ordering items and services from entities with which they have a financial arrangement.

These laws contain many ambiguities and uncertainties about their scope. As networks and integrated delivery systems are organized, particular attention must be paid to ensure that arrangements are in compliance.

## THE "STARK" SELF-REFERRAL LAW

The federal statute of most direct concern is the "Stark" law,[13] which is named after its principal congressional proponent. In essence, the law prohibits a physician from referring patients to, or ordering services from, an entity in which the physician (or immediate family member) has an ownership interest or with which he or she has a compensation arrangement unless one of the exceptions is satisfied. The law pertains to the following "designated health services": clinical laboratory services, physical and occupational therapy services, radiology and radiation therapy services, durable medical equipment, parenteral and enteral nutrition services, prosthetics and orthotics, home health services, outpatient prescription drugs, and inpatient and outpatient hospital services. It applies to Medicare and Medicaid patients.

**In-Office Ancillary Services.** Although there are many exceptions that can apply under the Stark law, a few govern most situations. An important exception is that for in-office ancillary services. Under this exception, a physician or a group practice can furnish laboratory, radiology, and other services if the services are supervised by a physician in the group and the services are provided in a building in which unrelated physician services are also provided. This prohibits, for example, a freestanding computed tomography center but allows a practice to offer such services in the same building in which it conducts office visits.

With the exception of infusion pumps, durable medical equipment and parenteral and enteral nutrition services may no longer be provided by physicians to Medicare and Medicaid patients. Patients must be referred to a supplier that is not affiliated with the physician.

To take advantage of the exception for in-office ancillary services, a group practice must meet the statutory definition of a group practice. The primary criteria in the definition are that services must be billed under a group billing number, and physicians in the group cannot be compensated based on the volume or value of referrals within the group.

**Personal Service Arrangements.** Another of the exceptions covers personal service arrangements between a physician and another entity. For example, if a physician is a part-time medical director for a home health agency, he or she could refer patients to the agency only if the terms of this exception are met. Under the exception, there must be a written agreement between the parties with a term of at least 1 year and covering all the services provided by the physician. The key financial standards require that the compensation must be set in advance, cannot exceed the fair market value, and ordinarily cannot take into account the volume or value of referrals between the parties.

**Other Issues.** The Stark law is notorious for its complexity, and this complexity is complicated by various interpretations that the government has proposed but not yet finalized. For example, despite the statutory exception allowing physicians to furnish infusion pumps to their patients, HCFA has proposed that this be interpreted as applying only to pumps that are implanted in a physician's office. As another example, the requirement for physician supervision of designated health services has been interpreted as a requirement that, except for lunch breaks and emergencies, a physician must be present in the office whenever a laboratory test is being performed or another designated health service is being furnished.

This complicated and dubious regulatory regimen has caused even Congressman Stark to question whether revisions need to be made. The law has not yet imposed major impediments to the practice of oncology, although implementation of some of the proposed interpretations could, at a minimum, result in serious inconveniences.

## ANTIKICKBACK STATUTE

Another federal "fraud and abuse" law is the antikickback statute.[14] This law, which is also complex, in general prohibits any form of "remuneration" to induce referrals for, or purchases of, health care services if those services will be paid for under Medicare, Medicaid, or certain other federally funded programs. A number of states have analogous laws that cover all payers.

The term *remuneration* is given a broad interpretation, and the law may apply to situations that do not obviously involve remuneration, such as investments. The antikickback statute contains several exceptions, and additional "safe harbors" have been established by regulation.

The typical situation in which the antikickback statute may become relevant is in connection with joint ventures and similar arrangements among providers. These arrangements should be carefully scrutinized for compliance with this law.

## Conclusion

Dramatic changes are occurring in the economic sphere of medical practice. The increased use of managed care, the development of new payment methods in the fee-for-service sector, and the rise of large networks and integrated delivery systems will substantially alter the financial incentives and risks and the economic structure in which oncology is practiced. These changes bear the close attention of all practitioners and other providers.

## SUGGESTION FOR ADDITIONAL READING

Hewitt M, Simone JV, eds. Ensuring quality cancer care: National Cancer Policy Board, Institute of Medicine and National Research Council, 1999;256 pp. (see http://www.nap.edu/catalog/6467.html)

## REFERENCES

1. Medicare Carriers Manual, section 2050.5(D).
2. Section 1881(t)(2) of the Social Security Act; United States Code, title 42, section 1395x(t)(2).

3. Section 1927(d)(4) of the Social Security Act; United States Code, title 42, section 1396r-8(d)(4).
4. Medicare Carriers Manual, section 2050.5(B).
5. Medicare Carriers Manual, section 2050.3.
6. Medicare Carriers Manual, section 2100.5.
7. Testimony of Susan Gleeson, Executive Director, Medical and Quality Management, Blue Cross and Blue Shield Association, before the Committee on Finance, United States Senate, March 3, 1994.
8. Health Care Financing Administration. Medicare program; criteria and procedures for making medical services coverage decisions that relate to health care technology. Federal Register 1989;54:4302–18.
9. Statement of Thomas Ault, Director, Bureau of Policy Development, Health Care Financing Administration.
10. Hsiao WC, Braun P, Yntema D, Becker ER. Estimating physicians' work for a resource-based relative-value scale. N Engl J Med 1988;319:835–41.
11. Hsiao WC, Braun P, Dunn D, Becker ER. Resource-based relative values. JAMA 1988;260:2347–53.
12. Wennberg JE, Goodman DC, Nease RF, Keller RB. Finding equilibrium in U.S. physician supply. Health Affairs (Summer) 1993;12:89–103.
13. United States Code, title 42, section 1395nn.
14. United States Code, title 42, section 1320a-7b(b).

# CHAPTER 33

# ETHICAL ISSUES IN CANCER TREATMENT

- PAUL SCHNEIDER

Medical ethics is best understood as a process through which one may comment on and understand medical science's appropriate role in the treatment of patients. By nature, it allows definitions of the appropriate interactions of the physician with patients, society, commerce, and research. Its topics are a function of extant medical science, philosophy, and society's interests and values at large.

Although it is true that the concepts of beneficence and nonmaleficence were already defined in antiquity, no guiding principles for the ethics of medical research existed until the Nuremburg Code of 1947.[1] Preliminary attempts have been made at codifying the conduct of human fetal tissue transplantation research,[2] but no full consensus has yet emerged. Indeed, one may observe that the true consolidation of ethical principles in medicine lags at least decades behind the cutting edge of medical enterprise. It is this need to place the science of medicine into human and moral context that is the raison d'être of modern bioethics.

Unfortunately, retrospective recognition of our great failures as a profession is all too often necessary prior to consensus. In this regard, the Tuskegee study[3] and Nazi medical experimentation[4] can be viewed as tragic events that successfully focused society's and medicine's efforts on the need to create principles by which such betrayals of our patients could be prevented. Yet, although many of the great lessons in bioethics are learned retrospectively, and at the macro level, they must be applied at the micro level and in real time. The physician skilled in the application of medical ethics recognizes conflict where it exists in the provision of health care and attempts to resolve it as part of his or her role. To resolve a conflict, it must first be dissected and viewed with scrutiny. This process requires objectivity and a willingness to rise above the fray to examine a conflict's causes and potential resolutions. One helpful model is the Jonsen-Siegler method of case analysis.[5] In practice, this role is frequently delegated to the bioethics committee, a useful tool for any health care provider when conflict arises.

Bioethics committees are mandated structures in almost all health care environments. They are multidisciplinary and must include members from outside the hospital environ-

ment. Community participants as varied as clergy, patient rights organization representatives, and volunteer retirees may sit on a hospital committee. Within the health care environment, social workers, psychologists, nutritionists, pharmacists, nurses, administrators, and various types of physicians are all valued members. This group creates a synergy in which solutions may arise where none could be envisioned by the individual. Moreover, the committee is generally available to consult with the general health care community, including patients, families, and all sorts of health care professionals. Specifically, ethics committees attempt to understand conflicts as functions of multiple potential parameters. These may include issues of beneficence and nonmaleficence, justice, fair distribution of scarce medical resources, patient autonomy versus medical paternalism, legal factors, surrogate decision-making, informed consent, and advance directives. Using the scenario of the cancer patient as a specific example throughout, this chapter discusses some of the preceding issues in depth.

## Informed Consent

The practice of informed consent has become standard not only for its originally intended purpose—entry of a human subject into research—but also for the routine provision of procedures in medicine. Differentiation must be made between informed consent—the appropriately informed and voluntary consent of a competent individual to participate in medical treatment—and implied consent—the consent that we assume any competent, concerned adult would naturally give for medical treatment in similar circumstances. When, then, is the use of one more appropriate than the other? Standards vary institutionally and also leave room for some judgment. Generally, procedures as benign as phlebotomy require only implied consent, that is, an average competent patient should already understand that the risks of phlebotomy are few and the potential benefits large, and that these do not need to be expressly examined with the patient.

However, a trigger-point injection, while technically similar, carries risks that the average patient may not intuitively understand, for example, sterile abscess formation or tendon rupture. Therefore, this procedure, although performed routinely with only implied consent, should really require informed consent. This has come to be known as the *reasonable person standard*.[6] This means that the amount of information sufficient to make a consent "informed" is that which a "reasonable person" would want to know in making the decision. Possible alternative treatments or procedures, or both, must also be explored with the patient to make a consent truly informed. Consensus holds that it is acceptable to recommend one treatment over others, even to try to persuade a patient in one direction, as long as the physician has discussed the procedure and alternatives with the patient.

The informed consent process requires that the patient be able to comprehend the decision-making process at least to the level required to appreciate both the risks and benefits of the proposed action and, conversely, the lack of same. When patients cannot demonstrate this, they are said to lack decision-making capacity, the medical equivalent of the legal concept of incompetence. In difficult cases, or when mental illness complicates this analysis, psychiatric consultation should be obtained.

When patients lack decision-making capacity for elective treatments or procedures, or both, physicians are bound to look for any advance directives the patient might have executed previously. A living will may actually outline the treatment decision being pondered and give the patient's a priori feelings about it. When available and valid, living wills must be respected. If executed, a durable power of attorney for health care (DPA-HC) is the next most important document. The person appointed therein becomes, by definition, the surrogate decision-maker for health care, to supersede but not necessarily completely exclude family and friends. When a DPA-HC has not been executed, rules vary from state to state and hospital to hospital regarding the specific prioritization of relatives; local policies should be consulted. By consensus, good friends frequently make better surrogates than distant relatives and should not be excluded from decision-making. A surrogate must demonstrate the decision-making capacity that the patient lacked and must be willing to accept the responsibility. It cannot be forced on anyone, even a spouse. Surrogates are generally "allowed" to make decisions that are not in the patient's *physiologic* best interest as long as they can provide rationale for why they are in the patient's *overall* best interest, which may also include social, spiritual, or, potentially, even economic factors. However, when surrogates show disregard for the patient's best welfare, or prioritize others' welfare above that of the patient in the decision-making process, legal counsel should be sought regarding removing surrogacy from those individuals.

Regarding chemotherapy, good informed consent practice requires an honest explanation of possible alternative therapies, expected probabilities of "cure" and palliation, and the likelihood of the most frequent toxicities. Not every possible toxicity need be mentioned, as the Texas Medical Disclosure Panel has elucidated for surgical procedures.[7] Likewise, therapies that are not considered part of mainstream allopathic medicine, for example, herbs and chiropractic, do not need to be offered or discussed.

Specifically, then, if there are several reasonable therapeutic routes for a patient's coordinated multimodality cancer care, they must be laid out and explained and the patient offered some choice in the matter. In explaining these alternatives, medical specifics must be discussed—again, to the degree that a reasonable person would want to know. In the age of medical consumerism and the Internet, the reasonable person standard is an ever-increasing one. Moreover, if a sophisticated patient wants to have a more detailed explanation than his or her cohort, it is incumbent on the medical community to rise to the demand, within reason. In one case, the court held that a medical oncologist was negligent in the treatment of a patient's pancreatic cancer for not discussing the specific likelihood of success of the therapy.

## Life Support

In the broadest sense, life support is any and all supportive medical interventions, the absence of which leads proximately to death. Mechanical ventilation and advanced cardiac life support qualify as such. Most authorities also agree that hemodialysis, artificial nutrition and hydration, and transfusion qualify in many but not all cases. Philosophically, although the procedures may vary in invasiveness, cost, and tolerability, they are all medical technologies that do not exist in the natural state and thus are to various extents treatments.

Treatments, by definition, are subject to discussion in the context of the physician-patient relationship. It is in this context that life support is best viewed. In this circumstance, because of the gravity of not pursuing life support, U.S. society has clearly spoken through the Patient Self-Determination Act of 1990. This federal law ensures that all patients in hospital, long-term care, managed care, and hospice settings are guaranteed the right to express their desires in regard to life support within 24 hours of admission.[8] More broadly, the law actually mandates that the patient has the right to execute a DPA-HC and a living will and to decide their code status (e.g., do not resuscitate [DNR]).

Patients "draw the line" of intolerable disease and intolerable treatment in different places. Almost all patients feel that lifelong intensive care unit care is unacceptable. Chief among its indignities is mechanical ventilation. Most feel that if this intervention can be limited to a short-term trial, or in the long-term to certain hours (e.g., night-time hours only), it is more palatable. Hence, by this logic, most patients find three-times-a-week hemodialysis or night-time chronic ambulatory peritoneal dialysis acceptable but would not accept permanent, around-the-clock dialysis (hypothetically). This is essentially a quality of life argument. Most patients' ideas of what constitutes an unacceptable quality of life converge on permanent, highly invasive, potentially painful care.

The decision to initiate life support is a complicated one for patients, physicians, families, and other surrogate decision makers. By nature, it is highly personal, even idiosyncratic, and tinted by emotionality that touches on the actual decision to varying degrees from person to person, sometimes confounding our efforts to understand it. It is the evaluation of this uniqueness that is at the heart of the ethical principle of patient autonomy, the element that weighs most heavily on modern ethical case analysis.

Does informed consent or implied consent apply to the initiation of life support? It is easy to recognize that both do. Clearly trauma care and emergency services to unconscious patients both rest squarely on implied consent. Similarly, resuscitation of hospitalized patients with relatively minor medical-surgical illnesses and sudden decompensation or death is ethically accepted and demanded universally. The situation changes dramatically when chronic illness, poor prognosis, old age, or other factors complicate the decision. In such cases, which make up the bulk of internal medicine and medical oncology practice, consent for life support should not properly be assumed but should be discussed with the patient or surrogate, or both, in the context of overall health care plans. As a matter of general principle, it is easier for patients to discuss this subject as a function of their desires for the direction of their total future care mode than as an isolated decision. To rephrase, it is both easier and more appropriate for many patients to verbalize that they want to pursue palliative care than that they want to be considered DNR. Although the correlations between cure mode care (aggressive therapy) and full code and palliative mode care and DNR are not perfect, they are strong and serve as the most appropriate milieu in which to understand the wishes of our patients.

Regarding the termination of life support, analogously, this is best understood as the termination of a medical treatment. However, it is a decision never to be made lightly or without consultation with nurses, allied health personnel, families, hospital policy and, usually, ethics committees. The chief goals in such cases are to understand prognosis, the positions of all parties involved, the relevant law, and hospital policy and to attempt to achieve consensus of thought among all involved. Lastly, it is incumbent on the involved decision makers to help arrange appropriate palliative care if death is not imminent. With the legalization of physician-assisted suicide in some states, many physicians have become fearful that their patients may request it. It is clear though that the switch from cure to palliative care mode and the decision to terminate life support far outnumber situations in which patients request help in suicide.

The law has repeatedly upheld the rights of patients and surrogate decision makers to terminate mechanical ventilation, intravenous fluids, and artificial nutrition. The provider who continues such therapies against the wishes of the patient or surrogate, or both, treads on thin ice in the current environment and should do so only when there is evidence that the surrogacy is invalid or should be so.

## Medical Research

Paramount in the ethics of medical research is the separation of physician-scientist role from physician-healer role.[9] It is clear that most commonly patients seek a physician's advice for their expertise in medical treatment. When going to an academic medical center, patients may expect increased medical expertise but not necessarily to be entered into medical research as part of that. It is because of the inherent inequity in the physician-patient relationship and the vulner-

able nature of the patient's position that specific disclosure of research intent must be made. The Helsinki Declaration of 1964 and its subsequent World Medical Assembly amendments[10] have specifically addressed the subject of medical research combined with professional care (clinical research). Its six principles in this area are as follows:

1. In the treatment of the sick person, the doctor must be free to use a new diagnostic and therapeutic measure if in his or her judgment it offers hope of saving life, reestablishing health or alleviating suffering.

2. The potential benefits, hazards, and discomforts of a new method should be weighed against the advantages of the best current diagnostic and therapeutic methods.

3. In any medical study, every patient—including those of a control group, if any—should be assured of the best proven diagnostic and therapeutic method.

4. The refusal of the patient to participate in a study must never interfere with the doctor-patient relationship.

5. If the doctor considers it essential not to obtain informed consent, the specific reasons for this proposal should be stated in the experimental protocol for transmission to the independent committee.

6. The doctor can combine medical research with professional care, the objective being the acquisition of new medical knowledge, only to the extent that medical research is justified by its potential diagnostic or therapeutic value for the patient.

It is clear that to fulfill the preceding principles when clinical care and research must coexist, care must take priority. It is for this reason that if one individual is to serve as both physician-scientist and physician-healer to patients, it is incumbent on that individual to safeguard the patient's health and welfare vigorously at all times. This may be aided by always remembering whether an individual visit is care driven or research driven and placing the patient's needs at top priority. The Belmont Report of 1979 further addressed this problem. It is the result of Congress' empowering the National Commission for the Protection of Human Subjects of Biomedical and Behavioral Research to make recommendations to the Secretary of Health, Education, and Welfare regarding ethical principles and guidelines for the protection of human subjects of research. The panel published specific recommendations in the areas of research on the human fetus, children, and prisoners and on the functions of institutional review boards (IRBs). Also published were specifics on the applications of informed consent, assessment of risks and benefits, and selection of subjects in research involving human subjects. This last document urges physician investigators to apply social justice in the choice of human subjects, as follows.[11]

Some populations, especially institutionalized ones, are already burdened in many ways by their infirmities and environments. When research is proposed that involves risks and does not include a therapeutic component, other less burdened classes of persons should be called upon first to accept these risks of research, except where the research is directly related to the specific conditions of the class involved. Also, even though public funds for research may often flow in the same directions as public funds for health care, it seems unfair that populations dependent on public health care constitute a pool of preferred research subjects if more advantaged populations are likely to be the recipients of the benefits. One special instance of injustice results from the involvement of vulnerable subjects. Certain groups, such as racial minorities, the economically disadvantaged, the very sick, and the institutionalized may continually be sought as research subjects, owing to their ready availability in settings where research is conducted. Given their dependent status and their frequently compromised capacity for free consent, they should be protected against the danger of being involved in research solely for administrative convenience, or because they are easy to manipulate as a result of their illness or socioeconomic condition.

In the areas of IRBs, fetuses, children, and prisoners, many of the panel's recommendations were later codified into official regulations applying to all federally funded research in the United States. Extremely detailed, specific policies apply to IRB membership, functions, and operations; review of research; criteria for approval of research; empowerment of the IRB to suspend or terminate research; and record keeping.[12]

## Professionalism

No longer satisfied to leave physician behavior completely to individual judgment, several societies in U.S. medicine have issued codes of ethical conduct. In this regard, The American College of Physicians (ACP) has now issued the fourth edition of its ethics manual,[13] which is available free on the Internet at http://www.acponline.org/journals/annals/o1apr98/ethicman.htm. In addition to the topics discussed previously, the emphasis has been toward the codification of professionalism. Specific areas of note include confidentiality, the medical record, medical risk to physician and patient, alternative therapies, disability certification, sexual contact between physician and patient, organ donation, managed care, financial conflicts of interest, physician strikes, the relationship of attending to resident, the impaired physician, and scientific publication.

## Conflict of Interest

When physicians' financial interests (directly or indirectly related to patient care) conflict with medically appropriate care, ethical conflict exists. The ACP ethics manual specifically calls unethical, "a fee paid to one physician by another for the referral of a patient, historically known as fee-splitting." In this same category of conduct lies kickbacks from manufacturers of drugs or medical supplies. Likewise, physicians are not to refer patients to facilities at which they have invested and do not directly provide care. Finally, advertising that is "unsubstantiated, false, deceptive, or misleading, including statements that mislead by omitting necessary information is wrong and unacceptable behavior for physicians."

The manual cautions against but does not prohibit other financial arrangements. Within the context of its cautionary

tone, self-scrutiny for even the appearance of conflict of interest and patient or public disclosure, or both, are strongly recommended. The manual provides additional guidance, as follows: "Physicians may, however, invest in or own health care facilities when capital funding and necessary services are provided that would otherwise not be made available . . ." and "Physicians may invest in publicly traded securities." "The acceptance of individual gifts, hospitality, trips, and subsidies of all types from the health care industry by an individual physician is strongly discouraged."

All matters of professionalism in medicine, of paramount importance—second only to the primacy of the physician-patient relationship—is the public trust in medicine. Keeping these two goals in mind is sure to guide any physician in the right direction when contemplating a conflict of interest issue.

## SUGGESTION FOR ADDITIONAL READING

Anonymous. Ethics manual. 4*th* ed. Ann Intern Med 1998;128:576–94.

## REFERENCES

1. The Nuremberg Code. In: Jonsen AR, Veatch RM, Walters L, eds. Source book in bioethics: a documentary history. Washington, D.C.: Georgetown University Press, 1998:11.
2. Human Fetal Tissue Transplantation Research Panel: National Institutes of Health, 1988. In: Jonsen AR, Veatch RM, Walters L, eds. Source book in bioethics: a documentary history. Washington, D.C.: Georgetown University Press, 1998:103.
3. Final report of the Tuskegee Syphilis Study Ad Hoc Advisory Panel. In: Jonsen AR, Veatch RM, Walters L, eds. Source book in bioethics: a documentary history. Washington, D.C.: Georgetown University Press, 1998:76.
4. Lifton RJ. The Nazi doctors: medical killing and the psychology of genocide. New York: Basic Books, 1986.
5. Jonsen RJ, Siegler M, Winslade WJ. Clinical ethics: a practical approach to ethical decisions in clinical medicine. 2*nd* ed. New York: Macmillan, 1986.
6. Canterbury v. Spence, 464 F. 2D 772 (1972). In: Jonsen AR, Veatch RM, Walters L, eds. Source book in bioethics: a documentary history. Washington, D.C.: Georgetown University Press, 1998:484.
7. Schiffman MA. Oncology patients. In: Sanbar SS, Gibofsky A, Firestone MH, LeBlang TR, eds. Legal medicine. 3*rd* ed. St. Louis, CV Mosby, 1995:497.
8. Clarke DB. The patient self-determination act. In: Monagle JF, Thomasma DC, eds. Health care ethics: critical issues. Gaithersburg, Md.: Aspen, 1994:93.
9. Emanuel EJ, Patterson WB: Ethics of randomized clinical trials. J Clin Oncol 1998;16:365–71.
10. Declaration of Helsinki: Recommendations guiding medical doctors in biomedical research involving human subjects. In: Jonsen AR, Veatch RM, Walters L, eds. Source book in bioethics: a documentary history. Washington, D.C.: Georgetown University Press, 1998:13.
11. The Belmont Report: ethical principles and guidelines for the protection of human subjects of research. In: Jonsen AR, Veatch RM, Walters L, eds. Source book in bioethics: a documentary history. Washington, D.C.: Georgetown University Press, 1998:13.
12. Federal Register 46FR 8386, January 26, 1981.
13. Anonymous. Ethics manual. 4*th* ed. Ann Intern Med 1998;128:576–94.

# CHAPTER 34

# INTEGRATIVE MEDICINE

• JACOB ZIGHELBOIM

Revolutionary developments in the diagnosis and treatment of cancer have not been matched by a similar understanding of the patient's experience. Although molecular and cell biology, immunology, clinical oncology, and medical therapeutics have advanced dramatically, the psychosocial and spiritual concerns of the patient have not received the same level of attention.

From a scientific standpoint, we have progressed significantly. The elucidation of the molecular basis for the oncogenic process already allows us to detect mutations in individuals with familial histories of cancer,[1] to develop more sensitive means of detecting cancer cells,[2] and to diagnose more precisely.[3] These advances also hold the promise of new cancer therapies that are more specific (targeting genetic abnormalities), more effective, and less damaging to normal tissues.[4, 5]

Paradoxically, these dramatic advances in our ability to diagnose and treat cancer have not been complemented with a comparable understanding of the patient's experience of cancer. The dichotomy in progress is not surprising, but it reflects a divergence in focus between empirical science, which is the foundation of Western medicine, and human experience, a reality immediate to us all.[6]

For biomedical scientists, cancer is primarily a disorder of cell proliferation and maturation induced by mutations in the cell's genetic code. These mutations determine the phenotypic characteristics of cancer cells and are responsible for the clinical and biochemical features of the disease. For individuals with cancer, however, the disease is also a cognitive event, one that evokes not only intense emotions but also disturbing questions about the meaning, quality, and length of life; the capacity to overcome the rigors of illness and treatment; financial solvency; and much more. In addition, although patients and physicians are equally invested in seeing the disease eradicated and cured, the former often find themselves searching alone for psychosocial, spiritual, and body-mind resources to integrate the complex experience unleashed by their medical diagnoses.

This divergence in focus is detrimental to the care of the oncology patient and must be quickly remedied. Oncologists who explore their patients' cancer experiences discover promptly that addressing and even curing physical cancer does not resolve the existential challenges the disease evokes. Indeed, they encounter in their daily practices persons who have been cured from clinical cancer but who, nonetheless, feel overwhelmed by their emotional concerns about the disease. These are individuals who are often paralyzed by the fear of recurrence and oppressed by the reality that their lives are forever uncertain, a reality no reputable physician can categorically dismiss. These individuals cannot follow physicians' orders and "go on and have a good life," despite their good fortune of having no clinical or biochemical evidence of cancer.

## Need for a New Approach

Just as the elucidation of the molecular basis of tumorigenesis reveals cancer to be a complex, multistep process,[7, 8] so has the clinicians' involvement with cancer patients and their families exposed the multidimensionality and complexity of the cancer experience.

The cancer experience may be described as the sum total of all the thoughts, feelings, images, and actions that follow the cognition of cancer. The integration of this experience into oncologic practice requires an expansion of our understanding of what cancer is and what it does to our patients. Furthermore, integration requires our acceptance of a greater level of responsibility in assisting the patient and family. The complexity of the task demands from medical practitioners a set of psychosocial skills and resources not provided by traditional training programs. Complementary programs of instruction and experiential learning must be created to prepare physicians for this critical dimension of care.

Our understanding of the complexity of the cancer experience has also been spurred by developments in cognitive science[6, 9] and neuroscience,[10, 11] psychoneuroimmunology,[12, 13] psychology,[14, 15] and the social sciences,[16, 17] all of which reveal human beings as creative and resourceful creatures capable of contributing to their recovery from illness[18] and as living entities whose thought, affects, attitudes, and behaviors have a significant impact on their bodily events.[12, 19, 20] This type of information challenges the mechanistic-reductionistic conception of human life and demands a more encompassing point of view—integrative oncology.

## Integrative Oncology

Integrative oncology is a novel form of medical theory and practice that views cancer not just as an accumulation of genetically transformed, immature cells that disturb the body's economy but also as the sum total of the feelings, thoughts, images, and actions evoked by the awareness of cancer—not only in those afflicted with the disease but also in their loved ones. This understanding of cancer ensures that the complexity of the condition is properly acknowledged and the best resources for recovery and healing present within the human community are optimally used.

The uniqueness of the integrative oncology approach to cancer is illuminated by a report by Schwartz and Russek in which they describe eight different views of nature, each world view generating a unique perspective on physical and biologic reality and, hence, on the nature of health and illness (Table 34–1).[21]

When all eight world views are applied to the understanding and management of the oncologic process, they give rise to a more comprehensive and dynamic model of patient care. Such a larger perspective creates a more effective practice, one based on a multilayered understanding of nature and humanity. Integrative oncology meets individuals with cancer in such a comprehensive fashion, offering a complementary and unique approach to the care of patients and their families.

By contrast, conventional oncology *understands and treats* cancer from the perspective of only the first two world views. Formistically (world hypothesis No. 1) it *catalogues* cancer biologically as a malady of genes whose cells are classified according to their molecular, biochemical, and immunologic features, as well as by location in the physical body (stage of disease). Mechanistically (world hypothesis No. 2), it investigates the cause-and-effect relationships responsible for the causation of the illness, its clinical and biochemical features, and its natural history.

Conventional oncology thus largely reflects the perspectives that biomedical science has adopted for the study of disease, but unfortunately it does not reflect the perspective of those afflicted with the illness. The formistic and mechanistic points it espouses view reality as objective—out *there* (or inside the body) and independent of those who observe and examine it. This way of perceiving reality is valuable when addressing the formal and mechanical features of the cancerous condition, but it is inadequate when addressing cancer as a human experience. Abstracted from the psychosocial and spiritual realities of patients, conventional

oncology frequently fails to help and comfort the individuals it addresses. Moreover, its disregard for the capacity of human beings to participate actively in self-repair and healing processes precludes patients from making the highest possible contributions to their own recovery and well-being.

The moment we can acknowledge, however, that there are other meaningful ways of viewing oncologic disease, we have included the third view of reality—No. 3, contextual—and opened medicine to exploring and eventually integrating the experience of cancer with all its complex richness and potentialities. Contextual medical awareness adds a focus of attention to the perceptions and needs of the individuals experiencing the disease as well as those who love them or care for them professionally.

In addition, when human beings are viewed only as complex machine-like creatures—mechanical entities whose attributes and functions can be adequately deduced merely from knowing their component parts—we can easily overlook the remarkable properties that have evolved in them as a result of their increased material complexity.[10] These properties can be uncovered only when approaching them as total organisms (No. 4—the organismic world view). When doing so, human beings are perceived as irreducible wholes capable of reflective consciousness, will, love and compassion, self-repair, creativity, and imagination. When confronted with a serious illness, these human organisms are expected to mount body-mind responses that may include physiologic, behavioral, and even structural changes, all aimed at overcoming the threat that the illness poses to their survival. In fact, the impulse to survive, which is present even in the most primitive unicellular organisms, is a manifestation of a nonreducible, global property that all living creatures seemingly possess.

We must attend to the total effort—biologic, psychological, and social—that such complex organisms make to overcome cancer and its diverse manifestations. Using novel interventions that promote self-repair, regeneration, and psychosocial rehabilitation is one of the ways the organismic viewpoint contributes to the professional care of the oncology patient.

The inclusion of the organismic world view within the purview of oncologic care also reveals how our mental attributes (the higher levels of organization of the body's economy) may contribute to the causation and recovery from an illness.[20]

We can now clarify and determine how the many dimensions of mind (e.g., consciousness, feelings, attitude, and psychological conditionings) contribute to either the development or resolution of the cancer condition.[19] Doing so, we have added a perspective to oncology—that of implicit process (the fifth world view), which addresses the unconscious forces and patterns of behavior and thought that influence and help determine how cancer develops and evolves. Within this perspective, we find placebo and nocebo (defined as remembered illness, placebo's negative counterpart) effects,[18, 22] as well as diverse types of belief systems that influence our responses to cancer and our survival.[23]

Acknowledging this reality supports the inclusion into oncologic practice of programs of psychological deconditioning aimed at neutralizing noxious beliefs, as well as programs that raise and sustain hope and that may trigger physiologic responses favoring recovery.

*Table 34–1.* **Eight World Hypotheses**

| World Hypothesis (WH) | Description |
| --- | --- |
| WH1 Formistic | All structures and functions exist as separate categories |
| WH2 Mechanistic | All effects have causes that precede them |
| WH3 Contextual | All structures and functions exist in context and are relative |
| WH4 Organismic | All structures and functions reflect organizations of interactive relationships—parts interact and become whole systems |
| WH5 Implicit process | All systems involve invisible processes of information-energy-matter that interact over time |
| WH6 Circular causality | All systems involve the circulation of information-energy-matter that interact and change dynamically over time |
| WH7 Creative unfolding | All systems reflect flexible orders, express plans, and serve multiple purposes |
| WH8 Integrative diversity | All phenomena in nature reflect complex interconnected, integrated orders of diverse processes |

Integrative oncology also acknowledges the existence in our bodies of interacting systems of matter, energy, and information that allow knowledge to be stored in our cellular systems and to be used for homeostatic purposes (the sixth world view—circular causality). Feedback mechanisms and memory processes in our immune systems and brains fall within the category of circular causality. Awareness of this level of biopsychological reality alerts us to the existence of natural responses that support wellness and health as well as to the health-inductive and -transformative power that human beings who have overcome cancer and healed their lives can have on those just beginning the cancer process. The use of group work to facilitate recovery from cancer, including the amplification of the beneficial effects of conventional therapies, falls within the compass of this world view.[24, 25] It is clear that the positive experience of others can reinforce our sense of competency and power and help us handle future challenges with more equanimity and strength, thereby changing the way cancer affects our lives both biologically and qualitatively.

By including the seventh world view—creative unfolding—in oncologic practice, we become aware of the possible intentionality, meaning, and growth-promoting effects of the cancer condition. We can now acknowledge the evolutionary pressure that the patient's cognition of cancer exerts on the psyche and how this pressure may force a new differentiation of mind that brings a sense of general coherence to the patient's life,[26–28] along with new ways of perceiving, mentally organizing, and actively responding to outer and inner environments.

From the perspective of this seventh hypothesis, health is the product of a dynamic process of growth and change, and healing is the way to reinforce and sustain this flexible plan. Cancer, like all disease, thus becomes an opportunity to exercise and unfold the innate healing mechanisms available to all human beings. Healing work and natural processes are invested in promoting the positive resolution of all physical manifestations of cancer but do not demand or depend on this. A person involved in healing work and processes may find balance, equilibrium, and harmony, even when facing clinical situations that are not fully reversible. In the final analysis, the greatest intention of healing work, whether deliberate or unconscious, is to help patients find pathways that allow them to face the truth of their circumstance without experiencing unbearable suffering. In clinical healing work, integrative oncologists try to help individuals become fully attuned with their physical, psychological, and spiritual realities. Here the emphasis is not just on the disease and its eradication but on living one's life to the fullest, even in periods when illness is present and medical science cannot effectively reverse its course.

Obviously, physicians' deliberate exploration of the meanings that a disease may have for a patient does not entitle them to overlay their own beliefs and prejudices on patients' experiences. To suggest, for example, that cancer has occurred as a retribution for the person's lifestyle or as something the patient has "chosen" to manifest is inappropriate and cruel. The attribution of a particular meaning must be part of an all-out effort to understand and align ourselves with nature—the world as it is—and not as an opportunity to create an infantile, moralistic, or prejudicial way of looking at life.

The eighth world view—integrative diversity—acknowledges the human search for wholeness and a world view that contributes to healthy understanding and action. More important, it implies a theory of health and disease that explains and integrates all facets of the cancer condition. This world view or hypothesis encourages us to develop a system of care that is comprehensive, dynamic, and coherent—one that allows all the viewpoints described thus far to be effectively harmonized in our care of the oncology patient.

## Some Specific Clinical Functions of an Integrative Oncology Program

### PROVIDE STATE-OF-THE-ART DIAGNOSTIC AND THERAPEUTIC SERVICES IN AN ENVIRONMENT THAT IS CARING AND SUPPORTIVE OF INDIVIDUALS EXPERIENCING LIFE-THREATENING ILLNESS

Integrative oncology provides patients with the most advanced resources that biomedical science can offer in the context of an environment of care where they are free to express their feelings and opinions without fear of critical judgment or emotional or physical abandonment. Feelings of safety, validation, support, compassion, and love are important ingredients for health, maturation, and personal growth; without them the work of healing is compromised and frequently aborted.

### PROVIDE MEDICAL COUNSELING

Medical counseling helps individuals with cancer be more knowledgeable about their medical conditions and about the therapeutic alternatives available to them. Borrowing from Antonovsky,[28] it helps them make their disease "comprehensible." When a person's medical condition makes sense, his or her fears diminish and confidence heightens. Persons who are less scared of cancer feel more stable and tend to make better choices. Too often, the therapeutic choices faced by individuals with neoplastic disease involve treatments whose benefits are unknowable and whose negative effects on the patient's body can be far-reaching. In such circumstances, quality-of-life issues are as relevant as concerns about length of survival. Although much of the decision-making faced by individuals with cancer can rely on objective information, other facets of the process depend on subjective knowledge. Such knowledge is often less accessible to many persons and therefore is one area that integrative oncologists aim to help access and support.

Most individuals suffering from neoplastic disease want to feel that they have participated actively and responsibly in its resolution, regardless of how the disease ultimately unfolds. In the end, they want to believe that fear and psychospiritual dysfunction were not the determining forces dictating their fate.

### PROVIDE PSYCHOSPIRITUAL DECONDITIONING

An integrative oncology program helps those affected by cancer break the negative mindset associated with their diagnosis. This mindset promotes emotions of fear, uncertainty, and dejection, together with a strong belief that the condition is incurable. Integrative oncologists help their patients become empowered—to be human beings able to find constructive ways to handle life-threatening challenges. Persons who think of themselves mainly as "patients" are usually expecting others to resolve their difficulties. Often they are not active or even participatory at times, and they contradict the premise that afflicted individuals know what is best for them and that education, information, and effective guidance are important.

Integrative oncologists function more like teachers and guides than as authoritative figures responsible for the resolution of their patients' medical crises. Unfortunately, the traditional physician-patient relationship too often has the quality of a parent-child dyad, locking the afflicted person in a state of powerlessness. However, it is neither necessary nor helpful to the ill person to promote attitudes of victimization, hopelessness, or helplessness. On the contrary, the involvement of patients in the resolution of the disease processes provides an outlet for their creative energies and thereby helps them overcome the sense of defeat that may otherwise overcome them.

By emphasizing the patient's natural capacity for self-healing, integrative oncologists attempt to counteract the mental distortion and confusion that learned helplessness produces. The notion that patients are mere bystanders to the medical crises and challenges they experience is inaccurate and harmful. From the initial visit to an integrative oncology program, patients learn that deep within their anatomic structures are self-repairing mechanisms coming into action to help their bodies regain balance and thereby health.

## PROVIDE OPPORTUNITIES FOR EXPERIENTIAL LEARNING

Encountering neoplastic disease often raises challenges that call for new understandings, resources, and tools, and it can force us into a quest for greater inner strength, wisdom, and spiritual meaning. Through experiential individual and group work, integrative physicians offer individuals who have been thrust into this quest opportunities to gather the wisdom and understanding they desperately seek. Physicians make available experiences that promote learning about the inner workings of the psychospiritual body (such as dream work, meditation, active imagination, and artistic expression) as well as help clarify the principles that sustain health and well-being.[20] These experiences, deeply moving and illuminating, need to be guided by persons who themselves have been and are involved in similar quests. Guiding others on this type of journey requires a lived understanding of the questing process, in addition to knowledge and the skills acquired from medical and oncologic training. We need experiences of our own that qualify us as guides to those venturing into these uncharted territories. Persons who have experienced processes of deep introspection and consciousness expansion tend to emerge with a broader and richer perspective of reality, a better sense of human capacities and limitations, and the alternatives and options for recovery. Patients guided by such individuals typically become less afraid to live and tend to appreciate and participate

more actively in the life they do have, regardless of its ultimate length.

## The Place of Alternative Medicine Within the Framework of an Integrative Oncology Program

Integrative oncology's attitude toward all mechanical phenomena (world hypotheses Nos. 1 and 2) associated with cancer is totally conventional, advocating the use of the scientific method for evaluating all pertinent information. All diagnostic procedures; physical, chemical, and biologic treatments; and any other intervention recommended for the treatment and cure of cancer must be assessed in the light of reliable scientific knowledge. Although integrative oncology is indeed open to every possible avenue of oncologic care, it demands from those promoting "alternative" approaches more than just the testimonies of those who receive such treatments—objectifiable hypotheses verified by qualified independent observers are essential.

### TYPES OF UNCONVENTIONAL TREATMENTS

In a chapter on alternative cancer treatments published in *Alternative Medicine*,[29] the authors identify four basic types of therapies: biopharmaceutical, immune-enhancing, metabolic, and herbal.

Biopharmaceutical therapies are those that aim to balance the body's biochemical functioning using nontoxic, naturally derived compounds. Included in this category of treatment are antineoplastons, hydrazine sulfate, shark cartilage, high-dose vitamins, laetrile, and compound 714x (nitrogen-rich camphor). Of all these compounds, the antineoplastons, developed by Burzynsky,[30] have the better-defined track record. These are short-chain peptides alleged to inhibit cancer cell growth and to influence the progression of malignant brain tumors and other types of solid tumors. To date, however, no clinical trials confirming these claims have been reported.

Immune-enhancing therapies are based on the premise that poor nutrition and exposure to environmental pollutants and natural toxins cripple the immune systems of cancer patients, causing the development of cancer. The intention of these therapies is to restore the patient's immune system by administering nontoxic compounds that stimulate immune cell function. Examples of immune-enhancing therapies are the ones proposed by Drs. Burton and Livingston. Burton's treatment consists of injecting patients with blood-borne proteins that presumably modulate immune rejection mechanisms. The Livingston treatment attempts to restore the patient's immune system (presumably damaged by a cancer-causing bacterium) with a diet of vegetarian raw foods, nutritional supplements, and a vaccine prepared from a culture of the patient's own cancer-causing bacteria.

Metabolic therapies aim to rebuild and revitalize all the body's life-sustaining functions, thus eliminating the conditions that caused the appearance of the cancer in the first place. These goals are accomplished by offering patients programs that combine nutritional supplements, colonics to detoxify the body, and enzyme therapy to stimulate immune and other defense systems. Among these therapies are Gerson's, Kelley's, and Revici's.

Finally, herbal therapies attempt to take advantage of natural products in herbs that inhibit cancer cell growth. This type of treatment is prevalent in China and is now gaining in popularity in the United States.

Despite the abundance of alternative cancer treatments, their premises have never been reliably and objectively established. For example, there is no proof that the biochemical or immune functions in cancer patients are significantly perturbed. Similarly, there is only limited evidence that a bacterium[31] (*Helicobacter pylori* and gastric lymphoma) may be involved in the causation or pathogenesis of cancer, and there is no evidence that cancer patients' tissues contain high levels of pollutants and toxins capable of producing oncogenic transformation. The proponents of alternative treatments have also failed to demonstrate that the effects they attribute to their treatments actually happen at the cell or biochemical level. Thus, at this juncture we cannot recommend any of these alternative treatments wholeheartedly to our patients.

We are aware, however, of patients' needs for *hope and reassurance,* particularly those whose cancers seem incapable of being cured by traditional methods. These needs often override all rational considerations and logical thinking, driving many cancer patients to try unproven alternative treatments. In a survey conducted in 1990, about a third of all American adults were found to have used at least one form of alternative medical treatment. Of the respondents, 3% were using these types of treatment to control their cancers.[32]

Cassileth and coworkers[33] found that patients who seek alternative cancer treatments are often well educated, belong to the middle-upper socioeconomic class, and have conditions that are not beyond cure or effective palliation by conventional methods. Danielson and colleagues,[34] while investigating cancer patients' use of alternative cancer treatments, identified a variety of factors that motivate them to explore these treatments. They noted that fear, ignorance, misinformation, feelings of hopelessness, and peer pressure from family and friends encouraged patients to use alternative cancer treatments.

Traditional oncologists have by and large failed to address these critical issues. It would be unwise for oncologists to continue ignoring the feelings of empowerment and sense of control that those who undertake alternative treatments often report. Moreover, the fact that many of the alternative treatments have only mild or no side effects contributes to the patients' maintenance of a sense of positive healthfulness. When patients receiving alternative cancer treatments develop clear-cut evidence of clinical progression, they will often argue that had they not been on the alternative program their condition would have been much worse. Although it is easy to dismiss these statements as nonsensical, in doing so we can fail to understand their underlying meaning or the desperation that motivated them.

We must understand that the consumption of "alternative oncologic care" often exposes the patient's feeling of emptiness and significant dissatisfactions with the way oncologists usually approach the patient with cancer. We should not continue denying this reality and pretend that there is no problem or that it will be solved when traditional medicine eventually cures all human cancers. The body of knowledge given to us from both conventional science and lived human experience already contains enough pharmacologic, biologic, psychological, and social information and resources to enable us to validate cancer patients' needs and hopes and assure them that they have access to resources for recovery and healing. For example, studies by Bonavida and colleagues[35] suggest that tumor cell lines and fresh tumor explants resistant to immune-mediated cell killing become sensitive when exposed to subtoxic doses of chemotherapeutic drugs in vitro. Similarly, these same investigators have shown that tumor cell resistance to chemotherapeutic agents can be overcome by exposing the resistant cells to small, sometimes minute, amounts of human lymphokines. These observations merit clinical investigation and may well lead to therapeutic approaches that are biologically useful while causing minimal side effects to the patients. Also, a variety of body-mind techniques (visualization, guided affective imagery, deep relaxation, group psychotherapy and support) seem to influence immune system function and could also assist in the treatment of cancer patients at different stages of their illness. Interventions such as these may mitigate the use of alternative cancer treatments and satisfy the medical and psychological needs expressed by the patients we have agreed to assist.

## How Integrative Oncology Approaches the Cancer Patient at Principal Points in the Course of Oncologic Disease

The integrative oncologist's global approach to individuals with cancer is comprehensive and humane over the entire course of illness. The intention is to attend to both the experiential dimensions of the cancer condition and its physical manifestations. At particular stages of treatment, however, the integrative practitioner will also use more particular approaches.

### AT THE TIME OF DIAGNOSIS

During this stage of oncologic care the primary goals of the integrative program are to

- Provide patients with state-of-the-art diagnostic and therapeutic recommendations regarding their cancers
- Help them overcome the fear and distress that the diagnosis of cancer may have produced
- Educate them about the meaning of the diagnostic and therapeutic options presented to them and help them with the inner psychological processes of decision-making
- Offer support, guidance, and psychospiritual assistance to the patient and his or her family

### DURING THE ADMINISTRATION OF TREATMENT

Once the patient has decided on a course of treatment, the integrative program offers a series of services to reduce or prevent the side effects associated with the selected therapeutic interventions. These services include nutritional counseling; teaching body-mind techniques that reduce fear, stress, and side effects (such as nausea and vomiting); and psychological counseling for the patient and the family, in particular for the healthy spouse.

## ONCE TREATMENT HAS BEEN COMPLETED

After the completion of treatment (especially when the treatment was given with curative intent), patients tend to manifest one of the following two psychological reactions: (1) they dismiss their diagnosis as a fluke, put it behind them, and proceed as if nothing had happened or (2) face a period of uncertainty and confusion during which they experience an unexpected outburst of emotion and distress.

Starting with the initial diagnosis, patients endure a period of intense interaction with the health professionals caring for them, during which a great deal of their energy and attention is required. They may undergo additional diagnostic testing (including invasive procedures), be asked to make difficult therapeutic decisions, and ultimately cope with the effects of the treatment or treatments chosen. Denial and emotional numbness often prevail in them and in their family members. Such defensive psychological reactions are often helpful to patients and need to be respected. Once such defenses subside, however, the emotional and psychological effects of the cancer process demand practitioners' attention. During this third stage patients often feel unsettled, uncertain, confused, and in need of effective psychosocial interventions and rehabilitation.

One often ignored source of patient distress is the frequent perception that when medical treatment is finished, "nothing more" is being done for their cancers. The physicians who were active participants in their recovery now apparently have nothing more to accomplish.

"What if the treatment did not kill all my cancer cells?" This and similar disturbing questions flood patients' minds and require proper attention. Oncologists must maintain open lines of communication with patients and with patients' families, and all concerned need encouragement to express their fears, needs, and beliefs at all times.

During clinical remission, individuals with cancer often search for meaningful ways to sustain their recovery and avoid recurrence. Integrative oncologists offer these patients programs that enhance health and foster recovery from illness. Such programs are based on the insights we are gaining from psychoneuroimmunology, behavioral medicine, and psychology, and also from lived human experience.

This period of clinical stability is also a good time to approach family members about genetic counseling. The genetic counselor often works best with mental health professionals equipped to handle psychosocial issues raised by genetic information, thus ensuring that everyone receives all the support and guidance required.

## DEVELOPING A STRATEGY FOR THE FUTURE

When patients are well is also an auspicious time to encourage them to become educated about resources and facilities available to treat their disease should it recur in the future. Knowing the biologic and psychological meanings of recur-

rence, and how to access needed medical resources wherever they may be, gives many persons a sense of security and power, obviating hasty decisions during a future time of crisis.

## STRATEGY AT THE TIME OF FIRST RECURRENCE

After diagnosis and primary treatment, a substantial number of patients succeed in diminishing their concerns and thus bypass the emotional and spiritual consequences of having had the disease. Once a recurrence takes place, however, denial is not feasible any longer, and fear and other overwhelming feelings occupy the patient's mind. The patient now knows that the physicians' estimates of outcome are just that and are not exact predictions. At this time they also see that negative diagnostic tests cannot fully rule out the presence of cancer cells. Patients who felt trust in their doctors and themselves now feel uncertain and vulnerable to unpredictable events.

Whole belief systems can now collapse under the weight of emerging clinical evidence. Psychological denial or blissful innocence breaks, and the initial cancer episode can no longer be dismissed merely as a one-time fluke in an otherwise steady life.

It is at this time that one of the most critical aspects of healing work can take place. During this stage, patients enter what I have called a "no man's land of uncertainty," a psychospiritual desert where they feel lost, confused, and forsaken. Both experienced integrative oncologists and patients who have traversed this stage successfully can be of great help to those who have newly entered it. These sufferers need a warm, supportive, and reassuring person to guide them through this difficult stage of the journey and help them emerge stronger and more resourceful, no matter what their eventual physical end may be.

Any recurrence is a dreadful experience, but all recurrences do not have the same clinical significance. Certain factors bear significantly on clinical evolution and on what can or needs to be done therapeutically, for example, the number of recurrence sites detected, the associated clinical manifestations, and the length of time between the completion of primary therapy and recurrence.

Patients need to distinguish between fantasies of what the recurrence will do to their lives and what factual information about their medical condition allows them to reasonably predict. Avoiding the creation of negative mental sets, self-conditioned responses, and self-fulfilling prophecies is critical at this stage.

Although chances for cure are less after recurrence, they are certainly not nil. Because we cannot anticipate a priori which patient will be cured of recurrence or live for many years after its detection, it behooves us to encourage all our patients to consider themselves belonging to this survival group of patients until such time that positive possibilities become manifestly unlikely.

It is also important to help patients recognize that cancer is a highly heterogeneous disease: In some patients it has a slow unfolding, one that may take years and even decades to complete. Patients in this category need to be treated differently from those whose cancers grow faster and have more pernicious, immediate effects on the body's functions.

## STRATEGIES DURING DISEASE PROGRESSION OR WHEN THERE HAVE BEEN SEVERAL RECURRENCES

Patients whose cancers have recurred more than once or whose disease is progressing despite treatment urgently need an awareness of newly emerging therapeutic resources as well as effective psychosocial support. This is a time when families need reassurance and direct guidance and when patients need hard-headed encouragement to maintain vitality in their hopes and desires.

During this stage, considerations of issues such as quality of life and patients' total needs are as relevant as those biomedical interventions suggested from the results of diagnostic tests. For example, the treatment needs of patients with widely metastatic cancer that has progressed after several chemotherapeutic interventions with the patients remaining relatively asymptomatic are different from those of patients with a lesser tumor burden but who are more symptomatic and functionally impaired. Patients should have the freedom to participate in the choice of treatment and not feel compelled to participate in studies that may either have no significance for them or may further diminish the quality or length of their lives, or both.

## PREPARATION FOR DEATH

For integrative oncologists, death is an integral part of the life cycle and not something to negate or reject at all costs. Although integrative oncologists are deeply invested in preventing and delaying "untimely" death, they are also prepared to engage the death process once it arrives. Among the greatest fears voiced by cancer patients facing death is the fear of alienation and abandonment. Patients fear that as their physical illness progresses, physicians will distance themselves from them and eventually desert them. In addition, they are equally concerned that family members and other loved ones will grow distant, treating them only as ill persons and creating barriers to intimate communication and communion.

A stated goal of an integrative program is to offer support and service to individuals with cancer from the beginning to the completion of their journey. Part of the service is teaching family members and patients how to remain intimate throughout the experience. Regardless of how advanced an illness may be and how little medical science can do to reverse its inexorable progression, there is always love, caring, and support that we can share with our patients and with each other. Understanding this capacity helps patients and physicians alike to overcome the helplessness that often descends on them during the final stages of patients' lives. Reassuring individuals that they will not be emotionally abandoned regardless of their clinical condition is the final function of an integrative program, and one it must address with total devotion and dedication.

## Toward an Oncology of the 21st Century

Integrative oncology is still in its embryonic state. Few oncologists currently practice it, and its foundational basis is not yet part of traditional oncologic training. It is clear, however, that the increasing knowledge and understanding of our biologic, psychological, sociologic, and spiritual foundations will make it impossible for us to continue practicing an oncologic discipline that remains abstract and separate from this challenging knowledge.

Although integrative oncology is still in its developmental stages, there is little doubt that its paradigmatic construct integrates the complexity and multidimensionality of the cancer condition. In my estimation, integrative oncology is the oncology of the 21st century, invested in restoring to healthfulness not only the body but also the mind of those who suffer from oncologic illness. By acknowledging and validating the complexity and uniqueness of each human being, integrative oncology helps individuals with cancer achieve their highest potential for psychophysical wellness.

## SUGGESTIONS FOR ADDITIONAL READING

Cunningham AJ. Mind-body research in psychooncology: what directions will be most useful? Adv Mind Body Med 1999;15:252–5.

Spiegel D. Embodying the mind in psychooncology research. Adv Mind Body Med 1999;15:267–73.

Micozzi MS, ed. Fundamentals of complementary and alternative medicine. Foreword by C. Everett Koop. New York: Churchill Livingstone, 1996:xvii.

Jacobson JS, Workman SB, Kronenberg F. Research on complementary/alternative medicine for patients with breast cancer: a review of the biomedical literature. J Clin Oncol 2000;18:668–83.

Cassileth BR. Complementary and alternative cancer medicine. J Clin Oncol 1999;17:11 Suppl:44–52.

American Society of Clinical Oncology. The physician and unorthodox cancer therapies (ASCO special article). J Clin Oncol 1997;15:401–6.

Kaptchuk TJ. More on alternative medicine. Ann Intern Med 2000;132:675. letters.

## REFERENCES

1. National Advisory Council for Human Genome Research. Statement on use of DNA testing for presymptomatic identification of cancer risk. JAMA 1994;27:785.
2. Vogelstein B, Fearon ER, Hamilton SR, et al. Genetic alterations during colorectal tumor development. N Engl J Med 1988;319:525–32.
3. Allan SM, Dean C, Fernando I, et al. Radioimmunolocalization in breast cancer using the gene product of c-erbB2 as the target antigen. Br J Cancer 1993;67:706–12.
4. Wagner RF. Gene inhibition using antisense oligodeoxynucleotides. Nature 1994;372:333–5.
5. Rosenfeld MD, Curiel DT. Gene therapy strategies for novel cancer therapeutics. Curr Opin Oncol 1996;8:72–77.
6. Varela FJ, Thompson E, Rosch E. The embodied mind. Cambridge, Mass: MIT Press, 1991:15–33.
7. Vogelstein B, Kinzler K. The multistep nature of cancer. Trends Genet 1993;9:138–41.
8. Weinberg RA, Hanahan D. The molecular pathogenesis of cancer. In: Bishop JM, Weinberg RA, eds. Molecular oncology. New York: Scientific American, 1996:179–204.
9. Dennet DC. Toward a cognitive theory of consciousness. In: Dennet DC, ed. Brainstorms. Cambridge, Mass: MIT Press, 1978.
10. Von Uexkull T, Geigges W, Hermann JM. The principle of teleologic coherence and harmony of purpose exists at every level of integration in the hierarchy of living systems. Advances 1993;9:50–63.
11. Damasio AR. Descartes' error. New York: Avon Books, 1994:205–22.
12. Bovbjerg D, Cohen N, Ader R. The central nervous system and learning: a strategy for immune regulation. Immunol Today 1982;3:287–91.
13. Pelletier KR, Herzing DL. Psychoneuroimmunology: toward a mind-body model. Advances 1989;5:27–56.
14. Friedman M, Roseman RM. Association of specific overt behavior pattern with blood and cardiovascular findings. JAMA 1959;169:1286–96.

15. Mechanic D. Illness behavior, social adaptations, and the management of illness. J Nerv Ment Dis 1977;165:79–87.
16. Berkman LF, Syme SL. Social networks, host resistance, and mortality: a nine-year follow-up study of Alameda County residents. Am J Epidemiol 1979;109:186–204.
17. Goodwin JS, Hunt WC, Key CR, Samet JM. The effects of marital status on stage, treatment, and survival of cancer patients. JAMA 1987;258:3125–30.
18. Benson H, Epstein MD. The placebo effect: a neglected asset in the care of patients. JAMA 1975;232:1225–7.
19. Cunningham AJ. The influence of mind on cancer. Can Psychol 1985;26:13–29.
20. Cunningham AJ. Information and health in the many levels of man. Advances 1986;3:32–45.
21. Schwartz GE, Russek LG. The challenge of one medicine: theories of health and eight world hypotheses. Advances 1997;13:7–23.
22. Engel G. Sudden and rapid death during psychological stress. Ann Intern Med 1971;74:771–82.
23. Phillips DP, Ruth TE, Wagner LM. Psychology and survival. Lancet 1993;342:1142–5.
24. Spiegel D, Bloom J, Kraemer HC, et al. Effect of psychosocial treatment on survival of patients with metastatic breast cancer. Lancet 1989;2:889–91.
25. Fawzy FI, Kemeny ME, Fawzy NW, et al. A structured psychiatric intervention for cancer patients. II: Changes over time in immunological measures. Arch Gen Psychiatry 1990;47:729–35.
26. Antonovsky A. A call for a new question—salutogenesis—and a proposed answer—the sense of coherence. J Prevent Psychiatry 1984;2:1–13.
27. Antonovsky A, Sagy S. The development of a sense of coherence and its impact on responses to stress situation. J Soc Psychol 1986;126:213–25.
28. Antonovsky A. Unraveling the mystery of health. San Francisco: Jossey-Bass, 1987.
29. The Burton Goldberg Group, Strohecker J, ed. Alternative medicine. Puyallup, Wash.: Future Medicine, 1994:556–88.
30. Burzynsky S. Synthetic antineoplastons and analogues. Drugs Future 1986;11:679.
31. Parsonnet J, Hansen S, Rodriguez L, et al. *Helicobacter pylori* infection and gastric lymphoma. N Engl J Med 1994;330:1267–71.
32. Eisenberg DM, Kessler RC, Foster C, et al. Unconventional medicine in the United States. N Engl J Med 1993;328:246–52.
33. Cassileth BR, Lusk E, Strouss TE, et al. Contemporary unorthodox treatments in cancer medicine. Ann Intern Med 1984;101:105–12.
34. Danielson KJ, Stewart DE, Lippert GP. Unconventional cancer remedies. Can Med Assoc J 1988;138:1005–11.
35. Bonavida B, Safrit J, Morimoto H, et al. Cross resistance and implications in gene therapy. Oncol Rep 1997;4:201–5.

# PART

# VIII

# BREAST CANCER

- CHARLES M. HASKELL

**B**reast cancer is the most common malignant neoplasm in women worldwide.[1] This situation is also true in the United States; the American Cancer Society (ACS) estimated that 175,000 new cases of invasive breast cancer would occur in women during 1999.[2] This number represents an annual incidence in 1999 of about 110 new cases per 100,000. The lifetime risk of breast cancer in the United States is about one case for every eight women (12.5% projected over a life span of >95 years). Overall, breast cancer makes up 29% of all cancer in U.S. women. The ACS states that the incidence rate of breast cancer in women had been increasing at a rate of about 4% per year in the 1980s, but the rate has stabilized in the 1990s. The ACS also estimated that there would be about 1300 new cases of breast cancer in men during 1999.

The ACS estimated there would be 43,700 deaths in women and 400 deaths in men from breast cancer in the United States during 1999.[2] The annual mortality rate from breast cancer in the 1980s remained stable at about 27 deaths per 100,000 despite improvements in medical management.[3] More recent data from the ACS shows a declining mortality rate during 1991 through 1995, with the largest decreases in younger women.[2]

Geographic variations in breast cancer incidence and survival have been reported in the United States, with a higher mortality rate in the Northeast and a lower rate in the South. These differences are unexplained, with one study suggesting they may be due to differences in cancer control practices,[4] whereas another group postulates the differences are explained by an uneven distribution of known breast cancer risk factors in different geographic areas.[5]

Two factors that have probably contributed to the improvement in survival are as follows: First, screening mammography reduces the mortality of breast cancer by 30% in women older than age 50, and mammography is now widely used in the preoperative assessment and follow-up of patients with breast cancer. Second, systemic adjuvant therapy decreases the annual risk of recurrence and increases the disease-free survival of patients at sufficient risk of recurrence to justify its use. Advances that are unrelated to survival but that improve the quality of life of women with breast cancer are also important. Examples are breast conservation and reconstruction.

The most exciting advances have come in understanding the molecular biology and genetics of breast cancer. Discovering genetic alterations that lead to breast cancer and developing strategies to exploit them will usher in the next decade of breast cancer research and treatment.

This chapter starts with a section that summarizes the natural history of breast cancer, including etiology, molecular pathogenesis, epidemiology and risk factors, biology, classification (pathology), diagnosis, staging, and prognosis. This section is followed by sections on the treatment of carcinoma in situ, local control with surgery and reconstruction, local control with radiation therapy, the treatment of metastatic disease, and adjuvant therapy. The chapter concludes with a section summarizing the authors' approach to the integration of treatment modalities for specific patients and selected clinical problems.

## REFERENCES

1. Pisani P, Parkin DM, Ferlay J. Estimates of the worldwide mortality from eighteen major cancers in 1985: implications for prevention and projections of future burden. Int J Cancer 1993;55:891–903.
2. American Cancer Society. Cancer Facts and Figures—1999. Atlanta: American Cancer Society, 1999.
3. Marshall E. The politics of breast cancer. Science 1993;259:616–7.
4. Goodwin JS, Freeman JL, Freeman D, Nattinger AB. Geographic variations in breast cancer mortality: do higher rates imply elevated incidence or poorer survival? Am J Public Health 1998;88:458–60.
5. Laden F, Spiegelman D, Neas LM, et al. Geographic variation in breast cancer incidence rates in a cohort of U.S. women. J Natl Cancer Inst 1997;89:1373–8.

# CHAPTER 35

# BREAST CANCER

.........................................

## NATURAL HISTORY AND PRETREATMENT ASSESSMENT

- Linnea I. Chap • Sanford H. Barsky
- Lawrence W. Bassett • Charles M. Haskell

### ETIOLOGY AND MOLECULAR PATHOGENESIS

The molecular pathogenesis of breast cancer involves genetic alterations of breast epithelial cell DNA resulting in progressively more invasive and malignant somatic cells.[1, 2] The process is probably initiated by a variety of carcinogens, including chemicals,[3] radiation,[4] and possibly retroviruses,[5, 6] and it can be promoted by many physiologic and environmental factors. Evidence also exists for breast cancer susceptibility genes that account for a minority of breast cancer cases. The disease is clearly the result of a complex, poorly understood multistep process. This schema will be refined in the future through detailed studies of new models of breast cancer pathogenesis.[7]

Breast cancer usually arises in women as a sporadic event. Generally, there is no family history of the disease, but other, more subtle, risk factors may be present. This section reviews the cause, molecular pathogenesis, epidemiology (risk factors), and biology of breast cancer. It also summarizes the clinical information needed for formulating a plan of therapy.

Breast cancer develops in genetically altered cells of the ductal lobular unit, mainly through a multistep series of genetic alterations. Some genetic alterations involving susceptibility genes may also be inherited. The most important and best-established genes involved in this process are the *BRCA1* gene and the p53 gene found on chromosome 17 (Fig. 35–1) and the *BRCA2* gene found on chromosome 13. For men, the androgen receptor gene has been implicated as a causative factor. Using the techniques of molecular genetics, it has been found that other genes may also be involved in some patients. Some of these genes are altered by mutation, others by amplification or rearrangement, and still others by loss or deletion. Table 35–1 summarizes the results of one large study of patients with familial breast cancer that illustrates the wide variety of potential genetic loci involved. Some of these are likely to be involved in the initiation or early promotion of breast cancer (*BRCA1*, *BRCA2*, and p53 for women and the androgen receptor for men). Other changes are probably not involved in initiation or early promotion but may play a role in the amplification and later promotion of these earlier genetic alterations. This subject is discussed further in the section on the biology of breast cancer.

***BRCA1.*** The breast cancer susceptibility gene *BRCA1* is located in a region of chromosome 17q21 known as

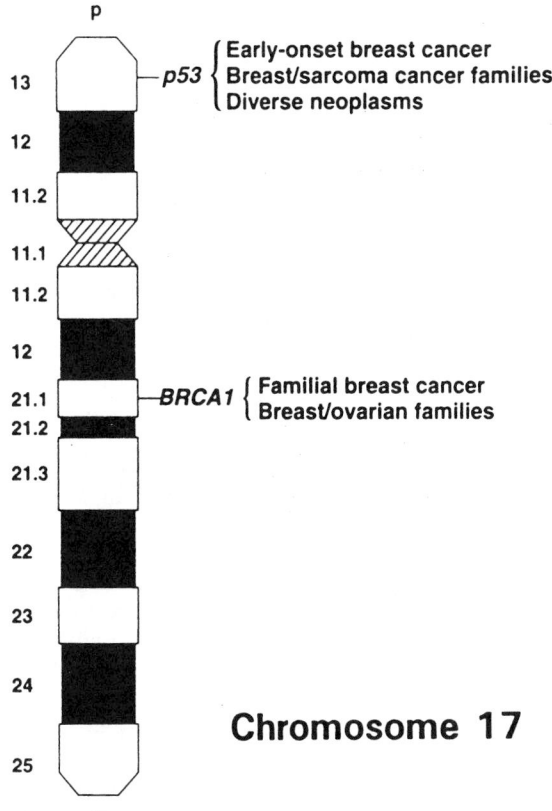

**Figure 35–1.** Human chromosome 17.

*D17S855.*[8] It is an autosomal dominant gene that codes for a suppressor protein of 1863 amino acids. This protein contains a zinc finger domain, but it is otherwise distinct from other known proteins. Its precise physiologic function is currently unknown, but it appears to act as a tumor suppressor gene. A number of mutations in this gene have been identified in patients with familial breast and ovarian cancer.[8, 9] The pattern of mutation suggests that *BRCA1* is of etiologic significance in patients with familial breast and ovarian cancer, but its actual role is unknown.[9] Data from the Breast Cancer Linkage Consortium predicted that inheritance of this gene conferred a 63% risk of ovarian cancer by age 70 and an 85% risk of breast cancer by age 80.[10]

***BRCA2.*** Shortly after the *BRCA1* gene was isolated, the

*Table 35–1.* **Genetic Factors in Familial Breast Cancer**

| Genetic Locus | Chromosomal Location | Approximate Frequency (%) |
|---|---|---|
| *BRCA1* | 17q | 29 |
| p53 | 17p | 25 |
| Androgen receptor | X | ? |
| ? | Distal 17p | 16 |
| ? | Distal 17q | 5–40 |
| ? | 8p | 42 |
| ? | 16q | 24 |
| ? | 19p | 36 |
| ? | 22q | 21 |

An additional candidate suppressor gene has been identified at 13q12-q13 (*BRCA2*), but its frequency is uncertain at the time of this writing (Schott DR, et al. Cancer Res 1994;54:1393).

Data from Lindblom A, Skoog L, Rotstein S, et al. Loss of heterozygosity in familial breast carcinomas. Cancer Res 1993;53:4356–61, and from Lindblom A, Skoog L, Andersen TI, et al. Four separate regions on chromosome-17 show loss of heterozygosity in familial breast carcinomas. Hum Genet 1993;91:6–12.

*BRCA2* gene was described.[11] This breast cancer susceptibility gene is located in a 6-cM region of chromosome 13q12–13[12] and, similar to *BRCA1*, appears to function as a tumor suppressor gene. Initial data, based on high-risk families, reported the risk of breast cancer in women with *BRCA2* to be 87% by age 80. The initial risk estimates, however, for *BRCA1* and for *BRCA2*, may have been overestimates and not applicable to all patient subsets with either of these genetic mutations (see later).

**p53.** p53 is a tumor suppressor gene with putative roles in DNA replication, transcription, and cell cycle control. It inhibits transformation of cells by *myc* and *ras*, both of which are well-established oncogenes. Somatic alterations of p53 may occur by either deletions or point mutations. This alteration leads to an abnormal accumulation of complexes of abnormal p53 with wild-type p53 in the cytoplasm. This abnormal accumulation prevents p53 from entering the nucleus and regulating transcription. These effects are termed *dominant negative* and explain why only one allele of p53 needs to be altered instead of the traditional two alleles for a classic tumor-suppressor mechanism.[13] The high frequency of p53 mutations in one series was interpreted as supporting an important role for chemical carcinogenesis in the cause of breast cancer.[14] Certain familial syndromes also involve this gene, especially the Li-Fraumeni syndrome, in which mutations in p53 are inherited (see subsequent discussion).

**Androgen Receptor.** The androgen receptor is normally controlled by a gene on the X chromosome. Two brothers with breast cancer had a constitutional mutation in the androgen receptor gene,[15] and mutations have been found in two other patients with male breast cancer.[16] These findings support, but do not completely prove, a role for the androgen receptor gene in the pathogenesis of male breast cancer. Whether or not this gene is involved in the cause of female breast cancer is unknown.

**HER-2/neu.** HER-2/neu, a member of the class I growth factor–receptor tyrosine kinase family, is amplified and overexpressed in up to 30% of all breast cancers, including both precancerous (ductal carcinoma in situ [DCIS]) and invasive carcinomatous epithelium.[17] The genetic abnormality is not inherited but acquired, and is thought to confer aggressive biology and refractoriness to chemotherapy. Translational research initiatives have targeted this gene with monoclonal antibodies, as discussed later in this chapter.

## EPIDEMIOLOGY AND RISK FACTORS

A variety of interrelated genetic, environmental, hormonal, sociobiologic, and physiologic factors exert an influence on the development of breast cancer. We discuss the most important of these risk factors individually. Of women with breast cancer, 70 to 80% have no apparent risk factors for the disease. These patients are considered to have *sporadic* breast cancer.

**Heredity.** When the genetic basis of breast cancer is fully clarified, it will be possible to determine whether or not any given woman has a genetic predisposition to the disease. Until then, counseling women about genetic risk must be based on the following epidemiologic observations. A woman with a first-degree relative with breast cancer is about two to three times more likely to develop the disease than a woman with a negative family history. This average figure is inappropriate for individual counseling, however, because this group includes at least three subgroups with different risks of breast cancer. About 5 to 8% of families with breast cancer have a truly hereditary form of the disease. These patients tend to develop breast cancer at a much younger age than sporadic cases and have a higher incidence of bilateral disease. In some patient subsets, there may also be an association with other tumors, such as colon, prostate, ovarian, sarcoma, and endometrial cancer. First-degree relatives of patients from this group have at least a 50% risk of breast cancer, and some studies suggest that the risk may exceed 90% for some patients of high-risk families by age 85. For a second group of families, the risk is intermediate (about 30%). This intermediate risk is probably because of higher than normal exposure to the environmental factors that contribute to the risk of breast cancer in all women. These women may not have inherited the actual genetic alteration for breast cancer susceptibility, but they may have inherited a genetic propensity for a risk factor for breast cancer. An example is a genetic propensity to have an early first menstrual period. Another example may be related to body fat distribution, with a high waist/hip ratio leading to a higher risk of breast cancer, especially for women with a strong family history of the disease.[18] Obesity itself is a modest risk factor for breast cancer. In a final group, the risk is identical to that of the general population—about 12% over a lifetime projected to age 110 years. Table 35–2 provides a guide to assessing breast cancer risk for individual women based on familial risk factors.[19] These include the age of the woman at risk and the age, laterality (unilateral vs. bilateral), and menopausal status of the relatives with breast cancer. An alternative model for the prediction of individual breast cancer risk has been published by Gail and associates.[20] This model is fairly good at predicting the individual risk of breast cancer in women older than age 50 participating in programs of breast cancer screening with mammography, but the model overestimates the risk for younger women.[21]

There are several well-defined hereditary syndromes involving breast cancer. They are potentially important in differential diagnosis and family counseling.

*Table 35–2.* **Lifetime Risks of Breast Cancer for Women with Selected Family Histories of Breast Cancer**

| Affected Relatives | Clinical Features | Risk |
|---|---|---|
| Mother* | Pre | 0.18–0.27 |
| | Post | 0.18–0.27 |
| Sister | Pre/bil | 0.56 |
| | Pre/uni | 0.08 |
| | Post/uni | 0.18 |
| Mother and sister | Both pre, 1 bil | 0.51 |
| | Both pre, uni | 0.33 |
| | 1 Pre, 1 post, 1 bil | 0.23 |
| | Both post, 1 bil | 0.28 |
| | 1 Pre, 1 post, both uni | 0.10 |
| | Both post, both uni | 0.05 |
| Two sisters | Both pre, 1 bil | 0.50 |
| | Both pre, both uni | 0.18 |
| | 1 Pre, 1 post, 1 bil | 0.11 |
| | 1 Pre, 1 post, both uni | 0.08 |
| | Both post, both uni | 0.05 |
| Mother and grandmother | Both pre/1 pre, 1 post/both post | 0.27 |
| Mother and aunt | Both pre/1 pre, 1 post/both post | 0.14 |

*We estimate the risk of subsequent breast cancer to be 0.5 for a woman whose mother has premenopausal, bilateral breast cancer.

Pre, premenopausal; post, postmenopausal; bil, bilateral; uni, unilateral.

From Williams WR, Osborne MP. Familial aspects of breast cancer: an overview. In: Harris JR, et al, eds. Breast diseases. Philadelphia: JB Lippincott, 1987:115.

***Hereditary Breast and Ovarian Cancer Syndrome.*** Most patients with hereditary breast and ovarian cancer are thought to have a mutation of the *BRCA1* or *BRCA2* genes.[22] In one study of 33 families with evidence of linkage to *BRCA1*, the lifetime risk of breast cancer was 87% by age 70.[23] The cumulative risk of ovarian cancer in this study was 44% by age 70. The relative risk (RR) of colon cancer (RR, 4.11) and of prostate cancer (RR, 3.33) was also increased in these families. In another study of 98 such patients, the group was characterized by breast cancer of no special type, but there was a high frequency of aneuploidy and high S-phase fraction, and patients were younger than normally seen for groups of patients with breast cancer.[24] Despite these characteristics, which would be expected to confer a poor prognosis, these patients had a better prognosis than other patients with familial breast cancer.

As initially described with *BRCA1*, in some kindreds, the presence of the *BRCA2* susceptibility allele conferred more than a 90% lifetime risk of breast cancer as well as an increased susceptibility to ovarian cancer.[25, 26] An increased frequency of male breast cancer also has been observed in *BRCA2*-linked breast cancer families.[22, 27] In several ethnic groups, an increased prevalence of *BRCA1* or *BRCA2*, or both, has been demonstrated. In Ashkenazi Jews, for example, 1 in 44 carry a *BRCA1* or *BRCA2* mutation.[28–30] This high prevalence has led to considerable study of breast cancer in Ashkenazi Jews. In the Washington D.C. Area Ashkenazi Study (WAS), Ashkenazian women having either the *BRCA1* or *BRCA2* mutation had a 56% chance of developing breast cancer and a 16% chance of developing ovarian cancer by age 70.[31] In an Icelandic population–based study, the risk of breast cancer in patients with *BRCA* mutation was found to be 37.2% by age 70.[32]

The risk estimations just described are lower than those estimated by the Breast Cancer Linkage Consortium. The variation in risk may be secondary to variable gene pene-trance and other unidentified factors. Overall, it appears that the risk of breast cancer associated with mutation of the *BRCA1* or *BRCA2* gene ranges from 40 to 85%. These high-risk families are candidates for aggressive screening, prevention trials, and possibly prophylactic surgery (see later).

***Li-Fraumeni or SBLA Syndrome.*** This rare autosomal-dominant syndrome predisposes individuals to breast cancer and to a variety of other malignancies. These include soft tissue sarcomas (S), brain tumors (B), leukemias and lung cancer (L), and adrenocortical tumors (A).[33, 34] Variants of the Li-Fraumeni syndrome probably exist, as illustrated by an increased risk of breast cancer in the mothers of children with osteosarcoma and chondrosarcoma in one study.[35] The genetic basis of this syndrome probably resides in inherited mutations in one p53 suppressor allele.

***Other Familial Syndromes.*** Cowden's syndrome is a rare disorder characterized by hamartomatous lesions of the oral cavity and skin. In one review, 74% of the patients with this disease had breast cancer.[36] *Muir's syndrome* is a rare autosomal dominant disorder characterized by multiple skin tumors (usually involving sebaceous glands) with polyps and adenocarcinomas, primarily of the large bowel, small intestine, and stomach.[37] The sebaceous neoplasms associated with this syndrome may arise in the breast, but there is no compelling evidence that this syndrome is associated with an increased risk of the usual types of breast cancer.

There is a final group of syndromes of uncertain importance. This group is based on the aggregation of breast cancer with a variety of other malignant disorders. It is possible that an inherited breast cancer susceptibility gene is pleiotropic for other tumors as well. Examples of this association include clusters of breast cancer with melanoma,[38, 39] meningioma,[40, 41] and osteosarcoma.[42] Inactivation or structural rearrangement of the retinoblastoma gene may contribute to these multiple cancers.[43, 44] There also may be an association with the gene for ataxia-telangiectasia.[45]

**Age.** Advancing age has an enormous impact on the incidence of breast cancer. The older a woman, the higher her risk of developing breast cancer (Table 35–3). The reason for this striking finding is not totally clear but most likely relates to the requirement for multiple somatic mutations (multiple hits) for the genes of breast cancer. This phenome-

*Table 35–3.* **Risk of Developing Breast Cancer**

| By Age (yr) | Risk |
|---|---|
| 25 | 1 in 19,608 |
| 30 | 1 in 2525 |
| 35 | 1 in 622 |
| 40 | 1 in 217 |
| 45 | 1 in 93 |
| 50 | 1 in 50 |
| 55 | 1 in 53 |
| 60 | 1 in 24 |
| 65 | 1 in 17 |
| 70 | 1 in 14 |
| 75 | 1 in 11 |
| 80 | 1 in 10 |
| 85 | 1 in 9 |
| Ever | 1 in 8 |

Data from National Cancer Institute, reported in Science 1993;259:618.

non probably contributes to the increasing incidence of breast cancer in the United States as the population becomes increasingly older.

### Environmental Factors

*Diet.* The incidence rates and mortality rates for breast cancer vary widely around the world. Studies of migrating populations point to the importance of environmental factors in the cause of breast cancer, especially dietary factors.[46-48] For example, women in Japan have a low incidence of breast cancer, but when they move to the United States the rate increases. It goes up even further in their daughters. This increased incidence may be secondary to dietary factors, such as low fat or high soy intake diet, but the cause of this increase is uncertain. High soy consumption in native Asians has been associated with a reduced risk of breast cancer.[49, 50] Additionally the administration of soy constituents to rodent cancer models and human breast cancer lines has an inhibitory effect.[51] In humans, the risk of breast cancer is increased by obesity. In animal studies, it is not clear whether it is dietary fat or just calories. Caloric restriction markedly reduces the development of breast cancer in rats, regardless of fat intake.[52] Well-nourished girls start menstruating at an early age. High dietary fat intake by these girls at puberty may be more carcinogenic than the same high-fat diet in an adult. Diets high in total and saturated fat content have been of special concern as well as obesity and a high caloric intake. Several reports, however, question the importance of a high-fat diet in the cause of this disease.[53-57] An important study of the lifestyle of nurses does not support a role for fat intake as a risk factor in adults.[58] Fat intake may be important, but proof of a role for fat in causing human breast cancer requires appropriate randomized clinical trials. Such trials include one in Toronto[59] and those supported by the National Cancer Institute.[60]

Potentially protective dietary factors include the intake of vitamins A, C, and E, although a large prospective study of these vitamins failed to demonstrate any protective value from the intake of large doses of these vitamins.[61] Beta-carotene may exert a protective effect, as suggested by the Nurses Health Study. A case-control study from Australia found that the risk of breast cancer was reduced by eating a high-fiber diet.[62]

*Alcohol.* Alcohol appears to increase the risk of breast cancer. In a meta-analysis of the available data in 1988, the RR of a daily intake of 24 g (1 oz) of absolute alcohol compared with no alcohol ranged from 1.4 to 1.7.[63] A more recent study found a RR of 2.1.[64] The available data support an association between alcohol consumption and breast cancer, but it is modest and does not prove a causal relationship.

*Miscellaneous Carcinogens.* Passive exposure to cigarette smoke and possibly other environmental carcinogens may increase the risk of breast cancer.[65] Radiation is carcinogenic, especially when exposure is high and occurs at an early age. For example, women who receive radiation therapy for chest acne and women with scoliosis who receive multiple diagnostic radiographs around puberty develop breast cancer at an increased rate. Radiation therapy for benign breast disease nearly doubled the rate of breast cancer in a large Swedish study.[4] Higher levels of chlorinated compounds were found in the fat of women with breast cancer than in controls in one study.[66] A small study from New York confirmed this finding,[67] but a subsequent major study from the San Francisco Bay area provided substantial evidence against this hypothesis.[68] Genotoxic carcinogen exposure is suggested by studies of p53 mutations in various tumors,[69] but the weight of evidence at present does not support a major role for chemical carcinogens in the cause of breast cancer.

**Endocrine Factors.** Hormonal regulation of the breast is important in the development of breast cancer. Early pregnancy and early oophorectomy lower the incidence of this neoplasm, whereas late menopause and early menarche increase the incidence. An early therapeutic or spontaneous abortion appears to increase the risk, as long as it is before the first pregnancy. Nulliparous women (including nuns and many lesbians) have a higher risk of breast cancer. Women with a late first pregnancy have a higher risk of breast cancer, however, than women who have never been pregnant at all. These anomalous findings suggest that hormones may function differently during pregnancy. For example, the hormones of pregnancy may protect a normal cell against the initiation of genetic damage, but they may act as promotional agents for cells already initiated. Attempts to define and quantify the endocrine factors that promote or contribute to breast cancer have proved difficult, however. There is no clear-cut pattern of hormonal imbalance that explains the high incidence of this disease in women in general. Differences in estriol excretion in women have been associated with an increased risk of breast cancer, but this may be a spurious association resulting from alterations in steroid metabolism that are secondary to age, the use of oral contraceptives, sampling errors related to menstruation, or other unknown factors.[70] Another hypothesis relates to a potential long-term effect of a first pregnancy on the secretion of prolactin.[71] This hypothesis, too, requires further study before acceptance as a modulating endocrine factor.

The risk of breast cancer from the use of exogenous hormones is uncertain. Diethylstilbestrol (DES) exposure during pregnancy increases the risk of breast cancer.[72] Oral contraceptives do not appear to increase the risk of breast cancer in most women. A meta-analysis of 27 epidemiologic studies, however, suggests that these agents may increase the risk of breast cancer minimally in some subgroups. Specifically the risk increases slightly for women younger than age 45, nulliparous women, and women using these agents for more than 8 years.[73] In another study, the risk was increased for women using oral contraceptives for more than 10 years before their first pregnancy, and several studies suggest that the use of oral contraceptives in the early teenage years may increase the risk of subsequent breast cancer.[74-77] The development of a contraceptive that would help prevent breast and ovarian cancer while suppressing ovulation is a high research priority.

Postmenopausal estrogen replacement may affect the incidence of breast cancer in a dose-related fashion. Some studies have suggested that estrogen, particularly given in high dosage, increases the risk of subsequent breast cancer.[78-80] Several other studies suggest that estrogen given in low doses to relieve menopausal symptoms probably does not increase the incidence of breast cancer, unless given for more than 10 years.[81-85] A meta-analysis of 51 studies of 52,705 women with breast cancer showed a 31% increase in breast cancer for users of long-term hormone replacement therapy (HRT).[86] In two large cohorts, one of Swedish women[87] and another the Nurses Health Study,[88] both showed an approximately 40% increase in breast cancer risk for women who took hormones for more than 10 years. The issue of HRT use and breast cancer risk is being addressed further by the Women's Health Initiative, a multicenter randomized trial comparing HRT with placebo in 27,500 postmenopausal women.[89]

The association between lactation and the risk of breast cancer is uncertain. A large multicenter case-control study found a reduced risk of premenopausal breast cancer in women who lactated, but there was no effect on postmenopausal breast cancer.[90] Risk was related to the duration of lactation, with a reduction of risk of 11% for 4 to 12 months of breast-feeding and a reduction of nearly 25% for lactation lasting 24 months or longer. Reanalysis of a large international case-control study by menopausal status, however, found no significant effect of lactation in premenopausal and postmenopausal women.[91]

**Benign Breast Disease.** Benign breast disease may be a risk factor for subsequent breast cancer. Some studies have shown that a previous breast biopsy increases the subsequent risk of breast cancer regardless of the pathology, whereas others have shown only an increased risk with proliferative disease, particularly the presence of atypia. Clinical or mammographic *fibrocystic disease or change* has no greater subsequent risk. This problem is discussed further in the section on pathology.

**Prior Treatment for Cancer.** Children and young adults cured of cancer by aggressive combined-modality therapy are subject to an increased incidence of delayed neoplasms. Initially, this incidence was limited to acute leukemia, but breast cancer has also become a potentially serious problem for these patients. This situation is particularly true of young patients treated with combined-modality therapy for Hodgkin's disease.[92, 93]

**Emotional Factors.** The available evidence suggests that emotional factors play no causative role in breast cancer.[94] For example, in one case-control study, there were no differences in life stresses between women in general and breast cancer patients.[95] In a prospective study, depression was equally common among women who did and did not develop subsequent breast cancer.[96]

## BIOLOGY

**Oncogenes and Growth Factors.** Abnormalities of oncogene expression probably influence the cancer cell through specific growth factors or growth factor receptors. This influence can occur either by an autocrine mechanism involving only the cancer cell or through a paracrine mechanism involving adjacent stromal cells. In addition to estrogen and progesterone, numerous growth factors influence the growth of the breast cancer cell. This influence is illustrated by evidence implicating the in vivo amplification and rearrangement of the c-*myc93* and the c-*erb*B-2 (HER-2/*neu*) oncogenes in breast cancer.[97, 98] Breast cancer also may be associated with mutations in the H-*ras*-1 minisatellite locus, which is just downstream from the proto-oncogene H-*ras*-1.[99] Other examples of important growth factors (which have specific receptors on the breast cancer cell membrane) include transforming growth factor-α and transforming growth factor-β, insulin-like growth factors I and II, epidermal growth factor,[100, 101] somatostatin receptors,[102] and retinoic acid receptors.[103] Figure 35–2 illustrates selected growth regulatory pathways involving the breast cancer cell.

**Estrogen and Progesterone Receptors.** The demonstration of hormone responsiveness in mammary carcinomas in 1896 led to the important principle that neoplasms retain some of the differentiated functions of the tissue of origin. Endocrine organ ablation and hormonal manipulation have been widely used in the treatment of metastatic breast cancer. Steroid hormone action depends on specific binding to high-affinity intracellular receptors that have great specificity for the hormone.[104] Binding to defective hormone receptors may prevent a response to hormonal therapy.[105]

The importance of hormone-receptor interactions in clinical medicine is discussed in Chapter 8 and a subsequent section of this chapter (Systemic Treatment for Metastatic Breast Cancer), as well as in a general review article.[106] Quantifying the expression of receptors for estrogen and progesterone is now standard practice for all patients with primary breast cancer. Receptor measurements can be performed by immunohistochemistry or one of several biochemical methods.[107] Immunohistochemistry is preferable in women taking hormonal therapy, and it is generally more

**Figure 35–2.** Schema depicting possible growth regulatory pathways in human cancer. IGF, insulin-like growth factor; EGF, epidermal growth factor; ER, estrogen receptor; TGF, transforming growth factor; PDGF, platelet-derived growth factor. (From Osborne CVK. Autocrine and paracrine growth regulation of breast cancer: clinical implications. Breast Cancer Res Treat 1990;15:5.)

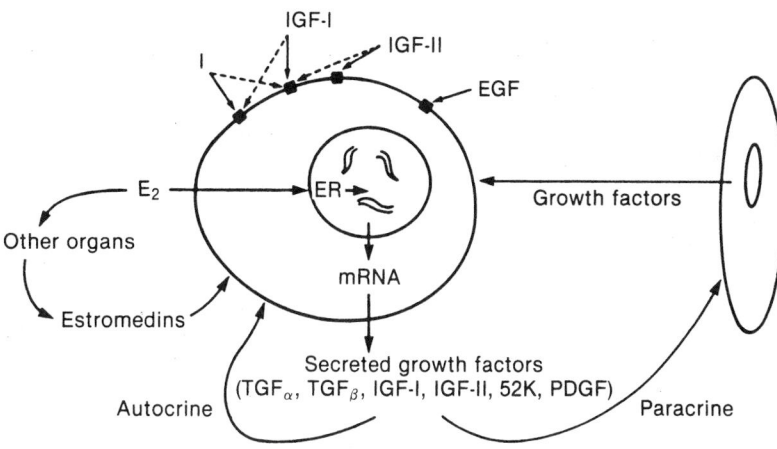

convenient for pathologists. Biochemical studies remain the standard approach in some institutions, however, because most of the studies correlating the response of patients to hormonal therapy and the role of receptors in determining prognosis were performed in the past using biochemical methods. The relative value of biochemical and immunohistochemical techniques, particularly for progesterone receptors, continues to be an area of active research.

**Tumor Doubling Time.** The concept of the tumor doubling time (TDT) is useful in estimating the duration of the preclinical stage of breast cancer and in understanding the clinical course of the disease. The TDT is a function of many variables (e.g., rate of cell division, proportion of cells actively dividing, rate of cell death, proportion of tumor composed of cells as opposed to fibrotic tissue, intermitotic interval, tumor burden, desquamation, dormancy, and effects of therapy). Because of these many variables, the TDTs of breast cancer are extremely heterogeneous.

It makes a difference whether the TDT is measured in early breast cancer or in late breast cancer. In a comprehensive review, Shackney and associates[108] reported a mean TDT of 25 days for early breast cancer. The TDT in patients with late breast cancer was much longer—129 days (Fig. 35–3). The difference in mean TDT in early and late breast cancer was statistically significant ($p<0.0001$), providing convincing documentation of growth retardation in advanced human tumors (so-called gompertzian growth, as discussed by Norton[109] and as illustrated in Figs. 1–5 and 8–10).

The use of the TDT to estimate the duration of preclinical breast cancer can be illustrated by a simple example. A 1-cm *early* breast cancer contains $10^9$ cells and has already undergone 30 of the 40 doublings that occur before the woman's death. The TDTs in Figure 35–3 of primary breast cancer vary from 3 to 250 days for early lesions, with a mean of 25 days. Multiplying these values by 30 doublings, we see that the average time for a single breast cancer cell to grow to be a 1-cm early breast cancer is 2 years. The range in this period varies between 90 days and 21 years. A comparable calculation using the TDT values for *late* breast cancer would be an average of 10.6 years. For comparison, Speer and coworkers[110] have used another model of breast cancer growth that estimates the average preclinical duration of breast cancer to be about 8 years.

The natural history of breast cancer suggests that it is an acute or chronic disease, depending on the TDT.[111] Kusama and colleagues[112] found a direct correlation between the TDT and the duration of survival after radical mastectomy. Galante and associates[113] prospectively correlated TDT with survival and showed a good correlation between growth rate and survival in patients with three or more positive lymph nodes; in contrast, no significant differences were found among slow-growing tumors in women with varying degrees of axillary lymph node involvement. The importance of the TDT is even easier to illustrate in patients who receive no therapy at all. In one study, the average survival from first symptoms was 40 months in 100 untreated patients.[114] The median survival was 2.5 years; 22% of the patients were alive at the end of 5 years, and 5% were alive at 10 years. *Chronic* forms of breast cancer result from tumors with the longest TDTs. In contrast, about 20% of untreated patients survive less than 1 year from the first symptoms, and this fraction represents those with more rapid TDTs.

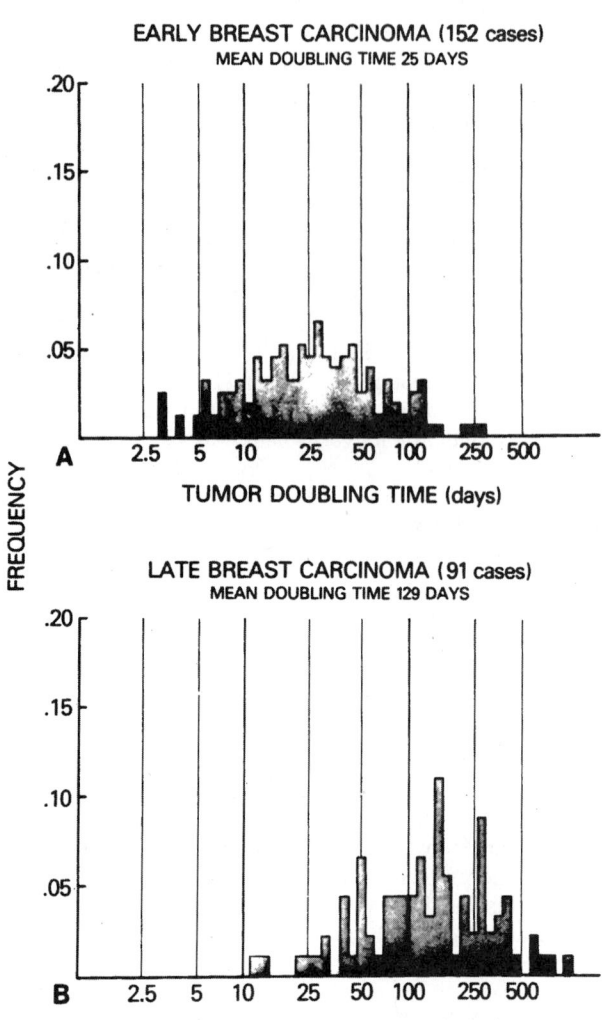

**Figure 35–3.** Tumor doubling time distributions in breast carcinoma. *A*, Early breast carcinoma. *B*, Late breast carcinoma. (From Shackney SE, et al. Growth rate patterns of solid tumors and their relation to responsiveness to therapy—an analytical review. Ann Intern Med 1978;89:107.)

**Flow Cytometry.** Flow cytometry allows an assessment of several biologic characteristics of breast cancer tissue.[115] One of the most important uses of flow cytometry is to determine the percentage of cells in S phase.[116–118] This percentage reflects the growth fraction of the tumor as well as the TDT. Flow cytometry can also show whether the tumor is predominantly composed of diploid cells or whether significant aneuploidy exists. Numerous retrospective studies suggest that aneuploidy may be associated with a poor prognosis. This association is especially true of patients with a high percentage of cells in S phase.[119] Prospective trials using flow cytometry as a prognostic factor, however, are not as convincing (see discussion under prognosis). Flow cytometry can be performed on formalin-fixed tissue so that it is relatively easy to perform this test retrospectively for investigational purposes. The value of flow cytometry would be enhanced if it could be adapted to include the measurement of hormone receptors.

**Breast Cancer as a Systemic Disease.** In many women, breast cancer is a systemic disease at the time of first diagnosis, that is, cancer cells have been shed during the preclinical phase of tumor growth.[120] In the past, most physicians believed that breast cancer universally spreads from the primary tumor to the lymph nodes then to distant sites (Halsted's model). Now it is clear that breast cancer can bypass lymph nodes and spread directly to the bloodstream. Breast cancer can present as a metastasis without any evidence of a primary tumor (systemic model).

The concept of breast cancer as a systemic disease is not new. In 1896, Beatson[121] suggested that "the tumor in the breast is only a local manifestation of a blood affection." Subsequently, Mueller and Jeffries[122] reported that 80 to 85% of all women who die after developing breast cancer die of the breast cancer and that the rate of dying is constant 15 years following operation. If breast cancer were truly a localized disease susceptible to cure, one would expect the survival curve eventually to be parallel to that of the normal population or at least to show a plateau.[123, 124] If this plateau occurs at all, it does so in only a small fraction of patients, even after 15 years of follow-up.[125-127]

Mueller[128] has shown that the rate of dying is different for patients with and without positive axillary lymph node involvement at the time of surgery. This difference implies that stage II breast cancer is not merely a later version of stage I disease resulting from a delay in diagnosis (lead-time bias). The differences in the annual rates of dying for the two stages of breast cancer suggest that they are different variants of breast cancer.

Microscopic or histologic cancer does not always progress to clinical cancer, and even advanced breast cancer may rarely undergo spontaneous regression.[129] Three clinical observations support this view. First, pathologists frequently find evidence of multiple lesions in the breast, but finding two or more clinically apparent breast tumors is rare.[130] Second, in women with proven breast cancer in one breast, the incidence of clinically apparent cancer developing in the opposite breast is much lower than the incidence of histologic cancer detected by *mirror image* biopsy, prophylactic mastectomy, or autopsy. Finally, the frequency of tumor growth in untreated axillary nodes is much lower than would be expected based on the frequency of regional node involvement in patients undergoing radical mastectomy.[131, 132]

These studies support the view that many breast carcinomas metastasize before diagnosis of the primary lesion and that the exponential recurrence rate of breast cancer for the ensuing 15 years is a function of tumor dormancy[133] or the random distribution of different TDTs among these metastatic lesions,[125] or both. Some studies suggest that about 30 to 50% of breast carcinomas are truly localized and completely eradicable by local means. These patients are cured of breast cancer, although they probably cannot be identified as such for at least 15 years following initial therapy.[125] Hellman[134] has proposed a new model of breast cancer (the *spectrum* model) that accommodates this growing awareness of a curable population of patients treated solely with local-regional therapy.

Although there is some evidence that rare patients with widely metastatic breast cancer may be cured with chemotherapy,[135] there is wide agreement that chemotherapy is more likely to cure patients with micrometastatic breast cancer. With the ascendancy of the systemic disease model of breast cancer, systemic chemotherapy is now widely used as part of the initial management of breast cancer. This is known as *adjuvant* therapy, and it is the most important use of chemotherapy in patients with breast cancer at this time (see the section Adjuvant Treatment of Breast Cancer).

## CLASSIFICATION (PATHOLOGY)

Most breast cancers are invasive adenocarcinomas arising from the ductal lobular epithelial unit.[130] Table 35–4 lists the relative incidence, some clinical features, and survival data for the various forms of breast cancer.[136]

Most patients have infiltrating ductal carcinomas (*duct carcinomas with productive fibrosis* in Table 35–4). A few patients have the classic form of infiltrating lobular carcinoma, which carries the same prognosis as infiltrating ductal carcinoma. Other histologic subtypes of breast cancer are rare, but their identification can be important in planning treatment. Specifically, one can identify a group of highly unfavorable and a group of highly favorable carcinomas that require special consideration,[137] and a variety of rare mesenchymal tumors can occur that raise yet other problems in management. Also to be discussed in this section are the various forms of noninvasive and benign breast diseases.

**Unfavorable Histologic Subtypes.** Several forms of breast cancer are especially aggressive and usually require individualized management that may differ from the treatment of the more common forms of breast cancer.

*Table 35–4.* **Comparison of Histologic Types of Infiltrating Breast Carcinoma***

| Histologic Type | % of Total | Average Age (yr) | Average Size (cm) | % of Node Involvement | Median Survival of Treatment Failures (yr) | % of Crude Survival 5 yr | % of Crude Survival 10 yr |
|---|---|---|---|---|---|---|---|
| Duct carcinomas with productive fibrosis | 78.1 | 50.7 | 3.1 | 60 | 3.75 | 54 | 38 |
| Lobular carcinoma | 8.7 | 53.8 | 3.5 | 60 | 3.25 | 50 | 32 |
| Medullary | 4.3 | 49.0 | 3.4 | 44 | 2.25 | 63 | 50 |
| Colloid | 2.6 | 49.7 | 3.8 | 32 | 4.3 | 73 | 59 |
| Comedocarcinomas | 4.6 | 48.6 | 3.9 | 32 | 2.7 | 73 | 58 |
| Papillary | 1.2 | 51.9 | 3.4 | 17 | 5 | 83 | 56 |

*Derived from a long-term follow-up study of 1458 patients with infiltrating breast carcinomas, all of whom were treated with radical mastectomy at the Memorial Hospital or James Ewing Hospital between 1940 and 1943. The histologies and statistical analyses were done by Drs. J Berg and GF Robbins, as reported in 1968 by McDivitt, et al. In: Atlas of Tumor Pathology, Second Series, Fascicle 2. Washington, D.C.: Armed Forces Institute of Pathology, 1967.

***Inflammatory Carcinoma.*** This form of breast cancer is highly malignant based on histopathologic and immunohistochemical characteristics.[138] It is characterized by erythema and edema in the skin overlying the breast; these are secondary to extensive dermal lymphatic spread.[139, 140] The diagnosis should be made on both the clinical and the microscopic appearance. Treatment requires a multimodality approach, as discussed in the section Treatment by Stage of Disease and Special Problems.

***Signet Ring Carcinoma.*** This is an extremely aggressive subtype of poorly differentiated ductal and pleomorphic lobular carcinoma.[141] These tumors show an unusual metastatic pattern with a strong propensity to involve serosal surfaces, leading to syndromes mimicking gastrointestinal disease or retroperitoneal fibrosis. Histologically, the tumor stroma contains a diffuse infiltrate of individual epithelial cells with basophilic or clear cytoplasm containing mucin. In signet ring cell poorly differentiated ductal carcinomas, the mucin displaces the nucleus, causing it to become crescentic in shape. In signet ring pleomorphic lobular carcinomas, the nucleus, although displaced, is not deformed. These signet ring cells make up at least 20% of the tumor.

***Metaplastic Carcinomas (Carcinosarcomas or Malignant Mixed Tumors).*** Carcinomas of this type contain varying amounts of malignant spindle cell differentiation.[142] There may be malignant cartilage or osteoid present, and some authors consider these tumors to occur along a spectrum from relatively benign to highly malignant.[143] These tumors are usually large at initial diagnosis, and they grow rapidly. Despite this large size and rapid growth, however, axillary lymph node involvement is rare. Nevertheless, regardless of the stage of disease at presentation, the prognosis is poor, and survival usually does not exceed 35% at 5 years.

**Favorable Histologic Types.** There is a striking preponderance of certain rare histologic subtypes of breast cancer among long-term survivors of the disease.[144, 145] In 767 node-negative patients treated with surgery alone at Memorial Sloan-Kettering Cancer Center, Rosen and colleagues[146] found that typical medullary, mucinous, papillary, tubular, and adenocystic carcinomas had much better prognoses than other forms of invasive adenocarcinoma. Except for medullary carcinomas, this improved prognosis probably relates to the relatively long TDTs for these tumors as determined by thymidine labeling indices.[147] The good prognosis of typical medullary carcinomas, despite high labeling indices and the usual absence of estrogen receptors, is unexplained.[148] One possibility is that the immunocompetent cells that infiltrate this tumor are activated and play a suppressive role.[149] Another possibility is that medullary carcinomas, although rapidly dividing, do not exhibit the full-blown invasive phenotype. A variant of medullary carcinoma termed *atypical medullary carcinoma* has been recognized, exhibiting a more invasive pattern of growth and more aggressive clinical behavior.

***Mesenchymal Tumors.*** A variety of true sarcomas and lymphomas can occur in the breast.[150] Cystosarcoma phylloides is a rare variant of this group of tumors that has a relatively good prognosis.[150] These tumors are usually large at initial diagnosis, and they grow rapidly. Despite this large size and rapid growth, however, axillary lymph node involvement is rare.

**Noninvasive, In Situ Carcinomas.** Two major patterns of in situ carcinoma are recognized: ductal carcinoma and lobular carcinoma. DCIS was considered rare in the past but with modern mammography is considered much more common. DCIS is discussed in detail in the next section In Situ Breast Cancer. Lobular carcinoma in situ (LCIS) is actually a marker of malignancy; it, too, is discussed in the section In Situ Breast Cancer. DCIS is a malignant lesion. It is classically subclassified into two histologic groups: comedo and noncomedo. Both groups are further subclassified.[151] These lesions can vary in size and appearance, and occasionally microinvasion occurs. All these factors may be considered in clinical management, as discussed further in the section In Situ Breast Cancer.

**Benign and Premalignant Breast Lesions.** The terminology applied to benign and premalignant lesions of the breast is evolving, primarily because of controversy about their malignant potential. Haagensen[152] reviewed the experience with these lesions at Columbia University and published a working classification of benign breast lesions. Of the 10 lesions in this classification system, only gross cystic disease, multiple intraductal papillomas, and lobular neoplasia (more commonly known as *LCIS*) were considered premalignant. Contemporary studies suggest that only lesions with epithelial proliferation or atypia (hyperplasia, atypical ductal hyperplasia, papillomatosis, LCIS) are prone to malignancy.[153] This view is reflected in the consensus statement developed by the College of American Pathologists (Table 35–5).[154]

## CLINICAL FEATURES AND DIAGNOSIS

The diagnosis of breast cancer is undergoing an enormous shift. In the past, 80% of all breast cancers were detected

***Table 35–5.*** **Relative Risk for Invasive Breast Carcinoma Based on Pathologic Examination of Benign Breast Tissue\***

*No Increased Risk*

Adenosis, sclerosing or florid
Apocrine metaplasia
Cysts, macro and/or micro
Duct ectasia
Fibroadenoma
Fibrosis
Hyperplasia, mild†
Mastitis (inflammation)
Periductal mastitis
Squamous metaplasia

*Slightly Increased Risk (1.5–2 times)*

Hyperplasia, moderate or florid, solid or papillary
Papilloma with fibrovascular core

*Moderately Increased Risk (5 times)*

Atypical hyperplasia (borderline lesion)
    Ductal
    Lobular

\*Consensus Statement of the College of American Pathologists developed at a meeting in New York, October 3 to 5, 1985, published in Arch Pathol Lab Med 1986;110:171–3. Each risk group in the table refers to the risk in a woman with the biopsy finding specified compared with the risk for invasive breast carcinoma in a comparable woman who has had no breast biopsy.

†Ducts or ductules (lobules) with an epithelial lining no more than two cells deep are normal. *Mild hyperplasia* exists when the epithelium is greater than two but not more than four cells deep. *Moderate* and *florid hyperplasia* refer to more extensive degrees of epithelial proliferation.

initially by the woman herself. Now, increasingly, the disease is initially found by screening. Common symptoms of breast cancer other than an abnormal mammogram include a painless, persistent dominant lump; a persistent thickening or dimpling of the skin; nipple retraction; and spontaneous unilateral nipple discharge. The cancer is most often a hard mass with an irregular border, but it may present as an area of thickening in what appears to be a physiologic nodularity of the breast. Fixation of the cancer to the skin or pectoral fascia, skin edema or ulceration, satellite nodules, and the presence of large axillary metastases are all signs of more advanced breast cancer. These are all less frequent than in the past.[155]

The accuracy of diagnosing a breast cancer on physical examination increases as the patient's age increases. The diagnostic accuracy in premenopausal women is 30%. Because of the inaccuracy of clinical diagnosis, any woman with a dominant mass in her breast should undergo biopsy or aspiration of the mass. If there is a palpable lump, fine-needle aspiration or core biopsy can be performed. This is performed in the physician's office or clinic with local anesthesia. The results are often definitive and allow the physician to proceed directly with treatment. There is a false-negative rate to these procedures, and it is important that one always follow the rule of concordance, that is, the mammogram, clinical impression, and cytologic features must be concordant. If there is any question, an open biopsy is indicated. For mammographic lesions, there is also the availability of noninvasive techniques for diagnosis. Both fine-needle aspirations and core biopsies can be performed under stereotactic guidance. Biomarkers, including estrogen receptors, and flow cytometry can be determined using either fine-needle aspiration or core biopsy specimens if needed.[156]

**Mammography.** Mammography is an extremely useful tool in the detection and diagnosis of breast cancer. Since the first report on mammography in the United States in the 1930s, mammography has undergone striking technologic improvements that have increased its sensitivity and accuracy.[157] Quality assurance procedures also have played an important role in improving mammography in the United States.[158] The Mammography Quality Standards Act was passed by Congress in 1992 and implemented by the U.S. Food and Drug Administration (FDA) on October 1, 1994 to ensure that mammography was of high quality at all facilities. Standardized reporting has been developed to improve the communication of the results of mammography and appropriate management recommendations.[159] Clinicians who refer women for mammography should become familiar with the standardized terminology used in mammography reporting today. Standardized terminology is used in this discussion of mammography and other breast imaging.

Mammography should be separated into two basic types: screening mammography and diagnostic mammography.[160] *Screening mammography* is used for the detection of unexpected breast cancer in asymptomatic women. Screening mammography is the only method proved effective in reducing mortality from breast cancer.[161, 162] The screening examination uses a two-view depiction of each breast to make a binary decision: (1) The examination is normal or (2) the examination is abnormal. If normal, the woman has her next mammography at the routine screening interval, usually in 1 year. If abnormal, the patient has a further diagnostic work-up or biopsy. Mammographic screenings that show abnormalities that turn out to be benign by further diagnostic work-up or biopsy are frequently referred to as *false positives*. Much has been made of the adverse effects of these false-positive examinations in terms of morbidity.[163] Most false-positive examinations are resolved by the diagnostic work-up, consisting of additional mammographic views or ultrasonography, or both.[164] These diagnostic work-ups for abnormal screening examinations result in anxiety and health care costs; however, the adverse effects of biopsies performed for benign mammographic abnormalities are of greater concern. Current radiology literature recommends a positive biopsy rate (yield of carcinoma) of 25 to 40%.[165] This positive biopsy yield is currently thought to provide the best balance between detecting as many cancers as possible and reducing the number of unnecessary biopsies that are performed. One study showed that the cancer yield for biopsies for impalpable, mammographically detected abnormalities was not significantly higher than for palpable abnormalities.[166] The cancers, however, detected on mammography were smaller, less likely to involve the axillary nodes, and more likely to be *minimal* or noninvasive.

In the detection of breast cancer, mammography has a sensitivity of 85 to 90%.[167] The age at which screening should begin is controversial. The American Cancer Society currently recommends that asymptomatic women begin screening with annual mammograms at age 40.[168] Indications for initiating screening mammography in younger women include a strong family history of breast cancer or a previous diagnosis of breast cancer. The age for discontinuing screening is uncertain, but one reasonable guideline is to take into account the woman's general health status to determine the practical benefits of screening on an individual basis, rather than generalizing.

*Diagnostic mammography*, sometimes called *consultative* or *problem-solving* mammography, is performed to evaluate the breasts of patients with an abnormal screening examination or a clinical abnormality, such as a palpable lump or nipple discharge. If the diagnostic examination is being performed after an abnormal screening mammography, the diagnostic work-up could include additional mammographic projections, such as magnification views. In addition to further mammographic views, ultrasonography is an important adjunctive imaging modality for the evaluation of some abnormal screening and clinical findings.

The diagnostic examination is usually tailored for the individual patient's specific screening abnormality or clinical finding.[169] If the diagnostic examination is being performed for a clinical abnormality and screening has not been performed, the examination usually begins with the routine two-view screening. A radiopaque BB is superimposed directly on the palpable finding before taking the films, however. On the mammograms, the BB indicates the exact location of any palpable findings (Fig. 35–4). The interpreting physician should be on site during the performance of diagnostic mammography. Mammography is an important diagnostic tool for women with breast symptoms because it can define the nature of many breast abnormalities and their extent, and it can detect unexpected malignancy, including multifocal disease (Fig. 35–5). These diagnostic capabilities often have significant implications for therapy.

For women older than age 30, diagnostic mammography

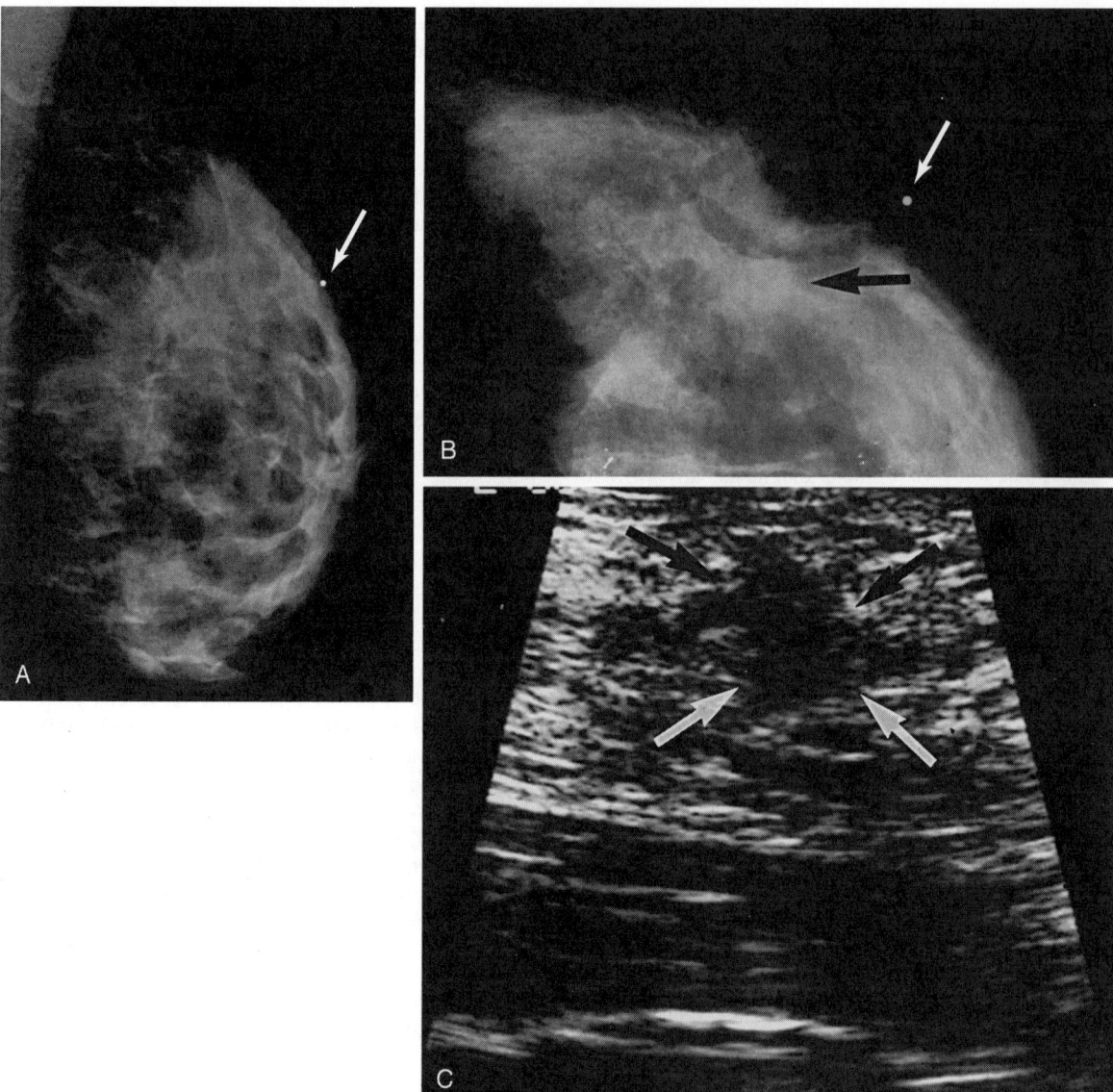

**Figure 35–4.** Evaluation of palpable mass. The patient felt a mass in the upper outer left breast. *A,* Mediolateral oblique view shows a metallic marker ("BB") placed over the site of the mass, but there are no definite abnormalities. *B,* Close-up shows a subtle architectural distortion *(arrow)* that would not have been noticed without the BB. *C,* Ultrasonography over this area revealed an irregular mass *(arrows)* with low-level internal echoes. The findings are highly suggestive of malignancy. Biopsy revealed infiltrating ductal carcinoma.

should be performed even when a biopsy is planned for a palpable breast lump. The purpose of mammography is not to defer a biopsy of a suspicious clinical finding. Rather the purpose of mammography before the scheduled biopsy is to (1) define better the nature of the palpable abnormality, (2) detect unexpected lesions in the ipsilateral (multifocal or multicentric carcinoma) or contralateral breast, and (3) identify an extensive intraductal component of a palpable invasive carcinoma.

***Standardized Reporting and Terminology.*** The American College of Radiology Breast Imaging Reporting and Data System (BI-RADS) was devised to standardize mammography reports and the terminology used to describe mammographic findings, reduce confusing interpretations, and facilitate outcome monitoring.[170] In addition to standardized terms to describe abnormalities, the standardized mammography report includes an *overall* assessment of the probability of

malignancy at the end of the report. There are six possible assessment categories, and each of these categories is associated with a specific management recommendation (Table 35–6). Category *0* is reserved for cases in which additional imaging work-up is needed. Once the imaging is completed, the case is assigned one of five final assessment categories. The final assessment eliminates any potential misunderstanding by the referring health care provider as to the most significant findings and the management recommendations. Classifying examinations into five distinct categories also facilitates follow-up and tracking responsibilities for the referring health care provider and the mammography facility.

***Breast Tissue Composition.*** There is a wide range in the appearance of the normal breast on mammography. The breast tissue composition, which can range from almost all fat to extremely dense fibroglandular tissue, directly affects the sensitivity of mammography. Because breast cancers are

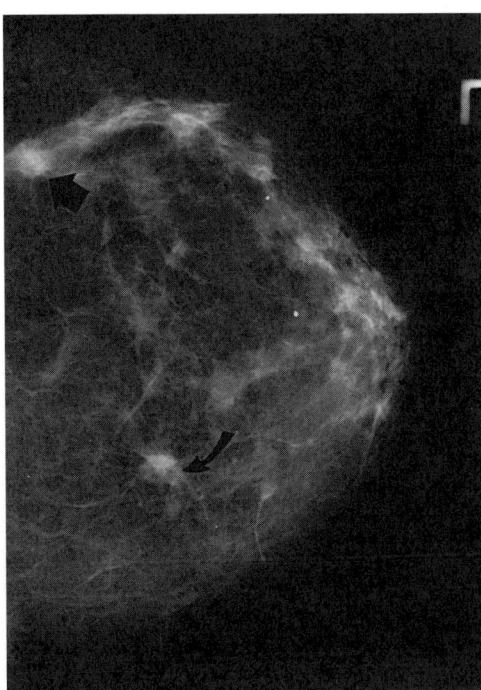

**Figure 35–5.** Multicentric carcinoma. The patient felt a lump in the outer hemisphere of the breast. A round, ill-defined, dense mass *(arrow)* was seen at the site of the palpable abnormality. The spiculated mass *(curved arrow)* in the inner aspect of the breast was identified on mammograms performed before biopsy.

radiodense, radiolucent fat (dark gray to black on mammograms) provides an excellent background in which to detect small cancers, but dense fibroglandular tissue (white on mammograms) can obscure breast cancers. In the standardized mammography report, the breast tissue composition is divided into four types: (1) almost entirely fat, (2) mostly fatty with scattered islands of fibroglandular densities, (3) heterogeneously dense, which may lower the sensitivity of mammography, or (4) extremely dense, which lowers the sensitivity of mammography. Although young women tend to have more fibroglandular tissue than older women, there is a wide variation in breast tissue density among women of

the same age. Some young women have almost completely fatty breasts, and some older women have extremely dense breasts.

***Abnormal Mammographic Findings.*** Masses and calcifications are the most common abnormalities encountered on mammograms, and the radiographic features of these abnormalities are important clues to their cause. Other abnormalities include a new or evolving density, asymmetric distribution of the fibroglandular tissue between the breasts, and architectural distortion.

• *Masses.* Masses are described by their shape, margins, and density. The *shape* can be round, oval, lobulated, or irregular (Fig. 35–6). Oval and round masses are usually benign. An irregular shape suggests a greater likelihood of malignancy. Of all the features, the *margins* of a mass are the most reliable indicator of the probability of malignancy. Margins can be circumscribed, microlobulated, obscured, indistinct, or spiculated. *Circumscribed* margins favor a benign cause, and the likelihood of malignancy for a circumscribed mass is low, probably less than 2%.[171] If it is proved to be a simple cyst by ultrasonography, no further work-up is needed. If solid, magnification mammography may be required to confirm that all of the margins of a solid mass are circumscribed. Multiple circumscribed masses almost always indicate a benign finding, usually cysts, fibroadenomas, or benign intramammary lymph nodes, and routine follow-up in 1 year is usually sufficient. *Microlobulated* margins (multiple tiny undulations) are unusual, but they increase the possibility of malignancy. The margin of a mass may be *obscured* by

*Table 35–6.* **Mammography Final Assessment Categories**

| Category | Final Assessment | Findings, Recommendation |
|---|---|---|
| 0 | Incomplete | Additional work-up is indicated. This could include mammography views or ultrasonography. |
| 1 | Negative | There is nothing to comment on. Routine screening. |
| 2 | Benign finding | A definitely benign finding. Routine screening. |
| 3 | Probably benign finding | High probability of benignity. Short-term follow-up recommended to establish stability. |
| 4 | Suspicious abnormality | Not characteristic but has reasonable probability of malignancy. Biopsy should be considered. |
| 5 | Highly suggestive of malignancy | High probability of malignancy. Appropriate action should be taken. |

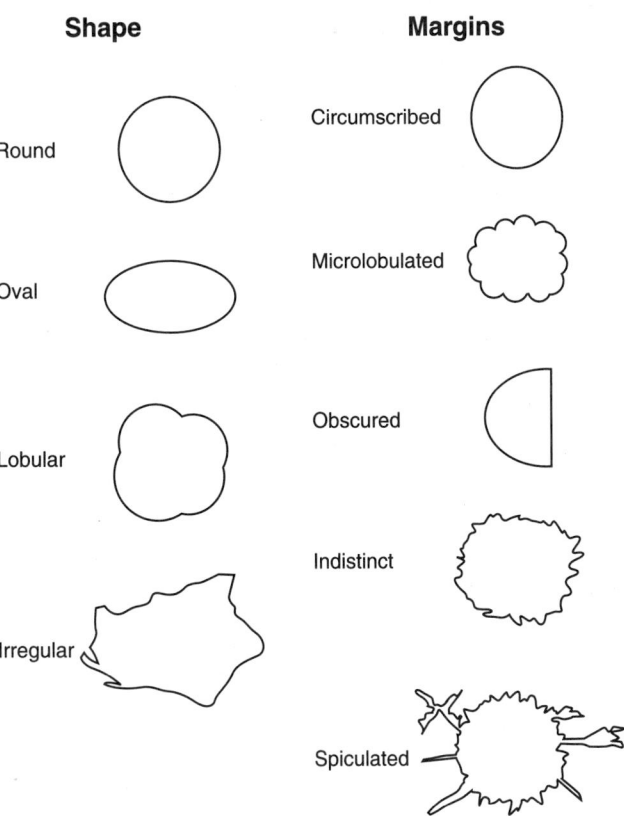

**Figure 35–6.** Masses: terminology for shapes and margins.

fibroglandular tissue of similar density so that a definite determination cannot be made. *Indistinct* or ill-defined margins are suspicious for malignancy. A mass with *spiculated* margins has fine lines (spicules) radiating from its border, a finding that is highly suggestive of malignancy. An area of spiculation without any associated mass is called an *architectural distortion.*[172] Such distortion could represent a manifestation of malignancy, a benign radial scar, or previous surgery. The *density* of a mass also provides a clue as to its cause. In general, benign masses tend to be lower in density, equal to or less than normal tissue. Malignant masses tend to have high radiodensity compared with benign masses or surrounding normal breast tissue. The density of a mass, however, is not always a reliable sign as to whether it is benign or malignant.[173]

• *Calcifications.* Calcifications are divided into three general categories: (1) typically benign, (2) intermediate, and (3) higher probability of malignancy. *Typically benign* calcifications can usually be definitively characterized by their mammographic features. Examples of typically benign calcifications are skin (dermal), vascular, coarse, large rod-like, round, eggshell, and milk-of-calcium types (Fig. 35–7A). *Intermediate* calcifications are tiny, amorphous, and indistinct, making more specific characterization difficult (Fig. 35–7B). *Higher probability of malignancy* calcifications include those that are pleomorphic or fine, linear, and branching (see Fig. 35–7B). The distribution of calcifications is another feature indicating whether they are more likely benign or malignant. *Grouped* or *clustered* calcifications, which include more than five in a small area (<2 cm³), can be benign or malignant. A *linear* distribution of a cluster of calcifications suggests malignancy. A *segmental* distribution, meaning in a duct and its branches, also suggests malignancy but more extensive. A *regional* distribution involves a larger volume of breast tissue, not necessarily in a ductal distribution, a distribution that can be benign or malignant. A *diffuse or scattered* distribution of calcifications randomly in both breasts is considered benign.

• *Invasive cancer with extensive intraductal component.* Invasive tumors are classified as having an extensive intraductal component (EIC+) if they are predominately intraductal with small areas of invasion or if they are primarily invasive with one of the following: (1) DCIS fills nonobliterated ducts within the invasive cancer, or (2) there is DCIS in the tissue adjacent to the invasive tumor (Fig. 35–8).[174] The significance of EIC+ on mammography is that it suggests a malignancy with greater likelihood of local recurrence if vigorous efforts are not made to identify its full extent and excise it completely.[175] Mammography plays an important role in the management of EIC+ tumors. Mammographic wire localization is essential before the surgical excision to ensure that the location of the extensive calcifications is identified for the surgeon. Bracketing, the use of multiple wires to delineate the extent of the calcifications before surgery, is recommended if the calcifications are extensive.[176] Specimen radiography should be performed to determine whether removal of calcifications is complete. Specimen radiography, however, cannot accurately predict whether all intraductal carcinoma has been removed, and histologic evaluation of the specimens is critical.[177] The complex branching of the breast ductal system can lead to errors at histologic evaluation of the margins. It is important that cases with extensive DCIS manifested by calcifications have mammography performed after surgery and before initiation of radiotherapy to identify any residual malignant calcifications (Fig. 35–9).[178] To minimize possible discomfort associated with

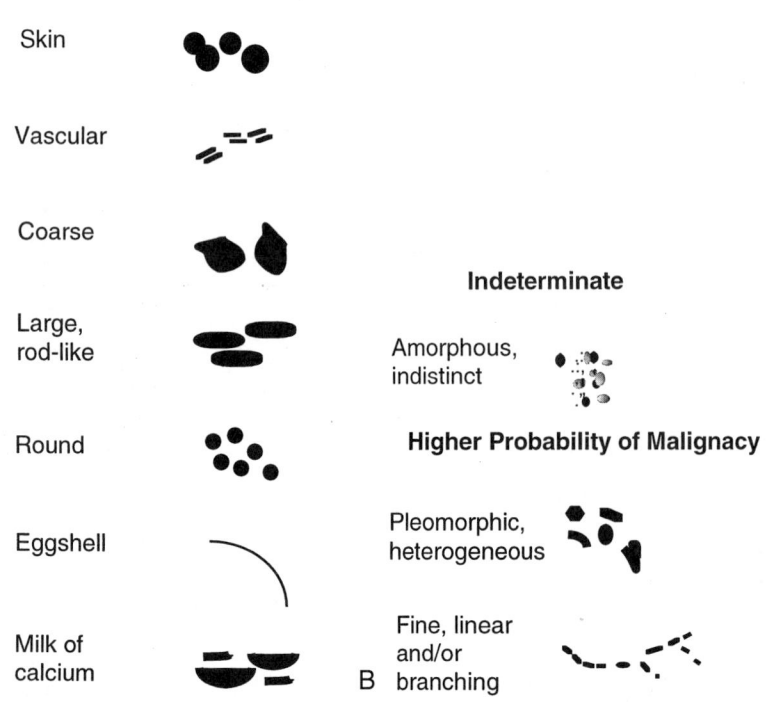

**Figure 35–7.** Calcifications. *A,* Typically benign. *B,* Indeterminate and higher probability of malignancy.

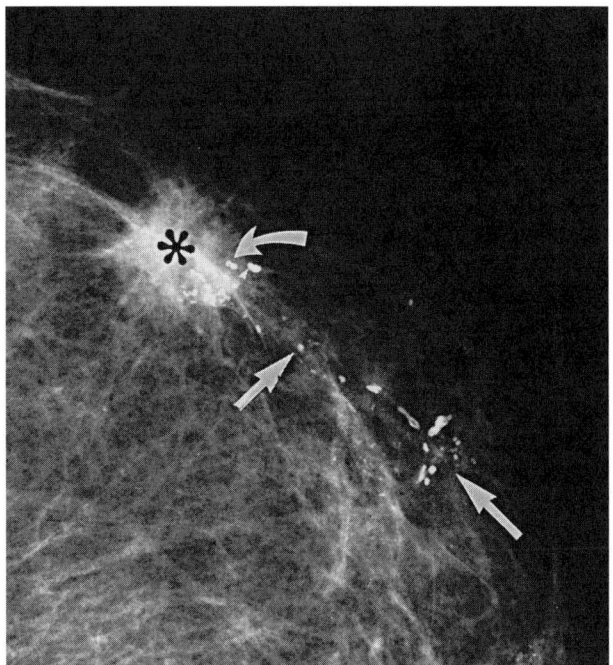

**Figure 35–8.** Extensive intraductal component. There is an irregular, spiculated mass *(asterisk),* which is highly suggestive of malignancy. There is an extensive intraductal component, manifested by pleomorphic calcifications within *(curved arrow)* and adjacent to the mass *(arrows).* The mass was palpable and easily excised, but complete excision of the calcifications is required to avoid tumor recurrence. This excision requires presurgical bracketing of the full extent of the calcifications with at least two hook wires. Evidence of successful excision before beginning radiography requires (1) clear margins at histologic evaluation of the excised tissue and (2) preradiotherapy mammograms that show no residual calcifications.

employing magnification techniques (Fig. 35–10). If the preradiotherapy mammograms disclose residual calcifications, re-exision is performed even if the margins were clear histologically. If the residual calcifications are extensive or distant from the surgical cavity, wire localization of the calcifications may be needed to ensure excision.

- *Other mammographic signs of breast carcinoma.* In addition to masses and calcifications, breast cancer may be manifested by a new or evolving density, architectural distortion (Fig. 35–11), or bilaterally asymmetric breast tissue. These *other signs* or *subtle signs* have been reported to be the only evidence of malignancy in 20% of mammographically detected cancers.[179]

**Ultrasonography.** Ultrasonography is the most important imaging adjunct to mammography. The most common indication for sonography is to determine whether a solitary circumscribed mass is cystic or solid.[180] Cysts are characterized by round to oval shape, anechoic interior, and posterior echo enhancement (Fig. 35–12). Improvements in ultrasonography technology, including the introduction of higher-resolution transducers and imaging protocols tailored for the breast, have led to a renewed interest in expanding the role of ultrasonography for the evaluation of breast diseases. One important area of progress has been the development of reliable ultrasonographic criteria for differentiating benign versus malignant solid masses.[181] Benign solid masses characteristically have an oval shape, with a width on the plane of the breast greater than the anterior to posterior diameter, circumscribed margins, and homogeneous internal echoes (Fig. 35–13). Malignant masses characteristically have an irregular shape, ill-defined margins, and heterogeneous inter-

mammographic compression, pretherapy mammograms are performed just before initiation of radiotherapy, usually 3 to 5 weeks after surgery. The pretherapy mammography is optimized by placing a wire over the surgical site and

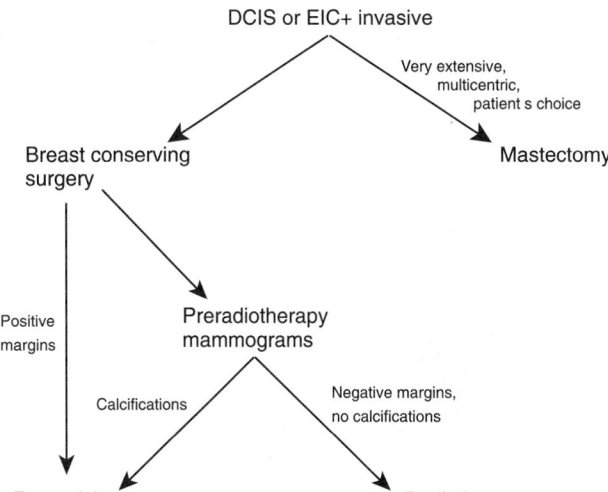

**Figure 35–9.** Imaging management of extensive ductal carcinoma in situ calcifications. DCIS, ductal carcinoma; EIC +, extensive intraductal component.

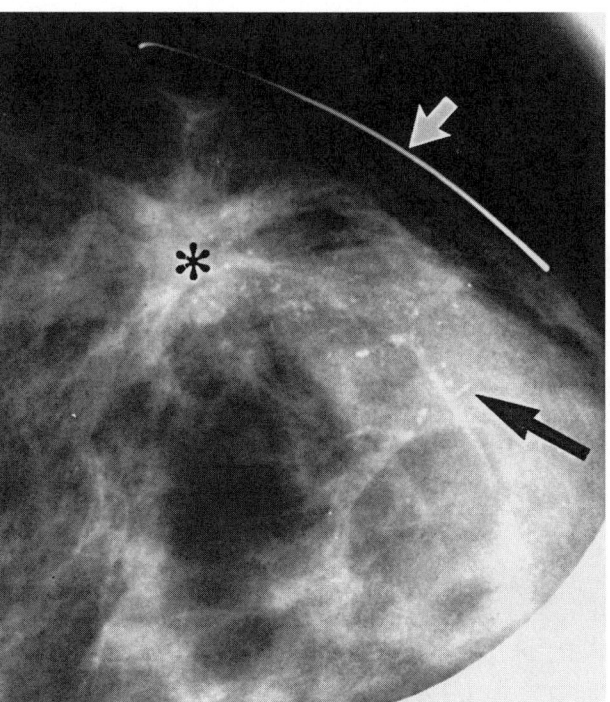

**Figure 35–10.** Postsurgery, preradiotherapy mammograms, performed directly over the surgical site 5 weeks after lumpectomy for ductal carcinoma in situ. The site of the skin incision was marked by a wire *(white arrow).* Residual ductal carcinoma in situ calcifications *(black arrow)* extend several centimeters from the surgical bed *(asterisk).*

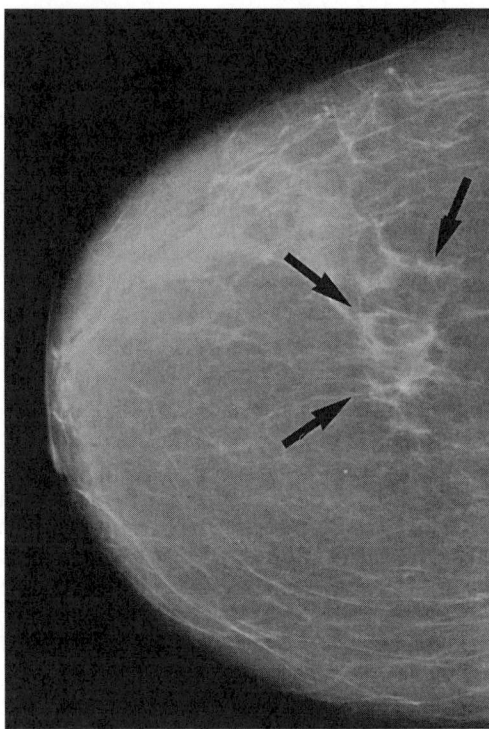

**Figure 35–11.** Invasive carcinoma manifested on mammography by an architectural distortion *(arrows)*.

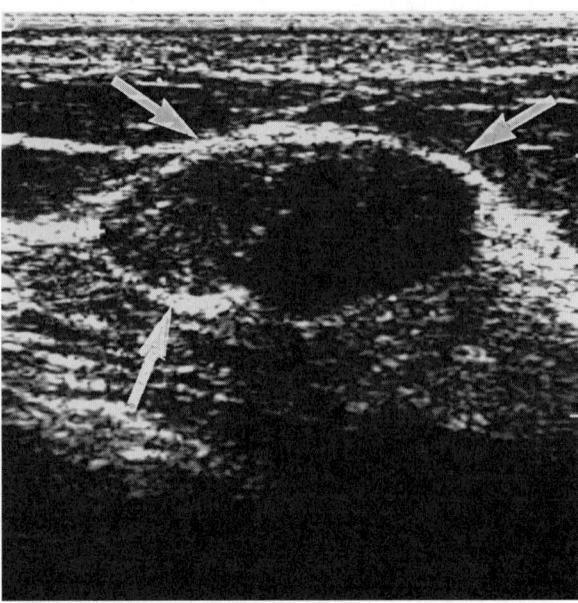

**Figure 35–13.** Fibroadenoma, example of ultrasonography of a benign mass. The mass is oval, with width greater than anterior-to-posterior diameter, circumscribed margins with a highly echogenic pseudocapsule *(arrows)*, and relatively homogeneous interior echoes.

nal echoes (Fig. 35–14). As with physical examination and mammography, however, carcinomas may have a wide range of shapes, margins, and tissue composition.

In the past, ultrasonography has not been successful as a method to *screen* for occult multicentric or bilateral disease in women with a mammographically or clinically evident breast carcinoma.[182] Improvements in ultrasonography, however, and some reports have renewed interest in the use of sonography for searching for multicentric disease or evaluating the whole breast.[183] These newer roles for ultrasonography have not yet been widely accepted.[184]

**Imaging-Guided Interventional Procedures.** A variety of interventional procedures are guided by imaging. These include needle aspiration of a mammographically detected cyst, fine-needle aspiration cytology, core needle biopsy, and prebiopsy needle localization of nonpalpable lesions before excision. Ductography can be employed to determine the

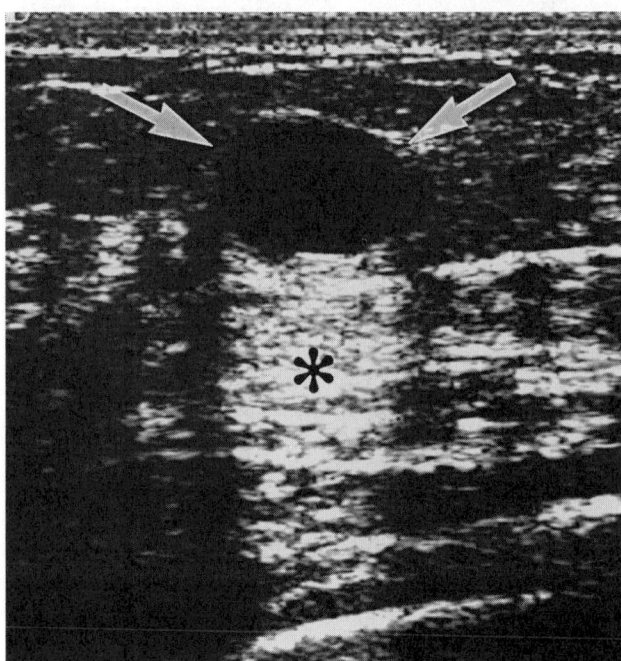

**Figure 35–12.** Ultrasonography of simple cyst. The cyst *(arrows)* shows an oval shape, absence of interior echoes, and increase in echoes posteriorly *(asterisk)*.

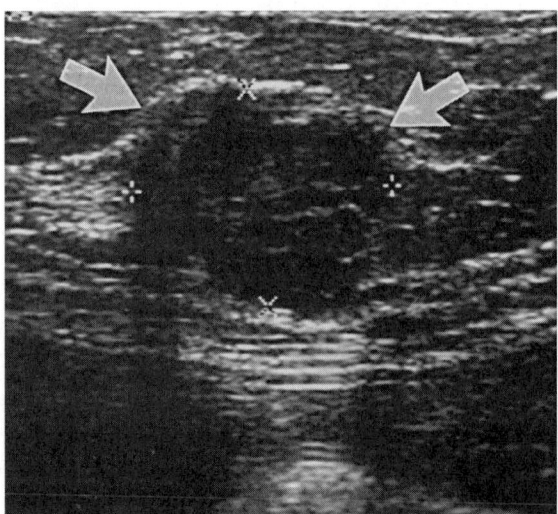

**Figure 35–14.** Invasive carcinoma, example of ultrasonographic features of a malignant mass. The shape is irregular, with numerous lobulations; the margins are ill-defined; and the internal echoes are heterogeneous.

cause of persistent unilateral bloody or serous nipple discharge.

***Imaging-Guided Needle Biopsy.*** It is estimated that 500,000 to 1 million breast biopsies are performed each year in the United States.[164] This translates to 400,000 to 700,000 benign breast biopsies. In addition to tremendous costs, biopsies with false-positive results lead to unnecessary morbidity and are a barrier to women participating in breast cancer screening projects.[163] Imaging-guided needle biopsy offers an attractive alternative to surgical biopsy for mammographically detected abnormalities. Needle biopsy is generally less expensive than surgery, results in less morbidity, and leaves no scar. Is it accurate enough to replace surgery? In Europe, fine-needle aspiration cytology has reduced the costs of screening programs by greatly reducing the number of excisional biopsies.[185] Although fine-needle aspiration cytology has not been as successful in the United States, core needle biopsy of the breast has gained wide acceptance.[186]

Needle biopsy of occult lesions can be guided by stereotactic mammography or ultrasonography. The modality chosen to guide the needle biopsy depends on the following: (1) which best depicts the abnormality, (2) the location of the lesion within the breast, and (3) the operator's preferences. Stereotaxis uses the principle of triangulation to ascertain the exact location of an abnormality based on the shift in its position observed on two images taken at different angles off of the midline.[187] Stereotactic equipment includes add-on devices that are mounted on mammography units and dedicated stereotactic biopsy tables. Ultrasonography is an excellent method for guiding needle biopsy procedures for breast masses that can be seen on ultrasonography.[188] An advantage of ultrasonography-guided intervention is that it allows for *real-time* imaging during the procedure.

***Ductography (Galactography).*** Ductography is the injection of contrast medium into the lactiferous ducts in an attempt to determine preoperatively the nature, location, and extent of lesions causing serous or bloody discharge. A bloody or serous discharge from the nipple may be caused by an intraductal papilloma (Fig. 35–15), fibrocystic changes, duct ectasia, or carcinoma. Although the discharge is usually associated with benign conditions, approximately 15% are secondary to carcinoma.[189] Ductography is not useful for cases with discharge from multiple orifices or with milky or greenish discharge. During the procedure, the duct that is discharging is cannulated, and a small volume of water-soluble contrast material is injected. Mammograms are then taken in two projections (see Fig. 35–15). When a filling defect is shown, the ductogram may be repeated shortly before surgery using a mixture of methylene blue dye and contrast material. The blue dye identifies the abnormal duct, and the contrast medium verifies that the duct contains the filling defect. Only half the carcinomas shown by filling defects on ductography are evident on conventional mammograms, and cytology is even more unreliable in identifying malignant cells in the fluid from these cancers.

### Other Breast Imaging Technologies

***Digital Mammography.*** This technology records the radiographic image electronically in a digital format rather than directly on film.[190] The image is kept in a digital format in a computer and can be displayed on a fluorescent monitor or transferred to a hard-copy film. It is hoped that digital mammography will eventually solve many of the problems

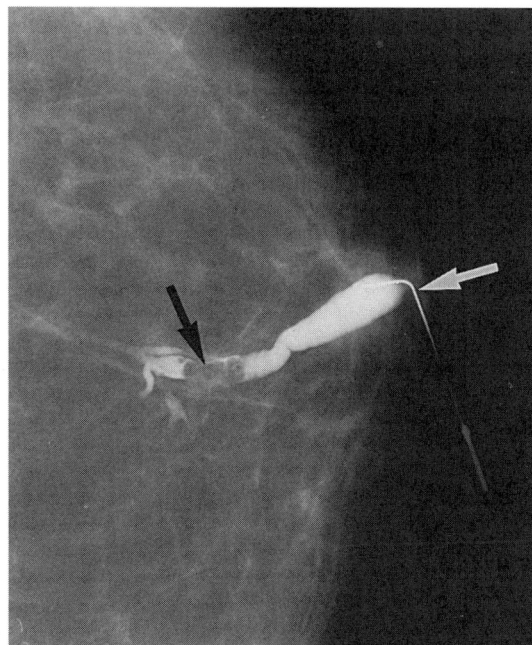

**Figure 35–15.** Ductogram of patient with unilateral, persistent, bloody discharge. The ductogram needle *(white arrow)* has been used to cannulate the orifice of the duct, and contrast material has been injected. The filling defect *(black arrow)* could represent a papilloma, epithelial proliferation (fibrocystic change), or carcinoma. Biopsy revealed benign papilloma.

inherent in film mammography, such as limited contrast, film storage, and lost films. Additional potential advantages of digital mammography involve the ability to adjust image quality on the display monitor, to facilitate computer-aided detection and diagnosis, and to transmit the images over long distances (teleradiography).[191] Currently, digital mammography is used for stereotactic biopsies, in which immediate access to images is desirable. Although digital mammography has many potential advantages, there are disadvantages, such as its anticipated high cost, inadequate resolution of current viewing monitors, and limited image storage capacity.

***Breast Magnetic Resonance Imaging.*** The first reports on magnetic resonance imaging (MRI) for the evaluation of breast cancer were published in the mid-1980s and were focused on breast tissue characterization using T1-weighted and T2-weighted images.[192] These early investigations were disappointing. In 1986, Heywang and colleagues[193] first applied the use of MRI contrast agents to improve differentiation of benign from malignant lesions. The results were encouraging, with most malignant tumors showing enhancement, whereas most benign breast lesions did not. Several other investigators have confirmed the value of MRI with contrast agents.[194] Clinical investigations show a range of sensitivities from 88 to 100%.[195] The specificity of MRI may be relatively low, however, because many benign lesions show contrast enhancement. The potential advantages of MRI of the breast include (1) no ionizing radiation; (2) no limitations from breast density; (3) ability to localize lesions seen on only one mammographic projection; (4) better characterization of lesions as benign or malignant; (5) improved evaluation of the extent of tumors, including multiple foci;

and (6) surveillance of the postlumpectomy breast, which can be difficult to evaluate mammographically.

*Radionuclide Imaging.* Another area of active investigation involves radionuclide scanning of the breast after the injection of radionuclide-labeled substances that concentrate in breast tumors. For example, tumor uptake has been identified on positron emission tomography after the injection of fluorine-18 2-deoxy-2-fluoro-D-glucose.[196] This agent also accumulates in axillary nodes, potentially indicating nodal status without surgery. Other investigators are scanning the breasts after the injection of technetium 99m sestamibi.[197] The high negative predictive value of this agent could make it an important adjunct to mammography by potentially reducing the number of biopsies performed for benign findings. Other studies have shown low sensitivity for breast scintigraphy in the detection of lesions found only on mammography and less than 1 cm in diameter[198] and a lower breast cancer detection sensitivity (83%) for detecting breast cancer when compared with MRI (96%).[199]

**Metastatic Disease.** The natural history of breast cancer may include metastasis to any organ, and 85% of fatal cases have involvement of bone, lung, or liver.[200] If any one of these three sites is involved, the likelihood of other organ involvement increases markedly. With the expanded use of chemotherapy, there has been a rising frequency of sites that were formerly less common, including the remaining breast, lymph nodes, retroperitoneum, pleura, endobronchial region, and central nervous system (especially the meninges). Among autopsied patients, 50% of patients die of the malignant process itself, about 25% of infection, 10% of hemorrhage, and 15% of other causes (especially cardiopulmonary disease). The reader interested in further details about the natural history of breast cancer may consult articles on breast cancer involving the brain,[201, 202] pituitary[203] (with diabetes insipidus), eye,[204] cranial nerves,[205] meninges,[206] pleura,[207] pericardium,[208] endobronchial component of lung,[209] bone marrow,[210, 211] and stomach[212] (linitis plastica).

The most common metabolic complication of breast cancer is hypercalcemia, which has been reported to occur in about 9% of patients.[213] This complication is usually ascribed to bone destruction by tumor, but it may also result from the elaboration of humoral factors by the tumor, as discussed in Chapter 18. In one series of 24 hypercalcemic patients with breast cancer, 92% had biochemical evidence of bone destruction, and histologic proof of tumor cell–mediated bone destruction was found in 54%. In addition, 42% of the overall group had increased blood levels of one or more humoral factors, including parathyroid hormone–related protein, prostaglandin $E_2$, or interleukin-1.[214]

Because of the importance of metastasis in this disease as well as the diversity of available systemic therapies, there has been interest in identifying biochemical markers of disease activity. Serial measurements of serum calcium and alkaline phosphatase[215] are of established value for patients with known metastatic disease. Several studies suggest that serial measurements of carcinoembryonic antigen (CEA) may be useful in assessing the response of some patients to chemotherapy.[216–219] Because CEA has no role in the diagnosis or staging of breast cancer, we do not recommend its routine measurement in newly diagnosed patients. It may, however, be useful in following patients with advanced disease who have markedly elevated blood levels, especially in patients with metastatic disease to bone.[220] The role of other potential tumor markers is less well established, although some data suggest that CA 549[221] or CA 27.29[222–224] may be useful replacements or adjuncts to CEA.

## Role of Imaging in the Follow-up and Staging of Women with Breast Cancer

*Follow-up of the Conservatively Treated Breast.* Follow-up evaluation after initial treatment with breast conservation surgery depends on the original mammographic findings. For women with DCIS manifested by extensive calcifications, mammography should be performed before radiotherapy to identify any residual calcifications (see Fig. 35–9). Otherwise, the traditional recommendation after lumpectomy and radiotherapy is for mammograms of the treated breast to be performed at 6-month intervals for 2 years and annually thereafter.[225] The importance of 6-month interval mammography is not universally accepted, and more clinical studies are needed to determine whether annual mammography would be just as effective.[226]

*Follow-up After Mastectomy.* For patients who are treated with mastectomy, imaging follow-up involves annual mammography of the contralateral breast. Mammography of the mastectomy site is not believed to have clinical utility because it does not increase the detection of locally recurrent disease.[227]

*Evaluation for Metastases from Breast Cancer.* The most common sites for distant metastases from breast carcinoma are the skeleton, lungs, liver, and brain.[228] Several imaging examinations are available that can potentially identify metastases to these organs. Surveys of patients with breast cancer indicate that most patients with breast cancer prefer an intensive follow-up to detect asymptomatic disease, including metastases.[229] Surveys indicate that the physicians that care for breast cancer patients also favor intensive surveillance programs of asymptomatic patients.[230] For purposes of cost-effectiveness, however, there should be a reasonable anticipated yield and an expected effect on patient management and outcome when imaging examinations are ordered on asymptomatic breast cancer patients.

Several large population-based studies have failed to show that metastatic work-ups for stage I or stage II breast cancer are cost-effective because of the low yield of the examination as well as a lack of a proven effect on management or survival.[231–233] Our current policy is to limit imaging work-ups for metastatic disease to women with stage III carcinoma (in which the tumor is >5 cm with movable ipsilateral positive axillary nodes, the invasive tumor is associated with positive ipsilateral axillary nodes fixed one to another or to other structures, or the tumor has direct extension to the chest wall or skin).[234] These women receive a bone scan, chest radiography, and imaging of the liver if liver function test results are abnormal.

- *Skeletal metastases.* Radionuclide scanning is more effective than conventional radiography for the detection of skeletal metastases because of its higher sensitivity and ability to survey the entire skeleton.[235] Despite a low yield in asymptomatic women with stage I or stage II breast carcinoma, many clinicians have recommended *baseline* bone scans for comparison with subsequent scans if patients develop symptoms.[236] Routine bone scans are unlikely to be useful in stage I or stage II disease because

(1) few patients convert to positive scans, and (2) clinical trials indicate that earlier detection of metastases does not reduce overall mortality.[237] In addition, many false-positive scans are encountered when screening for metastases in asymptomatic patients.[238] If radionuclide bone scans are not definitive for metastases, radiographs of areas of abnormal isotope accumulation should be obtained for correlation. If radionuclide and radiographic findings are indeterminate, MRI is usually definitive.[239]

- *Lung metastases.* Conventional chest radiography is the most reasonable approach for detection of unsuspected lung metastases, as a baseline for monitoring, and for routine follow-up.[240] Signs of metastatic breast carcinoma include pulmonary nodules, adenopathy, lymphangitic spread, and pleural masses or effusions. High-resolution computed tomography (CT) is the method of choice to evaluate equivocal findings on chest radiography and to identify additional nodules in positive cases.[241] Despite its relatively low cost, routine chest radiography has not been proved to be effective, largely because of the low yield in stage I disease. Another problem is that false-positive chest radiographs can lead to expensive diagnostic work-ups.[242]

- *Liver metastases.* Although liver metastases are not as common as lung or bone metastases, the appearance of liver metastases is associated with the worst prognosis. Both radionuclide scanning and ultrasonography have been employed to detect liver metastases. To be detected reliably by technetium 99m sulfur colloid liver scans, metastases generally must be greater than 2 cm in size.[243] Ultrasonography can also identify liver metastases 2 cm or larger and can be used to localize these lesions for biopsy or fine-needle aspiration cytology.[244] Large randomized controlled studies, however, have failed to show a benefit from screening for liver metastases with ultrasonography. CT and MRI are more sensitive in the detection of liver metastases than radionuclide imaging or ultrasonography.[245] CT scans of the liver should be obtained before and after intravenous contrast injection because some breast metastases may show up on one but not the other of these examinations. There is no evidence in the literature that routine imaging of the liver with either CT or MRI has clinical utility in asymptomatic patients with breast carcinoma.

- *Brain metastases.* Few patients have brain metastases at the time of breast cancer diagnosis, especially when the tumor is detected at stage I or II.[246] In CT examinations, brain metastases may be nodular or ring-shaped, single or multiple; are usually associated with extensive edema; and show varying amounts of enhancement with intravenous contrast agents.[247] A review of breast cancer patients at all stages who had radionuclide scanning and CT scanning failed to identify brain metastases in the absence of neurologic symptoms.[248] Because of its greater sensitivity, MRI has largely replaced CT for the detection and evaluation of brain lesions.[249] Contrast-enhanced MRI further increases the number of suspected cerebral metastases that can be detected.[246] Contrast-enhanced MRI also has been shown to be superior to double-dose delayed CT for detection of brain metastases.[250] Despite these improvements in the sensitivity of imaging modalities for the detection of cerebral metastases, there are no studies supporting the usefulness of routine imaging with any modality for the detection of cerebral metastases in asymptomatic women with breast carcinoma.

## STAGING

Once a histopathologic diagnosis of breast cancer has been made, it is critical to establish the clinical stage of the disease. The clinical staging system developed at Columbia University by Haagensen[155] was widely used for many years, but it has been supplanted by the TNM (tumor-node-metastasis) system of the American Joint Committee on Cancer (AJCC) and the International Union Against Cancer.[251] A major advantage of the TNM system is that it lends itself to clinical staging (cTNM) before definitive surgical or radiation therapy as well as pathologic staging (pTNM) using the results of the histologic examination of resected tissue. A major disadvantage of the current TNM system is that it uses T and N categories that are of questionable relevance. For example, the prognosis of node-negative patients with tumors of 2 to 3 cm is distinctly better than the prognosis of patients with 3- to 5-cm lesions, whereas both are technically T2 lesions by the TNM system.[146] Similarly, there is a continuous gradient of risk of recurrence with increasing numbers of axillary lymph nodes, from 0 to more than 13.

Table 35–7 presents the current TNM system and stage groupings. A variant of the TNM system that we use at times in this book is to give T and N values as absolute numbers. For example, a 3-cm lesion with five positive lymph nodes of 12 nodes sampled would be identified as a *T = 3 cm, N = 5/12 lesion*.

The extent of the preoperative or preradiation therapy evaluation depends on the initial clinical stage of the patient. In patients with clinical stage I or stage II disease and no symptoms of metastases, a chest radiograph, mammogram, complete blood count, and screening blood chemistry panel are sufficient. These patients do not routinely need a bone scan[252, 253] or liver scan.[254, 255] In patients with clinical stage III or stage IV disease or high-risk stage II (>10 involved lymph nodes), a bone scan and an abdominal CT scan are recommended as well as any other test that is required to define the meaning of symptoms. A bone marrow biopsy is generally unnecessary, unless the patient has unexplained bone marrow dysfunction.

## PROGNOSIS

The most important guide to prognosis for patients with invasive breast cancer is the pathologic TNM stage of the disease (see Table 35–7). Table 35–8 provides an approximate guide to prognosis for patients with infiltrating ductal and lobular carcinomas who have had sufficient surgery to determine their pathologic TNM stage.

The survival results in Table 35–7 are only approximate, in part because of dramatic changes in the patterns of practice, making predictions difficult. The AJCC staging system does not deal adequately with the important variable of the number of involved lymph nodes in the axilla. The importance of this variable is reflected in Table 35–8, which provides more detailed information on the relationship between recurrence rates at 10 years and the precise number

*Table 35–7.* **TNM System for Clinical or Pathologic Staging of Breast Cancer**

*Primary Tumor (T)\**

| | |
|---|---|
| TX | Primary tumor cannot be assessed |
| T0 | No evidence of primary tumor |
| Tis | Carcinoma in situ: intraductal carcinoma, lobular carcinoma in situ, or Paget's disease of the nipple with no tumor† |
| T1 | Tumor 2 cm or less in greatest dimension |

| | | |
|---|---|---|
| | T1mic | Microinvasion 0.1 cm or less in greatest dimension |
| | T1a | Tumor more than 0.1 but not more than 0.5 cm in greatest dimension |
| | T1b | Tumor more than 0.5 cm but not more than 1 cm in greatest dimension |
| | T1c | Tumor more than 1 cm but not more than 2 cm in greatest dimension |

| | |
|---|---|
| T2 | Tumor more than 2 cm but not more than 5 cm in greatest dimension |
| T3 | Tumor more than 5 cm in greatest dimension |
| T4 | Tumor of any size with direct extension to (a) chest wall or (b) skin, only as described below |

| | | |
|---|---|---|
| | T4a | Extension to chest wall |
| | T4b | Edema (including peau d'orange) or ulceration of the skin of the breast or satellite skin nodules confined to the same breast |
| | T4c | Both (T4a and T4b) |
| | T4d | Inflammatory carcinoma |

*Regional Lymph Nodes (N)*

| | |
|---|---|
| NX | Regional lymph nodes cannot be assessed (e.g., previously removed) |
| N0 | No regional lymph node metastasis |
| N1 | Metastasis to movable ipsilateral axillary lymph node(s) |
| N2 | Metastasis to ipsilateral axillary lymph node(s) fixed to one another or to other structures |
| N3 | Metastasis to ipsilateral internal mammary lymph node(s) |

*Pathologic Classification (pN)*

| | |
|---|---|
| pNX | Regional lymph nodes cannot be assessed (e.g., previously removed or not removed for pathologic study) |
| pN0 | No regional lymph node metastasis |
| pN1 | Metastasis to movable ipsilateral axillary lymph node(s) |

| | | |
|---|---|---|
| | pN1a | Only micrometastasis (none larger than 0.2 cm) |
| | pN1b | Metastasis to lymph node(s), any larger than 0.2 cm |

| | | |
|---|---|---|
| | pN1bi | Metastasis in 1 to 3 lymph nodes, any more than 0.2 cm and all less than 2 cm in greatest dimension |
| | pN1bii | Metastasis to 4 or more lymph nodes, any more than 0.2 cm and all less than 2 cm in greatest dimension |
| | pN1biii | Extension of tumor beyond the capsule of a lymph node metastasis less than 2 cm in greatest dimension |
| | pN1biv | Metastasis to a lymph node 2 cm or more in greatest dimension |

| | |
|---|---|
| pN2 | Metastasis to ipsilateral axillary lymph nodes that are fixed to one another or to other structures |
| pN3 | Metastasis to ipsilateral internal mammary lymph node(s) |

*Distant Metastasis (M)*

| | |
|---|---|
| MX | Distant metastasis cannot be assessed |
| M0 | No distant metastasis |
| M1 | Distant metastasis (includes metastasis to ipsilateral supraclavicular lymph node[s]) |

*Stage Grouping*

| | | | |
|---|---|---|---|
| Stage 0 | Tis | N0 | M0 |
| Stage I | T1‡ | N0 | M0 |
| Stage IIA | T0 | N1 | M0 |
| | T1‡ | N1§ | M0 |
| | T2 | N0 | M0 |
| Stage IIB | T2 | N1 | M0 |
| | T3 | N0 | M0 |
| Stage IIIA | T0 | N2 | M0 |
| | T1‡ | N2 | M0 |
| | T2 | N2 | M0 |
| | T3 | N1 | M0 |
| | T3 | N2 | M0 |
| Stage IIIB | T4 | Any N | M0 |
| | Any T | N3 | M0 |
| Stage IV | Any T | Any N | M1 |

\*Definitions for classifying the primary tumor (T) are the same for clinical and for pathologic classification. If measurements are made by physical examination, use only the major headings for T1, T2, and T3 lesions. If other measurements are used, such as mammographic or pathologic measurements, the subsets of T1 can be used.

†Paget's disease associated with a tumor is classified according to the size of the tumor.

‡T1 includes T1mic.

§The prognosis of patients with N1a is similar to that of patients with pN0.

*Table 35–8.* **Prognosis of Patients with Breast Cancer by pTNM Stage**

| | Approximate Survival* (%) | | Approximate Cure Rate§ |
|---|---|---|---|
| | 5 yr† | 10 yr‡ | (%) |
| 0 | >98 | ~90 | — |
| I | 95 | 65 | 54 ± 3 |
| IIA | 85 | 55 | 27 ± 1 |
| IIB | 70 | 45 | |
| IIIA | 52 | 40 | 19 ± 2 |
| IIIB | 50 | 20 | |
| IV | 17 | 5 | 2 ± 1 |
| Overall | | | 35 ± 1 |

*Estimates of survival are based on our assessment of the literature, with particular emphasis on data identified for each column of the table.

†Based on data from Beahrs OH, et al, eds. American Joint Committee on Cancer: Manual for Staging of Cancer. 4th ed. Philadelphia: JB Lippincott, 1992:151.

‡Based on data from Harris JR, Henderson IC. In: Harris JR, et al, eds. Breast diseases. Philadelphia: JB Lippincott, 1987:233.

§Based on an analysis of 14,731 women with breast cancer from Norway (Rutqvist LE, et al. Cancer 1984;53:1793).

of involved axillary lymph nodes. The number of nodes involved is increasingly used to define groups of patients with high-risk disease and a need for especially aggressive adjuvant therapy. A commonly employed cutoff is 10 positive nodes[256]; patients with numbers in excess of this are widely considered to be candidates for clinical trials of high-dose chemotherapy followed by stem cell support or autologous bone marrow transplantation, or both.

A critical factor in estimating prognosis and establishing a treatment plan is the presence or absence of comorbid diseases. In one study, patients with three or more of seven selected comorbid conditions had a 20-fold higher rate of mortality from causes other than breast cancer.[257]

**Prognostic Factors Related to Local Control.** The most important prognostic factor is tumor stage by the TNM system. In addition to the stage of disease, several other factors should be considered in assessing prognosis and choosing local therapy. Tumor characteristics that seem to predict for a higher probability of local recurrence include multicentric involvement of the breast,[258, 259] the presence of an extensive intraductal component in the breast tumor (as a risk factor for recurrence after segmental mastectomy and radiation therapy),[260] and vascular or lymphatic invasion (as a risk factor for total mastectomy).[262] The number of positive nodes is also critical, as illustrated in Table 35–9.

*Table 35–9.* **Ten-Year Treatment Failure Rates as a Function of the Number of Axillary Lymph Nodes Involved at the Time of Initial Treatment**

| Positive Nodes (No.) | Treatment Failure (%) |
|---|---|
| 0 | 20 |
| 1–3 | 47 |
| 4–6 | 59 |
| 7–12 | 69 |
| ≥13 | 87 |

From Fisher ER, et al. Pathologic findings from the National Surgical Adjuvant Project for Breast Cancer. Cancer 1984;53:712.

**Prognostic Factors for the Development of Systemic Disease.** Tumor factors that seem especially important in predicting a poor prognosis from subsequent metastatic disease include the absence of hormone receptors,[261–263] poorly differentiated histology (especially a high nuclear grade),[264] and tumor invasion of lymphatics, nerves, or venous vascular channels.[265, 266] Retrospective studies of the prognostic importance of a high tumor labeling index or high percentage of cells in S phase determined by flow cytometry[267] and aneuploidy (as opposed to diploidy) as found by flow cytometry[115, 268–270] have suggested that these are useful as well. Prospective studies have been less convincing, however. In one large study involving two prospective randomized clinical trials of adjuvant therapy, DNA ploidy and percent S phase determinations in node-positive patients were not useful.[271] Similar negative or equivocal results have been reported in a large retrospective study by the National Surgical Adjuvant Breast Project (NSABP).[272] Overexpression of the HER-2/*neu* oncogene has been found to correlate with a worse prognosis, particularly in patients with lymph node involvement.[273, 274] The search for new and more useful prognostic factors continues.

An enormous number of other prognostic factors have been identified, many of which are the subject of ongoing trials. Examples include tumor angiogenesis,[275, 276] tumor microvessel density,[277] immunolabeling of proliferating cell nuclear antigen,[278] measuring the level of p53,[279, 280] cathepsin D and pro-cathepsin D levels (with some studies positive[281] and others negative[282]), high expression of the gene for heat-shock protein,[283] tissue levels of urokinase and its inhibitor plasminogen activator inhibitor-1,[284] the expression of transforming growth factors in tumor tissue,[285] nm23 (a potential marker of metastatic potential),[286, 287] the levels of cyclic adenosine monophosphate–binding proteins,[288] the presence of cyclin E,[289] the timing of mastectomy in regard to the menstrual cycle,[290–292] the presence of obesity as a poor prognostic factor,[293] and tumor necrosis in the primary tumor (defined as confluent cell death in areas of invasive cancer).[294] Several groups have attempted to use the available prognostic variables to develop a prognostic index,[295–297] but these indices are rarely used.

Some of these prognostic factors have been used in identifying patients with node-negative disease who are at sufficiently high risk of recurrent disease to justify the use of adjuvant chemotherapy (see sections Adjuvant Treatment and Treatment by Stage of Disease and Special Problems). The wisdom of such aggressive therapy is contingent on many factors, including the patient's age and general physiologic condition. The patient's menopausal status is also important in assessing the role of the available forms of systemic therapy, especially in patients with advanced or recurrent disease.

**Prognostic Factors and the Choice of Systemic Therapy.** In addition to predicting the risk of recurrence, prognostic factors may be useful in selecting specific forms of systemic therapy. The best example of this is the use of hormone receptors to predict the potential value of endocrine manipulation. A newer example of this concept involves the HER-2/*neu* oncogene. In a study of adjuvant chemotherapy with doxorubicin, amplification of the HER-2/*neu* oncogene was associated with markedly improved survival.[298] More study of this observation is needed. Further discussion of this topic appears in the section Adjuvant Treatment.

**Prognosis After Local Recurrence.** The goal of treatment for patients in whom disease recurs locally without evidence of systemic disease remains cure by local-regional means. Patients with noninvasive or only focally invasive recurrent disease after conservation therapy have an excellent prognosis, whereas patients with invasive disease do more poorly. In one series, none of 24 patients with noninvasive disease had subsequent recurrence, whereas the relapse rate was 52% in patients with invasive recurrent disease.[299]

**Prognosis After Systemic Recurrence.** The goal of treatment for patients who have recurrence of systemic disease is palliation. The overall median survival of such patients is short; for example, it was 26 months in a series from Miami[300] and 28 months at a major center in the Netherlands.[301] Patients with visceral metastases died much sooner than did those with bone or soft tissue involvement (median survivals, 16 vs. 34 vs. 41 months).

## RISK REDUCTION AND PREVENTION

**Chemoprevention.** Chemoprevention is an area of intense research in women at high risk for developing breast cancer. Most notable has been the study of tamoxifen. Based on earlier studies[302, 303] that demonstrated a statistically lower risk of contralateral breast cancer in women treated with tamoxifen, the NSABP initiated a trial in 1992 with tamoxifen in high-risk women.[304] Eligible women were those older than age 60 and patients 35 to 59 with a 5-year predicted risk of breast cancer greater than 1.66% or a history of LCIS. Women (n = 13,388) were randomized to tamoxifen 20 mg/day or placebo. At a median follow-up of 54.6 months, tamoxifen was found to lower the risk of breast cancer by 49% and noninvasive disease by 50%, across all age groups. Two European studies[305, 306] have been published that do not support the NSABP findings. Both of these studies, however, were much smaller; the studies had fewer breast cancer events; and, among other differences, the women had different risks.

Raloxifene is a selective estrogen receptor modulator (SERM) that has been associated with a reduced incidence of breast cancer in postmenopausal women treated for osteoporosis.[307] The next NSABP prevention trial, P-2, will compare the toxicities and benefits of tamoxifen with raloxifene.

In 1987, a study was initiated with a retinoid, fenretinide, to evaluate efficacy in terms of breast cancer reduction.[308]

**Prophylactic Mastectomy.** Prophylactic mastectomy has been an option for women at high risk of developing breast cancer, but relatively minimal data have been available regarding its long-term efficacy. Concern has focused on the inability to remove completely all of the breast tissue[309] and cases of local recurrence after prophylactic mastectomies.[310–312] A retrospective analysis was published[313] examining women with a family history of breast cancer who underwent prophylactic surgery at the Mayo Clinic between 1960 and 1993. Risk assessment for these women was based on the Gail model,[20] and the control group was the patients' sisters. Overall, with a median follow-up of 14 years, prophylactic mastectomy was associated with approximately a 90% reduction in the incidence of breast cancer. The authors

appropriately point out, however, the importance of individual counseling and risk assessment with patients who are considering this surgery.

## SUGGESTIONS FOR ADDITIONAL READING

Eeles RA. Screening for hereditary cancer and genetic testing, epitomized by breast cancer. Eur J Cancer 1999;35:1954–62.
Gail MH, Costantino JP, Bryant J, et al. Weighing the risks and benefits of tamoxifen treatment for preventing breast cancer. J Natl Cancer Inst 1999;91:1829–46.
Glass EC, Essner R, Giuliano AE. Sentinel node localization in breast cancer. Semin Nucl Med 1999;29:57–68.
Hughes KS, Papa MZ, Whitney T, McLellan R. Prophylactic mastectomy and inherited predisposition to breast carcinoma. Cancer 1999;86:11:Suppl:2502–16.
Lakhani SR. The transition from hyperplasia to invasive carcinoma of the breast. J Pathol 1999;187:272–8.
Richards MA, Westcombe AM, Love SB, et al. Influence of delay on survival in patients with breast cancer: a systematic review. Lancet 1999;86:11:Suppl:2502–16.
Yarbro JW, Page DL, Fielding LP, et al. American Joint Committee on Cancer prognostic factors consensus conference. Cancer 1999;86:2436–46.

## REFERENCES

1. Wazer DE, Band V. Molecular and anatomic considerations in the pathogenesis of breast cancer. Radiat Oncol Invest 1999;7:1–12.
2. Porter DE, Steel CM. Recent advances in the genetics of heritable breast cancer. Dis Markers 1993;11:11-21.
3. Russo J, Calaf G, Russo IH. A critical approach to the malignant transformation of human breast epithelial cells with chemical carcinogens. Crit Rev Oncog 1993;4:403–17.
4. Mattsson A, Rudén BI, Hall P, et al. Radiation-induced breast cancer: long-term follow-up of radiation therapy for benign breast disease. J Natl Cancer Inst 1993;85:1679–85.
5. Al-Sumidaie AM, Leinster SJ, Hart CA, et al. Particles with properties of retroviruses in monocytes from patients with breast cancer. Lancet 1988;1:5–9.
6. Faff O, Murray AB, Schmidt J, et al. Retrovirus-like particles from the human T47D cell line are related to mouse mammary tumour virus and are of human endogenous origin. J Gen Virol 1992;73:1087–97.
7. Miller FR, Soule HD, Tait L, et al. Xenograft model of progressive human proliferative breast disease. J Natl Cancer Inst 1993;85:1725–32.
8. Miki Y, Swensen J, Shattuck-Eidens D, et al. Isolation of BRCA1, the 17q-linked breast and ovarian cancer susceptibility gene. Science 1994;266:66–71.
9. Futreal PA, Liu Q, Shattuck-Eidens D, et al. BRCA1 mutations in primary breast and ovarian carcinomas. Science 1994;266:120–2.
10. Easton DF, Bishop DT, Ford D, Crockford GP. Genetic linkage analysis in familial breast and ovarian cancer: results from 214 families. The Breast Cancer Linkage Consortium. Am J Hum Genet 1993;52:678–701.
11. Wooster R, Bignell G, Lancaster J, et al. Identification of the breast cancer susceptibility gene BRCA2. Nature 1995;378:789–92.
12. Wooster R, Neuhausen SL, Mangion J, et al. Localization of a breast cancer susceptibility gene, BRCA2, to chromosome 13q12–13. Science 1994;265:2088–90.
13. Hollstein M, Sidransky D, Vogelstein B, Harris CC. p53 mutations in human cancers. Science 1991;253:49–53.
14. Coles C, Condie A, Chetty U, et al. p53 mutations in breast cancer. Cancer Res 1992;52:5291–8.
15. Wooster R, Mangion J, Eeles R, et al. A germline mutation in the androgen receptor gene in two brothers with breast cancer and Reifenstein syndrome. Nat Genet 1992;2:132–4.
16. Poujol N, Lobaccaro JM, Chiche L, et al. Functional and structural analysis of R607Q and R608K androgen receptor substitutions associated with male breast cancer. Mol Cell Endocrinol 1997;130:43–51.
17. Pauletti G, Godolphin W, Press MF, Slamon DJ. Detection and quanti-

tation of HER-2/*neu* gene amplification in human breast cancer archival material using fluorescence in situ hybridization. Oncogene 1996;13:63–72.

18. Sellers TA, Kushi LH, Potter JD, et al. Effect of family history, body-fat distribution, and reproductive factors on the risk of postmenopausal breast cancer [erratum 1992;327:1612]. N Engl J Med 1992;326:1323–9.

19. Williams WR. In: Harris JR, ed. Breast diseases. Philadelphia: JB Lippincott, 1987:109.

20. Gail MH, Brinton DP, Corle DK, et al. Projecting individualized probabilities of developing breast cancer for white females who are being examined annually. J Natl Cancer Inst 1989;81:1879–86.

21. Spiegelman D, Colditz GA, Hunter D, Hertzmark E. Validation of the Gail et al. model for predicting individual breast cancer risk. J Natl Cancer Inst 1994;86:600–7.

22. Narod SA, Ford D, Devilee P, et al. An evaluation of genetic heterogeneity in 145 breast-ovarian cancer families. Breast Cancer Linkage Consortium. Am J Hum Genet 1995;56:254–64.

23. Ford D, Easton DF, Bishop DT, et al. Risks of cancer in *BRCA1*-mutation carriers. Breast Cancer Linkage Consortium. Lancet 1994;343:692–5.

24. Lynch HT, Marcus J, Watson P, Page D. Distinctive clinicopathologic features of *BRCA1*-linked hereditary breast cancer. Proc ASCO 1994;13:56. abstract 27.

25. Ottman R, Pike MC, King MC, Henderson BE. Practical guide for estimating risk for familial breast cancer. Lancet 1983;2:556–8.

26. Schwartz AG, King MC, Belle SH, et al. Risk of breast cancer to relatives of young breast cancer patients. J Natl Cancer Inst 1985;75:665–8.

27. Akashi-Tanaka S, Fukutomi T, Fukami A, Fujiki T. Male breast cancer in patients with a family history of breast cancer. Surg Today 1996;26:975–9.

28. Oddoux C, Struewing JP, Clayton CM, et al. The carrier frequency of the *BRCA2* 6174delT mutation among Ashkenazi Jewish individuals is approximately 1%. Nat Genet 1996;14:188–90.

29. Roa BB, Boyd AA, Volcik K, Richards CS. Ashkenazi Jewish population frequencies for common mutations in *BRCA1* and *BRCA2*. Nat Genet 1996;14:185–7.

30. Struewing JP, Abeliovich D, Peretz T, et al. The carrier frequency of the *BRCA1* 185delAG mutation is approximately 1% in Ashkenazi Jewish individuals. Nat Genet 1995;11:198–200.

31. Struewing JP, Hartge P, Wacholder S, et al. The risk of cancer associated with specific mutations of *BRCA1* and *BRCA2* among Ashkenazi Jews. N Engl J Med 1997;336:1401–8.

32. Thorlacius S, Struewing JP, Hartge P, et al. Population-based study of risk of breast cancer in carriers of *BRCA2* mutation. Lancet 1998;352:1337–9.

33. Li FP, Fraumeni JF Jr. Rhabdomyosarcoma in children: epidemiologic study and identification of a familial cancer syndrome. J Natl Cancer Inst 1969;43:1365–73.

34. Li FP, Fraumeni JF Jr, Mulvihill JJ, et al. A cancer family syndrome in twenty-four kindreds. Cancer Res 1988;48:5358–62.

35. Hartley AL, Birch JM, Marsden HB, Harris M. Breast cancer risk in mothers of children with osteosarcoma and chondrosarcoma. Br J Cancer 1986;54:819–23.

36. Schrager CA, Schneider D, Gruener AC, et al. Clinical and pathological features of breast disease in Cowden's syndrome: an underrecognized syndrome with an increased risk of breast cancer. Hum Pathol 1998;29:47–53.

37. Schwartz RA, Torre DP. The Muir-Torre syndrome: a 25-year retrospect. J Am Acad Dermatol 1995;33:90–104.

38. Barnes N, Young C. The expression of p53 in patients with coexistent breast carcinoma and malignant melanoma. Clin Oncol (R Coll Radiol) 1996;8:185–6.

39. Padmore RF, Lara JF, Ackerman DJ, et al. Primary combined malignant melanoma and ductal carcinoma of the breast: a report of two cases. Cancer 1996;78:2515–25.

40. Mehta D, Khatib R, Patel S. Carcinoma of the breast and meningioma: association and management. Cancer 1983;51:1937–40.

41. Jacobs DH, McFarlane MJ, Holmes FF. Female patients with meningioma of the sphenoid ridge and additional primary neoplasms of the breast and genital tract. Cancer 1987;60:3080–2.

42. Russo CL, McIntyre J, Goorin AM, et al. Secondary breast cancer in patients presenting with osteosarcoma: possible involvement of germline p53 mutations. Med Pediatr Oncol 1994;23:354–8.

43. Nielsen NH, Emdin SO, Cajander J, Landberg G. Deregulation of cyclin E and D1 in breast cancer is associated with inactivation of the retinoblastoma protein. Oncogene 1997;14:295–304.

44. Lee EY, Bookstein R, Lee WH. Role of the retinoblastoma gene in the oncogenesis of human breast carcinoma. Cancer Treat Res 1991;53:23–44.

45. Gatti RA, Berkel I, Boder E, et al. Localization of an ataxia-telangiectasia gene to chromosome 11q22–23. Nature 1988;336:577–80.

46. Armstrong B, Doll R. Environmental factors and cancer incidence and mortality in different countries, with special reference to dietary practices. Int J Cancer 1975;15:617–31.

47. Rohan TE, Bain CJ. Diet in the etiology of breast cancer. Epidemiol Rev 1987;9:120–45.

48. Ziegler RG, Hoover RN, Pike MC, et al. Migration patterns and breast cancer risk in Asian-American women. J Natl Cancer Inst 1993;85:1819–27.

49. Wu AH, Ziegler RG, Nomura AM, et al. Soy intake and risk of breast cancer in Asians and Asian Americans. Am J Clin Nutr 1998;68:6 Suppl:1437S–43S.

50. Messina MJ, Persky V, Setchell KD, Barnes S. Soy intake and cancer risk: a review of the in vitro and in vivo data. Nutr Cancer 1994;21:113–31.

51. Barnes S. The chemopreventive properties of soy isoflavonoids in animal models of breast cancer. Breast Cancer Res Treat 1997;46:169–79.

52. Bunk B, Zhu P, Klinga K, et al. Influence of reducing luxury calories in the treatment of experimental mammary carcinoma. Br J Cancer 1992;65:845–51.

53. Jones DY, Schatzkin A, Green SB, et al. Dietary fat and breast cancer in the National Health and Nutrition Examination Survey I Epidemiologic Follow-up Study. J Natl Cancer Inst 1987;79:465-71.

54. Mezzetti M, La Vecchia C, Decarli A, et al. Population attributable risk for breast cancer: diet, nutrition, and physical exercise. J Natl Cancer Inst 1998;90:389–94.

55. Goodwin PJ, Boyd NF. Critical appraisal of the evidence that dietary fat intake is related to breast cancer risk in humans. J Natl Cancer Inst 1987;79:473–85.

56. Mills PK, Annegers JF, Phillips RL. Animal product consumption and subsequent fatal breast cancer risk among Seventh-day Adventists. Am J Epidemiol 1988;127:440–53.

57. van den Brandt PA, van't Veer P, Goldbohm RA, et al. A prospective cohort study on dietary fat and the risk of postmenopausal breast cancer. Cancer Res 1993;53:75–82.

58. Colditz GA. Epidemiology of breast cancer: findings from the Nurses' Health Study. Cancer 1993;71:4 Suppl:1480–9.

59. Boyd NF, Cousins M, Beaton M, et al. Clinical trial of low-fat, high-carbohydrate diet in subjects with mammographic dysplasia: report of early outcomes. J Natl Cancer Inst 1988;80:1244–8.

60. Prentice RL, Kakar F, Hursting S, et al. Aspects of the rationale for the Women's Health Trial. J Natl Cancer Inst 1988;80:802–14.

61. Hunter DJ, Manson JE, Colditz GA, et al. A prospective study of the intake of vitamins C, E, and A and the risk of breast cancer. N Engl J Med 1993;329:234–40.

62. Baghurst PA, Rohan TE. High-fiber diets and reduced risk of breast cancer. Int J Cancer 1994;56:173–6.

63. Longnecker MP, Berlin JA, Orza MJ, Chalmers TC. A meta-analysis of alcohol consumption in relation to risk of breast cancer. JAMA 1988;260:652–6.

64. Tseng M, Weinberg CR, Umbach DM, Longnecker MP. Calculation of population attributable risk for alcohol and breast cancer (United States). Cancer Causes Control 1999;10:119–23.

65. Horton AW. Indoor tobacco smoke pollution: a major risk factor for both breast and lung cancer. Cancer 1988;62:6–14.

66. Djordjevic MV, Hoffmann D, Fan J, et al. Assessment of chlorinated pesticides and polychlorinated biphenyls in adipose breast tissue using a supercritical fluid extraction method. Carcinogenesis 1994;15:2581–5.

67. Wolff MS, Toniolo PG, Lee EW, et al. Blood levels of organochlorine residues and risk of breast cancer. J Natl Cancer Inst 1993;85:648–52.

68. Krieger N, Wolff MS, Hiatt RA, et al. Breast cancer and serum organochlorines: a prospective study among white, black, and Asian women. J Natl Cancer Inst 1994;86:589–99.

69. Biggs PJ, Warren W, Venitt S, Stratton MR. Does a genotoxic carcinogen contribute to human breast cancer? The value of mutational spectra in unravelling the aetiology of cancer. Mutagenesis 1993;8:275–83.

70. Cole P, Cramer D, Yen S, et al. Estrogen profiles of premenopausal women with breast cancer. Cancer Res 1978;38:745–8.

71. Musey VC, Collins DC, Musey PI, et al. Long-term effect of a first pregnancy on the secretion of prolactin. N Engl J Med 1987;316:229–34.

72. Colton T, Greenberg ER, Noller K, et al. Breast cancer in mothers prescribed diethylstilbestrol in pregnancy: further follow-up. JAMA 1993;269:2096–100.

73. Rushton L, Jones DR. Oral contraceptive use and breast cancer risk: a meta-analysis of variations with age at diagnosis, parity and total duration of oral contraceptive use. Br J Obstet Gynaecol 1992;99:239–46.

74. Pike MC, Henderson BE, Krailo MD, et al. Breast cancer in young women and use of oral contraceptives: possible modifying effect of formulation and age at use. Lancet 1983;2:926–30.

75. Oral-contraceptive use and the risk of breast cancer. N Engl J Med 1987;316:162–4.letter.

76. McPherson K, Vessey MP, Neil A, et al. Early oral contraceptive use and breast cancer: results of another case-control study. Br J Cancer 1987;56:653–60.

77. Ursin G, Ross RK, Sullivan-Halley J, et al. Use of oral contraceptives and risk of breast cancer in young women. Breast Cancer Res Treat 1998;50:175–84.

78. Hoover R, Gray LA Sr, Cole P, MacMahon B. Menopausal estrogens and breast cancer. N Engl J Med 1976;295:401–5.

79. Greenberg ER, Barnes AB, Resseguie L, et al. Breast cancer in mothers given diethylstilbestrol in pregnancy. N Engl J Med 1984;311:1393–8.

80. Brinton LA, Hoover R, Fraumeni JF Jr. Menopausal oestrogens and breast cancer risk: an expanded case-control study. Br J Cancer 1986;54:825–32.

81. Rohan TE, McMichael AJ. Non-contraceptive exogenous oestrogen therapy and breast cancer. Med J Aust 1988;148:217–21.

82. Horwitz RI, Stewart KR. Effect of clinical features on the association of estrogens and breast cancer. Am J Med 1984;76:192–8.

83. Kaufman DW, Miller DR, Rosenberg L, et al. Noncontraceptive estrogen use and the risk of breast cancer. JAMA 1984;252:63–7.

84. Hulka BS. Replacement estrogens and risk of gynecologic cancers and breast cancer. Cancer 1987;60:Suppl:1960–4.

85. Kaufman DW, Palmer JR, de Mouzon J, et al. Estrogen replacement therapy and the risk of breast cancer: results from the case-control surveillance study. Am J Epidemiol 1991;134:1375–85; discussion 1396–401.

86. Collaborative Group on Hormone Factors in Breast Cancer. Breast cancer and hormone replacement therapy: collaborative reanalysis of data from 51 epidemiological studies of 52,705 women with breast cancer and 108,411 women without breast cancer. Lancet 1997;350:1047–59.

87. Persson I, Yuen H, Bergkvist L, et al. Cancer incidence and mortality in women receiving estrogen and estrogen-progestin replacement therapy: long term follow-up of a Swedish cohort. Int J Cancer 1996;67:327–32.

88. Grodstein F, Stamfer MJ, Colditz GA, et al. The use of estrogens and progestins and the risk of breast cancer in postmenopausal women. N Engl J Med 1997;336:1769–75.

89. The Women's Health Initiative Study Group. Design of the Women's Health Initiative clinical trial and observational study. Control Clin Trials 1998;19:61–109.

90. Newcomb PA, Storer BE, Longnecker MP, et al. Lactation and a reduced risk of premenopausal breast cancer. N Engl J Med 1994;330:81–7.

91. Stuver SO, Hsieh CC, Betone E, Trichopoulos D. The association between lactation and breast cancer in an international case-control study: a re-analysis by menopausal status. Int J Cancer 1997;71:166–9.

92. Yahalom J, Petrek JA, Biddinger PW, et al. Breast cancer in patients irradiated for Hodgkin's disease: a clinical and pathologic analysis of 45 events in 37 patients. J Clin Oncol 1992;10:1674–81.

93. Hancock SL, Tucker MA, Hoppe RT. Breast cancer after treatment of Hodgkin's disease. J Natl Cancer Inst 1993;85:25–31.

94. Barraclough J, Pinder P, Cruddas M, et al. Life events and breast cancer prognosis. Br Med J 1992;304:1078–81.

95. Priestman TJ, Priestman SG, Bradshaw C. Stress and breast cancer. Br J Cancer 1985;51:493–8.

96. Hahn RC, Petitti DB. Minnesota Multiphasic Personality Inventory–rated depression and the incidence of breast cancer. Cancer 1988;61:845–8.

97. Slamon DJ, Clark GM, Wong SG, et al. Human breast cancer: correlation of relapse and survival with amplification of the HER-2/neu oncogene. Science 1987;235:177–82.

98. Tandon A, Clark G, Ullrich A, et al. Overexpression of the HER-2/neu oncogene predicts relapse and survival in stage II human breast cancer. Proc ASCO 1988;7:14.

99. Krontiris TG, Devlin B, Karp DD, et al. An association between the risk of cancer and mutations in the HRAS1 minisatellite locus. N Engl J Med 1993;329:517–23.

100. Osborne CK. Receptors. In: Harris JR, ed. Breast diseases. Philadelphia: JB Lippincott, 1987:210–32.

101. Lippman ME. Hormones and cancer 3. Prog Cancer Res Ther 1988;35:203.

102. Reubi JC, Laissue J, Krenning E, Lamberts SW. Somatostatin receptors in human cancer: incidence, characteristics, functional correlates and clinical implications. J Steroid Biochem Mol Biol 1992;43:27–35.

103. Roman SD, Clarke CL, Hall RE, et al. Expression and regulation of retinoic acid receptors in human breast cancer cells. Cancer Res 1992;52:2236–42.

104. Jensen EV. Hormone dependency of breast cancer. Cancer 1981;47:2319–26.

105. Raam S, Robert N, Pappas CA, Tamura H. Defective estrogen receptors in human mammary cancers: their significance in defining hormone dependence. J Natl Cancer Inst 1988;80:756–61.

106. Thorpe SM. Estrogen and progesterone receptor determinations in breast cancer: technology, biology and clinical significance. Acta Oncol 1988;27:1–19.

107. Aziz DC. Quantitation of estrogen and progesterone receptors by immunocytochemical and image analyses. Am J Clin Pathol 1992;98:105–11.

108. Shackney SE, McCormack GW, Cuchural GJ Jr. Growth rate patterns of solid tumors and their relation to responsiveness to therapy: an analytical review. Ann Intern Med 1978;89:107–21.

109. Norton L. A Gompertzian model of human breast cancer growth. Cancer Res 1988;48:Pt 1:7067–71.

110. Speer JF, Petrosky VE, Retsky MW, Wardwell RH. A stochastic numerical model of breast cancer growth that simulates clinical data. Cancer Res 1984;44:4124–30.

111. Spratt JS Jr, Kaltenbach ML, Spratt JA. Cytokinetic definition of acute and chronic breast cancer. Cancer Res 1977;37:226–30.

112. Kusama S, Spratt JS Jr, Donegan WL, et al. The cross rates of growth of human mammary carcinoma. Cancer 1972;30:594–9.

113. Galante E, Gallus G, Guzzon A, et al. Growth rate of primary breast cancer and prognosis: observations on a 3- to 7-year follow-up in 180 breast cancers. Br J Cancer 1986;54:833–6.

114. Deland EM. Surg Gynecol Obstet 1927;44:264.

115. Merkel DE, Dressler LG, McGuire WL. Flow cytometry, cellular DNA content, and prognosis in human malignancy. J Clin Oncol 1987;5:690–703.

116. Dressler LG, Seamer L, Owens MA, et al. Evaluation of a modeling system for S-phase estimation in breast cancer by flow cytometry. Cancer Res 1987;47:5294–302.

117. Dressler LG, Seamer LC, Owens MA, et al. DNA flow cytometry and prognostic factors in 1331 frozen breast cancer specimens. Cancer 1988;61:420–7.

118. Meyer JS, Coplin MD. Thymidine labeling index, flow cytometric S-phase measurement, and DNA index in human tumors: comparisons and correlations. Am J Clin Pathol 1988;89:586–95.

119. Hedley DW, Clark GM, Cornelisse CJ, et al. Consensus review of the clinical utility of DNA cytometry in carcinoma of the breast: report of the DNA Cytometry Consensus Conference. Cytometry 1993;14:482–5.

120. Fisher B. Laboratory and clinical research in breast cancer—a personal adventure. The David A. Karnofsky memorial lecture. Cancer Res 1980;40:3863–74.

121. Beatson GT. Lancet 1896;2:104.

122. Mueller CB, Jeffries W. Cancer of the breast: its outcome as measured by the rate of dying and causes of death. Ann Surg 1975;182:334–41.

123. Baum M. The curability of breast cancer. Br Med J 1976;1:439–42.

124. Haybittle JL. Commentaries on Research in Breast Disease 1983;3:181.

125. Allan E. Breast cancer: the error of the exponential. Eur J Cancer 1978;14:1389–93.

126. Rutqvist LE, Wallgren A, Nilsson B. Is breast cancer a curable disease? A study of 14,731 women with breast cancer from the Cancer Registry of Norway. Cancer 1984;53:1793–800.

127. Ciatto S, Bonardi R. Is breast cancer ever cured? Follow-up study of 5623 breast cancer patients. Tumori 1991;77:465–7.

128. Mueller CB. Stage II breast cancer is not simply a late stage I. Surgery 1988;104:631–8.

129. Lewison EF. Spontaneous regression of breast cancer. Prog Clin Biol Res 1977;12:47–53.

130. Fisher ER, Gregorio RM, Fisher B, et al. The pathology of invasive breast cancer: a syllabus derived from findings of the National Surgical Adjuvant Breast Project (protocol no. 4). Cancer 1975;36:1–85.

131. Fisher B, Montague E, Redmond C, et al. Comparison of radical mastectomy with alternative treatments for primary breast cancer: a first report of results from a prospective randomized clinical trial. Cancer 1977;39:Suppl:2827–39.

132. Management of early cancer of the breast: report on an international multicentre trial supported by the Cancer Research Campaign. Br Med J 1976;1:1035–8.

133. Demicheli R, Terenziani M, Valagussa P, et al. Local recurrences following mastectomy: support for the concept of tumor dormancy. J Natl Cancer Inst 1994;86:45–8.

134. Hellman S. Karnofsky Memorial Lecture. Natural history of small breast cancers. J Clin Oncol 1994;12:2229–34.

135. McBride CM, Brown BW, Thompson JR, et al. Can patients with breast cancer be cured of their disease? A sample of the M.D. Anderson Hospital experience. Cancer 1983;51:938–45.

136. McDivitt RW. In: Atlas of tumor pathology, second series, fascicle 2. Washington, D.C.: Armed Forces Institute of Pathology, 1967.

137. Gallager HS. Pathologic types of breast cancer: their prognoses. Cancer 1984;53:Suppl:623–9.

138. Charpin C, Bonnier P, Khouzami A, et al. Inflammatory breast carcinoma: an immunohistochemical study using monoclonal anti-pHER-2/neu, pS2, cathepsin, ER and PR. Anticancer Res 1992;12:591–7.

139. Ellis DL, Teitelbaum SL. Inflammatory carcinoma of the breast: a pathologic definition. Cancer 1974;33:1045–7.

140. Lucas FV, Perez-Mesa C. Inflammatory carcinoma of the breast. Cancer 1978;41:1595–605.

141. Merino MJ, Livolsi VA. Signet ring carcinoma of the female breast: a clinicopathologic analysis of 24 cases. Cancer 1981;48:1830–7.

142. Kaufman MW, Marti JR, Gallager HS, Hoehn JL. Carcinoma of the breast with pseudosarcomatous metaplasia. Cancer 1984;53:1908–17.

143. Christensen L, Schiødt T, Blichert-Toft M. Sarcomatoid tumours of the breast in Denmark from 1977 to 1987: a clinicopathological and immunohistochemical study of 100 cases. Eur Cancer 1993; 29A:1824–31.

144. Pathology of breast cancers in long-term survivors. Lancet 1985;2:758–9. editorial.

145. Dixon JM, Page DL, Anderson TJ, et al. Long-term survivors after breast cancer. Br J Surg 1985;72:445–8.

146. Rosen PP, Groshen S, Kinne DW, Norton L. Factors influencing prognosis in node-negative breast carcinoma: analysis of 767 T1N0M0/T2N0M0 patients with long-term follow-up. J Clin Oncol 1993;11:2090–100.

147. Meyer JS. Cell kinetics in selection and stratification of patients for adjuvant therapy of breast carcinoma. NCI Monogr 1986;1:25–8.

148. Pedersen L, Holck S, Schiødt T. Medullary carcinoma of the breast. Cancer Treat Rev 1988;15:53–63.

149. Tanaka H, Hori M, Ohki T. High endothelial venule and immunocompetent cells in typical medullary carcinoma of the breast. Virchows Arch A Pathol Anat Histopathol 1992;420:253–61.

150. Reynolds J, Mies C, Daly JM. Mesenchymal infiltrating tumors. In: Bland KI, ed. The breast—comprehensive management of benign and malignant diseases. Philadelphia: WB Saunders, 1991:210.

151. Lagios MD, Margolin FR, Westdahl PR, Rose MR. Mammographically detected duct carcinoma in situ: frequency of local recurrence following tylectomy and prognostic effect of nuclear grade on local recurrence. Cancer 1989;63:618–24.

152. Haagensen CD. Breast carcinoma—risk and detection. Philadelphia: WB Saunders, 1981.

153. Dupont WD, Page DL. Risk factors for breast cancer in women with proliferative breast disease. N Engl J Med 1985;312:146–51.

154. Coll Am Pathol. Is 'fibrocystic disease' of the breast precancerous? Arch Pathol Lab Med 1986;110:171–3.

155. Haagensen CD. Diseases of the breast. 3rd ed. Philadelphia: WB Saunders, 1986.

156. Martelli G, Daidone MG, Mastore M, et al. Combined analysis of ploidy and cell kinetics on fine-needle aspirates from breast tumors. Cancer 1993;71:2522–7.

157. Bassett LW. In: Haus AG, ed. RSNA categorical course in physics syllabus. Oak Brook, Ill.: Radiological Society of North America, 1994:9.

158. American College of Radiology Committee on Quality Assurance in Mammography. Mammography quality control. Reston, Va.: American College of Radiology, 1992:57.

159. American College of Radiology. Breast imaging reporting and data system (BI-RADS). III ed. Reston, Va.: American College of Radiology, 1998.

160. Bassett LW. Quality determinants of mammography. Rockville, Md.: Agency for Health Care Policy and Research, Public Health Service, U.S. Department of Health and Human Services, 1994.

161. Chu KC, Smart CR, Tarone RE. Analysis of breast cancer mortality and stage distribution by age for the Health Insurance Plan clinical trial. J Natl Cancer Inst 1988;80:1125–32.

162. Tabar L, Fagerberg G, Chen HH, et al. Efficacy of breast cancer screening by age: new results from the Swedish Two-County Trial. Cancer 1995;75:2507–17.

163. Howard J. Using mammography for cancer control: an unrealized potential. CA Cancer J Clin 1987;37:33–48.

164. Hall FM, Storella JM, Silverstone DZ, Wyshak G. Nonpalpable breast lesions: recommendations for biopsy based on suspicion of carcinoma at mammography. Radiology 1988;167:353–8.

165. Linver MN, Osuch JR, Brenner RJ, Smith RA. The mammography audit: a primer for the mammography quality standards act (MQSA). AJR Am J Roentgenol 1995;165:19–25.

166. Bassett LW, Liu TH, Giuliano AE, Gold RH. The prevalence of carcinoma in palpable vs impalpable, mammographically detected lesions. AJR Am J Roentgenol 1991;157:21–4.

167. Linver MN. The medical audit: statistical basis of clinical outcomes analysis. In: Bassett LW, ed. Diagnosis of diseases of the breast. Philadelphia: W.B. Saunders, 1997:127–40.

168. Leitch AM, Dodd GD, Costanza M, et al. American Cancer Society guidelines for the early detection of breast cancer: update 1997. CA Cancer J Clin 1997;47:150–3.

169. American College of Radiology. Standards for the performance of diagnostic mammography and problem-solving breast evaluation. Reston, Va.: American College of Radiology, 1994.

170. American College of Radiology. Breast imaging reporting and data system. Reston, Va.: American College of Radiology, 1998.

171. Sickles EA. Nonpalpable, circumscribed, noncalcified solid breast masses: likelihood of malignancy based on lesion size and age of patient. Radiology 1994;192:439–42.

172. Sickles EA. The subtle and atypical mammographic features of invasive lobular carcinoma. Radiology 1991;178:25–6.

173. Jackson VP, Dines KA, Bassett LW, et al. Diagnostic importance of the radiographic density of noncalcified breast masses: analysis of 91 lesions. AJR Am J Roentgenol 1991;157:25–8.

174. Holland R, Hendriks JH, Vebeek AL, et al. Extent, distribution, and mammographic/histological correlations of breast ductal carcinoma in situ. Lancet 1990;335:519–22.

175. Boyages J, Recht A, Connolly J, et al. Factors associated with local recurrence as a first site of failure following the conservative treatment of early breast cancer. Recent Results Cancer Res 1989;115:92–102.

176. Stomper PC, Margolin FR. Ductal carcinoma in situ: the mammographer's perspective. AJR Am J Roentgenol 1994;162:585–91.

177. Graham RA. The efficacy of specimen radiography in evaluating the surgical margins of impalpable breast carcinoma. AJR Am J Roentgenol 1994;162:33.

178. Lagios MD, Westdahl PR, Margolin FR, Rose MR. Duct carcinoma in situ: relationship of extent of noninvasive disease to the frequency of occult invasion, multicentricity, lymph node metastasis, and short-term treatment failures. Cancer 1982;50:1309–14.

179. Sickles EA. Mammographic features of 300 consecutive nonpalpable breast cancers. AJR Am J Roentgenol 1986;146:661–3.

180. Hilton S, Leopold GR, Olson LK, Willson SA. Real-time breast sonography: application in 300 consecutive patients. AJR Am J Roentgenol 1986;147:479–86.

181. Stavros AT, Thickman D, Rapp CL, et al. Solid breast nodules: use of sonography to distinguish between benign and malignant lesions. Radiology 1995;196:123–34.

182. Sickles EA, Filly RA, Callen PW. Breast cancer detection with sonography and mammography: comparison using state-of-the-art equipment. AJR Am J Roentgenol 1983;140:843–5.

183. Kolb TM, Lichy J, Newhouse JH. Occult cancer in women with dense

breasts: detection with screening US—diagnostic yield and tumor characteristics. Radiology 1998;207:191–9.

184. Jackson VP. The current role of ultrasonography in breast imaging. Radiol Clin North Am 1995;33:1161–70.

185. Azavedo E, Svane G, Auer G. Stereotactic fine-needle biopsy in 2594 mammographically detected non-palpable lesions. Lancet 1989; 1:1033–6.

186. Bassett L, Winchester DP, Caplan RB, et al. Stereotactic core-needle biopsy of the breast: a report of the Joint Task Force of the American College of Radiology, American College of Surgeons, and College of American Pathologists. CA Cancer J Clin 1997;47:171–90.

187. Parker SH, Lovin JD, Jobe WE, et al. Stereotactic breast biopsy with a biopsy gun. Radiology 1990;176:741–7.

188. Fornage BD, Coan JD, David CL. Ultrasound-guided needle biopsy of the breast and other interventional procedures. Radiol Clin North Am 1992;30:167–85.

189. Tabár L, Dean PB, Péntek Z. Galactography: the diagnostic procedure of choice for nipple discharge. Radiology 1983;149:31–8.

190. Feig SA. Digital imaging. In: Bassett LW, ed. Diagnosis of diseases of the breast. Philadelphia: WB Saunders, 1997:197.

191. Williams MB, Fajardo LL. Digital mammography: performance considerations and current detector designs. Acad Radiol 1996;3:429–37.

192. Turner DA, Alcorn FS, Adler YT. Nuclear magnetic resonance in the diagnosis of breast cancer. Radiol Clin North Am 1988;26:673–87.

193. Heywang SH, Hahn D, Schmidt H, et al. MR imaging of the breast using gadolinium-DTPA. J Comput Assist Tomogr 1986;10:199–204.

194. Harms SE, Flamig DP, Hesley KL, et al. MR imaging of the breast with rotating delivery of excitation off resonance: clinical experience with pathologic correlation. Radiology 1993;187:493–501.

195. Lewis-Jones HG, Whitehouse GH, Leinster SJ. The role of magnetic resonance imaging in the assessment of local recurrent breast carcinoma. Clin Radiol 1991;43:197–204.

196. Adler LP, Crowe JP, al-Kaisi NK, Sunshine JL. Evaluation of breast masses and axillary lymph nodes with [F-18] 2-deoxy-2-fluoro-D-glucose PET. Radiology 1993;187:743–50.

197. Khalkhali I, Cutrone JA, Mena IG, et al. Scintimammography: the complementary role of Tc-99m sestamibi prone breast imaging for the diagnosis of breast carcinoma. Radiology 1995;196:421–6.

198. Maffioli L, Agresti R, Chiti A, et al. Prone scintimammography in patients with non-palpable breast lesions. Anticancer Res 1996;16:1269–73.

199. Helbich TH, Becherer A, Trattnig S, et al. Differentiation of benign and malignant breast lesions: MR imaging versus Tc-99m sestamibi scintimammography. Radiology 1997;202:421–9.

200. Lee YT. Breast carcinoma: pattern of metastasis at autopsy. J Surg Oncol 1983;23:175–80.

201. DiStefano A, Yong Yap Y, Hortobagyi GN, Blumenschein GR. The natural history of breast cancer patients with brain metastases. Cancer 1979;44:1913–8.

202. Paterson AH, Agarwal M, Lees A, et al. Brain metastases in breast cancer patients receiving adjuvant chemotherapy. Cancer 1982; 49:651–4.

203. Yap HY, Tashima CK, Blumenschein GR, Eckles N. Diabetes insipidus and breast cancer. Arch Intern Med 1979;139:1009–11.

204. Ratanatharathorn V, Powers WE, Grimm J, et al. Eye metastasis from carcinoma of the breast: diagnosis, radiation treatment and results. Cancer Treat Rev 1991;18:261–76.

205. Hall SM, Buzdar AU, Blumenschein GR. Cranial nerve palsies in metastatic breast cancer due to osseous metastasis without intracranial involvement. Cancer 1983;52:180–4.

206. Marcus FS, Dandolos EM, Friedman MA. Meningeal carcinomatosis in breast cancer presenting as central hypoventilation: a case report with a brief review of the literature. Cancer 1981;47:982–4.

207. Fentiman IS, Rubens RD, Hayward JL. The pattern of metastatic disease in patients with pleural effusions secondary to breast cancer. Br J Surg 1982;69:193–4.

208. Almagro UA, Caya JG, Remeniuk E. Cardiac tamponade due to malignant pericardial effusion in breast cancer: a case report. Cancer 1982;49:1929–33.

209. Albertini RE, Ekberg NL. Endobronchial metastasis in breast cancer. Thorax 1980;35:435–40.

210. Leland J, MacPherson B. Hematologic findings in cases of mammary cancer metastatic to bone marrow. Am J Clin Pathol 1979;71:31–5.

211. Dearnaley DP, Ormerod MG, Sloane JP, et al. Detection of isolated mammary carcinoma cells in marrow of patients with primary breast cancer. J R Soc Med 1983;76:359–64.

212. Cormier WJ, Gaffey TA, Welch JM, et al. Linitis plastica caused by metastatic lobular carcinoma of the breast. Mayo Clin Proc 1980;55:747–53.

213. Hickey RC, Samaan NA, Jackson GL. Hypercalcemia in patients with breast cancer: osseous metastases, hyperplastic parathyroid tissue, or pseudohyperparathyroidism? Arch Surg 1981;116:545–52.

214. Francini G, Petrioli R, Maioli E, et al. Hypercalcemia in breast cancer. Clin Exp Metastasis 1993;11:359–67.

215. White DR, Maloney JJ 3d, Muss HB, et al. Serum alkaline phosphatase determination: value in the staging of advanced breast cancer. JAMA 1979;242:1147–9.

216. Horn Y, Hacohen D, Zeidman JL, et al. Carcinoembryonic antigen and interferon as tumor markers in breast cancer. J Surg Oncol 1983;22:254–6.

217. Silva JS, Leight GS, Haagensen DE Jr. Quantitation of response to therapy in patients with metastatic breast carcinoma by serial analysis of plasma gross cystic disease fluid protein and carcinoembryonic antigen. Cancer 1982;49:1236–42.

218. Falkson HC, Falkson G, Portugal MA, et al. Carcinoembryonic antigen as a marker in patients with breast cancer receiving postsurgical adjuvant chemotherapy. Cancer 1982;49:1859–65.

219. Mughal AW, Hortobagyi GN, Fritsche HA, et al. Serial plasma carcinoembryonic antigen measurements during treatment of metastatic breast cancer. JAMA 1983;249:1881–6.

220. Beard DB, Haskell CM. Carcinoembryonic antigen in breast cancer: clinical review. Am J Med 1986;80:241–5.

221. Beveridge RA, Chan DW, Bruzek D, et al. A new biomarker in monitoring breast cancer: CA 549. J Clin Oncol 1988;6:1815–21.

222. Kallioniemi OP, Oksa H, Aaran RK, et al. Serum CA 15–3 assay in the diagnosis and follow-up of breast cancer. Br J Cancer 1988;58:213–5.

223. Geraghty JG, Coveney EC, Sherry F, et al. CA 15–3 in patients with locoregional and metastatic breast carcinoma. Cancer 1992;70:2831–4.

224. Rubach M, Szymendera JJ, Kaminska J, Kowalska M. Serum Ca 15.3, CEA and ESR patterns in breast cancer. Int J Biol Markers 1997;12:168–73.

225. Mendelson EB. Evaluation of the postoperative breast. Radiol Clin North Am 1992;30:107–38.

226. Orel SG, Troupin RH, Patterson EA, Fowble BL. Breast cancer recurrence after lumpectomy and irradiation: role of mammography in detection. Radiology 1992;183:201–6.

227. Fajardo LL, Roberts CC, Hunt KR. Mammographic surveillance of breast cancer patients: should the mastectomy site be imaged? AJR Am J Roentgenol 1993;161:953–5.

228. Jain S, Fisher C, Smith P, et al. Patterns of metastatic breast cancer in relation to histological type. Eur J Cancer 1993;29A:2155–7.

229. Muss HB, Tell GS, Case LD, et al. Perceptions of follow-up care in women with breast cancer. Am J Clin Oncol 1991;14:55–9.

230. Loomer L, Brockschmidt JK, Muss HB, Saylor G. Postoperative follow-up of patients with early breast cancer: patterns of care among clinical oncologists and a review of the literature. Cancer 1991;67:55–60.

231. Rosselli Del Turco M, Palli D, Cariddi A, et al. Intensive diagnostic follow-up after treatment of primary breast cancer: a randomized trial. National Research Council Project on Breast Cancer follow-up. JAMA 1994;271:1593–7.

232. GIVIO Investigators. Impact of follow-up testing on survival and health-related quality of life in breast cancer patients: a multicenter randomized controlled trial. The GIVIO Investigators. JAMA 1994;271:1587–92.

233. Ciatto S, Pacini P, Azzini V, et al. Preoperative staging of primary breast cancer: a multicentric study. Cancer 1988;61:1038–40.

234. AJCC manual for staging cancer. 4th ed. Philadelphia: JB Lippincott, 1992:149.

235. O'Mara RE. Bone scanning in osseous metastatic disease. JAMA 1974;229:1915–7.

236. Khansur T, Haick A, Patel B, et al. Evaluation of bone scan as a screening work-up in primary and local-regional recurrence of breast cancer. Am J Clin Oncol 1987;10:167–70.

237. Coleman RE, Rubens RD, Fogelman I. Reappraisal of the baseline bone scan in breast cancer. J Nucl Med 1988;29:1045–9.

238. McNeil BJ, Pace PD, Gray EB, et al. Preoperative and follow-up bone scans in patients with primary carcinoma of the breast. Surg Gynecol Obstet 1978;147:745–8.

239. Bassett LW, Giuliano AE, Gold RH. Staging for breast carcinoma. Am J Surg 1989;157:250–5.

240. Loprinzi CL. It is now the age to define the appropriate follow-up of primary breast cancer patients. J Clin Oncol 1994;12:881–3.
241. Schaner EG, Chang AE, Doppman JL, et al. Comparison of computed and conventional whole lung tomography in detecting pulmonary nodules: a prospective radiologic-pathologic study. AJR Am J Roentgenol 1978;131:51–4.
242. Vestergaard A, Herrstedt J, Thomsen HS, et al. The value of yearly chest x-ray in patients with stage I breast cancer. Eur J Cancer Clin Oncol 1989;25:687–9.
243. Bernardino ME, Thomas JL, Barnes PA, Lewis E. Diagnostic approaches to liver and spleen metastases. Radiol Clin North Am 1982;20:469–85.
244. Yeh HC, Rabinowitz JG. Ultrasonography and computed tomography of the liver. Radiol Clin North Am 1980;18:321–38.
245. Ferrucci JT. Leo J. Rigler lecture. MR imaging of the liver. AJR Am J Roentgenol 1986;147:1103–16.
246. Russell EJ, Geremia GK, Johnson CE, et al. Multiple cerebral metastases: detectability with Gd-DTPA–enhanced MR imaging. Radiology 1987;165:609–17.
247. Bentson JR, Steckel RJ, Kagan AR. Diagnostic imaging in clinical cancer management: brain metastases. Invest Radiol 1988;23:335–41.
248. Khansur T, Haick A, Patel B, et al. Preoperative evaluation with radionuclide brain scanning and computerized axial tomography of the brain in patients with breast cancer. Am J Surg 1988;155:232–4.
249. Brant-Zawadzki M. MR imaging of the brain. Radiology 1988;166:Pt 1:1–10.
250. Davis PC, Hudgins PA, Peterman SB, Hoffman JC Jr. Diagnosis of cerebral metastases: double-dose delayed CT vs contrast-enhanced MR imaging. AJNR Am J Neuroradiol 1991;12:293–300.
251. Beahrs OH, ed. American Joint Committee on Cancer: manual for staging of cancer. 4th ed. Philadelphia: JB Lippincott, 1992:149.
252. Lee Y-TN. Bone scanning in patients with early breast carcinoma: should it be a routine staging procedure? Cancer 1981;47:486–95.
253. Pupi A, Castagnoli A, Rosselli Del Turco M, et al. The role of whole body scan and skeletal radiography in the preoperative staging of breast cancer. Tumori 1981;67:231–4.
254. Wiener SN, Sachs SH. An assessment of routine liver scanning in patients with breast cancer. Arch Surg 1978;113:126–7.
255. Brar HS, Sisley JF, Johnson RH Jr. Value of preoperative bone and liver scans and alkaline phosphatase in the evaluation of breast cancer patients. Am J Surg 1993;165:221–4.
256. Buzdar AU, Kau SW, Hortobagyi GN, et al. Clinical course of patients with breast cancer with ten or more positive nodes who were treated with doxorubicin-containing adjuvant therapy. Cancer 1992;69:448–52.
257. Satariano WA, Ragland DR. The effect of comorbidity on 3-year survival of women with primary breast cancer. Ann Intern Med 1994;120:104–10.
258. Holland R, Veling SH, Mravunac M, Hendriks JH. Histologic multifocality of Tis, T1–2 breast carcinomas: implications for clinical trials of breast-conserving surgery. Cancer 1985;56:979–90.
259. Fisher ER, Sass R, Fisher B, et al. Pathologic findings from the National Surgical Adjuvant Breast Project (protocol 6): II. relation of local breast recurrence to multicentricity. Cancer 1986;57:1717–24.
260. Kurtz JM. Factors influencing the risk of local recurrence in the breast. Eur J Cancer 1992;28:660–6.
261. Kinne DW, Ashikari R, Butler A, et al. Estrogen receptor protein in breast cancer as a predictor of recurrence. Cancer 1981;47:2364–7.
262. Samaa NA, Buzdar AU, Aldinger KA, et al. Estrogen receptor: a prognostic factor in breast cancer. Cancer 1981;47:554–60.
263. Shek LL, Godolphin W, Spinelli JJ. Oestrogen receptors, nodes and stage as predictors of post-recurrence survival in 457 breast cancer patients. Br J Cancer 1987;56:825–9.
264. Fisher ER. Prognostic and therapeutic significance of pathological features of breast cancer. NCI Monogr 1986;1:29–34.
265. Rosen PP, Saigo PE, Braun DW Jr, et al. Predictors of recurrence in stage I (T1N0M0) breast carcinoma. Ann Surg 1981;193:15–25.
266. Atiba J, Coppin C, Ragaz J, et al. Clinical significance of lymphatic, vascular or neural invasion in node negative breast cancer. Proc ASCO 1988;7:12.
267. Meyer JS. Cell kinetics in selection and stratification of patients for adjuvant therapy of breast carcinoma. NCI Monogr 1986;1:25–8.
268. Kallioniemi OP, Blanco G, Alavaikko M, et al: Improving the prognostic value of DNA flow cytometry in breast cancer by combining DNA index and S-phase fraction: a proposed classification of DNA histograms in breast cancer. Cancer 1988;62:2183–90.
269. Feichter GE, Mueller A, Kaufmann M, et al. Correlation of DNA flow cytometric results and other prognostic factors in primary breast cancer. Int J Cancer 1988;41:823–8.
270. Fallenius AG, Franzén SA, Auer GU. Predictive value of nuclear DNA content in breast cancer in relation to clinical and morphologic factors: a retrospective study of 227 consecutive cases. Cancer 1988;62:521–30.
271. Witzig TE, Ingle JN, Schaid DJ, et al. DNA ploidy and percent S-phase as prognostic factors in node-positive breast cancer: results from patients enrolled in two prospective randomized trials. J Clin Oncol 1993;11:351–9.
272. Fisher B, Gunduz N, Costantino J, et al. DNA flow cytometric analysis of primary operable breast cancer: relation of ploidy and S-phase fraction to outcome of patients in NSABP B-04. Cancer 1991;68:1465–75.
273. Slamon DJ, Clark GM, Wong SG, et al. Human breast cancer: correlation of relapse and survival with amplification of the Her-2/neu oncogene. Science 1987; 235:177–82.
274. Gusterson BA, Gelber RD, Goldhirsch A, et al. Prognostic importance of c-erbB-2 expression in breast cancer. International Ludwig Breast Cancer Study Group. J Clin Oncol 1992;10:1049–56.
275. Weidner N, Folkman J, Pozza F, et al. Tumor angiogenesis: a new significant and independent prognostic indicator in early-stage breast carcinoma. J Natl Cancer Inst 1992;84:1875–87.
276. Toi M, Kashitani J, Tominaga T. Tumor angiogenesis is an independent prognostic indicator in primary breast carcinoma. Int J Cancer 1993;55:371–4.
277. Gasparini G, Weidner N, Bevilacqua P, et al. Tumor microvessel density, p53 expression, tumor size, and peritumoral lymphatic vessel invasion are relevant prognostic markers in node-negative breast carcinoma. J Clin Oncol 1994;12:454–66.
278. Aaltomaa S, Lipponen P, Syrjänen K. Proliferating cell nuclear antigen (PCNA) immunolabeling as a prognostic factor in axillary lymph node negative breast cancer. Anticancer Res 1993;13:533–8.
279. Silvestrini R, Benini E, Daidone MG, et al. p53 as an independent prognostic marker in lymph node-negative breast cancer patients. J Natl Cancer Inst 1993;85:965–70.
280. Allred DC, Clark GM, Elledge R, et al. Association of p53 protein expression with tumor cell proliferation rate and clinical outcome in node-negative breast cancer. J Natl Cancer Inst 1993;85:200–6.
281. Brouillet JP, Spyratos F, Hacene K, et al. Immunoradiometric assay of pro-cathepsin D in breast cancer cytosol: relative prognostic value versus total cathepsin D. Eur J Cancer 1993;29A:1248–51.
282. Ravdin PM, Tandon AK, Allred DC, et al. Cathepsin D by Western blotting and immunohistochemistry: failure to confirm correlations with prognosis in node-negative breast cancer. J Clin Oncol 1994;12:467–74.
283. Jameel A, Skilton RA, Campbell TA, et al. Clinical and biological significance of HSP89 alpha in human breast cancer. Int J Cancer 1992;50:409–15.
284. Jänicke F, Schmitt M, Pache L, et al. Urokinase (uPA) and its inhibitor PAI-1 are strong and independent prognostic factors in node-negative breast cancer. Breast Cancer Res Treat 1993;24:195–208.
285. Murray PA, Barrett-Lee P, Travers M, et al. The prognostic significance of transforming growth factors in human breast cancer. Br J Cancer 1993;67:1408–12.
286. Liotta LA. Cancer cell invasion and metastasis. Sci Am 1992;266:54–9, 62–3.
287. Steeg PS, de la Rosa A, Flatow U, et al. Nm23 and breast cancer metastasis. Breast Cancer Res Treat 1993;25:175–87.
288. Miller WR, Hulme MJ, Cho-Chung YS, Elton RA. Types of cyclic AMP binding proteins in human breast cancers. Eur J Cancer 1993;29A:989–91.
289. Keyomarsi K, O'Leary N, Molnar G, et al. Cyclin E, a potential prognostic marker for breast cancer. Cancer Res 1994;54:380–5.
290. Senie RT, Rosen PP, Rhodes P, Lesser ML. Timing of breast cancer excision during the menstrual cycle influences duration of disease-free survival. Ann Intern Med 1991;115:337–42.
291. Gnant MF, Seifert M, Jakesz R, et al. Breast cancer and timing of surgery during menstrual cycle: a 5-year analysis of 385 pre-menopausal women. Int J Cancer 1992;52:707–12.
292. McGuire WL, Hilsenbeck S, Clark GM. Optimal mastectomy timing. J Natl Cancer Inst 1992;84:346–8.
293. Bastarrachea J, Hortobagyi GN, Smith TL, et al. Obesity as an adverse prognostic factor for patients receiving adjuvant chemotherapy for breast cancer. Ann Intern Med 1994;120:18–25.

294. Gilchrist KW, Gray R, Fowble B, et al. Tumor necrosis is a prognostic predictor for early recurrence and death in lymph node–positive breast cancer: a 10-year follow-up study of 728 Eastern Cooperative Oncology Group patients. J Clin Oncol 1993;11:1929–35.

295. Fuster E, Garcia-Vilanova A, Narbona B, et al. A statistical approach to an individualized prognostic index (IPI) for breast cancer survivability. Cancer 1983;52:728–36.

296. Hortobagyi GN, Smith TL, Legha SS, et al. Multivariate analysis of prognostic factors in metastatic breast cancer. J Clin Oncol 1983;1:776–86.

297. Aaltomaa S, Lipponen P, Eskelinen M, et al. Predictive value of a morphometric prognostic index in female breast cancer. Oncology 1993;50:57–62.

298. Muss HB, Thor AD, Berry DA, et al. C-erbB-2 expression and response to adjuvant therapy in women with node-positive, early breast cancer. N Engl J Med 1994;330:1260–66.

299. Abner AL, Recht A, Eberlein T, et al. Prognosis following salvage mastectomy for recurrence in the breast after conservative surgery and radiation therapy for early-stage breast cancer. J Clin Oncol 1993;11:44–8.

300. Vogel CL, Azevedo S, Hilsenbeck S, et al. Survival after first recurrence of breast cancer: the Miami experience. Cancer 1992;70:129–35.

301. Koenders PG, Beex LV, Kloppenborg PW, et al. Human breast cancer: survival from first metastasis. Breast Cancer Study Group. Breast Cancer Res Treat 1992;21:173–80.

302. Rutqvist LE, Cedermark B, Glas U, et al. Contralateral primary tumors in breast cancer patients in a randomized trial of adjuvant tamoxifen therapy. J Natl Cancer Inst 1991;83:1299–306.

303. Fisher B, Costantino J, Redmond C, et al. A randomized clinical trial evaluating tamoxifen in the treatment of patients with node-negative breast cancer who have estrogen-receptor–positive tumors. N Engl J Med 1989;320:479–84.

304. Fisher B, Costantino J, Wickerham D, et al. Tamoxifen for prevention of breast cancer: report of the National Surgical Adjuvant Breast and Bowel Project P-1 Study. J Natl Cancer Inst 1998;90:1371–88.

305. Veronesi U, Maisonneuve P, Costa A, et al. Prevention of breast cancer with tamoxifen: preliminary findings from the Italian randomised trial among hysterectomized women. Italian Tamoxifen Prevention Study. Lancet 1998;352:93–7.

306. Powles T, Eeles R, Ashley S, et al. Interim analysis of the incidence of breast cancer in the Royal Marsden Hospital tamoxifen randomised chemoprevention trial. Lancet 1998;352:98–101.

307. Cummings SR, Norton L, Eckert S, et al. Raloxifene reduces the risk of breast cancer and may decrease the risk of endometrial cancer in post-menopausal women: two-year findings from the Multiple Outcomes of Raloxifene Evaluation (MORE) trial. Proc ASCO 1998;17:2a.

308. De Palo G, Camerini T, Marubini E, et al. Chemoprevention trial of contralateral breast cancer with fenretinide: rationale, design, methodology, organization, data management, statistics and accrual. Tumori 1997;83:884–94.

309. Hicken NF. Mastectomy: clinical pathologic study demonstrating why most mastectomies result in incomplete removal of mammary gland. Arch Surg 1940;40:6–14.

310. Ziegler LD, Kroll SS. Primary breast cancer after prophylactic mastectomy. Am J Clin Oncol 1991;14:451–4.

311. Eldar S, Meguid MM, Beatty JD. Cancer of the breast after prophylactic subcutaneous mastectomy. Am J Surg 1984;148:692–3.

312. Pennisi VR, Capozzi A. Subcutaneous mastectomy data: a final statistical analysis of 1500 patients. Aesthetic Plastic Surg 1989;13:15–21.

313. Hartmann LC, Schaid DJ, Woods JE, et al. Efficacy of bilateral prophylactic mastectomy in women with a family history of breast cancer. N Engl J Med 1999;340:77–84.

......................................

# IN SITU BREAST CANCER

• Helena R. Chang • Chia Soo • Sanford H. Barsky

## Overview of Ductal Carcinoma In Situ and Lobular Carcinoma In Situ

DCIS and LCIS were first described by Foote and Stewart[1, 2] as two distinct pathologic entities in the 1940s. DCIS and LCIS were viewed as variants of invasive breast disease, and the initial treatment for both was mastectomy. Since then, clinicians have recognized that in addition to being pathologically distinct, DCIS and LCIS are two distinct clinical entities with different natural histories. DCIS is broadly viewed as a premalignant lesion with the potential to progress to invasive breast cancer in the same breast, whereas LCIS is considered a marker of increased cancer risk in either breast. In the last 25 years, an increased incidence of DCIS and, to a lesser extent, LCIS has been seen primarily as a result of an increase in screening mammography and liberal biopsy of suspicious breast lesions.[3] Mammographic detection of earlier, smaller, and more frequent DCIS lesions and the success of breast conservation surgery for treating invasive cancer have challenged the necessity of mastectomy for DCIS. Research on the subject in the 1990s focused on optimizing local treatment of DCIS. In the future, studies exploring the molecular mechanisms for confining DCIS are likely to stimulate development of therapeutic strategies for preventing DCIS progression. Other preventive regimens, such as chemoprevention and lifestyle, may reduce the incidence of preinvasive and invasive breast cancer.

## Ductal Carcinoma In Situ

### EPIDEMIOLOGY

**Risk Factors.** The risk factors for DCIS are similar to those for invasive breast carcinoma. Kerlikowske and associates[4] reported an increased risk for DCIS in all patients 30 years old or older who had a first-degree relative with breast cancer (odds ratio [OR], 2.4 [95% confidence interval (CI), 1.1 to 4.9] for ages 30 to 49; OR, 2.2 [95% CI, 1 to 4.2] for age ≥50).[4] Nulliparity or birth of first child at age 30 or older increased the risk for DCIS in women who were 50 or older (OR, 2.3 [95% CI, 1.3 to 3.8]) but not in women ages 30 to 49. Atypical ductal hyperplasia (ADH) also presents as a risk marker for DCIS. In a series of image-guided core biopsies of 510 mammographically identified lesions, ADH was identified and surgical excision performed in 21 of these cases, of which 7 (33.3%) indicated DCIS.[5] Ringberg and colleagues[6] found that in 36 cases of women with DCIS, 7 (19%) developed DCIS in the contralateral breast, suggesting a predisposed risk in the other breast.

**Incidence.** The incidence of DCIS in autopsy studies of

asymptomatic women has varied from 0 to 14.5[7] and likely reflects differences in race, age, and specimen sampling methods among the studies (Table 35–10). Bartow and coworkers[10] have suggested that DCIS may be more common in white than in Hispanic or Native American populations. DCIS represented only 2% of all breast cancers in the premammography era and usually presented with late clinical symptoms, such as abnormal nipple discharge or a palpable mass.[17] With the onset of mammographic screening, DCIS now comprises 10 to 40% of all newly diagnosed breast cancers in women and 4 to 10% of male breast malignancies.[7, 18] Analysis of the National Cancer Institute's Surveillance, Epidemiology, and End Results (SEER) program from 1973 to 1992 revealed that more than 23,000 cases of DCIS are diagnosed in American women each year and that 10,000 breasts are removed as a consequence.[19] The number of DCIS diagnosed cases has increased by 200% since the widespread use of mammography in the 1980s.[19]

The average age of women with DCIS is the mid-50s, which is approximately 10 years younger than the average for women with invasive breast cancer.[20, 21] Additional screening mammography data on younger women show a relatively higher incidence of DCIS in women younger than age 50; DCIS represents 46.6% of all breast cancers in these women, as opposed to 36.6% in women older than age 50.[22] The clinical significance of mammographically detected DCIS is unclear, and several studies suggest that subclinical DCIS is common. For example, the report of Nielsen and colleagues[15] on 110 medicolegal autopsies on women between the ages of 20 and 54 found a 15% prevalence of DCIS (four to five times greater than the number of invasive breast cancers expected to develop over a 20-year period). Similarly, Alpers and Wellings[8] observed that 48% of women with invasive unilateral breast cancer who underwent prophylactic mastectomy of the contralateral breast had DCIS in the contralateral breast. Because only about 12.5% of women with a history of breast carcinoma develop invasive contralateral breast cancer after 20 years of follow-up, the authors suggested that not all cases of DCIS progress to invasive cancer. This suggestion raises the question as to whether current therapeutic strategies for DCIS would be overtreatment for a subset of women with DCIS that would have remained subclinical in the premammographic era.[23]

Current knowledge of DCIS is not sufficient to allow accurate prediction of the factors that correlate with the progression of DCIS to invasive disease.

## PATHOLOGY

**Classification.** Traditional DCIS classification is based on the architectural pattern of comedo versus noncomedo histologic type. The noncomedo subtype is further divided into cribriform, micropapillary, papillary, and solid forms, depending on histologic architecture. Comedo DCIS is often associated with high nuclear grade, frequent mitoses, and central necrosis within the ductal lumen.[24] Partial calcification of the necrotic debris results in the typical branching-linear pattern seen on mammograms.[24] Biologically, comedo DCIS is associated with a greater degree of microinvasion and a higher risk of local recurrence after simple excision.[25] The dual classification system for DCIS, however, is too simplistic. Essentially any architectural subtype can present with any nuclear grade, and low-grade lesions can also present with necrosis.[26] Frequently a single biopsy specimen contains different architectural subtypes.[26] Although the histologic subtypes of DCIS may be agreed on by most pathologists, low-grade DCIS can be difficult to distinguish from ductal hyperplasia with or without atypia.[27, 28] Standardized criteria help to minimize interobserver variability.

Because not all cases of DCIS progress to invasive disease, much interest has been focused on identifying specific factors that prognosticate invasion. At least six different pathologic classification systems for DCIS have been proposed.[29, 30] Each attempts to correlate certain features, such as nuclear grade, degree of necrosis, and architectural pattern, with clinical outcomes in terms of local recurrence and risk of invasive carcinoma after local excision with or without radiation. The validity of these classification schemes with regard to interobserver reproducibility and prediction of clinical outcomes has not yet been tested in large prospective studies, however.[7]

Studies using the Van Nuys classification system suggested a modified classification system for DCIS. It defines three distinct groups of patients: (1) non–high-grade DCIS without comedo-type necrosis, (2) non–high-grade DCIS

*Table 35–10.* Incidence of Ductal Carcinoma In Situ in Asymptomatic Women at Autopsy

| Study | Age (years) at Autopsy | | Patients (*n*) | Incidence of DCIS (*n*[%]) |
|---|---|---|---|---|
| | RANGE | MEAN | | |
| Alpers and Wellings[8] | NR | 15–99 | 101 | 11 (10.9) |
| Andersen et al[9] | NR | NR | 83 | 11 (13.2) |
| Bartow et al[10] | 37 | 15–98 | 519 | 1 (0.2) |
| Bhathal et al[11] | 60 | 15–97 | 207 | 25 (12.1) |
| Frantz et al[12] | NR | 13–88 | 225 | 0 (0.0) |
| Kramer and Rush[13] | NR | >70 | 70 | 4 (5.7) |
| Nielsen et al[14] | 67 | 22–89 | 77 | 11 (14.3) |
| Nielsen et al[15] | 39 | 20–54 | 110 | 16 (14.5) |
| Rush and Kramer[16] | 78 | >70 | 20 | 2 (10.0) |
| All studies | | | 1412 | 81 (5.7) |

DCIS, ductal carcinoma in situ; NR, not reported.
Modified from Delaney G, et al. Ductal carcinoma in situ: Part I. definition and diagnosis. Aust N Z J Surg 1997;67:81–93. Based on work at the New South Wales Breast Cancer Institute.

with comedo-type necrosis, and (3) high-grade DCIS with or without comedo-type necrosis.[31] Silverstein and Lagios[26] have shown that nuclear grade, tumor size, and margin width were all significant predictors of local recurrence in DCIS patients. From this study, they devised the Van Nuys Prognostic Index, which assigns lesions a score from 1 to 3 for each of three factors (tumor size, margin width, and pathologic classification), based on the Van Nuys classification system.[26] Support for the Van Nuys classification system was shown by Douglas-Jones and associates,[29] who reported low interobserver variability and apparent correlation with disease-free survival.

**Tumor Size and Margin Width.** In addition to different classification systems for DCIS, there are also several methods to determine the size and margin status of DCIS.[30] Methods for determining tumor size range from clinical palpation and mammograms to macroscopic or microscopic examination.[30] Optimally, serial uniform sections are formed from the resected DCIS specimen, and the size is estimated microscopically because the extent of DCIS may be underestimated by clinical examination and mammography.[32] This approach, however, may not be feasible for large or diffuse DCIS lesions.

The clearance of surgical margins critically affects the outcome of DCIS treatment. The definition of what constitutes a clear margin varies from series to series, however. In the NSABP B-17 trial, a margin was regarded as clear when the tumor was not transected.[25] Others have defined negative margins as being greater than 1 to 2 mm away from the tumor.[33, 34] Holland and coworkers[33] determined that ipsilateral recurrence was primarily related to margin status. In their series of 129 women who underwent local excision of DCIS, only 2 of 101 (2%) who had clear margins (DCIS >1 mm from nearest margin of excision) experienced recurrence, whereas 10 of 28 (36%) women with close margins (DCIS ≤1 mm from resection margin) experienced recurrence. In a subset of 24 women with DCIS who were treated at the University of California Los Angeles (UCLA) by excision alone, 4 of 19 (21%) patients with negative margins (>2 mm) experienced recurrence, whereas 2 of 5 women (40%) with close (≤2 mm) or positive margins experienced recurrence over a median follow-up of 100 months.[35] In this study, the negative margin was defined as either no residual DCIS found in the re-excision specimen or the margin exceeding 2 mm, with normal intervening duct between the DCIS and the closest margin.

Ideally, when excision alone is selected for treatment, a minimal excision margin of 10 mm for DCIS is required.[26, 33] Cavity shavings[33] and frozen sections have not been useful in determining adequate excision, owing to sampling error.[36] Imprint cytology is another modality that may be helpful for intraoperative determination of lumpectomy margins.[37]

**Multifocal or Multicentric.** *Multifocal* and *multicentric* are two terms that have been variably defined and interchangeably used in the literature, contributing to the confusion as to whether DCIS is multifocal or multicentric. *Multifocal* refers to an additional focus of disease within the same quadrant as the primary tumor, whereas *multicentric* refers to disease foci in a different quadrant from the primary tumor.[7] A 15 to 78% incidence of multicentricity has been cited in the literature, but the true incidence is probably lower.[7] The definitive study of Holland and colleagues[38] involving serial sections of mastectomy specimens showed that 81 of 82 (99%) specimens had contiguous growth. Quadrant-based definitions of multifocality and multicentricity are problematic, in that they do not distinguish contiguous from discontiguous growth and do not take into account the variability in breast size and contour. Currently, DCIS is largely viewed as a unicentric rather than multicentric disease. Multicentricity, however, may be more common in larger[39] and macropapillary-type lesions.[40]

**Origin and Natural History.** Although the origin of DCIS is not completely understood, work suggests that there may be a continuum between ADH, DCIS, and invasive carcinoma.[41] Lennington and coworkers[41] suggest that DCIS may develop from a central focus of ADH and expand peripherally. At the molecular level, there is also support for the view that DCIS is a precursor lesion of invasive breast carcinoma.[42] Gupta and associates[43] have shown that increased in situ dysplasia does not necessarily occur before the development of stromal invasion, and well-differentiated DCIS may give rise to low-grade invasive breast carcinoma, with a better long-term clinical outcome. Taken together, the evidence suggests that DCIS may originate from ADH, with eventual progression to invasive cancer. The biomolecular characteristics of the initial DCIS lesion may predict the aggressiveness of the invasive carcinoma.[43, 44] The current challenge in DCIS studies is to determine which lesions will stay dormant and which will expand to extensive in situ disease or progress to invasive carcinoma, providing guidance in choosing the best course of treatment.[45]

The treatment of DCIS has been mastectomy; its natural history has not been well characterized. The only data available on the natural history of DCIS stem from a report of symptomatic lesions in 123 women, which were initially mistaken for benign disease by breast biopsy and not treated further.[45–49] Approximately 14 to 53% of these women developed invasive disease over a mean follow-up of 9.7 to 30 years.[45–49] In one study, the calculated overall risk of developing invasive carcinoma for these women was nine times that of the general population over a 30-year period (95% CI, 4.7 to 17).[45] These studies have been criticized for their small numbers, selection bias, predominance of noncomedo-type pathology, inclusion of patients with microinvasion, and the presence of palpable disease (presumably from larger tumors that would have a higher likelihood for microinvasion).[7]

**Molecular Mechanisms of Ductal Carcinoma In Situ Development.** DCIS of the breast is a disease that behaves more aggressively than any other organ type of carcinoma in situ. Although DCIS is not a life-threatening disease, it clearly is a serious breast malignancy. DCIS can be extensive, even throughout entire ductal systems, and appears either as multiple discrete foci or as a continuous network of involved ducts.[50] Despite surgical treatment targeted to complete extirpation, DCIS often recurs. This clinical behavior is not that of an in situ or localized disease process.

Genetic information has shed additional light on the DCIS process. Polymerase chain reaction clonality studies exploiting X-linked inactivation genes, including the human androgen receptor gene (*HUMARA*),[51] the human phosphoglycerate kinase gene (*PGK*),[52] and the human hypoxanthine phosphoribosyl transferase gene (*HPRT*),[53] and their resulting methylation alterations have shown that DCIS is a monoclonal process.[54] Additionally, in comparative studies with concomitant invasive carcinoma, identical genetic markers are present in both phases.[55, 56] For example, there is a strong correlation of S phase; Ki-67; ploidy; presence or absence of estrogen receptor (ER), progesterone receptor (PR), or HER-2/*neu* amplification; epidermal growth factor receptor overexpression; and p53 alterations in DCIS compared with respective values in invasive carcinoma within a given case. This correlation suggests that DCIS and invasive breast carcinoma are biologically and genetically similar, if not identical.

Most studies examining loss of heterozygosity at key genomic loci and gains and losses of genetic information through comparative genomic hybridization have demonstrated that DCIS, similar to invasive cancer, is a disease of genetic instability. Common allelic losses present within DCIS and its invasive counterpart in the same individual confirm that the invasive carcinoma arises from the DCIS clone.[57] These studies of loss of heterozygosity and comparative genomic hybridization, however, have failed to reveal any additional genetic alterations within the invasive carcinoma, suggesting that the DCIS cell already possesses all of the necessary genetic alterations required for invasion and metastasis.[58–61]

DCIS, similar to invasive cancer, has also been observed to stimulate angiogenesis, producing *bursts* of new blood vessel formation within the stroma directly outside of the ducts involved in DCIS.[62] The only difference between DCIS and invasive carcinoma is that the former process is confined to the ductal system by the basement membrane. DCIS, nevertheless, often spreads uncontrollably within this system, and recurs with high frequency. This is not the biology of a typical in situ disease process.

Data generated by our laboratory have suggested that the determinants of the progression of DCIS to invasive cancer are epigenetic rather than genetic. These determinants consist of strong paracrine regulation by neighboring myoepithelial cells. Because of their close proximity, myoepithelial cells would be anticipated to exert important paracrine influences on DCIS progression. Myoepithelial cells of the breast differ from luminal ductal and acinar epithelial cells in many ways, in that they lack expression of the common hormonal receptor, ER, and its responsive genes, such as PR; myoepithelial cells lie next to the basement membrane and contribute to the synthesis of that structure; myoepithelial cells rarely transform or proliferate, but when they do, they give rise to only low-grade benign neoplasms.[63] Myoepithelial cells ubiquitously surround normal ducts, benign glandular proliferations such as adenosis, and malignant intraductal proliferations (e.g., DCIS). Sternlicht and colleagues[64, 65] have established immortalized myoepithelial cell lines and transplantable xenografts from benign human myoepitheliomas of the salivary gland (HMS-1, HMS-X; HMS-3, HMS-3X), breast (HMS-4), and bronchus (HMS-6, HMS-6X). These cell lines and xenografts express myoepithelial markers identical to those of normal myoepithelial cells in situ and display an essentially normal diploid karyotype. Myoepithelial cell lines and xenografts and myoepithelial cells in situ constitutively express high amounts of proteinase and angiogenesis inhibitors, including tissue inhibitor of metalloproteinases (TIMP-1), protease nexin-II, α1-antitrypsin, an unidentified 31- to 33-kd trypsin inhibitor, thrombospondin-

1, soluble basic fibroblast growth factor receptors, and maspin.[66] These human myoepithelial cell lines inhibit both ER-positive and ER-negative breast carcinoma cell invasion and endothelial migration and proliferation (angiogenesis) in vitro. These cell lines also inhibit breast carcinoma proliferation in vitro through induction of breast carcinoma cell G2-M arrest and apoptosis[67]; the latter phenomenon occurs in situ in DCIS.[68] On the basis of immunoprecipitation studies, maspin secreted by myoepithelial cells is the major effector molecule, which inhibits invasion, and thrombospondin-1 is a major angiogenic inhibitor. Myoepithelial cell–released nitric oxide appears to be the major effector molecule, which inhibits breast carcinoma cell proliferation through its induction of apoptosis.[69] These cumulative studies suggest that DCIS is cancer of the breast in the true genetic, biologic, and clinical sense of the word but is limited to the confines of the ductal system by myoepithelial cells.

## DIAGNOSIS

**Clinical Presentation.** Before the introduction of widespread mammographic screening, most cases of DCIS presented with advanced signs and symptoms, including nipple discharge, a palpable mass, and Paget's disease.[70, 71] Since the institution of routine mammography screening, there has been a substantial increase in the incidence of largely asymptomatic DCIS. Most cases of DCIS are found as nonpalpable mammographic findings.

**Radiographic Characteristics.** The different histologic subtypes of DCIS frequently have characteristic mammographic appearances.[72] Poorly differentiated DCIS (e.g., comedo type) frequently presents with linear and branching (casting) calcifications.[72, 73] In contrast, well-differentiated DCIS is associated with clusters of fine granular calcifications.[73] The correlation between mammographic appearance and the predominant histologic subtype is not absolute, however, especially because DCIS often presents with mixed histologic subtypes.[74] DCIS can also present with mammographic signs other than microcalcifications, such as asymmetry, dilated retroareolar ducts, ill-defined rounded tumors, focal architectural distortion, subareolar mass, and developing density.[75] Although in the past mammography frequently underestimated the size of DCIS, state-of-the-art mammography, including magnification views, can reduce this error in more than 80% of the cases.[73]

The role for MRI in DCIS is unclear. MRI may be useful as an adjunct to mammography in determining tumor extent and presence of invasion. Typically, pure DCIS presents as a clumped enhancement pattern on rotating delivery of excitation-off resonance (RODEO) MRI, whereas DCIS with microinvasion and invasive ductal carcinoma with extensive intraductal component can be associated with a spiculated enhancement pattern.[76] Others have suggested a limited role of MRI in detection of microinvasion in DCIS.

**Biopsy.** Once a suspicious breast abnormality is detected by breast examination or mammography, the next step is tissue diagnosis to rule out or confirm malignancy. Palpable lesions can be pathologically examined by fine-needle aspiration, core biopsy, or surgical biopsy. Nonpalpable lesions can be biopsied stereotactically, occasionally with ultrasonographic guidance. Fine-needle aspiration cannot distinguish

DCIS from invasive carcinoma or ADH.[77] Kerin and associates,[78] in a series of 1500 consecutive fine-needle aspiration cytology specimens, found fine-needle aspiration to be unreliable in patients with invasive carcinomas of less than 1 cm in diameter and for the detection of DCIS and LCIS. The primary shortcoming of fine-needle aspiration is that cytology alone, devoid of histologic context, cannot exclude invasion.

Core biopsies can confirm with high accuracy the presence of invasion or benign disease within a particular sample.[79] A tissue diagnosis of invasive carcinoma by core biopsy is sufficient to proceed with definitive therapy[80]; invasive carcinoma, however, cannot be excluded by core biopsy alone. Core biopsy with a finding of cellular atypia should be followed with open excisional biopsies to exclude the presence of malignancy.[81]

## TREATMENT

Before the widespread use of screening mammography, DCIS was a clinical rarity that was routinely treated by mastectomy. This choice was based on the frequent large size of DCIS at presentation and on the belief that DCIS was largely a multifocal disease. The success of treating invasive carcinoma by breast-conserving therapy and the diagnosis of smaller DCIS lesions by screening mammography has challenged the need for mastectomy for all DCIS lesions.[82]

**Total Mastectomy.** Total mastectomy is effective treatment for DCIS and is the standard by which other therapeutic modalities are measured. A review of 1640 patients in 23 studies who underwent mastectomy with variable follow-up periods showed that 23 (1.4%) had local recurrence of disease, with 83% of the recurrences being invasive carcinoma (Table 35–11). We observed one invasive recurrence (3.8%) in a series of 26 DCIS patients treated with mastectomy at UCLA, with a follow-up of 100 months.[35] At UCLA, simple mastectomy was reserved for patients with recurrent DCIS or those who could not be treated by a less extreme procedure because of the extent of the disease. Generally a prophylactic mastectomy on the contralateral side is not necessary because there is only a 5 to 10% incidence of synchronous and metachronous malignancy.[104] Although the overall focus for DCIS treatment has shifted away from mastectomy, there are still situations associated with a high risk of local-regional recurrence (e.g., large tumor size, comedo histology, inability to obtain clear margins, extensive disease, young age), for which total mastectomy is advised.[105] Subcutaneous mastectomy is not recommended because it is associated with high recurrence rates of 50%.[95] For a patient with diffuse disease, even total or modified radical mastectomy does not guarantee total disease eradication.[106]

**Lumpectomy.** Although mastectomy may overtreat many

*Table 35–11.* **Risk for Recurrence After Mastectomy for Ductal Carcinoma In Situ**

| Study | Patients (n) | Median Follow-up (mo) | Patients with Local Recurrence | |
|---|---|---|---|---|
| | | | TOTAL TUMORS (NONINVASIVE + INVASIVE) (n[%]) | INVASIVE TUMORS ONLY (n) |
| Ashikari et al[83] | 111 | 12–120* | 2 (2) | 2 |
| Arnesson et al[84] | 28 | 77 | 0 (0) | 0 |
| Bellamy et al[40] | 99 | 60 | 4 (4) | 1 |
| Brown et al[85] | 40 | NR | 0 (0) | 0 |
| Carpenter et al[86] | 10 | 55 | 0 (0) | 0 |
| Cataliotti et al[87] | 103 | 128 | 3 (3) | 3 |
| Ciatto et al[88] | 210 | 65† | 3 (1) | 1 |
| Cutuli et al[89] | 34 | 82 | 1 (3) | 1 |
| Farrow[90] | 181 | NR | 2 (1) | 2 |
| Fisher et al[91] | 27 | 39 | 0 (0) | 0 |
| Kinne et al[92] | 101 | 138 | 0 (0) | 0 |
| Lagios et al[39] | 53 | 44 | 3 (6) | 3 |
| Millis and Thynne[93] | 20 | 24–180* | 0 (0) | 0 |
| Montague[94] | 134 | NR | 1 (1) | 1 |
| Price et al[95] | 16 | 108 | 1 (6) | 1 |
| Schuh et al[96] | 52 | 65† | 0 (0) | 0 |
| Silverstein et al[97] | 98 | 60 | 1 (1) | 1 |
| Sunshine et al[98] | 74 | >120* | 0 (0) | 0 |
| Temple et al[99] | 9 | 72 | 0 (0) | 0 |
| von Rueden and Wilson[100] | 45 | NR | 0 (0) | 0 |
| Warneke et al[101] | 75 | 43† | 1 (1) | 1 |
| Westbrook and Gallager[102] | 60 | NR | 1 (1) | 2 |
| All studies | 1640 | | 23 (1.4) | 19 (83% of recurrences) |

*Range.
†Mean.
NR, not reported.
Modified from Delaney G, et al. Ductal carcinoma in situ. Part 2. treatment. Aust N Z J Surg 1997;67:157–65. Based on work performed at the New South Wales Breast Cancer Institute.

cases of DCIS, lumpectomy alone may result in undertreatment. In 19 studies of 1056 patients who underwent breast-conserving surgery alone, there were 244 (23%) recurrences, of which 110 (45%) were invasive (Table 35–12). The recurrence rate of DCIS and invasive cancer is consistently high after excision alone. However, many of these earlier studies had what is now considered to be inadequate margins for local DCIS control; some of the local recurrences are believed to be a manifestation of the residual disease.[116, 117] Silverstein and associates[116] showed that 43% of locally excised DCIS with clear margins (>1 mm) have evidence of residual disease at mastectomy. Silverstein and Lagios[26] defined a small subset of DCIS lesions with favorable histology, tumor grade, size, and margin status that may be treated by lumpectomy alone, with relatively low recurrence rates. In our experience at UCLA, 4 of 19 patients (21%) with DCIS treated by local surgery alone experienced recurrence within a median follow-up of 8 years.[35] All these patients had noncomedo DCIS, clear (>2 mm) margins, and calcification-free postoperative mammograms. Local excision alone for DCIS may still be associated with a higher rate of recurrence, and its role in definitive DCIS management remains uncertain.

**Lumpectomy and Radiation.** Successful application of breast conservation surgery to invasive disease challenges the practice of mastectomy for DCIS. A direct transfer of an effective local treatment for invasive breast carcinoma into successful treatment for DCIS is overly simplistic, however. Table 35–13 summarizes the data from 23 studies, in which 1518 patients underwent local DCIS excision, followed by radiation. Of these patients, 137 (9%) experienced recur-

rence, with invasive disease in 49% of these recurrences. The recurrence rate is significantly reduced when compared with the outcomes from surgical excision alone, although the percentage of invasive disease is relatively unchanged. Longer follow-up in many studies is needed to show that radiation actually prevents rather than merely delays recurrence. Shorter term studies quote a 5-year actuarial recurrence rate of 4 to 11%,[112, 118, 123, 125–128, 130] whereas 15-year actuarial studies report a local failure rate of 19%,[131] which approaches the recurrence rate for lumpectomy alone and signifies the importance of adequate follow-up. Over a 100-month follow-up period at UCLA, we found local recurrence rates after lumpectomy with radiation (4.2% recurrence in 23 patients) to be equivalent to mastectomy (4.2% recurrence in 24 patients) provided that surgical margins were clear at initial lumpectomy.[35] Studies with higher recurrence rates after lumpectomy with radiation may reflect inadequate tumor margins and a significant amount of residual disease at the site of excision.

Several studies have suggested that for high-grade DCIS, the addition of radiation appeared only to delay rather than prevent recurrence.[97, 121, 132] In contrast, for low-grade to intermediate-grade DCIS, Lagios and Silverstein[133] showed in a nonrandomized study that radiation conveyed no demonstrable benefit over excision alone on recurrence. These results, however, are not supported by data from the NSABP B-17 trials, which showed that radiation reduced the recurrence rate from 17.2 to 6.8% for high-grade lesions and from 11 to 3.2% for low-grade lesions over a 48-month mean follow-up period.[25] The current consensus is that radiation can delay and possibly reduce the number of invasive

*Table 35–12.* **Risk for Recurrence After Lumpectomy Alone for Ductal Carcinoma In Situ**

| Study | Patients (*n*) | Median Follow-up (mo) | Patients with Local Recurrence | |
|---|---|---|---|---|
| | | | TOTAL TUMORS (NONINVASIVE + INVASIVE) (*n* [%]) | INVASIVE TUMORS ONLY (*n*) |
| Arnesson et al[84] | 38 | 60 | 5 (13) | 2 |
| Baird et al[107] | 30 | 43* | 4 (13) | 1 |
| Bellamy et al[40] | 31 | 60 | 10 (32) | 5 |
| Carpenter et al[86] | 28 | 38 | 5 (18) | 1 |
| Cataliotti et al[87] | 46 | 70 | 5 (11) | 5 |
| Farrow[90] | 25 | NR | 5 (20) | 0 |
| Fisher et al[108] | 21 | 83* | 9 (43) | 5 |
| Fisher et al[109] | 403 | 90* | 104 (26) | 53 |
| Gallagher et al[110] | 13 | 100 | 5 (38) | 3 |
| Graham et al[111] | 37 | 97 | 14 (38) | 7 |
| Kuske et al[112] | 7 | 48 | 3 (43) | 1 |
| Lagios et al[113] | 79 | 44 | 8 (10) | 4 |
| Millis and Thynne[93] | 8 | 24–180† | 2 (25) | 0 |
| Ottesen et al[114] | 112 | 53 | 25 (22) | 5 |
| Price et al[95] | 35 | 108 | 22 (63) | 12 |
| Schwartz et al[115] | 72 | 49* | 11 (15) | 3 |
| Silverstein et al[97] | 26 | 19 | 2 (8) | 1 |
| Temple et al[99] | 17 | 72* | 2 (12) | 1 |
| Warneke et al[101] | 28 | 43* | 3 (11) | 1 |
| All studies | 1056 | | 244 (23) | 110 (45% of recurrences) |

*Mean.
†Range.
NR, not reported.
Modified from Delaney G, et al. Ductal carcinoma in situ. Part 2. treatment. Aust N Z J Surg 1997;67:157–65. Based on work performed at the New South Wales Breast Cancer Institute.

*Table 35–13.* **Risk for Recurrence After Lumpectomy and Radiation for Ductal Carcinoma In Situ**

| Study | Patients (*n*) | Median Follow-up (mo) | Patients with Local Recurrence TOTAL TUMORS (NONINVASIVE + INVASIVE) (*n* [%]) | INVASIVE TUMORS ONLY (*n*) |
|---|---|---|---|---|
| Baird et al[107] | 8 | 43* | 2 (25) | 1 |
| Bornstein et al[118] | 38 | 81 | 7 (18) | 4 |
| Bullock et al[119] | 43 | 62 | 3 (7) | 1 |
| Cataliotti et al[87] | 34 | 50 | 3 (9) | 3 |
| Cutuli et al[89] | 34 | 56 | 3 (9) | 1 |
| Fisher et al[108] | 27 | 83* | 2 (7) | 1 |
| Fisher et al[109] | 411 | 90* | 47 (11) | 17 |
| Fourquet et al[120] | 67 | 104 | 7 (10) | 5 |
| Fowble[121] | 46 | 35 | 2 (4) | NR |
| Fowble et al[34] | 110 | 64 | 3 (3) | 3 |
| Hiramatsu et al[122] | 76 | 74 | 7 (9) | 4 |
| Kurtz et al[123] | 43 | 61 | 3 (7) | 3 |
| Kuske et al[112] | 70 | 48 | 3 (4) | 3 |
| McCormick et al[124] | 54 | 36 | 10 (19) | 3 |
| Montague[94] | 34 | NR | 1 (3) | 1 |
| Ray et al[125] | 58 | 61 | 5 (9) | 1 |
| Recht et al[126] | 40 | 44 | 4 (10) | 2 |
| Silverstein et al[97] | 103 | 63 | 10 (10) | 5 |
| Solin et al[127] | 51 | 68 | 5 (10) | 2 |
| Stotter et al[128] | 44 | 92 | 4 (9) | 4 |
| Warneke et al[101] | 21 | 43* | 0 | 0 |
| White et al[129] | 52 | 68 | 3 (6) | 1 |
| Zafrani et al[130] | 54 | 55 | 3 (6) | 1 |
| All studies | 1518 | | 137 (9) | 66 (49% of recurrences) |

*Mean.
NR, not reported.
Modified from Delaney G, et al. Ductal carcinoma in situ. Part 2. treatment. Aust N Z J Surg 1997;67:157–65.

recurrences after lumpectomy for DCIS. Whether radiation therapy can be stratified to different subtypes of DCIS or affect survival remains to be determined.

**Randomized Trials.** In contrast to breast carcinoma, the treatment for DCIS has not evolved systematically, and its optimal management is still being debated. Other than the NSABP B-06 trial, there are no data from randomized trials directly comparing the three treatment options of mastectomy versus lumpectomy versus lumpectomy and radiation. Table 35–14 summarizes the ongoing randomized studies specific for DCIS. Of these, only the NSABP B-17 trial

*Table 35–14.* **Summary of Randomized Ductal Carcinoma In Situ Studies**

| Study | Randomization Arms After Lumpectomy |
|---|---|
| NSABP (National Surgical Adjuvant Breast and Bowel Project) B-17 | No radiation vs. radiation |
| EORTC (European Organization for Research on Treatment of Cancer) 10853 | No radiation vs. radiation |
| DBGG 89-IS (Denmark) | No radiation vs. radiation |
| Sweden | No radiation vs. radiation |
| Germany | No radiation vs. radiation |
| UKCCCR-DCIS, CRC-PHASE-III-90001 (United Kingdom) | No radiation vs. radiation vs. tamoxifen vs. radiation-tamoxifen |
| NSABP B-24 | Radiation vs. radiation-tamoxifen |

has been completed. This trial sought to determine whether radiation was effective in preventing DCIS recurrence after lumpectomy.[108, 109] The latest NSABP B-17 results show that after a mean follow-up of 90 months, 104 (26%) of 403 women who underwent lumpectomy alone experienced recurrence, whereas 47 of 411 (11%) women who underwent lumpectomy and radiation experienced recurrence.[109] The proportion of invasive tumor recurrence was greater in the nonirradiated group (51% vs. 36%).

The NSABP B-06 study was designed to randomize patients with early invasive cancer to mastectomy versus lumpectomy with or without radiation.[137] A subset of 76 patients was found, after a later pathologic review, to have DCIS alone. After a mean follow-up of 83 months, 9 of 21 who had local excision alone recurred, 2 of 27 who had excision and radiation recurred, and 0 of 28 who had mastectomy recurred.[138] Overall, this trial was flawed by small study numbers, relatively large tumor sizes (2.2 cm ± 1.3 cm), and ambiguity over margin status. In addition, although no significant difference in cause-specific survival was observed, the short follow-up precludes any solid conclusions about survival to be drawn from the B-06 trial.

NSABP B-17, a large prospective randomized study, was designed to compare the outcomes of women with DCIS who were treated by wide excision alone or wide excision plus irradiation. Although this trial showed that radiation appeared to reduce the risk for invasive and noninvasive recurrence,[134] it has been criticized for its definition of clear margins, inadequacy of size measurements, and lack of pathologic subset analysis.[135] The B-17 trial has not definitively answered the question of whether radiotherapy is of value (see Table 35–14).[136]

In contrast to invasive carcinoma, antiestrogens, such as tamoxifen, are of unclear benefit in the management of DCIS because their success depends on the expression of estrogen receptors by DCIS.[139–141] Preliminary results from the NSABP B-24 trial on the role of tamoxifen in DCIS indicate that tamoxifen may reduce recurrence further after excision and radiation. Another study (UKCCCR-DCIS, CRC-PHASE-III-90001) is under way in the United Kingdom. Longer term follow-up is required before the efficacy of tamoxifen treatment can be evaluated. HER-2/*neu* oncogene overexpression is observed in many comedo-type DCIS lesions.[142, 143] Monoclonal antibodies against the HER-2/neu protein or other pharmacologically active agents targeting the HER-2/neu peptide may play a future role in DCIS therapy.

**Axillary Dissection.** Because DCIS is a preinvasive lesion, axillary lymph node dissection is not indicated.[144] Larger sized DCIS lesions and comedo-type DCIS, however, may have an increased risk for microinvasion and axillary metastases. Lagios[145] determined that occult invasion was present in 48% of DCIS specimens of greater than 55 mm. Intraoperative lymphatic mapping and selective sentinel lymphadenectomy is gaining increased acceptance in the management of invasive breast cancer and may play a future role in the management of large high-grade DCIS lesions.[146]

**Survival.** Survival rates for DCIS patients are excellent. Most studies cite cause-specific survivals ranging from 97 to 100% with median follow-ups of 5 to 10 years.[34, 131] No significant differences in cause-specific survival have been observed between mastectomy versus lumpectomy and radiation[147] and mastectomy versus lumpectomy with or without radiation.[148] Hillner and colleagues[148] used a Markov decision analysis model to show that mastectomy gave a slightly better (0.7%) actuarial survival over lumpectomy with breast irradiation after 20 years of follow-up.

## SPECIFIC PREDICTORS FOR RECURRENCE

The recognition of DCIS heterogeneity and the detection of earlier smaller DCIS lesions by mammography have increased the complexity of DCIS treatment. Although mastectomy was once the therapy of choice, there is now evidence that breast conservation surgery may be an alternative for most DCIS lesions. The current challenge in DCIS therapy is to tailor the treatment to the specific characteristics of the lesion. Various factors, such as lesion size, histology and nuclear grade, and margin status, have all been advocated to predict treatment outcome. Additional prognosticators may further refine knowledge in optimizing the treatment of DCIS.

**Size.** Patients with larger sized DCIS lesions are at increased risk for recurrence after breast conservation surgery because of the inability to achieve clear margins or the increased risk of microinvasion, or both. Silverstein and coworkers[116] determined that larger tumor size is a significant predictor of initial margin involvement and residual DCIS. In addition, Lagios[145] showed that size (>55 mm) correlates

with the incidence of microinvasion and is a risk factor for subsequent invasive recurrence.

**Histology and Nuclear Grade.** Many studies have reported an increased risk of local recurrence with comedo necrosis and high nuclear grade.[113, 115, 149] Longer follow-up studies, however, have not shown a significant increase in recurrence rates for comedo DCIS or high-grade lesions.[131]

**Margin Status.** The presence of clear margins may be the most important prognostic indicator.[26, 35] Most recurrences occur near previous excision sites, suggesting inadequate excision rather than a separate recurrence.[34, 89] Holland and associates[33] showed that ipsilateral recurrence is primarily a consequence of inadequate margin.

**Van Nuys Prognostic Index.** Silverstein and associates[31] have proposed the Van Nuys classification system and the Van Nuys Prognostic Index, based on tumor size, margin width, and pathologic classification.[26, 150] The validity of this system is yet to be confirmed by a longer follow-up and independent observations from other prospective studies.

## MANAGEMENT OF RECURRENCE

**Surveillance.** Mammography is highly sensitive in detection of local recurrences.[151] Of new calcifications for which biopsy specimens were obtained after lumpectomy and radiation, 58% were shown to be recurrent DCIS or invasive disease.[152]

**Treatment.** Approximately half of all DCIS recurrences are invasive cancer (see Tables 35–11, 35–12, and 35–13). Most patients, however, can be salvaged with mastectomy. In selected cases, further lumpectomy has resulted in high rates (84 to 100%) of cause-specific survival.[101, 153, 154]

## Lobular Carcinoma In Situ

### EPIDEMIOLOGY

Because LCIS is undetectable by clinical or radiographic examination, it usually presents as an incidental pathologic finding in women undergoing breast biopsy for other reasons.[155] The true incidence of LCIS is unknown. The only information on the incidence of LCIS comes from biopsy and autopsy studies, with ranges of 0 to 3.6%.[155] These studies, however, are biased toward women with underlying breast pathology and older women.[155] The risk factors for LCIS are unclear, but hormonal status may play a role because LCIS appears to be more common in premenopausal women,[156] although no association between LCIS and exogenous estrogen use in postmenopausal women has been found.[157] Age rather than hormones may govern the onset of LCIS.

### PATHOLOGY

LCIS is generally believed to be a marker of increased risk for subsequent invasive carcinoma rather than a precursor lesion to invasive disease, although there is evidence to suggest that LCIS may be a precursor to invasive lobular carcinoma.[158, 159] More than half the invasive breast carcinomas, after a diagnosis of LCIS, are ductal rather than lobular in nature and can occur anywhere in either breast, regardless of the location of the original LCIS biopsy site.[160, 161] From a pathologic standpoint, LCIS tends to be ER and PR positive,[159] multicentric, and bilateral (90%).[162]

The risk for invasive cancer after a diagnosis of LCIS on biopsy depends on (1) the duration of follow-up (invasive disease may develop 25 years later),[163] (2) age (risk decreases with increasing age at diagnosis),[164] and (3) the presence of benign proliferative breast changes and positive family history for breast cancer.[165] Several studies have determined that the presence of LCIS results in a 7-fold to 12-fold RR over the general population for invasive breast cancer in both breasts.[158, 163, 164] This risk is roughly equal to that for women whose mothers had bilateral breast cancer before menopause. With sufficient follow-up after biopsy, approximately 20 to 25% of women with LCIS develop invasive cancer.[166]

## TREATMENT

Both breasts must be treated as a single entity when considering treatment options for LCIS because the risk for invasive disease is equal bilaterally. The treatment options include observation,[167] bilateral mastectomy,[168] or antihormonal therapy.[155] Ipsilateral mastectomy and contralateral mirror image biopsy have largely fallen out of favor as treatment options, but routine contralateral breast biopsy is practiced at some institutions.[169] There is no role for axillary dissection in treatment of LCIS. Current trials are under way to evaluate the efficacy of tamoxifen in treatment of LCIS.

## ACKNOWLEDGMENT

The authors thank Melanie Moorehead for help in the preparation of this manuscript.

## REFERENCES

1. Foote FWJ, Stewart FW. A histologic classification of carcinoma of the breast. Surgery 1946;19:74–9.
2. Foote FWJ, Stewart FW. Lobular carcinoma in situ: a rare form of mammary carcinoma. Am J Pathol 1941;17:491–5.
3. Frykberg ER, Bland KI. Management of in situ and minimally invasive breast carcinoma. World J Surg 1994;18:45–57.
4. Kerlikowske K, Barclay J, Grady D, et al. Comparison of risk factors for ductal carcinoma in situ and invasive breast cancer. J Natl Cancer Inst 1997;89:76–82.
5. Moore MM, Hargett CW, Hanks JB, et al. Association of breast cancer with the finding of atypical ductal hyperplasia at core breast biopsy. Ann Surg 1997;225:726–31.
6. Ringberg A, Palmer B, Linell F, et al. Bilateral and multifocal breast carcinoma: a clinical and autopsy study with special emphasis on carcinoma in situ. Eur J Surg Oncol 1991;17:20–9.
7. Delaney G, Ung O, Bilous M, et al. Ductal carcinoma in situ: Part I. definition and diagnosis. Aust N Z J Surg 1997;67:81–93.
8. Alpers CE, Wellings SR. The prevalence of carcinoma in situ in normal and cancer-associated breasts. Hum Pathol 1985;16:796–807.
9. Andersen J, Nielsen M, Christensen L. New aspects of the natural history of in situ and invasive carcinoma in the female breast: results from autopsy investigations. Verh Dtsch Ges Pathol 1985;69:88–95.
10. Bartow SA, Pathak DR, Black WC, et al. Prevalence of benign, atypical, and malignant breast lesions in populations at different risk for breast cancer: a forensic autopsy study. Cancer 1987;60:2751–60.
11. Bhathal PS, Brown RW, Lesueur GC, Russell IS. Frequency of benign and malignant breast lesions in 207 consecutive autopsies in Australian women. Br J Cancer 1985;51:271–8.
12. Frantz VK, Pickren JW, Melcher GW. Incidence of chronic cystic disease in so called normal breasts: a study based on 225 post-mortem examinations. Cancer 1951;762–83.
13. Kramer WM, Rush BF Jr. Mammary duct proliferation in the elderly: a histopathologic study. Cancer 1973;31:130–7.
14. Nielsen M, Jensen J, Andersen J. Precancerous and cancerous breast lesions during lifetime and at autopsy: a study of 83 women. Cancer 1984;54:612–5.
15. Nielsen M, Thomsen JL, Primdahl S, et al. Breast cancer and atypia among young and middle-aged women: a study of 110 medicolegal autopsies. Br J Cancer 1987;56:814–9.
16. Rush BF, Kramer WM. Proliferative histologic changes and occult carcinoma in the breast of the aging female. Surg Gynecol Obstet 1963;117:425–32.
17. Rosner D, Bedwani RN, Vana J, et al. Noninvasive breast carcinoma: results of a national survey by the American College of Surgeons. Ann Surg 1980;192:139–47.
18. Camus MG, Joshi MG, Mackarem G, et al. Ductal carcinoma in situ of the male breast. Cancer 1994;74:1289–93.
19. Ernster VL, Barclay J, Kerlikowske K, et al. Incidence of and treatment for ductal carcinoma in situ of the breast. JAMA 1996;275:913–8.
20. Wazer DE, Gage I, Homer MJ, et al. Age-related differences in patients with nonpalpable breast carcinomas. Cancer 1996;78:1432–7.
21. Ciatto S, Grazzini G, Iossa A, et al. In situ ductal carcinoma of the breast—analysis of clinical presentation and outcome in 156 consecutive cases. Eur J Surg Oncol 1990;16:220–4.
22. Evans WP III, Starr AL, Bennos ES. Comparison of the relative incidence of impalpable invasive breast carcinoma and ductal carcinoma in situ in cancers detected in patients older and younger than 50 years of age. Radiology 1997;204:489–91.
23. Jatoi I, Baum M. Mammographically detected ductal carcinoma in situ: are we overdiagnosing breast cancer? Surgery 1995;118:118–20.
24. Fonseca R, Hartmann LC, Petersen IA, et al. Ductal carcinoma in situ of the breast. Ann Intern Med 1997;127:1013–22.
25. Fisher ER, Costantino J, Fisher B, et al. Pathologic findings from the National Surgical Adjuvant Breast Project (NSABP) Protocol B-17: intraductal carcinoma (ductal carcinoma in situ). The National Surgical Adjuvant Breast and Bowel Project Collaborating Investigators. Cancer 1995;75:1310–9.
26. Silverstein MJ, Lagios MD. Use of predictors of recurrence to plan therapy for DCIS of the breast. Oncology 1997;11:393–406.
27. Sloane JP, Ellman R, Anderson TJ, et al. Consistency of histopathological reporting of breast lesions detected by screening: findings of the U.K. National External Quality Assessment (EQA) Scheme. U.K. National Coordinating Group for Breast Screening Pathology. Eur J Cancer 1994;30A:1414–9.
28. Rosai J. Borderline epithelial lesions of the breast. Am J Surg Pathol 1991;15:209–21.
29. Douglas-Jones AG, Gupta SK, Attanoos RL, et al. A critical appraisal of six modern classifications of ductal carcinoma in situ of the breast (DCIS): correlation with grade of associated invasive carcinoma. Histopathology 1996;29:397–409.
30. The Consensus Conference Committee. Consensus Conference on the classification of ductal carcinoma in situ. Cancer 1997;80:1798–1802.
31. Silverstein MJ, Poller DN, Waisman JR, et al. Prognostic classification of breast ductal carcinoma-in-situ. Lancet 1995;345:1154–7.
32. Coombs JH, Hubbard E, Hudson K, et al. Ductal carcinoma in situ of the breast: correlation of pathologic and mammographic features with extent of disease. Am Surg 1997;63:1079–83.
33. Holland PA, Gandhi A, Knox WF, et al. The importance of complete excision in the prevention of local recurrence of ductal carcinoma in situ. Br J Cancer 1998;77:110–4.
34. Fowble B, Hanlon A, Fein DA, et al. Results of conservative surgery and radiation for mammographically detected ductal carcinoma in situ (DCIS). Int J Radiat Oncol Biol Phys 1997;38:949–57.
35. Weng E, Juillard G, Parker R, et al. Outcomes and factors impacting local recurrence of ductal carcinoma in situ (DCIS). 2000 (in press).
36. Cheng L, Al-Kaisi NK, Liu AY, Gordon NH. The results of intraoperative consultations in 181 ductal carcinomas in situ of the breast. Cancer 1997;80:75–9.

37. Cox CE, Hyacinthe M, Gonzalez RJ, et al. Cytologic evaluation of lumpectomy margins in patients with ductal carcinoma in situ: clinical outcome. Ann Surg Oncol 1997;4:644–9.

38. Holland R, Hendriks JH, Vebeek AL, et al. Extent, distribution, and mammographic/histological correlations of breast ductal carcinoma in situ. Lancet 1990;335:519–22.

39. Lagios MD, Westdahl PR, Margolin FR, Rose MR. Duct carcinoma in situ: relationship of extent of noninvasive disease to the frequency of occult invasion, multicentricity, lymph node metastases, and short-term treatment failures. Cancer 1982;50:1309–14.

40. Bellamy CO, McDonald C, Salter DM, et al. Noninvasive ductal carcinoma of the breast: the relevance of histologic categorization. Hum Pathol 1993;24:16–23.

41. Lennington WJ, Jensen RA, Dalton LW, Page DL. Ductal carcinoma in situ of the breast: heterogeneity of individual lesions. Cancer 1994;73:118–24.

42. James LA, Mitchell EL, Menasce L, Varley JM. Comparative genomic hybridization of ductal carcinoma in situ of the breast: identification of regions of DNA amplification and deletion in common with invasive breast carcinoma. Oncogene 1997;14:1059–65.

43. Gupta SK, Douglas-Jones AG, Fenn N, et al. The clinical behavior of breast carcinoma is probably determined at the preinvasive stage (ductal carcinoma in situ). Cancer 1997;80:1740–5.

44. Leal CB, Schmitt FC, Bento MJ, et al. Ductal carcinoma in situ of the breast: histologic categorization and its relationship to ploidy and immunohistochemical expression of hormone receptors, p53, and c-erbB-2 protein. Cancer 1995;75:2123–31.

45. Betsill WL Jr, Rosen PP, Lieberman PH, Robbins GF. Intraductal carcinoma: long-term follow-up after treatment by biopsy alone. JAMA 1978;239:1863–7.

46. Rosen PP, Braun DW Jr, Kinne DE. The clinical significance of pre-invasive breast carcinoma. Cancer 1980;46:919–25.

47. Page DL, Dupont WD, Rogers LW, Landenberger M. Intraductal carcinoma of the breast: follow-up after biopsy only. Cancer 1982;49:751–8.

48. Page DL, Dupont WD, Rogers LW, et al. Continued local recurrence of carcinoma 15–25 years after a diagnosis of low grade ductal carcinoma in situ of the breast treated only by biopsy. Cancer 1995;76:1197–200.

49. Eusebi V, Feudale E, Foschini MP, et al. Long-term follow-up of in situ carcinoma of the breast. Semin Diagn Pathol 1994;11:223–35.

50. Silverstein MJ. Ductal carcinoma in situ of the breast. Baltimore: Williams & Wilkins, 1997.

51. Busque L, Zhu J, Dehart D, et al. An expression based clonality assay at the human androgen receptor locus (HUMARA) on chromosome X. Nucleic Acids Res 1994;22:697–8.

52. Gilliland DG, Blanchard KL, Levy J, et al. Clonality in myeloproliferative disorders: analysis by means of the polymerase chain reaction. Proc Natl Acad Sci U S A 1991;88:6848–52.

53. Sternlicht M, Mirell C, Safarians S, Barsky SH. A novel strategy for the investigation of clonality in precancerous disease states and early stages of tumor progression. Biochem Biophys Res Commun 1994;199:511–8.

54. Noguchi S, Motomura K, Inaji H, et al. Clonal analysis of predominately intraductal carcinoma and precancerous lesions of the breast by means of polymerase chain reaction. Cancer Res 1994;54:1849–53.

55. Van de Vijver M, Peterse J, Mooi W, et al. Neu-protein overexpression in breast cancer. N Engl J Med 1988;319:1239–45.

56. Meyer JS. Cell kinetics of histologic variants of in situ breast carcinoma. Breast Cancer Res Treat 1986;7:171–80.

57. Zhuang Z, Merino MJ, Chuaqui R, et al. Identical allelic loss on chromosome 11q13 in microdissected in situ and invasive human breast cancer. Cancer Res 1995;55:467–71.

58. James LA, Mitchell EL, Menasce L, Varley JM. Comparative genomic hybridisation of ductal carcinoma in situ of the breast: identification of regions of DNA amplification and deletion in common with invasive breast carcinoma. Oncogene 1997;14:1059–65.

59. Chen T, Sahin A, Aldaz CM. Deletion map of chromosome 16q in ductal carcinoma in situ of the breast: refining a putative tumor suppressor gene region. Cancer Res 1996;56:5605–9.

60. Bose S, Wang SI, Terry MB, et al. Allelic loss of chromosome 10q23 is associated with tumor progression in breast carcinomas. Oncogene 1998;17:123–7.

61. Kuukasjarvi T, Tanner M, Pennanen S, et al. Genetic changes in intraductal breast cancer detected by comparative genomic hybridization. Am J Pathol 1997;150:1465–71.

62. Weidner N, Folkman J, Pozza F, et al. Tumor angiogenesis: a new significant and independent prognostic indicator in early-stage breast carcinoma. J Natl Cancer Inst 1992;84:1875–87.

63. Sternlicht MD, Barsky SH. The myoepithelial defense: a host defense against cancer. Med Hypotheses 1997;48:37–46.

64. Sternlicht MD, Safarians S, Calcaterra TC, Barsky SH. Establishment and characterization of a novel human myoepithelial cell line and matrix-producing xenograft from a parotid basal cell adenocarcinoma. In Vitro Cell Dev Biol 1996;32:550–63.

65. Sternlicht MD, Safarians S, Rivera SP, Barsky SH. Characterizations of the extracellular matrix and proteinase inhibitor content of human myoepithelial tumors. Lab Invest 1996;74:781–96.

66. Sternlicht MD, Kedeshian P, Shao ZM, et al. The human myoepithelial cell is a natural tumor suppressor. Clin Cancer Res 1997;3:1949–58.

67. Shao ZM, Nguyen M, Alpaugh ML, et al. The human myoepithelial cell exerts antiproliferative effects on breast carcinoma cells characterized by p21$^{WAF1/CIP1}$ induction, G2/M arrest and apoptosis. Exp Cell Res 1998;241:394–403.

68. Bodis S, Siziopikou KP, Schnitt SJ, et al. Extensive apoptosis in ductal carcinoma in situ of the breast. Cancer 1996;77:1831–5.

69. Shao ZM, Barsky SH. The anti-invasive phenotype of breast myoepithelial cells is hormonally regulated. 3rd Annual Multidisciplinary Symposium on Breast Disease, Amelia Island, Fla., 1998.

70. Dershaw DD, Abramson A, Kinne DW. Ductal carcinoma in situ: mammographic findings and clinical implications. Radiology 1989;170:411–5.

71. Dixon AR, Galea MH, Ellis IO, et al. Paget's disease of the nipple. Br J Surg 1991;78:722–3.

72. Bassett LW. Mammographic analysis of calcifications. Radiol Clin North Am 1992;30:93–105.

73. Holland R, Hendriks JH. Microcalcifications associated with ductal carcinoma in situ: mammographic-pathologic correlation. Semin Diagn Pathol 1994;11:181–92.

74. Stomper PC, Connolly JL. Ductal carcinoma in situ of the breast: correlation between mammographic calcification and tumor subtype. AJR Am J Roentgenol 1992;159:483–5.

75. Ikeda DM, Andersson I. Ductal carcinoma in situ: atypical mammographic appearances. Radiology 1989;172:661–6.

76. Soderstrom CE, Harms SE, Copit DS, et al. Three-dimensional RODEO breast MR imaging of lesions containing ductal carcinoma in situ. Radiology 1996;201:427–32.

77. Abendroth CS, Wang HH, Ducatman BS. Comparative features of carcinoma in situ and atypical ductal hyperplasia of the breast on fine-needle aspiration biopsy specimens. Am J Clin Pathol 1991;96:654–9.

78. Kerin MJ, McAnena OJ, Waldron RP, et al. Diagnostic pitfalls of fine needle aspiration cytology for breast disease. Ir Med J 1993;86:100–1.

79. Liberman L, Dershaw DD, Rosen PP, et al. Stereotaxic core biopsy of breast carcinoma: accuracy at predicting invasion. Radiology 1995;194:379–81.

80. Frayne J, Sterrett GF, Harvey J, et al. Stereotactic 14 gauge core-biopsy of the breast: results from 101 patients. Aust N Z J Surg 1996;66:585–91.

81. Bauer RL, Sung J, Eckhert KH Jr, et al. Comparison of histologic diagnosis between stereotactic core needle biopsy and open surgical biopsy. Ann Surg Oncol 1997;4:316–20.

82. Talamonti MS. Management of ductal carcinoma in situ. Semin Surg Oncol 1996;12:300–13.

83. Ashikari R, Hajdu SI, Robbins GF. Intraductal carcinoma of the breast (1960–1969). Cancer 1971;28:1182–7.

84. Arnesson LG, Smeds S, Fagerberg G, Grontoft O. Follow-up of two treatment modalities for ductal cancer in situ of the breast. Br J Surg 1989;76:672–5.

85. Brown PW, Silverman J, Owens E, et al. Intraductal "noninfiltrating" carcinoma of the breast. Arch Surg 1976;111:1063–7.

86. Carpenter R, Boulter PS, Cooke T, Gibbs NM. Management of screen detected ductal carcinoma in situ of the female breast. Br J Surg 1989;76:564–7.

87. Cataliotti L, Distante V, Ciatto S, et al. Intraductal breast cancer: review of 183 consecutive cases. Eur J Cancer 1992;28A:917–20.

88. Ciatto S, Bonardi R, Cataliotti L, Cardona G. Intraductal breast carcinoma: review of a multicenter series of 350 cases. Coordinating Center and Writing Committee of FONCAM (National Task Force for Breast Cancer), Italy. Tumori 1990;76:552–4.

89. Cutuli B, Teissier E, Piat JM, et al. Radical surgery and conservative treatment of ductal carcinoma in situ of the breast. Eur J Cancer 1992;28:649–54.

90. Farrow JH. Current concepts in the detection and treatment of the earliest of the early breast cancers. Cancer 1970;25:468–77.
91. Fisher ER, Sass R, Fisher B, et al. Pathologic findings from the National Surgical Adjuvant Breast Project (protocol 6): I. intraductal carcinoma (DCIS). Cancer 1986;57:197–208.
92. Kinne DW, Petrek JA, Osborne MP, et al. Breast carcinoma in situ. Arch Surg 1989;124:33–6.
93. Millis RR, Thynne GS. In situ intraduct carcinoma of the breast: a long term follow-up study. Br J Surg 1975;62:957–62.
94. Montague ED. Conservation surgery and radiation therapy in the treatment of operable breast cancer. Cancer 1984;53:700–4.
95. Price P, Sinnett HD, Gusterson B, et al. Duct carcinoma in situ: predictors of local recurrence and progression in patients treated by surgery alone. Br J Cancer 1990;61:869–72.
96. Schuh ME, Nemoto T, Penetrante RB, et al. Intraductal carcinoma: analysis of presentation, pathologic findings, and outcome of disease. Arch Surg 1986;121:1303–7.
97. Silverstein MJ, Cohlan BF, Gierson ED, et al. Duct carcinoma in situ: 227 cases without microinvasion. Eur J Cancer 1992;28:630–4.
98. Sunshine JA, Moseley HS, Fletcher WS, Krippaehne WW. Breast carcinoma in situ: a retrospective review of 112 cases with a minimum 10 year follow-up. Am J Surg 1985;150:44–51.
99. Temple WJ, Jenkins M, Alexander F, et al. Natural history of in situ breast cancer in a defined population. Ann Surg 1989;210:653–7.
100. von Rueden DG, Wilson RE. Intraductal carcinoma of the breast. Surg Gynecol Obstet 1984;158:105–11.
101. Warneke J, Grossklaus D, Davis J, et al. Influence of local treatment on the recurrence rate of ductal carcinoma in situ. J Am Coll Surg 1995;180:683–8.
102. Westbrook KC, Gallager HS. Intraductal carcinoma of the breast: a comparative study. Am J Surg 1975;130:667–70.
103. Delaney G, Ung O, Cahill S, et al. Ductal carcinoma in situ. Part 2: treatment. Aust N Z J Surg 1997;67:157–65.
104. Frykberg ER, Ames FC, Bland KI. Current concepts for management of early (in situ and occult invasive) breast carcinoma. In: Bland KI, Copeland EM, eds. The breast: comprehensive management of benign and malignant diseases. Philadelphia: WB Saunders, 1991:731.
105. Frykberg ER, Masood S, Copeland EM, Bland KI. Ductal carcinoma in situ of the breast. Surg Gynecol Obstet 1993;177:425–40.
106. Lagios MD. Duct carcinoma in situ: controversies in diagnosis, biology, and treatment. Breast J 1995;1:68–78.
107. Baird RM, Worth A, Hislop G. Recurrence after lumpectomy for comedo-type intraductal carcinoma of the breast. Am J Surg 1990;159:479–81.
108. Fisher B, Costantino J, Redmond C, et al. Lumpectomy compared with lumpectomy and radiation therapy for the treatment of intraductal breast cancer. N Engl J Med 1993;328:1581–6.
109. Fisher B, Dignam J, Wolmark N, et al. Lumpectomy and radiation therapy for the treatment of intraductal breast cancer: findings from National Surgical Adjuvant Breast and Bowel Project B-17. J Clin Oncol 1998;16:441–52.
110. Gallagher WJ, Koerner FC, Wood WC. Treatment of intraductal carcinoma with limited surgery: long-term follow-up. J Clin Oncol 1989;7:376–80.
111. Graham MD, Lakhani S, Gazet JC. Breast conserving surgery in the management of in situ breast carcinoma. Eur J Surg Oncol 1991;17:258–64.
112. Kuske RR, Bean JM, Garcia DM, et al. Breast conservation therapy for intraductal carcinoma of the breast. Int J Radiat Oncol Biol Phys 1993;26:391–6.
113. Lagios MD, Margolin FR, Westdahl PR, Rose MR. Mammographically detected duct carcinoma in situ: frequency of local recurrence following tylectomy and prognostic effect of nuclear grade on local recurrence. Cancer 1989;63:618–24.
114. Ottesen GL, Graversen HP, Blichert-Toft M, et al. Ductal carcinoma in situ of the female breast: short-term results of a prospective nationwide study. The Danish Breast Cancer Cooperative Group. Am J Surg Pathol 1992;16:1183–96.
115. Schwartz GF, Finkel GC, Garcia JC, Patchefsky AS. Subclinical ductal carcinoma in situ of the breast: treatment by local excision and surveillance alone. Cancer 1992;70:2468–74.
116. Silverstein MJ, Gierson ED, Colburn WJ, et al. Can intraductal breast carcinoma be excised completely by local excision? Clinical and pathologic predictors. Cancer 1994;73:2985–9.
117. Holland R, Connolly JL, Gelman R, et al. The presence of an extensive intraductal component following a limited excision correlates with prominent residual disease in the remainder of the breast. J Clin Oncol 1990;8:113–8.
118. Bornstein BA, Recht A, Connolly JL, et al. Results of treating ductal carcinoma in situ of the breast with conservative surgery and radiation therapy. Cancer 1991;67:7–13.
119. Bullock CG, Magnant C, Ayoob M, et al. The utility of conservative surgery and radiation therapy in ductal carcinoma in situ. Int J Radiat Oncol Biol Phys 1993;27:Suppl 1:268. abstract.
120. Fourquet A, Zafrani B, Campana F, et al. Breast-conserving treatment of ductal carcinoma in situ. Semin Radiat Oncol 1992;2:116–24.
121. Fowble B. Intraductal noninvasive breast cancer: a comparison of three local treatments. Oncology 1989;3:51–8.
122. Hiramatsu H, Bornstein BA, Recht A, et al. Outcome and risk factors for local failure after conservative surgery and radiotherapy for ductal carcinoma in situ. Int J Radiat Oncol Biol Phys 1994;30:Suppl 1:153. abstract.
123. Kurtz JM, Jacquemier J, Torhorst J, et al. Conservation therapy for breast cancers other than infiltrating ductal carcinoma. Cancer 1989;63:1630–5.
124. McCormick B, Rosen PP, Kinne D, et al. Duct carcinoma in situ of the breast: an analysis of local control after conservation surgery and radiotherapy. Int J Radiat Oncol Biol Phys 1991;21:289–92.
125. Ray GR, Adelson J, Hayhurst E, et al. Ductal carcinoma in situ of the breast: results of treatment by conservative surgery and definitive irradiation. Int J Radiat Oncol Biol Phys 1994;28:105–11.
126. Recht A, Danoff BS, Solin LJ, et al. Intraductal carcinoma of the breast: results of treatment with excisional biopsy and irradiation. J Clin Oncol 1985;3:1339–43.
127. Solin LJ, Fowble BL, Schultz DJ, et al. Definitive irradiation for intraductal carcinoma of the breast. Int J Radiat Oncol Biol Phys 1990;19:843–50.
128. Stotter AT, McNeese M, Oswald MJ, et al. The role of limited surgery with irradiation in primary treatment of ductal in situ breast cancer. Int J Radiat Oncol Biol Phys 1990;18:283–7.
129. White J, Levine A, Gustafson G, et al. Outcome and prognostic factors for local recurrence in mammographically detected ductal carcinoma in situ of the breast treated with conservative surgery and radiation therapy. Int J Radiat Oncol Biol Phys 1995;31:791–7.
130. Zafrani B, Fourquet A, Vilcoq JR, et al. Conservative management of intraductal breast carcinoma with tumorectomy and radiation therapy. Cancer 1986;57:1299–1301.
131. Solin LJ, Kurtz J, Fourquet A, et al. Fifteen-year results of breast-conserving surgery and definitive breast irradiation for the treatment of ductal carcinoma in situ of the breast. J Clin Oncol 1996;14:754–63.
132. Solin LJ, Recht A, Fourquet A, et al. Ten-year results of breast-conserving surgery and definitive irradiation for intraductal carcinoma (ductal carcinoma in situ) of the breast. Cancer 1991;68:2337–44.
133. Lagios MD, Silverstein MJ. Ductal carcinoma in situ: the success of breast conservation therapy: a shared experience of two single institutional nonrandomized prospective studies. Surg Oncol Clin N Am 1997;6:385–92.
134. Fisher B, Anderson S, Redmond CK, et al. Reanalysis and results after 12 years of follow-up in a randomized clinical trial comparing total mastectomy with lumpectomy with or without irradiation in the treatment of breast cancer. N Engl J Med 1995;333:1456–61.
135. Page DL, Lagios MD. Pathologic analysis of the National Surgical Adjuvant Breast Project (NSABP) B-17 Trial: unanswered questions remaining considering current concepts of ductal carcinoma in situ. Cancer 1995;75:1219–22.
136. Recht A, van Dongen JA, Fentiman IS, et al. Third meeting of the DCIS Working Party of the EORTC (Fondazione Cini, Isola S. Giorgio, Venezia, 28 February 1994)—Conference report. Eur J Cancer 1994;30A:1895–1900.
137. Fisher B, Redmond C, Poisson R, et al. Eight-year results of a randomized clinical trial comparing total mastectomy and lumpectomy with or without irradiation in the treatment of breast cancer. N Engl J Med 1989;320:822–8.
138. Fisher ER, Leeming R, Anderson S, et al. Conservative management of intraductal carcinoma (DCIS) of the breast. Collaborating NSABP investigators. J Surg Oncol 1991;47:139–47.
139. Bur ME, Zimarowski MJ, Schnitt SJ, et al. Estrogen receptor immunohistochemistry in carcinoma in situ of the breast. Cancer 1992;69:1174–81.

140. Chaudhuri B, Crist KA, Mucci S, et al. Distribution of estrogen receptor in ductal carcinoma in situ of the breast. Surgery 1993;113:134–7.
141. Holland PA, Knox WF, Potten CS, et al. Assessment of hormone dependence of comedo ductal carcinoma in situ of the breast. J Natl Cancer Inst 1997;89:1059–65.
142. Allred DC, Clark GM, Molina R, et al. Overexpression of HER-2/neu and its relationship with other prognostic factors change during the progression of in situ to invasive breast cancer. Hum Pathol 1992;23:974–9.
143. Brower ST, Ahmed S, Tartter PI, et al. Prognostic variables in invasive breast cancer: contribution of comedo versus noncomedo in situ component. Ann Surg Oncol 1995;2:440–4.
144. Pandelidis SM, Peters KL, Walusimbi MS, et al. The role of axillary dissection in mammographically detected carcinoma. J Am Coll Surg 1997;184:341–5.
145. Lagios MD. Duct carcinoma in situ: biological implications for clinical practice. Semin Oncol 1996;23:6–11.
146. Giuliano AE, Kirgan DM, Guenther JM, Morton DL. Lymphatic mapping and sentinel lymphadenectomy for breast cancer. Ann Surg 1994;220:391–8.
147. Silverstein MJ, Barth A, Poller DN, et al. Ten-year results comparing mastectomy to excision and radiation therapy for ductal carcinoma in situ of the breast. Eur J Cancer 1995;31A:1425–7.
148. Hillner BE, Desch CE, Carlson RW, et al. Trade-offs between survival and breast preservation for three initial treatments of ductal carcinoma-in-situ of the breast. J Clin Oncol 1996;14:70–7.
149. Solin LJ, Yeh IT, Kurtz J, et al. Ductal carcinoma in situ (intraductal carcinoma) of the breast treated with breast-conserving surgery and definitive irradiation: correlation of pathologic parameters with outcome of treatment. Cancer 1993;71:2532–42.
150. Silverstein MJ, Lagios MD, Craig PH, et al. A prognostic index for ductal carcinoma in situ of the breast. Cancer 1996;77:2267–74.
151. Liberman L, Van Zee KJ, Dershaw DD, et al. Mammographic features of local recurrence in women who have undergone breast-conserving therapy for ductal carcinoma in situ. AJR Am J Roentgenol 1997;168:489–93.
152. Solin LJ, Fowble BL, Troupin RH, Goodman RL. Biopsy results of new calcifications in the postirradiated breast. Cancer 1989;63:1956–61.
153. Solin LJ, Fourquet A, McCormick B, et al. Salvage treatment for local recurrence following breast-conserving surgery and definitive irradiation for ductal carcinoma in situ (intraductal carcinoma) of the breast. Int J Radiat Oncol Biol Phys 1994;30:3–9.
154. Silverstein MJ, Lagios MD, Martino S, et al. Outcome after invasive local recurrence in patients with ductal carcinoma in situ of the breast. J Clin Oncol 1998;16:1367–73.
155. Gump FE. Lobular carcinoma in situ: pathology and treatment. Surg Clin North Am 1990;70:873–83.
156. Ringberg A, Andersson I, Aspegren K, Linell F. Breast carcinoma in situ in 167 women—incidence, mode of presentation, therapy and follow-up. Eur J Surg Oncol 1991;17:466–76.
157. Rosen PP, Senie RT, Farr GH, et al. Epidemiology of breast carcinoma: age, menstrual status, and exogenous hormone usage in patients with lobular carcinoma in situ. Surgery 1979;85:219–24.
158. Ottesen GL, Graversen HP, Blichert-Toft M, et al. Lobular carcinoma in situ of the female breast: short-term results of a prospective nationwide study. The Danish Breast Cancer Cooperative Group. Am J Surg Pathol 1993;17:14–21.
159. Fisher ER, Costantino J, Fisher B, et al. Pathologic findings from the National Surgical Adjuvant Breast Project (NSABP) Protocol B-17: five-year observations concerning lobular carcinoma in situ. Cancer 1996;78:1403–16.
160. Haagensen CD, Bodian C, Haagensen DE Jr. Lobular neoplasia (lobular carcinoma in situ). In: Breast cancer: risk and detection. Philadelphia: WB Saunders, 1981:238.
161. Fisher ER, Fisher B. Lobular carcinoma of the breast: an overview. Ann Surg 1977;185:377–85.
162. Rosen PP. Lobular carcinoma in situ and intraductal carcinoma of the breast. Monogr Pathol 1984;25:59–105.
163. Haagensen CD, Lane N, Lattes R, Bodian C. Lobular neoplasia (so-called lobular carcinoma in situ) of the breast. Cancer 1978;42:737–69.
164. Page DL, Kidd TE Jr, Dupont WD, et al. Lobular neoplasia of the breast: higher risk for subsequent invasive cancer predicted by more extensive disease. Hum Pathol 1991;22:1232–9.
165. Bodian CA, Perzin KH, Lattes R. Lobular neoplasia: long term risk of breast cancer and relation to other factors. Cancer 1996;78:1024–34.
166. Gump FE. Lobular carcinoma in situ (LCIS): pathology and treatment. J Cell Biochem 1993;17G:Suppl:53–8.
167. Carson W, Sanchez-Forgach E, Stomper P, et al. Lobular carcinoma in situ: observation without surgery as an appropriate therapy. Ann Surg Oncol 1994;1:141–6.
168. Goldschmidt RA, Victor TA. Lobular carcinoma in situ of the breast. Semin Surg Oncol 1996;12:314–20.
169. Cody HS 3rd. Routine contralateral breast biopsy: helpful or irrelevant? Experience in 871 patients, 1979–1993. Ann Surg 1997;225:370–6.

# LOCAL TREATMENT WITH SURGERY

• Helena R. Chang

The surgical management of breast cancer has undergone continuous evolution since the 1980s with respect to types of surgery based on understanding of the disease. Nonetheless, surgery remains the primary therapeutic modality for early and locally advanced breast cancer. This section discusses the current issues surrounding the surgical management of breast cancer with respect to issues of breast and axillary management.

## PRESENTATION

Breast cancer typically occurs in perimenopausal and post-menopausal women. Approximately 50% of patients with breast cancer are diagnosed after age 60. Patients may present with a breast or axillary mass (or both), nipple discharge or retraction, skin dimpling, an eczematous nipple, breast pain, or inflammatory changes. With increased acceptance of breast cancer screening, many women now present with asymptomatic mammographic findings. The frequent radiographic signs for breast cancer are a spiculated mass, asymmetric density, architectural distortion, and microcalcifications that are suspicious in appearance, worsening during two consecutive studies, or associated with a mass.

## DIAGNOSIS

The initial breast cancer diagnosis can be made by histologic or cytologic studies. Patients who present with a mass may undergo fine-needle aspiration for cytology, or they may undergo a biopsy by core needle or surgical removal. Patients with nonpalpable suspicious microcalcifications may undergo stereotactic core biopsy. A nonpalpable breast mass can be approached by ultrasound-guided or stereotactic core biopsy as a nonoperative procedure. When surgery is indicated, all nonpalpable breast lesions require preoperative wire localization and radiographs of the specimens to guide and confirm an accurate removal.

Histologically, breast cancers are divided into malignancies of the epithelial cells lining the ducts and lobules and nonepithelial cells of the stroma, with the former as the dominant type of breast cancer. These carcinomas are further divided into *in situ* and *infiltrating* types. In situ carcinomas are confined within the basement membrane. LCIS is an abnormal proliferation of the lobular and acinar cells, which typically do not cause ductal expansion and frequently are not palpable. LCIS does not have characteristic mammographic findings. LCIS is usually diagnosed as an incidental finding. DCIS is frequently present as suspicious microcalcifications seen on mammography and less frequently as a palpable abnormality. These microcalcifications are usually the result of central necrosis of tumor cells within the ducts. An important aspect of DCIS is its tendency to be multifocal (disease within the same quadrant) and sometimes multicentric (disease found in other quadrants of the same breast). Extensive multifocal presentation or multicentric distribution may make breast conservation treatment impossible.

## STAGING

Breast cancers are staged clinically and pathologically. Clinical staging is highly inaccurate with respect to tumor size and nodal involvement. Because of the inadequacy of clinical staging, pathologic staging for nonmetastatic breast cancer is required to determine prognosis and to guide adjuvant chemotherapy. The current staging system published by the AJCC is based on the TNM system.

## SURGICAL TREATMENT

The two major operations for early invasive breast cancer are the modified radical mastectomy (MRM) and breast conservation treatment (BCT). The following discussion describes the historical development of these techniques, the current operative techniques, choice of procedures, and their respective potential complications.

**History.** The changes in surgical management of invasive breast cancer have paralleled the understanding of its mode of spread. In 1894, Halsted[1] reported a low local recurrence rate of 6% and 3-year survival rate of 45% in patients he treated by radical mastectomy. Radical mastectomy was developed based on an assumption that breast cancer spreads in an orderly fashion from breast to axillary lymph nodes before hematogenous metastasis. It involved removal of the breast, pectoralis major and minor muscles, and axillary nodes levels I through III. Because the success of locally controlling breast cancer by radical mastectomy exceeded other operations of his time, it became the operation of choice for invasive breast cancer throughout the early 20th century.

Subsequently the radical mastectomy underwent several modifications with more radical approaches; however, despite its success at decreasing local recurrence, it did not affect overall survival. Halsted noted that 23% of node-negative patients who were presumably cured of all local-regional disease eventually died of disease.

The radical mastectomy was succeeded by the MRM that was described by Patey and Dyson[2, 3] of London's Middlesex hospital in 1948. This modification spared the pectoralis major muscle from the previous radical mastectomy. The change reflected the recognition that the treatment failures from the radical mastectomy were frequently systemic rather than local. The more conservative MRM continued to evolve as Auchincloss of the Columbia Presbyterian Hospital further proposed to spare the pectoralis minor.[4, 5] In 1980, the National Institutes of Health consensus conference adopted the MRM as an acceptable alternative to the radical mastectomy. The MRM remains the most common surgical procedure for breast cancer.[6]

As the biology of breast cancer became better understood, the need for mastectomy was further questioned and prompted another modification in surgical treatment: BCT. BCT involves lumpectomy, axillary dissection, and breast radiation therapy. Multiple randomized clinical trials have been conducted comparing outcomes in MRM versus BCT, showing no difference in survival between the two operations.[7–13] In 1996, the National Cancer Institute consensus conference on the treatment of early-stage breast cancer concluded that "BCT is an appropriate method of primary therapy for the majority of women with stage I and II breast cancer. It is preferable because it provides survival equivalence to total mastectomy and axillary dissection while preserving the breast."[14] The 20th century has seen a continued evolution in the understanding of breast cancer spread, which leads to surgical procedures that are not only more sound biologically, but also less morbid.

**Modified Radical Mastectomy.** The most commonly used MRM involves removal of the breast, including the nipple-areolar complex and axillary nodes.[15] The pectoralis major and minor muscles are preserved. The axillary nodal dissection is frequently limited to levels I and II. The procedure is performed via an elliptical skin incision encompassing the biopsy scar and nipple-areolar complex. The skin flaps are developed superiorly to clavicle, inferiorly to rectus sheath, medially to sternal border, and laterally to latissimus dorsi. The breast and the pectoralis major fascia are removed from the pectoralis major muscle in a medio-superior to lateroinferior direction. The nodes are removed by retracting the pectoralis major and the pectoralis minor medially and anteriorly to allow the exposure of axillary vein. The axillary content below axillary vein and at the level behind the pectoralis muscles is removed en bloc with the breast. The long thoracic nerve innervating the serratus anterior muscles is preserved. Damage to this nerve can result in the *winged scapula* and diminished shoulder strength. Laterally the thoracodorsal nerve supplying the latissimus dorsi muscle is preserved. Once the specimen is removed, two soft Silastic tube drains are placed. One drain is placed along the chest wall and the other in the axilla. These drains are placed to prevent seroma formation. The drains are frequently removed 1 week postoperatively when their output has decreased to less than 30 to 50 ml a day.

**Complications.** The potential complications following MRM are few and infrequent. Early complications of MRM include wound infection, skin flap necrosis, and seroma formation. Seromas may involve the skin flaps at the chest wall or the axilla after removal of the closed suction drains. These seromas can be treated with percutaneous aspiration. Rarely, persistent seromas require replacement of closed suction drains.

Late complications include lymphedema of the arm as well as postmastectomy pain. The incidence of lymphedema is 10 to 20%. The combination of axillary dissection and irradiation predisposes patients to lymphedema of the arm. It is generally recommended to avoid heavy lifting, venipuncture, constrictive pressure of the arm and hand as well as soft tissue infection at the involved arm or chest wall to minimize the risk of developing lymphedema. Persistent postmastectomy pain of chest wall and axilla is usually associated with neuroma formation of sensory cutaneous nerves divided during dissection.

### Breast Conservation Surgery

*Patient Selection.* Lumpectomy and axillary dissection has become the preferred method of surgical management of stage I and II breast cancer.[16] Important considerations of breast conservation surgical technique include placement of the incision site, achieving tumor-free margins, and adequate axillary dissections. Most important to breast conservation surgery is proper patient selection. Factors that affect the choice of surgery are outlined as follows:

- *Tumor size.* In general, tumors greater than 5 cm are not amenable to BCT, and MRM is recommended. Similarly the same concept applies for tumors that are disproportionately large in relation to the size of the breast.
- *Tumor location.* Tumors that are retronipple or subareolar may result in a compromised cosmetic appearance, which sometimes renders the tumor less suitable for BCT.
- *Multicentric cancers.* Tumors in different quadrants of the breast or at least 3 cm apart may compromise the cosmesis and local control of the disease. Such tumors may be better treated with MRM.
- *Persistent tumor involvement of tumor margins despite multiple excisions.* MRM is preferred because of the wide spread of the disease within the breast.
- Extensive DCIS in an invasive cancer or diffuse suspicious microcalcifications are associated with a higher incidence of local failure, particularly in young women (≤35 years). Dense breasts on mammography associated with young women may also make follow-up difficult.
- Pregnancy and previous irradiation treatment to the breast are absolute contraindications for postlumpectomy radiation. These patients should be treated with MRM instead of BCT.

*Techniques of Breast Conservation Surgery.* Important aspects to consider in performing lumpectomy are making the proper incision and obtaining adequate tumor-free margins. Curvilinear skin incisions in the direction of Langer's lines are preferred in general. The incision should be placed adjacent to the cancer and can be incorporated into the subsequent mastectomy incision if necessary. In cases of re-

excision for positive margins, the scar and the previous lumpectomy cavity are removed as one specimen. With respect to obtaining proper margins, at least 1 cm of normal tissue around the tumor should be provided. Once the specimen is excised, it is important to orient the specimen for histologic analysis. Commonly, short and long stitches are placed in the superior and lateral edges.

Axillary dissection is a part of breast conservation surgery. It differs from MRM in that it is performed through a separate skin incision in the axilla. It is usually placed just caudad to the axillary hairline in a curvilinear fashion along Langer's skin lines. Similar to the MRM, the axillary dissection is frequently limited to levels I to II, with the pectoralis muscles preserved. The boundaries of the dissection are also the same with the apical dissection at the medial edge of the pectoralis minor, and laterally, dissection is completed at the latissimus dorsi muscle. The long thoracic and thoracodorsal nerves are preserved. An axillary drain is left for 5 to 7 days to prevent seroma formation.

## AXILLARY MANAGEMENT

Axillary lymph node dissection has been part of the surgical treatment of breast cancer for the following reasons: (1) to allow proper staging, (2) to provide useful prognostic information, (3) to guide for subsequent treatment, and (4) to increase potential therapeutic gain. Axillary lymph node dissection is recommended for all patients with invasive cancer. In the absence of grossly involved high axillary nodes, level I and II dissection is considered optimal. Selective arguments to support the inclusion of level II lymph node dissection as part of the nodal removal are summarized as follows:

- Studies have shown that the accuracy of pathologic staging of lymph nodes depends on the number of lymph nodes that are removed and examined. A minimum of 10 nodes should be retrieved to ensure accurate pathologic staging of the axilla. Axillary dissection, including levels I and II, provides a sufficient number of lymph nodes for pathologic evaluation.[17, 18]
- Skip metastasis identified in level III is rare (1 to 3%)[19]; however, the incidence is relatively high for level II (approximately 15%). Axillary dissection of less than level I and II removal results in a significant chance of downstaging the disease and retention of metastatic lymph nodes.
- In the absence of extracapsular tumor extension or numerous nodal metastases, level I and II axillary dissection provides adequate regional control. When the combination of axillary dissection and radiation is needed, it is less morbid if dissection does not include level III.
- There may be survival benefits in the subset of patients who have only microscopic nodal metastases that are completely removed as part of the level I and II dissection.[20]
- There has been increasing difficulty in justifying the practice of routine axillary dissection. The trend of surgery is moving toward minimal invasiveness and maximal function preservation. The challenge is to apply axillary dissection only to patients with metastatic nodes. The breast cancer size on presentation has been progressively smaller

because of the widespread usage of screening mammography. The probability of nodal involvement diminishes as the tumor size decreases.

Axillary dissection has been suggested in controlling regional disease. Although NSABP B-04 showed an equivalent survival among women who had axillary dissection as part of the initial surgical treatment or delayed axillary dissection when axillary nodes became clinically suspicious, one third of the women in the latter group actually had partial axillary nodes removed. Even so, 20% of women in the observed group subsequently required nodal dissection for grossly metastatic nodes. Success of the salvage therapy in these women was reportedly low.[21] A retrospective review of the National Cancer Data Base (NCDB) of 47,944 stage I and 23,283 stage II breast cancers revealed a more frequent omission of axillary dissection in women with small breast cancer, low-grade cancer, elderly age, and low socioeconomic class. The 10-year survival rate was superior in stage I women treated with partial mastectomy and axillary dissection (85%) when compared with women with comparable clinical stage without axillary dissection (66%). Adding radiation and adjuvant chemotherapy to women in the latter group did not improve survival rate (58%).[22]

Surgeons have re-evaluated operative approaches toward nodal staging. Attempts have been made to develop a model for women with small cancer in whom the risk of nodal metastasis is minimal, with the intent of sparing them axillary dissection. Using a risk profile of the individual's age, tumor size, and differentiation, elderly women with T1a (<0.5 cm) and well-differentiated breast cancer carried a risk of 7% for nodal metastasis. This risk is in contrast to 37% of young women (≤40 years) with T1b (<1 cm but >0.5 cm) and less well differentiated tumors having nodal metastases.[23] This risk profile may facilitate a selective approach to axillary dissection in some women. Applicability of these risk factors has been further evaluated to predict cancer-related death. The thought was it could serve as a surrogate of nodal information. In a multivariate analysis of 2153 patients with 1-cm breast cancer, none of these factors was found to be of equivalent value to nodal staging.[24] The lymph node status remains critical in assessing patient prognosis and in guiding the choice of adjuvant systemic treatment.

Although data still suggest benefit from axillary dissection, including early-stage breast cancer, this procedure is morbid and unnecessary for many women with breast cancer. Before an improved classification can be used to replace the current TNM staging, effort should be directed toward selectively performing axillary node dissection only in those with nodal metastasis. Sentinel lymph node (SLN) mapping may be an ideal approach for select patients who require conventional lymphadenectomy. The rationale of SLN mapping is that each breast cancer has its unique lymph node draining preference. The SLNs represent the first draining nodes that are most likely to be involved in tumor metastasis. When SLNs are free of cancer, it is assumed that the remaining lymph nodes are not involved by metastasis. The goal of SLN mapping is to develop a minimally invasive procedure with least morbidity and a maximally predictive value for nodal metastasis.

SLN mapping can be achieved by injecting radiolabeled tracers[25–27] or vital dye[28, 29] that are primarily taken up by the particular lymphatics of a cancer and trapped in the SLNs for a variable period.[30, 31] The preferred radiocolloid agent is technetium 99m sulfur colloid (filtered or nonfiltered). These SLNs can be located either by a hand-held gamma counter or by visible blue dye.

The technique that has been adopted by the Revlon/UCLA Breast Center for localizing SLNs consists of preoperative injection of either 1 mCi of technetium 99m sulfur colloid at least 2 hours before surgery or 2 mCi of nonfiltered technetium 99m sulfur colloid the night before surgery, with or without intraoperative injection of isosulfan blue (Lymphazurin) (3 to 6 ml) 5 to 10 minutes before axillary incision. Lymphoscintigraphy immediately before surgery may be helpful, particularly for inner-quadrant lesions; however, it is not essential. Before skin incision and using a hand-held gamma counter, the radioactivity at the injection site, upper arm area and ipsilateral axilla, and supraclavicular, infraclavicular, and second through fourth intercostal areas are scanned individually and recorded. If the radioactivity is localized in the axilla, the area with the most intense radioactivity is marked for incision. When isosulfan blue is given, a lesion at the upper-outer quadrant requires less dye and a shorter waiting period before axillary incision than those in the inner quadrants. A primary breast cancer adjacent to the axilla frequently needs to be removed before mapping the SLNs because of the high radioactivity in the background. The incision for the SLN removal in axilla is typically small and is carried deeply to the node-bearing area. The blue lymphatics that lead to the blue nodes are first identified, and the hand-held gamma counter is used to search the axilla level I and II. Both the highly radioactive (high-count) nodes and blue lymph nodes are removed, and the ex vivo count of each lymph node is recorded. A complete removal of the SLNs is confirmed by a minimal residual radioactivity in the axillary wound that approaches the background count.

Several important questions regarding the application of SLN mapping need to be addressed before accepting this procedure as a possible alternative to axillary lymph node dissection:

1. *What is the rate of identifying SLNs in the axilla?* The detection rate of SLNs in the axilla is high, with most reports showing a detection rate of 90% or higher. The SLNs are more likely to be in the axilla than in the internal mammary chain, even when the primary cancer is in inner quadrants. Previous wide excision, elderly age, and obesity have been associated with lower detection rates.

2. *What is the false-negative prediction rate of SLNs when compared with axillary dissection?* The false-negative prediction or skip metastases made by SLNs is approximately 5% or less,[26, 31, 32] which is acceptable to most physicians and patients.

3. *What is the clinical significance of micrometastasis detected in the SLNs by the immunohistochemical staining or polymerase chain reaction techniques?* More thorough pathologic examination of SLNs is made possible because fewer lymph nodes need to be examined. This change in practice leads to an increased detection of micrometastasis

in the SLNs. The clinical significance of upstaging nodal metastasis is unclear at present. The recommendation regarding subsequent full axillary dissection or adjuvant chemotherapy in patients with micrometastasis in SLNs detected by either immunohistochemical staining or polymerase chain reaction requires a better understanding of its natural history.

In addition to SLN mapping, other noninvasive techniques, such as positron emission tomography as well as antibody-mediated lymphoscintigraphy, have been investigated for axillary staging. The use of positron emission tomography scan in detecting breast cancer has been described by Auril and colleagues.[33] In this study, breast cancer patients with clinically negative axillae underwent intravenous injection of a radiolabeled glucose analogue, followed by a total-body positron emission tomography scan. The positron emission tomography scan findings were compared with pathologic nodal staging. The authors reported a 79% overall sensitivity of this technique. The sensitivity increased to 94% if primary breast tumors were limited to tumors greater than 2 cm. The reported specificity was 96% overall and 100% when limited to primary tumors of 2 cm or bigger. Positron emission tomography imaging for large breast cancer may not only provide information regarding nodal status, but also possible distant metastasis.

Another technology, immune lymphoscintigraphy, involves the subcutaneous injection of radiolabeled mouse monoclonal antibody against a breast cancer antigen. The radioactivity localized in the axilla by a hand-held gamma probe indicates nodal metastasis. This technique has been reported with a sensitivity of 86% and specificity of 97%.[34] When coupled with preoperative clinical assessment, sensitivity was improved to 100%; however, the specificity was low. In the future, cancer-directed imagings coupled with other clinical and pathologic markers of the primary breast cancer may replace the need for surgical removal of lymph nodes for staging.

## CONCLUSIONS

BCT and MRM are the two accepted surgical operations for early-stage breast cancer, with BCT as the preferred operation when possible. With respect to axillary management, current standards recommend a level I to II axillary lymph node dissection for prognostic information, to guide adjuvant treatment, and for improved local-regional control. A growing body of literature exists questioning the need for a routine level I to II dissection. SLN mapping may spare node-negative women from a formal axillary dissection. In the future, better characterization of primary tumors may provide sufficient prognostic information that can guide adjuvant therapy. Tumor-specific imagings may make it possible to achieve selective axillary management.

## ACKNOWLEDGMENT

The author thanks Melanie Moorehead for help in the preparation of this manuscript.

## REFERENCES

1. Halsted WS. The results of radical operations for the cure of cancer of the breast. Tr Am SA 1907;25:61–79.
2. Patey DH, Dyson WH. The prognosis of carcinoma of the breast in relation to the type of operation performed. Br J Cancer 1948;2:7–13.
3. Patey DH. A review of 146 cases of carcinoma of the breast operated on between 1930 and 1943. Br J Cancer 1967;21:260–9.
4. Madden JL. Modified radical mastectomy. Surg Gynecol Obstet 1965;121:1221–30.
5. Madden JL, Kandalaft S, Bourque RA. Modified radical mastectomy. Ann Surg 1972;175:624–34.
6. Morrow M. Local management of primary breast cancer. Cancer Control 1997;4:201–24.
7. Fisher B, Redmond C, Poisson R, et al. Eight-year results of a randomized clinical trial comparing total mastectomy and lumpectomy with or without irradiation in the treatment of breast cancer. N Engl J Med 1989;320:822–8.
8. Veronesi U, Banfi A, Del Vecchio M, et al. Comparison of Halsted mastectomy with quadrantectomy, axillary dissection, and radiotherapy in early breast cancer: long-term results. Eur J Cancer Clin Oncol 1986;22:1085–9.
9. Sarrazin D, Le MG, Arriagada R, et al. Ten-year results of a randomized trial comparing a conservative treatment to mastectomy in early breast cancer. Radiother Oncol 1989;14:177–84.
10. Blichert-Toft M. Danish randomized trial comparing breast conservation with mastectomy in mammary carcinoma. Br J Cancer 1990;62:Suppl 12:15.
11. Bader J, Lippman ME, Swain SM, et al. Preliminary report of the NCI early breast cancer study: a prospective randomized trial comparison of lumpectomy and radiation to mastectomy for stage I and II breast cancer. Int J Radiat Oncol Biol Phys 1987;13:Suppl:160.
12. Glastein E, Strauss K, Lichter A, et al. Results of the NCI early breast cancer trial. Proceedings of the NIH Consensus Development Conference, June 18–21, 1990:32.
13. Fisher B, Anderson S, Redmond CK, et al. Reanalysis and results after 12 years of follow-up in a randomized clinical trial comparing total mastectomy with lumpectomy with or without irradiation in the treatment of breast cancer. N Engl J Med 1995;333:1456–61.
14. Nixon AJ, Troyan SL, Harris JR. Option in the local management of invasive breast cancer. Semin Oncol 1996;23:453–63.
15. Bland KI, Chang HR, Copeland EM. Modified radical mastectomy and total mastectomy in the breast. In: Bland KI, Copeland EM, eds. The breast: comprehensive management of benign and malignant diseases. 2nd ed. Philadelphia: WB Saunders, 1998:881.
16. Chang HR, Bland KI. Local management of breast cancer. In: Rakel RE, ed. Conn's current therapy. Philadelphia: WB Saunders, 1996:1029.
17. Fisher B, Bauer M, Margolese R, et al. Five-year results of a randomized clinical trial comparing total mastectomy and segmental mastectomy with or without radiation in the treatment of breast cancer. N Engl J Med 1985;312:665–73.
18. Veronesi U, Rilke F, Luine A, et al. Distribution of axillary metastases by level of invasion. Cancer 1987;59:682–7.
19. Rosen PP, Lesser ML, Kinne DW, Bettie FJ. Discontinuous or "skip" metastases in breast carcinoma analysis of 1228 axillary dissections. Ann Surg 1983;197:276–83.
20. Harris JR, Osteen RT. Patients with early breast cancer benefit from effective axillary treatment. Breast Cancer Res Treat 1985;5:17–21.
21. Recht A, Pierce SM, Abner A, et al. Regional nodal failure after conservative surgery and radiotherapy for early stage breast carcinoma. J Clin Oncol 1991;9:988–96.
22. Bland KI, Scott-Conner CEH, Menck H, Winchester DP. Axillary dissection in breast-conserving surgery for stage I and II breast cancer: A national cancer data base study of patterns of omission and implications for survival. J Am Coll Surg 1999;186:562–9.
23. Mustafa IA, Cole B, Wanebo HJ, et al. The impact of histology on nodal metastasis in minimal breast cancer. Arch Surg 1997;132:384–91.
24. Mustafa IA, Cole B, Wanebo HJ, et al. Prognostic analysis of survival in small breast cancers. J Am Coll Surg 1998;186:562–9.
25. Krag D, Weaver D, Ashikaga T, et al. The sentinel lymph node in breast cancer—a multicenter validation study. N Engl J Med 1998;339:941–6.
26. Offodile R, Hoh C, Barsky SH, et al. Minimally invasive breast carcinoma staging using lymphatic mapping with radiolabeled dextran. Cancer 1998;82:1704–8.

27. Krag DN, Ashikaga T, Harlow SP, Weaver DL. Development of sentinel node targeting technique in breast cancer patients. Breast 1998;4:67–74.
28. Giuliano AE, Kirgan DM, Guenther JM, Morton DL. Lymphatic mapping and sentinel lymphadenectomy for breast cancer. Ann Surg 1994;220:391–8.
29. Giuliano AE, Dale PS, Turner RR, et al. Improved axillary staging of breast cancer with sentinel lymphadenectomy. Ann Surg 1995;222:394–9.
30. Cox CE, Pendas S, Cox JM, et al. Guidelines for sentinel node biopsy and lymphatic mapping of patients with breast cancer. Ann Surg 1998;227:645–51.
31. Albertini JJ, Lyman GH, Cox C, et al. Lymphatic mapping and sentinel node biopsy in the patient with breast cancer. JAMA 1996;276:1818–22.
32. Reintgen D, Emmanuella J, Lyman GH, et al. The role of selective lymphadenectomy in breast cancer. Cancer Control 1997;4:211–9.
33. Auril N, Dose J, Janich F, et al. Assessment of axillary lymph node involvement in breast cancer patients with positron emission tomography using radiolabeled 18 fluoro-2-deoxy-D glucose. J Natl Cancer Inst 1996;88:1204–9.
34. Tjandra JJ, Russell IS, Collins JP, et al. Immunolymphatic scintigraphy for dissection of lymph node metastases from breast cancer. Cancer Res 1989;49:1600–8.

......................................

# SURGICAL RECONSTRUCTION

• William W. Shaw

The trend toward less disfiguring mastectomy and breast conservation surgery has reduced considerably the fear of mutilation associated with the diagnosis and treatment of breast cancer. For oncologic reasons and personal preference, however, many women are still candidates for mastectomy. Although the female breast is not essential for survival or indispensable for any biologic function after child rearing, its absence may cause significant functional and emotional problems (Table 35–15). Because of the personal suffering and compromised quality of life, surgical reconstruction should be considered in all suitable patients. It should not be considered a frivolous cosmetic procedure.

## METHODS AND APPLICATIONS OF BREAST RECONSTRUCTION

**Historical Considerations.** In the early part of the 20th century, several multistage reconstructions were described using tube flaps from the abdomen or opposite breast.[1] The breast mound created was generally inadequate, and the results were marginal by today's standards.

In 1963, Cronin and Bauer, working with Dow Corning, developed the first silicone breast implant, a round outer silicone envelope containing viscous silicone gel.[2] When placed in a subcutaneous or submuscular pocket, this instantly produced a reasonable breast mound. Many different implant designs have been marketed over the years. Also, to overcome the problem of skin tightness and to provide better coverage over the implant, several flap techniques were described, such as local flaps, omentum, or latissimus dorsi muscle flaps. In 1982, Radovan[3] introduced the concept of tissue expansion with a reinjectable saline implant and added more control of the skin envelope over the implant. The results of implant reconstructions, however, were not always consistent owing to the unpredictable foreign body reaction and the deforming capsular contracture. Also, there were increasing concerns over the potential problems of silicone leakage, implant rupture, and possible systemic symptoms. In 1993, the FDA issued a moratorium on the use of the standard gel-filled implants. Such implants are now available only under an experimental protocol for breast reconstruction and for replacement of ruptured implants. Saline-filled implants, however, are still available.

In 1976, Fujino and colleagues[4] described a superior gluteal free flap for breast reconstruction without silicone implants, initiating the era of autologous tissue reconstruction. Hartrampf and colleagues[5] described the use of pedicled rectus abdominis muscle and lower abdominal skin to achieve superb results in breast reconstruction. Subsequently, this procedure has increasingly been done as a microvascular free flap because of the improved blood supply and the

*Table 35–15.* **Functional and Emotional Problems After Mastectomy**

Pain
  Chest wall pain or discomfort
  Shoulder or back discomfort from breast asymmetry
  Tightness and restriction of shoulder, especially after radiation therapy
Problems with external prostheses
  Heaviness
  Folliculitis
  Displacement
  Limitations in choice of clothing and physical activity
Emotional problems
  Feeling disfigured or maimed
  Fear of loss of feminine attractiveness and rejection
  Painful reminder of cancer and threat of death

*Table 35–16.* **Options in Breast Reconstruction**

| Method | Ideal Patients |
| --- | --- |
| Silicone implant (with tissue expander if needed) | Good skin with intact pectoralis minor muscle |
|  | Elderly and poor-risk patient |
|  | Young mother with limited time |
| Pedicled latissimus dorsi muscle and back skin as fleur-de-lis flap without implant | Loose back skin with generous fat |
|  | Smaller breast |
| TRAM flap, pedicled or free | Patient unsuitable for TRAM flap |
|  | Moderately built woman with 2–4 cm of abdominal fat (this is true of 80% of patients) |
| Other free flaps: gluteus, tensor fascia lata | Thin abdomen |
|  | TRAM failure |

TRAM, transverse rectus abdominis myocutaneous.

reduced muscle function loss.[6] Other methods of autologous reconstruction included the omentum, a trilobed latissimus dorsi flap (fleur-de-lis flap), the tensor fascia lata free flap, and other free flaps.[7] The more extensive surgery and donor scars are well justified by the permanent and remarkably realistic results achieved. These methods are now routinely used for a variety of reconstructive situations.

**Current Methods of Breast Reconstruction.** The relative indications of the various methods of breast reconstruction are summarized in Table 35–16. Our experience at the UCLA Breast Center has shown that about 80% of patients are suitable for the transverse rectus abdominis myocutaneous free flap technique. It is also our reconstruction of choice. It is an excellent method for immediate reconstruction. The thoracodorsal vessels are already exposed, and the flap is raised simultaneously with the mastectomy (Fig. 35–16). When the abdomen is too thin with insufficient bulk, the superior gluteal free flap is the next choice (Fig. 35–17). For patients with significant anesthetic risks or reluctance over the magnitude of the flap operations, tissue expanders and later implant placement are used.

There is no single perfect method that fits every patient. Each reconstruction should be customized based on the patient's risk factors, reconstructive needs, and availability of donor tissues. The patient must also understand the pros and cons of the different options. For instance, when choosing a simpler implant reconstruction, the patient must accept some aesthetic limitations and the possibility of later implant complications or the need for additional surgical correction. Selecting a permanent reconstruction with the patient's own tissues would require more extensive initial surgery and the acceptance of its attendant risks. In nearly all patients, however, a reasonable reconstruction can be achieved.

## APPLICATIONS OF BREAST RECONSTRUCTION

Breast reconstruction is indicated whenever there is potential disfigurement of the breast or loss of chest wall coverage. The common reconstructive solutions for the different situations are summarized in Table 35–17. An autologous tissue reconstruction may be an essential part of the local breast cancer treatment in certain circumstances. These can be summarized as presented in the following sections.

*Table 35–17.* **Reconstructive Problems and Possible Solutions**

| Problems | Solutions |
| --- | --- |
| Lumpectomy with deformity | Contralateral reduction or latissimus flap augmentation |
| Mastectomy reconstruction (immediate or delayed) | Flaps (TRAM, gluteus) or implant/expanders |
| Bilateral mastectomies | Bilateral TRAM flaps or implants |
| Lumpectomy with recurrence | Mastectomy with immediate flap |
| Chest wall recurrence | Resection and immediate flap (Latissimus free TRAM or gluteus) |
| Radiation necrosis | Resection and immediate flap (Latissimus free TRAM or tensor) |

TRAM, transverse rectus abdominis myocutaneous.

**Mastectomy for Recurrence After Previous Lumpectomy and Radiation.** The breast skin is often stiff from radiation in these patients, and the amount of skin excision needed may be substantial. Primary closure or reconstruction with implants would be difficult and associated with a high incidence of failure. Immediate reconstruction with a flap allows for comfortable wound closure and good aesthetic results.

**Radiation Necrosis or Brachial Plexus Neuropathy.** When ribs or sternum is exposed because of radiation damage to the skin and soft tissues, wide debridement and skin excision are needed to prevent progressive infection and necrosis. Also, in cases of pain and brachial plexus neuropathy from radiation to the axilla, neurolysis and excision of constricting dense scar may be indicated. In both situations, the local skin is generally compromised and insufficient to provide coverage. Wound breakdown and infection may ensue. Instead, healthy, well-vascularized tissue from the back or elsewhere should be transplanted into the wound to achieve reliable primary healing.

**Palliative Resections for Control of Local Recurrence.** Skin recurrences involving large areas of chest wall may require wide resection for palliation to avoid the miserable outcome of a foul-smelling, necrotizing lesion. Wide resection and immediate flap reconstruction can achieve effective local palliation (Fig. 35–18).

**Salvage After Failed Implant Reconstructions.** The possibility of a poor cosmetic result, pain, infection, or loss of an implant is inherent to silicone implant breast reconstruction. In cases of repeated implant failures or unsuitable local skin conditions, autologous tissue replacement of the implant is an invaluable alternative for these greatly distressed patients.

**Deformity After Lumpectomy and Radiation.** Asymmetry or localized tissue deficiency may result from lumpectomy and radiation. If there is generous breast tissue in the opposite breast, a reduction or mastopexy may be sufficient to achieve symmetry. Other times, the localized depression can be corrected with a latissimus dorsi myocutaneous flap or scapular skin flap from the adjacent back.

## CONCLUSION

Patients who require an MRM for local control as well as those who choose this procedure for personal reasons should be offered consultation with a surgeon trained in the specialized techniques of reconstructive surgery. The goal of such reconstruction is to provide a lasting mound of tissue with an acceptable shape, form, and consistency that is reasonably symmetric with that of the opposite breast. In the past, this reconstruction was usually accomplished by the use of a silicone implant. Silicone implants have been associated with a variety of complications, however, including possible rheumatologic problems, and their use has dramatically declined.[8] The optimal approach now involves the use of the patient's own tissues using one of several techniques of transplantation. An example of such an approach involving a transverse rectus abdominis muscle flap is shown in Figure 35–16. The increasing acceptance of immediate reconstruction with flaps has greatly improved the overall rehabilitation of patients and the effectiveness of surgical treatment of

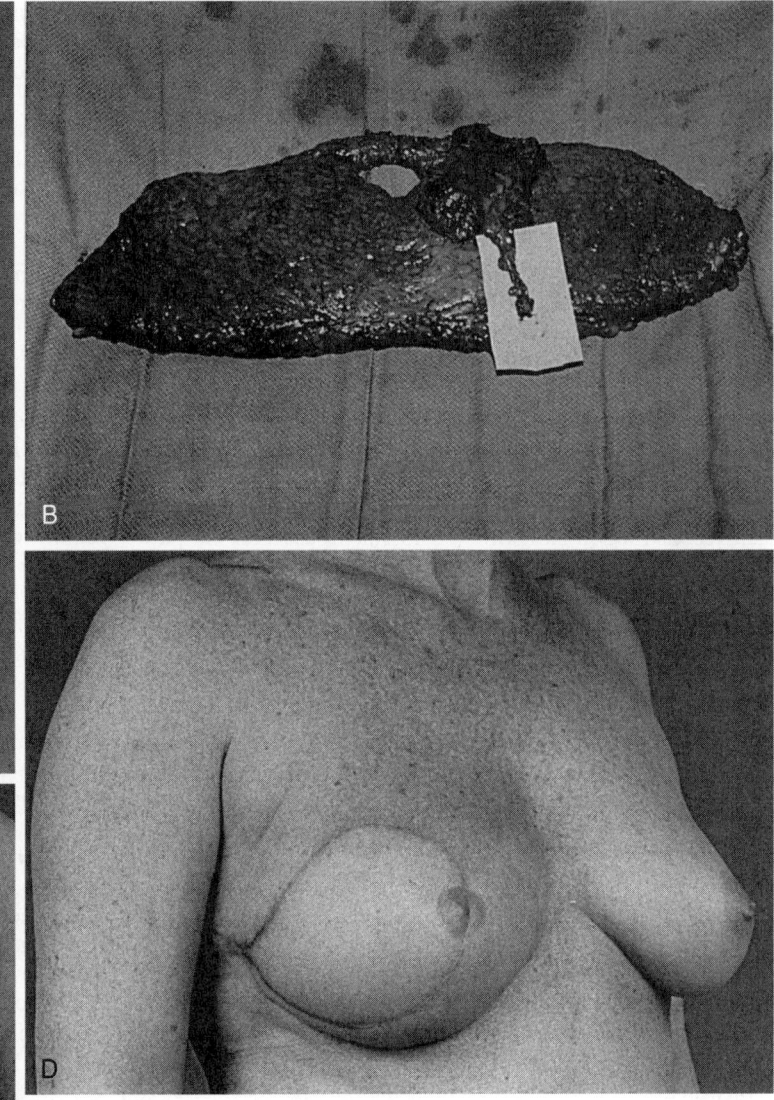

**Figure 35–16.** Immediate reconstruction with a transverse rectus abdominis myocutaneous (TRAM) free flap after a right modified radical mastectomy. *A*, Preoperative marking of the patient with attention to the location of the left inferior epigastric artery and vein. *B*, Undersurface of the abdominal flap showing the small cuff of muscle and the long vascular pedicle. Anastomoses were then made to the thoracodorsal vessels. *C* and *D*, Reconstructed breast and the abdominal donor scar 7 months later. The patient underwent an outpatient reconstruction of the nipple 3 months earlier.

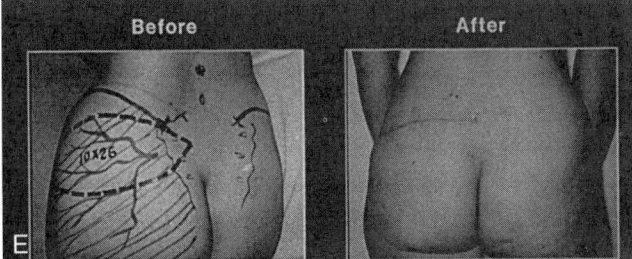

**Figure 35–17.** Delayed reconstruction with a gluteal free flap. *A,* Preoperative chest marking. *B,* The superior mammary vessels. *C,* One month postoperatively. *D,* Appearance at 8 months. The patient underwent a revision of the breast mound and nipple reconstruction at 3 months. *E,* Buttock donor scar.

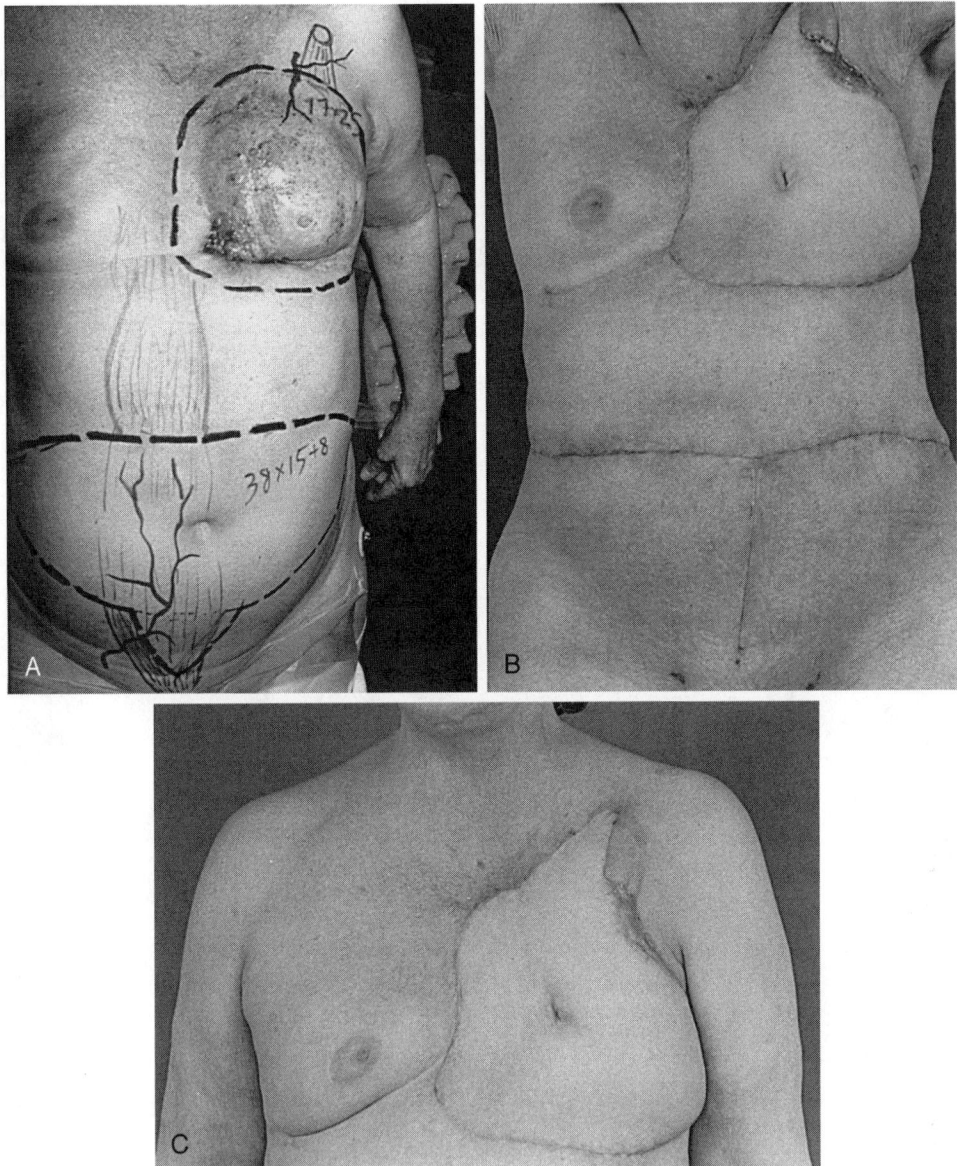

**Figure 35–18.** Patient treated with a transverse rectus abdominis myocutaneous (TRAM) flap for recurrent carcinoma after previous mastectomy and implant reconstruction. Multiple fungating, ulcerating lesions are present. *A,* Preoperative markings. Note the wide skin excision and the large TRAM flap design. *B* and *C,* One month after wide excision, removal of implant, and reconstruction with a TRAM flap. The vascular anastomoses were made to the thoracoacromial vessels.

breast cancer. The ability to provide satisfactory surgical reconstruction for a variety of situations is now an essential part of comprehensive breast cancer care.

## SUGGESTIONS FOR ADDITIONAL READING

Slavin SA, Love SM, Goldwyn RM. Recurrent breast cancer following immediate reconstruction with myocutaneous flaps. Plast Reconstr Surg 1994;93:1191–204. *Data from 161 patients showed the safety and efficacy of this approach to management.*

Janowsky EC, Kupper LL, Hulka BS. Meta-analysis of the relation between silicone breast implants and the risk of connective-tissue diseases. N Engl J Med 2000;342:781–90.

Shaw WW. Superior gluteal free flap breast reconstruction. Clin Plast Surg 1998;25:267–74.

Khouri RK, Ahn CY, Salzhauer MA, et al. Simultaneous bilateral breast reconstruction with the transverse rectus abdominus musculocutaneous free flap. Ann Surg 1997;226:25–34.

Takeishi M, Shaw WW, Ahn CY, Borud LJ. TRAM flaps in patients with abdominal scars. Plast Reconstr Surg 1997;99:713–22.

## REFERENCES

1. Davis JS. Plastic surgery: principles and practice. Philadelphia: Blakiston, 1919.
2. Cronin TD, Upton J, McDonough JM. Reconstruction of the breast after mastectomy. Plast Reconstr Surg 1977;59:1–14.
3. Radovan C. Tissue expansion in soft-tissue reconstruction. Plast Reconstr Surg 1984;74:482–92.
4. Fujino T, Harashina T, Enomoto K. Primary breast reconstruction after a standard radical mastectomy by a free flap transfer: case report. Plast Reconstr Surg 1976;58:371–4.
5. Hartrampf CR, Scheflan M, Black PW. Breast reconstruction with a transverse abdominal island flap. Plast Reconstr Surg 1982;69:216–25.
6. Shaw WW. Microvascular free flap breast reconstruction. Clin Plast Surg 1984;11:333–41.
7. Shaw WW, Ahn CY. Microvascular free flaps in breast reconstruction. Clin Plast Surg 1992;19:917–26.
8. Bridges AJ, Vasey FB. Silicone breast implants: history, safety, and potential complications. Arch Intern Med 1993;153:2638–44.

···········································

# RADIATION THERAPY

• Robert G. Parker

Ionizing radiations have been used in the curative and palliative treatment of patients with breast cancer since shortly after the discovery of x-rays by Roentgen in 1895.[1] In January 1896, a patient with breast cancer was apparently referred to Grubbé, a medical student in Chicago, because a physician noted damage to Grubbé's hands consequent to testing Crookes' tubes and wondered whether the mysterious, invisible rays would damage the cancer.[2] Since then, there has been a continuing evolution of indications for use until, currently, radiation therapy has major roles in conservation management after excision of the primary tumor, in multimodality treatment of locally extensive tumors including inflammatory carcinomas, as an adjuvant to mastectomy, and as an effective palliative agent.

## BREAST CONSERVATION MANAGEMENT

There is abundant evidence that for many breast cancers, local-regional tumor control and tumor-free survival are as good after limited surgery (wide excision, tylectomy, lum-

pectomy, segmental resection) plus irradiation of the breast and occasionally the regional lymph nodes plus chemotherapy as following radical mastectomy or MRM plus appropriate adjuvant treatment.[3–14] A conclusion of a 1991 National Institutes of Health Consensus Conference[15] was that BCT was preferable because a comfortable, cosmetically acceptable breast can be preserved without lessening of tumor control. Nevertheless, in many instances, the patient is not given a choice of treatment. It has been documented that in some places in the United States, the frequency of MRM for patients eligible for BCT has been increasing.[16]

BCT was advocated by a surgeon, Keynes, in 1924[3] and was soon supported by pioneer radiation oncologists.[4, 6] Although many reports[4–10, 17–21] claimed that BCT was as effective as MRM (Table 35–18), more convincing evidence was supplied by prospective randomized trials from Milan,[11] the Institut Gustave Roussy,[12] and the NSABP[13] (Table 35–19). In the Milan study,[11] radical mastectomy was compared with quadrant resection plus axillary dissection followed by irradiation of breast to 50 Gy. Only patients with primary cancers less than 2 cm in greatest dimension, not centrally

*Table 35–18.* **Limited Surgery and Radiation Therapy, Uncontrolled Retrospective Studies**

| | Stage I Survival (%) | | | Stage II Survival (%) | | |
|---|---|---|---|---|---|---|
| Reference | NO. PATIENTS | 5 yr | 10 yr | NO. PATIENTS | 5 yr | 10 yr |
| Mustakallio (1954)[4] | 127 | 84 | 72 | — | — | — |
| Peters (1954)[9] | 145 | 84 | 71 | — | — | — |
| Calle et al (1978)[10] | 120 | 85 | 75 | 203 | 77 | 54 |
| Bedwinek et al (1980)[17] | 102 | 83 | — | 132 | 67 | — |
| Clark et al (1982)[18] | 312 | 83 | 63 | 144 | 71 | 62 |
| Romsdahl et al (1983)[19] | 103 | 86 | 78 | — | — | — |
| Kurtz et al (1987)[20] | 170 | — | 80 | 130 | — | 76 |
| Solin et al (1988)[21] | 252 | 97 | — | 300 | 87 | — |

*Table 35–19.* Breast Conservation Surgery Compared with Radical Mastectomy, Clinical Trials with Randomization of Patients

| Reference | Limited Surgery + Radiation Therapy Survival (%) | | | | Radical Mastectomy + Radiation Therapy Survival (%) | | | |
|---|---|---|---|---|---|---|---|---|
| | NO. PATIENTS | STAGE | 5 yr | 8 yr | NO. PATIENTS | STAGE | 5 yr | 8 yr |
| Sarrazin et al (Institute Gustave-Roussy)[12] | 88 | I/II | 95 | — | 91 | I/II | 91 | — |
| Fisher et al (NSABP)[13] | 396 | I | 92 | — | 362 | I | 82 | — |
| | 229 | II | 75 | — | 224 | II | 66 | — |
| Veronesi et al (Milan)[11] | 352 | I | 90 | 85 | 349 | I | 90 | 83 |

located, and without palpable axillary adenopathy were included. In the NSABP study (B-06),[13] patients were entered if their primary tumors were 4 cm in greatest dimension or smaller and not centrally located; there was no tumor involvement of the skin or nipple; and their axillary nodes, when palpable, were not *fixed.* In this study, wide excision of the primary tumor, by segmental resection or lumpectomy, required tumor-free margins in the removed breast tissue. Radical mastectomy was compared with local removal of the primary tumor with or without postoperative irradiation. Although there was no significant difference in overall or disease-free survival among the three groups, patients with only segmental resection plus axillary dissection had more frequent local recurrences than those in the other two groups. All patients with tumor in axillary lymph nodes received chemotherapy. The highest survival in this group was in patients treated with limited surgery and postoperative irradiation.

BCT should proceed only after the surgeon, radiation oncologist, medical oncologist, and mammographer have agreed that such treatment is reasonable and the patient understands all treatment options and selects conservation management. The medical decision is based on size of the primary tumor related to breast size; histology of the tumor; local findings, such as skin involvement by tumor or fixation of the tumor to the chest wall; tumor involvement of the nipple; and presence of widespread microcalcifications in the breast.

Although previous studies have limited tumors to 4 cm[13] or 2 cm[11] in greatest dimension, there is evidence that larger primary tumors are as effectively controlled as smaller lesions if the excision is complete with tumor-free margins in the resected specimen.[22, 23] As the primary tumor becomes large in proportion to the remaining breast, however, the cosmesis after resection may not be acceptable.

Contraindications to BCT involving postoperative irradiation are relative and include widespread microcalcifications not removable by wide excision or segmental resection; a large tumor in a small breast, making cosmesis unacceptable to the patient; a breast large enough to make daily reproducible positioning for irradiation unlikely; fixation of the tumor to the overlying skin or underlying chest wall; collagen-vascular disease predictive for an intolerable normal tissue radiation reaction; a patient preference for surgery or an antiradiation phobia; and nonavailability of professional competence. Most patients who understand and desire BCT and have tumors that are completely resectable with a resultant acceptable cosmesis are candidates for such treatment.

The success of BCT depends on the surgeon's interest, advocacy, and ability. Inasmuch as the *gatekeeper* for the care of most patients with breast cancer is a surgeon, treatment options can be unevenly presented with a bias toward mastectomy. Cosmesis depends on the surgeon's skill in completely excising the primary tumor with minimal distortion of the breast. Usually this excision can be accomplished with less than a quadrant resection (a quadrant can be a quarter of the breast in various orientations, i.e., 12 o'clock to 3 o'clock or 11 o'clock to 2 o'clock). The axillary dissection should be performed through a separate incision. If a drain is used, it should be exteriorized anterior to the midaxillary line so that this site can be included in the standard radiation treatment volume.

In many patients selecting conservation management with irradiation, adjuvant chemotherapy is used. Indications for such use are described elsewhere in this book. The effects of these drugs and ionizing radiations are additive, as reviewed in Chapter 7. The combination of cyclophosphamide, methotrexate, and 5-fluorouracil (CMF) can be administered concurrently with the radiation therapy,[11] although sometimes methotrexate is reduced or withheld.[24] Doxorubicin and ionizing radiations have been used consecutively, rather than concurrently, because of a concern about increased normal tissue radiation reactions. Usually, based on a substantial risk of systemic dissemination of tumor as well as a *recall* radiation phenomenon, the doxorubicin has been used first. The concurrent use of full doses of CMF or doxorubicin or tamoxifen[25, 26] has been correlated with a lesser cosmetic result.

With limitations of current knowledge, irradiation of the entire breast is recommended following complete excision of the primary tumor, if it is infiltrating carcinoma. This recommendation is based on evidence, such as from the NSABP B-06 study,[13] that local recurrence after complete excision alone approaches 40% in 8 years and that irradiation reduces this frequency to less than 10%. Postoperative irradiation of the breast after complete excision of DCIS or LCIS is less well defined, although the local recurrence at 4 years was less in the irradiated compared with the unirradiated breasts in one study.[27]

The radiations are delivered to the breast through opposing tangential fields, which include the underlying chest wall with a small *rim* of lung, in daily increments of 1.8 to 2 Gy to a total of 45 to 50 Gy. The objective of this treatment is control of clinically imperceptible tumor cells in the postoperative breast. Inasmuch as most local failures are at the primary excision site, even if the margins were judged to be tumor-free, a boost dose of 10 to 20 Gy is usually delivered to that site. This may be done with a beam of high-energy electrons (6 to 15 MeV), photons, or an interstitial implant of radioactive isotopes, usually iridium 192. The volume of this boost should be generous and include more than the excision scar and immediately underlying tissue.

Indications for irradiation of the regional lymphatics remain unsettled. There is evidence from postmastectomy studies that radiation therapy can decrease problems caused by metastases to the chest wall or regional nodes and can influence survival favorably.[28, 29] Decision making should be based on evidence obtained by a partial axillary dissection (6 to 10 nodes, lower and middle axilla). *Complete* axillary dissection to the axillary vein is usually unnecessary and contributes to the development of edema of the ipsilateral upper limb. If metastases are identified in axillary nodes, especially if tumor extends through the capsule of a node, the ipsilateral axillary and infraclavicular and supraclavicular nodes are usually irradiated regardless of the primary tumor site within the breast. Some radiation oncologists also irradiate the ipsilateral internal mammary nodes wherever the axillary nodes are tumor bearing. Others hesitate to irradiate the internal mammary nodes, unless the primary tumor is in the medial or central breast, especially when axillary nodes contain metastases. Restraint from irradiating the internal mammary nodes is based on the belief that such involvement is a harbinger of problems from systemic rather than local-regional disease.

Of patients, 80 to 90% judge the cosmetic result of conservation treatment with irradiation to be good to excellent.[30] Physicians judge the results more harshly. Cosmesis is related to primary tumor size compared with breast size, amount of normal tissue removed (quadrant resection vs. wide resection), surgical technique (separate limited incisions), preservation of the nipple-areola, radiation therapy technique (total dose, dose increment size, dose distribution), and use of adjuvant chemotherapy.

For patients suffering local recurrences after BCT, 5-year disease-free survival rates of 76% have been reported following further treatment (Table 35–20),[31] in contrast to patients with local-regional recurrences following mastectomy, when the tumor-free survival is lower. Good results have been reported after a second breast-conserving resection without postoperative irradiation, however.[33] Five-year survival rates after salvage surgery have been reported at 71% for those originally with stage I cancer with no axillary tumor involvement at time of salvage and 37% for those with tumor in axillary nodes at that time.[33]

The expected acute side effects of irradiation of the breast and regional nodes are a mild erythematous skin reaction, most intense under the breast, in the axilla, and behind the clavicle, and mild edema of the breast with skin thickening. Some patients complain of tiredness. The skin reaction heals within a few weeks, although some *bronzing* may persist for a few months. The edema should subside within a few months, although skin thickening can be detected mammographically for many months.[34] When the breast is irradiated with tangential beams, the rim of lung adjacent to the anterior thoracic wall that is included eventually develops fibrosis, which is rarely symptom producing. Rarely, fractures in the irradiated anterior ribs have been reported.[35] Although part of the heart may be irradiated in treatment of the left internal mammary nodes, use of electron beams can reduce the total dose and the risk of damage to the heart. In one study, no permanent cardiac damage was detected.[36] Other, rarely reported (<1%) long-term complications include severe breast fibrosis, ulceration, and brachial plexopathy.[37] Usually these complications have followed deviations from standard techniques. The risk of ipsilateral upper limb edema varies with the extent of surgery[38] and the radiotherapy techniques.[39] When such limb edema occurs, often a full axillary dissection has been followed by irradiation of the entire axilla to a high dose. Although radiation carcinogenesis in the opposite breast is a concern, in clinical practice, the frequency has not exceeded that in patients treated by mastectomy without irradiation.[40]

An important component of BCT is close long-term follow-up of the patient. This follow-up includes periodic mammography by an experienced radiologist. Dense breast tissue, which obscures microcalcifications, may hinder evaluation and make necessary follow-up examinations uncertain. Involved physicians must understand postirradiation changes and distinguish them from recurrent cancer. Otherwise the symptoms and signs of recurrence may be the same as for the initial diagnosis of cancer. Biopsy of this irradiated tissue should be done with discretion.[32] The diagnosis of recurrent or persistent tumor is important, however, because treatment, usually by mastectomy, is potentially curative.

## MANAGEMENT OF PATIENTS WITH DUCTAL CARCINOMA IN SITU AND LOBULAR CARCINOMA IN SITU

Since the 1970s, intraductal (noninvasive) breast cancer has become well defined.[41] The diagnosis of DCIS and LCIS has increased in frequency secondary to the widespread use of mammography. Of all diagnosed breast cancers, 40% have been reported as DCIS.[42]

The best management of these tumors remains controversial. These noninvasive breast cancers, especially lobular lesions, were previously treated by mastectomy even though BCT was well established for invasive ductal and lobular cancers. Although, intuitively, there must be a subset of patients who do not need postexcision breast irradiation, this group has not been identified. The randomized clinical trial

*Table 35–20.* **Results of Treatment of Local-Regional Recurrence Following Conservation Treatment**

| Reference | No. Patients | Study Dates | 5-yr Survival (%) |
|---|---|---|---|
| Montague et al (M.D. Anderson Cancer Center)[23] | 16 | 1955–80 | 67 |
| Kurtz et al (Cancer Institute Marseilles)[33] | 147 | 1960–71 | 51 |
| Calle et al (Institut Curie, Paris)[31] | 25 | 1960–78 | 76 |

NSABP B-17[43] produced data that postoperative radiation therapy reduced noninvasive local recurrences from 13.4 to 8.2% and invasive recurrences from 13.4 to 3.9%. Lagios and colleagues[44] proposed criteria to treat DCIS with excision alone. These criteria were DCIS detected by microcalcifications on mammography, tumor size less than 2.5 cm in greatest dimension, histologic confirmation of noncomedo tumor, excision with tumor-free margins, postoperative mammograms confirming that there are no residual microcalcifications, health favorable for clinical and mammographic evaluations, and patient understanding of risks. At UCLA, an additional requirement has been that no tumor could be identified in the re-excision specimen.[45] At UCLA, currently all patients with comedo histology receive postexcision irradiation of the entire breast. Although the results reported by Lagios and colleagues[44] have been favorable, local recurrence rates of 30% in 44 months have been reported.[46] Inasmuch as correctly diagnosed in situ cancers do not metastasize, axillary dissection should not be included.[47]

## RADIATION THERAPY AFTER RADICAL OR MODIFIED RADICAL MASTECTOMY

Although in the past many patients received local-regional radiation therapy following radical mastectomy (MRM), such use has become controversial[48] and infrequent[49] (treatment of patients with metastases to axillary nodes: 50% in 1972 and 25% in 1981). In large part, this change in policy was based on the assumption that chemotherapy would be effective against distant metastases and local-regional recurrences. The success of chemotherapy in the prevention of chest wall and regional lymph node recurrences in *high-risk* patients has not been documented, however.[50, 51] Consequently, in addition to systemic chemotherapy, it is prudent to irradiate the chest wall and regional lymphatics in some of these patients.[52] Fletcher[53] identified subsets of patients at risk for local-regional recurrences as a basis for elective irradiation: peripheral lymphatics and chest wall if more than 20% of the axillary nodes contained tumor regardless of the size or site of the primary tumor; chest wall if the primary tumor was larger than 5 cm, tumor involved the margins of resection, perineural or vascular spaces were extensively invaded, or grave signs, such as fixation to the chest wall or involvement of skin, were present.

Postmastectomy radiation therapy should be measured by its effectiveness in reducing tumor regrowth on the chest wall or in the peripheral lymphatics. In prospective randomized studies from Oslo[54] and Stockholm,[29, 54, 55] evidence was provided that local-regional recurrences can be reduced. Survival benefit in these studies was small. In the Oslo II study, however, 47 patients with central or medial primary tumors had a 20% survival advantage. Likewise, a report from Institut Gustave Roussy[56] indicated a survival benefit for patients with central or medial primary tumors when the internal mammary nodes were irradiated or resected.

Some authorities advocate withholding irradiation of the chest wall and regional lymphatics until local-regional recurrences appear in the few patients reflecting high-risk factors. Such gross recurrences are controlled in only about half of these patients,[57] however, and the clinical consequences of tumors progressing on the chest wall with ulceration and infection, axillary venous and lymphatic obstruction, or brachial plexopathy are morbid.

Inasmuch as patients receiving postmastectomy radiation therapy also are at high risk for distant metastases, chemotherapy is likely to be used. Although CMF and chest wall irradiation are tolerated when used concurrently, consecutive administration, usually with initial chemotherapy, especially when doxorubicin is included, has been the most frequent program.[58]

## PREOPERATIVE RADIATION THERAPY

Following Baclesse's demonstration in the 1930s[59] that when breast cancers in 21 patients were irradiated to at least 5000 roentgens over 8 to 13 weeks no tumor was found in 7 of the specimens and marked morphologic changes were noted in 12 others, there was some curiosity about preoperative breast irradiation. Current use in many institutions is limited to breast cancers that are questionably resectable or have been *disturbed*, such as those with extensive postbiopsy ecchymoses.[60] A few reports have claimed improved tumor-free survival, decreased local recurrences,[61] and fewer tumor-bearing axillary nodes[62] in patients preoperatively irradiated for clinical stages II and III breast cancers.

Although primary surgical treatment for patients with clinical stage III disease often is futile,[63] and radiation therapy also may be comparably ineffective,[64] mastectomy after irradiation apparently increases the frequency of local tumor control[65] and survival.[66]

## LOCALLY ADVANCED BREAST CANCER

The term *locally advanced breast cancer* includes a heterogeneous group of tumors with variable biologic behavior, ranging from tumors that become rapidly widespread and fatal to slowly progressive tumors that remain local-regional for prolonged periods. Generally, these cancers include all patients with TNM stage III tumors.[67–69] Some of these cancers are initially resectable, whereas others are not. It has been established that this group may compose 20% of all patients with breast cancer at the time of diagnosis.[69] Some of these patients survived even before the institution of *modern* treatment, with 17% remaining tumor free at 20 years in one report.[70]

On the basis of objectives of reducing tumor bulk and eradicating micrometastatic cancer cells, chemotherapy has become integrated with surgery and radiation therapy in potentially curative treatment. This has been called *primary chemotherapy*.[71] Most studies have included induction chemotherapy before local treatment with surgery or irradiation, or both.[67] Radiation therapy has been used with chemotherapy as preoperative induction,[72] as definitive treatment,[73, 74] or as a postoperative adjuvant.[74] Such programs have resulted in complete response rates of 58[75] to 100%,[73] 5-year disease-free survival rates of 20[76] to 47%,[77, 78] and local recurrence rates of 13[75, 76] to 38%.[76]

Radiation therapy alone has produced local tumor control rates of 19[78] to 100%,[79] with 5-year survival rates of 10[80] to 59%.[81] The local-regional success of such primary irradiation is inversely related to the size of the tumor and directly related to the total dose. Doses as high as 80 to 100 Gy have been used with consequent severe sequelae, such as marked fibrosis, noted in 20 to 25% of cases.[82, 83]

Moderate total doses of 45 to 50 Gy in 25 fractions in 5 weeks, plus a boost of 10 to 15 Gy to high-risk sites, can be used preoperatively or postoperatively with total mastectomy with at least as good results and fewer sequelae.[84] Tapley and Montague[85] reported chest wall tumor control in 88% of patients with tumor-involved axillary nodes or with primary tumors larger than 5 cm with the grave signs defined by Haagensen.

Inflammatory breast cancer was described by Lee and Tannenbaum in 1924.[86] Clinical features include an enlarged, warm, edematous painful breast with reddened skin and nipple retraction. Often a mass cannot be defined.[87] These presenting clinical findings have been called *primary inflammatory carcinoma*,[88] with a secondary type involving inflammatory signs in a breast with a defined cancer. Tumor invasion of the dermal lymphatics has been noted in many, but not all, of these patients, provoking an argument about whether inflammatory carcinoma is a clinical or pathologic entity. In a review of SEER data, patients with only clinical features (3-year survival rate, 60%) and those with only pathologic features (3-year survival rate, 52%) had better survival rates than patients with both clinical and pathologic features (3-year survival rate, 34%).[89]

Inflammatory carcinoma is classified T4, stage IIIB in the TNM system.[90] Many of these patients have palpable axillary adenopathy, and nearly all have microscopic tumor in these nodes.[87] Identified metastatic spread at the time of diagnosis is frequent in these patients (17[87] to 36%[89]).

Neither primary radical mastectomy[91] nor radiation therapy[92] has been successful in many patients, and their combined use has not resulted in much improvement.[93] Consequently, multidrug chemotherapy has become a mainstay of treatment.

## PALLIATIVE RADIATION THERAPY

Radiation therapy is effective in the relief or avoidance of the symptoms and signs of metastases from breast cancer to many different anatomic sites. Many patients with breast cancer ultimately need such treatment.[94] The initial step is evaluation of the specific problem in relation to the patient's general status. If rehabilitation and a reasonably long life expectancy are likely, high-dosage irradiation, protracted to avoid sequelae, may be reasonable. If the patient is near death, withholding irradiation and substitution of a simpler treatment may be in order. Patient inconvenience and acute treatment-induced reactions must be minimized.

The most common problem is metastases to bone causing pain or threatening structural integrity. Breast cancer accounts for about one half of bony metastases.[95, 96] Using a range of schedules from 9 Gy in a single increment to 30 Gy in 10 increments, Tong and associates[97] reported an 82% total response rate. Response is usually rapid (60% within 7 days)[96] and long-lasting (70% without relapse until death).[97] Pathologic fracture threatens to immobilize patients during their shortened life expectancy. Attention to risk factors may avoid such catastrophes. For example, if there is a lytic lesion of 2 cm or larger in the proximal femur or 50% of

the cortex of a long bone is compromised, surgical fixation before local irradiation is warranted. Because the initial response to irradiation is hyperemia and osteoporosis, with structural weakening at 2 to 3 weeks after irradiation, this is the period of highest risk for fracture.[98] Management of patients with fractures involving tumor-involved, weight-bearing bones requires surgical fixation before irradiation. Although radiation therapy may interfere with the normal healing mechanism,[98] uncontrolled tumor is likely to prevent healing. For patients suffering pain from widespread bony metastases, single-dose hemibody irradiation of 6 to 8 Gy to the upper body and 8 to 10 Gy to the lower body (after medications such as steroids and antinausea drugs) has resulted in total response rates of 80[99] to 100%[100] within a short time (50% within 48 hours and 80% within 7 days).[101]

Multiple brain metastases are an indication for whole-brain irradiation, with objectives of arresting or even reversing recently appearing neurologic deficits and relieving increased intracranial pressure and headache. Most *single metastases* may be treated with radiosurgery. Metastases to the meninges can also cause serious morbidity. A response to systemic steroids provides rapid relief and predicts for the success of slower acting irradiation. Response rates of 75 to 85%[102, 103] have followed a range of doses (10 Gy in one increment to 40 Gy in 3 to 4 weeks).[104]

Spinal cord compression is usually an oncologic emergency. Breast cancer is the primary tumor in 25% of these situations.[105] Cord compression may result from extension of tumor through intervertebral foramina, from vertebral bodies, or from intramedullary metastases.[106] Treatment has often been with surgical decompression (laminectomy). The addition of postoperative irradiation has provided better motor recovery[105] with less chance for local recurrence.[107] In one study, laminectomy plus postoperative irradiation was no better than irradiation alone.[108] Recovery for paraplegic patients only follows paralysis of short duration.[109]

Metastases to the choroid are usually associated with widespread metastases but may be the first clinical indication of distant spread of tumor in 30% of patients with breast cancer.[110] In 40% of patients, the metastases are bilateral.[111] Uncontrolled tumor is likely to cause blindness, from retinal detachment, or glaucoma from obstruction of the iris angle.[112] Of these patients, 50% have complete disappearance of symptoms after irradiation.[113] Another third have a partial response or at least stabilization of signs and symptoms.[113]

Patients with untreated metastases to the liver have a median survival of 75 days, with less than 10% living for 12 months.[114] Irradiation of the entire liver for multiple metastases is limited by normal tissue tolerance (25 Gy at 2 Gy per day).[115] Limited treatment has resulted in lessening of the signs and symptoms of pain, nausea, fever, ascites, and jaundice in less than a third of patients.[116] Other problems, such as metastases to the skin or ribs, can be treated for relief of signs and symptoms as they arise.

## SUGGESTIONS FOR ADDITIONAL READING

Cuzick J, Stewart H, Rutqvist L, et al. Cause-specific mortality in long-term survivors of breast cancer who participated in trials of radiotherapy. J Clin Oncol 1994;12:447–53. *A reduced number of deaths in patients receiving radiation therapy for primary breast cancer led the authors to conclude that radiation therapy may accomplish more than local control in this setting.*

Pierce LJ, Lichter AS. Postmastectomy radiotherapy: more than local regional control. J Clin Oncol 1994;12:444–6.

## REFERENCES

1. Roentgen WC. Zwaite Mitteilung 1896;March 9:132.
2. Grubbé EH. Priority in the therapeutic use of x-rays. Radiology 1933;21:156–62.
3. Keynes G. The treatment of primary carcinoma of the breast with radium. Acta Radiol 1929;10:393–402.
4. Mustakallio SJ. Conservative treatment of breast carcinoma: review of 25-year follow-up. Clin Radiol 1972;23:110–16.
5. Porritt A. Early carcinoma of the breast. Br J Surg 1965;51:214–6.
6. Peters MV. Carcinoma of the breast: stage II—radiation range: wedge resection and irradiation: an effective treatment in early breast cancer. JAMA 1967;200:134–5.
7. Cope O. Breast cancer: has the time come for a less mutilating treatment? Psychiatry Med 1971;2:263–9.
8. Montague ED, Gutierrez AE, Barker JL, et al. Conservation surgery and irradiation for the treatment of favorable breast cancer. Cancer 1979;43:1058–61.
9. Peters MV. Wedge resection and irradiation: an effective treatment in early breast cancer. JAMA 1967;200:144–45.
10. Calle R, Pilleron JP, Schlienger P, Vilcoq JR. Conservative management of operable breast cancer: ten years experience at the Foundation Curie. Cancer 1978;42:2045–53.
11. Veronesi U, Saccozzi R, Del Vecchio M, et al. Comparing radical mastectomy with quadrantectomy, axillary dissection, and radiotherapy in patients with small cancers of the breast. N Engl J Med 1981;305:6–11.
12. Sarrazin D, Lê M, Rouëssé J, et al. Conservative treatment versus mastectomy in breast cancer tumors with macroscopic diameter of 20 millimeters or less: the experience of the Institut Gustave-Roussy. Cancer 1984;53:1209–13.
13. Fisher B, Bauer M, Margolese R, et al. Five-year results of a randomized clinical trial comparing total mastectomy and segmental mastectomy with or without radiation in the treatment of breast cancer. N Engl J Med 1985;312:665–73.
14. Calle R, Vilcoq JR, Zafrani B, et al. Local control and survival of breast cancer treated by limited surgery followed by irradiation. Int J Radiat Oncol Biol Phys 1986;12:873–8.
15. NIH consensus conference. Treatment of early-stage breast cancer. JAMA 1991;265:391–5.
16. Lazovich DA, White E, Thomas DB, Moe RE: Underutilization of breast-conserving surgery and radiation therapy among women with stage I or II breast cancer. JAMA 1991;266:3433–8.
17. Bedwinek JM, Brady L, Perez CA, et al. Irradiation as the primary management of stage I and II adenocarcinoma of the breast: analysis of the RTOG breast registry. Cancer Clin Trials 1980;3:11–8.
18. Clark RM, Wilkinson RH, Mahoney LJ, et al. Breast cancer: a 21 year experience with conservative surgery and radiation. Int J Radiat Oncol Biol Phys 1982;8:967–79.
19. Romsdahl MM, Montague ED, Ames FC, et al. Conservation surgery and irradiation as treatment for early breast cancer. Arch Surg 1983;118:521–8.
20. Kurtz JM, Amalric R, Delouche G, et al. The second ten years: long-term risks of breast conservation in early breast cancer. Int J Radiat Oncol Biol Phys 1987;13:1327–32.
21. Solin LJ, Fowble L, Martz KL, Goodman RL. Definitive irradiation for early stage breast cancer: the University of Pennsylvania experience. Int J Radiat Oncol Biol Phys 1988;14:235–42.
22. Khanna MM, Mark RJ, Silverstein MJ, et al. Breast conservation management of breast tumors 4 cm or larger. Arch Surg 1992;127:1038–43.
23. Montague ED, Ames FC, Schell SR, Romsdahl MM. Conservation surgery and irradiation as an alternative to mastectomy in the treatment of clinically favorable breast cancer. Cancer 1984;54:11 Suppl:2668–72.
24. Glick JH, Fowble BL, Haller DG, et al. Integration of full-dose adjuvant chemotherapy with definitive radiotherapy for primary breast cancer: four-year update. NCI Monogr 1988;6:297–301.
25. Abner AL, Recht A, Vicini FA, et al. Cosmetic results after surgery, chemotherapy, and radiation therapy for early breast cancer. Int J Radiat Oncol Biol Phys 1991;21:331–8.
26. Wazer DE, DiPetrillo T, Schmidt-Ullrich R, et al. Factors influencing cosmetic outcome and complication risk after conservative surgery and radiotherapy for early-stage breast carcinoma. J Clin Oncol 1992;10:356–63.
27. Fisher B, Costantino J, Redmond C, et al. Lumpectomy compared with lumpectomy and radiation therapy for the treatment of intraductal breast cancer. N Engl J Med 1993;328:1581–6.
28. Fletcher GH, McNeese MD, Oswald MJ. Long-range results for breast cancer patients treated by radical mastectomy and postoperative radiation without adjuvant chemotherapy: an update. Int J Radiat Oncol Biol Phys 1989;17:11–4.
29. Høst H, Brennhovd IO, Loeb M. Postoperative radiotherapy in breast cancer—long-term results from the Oslo study. Int J Radiat Oncol Biol Phys 1986;12:727–32.
30. Beadle GF, Silver B, Botnick L, et al. Cosmetic results following primary radiation therapy for early breast cancer. Cancer 1984;54:2911–8.
31. Calle R, Vilcoq JR, Zafrani B, et al. Local control and survival of breast cancer treated by limited surgery followed by irradiation. Int J Radiat Oncol Biol Phys 1986;12:873–8.
32. Harris JR, Recht A, Amalric R, et al. Time course and prognosis of local recurrence following primary radiation therapy for early breast cancer. J Clin Oncol 1984;2:37–41.
33. Kurtz JM, Spitalier JM, Amalric R. Results of salvage surgery for local failure following conservative therapy of operable breast cancer. Front Radiat Ther Oncol 1983;17:84–90.
34. Bassett LW. Mammography and ultrasound in breast cancer detection. New York: Grune & Stratton, 1982.
35. Montague ED, Paulus DD, Schell SR. Selection and follow-up of patients for conservation surgery and irradiation. Front Radiat Ther Oncol 1983;17:124–30.
36. Loeffler JS, Goldberg ID, Risser TA, et al. Non-invasive cardiac evaluation after definitive radiation therapy for carcinoma of the breast. Int J Radiat Oncol Biol Phys 1985;11:Suppl 1:103.abstract.
37. Delouche G, Bachelot F, Premont M, Kurtz JM. Conservation treatment of early breast cancer: long term results and complications. Int J Radiat Oncol Biol Phys 1987;13:29–34.
38. Larson D, Weinstein M, Goldberg I, et al. Edema of the arm as a function of the extent of axillary surgery in patients with stage I–II carcinoma of the breast treated with primary radiotherapy. Int J Radiat Oncol Biol Phys 1986;12:1575–82.
39. Dewar JA, Sarrazin D, Benhamou E, et al. Management of the axilla in conservatively treated breast cancer: 592 patients treated at Institut Gustave-Roussy. Int J Radiat Oncol Biol Phys 1987;13:475–81.
40. Parker RG, Grimm P, Enstrom JE. Contralateral breast cancers following treatment for initial breast cancers in women. Am J Clin Oncol 1989;12:213–6.
41. McDivitt RN, Stewart FW, Bey JW. Tumors of the breast. An Atlas of tumor pathology. Washington, D.C.: Armed Forces Institute of Pathology, 1968:29.
42. Schnitt SJ, Silen W, Sadowsky NL, et al. Ductal carcinoma in situ (intraductal carcinoma) of the breast. N Engl J Med 1988;318:898–903.
43. Fisher B, Dignam J, Wolmark N, et al. Lumpectomy and radiation therapy for the treatment of intraductal breast cancer: findings from National Surgical Adjuvant Breast and Bowel Project B-17. J Clin Oncol 1998;16:441–52.
44. Lagios MD, Margolin FR, Westdahl PR, et al. Mammographically detected duct carcinoma in situ: frequency of local recurrence following tylectomy and prognostic effect of nuclear grade on local recurrence. Cancer 1989;63:618–24.
45. Love SM, Parker B, Imes M, et al. Practice guidelines for breast cancer. Cancer J Sci Am 1996;2:501–21.
46. Delaney G, Ung O, Cahill S, et al. Ductal carcinoma in situ: Part 2. treatment. Aust N Z J Surg 1997;67:157–65.
47. Parker RG, Berkbigler D, Rees K, et al. Axillary node dissection in ductal carcinoma in situ. Am J Clin Oncol 1998;21:109–10.
48. Lipsett MB. Postoperative radiation for women with cancer of the breast and positive axillary lymph nodes: should it continue? N Engl J Med 1981;304:112–4.
49. Wilson RE, Donegan WL, Mettlin C, et al. The 1982 national survey

50. Bonadonna G, Valagussa P, Rossi A, et al. Ten-year experience with CMF-based adjuvant chemotherapy in resectable breast cancer. Breast Cancer Res Treat 1985;5:95–115.

51. Stefanik D, Goldberg R, Byrne, P, et al. Local-regional failure in patients treated with adjuvant chemotherapy for breast cancer. J Clin Oncol 1985;3:660–5.

52. Fowble B, Gray R, Gilchrist K, et al. Identification of a subgroup of patients with breast cancer and histologically positive axillary nodes receiving adjuvant chemotherapy who may benefit from postoperative radiotherapy. J Clin Oncol 1988;6:1107–17.

53. Fletcher GH. Textbook of radiotherapy. 3rd ed. Philadelphia: Lea & Febiger, 1980.

54. Wallgren A, Arner O, Bergström J, et al. Radiation therapy in operable breast cancer: results from the Stockholm trial on adjuvant radiotherapy. Int J Radiat Oncol Biol Phys 1986;12:533–7 and 1987;13:149.

55. Rutqvist LE, Cedermark B, Glas U, et al. Radiotherapy, chemotherapy, and tamoxifen as adjuncts to surgery in early breast cancer: a summary of three randomized trials. Int J Radiat Oncol Biol Phys 1989;16:629–39.

56. Tubiana M, Arriagada R, Sarrazin D. Human cancer natural history, radiation induced immunodepression and post-operative radiation therapy. Int J Radiat Oncol Biol Phys 1986;12:477–85.

57. Montague ED, Fletcher GH. The curative value of irradiation in the treatment of nondisseminated breast cancer. Cancer 1980;46:Suppl:995–8.

58. Muss HB. Adjuvant irradiation following mastectomy: where are we? J Clin Oncol 1987;5:1500–1.

59. Baclesse F. Roentgen therapy as the sole method of treatment of cancer of the breast. Am J Roentgenol 1949;62:311–18.

60. Rodger A, Montague ED, Fletcher G. Preoperative or postoperative irradiation as adjunctive treatment with radical mastectomy in breast cancer. Cancer 1983;51:1388–92.

61. Wallgren A, Arner O, Bergström J, et al. The value of preoperative radiotherapy in operable mammary carcinoma. Int J Radiat Oncol Biol Phys 1980;6:287–90.

62. Strender LE, Wallgren A, Arndt J, et al. Adjuvant radiotherapy in operable breast cancer: correlation between dose in internal mammary nodes and prognosis. Int J Radiat Oncol Biol Phys 1981;7:1319–25.

63. Stoker TA. The place of surgical excision in the management of locally advanced breast cancer. Cancer Treat Rev 1974;1:27–37.

64. Harris JR, Sawicka J, Gelman R, Hellman S. Management of locally advanced carcinoma of the breast by primary radiation therapy. Int J Radiat Oncol Biol Phys 1983;9:345–9.

65. Bedwinek J, Rao DV, Perez C, et al. Stage III and localized stage IV breast cancer: irradiation alone vs irradiation plus surgery. Int J Radiat Oncol Biol Phys 1982;8:31–6.

66. Zucali R, Uslenghi C, Kenda R, Bonadonna G. Natural history and survival of inoperable breast cancer treated with radiotherapy and radiotherapy followed by radical mastectomy. Cancer 1976;37:1422–31.

67. Booser DJ, Hortobagyi GN. Treatment of locally advanced breast cancer. Semin Oncol 1992;19:278–85.

68. Swain SM, Lippman ME. Locally advanced breast cancer. In: Bland KI, ed. The breast—comprehensive management of benign and malignant diseases. Philadelphia: WB Saunders, 1991:843.

69. Dorr FA, Bader J, Friedman MA. Locally advanced breast cancer: current status and future directions. Int J Radiat Oncol Biol Phys 1989;16:775–84.

70. Ferguson DJ, Meier P, Karrison T, et al. Staging of breast cancer and survival rates: an assessment based on 50 years of experience with radical mastectomy. JAMA 1982;248:1337–41.

71. Wolff AC, Davidson NE. Primary systemic therapy in breast cancer. J Clin Oncol 2000;18:1558–69.

72. Piccart MJ, de Valeriola D, Paridaens R, et al. Six-year results of a multimodality treatment strategy for locally advanced breast cancer. Cancer 1988;62:2501–6.

73. Jacquillat C, Baillet F, Weil M, et al. Results of a conservative treatment combining induction (neoadjuvant) and consolidation chemotherapy, hormonotherapy, and external and interstitial irradiation in 98 patients with locally advanced breast cancer (IIIA–IIIB). Cancer 1988;61:1977–82.

74. Morrow M, Braverman A, Thelmo W, et al. Multimodal therapy for locally advanced breast cancer. Arch Surg 1986;121:1291–6.

75. Perloff M, Lesnick GJ, Korzun A, et al. Combination chemotherapy with mastectomy or radiotherapy for stage III breast carcinoma: a Cancer and Leukemia Group B study. J Clin Oncol 1988;6:261–9.

76. Valagussa P, Bonnadonna G, Veronisi U. Patterns of relapse and survival following radical mastectomy. Cancer 1978;41:1170–8.

77. Hortobagyi GN, Ames FC, Buzdar AU, et al. Management of stage III primary breast cancer with primary chemotherapy, surgery, and radiation therapy. Cancer 1988;62:2507–16.

78. Rubens RD, Armitage P, Winter PJ, et al. Prognosis in inoperable stage III carcinoma of the breast. Eur J Cancer 1977;13:805–11.

79. Alderman SJ. Combination teletherapy and iridium implantation in the treatment of locally advanced breast cancer. Cancer 1976;38:1936–8.

80. Bruckman JE, Harris JR, Levene MB, et al. Results of treating stage III carcinoma of the breast by primary radiation therapy. Cancer 1979;43:985–93.

81. Fletcher GH. Clinical dose response curves of human malignant epithelial tumours. Br J Radiol 1973;46:151.

82. Bedwinek J, Rao DV, Perez C, et al. Stage III and localized stage IV breast cancer: irradiation alone vs irradiation plus surgery. Int J Radiat Oncol Biol Phys 1982;8:31–6.

83. Spanos WJ Jr, Montague ED, Fletcher GH. Late complications of radiation only for advanced breast cancer. Int J Radiat Oncol Biol Phys 1980;6:1473–6.

84. Montague ED. Radiation management of advanced breast cancer. Int J Radiat Oncol Biol Phys 1978;4:305–7.

85. Tapley ND, Montague ED. Elective irradiation with the electron beam after mastectomy for breast cancer. AJR Am J Roentgenol 1976;126:127–34.

86. Lee BJ, Tannenbaum NE. Inflammatory carcinoma of the breast. Surg Gynecol Obstet 1924;39:580–95.

87. Haagensen CD. Diseases of the breast. 2nd ed. Philadelphia: WB Saunders, 1971:576.

88. Taylor GW, Meltzer A. Inflammatory carcinoma of the breast. Am J Cancer 1938;33:33–49.

89. Levine PH, Steinhorn SC, Ries LG, Aron JL. Inflammatory breast cancer: the experience of the surveillance, epidemiology, and end results (SEER) program. J Natl Cancer Inst 1985;74:291–7.

90. Beahrs OH, et al, eds. American Joint Committee on Cancer. Manual for staging of cancer. 2nd ed. Philadelphia: JB Lippincott, 1983.

91. Bozzetti F, Saccozzi R, De Lena M, Salvadori B. Inflammatory cancer of the breast: analysis of 114 cases. J Surg Oncol 1981;18:355–61.

92. Wang CC. Management of inflammatory carcinoma of the breast. Int J Radiat Oncol Biol Phys 1978;4:709–10.

93. Perez CA, Presant C, Philpott G, Ratkin G. Phase I–II study of concurrent irradiation and multi-drug chemotherapy in advanced carcinoma of the breast: a pilot study by the Southeastern Cancer Study Group. Int J Radiat Oncol Biol Phys 1979;5:1329–33.

94. Thomas P. Radiotherapy of metastases of mammary carcinoma. Radiol Clin 1976;45:306–13.

95. Schocker JD, Brady LW. Radiation therapy for bone metastasis. Clin Orthop 1982;169:38–43.

96. Trodella L, Ausili-Cefaro G, Turriziani A, et al. Pain in osseous metastases: results of radiotherapy. Pain 1984;18:387–96.

97. Tong D, Gillick L, Hendrickson FR. The palliation of symptomatic osseous metastases: final results of the study by the Radiation Therapy Oncology Group. Cancer 1982;50:893–9.

98. Bonarigo BC, Rubin P. Nonunion of pathologic fracture after radiation therapy. Radiology 1967;88:889–98.

99. Fitzpatrick PJ, Garrett PG. Metastatic breast cancer: ovarian ablation with lower half-body irradiation. Int J Radiat Oncol Biol Phys 1981;7:1523–6.

100. Bartelink H, Battermann J, Hart G. Half body irradiation. Int J Radiat Oncol Biol Phys 1980;6:87–90.

101. Salazar OM, Rubin P, Hendrickson FR, et al. Single-dose half-body irradiation for palliation of multiple bone metastases from solid tumors: final Radiation Therapy Oncology Group report. Cancer 1986;58:29–36.

102. West J, Maor M. Intracranial metastases: behavioral patterns related to primary site and results of treatment by whole brain irradiation. Int J Radiat Oncol Biol Phys 1980;6:11-5.

103. Chu FCH, Hilaris BB. Value of radiation therapy in the management of intracranial metastases. Cancer 1961;14:577–81.

104. Coia LR. The role of radiation therapy in the treatment of brain metastases. Int J Radiat Oncol Biol Phys 1992;23:229–38.

105. Wright RL. Malignant tumors in the spinal epidural space: results of surgical treatment. Am Surg 1963;157:227–31.

106. Winkelman MD, Adelstein DJ, Karlins NL. Intramedullary spinal cord metastasis: diagnostic and therapeutic considerations. Arch Neurol 1987;44:526–31.
107. White WA, Patterson RH Jr, Bergland RM. Role of surgery in the treatment of spinal cord compression by metastatic neoplasm. Cancer 1971;27:558–61.
108. Young RF, Post EM, King GA. Treatment of spinal epidural metastases: randomized prospective comparison of laminectomy and radiotherapy. J Neurosurg 1980;53:741–8.
109. Makin WP. Treatment of spinal cord compression due to malignant disease. Br J Radiol 1988;61:715. abstract.
110. Maor M, Chan RC, Young SE. Radiotherapy of choroidal metastases: breast cancer as primary site. Cancer 1977;40:2081–6.
111. Dobrowsky W. Treatment of choroid metastases. Br J Radiol 1988;61:140–2.
112. Glassburn JR, Klionsky M, Brady LW. Radiation therapy for metastatic disease involving the orbit. Am J Clin Oncol 1984;1:145–8.
113. Chu FC, Huh SH, Nisce LZ, Simpson LD. Radiation therapy of choroid metastasis from breast cancer. Int J Radiat Oncol Biol Phys 1977;2:273–9.
114. Jaffe BM, Donegan WL, Watson F, Spratt JS Jr. Factors influencing survival in patients with untreated hepatic metastases. Surg Gynecol Obstet 1968;127:1–11.
115. Wharton JT, Delclos L, Gallager S, Smith JP. Radiation hepatitis induced by abdominal irradiation with the cobalt 60 moving strip technique. Am J Roentgenol Radium Ther Nucl Med 1973;117:73–80.
116. Borgelt BB, Gelber R, Brady LW, et al. The palliation of hepatic metastases: results of the Radiation Therapy Oncology Group pilot study. Int J Radiat Oncol Biol Phys 1981;7:587–91.

# SYSTEMIC TREATMENT FOR METASTASES

• Linnea I. Chap • Charles M. Haskell

Most women with breast cancer receive systemic therapy at some point in the course of their disease. This therapy may consist of endocrine manipulation or cytotoxic chemotherapy, or both. The goals of therapy vary from palliation to cure, depending on a wide variety of factors. This section reviews palliative chemotherapy and endocrine therapy for patients with metastatic breast cancer as well as the use of these modalities given with curative intent for patients with less advanced disease (*adjuvant therapy*).

## PRINCIPLES OF SYSTEMIC TREATMENT

Endocrine manipulation and cytotoxic chemotherapy represent the two major classes of systemic therapy used in the treatment of metastatic breast cancer. Immunotherapy is currently investigational. Because of the concept of tumor cell heterogeneity and the principles of combination chemotherapy, some clinicians use chemotherapy and endocrine therapy together. Particularly in patients with metastatic disease, however, there are many advantages to using them separately in a sequential manner. The quality of life during a remission induced by endocrine manipulation is usually superior to that seen with cytotoxic chemotherapy, and the duration of response may extend for many years. If chemotherapy is postponed too long in a fruitless attempt to obtain a response with endocrine therapy, however, chemotherapy may be less effective and less well tolerated.[1] When the two modalities are combined, one cannot differentiate which modality has conferred benefit. The use of some forms of endocrine manipulation may interfere with the successful use of chemotherapy.[2–5] Little is known about the biochemical and cytokinetic interactions of chemotherapy and hormonal therapy, and, with such precise information lacking, their use in combination remains empirical and of uncertain value. The key question is how to distinguish between the patient with metastatic disease who should receive chemotherapy initially and the patient who should be treated with endocrine manipulation.

## CHOOSING BETWEEN ENDOCRINE MANIPULATION AND CHEMOTHERAPY

Choosing therapy for a patient with metastatic breast cancer requires an understanding of the natural history of the disease and a careful evaluation of the individual patient. The hormone receptor status of the patient's tumor is of paramount importance. It is widely accepted that endocrine therapy is unlikely to benefit a patient with breast cancer tissue that lacks hormone receptor proteins. This fact is illustrated in Table 35–21, which gives data on the frequency of response to various forms of endocrine manipulation for patients with various combinations of ERs and PRs.

There is a correlation between the quantitative level of ERs and the clinical response to hormonal manipulation. In general, about 50 to 60% of premenopausal women and 60 to 75% of postmenopausal women with breast cancer have positive ERs.[7] The frequency and concentration of ERs increase in the order of perimenopausal, premenopausal, and postmenopausal periods. This increase correlates with the observation that endocrine manipulation tends to be more useful in postmenopausal patients of advanced age than in the premenopausal age group. For example, estrogen treatment is more effective in women who are more than 5 years postmenopausal than in younger women,[8] and the response rate to adrenalectomy is higher in postmenopausal women than in premenopausal or perimenopausal women.[9] If treatment is based on hormone receptor assays, the rate of hor-

*Table 35–21.* **Hormone Receptors and Response to Endocrine Therapy**

| Receptor Status | No. Patients | Response Rate (%) |
|---|---|---|
| ER − PgR − | 96 | 10 |
| ER − PgR + | 12 | 33 |
| ER + PgR − | 132 | 34 |
| ER + PgR + | 159 | 74 |

ER, estrogen receptor; PgR, progesterone receptor.
From Lippman M. Steroid hormone receptors and mechanisms of growth regulation of human breast cancer. In: Lippman M, ed. Diagnosis and management of breast cancer. Philadelphia: WB Saunders, 1988:337.

monal response between premenopausal and postmenopausal women is nearly the same. In either case, 50 to 60% response rates are seen in patients with hormone receptor–positive tumors, and only 5 to 10% response rates are found in those with hormone receptor–negative tumors.

In addition to the hormone receptor status of a tumor, a variety of other factors may affect the choice of therapy. These include (1) the disease-free interval; (2) the sites of metastatic disease; (3) the age, performance status, and hematologic status of the patient; and (4) the response to previous therapy. It is widely recognized that a short disease-free interval (<1 year) between primary treatment and subsequent metastatic disease is associated with rapidly growing disease. These patients tend to respond poorly to hormonal manipulation, but the more rapid tumor growth may allow some degree of control by cytotoxic chemotherapy. Conversely a disease-free interval greater than 36 months has been reported to be one of the most significant predictors for tumor responsiveness to hormonal therapy.[10]

The sites of metastatic disease may also influence the choice of systemic treatment. For example, patients with metastatic disease restricted to the skeleton often have an indolent course. Metastatic disease in the soft tissues, skin, regional lymph nodes, pleural cavity, or bone tends to respond better to endocrine manipulation than does involvement of the abdominal or thoracic viscera or the brain. For this reason, trials of hormonal therapy in patients with unknown ER and PR status may be justified for patients with soft tissue or bone metastases but are less likely to be useful in treating patients with advanced visceral disease. Some forms of visceral involvement (such as extensive liver or pulmonary lymphangitic disease) so rarely respond to endocrine manipulation that immediate chemotherapy is usually necessary.

The importance of age in choosing treatment is somewhat controversial. Some authorities decry the use of minimal treatment in elderly patients.[11, 12] Nevertheless, several studies suggest that elderly patients may benefit from the use of less aggressive treatment. Two examples serve to illustrate this point. First, in a randomized trial of combination chemotherapy compared with tamoxifen in patients older than age 65, survival rates tended to favor tamoxifen as the initial treatment, even for elderly patients lacking hormonal receptors.[13] Second, two randomized clinical trials of mastectomy versus tamoxifen for patients with primary breast cancer have been conducted in the United Kingdom.[14, 15] Local control was better in one of the two trials for mastectomy, but neither trial found a significant difference in survival between the two treatments. These studies have generated a vigorous debate but suggest that conservative therapy with tamoxifen alone is an option in selected elderly patients with primary breast cancer. If other factors suggest a need for chemotherapy, the older patient can frequently tolerate cytotoxic therapy. In a review of five trials for metastatic disease, the response rate was not statistically different for patients 70 years and older.[16] There was no difference in time to progression or survival for older patients, and performance status was the best predictor of response. The older patients were less likely to have gastrointestinal side effects but had a higher incidence of severe neutropenia.

A previous response to oophorectomy or other hormonal manipulations may be useful in predicting a response to other forms of hormonal or ablative therapy. Conversely, a history of adjuvant therapy in the recent past in a patient with metastatic disease is associated with a poor response to subsequent endocrine therapy.[17–19] One mechanism of such resistance is the acquisition of the multiple drug resistance phenotype (mdr phenotype) following either tamoxifen or chemotherapy. The treatment of relapse after adjuvant systemic treatment has been reviewed for the reader interested in further discussion of this important topic.[20]

A few studies have attempted to correlate tumor responsiveness to hormonal therapy with HER-2/*neu* oncogene expression and have reported conflicting results. An intergroup study evaluated 205 patients with ER-positive breast cancer for HER-2/*neu* expression by immunohistochemistry. The patients all received tamoxifen as first-line therapy for metastatic disease. HER-2/*neu* positivity bore no prognostic significance with regard to response rate, time to failure, or survival.[21] Other studies, measuring circulating levels for the extracellular domain of the HER-2/*neu* oncogene, have found that ER-positive patients are less likely to respond to hormonal treatment.[22, 23] Until further prospective investigation, using standardized methodology, it may be premature to use HER-2/*neu* expression in making treatment decisions regarding hormonal therapy.

## ENDOCRINE MANIPULATION

Before discussing the details of endocrine manipulation, several guidelines are presented. First, only one course of endocrine therapy is employed at a time. There is no evidence that combining endocrine agents improves survival, and combination hormonal therapy is associated with additive toxicity. Combined therapy complicates the evaluation of response to any particular individual agent. This guideline does not preclude the addition of other essential therapy, such as the use of radiation therapy to palliate an area of metastatic disease in the bone, brain, or elsewhere.

Second, therapy is changed only if disease is advancing and not, as a rule, if it is static. This is because the survival of a patient with stable disease appears to be the same as that of a patient who achieves a partial or even a complete response from endocrine therapy.[24–27] This situation is in marked contrast to some other diseases, such as the high-grade malignant lymphomas, in which only complete responses have a clinically important impact on prognosis. It can be extremely difficult to evaluate some areas of metastatic disease. An important example of this is the evaluation of destructive or osteoblastic bone metastases. Such lesions are notoriously difficult to evaluate and rarely show evidence of healing. In this case, the development of new lesions may be the best indicator of disease progression and the need for a change in therapeutic strategy. In evaluating new lesions found by bone scan, however, it is important to differentiate between a good response to therapy with bone healing and progressive disease with bone destruction. This differential diagnosis generally requires a correlation of all new bone scan abnormalities with plain radiographs, possibly supplemented by observing serial levels of the serum CEA level or Ca 27.29 (or other marker, if available).

Third, a patient with slowly progressive disease being treated with endocrine manipulation can usually be observed for a period off treatment before changing therapy. This practice is to ascertain whether or not the patient has a *remission of withdrawal* before a new treatment program is started. This situation is most likely to occur in patients who have had a beneficial effect from estrogen therapy,[28] but it has also been reported after the use of tamoxifen and megestrol acetate.[29, 30] This guideline is inappropriate for patients with rapidly advancing disease or those with involvement of vital organs.

Finally, contraceptive pills are contraindicated in the young patient because they introduce another hormonal variable and, in some instances, may cause exacerbation of disease.[31] Barrier contraception should be recommended, especially for patients taking tamoxifen, because of potential embryotoxicity.

The precise choice of endocrine therapy varies with the menopausal status of the patient. It may consist of a surgical procedure or any of several hormonal agents (Table 35–22). The initial choice of endocrine manipulation is commonly called *primary* hormonal manipulation, whereas subsequent manipulation is called *secondary* or *tertiary* therapy.[9]

**Premenopausal Patients.** Patients who are menstruating or within 1 year of their last menstrual period are considered premenopausal.

*Primary Endocrine Manipulation.* Bilateral oophorectomy was the usual initial therapy in premenopausal women who were candidates for endocrine therapy.[32–34] Oophorectomy is presumed to work by the elimination of ovarian hormones, including estrogen, progesterone, and androgens, all of which may stimulate the growth of breast cancer. Bilateral oophorectomy causes an objective regression in about one third of all premenopausal women (range, 15 to 56%), but this response rate can be doubled by excluding patients who have ER-negative tumors. Responses generally last 9 to 15 months; the longest response on record is 18 years.[35]

If the patient is an acceptable operative risk, surgical castration is preferable to ovarian radiation because it acts rapidly, results in a more complete reduction in hormone levels, and does not compromise bone marrow areas that may be needed during later cytotoxic chemotherapy. Using modern endoscopic surgery, this is a relatively simple procedure. Hysterectomy is not necessary in these patients, and they should not be given postoperative estrogen to relieve attendant menopausal symptoms. Other measures to control vascular instability may be considered, such as the administration of megestrol acetate, clonidine, or the ergot alkaloids. Poor-risk patients or those who refuse surgical oophorectomy may undergo radiation ablation with 15 Gy given over 5 days, delivered to the pelvis.[34] Another approach is to perform a medical oophorectomy using a luteinizing hormone–releasing hormone (LHRH) agonist or gonadotropin-releasing hormone (GnRH) agonist, such as leuprolide or goserelin (Zoladex).[36] It is generally held that oophorectomy is not useful in patients who are more than 1 year past menopause,[37, 38] although not all authors agree with this view.[33]

Many clinicians (and nearly all patients) prefer to use tamoxifen as the primary form of endocrine manipulation in premenopausal patients. Pritchard and coworkers,[39] in a small phase II trial of 42 patients, reported a 32% response rate for unselected patients and a 44% response rate for patients with hormone receptor–positive tumors. Similar results have been reported by others,[40–43] and the response duration with tamoxifen appears to be similar to that seen with oophorectomy. There have been two randomized clinical trials comparing tamoxifen with bilateral oophorectomy,

*Table 35–22.* **Hormonal Agents Used for Advanced Breast Cancer**

| Agent | Class | Dose and Schedule of Administration and Selected References* |
|---|---|---|
| *Commercially available agents approved by the FDA for the treatment of breast cancer* | | |
| Tamoxifen (Nolvadex) | Antiestrogen | 20 mg PO once daily |
| Megestrol acetate (Megace) | Progestin | 40 mg PO 4 times daily |
| Diethylstilbestrol | Estrogen | 5 mg PO 3 times daily |
| Fluoxymesterone (Halotestin) | Androgen | 10–40 mg PO daily (divided dose) |
| Methyltestosterone | Androgen | 50–200 mg PO daily (divided dose) |
| Testolactone (Teslac) | Androgen (?) | 250 mg PO 4 times daily |
| Toremifene (Fareston) | Antiestrogen | 60 mg PO once daily |
| Letrozole (Femara) | Selective aromatase inhibitor | 2.5 mg PO once daily |
| Anastrozole (Arimidex) | Selective aromatase inhibitor | 1 mg PO once daily |
| Goserelin (Zoladex) | GnRH agonist analogue | 3.6 mg SC once monthly |
| *Commercially available agents not specifically approved by the FDA for the treatment of breast cancer, but use in breast cancer is under investigation or is supported by some authorities and by articles in the medical literature* | | |
| Leuprolide (Lupron Depot) | LHRH agonist analogue | 7.5 mg depot IM once monthly‡ |
| Aminoglutethimide (Cytadren) | Aromatase inhibitor | 250 mg PO 4 times daily with hydrocortisone†§ |
| Medroxyprogesterone acetate (Depo-Provera) | Progestin | Investigational doses of 1–1.5 g daily by the IM route[183] |
| Flutamide | Antiandrogen | Di Monaco[184] |
| Octreotide acetate (Sandostatin) | Somatostatin analogue | Weckbecker[185]; Pollak[186] |

*Authorities recognized by the Health Care Finance Authority, which is responsible for Medicare payments in the United States, are as identified below. Approval of each drug for the treatment of breast cancer is indicated by the presence of the appropriate footnote designation.
†AMA Drug Evaluations. The American Medical Association, Division of Drugs and Toxicology, 535 N. Dearborn Street, Chicago, IL 60610.
‡AHFS Drug Information. American Society of Hospital Pharmacists, Inc., 4630 Montgomery Avenue, Bethesda, MD 20814.
§USP DI. The United States Pharmacopeial Convention, Inc., 12601 Twinbrook Parkway, Rockville, MD 20852.
FDA, Food and Drug Administration; GnRH, gonadotropin-releasing hormone; LHRH, luteinizing hormone–releasing hormone; SC, subcutaneously; IM, intramuscularly.

in which no significant difference in survival or response could be seen between the two forms of treatment.[44, 45] There is controversy, however, about whether a response to tamoxifen predicts the subsequent value of other forms of endocrine manipulation.[39, 41, 46] On the basis of the available evidence, it appears that an initial failure of tamoxifen does not preclude the possibility of a subsequent response to castration.[43, 44, 47–49] There is no evidence that combining ovarian ablation with tamoxifen is superior to either therapy alone.

*Secondary Endocrine Manipulation.* Patients who fail to respond to oophorectomy or tamoxifen are usually considered candidates for systemic chemotherapy, unless indolent disease and high levels of hormonal receptors in the tumor suggest that another trial of endocrine treatment is reasonable. Patients who respond to oophorectomy or tamoxifen and then experience relapse may be considered for a variety of endocrine treatments.[9, 37] Tamoxifen is generally employed in patients who relapse after an oophorectomy because of its relative safety and ease of use. Alternatively, other hormones may be used (notably megestrol acetate[50–54] or, less frequently, an androgen[55]), or one may choose an endocrine-ablative approach to therapy. In the past, this ablation was primarily achieved by either an adrenalectomy or a hypophysectomy,[56] but now this can be achieved medically by the use of an aromatase inhibitor, such as aminoglutethimide (Cytadren)[57–60] or one of the more recently approved selective aromatase inhibitors (see later). The results of medical adrenalectomy with aminoglutethimide appear to be equivalent to those of surgical ablation but without the risks of surgery and the creation of irreversible adrenal suppression. Consequently, at present, surgical ablation is never recommended.

Numerous groups are exploring the use of various hormones used together as combination hormonal therapy, and newer hormones (such as the LHRH and GnRH agonists) are being tested for use. The relative value of these new agents and combinations is currently unclear, as are precise guidelines for selecting among the currently available hormones in patients with hormonally responsive tumors. The limited crossover studies available suggest that patients with slowly progressive disease may be sequentially treated with any of several hormonal agents as long as they continue to respond.[61]

**Postmenopausal Patients.** Patients whose last menstrual period occurred more than 1 year before the development of metastatic breast cancer are generally considered postmenopausal.

*Primary Endocrine Manipulation.* The treatment of choice for postmenopausal women with ER-positive metastatic breast cancer is tamoxifen.[62–65] This appears to be the case for patients who had received a short course of tamoxifen as adjuvant therapy as well as for patients with no prior endocrine treatment.[66] The response rate in these treated women is approximately 50%, with a duration of response of 12 to 15 months. The usual dose of tamoxifen is 20 mg once daily. Despite anecdotal reports to the contrary,[67] there is little to be gained with higher doses, either initially or at the time of disease progression.[68–70] Toremifene (Fareston) was approved in 1997 by the FDA for the first-line treatment of postmenopausal women with estrogen-positive or unknown metastatic breast cancer. The drug is structurally

similar to tamoxifen, differing only by a single chlorine atom. In phase II and III clinical trials, it appears to be of comparable efficacy and tolerability as tamoxifen and is an acceptable alternative in this setting.[71, 72]

*Secondary Endocrine Manipulation.* Postmenopausal patients who respond to tamoxifen and subsequently experience relapse are candidates for secondary endocrine manipulation. In the past, megestrol acetate[51, 73, 74] was frequently chosen at this point or aminoglutethimide as a reasonable alternative. Given the favorable toxicity profiles of the newer selective aromatase inhibitors, such as letrozole[75] and anastrozole,[76] however, one of these agents should be considered for second-line therapy. Both these drugs are FDA approved for the treatment of postmenopausal metastatic breast cancer and do not require corticosteroid supplementation. DES or an androgen may subsequently be considered, but these are generally avoided because of toxicity.[77] The doses, mechanisms of action, and toxicities of these drugs are given in Chapter 10. As discussed previously for premenopausal patients, combination hormonal therapy is currently investigational.

*Investigational Endocrine Therapy.* A variety of new hormonal agents are under investigation. Some of these agents are SERMs, designed with the hope that more effective and less toxic antiestrogen therapy can be used. New LHRH and GnRH agonists are being studied, oriented toward the induction of a medical oophorectomy. Studies are also readdressing the utility of combined hormonal therapy, such as the combination of tamoxifen and a selective aromatase inhibitor.

## CHEMOTHERAPY

Candidates for palliative, nonhormonal chemotherapy include patients with disseminated breast cancer who fail to maintain a response to hormonal manipulation, patients with rapidly advancing and widespread disease (especially in the liver or lungs), and symptomatic patients with metastatic tumors that lack hormone receptors. Patients with metastatic breast cancer who are treated with chemotherapy often receive several drugs in combination rather than single-agent chemotherapy. Because chemotherapy is rarely, if ever, curative in patients with advanced disease, the precise use of this modality is controversial. Specific controversies are addressed subsequently.

**Duration of Therapy.** Chemotherapy can be given as *induction therapy* over a finite period, followed either by continuous *maintenance* chemotherapy or a period of observation off treatment.[78] One trial of 18 versus 6 months of chemotherapy found a survival advantage with 18 months of chemotherapy.[79] Two other trials comparing short-term and continuous chemotherapy found no survival difference, but continuous therapy was associated with better quality of life in one study,[80] and in another it was associated with a longer progression-free interval.[81] We are aware of only one formal trial of induction therapy followed by attempted reinduction treatment in patients who progress after a period of observation.[82] The response rate to reinduction was 18%, the time to treatment failure was 3 months, and toxicity was high. On the basis of the available literature and our personal experience, we usually encourage the patient to remain on chemotherapy indefinitely once it is started, presuming the disease is under reasonable control. It is not unreasonable, however, to offer the patient *treatment-free* holidays. For patients who achieve an excellent response to initial chemotherapy, consideration can be given to *maintenance* hormonal therapy (e.g., tamoxifen) if they are hormone receptor positive and have not previously done poorly with such therapy. Another option is an arbitrary number of cycles of chemotherapy (e.g., four to six after a complete remission is attained).

**Dose Intensity.** Response rates in metastatic breast cancer correlate well with dose intensity, but it has been difficult to prove that higher response rates result in improved overall survival.[78, 83–85] This difficulty may relate to a high rate of intrinsic drug resistance in metastatic breast cancer and the relatively small number of complete responses seen with chemotherapy, even with high-dose therapy. Because of laboratory studies and a strong theoretical basis for predicting improved survival with more dose-intense therapy, this represents an area of active investigation.[86] Approaches to increasing dose intensity for breast cancer include the use of growth factors (such as granulocyte colony–stimulating factor); autologous bone marrow transplantation (ABMT), either alone or with peripheral stem cell support; and the use of high-dose sequential single-agent therapy in lieu of combination chemotherapy. High-dose therapy is accompanied by a relatively high risk of toxicity, and there is no proof at present that it cures metastatic breast cancer or results in long-term disease control. Further discussion on ABMT follows later in this section.

**Choice of Agents.** In the sections that follow, we review the available single agents, combination chemotherapy as first-line treatment of metastatic disease, chemotherapy for patients who relapse after chemotherapy, combined chemotherapy and endocrine therapy, dose-intense therapy with ABMT, and immunotherapy. Recommendations for the treatment of specific groups of patients are discussed further in the section Treatment by Stage of Disease and Special Problems.

**Single Agents.** Doxorubicin (Adriamycin), paclitaxel (Taxol), docetaxel (Taxotere), several alkylating agents (including classic agents such as cyclophosphamide and nonclassic agents such as cisplatin), methotrexate, and 5-fluorouracil (5-FU) are considered to be active single agents in the treatment of metastatic breast cancer (Table 35–23). Lesser degrees of activity have also been seen with mitoxantrone, mitomycin, low-dose oral etoposide (but not intravenous etoposide), vinorelbine, vinblastine, vincristine, and gemcitabine. Single-agent responses are only rarely complete, and the median duration of response varies between 4 and 6 months. The standard doses and schedules of administration for these drugs are given in Chapter 10. Experimental schedules and dose-intense protocols for doxorubicin,[87, 88] mitoxantrone,[89] vincristine,[90] and vinblastine[91, 92] have been reported, but none of these approaches is standard therapy. There is continued interest, however, in two unusual schedules of administration for two of the most useful single agents. There is growing evidence that continuous-infusion 5-FU may be effective in patients who have previously become resistant to standard bolus therapy.[93, 94] The FDA approved capecitabine (Xeloda)[95] for the treatment of metastatic breast cancer in patients previously treated with doxo-

*Table 35–23.* **Single-Agent Chemotherapy for Metastatic Breast Cancer\***

| Drug | No. Patients | Response Rate (%) |
|---|---|---|
| *Antibiotics* | | |
| Doxorubicin[187–192] | 672 | 37 |
| Idarubicin[193] | 121 | 26 |
| Mitoxantrone[192–194] | 859 | 19 |
| Mitomycin[195] | 394 | 19 |
| *Alkylating Agents* | | |
| Cisplatin (first line)[196, 197] | 74 | 49 |
| Mechlorethamine[187, 188] | 92 | 35 |
| Cyclophosphamide[187, 188] | 529 | 34 |
| Ifosfamide[198] | 341 | 34 |
| Carboplatin (first line)[199] | 85 | 31 |
| Thiotepa[187, 188] | 162 | 30 |
| Melphalan[187, 188] | 86 | 23 |
| Carmustine[187, 188] | 76 | 21 |
| Chlorambucil[187, 188] | 54 | 20 |
| Cisplatin (second line)[200–202] | 174 | 20 |
| *Antimetabolites* | | |
| Methotrexate[187, 188] | 356 | 34 |
| Fluorouracil with leucovorin[203–206] | 197 | 30 |
| Fluorouracil[187, 188] | 1236 | 26 |
| Capecitabine (third line)[95, 207] | 43 | 26 |
| *Other* | | |
| Paclitaxel[120, 208, 209] | 128 | 45 |
| Docetaxel (second line)[121] | 161 | 45 |
| Etoposide (second line, long-term PO)[210, 211] | 61 | 31 |
| Vinblastine[187, 188, 212] | 118 | 22 |
| Vincristine[187, 188, 212] | 241 | 20 |
| Vinorelbine[213, 214] | — | — |
| Epirubicin[189, 190, 193, 215–218] | — | — |
| Gemcitabine[219] | 44 | 25 |
| Irinotecan[220] | 65 | 23 |

\*Response rates are for combined complete and partial responses. Older drugs may have been tested in previously untreated patients, whereas most of the newer drugs have been tested only in patients with extensive prior therapy (exceptions are noted). Commercially available drugs with response rates of 15% or less are as follows: etoposide (as first-line or second-line intravenous therapy); mercaptopurine, plicamycin, lomustine, hydroxyurea, altretamine, cytarabine, bleomycin, dacarbazine, carboplatin (second line), estramustine, teniposide, dactinomycin, thioguanine, procarbazine, trimetrexate, and streptozocin.

rubicin and paclitaxel. The drug is an oral analogue of 5-FU with comparable efficacy to intravenous administration of the latter. There has been a growing experience with the weekly administration of doxorubicin in elderly and frail patients, especially following the failure of combination chemotherapy.[96–98] Although further study of these techniques is needed, they may prove useful in selected patients.

Older reports of cancer chemotherapy have not used consistent response criteria, and many drugs have been tested in patients who have been extensively pretreated with chemotherapy. The response rates given in Table 35–23 should be taken as approximations. The importance of this problem has been reviewed.[99]

**First-Line Combination Chemotherapy.** Because of the success of combination chemotherapy in treating acute leukemia, Hodgkin's disease, and a variety of childhood tumors, it was natural that combination chemotherapy should be tested extensively in metastatic breast cancer. Although the first report of successful combination chemotherapy in breast cancer was published in 1963 by Greenspan,[100] it was only with the report of Cooper[101] in 1969 describing the use of a cyclophosphamide, methotrexate, 5-FU, vincristine, and prednisone (CMFVP) regimen that combination chemotherapy became a widely accepted approach to management. A variety of modifications of Cooper's regimen have been tried, as summarized in Table 35–24.

Nearly all these regimens have been associated with an antitumor response rate of about 50%. These responses may be complete, and they commonly last about 9 to 12 months. Patients who respond to treatment live a median of two to three times as long as those who fail to respond, and some patients have responses that last many years. Combination chemotherapy appears to be superior to single-agent treatment in terms of overall response rates, the frequency of complete remissions, and the impact of treatment on survival. In the few studies that directly compare combination chemotherapy with single-agent treatment, this conclusion is confirmed,[102–104] although contradictory results exist.[105–107] One of the biggest problems in assessing the relative value of combination chemotherapy and single-agent chemotherapy relates to the adequacy of the single-agent treatment employed in early studies. Most of these studies used relatively ineffective single agents in relatively low doses. In trials with single-agent doxorubicin given in higher doses, the apparent superiority of combination chemotherapy is less clear.[108–110]

One randomized study compared single-agent weekly epirubicin followed by single-agent mitomycin with combination cyclophosphamide, epirubicin, and 5-FU followed by mitomycin and vinblastine as first-line and second-line therapies.[111] No significant difference was found in the time to progression or survival between the two arms. The single-agent arm, however, experienced less toxicity and better quality of life. There is great interest in the potential value of high-dose single-agent therapy as a way of giving more dose-intense treatment, both in the setting of advanced disease and in adjuvant therapy.

Subsequent to CMFVP, two other groups of combination chemotherapy regimens were developed. The first and most important group uses doxorubicin, whereas the other group includes a wide variety of miscellaneous regimens that have usually been studied as possible salvage regimens for patients who develop resistance to CMF. Several randomized trials have demonstrated improved response rates with CAF (cyclophosphamide, doxorubicin [Adriamycin], 5-FU) versus

CMF but with little to no impact on overall survival.[112–114] Various alternative combination regimens have been examined as first-line therapy, including the substitution of mitoxantrone (Novantrone) for doxorubicin in CAF, with corresponding response rates of 29% versus 37% (CNF (cyclophosphamide, Novantrone [mitoxantrone], fluorouracil) vs. CAF).[115] The combination of a taxane (paclitaxel or docetaxel) with doxorubicin has shown response rates of 90% in chemotherapy-naive patients but to date has not affected survival and may increase the risk of cardiotoxicity.[116–119]

Despite the widespread use of a variety of combination regimens, few are unequivocally superior to the others and have only rarely been directly compared in randomized trials. One can rank the various regimens by response rates, but this single parameter hardly does justice to estimating the value of the different approaches. The details of prior therapy, the presence or absence of various prognostic factors, and the impact of treatment on overall survival are also important considerations. None of the available regimens can be considered ideal because none of them cures metastatic breast cancer, and they are all highly toxic regimens. Nevertheless, combination chemotherapy is a cornerstone of the modern management of metastatic breast cancer, and these regimens are potentially even more valuable when used for the treatment of micrometastatic disease (see discussion of adjuvant chemotherapy later).

## SALVAGE CHEMOTHERAPY

Patients who do not respond to a first-line combination chemotherapy regimen or respond and subsequently relapse are candidates for second-line regimens or one of several single agents. This is often called *salvage chemotherapy*. A variety of regimens have been tried for this purpose (Table 35–25). Because of the variability of prior treatment with doxorubicin, these regimens are separated into two groups: those with and those without doxorubicin in the combination. In general, salvage regimens containing doxorubicin are not used in patients with prior doxorubicin therapy.

Patients naive to doxorubicin can be offered the drug in combination or as a single agent. For patients who have received prior doxorubicin therapy, a taxane is the next agent of choice. Paclitaxel and docetaxel have reported response rates between 30 and 60% in patients previously treated with doxorubicin.[120, 121]

## CHEMOTHERAPY PLUS ENDOCRINE MANIPULATION

There has been substantial interest in testing combinations of various cytotoxic drugs with endocrine manipulation because of tumor cell heterogeneity and the established principles of combination chemotherapy calling for the use of non–cross-resistant drugs with different mechanisms of action (see Chapter 8). Most of the early trials addressing this question involved relatively small numbers of patients, did not take into account the hormone receptor status of the tumors, and emphasized an analysis of initial response rates rather than the effect of treatment on survival. Many of the

*Table 35–24.* **Combination Chemotherapy Regimens Based on the Drugs of the Cooper Regimen Used as First-Line Chemotherapy for Patients with Metastatic Breast Cancer**

| Drug Combination | No. Patients | Response Rate (% CR + PR) |
|---|---|---|
| CMFP[221, 222] | 208 | 64 |
| CMF[222–226] | 324 | 50 |
| CMFVP[227–229] | 719 | 49 |
| CMFV[228–230] | 226 | 42 |

CR, complete response; PR, partial response (≥50% reduction); C, cyclophosphamide; M, methotrexate; F, 5-fluorouracil; P, prednisone; V, vincristine.

*Table 35–25.* Combination Chemotherapy Regimens for the Salvage Treatment of Metastatic Breast Cancer After the Use of One or More Other Regimens of Chemotherapy*

| Drug Combination | No. Patients | Response Rate (%) |
|---|---|---|
| *Regimens Containing Doxorubicin (Doxo)* | | |
| Doxo + mitomycin + vincristine[231] | 15 | 73 |
| Doxo + mitomycin[232, 233] | 95 | 44 |
| Doxo + etoposide[234, 235] | 58 | 38 |
| Doxo + vinblastine[236, 237] | 65 | 37 |
| Doxo + fluorouracil + vincristine (Oncovin), + mitomycin (FOAM)[238] | 82 | 35 |
| Doxo + mitomycin + vinblastine[239] | 27 | 33 |
| Doxo + vincristine[232] | 142 | 29 |
| Doxo + mitoxantrone[240] | 28 | 14 |
| *Regimens Without Doxorubicin* | | |
| Cyclophosphamide + mitoxantrone + fluorouracil + leucovorin[241] | 38 | 55 |
| Cisplatin + fluorouracil (infusion)[242] | 24 | 50 |
| Cyclophosphamide + etoposide[243] | 27 | 41 |
| Mitomycin + etoposide[244] | 25 | 40 |
| Mitoxantrone + methotrexate + fluorouracil[245] | 48 | 38 |
| Cisplatin + fluorouracil[246, 247] | 47 | 38 |
| Vinblastine + mitoxantrone[248, 249] | 96 | 38 |
| Mitoxantrone + fluorouracil + leucovorin ± cyclophosphamide[250–252] | 123 | 37 |
| Fluorouracil + dacarbazine + carmustine + prednisolone[253] | 60 | 37 |
| Mitomycin + fluorouracil + leucovorin[254] | 41 | 37 |
| Methotrexate + mitoxantrone + mitomycin[255] | 51 | 30 |
| Vinblastine + mitomycin[256–258] | 127 | 28 |
| Methotrexate + mitoxantrone[255] | 54 | 26 |
| Methotrexate + fluorouracil + leucovorin[259, 260] | 55 | 25 |
| Vinblastine + methotrexate[261] | 74 | 23 |
| Vinblastine + methotrexate + leucovorin[261] | 75 | 23 |
| Ifosfamide + etoposide[262] | 44 | 22 |
| Cisplatin + etoposide[271] | 206 | 20 |
| Ifosfamide + carboplatin + etoposide (ICE)[264] | 93 | 20 |
| Ifosfamide + methotrexate + fluorouracil[265] | 51 | 20 |
| Mitoxantrone + vinblastine[266] | 115 | 18 |
| Mitoxantrone + mitomycin ± methotrexate[267] | 33 | 15 |
| Carboplatin + etoposide[263, 269] | 64 | 14 |
| Carboplatin + fluorouracil + leucovorin[268] | 29 | 10 |
| Cisplatin + cytarabine[270] | 44 | 7 |

*This table is limited to representative regimens involving drugs that are commercially available in the United States.

early trials contained statistical flaws and were reported in the literature with minimal follow-up time. This problem is illustrated by the differences between survival reported initially and finally in a study conducted at the Mayo Clinic.[122, 123] Most of these early trials involved the mere addition of endocrine therapy to chemotherapy, without concern for potential schedule dependency. An exception was a study by Allegra,[124] in which a high response rate was reported with treatment involving tamoxifen given orally for 10 days, followed by estrogen (Premarin) in a physiologic dose for 4 days, followed by sequential methotrexate, 5-FU, and citrovorum factor rescue. Attempts to replicate this finding have been unsuccessful.[125]

The critical test of the value of chemohormonal therapy is the impact of such treatment on survival. Table 35–26 summarizes the results of 19 randomized clinical trials that address this question. On the basis of the results summarized in Table 35–26, plus the results of several publications suggesting that pharmacologic doses of some hormones may antagonize the effects of cytotoxic chemotherapy,[2–5, 126] the combined use of endocrine therapy and cytotoxic chemotherapy in patients with advanced breast cancer is of unproved value. This field needs considerable experimental work to place it on a rational footing.

## AUTOLOGOUS BONE MARROW AND STEM CELL TRANSPLANTATION

Autologous bone marrow and, more recently, autologous peripheral stem cells have been used as a means to deliver high-dose chemotherapy (HDC) to patients with metastatic breast cancer. Results from several centers have suggested a 25% 5-year disease-free survival rate.[127] The patients included in these studies, however, are a fairly select group of patients. They are typically young (<55 years), are in otherwise excellent health, and have had a complete or partial response to conventional chemotherapy. There have been two published randomized trials of HDC versus conventional therapy. The first was reported in 1995 from the University of Witwatersrand in South Africa,[128] but it was subsequently discredited because the data were fraudulent. The second trial was conducted by the Philadelphia group, which found no benefit from the higher doses of chemotherapy employed

*Table 35–26.* Randomized Clinical Trials Comparing Chemotherapy Alone and Chemohormonal Therapy for Metastatic Breast Cancer

| Reference | Treatment | No. Patients | Median Survival of Chemotherapy vs. Chemohormonal Therapy |
|---|---|---|---|
| Brunner et al[272] | CMFVP ± oophorectomy | 52* | 13.2 vs. 19.9 (NSD) |
| Brunner et al[272] | CMFVP ± diethylstilbestrol | 96 | 19.2 vs. 26.7 (NSD) |
| Rubens et al[273] | AV/CMF ± norethisterone | 69 | 15.0 vs. 8.0 (NSD) |
| Tormey et al[274] | DA ± tamoxifen | 122 | 9.0 vs. 11.3 (NSD) |
| Cocconi et al[275] | CMF ± tamoxifen | 133 | 27.8 vs. 19.5 (NSD) |
| CALGB[276] | CAF ± tamoxifen | 451 | NSD |
| Viladiu et al[277] | CMF ± tamoxifen or medroxyprogesterone | 98 | 22.5 vs. 24.7 (NSD) 22.5 vs. 21.7 (NSD) |
| Mouridsen et al[278] | CMF ± tamoxifen | 220 | 19 vs. 24 (NSD) |
| Kiang et al[279] | CF ± diethylstilbestrol | 31* | 16 vs. 16 (NSD) |
| ANZBCTG[280] | AC ± tamoxifen | 226 | 18 vs. 20 (NSD) |
| Krook et al[281] | CFP ± tamoxifen | 125 | 18 vs. 13 (NSD) |
| Falkson et al[282] | CAF ± oophorectomy | 131* | NSD |
| Jouve et al[283] | CAVF/Mtx, VM-26, Mmc ± tamoxifen | 223 | NSD |
| Conte et al[284] | CEF ± diethylstilbestrol | 117 | NSD |
| NCI[285, 286] | CAMF ± tamoxifen + Premarin | 110 | NSD |
| Elomaa et al[287] | Doxorubicin ± medroxyprogesterone | 43 | NSD |
| Gundersen et al[288] | FuMc or VAC ± medroxyprogesterone | 142† | 9 vs. 13 ($p > 0.05$) |
| Ingle et al[289] | CMF ± estrogen recruitment | 165 | NSD |
| Paridaens et al[290] | FAC aminoglutethimide/oophorectomy ± estrogen recruitment | 154 | NSD |

*Premenopausal patients only.

†Patients were hormone receptor negative; survival was shorter with medroxyprogesterone acetate, even though response rates were higher with chemoendocrine therapy.

NSD, no significant difference ($p > 0.05$); drug abbreviations given in Appendix C.

with transplantation.[291] HDC with stem cell support for patients with documented metastatic disease is of unproved benefit.

## CLINICAL USE OF SELECTED REGIMENS

The most widely employed regimens of combination chemotherapy are summarized in Table 35–27 for reference. These are discussed here briefly.

**CMF and CMFP.** The most widely used variations of the CMFVP regimen are the CMF and CMFP regimens developed by Canellos and associates (see Tables 35–24 and 35–27). These two combinations were modeled after the highly successful MOPP (mechlorethamine, vincristine [Oncovin], procarbazine, prednisone) regimen for Hodgkin's disease, which was also developed at the National Cancer Institute (see Chapter 87). As with the MOPP regimen, two drugs are given intravenously on days 1 and 8, with either one or two other drugs given orally for 2 weeks, followed by a 2-week rest period. The CMF regimen can be given almost indefinitely provided that the patient continues to respond to therapy. Some physicians have used prednisone with CMF because of improved treatment tolerance, although long-term use of prednisone should be avoided because it causes iatrogenic Cushing's syndrome. The value of prednisone in this regimen has been established, despite its toxicity, by a randomized trial in patients with metastatic breast cancer.[129, 130] The various forms of short-term toxicity seen with CMF are summarized in Table 35–28.

The doses of CMF chemotherapy are modified on the basis of the patient's age and the functional status of the bone marrow, liver, and kidney. Specifically, women younger than age 60 with normal blood counts, normal liver and kidney function, no previous cytotoxic chemotherapy, and minimal radiation therapy receive full doses. Methotrexate is omitted in the face of azotemia. Drug doses are initially reduced by one third to one half for women older than 70 to 75 years, for jaundice or liver dysfunction, or for grade 1 or 2 bone marrow toxicity, as defined in Chapter 8 and Appendix B. Chemotherapy is withheld for grade 3 or 4 bone marrow depression or serious gastrointestinal dysfunction.

**Intravenous CMF.** This regimen can be used in one of two forms: as intravenous injections every 3 weeks or on a day 1 and 8 schedule repeated every 4 weeks. The *every 3 week* schedule is not as effective as oral CMF in the treatment of metastatic breast cancer,[131] but it is in common use in the adjuvant setting. The day 1 and 8 schedule was developed, in part, because of concern about the efficacy of the 3-week schedule, but it has never been directly compared with classic oral CMF. Both schedules of intravenous CMF have the advantage of ensuring patient compliance because all of the drugs are given intravenously. The spectrum of toxicity is similar between the two regimens of intravenous CMF and that of oral CMF.

**AC.** This regimen (doxorubicin [Adriamycin] and cyclophosphamide) was initially developed at the University of Arizona as an intravenous injection of doxorubicin in a dose of 40 mg/m² on day 1 of each cycle, followed by 4 days of oral cyclophosphamide in a dose of 200 mg/m²/day given on days 3, 4, 5, and 6, with repeat cycles every 21 to 28 days, depending on tolerance. Once the total dose of doxorubicin reaches 450 mg/m², the patient is converted to a CMF maintenance regimen. This regimen is easy to use in the outpatient setting, and its efficacy is roughly similar to that of CMF. The spectrum of toxicity is similar to that of CMF except for nearly complete alopecia in most patients as well as the risk of cardiac toxicity. It requires the use of

*Table 35–27.* **Selected Combination Chemotherapy Regimens for the Adjuvant Treatment of Breast Cancer**

| Regimen | Cytotoxics | Dosage and Frequency |
|---|---|---|
| CMF—Classic | Cyclophosphamide<br>Methotrexate<br>5-Fluorouracil | $100$ mg/m$^2$ PO on days 1–14<br>$40$ mg/m$^2$ IV on days 1 and 8<br>$600$ mg/m$^2$ IV on days 1 and 8<br>*Repeat every 28 days for 6 cycles* |
| CMF—Contemporary | Cyclophosphamide<br>Methotrexate<br>5-Fluorouracil | $600$ mg/m$^2$ IV on day 1<br>$40$ mg/m$^2$ IV on day 1<br>$600$ mg/m$^2$ IV on day 1<br>*Repeat every 21 days for 9–12 cycles* |
| CAF | Cyclophosphamide<br>Adriamycin<br>5-Fluorouracil | $600$ mg/m$^2$ IV on day 1<br>$60$ mg/m$^2$ IV on day 1<br>$600$ mg/m$^2$ IV days 1 and 8<br>*Repeat every 21 days for 6 cycles* |
| FAC | 5-Fluorouracil<br>Adriamycin<br>Cyclophosphamide | $500$ mg/m$^2$ IV on days 1 and 8<br>$50$ mg/m$^2$ IV on day 1<br>$500$ mg/m$^2$ on day 1<br>*Repeat every 21 days for 6 cycles* |
| FEC | 5-Fluorouracil<br>Epirubicin<br>Cyclophosphamide | $600$ mg/m$^2$ IV on day 1<br>$100$ mg/m$^2$ IV on day 1<br>$600$ mg/m$^2$ IV on day 1<br>*Repeat every 21 days for 6 cycles* |
| CEF | Cyclophosphamide<br>Epirubicin<br>5-Fluorouracil | $75$ mg/m$^2$ PO on days 1–4<br>$60$ mg/m$^2$ IV on days 1 and 8<br>$500$ mg/m$^2$ IV on days 1 and 8<br>*Repeat every 28 days for 6 cycles* |
| AC | Adriamycin<br>Cyclophosphamide | $60$ mg/m$^2$ IV on day 1<br>$600$ mg/m$^2$ IV on day 1<br>*Repeat every 21 days for 4 cycles* |
| AC→T | Adriamycin<br>Cyclophosphamide<br><br>Taxol | $60$ mg/m$^2$ IV on day 1<br>$600$ mg/m$^2$ IV on day 1<br>*Repeat every 21 days for 4 cycles*<br>$175$ mg/m$^2$ IV on day 1<br>*Repeat every 21 days for 4 cycles* |
| A→CMF | Adriamycin<br><br>CMF | $75$ mg/m$^2$ IV on day 1<br>*Repeat every 21 days for 4 cycles*<br>As above, every 3 weeks for 8 cycles |

oral cyclophosphamide, however, which is poorly tolerated by some patients. Given the availability of modern antiemetic therapy, most clinicians prefer to give all chemotherapeutic agents intravenously. The regimen in Table 35–27 gives a contemporary version of the AC regimen, as used by the NSABP in their studies of adjuvant chemotherapy. This regimen has been studied by the NSABP in comparison with two other AC regimens using higher doses of cyclophosphamide.[132] A preliminary analysis of the results of this study suggests that dose intensification of cyclophosphamide in this regimen does not improve the results of treatment in the adjuvant setting.

**FAC and CAF.** The FAC (5-FU, doxorubicin, cyclophosphamide) regimen was developed at the University of Texas, M.D. Anderson Hospital, by Gottlieb. Several variations of this regimen have subsequently been developed, such as the CAF regimen that has been widely studied by the Cancer and Leukemia Group B.[133] The precautions and limitations of the FAC and CAF regimens are similar to those described previously for the AC regimen.

**A→CMF.** The Milan group has developed a new combination for adjuvant therapy in patients with four or more positive lymph nodes.[109, 110] This regimen was designed to maximize the dose intensity of doxorubicin by using it as a

single agent with subsequent intravenous CMF to consolidate the benefit of doxorubicin. This regimen has proved effective in the adjuvant setting and is a prototype for newer studies of sequential single-agent chemotherapy in the adjuvant setting and for patients with advanced disease.

**Choosing a Chemotherapy Strategy.** The relative efficacy, safety, and tolerance of the various CMF and doxorubicin-containing regimens appear similar, although some authorities voice strong preferences for one or another regimen. Several trials have demonstrated a 10 to 20% higher response rate to doxorubicin-containing regimens with an increase in median survival from 14 to 18 months and an increase in median time to treatment failure from 5 to 7 months.[134] Although the latter benefits are modest, these benefits along with the improvements in antiemetic therapy favor a doxorubicin-containing regimen as the first choice of therapy. CMF is an acceptable alternative, however, for patients who are chemotherapy naive or who received prior CMF in the adjuvant setting with a disease-free interval of greater than 1 to 2 years. For patients who have received doxorubicin for prior adjuvant therapy, a taxane is generally prescribed as first-line therapy. When paclitaxel was administered as first-line therapy, an overall response rate of 62% was achieved with 12% of the patients achieving a complete

*Table 35–28.* **Toxicity of CMF Chemotherapy\***

| Symptom or Side Effect | CMF(P)†(%) |
|---|---|
| Fatigue | 96 |
| Nausea | 88 |
| Leukopenia | |
| 2500–3999/ml | 67 |
| <2500/ml | 4 |
| Nervousness/irritability | 62 |
| Thrombocytopenia | |
| 75,000–129,000/ml | 57 |
| <75,000/ml | 14 |
| Alopecia | 40–55 |
| Amenorrhea | 54 |
| Cystitis | 28 |
| Changes in weight or appetite | 28 |
| Flu-like symptoms | 28 |
| Vomiting | 28 |
| Conjunctivitis | 25 |
| Musculoskeletal pain | 8 (14–20) |
| Cushingoid appearance | (7–10) |
| Hypertension | (3) |
| Deep vein thrombosis | 0.5–3 |
| Cardiotoxicity | 0 |

\*Combined results of short-term toxicity for CMF (cyclophosphamide, methotrexate, fluorouracil) given in the adjuvant setting, as reported from Milan (Bonadonna G, Brusamolino E, Valagussa P, et al. Combination chemotherapy as an adjuvant treatment in operable breast cancer. N Engl J Med 1976;294:405–10) and University of California Los Angeles (Meyerowitz BE, Sparks FC, Spears IK. Adjuvant chemotherapy for breast carcinoma: psychosocial implications. Cancer 1979;43:1613–8).

†Values in parentheses are for CMF given with prednisone (P) (NCI Monogr 1986;1:75).

remission.[135] At present, none of these regimens is ideal, and their selection should be individualized outside the confines of a clinical trial. In rare patients with multiple medical problems, sequential single-agent therapy is a reasonable alternative.

Patients who do not respond to first-line chemotherapy or who respond and then progress are candidates for second-line treatment. In most cases, we use sequential single agents given with palliative intent, depending on the details of prior therapy. For patients who fail anthracycline therapy in the metastatic setting, a taxane is generally the next agent of choice. The relative usefulness of the commercially available single agents as salvage agents can be ranked as follows, and in most cases we use them in sequence (unless earlier resistance to the agent has been established by failure of a drug combination using the respective agents): doxorubicin, paclitaxel or docetaxel, 5-FU (usually given with leucovorin or as a continuous infusion) or capecitabine, vinorelbine, mitomycin or gemcitabine. The response rates to these drugs in previously treated patients varies from 10 to 40%. There is no evidence that any of these regimens truly differ in efficacy. If the decision has been made to continue treatment for palliation, the physician must consider the various toxicities of these agents. Whenever possible, these patients should be considered for a clinical trial. We generally do not use cisplatin and carboplatin as salvage therapy because their activity in breast cancer is modest in previously treated patients. These two agents are more widely used in high dosage as part of investigational dose-intense regimens. The potential role of monoclonal antibody treatment (e.g., trastuzumab [Herceptin]) combined with chemotherapy is discussed subsequently.

Patients who do not respond to chemotherapy may be considered for an additional trial of hormonal therapy, such as a selective aromatase inhibitor or megestrol acetate. Elderly patients or those with serious organ dysfunction that makes combination chemotherapy unsafe may be candidates for single-agent chemotherapy for initial, first-line chemotherapy. In this latter setting, treatment is generally initiated with doxorubicin, vinorelbine, or capecitabine. When doxorubicin is used in this setting, it is often given weekly in low dosage (10 to 15 mg/m$^2$ intravenous bolus).

Whichever regimen is chosen, it is important to remember that chemotherapy is being given to these patients with palliative, not curative, intent. Consequently, asymptomatic patients with chronic and only slowly progressive disease may benefit more from the avoidance of chemotherapy than from its use. Chemotherapy is not to be used as a placebo in settings in which benefit is unlikely.

## IMMUNOTHERAPY

A host immune response to breast cancer is suggested by the natural history of the disease and by the observation that lymphoid infiltration of the primary tumor correlates with an improved survival rate.[136, 137] Antibody to tumor-associated antigens has also been shown to correlate with the survival rate,[137] and circulating levels of a mammary tumor antigen have been reported to vary according to the clinical course of the disease.[138, 139] The true role of the immune system in the development and treatment of breast cancer is unclear.[136, 140]

Despite these uncertainties, many different forms of immunotherapy (or biologic response modifiers) have been studied for their potential therapeutic value (alone or with traditional systemic therapy) in adjuvant and advanced disease settings.[141] Examples of tested agents include levamisole,[142] bacillus Calmette-Guérin (BCG),[143–147] the methanol-extracted residue of BCG (MER),[148] *Corynebacterium parvum*,[149, 150] the streptococcal preparation OK-432,[151] vitamin D analogues,[152, 153] ditiocarb,[154] monoclonal antibodies (alone,[155–159] with an immunotoxin,[160–162] with interferon,[163] with interleukin-2,[164] or with chemotherapy[165]), interleukin-2,[166] interleukin-2–cultured lymphocytes,[167] tumor necrosis factor,[168] and interferons (see reference 169 for a review of the older literature).[169, 170]

Despite considerable promise, no form of immunotherapy has been accepted to date as an effective systemic therapy for this disease, and the meta-analysis of immunotherapy in the adjuvant setting performed by the Early Breast Cancer Trialists' Collaborative Group (EBCTCG) found no significant benefit for immunotherapy as an adjuvant treatment. Revolutionary advances in molecular oncology are likely to change this conclusion in the near future.

**Monoclonal Antibody Therapy.** Trastuzumab was approved by the FDA for clinical use in the treatment of metastatic breast cancer overexpressing the HER-2/*neu* oncogene. The drug is a humanized monoclonal antibody directed at the extracellular domain of the HER-2/*neu* growth factor receptor. The clinical trials have primarily been limited to patients with 2 to 3+ overexpression (on a scale of 0 to 3+). Based on in vitro data suggesting synergy of trastuzumab with cisplatin, a phase II study of this combination was carried out in relatively heavily pretreated patients with progressive disease. An overall response rate of 24.3% was reported.[171] A large phase III randomized trial[172] then compared first-line chemotherapy with or without Herceptin (H). Patients were treated with AC or taxol (T), if previously treated with doxorubicin in the adjuvant setting. The response rates were significantly higher in the combination groups: AC versus AC + H, 42.1% versus 64.9%, and T versus T + H, 25% versus 57.3%. An increased incidence of grade 3 to 4 cardiotoxicity of 18% was observed with AC + H versus 3% with AC alone. In the largest single-agent study of trastuzumab in patients previously treated with chemotherapy,[173] the investigator-determined overall response rate was 21% and stable disease in 30% with a median duration of response of 8.4 months.

For patients with 2 to 3 + overexpression of HER-2/*neu*, the addition of trastuzumab to chemotherapy is an attractive option. Chemotherapeutic agents to consider include a taxane, carboplatin or cisplatin, or an anthracycline. Caution must be used, however, with the addition of an anthracycline in terms of potential cardiotoxicity. Given the favorable toxicity profile of trastuzumab alone, it is a reasonable single-agent salvage therapy or first-line therapy for patients with comorbid conditions. It is not currently known what the activity of trastuzumab is in patients with 1 + overexpression.

## ADJUNCTIVE THERAPIES

**Bisphosphonates.** Skeletal complications of bone metastases (hypercalcemia, pathologic fractures, pain, and spinal cord compression) result in considerable morbidity in breast cancer. In a large study of patients who received chemotherapy alone, the average rate of skeletal events was 3.5/year.[174] Multiple studies have clearly shown that the skeletal complications in breast cancer can be reduced by the concomitant long-term use of bisphosphonate treatment. Two of these studies[175, 176] used oral clodronate and four more studies used intravenous pamidronate (Aredia).[177–180] Most of these studies required the presence of at least one lytic lesion. Pamidronate is the most widely used bisphosphonate in the United States, administered on a monthly basis. Additional palliative measures for localized bone pain include external-beam radiotherapy and radiopharmaceuticals, such as strontium 89[181] and samarium 153.[182]

## SUMMARY

Chemotherapy, endocrine therapy, and combinations of these approaches have proved useful in the management of metastatic breast cancer, but numerous questions on their optimal use remain. New drugs and approaches to therapy tested in well-designed clinical trials are needed to resolve many of the unanswered questions about systemic therapy. It is hoped that physicians and patients will continue to support clinical trials as the most rational way of improving therapy for patients with breast cancer.

In patients who are not participating in a clinical trial, we prefer to choose a strategy of therapy that emphasizes either endocrine manipulation or systemic chemotherapy. The spe-

cific choice of therapy depends on patient factors (such as age, menopausal status, prior therapy, and the presence or absence of comorbid diseases) as well as tumor factors (such as the presence or absence of hormone receptors, HER-2/*neu* expression, and the specific areas of organ involvement by tumor).

## SUGGESTIONS FOR ADDITIONAL READING

Miller KD, Sledge GW Jr. The role of chemotherapy for metastatic breast cancer. Hematol Oncol Clin North Am 1999;13:415–34.

Costanza ME, Weiss RB, Henderson IC, et al. Safety and efficacy of using a single agent or a phase II agent before instituting standard combination chemotherapy in previously untreated metastatic breast cancer patients: report of a randomized study—Cancer and Leukemia Group B 8642. J Clin Oncol 1999;17:1397–406.

McLachlan SA, Pintilie M, Tannock IF. Third line chemotherapy in patients with metastatic breast cancer: an evaluation of quality of life and cost. Breast Cancer Res Treat 1999;54:213–23.

Stadtmauer EA, O'Neill A, Goldstein LJ, et al, for the Philadelphia Bone Marrow Transplant Group. Conventional-dose chemotherapy compared with high-dose chemotherapy plus autologous hematopoietic stem-cell transplantation for metastatic breast cancer. N Engl J Med 2000;342:1069–76.

Rowlings PA, Williams SF, Antman KH, et al. Factors correlated with progression-free survival after high-dose chemotherapy and hematopoietic stem cell transplantation for metastatic breast cancer. JAMA 1999;282:1335–43.

Hillner BE, Ingle JN, Berenson JR, et al, for the American Society of Clinical Oncology Bisphosphonates Expert Panel. ASCO special article. American Society of Clinical Oncology Guideline on the Role of Bisphosphonates in Breast Cancer. J Clin Oncol 2000;18:1378–91.

## REFERENCES

1. Priestman T, Baum M, Jones V, Forbes J. Comparative trial of endocrine versus cytotoxic treatment in advanced breast cancer. Br Med J 1977;1:1248–50.
2. Fisher B, Redmond C, Brown A, et al. Influence of tumor estrogen and progesterone receptor levels on the response to tamoxifen and chemotherapy in primary breast cancer. J Clin Oncol 1983;1:227–41.
3. Osborne CK, Boldt DH, Clark GM, Trent JM. Effects of tamoxifen on human breast cancer cell cycle kinetics: accumulation of cells in early G1 phase. Cancer Res 1983;43:3583–5.
4. Lippman ME. Efforts to combine endocrine and chemotherapy in the management of breast cancer: do two and two equal three? Breast Cancer Res Treat 1983;3:117–27.
5. Woods KE, Randolph JK, Gewirtz DA. Antagonism between tamoxifen and doxorubicin in the MCF-7 human breast tumor cell line. Biochem Pharmacol 1994;47:1449–52.
6. Osborne CK. Receptors. In: Harris I, et al, eds. Breast diseases. Philadelphia: JB Lippincott, 1991:301.
7. Lippman M. Steroid hormone receptors and mechanisms of growth regulation of human breast cancer. In: Lippman M, ed. Diagnosis and management of breast cancer. Philadelphia: WB Saunders, 1988:334.
8. Kiang DT, Kennedy BJ. Factors affecting estrogen receptors in breast cancer. Cancer 1977;40:1571–6.
9. Kennedy BJ. Hormonal therapies in breast cancer. Semin Oncol 1974;1:119–30.
10. Brufman G. Prognostic factors affecting response to aminoglutethimide in advanced breast cancer. Anticancer Res 1993;13:1235.
11. Greenfield S, Blanco DM, Elashoff RM, Ganz PA. Patterns of care related to age of breast cancer patients. JAMA 1987;257:2766–70.
12. Amsterdam E, Birkenfeld S, Gilad A, Krispin M. Surgery for carcinoma of the breast in women over 70 years of age. J Surg Oncol 1987;35:180–3.
13. Taylor SG 4th, Gelman RS, Falkson G, Cummings FJ. Combination chemotherapy compared to tamoxifen as initial therapy for stage IV breast cancer in elderly women. Ann Intern Med 1986;104:455–61.
14. Gazet JC, Markopoulos C, Ford HT, et al. Prospective randomised

trial of tamoxifen versus surgery in elderly patients with breast cancer. Lancet 1988;1:679–81.

15. Robertson JFR, Todd JH, Ellis IO, et al. Comparison of mastectomy with tamoxifen for treating elderly patients with operable breast cancer. Br Med J 1988;297:511–4.

16. Christman K, Muss HB, Case LD, Stanley V. Chemotherapy of metastatic breast cancer in the elderly. The Piedmont Oncology Association experience. see comment. JAMA 1992;268:57–62.

17. Bitran JD, Desser RK, Shapiro CM, et al. Response to secondary therapy in patients with adenocarcinoma of the breast previously treated with adjuvant chemotherapy. Cancer 1983;51:381–4.

18. Wendt AG, Jones SE, Salmon SE. Salvage treatment of patients relapsing after breast cancer adjuvant chemotherapy. Cancer Treat Rep 1980;64:269–73.

19. Ahmann FR, Jones SE, Moon TE. The effect of prior adjuvant chemotherapy on survival in metastatic breast cancer. J Surg Oncol 1988;37:116–22.

20. Rubens RD, Bajetta E, Bonneterre J, et al. Treatment of relapse of breast cancer after adjuvant systemic therapy—review and guidelines for future research. Eur J Cancer 1994;30A:106–11.

21. Elledge RM, Green S, Ciocca D, et al. HER-2 expression and response to tamoxifen in estrogen receptor–positive breast cancer: a Southwest Oncology Group study. Clin Cancer Res 1998;4:7–12.

22. Yamauchi H, O'Neill A, Gelman R, et al: Prediction of response to antiestrogen therapy in advanced breast cancer patients by pretreatment circulating levels of extracellular domain of the extracellular domain of the HER-2/NEU protein. J Clin Oncol 1997;15:2518–25.

23. Leitzel K, Teramoto Y, Konrad K, et al. Elevated serum c-ERB-2 antigen levels and decreased response to hormone therapy of breast cancer. J Clin Oncol 1995;13:1129–35.

24. Henderson IC. Chemotherapy for advanced disease. In: Harris JR, et al, eds. Breast diseases. Philadelphia: JB Lippincott, 1987:428.

25. Petru E, Schmähl D. No relevant influence on overall survival time in patients with metastatic breast cancer undergoing combination chemotherapy. J Cancer Res Clin Oncol 1988;114:183–5.

26. Paterson AH, Cyr M, Szafran O, et al. Response to treatment and its influence on survival in metastatic breast cancer. Am J Clin Oncol 1985;8:283–92.

27. Patel JK, Nemoto T, Vezeridis M, et al. Does more intense palliative treatment improve overall survival in metastatic breast cancer patients? Cancer 1986;57:567–70.

28. Baker LH, Vaitkevicius VK. Reevaluation of rebound regression in disseminated carcinoma of the breast. Cancer 1972;29:1268–71.

29. Howell A, Dodwell DJ, Anderson H, et al. Response after withdrawal of tamoxifen and progestogens in advanced breast cancer. Ann Oncol 1992;3:611–17.

30. Stein W 3d, Hortobagyi GN, Blumenschein GR. Response of metastatic breast cancer to tamoxifen withdrawal: report of a case. J Surg Oncol 1983;22:45–6.

31. Longman SM, Buehring GC. Oral contraceptives and breast cancer: in vitro effect of contraceptive steroids on human mammary cell growth. Cancer 1987;59:281–7.

32. Veronesi U, Pizzocaro G, Rossi A. Oophorectomy for advanced carcinoma of the breast. Surg Gynecol Obstet 1975;141:569–70.

33. Peetz ME, Awrich AE, Moseley HS, et al. Results of oophorectomy by menstrual and estrogen receptor states in patients with metastatic breast cancer. Am J Surg 1981;141:554–8.

34. Lees AW, Giuffre C, Burns PE, et al. Oophorectomy versus radiation ablation of ovarian function in patients with metastatic carcinoma of the breast. Surg Gynecol Obstet 1980;151:721–4.

35. Mecklenburg RS, Lipsett MB. Disappearance of metastatic breast cancer after oophorectomy. N Engl J Med 1973;289:845–6.

36. Bajetta E, Celio L, Zilembo N, et al. Ovarian function suppression with the gonadotrophin-releasing hormone (GnRH) analogue goserelin in premenopausal advanced breast cancer. Tumori 1994;80:28–32.

37. Henderson IC, Canellos GP. Cancer of the breast: the past decade (first of two parts). N Engl J Med 1980;302:17–30.

38. Barlow JJ, Emerson K Jr, Saxena BN. Estradiol production after ovariectomy for carcinoma of the breast. N Engl J Med 1969; 280:633–7.

39. Pritchard KI, Thomson DB, Myers RE, et al. Tamoxifen therapy in premenopausal patients with metastatic breast cancer. Cancer Treat Rep 1980;64:787–96.

40. Manni A, Pearson OH. Antiestrogen-induced remissions in premenopausal women with stage IV breast cancer: effects on ovarian function. Cancer Treat Rep 1980;64:779–85.

41. Hoogstraten B, Fletcher WS, Gad-el-Mawla N, et al. Tamoxifen and oophorectomy in the treatment of recurrent breast cancer: a Southwest Oncology Group study. Cancer Res 1982;42:4788–91.

42. Margreiter R, Wiegele J. Tamoxifen (Nolvadex) for premenopausal patients with advanced breast cancer. Breast Cancer Res Treat 1984;4:45–8.

43. Planting AS, Alexieva-Figusch J, Blonk-van der Wijst J, van Putten WL. Tamoxifen therapy in premenopausal women with metastatic breast cancer. Cancer Treat Rep 1985;69:363–8.

44. Ingle JN, Krook JE, Green SJ, et al. Randomized trial of bilateral oophorectomy versus tamoxifen in premenopausal women with metastatic breast cancer. J Clin Oncol 1986;4:178–85.

45. Buchanan RB, Blamey RW, Durrant KR, et al. A randomized comparison of tamoxifen with surgical oophorectomy in premenopausal patients with advanced breast cancer. J Clin Oncol 1986;4:1326–30.

46. Kalman AM, Thompson T, Vogel CL. Response to oophorectomy after tamoxifen failure in a premenopausal patient. Cancer Treat Rep 1982;66:1867–8.

47. Sawka CA, Pritchard KI, Paterson AH, et al. Role and mechanism of action of tamoxifen in premenopausal women with metastatic breast carcinoma. Cancer Res 1986;46:3152–6.

48. Hartley JW, Wong J, Fletcher WS. Response of advanced breast cancer to total endocrine ablation after exacerbation on tamoxifen: results in seven patients and possible mechanism of action. J Surg Oncol 1987;34:182–7.

49. Legha SS. Tamoxifen in the treatment of breast cancer. Ann Intern Med 1988;109:219–28.

50. Sedlacek SM. An overview of megestrol acetate for the treatment of advanced breast cancer. Semin Oncol 1988;15:Suppl 1:3–13.

51. Muss HB, Wells HB, Paschold EH, et al. Megestrol acetate versus tamoxifen in advanced breast cancer: 5-year analysis—a phase III trial of the Piedmont Oncology Association. J Clin Oncol 1988;6:1098–106.

52. Blackledge GR, Latief T, Mould JJ, et al. Phase II evaluation of megestrol acetate in previously treated patients with advanced breast cancer: relationship of response to previous treatment. Eur J Cancer Clin Oncol 1986;22:1091–4.

53. Aisner J, Tchekmedyian NS, Moody M, Tait N. High-dose megestrol acetate for the treatment of advanced breast cancer: dose and toxicities. Semin Hematol 1987;24:Suppl 1:48–55.

54. Canney PA, Priestman TJ, Griffiths T, et al. Randomized trial comparing aminoglutethimide with high-dose medroxyprogesterone acetate in therapy for advanced breast carcinoma. J Natl Cancer Inst 1988;80:1147–51.

55. Manni A, Arafah BM, Pearson OH. Androgen-induced remissions after antiestrogen and hypophysectomy in stage IV breast cancer. Cancer 1981;48:2507–9.

56. Wells SA Jr, Santen RJ. Ablative procedures in patients with metastatic breast carcinoma. Cancer 1984;53:Suppl:762–5.

57. Allison RW, Furnival CM, Lee JF, Roberts SJ. Response to aminoglutethimide after tamoxifen therapy in advanced breast cancer. Med J Aust 1982;1:44–5.

58. Buzdar AU, Powell KC, Blumenschein GR. Aminoglutethimide after tamoxifen therapy in advanced breast cancer: M.D. Anderson Hospital experience. Cancer Res 1982;42:Suppl:3448s–50s.

59. Wells SA Jr, Worgul TJ, Samojlik E, et al. Comparison of surgical adrenalectomy to medical adrenalectomy in patients with metastatic carcinoma of the breast. Cancer Res 1982;42:Suppl:3454s–7s.

60. Santen RJ, Worgul TJ, Samojlik E, et al. A randomized trial comparing surgical adrenalectomy with aminoglutethimide plus hydrocortisone in women with advanced breast cancer. N Engl J Med 1981;305:545–51.

61. Harvey HA, Lipton A, White DS, et al. Cross-over comparison of tamoxifen and aminoglutethimide in advanced breast cancer. Cancer Res 1982;42:Suppl:3451s–3s.

62. Bono A, Fariselli G, Bettoni I, et al. Tamoxifen therapy in advanced breast cancer with positive estrogen receptors in postmenopausal women. Tumori 1982;68:143–7.

63. Pearson OH, Manni A, Arafah BM. Antiestrogen treatment of breast cancer: an overview. Cancer Res 1982;42:Suppl:3424s–9s.

64. Beex L, Pieters G, Smals A, et al. Tamoxifen versus ethinyl estradiol in the treatment of postmenopausal women with advanced breast cancer. Cancer Treat Rep 1981;65:179–85.

65. Matelski H, Greene R, Huberman M, et al. Randomized trial of estrogen vs. tamoxifen therapy for advanced breast cancer. Am J Clin Oncol 1985;8:128–33.

66. Muss HB, Smith LR, Cooper MR. Tamoxifen rechallenge: response to tamoxifen following relapse after adjuvant chemohormonal therapy for breast cancer. J Clin Oncol 1987;5:1556–8.

67. Manni A, Arafah BM. Tamoxifen-induced remission in breast cancer by escalating the dose to 40 mg daily after progression on 20 mg daily: a case report and review of the literature. Cancer 1981;48:873–5.

68. Rose C, Theilade K, Boesen E, et al. Treatment of advanced breast cancer with tamoxifen: evaluation of the dose-response relationship at two dose levels. Breast Cancer Res Treat 1982;2:395–400.

69. Stewart JF, Minton MJ, Rubens RD. Trial of tamoxifen at a dose of 40 mg daily after disease progression during tamoxifen therapy at a dose of 20 mg daily. Cancer Treat Rep 1982;66:1445–6.

70. Goldhirsch A, Joss RA, Leuenberger U, et al. An evaluation of tamoxifen dose escalation in advanced breast cancer. Am J Clin Oncol 1982;5:501–3.

71. Vogel CL. Phase II and III clinical trials of toremifene for metastatic breast cancer. Oncology 1998;12:Suppl 5:9–13.

72. Buzdar AU, Hortobagyi GN. Tamoxifen and toremifene in breast cancer: comparison of safety and efficacy: see comments. J Clin Oncol 1998;16:348–53.

73. Johnson PA, Bonomi PD, Anderson KM, et al. Progesterone receptor level as a predictor of response to megestrol acetate in advanced breast cancer: a retrospective study. Cancer Treat Rep 1983;67:717–20.

74. Alexieva-Figusch J, van Gilse HA, Hop WC, et al. Progestin therapy in advanced breast cancer: megestrol acetate—an evaluation of 160 treated cases. Cancer 1980;46:2369–72.

75. Dombernowsky P, Smith I, Falkson G, et al. Letrozole, a new oral aromatase inhibitor for advanced breast cancer: double-blind randomized trial showing a dose effect and improved efficacy and tolerability compared with megestrol acetate. J Clin Oncol 1998;16:453–61.

76. Buzdar A, Jonat W, Howell A, et al. Anastrozole, a potent and selective aromatase inhibitor, versus megestrol acetate in postmenopausal women with advanced breast cancer: results of overview analysis of two Phase III trials. J Clin Oncol 1996;14:2000–11.

77. Henderson IC. Endocrine therapy in metastatic breast cancer. In: Harris JR, Hellman S, Henderson IC, Kinne DW (eds). Breast diseases. Philadelphia: JB Lippincott, 1987:398–428.

78. Clavel M, Catimel G. Breast cancer: chemotherapy in the treatment of advanced disease. Eur J Cancer 1993;29A:598–604.

79. Ejlertsen B, Pfeiffer P, Pedersen D, et al. Decreased efficacy of cyclophosphamide, epirubicin and 5-fluorouracil in metastatic breast cancer when reducing treatment duration from 18 to 6 months. Eur J Cancer 1993;29A:527–31.

80. Coates A, Bebski V, Stat M, et al. Improving the quality of life during chemotherapy for advanced breast cancer: a comparison of intermittent and continuous treatment strategies. N Engl J Med 1987;317:1490.

81. Muss HB, Case LD, Richards F 2d, et al. Interrupted versus continuous chemotherapy in patients with metastatic breast cancer. The Piedmont Oncology Association. see comments. N Engl J Med 1991;325:1342–8.

82. Falkson G, Gelman R, Glick J, et al. Reinduction with the same cytostatic treatment in patients with metastatic breast cancer: an Eastern Cooperative Oncology Group study. J Clin Oncol 1994;12:45–9.

83. Focan C, Andrien JM, Closon MT, et al. Dose-response relationship of epirubicin-based first-line chemotherapy for advanced breast cancer: a prospective randomized trial. J Clin Oncol 1993;11:1253–63.

84. Hryniuk W, Bush H. The importance of dose intensity in chemotherapy of metastatic breast cancer. J Clin Oncol 1984;2:1281–88.

85. Bastholt L, Dalmark M, Gjedde SB, et al. Dose response relationship of epirubicin in the treatment of postmenopausal patients with metastatic breast cancer: a randomized study of epirubicin at four different dose levels performed by the Danish Breast Cancer Cooperative Group. J Clin Oncol 1996;14:1146–55.

86. Sledge GW Jr, Antman KH. Progress in chemotherapy for metastatic breast cancer. Semin Oncol 1992;19:317–32.

87. Legha SS, Benjamin RS, Mackay B, et al. Adriamycin therapy by continuous intravenous infusion in patients with metastatic breast cancer. Cancer 1982;49:1762–6.

88. Jones RB, Holland JF, Bhardwaj S, et al. A phase I–II study of intensive-dose Adriamycin for advanced breast cancer. J Clin Oncol 1987;5:172–7.

89. Shpall EJ, Jones RB, Holland JF, et al. Intensive single-agent mitoxantrone for metastatic breast cancer. J Natl Cancer Inst 1988;80:204–8.

90. Jackson DV, White DR, Spurr CL, et al. Moderate-dose vincristine infusion in refractory breast cancer. Am J Clin Oncol 1986;9:376–8.

91. Giaccone G, Bagatella M, Bertetto O, et al. Phase II study of divided-dose vinblastine in advanced breast cancer patients. Cancer Chemother Pharmacol 1988;21:65–7.

92. Fraschini G, Fleishman G, Charnsangavej C, et al. Continuous 5-day infusion of vinblastine for percutaneous hepatic arterial chemotherapy for metastatic breast cancer. Cancer Treat Rep 1987;71:1001–5.

93. Hansen R, Quebbeman E, Beatty P, et al. Continuous 5-fluorouracil infusion in refractory carcinoma of the breast. Breast Cancer Res Treat 1987;10:145–9.

94. Cameron DA, Gabra H, Leonard RC. Continuous 5-fluorouracil in the treatment of breast cancer. Br J Cancer 1994;70:120–4.

95. O'Reilly SM, Moiseyenko V, Talbot DC, et al. A randomized phase II study of Xeloda (capecitabine) vs paclitaxel in breast cancer patients failing previous anthracycline therapy. Proc Am Clin Oncol 1998;17:A627.

96. Weiss AJ. Studies on cardiotoxicity and antitumor effect of doxorubicin administered weekly. Cancer Treat Symp 1984;3:91–4.

97. Scheithauer W, Zielinksi C, Ludwig H. Weekly low dose doxorubicin monotherapy in metastatic breast cancer resistant to previous hormonal and cytostatic treatment. Breast Cancer Res Treat 1985;6:89–93.

98. Milano G, Cassuto-Viguier E, Fischel JL, et al. Doxorubicin weekly low dose administration: in vitro cytotoxicity generated by the typical pharmacokinetic profile. Eur J Cancer 1992;28A:1881–5.

99. Davis HL Jr, Multhauf P, Klotz J. Comparisons of Cooperative Group evaluation criteria for multiple-drug therapy for breast cancer. Cancer Treat Rep 1980;64:507–17.

100. Greenspan EM. Combination chemotherapy for advanced mammary carcinoma: a twelve-year experience. Mt Sinai J Med 1972;39:435–46.

101. Cooper RG. Combination chemotherapy in hormone-resistant breast cancer. Proc AACR 1969;10:15.

102. Canellos GP, Pocock SJ, Taylor SG 3d, et al. Combination chemotherapy for metastatic breast carcinoma: prospective comparison of multiple drug therapy with L-phenylalanine mustard. Cancer 1976;38:1882–6.

103. Smalley RV, Murphy S, Huguley CM Jr, Bartolucci AA. Combination versus sequential five-drug chemotherapy in metastatic carcinoma of the breast. Cancer Res 1976;36:Pt 1:3911–6.

104. Mouridsen HT, Palshof T, Brahm M, Rahbek I. Evaluation of single-drug versus multiple-drug chemotherapy in the treatment of advanced breast cancer. Cancer Treat Rep 1977;61:47–50.

105. Chlebowski RT, Irwin LE, Pugh RP, et al. Survival of patients with metastatic breast cancer treated with either combination or sequential chemotherapy. Cancer Res 1979;39:4503–6.

106. Baker LH, Vaughn CB, al-Sarraf M, et al. Proceedings: evaluation of combination vs. sequential cytotoxic chemotherapy in the treatment of advanced breast cancer. Cancer 1974;33:513–8.

107. Gundersen S, Kvinnsland S, Klepp O, et al. Weekly Adriamycin versus VAC in advanced breast cancer: a randomized trial. Eur J Cancer Clin Oncol 1986;22:1431–4.

108. Jones RB, Holland JF, Bhardwaj S, et al. A phase I–II study of intensive-dose Adriamycin for advanced breast cancer. J Clin Oncol 1987;5:172–7.

109. Bonadonna G, Valagussa P, Brambilla C, et al. Adjuvant and neoadjuvant treatment of breast cancer with chemotherapy and/or endocrine therapy. Semin Oncol 1991;18:515–24.

110. Buzzoni R, Bonadonna G, Valagussa P, Zambetti M. Adjuvant chemotherapy with doxorubicin plus cyclophosphamide, methotrexate, and fluorouracil in the treatment of resectable breast cancer with more than three positive axillary nodes. J Clin Oncol 1991;9:2134–40.

111. Juensuu H, Hollik K, Heikkinen M, et al. Combination chemotherapy versus single-agent therapy as first- and second-line treatment in metastatic breast cancer: a prospective randomized trial. J Clin Oncol 1998;16:3720–30.

112. Tormey DC, Weinberg VE, Leone LA, et al. A comparison of intermittent vs continuous and of Adriamycin vs methotrexate 5-drug chemotherapy for advanced breast cancer. Am J Clin Oncol 1984;7:231–9.

113. Smalley RV, Lefante J, Bartolucci A, et al. A comparison of cyclophosphamide, Adriamycin, and 5-fluorouracil (CAF) and cyclophosphamide, methotrexate, 5-fluorouracil, vincristine, and prednisone (CMFVP) in patients with advanced breast cancer. Breast Cancer Res Treat 1983;3:209–20.

114. A'Hern RP, Smith IE, Ebbs SR, et al. Chemotherapy and survival in advanced breast cancer: the inclusion of doxorubicin in Cooper type regimens. Br J Cancer 1993;67:801–5.

115. Bennett JM, Muss HB, Doroshow JH, et al. A randomized multicenter

trial comparing mitoxantrone, cyclophosphamide and fluorouracil with doxorubicin, cyclophosphamide, and fluorouracil in the therapy of metastatic breast cancer. J Clin Oncol 1998;6:1611.

116. Gianni L. Paclitaxel plus doxorubicin in metastatic breast cancer: the Milan experience. Oncology 1998;12:Suppl 1:13–5.

117. Dieras V, Fumoleau P, Kalla S, et al. Docetaxel in combination with doxorubicin or vinorelbine. Eur J Cancer 1997;33:Suppl 7:S20–2.

118. Dieras V. Review of docetaxel/doxorubicin combination in metastatic breast cancer. Oncology 1997;11:Suppl 8:31–3.

119. Schwartsmann G, Mans DR, Menke CH, et al. A phase II study of doxorubicin/paclitaxel plus G-CSF for metastatic breast cancer. Oncology 1997;11:Suppl 3:24–9.

120. Homes F, Wallers R, Theriault R, et al. Phase II trial of Taxol, an active drug in the treatment of metastatic breast cancer. J Natl Cancer Inst 1991;83:1797–1805.

121. Ravdin PM. Docetaxel (Taxotere) for the treatment of anthracycline-resistant breast cancer. Semin Oncol 1997;24:Suppl 10:S10–21.

122. Ahmann DL, O'Connell MJ, Hahn RG, et al. An evaluation of early or delayed adjuvant chemotherapy in premenopausal patients with advanced breast cancer undergoing oophorectomy. N Engl J Med 1977;297:356–60.

123. Ahmann DL, Green SJ, Bisel HF, et al. An evaluation of early or delayed adjuvant chemotherapy in premenopausal patients with advanced breast cancer undergoing oophorectomy: a later analysis. Am J Clin Oncol 1982;5:355–8.

124. Allegra JC. Methotrexate and 5-fluorouracil following tamoxifen and Premarin in advanced breast cancer. Semin Oncol 1983;10:Suppl 2:23–8.

125. Paridaens R, Heuson JC, Julien JP, et al. Assessment of estrogenic recruitment before chemotherapy in advanced breast cancer: a double-blind randomized study. European Organization for Research and Treatment of Cancer Breast Cancer Cooperative Group. J Clin Oncol 1993;11:1723–8.

126. Hug V, Hortobagyi GN, Drewinko B, et al. Tamoxifen citrate counteracts the antitumor effects of cytotoxic drugs in vitro. J Clin Oncol 1985;3:1672–7.

127. Myers SE, Williams SF. Role of high-dose chemotherapy and autologous stem cell support in the treatment of breast cancer. Hematol Oncol Clin North Am 1993;7:631–45.

128. Bezwoda WR, Seymour L, Dansey RD. High-dose chemotherapy with hematopoietic rescue as primary treatment for metastatic breast cancer: a randomized trial. J Clin Oncol 1995;13:2483–9.

129. Tormey D, Gelman R, Falkson G. Prospective evaluation of rotating chemotherapy in advanced breast cancer. An Eastern Cooperative Oncology Group trial. Am J Clin Oncol 1983;6:1–18.

130. Tormey DC, Weinberg VE, Holland JF, et al. A randomized trial of five and three drug chemotherapy and chemoimmunotherapy in women with operable node positive breast cancer. J Clin Oncol 1983;1:138–45.

131. Englesman E, Klijn JC, Rubens RD, et al. "Classical" CMF versus a 3-weekly intravenous CMF schedule in postmenopausal patients with advanced breast cancer. An EROTC Breast Cancer Co-operative Group Phase III trial (10808). Eur J Cancer 1991;27:966–70.

132. Dimitrov N, Anderson S, Fisher B, et al. Dose intensification and increased total dose of adjuvant chemotherapy for breast cancer (BC): findings from NSABP B-22. Proc ASCO 1994;13:64.

133. Aisner J, Weinberg V, Perloff M, et al. Chemotherapy versus chemoimmunotherapy (CAF v CAFVP v CMF each ± MER) for metastatic carcinoma of the breast: a CALGB study. Cancer and Leukemia Group B. J Clin Oncol 1987;5:1523–33.

134. Harris JR, Lippman ME, Morrow M, Hellman S. Diseases of the breast. Philadelphia: Lippincott-Raven, 1996:674.

135. Reichman B, Seidman A, Crown J, et al. Paclitaxel and recombinant human granulocyte colony-stimulating factor as initial chemotherapy for metastatic breast cancer. J Clin Oncol 1993;11:1943–51.

136. Nathanson L. Immunology and immunotherapy of human breast cancer. Cancer Immunol Immunother 1977;2:209–24.

137. Sparks FC, Wile AG, Ramming KP, et al. Immunology and adjuvant chemoimmunotherapy of breast cancer. Arch Surg 1976;111:1057–62.

138. Stacker SA, Thompson CH, Sacks NP, et al. Detection of mammary serum antigen in sera from breast cancer patients using monoclonal antibody 3E1.2. Cancer Res 1988;48:Pt 1:7060–6.

139. Springer GF, Desai PR, Tegtmeyer H, et al. Pancarcinoma T/Tn antigen detects human carcinoma long before biopsy does and its vaccine prevents breast carcinoma recurrence. Ann N Y Acad Sci 1993;690:355–7.

140. Harris JE. The immunology of malignant disease. 2nd ed. St Louis: CV Mosby, 1976:480.

141. Sparano JA, O'Boyle K. The potential role for biological therapy in the treatment of breast cancer. Semin Oncol 1992;19:333–41.

142. DeBrabander M, DeCrée J, Vandebroek J, et al. Levamisole in the treatment of cancer: anything new? Anticancer Res 1992;12:177–87.

143. Senn H, Jungi WF, Amgwerd R. Chemo(immuno)therapy with LMF + BCG in node-negative and node-positive breast cancer. In: Salmon SE, ed. Adjuvant therapy of cancer III. New York: Grune & Stratton, 1981:385–93.

144. Buzdar AU, Blumenschein GR, Smith TL, et al. Adjuvant chemotherapy with fluorouracil, doxorubicin, and cyclophosphamide, with or without Bacillus Calmette-Guérin and with or without irradiation in operable breast cancer: a prospective randomized trial. Cancer 1984;53:384–9.

145. Pearson OH, Hubay CA, Marshall JS, et al. Adjuvant endocrine therapy, cytotoxic chemotherapy, and immunotherapy in stage-II breast cancer: five-year results. Breast Cancer Res Treat 1983;3:Suppl:S61–8.

146. Giuliano AE, Sparks FC, Patterson K, et al. Adjuvant chemo-immunotherapy in stage II carcinoma of the breast. J Surg Oncol 1986;31:255–9.

147. Sparks FC, Pardridge D, Wile A, et al. Immunotherapy of human breast cancer with BCG and viable and irradiated tumor cell vaccines. In: Crispen RG, ed. Neoplasm immunity: solid tumor therapy. Chicago: Franklin Institute Press, 1977:179–88.

148. Aisner J, Weinberg V, Perloff M, et al. Chemotherapy versus chemoimmunotherapy (CAF v CAFVP v CMF each ± MER) for metastatic carcinoma of the breast: a CALGB study. Cancer and Leukemia Group B. J Clin Oncol 1987;5:1523–33.

149. Pinsky C, DeJager R, Wittes R, et al. *Corynebacterium parvum* as adjuvant to combination chemotherapy in patients with advanced breast cancer. In: Crispen RG, ed. Neoplasm immunity: solid tumor therapy. Chicago: Franklin Institute Press, 1977:145–51.

150. Haskell CM, Ossorio R, Sarna G. Cyclophosphamide, methotrexate and 5-fluorouracil with and without *Corynebacterium parvum* in the treatment of metastatic breast cancer. In: Crispen RG, ed. Neoplasm immunity: solid tumor therapy. Chicago: Franklin Institute Press, 1977:153–60.

151. Kan N, Kodama H, Hori, T, et al. Intrapleural adaptive immunotherapy for breast cancer patients with cytologically-confirmed malignant pleural effusions: an analysis of 67 patients in Kyoto and Shiga Prefecture, Japan. Breast Cancer Res Treat 1993;27:203–10.

152. Colston KW, Mackay AG, James SY, et al. EB1089: a new vitamin D analogue that inhibits the growth of breast cancer cells in vivo and in vitro. Biochem Pharmacol 1992;44:2273–80.

153. Bower M, Colston KW, Stein RC, et al. Topical calcipotriol treatment in advanced breast cancer [published erratum appears in Lancet 1991;337(8757):1618]. see comments. Lancet 1991;337:701–2.

154. Dufour P, Lang JM, Giron C, et al. Sodium ditiocarb as adjuvant immunotherapy for high risk breast cancer: a randomized study. Biotherapy 1993;6:9–12.

155. Ceriani RL, Blank EW, Peterson JA. Experimental immunotherapy of human breast carcinomas implanted in nude mice with a mixture of monoclonal antibodies against human milk fat globule components. Cancer Res 1987;47:532–40.

156. Weiner LM, Holmes M, Adams GP, et al. A human tumor xenograft model of therapy with a bispecific monoclonal antibody targeting c-erbB-2 and CD16. Cancer Res 1993;53:94–100.

157. Xu F, Lupu R, Rodriguez GC, et al. Antibody-induced growth inhibition is mediated through immunochemically and functionally distinct epitopes on the extracellular domain of the c-erbB-2 (HER-2/neu) gene product p185. Int J Cancer 1993;53:401–8.

158. Sugiyama Y, Aihara M, Shibamori M, et al. In vitro anti-tumor activity of anti-c-erbB-2 × anti-CD3 epsilon bifunctional monoclonal antibody. Jpn J Cancer Res 1992;83:563–7.

159. Schnürch HG, Stegmüller M, Vering A, et al. Growth inhibition of xenotransplanted human carcinomas by a monoclonal antibody directed against the epidermal growth factor receptor. Eur J Cancer 1994;30A:491–6.

160. Bjorn MJ, Smith HS, Dairkee SH. Response of primary human mammary tumor cell cultures to a monoclonal antibody-recombinant ricin A chain immunotoxin. Cancer Immunol Immunother 1988;26:121–4.

161. LeMaistre CF, Edwards DP, Krolick KA, McGuire WL. An immunotoxin cytotoxic for breast cancer cells in vitro. Cancer Res 1987;47:730–4.

162. Rodríguez GC, Boente MP, Berchuck A, et al. The effect of antibodies and immunotoxins reactive with HER-2/neu on growth of ovarian and breast cancer cell lines. Am J Obstet Gynecol 1993;168:Pt 1:228–32.

163. Ozzello L, De Rosa CM, Blank EW, et al. The use of natural interferon alpha conjugated to a monoclonal antibody antimammary epithelial mucin (Mc5) for the treatment of human breast cancer xenografts. Breast Cancer Res Treat 1993;25:265–76.

164. Ziegler LD, Palazzolo P, Cunningham J, et al. Phase I trial of murine monoclonal antibody L6 in combination with subcutaneous interleukin-2 in patients with advanced carcinoma of the breast, colorectum, and lung. J Clin Oncol 1992;10:1470–8.

165. Hancock MC, Langton BC, Chan T, et al. A monoclonal antibody against the c-erbB-2 protein enhances the cytotoxicity of cis-diamminedichloroplatinum against human breast and ovarian tumor cell lines. Cancer Res 1991;51:4575–80.

166. Spicer DV, Kelley A, Herman R, et al. Low-dose recombinant interleukin-2 and low-dose cyclophosphamide in metastatic breast cancer. Cancer Immunol Immunother 1992;34:424-6.

167. Yamasaki S, Kan N, Mise K, et al. Cellular interaction against autologous tumor cells between IL-2–cultured lymphocytes and fresh peripheral blood lymphocytes in patients with breast cancer given immunochemotherapy. Biotherapy 1993;6:63–71.

168. Budd GT, Green S, Baker LH, et al. A Southwest Oncology Group phase II trial of recombinant tumor necrosis factor in metastatic breast cancer [published erratum appears in Cancer 1992;69(11):2866]. Cancer 1991;68:1694–5.

169. Repetto L, Venturino A, Simoni C, et al. Interferons in the treatment of advanced breast cancer. J Biol Regul Homeost Agents 1993;7:109–14.

170. Reed MJ, Topping L, Coldham NG, et al. Control of aromatase activity in breast cancer cells: the role of cytokines and growth factors. J Steroid Biochem Mol Biol 1993;44:589–96.

171. Pegram M, Lipton A, Pitras R, et al. A Phase II study of receptor-enhanced chemosensitivity using recombinant humanized anti-p185 HER-2/neu monoclonal antibody plus cisplatin in patients with HER-2/neu overexpressing metastatic breast cancer refractory to chemotherapy treatment. J Clin Oncol 1998;16:2659–71.

172. Slamon D, Leyland-Jones B, Shak S, et al. Addition of Herceptin to first line chemotherapy for HER-2 overexpressing metastatic breast cancer markedly increases anticancer activity: a randomized, multinational controlled Phase III trial. Proc Am Soc Clin Oncol 1998;17:A98.

173. Cobleigh MA, Vogel CL, Tripathy D, et al. Efficacy and safety of Herceptin (humanized anti-HER 2 antibody) as a single agent in 222 women with HER-2 overexpression who relapsed following chemotherapy for metastatic breast cancer. Proc Am Soc Clin Oncol 1998;17:A97.

174. Hortobagyi GN, Theriault RL, Porter L, et al. Efficacy of pamidronate in reducing skeletal complications in patients with breast cancer and lytic bone metastases. N Engl J Med 1996;335:1785–91.

175. Paterson AHG, Powles TJ, Kanis JA, et al. Double blind controlled trial of clodronate in patients with bone metastases from breast cancer. J Clin Oncol 1993;11:59–65.

176. van Holten-Verzantvoort AT, Bijvoet OLM, et al. Reduced morbidity from skeletal metastases in breast cancer patients during long term bisphosphonate (APD) treatment. Lancet 1987;2:983–85.

177. Hortobagyi GN, Theriault RL, Lipton A, et al. Long-term prevention of skeletal complications of metastatic breast cancer with pamidronate. J Clin Oncol 1998;16:2038–44.

178. Hultborn R, Ryden S, Gunderson S, et al. Efficacy of pamidronate on skeletal complications from breast cancer metastases: a randomized prospective double-blind placebo-controlled trial. Acta Oncol 1996;35:73–4.

179. Conte PF, Mauriac L, Calabresi F, et al. Delay in progression of bone metastases treated with intravenous pamidronate: results from a multicenter randomized controlled trial. J Clin Oncol 1996;14:2552–9.

180. Lipton A, Theriault R, Leff R, et al. Long term reduction of skeletal complications in breast cancer patients with osteolytic bone metastases receiving hormone therapy, by monthly 90 mg pamidronate (Aredia) infusions. Proc Am Soc Clin Oncol 1997;19:A152.

181. Robinson RG, Preston DF, Baxter KG, et al. Clinical experience with strontium-89 in prostatic and breast cancer patients. Semin Oncol 1993;20:Suppl 2:44–8.

182. Resche I, Chatal JF, Pecking A, et al. A dose-controlled study of 153 Sm-ethylenediaminetetramethylenephosphate (EDTMP) in the treatment of patients with painful bone metastases. Eur J Cancer 1997;33:1583–91.

183. Lundgren S. Progestins in breast cancer treatment: a review. Acta Oncol 1992;31:709–22.

184. DiMonaco M, Brignardello E, Leonardi L, et al. Inhibitory effect of hydroxyflutamide plus tamoxifen on oestradial-induced growth of MCF-7 breast cancer cells. J Cancer Res Clin Oncol 1995;121:710–4.

185. Weckbecker G, Liu R, Tolcsvai L, Bruns C. Antiproliferative effects of the somatostatin analogue octreotide (SMS 201–995) on ZR-75-1 human breast cancer cells in vivo and in vitro. Cancer Res 1992;52:4973–8.

186. Pollak M, Gallant K, Poisson R, Harris A. Potential role for somatostatin analogues in breast cancer: rationale and description of an ongoing trial. Metabolism 1992;41:Suppl 2:119–20.

187. Broder L, Tormey DC. Combination chemotherapy of carcinoma of the breast. Cancer Treat Rev 1974;1:183–203.

188. Carbone PP, Tormey DC. Combination chemotherapy for advanced disease. In: McGuire WL, ed. Breast cancer: advances in research and treatment: current approaches to therapy. Vol. 1. New York: Plenum Publishing, 1977:165–215.

189. Perez DJ, Harvey VJ, Robinson BA, et al. A randomized comparison of single-agent doxorubicin and epirubicin as first-line cytotoxic therapy in advanced breast cancer. J Clin Oncol 1991;9:2148–52.

190. Gasparini G, Dal Fior S, Panizzoni GA, et al. Weekly epirubicin versus doxorubicin as second line therapy in advanced breast cancer: a randomized clinical trial. Am J Clin Oncol 1991;14:38–44.

191. Richards MA, Hopwood P, Ramirez AJ, et al. Doxorubicin in advanced breast cancer: influence of schedule on response, survival and quality of life. Eur J Cancer 1992;28A:1023–8.

192. Cowan JD, Neidhart J, McClure S, et al. Randomized trial of doxorubicin, bisantrene, and mitoxantrone in advanced breast cancer: a Southwest Oncology Group study. J Natl Cancer Inst 1991;83:1077–84.

193. Henderson IC. Chemotherapy for advanced disease. In: Harris JR, ed. Breast diseases. Philadelphia: JB Lippincott, 1987:428–79.

194. Dixon AR, Jackson L, Chan S, et al. A randomised trial of second-line hormone vs single agent chemotherapy in tamoxifen resistant advanced breast cancer. Br J Cancer 1992;66:402–4.

195. Hortobagyi GN. Mitomycin: its evolving role in the treatment of breast cancer. Oncology 1993;50:Suppl 1:1–8.

196. Smith IE, Talbot DC. Cisplatin and its analogues in the treatment of advanced breast cancer: a review [published erratum appears in Br J Cancer 1992;66(2):419]. see comments. Br J Cancer 1992;65:787–93.

197. Willemse P, Sleijfer DT, Mulder NH, de Vries EG. Cisplatin in breast cancer. Br J Cancer 1993;67:638. letter; comment.

198. Hortobagyi GN. Activity of ifosfamide in breast cancer. Semin Oncol 1992;19:Suppl 12:36–41.

199. O'Brien ME, Talbot DC, Smith IE. Carboplatin in the treatment of advanced breast cancer: a phase II study using a pharmacokinetically guided dose schedule. J Clin Oncol 1993;11:2112–7.

200. Fraschini G, Fleishman G, Yap HY, et al. Percutaneous hepatic arterial infusion of cisplatin for metastatic breast cancer. Cancer Treat Rep 1987;71:313–5.

201. Martino S, Samal BA, Singhakowinta A, et al. A phase II study of cis-diamminedichloroplatinum II for advanced breast cancer: two dose schedules. J Cancer Res Clin Oncol 1984;108:354–6.

202. Bajorin D, Bosl GJ, Fein R. Phase I trial of escalating doses of cisplatin in hypertonic saline. J Clin Oncol 1987;5:1589–93.

203. Marini G, Simoncini E, Zaniboni A, et al. 5-Fluorouracil and high-dose folinic acid as salvage treatment of advanced breast cancer: an update. Oncology 1987;44:336-40.

204. Margolin KA, Doroshow JH, Akman SA, et al. Effective initial therapy of advanced breast cancer with fluorouracil and high-dose, continuous infusion calcium leucovorin. J Clin Oncol 1992;10:1278–83.

205. Loprinzi CL, Ingle JN, Schaid DJ, et al. 5-Fluorouracil plus leucovorin in women with metastatic breast cancer: a phase II study. Am J Clin Oncol 1991;14:30–2.

206. Margolin KA, Green S, Osborne K, et al. Phase II trial of 5-fluorouracil and high-dose folinic acid as first- or second-line therapy for advanced breast cancer. Am J Clin Oncol 1994;17:175–80.

207. Ault A. FDA panel approves new breast cancer pill for therapy failures. Lancet 1998;351:962.

208. Seidman AD, Norton L, Reichman BS, et al. Preliminary experience with paclitaxel (Taxol) plus recombinant human granulocyte colony-stimulating factor in the treatment of breast cancer. Semin Oncol 1993;20:Suppl 3:40–5.

209. Reichman BS, Seidman AD, Crown JP, et al. Paclitaxel and recombi-

nant human granulocyte colony-stimulating factor as initial chemotherapy for metastatic breast cancer. J Clin Oncol 1993;11:1943–51.

210. Palombo H, Estapé J, Viñolas N, et al. Chronic oral etoposide in advanced breast cancer. Cancer Chemother Pharmacol 1994;33:527–9.

211. Martín M, Lluch A, Casado, A, et al. Clinical activity of chronic oral etoposide in previously treated metastatic breast cancer. see comments. J Clin Oncol 1994;12:986–91.

212. Yau JC, Yap YY, Buzdar AU, et al. A comparative randomized trial of vinca alkaloids in patients with metastatic breast carcinoma. Cancer 1985;55:337–40.

213. Romero A, Rabinovich MG, Vallejo CT, et al. Vinorelbine as first-line chemotherapy for metastatic breast carcinoma. J Clin Oncol 1994;12:336–41.

214. Fumoleau P, Delgado FM, Delozier T, et al. Phase II trial of weekly intravenous vinorelbine in first-line advanced breast cancer chemotherapy. J Clin Oncol 1993;11:1245–52.

215. Barni S, Archili C, Lissoni P, et al. A weekly schedule of epirubicin in pretreated advanced breast cancer. Tumori 1993;79:45–8.

216. Neri B, Pacini P, Algeri R, et al. Conventional versus high-dose epidoxorubicin as single agent in advanced breast cancer. Cancer Invest 1993;11:106–12.

217. Barni S. A weekly schedule of epirubicin in pretreated advanced breast cancer. Tumori 1993;79:45.

218. A prospective randomized trial comparing epirubicin monochemotherapy to two fluorouracil, cyclophosphamide, and epirubicin regimens differing in epirubicin dose in advanced breast cancer patients. The French Epirubicin Study Group. J Clin Oncol 1991;9:305–12.

219. Carmichael J, Walling J. Phase II activity in gemcitabine in advanced breast cancer. Semin Oncol 1996;2315:5 Suppl 10:77–81.

220. Taguchi T, Tominaga T, Ogawa M, et al. A late phase II study of CPT-11 (Irinotecan) in advanced breast cancer. CPT-11 Study Group of Breast Cancer. Gan To Kagaku Ryoho 1994;21:1017–24.

221. Tormey D, Gelman R, Falkson G. Prospective evaluation of rotating chemotherapy in advanced breast cancer. An Eastern Cooperative Oncology Group trial. Am J Clin Oncol 1983;6:1–18.

222. Carmo-Pereira J, Costa FO, Henriques E, Ricardo JA. Advanced ovarian carcinoma: a prospective and randomized clinical trial of cyclophosphamide versus combination cytotoxic chemotherapy (Hexa-CAF). Cancer 1981;48:1517.

223. Tormey DC, Lippman ME, Edwards BK, Cassidy JG. Evaluation of tamoxifen doses with and without fluoxymesterone in advanced breast cancer. Ann Intern Med 1983;98:139–44.

224. Muss HB, Richards F 2d, Jackson DV, et al. Vincristine, doxorubicin, and cyclophosphamide versus low-dose intravenous cyclophosphamide, methotrexate, and 5-fluorouracil in advanced breast cancer: a randomized trial of the Piedmont Oncology Association. Cancer 1982;50:2269–74.

225. Biran S, Brufman G. Cyclic combination chemotherapy for metastatic breast cancer: comparison of two CMF schedules. Oncology 1981;38:257–9.

226. Tormey DC, Weinberg VE, Holland JF, et al. A randomized trial of five and three drug chemotherapy and chemoimmunotherapy in women with operable node positive breast cancer. J Clin Oncol 1983;1:138–45.

227. Cooper RG. Combination chemotherapy in hormone-resistant breast cancer. Proc AACR 1969;10:15.

228. Carter SK. Integration of chemotherapy into combined modality treatment of solid tumors. VII: adenocarcinoma of the breast. Cancer Treat Rev 1976;3:141–74.

229. Smalley RV, Lefante J, Bartolucci A, et al. A comparison of cyclophosphamide, Adriamycin, and 5-fluorouracil (CAF) and cyclophosphamide, methotrexate, 5-fluorouracil, vincristine, and prednisone (CMFVP) in patients with advanced breast cancer. Breast Cancer Res Treat 1983;3:209–20.

230. CMEA Cooperative Treatment Group. Clinical controlled trial in advanced breast cancer: CMFV (cyclophosphamide, methotrexate, fluorouracil, vincristine) versus CD (carminomycin, dibromodulcitol). Neoplasma 1982;29:741–47.

231. Oster MW, Park Y. Vincristine, Adriamycin, and mitomycin (VAM) therapy for previously treated breast cancer: a preliminary report. Cancer 1983;51:203–5.

232. Harris MA, Byrne PJ, Smith FP, et al. Treatment of advanced breast cancer with two doxorubicin-containing regimens. Am J Clin Oncol 1984;7:51–8.

233. Creech RH, Dayal H, Catalano RB, et al. Combination doxorubicin-mitomycin therapy for hormonal and CMF-refractory metastatic breast cancer. Proc ASCO 1984;3:126.

234. Vaughn CB, Maniscalco-Greb E, Lockhard C. VP-16 and Adriamycin in patients with advanced breast cancer. Am J Clin Oncol 1982;5:505–9.

235. Konits PH, Van Echo DA, Aisner J, et al. Doxorubicin plus VP-16-213 for the treatment of refractory breast carcinoma. Am J Clin Oncol 1982;5:515–9.

236. Tannir N, Yap HY, Hortobagyi GH, et al. Sequential continuous infusion with doxorubicin and vinblastine: an effective chemotherapy combination for patients with advanced breast cancer previously treated with cyclophosphamide, methotrexate, 5-FU, vincristine, and prednisone. Cancer Treat Rep 1984;68:1039–41.

237. Yap HY, Blumenschein GR, Barnes B, et al. Sequential combinations of continuous infusion Adriamycin and vinblastine in patients with metastatic breast cancer. Proc ASCO 1982;1:78.

238. Friedman MA, Marcus FS, Cassidy MJ, et al. 5-Fluorouracil + Oncovin + Adriamycin + mitomycin C (FOAM): an effective program for breast cancer, even for disease refractory to previous chemotherapy. A Northern California Oncology Group (NCOG) study. Cancer 1983;52:193–7.

239. Luikart SD, Witman GB, Portlock CS. Adriamycin (doxorubicin), vinblastine, and mitomycin C combination chemotherapy in refractory breast carcinoma. Cancer 1984;54:1252–5.

240. Bontenbal M, Planting AS, Rodenburg CJ, et al. Weekly low-dose mitoxantrone plus doxorubicin as second-line chemotherapy for advanced breast cancer. Breast Cancer Res Treat 1992;21:133–8.

241. Aitini E, Cavazzini G, Cantore M, et al. A phase II study of 5-fluorouracil and high-dose folinic acid in combination with cyclophosphamide and mitoxantrone for advanced breast cancer. Eur J Cancer 1992;28A:1968–70.

242. Bitran JD, Kozloff MF, Desser RK. Platinol (CDDP) and continuous intravenous infusion 5-fluorouracil in refractory stage IV breast cancer: a phase II study. Cancer Invest 1990;8:335–8.

243. Estapé J, Cirera L, Millá A, Doncel F. VP16-213 and cyclophosphamide in advanced breast cancer: a phase II study. Cancer Chemother Pharmacol 1983;10:154–7.

244. Menichetti ET, Silva RR, Tummarello D, et al. Etoposide and mitomycin-C in pretreated metastatic breast cancer. Tumori 1989;75:473–4.

245. Bezwoda WR, Hesdorffer CS. Mitoxantrone, methotrexate, and 5-fluorouracil combination chemotherapy as first-line treatment in stage IV breast cancer. Cancer 1986;57:218–21.

246. Bitran JD, Desser RK, Kozloff MF. Platinol and continuous infusion 5-fluorouracil in refractory stage IV breast cancer. Breast Cancer Res Treat 1988;12:149.

247. Amoroso D, Pronzato P, Bertelli G, et al. Cisplatin and 5-fluorouracil in refractory breast cancer patients: a phase II study. Breast Cancer Res Treat 1988;11:269–71.

248. Mann G, Yap HY, Blumenschein GR, et al. A trial of vinblastine (VLB) and mitoxantrone (M) in the treatment of advanced breast carcinoma (BC). Proc ASCO 1983;2:108.

249. Cruciani G, Tienghi A, Fiorentini G, et al. Mitoxantrone (M) and vinblastine (V) in the treatment of advanced breast cancer. Tumori 1990;76:196–8.

250. Swain SM, Honig SF. Mitoxantrone, 5-FU, and leucovorin in breast cancer. Med Pediatr Oncol 1994;22:370–4.

251. Wils JA. Mitoxantrone, leucovorin and high-dose infusional 5-fluorouracil: an effective and well-tolerated regimen for the treatment of advanced breast cancer. Eur J Cancer 1993;29A:2106–8.

252. Mammoliti S, Merlini L, Caroti C, Gallo L. Mitoxantrone, 5-fluorouracil and levo-leucovorin as salvage treatment in advanced breast cancer patients. Eur J Cancer 1994;30A:248–9. letter.

253. Cufer T, Kolaric K, Cervek J, Cerar O. Combination of 5-fluorouracil, imidazole carboxamide, BCNU and prednisolone (FIB-P) as a salvage chemotherapy in heavily pretreated breast cancer patients. Tumori 1992;78:26–31.

254. Francini G, Petrioli R, Aquino A, Gonnelli S. Advanced breast cancer treatment with folinic acid, 5-fluorouracil, and mitomycin C. Cancer Chemother Pharmacol 1993;32:359–64.

255. Stein RC, Bower M, Law M, et al. Mitozantrone and methotrexate chemotherapy with and without mitomycin C in the treatment of advanced breast cancer: a randomised clinical trial. Eur J Cancer 1992;28A:1963–5.

256. Garewal HS, Brooks RJ, Jones SE, Miller TP. Treatment of advanced breast cancer with mitomycin C combined with vinblastine or vindesine. J Clin Oncol 1983;1:772–5.

257. Perrone F, De Placido S, Carlomagno C, et al. Chemotherapy with mitomycin C and vinblastine in pretreated metastatic breast cancer. Tumori 1993;79:254–7.

258. Sedlacek SM. First-line and salvage therapy of metastatic breast cancer with mitomycin/vinblastine. Oncology 1993;50:Suppl 1:16–21.

259. Gewirtz AM, Cadman E. Preliminary report on the efficacy of sequential methotrexate and 5-fluorouracil in advanced breast cancer. Cancer 1981;47:2552–5.

260. Perrault DJ, Erlichman C, Hasselback R, et al. Sequenced methotrexate (MTX) and 5-fluorouracil (5FU) in refractory metastatic breast cancer: a phase II study. Proc ASCO 1983;2:100.

261. Hortobagyi GN, Yap HY, Blumenschein GR, et al. Phase II evaluation of vinblastine, methotrexate, and calcium leukovorin rescue in patients with refractory metastatic breast cancer. Cancer 1983;51:769–72.

262. Manegold C, Worst P, Bickel J, et al. Ifosfamide/etoposide and mesna uroprotection in advanced breast cancer. Cancer Chemother Pharmacol 1990;26:Suppl:S87–90.

263. Fountzilas G, Skarlos D, Theoharis D, et al. Carboplatin and oral etoposide in the treatment of patients with advanced breast cancer refractory to anthracyclines. Tumori 1993;79:389–92.

264. Fields KK, Zorsky PE, Hiemenz JW, et al. Ifosfamide, carboplatin, and etoposide: a new regimen with a broad spectrum of activity. J Clin Oncol 1994;12:544–52.

265. Becher R, Höfeler H, Kloke O, et al. Ifosfamide, methotrexate and 5-fluorouracil for pretreated advanced breast cancer. Oncology 1991;48:459–63.

266. Fraschini G, Yap HY, Mann G, et al. Chemotherapy with mitoxantrone in combination with continuous infusion vinblastine for metastatic breast cancer. Cancer 1987;60:1724–8.

267. Barone C, Astone A, Cassano A, et al. Salvage chemotherapy with mitoxantrone and mitomycin with or without methotrexate in advanced breast cancer. Anticancer Drugs 1992;3:471.

268. Pai LH, Swain SM, Venzon DJ, et al. Therapy of patients with metastatic breast cancer with 5-fluorouracil, leucovorin and carboplatin. Anticancer Drugs 1992;3:463.

269. Barker LJ, Jones SE, Savin MA, Mennel RG. Phase II evaluation of carboplatin and VP-16 for patients with metastatic breast cancer and only one prior chemotherapy regimen. Cancer 1993;72:771–3.

270. Oster MW, Schilsky RL, Faraggi D, et al. Cytosine arabinoside and cisplatin for advanced breast cancer: a phase II study of the Cancer and Leukemia Group B. Cancer 1991;68:1696–8.

271. Nichols CR. Role of etoposide in treatment of breast cancer. Semin Oncol 1992;19:6 Suppl 13:67–71.

272. Brunner KW, Sonntag RW, Alberto P, et al. Combined chemo- and hormonal therapy in advanced breast cancer. Cancer 1977;39:Suppl:2923–33.

273. Rubens RD, Begent RH, Knight RK, et al. Combined cytotoxic and progestogen therapy for advanced breast cancer. Cancer 1978;42:1680–6.

274. Tormey DC, Falkson G, Crowley J, et al. Dibromodulcitol and Adriamycin ± tamoxifen in advanced breast cancer. Am J Clin Oncol 1982;5:33–9.

275. Cocconi G, De Lisi V, Boni C, et al. Chemotherapy versus combination of chemotherapy and endocrine therapy in advanced breast cancer: a prospective randomized study. Cancer 1983;51:581–8.

276. Perry MC, Kardinal CG, Korzun AH, et al. Chemohormonal therapy in advanced carcinoma of the breast. Cancer and Leukemia Group B protocol 8081. J Clin Oncol 1987;5:1534–45.

277. Viladiu P, Alonso MC, Avella A, et al. Chemotherapy versus chemotherapy plus hormonotherapy in postmenopausal advanced breast cancer patients: a randomized trial. Cancer 1985;56:2745–50.

278. Mouridsen HT, Rose C, Engelsman E, et al. Combined cytotoxic and endocrine therapy in postmenopausal patients with advanced breast cancer: a randomized study of CMF vs CMF plus tamoxifen. Eur J Cancer Clin Oncol 1985;21:291–9.

279. Kiang DT, Gay J, Goldman A, Kennedy BJ. A randomized trial of chemotherapy and hormonal therapy in advanced breast cancer. N Engl J Med 1985;313:1241–6.

280. Anonymous. A randomized trial in postmenopausal patients with advanced breast cancer comparing endocrine and cytotoxic therapy given sequentially or in combination. The Australian and New Zealand Breast Cancer Trials Group, Clinical Oncology Society of Australia. J Clin Oncol 1986;4:186–93.

281. Krook JE, Ingle JN, Green SJ, et al. Randomized clinical trial of cyclophosphamide, 5-FU, and prednisone with or without tamoxifen in postmenopausal women with advanced breast cancer. Cancer Treat Rep 1985;69:355–61.

282. Falkson G, Gelman RS, Tormey DC, et al. Treatment of metastatic breast cancer in premenopausal women using CAF with or without oophorectomy: an Eastern Cooperative Oncology Group study. J Clin Oncol 1987;5:881–9.

283. Jouve M, Palangie T, Garcia-Giralt E, et al. [Metastatic breast cancer: controlled trial of chemotherapy with and without hormones]. Bull Cancer 1984;71:432–41.

284. Conte PF, Pronzato P, Rubagotti A, et al. Conventional versus cytokinetic polychemotherapy with estrogenic recruitment in metastatic breast cancer: results of a randomized cooperative trial. J Clin Oncol 1987;5:339–47.

285. Lippman ME, Cassidy J, Wesley M, Young RC. A randomized attempt to increase the efficacy of cytotoxic chemotherapy in metastatic breast cancer by hormonal synchronization. J Clin Oncol 1984;2:28–36.

286. Davidson NE, Lippman ME. Stimulation of breast cancer with estrogens: how much clinical value? Eur J Cancer Clin Oncol 1987;23:897–900.

287. Elomaa I, Blomqvist C, Rissanen P, Mäntylä M. Weekly low-dose doxorubicin with or without high-dose medroxyprogesterone acetate as secondary treatment in metastatic breast cancer—a randomized trial. Acta Oncol 1988;27:297–9.

288. Gundersen S, Kvinnsland S, Klepp O, et al. Chemotherapy with or without high-dose medroxyprogesterone acetate in oestrogen-receptor–negative advanced breast cancer. Norwegian Breast Cancer Group. Eur J Cancer 1992;28:390–4.

289. Ingle JN, Foley JF, Mailliard JA, et al. Randomized trial of cyclophosphamide, methotrexate, and 5-fluorouracil with or without estrogenic recruitment in women with metastatic breast cancer. Cancer 1994;73:2337–43.

290. Paridaens R, Heuson JC, Julien JP, et al. Assessment of estrogenic recruitment before chemotherapy in advanced breast cancer: a double-blind randomized study. European Organization for Research and Treatment of Cancer Breast Cancer Cooperative Group. J Clin Oncol 1993;11:1723–8.

291. Stadtmauer EA, O'Neill A, Goldstein LJ, et al (for the Philadelphia Bone Marrow Transplant Group). Conventional-dose chemotherapy compared with high-dose chemotherapy plus autologous hematopoietic stem-cell transplantation for metastatic breast cancer. N Engl J Med 2000;342:1069–76.

# ADJUVANT TREATMENT OF BREAST CANCER

• Steven J. Tucker • Linnea I. Chap • Charles M. Haskell

The concept of breast cancer as a systemic disease, plus the availability of systemic therapies that are moderately effective against advanced breast cancer, led to the use of systemic therapy as an adjunct to surgery or radiation therapy in patients with primary breast cancer. The use of chemother-

apy, endocrine therapy, or both in the phase immediately following primary treatment is called *adjuvant therapy*. When it is used before local therapy, it is called *primary* or *neoadjuvant* chemotherapy.

The theoretical rationale for adjuvant treatment has been

discussed in Chapters 1 and 8. In the subsequent discussion, the results of adjuvant chemotherapy, endocrine therapy, and chemoendocrine therapy are summarized. Specific recommendations for integrating adjuvant therapy into a plan of management for specific groups of patients is presented in the section Treatment by Stage of Disease and Special Problems.

## HISTORICAL PERSPECTIVE

The earliest studies of adjuvant chemotherapy for breast cancer were performed between 1955 and 1970 and consisted of single perioperative courses of chemotherapy given with the goal of eradicating circulating tumor cells in the bloodstream. The two most important trials from this period were the thiotepa trial conducted by the NSABP[1] and a Scandinavian trial with cyclophosphamide conducted by Nissen-Meyer and colleagues.[2] These studies suggested a role for adjuvant chemotherapy in patients with carcinoma of the breast, but neither was definitive. Subsequent studies, such as the NSABP B-05,[3] which compared L-phenylalanine mustard with placebo and the initial Milan CMF trial,[4] which compared combination chemotherapy with a surgery-alone control group, showed that early relapse could be delayed by chemotherapy. After the success of the NSABP and the Milan trials, the use of placebo or observation-only control groups was abandoned in the study of adjuvant therapy. Follow-up reports of the Milan CMF trial continue to show relapse-free survival and overall survival benefits compared with no treatment at a median of 19.4 years. The benefits in

overall survival and relapse-free survival were limited to premenopausal patients and possibly due to the induction of amenorrhea. The lack of observed benefit in older women was likely due to lower chemotherapy doses being given. CMF has remained the standard of care for node-positive carcinoma of the breast.

**Early Breast Cancer Trialists' Collaborative Group.** In 1992, the EBCTCG, located at Oxford University, released their landmark meta-analysis of breast cancer adjuvant trials; this was updated in 1998.[5, 6] The initial overview supported the benefit of chemotherapy in premenopausal women with both node-negative and node-positive disease and suggested there may be a benefit in postmenopausal women as well. The 1998 overview confirmed the benefit of adjuvant polychemotherapy for both premenopausal and postmenopausal women and in women with node-negative and node-positive disease. The meta-analysis also showed that longer duration of chemotherapy was not found to confer any more benefit than a few months of chemotherapy. The 1998 overview involved approximately 18,000 women in 47 trials of prolonged polychemotherapy versus no chemotherapy, 6000 women in 11 trials of shorter versus longer duration of therapy, and approximately 6000 women in 11 trials comparing anthracycline-containing regimens versus CMF. The results, summarized in Table 35–29, are as follows. For recurrence, polychemotherapy produced proportional reductions among women younger than 50 (35% ± 4 reduction; $p < 0.00001$) and among those age 50 to 69 (20% ± 8; $p < 0.00001$). For mortality, the reductions were significant among women younger than 50 (27% ± 5; $p < 0.00001$) and among those age 50 to 69 (11% ± 3; $p < 0.0001$). Table

*Table 35–29.* Meta-Analysis of Polychemotherapy for Early Breast Cancer*

| | No. Patients | Typical Reduction (% ± SD) in Annual Odds of | |
| --- | --- | --- | --- |
| | | RECURRENCE AS FIRST EVENT | DEATH FROM ANY CAUSE |
| Total polychemotherapy | 18,788 | 23.5 ± 2 | 15.3 ± 2 |
| CMF alone | 8150 | 24 ± 3 | 14 ± 4 |
| CMF with extra cytotoxic drugs | 3218 | 20 ± 5 | 15 ± 5 |
| Other polychemotherapy | 7420 | 25 ± 4 | 17 ± 4 |
| Subdivided by age at randomization | | | |
| <40 | 1369 | 37 ± 7 | 27 ± 8 |
| 40–49 | 3160 | 34 ± 5 | 27 ± 5 |
| 50–59 | 6773 | 22 ± 4 | 14 ± 5 |
| 60–69 | 6807 | 18 ± 4 | 8 ± 4 |
| Estrogen Receptor (ER) status | | | |
| ER poor, age <50 | 1398 | 40 ± 7 | 35 ± 9 |
| ER unknown, age <50 | 2027 | 30 ± 6 | 23 ± 6 |
| ER positive, age <50 | 1115 | 33 ± 8 | 20 ± 10 |
| ER poor, age 50–69 | 3240 | 30 ± 5 | 17 ± 6 |
| ER unknown, age 50–69 | 3607 | 18 ± 4 | 11 ± 5 |
| ER positive, age 50–69 | 6793 | 18 ± 4 | 9 ± 5 |
| Longer vs. shorter treatment | 6154 | 7 ± 4 | −1% ± 5 |
| Anthracycline regimen vs. CMF | 6850 | 12 ± 4 | 11 ± 5 |

*The annual odds of death is the probability of dying during a year divided by the probability of surviving the year, and the ratio of the odds (called *odds ratio*) for the treatment group relative to the control group is a measure of whether the treatment reduces mortality. An odds ratio of 1.0 indicates equivalent outcomes for treatment and control groups, whereas an odds ratio < 1.0 indicates a reduction in the odds of death for the treatment group; 100 × (1.0 − estimated odds ratio) gives the percent reduction in annual odds of death. For all practical purposes, estimates of the reduction in the annual odds of death can be interpreted as estimates of the relative reduction in the annual risk or probability of an event. This is because individual patient data are used in the log-rank procedure to combine multiple estimates of the odds of an event calculated over short time intervals for which the probability of surviving is close to 1.

CMF, cyclophosphamide, methotrexate, fluorouracil.

Data from Early Breast Cancer Trialists' Collaborative Group. Polychemotherapy for early breast cancer: an overview of the randomised trials. Lancet 1998;352:930.

*Table 35–30.* **Absolute Risk Reductions with Chemotherapy During 5 and 10 Years of Follow-up from the 1998 Early Breast Cancer Trialists'
Collaborative Group Overview**

| | Lymph Node Negative | | | Lymph Node Positive | | |
|---|---|---|---|---|---|---|
| | CONTROL (%) | CHEMOTHERAPY (%) | ABSOLUTE RISK REDUCTION (%) | CONTROL (%) | CHEMOTHERAPY (%) | ABSOLUTE RISK REDUCTION (%) |
| Age <50 | | | | | | |
| 5-yr RFS | 65.9 | 75.3 | 9.4 | 41.9 | 57.1 | 15.2 |
| 10-yr RFS | 58.0 | 68.3 | 10.3 | 32.2 | 47.6 | 15.4 |
| 5-yr OS | 83.5 | 86.5 | 3.0 | 61.8 | 68.6 | 6.8 |
| 10-yr OS | 71.9 | 77.6 | 5.7 | 41.4 | 53.8 | 12.4 |
| Age 50–69 | | | | | | |
| 5-yr RFS | 70.3 | 76.6 | 6.3 | 53.3 | 60.0 | 6.7 |
| 10-yr RFS | 59.9 | 65.6 | 5.7 | 38.0 | 43.4 | 5.4 |
| 5-yr OS | 81.4 | 85.3 | 3.9 | 68.7 | 70.8 | 2.1 |
| 10-yr OS | 64.8 | 71.2 | 6.4 | 46.3 | 48.6 | 2.3 |

RFS, recurrence-free survival; OS, overall survival.
From Early Breast Cancer Trialists' Collaborative Group. Polychemotherapy for early breast cancer: an overview of randomised trials. Lancet 1998;352:930–42.

35–30 summarizes the absolute risk reductions subdivided by age and nodal status. Proportional reductions in risk were similar in node-negative and node-positive disease regardless of age. Recurrence reductions occurred chiefly in the first 5 years of follow-up, whereas reductions in mortality grew throughout the first 10 years.

Improved 10-year survival was seen in all groups regardless of nodal status. For node-negative women younger than age 50, 10-year survival improved from 71 to 78%, and for node-positive women younger than age 50, 10-year survival improved from 42% to 53%. In women age 50 to 69, smaller absolute benefits were seen, changing 10-year survival of 67 to 69% for node-negative patients and of 46 to 49% for node-positive patients. Age-specific benefits were seen in ER-negative and ER-positive disease. The benefit was twice as large in ER-negative women aged 50 to 59 compared with ER-positive women. Anthracycline-containing regimens, compared with CMF, produced an absolute benefit on mortality (69% vs. 72%), but this result, as suggested by the EBCTCG, may be selected for bias and premature. Lastly, direct comparisons of longer versus shorter duration of chemotherapy did not show any benefit with greater than 3 to 6 months of therapy.

The success of the overview process was possible because physicians and patients were willing to participate in randomized clinical trials of adjuvant therapy. Such trials are indispensable to medical progress in this field. In describing the benefits of adjuvant therapy to patients, a physician can use the reduction in the annual odds of recurrence or death, as given in Table 35–29. This reduction can be misleading, however, because the benefits of adjuvant therapy are highly dependent on each patient's risk of recurrence or death. Because these figures are interdependent, Table 35–30 provides another way of estimating benefit.

## PROGNOSTIC FACTORS

As demonstrated by the EBCTCG, all patients regardless of age and nodal status benefit from adjuvant therapy. Before choosing the kind of adjuvant therapy to be delivered, how-

ever, many patient factors need to be evaluated: an estimation of the patient's risk of recurrence and survival based on known prognostic factors, an estimation of the benefit of therapy in terms of absolute risk reduction of relapse and death, and an estimation of the toxicity associated with therapy. Historically the most important prognostic factors have been the number of involved axillary lymph nodes,[7] primary tumor size,[8] histologic grade,[9–12] and the hormone receptor status.[13, 14]

Overexpression or amplification of the HER-2/*neu* proto-oncogene has been associated with a poor prognosis in patients regardless of nodal status or hormone receptor status.[15, 16] These reports confirm most retrospective analyses performed previously. The prospective studies show HER-2/*neu* amplification to be an independent predictor of poor disease-free survival regardless of tumor size, grade, or ER status. This genetic marker is now exploited as targeted therapy by the monoclonal antibody trastuzumab. Phase II and III study rates in heavily pretreated patients with advanced disease have shown improved response[17] and improved disease-free survival and time to progression when trastuzumab is given with chemotherapy.[18, 19]

Many other important prognostic factors are still under investigation (Table 35–31). A high S-phase fraction has been associated with a poor prognosis.[20] The microvessel count, an indirect measure of angiogenesis, has also been

*Table 35–31.* **Prognostic Factors in Breast Cancer**

*Conventional*

| | |
|---|---|
| Tumor size | Hormone receptor status |
| Nodal status | HER-2/*neu* overexpression |
| Histologic grade | Lymphatic and vascular invasion |

*Investigational*

| | |
|---|---|
| S phase fraction | p53 protein |
| Ki-67 | Cathepsin-D |
| Ploidy | Stomelysin-3 |
| Thymidylate synthetase | Microvessel count |
| Epidermal growth factor receptor | *nm23* |
| | MDR1 |

associated with a poorer prognosis in breast cancer.[21] No one factor in node-negative breast cancer has enough utility to categorize patients at this time. For this reason, some authors have proposed modeling of several markers to accomplish this. These models[22, 23] frequently include tumor size, nodal status, histologic grade, S phase, and ER status to stratify patients into high and low risk.

## CHOOSING ADJUVANT CHEMOTHERAPY REGIMENS

The Oxford meta-analysis clearly showed that polychemotherapy is effective at prolonging survival and delaying relapse regardless of menopausal status, axillary nodal status, or hormonal status of the tumor. The power of the meta-analysis in showing overall benefit does not extend to defining the relative value of different chemotherapy regimens. Table 35–32 provides a general framework of indications for adjuvant chemotherapy in breast cancer. At present, a variety of regimens can be considered reasonable, and this is an area of active investigation (see Table 35–27). A number of questions must be considered in choosing adjuvant chemotherapy.

The first issue relates to choosing which of several regimens is optimal, in terms of risk and benefit. The CMF regimen probably has been the most widely used regimen of adjuvant chemotherapy in the United States. Since the 1980s, this regimen has undergone numerous modifications from its original formulation. We advocate use of one of the original CMF schedules using a day 1 and day 8 infusion schedule with either oral or intravenous cyclophosphamide, which have been tested in randomized, controlled trials. Another popular regimen is to use CMF every 3 weeks for eight to nine cycles over a 6-month period. There are no randomized, controlled data to support the use of this abbreviated CMF regimen. Currently, many clinicians have switched to the use of a doxorubicin-containing regimen, such as FAC, CAF, or AC. Numerous randomized clinical trials have been conducted or are ongoing and suggest a benefit with the administration of anthracycline-containing chemotherapy regimens.[24–28] Anthracycline-containing regimens appear to improve disease-free survival, relapse-free survival, and overall survival, although the absolute benefits appear to be limited as demonstrated in the Oxford overview. Additionally, some studies have not found a significant benefit for anthracyclines over CMF,[29–31] but no trials have shown CMF to be superior to the anthracycline regimens. The bulk of the data favoring anthracyclines are in premenopausal women and younger postmenopausal women.

The second issue has to do with the duration of adjuvant treatment. The Milan Group[32] has shown that 6 months of classic CMF (day 1 and day 8 dosing) is equivalent to 12 months of CMF treatment so that 6 months of treatment has become the usual duration of treatment outside of a clinical trial. Shorter duration of chemotherapy may be adequate, especially for trials using anthracycline-based regimens, as shown by several clinical trials involving 12 to 18 weeks of adjuvant therapy. Fisher and coworkers have shown that four cycles of AC are comparable with 6 months of classic CMF.[30] Six cycles of CAF or FAC appear to be equivalent to four cycles of AC. Perioperative chemotherapy, such as that given in the original adjuvant chemotherapy trials in the 1960s, appears to be inferior to the use of a full 6 months of treatment.[33]

A third question has to do with the dose intensity of adjuvant chemotherapy. Hryniuk[34] has proposed that inadequate dose intensity is a major reason for treatment failure in breast cancer. The importance of dose intensity was confirmed in a large trial conducted by the Cancer and Leukemia Group B (CALGB), in which patients were randomized to receive one of three dose levels of CAF.[35] The highest (C, 600 mg/m$^2$; A, 60 mg/m$^2$; F, 600 mg/m$^2$; four cycles) and intermediate (C, 400 mg/m$^2$; A, 40 mg/m$^2$; F, 400 mg/m$^2$; six cycles) doses had clearly better disease-free survival (75% vs. 64%; $p<0.001$) and overall survival (92% vs. 84%; $p=0.004$) than the lowest dose regimen, but the difference between the two highest levels was not significant. Two caveats to this study were (1) the high-dose arm actually contained conventional doses of A and C and (2) patients whose tumors overexpressed HER-2/*neu* protein had an improved survival with higher doses of A. In direct contrast, NSABP B-22 and NSABP B-25, which intensified cyclophosphamide over a fourfold range with a steady dose of doxorubicin did not show any advantages in overall survival or disease-free survival for the intensified arms.[36] Additionally, preliminary results from CALGB 93-44, which compared three dose levels of doxorubicin, found no difference in disease-free survival and overall survival at the 18-month follow-up point.[37] Henderson and colleagues[38] reviewed the question of dose intensity in breast cancer and concluded that small, or even moderate, reductions in drug dose for appropriate reasons would probably not compromise the survival of patients with either early or metastatic disease. This would be true, however, only if an adequately dose-intense regimen has been chosen in the first place.

A newer concept, proposed by Norton,[39] is that of dose density, which is defined as administration of full doses of chemotherapy over short periods (weekly or biweekly) in a sequential manner. Results from metastatic disease[40, 41] have

*Table 35–32.* **Selection of Appropriate Adjuvant Therapy**

| | Tamoxifen × 5 yr | | Chemotherapy | |
|---|---|---|---|---|
| **Estrogen Receptor** | NODE (−) | NODE (+) | NODE (−) | NODE (+) |
| Negative | No | No | Yes | Yes |
| Positive, low risk | Yes | Yes | No | Yes |
| Positive, high risk | Yes | Yes | Yes | Yes |

High-risk tumors contain at least one of the following: >1 cm, estrogen receptor negative, Her-2/*neu* overexpression, poorly differentiated tumor, high S phase.

been encouraging and the approach is now proposed for the adjuvant setting. Currently a regimen of doxorubicin 80 mg/$m^2$ every 2 weeks for three cycles, paclitaxel 200 mg/$m^2$ every 2 weeks for three cycles, and cyclophosphamide 3 g/$m^2$ every 2 weeks for three cycles is being compared with HDC with peripheral stem cell support in patients with four to nine positive axillary nodes. There is currently a great deal of controversy over the use of HDC for patients at high risk of relapse with several randomized trials still ongoing.

Initial enthusiasm for HDC was based on a single-institution study at Duke University,[42] in which 85 patients with breast cancer who had 10 or more involved axillary lymph nodes received four cycles of CAF, which was followed by HDC with cisplatin, cyclophosphamide, and carmustine. At the median follow-up of 5 years, event-free survival was 71%, and overall survival was 78%. This outcome appeared significantly superior to historical age-matched and stage-matched controls receiving conventional chemotherapy. A randomized phase II trial of 97 patients with extensive axillary node metastases compared four courses of an anthracycline regimen with or without HDC and peripheral stem cell support[43] and did not report encouraging results. At a median follow-up of 49 months, the 4-year overall survival and recurrence-free survival for all patients were 75% and 54%, respectively. There were no significant differences between the patients in the standard arm and the HDC arm. Additionally, investigators have shown that meeting criteria for inclusion in HDC trials is an independent indicator of good prognosis in patients with greater than 10 positive lymph nodes.[44] Until larger randomized trials are completed and reported, the routine use of HDC cannot be recommended in the adjuvant setting.

The last issue is how to incorporate newer agents, such as taxanes, into the adjuvant chemotherapy setting. As a result of their success as single agents in patients with metastatic breast cancer,[45, 46] there are currently several ongoing randomized trials of paclitaxel and docetaxel in the adjuvant setting. Only one randomized trial in the adjuvant setting has been reported, but the results are preliminary based on a median follow-up of only 18 months. In that trial, CALGB 93-44, patients were randomized to three dose levels of doxorubicin and cyclophosphamide with or without paclitaxel. The addition of paclitaxel improved disease-free survival from 86 to 90% ($p = 0.0077$) and overall survival from 86 to 97% ($p = 0.0390$). NSABP-28 is a study of 3060 patients with node-positive cancer who were randomized to four cycles of AC with or without paclitaxel. This study closed in 1998, and the results are expected in 2001. Three other large randomized trials were planned to open in 1999,

including AC versus AT (docetaxel) in high-risk patients with one to three positive nodes; NSABPB-30, which randomizes between four cycles of AT, four cycles of ATC, and four cycles of AC followed by four cycles of T; and CALGB 97-44 (currently open), which is randomizing patients to ATC administered sequentially as single agents every 21 days versus AC every 21 days for four cycles followed by paclitaxel every 21 days for four cycles. These trials, along with many others under way, should help delineate the role of taxanes in the adjuvant setting.

## RISKS OF ADJUVANT CHEMOTHERAPY

**Short-Term Toxicity.** The toxic side effects of classic CMF chemotherapy occurring during the period of active treatment are summarized in Table 35–28. The side effects of the doxorubicin-containing regimens are similar except that nearly all patients develop alopecia with the use of doxorubicin. Thromboembolic phenomena are also known to occur at a slightly increased frequency (2% vs. 0.6% in a randomized trial of perioperative FAC chemotherapy vs. no chemotherapy).[47] Taxanes have a different risk profile that includes anaphylaxis, alopecia, and peripheral neuropathy.

**Delayed Toxicity.** The most important delayed complications of these regimens are acute leukemia and cardiac dysfunction. The best data on leukemia are those of the NSABP (Table 35–33). This experience suggests that the risk of leukemia is increased by the use of adjuvant chemotherapy, although this risk appears minimal. The risk of delayed leukemia in patients receiving CMF in Milan has been negligible.[48]

Anthracycline-based chemotherapy is associated with a substantial risk of delayed cardiac toxicity that is not seen with CMF.[49] The experience from Milan suggests that this cardiac risk is increased even further in patients receiving radiation therapy to the left side of the chest (Table 35–34).[50] According to a review of anthracycline-induced cardiotoxicity,[51] the risk of congestive heart failure is 0.14% at total doses less than 400 mg/$m^2$ but increases to 7% at 550 mg/$m^2$ and to 18% at a dose of 700 mg/$m^2$. Proposed risk factors for anthracycline toxicity include higher rates of drug administration, mediastinal radiation, advanced age, female sex, pre-existing heart disease, and hypertension. Excess cardiac toxicity—congestive heart failure—has also been shown in patients treated with anthracyclines and trastuzumab. The rate of cardiac toxicity was 15 to 25% in the phase III clinical trial of trastuzumab in patients who received doxorubicin,[19] and it is currently not encouraged in combina-

*Table 35–33.* **Risk of Acute Leukemia in Patients Treated with Adjuvant Chemotherapy**

| Adjuvant Treatment | No. Patients | Observed Risk | Expected Risk | Relative Risk |
|---|---|---|---|---|
| None | 2068 | 3 | 1.94 | 1.5 |
| Radiation therapy | 1116 | 6 | 0.99 | 6.1* |
| Chemotherapy | 5299 | 27 | 2.45 | 11.0† |

*$p < 0.05$.
†$p < 0.01$.
From Fisher B, Rockette H, Fisher ER, et al. Leukemia in breast cancer patients following adjuvant chemotherapy or postoperative radiation: the NSABP experience. J Clin Oncol 1985;3:1640–58.

*Table 35–34.* **Delayed Cardiac Toxicity from Adjuvant Chemotherapy***

| Group | CHF (%) | ST-T Wave Changes (%) | Other Abnormalities (%) |
|---|---|---|---|
| CMF | 0 | 2.7 | 6.4 |
| No chemotherapy | 0 | 3.7 | 11.1 |
| CMF + doxorubicin | 0.8 | 3.8 | 6.8 |
| Radiation to left breast | 1.6 | 9.7 | 12.4 |

*A total of 825 patients were treated with adjuvant doxorubicin between 12/80 and 7/90 with a median follow-up of 80 months. There were two deaths from CHF at 32 and 86 months.

CHF, congestive heart failure; CMF, cyclophosphamide, methotrexate, fluorouracil.

From Valagussa P, Zambetti M, Biasi S, et al. Cardiac effects of adjuvant chemotherapy in operable breast cancer. Proc ASCO 1993;12:61.

tion. Taxanes may have a similar adverse cardiac profile when used in combination with Herceptin.

Another form of delayed toxicity from chemotherapy is difficult to assess at this point—the potential for increasing drug resistance in patients who experience recurrence. Specifically, there is some evidence that patients given adjuvant chemotherapy whose disease later recurs are likely to die more quickly than are patients who were not given adjuvant therapy. For example, the median survival after recurrence for patients treated with CMF in the initial trial in Milan was 23 months, compared with 33 months for patients whose disease recurred in the observation-alone control group. Similar findings have been reported from Tucson[52] following adjuvant chemotherapy with doxorubicin and cyclophosphamide. One possible explanation for a poor response to chemotherapy after adjuvant therapy with tamoxifen relates to the concurrent acquisition of tamoxifen resistance and the mdr phenotype in many patients (see Chapter 8).

Despite the many risks of adjuvant chemotherapy, the overall quality of life of patients receiving adjuvant therapy, compared with that of patients randomized to observation alone in clinical trials, has been excellent. The Ludwig Institute for Cancer Research in Europe has done an especially good job of considering this concern and has developed a new way of defining quality of life for such patients. Called *TWIST*, it refers to the time without symptoms or toxicity in clinical trials.[53, 54] These investigators have found that despite prolonged treatment, the benefits of adjuvant chemotherapy include an improved duration of quality life, not just a prolongation of life, as a result of receiving toxic therapy.

## ADJUVANT ENDOCRINE MANIPULATION

Two major forms of endocrine therapy have been widely studied as adjuvant therapy. The first is ovarian ablation in premenopausal patients, either by surgical means (oophorectomy) or by the use of pelvic radiation therapy. The second is tamoxifen for premenopausal and postmenopausal patients.

**Ovarian Ablation.** Early studies in premenopausal patients conducted without the benefit of hormone-receptor measurements showed delayed recurrence but no improvement in overall survival with oophorectomy. This conclusion was challenged by two Canadian studies, one involving surgical oophorectomy and the other radiation-induced ovarian ablation supplemented with prednisone.[55, 56] The updated meta-analysis from the EBCTCG shows that ovarian ablation significantly improves long-term survival in the absence of chemotherapy in premenopausal patients (Table 35–35).[57] This report of 12 trials with 15 years of follow-up involving 2102 women younger than 50 reported improved overall survival (52.4% vs. 46.1%; $p = 0.001$) and recurrence-free survival (45% vs. 39%; $p = 0.0007$), and this benefit was seen in node-negative and node-positive patients. No conclusions could be drawn about the role of ablation plus chemotherapy because of small sample sizes. Among 1354 women aged 50 or older at randomization, no benefit in overall survival or recurrence-free survival was seen. There are some concerns about the use of ovarian ablation. First, the use of adjuvant pelvic radiation poses the risk of damaging

*Table 35–35.* **Meta-Analysis of Ovarian Ablation in Early Breast Cancer, Among Women Aged Younger than 50 at Randomization***

| | No. Patients | Typical Reduction (% ± SD) in Annual Odds of | |
|---|---|---|---|
| | | RECURRENCE AS FIRST EVENT | DEATH FROM ANY CAUSE |
| Ovarian ablation alone | 1295 | 25 ± 7 | 24 ± 7 |
| Ovarian ablation + chemotherapy | 933 | 10 ± 9 | 8 ± 10 |
| All patients | 2228 | 18.5 ± 5.5 | 18.4 ± 5.7 |

| | Absolute Reductions in Recurrence-Free Survival and Overall Survival | | | |
|---|---|---|---|---|
| | RFS (%) | | OS (%) | |
| | *Control* | *Ablation* | *Control* | *Ablation* |
| 5-yr follow-up | 56 | 62.8 | 69.0 | 74.2 |
| 10-yr follow-up | 45.3 | 51.7 | 54.4 | 60 |
| 15-yr follow-up | 39 | 45.0 | 46.1 | 52.4 |

*See Table 35–29 for a description of the statistical procedures involved.

RFS, recurrence-free survival; OS, overall survival.

Data from Early Breast Cancer Trialists' Collaborative Group. Overview ablation in early breast cancer: overview of the randomised trials. Lancet 1996;348:1189–96.

the pelvic bone marrow, which may compromise subsequent chemotherapy. Second, the use of surgical oophorectomy in the adjuvant setting places the patient at risk for all of the problems of general anesthesia and pelvic surgery at a time when she is otherwise well and free of symptoms. This problem now is of less concern thanks to the availability of endoscopic oophorectomy in most parts of the United States. Nevertheless, in the United States, surgical ovarian ablation is much less widely used than in Europe because most American physicians prefer the use of tamoxifen for these patients, as discussed subsequently. Alternatively, medical oophorectomy is of increasing interest as achieved with a LHRH or GnRH agonist, such as leuprolide (Lupron) or goserelin.

**Tamoxifen.** Numerous studies in many thousands of patients have firmly established tamoxifen as an effective adjuvant therapy. In 1998, the EBCTCG published an updated overview of randomized trials of adjuvant tamoxifen therapy among women with early breast cancer.[58] The overview included 55 trials involving more than 37,000 women, which combined represents 87% of the worldwide evidence on tamoxifen. Table 35–36 summarizes the effect of adjuvant tamoxifen on recurrence and mortality as a function of age, hormone receptor status, and the presence or absence of axillary node involvement by tumor as reported by the Oxford group.

The overview indicates the importance of hormone-receptor measurement as a determinant of the response to treatment. Although the analysis overwhelmingly confirms the benefits of tamoxifen regardless of menopausal or nodal status, it also shows the use of adjuvant tamoxifen in hormone receptor–negative patients to be without overall benefit. In ER-positive women, the proportional recurrence reduction was 50% (standard deviation ± 4), and the mortality reduction was 28% ± 5). These benefits were also seen in node-negative patients with a proportional recurrence reduction of 49% ± 4) and mortality reduction of 25% ± 5). In contrast to prior studies, a significant proportional recurrence reduction was also seen in women younger than age 40 (54% ± 13]) and women aged 40 to 49 (41% ± 10]).

Duration of therapy with tamoxifen has always been controversial, and the Oxford overview supplies strong indirect evidence in support of 5 years of therapy. This support was manifest in proportional reduction in recurrence (47% [SD, 3]) and mortality (26% [SD, 4]). Direct evidence from randomized clinical trials favors 5 years over 2 years of adjuvant tamoxifen therapy.[59, 60] Randomized trials of 10 years versus 5 years of adjuvant tamoxifen have not shown a relapse or survival advantage for longer duration.[61, 62]

The additional risks and benefits of tamoxifen therapy are well known.[63] These benefits include reductions in serum cholesterol, low-density lipoprotein, and an overall reduction in deaths from cardiovascular causes (deaths before relapse). In postmenopausal women, tamoxifen increases axial skeleton bone density and stabilizes bone density in the appendicular skeleton. The induction of menopausal symptoms and the increased risk of thromboembolic events, including pulmonary embolus, deep venous thrombosis, and cerebrovas-

*Table 35–36.* **Meta-Analysis of 5 Years of Adjuvant Tamoxifen in Early Breast Cancer***

| | No. Patients | Typical Reduction (% ± SD) in Annual Odds of | |
| --- | --- | --- | --- |
| | | RECURRENCE AS FIRST EVENT | DEATH FROM ANY CAUSE |
| Estrogen receptor (ER) status | | | |
| ER poor | 922 | 6 ± 11 | −3 ± 11 |
| ER unknown | 1558 | 37 ± 8 | 21 ± 9 |
| ER positive | 5896 | 50 ± 4 | 28 ± 5 |
| Subtotal | 8349 | 43 ± 3 | 23 ± 4 |
| Lymph node status | | | |
| Node negative | 5217 | 49 ± 4 | 25 ± 5 |
| Node positive | 2210 | 43 ± 5 | 28 ± 6 |
| Subtotal | 7427 | 47 ± 3 | 26 ± 4 |
| All patients regardless of duration of adjuvant tamoxifen therapy | 37,099 | 26.4 ± 1.5 | 14.5 ± 1.7 |

| | Absolute Reductions in Recurrence-Free Survival and Overall Survival | | | |
| --- | --- | --- | --- | --- |
| | RFS (%) | | OS (%) | |
| | *Control* | *Tamoxifen* | *Control* | *Tamoxifen* |
| At 5-yr follow-up | | | | |
| Lymph node negative | 74.9 | 87.4 | 88.3 | 91.8 |
| Lymph node positive | 58.3 | 75.6 | 74.2 | 80.1 |
| At 10-yr follow-up | | | | |
| Lymph node negative | 64.3 | 79.2 | 73.3 | 78.9 |
| Lymph node positive | 44.5 | 59.7 | 50.5 | 61.4 |

*See Table 35–29 for a description of the statistical procedures involved. Absolute risk reductions have excluded patients with ER-poor disease.
RFS, recurrence-free survival; OS, overall survival.
Data from Early Breast Cancer Trialists' Collaborative Group. Tamoxifen for early breast cancer: an overview of the randomised trials. Lancet 1998;351:1451–67.

cular accidents, may offset these benefits. The most well-known risk of tamoxifen is the increased possibility of endometrial cancer. The 1998 tamoxifen overview found a RR of 2.58 for endometrial cancer as compared with population-based rates of endometrial cancer. Nearly all cases reported occurred in postmenopausal women and were of low stage and grade. According to the 1998 EBCTCG overview, the reduction in the incidence of contralateral breast cancer (approximately 50%) is about twice as large as the increase in the incidence of endometrial cancer.

## ADJUVANT CHEMOTHERAPY PLUS TAMOXIFEN

The EBCTCG tamoxifen overview confirms prior studies that showed a decrease in recurrence and improved survival in patients whose tumors are ER positive with tamoxifen plus chemotherapy versus chemotherapy alone. Chemotherapy plus tamoxifen decreased the annual odds of recurrence by 52% and the annual odds of dying by 47% when compared with chemotherapy alone. Individual randomized trials have also confirmed the benefits of tamoxifen plus chemotherapy over chemotherapy alone for patients whose tumors are ER positive. NSABP B-16 showed that AC plus tamoxifen was superior to AC alone with reductions in recurrence rate (32%) and mortality rate (26%).[64] This result was confirmed by two large randomized trials, NSABP B-20 and the International Breast Cancer Study Group, in which chemotherapy plus tamoxifen reduced the RR of recurrence and mortality compared with tamoxifen alone.[65, 66] The benefits were most pronounced in women age 49 or younger but extended to patients 50 or older. There was also a lower incidence of ipsilateral breast tumor recurrence in patients treated with lumpectomy and breast radiation.

These direct and indirect pieces of evidence support the use of chemoendocrine therapy in the adjuvant treatment of breast cancer. All patients with ER-positive tumors, regardless of nodal status, should be offered tamoxifen therapy. The difficulty lies in identifying which ER-positive, node-negative patients would benefit from the addition of chemotherapy to tamoxifen.

## SUMMARY AND PROSPECTS FOR THE FUTURE

The overall results of adjuvant therapy support the hypothesis that breast cancer is a systemic disease from the outset in a substantial number of patients with operable invasive breast cancer. The meta-analysis of randomized clinical trials performed by the EBCTCG establishes an important role for adjuvant therapy in prolonging the lives of these patients. Independent evidence of a survival benefit from adjuvant therapy comes from an epidemiologic study in British Columbia.[67] There is also evidence that adjuvant therapy decreases the risk of local recurrence in patients treated with lumpectomy and radiation therapy.[68] The results are still modest, however, in terms of clinical benefit, and further research is needed to improve on current results. Investigators in Toronto have shown that many oncologists exaggerate the potential benefits of such therapy and that at least some women would choose to forego therapy if given realistic and accurate information.[69] It is hoped that the information in Tables 35–29 and 35–30 will prove useful to oncologists and their patients in dealing realistically with this concern. Specific recommendations for the use of adjuvant therapy outside the setting of clinical trials are given in the next section.

## SUGGESTIONS FOR ADDITIONAL READING

Wolff AC, Davidson NE. Primary systemic therapy in operable breast cancer. J Clin Oncol 2000;18:1558–69.
Peters WP, Dansey RD, Klein JL, Baynes RD. High-dose chemotherapy and peripheral blood progenitor cell transplantation in the treatment of breast cancer. Oncologist 2000;5:1–13.

## REFERENCES

1. Fisher B, Ravdin RG, Ausman RK, et al. Surgical adjuvant chemotherapy in cancer of the breast: results of a decade of cooperative investigation. Ann Surg 1968;168:337–56.
2. Nissen-Meyer R, Kjellgren K, Mansson B. Adjuvant chemotherapy in breast cancer. Recent Results Cancer Res 1982;80:142–8.
3. Fisher B, Carbone P, Economou SG, et al. L-Phenylalanine mustard (L-PAM) in the management of primary breast cancer: a report of early findings. N Engl J Med 1975;292:117–22.
4. Bonadonna G, Brusamolino E, Valagussa P, et al. Combination chemotherapy as an adjuvant treatment in operable breast cancer. N Engl J Med 1976;294:405–10.
5. Group EBCTC. Systemic treatment of early breast cancer by hormonal, cytotoxic, or immune therapy: 133 randomised trials involving 31,000 recurrences and 24,000 deaths among 75,000 women. Early Breast Cancer Trialists' Collaborative Group. Lancet 1992;339:71–85.
6. Group EBCTC. Polychemotherapy for early breast cancer: an overview of the randomised trials. Early Breast Cancer Trialists' Collaborative Group. Lancet 1998;352:930–42.
7. Nemoto T, Vana J, Bedwani RN, et al. Management and survival of female breast cancer: results of a national survey by the American College of Surgeons. Cancer 1980;45:2917–24.
8. Koscielny S, Tubiana M, Le MG, et al. Breast cancer: relationship between the size of the primary tumour and the probability of metastatic dissemination. Br J Cancer 1984;49:709–15.
9. Shetty MR, Reiman HM Jr. Tumor size and axillary metastasis, a correlative occurrence in 1244 cases of breast cancer between 1980 and 1995. Eur J Surg Oncol 1997;23:139–41.
10. Simpson JF, Page DL. The role of pathology in premalignancy and as a guide for treatment and prognosis in breast cancer. Semin Oncol 1996;23:428–35.
11. Neville AM, Bettelheim R, Gelber RD, et al. Factors predicting treatment responsiveness and prognosis in node-negative breast cancer. The International (Ludwig) Breast Cancer Study Group. J Clin Oncol 1992;10:696–705.
12. Ketterhagen JP, Quackenbush SR, Haushalter RA. Tumor histology as a prognostic determinant in carcinoma of the breast. Surg Gynecol Obstet 1984;158:120–3.
13. Fisher B, Redmond C, Brown A, et al. Influence of tumor estrogen and progesterone receptor levels on the response to tamoxifen and chemotherapy in primary breast cancer. J Clin Oncol 1983;1:227–41.
14. 1997 update of recommendations for the use of tumor markers in breast and colorectal cancer. Adopted on November 7, 1997 by the American Society of Clinical Oncology. J Clin Oncol 1998;16:793–5.
15. Press MF, Bernstein L, Thomas PA, et al. HER-2/neu gene amplification characterized by fluorescence in situ hybridization: poor prognosis in node-negative breast carcinomas. J Clin Oncol 1997;15:2894–904.
16. Andrulis IL, Bull SB, Blackstein ME, et al. Neu/erbB-2 amplification identifies a poor-prognosis group of women with node-negative breast cancer. Toronto Breast Cancer Study Group. J Clin Oncol 1998;16:1340–9.
17. Baselga J, Norton L, Albanell J, et al. Recombinant humanized anti-HER2 antibody (Herceptin) enhances the antitumor activity of paclitaxel and doxorubicin against HER2/neu overexpressing human breast cancer xenografts. Cancer Res 1998;58:2825–31.

18. Pegram MD, Lipton A, Hayes DF, et al. Phase II study of receptor-enhanced chemosensitivity using recombinant humanized anti-p185HER2/neu monoclonal antibody plus cisplatin in patients with HER2/neu-overexpressing metastatic breast cancer refractory to chemotherapy treatment. J Clin Oncol 1998;16:2659–71.

19. Slamon DJ, Leyland-Jones B, Shak S, et al. Addition of Herceptin (humanized anti-HER2 antibody) to first-line chemotherapy for HER2 overexpressing metastatic breast cancer (HER2+/MBC) markedly increases anticancer activity: a randomized, multinational controlled phase III trial. Proc ASCO 1998;17:377a.

20. Clark GM, Mathieu MC, Owens MA, et al. Prognostic significance of S-phase fraction in good-risk, node-negative breast cancer patients. J Clin Oncol 1992;10:428–32.

21. Bevilacqua P, Barbareschi M, Verderio P, et al. Prognostic value of intratumoral microvessel density, a measure of tumor angiogenesis, in node-negative breast carcinoma—results of a multiparametric study. Breast Cancer Res Treat 1995;36:205–17.

22. Haybittle JL, Blamey RW, Elston CW, et al. A prognostic index in primary breast cancer. Br J Cancer 1982;45:361–6.

23. Clark GM, Hilsenbeck SG, Ravdin PM, et al. Prognostic factors: rationale and methods of analysis and integration. Breast Cancer Res Treat 1994;32:105–12.

24. Coombes RC, Bliss JM, Wils J, et al. Adjuvant cyclophosphamide, methotrexate, and fluorouracil versus fluorouracil, epirubicin, and cyclophosphamide chemotherapy in premenopausal women with axillary node-positive operable breast cancer: results of a randomized trial. The International Collaborative Cancer Group. J Clin Oncol 1996;14:35–45.

25. Tormey DC, Gray R, Abeloff MD, et al. Adjuvant therapy with a doxorubicin regimen and long-term tamoxifen in premenopausal breast cancer patients: an Eastern Cooperative Oncology Group trial. J Clin Oncol 1992;10:1848–56.

26. Levine MN, Bramwell VH, Pritchard KI, et al. Randomized trial of intensive cyclophosphamide, epirubicin, and fluorouracil chemotherapy compared with cyclophosphamide, methotrexate, and fluorouracil in premenopausal women with node-positive breast cancer. National Cancer Institute of Canada Clinical Trials Group. J Clin Oncol 1998;16:2651–8.

27. Hutchins L, Green S, Ravdin P, et al. CMF versus CAF with and without tamoxifen in high-risk node-negative breast cancer patients and a natural history follow-up study in low-risk node-negative patients: first results of intergroup trial INT 0102. Proc ASCO 1998;17:1a.

28. Fisher B, Redmond C, Wickerham DL, et al. Doxorubicin-containing regimens for the treatment of stage II breast cancer: the National Surgical Adjuvant Breast and Bowel Project experience. J Clin Oncol 1989;7:572–82.

29. Mauriac L, Durand M, Chauvergne J, et al. Randomized trial of adjuvant chemotherapy for operable breast cancer comparing i.v. CMF to an epirubicin-containing regimen. Ann Oncol 1992;3:439–43.

30. Fisher B, Brown AM, Dimitrov NV, et al. Two months of doxorubicin-cyclophosphamide with and without interval reinduction therapy compared with 6 months of cyclophosphamide, methotrexate, and fluorouracil in positive-node breast cancer patients with tamoxifen-nonresponsive tumors: results from the National Surgical Adjuvant Breast and Bowel Project B-15. J Clin Oncol 1990;8:1483–96.

31. Moliterni A, Bonadonna G, Valagussa P, et al. Cyclophosphamide, methotrexate, and fluorouracil with and without doxorubicin in the adjuvant treatment of resectable breast cancer with one to three positive axillary nodes. J Clin Oncol 1991;9:1124–30.

32. Bonadonna G, Valagussa P, Rossi A, et al. Ten-year experience with CMF-based adjuvant chemotherapy in resectable breast cancer. Breast Cancer Res Treat 1985;5:95–115.

33. Group TLBCS. Combination adjuvant chemotherapy for node-positive breast cancer: inadequacy of a single perioperative cycle. The Ludwig Breast Cancer Study Group. N Engl J Med 1988;319:677–83.

34. Hryniuk WM. More is better. J Clin Oncol 1988;6:1365–7.

35. Wood WC, Budman DR, Korzun AH, et al. Dose and dose intensity of adjuvant chemotherapy for stage II, node-positive breast carcinoma. N Engl J Med 1994;330:1253–9 and 331:139.

36. Fisher B, Anderson S, Wickerham DL, et al. Increased intensification and total dose of cyclophosphamide in a doxorubicin-cyclophosphamide regimen for the treatment of primary breast cancer: findings from National Surgical Adjuvant Breast and Bowel Project B-22. J Clin Oncol 1997;15:1858–69.

37. Henderson IC, Berry D, Demetri G, et al. Improved disease-free (DFS) and overall survival (OS) from the addition of sequential paclitaxel (T) but not from the escalation of doxorubicin (A) dose level in the adjuvant chemotherapy of patients (PTS) with node-positive primary breast cancer (BC). Proc ASCO 1998;17:390a.

38. Henderson IC, Hayes DF, Gelman R. Dose-response in the treatment of breast cancer: a critical review. J Clin Oncol 1988;6:1501–15.

39. Norton L. Kinetic concepts in the treatment of breast cancer. Recent Results Cancer Res 1993;127:1–6.

40. Hudis CA, Seidman AD, Baselga J, et al. Sequential adjuvant therapy with doxorubicin/paclitaxel/cyclophosphamide for resectable breast cancer involving four or more axillary nodes. Semin Oncol 1995;22:18–23.

41. Hudis C. New approaches to adjuvant chemotherapy for breast cancer. Pharmacotherapy 1996;16:88S–93S.

42. Peters WP, Ross M, Vredenburgh JJ, et al. High-dose chemotherapy and autologous bone marrow support as consolidation after standard-dose adjuvant therapy for high-risk primary breast cancer. J Clin Oncol 1993;11:1132–43.

43. Rodenhuis S, Richel DJ, van der Wall E, et al. Randomised trial of high-dose chemotherapy and haemopoietic progenitor-cell support in operable breast cancer with extensive axillary lymph-node involvement. Lancet 1998;352:515–21.

44. Garcia-Carbonero R, Hidalgo M, Paz-Ares L, et al. Patient selection in high-dose chemotherapy trials: relevance in high-risk breast cancer. J Clin Oncol 1997;15:3178–84.

45. Holmes FA, Walters RS, Theriault RL, et al. Phase II trial of taxol, an active drug in the treatment of metastatic breast cancer. J Natl Cancer Inst 1991;83:1797–805.

46. Valero V, Holmes FA, Walters RS, et al. Phase II trial of docetaxel: a new, highly effective antineoplastic agent in the management of patients with anthracycline-resistant metastatic breast cancer. J Clin Oncol 1995;13:2886–94.

47. Clahsen PC, van de Velde CJ, Julien JP, et al. Thromboembolic complications after perioperative chemotherapy in women with early breast cancer: a European Organization for Research and Treatment of Cancer Breast Cancer Cooperative Group study. J Clin Oncol 1994;12:1266–71.

48. Valagussa P, Moliterni A, Zambetti M, Bonadonna G. Long-term sequelae from adjuvant chemotherapy. Recent Results Cancer Res 1993;127:247–55.

49. Ryberg M, Nielsen D, Skovsgaard T, et al. Epirubicin cardiotoxicity: an analysis of 469 patients with metastatic breast cancer. J Clin Oncol 1998;16:3502–8.

50. Valagussa P, Zambetti M, Biasi S, et al. Cardiac effects following adjuvant chemotherapy and breast irradiation in operable breast cancer. Ann Oncol 1994;5:209–16.

51. Shan K, Lincoff AM, Young JB. Anthracycline-induced cardiotoxicity. Ann Intern Med 1996;125:47–58.

52. Ahmann FR, Jones SE, Moon TE. The effect of prior adjuvant chemotherapy on survival in metastatic breast cancer. J Surg Oncol 1988;37:116–22.

53. Gelber RD, Goldhirsch A. A new endpoint for the assessment of adjuvant therapy in postmenopausal women with operable breast cancer. J Clin Oncol 1986;4:1772–9.

54. Gelber RD, Cole BF, Goldhirsch A, et al. Adjuvant chemotherapy plus tamoxifen compared with tamoxifen alone for postmenopausal breast cancer: meta-analysis of quality-adjusted survival. Lancet 1996;347:1066–71.

55. Bryant AJ, Weir JA. Prophylactic oophorectomy in operable instances of carcinoma of the breast. Surg Gynecol Obstet 1981;153:660–4.

56. Meakin JW, Allt WE, Beale FA, et al. Ovarian irradiation and prednisone following surgery and radiotherapy for carcinoma of the breast. Breast Cancer Res Treat 1983;3:Suppl:S45–8.

57. Group EBCTC. Ovarian ablation in early breast cancer: overview of the randomised trials. Early Breast Cancer Trialists' Collaborative Group. Lancet 1996;348:1189–96.

58. Group EBCTC. Tamoxifen for early breast cancer: an overview of the randomised trials. Early Breast Cancer Trialists' Collaborative Group. Lancet 1998;351:1451–67.

59. Group SBCC. Randomized trial of two versus five years of adjuvant tamoxifen for postmenopausal early stage breast cancer. Swedish Breast Cancer Cooperative Group. J Natl Cancer Inst 1996;88:1543–9.

60. Preliminary results from the cancer research campaign trial evaluating tamoxifen duration in women aged fifty years or older with breast cancer. Current Trials Working Party of the Cancer Research Campaign Breast Cancer Trials Group. J Natl Cancer Inst 1996;88:1834–9 and 1997;89:590.

61. Fisher B, Dignam J, Bryant J, et al. Five versus more than five years of tamoxifen therapy for breast cancer patients with negative lymph nodes and estrogen receptor–positive tumors. J Natl Cancer Inst 1996;88:1529–42.
62. Office SCT. Adjuvant tamoxifen in the management of operable breast cancer: the Scottish Trial. Report from the Breast Cancer Trials Committee, Scottish Cancer Trials Office (MRC), Edinburgh. Lancet 1987;2:171–5.
63. Osborne CK. Tamoxifen in the treatment of breast cancer. N Engl J Med 1998;339:1609–18.
64. Fisher B, Redmond C, Legault-Poisson S, et al. Postoperative chemotherapy and tamoxifen compared with tamoxifen alone in the treatment of positive-node breast cancer patients aged 50 years and older with tumors responsive to tamoxifen: results from the National Surgical Adjuvant Breast and Bowel Project B-16. J Clin Oncol 1990;8:1005–18.
65. Fisher B, Dignam J, Wolmark N, et al. Tamoxifen and chemotherapy for lymph node-negative, estrogen receptor–positive breast cancer. J Natl Cancer Inst 1997;89:1673–82.
66. Group EBCTC. Effectiveness of adjuvant chemotherapy in combination with tamoxifen for node-positive postmenopausal breast cancer patients. International Breast Cancer Study Group. J Clin Oncol 1997;15:1385–94.
67. Olivotto IA, Bajdik CD, Plenderleith IH, et al. Adjuvant systemic therapy and survival after breast cancer [see comments]. N Engl J Med 1994;330:805–10.
68. Haffty BG, Wilmarth L, Wilson L, et al. Adjuvant systemic chemotherapy and hormonal therapy: effect on local recurrence in the conservatively treated breast cancer patient. Cancer 1994;73:2543–8.
69. Rajagopal S, Goodman PJ, Tannock IF. Adjuvant chemotherapy for breast cancer: discordance between physicians' perception of benefit and the results of clinical trials. J Clin Oncol 1994;12:1296–304.

......................................

# TREATMENT BY STAGE OF DISEASE AND SPECIAL PROBLEMS

• Steven J. Tucker • Linnea I. Chap • Charles M. Haskell

## BACKGROUND

The treatment of breast cancer is in a constant state of flux, and clinical recommendations must be made in the context of the results of current therapeutic research. Eligible patients should be encouraged to participate in clinical trials, which will answer important therapeutic questions while they receive state-of-the-art treatment. Some experienced physicians, including ourselves, may disagree about the management of individual patients. Each patient is unique, with a distinct socioeconomic and psychological background, spectrum of associated organ dysfunctions, and stage of disease. The tumor is also distinctive, in terms of the rate of tumor growth and the areas of dominant disease. The experienced physician individualizes therapy when it is appropriate; nevertheless, it is useful to have a generalized approach to treatment as a point of reference. This section briefly sketches such an approach. It draws heavily on practice guidelines developed for the UCLA Breast Center. Figures 35–19 to 35–21 and Tables 35–32 and 35–37 provide summaries of the UCLA Breast Center guidelines for local control, adjuvant therapy, and combined-modality therapy for patients with stage IIIA and IIIB disease.

## CARCINOMA IN SITU

Carcinoma in situ is considered in detail in the section In Situ Breast Cancer. The two major forms of carcinoma in situ are managed differently.

**Ductal Carcinoma In Situ.** The key to managing DCIS is careful clinical, mammographic, and histologic evaluation. At the UCLA Breast Center, we treat small (<2.5 cm) DCIS lesions with clean margins by wide excision. Most of these patients are offered postoperative radiation, although exception is made for disease of low-grade histology and low volume (e.g., <1 to 2 cm). Larger lesions (2.5 to 5 cm) and those that have close or dirty margins are treated with wide excision and radiation therapy or total mastectomy if BCT is not technically feasible. Lesions larger than 5.0 cm are treated by total mastectomy without axillary dissection.

**Lobular Carcinoma In Situ.** The treatment of LCIS is highly dependent on patient preference. Among the options are close follow-up with physical examination every 6 months and yearly mammograms, bilateral total mastectomies, or participation in a chemoprevention trial (such as the tamoxifen trial, discussed subsequently). At present, our preference is for close follow-up for most patients rather than mastectomy.

## STAGES I AND II

A generalized approach to local control, developed by physicians in the UCLA Breast Center, is summarized in Figure 35–13.

**Local Control with Surgery.** Primary operable breast cancer may be treated surgically by total mastectomy or a less radical procedure (wide local excision or segmental mastectomy with total gross removal) followed by radiation therapy. If a total mastectomy is used, we usually recommend immediate reconstruction as well. An axillary lymph node dissection (at least levels 1 and 2) is performed whether the patient is treated with a total mastectomy or a partial mastectomy,[1] although the necessity of this procedure is questioned by some authorities.[2]

The patient is encouraged to take an active part in deciding between these alternatives. In some cases, there are medical indications for preferring one surgical procedure over another. For example, we recommend a MRM for patients with tumors that are multiple or too large for a good cosmetic result by segmental mastectomy. This includes patients with small breasts. The extent of subsequent surgery is also influenced by the status of surgical margins achieved after excision or segmental mastectomy.[3] Patients with clean margins do not require additional surgery but do receive radiation therapy. Patients with close margins receive a balanced discussion of the options. Patients with infiltrating ductal carcinoma are usually treated with radiation therapy and no further surgical resection, whereas those with extensive intraductal carcinoma or infiltrating lobular carcinoma

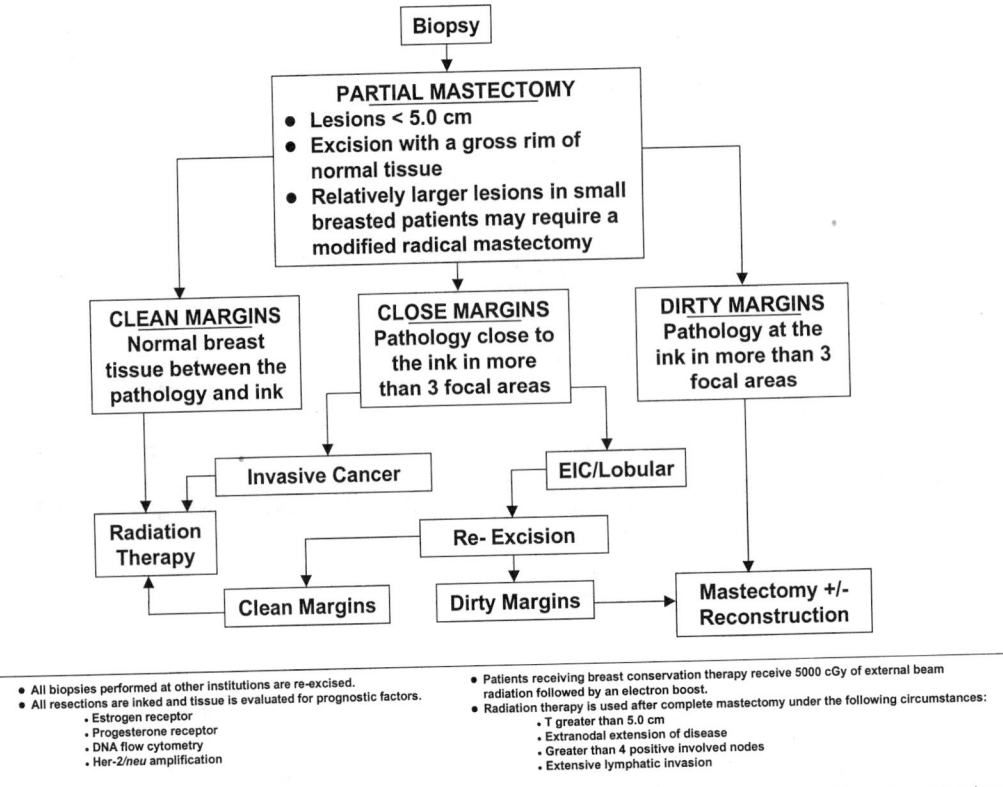

• All biopsies performed at other institutions are re-excised.
• All resections are inked and tissue is evaluated for prognostic factors.
  • Estrogen receptor
  • Progesterone receptor
  • DNA flow cytometry
  • Her-2/neu amplification

• Patients receiving breast conservation therapy receive 5000 cGy of external beam radiation followed by an electron boost.
• Radiation therapy is used after complete mastectomy under the following circumstances:
  • T greater than 5.0 cm
  • Extranodal extension of disease
  • Greater than 4 positive involved nodes
  • Extensive lymphatic invasion

**Figure 35–19.** Local control of primary breast cancer as practiced at the UCLA/Revlon Breast Center. All biopsies performed at other institutions are re-excised. All resections are inked, and tissue is sent for estrogen and progesterone receptor measurements, DNA flow cytometry, and assessment of HER-2/*neu* amplification. All women with invasive cancer have a level 1 and level 2 axillary dissection. Patients treated with breast conservation receive 50 Gy of external-beam radiation therapy followed by an electron boost. Radiation therapy is also used after total mastectomy for the following groups of patients: T greater than 5 cm; extranodal extension of disease; more than four positive nodes or extensive lymphatic invasion. A modified radical mastectomy is performed for lesions less than 5 cm. EIC, extranodal intraductal component.

are considered for re-excision or mastectomy, depending on the extent of disease. Patients with continued involvement of the surgical margins at re-excision are usually treated with a total mastectomy, although an additional re-excision may be offered if cosmetically feasible.

**Local Control with Radiation Therapy.** Patients treated with BCT are treated with 50 Gy of external-beam radiation followed by an electron boost to the tumor bed. After a total mastectomy with lymph node dissection, radiation therapy is also recommended for women with T3 lesions, extranodal extension of tumor, extensive lymphatic invasion within the tumor, or four or more positive lymph nodes.

**Control of Possible Systemic Micrometastases.** After the pathologic stage of the disease has been determined by a lymph node dissection, patients are informed of their RRs of local and distant recurrence and the possible role of adjuvant therapy in modifying those risks. Patients are encouraged to participate in one of the available clinical trials of adjuvant treatment. Those who refuse enrollment in a clinical trial but are willing to undergo systemic therapy based on our assessment of the available literature are treated under the guidelines summarized in Table 35–37 and Figure 35–20. These guidelines are based on tumor size and the actual number of involved lymph nodes, rather than the usual pTNM system. This information may be indicated by the use of *T = and N = categories,* which refer to the

greatest diameter of the tumor (e.g., T = 3 cm shows a 3-cm tumor) and the number of axillary lymph nodes (e.g., N = 4/10 indicates four positive lymph nodes of 10 nodes sampled).

*Node-Negative Women with a Low Risk of Micrometastases.* Patients with DCIS of any size, node-negative patients with invasive tumors of special types (tubular, papillary, mucinous, colloid, and typical medullary types) and a T less than 2 cm, and patients with the more usual forms of invasive breast cancer with favorable prognostic factors and a T less than 0.5 cm are not candidates for adjuvant therapy. These patients have little risk of developing metastatic disease. Tamoxifen may be considered as adjuvant therapy, particularly if the ER is positive or the patient is concerned with decreasing the risk of contralateral breast disease.

Patients with invasive tumors between T greater than 0.5 cm and T less than 1 cm and of the usual histologic types currently represent a treatment controversy. Patients in this group whose tumors are hormone receptor positive would be candidates for adjuvant therapy with tamoxifen. Conversely, hormone receptor negativity in these patients represents an independent adverse prognostic factor, and these patients may have some, albeit small, benefit from adjuvant chemotherapy. Even though the risk of metastatic disease is low in these patients, an exhaustive, balanced discussion of the potential risks and benefits of adjuvant therapy is required

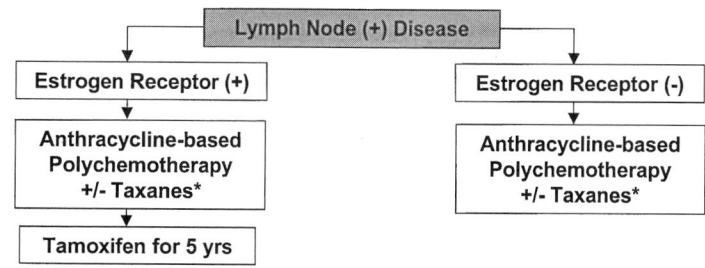

*Sequential Taxane use generally recommended for >3(+) lymph nodes and/or estrogen receptor(-)

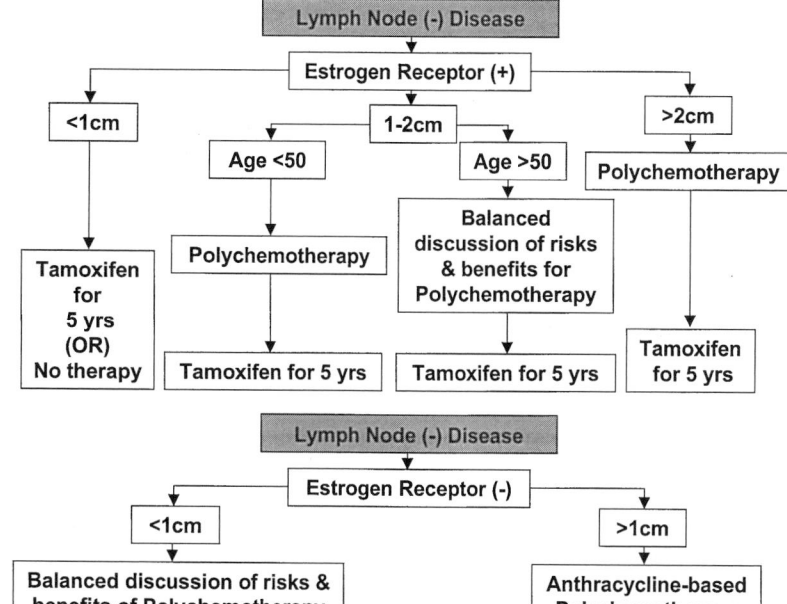

**Figure 35–20.** UCLA/Revlon Breast Center approach to the use of adjuvant therapy in patients with operable breast cancer. The A → CMF regimen refers to the every-3-week doxorubicin × 4 followed by IV CMF × 8 regimen.

When appropriate, all patients should be enrolled in clinical trials evaluating adjuvant therapy.
Anthracycline-based polychemotherapy is favored if tumors are: 1) Her-2/*neu* overexpressing 2) ≥ 2 cm  3) 1-2 cm with ≥1 poor prognostic feature.

in such cases. Additionally, tamoxifen is recommended to hormone receptor–positive patients in light of the additional beneficial effects in decreasing the incidence of contralateral breast cancer.

Patients with invasive tumors of the usual histologic types (T >1 to <2 cm) and favorable prognostic features (specifically, positive for hormone receptors) and patients with special types as listed (T >2 to <3 cm) have a slightly higher risk of metastatic disease (about 15%). This risk can be reduced, usually by one third, with the use of adjuvant therapy, which should be discussed with all patients. Patients whose tumors express hormone receptors should be encouraged to undergo 5 years of tamoxifen for primary adjuvant endocrine therapy as well as prevention of contralateral primary breast cancer.

***Node-Negative Women with a High Risk of Micrometastases.*** This group includes all node-negative women with the usual invasive tumors measuring between 2 and 5 cm as well as those with smaller tumors (T1c or T >1 to <2 cm) and unfavorable tumor characteristics. These women have a lifetime risk of metastases of 30 to 50% and are likely to benefit from systemic therapy. We recommend adjuvant chemotherapy for these high-risk, node-negative patients. Most of the contemporary clinical trials for patients in this

group use one of several doxorubicin-containing regimens (AC or CAF), described further in more detail in previous sections of this chapter. Alternatively, in the nontrial setting, classic CMF is a reasonable choice. Patients whose tumors overexpress the HER-2/*neu* oncogene are more likely to benefit from an anthracycline-containing regimen than CMF. Advanced patient age has been used as a relative contraindication for adjuvant chemotherapy. Rather than chronologic age, we suggest the use of functional status as the major determinant for initiation of adjuvant chemotherapy in older patients. Postmenopausal patients with pT2 N0 M0 (T >2 to 5 cm) carcinomas with otherwise favorable prognostic factors (including the presence of hormone receptors) may be managed with combined chemohormonal therapy or adjuvant tamoxifen alone. The duration of tamoxifen therapy should extend for 5 years.[4] It is unclear whether the tamoxifen should be given concurrently with chemotherapy or following chemotherapy if adjuvant chemotherapy is employed.

For node-negative breast cancer with a high risk of micrometastases, initiation of adjuvant therapy is recommended for all highly functional patients regardless of age. Patients whose tumors are clearly less than 0.5 cm should not undergo adjuvant chemotherapy, whereas patients whose tu-

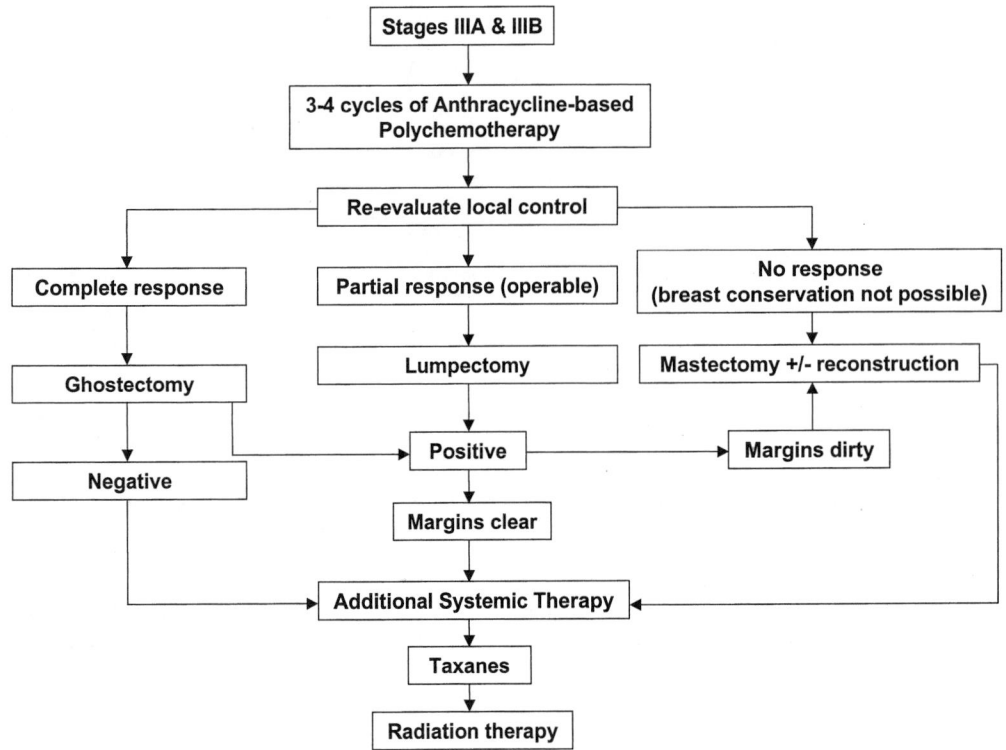

**Figure 35–21.** Approach to patients with locally advanced disease used at the UCLA/Revlon Breast Center.

mors are between 0.5 and 1 cm need careful risk assessment. Generally, endocrine therapy with tamoxifen should be employed in all patients whose tumors express hormone receptors for potential adjuvant benefits as well as the benefits of contralateral breast cancer prevention.

***Node-Positive Patients.*** Adjuvant chemotherapy is clearly indicated for node-positive patients. The intensity of the adjuvant regimen is a function of risk, usually determined by the size of the primary tumor and number of involved axillary lymph nodes. In the UCLA Breast Center, patients

*Table 35–37.* **Summary of the Role of Adjuvant Therapy in Patients with Invasive Breast Cancer***

| Patient Characteristics (T = tumor size in cm) (N = number of nodes involved) | Lifetime Risk of Metastasis (approx. %) | Survival Benefit of Adjuvant Therapy (approx. %)* | Recommended Adjuvant Therapy |
|---|---|---|---|
| Special histology (T <2 cm, N=0) Tubular Papillary Mucinous Colloid Typical medullary | <5 | 0 | None |
| Routine histology (T ≤0.5 cm, N=0) Favorable prognostic factors | <10 | <2 | None |
| Routine histology (T >0.5 cm ≤1.0 cm, N=0) Favorable prognostic factors | <10 | <2 | None |
| Routine histology (T >0.5 cm ≤1.0 cm, N=0) Unfavorable prognostic factors | <10 | Unknown | Tamoxifen for ER(+) patients Balanced discussion of polychemotherapy for ER(−) patients |
| Special histology (T <2 cm ≤3, N=0) | 15 | 3 | Tamoxifen for ER(+) patients |
| Routine histology (T >1 cm ≤2 cm, N=0) | 30 | 9 | Polychemotherapy + tamoxifen or tamoxifen alone |
| Routine histology (T >2 cm ≤5 cm, N=0) | 40–50 | 12–15 | Polychemotherapy + tamoxifen |
| Routine histology (T ≤5 cm, N=1–3) | 40–50 | 12–15 | Polychemotherapy + tamoxifen |
| Routine histology (T ≤5 cm, N=4–10) | 60–70 | 18–21 | Polychemotherapy + tamoxifen |
| Routine histology (T ≤5 cm, N > 10) | 70–90 | 21–27 | Polychemotherapy + tamoxifen |
| Inflammatory breast cancer | >90 | 27 | Polychemotherapy + tamoxifen |

*These approximations are based on the estimation of the overall odds of dying according to the Oxford Overview of Polychemotherapy. The overall odds of dying are improved by approximately 20% for tamoxifen and 30% for polychemotherapy. It is assumed that adjuvant therapy reduces the odds of death and the development of metastatic disease in an equivalent fashion.

with positive axillary nodes are treated with adjuvant combination chemotherapy. Classic CMF or a doxorubicin-based regimen is employed to treat patients with one to three positive nodes. Data now indicate, however, that there may be limited clinical benefit with CMF therapy for tumors that overexpress the HER-2/*neu* oncogene. The benefits of adjuvant therapy in these patients are maintained when doxorubicin-based treatment is employed. An anthracycline regimen is preferred in these patients as well as in patients with other adverse prognostic factors (e.g., poorly differentiated histology, lymphovascular invasion, or hormone receptor negativity). Patients are generally treated with four cycles of AC or six cycles of CAF. For patients with 4 to 9 nodes involved, options include six cycles of CAF or sequential therapy with four cycles of AC followed by four cycles of a taxane or the Milan A→CMF regimen (doxorubicin followed by intravenous CMF), as described by Buzzoni and colleagues.[5] There is also a national randomized trial studying high-dose chemotherapy with autologous stem cell support for patients with 4 to 9 lymph nodes involved. Patients with more than 10 positive nodes are counseled regarding HDCT with autologous stem cell support versus other aggressive therapies, such as sequential dose-intense therapy with growth factor support. Currently, high-dose regimens should be administered only in the setting of a clinical study.

All node-positive patients with positive hormone receptors should receive 5 years of tamoxifen therapy as well. The benefits on recurrence and contralateral prevention are summarized in the previous section of this chapter.

**Timing of Adjuvant Therapy and Radiation Therapy.** Patients who are to receive adjuvant tamoxifen are usually started on therapy within a few days or weeks of their definitive therapy. The timing of radiation therapy and chemotherapy is controversial. Cogent arguments can be posed for using either modality first, and some investigators prefer to use them together or to sandwich radiation therapy between courses of chemotherapy. Delaying chemotherapy has been reported to diminish its effectiveness in eradicating micrometastatic disease, whereas delaying radiation therapy has been reported to increase the local failure rate and to decrease relapse-free survival.[6, 7] Other investigators have found no increase in local-regional failure or survival by delaying radiation therapy until the completion of adjuvant chemotherapy.[8] In practical terms, we generally employ concomitant radiation therapy for patients receiving CMF chemotherapy and employ sequential radiation therapy for patients who are receiving doxorubicin-based chemotherapy.

## STAGES IIIA AND IIIB

Stage IIIA disease is technically operable but carries a high risk of early relapse. Stage IIIB disease is considered technically inoperable, but preoperative chemotherapy can reduce the size of the tumor in some patients so that surgical resection is possible. Combined-modality therapy is needed for both of these groups of patients, although the optimal program is uncertain.[9–12] The approach used at the UCLA Breast Center is summarized in Figure 35–15. For some patients with tumors only slightly greater than 5 cm, immediate surgical resection may be reasonable. We generally treat patients who have locally advanced breast cancer with four

cycles of doxorubicin-based chemotherapy (usually CAF or AC), regardless of the distinction between IIIA and IIIB. This therapy is followed by surgical resection if possible (either a segmental resection or total mastectomy, depending on lesion size, plus a lymph node dissection) and postoperative radiation therapy. Postoperatively, patients are treated with two or three additional cycles of anthracycline-based therapy or four cycles of a taxane.

Patients with positive hormone receptors are treated with tamoxifen at the conclusion of chemotherapy. In our view, surgical resection of the tumor is important for these patients, even if the tumor responds completely to chemotherapy. This resection is sometimes referred to as *ghostectomy,* but these lesions may contain viable tumor, and local control is improved by this surgical procedure.

## INFLAMMATORY CARCINOMA OF THE BREAST

The initial management of localized inflammatory breast cancer is combination chemotherapy.[13–16] Anthracycline-based regimens are commonly used, and some now employ anthracyclines plus taxanes as first-line treatment in inflammatory breast carcinoma.[17] This treatment is followed by radiation therapy and additional courses of chemotherapy. In patients showing a response to chemotherapy and radiation therapy, surgical resection should be performed if possible.[9, 18–20] Tamoxifen is used for at least 5 years after completion of local-regional therapy and adjuvant chemotherapy in patients who are hormone receptor positive.

## STAGE IV

**Metastatic Disease.** Patients with metastatic breast cancer to distant sites and those who experience distant relapse after adjuvant treatment are treated with palliative intent by endocrine manipulation or chemotherapy. In brief, patients with positive hormone receptors and nonvisceral disease are treated initially with endocrine manipulation. For premenopausal patients, this treatment starts with tamoxifen or occasionally medical oophorectomy with a LHRH-GnRH agonist. Surgical oophorectomy is rarely performed in the United States for this condition. For postmenopausal patients, initial endocrine therapy is with tamoxifen. Traditionally, megestrol acetate has been a good second-line choice of endocrine therapy for premenopausal and postmenopausal patients. The newer selective aromatase inhibitors (letrozole and anastrozole) have a generally more favorable side-effect profile, however, and are usually the preferred second-line agents today. For patients who are candidates for chemotherapy because of failure on hormonal management or the presence of life-threatening visceral disease (especially liver and lymphangitic pulmonary metastases), chemotherapy can be initiated with classic CMF, a doxorubicin-containing regimen, a single-agent taxane, or oral chemotherapy with 5-FU–related drugs. This topic is discussed further in the section Systemic Treatment for Metastatic Breast Cancer.

## RECURRENT LOCAL-REGIONAL BREAST CANCER

**Recurrence After Conservation Therapy.** Patients treated with conservation therapy (segmental mastectomy plus radiation therapy) who experience recurrence are usually treated with a total mastectomy.[21] Patients with noninvasive or only focally invasive recurrent disease have a good prognosis. In one series, 0 of 24 patients with this problem had a subsequent relapse.[22] In the same series, patients with invasive recurrent disease had a substantial (52%) relapse rate, which argues for aggressive combined-modality therapy for these patients.

**Stage IV, No Evidence of Disease.** Patients who experience recurrence in the skin of the chest wall as the only site and who undergo resection of all apparent disease have stage IV disease by definition, but they have *no evidence of disease* (NED). The management of these patients is controversial. On one extreme, highly aggressive systemic chemotherapy may be coupled with local radiation therapy, and, on the other extreme, the patient may be placed on hormonal therapy and followed closely for recurrence without further local therapy. A randomized study comparing these two strategies has never been performed to our knowledge. In general, we tend to treat these patients with radiation therapy and to individualize the use of systemic therapy. In younger patients, we tend to use multiagent chemotherapy followed by tamoxifen if the tumor contains hormone receptors. For older patients, we tend to use tamoxifen alone.

## FOLLOW-UP STUDIES

Because patients with breast cancer are at risk for both new primary breast cancer and recurrence, a program of regular follow-up should be started at the completion of primary treatment. Guidelines for such follow-up vary among institutions; the approach used in the UCLA Breast Center is as follows. Patients who are treated with BCT have a mammogram before starting radiation therapy. The mammogram is repeated within 6 to 8 weeks of completing radiation therapy, every 6 months for 2 years, then yearly. Mammograms of the contralateral breast are obtained yearly in patients treated with a MRM. Patients are examined by their physician every 6 months for 5 years and yearly after that. Blood chemistry values, tumor marker measurements, chest radiographs,[23] bone and liver scans, or CT scans are not requested on a routine basis. This strategy is based on the fact that making an earlier diagnosis of distant metastatic disease does not improve survival or the patient's quality of life. It is important to distinguish early diagnosis of metastasis from early diagnosis of local-regional breast cancer. Our approach is strongly oriented toward the latter concern. Because patients expect extensive testing after treatment for breast cancer, this emphasis on the history and physical examination must be explained to the patient to avoid the appearance of inadequate concern for *early diagnosis.*[24]

Routine screening studies for other primary malignancies should be performed according to the patient's age and the physician's assessment of overall risk (see Chapter 5). Lurie and colleagues[25] have found that women are more likely to undergo screening with Papanicolaou's smears and mammograms if they see female rather than male physicians. The oncologist and general physician should be careful not to allow such sex-oriented bias to influence the quality of care provided these patients.

## PSYCHOLOGICAL FACTORS AND REHABILITATION

The ACS, through its Reach to Recovery program,[26] has pioneered in efforts to help women who have had mastectomies adjust to their altered body images. The ACS program may be helpful to women receiving a variety of forms of primary treatment, including lesser degrees of surgery with radiation therapy. Patients with newly diagnosed breast cancer should be informed of this excellent resource.

There is a growing appreciation of the short-term rehabilitation needs of patients with newly diagnosed breast cancer. These are discussed in Chapter 23 and in an article by Schag and colleagues.[27] The most common problems in this group of patients are physical and psychological. Specifically, patients undergoing total mastectomy and axillary dissection are especially troubled by problems of body image and finding appropriate clothing, whereas patients with segmental resection and radiation therapy have more difficulty with disruption of recreation and social activities.

The psychological impact of mastectomy versus segmental resection has been studied by several investigators. Most studies have shown no significant difference in psychological adjustment between the two forms of therapy.[28] We are aware of only one psychological assessment of patients in a randomized clinical trial of these two forms of treatment, however. In this study by Kemeny and colleagues,[29] the psychosexual adaptation and fears of cancer recurrence were significantly better in the patients randomized to receive segmental resection. The authors concluded that segmental resection was a better option for women with breast cancer and that its use was associated with a better quality of life.

A sensible and attentive approach is critical in trying to assess the patient's emotional resources in dealing with the problem of breast surgery. Most patients do adjust; however, the speed of this adjustment may be influenced by attentive and sensitive physicians.[30]

## AGEISM IN BREAST CANCER TREATMENT

One should never ignore the physiologic age of the patient in choosing therapy. Some physicians, however, appear to neglect older patients with breast cancer solely because of their chronologic age. This neglect may take the form of avoiding adjuvant therapy or ignoring the potential value of BCT in the older patient. Such neglect may be referred to as *ageism.* As the population ages and as treatment regimens become more aggressive and toxic, it is vital to consider physiologic age and functional status rather than chronologic age in treatment planning. It is also important to address issues of cost versus benefit[31] and quality of life.[32] It is hoped that future trials will provide better guidance on these matters and yield practical guidelines for management.[33]

## PROPHYLACTIC MASTECTOMY WITH RECONSTRUCTION

Some women with a high risk of developing breast cancer find the uncertainty overwhelming. For such patients, a prophylactic procedure has considerable appeal. There are several theoretical and practical reasons to avoid *prophylactic mastectomy.* On a theoretical level, it is probably necessary to eliminate totally all breast tissue to eliminate the risk of breast cancer. Experimental data in animals suggest that the risk of carcinogenesis may be increased when the volume of target breast tissue is reduced but not eradicated.[34] On a practical level, even a total mastectomy leaves some breast tissue behind, and an operation known as *subcutaneous mastectomy* leaves considerable breast tissue. This operation proved to be highly morbid in one series, with an unsatisfactory cosmetic outcome in many patients.[35] Simply stated, prophylactic mastectomy does not guarantee the prevention of breast cancer.[36–39] Despite these considerations, one retrospective analysis of the efficacy of prophylactic mastectomy in women with a family history of breast cancer showed a significant reduction in the incidence of breast cancer when compared with sisters of the probands and when compared with the Gail model.[40]

At present, prophylactic mastectomy is recommended infrequently.[41] Primary situations in which prophylactic mastectomy is a reasonable option include (1) women who have developed unilateral breast cancer and who are likely to develop a contralateral breast primary based on their being members of a family with a hereditary breast cancer syndrome,[42, 43] (2) women without invasive breast cancer but who have positive genetic testing or a family pedigree consistent with a familial syndrome,[41] and (3) women with LCIS.[44] Women with these conditions may be offered total mastectomies with reconstruction for prophylaxis. They should also be offered psychological counseling before and after the procedure because the anxiety of possibly developing breast cancer will be replaced with the certainty of an altered body image and the morbidity of several major operative procedures.

We do not recommend prophylactic mastectomies for patients with sporadic forms of invasive breast cancer. The risk of recurrent disease from the documented primary lesion is generally of greater concern than the likelihood of a new sporadic breast primary.

## SILICONE IMPLANTS

There is increasing concern about possible rheumatic disease in patients who have received a silicone breast implant.[45–48] Silicone can leak from implants and migrate to distant sites, and there is evidence of cellular and humoral immune responses to silicone. In one autopsy study of women with apparently intact silicone implants, extracapsular spread of silicone was found in all of the patients to at least some degree.

Causality has not been proved. One well-cited case-control study of rheumatic disorders in implant patients compared with a control group found no significant difference in the incidence of any disorder, with the possible exception of morning stiffness.[49] A review of meta-analyses of all the case-control and cohort studies found no evidence for causation of rheumatic disease.[50] Given the high likelihood of spread and the low likelihood of silicone-induced disease, we generally use diagnostic studies searching for such leakage only sparingly and only if the results of the study would be used to alter therapy. In such circumstances, MRI is the most effective modality for showing the presence or absence of leakage.[51] Most patients, however, can be managed without MRI or other expensive imaging modality. As for removal of silicone implants, we approach these patients on an individualized basis.

The issue is now before the courts. A class action suit was settled by three manufacturers of implants by establishing a fund of $4.2 billion to compensate women with implants who acquired one or more of eight specified disorders. This settlement was approved on April 1, 1994, and it was joined 2 weeks later by an additional four implant manufacturers.[52] As for patients considering such implants, a national survey suggests that many patients benefit from implants, but many of these same patients would probably refuse a silicone implant given the current state of concern about safety.[53]

## BILATERAL BREAST CANCER

The earlier the age of diagnosis and the stronger the patient's family history of breast cancer, the higher is the risk of bilaterality. In one study of 556 patients,[54] the probabilities to the 19th year of developing an additional primary breast cancer for premenopausal patients with breast cancer and a strong family history was 35 to 38%, whereas for postmenopausal patients it ranged from 11 to 26%. The importance of the family history to the problem of bilateral breast cancer was discussed in detail earlier in the section Natural History and Pretreatment Assessment.

Although bilateral breast cancer occurs most commonly in the context of a strong family history of the disease, it occasionally occurs as an isolated event.[55–59] When this happens, it appears to have an adverse impact on prognosis, similar to that of finding positive axillary lymph node involvement.[60] The prognosis for patients with bilateral breast cancer given adjuvant chemotherapy, however, is essentially identical to that of patients with similarly staged unilateral disease.[61]

Asynchronous bilateral breast cancer is not unusual, and it carries a less serious prognosis than does the synchronous form of the disease. For this reason, a woman who has had unilateral breast cancer should have careful lifelong follow-up with close attention to the possible development of a new primary tumor in the remaining breast. The likelihood of developing cancer in the contralateral breast after mastectomy is about 13%.[54] This risk is not increased by the use of radiation therapy as primary management.[58, 62]

## TX N1–2 M0 BREAST CANCER

Patients who present with a palpable axillary mass that proves to be an adenocarcinoma with no obvious breast primary are treated as having primary breast cancer, rather than metastatic cancer of unknown primary origin. In the past, these women were usually managed with a total mastectomy, but conservative therapy with radiation and close follow-up is considered reasonable for fully informed patients. In limited reports, the overall survival results of total mastectomy and breast-conserving radiation therapy without further breast resection appear to be about the same.[63] Currently, there is good evidence for the use of MRI and positron emission tomography to help guide appropriate local control.[64, 65] All patients who present with occult axillary pathology in the absence of a palpable abnormality and unremarkable mammography should undergo individualized evaluation employing any necessary imaging, including MRI, positron emission tomography, and ultrasound.

## LYMPHEDEMA

About 5 to 10% of women develop severe lymphedema after total mastectomy with axillary dissection. Lymphedema is one of the most important complications of mastectomy with axillary dissection because it may cause physical discomfort, debility, and disfigurement and may result in cellulitis, lymphangitis, and, rarely, lymphangiosarcoma (Treves' syndrome).[66]

It was previously believed that the risk of lymphedema is increased in the presence of older age, obesity, and postoperative wound complications and possibly by splitting the pectoralis minor muscle during the axillary dissection in patients treated with conservative surgery.[67] An overview of published studies showed, however, that the two most significant risk factors for the development of lymphedema are the extent of axillary surgery and high doses of postoperative radiotherapy.[68] In patients who receive postoperative radiation therapy to the axilla, there is a direct relationship between the frequency and severity of lymphedema and the extent of the axillary dissection. In a series from Boston, for example, lymphedema occurred as follows: no axillary dissection, 4%; axillary sampling only, 5%; low axillary dissection only, 8%; and full axillary dissection, 37%.[69] The only other factors that Rockson[68] identified as possible precipitating causes were increased airplane travel and hypertension.

The best treatment of lymphedema is its prevention. In addition to the factors discussed earlier, patients should be instructed in the principles of good hand and arm hygiene and should receive postoperative help with hand and arm exercises, as reviewed by the ACS Lymphedema Workgroup.[80] In patients who develop chronic lymphedema later, one should consider the possibility of vascular thrombosis and recurrent tumor as causes. Treatment measures for chronic lymphedema include the use of arm elevation, an elastic sleeve or stocking, or a compression pump and manual lymphatic drainage for severe cases. Ultrasonography has been used, but its benefit is equivocal.[70] Patients should be counseled to avoid weight gain because this is a negative prognostic factor for the control of lymphedema.[71, 72] Patients should also be counseled to seek medical attention promptly at any sign of local infection. Rarely, severe lymphedema may benefit from one of several operative procedures.[73–75]

Previously, patients with lymphedema had been counseled in the use of coumarin as an effective means of reduction of lymphedema. Well-controlled clinical trials have now shown no benefit to this treatment option.[76] Currently, aggressive physiotherapy remains the standard of care in the treatment of lymphedema. An excellent overview of the predisposition, evaluation, diagnosis, and treatment of lymphedema is presented by the ACS Lymphedema Workshop.[77–81]

## LYMPHANGIOSARCOMA

Lymphangiosarcoma is a rare complication of lymphedema that was first reported by Stewart and Treves in 1948.[82] It occurs after mastectomy-induced lymphedema with a frequency of 0.03 to 0.8% in different series.[83]

The lesion usually presents after a delay of 5 to 25 years as an ecchymotic or swollen area or both in the arm of a patient with postmastectomy lymphedema.[66] The ecchymotic area usually becomes ulcerated, and chest wall satellite lesions appear within 1 year. Biopsy reveals typical malignant endothelial cells in the stroma against the background of chronic lymphedema. Subsequent metastatic spread is common.

The median survival for patients treated by forequarter amputation has previously been reported as 1.33 years[82]; however, current 5-year survival rates range from about 25 to 30%.[84] Current therapy includes the use of doxorubicin and ifosfamide-based chemotherapy, as used for other soft tissue sarcomas (see Chapter 83).

## PREGNANCY

Pregnancy at an early age reduces a woman's risk of breast cancer, whereas delayed pregnancy after age 30 seems to increase the risk of breast cancer. The prognosis for women younger than age 35 is worse than that for older women, and the differences are not completely explained by differences in prognostic factors.[85] These facts have contributed to making the role of pregnancy in breast cancer intriguing and controversial. The management of breast cancer in the pregnant patient and the question of later pregnancy in patients who have completed primary treatment for breast cancer are also controversial.[86–88] No firm, unequivocal recommendations can be made in this difficult area, but some of the facts that patients and physicians should consider in individualizing therapy are discussed next. Pregnancy and the cancer patient are discussed further in Chapter 27.

**Pregnant Patient with Breast Cancer.** Numerous case-control and retrospective studies of pregnancy-associated breast cancer have been published, and the results are variable. Bonnier and colleagues[89] found that pregnancy-associated breast cancer was associated with an increased frequency of inflammatory breast cancer, increased size of tumors at presentation, and more frequent findings of negative hormone receptors when compared with a control group. A large case-control analysis at Memorial Sloane-Kettering found that for stages I and II, disease-free survival and overall survival were not compromised by pregnancy, but that patients with stage III pregnancy-associated breast cancer did significantly worse than matched controls.[90] Other authors who have studied this question have found no difference in outcomes when strict attention is paid to age-matched and stage-matched controls.[85, 91] The most likely explanation for the variability in these studies is delays in diagnosis. This difference of opinion can be resolved only by additional study with particular attention to the multitude of risk factors that can influence prognosis, especially time of diagnosis. It is important to treat these patients with a multidisciplinary approach involving medical oncology, surgical oncology, obstetrics, and radiation therapy as indicated by the stage of disease at presentation. The patient may raise the question of whether or not to abort the fetus. Patient survival has not been shown to be improved with termination of pregnancy,[92–95] and pregnancy termination

*Breast Cancer* **593**

may possibly harm the patient.[96] Generally, radiation therapy, as necessary by stage and treatment plan, is delayed until after delivery of the fetus.[97]

**Pregnancy After Breast Cancer.** There is a short-term increase in the risk of breast cancer after a full-term pregnancy,[98] but there does not appear to be any long-term risk from subsequent pregnancy. Breast cancer is not in itself a contraindication to subsequent pregnancy.[99] Specific caveats for breast cancer survivors interested in becoming pregnant include the following: (1) Infertility after breast cancer treatment is directly proportional to patient age and the use and dose of alkylating agents, (2) there appears to be no increase in birth defects in children whose parents were exposed to chemotherapy earlier in life, (3) milk production of the irradiated breast is likely to be limited, and (4) adjuvant tamoxifen therapy has adverse effects on pregnancy in vivo and in laboratory animals. No reports exist on the effects of tamoxifen on human pregnancy.[88] In general, it is recommended that patients wait at least 2 years after treatment before attempting to become pregnant.[100]

## MALE BREAST CANCER

Cancer of the breast is a rare disease in men. It composes less than 1% of all breast carcinomas and less than 1.5% of all malignant tumors in men. A family history of breast cancer is frequently found in men with breast cancer, and most of these are now known to be associated with germline mutations in *BRCA2*.[101–103] The only other known predisposing factors are Klinefelter's syndrome[104] and radiation exposure.[105] Gynecomastia does not appear to be associated with increased risk of male breast cancer, but the histologic changes of gynecomastia are frequently present in male breast cancer specimens.[106, 107] The role of the hormonal milieu, either hyperestrogenic or hypoandrogenic, may also play a role in development of male carcinoma of the breast. There is a high frequency of ER and PR positivity in male breast cancer tissue,[108] and there is an inverse relationship between age and receptor positivity. The disease also mimics female breast cancer in the histologic appearance, the clinical presentation, and the tendency to metastasize to bone. LCIS and infiltrating lobular carcinomas are exceedingly rare in the presentation of male breast cancer.[106, 109] Staging of male breast cancer is identical to that in women.

Therapy for local control usually involves MRM. Breast conservation is rarely feasible given the size of the male breast and the location of the tumor. These procedures are usually combined with an axillary lymph node dissection. These patients are treated with a multidisciplinary approach similar to their female counterparts.

Systemic control is frequently with tamoxifen given the high percentage of patients with positive hormone receptors. Administration of tamoxifen in the adjuvant setting for male breast cancer has been shown to improve overall survival when compared with historical controls.[110, 111] In fact, most forms of hormonal manipulation from castration, either surgical or medical, to androgen therapy provide clinical benefit in these patients.[112–114] Following the lead from female breast cancer, T2 and N1 positive lesions can be treated with adjuvant systemic chemotherapy. There have been no randomized clinical trials of adjuvant therapies in male breast

cancer, but the paradigm as well as outcomes appear to be similar.

Based on these considerations, we recommend that men with breast cancer be managed in a manner analogous to women with breast cancer. The concentration of ERs and PRs in tumor tissue should be assessed. Patients with metastatic ER-positive tumors or with slowly growing disease that is limited to soft tissues, nodes, or bones should initially be treated with endocrine manipulation. This treatment is usually with tamoxifen, although orchiectomy, DES, or a LHRH agonist are reasonable alternatives. Overall, tamoxifen tends to be less well tolerated in men than women with loss of libido as a frequent complaint.[115] The indications for combination chemotherapy are the same as those for female breast cancer. Reviews are available for more detailed discussions of this entity.[116, 117]

## SUGGESTIONS FOR ADDITIONAL READING

Armstrong K, Eisen A, Weber B. Assessing the risk of breast cancer. N Engl Med 2000;342:564–71.

Fisher B, Powles TJ, Pritchard KJ. Tamoxifen for the prevention of breast cancer. Eur J Cancer 2000;36:142–50.

Bostick PJ, Giuliano AE. Vital dyes in sentinel node localization. Semin Nucl Med 2000;30:18–24.

Fisher B. From Halsted to prevention and beyond: advances in the management of breast cancer during the twentieth century. Eur J Cancer 1999;35:1963–73.

Jacobson JS, Workman SB, Kronenberg F. Research on complementary/alternative medicine for patients with breast cancer: a review of the biomedical literature. J Clin Oncol 2000;18:668–83.

## REFERENCES

1. Siegel BM, Mayzel KA, Love SM. Level I and II axillary dissection in the treatment of early-stage breast cancer: an analysis of 259 consecutive patients. Arch Surg 1990;125:1144–7.
2. Lin PP, Allison DC, Wainstock J, et al. Impact of axillary lymph node dissection on the therapy of breast cancer patients. J Clin Oncol 1993;11:1536–44.
3. Anscher MS, Jones P, Prosnitz LR, et al. Local failure and margin status in early-stage breast carcinoma treated with conservation surgery and radiation therapy. Ann Surg 1993;218:22–8.
4. Tamoxifen for early breast cancer: an overview of the randomised trials. Early Breast Cancer Trialists' Collaborative Group [see comments]. Lancet 1998;351:1451–67.
5. Buzzoni R, Bonadonna G, Valagussa P, Zambetti M. Adjuvant chemotherapy with doxorubicin plus cyclophosphamide, methotrexate, and fluorouracil in the treatment of resectable breast cancer with more than three positive axillary nodes. J Clin Oncol 1991;9:2134–40.
6. Buchholz TA, Austin-Seymour MM, Moe RE, et al. Effect of delay in radiation in the combined modality treatment of breast cancer [see comments]. Int J Radiat Oncol Biol Phys 1993;26:23–35.
7. Recht A, Come SE, Gelman RS, et al. Integration of conservative surgery, radiotherapy, and chemotherapy for the treatment of early-stage, node-positive breast cancer: sequencing, timing, and outcome [see comments]. J Clin Oncol 1991;9:1662–7.
8. Buzdar AU, Kau SW, Smith TL, et al. The order of administration of chemotherapy and radiation and its effect on the local control of operable breast cancer. Cancer 1993;71:3680–4.
9. Booser DJ, Hortobagyi GN. Treatment of locally advanced breast cancer. Semin Oncol 1992;19:278–85.
10. Kling KM, Ostrzega N, Schmit P. Breast conservation after induction chemotherapy for locally advanced breast cancer. Am Surg 1997;63:861–4.
11. Veronesi U, Bonadonna G, Zurrida S, et al. Conservation surgery after primary chemotherapy in large carcinomas of the breast [see comments]. Ann Surg 1995;222:612–8.

12. Semiglazov VF, Topuzov EE, Bavli JL, et al. Primary (neoadjuvant) chemotherapy and radiotherapy compared with primary radiotherapy alone in stage IIb–IIa breast cancer. Ann Oncol 1994;5:591–5.

13. Jaiyesimi IA, Buzdar AU, Hortobagyi G. Inflammatory breast cancer: a review. J Clin Oncol 1992;10:1014–24.

14. Honkoop AH, Wagstaff J, Pinedo HM. Management of stage III breast cancer. Oncology 1998;55:218–27.

15. Ueno NT, Buzdar AU, Singletary SE, et al. Combined-modality treatment of inflammatory breast carcinoma: twenty years of experience at M.D. Anderson Cancer Center. Cancer Chemother Pharmacol 1997;40:321–9.

16. Fleming RY, Asmar L, Buzdar AU, et al. Effectiveness of mastectomy by response to induction chemotherapy for control in inflammatory breast carcinoma. Ann Surg Oncol 1997;4:452–61.

17. Hortobagyi GN, Holmes FA, Ibrahim N, et al. The University of Texas M.D. Anderson Cancer Center experience with paclitaxel in breast cancer. Semin Oncol 1997;24:S30–3.

18. Chollet P, Charrier S, Brain E, et al. Clinical and pathological response to primary chemotherapy in operable breast cancer. Eur J Cancer 1997;33:862–6.

19. Buzdar AU, Montague ED, Barker JL, et al. Management of inflammatory carcinoma of breast with combined modality approach—an update. Cancer 1981;47:2537–42.

20. Valagussa P, Zambetti M, Bignami P, et al. T3b-T4 breast cancer: factors affecting results in combined modality treatments. Clin Exp Metastasis 1983;1:191–202.

21. Kennedy MJ, Abeloff MD. Management of locally recurrent breast cancer [see comments]. Cancer 1993;71:2395–409.

22. Abner AL, Recht A, Eberlein T, et al. Prognosis following salvage mastectomy for recurrence in the breast after conservative surgery and radiation therapy for early-stage breast cancer. J Clin Oncol 1993;11:44–8.

23. Moskovic E, Parsons C, Baum M. Chest radiography in the management of breast cancer. Br J Radiol 1992;65:30–2.

24. Muss HB, Tell GS, Case LD, et al. Perceptions of follow-up care in women with breast cancer. Am J Clin Oncol 1991;14:55–9.

25. Lurie N, Slater J, McGovern P, et al. Preventive care for women: does the sex of the physician matter? see comments. N Engl J Med 1993;329:478–82.

26. Wiesenthal M. Reach-to-Recovery Program of the American Cancer Society. Cancer 1984;53:825–7.

27. Schag CA, Ganz PA, Polinsky ML, et al. Characteristics of women at risk for psychosocial distress in the year after breast cancer. J Clin Oncol 1993;11:783–93.

28. Pozo C, Carver CS, Noriega V, et al. Effects of mastectomy versus lumpectomy on emotional adjustment to breast cancer: a prospective study of the first year postsurgery. J Clin Oncol 1992;10:1292–8.

29. Kemeny MM, Wellisch DK, Schain WS. Psychosocial outcome in a randomized surgical trial for treatment of primary breast cancer. Cancer 1988;62:1231–7.

30. Frankel MR. Breast cancer—a woman's perspective. West J Med 1988;149:723–5.

31. Desch CE, Hillner BE, Smith TJ, Retchin SM. Should the elderly receive chemotherapy for node-negative breast cancer? A cost-effectiveness analysis examining total and active life-expectancy outcomes. J Clin Oncol 1993;11:777–82.

32. Ganz PA, Lee JJ, Sim MS, et al. Exploring the influence of multiple variables on the relationship of age to quality of life in women with breast cancer. J Clin Epidemiol 1992;45:473–85.

33. Silliman RA, Balducci L, Goodwin JS, et al. Breast cancer care in old age: what we know, don't know, and do. J Natl Cancer Inst 1993;85:190–9.

34. Wong JH, Jackson CF, Swanson JS, et al. Analysis of the risk reduction of prophylactic partial mastectomy in Sprague-Dawley rats with 7,12-dimethylbenzanthracene-induced breast cancer. Surgery 1986;99:67–71.

35. Slade CL. Subcutaneous mastectomy: acute complications and long-term follow-up. Plast Reconstr Surg 1984;73:84–90.

36. Ziegler LD, Kroll SS. Primary breast cancer after prophylactic mastectomy [clinical conference]. Am J Clin Oncol 1991;14:451–4.

37. Eldar S, Meguid MM, Beatty JD. Cancer of the breast after prophylactic subcutaneous mastectomy. Am J Surg 1984;148:692–3.

38. Kieback DG, Kieback CC. Advanced breast cancer after subcutaneous mastectomy and immediate prosthetic reconstruction for benign breast disease—a rare observation and a diagnostic problem. Breast Cancer Res Treat 1986;7:119–20. letter.

39. Goodnight JE Jr, Quagliana JM, Morton DL. Failure of subcutaneous mastectomy to prevent the development of breast cancer. J Surg Oncol 1984;26:198–201.

40. Hartmann L, Schaid D, Woods J, et al. Efficacy of bilateral prophylactic mastectomy in women with a family history of breast cancer. N Engl J Med 1999;340:77–84.

41. Eisen A, Rebbeck R, Wood WC, Weber BL. Prophylactic surgery in women with a hereditary predisposition to breast and ovarian cancer. J Clin Oncol 2000;18:1980–85.

42. Schaid DJ. Re: probability of carrying a mutation of breast-ovarian cancer gene *BRCA1* based on family history [comment]. J Natl Cancer Inst 1997;89:1632–4. letter.

43. Berry DA, Parmigiani G, Sanchez J, et al. Probability of carrying a mutation of breast-ovarian cancer gene *BRCA1* based on family history [see comments]. J Natl Cancer Inst 1997;89:227–38.

44. Morrow M, Schnitt S. Lobular carcinoma in situ. In: Harris J, Lippman M, Morrow M, Hellman S, eds. Diseases of the breast. Philadelphia: Lippincott-Raven, 1996:369.

45. Nyren O, Yin L, Josefsson S, et al. Risk of connective tissue disease and related disorders among women with breast implants: a nationwide retrospective cohort study in Sweden [see comments]. Br Med J 1998;316:417–22.

46. Edworthy SM, Martin L, Barr SG, et al. A clinical study of the relationship between silicone breast implants and connective tissue disease [see comments]. J Rheumatol 1998;25:254–60.

47. Hennekens CH, Lee IM, Cook NR, et al. Self-reported breast implants and connective-tissue diseases in female health professionals: a retrospective cohort study [see comments] [published erratum appears in JAMA 1998;279(3):198]. JAMA 1996;275:616–21.

48. Hirmand H, Latrenta GS, Hoffman LA. Autoimmune disease and silicone breast implants. Oncology (Huntingt) 1993;7:17–24.

49. Gabriel SE, O'Fallon WM, Kurland LT, et al. Risk of connective-tissue diseases and other disorders after breast implantation [see comments]. N Engl J Med 1994;330:1697–702.

50. Janowsky EC, Kupper LL, Hulka BS. Meta-analyses of the relation between silicone breast implants and the risk of connective-tissue disease. N Engl J Med 2000;342:781–90.

51. Ahn CY, Shaw WW, Narayanan K, et al. Definitive diagnosis of breast implant rupture using magnetic resonance imaging [see comments]. Plast Reconstr Surg 1993;92:681–91.

52. Angell M. Do breast implants cause systemic disease? Science in the courtroom [editorial; comment] [see comments]. N Engl J Med 1994;330:1748–9.

53. Winer EP, Fee-Fulkerson K, Fulkerson CC, et al. Silicone controversy: a survey of women with breast cancer and silicone implants [see comments]. J Natl Cancer Inst 1993;85:1407–11.

54. Anderson DE, Badzioch MD. Bilaterality in familial breast cancer patients. Cancer 1985;56:2092–8.

55. Harris RE, Lynch HT, Guirgis HA. Familial breast cancer: risk to the contralateral breast. J Natl Cancer Inst 1978;60:955–60.

56. Kruse CA, Wagner DE. An evaluation of bilateral breast carcinoma: simultaneous and sequential lesions. West J Med 1976;124:187–90.

57. Kesseler HJ, Grier WR, Seidman I, McIlveen SJ. Bilateral primary breast cancer. JAMA 1976;236:278–80.

58. Schell SR, Montague ED, Spanos WJ Jr, et al. Bilateral breast cancer in patients with initial stage I and II disease. Cancer 1982;50:1191–4.

59. Fisher ER, Fisher B, Sass R, Wickerham L. Pathologic findings from the National Surgical Adjuvant Breast Project (Protocol No. 4): XI. bilateral breast cancer. Cancer 1984;54:3002–11.

60. Tulusan AH, Ronay G, Egger H, Willgeroth F. A contribution to the natural history of breast cancer: V. bilateral primary breast cancer: incidence, risks and diagnosis of simultaneous primary cancer in the opposite breast. Arch Gynecol 1985;237:85–91.

61. Berte E, Buzdar AU, Smith TL, Hortobagyi GN. Bilateral primary breast cancer in patients treated with adjuvant therapy. Am J Clin Oncol 1988;11:114–8.

62. Hankey BF, Curtis RE, Naughton MD, et al. A retrospective cohort analysis of second breast cancer risk for primary breast cancer patients with an assessment of the effect of radiation therapy. J Natl Cancer Inst 1983;70:797–804.

63. Baron PL, Moore MP, Kinne DW, et al. Occult breast cancer presenting with axillary metastases: updated management. Arch Surg 1990;125:210–4.

64. Scoggins CR, Vitola JV, Sandler MP, et al. Occult breast carcinoma presenting as an axillary mass. Am Surg 1999;65:1–5.

65. Block EF, Meyer MA. Positron emission tomography in diagnosis of occult adenocarcinoma of the breast. Am Surg 1998;64:906–8.
66. Stewart NJ, Pritchard DJ, Nascimento AG, Kang YK. Lymphangiosarcoma following mastectomy. Clin Orthop 1995;320:135–41.
67. Pezner RD, Patterson MP, Hill LR, et al. Arm lymphedema in patients treated conservatively for breast cancer: relationship to patient age and axillary node dissection technique. Int J Radiat Oncol Biol Phys 1986;12:2079–83.
68. Rockson SG. Precipitating factors in lymphedema: myths and realities. Cancer 1998;83:2814–6.
69. Larson D, Weinstein M, Goldberg I, et al. Edema of the arm as a function of the extent of axillary surgery in patients with stage I–II carcinoma of the breast treated with primary radiotherapy. Int J Radiat Oncol Biol Phys 1986;12:1575–82.
70. Balzarini A, Pirovano C, Diazzi G, et al. Ultrasound therapy of chronic arm lymphedema after surgical treatment of breast cancer. Lymphology 1993;26:128–34.
71. Bertelli G, Venturini M, Forno G, et al. An analysis of prognostic factors in response to conservative treatment of postmastectomy lymphedema. Surg Gynecol Obstet 1992;175:455–60.
72. Segerstrom K, Bjerle P, Graffman S, Nystrom A. Factors that influence the incidence of brachial oedema after treatment of breast cancer. Scand J Plast Reconstr Surg Hand Surg 1992;26:223–7.
73. Savage RC. The surgical management of lymphedema. Surg Gynecol Obstet 1984;159:501–8.
74. Kambayashi J, Ohshiro T, Mori T. Appraisal of myocutaneous flapping for treatment of postmastectomy lymphedema: case report. Acta Chir Scand 1990;156:175–7.
75. Brorson H, Svensson H. Complete reduction of lymphoedema of the arm by liposuction after breast cancer. Scand J Plast Reconstr Surg Hand Surg 1997;31:137–43.
76. Loprinzi CL, Kugler JW, Sloan JA, et al. Lack of effect of coumarin in women with lymphedema after treatment for breast cancer [see comments]. N Engl J Med 1999;340:346–50.
77. Candeira M, Schuch W, Greiner L, et al. American Cancer Society Lymphedema Workshop: Workgroup V: collaboration and advocacy. Cancer 1998;83:2888–90.
78. Leitch AM, Meek AG, Smith RA, et al. American Cancer Society Lymphedema Workshop. Workgroup I: treatment of the axilla with surgery and radiation—preoperative and postoperative risk assessment. Cancer 1998;83:2877–9.
79. Walley DR, Augustine E, Saslow D, et al. American Cancer Society Lymphedema Workshop. Workgroup IV: lymphedema treatment resources—professional education and availability of patient services. Cancer 1998;83:2886–7.
80. Rockson SG, Miller LT, Senie R, et al. American Cancer Society Lymphedema Workshop. Workgroup III: diagnosis and management of lymphedema. Cancer 1998;83:2882–5.
81. Runowicz CD, Passik SD, Hann D, et al. American Cancer Society Lymphedema Workshop. Workgroup II: patient education—pre- and posttreatment. Cancer 1998;83:2880–1.
82. Stewart FW, Treves N. Lymphangiosarcoma in postmastectomy lymphedema: a report of six cases in elephantiasis chirurgica. Cancer 1948;1:64–81.
83. Mark RJ, Poen J, Tran LM, et al. Postirradiation sarcomas: a single-institution study and review of the literature. Cancer 1994;73:2653–62.
84. Brady MS, Garfein CF, Petrek JA, Brennan MF. Post-treatment sarcoma in breast cancer patients. Ann Surg Oncol 1994;1:66–72.
85. Nixon AJ, Neuberg D, Hayes DF, et al. Relationship of patient age to pathologic features of the tumor and prognosis for patients with stage I or II breast cancer. J Clin Oncol 1994;12:888–94.
86. Berry DL, Theriault RL, Holmes FA, et al. Management of breast cancer during pregnancy using a standardized protocol. J Clin Oncol 1999;17:855–61.
87. Sorosky JI, Scott-Conner CE. Breast disease complicating pregnancy. Obstet Gynecol Clin North Am 1998;25:353–63.
88. Collichio FA, Agnello R, Staltzer J. Pregnancy after breast cancer: from psychosocial issues through conception. Oncology (Huntingt) 1998;12:759–65, 769.
89. Bonnier P, Romain S, Dilhuydy JM, et al. Influence of pregnancy on the outcome of breast cancer: a case-control study. Société Française de Senologie et de Pathologie Mammaire Study Group. Int J Cancer 1997;72:720–7.
90. Anderson BO, Petrek JA, Byrd DR, et al. Pregnancy influences breast cancer stage at diagnosis in women 30 years of age and younger. Ann Surg Oncol 1996;3:204–11.
91. Ezzat A, Raja MA, Berry J, et al. Impact of pregnancy on non-metastatic breast cancer: a case control study. Clin Oncol 1996;8:367–70.
92. Hubay CA, Barry FM, Marr CC. Pregnancy and breast cancer. Surg Clin North Am 1978;58:819–31.
93. Ribeiro G, Jones DA, Jones M. Carcinoma of the breast associated with pregnancy. Br J Surg 1986;73:607–9.
94. Nugent P, O'Connell TX. Breast cancer and pregnancy. Arch Surg 1985;120:1221–4.
95. Barnavon Y, Wallack MK. Management of the pregnant patient with carcinoma of the breast. Surg Gynecol Obstet 1990;171:347–52.
96. Ownby HE, Martino S, Roi LD, et al. Interrupted pregnancy as an indicator of poor prognosis in T1, 2, N0, M0 primary breast cancer. Breast Cancer Res Treat 1983;3:339–44.
97. Mayr NA, Wen BC, Saw CB. Radiation therapy during pregnancy. Obstet Gynecol Clin North Am 1998;25:301–21.
98. Bruzzi P, Negri E, La Vecchia C, et al. Short term increase in risk of breast cancer after full term pregnancy. Br Med J 1988;297:1096–8.
99. Danforth DN Jr. How subsequent pregnancy affects outcome in women with a prior breast cancer. Oncology (Huntingt) 1991;5:23–30.
100. Petrek JA. Pregnancy safety after breast cancer. Cancer 1994;74:528–31.
101. Couch FJ, Farid LM, DeShano ML, et al. *BRCA2* germline mutations in male breast cancer cases and breast cancer families. Nat Genet 1996;13:123–5.
102. Haraldsson K, Loman N, Zhang QX, et al. *BRCA2* germ-line mutations are frequent in male breast cancer patients without a family history of the disease. Cancer Res 1998;58:1367–71.
103. Thorlacius S, Tryggvadottir L, Olafsdottir GH, et al. Linkage to *BRCA2* region in hereditary male breast cancer. Lancet 1995;346:544–5.
104. Jackson A, Muldal S, Ockey C, et al. Carcinoma of the male breast in association with Klinefelter syndrome. Br Med J 1965;1:223.
105. Eldar S, Nash E, Abrahamson J. Radiation carcinogenesis in the male breast. Eur J Surg Oncol 1989;15:274–8.
106. Heller KS, Rosen PP, Schottenfeld D, et al. Male breast cancer: a clinicopathologic study of 97 cases. Ann Surg 1978;188:60–5.
107. Axelsson J, Andersson A. Cancer of the male breast. World J Surg 1983;7:281–7.
108. Friedman MA, Hoffman PG Jr, Dandolos EM, et al. Estrogen receptors in male breast cancer: clinical and pathologic correlations. Cancer 1981;47:134–7.
109. Borgen PI, Wong GY, Vlamis V, et al. Current management of male breast cancer: a review of 104 cases. Ann Surg 1992;215:451–9.
110. Ribeiro G, Swindell R. Adjuvant tamoxifen for male breast cancer (MBC). Br J Cancer 1992;65:252–4.
111. Hortobagyi GN, DiStefano A, Legha SS, et al. Hormonal therapy with tamoxifen in male breast cancer. Cancer Treat Rep 1979;63:539–41.
112. Doberauer C, Niederle N, Schmidt CG. Advanced male breast cancer treatment with the LH-RH analogue buserelin alone or in combination with the antiandrogen flutamide. Cancer 1988;62:474–8.
113. Stephens RL, Muggia FM. Breast cancer in men: report illustrating the value of endocrine ablation. Am J Med 1974;57:679–82.
114. Neifeld JP, Meyskens F, Tormey DC, Javadpour N. The role of orchiectomy in the management of advanced male breast cancer. Cancer 1976;37:992–5.
115. Anelli TF, Anelli A, Tran KN, et al. Tamoxifen administration is associated with a high rate of treatment-limiting symptoms in male breast cancer patients. Cancer 1994;74:74–7.
116. Williams WL Jr, Powers M, Wagman LD. Cancer of the male breast: a review. J Natl Med Assoc 1996;88:439–43.
117. Ravandi-Kashani F, Hayes TG. Male breast cancer: a review of the literature. Eur J Cancer 1998;34:1341–7.

# IX

# NEOPLASMS OF THE LUNG, PLEURA, AND MEDIASTINUM

# CHAPTER 36

# NON–SMALL CELL LUNG CANCER

• ROBERT A. FIGLIN • ROBERT B. CAMERON •
• ANDREW T. TURRISI, III

## Natural History

### ETIOLOGY AND EPIDEMIOLOGY

Cancers of the lung continue to be a major health problem in the United States. The incidence and mortality rates of these tumors are excessive and, although declining modestly in men, continue to increase in women.[1] The estimated number of lung cancer cases in the United States for 1998 is 171,500 (91,400 men and 80,100 women), whereas the estimated number of deaths is 160,100 (93,100 men and 67,000 women). Lung cancers are estimated to account for 14% of cancer incidence (15% in men and 13% in women) and 28% of cancer mortality (32% in men and 25% in women) in 1998 (excluding nonmelanomatous skin lesions and carcinoma in situ of the uterine cervix). Lung cancer in women is now the leading cause of cancer mortality (25% for lung cancer, 16% for breast cancer). Black men have an increased incidence of lung cancer, especially when diagnosed before the age of 54, whereas lung cancer incidence rates for black and white women appear equal. Black patients have a shorter survival than whites, and the death rate is 45% higher for blacks than for nonminority men.[2] Survival prognosis is also associated with socioeconomic status.

The control of lung cancer is a formidable problem. The identification of tobacco smoking as a major etiologic factor has been reviewed by Wynder and Hoffmann,[3] Bartecchi and colleagues,[4] and the U.S. Surgeon General.[5] It is estimated that tobacco smoking is the cause of 90% of all lung cancer deaths and 30 to 40% of deaths from cancer in general. Currently, 46.3 million adults (25.7% of the population) are smokers. The prevalence is highest among persons 25 to 44 years.[6]

This strong relationship suggests that control of this disease might be improved more effectively by preventive rather than by therapeutic advances. Although attempts to modify American smoking habits through education have resulted in decreased smoking prevalence since the 1950s, prevalence is still substantial, and per capita cigarette consumption is similar to that in 1952. Although it is possible that attempts to decrease tobacco carcinogenicity through filters have had or will have some effect, this effect is not likely to be substantial,[7–10] and lung cancer remains largely a smoker's disease. Lung cancer accounted for 29% of the more than 415,000 deaths attributed to smoking in the United States in 1990.[11] The risk of lung cancer increases by smoking cigars or a pipe, and this risk appears to be related to inhalation practices.[12] Smokeless tobacco, such as chewing tobacco or snuff, is carcinogenic for the upper aerodigestive tract but does not increase the risk for lung cancer.[13] Passive inhalation of tobacco smoke at home or in the workplace is associated with an increased risk of lung cancer.[14–16] It is suggested that approximately 17% of lung cancer among nonsmokers can be attributed to high levels of exposure to cigarette smoke during childhood and adolescence.[17] Denissenko and associates[18] mapped the distribution of benzo-[a]-pyrene diol epoxide (BPDE) adducts along exons of p53 in BPDE-treated HeLa cells and bronchial epithelial cells, noting selective adduct formation at codons 157, 248, and 273. These data provided the first direct link between tobacco smoke and lung cancer mutations.

Other important risk factors for lung cancer include exposure to asbestos, radon progeny, and carcinogens that may be found in the workplace. The relative risk of developing lung cancer from asbestos is approximately 1.4 to 2.6 and may account for 4000 to 6000 lung cancer deaths per year in the United States.[19, 20] Radon exposure in uranium miners may increase the lung cancer risk of all cell types in a dose-responsive manner.[21–23] The role of radon exposure in the home, with the subsequent risk of lung cancer development, remains open to further analysis.[24–26] Carcinogens in the workplace may interact with smoking to increase lung cancer risk,[27] including chloromethyl ether in chemical workers,[28] cadmium in nickel-cadmium battery plants,[29] arsenic,[30] chromate,[31] hexavalent chromium (masons),[32] formaldehyde,[33] and terpenes (wood industry).[34]

There may be genetic[35] or familial[36] risk factors. A biochemical risk factor—the inducibility of aryl hydrocarbon hydroxylase—has been reported.[37, 38] An association between lung cancer and certain systemic diseases (sarcoidosis, scleroderma, and interstitial fibrosis) has been noted. A threefold increased risk of lung cancer was found in patients with sarcoidosis,[39] and an increased risk of adenocarcinoma (particularly of bronchioloalveolar cell carcinoma) has been seen in patients with scleroderma. These associations may relate to the existence of *scar carcinomas*, lung cancers arising in pulmonary scars (e.g., resulting from tuberculosis, pneumonia, infarction, and pneumoconiosis).[40] Chronic obstructive pulmonary disease increases the risk for the development of lung cancer in proportion to the degree of airways obstruction. Among cigarette smokers, the presence of airways obstruction was more of an indicator for the subsequent development of lung cancer than was age or the level of smoking.[41, 42] A case-control study in women has suggested an association between estrogen replacement therapy and the risk of adenocarcinoma, even when adjusted for smoking.[43] If confirmed in a larger database, this finding would have important public health implications.

Increased susceptibility to lung cancer has been retrospectively linked to deficiencies of vitamin A, vitamin E, beta-carotene, and zinc.[44, 45] Beta-carotene may have a potential role as a protective agent,[46] whereas vitamin A intake has been shown to be inversely correlated with lung cancer risk, especially among cigarette smokers.[47] A randomized, double-blind, placebo-controlled primary prevention trial with α-tocopherol, beta-carotene, or both failed to reduce the incidence of lung cancer among male smokers after 5 to 8 years of dietary supplementation.[48]

## MOLECULAR BIOLOGY OF LUNG CANCER

Advances in cancer research have elucidated many of the molecular events involved in the pathogenesis of lung cancer. Studies in animal models have led to the understanding that carcinogenesis is a multistage process involving carcinogen-induced genetic damage that leads to activation of proto-oncogenes or inactivation of tumor-suppressor genes, or both. As a result of this process, susceptible cells may gain a selective growth advantage and undergo clonal expansion and metastasis. Lung cancer represents cells with multiple genetic abnormalities that provide the behavioral phenotype characteristic of malignancy (e.g., invasiveness, dedifferentiation, abnormal response to growth factors and regulators, and metastasis). A few of the more important genetic abnormalities characteristic of lung cancer are briefly described here; more detailed discussions concerning lung cancer carcinogenesis and molecular biology are the subject of excellent reviews.[49–51]

Genetic damage resulting from carcinogens may be complex and involve multiple chromosomes, deletions, translocations, double minutes, and homogeneously staining regions and aneuploidy. Whang-Peng and colleagues in 1982[52] described the 3p deletion, which was believed to be specific for small cell lung carcinoma (SCLC) but has since been described in non–small cell lung carcinoma (NSCLC) biopsy samples and cell lines.[53–55] Further studies have confirmed the presence of 3p deletions in virtually all SCLC tumors and approximately 50% of NSCLC tumors.[56] Candidate molecules located on 3p include the proto-oncogene c-*raf*-1,[57] the β-retinoic acid receptor–like gene Hap-1,[58] the protein tyrosine phosphatase-α gene,[59] and the von Hippel–Lindau tumor-suppressor gene.[60]

Genetic data indicate that chromosomal deletions tend to affect certain chromosomes more often than others. The heterogeneity and complex abnormalities suggest multiple potential proto-oncogene, growth factor, and tumor-suppressor interactions. Of note are the significantly frequent aberrations of chromosomes 13 and 17 involving regions containing the tumor-suppressor genes Rb and p53.[61] The details concerning proto-oncogene activation, growth factor receptor changes, and tumor-suppressor gene deactivation are not clearly understood. The importance of several genetic alterations has been established for lung cancer, however. These include the *myc*, *ras*, and *jun* families; various growth factor receptor genes; and the tumor-suppressor genes Rb and p53.

*myc*. The *myc* family consists of at least six functional members plus a pseudogene that are nuclear phosphoproteins important in the regulation of the cell cycle.[62] c-*myc*, L-*myc*, and N-*myc* amplifications have been described in lung cancer in SCLC[63, 64] as well as NSCLC cell lines.[65] In NSCLC, it appears that activated oncogenes other than the *myc* family are more important, although one study suggested that variant L-*myc* transcripts detected by restriction fragment-length

polymorphism may be associated with a higher frequency of distant metastases.[66]

*ras*. The *ras* family includes three well-characterized genes that have been associated with human cancers: H-*ras*, K-*ras*, and N-*ras*.[67] These genes code for closely related guanosine diphosphate (GDP) and guanosine triphosphate (GTP) binding proteins that have GTPase activity and are thought to play a role in the transduction of growth signals. Occurrences of lung adenocarcinomas in inbred or transgenic mice are closely associated with aberrant K-*ras* genes.[68] Subsequent screening of biopsy specimens has revealed a high frequency of codon 12 mutations in adenocarcinoma, with few or no mutations in other codons or in H-*ras* or N-*ras* genes. K-*ras* mutations exhibited a striking specificity for adenocarcinoma ($p < 0.001$, chi-squared test).

Retrospective analysis of DNA isolated from paraffin-embedded tumor material screened for *ras* mutations was performed in 69 patients with lung adenocarcinoma for whom complete resection of the tumor was possible. The K-*ras* codon 12 point mutation was a strong, unfavorable, independent prognostic factor for disease-free and overall survival.[69] In a second study,[70] 244 patients with stage I NSCLC were molecular pathologically staged. p53 expression, K-*ras* codon 12 mutation, and absence of H-*ras* p21 expression were among nine independent predictors of recurrence.

**Transcription Factors and Other Proto-Oncogenes.** Other proto-oncogenes have been studied in relation to growth factor signals. The oncogene *jun* is one of the proteins making up AP-1, a complex that regulates transcription and has been associated with tumor promotion induced by phorbol esters.[71] *jun*-A and *jun*-B are expressed in high levels in normal lung; may autoregulate their own expression; and may give rise to immortalized cell lines when cotransfected with other oncogenes, such as *myc* or *ras*.[72] Virtually all lung cancer cell lines express high levels of *jun*-B, whereas about one quarter express high levels of *jun*-A. The *jun* family of oncogenes may be important in transcription of genes related not only to growth but also to normal bronchial epithelial function or differentiation, or both. Chromosome deletion mutations, such as those involving 3p or the tumor-suppressor genes p53 or Rb, may release bronchial epithelium from growth control of differentiation signals triggered by genes transcribed by *jun*.[68]

**Rb and p53.** The retinoblastoma (Rb) gene is the best-studied example of a tumor-suppressor gene.[73] This gene was first described in patients with familial retinoblastoma. Structural abnormalities in the Rb gene have been identified in approximately 20% of SCLC cell lines, and absent Rb mRNA occurs in 60% of the SCLC cell lines and 75% of the carcinoid cell lines. A lower frequency of gene inactivation is seen in NSCLC, which ranges from 15 to 50% in various series.[74]

The tumor-suppressor gene p53 is located at 17p13, a region that is frequently the target for loss of heterozygosity in a variety of malignancies. Alterations described in p53 occur in approximately 50% of lung cancer cell lines and include homozygous deletions, DNA rearrangements, and point or small mutations. Studies of transgenic mice carrying a mutant p53 gene have shown a high incidence of lung cancers as well as bone and lymphoid tumors.[75]

These data suggest that the loss of the tumor-suppressor

genes Rb and p53 may be important in the pathogenesis of human lung cancer. It is also likely that there is a requirement for a *two-hit* gene inactivation in tumor-suppressor alleles in addition to a concurrent activation of one or more proto-oncogenes. Mutations of p53 and Rb have been associated with a poor prognosis in NSCLC patients.[76-78] The pathogenesis of human lung cancer is a complex and multistep process involving proto-oncogenes, tumor-suppressor genes, and growth factor activation. A possible sequence of events is illustrated in Table 36–1.

## CLASSIFICATION

In an attempt to standardize the histologic typing of lung tumors, a committee of the World Health Organization developed a classification system that has proved reliable and reproducible and has been accepted, with or without minor modifications, by most pathologists and oncologists. Table 36–2 presents the 1999 modified version of the standard classification system for lung cancer developed by the World Health Organization. A survey of several major series suggests that most lung cancers fall into the first four categories in that schema: (1) squamous cell carcinoma, which constitutes 35 to 71% of cases; (2) SCLC, which constitutes 12 to 25% of cases and is discussed in a separate chapter (Chapter 37); (3) adenocarcinoma, which constitutes 9 to 29% of cases; and (4) large cell carcinoma, which constitutes 3 to 16% of cases. There is evidence that adenocarcinoma of the lung is increasing in relative and absolute prevalence, particularly in women.[79, 80]

Squamous cell carcinomas are derived from bronchial epithelium. They tend to be centrally located and locally invasive, and they are less likely to have distant metastases than are other histologic types. Nearly half of superior sulcus

**Table 36–1.** Possible Sequence of Events in the Pathogenesis of Human Lung Cancer

Carcinogens + inherited factors
Multiple chromosomal alterations
Activation of proto-oncogenes
c-*jun* AP-I regulates transcription and mediates tumor promotion
   c-*ras*
   c-*raf*-1
Deletion of tumor suppressor genes
   Rb
   p53
Activation of growth factor production
Tumor promotion
   Activation of proto-oncogenes of importance for the differentiation of:
   SCLC
      c-*src*
      c-*myb*
      L-*myc*
   NSCLC
      C-sis
         c-*erb*B2
         c-*fos*
Activation of c-*myc*
Manifest lung cancer with metastasis

SCLC, small cell lung cancer; NSCLC, non–small cell lung cancer.
From Bergh JC. Gene amplification in human lung cancer. The *myc* family genes and other proto-oncogenes and growth factor genes. Am Rev Respir Dis 1990;142:6Pt.2:S20–6.

**Table 36–2.** 1999 WHO Histologic Classification of Malignant Epithelial Lung Tumors

Squamous cell carcinoma
  Variants
  Papillary
  Clear cell
  Small cell
  Basaloid
Small cell carcinoma
  Variant
  Combined small cell carcinoma
Adenocarcinoma
  Acinar
  Papillary
  Bronchioloalveolar carcinoma
    Nonmucinous (Clara cell/type II pneumocyte type)
    Mucinous (Goblet cell type)
    Mixed mucinous and nonmucinous or indeterminate
  Solid adenocarcinoma with mucin formation
  Adenocarcinoma with mixed subtypes
    Variants
    Well-differentiated fetal adenocarcinoma
    Mucinous (colloid) adenocarcinoma
    Signet ring adenocarcinoma
    Clear cell adenocarcinoma
Large cell carcinoma
  Variants
  Large cell neuroendocrine carcinoma
    Combined large cell neuroendocrine carcinoma
  Basaloid carcinoma
  Lymphoepithelioma-like carcinoma
  Clear cell carcinoma
  Large cell carcinoma with rhabdoid phenotype
Adenosquamous carcinoma
Carcinomas with pleomorphic, sarcomatoid, or sarcomatous elements
  Carcinomas with spindle or giant cells, or both
    Pleomorphic carcinoma
    Spindle cell carcinoma
    Giant cell carcinoma
  Carcinosarcoma
  Pulmonary blastoma
  Other
Carcinoid tumor
  Typical carcinoid
  Atypical carcinoid
Carcinomas of salivary gland type
  Mucoepidermoid carcinoma
  Adenoid cystic carcinoma
  Others
Unclassified carcinoma

From Koss M. In: Travis WD, Colby TV, Corrin B, et al. World Health Organization Pathology Panel: World Health Organization. Histological typing of lung and pleural tumors. International histological classification of tumors. 3rd ed. Heidelberg: Springer Verlag, 1999.

(*Pancoast*) tumors are of this histologic type.[81] Of the four major histologic types, these are the most likely to be resectable, and, accordingly, they are associated with the best prognosis. Squamous cell cancers may constitute a greater proportion of lung cancers in elderly patients than in younger patients. The relationship of the degree of differentiation of squamous cell tumors to survival is not clear. Advances in the flow cytometric evaluation of lung tumors suggest that DNA ploidy is a strong and independent prognostic factor in patients with all types of NSCLC. Patients with tumors characterized by aneuploidy and a high proliferative index have significantly shorter survival than patients whose tumors are diploid with low proliferative activity.[81] Flow cytometric evaluation of tumors has become a useful adjunct to the standard pathologic evaluation of these tumors.

Karyotypic abnormalities may occur in NSCLC. These tend to be multiple but commonly involve chromosome 7.[82]

Adenocarcinomas of the lung may arise from bronchioloalveolar epithelium or from mucous glands. They tend to be peripheral, small, and confined to one lobe. Tobacco exposure, chronic interstitial pulmonary disease, pulmonary scars, and fibrosis may predispose to this tumor type. Scar carcinomas are likely but not certain to be adenocarcinomas. Adenocarcinomas frequently involve the pleura and often metastasize to the scalene nodes. Women are likely to have adenocarcinomas. Bronchioloalveolar carcinoma, along with bronchogenic types (acinar and papillary), are included in this category. The bronchioloalveolar type of carcinoma usually arises peripherally as a unicentric lesion and may be related to pre-existent scars. It may rise from Clara cells (nonciliated bronchiolar epithelial cells). Although this type of carcinoma tends to metastasize by aerogenous spread, particularly when mucinous, resulting in multiple metastatic pulmonary nodules, the early diagnosis of limited disease may lead to surgical cure.[83–85] A viral cause for bronchioloalveolar carcinoma is postulated. Jaagsiekte or pulmonary adenomatosis in sheep is similar to bronchioloalveolar carcinoma in humans.[86–88] It is causally linked to a retrovirus with documented sheep-to-sheep transmission. Reports of sheep farmers developing diffuse bronchioloalveolar carcinoma have been published, but no sheep-to-human transmission is documented.[89] The role of tobacco in bronchioloalveolar carcinoma is controversial. Tobacco smoking is a strong risk factor for each of the four major histologic types of lung cancer, but the relationship is least strong for adenocarcinoma, and it is this histologic type that the nonsmoker who develops lung cancer is likely to have.

Large cell carcinoma of the lung may be peripheral or central and is often bulky. Giant cell and clear cell carcinomas are included in this category. Causative factors are similar to those for adenocarcinoma, and the histologic distinction between them is sometimes unclear. One subset consists of NSCLC, frequently classified as large cell, that expresses neuroendocrine features (i.e., chromogranin A, Leu-7 antigen, high L-dopa decarboxylase levels, and neuron-specific enolase). This variety may constitute 10 to 20% of all NSCLCs and has a more favorable response to chemotherapy.[90]

Other, less common histologic types of tumors are also listed in Table 36–2. Adenosquamous carcinoma accounts for 1 to 3% of diagnoses at initial biopsy and perhaps more (5%) at autopsy. Other *mixed* tumors may also occur.

Bronchial carcinoid tumors compose less than 1% of lung tumors. They, similar to SCLCs, may be related to Kulchitsky-type cells. The epidemiologic pattern of these tumors differs from that of SCLC, however, making the relationship between the two unclear. This finding is consistent with SCLC being derived from a pluripotent pulmonary cell but carcinoid being derived from a Kulchitsky cell. Although bronchial carcinoid tumors have previously been classified by some as *bronchial adenomas*, they are frequently invasive and metastasize.[91, 92] Histologic criteria do not predict well for malignant behavior. These tumors tend to be central, with most occurring in the main, lobar, or segmental bronchi and presenting with local obstructive symptoms (cough, wheeze, dyspnea, and hemoptysis). When they are peripheral, they tend to be silent or to present with hemoptysis. The elevation of 5-hydroxyindoleacetic acid may occur with or without carcinoid syndrome. The treatment of choice for resectable carcinoids of the lung is surgery, with the 5-year survival rate for local-regional disease in the 60 to 80% range.[92] When distant metastases are present, the 5-year survival rate has been estimated at 11%.

Bronchial gland tumors (adenoid cystic and mucoepidermoid carcinomas) are less frequent than carcinoid tumors, but, similar to carcinoids, they may behave malignantly. The lesions tend to present with bronchial obstruction. The adenoid cystic tumor is likely to be infiltrative and locally invasive, whereas the mucoepidermoid carcinoma may be pedunculated.[93] Surgery is the treatment of choice, but frequently the disease is unresectable or fails to respond to surgery. Pulmonary blastomas are rare tumors, histologically similar to fetal lung, and are frequently metastatic and aggressive.

Unclassified tumors cannot be discussed homogeneously, and secondary metastatic tumors vary with the primary. It is sometimes difficult to distinguish metastatic from primary lung cancer, particularly if the histologic type is adenocarcinoma. Anatomic features (endobronchial vs. nonendobronchial, solitary vs. multiple, presence of ipsilateral hilar or mediastinal nodes vs. absence) may be useful in distinguishing primary from metastatic tumors. Special studies (e.g., immunoperoxidase for specific antigens, β-human chorionic gonadotropin, alpha-fetoprotein) may be useful in selected difficult cases.

## CLINICAL FEATURES AND DIAGNOSIS

Attempts have been made to *screen* persons at high risk for lung cancer in an effort to improve disease curability and patient survival by early diagnosis. The Philadelphia Pulmonary Neoplasm Research Project enrolled more than 6000 men age 45 or older in a program of screening chest radiographs every 6 months. They found 84 cases of lung cancer at the first visit (prevalence cases), and 121 cases were subsequently diagnosed (incidence cases). In the incidence cases, the 5-year survival rate was only 8% (12% in fully compliant patients who had a negative chest radiograph within 6 months of diagnosis).

Trials involving screening high-risk patients more aggressively have been ongoing at other centers.[94–102] These are summarized in Table 36–3. In general, these studies use chest radiography once to three times a year along with sputum cytology three times a year in smoking men older than 45 years. They showed similar prevalence rates (5.5 to 8.3/1000) and incidence rates (3 to 5.5/1000/year), and intensive screening generally led to more frequent early-stage diagnosis than in control groups. Early diagnosis was mainly seen in squamous carcinoma and adenocarcinoma. Cytology was less useful than radiography for diagnosis but did have some independent yield. These studies showed that chest radiography and sputum cytology complemented one another, with 7 to 20% of cases detected by both methods. Although these studies provided no justification for large-scale screening of persons at high risk, the detection of early lung cancer in some patients, with concomitantly improved 5-year survival rates, may provide justification for screening in individually selected patients.

*Table 36–3.* **Screening of Lung Cancer**

| | Mayo Clinic[95, 96, 100] | Memorial Sloan-Kettering[97, 101, 102] | Johns Hopkins[98, 99] |
|---|---|---|---|
| *Screening* | CXR, sputum every 4 mo vs. control (optional yearly CXR) | CXR yearly Å sputum cytology every 4 mo | CXR yearly Å sputum cytology every 4 mo |
| *Prevalence* | 8.3/1000 | 5.5/1000 | 7/1000 |
| *Incidence* | 4.9/1000 yr; overall 5.5/1000/yr screened | 3/1000/yr | 4–5/1000/yr |
| *Early Disease* | Resectable incidence cases: 46% screened; 32% control | Overall results, stage I incidence and prevalence cases: 38% | 56% prevalence case and >45% incidence cases resectable for cure |
| *Mortality* | Incidence cases 5-yr survival: 40% (3.2/1000/yr) screened, 15% (3.0/1000/yr) control | 5-year survival (all cases): >90% stage I, >5% stage II/III | 3.8/1000/yr with cytology; 3.8/1000/yr without cytology |

CXR, chest radiograph.

Tockman[103] evaluated the sensitivity and specificity of monoclonal antibodies to antigens present on SCLCs and NSCLCs by using preserved sputum specimens from individuals who participated in the Johns Hopkins Lung Project. Of the 626 sputum specimens that showed moderate (or greater) atypia, 69 were randomly selected for a blinded monoclonal antibody immunostaining protocol. The antibodies were nonreactive in 88% of the specimens that did not progress to lung cancer. Positive staining could be shown in 14 of 22 patients who eventually progressed to cancer. All of the true-positive results were collected 24 months in advance of the diagnosis, however, as compared with the eight false-negative results that were collected an average of 57 months preceding the diagnosis. Subsequent specimens obtained approximately 26 months before cancer from participants who were originally considered to have false-negative results stained positively. This change improved the sensitivity to 91% among specimens collected an average of 2 years in advance of the clinical appearance of lung cancer. Evidence suggests that oncogene mutations (*ras* or p53) may also be detectable and precede sputum diagnosis of lung cancer.[104] The use of monoclonal antibodies to screen sputum in patients at high risk for developing lung cancer is currently the subject of a large multicenter clinical trial.

Tockman and coworkers[105] have shown that hnRNP $A_2/B_1$, an RNA binding protein, is upregulated in pulmonary cancers. Using archived preneoplastic sputum samples, hnRNP $A_2/B_1$ overexpression was detected. This test identified preclinical cancer more accurately than cytomorphology. In an ongoing prospective study of Yunnan tin miners at high risk for developing lung cancer, upregulation of hnRNP $A_2/B_1$ in the sputum in 69 of 94 primary lung cancers was detected compared with 10 primary lung cancers being detected cytologically. Sputum from resected stage I patients showed upregulation of hnRNP $A_2/B_1$ in 32 of 42 specimens, compared with cytologic changes found in only one patient, and accurately predicted outcome. These studies predicted that 69% of the miners and 67% of resected stage I patients with elevated hnRNP $A_2/B_1$ would develop lung cancer as compared with background. The upregulation of hnRNP $A_2/B_1$ is an early finding. The accuracy of this test appears similar to that of the prostate-specific antigen test used for prostate cancer screening.

The utility of mobile spiral computed tomography (CT) of the chest has also been assessed. In 1996, 5843 individuals in Japan age 40 to 74 years underwent chest radiography, cytologic sputum assessment, and spiral CT of the chest.[106] Nineteen patients were diagnosed with lung cancer, of which 18 were surgically confirmed. In 4 of 19 patients, CT and chest radiography revealed an abnormality. Of these patients, 16 had stage I disease, and the remainder had stage IV disease. The detection rate for CT screening was 0.48% (19 of 3967), compared with a 0.03 to 0.05% detection rate for chest radiography and sputum cytology screening previously performed in the same area. The authors found a 10-fold increase in the detection rate for lung cancer, many of which were at an early stage.

Although the diagnosis of asymptomatic patients may occur with routine screening, greater than 90% of patients with lung cancer are symptomatic at the time of presentation. Symptoms may be classified as local (direct effects of local tumor related to site), metastatic (direct effects of metastatic tumor related to site), or systemic (indirect effects of tumor not directly related to site).

Local effects of lung cancer and estimates of their frequency at presentation are shown in Table 36–4. Central lesions frequently cause cough, hemoptysis, and dyspnea. They also may cause hoarseness, dysphagia, wheezing, and symptoms resulting from superior vena cava obstruction or pericardial involvement. Peripheral lesions may be more common than central lesions. They frequently do not cause local symptoms, but they may cause cough, chest pain, and dyspnea because of pleural effusion or restrictive changes. New or increased chronic cough or expectoration in an older male smoker may herald the appearance of lung cancer.

Distant effects relate to the frequent sites of distant metas-

*Table 36–4.* **Local Effects of Lung Cancer at Presentation**

| Symptom or Sign | Frequency (%) |
|---|---|
| Cough/hemoptysis | 70/40 |
| Dyspnea | 40 |
| Chest pain | 35 |
| Hoarseness | 5 |
| Effects of superior vena caval obstruction | 5 |
| Wheezing | |
| Pericardial effusion | 2 |
| Effects of brachial plexus compression or Horner's syndrome | Rare |

*Table 36-5.* **Metastatic Effects of Lung Cancer at Presentation**

| Symptom or Sign | Frequency (%) |
|---|---|
| Bone pain/hepatomegaly | 25/20 |
| Lymphadenopathy | 20 |
| Neurologic manifestations of intracranial metastases | 5–10 |

tases. Table 36–5 reflects the tendency for tumors to spread to bone, liver, lymph nodes, and brain. The frequency of those manifestations at presentation is variable.

Systemic effects are listed in Table 36–6. These include endocrine and nonendocrine manifestations of disease. Endocrine manifestations of bronchogenic carcinoma have been extensively reviewed.[107] It has been estimated that 10% of patients with lung cancer have clinical manifestations of ectopic hormone production. Biochemical evidence of ectopic hormone production may be more common. Hypercalcemia may be found in more than 10% of patients with advanced lung cancer. This finding is most prevalent in squamous cell and large cell carcinomas and may or may not be related to lytic bone lesions. Parathyroid hormone–related protein, partially homologous to but distinct from parathyroid hormone, is the common cause of this phenomenon in patients without bone metastases.[108] Constitutional symptoms, neurologic syndromes, cutaneous changes, skeletal changes, and thrombotic events are prominent among nonendocrine systemic manifestations. They are detailed in Table 36–6.

In the patient who is evaluated because of symptoms or in asymptomatic screened patients, radiographic abnormalities

*Table 36-6.* **Systemic Effects of Bronchogenic Carcinoma**

Constitutional
    Weight loss
    Anorexia
    Weakness
    Fever
Neurologic
    Autonomic overactivity (Horner's syndrome)
    Corticocerebellar degeneration
    Spinal-cerebellar degeneration
    Carcinomatous myopathies (including Eaton-Lambert syndrome)
    Carcinomatous neuropathy
    Polymyositis
Cutaneous
    Acanthosis nigricans
    Dermatomyositis
    Scleroderma
    Tylosis
Skeletal
    Clubbing
    Hypertrophic pulmonary osteoarthropathy
Vascular coagulation
    Thrombophlebitis
    Disseminated intravascular coagulation
    Nonbacterial thrombotic endocarditis
Endocrine
    Antidiuretic hormone secretion
    Hypercalcemia (parathyroid hormone–related protein)
    Adrenocorticotropic hormone
    Gynecomastia
    Melanocyte-stimulating hormone

may suggest the diagnosis of lung cancer. Radiographic findings that are suggestive of malignancy include a new or enlarged pulmonary nodule (particularly if the outline is regular or notched and if calcium is absent), an enlarged hilar shadow, a rapidly increasing or nodular infiltrative lesion, unresolved pneumonia, localized atelectasis or emphysema, and bronchostenosis.[109] Squamous cell carcinoma may also be infrequently peripheral (31%), and it tends to be large when it is peripheral. It is commonly associated with hilar prominence (40%) and is frequently associated with bronchial obstruction (53%). Cavitation is not rare in squamous cell carcinoma (22%), in contrast to other histologic types ($\leqq$6%). Adenocarcinoma and large cell carcinoma are frequently peripheral and usually less than 4 cm in diameter (72% and 64%, respectively). An excellent review documents current radiographic presentations, diagnosis, and staging.[109]

In a patient with an abnormal chest radiograph that is suspicious for tumor, it is important to diagnose or exclude malignancy. Cytologic examination of expectorated sputum is a noninvasive procedure that may be diagnostic. Freshly processed samples of early morning sputum are best. Optimal yield results from a series of separate sputum samples collected on 5 consecutive days. Expectoration of sputum may be enhanced by manual or mechanical percussion or by aerosol induction.

If adequate sputum is not produced or is nondiagnostic, endoscopy may be rewarding, particularly for relatively central lesions. The fiberoptic bronchoscope allows visualizing and sampling some lesions beyond the central hilar regions and is generally well tolerated. Bronchoscopy can provide visualization and biopsy of endobronchial lesions, differential washings of bronchi, aspiration and brushings from various areas, and transbronchial biopsy of peribronchial lesions. It may also stimulate the production of good expectorated sputum samples. In a patient with a normal chest radiograph but a positive sputum cytologic finding or other suggestion of bronchogenic carcinoma, this technique may allow the identification and localization of an occult carcinoma. A positive finding on cytopathologic examination of sputum or bronchial washing is reliable for the diagnosis of malignancy (98%) and reasonably good (75%) for identifying cell type. It is important to realize, however, that a positive sputum cytologic finding rarely may be due to aspirated tumor cells shed from a head and neck malignancy.

In tumors that are too peripherally located for bronchoscopic diagnosis, transthoracic needle aspiration, or biopsy, usually performed under fluoroscopy, may provide a diagnosis. In reported series, the accuracy of this technique for malignant lesions has been estimated to be 74 to 96%. Pleural or pericardial fluid aspiration, mediastinoscopy or parasternal mediastinotomy, and scalene or supraclavicular node biopsies may be appropriate for individual cases.

In some patients, the techniques just described are not diagnostic, and a thoracotomy may be necessary. The decision as to when or if thoracotomy should be done must be individualized on the basis of a number of variables, including the radiographic appearance of the lesion, the growth rate of the lesion, the patient's age, the prevalence of locally endemic fungal infections, and the response to antituberculosis or antifungal therapy. Slow growth rate, small size, and calcification do not exclude malignancy, and a large proportion of coin lesions are malignant. Other imaging techniques for the characterization of coin lesions include [$^{18}$F]2-fluoro-2-deoxy-D-glucose (FDG) positron emission tomography (PET). The use of FDG-PET for the diagnosis of coin lesions is growing.[110, 111] FDG-PET is based on localizing tumors by their higher rates of glucose use. The specificity is compromised by increased FDG uptake in active tuberculosis, histoplasmosis, or abscess, but its overall accuracy seems to warrant its continued usage.[112] In general, in a patient with a coin lesion that is undiagnosed after other diagnostic studies, thoracotomy should be strongly considered because of the significant chance of malignancy and the high cure rate for these carcinomas when diagnosed early.

Although carcinoembryonic antigen levels and other marker substances are frequently elevated in all histologic types of lung cancer, these tests are not sensitive or specific enough to be of great clinical use in screening or diagnosis. In patients screened for lung cancer with sputum cytology and radiographs, positive cytologic results but a normal chest radiograph may be found. In such patients, a careful head and neck examination should be done to exclude carcinoma of the larynx, pharynx, and nasopharynx. If findings in such an examination are negative, fiberoptic bronchoscopy may be effective in localizing otherwise occult pulmonary tumors. Experimental techniques, using hematoporphyrin derivatives and fluorescent bronchoscopy, may also be helpful.

## STAGING

Because there is significant morbidity and mortality associated with the surgical treatment of lung cancer, it is important to identify and to exclude from primary surgical therapy patients who would not benefit from attempts at resection. Studies that identify distant and local disease and a staging system that organizes such information into categories of prognostic and therapeutic importance are useful in planning and evaluating the efficacy of therapy.

Most patients with lung cancer are not curable. Five-year survivorship for all patients is less than 10%. For surgically treated patients, it has been in the 20 to 50% range but has varied with selection criteria. Improved staging techniques may decrease the number of surgically treated patients and result in improved survival figures for the more select group. A frequent cause of treatment failure is nonresectable or residual disease, both local and distant. The tumors in many patients may exhibit evidence of nonresectability at a preliminary clinical investigation. Estimates of the percentage of patients whose disease is not resectable at presentation vary with criteria for resectability and patterns of referral, but probably only 20 to 35% of lung carcinomas are resectable.[113–116]

One criterion for nonresectability is the presence of distant metastases. If such metastases are present and detectable, they should not be overlooked in a patient for whom surgery is otherwise planned. Approximately half of the patients who have inoperable cancers at presentation may have distant metastases. Frequent sites of these metastases include bone, thorax (contralateral lung, mediastinum, and pericardium), skin and peripheral lymph nodes, liver, and brain. The frequency of distant metastases at initial diagnosis varies in relation to histologic cell type and diagnostic techniques used for staging.

A possible exception to the policy of not resecting a lung cancer if a distant metastasis is present is the patient with a resectable primary (non–small cell) and a resectable solitary brain metastasis. Uncontrolled studies have suggested meaningful palliation and occasional long-term survival with resection of the primary tumor and the brain metastasis (plus radiation to the brain).

In autopsy studies, distant metastases are common. The frequency of sites of distant metastases at autopsy varies in relation to histologic cell type. Common sites include lymph nodes, liver, adrenal gland, brain, bone, pleura, kidney, pancreas, heart, and pericardium.

Lung cancer is frequently a disseminated disease. The limited 5-year survivorship in patients who have undergone resection for the disease suggests that it is common for nonresectable disease to be undetectable or undetected before surgical attempts at cure. Supportive evidence is found in the work of Matthews and associates,[117] who have reviewed autopsy findings in patients who died within 30 days of a *curative* surgical resection of lung cancer. They found persistent disease in 35% of those patients. Metastases were predominantly distant in patients with histologic types other than squamous cell carcinoma, and they were equally distant and local in patients with squamous cell carcinomas. Frequent sites of distant metastases included adrenal glands, liver, lymph nodes, brain (particularly SCLC and adenocarcinoma), bone, kidney, and lung.

It is reasonable to attempt to evaluate patients with potentially operable disease to ensure that no detectable distant metastases preclude surgical therapy. In addition to history, physical examination, screening chemistries, and chest radiography, other diagnostic studies have been used for the staging of patients with lung cancer. Because the liver, pancreas, and adrenal glands are frequent sites of metastatic tumor involvement, the investigation of those organs may be appropriate. In most institutions, the computed tomographic scan is extended inferiorly to include the adrenal glands and the superior portion of the liver.

Hepatic involvement may be suspected from physical findings or screening chemistries. Detectable metastases are almost always associated with an elevated alkaline phosphatase level, but abnormal results of that test as well as tests for levels of bilirubin and serum glutamic-oxaloacetic transaminase are not specific, and false-positive elevations may be more frequent than true-positive elevations.

CT of the abdomen compares favorably with radioisotopic liver scan as a test of hepatic involvement with lung cancer and offers the advantage of surveying abdominal organs other than the liver as well.[118] Although cost-effectiveness of abdominal CT in the otherwise stage I patient is not well defined, the yield of this test may be appreciable, particularly in SCLC. It is reasonable to use this modality to stage all patients with NSCLC who have abdominal symptoms, weight loss, or performance status (PS).

Bone involvement is frequently detectable with noninvasive staging. Bone scans are often positive (46%), even in patients who have otherwise limited disease (32%). Radiographic bone surveys also have an appreciable yield; lesions are primarily lytic but may be blastic. The value of bone scans in asymptomatic patients is unproved and should be reserved for the symptomatic patient with an abnormal alkaline phosphatase but not of liver origin. CT of the brain with intravenous contrast administration is the test of choice in patients either with symptoms or in whom the clinician wants to rule out central nervous system metastasis. Bone marrow examination is a useful staging procedure in SCLC (about 24% positive), but it is not of great value in NSCLC. Immunocytologic detection of bone marrow micrometastases in operable NSCLC remains investigative.[119]

Unresectable local disease, similar to distant metastases, may be a cause of surgical failure. Mediastinoscopy is a safe, effective diagnostic technique that may show otherwise occult mediastinal tumor in a significant number of patients with lung cancer.[120–122] The prognostic implications of mediastinal node tumor and the procedure itself are discussed further in the next section. Scalene node biopsy is another technique for evaluation of regional disease. Although this biopsy technique may be of value in a patient with palpable nodes, it has a considerably lower yield than mediastinoscopy if the nodes are not palpable.

Chest CT as a staging tool has become the standard in the work-up of a patient with lung cancer. Its use must be individualized, and the technique is incapable of giving a histologic diagnosis of tumor extent. Mediastinal disease sufficient to contraindicate surgery may be detectable by other means, and modestly enlarged mediastinal nodes detected by CT may be reactive or may be malignant but resectable. Magnetic resonance imaging (MRI) is not superior to chest CT.[123] To attempt to evaluate patients more thoroughly, some newer imaging modalities are being employed. To compare the accuracy of CT and PET in local-regional lymph node staging, 68 patients underwent CT, PET, and surgical staging.[124] Surgical staging data were available for 690 lymph node samples. CT correctly identified nodal stage in 40 of 68 patients (59%), with understaging in 12 patients and overstaging in 16 patients. PET plus CT was accurate in 59 patients (87%), with understaging in 5 patients and overstaging in 4 patients. For N2/N3 disease, the sensitivity, specificity, and accuracy of CT were 75%, 63%, and 68%, respectively. For PET plus CT, they were 93%, 95%, and 94%, respectively. CT plus PET appears to be significantly more accurate than CT alone. The high negative predictive value of mediastinal PET may reduce the need for mediastinoscopy.[124]

A recommended approach toward diagnostic *staging studies* is provided in Table 36–7. Multiple staging systems have been devised for the categorization of disease patterns in patients with lung cancer. The system devised by the Task Force on Lung Cancer of the American Joint Committee for Cancer (AJCC) Staging and End Results Reporting classifies disease as to characteristics of T (primary tumor), N (regional lymph nodes), and M (distant metastases), then defines stage on the basis of the TNM patterns, defining criteria for assigning TNM categories and stages for lung carcinomas such that each group has similar life expectancy.

The revised International System for Staging Lung Cancer is presented in Tables 36–8 and 36–9.[125, 126] Subsets of patients are combined according to TNM descriptors into stages, each having similar treatment options and survival expectations. Stage I has been split into stages IA and IB. Stage II has now been divided into IIA and IIB with the patient group T3 N0 M0 being moved to the IIB category because of their improved survival compared with other stage III patients. Fifty-five percent of patients with pT1 N1 M0 lesion (stage IIA) are expected to survive 5 years or more following complete resection versus a 39% survival for patients with pT2 N1 M0 and a 38% survival for patients with a pT3 N0 M0 lesion (stage IIB). Stage IIIA patients now comprise T3 N1 M0, T1 N2 M0, T3 N2 M0. Clinically staged T3 N1 M0 tumors have a 9% 5-year survival compared with 13% for the remainder of the subsets in the group. Of the N2 group, 72% are accounted for by the cT2 N2 M0 category, 22% by cT3 N2 M0, and 6% by T1 N2 M0. For stages IIIB and IV, the classification is unchanged. The presence of satellite tumors in the primary tumor lobe should be classified as T4, whereas intrapulmonary ipsilateral metastasis in a nonprimary lobe is classified as M1. Urschel and colleagues[127] retrieved 11 articles from the literature in which 568 patients with satellite nodules underwent resection of the primary and satellite nodules. The 5-year actuarial survival was 20%, with the 5-year survival being better if the satellite nodules were in the primary lobe.[127] This survival is clearly better than that for T4 lesions, raising the question of whether the T4 designation is accurate. Satellite nodules in ipsilateral nonprimary lobes, however, share metastatic mechanisms and have survival results consistent with M1 stage disease. *All of the studies described in the treatment section have used the old staging system.*[128, 129] When the TNM definitions and stage grouping rules are applied to the database, the end results shown in Table 36–10 are obtained.

## PROGNOSIS

With the AJCC staging system applied before the era of accurate intraoperative staging, the 18-month survival rate for subsets of clinically staged patients with stage I disease was in the 49 to 65% range. For patients with stage III disease, it ranged from 4 to 15% (excluding 24% for patients with T3N0M0 lesions, including superior sulcus tumors), approximately 10 to 15% for stage III, M0 disease and 8% for stage III, M1 disease. More recent data in pathologically (p), surgically staged patients demonstrate 5-year survival rates as follows: pIA, 67%; pIB, 57%; pIIA, 55%; pIIB, 39%; pIIIA, 23%; cIIIB, 5%; cIV, 1%.[125] Survival experience by TNM subset and histologic cell type may vary in surgically staged patients. Comparing 5-year survival rates of squamous cell carcinoma with adenocarcinoma, following surgical resection, reveals superior survival for squamous

---

***Table 36–7. Recommended Staging Work-up***

History, including performance status and evaluation of weight loss
Physical examination
Screening chemistries, blood count, urinalysis
Chest radiography
CT and PET scanning
Bone scan with radiographs of abnormal areas
Mediastinoscopy at the time of surgery if tumor otherwise resectable
   (optional for small, well-differentiated peripheral lesions with
   negative mediastinal and hilar tomography, PET)
Upper abdominal CT (suggested before surgical resection)

PET, positron emission tomography.

*Table 36–8.* **TNM Definitions in the Revised International Staging System for Lung Cancer**

*Primary Tumor (T)*

| | |
|---|---|
| TX | Primary tumor cannot be assessed, or tumor proved by the presence of malignant cells in sputum or bronchial washings but not visualized by imaging or bronchoscopy |
| T0 | No evidence of primary tumor |
| Tis | Carcinoma in situ |
| T1 | Tumor ≤3 cm in greatest dimension, surrounded by lung or visceral pleura, without bronchoscopic evidence of invasions more proximal than the lobar bronchus* (e.g., not in the main bronchus) |
| T2 | Tumor with any of the following features of size or extent:<br>>3 cm in greatest dimension<br>Involves main bronchus, ≥2 cm distal to the carina<br>Invades the visceral pleura<br>Associated with atelectasis or obstructive pneumonitis that extends to the hilar region but does not involve the entire lung |
| T3 | Tumor of any size that directly invades any of the following: chest wall (including superior sulcus tumors), diaphragm, mediastinal pleura, parietal pericardium; or tumor in the main bronchus <2 cm distal to the carina but without involvement of the carina; or associated atelectasis or obstructive pneumonitis of the entire lung |
| T4 | Tumor of any size that invades any of the following: mediastinum, heart, great vessels, trachea, esophagus, vertebral body, carina; or tumor with a malignant pleural or pericardial effusion† or with satellite tumor nodules within the ipsilateral primary-tumor lobe of the lung |

*Regional Lymph Nodes (N)*

| | |
|---|---|
| NX | Regional lymph nodes cannot be assessed |
| N0 | No regional lymph node metastasis |
| N1 | Metastasis to ipsilateral peribronchial and/or ipsilateral hilar lymph nodes and intrapulmonary nodes involved by direct extension of the primary tumor |
| N2 | Metastasis to ipsilateral mediastinal and/or subcarinal lymph nodes |
| N3 | Metastasis to contralateral mediastinal, contralateral hilar, ipsilateral or contralateral scalene, or supraclavicular lymph nodes |

*Distant Metastasis (M)*

| | |
|---|---|
| MX | Presence of distant metastasis cannot be assessed |
| M0 | No distant metastasis |
| M1 | Distant metastasis present‡ |

*The uncommon superficial tumor of any size with its invasive component limited to the bronchial wall, which may extend proximal to the main bronchus, is also classified T1.

†Most pleural effusions associated with lung cancer are due to tumor. There are a few patients, however, in whom multiple cytopathologic examinations of pleural fluid show no tumor. In these cases, the fluid is nonbloody and is not an exudate. When these elements and clinical judgment dictate that the effusion is not related to the tumor, the effusion should be excluded as a staging element, and the patient's disease should be staged T1, T2, or T3. Pericardial effusion is classified according to the same rules.

‡Separate metastatic tumor nodules in the ipsilateral nonprimary-tumor lobes of the lung also are classified M1.

From Mountain CF. Revisions in the International System for Staging Lung Cancer. Chest 1997;111:1710–17.

*Table 36–9.* **Stage Grouping of TNM Subsets* in the Revised International System of Lung Cancer Staging**

| Stage | TNM Subset |
|---|---|
| 0 | Carcinoma in situ |
| IA | T1 N0 M0 |
| IB | T2 N0 M0 |
| IIA | T1 N1 M0 |
| IIB | T2 N1 M0 |
| | T3 N0 M0 |
| IIIA | T3 N1 M0 |
| | T1 N2 M0 |
| | T2 N2 M0 |
| | T3 N2 M0 |
| IIIB | T4 N0 M0 |
| | T4 N1 M0 |
| | T4 N2 M0 |
| | T1 N3 M0 |
| | T2 N3 M0 |
| | T3 N3 M0 |
| | T4 N3 M0 |
| IV | Any T Any N M1 |

*Staging is not relevant for occult carcinoma, designated TXN0M0.

From Mountain C. Revisions in the International System for Staging Lung Cancer. Chest 1997;111:1710–17.

stage for stage to that in patients staged clinically. This superiority does not imply a therapeutic benefit to surgical staging. Patients who previously had occult mediastinal disease and were staged clinically as stage I or stage II may now be staged surgically as stage III. This phenomenon results in the placement of stage I and stage II disease in

*Table 36–10.* **Clinical and Surgical Pathologic Stage***

| | Months After Treatment (Cumulative Percent Surviving) | | | | |
|---|---|---|---|---|---|
| | 12 (%) | 24 (%) | 36 (%) | 48 (%) | 60 (%) |
| *cStage†* | | | | | |
| cIA (*n* = 687) | 91 | 79 | 71 | 67 | 61 |
| cIB (*n* = 1189) | 72 | 54 | 46 | 41 | 38 |
| cIIA (*n* = 29) | 79 | 49 | 38 | 34 | 34 |
| cIIB (*n* = 357) | 59 | 41 | 33 | 26 | 24 |
| cIIIA (*n* = 511) | 50 | 25 | 18 | 14 | 13 |
| cIIIB (*n* = 1030) | 34 | 13 | 7 | 6 | 5 |
| cIV (*n* = 1427) | 19 | 6 | 2 | 2 | 1 |
| *pStage‡* | | | | | |
| pIA (*n* = 511) | 94 | 86 | 80 | 73 | 67 |
| pIB (*n* = 549) | 87 | 76 | 67 | 62 | 57 |
| pIIA (*n* = 76) | 89 | 70 | 66 | 61 | 55 |
| pIIB (*n* = 375) | 73 | 56 | 46 | 42 | 39 |
| pIIIA (*n* = 399) | 64 | 40 | 32 | 26 | 23 |

*Overall comparison: *p*<0.05.

†Percentage distribution of cell types: adenocarcinoma, 47.2% (2466/5230); squamous cell carcinoma, 33.9% (1773/5230); large cell carcinoma, 3.1% (163/5230); small cell carcinoma, 11.9% (624/5230); NOS (carcinoma not specified), 3.9% (204/5230).

‡Percentage distribution of cell types: adenocarcinoma, 53.0% (1012/1910); squamous cell carcinoma, 41.6% (794/1910); large cell carcinoma, 3.6% (68/1910); NOS (carcinoma not specified), 1.9% (36/1910).

From Mountain C. Revisions in the International System for Staging Lung Cancer. Chest 1997;111:1710–17.

cell carcinoma in the T1 N0, T1 N1, and T2 N1 subsets (T1 N0, 83% vs. 69%, *p*=0.02; T1 N1, 75% vs. 52%, *p*=0.04; T2 N1, 53% vs. 25%, *p*=0.01).[130, 131]

Survivorship in patients surgically staged appears superior

smaller but more favorable categories. Stage III prognosis may also be improved by the inclusion of patients who without surgical staging would have been classified as stage I. Although survival may appear to be improved in all stages of disease, much of this improvement may be due to a shift of patients from (clinical) stages I and II to (pathologic) stage III.[125] As a subgroup, patients with N2 disease who undergo resection have a varied outcome. Vansteenkiste and associates[132] reported an analysis of 18 series in the literature to determine if any clinical prognostic factors could be identified. The absence of preoperative evidence of N2 disease was a favorable factor. The extent of surgery, lobectomy versus pneumonectomy, did not have a significant effect on outcome. The histopathologic tumor type favors squamous cell carcinoma, with these patients generally doing better than those with other cell types. In all of the series, the extent of the primary tumor (lower T stage) was associated with a survival advantage. In addition, patients with only one mediastinal lymph node station involved had a better prognosis, whereas metastasis to the subcarinal lymph nodes portended a poorer prognosis. These analyses are all hampered by the limited number of patients enrolled in the studies, necessitating pooling of data.

Molecular analysis may be an important adjunct for accurate staging. A study of 244 stage I NSCLC patients treated at the Brigham and Women's Hospital investigated the effects of demographics, surgical extent, pathologic features, and molecular factors on cancer-free survival.[133] The molecular analysis consisted of immunohistochemical staining for *erb*-B2, *ras*-p21, p53, Rb, *bcl-2*, and blood group A antigen and polymerase chain reaction and sequence analysis for k-*ras* codon 12. p53 positivity was associated with a decreased cancer-free survival in univariate analysis ($p = 0.018$). Stepwise multivariate analysis identified solid mucin-producing adenocarcinoma tumor, lymphatic invasion, p53 expression, tumor dimension 4 cm or greater, k-*ras* mutation, and H-*ras*-p21 negativity as influencing cancer-free survival. This study did not find any correlation with abnormalities of Rb, *bcl-2*, or *erb*-B2, which have been reported in other studies.

Perioperative risk may be greater in men than in women; may increase with age, particularly with men aged 80 years or older; may be greater in right-sided than in left-sided pneumonectomy; and may be greater in pneumonectomy than in lobectomy patients.[134, 135] Various studies suggest that perioperative blood transfusions may increase the likelihood of treatment failure in surgically resected patients.[136, 137] Neuroendocrine markers and carcinoembryonic antigen were not found to be of prognostic significance in patients with resected stage I and stage II NSCLC.[138]

For patients with inoperable or nonresectable disease, PS is strongly correlated with survival duration. The assessment of PS by the Karnofsky performance scale (see Chapter 8)[139] or by similar scales has been shown to correlate strongly with survival.[140, 141] The median survival rate for placebo-treated patients with extensive disease ranged from 5 weeks (SCLC) to 11 weeks (large cell carcinoma). For limited disease, the median survival rate ranged from 11.7 weeks (SCLC) to 22.4 weeks (large cell carcinoma). Within limited and extensive groups, however, survival was more closely related to PS than to histologic type. In extensive disease, the median survival rate varied from 2 weeks (Karnofsky PS 30) to 7 weeks (PS 50) to 25 weeks (PS 100). For limited disease, the median survival rate varied from 7 weeks (PS 30) to 28 weeks (PS 100). Other factors correlating with poor prognosis in patients with nonresectable disease include the presence of weight loss in the 6 months before diagnosis and, of lesser importance, brain metastases, patient age of more than 70 years, and hepatic metastases.

The natural history of untreated advanced lung cancer (nonresectable or recurring after resection) has been addressed by the studies by the Veterans Administration of placebo-treated groups (survival figures discussed earlier)[142] and by earlier studies of untreated patients.[143–148] In a controlled trial[149] of chemotherapy for advanced NSCLC (discussed further subsequently), median survival in the supportive care–alone group was 17 weeks, with 1-year survival roughly 10%. This group consisted of 50 evaluable patients, 90% with extensive disease and 40% with an Eastern Cooperative Oncology Group (ECOG) PS of 2 (60% PS 0 or PS 1).

Multiple factors are of prognostic significance in resectable and nonresectable cancers. The accurate assessment of prognosis may be based on the patient's age, sex, symptom status, PS, weight loss, comorbid diseases, tumor histologic type, tumor location, tumor size, characteristics of regional and distant metastases, and therapy. The impact of therapeutic regimens on survivorship is difficult to evaluate unless the pertinent prognostic factors of the treatment group are defined.

## Treatment

### SURGERY

Although surgical resection is the preferred treatment for lung cancer, only a few patients with this disease are eligible for this mode of therapy. The development of improved techniques for earlier detection and the development of more effective adjuvant therapy, however, may increase the percentage of candidates for resection of curative intent.

The surgical management of patients with bronchogenic carcinoma begins in the preoperative period with careful assessment and staging. To optimize treatment and to estimate prognosis, it is useful to identify the extent of the disease carefully by preoperative and intraoperative staging. This staging may facilitate an appropriate surgical resection and allow postoperative treatment to be tailored to the needs of the patients.

**Preoperative Assessment.** Distant metastatic disease, including dissemination to the supraclavicular lymph nodes, is a contraindication to pulmonary resection for cure. Although disease metastatic to the mediastinum is commonly technically unresectable (e.g., by virtue of involvement of the great vessels), when it is technically resectable (commonly ipsilateral and intranodal), the presence of mediastinal disease should not be a contraindication to resection. Figure 36–1 summarizes the 5-year survival rates for patients with N2 disease who have undergone careful pathologic staging and complete surgical resection. Patients with T1 lesions, squamous histology, and no CT evidence of adenopathy probably do not require this procedure because the incidence of nodal involvement is probably less than 10%; however,

## CLINICAL

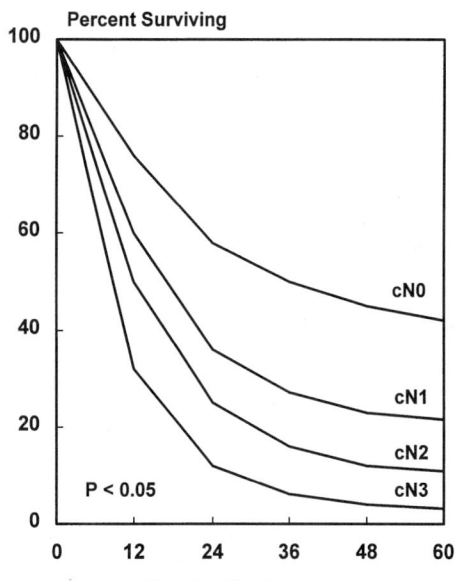

## SURGICAL

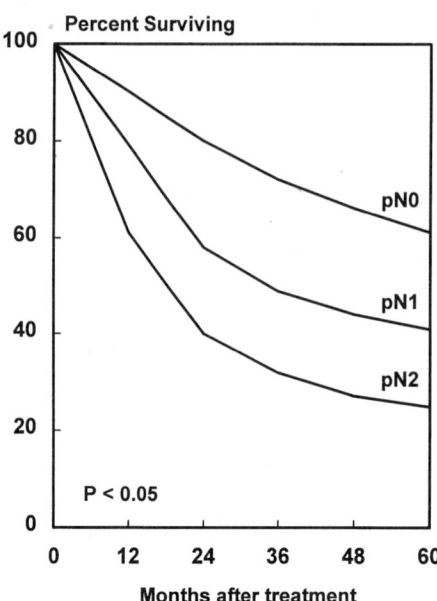

**Figure 36–1.** *Left,* Cumulative survival according to clinical estimates of the extent of regional lymph node involvement, the cN classification. *Right,* Cumulative survival according to clinical estimates of the extent of regional lymph node involvement, determined from pathologic examination of resected specimens, the pN classification. (From Mountain CF, Dressler C. Regional lymph node classification for lung cancer staging. Chest 1997;111:1718–23.)

in stage I patients with central lesions or adenocarcinoma histology and in patients with clinical stage II disease, it is worthwhile to exclude mediastinal metastases, particularly because (1) there are numerous reports showing an 18% or greater false-negative rate based on CT scans, and (2) prospective trials have shown a significant benefit to preoperative induction chemotherapy in patients with N2 (see later).[120]

Pleural effusion containing malignant cells is a contraindication to pulmonary resection. Pulmonary resection is rarely possible in patients with cytologically negative effusions, however, and they may have prolonged survival. Although such patients exist, most lung cancer patients with negative cytology and ipsilateral effusions have pleural disease, and survival of patients with positive and negative cytology may be indistinguishable. The presence of chest wall involvement that does not involve the vertebral bodies or the sternum is not a contraindication to surgery. Recurrent laryngeal nerve paralysis on the side of the tumor is considered an absolute contraindication to pulmonary resection. Superior vena caval obstruction secondary to tumor is considered a contraindication to curative resection, although technically in some instances resection of the superior vena cava may be feasible.

The involvement of the main stem bronchi within 2 cm of the carina is a contraindication to resection because it is difficult to obtain an adequate surgical margin with these tumors. In some radiosensitive tumors that are close to the carina, an occasional prolonged survival can be obtained by use of a combination of preoperative radiation therapy and surgery. A repeated biopsy following radiation therapy that reveals no evidence of tumor within 2 cm of the carina indicates that an adequate surgical resection may be feasible. Problems with bronchial stump healing may occur, however, if high-dose radiotherapy is given.

The involvement of the phrenic nerve or diaphragm is not an absolute contraindication to pulmonary resection, although a poorer prognosis is indicated. Occasionally resection of these structures, with adequate margins, results in a

prolonged survival rate. The involvement of the chest wall, phrenic nerve, or diaphragm does not contraindicate resection. The diaphragm can be resected and reconstituted with prosthetic material, as can the chest wall. All cell types of lung cancer, including infrequent cases of SCLC, are amenable to surgical resection when in the appropriate stage.

The preoperative assessment should identify patients who are not surgical candidates by virtue of comorbid disease (e.g., recent myocardial infarction, other lethal malignancy) or impaired pulmonary function. Preoperative pulmonary function studies showing 1-second forced expiratory volume levels less than 40% of predicted or a maximal ventilatory volume level less than 50% of predicted generally contraindicate resection, as would an arterial carbon dioxide partial pressure greater than 45 mm Hg. This is a rough guideline, however, which should not be interpreted as implying that pulmonary resection would be tolerated in patients marginally or moderately surpassing these pulmonary functions. Assessment of the safety of pulmonary resection in difficult cases may vary with the extent of required surgery and may require more extensive pulmonary evaluation preoperatively. The functional capacity of the cardiorespiratory system can account for three fourths of postoperative morbidity and mortality. Cardiac complications cause about 20% of postoperative deaths, and a history of cardiac disease doubles the risk of major morbidity (18% vs. 9%). A preoperative electrocardiogram is mandatory as well as specialized testing in higher risk patients.

**Surgical Staging.** Because the presence or absence of lymph node metastases and the location of lymph node involvement are of prognostic importance, the determination of lymph node spread by mediastinoscopy is useful in the preoperative evaluation of patients. Surgical staging via mediastinoscopy helps to determine resectability and to avoid unnecessary thoracotomy.

There is no uniformity of opinion regarding the indications for mediastinoscopy before pulmonary resection. The diagnostic yield of this procedure is 10 to 75% and varies considerably with the histologic type of the tumor, the size and location of the primary tumor, and the extent of the disease as revealed by noninvasive studies. The incidence of positive findings on mediastinoscopy depends on patient selection. Patients with advanced disease and those with more undifferentiated tumors have a higher incidence of positive findings. Although some surgeons recommend routine cervical mediastinal exploration before thoracotomy and others use it infrequently, the development of mediastinoscopy has decreased the incidence of patients with unresectable disease having to undergo thoracotomy.[120–122] Patients who have negative findings on cervical mediastinal exploration have an incidence of unresectability at the time of thoracotomy of less than 15%. However, many surgeons believe that not all patients with bronchogenic carcinoma require mediastinal exploration preoperatively. Patients with well-differentiated peripheral carcinomas and a normal mediastinum on a CT scan, radiograph, and PET have a low incidence of positive mediastinal node involvement. Most surgeons recommend that cervical mediastinal exploration be employed in patients with a diagnosis of undifferentiated carcinoma and in those who have central lesions. Usually routine cervical mediastinoscopy is not performed for peripheral well-differentiated tumors when there is no evidence of abnormality of the mediastinum on chest radiography, CT, and PET.

Mediastinoscopy is especially indicated when radiographs show mild mediastinal abnormalities in a patient with an otherwise resectable cancer. It is also useful in the elderly patient or in a patient with severe cardiovascular or pulmonary disease for whom a thoracotomy carries a high risk. Some patients have enlarged mediastinal and hilar nodes secondary to hyperplasia with no tumor involvement. Some forms of mediastinal tumor are resectable. All of these patients would be inappropriately denied curative resection if the cancer was deemed unresectable without a cervical mediastinal exploration being performed.

Mediastinal exploration can be performed by a cervical or a parasternal incision. In the cervical approach, a small incision is made in the lower neck over the trachea, and a plane of dissection is established just anterior to the trachea and deep to the innominate vessels. Through this approach, the right and left paratracheal lymph nodes can be carefully evaluated, and in most instances, the carinal nodes as well as the right and left main stem bronchial lymph nodes can be biopsied. The azygos lymph nodes on the right side can also be evaluated through this approach. The parasternal approach is performed through a vertical or transverse incision over the second or third costal cartilage on the right or left side. A small portion of rib and costal cartilage can be removed, and the perihilar areas can be evaluated more thoroughly than from the cervical approach. The parasternal approach is commonly indicated for left-sided lesions because the presence of the aortic arch prevents an adequate evaluation of the distal left main stem bronchus from a cervical approach. Juxtahilar lesions are more easily evaluated through the parasternal approach than through the cervical approach. The routine use of scalene lymph node biopsy is not recommended because the yield is low unless the lymph nodes are palpable.

**Surgical Resection.** A wide variety of operations has been used in the surgical treatment of this disease since the initial report of a successful pneumonectomy for lung cancer in 1933.[150] Lobectomy has been the most widely used operation during this time, but the need for pneumonectomy varies between 10 and 55%. Since the 1980s, there has been increasing interest in the use of conservative resections—the minimal operation encompassing all the known areas of disease. This trend reflects the major surgical objective of conserving pulmonary tissue and pulmonary function. Minimal surgery has been facilitated by increased use of careful intraoperative staging, including the evaluation of frozen sections of biopsy specimens of surgical margins and lymph nodes obtained at the time of surgery. This kind of intraoperative staging has allowed the use of wedge resections, segmental resections, sleeve lobectomies, or more aggressive resections, including the chest wall and diaphragm, the lower roots of the brachial plexus in superior sulcus tumors, and parts of the left atrium in selected patients.

**Limited Resection Versus Lobectomy and Pneumonectomy.** Uncontrolled studies have suggested that more limited resections might produce equivalent results to more radical procedures, such as lobectomy and pneumonectomy. This question was addressed by the Lung Cancer Study Group (LCSG) in a randomized trial in stage I patients. Patients were randomized intraoperatively to a limited wedge or segmental resection versus standard lobectomy. Results showed that local-regional recurrence rates tripled with limited resection (0.022, 0.044, and 0.086 person/year for lobectomy, segmentectomy, and wedge resection, respectively). The overall cancer-related death rate was increased 50% with limited resections.[151] This increase has been confirmed by others.[152] There was no difference in postoperative pulmonary function between the two groups. Lobectomy and pneumonectomy are currently recommended, whenever possible. Limited resections, however, are still superior to other alternatives in patients with marginal pulmonary reserve.

**Pancoast and Other Superior Sulcus Tumors.** T3 tumors that occur at the thoracic apex constitute an important subset of patients with NSCLC. Classically, Pancoast tumors involve the apex of the lung; invade the first and second ribs posteriorly; involve the lower brachial plexus nerve roots (T1 and C8), producing pain that radiates down the inner aspect of the arm and forearm; often involve the stellate ganglion, causing a Horner's syndrome; and frequently exhibit a squamous histology. Anterior-superior sulcus tumors involve the apex of the lung, invade the first and second ribs anteriorly, involve the subclavian vein and artery, and cause primarily chest wall pain. Radiologic evaluation includes a computed tomographic scan and an MRI scan, particularly if involvement of the vascular structures is suspected. Although bone scans are often obtained that show local rib destruction, they usually do not show distant metastases and in most cases are unnecessary. Results from treatment of Pancoast and other superior sulcus tumors were dismal until Paulson[153] and Shaw and coworkers[154] described the use of preoperative radiation therapy, resulting in a 5-year survival of 31%. These results have not changed. It is imperative that patients initially undergo mediastinoscopy before therapy because a small group of these patients show mediastinal lymph node metastases that carry an extremely poor prognosis and are a contraindication to surgical resection. Following this, radiation therapy is initiated either in 30-Gy fractions over 2 weeks or in 20-Gy fractions over 4 weeks.[155] Resection is carried out 3 to 4 weeks later and includes en bloc removal of the upper lobe, involved ribs and transverse spinal processes, dorsal sympathetic chain, and lower trunk of the brachial plexus, if necessary. As in other stage II tumors, a complete mediastinal lymph node dissection is recommended. With this approach, 21 to 90% of tumors can be completely resected.[156, 157]

The prognosis following perioperative radiation and complete surgical resection has not changed since Shaw and Paulson first described this approach. Poor prognostic factors that have been identified include N2 disease, incomplete resection, and the use of wedge resection instead of lobectomy.[158]

**Results of Surgical Resection.** The survival rate after surgical resection of (resectable) NSCLC is directly related to the histologic type and the TNM classification or the stage of the disease (see Table 36-10 and Fig. 36-1). Patients with stage I carcinoma of the lung in whom careful surgical staging has been performed can anticipate an excellent 5-year survival rate. As Table 36–10 and Figure 36–1 indicate, patients with T1 N0, T2 N0, or T1 N1 lesions have a favorable prognosis after pulmonary resection. The survival rates diminish in stage II and stage III resectable lung cancer. The presence of mediastinal lymph node involvement, regardless of the cell type, is associated with a lower 5-year survival rate after surgical resection, but it may be improved in the subset of patients with resectable disease.[159]

To assess modern mortality rates following resection for lung cancer, the LCSG analyzed the 30-day operative mortality at participating institutions from 1979 through 1981.[160] During these 3 years, 2220 resections for lung cancer were done in 12 institutions from five contributing LCSG centers. There were 1508 lobectomies, 569 pneumonectomies, and 143 lesser resections. The operative mortality was calculated for each type of resection and for different age groups.

Overall operative mortality for the 2220 resections was 3.7%. The operative mortality for segmental or wedge resection was 1.4%, for lobectomy 2.9%, and for pneumonectomy 6.2%. The mortality rates increased with age, increasing from 1.3% in patients younger than 50 years to 8.1% in patients older than 80. It was revealing, nonetheless, that 85 patients older than 70 years underwent pneumonectomy with a low operative mortality of 5.9%. Mortality rates in other series may be higher, as a function of patient selection or treatment-related factors.[161–163]

**Occult Non–Small Cell Lung Cancer (TX N0 M0).** Lung cancer that is diagnosed by cytologic examination of sputa samples but associated with normal findings on chest imaging studies is considered *occult* lung cancer. Most of these tumors are proximal squamous cell carcinomas. With widespread use of flexible bronchoscopy, the advent and increasing resolution of CT scans, and the introduction of new technologies (e.g., MRI, PET), the incidence of truly occult lung carcinoma has become rare. One third of patients thought to have occult lung cancer are found to have a primary tumor in the head and neck region that explains the cytologic findings.[164] A thorough upper aerodigestive tract examination is mandatory in these patients. Developments in lung cancer screening, including the generation of new monoclonal antibodies that detect specific malignant changes on exfoliated cells in sputa and the use of the lung imaging fluorescence endoscope bronchoscopy, which detects au-

tofluorescence of malignant and premalignant cells using a helium-cadmium (442 nm) laser, may increase the incidence of new occult lung cancers detected.[165, 166] In cases of true occult lung cancer, a systematic and meticulous sampling of cytologic specimens obtained by brushing and washing each individual segmental bronchus is necessary, taking great care to avoid cross-contamination of specimens from neighboring bronchi. Repeated positive findings (on at least two different occasions) from the same bronchus is enough evidence to warrant definitive treatment.

Treatment of occult lung carcinoma generally has been limited to surgical resection of the involved portion of the lung. This treatment usually necessitates lobectomy or pneumonectomy, although segmentectomy is occasionally possible. Other forms of therapy have been reported, however.[167] Successful treatment of occult and early lung cancers with a combination of external beam radiation and iridium 192 endobronchial brachytherapy has been reported.[167] Japanese investigators also have produced impressive results with photodynamic therapy (PDT) using photofrin as a photosensitizing agent and either an argon or excimer dye laser as the light source.[168] Finally, a report using transbronchoscopic electrocautery has shown some promise.[169] These latter treatments have been developed primarily as an alternative to surgical resection for patients who are not surgical candidates, but if early success rates are substantiated, one or more of these therapies may replace surgery as the treatment of choice for these lesions.

Survival of patients treated for occult lung carcinoma is generally high. Following surgical resection, recurrences are rare, but second primary lung cancers develop in many patients. Five-year survival in patients treated with external-beam irradiation and endobronchial brachytherapy has been reported to exceed 85%.[167] Although PDT also has a high clinical complete response rate, with all 30 lesions in 26 patients responding in one report, only 5 of 15 lesions (33%) treated surgically following PDT were confirmed to have a pathologic complete response.[170] Electrocautery also has an impressive clinical complete response rate of 12 of 15 lesions (80%) in 10 of 13 patients (77%); however, histologic confirmation and long-term survival data are lacking.[169]

## RADIATION THERAPY

Radiotherapy in the management of lung cancer may be used with curative or palliative intent. We use palliative radiotherapy for patients who exhibit distressing symptoms and signs caused by the primary tumor or metastatic lesions. Palliative radiotherapy uses brief, intense courses of treatment intended to relieve symptoms rapidly for patients with short life expectancy. For definitive or curative treatment, the radiation may be administered by itself, as a single modality, or as part of a multimodality approach with surgery, chemotherapy, and immunotherapy. The radiation therapy goals should be based on a careful clinical evaluation, including staging and the histologic diagnosis. The recommended pretherapy staging work-up has been summarized in Table 36–7.

Few objective facts support the use of radiotherapy in asymptomatic, unresectable, or inoperable lung cancer. Technical improvements have made delivery of radiotherapy to deeply located tumors rather easy. Subsequent to the ortho-voltage and cobalt 60 era, the peak radiotherapy dose is absorbed beneath the skin surface so that erythema rarely, if ever, causes limitation of dose. Despite surrounding skin toxicity, the tolerance of other normal tissue limits most of the dose schemes in thoracic radiotherapy. Spinal cord tolerance, in particular, dictates total and daily dose. Reports of myelopathy at doses less than 50 Gy in 5 weeks are rare but have limited the dose used in an attempt to prevent the complication of radiation-induced myelopathy.

Other normal tissues, the esophagus acutely and the heart and lungs in the subacute and late periods, are more likely to be the dose-limiting structures for higher doses of radiotherapy. For the most part, the tolerances of these organs are based on animal models and extrapolations from other diseases but rarely are based on data derived from patients with lifelong smoking habits. At a dose of 40 Gy to the heart, 5% of patients develop coronary or pericardial disease.[171] Because this estimate is derived from younger patients with Hodgkin's disease, it is unclear how to extrapolate these observations to older patients who have lifelong cigarette habits. Although intuition might suggest that these patients would have less tolerance, there is a surprising lack of data for heart tolerance or late effects. This lack may be due more to the limited duration of survival for the group of patients subjected to definitive irradiation. Many of these patients succumb to the disease or comorbid conditions before the chronic radiotherapy toxicity might be manifested. Hypoxic, poorly vascularized, elderly normal tissues, however, may tolerate more radiation than the same tissues from younger Hodgkin's disease patients with pristine hearts and lungs. There are, for instance, no data concerning the tolerance of coronary artery bypass grafts to subsequent lung irradiation. Pericardial toxicity, the other commonly recognized risk in Hodgkin's disease, is rarely found. Cardiac valves and the myocardium itself are tolerant to even high doses of thoracic irradiation.

Lung data for tolerance are based on whole-lung irradiation either in the pediatric population, in which whole-lung therapy was once used more commonly in Wilms' tumors and Ewing's sarcoma, or in rodent models under experimental conditions. Tolerance of partial organ irradiation is not clearly defined, particularly for patients exposed to lifelong tobacco addiction. Today, investigators in this field are assessing innovations in radiotherapy treatment planning, dosimetry, beam placement, dose, volume, fractionation, and the role of radiation therapy and the role of other modalities in the subsets of patients not selected to be eligible for curative surgical approaches.

Radiotherapy requires technical sophistication, which has improved over the decades. Advances in the delivery of radiotherapy allow higher doses to be administered without injury to the skin. Simulators, treatment planning systems, and dosimetry have allowed clinicians to provide a better distribution of the radiotherapy, a more homogeneous tumor dose, and distribution of lower, less injurious doses of radiotherapy to the surrounding normal tissues. Tumors can receive larger doses than the more delicate neighboring tissues and organs. In contrast to the dose of many chemotherapeutic agents, the proper dose of radiotherapy has not been determined by formal dose-escalation methodology but rather

from analogous dose and volume limits in other diseases. For lung cancer, this situation has limited the tumor doses used.

In addition to dose, the issue of irradiation volume is crucial for local control and is likely to be influential or even dominant in the frequency of pulmonary toxicity. Based on the Halsted hypothesis articulated for breast cancer, which suggests orderly spread of cancer from the primary to regional lymphatics, inclusion of mediastinal, hilar, and supraclavicular lymphatics has been the mainstream practice of thoracic radiotherapy. The frequent finding of nodes supported this practice for patients brought to thoracotomy. These techniques treat regional lymphatics in the contralateral hilar and scalene or supraclavicular nodal regions, and surgeons for curative therapy never dissected these nodal regions. These nodal inclusions cause larger volumes of innocent normal esophagus and lungs to treat clinically uninvolved nodes. Although treatment of these clinically negative nodes has become the normal practice, the hypothesis that the treatment of uninvolved nodal tissue improves survival or local control has never been tested. The downside of this practice is that these larger volumes limit the total dose to gross tumor or subject the normal tissues to toxicity, particularly when blended with chemotherapy. Today, investigators are deviating from this practice and conducting studies with more limited volumes and increasing the total doses to the tumor. The question of elective treatment of nodal stations that are either clinically negative or normal sized on CT seems to be more accepted and commonly used. Clinical trials are needed to show that the resultant larger doses improve local control or at least do not lead to unacceptable toxicity.

Fractionation, the division of the total doses into daily or more frequent segments, provides another thoracic radiotherapy variable. As practiced from the beginning of the 20th century, radiotherapy has been administered once each day, Monday to Friday. Only more recently has the community begun to explore multiple daily fraction schedules, including some that treat through weekends. With a smaller dose separated by a minimum of 4 hours, today usually 6 to 8 hours allows for repair between fractions of the damage. A smaller dose, less than the 1.8- to 2.0-Gy standard fractions, causes a higher frequency of late effects to normal tissue. Providing more radiation to the tumor in a short period of time may lead to better tumor control by eliminating an aggressively repopulating clone of cells, which grow between fractions with longer intervals. These hypotheses have fueled the radiotherapy community's disquiet about split-course treatment and hypofractionation using larger daily dose and planned gaps to allow for repair of acute effects to normal tissue and reoxygenation. Using smaller fractions of radiation exposure to normal tissues reduces the truly debilitating late effects, such as radiation pneumonitis and fibrosis or esophageal stricture. Allowing treatment interruptions for acute toxicity (lowered blood counts, esophageal discomfort) or planning breaks in therapy to allow for these reactions to subside has been shown to decrease beneficial outcomes.[172]

When radiotherapy and chemotherapy are used in patient treatment, the scheduling of the modalities must be described. *Concurrent treatment* indicates that both modalities are given at the same time. *Sequential therapy* gives one modality before the other without overlap. *Alternating mo-*

*dalities* describes a method of attempting to use both modalities in full dose, within the same period of weeks, but with alternating chemotherapy and radiotherapy weeks, which causes gaps in the radiotherapy. One can blend the local modality early in the course of therapy or delay it until later in the course. Dose, volume, fractionation, timing, and integration are definable variables that may influence beneficial and negative effects of therapy.

**Treatment Planning and Dosimetry Advances.** Computers, as used in imaging (CT and MRI), provide new capability to reconstruct solid structures from planar images. Dose can be recorded for each voxel of normal tissue and tumor so that cumulative dose information for organs and target volumes treated can be collected and analyzed. This approach allows collection of information about the part of organs receiving doses and the remainder of the organ that is spared treatment. These data promise to provide tolerances to percentage of the sensitive organ treated. In the past, we spoke of organ tolerance but could not prove with data if the tolerance was greater if portions of the organ were protected from radiation exposure. Absorbed doses in tissue require information about the stopping power of the tissue traversed by the entering beams. CT provides the *Hounsfield numbers*, which record the matrix of dose absorbed corrected by the density of the tissue traversed. With this information, we have the ability to determine correctly the stopping ability of the tissue for each patient: Those with hyperaerated, emphysematous lungs allow less radiation to be absorbed, so more penetrates. Those with metallic objects, bones, or consolidated lung absorb more radiation than normally aerated lungs. Before CT planning methods, doses were prescribed to depths or points that assumed water density of the traversed tissue regardless of whether it was aerated lung or bony tissue.

Analytic and perceptual tools, such as dose-volume histograms and beam's-eye views, have revolutionized dosimetry and treatment planning. The technical improvements introduced by integrating these ideas provide new ways to administer and record dose to targets and to avoid dosing structures that formerly limited the tumor treatment. Mathematical models propose methods to predict normal tissue complication and tumor control probabilities.[173–175] Dose can be displayed and an array of competing plans compared by analysis of proportional doses to organs (dose-volume histogram); target coverage and normal tissue sparing can be visualized using computer graphics displaying the target and distinguishing it from the identified crucial normal tissue by use of the beam's-eye view display. This approach provides a perspective similar to being able to peer through the patient with x-ray vision from the radiation source. This *virtual* accomplishment allows the use of beams from angles that were never considered before because one could not appreciate that the target was covered or a sensitive normal tissue either in or outside the field of treatment. With these three-dimensional capabilities, clinicians can be assured that tumor targets are well covered and normal tissues are excluded if desired, and we can even be sure of what margin we have added. This approach offers the tools for formal dose-escalation studies. These can be carried out to determine if larger doses can produce better control rates than in the past. These theories acknowledge that doses and volumes are interrelated, and the larger volumes employed to treat lymph node structures at risk potentially impair the ability to increase dose. The downside of not treating nodes is the potential problem of relapse in these structures leading to failure to cure or local failure. Because the doses to structures are more precisely defined, however, retreatment and field junctions, which can overlap doses, may now be accomplished, if not more safely, more secure in the knowledge of what is being done. These tools provide a means to rediscover the toxicity and efficacy of thoracic radiotherapy in lung cancer. At the same time, this approach provides baseline information to integrate radiotherapy into multimodal approaches as needed for the different stages of lung cancer.

Radiotherapy, similar to surgery, is a local form of therapy. It can eliminate cancer cells but may injure or destroy normal tissues if they are treated to a cancer-killing dose. Treatment needs to focus the high dose to the target region, where there are high prospects of cancer. To hit the target region and to distribute the lower, repairable, less toxic doses to adjacent normal tissues, we need to aim beams more precisely. Rapidly dividing cells tend to be more prone to cell death than quiescent, resting cells. Finding a window of opportunity to kill cancer cells differentially has proved elusive. Radiotherapy has been found useful for all histologic types and in all stages of lung cancer. Radiotherapy has been applied in cases considered unfit for surgery, in cases preoperatively, in cases postoperatively, and in cases in which resectability was thought to be impossible or ill advised. Comparison between studies that employed surgery and those that employed radiotherapy commonly show advantages to surgery. No randomized prospective trials have been done, however. Because the standard radiotherapy doses (60 Gy) produce no better than 50% local control, a test between surgery or radiotherapy has been considered neither ethical nor feasible. A modern study of well-staged patients comparing thoracic radiotherapy alone or *benchmark* radiotherapy, with best supportive care, is lacking.

Two studies have suggested improvements in survival after thoracic radiotherapy as opposed to *expectant* management. Leddy and Moersch[176] reported no 1-year survivors in 125 patients who received no anticancer treatment. In a matched group of 125 patients, 20% survived for at least 1 year after receiving thoracic radiotherapy.[176] In the 1960s, Wolf and colleagues[177] from a Veterans Administration Cooperative study reported improved median and 1-year survival in 554 patients with localized lung cancer randomized to receive 40 to 50 Gy versus observation without definitive radiotherapy management. The treated group had 18% surviving after 1 year as opposed to 14% in the observation group. These studies are flawed by inclusion of small cell histology, primitive radiotherapy equipment and technique, limited staging studies by today's standards, and inclusion of poor PS patients. Nevertheless, these dated facts suggest that observation is inferior to intervention.

The adoption of the Mountain staging system, designed with surgical therapy in mind, has been difficult to apply prospectively for nonsurgical therapy. The system has been modified to a minor degree.[125, 126] The distinction between stages IIIA and IIIB has been investigated. A Fox Chase report looked back at results obtained from retrospectively characterized stage IIIA versus IIIB patients treated by definitive radiotherapy averaging a dose of 59 Gy. The median survival and 2- and 5-year survivals were not different by stage.[178] The new adaptation of the staging system has been critiqued, particularly for missing the opportunity to classify any pleural effusion as an M1 lesion. Subclassifications of the IIIA category need definition for which patients have potential for benefit with surgical therapy and which do not.

**Radiotherapy as Primary Therapy.** Despite the selection of the most favorable patients for surgery, some patients refuse operations, and others are unfit for surgery because of poor pulmonary function or other underlying comorbid medical problems. Poor pulmonary function is the most likely cause of rejection for surgical therapy, but other comorbid medical conditions, such as heart disease, liver failure, renal failure, prior surgery, and poor overall condition (poor PS), have all been cited as justification to deny surgery. Formerly, implications about the effectiveness of radiotherapy in early-stage disease rested solely on the Hilton report about patients treated in the 1950s.[179] This series used orthovoltage treatments of uncertain and varied dose and volume. More recently, a handful of reports disclosed median survivals ranging from 17 to 32 months and 2- to 3-year survival of 19 to 60% and 5-year survival 6 to 38% with radiotherapy (Table 36–11).[180–189] Subsets with small-volume disease and higher doses may provide survival figures comparable to those of surgery for similarly staged patients. Some of these reports used quite limited fields, eliminating mediastinal nodal irradiation. Tumor size seems to be an important variable. The reports vary with the cutoff point, but larger (>3 to 5 cm) tumors tend to fare worse. Although there is a likely bias about dose selection, the higher dose patients seemed to respond and survive longer than those treated to lower doses. It is likely that larger doses may be required to increase local control. Especially for patients with limited pulmonary reserve, reduced volumes may lead to improved local control without compromising survival, but it is possible that nodal relapse might ensue, leading to poorer survival. More data about patterns of failure, particularly when regional nodes are not treated, and complications in patients with limited pulmonary function would be useful.

**Dose and Fractionation Issues.** Despite an occasional report with slightly higher or lower 5-year survival figures, external radiotherapy to 60 Gy produces about 5% 5-year survival.[190] The Radiotherapy Oncology Group (RTOG)

**Table 36–11. Results of Radiotherapy in Early-Stage Lung Cancer**

| Author | No. Patients | Dose (Gy) | Median Survival Time (mo) | Survival 2–3 yr (%) | Survival 5 yr (%) |
|---|---|---|---|---|---|
| Dosoretz et al.[180] | 152 | 50–70 | 17 | 40 | 10 |
| Graham et al.[181] | 103 | 60 | N/A | 35 | 14 |
| Hilton[179] | 38 | Unknown | 27 | 59 | 38 |
| Haffy et al.[182] | 43 | 54–59* | 28 | 60 | 21 |
| Kaskowitz et al.[183] | 53 | 63.2 | 24 | 19 | 6 |
| Krol et al.[184] | 108 | 60–65 | 24 | 31 | 15 |
| Noordijk et al.[185] | 50 | 60 | 25 | 56 | 16 |
| Sandler et al.[186] | 77 | 60 | 20 | 30 | 10 |
| Sibley[187] | 141 | 64 | N/A | 24 | 13 |
| Talton et al.[188] | 77 | 60 | 17 | 36 | 17 |
| Zhang et al.[189] | 44 | 55–70* | >36 | >55 | 32 |

*Mean or median dose.
N/A, not available.

**Table 36–12. Intrathoracic Tumor Control, Complete Response Rates, and Survival in Stage III Non–Small Cell Lung Cancer Treated with Radiotherapy Alone (RTOG 73-01)**

| Total Dose (Schedule) | No. Patients | No. Locally Controlled* (%) | CR (%) | % Survival 2 yr | % Survival 3 yr |
|---|---|---|---|---|---|
| 40 Gy (split-course) | 97 | 54 (56) | 10/97 (10) | 12 | 6 |
| 40 Gy (continuous) | 103 | 49 (48) | 19/103 (18) | 12 | 6 |
| 50 Gy (continuous) | 91 | 53 (58) | 21/91 (23) | 17 | 10 |
| 60 Gy (continuous) | 85 | 57 (67)† | 21/85 (25) | 20 | 5 |

*Defined as overall control within the irradiated lung at 3 years.
†*p* = 0.02 (60 Gy vs. ≤50 Gy).
Cr, complete response.
Data from Perez CA, Pajak TF, Rubin R. Long-term observations of the patterns of failure in patients with unresectable non-oat cell carcinoma of the lung treated with definitive radiotherapy: report by the Radiation Therapy Oncology Group. Cancer 1987;59:1874–81.

1973 study compared split-course thoracic radiotherapy (40 Gy over 4 to 5 weeks) with three successively higher continuous-course doses (40, 50, or 60 Gy). The split-course regimen, 20 Gy administered over 1 week, followed by a 2- to 3-week break, then an additional 20 Gy, was widely accepted as comparable therapy.[191] This study included 383 patients with medically inoperable stages I, II, and III disease and patients with mediastinal or chest wall invasion, supraclavicular lymph node involvement, or both. The study predated the CT scan era, and surgical staging was not required. Technically, megavoltage equipment irradiated all patients, but simulation of fields was not required. Table 36–12 displays the local control, complete response rate, and 2- and 3-year survival from this large series. Only the response rate was significantly improved by higher doses; the survival curves overlap at 5 years.

Table 36–13 shows a variety of results from the 1960s through the modern era from selected series using radiotherapy alone for locally advanced NSCLC. The doses during the earlier part of this era did not exceed 60 Gy. The Veterans

**Table 36–13. Radiotherapy for Locally Advanced Non–Small Cell Lung Cancer**

| Institution | No. Patients | Dose (Course) Gy | Survival MEDIAN (mo.) | Survival 2 yr (%) | Survival 5 yr (%) |
|---|---|---|---|---|---|
| VA[177, 264] | 240 | 0 | 4 | — | — |
| | 302 | 45 | 5 | — | — |
| RTOG[191] | 97 | 40 (s) | 9.2 | 10 | 5 |
| | 103 | 40 (c) | 10.6 | 10 | 5 |
| | 91 | 50 (c) | 10.8 | 20 | 5 |
| | 85 | 60 (c) | 11.5 | 25 | 5 |
| Fox Chase[178] | 166 IIIA | 59 (c/s) | 9.4 | 17 | <10 |
| | 140 IIIB | 59 (c/s) | 9.8 | 18 | <10 |
| RTOG[192] | 83 | 60 (c) | 9.2 | 16 | — |
| | 172 | 64.8 (h) | 6.3 | 14 | — |
| | 220 | 69.6 (h) | 10.0 | 20 | — |
| | 221 | 74.4 (h) | 8.7 | 15 | — |
| | 207 | 79.2 (h) | 10.5 | 20 | — |

c, continuous; s, split; h, hyperfractionated.

Administration study shows modest but significant advantage to treatment versus observation. Most (75 to 80%) patients manifest distant metastasis. The RTOG dose-seeking pilot study used doses ranging from 64.8 to 79.2 Gy.[192] These doses were administered using an altered fractionation method known as *hyperfractionation*. This method uses two small doses each day with 4 to 6 hours between each administration. Its purpose is to reduce late effect injury to normal tissue, but it does increase the total dose. Despite increasing the total dose in this phase I pilot study, 2-year survival was 10 to 25%. The unacceptably poor 5-year survival has led many radiation oncologists to seek other strategies (i.e., higher doses).

An alternative altered fraction scheme to hyperfractionation is accelerated radiotherapy, which provides dose intensification of the radiotherapy by giving more frequent fractions and reducing the time. These schedules intend to attack a rapidly proliferating clone of cells. These schedules are limited, however, in total dose and fraction size by acute reactions. The multiple fractions are intended to provide reduction in late effects. Saunders and colleagues[193] at Mt. Vernon Hospital in the United Kingdom have reported their results from a randomized trial. The unique aspect of the Mt. Vernon trial is its use of uninterrupted thoracic radiotherapy treatment delivered in a short time, 12 days. This group delivered radiotherapy three times each day with an approximately 8-hour interval between treatments, 7 days per week, and compared it with 60 Gy given in conventional fashion. Although the total dose appears modest (54 Gy), the biologic effect of this dose given in only 12 days is likely similar to the 69.6 Gy given in 1.2-Gy fractions (hyperfractionated) or the 60 Gy in standard schedules.[194] Table 36–14 provides some comparisons with some dose-altered and dose-escalated trials.

**Dose Escalation and Standard Fractionation.** Hazuka and associates[195] published the retrospective, high-dose, mostly three-dimensionally applied treatment from the University of Michigan. In contrast to the similarly retrospective observations from Fox Chase,[191] there was a significant difference favoring improved survival for the IIIA patients versus those classified as IIIB. Cox and associates[192] provide similar and confirmatory data. Patients treated to higher doses in standard fraction survived significantly longer than those receiving lower doses (albeit still higher than the standard doses). Because these were retrospective analyses, the inference that dose influenced survival and local control has led to a formal dose-escalation study in attempts to control for volume of irradiation using three-dimensional treatment planning. We suspected that smaller volume disease might have been treated to higher total doses (not found when reanalyzed); the confirmatory study testing simultaneously for dose and volume will provide clearer data. Doses may be different for increasing volumes treated. Also, because the adverse effects of these higher doses on normal tissues have not been tested, the Michigan investigators are proceeding cautiously with limits based on volumes of normal lung, heart, esophagus, and spinal cord. The facts from this study are intended to provide guidelines for radiotherapy doses when combination therapy is used. Graham and colleagues[171] showed that tumors less than or equal to 70 cm³ are influenced markedly by dose, but larger tumors are not influenced in terms of response or survival by dose. They found that lung toxicity was related to volume of irradiation. When more than 20% of normal lung was necessary to treat the tumor, frequency of lung toxicity rose precipitously.[171]

Radiotherapy, similar to surgery, is a local treatment modality. Local control may measure how effective the local therapy is. It is a difficult end point and can be hard to define clinically without invasive procedures. NSCLCs do not disappear as completely or as quickly as SCLCs or

*Table 36–14.* **Selected Studies of Altered Radiation Therapy Fractionation Approaches and Dose Escalation in Locally Advanced Non–Small Cell Lung Cancer**

| Author | No. Patients | Total Dose (Gy) | No. Fractions/Dose per Fraction (Gy) | MST (mo.) | 2-yr Survival (%) | Remarks |
|---|---|---|---|---|---|---|
| *Hyperfractionation* | | | | | | |
| Cox et al.[192] | 83 | 60 | 50/1.2* | 9.2 | 16 | For PS 0–1, 5% weight loss, no N3 nodes; superior survival for 69.6 Gy arm and above (*p* = 0.02) |
| | 127 | 64.8 | 54/1.2* | 6.3 | 14 | |
| | 220 | 69.6 | 58/1.2* | 10.0 | 20 | |
| | 221 | 74.4 | 62/1.2* | 8.7 | 15 | |
| | 207 | 79.2 | 66/1.2* | 10.5 | 20 | |
| *Accelerated* | | | | | | |
| Saunders et al[193] | 62 | 50.4–54 | 36/1.4–1.5† | ~15 | 34 | Survival superior than historical control (*p* = 0.004) |
| *Dose Escalation* | | | | | | |
| Hazuka et al[195] | 91 | 60–74 | 30–40/1.8–2.0 | 17.5 | 38 | CT-based radiation treatment planning |
| Emami et al[266] | 23 | Up to 70 | 35/2.0 | 18 | 45 (25‡) | PS 0–1, <5% weight loss |

*BID.
†TID.
‡Three-year survival.
MST, median survival time; PS, performance status.

lymphomas. The true complete response rates are modest. The starting point for local control may not necessarily be a pristine, complete response but something less than that. Sometimes the measure may be *time to local progression*, which reflects the difficulty in defining local control when complete response cannot be ensured. For the most part, local control evaluations are determined from images: chest radiographs, CT scans, and MRI scans. Although early responses show definite regression or stabilization, with time, the normal lung's response shows increased density and later scar and fibrosis. Distinguishing this response from progression cannot always be as precise as clinicians might like.

In contrast to the local control rates of 50 to 60% reported in the RTOG 73-01 trial,[191] the study of Arriagada and colleagues[196] using squamous and large cell lung cancers, treated with radiotherapy alone or with neoadjuvant chemotherapy, reported only a 17% local control rate at 1 year following the delivery of 65 Gy in 26 fractions over 45 days (given by continuous-course therapy). In this trial, patients were defined as locally controlled only if they had a complete clinical, radiographic, and histologic response by repeat bronchoscopy.[196] This definition emphasized how poor local control can be with conventional chest radiotherapy when strict definitions are applied.[177] The inability to control NSCLC locally may, in part, be from an insufficient radiation dose to large bulky disease. Although improvement in survival may be the ultimate goal, reduction in local failure is a reasonable end point to assess the contribution of thoracic radiotherapy in lung cancer treatment. New approaches are needed to allow the safe delivery of higher tumor doses.

**Preoperative Irradiation.** Preoperative irradiation was introduced in an attempt to (1) reduce the high incidence of local spread of the tumor and increase the resectability rate, (2) decrease the incidence of tumor spread to the regional lymphatics, (3) decrease the possibility of tumor spread during the surgical procedure, and (4) decrease the incidence of postsurgical recurrence. Preoperative radiotherapy continues to be used in the treatment of superior sulcus tumors. Mallams and colleagues,[197] using a 30- to 35-Gy tumor dose in 10 to 15 treatments over 19 days, followed by surgical resection 4 weeks later, showed increases in resectability and survival rates. Hilaris and coworkers[198] with the use of preoperative radiotherapy and interstitial implants reported similar favorable results. This report must be balanced with a report by Komaki and associates.[199] In their 36 patients with superior sulcus tumors treated by radiation therapy alone, the 5-year survival rate was 23%.

Although preoperative therapy remains a common prescription for superior pulmonary sulcus tumors, its use in other situations has been curtailed. In a randomized trial of preoperative radiotherapy or immediate surgery in 339 operable patients with NSCLC, Shields[200] showed that the resectability rate was slightly less in the preoperative group (51% vs. 53%). Survival was shortened by the addition of radiation, and survival shortening was dose related. The results of a National Cancer Institute study[201] in 568 patients randomized to receive either immediate surgery or 40 to 50 Gy preoperative radiation showed no difference in resectability (61% vs. 64%), more postoperative complications, and no difference in survival or local or distant relapse rates. At this time, it appears that preoperative radiotherapy is indi-

cated only for patients with superior sulcus tumors or as part of combined modality therapy in stage IIIA patients.

**Postoperative Radiotherapy.** A rationale for postoperative radiotherapy has been the considerable incidence of persistent local disease that is found in patients who have had surgical resection for cure. In a retrospective study of 202 patients who died within 30 days after a curative pulmonary resection, Matthews and colleagues[117] found that 73 patients (35%) had persistent disease. The addition of postoperative radiotherapy has improved the survival rate in some uncontrolled series.[202, 203]

Few trials have addressed the value of postoperative radiation therapy in node-positive patients. The LCSG compared postoperative radiation therapy with no further treatment in surgically staged patients with resected stage II and stage III squamous carcinoma of the lung.[204] Greater than 95% of the 210 patients in this trial had regional lymph node involvement by tumor. For patients with N2 stations positive, postoperative radiation therapy reduced the rate of local recurrence (3% with radiation therapy and 35% without radiation therapy). Despite the improved local control, there was no difference in survival between the groups regardless of thoracic radiotherapy. An overview of published and nonpublished trials concerning postoperative radiotherapy has clarified the role of postoperative therapy.[205] This meta-analysis reviewed mostly European trials but provides some clear guidelines about which patients are not benefited and possibly harmed by postoperative therapy. All patients with N0 and N1 nodes were found to have more chance of harm than benefit with postoperative therapy. Making these results a little less reliable was a treatment prescription to 60 Gy and the inclusion of cobalt 60 equipment. The prospect of benefit in these patients seems slim. The benefit of postoperative therapy for patients with N2 nodes was not proved, but the prospect of benefit seemed more likely.

Prophylactic cranial irradiation offers a potential remedy for this problem. There has been controversy in the treatment of small cell and non–small cell cancer patients because of the possibility of late effects caused by the treatment.

Brain metastases are a postmortem finding in nearly half of the patients with SCLC and nonsquamous NSCLC of the lung.[206, 207] The brain is a common site of initial treatment failure and may be the only site of disease outside the thorax.[208–212] An overview has established an approximately 5% survival advantage for SCLC patients in complete remission treated with prophylactic cranial irradiation as opposed to those observed.[213] A British Medical Research Council trial suggested that higher doses were associated with fewer relapses intracranially, but there was not a dose-response relationship to survival.[214] In this trial, more relapses were observed with single doses (8 Gy) and lower doses (<2400 Gy). A French trial, despite the use of 3 Gy fractions to a total dose of 30 Gy, detected no significant neurologic consequences on psychometrics or imaging for patients tested 2 to 3 years after diagnosis.[215] An enduring concern about prophylactic cranial irradiation–induced dementia has largely been eliminated by these trials,[213–215] which found no excess in neurotoxicity in the randomized trials. One report, however, continues to find evidence of abnormal test results after prophylactic cranial irradiation.[216]

Figlin and coworkers,[208] reporting for the LCSG, analyzed the risk of intracranial recurrence of cancer in 1532 patients who were surgically treated for stage I, II, or III NSCLC. Of these patients, 104 (6.8%) had documented first recurrences involving the brain, including 98 patients (6.4%) in whom the brain was the sole site of first recurrence. Sixty patients (3.9%) had only intracranial involvement at the time of death. Prognostic variables that had a significant effect on the time to recurrence in the brain were the histologic features of the carcinoma (patients with nonsquamous cell cancer were more at risk than those with squamous cell cancer), the T1 N1/T2 N0 and T2 N1 staging subsets, and initial weight loss of more than 10%. Figlin and coworkers[208] concluded that prophylactic cranial irradiation would at best benefit only a small subset of patients and is not indicated in patients who have undergone complete resection for NSCLC.

Palliative treatment is indicated to relieve distressing symptoms caused by the presence of primary tumor or metastatic disease. It may also be indicated to prevent the occurrence of such symptoms and signs. For example, radiographic evidence of a substantial metastatic lytic lesion in the femur without symptoms is an indication for palliative radiotherapy to prevent a pathologic fracture. Although durable control of pain and relief of symptoms can be achieved with radiotherapy, the optimal course of therapy is not defined. Data suggest that shorter fractionation schemes, in some cases as few a one fraction, can relieve symptoms as well and as long as longer courses.[209]

## COMBINED-MODALITY APPROACHES TO STAGE III NON–SMALL CELL LUNG CANCER

Long-term disease control in patients with stage III NSCLC requires eradication of obvious local-regional macroscopic disease and undocumented but usually disseminated micrometastases. Radiation alone, using current standard doses and schedules, fails to sterilize the local-regional disease in most treated patients. Available single agents and chemotherapy combinations (see the following discussion) produce partial or complete responses in only a few NSCLC patients treated for stage IV disease. The same chemotherapy induces more frequent responses in stage III patients, however.

Initial (induction) chemotherapy in stage III patients produced local-regional disease regression in 30 to more than 75% of patients in selected series (Table 36–15). The role of sequential chemotherapy and radiotherapy, concurrent

*Table 36–15.* **Induction Chemotherapy in Stage III Non–Small Cell Lung Cancer**

| Author | No. Patients | Drugs | CR + PR (%) |
|---|---|---|---|
| Martini et al[217] | 136 | MVP | 77 |
| Burkes et al[218] | 39 | MVP | 68 |
| Bitran et al[219] | 20 | VP-16, VIND, P | 70 |
| Vokes et al[220] | 27 | VP-16, VIND, P | 48 |
| Skarin et al[221] | 32 | CAP | 53 |
| Cullen[222] | 81 | M, IFEX, P | 54 |
| Le Chevalier et al[223, 224] | 33, 165 | VIND, CCNU, C, P | 42, 27 |
| Dillman et al[225] | 78 | VP | 36 |

M, mitomycin C; V, vinblastine; P, cisplatin; VP-16, etoposide; VIND, vindesine; C, cyclophosphamide; A, Adriamycin (doxorubicin); IFEX, ifosfamide; CCNU, lomustine.

chemotherapy and radiotherapy, or chemotherapy with or without radiotherapy followed by definite surgery is the focus of the following paragraphs.

In a study conducted by the Southeastern Cancer Study Group (SECSG), 319 stage IIIA and IIIB patients were randomized to radiotherapy alone (60 Gy given over 6 weeks), vindesine alone (3 mg/m$^2$ weekly), or the combination of the same radiotherapy and chemotherapy. Crossover between arms was allowed, with 44% crossing over from vindesine to radiotherapy and 27% crossing over from radiotherapy to vindesine.[226] All patients received treatments with megavoltage equipment using modern techniques. Treatment planning and simulation was not required in this trial. No difference in median survivals (radiotherapy alone, 8.6 months; radiotherapy plus vindesine, 9.4 months; vindesine alone, 10.1 months; $p = 0.58$) or long-term survivals (5-year survivals were 3%, 3%, and 1%; $p = 0.56$) was observed among the three arms. Because the groups were crossed over to other arms at the time of progression, the vindesine group represents a *delayed* radiotherapy arm, and the results achieved in this study are compatible with those in RTOG 73-01 and the historical radiotherapy series. The SECSG results could also be interpreted as showing that the simultaneous combination of vindesine (a marginally active agent in NSCLC) plus thoracic radiotherapy is no better than thoracic radiotherapy alone.

Because of lackluster results with radiotherapy alone or even combined with marginally effective chemotherapy, surgery and chemotherapy are advocated for patients with stage III disease. Many stage III patients, however, do not benefit from surgery because of (1) tumor invasion into unresectable structures (T4); (2) extensive peritracheal involvement or subcarinal lymph node involvement, or both—bulky, multilevel, or extracapsular N2 disease; or (3) involvement of contralateral mediastinal or hilar lymph nodes (N3), which is a relatively infrequent (<10%) presentation. Other stage III patients with technically resectable tumors may be poor surgical candidates because of underlying severe cardiovascular or pulmonary diseases (medically inoperable).

Randomized clinical trials evaluating combined chemoradiotherapy approaches are now complete but provide contradictory results. Although the role of surgery as part of combined-modality therapy in unresectable stage III patients is being studied, at present no randomized comparative phase III data regarding survival or toxicity have been published for patients managed with surgery after induction chemotherapy or chemoradiotherapy. Control groups may include chemoradiotherapy, radiotherapy, or surgery without pretreatment.

A rationale for combining chemotherapy with radiotherapy in locally advanced NSCLC is the high frequency of distant metastasis in this set of patients and the poor outcomes with standard thoracic radiotherapy. The aim of combined chemoradiotherapy is to decrease the incidence of distant metastases and to improve local control of the primary tumor. At the same time, an unacceptable increase in toxicity needs to be avoided. Chemotherapy can be combined with radiotherapy by one of the following tactics: (1) sequential administration, (2) concurrent administration, or (3) rapid alternation of both modalities. With sequential therapy, one modality is given first, followed by the other.

Sequential therapy avoids interaction between modalities,

which is perhaps its principal advantage. This advantage is particularly true if the chemotherapy and radiotherapy have overlapping toxicities, such as the lung for mitomycin and lomustine (CCNU) and the esophagus for doxorubicin and 5-fluorouracil. The term *induction* (or a variety of synonyms, including *neoadjuvant, protoadjuvant, primary,* or *up-front*) *chemotherapy* has been used to describe the delivery of chemotherapy before the definitive treatment. The main idea is that the radiation therapy or surgery may alter the efficacy of chemotherapy. Giving chemotherapy first provides an opportunity to deliver drugs before the vascularity has been compromised by sclerosing radiotherapy or truncating surgery. In some cases, this approach may decrease the size or the invasiveness of the primary tumor before radiotherapy or surgery. Chemotherapy offers the prospect of sterilizing distant occult metastases. The local therapies, surgery and radiotherapy, destroy or remove cells potentially resistant to chemotherapy.

At present, the up-front use of chemotherapy continues to command attention, but its precise role requires further definition. If the chemotherapy is given after the radiotherapy, the term *adjuvant* is used. The advantage of this sequencing is that the local treatment is directed first to the primary site. A disadvantage is the delay, which may permit growth of subclinical disease while awaiting the administration of systemic therapy. It is not clear that neoadjuvant uses of chemotherapy or radiotherapy improve resectability.

Concurrent therapy delivers both modalities together without delay and offers the prospect for chemotherapy and radiotherapy to influence each other's effectiveness. An advantage of this timing is that the chemotherapy can sensitize cells, preparing them for more efficient cell killing by radiotherapy. By killing cells, the chemotherapy may reduce the hypoxic, more radioresistant components of the tumor. Radiotherapy potentially can kill the chemoresistant clone of cells. Finally the cell kill caused by radiotherapy improves vascular access for the delivery of subsequent chemotherapy. Ideally, these enhanced effects would be confined to tumor cells. Concurrent therapy potentiates normal tissue toxicity. A therapeutic gain occurs when there is less potentiation of the effects on normal tissues than effects against tumor. Clinical trials are always charged with identifying the relative merits of the combinations. As the SECSG study shows, ineffective chemotherapy used concurrently produces little benefit.[226]

A third method of integration of modalities is the rapid alternation of chemotherapy with radiotherapy—the alternating method. With this method, the chemotherapy and radiotherapy are administered on alternate weeks but not concurrently. Each modality is commonly applied on alternating weeks. This approach allows time for recovery from the acute toxic effects of each modality. The main advantage of this sequencing is that the chemotherapy is started without delay and given with the usual scheduling of about one cycle every 4 weeks. A disadvantage is the administration of radiotherapy as split courses to interdigitate chemotherapy; a split course leads to poorer local control and increased risks of late effects.[172] This method was actively investigated in the late 1980s but is receiving much less attention today.

Clinical trials employing these combined chemoradiotherapy strategies have been conducted in unresectable stage III NSCLC. The concomitant administration of chemotherapy

and radiotherapy is feasible, but tolerance may depend on the agents used. What seems to be a particularly advantageous interaction results with the use of cisplatin, which has been used as a radiosensitizer and a systemic agent. Randomized studies comparing the sequential and the concurrent combined-modality approaches versus *benchmark* radiotherapy have been conducted worldwide. In contrast, fewer studies have been performed using the rapid alternating concept in NSCLC, at least as definitive therapy.

## SEQUENTIAL ADMINISTRATION OF COMBINED CHEMORADIOTHERAPY: RESULTS OF RANDOMIZED STUDIES

Several large (>100 patients per trial) randomized phase III trials have compared sequentially delivered chemotherapy plus radiotherapy with radiotherapy alone; the outcomes of these trials are summarized in Table 36–16. Only two trials failed to include cisplatin as an agent in the combined modality regimen.

The earliest randomized effort was reported from Finland. Mattson and colleagues[230] randomized 238 patients with inoperable NSCLC. This series included patients with medically inoperable stages I and II as well as unresectable stage III patients. Supraclavicular node-positive patients were excluded from this trial. Treatment consisted of thoracic radiotherapy given as 55 Gy, using a split-course regimen. The trial randomized patients to up-front chemotherapy employing CAP or observation.[230] The CAP regimen is cyclophosphamide (Cytoxan) 400 mg/m$^2$, doxorubicin (Adriamycin) 40 mg/m$^2$, and platinum (cisplatin) 40 mg/m$^2$. These doses are modest, particularly the cisplatin dose. Although many advocate for higher-dose cisplatin, the optimal dose is not agreed on. Doses greater than 100 mg/m$^2$ are associated with more toxicity and better response but not necessarily better survival. Two cycles of CAP were given before thoracic radiotherapy, one cycle was given during the rest interval of the split-course radiotherapy, and six cycles were given after the local therapy.

No significant differences between the radiotherapy-alone and the combined-modality groups occurred with respect to overall response rates (44% and 49%), complete response rates (11% and 15%), median duration of response (9.1 months and 10.5 months), local failure (31% and 20%), distant progression (23% and 20%), and median survival (10.2 months and 10.6 months). When the survival analysis was confined to stage III patients only, however, the difference was of borderline significance ($p = 0.05$) in favor of the combined regimen.[232] Early discontinuation of chemotherapy was common so that only 31 and 12% of randomized patients received all nine cycles of CAP, respectively.

The Cancer and Leukemia Group B (CALGB) trial of Dillman and associates[225] was the first to report improved survival from chemotherapy before standard 60-Gy thoracic radiotherapy. The CALGB trial used cisplatin (100 mg/m$^2$ on days 1 and 29) and vinblastine (5 mg/m$^2$ on days 1, 8, 15, 22, and 29) for two cycles followed by thoracic radiotherapy (60 Gy given continuously as 30 fractions over 6 weeks). This therapy was compared with the same chest radiotherapy without the antecedent chemotherapy. A total of 155 eligible stage III patients with an ECOG PS of 0 to

*Table 36–16.* **Randomized Trials of Radiotherapy Alone Versus Combined Chemotherapy with Radiotherapy in Locally Advanced Non–Small Cell Lung Cancer**

| | | Treatment | | MST | % Survival | | | |
|---|---|---|---|---|---|---|---|---|
| Author | No. Patients | CHEMOTHERAPY | RT (Gy) | (mo.) | 1 yr | 2 yr | 3 yr | *p* Value |
| *Neoadjuvant Administration* | | | | | | | | |
| Dillman et al.[225, 227] | 78 | PV | 60 C | 13.8 | 55 | 26 | 23 | |
| | 77 | | 60 C | 9.7 | 40 | 13 | 11 | 0.0066 |
| Le Chevalier et al.[224, 228] | 176 | VCPC | 65 C | 12 | 50 | 21 | 11 | |
| | 177 | | 65 C | 10 | 41 | 14 | 5 | 0.02 |
| Mira et al.[229] | 109 | FOMi/CAP | 58 C | 9.1 | NR | | | |
| | 117 | | 58 C | 9.2 | NR | | | NS |
| Mattson et al.[230] | 119 | CAP | 55 S | 10.9 | 42 | 19 | 6 | |
| | 119 | | 55 S | 10.2 | 41 | 17 | 8 | NS* |
| Morton et al.[265] | 56 | MACC | 60 C | 10.3 | 46 | 21 | | |
| | 58 | | 60 C | 10.4 | 45 | 16 | | NS |
| Trovò et al.[231] | 49 | CAMP | 45 C | 10 | 35 | 16 | 10 | |
| | 62 | | 45 C | 11.7 | 50 | 19 | 13 | NS |

\**p* = 0.046 for stage III patients only.

PV, cisplatin, vinblastine; VCPC, vindesine, cyclophosphamide, cisplatin, lomustine; CAP, cyclophosphamide, doxorubicin, cisplatin; MACC, methotrexate, doxorubicin, cyclophosphamide, lomustine; CAMP, cyclophosphamide, doxorubicin, methotrexate, procarbazine; FOMi/CAP, 5-fluorouracil, vincristine, mitomycin/cyclophosphamide, doxorubicin, cisplatin; P, cisplatin; RT, radiation therapy; MST, median survival time; C, continuous course; S, split course; NR, not reported; NS, not significant.

1, a weight loss of less than 5%, and no supraclavicular nodes were entered into this study. The study was intended to accrue nearly twice this number, but early stopping rules were applied when significant differences were found. Although the response rates and failure patterns were not significantly different between the two groups, the median survival was improved by 4 months (13.8 vs. 9.7 months). The 2- and 3-year survival rates were doubled (26% and 23% vs. 13% and 11%) by the experimental protoadjuvant treatment. Despite an excessive number of early deaths in the radiotherapy arm (14 vs. 4), an analysis that excluded these 18 deaths still showed a trend toward better survival for patients who received induction chemotherapy (*p* = 0.059).[225] This trial has been updated.[227] With a minimum follow-up of more than 5 years, survival remains significantly better in the combined-modality group when compared with radiotherapy alone: 54% versus 40% at 1 year, 26% versus 13% at 2 years, 24% versus 10% at 3 years, and 19% versus 7% at 4 and 5 years. Median survival continues to favor combined thoracic radiotherapy and priming chemotherapy (13.7 vs. 9.6 months, *p* = 0.01). Now, with follow-up beyond 4 years, there are 12 survivors in the combined-modality group but only 4 in the radiotherapy-alone group.

## CONCURRENT ADMINISTRATION OF COMBINED CHEMORADIOTHERAPY: RESULTS OF RANDOMIZED STUDIES

Modern phase III studies have compared concurrent cisplatin combined-modality therapy with thoracic radiotherapy alone (Table 36–17). The combined concurrent chemoradiotherapy arm consisted of single-agent cisplatin given daily at 6 mg/m², weekly at 15 mg/m² or 30 mg/m², or on an every-3-week schedule at 70 mg/m² on days 1, 22, and 43 concurrently with continuous-course or split-course chest radiotherapy.

In the largest of these studies, the European Organization for Research and Treatment of Cancer (EORTC) conducted a randomized phase III three-arm trial looking at the effect of concurrent cisplatin in two schedules. The trial used European-style split-course thoracic radiotherapy alone at 55 Gy (30 Gy in 10 fractions followed by a 3- to 4-week rest period, followed by an additional 25 Gy in 10 fractions). To this radiotherapy schedule, concurrent daily cisplatin (6 mg/m²) before fractionated daily chest radiotherapy or weekly cisplatin (30 mg/m²) was given on the first day of each treatment week.[233] From 20 centers, 331 patients with inoperable stage I, II, or III NSCLC were enrolled in this study. The addition of daily cisplatin to the treatment radiotherapy significantly improved the survival compared with chest radiotherapy alone (*p* = 0.009). The survival rate in the daily cisplatin arm was 54% at 1 year, 26% at 2 years, and 16% at 3 years, as compared with 46%, 13%, and 2% in the thoracic radiotherapy-alone arm. Survival in the weekly cisplatin arm was intermediate (44% at 1 year, 19% at 2 years, and 13% at 3 years) and not significantly different from either of the other two treatment arms. As opposed to the reduced distant metastases from the French sequential randomized study,[224, 228] the improved survival here resulted from improved local tumor control. Survival without local recurrence at 1 and 2 years was 59% and 31% in the daily cisplatin plus radiotherapy arm as compared with 41% and 19% in the radiotherapy-alone arm (*p* = 0.003). The difference was not statistically significant (*p* = 0.15) between the weekly cisplatin plus radiotherapy arm and the radiotherapy-alone arm. An actuarial analysis of the time to distant metastasis showed that there was no difference among the three different treatment groups (*p* = 0.37 overall). The significant survival advantage found for patients treated with concurrent daily low-dose cisplatin and radiotherapy seems to be due to a reduction or delay in local tumor failure.

As shown in Table 36–17, not all concurrent trials have resulted in positive outcomes. Combined daily low-dose cisplatin and concurrent radiotherapy was also evaluated in

*Table 36–17.* **Phase III Trials of Concurrent Chemoradiotherapy Versus Radiotherapy Alone in Stage III Non–Small Cell Lung Cancer**

| Author | No. Patients | Treatment | | MST (mo.) | % Survival | | | p Value |
|---|---|---|---|---|---|---|---|---|
| | | CHEMOTHERAPY | RT (Gy) | | 1 yr | 2 yr | 3 yr | |
| *Concurrent Administration of Cisplatin* | | | | | | | | |
| Ansari[232] | 90 | P days 1, 22, 43 | 60 C | 8.1 | 35 | 15 | | |
| | 93 | | 60 C | 9.5 | 40 | 9 | | NS |
| Schaaks-Koning et al.[233] | 107 | P daily | 55 S | NR | 54 | 26 | 16 | |
| | 110 | P wkly | 55 S | NR | 44 | 19 | 13 | |
| | 114 | | 55 S | NR | 46 | 13 | 2 | 0.009 |
| Soresi et al.[234] | 45 | P wkly | 50.4 | 9.4 | 36 | 14 | 7 | NS |
| | 50 | | 50.4 | 8.6 | 31 | 13 | 5 | |
| Trovò et al[231] | 86 | P daily | 45 C | NR | 50 | 17 | | |
| | 83 | | 45 C | NR | 41 | 20 | | NS |

P, cisplatin; RT, radiation therapy; MST, median survival time; C, continuous course; S, split course; NR, not reported; NS, not significant.

a randomized phase III Italian trial.[235] In this trial, 173 patients with unresectable stage III disease (ipsilateral supraclavicular nodes without pleural effusions were eligible) were randomized to receive daily cisplatin (6 mg/m$^2$) about 1 hour before each radiotherapy fraction plus radiotherapy (45 Gy in 15 daily fractions, 5 fractions per week) or the same thoracic radiotherapy without chemotherapy. Although the median time to progression was slightly longer in the daily cisplatin arm (14.2 vs. 10.6 months, $p = 0.237$), all survival results were nearly identical. The median survival and 2-year survival rates were 9.7 months and 17% in the daily cisplatin and radiotherapy arm versus 10.3 months and 20% in the thoracic radiotherapy arm ($p = 0.89$). No difference was noted in the pattern of relapse between the two treatment groups. Similarly, two other randomized studies failed to show benefit with the addition of cisplatin chemotherapy, given weekly (15 mg/m$^2$) or every 3 weeks, on days 1, 22, and 43 (70 mg/m$^2$), with thoracic radiotherapy of 50.4 Gy and 60 Gy.[232, 233] The negative studies presented could be criticized for the way the cisplatin and radiotherapy were sequenced in two studies[232, 234] and the relatively low total radiation dose (50 to 60 Gy) that was delivered in another study.

Three large prospective randomized trials have now shown that radiotherapy plus a cisplatin-containing regimen or cisplatin alone improves survival as compared with standard thoracic radiotherapy. The benefit results in a modest 2- to 3-month increase in the median survival and a doubling of the 2- and 3-year survivals; however, both are less than 50%. A confirmatory intergroup trial will be presented soon, and a planned meta-analysis of all completed randomized trials may clarify these issues. In two of the positive studies, the chemotherapy was combined sequentially as a neoadjuvant to the thoracic radiotherapy, and in the other study, daily cisplatin was given concurrently with split-course chest irradiation. In the French sequential study, the survival improvement was attributed to a delay in the appearance of distant metastasis; sequentially delivered chemotherapy did not affect local control. Conversely, in the EORTC trial, the increased survival was due to improved local control or a delay in local failure. Low-dose daily cisplatin did not influence the distant metastasis rate. Although the use of combined chemoradiotherapy described previously produced a

statistically significant survival prolongation in the three trials, its overall impact on survival improvement can be considered modest at best. Improved control of local and distant disease remains a formidable challenge. Further improvements in the nonoperative therapy of stage III NSCLC await the development of newer systemic agents, better delivery of chest radiotherapy, and optimal ways to combine these therapies.

## NEOADJUVANT CHEMOTHERAPY OR CHEMORADIOTHERAPY IN STAGE IIIA (N2) NON–SMALL CELL LUNG CANCER

Stage IIIA patients who have ipsilateral mediastinal lymph node (N2) involvement represent a therapeutic challenge because they have advanced local tumors that may be only marginally resectable. The results of resection alone in this group of patients are poor. Martini and Flehinger[235] reported that among 706 patients with N2 disease, only 151 (21%) were completely resectable. Of the 151 resected patients, 119 were suspected of having only N0 or N1 disease based on radiographic and bronchoscopic findings, but microscopic N2 disease was detected in the resected specimens. The 5-year survival rates of patients who had microscopic N2 disease and clinically detected N2 disease were 34 and 9%, respectively. This study raises the question of whether or not surgery alone is of value in all patients who have stage IIIA (N2) NSCLC, especially in those who have clinical N2 disease in which similar survival rates have been noted with radiotherapy alone.

Neoadjuvant chemotherapy or chemoradiotherapy used to downstage primary tumors and facilitate resection and to obtain early and increased control of systemic disease is being tested as an important step in developing a multimodality approach for stage IIIA (N2) NSCLC. Neoadjuvant therapies have been used in either sequential or concurrent study designs. Although this concept is being practiced more often, the results remain preliminary because all the trials have been single-arm phase II pilot studies or inadequately powered, small randomized trials. The randomized trials comparing multimodal management with standard therapy have not been completed.

The results of these pilot trials (Table 36–18) of neoadjuvant chemotherapy and chemoradiotherapy have differed in several ways, including study design, extent of staging evaluation, and eligibility for surgical resection.[236–246] The results have shown substantially higher overall response rates with preoperative therapies, and in 15 to 23% of patients, histologic complete remission has been achieved. These patients seem to have a prolonged long-term survival. The resectability rates have been high, with median survival ranging from 9 to 22 months. The differences in resectability rates and median survival rates may be accounted for by patient selection factors, lack of precise staging, stratification for prognostic variables, and variations in study design. Intensive neoadjuvant studies have been feasible in the cooperative group setting, and their results are comparable with single institutional trials.

A study conducted by the Southwest Oncology Group (SWOG) in patients with stage IIIA and IIIB NSCLC is a good example.[239, 240] The SWOG published a report of a 25-institution, phase II trial, conducted with stringent staging criteria based on CT scanning and mediastinoscopy. The patients in the trial were treated with concurrent chemotherapy (two cycles of cisplatin and etoposide) and 45 Gy of chest radiotherapy and were evaluated and restaged 2 to 4 weeks after the completion of induction treatment. All patients went to thoracotomy, unless they had evidence of locally progressive tumor or distant metastases. Based on the first 75 eligible patients for whom survival data are relatively mature, the results showed the following:

1. The induction therapy was well tolerated.
2. Ninety-one percent of patients were eligible for resection.
3. Eighty-four percent of patients underwent thoracotomy.
4. Seventy-three percent of patients had a complete resection.

5. One third of the patients required a complex resection, such as lobectomy plus chest wall or vertebral body resection.
6. Of 53 patients for whom complete pathologic data were available, 21% had no residual tumor, and 30% had rare microscopic foci of residual cancer.

The 2-year survival for patients with both stage IIIA and IIIB disease is 40%, significantly better than survival among historical control patients. A phase III randomized intergroup trial—RTOG 9309—is currently under way and will help in understanding the role of surgery when added to chemoradiotherapy. These results argue in favor of a multimodality approach for the management of patients who have stage IIIA (N2) disease, and the data are sufficiently intriguing to support larger cooperative group attempts at randomized trials to determine definitively if combined-modality treatment is associated with improved survival.

A randomized study compared preoperative chemotherapy plus surgery with surgery alone in 60 patients with surgically resectable stage IIIA NSCLC.[245] Patients received either surgery alone or three courses of chemotherapy followed by surgery. All patients received mediastinal radiation after surgery. The rates of recurrence (56% vs. 74%), disease-free survival (20 vs. 5 months), and overall survival (26 vs. 8 months) favored the chemotherapy plus surgery group. The M.D. Anderson group in a comparable group of patients treated with a slightly different chemotherapy regimen has reported nearly identical results.[246]

Randomized trials should continue to evaluate each component of this multimodality approach involving chemotherapy, radiotherapy, and surgery. Is chemotherapy of value in stage IIIA (N2) disease? Does surgery play a role in improving survival and in what patient population? Large-scale randomized trials need to be designed to answer these questions, and these trials can be performed only in the cooperative group setting.

*Table 36–18.* **Results of Phase II-III Trials Using Chemotherapy or Combined-Modality Therapy with Surgical Resection for Stage III Non–Small Cell Lung Cancer**

| Author | Stage Treated | Induction Regimen | No. Patients | RR (%) | Resectability (%) | Operative Mortality (%) | Median Survival (mo.) | Overall Survival |
|---|---|---|---|---|---|---|---|---|
| Eagan et al[236] | IIIA | CAP | 39 | 51 | 49 | 0 | 15 | 10% at 2 yr |
| Faber et al[237] | IIIA (includes T3N0) | CDDP, 5FU | 64 | 88 | 48 | 5 | 22 | 40% at 3 yr |
| | Selected IIIB | CDDP, 5FU ± VP-16 | 66 | 44 | | | | |
| Weiden et al[238] | IIIA Selected IIIB | CDDP, 5FU | 85 | 56 | 52 | 0 | 13 | 22% at 2 yr |
| Albain et al,[239] Rusch et al[240] | IIIA (T1–3, N2) IIIB (T4 or N3) | CDDP, VP-16 | 75 | 69 | 73 | 6 | 17 | 40% at 2 yr |
| Bitran et al[241] | IIIA | CDDP, VP-16 Vindesine | 23 | 70 | 35 | 0 | 9 | 34% at 1 yr |
| Martini et al,[242] Gralla[243] | IIIA | VP or MVP | 58 | 62 | 57 | 3 | 19.5 | 34% at 3 yr |
| Burkes et al[244] | IIIA | MVP | 35 | 68 | 60 | 9 | >14.6 | N/A |
| Rosel et al[245] | IIIA | IMP vs. surgery | 30 | 60 | 85 | 9 | 26 | 25% at 2 yr |
| | | | 30 | — | 90 | 7 | 8 | 0% at 2 yr |
| Roth et al[246] | IIA | CEP vs. surgery | 26 | 35 | 61 | 0 | 64 | 56% at 3 yr |
| | | | 32 | | 66 | 6 | 11 | 15% at 3 yr |

CAP, cyclophosphamide, Adriamycin, and cisplatin; CDDP, cisplatin; 5-FU, fluorouracil; VP-16, etoposide; VP or MVP, vinblastine, cisplatin, mitomycin; IMP, ifosfamide, mitomycin, cisplatin; CEP, cyclophosphamide, etoposide, cisplatin; RR, response rate; N/A, not stated.

## CHEMOTHERAPY FOR ADVANCED DISEASE

Early studies of alkylating agents in lung cancer showed that they impaired survival, and no single agent was found to produce a response rate exceeding 20% in stage IV NSCLC.[247, 248] This low rate created considerable pessimism for treating NSCLC patients with chemotherapy. Studies indicate that newer chemotherapeutic agents prolong survival and alleviate symptoms in all stages of lung cancer, such that all NSCLC patients, with the exception of those with poor performance status (PS 3 to 4), should be offered modern chemotherapy.

The survival of patients with advanced (stage IV) NSCLC is extremely poor. Best supportive care measures, including palliative radiotherapy, produce median survivals of 16 to 17 weeks, and only 10 to 15% of patients are alive at 1 year.[248–250] Before the 1990s, no single drug or drug combination had been proved to improve survival or quality of life in advanced NSCLC. Multiple randomized trials were conducted in the 1980s and early 1990s that compared best supportive care with chemotherapy using cisplatin-based combinations. Meta-analysis of these trials proved that the cisplatin-based therapy improved the survival of these patients, although the benefits were modest.[248–250] On average, the median survival of the cisplatin-treated patients improved by 10 weeks (from 16 to 26 weeks), and the 1-year survival rate improved by 10% (from 15 to 25%). Randomized trials also showed that cisplatin combinations were superior to single-drug therapy. The completed randomized trials showed that cisplatin-based combinations also improve quality of life. On the basis of these randomized studies and meta-analyses, the American Society of Clinical Oncology's NSCLC guidelines include the recognition that chemotherapy can prolong the survival of patients with advanced NSCLC.[251] Retrospective analysis of the SWOG experience showed that cisplatin-based chemotherapy improved survival of advanced NSCLC patients with any PS, but the survival gains were much more striking in patients with good PS.[252]

Table 36–19 summarizes the phase I and II studies of six new chemotherapeutic agents that have been approved by the U.S. Food and Drug Administration for various indications over the past 2 years. These agents include two taxanes, paclitaxel and docetaxel; two topoisomerase I inhibitors, irinotecan and topotecan; a novel antimetabolite, gemcitabine; and a novel vinca alkaloid, vinorelbine. As shown in Table 36–19, five of the new agents, with the exception of topotecan, produced an objective response rate of 20% or higher, and at least 100 patients were available for response analysis. These studies were conducted in patients with good PS only. The median survival in these studies averaged about 40 weeks, which is longer than with any previously reported single agent and longer than with the best previously reported cisplatin combination studies.

The activity of these new agents makes it logical to combine them with other standard therapies, especially the platinum compounds. In all instances, the combination of one of these new agents with cisplatin or carboplatin led to higher response rates than those reported for either agent alone. Median and 1-year survival rates also were generally higher. Table 36–20 summarizes the results of phase II trials combining these new agents with cisplatin and carboplatin.

A phase III trial comparing gemcitabine plus cisplatin with etoposide plus cisplatin revealed a 40.6% response rate for gemcitabine plus cisplatin versus a 21.9% response for the etoposide plus cisplatin combination.[253] The cisplatin-gemcitabine combination had a significant delay in time to disease progression—6.9 months versus 4.3 months for the cisplatin plus etoposide combination. There was no impairment of quality of life. Survival time was 8.7 months for the gemcitabine plus cisplatin arm and 7.2 months for the etoposide plus cisplatin arm, although the study was not sufficiently powered to show a difference in survival. The toxicity profiles for the drugs in each arm were similar.

In a randomized phase III study conducted by SWOG comparing cisplatin with cisplatin plus vinorelbine, response rates of 12% and 26% were observed.[254] The 1- and 2-year survivals for the cisplatin arm are 20% and 6%, compared with 36% and 12% for the cisplatin plus vinorelbine arm, demonstrating the superiority of the combination. Similarly a phase III trial comparing cisplatin with cisplatin plus gemcitabine revealed 31% versus 9.1% response rate in favor of the combination with an interim survival analysis favoring the combination (8.7 months vs. 7.6 months).[255]

Although there are few studies that specifically report on quality of life rather than objective response rates, all studies show symptom relief for most patients. A randomized study conducted in the United Kingdom showed an improved quality of life and prolonged survival for patients receiving a cisplatin-based combination regimen.[256] In the EORTC randomized study that compared paclitaxel plus cisplatin with teniposide plus cisplatin, the former combination was associated with a superior quality of life.[257]

*Table 36–19.* **Single-Agent Activity of New Chemotherapeutic Agents for Non–Small Cell Lung Cancer**

| Agent | No. Patients | Total CR + PR | Median Survival* | 1-yr Survival (%) |
|---|---|---|---|---|
| Paclitaxel | 317 | 84 (26%) | 37.3 (24–56) | 41 |
| Docetaxel | 300 | 77 (26%) | 41 (27–48) | 52 |
| Vinorelbine | 621 | 126 (20%) | 32.5 (29–40) | 24 |
| Gemcitabine | 572 | 122 (21%) | 40.6 (31–49) | 39 |
| Irinotecan | 138 | 37 (27%) | 35 (27–42) | NR |
| Topotecan | 119 | 15 (13%) | 38 (33–40) | 35 |

*Average median survival in weeks (range).

CR, complete response; PR, partial response; NR, not reported.

From Bunn PA, Kelly K. New chemotherapeutic agents prolong survival and improve quality of life in non small cell lung cancer: a review of the literature and future directions. Clin Cancer Res 1998;5:1087–100.

*Table 36–20.* **Phase II Studies of New Drugs plus Cisplatin or Carboplatin**

| Agent | No. Patients | Total CR + PR (%) | Median Survival (wk) | 1-yr Survival (%) |
|---|---|---|---|---|
| Vinorelbine + cisplatin | 328 | 135 (41%) | 38 | 35–40 |
| Paclitaxel + cisplatin | 286 | 121 (42%) | 42 | 36 |
| Paclitaxel + carboplatin | 333 | 137 (46%) | 38 | 40 |
| Docetaxel + cisplatin | 255 | 88 (35%) | 35 | 58 |
| Gemcitabine + cisplatin | 245 | 114 (47%) | 57 | 61 |
| Irinotecan + cisplatin | 185 | 81 (44%) | 34 | NR |
| Topotecan + cisplatin | 22 | 3 (22%) | 32 | 26 |

CR, complete response; PR, partial response; NR, not reported.
From Bunn PA, Kelly K. New chemotherapeutic agents prolong survival and improve quality of life in non small cell lung cancer: a review of the literature and future directions. Clin Cancer Res 1998;5:1087–100.

## ECONOMIC ISSUES IN LUNG CANCER

Lung cancer represents 2% of all health care costs and about 20% of all cancer care costs in the United States.[258] This cost constitutes about $8 billion to the American health care system.[259] Evans and coworkers[259] using a lung cancer cost model have reported that the total health care costs to the Canadian system for patients with NSCLC treated with radiation only was $14,110 versus $12,474 for surgery alone versus $17,889 for surgery plus radiation therapy (1988 Canadian dollars). Management of localized NSCLC cost $18,691 (Canadian dollars). For all stages of disease, hospitalization was the major cost. Despite growing evidence that combined-modality therapy and combination chemotherapy induce remissions and prolong survival, many patients with lung cancer do not have an opportunity to pursue these therapies. Although economic data show the cost-effectiveness of these strategies, the reluctance to offer these interventions to patients still remains. Evans and coworkers[259] showed that this reluctance may, in part, be due to the absolute cost of introducing new treatments. Standard radiation therapy for stages IIIA and IIIB disease is estimated to cost $16,086 and $13,391 (Canadian dollars). When patients relapse, diagnostic work-up ($2141 Canadian dollars) and supportive or palliative care ($17,575 Canadian dollars) increase costs significantly.[260] Assuming relapse will occur, the average cost to care for a patient with stage IIIA lung cancer is $34,595 (Canadian dollars) versus $31,928 (Canadian dollars) for stage IIIB lung cancer. Evaluating the cost-effectiveness of the combined-modality strategies in patients with stage III disease, the costs associated with neoadjuvant therapy for stage IIIA and combined-modality therapy for stage IIIB are acceptable.[260]

For advanced NSCLC, data on economic costs are derived from Canadian studies, which compared best supportive care with two cisplatin regimens.[261] Best supportive care costs ($8595, 1984 Canadian dollars) were for a median survival of 17 weeks. Costs of the two chemotherapy arms were $7645 and $12,232, respectively, with a median survival of 33 weeks for the higher cost arm. The extra costs were $3637 for 16 additional weeks of life, which calculates into $11,820 per year of added life. For vinorelbine and cisplatin, the cost-effectiveness per year gained was $17,700.[262] In comparing the cost of treating patients with gemcitabine versus cisplatin plus etoposide, the gemcitabine therapy was less expensive, saving $1500 to $7000 per cycle.[263]

Although the costs of therapy for NSCLC are well within the range of other accepted medical therapies, efforts to reduce tobacco use should be vigorously pursued. Reducing tobacco consumption would likely be associated with enhanced quality of life and a net economic benefit.

## SUPPORTIVE CARE

Patients with lung cancer are frequently in need of emotional as well as medical supportive care. Successful sources of support include physicians, nurses, social workers, psychologists, and psychiatrists. Hospices and specialized units may also provide care for dying patients.

Specific problems frequently arising in cancer patients include coping with death and dying; maintaining quality of life until and through the dying period; dealing with feelings of helplessness, anger, depression, loss of self-esteem, and guilt (e.g., regarding smoking history); dealing with rejection and pity from peers and employers; preparing financially for medical care; settling financial affairs and preparing for the family's well-being; coping with pain and dyspnea; and dealing with the side effects and risk of therapy.

It is important to deal with both the patient and the family and to handle matters in an understanding manner, protecting patient dignity, assuaging guilt, and giving permission to be ill. Honesty is critically important, but the maintenance of some hope (of worthwhile quality, if not quantity, of life) is also essential. Education regarding the illness and therapy may be helpful. A full discussion of the management of these problems is beyond the scope of this chapter. Emotional supportive care is discussed more fully in Chapters 24 and 25.

## SUMMARY OF TREATMENT BY STAGE OF DISEASE

Having discussed at length the potential contributions of surgery, radiation therapy, and chemotherapy to the management of NSCLC, we now address the question of integrating therapy for specific groups of patients. These recommendations should be considered as guidelines, not rules, and the care of each patient should be individualized, taking into account factors such as the patient's age, general state of health, cardiopulmonary status, psychosocial status, and personal system of values. No matter what therapy is undertaken, it must be consistent with the needs of the individual patient. In 1997, the Board of Directors of the American Society of Clinical Oncology adopted a set of practice guidelines for patients with surgically unresectable stage III-IV NSCLC.[251]

Patients with NSCLC are staged as shown in Table 36–7. Our recommendations for the management of patients with resected NSCLC are as follows.

**Stage I Disease.** The treatment of operable stage I NSCLC is surgical resection of the primary tumor accompanied by careful intraoperative staging of the intrapulmonary, hilar, and ipsilateral mediastinal lymph nodes. This therapy is curative in more than 60 to 70% of patients with pathologic stage I disease. Inoperable stage I disease should receive radiotherapy with curative intent. The use of chemotherapy in the high-risk stage I patient (IB) should take place in a clinical trial.

**Stage II Disease.** Patients with positive intrapulmonary or hilar lymph nodes at the time of surgical resection (N1 disease) are at increased risk for recurrence compared with patients with stage I disease. Although 40 to 50% of these patients are potentially cured, the increased risk of recurrence is sufficiently high to warrant experimental preoperative and postoperative therapy in properly controlled trials.

**Stage IIIA Disease.** The management of this group of patients is difficult and is heavily influenced by the skill and experience of the thoracic surgeon. In general, surgical resection is indicated if possible. The value of either preoperative or postoperative adjuvant chemotherapy with or without radiotherapy remains to be proved unequivocally by appropriate randomized trials. We do not usually treat these patients with postoperative radiation therapy, although this remains an option used at many centers.

**Stage IIIB Disease.** These patients have regionally advanced disease not amenable to surgical resection with curative intent. We advise multimodality therapy, consisting of concurrent chemotherapy plus radiotherapy or sequential chemotherapy plus radiotherapy. Attempts at downstaging using concomitant chemotherapy with or without radiotherapy before surgical resection remain unproved and should be performed within the context of an experimental trial. If there is any group for which combined-modality experimental therapy is indicated, this is the group.

**Stage IV Disease.** Patients with disseminated disease who are of good PS have improved survival with the use of combination chemotherapy; however, this must be balanced by the toxicity and altered quality of life brought with its use. No single-combination regimen has been shown to be superior over others. Combination chemotherapy would be continued as tolerated in responders but discontinued in those who have progressive disease or intolerance to therapy. Patients of poor PS may be better treated with supportive care only. Palliative radiation therapy would be given for brain metastases and as needed for symptomatic metastases in other sites. Experimental therapy remains an option in previously untreated patients.

## SUGGESTIONS FOR ADDITIONAL READING

Reif AE, Heeren T. Consensus on synergism between cigarette smoke and other environmental carcinogens in the causation of lung cancer. Adv Cancer Res 1999;76:161–86.

Lam S, Shibuya H. Early diagnosis of lung cancer. Clin Chest Med 1999;20:53–61.

Coleman RE. PET in lung cancer. J Nucl Med 1999;40:814–20.

Ruckdeschel JC, Gridelli C, Perrone F, et al. Are platinum compounds mandatory in the treatment of metastatic non-small cell lung cancer? Eur J Cancer 1998;34:1993–9.

Livingston RB. Combined modality therapy of lung cancer. Clin Cancer Res 1997;3:12 Pt 2:2638–47.

Virgo KS, Johnson FE, Naunheim KS. Follow-up of patients with thoracic malignancies. Surg Oncol Clin North Am 1999;8:355–69.

Davey P. Brain metastases. Curr Probl Cancer 1999;23:59–98.

## REFERENCES

1. Landis SH, Murray T, Bolden S, Wingo PA. Cancer statistics, 1998. CA Cancer J Clin 1998;48:6-29, 192.
2. Ries LG, Pollack ES, Young J Jr. Cancer patient survival: Surveillance, Epidemiology, and End Results Program, 1973–79. J Natl Cancer Inst 1983;70:693–707.
3. Wynder EL, Hoffmann D. Tobacco and health: a societal challenge. N Engl J Med 1979;300:894–903.
4. Bartecchi CE, MacKenzie TD, Schrier RW. The human costs of tobacco use. N Engl J Med 1994;330:907–12.
5. U.S. Surgeon General. Reducing the health consequences of smoking: 25 years of progress. Washington, D.C.: U.S. Government Printing Office, 1989.
6. MMWR Morb Mortal Wkly Rep 1993;42:230.
7. Benowitz NL, Hall SM, Herning RI, et al. Smokers of low-yield cigarettes do not consume less nicotine. N Engl J Med 1983;309:139–42.
8. Wynder EL, Kabat GC. The effect of low-yield cigarette smoking on lung cancer risk. Cancer 1988;62:1223–30.
9. Lenfant C. Are "low-yield" cigarettes really safer? N Engl J Med 1983;309:181–2.
10. Benowitz NL, Jacob P 3d, Kozlowski LT, Yu L. Influence of smoking fewer cigarettes on exposure to tar, nicotine, and carbon monoxide. N Engl J Med 1986;315:1310–3.
11. MMWR Morb Mortal Wkly Rep 1993;42:645.
12. Lubin JH, Richter BS, Blot WJ. Lung cancer risk with cigar and pipe use. J Natl Cancer Inst 1984;73:377–81.
13. Connolly GN, Winn DM, Hecht SS, et al. The reemergence of smokeless tobacco. N Engl J Med 1986;314:1020–7.
14. Stockwell HG, Goldman AL, Lyman GH, et al. Environmental tobacco smoke and lung cancer risk in nonsmoking women. J Natl Cancer Inst 1992;84:1417–22.
15. Garfinkel L, Auerbach O, Joubert L. Involuntary smoking and lung cancer: a case-control study. J Natl Cancer Inst 1985;75:463–9.
16. Boyle P. The hazards of passive- and active-smoking. N Engl J Med 1993;328:1708–9.
17. Janerich DT, Thompson WD, Varela LR, et al. Lung cancer and exposure to tobacco smoke in the household. N Engl J Med 1990;323:632–6.
18. Denissenko MF, Pao A, Tang M, et al. Preferential formation of benzo[a]pyrene adducts at lung cancer mutational hotspots in p53. Science 1996;274:430–2.
19. Kolonel LN, Yoshizawa CN, Hirohata T, Myers BC. Cancer occurrence in shipyard workers exposed to asbestos in Hawaii. Cancer Res 1985;45:3924–8.
20. Hodgson JT, Jones RD. Mortality of asbestos workers in England and Wales 1971–81. Br J Ind Med 1986;43:158–64.
21. Saccomanno G, Yale C, Dixon W, et al. An epidemiological analysis of the relationship between exposure to Rn progeny, smoking and bronchogenic carcinoma in the U-mining population of the Colorado Plateau—1960–1980. Health Phys 1986;50:605–18.
22. Harley N, Samet JM, Cross FT, et al. Contribution of radon and radon daughters to respiratory cancer. Environ Health Perspect 1986;70:17–21.
23. Howe GR, Nair RC, Newcombe HB, et al. Lung cancer mortality (1950–80) in relation to radon daughter exposure in a cohort of workers at the Eldorado Beaverlodge uranium mine. J Natl Cancer Inst 1986;77:357–62.
24. Samet JM, Marbury MC, Spengler JD. Health effects and sources of indoor air pollution: Part II. Am Rev Respir Dis 1988;137:221–42.
25. Logue J. MMWR Morb Mort Wkly Rep 1985;34:657.

26. Samet JM, Nero AV Jr. Indoor radon and lung cancer. N Engl J Med 1989;320:591–4.
27. Steenland K, Thun M. Interaction between tobacco smoking and occupational exposures in the causation of lung cancer. J Occup Med 1986;28:110–8.
28. Maher KV, DeFonso LR. Respiratory cancer among chloromethyl ether workers. J Natl Cancer Inst 1987;78:839–43.
29. Peters JM, Thomas D, Falk H, et al. Contribution of metals to respiratory cancer. Environ Health Perspect 1986;70:71–83.
30. Chen CJ, Chuang YC, You SL, et al. A retrospective study on malignant neoplasms of bladder, lung and liver in blackfoot disease endemic area in Taiwan. Br J Cancer 1986;53:399–405.
31. Nishiyama H, Yano H, Nishiwaki Y, et al. Lung cancer in chromate workers—analysis of 11 cases. Jpn J Clin Oncol 1985;15:489–97.
32. Rafnsson V, Jóhannesdóttir SG. Mortality among masons in Iceland. Br J Ind Med 1986;43:522–5.
33. Nelson N, Levine RJ, Albert RE, et al. Contribution of formaldehyde to respiratory cancer. Environ Health Perspect 1986;70:23–35.
34. Kauppinen TP, Partanen TJ, Nurminen MM, et al. Respiratory cancers and chemical exposures in the wood industry: a nested case-control study. Br J Ind Med 1986;43:84–90.
35. Joishy SK, Cooper RA, Rowley PT. Alveolar cell carcinoma in identical twins: similarity in time of onset, histochemistry, and site of metastasis. Ann Intern Med 1977;87:447–50.
36. Tokuhata GK, Lilenfeld AM. Familial aggregation of lung cancer in humans. J Natl Cancer Inst 1986;76:217–22.
37. Bartsch H, Petruzzelli S, De Flora S, et al. Carcinogen metabolism in human lung tissues and the effect of tobacco smoking: results from a case-control multicenter study on lung cancer patients. Environ Health Perspect 1992;98:119–24.
38. Bartsch H, Hietanen E, Petruzzelli S, et al. Possible prognostic value of pulmonary AH-locus-linked enzymes in patients with tobacco-related lung cancer. Int J Cancer 1990;46:185–8.
39. Brincker H. The incidence of malignant tumors in patients with respiratory sacroidosis. Br J Cancer 1974;29:247.
40. Bakris GL. Pulmonary scar carcinoma: a clinicopathologic analysis. Cancer 1983;52:493.
41. Tockman MS, Anthonisen NR, Wright EC, Donithan MG. Airways obstruction and the risk for lung cancer. Ann Intern Med 1987;106:512–8.
42. Skillrud DM, Offord KP, Miller RD. Higher risk of lung cancer in chronic obstructive pulmonary disease: a prospective, matched, controlled study. Ann Intern Med 1986;105:503–7.
43. Taioli E, Wynder EL. Re: endocrine factors and adenocarcinoma of the lung in women. J Natl Cancer Inst 1994;86:869–70.
44. Atukorala S, Basu TK, Dickerson JW, et al. Vitamin A, zinc and lung cancer. Br J Cancer 1979;40:927–31.
45. Menkes MS, Comstock GW, Vuilleumier JP, et al. Serum beta-carotene, vitamins A and E, selenium, and the risk of lung cancer. N Engl J Med 1986;315:1250–4.
46. Colditz GA, Stampfer MJ, Willett WC. Diet and lung cancer: a review of the epidemiologic evidence in humans. Arch Intern Med 1987;147:157–60.
47. Bond GG, Thompson FE, Cook RR. Dietary vitamin A and lung cancer: results of a case-control study among chemical workers. Nutr Cancer 1987;9:109–21.
48. The Alpha-Tocopherol, Beta Carotene Cancer Prevention Study Group. The effect of vitamin E and beta carotene on the incidence of lung cancer and other cancers in male smokers. N Engl J Med 1994;330:1029–35.
49. Richardson GE, Johnson BE. The biology of lung cancer. Semin Oncol 1993;20:105–27.
50. Gazdar AF. Molecular markers for the diagnosis and prognosis of lung cancer. Cancer 1992;69:Suppl:1592–9.
51. Salgia R, Skarin AT. Molecular abnormalities in lung cancer. J Clin Oncol 1998;16:1207–17.
52. Whang-Peng J, Kao-Shan CS, Lee EC, et al. Specific chromosome defect associated with human small-cell lung cancer; deletion 3p(14–23). Science 1982;215:181–2.
53. Brauch H, Johnson B, Hovis J, et al. Molecular analysis of the short arm of chromosome 3 in small-cell and non-small-cell carcinoma of the lung. N Engl J Med 1987;317:1109–13.
54. Kok K, Osinga J, Carritt B, et al. Deletion of a DNA sequence at the chromosomal region 3p21 in all major types of lung cancer. Nature 1987;330:578–81.
55. Naylor SL, Johnson BE, Minna JD, Sakaguchi AY. Loss of heterozygosity of chromosome 3p markers in small-cell lung cancer. Nature 1987;329:451–4.
56. Otterson G, Lin A, Kay F. Genetic etiology of lung cancer. Oncology 1992;6:97–104, 107.
57. Graziano S, Pfeifer A, Testa J, et al. Involvement of the RAF1 locus, at band 3p25, in the 3p deletion of small-cell lung cancer. Genes Chromosomes Cancer 1991;3:282–92.
58. Croce C. Genetic approaches to the study of the molecular basis of human cancer. Cancer Res 1991;51:Suppl:5015S–8S.
59. LaForgia S, Morse B, Levy J, et al. Receptor protein-tyrosine phosphatase gamma is a candidate tumor suppressor gene at human chromosome region 3p21. Proc Natl Acad Sci U S A 1991;86:5036–40.
60. Latif F, Tory K, Gnarra J, et al. Identification of the von-Hippel-Lindau disease tumor suppressor gene. Science 1993;260:1317–20.
61. Takahashi T, Nau MM, Chiba I, et al. p53: a frequent target for genetic abnormalities in lung cancer. Science 1989;246:491–4.
62. Alt FW, DePinho R, Zimmerman K, et al. The human myc gene family. Cold Spring Harb Symp Quant Biol 1986;51:Pt 2:931–41.
63. Little, CD, Nau MM, Carney DN, et al. Amplification and expression of the c-myc oncogene in human lung cancer cell lines. Nature 1983;306:194–6.
64. Gazdar AF, Carney DN, Nau MM, Minna JD. Characterization of variant subclasses of cell lines derived from small cell lung cancer having distinctive biochemical, morphological, and growth properties. Cancer Res 1985;45:2924–30.
65. Saksela K, Bergh J, Lehto VP, et al. Amplification of the c-myc oncogene in a subpopulation of human small cell lung cancer. Cancer Res 1985;45:1823–7.
66. Kawashima K, Shikama H, Imoto K, et al. Close correlation between restriction fragment length polymorphism of the L-MYC gene and metastasis of human lung cancer to the lymph nodes and other organs. Proc Natl Acad Sci U S A 1988;85:2353–6.
67. Bos JL. ras oncogenes in human cancer: a review. Cancer Res 1989;49:4682–9 and 1990;50:1352.
68. Ryan J, Barker PE, Nesbitt MN, Ruddle FH. KRAS2 as a genetic marker for lung tumor susceptibility in inbred mice. J Natl Cancer Inst 1987;79:1351–7.
69. Slebos RJC, Kibbelaar RE, Dalesio O, et al. K-ras oncogene activation as a prognostic marker in adenocarcinoma of the lung. N Engl J Med 1990;323:561–5.
70. Kwiatowksi D, Harpole Jr D, Godleski J, et al. Molecular pathologic substaging in 244 stage i non-small cell lung cancer patients: clinical implications. J Clin Oncol 1998;16:2468–77.
71. Bohmann D, Bos TJ, Admon A, et al. Human proto-oncogene c-jun encodes a DNA binding protein with structural and functional properties of transcription factor AP-1. Science 1987;238:1386–92.
72. Minna JD, Schütte J, Viallet J, et al. Transcription factors and recessive oncogenes in the pathogenesis of human lung cancer. Int J Cancer 1989;4:Suppl:32–4.
73. Klein G. The approaching era of the tumor suppressor genes. Science 1987;238:1539.
74. Nau MM, Brooks BJ, Battey J, et al. L-myc, a new myc-related gene amplified and expressed in human small cell lung cancer. Nature 1985;318:69–73.
75. Lavigueur A, Maltby V, Mock D, et al. High incidence of lung, bone, and lymphoid tumors in transgenic mice overexpressing mutant alleles of the p53 oncogene. Mol Cell Biol 1989;9:3982–91.
76. Ebina M, Steinberg SM, Mulshine JL, Linnoila RI. Relationship of p53 overexpression and up-regulation of proliferating cell nuclear antigen with the clinical course of non-small cell lung cancer. Cancer Res 1994;54:2496–503.
77. Mitsudomi T, Oyama T, Kusano T, et al. Mutations of the p53 gene as a predictor of poor prognosis in patients with non-small-cell lung cancer. J Natl Cancer Inst 1993;85:2018–23.
78. Xu HJ, Quinlan DC, Davidson AG, et al. Altered retinoblastoma protein expression and prognosis in early-stage non-small-cell lung carcinoma. J Natl Cancer Inst 1994;86:695–9.
79. Linnoila I. Pathology of non-small cell lung cancer: new diagnostic approaches. Hematol Oncol Clin North Am 1990;4:1027.
80. Wu A. Secular trends in histologic types of lung cancer. J Natl Cancer Inst 1986;77:53.
81. Paulson DL. Superior sulcus tumors: results of combined therapy. N Y State J Med 1971;71:2050–7.
82. Lee JS. Involvement of chromosome 7 in primary lung tumor. Cancer Res 1987;47:6349.

83. Auerbach O, Garfinkel L. The changing pattern of lung adenocarcinoma. Cancer 1991;68:1973–7.
84. Ikeda T, Kurita Y, Inutsuka S, et al. The changing pattern of lung cancer by histologic type: a review of 1151 cases from a university hospital in Japan. 1970–1989. Lung Cancer 1991;7:157–64.
85. Barsky SH, Cameron R, Osann KE, et al. Rising incidence of bronchioloalveolar lung carcinoma and its clinicopathologic features. Cancer 1994;73:1163–70.
86. Bonne C. Morphological resemblance of pulmonary adenomatosis (jaagsiekte) in sheep and certain cases of cancer of the lung in man. Am J Cancer 1939;35:491–501.
87. Nobel TA, Perk K. Bronchioloalveolar cell carcinoma: animal model: pulmonary adenomatosis of sheep, pulmonary carcinoma of sheep (jaagsiekte). Am J Pathol 1978;90:783–6.
88. Perk K, Hod I. Sheep lung carcinoma: an endemic analogue of a sporadic human neoplasm. J Natl Cancer Inst 1982;69:747–79.
89. Heiman HL, Samuel E. Pulmonary adenomatosis: case report. S Afr Med J 1953;29:934–5.
90. Graziano S. The use of neuroendocrine immunoperoxidase markers to predict chemotherapy response in patients with non-small-cell lung cancer. J Clin Oncol 1989;7:1398.
91. Smith RA. Bronchial carcinoid tumours. Thorax 1969;24:43–50.
92. Godwin JD II. Carcinoid tumors: an analysis of 2,837 cases. Cancer 1975;36:560.
93. Yousem SA. Mucoepidermoid tumors of the lung. Cancer 1987;60:1346.
94. Weiss W, Boucot KR, Seidman H. The Philadelphia Pulmonary Neoplasms Research Project. Clin Chest Med 1982;3:243–56.
95. Sanderson DR. Screening (lung cancer). Chest 1986;89:4 Suppl:324S–6S.
96. Fontana RS, Sanderson DR, Taylor WF, et al. Early lung cancer detection: results of the initial (prevalence) radiologic and cytologic screening in the Mayo Clinic study. Am Rev Respir Dis 1984;130:561–5.
97. Melamed MR, Flehinger BJ, Zaman MB, et al. Detection of true pathologic stage I lung cancer in a screening program and the effect on survival. Cancer 1981;47:Suppl:1182–7.
98. Tockman MS. Lung cancer screening. Chest 1986;89:4 Suppl:324S–6S.
99. Frost JK, Ball WC Jr, Levin ML, et al. Early lung cancer detection: results of the initial (prevalence) radiologic and cytologic screening in the Johns Hopkins study. Am Rev Respir Dis 1984;130:549–54.
100. Muhm JR, Miller WE, Fontana RS, et al. Lung cancer detected during a screening program using four-month chest radiographs. Radiology 1983;148:609–15.
101. Martini N. Results of Memorial Sloan-Kettering lung project. Recent Results Cancer Res 1982;82:174–8.
102. Woolner LB, Fontana RS, Sanderson DR, et al. Mayo Lung Project: evaluation of lung cancer screening through December 1979. Mayo Clin Proc 1981;56:544–55.
103. Tockman MS. Sensitive and specific monoclonal antibody recognition of human lung cancer antigen on preserved sputum cells: a new approach to early lung cancer detection. J Clin Oncol 1988;6:1685.
104. Mao L, Hruban RH, Boyle JO, et al. Detection of oncogene mutations in sputum precedes diagnosis of lung cancer. Cancer Res 1994;54:1634–7.
105. Tockman MS, Mulshine JL, Piantadosi S, et al. Prospective detection of preclinical lung cancer: results from two studies of heterogeneous nuclear ribonucleoprotein A2/B1 overexpression. Clin Cancer Res 1997;3:2237–46.
106. Sone S, Takashima S, Li F, et al. Mass screening for lung cancer with mobile spiral computed tomography scanner. Lancet 1998;351:1242–5.
107. Gropp C, Havemann K, Scheuer A. Ectopic hormones in lung cancer patients at diagnosis and during therapy. Cancer 1980;46:347.
108. Barnes DM. New tumor factor may disrupt calcium levels. Science 1987;237:363–4.
109. Heelan R. Lung cancer imaging: primary diagnosis, staging, and local recurrence. Semin Oncol 1991;18:87–98.
110. Weber W, Romer W, Zeigler SI. Clinical value of F-18 FDG PET in solitary pulmonary nodules. J Nucl Med 1995;36:775.
111. Gupta NC, Maloof J, Gunel E. Probability of malignancy in solitary pulmonary nodules using fluorine-18-PDG and PET. J Nucl Med 1996;37:943–8.
112. Gambhir SS, Sheperd JE, Shah BD, et al. Analytical decision model for the cost-effective management of solitary pulmonary nodules. J Clin Oncol 1998;16:2113–25.
113. Lince L. Carcinoma of the lung: a comparative series of 687 cases. Arch Surg 1971;102:103.
114. Hyde L, Wolf J, McCracken S, Yesner R. Natural course of inoperable lung cancer. Chest 1973;64:309–12.
115. Overholt RH. Primary cancer of the lung: a 42-year experience. Ann Thorac Surg 1975;20:511.
116. Benfield JR. Current and future concepts of lung cancer. Ann Intern Med 1975;83:93–106.
117. Matthews MJ, Kanhouwa S, Pickren J, Robinette D. Frequency of residual and metastatic tumor in patients undergoing curative surgical resection for lung cancer. Cancer Chemother Rep 1973;4:Pt 3:63–7.
118. White CS, Templeton PA, Belani CP. Imaging in lung cancer. Semin Oncol 1993;20:142–52.
119. Kristensen S, Asaby C, Nielsen SM. Mediastinal staging of lung cancer: is mediastinoscopy still essential? Dan Med Bull 1995;42:192–4.
120. Izbicki JR, Passlick B, Karg O. Impact of radical systematic mediastinal lymphadenectomy on tumor staging in lung cancer. Ann Thorac Surg 1995;59:209–14.
121. Martini N. Mediastinal lymph node dissection for lung cancer: the Memorial experience. Chest Surg Clin N Am 1995;5:189–203.
123. Webb WR, Gatsonis C, Zerhouni EA, et al. CT and MR imaging in staging non-small cell bronchogenic carcinoma: report of the Radiologic Diagnostic Oncology Group. Radiology 1991;178:705–13.
124. Vansteenkiste JF, Stroobants SG, DeLeyn PR, et al. Lymph node staging in non small-cell lung cancer with FDG-PET scan: a prospective study on 690 lymph node stations from 68 patients. J Clin Oncol 1998;16:2142–9.
125. Mountain C. Revisions in the International System for Staging Lung Cancer. Chest 1997;111:1710–7.
126. Mountain C, Dresler C. Regional lymph node classification for lung cancer staging. Chest 1997;111:1718–23.
127. Urschel JD, Urschel DM, Anderson TM, et al. Prognostic implications of pulmonary satellite nodules: are the 1997 staging revisions appropriate? Lung Cancer 1998;21:83–7.
128. Mountain CF. A new international staging system for lung cancer. Chest 1986;89:Suppl:225S–33S.
129. Mountain CF. Revisions in the International System for Staging Lung Cancer. Chest 1997;111:1710–7.
130. Naruke T, Goya T, Tsuchiya R, Suemasu K. Prognosis and survival in resected lung carcinoma based on the new international staging system. J Thorac Cardiovasc Surg 1988;96:440–7 and 1989;97:350.
131. Mountain CF, Lukeman JM, Hammar SP, et al. Lung cancer classification: the relationship of disease extent and cell type to survival in a clinical trials population. J Surg Oncol 1987;35:147–56.
132. Vansteenkiste JF, De Leyn PR, Deneffe GJ, et al. Clinical prognostic factors in surgically treated stage IIIA-N2 non-small cell lung cancer: analysis of the literature. Lung Cancer 1998;19:3–13.
133. Kwiatkowski DJ, Harpole DH Jr, Godleski J, et al. Molecular pathologic substaging in 244 stage I non-small-cell lung cancer patients: clinical implications. J Clin Oncol 1998;16:2468–77.
134. Ginsberg RJ, Hill LD, Eagan RT, et al. Modern thirty-day operative mortality for surgical resections in lung cancer. J Thorac Cardiovasc Surg 1983;86:654–8.
135. Nagasaki F, Flehinger BJ, Martini N. Complications of surgery in the treatment of carcinoma of the lung. Chest 1982;82:25–9.
136. Piantadosi S. The adverse effect of blood transfusion in lung cancer. Chest 1992;102:6–8.
137. Pena CM, Rice TW, Ahmad M, Medendorp SV. Significance of perioperative blood transfusions in patients undergoing resection of stage I and II non-small-cell lung cancers. Chest 1992;102:84–8.
138. Graziano SL, Tatum AH, Newman NB, et al. The prognostic significance of neuroendocrine markers and carcinoembryonic antigen in patients with resected stage I and II non small cell lung cancer. Cancer Res 1994;54:2908–13.
139. Karnofsky DA, Burchenal JH. The clinical evaluation of chemotherapeutic agents in cancer. In: MacLeod CM, ed. Evaluation of chemotherapeutic agents. New York: Columbia University Press, 1949:192–205.
140. Stanley KE. Prognostic factors for survival in patients with inoperable lung cancer. J Natl Cancer Inst 1980;65:25.
141. Zelen M. Preliminary report on the treatment of nonresectable cancer of the lung. Cancer Chemother Rep 1973;4:Suppl 3:31.

142. Wolf J. Controlled studies of the therapy of nonresectable cancer of the lung. Ann Thorac Surg 1965;1:25–32.
143. Ariel IM, Avery EE, Kanter L, et al. Primary carcinoma of the lung: a clinical study of 1205 cases. Cancer 1950;3:229–39.
144. Burford TH, Center S, Ferguson TB, Spjut HJ. Results in the treatment of bronchogenic carcinoma: an analysis of 1,008 cases. J Thorac Surg 1958;36:316–24.
145. Buchberg A, Lubliner R, Rubin EH. Carcinoma of the lung: duration of life in individuals not treated surgically. Dis Chest 1951;20:257–72.
146. Boyd DP, Smedal MI, Kirtland HB Jr, et al. Carcinoma of the lung—a report of 403 cases. J Thorac Surg 1954;28:392–408.
147. Ochsner A, Ochsner A Jr, H'Doubler C, Blalock J. Bronchogenic carcinoma. Dis Chest 1960;37:1–12.
148. Garland LH, Sisson MA. The results of radiotherapy of bronchial cancer. Radiology 1956;67:48–62.
149. Rapp E, Pater JL, Willan A, et al. Chemotherapy can prolong survival in patients with advanced non-small-cell lung cancer—report of a Canadian multicenter randomized trial. J Clin Oncol 1988;6:633–41.
150. Graham EA, Singer JJ. Successful removal of an entire lung for carcinoma of the bronchus. JAMA 1933;101:1371–4.
151. Ginsberg RJ, Rubenstein LV. Randomized trial of lobectomy versus limited resection for T1N0 non-small cell lung cancer. Lung Cancer Study Group. Ann Thorac Surg 1995;60:615–22.
152. Warren WH, Faber LP. Segmentectomy vs. lobectomy in patients with stage I pulmonary carcinoma: five year survival and patterns of intrathoracic recurrence. J Thorac Cardiovasc Surg 1994;107:1087.
153. Paulson DL. Combined preoperative irradiation and extended resection for carcinoma in the superior pulmonary sulcus. In: Bonica JJ, Lindblom U, Iggo A, et al, eds. Advances in pain research and therapy. New York: Raven Press, 1982:47.
154. Shaw RR, Paulson DL, Kee JL Jr. Treatment of the superior sulcus tumor by irradiation follwed by resection. Ann Surg 1961;154:29.
155. Hilaris BS, Martini N. Multimodality therapy of superior sulcus tumors. In: Bonica JJ, Lindblom U, Iggo A, et al, eds. Advances in pain research and therapy. New York: Raven Press, 1982:113.
156. Hilaris BS, Martini N, Wong GY, et al. Treatment of superior sulcus tumor (Pancoast tumor). Surg Clin North Am 1987;67:965–77.
157. Paulson DL. The "superior sulcus" lesion. In: Delarue NC, Eschapasse H, eds. International trends in general thoracic surgery. Philadelphia: WB Saunders, 1985:121.
158. Dartevelle TG, Chapelier AR, Macchiarini P, et al. Anterior transcervical-thoracic approach for radical resection of lung tumors invading the thoracic inlet. J Thorac Cardiovasc Surg 1993;105:1025.
159. Mountain CF. Surgery for stage IIIa-N2 non-small cell lung cancer. Cancer 1994;73:2589–98.
160. Ginsberg RJ, Hill LD, Eagan RT. Modern thirty-day operative mortality for surgical resections in lung cancer. J Thorac Cardiovasc Surg 1983;86:654–8.
161. Romano PS, Mark DH. Patient and hospital characteristics related to in-hospital mortality after lung cancer resection. Chest 1992;101:1332–7.
162. Deslauriers J, Ginsberg RJ, Dubois P, et al. Current operative morbidity associated with elective surgical resection for lung cancer. Can J Surg 1989;32:335–9.
163. Nagasaki F, Flehinger BJ, Martini N. Complications of surgery in the treatment of carcinoma of the lung. Chest 1982;82:25–9.
164. Martini N, Melamed MR. Occult carcinoma of the lung. Ann Thorac Surg 1980;30:215–23.
165. Tockman MS, Erozan YS, Gupta PK, et al. The early detection of second primary lung cancers by sputum immunostaining. Chest 1994;106:Suppl:385S–90S.
166. Lam S, MacAulay C, Hung J, et al. Detection of dysphagia and carcinoma in situ with a lung imaging fluorescence endoscope device. J Thorac Cardiovasc Surg 1993;105:1035–40.
167. Morita K. Recent advances in radiation therapy for non-small cell lung cancer. Nippon Kyobu Geka Gakkai Zasshi 1996;34:Suppl:103–6.
168. Kawate KH, Kinoshita K, Yamamoto H, et al. Photodynamic therapy of early-stage lung cancer. Ciba Found Symp 1989;146:183–94.
169. van Boxem TJ, Venmans BJ, Schramel FM, et al. Radiographically occult lung cancer treated with fiberoptic bronchoscopic electrocautery: a pilot study of a simple and inexpensive technique. Eur Respir J 1998;11:169–72.
170. Kato H, Kawate N, Kinoshita K, et al. Photodynamic therapy of early-stage lung cancer. Ciba Found Symp 1989;146:183–94.
171. Graham MV, Purdy JA, Harms W, et al. Survival and prognostic factors of non–small cell lung cancer (NSCLC) patients treated with definitive three-dimensional (3D) radiation therapy. Int J Radiat Oncol Biol Phys 1998;42:Suppl 1:166.
172. Cox JD, Pajak TF, Asbell S, et al. Interruptions of high-dose radiation therapy decrease long-term survival of favorable patients with unresectable non-small cell carcinoma of the lung: analysis of 1244 cases from 3 Radiation Therapy Oncology Group (RTOG) trials. Int J Radiat Oncol Biol Phys 1993;27:493–8.
173. Lyman JT. Complication probability as assessed from dose-volume histograms. Radiat Res 1985;8:Suppl:S13–9.
174. Kutcher GJ, Burman C. Calculation of complication probability factors for non-uniform normal tissue irradiation: the effective volume method. Int J Radiat Oncol Biol Phys 1989;16:1623–30.
175. Burman C, Kutcher GJ, Emami B, Goitein M. Fitting of normal tissue tolerance data to an analytic function. Int J Radiat Oncol Biol Phys 1991;21:123–35.
176. Leddy ET, Moersch HJ. Roentgen therapy for bronchogenic carcinoma. JAMA 1940;115:2239–42.
177. Wolf J, Patno ME, Roswit B, D'Esopo N. Controlled study of survival of patients with clinically inoperable lung cancer treated with radiation therapy. Am J Med 1966;40:360–7.
178. Curran WJ Jr, Stafford PM. Lack of apparent difference in outcome between clinically staged IIIA and IIIB non-small-cell lung cancer treated with radiation therapy. J Clin Oncol 1990;8:409–15.
179. Hilton G. Present position relating to cancer of the lung: results with radiotherapy alone. Thorax 1960;15:17–8.
180. Dosoretz DE, Katin MJ, Blitzer PH, et al. Radiation therapy in the management of medically inoperable carcinoma of the lung: results and implications for future treatment strategies. Int J Radiat Oncol Biol Phys 1992;24:3–9.
181. Graham PH, Gebski VJ, Langlands AO. Radical radiotherapy for early nonsmall cell lung cancer. Int J Radiat Oncol Biol Phys 1995;31:261–6.
182. Haffty BG, Goldberg NB, Gerstley J, et al. Results of radical radiation therapy in clinical stage I, technically operable non-small cell lung cancer. Int J Radiat Oncol Biol Phys 1988;15:69–73.
183. Kaskowitz L, Graham MV, Emami B, et al. Radiation therapy alone for stage I non-small cell lung cancer. Int J Radiat Oncol Biol Phys 1993;27:517–23.
184. Krol AD, Aussems P, Noordijk EM, et al. Local irradiation alone for peripheral stage I lung cancer: could we omit the elective regional nodal irradiation? Int J Radiat Oncol Biol Phys 1996;34:297–302.
185. Noordijk EM, v d Poest Clement E, Hermans J, et al. Radiotherapy as an alternative to surgery in elderly patients with resectable lung cancer. Radiother Oncol 1988;13:83–9.
186. Sandler HM, Curran WJ Jr, Turrisi AT 3d. The influence of tumor size and pre-treatment staging on outcome following radiation therapy alone for stage I non-small cell lung cancer. Int J Radiat Oncol Biol Phys 1990;19:9–13.
187. Sibley GS. Radiotherapy for patients with medically inoperable stage I nonsmall cell lung carcinoma: smaller volumes and higher doses—a review. Cancer 1998;82:433–8.
188. Talton BM, Constable WC, Kersh CR. Curative radiotherapy in non-small cell carcinoma of the lung. Int J Radiat Oncol Biol Phys 1990;19:15–21.
189. Zhang HX, Yin WB, Zhang LJ, et al. Curative radiotherapy of early operable non-small cell lung cancer. Radiother Oncol 1989;14:89–94.
190. Katz HR, Alberts RW. A comparison of high-dose continuous and split-course irradiation in non-oat-cell carcinoma of the lung. Am J Clin Oncol 1983;6:445–57.
191. Perez CA, Pajak TF, Rubin P. Long-term observations of the patterns of failure in patients with unresectable non-oat cell carcinoma of the lung treated with definitive radiotherapy: report by the Radiation Therapy Oncology Group. Cancer 1987;59:1874–81.
192. Cox JD, Azarnia N, Byhardt RW, et al. A randomized phase I/II trial of hyperfractionated radiation therapy with total doses of 60.0 Gy to 79.2 Gy: possible survival benefit with greater than or equal to 69.6 Gy in favorable patients with Radiation Therapy Oncology Group stage III non-small-cell lung carcinoma: report of Radiation Therapy Oncology Group 83-11. J Clin Oncol 1990;8:1543–55.
193. Saunders M, Dische S, Barrett A, et al. Continuous hyperfractionated accelerated radiotherapy (CHART) versus conventional radiotherapy in non-small-cell lung cancer: a randomised multicentre trial. CHART Steering Committee. Lancet 1997;350:161–5.
194. Turrisi AT. Considerations on radiotherapy dose intensity for limited small cell lung cancer. Lung Cancer 1994;10:Suppl 1:S167-73.

195. Hazuka MB, Turrisi AT 3d, Lutz ST, et al. Results of high-dose thoracic irradiation incorporating beam's eye view display in non-small cell lung cancer: a retrospective multivariate analysis. Int J Radiat Oncol Biol Phys 1993;27:273–84.

196. Arriagada R, Le Chevalier T, Quoix E, et al. ASTRO (American Society for Therapeutic Radiology and Oncology) plenary: effect of chemotherapy on locally advanced non-small cell lung carcinoma: a randomized study of 353 patients. GETCB (Groupe d'Etude et Traitement des Cancers Bronchiques), FNCLCC (Féderation Nationale des Centres de Lutte contre le Cancer) and the CEBI trialists. Int J Radiat Oncol Biol Phys 1991;20:1183–90.

197. Mallams JT, Paulson DL, Collier RE, Shaw RR. Presurgical irradiation in bronchogenic carcinoma, superior sulcus type. Radiology 1964;82:1050–4.

198. Hilaris BS, Martini N, Luomanen RK, et al. The value of preoperative radiation therapy in apical cancer of the lung. Surg Clin North Am 1974;54:831–40.

199. Komaki R, Roh J, Cox JD, Lopes da Conceicao A. Superior sulcus tumors: results of irradiation of 36 patients. Cancer 1981;48:1563–8.

200. Shields TW. Preoperative radiation therapy in the treatment of bronchial carcinoma. Cancer 1972;30:1388–94.

201. Warram J. Preoperative irradiation of cancer of the lung: final report of a therapeutic trial: a collaborative study. Cancer 1975;36:914–25.

202. Green N, Kurohara SS, George FW 3rd, Crews QE Jr. Postresection irradiation for primary lung cancer. Radiology 1975;116:405–7.

203. Kirsh MM, Sloan H. Mediastinal metastases in bronchogenic carcinoma: influence of postoperative irradiation, cell type, and location. Ann Thorac Surg 1982;33:459–63.

204. Effects of postoperative mediastinal radiation on completely resected stage II and stage III epidermoid cancer of the lung. The Lung Cancer Study Group. N Engl J Med 1986;315:1377–81.

205. Postoperative radiotherapy in non-small-cell lung cancer: systematic review and meta-analysis of individual patient data from nine randomised controlled trials. PORT Meta-analysis Trialists Group. Lancet 1998;352:257–63.

206. Bunn PA Jr, Nugent JL, Matthews MJ. Central nervous system metastases in small cell bronchogenic carcinoma. Semin Oncol 1978;5:314–22.

207. Cox JD, Yesner RA. Adenocarcinoma of the lung: recent results from the Veterans Administration Lung Group. Am Rev Respir Dis 1979;120:1025–9.

208. Figlin RA, Piantadosi S, Feld R. Intracranial recurrence of carcinoma after complete surgical resection of stage I, II, and III non-small-cell lung cancer. N Engl J Med 1988;318:1300–5.

209. Nielsen OS, Bentzen SM, Sandberg E, et al. Randomized trial of single dose versus fractionated palliative radiotherapy of bone metastases. Radiother Oncol 1998;47:233–40.

210. Cox JD, Yesner R, Mietlowski W, Petrovich Z. Influence of cell type on failure pattern after irradiation for locally advanced carcinoma of the lung. Cancer 1979;44:94–8.

211. Martini N, Beattie EJ Jr: Results of surgical treatment in Stage I lung cancer. J Thorac Cardiovasc Surg 1977;74:499–505.

212. Feld R, Rubinstein LV, Weisenberger TH. Sites of recurrence in resected stage I non-small-cell lung cancer: a guide for future studies. J Clin Oncol 1984;2:1352–8.

213. Arriagada R, Auperin A, Pignon JP, et al. Prophylactic cranial irradiation overview in patients with small cell lung cancer in complete remission. Proc Am Soc Clin Oncol 1998;17:457a.

214. Gregor A, Cull A, Stephens RJ, et al. Prophylactic cranial irradiation is indicated following complete response to induction therapy in small cell lung cancer: results of a multicentre randomised trial. United Kingdom Coordinating Committee for Cancer Research (UKCCCR) and the European Organization for Research and Treatment of Cancer (EORTC). Eur J Cancer 1997;33:1752–8.

215. Arriagada R, Le Chevalier T, Borie F, et al. Prophylactic cranial irradiation for patients with small-cell lung cancer in complete remission. J Natl Cancer Inst 1995;87:183–90.

216. Ahles TA, Silberfarb PM, Herndon J 2nd: Psychology and neuropsychologic functioning of patients with limited small-cell lung cancer treated with chemotherapy and radiation therapy with or without warfarin: a study by the Cancer and Leukemia Group B. J Clin Oncol 1998;16:1954–60.

217. Martini N, Kris MG, Flehinger BJ, et al. Preoperative chemotherapy for stage IIIa (N2) lung cancer: the Sloan-Kettering experience with 136 patients. Ann Thorac Surg 1993;55:1365–73.

218. Burkes RL, Ginsberg RJ, Shepherd FA, et al. Induction chemotherapy with mitomycin, vindesine, and cisplatin for stage III unresectable non-small-cell lung cancer: results of the Toronto Phase II Trial. J Clin Oncol 1992;10:580–6.

219. Bitran JD, Golomb HM, Hoffman PC, et al. Protochemotherapy in non-small cell lung carcinoma: an attempt to increase surgical resectability and survival: a preliminary report. Cancer 1986;57:44–53 and 58:1377.

220. Vokes EE, Bitran JD, Hoffman PC, et al: Neoadjuvant vindesine, etoposide, and cisplatin for locally advanced non-small cell lung cancer: final report of a phase 2 study. Chest 1989;96:110–3.

221. Skarin A, Jochelson M, Sheldon T, et al. Neoadjuvant chemotherapy in marginally resectable stage III M0 non-small cell lung cancer: long-term follow-up in 41 patients. J Surg Oncol 1989;40:266–74.

222. Cullen MH, Ferry D, Souhami RL, et al. A randomised trial of chemotherapy plus radiotherapy versus radiotherapy alone in localised non-small cell lung cancer: preliminary report. Lung Cancer 1991;7:Suppl:164.

223. Le Chevalier T, Arriagada R, Baldeyrou P, et al. Combined chemotherapy (vindesine, lomustine, cisplatin, and cyclophosphamide) and radical radiotherapy in inoperable nonmetastatic squamous cell carcinoma of the lung. Cancer Treat Rep 1985;69:469–72.

224. Le Chevalier T, Arriagada R, Quoix E, et al. Radiotherapy alone versus combined chemotherapy and radiotherapy in nonresectable non-small-cell lung cancer: first analysis of a randomized trial in 353 patients. J Natl Cancer Inst 1991;83:417–23.

225. Dillman RO, Seagren SL, Propert KJ, et al. A randomized trial of induction chemotherapy plus high-dose radiation versus radiation alone in stage III non-small-cell lung cancer. N Engl J Med 1990;323:940–5.

226. Johnson DH, Einhorn LH, Bartolucci A, et al. Thoracic radiotherapy does not prolong survival in patients with locally advanced, unresectable non-small cell lung cancer. Ann Intern Med 1990;113:33–8.

227. Dillman RO, Seagren SL, Herdon J, Green MR. Randomized trial of induction chemotherapy plus radiation therapy vs. RT alone in stage III non-small-cell lung cancer (NSCLC): five year follow up of CALGB. Proc ASCO 1993;12:329.

228. Le Chevalier T, Arriagada R, Tarayre M, et al. Significant effect of adjuvant chemotherapy on survival in locally advanced non-small-cell lung carcinoma. J Natl Cancer Inst 1992;84:58.

229. Mira JG, Miller TP, Crowley JJ. Chest irradiation (RT) vs. chest RT + chemotherapy + prophylactic brain RT in localized non small cell lung cancer: a SWOG randomized study. Int J Radiat Oncol Biol Phys 1990;19:Suppl:145.

230. Mattson K, Holsti LR, Holsti P, et al. Inoperable non-small cell lung cancer: radiation with or without chemotherapy. Eur J Cancer Clin Oncol 1988;24:477–82.

231. Trovò MG, Minatel E, Veronesi A, et al. Combined radiotherapy and chemotherapy versus radiotherapy alone in locally advanced epidermoid bronchogenic carcinoma: a randomized study. Cancer 1990;65:400–4.

232. Ansari R, Tokar SR, Fisher W, et al. A phase III study of thoracic irradiation with or without concomitant cisplatin in locoregional unresectable non-small cell lung cancer (NSCLC): a Hoosier Oncology Group protocol. Proc Am Soc Clin Oncol 1991;10:241.

233. Schaake-Koning C, van den Bogaert W, Dalesio O, et al. Effects of concomitant cisplatin and radiotherapy on inoperable non-small-cell lung cancer. N Engl J Med 1992;326:524–30.

234. Soresi E, Clerici M, Grilli R, et al. A randomized clinical trial comparing radiation therapy v radiation therapy plus cis-dichlorodiammine platinum (II) in the treatment of locally advanced non-small cell lung cancer. Semin Oncol 1988;15:Suppl 7:20–5.

235. Martini N, Flehinger BJ. The role of surgery in N2 lung cancer. Surg Clin North Am 1987;67:1037–49.

236. Eagan RT, Ruud C, Lee RE, et al. Pilot study of induction therapy with cyclophosphamide, doxorubicin, and cisplatin (CAP) and chest irradiation prior to thoracotomy in initially inoperable stage III M0 non-small cell lung cancer. Cancer Treat Rep 1987;71:895–900.

237. Faber LP, Kittle CF, Warren WH, et al. Preoperative chemotherapy and irradiation for stage III non-small cell lung cancer. Ann Thorac Surg 1989;47:669–75.

238. Weiden PL, Piantadosi S. Preoperative chemotherapy (cisplatin and fluorouracil) and radiation therapy in stage III non-small-cell lung cancer: a phase II study of the Lung Cancer Study Group. J Natl Cancer Inst 1991;83:266–73.

239. Albain KS, Rusch VW, Crowley JJ, et al. Concurrent cisplatin/etoposide plus chest radiotherapy followed by surgery for stages IIIA (N2) and IIIB non-small-cell lung cancer: mature results of Southwest Oncology Group phase II study 8805. J Clin Oncol 1995;13:1880–92.

240. Rusch VW, Albain KS, Crowley JJ, et al. Surgical resection of stage IIIA and stage IIIB non-small-cell lung cancer after concurrent induction chemoradiotherapy: a Southwest Oncology Group trial. J Thorac Cardiovasc Surg 1993;105:97–104.

241. Bitran JD, Golomb HM, Hoffman PC, et al. Protochemotherapy in non-small cell lung carcinoma: an attempt to increase surgical resectability and survival: a preliminary report. Cancer 1986;57:44–53 and 58:1377.

242. Martini N, Kris MG, Gralla RJ, et al. The effects of preoperative chemotherapy on the resectability of non-small cell lung carcinoma with mediastinal lymph node metastases (N2 M0). Ann Thorac Surg 1988;45:370–9.

243. Gralla RJ. Preoperative and adjuvant chemotherapy in non-small cell lung cancer. Semin Oncol 1988;15:8–12.

244. Burkes R, Ginsberg R, Shepherd M, et al. Neo-adjuvant trial with MVP (mitomycin-C + vindesine + cis-platin) chemotherapy for stage III (T1–3, N2 M0) unresectable non-small cell lung cancer (NSCLC). Proc ASCO 1989;8:221.

245. Rosell R, Gómez-Codina J, Camps C, et al. A randomized trial comparing preoperative chemotherapy plus surgery with surgery alone in patients with non-small-cell lung cancer. N Engl J Med 1994;330:153–8.

246. Roth JA, Fossella F, Komaki R, et al. A randomized trial comparing perioperative chemotherapy and surgery with surgery alone in resectable stage IIIA non-small-cell lung cancer. J Natl Cancer Inst 1994;86:673–80.

247. Ihde DC. Chemotherapy of lung cancer. N Engl J Med 1992;327:1434–41.

248. Soquet PJ, Chauvin F, Boissel JP, et al. Polychemotherapy in advanced non-small cell lung cancer: a meta-analysis. Lancet 1993;342:19–21.

249. Non-small Cell Lung Cancer Collaborative Group. Chemotherapy in non-small cell lung cancer: meta-analysis using updated data on individual patients from 52 randomized clinical trials. Br Med J 1995;311:899–909.

250. Marino P, Pampallona S, Preatoni A, et al. Chemotherapy *versus* supportive care in advanced non-small cell lung cancer: results of a meta-analysis of the literature. Chest 1994;106:861–5.

251. American Society of Clinical Oncology. Special article: clinical practice guidelines for treatment of unresectable non-small cell lung cancer. J Clin Oncol 1997;15:2996–3018.

252. Albain KS, Crowley JJ, LeBlane M, et al. Survival determinants in extensive stage non-small cell lung cancer: the Southwest Oncology Group experience. J Clin Oncol 1991;9:1618–26.

253. Cardenal F, Lopez-Cabrerizo MP, Anton A, et al. Randomized Phase III study of gemcitabine-cisplatin versus etopside-cisplatin in the treatment of locally advanced or metastatic non-small-cell lung cancer. J Clin Oncol 1999;17:12–8.

254. Wozniak AJ, Crowley JJ, Balcerzak SP, et al. Randomized trial comparing cisplatin with cisplatin plus vinorelbine in the treatment of advanced non-small-cell lung cancer: a Southwest Oncology Group study. J Clin Oncol 1998;16:2459–65.

255. Sandler J, Nemunaitis J, Dehham C, et al. Phase III study of cisplatin (C) with or without gemcitabine (G) in patients with advanced non-small cell lung cancer (NSCLC). Proc ASCO 1998;17:1747.

256. Billingham LJ, Cullen MH, Woods J, et al. Mitomycin, ifosfamide and cisplatin in non-small cell lung cancer: results of a randomized trial evaluating palliation and quality of life. Lung Cancer 1997;18:Suppl 1:9.

257. Giaccone G, Ted AW, Splinter CD, et al. Randomized study of paclitaxel-cisplatin versus cisplatin-teniposide in patients with advanced non-small-cell lung cancer. J Clin Oncol 1998;16:2133–41.

258. Desch CE, Hillner BE, Smith TJ. Economic considerations in the care of lung cancer patients. Curr Opin Oncol 1996;8:126–32.

259. Evans WK, Will BP, Berthelot JM, et al. Estimating the cost of lung cancer diagnosis and treatment in Canada: the POHEM model. Can J Oncol 1995;5:408–19.

260. Evans WK, Will BP, Berthelot JM, et al. Cost of combined modality interventions for stage III non-small-cell lung cancer. J Clin Oncol 1997;15:3038–48.

261. Jaakinainen L, Goodwin PJ, Pater L, et al. Counting the costs of chemotherapy in a National Cancer Institute of Canada randomized trial in non-small cell lung cancer. J Clin Oncol 1990;13:1301–9.

262. Smith TJ, Hillner BE, Neighbors DM, et al. Economic evaluation of a randomized clinical trial comparing vinorelbine, vinorelbine plus cisplatin and vindesine plus cisplatin. J Clin Oncol 1995;13:2166–73.

263. Copley-Merriman C, Corral J, King K, et al. Economic value of gemcitabine compared to cisplatin and etoposide in non-small cell lung cancer. Lung Cancer 1996;14:45–61.

264. Pedersen AG, Kristjansen PE, Hansen HH. Prophylactic cranial irradiation and small cell lung cancer. Cancer Treat Rev 1988;15:85–103.

265. Morton RF, Jett JR, McGinnis WL, et al. Thoracic radiation therapy alone compared with combined chemoradiotherapy for locally unresectable non-small cell lung cancer: a randomized, phase III trial. Ann Intern Med 1991;115:681–6.

266. Emami B, Graham M, Lockett MA. High dose conventional fractionation radiation therapy in unresectable non-small cell lung cancer: patients with good prognostic factors. Lung Cancer 1991;7:Suppl:89.

## CHAPTER 37

# SMALL CELL CARCINOMA OF THE LUNG

• ULRIK LASSEN • HEINE H. HANSEN

The management of patients with small cell lung cancer (SCLC) has undergone pronounced changes since 1970. Before 1970, surgery and radiotherapy were the most common forms of treatment, but these local methods rarely result in long-term control when used as a single treatment modality. An appreciation of the frequency and extent of metastases, coupled with the sensitivity of SCLC to a variety of chemotherapeutic agents, has led to the present emphasis on the central role of systemic chemotherapy. These changes have resulted in a fivefold increase in median survival and a long-term disease-free survival of more than 3 years in 5 to 10% of patients with SCLC as a whole and in 15 to 20% of patients presenting with a limited extent of disease and other favorable prognostic factors.[1, 2] Even though considerable progress has been achieved, there is still no standardized treatment for SCLC. Work is being carried out in many centers and in national and international groups to expand knowledge of the special biologic features and treatment of SCLC, in the hope that it will become more readily curable. This chapter discusses the present range of therapeutic options based on the literature, including the vast amount of data presented at the Eighth World Congress on Lung Cancer in Dublin 1997.[3] Etiologic and epidemiologic aspects of SCLC are covered in Chapter 36.

## Natural History

### HISTOPATHOLOGY

The prognostic value of the histopathologic subclassification of SCLC according to the World Health Organization (WHO) classification of 1981[4] is somewhat confusing, and there is disagreement regarding the prognostic impact of the various subtypes, such as oat cell and intermediate-type carcinoma. This disagreement may reflect a lack of consistency in the different pathologic findings rather than a genuine difference in the biology of the various subtypes. An especially poor prognosis has been demonstrated for patients with small cell carcinoma characterized before treatment as tumors with small cell and large cell components.[5] These tumors have been difficult to classify, and this was one of the reasons for the International Association for the Study of Lung Cancer (IASLC) proposal for a new classification.[6] In this revised system, tumors are categorized into three groups: (1) pure small cell carcinoma, (2) small cell and large cell, and (3) combined tumors with SCLC components. This simpler recommendation avoids former inconsistencies and takes into account the present knowledge of prognostic factors. Accordingly the term *small cell carcinoma* is recommended for all SCLC tumors that have no non–small cell

elements and include the neoplastic cell with oval, round, or fusiform nuclei in which the chromatin is diffusely distributed in a stripped pattern, most nucleoli being small and indistinct, with scanty cytoplasm. The cell borders are indistinct, being arranged in clusters, cords, sheets, or trabeculae. These features of pure small cell carcinoma are seen in more than 90% of untreated SCLC and correspond to the classic SCLC cell line. The second subtype of SCLC is the mixed small cell and large cell carcinoma containing subpopulations of cells resembling large cell carcinoma. A characteristic finding consists of prominent, frequent eosinophilic nucleoli with a paranucleolar halo. The chromatin pattern may be finely granulated and the diameter of the nuclei large, with varying amounts of cytoplasm. Four to 6% of untreated cases of SCLC are mixed small cell and large cell carcinomas that correspond to the variant SCLC cell lines. The third SCLC subtype is another variant of combined small cell carcinoma, in which the pure small cell component is combined with squamous carcinoma or adenocarcinoma of the lung. Less than 1% of untreated SCLC falls into this group.[7]

## BIOLOGY

The development of various media for culturing cell lines of SCLC has resulted in major advances in the understanding of the biologic properties of this tumor. The cell lines can be subdivided into classic or variant types.[8] The classic cell line corresponds to the pure small cell carcinoma. Characteristic findings are long doubling time (>50 hours), poor cloning ability, and the typical appearance of a scanty cytoplasm, nuclear molding, and inconspicuous nucleoli. The classic cell line usually exerts a high expression of neuroendocrine markers, such as BB-isoenzymes of creatine kinase, L-dopa-decarboxylase (DDC), bombesin–gastrin releasing polypeptide (GRP), chromogranin A, neural cell adhesion molecule (NCAM), and neuron-specific enolase (NSE). Other neuroendocrine features include synaptophysin and Leu-7. In contrast, the variant cell lines have lower contents of DDC and bombesin-GRP, have a shorter doubling time (<30 hours), and resemble large cell undifferentiated carcinoma with more cytoplasm and prominent nucleoli. The variant cell lines are radioresistant and often have substantial amplification of the C-*myc* gene.[8] Retrospective studies have shown a shorter survival in patients from whom variant cell lines were established,[9] but a study of patients with limited disease showed no adverse prognosis of variant morphology compared with the classic type.[10] Many polypeptide hormones probably act as autocrine growth factors. Bombesin-GRP is a potent growth factor for SCLC, and epidermal growth factor, insulin-like growth factor I, and transferrin are also important growth factors and act as mitogens in various cell types. Transforming growth factor (TGF) is nonmitogenous, and the expression of TGF-receptor seems to influence growth suppression by TGF-β.[11]

Many chromosome abnormalities have been observed in SCLC, and the clinical emergence of lung cancer may precede 10 to 20 genetic mutations. The changes cover translocations, activation or mutation of dominant oncogenes, or loss or mutation of tumor-suppressor genes.[12] The most common change is deletion on the short arm of chromosome 3p, which is found in more than 90% of SCLC cell lines. Three suppressor genes on chromosome 3p have been suggested to contribute to the malignant transformation, but the sequence has not been fully identified.[13] The gene coding for p53, which is present on chromosome 17p, is mutated in almost 100% of SCLCs and in approximately 50% of non-SCLCs.[8] Normally, p53 regulates normal proliferation and may induce apoptosis in response to DNA damage, but the mutated form may stimulate proliferation and inhibit apoptosis and act as a dominant oncogene.[12] The retinoblastoma gene (Rb) is located on chromosome 13q14, and structural changes have been observed in 70% of SCLC cell lines. Rb acts by suppressing the transition from the $G_1$ phase to the S phase, and absent expression may lead to uncontrolled proliferation.[12]

Oncogene mutations in SCLC are predominantly among the *myc* family, the most frequent abnormality being overexpression without amplification.[14] This overexpression is seen late in the natural history of SCLC, mainly in relapsed patients, and may correlate negatively with survival.[12]

Flow cytometry analysis of fresh tumors and permanent cell lines has shown considerable DNA and chromosomal heterogeneity in SCLC.[15-17] No relationship between the degree of aneuploidy and survival has been observed, however.[17] This is in contrast to the situation in lymphomas, leukemias, and multiple myeloma.

## STAGING

The recognition of SCLC as a systemic disease has rendered the anatomic staging of patients less important as the basis of treatment outside an experimental setting. To assess prognosis and compare results from different trials, staging procedures are still important, although it is now evident that patients can be stratified into distinct prognostic groups on the basis of biochemical evaluation, including lactate dehydrogenase (LDH) and alkaline phosphatase levels, in combination with other descriptive data.[18-25] The anatomic stage is an important guideline in deciding whether to apply additional local treatment, such as radiotherapy or surgery, as part of the overall treatment plan. The TNM system as recommended by the Union Internationale Contre le Cancer (UICC) has not traditionally been considered well suited for SCLC because more than 95% of the patients would be classified in the worst stages. Modification of the TNM system[26] has changed the situation, and two systems are now available for staging SCLC patients: (1) the classic VA Lung Cancer Study Group (VALG) system of *limited* or *extensive* disease and (2) the revised TNM system (see Tables 36–8 and 36–9). In the VALG system, the classification of patients with contralateral mediastinal or supraclavicular nodes and

of patients with ipsilateral pleural effusions has not been uniformly handled by different investigators.

**Limited Disease.** The limited disease classification includes patients with disease restricted to one hemithorax with regional lymph node metastases, including hilar, ipsilateral, and contralateral mediastinal and supraclavicular nodes. Patients with ipsilateral pleural effusion are included, regardless of whether the cytologic study results are positive or negative. Inclusion of the contralateral nodes in the mediastinum and the supraclavicular region was decided on because the prognostic influence of these metastatic sites is less than that of distant metastases and because the revised TNM system groups these patients in stage III and not stage IV. Stages I to III of the revised TNM offer a subdivision of the limited disease category, which may be useful when local treatment modalities are evaluated.

**Extensive Disease.** The extensive disease classification includes all patients with disease sites not eligible for the limited stage, and this category is equivalent to stage IV of the TNM system. Detailed staging procedures are given in Table 37–1. The assessment should be repeated after treatment to evaluate the response and when additional treatment is being considered, such as prophylactic cranial irradiation.

*Table 37–1.* **Recommendation of Staging Procedures in Small Cell Lung Cancer**

| | Clinical Practice | | |
| --- | --- | --- | --- |
| | LOCAL TREATMENT MODALITY CONSIDERED | | Clinical Trial |
| **Procedure** | *No* | *Yes* | |
| *General Procedures* | | | |
| Physical examination | + | + | + |
| Blood counts | + | + | + |
| Serum biochemistry | + | + | + |
| Cytologic or histologic documentation of SCLC | + | + | + |
| *Procedures for Local Disease* | | | |
| Chest radiography | + | + | + |
| Chest CT | − | − | +* |
| Bronchoscopy | − | − | +† |
| Mediastinoscopy | − | − | +‡ |
| Cytology of effusion | − | − | + |
| Cytology of supraclavicular node | − | − | +§ |
| *Procedures for Distant Disease* | | | |
| Bone scan | − | +‖ | + |
| Bone radiography | − | +¶ | +¶ |
| Ultrasonography or abdominal CT | − | +‖ | + |
| Fine-needle aspiration and biopsy | − | +‖ | +§ |
| Bone marrow aspiration and biopsy | − | +‖ | + |
| Brain CT and MRI | − | +‖ | + |

*Especially for trials of limited disease.

†If bronchoscopy is anticipated at restaging, surgery for limited disease is necessary or diagnosis cannot be obtained.

‡Only if needed by the surgeon for preoperative work-up.

§If findings are doubtful and establishment of a positive finding affects treatment.

‖If one test is positive, further evaluation can be discontinued.

¶Only in areas of increased uptake on bone scan.

SCLC, small cell lung cancer; CT, computed tomography; MRI, magnetic resonance imaging.

Restaging should include a re-evaluation of all abnormal pretreatment findings. Magnetic resonance imaging (MRI) has in many centers replaced computed tomography (CT) for diagnosis of brain metastases because of higher accuracy.[27] Positron emission tomography (PET) for detection of distant metastases is under investigation.[28] The diagnosis of bone marrow metastases—which can be missed by conventional histologic techniques—can be made by culture techniques, discontinuous gradient sedimentation, staining with monoclonal antibodies, and MRI.[29, 30] The impact of the results of these investigations on staging and prognosis remains to be defined. Biologic markers in serum, such as NSE and chromogranin, are still being investigated[31] and are not yet used routinely in the clinic.

## PROGNOSTIC FACTORS

With current therapeutic options, it is important to define the objective of treatment before initiating therapy. In elderly patients and in those with an adverse prognosis, palliation may be the most important and realistic objective, whereas in other patients, long-term survival or cure is the ultimate goal, despite the more pronounced toxicity associated with treatment. Accordingly, it is important to evaluate patients carefully with respect to the main prognostic factors before starting treatment. Some of the most important prognostic factors are listed in Table 37–2. The two key factors are pretreatment performance status and extent of disease. LDH is also an important prognostic factor with impact on overall survival and fatal toxic complications.[32] With regard to age and sex, several studies have reported that patients younger than age 60 do better than those older than 60, and women appear to have a better prognosis than men. It has been suggested that the superior survival of the female gender is due to a more aggressive (myelotoxic) treatment of young female patients, but Wolf and colleagues[23] were not able to find differences in leukocyte nadirs between male and female patients. With regard to the impact of anatomic stage on survival, bone marrow metastases and central nervous system (CNS) involvement per se result in a poor prognosis.

## Chemotherapy of Small Cell Lung Cancer

The main treatment modality for SCLC is chemotherapy. The ideal therapeutic goal in SCLC is to achieve the highest

*Table 37–2.* **Prognostic Factors in Small Cell Lung Cancer**

Stage, limited vs. extensive disease
Performance status
Sex*
Age
Histologic subclassification†
Bone marrow metastases
Liver metastases
Central nervous system involvement
Blood biochemistry, especially lactate dehydrogenase levels

*The prognostic impact of the patient's sex seems to have lessened along with the increase in incidence of small cell lung cancer in women.
†The prognosis is especially poor if large cell elements are observed.

*Table 37–3.* **Cytotoxic Drugs for Small Cell Lung Cancer**

| | |
|---|---|
| Alkylating agents | Epipodophyllotoxin |
|   Cyclophosphamide |   derivatives |
|   Ifosfamide |   Etoposide |
|   Hexamethylmelamine |   Teniposide |
|   Lomustine | Platinum analogues |
| *Vinca* alkaloids |   Cisplatin |
|   Vincristine |   Carboplatin |
|   Vindesine | Miscellaneous |
| |   Doxorubicin |
| |   Methotrexate |

long-term disease-free survival (*cure*) with the lowest possible morbidity. This ambition is still far from being realized despite the fact that many antineoplastic agents have been shown to have antitumor activity in SCLC and produce initial responses in 90% of patients when used in combination.

The cytostatic treatment of SCLC is constantly subjected to changes and refinements. During the 1970s, the median survival period was prolonged fourfold to fivefold, and possible cure was obtained in 5 to 10% of all patients.[126] No major additional improvement has been observed in extensive disease since then,[33] but a vast amount of work has consolidated the early results. Many agents have exhibited antitumor activity (Table 37–3), and since the mid-1990s many new agents with different modes of actions have been added.[34] Most studies have included compounds, such as etoposide, teniposide, vincristine, cyclophosphamide, ifosfamide, doxorubicin, chloroethyl-cyclohexyl-nitrosourea (CCNU), cisplatin, carboplatin, and methotrexate. Among the most commonly used combinations are the following:

1. Epipodophyllotoxins (etoposide or teniposide) and platinum compounds (cisplatin or carboplatin) (*EP*)
2. Doxorubicin (Adriamycin), cyclophosphamide, and etoposide (*ACE*)
3. Cyclophosphamide, doxorubicin (Adriamycin), and vincristine (*CAV*)

Examples of these regimens, including scheduling and doses, are shown in Table 37–4.

There has been a tendency to include etoposide or teniposide in the initial treatment because studies have shown that combinations with these agents are superior to those without.[35, 36] For some time, it was considered evident that

*Table 37–4.* **Commonly Used Regimens for Small Cell Lung Cancer**

| Agent | Regimen |
|---|---|
| Etoposide | 80 mg/m² IV daily on days 1–3 q 3 wk |
| Cisplatin | 80 mg/m² IV q 3 wk, day 1 |
|   or | |
| Carboplatin | AUC 6 day 1 |
| Ifosfamide | 5000 mg/m² day 1 q 3 wk |
| Carboplatin | 300 mg/m² day 1 q 3 wk |
| Etoposide | 120 mg/m² IV daily on days 1–3 q 3 wk |
| Cyclophosphamide | 1500 mg/m² IV q 3 wk |
| Doxorubicin | 40 mg/m² IV q 3 wk |
| Vincristine | 2 mg IV q 3 wk |

IV, intravenous; AUC, area under the curve.

drug combinations with three or four drugs were superior to single-agent therapy. This belief is based on theoretical considerations as well as clinical investigations. Other results indicate that epipodophyllotoxins, in a two-drug combination with cisplatin, are as effective as multidrug combinations in producing initial responses.[37] Carboplatin has shown levels of activity similar to these of cisplatin and may have a more favorable toxicity profile and easier administration.[36, 38, 39]

Combination regimens result in a response rate greater than 80% for both stages of SCLC. A complete response is produced in 30 to 40% of patients with limited disease and in more than 15 to 20% of those with extensive disease.

For unselected patients, the median survival for patients with limited disease should be greater than 12 to 14 months provided that an adequate staging procedure has been completed; median survival for patients with extensive disease is usually 8 months or more. An evaluation of treatment-associated toxicity is essential, and fatal toxicity of more than 5% is considered unacceptable. Experience suggests that the regimens including epipodophyllotoxins and platinum improve response rates and median survival at the expense of increased toxicity, including toxic deaths.[32]

Treatment of elderly patients and patients with a poor performance status is often associated with increased toxicity.[32] Intensive combination chemotherapy is not feasible in these categories of patients, and less aggressive regimens are required. The use of intravenous etoposide or teniposide alone has shown significant activity.[40] This treatment can be administered entirely on an outpatient basis with minimal mortality and morbidity.[41] Studies of prolonged schedules of oral etoposide have shown clinically useful activity in patients in whom standard administration fails,[42] but two British randomized studies have compared first-line single-agent oral etoposide with multiagent intravenous chemotherapy in patients with adverse prognostic factors based on performance status and disease extent. Both these studies concluded that single-agent oral etoposide is inferior to intravenous combination chemotherapy.[43, 44] These studies did not answer whether this difference was the result of the number of agents used or the route of administration.

The changes in staging procedures may have led to a *stage-migration effect*,[45] and one should be careful when comparing data from the late 1980s with those obtained in the 1970s because important changes in staging procedures have taken place. These changes may have enlarged the extensive disease group and diminished the limited disease group. Treatment results for groups analyzed individually might show an improvement, although the overall results would be unchanged.[46]

Survival beyond 5 years is achieved in 10 to 20% of patients with limited disease and in 3 to 5% of those with extensive disease, although these results depend on selection criteria.[1, 2] In large national studies, which are more representative of the patient population as a whole than cooperative group studies, the results are less encouraging. For instance, studies from England, Denmark, and Italy show 5-year survival rates of only 4% and 2 to 3%, respectively.[25, 47, 48] Relapses are seen as late as 11 years after initiation of treatment.[49] A variety of issues about the cytostatic treatment of SCLC are under investigation concerning (1) improvement of treatment efficacy, (2) reduction of the toxicity associated with the treatment, and (3) treatment of special clinical conditions, including CNS disease, paraneoplastic syndromes, and superior vena cava syndrome. The approaches to improve the outcome include the following options:

1. Alternating *non–cross-resistant* chemotherapy
2. Intensive high-dose chemotherapy with or without growth factors or bone marrow support or transplantation
3. New schedules of drug administration
4. Incorporation of new agents with high activity into the combination chemotherapy regimens
5. Gene therapy and anti-invasive or antiangiogenic modifiers

## ALTERNATING CHEMOTHERAPY

Resistant clones of SCLC cells, which develop at the time of diagnosis or during chemotherapy, are the reason for treatment failure in most patients. Evidence associating clonal heterogeneity and clinical resistance has come from clinical studies and from permanent cell lines and human xenografts. Goldie and Coldman[50, 51] have described a simple mathematical model based on the probabilistic nature of spontaneously arising resistant clones. Review of 13 randomized phase III trials of alternating versus sequential combination chemotherapy provides no convincing evidence to suggest a clinically important advantage of alternating use of different non–cross-resistant combinations of various cytostatic agents over existing regimens.[52–64] Trials comparing EP versus CAV versus alternation with these two regimens (EP-CAV) have had conflicting results. Roth and coworkers[54] found no difference in response rates and survival, whereas Fukuoka and associates[64] found increased overall response rates and increased median survival in patients with limited disease treated with the alternating approach.

## DOSE INTENSIFICATION

Most large studies addressing dose intensity have been retrospective, and only a few randomized trials have investigated this issue in SCLC. A meta-analysis addressed to intended dose intensity over the first two cycles of chemotherapy (6 weeks) was made in 1991 by Klasa and colleagues.[65] For limited and extensive disease, few correlations between dose intensity and outcome have been observed. Because of the heterogeneity of the rather small patient population, however, no firm conclusions can be derived from this meta-analysis.

Colony-stimulating factors (CSFs) are known to reduce hematologic toxicity by stimulating proliferation and differentiation of hematopoietic stem cells. In several studies, granulocyte colony–stimulating factors (G-CSFs) have been able to accelerate neutrophil recovery in patients with SCLC, and two large randomized trials using G-CSFs have shown a decrease in febrile episodes with less hospitalization and higher neutrophil counts when G-CSF was applied together with intensive chemotherapy. No impact on response rate, response duration, or median survival was observed.[66, 67]

Studies have succeeded in increasing dose intensity of CODE (cisplatin, vincristine [Oncovin], doxorubicin, and etoposide) by a factor of 2 in extensive-stage SCLC, resulting in improved complete response rates and increased toxicity but no impact on survival.[68, 69] In other studies, the use of hematopoietic growth factors did not result in increasing dose intensity.[67] Preliminary data from a British study in which the dose intensity of ACE was increased by a factor of 1.3 seem to indicate improved survival,[70] however, and another European randomized trial with V-ICE (vincristine, ifosfamide, cisplatin, and etoposide) also demonstrated a significant survival benefit by dose intensification.[71]

Several phase II studies of high-dose chemotherapy with autologous bone marrow transplantation have been performed as another method of dose intensification but without definite evidence of improved overall survival. Further studies are needed to exploit the potential value of intensification of chemotherapy as a part of the initial treatment or in terms of late intensification.

## DURATION OF TREATMENT

The toxicity of maintenance chemotherapy, including an increased appearance of secondary leukemias and decreased quality of life, led to a tendency to shorten the duration of treatment in the early 1980s. At that time, treatment was often scheduled to last 12 to 18 months. When SCLC responds to chemotherapy, the maximal response is usually achieved within the first three courses. Because of side effects, it is preferable to continue treatment no longer than necessary, and several phase III trials have focused on this issue. Two large British studies showed a modest survival benefit from maintenance chemotherapy after four to six courses,[72, 73] whereas a large phase III trial from the European Organization for Research and Treatment of Cancer (EORTC) concluded that prolonged chemotherapy does not increase the chance of survival.[74] In this trial, patients were randomly assigned to either 5 or 12 cycles of combination chemotherapy. Even though the maintenance arm had a progression-free survival of 2 months longer than the follow-up arm, there was no difference in overall survival. In the Third IASLC Workshop on SCLC in 1989, the consensus was that six to eight cycles of chemotherapy is an acceptable standard.[75] This number corresponds to a total treatment duration of 5 to 8 months. Results of a randomized trial from the European Lung Cancer Working Party have not affected this consensus, despite the fact that initial responders receiving maintenance therapy had an increased progression-free survival period. In this study, the maintenance regimen was different from the induction regimen, and the result probably reflects the effect of second-line therapy.[76]

Maintenance treatment with biologic response modifiers, such as interferons, has been studied in patients who responded to induction chemotherapy. Small randomized trials have yielded conflicting results with respect to response, progression-free survival, and overall survival.[77–80] Treatment with interferon is associated with significantly higher grade III and IV hematologic and nonhematologic toxicity, and such treatment is still considered experimental.

Antiaggregants, such as aspirin or warfarin, have been proposed to regulate SCLC cell growth and metastatic potential.[81, 82] At present, anticoagulants have no place in the therapy of SCLC. An initial small randomized trial suggested a possible survival benefit from adding warfarin to chemotherapy,[83] but subsequent larger trials[84] failed to detect any survival benefit.

## SECOND-LINE TREATMENT

Even though response rates to initial chemotherapy are high, most patients eventually develop progressive disease. Local recurrence occurs frequently, and if the patient has not previously received radiotherapy, thoracic irradiation is the treatment of choice.[1, 85] Patients with primary resistance to regimens containing multiple cytotoxic agents active against SCLC rarely respond to second-line chemotherapy. With a chemotherapy-free interval of more than 6 months before relapse, however, patients occasionally benefit from reinduction using primary chemotherapy, treatment with cisplatin and etoposide, or other non–cross-resistant regimens.[86] Response rates have been 29 to 75%, but the responses have been of short duration, usually 2 to 4 months.[87] Long-term, daily, low-dose oral etoposide given in a prolonged 21-day schedule has produced a response rate of 48%.[42] In a randomized trial including 211 patients comparing topotecan and CAV as second-line treatment in relapsed patients who achieved an initial response to first-line chemotherapy, partial responses were 25% and 15%, suggesting that topotecan as second-line treatment is at least as effective as CAV. No difference in survival was detected between the two regimens.[88]

## DRUG DEVELOPMENT

**New Drugs.** The most active of the new drugs tested in the 1980s include carboplatin[38] and the epipodophyllotoxin derivatives VP-16 (etoposide) and VM-26 (teniposide). Teniposide has proved highly active, with a response rate of 90% in untreated patients with SCLC.[89] The marked difference in response rates observed for teniposide in untreated (90%) and previously treated (18%) patients is important.[90] This difference reveals that there are major methodologic problems in the design and execution of clinical phase II trials with new agents for a highly chemosensitive tumor (see later). Epipodophyllotoxins are now included in most first-line combination regimens.

**Phase II Study Design.** Traditionally, phase II studies have been conducted in patients in whom primary treatment has failed. This approach involves the risk that valuable agents may be discarded if tested only in such patients. The active agent etoposide was missed when first tested in previously treated patients, whereas a subsequent trial by the same group of investigators in untreated patients produced an extremely high response rate. Similar experience has been obtained with carboplatin. The strategic problems are not settled by this trend because although highly active drugs might not be identified when tested in previously treated patients, untreated patients enrolled in phase II trials may receive an inactive phase II agent and no further therapy and subsequently have a short survival. In a randomized trial, however, patients who failed to respond to the investigational drug menogaril were switched to CAV.[91] Despite the low response rate to menogaril (5%), the overall survival was similar for the two patient groups. This study suggests that overall survival is not affected negatively by a short period of administration of an investigational agent.

The design and monitoring of trials should be aimed at minimizing possible adverse consequences as well as identifying active agents. Previously treated patients may still be included in phase II trials when the threshold for further study is greater than 10% activity and not the conventional 20%. Studies with a lower threshold of activity require more patients to establish that an agent is inactive.

In the 1990s, several new agents showed significant activity in previously treated and relapsing patients with SCLC.[34] The antineoplastic agents with demonstrable activity in small cell carcinoma are shown in Table 37–5.

Topotecan has been the most extensively studied single agent with 292 patients included in phase II studies.[92–94] EORTC studied 101 previously treated patients, with a distinction between sensitive patients, who responded to prior chemotherapy, and refractory patients, who did not respond or relapsed less than 3 months after first-line therapy. In the sensitive group, an objective response rate of 38% was achieved, including 13% complete remissions. In the refractory group, the response rate was 6%, including one complete response.[92] It is hoped that ongoing phase II studies of combinations of topotecan and platinum derivatives will determine the role of topotecan in first-line combinations. According to phase I studies, the toxicity is schedule dependent.

Irinotecan (CPT-11) has resulted in significant responses in previously treated patients. Two phase II studies with a total of 50 patients achieved a 28% response rate.[95, 96]

Paclitaxel has been studied only as a single agent in two phase II studies with previously untreated patients. Objective response rates ranged from 34 to 68%.[97, 98] This compound has been studied more extensively in combination with platinum and etoposide. Hainsworth and colleagues[99] achieved more than 90% tumor reduction in 91% of 72 patients included; among 41 patients with limited disease, 71% had a complete response.

Docetaxel has been evaluated in one study with 14 previously untreated patients. The objective response rate was 8%,[100] and in a study with previously treated patients it was 25%.[101] Another new agent, gemcitabine, which has been extensively tested in non-SCLC, has been evaluated in only one phase II trial including 26 previously untreated patients;

an objective response rate of 27% was achieved.[102] Finally, vinorelbine has been evaluated in previously treated SCLC patients resulting in a response rate of 17%.[103–105]

## CHEMOTHERAPY FOR SPECIAL CLINICAL SITUATIONS

Chemotherapy is used increasingly for special clinical situations, including CNS metastases, spinal cord compression, superior vena cava syndrome, and paraneoplastic syndromes.

**Central Nervous System Metastases.** The management of primary CNS involvement at the start of systemic treatment generally includes concomitant radiotherapy because most cytostatic agents are presumed not to penetrate sufficiently into brain metastases. Some studies have questioned this therapeutic approach[106] because patients with CT–verified brain metastases from the start of treatment apparently do as well *without* —at least initially— as *with* irradiation, provided chemotherapy is given initially. Complete responses demonstrated by CT of the brain and subsequent neurologic improvement after induction chemotherapy suggest that initial brain metastases respond as frequently as do metastatic SCLC tumors in other sites. In a review of 71 patients in eight clinical trials, 76% responded to chemotherapy for brain metastases when given at the time of diagnosis.[107] The precise impact of these observations on the overall management of SCLC awaits prospective analysis of large groups of patients.

The results of treatment of leptomeningeal carcinomatosis are generally disappointing. These poor results may be partially due to the frequent occurrence of concurrent multiple metastases. The poor prognosis of these patients, along with the lack of reliable objective parameters to monitor treatment outcome, makes the evaluation of various approaches difficult. Intrathecal methotrexate remains the most widely used therapy, and information on the use of other cytostatic agents is sparse. Intravenous high-dose etoposide has also been used with some effect but with considerable systemic toxicity.[108]

**Spinal Cord Compression.** During the natural history of SCLC, approximately 3% of patients develop spinal cord compression.[109] Because of the often disabling symptoms, acute therapy, either radiotherapy or laminectomy, should always be initiated. The role of steroids is controversial, but according to one randomized trial, the use of high-dose

*Table 37–5.* **New Active Agents in Small Cell Lung Cancer**

| Agent | Previously Untreated | Previously Treated | Response Rate (%) | 95% Confidence Interval | Reference |
|---|---|---|---|---|---|
| Camptothecin | 8 | | 50 | 16–84 | 95 |
| (CPT-11) | | 50 | 28 | 16–42 | 96 |
| Topotecan | 48 | | 40 | 1–32 | 94 |
| | | 292 | 17 | 13–22 | 92, 93 |
| Gemcitabine | 26 | | 27 | 12–48 | 102 |
| | | 0 | | | |
| Docetaxel | 14 | | 8 | 0–34 | 100 |
| (Taxotere) | | 28 | 25 | 11–45 | 101 |
| Paclitaxel | 69 | | 38 | 26–50 | 97, 98 |
| (Taxol) | | 0 | | | |
| Vinorelbine | 0 | | | | |
| (Navelbine) | | 49 | 17 | 5–28 | 104, 105 |

steroids for 3 days, followed by tapering, results in a significant effect on gait function preservation.[110] At present, steroids are recommended during radiotherapy for spinal cord compression.

**Superior Vena Cava Obstruction.** Radiotherapy was once considered essential when superior vena cava syndrome was part of the initial presentation. Subsequent studies have shown that systemic chemotherapy alone in almost all cases produces sufficient relief from this condition, with no additional benefit obtained from mediastinal irradiation.[111, 112] The effect of chemotherapy is usually observed within a few days; if not, palliative radiotherapy is recommended (e.g., 10 Gy in 1 fraction or 30 Gy in 3 to 10 fractions).

**Paraneoplastic Syndromes.** The palliation of symptoms related to paraneoplastic syndromes, such as the syndrome of inappropriate antidiuretic hormone, depends almost entirely on the overall response to systemic therapy. Hyponatremia at the time of diagnosis is an especially poor prognostic factor, and symptomatic treatment is fluid restriction.

## Local-Regional Therapy

### THORACIC RADIOTHERAPY

The role of thoracic irradiation in patients with limited disease is incompletely defined. Radiotherapy significantly decreases the rate of local recurrence, but the impact of radiotherapy on survival has been widely debated for years. A number of randomized trials has failed to show a significant survival increase with chemotherapy plus thoracic irradiation versus chemotherapy alone,[113–116] whereas other randomized trials have shown survival benefits.[117–119] Combined-modality therapy is usually associated with acute and chronic toxicity, such as pneumonitis, pulmonary fibrosis, esophagitis, and toxic cardiac effects.[120] This toxicity impeded the widespread use of combined-modality treatment until 1991, when two published meta-analyses of studies of more than 2000 patients with limited disease showed a survival benefit of thoracic radiotherapy. The 2-year and 3-year survival rates were significantly improved by approximately 5% by adding radiotherapy to chemotherapy.[121, 122]

Several methods of integrating thoracic irradiation and chemotherapy have been used in SCLC; the optimal timing, fractionation, and dose remain to be settled.[120] The results of the sequential approach have been disappointing,[113, 114, 116] whereas the results from applying hyperfractionation and rapid alternation of combined-modality treatment are more encouraging.[118, 119] In a trial including 308 patients with limited disease, early administration of radiotherapy was found to yield a better survival than late or consolidative radiotherapy.[123] An EORTC study compared alternating radiotherapy with sequential radiotherapy and failed to detect any survival differences,[124] whereas a study published by Jeremic and coworkers[125] compared initial versus late hyperfractionated radiotherapy. This study favored the early arm but included only a few patients. In contrast, a Danish randomized study compared initial versus late sequential radiotherapy and failed to detect any survival difference.[126] Based on radiobiologic experience from squamous cell head and neck cancer, early hyperfractionated radiotherapy may

be the optimal method, but firm conclusions cannot be drawn from the available randomized trials. Two randomized trials have addressed this issue. The final report of the intergroup 0096 trial concluded that twice-daily radiotherapy administered concomitant with cisplatin and etoposide yielded a significant survival benefit compared with once-daily radiotherapy.[127] In contrast, a study by Bonner and associates[128] found no survival benefit from hyperfractionation. The data from these studies cannot easily be interpreted because they address different issues. The intergroup 0096 study addressed concomitant chemoradiotherapy, whereas the study by Bonner and associates[128] addressed sequential chemoradiotherapy. More recent randomized trials have all tried to clarify the optimal dose, timing, and fractionation for thoracic radiotherapy in limited SCLC. These issues remain to be settled with respect to the concomitant use of cytotoxic agents, especially doxorubicin, which results in increased toxicity in the form of esophagitis and cardiac and pulmonary damage. It appears that other combinations, such as cisplatin-etoposide regimens, can more easily be integrated with concurrent hyperfractionated radiotherapy, with less toxicity and perhaps more efficacy.[127] Future studies should be aimed at exploring the optimal integration of combinations with the new active drugs and thoracic irradiation.

### PROPHYLACTIC CRANIAL IRRADIATION

Cranial metastasis is common among patients with SCLC. At the time of diagnosis, 10% of patients have subclinical brain metastases, and 20% develop brain metastases during treatment. Brain metastases are present in 50% at autopsy, and 10% of complete responders develop brain metastases as the sole site of recurrence.[75, 129] Prophylactic cranial irradiation is effective in reducing the frequency of clinically detected brain metastases, but randomized trials have not been able to show significant survival benefits.[75] Prophylactic cranial irradiation has some late neurologic complications, such as leukoencephalopathy and neuropsychological impairment, and its use has been extensively debated.[130] An overview of seven randomized trials of prophylactic cranial irradiation found a statistically significant survival benefit from prophylactic cranial irradiation among patients in complete remission, for patients with initial limited and extensive disease.[131] The reduction in mortality was 16% compared with the controls, corresponding with a 5.4% 3-year survival increase from 15.3 to 20.7%. A total dose of 20 to 40 Gy given in fractions of no more than 2 to 2.5 Gy, delayed until chemotherapy is completed, is considered less toxic than previously applied schedules.[130]

### SURGERY

Patients with limited SCLC (TNM stages I and II) have been effectively managed by initial surgery and postoperative chemotherapy. Five-year survival rates of 36 to 38% have been reported,[132, 133] but less than 5% of all patients with small cell carcinoma present with these stages. A retrospective analysis of operable patients with SCLC disclosed no advantage of surgery before chemotherapy compared with chemotherapy alone.[134] Surgery in patients with a striking response to chemotherapy or irradiation is being explored at various centers. The therapeutic role of this approach is uncertain. An Eastern Cooperative Oncology Group (ECOG) trial randomized 146 patients with complete or partial response after chemotherapy. Seventy patients were randomized to surgery, and all received radiotherapy. The resectability rate was 83%, and no difference in median survival was observed.[135] Surgical resection of residual disease after chemotherapy is not recommended outside clinical trials.

## Future Prospects

Despite multiple clinical trials in SCLC, the efficacy of treatment has reached a plateau with modest improvements since 1980. Cure is extremely rare, especially in the case of extensive disease, with 5-year survival rates of approximately 2%.[25] Long-term survivors continue to show considerable mortality and morbidity rates as a result of late relapses, second malignancies, and cardiopulmonary diseases.[25, 47]

Although irradiation and surgery may contribute to disease control and may extend survival in individual cases, progress in treatment of this highly aggressive malignant tumor will ultimately depend on the development of more effective and selective systemic treatments. Emphasis should be focused on the establishment of valid screening systems for preclinical testing of new cytostatic or biologic agents, including an appropriate approach to clinical testing of such therapies.

It is also important to pursue treatment strategies that focus on the palliative effects of therapy, including quality of life studies. Contemporary investigations have clearly shown a positive treatment effect on quality of life.[85] With the increasing size of the elderly population and with economic restrictions on the health care system in general, cost-benefit issues should also be the subject of future studies in SCLC.

In line with the growing understanding of the biologic properties of SCLC, new strategies for treatment are under development. This includes studies of chemoprevention and early detection. The use of growth factors and the biologic manipulation of specific genes allow opportunities to suppress or stimulate genes regulating tumor growth or dissemination. Antiangiogenic and antimetastatic therapy with antagonists against endothelial proliferation and metallomatrix-protease-inhibitors are now being evaluated in phase II and III studies as are monoclonal antibodies for diagnostic and therapeutic use.

## SUGGESTIONS FOR ADDITIONAL READING

Kristensen CA, Jensen PB, Poulsen HS, et al. Small cell lung cancer: biological and therapeutic aspects. Crit Rev Oncol Hematol 1996;22:27–60.

Salgia R, Skarin AT. Molecular abnormalities in lung cancer. J Clin Oncol 1998;16:1207–17.

Edelman MJ, Gandara DR. Small cell lung cancer: current status of new chemotherapeutic agents. Crit Rev Oncol Hematol 1998;27:211–28.

## REFERENCES

1. Hansen HH. Management of small-cell cancer of the lung. Lancet 1992;339:846–9.
2. Kristensen CA, Jensen PB, Poulsen HS, et al. Small cell lung cancer: biological and therapeutic aspects. Crit Rev Oncol Hematol 1996;22:27–60.
3. 8th World Conference on Lung Cancer, Dublin, Ireland. Lung Cancer 1997;18:Suppl 1:1–268. abstracts.
4. World Health Organization. The World Health Organization histological typing of lung cancer: second edition. Am J Clin Oncol 1982;77:123.
5. Carney DN, Gazdar AF, Bepler G, et al. Establishment and identification of small cell lung cancer cell lines having classic and variant features. Cancer Res 1985;45:2913–23.
6. Hirsch FR, Matthews MJ, Aisner S, et al. Histopathologic classification of small cell lung cancer. Cancer 1988;62:973–7.
7. Hirsch FR, Østerlind K, Hansen HH. The prognostic significance of histopathologic subtyping of small cell carcinoma of the lung according to the classification of the World Health Organization. Cancer 1983;52:2144–50.
8. Carney DN. Biology of small-cell lung cancer. Lancet 1992;339:843–9.
9. Stevenson HC, Gazdar AF, Linnoila RI, et al. Lack of relationship between in vitro tumor cell growth and prognosis in extensive-stage small-cell lung cancer. J Clin Oncol 1989;7:923–31.
10. Aisner SC, Turrisi AT, Kim K, et al. Incidence and clinical significance of variant morphology (small cell/large cell subtype) in limited small cell lung cancer: a prospective analysis of an intergroup ECOG, RTOG and SWOG study. Proc ASCO 1998;17:458. abstract.
11. Nørgaard P, Damhuis RAM, Rygaard K, et al. Growth suppression by transforming growth factor β1 of human small-cell lung cancer cell lines is associated with expression of the type II receptor. Br J Cancer 1994;69:802–8.
12. Salgia R, Skarin AT. Molecular abnormalities in lung cancer. J Clin Oncol 1998;16:1207–17.
13. Minna JD. The molecular biology of lung cancer pathogenesis. Chest 1993;103:s449–s56.
14. Richardson GE, Johnson BE. The biology of lung cancer. Semin Oncol 1993;20:105–27.
15. Vindeløv LL, Hansen HH, Gersel A, et al. Treatment of small-cell carcinoma of the lung monitored by sequential flow cytometric DNA analysis. Cancer Res 1982;42:2499–505.
16. Vindeløv LL, Hansen HH, Christensen IJ, et al. Clonal heterogeneity of small-cell anaplastic carcinoma of the lung demonstrated by flow-cytometric DNA analysis. Cancer Res 1980;40:4295–300.
17. Bunn PA, Carney DN, Gazdar AF, et al. Diagnostic and biological implications of flow cytometric DNA content analysis in lung cancer. Cancer Res 1983;43:5026–32.
18. Cerny T, Blair V, Anderson H, et al. Pretreatment prognostic factors and system in 407 small-cell lung cancer patients. Int J Cancer 1987;39:146–9.
19. Cohen MH, Makuch R, Johnston-Early A, et al. Laboratory parameters as an alternative to performance status in prognostic stratification of patients with small cell lung cancer. Cancer Treat Rep 1981;65:187–95.
20. Sagman U, Feld R, DeBoer G, et al. Small cell carcinoma of the lung—derivation of a prognostic index. Clin Invest 1986;27:189.
21. Souhami RL, Bradbury I, Geddes DM, et al. Prognostic significance of laboratory parameters measured at diagnosis in small cell carcinoma of the lung. Cancer Res 1985;45:2878–82.
22. Vincent MD, Ashley SE, Smith IE. Prognostic factors in small cell lung cancer: a simple prognostic index is better than conventional staging. Eur J Cancer Clin Oncol 1987;23:1589–99.
23. Wolf M, Holle R, Hans K, et al. Analysis of prognostic factors in 766 patients with small cell lung cancer (SCLC): the role of sex as a predictor for survival. Br J Cancer 1991;63:986–92.
24. Østerlind K, Ihde DC, Ettinger DS, et al. Staging and prognostic factors in small cell carcinoma of the lung. Cancer Treat Rep 1983;67:3–8.
25. Lassen U, Østerlind K, Hansen M, et al. Long-term survival in small-cell lung cancer: posttreatment characteristics in patients surviving 5 to 18 + years—an analysis of 1714 consecutive patients. J Clin Oncol 1995;13:1215–20.
26. Mountain CF. Staging of lung cancer: the new international system. Lung Cancer 1987;3:4–11.

27. Sze G, Shin J, Krol G, et al. Intraparenchymal brain metastases: MR imaging versus contrast-enhanced CT. Radiology 1988;168:187–94.

28. Davis WK, Boyko OB, Hoffman JM, et al. [18-F]2-Fluoro-2-deoxy-glucose-positron emission tomography correlation of gadolinium-enhanced MR imaging of central nervous system neoplasia. AJNR Am J Neuroradiol 1993;14:515–23.

29. Beiske K, Myklebust AT, Aamdal S, et al. Detection of bone marrow metastases in small cell lung cancer patients: comparison of immuno-logic and morphologic methods. Am J Clin Pathol 1992;141:531–8.

30. Jelinek JS, Redmond J, Perry JJ, et al. Small cell lung cancer: staging with MR imaging. Radiology 1990;177:837–42.

31. Jørgensen LGM, Østerlind K, Cooper EH. Serum neuron specific enolase (NSE) is determinant of response in small cell lung cancer (SCLC). Br J Cancer 1992;66:594–8.

32. Lassen UN, Østerlind K, Hirsch FR, et al. Toxic death during chemo-therapy for small cell lung cancer: a confounder of improved outcome in chemotherapy trials. Br J Cancer 1999;79:515–9.

33. Lassen UN, Hirsch FR, Østerlind K, et al. Outcome of combination chemotherapy in extensive stage small-cell lung cancer: any treatment related progress? Lung Cancer 1998;20:151–60.

34. Edelman MJ, Gandara DR. Small cell lung cancer: current status of new chemotherapeutic agents. Crit Rev Oncol Hematol 1998;27:211–28.

35. Hirsch FR, Hansen HH, Hansen M, et al. The superiority of combina-tion chemotherapy including etoposide based on in vivo small-cell lung cancer: a randomized trial of 288 consecutive patients. J Clin Oncol 1987;5:585-91.

36. Lassen U, Kristjansen PEG, Østerlind K, et al. Superiority of cisplatin or carboplatin in combination with teniposide and vincristine in the induction chemotherapy of small-cell lung cancer: a randomized trial with 5 years follow up. Ann Oncol 1996;7:365–71.

37. Roed H, Vindeløv LL, Christensen IJ, et al. The cytotoxic activity of cisplatin, carboplatin and teniposide alone and combined determined by four human small cell lung cancer cell lines by the clonogenic assay. Eur J Cancer Clin Oncol 1989;24:247–53.

38. Gatzemeier U, Hossfeld DK, Neuhauss R, et al. Phase II and III studies with carboplatin in small cell lung cancer. Semin Oncol 1992;19:28–36.

39. Kosmidis PA, Samantas E, Fountzilas G, et al. Cisplatin/etoposide versus carboplatin/etoposide chemotherapy and irradiation in small cell lung cancer: a randomized phase III study. Semin Oncol 1994;21:23–30.

40. Bork E, Ersbøll J, Dombernowsky P, et al. Teniposide and etoposide in previously untreated small cell lung cancer: a randomized study. J Clin Oncol 1991;9:1627–31.

41. Carney DN, Byrne A. Etoposide in the treatment of elderly/poor-prognosis patients with small-cell lung cancer. Cancer Chemother Pharmacol 1994;34:s96–s100.

42. Johnson DH, Greco FA, Strupp J, et al. Prolonged administration of oral etoposide in patients with relapsed or refractory small-cell lung cancer: a phase II trial. J Clin Oncol 1990;8:1613–7.

43. Souhami RL, Spiro SG, Rudd RM, et al. Five-day oral etoposide treatment for advanced small-cell lung cancer: randomized comparison with intravenous chemotherapy. J Natl Cancer Inst 1997;89:577–80.

44. Girling DJ, Thatcher N, Clark PI, et al. Comparison of oral etoposide and standard multidrug intravenous chemotherapy for small cell lung cancer: a stepped multicentre randomised trial. Lancet 1996;348:563–6.

45. Dearing MP, Steinberg SM, Phelps R, et al. Outcome of patients with small-cell lung cancer: effect of changes in staging procedures and imaging technology on prognostic factors over 14 years. J Clin Oncol 1990;8:1042–9.

46. Feinstein AR, Sosin DM, Wells CK. The Will Rogers phenomenon: stage migration and new diagnostic techniques as a source of mis-leading statistics for survival in cancer. N Engl J Med 1985;312:1604–8.

47. Souhami RL, Law K. Longevity in small cell lung cancer. Br J Cancer 1990;61:584–9.

48. Rosti G, Donadio M, Crinò L, et al. Long survivers in small cell lung cancer (SCLC): Italian report on 3245 cases. Lung Cancer 1991;10:268. abstract.

49. Niiranen A. Long-term survival in small-cell carcinoma of the lung. Eur J Cancer Clin Oncol 1988;24:749–52.

50. Goldie JH, Coldman AJ. A mathematic model for relating the drug sensitivity of tumors to their spontaneous mutation rate. Cancer Treat Rep 1979;63:1727–33.

51. Goldie JH. Arguments supporting the concept of non-cross-resistant combinations of chemotherapy. Cancer Invest 1994;12:324–8.

52. Østerlind K, Sörenson S, Hansen HH, et al. Continuous *versus* alter-nating combination chemotherpy for advanced small cell carcinoma of the lung. Cancer Res 1983;43:6085–9.

53. Pedersen AG, Østerlind K, Vindeløv LL. Alternating or continuous chemotherapy of small cell lung cancer: a three armed randomized trial. Proc ASCO 1987;6:187. abstract.

54. Roth BJ, Johnson DH, Einhorn LH, et al. Randomized study of cyclophosphamide, doxorubicin, and vincristine versus etoposide and cisplatin versus alternation of these two regimens in extensive small-cell-lung cancer: a phase II trial of the Southeastern Cancer Study Group. J Clin Oncol 1992;10:282–91.

55. Smith AP, Anderson G, Chapell G, et al. Does the substitution of cisplatin in a standard four drug regimen improve survival in small cell carcinoma of the lung. Thorax 1991;46:172–4.

56. Evans WK, Feld R, Murray N, et al. Superiority of alternating non-cross-resistant chemotherapy in extensive small cell lung cancer: a multicenter, randomized clinical trial by the National Cancer Institute of Canada. Ann Intern Med 1987;107:451–8.

57. Ettinger DS, Finkelstein DM, Abeloff MD, et al. A randomized comparison of standard chemotherapy versus alternating chemother-apy and maintenance versus no maintenance therapy for extensive-stage small-cell lung cancer: a phase III study of the Eastern Coopera-tive Oncology Group. J Clin Oncol 1990;8:230–40.

58. Feld R, Evans WK, Coy P, et al. Canadian multicentre randomized trial comparing sequential and alternating administration of two non-cross-resistant chemotherapy combinations in patients with limited small-cell carcinoma of the lung. J Clin Oncol 1987;5:1401–9.

59. Havemann K, Wolf M, Holle R, et al. Alternating versus sequential chemotherapy in small cell lung cancer: a randomized German multicenter trial. Cancer 1987;59:1072–82.

60. Daniels JR, Chak LY, Sikic BI, et al. Chemotherapy of small-cell carcinoma of the lung: a randomized comparison of alternating and sequential combination chemotherapy programs. J Clin Oncol 1984;2:1192–9.

61. Goodman GE, Crowley JJ, Blasko JC, et al. Treatment of limited small-cell lung cancer with etoposide and cisplatin alternating with vincristine, doxorubicin and cyclophosphamide versus concurrent eto-poside, vincristine, doxorubicin and cyclophosphamide and chest ra-diotherapy: a Southwest Oncology Group Study. J Clin Oncol 1990;8:39–47.

62. Wolf M, Prithch M, Drings P, et al. Cyclic-alternating versus response-oriented chemotherapy in small-cell lung cancer: a German multicen-ter randomized trial of 321 patients. J Clin Oncol 1991;9:614–24.

63. Wampler GL, Heim WJ, Ellison NM, et al. Comparison of cyclophos-phamide, doxorubicin, and vincristine with an alternating regimen of methotrexate, etoposide and cisplatin/cyclophosphamide, doxorubicin, and vincristine in the treatments of extensive-disease small-cell lung carcinoma: a Midatlantic Oncology Program Study. J Clin Oncol 1991;9:1438–45.

64. Fukuoka M, Furuse K, Saijo N, et al. Randomized trial of cyclophos-phamide, doxorubicin, and vincristine versus cisplatin and etoposide versus alternation of these regimens in small-cell lung cancer. J Natl Cancer Inst 1991;83:855–61.

65. Klasa RJ, Murray N, Coldman AJ. Dose-intensity meta-analysis of chemotherapy regimens in small-cell carcinoma of the lung. J Clin Oncol 1991;9:499–508.

66. Crawford J, Ozer H, Stoller R, et al. Reduction by granulocyte colony-stimulating factor of fever and neutropenia induced by chemotherapy in patients with small-cell cancer. N Engl J Med 1991;325:164–70.

67. Pujol J-L, Douillard JY, Rivière A, et al. Dose intensity of a four drug chemotherapy regimen with or without recombinant human granulo-cyte colony stimulating factor in small cell lung cancer. J Clin Oncol 1997;15:2082–9.

68. Murray N, Livingston RB, Shepard FA, et al. A randomized study of CODE plus thoracic irradiation versus alternating CAV/EP for exten-sive stage small cell lung cancer (ESCLC). Proc ASCO 1997;16:456. abstract.

69. Furuse K, Fukuda M, Nishiwaki Y, et al. Phase III study of intensive weekly chemotherapy with recombinant human granulocyte colony-stimulating factor versus standard chemotherapy in extensive-disease small-cell lung cancer. J Clin Oncol 1998;16:2126–32.

70. Thatcher N, Sambrook NRJ, Qian W, et al. Dose intensification (DI)

with G-CSF improves survival in small cell lung cancer (SCLC): results of a randomized trial. Proc ASCO 1998;17:456. abstract.

71. Steward WP, von Pawel J, Gatzemeier U, et al. Effects on granulocyte-macrophage colony-stimulating factor and dose intensification of V-ICE chemotherapy in small cell lung cancer: a prospective randomized study of 300 patients. J Clin Oncol 1998;16:642–50.

72. Bleehen NM, Fayers PM, Girling DJ, et al. Controlled trial of twelve versus six courses of chemotherapy in the treatment of small-cell lung cancer. Br J Cancer 1989;59:584–90.

73. Spiro SG, Souhami RL, Geddes DM, et al. Duration of chemotherapy in small cell lung cancer: a Cancer Research Campaign trial. Br J Cancer 1989;59:578–83.

74. Giaccone G, Dalesio O, Mcvie JG, et al. Maintenance chemotherapy in small-cell lung cancer: long-term results of a randomized trial. J Clin Oncol 1993;11:1230–40.

75. Pedersen AG, Bishop J, Bleehen NM, et al. Management of CNS metastases in small cell lung cancer: a consensus report. Lung Cancer 1989;5:140–2.

76. Sculier J-P, Paesmans M, Bureau G, et al. Randomized trial comparing induction chemotherapy versus induction chemotherapy followed by maintenance chemotherapy in small cell-lung cancer. J Clin Oncol 1996;14:2337–44.

77. Mattson K, Niiranen A, Ruotsalainen T, et al. Interferon maintenance therapy for small cell lung cancer: improvement in long-term survival. J Interferon Cytokine Res 1997;17:103–5.

78. Jett JR, Maksymiuk AW, Su JQ, et al. Phase III trial of recombinant interferon gamma in complete responders with small-cell lung cancer. J Clin Oncol 1994;12:2321–6.

79. Prior C, Oroszy S, Oberaigner W, et al. Adjunctive interferon-α-2c in stage III/IV small cell lung cancer: a phase III trial. Eur Respir J 1997;10:392–6.

80. Zarogoulidis K, Ziogas E, Papagiannis A, et al. Interferon alpha-2a and combined chemotherapy as first line treatment in SCLC patients: a randomized trial. Lung Cancer 1996;15:197–205.

81. Mehta P. Potential role of platelets in the pathogenesis of tumor metastasis. Blood 1998;63:55–63.

82. Wojtukiewicz MZ, Zacharski LR, Memoli VA, et al. Abnormal regulation of coagulation/fibrinolysis in small cell carcinoma of the lung. Cancer 1990;65:481–5.

83. Zacharski LR, Henderson WG, Rickles FR. Effect of warfarin on survival in small cell carcinoma of the lung. JAMA 1998;245:831–5.

84. Chahinian AP, Propert KJ, Ware JH, et al. A randomized trial of anticoagulation with warfarin and of alternating chemotherapy in extensive small-cell lung cancer. J Clin Oncol 1989;7:993–1002.

85. Bergman B, Sullivan M, Sørenson S. Quality of life during chemotherapy for small cell lung cancer. Acta Oncol 1991;30:947–56.

86. Chute JP, Kelley MJ, Venzon D, et al. Retreatment of patients surviving cancer-free 2 or more years after initial treatment of small cell lung cancer. Chest 1996;110:165–70.

87. Andersen M, Kristjansen PEG, Hansen HH. Second-line chemotherapy in small cell lung cancer. Cancer Treat Rev 1990;17:427–36.

88. Schiller J, von Pawel J, Shepard FA, et al. Topotecan versus cyclophosphamide, doxorubicin and vincristine for the treatment of patients with recurrent small cell lung cancer: a phase III study. Proc ASCO 1998;17:456. abstract.

89. Bork E, Hansen M, Dombernowsky P, et al. Teniposide [VM-26], an overlooked highly active agent in small-cell lung cancer: results of a phase II trial in untreated patients. J Clin Oncol 1986;4:524.

90. Giaccone G, Danadie M, Bonardi GM, et al. Teniposide in the treatment of small-cell lung cancer: the influence of prior chemotherapy. J Clin Oncol 1988;6:1264–70.

91. Ettinger DS, Finkelstein DM, Abeloff MD. Justification for evaluating new anticancer drugs in selected untreated patients with extensive-stage small-cell lung cancer: an Eastern Cooperative Oncology Group randomized study. J Natl Cancer Inst 1992;84:1077–84.

92. Ardizzoni A, Hansen HH, Dombernowsky P, et al. Topotecan, a new active drug in the second-line treatment of small-cell lung cancer: a phase II trial in patients with refractory and sensitive disease. J Clin Oncol 1997;15:2090–6.

93. Perez-Soler R, Glisson BS, Lee JS, et al. Treatment of patients with small-cell lung cancer refractory to etoposide and cisplatin with the topoisomerase I poison topotecan. J Clin Oncol 1996;14:2785–90.

94. Schiller J, Kim K, Hutson P, et al. Phase II study of topotecan in patients with extensive-stage small cell carcinoma of the lung: an Eastern Cooperative Oncology Group trial. J Clin Oncol 1996;14:2345–52.

95. Masuda N, Fukuoka M, Kusunoki Y, et al. CPT-11: a new derivative of camptothecin for the treatment of refractory or relapsed small-cell lung cancer. J Clin Oncol 1992;10:1225–9.

96. Negoro S, Fukuoka M, Niitani H, et al. Phase II study of CPT-11, a new camptothecin derivative in small cell lung cancer. Proc ASCO 1991;10:241. abstract.

97. Ettinger DS, Finkelstein DM, Sarma R, et al. Phase II study of paclitaxel in patients with extensive-disease small-cell lung cancer: an Eastern Cooperative Oncology Group study. J Clin Oncol 1995;13:1431–5.

98. Kirschling RJ, Jung S-H, Jett JR. A phase II trial of taxol and G-CSF in previously untreated patients with extensive-stage small cell lung cancer. Proc ASCO 1994;13:326. abstract.

99. Hainsworth JD, Gray JR, Stoup SL, et al. Paclitaxel, carboplatin, and extended schedule etoposide in the treatment of small-cell lung cancer: comparison of sequential phase II trials using different dose-intensities. J Clin Oncol 1997;15:3463–70.

100. Latreille J, Cormier Y, Martins H, et al. Phase II study of docetaxel in patients with previously untreated extensive small cell lung cancer. Invest New Drugs 1996;13:342–5.

101. Smyth J, Smith IE, Sessa C, et al. Activity of docetaxel in small cell lung cancer. Eur J Cancer 1994;30A:1058–60.

102. Cormier Y, Eisenhauer EA, Muldal A, et al. Gemcitabine is an active new agent in previously untreated extensive small cell lung cancer: a study of the National Cancer Institute of Canada Clinical Trial. Ann Oncol 1994;5:283–5.

103. Higano CS, Crowley JJ, Veith RV, et al. A phase II trial of intravenous vinorelbine in previously untreated patients with extensive small cell lung cancer, a SWOG study. Invest New Drugs 1997;15:153–6.

104. Furuse K, Kubota K, Kawahara M, et al. Phase II study of heavily previously treated small cell lung cancer. Japanese Lung Cancer Vinorelbine Study Group. Oncology 1996;53:169–72.

105. Jassem J, Karnicka-Mlodkowska H, van Pottensberghe C, et al. Phase II study of vinorelbine in previously treated small cell lung cancer patients. EORTC Lung Cancer Cooperative Group. Eur J Cancer 1993;29A:1720–2.

106. Kristjansen PEG, Sørensen PS, Hansen MS, et al. Prospective evaluation of the effect on initial brain metastases from small cell lung cancer of platinum-etoposide based induction chemotherapy followed by an alternating multidrug regimen. Ann Oncol 1993;4:579–83.

107. Kristensen CA, Kristjansen PEG, Hansen HH. Systemic chemotherapy of brain metastases from small-cell lung cancer: a review. J Clin Oncol 1992;10:1498–1502.

108. Postmus PE, Sleijfer DTh, Haaxma-Reiche H. Chemotherapy for central nervous system metastases from small cell lung cancer: a review. Lung Cancer 1989;5:254–63.

109. Pedersen AG, Bach F, Melgaard B. Frequency, diagnosis and prognosis of spinal cord compression in small cell bronchogenic carcinoma: a review of 817 consecutive patients. Cancer 1985;55:1818–22.

110. Sørensen PS, Helweg-Larsen S, Mouridsen H, et al. Effect of high-dose dexamethasone in carcinomatous metastatic spinal cord compression treated with radiotherapy: a randomized trial. Eur J Cancer 1994;30A:22–7.

111. Kane RC, Cohen MH. Superior vena caval obstruction due to small-cell anaplastic lung carcinoma: response to chemotherapy. JAMA 1976;235:1717–8.

112. Dombernowsky P, Hansen HH. Combination chemotherapy in the management of superior vena caval obstruction in small-cell anaplastic carcinoma of the lung. Acta Med Scand 1978;204:513–6.

113. Østerlind K, Hansen HH, Hansen HS, et al. Chemotherapy *versus* chemotherapy plus irradiation in limited small cell lung cancer: results of a controlled trial with 5 years follow-up. Br J Cancer 1986;54:7–17.

114. Souhami RL, Geddes DM, Spiro SG, et al. Radiotherapy in small cell lung cancer of the lung treated with combination chemotherapy: a controlled trial. Br Med J 1984;288:1643–6.

115. Johnson DH, Bass D, Einhorn LH, et al. Combination chemotherapy with or without thoracic radiotherapy in limited-stage small-cell lung cancer: a randomized trial of the Southeastern Cancer Study Group. J Clin Oncol 1993;11:1223–9.

116. Kies MS, Mira J, Crowley JJ, et al. Multimodal therapy for limited small-cell lung cancer: a randomized study of induction combination chemotherapy with or without thoracic radiation in complete responders. J Clin Oncol 1987;5:592–600.

117. Perez CA, Einhorn LH, Oldham RK, et al. Randomized trial of radiotherapy to the thorax in limited small cell carcinoma of the lung

treated with multiagent chemotherapy and elective brain irradiation: a preliminary report. J Clin Oncol 1984;2:1200–8.

118. Perry MC, Eaton WL, Propert KJ, et al. Chemotherapy with or without radiation therapy in limited small-cell carcinoma of the lung. N Engl J Med 1987;316:912–8.

119. Bunn PA, Lichter AS, Makuch RW, et al. Chemotherapy alone or chemotherapy with chest radiation in limited small cell lung cancer. Ann Intern Med 1987;106:655.

120. Wagner H. Thoracic irradiation of limited small cell lung cancer: have we defined the optimal dose time and fractionation? Lung Cancer 1997;17:Suppl 1:s137–s48.

121. Pignon J-P, Arriagada R, Ihde DC, et al. A meta-analysis of thoracic radiotherapy for small cell lung cancer. N Engl J Med 1992;327:1618–24.

122. Warde P, Payne D. Does thoracic irradiation improve survival and local control in limited-stage small-cell carcinoma of the lung? A meta-analysis. J Clin Oncol 1992;10:890–5.

123. Murray N, Coy P, Pater JL, et al. Importance of timing for thoracic irradiation in the combined modality treatment of limited-stage small-cell lung cancer. J Clin Oncol 1993;11:336–44.

124. Gregor A, Drings P, Burghouts J, et al. Randomized trial of alternating versus sequential radiotherapy/chemotherapy in limited disease patients with small cell lung cancer: a EORTC study. J Clin Oncol 1997;15:2840–9.

125. Jeremic B, Shibamoto Y, Acimovic L, et al. Initial versus late accelerated hyperfractionated radiotherapy and concurrent chemotherapy in limited small-cell lung cancer: a randomized study. J Clin Oncol 1997;15:893–900.

126. Work E, Nielsen OS, Bentzen SM, et al. Randomized study of initial versus late chest irradiation combined with chemotherapy in limited-stage small-cell lung cancer. J Clin Oncol 1997;15:3030–7.

127. Turrisi AT 3rd, Kim K, Blum R, et al. Twice-daily compared with once-daily thoracic radiotherapy in limited small-cell lung cancer treated concurrently with cisplatin and etoposide. N Engl J Med 1999;340:265–71.

128. Bonner JA, Sloan JA, Shanahan TG, et al. Phase III comparison of twice-daily split-course irradiation versus once-daily irradiation for patients with limited stage small-cell lung carcinoma. J Clin Oncol 1999;17:2681–91.

129. Nugents JL, Bunn PA, Matthews MJ, et al. CNS metastases in small-cell bronchogenic carcinoma: increasing frequency and changing pattern with lengthening survival. Cancer 1979;44:1885–93.

130. Kristjansen PEG, Kristensen CA. The role of prophylactic cranial irradiation in the management of small cell lung cancer. Cancer Treat Rev 1993;19:3–16.

131. Arriagada R, Auperin A, Pignon J-P, et al. Prophylactic cranial irradiation overview in patients with small cell lung cancer in complete remission. Proc ASCO 1998;17:457. abstract.

132. Shields TW, Higgins GA, Matthews MJ, et al. Surgical resection in the management of small cell carcinoma of the lung. J Thorac Cardiovasc Surg 1982;84:481–8.

133. Macchiarini P, Hardin M, Basolo F, et al. Surgery plus adjuvant chemotherapy for T1-3N0M0 small-cell lung cancer. Am J Clin Oncol 1991;14:218–24.

134. Østerlind K, Hansen M, Hansen HH, et al. Influence of surgical resection prior to chemotherapy on the long-term results in small cell lung cancer: a study of 150 operable patients. Eur J Cancer Clin Oncol 1986;22:589–93.

135. Lad T, Piantadosi S, Thomas P, et al. A prospective randomized trial to determine the benefit of surgical resection of residual disease following response of small cell lung cancer to combination chemotherapy. Chest 1994;106:Suppl 6:320s–3s.

# CHAPTER 38

# PLEURAL MESOTHELIOMA

• VALERIE W. RUSCH • ROBERT FIGLIN

Mesothelioma is a primary cancer of the pleura that is generally classified as localized or diffuse. It should be distinguished from the entity previously known as *benign mesothelioma* and now called *benign fibrous tumor of the pleura*, which presents as a solitary, pedunculated mass arising from the visceral pleura. This entity is clinically and histologically distinct from malignant mesothelioma and is cured by surgical excision.[1] *Localized* malignant mesotheliomas are fibrosarcomatous in histologic appearance,[2] rarely spread around the pleural cavity, and are potentially curable by surgical resection.[3] Although they may exhibit varying degrees of sarcomatoid histology, *diffuse* malignant mesotheliomas are fundamentally epithelial tumors. They arise unilaterally, involve all pleural surfaces, and are difficult and controversial in terms of their overall management.[4]

## Natural History

### ETIOLOGY AND EPIDEMIOLOGY

Diffuse malignant mesotheliomas are clearly related to asbestos exposure, whereas localized malignant mesotheliomas are not. Diffuse malignant mesothelioma is an uncommon tumor, but its incidence is rising because of widespread industrial use of asbestos during the 1940s and 1950s.[5] The annual incidence of diffuse malignant mesothelioma is approximately 15 per 1 million in white men and 2 per 1 million in white women. It has been calculated that the incidence in the United States will continue to rise until after the year 2000, with between 3600 and 4200 new cases per year.[6]

The relationship between asbestos exposure and diffuse malignant mesothelioma was first established in 1960 by Wagner and colleagues.[7] Their work also documented that the latency period between exposure to asbestos and the development of mesothelioma usually exceeds 20 years. Individuals exposed during the World War II era and thereafter up into the 1960s, when asbestos was frequently used in shipbuilding industries, are only now developing malignant mesothelioma. An estimated 4 million Americans have been heavily exposed to asbestos. The major occupational exposures are seen in individuals engaged in the building and repair of ships, in the construction industry, and in automobile maintenance.[8]

Asbestos consists of a family of silicate fibers that are widely distributed in nature. Although inert chemically, asbestos is a potent carcinogen. Asbestos enters the body predominantly via the respiratory tract, with certain physical properties allowing the fibers to penetrate and remain in the lungs, enhancing their carcinogenicity. These properties include narrow width, increased length/width ratio, and chemical stability.[9, 10] Asbestos fibers have two configurations: amphibole (crocidolite, amosite) and serpentine (chrysotile). The type of asbestos used can affect the risk of subsequent disease. Chrysotile asbestos is now used in the United States, although significant amounts of amphiboles have been used in the past.[11] In general, crocidolite, amosite, and chrysotile, in decreasing order of potency, induce mesothelioma in humans, whereas most other asbestos fibers are only weakly pathogenic.[12] Chrysotile asbestos, however, is frequently contaminated with small amounts of tremolite or amosite. Exposure to amphibole fibers can occur even in industries that use only chrysotile asbestos.[13] Asbestos-related disease is not limited to diffuse malignant mesothelioma: Pulmonary fibrosis, lung cancer, and other malignancies are increased in patients exposed to asbestos. The risk of developing mesothelioma appears unrelated to previous smoking. This situation is in stark contrast to the apparently synergistic interaction between asbestos and tobacco in causing lung cancer.[14] The clustering of malignant mesothelioma within families has been reported. One study has shown that the age at which these mesotheliomas occur, their site and histologic pattern, and the asbestos fiber burden are similar to the characteristics of mesothelioma seen in the nonfamilial setting.[15]

Not all mesotheliomas are associated with asbestos exposure, and only a few individuals exposed to asbestos develop mesothelioma. Reports suggest the presence of simian virus 40 (SV40) in malignant mesothelioma.[16–18] A multi-institutional study to verify these findings reported (1) SV40 sequences and SV40 large T antigen expression in 83% of mesotheliomas tested and (2) electron microscopy demonstrating asbestos fibers in 71% of all tissues available for analysis.[19] The relationship of SV40 and asbestos acting as two carcinogens requires further study.

## PATHOLOGY

Although they are fundamentally epithelial tumors, diffuse malignant mesotheliomas tend to differentiate toward either an epithelioid or sarcomatoid histology.[20] Depending on whether the tumor contains elements of both, mesotheliomas are classified as pure epithelial, mixed epithelial and fibrosarcomatous, pure fibrosarcomatous, or desmoplastic. Pure epithelial tumors are the most common form, accounting for more than half of all mesotheliomas.[21] The pathologic diagnosis of mesothelioma and its differentiation from other tumors involving the pleura are facilitated by the routine use of immunohistochemical and ultrastructural techniques.[22] Mesotheliomas characteristically do not stain for antibodies to carcinoembryonic antigen, whereas adenocarcinomas almost invariably do.[23, 24] The microvilli in mesotheliomas are long, thin, and multiply branched. Warhol and colleagues[25, 26] suggest that a length/diameter ratio of more than 10 helps to distinguish mesotheliomas from adenocarcinomas. Although the histologic diagnosis of mesothelioma can be difficult, the combination of typical ultrastructural features as seen by electron microscopy and the characteristic patterns of histochemical and immunohistochemical staining makes a definitive tissue diagnosis of malignant mesothelioma possible in most patients.

## CLINICAL FEATURES AND DIAGNOSIS

Mesothelioma usually develops in the 50s and 60s and is more common in men.[4, 27] More than half of patients with mesothelioma give a history of definite exposure to asbestos. The incidence of the disease among the asbestos-exposed population increases in proportion to the number of years that have elapsed since first exposure,[6] with most cases occurring after a latent interval of 30 to 40 years.[28] The most common presenting symptom of pleural mesothelioma is pain or shortness of breath, or both.[29, 30] The diagnosis of mesothelioma should be suspected on clinical grounds whenever a patient who has been exposed to asbestos more than 15 years previously presents with an otherwise unexplained pleural effusion or with unilateral pleural thickening.[31] Systemic complaints of fatigue, weight loss, anorexia, and malaise are common. Shortness of breath occurs during the early stages of disease when the pleural space is free and a pleural effusion is present. Chest pain develops during the more advanced stages of disease after the tumor has become confluent, obliterating the pleural space and encasing the lung and chest wall. Infiltration of the intercostal spaces and chest wall muscles occurs with locally advanced malignant mesothelioma and causes excruciating pain that can be difficult to control, even with high-dose opiates. Because the symptoms associated with the early stages of disease are insidious and nonspecific, diagnosis is often delayed for 3 to 6 months.[31, 32]

No laboratory findings are specific for the diagnosis of mesothelioma. Thrombocytosis or an elevated CA-125 occurs in 20 to 30% of patients.[32] The radiographic presentation of mesothelioma is also nonspecific. Early-stage disease is characterized by a pleural effusion with minimal pleural thickening and irregularity. As the disease progresses, the pleura becomes thicker and more irregular, and large pleural masses are sometimes present. The pleural effusion becomes loculated, then disappears as the pleural space fuses. In the final stages of disease, tumor invades throughout the pericardium and diaphragm and into the chest wall. Rib destruction is an occasional finding. Pleural plaques, indicative of asbestos exposure, may be seen on the contralateral parietal or diaphragmatic pleura. Ascites, contralateral pleural effusion, pericardial effusion, or contralateral pulmonary nodules are seen in patients with end-stage disease when the tumor has metastasized.[33–37]

The clinical and radiographic presentations of malignant mesothelioma are indistinguishable from those of metastatic disease involving the pleura, particularly metastatic adenocarcinoma. The diagnosis is based on pathologic findings, which require an invasive procedure. In choosing the best approach, it should be remembered that mesothelioma spreads along needle tracks and that a significant proportion of patients develop tumor nodules at the site of pleural biopsy.[27, 30] An evaluation of the success rate of various diagnostic procedures in 140 patients revealed that a definitive diagnosis was achieved in none of 80 patients via cytologic studies, in 21% via closed pleural biopsy, and in 54% via trephine pleural biopsy.[30] Almost all patients can be reliably diagnosed by thoracoscopy, however, a minimally invasive surgical procedure. In a study of 137 patients in whom complete endoscopic inspection was possible, diagnosis was achieved by thoracoscopy in 98%, fluid cytology in 26%, and needle biopsy in 21%.[38, 39] When a diagnosis of mesothelioma is suspected, the surgeon should alert the pathologist so that the pleural biopsy specimens can be placed in the appropriate fixatives for immunohistochemistry and electron microscopy.

## STAGING

The pathologic staging of mesothelioma is defined by the presence of the parietal pleura acting as an anatomic barrier to the spread of disease in the early stage.[31] Direct invasion of mediastinal structures, penetration of the diaphragm with peritoneal involvement, and chest wall invasion occur late in the course of the disease.[4, 27] Mediastinal lymph node involvement is a common finding at autopsy and may occur in 50% of patients with early-stage disease suitable for surgical resection.[32, 40]

Hematogenous spread of tumor is a late occurrence and a common finding at autopsy.[32] The organs most often involved are the peritoneum or intra-abdominal viscera and the opposite lung, but organs as diverse as the brain, spinal cord, prostate, and thyroid may also be involved at autopsy.[41, 42]

Despite the routine use of computed tomography (CT), it is often difficult to determine the tumor stage accurately until thoracotomy has been performed. The most difficult areas to evaluate are the diaphragm and the chest wall.[43] Magnetic resonance imaging (MRI) has been investigated as a way to image these areas more accurately. MRI has not proved significantly more accurate than CT, however, which remains the standard imaging study.[44] Equivocal findings of transdiaphragmatic extension on CT or MRI are best investigated by laparoscopy.[45]

Because hematogenous spread is rare in early-stage disease,[46] routine evaluation with radioisotopic scanning is not recommended in patients who otherwise appear to be candidates for surgical resection. The role of positron emission tomography scanning is undefined. A report suggests that it may help distinguish between malignant and benign pleural disease.[47] The ability of positron emission tomography to stage the extent of local-regional or distant extent of disease in malignant mesothelioma needs to be evaluated.

Since the 1970s, several staging systems have been proposed for malignant mesothelioma, none of which was universally accepted or validated by clinicopathologic correlation. Despite its vague descriptions of T and N status, the staging system proposed by Butchart and colleagues[48] in 1976 was the one most widely used (Table 38–1). More recently, the International Mesothelioma Interest Group, a group of clinicians and researchers with expertise in malignant mesothelioma, reviewed the information currently available on the natural history of malignant mesothelioma and developed a new staging system.[49] This is now the most widely accepted system and can be applied to the radio-

**Table 38–1.** Initial Butchart Clinical Staging System for Malignant Mesothelioma

| | |
|---|---|
| Stage I | Tumor confined within the capsule of the parietal pleura (i.e., involving only ipsilateral pleura, lung diaphragm, and *external* surface of pericardium within the pleural reflection) |
| Stage II | Tumor invading chest wall or mediastinal tissues or structures (e.g., esophagus, trachea, great vessels) |
| Stage III | Tumor *penetrating* diaphragmatic muscle to involve peritoneum or the retroperitoneal space<br>Tumor *penetrating* pericardium to involve its *internal* surface or to involve the heart<br>Involvement of the opposite pleura<br>Lymph node involvement outside the chest |
| Stage IV | Distant blood-borne metastases |

From Butchart EG. Pleuropneumectomy in the management of diffuse malignant mesothelioma of the pleura. Thorax 1976;31:15–24.

graphic, clinical, and pathologic staging of mesothelioma (Table 38–2).

## PROGNOSIS

Factors influencing the prognosis of patients with malignant mesothelioma are still incompletely defined. Cell type and stage are the most important prognostic factors in reported clinical series. Purely epithelial mesothelioma carries an improved survival rate compared with the sarcomatoid or mixed variants.[50–53] Other factors associated with improved prognosis include female gender, a good performance status, absence of chest pain, an interval of more than 6 months from the onset of symptoms, and a normal platelet count.[32, 54] The improved survival of women may be due to the more common occurrence of the purely epithelial pathologic subtype. Other purported prognostic factors, such as performance status and chest pain, are merely the clinical manifestations of tumor stage. The median survival of untreated patients is directly linked to stage and tumor histology and ranges from 6 to 12 months for patients with stage IV disease to 22 months for patients with stage IA tumors.[20, 39, 40, 52]

## Treatment

### SURGERY

Surgery has three major roles in malignant mesothelioma: diagnosis, palliation, and therapeutic resection. Having already discussed the utility of surgery in the diagnosis of mesothelioma, we now turn our attention to the other two roles.

Pleurectomy and extrapleural pneumonectomy are the procedures with which there is the greatest experience,[31, 40, 48, 54–56] but there is continued disagreement over the relative benefit of these two operations. Pleurectomy-decortication, in which the pleura is removed but the lung is left in place, carries an operative mortality of less than 2% but can lead to complete resection of all gross tumor only in patients who

*Table 38–2.* **New International Staging System for Diffuse Malignant Pleural Mesothelioma (IMIG)**

*T—Tumor*

T1

T1a     Tumor limited to the ipsilateral parietal ± mediastinal ± diaphragmatic pleura
       *No involvement of the visceral pleura*

T1b     Tumor involving the ipsilateral parietal ± mediastinal ± diaphragmatic pleura
       *Tumor also involving the visceral pleura*

T2       Tumor involving each of the ipsilateral pleural surfaces (parietal, mediastinal, diaphragmatic, and visceral pleura) with at
           least one of the following features:
           Involvement of diaphragmatic muscle
           Extension of tumor from visceral pleura into the underlying pulmonary parenchyma

T3       Describes locally advanced but *potentially resectable* tumor
           Tumor involving all of the ipsilateral pleural surfaces (parietal, mediastinal, diaphragmatic, and visceral pleura) with at
           least one of the following features:
           Involvement of the endothoracic fascia
           Extension into the mediastinal fat
           Solitary, completely resectable focus of tumor extending into the soft tissues of the chest wall
           Nontransmural involvement of the pericardium

T4       Describes locally advanced *technically unresectable* tumor
           Tumor involving all of the ipsilateral pleural surfaces (parietal, mediastinal, diaphragmatic, and visceral pleura) with at
           least one of the following features:
           Diffuse extension or multifocal masses of tumor in the chest wall, with or without associated rib destruction
           Direct transdiaphragmatic extension of tumor to the peritoneum
           Direct extension of tumor to the contralateral pleura
           Direct extension of tumor to mediastinal organs
           Direct extension of tumor into the spine
           Tumor extending through to the internal surface of the pericardium

*N—Lymph nodes*

NX     Regional lymph nodes cannot be assessed
N0     No regional lymph node metastases
N1     Metastases in the ipsilateral bronchopulmonary or hilar lymph nodes
N2     Metastases in the subcarinal or the ipsilateral mediastinal lymph nodes including the ipsilateral internal mammary nodes
N3     Metastases in the contralateral mediastinal, contralateral internal mammary, ipsilateral or contralateral supraclavicular
        lymph nodes

*M—Metastases*

MX     Presence of distant metastases cannot be assessed
M0     No distant metastasis
M1     Distant metastasis present

Stage Grouping

| | | | |
|---|---|---|---|
| Stage I | | | |
| Ia | $T_{1a}$ | $N_0$ | $M_0$ |
| Ib | $T_{1b}$ | $N_0$ | $M_0$ |
| Stage II | $T_2$ | $N_0$ | $M_0$ |
| Stage III | Any $T_3$ | Any $N_1$ | $M_0$ |
| | | Any $N_2$ | |
| Stage IV | Any $T_4$ | Any $N_3$ | Any $M_1$ |

From Rusch VW. The International Mesothelioma Interest Group. A proposed new international TNM staging system for malignant pleural mesothelioma. Chest 1995;108:1122–28.

have early disease.[41, 57] Extrapleural pneumonectomy (also termed *pleuropneumonectomy*) is associated with a mortality rate of 5 to 15% but can effectively remove all tumor in patients with extensive visceral pleural or locally advanced disease. The higher operative risk is related to the en bloc removal of the lung along with the pleura, pericardium, and diaphragm but can be kept in the range of 5 to 7% mortality in the hands of experienced surgeons.[43, 56, 58–63] Randomized trials comparing these two operations are not possible because of the small numbers of patients involved and the clear difference in operative mortality. Information suggests that survival is more closely linked to tumor histology and stage than to the type of resection performed.[61] Because of the anatomic location of the tumor, surgical resection can lead to complete resection of all *gross* tumor only. Residual microscopic disease, almost certainly present no matter what type of operation is performed, must be treated with some other modality.

Palliative surgery is often used in mesothelioma because of its potential to relieve symptoms and improve quality of life. It can be used in patients not fit for pleuropneumonectomy and in those with advanced disease. The aims of palliative surgery are prevention of recurrent effusion, amelioration of the discomfort and respiratory embarrassment produced by tumor bulk, and prevention of pain caused by chest wall involvement as the disease progresses. Palliative surgery can be accomplished by parietal pleurectomy, with or without decortication of the lung, or by thoracoscopy with talc pleurodesis if the underlying lung can still expand fully.[32] An extensive review by Butchart[31] of the utility of palliative surgery in the management of malignant mesothelioma provides additional details.

## RADIATION THERAPY

The true role of radiation therapy as either definitive or palliative treatment of mesothelioma remains undefined. External-beam radiotherapy has been used in uncontrolled studies,[64, 65] but there is little evidence that hemithorax radiation alone prolongs survival in most patients, although relief of symptoms may occur with total doses greater than 40 Gy.[65–69] A significant barrier to the effective use of external-beam radiation is the intolerance of the lung and mediastinal organs to doses of radiation that might be tumoricidal. These problems are illustrated by the experience at Memorial Sloan-Kettering Cancer Center, in which 105 patients received postoperative external-beam radiation with or without intraoperative brachytherapy after pleurectomy-decortication. Although a favorable subset of patients with epithelial histology who underwent surgical removal of all gross tumor experienced a median survival of 22.5 months, the median survival for the entire group of patients was only 12.5 months. Local recurrence was the most common form of relapse, and radiation pneumonitis or pericarditis occurred in 20% of patients.[55, 69, 70]

Adjuvant postoperative radiation is frequently used after extrapleural pneumonectomy. A report indicates that low-dose radiation (<40 Gy) is not effective in preventing local recurrence.[71] The use of high-dose adjuvant hemithoracic radiation (54 Gy) after extrapleural pneumonectomy is currently being investigated in a prospective clinical trial at Memorial Sloan-Kettering Cancer Center.

Boutin and associates[72] have reported the use of short-course, high dose per fraction radiation (700 Gy daily for 3 days) to the chest wall after thoracoscopy. A small randomized trial shows that this regimen effectively prevents the development of tumor implants in the chest wall incisions.

There are anecdotal reports of prolonged survival after intrapleural instillation of radiocolloids.[73] Some of these patients also received external-beam radiotherapy. It is not clear whether intracavitary radiation provides any real benefit beyond that supplied by standard external-beam radiotherapy.

## CHEMOTHERAPY

Detorubicin, high-dose methotrexate, and edatrexate appear to have the highest single-agent activity against malignant mesothelioma.[74] Response rates of 10 to 20% have been reported with doxorubicin, epirubicin, mitomycin, cyclophosphamide, ifosfamide, cisplatin, and carboplatin.[74, 75] Reported response rates vary widely from institution to institution and are often the results of small series, publication bias, and patient selection but are in the range of 10 to 20%.[74–76]

Combination chemotherapy has been evaluated in cooperative group trials, but these trials have not shown a consistently greater response rate than single-agent trials. A Sarcoma Intergroup study reported by Samson and coworkers[77] compared cyclophosphamide and doxorubicin with or without dacarbazine (DTIC) in 76 fully evaluable patients with advanced-stage mesothelioma. A response rate of 12% was documented, with no significant difference in response duration or survival between treatment groups. A randomized trial by the Cancer and Leukemia Group B (CALGB) com-

paring cisplatin and doxorubicin with cisplatin and mitomycin found response rate, time to treatment failure, and survival rate to be similar to those for cisplatin and mitomycin.[78] Currently, combination chemotherapy does not have clearly demonstrable superiority to single-agent chemotherapy and can be recommended for the treatment of advanced mesothelioma only in the context of an investigational setting.

Intracavitary chemotherapy in malignant mesothelioma is theoretically attractive because it may expose the tumor to high concentrations of drug while sparing normal tissues from drug-related systemic toxicity. Intracavitary cisplatin and doxorubicin therapy has been attempted in this population, with preliminary results showing some minor activity.[79–81] The major theoretical obstacle to tumor control by this route is the shallow depth of free-surface drug diffusion, with the result that this therapy may be useful only in selected patients with early-stage disease or in combination with surgical resection of all gross tumor.

## NEWER TREATMENT MODALITIES

The use of immunotherapy, particularly gamma interferon administered intrapleurally, has been investigated in Europe. In a phase II trial involving 81 patients, Boutin and associates[82] reported an objective response rate of 16% and a median survival of 10 months after 16 doses of intrapleural human gamma interferon. The efficacy of this approach, similar to that of intrapleural chemotherapy, is probably influenced by dispersion of drug throughout the pleural space and the depth of penetration of intrapleural drug into tumor.

The use of photodynamic therapy after surgical resection has been investigated in a phase I trial at the National Cancer Institute. Preliminary data regarding toxicity and feasibility were promising enough to warrant extension of this approach into a phase II trial.[83] It is unclear, however, how effective this photodynamic therapy is in preventing local tumor recurrence. Intrapleural adenovirus-mediated gene transfer is being investigated for the therapy of early mesotheliomas. The feasibility of this novel treatment is currently being evaluated in phase I clinical trials.[84–86]

## COMBINED-MODALITY THERAPY

Combined-modality treatment has been investigated at several institutions. As mentioned previously, the combination of pleurectomy-decortication, with or without intraoperative brachytherapy (iodine 125 or iridium 102), followed by external-beam radiotherapy has been used at Memorial Sloan-Kettering Cancer Center. Although prolonged survival has been observed in highly selected patients, overall results have been disappointing with respect to overall survival and local control.[55, 69] At the Dana Farber Cancer Center, extrapleural pneumonectomy followed by combination chemotherapy (cyclophosphamide, doxorubicin, and cisplatin) and limited-field radiotherapy has led to a median survival of 21 months and an overall 5-year survival of 22%. This favorable outcome was not observed in patients with mixed cellularity or fibrosarcomatous histology tumors or with involved mediastinal lymph nodes, and it is unclear how much chemotherapy contributes to overall survival in this setting.[40, 62]

## SUMMARY OF TREATMENT

There is still no standard therapy for pleural mesothelioma at any stage of disease. Complete surgical resection of gross tumor combined with adjuvant radiation, with or without chemotherapy, appears to prolong survival in carefully selected patients, but it is still hard to assess reported results because of the paucity of well-designed prospective studies based on careful pretreatment staging. Only through well-designed multidisciplinary clinical trials will the prognosis of malignant mesothelioma be improved.

## SUGGESTIONS FOR ADDITIONAL READING

Antman K, Aisner J, eds. Asbestos-related malignancy. Orlando: Grune & Stratton, 1987.

Rusch VW. Diffuse malignant mesothelioma. In: Shields TW, ed. General thoracic surgery. 4th ed. Baltimore: Williams & Wilkins, 1994.

## REFERENCES

1. Okike N, Bernatz PE, Woolner LB. Localized mesothelioma of the pleura: benign and malignant variants. J Thorac Cardiovasc Surg 1978;75:363–72.
2. Briselli M, Mark EJ, Dickersin R. Solitary fibrous tumors of the pleura: eight new cases and review of 360 cases in the literature. Cancer 1981;47:2678–89.
3. England DM, Hochholzer L, McCarthy MJ. Localized benign and malignant fibrous tumors of the pleura: a clinicopathologic review of 223 cases. Am J Surg Pathol 1989;13:640–58.
4. Antman KH. Clinical presentation and natural history of benign and malignant mesothelioma. Semin Oncol 1981;8:313–20.
5. McDonald JC, McDonald AD. Epidemiology of mesothelioma from estimated incidence. Prev Med 1977;6:426–42.
6. Walker AM, Loughlin JE, Friedlander ER, et al. Projections of asbestos-related disease 1980–2009. J Occup Med 1983;25:409–25.
7. Wagner JC, Slegg CA, Marchand P. Diffuse pleural mesotheliomas and asbestos exposure in Northwestern Cape Province. Br J Ind Med 1960;17:260–71.
8. Lemen RA, Dement JM, Wagoner JK. Epidemiology of asbestos-related diseases. Environ Health Perspect 1980;34:1–11.
9. Stanton MF, Laynard M, Tegeris A, et al. Carcinogenicity of fibrous glass: pleural response in the rat in relation to fiber dimension. J Natl Cancer Inst 1977;58:587–603.
10. Lee KP, Barras CE, Griffith FD, Waritz RS. Pulmonary response and transmigration of inorganic fibers by inhalation exposure. Am J Pathol 1981;102:314–23.
11. Craighead JE, Mossman BT. The pathogenesis of asbestos-associated diseases. N Engl J Med 1982;306:1446–55.
12. Becklake MR. Asbestos-related diseases of the lung and other organs: their epidemiology and implications for clinical practice. Am Rev Respir Dis 1976;114:187–227.
13. McDonald AD, McDonald JC. Epidemiology of malignant mesothelioma. In: Antman K, Aisner J, eds. Asbestos-related malignancy. Orlando: Grune & Stratton, 1987:31–55.
14. Selikoff IJ, Churg J, Hammond EC. Relation between exposure to asbestos and mesothelioma. N Engl J Med 1965;272:560–5.
15. Lynch HT, Katz D, Marvicka SE. Familial mesothelioma: review and family study. Cancer Genet Cytogenet 1985;15:25–35. abstract.
16. Carbone M, Pass HI, Rizzo P, et al. Simian virus 40-like DNA sequences in human mesothelioma. Oncogene 1994;9:1781–90.
17. Carbone M, Rizzo P, Grimley PM, et al. Simian virus-40 large-T antigen binds p53 in human mesothelioma. Nat Med 1997;3:908–12.
18. Galateau-Salle F, Bidget P, Iwatsubo Y, et al. SV40 like DNA in pleural mesothelioma, brochopulmonary carcinoma, and non-malignant pulmonary diseases. J Pathol 1998;184:252–7.
19. Testa JR, Carbone M, Hirvonen A, et al. A multi-institutional study confirms the presence and expression of Simian virus 40 in human malignant mesotheliomas. Cancer Res 1998;58:4505–9.
20. Donna A, Betta PG. Mesodermomas: a new embryological approach to primary tumours of coelomic surfaces. Histopathology 1981;5:31–44.
21. Legha SS, Muggia F. Pleural mesothelioma: clinical features and therapeutic implications. Ann Intern Med 1977;87:613–21.
22. Warhol MJ. Electron microscopy in the diagnosis of mesothelioma with routine biopsy, needle biopsy, and fluid cytology. In: Antman K, Aisner J, eds. Asbestos-related malignancy. Orlando: Grune & Stratton, 1987:201–21.
23. Schlegel R, Banks-Schlegel S, McLeod JA, Pinkus GS. Immunoperoxidase localization of keratin in human neoplasms: a preliminary survey. Am J Pathol 1980;101:41–50.
24. Gibbs AR, Harach R, Wagner JC, Jasani B. Comparison of tumour markers in malignant mesothelioma and pulmonary adenocarcinoma. Thorax 1985;40:91–5.
25. Warhol MJ, Hickey WF, Corson JM. Malignant mesothelioma: ultrastructural distinction from adenocarcinoma. Am J Surg Pathol 1982;6:307–14.
26. Kwee WS, Veldhuizen RW, Golding RP, et al. Histologic distinction between malignant mesothelioma, benign pleural lesions and carcinoma metastasis: evaluation of the application of morphometry combined with histochemistry and immunostaining. Virchows Archiv 1982;297:287–99.
27. Elmes PC, Simpson MJC. The clinical aspects of mesothelioma. QJM 1976;45:427–49.
28. Selikoff IJ, Hammond EC, Seidman H. Latency of asbestos disease among insulation workers in the United States and Canada. Cancer 1980;46:2736–40.
29. Law MR, Hodson ME, Heard BE. Malignant mesothelioma of the pleura: relation between histological type and clinical behaviour. Thorax 1982;37:810–5.
30. Law MR, Hodson ME, Turner-Warwick M. Malignant mesothelioma of the pleura: clinical aspects and symptomatic treatment. Eur J Respir Dis 1984;65:162–8.
31. Butchart EG. Surgery of mesothelioma of the pleura. In Roth JA, Ruckdeschel JC, Weisenburger TH, eds. Thoracic oncology. Philadelphia: WB Saunders, 1989:566–83.
32. Ruffie R, Feld R, Minkin S, et al. Diffuse malignant mesothelioma of the pleura in Ontario and Quebec: a retrospective study of 332 patients. J Clin Oncol 1989;7:1157–68.
33. Kreel L. Computed tomography in mesothelioma. Semin Oncol 1981;8:302–12.
34. Grant DC, Seltzer SE, Antman KH, et al. Computed tomography of malignant pleural mesothelioma. J Comput Assist Tomogr 1983;7:626–32.
35. Rabinowitz JG, Efremidis SC, Cohen B, et al. A comparative study of mesothelioma and asbestosis using computed tomography and conventional chest radiography. Radiology 1982;144:453–60.
36. Heller RM, Janower ML, Weber AL. The radiological manifestations of malignant pleural mesothelioma. AJR Am J Roentgenol 1970;108:53–9.
37. Katz D, Kreel L. Computed tomography in pulmonary asbestosis. Clin Radiol 1979;30:207–13.
38. Boutin C, Rey F. Thoracoscopy in pleural malignant mesothelioma: a prospective study of 188 consecutive patients: Part 1. diagnosis. Cancer 1993;72:389–93.
39. Boutin C, Rey F, Gouvernet J, et al. Thoracoscopy in pleural malignant mesothelioma: a prospective study of 188 consecutive patients: Part 2. prognosis and staging. Cancer 1993;72:394–404.
40. Sugarbaker DJ, Strauss GM, Lynch TJ, et al. Node status has prognostic significance in the multimodality therapy of diffuse, malignant mesothelioma. J Clin Oncol 1993;11:1172–8.
41. Walters KL, Martinez AJ. Malignant fibrous mesothelioma: metastatic to brain and liver. Acta Neuropathol (Berl) 1975;33:173–7.
42. Roberts GH. Distant visceral metastases in pleural mesothelioma. Br J Dis Chest 1976;70:246–50.
43. Rusch VW, Godwin JD, Shuman WP. The role of computed tomography scanning in the initial assessment and the follow-up of malignant pleural mesothelioma. J Thorac Cardiovasc Surg 1988;96:171–7.
44. Heelan RT, Rusch VW, Begg CB, et al. Staging of malignant pleural mesothelioma: comparison of CT and MR imaging for staging. Am J Radiol 1999;172:1039–1047.

45. Conlon KC, Rusch VW, Gillern S. Laparoscopy: an important tool in the staging of malignant pleural mesothelioma. Ann Surg Oncol 1996;3:489–94.
46. Nauta RJ, Osteen RT, Antman KH, Koster JK. Clinical staging and the tendency of malignant pleural mesotheliomas to remain localized. Ann Thorac Surg 1982;34:66–70.
47. Bénard F, Sterman D, Smith RJ, et al. Metabolic imaging of malignant pleural mesothelioma with fluorodeoxyglucose positron emission tomography. Chest 1998;114:713–22.
48. Butchart EG, Ashcroft T, Barnsley WC, Holden MP. Pleuropneumonectomy in the management of diffuse malignant mesothelioma of the pleura: experience with 29 patients. Thorax 1976;31:15–24.
49. Rusch VW, The International Mesothelioma Interest Group. A proposed new international TNM staging system for malignant pleural mesothelioma. Chest 1995;108:1122–8.
50. Chahinian AP, Pajak TF, Holland JF, et al. Diffuse malignant mesothelioma: prospective evaluation of 69 patients. Ann Intern Med 1982;96:Part 1:746–55.
51. Antman KH, Shemin R, Ryan L, et al. Malignant mesothelioma: prognostic variables in a registry of 180 patients, the Dana-Farber Cancer Institute and Brigham and Women's Hospital experience over two decades, 1965–1985. J Clin Oncol 1988;6:147–53.
52. Adams VI, Unni KK, Muhm JR, et al. Diffuse malignant mesothelioma of pleura: diagnosis and survival in 92 cases. Cancer 1986;58:1540–51.
53. Alberts AS, Falkson G, Goedhals L, et al. Malignant pleural mesothelioma: a disease unaffected by current therapeutic maneuvers. J Clin Oncol 1988;6:527–35.
54. Rusch VW, Piantadosi S, Holmes EC. The role of extrapleural pneumonectomy in malignant pleural mesothelioma. J Thorac Cardiovasc Surg 1991;102:1–9.
55. McCormack PM, Nagasaki F, Hilaris BS, Martini N. Surgical treatment of pleural mesothelioma. J Thorac Cardiovasc Surg 1982;84:834–42.
56. Sugarbaker DJ, Heher EC, Lee TH, et al. Extrapleural pneumonectomy, chemotherapy, and radiotherapy in the treatment of diffuse malignant pleural mesothelioma. J Thorac Cardiovasc Surg 1991;102:10–5.
57. Martini N, Bains MS, Beattie Jr EJ. Indications for pleurectomy in malignant effusion. Cancer 1975;35:734–8.
58. Wörn H. Moglichkeiten und ergebnisse der chirurgischen behandlung des malignen pleuramesothelioms. Thoraxchirurgie Vaskulare Chirurgie 1974;22:391.
59. DeLaria GA, Jensik R, Faber LP, Kittle CF. Surgical management of malignant mesothelioma. Ann Thorac Surg 1978;26:375–82.
60. Bamler KJ, Maassen W. Uber die Verteilung der benignen und malignen Pleuraturmoren im Krankengut einer lungenchirurgischen Klinik mit besonderer Berucksichtigung des malignen Pleuramesothelioms und seiner radikalen Behandlung einschliesslich der Ergebnisse des Zwerchfellersatzes mit konservierter Dura mater. Thoraxchirurgie Vaskulare Chirurgie 1974;22:386–91.
61. Rusch VW, Venkatraman E. The importance of surgical staging in the treatment of malignant pleural mesothelioma. J Thorac Cardiovasc Surg 1996;111:815–26.
62. Sugarbaker DJ, Garcia JP, Richards WG, et al. Extrapleural pneumonectomy in the multimodality therapy of malignant pleural mesothelioma: results in 120 consecutive patients. Ann Surg 1996;224:288–96.
63. Allen KB, Faber LP, Warren WH. Malignant pleural mesothelioma: extrapleural pneumonectomy and pleurectomy. Chest Surg Clin N Am 1994;4:113–26.
64. Eschwège F, Schlienger M. La radiotherapie des mesotheliomes pleuraux malins: a propos de 14 cas irradies a doses elevees. J Radiol 1973;54:255–9.
65. Gordon Jr W, Antman KH, Greenberger JS, et al. Radiation therapy in the management of patients with mesothelioma. Int J Radiat Oncol Biol Phys 1982;8:19–25.
66. Law MR, Gregor A, Hodson ME, et al. Malignant mesothelioma of the pleura: a study of 52 treated and 64 untreated patients. Thorax 1984;39:255–9.
67. Briney WF. Treatment of pleural mesothelioma. JAMA 1974;229:141. letter.
68. Vogelzang NJ, Schultz SM, Iannucci AM, Kennedy BJ. Malignant mesothelioma: the University of Minnesota experience. Cancer 1984;53:377–83.
69. Hilaris BS, Dattatreyudu N, Kwong E, et al. Pleurectomy and intraoperative brachytherapy and postoperative radiation in the treatment of malignant pleural mesothelioma. Int J Radiat Oncol Biol Phys 1984;10:325–31.
70. Mychalczak BR, Nori D, Armstrong JG, et al. Results of treatment of malignant pleural mesothelioma with surgery, brachytherapy, and external beam irradiation. Endocurie Hypertherm Oncol 1989;5:245. abstract.
71. Baldini EH, Recht A, Strauss GM, et al. Patterns of failure after trimodality therapy for malignant pleural mesothelioma. Ann Thorac Surg 1997;63:334–8.
72. Boutin C, Rey F, Viallat J-R. Prevention of malignant seeding after invasive diagnostic procedures in patients with pleural mesothelioma: a randomized trial of local radiotherapy. Chest 1995;108:754–8.
73. Reichert R, Sherman CD. Prolonged survival in diffuse pleural mesothelioma treated with Au$^{198}$. Cancer 1959;17:799–805.
74. Tiong Ong S, Vogelzang NJ. Chemotherapy in malignant pleural mesothelioma: a review. J Clin Oncol 1996;14:1007–17.
75. Krarup-Hansen A, Hansen HH. Chemotherapy in malignant mesothelioma: a review. Cancer Chemother Pharmacol 1991;28:319–30.
76. Vogelzang NJ. Malignant mesothelioma: diagnostic and management strategies for 1992. Semin Oncol 1992;19:4 Suppl 11:64–71.
77. Samson MK, Wasser LP, Borden EC, et al. Randomized comparison of cyclophosphamide, imidazole, carboxamide, and Adriamycin versus cyclophosphamide and Adriamycin in patients with advanced stage malignant mesothelioma: a Sarcoma Intergroup study. J Clin Oncol 1987;5:86–91.
78. Chahinian AP, Antman K, Goutsou M, et al. Randomized phase II trial of cisplatin with mitomycin or doxorubicin for malignant mesothelioma by the Cancer and Leukemia Group B. J Clin Oncol 1993;11:1559–65.
79. Chahinian AP, Norton L, Holland JF, et al. Experimental and clinical activity of mitomycin C and cis-Diamminedichloroplatinum in malignant mesothelioma. Cancer Res 1984;44:1688–92.
80. Markman M, Cleary S, Pfeifle CE, Howell SB. Cisplatin administered by the intracavitary route as treatment for malignant mesothelioma. Cancer 1986;58:18–21.
81. Mintzer DM, Kelsen D, Frimmer D, et al. Phase II trial of high-dose cisplatin in patients with malignant mesothelioma. Cancer Treat Rep 1985;69:711–2.
82. Boutin C, Viallat J-R, Van Zandwijk N, et al. Activity of intrapleural recombinant gamma-interferon in malignant mesothelioma. Cancer 1991;67:2033–7.
83. Pass HI, DeLaney TF, Tochner Z, et al. Intrapleural photodynamic therapy: results of a phase I trial. Ann Surg Oncol 1994;1:28–37.
84. Hwang HC, Smythe WR, Elshami AA, et al. Gene therapy using adenovirus carrying the herpes simplex-thymidine kinase gene to treat in vivo models of human malignant mesothelioma and lung cancer. Am J Respir Cell Mol Biol 1995;13:7–16.
85. Albelda SM. Gene therapy for lung cancer and mesothelioma. Chest 1997;111:Suppl:114S–49S.
86. Takita H, Dougherty TJ. Intracavitary photodynamic therapy for malignant pleural mesothelioma. Semin Surg Oncol 1995;11:368–71.

# CHAPTER 39

# MEDIASTINAL TUMORS

• JOHN D. HAINSWORTH • F. ANTHONY GRECO

The mediastinum is frequently involved by malignant tumors, although in most cases the involvement represents metastatic spread to mediastinal lymph nodes. However, a wide variety of relatively uncommon primary tumors arise in the mediastinum. Approximately two thirds of all primary mediastinal tumors are benign, and surgical removal is usually curative.[1, 2] The malignant tumors that occur in the mediastinum are uncommon, but effective treatment is available for some of these tumors. Treatable tumors in this group include Hodgkin's disease, non-Hodgkin's lymphomas, germ cell tumors, malignant thymomas, and poorly differentiated carcinoma. The treatment of lymphomas is dealt with in Part XX; in this chapter, other primary malignant tumors arising in the mediastinum are discussed.

The mediastinum has traditionally been subdivided into anterior, middle, and posterior compartments, as shown in Figure 39–1. Although there is considerable overlapping, these anatomic divisions are helpful in the differential diagnosis of mediastinal tumors. The anterior mediastinum is most frequently involved with malignant tumors, including lymphomas, thymomas, germ cell tumors, and thyroid tumors. The middle mediastinum is a rare site for the origin of primary mediastinal tumors, although occasional lymphomas arise in this area. Tumors arising in the posterior mediastinum include neurogenic tumors and soft tissue sarcomas. The frequency and distribution of various mediastinal tumors in one large reported series are outlined in Table 39–1.

Most patients with primary mediastinal tumors come to medical attention because of the development of local symptoms or as a result of an asymptomatic lesion being found on a routine chest radiograph. Local symptoms are generally caused by compression or invasion of adjacent structures and can include substernal chest pain, dyspnea, cough, or dysphagia. Less frequently, superior vena cava syndrome is the presenting manifestation. Symptomatic patients more often have malignant tumors.

Initial evaluation should narrow the differential diagnosis and determine the appropriate biopsy approach. The previously difficult problem of excluding a vascular lesion (e.g., an aortic aneurysm) has been greatly simplified by the use of computed tomography (CT). This test should be routinely employed to delineate the extent and location of the mediastinal tumor, as well as to better evaluate the lung fields. All patients should undergo a careful physical examination, particularly to exclude peripheral adenopathy, which would provide a more accessible site for biopsy. In addition, CT of the abdomen should be performed before the biopsy. In young men, serum levels of alpha-fetoprotein (AFP) and human chorionic gonadotropin (hCG) should be measured. If staging evaluation reveals metastatic tumor, a biopsy specimen should be obtained from the most accessible tumor site.

Options for biopsy of mediastinal masses include fine-needle aspiration, mediastinoscopy, limited thoracotomy, and full thoracotomy with resection. The biopsy technique should depend on the location of the mediastinal tumor as well as on the suspected diagnosis based on prebiopsy evaluation. Although fine-needle aspiration biopsy is often the least invasive procedure available, the small amount of tissue obtained can limit optimal pathologic evaluation of poorly differentiated tumors. Several primary mediastinal tumor types (e.g., lymphoma, germ cell tumor, carcinoma) have poorly differentiated histology, particularly in younger patients; definitive diagnosis of these tumors often requires open biopsy. In patients with large unresectable tumors, biopsy should be achieved with the least invasive technique, usually mediastinoscopy or limited parasternal incision. However, in patients with small tumors that are potentially resectable, the most appropriate approach is usually a full thoracotomy or a median sternotomy with planned tumor resection.

Most of this chapter is devoted to a discussion of primary mediastinal germ cell tumors and malignant thymomas. In addition, poorly differentiated carcinomas of the mediasti-

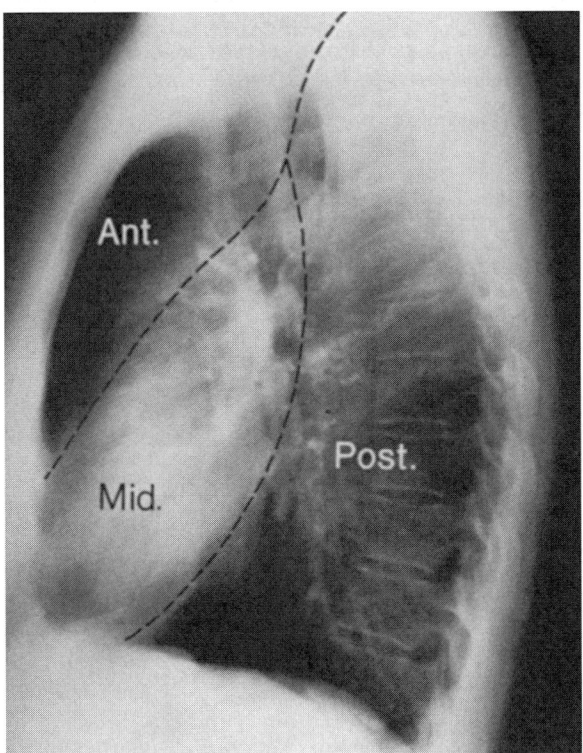

**Figure 39–1.** Normal lateral chest radiograph indicating the anatomic compartments of the mediastinum.

*Table 39–1.* **Anatomic Location of Primary Mediastinal Cysts and Neoplasms**

| Type of Lesion | Percentage |
|---|---|
| *Anterosuperior Mediastinum (N = 215; 54%)* | |
| Thymic neoplasms | 30 |
| Lymphomas | 20 |
| Germ cell | 18 |
| Carcinoma | 13 |
| Cysts | 7 |
| Mesenchymal neoplasms | 5 |
| Endocrine | 5 |
| Other | 2 |
| *Middle Mediastinum (N = 82; 20%)* | |
| Cysts | 60 |
| Lymphomas | 21 |
| Mesenchymal neoplasms | 9 |
| Carcinoma | 7 |
| Other | 3 |
| *Posterior Mediastinum (N = 103; 26%)* | |
| Neurogenic | 53 |
| Cysts | 34 |
| Mesenchymal neoplasms | 9 |
| Endocrine | 2 |
| Other | 2 |

From Davis RD, Oldham HN Jr, Sabiston DC Jr. Primary cysts and neoplasms of the mediastinum: recent changes in clinical presentation, methods of diagnosis, management, and results. Ann Thorac Surg 1987;44:229.

This table was based on a review of 400 cases seen at Duke University Medical Center between 1930 and 1986. Esophageal, pulmonary, and metastatic tumors were excluded. As a supplement to this table, the differential diagnosis of mediastinal lesions should also include the following entities, with their mediastinal location identified as anterior (A), middle (M), or posterior (P): chemodectoma (A), lymphadenopathy due to inflammation or sarcoidosis (M), cylindroma (A); chordoma (A, P); fibroma-fibrosarcoma (P, A); myxoma (P); xanthogranuloma (P); lymphangioma (A); thyroid goiters and endocrine tumors of the thyroid (A, P) or parathyroid glands (A); a variety of cystic lesions, including pericardial cysts (A, M), bronchogenic cysts (M, P), enteric-esophageal cysts (P), thymic cysts (A), thoracic duct cysts (P), and meningoceles (P); hiatal hernia (M, P); hernia of Morgagni (A); and aortic aneurysm (M, P). Subclassifications of thymic neoplasms, germ cell tumors, lymphomas, and neurogenic tumors are given in the text and accompanying tables.

num and neurogenic tumors of the posterior mediastinum are briefly discussed.

# Mediastinal Germ Cell Tumors

Mediastinal germ cell tumors are now recognized as a distinct biologic and clinical entity. Although they are rare, it is important to recognize them; they occur predominantly in young males and are often curable with appropriate treatment. These tumors can be grouped into three general categories: benign teratomas, pure seminomas, and malignant nonseminomatous germ cell tumors.

## BENIGN TERATOMA OF THE MEDIASTINUM

Benign teratoma of the mediastinum (*dermoid* tumor) is a rare neoplasm that accounts for only 3 to 12% of mediastinal tumors.[2] These tumors most frequently occur in young adults, but cases in patients from 7 months to 65 years have been reported. The incidence in males and females is approximately equal.[3] No predisposing conditions or associated abnormalities have been described.

## Pathology

The pathologic appearance of benign mediastinal teratoma is identical to that of benign teratomas arising in the more common ovarian location. Grossly, these tumors are well encapsulated and are composed either of a single large cystic cavity or of several smaller intercommunicating cystic spaces. Mature ectodermal, mesodermal, and endodermal tissue from germ cell layers is typically present. The ectodermal component is usually predominant (i.e., skin, neural tissue, pilosebaceous tissue), hence, the term *dermoid tumors*.[7]

## Clinical Features

Benign teratomas of the mediastinum are slow-growing tumors, 95% of which arise in the anterior mediastinum; the remainder are found in the posterior mediastinum.[6] In contemporary series, approximately half the patients are asymptomatic when these tumors are detected by routine chest radiography.[3] Substernal chest pain and dyspnea are the most common symptoms. Cough productive of hair or sebum is a rare but pathognomonic symptom of this disease that occurs with tumor rupture into the tracheobronchial tree.

These tumors are usually large at the time of diagnosis and appear well encapsulated on the chest radiograph. Calcification within the tumor is seen in approximately 25% of patients; occasionally, definitive diagnosis can be made by observing teeth within the tumor.

Laboratory evaluation is usually normal in these patients; in particular, serum levels of β-hCG and AFP are always normal.

## Treatment

Surgical excision is the treatment of choice for benign teratoma of the mediastinum. Median sternotomy is the preferred approach, although successful resection can also be achieved via a thoracotomy incision. Because of the large size of the tumor and frequent invasion of adjacent structures, surgical resection may be difficult. Adjacent mediastinal structures that are sometimes involved include pericardium, lung, great vessels, thymus, chest wall, hilar structures, and diaphragm.[3] In 10 to 15% of patients, resection of adjacent structures (e.g., via pericardiectomy or lobectomy) is necessary for complete tumor resection. Other modalities, such as radiation therapy and chemotherapy, have no role in the treatment of benign teratoma.

Tumor recurrence is rare after complete surgical resection.[3] Prolonged survival has also been reported in patients who undergo subtotal tumor resection because of involvement of adjacent vital mediastinal structures. In recent years, improved surgical technique and earlier diagnosis of these tumors has resulted in a high rate of complete resection and negligible mortality.

## MALIGNANT MEDIASTINAL GERM CELL TUMORS (PURE SEMINOMAS AND MALIGNANT NONSEMINOMATOUS GERM CELL TUMORS)

### Etiology and Pathogenesis

Mediastinal germ cell tumors are thought to arise from primitive rests of totipotential cells that either become detached early in embryogenesis or fail to migrate appropriately during development.[4, 5] However, these hypotheses are unproved. Substantial evidence now indicates that these tumors indeed arise in the mediastinum, rather than representing metastases from unsuspected testicular primary tumors.[6, 7]

### Epidemiology

Malignant mediastinal germ cell tumors are uncommon and represent only 3 to 10% of tumors originating in the mediastinum.[1, 2, 8] They are much less common than germ cell tumors of the testes and account for 1 to 5% of all germ cell neoplasms in males.[9, 10] However, it is likely that some of these tumors are not recognized because of their poorly differentiated histologic appearance. Young men with poorly differentiated carcinoma in the mediastinum often respond dramatically to chemotherapy for germ cell tumor.[11, 12] Molecular genetic analysis has demonstrated the i(12p) chromosomal abnormality specific for germ cell tumors in some such patients after all other pathologic studies were nondiagnostic.[13] The clinician should therefore consider the possibility of an unrecognized germ cell tumor in all young men with poorly differentiated carcinoma or poorly differentiated neoplasm in the mediastinum.

Most malignant mediastinal germ cell tumors occur in males between 20 and 35 years. They have rarely been reported in women, but there is a strong association between mediastinal nonseminomatous germ cell tumors in men and Klinefelter's syndrome.[14, 15] In one series, 4 (18%) of 22 consecutive patients with mediastinal germ cell tumors had Klinefelter's syndrome, and a fifth patient had clinical features without karyotypic confirmation.[15] The average age of patients with Klinefelter's syndrome who develop mediastinal germ cell tumors is approximately 18 years, which is 10 years younger than the median age of patients who develop these tumors in the absence of Klinefelter's syndrome. The explanation for this peculiar association is unknown, but it is reasonable to assume that the chromosomal abnormality plays a causative role.

### Pathology

Malignant mediastinal germ cell tumors exhibit the same range of histologic subtypes seen in testicular germ cell tumors; however, the relative incidence of the various histologic types differs. Approximately one third of mediastinal germ cell tumors are pure seminomas, and the remaining two thirds have various nonseminoma histologies. In a group of 372 patients reviewed at the Armed Forces Institute of Pathology, the following incidences of nonseminoma histologic types were reported: teratocarcinoma, 41%; endodermal sinus (yolk sac) tumor, 35%; choriocarcinoma, 7%; embryonal carcinoma, 6%; mixed histologic types, 11%.[16] Non–germ cell components (usually sarcoma or epithelial

carcinoma) were found in 26 (58%) of 45 teratocarcinomas. The pathologic features of mediastinal germ cell tumors therefore differ from those of testicular tumors in the following ways: (1) pure endodermal sinus tumor is rare in the testis and relatively common in the mediastinum, (2) embryonal carcinoma is uncommon in the mediastinum, and (3) non–germ cell elements are more frequent in mediastinal germ cell tumors.

### Clinical Features

Malignant mediastinal germ cell tumors are usually large at the time of diagnosis, and local symptoms are present in most patients. The clinical features of pure seminomas and tumors containing nonseminomatous elements are discussed separately, but considerable overlap is seen in their clinical characteristics.

**Seminoma.** Pure seminomas are relatively slow growing compared with other germ cell tumors, and they can reach a large size in the mediastinum before causing symptoms. Twenty to 30% of these tumors are asymptomatic when detected by routine chest radiographs.[17] Signs and symptoms are nonspecific and are typical of those seen with other slowly expanding mediastinal tumors. Systemic symptoms are uncommon, although some patients may experience weight loss or easy fatigability. Symptoms related to metastatic lesions are uncommon at diagnosis. Current staging techniques, including CT, show that approximately 30 to 40% of patients have tumor localized to the mediastinum.[18] The lungs and other intrathoracic structures are the most common metastatic sites and are often detected only by CT. Osseous metastases are the most frequently recognized metastatic sites outside the chest. The retroperitoneum is an uncommon site of metastasis in patients with mediastinal seminoma, in contrast to the common involvement of this area in patients with testicular primary tumors.[7, 18]

The radiographic appearance of primary mediastinal seminoma does not allow its distinction from other mediastinal tumors. CT of the chest typically shows a large, homogeneous anterior mediastinal mass obliterating the fat planes surrounding the mediastinal vascular structures.

Serum levels of hCG are elevated in approximately 10% of patients with mediastinal seminoma.[18] These elevations are usually low (<100 mIU/ml); higher levels of hCG should suggest the presence of nonseminomatous elements. The serum AFP level is always normal in pure mediastinal seminoma; elevation of this marker indicates the presence of nonseminomatous elements, regardless of the histologic findings. Serum lactate dehydrogenase levels are elevated in most patients with mediastinal seminoma.

**Nonseminomatous Germ Cell Tumors.** As a group, nonseminomatous tumors grow more rapidly than do pure seminomas. These tumors are rarely asymptomatic at the time of diagnosis. They frequently produce symptoms by compressing or invading adjacent mediastinal structures. However, in contrast to pure seminomas, 85 to 95% of patients with nonseminomatous neoplasms have at least one site of metastatic disease at diagnosis, and presenting symptoms are often due to metastatic lesions.[19–21] Common sites of metastases include lung, pleura, lymph nodes (supraclavicular, retroperitoneal), and liver. Gynecomastia is occasionally present in patients with high serum levels of β-hCG. Constitutional symptoms, including weight loss, fever, and weakness, are common. Neoplasms with elements of choriocarcinoma have a marked hemorrhagic tendency, and these patients may present with catastrophic events related to hemorrhage at a metastatic site.

Features seen on chest radiography do not differ significantly from those of mediastinal seminoma. CT usually shows an inhomogeneous mass with multiple areas of hemorrhage and necrosis, as opposed to the usually homogeneous appearance of mediastinal seminomas. Approximately 90% of patients have elevated levels of β-hCG or AFP, or both.[19, 21]

The unique association between mediastinal nonseminomatous germ cell tumors and a variety of hematologic malignant conditions has been well established.[22] Although the frequency of this association has not been defined in prospective studies, it may be as high as 10%. Several hematologic malignancies have been reported, including acute nonlymphocytic leukemia, acute lymphocytic leukemia, erythroleukemia, myelodysplastic syndromes, and malignant histiocytosis. Most patients developed the hematologic malignancies subsequent to the diagnosis of mediastinal germ cell tumor, but usually within 24 months. These hematologic neoplasms appear to arise from clones of malignant lymphoblasts or myeloblasts contained within the mediastinal germ cell tumor. Foci of lymphoblasts have been recognized in several mediastinal germ cell tumors.[23, 24] More important, several patients have been found to have an identical chromosomal abnormality (an isochromosome of the short arm of chromosome 12) in neoplastic cells from the mediastinal germ cell tumor and also in the hematologic neoplasm, suggesting a common origin.[24, 25] This karyotypic abnormality has been identified as a specific cytogenetic marker in extragonadal and testicular germ cell tumors.[26] The cause of the specific association between mediastinal nonseminomatous germ cell tumors (rather than all germ cell tumors) and hematologic neoplasia is unexplained.

Rarely, other syndromes, including idiopathic thrombocytopenia, hemophagocytic syndrome, and systemic mast cell disease, have been associated with mediastinal germ cell tumors.[27–29] These syndromes have been refractory to treatment, and their cause is unknown.

## Pretreatment Evaluation

The diagnosis of mediastinal germ cell tumor should be considered in all young males who have a mediastinal mass. The approach to initial work-up and staging has been outlined previously; prebiopsy determination of serum hCG and AFP levels is critical in these patients. If metastases are present, biopsy of the most accessible area is recommended, since surgical therapy does not play an initial role in treatment, and rapid initiation of systemic therapy is important. Very high levels of AFP or hCG are diagnostic of nonseminomatous germ cell tumors; biopsy is not necessary in these patients, and systemic treatment should begin immediately.

In patients with tumors that are seemingly localized to the mediastinum, the biopsy technique should be determined by the extent and location of tumor as seen on CT. In patients with tumors that are obviously unresectable owing to involvement of vital mediastinal structures or other intrathoracic spread, mediastinoscopy or parasternal incision is the biopsy method of choice. Thoracotomy with attempted complete resection is sometimes indicated if standard criteria suggest that the tumor is resectable.

## Treatment

The treatment and prognosis of pure mediastinal seminoma and mediastinal germ cell tumors with nonseminomatous histologic aspects differ and are therefore discussed separately.

**Seminoma.** Reports documenting curative surgical resection of pure mediastinal seminoma appeared as early as the 1950s.[30] However, complete resection is possible in a few patients only. In contemporary series, staging evaluation, including chest tomography, has demonstrated metastases in more than 50% of patients with mediastinal seminoma. Therefore, the possibility of complete surgical resection exists in less than 25% of patients and is probably limited to those in whom an asymptomatic mediastinal mass is found on routine chest radiography. Even after "complete" surgical resection, some patients have local recurrence[31]; therefore, surgical treatment should never be used as the sole therapeutic modality.

Pure mediastinal seminomas share the exquisite radiosensitivity of testicular seminoma, and primary radiotherapy is often curative in this disease. Although most reported series have contained fewer than 20 patients treated with varying radiotherapeutic techniques, approximately 60% of patients achieved long-term disease-free survival.[18, 32, 33] Most treatment failures were due to the appearance of distant metastases, rather than inadequate local tumor control. Specific recommendations for radiation therapy dosage and technique are based on the much larger experience in the treatment of metastatic testicular seminoma. Most authors recommend 35 to 50 Gy delivered over 6 weeks by external-beam megavoltage irradiation to a shaped mediastinal field, including both supraclavicular areas.[32, 33] Routine irradiation of the retroperitoneum is unnecessary. The benefit of surgical debulking before definitive radiation therapy is doubtful. Unless complete tumor resection can be accomplished, extensive mediastinal procedures should be avoided because they delay the use of more effective forms of treatment.

Highly effective systemic combination chemotherapy now offers an additional option for the treatment of pure mediastinal seminoma. A large experience in advanced testicular seminoma indicates that intensive cisplatin-based regimens are at least as active against seminoma as they are against nonseminomatous germ cell tumors. Table 39–2 summarizes the experience with optimal cisplatin-based combination regimens in the treatment of pure mediastinal seminoma. Even though many patients have bulky tumors or metastatic disease, or both, a large majority are cured with treatment. Chemotherapy is equally effective in pure mediastinal seminoma and advanced testicular seminoma. In one nonrandomized study comparing initial chemotherapy and initial radiation therapy, 5 of 9 patients treated initially with radiation therapy remained disease free, compared with 10 of 11 patients receiving initial chemotherapy.[18] Similar excellent results with chemotherapy were seen in the Southeastern Cancer Study Group, in which 7 of 9 patients achieved complete response and long-term survival with chemotherapy, even after previous radiation therapy.[34] Therefore,

*Table 39–2.* Mediastinal Seminoma: Results of Treatment with Cisplatin-Based Combination Chemotherapy

| Series | Year | NO. OF PATIENTS | TREATMENT REGIMENS | NO. OF COMPLETE RESPONSES (%) | NO. OF DISEASE-FREE SURVIVORS >24 mo (%) |
|---|---|---|---|---|---|
| Hainsworth et al[19] | 1982 | 4* | PVB | 3 (75) | 3 (75) |
| Jain et al[18] | 1984 | 11 | VAB-6, PVB, CP | 10 (91) | 10 (91) |
| Logothetis et al[20] | 1985 | 4 | CP, CISCA II | 4 (100) | 4 (100) |
| Loehrer et al[34] | 1987 | 9* | PVB, BEP | 8 (89) | 7 (78) |
| Bukowski et al[35] | 1993 | 8 | PVB/EBAP | 5 (63) | 4 (50) |
| Delgado et al[36] | 1993 | 16 | VAB-6, BEP, PVB | 15 (94) | 10 (63) |
| Goss et al[37] | 1994 | 8 | BEP | 8 (100) | 8 (100) |
| Mencel et al[38] | 1994 | 19 | VAB-6, EP | 19 (100) | 19 (100) |
| Gerl et al[39] | 1996 | 4* | VIP, EIP | 4 (100) | 4 (100) |
| *Total* | | 83 | | 76 (92) | 69 (83) |

*Some patients had received prior radiation therapy.

PVB, cisplatin, vinblastine, bleomycin; VAB-6, multidrug regimen developed at Memorial Sloan-Kettering; CP, cyclophosphamide, cisplatin; CISCA II, multidrug regimen developed at M.D. Anderson; BEP, bleomycin, etoposide, cisplatin; EBAP, etoposide, bleomycin, doxorubicin, cisplatin; VIP, vinblastine, ifosfamide, cisplatin.

sufficient evidence exists to allow recommendation of cisplatin-based combination chemotherapy, rather than radiation therapy, as initial therapy for most patients with mediastinal seminoma.

After therapy, many patients with bulky mediastinal seminoma have residual radiographic abnormalities. In most patients, these masses represent dense scirrhous reaction rather than viable seminoma or benign teratoma.[40, 41] Surgical resection is often difficult and risky in these individuals. In one series, residual masses greater than 3 cm in diameter were associated with a higher incidence of residual active seminoma[41]; other investigators have not verified this observation.[40] Patients with small residual masses (<3 cm) should be followed without biopsy; larger masses should either be biopsied or followed closely, with early biopsy of any enlarging tumor mass.

In summary, most patients with pure mediastinal seminoma are curable with appropriate therapy. Patients with small tumors (usually asymptomatic) that appear resectable should either have complete excision followed by radiation therapy or receive radiation therapy alone. Radical debulking procedures for patients with extensive mediastinal involvement are contraindicated. All other patients should receive

initial cisplatin-based chemotherapy. Although the optimal chemotherapy regimen for mediastinal seminoma is not defined, the use of four courses of BEP (bleomycin, etoposide, and cisplatin), as recommended for poor-prognosis testicular germ cell tumors (see Chapter 54), is our regimen of choice. The unusual patient who does not achieve complete remission or relapses after first-line therapy should be considered for high-dose salvage chemotherapy, as discussed in Chapter 54.

**Nonseminomatous Germ Cell Tumors.** Before the development of effective combination chemotherapy, the results of treatment of mediastinal nonseminomatous germ cell tumors were dismal. In a 1975 review of the literature, no long-term survivors among the 85 patients were reported.[41] These tumors not only are almost always metastatic at the time of diagnosis but also are relatively resistant to radiation therapy.

Intensive cisplatin-based combination chemotherapy now provides curative treatment for a sizable percentage of patients with nonseminomatous mediastinal germ cell tumors. When intensive cisplatin-based regimens are used, the long-term survival rate is approximately 40% (Table 39–3). This

*Table 39–3.* Nonseminomatous Mediastinal Germ Cell Tumors: Results of Treatment with Cisplatin-Based Combination Chemotherapy

| Series | Year | No. of Evaluable Patients | Chemotherapy Treatment Regimen | No. of Complete Responders (%) | Long-Term (>24 mo) Disease-Free Survival (%) |
|---|---|---|---|---|---|
| Funes et al[42] | 1981 | 13 | PVB | 6 (46) | 5 (38) |
| Hainsworth et al[19] | 1982 | 12 | PVB ± A | 7 (58) | 7 (58) |
| Logothetis et al[20] | 1985 | 11 | CISCA II, CISCA/VB IV | NA | 4 (36) |
| Kay et al[43] | 1987 | 11 | PVB, BEP | 7 (64) | 5 (45) |
| Nichols et al[44] | 1990 | 31 | PVB ± A, BEP | 18 (58) | 13 (42) |
| Bukowski et al[35] | 1993 | 16 | PVB/EBAP | 13 (81) | 9 (56) |
| Dulmet et al[45] | 1993 | 14 | PVB | 8 (57) | 6 (43) |
| Delgado et al[36] | 1993 | 40 | VAP-6, PVB, BEP | 15 (38) | 14 (35) |
| Goss et al[37] | 1994 | 15 | VAB-6, PVB, BEP | 8 (53) | 7 (47) |
| Gerl et al[39] | 1996 | 12 | PVB, BEP, ECBC | 8 (67) | 6 (50) |
| Fizazi et al[46] | 1998 | 29 | VAB-6, PVeVB, PVB, BEP | 19 (66) | 10 (34) |
| *Total* | | 204 | | 109 (53) | 86 (42) |

PVB (Einhorn regimen): cisplatin, vinblastine, bleomycin; A, Adriamycin; CISCA regimens, multidrug regimens developed at M.D. Anderson; VAB-6, multidrug regimen developed at Memorial Sloan-Kettering; BEP, bleomycin 30 units weekly, etoposide 100 mg/m² IV × 5 days, cisplatin 20 mg/m² IV × 5 days; ECBC, etoposide, cisplatin, bleomycin, cyclophosphamide; PVeVB, cisplatin, etoposide, vinblastine, bleomycin; NA, not available.

survival rate is comparable to that reported for far-advanced (poor-prognosis) testicular nonseminomatous germ cell tumors. However, reviews of survival and prognostic factors have suggested that inherent biologic differences between mediastinal and testicular germ cell tumors may also play a role in determining the relatively low cure rate.[47]

After completion of four courses of combination chemotherapy, further management should parallel that recommended for patients with nonseminomatous testicular tumors. Patients with complete response (i.e., normal serum tumor markers and normal radiographic results) should undergo chest radiography and serum tumor marker determinations monthly during the first year after therapy and every 2 months during the second year. Patients with elevated tumor markers at the completion of chemotherapy have residual active tumor and should receive further chemotherapy. Salvage regimens are discussed in Chapter 54, but the cure rate from salvage regimens for extragonadal tumors has been low. Patients with normal serum tumor marker levels and residual radiographic abnormalities should be considered for surgical resection. This approach is also described in Chapter 54. In this setting, 60 to 70% of patients have necrotic tumor or benign teratoma and no evidence of active malignancy. If viable germ cell carcinoma is present but is completely resected, two additional courses of chemotherapy should be administered. The presence of non–germ cell elements (sarcoma, carcinoma) portends a poor prognosis, even if complete resection can be accomplished. These histologic types are refractory to germ cell chemotherapy regimens; such patients should receive either investigational treatment or symptomatic care alone. Figure 39–2 summarizes the management of patients with mediastinal nonseminomatous germ cell tumors after completion of initial chemotherapy.

At present, the treatment approach for mediastinal nonseminomatous tumors should be the same regardless of the specific histologic appearance. Contrary to early reports, the outcome for patients with pure endodermal sinus tumor is probably similar to that for patients with other nonseminomatous appearances on histologic examination.[20] The rarity of these patients makes definitive statements difficult. Similarly, pure choriocarcinoma of the mediastinum has been considered by some to have a poor prognosis,[19] but only a few patients with this condition have been reported.

# Thymoma

## EPIDEMIOLOGY AND PATHOGENESIS

Thymomas are uncommon, slow-growing tumors that usually arise in adults between 40 and 60 years. The occurrence in males and females is approximately equal. Thymomas are rare in individuals less than 20 years.[48] Almost all are in the superior portion of the anterior mediastinum, in the usual location of the thymus gland. Occasionally, they occur in ectopic locations such as the middle or posterior mediastinum, pleura, or head and neck.

Thymomas originate from the epithelium of the thymus. Many of these tumors contain prominent lymphocytic elements (hence, the previously common term *lymphoepithelioma),* but immunophenotyping studies of these lymphocytes show a polytypic population containing B and T cells. The cause of thymoma is unknown, although several cases of poorly differentiated thymoma have been associated with Epstein-Barr virus infections.[49, 50]

## NATURAL HISTORY

### Pathology

Several classifications of thymomas have been devised based on the histopathologic characteristics of these tumors. The simplest classification identifies three types of thymomas, based on the predominant cell seen on light microscopic examination. If more than two thirds of the tumor consists of lymphocytes or epithelial cells, it is classified as *lymphocytic* or *epithelial,* respectively.[51, 52] If the two cell types

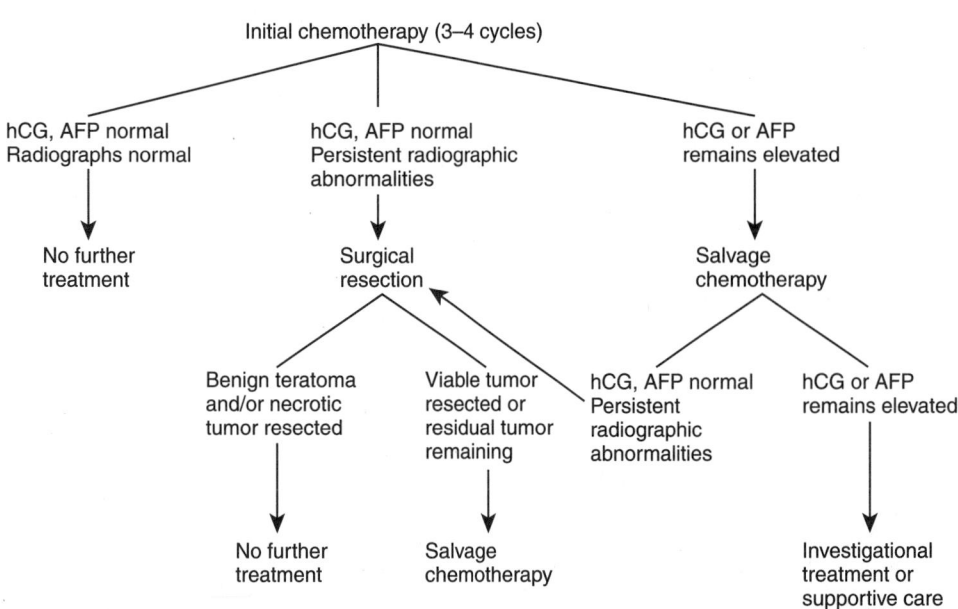

Figure 39–2. Management of nonseminomatous mediastinal germ cell tumors after completion of initial chemotherapy. hCG, human chorionic gonadotropin; AFP, alpha-fetoprotein. (Modified from Hainsworth JD, Greco FA. Mediastinal germ cell neoplasms. In: Roth JA, Ruckdeschel JC, Weisenburger H, eds. Thoracic Oncology. Philadelphia: WB Saunders, 1989:486.)

occur in approximately equal numbers, the tumor is called *mixed* or *lymphoepithelial.* Thymomas that are predominantly lymphocytic are often difficult to distinguish histologically from hematologic neoplasms, particularly Hodgkin's disease and non-Hodgkin's lymphoma. All thymomas have a relatively low mitotic rate, and histologic subtype is not an important prognostic feature.[51]

Although thymomas have been traditionally separated into benign and malignant categories, a reliable distinction cannot be made on the basis of either histopathologic or electron microscopic findings. Some thymomas show evidence of invasion through the capsule and are definitely malignant. However, even noninvasive thymomas should be considered potentially invasive if untreated and should be staged in the traditional manner of malignant tumors.

Unlike most other malignant tumors, hematogenous metastases are uncommon with thymoma. Involvement of regional lymph nodes is also uncommon. The most common metastatic sites are the pleura and pericardium. Tumor implants in these sites are thought to result from shedding of tumor cells from the primary thymoma.

## Clinical Presentation

In 30 to 40% of patients, thymoma is asymptomatic when diagnosed by a routine chest radiograph. Local symptoms are caused by compression or invasion of mediastinal structures. Chest pain and cough are seen most frequently; other symptoms such as dysphagia, superior vena cava syndrome, and dyspnea are less common. Although rarely occurring in children and young adults, thymomas are more aggressive in this age group and more frequently present with local symptoms.[53]

The most striking clinical manifestations of thymoma are the various paraneoplastic syndromes that can be anticipated in at least half the patients with this tumor. Myasthenia gravis is by far the most common associated syndrome, occurring in 40 to 50% of patients with thymoma. Table 39–4 lists the wide variety of autoimmune or immune phenomena associated with thymoma. In addition to these immunologic disorders, approximately 10% of patients with thymoma have a second malignancy, and 5% have a coexisting endocrine disorder.[54] The most common autoimmune disorders are discussed separately.

**Myasthenia Gravis.** This disease is caused by an abnormality of neuromuscular transmission resulting from autoimmune destruction of the acetylcholine receptors in the postsynaptic villi of voluntary muscle. The major symptoms of patients with this disease are weakness and fatigue; the typical electromyographic finding consists of progressive decrements in muscle action potential with repetitive stimulation. The relationship of thymic abnormalities and myasthenia gravis was first suspected when thymic lymphoid hyperplasia and germinal centers were found in 70 to 75% of patients with myasthenia gravis.[55] Fifteen percent of patients developing myasthenia have either gross or microscopic thymoma; however, the relationship of thymic abnormalities to the development of myasthenia gravis remains unexplained.

Patients with myasthenia gravis and associated thymoma are older than myasthenic patients without thymoma. In addition, the prognosis of the myasthenia in these patients is relatively poor, because improvement in muscle strength after thymectomy occurs in only 25 to 40%. This contrasts with the 40 to 60% response rate expected in patients without thymoma. Thymomas tend to be smaller and more frequently noninvasive in patients with associated myasthenia, perhaps as a result of earlier detection. If surgery is to be attempted in a patient with myasthenia gravis and thymoma, it is important that all thymic tissue, not only the thymoma, be removed. Residual normal thymus tissue, as well as regrowth of the thymoma, has been associated with persistence of myasthenic symptoms.[56]

**Pure Red Cell Aplasia.** Pure red cell aplasia is found in 5% of patients with thymoma and is considered an autoimmune disorder. One third to one half of patients with red cell aplasia have coexistent thymomas, although the relationship between these two illnesses is not well understood.[57, 58] Bone marrow examination shows a lack of erythrocyte precursors, with normal platelet and leukocyte elements. When red cell aplasia is associated with thymoma, other cytopenias coexist in up to one third of patients. Thymectomy corrects the anemia in approximately 25% of patients.

**Hypogammaglobulinemia.** Five to 10% of patients with thymoma develop hypogammaglobulinemia; more than one third of these individuals also have red cell aplasia. Combined hormonal and cellular immunodeficiencies exist, and bronchopulmonary infections and diarrhea are the most common presenting manifestations.[59] The immune deficiencies rarely improve after thymectomy.[60]

## Diagnosis

Most thymomas can be seen on routine chest radiography, and since they are in the anterior mediastinum, they are often best viewed on the lateral film (Fig. 39–3). CT of the chest provides important additional information about the size, location, and potential resectability of these tumors (Fig. 39–4). Some small thymomas can be seen only on CT, which should be performed in all patients with myasthenia gravis or pure red cell aplasia of uncertain cause. Preoperative evaluation of large thymomas should also include angiography to define tumor invasion or compression of the great vessels or heart.

When a thymoma is suspected and the preoperative evaluation suggests a resectable tumor, limited biopsy via mediastinoscopy or parasternal exploration is not indicated. Instead, the patient should undergo median sternotomy or thoracotomy for attempted definitive resection. In the unusual patient with extensive mediastinal tumor or metastatic spread that precludes resection, a more limited procedure to obtain diagnostic tissue is the best initial approach.

*Table 39–4.* **Immunologic Disorders Associated with Thymomas**

| | |
|---|---|
| Myasthenia gravis | Rheumatoid arthritis |
| Cytopenias | Thyroiditis |
|   Red cell aplasia | Sjögren's syndrome |
|   Thrombocytopenia | Dermatomyositis |
|   Hemolytic anemia | Scleroderma |
|   White cell aplasia | Takayasu's syndrome |
|   Combined cytopenias | Sarcoidosis |
| Hypogammaglobulinemia | Chronic ulcerative colitis |
| Polymyositis | Regional enteritis |
| Systemic lupus erythematosus | Pernicious anemia |

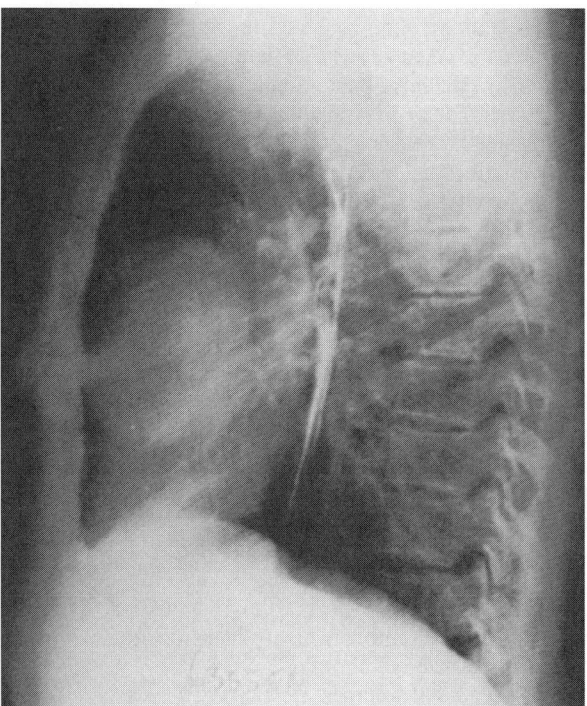

**Figure 39–3.** Lateral chest radiograph showing a large, lobulated, discrete mass in the right mediastinum: the classic appearance of a thymoma.

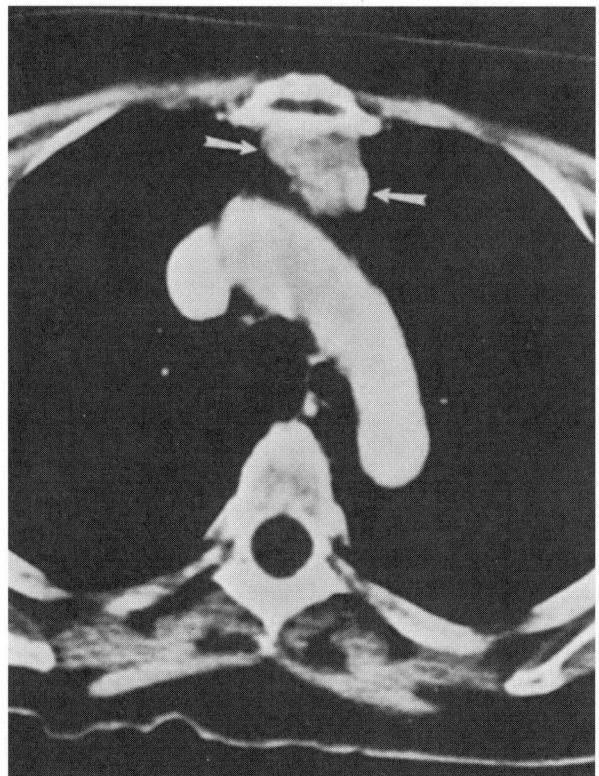

**Figure 39–4.** Computed tomographic scan with contrast material shows an encapsulated thymoma. (From Batra P, Hermann C Jr, Mulder D. Mediastinal imaging in myasthenia gravis: correlation of chest radiography, CT, MR, and surgical findings. AJR 1987;148:515–19. © 1987, American Roentgen Ray Society.)

## Staging

Staging of thymoma should be based on the anatomic extent of involvement, as determined clinically and histopathologically. Defining the extent of local, regional, and distant involvement is much more meaningful than classifying these tumors as either benign or malignant. The staging system in common use was introduced by Masaoka and colleagues in 1981[61] and is outlined in Table 39–5.

## TREATMENT

### Surgery

Complete resection is the best treatment for thymoma. If a thymoma is encapsulated (stage I), complete resection can be accomplished by removing the entire thymus without disturbing the integrity of the capsule. This procedure is curative in more than 98% of patients with stage I thymoma.[62]

In patients with invasive thymoma (stage II or III), radical surgical procedures are indicated to accomplish complete tumor resection. Adjacent pleura, pericardium, diaphragm, and lung should be resected if these structures are involved. Lobectomy or pneumonectomy may be required, depending on the extent of tumor involvement. Occasionally, resection of the great vessels with prosthetic patches is required for complete tumor resection. Every effort should be made to spare the phrenic nerves because diaphragmatic paralysis can be disastrous, particularly in patients with associated myasthenia gravis. When extensive tumor involvement precludes complete resection, subtotal resection is indicated because some of these patients have prolonged survival after additional therapy.

Most thymomas are best resected through a median sternotomy incision. Occasionally, if the tumor is dominant in one of the thoracic cavities, resection through a standard right or left thoracotomy incision is preferable. Other approaches, particularly the bilateral submammary incision, are to be discouraged because they provide less adequate exposure and may preclude radical excision of invasive thymoma.

Patients with thymoma and myasthenia gravis present challenging intraoperative and perioperative management problems. Optimal management often requires collaboration among the surgeon, the neurologist, and the anesthesiologist. In patients whose myasthenia is inadequately controlled with pyridostigmine preoperatively, plasmapheresis is sometimes required to improve strength temporarily. Endotracheal intu-

*Table 39–5.* **Staging System for Thymoma**

| Stage | Definition | Proportion of Cases (%) |
|-------|-----------|--------------------------|
| I | No capsular invasion | 40 |
| IIA | Microscopic capsular invasion | 14 |
| IIB | Macroscopic capsular invasion | 14 |
| III | Invasion by direct extension into surrounding tissues (e.g., lung, pericardium, great vessels) | 34 |
| IVA | Pleural or pericardial implants | 9 |
| IVB | Lymphogenous or hematogenous metastasis | 3 |

bation should be accomplished without the use of paralyzing agents in these patients. Postoperative problems are common and are mostly related to pulmonary complications; weaning from the ventilator may be difficult in patients with severe myasthenia. Despite these difficulties, careful management has resulted in a marked decrease in mortality rates, approximately 6% in contemporary series.[63]

## Radiation Therapy

After resection of encapsulated (stage I) thymoma, the risk of recurrence is 2% or less, and therefore no additional therapy is recommended.[62]

All patients with invasive thymoma should receive postoperative irradiation, even when "complete" resection is accomplished.[64, 65] In a retrospective review of the literature, the recurrence rate for invasive thymoma after total resection alone was 28%; this dropped to only 5% if postoperative radiation therapy was added.[66]

Radiation therapy is curative in some patients even when incomplete tumor resection has been accomplished. For optimal results, the surgeon should delineate the extent of the resected tumor and thymus with metallic clips and should clearly demarcate areas of incomplete tumor resection. The recurrence rate after radiation therapy is increased in patients who have had incomplete tumor resection or biopsy alone; Curran and colleagues reported a 21% recurrence rate in this group.[66]

Although the optimal radiation therapy fields and doses for the treatment of stages II and III thymomas have not been well defined, a dose of 45 to 50 Gy as used for other epithelial malignancies seems appropriate. If feasible, doses up to 60 Gy should be used for areas of gross residual disease. Postoperative radiation therapy fields should encompass the entire mediastinum, including the low mediastinum, because local drop metastases have been noted in this area. A shrinking field technique with CT-directed treatment planning should be used to keep the radiation dose to the lungs and spinal cord within accepted tolerance limits.

## Chemotherapy

Experience with chemotherapy for thymoma is limited because most patients with this uncommon tumor are adequately treated with surgical excision, with or without radiation therapy. Until the late 1990s, most patients given chemotherapy had metastatic disease or locally recurrent tumors after primary therapy. However, results of chemotherapy given before definitive resection or radiation therapy have been reported in a few patients with large, locally invasive thymomas.

In the past, high-dose corticosteroids were reported to be effective in the treatment of thymoma. Most of these responses were partial, with rapid regrowth of tumor after completion of treatment. It is likely that these "responses" were due to the lympholytic effect of corticosteroids on the nonmalignant, lymphocytic component of the tumor. The fact that all such responses were in thymomas with lymphoid or mixed histologic subtypes supports this hypothesis.

Several combination chemotherapy regimens have shown activity against malignant thymoma; the optimal regimen is currently unknown. The results of combination chemotherapy in metastatic or recurrent thymomas are summarized in Table 39–6. Contemporary interest has focused on cisplatin-containing regimens, since cisplatin has produced complete responses when used as a single agent. Although reported series are rather small, it is clear that a majority of patients have responses to treatment and that complete responses are achieved in approximately one third of patients. Long-term disease-free survival has been documented in a minority (10 to 20%) of patients in several reports; because many of these patients were followed for more than 5 years, it is reasonable to assume that chemotherapy is curative in a small percentage of patients with advanced thymoma.

A role for combination chemotherapy has also been suggested in the initial combined-modality treatment of locally advanced (stage III) thymoma. In an Intergroup trial, 26 patients with locally unresectable thymoma received two to four courses of cisplatin, doxorubicin, and cyclophosphamide followed by 54 Gy to the primary tumor and regional lymph nodes.[76] Most patients had large tumors that had not been amenable to debulking at thoracotomy. Five patients (19%) had complete responses and 11 (42%) had partial responses to chemotherapy; the median survival was 93 months. Macchiarini and associates had previously reported 7 patients treated with chemotherapy (cisplatin, epirubicin,

*Table 39–6.* **Results of Chemotherapy for Advanced or Recurrent Thymoma**

| Series | No. of Patients | Treatment Regimen | Response Rate (%) | Complete Response Rate (%) | No. of Patients Disease Free >24 mo (%) |
|---|---|---|---|---|---|
| *Non-Cisplatin–Containing Regimens* | | | | | |
| Evans et al[67] | 5 | CV/Pro/Pred | 80 | 0 | 1 (20) |
| Daugaard et al[68] | 9 | CVL/Pred | 56 | 44 | 0 |
| Kosmidis et al[69] | 5 | CAV | 100 | 40 | 2 (40) |
| Goldel et al[70] | 12 | CAV/Pred, CV/Pro/Pred, CV/Pred | NA | 42 | 3 (25) |
| *Cisplatin-Containing Regimens* | | | | | |
| Chahinian et al[71] | 5 | BAP/Pred | 40 | 0 | 0 |
| Loehrer et al[72] | 30 | CAP | 50 | 10 | 4* (13) |
| Fornasiero et al[73] | 37 | CAVP | 92 | 43 | 10 (27) |
| Park et al[74] | 17 | CAP ± Pred | 64 | 35 | NA |
| Giaccone et al[75] | 16 | EP | 56 | 31 | 4 (25) |

*Two patients had resection of residual disease after partial response to chemotherapy.
C, cyclophosphamide; V, vincristine; Pro, procarbazine; Pred, prednisone; L, lomustine; A, doxorubicin; B, bleomycin; P, cisplatin; E, etoposide; NA, not available.

etoposide) followed by resection and local radiation therapy; the projected 2-year survival was 80%.[77] Although not definitive, these results suggest improved results over local treatment modalities alone.

### Integration of Treatment Modalities

With optimal treatment, most patients with thymoma can be cured, and all patients should be approached with this intent. Treatment should be based on stage and resectability of tumor.

**Stage I.** These patients are treated with surgical resection, and subsequent recurrence is rare. No adjunctive radiation therapy or chemotherapy is indicated.

**Stage II or Stage III.** At present, standard therapy for these patients involves a radical surgical procedure, with complete or subtotal tumor removal. Patients with complete resection or minimal residual disease should receive postoperative radiation therapy. Patients with unresectable tumors and those who have gross thymoma remaining after debulking surgery should receive chemotherapy followed by radiation therapy. Results with preoperative chemotherapy are promising, but too few patients have been reported to establish this approach as standard treatment.

**Stage IV.** Although most of these patients have incurable disease, a trial of combination chemotherapy is warranted in most because complete response and long-term disease-free survival can be achieved in a minority. The optimal chemotherapy regimen remains undefined, but most complete responders and long-term survivors have received cisplatin-containing regimens.

### Poorly Differentiated Carcinoma of the Mediastinum

Occasionally, biopsy of a mediastinal mass reveals a poorly differentiated carcinoma. Often, these patients are suspected to have metastatic lung cancer with an undetected primary lesion, and palliative radiotherapy alone is considered for treatment. An extensive discussion of poorly differentiated carcinoma of unknown primary site is beyond the scope of this chapter, but this brief section is included because some of these patients have highly responsive neoplasms.

We previously reported the results of cisplatin-based chemotherapy in a group of 220 patients with poorly differentiated carcinoma of unknown primary site.[78] The tumor location in 43 of these patients was predominantly in the mediastinum. The median age of these patients was 38 years. Thirty-two patients had other metastatic sites in addition to the mediastinum, and serum hCG and AFP levels were normal in all but 5 patients. Thirteen patients (30%) had complete response to cisplatin-based combination regimens as used in the treatment of germ cell tumors; 7 of these patients (16%) had long-term disease-free survival.

The identity of the responsive tumors in this group remains unclear. However, it is likely that at least some of these patients had histologically unrecognizable mediastinal germ cell tumors. One article reported a group of similar patients in whom molecular genetic analysis identified the i(12p) chromosomal abnormality specific for germ cell tu-

mors.[13] Other patients in this group had poorly differentiated neuroendocrine tumors, which have proved highly responsive to cisplatin-based chemotherapy regimens.[79] The primary site and identity of these tumors remain unknown. Finally, some of these patients may have had "thymic carcinoma," described as high-grade epithelial tumors arising in the mediastinum and postulated to arise within the thymus. However, these tumors bear little relation to typical thymomas, since they grow rapidly, metastasize widely, and respond poorly to local treatment modalities.

Although the histogenesis of poorly differentiated carcinoma in the mediastinum is often uncertain, patients should receive careful pathologic evaluation to identify treatable neoplasms such as anaplastic lymphomas, germ cell tumors, and neuroendocrine tumors. Serum hCG and AFP levels should be measured in all young males with these tumors. An empirical trial of cisplatin-based combination chemotherapy, as recommended for mediastinal germ cell tumors, should be considered.

### Tumors of the Posterior Mediastinum

Most primary tumors of the posterior mediastinum are neurogenic in origin, arising from the sympathetic and intercostal nerves in this area. In one large review, these tumors made up 24% of all mediastinal tumors.[80] Approximately 80% of these tumors are benign.[81] Neurogenic tumors may be divided into two groups, depending on their origin from either the nerve sheath or nerve cells. Tumors of the nerve sheath include neurofibromas, neurilemomas, and neuroblastomas.

Neurogenic tumors are usually found in the posterior costovertebral gutter and are usually asymptomatic when detected by routine chest radiography. However, some tumors can cause symptoms by compression of adjacent nerves or by invasion into adjacent pleura or vertebral bodies. Occasionally, extension through intervertebral foramina can cause neurologic symptoms. Prompt evaluation of these symptoms with either myelography or magnetic resonance imaging is important to prevent or minimize neurologic complications.

#### NEUROFIBROMA

Neurofibromas are almost always benign and typically surround all the nerve components (axon, sheath cell, and connective tissue). Symptoms of nerve entrapment or spinal cord compression may be present; however, these lesions are usually found incidentally on chest radiography. Neurofibromas can occur in all age groups, and sex distribution is equal. On chest radiography, these tumors appear to have a narrow base and usually form an acute angle with the mediastinum. The treatment of choice is complete resection, and prognosis after surgical excision is excellent, even if the tumor is incompletely removed. Removal of tumors with extension through the intervertebral foramina ("dumbbell" tumors) requires a combined procedure, with resection of the intraspinal portion of the tumor first. Radiation therapy and chemotherapy are not indicated.

## NEURILEMOMA (SCHWANNOMA)

Neurilemoma is the most common neurogenic tumor, is usually benign, and arises from nerve sheath cells. Most patients are asymptomatic, but a few have vague back pain or mild osteoarthropathy. Calcification within these tumors may be seen radiographically but is not indicative of invasiveness and is not prognostically significant. Most tumors are encapsulated and solitary, and treatment involves surgical resection as described for neurofibromas. The prognosis after resection is excellent, with only rare local recurrences. Adjuvant therapy with radiation or chemotherapy is not indicated.

## NEUROSARCOMA (MALIGNANT SCHWANNOMA)

Microscopically, neurosarcomas have similarities to both neurofibromas and neurilemomas and may represent malignant "degeneration" of these tumors. Most patients are older than age 50 and present with pain caused by invasion of adjacent structures. Occasionally, these tumors have been associated with symptomatic hypoglycemia. Because of local invasion, complete surgical excision is difficult, and local recurrence is common. Patients with recurrent or metastatic disease should be treated according to the guidelines for soft tissue sarcomas (see Chapter 83). Prognosis is poor for these patients.

## GANGLIONEUROMA

Ganglioneuromas are benign tumors that originate from the sympathetic chain and are the most common neurogenic tumor in children.[80] In children, ganglioneuromas are usually asymptomatic, but adults often present with hypertension secondary to catecholamine production. Surgical excision is the treatment of choice and is usually easily accomplished. Recurrence after complete resection is rare.

## NEUROBLASTOMA

Neuroblastomas are reviewed in Chapter 79. The prognosis of intrathoracic neuroblastoma is better than that of neuroblastoma arising in the abdomen.

## GANGLIONEUROBLASTOMA

Ganglioneuroblastomas contain immature sympathetic nerve tissue and mature ganglion cells and have a biologic behavior between that of the benign ganglioneuroma and the highly malignant neuroblastoma. Occasionally, these tumors are found in the posterior mediastinum. Some secrete vanillylmandelic acid. The cure rate after complete resection is high; however, patients presenting with disseminated disease have a uniformly poor prognosis. Ganglioneuroblastomas are rare in adults.

## NEURAL CREST TUMORS (PHEOCHROMOCYTOMA, PARAGANGLIOMA, CHEMODECTOMA, AND AORTIC BODY TUMOR)

Surgical excision is the treatment of choice for neural crest tumors, which occasionally occur in the posterior mediastinum.

## SUGGESTIONS FOR ADDITIONAL READING

Moran CA, Suster S. Primary germ cell tumors of the mediastinum. Cancer 1997;80:681–90. *This article reviews the pathologic features of mediastinal germ cell tumors in a large series of patients from the AFIP.*

Mencel PJ, Motzer RJ, Mazumder M, et al. Advanced seminoma: treatment results, survival, and prognostic factors in 142 patients. J Clin Oncol 1994;12:120–6. *This article discusses a large single-institution series documenting the excellent results of initial chemotherapy in mediastinal seminoma.*

Toner GC, Geller NL, Lin SY, Bosl GJ. Extragonadal and poor risk nonseminomatous germ cell tumors: survival and prognostic features. Cancer 1991;67:2049–57. *This is a review of treatment results and a comparison of mediastinal and testicular germ cell tumors with respect to biology, histology, and prognostic factors.*

Loehrer PJ Sr, Chen M, Kim K, et al. Cisplatin, doxorubicin, and cyclophosphamide plus thoracic radiation therapy for limited-stage unresectable thymoma: an Intergroup trial. J Clin Oncol 1997;15:3093–9. *Intergroup results document the role of combined-modality treatment for locally unresectable thymoma.*

## REFERENCES

1. Davis RD, Oldham HN Jr, Sabiston DC Jr. Primary cysts and neoplasms of the mediastinum: recent changes in the clinical presentation, methods of diagnosis, management, and results. Ann Thorac Surg 1987;44:229–37.
2. Rubush JL, Gardner IR, Boyd WC, et al. Mediastinal tumors: review of 186 cases. J Thorac Cardiovasc Surg 1973;65:216–22.
3. Lewis BD, Hurt RD, Payne WS, et al. Benign teratomas of the mediastinum. J Thorac Cardiovasc Surg 1983;86:727–31.
4. Schlumberger HG. Teratoma of anterior mediastinum in a group of military age: study of 16 cases and review of theories of genesis. Arch Pathol 1946;41:398–444.
5. Friedman NB. The comparative morphogenesis of extragenital and gonadal teratoid tumors. Cancer 1951;4:265–76.
6. Oberman HA, Libcke JH. Malignant germinal neoplasms of the mediastinum. Cancer 1964;17:498–507.
7. Luna MA, Valenzuela-Tamariz J. Germ-cell tumors of the mediastinum: postmortem findings. Am J Clin Pathol 1976;65:450–4.
8. Hodge J, Aponte G, McLaughlin E. Primary mediastinal tumors. J Thorac Surg 1959;37:730–44.
9. Collins DH, Pugh RCB. Classification and frequency of testicular tumors. Br J Urol 1964;36:Suppl:1–11.
10. Nichols CR. Mediastinal germ cell tumors: clinical features and biologic correlates. Chest 1991;99:472–9.
11. Richardson RL, Schoumacher RA, Fer MF, et al. The unrecognized extragonadal germ cell cancer syndrome. Ann Intern Med 1981;94:181–6.
12. Fox FM, Woods RL, Tattersall MHN. Undifferentiated carcinoma in young men: the atypical teratoma syndrome. Lancet 1979;1:1316–8.
13. Motzer RJ, Rodriguez E, Reuter VE, et al. Molecular and cytogenetic studies in the diagnosis of patients with poorly differentiated carcinomas of unknown primary site. J Clin Oncol 1995;13:274–82.
14. Turner AR, MacDonald RN. Mediastinal germ cell cancers in Klinefelter's syndrome. Ann Intern Med 1981;94:279.
15. Nichols CR, Heerema NA, Palmer C, et al. Klinefelter's syndrome associated with mediastinal germ cell neoplasms. J Clin Oncol 1987;5:1290–4.
16. Moran CA, Suster A. Primary germ cell tumors of the mediastinum. I: Analysis of 372 cases with special emphasis on teratomatous lesions and a proposal for histopathologic classification and clinical staging. Cancer 1997;80:681–90.
17. Polansky SM, Barwick KW, Ravin CE. Primary mediastinal seminoma. Am J Radiol 1979;132:17–21.
18. Jain KK, Bosl GJ, Bains MS, et al. The treatment of extragonadal seminoma. J Clin Oncol 1984;2:820–7.
19. Hainsworth JD, Einhorn LH, Williams SD, et al. Advanced extragonadal germ cell tumors: successful treatment with combination chemotherapy. Ann Intern Med 1982;97:7–11.
20. Logothetis CJ, Samuels ML, Selig DE, et al. Chemotherapy of extragonadal germ cell tumors. J Clin Oncol 1985;3:316–25.
21. Israel A, Bosl GJ, Golbey RB, et al. The results of chemotherapy for

extragonadal germ cell tumors in the cisplatin era: the Memorial Sloan-Kettering Cancer Center experience (1975 to 1982). J Clin Oncol 1985;3:1073–1078.

22. Nichols CR, Roth B, Heerema N, et al. Hematologic neoplasia associated with primary mediastinal germ cell tumors: an update. N Engl J Med 1990;322:1425–9.

23. Larsen M, Evans WK, Shepherd FA, et al. Acute lymphoblastic leukemia: possible origin from a mediastinal germ cell tumor. Cancer 1984;53:441–4.

24. Orazi A, Neiman RS, Ulbright TM, et al. Hematopoietic precursor cells within the yolk sac tumor component are the source of secondary hematopoietic malignancies in patients with mediastinal germ cell tumors. Cancer 1993;71:3873–81.

25. Ulbright TM, Loehrer PJ, Roth LM, et al. The development of non-germ cell malignancies within germ cell tumors: a clinicopathologic study of 11 cases. Cancer 1984;54:1824–33.

26. Bosl GJ, Dmitrovsky E, Reuter V, et al. i(12p): a specific karyotypic abnormality in germ cell tumors. abstract. Proc Am Soc Clin Oncol 1989;8:131.

27. Garnick MB, Griffin JD. Idiopathic thrombocytopenia in association with extragonadal germ cell cancer. Ann Intern Med 1983;98:926–7.

28. Myers TJ, Kessimian N, Schwartz S. Mediastinal germ cell tumor associated with the hemaphagocytic syndrome. Ann Intern Med 1988;109:504–5.

29. Chariot P, Monnet I, LeLong F, et al. Systemic mast cell disease associated with primary mediastinal germ cell tumor. Am J Med 1991;90:381–5.

30. Lattes R. Thymoma and other tumors of thymus: analysis of 107 cases. Cancer 1962;15:1224–60.

31. Woolner LB, Jamplis RW, Kirklin JW. Seminoma (germinoma) apparently primary in anterior mediastinum. N Engl J Med 1955;252:653–7.

32. Hurt RD, Bruckman JE, Farrow GM, et al. Primary anterior mediastinal seminoma. Cancer 1982;49:1658–63.

33. Bush SE, Martinez A, Bagshaw MA. Primary mediastinal seminoma. Cancer 1981;48:1877–82.

34. Loehrer PJ, Birch R, Williams SD, et al. Chemotherapy of metastatic seminoma: the Southeastern Cancer Study Group experience. J Clin Oncol 1987;5:1212–20.

35. Bukowski RM, Wolf M, Kulander BG, et al. Alternating combination chemotherapy in patients with extragonadal germ cell tumors. Cancer 1993;71:2631–38.

36. Delgado FG, Tjulandin SA, Garin AM. Long-term results of treatment in patients with extragonadal germ cell tumours. Eur J Cancer 1993;29A:1002–05.

37. Goss PE, Schwertfeger L, Blackstein ME, et al. Extragonadal germ cell tumors: a 14-year Toronto experience. Cancer 1994;73:1971–9.

38. Mencel PJ, Motzer RJ, Mazumdar M, et al. Advanced seminoma: treatment results, survival, and prognostic factors in 142 patients. J Clin Oncol 1994;12:120–6.

39. Gerl A, Clemm C, Lamerz R, Wilmanns W. Cisplatin-based chemotherapy of primary extragonadal germ cell tumors: a single-institution experience. Cancer 1996;77:526–32.

40. Schultz SM, Einhorn LH, Conces DJ, et al. Management of post-chemotherapy residual mass in patients with advanced seminoma: Indiana University experience. J Clin Oncol 1989;7:1497–1503.

41. Puc HS, Heelan R, Mazumdar M, et al. Management of residual mass in advanced seminoma: results and recommendations from the Memorial Sloan-Kettering Cancer Center. J Clin Oncol 1996;14:454–60.

42. Funes HC, Mendez M, Alonso E, et al. Mediastinal germ cell tumors treated with cisplatin, bleomycin, and vinblastine (PVB). abstract. Proc Am Assoc Cancer Res 1981;22:474.

43. Kay PH, Wells FC, Goldstraw P. A multi-disciplinary approach to primary nonseminomatous germ cell tumors of the mediastinum. Ann Thorac Surg 1987;44:578–82.

44. Nichols CR, Saxman S, Williams SD, et al. Primary mediastinal nonseminomatous germ cell tumors: a modern single-institution experience. Cancer 1990;65:1641–6.

45. Dulmet EM, Macchiarini P, Suc B, Verley JM. Germ cell tumors of the mediastinum: a 30-year experience. Cancer 1993;72:1894–1901.

46. Fizazi K, Culine S, Droz JP, et al. Primary mediastinal nonseminomatous germ cell tumors: results of modern therapy including cisplatin-based chemotherapy. J Clin Oncol 1998;16:725–32,.

47. Toner GC, Geller NL, Lin SY, Bosl GJ. Extragonadal and poor risk nonseminomatous germ cell tumors: survival and prognostic features. Cancer 1991;67:2049–57.

48. Bergh NP, Gatzinsky P, Larsson S, et al. Tumors of the thymus and thymic region. I: Clinicopathological studies on thymomas. Ann Thorac Surg 1978;25:91–8.

49. Dimery IW, Lee JS, Blick M, et al. Association of the Epstein-Barr virus with lymphoepithelioma of the thymus. Cancer 1988;61:2475–80.

50. Leyvraz S, Henle W, Chahinian AP, et al. Association of Epstein-Barr virus with thymic carcinoma. N Engl J Med 1985;312:1296–9

51. Walker AN, Mills SE, Fechner RE. Thymomas and thymic carcinomas. Semin Diagn Pathol 1990;7:250–65.

52. Lewis JE, Wick MR, Scheithauer BW, et al. Thymoma: a clinicopathologic review. Cancer 1987;60:2727–43.

53. Whittaker LD, Lynn HB. Mediastinal tumors and cysts in the pediatric patient. Surg Clin North Am 1973;53:893–904.

54. Souadjian JV, Enriques P, Silverstein MN, et al. The spectrum of disease associated with thymoma. Arch Intern Med 1974;134:374–9.

55. Alpert LI, Papatestas A, Kark A, et al. A histological reappraisal of the thymus gland in myasthenia gravis. Arch Pathol 1971;91:55–61.

56. Rosenberg M, Jauregui WO, DeVega ME, et al. Recurrence of thymic hyperplasia after thymectomy in myasthenia gravis: its importance as a cause of failure of surgical treatment. Am J Med 1983;74:78–82.

57. Hirst E, Robertson TI. The syndrome of thymoma and erythroblastopenic anemia. Medicine 1967;46:225–64.

58. Masaoka A, Hashimoto T, Shibata K, et al. Thymomas associated with pure red cell aplasia. Cancer 1989;64:1872–8.

59. Fox MA, Lynch DA, Make BJ: Thymoma with hypogammaglobulinemia (Good's syndrome): an unusual case of bronchiectasis. Am J Roentgenol 1992;158:1229–30.

60. Rogers BHG, Manaligod JR, Blazek WV. Thymoma associated with pancytopenia and hypogammaglobulinemia. Am J Med 1968;44:154–64.

61. Masaoka A, Monden Y, Nakahara K, et al. Follow-up study of thymomas with special reference to their clinical stages. Cancer 1981;48:2485–93.

62. Fechner RE. Recurrence of noninvasive thymomas. Cancer 1969;23:1423–7.

63. Wilkins EW, Grillo HL, Scannell JG, et al. Role of staging in prognosis and management of thymoma. Ann Thorac Surg 1991;51:888–92.

64. Penn CR, Hope-Stone HF. The role of radiotherapy in the management of malignant thymoma. Br J Surg 1972;59:533–9.

65. Nakahara K, Ohno K, Hashimoto J, et al. Thymoma: results with complete resection and adjuvant post-operative irradiation in 141 consecutive patients. J Thorac Cardiovasc Surg 1988;95:1041–47.

66. Curran WJ, Kornstein MJ, Brooks JJ, et al. Invasive thymoma: the role of mediastinal irradiation following complete or incomplete surgical resection. J Clin Oncol 1988:1722–7.

67. Evans WK, Thompson DM, Simpson WJ, et al. Combination chemotherapy in invasive thymoma: role of COPP. Cancer 1980;46:1523–7.

68. Daugaard G, Hansen HH, Rorth M. Combination chemotherapy for malignant thymoma. Ann Intern Med 1983;99:189–90.

69. Kosmidis PA, Iliopoulos E, Pentea S. Combination chemotherapy with cyclophosphamide, Adriamycin, and vincristine in malignant thymoma and myasthenia gravis. Cancer 1988;61:1736–40.

70. Goldel N, Boning L, Fredrik A, et al. Chemotherapy of invasive thymoma—a retrospective study of 22 cases. Cancer 1989;63:1493–1500.

71. Chahinian AP, Holland JF, Bhardwaj S. Chemotherapy for malignant thymoma. Ann Intern Med 1983;99:736.

72. Loehrer PJ Sr, Kim K, Aisner SC, et al. Cisplatin plus doxorubicin plus cyclophosphamide in metastatic or recurrent thymoma: final results of an Intergroup trial. J Clin Oncol 1994;12:1164–8.

73. Fornasiero A, Daniele O, Ghiotto C, et al. Chemotherapy for invasive thymoma: a 13-year experience. Cancer 1991;68:30–3.

74. Park HS, Shin DM, Lee JS, et al. Thymoma: a retrospective study of 87 cases. Cancer 1994;73:2491–8.

75. Giaccone G, Ardizzoni A, Kirkpatrick A, et al. Cisplatin and etoposide combination chemotherapy for locally advanced or metastatic thymoma: a phase II study of the European Organization for Research and Treatment of Cancer. Lung Cancer Cooperative Group. J Clin Oncol 1996;14:814–20.

76. Loehrer PJ Sr, Chen M, Kim K, et al. Cisplatin, doxorubicin, and cyclophosphamide plus thoracic radiation therapy for limited-stage unresectable thymoma: an Intergroup trial. J Clin Oncol 1997;15:3093–9.

77. Macchiarini P, Chella A, Ducci F, et al. Neoadjuvant chemotherapy, surgery, and postoperative radiation therapy for invasive carcinoma. Cancer 1991;68:706–13.
78. Hainsworth JD, Johnson DH, Greco FA. Cisplatin-based combination chemotherapy in the treatment of poorly differentiated carcinoma and poorly differentiated adenocarcinoma of unknown primary site: results of a 12-year experience. J Clin Oncol 1992;10:912–22.
79. Hainsworth JD, Johnson DH, Greco FA. Poorly differentiated neuroendocrine carcinoma of unknown primary site: a newly recognized clinicopathologic entity. Ann Intern Med 1988;109:364–72.
80. Oldham HN Jr. Mediastinal tumors and cysts. Ann Thorac Surg 1971;11:246–75.
81. Silverman NA, Sabiston DC Jr. Primary tumors and cysts of the mediastinum. Curr Probl Cancer 1977;2:1–55.

# PART

# X

# NEOPLASMS OF THE GASTROINTESTINAL SYSTEM

- CHARLES M. HASKELL

Malignancies of the gastrointestinal system constitute a tremendous health problem throughout the world. In the United States, nearly one fourth of the annual cancer mortality rate can be attributed to malignancies of gastrointestinal origin. In 1999, 226,300 of the 1,221,800 new cancers and 131,000 of the 563,100 deaths from cancer in the United States were predicted to be the result of gastrointestinal tract malignancies by the American Cancer Society.[1] The annual U.S. incidence and mortality rates and 5-year relative survival rates for both sexes and all races are given in the accompanying table.[2] The data are age adjusted to the 1970 U.S. standard population. Regular updates of these data can be obtained from the web site of the Surveillance, Epidemiology, and End Results (SEER) program of the National Cancer Institute.

Common themes are apparent in the molecular pathogenesis and management of this large group of human neoplasms. Most of the tumors of the gastrointestinal tract are adenocarcinomas or squamous cell carcinomas. They all arise by the process of multistage carcinogenesis, which is being clarified by the techniques of molecular biology. Most gastrointestinal tumors are asymptomatic for long periods, resulting in far-advanced, incurable disease at diagnosis. These facts support the development of improved prevention and early diagnosis strategies. This development includes screening by looking for occult blood in stool samples from asymptomatic individuals, expanded availability of flexible sigmoidoscopy and colonoscopy, and development of more sensitive and specific tumor markers (especially molecular markers).

Surgery is the cornerstone of management for most gastrointestinal neoplasms, and this is especially true of the various adenocarcinomas that involve these organs. Chemotherapy and radiation therapy are of increasing importance in management, however. Several examples of such combined-modality therapy can be cited. Combined radiation therapy and chemotherapy has become the mainstay of curative treatment for epidermoid carcinoma of the anus and palliative therapy for esophageal cancer. Chemotherapy, radiation therapy, and surgery now constitute standard components of management for patients with stage II or III rectal cancer in the United States. Clinical trial results have shown improved survival with limited cost from the use of adjuvant chemotherapy after surgery in patients with stage III colon cancer. These advances have been established by large, randomized clinical trials, which are now the standard way of estab-

**Age-Adjusted SEER Incidence and U.S. Mortality Rates and 5-Year Relative Survival Rates for Cancer of the Digestive System for Both Sexes and All Races**

| Site | Annual Incidence (1992–1996) (New cases/100,000) | Annual Mortality (1992–1996) (Deaths/100,000) | Relative Survival (1989–1995) (% alive at 5 years) |
|---|---|---|---|
| Digestive system as a whole | 73.2 | 39.1 | 43.1 |
| Esophagus | 3.9 | 3.6 | 12.3 |
| Stomach | 7.0 | 4.2 | 21.1 |
| Small intestine | 1.3 | 0.3 | 49.0 |
| Colon and rectum | 44.3 | 17.5 | 61.0 |
| Colon | 31.9 | — | 61.6 |
| Rectum | 12.4 | — | 59.5 |
| Anus, anal canal, anorectum | 1.0 | 0.1 | 59.6 |
| Liver | 3.1 | 2.8 | 5.7 |
| Intrahepatic bile ducts | 0.6 | 0.6 | 2.8 |
| Gallbladder | 1.0 | 0.6 | 13.7 |
| Other biliary | 1.1 | 0.5 | 17.0 |
| Pancreas | 8.9 | 8.4 | 4.1 |
| Retroperitoneum | 0.4 | 0.1 | 47.0 |
| Peritoneum, omentum, and mesentery | 0.4 | 0.1 | 28.3 |
| Other digestive organs | 0.3 | 0.1 | 2.6 |

SEER, Surveillance, Epidemiology, and End Results.

lishing the value of new treatments for cancer. The ensuing chapters focus on current aspects of epidemiology, etiology, molecular pathogenesis, diagnosis, staging, prognosis, and treatment of gastrointestinal malignancies, with an emphasis on the integration of therapeutic modalities in the management of patients.

## REFERENCES

1. Landis SH, Murray T, Bolden S, Wingo PA. Cancer statistics, 1999. CA Cancer J Clin 1999;49:8–31.
2. SEER Cancer Statistics Review 1973–1996. (See http://www-seer.ims.nci.nih.gov.)

# ESOPHAGUS

......................................

# NATURAL HISTORY AND STAGING OF ESOPHAGEAL CANCER

• Carol Nishikubo  • Charles M. Haskell

## EPIDEMIOLOGY

Esophageal carcinoma is the sixth most commonly diagnosed malignancy in the United States with more than 12,000 new cases diagnosed annually, accounting for more than 10,000 deaths. Men are more commonly affected than women by a ratio of 2 to 3:1,[1] and the median age at diagnosis is 65 years. Esophageal cancer is more common in certain parts of the world, with an increased incidence seen in China, South Africa, Russia, northern Italy, and Iran.[2, 3] The risk of esophageal cancer in descendants of immigrants from these countries to countries where a lower incidence of esophageal cancer is seen approaches that of the country of destination, suggesting a role for environmental or dietary factors.[4] Hereditary factors may also contribute to development of these malignancies in certain areas of the world, especially in China. An increased incidence of esophageal neoplasms is also seen in certain genetic disorders, such as the Li-Fraumeni syndrome and tylosis palmaris et plantaris.

Socioeconomic factors have been implicated in the cause of esophageal malignancies. Esophageal cancer is more common in urban areas of the United States and in individuals in the low-income and middle-income tertiles than in the high-income group. Certain occupations are more frequently associated with development of esophageal cancer, including construction workers, outdoor laborers, waiters, bartenders, and metal workers. Many centers have reported an increase in the incidence of esophageal adenocarcinoma relative to squamous cell histology.[5] This phenomenon is not seen uniformly,[6] and the reason for the shift in histologic type is unclear.

## ETIOLOGY

A possible role of viral agents in the development of esophageal malignancies has been debated. Some areas of the world, such as South Africa, Sweden, and China, report a 50% incidence of human papillomavirus detected in esophageal carcinomas.[7, 8] Other series, however, from Slovenia, Italy, France, Japan, China, and the United States have reported only low rates (0 to 8%) of detection.[9–14]

The role of dietary factors has been analyzed in many studies. Some studies have implicated pickled vegetables, most likely from N-nitroso compounds, in the predisposition to develop esophageal malignancies.[15] Several studies have found that increased intake of vegetables and citrus fruits is protective,[16, 17] whereas ingestion of red meat may confer a slightly increased risk.[18] Butter, oils, and fats may be associated with development of esophageal cancer, especially adenocarcinoma.[16, 19] A case-control study conducted at Memorial Sloan-Kettering Cancer Center showed a significantly decreased risk associated with diets high in fiber, lutein, niacin, vitamin $B_6$, iron, and zinc.[20]

Smoking and alcohol use have been implicated in the development of esophageal tumors.[21] As opposed to the risk of alcohol use seen with other aerodigestive tumors, however, the increased risk seen in current drinkers may rapidly decrease after they stop drinking.[22] A study showed an increased risk of squamous cell carcinoma of the esophagus in women treated with radiation therapy for breast cancer, especially in the inner half of the breast.[23] Some studies have also found that aspirin and nonsteroidal anti-inflammatory drug (NSAID) users have a twofold protective effect in development of esophageal and noncardia gastric carcinomas.[21, 24] Whether NSAIDs or aspirin can be used in the prevention of esophageal cancer remains questionable.

Certain conditions are known to predispose patients to develop esophageal tumors. An increased incidence of adenocarcinoma—100 times that of the general population in some series—is observed in patients with Barrett's esophagus (presence of intestinalized mucosa in the lower esophagus).[25] Achalasia (a motility disorder characterized by aperistalsis and failure of the lower esophageal sphincter to relax on swallowing) is associated with a 7-fold to 16-fold increase in the risk of squamous cell carcinoma.[26, 27] The Plummer-Vinson syndrome, characterized by achlorhydria, iron deficiency, and esophageal webs, carries an increased risk of upper esophageal (i.e., cervical and postcricoid) squamous cell tumors.[28] Other mechanical injuries to the esophagus, such as lye burns and reflux esophagitis, also carry an increased risk of development of malignancy.[29–31] Certain genetic disorders carry an increased risk of development of esophageal malignancies, as mentioned previously.

## BIOLOGY

Esophageal cancer likely develops as a result of a series of genetic alterations, at least in some patients. A multistep progression of genetic mutations has been described in the progression of Barrett's metaplasia to dysplasia to adenocarcinoma in some series.[32] This sequence of genetic events is less well characterized but is similar to that described in the progression from adenomatous polyp to colon adenocarcinoma. p53 overexpression has been described in several studies[32, 33] as occurring with increased frequency as lesions progress from normal to dysplastic to carcinomatous. Other chromosomal abnormalities involving the long arms of chromosomes 18 and 5 and the short arm of chromosome 11 have also been described.[32–34]

## PATHOLOGY

More than half of all esophageal tumors arise in the lower third of the esophagus or at the gastroesophageal junction, whereas a quarter develop in the middle third. Gastroesophageal junction tumors are most often adenocarcinomas, whereas squamous cell tumors predominate in the remainder of the esophagus.[35–37] Less than 1% of esophageal tumors are of other histologic types, such as carcinosarcoma, lymphoma, adenoid cystic carcinoma, leiomyosarcoma, small cell carcinoma, or melanoma.

Spread of esophageal carcinoma is by way of the abundant lymphatics found in the mucosa and submucosa, by hematogenous spread, and by direct extension. The esophagus lacks a serosal surface, perhaps allowing earlier spread of the disease to contiguous organs of the mediastinum, such as the trachea, left mainstem bronchus, and neurovascular structures including the recurrent laryngeal nerve, aorta, and carotid artery. Lymph node involvement reflects the level at which the tumor develops. Cervicoesophageal cancers spread to the anterojugular and supraclavicular nodes. The mediastinal and subdiaphragmatic nodes are involved in thoracoesophageal tumors, whereas gastroesophageal junction tumors drain to the celiac, gastric, pancreatic, and periaortic lymph nodes. Between 60 and 90% have involvement of lymphatics at the time of diagnosis or early in the course of disease, as shown in autopsy series.[38] The likelihood of metastatic disease increases with increased depth of lesion, lymph node involvement, and longer length of the tumor. For tumors greater than 5 cm in length, only 10% are localized at presentation, with distant metastases detectable in 75% of these patients. The most common sites of spread are lymph nodes (abdominal [45%], cervical or supraclavicular [18%]), liver (35%), lung (20%), bone (9%), and adrenal gland (5%). Metastases to the peritoneum, brain, stomach, pancreas, pleura, skin or body wall, pericardium, and spleen also occur.[39]

## CLINICAL FEATURES AND DIAGNOSIS

Symptomatic esophageal cancers are usually too far advanced to be highly curable. The primary symptoms of esophageal cancer are dysphagia and weight loss. Dysphagia is usually painless and progressive, with patients initially noting difficulty swallowing solid food and then developing difficulty swallowing liquids as well. The dysphagia is usually due to a mechanical obstruction or a circumferential constriction of the lumen of the esophagus by the mass. Patients presenting with dysphagia of solids and liquids from the onset are more likely to have a motility disorder, but an esophageal malignancy should not be excluded based on this history alone.

Dyspepsia, especially ongoing despite treatment with ant-

acids or $H_2$ blockers, should arouse suspicion for an underlying neoplasm. Hypercalcemia develops in 25% of patients with esophageal neoplasms, although bone metastases are seen in only 10 to 15% of cases.[39–41] The hypercalcemia is a paraneoplastic process mediated by parathyroid hormone–related protein, which is produced by the tumor.[42]

Radiographic studies including a barium swallow are abnormal in 90% of cases. The typical finding is an irregular, ragged mucosa with luminal narrowing. Prestenotic dilatation of the esophagus is usually present above benign, but not above malignant, obstructive lesions. It has been reported that double-contrast studies may be of value in early lesions.[43] Histologic diagnosis is required, with a biopsy specimen or, less frequently, a cytologic specimen to establish a firm diagnosis. This is usually obtained at the time of diagnostic endoscopy.

## SCREENING

There is considerable debate over the benefit of screening procedures in high-risk individuals. Detecting early-stage disease would lead to higher cure rates. In one Japanese study, 237 patients found to have early stage I esophageal carcinoma by cytologic examination had 5- and 10-year survival rates of 86 and 56%, respectively, following surgery.[44] In a study of 1471 patients in China, 2% were found to have cancer by cytologic screening.[45] In a Japanese study of alcoholics admitted to the hospital for treatment of alcohol-related disease, 629 patients underwent endoscopy and mucosal iodine staining. Biopsy specimens were obtained of any unstained areas, and patients underwent mucosal resection if the biopsy specimen was positive with no lymphadenopathy by computed tomography (CT). Of those patients, 162 underwent biopsy (25.8%), and 21 were found to have squamous cell carcinoma (3.3%).[46] Seventeen of these patients underwent mucosal resection, and two had a more extensive surgical procedure. The benefits of these screening procedures in populations that are not at an increased risk are questionable.

Barrett's esophagus is associated with an increased risk of developing adenocarcinoma of the esophagus. A study of endoscopic surveillance done every 17 months in 149 patients with Barrett's esophagus resulted in detection of seven malignancies.[47] A cost analysis of endoscopy in these patients showed that the cost of screening was comparable to that spent on screening mammography, and the cost per year of life saved was much lower for the endoscopic surveillance than for the mammography. Endoscopic surveillance may be warranted in this group of patients. For patients with Barrett's esophagus with high-grade dysplasia, 43% have been found to have adenocarcinoma at resection,[48] and prophylactic esophagectomy should be considered for this group of patients.

## STAGING AND PROGNOSIS

Patients with carcinoma of the esophagus are staged according to the TNM system developed jointly by the American Joint Committee on Cancer and the International Union Against Cancer (Table 40–1). This staging may be done

**Table 40–1. Staging of Esophageal Cancer: TNM Classification**

*Primary Tumor (T)*

| | |
|---|---|
| Tx | Primary tumor cannot be assessed |
| T0 | No evidence of primary tumor |
| Tis | Carcinoma in situ |
| T1 | Tumor invades lamina propria or submucosa |
| T2 | Tumor invades muscularis propria |
| T3 | Tumor invades adventitia |
| T4 | Tumor invades adjacent structures |

*Regional Lymph Nodes (N)*

| | |
|---|---|
| Nx | Regional lymph nodes cannot be assessed |
| N0 | No regional lymph node metastasis |
| N1 | Regional lymph node metastasis |

*Distant Metastasis (M)*

| | |
|---|---|
| Mx | Distant metastasis cannot be assessed |
| M0 | No distant metastasis |
| M1 | Distant metastasis |

Tumors of lower thoracic esophagus:

| | |
|---|---|
| M1a | Metastasis in celiac lymph nodes |
| M1b | Other distant metastases |

Tumors of the midthoracic esophagus:

| | |
|---|---|
| M1a | Not applicable |
| M1b | Nonregional lymph nodes and/or other distant metastasis |

Tumors of the upper thoracic esophagus:

| | |
|---|---|
| M1a | Metastasis in cervical nodes |
| M1b | Other distant metastases |

*Stage Grouping*

| | | | |
|---|---|---|---|
| Stage 0 | Tis | N0 | M0 |
| Stage I | T1 | N0 | M0 |
| Stage IIA | T2 | N0 | M0 |
| | T3 | N0 | M0 |
| Stage IIB | T1 | N1 | M0 |
| | T2 | N1 | M0 |
| Stage III | T3 | N1 | M0 |
| | T4 | Any | M0 |
| Stage IV | Any T | Any N | M1 |
| Stage IVA | Any T | Any N | M1a |
| Stage IVB | Any T | Any N | M1b |

Used with the permission of the American Joint Committee on Cancer (AJCC), Chicago, Illinois. The original source for this material is the AJCC Cancer Staging Manual, 5th edition (1997) published by Lippincott-Raven Publishers, Philadelphia, Pennsylvania.

using clinical criteria alone (cTNM) or after a pathologist examines the resected specimen (pTNM).

Staging evaluation should include a computed tomographic scan of the chest and upper abdomen, including the liver, adrenal glands, and upper abdominal lymph nodes; bronchoscopy for all patients with tumors above the gastroesophageal junction; and esophageal ultrasonography, if available. The role of measuring serum markers is debatable.

The role of CT in staging esophageal cancer is to determine the extent of local spread of the disease and to examine the abdomen for evidence of distant metastases. The accuracy of the examination, however, especially in determining the extent of local disease, is limited. Endoscopic ultrasonography is increasingly used as a more accurate tool in predicting the T and N stages of disease. Even this procedure, however, shows a variable (59 to 89%) accuracy in determining T stage and a 70 to 80% accuracy at predicting N

stage.[49–51] In one small series of 26 patients, laparoscopic or thoracoscopic surgical staging with lymph node sampling was found to be more sensitive than endoscopic ultrasonography in detecting lymph node involvement.[52]

Bronchoscopy to determine the presence or absence of tracheobronchial tree involvement is mandatory for lesions above the gastroesophageal junction. Approximately one third of patients show either impingement or infiltration of the trachea by this technique.[53] Infiltration, especially, is associated with a high incidence of subsequent tracheoesophageal fistula. Such patients may require palliative resection to avoid fistula formation, even though there is little chance of cure. Whenever palpable, clinically suspicious cervical nodes are present, a biopsy is indicated.

The use of serum tumor markers either in detecting or monitoring the course of esophageal tumors is limited. Carcinoembryonic antigen (CEA) levels are elevated in about 70% of cases.[54] The CA-50 level is increased in about 40% of cases of squamous cell carcinoma.

Clinical staging is usually inadequate for planning treatment. The sensitivity and specificity of CT and of endoscopic ultrasonography are too limited to use as an absolute determinant of who is or is not a candidate for a curative resection, especially in assessing locally advanced disease. A patient should not be excluded from potentially curative resection based on clinical staging by CT scan or endoscopic ultrasonography.

The pTNM classification is a far more accurate guide to prognosis than cTNM. In the Far East, the 5-year survival for the pTNM stages is as follows: stage I, 83%; stage II, 46%; stage III, 26%; and stage IV, 7%.[55] In the United States, the results of treatment have not been as good, with 5-year survival rates typically in the 5 to 11% range.

In addition to stage, several aspects of tumor biology are associated with a poor prognosis, including a poor histopathologic grade, aneuploidy of DNA by DNA histogram or flow cytometry, overexpression of cyclin D1 mRNA,[56] expression of vasculoendothelial growth factor,[57] mutation of p53,[58–60] and a high score on the argyrophilic nucleolar organizer regions test (AgNOR number). Aneuploidy especially has been linked to the prognosis for patients with Barrett's columnar epithelium.[61] The presence of aneuploidy predicts for at least a 50% incidence of subsequent invasive cancer and is an indication for intensive screening or immediate surgical resection. Expression of *bcl-2* in squamous cell carcinomas has been associated with longer survival and negative lymph node status.[62]

## REFERENCES

1. Daly JM, Karnell LH, Menck HR. National Cancer Data Base Report on esophageal carcinoma. Cancer 1996;78:1820–8.
2. Yang CS. Research on esophageal cancer in China: a review. Cancer Res 1980;40:2633–44.
3. Giarelli L, Silvestri F, Ferlito A, et al. Observations on the epidemiology of oesophageal carcinoma in the province of Trieste. Clin Otolaryngol 1980;5:13–21.
4. Thomas DB, Karagas MR. Cancer in first and second generation Americans. Cancer Res 1987;47:5771–6.
5. Yang PC, Davis S. Incidence of cancer of the esophagus in the US by histologic type. Cancer 1988;61:612–7.
6. Sharma VK, Chockalingam H, Hornung CA, et al. Changing trends in esophageal cancer: a fifteen year experience in a single center. Am J Gastroenterol 1998;93:702–5.

7. Han C, Qiao G, Hubbert NL, et al. Serologic association between human papillomavirus type 16 infection and esophageal cancer in the Shaanxi Province, China. J Natl Cancer Inst 1996;88:1467–71.

8. Dillner J, Knekt P, Schiller JT, et al. Prospective seroepidemiological evidence that human papillomavirus type 16 infection is a risk factor for oesophageal squamous cell carcinoma. Br Med J 1995;311:1346.

9. Suzuk L, Noffsinger AE, Hui YZ, et al. Detection of human papilloma virus in esophageal squamous cell carcinoma. Cancer 1996;78:704–10.

10. Rugge M, Bovo D, Busatto G, et al. p53 alterations but no human papillomavirus infection in preinvasive and advanced squamous esophageal cancer in Italy. Cancer Epidemiol Biomarkers Prev 1997;6:171–6.

11. Poljak M, Cerar A, Seme K. Human papillomavirus infection in esophageal carcinomas: a study of 121 lesions using multiple broad-spectrum polymerase chain reactions and literature review. Hum Pathol 1998;29:266–71.

12. Lam KY, He D, Ma L, et al. Presence of human papillomavirus in esophageal squamous cell carcinomas of Hong Kong Chinese and its relationship with p53 gene mutation. Hum Pathol 1997;28:657–63.

13. Benamouzig R, Jullian E, Chang F, et al. Absence of human papillomavirus DNA detected by polymerase chain reaction in French patients with esophageal carcinoma. Gastroenterology 1995;109:1876–81.

14. Akutsu N, Shirasawa H, Nakano K, et al. Rare association of human papillomavirus DNA with esophageal cancer in Japan. J Infect Dis 1995;171:421–8.

15. Cheng KK, Day NE, Duffy SW, et al. Pickled vegetables in the aetiology of oesophageal cancer in Hong Kong Chinese. Lancet 1992;339:1314–8.

16. Tzonou A, Lipworth L, Garidou A, et al. Diet and risk of esophageal cancer by histologic type in a low-risk population. Int J Cancer 1996;68:300–4.

17. Cheng KK, Duffy SW, Day NE, et al. Oesophageal cancer in never smokers and never drinkers. Int J Cancer 1995;60:820–2.

18. Ward MH, Sinha R, Heineman EF, et al. Risk of adenocarcinoma of the stomach and esophagus with meat cooking method and doneness preference. Int J Cancer 1997;71:14–9.

19. Launoy G, Milan C, Day NE, et al. Diet and squamous-cell cancer of the oesophagus: a French multicentre case-control study. Int J Cancer 1998;76:7–12.

20. Zhang ZF, Kurtz RC, Yu GP, et al. Adenocarcinomas of the esophagus and gastric cardia: the role of diet. Nutr Cancer 1997;27:298–309.

21. Funkhouser EM, Sharp GB. Aspirin and reduced risk of esophageal cancer. Cancer 1995;76:1116–9.

22. Cheng KK, Duffy SW, Day NE, et al. Stopping drinking and risk of oesophageal cancer. Br Med J 1995;310:1094–7.

23. Ahsan H, Neugut AI. Radiation therapy for breast cancer and increased risk for esophageal carcinoma. Ann Intern Med 1998;128:114–7.

24. Farrow DC, Vaughan TL, Hansten PD, et al. Use of aspirin and other nonsteroidal anti-inflammatory drugs and risk of esophageal and gastric cancer. Cancer Epidemiol Biomarkers Prev 1998;7:97–102.

25. Riddell RH, Path FRC. Early detection of neoplasia of the esophagus and gastroesophageal junction. Am J Gastroenterol 1996;91:853–62.

26. Streitz FM Jr, Ellis FH Jr, Gibb SP, et al. Achalasia and squamous cell carcinoma of the esophagus: analysis of 241 patients. Ann Thorac Surg 1995;59:1604–9.

27. Sandler RS, Nyren O, Ekbom A, et al. The risk of esophageal cancer in patients with achalasia. JAMA 1995;274:1359–62.

28. Jacobs A. Anaemia and post-cricoid carcinoma. Br J Cancer 1961;15:736–44.

29. Hopkins RA, Postlethwait RW. Caustic burns and carcinoma of the esophagus. Ann Surg 1981;194:146–8.

30. Michel JO, Olsen AM, Dockerty MB. The association of diaphragmatic hiatal hernia and gastroesophageal carcinoma. Surg Gynecol Obstet 1967;124:583–9.

31. Shafer RB. Adenocarcinoma in Barrett's columnar-lined esophagus. Arch Surg 1971;103:411–3.

32. Wu T, Watanabe T, Heitmiller R, et al. Genetic alterations in Barrett's esophagus and adenocarcinomas of the esophagus and esophagogastric junction region. Am J Pathol 1998;153:287–94.

33. Parenti AR, Rugge M, Frizzera E, et al. p53 overexpression in the multistep process of esophageal carcinogenesis. Am J Surg Pathol 1995;19:1418–22.

34. Moskaluk CA, Rumpel CA. Allelic deletion in 11p15 is a common occurrence in esophageal and gastric adenocarcinoma. Cancer 1998;83:232–9.

35. Raphael HA, Ellis FH Jr, Dockerty MB. Primary adenocarcinoma of the esophagus: 18-year review and review of literature. Ann Surg 1966;164:785–96.

36. Gunnlaugsson GH, Wychulis AR, Roland C, et al. Analysis of the records of 1,657 patients with carcinoma of the esophagus and cardia of the stomach. Surg Gynecol Obstet 1970;130:997–1005.

37. Sanderson DR. In: Payne WS, ed. The esophagus. Philadelphia: Lea & Febiger, 1974.

38. Kelsen D, Atiq OT. Therapy of upper gastrointestinal tract cancers. Curr Probl Cancer 1991;15:235–94.

39. Quint LE, Hepburn LM, Francis IR, et al. Incidence and distribution of distant metastases from newly diagnosed esophageal carcinoma. Cancer 1995;76:1120–5.

40. Mann NS, Sachdev AJ. Carcinoma of the esophagus and hypercalcemia. Am J Gastroenterol 1977;67:135–40.

41. Giuli R, Gignoux M. Treatment of carcinoma of the esophagus: retrospective study of 2,400 patients. Ann Surg 1980;192:44–52.

42. Tachimori Y, Watanabe H, Kato H, et al. Hypercalcemia in patients with esophageal carcinoma: the pathophysiologic role to parathyroid hormone-related peptide. Cancer 1991;68:2625–9.

43. Itai Y, Kogure T, Okuyama Y, et al. Superficial esophageal carcinoma: radiological findings in double contrast studies. Radiology 1978;126:597–601.

44. Huang GJ. Early detection and surgical treatment of esophageal carcinoma. Surg Today 1981;1:399–405.

45. Shen O, Liu SF, Dawsey SM, et al. Cytologic screening for esophageal cancer: results from 12,877 subjects from a high-risk population in China. Int J Cancer 1993;54:185–8.

46. Yokoyama A, Ohmori T, Makuuchi H, et al. Successful screening for early esophageal cancer in alcoholics using endoscopy and mucosa iodine staining. Cancer 1995;76:928–34.

47. Streitz JM Jr, Ellis FH Jr, Tilden RL, et al. Endoscopic surveillance of Barrett's esophagus: a cost-efficacy comparison with mammographic surveillance for breast cancer. Am J Gastroenterol 1998;93:911–5.

48. Heitmiller RF, Redmond M, Hamilton SR. Barrett's esophagus with high grade dysplasia: an indication for prophylactic esophagectomy. Ann Surg 1996;224:66–71.

49. Van Dam J. Endosonographic evaluation of the patient with esophageal cancer. Chest 1997;112:184S–90S.

50. Pham T, Roach E, Falk GL, et al. Staging of oesophageal carcinoma by endoscopic ultrasound: preliminary experience. Aust N Z J Surg 1998;68:209–12.

51. Hiele M, De Leyn P, Schurmans P, et al. Relation between endoscopic ultrasound findings and outcome of patients with tumors of the esophagus or esophagogastric junction. Gastrointest Endosc 1997;45:381–6.

52. Luketich JD, Schauer P, Landreneau R, et al. Minimally invasive surgical staging is superior to endoscopic ultrasound in detecting lymph node metastases in esophageal cancer. J Thorac Cardiovasc Surg 1997;114:817–23.

53. Choi TK, Siu KF, Lam KH, et al. Bronchoscopy and carcinoma of the esophagus I and II. Am J Surg 1984;147:757–62.

54. Alexander JC Jr, Chretien PB, Dellon AL, et al. CEA levels in patients with carcinoma of the esophagus. Cancer 1978;42:3 Suppl:1492–7.

55. Huang GJ, Zhang DW, Wang GQ, et al. Surgical treatment of carcinoma of the esophagus: report of 1,647 patients. Chin Med J 1981;94:305–7.

56. Naitoh H, Shibata J, Kawaguchi A, et al. Overexpression and localization of cyclin D1 mRNA and antigen in esophageal cancer. Am J Pathol 1995;146:1161–9.

57. Inoue K, Ozeki Y, Suganuma T, et al. Vascular endothelial growth factor expression in primary esophageal squamous cell carcinoma: association with angiogenesis and tumor progression. Cancer 1997;79:206–13.

58. Ribeiro U, Findelstein DS, Safatle-Ribeiro AV, et al. P53 sequence analysis predicts treatment response and outcome of patients with esophageal carcinoma. Cancer 1998;83:7–18.

59. Lam KY, Tsao SW, Zhang D, et al. Prevalence and predictive value of p53 mutation in patients with oesophageal squamous cell carcinomas: a prospective clinico-pathological study and survival analysis of 70 patients. Int J Cancer 1997;74:212–9.

60. Uchino S, Saito T, Inomata M, et al. Prognostic significance of p53 mutation in esophageal cancer. Jpn J Clin Oncol 1996;26:287–92.

61. Krishnadath KK, Tilanus HW, van Blankenstein M, et al. Accumulation of genetic abnormalities during neoplastic progression in Barrett's esophagus. Cancer Res 1995;55:1971–6.

62. Ohbu M, Saegusa M, Kobayashi N, et al. Expression of bcl-2 protein in esophageal squamous cell carcinomas and its association with lymph node metastases. Cancer 1997;79:1287–93.

# SURGERY FOR ESOPHAGEAL CANCER

• Kenneth P. Ramming

## PHILOSOPHY OF SURGICAL MANAGEMENT

The task of the surgeon in esophageal cancer, as for all gastrointestinal malignancies, is to excise the lesion and the regional metastases totally and to re-establish intestinal continuity whenever possible. This surgery is undertaken with curative intent, although the advanced stages of disease that are commonly seen in the United States and Europe make cure uncommon. Cure is more likely in Asian countries, where early esophageal cancer is more commonly diagnosed.[1, 2] The more realistic goal of palliation becomes the primary objective in most cases. Because of the limited effectiveness of other modalities, poor prognostic signs (such as significant node involvement outside the field of resection), which might dictate lesser procedures in other neoplasms (although not necessarily curative), often do not preclude major surgery in cancer of the esophagus. The goal of surgery is most often to prolong and improve the quality of life through nutrition and the ability to handle oral secretions.

## PREPARATION BEFORE SURGERY

A high incidence of chronic pulmonary disease is present in patients with esophageal carcinoma. Although this pulmonary disease is often caused by the long-term use of tobacco, chronic aspiration pneumonia is not infrequent. Almost all patients are nutritionally depleted. Dehydration is common. The red cell mass is frequently low, although the patient's hematocrit might be deceptively high because of the general reduction of circulating blood volume.

Although prolonged periods of preoperative preparation cannot be justified in a disease in which survival is often short, severely debilitated patients may benefit from brief but intensive in-hospital preoperative treatment. This treatment includes meticulous pulmonary toilet and instruction in postoperative pulmonary supportive methods. Blood volume, fluid, and electrolyte balance should be normal; this usually requires the infusion of colloid and blood. Hyperalimentation by the parenteral route has been reported to be beneficial. It is our opinion, however, that preoperative nutritional supplementation delays surgery unnecessarily and does not decrease operative mortality rates.

The surgeon must be prepared to deal with any contingency, such as the necessity to excise or mobilize the great vessels, pericardium, or lung to achieve removal of the tumor. An operative plan that includes options for logical alterations in technique for the various possible anatomic findings greatly reduces surprise, anxiety, and poor judgment at the operating table if local extension should be encountered.

## SURGERY FOR LOWER AND MIDTHORACIC ESOPHAGEAL CANCER

The combined abdominal–right thoracotomy approach is the procedure of choice for lower and midthoracic esophageal lesions (Fig. 40–1). The patient is placed in the oblique position, with the right side of the chest at about an 80-degree angle and the abdomen torqued to the left. Exposure is greatly facilitated by keeping the patient's right arm free, preparing it in a sterile wrap, and positioning it as necessary during the procedure. This positioning allows simultaneous exposure of the abdomen and chest. Laparotomy is performed, and the stomach is mobilized. We favor a bilateral subcostal incision. The use of a double-lumen endotracheal tube enables the right lung to be deflated, facilitating exposure and minimizing retractor-induced lung contusion. The esophagus is mobilized through a right thoracotomy incision. When all mobilization is complete and the tumor is free, the stomach is advanced into the chest and is divided with a staple line. The esophagus is then divided, usually at the level of the azygos vein. An end-to-side esophagogastric tube anastomosis is performed with double-layer 3–0 Maxon sutures or with the EEA stapling device. The advantages of this approach are that a large length of esophagus can be resected and the anastomosis can be constructed without anatomic confinement.

Some surgeons prefer a left thoracoabdominal incision

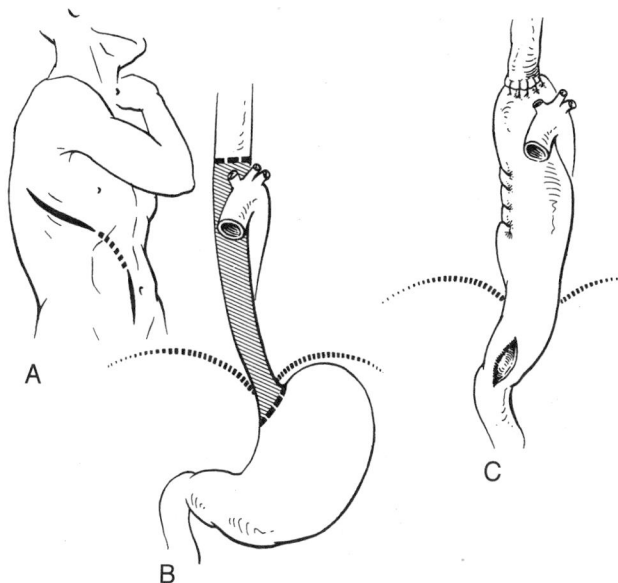

**Figure 40–1.** Technique of esophagogastrectomy and esophagogastrostomy for carcinoma of the thoracic esophagus. *A,* Right thoracotomy and upper abdominal incision *(dotted lines). B,* Extent of esophageal resection *(shaded area). C,* Completed esophagogastrostomy and pyloromyotomy. (From Ellis FH Jr. Treatment of carcinoma of the esophagus and cardia. Mayo Clin Proc 1960;35:653–63.)

for low-lying lesions close to the gastroesophageal junction. The disadvantage of this approach is that the diaphragm is divided, and sometimes the anastomosis has to be constructed at a difficult angle because of the proximity of the beating heart. Transhiatal esophagectomy is another alternative procedure, as described subsequently.

## SURGERY FOR UPPER ESOPHAGEAL LESIONS

When possible, right thoracotomy and esophagogastrectomy, as described, are used. For high thoracic lesions in which the superior margin must be at the low cervical esophagus, however, colon interposition may be preferable. In this procedure, a segment of colon and its blood supply are isolated by preservation of one nutrient vessel and the corresponding marginal artery. Figure 40–2 shows this procedure in schematic form.

In palliative procedures, it is not necessary to open the chest. Simple blunt substernal dissection from the abdominal and cervical incisions safely creates a channel through which a colonic segment can be passed. Ascending, transverse, or descending colon segments can be so interposed, as anatomy and preference dictate. Our preference under ideal circumstances is to mobilize the descending colon based on the left colic artery.

Clinical maneuvers that are necessary for the success of this procedure include preoperative arteriography to ensure that appropriate vascular anatomy to the colon exists, resection of the sternoclavicular angle to prevent constriction or venous obstruction of the distal colonic segment, and the necessary arterial clamping and evaluations before resection

of the colon to ensure an adequate blood supply to the transposed colon segment that was chosen.

The advantage of this procedure is that it preserves maximal length of esophagus. Disadvantages include long operative time, the demand for technical expertise and experience, and a certain percentage of failures of the cervical anastomosis, usually because of compromised vascularity. The use of stapling devices to fashion gastric conduits reduces operative time. Circular staples at the site of the anastomosis, however, can result in strictures that cannot be dilated.

## TRANSHIATAL ESOPHAGECTOMY

First described by Turner in 1933 and later reintroduced by Orringer, Kirk, and Akiyama in the 1970s, transhiatal esophagectomy involves blunt dissection of the esophagus from its bed without thoracotomy (Fig. 40–3).[3, 4] The popularity of the procedure increased in the 1990s primarily because of its perceived safety and results equivalent to other procedures. Many authors advocate this procedure whenever possible for resectable esophageal carcinoma provided that an assessment of the tumor through the diaphragmatic hiatus does not indicate invasion of contiguous structures that would preclude a transhiatal dissection.

A combined thoracic and abdominal operation may cause respiratory insufficiency in a debilitated patient because of postoperative incisional pain and the inability to breathe deeply, resulting in dependence on mechanical ventilatory assistance and a high risk of death from pneumonia. The combined procedure also is susceptible to leaks and disruption of the intrathoracic anastomosis, which is the most dreaded complication of the procedure. This complication commonly results in mediastinitis and sepsis, which is fatal in about 50% of cases. Additional disadvantages of intrathoracic esophageal reconstruction include inadequate relief of dysphagia resulting from either anastomotic tumor recurrence in the suture line or the development of reflux esophagitis above the anastomosis. Transhiatal esophagectomy prevents these complications because the anastomosis is not buried deeply in the chest, and the lack of a thoracotomy reduces the risk of mandatory, prolonged mechanical ventilatory assistance in debilitated patients.

Regardless of the level of the tumor, transhiatal esophagectomy involves resection of the entire thoracic esophagus, being replaced whenever possible with the stomach, which is anastomosed to the remaining cervical esophagus above the level of the clavicles. This procedure is performed through an abdominal and a cervical incision. The thoracic esophagus is resected through the diaphragmatic hiatus and the neck. The stomach is mobilized, appropriate vessels are divided and preserved, and a pyloromyotomy and feeding jejunostomy are performed. The entire thoracic esophagus from the level of the clavicles to the cardia is resected (see Figs. 40–2 and 40–3).

In performing this procedure, accessible cervical, intrathoracic, and intra-abdominal lymph nodes are sampled for staging, but no attempt is made to undertake a therapeutic lymph node dissection. The advantages of transhiatal esophagectomy are as follows: (1) A thoracotomy is not performed, avoiding the ventilatory complications; (2) there is no intrathoracic anastomosis, avoiding the complication of an anas-

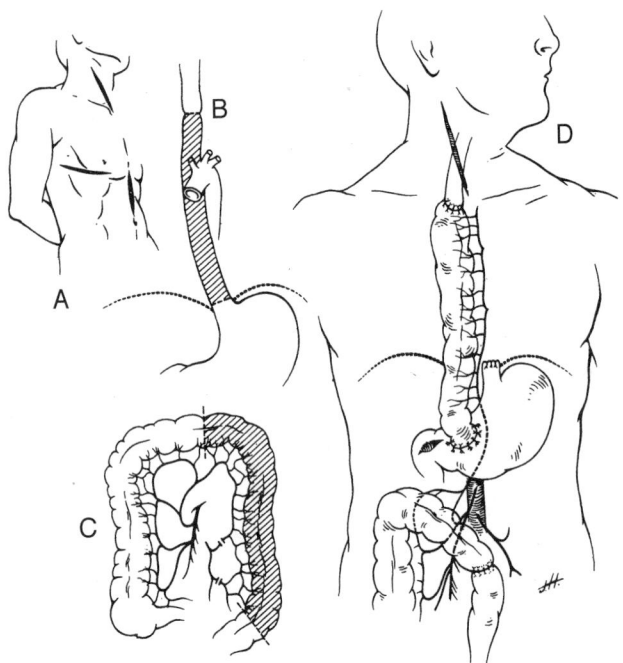

**Figure 40–2.** Esophagectomy with interposition of left colon. *A*, Incision. A left cervical incision is preferred by many surgeons. *B*, Extent of esophageal resection *(shaded area)*. *C*, Mobilization of descending colon. *D*, Completed operation. (From Ellis FH Jr. The esophagus. In: Davis L, ed. Christopher's textbook of surgery. 9th ed. Philadelphia: WB Saunders, 1968:637.)

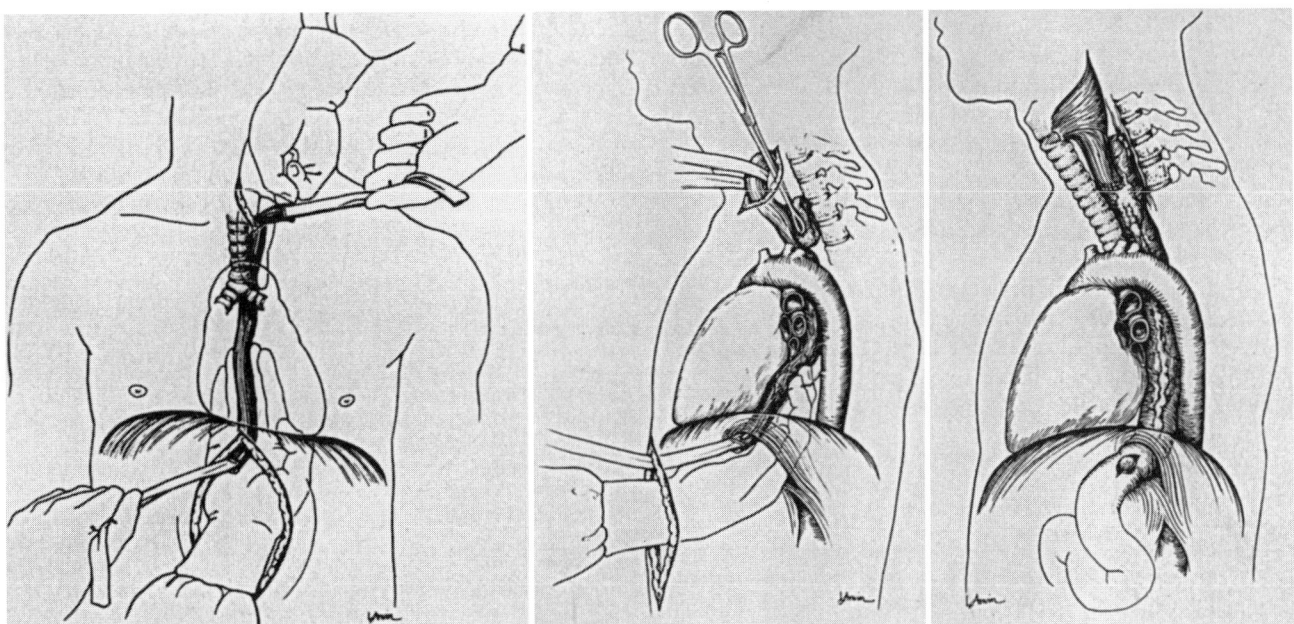

**Figure 40–3.** Transhiatal dissection of the lower esophagus is performed through the diaphragm using an abdominal incision. The upper thoracic esophagus is mobilized through a limited cervical incision. Penrose drains around either end of the esophagus provide traction during the procedure. Blunt dissection is performed from below using the surgeon's hand; it is accomplished from above with a *sponge-on-a-stick* inserted through the cervical incision. After a transhiatal esophagectomy and pyloromyotomy, the stomach is mobilized through the posterior mediastinum, and the fundus is sutured to the cervical prevertebral fascia. An end-to-side esophagogastrostomy is performed to complete the procedure. (From Orringer MB, Sloan H. Esophagectomy without thoracotomy. J Thorac Cardiovasc Surg 1978;76:644–5.)

tomotic leak in an inaccessible anatomic area; and (3) gastroesophageal reflux seldom occurs, avoiding reflux esophagitis above the anastomosis.

Critics of transhiatal esophagectomy are concerned about the limited exposure of the intrathoracic esophagus and its blood supply during the procedure, which is accompanied by a risk of uncontrollable hemorrhage. They are also concerned about the inadequacy of mediastinal lymph node dissections for complete staging and for potential cure. When the results of this procedure are compared with a combined thoracoabdominal approach, including en bloc dissection of contiguous lymph node–bearing tissues, no significant difference in 3-year survival rates was apparent in series reported by Skinner[5] and Orringer.[3]

## SURGERY FOR THE CERVICAL ESOPHAGUS

Except for low-lying lesions at the thoracocervical junction that may be amenable to colon interposition, we usually treat cervical cancers with radiation therapy. Several operations have been successfully used, however, such as the Wookey[6] procedure, which creates a pharyngeal tube linked with skin inside and outside for establishing esophageal continuity. These procedures are usually performed after pharyngectomy and laryngectomy. Their main disadvantage is the necessity for multiple, lengthy staged manipulations before the formation of the tube in a patient who often has had extensive surgery or radiation, or both, in that area.

Probably the only surgical procedure that offers the possibility of cure in this difficult area is pharyngolaryngoesophagectomy. This complex operation can be used when invasion of the trachea is present.[7] The use of free jejunal grafts (i.e.,

segments of jejunum resected with their vascular supply, transposed to the cervical area, and then revascularized by microvascular techniques to arterial and venous sources in the neck) has been reported as a method of re-establishing esophageal continuity following resection for cancer.[8] Hundreds of these procedures have been performed, and they now constitute the best available surgical approach to esophageal cancer in this difficult anatomic region.[9]

## PALLIATIVE PROCEDURES

In patients with advanced disease, extensive local unresectable tumor with obstruction, or complications such as tracheoesophageal fistula, palliative bypass without resection may be indicated. Orringer[10] has advocated substernal bypass using the stomach while simply excluding the unresected esophagus. Heimlich and Winfield[11] proposed a gastric tube fashioned from the greater curvature of the stomach to provide a similar bypass. Griffen and coworkers[12] have advocated using the reverse gastric tube in all patients who have carcinoma of the esophagus. Esophagectomy without thoracotomy has also been reported.[13] Steiger and colleagues[14] reported 54 patients with far-advanced carcinoma of the esophagus in whom no attempt was made to resect the lesion while gastric or colonic bypass was performed. The operative mortality rate was 7.5%, and the average survival was 5 months. Osborne and associates[15] reported a good functional result in 78% and a 3-year survival rate of 32% in 40 consecutive cases treated with colon interposition.

Other nonresectional procedures have also been documented. Atkinson and Ferguson[16] used fiberoptic endoscopy, preliminary dilatation, and Celestin tube insertion in 13 patients. One death resulted from the procedure. Palliative pulsion intubation has also been reported by Haffejee and Angorn[17] and others.[18, 19] Kairaluoma and colleagues[20] used a Celestin tube intubation on 108 patients, with a hospital mortality rate of 16%. This latter experience has been more consistent with our observations (i.e., high mortality or morbidity from insertion of the tube itself, usually from esophageal perforation). We have not been impressed by the degree of palliation obtained, noting frequent blockage or dislodgment of the tube, and we no longer use prosthetic stents of any type. Virkkula and coworkers[21] have reported the use of a reversed pectoralis skin pedicle flap and free skin grafts to create an extrathoracic conduit from esophagus to stomach. Robinson and colleagues[22] advocate a substernal gastric bypass technique.

## SURGICAL RESULTS

The 5-year survival rate after surgery for carcinoma of the esophagus averaged 6% over a 35-year period, with an operative mortality rate of 28% (Table 40–2). If one considers the results of reports from 1983 to 1988 in Table 40–2, however, the 5-year survival rate averaged 28%, and the operative mortality rate averaged 11%. Even more impressive are the results from Akiyama's service in Tokyo.[2] As reported by Khoury,[23] the operative mortality rate has been 1.7% for squamous cell carcinoma of the esophagus, and 36% of the patients are alive at 5 years. These excellent results are especially impressive considering that more than half of the resections are in patients with advanced disease. These improved statistics are probably the result of more appropriate patient selection criteria, the use of preoperative hyperalimentation, better postoperative care (mainly respiratory support[24]), and the use of more refined surgical techniques (such as en bloc resections and staged procedures in some patients).[25] Despite such advances, these overall results

*Table 40–2.* **Results of Surgical Treatment of Cancer of the Esophagus***

| First Author (Year) | Resections (No.) | Operative Mortality (%) | 5-Year Survival (%) |
|---|---|---|---|
| Earlam (1980) | ~32,675† | 29 ± 16 | 4 ± 3 |
| Giuli (1980) | 2400 | 30 | 14 |
| Schuchmann (1980) | 46 | 22 | 14.3 |
| Hiebert (1981) | 139 | 28 | 3 |
| Lam (1981) | 885 | 41 | 18 |
| Huang (1981) | 1367 | 4 | 30‡ |
| Borst (1981) | 125 | 17 | 10 |
| Skinner (1983) | 199 | 10 | 21 |
| Akiyama (1984) | 295 | 1.7 | 34.7 |
| Goldfaden (1986) | 72 | 11 | ~18 |
| Giuli (1986) | 790 | 14.7 | — |
| Desa (1988) | 21 | 14.3 | 9.5 |
| Results overall | 38,934 | 28 | 6 |
| Results for 1983–1988 trials | 1297 | 11 | 28 |

*Five-year survival of patients undergoing resection.
†Pre-1980, 30-year review of the results from multiple centers.
‡Early case detection included.

are still far from satisfactory. We agree with others that surgery should be performed in all cases in which the tumor is potentially resectable[26-32] provided that the patient has access to a center and treatment team with sufficient experience and skill to undertake this difficult form of cancer surgery. Neoadjuvant or adjuvant therapy may improve survival duration in resectable patients. These approaches are discussed in the following sections.

## REFERENCES

1. Nabeya K, Hanaoka SL, Nyumura T. What is the ideal treatment for early esophageal cancer? Endoscopy 1993;25:670–1.
2. Akiyama H. Surgery for cancer of the esophagus. Baltimore: Williams & Wilkins, 1990.
3. Orringer MB. Transhiatal esophagectomy without thoracotomy for carcinoma of the thoracic esophagus. Ann Surg 1984;200:282–8.
4. Orringer MB, Sloan H. Esophagectomy without thoracotomy. J Thorac Cardiovasc Surg 1978;76:644–5.
5. Skinner DB. En bloc resection for neoplasms of the esophagus and cardia. J Thorac Cardiovasc Surg 1983;85:59–71.
6. Wookey H. The surgical treatment of carcinoma of the hypopharynx and the oesophagus. Br J Surg 1948;35:249–66.
7. Lam KH, Wong J, Lim ST, Ong GB. Surgical treatment of carcinoma of the hypopharynx and cervical oesophagus. Ann Acad Med Singapore 1980;9:317–22.
8. Chang TS, Hwang OL, Wang-Wei. Reconstruction of esophageal defects with microsurgically revascularized jejunal segments: a report of 13 cases. J Microsurg 1980;2:83–94.
9. Omura K, Misaki T, Watanabe Y, et al. Reconstruction with free jejunal autograft after pharyngolaryngoesophagectomy. Ann Thorac Surg 1994;57:112–8.
10. Orringer M. Multimodality therapy for esophageal carcinoma. Chest 1993;103:Suppl:S406–9.
11. Heimlich HJ, Winfield JM. The use of a gastric tube to replace or bypass the esophagus. Surgery 1955;37:549–59.
12. Griffen WO Jr, Daugherty ME, McGee EM, Utley JR. Unified approach to carcinoma of the esophagus. Ann Surg 1976;183:511–6.
13. Tryzelaar JF, Neptune WB, Ellis FH Jr. Esophagectomy without thoracotomy for carcinoma of the esophagus. Am J Surg 1982;143:486–9.
14. Steiger Z, Nickel WO, Wilson RF, Arbulu A. Improved surgical palliation of advanced carcinoma of the esophagus. Am J Surg 1978;135:782–4.
15. Osborne MP, Griffiths JD, Shaw HJ. Colon transposition in the management of upper gastrointestinal cancer. Cancer 1982;50:2235–42.
16. Atkinson M, Ferguson R. Fibreoptic endoscopic palliative intubation of inoperable oesophagogastric neoplasms. Br Med J 1977;1:266–7.
17. Haffejee AA, Angorn IB. Oral alimentation following intubation for esophageal carcinoma. Ann Surg 1977;186:759–61.
18. Bennett JR. Intubation of gastro-oesophageal malignancies: a survey of current practice in Britain, 1980. Gut 1981;22:336–8.
19. Jones DB, Davies PS, Smith PM. Endoscopic insertion of palliative oesophageal tubes in oesophagogastric neoplasms. Br J Surg 1981;68:197–8.
20. Kairaluoma MI, Jokinen K, Kärkölä P, Larmi TK. Celestin tube palliation of unresectable esophageal carcinoma. J Thorac Cardiovasc Surg 1977;73:783–6.
21. Virkkula L, Eerola S, Appelqvist P. Repair of stricture and fistula of the antethoracic oesophagogastrostoma using a reversed pectoralis skin flap. Scand J Thorac Cardiovasc Surg 1977;11:67–9.
22. Robinson JC, Isa SS, Spees EK, et al. Substernal gastric bypass for palliation of esophageal carcinoma: rationale and technique. Surgery 1982;91:305–11.
23. Khoury GA. Oesophageal surgery under Akiyama. Lancet 1989;1:91–2.
24. Imamura M, Yanagibashi K, Tobe T, et al. Transthoracic resection of esophageal cancer in patients with pulmonary dysfunction. Ann Surg 1988;208:601–5.
25. Nishi M, Hiramatsu Y, Hioki K, et al. Risk factors in relation to postoperative complications in patients undergoing esophagectomy or gastrectomy for cancer. Ann Surg 1988;207:148–54.
26. Schuchmann GF, Heydorn WH, Hall RV, et al. Treatment of esophageal

carcinoma: a retrospective review. J Thorac Cardiovasc Surg 1980;79:67–73.
27. Ellis FH. Esophagogastrectomy for carcinoma: technical considerations based on anatomic location of lesion. Surg Clin North Am 1980;60:265–79.
28. Heck HA Jr, Rossi NP. Esophageal and gastroesophageal junction carcinoma: an evolved philosophy of management. Cancer 1980;46:1873–8.
29. Molina JE, Lawton BR, Myers WO, Humphrey EW. Esophagogastrec-
tomy for adenocarcinoma of the cardia: ten years' experience and current approach. Ann Surg 1982;195:146–51.
30. Hoffmann TH, Kelley JR, Grover FL, Trinkle JK. Carcinoma of the esophagus: an aggressive one-stage palliative approach. J Thorac Cardiovasc Surg 1981;81:44–9.
31. Skinner DB, Ferguson MK, Soriano A, et al. Selection of operation for esophageal cancer based on staging. Ann Surg 1986;204:391–401.
32. Hennessy TP. Choice of treatment in carcinoma of the oesophagus. Br J Surg 1988;75:193–4.

# RADIATION THERAPY FOR ESOPHAGEAL CARCINOMA

• Luu M. Tran

The primary treatment for esophageal carcinoma has traditionally been surgery, especially for lesions of the middle and lower third of the esophagus. Survival rates and local-regional control following surgery, however, depend on the degree of tumor extension, and only 20% of patients diagnosed have carcinoma limited to the esophagus (T1–T2 N0).[1] In these cases, when the tumors do not extend outside the muscularis propria, the 5-year survival can be 80%.[2] Surgical resection is less successful, however, in the remaining 80% whose tumors extend to the esophageal wall (T3) or regional lymph nodes (N1). In these cases, the 5-year survival rate is 7 to 28%, with local recurrence of 20 to 35%.[3, 4] In the presence of invasive esophageal cancer, radiation therapy has been used either as the primary treatment for unresectable tumors or as an adjunct to surgery. Since the late 1970s, radiation therapy has increasingly been combined with chemotherapy, and several trials of nonsurgical combined-modality therapy (CMT) have shown survival rates comparable to surgery.

We discuss the role of radiation therapy in the treatment of esophageal carcinoma, particularly within the context of prospective randomized trials that included radiation therapy alone, preoperative or postoperative radiation therapy, and a nonsurgical approach with chemoradiation (CMT).

## RADIATION TECHNIQUES

The patient is set up in the supine position, which is especially important for lesions in the cervical esophagus. The radiation fields include all gross disease and adjacent nodal areas at risk. The field borders extend at least 5 cm above and below the gross tumor borders, within a 2-cm lateral margin. If the tumor extends above the level of the carina, the superior border should include the supraclavicular fossa. For lesions in the lower half of the esophagus, the inferior border should include the celiac nodes.

Anterior and posterior (anteroposterior and posteroanterior) portals are commonly used during the first 40 Gy, and lateral or oblique fields are used for the remaining fractions to boost the primary tumor with limited margins to the desired dose. Patients should be treated with high-energy photons ($\geq 4$ MV) delivering 1.8 Gy/day, 5 days per week. The total radiation dose ranges from preoperative treatment of 45 Gy in 5 weeks to primary therapy of 66 Gy in 7 weeks.

If the total dose exceeds 45 Gy, CT treatment planning or three-dimensional conformal therapy would be helpful. A variety of adjunctive devices are used to limit the doses to the spinal cord ($<45$ Gy), the lung ($<18$ Gy), and the heart ($<30$ Gy), such as the Cerrobend block, multileaf collimators, compensator filters, and wedges.

## TREATMENT RESULTS FOR RESECTABLE TUMORS

**Preoperative Radiation Therapy.** One benefit of using preoperative radiation in treatment of esophageal carcinoma is that it can sterilize cells at the margins of resection and reduce the tumor volume, improving resectability. Studies do not support its routine use, however. There are five phase III randomized trials[5–9] that evaluate the results of preoperative radiation versus surgery alone in the treatment of resectable carcinoma (mainly squamous cell) of the esophagus; the trials used different doses and fractionation schemes. We review only studies using conventional techniques and adequate intervals between radiation and surgery.

Nygaard and colleagues[5] compared surgery alone with three different preoperative treatments: (1) 35 Gy radiation therapy, (2) 35 Gy plus chemotherapy (cisplatin-bleomycin) followed by surgery, or (3) chemotherapy. The study enrolled 186 patients with squamous cell carcinoma of the esophagus. The 3-year survival was significantly higher in the pooled groups receiving radiation therapy compared with the pooled groups not receiving radiation therapy (19% vs. 6%, $p = 0.009$). There was no survival advantage for the group treated with preoperative chemotherapy compared with those not receiving chemotherapy. This trial used low doses of radiation therapy and enrolled a relatively small sample size, making it difficult to form conclusions regarding neoadjuvant treatment.

Wang and coworkers[6] from the Cancer Institute of China reported the results of another preoperative trial that randomized 206 patients. The preoperative dose was 40 Gy in eight fractions, and the interval between radiation and surgery was 2 to 4 weeks. Local recurrence was lower in the radiation group than in the surgery-only group (4% vs. 3%), but there was no survival advantage between the two groups (35% vs. 30%).

Gignoux and associates[7] reported another trial from the European Organization for Research and Treatment of Cancer (EORTC). The study randomized 229 patients with squamous cell carcinoma; half were treated with surgery alone, and the other half received preoperative radiation 33 Gy in 10 fractions. The interval between radiation therapy and surgery was only 8 days. There was a significant decrease in local failure rate treated with preoperative radiation (33% vs. 21%). There was no difference in the 5-year survival and resectability between the two groups.

These randomized trials do not support the routine use of preoperative radiation therapy. No statistically significant difference in median survival (4 to 12 months), 5-year survival (6 to 12%), resectability, or operative mortality has been shown in this setting. One explanation could be that most of these trials used suboptimal, unconventional techniques that resulted in unacceptable mortality. Also, the short interval between radiation and surgery does not allow tumors adequate time for maximal downstaging.

**Preoperative Chemoradiation.** Subsequent to these poor results with preoperative radiation therapy, several institutions studied the combination of preoperative radiation therapy plus chemotherapy. In the 1970s, pilot studies from Wayne State University[10] investigated the use of low doses of radiation therapy (30 Gy in 15 fractions) plus 5-fluorouracil (5-FU) and platinum followed by esophagectomy 4 to 6 weeks later. Resectability, median survival, and 2-year survival were 60 to 80%, 12 to 19 months, and 15 to 40%, respectively. This regimen was further studied in national trials by Southwest Oncology Group/Radiation Therapy Oncology Group (SWOG/RTOG). Poplin and colleagues[11] reported median survival of 12 months and a 2-year survival rate of 28% in 113 patients with resectable esophageal cancer. The pathologic complete response in this series was 17%. This combination study failed to show an overall or median survival greater than that attained from surgery alone or radiation therapy alone. Several pilot studies have used a moderate dose of radiation (45 to 50 Gy) concurrent with platinum-based chemotherapy. Using this approach, the University of Michigan[12] reported that 43 patients (22 with squamous cell carcinoma and 21 with adenocarcinoma) were treated with chemotherapy (continuous infusion of platinum and vinblastine [Velban]) and concurrent radiation therapy. The first 20 patients received 2.5-Gy fractions, 5 days per week to a total dose of 37.5 Gy over 3 weeks. Subsequent patients received 1.5 Gy twice a day, 5 days per week to a total dose of 45 Gy over 3 weeks. This combination therapy was followed by transhiatal esophagectomy 21 days later. The operability rate was 95%, the resectability rate was 84%, and the pathologic complete response was 24%. Patients who achieved a pathologic complete response had a median survival of 70 months and a 5-year survival rate of 60%, whereas those without a pathologic complete response had a lower median survival of 26 months and a lower 5-year survival of 26%. Forastiere and coworkers[13] from Johns Hopkins evaluated the results of 50 patients with resectable esophageal cancer treated with a similar regimen. Radiation therapy was 44 Gy using standard fractionation and given concurrent with cisplatin-based chemotherapy. With a median follow-up of 23 months, the estimated 2-year survival was 52%, and pathologic complete response was 42%. The toxicity was much less than in the previous twice-a-day regimen. A group[14] at Nashville, Tennessee, has reported results of preoperative chemotherapy (paclitaxel, carboplatin,

5-FU) and radiation therapy (45 Gy with standard fractionation) for 22 patients with stage II to stage III resectable esophageal cancer. Surgical resection was planned 4 to 6 weeks after completion of therapy. Thirteen of 22 patients were able to undergo surgical resection. Of these, 9 had a pathologic complete response (69%), and 2 patients had only microscopic residual disease.

Six randomized trials (Table 40–3)[4, 15–19] compared preoperative CMT with surgery alone in resectable tumors. Three of these studies used sequential CMT, whereas three used concomitant CMT. As previously mentioned, the study by Nygaard and colleagues[5] had suggested that preoperative radiation may have a beneficial effect on survival.

A study from the University of Michigan[15] randomized 100 patients between two groups: surgery alone versus preoperative chemoradiation (5-FU, platinum, and vinblastine concurrent with 45 Gy at 1.5 Gy twice a day). Transhiatal esophagectomy was performed on all patients. After several years of follow-up, there was a survival advantage favoring the trimodality group (3-year survival of 32% as compared with 15% for the surgery-alone group, $p = 0.04$).

An EORTC trial[16] randomized 257 patients in two groups: surgery alone versus preoperative CMT (cisplatin for two courses concomitant with split-course radiation therapy using 18.5 Gy in five fractions per course). Median follow-up 2.8 years later indicated no difference between the two groups with respect to median survival, but the mortality and resection rates were higher in the group receiving CMT. This trial was criticized for three shortcomings: a low radiation dose, a high dose per fraction over short periods, and a low dose of chemotherapy.

Walsh and associates[17] reported data from a trial of 113 Irish patients with esophageal adenocarcinoma. The patients were randomized between surgery alone versus CMT (5-FU and cisplatin in weeks 1 and 6 concurrent with 40 Gy in 15 fractions) followed by surgery. With the neoadjuvant chemoradiation, the authors observed a pathologic complete response rate of 25%. The 3-year survival rate was five times higher for the CMT group—32% compared with 6% for the surgery-alone group ($p = 0.01$). The survival rate (6%) in the latter group is unusually low compared with other surgical series.[1–3]

Le Prise and colleagues[18] evaluated the treatment results of 86 patients with localized esophageal cancer. They were randomized between surgery alone versus preoperative, sequential chemotherapy (5-FU and cisplatin) followed by radiation therapy (20 Gy in 10 fractions) and chemotherapy again. The median survival was the same at 10 months, which is similar to that of historical controls.

Most of these randomized trials, with few exceptions, have proved that preoperative CMT does not improve overall survival. They have demonstrated a high pathologic complete response rate, however, which can be obtained with modest doses of radiation and concurrent chemotherapy. Additional research with phase III trials is warranted because the combination of surgery and radiation therapy may offer an increased chance of local control.

**Postoperative Radiation Therapy.** Postoperative radiation therapy is recommended for patients with positive surgical margins, lymph node involvement, gross residual disease, or invasion through the entire esophageal wall. The advantage of a postoperative radiation therapy approach is that it

***Table 40–3.*** **Randomized Trials of Preoperative Chemoradiotherapy Versus Surgery Alone**

| Series | Location | Patients (No.) | Radiation | Chemotherapy | Surgery | Median Survival (mo) | Actuarial Survival |
|---|---|---|---|---|---|---|---|
| Nygaard (1992) | Scandinavia II | 41 | | | S alone | | 9% (3 yr) NS |
| | | 50 | 35 Gy/20 frs | Cisplatin + bleomycin × 2 cycles | S | | 3% (3 yr) |
| Apinop (1994) | Thailand | 34 | | | S alone | 7 | 10% (5 yr) NS |
| | | 35 | 40 Gy | Cisplatin + 5-FU | S | 10 | 24% (5 yr) |
| Urba (1997) | University of Michigan | 50 | | | S alone | 18 | 39% (2 yr) NS |
| | | 50 | 45 Gy (BID) | Cisplatin + 5-FU + vinblastine | S | 17 | 42% (2 yr) |
| Le Prise (1994) | Rennes | 45 | | | S alone | | 14% (3 yr) NS |
| | | 41 | 20 Gy/10 frs | Cisplatin + 5-FU | S | | 19% (3 yr) |
| Bossett (1994) | EORTC 40881 | 139 | | | S | 19 | 25% (5 yr) NS |
| | | 143 | 18.5 Gy × 2 | Cisplatin | S | 19 | 25% (5 yr) |
| Walsh (1996) | Dublin | 55* | | | S alone | 11 mo | 6% (3 yr) p = .01 |
| | | 58* | 40 Gy/3 wk | 5-FU + cisplatin | | 16 mo | 32% (3 yr) |

*Patients limited to cases of adenocarcinoma.
frs, fractions; S, surgery; NS, not significant; 5-FU, 5-fluorouracil.

permits more accurate staging selection. The disadvantage from a radiation standpoint is that the stomach has a low tolerance to radiation; when it lies within the target volume, the dose must be limited to 45 to 50 Gy. Another disadvantage is that a larger volume of normal tissue (from the upper esophagus to the diaphragm) may be irradiated, increasing the risk of debilitating morbidity.

A few studies have evaluated the role of radiation therapy alone (without chemotherapy) as an adjuvant treatment following esophagectomy. These nonrandomized trials[20–23] do not allow firm conclusions about the value of this approach. Kasai and associates[20] found that postoperative radiation 60 Gy over 6 weeks decreased local-regional recurrence rates when compared with nonirradiated patients. The use of postoperative radiation therapy showed an improvement in 5-year survival only in the group with negative nodes (88% vs. 27%).

Three other prospective, randomized trials evaluated postoperative radiation therapy. Teniere and colleagues[21] from the French University Association reported a study of 221 patients with squamous cell carcinoma of the middle to lower third of the esophagus undergoing curative resection. They were randomized to surgery alone or postoperative radiation (45 to 50 Gy at 1.8-Gy fractions). In the node-negative patients, local failure significantly decreased with the adjuvant radiation therapy compared with surgery alone (10% vs. 35%). The survival rate was the same at 19% in both groups.

Fok and coworkers[22] from Queen Mary Hospital, Hong Kong, reported their experience of 130 patients with both squamous cell carcinoma and adenocarcinoma who underwent surgery and were then randomized to no treatment or to adjuvant radiation treatment (49 to 52 Gy at 3.5 Gy per fraction with three fractions per week). Within these two groups, 60 had curative resection. The addition of radiation therapy in the curative resection group provided no significant decrease in local failure (10% vs. 13%). Subset analysis, however, noted that adjuvant radiation therapy did show a decrease of local recurrence in patients with gross residual disease (46% vs. 20%). Overall the median survival was worse in the radiation therapy group (8.7 months vs. 5 months, p = 0.02) than in the surgery-only group. This study was criticized for the complications of radiation (high dose per fraction) and metastatic disease.

Iizuka and colleagues[23] reported the results of 258 patients with squamous cell carcinoma treated with curative resection. They were randomized between surgery plus postoperative chemotherapy (cisplatin and vindesine) versus surgery plus postoperative radiation therapy (50 Gy in 5 weeks). There was no significant difference in survival or local recurrence between the two groups.

Based on these randomized studies, the use of postoperative radiation therapy alone is not clearly defined. Results of adjuvant postoperative radiation therapy in patients with completely resected tumors (T1–T2 N0) are largely negative. So far, no retrospective studies have shown a survival benefit from adjuvant therapy after surgical resection for locally advanced (T3–T4 N1) disease. Although adjuvant therapy may reduce the rate of local failure, it has not resulted in improvement of overall survival. Radiation therapy should be reserved for patients with positive surgical margins, and the treatment technique should be carefully planned to avoid debilitating morbidity.

## RADIATION THERAPY ALONE VERSUS COMBINED CHEMORADIOTHERAPY WITHOUT SURGERY

Approximately 50% of patients are not candidates for curative resection because their lesions are medically inoperable or they have clinically locally advanced tumors. In such cases in the past, radiation therapy alone was used mainly for palliation of dysphagia and malnutrition, with favorable results.[24] Recurrence results have been poor, however, with median survivals of 6 to 12 months and 3-year survivals of less than 10%.[25] With radiation therapy alone, the most frequent site of failure is the primary site at 86%.[24, 26] Distant failure can be 36 to 50% based on retrospective data.[26] Several studies have added chemotherapy to radiation therapy in an attempt to improve these results. This concept of treatment combining radiation with chemotherapy either alone or with esophagectomy has been used since the 1980s. The first nonrandomized study was from Wayne State University,[27] which showed that the combination of radiation therapy with chemotherapy (5-FU, mitomycin, or cisplatin) induced a pathologic complete response in local-regional disease. At the Fox Chase Cancer Center, Coia and associ-

ates[28] reported the results of 90 patients (both squamous cell carcinoma and adenocarcinoma), of whom 57 had stages I and II disease. Patients were treated with concurrent radiation, 50 to 60 Gy, and chemotherapy with 5-FU and mitomycin C. For stage I disease, the local control was 100% and overall survival 73% at 5 years. Combined stage I and stage II patients have local failure rates of 25% and actuarial survival of 30% at 5 years. There was no difference in survival between patients with squamous cell carcinoma and adenocarcinoma.

Poplin and coworkers[29] reported the results of a SWOG trial of 32 patients with squamous cell carcinoma and adenocarcinoma. They were treated using 50 Gy concomitant with 5-FU and cisplatin (two cycles followed by two additional cycles after completion of radiation). Surgery was used only for patients with residual local disease. Complete response was seen in 44% of patients. The median survival and 1-year survival were 20 months and 59%, respectively. The toxicity was severe, with four deaths noted.

Four randomized trials compared radiation therapy alone with combined chemoradiation (Table 40–4). Herskovic and colleagues[30, 31] reported an RTOG trial in 121 patients with squamous cell carcinoma or adenocarcinoma of the esophagus, in which the patients were randomized between radiation therapy alone (64 Gy) and CMT (50 Gy with two cycles of 5-FU and cisplatin given concurrently and two afterward). Median follow-up of 5 years showed a significant difference in median survival between the two treatment groups: 9 months for the radiation-alone group compared with 12.5 months for the CMT group. None of the radiation therapy–alone group survived at 5 years, compared with a 30% survival rate in the CMT group. The local failure rates were high in both groups: 44% (27 of 61) for the CMT group compared with 65% (39 of 60) in the radiation therapy–alone group. This randomized trial established the role of combined therapy—radiation therapy and chemotherapy (5-FU and cisplatin)—as a standard of care in unresectable esophageal cancers.

Roussel and associates[32] reported an EORTC trial in

*Table 40–4.* **Randomized Trials of Radiation Alone Versus Chemoradiotherapy**

| Series | Patients (No.) | Radiation | Chemotherapy | Local Failure (%) | Median Survival (mo) | Survival (%) |
|---|---|---|---|---|---|---|
| RTOG (Al-Saraf, 1997) | | | | | | |
| | 62 | 64 Gy/6 wk | | 68 | NA | 0 at 5 yr p = .0001 |
| | 61 | 50 Gy/5 wk | 5-FU + cisplatin | 45 | NA | 27 at 5 yr |
| EORTC (Roussel, 1988) | 69 | 56 Gy/6 wk | | NA | NA | 6 (3 yr) |
| | 75 | 56 Gy/6 wk | Methotrexate | NA | NA | 12 (3 yr) |
| ECOG (Sischy, 1990) | 117 | 60 Gy/6 wk (option of surgery after 40 Gy) | | NA | 9 | 12 (2 yr) |
| | | 60 Gy/6 wk | 5-FU + mitomycin | NA | p = .03 15 | 30 (2 yr) |
| Araujo (1991) | 31 | 50 Gy/5 wk | | 84 | NA | 6 (5 yr) |
| | 28 | 50 Gy/5 wk | 5-FU + mitomycin + bleomycin | 61 | NA | 16 (5 yr) |

5-FU, 5-fluorouracil; NA, not available.

which single-agent methotrexate plus 56 Gy was compared with a control group of radiation therapy alone. The two groups showed similar rates of response and survival. This poor result in the combination group could be from inadequate chemotherapy with subcutaneous methotrexate.

In the 1990s, Sischy and coworkers[33] reported an Eastern Cooperative Oncology Group (ECOG) trial in which 130 patients with squamous cell carcinoma were randomized between radiation therapy (40 Gy) alone versus concurrent CMT (40 Gy with 5-FU and mitomycin C). There was an option for surgery after 40 Gy (nonrandomized). Those who did not have surgery received an additional 20 Gy. A survival advantage was observed in the CMT group (15 months vs. 9 months), and the 2-year survivals were also more than double (30% vs. 12%). These results might have been influenced by the option of surgery in some patients.

Araujo and associates[34] from Brazil randomized 59 patients with squamous cell carcinoma of the esophagus to either radiation therapy alone, 50 Gy, versus CMT (50 Gy concurrent with 5-FU and mitomycin C, bleomycin). There was no statistical difference in response, and survival rates between the two groups were as follows: The 1-, 2-, and 3-year survival rates for the radiation therapy–alone arm were 55, 22, and 6%, respectively, versus 64, 38, and 16%, respectively, in the CMT group ($p = 0.16$). The poor outcome of the study could be the result of a small sample size or inadequate chemotherapy because only one cycle was used.

CMT is better than radiation alone. The 5-year survival rate appears to be similar (10 to 30%) compared with surgical series, however.[1-3] This nonsurgical approach to esophageal carcinoma is the treatment of choice for patients with medically inoperable disease or who have locally advanced (T3 N1) disease. Still the local failure is high (44%) and continues to be the dominant cause of mortality in esophageal carcinoma. New approaches have emerged in an attempt to maximize the cure rates, including multimodality therapy, dose acceleration, and neoadjuvant chemotherapy.

## PALLIATIVE TREATMENT

Patients with advanced-stage disease are usually treated palliatively with radiation, with or without chemotherapy. Radiation relieves dysphagia, which is the predominant presenting symptom of esophageal cancer, in 70 to 90% of patients within 1 month of the initiation of treatment.[25, 35] In most cases, radiation therapy also provides symptomatic relief from bone, liver, and brain metastases. Radiation also can be used as a salvage approach for patients whose disease recurs following surgery. In addition to external-beam therapy, laser surgery and intraluminal brachytherapy have been beneficial for treating patients with stenosis.

## NEWER MODALITIES

Intraluminal brachytherapy offers the advantage of increasing the radiation dose while protecting adjacent dose-limiting structures, such as the heart, lung, and spinal cord. It has been used as a sole treatment for early esophageal carcinoma, but currently it has been used primarily as a boost after external-beam therapy. It can be delivered by high dose rate or low dose rate. Several retrospective studies[36-38] using brachytherapy combined with external-beam radiation therapy plus chemotherapy have claimed improvement in local control and swallowing ability. In the RTOG 92-07 trial,[30] intraluminal brachytherapy (15 Gy in three fractions) with iridium 192 was used as a boost after 50 Gy external-beam therapy plus 5-FU and cisplatin. Treatment morbidity was 14%, with two deaths resulting from fistulas. Based on this finding, the authors urged extreme caution in employing brachytherapy as a boost following external-beam therapy.

In 1997, the American Brachytherapy Society[39] developed guidelines for the use of brachytherapy in patients with esophageal carcinoma under the following conditions: when the primary tumor is less than 10 cm in length, is confined to the esophageal wall, and lacks lymph node involvement or systemic disease. Brachytherapy should follow external-beam therapy and should not be given concurrent with chemotherapy.

Another way to increase the control rate is to use more than one daily fraction in doses smaller than conventional fractions (1.8 or 2 Gy). This theory is based on the concept that repopulation of surviving cells during fractionated radiation could be a major cause of failure. To overcome this repopulation effect, hyperfractionation or accelerated fractionation has been used in various tumor sites, mainly in head and neck tumors. In a preoperative setting, the University of Michigan[15] used accelerated fractionation, 1.5 Gy twice a day to 45 Gy, and reported acceptable morbidity. Also, Nishimura and colleagues[40] from Kyoto University evaluated the results of 88 patients with esophageal cancer treated with conventional fractionation (1.7 Gy/day, five fractions per week) or accelerated fractionation (1.5 Gy twice a day, 6-hour intervals). The local recurrence rate with accelerated fractionation was significantly less than with conventional fractionation (53% vs. 78%, $p < 0.05$). Twice-a-day fractionation produced a high incidence of esophageal stenosis, however.[41] Accelerated fractionation has shown a lower incidence of local recurrence, but it may also be more toxic than standard fractionation.

## REFERENCES

1. Ellis FH Jr, Heatley GJ, Krasna MJ, et al. Esophagectomy for carcinoma of the esophagus and cardia: a comparison of findings and results after standard resection in three consecutive 8-year intervals with improving staging criteria. J Thorac Cardiovasc Surg 1997;113:836–46.
2. Roth JA, Putnam JB Jr. Surgery for cancer of the esophagus. Semin Oncol 1994;21:453–61.
3. Altorki NK, Giraldi L, Skinner DB. En bloc esophagectomy improves survival for stage III esophageal cancer. J Thorac Cardiovasc Surg 1997;114:948–55.
4. Earlam R, Cunha-Melo JR. Oesophageal squamous cell carcinoma: I. A critical review of surgery. Br J Surg 1980;67:381–90.
5. Nygaard K, Hagen S, Hansen. HS, et al. Preoperative radiotherapy prolongs survival in operable esophageal carcinoma: a randomized, multicenter study of preoperative radiotherapy and chemotherapy (the second Scandinavian Trial in Esophageal Cancer). World J Surg 1992;16:1104–10.
6. Wang M, Gu XZ, Yin WB, et al. Randomized clinical trial on the combination of preoperative irradiation and surgery in the treatment of esophageal carcinoma: report on 206 patients. Int J Radiat Oncol Biol Phys 1989;16:325–7.
7. Gignoux M, Roussel A, Paillot B, et al. The value of preoperative radiotherapy in esophageal cancer: results of a study of the E.O.R.T.C. World J Surg 1987;11:426–32.

8. Launois B, Delarue D, Campion JP, Kerbaol M. Preoperative radiotherapy for carcinoma of the esophagus. Surg Gynecol Obstet 1981;153:690–2.
9. Arnott SJ, Duncan W, Kerr GR, et al. Low dose pre-operative radiotherapy for carcinoma of the esophagus: results of a randomized clinical trial. Radiother Oncol 1992;24:108–13.
10. Leichman L, Steiger Z, Seydel HG, Vaitkevicius VK. Combined preoperative chemotherapy and radiation therapy for cancer of the esophagus: the Wayne State University, Southwest Oncology Group and Radiation Therapy Oncology Group experience. Semin Oncol 1984;11:178–85.
11. Poplin E, Fleming T, Leichman L, et al. Combined therapies for squamous-cell carcinoma of the esophagus, a Southwest Oncology Group Study (SWOG 8037). J Clin Oncol 1987;5:622–8.
12. Forastiere A, Orringer MB, Perez-Tamayo C, et al. Concurrent chemotherapy and radiation therapy followed by transhiatal esophagectomy for local-regional cancer of the esophagus. J Clin Oncol 1990;8:119–27.
13. Forastiere AA, Heitmiller R, Lee DJ, et al. A four-week intensive preoperative chemoradiation program for locoregional cancer of the esophagus. Proc ASCO 1994;13:195.
14. Meluch A, Hainsworth JD, Thomas M, et al. Preoperative therapy with pacitaxel, carbo, 5-FU, and radiation yields 69 percent pathologic complete response rate in the treatment of local esophageal carcinoma. Proc ASCO 1997;16:261a.
15. Urba S, Orringer M, Turrisi A, et al. A randomized trial comparing surgery to preoperative concomitant chemoradiation plus surgery in patients with resectable esophageal cancer—updated analysis. Proc ASCO 1997;16:277a. abstract.
16. Bossett J, Gignoux M, Triboulet J, et al. Randomized phase III clinical trial comparing surgery alone versus preoperative combined radiochemotherapy in stage I–II epidermoid carcinoma of the thoracic esophagus: preliminary analysis, a study of the French group. Proc ASCO 1994;13:197.
17. Walsh TN, Noonan N, Hollywood D, et al. A comparison of multimodal therapy and surgery for esophageal adenocarcinoma. N Engl J Med 1996;225:462–7.
18. Le Prise E, Etienne P, Meunier B, et al. A randomized study of chemotherapy, radiation therapy, and surgery versus surgery for localized squamous cell carcinoma of the esophagus. Cancer 1994;73:1779–84.
19. Apinop C, Puttisak P, Preecha N. A prospective study of combined therapy in esophageal cancer. Hepatogastroenterology 1994;41:391–3.
20. Kasai M, Mori S, Watanabe T. Follow-up results after resection of thoracic esophageal cancer. World J Surg 1978;2:543–51.
21. Teniere P, Hay JM, Fingerhut A, Fagniez PL. Postoperative radiation therapy does not increase survival after curative resection for squamous cell carcinoma of the middle and lower esophagus as shown by a multicenter controlled trial. French University Association for Surgical Research. Surg Gynecol Obstet 1991;173:123–30.
22. Fok M, Sham JS, Choy D, et al. Postoperative radiotherapy for carcinoma of the esophagus: a prospective, randomized controlled study. Surgery 1993;113:138–47.
23. Iizuka T, Ide H, Kakegawa T, et al. Preoperative radioactive therapy for esophageal carcinoma: randomized evaluation trial in eight institutions. Chest 1988;93:1054–8.
24. Langer M, Choi NC, Orlow E, et al. Radiation therapy alone or in combination with surgery in the treatment of carcinoma of the esophagus. Cancer 1986;58:1208–13.
25. Earlam R, Cunha-Melo JR: Oesophageal squamous cell carcinoma: II. A critical review of radiotherapy. Br J Surg 1980;67:457–61.
26. Smalley SR, Gunderson LL, Reddy EK, Williamson S. Radiotherapy alone in esophageal carcinoma: current management and future directions of adjuvant, curative and palliative approaches. Semin Oncol 1994;21:467–73.
27. Leichman L, Steiger Z, Seydel HG, et al. Preoperative chemotherapy and radiation therapy for patients with cancer of the esophagus: a potentially curative approach. J Clin Oncol 1984;2:75–9.
28. Coia LR, Engstrom PF, Paul AR, et al. Long-term results of infusional 5-FU, mitomycin C, and radiation: a primary management of esophageal cancer. Int J Radiat Oncol Biol Phys 1991;20:29–36.
29. Poplin E, Jacobson J, Herskovic A, et al. Evaluation of multimodality treatment of locoregional esophageal carcinoma by SWOG Group 9060. Cancer 1996;78:1851–6.
30. Herskovic A, Martz K, al-Sarraf M, et al. Combined chemotherapy and radiotherapy compared with radiotherapy alone in patients with cancer of the esophagus. N Engl J Med 1992;326:1593–8.
31. al-Sarraf M, Martz K, Herskovic A, et al. Progress report of combined chemoradiotherapy versus radiotherapy alone in patients with esophageal cancer: an intergroup study. J Clin Oncol 1997;15:277–84, 866.
32. Roussel A, Jacob JH, Haegele P, et al. Controlled clinical trial for the treatment of patients with inoperable esophageal carcinoma: a study of EORTC Gastrointestinal Tract Cancer Cooperative Group. Recent Results Cancer Res 1988;110:21–30.
33. Sischy B, Ryan L, Haller D, et al. Interim report of EST-1282 Phase III protocol for the evaluation of combined modalities in the treatment of patients with carcinoma of the esophagus, stage II and I. Proc ASCO 1990;9:105.
34. Araujo CM, Souhami L, Gil RA, et al. A randomized trial comparing radiation therapy versus concomitant radiation therapy and chemotherapy in carcinoma of the thoracic esophagus. Cancer 1991;67:2258–61.
35. Hancock SL, Glatstein E. Radiation therapy of esophageal cancer. Semin Oncol 1984;11:144–58.
36. Caspers R, Zwinderman A, Griffioen G, et al. Combined external beam and low dose rate intraluminal radiotherapy in oesophageal cancer. Radiother Oncol 1993;27:7–12.
37. Hyden EC, Langholz B, Tilden T, et al. External beam and intraluminal radiotherapy in the treatment of carcinoma of the esophagus. J Thorac Cardiovasc Surg 1988;96:237–41.
38. Hishikawa Y, Kurisu K, Taniguchi M, et al. High dose rate intraluminal brachytherapy for esophageal cancer: 10 year experience in Hyogo College of Medicine. Radiother Oncol 1991;21:107–14.
39. Gaspar L, Nag S, Herskovic A, et al. American Brachytherapy Society (ABS) consensus guidelines for brachytherapy of esophageal cancer. Int J Radiat Oncol Biol Phys 1997;38:127–32.
40. Nishimura Y, Ono K, Tsutsui K, et al. Esophageal cancer treated with radiotherapy: impact of total treatment time and fractionation. Int J Radiat Oncol Biol Phys 1994;30:1099–105.
41. Kikuchi Y. [Study on clinical application of multiple fractions per day radiation therapy with concomitant boost technique for esophageal cancer]. Hokkaido Igaku Zasshi 1993;68:537–56.

····································

# CHEMOTHERAPY FOR ESOPHAGEAL CANCER

• Carol Nishikubo • Charles M. Haskell

## SINGLE-AGENT CHEMOTHERAPY

There is no established role for single-agent chemotherapy in the management of esophageal carcinoma, including both adenocarcinomas and squamous cell carcinomas, which are generally treated in an identical fashion. Relatively few drugs are active against esophageal cancer (Table 40–5), and responses tend to be of short duration.[1-8] Single-agent chemotherapy is not recommended as first-line therapy for esophageal cancer except in the setting of a clinical trial of a new investigational agent.

## COMBINATION CHEMOTHERAPY

The precise role of combination chemotherapy and the optimal agents remains a matter of controversy in treating esoph-

*Table 40–5.* **Single Agents with Greater than 20% Response Rates in Esophageal Cancer**

| Agent | Response Rate (% CR + PR) |
|---|---|
| 5-Fluorouracil | 42 |
| Methotrexate | 34 |
| Paclitaxel | 28–34 |
| Cisplatin | 8–32 |
| Mitomycin | 26 |

CR, complete response; PR, partial response.
Data from references 1–8.

ageal malignancies. Table 40–6 summarizes the results of treatment with combination chemotherapy regimens in patients with measurable disease.[2, 5, 9–25] The combination of cisplatin and 5-FU with or without an anthracycline is one of the more commonly used regimens. Typical doses are 100 mg/m² of cisplatin intravenously on day 1 with 1000 mg/m²/day of 5-FU by continuous infusion on days 1 to 5, with the cycle being repeated every 3 weeks. Early data adding paclitaxel as another component of therapy have been encouraging, with high response rates[26] and high 1-year actuarial survival rates of 82%,[27] but follow-up on these patients has typically been short.

## COMBINED-MODALITY THERAPY

**Neoadjuvant Therapy for Operable Disease.** Studies of neoadjuvant chemotherapy or chemoradiotherapy followed by definitive surgery or radiation therapy have shown high response rates to initial treatment but a less definitive impact on overall survival.[28–45] The only study[42] showing a survival advantage in the CMT arm has been criticized for the low survival rates in the surgery-alone arm, the lack of the use of endoscopic ultrasonography for staging, and the lack of routine CT for staging.[43] Neoadjuvant chemoradiotherapy is discussed further in the preceding subchapter Radiation

Therapy for Esophageal Carcinoma. Randomized clinical trials of surgery alone versus preoperative, neoadjuvant chemotherapy alone are summarized in Table 40–7.[31, 34, 35, 39, 46–50]

**Postoperative Adjuvant Chemotherapy.** Studies examining the role of adjuvant chemotherapy or chemoradiotherapy following surgery have been disappointing. Nonrandomized studies have not shown a difference in survival in patients treated with adjuvant therapy compared with historical controls of patients treated with primary therapy alone.[51] Table 40–8 summarizes the results of randomized trials comparing surgery (alone or with postoperative radiation therapy) with surgery followed by chemotherapy.[52–54] These studies showed no benefit from the use of postoperative adjuvant chemotherapy with cisplatin-based combinations.

**Unresectable, Locally Advanced Esophageal Carcinoma.** Several studies have shown that preoperative chemotherapy or chemoradiotherapy can convert inoperable disease to operable disease.[55–61] Survival in some of these studies compares favorably with historical controls[56, 61]; however, there is no prospective randomized, controlled study that shows a survival advantage to this course of treatment.[37] Studies of CMT compared with CMT followed by surgery have shown no definite benefit to the addition of surgery after chemoradiotherapy,[62] although this remains to be proved in a large, randomized, prospective trial.

CMT with chemotherapy and radiation therapy is generally thought to be superior to either modality alone for palliation of symptoms and survival for patients with unresectable, locally advanced disease.[63–65] Carboplatin has been inferior in some studies in terms of survival compared with studies using cisplatin-based combinations,[66] although there has not been a direct comparison in a phase III trial of these agents.

## IMMUNOTHERAPY

Immunotherapy with a variety of agents has been increasingly studied in patients with cancer of the esophagus. Some of the more encouraging results have been seen with OK432.

*Table 40–6.* **Combination Chemotherapy for Esophageal Cancer**

| Drugs | Patients (No.) | Response (%) | Reference |
|---|---|---|---|
| Cisplatin + methotrexate | 42 | 76 | 3 |
| Cisplatin + fluorouracil + methotrexate | 34 | 71 | 9 |
| Cisplatin + vincristine + methotrexate + leucovorin | 28 | 68 | 10 |
| Cisplatin + fluorouracil + bleomycin | 38 | 61 | 5 |
| Cisplatin + epirubicin + fluorouracil (CI) | 235 | 61 | 11 |
| Cisplatin + fluorouracil | 229 | 52 | 5, 12, 13, 46 |
| Cisplatin + doxorubicin + etoposide | 26 | 50 | 14 |
| Cisplatin + fluorouracil + etoposide | 35 | 49 | 15 |
| Cisplatin (high dose) + etoposide | 27 | 48 | 16 |
| Cisplatin + etoposide | 73 | 48 | 17 |
| Cisplatin + mitomycin + bleomycin | 53 | 45 | 18 |
| Cisplatin + epirubicin + fluorouracil | 137 | 45 | 19 |
| Cisplatin + fluorouracil (CI) + allopurinol | 37 | 35 | 20 |
| Cisplatin + fluorouracil + doxorubicin | 21 | 33 | 21 |
| Cisplatin + methotrexate + bleomycin | 41 | 32 | 22 |
| Fluorouracil + interferon-α | 60 | 27 | 23, 24 |
| Cisplatin + bleomycin | 115 | 26 | 5 |
| Cyclophosphamide + doxorubicin | 24 | 25 | 25 |

CI, continuous infusion.

*Table 40–7.* **Randomized Trials of Preoperative Chemotherapy for Esophageal Cancer**

| Reference | Location or Group | Accrual Period | Treatment | Patients (No.) | Resectability Rate (%) | Mortality Rate (%) | Median Survival (mo) | Survival | Significance (p) |
|---|---|---|---|---|---|---|---|---|---|
| Roth et al[34] | U.S. | 1982–1986 | Surgery alone | 20 | — | — | 9 | 5% at 3 yr | |
| | | | Cisplatin + bleomycin + vindesine → surgery | 19 | — | — | 9 | 25% at 3 yr | NS |
| Nygaard et al[46] | Scandinavia II | 1983–1988 | Surgery alone | 41 | 69 | 13* | | 9% at 3 yr | |
| | | | Cisplatin + bleomycin → surgery | 50 | 58 | 15* | | 3% at 3 yr | NS |
| Schlag[35] | Germany | | Surgery alone | 24 | 79 | (14)†‡ | 8 | 25% at 1 yr | |
| | | | 5-FU + cisplatin → surgery | 22 | 61 | (24)†‡ | 5 | 18% at 1 yr | NS |
| Maipang et al[47] | Thailand | 1988–1990 | Surgery alone | 22 | — | — | 17 | 36% at 3 yr | |
| | | | Cisplatin + bleomycin + vinblastine → surgery | 24 | — | — | 17 | 31% at 3 yr | NS |
| Ancona et al[48] | Padua | | Surgery alone | 43 | 86 | 5† | | | |
| | | | 5-FU + cisplatin → surgery | 35 | 78 | 7† | | | |
| Law et al[39] | Hong Kong | 1989–1995 | Surgery alone | 73 | 95 | 9† | 13 | 31% at 2 yr | |
| | | | 5-FU + cisplatin → surgery | 74 | 89 | 8† | 17 | 44% at 2 yr | NS |
| Kelsen et al[49] | Intergroup 113 | | Surgery alone | 221 | 66 | — | 17 | 40% at 2 yr | |
| | | | 5-FU + cisplatin → surgery | 202 | 65 | — | 16 | 38% at 2 yr | NS |
| Kok et al[50] | Rotterdam | 1990–1996 | Surgery alone | 74 | 85 | — | 11 | | |
| | | | Cisplatin + etoposide → surgery | 74 | 85 | — | 9 | | 0.002 |

*30-day mortality rate.
†Hospital mortality rate.
‡Randomized plus nonrandomized patients.
NS, not significant; 5-FU, 5-fluorouracil.
Modified from Lehnert T. Multimodal therapy for squamous carcinoma of the oesophagus. Br J Surg 1999;86:727–39.

This agent is thought to exert its effect by stimulation of T-killer cells, natural killer cells, and neutrophils. In a pilot study of 73 patients (18.6% T1, 34.3% T2–T3, 47.1% T4) treated with radiation therapy and endoscopic administration of OK432, 49 patients had a complete response and 21 had a partial response.[67] Overall survival was 20.8% at 5 years; 5-year survival in the complete responders was 44.9% as compared with the partial responders, none of whom lived more than 2 years.

Another agent thought to improve host immune function, protein-bound polysaccharide K (PSK), has been studied in a randomized trial of postoperative chemoradiation therapy alone versus chemoradiation therapy plus PSK.[68] This study showed no difference in survival between the two groups.

Interferon alfa has been used in combination with chemotherapy in phase II studies of patients with advanced disease with a 50% response rate,[69] with median survival in these patients of 33 weeks. Other studies have shown high response rates[70] of 65% but median survival rates of only 8 to 9 months.

## PHOTODYNAMIC THERAPY

The role of photodynamic therapy in early-stage and precancerous lesions has been increasingly studied. Typically a photosensitizing agent is administered intravenously 1 to 2 days before phototherapy. The photosensitizer accumulates in the tumor cells, making them more susceptible to damage by laser therapy at certain wavelengths.

A small study was conducted in 32 patients with Barrett's esophagus[71] with either high-grade dysplasia (10 patients) or cancer confined to the mucosa (22 patients) treated with 5-aminolevulinic acid as a photosensitizer followed by dye laser therapy at a 635-nm wavelength at a dose of 150 J/cm$^2$. Treatment resulted in 100% eradication of the dysplastic lesions and elimination of 77% (17 of 22) of the mucosal tumors, although follow-up was short (9.9 months). All tumors less than or equal to 2 mm in thickness were ablated. There was no associated mortality or morbidity.

In a study of photodynamic therapy treating patients in whom prior therapy had failed or who were ineligible for other treatment, overall survival was 6.3 months.[72] In a large retrospective study of 123 patients who were not surgical candidates and were treated with photodynamic therapy, 87% achieved a complete response with a 5-year survival of 25%. No difference was observed in patients receiving chemotherapy or radiation therapy in addition to the photodynamic therapy.[73]

## HYPERTHERMIA

Treatment of esophageal malignancies with hyperthermia has been used largely in combination with chemotherapy

**Table 40–8.** Randomized Clinical Trials of Postoperative Chemotherapy for Esophageal Carcinoma

| Reference | Location or Group | Accrual Period | Stage | Treatment | Patients (No.) | Median Survival (mo) | Survival | Significance (p) |
|---|---|---|---|---|---|---|---|---|
| JEOG[52] | Japan | 1985–1987 | I–IV | Surgery + 50 Gy | 128 | NA | 50% at 3 yr | |
| | | | | Surgery + vindesine + cisplatin | 130 | NA | 52% at 5 yr | NS |
| Pouliquen et al[53] | France | 1987–1992 | IIb–III | Surgery alone | 38 | 20 | 17% at 5 yr | |
| | | | | Surgery + 5-FU + cisplatin | 24 | 20 | 10% at 5 yr | NS |
| Ando et al[54] | Japan (JEOG) | 1988–1991 | I–IV | Surgery alone | 100 | NA | 45% at 5 yr | |
| | | | | Surgery + vindesine + cisplatin | 105 | NA | 48% at 5 yr | NS |

JEOG, Japanese Esophageal Oncology Group; NA, not available; NS, not significant.
Modified from Lehnert T. Multimodal therapy for squamous carcinoma of the oesophagus. Br J Surg 1999;86:727–39.

and chemoradiotherapy. Hyperthermia combined with chemoradiotherapy has been used preoperatively to convert inoperable tumors to operable ones.[74] Trials comparing chemoradiotherapy alone to chemoradiotherapy with the addition of hyperthermia suggest a possible increase in long-term survival, with 3-year survival rates of 50% in the hyperthermia arm versus 24% in the chemoradiotherapy arm.[75] Studies of hyperthermia combined with chemoradiotherapy in a neoadjuvant setting also suggest a possible long-term survival advantage to the hyperthermia arm.[76] Further studies are needed to define the potential role of hyperthermia outside the setting of a clinical trial.

## REFERENCES

1. Ezdinli EZ, Gelber R, Desai DV, et al. Chemotherapy of advanced esophageal carcinoma: Eastern Cooperative Oncology Group experience. Cancer 1980;46:2149–53.
2. Lokich JJ, Shea M, Chaffey J. Sequential infusional 5-fluorouracil followed by concomitant radiation for tumors of the esophagus and gastroesophageal junction. Cancer 1987;60:275–9.
3. Advani SH, Saikia TK, Swaroop S, et al. Anterior chemotherapy in esophageal cancer. Cancer 1985;56:1502–6.
4. Ajani JA, Ilson DH, Daugherty K, et al. Activity of taxol in patients with squamous cell carcinoma and adenocarcinoma of the esophagus. J Natl Cancer Inst 1994;86:1086–91.
5. Kelsen D, Atiq OT. Therapy of upper gastrointestinal tract cancers. Curr Probl Cancer 1991;15:235–94.
6. Desai PB, Borges EJ, Vohra VG, et al. Carcinoma of the esophagus in India. Cancer 1969;23:979–89.
7. Whittington RM, Close HP. Clinical experience with mitomycin C. Cancer Chemother Rep 1970;54:195–8.
8. Engstrom PF, Lavin PT, Klaassen DJ. Phase II evaluation of mitomycin C and cisplatin in advanced esophageal carcinoma. Cancer Treat Rep 1983;67:713–5.
9. Lester EP, Pate JW, Memula NG, et al. Esophageal carcinoma: results of initial chemotherapy with methotrexate, leucovorin, cisplatinum, and 5-fluorouracil. Proc ASCO 1990;9:115.
10. Resbeut M, Le Prise-Fleury E, Ben-Hassel M, et al. Squamous cell carcinoma of the esophagus: treatment by combined vincristine, methotrexate and folinic acid rescue and cisplatin before radiotherapy. Cancer 1985;56:1246–50.
11. Bamias A, Hill ME, Cunningham D, et al. Epirubicin, cisplatin, and protracted venous infusion of 5-fluorouracil for esophagogastric adenocarcinoma: response, toxicity, quality of life and survival. Cancer 1996;77:1978–85.
12. Carey RW, Hilgenberg AD, Choi NC, et al. A pilot study of neoadjuvant chemotherapy with 5-fluorouracil and cisplatin with surgical resection and postoperative radiation therapy and/or chemotherapy in adenocarcinoma of the esophagus. Cancer 1991;68:489–92.
13. Ajani JA, Ryan B, Rich TA, et al. Prolonged chemotherapy for localised squamous carcinoma of the oesophagus. Eur J Cancer 1992;28A:880–4.
14. Ajani JA, Roth JA, Ryan MB, et al. Intensive preoperative chemother-
apy with colony stimulating factor for resectable adenocarcinoma of the esophagus or gastroesophageal junction. J Clin Oncol 1993;11:22–8.
15. Ajani JA, Roth JA, Ryan B, et al. Evaluation of pre and post operative chemotherapy for resectable adenocarcinoma of the esophagus or gastroesophageal junction. J Clin Oncol 1990;8:1231–8.
16. Spiridonidis CH, Laufman LR, Jones JJ, et al. A phase II evaluation of high dose cisplatin and etoposide in patients with advanced esophageal adenocarcinoma. Cancer 1996;78:2070–7.
17. Kok TC, Van der Gaast A, Dees J, et al. Cisplatin and etoposide in oesophageal cancer: a phase II study. Br J Cancer 1996;74:980–4.
18. Lad TE, Kukla LJ, Haas AJ, et al. Multimodality treatment of squamous cell carcinoma of the esophagus. Proc ASCO 1983;2:115.
19. Webb A, Cunningham D, Scarffe JH, et al. Randomized trial comparing epirubicin, cisplatin and fluorouracil versus fluorouracil, doxorubicin and methotrexate in advanced esophagogastric cancer. J Clin Oncol 1997;15:261–7.
20. De Besi P, Sileni VC, Salvagno L, et al. Phase II study of cisplatin, 5-fluorouracil, and allopurinol in advanced esophageal cancer. Cancer Treat Rep 1986;70:909–10.
21. Gisselbrecht C, Calvo F, Mignot L, et al. Fluorouracil (F), adriamycin (A), and cisplatin (P) (FAP): combination chemotherapy of advanced esophageal carcinoma. Cancer 1983;52:974–7.
22. Vogl SE, Greenwald E, Kaplan BH. Effective chemotherapy for esophageal cancer with methotrexate, bleomycin and cis-diamminedichloroplatinum II. Cancer 1981;48:2555–8.
23. Kelsen D, Lovett D, Wong J, et al. Interferon alfa-2a and fluorouracil in the treatment of patients with advanced esophageal cancer. J Clin Oncol 1992;10:269–74.
24. Wadler S, Fell S, Haynes H, et al. Treatment of carcinoma of the esophagus with 5-fluorouracil and recombinant alfa-2a-interferon. Cancer 1993;71:1726–30.
25. Nicolaou N, Conlan AA. Cyclophosphamide, doxorubicin and celestin intubation for inoperable oesophageal carcinoma. S Afr Med J 1982;61:428–31.
26. Ilson DH, Ajani J, Bhalla K, et al. Phase II trial of paclitaxel, fluorouracil and cisplatin in patients with advanced carcinoma of the esophagus. J Clin Oncol 1998;16:1826–34.
27. Belani CP, Luketich JD, Landreneau RJ, et al. Efficacy of cisplatin, 5-fluorouracil and paclitaxel regimen for carcinoma of the esophagus. Semin Oncol 1997;24:Suppl 19:S19-89–92.
28. Kun LE, Toohill RJ, Holoye PY, et al. A randomized study of adjuvant chemotherapy for cancer of the upper aerodigestive tract. Int J Radiat Oncol Biol Phys 1986;12:173–8.
29. Andersen AP, Berdal P, Edsmyr F, et al. Irradiation, chemotherapy and surgery in esophageal cancer: a randomized clinical study: the first Scandinavian trial in esophageal cancer. Radiother Oncol 1984;2:179–88.
30. Hatlevoll R, Hagen S, Hansen HS, et al. Bleomycin/cis-platin as neoadjuvant chemotherapy before radical radiotherapy in localized, inoperable carcinoma of the esophagus: a prospective randomized multicentre study: the second Scandinavian trial in esophageal cancer. Radiother Oncol 1992;24:114–6.
31. Kelsen DP, Minsky B, Smith M, et al. Preoperative therapy for esophageal cancer: a randomized comparison of chemotherapy versus radiation therapy. J Clin Oncol 1990;8:1352–61.
32. Roussel A, Bleiberg H, Dalesio O, et al. Palliative therapy of inoperable oesophageal carcinoma with radiotherapy and methotrexate: final re-

sults of a controlled clinical trial. Int J Radiat Oncol Biol Phys 1989;16:67–72.

33. Araujo CM, Souhami L, Gil RA, et al. A randomized trial comparing radiation therapy versus concomitant radiation therapy and chemotherapy in carcinoma of the thoracic esophagus. Cancer 1991;67:2258–61.

34. Roth JA, Pass HI, Flanagan MM, et al. Randomized clinical trial of preoperative and postoperative adjuvant chemotherapy with cisplatin, vindesine, and bleomycin for carcinoma of the esophagus. J Thorac Cardiovasc Surg 1988;96:242–8.

35. Schlag PM. Randomized trial of preoperative chemotherapy for squamous cell cancer of the esophagus. The Chirurgische Arbeitsgemeinschaft für Onkologie der deutschen Gesellschaft für Chirurgie Study Group. Arch Surg 1992;127:1446–50.

36. Le Prise E, Etienne PL, Meunier B, et al. A randomized study of chemotherapy, radiation therapy and surgery versus surgery for localized squamous cell carcinoma of the esophagus. Cancer 1994;73:1779–84.

37. Burmeister BH, Denham JW, O'Brien M, et al. Combined modality treatment for esophageal carcinoma: preliminary results from a large Australasian multicenter study. Int J Radiat Oncol Biol Phys 1995;32:997–1006.

38. Bosset JF, Gignoux M, Triboulet JP, et al. Chemoradiotherapy followed by surgery compared with surgery alone in squamous-cell cancer of the esophagus. N Engl J Med 1997;337:161–7.

39. Law S, Fod M, Chow S, et al. Preoperative chemotherapy versus surgical therapy alone for squamous cell carcinoma of the esophagus: a prospective randomized trial. J Thorac Cardiovasc Surg 1997; 114:210–17.

40. al-Sarraf M, Martz K, Herskovic A, et al. Progress report of combination chemoradiotherapy versus radiotherapy alone in patients with esophageal cancer: an intergroup study. J Clin Oncol 1997;15:277–84.

41. Sischy B, Ryan L, Haller D, et al. Interim report of EST 1282 Phase III protocol for the evaluation of combined modalities in the treatment of patients with carcinoma of the esophagus. Proc ASCO 1990;9:105.

42. Walsh TN, Noonan N, Hollywood D, et al. A comparison of multimodal therapy and surgery for esophageal adenocarcinoma. N Engl J Med 1996;335:462–7.

43. Wilke H, Fink U. Multimodal therapy for adenocarcinoma of the esophagus and esophagogastric junction. N Engl J Med 1996;335:509–10. editorial.

44. Estes NC, Stauffer J, Romberg M, et al. Squamous cell carcinoma of the esophagus. Am Surg 1996;62:573–6.

45. Minsky BD, Neuberg D, Kelsen DP, et al. Final report of Intergroup Trial 0122 (ECOG PE-289, RTOG 90-12): phase II trial of neoadjuvant chemotherapy plus concurrent chemotherapy and high-dose radiation for squamous cell carcinoma of the esophagus. Int J Radiat Oncol Biol Phys 1999;43:517–23.

46. Nygaard K, Hagen S, Hansen HS, et al. Pre-operative radiotherapy prolongs survival in operable esophageal carcinoma: a randomized, multicenter study of pre-operative radiotherapy and chemotherapy: the second Scandinavian trial in esophageal cancer. World J Surg 1992;16:1104–10.

47. Maipang T, Vasinanukorn P, Petpichetchian C, et al. Induction chemotherapy in the treatment of patients with carcinoma of the esophagus. J Surg Oncol 1994;56:191–7.

48. Ancona E, Ruol A, Chiarion-Sileni V, et al. Studio prospettico randomizzato di chemioterapia neoadjuvante versus sola chirurgia nel cancro operabile (T2–3, ongi N, M0) dell'esophago. Acta Chir Ital 1995;51:308–17.

49. Kelsen DP, Ginsberg R, Qian C, et al. Chemotherapy followed by operation versus operation alone in the treatment of patients with localized esophageal cancer: a preliminary report of Intergroup study 113 (RTOG 89-11). Proc ASCO 1997;17:982.

50. Kok TC, van Lanschot J, Siersema PD, et al. Neoadjuvant chemotherapy in operable squamous cell cancer: final report of a phase III multicenter randomised trial. Proc ASCO 1997;17:984.

51. Mukaida H, Hirai T, Yamashita Y, et al. Clinical evaluation of adjuvant chemoradiotherapy with CDDP, 5-FU, and VP-16 for advanced esophageal cancer. Nippon Kyobu Geka Gakkai Zasshi 1998;46:11–7.

52. Japanese Esophageal Oncology Group. A comparison of chemotherapy and radiotherapy as adjuvant therapy to surgery for esophageal carcinoma. Chest 1993;104:203–7.

53. Pouliquen X, Levard H, Hay JM, et al. 5-Fluorouracil and cisplatin therapy after palliative surgical resection of squamous cell carcinoma of the esophagus: a multicenter randomized trial. Ann Surg 1996;223:127–33.

54. Ando N, Iizuka T, Kakegawa T, et al. A randomized trial of surgery with and without chemotherapy for localized squamous carcinoma of the thoracic esophagus: the Japan Clinical Oncology Group study. J Thorac Cardiovasc Surg 1997;114:205–9.

55. Naunheim KS, Petruska PJ, Roy TS, et al. Multimodality therapy for adenocarcinoma of the esophagus. Ann Thorac Surg 1995;59:1085–91.

56. Vogel SB, Mendenhall WM, Sombeck MD, et al. Downstaging of esophageal cancer after preoperative radiation and chemotherapy. Ann Surg 1995;221:685–95.

57. Plukker JTM, Sleijferz DT, Verschueren RCJ, et al. Neoadjuvant chemotherapy with carboplatin, 4-epiadriamycin and teniposide (CET) in locally advanced cancer of the cardia and lower oesophagus: a phase II study. Anticancer Res 1995;15:2357–62.

58. Melcher AA, Mort D, Maughan TS. Epirubicin, cisplatin and continuous infusion 5-FU (ECF) as neoadjuvant chemotherapy in gastro-oesophageal cancer. Br J Cancer 1996;74:1651–4.

59. Ohwada S, Nakamura S, Izumi M, et al. Neoadjuvant chemotherapy with etoposide, leucovorin, 5-FU and cisplatin for advanced esophageal squamous cell carcinoma. Jpn J Clin Oncol 1995;25:79–85.

60. Ganem G, Dubray B, Raoul Y, et al. Concomitant chemoradiotherapy followed, where feasible, by surgery for cancer of the esophagus. J Clin Oncol 1997;15:701–11.

61. Ancona E, Ruol A, Castoro C, et al. First-line chemotherapy improves the resection rate and long-term survival of locally advanced (T4, any N, M0) squamous cell carcinoma of the thoracic esophagus: final report on 163 consecutive patients with 5-year follow-up. Ann Surg 1997;226:714–24.

62. Algan O, Coia LR, Keller SM, et al. Management of adenocarcinoma of the esophagus with chemoradiation alone or chemoradiation followed by esophagectomy: results of sequential nonrandomized phase II studies. Int J Radiat Oncol Biol Phys 1995;32:753–61.

63. Sakai K, Inakoshi H, Sueyama H, et al. Concurrent radiotherapy and chemotherapy with protracted continuous infusion of 5-FU in inoperable esophageal squamous cell carcinoma. Int J Radiat Oncol Biol Phys 1995;31:921–7.

64. Reddy SP, Lad T, Mullane M, et al. Radiotherapy alone compared with radiotherapy and chemotherapy in patients with squamous cell carcinoma of the esophagus. Am J Clin Oncol 1995;18:376–81.

65. Herskovic A, Martz K, Al-Sarraf M, et al. Combined chemotherapy and radiotherapy compared with radiotherapy alone in patients with cancer of the esophagus. N Engl J Med 1992;326:1593–8.

66. Urba SG, Turrisi AT. Split course accelerated radiation therapy combined with carboplatin and 5-FU for palliation of metastatic or unresectable carcinoma of the esophagus. Cancer 1995;75:435–9.

67. Mukai M, Kubota S, Morita S, et al. A pilot study of combination therapy of radiation and local administration of OK432 for esophageal cancer. Cancer 1995;75:2276–80.

68. Ogoshi K, Satou H, Isono K, et al. Immunotherapy for esophageal cancer: a randomized trial in combination with radiotherapy and radiochemotherapy. Am J Clin Oncol 1995;18:216–22.

69. Ilson DH, Sirott M, Saltz L, et al. A phase II trial of interferon alpha-2A, 5-FU and cisplatin in patients with advanced esophageal carcinoma. Cancer 1995;75:2197–202.

70. Wadler S, Haynes H, Beitler JJ, et al. Phase II clinical trial with 5-FU, recombinant IFN-α-2b and cisplatin for patient with metastatic or regionally advanced carcinoma of the esophagus. Cancer 1996;78:30–4.

71. Gossner L, Stolte M, Sroka R, et al. Photodynamic ablation of high-grade dysplasia and early cancer in Barrett's esophagus by means of 5-aminolevulinic acid. Gastroenterology 1998;114:448–55.

72. McCaughan JS Jr, Ellison EC, Guy JT, et al. Photodynamic treatment for esophageal malignancy: a prospective 12 year study. Ann Thorac Surg 1996;62:1005–10.

73. Sibille A, Lambert R, Souquet JC, et al. Long term survival after photodynamic therapy for esophageal cancer. Gastroenterology 1995;108:337–44.

74. Sakamoto T, Katoh H, Shimizu T, et al. Clinical results of treatment of advanced esophageal carcinoma with hyperthermia in combination with chemoradiotherapy. Chest 1997;112:1487–93.

75. Kitamura K, Kuwano H, Watanabe M, et al. Prospective randomized study of hyperthermia combined with chemoradiotherapy for esophageal carcinoma. J Surg Oncol 1995;60:55–8.

76. Kuwano H, Sumiyoshi K, Watanabe M, et al. Preoperative hyperthermia combined with chemotherapy and irradiation for the treatment of patients with esophageal carcinoma. Tumori 1995;81:18–22.

# TREATMENT OF ESOPHAGEAL CANCER BY STAGE OF DISEASE

• Carol Nishikubo • Charles M. Haskell

## OVERVIEW OF TREATMENT

The optimal management of esophageal cancer depends on the expertise of a variety of specialists. Commonly the diagnosis is established by a gastroenterologist, who performs the initial esophagoscopy and biopsy. When the patient presents with obstructive symptoms, initial therapy may involve endoscopic dilatation, with or without the placement of a stent,[1, 2] or endoscopic laser therapy.[3–6] These techniques may be repeated for palliation, as needed. When laser therapy is chosen, the procedure is usually done under intravenous sedation. The best results may be expected in patients with inoperable exophytic mucosal tumors less than 5 cm in length, especially in a straight part of the midesophagus. Because it is often difficult to identify the esophageal lumen in these patients, treatment is often spread over several sessions, letting necrotic tissue slough before retreating. There is a small risk of perforation, and the mortality rate for the procedure itself appears to be about 5%. Most important, palliation is immediate in most patients. Endoscopic therapy is likely to play an increasing role in the management of this disease.[7]

Definitive management decisions for patients with invasive esophageal cancer involve the use of surgery, radiation therapy, chemotherapy, or some combination of these modalities. When possible, we advise that patients with esophageal cancer be offered the opportunity to participate in a clinical trial that provides state-of-the-art treatment while serving to advance the field of oncology by addressing important management questions. Table 40–9[8] lists some of these clinical trials; the PDQ database at the U.S. National Cancer Institute provides a further listing that is updated continuously to reflect the normal completion and creation cycle for such studies.

## PREINVASIVE CANCER

The management of Barrett's columnar epithelium and preinvasive lesions of the esophagus involves close follow-up by a gastroenterologist. Surveillance endoscopy may be indicated at 1- to 2-year intervals, especially for patients with dysplastic changes. Patients with high-grade dysplasia or aneuploidy are at sufficiently high risk of developing invasive cancer to justify either aggressive, frequent screening or possibly a prophylactic esophagectomy.

## INVASIVE CANCER

**Stage I and Stage II.** Surgical resection is the mainstay of therapy for limited-stage tumors of the thoracic esophagus and gastroesophageal junction, although many clinicians

*Table 40–9.* **Investigational Trials of Neoadjuvant or Adjuvant Therapy for Esophageal Carcinoma**

| Location or Group and Study Number | Stage | Treatment |
|---|---|---|
| Japanese Esophageal Oncology Group | | Surgery alone vs. surgery + 5-FU + cisplatin |
| Italian Study CNR-012809 | II–III | Surgery alone vs. surgery + 5-FU + cisplatin |
| French Association for Surgical Research | | Surgery alone vs. surgery + 44 Gy + 5-FU + cisplatin |
| International Organisation for Statistical Studies of Diseases of the Oesophagus | | Surgery alone vs. surgery + RT vs. surgery + cisplatin + vindesine + bleomycin |
| Medical Research Council, U.K. (OE-02) | | Surgery alone vs. surgery + 5-FU + cisplatin |
| Hong Kong | | Surgery alone vs. preoperative chemoradiotherapy → surgery |
| U.S. (CALGB 9871) | T1–3NxM0 | Surgery alone vs. 50 Gy RT + 5-FU + cisplatin + surgery |
| Australia | Resectable | Surgery alone vs. 35 Gy RT + 5-FU + cisplatin → surgery |
| France (FFCD 9102) | III | 30 Gy + 5-FU + cisplatin vs. 30 Gy + 5-FU + cisplatin + surgery |
| Germany | T3–4NxM0 | 40 Gy + cisplatin + 5-FU/FA + etoposide + surgery vs. 65–68 Gy + cisplatin + 5-FU + etoposide |
| U.S. (INT-0123 or RTOG-9405) | T1–4NxM0 | High-dose radiotherapy + 5-FU + cisplatin vs. conventional-dose radiotherapy + 5-FU + cisplatin |

5-FU, 5-fluorouracil; RT, radiotherapy; FA, folinic acid.
Modified from Lehnert T. Multimodal therapy for squamous carcinoma of the oesophagus. Br J Surg 1999;86:727–39.

consider chemoradiotherapy an acceptable alternative.[9] This is true for squamous cell carcinomas and adenocarcinomas. Primary treatment for tumors of the cervical esophagus may be radiation therapy or surgery. The role of neoadjuvant chemotherapy, radiation therapy, or chemoradiotherapy is unproved in terms of improving survival, although neoadjuvant therapy can make surgery feasible in selected patients.

**Stage III.** Chemoradiotherapy is indicated for most patients with regionally advanced esophageal cancer, as outlined in Table 40–10.[10] Other approaches to palliation are described in the overview section. Surgical resection is reserved for the rare patient in whom palliation cannot be achieved by any other means.

**Stage IV.** Metastatic tumors are usually treated with combination chemotherapy including cisplatin and 5-FU along with palliative radiation therapy or surgical therapy to manage obstruction or bony metastases. Hyperthermia, photodynamic therapy, and immunotherapy are areas of interest but are currently limited to the setting of clinical trials. These patients may be candidates for nutritional support, as discussed in Chapter 21.

## SUGGESTIONS FOR ADDITIONAL READING

Morales TG, Sampliner RE. Barrett's esophagus: update on screening, surveillance, and treatment. Arch Intern Med 1999;159:1411–6.

Kozarek RA. Complications and lessons learned from 10 years of expandable gastrointestinal prostheses. Dig Dis 1999;17:14–22.

Casale V, Lapenta R, Gigliozzi A, Villotti G. Endoscopic palliative therapy in neoplastic diseases of the esophagus. J Exp Clin Cancer Res 1999;18:63–7.

Ellis FH Jr. Standard resection for cancer of the esophagus and cardia. Surg Oncol Clin North Am 1999;8:279–94.

Coia LR, Minsky BD, John MJ, et al. Patterns of care study decision tree and management guidelines for esophageal cancer. American College of Radiology. Radiat Med 1998;16:321–7.

Flood WA, Forastiere AA. Esophageal cancer. Cancer Treat Res 1998;98:1–40.

Lehnert T. Multimodal therapy for squamous carcinoma of the oesophagus. Br J Surg 1999;86:727–39.

*Table 40–10.* **Chemoradiotherapy for Esophageal Cancer**

| Modality | Dose and Schedule of Administration |
|---|---|
| Radiation therapy | 10 Gy/wk $\times$ 5 wk (50-Gy total dose) starting day 1 |
| Chemotherapy | Cisplatin 75 mg/m$^2$ IV with hydration and mannitol on day 1 |
| | 5-FU 1000 mg/m$^2$ daily $\times$ 4 by continuous IV infusion starting day 1 |
| | Two cycles of chemotherapy are given during RT at 4-wk intervals |
| | Two cycles of chemotherapy are given after RT at 3-wk intervals |

5-FU, 5-fluorouracil; IV, intravenously; RT, radiotherapy.
From Al-Sarraf M, Martz K, Herskovic A, et al. Progress report of combined chemoradiotherapy versus radiotherapy alone in patients with esophageal cancer: an intergroup study. J Clin Oncol 1997;15:277–384.

## REFERENCES

1. Knyrim K, Wagner HJ, Bethge N, et al. A controlled trial of an expansile metal stent for palliation of esophageal obstruction due to inoperable cancer. N Engl J Med 1993;329:1302–7.
2. Boyce HW Jr. Stents for palliation of dysphagia due to esophageal cancer. N Engl J Med 1993;329:1345–6.
3. Spinelli P, Cerrai FG, Dal Fante M, et al. Endoscopic treatment of upper gastrointestinal tract malignancies. Endoscopy 1993;25:675–8.
4. Maunoury V, Brunetaud JM, Cochelard D, et al. Endoscopic palliation for inoperable malignant dysphagia: long term follow up. Gut 1992;33:1602–7.
5. Barr H, Krasner N. Prospective quality of life analysis after palliative photoablation for the treatment of malignant dysphagia. Cancer 1991;68:1660–4.
6. Loizou LA, Rampton D, Atkinson M, et al. A prospective assessment of quality of life after endoscopic intubation and laser therapy for malignant dysphagia. Cancer 1992;70:386–91.
7. Pritikin J, Weinman D, Harmatz A, et al. Endoscopic laser therapy in gastroenterology. West J Med 1992;157:48–54.
8. Lehnert T. Multimodal therapy for squamous carcinoma of the oesophagus. Br J Surg 1999;86:727–39.
9. Coia LR, Minsky BD, John MJ, et al. Patterns of care study decision tree and management guidelines for esophageal cancer. American College of Radiology. Radiat Med 1998;16:321–7.
10. Al-Sarraf M, Martz K, Herskovic A, et al. Progress report of combined chemoradiotherapy versus radiotherapy alone in patients with esophageal cancer: an Intergroup Study. J Clin Oncol 1997;15:277–84.

# CHAPTER 41

# STOMACH

# NATURAL HISTORY, DIAGNOSIS, AND STAGING OF GASTRIC CANCER

• Carol Nishikubo • Charles M. Haskell

## EPIDEMIOLOGY

The incidence of gastric cancer is variable in different parts of the world, and treatment and prognosis vary depending on geographic area. The incidence in Japan is extremely high, where there are 75 to 100 new cases per 100,000 persons per year.[1] These tumors are often seen at an earlier stage than cancers diagnosed in Western countries such as the United States; the prognosis of gastric malignancy diagnosed in Japan may reflect the less advanced nature of the disease, with survival rates generally higher than those seen in the United States. Other areas of high prevalence include Chile and Scandinavia. In contrast, the incidence of gastric cancer in the United States is 7 cases per 100,000 population; it is the 10th most common cause of cancer death in the United States.[2]

Although the overall incidence of gastric cancer in the United States is low, it should be noted that the time trends of incidence are possibly changing. With the increased availability of refrigeration in the United States, there was an initial decline in the incidence of gastric cancer after 1950.[3] More recently, however, there appears to be an increase in the incidence of adenocarcinomas of the distal esophagus and cardia of the stomach.[4] This apparent increase is unexplained.

Gastric cancers affect older men more commonly, with a peak incidence seen in the 60s.[4] The male/female risk ratio is 1.5:1, and the disease is more common in nonwhites than in whites. As mentioned previously, different countries observe different rates of cancer, but migrants to other countries develop the risk of the country to which they move so that Japanese individuals who move to the United States have a risk similar to that seen in the United States. This phenomenon is probably mainly due to dietary changes.[5] Genetic factors, however, also play a role, with relatives of patients with gastric carcinoma having an increased risk of developing cancer themselves. Patients with familial adenomatous polyposis also have a risk approximately three times higher than that of the general population of developing gastric cancer.[6] Certain blood group antigens have also been associated with gastric cancer, with the incidence highest in persons with blood type A and lowest in persons with blood type O.

## ETIOLOGY

Dietary factors affecting the risk of developing gastric cancer have been extensively examined. Salted or smoked fish, pickled vegetables, and well-cooked meats have been commonly cited as contributory.[7–9] Fruit and fiber have been found to be protective,[10–12] the former probably through the vitamin C content. Vitamin C is thought to protect against some of the mutagens present especially in smoked foods, and it has been suggested that it may decrease growth of *Helicobacter pylori* as a mechanism of decreasing cancer risk.[13] Ingestion of fats and butter and, in some studies, caloric intake also increased the risk of developing gastric tumors.[10, 11] Foods high in carbohydrate content, such as pastas, pastries, and bread, have also been associated with an increased risk.[10, 12] Some studies have suggested an association of gastric cancer with nitrate levels found in the drinking water[14]; however most have found no association.[15, 16]

Tobacco use is associated with a twofold increase in the risk of developing gastric cancer in some series.[17, 18] Certain occupations, such as nickel plating, may also have an increased risk,[19] as may iron and steel work,[20] coal mining, occupations with exposure to mineral and metal dust, woodworking, and farming.[21]

Aspirin use and use of nonsteroidal anti-inflammatory drugs have been associated with a decreased risk of developing esophageal cancer and noncardia gastric carcinomas.[22]

Certain medical conditions are associated with an increased risk of development of gastric tumors. Pernicious anemia and peptic ulcer disease (especially gastric ulcer)[23–25] are perhaps the most commonly described; however, some authors have found an increased risk with hypertension (twofold increase in tumors of the gastric cardia) and iron deficiency (fourfold increase in tumors affecting all parts of the stomach).[26] Pernicious anemia is associated with an increased risk of developing gastric adenocarcinoma. The proposed mechanism of this increased risk is that patients with pernicious anemia have a higher production of *N*-nitroso compounds in the stomach, which are carcinogenic. Some studies have found a 50-fold increase in mean nitrite concentration in the gastric juice from patients with pernicious anemia compared with age-matched controls.[27]

It has been debated whether medications or conditions that cause hypochlorhydria may also confer an increased risk of gastric cancer by this same increase in gastric nitrate concentration.[28] Medications such as $H_2$ antagonists induce hypochlorhydria in the stomach, and some authors have suggested that they may directly induce carcinogen production. It is difficult to separate this risk, however, from the risk associated with peptic ulcer disease and specifically *H. pylori* infection, which is discussed subsequently.

The association of *H. pylori* with MALTomas has been fairly well characterized, and the fact that eradication of the bacteria often results in resolution of the cancer has led to general acceptance of a causative role for the bacteria in that disease.[29] The detection of *H. pylori*, especially the cag A + strain, in cases of gastric cancer has been described in several patient series from around the world.[30–33] A large meta-analysis of 19 studies involving 2491 patients and 3959 controls showed an overall odds ratio of 1.92 for gastric cancer in *H. pylori*–infected patients.[34] There is also some evidence that treatment of *H. pylori* decreases the risk of developing a carcinoma. In one series of 132 patients with early gastric cancer (EGC), 65 were treated for *H. pylori* infection and 67 were not. None of the patients treated for infection developed new EGC lesions, whereas six patients (9%) in the untreated group developed new EGC lesions within 2 years of follow-up.[35] There is a discrepancy, however, in terms of the geographic and sex distribution of gastric cancer not matching the pattern of *H. pylori* infection. Some authors have implicated the bacteria in causing the initial chronic inflammation but not the subsequent development of carcinoma.[36]

Infections with other microbes have been suggested as having a causative role in developing gastric cancer as well. The Epstein-Barr virus has been detected in some studies more frequently in patients with gastric cancer than in normal controls.[37] Other groups have found low levels of expression in gastric cancer in 1 to 9% of cases.[38–42] One study found that despite low levels of detecting the virus, the malignant cells expressed EBNA-1, whereas the surrounding normal tissue did not, suggesting integration of at least part of the viral genome into the malignant clone but not into normal tissue.[39]

## BIOLOGY

**Molecular Pathogenesis.** Correa[43] has developed a model of human gastric carcinogenesis that incorporates the known epidemiologic data. This model involves a sequence starting with nonspecific mucosal injury (from aging, alcohol, autoimmune factors, or other events). Genetic or nutritional factors may then impede mucosal repair, causing chronic gastritis and the subsequent proliferation of intraluminal bacteria. Bacterial nitrate reductases would then convert dietary nitrates to nitrites, which could react with any number of substances to produce nitrosamines. A sequence of atrophy, intestinal metaplasia, dysplasia, carcinoma in situ, and ultimately invasive carcinoma would follow. This pathogenetic sequence has not been proved, but it is consistent with the epidemiologic findings.

A wide variety of receptors, enzymes, and other biologic materials have been found in gastric carcinoma tissue. Their role in molecular carcinogenesis is unclear. Examples include pepsinogen II,[44] estrogen and progesterone receptors,[45] human epidermal growth factor,[46] the p21 product of the *ras* oncogene,[47] the MAGE gene product,[48, 49] the vascular cell adhesion molecule-1 (VCAM-1), the intracellular cell adhesion molecule-1 (ICAM-1),[50] and abnormalities of c-*erb*B2 (HER-2/*neu*).[51–53] Mutations in the p53 tumor-suppressor gene are also common in gastric cancer.[51, 54]

**Pathophysiology.** The stomach is a hollow organ with the thickest wall and greatest lumen diameter of any structure within the gastrointestinal tract. It is likely that lesions developing in the stomach attain a large size and are present for long periods before diagnosis. Although cancers may occur anywhere in the stomach, most develop in the pyloric and antral regions, particularly along the lesser curvature. In a study of more than 5000 gastric carcinomas, 51% were found to involve the pylorus and antrum; 18%, the lesser curvature; 21%, the body; 7%, the cardia; and 3%, the greater curvature. Benign ulcers, which frequently mimic gastric cancer, rarely appear on the greater curvature.[55]

Gastric cancer spreads in typical patterns: by continuity on the mucosal surface, infiltrating the gastric wall and sometimes resulting in widespread scirrhous infiltration (linitis plastica), or by direct extension outside the stomach, involving adjacent organs such as the omentum, liver, pancreas, and colon. Nodal metastases involve the inferior gastric, subpyloric, and celiac axis nodes when the neoplasm begins in the distal stomach. Pancreatic, splenic, pericardial, and superficial diaphragmatic nodes are most often involved with proximal lesions. Vascular spread most commonly involves the liver and is noted in about 30% of patients coming to operation.

A classic finding in advanced gastric cancer is involvement of the left supraclavicular node (Virchow's node or the sentinal node), indicating spread through the thoracic duct. Gastric cancer also spreads by transperitoneal extension, and it may present as a metastasis to the ovaries (Krukenberg's tumor)[56] or to the pouch of Douglas (rectal shelf metastasis). Pulmonary, osseous, adrenal, and cutaneous metastases are common in the later stages of the disease.[57–59] Central nervous system involvement is unusual.

## PATHOLOGY AND CLASSIFICATION

Of tumors arising in the stomach, 95% are adenocarcinomas, although lymphomas, sarcomas, and other rare tumors occur.[57, 59, 60] Adenocarcinoma usually presents as an ulcer

(75%) but may also present as a polypoid mass (10%), a diffuse scirrhous lesion (10%), or a superficial mucosal lesion (5%). About 2% of cases present with multiple primary sites.

The degree of differentiation in carcinoma of the stomach affects prognosis, as does the stage. Broder's classification has been employed to quantify the differentiation of these lesions, grade 1 being well-differentiated lesions and grade 4 highly anaplastic lesions.[61]

The most widely used international classification of gastric carcinomas is that of Laurén.[62] This system, which is the one recommended by the American Joint Committee on Cancer, differentiates between intestinal and diffuse carcinomas. The intestinal (well-differentiated) type has a better prognosis. It is the most common type found in Japan and is frequently found in association with intestinal metaplasia.[63]

EGC is defined by a T1 lesion of three morphologic types: type I, polypoid or mass-like; type II, superficial with only minor elevation or depression; and type III, cancer associated with a gastric ulcer.[64, 65] EGCs may be large (10 cm in diameter), have any degree of differentiation, and may have associated regional lymph node involvement without markedly changing the prognosis. In Japan, nearly all patients with EGC who undergo gastrectomy are cured.[66, 67] This lesion has also been shown to be highly curable in the United States and Europe, although late recurrences are more common than in patients from Japan,[68, 69] perhaps because of the extent of the lymph node dissection carried out during the surgery.

## CLINICAL FEATURES

Vague epigastric discomfort is the most common presenting symptom, followed by anorexia, early satiety, eructation, weight loss, weakness, and dysphagia or obstruction. Hematemesis is uncommon and should suggest another diagnosis, either benign (ulcer, gastritis) or another malignancy (leiomyosarcoma). Pain is a common first symptom and has been reported in 85% of patients by the time of diagnosis. Pain may be similar to that experienced with peptic ulcer disease and may be relieved by food or antacids. Continual pain, however, generally suggests tumor involvement outside the stomach wall. Substernal or precordial pain may also be associated with tumors of the cardia.[70]

A variety of paraneoplastic syndromes have been reported with gastric carcinoma.[71] The most common are (1) skin complaints, including acanthosis nigracans, dermatomyositis, circinate erythemas, and pemphigoid; (2) central nervous system problems, including dementia and cerebellar ataxia; (3) thrombophlebitis; and (4) ectopic peptide hormone syndromes, such as Cushing's syndrome or the carcinoid syndrome. A seronegative synovitis with edema has also been described.[72]

## DIAGNOSIS

Any patient experiencing persistent gastrointestinal complaints despite attempts at medical management should have a thorough evaluation of the gastrointestinal tract. Screening strategies for asymptomatic patients have been proposed, especially in high-incidence areas, but in countries where the incidence is lower, such as the United States, there has been no recommendation for the screening of the general population.

**Radiographic Studies.** Barium swallow with air contrast plus an upper gastrointestinal series has been the traditional radiologic study to detect gastric carcinoma. Findings suggestive of a gastric neoplasm include a constant filling defect in the normal outline of the stomach, loss of flexibility and distensibility, or an alteration in the relief pattern of the mucosal folds, with or without ulceration.

Differentiation between malignant and benign ulcers is frequently difficult. The characteristic malignant ulcer crater lies in a mass and does not extend beyond the boundaries of the gastric wall. The mucosal folds do not radiate toward the center of the crater but instead remain with their usual contour up to and beyond the ulcer. Malignant ulcers are usually larger than 1 cm, and on fluoroscopy the surrounding gastric wall is rigid. Benign ulcers often penetrate beyond the limit of the stomach wall, there is often no surrounding tumor, and the rugal folds radiate outward from the center of the crater.

**Endoscopy.** Endoscopy by itself without biopsy and cytologic and radiographic studies is not sufficiently reliable in establishing a diagnosis of gastric carcinoma. In one series of 1005 patients examined by endoscopy alone, an incorrect interpretation was made in 7% of cases, and no conclusion was possible in another 8%.[73] Endoscopic ultrasonography is being used increasingly to provide preoperative staging information on the extent of tumor invasion of the stomach and may be useful in determining which patients could potentially benefit from neoadjuvant therapy.

**Exfoliative Cytology.** Exfoliative cytology is best used in conjunction with endoscopy and biopsy. Alone, it has an accuracy rate of approximately 85%,[74, 75] but this rate increases to 95% when combined with biopsy.[75]

**Tumor Markers.** Serum levels of CEA, CA 19-9, alpha-fetoprotein, and other tumor markers can be elevated in patients with gastric carcinoma. Their value in the diagnosis and management of disease, however, is not well established.

**Follow-up for Previous Gastrectomy Patients.** There has been considerable controversy over the risk of stomach cancer among patients surgically treated for peptic ulcer disease. An association was initially reported by Balfour[76] in 1922. Osnes and coworkers[77] subsequently found 43 patients with gastric carcinoma in a series of 830 consecutive routine gastroscopies. Thirteen of these patients had previously undergone Billroth operations for ulcer disease, which was considered a disproportionately high frequency. All patients were symptomatic. Multiple biopsy specimens and brush cytology from the entire gastrojejunal anastomosis were responsible for detecting these early cancers. Similar results have been published by Domellof and Janunger,[78] Schrumpf and associates,[79] and Farrands and coworkers.[80] In an autopsy study using matched retrospective controls, however, only 9 of 464 patients dying of gastric cancer had undergone previous partial gastrectomy, whereas the respective number among the controls without gastric cancer was 5.[81] Studies from the Mayo Clinic,[82, 83] Denmark,[84] and Sweden[85] found similar gastric cancer prevalence rates in controls as in patients with prior surgical therapy for benign ulcer disease. The Swedish study, however, identified an increase in the risk of developing gastric cancer in the few patients who underwent partial gastrectomy for benign ulcer disease before age 50 provided that they lived at least 20 years. Greene[86] published a study of 145 patients who underwent annual endoscopic screening after resection for benign gastric disease. Thirteen patients were diagnosed with cancer, all of whom were clinically asymptomatic and all of whom were resected for cure. Based on these data, annual screening was recommended for patients following resection for benign disease, especially those who survived for more than 20 years after resection.

## STAGING

**Staging Systems.** The staging system for gastric cancer used in the United States is the International TNM system developed by the American Joint Committee on Cancer and the International Union Against Cancer (Table 41–1).[87] As with an earlier version of the TNM system, it is based on the fact that prognosis in gastric cancer is influenced by the degree of penetration into the stomach wall by the primary lesion, the involvement of regional lymph nodes, and the presence of distant metastases. The size or location of the primary tumor is considered to be less important, and the histopathologic grade of the carcinoma has not been included as a separate prognostic variable.

The International TNM staging system is useful in identifying groups of patients with different prognoses. It does not include prognostic information considered important by investigators in Japan. Specifically, it does not include information about the extent of lymph node involvement as a function of the primary site of disease, and it ignores the extent of lymph node dissection as a prognostic variable. Of the two considerations, the extent of resection is probably the more important variable. In a large study from Japan, the number of metastatic nodes was a better guide to prognosis than nodal stage based on the location of nodes relative to the primary lesion.[88]

Japanese investigators have developed their own staging system incorporating information on serosal invasion, peritoneal metastases, and lymph node involvement based on the anatomic site of the primary tumor.[89] Five-year survival results by TNM stage of disease in the United States and Japan as well as 5-year survival results in Japan according to the Japanese staging system are given in Table 41–2.[90] The superior survival results reported from Japan are unexplained, although one study comparing the findings of Japanese pathologists staging gastric cancer with the findings of pathologists from Western countries suggests a difference in the definition of what constitutes a neoplastic versus a dysplastic or early neoplastic lesion.[91] Japanese investigators consider the differences to be largely due to the more extensive lymph node dissections that are routinely used in Japan. Attempts to validate this explanation in patients in the United States and Europe with a randomized surgical trial of standard gastrectomy versus gastrectomy with an extended lymph node dissection have been fraught with problems, and the issue remains unresolved.[92] Further discussion of this important topic can be found in reviews by Thompson and colleagues[93] and Rothenberg and associates.[90]

**Pretreatment Staging Studies.** The extent of preopera-

*Table 41–1.* **Staging of Gastric Cancer**

*Primary Tumor (T)*

TX   Primary tumor cannot be assessed
T0   No evidence of primary tumor
TIS  Carcinoma in situ: intraepithelial tumor without invasion of lamina propria
T1   Tumor invades lamina propria or submucosa
T2   Tumor invades muscularis propria or subserosa*
T3   Tumor penetrates serosa (visceral peritoneum) without invasion of adjacent structures**, ***
T4   Tumor invades adjacent structures**, ***

*Regional Lymph Nodes (N)*

NX   Regional lymph node(s) cannot be assessed
N0   No regional lymph node metastasis
N1   Metastasis in 1 to 6 regional lymph nodes
N2   Metastases in 7 to 15 regional lymph nodes
N3   Metastases in more than 15 regional lymph nodes

*Distant Metastasis (M)*

MX   Distant metastasis cannot be assessed
M0   No distant metastasis
M1   Distant metastasis

*Stage Grouping*

| | | | |
|---|---|---|---|
| Stage 0 | Tis | N0 | M0 |
| Stage IA | T1 | N0 | M0 |
| Stage IB | T1 | N1 | M0 |
| | T2 | N0 | M0 |
| Stage II | T1 | N2 | M0 |
| | T2 | N1 | M0 |
| | T3 | N0 | M0 |
| Stage IIIA | T2 | N2 | M0 |
| | T3 | N1 | M0 |
| | T4 | N0 | M0 |
| Stage IIIB | T3 | N2 | M0 |
| Stage IV | T4 | N1 | M0 |
| | T1 | N3 | M0 |
| | T2 | N3 | M0 |
| | T3 | N3 | M0 |
| | T4 | N2 | M0 |
| | T4 | N3 | M0 |
| | Any T | Any N | M1 |

*Note:* A tumor may penetrate the muscularis propria with extension into the gastrocolic or gastrohepatic ligaments, or into the greater or lesser omentum without perforation of the visceral peritoneum covering these structures. In this case, the tumor is classified T2. If there is perforation of the visceral peritoneum covering the gastric ligaments or the omentum, the tumor should be classified T3.

**Note:* The adjacent structures of the stomach include the spleen, transverse colon, liver, diaphragm, pancreas, abdominal wall, adrenal gland, kidney, small intestine, and retroperitoneum.

***Note:* Intramural extension to the duodenum or esophagus is classified by the depth of greatest invasion in any of these sites, including stomach.

Used with permission of the American Joint Committee on Cancer (AJCC®), Chicago, Illinois. The original source for this material is the AJCC® Cancer Staging Manual, 5th edition (1997) published by Lippincott-Raven Publishers, Philadelphia, Pennsylvania.

tive staging studies in patients with biopsy-proven gastric cancer is controversial. Symptoms or signs suggestive of metastatic disease should be carefully assessed with the appropriate studies because they may alter the extent of the surgical therapy. Preoperative tests typically employed include a complete blood count, liver function tests, serum CEA level, chest radiography, and an abdominal computed tomography (CT) scan. A bone scan is indicated if the serum alkaline phosphatase level is elevated or there are skeletal symptoms, and plain film correlation is obtained of painful areas or areas of increased radionuclide uptake.

*Table 41–2.* **Five-Year Survival Based on Stage of Disease**

| Stage | U.S. (%) | Japan (%) |
|---|---|---|
| I | 52 | 30 |
| II | 30 | 70 |
| III | 15 | 36 |
| IV | 5 | 11 |

An abdominal CT scan can be useful but should not be used as the sole modality of determining surgical resectability.[94, 95] In a study conducted by Cook and colleagues,[96] 37 patients with biopsy-proven gastric adenocarcinoma were evaluated with CT before surgical resection. Nineteen (51%) were found to have more extensive disease than predicted, whereas three of six patients thought to have widespread disease by CT were found at surgery to have disease confined to the stomach or regional nodes. The computed tomographic scan was as likely to be incorrect as correct in predicting the extent of disease.

**Post-Treatment Follow-up Studies.** Frequent follow-up evaluations of patients after definitive therapy are usually not indicated outside the setting of a clinical trial. With the possible exception of patients with more extensive forms of EGC, in which subsequent recurrence may still be resectable, recurrent disease generally cannot be resected for cure.[97] In the absence of symptoms, only minimal follow-up studies are needed. Close follow-up with endoscopy, serum tumor marker studies, chest radiographs, and other expensive tests in the absence of symptoms is unlikely to influence the patient's survival or quality of life.

## PROGNOSIS

Overall, survival in gastric carcinoma is poor. In a large review involving more than 20,000 cases, the 5-year survival rate was 8%.[98] The most important prognostic variable is the TNM stage of disease as determined pathologically (pTNM). In one large retrospective study conducted in Japan, tumors of the gastric cardia had a worse prognosis than did tumors arising in other parts of the stomach.[99] Setala and coworkers,[100] in a series of 321 patients, found that tumors arising in the proximal third of the stomach had a worse prognosis than those arising more distally.

The American Joint Committee on Cancer recommends that gastric adenocarcinomas be classified using the Laurén system as intestinal, diffuse, or mixed. The prognosis is worse for the diffuse type.[101, 102]

Studies of outcome for patients with gastric carcinoma have identified other factors that may have prognostic significance. Factors such as absence of dysphagia, absence of an abdominal mass, and lack of weight loss[103] have been associated with a better prognosis. Some studies have also observed a trend toward better survival in tumors that are *bcl-2* positive.[104] In Japan, extended resections are considered essential to achieve the best possible survival results. Aneuploidy has been associated with a poor-prognosis group,[105, 106] as has CD44 expression[107–109] and c-*erb*B2 expression.[53]

For patients who present with advanced disease that is

not surgically resectable, the presence of liver metastases, serum bilirubin level, presence of ascites, tumor mass, and weight loss are associated with a more rapidly progressive course.[110] Tumor marker levels, such as CEA, CA 19-9, CA 50, and CA 72-4, have not been consistently shown to be predictive of the course of disease, although some series have shown an association.[111, 112]

# REFERENCES

1. Munoz N, Franceschi S. Epidemiology of gastric cancer and perspectives for prevention. Salud Publica Mex 1997;39:318–30.
2. SEER Cancer Statistics Review 1973–1996. (See http://www-seer.ims.nci.nih.gov)
3. Fuchs CS, Mayer RJ. Gastric carcinoma. N Engl J Med 1995;333:32–41.
4. Devesa SS, Blot WJ, Fraumeni JF Jr. Changing patterns in the incidence of esophageal and gastric carcinoma in the United States. Cancer 1998;83:2049–53.
5. Weisburger JH, Marquardt H, Mower HF, et al. Inhibition of carcinogenesis: vitamin C and the prevention of gastric cancer. Prev Med 1980;9:352–61.
6. Wallace MH, Phillips RK. Upper gastrointestinal disease in patients with familial adenomatous polyposis. Br J Surg 1998;85:742–50.
7. Dungal N, Sigurjonsson J. Gastric cancer and diet: a pilot study in dietary habits in two districts differing markedly in respect of mortality from gastric cancer. Br J Cancer 1967;21:270–6.
8. Erkisi M, Colakoglu S, Koksal F, et al. Relationship of *Helicobacter pylori* infection to several malignant and non-malignant gastrointestinal diseases. J Exp Clin Cancer Res 1997;16:289–93.
9. Ward MH, Sinha R, Heineman EF, et al. Risk of adenocarcinoma of the stomach and esophagus with meat cooking method and doneness preference. Int J Cancer 1997;71:14–9.
10. Harrison LE, Zhang ZF, Karpeh MS, et al. The role of dietary factors in the intestinal and diffuse histologic subtypes of gastric adenocarcinoma. Cancer 1997;80:1021–8.
11. Munoz SE, Ferraroni M, La Vecchia C, et al. Gastric cancer risk factors in subjects with family history. Cancer Epidemiol Biomarkers Prev 1997;6:737–40.
12. Pobel D, Riboli E, Cornee J, et al. Nitrosamine, nitrate and nitrite in relation to gastric cancer: a case control study in Marseille, France. Eur J Epidemiol 1995;11:67–73.
13. Zhang HM, Wakisaka N, Maeda O, et al. Vitamin C inhibits the growth of a bacterial risk factor for gastric carcinoma: *Helicobacter pylori*. Cancer 1997;80:1897–1903.
14. Yang CY, Cheng MF, Tsai SS, et al. Calcium, magnesium and nitrate in drinking water and gastric cancer mortality. Jpn J Cancer Res 1998;89:124–30.
15. Barrett JH, Parslow RC, McKinney PA, et al. Nitrate in drinking water and the incidence of gastric, esophageal and brain cancer in Yorkshire, England. Cancer Causes Control 1998;9:153–9.
16. van Loon AJ, Botterweck AA, Goldbohm RA, et al. Intake of nitrate and nitrite and the risk of gastric cancer: a prospective cohort study. Br J Cancer 1998;78:129–35.
17. Gammon MD, Schoenberg JB, Ahsan H, et al. Tobacco, alcohol and socioeconomic status and adenocarcinomas of the esophagus and gastric cardia. J Natl Cancer Inst 1997;89:1277–84.
18. Gajalakshmi CK, Shanta V. Lifestyle and risk of stomach cancer: a hospital-based case-control study. Int J Epidemiol 1996;25:1146–53.
19. Pang D, Burges DC, Sorahan T. Mortality study of nickel platers with special reference to cancers of the stomach and lung, 1945–93. Occup Environ Med 1996;53:714–17.
20. Xu Z, Brown LM, Pan GW, et al. Cancer risks among iron and steel workers in Anshan, China: Part II. case-control studies of lung and stomach cancer. Am J Ind Med 1996;30:7–15.
21. Cocco P, Ward MH, Buiatti E. Occupational risk factors for gastric cancer: an overview. Epidemiol Rev 1996;18:218–34.
22. Farrow DC, Vaughan TL, Hansten PD, et al. Use of aspirin and other nonsteroidal anti-inflammatory drugs and risk of esophageal and gastric cancer. Cancer Epidemiol Biomarkers Prev 1998;7:97–102.
23. Molloy RM, Sonnenberg A. Relation between gastric cancer and previous peptic ulcer disease. Gut 1997;40:247–52.
24. LaVecchia C, Braga C, Negri E, et al. Risk of stomach cancer in patients with gastric or duodenal ulcer. Eur J Cancer Prev 1997;6:20–3.
25. Hansson LE, Nyren O, Hsing AW, et al. The risk of stomach cancer in patients with gastric or duodenal ulcer disease. N Engl J Med 1996;335:242–9.
26. Zhang ZF, Kurtz RC, Sun M, et al. Adenocarcinomas of the esophagus and gastric cardia: medical conditions, tobacco, alcohol and socioeconomic factors. Cancer Epidemiol Biomarkers Prev 1996;5:761–8.
27. Ruddell WS, Bone ES, Hill MJ, et al. Pathogenesis of gastric cancer in pernicious anemia. Lancet 1978;1:521–3.
28. Colin-Jones DG, Langman MH, Lawson DH, et al. Cimetidine and gastric cancer: preliminary report from post-marketing surveillance study. Br Med J 1982;285:1311–3.
29. Wotherspoon AD, Doglioni C, Diss TC, et al. Regression of primary low-grade B-cell gastric lymphoma of mucosa-associated lymphoid tissue type after eradication of *Helicobacter pylori*. Lancet 1993;342:575–7.
30. Shimoyama T, Fukuda S, Tanaka M, et al. CagA seropositivity associated with development of gastric cancer in a Japanese population. J Clin Pathol 1998;51:225–8.
31. Siman JH, Forsgren A, Berglund G, et al. Association between *Helicobacter pylori* and gastric cancinoma in the city of Malmo, Sweden: a prospective study. Scand J Gastroenterol 1997;32:1215–21.
32. Parsonnet J, Friedman GD, Vandersteen DP, et al. *Helicobacter pylori* infection and the risk of gastric carcinoma. N Engl J Med 1991;325:1127–31.
33. Parsonnet J, Friedman GD, Orentreich N, et al. Risk for gastric cancer in people with CagA positive or CagA negative *Helicobacter pylori* infection. Gut 1997;40:297–301.
34. Huang JQ, Sridhar S, Chen Y, et al. Meta-analysis of the relationship between *Helicobacter pylori* seropositivity and gastric cancer. Gastroenterology 1998;114:1169–79.
35. Uemura N, Mukai T, Okamoto S, et al. Effect of *Helicobacter pylori* eradication on subsequent development of cancer after endoscopic resection of early gastric cancer. Cancer Epidemiol Biomarkers Prev 1997;6:639–42.
36. Crespi M, Citarda F. *Helicobacter pylori* and gastric cancer: what is the real risk? Gastroenterologist 1998;6:16–20.
37. Shibata D, Weiss LM. Epstein-Barr virus associated gastric adenocarcinoma. Am J Pathol 1992;140:769–74.
38. Rowlands DC, Ito M, Mangham DC, et al. Epstein-Barr virus and carcinomas: rare association of the virus and gastric adenocarcinomas. Br J Cancer 1993;68:1014–9.
39. Imai S, Koizumi S, Sugiura M, et al. Gastric carcinoma: monoclonal epithelial malignant cells expressing Epstein-Barr virus latent infection protein. Proc Natl Acad Sci U S A 1994;91:9131–5.
40. Qiu K, Tomita Y, Hashimoto M, et al. Epstein-Barr virus in gastric carcinoma in Suzhou, China and Osaka, Japan: association with clinico-pathologic factors and HLA subtype. Int J Cancer 1997;71:155–8.
41. Yanai H, Nishikawa J, Mizugaki Y, et al. Endoscopic and pathologic features of Epstein-Barr virus associated gastric carcinoma. Gastrointest Endosc 1997;45:236–42.
42. Galetsky SA, Tsvetnov VV, Land CE, et al. Epstein-Barr virus associated gastric cancer in Russia. Int J Cancer 1997;73:786–9.
43. Correa P. Human gastric carcinogenesis: a multistep and multifactorial process—First American Cancer Society Award Lecture on cancer epidemiology and prevention. Cancer Res 1992;52:6735–40.
44. Fiocca R, Cornaggia M, Villani L, et al. Expression of pepsinogen II in gastric cancer: its relationship to local invasion and lymph node metastases. Cancer 1988;61:956–62.
45. Tokunaga A, Nishi K, Matsukura N, et al. Estrogen and progesterone receptors in gastric cancer. Cancer 1986;57:1376–9.
46. Tahara E, Sumiyoshi H, Hata J, et al. Human epidermal growth factor in gastric carcinoma as a biologic marker of high malignancy. Jpn J Cancer Res 1986;77:145–52.
47. Czerniak B, Herz F, Koss LG, et al. ras oncogene p21 as a tumor marker in the cytodiagnosis of gastric and colonic carcinomas. Cancer 1987;60:2432–6.
48. Li J, Yang Y, Fujie T, et al. Expression of the MAGE gene family in human gastric carcinoma. Anticancer Res 1997;17:3559–63.
49. Katano M, Nakamura M, Morisaki T, et al. Melanoma antigen-encoding gene-1 expression in invasive gastric carcinoma: correlation with stage of disease. J Surg Oncol 1997;64:195–201.
50. Velikova G, Banks RE, Gearing A, et al. Circulating soluble adhesion

molecules E-cadherin, E-selectin, intercellular adhesion molecule-1 (ICAM-1) and vascular cell adhesion molecule-1 (VCAM-1) in patient with gastric cancer. Br J Cancer 1997;76:1398–1404.

51. Wu MS, Shun CT, Sheu JC, et al. Overexpression of mutant p53 and c-erbB-2 proteins and mutations of the p15 and p16 genes in human gastric carcinoma: with respect to histologic subtypes and stages. J Gastroenterol Hepatol 1998;13:305–10.
52. Yonemura Y, Ninomiya I, Tsugawa K, et al. Prognostic significance of c-erbB-2 gene expression in the poorly differentiated type of adenocarcinoma of the stomach. Cancer Detect Prev 1998;22:139–46.
53. Orita H, Maehara Y, Emi Y, et al. c-erbB-2 expression is predictive for lymphatic spread of clinical gastric carcinoma. Hepatogastroenterology 1997;44:294–8.
54. Gomyo Y, Ikeda M, Osaki M, et al. Expression of p21 (waf1/cip1/sdi1), but not p53 protein, is a factor in the survival of patients with gastric carcinoma. Cancer 1997;79:2067–72.
55. Berkson J. In: ReMine WH, ed. Cancer of the stomach. Philadelphia: WB Saunders, 1964.
56. Holtz F, Hart WR. Krukenberg tumors of the ovary: a clinicopathologic analysis of 27 cases. Cancer 1982;50:2438–47.
57. Moertel CG. The stomach. In: Holland JF, Frei E III, eds. Cancer medicine. 2nd ed. Philadelphia: Lea & Febiger, 1982:1760–74.
58. Grage TB, Ferguson RM, Simmons RL. Gastrointestinal tract cancer. In: Horton J, Hill GJ II, eds. Clinical oncology. Philadelphia: WB Saunders, 1977:244–318.
59. Macdonald JS, Gunderson LL, Cohn I Jr. Cancer of the stomach In: DeVita VT Jr, Hellman S, Rosenberg SA, eds. Cancer: principles and practice of oncology. Philadelphia: JB Lippincott, 1982:534–62.
60. Moertel CG. Multiple primary malignant neoplasms. New York: Springer-Verlag, 1966.
61. Moertel CG. Advanced gastrointestinal cancer: clinical management and chemotherapy. New York: Harper & Row, 1969.
62. Laurén P. The two histological main types of gastric carcinoma: diffuse and so-called intestinal-type: an attempt at a histo-clinical classification. Acta Pathol Microbiol Scand 1965;64:31–49.
63. Matsukura N, Suzuki K, Kawachi T, et al. Distribution of marker enzymes and mucin in intestinal metaplasia in human stomach and relation to complete and incomplete types of intestinal metaplasia in minute gastric carcinomas. J Natl Cancer Inst 1980;65:231–40.
64. Green PH, O'Toole KM. Early gastric cancer. Ann Intern Med 1982;97:272–3.
65. O'Brien MJ, Burakoff R, Robbins EA, et al. Early gastric cancer: clinicopathologic study. Am J Med 1985;78:195–202.
66. Yamazaki H, Oshima A, Murakami R, et al. A long term follow up study of patients with gastric cancer detected by mass screening. Cancer 1989;63:613–7.
67. Sano T, Sasako M, Kinoshita T, et al. Recurrence of early gastric cancer: follow up of 1475 patients and review of the Japanese literature. Cancer 1993;72:3174–8.
68. Green PH, O'Toole KM, Slonim D, et al. Increasing incidence and excellent survival of patients with early gastric cancer: experience in a United States medical center. Am J Med 1988;85:658–61.
69. Guadagni S, Reed PI, Johnston BJ, et al. Early gastric cancer: follow-up after gastrectomy in 159 patients. Br J Surg 1993;80:325–8.
70. Longmire WB Jr. Carcinoma of the stomach. In: Sabiston DC Jr, ed. Davis-Christopher textbook of surgery. Philadelphia: WB Saunders, 1977.
71. Tabbarah HJ. Gastrointestinal tract cancers. In: Casciato DA, Lowitz BB, eds. Manual of clinical oncology. 3rd ed. Boston: Little, Brown, 1995:150.
72. Tada Y, Sato H, Yoshizawa S, et al. Remitting seronegative symmetrical synovitis with pitting edema associated with gastric carcinoma. J Rheumatol 1997;24:974–5.
73. Dekker W, Tytgat GN. Diagnostic accuracy of fiber-endoscopy in the detection of upper intestinal malignancies: a follow-up analysis. Gastroenterology 1977;73:710–4.
74. Pilotti S, Rilke F, Clemente C, et al. The cytologic diagnosis of gastric carcinoma related to the histologic type. Acta Cytol 1977;21:48–59.
75. Tamura K, Masuzawa M, Akiyama T, et al. Touch smear cytology for endoscopic diagnosis of gastric carcinoma. Am J Gastroenterol 1977;67:463–7.
76. Balfour DC. Factors influencing the life expectancy of patients operated on for gastric ulcer. Ann Surg 1922;76:405–8.
77. Osnes M, Lotveit T, Myren J, et al. Early gastric carcinoma in patients with a Billroth II partial gastrectomy. Endoscopy 1977;9:45–9.

78. Domellof L, Janunger KG. The risk for gastric carcinoma after partial gastrectomy. Am J Surg 1977;134:581–4.
79. Schrumpf E, Serck-Hanssen A, Stadaas J, et al. Mucosal changes in the gastric stump 20–25 years after partial gastrectomy. Lancet 1977;2:467–9.
80. Farrands PA, Blake JR, Ansell ID, et al. Endoscopic review of patients who have had gastric surgery. Br Med J 1983;286:755–8.
81. Kivilaakso E, Hakkiluoto A, Kalima TV, et al. Relative risk of stump cancer following partial gastrectomy. Br J Surg 1977;64:336–8.
82. Schafer LW, Larson DE, Melton LJ III, et al. The risk of gastric carcinoma after surgical treatment for benign ulcer disease: a population-based study in Olmsted County, Minnesota. N Engl J Med 1983;309:1210–3.
83. Thiruvengadam R, Hench V, Melton LJ III, et al. Cancer of the nongastric hollow organs of the gastrointestinal tract after gastric surgery. Arch Intern Med 1988;148:405–7.
84. Fischer AB, Graem N, Jensen OM. Risk of gastric cancer after Bilroth II resection for duodenal ulcer. Br J Surg 1983;70:552–4.
85. Lundegardh G, Adami HO, Helmick C, et al. Stomach cancer after partial gastrectomy for benign ulcer disease. N Engl J Med 1988;319:195–200.
86. Greene FL. Management of gastric remnant carcinoma based on the results of a 15 year endoscopic screening program. Ann Surg 1996;223:701–8.
87. Fleming ID, Cooper JS, Henson DE, et al, eds. Manual for staging of cancer of the American Joint Committee on Cancer. 5th ed. Philadelphia: JB Lippincott, 1997:75.
88. Ichikura T, Tomimatsu S, Okusa Y, et al. Comparison of the prognostic significance between the number of metastatic lymph nodes and nodal stage based on their location in patients with gastric cancer. J Clin Oncol 1993;11:1894–900.
89. Kajitani T. The general rules for the gastric cancer study in surgery and pathology: part I and II. Jpn J Surg 1981;11:127–45.
90. Rothenberg ML, Fukushima M, Coltman CA Jr. Gastric and esophageal cancers: perspectives from a U.S.-Japan meeting. J Cancer Res Clin Oncol 1994;120:747–53.
91. Schlemper RJ, Itabashi M, Kato Y, et al. Differences in diagnostic criteria for gastric carcinoma between Japanese and Western pathologists. Lancet 1997;349:1725–9.
92. Bunt AM, Hermans J, Boon MC, et al. Evaluation of the extent of lymphadenectomy in a randomized trial of Western versus Japanese type surgery in gastric cancer. J Clin Oncol 1994;12:417–22.
93. Thompson GB, van Heerden JA, Sarr MG. Adenocarcinoma of the stomach: are we making progress? Lancet 1993;342:713–8.
94. Kim JJ, Jung HC, Song IS, et al. Preoperative evaluation of the curative resectability of gastric cancer by abdominal computed tomography and ultrasonography: a prospective comparison study. Korean J Intern Med 1997;12:1–6.
95. Stell DA, Carter CR, Stewart I, et al. Prospective comparison of laparoscopy, ultrasonography and computed tomography in the staging of gastric cancer. Br J Surg 1996;83:1260–2.
96. Cook AO, Levine BA, Sirinek KR, et al. Evaluation of gastric adenocarcinoma: abdominal computed tomography does not replace celiotomy. Arch Surg 1986;121:603–6.
97. Huguier M, Houry S, Lacaine F. Is the follow-up of patients operated on for gastric carcinoma of benefit to the patient? Hepatogastroenterology 1992;39:14–6.
98. Dupont BJ Jr, Cohn I Jr. Gastric adenocarcinoma. Curr Probl Cancer 1980;4:1–46.
99. Kajiyama Y, Tsurumaru M, Udagawa H, et al. Prognostic factors in adenocarcinoma of the gastric cardia: pathologic stage analysis and multivariate regression analysis. J Clin Oncol 1997;15:2015–21.
100. Setala LP, Kosma VM, Mann S, et al. Prognostic factors in gastric cancer: the value of vascular invasion, mitotic rate and lymphoplasmacytic infiltration. Br J Cancer 1996;74:766–72.
101. Hermanek P. Clinical significance of histologic classification in accordance with Lauren as an addition to pTNM. Scand J Gastroenterol 1987;22:Suppl 133:31–2.
102. Viste A, Eide GE, Halvorsen K, et al. Lauren's histologic classification and ABO blood group as prognostic factors for patients with stomach carcinoma. Scand J Gastroenterol 1987;22:Suppl 133:49–50.
103. Sanchez-Bueno F, Garcia-Marcilla JA, Perez-Flores D, et al. Prognostic factors in a series of 297 patients with gastric adenocarcinoma undergoing surgical resection. Br J Surg 1998;85:255–60.

104. Inada T, Kikuyama S, Ichikawa A, et al. Bcl-2 expression as a prognostic factor of survival of gastric carcinoma. Anticancer Res 1998;18:2003–10.
105. Hirose K, Iida A, Yamaguchi A, et al. Prognostic value of DNA ploidy and proliferative cell nuclear antigen in gastric cancer. Oncology 1998;55:300–6.
106. Rugge M, Sonego F, Panozzo M, et al. Pathology and ploidy in the prognosis of gastric cancer with no extranodal metastases. Cancer 1994;73:1127–33.
107. Yamamichi K, Uehara Y, Kitamura N, et al. Increased expression of CD44v6 mRNA significantly correlates with distant metastases and poor prognosis in gastric cancer. Int J Cancer 1998;79:256–62.
108. Mayer B, Jauch KW, Gunthert U, et al. De-novo expression of CD44 and survival in gastric cancer. Lancet 1993;342:1019–22.

109. Guo YJ, Liu G, Wang X, et al. Potential use of soluble CD44 in serum as an indicator of tumor burden and metastasis in patients with gastric or colon cancer. Cancer Res 1994;54:422–6.
110. Bedikian AY, Chen TT, Kankhanian N, et al. The natural history of gastric cancer and prognostic factors influencing survival. J Clin Oncol 1984;2:305–10.
111. Reiter W, Stieber P, Reuter C, et al. Prognostic value of preoperative serum levels of CEA, Ca19-9 and CA72-4 in gastric carcinoma. Anticancer Res 1997;17:2903–6.
112. Sakamoto J, Nakazato H, Teramukai S, et al. Association between preoperative plasma CEA levels and the prognosis of gastric cancer following curative resection. Tumor Marker Committee, Japanese Foundation for Multidisciplinary Treatment of Cancer, Tokyo, Japan. Surg Oncol 1996;5:133–9.

..........................................

# SURGERY FOR GASTRIC NEOPLASMS

• Kenneth P. Ramming

Since the first successful partial gastrectomy by Billroth in 1881, surgical removal of gastric cancer has been the only known successful treatment of this disease. It has been demonstrated that the routine use of total gastrectomy has failed to yield a better 5-year survival rate than subtotal gastrectomy, and the immediate mortality rate and side effects are greater.[1] The location and size of the tumor dictate the type of operation to be performed.

A 6-cm margin of grossly uninvolved normal stomach wall has been recommended by several authorities.[2] For proximal lesions at the gastroesophageal junction and the cardia, we prefer proximal gastrectomy and resection of the involved esophagus. For lesions in the distal gastric segment, a subtotal gastric resection is usually performed, as illustrated in Figure 41–1. If there is infiltration proximally or if a large cancer of the midgastric segment is encountered,

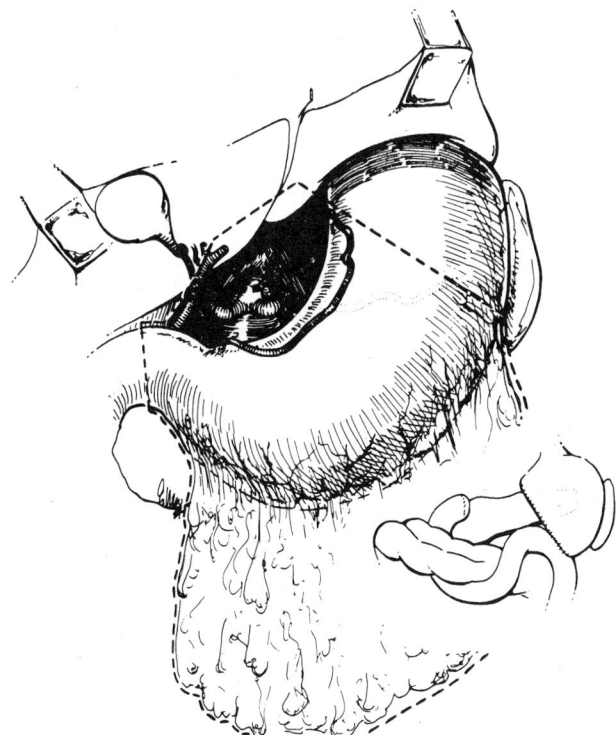

**Figure 41–1.** Extent of resection margins of radical subtotal gastrectomy for distal gastric carcinoma. Inset on the lower right shows the appearance after anastomoses have been performed. (From Macdonald JS, Cohn I Jr, Gunderson LL. Cancer of the stomach. In: DeVita VT, Hellman S, Rosenberg SA, eds. Principles and Practice of Oncology. 2nd ed. Philadelphia: JB Lippincott, 1985:673.)

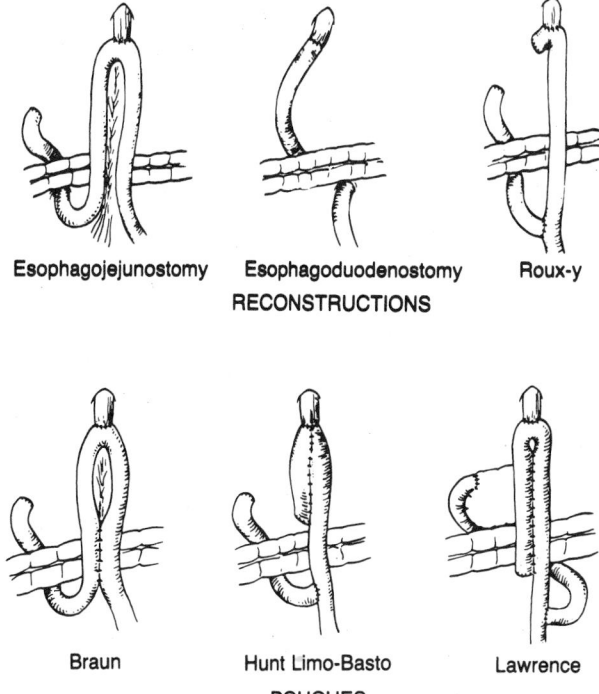

**Figure 41–2.** Variations in the types of reconstruction possible after total gastrectomy, with examples of gastric reservoir pouches that can be used to increase the capacity of the substitute stomach after a total gastrectomy. (From Macdonald JS, Cohn I Jr, Gunderson LL. Cancer of the stomach. In: DeVita VT, Hellman S, Rosenberg SA, eds. Principles and Practice of Oncology. 2nd ed. Philadelphia: JB Lippincott, 1985:673.)

total gastrectomy may be required because adequate margins on either side would not be attained with anything less. The surgical options for reconstruction and examples of gastric reservoir pouches that can be used to increase the capacity of the substitute stomach after a total gastrectomy are illustrated in Figure 41–2.

Direct invasion of contiguous organs, such as liver or pancreas, should not be a deterrent to resection if partial removal of these organs is feasible and safe. There are recorded instances of patients with contiguous organ involvement who have been cured.

Reconstruction in partial gastrectomy is usually by gastroduodenostomy (Billroth I) when possible but more often by gastrojejunostomy (Billroth II) because the amount of resected stomach often is of insufficient length to allow gastroduodenostomy. The construction of these anastomoses and the division of the stomach are greatly facilitated by the use of stapling devices. The position of the efferent and afferent limbs with respect to the colon is determined by the preference of the surgeon. We prefer a retrocolic anastomosis. For re-establishing intestinal continuity in cases of total gastrectomy, we have not favored the construction of intestinal pouches but prefer that a jejunal loop be brought up and an end-to-side esophageal-jejunal anastomosis be constructed with an end-to-side Roux-en-Y jejunojejunostomy fashioned distally to provide flow of bile and pancreatic secretions.

The results of surgery for gastric carcinoma are directly related to the stage of the cancer when first seen. Representative results of surgery have been reported by Dupont and associates.[3] In their series of 1497 patients, the operability rate was 82%, and the resectability rate was 48%. The 5-year survival rates were 22% after radical subtotal gastrectomy, 30% for localized disease, 2% after esophagogastrectomy, and 7.4% overall for the 48% of patients with resectable tumors.

The postoperative complications and mortality after surgery for gastric cancer have been reviewed in detail by Viste and coworkers[4] from Norway. In a series of 1010 consecutive patients participating in a prospective trial, 28% of the patients had one or more complications (usually pneumonia, thromboembolism, or cardiac problems). The postoperative mortality rate for resected patients was 8%, with a range from 7% for distal resections to 16% for proximal resections.

## REFERENCES

1. Shiu MH, Moore E, Sanders M, et al. Influence of the extent of resection on survival after curative treatment of gastric carcinoma. Arch Surg 1987;122:1347–51.
2. Bozzetti F, Bonfanti G, Bufalino R, et al. Adequacy of margins of resection in gastrectomy for cancer. Ann Surg 1982;196:685–90.
3. Dupont JB Jr, Lee JR, Burton GR, Cohn I Jr. Adenocarcinoma of the stomach: review of 1,497 cases. Cancer 1978;41:491–7.
4. Viste A, Haùgstvedt T, Eide GE, et al. Postoperative complications and mortality after surgery for gastric cancer. Ann Surg 1988;207:7–13.

............................................

# RADIATION THERAPY FOR GASTRIC CARCINOMA

• Luu M. Tran • Charles M. Haskell

Although surgery remains the mainstay of treatment of patients with gastric carcinoma, the 5-year survival rate in Western countries is poor. These cancers usually present with locally advanced disease, wherein curative resections are possible in only 50 to 60% of patients. Based on the failure data from University of Minnesota[1] and Massachusetts General Hospital,[2] the rate of local recurrence approaches 40%, even in patients in whom a complete resection was performed. Using the data on recurrence patterns after surgery alone, adjuvant therapy may be considered following complete surgical resection.

To date, single-modality adjuvant treatment with either radiation therapy or chemotherapy has not had a meaningful impact on survival. Several studies using 5-fluorouracil (5-FU)–based chemotherapy in combination with radiation therapy as an adjuvant treatment have suggested a positive outcome on local recurrence and, occasionally, survival.[3–9] Radiation therapy also has been used for locally advanced, unresectable disease and in 40 to 70% of the cases[6] can provide symptomatic relief of pain, bleeding, and obstruction.

## RADIATION TECHNIQUES

When radiation therapy is used, the irradiated area typically covers the gastric bed and adjacent lymphatic drainage with adequate margins. Because the gastric fundus usually extends posteriorly to the pancreas and the retroperitoneal tissues, the radiation fields are generally anterior and posterior (anteroposterior or posteroanterior). Lateral fields are not advisable because using these portals may increase the dose to both kidneys. Superiorly the field extends from above the diaphragm at the level of T8–T9 to the level of L3 inferiorly, including the entire gastric bed in the left upper quadrant, the paragastric and para-aortic nodes bilaterally, and the celiac axis in the right upper quadrant. Three-dimensional conformal radiation therapy, Cerrobend custom blocking, and small bowel contrast enhancement are helpful to determine the tumor volume and to spare as much dose to small bowel, heart, liver, and kidneys as possible. The spinal cord dose should not exceed 45 Gy, and kidneys should receive no more than 18 Gy. The total dose to the tumor is limited to 45 to 50.4 Gy over 5 weeks at 1.8 Gy/day with high-energy (6 to 18 MV) photons.

## RESULTS

**Postoperative Radiation Therapy and Chemotherapy After Curative Resection.** Postoperative radiation with 5-FU–based chemotherapy has been used extensively for patients whose tumors involve the serosa, regional lymph nodes, or resection margins after curative resection.[3-9] This combined approach has been shown in several trials (Table 41–3) to sterilize residual disease and decrease the local recurrence rate for these patients from about 55 to 35%. However, it has been difficult to prove a survival benefit from combined-modality therapy. Because of ambiguous survival results from older clinical trials, the role of CMT in prolonging survival has been addressed in a large Intergroup trial (INT-0116).[9] More than 600 patients with stage IB to stage IV disease (excluding patients with positive surgical margins, visceral metastases, or noncontiguous lymphatic metastases) were registered and randomized after potentially curative gastric resections. One group was followed without further treatment, whereas the other received CMT. The CMT consisted of initial therapy with bolus 5-fluorouracil and leucovorin given daily for 5 days, followed by 45 Gy of radiation therapy given with two concurrent cycles of bolus 5-fluorouracil and leucovorin, followed by additional chemotherapy after the completion of radiation therapy. An important part of this trial was careful review of the proposed radiation ports by a central reference center. This central review resulted in a revision of the radiation treatment plan in more than a third of the patients. The major toxic side effects of treatment were severe bone marrow suppression (54%) and gastrointestinal toxicity (33%). There were three treatment-related deaths. Both overall survival and disease-free survival were improved about 50% in the group receiving CMT ($p = 0.01$) and regional failure was decreased substantially. The authors concluded that CMT should be considered the standard of care for patients with gastric cancer who are at high risk of recurrence after potentially curative resections, as practiced in the United States.

**Preoperative Radiation Therapy.** Few centers have used preoperative chemotherapy and radiation therapy to prevent local-regional relapse. Ajani and coworkers[10] reported the results of 19 patients treated with preoperative chemotherapy (continuous-infusion 5-FU, cisplatin) and radiation therapy (45 Gy in 25 fractions over 5 weeks). Eight patients have been resected. Of these, four had pathologic complete responses and one a partial response (>90% necrosis). Five of 18 (28%) of the patients had grade 4 treatment-related toxicities, but there have been no treatment-related deaths.

Three randomized trials exist on preoperative radiation therapy in potentially resectable gastric carcinoma. One trial from Russia[11] reported the results of 142 patients randomized to surgery alone and 139 patients randomized to receive preoperative 20-Gy gamma irradiation. Combined treatment appeared to improve 3- and 5-year survival and was not followed by higher complication rates. A second trial from Russia[12] compared surgery alone with preoperative radiation therapy (40 Gy in 10 fractions, three times a week) and inhalation of 8% oxygen. A 17% increase in resection rate was achieved with preoperative treatment, a doubling of survival after preoperative treatment, and there was no increase in complications or morbidity.

In the third trial, which is from the Lombardi Cancer Center[13] at Georgetown University, 293 patients were randomized into three treatment groups: surgery alone, preoperative radiation therapy (20 Gy in four fractions), and preoperative radiation plus hyperthermia. Preoperative radiation did not result in improvement of 3- and 5-year survival in comparison with surgery alone. Radiation plus hyperthermia followed by surgery produced a significant improvement, with a 3-year survival rate of 22% and a 5-year survival rate of 21%. In unresectable gastric carcinoma, radiation and hyperthermia preoperatively increased mean survival.

The results described previously indicate that preoperative

*Table 41–3.* **Radiation Therapy with or Without Chemotherapy for Gastric Carcinoma**

| Series | Patients (No.) | Treatment | Survival (%) | Local Failure (%) |
|---|---|---|---|---|
| Hallissey (1994)[3, 7] | | | | |
| | 138 | S + FAM | 19 (5 yr) | 19 |
| | 153 | S + 45 Gy | 12 (5 yr) | 10 |
| | 145 | S alone | 20 (5 yr) | 27 |
| Regine (1992)[4] | | | | |
| | 70 | S alone | 10 (5 yr) | 45 |
| | 17 | S + CM (FAM) | 19 (5 yr) | |
| | 13 | S + RT (45–50 Gy) | 22 (5 yr) | |
| | 20 | S + RT (45–50 Gy) + CM (FAM) | 24 (5 yr) | 19 |
| Moertel (1984)[5] | | | | |
| | 33 | S alone | 12 (5 yr) | 54 |
| | 29 | S + RT (37.5 Gy) + CM (FAM) | 20 (5 yr) | 39 |
| Dent (1988)[8] | | | | |
| | 35 | 20 Gy + 5-FU | 30 (2 yr) | |
| | 31 | S alone | 40 (2 yr) | |
| Abe (1991)[19] | | | | |
| | 20 (stage II) | S + IORT (28–35 Gy) | 84 (5 yr) | |
| | 11 (stage II) | S alone | 62 (5 yr) | |
| | 27 (stage IV) | S + IORT (28–35 Gy) | 15 (5 yr) | |
| | 18 (stage IV) | S alone | 0 | |
| Macdonald (2000)[9] | | | | |
| | 275 | S alone | 26 mo (median) | 72 |
| | 281 | S + 45 Gy + 5 FU/LV | 40 mo (median) | 10 |

S, surgery; FAM, fluorouracil doxorubicin (Adriamycin), mitomycin C; CM, chemotherapy; IORT, intraoperative radiation therapy; 5-FU/LV, 5-fluorouracil with leucovorin.

*Table 41–4.* **Chemoradiotherapy for Unresectable Gastric Cancer**

| Series | Patients (No.) | Treatment | Survival (%) |
|---|---|---|---|
| Moertel (1969)[14] | 23 | 35–40 Gy | 0 (5 yr) |
| | 25 | 35–40 Gy + 5-FU | 12 (5 yr) |
| GITSG (Schein, 1990)[16] | 45 | 25 Gy × 2 + 5-FU/meCCNU | 18 (4 yr) |
| | | 25 Gy × 2 | 6 (4 yr) |
| ECOG (Klaassen, 1985)[17] | 26 | 40 Gy + 5-FU, then weekly 5-FU | 37 (1 yr) |

5-FU, 5-fluorouracil; meCCNU, methyl-CCNU; GITSG, Gastrointestinal Tumor Study Group; ECOG, Eastern Cooperative Oncology Group.

chemoradiation therapy for gastric carcinoma can be performed safely and may have a favorable impact on resectability and survival. These studies, however, can be considered only as investigational, phase I trials. Additional multicenter trials are warranted for preoperative chemoradiation in patients with resectable and unresectable gastric carcinomas.

**Combined-Modality Therapy for Patients with Regionally Advanced Disease After Palliative Resection.** In patients undergoing palliative resection or biopsy alone, treatment options include chemotherapy or radiation therapy, or both. Most studies have been pilot studies involving small numbers of patients. Results of randomized trials of patients with locally advanced disease treated with combined-modality therapy are shown in Table 41–4.

In 1969, Moertel and associates[14] from the Mayo Clinic reported a phase III trial of 48 patients with locally unresectable gastric carcinoma. Patients were randomized to radiation (35 to 40 Gy) or radiation therapy plus 5-FU. None of the patients receiving radiation therapy alone survived long term, whereas 12% of the patients receiving both modalities survived 16 to 24 months. Based on the positive result obtained from this study as well as from other gastrointestinal carcinomas treated with the combination chemoradiation, the Gastrointestinal Tumor Study Group (GITSG)[15] designed a controlled clinical trial for locally advanced, unresectable gastric carcinoma. In this study, patients were randomized to receive chemotherapy (5-FU and methyl-CCNU) or split-course radiation therapy (50 Gy) plus chemotherapy. 5-FU was given on the first 3 days of radiation, followed by maintenance 5-FU and methyl-CCNU. Although early treatment-related mortality was higher in the combined arm, the 5-year survival was significantly higher in the combined-modality group (18 vs. 6%). Resection in patients with residual disease yielded better long-term survival rates than those whose cancers were not resected. In a subsequent GITSG[16] trial, doxorubicin was added to the chemotherapy regimen, and radiation therapy (50 Gy) was given continuously over 5 weeks. In contrast with the first study, there was no difference in survival between the chemotherapy arm and the combined chemoradiation arm.

In another study, Klaassen and colleagues[17] reported the results from an Eastern Cooperative Oncology Group (ECOG) study comparing 5-FU alone with 5-FU plus radiation in a randomized trial of 57 patients with locally unresectable gastric carcinoma. The investigators observed no difference in survival between the two groups.

In a third study, Bleiberg and associates[18] reported the results from the European Organization for the Research and Treatment of Cancer (EORTC) in 115 patients who underwent curative and palliative surgery for resectable gastric carcinoma. They were randomized to receive (1) radiation alone (55.5 Gy), (2) radiation in combination with short-term 5-FU, (3) long-term 5-FU, or (4) short-term and long-term 5-FU. The short-term 5-FU was given at a dosage of 575 mg/m$^2$ during the first 4 days of treatment. The long-term 5-FU was given at a dosage of 750 mg/m$^2$ every 2 weeks for 18 months. There was no survival advantage between the treatment groups, and the 5-year survival of the entire group was 22%. Among 22 patients with residual disease, the three who were still alive without evidence of disease progression had been treated with radiation therapy combined with 5-FU.

The results from these studies are discouraging, with local recurrence rates of 50 to 70%. This recurrence may be explained by suboptimal study design (split-course radiation therapy, small doses of radiation, and bolus injection of 5-FU). These regimens have theoretical and biologic disadvantages compared with modern regimens of continuous radiation and protracted venous infusion of 5-FU. Although no survival advantage has been proved, chemoradiation is capable of sterilizing residual disease after attempted curative resection. For patients with unresectable disease, there is a consensus that they are candidates for treatment with concurrent radiation therapy and 5-FU chemotherapy.

**Intraoperative Electron-Beam Therapy.** Even with the combined adjuvant chemoradiation following complete resection, the rate of local recurrence remains high (30%).[3, 4, 7] An alternative method of delivering high-dose radiation to the tumor bed is intraoperative electron-beam therapy (IORT), a technique that permits delivery of a high dose to the tumor bed while minimizing exposure to the surrounding normal tissue. IORT doses range from 10 to 20 Gy, and the toxicity has been acceptable.

For patients with locally advanced disease, combined external-beam irradiation plus chemotherapy or IORT has been shown to produce long-term survival in 10 to 20%.[19–21] Abe and colleagues[19] were the first to show the feasibility and efficacy in 14 patients with gastric cancers treated with IORT. Subsequent reports by Abe and colleagues[20] updated the Japanese experience in the management of gastric carcinoma with IORT. Of 211 patients in the study, 110 patients were randomized to receive surgery only, and 101 patients received surgery plus IORT. The IORT dose ranged from 28 Gy for microscopic disease to 35 Gy for macroscopic disease. Stage I outcome was not improved with IORT. Survival rates in patients with stage II and stage IV disease were improved with IORT, however. Sindelar and colleagues,[22] in a prospective randomized trial from the National Cancer Institute, compared gastrectomy and IORT (20 Gy) with gastrectomy plus conventional external-beam therapy. In terms of survival, the investigators showed no advantage of IORT over conventional radiation; however, both local and regional control were improved with IORT.

## REFERENCES

1. Gunderson LL, Sosin H. Adenocarcinoma of the stomach: areas of failure in a re-operation series (second or symptomatic look)—clinicopathologic correlation and implications for adjuvant therapy. Int J Radiat Oncol Biol Phys 1982;8:1–11.
2. Landry J, Tepper JE, Wood WC, et al. Patterns of failure following curative resection of gastric carcinoma. Int J Radiat Oncol Biol Phys 1990;19:1357–62.
3. Allum WH, Hallissey MT, Ward LC, Hockey MS. British Stomach Cancer Group: a controlled prospective, randomized trial of adjuvant chemotherapy or radiotherapy in resectable gastric cancer: interim report. Br J Cancer 1989;60:739–44.
4. Regine W, Mohiuddin M. Impact of adjuvant therapy on locally advanced adenocarcinoma of the stomach. Int J Radiat Oncol Biol Phys 1992;24:921–7.
5. Moertel CG, Childs DS, O'Fallon JR, et al. Combined 5-fluorouracil and radiation therapy as a surgical adjuvant for poor prognosis gastric carcinoma. J Clin Oncol 1984;2:1249–54.
6. Falkson G, Eden EB. A control clinical trial of fluorouracil and radiation therapy in stomach cancer. Med Pediatr Oncol 1976;2:111–7.
7. Hallissey MT, Dunn JA, Ward LC, Allum WH. The second British Stomach Cancer Group trial of adjuvant radiotherapy or chemotherapy in resectable gastric cancer: five-year follow-up. Lancet 1994;343:1309–12.
8. Dent DM, Madden MV, Price SK. Randomized comparison of R1 and R2 gastrectomy for gastric carcinoma. Br J Surg 1988;75:110–2.
9. Macdonald J, Smalley S, Benedetti JK, et al. Postoperative combined radiation and chemotherapy improves disease-free survival (DFS) and overall survival (OS) in resected adenocarcinoma of the stomach and GE junction. Proc Am Soc Clin Oncol 2000;19:1a.
10. Ajani JA, Mansfield P, Janjan N, et al. Preoperative chemoradiation therapy in patients with potentially resectable gastric carcinoma: a multi-institutional pilot. Proc ASCO 1998;17:283a.
11. Talaev M, Starinskii V, Kovalev B, et al. Results of combined treatment of the gastric antrum and gastric body. Vopr Onkol 1990;36:1485–8.
12. Kosse VA. Combined treatment of gastric cancer using hypoxic radiotherapy. Vopr Onkol 1990;36:1349–53.
13. Shchepotin IB, Evans SR, Chorny V, et al. Intensive preoperative radiotherapy with local hyperthermia for the treatment of gastric carcinoma. Surg Oncol 1994;3:37–44.
14. Moertel CG, Childs DS, Reitemeier RJ, et al. Combined 5-fluorouracil and supervoltage radiation therapy of locally unresectable gastrointestinal carcinoma. Lancet 1969;1:1865–7.
15. Schein PS, Smith FP, Woolley PV, Ahlgren JD. Current management of advanced and locally unresectable gastric carcinoma. Cancer 1982;50:Suppl:2590–6.
16. The Gastrointestinal Tumor Study Group. The concept of locally advanced gastric cancer: effect of treatment on outcome. Cancer 1990;68:2324–30.
17. Klaassen DJ, MacIntyre JM, Catton GE, et al. Treatment of locally unresectable cancer of the stomach and pancreas: a randomized comparison of 5-fluorouracil alone with radiation plus concurrent and maintenance 5-fluorouracil—an Eastern Cooperative Oncology Group study. J Clin Oncol 1985;3:373–8.
18. Bleiberg H, Goffin RK, Dalesio O, et al. Adjuvant radiotherapy and chemotherapy in resectable gastric cancer: a randomized trial of the gastro-intestinal tract cancer of the EORTC. Eur J Surg Oncol 1989;15:535–43.
19. Abe M, Takahashi M, Ono K, et al. Japan gastric trials in intraoperative radiation therapy. Int J Radiat Oncol Biol Phys 1988;15:1431–3.
20. Abe M, Shibamoto Y, Ono K, Takahashi M. Intraoperative radiation therapy for carcinoma of the stomach and pancreas. Front Radiat Ther Oncol 1991;25:258-69, 330–3.
21. Takahashi M, Abe M. Intra-operative radiotherapy for carcinoma of the stomach. Eur J Surg Oncol 1986;12:247–50.
22. Sindelar WF, Kinsella TJ, Tepper JE, et al. Randomized trial of intraoperative radiotherapy in carcinoma of the stomach. Am J Surg 1993;165:178–86.

......................................

# CHEMOTHERAPY FOR GASTRIC CANCER

• Carol Nishikubo • Charles M. Haskell

Chemotherapy is of marginal efficacy against gastric carcinomas. An antineoplastic effect has been repeatedly shown through the demonstration of objective, measurable responses to single agents and to various drug combinations. Most of the benefit is anecdotal, however, and limited to rare patients who do unexpectedly well with chemotherapy. This section reviews briefly the current role of this modality in the management of gastric carcinomas. Chemotherapy for gastric lymphomas and sarcomas is discussed elsewhere in this book.

## SINGLE-AGENT CHEMOTHERAPY

Table 41–5 shows chemotherapy agents that produce an objective response rate greater than 10%. No randomized, placebo-controlled studies have been conducted that show whether single-agent chemotherapy can prolong survival in patients with gastric carcinoma.

## COMBINATION CHEMOTHERAPY

5-FU–based combinations have been extensively studied in patients with gastric cancer (Table 41–6). Most commonly, 5-FU has been combined with an anthracycline and mitomycin C, methotrexate, platinum, or one of the nitrosoureas. In the past, the most popular combination in the United States was the FAM regimen, which in early studies showed a 42% response rate lasting for a median of 9 months.[1] The median survival for responding patients was 12.5 months, with 6 of 26 responding patients surviving longer than 2 years. These findings were significantly better than those of historic controls. Subsequent studies, however, directly comparing FAM with 5-FU alone showed no survival advantage and no advantage in terms of control of symptoms for the combination arm.[2] The toxicity of FAM was also considerable, with severe myelosuppression commonly seen and less often renal toxicity,[3] hemolytic anemia,[3–6] and hemolytic-uremic syndrome,[7] probably as a result of the mitomycin C.

Other regimens that do not incorporate 5-FU as one of

*Table 41–5.* Chemotherapy Agents with Single-Agent Activity in Gastric Cancer

| Drug | Activity (%) | Reference |
|---|---|---|
| Mitomycin C | 31 | 33–36 |
| Ftorafur | 26 | 37 |
| Paclitaxel (24-hr) | 24–31 | 38 |
| Doxorubicin | 23 | 39 |
| 5-Fluorouracil | 23 | 33, 34, 36, 40, 41 |
| Epirubicin | 22 | 42–45 |
| Etoposide (oral) | 21 | 46 |
| Hydroxyurea | 19 | 34 |
| Cisplatin | 17 | 37, 47, 48 |
| Chlorambucil | 17 | 34 |
| Docetaxel | 17 | 49 |
| Mechlorethamine | 16 | 49 |
| Altretamine | 15 | 37 |
| Decarbazine | 13 | 34 |
| Methotrexate | 10 | 34, 50 |

the components, such as EAP (etoposide, doxorubicin, and cisplatin), have also shown fairly high response rates but have significant toxicity.[8, 9] Combination regimens incorporating the taxanes are also being studied,[10] and there have been some promising studies conducted using oral UFT (tegafur) instead of 5-FU in combination with leucovorin, etoposide, and other agents.[11–14] Response rates have been in the 27 to 37% range with tolerable toxicity.

Randomized studies comparing treatment with chemotherapy with supportive care alone have shown an advantage in terms of survival (12.3 months vs. 3.1 months,[15] 8 months vs. 5 months[16]) and in terms of symptom control[16] favoring the chemotherapy arm. Randomized studies comparing single-agent chemotherapy with combination chemotherapy, however, have not shown an advantage to combination regimens.[2, 17–19] Some patients treated with combination chemotherapy live for prolonged periods. In a long-term follow-up study from Japan, 3% of patients with advanced gastric cancer treated with one of several different combination chemotherapy regimens survived longer than 5 years.[20]

For patients ineligible for or who choose not to participate in a clinical trial, chemotherapy has been shown to prolong survival and improve symptoms. Combination chemotherapy has not been shown in a randomized trial to be superior to single-agent 5-FU or 5-FU in combination with leucovorin. The latter is a reasonable alternative if the patient has a good performance status and desires chemotherapy.

## ADJUVANT COMBINED-MODALITY THERAPY

For patients with resected tumors involving the serosa, positive regional lymph nodes, or positive margins, radiation with or without chemotherapy can reduce the local recurrence rate from about 55 to 35% in randomized trials. Chemoradiotherapy also appears to improve overall survival, as demonstrated in a large intergroup trial (see discussion in previous subchapter on Radiation Therapy).[21]

Adjuvant chemotherapy alone is of uncertain benefit in the adjuvant setting. A trial from Spain published in 1999 found a survival benefit for adjuvant mitomycin and tegafur,[22] but most prior trials have not shown a survival advan-

tage from chemotherapy used as a single modality. For example, Tsavaris and coworkers[23] studied adjuvant chemotherapy versus placebo in a randomized, controlled study. Eighty-four patients participated; 42 received three cycles of 5-FU, epirubicin, and mitomycin C, whereas the other 42 had no postoperative chemotherapy. There was a trend toward improved survival in the adjuvant arm that was not statistically significant. Another larger study of 314 patients, 155 of whom received adjuvant FAM chemotherapy, showed no difference in overall survival, although the chemotherapy-treated patients had a longer time to progression.[24] A meta-analysis of 14 trials reported since 1980 did not find a survival benefit from adjuvant chemotherapy.[25]

Adjuvant intraperitoneal therapy has also been studied as a means of reducing peritoneal recurrences. One randomized study of mitomycin C in 50 patients conducted in Kyoto found a survival advantage in the mitomycin C–treated arm.[26] Cisplatin administered into the peritoneal cavity in the adjuvant setting has not been shown to improve survival in treated patients.[27] Better success has been achieved in combining adjuvant intraperitoneal therapy with neoadjuvant chemotherapy, described subsequently.

## COMBINED-MODALITY THERAPY FOR PATIENTS WITH REGIONALLY ADVANCED DISEASE

The optimal treatment for patients with unresectable, locally advanced disease remains unclear. Studies comparing combined-modality therapy with either radiation therapy or chemotherapy alone have shown variable results. Most have shown no difference in overall survival in patients treated with combined-modality therapy compared with single-modality therapy, but a few long-term survivors are seen in the combined-modality therapy arm.[28] A randomized study conducted by GITSG found that combined-modality therapy with radiation therapy, 5-FU, and semustine had an improved 5-year survival rate of 18% versus 6% in the radiation therapy–alone arm.[29] A subsequent study adding doxorubicin to the previous chemotherapy agents and comparing a combined-modality therapy arm with chemotherapy alone showed similar mean survival rates but a higher 3-year survival in the chemotherapy-alone arm.[29] Other studies, including an ECOG study comparing 5-FU alone with 5-FU plus radiation therapy, showed no difference in survival between the two groups.[30]

## NEOADJUVANT THERAPY

Several studies of patients treated with neoadjuvant chemotherapy followed by postoperative intraperitoneal chemotherapy have shown potential survival benefit to treated patients. In a trial conducted at the University of Southern California,[31] 59 patients with potentially resectable tumors were treated with two cycles of protracted-infusion 5-FU along with leucovorin and cisplatin. Postoperatively, patients received two cycles of intraperitoneal floxuridine and cisplatin. Fifty-six patients underwent surgery, with 40 patients (71%) resected for cure and 15 (27%) undergoing palliative surgery for stage IV disease; 1 patient died intraoperatively. With a median follow-up over 45 months, the calculated median

*Table 41–6.* **Combination Chemotherapy Trials***

| | Response Rate (%) | Reference |
|---|---|---|
| *Two-Drug Combinations* | | |
| 5-FU (CI)/Cisplat | 56 | 51 |
| 5-FU/Cisplat | 51 | 17 |
| 5′-Deoxy-5-fluorouridine/Cisplat | 50 | 52 |
| 5-FU/epi | 41 | 53 |
| 5-FU/carmustine | 32 | 54–58 |
| 5-FU/LV | 31 | 59, 60 |
| 5-FU/mitomycin | 31 | 61 |
| 5-FU (CI)/chromomycin A$_3$ | 29 | 62 |
| Mitomycin/triazinate | 27 | 63 |
| 5-FU/α-interferon | 25 | 64 |
| 5-FU (CI)/mitomycin | 24 | 65–68 |
| 5-FU/semustine | 19 | 69 |
| 5-FU/fluorometholone | 19 | 70 |
| 5-FU/cytarabine | 17 | 71 |
| Mitomycin/etoposide | 17 | 72 |
| 5-FU/cyclophosphamide | 16 | 73 |
| 5-FU/doxorubicin | 15 | 74, 75 |
| 5-FU (CI)/semustine | 14 | 65, 67, 76, 77 |
| Doxorubicin/mitomycin | 13 | 78 |
| Cisplat/etoposide | 11 | 79, 80 |
| *Three-Drug Combinations* | | |
| 5-FU (CI)/epi/Cisplat | 45–61 | 81, 82 |
| 5-FU/etoposide/LV (ELF) | 29–57 | 83–87 |
| 5-FU (CI)/epi/cisplat | 56 | 88 |
| 5-FU/LV/Cisplat | 52 | 89, 90 |
| 5-FU/LV/mitomycin | 47 | 91 |
| 5-FU/Cisplat/paclitaxel | 45 | 38 |
| 5-FU/epi/LV | 43 | 92, 93 |
| Cisplat/etoposide/doxorubicin (Adriamycin) (EAP) | 43 | 94–101 |
| 5-FU/epi/carmustine (FEB) | 42 | 102 |
| 5-FU/doxorubicin/carmustine | 41 | 103–105 |
| 5-FU/doxorubicin/cisplat (FAP) | 41 | 106–109 |
| 5-FU/doxorubicin/mitomycin (FAM) | 34 | 17, 75, 110–119 |
| Cisplat/epi/etoposide | 34 | 120 |
| 5-FU/mitomycin/cytarabine | 34 | 121–125 |
| 5-FU/LV/paclitaxel | 32 | 126 |
| 5-FU/doxorubicin/MTX | 26 | 127, 128 |
| 5-FU/doxorubicin/semustine (FAMe) | 25 | 113, 123, 124, 129, 130 |
| 5-FU/PALA/thymidine | 25 | 131 |
| 5-FU/semustine/ICRF-159 | 21 | 124 |
| Ftorafur/doxorubicin/mitomycin | 20 | 132 |
| FU/epi/mitomycin | 16 | 133 |
| *Combinations of Four or More Drugs* | | |
| 5-FU/Cisplat/epi/LV/G-CSF | 72 | 134 |
| 5-FU/LV/Cisplat/etoposide | 72 | 135 |
| 5-FU/LV/Cisplat/epi/etoposide | 71 | 136 |
| 5-FU/cisplat/epi/LV/glutathione/G-CSF | 62 | 137 |
| 5-FU/MTX/LV/epi/cisplat | 46 | 138 |
| 5-FU/doxorubicin/MTX/LV (FAMTX) | 40 | 9, 139–145 |
| 5-FU/doxorubicin/BCNU→FAM→XRT→FAM | 40 | 146 |
| 5-FU/doxorubicin/mitomycin/semustine | 39 | 147 |
| 5-FU/doxorubicin/mitomycin/LV | 38 | 148 |
| 5-FU/LV/doxorubicin/cisplat (FLAP) | 36 | 149 |
| 5-FU/doxorubicin/mitomycin/MTX | 29 | 150 |
| 5-FU/doxorubicin/mitomycin/chlorozotocin | 26 | 151 |
| 5-FU/doxorubicin/mitomycin/BCNU | 22 | 152 |
| 5-FU/doxorubicin/mitomycin/vincristine | 16 | 153 |
| 5-FU/doxorubicin/mitomycin/triazinate | 13 | 154 |

*Trials of at least 15 patients with ≥10% response.

5-FU, 5-fluorouracil; CI, continuous infusion; Cisplat, cisplatinum; epi, epirubicin; LV, leucovorin; MTX, methotrexate; G-CSF, granulocyte colony–stimulating factor; XRT, radiation therapy.

survival for all patients was longer than 4 years. In another phase II study[32] of neoadjuvant therapy for nonoperatively staged high-risk patients, 56 patients were treated with preoperative FAMTX (fluorouracil, Adriamycin, methotrexate [with leucovorin rescue]) with postoperative intraperitoneal cisplatin and 5-FU along with intravenous 5-FU. Median survival for this group was 15.3 months overall, with a median survival of 31 months in patients who underwent potentially curative resection at surgery. These encouraging data need to be confirmed in randomized, controlled trials.

# REFERENCES

1. Macdonald JS, Schein PS, Woolley PV, et al. 5-fluorouracil, doxorubicin and mitomycin (FAM) combination chemotherapy for advanced gastric cancer. Ann Intern Med 1980;93:533–6.
2. O'Connell MJ. Current status of chemotherapy for advanced pancreatic and gastric cancer. J Clin Oncol 1985;3:1032–9.
3. Karlin DA, Stroehlein JR. Rash, nephritis, hypertension and haemolysis in patient on 5-fluorouracil, doxorubicin and mitomycin. Lancet 1980;2:534–5.
4. Jones BG, Fielding JW, Newman CE, et al. Intravascular haemolysis and renal impairment after blood transfusion in two patients on long-term 5-fluorouracil and mitomycin. Lancet 1980;1:1275–7.
5. Lempert KD. Haemolysis and renal impairment syndrome in patients on 5-fluorouracil and mitomycin C. Lancet 1980;2:369–70.
6. Crocker J, Jones EL. Haemolytic-uraemic syndrome complicating long term mitomycin C and 5-fluorouracil therapy for gastric carcinoma. J Clin Pathol 1983;36:24–9.
7. Zimmerman SE, Smith FP, Phillips TM, et al. Gastric carcinoma and thrombotic thrombocytopenic purpura: association with plasma immune complex concentrations. Br Med J 1982;284:1432–4.
8. Lerner A, Gonin R, Steele GD, et al. Etoposide, doxorubicin and cisplatin chemotherapy for advanced gastric adenocarcinoma: results of a phase II trial. J Clin Oncol 1992;10:536–40.
9. Kelsen D, Atiq OT, Saltz L, et al. FAMTX versus etoposide, doxorubicin and cisplatin: a randomized assignment trial in gastric cancer. J Clin Oncol 1992;10:541–8.
10. Bokemeyer C, Hartmann JT, Lampe CS, et al. Paclitaxel and weekly 24-hour infusion of 5-fluorouracil/folinic acid in advanced gastric cancer. Semin Oncol 1997;24:6 Suppl 19:S19–96–100.
11. Kim YH, Shin SW, Kim BS, et al. A phase II trial: oral UFT and leucovorin in patients with advanced gastric carcinoma. Oncology 1997;11:119–23.
12. Gonzalez Baron M, Espinosa E, Feliu J, et al. The UFT/leucovorin/etoposide regimen for the treatment of advanced gastric cancer. Oncopaz Cooperative Group. Oncology 1997;11:9 Suppl 10:109–12.
13. Kim YH, Cheong SK, Lee JD, et al. Phase II trial of oral UFT and leucovorin in advanced gastric carcinoma. Am J Clin Oncol 1996;19:212–6.
14. Feliu J, Gonzalez Baron M, et al. Treatment of patients with advanced gastric carcinoma with the combination of eoposide and oral tegafur modulated by uracil and leucovorin: a phase II study of the ONCOPAZ cooperative group. Cancer 1996;78:211–6.
15. Pyrhonen S, Kuitunen T, Nyandoto P, et al. Randomised comparison of fluorouracil, epidoxorubicin and methotrexate (FEMTX) and supportive care with supportive care alone in patients with non-resectable gastric cancer. Br J Cancer 1995;71:587–91.
16. Glimelius B, Ekstrom K, Hoffman K, et al. Randomized comparison between chemotherapy plus best supportive care with best supportive care in advanced gastric cancer. Ann Oncol 1997;8:163–8.
17. Kim NK, Park YS, Heo DS, et al. A phase III randomized study of 5-fluorouracil and cisplatin versus 5-fluorouracil, doxorubicin and mitomycin C versus 5-fluorouracil alone in the treatment of advanced gastric cancer. Cancer 1993;71:3813–8.
18. Cullinan SA, Moertel CG, Wieand HS, et al. Controlled evaluation of three drug combination regimens versus fluorouracil alone for the therapy of advanced gastric cancer. North Central Cancer Treatment Group. J Clin Oncol 1994;12:412–6.
19. Estrada E, Lacave AJ, Valle M, et al. Methyl CCNU, 5-fluorouracil and Adriamycin (MeFA) as adjuvant chemotherapy in gastric cancer: 5 years of follow-up. Proc ASCO 1988;7:94.
20. Ohtsu A, Yoshida S, Miyata Y, Shimada Y. [Recent advances in chemotherapy for advanced gastric cancer: from the standpoint of survival advantages]. Gan To Kagaku Ryoho 1995;22:444–50.
21. Macdonald J, Smalley S, Benedetti JK, et al. Postoperative combined radiation and chemotherapy improves disease-free survival (DFS) and overall survival (OS) in resected adenocardinoma of the stomach and GE junction. Proc Am Soc Clin Oncol 2000;19:1a.
22. Cirera L, Balil A, Batiste-Alentorn E, et al. Randomized clinical trial of adjuvant mitomycin plus tegafur in patients with resected stage III gastric cancer. J Clin Oncol 1999;17:3810–5.
23. Tsavaris N, Tentas K, Kosmidis P, et al. A randomized trial comparing adjuvant fluorouracil, epirubicin and mitomycin with no treatment in operable gastric cancer. Chemotherapy 1996;42:220–6.
24. Lise M, Nitti D, Marchet A, et al. Prognostic factors in resectable gastric cancer: results of EORTC study number 40813 on FAM adjuvant chemotherapy. Ann Surg Oncol 1995;2:495–501.
25. Hermans J, Bonenkamp JJ, Boon MC, et al. Adjuvant therapy after curative resection for gastric cancer: meta-analysis of randomized trials. J Clin Oncol 1993;11:1441–7.
26. Hagiwara A, Takahashi T, Kojima O, et al. Prophylaxis with carbon-adsorbed mitomycin against peritoneal recurrence of gastric cancer. Lancet 1992;339:629–31.
27. Sautner T, Hofbauer F, Depisch D, et al. Adjuvant intraperitoneal cisplatin chemotherapy does not improve long-term survival after surgery for advanced gastric cancer. J Clin Oncol 1994;12:970–4.
28. Moertel CG, Childs DS Jr, Reitemeier RJ, et al. Combined 5-fluorouracil and supervoltage radiation therapy of locally unresectable gastrointestinal cancer. Lancet 1969;2:865–7.
29. Gastrointestinal Tumor Study Group. The concept of locally advanced gastric cancer: effect of treatment on outcome. Cancer 1990;66:2324–30.
30. Klaassen DJ, MacIntyre JM, Catton GE, et al. Treatment of locally unresectable cancer of the stomach and pancreas: a randomized comparison of 5-fluorouracil alone with radiation plus concurrent and maintenance 5-fluorouracil—an Eastern Cooperative Oncology Group study. J Clin Oncol 1985;3:373–8.
31. Crookes P, Leichman CG, Leichman L, et al. Systemic chemotherapy for gastric carcinoma followed by postoperative intraperitoneal therapy. Cancer 1997;79:1767–75.
32. Kelsen D, Karpeh M, Schwartz G, et al. Neoadjuvant therapy of high-risk gastric cancer: a phase II trial of preoperative FAMTX and postoperative intraperitoneal fluorouracil-cisplatin plus intravenous fluorouracil. J Clin Oncol 1996;14:1818–28.
33. Gupta S. Treatment of advanced gastric cancer with 5-FU versus mitomycin C. J Surg Oncol 1982;21:94–6.
34. Wasserman TH. Phase II trial summaries. Cancer Chemother Rep 1975;6:Part 3:399.
35. Comis RL, Carter SK. A review of chemotherapy in gastric cancer. Cancer 1974;34:1576–86.
36. Carter SK, Comis RL. Gastric cancer: current status of treatment. J Natl Cancer Inst 1977;58:567–78.
37. Wittes RE, Adrianza ME, Parsons R, et al. Compilation of phase II results with single antineoplastic agents. Cancer Treat Symp 1985;4:1–471.
38. Ajani JA. Treatment of patients with upper gastrointestinal carcinomas. Semin Oncol 1997;24:S19–72–6.
39. Wadler S, Green M, Muggia F. The role of anthracyclines in the treatment of gastric cancer. Cancer Treat Rev 1985;12:105–32.
40. Chlebowski RT, Paroly WS, Pugh RP, et al. Treatment of advanced gastric carcinoma with 5-fluorouracil: a randomized comparison of two routes of delivery. Cancer Treat Rep 1979;63:1979–81.
41. Moynihan T, Hansen R, Anderson T, et al. Continuous 5-fluorouracil infusion in advanced gastric carcinoma. Am J Clin Oncol 1988;11:461–4.
42. Scarffe JH, Kenny JB, Johnson RJ, et al. Phase II trial of epirubicin in gastric cancer. Cancer Treat Rep 1985;69:1275–7.
43. Kolaric K, Potrebica V, Cervek J. Phase II clinical trial of 4'epi-doxorubicin in metastatic solid tumor. J Cancer Res Clin Oncol 1983;106:148–52.
44. Ganzine F. 4'epi-doxorubicin, a new analogue of doxorubicin: a preliminary overview of preclinical and clinical data. Cancer Treat Rev 1983;10:1–22.

45. Cazap E, Estevez R, Bruno M, et al. Phase II trial of 4'epi-doxorubicin in locally advanced or metastatic gastric cancer. Tumori 1988;74:313–5.

46. Ajani JA, Dumas P. Evaluation of oral etoposide in patients with metastatic gastric carcinoma: a preliminary report. Semin Oncol 1992;19:6 Suppl 14:45–7.

47. Perry MC, Green MR, Mick R, et al. Cisplatin in patients with gastric carcinoma: a Cancer and Leukemia Group B phase II study. Cancer Treat Rep 1986;70:415–6.

48. Kantarjian H, Ajani JA, Karlin DA. Cis-diamminedichloroplatinum (II) chemotherapy for advanced adenocarcinoma of the upper gastrointestinal tract. Oncology 1985;42:69–71.

49. Einzig AI, Neuberg D, Remick SC, et al. Phase II trial of docetaxel (taxotere) in patients with adenocarcinoma of the upper gastrointestinal tract previously untreated with cytotoxic chemotherapy: the Eastern Cooperative Oncology Group (ECOG) results of protocol E1293. Med Oncol 1996;13:87–93.

50. Bruckner HW, Lokich JJ, Stablein DM. Studies of Baker's antifol, methotrexate, and razoxane in advanced gastric cancer: a Gastrointestinal Tumor Study Group report. Cancer Treat Rep 1982;66:1713–7.

51. Rougier PH, Oliveira J, Droz JP, et al. Cisplatin + five days continuous infusion 5-FU in advanced gastric cancer: preliminary results of a phase II trial. Proc Am Soc Clin Oncol 1988;7:106.

52. Koizumi W, Kurihara M, Sasai T, et al. A phase II study of combination therapy with 5'deoxy-5-fluorouridine and cisplatin in the treatment of advanced gastric cancer with primary foci. Cancer 1993;72:658–62.

53. Kolaric K, Potrebica V, Stanovnik M. Controlled phase III clinical study of 4-epi-doxorubicin + 5-fluorouracil versus 5-fluorouracil alone in metastatic gastric and rectosigmoid cancer. Oncology 1986;43:73–7.

54. Reitemeier RJ, Moertel CG, Hahn RG. Combination chemotherapy in gastrointestinal cancer. Cancer Res 1970;30:1425–8.

55. Kovach JS, Moertel CG, Schutt AJ, et al. Proceedings: a controlled study of combined 1,3-bis-(2-chloroethyl)-1-nitrosourea and 5-fluorouracil therapy for advanced gastric and pancreatic cancer. Cancer 1974;3:563–7.

56. Levi JA, Dalley DN, Aroney RS. Improved combination chemotherapy in advanced gastric cancer. Br Med J 1979;2:1471–3.

57. Jamieson GG, Gill PG. A prospective trial of 5-FU and BCNU in the treatment of advanced gastric cancer. Aust N Z J Surg 1981;51:16–9.

58. Schnitzler G, Queisser W, Heim ME, et al. Phase III study of 5-FU and carmustine versus 5-FU, carmustine and doxorubicin in advanced gastric cancer. Cancer Treat Rep 1986;70:477–9.

59. Machover D, Goldschmidt E, Chollet P, et al. Treatment of advanced colorectal and gastric adenocarcinomas with 5-fluorouracil and high dose folinic acid. J Clin Oncol 1986;4:685–96.

60. Arbuck SG, Douglass HO Jr, Trave F, et al. A phase II trial of 5-fluorouracil and high dose intravenous leucovorin in gastric carcinoma. J Clin Oncol 1987;5:1150–6.

61. Moertel CG, Lavin PT. Phase II–III chemotherapy studies in advanced gastric cancer. Eastern Cooperative Oncology Group. Cancer Treat Rep 1979;63:1863–9.

62. Saito T, Wakui A, Yokoyama M, et al. Combination chemotherapy for solid tumors using 5-fluorouracil, chromomycin-A, and prednisolone. Gann 1977;68:375–87.

63. O'Connell MJ, Schutt AJ, Moertel CG, et al. Phase II clinical trial of triazinate in combination with mitomycin C for patients with advanced gastric cancer. J Clin Oncol 1987;5:83–5.

64. Pazdur R, Ajani JA, Winn R, et al. A phase II trial of 5-fluorouracil and recombinant alpha-2a-interferon in previously untreated metastatic gastric carcinoma. Cancer 1992;69:878–82.

65. Buroker TR, Kim PN, Heilbrun L, Vaitkevicius V. 5-FU infusion with mitomycin C (MMC) vs. 5-FU infusion with methyl-CCNU (ME) in the treatment of advanced upper gastrointestinal cancer. Proc ASCO 1978;19:310.

66. Krauss S, Sonoda T. Treatment of metastatic gastrointestinal cancers with 5-fluorouracil and mitomycin C. Proc Am Assoc Cancer Res 1978;19:191.

67. Buroker T, Kim PN, Groppe C, et al. 5-FU infusion with mitomycin-C vs. 5-FU infusion with methyl-CCNU in the treatment of advanced upper gastrointestinal cancer: a Southwest Oncology Group study. Cancer 1979;44:1215–21.

68. Buroker TR, Kim PN, Baker LH, et al. Mitomycin-C alone and in combination with infused 5-fluorouracil to the treatment of disseminated gastrointestinal carcinomas. Med Pediatr Oncol 1978;4:35–42.

69. Wadler S, Green M, Muggia F. The role of anthracyclines in the treatment of gastric cancer. Cancer Treat Rev 1985;12:105–32.

70. Moertel CG. Cancer of the gastrointestinal tract: chemotherapy. JAMA 1974;228:1290–1.

71. Gailani S, Holland JF, Falkson G, et al. Comparison of treatment of metastatic gastrointestinal cancer with 5-fluorouracil (5-FU) to a combination of 5-FU with cytosine arabinoside. Cancer 1972;29:1308–13.

72. Tomirotti M, Lombardi F, Biasioli R, et al. Combination of mitomycin C + etoposide in advanced gastric carcinoma. Tumori 1985;71:371–3.

73. Chlebowski RT, Weiner JM, Silverberg I, et al. Cyclophosphamide plus 5-FU versus 5-FU alone in advanced gastric carcinoma. Oncology 1985;42:141–3.

74. Lacave A, Wils J, Bleiberg H, et al. An EORTC gastrointestinal group phase III evaluation of combinations of methyl-CCNU, 5-fluorouracil, and Adriamycin in advanced gastric cancer. J Clin Oncol 1987;5:1387–93.

75. Cullinan SA, Moertel CG, Fleming TR, et al. A comparison of three chemotherapeutic regimens in the treatment of advanced pancreatic and gastric carcinoma: fluorouracil vs. fluorouracil and doxorubicin vs. fluorouracil, doxorubicin and mitomycin. JAMA 1985;253:2061–7.

76. Kane RC, Cashdollar MR. Phase II trial of methyl CCNU plus five day fluorouracil infusion in advanced gastrointestinal adenocarcinoma. Proc ASCO 1977;18:313.

77. Krauss S, Sonoda T, Solomon A. Treatment of advanced gastrointestinal cancer with 5-fluorouracil and mitomycin C. Cancer 1979;43:1598–1603.

78. Dalley D, Erlichman C, Fine S. Treatment of advanced gastric carcinoma with mitomycin and doxorubicin. Cancer Treat Rep 1986;70:897–8.

79. Kelsen DP, Buckner J, Einzig A, et al. Phase II trial of cisplatin and etoposide in adenocarcinoma of the upper gastrointestinal tract. Cancer Treat Rep 1987;71:329–30.

80. Creagan ET, Richardson RL, Kovach JS. Pilot study of a continuous 5-day intravenous infusion of etoposide concomitant with cisplatin in selected patients with advanced cancer. J Clin Oncol 1988;6:1197–1201.

81. Webb A, Cunningham D, Scarffe JH, et al. Randomized trial comparing epirubicin, cisplatin and fluorouracil versus fluorouracil, doxorubicin, and methotrexate in advanced esophagogastric cancer. J Clin Oncol 1997;15:261–7.

82. Bamias A, Hill ME, Cunningham D, et al. Epirubicin, cisplatin and protracted venous infusion of 5-fluorouracil for esophagogastric adenocarcinoma: response, toxicity, quality of life and survival. Cancer 1996;77:1978–85.

83. Wilke H, Preusser P, Fink U, et al. New developments in the treatment of gastric carcinoma. Semin Oncol 1990;17:1 Suppl 2:61–70.

84. Gebbia V, Sciume C, Cannata G, et al. ELF regimen in advanced gastrointestinal malignancies—an analysis of its clinical effectiveness and toxicity. Int J Oncol 1994;4:411–5.

85. Au E, Koo WH, Tan EH, Ang PT. A phase II trial of etoposide, leucovorin and 5-fluorouracil (ELF) in patients with advanced gastric cancer. J Chemother 1996;8:300–3.

86. Macdonald JS, Havlin KA. Etoposide in gastric cancer. Semin Oncol 1992;19:6 Suppl 13:59–62.

87. Chiou TJ, Kung SP, Hsieh RK, et al. Treatment of advanced gastric cancer with a modified regimen of etoposide, leucovorin and 5-fluorouracil. Cancer Invest 1996;14:197–201.

88. Zaniboni A, Barni S, Labianca R, et al. Epirubicin, cisplatin, and continuous infusion 5-fluorouracil is an active and safe regimen for patients with advanced gastric cancer. Cancer 1995;76:1694–9.

89. Ychou M, Astre C, Rouanet P, et al. A phase II study of 5-fluorouracil, leucovorin and cisplatin (FLP) for metastatic gastric cancer. Eur J Cancer 1996;32A:1933–7.

90. Ychou M, Astre C, Rouanet P, et al. A phase II study of 5-fluorouracil, leucovorin and cisplatin (FLP) for metastatic gastric cancer. Eur J Cancer 1996;32A:1933–7.

91. Becouarn Y, Brunet R, Bussieres E, et al. 5-Fluorouracil, high-dose folinic acid and mitomycin C combination chemotherapy in advanced gastrointestinal adenocarcinomas: a pilot study. Oncology 1988;45:269–72.

92. Kornek G, Schulz F, Depisch D, et al. A phase I-II study of epirubicin,

5-fluorouracil, and leucovorin in advanced adenocarcinoma of the stomach. Cancer 1993;71:2177–80.

93. Neri B, Gemelli MT, Pantalone D, et al. Epidoxorubicin and high dose leucovorin plus 5-fluorouracil in advanced gastric cancer: a phase II study. Anticancer Drugs 1993;4:323–6.

94. Preusser P, Wilke H, Achterrath W, et al. Phase II study with the combination etoposide, doxorubicin and cisplatin in advanced measurable gastric cancer. J Clin Oncol 1989;7:1310–7.

95. Ridolfi R, Giunchi DC, Amadori M, et al. EAP in advanced gastric cancer. Eur J Cancer 1993;29A:1219–20.

96. Taguchi T. Combination chemotherapy with etoposide, adriamycin, and cisplatin (EAP) for advanced gastric cancer. Proc ASCO 1989;8:108.

97. Katz A, Gansl RC, Simon SD, et al. Phase II trial of etoposide (V), adriamycin (A), and cisplatinum (P) in patients with metastatic gastric cancer. Am J Clin Oncol 1991;14:357–8.

98. Kelsen D, Atiq OT, Saltz L, et al. FAMTX versus etoposide, doxorubicin and cisplatin: a randomized assignment trial in gastric cancer. J Clin Oncol 1992;10:541–8.

99. Haim N, Tsalik M, Robinson E. Treatment of gastric adenocarcinoma with the combination of etoposide, Adriamycin and cisplatin (EAP): comparison between two schedules. Oncology 1994;51:102–7.

100. Lerner A, Gonin R, Steele GD Jr, et al. Etoposide, doxorubicin and cisplatin chemotherapy for advanced gastric adenocarcinoma: result of a phase II trial. J Clin Oncol 1992;10:536–40.

101. Sparano JA, Schwartz EL, Salva KM, et al. Phase II trial of etoposide, doxorubicin (Adriamycin) and cisplatin (EAP regimen) in advanced gastric cancer. Am J Clin Oncol 1990;13:374–8.

102. Lopez M, Natali M, DiLauro L, et al. 5-Fluorouracil, epirubicin and BCNU (FEB) in advanced measurable gastric cancer. Am J Clin Oncol 1990;13:204–7.

103. Levi JA, Fox RM, Tattersall MH, et al. Analysis of a prospective randomized comparison of doxorubicin versus 5-fluorouracil, doxorubicin and BCNU in advanced gastric cancer: implications for future studies. J Clin Oncol 1986;4:1348–55.

104. Lopez M, DiLauro L, Papaldo P, et al. Treatment of advanced measurable gastric cancer with 5-fluorouracil, Adriamycin and BCNU. Oncology 1986;43:288–91.

105. Schnitzler G, Queisser W, Heim ME, et al. Phase III study of 5-FU and carmustine versus 5-FU, carmustine and doxorubicin in advanced gastric cancer. Cancer Treat Rep 1986;70:477–9.

106. Rougier P, Droz JP, Theodore C, et al. Phase II trial of combined 5-fluorouracil plus doxorubicin plus cisplatin (FAP regimen) in advanced gastric carcinoma. Cancer Treat Rep 1986;71:1301–2.

107. Epelbaum R, Haim N, Stein M, et al. Treatment of advanced gastric cancer with DDP (cisplatin), Adriamycin, and 5-fluorouracil (DAF). Oncology 1987;44:201–6.

108. Wagener DJ, Yap SH, Wobbes T, et al. Phase II trial of 5-fluorouracil, Adriamycin and cisplatin (FAP) in advanced gastric cancer. Cancer Chemother Pharmacol 1985;15:86–7.

109. Moertel CG, Rubin J, O'Connell MJ, et al. A phase II study of combined 5-fluorouracil, doxorubicin and cisplatin in the treatment of advanced upper gastrointestinal adenocarcinomas. J Clin Oncol 1986;4:1053–7.

110. Macdonald JS, Schein PS, Woolley PV, et al. 5-Fluorouracil, doxorubicin and mitomycin (FAM) combination chemotherapy for advanced gastric cancer. Ann Intern Med 1980;93:533–6.

111. Folman R, Magill GB, Pinsky C, Golbey RB. Chemoimmunotherapy with mitomycin, 5-FU and Adriamycin (MIFA) plus C parvum in advanced gastric carcinoma. Proc Am Assoc Cancer Res 1977;18:195.

112. Bitran JD, Desser RK, Kozloff MF, et al. Treatment of metastatic pancreatic and gastric adenocarcinomas with 5-fluorouracil, Adriamycin and mitomycin C (FAM). Cancer Treat Rep 1979;63:2049–51.

113. GITSG: A comparative clinical assessment of combination chemotherapy in the management of advanced gastric carcinoma. The Gastrointestinal Tumor Study Group. Cancer 1982;49:1362–6.

114. Haim N, Cohen Y, Honigman J, et al. Treatment of advanced gastric carcinoma with 5-fluorouracil, adriamycin and mitomycin C (FAM). Cancer Chemother Pharmacol 1982;8:277–80.

115. Fraschini P, Berretta G, Arnoldi E, et al: Confirmed activity of FAM polychemotherapy in advanced gastric carcinoma. Tumori 1983;69:59–64.

116. Vaughn CB, Chapman JL, Garland M, et al. The efficacy of 5-fluorouracil, mitomycin C and methyl CCNU in advanced gastrointestinal malignancy. Oncology 1981;38:129–33.

117. Ridolfi R, Casadei Giunchi D, Cortesi C, et al. A retrospective study of FAM regimen in 38 patients with advanced gastric cancer. Tumori 1984;70:375–9.

118. Rougier P, Droz JP, Spielmann M, et al. Treatment failure in gastric carcinoma with the association 5 fluoro-uracil (5 FU), doxorubicin (ADR), and mitomycin C (MMC). Bull Cancer (Paris) 1984;71:71–2.

119. Fornasiero A, Cartei G, Daniele O, et al. FAM2 regimen in disseminated gastric cancer. Tumori 1984;70:77–80.

120. Barone C, Cassano A, Astone A, et al. Association of epirubicin, etoposide and cisplatin in gastric cancer: a phase II study. Oncology 1991;48:353–5.

121. Ota K, Kurita S, Nishimura M, et al. Combination therapy with mitomycin C (NSC-26980), 5-fluorouracil (NSC-19893), and cytosine arabinoside (NSC-63878) for advanced cancer in man. Cancer Chemother Rep 1972;56:373–85.

122. DeJager RL, Magill GB, Golbey RB, et al. Combination chemotherapy with mitomycin C, 5-fluorouracil, and cytosine arabinoside in gastrointestinal cancer. Cancer Treat Rep 1976;60:1373–5.

123. O'Connell MJ, Moertel CG, Lavin PT. Adriamycin (A), 5-fluorouracil + mitomycin C + cytosine arabinoside (FMC), and 5-fluorouracil + Adriamycin + methyl CCNU (FAMe) in advanced gastric carcinoma. Proc ASCO 1978;19:343.

124. GITSG: Phase II-III chemotherapy studies in advanced gastric cancer. The Gastrointestinal Tumor Study Group. Cancer Treat Rep 1979;63:1871–6.

125. Cocconi G, DeLisi V, Di Blasio B. Randomized comparison of 5-FU alone or combined with mitomycin and cytarabine (MFC) in the treatment of advanced gastric cancer. Cancer Treat Rep 1982;66:1263–6.

126. Bokemeyer C, Hartmann JT, Lampe CS, et al. Paclitaxel and weekly 24-hour infusion of 5-fluorouracil/folinic acid in advanced gastric cancer. Semin Oncol 1997;24:6 Suppl 19:S19–96–100.

127. Muro H, Acuna LR, Castagnari A, et al. Sequential methotrexate, 5-fluorouracil (high dose), and doxorubicin for advanced gastric cancer. Cancer Treat Rep 1986;70:1333–4.

128. Wils J, Bleiberg H, Dalesio O, et al. An EORTC Gastrointestinal Group evaluation of the combination of sequential methotrexate and 5-fluorouracil combined with Adriamycin in advanced measurable gastric cancer. J Clin Oncol 1986;4:1799–1803.

129. Bunn PA Jr, Nugent JL, Ihde DC, et al. 5-fluorouracil, methyl-CCNU, Adriamycin and mitomycin C in the treatment of advanced gastric cancer. Cancer Treat Rep 1978;62:1287–93.

130. Lacave A, Wils J, Bleiberg H, et al. An EORTC Gastrointestinal Group phase III evaluation of combinations of methyl-CCNU, 5-fluorouracil, and adriamycin in advanced gastric cancer. J Clin Oncol 1987;5:1387–93.

131. Windschitl HE, O'Connell MJ, Wieand HS, et al. A clinical trial of biochemical modulation of 5-fluorouracil with N-phosphonoacetyl-L-aspartate and thymidine in advanced gastric and anaplastic colorectal cancer. Cancer 1990;66:853–6.

132. Woolley PV III, MacDonald JS, Smythe T, et al. A phase II trial of ftorafur, Adriamycin and mitomycin C (FAM II) in advanced gastric adenocarcinoma. Cancer 1979;44:1211–4.

133. Cascinu S, Latini L, Fedeli A, et al. The clinical impact of FEM regimen (5-fluorouracil, 4-epidoxorubicin and mitomycin C) in advanced gastric cancer patients. Anticancer Res 1995;15:2781–3.

134. Cascinu S, Fedeli A, Fedeli SL, et al. Intensive weekly chemotherapy for advanced gastric cancer using 5-fluorouracil, cisplatin, epi-doxorubicin, 6S-leucovorin and granulocyte-colony stimulating factor. Int J Oncol 1993;3:535–8.

135. Cheng AL, Yeh KH, Lin JT, et al. Cisplatin, etoposide, and weekly high-dose 5-fluorouracil and leucovorin infusion (PE-HDFL)—a very effective regimen with good patients' compliance for advanced gastric cancer. Anticancer Res 1998;18:1267–72.

136. Chi KH, Chao Y, Chan WK, et al. Weekly etoposide, epirubicin, cisplatin, 5-fluorouracil and leucovorin: an effective chemotherapy in advanced gastric cancer. Br J Cancer 1998;77:1984–8.

137. Cascinu S, Labianca R, Alessandroni P, et al. Intensive weekly chemotherapy for advanced gastric cancer using fluorouracil, cisplatin, epi-doxorubicin, 6S-leucovorin, glutathione, and filgrastim: a report from the Italian Group for the study of digestive tract cancer. J Clin Oncol 1997;15:3313–9.

138. Conroy T, Wils J, Paillot B, et al. Combination of 5-FU, high dose methotrexate, epirubicin and cisplatin (FEMTX-P protocol) in nonsur-

gical or locally recurrent metastatic gastric cancers. Bull Cancer (Paris) 1993;80:255–60.

139. Klein HO, Wickramanayake PD, Dieterle F, et al. Chemotherapy schedule for the management of metastasizing gastric cancers: methotrexate, Adriamycin and 5-fluorouracil. Dtsch Med Wochenschr 1982;107:1708–12.

140. Weh HJ, Platz D, Garbrecht M, et al. The results of a modified FAMeth chemotherapy protocol in metastatic stomach cancer. Dtsch Med Wochenschr 1989;114:1391–6.

141. Queisser W, Schnitzler G, Heim ME, et al. Prospective randomized study in advanced stomach cancer: comparison between combinations of 5-fluorouracil and carmustine with and without Adriamycin. Dtsch Med Wochenschr 1984;109:976–80.

142. Wils J, Bleiberg H, Dalesio O, et al. An EORTC gastrointestinal group evaluation of the combination of sequential methotrexate and 5-fluorouracil combined with Adriamycin in advanced measurable gastric cancer. J Clin Oncol 1986;4:1799–803.

143. Wils JA, Klein HO, Wagener DJ, et al. Sequential high dose methotrexate and fluorouracil combined with doxorubicin—a step ahead in the treatment of advanced gastric cancer: a trial of the European Organization for Research and Treatment of Cancer gastrointestinal tract cooperative group. J Clin Oncol 1991;9:827–31.

144. Murad AM, Santiago FF, Petroianu A, et al. Modern therapy with 5-fluorouracil, doxorubicin, and methotrexate in advanced gastric cancer. Cancer 1993;72:37–41.

145. Blijham G, Bleiberg H, Duez N, et al. An EORTC phase II study of sequential methotrexate-fluorouracil in locally advanced or metastatic gastric cancer. The EORTC gastrointestinal cancer cooperative group. Eur J Cancer 1990;26:63–5.

146. Bukowski RM, Theodors A, Purvis JP. Phase II trial of sequential chemotherapy and low-dose radiotherapy in advanced gastric adeno-

carcinoma. A Southwest Oncology Group pilot study. Am J Clin Oncol 1987;10:376–9.

147. Karlin DA, Stroehlein JR, Bennetts RW. Phase I–II study of the combination of 5-FU, doxorubicin, mitomycin, and semustine (FAMME) in the treatment of adenocarcinoma of the stomach, gastroesophageal junction and pancreas. Cancer Treat Rep 1982;66:1613–7.

148. Arbuck SG, Silk Y, Douglass HO Jr, et al. A phase II trial of 5-fluorouracil, doxorubicin, mitomycin C and leucovorin in advanced gastric carcinoma. Cancer 1990;65:2442–5.

149. Vaughn DJ, Meropol NJ, Holroyde C, et al. A phase II study of 5-fluorouracil, leucovorin, Adriamycin and cisplatin (FLAP) for metastatic gastric and gastroesophageal junction adenocarcinoma. Am J Clin Oncol 1997;20:242–6.

150. Anderson H, Scarffe JH, Ranson M, et al. MMAF for advanced gastric cancer. Eur J Cancer 1991;27:1234–8.

151. Gisselbrecht C, Smith FP, MacDonald JS, et al. The effect of sequential addition of the nitrosourea, chlorozotocin, to the FAM combination in advanced gastric cancer. Cancer 1983;51:1792–4.

152. De Lisi V, Cocconi G, Tonato M, et al. Randomized comparison of 5-FU alone or combined with carmustine, doxorubicin and mitomycin (BAFMI) in the treatment of advanced gastric cancer: a phase III trial of the Italian Clinical Research Oncology Group (GOIRC). Cancer Treat Rep 1986;70:481–5.

153. Haas C, Oishi N, McDonald B, et al. Southwest Oncology Group Phase II–III gastric study: 5-fluorouracil, Adriamycin, and mitomycin-C ± vincristine (FAM vs V-FAM) compared to chlorozotocin (CZT), *m*-AMSA, and dihydroxyanthracenedione (DHAD) with unimpressive differences. Proc ASCO 1983;2:122.

154. Ahlgren JD, Smith FP, Cazap E, et al. FAM (5-fluorouracil, doxorubicin and mitomycin) plus triazinate (FAM-T) in gastric carcinoma: a combined phase II trial of the mid-Atlantic Oncology Program and the Pan American Health Organization. Cancer Treat Rep 1987;71:419–20.

........................................

# TREATMENT OF GASTRIC CANCER BY STAGE OF DISEASE

• Carol Nishikubo • Charles M. Haskell

## STAGES I THROUGH III

The mainstay of treatment for local and regional gastric carcinoma is surgical resection when feasible. Some centers believe that the extent of lymph node dissection contributes to recurrence rates, although the curative value of more extended lymphadenectomies has not been proved. Contemporary studies suggest that more extended lymph node dissections serve to alter stage of disease without changing long-term outcome.

The role of adjuvant therapy following potentially curative resections is controversial, as discussed in prior subchapters. However, the standard of care for patients with stage IB–III tumors that have been resected with the techniques commonly used in North America and Europe should probably include postoperative chemoradiotherapy, as applied in Intergroup Study 0116. The doses and schedule of therapy for that study are given in Table 41–7. Several points deserve emphasis. First, nutritional support and monitoring of the patient is essential. Intergroup Study 0116 required that patients be able to sustain a caloric intake of at least 1500 calories/day or more to be eligible for chemoradiotherapy. Second, it must be emphasized that the use of this therapeutic protocol requires meticulous attention to the radiation ports used, since the anatomic landmarks for delineating the limits of radiation therapy are more difficult to

establish in the upper abdomen than in the pelvis. Third, a low rate of deaths from toxicity ($<1\%$) can be anticipated with this treatment program, even when given with meticulous care.

Although not tested in Intergroup Study 0116, it is reasonable to consider the treatment regimen described in Table 41–7 for patients with regionally advanced gastric cancer treated with a resection that is considered palliative because of positive surgical margins provided that there is no evidence of more distant metastases outside the limits of a reasonable radiation therapy field.

## STAGE IV

Palliative resection of the primary tumor appears to improve the quality of life and duration of survival, even in cases of advanced disease. Chemotherapy may be considered, but it is palliative at best, and long-term survival is rare. Combination chemotherapy for metastatic disease has not been proved superior to single-agent therapy in terms of survival rates, and combination chemotherapy is usually more toxic in terms of side effects. Radiation therapy may be indicated for the palliation of symptomatic disease not responsive to chemotherapy.

*Table 41–7.* **Combined Modality Therapy for Stages IB–III Gastric Cancer**

| Surgery and Supportive Care | Chemotherapy | Radiation Therapy (XRT) |
|---|---|---|
| The recommended surgical procedure is a radical subtotal (or total) gastrectomy with omentobursectomy and lymph node dissection | | |
| Postoperative or J-tube alimentation must exceed 1500 calories/day. Adjuvant therapy should start 3–6 wk after the day of surgery. | | |
| | Starting 3–6 wk after surgery, give 5-FU 425 mg/m$^2$/day IV bolus immediately after leucovorin 20 mg/m$^2$/day IV bolus for 5 days | |
| | 5-FU 400 mg/m$^2$/day and leucovorin 20 mg/m$^2$/day by IV bolus days 1–4 of week 1 of XRT and days 1–3 of week 5 of XRT | Four weeks after giving the first cycle of chemotherapy, start radiation therapy (45 Gy; 1.8 Gy/day; all treatment to be isocentric with a maximal field size of 400 cm$^2$) |
| | Starting 28–35 days after the completion of XRT, give 5-FU 425 mg/m$^2$/day and leucovorin 20 mg/m$^2$/day for 5 days and repeat this 5-day cycle 4 wk later for a total of two post-XRT courses | |

From Macdonald J, Smalley S, Benedetti JK, et al. Postoperative combined radiation and chemotherapy improves disease-free (DFS) and overall survival (OS) in resected adenocarcinoma of the stomach and GE junction. Proc Am Soc Clin Oncol 2000;19:1a.

## SUGGESTIONS FOR ADDITIONAL READING

Scheiman JM, Cutler AF. *Helicobacter pylori* and gastric cancer. Am J Med 1999;106:222–6.

Riddell RH, Iwafuchi M. Problems arising from Eastern and Western classification systems for gastrointestinal dysplasia and carcinoma: are they resolvable? Histopathology 1998;33:197–202.

Nevitt AW, Vida F, Kozarek RA, et al. Expandable metallic prostheses for malignant obstructions of gastric outlet and proximal small bowel. Gastrointest Endoscopy 1998;47:271–6.

Kozarek RA. Complications and lessons learned from 10 years of expandable gastrointestinal prostheses. Dig Dis 1999;17:14–22.

Roukos DH. Current advances and changes in treatment strategy may improve survival and quality of life in patients with potentially curable gastric cancer. Ann Surg Oncol 1999;6:46–56.

Whiting JL, Fielding JW. Radical surgery for early gastric cancer. Eur J Surg Oncol 1998;24:263–6.

Roukos DH. Extended lymphadenectomy in gastric cancer: when, for whom and why. Ann R Coll Surg Engl 1998;80:16–24.

Ajani JA. Chemotherapy for gastric carcinoma: new and old options. Oncology 1998;12:10 Suppl 7:44–7.

Karpeh MS, Kelsen DP. Combined modality therapy of gastric cancer. Surg Oncol Clin North Am 1997;6:741–7.

Toge T. Effectiveness of immunochemotherapy for gastric cancer: a review of the current status. Semin Surg Oncol 1999;17:139–43.

Kranenbarg EK, van de Velde CJ. Gastric cancer in the elderly. Eur J Surg Oncol 1998;24:384–90.

# CHAPTER 42

# SMALL INTESTINE

• CHARLES M. HASKELL • LUU M. TRAN • KENNETH P. RAMMING

## Natural History, Diagnosis, and Staging

### EPIDEMIOLOGY AND ETIOLOGY

**Incidence.** Small bowel tumors make up approximately 1.5% of all benign and malignant gastrointestinal neoplasms. About 4800 new cases of malignant small bowel tumors occurred in the United States in 1999, divided almost evenly between males (52%) and females (48%).[1] Approximately 1200 individuals were expected to die of the disease in the United States in 1999. The annual U.S. incidence of this tumor is about 1.3 cases per 100,000 population.[2] About one half of small bowel tumors are malignant. These tumors are much more common in some parts of the world, most notably in the Middle East and southern Mediterranean areas. The term *immunoproliferative small intestinal disease* (IPSID) has been applied to the small bowel lesions occurring in these geographic regions.

**Etiology.** The cause of small bowel neoplasms is unknown. Although the small bowel constitutes approximately 75% of the gastrointestinal tract and has an enormous mucosal surface that presumably is in constant contact with enteric carcinogenic substances, the incidence of neoplasms is much lower than that observed in other gastrointestinal organs. For example, there are about 12 gastric carcinomas and 46 rectal carcinomas for each small bowel malignancy.

Possible explanations for the rarity of small bowel disease, compared with neoplasms of the colon, in industrialized countries include differences between the two anatomic regions regarding bacterial flora, food composition, cell kinetics, levels of benzpyrene hydroxylase for detoxifying carcinogens, and quantitative secretion of IgA.[3] Several diseases have been reported to increase the incidence of small bowel carcinomas, including familial polyposis coli and Gardner's syndrome, Peutz-Jeghers syndrome, and regional enteritis (Crohn's disease). The best established of these risk factors are Crohn's disease and familial gastrointestinal cancer syndromes.[4] Risk factors for the development of small bowel lymphomas are somewhat different and include parasitic infections (especially with IPSID), immune deficiency states, and celiac disease.

**Molecular Genetics.** The available data suggest that the sequence of molecular-genetic changes that occur in colorectal cancer also explains the development of adenocarcinomas of the small bowel. Certain oncogenes appear to be consistently altered in both sites, including *erb*B2, K-*ras,* cyclin D1, and p53.[5] It is unclear, however, why these molecular changes occur so much less frequently in the small bowel than they do in the colon and rectum.

## PATHOLOGY

Table 42–1 shows the location and frequency of benign and malignant primary tumors of small bowel extracted from several large series.[6] It should be remembered that the most common malignant tumor of the small bowel is actually metastatic tumor from other organs—most frequently primary neoplasms of the ovary, stomach, and pancreas—as well as malignant melanoma. Most benign tumors of the

small bowel are undiagnosed in the lifetime of the patient and are discovered as incidental findings at the time of autopsy.

The carcinomatous lesion in the small intestine is characterized by a narrowed intestinal lumen, with an ulcerated mucosal surface. The histologic features are typical for adenocarcinoma of gastrointestinal origin, and the vast majority of these tumors produce mucin. Leiomyosarcomas arise in the smooth muscle of the intestine and are usually spheroid, firm, and vascular. Malignant lymphoma is often a rather rigid segment several centimeters long, with extension into the mesentery. Lymphomatous lesions are unlikely to cause complete obstruction but may lead to perforation. Malignant lymphomas of the bowel are discussed further in Chapters 88, 94, and 101. Carcinoid tumors are discussed in Chapter 71. Sarcomas are discussed in Chapter 83.

## CLINICAL COURSE AND DIAGNOSIS

Intermittent abdominal pain, which is usually vague and indistinct but is occasionally described as cramps, usually results from the partial bowel obstruction caused by these neoplasms and is the most common symptom.[7] Other clinical signs and symptoms of small bowel lesions, in decreasing order of frequency, include anorexia, nausea and vomiting, obstruction, bleeding, anemia, abdominal mass, weight loss, and, rarely, perforation. Only about 50% of small bowel neoplasms are diagnosed preoperatively; the remainder are diagnosed at laparotomy performed for the treatment of small bowel obstruction.[8]

Diagnosis is usually by physical examination, abdominal radiographs and, most often, barium contrast studies of the small bowel. Tumors of the terminal ileum that cause an ileocolic intussusception can usually be diagnosed by barium enema. Distal ileal adenocarcinomas, especially those that intermittently prolapse, can simulate Crohn's disease.

In the Middle East and developing Mediterranean areas, patients suspected of having IPSID should be considered for an upper intestinal fiberoptic endoscopic procedure. On the basis of the findings of a prospective study in Tunisia, in which endoscopic biopsies were diagnostic of lymphoma in 85% of cases, this procedure should be the first investigation in patients suspected of having this problem.[9] Endoscopy may also be useful in the early diagnosis and treatment of small bowel polyposis syndromes.[10]

## STAGING AND PROGNOSIS

The TNM staging system for small bowel tumors is presented in Table 42–2. Unlike the TNM staging system for colon cancer, there is no subdivision of the N category based on the number of lymph nodes involved with tumor. The T1 category also differs from that of colon cancer.

Survival is influenced by stage of disease, as shown in Figure 42–1. The overall 5-year relative survival rate for small bowel neoplasms in the United States is 49%.[2] Prognosis is also affected by the type of resection performed. In one series of 71 patients, the presence or absence of metastases and the resection status of the tumor were the only significant prognostic variables.[11] In this series, the overall

*Table 42–1.* **Primary Neoplasms of the Small Bowel**

| Neoplasm | Duodenum | Jejunum | Ileum | Total |
|---|---|---|---|---|
| *Malignant* | | | | |
| Adenocarcinoma | 92 | 90 | 28 | 210 |
| Lymphoma | 3 | 57 | 69 | 129 |
| Sarcoma | 15 | 23 | 33 | 71 |
| Miscellaneous | 1 | 4 | 4 | 9 |
| Subtotal | 111 | 174 | 134 | 419 |
| Carcinoid | 15 | 19 | 229 | 263 |
| *Benign* | | | | |
| Leiomyoma | 31 | 77 | 34 | 162 |
| Adenoma | 39 | 38 | 38 | 115 |
| Lipoma | 23 | 11 | 42 | 78 |
| Miscellaneous | 33 | 18 | 23 | 74 |
| Hemangioma | 3 | 39 | 21 | 63 |
| Neurofibroma | 2 | 6 | 3 | 11 |
| Lymphangioma | 0 | 2 | 4 | 6 |
| Fibroma | 0 | 2 | 2 | 4 |
| Fibromyoma | 0 | 1 | 0 | 1 |
| Subtotal | 133 | 194 | 187 | 514 |
| Grand total | | | | 1196 |

From Mason GR. In: Sabiston DC Jr, ed. Davis-Christopher Textbook of Surgery. 12th ed. Philadelphia: WB Saunders, 1981.

*Table 42–2.* **American Joint Committee on Cancer TNM Staging System for Small Intestine Neoplasm**

*Definition of TNM*

*Primary Tumor (T)*

| | |
|---|---|
| TX | Primary tumor cannot be assessed |
| T0 | No evidence of primary tumor |
| Tis | Carcinoma in situ |
| T1 | Tumor invades lamina propria or submucosa |
| T2 | Tumor invades muscularis propria |
| T3 | Tumor invades through the muscularis propria into the subserosa or into the nonperitonealized perimuscular tissue (mesentery or retroperitoneum) with extension 2 cm or less.* |
| T4 | Tumor perforates the visceral peritoneum, or directly invades other organs or structures (includes other loops of small intestine, mesentery, or retroperitoneum more than 2 cm, and the abdominal wall by way of the serosa; for the duodenum only, includes invasion of the pancreas). |

*Regional Lymph Nodes (N)*

| | |
|---|---|
| NX | Regional lymph nodes cannot be assessed |
| N0 | No regional lymph node metastasis |
| N1 | Regional lymph node metastasis |

*Distant Metastasis (M)*

| | |
|---|---|
| MX | Presence of distant metastasis cannot be assessed |
| M0 | No distant metastasis |
| M1 | Distant metastasis |

*Stage Grouping*

| | | | |
|---|---|---|---|
| Stage 0 | Tis | N0 | M0 |
| Stage I | T1 | N0 | M0 |
| | T2 | N0 | M0 |
| Stage II | T3 | N0 | M0 |
| | T4 | N0 | M0 |
| Stage III | Any T | N1 | M0 |
| Stage IV | Any T | Any N | M1 |

*\*Note:* The nonperitonealized perimuscular tissue is, for jejunum and ileum, part of the mesentery and, for the duodenum in areas where serosa is lacking, part of the retroperitoneum.

Used with the permission of the American Joint Committee on Cancer (AJCC®), Chicago, Illinois. The original source for this material is the AJCC Cancer Staging Manual, 5th edition (1997) published by Lippincott-Raven Publishers, Philadelphia, Pennsylvania.

5-year survival for patients with malignant small bowel neoplasms was 32%.

## Treatment

### SURGERY

The treatment of small intestine carcinomas is primarily by extended segmental resection. Frequently, particularly when the neoplasm is metastatic, there is extension of the malignant process beyond the scope of total surgical excision. A palliative procedure should be performed, however, to lessen the chance of obstruction, perforation, and hemorrhage. When palliative resections involve more than two areas of small bowel anastomosis, it is important not to use a stapling device. Repeated anastomoses with staples in the small bowel can interrupt peristalsis, leading to devastating, prolonged ileus. For carcinomas of the duodenum, a pancreatic-

oduodenectomy (modified Whipple procedure in which the pylorus is saved) may be necessary. When carcinomas of the terminal ileum are encountered, a right colectomy is usually part of the operative procedure. If malignant lymphoma is found, discrete focal disease is usually resected, and staging procedures are performed to determine the extent of intra-abdominal spread. These procedures include a sampling of intra-abdominal and periaortic nodes, a liver biopsy, and often a splenectomy.

### RADIATION THERAPY

There is no established role for radiation therapy for small bowel carcinomas. Few cases treated with radiation either primarily or in an adjuvant role have been reported in the literature.[12] The risk of adhesions resulting in intestinal obstruction limits the total dose to the small bowel to approximately 45 Gy given in 25 daily fractions. Doses in this range may be useful as a postoperative adjuvant treatment to decrease the chance of local recurrence in patients with retroperitoneal lesions that extend through the bowel wall or those with regional lymph node involvement. Unresectable disease is unlikely to be controlled with the moderate doses of radiation tolerated by the small bowel.

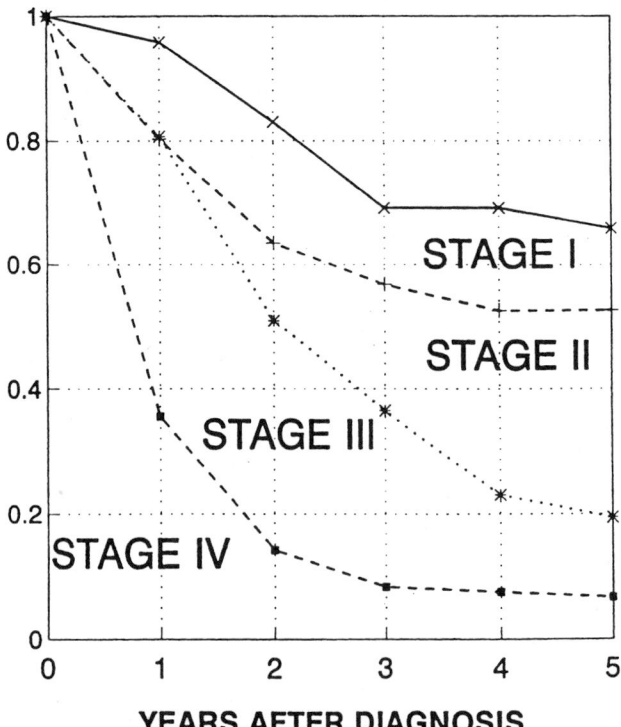

**SURVIVAL RATE**

STAGE I

STAGE II

STAGE III

STAGE IV

**YEARS AFTER DIAGNOSIS**

**Figure 42–1.** Relative survival rates according to stage of disease. Data based on 250 cases recorded in the Surveillance, Epidemiology, and End Results Program of the National Cancer Institute. Stage I includes 13 cases; stage II includes 77; stage III has 56; and stage IV has 104. (From Beahrs OH, Henson OH, Hutter RVP, Kennedy BJ, eds. The American Joint Committee on Cancer Manual on Staging. 4th ed. Philadelphia: JB Lippincott, 1992:70.)

## CHEMOTHERAPY

Adenocarcinomas of the small bowel are rare, and little has been published regarding the role of chemotherapy for this group of tumors. The results described in the available reviews suggest that chemotherapy is without value.[13] Our personal experience is consistent with this view, although it is impossible to define the true role of this modality on the basis of the available data. As a working approach to this problem, we and others suggest that palliative chemotherapy for this disease be the same as that used in colorectal carcinoma.[8]

Chemotherapy for other forms of small bowel tumor is described elsewhere in this book (Chapter 71, carcinoid tumors; Chapter 83, soft tissue sarcomas; Chapter 94, extranodal lymphomas).

## SUMMARY OF TREATMENT

**Carcinomas.** The mainstay of treatment is surgical resection. Radiation therapy has essentially no role in management, and chemotherapy is of uncertain value. There is interest in the use of metallic stents for the palliation of obstructive symptoms, but their value is less well established than is the case for cancer in other locations of the gastrointestinal tract.[14]

**Lymphomas and Sarcomas.** The management of these neoplasms is discussed in other chapters of this book.

## SUGGESTION FOR ADDITIONAL READING

Neugut AI, Marvin MR, Rella VA, Chabot JA. An overview of adenocarcinoma of the small intestine. Oncology 1997;11:529–36. *This is an excellent review of the differential diagnosis and management of primary tumors of the small intestine.*

## REFERENCES

1. Landis SH, Murray T, Bolden S, Wingo PA. Cancer statistics, 1999. CA Cancer J Clin 1999;49:8–31.
2. SEER Cancer Statistics Review 1973–1996 from http://www-seer.ims.nci.nih.gov.
3. Neugut AI, Jacobson JS, Suh S, et al. The epidemiology of cancer of the small bowel. Cancer Epidemiol Biomarkers Prev 1998;7:243–51.
4. Stemmermann GN, Goodman MT, Nomura AM. Adenocarcinoma of the proximal small intestine—a marker for familial and multicenter cancer? Cancer 1992;70:2766–71.
5. Arber N, Neugut AI, Weinstein IB, Holt P. Molecular genetics of small bowel cancer. Cancer Epidemiol Biomarkers Prev 1997;6:745–8.
6. Mason GR. Small bowel neoplasms. In: Sabiston DC Jr, ed. Davis-Christopher Textbook of Surgery. Philadelphia: WB Saunders, 1977;970.
7. Ashley SW, Wells SA Jr. Tumors of the small intestine. Semin Oncol 1988;15:116–28.
8. Neugut AI, Marvin MR, Rella VA, Chabot JA. An overview of adenocarcinoma of the small intestine. Oncology 1997;11:529–36.
9. Halphen M, Najjar T, Jaafoura H, et al. Diagnostic value of upper intestinal fiber endoscopy in primary small intestinal lymphoma. Cancer 1986;58:2140–5.
10. Rossini FP, Risio M, Pennazio M. Small bowel tumors and polyposis syndromes. Gastrointest Endosc Clin North Am 1999;9:93–114.
11. Brücher BL, Roder JD, Fink U, et al. Prognostic factors in resected primary small bowel tumors. Digest Surg 1998;15:42–51.
12. Kopelson G, Gunderson LL. Radiation therapy for small bowel carcinoma: report of three patients and review of the literature. Int J Radiat Oncol Biol Phys 1982;8:1055–7.
13. Jigyasu D, Bedikian AY, Stroehlein JR. Chemotherapy for primary adenocarcinoma of the small bowel. Cancer 1984;53:23–5.
14. Nevitt AW, Vida F, Kozarek RA, et al. Expandable metallic prostheses for malignant obstructions of gastric outlet and proximal small bowel. Gastrointest Endosc 1998;47:271–6.

# CHAPTER 43

# COLORECTAL CANCER

## NATURAL HISTORY, DIAGNOSIS, AND STAGING

• Charles M. Haskell

## EPIDEMIOLOGY AND ETIOLOGY

**Incidence.** Colorectal cancer is a major health problem in most affluent countries. In the United States, it is the fourth most frequent primary malignant neoplasm, with approximately 129,400 new cases and 56,600 deaths expected in 1999.[1] The incidence rates for colon cancer and rectal cancer in the United States are 31.9 and 12.4 cases per 100,000 population, respectively. The U.S. annual mortality rate for these two cancers combined is 17.5 deaths per 100,000 population.[2]

**Molecular Pathogenesis.** Colorectal cancer develops by a multistep process that can be influenced by numerous factors; some are hereditary, whereas others are environmental or acquired. The molecular events involved in this process are being clarified by elegant studies in many laboratories. Kinzler and Vogelstein[3] at Johns Hopkins have developed a model of carcinogenesis for colorectal cancer that has enjoyed wide acceptance (Fig. 43–1). This model accommodates many of the epidemiologic observations about risk factors summarized later in this chapter, including information about familial adenomatous polyposis (FAP) and hereditary nonpolyposis colorectal cancer (HNPCC), or Lynch syndrome types I and II.[4] Inherited predispositions to colo-

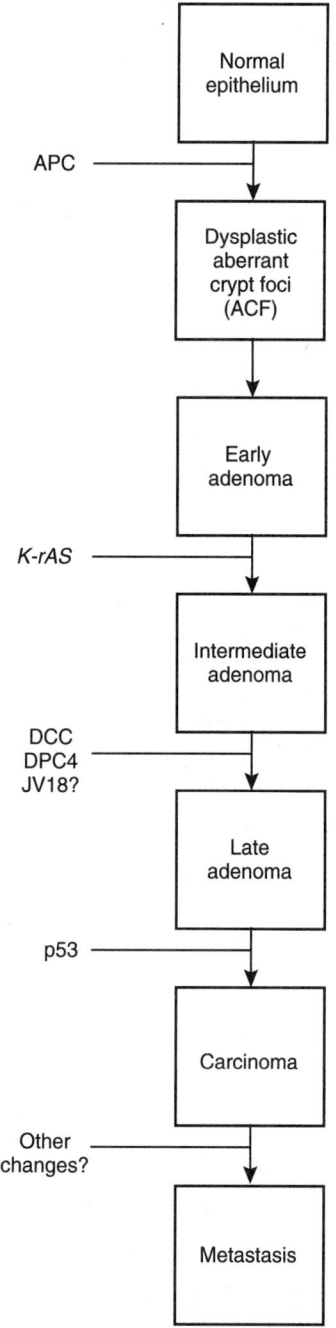

rectal cancer are the most important group of risk factors for developing the disease (Table 43–1).

Several features of this model warrant comment. Colorectal cancer arises in a sequential manner through a series of events during the progression of the disease from early adenoma to metastatic disease (as illustrated in Figs. 1–4 and 43–1 and discussed in Chapter 2). These steps are associated with particular morphologic and molecular abnormalities that involve the activation of oncogenes and the inactivation of tumor-suppressor genes.

Colorectal carcinogenesis can be summarized as follows: There may be inherited predispositions to colorectal cancer present, of which the best characterized are HNPCC and FAP. The latter is associated with germline mutations of the *APC* gene.[3] HNPCC is associated with abnormalities of many genes involved in DNA repair (*hMSH2, hMLH1, hPMS1, hPMS2*).[5] Most cases of colorectal cancer do not have a well-recognized inherited component; these are referred to as *sporadic* cases. Such cases result from a series of somatogenetic mutations, of which four genetic events have been described at the molecular level, including activation of *ras* oncogenes and inactivation of tumor-suppressor genes on chromosomes 5q (the *APC* gene), 17p (the p53 gene), and 18q (*DCC, DPC4,* and *JV18-1/MADR2*). The *APC* gene is especially important because it is responsible for the FAP syndrome, and it is present as a somatic mutation in more than 80% of sporadic colorectal neoplasms. Mutation of the *APC* gene appears to be the earliest genetic event in colorectal tumorigenesis, with the sequential occurrence of other mutations resulting in clonal expansion and progressive cellular disorganization. Overall, it appears to take at least

**Figure 43–1.** Molecular model of colorectal carcinogenesis. *APC* is the adenomatous polyposis gene on 5q that is mutated during carcinogenesis (influences early adenoma formation). K-*ras* is mutated in about 50% of cases (other oncogene mutations may include changes in *src, myc,* or HER-2/*neu*). *DCC* is the deleted in colorectal cancer suppressor gene found on chromosome 18q; *DPC4*, deleted in pancreatic cancer 4 gene; *JV18*, one of several smad genes, which influence the cell through the influence of transforming growth factor-β; and p53, a well-established suppressor gene on chromosome 17p. Other genes involved in this process in some patients include the *MCC* (mutated in colorectal cancer) gene on 5q and several genes associated with hereditary nonpolyposis cancer syndrome (Lynch syndromes I and II) (the *hMLH1* and *hMSH2* genes among others, which are involved in DNA repair). Carcinogenesis is associated with both the accumulation of these changes and the order in which changes occur. This is a rapidly evolving field, and the details of this model are subject to change. (From Kinzler KW, Vogelstein B. Colorectal tumors. In: Vogelstein B, Kinzler KW, eds. The genetic basis of human cancer. New York: McGraw-Hill, 1998:565.

**Table 43–1.** Inherited Predispositions to Colorectal Cancer

*Syndromes with Pre-existing Polyposis*

| | |
|---|---|
| Familial adenomatous polyposis | Colonic polyposis |
| Gardner's syndrome | Colonic polyposis in association with extracolonic lesions |
| Oldfield's syndrome | With sebaceous cysts |
| Turcot's syndrome | Malignant tumors of the central nervous system in association with polyposis of colon |
| Caroli's disease | Bile duct and renal anomalies |

*Syndromes with Pre-existing Hamartomatous Polyps*

| | |
|---|---|
| Peutz-Jeghers syndrome | Abnormal pigmentation on lips and buccal mucosa |
| Ruvalcaba-Myhre-Smith syndrome | Macrocephaly, pigmented macules on penis |
| Juvenile polyposis | Cystic hamartomatous polyps |
| Cowden's syndrome | Multiple hamartomatous lesions, primarily on mucocutaneous tissue |

*Syndromes Without Pre-existing Polyposis*

| | |
|---|---|
| Hereditary nonpolyposis colorectal cancer (Lynch type I and type II syndromes) | Few if any polyps, colorectal cancer tends to be site specific |
| Muir-Torre syndrome | Lynch type II syndrome with dermatologic lesions and laryngeal cancer |

From Scott RI, Müller H. Familial and genetic aspects of colorectal carcinogenesis. Eur J Cancer 1993;29A:2164. Copyright 1993, with kind permission from Elsevier Science Ltd, The Boulevard, Langford Lane, Kidlington, OX5 1GB, UK.

seven somatic mutations and decades for cases of sporadic colorectal cancer to evolve.

Carcinogenesis can be initiated by a variety of events or agents that can cause somatic mutations. A viral cause is possible, given studies showing cytomegalovirus in colon carcinoma tissue, but unproved. Exposure to radiation can initiate colorectal carcinogenesis.[6] Chemical carcinogens may initiate the process. Candidate chemicals include various protein metabolites, ammonia, volatile phenols, tryptophan, and N-nitroso compounds. Carcinogens may result from certain modes of cooking, particularly frying and grilling meat and fish. None of these is well established in humans as carcinogenic, however.

**Dietary Risk Factors for Carcinogenesis.** Global epidemiologic studies have revealed that colorectal cancer is much more prevalent in North America and most developed countries than in South American, African, and Asian countries. Studies of immigrants have shown that first-generation immigrants from low-incidence areas of colorectal carcinoma acquire a higher risk for this disease.[7] This change suggests that cancer of the large bowel can be caused, or at least promoted, by environmental factors. Of the many environmental factors studied to date, those related to diet appear to be the most important. Two major and several minor theories of dietary origin predominate, but none of these fully explains the available data. The first major theory relates to dietary fiber and the second to dietary fat. Given the importance of nutrition to health as well as the potential for cancer prevention if a dietary theory proves to be correct, the status of this topic is discussed briefly.

*Dietary Fiber.* Burkitt[8] pointed out the strong association between the low incidence of colorectal cancer and a diet high in fiber content, which results in rapid transit time and large bulk in the stools of the South African Bantu. He suggested that a rapid transit time reduces the time that carcinogens or their precursors are held in contact against the colonic mucosa. There is little evidence, however, that a decreased transit time reduces bacterial action on colon contents, and studies of populations with widely varying incidences of colon cancer show no differences in bowel transit times. The most compelling evidence against this hypothesis comes from a prospective study of 88,757 women, for whom no important protective effect from dietary fiber could be shown, and two prospective, randomized clinical trials that failed to support this hypothesis.[8a, 8b, 9]

*Dietary Fat.* A correlation between the intake of animal fat and large bowel cancer has been made in several studies. This is the most widely accepted association between diet and cancer, and the National Academy of Sciences has recommended that the diet of U.S. citizens be modified to contain less fat as a prudent preventive measure. Epidemiologic studies, however, have not provided unequivocal support for this association. Most cross-sectional correlation studies, but not all case-control studies, have shown a positive correlation between a high-fat and high-meat diet and an increased frequency of colon cancer.[7] The most sophisticated studies, which used precise methods for measuring the amount of fat and protein in the diet of study populations, have not shown the expected parallelism between large bowel cancer and fat and protein consumption.

*Dietary Sugar.* The elevated consumption of refined sugar has been noted as a possible causative factor in some populations with a high incidence of colon cancer,[10] but a positive correlation between intake of sugar and colon cancer is not uniform on a worldwide basis. Preliminary data suggest that glucose intolerance may correlate with an increased risk of colorectal cancer. Further studies to explore this relationship are warranted.[11]

*Alteration in Bowel Microflora.* Hill[12] postulated that the nature of the bacterial flora of the bowel can be determined by the diet and that diet provides a substrate for any bacteria-induced change of normal bowel contents to carcinogens. Because individuals living in areas with high incidences of colon cancer have high fecal concentrations of bile acids—both normal and degraded—Hill believed that the capacity of the bacteria to desaturate the bile acid nucleus might be an important factor in carcinogenesis.

Some investigators have noted changes in the microflora of subjects at high risk, whereas others have not found significant differences in fecal microflora of individuals consuming different diets. For instance, Goldberg and coworkers[13] compared the fecal microflora of Seventh Day Adventists, who have a low incidence of colon cancer and are often vegetarians, with individuals consuming a general Western diet. No statistically significant differences were identified between the fecal microflora of the two groups. It is possible that the induction or repression of bacterial enzymes can occur, which changes their metabolic activity—and possibly their carcinogenic potential—without appreciable changes in the actual number or types of bacteria that are present in the stool.

Because of the tremendous potential of bacteria for substrate alteration and subsequent carcinogenesis, most theories of dietary causes of colon cancer postulate a form of bacterial interaction at some stage of cancer development, although the precise mechanism is unclear. Research in this area is of particular interest because an active bacterial pathway to carcinogenesis, if identified, could possibly be blocked by appropriate treatment.

**Other Environmental Risk Factors.** Numerous factors have been linked to a higher risk of colon cancer, including beer drinking, asbestos exposure, low parity, a low serum cholesterol level, and prior cholecystectomy. The true role of these factors in carcinogenesis is unclear at present.

*Age.* The incidence of colon cancer begins to rise significantly after the age of 40 to 45 years and increases each decade thereafter by a factor of about 2 until it peaks at age 75 years.[14] This rise in incidence may result from the action of carcinogens on colonic cells over an increasing period. The risk is about the same for men and women older than age 40. When colon cancer occurs before the age of 40 years, it usually does so in conjunction with some of the other risk factors, especially familial ones.

*Polyps.* The incidence of colon cancer is higher in patients with colonic polyps, and the model of colorectal carcinogenesis shown in Figure 43–1 includes adenomas as a precursor to invasive malignancy. It seems logical to consider patients with adenomatous polyps or villous adenomas at increased risk for colon cancer because a large body of direct and indirect evidence suggests that most carcinomas, rather than arising de novo, evolve from adenomatous tissue. The evidence for this suggestion can be summarized as follows: First, about one third of operative specimens of colon cancer have at least one adenomatous polyp. Second, invasive cancer is frequently seen contiguous with adenomatous tissue. In some specimens, there is a spectrum of change from benign adenomatous tissue to atypia to focal cancer to invasive cancer. Third, as polyps grow, there is increasing cellular atypia and increasingly abnormal chromosome patterns similar to those seen in invasive cancer. Fourth, many adenomatous polyps seen in FAP, a well-documented premalignant state, are histologically similar to adenomas that occur as individual lesions. Finally, aggressive removal of adenomatous polyps by colonoscopy decreases the risk of death from colorectal cancer.

The effectiveness of prophylaxis (polypectomy) in reducing the incidence of colon cancer lends especially strong support to a link between polyps and cancer. Gilbertsen[15] reported a 25-year study of more than 100,000 proctosigmoidoscopies in 18,000 patients. Annual follow-up examinations were made, and the equivalent of 85,000 patient-years of experience was obtained. Whenever any polypoid lesion was encountered, it was removed. Statistically, 75 to 80 rectosigmoid cancers would have been expected to develop in this group, but only 11 occurred in these patients who had all polypoid lesions removed. Subsequently a large study of 1418 patients aggressively treated with colonoscopy and polypectomies confirmed the benefit of this treatment.[16]

A distinction must be drawn between hyperplastic and adenomatous polyps. Of 1000 colonic proliferations, about 900 are small, hyperplastic polyps, which are of little if any precancerous significance. Of the remaining 100, however, about 10 are large adenomas (>1 cm), and 1 of these 10 polyps contains a cancer. Although the overall incidence of cancer in polyps is about 1 in 1000, the incidence is high (10%) among large adenomas and becomes even higher when polyps greater than 2 cm or polyps of the villous type are encountered.[17]

**High-Risk Groups.** Among colorectal cancer patients at Memorial Sloan-Kettering Cancer Center, 3.6% of patients had a prior colorectal malignancy, and 1.9% had multiple colorectal primary tumors. Their risk for developing a subsequent primary colorectal cancer was 0.35% per year. The highest risk for a second colon cancer existed in patients whose initial lesions were in the cecum. The presence of adenomatous polyps in the resected specimen increased the risk of future colon cancer to six times that seen in the general population.[17]

Families with a high incidence of carcinoma in other anatomic sites, such as endometrium, ovary, and breast, have a greater than normal risk of malignancy (Lynch syndrome types). The risk of cancer of the colon in relatives of colon cancer patients is three times that noted in the normal population. The relatives of patients with multiple cancers of the colon not only have an increased risk of colon cancer but also are on average 5 to 10 years younger at diagnosis than other colon cancer patients. These families are considered to have HNPCC.

**Associated Diseases and Colon Cancer.** Almost all patients with FAP, a condition with an autosomal dominant mode of inheritance with 80% penetrance, develop colon cancer unless colectomy is performed (see Table 43–1).[18] Another high-risk group consists of patients with Gardner's syndrome, in which adenomatous polyps develop in the colon and are associated with soft tissue and lung tumors.[19] Patients with Turcot's syndrome (central nervous system tumors) or Oldfield's syndrome (extensive sebaceous cysts)

are at high risk to develop colon cancer. Peutz-Jeghers syndrome is occasionally associated with cancers of the stomach, ileum, and duodenum.[20] Patients with juvenile polyposis are also at high risk for cancer, and their relatives are more likely to develop adenomatous polyps and colon cancer.

Ulcerative colitis is frequently associated with the later development of colon cancer. When age is not considered, the likelihood of developing colon cancer is 5 to 10 times higher in colitis patients than in the general population. The risk begins to rise about 10 years after the onset of the disease, and it has been estimated to be 20 to 30% at 20 years. The risk doubles in patients in whom the onset of colitis occurs before age 25. In patients who develop colorectal cancers, the average age of cancer onset is earlier, and the cancers tend to be multicentric and often highly malignant. The cancers often develop during an asymptomatic period. Because of this high risk, patients with longstanding ulcerative colitis are usually advised to undergo prophylactic colectomy. For patients who refuse colectomy, vigorous surveillance that includes rectal biopsies to identify dysplastic changes is indicated. The patient should be informed that this approach is inferior to prophylactic colectomy.[21]

Granulomatous colitis, or Crohn's disease, is also generally thought to be premalignant, especially when the age of onset is before 21 years. The magnitude of risk is probably much less than that in ulcerative colitis.

## PREVENTION

The science of cancer prevention is in its infancy, as discussed in Chapter 4. The potential value of a low-fat diet in cancer prevention was discussed previously, although its value in preventing colorectal cancer is unproved. There is interest in the prevention of colorectal cancer using a wide variety of medications, vitamins, and minerals. These are of unproved value, as reflected in a negative randomized trial testing the ability of antioxidant vitamins to prevent the formation of colorectal polyps.[22] Clinical trials of chemoprevention are ongoing with wheat bran, retinol, calcium carbonate, piroxican, difluoromethylornithine, aspirin, omega-3 fatty acids, sulindac, beta-carotene, ascorbic acid, acarbose, and α-tocopherol.

## PATHOLOGY

Most primary malignant colorectal neoplasms are adenocarcinomas, but other neoplasms can occur (Table 43–2).[23–25] Lymphomas may arise from lymphoid tissue within the gut (see Chapter 94) and soft tissue sarcomas from mesodermal tissue within the gut (see Chapter 83). The rare occurrence of squamous cell carcinomas within the colon is less easily explained.[26] It has been proposed that most adenocarcinomas develop from a common endodermal stem cell and that a spectrum of tumors may arise, from the classic adenocarcinoma to the classic carcinoid tumor. The existence of a well-differentiated colonic adenocarcinoma containing large numbers of gastrointestinal neuroendocrine cells has been used to support this concept.[27] In this case, neurosecretory granules were confirmed by electron microscopy, and immunocytochemistry showed large numbers of cells containing serotonin with lesser numbers of cells containing a variety

*Table 43–2.* **World Health Organization Classification of Malignant Neoplasms of the Colon and Rectum**

I. Epithelial tumors
    A. Benign
        1. Adenoma
            a. Tubular (adenomatous polyp)
            b. Villous
            c. Tubulovillous
        2. Adenomatosis (adenomatous polyposis coli)
    B. Malignant
        1. Adenocarcinoma
        2. Mucinous adenocarcinoma
        3. Signet-ring cell carcinoma
        4. Squamous cell carcinoma
        5. Adenosquamous carcinoma
        6. Undifferentiated carcinoma
        7. Unclassified carcinoma
II. Carcinoid tumors
    A. Argentaffin
    B. Nonargentaffin
    C. Composite
III. Nonepithelial tumors
    A. Benign
        1. Leiomyoma
        2. Leiomyoblastoma
        3. Neurilemmoma (schwannoma)
        4. Lipoma
            Lipomatosis
        5. Vascular tumors
            a. Hemangioma
            b. Lymphangioma
        6. Others
    B. Malignant
        1. Leiomyosarcoma
        2. Others
IV. Hematopoietic and lymphoid neoplasms
V. Unclassified tumors
VI. Secondary tumors
VII. Tumor-like lesions
    A. Hamartomas
        1. Peutz-Jeghers polyp and polyposis
        2. Juvenile polyp and polyposis
    B. Heterotopia
        1. Gastric
    C. Hyperplastic (metaplastic) polyp
    D. Benign lymphoid polyp and polyposis
    E. Inflammatory polyp
    F. Colitis cystica profunda
    G. Endometriosis
VIII. Epithelial atypia in ulcerative colitis

Data from Morson BC, et al. Histological classification of tumours, No. 15: histological typing of intestinal tumours. Geneva: World Health Organization, 1976; and Sobin LH, et al. A coded compendium of the International Classification of Tumours. Geneva: World Health Organization, 1978:11.

of other neuroendocrine peptides. The histopathologic relationship between colorectal polyps and adenocarcinomas has been discussed previously in this chapter.

In the past, it was stated that one half of colorectal carcinomas could be diagnosed by digital examination of the rectum (8 cm) and two thirds by sigmoidoscopy (25 cm).[28] In more recent years, however, there has been a shift in the distribution of colon neoplasms to the more proximal colon. In one study of screening colonoscopy, 25% of patients with right-sided lesions would have been missed using flexible sigmoidoscopy alone (approximately 65 cm).[29]

A variety of histopathologic factors may influence prognosis. Annular lesions that narrow the bowel circumference lead to a shorter survival than do lesions that involve only a portion of bowel wall. The shape of the tumor may be significant. Nearly twice as many patients with polypoid or projecting growths survive 5 years compared with those with infiltrating growths. In general, the size of the tumor has less bearing on survival than nodal metastases. The precise location of nodal metastases can be important, with apical involvement conferring the worst prognosis. The location of the tumor has been of variable significance, although it is generally thought that tumors located in the ascending colon have a more favorable prognosis than those located in the descending colon.

Histologic features related to prognosis include grade of tumor; lymphatic, vascular, and perineural infiltration; and presence or absence of an inflammatory response. Infiltration of the tumor by eosinophils may represent an especially good prognostic sign. In histologic grading, as in the system of Broders,[30] most observers use a numbering system from 1 to 4, with larger numbers indicating less differentiation, or a series of modifying terms designating tumors as well, moderately, or poorly differentiated.[31] The percentage of cells showing differentiation or the arrangement of cells to form glandular structures or tubules is usually used as a criterion for differentiation. Poorly differentiated signet-ring cells and mucinous carcinomas carry a less favorable prognosis than do more differentiated neoplasms.

The character of the periphery or advancing margin of the tumor has been correlated with survival. A worse prognosis has been described in tumors with infiltrating margins as opposed to pushing margins. Lymphatic invasion in the absence of nodal metastases has not been of proven significance. Involvement of the perineural space, however, has definitely been related to local recurrence. Venous invasion by cancer cells is also a grave prognostic sign. Bowel wall and lymph node invasion are of utmost importance in colorectal cancer and are discussed in detail in the upcoming section on staging.

The inflammatory response of the regional lymphatics appears to be significant in determining prognosis. The presence of well-developed paracortical immunoblast proliferation and an associated sinus histiocytosis defined a group of patients with a particularly good 5-year survival regardless of the Dukes stage of the tumor—83% in contrast to 35% in those without significant numbers of paracortical immunoblasts.[31] Patients with only a paracortical immunoblastic response also did better. These observations suggest that the cellular immune response may have a favorable influence on prognosis in colon cancer.

Flow cytometry allows the quantitation of aneuploidy and growth rate, as reflected in the percentage of cells in S phase. Early studies of the technique suggested an independent prognostic importance for aneuploidy, which fits with expectations based on the role of histologic differentiation. More recent studies, however, have questioned the importance of measuring the DNA index. At present, the DNA index has not been established as an independent prognostic factor in this disease. The same is true of measurements of the many molecular markers described in the section on molecular pathogenesis.

## CLINICAL FEATURES AND DIAGNOSIS

The clinical features associated with colorectal carcinomas relate to tumor size and location. Large, exophytic, bulky tumors occur more commonly in the ascending colon, with its large diameter and fluid contents, and result in symptoms of abdominal pain, bleeding, and weight loss rather than obstruction. The pain is vague and dull and may be confused with gallbladder disease or peptic ulcer. Anemia may be present. In the descending colon, with its smaller diameter and semisolid or solid contents, tumors are more often infiltrating or annular and cause obstructive symptoms, changes in bowel habits, or bleeding. Gas pain, decrease in stool caliber, and increased use of laxatives are common.

The diagnosis of colorectal carcinomas, as in all malignancies, requires a high index of suspicion and diligent follow-up of all symptoms, especially in high-risk patients. The importance of early diagnosis cannot be overemphasized. A logical approach to early diagnosis is through routine screening tests in asymptomatic individuals. The two most widely used screening tools are tests for occult blood in the stool and screening flexible sigmoidoscopy. Both these tests are recommended by the American College of Physicians and the American Cancer Society on a regular basis, as discussed in Chapter 5 and the following paragraphs.

## SCREENING TESTS FOR ASYMPTOMATIC INDIVIDUALS

**Fecal Occult Blood Test.** In 1967, Greegor[32] developed a test for home use involving guaiac testing for occult blood. Subsequently, numerous poorly controlled studies suggested the test was efficacious, whereas subsequent prospective trials testing the true value of the test in screening were, to some extent, controversial or contradictory. Long-term follow-up is now available on three large, randomized clinical trials of fecal occult blood testing (FOBT) that clearly establish the efficacy of the technique (Table 43–3).[33–36] The earliest trial is from the University of Minnesota, where a prospective, randomized trial involving 46,551 participants showed a 33% decrease in the 18-year cumulative mortality from colorectal cancer with annual FOBT and a 21% reduction in mortality with testing every 2 years. The two European trials performed FOBT every 2 years and showed reduced mortality rates of 15% and 18%. Most authorities, but not all,[37] advocate the use of FOBT for widespread screening of asymptomatic, average-risk patients after the age of 50. The Department of Veterans Affairs, the American College of Physicians, and the Agency for Healthcare Policy all support annual FOBT. The American Cancer Society supports annual FOBT but only in association with the periodic use of flexible sigmoidoscopy.

The recommended test for screening asymptomatic subjects uses Hemoccult guaiac-impregnated paper.[35] Two samples are taken from each of three stool specimens, and the slides are developed within 3 days. Even if just one of the six slides is positive, further work-up is performed, as described subsequently for symptomatic patients. The advantages of this test include low cost, ease of performance, and a relatively low false-positive rate (1%). The ingestion of barium, iron, or laxatives does not adversely affect the quality of the test, although large amounts of vitamin C, a low concentration of stool hemoglobin, and intermittent bleeding can cause false-negative reactions. Some authorities recommend that the patient consume a diet high in fiber and

*Table 43–3.* Comparison of Trials of Fecal Occult Blood Testing for Colorectal Cancer Screening

| | Minneapolis, Minnesota[35, 36] | | Nottingham, England[34] | Funen, Denmark[23] |
|---|---|---|---|---|
| Frequency of FOBT (yr) | 1 | 2 | 2 | 2 |
| No. subjects | 46,551 | | 152,850 | 61,933 |
| Follow-up (yr) | 13 | 18 | 7.8 | 10 |
| Mortality reduction* (%) | 33 | 21 | 15 | 18 |

*The reduction of mortality was statistically significant in all three trials.
FOBT, fecal occult blood testing.

low in red meat for several days before the test, but others consider these preparations unnecessary. There is also controversy over what constitutes the optimal test conditions for FOBT—whether or not the sample should be rehydrated or tested without special treatment. It is likely that further technical improvements in the test will improve its usefulness in the future.

The major problem with this approach to early diagnosis in asymptomatic patients has been patient acceptance. In most studies, fewer than one third of the patients invited to participate have returned stool specimens for analysis. In one study conducted in a Veterans Hospital, patient compliance increased to 93% in a special clinic developed for this purpose and supervised by a nurse practitioner.[38] Even with special clinics, however, long-term compliance with annual testing is a problem in asymptomatic, low-risk patients.

**Flexible Sigmoidoscopy.** Flexible sigmoidoscopy is an important screening tool for asymptomatic, normal-risk patients. The American College of Physicians and the American Cancer Society recommend its use every 5 years after age 50 (see Chapter 5). In the United Kingdom, a trial has been proposed for screening the entire population at least once between the ages of 55 and 60 years.[39] Increasingly, this procedure is being taught to physicians specializing in general internal medicine so that it will become more widely available. The procedure can be taught to nurses, who can perform the procedure as accurately and safely as experienced gastroenterologists.[40] The procedure is also useful as a diagnostic test in the follow-up of accessible lesions identified by barium enema in symptomatic patients.

**Screening Recommendations for Asymptomatic, Average-Risk Patients.** Table 43–4 provides an overview of the

*Table 43–4.* Colorectal Cancer Screening Tests for Average-Risk Persons Beginning at Age 50*

| Test | Frequency of Repetition |
|---|---|
| FOBT | Yearly |
| Flexible sigmoidoscopy | 5 yr |
| Annual FOBT plus flexible sigmoidoscopy | 5 yr |
| Double-contrast barium enema | 5–10 yr |
| Colonoscopy | 10 yr |

*The American Cancer Society recommends all of these tests as options with the exception of FOBT alone. The Agency for Health Care Policy and Research considers all of these options acceptable. Not all health plans cover colonoscopy in average-risk patients, including Medicare.
FOBT, fecal occult blood testing.

commonly available screening tests for colorectal cancer in asymptomatic, average-risk patients. Many patients find it helpful to know that a variety of tests can be considered, some of which may be more acceptable to them than others. In general, Table 43–4 lists options in order of increasing cost, sensitivity, and specificity. The gold standard is colonoscopy, but it is not an option under many health insurance plans. In the Department of Veterans Affairs, the preferred option for screening in patients older than age 50 is annual FOBT plus flexible sigmoidoscopy every 5 years.

## DIAGNOSTIC STUDIES IN PATIENTS WITH POSITIVE FECAL OCCULT BLOOD TESTS AND IN HIGH-RISK ASYMPTOMATIC PATIENTS

Most authorities recommend that patients with positive FOBT have either a full colonoscopy or a flexible sigmoidoscopic examination and air-contrast barium enema. Aggressive screening is also indicated for patients with a family history of colorectal cancer, especially in patients with FAP and HNPCC. FAP is rare, but HNPCC may be present in 5% of colorectal cancer cases. Lacking genetic confirmation of the diagnosis of HNPCC, clinical criteria may be used to identify the patient for whom aggressive screening with a barium enema and flexible sigmoidoscopy or colonoscopy alone may be indicated (Table 43–5).[41]

**Barium Enema.** The full-column barium enema has been reported to miss one fifth to one fourth of all colon cancers and two fifths of all polypoid lesions. The double-contrast barium enema, however, detects almost all colonic lesions of at least 5 mm diameter. If a barium enema is used for screening, it is important to perform the study with air contrast. Contraindications include acute, severe, inflammatory bowel disease; suspected perforation; and recent bowel wall biopsy.

**Colonoscopy.** Depending on the risk of bowel disease, colonoscopy can be used without prior barium enema or following an air-contrast barium enema. Detected lesions are then biopsied or removed, or both. Colonoscopy and barium enema are complementary techniques, and their use together provides excellent diagnostic resolution in patients at high risk of colorectal cancer. Limitations of colonoscopy include failure to reach or examine fully the splenic flexure (10%), the hepatic flexure (15%), or the cecum (20%). Aggressive colonoscopy is indicated in patients with a proven diagnosis of colorectal cancer because synchronous lesions are not unusual, and these may be missed at the time of surgical exploration.[42]

Asymptomatic patients with well-documented occult blood in the stool and symptomatic patients should have a colonoscopic examination of the entire colon, even with

*Table 43–5.* **Amsterdam Criteria for Hereditary Nonpolyposis Colorectal Cancer**

≥3 relatives with colorectal cancer
1 affected case is a first-degree relative of the other 2
≥1 individual is <50 years of age
Colorectal cancer spans ≥2 generations
Familial adenomatous polyposis is excluded

From Vasen HFA, Mecklin J-P, Meera Khan P, Lynch HT. The International Collaborative Group on HNPCC. Dis Colon Rectum 1991;34:424–5.

normal sigmoidoscopic findings and normal or equivocal barium enemas. The importance of this examination is illustrated by the results of a series of colonoscopic examinations performed in 146 patients who had double-contrast barium enemas suggesting benign polypoid disease. Thirty-six patients (25%) did not have a neoplastic lesion at the suspected site. Seven of the 36 patients (19%) had unsuspected, benign polypoid adenomas elsewhere, and 4 patients (11%) had benign neoplastic lesions at the suspected area and unsuspected malignant lesions elsewhere. Of the remaining 110 patients who had neoplastic lesions correctly identified at the suspected site, 17 (15%) had either adenocarcinomas or neoplastic polyps with invasive cancer.

Colonoscopy is an essential procedure for the proper diagnosis, treatment, and surveillance of patients with nonfamilial colorectal polyps. The American College of Gastroenterology has issued a position paper on the subject giving detailed guidelines for the use of colonoscopy in these patients.[43] Table 43–6 summarizes the recommendations of the American College of Gastroenterology for reference.

Colonoscopy is an important part of surveillance in patients with colorectal cancer treated with curative intent. Although the frequency of colonoscopy in these patients is controversial, the procedure should be performed at least once after curative resections to rule out synchronous lesions and recurrent disease at the anastomosis.[44]

**Ultrasonography.** Traditional transabdominal ultrasonography is of minimal value in the evaluation of colonic diseases, but this procedure can be useful when augmented by the retrograde instillation of water into the colon.[45] This procedure is termed *hydrocolonic sonography*, and it permits a detailed evaluation of the structure of the bowel wall, permitting more precise preoperative staging. Technical limitations, however, make it inappropriate for use as the sole diagnostic study, especially in the lower rectum. Transrectal ultrasonography may also be useful in staging, especially for rectal cancer, but it has technical limitations. Further study is needed to define the role of ultrasonography in the management of colorectal cancer.

**Virtual Colonoscopy.** Thin-section, helical computed tomography (CT) using air contrast and glucagon bowel sedation has been reported to have efficacy similar to that of standard colonoscopy in the detection of polyps 6 mm or more in diameter.[46] Further study is needed to place this test in perspective relative to standard alternatives.

**Other Tests.** Stool cytologic techniques are well developed and accurate.[47] The necessity for meticulous, time-consuming bowel preparation and lavage has limited their applicability, however, and probably will continue to do so. Preoperative carcinoembryonic antigen (CEA) values often correlate with tumor burden and prognosis,[48] but CEA has no place in the diagnosis or screening of colorectal cancer. Other tumor markers are even less useful than CEA in the initial diagnosis of colorectal cancer. Immunoscintigraphy using radiolabeled antibodies directed against CEA or other colonic antigens (such as satumomab pendetide [OncoScint] directed against TAG-72) is of uncertain value in the initial management of colorectal cancer. Immunoscintigraphy may be more useful in patients with occult recurrent disease,[49] as discussed subsequently in the section on surgical treatment for recurrent cancer. Similarly, positron emission tomography scanning is proving to be useful in imaging occult areas of recurrent colorectal cancer in patients being considered

*Table 43–6.* **Summary of Guidelines from the American College of Gastroenterology for the Diagnosis, Treatment, and Surveillance of Patients with Nonfamilial Colorectal Polyps**

| | |
|---|---|
| Initial management | A. Most patients with polyps detected by barium enema or flexible sigmoidoscopy should undergo colonoscopy to excise the polyp and search for additional neoplasms |
| | B. The decision whether to perform colonoscopy for patients with polyps <0.5 cm in diameter must be individualized depending on the patient's age, comorbidity, and past history of colonic neoplasia |
| | C. Small polyps encountered during colonoscopy are usually examined by biopsy then destroyed by fulguration. Representative biopsy specimens are obtained when these small lesions are numerous |
| | D. When a small polyp is encountered during screening flexible sigmoidoscopy, it should be examined by biopsy to determine if it is an adenoma and may be an indication for colonoscopy. The balance of current evidence supports the recommendation that a hyperplastic polyp found during flexible sigmoidoscopy is not, by itself, an indication for subsequent colonoscopy |
| | E. A patient who has had successful colonoscopic excision of a large sessile polyp (≥2 cm) should undergo follow-up colonoscopy in 3 to 6 mo to determine if resection was complete. If residual polyp is present, it should be removed and the completeness of resection documented within another 3–6 mo interval. If complete resection is not possible after two to three examinations, the patient should usually be referred for surgical therapy |
| Malignant polyp | A. No further treatment is indicated after colonoscopic resection of a malignant polyp if the following criteria are fulfilled: |
| |   1. The polyp is considered completely excised by the endoscopist and is submitted in toto for pathologic examination |
| |   2. In the pathology laboratory, the polyp is fixed and sectioned so that it is possible to determine accurately the depth of invasion, grade of differentiation, and completeness of excision of the carcinoma |
| |   3. The cancer is not poorly differentiated |
| |   4. There is no vascular or lymphatic involvement |
| |   5. The margin of excision is not involved |
| | B. Patients with malignant polyps with favorable prognostic criteria should have follow-up colonoscopy in 3 mo to check for residual abnormal tissue at the polypectomy site, especially if the polyp was sessile. After one negative result of follow-up examination, the clinician can revert to standard surveillance, as is performed for patients with benign adenomas |
| | C. When a patient's malignant polyp has poor prognostic features, the relative risks of surgical resection should be weighed against the risk for death from metastatic cancer. The patient at high risk for morbidity and mortality from surgery should probably not have surgical resection. If a malignant polyp is located in that part of the low rectum that would require an abdominoperineal resection, local excision rather than a standard cancer resection is usually justified |
| Postpolypectomy surveillance | A. Complete colonoscopy should be performed at the time of polypectomy to detect and resect all synchronous adenomas. Additional clearing examinations may be required after resection of a large sessile adenoma or multiple adenomas to ensure complete resection |
| | B. Repeated colonoscopy to check for missed synchronous and for metachronous adenomas is performed in 3 yr for most patients with a single or only a few adenomas, provided they have had a high-quality initial clearing examination |
| | C. Selected patients with multiple adenomas or those who have had a suboptimal clearing examination might require colonoscopy at 1 and 4 yr |
| | D. After one negative 3 yr follow-up examination, subsequent surveillance intervals may be increased to 5 yr |
| | E. The presence of severe or high-grade dysplasia in a resected polyp does not per se modify recommendations A through D |
| | F. If complete colonoscopy is not feasible, flexible sigmoidoscopy followed by a double-contrast barium enema is an acceptable alternative |
| | G. Because patients undergoing resection of a single, small, tubular adenoma (<1 cm) may not have an increased subsequent risk for cancer, follow-up surveillance may not be indicated according to decision analysis of available data |
| | H. Follow-up surveillance should be discontinued when it appears unlikely that continued follow-up is capable of prolonging life expectancy |

From Bond JH, for the Practice Parameters Committee of the American College of Gastroenterology: Position paper. Polyp guideline: diagnosis, treatment, and surveillance for patients with nonfamilial colorectal polyps. Ann Intern Med 1993;119:836–43. Reproduced with permission.

for re-exploration.[50] Conventional tests, such as complete blood count, blood biochemical panel, chest radiograph, and abdominal CT, give information about the extent of disease that is necessary for appropriate surgical intervention. For patients with rectal cancer, magnetic resonance imaging (MRI) may be more useful than CT for defining the extent of the tumor.[51] Other biochemical, immunologic, and radiologic tests are of uncertain value in most cases.

## STAGING

The early Dukes pathologic staging system, which was introduced in 1932, separated colorectal malignancies into three groups. Lesions confined to the bowel wall and not penetrating the muscularis were designated *A*, lesions penetrating the muscularis into surrounding fat or adventitia were designated *B*, and lesions with positive lymph node involvement were designated *C*.[52] Numerous modifications of this system have subsequently been published, including the addition of a so-called Dukes D stage for patients with metastatic disease. Some of these variations are compared in Figure 43–2, and this subject has been critically reviewed by Zinkin.[53]

More recent efforts to develop a universally acceptable staging system for colorectal carcinoma have been those involving the TNM system of the International Union Against Cancer (UICC) and the American Joint Committee on Cancer (AJCC).[54] The TNM system has the advantage of being applicable to clinical-diagnostic staging before surgery as well as postsurgical resection pathologic staging, and it provides an opportunity to break entirely with the confusion

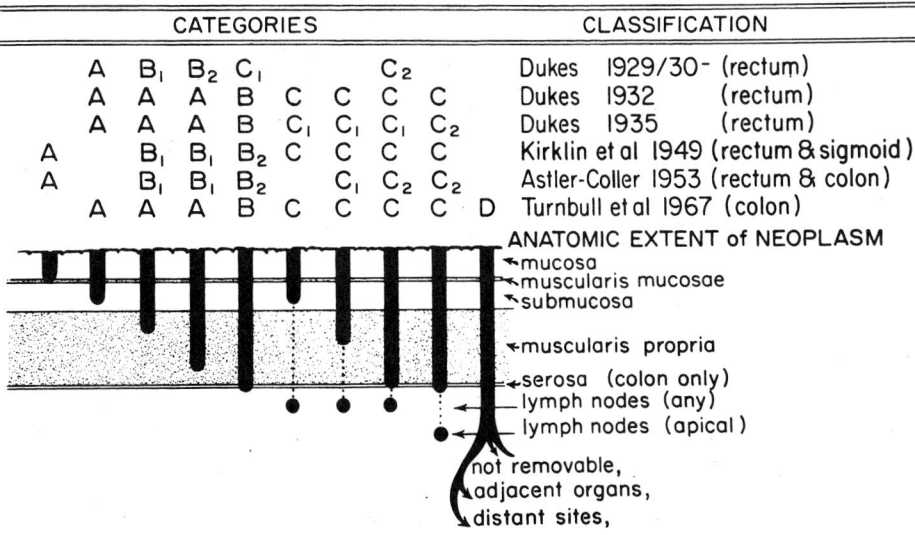

**Figure 43–2.** The evolution of the Dukes classification is shown, as are subsequent systems based on it. All except Turnbull's system are derived entirely from examination of the resected bowel. Not illustrated is the fact that the Dukes system included curative and palliative resections, and many of the class C cases would have qualified as stage D in the system of Turnbull. (From Donegan WL, DeCorse JJ. In: Enker WE, ed. Carcinoma of the colon and rectum. Chicago: Year Book Medical Publishers, 1978:55.)

created by the variations in the Dukes A, B, C system. For these reasons, the TNM system is becoming the standard system in the United States. The details of this system as well as a comparison with the Dukes stages appear in Table 43–7.

## PROGNOSIS

The most important guide to prognosis for patients with colorectal carcinoma is the stage of the disease. Figure 43–3 summarizes the survival results by stage from the

*Table 43–7.* **International TNM Staging System for Colorectal Carcinoma**

*Primary Tumor (T)*

| | |
|---|---|
| TX | Primary tumor cannot be assessed |
| T0 | No evidence of primary tumor |
| Tis | Carcinoma in situ: intraepithelial or invasion of lamina propria* |
| T1 | Tumor invades submucosa |
| T2 | Tumor invades muscularis propria |
| T3 | Tumor invades through the muscularis propria into the subserosa, or into nonperitonealized pericolic or perirectal tissues |
| T4 | Tumor directly invades other organs or structures, and/or perforates visceral peritoneum** |

*Regional Lymph Nodes (N)*

| | |
|---|---|
| NX | Regional lymph nodes cannot be assessed |
| N0 | No regional lymph node metastasis |
| N1 | Metastasis in 1 to 3 regional lymph nodes |
| N2 | Metastasis in 4 or more regional lymph nodes |

*Distant metastasis (M)*

| | |
|---|---|
| MX | Distant metastasis cannot be assessed |
| M0 | No distant metastasis |
| M1 | Distant metastasis |

*Stage Grouping*

| AJCC/UICC | | | | Dukes† |
|---|---|---|---|---|
| Stage 0 | Tis | N0 | M0 | — |
| Stage I | T1 | N0 | M0 | A |
| | T2 | N0 | M0 | — |
| Stage II | T3 | N0 | M0 | B |
| | T4 | N0 | M0 | — |
| Stage III | Any T | N1 | M0 | C |
| | Any T | N2 | M0 | — |
| Stage IV | Any T | Any N | M1 | — |

*\*Note:* Tis includes cancer cells confined within the glandular basement membrane (intraepithelial) or lamina propria (intramucosal) with no extension through the muscularis mucosae into the submucosa.

*\*\*Note:* Direct invasion in T4 includes invasion of other segments of the colorectum by way of the serosa; for example, invasion of the sigmoid colon by a carcinoma of the cecum.

†Dukes B is a composite of better (T3 N0 M0) and worse (T4 N0 M0) prognostic groups, as is Dukes C (any T N1 M0) and Any T N2 M0.

Used with the permission of the American Joint Committee on Cancer (AJCC®), Chicago, Illinois. The original source for this material is the AJCC® Cancer Staging Manual, 5th edition (1997) published by Lippincott-Raven Publishers, Philadelphia, Pennsylvania.

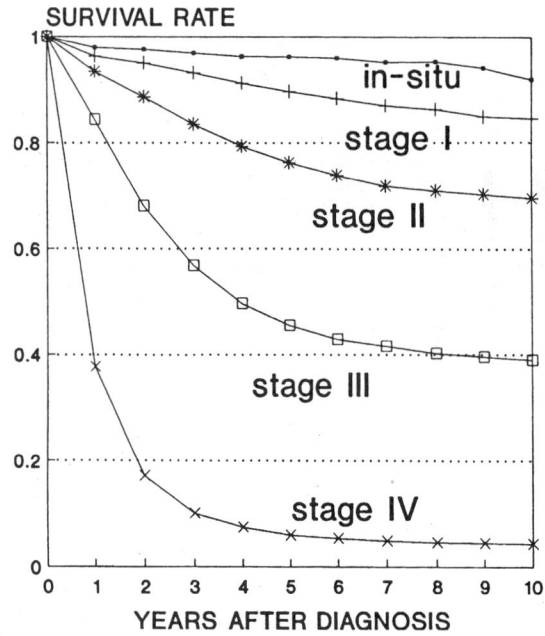

**Figure 43–3.** Relative survival rates based on 111,110 patients with colon cancer according to the stage of disease. Data are taken from the Surveillance, Epidemiology, and End Results Program of the National Cancer Institute for the years 1973–1987. Patients were staged according to the current TNM system. Stage 0 (in situ) includes 4841 patients; stage I, 19,623; stage II, 33,798; stage III, 29,615; and stage IV, 23,233. (From Beahrs OH, Henson DE, Hutter RVP, Kennedy BJ, eds. AJCC manual for staging of cancer. 4th ed. Philadelphia: JB Lippincott, 1992:76.)

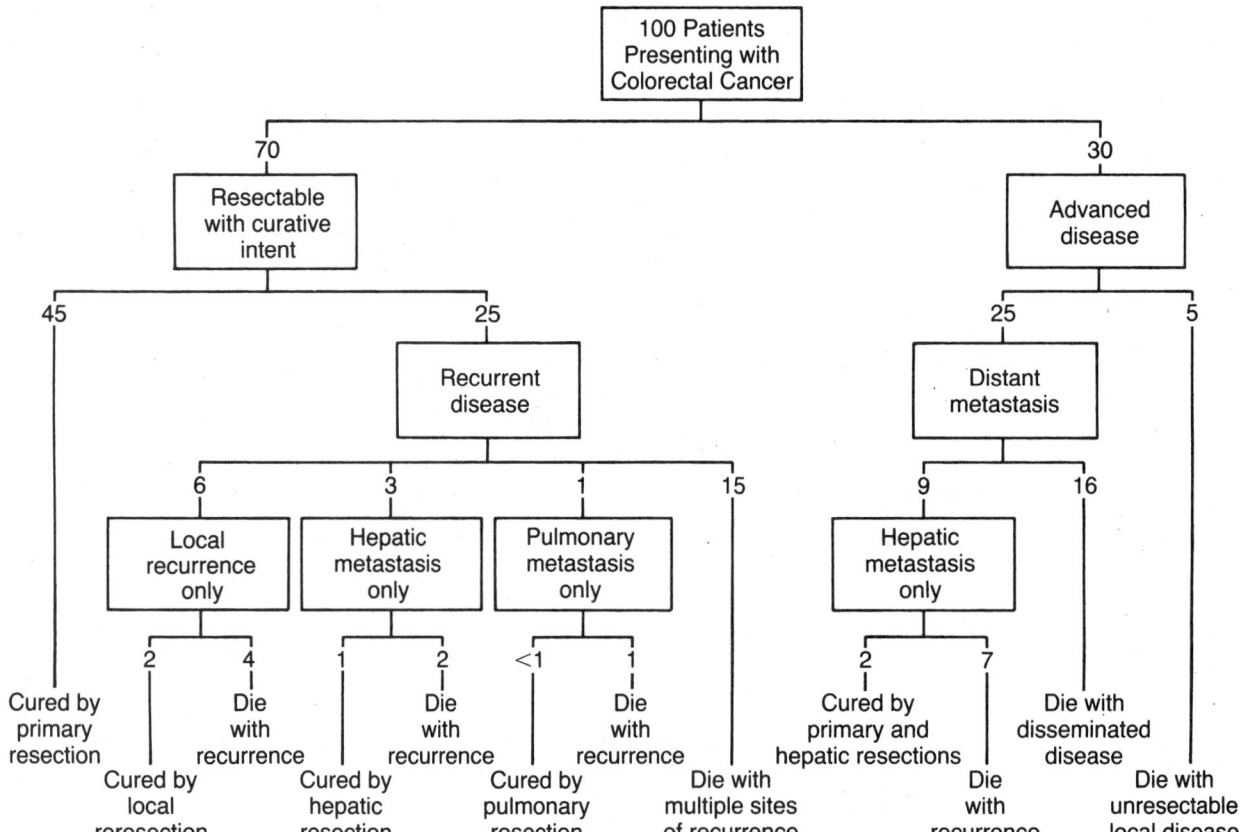

**Figure 43–4.** Patterns of failure in 100 patients presenting with large bowel cancer. (From August DA, Ottow RT, Sugarbaker PH. Clinical perspective of human colorectal cancer metastasis. Cancer Metastasis Rev 1984;3:303.)

Surveillance, Epidemiology and End Results program of the National Cancer Institute for the years 1973 through 1987. The 5-year overall relative survival rate for colorectal cancer in the United States is 61%.[2]

In addition to stage, various histologic features may be of prognostic importance (see previous discussion). The most important of these is tumor grade. From a review of 20,193 patients by the American College of Surgeons,[55] the 5-year survival rate was 57% and 54% for well-differentiated and moderately well-differentiated tumors but only 35% for poorly differentiated tumors. Overall, women had higher survival rates in this series than men, and white patients lived longer than blacks.

Molecular abnormalities may prove useful in estimating prognosis and choosing therapy in the future. For example, the p53 tumor-suppressor gene is altered in most colorectal carcinomas, and the precise pattern of alteration may have prognostic value. Specifically, lymphatic dissemination is highly correlated with *mutations* of p53, whereas hematogenous dissemination appears to be the result of the *absence* of the p53 gene.[56] Similarly, allelic loss of chromosome 18q has been associated with a poor prognosis in patients with stage II colon cancer.[57] If confirmed, these abnormalities might provide a new way of identifying patients who should receive systemic adjuvant therapy, even in the face of apparently limited disease.

There has been interest in the potential deleterious effects of perioperative blood transfusions in patients with colorectal cancer. Most studies now conclude that blood transfusion is not an independent prognostic factor in colorectal cancer,[58] although one study suggests that autologous blood transfusions may improve prognosis by decreasing the risk of postoperative infections.[59]

Another way to look at prognosis is by examining the patterns of failure of patients with colorectal cancer. August and coworkers[60] reviewed in detail the outcome of 100 patients with large bowel cancer seen at the National Cancer Institute. Figure 43–4 summarizes the results of that analysis, which illustrates the fact that recurrent disease does not necessarily portend death from cancer.

Median survival time is a more meaningful index of prognosis than 5-year survival rates for patients with advanced disease. Silverman and colleagues[61] provided guidelines to predicting median survival in such patients based on the extent of disease, age, sites of metastasis, and treatment performed. Kemeny and Braun[62] also studied the prognosis of patients with metastatic disease. They found that survival was significantly decreased by any of the following: abnormal serum lactate dehydrogenase (LDH), elevated level of CEA, a white blood cell count greater than $10,000/\mu l$, performance status less than 60 on the Karnofsky performance scale, and lung, as opposed to liver, metastasis. A similar analysis by Graf and colleagues[63] identified anemia, disease-free interval after initial surgery, and Karnofsky scale as important prognostic factors for patients with advanced disease.

## REFERENCES

1. Landis SH, Murray T, Bolden S, Wingo PA. Cancer statistics, 1999. CA Cancer J Clin 1999;49:8–31.
2. SEER Cancer Statistics Review 1973-1996. (See http://www.seer.ims.nci.nih.gov.)
3. Kinzler KW, Vogelstein B. Colorectal tumors. In: Vogelstein B, Kinzler KW, eds. The genetic basis of human cancer. New York: McGraw-Hill, 1998:565.
4. Lynch HT, Lemon SJ, Karr B, et al. Etiology, natural history, management and molecular genetics of hereditary nonpolyposis colorectal cancer (Lynch syndromes): genetic counseling implications. Cancer Epidemiol Biomarkers Prev 1997;6:987–91.
5. Boland CR. Hereditary nonpolyposis colorectal cancer. In: Vogelstein B, Kinzler KW, ed. The genetic basis of human cancer. New York: McGraw-Hill, 1998:333–46.
6. Sandler RS, Sandler DP. Radiation-induced cancers of the colon and rectum. Gastroenterology 1983;84:51–7.
7. Zaridze DG. Environmental etiology of large-bowel cancer. J Natl Cancer Inst 1983;70:389–400.
8. Burkitt DP. Epidemiology of cancer of the colon and rectum. Cancer 1971;28:3–13.
8a. Schatzkin A, Lanza E, Corle D, et al. Lack of effect of a low-fat, high-fiber diet on the recurrence of colorectal adenomas. N Engl J Med 2000;342:1149–55.
8b. Alberts DS, Martinez ME, Roe DJ, et al. Lack of effect of a high-fiber cereal supplement on the recurrence of colorectal adenomas. N Engl J Med 2000;342;1156–22.
9. Fuchs CS, Giovannucci EL, Colditz GA, et al. Dietary fiber and the risk of colorectal cancer and adenoma in women. N Engl J Med 1999;340:169–76.
10. Haenszel W, Berg JW, Segi M, et al. Large-bowel cancer in Hawaiian Japanese. J Natl Cancer Inst 1973;51:1765–79.
11. Schoen RE, Tangen CM, Kuller LH, et al. Increased blood gluose and insulin, body size, and incident colorectal cancer. J Natl Cancer Inst 1999;91:1147–54.
12. Hill MJ. Bacteria and the etiology of colonic cancer. Cancer 1974;34:815–8.
13. Goldberg MJ, Smith JW, Nichols RL. Comparison of the fecal microflora of Seventh-Day Adventists with individuals consuming a general diet: implications concerning colonic carcinoma. Ann Surg 1977;186:97–100.
14. Berg JS. Proceedings of the 2nd National Conference on Cancer of the Colon and Rectum. Bal Harbor, FL: American Cancer Society, September 1973.
15. Gilbertsen VA. Proctosigmoidoscopy and polypectomy in reducing the incidence of rectal cancer. Cancer 1974;34:Suppl:936–9.
16. Winawer SJ, Zauber AG, Ho MN, et al. Prevention of colorectal cancer by colonoscopic polypectomy. N Engl J Med 1993;329:1977–81.
17. Winawer SJ, Sherlock P: Detecting early colon cancer. Hosp Pract 1977;12:49–56.
18. Ross JE, Mara JE: Small bowel polyps and carcinoma in multiple intestinal polyposis. Arch Surg 1974;108:736–8.
19. Gardner EJ. A genetic and clinical study of intestinal polyposis, a predisposing factor for carcinoma of the colon and rectum. Am J Hum Genet 1951;3:167–76.
20. Jeghers H, McKusick VA, Katz KH. Generalized intestinal polyposis and melanin spots of the oral mucosa, lips and digits. N Engl J Med 1949;241:993–1005.
21. Bernstein CN, Shanahan F, Weinstein WM. Are we telling patients the truth about surveillance colonoscopy in ulcerative colitis? Lancet 1994;343:71–4.
22. Greenberg ER, Baron JA, Tosteson TD, et al. A clinical trial of antioxidant vitamins to prevent colorectal adenoma. N Engl J Med 1994;331:141–7.
23. Morson BC. Histological typing of intestinal tumors. In: Histological Classification of Tumors, No. 15. Geneva: World Health Organization, 1976.
24. Sobin LH. A coded compendium of the International Histological Classification of Tumors. Geneva: World Health Organization, 1978:11.
25. Cooper HS, Slemmer JR. Surgical pathology of carcinoma of the colon and rectum. Semin Oncol 1991;18:367–80.
26. Horne BD, McCulloch CF. Squamous cell carcinoma of the cecum: a case report. Cancer 1978;42:1879–82.
27. Ulich TR, Cheng L, Glover H, et al. A colonic adenocarcinoma with argentaffin cells: an immunoperoxidase study demonstrating the presence of numerous neuroendocrine products. Cancer 1983;51:1483–9.
28. Welch CE, Giddings WP. Carcinoma of colon and rectum: observations on Massachusetts General Hospital cases, 1937–48. N Engl J Med 1951;244:859–67.
29. Dinning JP, Hixson LJ, Clark LC. Prevalence of distal colonic neoplasia associated with proximal colon cancers. Arch Intern Med 1994;154:853–6.

30. Broders AC. Carcinoma: grading and practical application. Arch Pathol 1926;2:376–81.
31. Dukes CE. The relation of histology to spread in intestinal cancer. Br J Cancer 1950;4:59–62.
32. Greegor DH. Occult blood testing for detection of asymptomatic colon cancer. Cancer 1971;28:131–4.
33. Kronborg O, Fenger C, Olsen J, et al. Randomised study of screening for colorectal cancer with faecal-occult-blood test. Lancet 1996;348:1467–71.
34. Hardcastle JD, Chamberlain JO, Robinson MH, et al. Randomised controlled trial of faecal-occult-blood screening for colorectal cancer. Lancet 1996;348:1472–7.
35. Mandel JS, Bond JH, Church TR, et al. Reducing mortality from colorectal cancer by screening for fecal occult blood. N Engl J Med 1993;328:1365–71.
36. Mandel JS, Church TR, Ederer F, Bond JH. Colorectal cancer mortality: effectiveness of biennial screening for fecal occult blood. J Natl Cancer Inst 1999;91:434–7.
37. Towler B, Irwig L, Glasziou P, et al. A systematic review of the effects of screening for colorectal cancer using the faecal occult blood test, hemoccult. Br Med J 1998;317:559–65.
38. Sontag SJ, Durczak C, Aranha GV, et al. Fecal occult blood screening for colorectal cancer in a Veterans Administration Hospital. Am J Surg 1983;145:89–94.
39. Atkin WS, Cuzick J, Northover JMA, Whynes DK. Prevention of colorectal cancer by once-only sigmoidoscopy. Lancet 1993;341:736–40.
40. Maule WF. Screening for colorectal cancer by nurse endoscopists. N Engl J Med 1994;330:183–7.
41. Vasen HFA, Mecklin J-P, Meera Khan P, Lynch HT. The International Collaborative Group on HNPCC. Dis Colon Rectum 1991;34:424–5.
42. Dasmahapatra KS, Lopyan K. Rationale for aggressive colonoscopy in patients with colorectal neoplasia. Arch Surg 1989;124:63–6.
43. Bond JH, for the Practice Parameters Committee of the American College of Gastroenterology: Polyp guideline: diagnosis, treatment, and surveillance for patients with nonfamilial colorectal polyps. Ann Intern Med 1993;119:836–43.
44. Patchett SE, Mulcahy HE, O'Donoghue DP. Colonoscopic surveillance after curative resection for colorectal cancer. Br J Surg 1993;80:1330–2.
45. Limberg B. Diagnosis and staging of colonic tumors by conventional abdominal sonography as compared with hydrocolonic sonography. N Engl J Med 1992;327:65–9.
46. Fenlon HM, Nunes DP, Schroy PC III, et al. A comparison of virtual and conventional colonoscopy for the detection of colorectal polyps. N Engl J Med 1999;341:1496–503.
47. Gordon IL, Rypins EB, Wuerker RB, Jakowatz JJ. Cytologic detection of colorectal cancer after administration of oral lavage solution. Cancer 1991;68:106–10.
48. Gold P, Freedman SO. Specific carcinoembryonic antigens of the human digestive system. J Exp Med 1965;122:467–81.
49. Larson SM, Divgi CR, Scott AM. Overview of clinical radioimmunodetection of human tumors. Cancer 1994;73:832–5.
50. Valk PE, Abella-Columna E, Haseman MK, et al. Whole-body PET imaging with [18F]fluorodeoxyglucose in management of recurrent colorectal cancer. Arch Surg 1999;134:503-11.
51. Pema PJ, Bennett WF, Bova JG, Warman P. CT vs MRI in diagnosis of recurrent rectosigmoid carcinoma. J Comput Assist Tomogr 1994;18:256–61.
52. Dukes CE. The classification of cancer of the rectum. J Pathol Bacteriol 1932;35:323–32.
53. Zinkin LD. A critical review of the classifications and staging of colorectal cancer. Dis Colon Rectum 1983;26:37–43.
54. Fleming ID, Cooper JS, Henson DE, et al, eds. AJCC cancer staging manual. 5th ed. Philadelphia: Lippincott-Raven, 1997:83.
55. Mettlin C, Natarajan N, Mittelman A, et al. Management and survival of adenocarcinoma of the rectum in the United States: results of a national survey by the American College of Surgeons. Oncology 1982;39:265–73.
56. Goh HS, Chan CS, Khine K, Smith DR. p53 and behaviour of colorectal cancer. Lancet 1994;344:233–4.
57. Jen J, Kim H, Piantadosi S, et al. Allelic loss of chromosome 18q and prognosis in colorectal cancer. N Engl J Med 1994;331:213–21.
58. Busch ORC, Hop WCJ, Hoynck van Papendrecht MAW, et al. Blood transfusions and prognosis in colorectal cancer. N Engl J Med 1993;328:1372–6.
59. Heiss MM, Mempel W, Jauch K-W, et al. Beneficial effect of autologous blood transfusion on infectious complications after colorectal cancer surgery. Lancet 1993;342:1328–33.
60. August DA, Ottow RT, Sugarbaker PH. Clinical perspective of human colorectal cancer metastasis. Cancer Metastasis Rev 1984;3:303–24.
61. Silverman DT, Murray JL, Smart CR, et al. Estimated median survival times of patients with colorectal cancer based on experience with 9,745 patients. Am J Surg 1977;133:289–97.
62. Kemeny N, Braun DW Jr. Prognostic factors in advanced colorectal carcinoma: importance of lactic dehydrogenase level, performance status, and white blood cell count. Am J Med 1983;74:786–94.
63. Graf W, Bergstrom R, Pahlman L, Glimelius B. Appraisal of a model for prediction of prognosis in advanced colorectal cancer. Eur J Cancer 1994;30A:453–7.

# SURGERY

• Kenneth P. Ramming

The management of primary colorectal malignancies has been almost exclusively surgical since the advent of therapy for these diseases. Progressive improvement in surgical skills, aggressiveness, and patient preparation and support have increased operability and resectability, and operative mortality rates have declined. Resectability now approaches 90%, and mortality ranges from 2 to 10%, the lower figure reported by institutions with special interests in colorectal malignancies.

## OPERATIVE PRINCIPLES

The aims of surgery are to excise the primary lesion cleanly with adequate margins, to reconstitute continuity of the bowel whenever possible, and to avoid complications. The various routes of spread must be considered, including lymphatic, intramural, venous, implantation, and direct extension. Preoperative preparation includes appropriate clinical staging of the patient and preparation of the bowel with antibiotics.

Wide removal of the involved segment including lymphatic drainage areas, described by Rouvier in 1938 and Miles in 1908, is imperative. The standard treatment for tumors of the cecum and ascending colon is right colectomy, including a segment of the terminal ileum, the cecum, and the right half of the transverse colon, with the removal of the corresponding mesocolon at its base around the superior mesenteric artery to the takeoff of the middle colic vessels. Carcinomas of the splenic flexure or the descending or sigmoid colon are treated by excision of the distal transverse, descending, and sigmoid colon, along with the associated mesocolon excised to the aorta. For tumors of the sigmoid colon, some surgeons limit the proximal resection, excluding the transverse colon. For carcinomas in the upper part of the rectum, an anterior resection and reanastomosis can be performed if a 4- to 5-cm margin can be achieved. Below this, the anteroposterior resection generally has provided the best possibility for cure. See Figures 43–5 and 43–6 for a diagrammatic representation of resection methods for various colonic tumors.

By adhering to the most important surgical principle—total excision of draining lymphatics—adequate surgical margins of the bowel itself are ensured. The exception is in the low anterior resection, at which point the distal margin never approximates the proximal margin. Black[1] has shown by the examination of excised specimens that the intraluminal spread of cancer is short, less than 2 cm in most instances. In practice, however, the incidence of suture line recurrence following anterior resection, in which circumstance well-meaning surgeons may have the inclination to "fudge" the distal margins to preserve rectal function, far exceeds that for any other procedure; the frequently narrow margin obtained must have a direct bearing on this. The choice of operation for tumors of the upper and middle rectum depends on the evaluation of the pelvic configuration, the size and location of the tumor, and the skill and judgment of the surgeon in these procedures, including familiarity with newer techniques or *pull-through* procedures, the transsacral approach, and the concept of total mesorectal resection.[2]

A more subjective aspect of surgery, that is, the aggressiveness of the operative team, was addressed in a study by Péloquin.[3] An analysis was made of operations performed on more than 1200 patients by three small groups of surgeons. One group was extremely conservative, performing limited resections and frequently not removing all mesenteric nodes. The second was moderately aggressive, and the third was extremely aggressive, advocating initial vascular ligation and wide and even extended resections. When operative mortality, complications, and patient-group characteristics were compared, there was no difference between the surgical groups. Survival was better in every Dukes category in patients treated by the most aggressive group, however. This improved survival correlated best with the operability and resectability rate, which was highest for this group. In this series, the more aggressive the surgeons were in deciding to resect, the better were the results.

## ANTERIOR RESECTION OR ABDOMINOPERINEAL RESECTION

Quer and Mayo[4] showed that distal intramural spread of rectal cancer usually was restricted and that a margin of 2.5 cm of grossly normal wall was adequate. Grinnell,[5] however, showed that cancer cells could be found 4 cm distal to the tumor in more advanced cases. As mentioned earlier, Black[1] had also noted a generally short intraluminal spread of tumor distally. Most pathologists now agree that a 5-cm segment of normal rectum distal to the neoplasm is adequate.

Although Miles wrote that lymphatic spread took place upward, laterally, and downward, subsequent reviews of patients who usually have less advanced disease than that confronting Miles have shown that upward displacement is the most frequent type of spread. Nodal metastases distal to

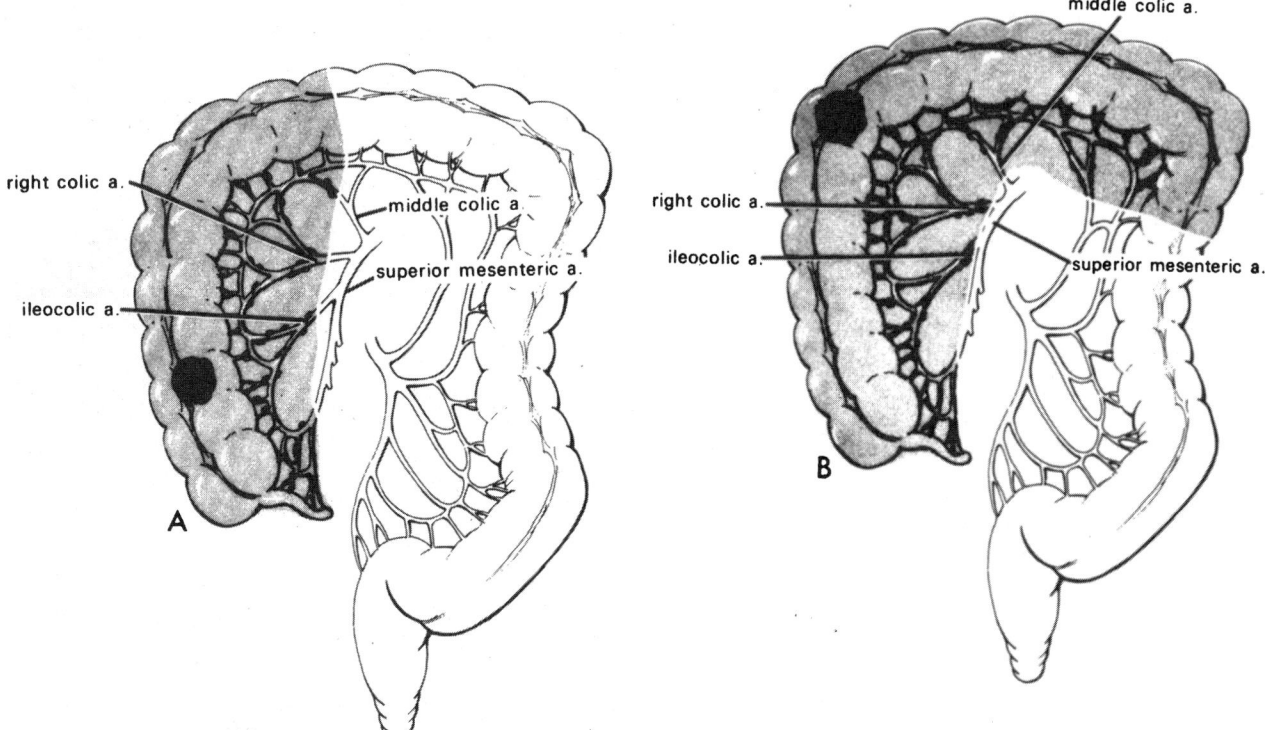

**Figure 43–5.** *A,* Extent of resection necessary for adenocarcinoma of the ascending colon, as dictated by potential sites of spread by way of the lymph nodes. *B,* Extended right colectomy suitable for lesions in the ascending colon, hepatic flexure, and transverse colon. (From Horton J, Hill GJ, eds. Clinical oncology. Philadelphia: WB Saunders, 1977:299.)

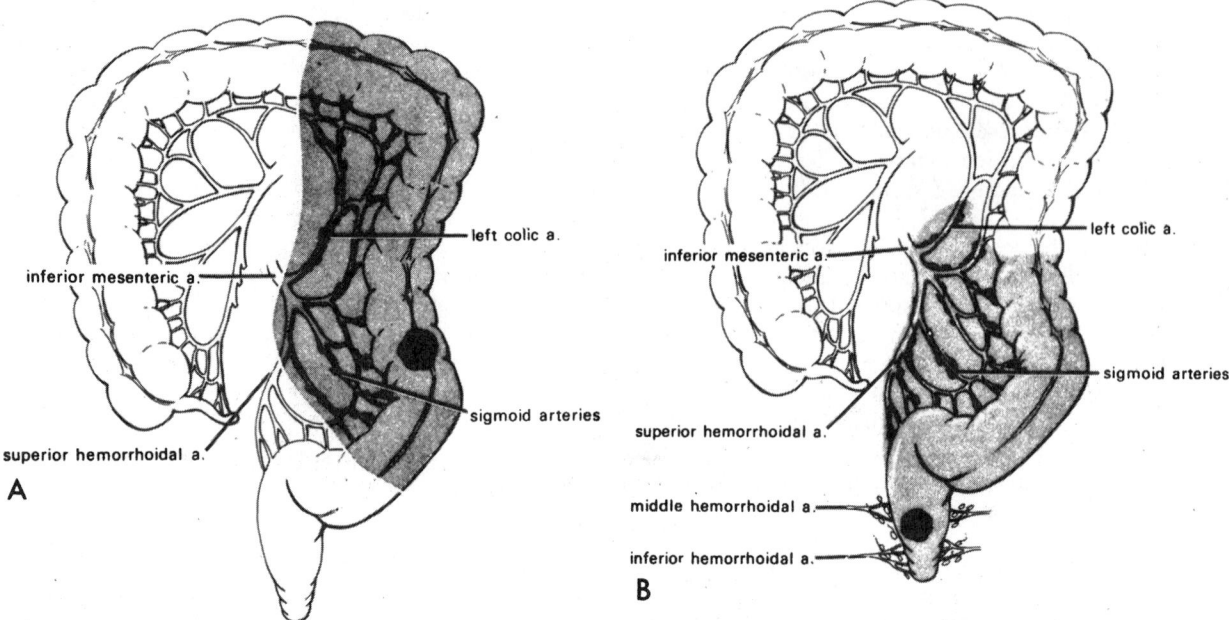

**Figure 43–6.** *A*, Left colectomy, suitable for malignancies involving the sigmoid colon, descending colon, and splenic flexure. *B*, Extent of combined abdominoperineal resection for tumors of the middle and lower rectum. (From Ellis FH Jr. Gastrointestinal tract cancer. In: Davis L, ed. Christopher's textbook of surgery. 9th ed. Philadelphia: WB Saunders, 1968:301.)

the primary cancer were noted in only 98 of 1500 abdominoperineal resection specimens examined by Goligher and coworkers.[6] Because most investigators now agree that spread is predominantly upward through superior hemorrhoidal and inferior mesenteric lymphatics, the decision to perform combined abdominoperineal resection or low anterior resection is determined primarily by the distance of the lower border of the cancer from the anus. The lateral pelvic extension of the two operations, both of which remove the upper lymphatic drainage areas, should be essentially the same.

Generally, tumors within 7 to 8 cm of the anal verge are treated by abdominoperineal resection, whereas those that are 12 cm or more from the anal verge are adequately treated with anterior resection. Lesions between 7 and 11 cm from the anal verge require the most judgment, and factors such as pelvic size, size of the lesion, and tumor differentiation must be considered. The narrow pelvises of many men can make low anterior resection hazardous. A general rule is that if the lesion is easily palpated with the examining finger, abdominoperineal resection is indicated. If the lesion can be brought to the level of the abdominal incision after mobilization of the rectum from the levator ani, an adequate resection may be performed. I have found that the use of the circumferential stapling device greatly facilitates the construction of a low-lying anastomosis.

If these principles are followed and patients are carefully chosen, the survival rates obtained from these operations are generally comparable. Survival achieved with these two procedures is noted in the large, representative series reported by Slanetz and colleagues.[7] There are no differences in operative mortality. Local recurrences have ranged from 7% for anterior resection to 18 to 21% for anteroposterior resection.[7] Women have fewer local recurrences in most series, and the higher the lesion, the less likely is recurrence.

## SPHINCTER-SPARING OPERATIONS

The case for operations that preserve the sphincter in patients with midrectal lesions derives from the opinion of many investigators that such lesions drain almost exclusively upward. An example is patients with advanced cancer in whom the hemorrhoidal vessels are choked by metastases. It would seem reasonable to design operations that would, in earlier cancers, achieve local control but preserve sphincter function. A brief description of some of these operations follows.

In the Kraske operation (an eponym many American physicians incorrectly associate with all transsacral rectal resections), a sacral colostomy was originally made. Later, transsacral resection and transanal anastomosis were performed. The operation was notorious for subsequent incontinence and anastomotic leak, and it did not contain the upward spread of cancer.

Later operations were designed to control local and upward spread of cancer as in the pull-through procedures of Babcock, Bacon, Black, Turnbull, and Cutait. These operations, which derive from the original work of Hochenegg, involve segmental rectal resection, preservation of an anal stump, and a sliding down of residual bowel with an attachment made between the stump and the advanced colon.

In the method of Bacon, the colon is pulled through a denuded anal canal. A short stump protrudes and is tied over a tube. Healing takes place between the serosa of the colon and the raw lining of the anal canal. The amputation of excessive bowel takes place in 10 days. This technique permits a low anastomosis but definitely compromises anal sensation, an important factor in continence. In the Black modification, the anal canal is left intact, and union takes place with the cut edge of the colon. Anastomosis disruption and retraction are the main risks. In the Turnbull-Cutait operation, the anorectal stump is inverted, the proximal colon is delivered through, and after 10 to 14 days the redundant bowel is amputated. Healing takes place by the union of the serosa of the colon and the serosa of the everted anorectal stump. This operation has the advantage of preserving sensation. The Maunsell-Weir operation is similar. The anorectum is everted, and the colon is delivered and sutured to the everted rectum through all layers immediately. The segment is then inverted, and a protecting colostomy is performed.

The role of these procedures in the surgical management of cancer is unsettled. Care must be taken not to compromise complete excision. These procedures are more appropriate for smaller lesions or in situations in which there are favorable technical considerations (i.e., a broad female pelvis). No matter what the procedure, some patients have wound complications, incontinence, pelvic infections, or necrosis. The fact that bladder and sexual functions are usually preserved in addition to sphincter function gives great impetus for the use of these procedures when appropriate.

Stearns[8] reported a cure rate with pull-through operations that was better than that for anteroposterior resection or anterior resection, although it was feasible in only 8% of the 495 patients reported. Bacon[9] reported a 53% 5-year survival rate in 778 pull-through operations for cancer, a rate identical to that obtained in 663 abdominoperineal procedures. The local recurrence rate was only 6.9% at the anocolonic anastomosis. Mann,[10] however, reported unacceptable operative mortality and morbidity for 61 pull-through procedures at St. Mark's Hospital in London and discouraged their use. The role of these intriguing procedures should become more clear as their use increases.

Localio and colleagues[11] have detailed the transsacral technique they have used in 175 patients with midrectal lesions. Their 15-year experience with this technique has been published, and the results are impressive. The 5-year survival rate for curative resections was 62.9% for patients treated with an anterior resection and 43.4% for patients treated with an abdominoperineal resection. The operative mortality rate was 2% for all three procedures. All the patients treated with the transsacral technique were continent, and in men erectile and orgasmic functions were uniformly preserved.

## ADDITIONAL SURGICAL CONSIDERATIONS AND SPECIAL TOPICS

**Laparoscopic Surgery.** Laparoscopic surgery is rapidly replacing many standard operative procedures on the gastrointestinal tract and associated organs.[12] Although the cost and technical expertise required for its performance are greater than with standard procedures, there may be savings in terms of total hospital costs. In one study, the mean operating time for laparoscopic left hemicolectomy was 170 minutes, and the average hospital stay was 3 to 8 days.[13] In another study, 33 of 40 patients had a successfully completed laparoscopic colectomy, although there was one postoperative death.[14] Laparoscopic techniques are clearly revolutionizing surgical procedures, but there are several potential problems when applied to patients with malignant disease. Laparoscopic surgery is a technique in rapid evolution. It is likely to play an increasing role in the management of colorectal cancer, as long as there is no compromise of

cancer surgical techniques, such as the resection of regional lymph nodes.

**Surgery for Obstruction and Perforation.** Complete intestinal obstruction occurs in 8 to 23% of patients with colorectal cancer. The predominant symptom is abdominal pain. Although a slowly growing annular carcinoma might be expected to cause a gradual onset of symptoms, obstruction frequently appears rapidly without any antecedent warning. Of 1556 cases of colorectal cancer reported from the Massachusetts General Hospital, the median duration of symptoms in obstructed patients was one quarter of that observed in nonobstructed patients.[15] Hypokalemia, hypochloremia, anemia, and hypoproteinemia were uncommon. The median preoperative interval was 12 hours. Of 124 patients in this series operated on for obstructing carcinoma, the overall mortality rate was 15%, and the postoperative complication rate was higher than that observed in elective colonic surgery. Of those resected for cure, however, 40% survived 5 years or more. When the obstructed patients who survived operation were analyzed by Dukes criteria and compared with patients from the same institution who underwent elective colonic surgery, the proportions of patients in the various Dukes categories did not differ significantly. The most important determinant of survival after successful emergency surgery is the pathologic stage of the lesion when first seen, just as in elective operations. This finding has been observed in other series and is encouraging because the significant difference between the groups (i.e., the operative mortality) continues to drop each year.

The addition of perforation to acute obstruction of the large bowel can increase the mortality rate greatly. Glenn and McSherry[16] noted a 31% operative mortality and a 7% 5-year survival rate in 29 patients with combined perforation and obstruction. Crowder and Cohn[17] reported that 42% of patients with proximal perforation of an obstructed colon died, and mortality rates of 100% have been reported.

The traditional surgical management for acutely obstructing colon cancer has been proximal diversion, followed by resection, then cecostomy or a diverting colostomy. Dissatisfaction with cecostomy and a recognition of the greater mortality rates inherent in right-sided obstructions (thin bowel leading to a greater degree of distention, perforation, and ischemia) led some authors to advocate primary resection of right-sided lesions. More than two thirds of obstructing lesions are distal to the transverse colon, however, and in these instances the classic three-stage surgical management has predominated. The rationale has been that only one of the three procedures is truly an emergency and that the last two can be done safely and electively on a colon that is prepared, defunctionalized, and empty. Theoretically, the manipulation of the tumor at more than one operation probably sends tumor cells into the circulation at a greater rate than that seen after one operation, however, and the disability from just one procedure is much less than that incurred in multiple operations. Fielding and Wells[18] compared the age-adjusted survival in 22 patients who underwent primary resections for obstructing colon cancer with 28 patients who underwent staged resections. The groups were similar in terms of tumor differentiation and Dukes stage. Survival was significantly better in the group that had primary resection. Bose and Sachdeva[19] have advocated emergency hemicolectomy in all cases of perforation, reasoning that the bowel is already decompressed and that the management of the complication of peritonitis as well as minimizing potential wound seeding is much better performed by primary resection. This viewpoint has been advocated by others.

The surgical management of acutely obstructed or perforated carcinoma of the colon, or both, must rest with the judgment and experience of the surgeon. The dilatation and viability of the bowel, the physical status of the patient, and the degree of contamination are all factors. A history of cancer, especially colorectal cancer, may also influence the decision. In the latter case, the potential quality of life of the patient with and without attempted surgical resection or diversion strongly influences the surgical decision. If the diverting colostomy must be used, consideration should be given to placing the colostomy as close to the lesion as possible to make the column of stool above the obstruction or leak, which is a source of potential contamination, as short as possible. The use of a cecostomy has been attended by many complications in most series, and unless absolutely necessary in unique situations, it should be avoided. Although the ideal preoperative randomized series comparing primary resectional therapy with the traditional staged management for obstructing colon cancer has not been (and probably never will be) performed, enough evidence is in the literature to suggest that resectional management with or without diversion is the treatment of choice.

**Extended Surgery for Colon Cancer.** Although the number of patients in whom extended surgery might have application is small, several observations should be kept in mind when extensive lesions are encountered and wider resections than conventional colectomy are contemplated. It has been established in several series that the size of the primary is not a determinant of regional metastases in large bowel cancer. Direct neoplastic extension into an adjacent organ is not a statistically more adverse prognostic sign than are one to five regional lymph node metastases, the latter being a situation in which conventional colectomy is performed uniformly without hesitation. The seemingly advanced colorectal tumor that has invaded another organ may bear favorable biologic characteristics, such as a tendency toward well-differentiated histologic appearance and an inflammatory response around the primary. A tumor of large size usually indicates that metastases have not occurred in the relatively long period of growth the tumor has taken to achieve such size. Metastases by way of the drainage routes of the invaded organ almost never occur.

Polk[20] reported 24 patients who underwent extended surgery, that is, colectomy and partial or total excision of at least one invaded organ. There was only one hospital death. Eight patients died of recurrent cancer, with a median survival of 28 months. Ten patients were alive and well at a median survival of 26 months, and the remainder were alive with disease or dead of other cancer at 33 to 41 months. An aggressive approach to locally advanced disease has been advocated by others. I do not consider invasion of the sacrum a contraindication to anteroposterior resection, and when used with an incontinuity sacral resection from the extended lithotomy position, it is feasible and safe. The fact that patients with large, locally advanced tumors might have tumors with biologically favorable characteristics, such as slow growth and late metastases, should encourage extended surgery with excision of invaded organs whenever possible.

**Suture Line Recurrence.** The incidence of suture line recurrence following colectomy has been reported to be 1.2 to 36%, with various incidences between. This subset of recurrent cancer deserves special attention because if locally recurrent disease is due to judgmental or technical errors at the time of surgery, the correction of these errors might be expected to lower the recurrence rate. Conversely, if local recurrence can be found before the widely disseminated stage, appropriately timed repeated surgical resection might be curative.[21]

Numerous theories to explain suture line recurrence have been advanced. One school of thought holds that the intact mucosa normally acts as a barrier to intraluminal tumor cells that are constantly shed from the tumor. As the suture passes through the bowel wall, it breaks this barrier and carries the viable tumor cells with it into the submucosal and muscularis layers, in which the proper nutritional milieu for tumor cell growth exists. The second theory is similar, suggesting that the inverted, raw, viable ends of the cut bowel serve as a hospitable environment onto which shed tumor cells can adhere and grow.

Another theory explains the suture line recurrence as a local metastasis resulting from tumor cells suspended in the fine reticular lymphatic system within the bowel wall. Although most of these cells die, some can become implanted at the site of resection at the point at which the lymphatic flow is obstructed. The most easily understood explanation for local recurrence is simply that the margin of resection is inadequate. Manson and colleagues[22] reported that the rate of recurrence is constant until a margin of 7 cm is reached. They found no recurrence with margins 7 cm or greater, although 5 cm is generally accepted as adequate, and other series suggest that a 7-cm margin is not necessary (see previous discussion on surgical principles). Two patients in one series failed to develop recurrent cancer, even though the distal margin was involved with tumor.[23]

In experimental models, a number of maneuvers have been devised to lower the incidence of local recurrence. A closed anastomosis, in which sutures do not enter the lumen of the bowel, has been shown to be superior to an open anastomosis. Devitalizing the cut ends of bowel has also been effective. The use of various intraluminal agents to kill viable tumor cells has been accompanied by lessened local recurrence. Cohn[24] carefully analyzed various measures to reduce local recurrence in an experimental model in which anastomoses were constructed in bowel that contained intraluminal tumor cells. Tumor implantation was not affected by bacteria in the peritoneal cavity, by use of the automatic stapler, or by irrigation with dimethyl sulfoxide, iodine, mechlorethamine, or saline. Suture line recurrences were reduced by the use of iodized sutures or a closed anastomosis, and peritoneal implants were reduced by irradiation, low-molecular-weight dextran irrigation, and clamping the lumen of the bowel close to the anastomosis.

Clinically, many maneuvers have been suggested to lower the incidence of recurrent cancer. Although few have been universally adopted, it is likely that more emphasis in this area could reduce recurrence. Logical and practical measures include wide local excision, intraluminal irrigation with a cytotoxic agent, avoidance of contamination and hemorrhage, cauterization of freshly cut bowel edges, and, particularly, prevention of laceration or injury to the bowel at any other site during the construction of the anastomosis. The adoption of the closed anastomosis technique, however effective in experimental preparations, is unlikely to occur. The use of iodized sutures, however, which has been effective experimentally and clinically in killing cancer cells that come into contact with it and which requires no modification of technique, probably should be more widespread. Postoperative radiation and chemotherapy are discussed in subsequent sections in this chapter.

**Second-Look Operation, Carcinoembryonic Antigen, and Immunoscintigraphy in Diagnosing Recurrence.** Local recurrence is an ominous finding. Greater than 90% of patients with this finding expired shortly in Welch and Donaldson's experience.[15] Taylor[25] found that 75% of patients with recurrent colorectal cancer died directly from complications of local recurrence. Aware of this finding, Griffen and associates[26] systematically reoperated on patients who were at high risk for recurrence 6 to 9 months after colectomy for colorectal cancer. Forty percent were found to have recurrence, and 14% eventually were rendered tumor free. The mortality rate initially reported with this study essentially negated the therapeutic benefit, however, and the concept of reoperation of all high-risk primary colon cancers did not gain wide acceptance.

Mackman and coworkers[27] employed second-look operations to assess the effectiveness of adjuvant 5-fluorouracil (5-FU) therapy. Recurrence was found in 10 of 60 patients, 5 of whom were made tumor free by resection. Later recurrence occurred in 3 of 50 patients with second-look procedures and in 2 of 5 patients who had been rendered tumor free by repeated resection. There was no operative mortality. When Gunderson and Sosin[28] analyzed the results of 75 patients who were found at reoperation to have recurrence after presumably curative colectomy, local recurrence or regional lymph node metastases, or both, were responsible for 50% of recurrences and were a component in 92%.

Routine reoperation subjects too many tumor-free patients to unnecessary surgery to be widely adopted. Yet the tendency for colorectal carcinoma to recur locally provides a possibility for significant surgical salvage if asymptomatic patients with recurrent cancer can be identified early in the course of their recurrence and be brought to prompt operation.

The use of immunologic markers of recurrence, such as the determination of the serum CEA level, makes it possible to choose patients more selectively who may benefit from reoperation. Although it was originally thought to be a relatively specific diagnostic indicator of gastrointestinal tumor, the blood CEA level, which measures antigen released by the tumor, was found to be variably positive in other disease states. Nevertheless, most studies suggest that it can be an important auxiliary tool for diagnosing recurrent tumor.

In general, the CEA usually declines to normal over the first 3 postoperative months, but in the presence of recurrence often rises weeks or months before recurrent disease is clinically evident. This is the time when surgical intervention is likely to be most beneficial. Although enthusiasm for this test has not been uniform, in many institutions the CEA level, along with other clinical diagnostic tests, has been instrumental in determining which patients will be subjected to reoperation. In a large meta-analysis, aggressive screening with the CEA test was associated with a 9% improvement in the 5-year survival rate compared with less aggressive follow-up.[29] Table 43–8 summarizes the results of some older studies using the CEA test as an indication for reoperation. Based on this information, I usually offer aggressive restaging studies and possible reoperation to patients with a steadily rising CEA level who are otherwise free of recurrence after primary treatment. If possible, restaging studies and reoperation should be undertaken before the CEA level is greater than about 11 ng/ml, based on the results reported by Martin and colleagues in Table 43–8.

A wide variety of potential tumor markers other than CEA are under study, including the measurement of immune complexes, a material known as *Tennessee antigen*, $\alpha_1$-acid glycoprotein, a variety of other acute-phase reactants, and many other antigens with variable similarities to CEA. None of these markers is clearly superior to CEA, and none is recommended for routine clinical use.

Numerous groups have studied the potential use of antibodies to CEA and related markers as carriers of drugs or radioactive chemicals in the diagnosis and treatment of colorectal carcinoma. The terms *immunoscintigraphy, radioimmunolocalization,* and *radioimmunodetection* have been applied to this methodology, and interest in this subject has

*Table 43–8.* Second-Look Procedures for Colon Cancer Based Only on CEA Elevations

| Investigator | No. Patients with Second-Look Laparotomy | No. Patients with Tumor Found at Laparotomy (%) | No. Patients with Curative Resection (%) | No. Patients with No Evidence of Disease |
|---|---|---|---|---|
| Wanebo[343] | 14 | 14 | 7 (50) | 4 at 12, 15, 22, & 7 mo |
| Martin[344] | 146 | 139 | 81 (55) | 64* |
| Attiyeh[345] | 32† | 33† | 16 (50) | 8 at 15 mo median follow-up |
| Steele[346] | 16‡ | 15 | 4 (27) | 2 at 13 and 24 mo |
| Evans[347] | 14§ | 11 | 1 (7) | Not given |
| Total | 222 | 212 (95) | 109 (49) | |

*Minimum follow-up for 64 patients with no evidence of disease is not given. Among 45 patients observed at least 5 years after second-look laparotomy, 14 (31%) were long-term survivors.

†Five patients had a third laparotomy for elevated CEA after a second-look procedure with resection of disease. There were 37 laparotomies. Of the four patients with negative laparotomies, three had recurrence 8, 10, and 23 months later, and one was disease free 53 months later.

‡One patient was disease free 32 months after negative laparotomy.

§Remaining patient(s) had negative laparotomy with follow-up not given.

From Bates SE, Longo DL: Use of serum tumor markers in cancer diagnosis and management. Semin Oncol 1987;14:102.

been heightened by a commercially available radiolabeled antibody to TAG-72 (satumomab pendetide [OncoScint], Knoll Pharmaceutical Company and Cytogen Corporation). This antibody is marketed for the determination of the extent and location of extrahepatic malignant disease in patients with known colorectal or ovarian cancer. A variant of immunoscintigraphy, termed *radioimmunoguided surgery*, involves the intraoperative detection of areas of radioactive antibodies. There are many technical limitations to the use of immunoscintigraphy, but the procedure holds promise. It is hoped that prospective trials will resolve the optimal use of this modality in the future. For now, I limit use of this technique to patients with occult recurrent disease that has resisted localization by all other available noninvasive tests.

An alternative imaging technique for these patients is positron emission tomography.[30] In my experience, this procedure has been useful in identifying occult areas of intraabdominal disease in patients being considered for re-exploration. When available, it is an excellent alternative to older forms of imaging, such as immunoscintigraphy with antibodies to CEA.

**Surgery for Metastatic Disease.** Although conventional logic might suggest that a localized therapeutic modality such as surgery is ill suited for the treatment of disseminated disease, many authors have shown that the judicious application of surgery for metastatic colon cancer can often prolong life and provide useful palliation. This is especially true of isolated liver and lung metastases, as discussed at length in Chapters 104 and 105.

**Palliative Surgery for Colorectal Cancer.** In the presence of multiple, unresectable, synchronous metastases that are found at the time of initial operation, the management of primary colon cancer still consists of resection of the primary in most patients. Although mortality is determined by the progression of the metastases, it has been shown in several series that those who undergo primary resection have a more favorable course. Nielson and coworkers[31] studied 103 such patients. Fifteen patients receiving no surgical treatment lived an average of only 6 weeks. Fifty patients who had laparotomy and a bypass procedure lived an average of 20 weeks, whereas 38 patients who had resection lived an average of 55 weeks. The duration of symptoms had been the same in all three groups. Resection prevented anemia, protein loss, obstruction, and pain but was contraindicated in the presence of ascites. Survival correlated inversely with the extent of metastases.

Cady and colleagues[32] also reported longer survival in patients who underwent resection compared with those receiving nonresectional therapy in a review of 169 patients with simultaneous liver metastases. Takaki and associates[33] have reviewed 78 palliative resections and concluded that resection in patients with local or distant metastases should be performed whenever feasible. After a review of 217 patients, Wanebo and coworkers[34] also strongly advise primary resection in patients with synchronous liver metastases. Other authors are less convinced of the benefits of this approach. This approach has been to resect the primary cancer and re-establish continuity of the bowel whenever possible. In addition, a hepatic artery infusion catheter may be placed at the time of surgery for constant infusion of 5-FU[35] (see Chapter 104).

**Patient Age and Survival.** Advanced age does not appear to be a major determinant of survival following surgery for colon cancer. Block and Enker[36] reported a survival rate of 57% in 111 patients older than age 70 following conventional surgery, compared with 61% in 1197 patients younger than age 70 during the years 1950 to 1965. The operative mortality in the octogenarians was 15% greater than that in the younger groups. Most complications were cerebrovascular or cardiovascular in origin. If death from operation was excluded, the 5-year survival rate was 67%.

The mean age for the diagnosis of colorectal cancer has been stated to be 67 to 69 years,[37] although analysis of ongoing studies suggests that the median age of onset might be lower. Colon cancer in the young is a much worse disease than in the old.[38] Most of the patients in Block and Enker's series were operated on more than 20 years ago, and it is likely that mortality would be somewhat lower with today's operative management. Adam and colleagues[39] reported 156 patients older than age 80 operated on for colorectal cancer. At 5 years, 22% were alive and well. Of these patients, 55% had Dukes stage C and stage D lesions. The 5-year survival for patients undergoing surgery for colorectal cancer of all ages was 22% during the same period. Although major abdominal surgery in the older population is associated with a higher mortality than in younger patients, the survival rates of those who recover from surgery are as good as, if not better than, those in the younger population. Advanced age does not justify withholding surgery, unless specific, identifiable contraindications are present.

**Alternatives to Conventional Surgery—Electrocoagulation and Local Excision.** The use of electrocoagulation in cancer of the rectum was advocated by Strauss and associates in 1935, and various reports of its use have since appeared by Pettit and Edgcomb, Swerdlow and Salvati, Crile and Turnbull, Madden and Kandalaft, and others. In this method of treatment, the patient is under spinal anesthesia, and the anus is dilated, the lesion is identified, and the entire area is cauterized and usually scraped. Ten to 12 days later, this process is repeated. In a series of 131 patients so treated, Madden and Kandalaft[40] used an average of 3.5 fulguration sessions per patient. Annular lesions were not treated, and only those within 10 cm of the anal verge, that is, below the peritoneal reflection, were considered amenable to cauterization.

The controversy that has always surrounded this modality stems from the claims of some of its advocates that this should be the primary method of treating rectal cancer rather than conventional surgical excision. This position is arrived at by comparing the 5-year survival rate of patients treated by electrocoagulation with that obtained in large surgical series in which anteroposterior resection was done. For instance, the 5-year survival rate in the series of Madden and Kandalaft[41] was 78%, which exceeds virtually all conventional surgical series, and complications and mortality were less. These data, however, were based on only 63 of 131 patients treated by cautery; the rest of the cases were not followed.

Because the incidence of local recurrence is relatively low following electrocoagulation, this modality must be considered effective in controlling localized cancer. The problem is that the procedure does not include regional lymph node removal, which is considered essential to appropriate cancer staging and treatment. Because the frequency of positive node involvement in large series of anteroposterior resection for rectal cancer is around 45 to 50%, good results from electrocoagulation could be presumed to result from the induction of a systemic response or from patient selection factors that are not operative in conventional series. Although it has been suggested in the past that electrocoagulation induces immunologic resistance to tumor, there is little, if any, evidence to support this. It is likely, however, that the cauterized lesions have more favorable characteristics, such as being small, earlier, polypoid, and noncircumferential, than those in large surgical series.

A prospective, controlled series to compare modalities will probably never be undertaken because by its nature the use of cautery prevents the staging necessary for such a clinical trial. The suggestion by Crile and Turnbull that fulguration be used first, and if it fails that anteroposterior resection be applied, is not appropriate because nodal or distant metastases can develop in the interval between inadequate cauterization and definitive surgery. In addition, the results of conventional surgery following electrocoagulation have been notably poor.[42]

Surgical excision, with the removal of regional lymph node–bearing tissue, remains the treatment of choice for primary cancer of the rectum. There are reports, however, in large surgical series by prominent surgeons that 2 to 3% of their patients were treated by cauterization. The usefulness of cautery as local therapy for advanced, symptomatic, metastatic, or inoperable rectal cancer is undeniable. There is probably a small subset of patients in whom it is applicable as primary treatment. The indications used by Turell[43] perhaps can be used to identify the patients who are well treated by fulguration. He has used cautery (1) in patients who have Dukes stage A and stage B carcinoma—small superficial lesions—especially when located on the posterior or lateral rectal walls; (2) in patients who represent poor surgical risks or who have advanced senility or concomitant serious systemic disorders, or both; (3) in blind or senescent institutionalized patients who are unable to care for themselves or cannot procure adequate care; (4) in patients who have bleeding from inoperable lesions or metastases; and (5) in patients who refuse conventional surgery. The use of local excision rather than conventional colectomy has also been described. This alternative to conventional surgery has been applied only to carefully selected patients. For instance, at St. Mark's Hospital in London, of 3999 operations done for colorectal cancer, only 143 were local excisions. The selection factors included completeness of excision, depth of spread into the bowel wall, and histologic grade of malignancy. Survival in these carefully selected patients, all of whom were followed a minimum of 5 years, was excellent.[44, 45] In selected patients with lesions less than 2 cm, local excision with radiation therapy has been found to provide local control with preservation of sphincter function.[46]

## REFERENCES

1. Black BM. Continence-preserving procedures in the treatment of carcinoma of the middle and upper parts of the rectum. Surg Gynecol Obstet 1954;99:497–9.
2. Poon RT, Chu KW, Ho JW, et al. Prospective evaluation of selective defunctioning stoma for low anterior resection with total mesorectal excision. World J Surg 1999;23:463-7.
3. Péloquin AB. Cancer of the colon and rectum: comparison of the results of three groups of surgeons using different techniques. Can J Surg 1973;16:28–34.
4. Quer EA, Mayo CW. Retrograde intramural spread of carcinoma of the rectum and rectosigmoid: a microscopic study. Surg Gynecol Obstet 1953;96:24–30.
5. Grinnell RS. Distal intramural spread of carcinoma of the rectum and rectosigmoid. Surg Gynecol Obstet 1954;99:421–30.
6. Goligher JC, Dukes CE, Bussey JR. Local recurrences after sphincter-saving excisions for carcinoma of the rectum and rectosigmoid. Br J Surg 1951;39:199–211.
7. Slanetz CA Jr, Herter FP, Grinnell RS. Anterior resection versus abdominoperineal resection for cancer of the rectum and rectosigmoid: an analysis of 524 cases. Am J Surg 1972;123:110–7.
8. Stearns MW Jr. The choice among anterior resection, the pull-through, and abdominoperineal resection of the rectum. Cancer 1974;34:suppl:969–71.
9. Bacon HE. Present status of the pull-through sphincter-preserving procedure. Cancer 1971;28:196–203.
10. Mann C. Results of 'pull-through' operations for carcinoma of the rectum. Proc R Soc Med 1972;65:976.
11. Localio SA, Eng K, Coppa GF. Abdominosacral resection for midrectal cancer: a fifteen-year experience. Ann Surg 1983;198:320–4.
12. Soper NJ, Brunt LM, Kerbl K. Laparoscopic general surgery. N Engl J Med 1994;330:409–19.
13. Rosin RD, ed. Minimal access medicine and surgery: principles and techniques. Oxford: Radcliffe Medical Press, 1993:279.
14. Monson JR, Darzi A, Carey PD, Guillou PJ. Prospective evaluation of laparoscopic-assisted colectomy in an unselected group of patients. Lancet 1992;340:831–3.
15. Welch JP, Donaldson GA. Management of severe obstruction of the large bowel due to malignant disease. Am J Surg 1974;127:492–9.
16. Glenn F, McSherry CK. Obstruction and perforation in colorectal cancer. Ann Surg 1971;173:983–92.
17. Crowder VH Jr, Cohn I Jr. Perforation in cancer of the colon and rectum. Dis Colon Rectum 1967;10:415–20.
18. Fielding LP, Wells BW. Large bowel obstruction: survival after curative resection for carcinoma. Proc R Soc Med 1973;66:683–4.
19. Bose SM, Sachdeva HS. Emergency hemicolectomy for perforation of the colon in association with carcinoma. Aust N Z J Surg 1972;42:156–8.
20. Polk HC Jr. Extended resection for selected adenocarcinomas of the large bowel. Ann Surg 1972;175:892–9.
21. Vassilopoulos PP, Yoon JM, Ledesma EJ, Mittelman A. Treatment of recurrence of adenocarcinoma of the colon and rectum at the anastomotic site. Surg Gynecol Obstet 1981;152:777–80.
22. Manson PN, Corman ML, Coller JA, Veidenheimer MC. Anastomotic recurrence after anterior resection for carcinoma: Lahey Clinic experience. Dis Colon Rectum 1976;19:219–24.
23. Flaherty RC, Sager GF. Suture line recurrence following resection of left colon carcinoma: Maine Medical Center experience. J Maine Med Assoc 1977;68:300–2.
24. Cohn I Jr. Cause and prevention of recurrence following surgery for colon cancer. Cancer 1971;28:183–9.
25. Taylor FW. Cancer of the colon and rectum: A study of routes of metastases and death. Surgery 1962;52:505–8.
26. Griffen WO Jr, Gilbertson VA, Wangensteen OH. The second-look operation for abdominal malignancies, 1948–1963. NCI Mongr 1964;15:267–76.
27. Mackman S, Ansfield FJ, Ramirez G, Curreri AR. A second look at the second operation in colonic cancer after the administration of fluorouracil. Am J Surg 1974;128:763–6.
28. Gunderson LL, Sosin H. Areas of failure found at reoperation (second or symptomatic look) following "curative surgery" for adenocarcinoma of the rectum: clinicopathologic correlation and implications for adjuvant therapy. Cancer 1974;34:1278–92.
29. Bruinvels DJ, Stiggelbout AM, Kievit J, et al. Follow-up of patients with colorectal cancer: a meta-analysis. Ann Surg 1994;219:174–82.
30. Valk PE, Abella-Columna E, Haseman MK, et al. Whole-body PET imaging with [18F]fluorodeoxyglucose in management of recurrent colorectal cancer. Arch Surg 1999;134:503–11.
31. Nielson J, Ib B, Jensen H-E. Carcinoma of the colon with liver metastases—operative indications and prognosis. Acta Chir Scand 1971;137:463–5.
32. Cady B, Monson DO, Swinton NW. Survival of patients after colonic

resection for carcinoma with simultaneous liver metastases. Surg Gynecol Obstet 1970;131:697–700.

33. Takaki HS, Ujiki GT, Shields TS. Palliative resections in the treatment of primary colorectal cancer. Am J Surg 1977;133:548–50.

34. Wanebo HJ, Semoglou C, Attiyeh F, Stearns MJ Jr. Surgical management of patients with primary operable colorectal cancer and synchronous liver metastases. Am J Surg 1978;135:81–5.

35. Ramming KP. The effectiveness of hepatic artery infusion in treatment of primary hepatobiliary tumors. Semin Oncol 1983;10:199–205.

36. Block GE, Enker WE. Survival after operations for rectal carcinoma in patients over 70 years of age. Ann Surg 1971;174:521–9.

37. Pratt CB, Rivera G, Shanks E, et al. Colorectal carcinoma in adolescents: implications regarding etiology. Cancer 1977;40:Suppl:2464–72.

38. O'Brien SE. Carcinoma of the colon in childhood and adolescence. Can Med Assoc J 1967;96:1217–9.

39. Adam YG, Calabrese C, Volk H. Colorectal cancer in patients over 80 years of age. Surg Clin North Am 1972;52:883–9.

40. Madden JL, Kandalaft S. Electrocoagulation in the treatment of cancer of the rectum: a continuing study. Ann Surg 1971;174:530–40.

41. Madden JL, Kandalaft S. Electrocoagulation in the treatment of cancer of the rectum. Surg Annu 1974;6:195–212.

42. Wanebo HJ, Quan SH. Failures of electrocoagulation of primary carcinoma of the rectum. Surg Gynecol Obstet 1974;138:174–6.

43. Turell R. Electrocoagulation of rectal cancer, colorectal adenomas, instrumentation, coloscopy, and biopsy: recapitulatory comments. Surg Clin North Am 1972;52:817–28.

44. Morson BC, Bussey HJ, Samoorian S. Policy of local excision for early cancer of the colorectum. Gut 1977;18:1045–50.

45. Lock MR, Cairns DW, Ritchie JK, Lockhart-Mummery HE. The treatment of early colorectal cancer by local excision. Br J Surg 1978;65:346-9.

46. Ramming KP, Juillard G, Parker R, Eilber F. Management of carcinoma of the rectum and anus without abdominoperineal resection. Am J Surg 1986;152:16–20.

·······································

# RADIATION THERAPY

• Luu M. Tran

Radiation therapy is almost never employed for patients with colon cancer and for patients with T1–T2 N0 rectal tumors with negative margins. Despite improvements in surgical technique, however, local recurrence remains the major pattern of relapse in patients with more advanced rectal lesions. In patients with tumor extension through the bowel wall or with nodal involvement (T3N+), about 50% recur locally after curative resection.[1, 2] In light of such data, adjuvant therapy with external-beam radiation therapy (EBRT) and chemotherapy following surgery has been studied in randomized trials. Adjuvant treatment has been shown in these trials to reduce local recurrence and improve survival.[3–5]

The 1990 National Institutes of Health conference on colorectal cancers recommended adjuvant EBRT and chemotherapy as standard treatment for T3 or node-positive rectal tumors.[6] Considerable controversy still exists regarding the sequencing of radiation and surgery. The European experience tends to favor the use of preoperative radiation, in contrast to several studies in the United States that favor the use of postoperative radiation in T3–T4 N+ rectal carcinoma. More recently, there has been an interest in radiation therapy as part of sphincter preservation (either postoperatively after local excision in T1–T2 tumors or preoperatively in distal T3 tumors near the dentate line). This section focuses mainly on randomized trials that have established the role of adjuvant radiation therapy and chemotherapy in resectable rectal tumors and as part of sphincter preservation in T3 or T1–T2 tumors as well as its role in locally advanced tumors of the rectum.

## RADIATION TECHNIQUES

Patients should be treated with modern radiation techniques, including treatment with megavoltage photon linear accelerators (>6 MV), using three-field (posterior, right and left lateral) or four-field (posterior and anterior, right and left lateral) techniques with fields treated daily (EBRT). The whole pelvic field covers the primary and lymphatic drainage with adequate margins. The superior border of the posterior and anterior (posteroanterior and anteroposterior) fields is at the L5–S1 junction. The inferior border depends on the location of the tumor and is usually set 3 cm distal to the tumor in the preoperative setting. When an abdominoperineal resection is performed, the inferior border should cover the perineal scar to at least 45 Gy. The lateral borders are 1 cm lateral to the pelvic rim. For the lateral fields, the superior and inferior borders are the same as posteroanterior and anteroposterior fields. Because the internal iliac chain is the first echelon of lymphatic drainage, the anterior border of the lateral fields is usually posterior to the pubic symphysis. This field spares a significant amount of normal structures in the pelvis, including the bladder, small bowel, or vagina in female patients. The posterior border is at least 1 cm behind the sacral bone. The boost fields can be three fields (posteroanterior, right and left lateral) or parallel opposed right and left lateral fields and should include the tumor bed with adequate margins. To minimize the toxicity of pelvic radiation, a small bowel series is performed during simulation, and shaped blocks are used to exclude small bowel from the fields. Another method of minimizing the dose to the small bowel is to treat in the prone position with the bladder full, which displaces the small bowel superiorly and anteriorly out of the field. Radiation therapy is delivered 5 days per week, with a standard fractionation of 1.8 Gy a day to a total dose of 45 Gy to the whole pelvis plus a 9-Gy boost to the tumor bed, provided that the dose to the small bowel does not exceed 50.4 Gy.

## TREATMENT RESULTS OF RESECTABLE RECTAL TUMORS

**Preoperative Radiation Therapy.** Preoperative radiation offers several advantages over postoperative radiation therapy. Preoperative therapy may decrease the risk of tumor seeding at surgery, and it uses smaller fields and total doses, which reduces the risk of chronic radiation enteritis. It may cause enough tumor regression in low-lying, large rectal carcinomas to permit a low anterior resection rather than an abdominoperineal resection. Two disadvantages of preoperative radiation therapy include the possibility of overtreating patients with early T1–T2 or M1 disease and the potential for increased surgical complications. Improved imaging techniques, however, such as endorectal ultrasonography and MRI, allow more accurate selection and reduce the likelihood that patients with early disease will receive treatment that may not be necessary.

In the 1970s, moderate doses of radiation therapy (either 5 Gy single dose or 20 to 25 Gy in five fractions) from two phase III preoperative randomized trials[7, 8] initially suggested a survival advantage in patients with positive nodes or in those undergoing abdominoperineal resection. This technique was largely abandoned when no benefit was observed in subsequent randomized trials.[9] Those trials, however, used suboptimal radiation therapy techniques with large field size and low total dosages with high doses per fraction that are now considered inappropriate. The Stockholm trial showed a higher incidence of perineal wound infections with these large doses. Long-term toxicity, such as small bowel obstruction, was lower in the preoperative group (5%) than in the postoperative group (11%).

Subsequently, several prospective randomized studies[10–14] using preoperative radiation therapy with adequate doses found a benefit for high-dose preoperative radiation compared with surgery alone. The local recurrence was reduced from 35% to 15% ($p = 0.02$) as reported by the Stockholm Rectal Study Group[13] and by the European Organization for Research and Treatment of Cancer (EORTC).[14]

Regarding the survival benefit of preoperative radiation, the results of retrospective series are conflicting. As previously mentioned, studies using low-dose preoperative radiation (<20 Gy) in the 1970s have not shown an impact on local recurrence or survival. One exception is the Swedish Rectal Cancer trial[15] published in 1997. These investigators conducted a prospective randomized trial using a short course of preoperative radiation therapy with high daily doses (25 Gy in five fractions) in 553 patients with resectable rectal carcinoma. After 9 years of follow-up, the rate of local recurrence was 11% (63 of 553) in the group that received preoperative radiation therapy and 27% (150 of 557) in the surgery-alone group ($p < 0.001$). The overall 5-year survival rate was 58% in the preoperative radiation group and 48% in the surgery-alone group ($p < 0.004$). There was no significant increase in morbidity in irradiated patients compared with nonirradiated patients (2% vs. 1%). So far, this is the only randomized trial of an intensive, short course of preoperative irradiation to show a survival advantage. The EORTC[16] reported a randomized study of 341 patients with rectal carcinoma assigned to receive preoperative 34.5 Gy of radiation at 2.3 Gy per fraction (which is radiobiologically equivalent to 45 Gy in standard fractionation) followed by surgery or to surgery alone. There was a borderline improvement in 5-year survival in favor of the preoperative group (69%) compared with the surgery-alone group (59%) ($p = 0.08$).

These preoperative trials used widely varying radiation techniques (including different field sizes, daily fraction doses, total doses, and intervals between radiation and surgery). Some used suboptimal radiation techniques, such as high doses per fraction and low total doses, which are known

to affect tumor sterilization rates adversely. This variation may explain the conflicting results of the randomized trials that have compared preoperative radiation with surgery alone. Based on the results of these trials, the 1996 Pattern of Care Rectal Cancer Committee[17] has now recommended 45 to 46.8 Gy to the whole pelvis followed by a boost to 50.4 Gy for patients who are selected to receive preoperative irradiation. Low total dose and high doses per fraction of preoperative radiation should not be used owing to poor local control and poor survival that result.

**Preoperative Radiation Therapy as Part of Sphincter Preservation.** Although an abdominoperineal resection with permanent colostomy remains the standard operation for tumors of distal rectum, data support the use of preoperative radiation therapy in the management of distal, large T3 rectal carcinomas as part of sphincter preservation. Preoperative radiation therapy can decrease the tumor volume and sometimes allow the surgeon to perform a low anterior resection instead of an abdominoperineal resection in low rectal cancer near the dentate line. Minsky and associates[18] from Memorial Sloan-Kettering Cancer Center reported the results of 29 patients with resectable tumors involving the distal half of the rectum treated with preoperative radiation therapy and coloanal anastomosis. The median distance from the anal verge was 4 cm (range, 3 to 7 cm) and would have required abdominoperineal resection. The whole pelvis received 46.8 Gy followed by a boost dose of 3.6 Gy to the tumor bed. With a median follow-up of 29 months, 24 of 29 patients (83%) were able to undergo a low anterior resection and coloanal anastomosis. The incidence of local failure as a component of failure was 23%, and the 4-year actuarial survival was 75%. Of the patients who underwent sphincter preservation, 77% had a good to excellent functional result.

Wagman and colleagues[19] from Memorial Sloan-Kettering Cancer Center have updated their results. A total of 35 patients with low-lying rectal cancer were treated with the same regimen. With a median follow-up of 56 months, 27 of 35 (77%) were able to undergo coloanal anastomosis, and 85% of them have good to excellent sphincter preservation. The 5-year actuarial disease-free and overall survivals were 60% and 64%, respectively. Marks and coworkers[20] from Thomas Jefferson University Hospital reported the results of 43 rectal cancer patients treated with radiation therapy (45 to 60 Gy for 4 to 6 weeks to the pelvis) followed by sphincter preservation surgery. The tumors were located at or below the 3-cm level. Local recurrence developed in 6 of 43 patients with a minimum of 2 years' follow-up. The authors concluded that sphincter preservation could be performed in cancer of the distal 3 cm of rectum if high-dose preoperative radiation therapy is administered.

Adjuvant radiation therapy plays an important role in the attempt for organ preservation in patients with large T3, low-lying tumor who would otherwise require abdominoperineal resection or in those who are medically inoperable or refuse colostomy. There are, however, few data regarding the use of this preoperative approach in T1–T2 low-lying rectal cancers as part of conservation management. Thomas Jefferson University Hospital[21] and Henri Mondor Hospital[22] have reported excellent results with the use of high-dose radiation (40 to 45 Gy for 5 weeks) followed in 4 to 8 weeks by full-thickness local excision in patients with T1–T2 rectal tumors in the lower third of the rectum. This approach has not gained widespread acceptance, however. Most clinicians prefer local excision as the primary treatment followed by adjuvant radiation therapy for early T1–T2 rectal cancers with the exception of small, superficial T1 lesions, in which local excision alone with negative margins appears to be an adequate treatment.

**Preoperative Chemoradiation.** Radiation therapy alone produces a moderate rate of local failure; several institutions,[23–27] especially in Europe, are now adding chemotherapy to radiation therapy for patients with clinically resectable rectal carcinoma in the preoperative setting (Table 43–9). The EORTC[28] presented the first preoperative randomized trials comparing chemoradiation and radiation alone in resectable rectal carcinoma. Because of insufficient doses of bolus 5-FU and suboptimal radiation techniques (34.5 Gy at 2.3 Gy/fraction, short interval between surgery and radiation therapy, large field size), the combined chemoradiation arm had no impact on survival (46% vs. 59% in the radiation therapy–alone arm, $p = 0.06$).

The ongoing EORTC randomized trial increases the preoperative EBRT dose to 45 Gy in standard fractionation. All patients in this four-arm study receive preoperative radiation therapy, as follows: (1) alone, (2) concomitant radiation therapy plus preoperative 5-FU and leucovorin, (3) radiation therapy plus postoperative 5-FU and leucovorin for four cycles, and (4) radiation therapy plus preoperative and postoperative 5-FU and leucovorin. This trial is examining the place of chemotherapy in the adjuvant, preoperative management of rectal carcinoma.

Several nonrandomized studies using preoperative 5-FU (either bolus or continuous infusion) and radiation therapy (dose 45 to 50.4 Gy) for resectable rectal carcinoma have achieved a local recurrence of 0 to 5%, and pathologic complete response rates of 9 to 29%.[21, 25] Based on these favorable results, the National Surgical Adjuvant Breast and Bowel Project (NSABP) has launched a phase III trial of preoperative versus postoperative chemoradiation in resectable rectal carcinoma (NSABP R-03).[29] In this trial, patients are randomized into two groups. The preoperative group received three cycles of 5-FU and leucovorin and 50.4 Gy 5.5 weeks before surgery followed by four additional cycles of 5-FU and leucovorin chemotherapy. The postoperative group received all radiation therapy and chemotherapy after surgery. Overall treatment-related toxicity was similar in both groups. There was evidence of tumor downstaging in the preoperative group, with 8% of patients having a pathologic complete response. The available results are only preliminary, so whether or not the preoperative arm will have any survival advantage awaits the completion of the study.

**Preoperative Chemoradiation for Sphincter Preservation in T3 Disease.** A potential advantage of using combined modalities preoperatively in the treatment of rectal cancer is that it allows conservative surgery of distal rectal cancer. Another advantage of preoperative chemoradiation is damaging malignant cells that may otherwise be spread to surrounding structures at the time of surgery. This approach became more popular in the 1990s. Grann and colleagues[23] obtained sphincter preservation in 85% (17 of 20) of T3 resectable rectal carcinoma patients treated with preoperative 5-FU and leucovorin and concurrent radiation therapy 50.4 Gy followed by postoperative bolus 5-FU and leucovorin.

Rich and colleagues[25] from M.D. Anderson Cancer Center reported similar results. Seventy-seven patients with T1–T3 resectable rectal carcinoma were treated with 45 Gy and concurrent infusion of 5-FU. Of patients with low rectal lesions, 68% were able to have a sphincter preservation procedure instead of an abdominoperineal resection. Valentini and coworkers[26] reported use of preoperative, combined radiation therapy 37.8 Gy with continuous infusion 5-FU and bolus mitomycin C for 83 patients with T3 resectable rectal carcinoma. The rate of sphincter preservation was 44%, and 9% of the patients had pathologic complete responses.

An interim analysis of the NSABP R-03 randomized trial[29] between preoperative and postoperative chemoradiation obtained only a 27% (6 of 22 patients) sphincter preservation rate in the preoperative chemoradiation arm. The reason for this poor rate of preservation is unclear and needs further evaluation.

The rates of sphincter preservation in the preoperative setting with chemoradiation from the aforementioned studies have been high, up to 85%. This regimen has been shown

*Table 43–9.* **Preoperative Chemoradiotherapy in Resectable Rectal Cancer**

| Series | Patients (No.) | Treatment | Sphincter Preservation (%) | Local Failure (%) | pCR (%) | Survival (%) |
|---|---|---|---|---|---|---|
| *Randomized* | | | | | | |
| EORTC[28] | | | | | | |
| RT + S | | 34.5 Gy/15 frcs | | | | 59 |
| RT + CM + S | | 34.5 Gy/15 frcs + 5-FU IV bolus × 4 days | | | | 46 |
| NSABP R-03[29] | 59 | 50.4 Gy + 5-FU/LV + postoperative 5-FU | 27 | NA | 8 | NA |
| *Nonrandomized* | | | | | | |
| Grann[23] | 32 | 50.4 Gy/5 wk + 5-FU/LV bolus postoperative 5-FU | 85 | 0 | 9 | 100 (2 yr) |
| Chari[24] | 43 | 45 Gy/5 wk + 2 × 5-FU bolus/cisplatinum | 14 | 5 | 27 | 93 (5 yr) |
| Rich[25] | 77 | 45 Gy/5 wk + CI 5-FU | 68 | 4 | 29 | 83 (3 yr) |
| Valentini[26] | 83 | 37.8 Gy/4 wk + CI 5-FU/mit-C | 44 | 10 | 9 | 75 (5 yr) |
| Stryker[27] | 30 | 50 Gy/5 wk + 5-FU/mit-C | | 4 | | 85 (5 yr) |

pCR, pathologic complete response; RT, radiation therapy; S, surgery; CM, chemotherapy; frcs, fractions; 5-FU, 5-fluorouracil; IV, intravenous; LV, leucovorin; NA, not available; CI, continuous infusion; mit-C, mitomycin C.

to decrease local recurrence and allow sphincter-preserving surgery in low-lying rectal carcinomas that previously had been managed with abdominoperineal resection. More information about the impact of preoperative combined-modality therapy on tumor response and sphincter preservation will derive from the results of the ongoing NSABP R-03 randomized trial.

**Postoperative Radiation Therapy for T3–T4 and Node-Positive Rectal Tumors.** Postoperative radiation therapy is commonly used in the United States for patients with disease extension through the rectal wall or positive lymph nodes. The advantage of postoperative radiation is the accurate pathologic staging of patients, which permits a better selection of which patients would benefit. About 30 to 50% of patients have pathologic stage T1–T2 M1 disease and are unlikely to benefit from adjuvant therapy. The disadvantage of postoperative radiation is the increased toxicity resulting from the larger volume of radiation, especially in patients who have had an abdominoperineal resection in which the perineal scar is included in the treatment field.

Using conventional radiation doses of 45 to 54 Gy, several retrospective studies[30–33] revealed that local recurrence decreased by 20% after postoperative radiation therapy in T3–T4 and N1–T2 M0 rectal carcinoma. The NSABP R-01 trial[5] compared adjuvant radiation with surgery alone in a randomized trial. They reported decreased local recurrence with adjuvant radiation (16% vs. 25%, $p = 0.06$). The Medical Research Council (MRC),[34] in another randomized trial, reported decreased local recurrence with the use of postoperative radiation therapy (21% vs. 34%, $p = 0.01$). Neither the NSABP trial nor the MRC trial showed a survival advantage. The EORTC[35] randomized trial failed to show any improvement in disease-free survival ($p = 0.81$) or local control ($p = 0.46$) when postoperative EBRT (46 Gy in standard fractionation) was given following resection of Dukes B and C rectal cancers.

**Postoperative Radiation Therapy Following Local Excision for Early T1–T2 Rectal Cancer.** For patients with small T1–T2 lesions in the distal rectum, there has been increasing interest in local excision as an alternative to abdominoperineal resection. Massachusetts General Hospital[36] reported a prospective trial of 20 patients (16 T1–T2 patients) with low rectal cancer who were treated with local excision followed by postoperative radiation therapy to the pelvis (45 Gy in 25 fractions). Patients with positive margins received an additional photon boost plus 5-FU. At a mean follow-up of 47 months, local control was achieved in all patients. Wagman and colleagues[37] reported the results of 39 patients with resectable, distal rectal cancer treated with local excision and postoperative radiation using 46.8 Gy to the whole pelvis followed by a boost dose of 3.6 to 10 Gy with or without 5-FU. With median follow-up of 37 months, the 5-year colostomy-free survival was 87%, and overall survival was 70%. The local failures were 0 of 6 for T1, 6 of 25 for T2, and 2 of 8 for T3 disease. Of those 8 patients with local recurrence, 5 were salvaged with abdominoperineal resection and were free of disease at the time of reporting. Valentini and associates[38] reported the local control and survival of 21 patients with T1–T2 middle and distal rectal cancer treated with transrectal excision and postoperative radiation therapy (44.6 Gy). With a median follow-up of 54 months, the 5-year actuarial recurrence-free survival

was 85%, and 5-year actuarial survival was 80.6%. Three patients developed local recurrence, and 1 was successfully salvaged with abdominoperineal resection.

These encouraging results of local excision plus radiation led investigators to study the addition of chemotherapy in an effort to reduce local recurrence further while preserving sphincter function. The results have been promising.[39, 40] For example, one trial[41] involved 113 patients with T1–T2 lesions treated with local excision with and without chemoradiation. Sixty patients with T1 disease received local excision only, and 53 patients with T2 disease were treated with EBRT using 54 Gy divided among 30 fractions and 5-FU starting 6 weeks following local excision. With a median follow-up of 24 months, only 2 of 113 patients experienced isolated local recurrence. Both patients underwent subsequent surgery and were alive at the time of reporting. These data support the view that in patients with superficial distal rectal cancer, sphincter preservation can be achieved with excellent local control without sacrifice of anal function.

**Postoperative Chemoradiation for T3–T4 and Node-Positive Rectal Tumors.** Because of the suboptimal results with postoperative radiation therapy alone, several randomized trials[3–5, 42, 43] began using postoperative radiation plus chemotherapy in patients with T3–4 and node-positive disease (Table 43–10). The results have been encouraging, showing decreased local recurrence and increased overall survival. In a Gastrointestinal Tumor Study Group (GITSG) trial,[4] patients with Dukes B or C lesions were assigned to one of four study arms: (1) surgery-alone control arm versus three postoperative adjuvant arms, (2) surgery with radiation therapy 40 to 48 Gy, (3) surgery with chemotherapy (5-FU plus MeCCNU), or (4) surgery combined with chemoradiation. Overall survival was significantly better in the combined chemoradiation group than among those who had no adjuvant treatment (54% vs. 27%, $p = 0.005$). Local recurrence was 24% in the control group compared with 27% in the chemotherapy arm, 20% in the radiation arm, and 11% in the chemoradiation arm. No apparent impact on local control was seen in the chemotherapy arm, but an apparent decrease in distant metastases was seen in patients who received chemotherapy. Local recurrence in the adjuvant radiation arm in this trial is still high, probably as a result of low radiation doses (40 to 48 Gy). This study, however, confirms that postoperative chemoradiation is superior to surgery alone.

The Mayo/North Central Cancer Treatment Group (NCCTG) conducted a randomized trial wherein patients received adjuvant radiation or chemoradiation.[43] The postoperative radiation dose was 50.4 Gy over 28 fractions in both arms; the chemotherapy was 5-FU and MeCCNU. There was a significant decrease in local recurrence in the chemoradiation arm (11%) compared with radiation alone (23%) ($p = 0.04$). Overall survival and disease-free survival were significantly better in the combined-modality arm (59% vs. 37%, $p = 0.002$ and 58% vs. 48%, $p = 0.025$). This NCCTG trial confirmed the effectiveness of adjuvant chemoradiation.

Intergroup trial INT 0114[44] is a four-arm study to determine whether combinations of 5-FU–based chemotherapy (leucovorin vs. levamisole vs. leucovorin plus levamisole) are better than 5-FU alone. The initial evaluation revealed no significant differences in survival or local control among the four arms, but the final analysis has not been published.

*Table 43–10.* Selected Randomized Trials of Postoperative Chemoradiotherapy for Rectal Carcinoma

| Institutions | Patients (No.) | Treatment | Local Failure (%) | Survival (%) |
|---|---|---|---|---|
| GITSG[4,42] | | | | |
| S alone | 58 | | 24 | 27 (5 yr) |
| S + RT | 50 | 40–48 Gy/4 wk | 20 | 46 (5 yr) |
| S + CM | 48 | 5-FU/methyl-CCNU | 27 | 46 (5 yr) |
| S + RT + CM | 46 | 40–44 Gy/4 wk + 5-FU/ methyl-CCNU (concurrent) | 11 | 54 (5 yr)* |
| NCCTG[43] | | | | |
| S + RT | 100 | 45–50.4 GY | 25 | 47 (5 yr) |
| S + RT + CM | 104 | 45–50.4 Gy + 5-FU/methyl- CCNU | 13.5* | 60 (5 yr)* |
| INT 0114[44] | | | | |
| 5-FU + RT | 421 | All patients in 4 arms received | 12 | 78 (3 yr) |
| 5-FU/LV + RT | 425 | RT (50.4–54 Gy/5 wk) | 9 | 80 (3 yr) |
| 5-FU/LEVAM + RT | 426 | sandwiched between 5- | 13 | 79 (3 yr) |
| 5-FU/LV/LEVAM + RT | 424 | FU–based chemotherapy | 9 | 79 (3 yr) |

*Difference significant at $p \leq 0.05$
S, surgery; RT, radiation therapy; CM, chemotherapy; 5-FU, 5-fluorouracil; LV, leucovorin; LEVAM, levamisole.

Based on the positive results of the randomized studies from NCCTG and GITSG, the National Cancer Institute in 1990 recommended that chemoradiation be used as standard adjuvant treatment for patients with T3–T4 N+ rectal tumors following surgery. Regarding the sequence of chemotherapy and radiation, the 1996 Patterns of Care Rectal Cancer Committee[17] recommended two cycles of 5-FU chemotherapy, then two cycles with radiation therapy, and then two more cycles of chemotherapy. Generally, EBRT involves a four-field pelvic technique, with delivery of 45 Gy in 25 fractions to the pelvis followed by a boost to 50.4 to 54 Gy depending on the amount of small bowel in the boost field.

**Treatment Results of Locally Advanced or Unresectable Tumors.** Locally advanced tumors of the rectum include tumors tethered or fixed to the pelvic side walls or sacrum, tumors infiltrating into visceral structures, and recurrent tumors after prior resection. Despite advances made in surgical techniques, 70% of these tumors recur locally after potential curative resection.[2, 45, 46] In the past, these patients were treated with palliative radiation alone, and the 5-year survival was expected to be no more than 10 to 15%.[47, 48] These poor results prompted the use of preoperative radiation therapy in an effort to improve resectability (Table 43–11). Willett and coworkers[49] from Massachusetts General Hospital reported the results of 117 patients treated with preoperative radiation therapy. The disease-free survival was significantly better in 13 patients who had pathologic complete response, compared with 104 patients who did not.

Chan and colleagues[50] from Alberta, Canada, reported a phase I–II study of preoperative concurrent radiation 40 Gy over 4 weeks and 5-FU–based chemotherapy plus mitomycin C in 46 patients. Surgery was performed 6 to 8 weeks later. After preoperative chemoradiation, 41 of 46 patients (89%) were able to undergo curative resection, with a 2-year local relapse rate of 16%. The author[51] subsequently modified the protocol and added postoperative radiation (18 Gy) plus similar chemotherapy, finding no local recurrence in this *sandwich* approach. Only two patients (7%) developed gastrointestinal complications.

Minsky and associates[52] designed a phase I trial studying concurrent preoperative radiation therapy 50.4 Gy plus two cycles of 5-FU (325 mg/m²) and low-dose leucovorin followed by surgery and 10 cycles of postoperative 5-FU and leucovorin. Chemotherapy and radiation therapy were begun concurrently on day 1. Of 24 patients enrolled, 23 underwent resection. Complete resection with negative surgical margins was achieved in all 23 cases (100%). The pathologic complete regression rate was 13% (3 of 23). In 1997, Minsky and associates[53] updated the results of two phase I dose escalation trials in 36 patients treated with neoadjuvant

*Table 43–11.* Preoperative Treatment of Locally Advanced, Unresectable Rectal Cancer

| Group | Patients (No.) | Treatment | Resectability (%) | Pathologic Complete Response (%) | Local Failure (%) | Survival (%) |
|---|---|---|---|---|---|---|
| Chan[50] | 46 | 40 Gy/4 wk + CI 5-FU + mit-C | 89 | 4 | 16 | 73 (2 yr) |
| Chan[51] | 27 | 40 Gy/4 wk + CI 5-FU postoperative 18 Gy + 5-FU (sandwich) | 100 | 15 | 0 | 73 (4 yr) |
| Minsky[53] | 36 | 5-FU/LV IV bolus × 2 + 50.4 Gy + postoperative 5-FU × 4 cycles | 97% with negative margins | 11 | 30 | 76 (6 yr) |
| Weinstein[54] | 37 | 45 Gy + IORT + PVI 5-FU + cisplatin | 84 | | 3 | 82 (5 yr) |

CI, continuous infusion; 5-FU, 5-fluorouracil; mit-C, mitomycin C; LV, leucovorin; IV, intravenous; IORT, electron-beam intraoperative radiation therapy; PVI, protracted venous infusion.

chemoradiation. The resectability rate with negative margins was 97%, and the pathologic complete response rate was 11%. Of the patients, 50% were able to undergo a sphincter preservation procedure.

Currently, preoperative chemoradiation in locally advanced rectal carcinoma appears to be more effective than radiation alone. About 75 to 80% of these patients are rendered completely resectable, with 5-year survival rates of 35 to 55%. Local recurrence, however, remains significant—20 to 30%. Distant metastases also occur at unacceptable rates. In an effort to decrease local and distant relapse, concurrent local and systemic treatments are being studied. These regimens employ continuous infusion 5-FU and leucovorin during radiation therapy. Weinstein and coworkers[54] used protracted infusion 5-FU plus concurrent radiation therapy (EBRT with or without electron-beam intraoperative radiation therapy [IORT]) and reported 97% local control in advanced rectal carcinoma. In the absence of a randomized trial, optimal treatment now seems to be preoperative radiation therapy plus concurrent 5-FU chemotherapy.

**Newer Approaches.** IORT is an investigative treatment. IORT boost doses of 10 to 20 Gy have been used with EBRT in several nonrandomized trials.[55–57] The data suggest decreased local recurrence. Willett and colleagues[55] reported a phase II trial of 42 patients with unresectable rectal carcinoma who were treated with preoperative EBRT plus IORT. Actuarial 5-year survival was 43%. In another Massachusetts General Hospital series,[56] the local, in-field recurrence rate was 43% for 17 non-IORT patients versus 0% for 16 IORT patients. Gunderson and coworkers[57] enrolled 113 patients with recurrent unresectable rectal disease in a phase II trial of preoperative radiation plus IORT. He reported a 37% local relapse rate (0% if negative margins). In contrast, Minsky and colleagues[53] reported a high recurrence rate in 5 patients treated with intraoperative brachytherapy compared with 30 patients who did not receive brachytherapy (40% vs. 10%). Because of the limited number of patients, selection bias, and the lack of randomized data, IORT and brachytherapy remain investigational.

# REFERENCES

1. Adloff M, Arnaud JP, Schloegel M, Thibaud D. Factors influencing local recurrence after abdominoperineal resection for cancer of the rectum. Dis Colon Rectum 1985;28:413–5.
2. Gunderson LL, Sosin H. Areas of failure found at reoperation (second or symptomatic look) following curative surgery for adenocarcinoma of the rectum. Cancer 1974;34:1278–92.
3. Gastrointestinal Tumor Study Group. Prolongation of the disease-free survival in surgically treated rectal carcinoma. N Engl J Med 1985;312:1465–72.
4. Gastrointestinal Tumor Study Group. Adjuvant therapy of colon cancer: results of a prospectively randomized trial. N Engl J Med 1984;310:737–43.
5. Fisher B, Wolmark N, Rockette H, et al. Postoperative adjuvant chemotherapy or radiation therapy for rectal cancer: results from NSABP protocol R-01. J Natl Cancer Inst 1988;80:21–9.
6. NIH Consensus Conference on adjuvant therapy for patients with colon and rectal cancer. JAMA 1990;264:1444–50.
7. Higgins G, Humphrey E, Dwight R, et al. Preoperative radiation and surgery for cancer of the rectum: Veterans Administration Surgical Oncology group Trial II. Cancer 1986;58:352–9.
8. Rider W, Palmer J, Mahoney L, Robertson CT. Preoperative irradiation in operable cancer of the rectum: report of the Toronto trial. Can J Surg 1977;20:335–8.
9. Cedermark B, Johansson H, Rutqvist LE, Wilking N. The Stockholm I trial of preoperative short term radiotherapy in operable rectal carcinoma: a prospective randomized trial. Stockholm Colorectal Cancer Study Group. Cancer 1995;75:2269–75.
10. Marsh PJ, James RD, Schofield PF. Adjuvant preoperative radiotherapy for locally advanced rectal carcinoma: results of a prospective, randomized trial. Dis Colon Rectum 1994;37:1205–14.
11. Gerard A, Berrod JL, Pene F, et al. Interim analysis of a phase III study on preoperative radiation therapy in resectable rectal carcinoma: trial of the Gastrointestinal Tract Cancer Cooperative Group of the European Organization for Research on Treatment of Cancer (EORTC). Cancer 1985;55:2375–9.
12. Cedermark B: The Stockholm II trial on preoperative short term radiotherapy in operable rectal carcinoma: a prospective randomized trial. Proc ASCO 1994;13:498.
13. Påhlman L, Glimelius B. Pre- or postoperative radiotherapy in rectal and rectosigmoid carcinoma: report from a randomized multicenter trial. Ann Surg 1990;211:187–95.
14. Frykholm GJ, Glimelius B, Påhlman L. Preoperative or postoperative irradiation in adenocarcinoma of the rectum: final treatment results of a randomized trial and an evaluation of late secondary effects. Dis Colon Rectum 1993;36:564–72.
15. Swedish Rectal Cancer Trial. Improved survival with preoperative radiotherapy in resectable rectal cancer. N Engl J Med 1997;336:980–7, 1539.
16. Gérard A, Buyse M, Nordlinger B, et al. Preoperative radiotherapy as adjuvant treatment in rectal cancer: final results of a randomized study of the European Organization for Research and Treatment of Cancer (EORTC). Ann Surg 1988;208:606–14.
17. Minsky B, Coia L, Haller D, et al. Treatment systems guidelines for primary rectal cancer from the 1996 Patterns of Care Study. Int J Radiat Oncol Biol Phys 1998;41:21–7.
18. Minsky B, Cohen A, Enker WE, Paty P. Sphincter preservation with preoperative radiation therapy and coloanal anastomosis. Int J Radiat Oncol Biol Phys 1995;31:553–9.
19. Wagman R, Minsky BD, Cohen AM, et al. Sphincter preservation in rectal cancer with preoperative radiation therapy and coloanal anastomosis: long term follow-up. Int J Radiat Oncol Biol Phys 1998;42:51–7.
20. Marks G, Mohiuddin M, Masoni L. The reality of radical sphincter preservation surgery for cancer of the distal 3 cm of rectum following high-dose radiation. Int J Radiat Oncol Biol Phys 1993;27:779–83.
21. Mohiuddin M, Regine W, Marks GJ, Marks JW. High dose preoperative radiation and the challenge of sphincter-preservation surgery for cancer of the distal 2 cm of the rectum. Int J Radiat Oncol Biol Phys 1998;40:569–74.
22. Despretz J, Otmezguine Y, Grimard L, et al. Conservative management of tumors of the rectum by radiotherapy and local excision. Dis Colon Rectum 1990;33:113–6.
23. Grann A, Minsky B, Cohen A, et al. Preliminary results of pre-operative 5FU, low dose leucovorin and concurrent radiation therapy for resectable T3 rectal cancer. Dis Colon Rectum 1997;40:515–22.
24. Chari RS, Tyler DS, Anscher MS. Preoperative radiation and chemotherapy in the treatment of adenocarcinoma of the rectum. Ann Surg 1995;221:778–87.
25. Rich TA, Skibber JM, Ajani JA, et al. Preoperative infusional chemoradiation therapy for stage T3 rectal cancer. Int J Radiat Oncol Biol Phys 1995;32:1025–9.
26. Valentini V, Coco C, Cellini N, et al. Preoperative chemoradiation for extraperitoneal T3 rectal cancer: acute toxicity, tumor response, and sphincter preservation. Int J Radiat Oncol Biol Phys 1998;40:1067–75.
27. Stryker SJ, Kiel KD, Rademaker A, et al. Preoperative chemoradiation for stage II and III rectal carcinoma. Arch Surg 1996;131:514–8.
28. Boulis-Wassif S, Gerard A, Loygue J, et al. Final results of a randomized trial on the treatment of rectal cancer with preoperative radiotherapy alone or in combination with 5FU, followed by radical surgery. Cancer 1984;53:1811–8.
29. Hyams D, Mamounas E, Petrelli N, et al. A clinical trial to evaluate the worth of preoperative multimodality therapy in patients with operable carcinoma of the rectum: a progress report of NSABP R-03. Dis Colon Rectum 1997;40:131–9.
30. Tepper JE, Cohen AM, Wood WC, et al. Postoperative radiation therapy of rectal cancer. Int J Radiat Oncol Biol Phys 1987;13:5–10.
31. Vigliotti A, Rich TA, Romsdahl MM, et al. Postoperative adjuvant radiotherapy for adenocarcinoma of the rectum and rectosigmoid. Int J Radiat Oncol Biol Phys 1987;13:999–1006.

32. Balslev I, Pedersen M, Teglbjaerg P, et al. Postoperative radiotherapy in Duke B and C carcinoma of the rectum and rectosigmoid: a randomized multicenter study. Cancer 1986;58:22–8.
33. Treurniet-Donker AD, van Putten WL, Wereldsma JC. Postoperative radiation therapy for rectal carcinoma: an interim analysis of a prospective randomized multicenter trial in the Netherlands. Cancer 1991;67:2042–8.
34. Medical Research Council Rectal Cancer Working Party. Randomised trial of surgery alone versus surgery followed by radiotherapy for mobile cancer of the rectum. Lancet 1996;348:1610–4.
35. Arnaud J, Nordlinger B, Bosset J, et al. Radical surgery and postoperative radiotherapy as combined treatment in rectal cancer: final results of a phase III study of the European Organization for Research and Treatment of Cancer. Br J Surg 1997;84:352–7.
36. Wood W, Willett C. Update of the Massachusetts General Hospital experience of combined local excision and radiotherapy for rectal cancer. Surg Oncol Clin North Am 1992;1:131.
37. Wagman R, Minsky BD, Cohen AM, et al. Conservative management of rectal cancer with local excision and postoperative adjuvant therapy. Int J Radiat Oncol Biol Phys 1999;44:841–6.
38. Valentini V, Morganti A, De Santis M, et al. Local excision and external beam radiotherapy in early rectal cancer. Int J Radiat Oncol Biol Phys 1996;35:759–64.
39. Fortunato L, Ahmad N, Yeung R, et al. Long term follow-up of local excision and radiation therapy for invasive rectal cancer. Dis Colon Rectum 1995;38:1193–9.
40. Wong CS, Stern H, Cummings BJ. Local excision and postoperative radiation therapy for rectal carcinoma. Int J Radiat Oncol Biol Phys 1993;25:669–75.
41. Steele G. Local excision of early rectal cancer. Hepatogastroenterology 1992;39:212–4.
42. Douglass HO Jr, Moertel CG, Mayer RJ. Survival after postoperative combination treatment of rectal cancer. N Engl J Med 1986;315:1294–5.
43. Krook JE, Moertel CG, Gunderson LL, et al. Effective surgical adjuvant therapy for high-risk rectal carcinoma. N Engl J Med 1991;324:709–15.
44. Tepper JE, O'Connell MJ, Petroni GR, et al. Adjuvant postoperative fluorouracil-modulated chemotherapy combined with pelvic radiation therapy for rectal cancer: initial results of Intergroup 0114. J Clin Oncol 1997;15:2030–9.
45. Pilipshen S, Heilweil M, Quan S, et al. Patterns of pelvic recurrence following definitive resection of rectal cancer. Cancer 1984;53:1354–62.
46. Rich T, Gunderson LL, Lew R, et al. Patterns of recurrence of rectal cancer after potentially curative resection. Cancer 1983;52:1317–29.
47. Moertel CG, Childs DS Jr, Reitemeier RJ, et al. Combined 5FU and supervoltage radiation therapy for locally unresectable gastrointestinal cancer. Lancet 1969;2:865–7.
48. Brierley JD, Cummings BJ, Wong A, et al. Adenocarcinoma of the rectum treated by radical external radiation therapy. Int J Radiat Oncol Biol Phys 1995;31:255–9.
49. Willett CG, Warland G, Hagan MP, et al. Tumor proliferation in rectal cancer following pre-operative irradiation. J Clin Oncol 1995;13:1417–24.
50. Chan A, Wong A, Langevin J, Khoo R. Preoperative concurrent 5FU infusion, mitomycin C and pelvic radiation therapy in tethered and fixed rectal carcinoma. Int J Radiat Oncol Biol Phys 1993;25:791–9.
51. Chan AK, Wong AO, Langevin JM, et al. "Sandwich" preoperative and postoperative combined chemotherapy and radiation in tethered and fixed rectal cancer: impact of treatment intensity on local control and survival. Int J Radiat Oncol Biol Phys 1997;37:629–37.
52. Minsky B, Cohen A, Enker W, et al. Preoperative 5FU, low dose leucovorin, and concurrent radiation therapy for rectal cancer. Cancer 1994;73:273–80.
53. Minsky B, Cohen A, Enker W, et al. Preoperative 5FU, low dose leucovorin, and radiation therapy for locally advanced and unresectable rectal cancer. Int J Radiat Oncol Biol Phys 1997;37:289–95.
54. Weinstein GD, Rich TA, Shumate CR. Preoperative infusional chemoradiation and surgery with or without an electron beam intraoperative boost for advanced primary rectal cancer. Int J Radiat Oncol Biol Phys 1995;32:197–204.
55. Willett CG, Shellito PC, Tepper E, et al. Intraoperative electron beam radiation therapy for primary locally advanced rectal and rectosigmoid carcinoma. J Clin Oncol 1991;9:843–9.
56. Willett CG, Shellito PC, Tepper JE, et al. Intraoperative electron beam radiation therapy for recurrent locally advanced rectal or rectosigmoid carcinoma. Cancer 1991;67:1504–8.
57. Gunderson LL, Nelson H, Martenson JA, et al. Intraoperative electron and external beam irradiation with or without 5FU and maximum surgical resection for previously unirradiated, locally recurrent colorectal cancer. Dis Colon Rectum 1996;39:1379–95.

......................................

# CHEMOTHERAPY

● Mace L. Rothenberg

Fluorinated pyrimidines have been the cornerstone of chemotherapy for colorectal cancer for decades. Previous editions of this book review this history in detail. Over the past several years, a number of important strides have been made to improve the effectiveness of systemic therapy in the treatment of colorectal cancer. These advances can be categorized as follows: (1) refinement of adjuvant therapy for locally advanced colon cancer, (2) optimization of 5-FU drug administration, (3) identification of new drugs with activity in advanced-stage colorectal cancer, and (4) identification of tumor characteristics that may predict response to therapy. Advances in the chemotherapy of colon cancer and rectal cancer are considered separately because chemotherapy is normally given without radiation therapy for colon cancer, and it is commonly given with radiation therapy in the United States for rectal cancer.

## COLON CANCER

**Adjuvant Therapy.** The impact of adjuvant 5-FU and levamisole in patients with stage III colon cancer was first demonstrated in the 1980s, and this combination has been in widespread use since that time.[1] Several randomized trials suggest that the combination of 5-FU and leucovorin is also effective in the adjuvant setting. The first of these trials, initiated before 5-FU and levamisole became established as standard treatment for stage III patients, showed that 6 months of 5-FU and leucovorin reduced 5-year tumor recurrences by 38% and reduced 5-year mortality rates by 30% compared with no postoperative adjuvant therapy in patients with stages II and III colon cancer.[2] A year of this combination also proved superior to adjuvant MOF chemotherapy (methyl-CCNU, vincristine [Oncovin], and 5-FU), with an improvement in 8-year relapse-free survival from 50 to 61% ($p<0.001$) and 8-year overall survival from 57 to 68% ($p=0.001$).[3, 4] These observations were followed by three large, cooperative studies to determine whether there were any differences between 5-FU biochemically modulated with leucovorin or levamisole, or both, and whether 4 to 6 months of therapy was as good as 10 to 12 months of therapy (Table 43–12).[5–7] Two complementary strategies were pursued in

*Table 43–12.* **Phase III Trials of Biochemical Modulation of 5-Fluorouracil in Locally Advanced Colon Cancer**

| Author or Group | No. Patients | 5-Fluorouracil | Leucovorin | Levamisole | Duration | 5-Yr Disease-Free Survival | 5-Yr Overall Survival (%) |
|---|---|---|---|---|---|---|---|
| O'Connell[5] | 222 | 450 mg/m² IVB QD × 5, then Q wk | — | 50 mg PO TID × 3 Q 2 wk | 6 mo | 58 | 60 $p<0.01$ |
| NCCTG | 223 | 370 mg/m² IVB QD × 5, then Q wk | 20 mg/m² IVB QD × 5, then Q wk | 50 mg PO TID × 3 Q 2 wk | 6 mo | 63 | 70 |
| | 220 | 450 mg/m² IVB QD × 5, then Q wk | — | 50 mg PO TID × 3 Q 2 wk | 12 mo | 63 | 68 |
| | 226 | 370 mg/m² IVB QD × 5, then Q wk | 20 mg/m² IVB QD × 5, then Q wk | 50 mg PO TID × 3 Q 2 wk | 12 mo | 57 | 63 |
| Wolmark[7] | 691 | 500 mg/m² IVB Q wk × 6, Q 8 wk | 500 mg/m² 2-hr IV Q wk × 6, Q 8 wk | — | 48 wk | 65 $p = 0.04$ | 74 |
| NSABP | 691 | 450 mg/m² IVB QD × 5, then Q wk | — | 50 mg PO TID × 3 Q 2 wk | 1 yr | 60 | 70 |
| | 696 | 500 mg/m² IVB Q wk × 6, Q 8 wk | 500 mg/m² 2-hr IV Q wk × 6, Q 8 wk | 50 mg PO TID × 3 Q 2 wk | 1 yr | 64 | 73 |
| Haller[6] | — | 500 mg/m² 1-hr IV Q wk × 6, Q 8 wk | 500 mg/m² 2-hr IV Q wk × 6, Q 8 wk | — | 8 mo | 59 | 65 |
| ECOG, SWOG, CALGB | — | 425 mg/m² IVB QD × 5, Q 4-5 wk | 20 mg/m² IVB QD × 5, Q 4-5 wk | — | 8 mo | 60 | 66 |
| Intergroup | — | 450 mg/m² IVB QD × 5, then Q wk | — | 50 mg PO TID × 3 Q 2 wk | 1 yr | 56 $p = 0.014$ | 63 $p = 0.0074$ |
| | — | 425 mg/m² IVB QD × 5, Q 4-5 wk | 20 mg/m² IVB QD × 5, Q 4-5 wk | 50 mg PO TID × 3 Q 2 wk | 8 mo | 60 | 67 |

IVB, intravenous bolus; IV, intravenous; NCCTG, North Central Cancer Treatment Group; NSABP, National Surgical Adjuvant Breast and Bowel Project; ECOG, Eastern Cooperative Oncology Group; SWOG, Southwest Oncology Group; CALGB, Cancer and Leukemia Group B; QD, daily; Q wk, weekly; TID, three times a day.

the development of the three-drug combinations used in these trials: (1) adding leucovorin to an established 5-FU plus levamisole schedule or (2) adding levamisole to an established 5-FU plus leucovorin regimen. These studies, which involved more than 6700 patients, showed that 6 months of 5-FU plus leucovorin is at least as good as 12 months of 5-FU plus levamisole in terms of disease-free and overall survival. The studies also showed that 6 months of 5-FU plus levamisole is not adequate adjuvant therapy and yields results inferior to these other strategies. As a result of these trials, 6 months of 5-FU plus leucovorin and 12 months of 5-FU plus levamisole can both be considered standard adjuvant therapy alternatives for patients with locally advanced colon cancer. The three-drug combinations showed no superiority over 6 months of 5-FU and leucovorin and are not recommended because of their increased toxicity.

The inclusion of patients with both stage II (Dukes stage B) and stage III (Dukes stage C) colon cancer in all three of these studies has done little to help resolve the debate over whether patients with stage II colon cancer should routinely receive adjuvant chemotherapy. Pooled analyses have not been successful in settling this controversy. When the results of four consecutive NSABP trials were analyzed together, they showed that patients with Dukes B colon cancer who were treated in each study with the superior treatment (chemotherapy in all four studies) had a 30% reduction in relative mortality risk compared with the group who received the inferior treatment (observation in two studies and chemotherapy in two studies).[8] When the results of five other randomized trials were analyzed by the International Multicentre Pooled Analysis of B2 Colon Cancer Trials (IMPACT B2) investigators, however, only a 12% improvement in event-free survival and 14% improvement in overall survival could be identified, neither of which was statistically significant.[9] As a result, there has been no resolution to the controversy over whether patients with stage II colon cancer should routinely receive postoperative adjuvant therapy.

Ideally, stage II patients at highest risk of tumor recurrence and death could be prospectively identified and given adjuvant therapy, while those at least risk could be spared exposure to unnecessary treatment. Certain molecular markers have been associated with poor outcome in this group of patients. One such candidate is allelic loss of chromosome 18q, the site of the deleted in colorectal cancer (*DCC*) gene. This abnormality has been identified by a number of independent laboratories as a negative prognostic factor for relapse-free and overall survival in patients with locally advanced colorectal cancer, and it retains its prognostic significance even in multivariate analysis.[10–12] Efforts are under way to determine whether this prognostic factor can also serve as a predictive factor (to identify patients most likely to benefit from adjuvant therapy). Another potential candidate as a predictive factor for response to therapy is thymidylate synthase, one of the primary targets through which 5-FU exerts its cytotoxic effect. In several studies of thymidylate synthase expression in patients with metastatic colorectal cancer, high thymidylate synthase levels in the primary tumor or metastases, or both, were associated with a reduced likelihood of response to therapy and shorter survival. This association is now being tested to determine if it holds true in patients with locally advanced disease.[13, 14] Other putative prognostic factors, such as p53 and *BAX* or CEA as detected

by polymerase chain reaction in regional lymph nodes,[15] have been found to correlate with outcome by some but not by others.[16]

**Regional Chemotherapy.** Although most colon cancer cells reach the liver by way of the portal vein, their growth primarily depends on hepatic arterial blood flow. Regional administration of chemotherapy to the liver through the hepatic artery has the theoretical advantage of exposing liver metastases to higher concentrations of drug than could be achieved through the intravenous route. Certain consistent characteristics have emerged from a meta-analysis of phase III trials comparing hepatic artery infusion (HAI) chemotherapy (usually floxuridine) with intravenous chemotherapy (usually 5-FU or floxuridine, without leucovorin) in patients with unresectable hepatic metastases. Objective response rates were significantly higher in the HAI-treated patients (41% vs. 14%, $p<10^{-10}$). This difference might be exaggerated because of the omission of leucovorin in the intravenous treatment arms. Although the meta-analysis calculated a 16-month median survival for HAI-treated patients and a 12.2-month median survival for intravenous chemotherapy–treated patients, a death hazard ratio of 0.81, this difference failed to achieve statistical significance ($p=0.14$). When these results are viewed from the perspective of the added risk of catheter-related complications and biliary toxicity of HAI-directed chemotherapy and the added expense of operative placement of an HAI catheter, HAI cannot be considered a standard treatment for patients with unresectable hepatic metastases from colorectal cancer.[17] Data suggest, however, that there may be an advantage to giving HAI with or without systemic chemotherapy as adjuvant therapy to patients with completely resected hepatic metastases. Patients treated with a combination of HAI floxuridine and dexamethasone plus systemic 5-FU and leucovorin had a 2-year overall survival rate of 86% following metastastectomy compared with 72% for patients who received systemic therapy alone ($p=0.03$).[18] However, the median survival was not significantly different between the two groups (72.2 vs. 59.3 months, respectively; log rank $p=0.21$). A smaller randomized study comparing HAI floxuridine plus systemic infusional 5-FU with no postoperative chemotherapy found a significant improvement in 3-year disease-free survival rate (58% vs. 34%, $p=0.04$) but no significant difference in overall survival.[19] In centers with experience in the placement and management of hepatic arterial catheters, HAI with or without systemic chemotherapy can be considered a treatment option for patients who have no evidence of disease following hepatic metastastectomy.

Early postoperative or perioperative administration of chemotherapy through the portal vein has the theoretical advantage of destroying tumor cells before their establishment and growth in the liver. Trials performed over three decades comparing portal vein infusions of 5-FU with no postoperative adjuvant therapy generated conflicting results, with some achieving a significant reduction in the rate of development of liver metastases without an improvement in survival, others showing no reduction of liver metastases while improving overall survival, and still others showing no beneficial effect at all.[20–22] Trials comparing portal vein infusion with or without systemic therapy with systemic therapy alone also fail to show any survival benefit to this method of regional chemotherapy.[23] Overall, portal vein infusion does not appear to offer any significant advantages over standard intravenous administration of adjuvant chemotherapy.

**Tumor Vaccines and Immunotherapy.** Immunologically based approaches have shown interesting preliminary data in the adjuvant treatment of colon cancer. Murine monoclonal antibody 17-1A, which recognizes a 34-kd glycoprotein on the cell membrane of epithelial cells, has been tested in a small randomized trial in patients with stage III (Dukes C) colon cancer and resulted in a 32% reduction in mortality rate and a 23% reduction in recurrence rate at 7 years of follow-up compared with a control arm of no postoperative adjuvant therapy. Confirmatory trials are under way in stage II (17-1A vs. observation) and stage III (5-FU plus leucovorin plus 17-1A) patients.[24, 25]

Another approach is active specific immunotherapy, which involves the use of the patient's own tumor to generate a long-term, cell-mediated immune response that is capable of eradicating subclinical metastases. Results from randomized studies have been conflicting, with two trials showing no substantial impact of active specific immunotherapy, whereas a third showed a significant reduction in tumor recurrences in patients with stage II or III colon cancer and an improvement in recurrence-free survival that was limited to stage II patients. No improvement in overall survival was reported in this small trial.[26]

### Treatment of Metastatic Colon Cancer

*Optimization of 5-Fluorouracil Drug Administration.* Even after four decades of clinical use, there is no consensus regarding the most effective way to administer 5-FU. There are three main areas of controversy: (1) Is 5-FU most effective when used alone or with a biochemical modifier? (2) Is 5-FU most effective when given by a bolus or infusional schedule? (3) Is 5-FU most effective when given by the systemic or liver-directed route?

*5-Fluorouracil Versus 5-Fluorouracil Plus Biochemical Modification.* Although most phase III trials and a meta-analysis have shown that objective response rates are doubled with the addition of leucovorin to 5-FU, this has not consistently translated into an improvement in overall survival, with some trials showing a significant survival advantage for the addition of leucovorin and others not. Reports of significant survival and quality of life advantages for 5-FU plus leucovorin from some of the early phase III trials led to the adoption of this combination as standard first-line therapy for patients with metastatic colorectal cancer in the United States.[27–29] Early phase III trials that compared the daily low-dose leucovorin for 5 days regimen (also known as the *Mayo Clinic* or *NCCTG* regimen) and the weekly 5-FU plus high-dose leucovorin regimen (also known as the *Roswell Park* or *RPMI* regimen) concluded that the two schedules were equally effective in terms of response rate, survival, and relief of tumor-related symptoms, but that the daily schedule was associated with fewer toxicity-related hospitalizations and was cheaper to administer than the weekly schedule.[30] Over the ensuing years, improvements in supportive care have reduced treatment-related toxicities and hospitalizations for both regimens, and the price of leucovorin has come down considerably. The toxicities associated with the weekly 5-FU plus leucovorin schedule are now considered more readily manageable than those associated with the daily regimen, leading many to consider the weekly

regimen the preferred choice.[31] The dose of leucovorin does not appear to be a factor in the clinical activity of the 5-FU plus leucovorin regimen in patients with advanced colorectal cancer, with low doses proving to be as effective as high doses in multiple phase III trials.[32, 33]

Methotrexate has been evaluated as a biochemical modulator for 5-FU because of its ability to inhibit purine synthesis through its inhibition of dihydrofolate reductase. This inhibition results in increased levels of phosphoribosylphosphate, which enhances the intracellular formation of 5-fluorodeoxyuridine monophosphate (F-dUMP) (which inhibits thymidylate synthase) and serves as a substrate for incorporation into RNA. Although individual phase III trials have yielded mixed results, a meta-analysis of randomized trials that compared single-agent 5-FU with sequential methotrexate and 5-FU identified a doubling of response rate and a small but statistically significant 13% risk reduction for death in patients treated with the biochemical modulation.[34] Trimetrexate, a methotrexate analogue that enters the cell independent of the reduced folate carrier and does not require polyglutamylation to inhibit dihydrofolate reductase, has been evaluated in combination with 5-FU and leucovorin and has resulted in encouraging response rates of 50% and median survival of 12.7 months in previously untreated patients.[35] One phase III trial has been completed and, in a preliminary analysis, did not show an improvement in disease-free survival with addition of trimetrexate to 5-FU and leucovorin.[36] A second trial has been completed, and the results are pending. With the data currently available, sequential therapy with methotrexate followed by 5-FU and leucovorin cannot be recommended as standard treatment for advanced colorectal cancer.

Interferons have shown synergistic cytotoxic effects with 5-FU with or without leucovorin in preclinical models, and response rates of 76% have been reported in phase II trials in patients with metastatic colorectal cancer. Phase III trials and a meta-analysis comparing 5-FU with or without leucovorin with or without alfa-interferon, however, have failed to show any consistent benefit for the addition of interferon to 5-FU–based chemotherapy in terms of higher response rates or improved survival. The one consistent effect that has been observed for interferon in this setting has been to increase the toxicity of the chemotherapy and to affect quality of life adversely.[37]

Two randomized trials have been performed to screen several biochemical modulation strategies for 5-FU (Table 43–13).[38, 39] Nine different 5-FU–based regimens evaluated variations on 5-FU dose, bolus versus infusional strategies, and modulation with leucovorin, phosphonacetyl-L-aspartate, or alfa-interferon. Both trials failed to identify any regimen that was associated with a substantial improvement in overall survival.

*5-Fluorouracil Bolus Versus Infusional Schedules.* When given as an intravenous bolus, 5-FU exerts its antitumor effect primarily through incorporation of 5-fluordeoxyuridine triphosphate into RNA. Given as a more prolonged intravenous infusion, thymidylate synthase inhibition appears to be the predominant site of action. Leucovorin contributes to more effective inhibition of thymidylate synthase through stabilization of binding of F-dUMP to thymidylate synthase, an enzyme critical to pyrimidine nucleotide synthesis.[40]

*Table 43–13.* Randomized Trials of Biochemical Modulation in Metastatic Colorectal Cancer

| Regimen | Response Rate (%) | Median Survival (mo) |
| --- | --- | --- |
| *SWOG Phase II Trial*[38] | | |
| 5-FU 500 mg/m² IVP QD × 5, Q 4–5 wk | 24 | 14 mo |
| Leucovorin 20 mg/m² IVP followed by 5-FU 425 mg/m² IVP QD × 5, Q 4–5 wk | 17 | 14 mo |
| Leucovorin 500 mg/m² 3-hr CIV followed by 5-FU 600 mg/m² IVP Q wk × 6, Q 8 wk | 14 | 13 mo |
| 5-FU 300 mg/m²/day CIV × 28 days, Q 35 days | 18 | 15 mo |
| 5-FU 200 mg/m²/day CIV × 28 days, Q 35 + leucovorin 20 mg/m² days 1, 8, 15, 22 | 19 | 14 mo |
| 5-FU 2600 mg/m² 24-hr CIV Q wk | 13 | 15 mo |
| PALA 250 mg/m² IV over 15 min day 1 + 5-FU 2600 mg/m² 24-hr CIV day 2 Q wk | 15 | 11 mo |
| *ECOG/CALGB Phase III Trial*[39] | | |
| 5-FU 2600 mg/m² 24-hr CIV Q wk | — | 15 mo |
| PALA 250 mg/m² day 1 + 5-FU 2600 mg/m² day 2 24-hr CIV Q wk | — | Not reported |
| Leucovorin 125 mg/m² PO Q hr × 4 followed by 5-FU 600 IV mg/m² Q wk | — | 13 mo |
| 5-FU 600 mg/m² + leucovorin 600 mg/m² IV Q wk | — | 14 mo |
| 5-FU 750 mg/m²/day 5-day CIV, followed by 5-FU 750 mg/m² Q wk + interferon alfa-2a 9 MU SC TIW | — | 15 mo |

5-FU, 5-fluorouracil; IVP, intravenous push; CIV, continuous intravenous infusion; SC, subcutaneously; MU, million units; TIW, three times a week.

Clinically the biggest differences between bolus and infusional schedules of 5-FU administration are (1) the severity and spectrum of toxicity, (2) the ability to deliver higher dose intensity with an infusional schedule, and (3) the requirement of a semipermanent catheter for prolonged infusions. Although most phase III trials in which 5-FU infusion has been directly compared with 5-FU bolus have failed to identify a survival advantage for the infusional approach, a meta-analysis of seven phase III trials identified a significantly higher response rate (22% vs. 14%, $p = 0.0002$) and longer median survival (12.1 months vs. 11.3 months, $p = 0.04$) for patients treated with infusional 5-FU.[41, 42] Despite the results of this meta-analysis, continuous-infusion 5-FU has not gained widespread popularity in the United States. Several factors have contributed to this situation: (1) the fact that the control arm in five of the seven trials included in this meta-analysis used bolus 5-FU alone, without leucovorin; (2) the added expense, inconvenience, and potential complications of a semipermanent intravenous catheter and ambulatory infusion pump, which may not justify the marginal improvement in survival; and (3) the identification of other active agents, such as irinotecan, that may enhance the effectiveness of front-line bolus 5-FU and leucovorin chemotherapy.

The actual delivery of *bolus* 5-FU has been the subject of a randomized trial.[43] Because 5-FU is metabolized so rapidly (plasma half-life is 8 to 15 minutes), small differences in infusion times may have a significant impact on clinical activity. In one phase III trial, bolus injection of 5-FU, defined as administration over 2 to 4 minutes, resulted in a significantly higher response rate (27% vs. 13%, $p = 0.92$) but not progression-free survival (5.5 months vs. 4.2 months, $p = 0.07$) or overall survival (9.5 months for both groups) in patients with metastatic colorectal cancer.

These insights into the potentially complementary mechanisms of action of 5-FU when given by different schedules prompted the development of so-called hybrid regimens that combine bolus and infusional 5-FU administration schedules. A few phase III trials have now compared bolus versus infusion versus combination approaches in patients with metastatic colorectal cancer. In one, a 5-FU bolus plus daily leucovorin for 5 days schedule (Mayo/NCCTG schedule) was compared with a 2-hour leucovorin infusion followed by a 5-FU bolus followed by a 22-hour 5-FU infusion schedule (termed the *de Gramont* or *LV5FU2* regimen).[44] Response rates (32.6% vs. 14.4%) and median progression-free survival (6.4 months vs. 5.1 months) were superior in the group receiving 5-FU by the de Gramont schedule. Differences in overall survival did not reach statistical significance (14.4 months vs. 13.2 months), however. Grade 3 to 4 toxicities, especially neutropenia, diarrhea, and mucositis, occurred less frequently using the hybrid schedule than with the daily for 5 days bolus schedule.

The most common toxicities of 5-FU depend on its schedule of administration. When given alone by bolus injection, myelosuppression, primarily in the form of neutropenia, is the predominant toxicity. When given as a bolus on a daily for 5 days basis with leucovorin, neutropenia, stomatitis, and to a lesser degree diarrhea are the most common toxicities. Diarrhea is the most common toxicity when 5-FU is given on a weekly basis in combination with high-dose leucovorin. Palmar-plantar erythrodysesthesia (also known as *hand-foot syndrome*), mucositis, and cerebellar ataxia are the most common toxicities of prolonged infusion schedules of 5-FU. The frequency and severity of these are also influenced by several other factors, including age, gender, performance status, drug clearance, and metabolism.[45] Several measures have been implemented to reduce the frequency and severity of these toxicities. Oral cooling, achieved by having the patient suck on ice chips while in the clinic, is one such maneuver that can significantly reduce the incidence of mucositis.[46]

***Oral Fluorinated Pyrimidines.*** Oral administration of 5-FU was abandoned because of an erratic pattern of absorption of drug through the gastrointestinal tract, which resulted in unpredictable and, in some cases, severe toxicity. The development of several novel analogues that are more completely and reliably absorbed through the gut has rekindled interest in the oral administration of fluorinated pyrimidines. Capecitabine is an oral 5-FU prodrug that undergoes succes-

*Table 43–14.* Randomized Trials of Oral Fluorinated Pyrimidines Versus Intravenous 5-Fluorouracil and Leucovorin in Metastatic Colorectal Cancer

| Regimen | RR (%) | Median Survival |
|---|---|---|
| *Twelves*[48] | | |
| Capecitabine 2500 mg/m²/day × 14 days, Q 21 days | 26.6 | 5.3 mo (PFS) |
| | $p = 0.013$ | |
| Leucovorin 20 mg/m² IVP followed by 5-FU 425 mg/m² IVP QD × 5, Q 4 wk | 17.9 | 4.8 mo (PFS) |
| *Cox*[49] | | |
| Capecitabine 2500 mg/m²/day × 14 days, Q 21 days | 23.2 | 4.4 mo (PFS) |
| | $p = 0.02$ | |
| Leucovorin 20 mg/m² IVP followed by 5-FU 425 mg/m² IVP QD × 5, Q 4 wk | 15.5 | 5.1 mo (PFS) |
| *Carmichael*[50] | | |
| UFT 300 mg/m²/day + leucovorin 90 mg/day × 28 days, Q 35 days | 11 | 12.2 mo |
| Leucovorin 20 mg/m² IVP followed by 5-FU 425 mg/m² IVP QD × 5, Q 5 wk | 9 | 11.9 mo |
| *Pazdur*[51] | | |
| UFT 300 mg/m²/day + leucovorin 75–90 mg/day × 28 days, Q 35 days | 12 | 12.4 mo |
| Leucovorin 20 mg/m² IVP followed by 5-FU 425 mg/m² IVP QD × 5, Q 4 wk | 15 | 13.4 mo |

IVP, intravenous push; PFS, progression-free survival; 5-FU, 5-fluorouracil; NR, not reported; UFT, tegafur and uracil.

sive activation in the liver and gastrointestinal tract and is converted into 5-FU within cells by the enzyme thymidine phosphorylase. Several studies have shown that thymidine phosphorylase expression is frequently higher in tumor cells than matched normal tissue, providing at least a theoretical basis for selectivity of this drug for cancer cells.[47] Preliminary reports from two phase III trials show slightly higher objective response rates and equivalent survival for patients with metastatic colorectal cancer treated with capecitabine compared with those treated with 5-FU and leucovorin given on a daily for 5 days basis (Table 43–14).[48, 49]

UFT combines tegafur and uracil in a molar ratio of 1:4 into a single tablet that is administered orally. Tegafur is a 5-FU prodrug that must be converted to 5-FU within the cell by thymidine phosphorylase. Uracil inhibits the catabolism of 5-FU through competitive inhibition of the intracellular catabolizing enzyme dihydropyrimidine dehydrogenase. Initial reports from two phase III trials comparing UFT and leucovorin with 5-FU and leucovorin given on a daily for 5 days schedule show equivalent response rates and survival.[50, 51] UFT with leucovorin and capecitabine represent reasonable therapeutic options to 5-FU and leucovorin for the first-line treatment of patients with metastatic colorectal cancer. Selection of therapy is likely to be driven by considerations of travel and convenience, cost, and differing toxicity profiles for each option.

***Identification of New Drugs with Activity in Advanced-Stage Colorectal Cancer.*** CPT-11 (irinotecan) is one of several water-soluble camptothecin analogues that target topoisomerase I, a nuclear enzyme involved in DNA replication and transcription. By stabilizing the topoisomerase I–DNA cleavable complex, CPT-11 converts topoisomerase I into a cellular poison. Collision of the replication fork with the stabilized cleavable complex converts the transient break in single-strand DNA to an irreparable double-strand break in DNA that ultimately results in cellular death through apoptosis.[52]

In patients with previously treated, progressive or rapidly recurrent colorectal cancer, irinotecan produces objective response rates ranging from 11 to 27% and median survival of 9 to 11 months. An additional 40 to 50% of patients experience disease stabilization.[53]

A phase III trial comparing irinotecan with best supportive care showed an improvement in median survival (9.2 months vs. 6.5 months, $p = 0.0001$) and quality of life for patients who received irinotecan.[54] A separate trial showed that patients treated with irinotecan survived longer than those given infusional 5-FU in this second-line setting (10.8 months vs. 8.5 months, $p = 0.035$) without any discernible sacrifice in quality of life.[55] These data support the use of irinotecan as standard second-line therapy in patients with recurrent or progressive colorectal cancer following first-line 5-FU–based therapy. The integration of irinotecan into first-line therapy has been evaluated in two phase III trials. In one phase III trial, the combination of irinotecan, 5-FU, and leucovorin administered on a weekly × 4 schedule, every 6 weeks was compared with a reference control regimen of 5-FU and leucovorin administered on a daily × 5 schedule (Mayo Clinic/NCCTG). A third arm, consisting of single-agent irinotecan, was included but was not part of the primary comparison of efficacy. This trial demonstrated significant improvement in objective response rate (39.4% vs. 20.8%, $p < 0.001$), progression-free survival (7 months vs. 4.3 months, $p = 0.004$), and median survival (14.8 months vs. 12.6 months, $p = 0.042$) in those patients treated with a combination of irinotecan, 5-FU, and leucovorin compared with those treated using 5-FU and leucovorin[56, 56a] (Table 43–15). Another phase III trial designed to address the same question using two regimens that are popular in Europe came to the same conclusion, demonstrating superiority of the irinotecan, 5-FU, and leucovorin combination in terms of objective response rate, progression-free survival, and median survival compared with 5-FU and leucovorin alone.[57] Taken together, these data provide strong support for the

*Table 43–15.* Phase III Trials of Irinotecan, 5-Fluorouracil, and Leucovorin as First-Line Treatment for Metastatic Colorectal Cancer

| Reference | Drug Dosages and Schedules | No. of Patients | RR (%) | Progression-Free Survival (mo) | Median Survival (mo) |
|---|---|---|---|---|---|
| Saltz[56a] | 5-FU 425 mg/m² IV bolus<br>Leucovorin 20 mg/m² IV bolus qd × 5, q 4 wk | 226 | 20.8 | 4.3 | 12.6 |
| | | | $p < 0.001$ | $p < 0.004$ | $p < 0.042$ |
| | Irinotecan 125 mg/m² IV over 90 min<br>5-FU 500 mg/m² IV bolus<br>Leucovorin 20 mg/m² IV bolus q wk × 4, q 6 wk | 231 | 39.4 | 7.0 | 14.8 |
| | Irinotecan 125 mg/m² IV over 90 min | 226 | 18.1 | 4.2 | 12.0 |
| Douillard[57] | Leucovorin 200 mg/m² IV over 2 hr<br>5-FU 400 mg/M² IV bolus<br>5-FU mg/m² IV 600 mg/m² IV over 22 hr qd × 2, q 2 wk<br>*or*<br>Leucovorin 500 mg/m² IV<br>5-FU 2600 mg/m² IV over 24 hr q wk | 187 | 21.9 | 4.4 | 14.1 |
| | | | $p = 0.005$ | $p < 0.001$ | $p = 0.031$ |
| | Irinotecan 180 mg/m² IV (day 1 only)<br>Leucovorin 200 mg/m² IV over 2 hr<br>5-FU 400 mg/m² IV bolus<br>5-FU mg/m² IV 600 mg/m² IV over 22 hr qd × 2, q 2 wk<br>*or*<br>Irinotecan 80 mg/m² IV<br>Leucovorin 500 mg/m² IV<br>5-FU 2300 mg/m² IV over 24 hr q wk | 198 | 34.8 | 6.7 | 17.4 |

IV, intravenously; qd, every day.

combination of irinotecan, 5-FU, and leucovorin to become the new standard of care for the front-line treatment of patients with metastatic colorectal carcinoma.

Oxaliplatin is a diaminocyclohexane platinum that is structurally and, to some extent, functionally distinct from cisplatin and carboplatin. Platinum-DNA adducts are formed faster with oxaliplatin (approximately 15 minutes) than with cisplatin (approximately 4 to 8 hours) or carboplatin (approximately 18 hours). The platinum-DNA adducts are bulkier and more hydrophobic than those formed by cisplatin or carboplatin. It is believed that these characteristics contribute to more effective inhibition of DNA synthesis by oxaliplatin and less efficient repair of these adducts by DNA excision-repair enzymes.[58]

As a single agent, oxaliplatin is associated with an objective response rate of approximately 10% in previously treated patients and 12 to 24% in previously untreated patients.[59–62] Greater interest has been generated by the activity observed when oxaliplatin is given in combination with 5-FU and leucovorin. In the salvage setting, response rates have ranged from 20 to 55%, with an additional 18 to 51% of patients achieving a best response of stable disease.[63] Median progression-free survival has varied from 6 to 10 months, and overall survival has ranged from 7 to 13 months. Response rates of 29 to 67% have been reported when oxaliplatin has been administered with 5-FU and leucovorin in patients with chemotherapy-naive colorectal cancer. The median survivals reported in these studies have been among the longest reported from any trials in this group of patients, ranging from 15 to 19 months.[64–67] Based on those observations and the high degree of activity seen with this combination when used as second-line chemotherapy, four phase III trials have been performed (Table 43–16).[64, 65, 68–70] Taken together, these four phase III trials offer tantalizing but inconsistent evidence of the activity of oxaliplatin as part of first-line chemotherapy for metastatic colorectal cancer. One can conclude from these trials that response rates are consis-

tently and substantially improved (roughly doubled) by the addition of oxaliplatin to 5-FU and leucovorin. Several important issues remain unresolved: (1) Why does the improved response rate not translate more consistently into improved survival? (2) Is the use of oxaliplatin as salvage therapy in patients who receive first-line 5-FU and leucovorin obscuring any survival benefit obtained through its use in first-line treatment? (3) Is there an advantage to using oxaliplatin as part of first-line treatment, or should its use be reserved for the time of relapse or progression? (4) What is the contribution of chronomodulation to the effectiveness and tolerability of oxaliplatin? It is anticipated that the answers to these questions will become available over the next several years and will help determine the optimal use of this drug in systemic treatment of colorectal cancer.

Raltitrexed is a selective thymidylate synthase inhibitor that can be administered on a convenient once every 3 weeks schedule. Although the results of initial phase III studies suggested therapeutic equivalence with 5-FU and leucovorin and led to regulatory approval in several countries, at least two phase III trials have shown inferior median survival for the raltitrexed-treated patients.[71–74] As a result, raltitrexed is not likely to become available as single-agent therapy for advanced colorectal cancer in the United States. Many other agents have undergone phase II evaluation in patients with advanced colorectal cancer. The results of those trials are summarized in Table 43–17.

## RECTAL CANCER

**Adjuvant Therapy.** Postoperative combined chemoradiotherapy has been the established standard adjuvant therapy for locally advanced rectal cancer since the 1990s. This combined-modality approach reduces local recurrence rates by more than 50% and reduces mortality rates by approximately 30 to 40% compared with no postoperative therapy.[75]

*Table 43–16.* Phase III Trials of Oxaliplatin, 5-Fluorouracil, and Leucovorin in Metastatic Colorectal Cancer

| Author | 5-FU | LV | Ox | No. Patients | RR (%) | SD (%) | PFS (mo) | MS (mo) |
|---|---|---|---|---|---|---|---|---|
| Lévi[66] | CI | CI | CI | 47 | 32 | 45 | 8 | 15 |
| | | | | | $p = 0.038$ | | $p = 0.19$ | $p = 0.03$ |
| | CM | CM | CM | 45 | 53 | 33 | 11 | 19 |
| Lévi[67] | CI | CI | CI | 93 | 29 | 40 | 5 | 17 |
| | | | | | $p = 0.003$ | | $p = $ NS | $p = $ NS |
| | CM | CM | CM | 93 | 51 | 30 | 6 | 16 |
| Giacchetti[68] | CM | CM | — | 100 | 16 | — | 6.1 | 19.9 |
| | | | | | $p < 0.001$ | | $p < 0.05$ | $p = $ NS |
| | CM | CM | CM | 100 | 53 | — | 8.7 | 19.4 |
| De Gramont[70, 70a] | B + CI | SI | — | 210 | 21.9 | — | 5.9 | 14.7 |
| | | | | | $p < 0.001$ | | $p = 0.0003$ | $p = $ NS |
| | B + CI | SI | SI | 210 | 49.0 | — | 8.1 | 15.9 |

5-FU, 5-fluorouracil; LV, leucovorin; Ox, oxaliplatin; RR, response rate; SD, stable disease rate; PFS, progression-free survival; MS, median survival; CI, continuous infusion; CM, chronomodulated; B, bolus; SI, short infusion.

Optimal administration appears to be two cycles of bolus 5-FU, followed by 5-FU by continuous infusion during radiation and then by two more cycles of bolus 5-FU.[76] Administration of the 5-FU by bolus instead of continuous infusion during the radiation yields inferior results. A large U.S. intergroup study determined that biochemical modulation of 5-FU chemotherapy with levamisole does not enhance survival in patients with stage II or III rectal cancer given postoperative adjuvant chemoradiotherapy.[77]

For several reasons, this approach is undergoing re-evaluation. First, approximately 20% of patients experience severe diarrhea or leukopenia, or both, as a result of postoperative

*Table 43–17.* Phase II Trials of New Drugs in Advanced Colorectal Cancer

| Drug | No. Patients | Prior Chemotherapy for Metastatic Disease | Response Rate (%) |
|---|---|---|---|
| Rhizoxin[84] | 18 | No | 0 |
| Doxifluridine + leucovorin (oral)[85] | 62 | No | 32 |
| | 28 | Yes (1) | 7 |
| | 18 | Yes (1 for adj) | 22 |
| Doxifluridine + L-leucovorin (IV)[86] | 63 | No | 41 |
| Doxifluridine + L-leucovorin (PO) | 67 | No | 15 |
| Doxifluridine[87] | 42 | No | 14 |
| Doxifluridine + leucovorin[88] | 34 | No | 35 |
| 9-Aminocamptothecin (72-hr CIV)[89] | 17 | No | 0 |
| 9-Aminocamptothecin (120-hr CIV)[90] | 17 | No | 0 |
| Endotoxin[91] | 27 | Yes (33%); no (67%) | 11 |
| Autologous activated macrophages[92] | 14 | Yes | 0 |
| EO9[93] | 25 | No | 0 |
| Octreotide[94] | 131 | No | 1.5 |
| Elsamitrucin[95] | 28 | No | 0 |
| Docetaxel[96] | 19 | No | 0 |
| Topotecan[97] | 48 | No | 4 |
| Topotecan + G-CSF[98] | 16 | Yes | 0 |
| Pyrazoloacridine[99] | 15 | No | 0 |
| CI-958[100] | 15 | Yes | 0 |
| Paclitaxel 120-hr CIV[101] | 14 | Yes | 0 |
| Mitonafide[102] | 16 | No | 0 |
| Edatrexate[103] | 12 | No | 0 |
| Trofosfamide[104] | 14 | Yes | 0 |
| Trimetrexate (Q 2 wk)[105] | 71 | No | 6 |
| Trimetrexate (QD × 5) | 29 | No | 0 |
| 13-cis-retinoic acid + interferon alfa-2a[106] | 16 | No | 0 |
| CI-980[107] | 14 | Yes (57%); No (43%) | 0 |
| Flavopiridol[108] | 10 | No | 0 |
| MTA (LY231514)[109] | 30 | Yes | 0 |
| MTA (LY231514)[110] | 39 | No | 16 |
| 5-FU + eniluracil[111] | 45 | No | 24 |

IV, intravenous; CIV, continuous intravenous infusion; G-CSF, granulocyte colony–stimulating factor; 5-FU, 5-fluorouracil; PO, orally.

combined-modality therapy. Second, modern surgical techniques, such as total mesorectal excision, may substantially reduce the risk of local recurrence from 25% to less than 10%. Lastly, preoperative radiation alone or combined-modality treatment of patients with T4 or large T3 tumors has allowed some patients to avoid an abdominoperineal resection and placement of a colostomy, which would have been required if those patients had undergone primary surgery followed by adjuvant therapy.

Preoperative therapy, in the form of chemoradiotherapy or radiotherapy alone, may have the advantage of causing fewer side effects than postoperative therapy and allowing sphincter-sparing surgery in 80 to 90% of patients with locally advanced tumors who would have required abdominoperineal resection if performed at the time of presentation.[78] Complete pathologic response appears to be more common in patients with locally advanced tumors who receive preoperative combined-modality therapy than in those who receive preoperative radiation alone, but randomized trials have not been performed, and there are insufficient data to determine whether this translates into a survival advantage.[79, 80] Randomized trials comparing preoperative versus postoperative therapy for patients with potentially resectable rectal cancer have been performed, but have been hampered by poor accrual. Preoperative therapy has the potential drawback of overtreating patients with stage I cancers.

Randomized trials of preoperative radiation followed by surgery versus surgery alone (without chemotherapy in either arm) have yielded conflicting results. Most have shown that preoperative radiation can reduce the size and stage of the tumors found at surgery, reduce the risk of local recurrence by approximately one-third, and improve disease-free survival by approximately one-quarter. Most failed to show a significant improvement in overall survival for the entire group treated but did identify subsets of patients who might be the subject for future studies. One randomized trial performed by the Swedish Rectal Cancer Group showed a substantial reduction in local recurrence rate (11% vs. 27%, $p<0.001$) and improvement in 5-year survival rate (58% vs. 48%, $p=0.004$) in patients who received neoadjuvant radiotherapy.[81, 82] Possible prognostic factors for locally advanced rectal cancer include age older than 60 years, distance from the anal verge of less than 6 cm, the number of involved lymph nodes (0 vs. 1 to 2 vs. ≥3), neural invasion, and depth of tumor penetration.[83]

## REFERENCES

1. Laurie JA, Moertel CG, Fleming TR, et al. Surgical adjuvant therapy of large-bowel carcinoma: an evaluation of levamisole and the combination of levamisole and fluorouracil. J Clin Oncol 1989;7:1447–56.
2. O'Connell MJ, Mailliard JA, Kahn MJ, et al. Controlled trial of fluorouracil and low-dose leucovorin given for 6 months as postoperative adjuvant therapy for colon cancer. J Clin Oncol 1997;15:246–50.
3. Wolmark N, Rockette H, Fisher B, et al. The benefit of leucovorin-modulated fluorouracil as postoperative adjuvant therapy for primary colon cancer: results from National Surgical Adjuvant Breast and Bowel Project protocol C-03. J Clin Oncol 1993;11:1879–87.
4. Mamounas E, Wieand S, Wolmark N, et al. Comparative efficacy of adjuvant chemotherapy in patients with Dukes' B versus Dukes' C colon cancer: results from four National Surgical Adjuvant Breast and Bowel Project adjuvant studies (C-01, C-02, C-03, and C-04). J Clin Oncol 1999;17:1349–55.
5. O'Connell MJ, Laurie JA, Kahn M, et al. Prospectively randomized trial of postoperative adjuvant chemotherapy in patients with high-risk colon cancer. J Clin Oncol 1998;16:295–300.
6. Haller DG, Catalano PJ, Macdonald JS, Mayer RJ. Fluorouracil, leucovorin, and levamisole adjuvant therapy for colon cancer: five-year final report of INT-0089. Proc ASCO 1998;17:256a.
7. Wolmark N, Rockette H, Mamounas E, et al. Clinical trial to assess the relative efficacy of fluorouracil and leucovorin, fluorouracil and levamisole, and fluorouracil, leucovorin, and levamisole in patients with Dukes' B and C carcinoma of the colon: results from National Surgical Adjuvant Breast and Bowel Project C-04. J Clin Oncol 1999;17:3553–9.
8. Mamounas E, Wieand S, Wolmark N, et al. Comparative efficacy of adjuvant chemotherapy in patients with Dukes' B versus Dukes' C colon cancer: results from four National Surgical Adjuvant Breast and Bowel Project adjuvant studies (C-01, C-02, C-03, C-04). J Clin Oncol 1999;17:1349–55.
9. International Multicentre Pooled Analysis of B2 Colon Cancer Trials (IMPACT B2) Investigators: Efficacy of adjuvant fluorouracil and folinic acid in B2 colon cancer. J Clin Oncol 1999;17:1356–63.
10. Ogunbiyi OA, Goodfellow PJ, Herfarth K, et al. Confirmation that chromosome 18q allelic loss in colon cancer is a prognostic factor. J Clin Oncol 1998;16:427–33.
11. Jen J, Kim H, Piantadosi S, et al. Allelic loss of chromosome 18q and prognosis in colorectal cancer. N Engl J Med 1994;331:213–21.
12. Shibata D, Reale MA, Lavin P, et al. The DCC protein and prognosis in colorectal cancer. N Engl J Med 1996;335:1727–32.
13. Leichman CG, Lenz H-J, Leichman L, et al. Quantitation of intratumoral thymidylate synthase expression predicts for disseminated colorectal cancer response and resistance to protracted-infusion fluorouracil and weekly leucovorin. J Clin Oncol 1997;15:3223–9.
14. Aschele C, Debernardis D, Casazza S, et al. Immunohistochemical quantitation of thymidylate synthase expression in colorectal cancer metastases predicts for clinical outcome to fluorouracil-based chemotherapy. J Clin Oncol 1999;17:1760–70.
15. Lieffers G-J, Cleton-Jansen A-M, van de Velde JH, et al. Micrometastases and survival in stage II colorectal cancer. N Engl J Med 1998;339:223–8.
16. Tortola S, Marcuello E, González I, et al. p53 and K-ras gene mutations correlate with tumor aggressiveness but are not of routine prognostic value in colorectal cancer. J Clin Oncol 1999;17:1375–81.
17. Meta-Analysis Group in Cancer. Reappraisal of hepatic arterial infusion in the treatment of nonresectable liver metastases from colorectal cancer. J Natl Cancer Inst 1996;88:252–8.
18. Kemeny N, Huang Y, Cohen A, et al. Hepatic arterial infusion of chemotherapy after resection of hepatic metastases from colorectal cancer. N Engl J Med 1999;341:2039–48.
19. Kemeny MM, Adak S, Lipsitz S, et al. Results of the intergroup (Eastern Cooperative Oncology Group and Southwest Oncology Group) prospective randomized study of surgery alone versus continuous infusion of FUDR and continuous systemic infusion of 5-FU after hepatic resection for colorectal liver metastases. Proc ASCO 1999;18:264a.
20. Nitti D, Wils J, Sahmoud T, et al. Final results of a Phase III clinical trial on adjuvant intraportal infusion with heparin and 5-fluorouracil in resectable colon cancer (EORTC GITCCG 1983–1987). Eur J Cancer 1997;33:1209–15.
21. Rougier P, Sahmoud T, Nitti D, et al. Adjuvant portal-vein infusion of fluorouracil and heparin in colorectal cancer: a randomised trial. Lancet 1998;351:1677–81.
22. James RD, on behalf of the AXIS Collaborators. Intraportal 5-FU and peri-operative radiotherapy in the adjuvant treatment of colorectal cancer—3681 patients randomized in the UK Coordinating Committee on Cancer Research AXIS trial. Proc ASCO 1999;18:264a.
23. Labianca R, Boffi L, Marsoni S, et al. A randomized trial of intraportal versus systemic versus intraportal and systemic chemotherapy in patients with resected Dukes B-C colon carcinoma. Proc ASCO 1999;18:264a.
24. Reithmüller G, Schneider-Gädicke E, Schlimok G, et al. Randomised trial of monoclonal antibody for adjuvant therapy of resected Dukes' C colorectal carcinoma. Lancet 1994;343:1177–83.
25. Reithmüller G, Holz E, Schlimok G, et al. Monoclonal antibody therapy for resected Dukes' C colorectal cancer: seven-year outcome of a multicenter randomized trial. J Clin Oncol 1998;16:1788–94.
26. Vermorken JB, Claessen AME, van Tinteren H, et al. Active specific

immunotherapy for stage II and stage III human colon cancer: a randomised trial. Lancet 1999;353:345–50.

27. Poon MA, O'Connell MJ, Moertel CG, et al. Biochemical modulation of fluorouracil: evidence of significant improvement in survival and quality of life in patients with advanced colorectal carcinoma. J Clin Oncol 1989;7:1407–17.

28. Borner M, Castiglione M, Bacchi M, et al. The impact of adding low-dose leucovorin to monthly 5-fluorouracil in advanced colorectal carcinoma: results of a Phase III trial. Ann Oncol 1998;7:535–41.

29. Advanced Colorectal Cancer Meta-Analysis Project. Modulation of fluorouracil by leucovorin in patients with advanced colorectal cancer: evidence in terms of response rate. J Clin Oncol 1992;10:896–903.

30. Buroker TR, O'Connell MJ, Wieand HS, et al. Randomized comparison of two schedules of fluorouracil and leucovorin in the treatment of advanced colorectal cancer. J Clin Oncol 1994;12:14–20.

31. Tomiak A, Vincent M, Kocha W, et al. Standard dose (Mayo regimen) 5-FU and folinic acid: prohibitive toxicity? Proc ASCO 1998;17:276a.

32. Jäger E, Heike M, Bernhard H, et al. Weekly high-dose leucovorin versus low-dose leucovorin combined with fluorouracil in advanced colorectal cancer: results of a randomized multicenter trial. J Clin Oncol 1996;14:2274–9.

33. Labianca R, Cascinu S, Frontini L, et al. High- versus low-dose levo-leucovorin as a modulator of 5-fluorouracil in advanced colorectal cancer: a "GISCAD" phase III study. Ann Oncol 1997;8:169–74.

34. Advanced Colorectal Cancer Meta-Analysis Project. Meta-analysis of randomized trials testing the biochemical modulation of fluorouracil by methotrexate in metastatic colorectal cancer. J Clin Oncol 1994;12:960–9.

35. Blanke CD, Kasimis B, Schein P, et al. Phase II study of trimetrexate, fluorouracil, and leucovorin for advanced colorectal cancer. J Clin Oncol 1997;15:915–20.

36. Punt CJA, Keizer HJ, Douma J, et al. Multicenter randomized trial of 5-fluorouracil and leucovorin with or without trimetrexate as first line treatment in patients with advanced colorectal cancer. Proc ASCO 1999;18:262a.

37 Raderer M, Scheithauer W. Treatment of advanced colorectal cancer with 5-fluorouracil and interferon-γ: an overview of clinical trials. Eur J Cancer 1995;31A:1002–8.

38. Leichman CG, Fleming TR, Muggia FM, et al. Phase II study of fluorouracil and its modulation in advanced colorectal cancer: a Southwest Oncology Group study. J Clin Oncol 1995;13:1303–11.

39. O'Dwyer PJ, Ryan LM, Valone FH, et al. Phase III trial of biochemical modulation of 5-fluorouracil by IV or oral leucovorin or by interferon in advanced colorectal cancer: an ECOG/CALGB Phase III trial. Proc ASCO 1996;15:207.

40. Sobrero AF, Aschele C, Bertino JR. Fluorouracil in colorectal cancer—a tale of two drugs: implications for biochemical modulation. J Clin Oncol 1997;15:368–81.

41. Rougier P, Paillot B, LaPlanche A, et al. 5-Fluorouracil continuous infusion compared with bolus administration: final results of a randomized trial in metastatic colorectal cancer. Eur J Cancer 1997;33:1789–93.

42. Meta-Analysis Group in Cancer. Efficacy of intravenous continuous infusion of fluorouracil compared with bolus administration in advanced colorectal cancer. J Clin Oncol 1998;16:301–8.

43. Glimelius B, Jakobsen A, Graf W, et al. Bolus injection (2–4 min) versus short-term (10–20 min) infusion of 5-fluorouracil in patients with advanced colorectal cancer: a prospective randomized trial. Eur J Cancer 1998;34:674–8.

44. De Gramont A, Vignoud J, Tournigand C, et al. Oxaliplatin with high-dose leucovorin and 5-fluorouracil 48-hour continuous infusion in pretreated metastatic colorectal cancer. Eur J Cancer 1997;33:214–9.

45. Meta-Analysis Group in Cancer. Toxicity of fluorouracil in patients with advanced colorectal cancer: effect of administration schedule and prognostic factors. J Clin Oncol 1998;16:3537–41.

46. Cascinu S, Fedeli A, Fideli SL, et al. Oral cooling (cryotherapy), an effective treatment for the prevention of 5-fluorouracil-induced stomatitis. Oral Oncol 1994;30B:234–6.

47. Miwa M, Ura M, Nishida M, et al. Design of a novel oral fluoropyrimidine carbamate, capecitabine, which generates 5-fluorouracil selectively in tumours by enzymes concentrated in human liver and cancer tissue. Eur J Cancer 1998;34:1274–81.

48. Twelves C, Harper P, Van Cutsem E, et al. A Phase III trial of Xeloda in previously untreated advanced/metastatic colorectal cancer. Proc ASCO 1999;18:263a.

49. Cox JV, Pazdur R, Thibault A, et al. A Phase III trial of Xeloda (capecitabine) in previously untreated advanced/metastatic colorectal cancer. Proc ASCO 1999;18:265a.

50. Carmichael J, Popiela T, Radstone D, et al. Randomized comparative study of ORZEL (oral uracil/tegafur—UFT) plus leucovorin versus parenteral 5-fluorouracil in patients with metastatic colorectal cancer. Proc ASCO 1999;18:264a.

51. Pazdur R, Douillard J-Y, Skillings JR, et al. Multicenter Phase III study of 5-fluorouracil or UFT in combination with leucovorin in patients with metastatic colorectal cancer. Proc ASCO 1999;18:263a.

52. Rothenberg ML. Topoisomerase I inhibitors: review and update. Ann Oncol 1997;8:837–55.

53. Rothenberg ML, Cox JV, DeVore RF, et al. A multicenter phase II trial of weekly irinotecan (CPT-11) in patients with previously treated colorectal cancer. Cancer 1999;85:786–95.

54. Cunningham D, Pyrhönen S, James RD, et al. Randomised trial of irinotecan plus supportive care versus supportive care alone after fluorouracil failure for patients with metastatic colorectal cancer. Lancet 1998;352:1413–8.

55. Rougier P, Van Cutsem E, Bajetta E, et al. Randomised trial of irinotecan versus fluorouracil by continuous infusion after fluorouracil failure in patients with metastatic colorectal cancer. Lancet 1998;352:1407–12.

56. Saltz LB, Locker PK, Pirotta N, et al. Weekly irinotecan, leucovorin, and fluorouracil is superior to daily × 5 leucovorin and 5-FU in patients with previously untreated metastatic colorectal cancer. Proc ASCO 1999;18:233a.

56a. Pharmacia & Upjohn. Irinotecan hydrochloride (CPT-11, Camptosar): Oncologic Drugs Advisory Committee Brochure, March 16, 2000, NDA No. 20-571, Suppl 9).

57. Douillard JY, Cunningham D, Roth AD, et al. Irinotecan combined with fluorouracil compared with fluorouracil alone as first-line treatment for metastatic colorectal cancer: a multicentre randomised trial. Lancet 2000;355:1041–7.

58. Raymond E, Faivre S, Woynarowski JM, Chaney SG. Oxaliplatin: mechanism of action and antineoplastic activity. Semin Oncol 1998;25:Suppl 5:4–12.

59. Becouarn Y, Ychou M, Ducreux M, et al. Oxaliplatin as first-line chemotherapy in metastatic colorectal cancer patients: preliminary activity/toxicity report. Proc ASCO 1997;16:229a.

60. Diaz-Rubio E, Sastre J, Zaniboni A. Oxaliplatin as single agent in previously untreated colorectal carcinoma patients: a phase II multicentric study. Ann Oncol 1998;9:105–8.

61. Machover D, Diaz-Rubio E, de Gramont A, et al. Two consecutive phase II studies of oxaliplatin for treatment of patients with advanced colorectal carcinoma who were resistant to previous treatment with fluoropyrimidines. Ann Oncol 1996;7:95–8.

62. Lévi F, Perpoint B, Garufi C, et al. Oxaliplatin activity against metastatic colorectal cancer: a phase II study of 5-day continuous infusion at circadian rhythm modulated rate. Eur J Cancer 1993;29A:1280–4.

63. de Gramont A, Bosset J-F, Milan C, et al. Randomized trial comparing monthly low-dose leucovorin and fluorouracil bolus with bimonthly high-dose leucovorin and fluorouracil bolus plus continuous infusion for advanced colorectal cancer: a French intergroup study. J Clin Oncol 1997;15:808–15.

64. Lévi F, Misset J-L, Brienza S, et al. A chronopharmacologic phase II clinical trial with 5-fluorouracil, folinic acid, and oxaliplatin using an ambulatory multichannel programmable pump: high antitumor effectiveness against metastatic colorectal cancer. Cancer 1992;69:893–900.

65. Lévi F, Dogliotti L, Perpoint B, et al. A multicenter phase II trial of intensified chronotherapy with oxaliplatin, 5-fluorouracil and folinic acid in patients with previously untreated metastatic colorectal cancer. Proc ASCO 1997;16:266a.

66. Lévi F, Zidani R, Vannetzel J-M, et al. Chronomodulated versus fixed-infusion-rate delivery of ambulatory chemotherapy with oxaliplatin, fluorouracil, and folinic acid (leucovorin) in patients with colorectal cancer metastases: a randomized multi-institutional trial. J Natl Cancer Inst 1994;86:1608–17.

67. Lévi F, Zidani R, Misset J-L. Randomised multicentre trial of chronotherapy with oxaliplatin, fluorouracil, and folinic acid in metastatic colorectal cancer. For the International Organization for Cancer Chronotherapy. Lancet 1997;350:681–6.

68. Giacchetti S, Perpoint B, Zidani R, et al. Phase III multicenter randomized trial of oxaliplatin added to chronomodulated fluorouracil-leucovorin as first-line treatment of metastatic colorectal cancer. J Clin Oncol 2000;18:136–47.

69. Giacchetti S, Brienza S, Focan C, et al. Contribution of second line oxaliplatin-chronomodulated 5-fluorouracil-folinic acid and surgery to survival in metastatic colorectal cancer patients. Proc ASCO 1998;17:273a.

70. De Gramont A, Figer A, Seymour M, et al. A randomized trial of leucovorin and 5-fluorouracil with or without oxaliplatin in advanced colorectal cancer. Proc ASCO 1998;17:257a.

70a. Sanofi-Synthelabo Research: Oncologic Drugs Advisory Committee Meeting briefing document of the effectiveness and safety of oxaliplatin in combination with 5-FU–based chemotherapy in the treatment of advanced colorectal cancer. 14 February 2000 (http://www.fda.gov/ohrms/dockets/ac/00/backgrd/3592b1cx.pdf).

71. Cunningham D, Zalcberg JR, Rath U, et al. Tomudex (ZD1694): results of a randomised trial in advanced colorectal cancer demonstrate efficacy and reduced mucositis and leucopenia. Eur J Cancer 1995;31A:1945–54.

72. Cocconi G, Cunningham D, Van Cutsem E, et al. Open, randomized, multicenter trial of raltitrexed versus fluorouracil plus high-dose leucovorin in patients with advanced colorectal cancer. J Clin Oncol 1998;16:2943–52.

73. Maughan TS, James RD, Kerr D, et al. Preliminary results of a multicentre randomised trial comparing 3 chemotherapy regimens (de Gramont, Lokich, and raltitrexed) in metastatic colorectal cancer. Proc ASCO 1999;18:262a.

74. Pazdur R, Vincent M. Raltitrexed (Tomudex) versus 5-fluorouracil and leucovorin in patients with advanced colorectal cancer: results of a randomized, multicenter, North American trial. Proc ASCO 1998;17:228a.

75. Krook JE, Moertel CG, Gunderson LL, et al. Effective surgical adjuvant therapy for high-risk rectal carcinoma. N Engl J Med 1991;324:709–15.

76. O'Connell MJ, Martenson JA, Wieand HS, et al. Improving adjuvant therapy for rectal cancer by combining protracted-infusion fluorouracil with radiation therapy after curative surgery. N Engl J Med 1994;331:502–7.

77. Tepper JE, O'Connell MJ, Petroni GR, et al. Adjuvant postoperative fluorouracil-modulated chemotherapy combined with pelvic radiation therapy for rectal cancer: initial results of Intergroup 0114. J Clin Oncol 1997;15:2030–9.

78. Minsky BD, Cohen AM, Enke WE, et al. Sphincter preservation with preoperative radiation therapy and coloanal anastomosis. Int J Radiat Oncol Biol Phys 1995;31:553–9.

79. Rich TA, Skipper JM, Ajani JA, et al. Preoperative infusional chemoradiation for stage T3 rectal cancer. Int J Radiat Oncol Biol Phys 1995;32:1025–9.

80. Minsky BD, Cohen AM, Kemeny N, et al. Enhancement of radiation-induced downstaging of rectal cancer by 5-FU and high-dose leucovorin chemotherapy. J Clin Oncol 1992;10:79–84.

81. Medical Research Council Rectal Cancer Working Party. Randomised trial of surgery alone versus surgery followed by radiotherapy for mobile cancer of the rectum. Lancet 1996;348:1610–4.

82. Swedish Rectal Cancer Trial. Improved survival with preoperative radiotherapy in resectable rectal cancer. N Engl J Med 1997;336:980–7.

83. Bognel C, Rekacewicz C, Mankarios H, et al. Prognostic value of neural invasion in rectal carcinoma: a multivariate analysis on 339 patients with curative resection. Eur J Cancer 1995;31A:894–8.

84. Kerr DJ, Rustin GJ, Kaye SB, et al. Phase II trials of rhizoxin in advanced ovarian, colorectal, and renal cancer. Br J Cancer 1995;72:1267–9.

85. Bajetta E, Colleoni M, Di Bartolomeo M, et al. Doxifluridine and leucovorin: an oral treatment combination in advanced colorectal cancer. J Clin Oncol 1995;13:2613–9.

86. Bajetta E, Di Bartolomeo M, Somma L, et al. Randomized phase II noncomparative trial of oral and intravenous doxifluridine plus levoleucovorin in untreated patients with advanced colorectal cancer. Cancer 1996;78:2087–93.

87. Falcone A, Pfanner E, Ricci S, et al. Oral doxifluridine in elderly patients with metastatic colorectal cancer: a multicenter Phase II study. Ann Oncol 1994;5:760–2.

88. Neri B, Gemelli MT, Pantalone D, et al. Results of leucovorin and doxifluridine oral regimen in the treatment of metastatic colorectal cancer. Anticancer Drugs 1998;9:599–602.

89. Pazdur R, Diaz-Canton E, Ballard WP, et al. Phase II trial of 9-aminocamptothecin administered as a 72-hour continuous infusion in metastatic colorectal carcinoma. J Clin Oncol 1997;15:2905–9.

90. Medgyesy D, Pazdur R, Dakhil S, et al. Phase II trial of 5-day continuous infusion of 9-amino camptothecin in advanced colorectal carcinomas. Proc ASCO 1998;17:296a.

91. Otto F, Schmid P, Mackensen A, et al. Phase II trial of intravenous endotoxin in patients with colorectal and non-small cell lung cancer. Eur J Cancer 1996;32A:1712–8.

92. Eymard JC, Lopez M, Cattan A, et al. Phase I/II trial of autologous activated macrophages in advanced colorectal cancer. Eur J Cancer 1996;32A:1905–11.

93. Dirix LY, Tonnesen F, Cassidy J, et al. EO9 Phase II study in advanced breast, gastric, pancreatic, and colorectal carcinoma by the EORTC early clinical studies group. Eur J Cancer 1996;32A:2019–2023.

94. Goldberg RM, Moertel CG, Wieand HS, et al. A phase III evaluation of a somatostatin analogue (octreotide) in the treatment of patients with asymptomatic advanced colon carcinoma. Cancer 1995;76:961–6.

95. Verweij J, Wanders J, Nielsen AL, et al. Phase II studies of elsamitrucin in breast cancer, colorectal cancer, non-small cell lung cancer, and ovarian cancer. Ann Oncol 1994;5:375–6.

96. Pazdur R, Lassere Y, Soh LT, et al. Phase II trial of docetaxel (Taxotere) in metastatic colorectal cancer. Ann Oncol 1994;5:468–70.

97. Macdonald JS, Benedetti JK, Modiano M, Alberts DS. Phase II evaluation of topotecan in patients with advanced colorectal cancer: a Southwest Oncology Group trial (SWOG-9241). Invest New Drugs 1997;15:357–9.

98. Rowinsky EK, Baker SD, Burks K, et al. High-dose topotecan with granulocyte-colony stimulating factor in fluoropyrimidine-refractory colorectal cancer: a Phase II and pharmacodynamic study. Ann Oncol 1998;9:173–80.

99. Zalupski MM, Philip PA, LoRusso P, Shields AF. Phase II study of pyrazoloacridine in patients with advanced colorectal carcinoma. Cancer Chemother Pharmacol 1997;40:225–7.

100. Shields AF, Philip PA, LoRusso PM, et al. Phase II study of CI-958 in colorectal cancer. Cancer Chemother Pharmacol 1999;43:162–4.

101. Ajani JA, Pazdur R, Duman P, Fairweather J. Phase II study of prolonged infusion of Taxol in patients with metastatic colorectal carcinoma. Invest New Drugs 1998;16:175–7.

102. Abad A, Gravalos C, Font A, et al. Phase II study of mitonafide in advanced and relapsed colorectal cancer. Invest New Drugs 1996;14:223–5.

103. Clamon GH, Riggs CE Jr, Dreicer R, Hohl RJ. Phase II trial of edatrexate in patients with metastatic colorectal cancer. Invest New Drugs 1996;13:359–61.

104. Strumberg D, Harstrick A, Klaassen U, et al. Phase II trial of continuous oral trofosfamide in patients with advanced colorectal cancer refractory to 5-fluorouracil. Anticancer Drugs 1997;8:293–5.

105. Brown TD, Fleming TR, Goodman PJ, et al. A randomized trial of two schedules of trimetrexate versus 5-fluorouracil in advanced colorectal cancer: a Southwest Oncology Group study. Anticancer Drugs 1995;6:219–23.

106. Pazdur R, Bready B, Ajani JA, et al. Phase II trial of isotretinoin and recombinant interferon alfa-2a in metastatic colorectal carcinoma. Am J Clin Oncol 1995;18:436–8.

107. Pazdur R, Meyers C, Diaz-Canton E, et al. Phase II trial of intravenous CI-980 (NSC 370147) in patients with metastatic colorectal carcinoma. Am J Clin Oncol 1997;20:573–6.

108. Bennett P, Mani S, O'Reilly S, et al. Phase II trial of flavopiridol in metastatic colorectal cancer: preliminary results. Proc ASCO 1999;18:277a.

109. Paulson R, Hainsworth J, Geyer C, et al. A Phase II trial of MTA (multitargeted antifolate, LY231514) in patients with 5-FU and irinotecan-refractory colorectal cancer. Proc ASCO 1999;18:297a.

110. John W, Picus J, Blanke C, et al. Activity of MTA (LY231514) in patients with advanced colorectal cancer—results from a Phase II study. Proc ASCO 1998;17:277a.

111. Mani S, Beck T, Chevlen E, et al. A Phase II open-label study to evaluate a 28-day regimen of oral 5-fluorouracil plus 776C85 for the treatment of patients with previously untreated metastatic colorectal cancer. Proc ASCO 1998;17:281a

# TREATMENT BY STAGE OF DISEASE

● Charles M. Haskell

Surgery is the cornerstone of management for colorectal cancer. It is used with curative intent in patients with resectable disease, and it is the most effective way of dealing with impending bowel obstruction in patients with unresectable tumors. Radiation therapy and chemotherapy are useful adjuncts to surgery, but their optimal use varies greatly among patients with different sites and stages of disease.

## STAGE I AND LOW-RISK STAGE II (T3 N0 M0) COLORECTAL CANCER

Patients with stage I and low-risk stage II disease are treated with surgical excision of the primary tumor. For patients with small, well-differentiated rectal lesions, local excision may be adequate.[1] Most of these patients, however, require a more complete resection, including the removal of the regional lymph nodes. There is a trend to preserve anal function wherever possible, although some patients still require an abdominoperineal resection. Postoperative radiation therapy, either alone or with chemotherapy, is not indicated for patients treated with a low anterior resection or abdominoperineal resection but should be considered for patients with rectal carcinomas treated with a limited local excision.[2]

## HIGH-RISK STAGE II (T4 N0 M0) AND STAGE III COLON CANCER

Patients with high-risk stage II and stage III disease are generally treated with an extensive surgical resection, including removal of regional lymph nodes. Adjuvant chemotherapy is also indicated for patients with stage III disease, although the choice of regimen is controversial.[3] The usual

*Table 43–18.* **Adjuvant Therapy for Stage III Colon Cancer***

*5-FU + Leucovorin × 6 mo (Mayo/NCCTG Regimen)[4–6]*

5-FU 425 mg/m² + leucovorin 20 mg/m² on days 1 through 5, both drugs given by rapid IV injection, repeated every 4–5 wk for 6 mo

*5-FU + Levamisole × 12 mo[7]*

5-FU 450 mg/m² by rapid IV injection, daily for 5 days, then weekly for 48 wk
Levamisole 50 mg orally 3 times daily for 3 days, every 2 wk for 1 yr

*Weekly 5-FU + Leucovorin × 12 mo (Roswell Park/NSABP Regimen)[8]*

Leucovorin 500 mg/m², given IV over 2 hr, with 5-FU 500 mg/m² given as an IV bolus injection 1 hour later, weekly during 6 of every 8 wk for 1 yr

*Drug regimens are started 3–5 weeks after surgery. All these regimens are potentially toxic and may occasionally be associated with toxicity-related mortality. Important details of drug administration are provided in the references cited. These regimens should be used only by clinicians experienced in the administration of cancer chemotherapy.
5-FU, 5-fluorouracil; IV, intravenous.

adjuvant treatment in the United States is a 6-month course of 5-FU plus low-dose leucovorin, as described in Table 43–18.[4, 5] Many clinicians consider the doses of 5-FU listed for the Mayo Clinic regimen in Table 43–18 to be excessively toxic.[6] As an alternative to this high-dose treatment, one can use a 12-month course of adjuvant weekly 5-FU plus biweekly levamisole,[7] a year of weekly 5-FU plus high-dose leucovorin,[8] or the de Gramont regimen described in the section Chemotherapy.

The use of adjuvant chemotherapy in patients with high-risk stage II disease is controversial.[9–11] The risks and potential benefits of such therapy should be discussed with the patient, although the weight of current evidence argues against the routine use of adjuvant therapy for patients with stage II disease unless complicated by obstruction or perforation of the bowel. Radiation therapy to the tumor bed may be considered for patients with primary tumors adherent to the peritoneum in a well-defined and treatable area, although there is no evidence that such treatment extends survival.[12]

## HIGH-RISK STAGE II (T4 N0 M0) AND STAGE III RECTAL CANCER

In the United States, most clinicians use combined-modality therapy for the management of patients with high-risk stage II and stage III disease. The optimal use of each modality is controversial and the subject of ongoing randomized clinical trials. Lacking definitive results from these trials, I usually base the timing and use of modalities on the judgment of the operating surgeon. If the surgeon believes the rectal lesion can be resected reasonably easily, surgical resection is undertaken, and subsequent management is tailored to the pathologic stage of disease. This management almost always includes a course of postoperative chemoradiotherapy using one of the regimens listed in Table 43–19.[13, 14, 17] If the surgeon has significant doubts about the resectability of the lesion, I usually proceed with preoperative (neoadjuvant) chemoradiotherapy, as described in Table 43–20.[15–17] This therapy is followed by surgical resection, if feasible, followed by additional chemotherapy for a total duration of chemotherapy of at least 6 months.

In many centers, particularly in Europe, the surgical resection is of the mesorectal type, which provides more complete surgical clearance of perirectal tissues than with traditional low anterior or abdominoperineal resections.[18] The role of postoperative radiation therapy in patients treated with this form of resection is uncertain.

## STAGE IV COLORECTAL CANCER

Patients with recurrent disease after initial surgical resection may benefit from resection of a local or metastatic recurrence.[19] This is particularly true of patients with recurrent

*Table 43–19.* **Adjuvant Therapy for Patients with High-Risk Pathologic Stage II or III Rectal Cancer***

| Study | Preradiation Chemotherapy | Chemoradiotherapy | Postradiation Chemotherapy |
|---|---|---|---|
| INT-0114[13] | 5-FU 425 mg/m$^2$/day, days 1–5, 29–33<br>Leucovorin 20 mg/m$^2$/day, days 1–5, 29–33 | RT 50.4–54 Gy/5 wk starting day 57 + 5-FU 400 mg/m$^2$/day, days 57–60, 85–88 + leucovorin 20 mg/m$^2$/day, days 57–60, 85–88 | 5-FU 380 mg/m$^2$/day, days 1–5, 29–33 + leucovorin 20 mg/m$^2$/day, days 1–5, 29–33 (begin 28 days after end of RT) |
| Mayo Clinic–NCCTG[14] | 5-FU 500 mg/m$^2$/day, days 1–5, 36–40 | RT 50.4–54 Gy/5 wk starting day 64 + 5-FU 225 mg/m$^2$/day as a continuous infusion throughout RT or 500 mg/m$^2$/day for 3 consecutive days during wk 1 and 5 of RT | 5-FU 450 mg/m$^2$/day, days 134–138 and 169–173 |
| NSABP R-03[17] | *Cycle 1:* Leucovorin 500 mg/m$^2$ over 2 hr IV, with 5-FU 500 mg/m$^2$ after 1 hr, days 1, 8, 15, 22, 29, and 36, followed by 21-day rest | *Cycles 2 and 3:* Leucovorin 20 mg/m$^2$ and 5-FU 325 mg/m$^2$ IV bolus days 1–5 and 29–33, given with 50.4 Gy/5 wk | *Cycles 4–7:* Same as cycle 1, to start 8 wk after the completion of RT |

*Drug regimens are started 3–5 weeks after surgery. All of these regimens are potentially quite toxic and may occasionally be associated with toxicity-related mortality. Important details of drug administration are provided in the references cited. These regimens should be used only by clinicians experienced in the administration of cancer chemotherapy.

5-FU, 5-fluorouracil; RT, radiation therapy; IV, intravenous.

disease in the liver, as discussed in Chapter 104.[20, 21] Palliative surgery or radiation therapy, or both, may also be used as needed for problems such as bowel obstruction or localized areas of painful tumor infiltration (e.g., bone metastases).

Patients with metastatic disease should be offered treatment with a fluoropyrimidine-based regimen, as discussed in the section Chemotherapy. Choosing a specific drug regimen may be influenced by a variety of patient-related factors, such as the patient's nutritional status, performance status, co-morbid conditions, and prior treatment (especially chemotherapy or chemoradiotherapy). Other factors may also be important in the decision-making process, such as the experience of the oncologist, the availability of supportive care services, the cost of the drugs, and the mature results of relevant clinical trials. Based on two preliminary reports at the time of this writing, the best front-line chemotherapy for metastatic colorectal cancer patients who have not received prior chemotherapy or chemoradiotherapy appears to be the combination of irinotecan, 5-fluorouracil, and leucovorin (see Table 43–15).[22, 23]

## POSTOPERATIVE FOLLOW-UP

Postoperative follow-up is primarily directed toward the early detection of recurrence amenable to salvage therapy and the identification of any missed areas of synchronous disease. Guidelines for follow-up are empirical and have not been critically tested in clinical trials.[24, 25] Lacking tested guidelines, I generally examine patients every 3 to 4 months for the first 2 years after surgery and then every 6 months from years 2 through 5; annual follow-up is recommended after 5 years. The frequency of diagnostic tests is controversial. I obtain a complete blood count, biochemical panel, and serum CEA (in patients with an elevated level of CEA preoperatively) at each visit. Colonoscopy is generally repeated about 1 year after surgery, looking for new or syn-

*Table 43–20.* **Preoperative (Neoadjuvant) Chemoradiotherapy for High-Risk Clinical Stage II and Stage III Patients with Rectal Cancer**

| Study | Representative Treatment Regimens | |
|---|---|---|
| | CHEMOTHERAPY | RADIATION THERAPY |
| Rich et al[15] | 5-FU 300 mg/m$^2$/day by continuous IV infusion concurrent with RT | 45 Gy/25 fractions/5 wk |
| Stryker et al[16] | 5-FU 1000 mg/m$^2$/day by continuous infusion days 1–5 and 28–32 and mitomycin C 10 mg/m$^2$ IV bolus day 1 of RT | 45–50 Gy over 5 wk, followed by surgery 4–8 wk later |
| NSABP R-03[17] | *Cycle 1:* Leucovorin 500 mg/m$^2$ over 2 hr IV with 5-FU 500 mg/m$^2$ after 1 hr, days 1, 8, 15, 22, 29, and 36, followed by 21-day rest<br>*Cycles 2 and 3:* Leucovorin 20 mg/m$^2$ and 5-FU 325 mg/m$^2$ IV bolus days 1, 2, 3, 4, 5 and 29, 30, 31, 32, and 33<br>*Cycles 4–7:* Same as cycle 1, to start 4 wk after surgical resection | 50.4 Gy/5 wk starting with the beginning of cycle 2. Surgical resection 8 wk after completion of RT |

5-FU, 5-fluorouracil; IV, intravenous; RT, radiation therapy.

chronous adenomatous polyps and any evidence of a suture line recurrence.[26, 27] Radiographic studies are obtained on an individual basis, depending on the patient's symptoms.[28] Further discussion of this topic can be found in the section on surgical therapy for recurrent disease and in the Recommended Colorectal Cancer Surveillance Guidelines of the American Society of Clinical Oncology.[29]

## SUGGESTIONS FOR ADDITIONAL READING

Gryfe R, Swallow C, Bapat B, et al. Molecular biology of colorectal cancer. Curr Probl Cancer 1997;21:233–300.

Lurie JD, Welch HG. Diagnostic testing following fecal occult blood screening in the elderly. J Natl Cancer Inst 1999;91:1641–6.

Havenga K, Enker WE, Norstein J, et al. Improved survival and local control after total mesorectal excision or D3 lymphadenectomy in the treatment of primary rectal cancer: an international analysis of 1411 patients. Eur J Surg Oncol 1999;25:368–74.

Vaughn DJ, Haller DG. The role of adjuvant chemotherapy in the treatment of colorectal cancer. Hematol Oncol Clin North Am 1997;11:699–719.

Bertino JR. Chemotherapy of colorectal cancer: history and new themes. Semin Oncol 1997;24:5 Suppl 18:S18-3–7.

Labianca R, Pancera G, Luporini G. Factors influencing response rates for advanced colorectal cancer chemotherapy. Ann Oncol 1996;7:901–6.

## REFERENCES

1. Gérard A, Pector JC, Ferreira J. Local excision as conservative treatment for small rectal cancer. Eur J Surg Oncol 1989;15:544–6.
2. Fortunato L, Ahmad NR, Yeung RS, et al. Long-term follow-up of local excision and radiation therapy for invasive rectal cancer. Dis Colon Rectum 1995;38:1193–9.
3. Slevin ML, Papamichael D, Rougier P, Schmoll HJ. Is there a standard adjuvant treatment for colon cancer? Eur J Cancer 1998;34:1652–63.
4. O'Connell MJ, Mailliard JA, Kahn MJ, et al. Controlled trial of fluorouracil and low-dose leucovorin given for 6 months as postoperative adjuvant therapy for colon cancer. J Clin Oncol 1997;15:246–50.
5. Buroker TR, O'Connell MJ, Wieand HS, et al. Randomized comparison of two schedules of fluorouracil and leucovorin in the treatment of advanced colorectal cancer. J Clin Oncol 1994;12:14–20.
6. Vincent M, Whiston F, Tomiak A. Mini-meta-analysis of toxicity of full dose Mayo regimen from two randomized controlled trials: a concern about dose. Proc ASCO 1999;18:242a.
7. Moertel CG, Fleming TR, Macdonald JS, et al. Fluorouracil plus levamisole as effective adjuvant therapy after resection of stage III colon carcinoma: a final report. Ann Intern Med 1995;122:321–6.
8. Wolmark N, Rockette H, Mamounas E, et al. Clinical trial to assess the relative efficacy of fluorouracil and leucovorin, fluorouracil and levamisole, and fluorouracil, leucovorin, and levamisole in patients with Dukes' B and C carcinoma of the colon: results from National Surgical Adjuvant Breast and Bowel Project C-04. J Clin Oncol 1999;17:3553–9.
9. Moertel CG, Fleming TR, Macdonald JS, et al. Intergroup study of fluorouracil plus levamisole as adjuvant therapy for stage II/Dukes' B2 colon cancer. J Clin Oncol 1995;13:2936–43.
10. Efficacy of adjuvant fluorouracil and folinic acid in B2 colon cancer. International Multicentre Pooled Analysis of B2 Colon Cancer Trials (IMPACT B2) investigators. J Clin Oncol 1999;17:1356–63.
11. Mamounas E, Wieand S, Wolmark N, et al. Comparative efficacy of adjuvant chemotherapy in patients with Dukes' B versus Dukes' C colon cancer: results from four National Surgical Adjuvant Breast and Bowel Project adjuvant studies (C-01, C-02, C-03, and C-04). J Clin Oncol 1999;17:1349–55.
12. Sargent D, Donohue J, Goldberg R, et al. A Phase III study of adjuvant radiation therapy, 5-fluorouracil, and levamisole versus 5-fluorouracil and levamisole in selected patients with resected, high risk colon cancer: initial results of Int 0130. Proc ASCO 1999;18:235a.
13. Tepper JE, O'Connell MJ, Petroni GR, et al. Adjuvant postoperative fluorouracil-modulated chemotherapy combined with pelvic radiation therapy for rectal cancer: initial results of intergroup 0114. J Clin Oncol 1997;15:2030–9.
14. O'Connell MJ, Martenson JA, Wieand HS, et al. Improving adjuvant therapy for rectal cancer by combining protracted-infusion fluorouracil with radiation therapy after curative surgery. N Engl J Med 1994;331:502–7.
15. Rich TA, Skibber JM, Ajani JA, et al. Preoperative infusional chemoradiation therapy for stage T3 rectal cancer. Int J Radiat Oncol Biol Phys 1995;32:1025–9.
16. Stryker SJ, Kiel KD, Rademaker A, et al. Preoperative "chemoradiation" for stages II and III rectal carcinoma. Arch Surg 1996;131:514–8.
17. Hyams DM, Mamounas EP, Petrelli N, et al. A clinical trial to evaluate the worth of preoperative multimodality therapy in patients with operable carcinoma of the rectum: a progress report of National Surgical Breast and Bowel Project Protocol R-03. Dis Colon Rectum 1997;40:131–9.
18. Havenga K, Enker WE, Norstein J, et al. Improved survival and local control after total mesorectal excision or D3 lymphadenectomy in the treatment of primary rectal cancer: an international analysis of 1411 patients. Eur J Surg Oncol 1999;25:368–74.
19. Goldberg RM, Fleming TR, Tangen CM, et al. Surgery for recurrent colon cancer: strategies for identifying resectable recurrence and success rates after resection. Eastern Cooperative Oncology Group, the North Central Cancer Treatment Group, and the Southwest Oncology Group. Ann Intern Med 1998;129:27–35.
20. Kemeny N, Cohen A, Huang Y, et al. Randomized study of hepatic arterial infusion and systemic chemotherapy versus systemic chemotherapy alone as adjuvant therapy after resection of hepatic metastases from colorectal cancer. Proc ASCO 1999;18:263a.
21. Kemeny MM, Adak S, Lipsitz S, et al. Results of the intergroup (Eastern Cooperative Oncology Group and Southwest Oncology Group) prospective randomized study of surgery alone versus continuous infusion of FUDR and continuous systemic infusion of 5-FU after hepatic resection for colorectal liver metastases. Proc ASCO 1999;18:264a.
22. Saltz LB, Locker PK, Pirotta N, et al: Weekly irinotecan, leucovorin, and fluorouracil is superior to daily ×5 leucorovin and 5-FU in patients with previously untreated metastatic colorectal cancer. Proc Am Soc Clin Oncol 1999;18:233a.
23. Douillard JY, Cunningham D, Roth AD, et al. Irinotecan combined with fluorouracil compared with fluorouracil alone as first-line treatment for metastatic colorectal cancer; a multicentre randomised trial. Lancet 2000;355:1041–7.
24. Steele G Jr. Standard postoperative monitoring of patients after primary resection of colon and rectum cancer. Cancer 1993;71:Suppl:4225–35.
25. Johnson FE, Virgo KS, eds. Cancer patients follow-up. St. Louis: CV Mosby, 1997.
26. Patchett SE, Mulcahy HE, O'Donoghue DP. Colonoscopic surveillance after curative resection for colorectal cancer. Br J Surg 1993;80:1330–2.
27. Barlow AP, Thompson MH. Colonoscopic follow-up after resection for colorectal cancer: a selective policy. Br J Surg 1993;80:781–4.
28. Scharling ES, Wolfman NT, Bechtold RE. Computed tomography evaluation of colorectal carcinoma. Semin Roentgenol 1996;31:142–53.
29. Desch CE, Benson AB III, Smith TJ, et al. Recommended colorectal cancer surveillance guidelines by the American Society of Clinical Oncology. J Clin Oncol 1999;17:1312–21.

# CHAPTER 44

## ANAL CANAL

........................................

## NATURAL HISTORY, DIAGNOSIS, AND STAGING

• Charles M. Haskell

In the past, abdominoperineal resection was the only potentially curative treatment for neoplasms of the anal canal. This procedure was associated with major morbidity and loss of bowel continuity. Today, combined-modality therapy with radiation therapy and chemotherapy provides the same cure rate but with preservation of bowel continuity in most patients. The success of combined-modality therapy for patients with epidermoid carcinoma of the anal canal provides a model for improving the results of treatment in other organs, and it has made the use of the abdominoperineal resection nearly obsolete as initial therapy.

### EPIDEMIOLOGY AND ETIOLOGY

**Incidence and Mortality Rates.** Based on Surveillance, Epidemiology, and End Results (SEER) data,[1] the annual incidence of neoplasms of the anus, anal canal, and anorectum is 1 per 100,000 in the United States. The relative frequency in males and females is now about the same (0.9 and 1.0 per 100,000, respectively). These neoplasms constitute 0.25% of all malignant neoplasms in the United States and 1.4% of all malignant neoplasms of the digestive system. The overall 5-year survival rate is 59.6%, whereas it is 54% in males and 63.5% in females.

**Risk Factors.** Anorectal disorders such as hemorrhoids, fissures, pruritus, and incontinence are common, whereas cancer of the anus is relatively rare.[2] There is a strong association between the diagnosis of benign anal lesions and the diagnosis of anal cancer, although a large Danish study did not consider the frequency sufficient to prove a causal link between the two.[3] Anal neoplasms compose about 2 to 3% of all malignancies of the bowel, with tumors of the anal canal being more frequent in women and perianal and rectal cancers more common in men.[4] The average age of these patients is 60 years,[4] although the average age may be somewhat younger in some subgroups of patients. For example, renal transplant recipients have a 100-fold increase in the incidence of carcinomas of the vulva and anus, with an average age of 37 years for females and 45 years for males.[5]

One of the most striking associations of anal cancer is with patients with acquired immunodeficiency syndrome (AIDS). The relative risk of anal cancer in homosexual men with AIDS has been reported to be 84.1 (95% confidence interval, 46.4 to 152).[6] This has resulted in a marked increase in the number of cases of anal carcinoma seen in men in urban centers.[7] Inflammatory bowel disease has been associ-

ated with an increased incidence of anal carcinoma. In one review, the relative incidence of anal cancer to all forms of colorectal cancer was 14%, compared with 1.4% in patients without inflammatory bowel disease.[8] There may be a hereditary component in some patients, as seen with two dizygotic twins who developed cloacogenic carcinoma of the anus almost simultaneously.[9]

### MOLECULAR PATHOGENESIS

The etiology and molecular pathogenesis of anal cancer are poorly defined but probably follow the process of multistep carcinogenesis that is unfolding for other malignant neoplasms, especially cervical cancer.[10] This process includes the formation of sequential steps of intraepithelial neoplasia before the development of invasive cancer.[11] It is likely that the initiation of this process is due to human papillomavirus infection[12] or infection with *Chlamydia trachomatis* and herpes simplex virus 2.[13–15] Promotion of carcinogenesis may be due to cigarette smoking[12, 16] or chronic irritation (as with inflammatory bowel disease), possibly augmented by states of immunosuppression (as seen with renal transplantation or AIDS).

The development of anal squamous neoplasia is strongly associated with aberrant expression of the *p53* oncogene.[17] Cytogenetic changes may be common during this process. For example, a study of eight cases of anal cancer, including one cloacogenic and seven squamous cell lesions, has been reported from Paris.[18] All the tumors had chromosomal abnormalities, the most consistent being recurrent deletions of chromosomes 11q and 3p. Further study is needed to define the details of this process.

### ANATOMIC CONSIDERATIONS

The terminology defining the anus and its anatomic subdivisions is confusing and varies among disciplines. The proximal margin of the anus is the anorectal ring, and the distal margin is the anal verge at the intersphincteric groove.[19] Some authorities subdivide this area into the anal canal and the anal margin; for the purposes of this discussion, the entire area is considered the anal canal. The perianal skin is not discussed in this chapter. This area of skin is managed the same as are other areas of skin (see Chapter 76).

## PATHOLOGY

The anus represents a blending of epithelial surfaces of soft tissues that can give rise to a variety of carcinomas and sarcomas, as noted in Figure 44–1. Thus adenocarcinomas and adenoacanthomas can arise from anal crypts and glands, or they may extend from a site of origin in the rectum; squamous cell carcinomas and malignant melanomas can arise from squamous epithelium of the anal canal; basal cell epitheliomas, Paget's disease, and Bowen's disease can arise from the perianal skin; and lymphomas and sarcomas can arise from the soft tissues.[20] Small cell carcinomas may also arise from neuroendocrine cells within the anus.[21]

Squamous cell cancers compose almost 90% of lesions in the area of the anus. Generally, they are poorly differentiated, and 20% have a basaloid appearance characterized by small basophilic cells. These have been designated *cloacogenic* or *transitional cell anal tumors* and may have an appearance similar to that of large bowel carcinomas.[22]

## CLINICAL FEATURES AND DIAGNOSIS

Early carcinoma of the anus often presents as a small nodule resembling a hemorrhoidal tag. As it increases in size, it becomes ulcerated and eventually may turn into an exophytic mass. Internally, it may extend beneath the intact rectal mucosa and become ulcerated farther above in the form of an apparently separate rectal tumor. Most arise in the anterior or posterior anal quadrants. Progressive growth can result in invasion of perianal skin, sphincter muscles, perirectal fat, prostate, bladder, cervix, and pelvic structures.[23] At the time of initial surgical treatment, 28 to 64% of patients are found to have involvement of perirectal or mesenteric nodes, and

up to 27% have inguinal node metastases.[24] Ten percent of patients may have hepatic metastases at the time of surgery.

Two of the first symptoms observed in carcinoma of the anus are pruritus and bleeding. Tenesmus and pain that is not relieved by defecation may become increasingly noticeable. These symptoms are indistinguishable from those of several common anorectal disorders, so the minimal evaluation of all patients with rectal symptoms is sigmoidoscopy.[2] Common constitutional symptoms, such as fever, weight loss, anemia, and weakness, are usually absent unless the lesion is far advanced. If the mass becomes large enough to obstruct the bowel lumen, severe constipation may result.

Tumor markers are of no established value in the diagnosis, staging, or follow-up of these neoplasms.[25] That includes the carcinoembryonic antigen test[26] and a test used by some investigators that involves a radioimmunoassay for a squamous cell carcinoma antigen.[27]

## STAGING

There are two staging systems for carcinomas of the anal canal. An international TNM system was published in 1988 and is given in Table 44–1 for reference purposes. It is based on the fact that prognosis is largely a function of the size and location of the tumor and extent of spread.[28, 29]

An alternative staging system has been developed by Papillon and coworkers[29] from Lyon, France. Since this system has commonly been used in many of the clinical trials discussed later in this chapter, we summarize it here briefly. It is primarily a clinical staging system based on an assessment of the primary tumor, as follows: T1, tumors less than 2 cm in diameter; T2, tumors between 2 and 4 cm; T3, tumors larger than 4 cm—these tumors are mobile, infiltrat-

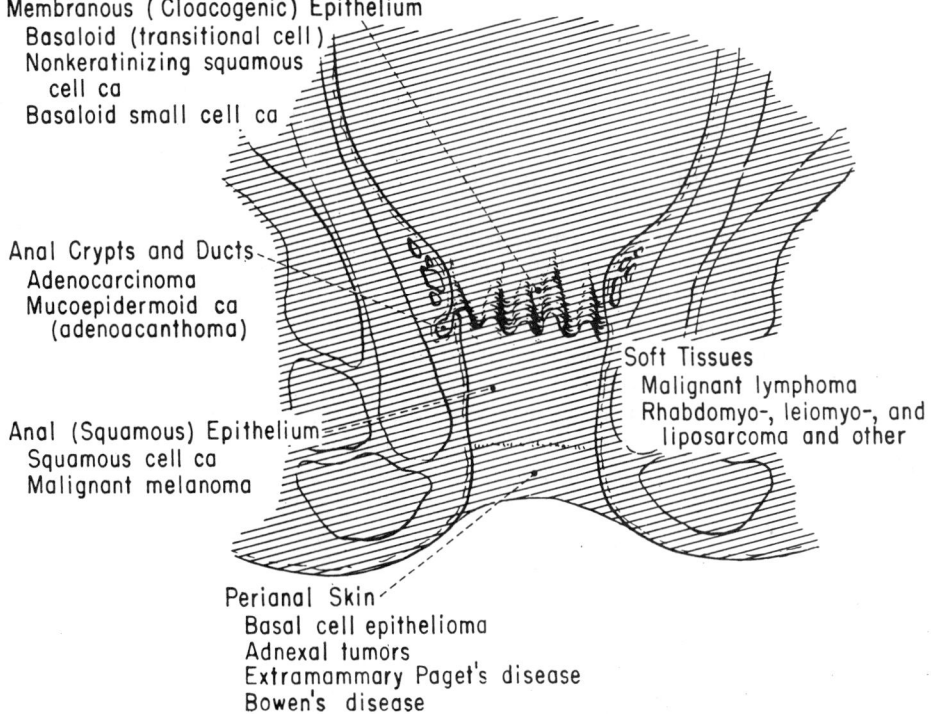

**Figure 44–1.** Malignant lesions originating from the various tissues in the area of the anus. (From Harrison EG Jr, Beahrs OH, Hill JR. Anal and perianal malignant neoplasms: pathology and treatment. Dis Colon Rectum 1966;9:255.)

Membranous (Cloacogenic) Epithelium
  Basaloid (transitional cell)
  Nonkeratinizing squamous
    cell ca
  Basaloid small cell ca

Anal Crypts and Ducts
  Adenocarcinoma
  Mucoepidermoid ca
    (adenoacanthoma)

Anal (Squamous) Epithelium
  Squamous cell ca
  Malignant melanoma

Soft Tissues
  Malignant lymphoma
  Rhabdomyo-, leiomyo-, and
    liposarcoma and other

Perianal Skin
  Basal cell epithelioma
  Adnexal tumors
  Extramammary Paget's disease
  Bowen's disease

*Table 44–1.* **TNM Staging for Carcinomas of the Anal Canal**

*Primary Tumor (T)*

| | |
|---|---|
| TX | Primary tumor cannot be assessed |
| T0 | No evidence of primary tumor |
| Tis | Carcinoma in situ |
| T1 | Tumor 2 cm or less in greatest dimension |
| T2 | Tumor more than 2 cm but not more than 5 cm in greatest dimension |
| T3 | Tumor more than 5 cm in greatest dimension |
| T4 | Tumor of any size invades adjacent organ(s), e.g., vagina, urethra, bladder (involvement of the sphincter muscle[s] alone is not classified as T4) |

*Regional Lymph Nodes (N)*

| | |
|---|---|
| NX | Regional lymph nodes cannot be assessed |
| N0 | No regional lymph node metastasis |
| N1 | Metastasis in perirectal lymph node(s) |
| N2 | Metastasis in unilateral internal iliac and/or inguinal lymph node(s) |
| N3 | Metastasis in perirectal and inguinal lymph nodes and/or bilateral internal iliac and/or inguinal lymph nodes |

*Distant Metastasis (M)*

| | |
|---|---|
| MX | Distant metastasis cannot be assessed |
| M0 | No distant metastasis |
| M1 | Distant metastasis |

*Stage Grouping*

| | | | |
|---|---|---|---|
| Stage 0 | Tis | N0 | M0 |
| Stage I | T1 | N0 | M0 |
| Stage II | T2 | N0 | M0 |
| | T3 | N0 | M0 |
| Stage IIIA | T1 | N1 | M0 |
| | T2 | N1 | M0 |
| | T3 | N1 | M0 |
| | T4 | N0 | M0 |
| Stage IIIB | T4 | N1 | M0 |
| | Any T | N2 | M0 |
| | Any T | N3 | M0 |
| Stage IV | Any T | Any N | M1 |

Used with the permission of the American Joint Committee on Cancer (AJCC®), Chicago, Illinois. The original source for this material is the AJCC® Cancer Staging Manual, 5th edition (1997) published by Lippincott-Raven Publishers, Philadelphia, Pennsylvania.

ing neither the vaginal mucosa nor two thirds of the anal circumference; T4a, tumors invading the vaginal mucosa or more than two thirds of the anal circumference; and T4b, tumors with extension to neighboring structures other than skin, rectum, and vaginal mucosa or fixed tumors.

Pathologic staging provides the most accurate prognostic information, but most patients are treated with radiation therapy or chemotherapy, or both, before the use of radical surgery is considered. Thus, clinical staging must suffice for initial treatment planning for most patients. This should generally include a complete history and physical examination, sigmoidoscopy, biochemical screening panel and blood count, chest radiograph, computed tomographic scan of the abdomen and pelvis, and careful examination of the anus and rectum (usually performed under general anesthesia). Endoscopic rectal ultrasonography is also useful in assessing the depth of tumor invasion, if it is available.[30] Endorectal magnetic resonance imaging is under investigation as an additional staging modality.[31]

With the advent of combined-modality therapy, the role of staging and other prognostic factors may be changing. Because nearly all patients are staged clinically, the precision that attends the use of pathologic or postsurgical staging does not exist.

## PROGNOSIS

The major prognostic factors are the histologic characteristics of the primary tumor and stage of disease (especially the size of the primary cancer, depth of penetration, and lymph node involvement). The importance of histologic appearance is emphasized by a review of 188 patients treated at the Mayo Clinic.[21] Essentially all the patients with only superficially invasive squamous cell lesions were cured by local excision, whereas survival following abdominoperineal resection decreased as the histologic type progressed from low-grade squamous cell to high-grade squamous cell to nonkeratinizing basaloid tumors. Among 13 patients with small cell anal carcinoma, only 1 patient survived 5 years, underlining the systemic nature of this disease. Malignant melanoma of the anal canal also carries a poor prognosis, with death from metastatic disease being common within 1 year.

The details of prognosis are presented in the discussions of surgery and radiation therapy. In general, local control and 3- to 5-year survival rates averaging 70 to 90% have been reported by several institutions using either radiation alone or radiation with concurrent chemotherapy. The local control rate of early (T1 to T2) tumors is 80 to 90% and of T3 to T4 lesions it is 50 to 70% with either technique. The

5-year survival for patients without metastatic disease is about 65% with combined-modality therapy.[33]

## REFERENCES

1. Website. SEER Cancer Statistics Review 1973–1996. (See http://www-seer.ims.nci.nih.gov.)
2. Lieberman DA. Common anorectal disorders. Ann Intern Med 1984;101:837–46.
3. Frisch M, Olsen JH, Bautz A, Melbye M. Benign anal lesions and the risk of anal cancer. N Engl J Med 1994;331:300–2.
4. Adam YG, Efron G. Current concepts and controversies concerning the etiology, pathogenesis, diagnosis, and treatment of malignant tumors of the anus. Surgery 1987;101:253–66.
5. Penn I. Cancers of the anogenital region in renal transplant recipients. Cancer 1986;58:611–6.
6. Melbye M, Coté TR, Kessler L, et al. High incidence of anal cancer among AIDS patients. Lancet 1994;343:636–9.
7. Tolmos J, Vargas HI, Lim S, Stamos M. A forty-year experience with anal carcinoma: changing trends and impact of multimodality therapy. Am Surg 1997;63:918–22.
8. Slater G, Greenstein A, Aufses AH Jr. Anal carcinoma in patients with Crohn's disease. Ann Surg 1984;199:348–50.
9. Jovanovic L, Babich M, Thomas K, et al. Simultaneous cloacogenic carcinoma in dizygotic twins. Cancer 1987;59:1233–5.
10. Melbye M, Sprøgel P. Aetiological parallel between anal cancer and cervical cancer. Lancet 1991;338:657–9.
11. Scholefield JH, Hickson WGE, Smith JHF, et al. Anal intraepithelial neoplasia: part of a multifocal disease process. Lancet 1992;340:1271–3.
12. Palefsky JM, Shiboski S, Moss A. Risk factors for anal human papillomavirus infection and anal cytologic abnormalities in HIV-positive and HIV-negative homosexual men. J Acquir Immune Defic Syndr 1994;7:599–606.
13. Daniell HW: Re: Causes of anal carcinoma. JAMA 1985;254:358.
14. Croxson T, Chabon AB, Rorat E, Barash IM. Intraepithelial carcinoma of the anus in homosexual men. Dis Colon Rectum 1984;27:325–30.
15. Daling JR, Weiss NS, Hislop TG, et al. Sexual practices, sexually transmitted diseases, and the incidence of anal cancer. N Engl J Med 1987;317:973–7.
16. Daling JR, Sherman KJ, Hislop TG, et al. Cigarette smoking and the risk of anogenital cancer. Am J Epidemiol 1992;135:180–9.
17. Ogunbiyi OA, Scholefield JH, Smith JHF, et al. Immunohistochemical analysis of p53 expression in anal squamous neoplasia. J Clin Pathol 1993;46:507–12.
18. Muleris M, Salmon R-J, Girodet J, et al. Recurrent deletions of chromosomes 11q and 3p in anal canal carcinoma. Int J Cancer 1987;39:595–8.
19. Leichman LP, Cummings BJ. Anal carcinoma. Curr Probl Cancer 1990;14:120–59.
20. Harrison EG Jr, Beahrs OH, Hill JR. Anal and perianal malignant neoplasms: pathology and treatment. Dis Colon Rectum 1966;9:255–67.
21. Boman BM, Moertel CG, O'Connell MJ, et al. Carcinoma of the anal canal—a clinical and pathologic study of 188 cases. Cancer 1984;54:114–25.
22. Klotz RG Jr, Pamukcoglu T, Souilliard DH. Transitional cloacogenic carcinoma of the anal canal: clinicopathologic study of three hundred seventy-three cases. Cancer 1967;20:1727–45.
23. Ackerman LV. Cancer. 4th ed. St. Louis: CV Mosby, 1970:526.
24. McConnell EM. Squamous carcinoma of the anus—a review of 96 cases. Br J Surg 1970;57:89–92.
25. Indinnimeo M, Reale MG, Cicchini C, et al. CEA, TPA, CA 19–9, SCC, and CYFRA at diagnosis and in the follow-up of anal canal tumors. Int Surg 1997;82:275–9.
26. Tanum G, Stenwig AE, Bormer OP, Tveit KM. Carcinoembryonic antigen in anal carcinoma. Acta Oncol 1992;31:333–5.
27. Petrelli NJ, Palmer M, Herrera L, Bhargava A. The utility of squamous cell carcinoma antigen for the follow-up of patients with squamous cell carcinoma of the anal canal. Cancer 1992;70:35–9.
28. Schraut WH, Wang CH, Dawson PJ, Block GE. Depth of invasion, location, and size of cancer of the anus dictate operative treatment. Cancer 1983;51:1291–6.
29. Papillon J, Mayer M, Montbarbon JF, et al. A new approach to the management of epidermoid carcinoma of the anal canal. Cancer 1983;51:1830–7.
30. Magdeburg B, Fried M, Meyenberger C. Endoscopic ultrasonography in the diagnosis, staging, and follow-up of anal carcinomas. Endoscopy 1999;31:359–64.
31. deSouza NM, Hall AS, Puni R, et al. High-resolution magnetic resonance imaging of the anal sphincter using a dedicated endoanal coil: comparison of magnetic resonance imaging with surgical findings. Dis Colon Rectum 1996;39:926–34.
32. Tanum G, Hannisdal E, Stenwig B. Prognostic factors in anal carcinoma. Oncology 1994;51:22–4.

# SURGERY

• Kenneth P. Ramming

The surgical management of neoplasms of the anal canal is governed by the location and histologic pattern of the lesion. Surgical biopsy plays a crucial role in initial diagnosis and, for patients with small, minimally invasive squamous cell carcinomas, local excision may be sufficient.[1, 2] If this approach is used, the resection should be complete enough to remove the tumor without entering it and to provide wide margins. Because these tumors often have considerable local invasion by the time they are diagnosed or treated, however, local excision is only rarely indicated. In fact, when surgery is indicated, most patients require an abdominoperineal resection. The 5-year survival rate of patients treated with an abdominoperineal resection ranges between 30% and 60%,[3–8] comparing favorably with patients receiving the same treatment for carcinoma of the rectum. However, there is increasing evidence that one can achieve much better results by using combined-modality therapy, with an emphasis on chemotherapy and radiation therapy. Thus, it is the rare patient today who requires such extensive surgery.

In the absence of clinically palpable inguinal nodes, there is little justification for inguinal lymphadenectomy. If the nodes are clinically involved, the prognosis is poor.[6] However, when there is an interval between the time of the resection of the primary lesion and the time that node dissection is required because of clinical involvement, a 5-year survival rate exceeding 60% has been reported.[7, 8]

## REFERENCES

1. Boman BM, Moertel CG, O'Connell MJ, et al. Carcinoma of the anal canal: a clinical and pathologic study of 188 cases. Cancer 1984;54:114–25.
2. Hohm WH, Jackman RJ. Anorectal squamous-cell carcinoma: conservative or radical treatment? JAMA 1964;188:241–4.
3. Harrison EG Jr, Beahrs OH, Hill JR. Anal and perianal malignant neoplasms: pathology and treatment. Dis Colon Rectum 1966;9:255–67.
4. Beahrs OH. Management of cancer of the anus. Janeway Lecture. AJR Am J Roentgenol 1979;133:790–5.

5. Sink JD, Kramer SA, Copeland DD, Seigler HF. Cloacogenic carcinoma. Ann Surg 1978;188:53–9.
6. Dillard BM, Spratt JS Jr, Ackerman LV, Butcher HR Jr. Epidermoid carcinoma of anal margin and canal. Arch Surg 1963;86:772–6.
7. Stearns MW Jr, Quan SH. Epidermoid carcinoma of the anorectum. Surg Gynecol Obstet 1970;131:953–7.
8. Welch JP, Malt RA. Appraisal of the treatment of carcinoma of the anus and anal canal. Surg Gynecol Obstet 1977;145:837–41.

......................................

# RADIATION THERAPY

• Luu M. Tran

The 1980s and 1990s saw a dramatic change in the management of anal carcinoma. In the past, the primary modality of treatment was abdominoperineal resection; now radiation therapy, either alone or in combination with chemotherapy, has become the initial treatment of choice. The obvious advantage of the nonsurgical approach includes preserving the anal sphincter and bowel continuity while sparing the morbidity and mortality of abdominoperineal resection. The surgical procedure, which results in permanent colostomy, is now reserved for patients with residual or recurrent carcinoma after treatment with primary chemoradiation therapy (CMT).

## RADIATION TECHNIQUES

Radiation techniques vary widely among treatment centers. The patient lies prone, and usually three or four portals are designed to cover the whole pelvis using high-energy photon beams. The posteroanterior and anteroposterior (PA/AP) portals encompass the pelvic lymph nodes, anus, and perineum. The L5–S1 junction is used as the upper border to cover the internal iliac and presacral lymph nodes. The inferior border should be about 3 cm from the primary tumor's inferior extent. The lateral borders are set wide enough to cover the medial inguinal lymph nodes except for superficial, T1, well-differentiated lesions. For the right-left (R-L) lateral portals, the superior and inferior borders match those of the PA-AP fields. The anterior border is posterior to the symphysis pubis, whereas the posterior border is at least 1 cm posterior to the bony sacrum. This initial pelvic field is coned down after approximately 36 Gy. Boost fields encompass the primary tumor with 2 to 3 cm margin.

The dose to the primary tumor depends on the tumor size and whether radiation therapy is delivered alone or in combination with chemotherapy. For patients receiving radiation therapy alone, the optimal dose is usually greater than 60 Gy. When radiation therapy is given concurrently with chemotherapy, the usual dosage is between 50.4 and 55.8 Gy for 5 to 6 weeks at a daily dose of 1.8 Gy per fraction depending on tumor size and clinical response. Elective bilateral inguinal lymph nodes are treated to 40 Gy. For clinically palpable inguinal lymph nodes, a boost dose of 10 to 15 Gy is delivered using electrons. Brachytherapy is not routinely used because of the risk of increased toxicity, for example, strictures, ulceration, and anal sphincter damage.

## RESULTS

**Radiation Therapy Alone.** Since the early 1960s, radiation therapy alone has been used to manage anal carcinoma.

The role of radiation alone is well established and has been documented in numerous studies, showing it to be effective for local control and survival. Institute Curie,[1] using cobalt teletherapy alone, reported 5-year disease-free survival rates of 68% for lesions less than 4 cm and 31% for lesions greater than 4 cm. Papillon and colleagues[2] reported 51% normal anal function and 65% overall survival for patients treated with split-course external-beam therapy and iridium implants. However, complications ranged from 5 to 15% and included proctitis, necrosis, incontinence, and anal strictures.[3]

The biggest series was reported by Touboul and coworkers[4] on 270 patients with anal canal cancer (stages T1 to T4) treated with radiation therapy alone. External-beam therapy was used in all but four patients, with the dose ranging from 40 to 45 Gy to the pelvis followed by an additional boost dose of 15 to 20 Gy external-beam irradiation or a 30-Gy interstitial implant. The overall anal conservation rate was 67%. The 10-year determinate survival for stage T1 disease was 86%; for T2 disease it was 82%; for T3 disease it was 57%; and for stage T4 disease it was 45%. The grade 3 complication rate requiring surgery was 27/270 (10%). Several other retrospective studies,[5–8] mainly from Europe, reported similar favorable results with radiation therapy alone, with more than 80% of patients maintaining anal preservation. The majority of these patients, however, required high-dose radiation therapy and interstitial implants.

In summary, these nonrandomized trials showed that radiation therapy was effective in achieving excellent local control and survival in patients with anal cancers. In tumors less than 4 cm, the cure rate can be as high as 90%, but for large tumors, the local control drops to 50%. However, when radiation is used alone, the required radiation dose is high, and complications requiring surgery, such as ulceration and anal stricture, range from 5 to 15%. Therefore, radiation therapy alone should be used for patients who refuse chemotherapy or for patients with human immunodeficiency virus infection who tolerate chemotherapy poorly.

**Combined Modality Therapy with Chemotherapy and Radiation.** Since the early 1990s, treatment using a combination of radiation and chemotherapy has replaced radiation therapy alone in the management of anal carcinoma. Most current treatment protocols are based on the regimen described in the 1970s by Nigro and colleagues,[9] who treated three patients with operable anal carcinoma with combination therapy. Following abdominoperineal resection, no tumor was found in the surgical specimens of two patients. In 1987, Nigro and colleagues[10] updated their experience, reporting on 28 patients with squamous cell carcinoma of the anal canal treated with preoperative chemoradiation: 30

Gy in 15 fractions, concurrently with continuous infusion (CI) 5-fluorouracil (5-FU), and bolus mitomycin C (Mit-C). Seven of the 12 patients underwent abdominoperineal resection and had no evidence of disease in the surgical specimen.

Using the same protocol, several others[11–14] reported significant response with tumor regression. Cummings and associates[11] from Princess Margaret Hospital reported a non-randomized experience of 192 patients with primary squamous cell carcinoma of the anal canal. The patients were treated in one of three ways: with radiation alone (45 to 55 Gy external-beam irradiation for 4 weeks), with radiation plus 5-FU/Mit-C, or with radiation and 5-FU only. Radiation alone controlled the primary tumor in 56% (32/57), radiation plus 5-FU/Mit-C controlled the primary in 86% (59/69), and radiation plus 5-FU controlled the primary tumor in 60% (39/65) of patients. The authors concluded that the most effective treatment protocols included the administration of Mit-C–5-FU concurrently with radiation.

In 1982, the Eastern Cooperative Oncology Group (ECOG)[12] initiated a study using CMT in 48 patients with stages T1 to T4 squamous cell carcinoma of the anal canal. Radiation therapy consisted of 40 Gy to the pelvis followed by a 10- to 13-Gy boost to the perineal area after a 2- to 3-week break. Chemotherapy was given concurrently with radiation therapy—specifically CI of 5-FU for 4 days and intravenous injection of Mit-C. Of the 46 patients evaluated for response, 34 (74%) had complete regression of the tumor. The freedom from local-regional recurrence at 7 years was 80%, and overall survival at 7 years was 53%.

Several randomized trials comparing radiation alone to radiation combined with chemotherapy are being conducted in Europe (Table 44–2). The first trial conducted by the United Kingdom Coordinating Committee for Cancer Research (UKCCCR)[15] studied 585 patients with squamous cell carcinoma of the anal margin and anal canal. Radiation therapy consisted of 45 Gy for 5 weeks, with or without a boost of 15 Gy with perineal external-beam irradiation or a 25-Gy interstitial implant, depending on the response of the tumor. Chemotherapy was given with 5-FU plus Mit-C in conjunction with radiation therapy in the CMT arm. After a median follow-up of 42 months, local-regional recurrence was observed in 101 (36%) of 283 patients treated with the combined approach and in 164 (59%) of 279 patients treated with radiation alone. Late morbidity was the same in both groups, but early morbidity was significantly more frequent in the combined arm. However, there was no overall survival advantage in either arm.

A phase III randomized European Organization for Research and Treatment of Cancer (EORTC) trial[16] reported results in 110 patients with stage T3 or T4 disease or positive lymph nodes. Patients were randomized between radiation therapy alone or CMT. Radiation therapy consisted of 45 Gy for 5 weeks with a daily dose of 1.8 Gy. After a rest period of 6 weeks, a boost of 15 to 20 Gy was given depending on the response of the tumor. Chemotherapy was given during radiation therapy with 5-FU infusion and single-dose Mit-C. The complete remission rate was better with the addition of chemotherapy: 54% with radiation alone versus 80% in the CMT arm. The survival rate and acute and late effects were the same in both groups.

Despite the success of CMT, the Radiation Therapy Oncology Group (RTOG) has reported local failure rates of 20 to 30% with radiation doses of 45 to 50 Gy, particularly with larger tumors.[14] Thus, the optimal dosage of radiation therapy plus chemotherapy has not been defined. In general, lower doses of chemotherapy require higher doses of radiation therapy and vice versa. When radiation (in doses of 30 Gy per 15 fractions to 40.8 Gy per 24 fractions) is combined with 5-FU/Mit-C, tumor clearance occurs in up to 90% of tumors 3 cm or smaller. For larger tumors (stages T3 to T4) or nodal metastases, a higher external-beam radiation therapy (EBRT) dose combined with an interstitial implant may be needed to eradicate the tumors; however, this treatment modality is inferior to the chemoradiation approach for most patients.

In 1992, the RTOG 92-08 trial[17] specifically addressed the issue of dose escalation in patients with anal cancers

*Table 44–2.* **Randomized Trials of Concurrent Chemoradiation for Carcinomas of the Anal Canal**

| Trials | Patients (No.) | Treatment RADIATION | Treatment CHEMOTHERAPY | Local-Regional Control (%) | Survival (%) | Morbidity (Grade 3) (%) |
|---|---|---|---|---|---|---|
| UKCCR[16] | | | | | | |
| RT alone | 285 | 45 Gy/20 frs ± boost with EBRT | | 39 | 3-yr OS: 58 3-year DFS: 61 | 38 |
| RT and CM | 292 | 45 Gy/20 frs ± 15 Gy boost with EBRT | CI of 5-FU and IV Mit-C | 61 | 3-year OS: 65 3-year DFS: 72 | 42 |
| EORTC[17] | 103 | | | | 5-year surv: 56 | |
| RT alone | | 45 Gy/5 wk ± 15 Gy boost with EBRT | | 54 $p = 0.02$ | | |
| RT and CM | | 45 Gy/5 wk ± 15 Gy boost with EBRT | CI of 5-FU and IV Mit-C | 80 | | |
| RTOG[19] | | | | | | |
| RT + 5-FU | 145 | 45–50.4 Gy/5 wk ± 9 Gy boost for salvage treatment | CI of 5-FU | 59 $p = 0.014$ | 4-year DFS: 51 $p = 0.003$ | 7 |
| RT + 5-FU/Mit-C | 146 | 45–50.4 Gy/5 wk ± 9 Gy boost for salvage treatment | CI of 5-FU and IV Mit-C | 71 | 4-year DFS: 73 | 23 |

RT, radiation therapy; CM, chemotherapy; CI, continuous infusion; DFS, disease-free survival; OS, overall survival; UKCCR, United Kingdom Coordinating Council for Cancer Research; EORTC, European Organization for Research on the Treatment of Cancer; RTOG, Radiation Therapy Oncology Group; Mit-C, mitomycin C; 5-FU, 5-fluorouracil; frs, fractions; EBRT, external-beam radiation therapy; IV, intravenous; surv, survival.

treated with CMT. Patients were treated with doses of 59.4 Gy in combination with 5-FU/Mit-C with a 2-week break at 36 Gy. The colostomy rates were high (30% at 2 years), similar to those in the groups treated with 45 Gy in continuous fashion. The RTOG is currently conducting a trial using the same dose of 59.4 Gy without a treatment break. The RTOG[18] also addressed the issue of whether or not mitomycin-C adds sufficient benefit to justify its toxic side effects. They reported the results of a phase III randomized trial of 310 patients receiving either radiation therapy plus 5-FU or radiation plus 5-FU/Mit-C. One hundred forty-five patients received 45 to 50.4 Gy of pelvic radiation therapy plus 5-FU, and 146 patients received radiation plus 5-FU/Mit-C. Patients showing residual disease on post-treatment biopsy results received a salvage regimen that consisted of an additional boost to the pelvis of 9 Gy, 5-FU, and cisplatin. Post-treatment biopsy results were positive in 15% of patients in the 5-FU arm versus 7.7% in the 5-FU/Mit-C arm. At 4 years, the colostomy-free survival was higher in the 5-FU/Mit-C (71% vs. 59%, $p = 0.014$). Subsequent 5-year results updated in abstract form[19] revealed that colostomy-free survival rates for stage T3 and T4 lesions were still higher in the 5-FU/Mit-C arm (55% vs. 48%, $p = 0.065$). They concluded that, despite greater toxicity, the use of Mit-C is justified, particularly in patients with large primary tumors.

Others have used cisplatin instead of Mit-C, basing their treatment on the favorable reports of cisplatin-based regimens in patients with epithelial carcinoma of the esophagus, head, and neck. Martenson and associates[20] reported a phase II trial of high-dose radiation (59.4 Gy), 5-FU, and cisplatin for 19 patients with advanced anal carcinoma. Radiation therapy was given in a split course after 36 Gy, and cisplatin was given on day 1 of radiation therapy, in conjunction with 5-FU on the first 4 days of radiation therapy. A second course of cisplatin was given after a 36-Gy dose of radiation. Overall, the response rate was 95% (68% with complete response, 26% with partial response, and 5% with stable disease). Fifteen patients had grade 3 toxicity or higher, with grade 4 in six patients and grade 5 in one. Doci and colleagues[21] reported the results of a phase II study of 35 patients with squamous cell carcinoma of the anal canal treated with combination 5-FU plus cisplatin concurrently with a radiation dose of 36 to 38 Gy to the pelvis, followed by an additional boost of 18 to 24 Gy to the perineal region.

Complete regression was noted in 33 patients (94%), and 9 patients with metastatic lymph nodes also had a complete response. Rich and colleagues[22] noted 85% local control at 5 years with radiation therapy plus 5-FU/cisplatin compared with 73% for those treated with 5-FU and radiation. Several other trials, mainly from Europe,[23, 24] have investigated the use of cisplatin/5-FU given either sequentially, concurrently, or alternating with radiation therapy, and obtained promising results (Table 44–3). Therefore, both 5-FU/Mit-C and 5-FU/cisplatin augment tumor control and survival after radiation therapy. So far, no randomized trial exists to determine whether cisplatin is better or worse than Mit-C in terms of control or toxicity. The results of such a trial would surely be welcome, as the toxicity spectrums of both drugs are different.

In 1996, the Pattern of Care Study (PCS) committee[25] recommended the concurrent combination of two cycles of 5-FU/Mit-C and EBRT for anal canal cancers. The 5-FU dose is administered by CI (1 g/m²/day for 4 days) and Mit-C (10 mg/m²) given by intravenous bolus. The EBRT doses range from 45 to 54.9 Gy for T1 to T2 lesions and 50 to 60 Gy for large T3 to T4 tumors.

## BRACHYTHERAPY

Interstitial implants alone have been used for early lesions that are unlikely to spread to regional lymph nodes. In the past, Papillon and Montbarbon[6] used mainly radium but abandoned this technique because of local reactions such as necrosis (25%) and poor local control. Combination CMT has yielded better local control and less morbidity and should be used for local-regional disease.

Combined interstitial implants and external-beam therapy has been used for treatment of locally advanced disease with good control; however, it produces a relatively high rate of complications.[1, 3, 8] Lagrange and colleagues[8] reported the experience of 33 patients treated with EBRT and implants. Four patients developed necrosis of the anal canal, two died of complications of general anesthesia, and one had radiation injury. The author concluded that this treatment is difficult to put into practice.

In a report from Scotland,[26] 79 patients with anal cancers were treated with an interstitial iridium 192 implant as a

*Table 44–3.* **Combined Radiation and Chemotherapy with 5-Fluorouracil and Cisplatin**

| Series | Patients (No.) | Radiation Therapy | Chemotherapy | Local Control (%) | Survival (%) |
|---|---|---|---|---|---|
| Martenson et al[20] | 19 | 59.4 Gy/33 frs (break after 36 Gy) | CI 5-FU (1000 mg/m²), cisplatin (75 mg/m²) | 95 | NA |
| Doci et al[21] | 35 | 38 Gy/4 wk | CI 5-FU (750 mg/m²), cisplatin (100 gm/m²) | 94 | 94 NED at 37 mo f/u |
| Rich et al[22] | 18 | 55 Gy/5 wk | CI 5-FU (300 mg/m²), cisplatin (4 mg/m²) | 85 | 94 (2-yr OS) |
| Peiffert et al[23] | 34 | 45 Gy/5 wk | CI 5-FU (800 mg/m²), cisplatin (80 mg/m²) | 96 | NA |
| Wagner et al[24] | 51 | 42 Gy/10 wk + implant | CI 5-FU (1000 mg/m²), cisplatin (25 mg/m²) | 92 | 75 (2-yr OS) |

CI, continuous infusion; NA, not available; NED, no evidence of disease; OS, overall survival; frs, fractions; f/u, follow-up; 5-FU, 5-fluorouracil.

boost following EBRT of 40 to 50 Gy for 5 weeks. Twelve patients received concurrent chemotherapy (5-FU/Mit-C). Anal sphincter preservation with local disease control was achieved in 56 patients (71%). Of the remaining 23 patients, 17 had local failure, and 6 had to undergo abdominoperineal resection or colostomy for treatment-related complications. Excellent results (92%) were achieved in stage T1 to T2 disease treated with primary external and interstitial implants. These response rates and local control and survival results have been reported by others[4, 24, 27, 28] At the University of California, Los Angeles, we usually deliver between 45 and 50.4 Gy to the pelvis in 5 weeks, followed by a boost with an iridium interstitial implant for an additional 15 Gy. So far, there have been no significant late side effects from this regimen.

We conclude that using interstitial implants as a boost following external-beam therapy can result in better local control. This approach results in a higher total dose, usually greater than 60 Gy; thus, there is a risk of increased late sequelae such as stricture, ulceration, or bleeding. Therefore, adding the interstitial implant should be carried out only by well-trained oncologists who have adequate experience with this technique.

## SALVAGE THERAPY

Despite the success rate with the use of CMT, there is local recurrence in 10 to 20% of patients, and the rate is even higher in T3 to T4 disease. Patients with recurrent disease need salvage treatment, but whether they should be treated with further chemoradiation or abdominoperineal resection is a subject of debate. To assess the role of salvage treatment in patients who have residual tumor following treatment, a phase III randomized trial by RTOG-ECOG[18] was undertaken in 310 patients who were randomized to receive either radiation therapy in a dose of 45 to 50.4 Gy and 5-FU or radiation and 5-FU/Mit-C. Patients with residual disease on post-treatment biopsy results were given salvage treatment of an additional 9 Gy and cisplatin, an approach that resulted in a 50% salvage rate. If disease persists 6 to 8 weeks after the first salvage treatment, abdominoperineal resection is recommended.[29] Based on the experience from Cummings and associates[11] and Nigro[30] suggesting that anal cancers regress slowly, sometimes up to a year after completion of treatment, several institutions now favor an 8-week waiting period before proceeding to salvage treatment. The 1996 PCS Committees[25] on anal cancer recommended salvage treatment with further chemoradiation (10 to 16 Gy plus 5-FU/cisplatin) in patients whose disease progresses after initial treatment. Abdominoperineal resection should be reserved only for patients whose disease recurred after the first salvage treatment or for those who received radiation therapy doses greater than 60 Gy.

## MORBIDITY

Since CMT has become the standard treatment for anal cancers, there has been a reduction in the risk of late reactions, such as stricture, ulceration, radiation necrosis, and fistula. The incidence of late reactions is about 5 to 15%

and usually occurs in patients treated with primary radiation and interstitial implants as a boost. Acute reactions with the combined chemoradiation can be severe, causing gastrointestinal disorders, leukopenia, mucositis, and skin reactions. A treatment break is sometimes required; however, these reactions are usually limited and can be managed with skin care medications, antidiarrhetics or antiemetics, and nutritional support.

## REFERENCES

1. Rousseau J, Mathieu G, Fenton J, et al. Résultats et complications de la radiothérapie des épithéliomas du canal anal. Étude de 128 cas traités de 1956 a 1970. Gastroenterol Clin Biol 1979;3:207–8.
2. Papillon J, Mayer M, Montbarbon JF, et al. A new approach to the management of epidermoid carcinoma of the anal canal. Cancer 1983;51:1830–7.
3. Eschwege F, Breteau N, Chavy A, et al. Complications de la radiothérapie transcutanée des épitheliomas du canal anal. Gastroenterol Clin Biol 1979;3:183–6.
4. Touboul E, Schienger M, Buffat L, et al. Epidermoid carcinoma of the anal canal: results of curative intent radiation therapy in a series of 270 patients. Cancer 1994;73:1569–79.
5. Svensson C, Goldman S, Friberg B. Radiation treatment of epidermoid cancer of the anus. Int J Radiat Oncol Biol Phys 1993;27:67–73.
6. Papillon J, Montbarbon JF. Epidermoid carcinoma of the anal canal: a series of 276 cases. Dis Colon Rectum 1987;30:324–33.
7. Doggett SW, Green JP, Cantril S. Efficacy of radiotherapy alone for limited squamous cell carcinoma of the anal canal. Int J Radiat Oncol Bio Phys 1988;15:1069–72.
8. Lagrange JL, Chauvel P, Francois E, et al. Conservative treatment of epidermoid cancer of the anal canal combining radiotherapy and curitherapy: experience at the Antoine-Lacassagne Center. Ann Gastroenterol Hepatol 1990;26:45–9.
9. Nigro ND, Vaitkevicius VK, Buroker T, et al. Combined therapy for cancer of the anal canal. Dis Colon Rectum 1981;24:73–5.
10. Nigro ND, Seydel HG, Considine B, et al. Combined preoperative and chemotherapy for squamous cell carcinoma of the anal canal. Cancer 1983;51:1826–9.
11. Cummings BJ, Keane TJ, O'Sullivan B, et al. Epidermoid anal cancer: treatment by radiotherapy alone or by radiation and 5-FU with or without mitomycin-C. Int J Radiat Oncol Biol Phys 1991;21:1115–25.
12. Martenson J, Lipsitz S, Lefkopoulou M, et al. Results of combined modality therapy for patients with anal canal (E7283): an Eastern Cooperative Study Group study. Cancer 1995;76:1731–6.
13. Leichman L, Nigro N, Vatitkevicius V, et al. Cancer of the anal canal: model for preoperative adjuvant combined modality therapy. Am J Med 1985;78:211–5.
14. Sischy B, Doggett R, Krall J, et al. Definite irradiation and chemotherapy for radiosensitization in management of anal carcinoma: interim report on RTOG study No 8314. J Natl Cancer Inst 1989;81:850–6.
15. United Kingdom Coordinating Committee for Cancer Research (UKCCCR) Anal Cancer Working Party. Epidermoid anal cancer: results from UKCCCR-randomized trial of radiotherapy alone versus radiotherapy, 5-FU, and mitomycin. Lancet 1996;348:1049–54.
16. Bartelink H, Roelofsen F, Eschwege F, et al. Concomitant radiotherapy and chemotherapy is superior to radiotherapy alone in the treatment of locally advanced anal cancer: results of a phase III randomized trial of the European Organization for Research and Treatment of Cancer Radiotherapy and Gastrointestinal Cooperative Groups. J Clin Oncol 1997;15:2040–9.
17. John M, Pajak T, Flam M et al. Dose escalation in chemoradiation for anal cancer: preliminary results of RTOG 92-08. Cancer J Sci Am 1996;2:205.
18. Flam MS, John M, Pajack T, et al. The role of mitomycin C in combination with 5-FU and radiotherapy and of salvage chemoradiation in the definitive non-surgical treatment of epidermoid carcinoma of the anal canal: results of a phase III randomized intergroup study. J Clin Oncol 1996;14:2527–39.
19. John M, Flam MS, Berkey J, et al. Five year results and analyses of a phase III randomized RTOG/ECOG chemoradiation protocol for anal cancer. Proc ASCO 1998;17:258a.

20. Martenson JA, Lipsitz SR, Wagner H Jr, et al. Initial results of a phase II trial of high dose radiation therapy, 5-FU, and cisplatin for patients with anal cancer (E4292): an Eastern Coopertive Oncology Group study. Int J Radiat Oncol Biol Phys 1996;35:745–9.
21. Doci R, Zucali R, La Monica G, et al. Primary chemoradiation therapy with fluorouracil and cisplatin for cancer of the anus: results in 35 consecutive patients. J Clin Oncol 1996;14:3121–5.
22. Rich TA, Ajani JA, Morrison WH, et al. Chemoradiation therapy for anal cancer: radiation plus continuous infusion of 5-fluorouracil with or without cisplatin. Radiother Oncol 1993;27:209–15.
23. Peiffert D, Seitz JF, Rougier P, et al. Preliminary results of a phase II study of high-dose radiation therapy and neoadjuvant plus concomitant 5-fluorouracil with CDDP chemotherapy for patients with anal cancer. A French cooperative study. Ann Oncol 1997;8:575–81.
24. Wagner JP, Mahe MA, Romestaing P, et al. Radiation therapy in the conservative treatment of carcinoma of the anal canal. Int J Radiat Oncol Biol Phys 1994;29:17–23.
25. PCS Consensus Committees. 1996 Decision trees and management guidelines. Semin Radiat Oncol 1997;7:163.
26. Sandhu AP, Symonds RP, Robertson AG, et al. Interstitial iridium-192 implantation combined with external radiotherapy in anal cancer: ten years' experience. Int J Radiat Oncol Biol Phys 1998;40:575–81.
27. Nigh SS, Smalley SR, Elman AJ, et al. Conservative therapy for anal carcinoma: an analysis of prognostic factors. Int J Radiat Oncol Biol Phys 1992;21:224. abstract.
28. Papillon J, Montbarbon JF, Gerard JP, et al. Interstitial curietherapy in the conservative treatment of anal and rectal cancers. Int J Radiat Oncol Biol Phys 1989;17:1161–9.
29. Ellenhorn JD, Enker WE, Quan SH. Salvage abdominoperineal resection following combined chemotherapy and radiotherapy for epidermoid carcinoma of the anus. Ann Surg Oncol 1994;1:105–10.
30. Nigro ND. Multi-disciplinary management of cancer of the anus. World J Surg 1987;11:446–51.

···········································

# CHEMOTHERAPY

• Charles M. Haskell

## SINGLE-AGENT CHEMOTHERAPY

Little is known about the use of single-agent chemotherapy used alone in the treatment of anal cancer. Anal carcinomas are clearly responsive to 5-FU, mitomycin C (Mit-C), and cisplatin, based on the studies on combined chemoradiotherapy reviewed in the section on Radiation Therapy. However, the role of other single agents is unclear. Scattered case reports exist of responses to lomustine,[1] semustine,[2] and doxorubicin,[3] but these drugs have no established place in the management of this group of tumors.

## COMBINATION CHEMOTHERAPY

As discussed in the section on Radiation Therapy, two combination chemotherapy regimens are of established efficacy in the treatment of anal cancer. Both use CI 5-fluorouracil for 4 to 5 days combined with either Mit-C or cisplatin. At present, 5-FU and Mit-C combined with radiation therapy is the standard regimen for primary chemoradiotherapy for this group of tumors. However, there is a growing interest in the use of induction courses of 5-FU and cisplatin before the use of chemoradiotherapy, and a number of studies demonstrate that the combination of cisplatin plus 5-FU is active.[4, 5] This has resulted in a number of studies using this combination, as summarized in Table 44–3.

## CHEMORADIOTHERAPY

Despite the paucity of data on the use of chemotherapy used alone, there is substantial experience using chemotherapy with radiation therapy in the initial management of this group of tumors. This approach to management was initiated by Nigro and colleagues[6] in three patients at Wayne State University, as discussed previously in this chapter. Their early experience was substantiated in a number of subsequent studies, and chemoradiotherapy is now standard therapy for this group of tumors, as discussed previously. Never-

theless, there are numerous questions about the most appropriate use of combined chemoradiotherapy.

There is a consensus that chemotherapy given with radiation therapy acts as a radiosensitizing agent that allows safer treatment. The risk of late radiation therapy complications is reduced, with anal radionecrosis or stricture being rare events with combined-modality therapy. However, acute radiation dermatitis is more severe with combined-modality therapy. Because of this, combined-modality therapy uses a lower total dose and often includes a treatment break as a formal part of the radiation therapy plan. The major complications of combined therapy are modest, as follows: leukopenia, thrombocytopenia, and anemia (about 50% of patients); gastrointestinal disorders, including nausea, vomiting, and diarrhea (40%); stomatitis and anal stricture or ulcers (13%).[7] In the nonrandomized experience at the Princess Margaret Hospital, local tumor control was achieved in 93% of patients with combined-modality therapy, compared with 60% with irradiation alone.[8]

Despite the success of combined chemotherapy and radiation therapy, questions abound about their optimal use. For example, the optimal dose and number of courses of 5-FU and Mit-C are undefined, as suggested by the range of schedules shown in Table 44–2. In general, lower doses of chemotherapy require higher doses of radiation therapy, and vice versa. A RTOG trial specifically addressed the issue of whether or not Mit-C adds sufficient benefit to justify its toxic side effects, with strong support for the importance of including Mit-C in the regimen.[9] It is unclear whether the optimal chemotherapy combination is 5-FU and Mit-C or 5-FU and cisplatin, or even combinations of both. Preliminary studies of 5-FU and cisplatin given with radiation therapy are promising (see Table 44–3), but a randomized comparison of cisplatin versus Mit-C in combined therapy has not been reported.[5, 10–14] All three drugs are being tested together in Europe against patients with advanced disease, but the results of these trials are unavailable. A phase II study in the United States by the Cancer and Leukemia Group B in patients with poor-risk anal cancer does suggest benefit from the initial use of 5-FU and cisplatin as induction therapy, followed by chemoradiotherapy using 5-FU and Mit-C.[15] Further study is needed to define the optimal use of these agents.

## REFERENCES

1. Moertel CG, Schutt AJ, Reitemeier RJ, Hahn RG. Therapy for gastrointestinal cancer with the nitrosoureas alone and in drug combination. Cancer Treat Rep 1976;60:729–32.
2. Zimm S, Wampler GL. Response of metastatic cloacogenic carcinoma to treatment with semustine. Cancer 1981;48:2575–6.
3. Fisher WB, Herbst KD, Sims JE, Critchfield CF. Metastatic cloacogenic carcinoma of the anus: sequential responses to Adriamycin and cis-dichlorodiammineplatinum(II). Cancer Treat Rep 1978;62:91–7.
4. Khater R, Frenay M, Bourry J, et al. Cisplatin plus 5-fluorouracil in the treatment of metastatic anal squamous cell carcinoma: a report of two cases. Cancer Treat Rep 1986;70:1345–6.
5. Wagner JP, Mahe MA, Romestaing P, et al. Radiation therapy in the conservative treatment of carcinoma of the anal canal. Int J Radiat Oncol Biol Phys 1994;29:17–23.
6. Nigro ND, Vaitkevicius VK, Considine B Jr. Combined therapy for cancer of the anal canal: a preliminary report. Dis Colon Rectum 1974;17:354–6.
7. Hussain M, al-Sarraf M. Anal carcinomas: new combined modality treatment approaches. Oncology 1988;2:42–8.
8. Cummings B, Keane T, Thomas G, et al. Results and toxicity of the treatment of anal canal carcinoma by radiation therapy or radiation therapy and chemotherapy. Cancer 1984;54:2062–8.
9. Flam M, John M, Pajak TF, et al. Role of mitomycin in combination with fluorouracil and radiotherapy, and of salvage chemoradiation in the definitive nonsurgical treatment of epidermoid carcinoma of the anal canal: results of a phase III randomized intergroup study. J Clin Oncol 1996;14:2527–39.
10. Byfield JE, Barone RM, Sharp TR, Frankel SS. Conservative management without alkylating agents of squamous cell anal cancer using cyclical 5-FU alone and x-ray therapy. Cancer Treat Rep 1985;67:709–12.
11. Roca E, Milano MC, Pennella E, et al. Medical treatment of 44 patients with anal canal carcinoma. Argentinian Intergroup for the treatment of Gastrointestinal tumors (IATTGI). Medicina 1995;55:243–8.
12. Tanum G. Treatment of relapsing anal carcinoma. Acta Oncol 1993;32:33–5.
13. Rich TA, Ajani JA, Morrison WH, et al. Chemoradiation therapy for anal cancer: radiation plus continuous infusion of 5-fluorouracil with or without cisplatin. Radiother Oncol 1993;27:209–15.
14. Díaz E, Young K, de La Rosa E. Cisplatin (CDP) and 5-fluorouracil (5FU) plus simultaneous radiotherapy (RT) for the treatment of epidermoid carcinoma of the anal region (ECAR). Proc ASCO 1993;12:190.
15. Meropol NJ, Niedzwiecki D, Shank B, et al. Combined-modality therapy of poor risk anal canal carcinonoma: a phase II study of the Cancer and Leukemia Group B (CALGB). Proc ASCO 1999;18:237a. abstract 909.

....................................

# TREATMENT BY STAGE OF DISEASE

• Charles M. Haskell

Treatment of anal carcinomas is strongly influenced by histologic type and the precise location of the lesion. Adenocarcinomas are generally treated in the same manner as is rectal cancer, as described in Chapter 43. Anorectal melanoma is generally treated surgically, with sphincter-saving therapy if possible because of the extremely poor prognosis and poor likelihood of cure from radical surgical therapy. Epidermoid carcinomas arising on perianal skin are treated like skin cancer arising in other areas, as discussed in Chapter 76. Epidermoid carcinomas of the anal canal and anal margin are treated as a function of stage of disease and the overall health of the patient.

Most patients presenting with anal carcinoma can be treated with curative intent and conservation of anal func-

*Table 44–4.* **Summary of Recommended Treatment for Carcinoma of the Anal Canal***

| T Stage | N Stage | Radiation Therapy† | Chemotherapy‡ |
|---|---|---|---|
| T0 | N0 | None (local excision alone) | None |
| T1 <1 cm | N0 | None (local excision alone) | None |
| T1 ≥1 cm | N0 | 45–54.9 Gy | None |
| T2 | N0 | 50–60 Gy | Yes |
| T3 | N0 | 50–60 Gy | Yes |
| T4 | N0 | 50–60 Gy | Yes |
| All | N1–N3 | 50–60 Gy | Yes |

*Specific recommendations involve the coordination of chemotherapy and radiation, as follows:

†Radiation therapy: The details of radiation therapy are discussed in the section on Radiation Therapy. The dose and schedule of radiation therapy varies with the size of the tumor, the planned doses of chemotherapy, and the general condition of the patient. Some centers use lower doses of radiation therapy for patients with small tumors. Some centers use lower doses of radiation therapy (30 Gy/15 fractions) for patients who are HIV-positive. (Data from Indinnimeo M, Ciccini C, Izzo P, Stazi A. Anal canal cancer diagnosis: usefulness of serum tumor markers. J Chemother 1997;9:121–2.)

‡Chemotherapy. Two chemotherapy regimens are commonly used. The best established of the two is the fluorouracil + mitomycin regimen, but some experienced oncologists prefer the fluorouracil + cisplatin regimen. Each is described briefly.

*Fluorouracil + mitomycin:* Mitomycin C (10 mg/m²) as a bolus on days 1 and 29 of radiation therapy. Fluorouracil (1000 mg/m²/day × 96 hr) is given as a continuous infusion starting on days 1 and 29 of radiation therapy. The second dose of mitomycin C should be delayed for thrombocytopenia (platelets <125,000) and may be omitted for HIV-positive patients and other patients who are in frail health. (For more information see the following: Tanum G, Tveit K, Karlsen KO, Hauer-Jensen M. Chemotherapy and radiation therapy for anal carcinoma; survival and late morbidity. Cancer 1991;67:2462–6; and Flam M, John M, Pajack TF, et al. Role of mitomycin in combination with fluorouracil and radiotherapy, and of salvage chemoradiation in the definitive nonsurgical treatment of epidermoid carcinoma of the anal canal: results of a phase III randomized intergroup study. J Clin Oncol 1996;14:2527–39.)

*Fluorouracil + cisplatin:* Fluorouracil (1000 mg/m²/day for 96 hr) by continuous infusion starting on days 1 and 21 of radiation therapy. Cisplatin (25 mg/m²) is given as an intravenous bolus injection daily on days 2 to 5 with hydration (see Appendix E) starting on days 1 and 21 of radiation therapy. Chemotherapy is given concurrently with radiation therapy, and it has been used in some patients as a separate course 3 wk before the initiation of chemoradiotherapy. (Data from Wagner J-P, Mahe MA, Romestaing P, et al. Radiation therapy in the conservative treatment of carcinoma of the anal canal. Int J Radiat Oncol Biol Phys 1994;29:17–23.)

tion. Although these goals may occasionally be met using surgery alone, nearly all patients are treated with chemoradiotherapy. Patients who relapse after combined-modality therapy may regain local control with an abdominoperineal resection, although long-term survival is unusual for this group of patients. Our general approach to treatment by stage of disease is summarized in Table 44–4.

## SUGGESTIONS FOR ADDITIONAL READING

Klas JV, Rothenberger DA, Wong WD, Madoff RD. Malignant tumors of the anal canal: the spectrum of disease, treatment, and outcomes. Cancer 1999;85:1686–93. *This article provides a good overview of the topic.*

Flam M, John M, Pajak TF, et al. Role of mitomycin in combination with fluorouracil and radiotherapy, and of salvage chemoradiation in the definitive nonsurgical treatment of epidermoid carcinoma of the anal canal: results of a phase III randomized intergroup study. J Clin Oncol 1996;14:2527–39. *This study demonstrates that mitomycin plus 5-FU is superior to 5-FU alone in the combined modality therapy of anal cancer.*

Svensson C, Goldman S, Friberg B, Glimelius B. Induction chemotherapy and radiotherapy in loco-regionally advanced epidermoid carcinoma of the anal canal. Int J Radiat Oncol Biol Phys 1998;41:863–7. *This is an excellent article on the use of cisplatin-based induction therapy before chemoradiotherapy in the management of anal cancer.*

Pocard M, Tiret E, Nugent K, et al. Results of salvage abdominoperineal resection for anal cancer after radiotherapy. Dis Colon Rectum 1998;41:1488–93. *Survival was poor for this group of patients treated with salvage surgery alone.*

Ryan DP, Compton CC, Mayer RJ. Carcinoma of the anal canal (medical progress). N Engl J Med 2000;342:792–8. *This an excellent review.*

# CHAPTER 45

# EXOCRINE PANCREAS

..............................

## NATURAL HISTORY, DIAGNOSIS, AND STAGING

• Charles M. Haskell

The natural history, diagnosis, and treatment of tumors of the pancreas are strongly influenced by histologic type. Tumors of the endocrine pancreas have unique biologic characteristics, and therapy is relatively effective, as discussed in Chapter 69. Neoplasms of the exocrine pancreas develop insidiously, and therapy is relatively ineffective. This group of patients has the lowest 5-year survival rate of all of the common human malignancies, and most patients die within a year. Treatment is nearly always palliative, and cure is highly unlikely.

## EPIDEMIOLOGY AND ETIOLOGY

**Incidence and Mortality Rates.** The American Cancer Society estimates that there will be 28,600 new cases of pancreatic cancer and 28,600 deaths from the disease in the United States in 2000.[1] This number represents 22% of all deaths from gastrointestinal malignancy in the United States. The annual incidence of pancreatic cancer in the Surveillance, Epidemiology, and End Results (SEER) database for the United States is 8.9 cases per 100,000 population.[2] The incidence of pancreatic carcinoma has increased almost 300% since 1950 and now exceeds the incidence of stomach cancer and cancer of the rectum.[3, 4] In the United States, the incidence of cancer of the pancreas is rising most rapidly in the nonwhite population.[5] Most patients range in age from 30 to 70 years, with the average age at the time that symptoms appear being about 56 years. The male/female ratio is about 1.3:1. The overall 5-year survival rate for the disease is 4.1%.[2]

The cause of pancreatic carcinoma is unknown, and the details of molecular pathogenesis are less completely defined than for colorectal cancer.[6] It is likely, however, that the process involves multiple steps, including cellular initiation, promotion, and conversion, resulting in multiple clones of malignant cells capable of invasion and metastasis. Factors that have been associated with the disease include heredity, cigarette smoking, a high-fat diet, prior peptic ulcer surgery, occupational exposure to 2-naphthylamine and benzidine or gasoline derivatives, chronic pancreatitis, diabetes mellitus, and alcoholism.[7] The available data on risk factors and molecular pathogenesis are reviewed here briefly.

**Heredity.** Hereditary factors may contribute to the cause of this disease.[8] Familial pancreatic cancer has been reported in a mother and daughter,[9] in three generations of the same family,[10] and as a coincident cancer with familial melanoma and retinoblastoma.[11] Pancreatic cancer can be a feature of cancer susceptibility syndromes associated with germline mutations in p16, *BRCA1*, *BRCA2*, and *APC*.[12, 13] Of patients with pancreatic cancer, 5 to 10% have first-degree relatives who develop pancreatic cancer.[12] Given these facts, family counseling should be considered for patients with pancreatic cancer.

**Cigarette Smoking.** One of the strongest associations that has been made is with cigarette smoking.[3, 14] Mortality rates from pancreatic carcinoma for cigarette smokers are approximately two to three times higher than those for non-smokers, and the rise of pancreatic carcinoma incidence parallels that of lung cancer. The risk of pancreatic cancer increases with increased amounts of smoking, and it decreases to baseline 10 to 15 years after smoking cessation.

Experimental pancreatic tumors can be induced by the administration of tobacco-specific nitrosamines in drinking water or by parenteral administration in animals.[7]

**Diet.** Experimentally, dietary fat and protein act as promoters of pancreatic carcinogenesis. In humans, an increased intake of protein appears to increase the risk of acquiring the disease.[15] Pancreatic cancer has been associated with coffee drinking,[16-18] and the roasting of coffee beans has been reported to form mutagens.[19] Subsequent studies, however, strongly refute any relationship between coffee drinking and pancreatic cancer.[20] A dietary basis for the cause of pancreatic cancer is tenuous at best.

**Chemical and Occupational Exposure.** Men employed in manufacturing occupations that use 2-naphthylamine or benzidine and men exposed to gasoline derivatives have a fivefold increase in the risk of pancreatic cancer.[7] Heavy exposure to dichlorodiphenyltrichloroethane (DDT) and related insecticides has also been associated with a fivefold increase in the risk of the disease.[21] One study suggests a possible link of pancreatic cancer with chlorinated water,[22] and another found a twofold increase in deaths from pancreatic cancer in female Vietnam veterans.[23] Excessive use of alcohol does not appear to be an important risk factor, unless the patient has developed pancreatitis.[24, 25]

**Pancreatitis and Diabetes Mellitus.** Pancreatitis has been associated with a marked increased risk of pancreatic cancer in one historical cohort study,[26] but most other studies suggest that the association is modest at best.[27] Diabetes mellitus also has been associated with an increased risk of the disease, but it is unclear whether this is of etiologic significance.

**Molecular Pathogenesis.** Although a cohesive model of pathogenesis has not yet been constructed, many of the oncogene and suppressor gene abnormalities reported in colorectal cancer have been seen in pancreatic cancer.[12, 13] Virtually all pancreatic cancers have inactivation of the p16 pathway, and most inactivate the transforming growth factor-β/*DPC4* and p53 tumor-suppressor pathways.[12, 28, 29] Other mutations have been described for Rb-1[30] and *DCC* (deleted in colorectal cancer gene),[31] and amplification of the HER-2/*neu* oncogene has been described.[32] K-*ras* mutations may be especially important,[13, 33, 34] so new drugs are being developed that target this oncogene. A variety of other tumor-suppressor genes have also been reported as abnormal in a small number of sporadic cases of pancreatic cancer, including *ALK-5*, *MKK4*, and *STK11* (the gene responsible for Peutz-Jeghers syndrome).[12] Further study is needed to place these observations into perspective. It is possible that unraveling this process will be facilitated by the use of model systems, such as the transgenic mouse.[35]

## PATHOLOGY

Carcinoma of the pancreas produces a hard, nodular, poorly defined enlargement of that portion of the gland from which it arises. Some authorities consider pancreatic cancer to be composed of nearly 20 different neoplasms, each with a specific treatment and different outcome.[36] The major histologic types of primary cancers of the pancreas are listed in Table 45–1.[37]

Adenocarcinomas of the pancreas are irregular, whitish

*Table 45–1.* **Cancers of the Pancreas by Histologic Cell Type**

| Cell Type | Occurrence (%) |
|---|---|
| Adenocarcinomas | |
| Ductal cell | 82 |
| Acinar cell | 13 |
| Anaplastic | 5 |
| Cystadenocarcinoma | Rare |
| Adenoacanthomas | Rare |
| Squamous cell carcinomas | Rare |
| Sarcomas | Rare |
| Solid and papillary neoplasms | Rare |

Modified from Moertel CG. Exocrine pancreas. In: Holland JF, Frei E III, eds. Cancer medicine. 2nd ed. Philadelphia: Lea & Febiger, 1982:1793.

masses that are often accompanied by fibrosis and surrounded by pancreatitis. These lesions can be multicentric in 38% of cases.[18] In most surgical series, 75% of these tumors are located in the head of the pancreas. These often cause fibrosis, duct obstruction, and pancreatitis after they reach a significant size. Invasion of the portal vein, superior mesenteric vein, and bile ducts is common. Carcinomas of the body and tail of the pancreas are usually found at autopsy, probably because these are often silent lesions in patients who die of other causes.[38] They may remain asymptomatic for long periods and present as large, palpable tumor masses frequently invading the surrounding structures of splenic artery and vein and the stomach.

The most frequent sites of metastases are the regional and periduodenal lymph nodes, the mesocolic and peripancreatic lymph nodes, and the nodes in the hilum of the liver. Other mesenteric, periaortic, or posterior mediastinal nodes may become involved as the disease progresses. Metastatic spread to the liver is seen almost invariably at the end stage of the disease, and direct peritoneal seeding of the abdominal cavity is common. Less common sites of metastases are lung and bone.

Contemporary studies of pancreatic pathology have focused on the histology of this neoplasm. Capella and coworkers[39] have made an ultrastructural study and classification of endocrine cells of the pancreas and have proposed seven different cell types that they believe may be the basis for a new cytologic classification. Tschang and colleagues[40] have described a pleomorphic carcinoma of the pancreas. This carcinoma is characterized by a noncohesive, sarcoma-like growth pattern with bizarre mononucleated and multinucleated giant cells. The clinical course in patients with this lesion is worse than with conventional adenocarcinoma. This pleomorphic, sarcoma-like cell architecture with a correspondingly poor prognosis has also been noted by others.[41] Webb[42] has described carcinomas of the pancreas that have a mixed cell type, and Sanfey and associates[43] have described a rare, potentially curable lesion known variously as *solid and papillary neoplasm* or *papillary-cystic neoplasm*. Cystadenocarcinoma of the pancreas is discussed at the end of this chapter as a distinct entity because of its unusual biology.

In an in vitro study, Wu and coworkers[44] purified and characterized a plasminogen activator secreted by cultured human pancreatic carcinoma cells that shared many properties with urokinase. This study is of interest because abnormal clotting states are frequently associated with carcinoma of the pancreas.

## CLINICAL FEATURES

The triad of symptoms usually observed in cancer of the head of the pancreas are pain, weight loss, and progressive jaundice. These symptoms are generally ill-defined and vague early in the course of disease, and conventional radiographic findings are often normal. The epigastric pain is often relieved by changes in posture, such as sitting up or bending forward. Diabetes mellitus is demonstrable in 20 to 40% of patients. Gastrointestinal tract hemorrhage is rare. Rarely the disease presentation may mimic acute pancreatitis.[45] Emotional disturbances characterized by depression, agitation, and anxiety have been reported in most patients.[46, 47]

Physical findings are usually few in patients with carcinomas of the tail and body of the pancreas. These lesions may achieve a large size and be palpable before the development of severe symptoms. Late in the course of the disease, ascites may become evident. The interval from the onset of symptoms until the death of the patient is usually 5 to 9 months. A variety of hematologic complications may occur, as reviewed in Chapter 13.

## DIAGNOSIS

There is no effective screening test for pancreatic cancer. Diagnosis in symptomatic patients may be approached differently by specialists from different disciplines, but the first step involves attempts to visualize or localize the tumor. Subsequently, diagnosis and rational management depend on obtaining appropriate tissue for a cytologic or histologic diagnosis. The commonly employed diagnostic tests for this disease are discussed here briefly.

**Pancreatic Imaging.** Computed tomography (CT) of the abdomen is the most commonly employed initial study for patients with suspected pancreatic disease in the United States.[48] It provides detailed anatomic information and is widely available. This study alone is sufficient to reach a diagnosis of pancreatic disease in about 75% of cases.[49] Ultrasonography can be used as an alternative, especially in the rapid differentiation of obstructive from nonobstructive jaundice. Magnetic resonance imaging plays little role in the diagnosis of pancreatic cancer.[7]

**Endoscopic Retrograde Cholangiopancreatography.** Endoscopic retrograde cholangiopancreatography (ERCP) has become the mainstay of differential diagnosis for complicated cases of carcinoma of the pancreaticobiliary junction.[50] Ampullary and duodenal carcinomas can usually be diagnosed by ERCP, and the procedure may identify encasement or obstruction of the pancreatic duct in patients with pancreatic cancer. Cytologic examination of cells from the pancreatic juice obtained during ERCP can be diagnostic. An investigational variant of this approach is to look for molecular diagnostic changes in the pancreatic juice. For example, the presence of the K-*ras* oncogene in pancreatic fluid was used to rule out pancreatitis in one small study.[51] ERCP rarely alters management when CT shows a definite mass.[52]

Its major role is in patients with a normal or atypical computed tomographic scan.

**Tumor Markers.** A variety of biochemical serum markers have been associated with pancreatic cancer, including serum amylase, immunoreactive elastase, carcinoembryonic antigen, carbohydrate antigen 19-9 (CA 19-9), CA-125, CA-50, CA-242, tissue polypeptide antigen, tissue polypeptide–specific antigen, and others. The most widely studied of these is CA 19-9.[7] High levels of CA 19-9 support a diagnosis of cancer, but it is not specific for pancreatic cancer. CA 19-9 serum levels decrease in patients with pancreatic cancer who undergo successful resections, but serum levels do not always correlate with tumor bulk, and patients with small tumors often have normal values. Even astronomical values do not ensure a diagnosis of cancer. In one case of benign biliary obstruction, the CA 19-9 level was 61,800 U/ml.[53] The CA 19-9 test is of marginal value in diagnosis and staging. The same conclusion applies to the other pancreatic markers. None of these has been consistently useful in the initial diagnosis or the subsequent staging of pancreatic cancer.[7] Combining multiple serum markers does not appreciably improve diagnostic accuracy.[54]

**Percutaneous Aspiration Cytology.** Cytologic diagnosis based on fine-needle aspirates of the pancreas is a safe, reliable procedure, with a reported sensitivity of 57 to 96% and virtually no false-positive results.[7] For example, a series by Dickey and colleagues[55] from Cleveland correctly diagnosed a primary tumor of the pancreas in 97.3% of patients from whom adequate tissue was obtained by one or two passes of a small needle. There was one false-negative and no false-positive results. The overall complication rate of fine-needle aspiration is low, but seeding can occur along the needle tract, and the rate of intraperitoneal spread may be increased after biopsy.[7] The procedure should be avoided in patients with apparently resectable lesions. The complication rate from intraoperative biopsy of the pancreas with a wedge biopsy or larger Vim-Silverman needle is much higher than that seen with percutaneous biopsy. Intraoperative biopsy by wedge biopsy or core needles has been associated with a 5 to 20% risk of hemorrhage, pancreatitis, fistula, or abscess and a reported 2 to 4% mortality rate.[49]

**Other Tests.** Endoscopic ultrasonography can image pancreatic tumors and lymph nodes directly through the gastrointestinal lumen.[56] Angiography can identify vascular signs of spread that would preclude a curative resection, such as infiltration of the portal vein by tumor. Immunoscintigraphy with radiolabeled antibodies has been tried in patients with pancreatic cancer.[7] Further studies of these newer methods are needed before their place in the diagnosis of pancreatic cancer can be established.

## STAGING AND PROGNOSIS

The international TNM system for staging pancreatic carcinomas is given in Table 45–2.[57] The system is less useful in pancreatic cancer than in most other tumors because it is difficult to assess the extent of local infiltration and regional nodal involvement in this disease.

Carcinoma of the exocrine pancreas is nearly always a fatal disease. Median survival by stage of disease in one study was as follows: stage I, 17 months; stage II, 10

**Table 45–2. TNM Staging for Carcinomas of the Exocrine Pancreas**

*Primary Tumor (T)*

| | |
|---|---|
| TX | Primary tumor cannot be assessed |
| T0 | No evidence of primary tumor |
| Tis | Carcinoma in situ |
| T1 | Tumor limited to the pancreas 2 cm or less in greatest dimension |
| T2 | Tumor limited to the pancreas more than 2 cm in greatest dimension |
| T3 | Tumor extends directly into any of the following: duodenum, bile duct, peripancreatic tissues |
| T4 | Tumor extends directly into any of the following: stomach, spleen, colon, adjacent large vessels |

*Regional Lymph Nodes (N)*

| | |
|---|---|
| NX | Regional lymph nodes cannot be assessed |
| N0 | No regional lymph node metastasis |
| N1 | Regional lymph node metastasis |
| pN1a | Metastasis in a single regional lymph node |
| pN1b | Metastasis in multiple regional lymph nodes |

*Distant Metastasis (M)*

| | |
|---|---|
| MX | Distant metastasis cannot be assessed |
| M0 | No distant metastasis |
| M1 | Distant metastasis |

*Stage Grouping*

| | | | |
|---|---|---|---|
| Stage 0 | Tis | N0 | M0 |
| Stage I | T1 | N0 | M0 |
| | T2 | N0 | M0 |
| Stage II | T3 | N0 | M0 |
| Stage III | T1 | N1 | M0 |
| | T2 | N1 | M0 |
| | T3 | N1 | M0 |
| Stage IVA | T4 | Any N | M0 |
| Stage IVB | Any T | Any N | M1 |

From Fleming ID, Cooper JS, Henson DE, et al, eds. AJCC cancer staging manual. 5th ed. Philadelphia: Lippincott-Raven, 1997:121.

months; stage III, 12 months; and stage IV, 6 months.[58] At the University of Chicago, the 3-year survival rate of 912 patients with pancreatic cancer was only 2.5%.[59] At the Memorial Sloan-Kettering Cancer Center, only 18% of patients were eligible for a possibly curative resection, with a 30-day operative mortality rate of 3.4%. The actuarial 5-year survival rate in patients who did not undergo resection was 0%, compared with 24% in patients who underwent resection.[60]

The patterns of failure after a potentially curative resection include local failure and metastatic involvement of the liver or peritoneal cavity. In one study of 36 patients, 19% experienced local failure only, whereas 73% had distant and local failure.[61] The most common sites of failure were in the liver (62%) and peritoneal cavity (42%).

In national chemotherapy and radiation therapy trials, the single factor that has consistently been of greatest prognostic importance is the performance status of the patient. The higher the level of performance, as determined by any of the commonly used systems, the better the response rate or survival rate, or both.

## REFERENCES

1. Landis SH, Murray T, Bolden S, Wingo PA. Cancer statistics, 1999. CA Cancer J Clin 1999;49:8–31.
2. SEER Cancer Statistics Review 1973–1996. (See http://www-seer.ims.nci.nih.gov.)
3. Benarde MA, Weiss W. A cohort analysis of pancreatic cancer, 1939–1969. Cancer 1977;39:1260–3.
4. Mack TM. Pancreas. In: Schottenfeld D, Fraumeni J, eds. Cancer epidemiology and prevention. Philadelphia: WB Saunders, 1982:638–67.
5. McKay FW, Hanson MR, Miller RW. Cancer mortality in the United States: 1950–1977. NCI Monogr 1982;59:1–475.
6. Friess H, Guo XZ, Nan BC, et al. Growth factors and cytokines in pancreatic carcinogenesis. Ann N Y Acad Sci 1999;880:110–21.
7. Warshaw AL, Fernández-del Castillo C. Pancreatic carcinoma. N Engl J Med 1992;326:455–65.
8. Lynch HT. Genetics and pancreatic cancer. Arch Surg 1994;129:266–8, 455.
9. Katkhouda N, Mouiel J. Pancreatic cancer in mother and daughter. Lancet 1986;2:747.
10. Ehrenthal D, Haeger L, Griffin T, Compton C. Familial pancreatic adenocarcinoma in three generations: a case report and a review of the literature. Cancer 1987;59:1661–4.
11. DerKinderen DJ, Koten JW, Den Otter W, et al. Retinoblastoma, melanoma, and pancreatic cancer. Lancet 1986;2:1335–6.
12. Goggins M, Kern SE, Offerhaus JA, Hruban RH. Progress in cancer genetics: lessons from pancreatic cancer. Ann Oncol 1999;10:Suppl 4:4–8.
13. Flanders TY, Foulkes WD. Pancreatic adenocarcinoma: epidemiology and genetics. J Med Genet 1996;33:889–98.
14. Mack TM, Yu MC, Hanisch R, Henderson BE. Pancreas cancer and smoking, beverage consumption, and past medical history. J Natl Cancer Inst 1986;76:49–60.
15. Farrow DC, Davis S. Diet and the risk of pancreatic cancer in men. Am J Epidemiol 1990;132:423–31.
16. MacMahon B, Yen S, Trichopoulos D, et al. Coffee and cancer of the pancreas. N Engl J Med 1981;304:630–3.
17. Cuckle HS, Kinlen LJ. Coffee and cancer of the pancreas. Br J Cancer 1981;44:760–1.
18. Nomura A, Stemmermann GN, Heilbrun LK. Coffee and pancreatic cancer. Lancet 1981;2:415.
19. Kosugi A, Nagao M, Suwa Y, et al. Roasting coffee beans produces compounds that induce prophage lambda in E. coli and are mutagenic in E. coli and S. typhimurium. Mutat Res 1983;116:179–84.
20. Conley CR, Scheithauer BW, van Heerden JA, Weiland LH. Diffuse intraductal papillary adenocarcinoma of the pancreas. Ann Surg 1987;205:246–9.
21. Garabrant DH, Held J, Langholz B, et al. DDT and related compounds and risk of pancreatic cancer. J Natl Cancer Inst 1992;84:764–71.
22. Ijsselmuiden CB, Gaydos C, Feighner B, et al. Cancer of the pancreas and drinking water: a population-based case-control study in Washington County, Maryland. Am J Epidemiol 1992;136:836–42.
23. Thomas TL, Kang HK, Dalager NA. Mortality among women Vietnam veterans, 1973–1987. Am J Epidemiol 1991;134:973–80.
24. Tønnesen H, Møller H, Andersen JR, et al. Cancer morbidity in alcohol abusers. Br J Cancer 1994;69:327–32.
25. Ghadirian P, Simard A, Baillargeon J. Tobacco, alcohol, and coffee and cancer of the pancreas: a population-based, case-control study in Quebec, Canada. Cancer 1991;67:2664–70.
26. Lowenfels AB, Maisonneuve P, Cavallini G, et al. Pancreatitis and the risk of pancreatic cancer. International Pancreatitis Study Group. N Engl J Med 1993;328:1433–7.
27. Ekbom A, McLaughlin JK, Karlsson BM, et al. Pancreatitis and pancreatic cancer: a population-based study. J Natl Cancer Inst 1994;86:625–7.
28. Zhang SY, Ruggeri B, Agarwal P, et al. Immunohistochemical analysis of p53 expression in human pancreatic carcinomas. Arch Pathol Lab Med 1994;118:150–4.
29. Redston MS, Caldas C, Seymour AB, et al. p53 mutations in pancreatic carcinoma and evidence of common involvement of homocopolymer tracts in DNA microdeletions. Cancer Res 1994;54:3025–33.
30. Ruggeri B, Zhang SY, Caamano J, et al. Human pancreatic carcinomas and cell lines reveal frequent and multiple alterations in the p53 and Rb-1 tumor-suppressor genes. Oncogene 1992;7:1503–11.
31. Simon B, Weinel R, Höhne M, et al. Frequent alterations of the tumor suppressor genes p53 and DCC in human pancreatic carcinoma. Gastroenterology 1994;106:1645–51.
32. Yamanaka Y, Friess H, Kobrin MS, et al. Overexpression of HER2/neu oncogene in human pancreatic carcinoma. Hum Pathol 1993;24:1127–34.

33. Motojima K, Urano T, Nagata Y, et al. Detection of point mutations in the Kirsten-ras oncogene provides evidence for the multicentricity of pancreatic carcinoma. Ann Surg 1993;217:138–43.
34. Hahn SA, Schmiegel WH. Recent discoveries in cancer genetics of exocrine pancreatic neoplasia. Digestion 1998;59:493–501.
35. Sandgren EP, Quaife CJ, Paulovich AG, et al. Pancreatic tumor pathogenesis reflects the causative genetic lesion. Proc Natl Acad Sci U S A 1991;88:93–7.
36. Wilentz RE, Hruban RH. Pathology of cancer of the pancreas. Surg Oncol Clin North Am 1998;7:43–65.
37. Moertel CG. Exocrine pancreas. In: Holland JF, Frei E III, eds. Cancer medicine. Philadelphia: Lea & Febiger, 1982:1793–1804.
38. Bell ET. Carcinoma of the pancreas: I. a clinical and pathologic study of 609 necropsied cases. II. the relation of carcinoma of the pancreas to diabetes mellitus. Am J Pathol 1957;33:499–523.
39. Capella C, Solcia E, Frigerio B, et al. The endocrine cells of the pancreas and related tumours: ultrastructural study and classification. Virchows Arch A Pathol Anat 1977;373:327–52.
40. Tschang TP, Garza-Garza R, Kissane JM. Pleomorphic carcinoma of the pancreas: an analysis of 15 cases. Cancer 1977;39:2114–26.
41. Alguacil-Garcia A, Weiland LH. The histologic spectrum, prognosis, and histogenesis of the sarcomatoid carcinoma of the pancreas. Cancer 1977;39:1181–9.
42. Webb JN. Acinar cell neoplasms of the exocrine pancreas. J Clin Pathol 1977;30:103–12.
43. Sanfey H, Mendelsohn G, Cameron JL. Solid and papillary neoplasm of the pancreas: a potentially curable surgical lesion. Ann Surg 1983;197:272–5.
44. Wu M, Arimura GK, Yunis AA. Purification and characterization of a plasminogen activator secreted by cultured human pancreatic carcinoma cells. Biochemistry 1977;16:1908–13.
45. Lin A, Feller ER. Pancreatic carcinoma as a cause of unexplained pancreatitis: report of ten cases. Ann Intern Med 1990;113:166–7.
46. Fras I, Litin EM, Pearson JS. Comparison of psychiatric symptoms in carcinoma of the pancreas with those in some other intra-abdominal neoplasms. Am J Psychiatry 1967;123:1553–62.
47. Holland JC, Silberfarb P, Feldman M, et al. Comparative assessment of depression in patients with advanced pancreatic and gastric cancer. Proc ASCO 1983;2:127.
48. Van Dyke JA, Stanley RJ, Berland LL. Pancreatic imaging. Ann Intern Med 1985;102:212–7.
49. Freeny PC, Marks WM, Ball TJ. Impact of high-resolution computed tomography of the pancreas on utilization of endoscopic retrograde cholangiopancreatography and angiography. Radiology 1982;142:35–9.
50. Liguory C, Lefebvre JF. Retrograde pancreatography: technical tips and spectrum of pathology. Gastrointest Endosc Clin N Am 1995;5:81–104.
51. Kondo H, Sugano K, Fukayama N, et al. Detection of point mutations in the K-ras oncogene at codon 12 in pure pancreatic juice for diagnosis of pancreatic carcinoma. Cancer 1994;73:1589–94.
52. Alvarez C, Livingston EH, Ashley SW, et al. Cost-benefit analysis of the work-up for pancreatic cancer. Am J Surg 1993;165:53–60.
53. Peterli R, Meyer-Wyss B, Herzog U, Tondelli P. CA19-9 has no value as a tumor marker in obstructive jaundice. Schweiz Med Wochenschr 1999;129:77–9.
54. Pasanen PA, Eskelinen M, Partanen K, et al. A prospective study of serum tumour markers carcinoembryonic antigen, carbohydrate antigens 50 and 242, tissue polypeptide antigen and tissue polypeptide specific antigen in the diagnosis of pancreatic cancer with special reference to multivariate diagnostic score. Br J Cancer 1994;69:562–5.
55. Dickey JE, Haaga JR, Stellato TA, et al. Evaluation of computed tomography guided percutaneous biopsy of the pancreas. Surg Gynecol Obstet 1986;163:497–503.
56. Rösch T, Braig C, Gain T, et al. Staging of pancreatic and ampullary carcinoma by endoscopic ultrasonography: comparison with conventional sonography, computed tomography, and angiography. Gastroenterology 1992;102:188–99.
57. Fleming ID, Cooper JS, Henson DE, et al, eds. AJCC cancer staging manual. 5th ed. Philadelphia: Lippincott-Raven, 1997:121.
58. Zerbi A, Balzano G, Bottura R, Di Carlo V. Reliability of pancreatic cancer staging classifications. Int J Pancreatol 1994;15:13–8.
59. Connolly MM, Dawson PJ, Michelassi F, et al. Survival in 1001 patients with carcinoma of the pancreas. Ann Surg 1987;206:366–73.
60. Geer RJ, Brennan MF. Prognostic indicators for survival after resection of pancreatic adenocarcinoma. Am J Surg 1993:165:68–73.
61. Griffin JF, Smalley SR, Jewell W, et al. Patterns of failure after curative resection of pancreatic carcinoma. Cancer 1990;66:56–61.

# SURGERY

- Kenneth P. Ramming

## CURATIVE OPERATIONS

Cancer of the pancreas may be more locally advanced at the time of diagnosis than any other gastrointestinal malignancy. This finding, combined with the fact that local invasion frequently affects vital structures to which surgical access is limited—such as the portal vein, vena cava, common bile duct, and liver—makes curative surgery formidable. For lesions of the head of the pancreas, radical pancreaticoduodenectomy (Whipple's procedure) is still the procedure of choice. In this operation, the distal stomach and the duodenum, the first portion of the jejunum, and the head and part of the body of the pancreas are resected en bloc. The bile duct is anastomosed end-to-side to the jejunal remnant, and the pancreatic remnant is anastomosed end-to-end or end-to-side with the jejunal remnant. A gastrojejunostomy is then performed. Most surgeons consider it essential to perform a vagotomy during this procedure because a well-recognized postoperative complication is upper gastrointestinal hemorrhage.

The most troublesome part of the procedure is the pancreaticojejunostomy, which has led some surgeons to advocate total pancreatectomy in most cases of radical pancreatic excision for carcinoma. Total pancreatectomy also has the advantage of preventing local recurrence of the tumor in the pancreatic remnant. The major disadvantage is varying degrees of exocrine insufficiency and permanent diabetes mellitus, with a continuing requirement for insulin therapy.[1]

Shiu[2] has reported an important technical innovation in the management of the pancreatic stump after pancreaticoduodenectomy (Fig. 45–1). This innovation involves the ligation of the pancreatic duct with an absorbable suture. By allowing the jejunal-pancreatic anastomosis to heal in the absence of amylase, anastomotic leaks are obviated. The polyglycolic acid suture melts by postoperative day 9 or 10, which can be determined by aspirating jejunal contents and measuring amylase. This innovation has largely eliminated one of the most serious complications of this potentially curative procedure.

Few surgeons achieve the excellent results reported by Aston and Longmire,[3] in which 31 patients underwent pancreaticoduodenectomy with no resulting operative deaths. Sato and colleagues[4] reported a study of 66 patients undergoing pancreaticoduodenectomy. The hospital mortality rate

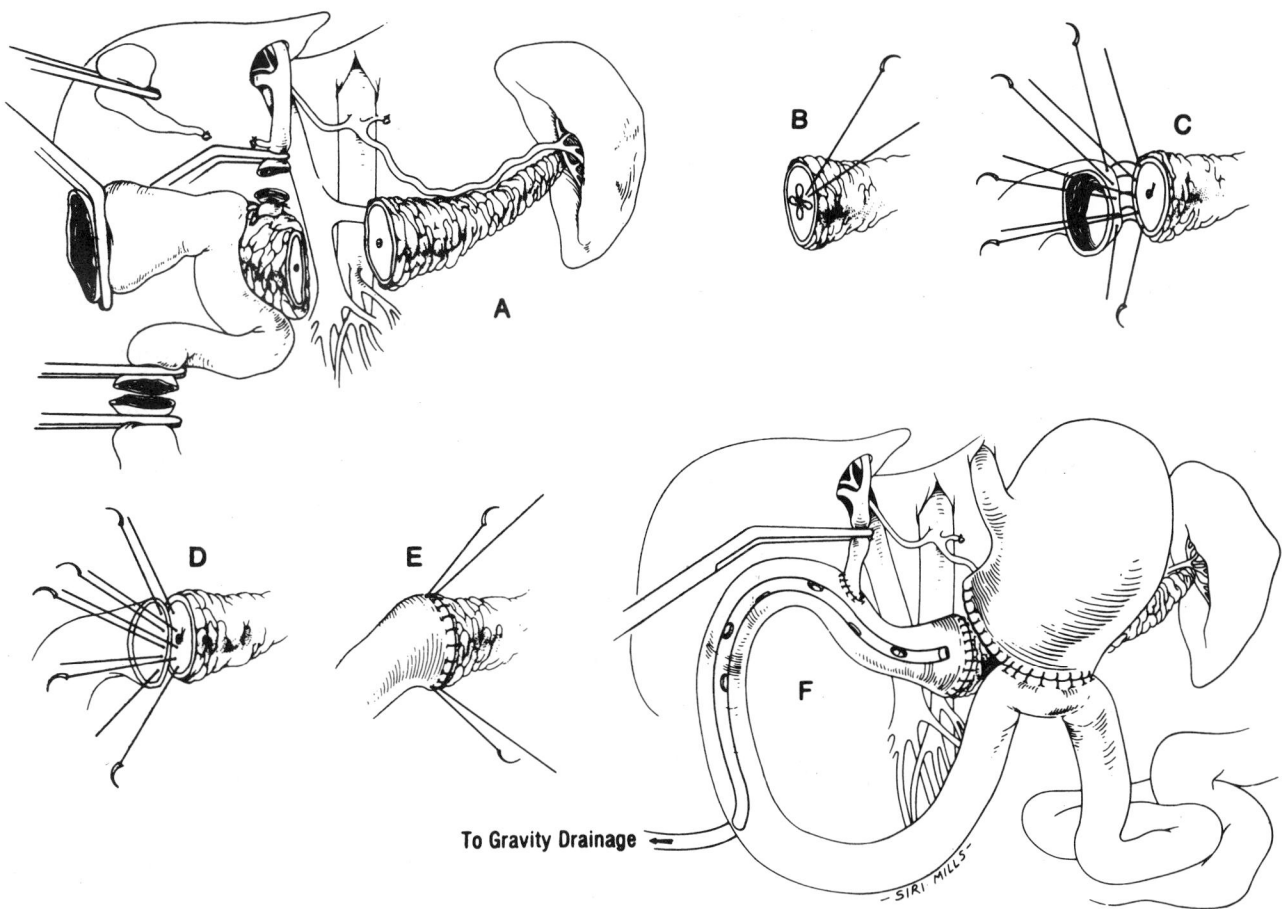

**Figure 45–1.** Management of the pancreatic stump after pancreaticoduodenectomy. *A*, The pancreas is divided with a scalpel at the selected site. *B*, The pancreatic duct is identified and occluded with a purse-string suture of 3–0 polyglycolic acid. *C* to *E*, The pancreatic stump is invaginated into the lumen of the jejunum by means of a pancreaticojejunal anastomosis, using two layers of 3–0 silk sutures. The inner layer unites the wall of the jejunum with the pancreatic capsule and subcapsular parenchyma. The outer layer pulls a cuff of the seromuscular coat of the jejunum over the pancreatic capsule, invaginating the stump. *F*, An 18F tube with side holes is used to drain bile and any pancreatic juice that may be present in the jejunum near the site of pancreaticojejunostomy. (From Shiu MH. Resection of pancreas without production of fistula. Surg Gynecol Obstet 1982;154:499.)

was 8%, and the 5-year survival rates were 8% in 20 patients with carcinoma of the head of the pancreas, 17% in 31 patients with carcinoma of the bile duct, and 38% in 15 patients with carcinoma of the ampulla of Vater. Fortner and associates[5] have advocated en bloc pancreatic, portal vein, and lymph node resection, with portal vein repair by end-to-end anastomosis without a graft. The 30-day mortality rate was 17%, and actuarial survival was 62% at 1 year, compared with a 36% 1-year survival rate for patients undergoing more conventional pancreaticoduodenectomy. Ihse and coworkers[6] considered total pancreatectomy to be superior to the conventional Whipple procedure in a review of 65 cases.

## PALLIATIVE OPERATIONS

Often, laparotomy or a prelaparotomy laparoscopy reveals that the pancreatic malignancy is not resectable for cure. Palliative procedures are often performed to treat obstructive jaundice and real or impending obstruction of the gastric outlet of the duodenum. Choledochojejunostomy and cholecystojejunostomy have been performed to relieve obstructive jaundice. I prefer the former with a Roux-en-Y loop of jejunum and a two-layer choledochojejunal anastomosis in either end-to-end or end-to-side fashion. If enlarged tumors of the head of the pancreas with duodenal obstruction are found, gastrojejunostomy should also be performed. The operations do not prolong survival but may well improve the quality of the remaining months of life.

Results and techniques that were used in large numbers of patients treated surgically for cure or palliation have been reported (see previous editions of this book and an excellent review by Warshaw and Fernández-del Castillo[7] for references). As with surgery for most other gastrointestinal malignancies, perioperative hyperalimentation has been shown to improve postoperative nutrition and function.[8] Weight loss is common in these patients, which is usually due to malabsorption related to pancreatic enzyme insufficiency.[9, 10] Significant palliation can be obtained in patients with moderate to severe malabsorption by the use of a pancreatic extract. Studies of chronic pancreatitis suggest that these patients should also receive supplemental fat-soluble vitamins (A, D, E, and K).[11]

An especially important goal of palliation at the time of surgery is the reduction of pain, but this goal is not always accomplished with the procedures described previously.

Alternative techniques are being explored, including the injection of the splenic nerve with phenol at the time of laparotomy[12] or combining such injections with pancreaticojejunostomy.[13]

## REFERENCES

1. Castellanos J, Manifacio G, Lillehei RC, Shatney CH. Total pancreatectomy for ductal carcinoma of the head of the pancreas: current status. Am J Surg 1976;131:595–8.
2. Shiu MH. Resection of pancreas without production of fistula. Surg Gynecol Obstet 1982;154:497–500.
3. Aston SJ, Longmire WP Jr. Pancreaticoduodenal resection: twenty years' experience. Arch Surg 1973;106:813–7.
4. Sato T, Saitoh Y, Noto N, Matsuno S. Follow-up studies of radical resection for pancreaticoduodenal cancer. Ann Surg 1977;186:581–8.
5. Fortner JG, Kim DK, Cubilla A, et al. Regional pancreatectomy: en bloc pancreatic, portal vein and lymph node resection. Ann Surg 1977;186:42–50.
6. Ihse I, Lilja P, Arnesjö B, Bengmark S. Total pancreatectomy for cancer: an appraisal of 65 cases. Ann Surg 1977;186:675–80.
7. Warshaw AL, Fernández-del Castillo C. Pancreatic carcinoma. N Engl J Med 1992;326:455–65.
8. Shils ME. Effects on nutrition of surgery of the liver, pancreas, and genitourinary tract. Cancer Res 1977;37:2387–94.
9. Perez MM, Newcomer AD, Moertel CG, et al. Assessment of weight loss, food intake, fat metabolism, malabsorption, and treatment of pancreatic insufficiency in pancreatic cancer. Cancer 1983;52:346–52.
10. Barkin JS, Kalser MH, Thomsen S, et al. Defect in assimilation following combined radiation and chemotherapy in patients with locally unresectable pancreatic carcinoma. Cancer 1982;50:2189–92.
11. Dutta SK, Bustin MP, Russell RM, Costa BS. Deficiency of fat-soluble vitamins in treated patients with pancreatic insufficiency. Ann Intern Med 1982;97:549–52.
12. Flanigan DP, Kraft RO. Continuing experience with palliative chemical splanchnicectomy. Arch Surg 1978;113:509–11.
13. Apalakis A, Dussault J, Knight M, Smith R. Relief of pain from pancreatic carcinoma. Ann R Coll Surg Engl 1977;59:401–3.

# RADIATION THERAPY

• Luu M. Tran

Pancreaticoduodenectomy is the standard procedure for carcinoma of the head of the pancreas. As a result of early extension beyond the pancreas, however, few patients (10%) are candidates for curative resection at diagnosis because most have locally advanced, unresectable disease at presentation. Even after curative resection, the outcome remains poor, with the 5-year survival less than 5% after Whipple's procedure alone[1]; local recurrence rates approach 75%.[2]

To improve outcome, adjuvant treatments, such as radiation therapy and chemotherapy, have been studied and have proved beneficial as adjuvant treatment and as primary management for unresectable disease. In addition to external-beam radiation therapy (EBRT), newer modalities, such as intraoperative electron-beam therapy (IORT), interstitial implant, or altered fractionation schedules, have been pursued in an attempt to decrease local recurrence and improve survival. Preoperative chemoradiation is under investigation.

## RADIATION TECHNIQUES

The target volume of EBRT includes the primary tumor site and the adjacent 3 to 5 cm of pancreatic tissue, the lymphatic drainage, and for tumors of the pancreatic head, the duodenum. Radiation fields encompass the pancreaticoduodenal, celiac, suprapancreatic, and porta hepatis lymph nodes. For lesions of the pancreatic body or tail, the field should also include the splenic hilar nodes. Contrast materials and three-dimensional conformal radiation therapy are helpful to determine the tumor volume as well as potential exposure to anatomic surrounding structures. Custom blocks with beam shaping are needed to limit the doses to small bowel, kidneys, spinal cord, and liver.

Patients should be treated with multiple three- or four-field technique using linear accelerators with high-energy photons. The upper border of the anteroposterior field is usually at the level of T10–T11 to cover the celiac nodes, and the lower border is usually at the level of L3. Lateral fields should set the superior and inferior borders the same as anteroposterior and posteroanterior fields. The posterior border is designed to include the para-aortic lymph nodes and to exclude both kidneys. The anterior border is shaped to provide adequate margins 2 to 3 cm beyond gross disease. The tumor volume is generally treated with 1.8 to 2 Gy/day, given 5 days per week over 4 to 6 weeks, to a total dose of 40 to 60 Gy.

## TREATMENT RESULTS FOR RESECTABLE TUMORS

**Adjuvant Treatment Following Resection.** In the management of pancreatic cancer, there have been no randomized trials to date designed to establish the role of primary radiation therapy alone, preoperative radiation therapy, intraoperative radiation therapy, or postoperative radiation therapy. In patients with resectable disease, there has been only one randomized, controlled trial of adjuvant therapy. In 1985, the Gastrointestinal Tumor Study Group (GITSG) protocol 9173[3, 4] randomized 43 patients following pancreaticoduodenectomy. They were randomized to surgery alone or 40 Gy split course with bolus injection of 5-fluorouracil (5-FU) on the first 3 days of radiation, followed by weekly maintenance 5-FU for 2 years. Overall 2-year survival with adjuvant therapy was 43% compared with 18% in the surgery-alone group. Five-year survivals were 18 and 7% ($p = 0.05$).

After this initial report, an additional 30 patients were given radiation therapy plus chemotherapy as the standard arm. Survival in this group was 18 months compared with only 10 months in the surgery-alone group. The local recurrence rate in this combined treatment group, however, remained high at 55%. So far, GITSG-9173 is the only randomized study that supports the effectiveness of adjuvant therapy for patients with resected pancreatic cancers.

The European Organization for Research and Treatment of Cancer (EORTC)[5] has completed a randomized study comparing adjuvant combined-modality therapy (CMT) (58 patients) with surgery alone (61 patients). The median and 2-year survival rates of the adjuvant group were 17 months and 37%, compared with 13 months and 23% for the surgery-alone group ($p = 0.099$). Several nonrandomized trials[6-8] from John Hopkins, the Eastern Cooperative Oncology Group (ECOG), and the Mayo Clinic (Table 45–3) provide further support for the use of adjuvant chemoradiation in patients with resectable pancreatic carcinoma.

Although CMT can decrease local recurrence and increase survival, intra-abdominal failure in the liver and peritoneal cavity remains as high as 60%. In hopes of reducing this high failure rate, further investigation is warranted to examine the benefits of aggressive systemic chemotherapy with continuous infusion of 5-FU and leucovorin, maintenance regimens, new radiation sensitizers (such as gemcitabine), IORT, or prophylactic whole-liver irradiation.

**Preoperative Chemoradiation.** As noted earlier, the local recurrence rates with surgery and adjuvant radiation therapy plus chemotherapy remain high. Several centers have used neoadjuvant radiation therapy plus chemotherapy before curative resection in patients with resectable disease (Table 45–4), with the goal being to improve local-regional control by facilitating a complete surgical resection and to prevent peritoneal seeding resulting from manipulation at the time of surgery. At laparotomy, about 25% of patients are found to have evidence of liver metastasis so that surgery is not performed, sparing these patients the potential morbidity associated with pancreaticoduodenectomy. A number of retrospective studies, mainly from M.D. Anderson Cancer Center, have employed this neoadjuvant preoperative approach in resectable pancreatic cancer.

Staley and colleagues[9] reported the results of 39 patients with operable pancreatic carcinoma treated with preoperative CMT (30 or 50.4 Gy EBRT and concomitant 5-FU before pancreaticoduodenectomy). IORT was given to the tumor bed before resection. At median follow-up of 11 months, 23 patients had died of disease, and there was one perioperative death. The liver was the most frequent site of failure and was a component of treatment failure in 53% of patients. Isolated local or peritoneal recurrences were documented in four (11%) patients. The median survival of 39 patients was 19 months, and the 4-year actuarial survival was 19%.

Spitz and associates[10] reported the results of 142 patients with localized adenocarcinoma of the head of the pancreas deemed resectable on the basis of radiographic images. Sixty patients were treated with curative intent using a multimodality approach involving either preoperative (41 patients) or postoperative chemoradiation (19 patients). Protocol-based preoperative chemoradiation consisted of 50.4 Gy (standard fractionation) or 30 Gy at 3 Gy per fraction combined with continuous-infusion 5-FU. Postoperative chemoradiation combined 50.4 Gy of EBRT and continuous infusion of 5-FU. At median follow-up of 19 months, no survival difference was seen between the groups. No patient who received preoperative chemoradiation experienced local recurrence, as opposed to 21% of 19 patients with the postoperative approach. Peritoneal (regional) recurrence occurred in 10 patients with the preoperative approach. No significant differences in toxicities were observed between groups.

ECOG[11] has initiated a phase II trial to examine the tolerance and efficacy of preoperative chemoradiation and surgical resection for patients with resectable adenocarcinoma of the pancreas. So far, 53 patients have been available for analysis. With a median follow-up of 52 months, 24 patients had resection, and their median survival was 16 months. Tumor progression was most frequent at metastatic sites: 33% of patients were found to have liver or peritoneal metastases (or both) at the time of laparotomy and were spared a major resection.

*Table 45–3.* **Adjuvant Therapy for Resectable Pancreatic Carcinoma**

| Series | Patients (No.) | Treatment RT | Treatment CM | Survival MEDIAN (mo) | Survival 2-yr (%) |
|---|---|---|---|---|---|
| GITSG[3] | | | | | |
| S + RT | 22 | 40 Gy/6 wk | | 11 | 18 |
| | | | | | $p = 0.05$ |
| S + RT ± CM | 21 | 40 Gy/6 wk | 5-FU (weekly bolus) | 21 | 43 |
| GITSG[4] | 30 | 40 Gy/6 wk | 5-FU (weekly bolus) | 18 | 46 |
| EORTC[5] | | | | | |
| S alone | 58 | | | 13 | 23 |
| | | | | | $p = 0.099$ |
| S + RT + CM | 61 | 40 Gy/6 wk | 5-FU (weekly bolus) No maintenance CM | 17 | 37 |
| NCI[26] | | | | | |
| S + EBRT | 16 | 50 Gy/5 wk | 5-FU | 12 | |
| S + IORT | 16 | 20 Gy | 5-FU | 12 | |
| Hopkins[6] | 56 | 45–50 Gy/5 wk | CI 5-FU | 20 | 39 |
| Univ. Penn. | 28 | 45–63 Gy | CI 5-FU/mitomycin C | 16 | 30 |
| Mayo[8] | 26 | 35–60 Gy | CI 5-FU | 23 | 48 |

RT, radiation therapy; CM, chemotherapy; S, surgery; 5-FU, 5-fluorouracil; EBRT, external-beam radiation therapy; IORT, electron-beam intraoperative radiation therapy; CI, continuous infusion.

*Table 45–4.* Preoperative Chemoradiation for Resectable and Unresectable Pancreatic Cancers

| Series | No. Patients | Treatment RADIATION THERAPY | CHEMOTHERAPY | Median Survival (mo) | Local-Regional Recurrence (%) | Resectability |
|---|---|---|---|---|---|---|
| *Resectable Tumors* | | | | | | |
| Spitz et al[10] | | | | | | |
|   Preoperative | 41 | 50.4/5 wk or 30 Gy/2 wk | CI 5-FU | 19 2-yr: 40% both | 10 (peritoneal) | |
|   Postoperative | 19 | 50.4 Gy/5 wk | CI 5-FU | 22 | 21 | |
| Staley et al[9] | 39 | 30–50 Gy EBRT + 10 Gy IORT | 5-FU | 19, 4-yr: 19% | 11 | |
| Hoffman et al[11] | 53 | 50.4 Gy/5 wk | CI 5-FU + Mit-C | 16 | | 24/53 (45%) |
| *Unresectable Tumors* | | | | | | |
| Jessup et al[20] | 23 | 50.4 Gy/5 wk | CI 5-FU | | | 10/23 (44%) |
| Coia et al[22] | 27 | 50.4 Gy/5 wk | 5-FU/Mit-C | 9, 3-yr: 19% | | 13/27 (50%) |
| Hoffman et al[18] | 34 | 50.4 Gy/5 wk | CI 5-FU + Mit-C | 33 | | 11/34 (33%) 10/11 patients had negative margins |
| Yeung et al[17] | 26 | 50 Gy/5 wk | 5-FU/Mit-C | 16% (5-yr) | | 10/18 (56%) Negative margins in all cases |
| Evans et al[19] | 28 | 50 gy + 10–20 Gy IORT | 5-FU | NA | | 17/28 (60%) Negative margins in 82% |

CI, continuous infusion; 5-FU, 5-fluorouracil; EBRT, external-beam radiation therapy; IORT, electron-beam intraoperative radiation therapy; Mit-C, mitomycin C.

Based on the results of these small, nonrandomized trials, it appears that preoperative chemoradiation is safe, is tolerable, and may increase resectability. To date, there has been no phase III randomized trial to confirm the benefit of neoadjuvant treatment.

## TREATMENT RESULTS FOR LOCALLY UNRESECTABLE PANCREATIC DISEASE

**Primary Chemoradiation Therapy.** GITSG-9273[12] was the first study using CMT for locally unresectable disease. In this three-arm study, 25 patients were randomized to radiation therapy alone (60 Gy), 31 patients to 60 Gy plus 5-FU, and 28 patients to 40 Gy plus 5-FU. Radiation therapy was given in split course (20 Gy with a 2-week break, followed by another 20 Gy). 5-FU was given with bolus injection 500 mg/m$^2$/day during the first 3 days of radiation therapy of each of the three courses followed by 2 years of weekly maintenance treatment. In the first phase of this study, a nearly twofold increase in median survival was observed in the CMT arms, 40 weeks each, compared with 22 weeks when using radiation therapy alone ($p<0.01$). A second phase of the study[13] compared median survival between two arms of CMT: The median survival of the 60 Gy plus 5-FU was 49 weeks, compared with only 36 weeks in the 40 Gy plus 5-FU arm ($p<0.1$) in those patients who were not bypassed. There was no difference in survival in the patients who were successfully bypassed. This study showed that chemoradiation was superior to radiation therapy alone for unresectable pancreatic carcinoma, the improvement in survival being more than twofold.

The latest GITSG[14] (GI-9283) trial was limited to patients with unresectable disease and tested the contribution of radiation therapy. Patients were treated with either combined radiation plus SMF (streptozotocin, mitomycin C, and 5-FU) chemotherapy or chemotherapy alone. In this study, the median survival for the CMT group was 42 weeks compared with 32 weeks for the chemotherapy-alone group ($p<0.02$).

Based on these studies, primary 5-FU–based chemotherapy plus radiation therapy emerged as standard treatment for locally unresectable pancreatic cancers. Klaassen and associates[15] from ECOG, however, failed to show a survival benefit to patients with unresectable disease between the group receiving 5-FU alone and the group receiving 5-FU plus radiation.

**Preoperative Chemoradiation.** Of the patients who present with nonmetastatic disease, only 10% have tumors considered surgically resectable because of tumor invading major viscera and vessels.[1] Preoperative chemoradiation has been used to convert these patients to resectable status. The first trial was from University of St. Louis,[16] where investigators administered 45 Gy over 5 weeks before exploratory laparotomy in 17 patients with locally advanced disease. Radical resection was successfully performed in six patients. Five were noted to have no gross disease at re-exploration laparotomy, and of these 5, 2 remained free of disease at 5 years, and 2 had relapsed. The results of the other retrospective trials[17–22] are shown in Table 45–4. Based on the experiences of these studies, the use of preoperative chemoradiation for patients with unresectable pancreatic cancers may result in downstaging and improvement in resectability. It is uncertain whether enhancing the resectability would increase overall survival.

## NEWER MODALITIES

With conventional EBRT, the local failure remains high even with the combination of radiation sensitizers. The main reason is the inability to deliver a tumoricidal dose of radiation because of the proximity of the dose-limited structures. To augment the action of radiation to the tumor, newer modalities have been used, such as IORT, brachytherapy, and three-dimensional conformal radiation therapy with radiation sensitizers via protracted venous infusion.

**Intraoperative Electron-Beam Therapy.** The anatomic relation of the pancreas to other organs prohibits the delivery of tumoricidal doses of EBRT and has prompted the use of IORT, which can be used either alone or more often in combination with EBRT 45 to 50 Gy over 5 weeks plus 5-FU–based chemotherapy. IORT is given with a single dose of electron-beam radiation ranging from 10 to 40 Gy to the tumor bed or to unresectable disease.

Significant data on the use of IORT are coming from Japan, where several investigators have noticed a substantial reduction in the incidence of local-regional recurrence. Abe and colleagues[23] using combined EBRT and IORT noted median survival of 12 months. Hiraoka and associates[24] reported 5-year survival of 29% in 16 patients treated with an extended pancreatectomy and IORT 30 Gy. Ozaki and coworkers[25] reported a 3-year survival of 53% for 16 patients treated with combined radical resection, IORT, and mitomycin C.

In the United States, the Mayo Clinic[26] has performed several studies using IORT in combination with EBRT and chemotherapy for resectable and unresectable pancreatic carcinomas. The investigators observed improvement in local control in those who were treated with combination of EBRT and IORT versus IORT alone.

In patients with resectable disease, reports on the role of IORT are relatively limited. The National Cancer Institute[27] randomized 24 patients with resectable pancreatic cancers to either 20 Gy IORT or 45 Gy EBRT. Both groups received concurrent 5-FU chemotherapy. All patients receiving postoperative radiation therapy alone developed local recurrence within 12 months compared with only 20% of those receiving IORT. The median disease-free survival was slightly better in the IORT group, 18 months compared with 12 months in the EBRT group ($p = 0.01$). The actuarial overall survival and morbidity in both groups were similar.

Several phase I and II trials[28–30] in patients with unresectable disease have used IORT in combination with EBRT with promising results. The National Cancer Institute[27] reported a prospective trial involving 23 patients with stage III unresectable pancreatic carcinoma. Patients in the experimental group received bypass surgery and postoperative IORT 25 Gy followed by EBRT to 50 Gy. Patients on the control arm received bypass and 60 Gy EBRT. Both groups received 5-FU–based chemotherapy. There was no difference in median survival (8 months in both groups). All patients were dead of disease within 18 months in the control arm and within 24 months in the IORT arm. Three IORT patients developed duodenal bleeding within 6 to 8 months following treatment.

The Radiation Therapy Oncology Group[31] initiated a phase I–II trial (85-05) for unresectable pancreatic carcinoma. Patients were treated with IORT 16.5 to 22 Gy and

postoperative EBRT 50 Gy plus 5-FU–based chemotherapy. Fifty-one patients were available for evaluation. The median survival was approximately 9 months, with 47 of 51 patients dead at the last analysis. This median survival is similar to the results obtained from EBRT and 5-FU.

Based on these trials, the combination of IORT and EBRT plus 5-FU has not resulted in improvement of survival for patients with locally advanced pancreatic carcinoma. Although there appears to be decreased local recurrence when IORT is added, peritoneal and hepatic metastasis continues to be a major problem. At this time, IORT cannot be recommended as part of standard treatment in locally advanced pancreatic carcinoma.

**Interstitial Implant.** Interstitial implant using radioisotope implantation at the time of surgery is another way of delivering high doses of radiation, while significantly sparing the adjacent structures. The most commonly used isotopes are iodine 125 and palladium 103. Doses range from 100 to 200 Gy. EBRT and chemotherapy are given following implantation, identical to the post-IORT regimen.

Mohiuddin and colleagues[32] from Thomas Jefferson University Hospital reported the results of 81 unresectable carcinomas of the pancreas treated with iodine implant, EBRT 50 to 55 Gy, and 5-FU and mitomycin C with or without CCNU (lomustine) chemotherapy. Iodine 125 was used to deliver 120 Gy over 1 year. The median survival was 13 months, and the 2-year survival was 22%. Local control was achieved in 71% of patients. By comparison, in 23 patients undergoing surgical resection alone, the medial survival was 12 months, with no patient surviving beyond 3 years. The authors concluded that the interstitial implant approach might achieve satisfactory local control and long-term survival in selected patients.

Memorial Sloan-Kettering Cancer Center[33] reported the results of 11 patients treated with palladium 103 implant during laparotomy. The median dose was 124 Gy. Four patients developed acute postoperative complications. Five of 11 (45%) patients were locally controlled as seen by computed tomographic scan. At median follow-up of 7 months, 10 of 11 patients had died of disease. The authors concluded that because there is no improvement in survival over conventional modalities, they do not recommend palladium as a component of treatment of unresectable pancreatic disease.

Based on these results with IORT and brachytherapy, there appears to be some modest decrease in local recurrence compared with EBRT alone. There is no survival benefit, however, because most patients eventually succumb from widespread metastatic disease during or after treatment.

**Protracted Venous Infusion of 5-Fluorouracil Combined with High-Dose Radiation Therapy.** Although conventional radiation therapy and bolus 5-FU have been shown to double the median survival in locally advanced pancreatic cancers, most patients eventually recur locally as well as distantly. Over the past several years, interest in the administration of radiation sensitizers through protracted venous infusion with high radiation therapy dose has increased steadily. Poen and colleagues[34] from Stanford University used protracted venous infusion 5-FU (225 mg/m$^2$) given concurrently with combined EBRT with or without IORT (61 Gy) in 30 patients with locally advanced pancreatic cancers. So far, all patients have tolerated the treatment well with no grade IV or V complications. Picus and associates[35] from the University of St. Louis reported a phase II trial of continuous-infusion 5-FU with three-dimensional conformal radiation therapy (50 to 54 Gy) in the adjuvant treatment of 20 patients with pancreatic cancers. With a median follow-up of 14 months, the recurrence rate was 55%, and the median survival of patients with positive lymph nodes or positive margins was projected to be 13 months. Rich and Evans,[36] Jessup and colleagues,[20] and Wittington and colleagues[37] have used similar regimens and have obtained promising results with acceptable toxicities.

## REFERENCES

1. Gudjonsson B. Cancer of the pancreas: 50 years of surgery. Cancer 1987;60:2284–303.
2. Griffin JF, Smalley SR, Jewell W, et al. Patterns of failure after curative resection of pancreatic carcinoma. Cancer 1990;66:56–61.
3. Kalser MH, Ellenberg SS. Pancreatic cancer: adjuvant combined radiation and chemotherapy following curative resection. Arch Surg 1985;120:899–903 and 1986;121:1045.
4. Gastrointestinal Tumor Study Group. Further evidence of effective combined radiation and chemotherapy following curative resection of pancreatic cancer. Cancer 1987;59:2006–10.
5. Klinkenbijl J, Sahmond T, van Pel R, et al. Radiotherapy and 5-FU after curative resection for cancer of the pancreas and peri-ampullary region: a phase III trial of the EORTC and GITCCG. Eur J Cancer 1997;33:S274.
6. Yeo C, Abrams RA, Grochow LB, et al. Pancreaticoduodenectomy for pancreatic adenocarcinoma: postoperative adjuvant chemoradiation improves survival: a prospective, single institution experience. Ann Surg 1997;225:621–33.
7. Whittington R, Bryer M, Haller D, et al. Adjuvant therapy of resected adenocarcinoma of the pancreas. Int J Radiat Oncol Biol Phys 1991;21:1137–43.
8. Foo ML, Gunderson L, Nagorney D, et al. Pattern of failure in grossly resected pancreatic ductal adenocarcinoma treated with adjuvant irradiation ± 5-FU. Int J Radiat Oncol Biol Phys 1993;26:483–9.
9. Staley C, Lee JE, Cleary K, et al. Preoperative chemoradiation, pancreaticoduodenectomy, and intraoperative radiation therapy for adenocarcinoma of the pancreatic head. Am J Surg 1996;171:118–24.
10. Spitz FR, Abbruzzese JL, Lee J, et al. Preoperative and postoperative chemoradiation strategies in patients with pancreaticoduodenectomy for adenocarcinoma of the pancreas. J Clin Oncol 1997;15:928–37.
11. Hoffman JP, Lipsitz S, Pisansky T, et al. Phase II trial of preoperative radiation therapy and chemotherapy for patients with localized, resectable adenocarcinoma of the pancreas: an Eastern Cooperative Oncology Group Study. J Clin Oncol 1998;16:317–23.
12. Gastrointestinal Tumor Study Group. A multi-institutional comparative trial of radiation therapy alone and in combination with 5FU for locally unresectable pancreatic cancer. Ann Surg 1979;189:205–8.
13. Moertel CG, Frytak S, Hahn RG, et al. Therapy of locally unresectable pancreatic carcinoma: a randomized comparison of high dose (6000 rads) radiation alone, moderate dose radiation (4000 rads + 5-fluorouracil), and high dose radiation + 5-fluorouracil. The Gastrointestinal Tumor Study Group. Cancer 1981;48:1705–10.
14. Gastrointestinal Tumor Study Group. Treatment of locally unresectable carcinoma of the pancreas: comparison of combined modality therapy (chemotherapy plus radiotherapy) to chemotherapy alone. J Natl Cancer Inst 1988;80:751–5.
15. Klaassen DJ, MacIntyre JM, Catton GE, et al. Treatment of locally unresectable cancer of the stomach and pancreas: a randomized comparison of 5-fluorouracil alone with radiation plus concurrent and maintenance 5-fluorouracil. An Eastern Cooperative Oncology Group Study. J Clin Oncol 1985;3:373–8.
16. Pilepich MV, Miller H. Preoperative irradiation in carcinoma of the pancreas. Cancer 1980;46:1945–9.
17. Yeung R, Weese J, Hoffman JP, et al. Neoadjuvant chemoradiation in pancreatic and duodenal carcinoma: a Phase II Study. Cancer 1993;72:2124–33.
18. Hoffman JP, Weese JL, Solin LJ. A pilot study of preoperative chemoradiation with localized adenocarcinoma of the pancreas. Am J Surg 1995;169:71–7.
19. Evans DB, Rich T, Byrd D, et al. Preoperative chemoradiation and pancreaticoduodenectomy for adenocarcinoma of the pancreas. Arch Surg 1992;127:1335–9.
20. Jessup JM, Steele G, Mayer RJ, et al. Neoadjuvant therapy for unresectable pancreatic adenocarcinoma. Arch Surg 1993;128:559–64.
21. Wanebo HJ, Vezeridis MP. Pancreatic carcinoma in perspective: a continuing challenge. Cancer 1996;78:580–91.
22. Coia L, Hoffman J, Scher R, et al. Preoperative chemoradiation for adenocarcinoma of the pancreas and duodenum. Int J Radiat Oncol Biol Phys 1994;30:161–7.
23. Abe M, Takahashi M, Yabumoto E, et al. Clinical experience with intraoperative radiotherapy of locally advanced cancers. Cancer 1980;45:40–8.
24. Hiraoka T, Uchino R, Kanemisty K, et al. Combination of intraoperative radiation with resection of cancer of the pancreas. Int J Pancreatol 1990;7:201–7.
25. Ozaki H, Kinoshira T, Kosuge T, et al. Effectiveness of multimodality treatment for resectable pancreatic cancer. Int J Pancreatol 1990;7:195–200.
26. Gunderson LL, Martin JK, Kvols LK, et al. Intraoperative and external beam irradiation ± 5-FU for locally advanced pancreatic cancer. Int J Radiat Oncol Biol Phys 1987;13:319–29.
27. Sindelar WF, Kinsella TJ. Randomized trial of intraoperative radiotherapy in resected carcinoma of the pancreas. Int J Radiat Oncol Biol Phys 1986;12:148.
28. Shibamoto Y, Manabe T, Baba N, et al. High dose, external beam and intraoperative radiotherapy in the treatment of resectable and unresectable pancreatic cancer. Int J Radiat Oncol Biol Phys 1990;19:605–11.
29. Zerbi A, Fossati V, Parolini D, et al. IORT adjuvant to resection in the treatment of the pancreatic cancer. Cancer 1994;73:2930–5.
30. Nishimura Y, Hosotani R, Shibamoto Y, et al. External and intraoperative radiotherapy for resectable and unresectable pancreatic cancer: analysis of survival rates and complications. Int J Radiat Oncol Biol Phys 1997;39:39–49.
31. Tepper J, Noyes D, Krall J, et al. Intraoperative radiation therapy of pancreatic cancer: a report of RTOG 85-05. Int J Radiat Oncol Biol Phys 1991;21:1145–9.
32. Mohiuddin M, Rosato F, Barbot D, et al. Long term results of combined modality treatment with iodine-125 implant for cancer of the pancreas. Int J Radiat Oncol Biol Phys 1992;23:305–11.
33. Raben A, Mychalczak B, Brennan MF, et al. Feasibility study of the treatment of primary unresectable cancer of the pancreas with $^{103}$Pd brachytherapy. Int J Radiat Oncol Biol Phys 1996;35:351–6.
34. Poen J, Collins H, Niederhuber J, et al. Chemo-radiotherapy for localized pancreatic cancer: increased dose intensity and reduced acute toxicity with concomitant radiotherapy and protracted venous infusion 5-fluorouracil. Int J Radiat Oncol Biol Phys 1998;40:93–9.
35. Picus J, Myerson R, Drebin S. A phase II trial of continuous infusion (CIV) 5-FU with 3D-conformal radiation in the adjuvant treatment of pancreatic, ampullary and biliary cancers. Proc ASCO 1998;17:266a.
36. Rich T, Evans D. Preoperative combined modality for pancreatic cancer. World J Surg 1995;19:264–9.
37. Whittington R, Neuberg D, Tester WJ, et al. Protracted IV fluorouracil infusion with radiation therapy in the management of localized pancreaticobiliary carcinoma: a phase I Eastern Cooperative Oncology Group Trial. J Clin Oncol 1995;13:227–32.

# CHEMOTHERAPY

• William Isacoff • Charles M. Haskell

## SINGLE-AGENT CHEMOTHERAPY

Using traditional criteria of antitumor response, advanced adenocarcinoma of the pancreas rarely responds to single-agent chemotherapy. Table 45–5 lists agents with aggregate combined complete and partial response rates of 20% or greater.[1] There is no strong evidence, however, that the responses recorded in Table 45-5 confer clinical benefit to the patient, in the sense of improved quality or duration of life.

The nucleoside analogue gemcitabine is not listed in Table 45–5 because its response rate is only about 11%.[2] There is considerable interest, however, in its use as a single agent or as a component of combination chemotherapy (see subsequent discussion) because of a randomized trial conducted by Burris and coworkers.[3] These investigators randomized 126 patients to receive either gemcitabine or 5-FU. The end points were survival and a nontraditional benefit they called a *clinical benefit response*, which was defined as a composite of pain control, Karnofsky performance status, and weight. Gemcitabine achieved a clinical benefit response in 24% of patients, whereas 5-FU achieved benefit in 5% of patients ($p = 0.0022$). Survival was also better with gemcitabine (median survival, 5.65 months) than for 5-FU (median survival, 4.41 months) ($p = 0.0025$). Both drugs appeared to be reasonably well tolerated, with similar profiles of toxicity. Largely as a result of this study, gemcitabine is marketed for the palliative treatment of advanced pancreatic carcinoma.

## ENDOCRINE THERAPY

Because of the presence of receptors for estrogen or progesterone, or both, in many cases of pancreatic cancer, several groups have studied the possible role of endocrine therapy. One case-control study found a survival benefit from the use of tamoxifen,[4] but randomized studies have shown no benefit from the use of tamoxifen.[5, 6] Similarly, other forms of hormonal therapy have proven ineffective. Octreotide acetate may be useful in treating some of the complications of pancreatic cancer and its treatment.[7] Its role as a directly cytotoxic agent is less clear.[8]

**Table 45–5. Single Agents with a Combined Complete and Partial Response Rate of 20% or Greater for Adenocarcinoma of the Exocrine Pancreas**

| Drug | Patients (No.) | Response Rate (% CR + PR) | References |
|---|---|---|---|
| Ifosfamide | 101 | 30 | 1 |
| 5-Fluorouracil | 236 | 29 | 1 |
| Mitomycin C | 53 | 21 | 1 |

CR, complete response; PR, partial response.

## COMBINATION CHEMOTHERAPY

**Historical Background.** Since the initial study by Reitemeier and colleagues[9] at the Mayo Clinic, there has been great interest in the use of combination chemotherapy in the treatment of pancreatic carcinoma. Table 45–6 summarizes the results of combination chemotherapy regimens without cisplatin or gemcitabine tested up until the mid-1990s.[1] The initial reports of most regimens proved overly optimistic, and none of these regimens emerged as superior to the rest. For example, the FAM regimen (5-FU, doxorubicin [Adriamycin], mitomycin) has given response rates varying from 2 to 40%, with a mean of 16%.[1] Early results with FAM plus streptozocin (S) were also much better than those reported subsequently. For example, a study by the Southwest Oncology Group found no difference in response rates or survival in patients randomized to receive the FAM-S combination or one of three different investigational single agents.[10]

Given the difficulties of assessing responses in pancreatic cancer, numerous studies have evaluated the survival of patients treated with combination chemotherapy or endocrine therapy.[11–19] In one small study,[12] a survival advantage was seen with combination chemotherapy compared with an untreated control group, whereas two larger studies showed no such survival advantage.[13, 20] Early reports tend to be optimistic (such as reported with the combination of 5-FU plus testolactone using a historical control group[18]), whereas definitive randomized trials show no advantage to the new combination (completing the example with 5-FU plus testolactone, a negative prospective trial was conducted by ECOG[19]). In our view, none of these older drug combinations is demonstrably superior to any other in the management of this disease.

**Table 45–6. Combination Chemotherapy Regimens Without Cisplatin Having Complete Plus Partial Response Rates Greater than 20% in Pancreatic Cancer**

| Drugs* | Patients (No.) | Response Rate (% CR + PR) | References |
|---|---|---|---|
| 5-FU + MMC + ADR + STZ | 37 | 54 | 1 |
| 5-FU + ACNU + MMC | 13 | 46 | 1 |
| 5-FU + ADR | 10 | 30 | 1 |
| 5-FU + vinblastine | 11 | 27 | 1 |
| Ftorafur + BCNU + ADR | 19 | 26 | 1 |
| 5-FU + PALA | 9 | 25 | 1 |
| 5-FU + MeCCNU + MMC | 22 | 22 | 1 |
| 5-FU + ADR + cisplatin | 29 | 21 | 1 |

*Abbreviations are given in Appendix C.
CR, complete response; PR, partial response.

*Table 45–7.* Cisplatin-Based Combination Chemotherapy for Advanced Pancreatic Cancer

| Drugs Added to Cisplatin | Patients (No.) | Response Rate (% CR + PR) | Median Survival (mo) | Alive at 1 yr (%) | References |
|---|---|---|---|---|---|
| 5-FU | 63 | 16 | 7.6 | 33 | 21 |
| 5-FU | 104 | 12 | NS | 17 | 22 |
| 5-FU | 20 | 50 | 11 | NS | 23 |
| 5-FU + leucovorin | 48 | 21 | 9.5 | 34.6 | 24 |
| 5-FU + ADR | 29 | 21 | 4 | NS | 25 |
| Gemcitabine | 22 | 36.4 | 7.4 | NS | 26 |
| Gemcitabine | 35 | 11.5 | 8.3 | NS | 27 |
| Gemcitabine | 32 | 31 | NS | NS | 28 |
| FU + epirubicin + gemcitabine | 39 | 69 | 8 + | NS | 29 |
| FU + leucovorin + epirubicin + etoposide + megestrol acetate | 24 | 18 | 6.2 | NS | 30 |
| Overall | 416 | 22 | | | |

CR, complete response; PR, partial response; 5-FU, 5-fluorouracil; ADR, Adriamycin (doxorubicin); NS, not stated.

**Cisplatin-Based Combination Chemotherapy.** There has been considerable interest in testing cisplatin-based combination chemotherapy regimens in advanced pancreatic cancer. Table 45–7 summarizes the use of these agents to date.[21-30] Many of these reports are preliminary, and the aggregate response rate of 22% is highly provisional. The impact of cisplatin-based chemotherapy on overall survival and quality of life has yet to be assessed.

**Gemcitabine-Based Combination Chemotherapy.** Despite the apparent activity of gemcitabine in the treatment of advanced pancreatic cancer, the use of gemcitabine in combination with other agents has been disappointing. Table 45–8 summarizes results with such combinations, which have achieved an aggregate response rate of only 17%.[31-35]

**Other Approaches.** As part of a phase II trial at the University of California Los Angeles (UCLA), Todd and colleagues[36] treated 38 patients with locally advanced adenocarcinoma of the pancreas with 5-FU 200 mg/m$^2$/day, given as a continuous intravenous infusion using an ambulatory pump; leucovorin calcium 30 mg/m$^2$, given as an intravenous bolus injection on day 1 and weekly thereafter; mitomycin C 10 mg/m$^2$ (each dose not to exceed 15 mg), as an intravenous bolus injection on day 1 and then every 6 weeks; and dipyridamole 75 mg orally four times daily. The overall response rate was 39%, with a median survival of 15.5 months. The 1-year survival was 70%. Of the 15 responding patients, 6 patients were thought to be successfully downstaged and met the eligibility criteria for a second-look exploration. Four were able to undergo a curative pancreaticoduodenectomy. As a result of the encouraging outcome of the initial 38 patients, this four-drug regimen has since been tested extensively in patients with advanced pancreatic cancer at UCLA. An additional 32 patients with locally advanced disease have been treated with this four-drug regimen. There were 12 additional partial responses, for an aggregate response rate of 37%. Five of these responding patients had significant tumor regression to allow reoperation and resection of the cancer. Thus far, 11 patients have undergone a second-look operation, with 9 having significant tumor regression resulting in resection with curative intent (Whipple's procedure). The median survival of the 9 patients undergoing surgery was greater than 30 months.

**Summary of Combination Chemotherapy.** Combination chemotherapy is of uncertain value in patients with advanced pancreatic cancer. In contrast to the survival advantage discussed previously with the combination of chemotherapy and radiation therapy, the data on survival with combination chemotherapy alone are provisional and unconvincing. We are encouraged by the results of the UCLA study discussed earlier, but further confirmation is needed before recommending the widespread use of this or any other regimen.

## ADJUVANT THERAPY

Chemoradiotherapy may be of some value, as discussed previously in the section Radiation Therapy. Chemotherapy

*Table 45–8.* Gemcitabine-Based Combination Chemotherapy Regimens for Pancreatic Carcinoma

| Drugs | Patients (No.) | Response Rate (% CR + PR) | Median Survival (mo) | Alive at 1 yr (%) | References |
|---|---|---|---|---|---|
| Gemcitabine + 5-FU | 23 | 19 | 5.5 | NS | 31 |
| Gemcitabine + 5-FU | 26 | 19.2 | 10.3 | NS | 32 |
| Gemcitabine + 5-FU + leucovorin | 48 | 19.1 | 8 | 38 | 33 |
| Gemcitabine + Taxotere (docetaxel) | 9 | 33 | NS | NS | 34 |
| Gemcitabine + Taxotere (docetaxel) | 27 | 7.4 | 7 | 22 | 35 |
| Overall | 133 | 17 | | | |

CR, complete response; PR, partial response; 5-FU, 5-fluorouracil; NS, not stated.

alone has only rarely been employed in the adjuvant setting, and it has not been tested in the neoadjuvant (preoperative) setting. A Norwegian study randomized 61 patients with pancreatic cancer to receive AMF (doxorubicin [Adriamycin], mitomycin C, 5-FU) or observation alone after radical pancreatic surgery.[37] The median survival in the chemotherapy group was 23 months compared with 11 months for the control group. The survival rates at 5 years were not significantly different. Chemotherapy may have postponed recurrent disease, but it did not contribute to a higher cure rate. A Japanese study of 158 patients randomized to receive postoperative mitomycin and 5-FU versus observation alone showed a 5-year survival rate of 11.5% with chemotherapy and 18% with observation alone.[38] Adjuvant chemotherapy alone is of unproven value in the treatment of pancreatic cancer.

## IMMUNOTHERAPY

There have been few studies of immunotherapy for patients with pancreatic carcinoma. Several oncofetal antigens have been associated with pancreatic carcinoma, but their biologic importance is uncertain.[39] Adjuvant immunotherapy studies have been limited. There have been some preliminary reports of immunotherapy using monoclonal antibodies to pancreatic antigens,[40, 41] but one monoclonal antibody tested in the adjuvant setting was ineffective.[42] A phase II study of the immunomodulator Virulizin showed no anticancer activity.[43] Immunotherapy remains an investigational modality in the treatment of pancreatic cancer.

## REFERENCES

1. Haskell C, Lavey RS, Ramming KP. Exocrine pancreas. In: Haskell CM, ed. Cancer treatment. 4th ed. Philadelphia: WB Saunders, 1995:502.
2. Casper ES, Green MR, Kelsen DP, et al. Phase II trial of gemcitabine (2′,2′-difluorodeoxycytidine) in patients with adenocarcinoma of the pancreas. Invest New Drugs 1994;12:29–34.
3. Burris HA III, Moore MJ, Andersen J, et al. Improvements in survival and clinical benefit with gemcitabine as first-line therapy for patients with advanced pancreas cancer: a randomized trial. J Clin Oncol 1997;15:2403–13.
4. Wong A, Chan A. Survival benefit of tamoxifen therapy in adenocarcinoma of pancreas: a case-control study. Cancer 1993;71:2200–3.
5. Bakkevold KE, Pettersen A, Arnesjo B, et al. Tamoxifen therapy in unresectable adenocarcinoma of the pancreas and the papilla of Vater. Br J Surg 1990;77:725–30.
6. Taylor OM, Benson EA, McMahon MJ. Clinical trial of tamoxifen in patients with irresectable pancreatic adenocarcinoma. The Yorkshire Gastrointestinal Tumour Group. Br J Surg 1993;80:384–6.
7. Buchler M, Friess H, Klempa I, et al. Role of octreotide in the prevention of postoperative complications following pancreatic resection. Am J Surg 1992;163:125–30.
8. Friess H, Buchler M, Ebert M, et al. Treatment of advanced pancreatic cancer with high-dose octreotide. Int J Pancreatol 1993;14:290–1.
9. Reitemeier RJ, Moertel CG, Hahn RG. Combination chemotherapy in gastrointestinal cancer. Cancer Res 1970;30:1425–8.
10. Bukowski RM, Fleming TR, Macdonald JS, et al. Evaluation of combination chemotherapy and phase II agents in pancreatic adenocarcinoma. A Southwest Oncology Group study. Cancer 1993;71:322–5.
11. Horton J, Gelber RD, Engstrom P, et al. Trials of single-agent and combination chemotherapy for advanced cancer of the pancreas. Cancer Treat Rep 1981;65:65–8.
12. Mallinson CN, Rake MO, Cocking JB, et al. Chemotherapy in pancreatic cancer: results of a controlled, prospective, randomised, multicentre trial. Br Med J 1980;281:1589–1.
13. Frey C, Twomey P, Keehn R, et al. Randomized study of 5-FU and CCNU in pancreatic cancer: report of the Veterans Administration Surgical Adjuvant Cancer Chemotherapy Study Group. Cancer 1981;47:27–31.
14. McCracken JD, Ray P, Heilbrun LK, et al. 5-Fluorouracil, methyl-CCNU, and radiotherapy with or without testolactone for localized adenocarcinoma of the exocrine pancreas: a Southwest Oncology Group study. Cancer 1980;46:1518–22.
15. Smith FP, Stablein D, Korsmeyer S, et al. Combination chemotherapy for locally advanced pancreatic cancer: equivalence to external beam irradiation and implication for future management. J Clin Oncol 1983;1:413–5.
16. Topham C, Glees J, Coombes RC. Comparison of single-agent epirubicin and 5-fluorouracil/epirubicin/mitomycin in patients with advanced adenocarcinoma of the pancreas. Oncology 1993;50:78–80.
17. Huguier M, Samama G, Testart J, et al. Treatment of adenocarcinoma of the pancreas with somatostatin and gonadoliberin (luteinizing hormone-releasing hormone). The French Associations for Surgical Research. Am J Surg 1992;164:348–53.
18. Waddell WR. Chemotherapy for carcinoma of the pancreas. Surgery 1973;74:420–9.
19. Moertel CG, Engstrom P, Lavin PT, et al. Chemotherapy of gastric and pancreatic carcinoma: a controlled evaluation of combinations of 5-fluorouracil with nitrosoureas and "lactones." Surgery 1979;85:509–13.
20. Andersen JR, Friis-Moller A, Hancke S, et al. A controlled trial of combination chemotherapy with 5-FU and BCNU in pancreatic cancer. Scand J Gastroenterol 1981;16:973–5.
21. Nicolson M, Webb A, Cunningham D, et al. Cisplatin and protracted venous infusion 5-fluorouracil (CF)-good symptom relief with low toxicity in advanced pancreatic carcinoma. Ann Oncol 1995;6:801–4.
22. Rougier P, Ducreux M, Douillard JY, et al. Efficacy of 5FU + cisplatin (FUP) compared to bolus 5FU (FU) in advanced pancreatic carcinoma (APC): a randomized trial from the French Anticancer Centers Digestive Group (FNLCCDG). Proc ASCO 1999;18:274a.
23. Charles A, Heider A, Steffens F, et al. 5-Fluorouracil/cisplatin in the treatment of advanced pancreatic cancer. Proc ASCO 1999;18:280a.
24. André T, Lotz JP, Bouleuc C, et al. Phase II trial of 5-fluorouracil, leucovorin and cisplatin for treatment of advanced pancreatic adenocarcinoma. Ann Oncol 1996;7:173–8.
25. Moertel CG, Rubin J, O'Connell MJ, et al. A phase II study of combined 5-fluorouracil, doxorubicin, and cisplatin in the treatment of advanced upper gastrointestinal adenocarcinomas. J Clin Oncol 1986;4:1053–7.
26. Philip PA, Zalupski M, Vaitkevicius VK, et al. Phase II study of gemcitabine and cisplatin in advanced or metastatic pancreatic cancer. Proc ASCO 1999;18:274a.
27. Heinemann V, Wilke H, Possinger K, et al. Gemcitabine and cisplatin in the treatment of advanced and metastatic pancreatic cancer. final results of a phase II study. Proc ASCO 1999;18:274a.
28. Colucci G, Riccardi F, Giuliani F, et al. Randomized trial of gemcitabine (GEM) alone or with cisplatin (CDDP) in the treatment of advanced pancreatic cancer (APC): a phase II multicenter study. Proc ASCO 1999;18:250a.
29. Villa E. PEF-G (cisplatin, epirubicin, 5-fluorouracil continuous infusion, gemcitabine): a new combination in advnced pancreatic adenocarcinoma. phase II study. Proc ASCO 1999;18:275a.
30. Liu JM, Chao Y, Tiu CM, et al. Biweekly continuous infusion chemotherapy (M-FLEEP) plus megestrol acetate for pancreatic cancer. Proc ASCO 1999;18:292a.
31. Rodríguez-Lescure A, Carrato A, Massutí B, García-Gómez J. Phase I–II study of gemcitabine (GEM) and weekly 48-hour continuous infusion of high dose 5-fluorouracil (5-FU) in advanced exocrine pancreatic cancer (APC). Proc ASCO 1999;18:298a.
32. Hidalgo M, Castellano D, Paz-Ares L, et al. Phase I–II study of gemcitabine and fluorouracil as a continuous infusion in patients with pancreatic cancer. J Clin Oncol 1999;17:585–92.
33. Louvet C, Hammel P, André R. Multicenter phase II study in advanced pancreatic adenocarcinoma patients treated with a combination of leucovorin, 5 FU bolus and infusion, and gemcitabine (FOLFUGEM regimen). Proc ASCO 1999;18:275a.
34. Jacobs AD, Otero H, Picozzi V, et al. Gemcitabine (G) and Taxotere (T) in patients with unresectable pancreatic carcinoma. Proc ASCO 1999;18:288a.

35. Kakolyris S, Stathopoulos G, Tsavaris N, et al. First line treatment with docetaxel (D) and gemcitabine (G) in patients with advanced pancreatic cancer: a multicenter phase II study. Proc ASCO 1999;18:250a.

36. Todd KE, Gloor B, Lane JS, et al. Resection of locally advanced pancreatic cancer after downstaging with continuous-infusion 5-fluorouracil, mitomycin-C, leucovorin, and dipyridamole. J Gastrointest Surg 1998;2:159–66.

37. Bakkevold KE, Arnesjo B, Dahl O, et al. Adjuvant combination chemotherapy (AMF) following radical resection of carcinoma of the pancreas and papilla of Vater—results of a controlled, prospective, randomised multicentre study. Eur J Cancer 1993;29A:698–703.

38. Amano H, Takada T, Kato H, et al. Five-year results of a randomized study of postoperative adjuvant chemotherapy for resected pancreaticobiliary carcinomas. Proc ASCO 1999;18:273a.abstract.

39. Warshaw AL, Fernandez-del Castillo C. Pancreatic carcinoma. N Engl J Med 1992;326:455–65.

40. Schulz G, Buchler M, Muhrer KH, et al. Immunotherapy of pancreatic cancer with monoclonal antibody BW 494. Int J Cancer 1988;2:89–94.

41. Buchler M, Kubel R, Malfertheiner P, et al. Immunotherapy of advanced pancreatic carcinoma with the monoclonal antibody BW 494. Dtsche Med Wochenschr 1988;113:374–80.

42. Buchler M, Friess H, Schultheiss KH, et al. A randomized controlled trial of adjuvant immunotherapy (murine monoclonal antibody 494/32) in resectable pancreatic cancer. Cancer 1991;68:1507–12.

43. Warner E, Weinroth J, Chang S, et al. Phase II trial of Virulizin in patients with pancreatic cancer: clinical and investigative medicine. Med Clin Exp 1994;17:37–41.

........................................

# TREATMENT BY STAGE OF DISEASE

• Charles M. Haskell

## LOCALIZED, RESECTABLE DISEASE

Patients with localized, resectable disease are usually treated surgically with the Shiu modification of Whipple's procedure (see Fig. 45–1). Total pancreatectomy is contraindicated because of unmanageable diabetes mellitus and a failure to provide a survival benefit over that achieved with a conventional Whipple's procedure. Postoperative treatment with radiation plus 5-FU is advocated because of the survival advantage conferred by this treatment in the randomized GITSG trial.[1] The total radiation dose should be 40 to 60 Gy given in 1.8- to 2-Gy daily fractions, either continuously or with treatment breaks of 2 weeks to allow recovery from nausea and fatigue. Chemotherapy with 5-FU is given as a continuous infusion or in an intravenous bolus dose of 500 mg/m$^2$ for 3 consecutive days once every 4 weeks during radiation. The 5-FU chemotherapy is continued following the completion of radiation therapy on a weekly schedule for 1 to 2 years of treatment.

## LOCALIZED, UNRESECTABLE DISEASE

A palliative bypass should be considered for patients having obstructive symptoms. We recommend that patients be treated with concomitant 5-FU and radiation therapy, based on the results of a randomized GITSG trial.[2] This randomized trial showed the superiority of this approach to chemotherapy alone. The optimal regimen has yet to be determined, but for now I usually use the treatment program described earlier for resectable pancreatic carcinoma. A variety of experimental approaches, including multiagent chemotherapy and intraoperative or interstitial radiation therapy, are also reasonable.

## ADVANCED DISEASE

Patients with advanced disease are candidates for palliative chemotherapy with gemcitabine. Alternatively, single-agent chemotherapy with 5-FU may be employed, as described in Chapters 10 and 43. Supportive care with nutrition and analgesics is also indicated, as discussed previously and in Chapters 21 and 22.

## PAPILLARY-CYSTIC CARCINOMA OF THE PANCREAS

Papillary-cystic neoplasms of the pancreas are rare lesions that present as cystic neoplasms filled with mucoid material in relatively young women.[3] The lining of the cysts is columnar epithelium with papillary formation and a low grade of neoplasia. The histogenesis of these tumors has been considered uncertain.[4] Two studies suggest, however, that these tumors may arise from endocrine cells within the pancreas. The first study found significant levels of estrogen and progesterone receptors in a single case of papillary-cystic pancreatic cancer.[5] The second study described two cases that were considered indistinguishable from islet cell carcinoma.[6]

The main reason for the special mention of these lesions is that patients with this tumor have much better prognoses after surgical treatment than do patients with conventional acinar adenocarcinoma. Although reported series are small, a 40 to 50% 5-year survival rate is not unrealistic following pancreaticoduodenectomy.[7, 8] Some authorities consider surgical resection of the involved portions of the pancreas to be adequate treatment.[9]

## SUGGESTIONS FOR ADDITIONAL READING

Warshaw AL, Fernández-del Castillo C: Pancreatic carcinoma. N Engl J Med 1992;326:455–65. *This article is an excellent review of pancreatic carcinoma.*

Brugge WR, van Dam J. Medical progress: pancreatic and biliary endoscopy. N Engl J Med 1999;341:1808–16.

Brentnall TA, Bronner MP, Byrd DR, et al. Early diagnosis and treatment of pancreatic dysplasia in patients with a family history of pancreatic cancer. Ann Intern Med 1999;131:247–55.

Sener SF, Fremgen A, Menck HR, Winchester DP. Pancreatic cancer: a report of treatment and survival trends for 100,313 patients diagnosed from 1985–1995, using the National Cancer Database. J Am Coll Surg 1999;189:1–7.

Huguier M, Mason NP. Treatment of cancer of the exocrine pancreas. Am J Surg 1999;177:257–65.

Gastrointestinal Tumor Study Group. Treatment of locally unresectable carcinoma of the pancreas: comparison of combined-modality therapy (chemotherapy plus radiotherapy) to chemotherapy alone. J Natl Cancer Inst 1988;80:751–5. *This randomized clinical trial establishes the superiority of combined-modality therapy over chemotherapy alone in the management of unresectable pancreatic cancer.*

Fisher BJ, Perera FE, Kocha W, et al. Analysis of the clinical benefit of 5-fluorouracil and radiation treatment in locally advanced pancreatic cancer. Int J Radiat Oncol Biol Phys 1999;45:291–5.

Go VLW, Dimagno EP, Gardner JD, et al. The pancreas: biology, pathobiology, and disease. New York: Raven Press, 1993. *This is an authoritative, comprehensive text on the full range of pancreatic disorders.*

## REFERENCES

1. Gastrointestinal Tumor Study Group. Further evidence of effective adjuvant combined radiation and chemotherapy following curative resection of pancreatic cancer. Cancer 1987;59:2006–10.
2. Gastrointestinal Tumor Study Group. Treatment of locally unresectable carcinoma of the pancreas: comparison of combined-modality therapy (chemotherapy plus radiotherapy) to chemotherapy alone. J Natl Cancer Inst 1988;80:751–5.
3. Bombi JA, Milla A, Badal JM, et al. Papillary-cystic neoplasm of the pancreas: report of two cases and review of the literature. Cancer 1984;54:780–4.
4. Morohoshi T, Kanda M, Horie A, et al. Immunocytochemical markers of uncommon pancreatic tumors: acinar cell carcinoma, pancreatoblastoma, and solid cystic (papillary-cystic) tumor. Cancer 1987;59:739–47.
5. Ladanyi M, Mulay S, Arseneau J, et al. Estrogen and progesterone receptor determination in the papillary cystic neoplasm of the pancreas: with immunohistochemical and ultrastructural observations. Cancer 1987;60:1604–11.
6. Yagihashi S, Sato I, Kaimori M, et al. Papillary and cystic tumor of the pancreas: two cases indistinguishable from islet cell tumor. Cancer 1988;61:1241–7.
7. Ilgren E, Tang CK, Thorbjarnarson B. Cystadenocarcinoma of pancreas. N Y State J Med 1976;76:548–50.
8. Shuman RL, Bouterie RL. Cystadenocarcinoma of the pancreas presenting as a splenic cyst. Surgery 1976;80:652–4.
9. Pezzi CM, Schuerch C, Erlandson RA, et al. Papillary-cystic neoplasm of the pancreas. J Surg Oncol 1988;37:278–85.

# CHAPTER 46

# LIVER

..................................

# NATURAL HISTORY, DIAGNOSIS, AND STAGING

• Charles M. Haskell

## ETIOLOGY AND EPIDEMIOLOGY

**Incidence and Mortality Data.** Hepatocellular carcinoma causes about 1 million deaths annually, with most of these occurring in the Far East and in sub-Saharan Africa.[1] In Mozambique, hepatocellular carcinoma is responsible for more than half of all cancer deaths in Shengaan men. Most cases in the Far East and Asia develop in men, and the disease follows a rapidly lethal course once it becomes symptomatic. In contrast, the disease is rare in the United States and Western Europe, with an annual U.S. incidence of about 3 cases per 100,000 population.[2, 3] There is only a modest male predominance in the West (3:1), and patients tend to survive somewhat longer than do patients in Asia and Africa. Even in the West, most patients with hepatocellular cancer die of the disease. The U.S. 5-year survival rate for hepatocellular cancer is only 5.7%.[3]

**Etiology.** There is an emerging consensus that hepatitis B virus (HBV) infection is the cause, either alone or in combination with other factors, in most cases worldwide. Hepatitis C virus (HCV) infection, although less common, is also strongly associated with the disease. The etiologic importance of hepatitis virus infection varies, however, between the regions of high and low incidence.[4] This variation relates to the frequency of HBV and HCV infection in different parts of the world and to a variety of other causative factors that may act alone or in combination with HBV to initiate or promote this tumor (Table 46–1). The most im-

portant of these factors and a model of molecular pathogenesis are discussed here briefly.

***Hepatitis Virus Infection.*** HBV and HCV infections, as well as infection with the hepatitis G virus, have been associated with the development of hepatocellular carcinoma.[5] Carriers of HBV have a 94-fold increased risk of hepatocellular carcinoma, and the viral genome has been found in most cases of hepatocellular carcinoma. The carriers of HCV are also at markedly increased risk of hepatocellular carcinoma.[6] There is a striking correlation between the incidence of hepatocellular carcinoma and the prevalence of HBV infection in different parts of the world. For example, in China and most of Southeast Asia, both of which are

***Table 46–1.*** **Conditions Predisposing to Hepatocellular Carcinoma**

Hepatitis B or C virus infection
   Chronic active hepatitis
   Macronodular cirrhosis
Cirrhosis due to or associated with
   Hemochromatosis
   $\alpha_1$-Antitrypsin deficiency
   Alcohol
   Acute intermittent porphyria
Chemical agents
   Aflatoxin
   Androgenic steroids
   Oral contraceptives
   Thorotrast

endemic areas for hepatocellular carcinoma, essentially 100% of adults have serologic evidence of HBV infection, and at least 10 to 15% are chronic virus carriers. The importance of HBV infection and cirrhosis in the cause of hepatocellular carcinoma is especially well shown in a prospective study of 22,107 Chinese men age 40 to 60 years conducted by Beasley and associates.[7, 8] The annual incidence of hepatocellular carcinoma in individuals with neither cirrhosis nor serologic evidence of prior HBV infection was 0.003%, compared with 0.5% and 2.4% in individuals with evidence of prior HBV infection either without or with cirrhosis. In other studies, the risk of developing hepatocellular carcinoma was even higher in patients with cirrhosis. In a study of 290 patients with hepatitis C infection, the annual cumulative risk of developing hepatocellular carcinoma was about 1% in patients without cirrhosis and 3 to 10% in those with cirrhosis, depending on the stage of cirrhosis and presence of causative cofactors.[9]

The likely pathway from viral hepatitis to hepatocellular carcinoma has been reviewed.[10] Figure 46–1 is an overview of the natural history of chronic HBV infection. In Asia, the predominant mode of HBV infection is perinatal, with about 90% of infants born to HBV carrier mothers developing the carrier state themselves. Chronic infection with HBV then proceeds through two distinct phases. First, there is a phase of active virus replication, leading to the accumulation of large amounts of replicative HBV DNA intermediates and the viral core antigen (HBcAg) in the liver. The host immune reaction to the virus is minimal during this period, but there is a high serum concentration of HBV DNA and hepatitis B

e antigen (HBeAg). Subsequently, after an average period of 20 to 30 years, the HBV infection enters its second phase. The HBeAg level decreases, and the infected person begins to produce T cells that recognize HBV-specific antigens. This production results in a full-fledged, cell-mediated immune response. The HBV-infected liver cells are killed, and the virus is cleared from the host. Although HBV does not replicate during this second phase, hepatitis B surface antigen (HBsAg) expression continues because the HBV genome is integrated into the host chromosome, and liver cells continue to produce copies of HBsAg. The liver displays residual lesions during this phase from previous damage sustained during the replicative phase of the virus. These patients are susceptible to cirrhosis, which develops at the rate of about 2% per year in the 40% of patients with severe lesions. The subsequent development of hepatocellular carcinoma in these patients results from a series of genetic and environmental insults (see Molecular Pathogenesis).

There has been some controversy about the importance of co-infection by two or more forms of hepatitis virus in the cause of hepatocellular carcinoma. Co-infection is common in these patients, but there is no compelling evidence that the combination of HCV and HBV is more carcinogenic than either alone.[11]

***Cirrhosis.*** Overall, about 80% of patients with hepatocellular carcinoma have cirrhosis. In geographic regions of high incidence, virtually all the cases of cirrhosis are of the macronodular variety, which is known to result from HBV infection.[4] Both micronodular and macronodular types of cirrhosis are seen in patients from geographic regions of low

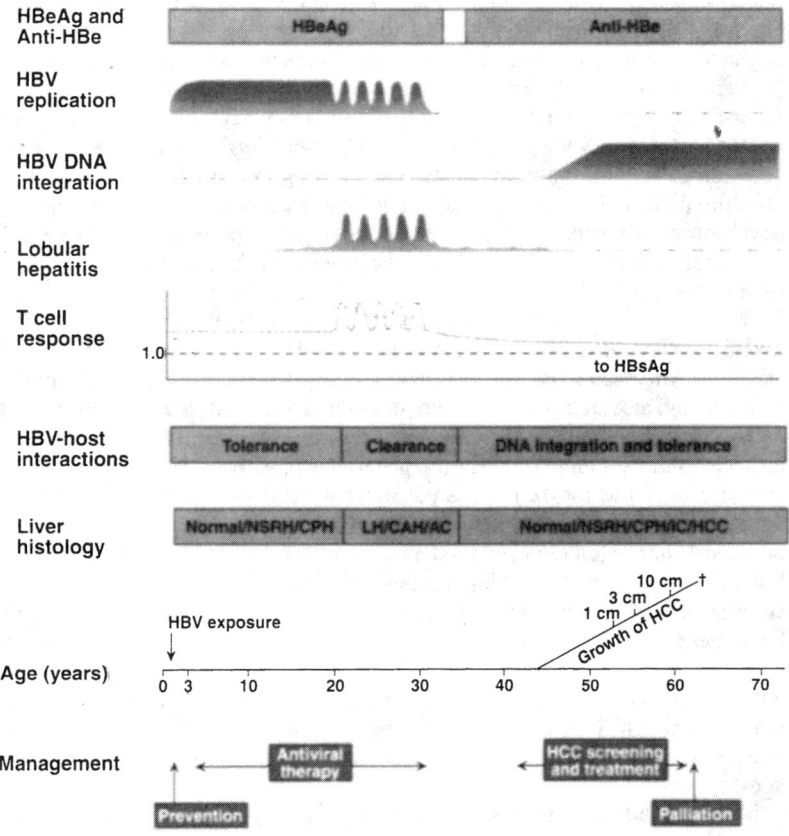

**Figure 46–1.** The natural history of chronic hepatitis B virus (HBV) infection. Further explanation of the figure is given in the text. Parameters that exist in minimal amounts or that contribute minimally to infection at a given time are indicated by dashed lines. NSRH, nonspecific reactive hepatitis; LH, lobular hepatitis; AC, active cirrhosis; CAH, chronic active hepatitis; CPH, chronic persistent hepatitis; HBIG, hepatitis B immune globulin; HCC, hepatocellular carcinoma; TAE, transcatheter arterial embolization for the treatment of HCC; C/T, chemotherapy for the treatment of HCC; †, death of the patient. (From Chen D-S. From hepatitis to hepatoma: lessons from type B viral hepatitis. Science 1993;262:369, copyright 1993 by the American Association for the Advancement of Science; modified from Cheb D-S. Natural history of chronic hepatitis B virus infection: new light on an old story. J Gastroenterol Hepatol 1993;8:470, Blackwell Scientific Publications.)

incidence. In the latter instance, other causes of cirrhosis are important as well. For example, it has been estimated that approximately 4% of all patients with cirrhosis eventually develop hepatocellular carcinoma.[12] The risk of hepatocellular carcinoma increases, however, when cirrhosis is related to several conditions. Specifically, the risk of hepatocellular carcinoma is about 10% in all cases of macronodular cirrhosis, 20% for untreated cases of hemochromatosis with cirrhosis, and 40% in cases of cirrhosis related to $\alpha_1$-antitrypsin deficiency.[13]

*Hepatotoxins.* Aflatoxins produced by *Aspergillus flavus* and related fungi are potent hepatic carcinogens in virtually all animals tested. These are major causative factors for the development of hepatocellular carcinoma in some parts of the world, particularly Africa, where the storage of food is a major problem,[14–16] and in some parts of China, where people drink pond ditch water contaminated by the blue-green algal toxin microcystin.[17]

A variety of other chemicals have been associated with hepatic cancer, although only rarely with hepatocellular carcinoma. Angiosarcomas have been associated with vinyl chloride and arsenic.[18] Thorium dioxide (Thorotrast) has been associated with sarcomas, hepatocellular carcinomas, and cholangiocarcinomas.[19] Hepatic adenomas have been associated with the long-term use of androgenic steroids, and there has been at least one case of hepatocellular carcinoma reported in a man who used anabolic steroids for body-building purposes.[20] Cases of hepatocellular carcinoma following the long-term use of oral contraceptives have been reported as well.[21] Alcohol abuse is modestly associated with hepatocellular carcinoma, but its use markedly increases the risk of hepatocellular carcinoma in patients with chronic HCV infection.[22] Alcohol use may also contribute to the development of especially aggressive forms of hepatocellular carcinoma.[23] Patients with cirrhosis or hepatitis who drink alcohol should be advised to abstain completely from the use of alcoholic beverages.

*Male Prevalence.* It is unclear why hepatocellular cancer is so much more common in men than in women. The usual explanation relates to differences in lifestyle, with a higher incidence of alcoholism in men than in women. There may also be differences in the metabolism of sex hormones in male versus female patients with alcoholic cirrhosis.[24]

*Other.* One study from Northern Italy found that the risk of hepatocellular carcinoma was increased by diabetes mellitus and decreased by a history of prior drug allergy.[25] Smoking cigarettes is a risk factor for the development of hepatocellular carcinoma.[26]

**Molecular Pathogenesis.** Hepatocellular carcinomas are genetically heterogeneous.[27] Initiation can probably occur with HBV or HCV infection or aflatoxin exposure, or both. The disease requires decades to evolve into a clinically apparent process, as shown in Figure 46–1. Promotion of this process occurs with the development of cirrhosis from alcohol or other hepatic toxins. Other promotional agents are less certain, but the composite result of these molecular insults involves changes in p53 suppressor gene function and the presence of viral X gene coding sequence changes.[28] In areas of the world where aflatoxin is the primary cause of hepatocellular carcinoma, such as Mozambique, the disease is associated with a high frequency of p53 mutations specifically related to aflatoxins (transversion of G7T in

codon 249 of the p53 tumor-suppressor gene[29]).[27] In patients with hepatocellular carcinoma developing in other parts of the world, p53 mutations are rare, but the frequent presence of viral X gene coding sequences suggests a possible interference in wild-type p53 function by the HBV gene.[27] Other changes that may be involved in hepatic carcinogenesis include the inactivation of the retinoblastoma gene,[30] overexpression of the c-*myc* gene,[31] and the loss of heterozygosity and other abnormalities identified by restriction landmark genomic scanning.[32]

The morphologic counterparts of hepatic carcinogenesis are not as well delineated as those for colorectal carcinoma. Both processes, however, involve sequential changes in morphologic appearance. For hepatic carcinogenesis, hepatic adenomatous hyperplasia serves as a preneoplastic lesion.[33] Chronic necrosis and inflammatory changes in the liver, in addition to cirrhosis, are commonly identified as precursor lesions.[34] Sequential morphologic changes occur during this process so that early lesions are well differentiated and later disease is poorly differentiated.[35]

Numerous other changes have been described in hepatocellular carcinomas, but their relationship to the sequence of carcinogenesis is uncertain. Some of these features can be listed. First, using flow cytometry, Saeter and colleagues[36] have shown that about one half of normal human hepatocytes are polyploid in DNA content and that human hepatocellular tumor growth is associated with a decreased tendency toward polyploidization, with a corresponding increase in diploid hepatocytes and increased cell division. Second, malignant hepatocytes can express a variety of receptor molecules, including glucocorticoid receptors,[37] various glycosphingolipids,[38] androgen receptors,[39, 40] ferritin,[41, 42] a novel thyroid hormone receptor,[43] and a new retinoic acid receptor.[44] These cells can also produce a relatively specific tumor marker commonly known as *alpha-fetoprotein* (AFP). The expression of the gene for AFP is regulated in a cell-autonomous fashion by malignant hepatocytes through one of two unlinked regulatory gene loci known as *raf*.[43] Finally, any discussion of pathogenesis must deal with the precise mechanism by which HBV and HCV infections cause cirrhosis and eventually hepatocellular carcinoma. The details of this process as it is currently understood have been reviewed.[1]

## PREVENTION

Given the importance of hepatitis virus infection to the cause of hepatocellular carcinoma and the availability of preventive measures for hepatitis as well as emerging treatments for chronic active hepatitis, there is great interest in programs of treatment that may prevent hepatocellular carcinoma. Specifically, lymphoblastoid interferon has been shown to improve liver function in patients with non-A, non-B hepatitis, so it could theoretically reduce the risk of hepatocellular carcinoma in this group of patients.[45] Several nonrandomized studies support the use of interferon in patients with hepatitis B or hepatitis C infection. For example, a study of interferon therapy in 419 patients with chronic active hepatitis C showed a reduced risk of hepatocellular carcinoma in patients whose hepatitis responded to the interferon therapy.[46] In another study from Japan, a retrospective cohort study of patients with chronic HCV infection, interferon therapy significantly reduced the risk of hepatocellular carcinoma, especially among virologic or biochemical responders to treatment.[47] Another study that suggests that a virologic response to interferon reduces the risk of hepatocellular carcinoma in these patients is that of Shindo and colleagues.[48] Randomized studies, however, have provided conflicting information. A randomized study of recombinant interferon alfa-2 in Chinese patients with chronic HBV infection was without benefit.[49] A randomized trial in patients with HCV infection showed improved liver function and a decreased incidence of hepatocellular carcinoma in patients treated with interferon.[50]

The most promising approach to prevention is through the prophylactic use of recombinant hepatitis B vaccine in individuals at high risk of the disease.[51, 52] In one study, immunization against HBV in the perinatal setting prevented chronic infections in about 85% of infants.[53] In Taiwan, universal vaccination of infants and children since 1984 has decreased the rate of children carrying HBsAg from greater than 10% to less than 2%.[10] This decrease has been associated with a significant decrease in the frequency of hepatocellular carcinoma in Taiwan (0.70 per 100,000 children in 1981 to 0.36 per 100,000 children in 1994, $p<0.01$).[54]

The rising incidence of hepatitis infection in the United States is a serious public health concern. Several groups have advocated screening for hepatitis infection with possible consideration of interferon therapy in individuals identified as carriers of HBV or HCV. Hepatitis C prevention and screening is discussed at length in an issue of *Morbidity and Mortality Weekly Report* from the Centers for Disease Control and Prevention devoted to this topic.[55]

## PATHOLOGY

Of primary hepatic cancers in adults, 90% arise in the hepatocellular parenchyma. Approximately 10% originate in the cells lining the bile ducts and are called *cholangiocarcinomas*. Rare types include hemangioepithelioma, Kupffer's cell sarcoma, hepatoblastoma, and mixed sarcomas. These rare lesions as well as primary osteosarcomas of the liver[56] and lymphomas[57–59] are not discussed in this chapter. Cholangiocarcinomas of the intrahepatic biliary system are discussed in Chapter 48.

Hepatocellular carcinoma presents as a soft vascular lesion in one of three major anatomic forms: (1) a solitary mass, (2) a primary mass but with surrounding satellite lesions in the liver tissue nearby, or (3) diffuse nodules throughout the liver without a recognizable primary lesion, suggesting a multifocal origin or rapid dissemination through intrahepatic vascular channels. Okuda and coworkers[60] have proposed that these three patterns should form the basis of a new classification system. In this system, they identify the three patterns as *expanding*, *spreading*, and *multifocal* forms of the disease. Kanai and colleagues[61] have proposed additional categories and subcategories of hepatocellular carcinoma, but the clinical value of these additional categories has yet to be substantiated by others.

The individual masses may be pale or even bile stained, but they are not fibrotic. The cholangiocarcinomas tend to be firm and fibrotic, and grossly they may resemble metastatic gastrointestinal carcinoma. Angiographically, hepatocellular carcinomas are hypervascular, whereas cholangiocarcinomas are relatively avascular. These patterns are apparent histologically as plentiful blood vessels in the former and sparse blood vessels in the latter. Intravascular tumor is frequently seen microscopically and grossly in hepatocellular carcinoma but not in cholangiocarcinoma. Ganjei and colleagues[62] have studied histochemical markers in liver tumors and have noted several patterns that may prove useful in the differential diagnosis of problem cases. Using antibodies to carcinoembryonic antigen (CEA) and a new erythropoiesis-associated antigen (ERY-1) on formalin-fixed tissue, they found that most patients with hepatocellular carcinoma tested positive for ERY-1 and negative for CEA. Most cholangiocarcinomas and metastatic lesions showed the opposite pattern. In these cases, CEA was usually positive and none of the patients tested positive for ERY-1.

There is a rare (about 1% of cases) histologic variant of hepatocellular carcinoma that is important to recognize. It is called *fibrolamellar hepatocellular carcinoma*, also known as *eosinophilic hepatocellular carcinoma with lamellar fibrosis* or *polygonal cell–type hepatocellular carcinoma with fibrous stroma*.[63–66] As suggested by its additional names, this variant has a distinctive histologic appearance, with a lamellar form of fibrosis separating individual hepatocytes and a peculiar polygonal cell that contains a highly eosinophilic cytoplasm. In contrast to the usual forms of hepatocellular carcinoma, this variant can have positive immunochemical staining for CEA.[67] Several other immunohistochemical stains have been reportedly positive as well, including fibrinogen, $\alpha_1$-antitrypsin, and copper. The importance of these tissue markers to the diagnosis of fibrolamellar carcinoma is uncertain, however. For example, it is now clear that copper and copper-binding proteins can be seen in a variety of liver tumors, so their presence is not diagnostic of fibrolamellar carcinoma.[68] The natural history and prognosis of fibrolamellar hepatocellular carcinoma also differ markedly from the usual varieties of this disease, as discussed subsequently.

The nomenclature of premalignant and early hepatocellular carcinoma has been addressed by a panel of expert pathologists.[69] After reviewing 23 nodular lesions, this multinational panel of five liver pathologists proposed a new nomenclature for early lesions that lack unequivocal signs of malignancy. These include the following two distinctions: (1) Benign nodules showing little histologic difference from cirrhotic nodules should be called *regenerative* or *macroregenerative*, and (2) nodules with atypical features not diagnostic of carcinoma should be called *borderline* lesions.

## CLINICAL COURSE AND DIAGNOSIS

The clinical presentation of hepatocellular carcinoma may be nonspecific, and a moderate number of cases in all series are discovered only at autopsy. Vague abdominal symptoms of epigastric pressure, discomfort, or fullness are common, but dull pain and a palpable mass or abdominal distention may be noted. Because of the propensity of hepatocellular carcinoma to invade veins, accelerated portal hypertension, ascites, and esophageal bleeding may herald development of the cancer. Occasional cases of intravascular growth may involve the inferior vena cava, right side of the heart, and pulmonary artery in a continuous cord of tumor, with a resulting dramatic, confusing, and lethal clinical course. Other telltale symptoms may include fever, ascites, acute abdominal pain and, occasionally, collapse and peritoneal signs from rupture and massive intra-abdominal hemorrhage.

In Africa and other high-incidence endemic areas, one half of eventual deaths may result from hemorrhage. Half of these are esophageal variceal hemorrhage, and the remainder are direct intra-abdominal hemorrhage from rupture of the tumor. A Japanese study indicated that in most cases of hepatocellular carcinoma with bleeding esophageal varices, patients had portal venous tumor invasion, and in the absence of such intravascular tumors, esophageal varices were less common and bleeding was infrequent.[70, 71]

Death can also ensue from liver failure, often with no extrahepatic extension of the cancer. When metastases do occur in patients with hepatocellular carcinoma, the following organs are most commonly involved: lung (44%), portal vein (35%), and portal lymph nodes (27%).[72] Compared with hepatocellular carcinoma, cholangiocarcinoma is less likely to involve the lung or portal vein but more likely to involve lymph nodes, peritoneum, bone, and bone marrow. The adrenal glands and brain are rare sites of involvement as well.[73, 74]

A high index of suspicion should be maintained in patients with cirrhosis who manifest unexpected clinical deterioration. Increased jaundice, the development of ascites, abdominal pain, weight loss, cachexia, fever, or a rapid increase in hepatic size may be observed. Sudden hypotension or abdominal pain, or both, may be observed in patients with rapid hemorrhage into the tumor mass or the peritoneal cavity. Numerous paraneoplastic syndromes have been associated with hepatocellular carcinoma, as listed in Table 46–2.[75]

**Diagnostic Imaging.** The imaging techniques that are used to detect hepatic neoplasms include ultrasonography, radionuclide liver scans, angiography, and computed tomography (CT). Ultrasonography is usually chosen as the initial imaging study in several clinical situations, including the new onset of ascites in a patient with cirrhosis of the liver (to rule out Budd-Chiari syndrome as well as hepatocellular carcinoma),[76] the evaluation of probable peliosis hepatis in a patient taking oral contraceptives,[77] and in combination with blood AFP levels to screen high-risk populations for hepatocellular carcinoma.[78, 79] In the setting of clinical prac-

tice, I usually obtain a computed tomographic scan of the abdomen as the initial imaging study when a liver neoplasm is suspected.[80] In most cases of operable hepatocellular carcinoma, the computed tomographic scan is the only imaging study required before surgical exploration.[81] In patients who are clearly inoperable, I usually proceed with a CT-guided fine-needle aspiration biopsy to establish a definitive histologic diagnosis. This procedure is usually safe despite the highly vascular nature of hepatocellular carcinoma.[82, 83] It is preferable, however, not to do a fine-needle biopsy in patients who are candidates for curative resections. Two cases of recurrent hepatocellular carcinoma 1 and 4 years after otherwise curative resections have been reported from London after this procedure, so this biopsy procedure should be used selectively.[84]

Four additional imaging procedures that I do not generally use deserve brief comment. Magnetic resonance imaging is of great interest as an imaging technique for hepatocellular carcinoma because it shows vascular structures well and avoids exposing the patient to radiation.[85–87] Intraoperative ultrasonography is reportedly useful in distinguishing regenerating liver nodules from small hepatocellular carcinomas during surgical exploration of the abdomen.[88] The third technique is dual-tracer scintigraphy and computer subtraction studies using technetium 99m sulfur colloid and gallium 67 citrate.[89] This procedure has a sensitivity of 96% and a specificity of 91% when used to diagnose hepatocellular carcinoma in patients likely to have the disease on a clinical basis (disease prevalence 20 to 60%). The final investigational diagnostic test is immunoscintigraphy with radiolabeled monoclonal antibodies to AFP.[90–92] All these procedures have their advocates, but I have yet to be convinced that they are as reliable and cost-effective as the use of a contrast-enhanced computed tomographic scan or ultrasonography.

**Tumor Markers.** The most important and characteristic tumor marker for hepatocellular carcinoma is AFP. It is a specific protein component of fetal serum that is also produced by hepatocellular carcinoma and germinal teratocarcinomas of the ovary and testis.[93] AFP has been successfully used in preliminary studies as a screening test for hepatocellular carcinoma in populations with a high risk of the disease.[94, 95] Less than 1% of adults with elevated AFP levels have had false-positive studies. Less than half of patients with hepatocellular carcinoma have increased AFP levels, however.[93] Some studies have also detected AFP in occasional normal adults and in patients with viral hepatitis, information that may tend to decrease the reliability of this diagnostic test.[96–100] It is possible that certain subfractions of AFP may be more useful in diagnosis. The fucosylation index of AFP is of particular interest because it may permit the earlier diagnosis of the disease in high-risk populations.[101] Studies of the diagnostic accuracy of AFP and related tumor markers are ongoing.[102, 103] At this time, however, the major value of the AFP test is in the follow-up of patients receiving active therapy. In this setting, a falling serum level of AFP correlates well with a response to treatment.[104] A more detailed discussion of the role of AFP in the diagnosis and treatment of hepatocellular carcinoma has been written by Bates and Longo.[105]

Many other tumor markers have been studied, most of which reflect the diverse constellation of proteins that are

*Table 46–2.* **Paraneoplastic Syndromes Associated with Hepatocellular Carcinoma**[75, 132–135]*

Erythrocytosis
Hypercalcemia
Hypercholesterolemia and hyperlipidemia
Gynecomastia (gonadotropin production)
Feminization
Hypoglycemia
Dysfibrinogenemia
Cryofibrinogenemia
Osteoporosis

*Porphyria cutanea tarda has been considered a paraneoplastic syndrome in patients with hepatocellular carcinoma by some authorities, whereas others doubt this relationship (see text for discussion). A variety of biologically active materials can be synthesized by normal liver, and many of these are elevated in patients with hepatocellular carcinoma. They are not listed here because they usually serve as tumor markers rather than as the basis for clinically apparent paraneoplastic syndromes.

normally synthesized in the liver. A partial list of these marker materials illustrates this point, as follows: clotting factor VII, protein C, protein S, and protein C inhibitor[106]; des-g-carboxy prothrombin[107, 108]; serum complement components[109]; single-chain factor X, prothrombin, and antithrombin III[110]; intestinal alkaline phosphatase isoenzyme and other variant alkaline phosphatases[111, 112]; carbohydrate antigen 19-9[113]; serum amino acid levels[114]; fibronectin[115]; serum vitamin $B_{12}$–binding proteins[116]; neurotensin[117, 118]; pseudouridine[119]; tissue polypeptide antigen[120]; serum ferritin[121]; transforming growth factor-$\alpha$[122]; serum secretory component (IgA);[123] and circulating endothelial growth factor.[124] Despite the promise that some of these potential tumor markers pose, at present there is no single serologic or immunologic test that is diagnostic for hepatocellular carcinoma, and a combination of diagnostic modalities must be used.

## STAGING AND PROGNOSIS

The American Joint Committee on Cancer TNM staging system for primary liver cancer is given in Table 46–3.[125] Vascular invasion, size, and the number of lesions are the essential elements of this system. In contrast to earlier versions of this system, cirrhosis is no longer included as a staging factor, although long-term survival is rare in patients with cirrhosis.[126] The TNM system is largely intended as a clinical staging system because most patients with hepatocellular carcinoma are not candidates for surgical resection.

Staging is largely irrelevant for most cases of hepatocellular carcinoma associated with HBV or HCV infection in Africa and the Pacific rim nations of Asia. The prognosis for this group of patients is abysmal. For example, the median survival in a series of 72 African patients was 1 month,[127] and in a series of 400 Japanese patients, the median survival was less than 3 months.[128] This rapidly fatal course is related to rapid tumor growth in symptomatic patients. In one study, the tumor doubling time for hepatocellular carcinoma was a few days.[126] Rare patients from the Far East have long-term survival, and there is a long latent period between viral infection and the onset of clinically apparent cancer. In a study from Taiwan, the 4-year actuarial survival rate for resected patients with *noninvasive* hepatocellular carcinoma was nearly 90%.[129]

Staging plays a larger role in the management of patients who develop hepatocellular carcinoma in the nonendemic areas of North America and western Europe. Long-term survival is possible in the small subset of patients who have resectable disease. Patients with the rare fibrolamellar variant of hepatocellular carcinoma have a relatively good prognosis. Wood and colleagues[130] compared the clinical characteristics and clinical courses of 15 patients with fibrolamellar carcinoma with 62 patients with other forms of hepatocellular carcinoma treated over the same period in Houston, Texas. Of patients, 47% with fibrolamellar carcinoma but only 10% with other forms of hepatocellular carcinoma had their tumors completely resected. Despite complete resections and the absence of cirrhosis, however, 5-year survival rates for the resected patients in the two groups were strikingly different. The 5-year survival rate was 45% for the resected patients with fibrolamellar carcinoma compared with 0% for the resected patients with other forms of hepatocellular carcinoma.

*Table 46–3.* **TNM Staging for Primary Neoplasms of the Liver (Including Intrahepatic Bile Ducts)**

*Primary Tumor (T)*

| | |
|---|---|
| TX | Primary tumor cannot be assessed |
| T0 | No evidence of primary tumor |
| T1 | Solitary tumor 2 cm or less in greatest dimension without vascular invasion |
| T2 | Solitary tumor 2 cm or less in greatest dimension with vascular invasion or multiple tumors limited to one lobe, none more than 2 cm in greatest dimension without vascular invasion, or a solitary tumor more than 2 cm in greatest dimension without vascular invasion |
| T3 | Solitary tumor more than 2 cm in greatest dimension with vascular invasion, or multiple tumors limited to one lobe, none more than 2 cm in greatest dimension, with vascular invasion, or multiple tumors limited to one lobe, any more than 2 cm in greatest dimension, with or without vascular invasion |
| T4 | Multiple tumors in more than one lobe or tumor(s) involve(s) a major branch of the portal or hepatic vein(s) or invasion of adjacent organs other than the gallbladder or perforation of the visceral peritoneum |

*Regional Lymph Nodes (N)*

| | |
|---|---|
| NX | Regional lymph nodes cannot be assessed |
| N0 | No regional lymph node metastasis |
| N1 | Regional lymph node metastasis |

*Distant Metastasis (M)*

| | |
|---|---|
| MX | Distant metastasis cannot be assessed |
| M0 | No distant metastasis |
| M1 | Distant metastasis |

*Stage Grouping*

| | | | |
|---|---|---|---|
| Stage I | T1 | N0 | M0 |
| Stage II | T2 | N0 | M0 |
| Stage IIIA | T3 | N0 | M0 |
| Stage IIIB | T1 | N1 | M0 |
| | T2 | N1 | M0 |
| | T3 | N1 | M0 |
| Stage IVA | T4 | Any N | M0 |
| Stage IVB | Any T | Any N | M1 |

Used with the permission of the American Joint Committee on Cancer (AJCC®), Chicago, Illinois. The original source for this material is the AJCC Cancer Staging Manual, 5th edition (1997) published by Lippincott-Raven Publishers, Philadelphia, Pennsylvania.

Falkson and colleagues[131] have evaluated a series of 432 patients with advanced hepatocellular carcinoma involved with investigational chemotherapy trials of the Eastern Cooperative Oncology Group. There were 301 North American and 131 South African patients, all of whom were evaluated and treated in a similar manner. Factors with the most significant adverse effect on survival were as follows: impaired performance status, male sex, older age, and disease symptoms (jaundice and reduced appetite). There was no apparent difference in survival between white and black patients within North America, but North American patients had longer survival than South African patients. The median survival of all patients in this study was 14 weeks, and only 13% of the patients were alive at 1 year.

## REFERENCES

1. Di Bisceglie AM, Rustgi VK, Hoofnagle JH, et al. NIH conference: hepatocellular carcinoma. Ann Intern Med 1988;108:390–401.

2. Young JL Jr, Percy CL, Asire AJ, et al. Cancer incidence and mortality in the United States, 1973–77. NCI Monogr 1981;57:1–187.

3. SEER Cancer Statistics Review 1973-1996. (See http://www-seer.ims.nci.nih.gov.)

4. Hepatocellular cancer: differences between high and low incidence regions. Lancet 1987;2:1183–4. editorial.

5. Yuan JM, Govindarajan S, Ross RK, Yu MC. Chronic infection with hepatitis G virus in relation to hepatocellular carcinoma among non-Asians in Los Angeles County, California. Cancer 1999;86:936–43.

6. Tsukuma H, Hiyama T, Tanaka S, et al. Risk factors for hepatocellular carcinoma among patients with chronic liver disease. N Engl J Med 1993;328:1797–1801.

7. Beasley RP, Hwang LY, Lin CC, Chien CS. Hepatocellular carcinoma and hepatitis B virus: a prospective study of 22 707 men in Taiwan. Lancet 1981;2:1129–33.

8. Beasley RP. Hepatitis B virus: the major etiology of hepatocellular carcinoma. Cancer 1988;61:1942–56.

9. Benvegnáu L, Alberti A. Risk factors and prevention of hepatocellular carcinoma in HCV infection. Dig Dis Sci 1996;41:12 Suppl:49S–55S.

10. Chen D-S. From hepatitis to hepatocellular carcinoma: lessons from Type B viral hepatitis. Science 1993;262:369–70.

11. Donato F, Boffetta P, Puoti M. A meta-analysis of epidemiological studies on the combined effect of hepatitis B and C virus infections in causing hepatocellular carcinoma. Int J Cancer 1998;75:347–54.

12. Higgins GK. In: Pack GT, Islami AH, eds. Tumors of the liver. New York: Springer-Verlag, 1970:15.

13. Berg NO, Eriksson S. Liver disease in adults with alpha-1-antitrypsin deficiency. N Engl J Med 1972;287:1264–7.

14. Enwonwu CO. The role of dietary aflatoxin in the genesis of hepatocellular cancer in developing countries. Lancet 1984;2:956–8.

15. Autrup H, Seremet T, Wakhisi J, Wasunna A. Aflatoxin exposure measured by urinary excretion of aflatoxin B1-guanine adduct and hepatitis B virus infection in areas with different liver cancer incidence in Kenya. Cancer Res 1987;47:3430–3.

16. Hadidane R, Roger-Regnault C, Bouattour H, et al. Correlation between alimentary mycotoxin contamination and specific diseases. Hum Toxicol 1985;4:491–501.

17. Yu SZ. Primary prevention of hepatocellular carcinoma. J Gastroenterol Hepatol 1995;10:674–82.

18. Tseng A. Primary hepatocellular carcinoma—recent advances and future prospects. Medical Staff Conference. West J Med 1985;143:503–7.

19. Ito Y, Kojiro M, Nakashima T, Mori T. Pathomorphologic characteristics of 102 cases of Thorotrast-related hepatocellular carcinoma, cholangiocarcinoma, and hepatic angiosarcoma. Cancer 1988;62:1153–62.

20. Overly WL, Dankoff JA, Wang BK, Singh UD. Androgens and hepatocellular carcinoma in an athlete. Ann Intern Med 1984;100:158–9.

21. Tao L-C. Oral contraceptive-associated liver cell adenoma and hepatocellular carcinoma. Cancer 1991;68:341–7.

22. Miyakawa H, Sato C, Izumi N, et al. Hepatitis C virus infection in alcoholic liver cirrhosis in Japan—its contribution to the development of hepatocellular carcinoma. Alcohol Alcohol 1993;28:Suppl 1A:85–90.

23. Kubo S, Kinoshita H, Hirohashi K, et al. High malignancy of hepatocellular carcinoma in alcoholic patients with hepatitis C virus. Surgery 1997;121:425–9.

24. Guéchot J, Peigney N, Ballet F, et al. Sex hormone imbalance in male alcoholic cirrhotic patients with and without hepatocellular carcinoma. Cancer 1988;62:760–2.

25. La Vecchia C, Negri E, D'Avanzo B, et al. Medical history and primary liver cancer. Cancer Res 1990;50:6274–7.

26. Chiba T, Matsuzaki Y, Abei M, et al. The role of previous hepatitis B virus infection and heavy smoking in hepatitis C virus infection. Am J Gastroenterol 1996;91:1195–203.

27. Unsal H, Yakicier C, Marcais C, et al. Genetic heterogeneity of hepatocellular carcinoma. Proc Natl Acad Sci U S A 1994;91:822–6.

28. Sirma H, Giannini C, Poussin K, et al. Hepatitis B virus X mutants, present in hepatocellular carcinoma tissue, abrogate both the antiproliferative and transactivation effects of HBx. Oncogene 1999;18:4848–59.

29. Aguilar F, Hussain SP, Cerutti P. Aflatoxin-B(1) induces the transversion of G → T in codon 249 of the p53 tumor suppressor gene in human hepatocytes. Proc Natl Acad Sci U S A 1993;90:8586–90.

30. Fujimoto Y, Hampton LL, Wirth PJ, et al. Alterations of tumor suppressor genes and allelic losses in human hepatocellular carcinomas in China. Cancer Res 1994;54:281–5.

31. Nishida N, Fukuda Y, Ishizaki K. Molecular aspects of hepatocarcinogenesis and their clinical implications. Int J Oncol 1994;4:615–22.

32. Nagai H, Ponglikitmongkol M, Mita E, et al. Aberration of genomic DNA in association with human hepatocellular carcinomas detected by 2-dimensional gel analysis. Cancer Res 1994;54:1545–50.

33. Takayama T, Makuuchi M, Hirohashi S, et al. Malignant transformation of adenomatous hyperplasia to hepatocellular carcinoma. Lancet 1990;336:1150–3.

34. Robinson WS. Molecular events in the pathogenesis of hepadenavirus-associated hepatocellular carcinoma. Annu Rev Med 1994;45:297–323.

35. Sugihara S, Nakashima O, Kojiro M, et al. The morphologic transition in hepatocellular carcinoma: a comparison of the individual histologic features disclosed by ultrasound-guided find-needle biopsy with those of autopsy. Cancer 1992;70:1488–92.

36. Saeter G, Lee CZ, Schwarze PE, et al. Changes in ploidy distributions in human liver carcinogenesis. J Natl Cancer Inst 1988;80:1480–5.

37. P'eng FK, Lui WY, Chang TJ, et al. Glucocorticoid receptors in hepatocellular carcinoma and adjacent liver tissue. Cancer 1988;62:2134–8.

38. Hiraiwa N, Iida N, Ishizuka I, et al. Monoclonal antibodies directed to a disulfated glycosphingolipid, SB1a (GgOse4Cer-II3IV3-bis-sulfate), associated with human hepatocellular carcinoma. Cancer Res 1988;48:6769–74.

39. Nagasue N, Yukaya H, Chang YC, et al. Active uptake of testosterone by androgen receptors of hepatocellular carcinoma in humans. Cancer 1986;57:2162–7.

40. Nagasue N, Kohno H, Chang YC, et al. Androgen and estrogen receptors in hepatocellular carcinoma and the surrounding liver in women. Cancer 1989;63:112–6.

41. Cohen C, Berson SD, Shulman G, Budgeon LR. Immunohistochemical ferritin in hepatocellular carcinoma. Cancer 1984;53:1931–5.

42. Zhou XD, DeTolla L, Custer RP, London WT. Iron, ferritin, hepatitis B surface and core antigens in the livers of Chinese patients with hepatocellular carcinoma. Cancer 1987;59:1430–7.

43. de Thé H, Marchio A, Tiollais P, Dejean A. A novel steroid thyroid hormone receptor-related gene inappropriately expressed in human hepatocellular carcinoma. Nature 1987;330:667–70.

44. Benbrook D, Lernhardt E, Pfahl M. A new retinoic acid receptor identified from a hepatocellular carcinoma. Nature 1988;333:669–72.

45. Jacyna MR, Brooks MG, Loke RHT, et al. Randomised controlled trial of interferon alfa (lymphoblastoid interferon) in chronic non-A non-B hepatitis. Br Med J 1989;298:80–2.

46. Imai Y, Kawata S, Tamura S, et al. Relation of interferon therapy and hepatocellular carcinoma in patients with chronic hepatitis C. Osaka Hepatocellular Carcinoma Prevention Study Group. Ann Intern Med 1998;129:94–9.

47. Yoshida H, Shiratori Y, Moriyama M, et al. Interferon therapy reduces the risk for hepatocellular carcinoma: national surveillance program of cirrhotic and noncirrhotic patients with chronic hepatitis C in Japan. IHIT Study Group. Inhibition of hepatocarcinogenesis by interferon therapy. Ann Intern Med 1999;131:174–81.

48. Shindo M, Ken A, Okuno T. Varying incidence of cirrhosis and hepatocellular carcinoma in patients with chronic hepatitis C responding differently to interferon therapy. Cancer 1999;85:1943–50.

49. Lok AS, Lai CL, Wu PC, Leung EK. Long-term follow-up in a randomised controlled trial of recombinant alpha 2-interferon in Chinese patients with chronic hepatitis B infection. Lancet 1988;2:298–302.

50. Nishiguchi S, Kuroki T, Nakatani S, et al. Randomised trial of effects of interferon-alpha on incidence of hepatocellular carcinoma in chronic active hepatitis C with cirrhosis. Lancet 1995;346:1051–5.

51. Hsu HM, Chen DS, Chuang CH, et al. Efficacy of a mass hepatitis B vaccination program in Taiwan: studies on 3464 infants of hepatitis B surface antigen-carrier mothers. JAMA 1988;260:2231–5.

52. The Gambia Hepatitis Intervention Study. The Gambia Hepatitis Study Group. Cancer Res 1987;47:5782–7.

53. Kane M. International Symposium on Viral Hepatitis and Liver Disease, Tokyo, May 1993.

54. Chang MH, Chen CJ, Lai MS, et al. Universal hepatitis B vaccination in Taiwan and the incidence of hepatocellular carcinoma in children. Taiwan Childhood Hepatocellular Carcinoma Study Group. N Engl J Med 1997;336:1855–9.

55. Recommendations for prevention and control of hepatitis C virus (HCV) infection and HCV-related chronic disease. MMWR Morb Mortal Wkly Rep 1998;47:1–39.

56. von Hochstetter AR, Hättenschwiler J, Vogt M. Primary osteosarcoma of the liver. Cancer 1987;60:2312–7.

57. Redondo C, Martin L, Cano AL, et al. Primary lymphoma of the liver treated with hepatic lobectomy and chemotherapy. Cancer 1987;60:736–40.

58. Ryan J, Straus DJ, Lange C, et al. Primary lymphoma of the liver. Cancer 1988;61:370–5.

59. DeMent SH, Mann RB, Staal SP, et al. Primary lymphomas of the liver: report of six cases and review of the literature. Am J Clin Pathol 1987;88:255–63.

60. Okuda K, Peters RL, Simson IW. Gross anatomic features of hepatocellular carcinoma from three disparate geographic areas: proposal of new classification. Cancer 1984;54:2165–73.

61. Kanai T, Hirohashi S, Upton MP, et al. Pathology of small hepatocellular carcinoma: a proposal for a new gross classification. Cancer 1987;60:810–9.

62. Ganjei P, Nadji M, Albores-Saavedra J, Morales AR. Histologic markers in primary and metastatic tumors of the liver. Cancer 1988;62:1994–8.

63. Edmonson HA. Tumors of the liver and intrahepatic bile ducts. Washington, D.C.: Armed Forces Institute of Pathology, 1958:90.

64. Ruffin MT IV. Fibrolamellar hepatocellular carcinoma. Ann Intern Med 1988;109:596–7.

65. Malondra AB, Picornell M, Pons JT, et al. European cases of fibrolamellar hepatocellular carcinoma. Ann Intern Med 1989;110:324.

66. Case records of the Massachusetts General Hospital. Weekly clinicopathological exercises. Case 35-1987: a 21-year-old woman with a hepatic mass after treatment for amenorrhea. N Engl J Med 1987;317:556–64.

67. Teitelbaum DH, Tuttle S, Carey LC, Clausen KP. Fibrolamellar carcinoma of the liver: review of three cases and the presentation of a characteristic set of tumor markers defining this tumor. Ann Surg 1985;202:36–41.

68. Guigui B, Mavier P, Lescs MC, et al. Copper and copper-binding protein in liver tumors. Cancer 1988;61:1155–8.

69. Ferrell LD, Crawford JM, Dhillon AP, et al. Proposal for standardized criteria for the diagnosis of benign, borderline, and malignant hepatocellular lesions arising in chronic advanced liver disease. Am J Surg Pathol 1993;17:1113–23.

70. Nagasue N, Inokuchi K, Kobayashi M, Saku M. Hepatoportal arteriovenous fistula in primary carcinoma of the liver. Surg Gynecol Obstet 1977;145:504–8.

71. Fortner JG, Kallum BO, Kim DK. Surgical management of hepatic vein occlusion by tumor: Budd-Chiari syndrome. Arch Surg 1977;112:727–8.

72. Lee YT, Geer DA. Primary liver cancer: pattern of metastasis. J Surg Oncol 1987;36:26–31.

73. Moertel CG. The liver. In: Holland JF, Frei E III, eds. Cancer medicine. Philadelphia: Lea & Febiger, 1973:1541–7.

74. Okuda K, Musha H, Nakajima Y, et al. Clinicopathologic features of encapsulated hepatocellular carcinoma: a study of 26 cases. Cancer 1977;40:1240–5.

75. Bhattacharya SK, Sealy WC. Paraneoplastic syndromes resulting from elaboration of ectopic hormones, antigens and bizarre toxins. Curr Probl Surg 1972;May:3–49.

76. Black M, Friedman AC. Ultrasound examination in the patient with ascites. Ann Intern Med 1989;110:253–5.

77. Foster JH. Evaluation of asymptomatic solitary hepatic lesions. Annu Rev Med 1988;39:85–93.

78. Tanaka S, Kitamura T, Ohshima A, et al. Diagnostic accuracy of ultrasonography for hepatocellular carcinoma. Cancer 1986;58:344–7.

79. Maringhini A, Cottone M, Sciarrino E, et al. Ultrasonography and alpha-fetoprotein in diagnosis of hepatocellular carcinoma in cirrhosis. Dig Dis Sci 1988;33:47–51.

80. LaBerge JM, Laing FC, Federle MP, et al. Hepatocellular carcinoma: assessment of resectability by computed tomography and ultrasound. Radiology 1984;152:485–90.

81. Clouse ME. Roentgenographic techniques for the diagnosis and management of liver tumors. Semin Oncol 1983;10:159–75.

82. Tao LC, Ho CS, McLoughlin MJ, et al. Cytologic diagnosis of hepatocellular carcinoma by fine-needle aspiration biopsy. Cancer 1984;53:547–52.

83. Bottles K, Cohen MB, Holly EA, et al. A step-wise logistic regression analysis of hepatocellular carcinoma: an aspiration biopsy study. Cancer 1988;62:558–63.

84. Evans GH, Harries SA, Hobbs KE. Safety of and necessity for needle biopsy of liver tumours. Lancet 1987;1:620.

85. Ebara M, Ohto M, Watanabe Y, et al. Diagnosis of small hepatocellular carcinoma: correlation of MR imaging and tumor histologic studies. Radiology 1986;159:371–7.

86. Titelbaum DS, Hatabu H, Schiebler ML, et al. Fibrolamellar hepatocellular carcinoma: MR appearance. J Comput Assist Tomogr 1988;12:588–91.

87. Lee VW, Allard JC, Weiss K, et al. Hepatocellular carcinoma imaging. J Surg Oncol 1988;38:244–9.

88. Hayashi N, Yamamoto K, Tamaki N. Metastatic nodules of hepatocellular carcinoma: detection with angiography, CT, and US. Radiology 1987;165:61–3.

89. Sostre S, Villagra D, Morales NE, Rivera JV. Dual-tracer scintigraphy and subtraction studies in the diagnosis of hepatocellular carcinoma. Cancer 1988;61:667–72.

90. Goldenberg DM, Goldenberg H, Higginbotham-Ford E, et al. Imaging of primary and metastatic liver cancer with 131I monoclonal and polyclonal antibodies against alphafetoprotein. J Clin Oncol 1987;5:1827–35.

91. Bergmann J-F, Lumbroso JD, Manil L. Radiolabelled monoclonal antibodies against alpha-fetoprotein for in vivo localization of human hepatocellular carcinoma by immunotomoscintigraphy. Eur J Nucl Med 1987;13:385–90.

92. Demangeat J-L, Manil L, Demangeat C, et al. Is anti-alphafetoprotein immunoscintigraphy a promising approach for the diagnosis of hepatocellular carcinoma? Implications of a quantitative study in 41 patients. Eur J Nucl Med 1988;14:612–20.

93. Abelev GI. Alpha-fetoprotein in ontogenesis and its association with malignant tumors. Adv Cancer Res 1971;14:295–358.

94. Heyward WL, Lanier AP, Bender TR, et al. Early detection of primary hepatocellular carcinoma by screening for alpha-fetoprotein in high-risk families: a case-report. Lancet 1983;2:1161–2.

95. Ellis JC. Screening for hepatocellular carcinoma: review and perspective. West J Med 1988;149:183–7.

96. Eleftheriou N, Heathcote J, Thomas HC, et al. Serum alpha-fetoprotein levels in patients with acute and chronic liver disease: relation to hepatocellular regeneration and development of primary liver cell carcinoma. J Clin Pathol 1977;30:704–8.

97. Kubo Y, Okuda K, Musha H, Nakashima T. Detection of hepatocellular carcinoma during a clinical follow-up of chronic liver disease: observations in 31 patients. Gastroenterology 1978;74:5780–2.

98. Chen D-S, Sung JL. Serum alphafetoprotein in hepatocellular carcinoma. Cancer 1977;40:779–83.

99. Phillips PJ, Rowland R, Reid DP, Coles ME. Alpha1-fetoprotein in the diagnosis of hepatocellular carcinoma: statistical and cost benefit aspects. J Clin Pathol 1977;30:1129–33.

100. Okuda K, Musha H, Nakajima Y, et al. Frequency of intrahepatic arteriovenous fistula as a sequela to percutaneous needle puncture of the liver. Gastroenterology 1978;74:1204–7.

101. Aoyagi Y, Suzuki Y, Isemura M, et al. The fucosylation index of alpha-fetoprotein and its usefulness in the early diagnosis of hepatocellular carcinoma. Cancer 1988;61:769–74.

102. Higashino K, Otani R, Kudo S, Yamamura Y. A fetal intestinal-type alkaline phosphatase in hepatocellular carcinoma tissue. Clin Chem 1977;23:1615–21.

103. Shimokawa Y, Okuda K, Kubo Y, et al. Serum glutamic oxalacetic transaminase/glutamic pyruvic transaminase ratios in hepatocellular carcinoma. Cancer 1977;40:319–24.

104. Buamah PK, James OF, Skillen AW, Harris AL. The value of tumour marker kinetics in the management of patients with primary hepatocellular carcinoma. J Surg Oncol 1988;37:161–4.

105. Bates SE, Longo DL. Use of serum tumor markers in cancer diagnosis and management. Semin Oncol 1987;14:102–38.

106. Fair DS, Marlar RA. Biosynthesis and secretion of factor VII, protein C, protein S, and the protein C inhibitor from a human hepatocellular carcinoma cell line. Blood 1986;67:64–70.

107. Liebman HA, Furie BC, Tong MJ, et al. Des-gamma-carboxy (abnormal) prothrombin as a serum marker of primary hepatocellular carcinoma. N Engl J Med 1984;310:1427–31.

108. Fujiyama S, Morishita T, Hashiguchi O, Sato T. Plasma abnormal prothrombin (des-gamma-carboxy prothrombin) as a marker of hepatocellular carcinoma. Cancer 1988;61:1621–8.

109. Chang WY, Chuang WL. Complements as new diagnostic tools of hepatocellular carcinoma in cirrhotic patients. Cancer 1988;62:227–32.

110. Fair DS, Bahnak BR. Human hepatocellular carcinoma cells secrete single chain factor X, prothrombin, and antithrombin III. Blood 1984;64:194–204.
111. Buamah PK, Skillen AW, Cassells-Smith AJ, et al. Intestinal alkaline phosphatase isoenzyme in patients with primary liver cancer during treatment with N10-propargyl 5, 8-dideazafolic acid (CB 3717). J Surg Oncol 1988;38:83–7.
112. Bukofzer S, Kew MC, Rowe P. The prevalence of variant alkaline phosphatase in hepatocellular carcinoma in southern African blacks. Cancer 1988;62:978–81.
113. Kew MC, Berger EL, Koprowski H. Carbohydrate antigen 19–9 as a serum marker of hepatocellular carcinoma: comparison with alpha-foetoprotein. Br J Cancer 1987;56:86–8.
114. Watanabe A, Higashi T, Sakata T, Nagashima H. Serum amino acid levels in patients with hepatocellular carcinoma. Cancer 1984;54:1875–82.
115. Glasgow JE, Colman RW. Fibronectin synthesized by a human hepatocellular carcinoma cell line. Cancer Res 1984;44:3022–8.
116. Buamah PK, James OF, Skillen AW, Harris AL. The value of tumour marker kinetics in the management of patients with primary hepatocellular carcinoma. J Surg Oncol 1988;37:161–4.
117. Collier NA, Weinbren K, Bloom SR, et al. Neurotensin secretion by fibrolamellar carcinoma of the liver. Lancet 1984;1:538–40.
118. Wood JR, Melia WM, Wood SM. Neurotensin and hepatocellular carcinoma. Lancet 1984;1:687.
119. Tamura S, Amuro Y, Nakano T, et al. Urinary excretion of pseudouridine in patients with hepatocellular carcinoma. Cancer 1986;57:1571–5.
120. Kew MC, Berger EL. The value of serum concentrations of tissue polypeptide antigen in the diagnosis of hepatocellular carcinoma. Cancer 1986;58:127–30.
121. Nagasue N, Yukaya H, Chang YC, Ogawa Y. Serum ferritin level after resection of hepatocellular carcinoma: correlation with alpha-fetoprotein level. Cancer 1986;57:1820–3.
122. Yeh Y-C, Tsai JF, Chuang LY, et al. Elevation of transforming growth factor alpha and its relationship to the epidermal growth factor and alpha-fetoprotein levels in patients with hepatocellular carcinoma. Cancer Res 1987;47:896–901.
123. Kew MC, Vincent C, Rossel M, Revillard JP. High serum levels of secretory component in hepatocellular carcinoma. Am J Med 1988;85:327–30.
124. Jinno K, Tanimizu M, Hyodo I, et al. Circulating vascular endothelial growth factor (VEGF) is a possible tumor marker for metastasis in human hepatocellular carcinoma. J Gastroenterol 1998;33:376–82.
125. Beahrs OH, ed. American Joint Committee on Cancer. Manual for staging of cancer. 4th ed. Philadelphia: JB Lippincott, 1992:89.
126. Tsuzuki T, Ogata Y, Iida S, et al. Long-term survival of patients with hepatocellular carcinoma combined with liver cirrhosis: report of two patients. Cancer 1985;55:2835–8.
127. Primack A, Vogel CL, Kyalwazi SK, et al. A staging system for hepatocellular carcinoma: prognostic factors in Ugandan patients. Cancer 1975;35:1357–64.
128. Liver Cancer Study Group of Japan. Primary liver cancers in Japan. Cancer 1980;45:2663–9.
129. Hsu H-C, Wu TT, Wu MZ, et al. Tumor invasiveness and prognosis in resected hepatocellular carcinoma: clinical and pathogenetic implications. Cancer 1988;61:2095–9.
130. Wood WJ, Rawlings M, Evans H, Lim CN. Hepatocellular carcinoma: importance of histologic classification as a prognostic factor. Am J Surg 1988;155:663–6.
131. Falkson G, Cnaan A, Schutt AJ, et al. Prognostic factors for survival in hepatocellular carcinoma. Cancer Res 1988;48:7314–8.
132. Kew MC, Fisher JW. Serum erythropoietin concentrations in patients with hepatocellular carcinoma. Cancer 1986;58:2485–8.
133. Ikeda T, Tozuka S, Hasumura Y, Takeuchi J. Prostaglandin-E-producing hepatocellular carcinoma with hypercalcemia. Cancer 1988;61:1813–4.
134. Larrañaga JR, Carreira J, Baquer A, Mardomingo P. Hepatoma-associated hyperlipidaemia type V with normal lipid values after removal of tumour. Lancet 1984;1:399–400.
135. Altman D. Hepatoma. West J Med 1980;132:514–20.

..........................................

# SURGERY

• Kenneth P. Ramming

## RESECTION

Surgical resection represents the only possibility for cure for hepatic carcinoma. Although most hepatic carcinomas have diffuse or multiple involvement of the liver precluding surgery, resection should be performed in every instance when anatomically feasible. A second resection may even be possible in selected patients who have a recurrence after an initial curative resection.[1, 2]

In most cases of potential resection, it is not necessary to have a preoperative tissue diagnosis. It is usually possible to make a decision about potential resectability based on minimal preoperative staging studies and a computed tomographic scan of the abdomen. Confirmation of the tissue diagnosis is usually easy to accomplish at the time of surgical exploration. In general, cirrhosis is not an absolute contraindication to surgical resection if the tumor is small and well localized, but the prognosis of the patient with cirrhosis is inferior to that of patients with normal liver function.[3] Elderly patients also tolerate surgery less well than younger patients, although age alone is not a contraindication to surgical resection.[4] Older patients and those with cirrhosis of the liver may do better with nonanatomic resections because these resections usually require a shorter operative

time and have fewer complications than those involving classic anatomic margins.

About a third of patients treated with partial hepatic resections live for 5 years after treatment (Table 46–4).[5–15] Most tumors are not suitable for surgical resection at the time that they are diagnosed.[16, 17] A discussion of the operative principles and techniques is beyond the scope of this book. These topics have been reviewed by Malt,[18] and excellent books on liver surgery have been produced by Tompkins[19] and Blumgart.[20]

## PALLIATIVE SURGICAL TECHNIQUES

**Hepatic Artery Ligation.** Hepatic artery ligation has been studied as a possible treatment for hepatocellular carcinoma, but it is rarely used at this time.[21]

**Transcatheter Arterial Embolization.** Transcatheter arterial embolization (TAE) with absorbable gelatin sponge (Gelfoam) may have a place when a spontaneous rupture of the tumor occurs.[22] Chen and colleagues[23] have treated three cases of hepatocellular carcinoma and spontaneous rupture with Gelfoam chemoembolization. All three patients underwent successful resections of tumor, two on day 5 and one

*Table 46–4.* **Surgical Resection for Hepatocellular Carcinoma**

| Center/Location | Patients (No.) | Patients with Cirrhosis (No.) | 30-Day Mortality Rate (%) | 1-Year Survival (%) | 3-Year Survival (%) | 5-Year Survival (%) |
|---|---|---|---|---|---|---|
| University of Pittsburgh[5] | 67 | — | 8 | 76 | 49 | 25 |
| Kanazawa, Japan[6] | 35 | 35 | 14 | 57* | — | — |
| Villejuif[7] | 35 | 35 | 14 | 62 | 22 | — |
| Cleveland Clinic[8] | 23 | — | 8 | — | 50 | 33 |
| Taiwan[9] | 120 | 55 | 4 | 55 | — | — |
| Keio University, Tokyo[10] | 119 | 80 | 9 | 80 | 47 | 39 |
| Tokyo University, Tokyo[11] | 94 | 71 | 11 | 73 | 42 | 25 |
| Toranomon Hospital, Tokyo[12] | 83 | 76 | 0 | — | — | — |
| Liver Group of Japan[13] | 222 | 153 | 27 | 33 | 20 | 12 |
| Mayo Clinic[14] | 87 | 26 | 9 | — | — | 27 |
| 1974 Liver Survey[15] | 109 | 23 | 21 | — | — | 34* |

*Cumulative survival expressed as a percentage of total patients. All other survival rates are actuarial survival rates in percent as calculated by the Kaplan-Meier method.

on day 10 after the hemorrhage. The use of TAE with chemotherapy is discussed further in a subsequent section.

**Intratumor Injection of Ethanol.** Percutaneous injections of alcohol into hepatocellular carcinomas, using ultrasonographic guidance, may be of palliative benefit in patients with one to three nodules less than 3 cm in diameter who are poor candidates for surgical resection.[24, 25] This procedure can also be used intraoperatively. The procedure involves the injection of 10 to 20 ml of sterile ethanol by ultrasonographic guidance three times weekly for 12 treatments. If the procedure is well tolerated, more than one nodule can be treated. Contrast-enhanced CT is used to evaluate the response to treatment. Enhancement of the tumor establishes the presence of residual viable tumor tissue. Complications include pain, fever, and intrahepatic or intraperitoneal hemorrhage. Survival results are fragmentary, and there are no fully controlled series. The largest study is a retrospective, case-control study from Italy comparing the outcome of 24 surgical patients and 77 alcohol-treated patients.[26] Log-rank test adjusted for strata showed no survival difference between the two groups ($p = 0.75$).

Overall, it appears that about two thirds of the patients treated with intratumor alcohol injections are alive at 3 years. This approach has never been compared with comparable palliative procedures in a randomized trial, but it has considerable appeal for selected patients.

**Cryosurgery.** Intraoperative cryosurgery with liquid nitrogen can be used to freeze nonresectable primary liver carcinomas.[27] This technique is being studied in Shanghai and reportedly confers considerable palliative benefit to pa-

tients without jaundice, ascites, or serious liver decompensation. Most of my experience with this technique has been in patients with metastatic lesions to the liver, which are discussed in Chapter 104.

## LIVER TRANSPLANTATION

Largely as a result of the successful use of cyclosporine to suppress immunologic rejection, liver transplantation for patients with end-stage liver disease is now a clinically viable option for selected patients (Table 46–5).[28–33] It has been used successfully in patients with extensive hepatic epithelioid hemangioendotheliomas,[34] a malignant soft tissue neoplasm derived from vascular tissue, as well as for primary hepatocellular carcinomas. For the latter, the most extensive experience has been reported from London by O'Grady and colleagues.[35] In their series of 93 patients with hepatocellular carcinoma undergoing orthotopic liver transplantation between 1968 and 1987, 50 patients had hepatocellular carcinoma (19 with cirrhosis, 31 without cirrhosis, including 7 with fibrolamellar hepatocellular carcinoma). Of these patients, 74% survived longer than 3 months, and one third of these cases did not recur. The longest survival in this group was 11.8 years post-transplantation, and three patients survived for more than 5 years.

The biggest problem with liver transplantation is the high frequency of subsequent recurrence of the tumor, usually in an area outside the liver. Rare cases of retransplantation have been reported,[36] but recurrent disease in this setting is a

*Table 46–5.* **Liver Transplantation for Hepatocellular Carcinoma**

| Center/Location | Patients (No.) | 30-Day Mortality Rate (%) | Recurrence Rate (%) | 1-Year Survival (%) | 3-Year Survival (%) | 5-Year Survival (%) |
|---|---|---|---|---|---|---|
| University of Pittsburgh[17] | 80 | 13 | 37 | 64 | 45 | 45 |
| London[18] | 50 | 23–32 | 65 | 42–48 | — | — |
| Birmingham, UK[19] | 21 | 38 | 29 | 45 | 21 | 21 |
| Hanover, Germany[20] | 87 | 13–24 | — | 55 | 30 | 20 |
| Boston[21] | 24 | 17 | 25 | 71 | 42 | — |
| UCLA[22] | 44 | 16 | 30 | 63 | 30 | 30 |

devastating problem. The procedure also carries a high emotional and economic cost to the patient and society. Busuttil and associates[37] have estimated the average cost per patient surviving 1 year after transplantation as $238,000 (1983 data). Given the high costs of this procedure, organ transplantation has engendered considerable debate about its proper place in modern treatment.[38] An extension of liver transplantation alone is liver transplantation as part of aggressive combined-modality therapy. This issue is discussed further in the section on chemotherapy.

The most appropriate role for liver transplantation for patients with hepatocellular carcinoma remains uncertain. It is a reasonable option for highly motivated patients with tumor restricted to the liver but with disease that cannot be safely removed by segmental resection.

## REFERENCES

1. Nagasue N, Yukaya H, Ogawa Y, et al. Second hepatic resection for recurrent hepatocellular carcinoma. Br J Surg 1986;73:434–8.
2. Kanematsu T, Matsumata T, Takenaka K, et al. Clinical management of recurrent hepatocellular carcinoma after primary resection. Br J Surg 1988;75:203–66.
3. Kanematsu T, Takenaka K, Matsumata T, et al. Limited hepatic resection effective for selected cirrhotic patients with primary liver cancer. Ann Surg 1984;199:51–6.
4. Yanaga K, Kanematsu T, Takenaka K, et al. Hepatic resection for hepatocellular carcinoma in elderly patients. Am J Surg 1988;155:238–41.
5. Iwatsuki S, Starzl TE. Personal experience with 411 hepatic resections. Ann Surg 1988;208:421–34.
6. Kinami Y, Takashima S, Miyazaki I. Hepatic resection for hepatocellular carcinoma associated with liver cirrhosis. World J Surg 1986;10:294–301.
7. Bismuth H, Houssin D, Ornowski J, Meriggi F. Liver resections in cirrhotic patients: a Western experience. World J Surg 1986;10:311–7.
8. Sesto ME, Vogt DP, Hermann RE. Hepatic resection in 128 patients: a 24-year experience. Surgery 1987;102:846–51.
9. Chen MF, Hwang TL, Jeng LB, et al. Hepatic resection in 120 patients with hepatocellular carcinoma. Arch Surg 1989;124:1025–8.
10. Tsuzuki T, Sugioka A, Ueda M, et al. Hepatic resection for hepatocellular carcinoma. Surgery 1990;107:511–20.
11. Nagao T, Inoue S, Goto S, et al. Hepatic resection for hepatocellular carcinoma: clinical features and long-term prognosis. Ann Surg 1987;205:33–40.
12. Ikeda K, Saitoh S, Tsubota A, et al. Risk factors for tumor recurrence and prognosis after curative resection of hepatocellular carcinoma. Cancer 1993;71:19–25.
13. Liver Cancer Study Group of Japan. Primary liver cancers in Japan. Cancer 1980;45:2663–9.
14. Nagorney DM, van Heerden JA, Ilstrup DM, Adson MA. Primary hepatic malignancy: surgical management and determinants of survival. Surgery 1989;106:740-8.
15. Foster JH, ed. Solid liver tumors. Philadelphia: WB Saunders, 1977:62.
16. Inouye AA, Whelan TJ Jr. Primary liver cancer: a review of 205 cases in Hawaii. Am J Surg 1979;138:53–61.
17. Wu MC, Zhang XH, Chen H, Wu BW. Experiences in 467 cases of hepatic resection. Acta Acad Med Wuhan 1983;3:1–7.
18. Malt RA. Surgery for hepatic neoplasms. N Engl J Med 1985;313:1591–6.
19. Tompkins RK, ed. Manual of liver surgery. New York: Springer-Verlag, 1981.
20. Blumgart LH, ed. Surgery of the liver and biliary tract. New York: Churchill Livingstone, 1988.
21. Niederhuber JE, Ensminger WD. Surgical considerations in the management of hepatic neoplasia. Semin Oncol 1983;10:135–47.
22. Hwang T-L, Chen MF, Lee TY, et al. Resection of hepatocellular carcinoma after transcatheter arterial embolization: reevaluation of the advantages and disadvantages of preoperative embolization. Arch Surg 1987;122:756–9.
23. Chen M-F, Jan YY, Lee TY. Transcatheter hepatic arterial embolization followed by hepatic resection for the spontaneous rupture of hepatocellular carcinoma. Cancer 1986;58:332–5.
24. Sheu J-C, Huang GT, Chen DS, et al. Small hepatocellular carcinoma: intratumor ethanol treatment using new needle and guidance systems. Radiology 1987;163:43–8.
25. Livraghi T, Salmi A, Bolondi L. Small hepatocellular carcinoma: percutaneous alcohol injection—results in 23 patients. Radiology 1988;168:313–7.
26. Perrone F, Ragone E, Mazzanti R, et al. Surgery and percutaneous ethanol injection as treatment of small hepatocellular carcinoma: a retrospective case-control CLIP study. Proc ASCO 1999;18:237a.
27. Zhou X-D, Tang ZY, Yu YQ, Ma ZC. Clinical evaluation of cryosurgery in the treatment of primary liver cancer: report of 60 cases. Cancer 1988;61:1889–92.
28. Yokoyama I, Todo S, Iwatsuki S, Starzl TE. Liver transplantation in the treatment of primary liver cancer. Hepatogastroenterology 1990;37:188–93.
29. O'Grady JG, Polson RJ, Rolles K, et al. Liver transplantation for malignant disease: results in 93 consecutive patients. Ann Surg 1988;207:373–9.
30. Ismail T, Angrisani L, Gunson BK, et al. Primary hepatic malignancy: the role of liver transplantation. Br J Surg 1990;77:983–7.
31. Pichlmayr R, Weimann A, Steinhoff G, Ringe B. Liver transplantation for hepatocellular carcinoma: clinical results and future aspects. Cancer Chemother Pharmacol 1992;31:Suppl:S157–61.
32. Haug CE, Jenkins RL, Rohrer RJ, et al. Liver transplantation for primary hepatic cancer. Transplantation 1992;53:376–82.
33. Farmer DG, Rosove MH, Shaked A, Busuttil RW. Current treatment modalities for hepatocellular carcinoma. Ann Surg 1994;219:236–47.
34. Marino IR, Todo S, Tzakis AG, et al. Treatment of hepatic epithelioid hemangioendothelioma with liver transplantation. Cancer 1988;62:2079–84.
35. O'Grady JG, Polson RJ, Rolles K, et al. Liver transplantation for malignant disease: results in 93 consecutive patients. Ann Surg 1988;207:373–9.
36. Klompmaker IJ, de Bruijn KM, Gouw AH, et al. Recurrence of hepatocellular carcinoma after liver retransplantation. Br Med J 1988;296:1445.
37. Busuttil RW, Goldstein LI, Danovitch GM, et al. Liver transplantation today. Ann Intern Med 1986;104:377–89.
38. Moore FD. The desperate case: CARE (costs, applicability, research, ethics). JAMA 1989;261:1483–4.

# RADIATION THERAPY

• Luu M. Tran

Surgery remains the only curative treatment for primary hepatocellular carcinoma and liver metastasis. Only 5% of patients are appropriate surgical candidates, however.[1] The role of whole-liver irradiation has been limited by the liver's relatively low normal tissue tolerance of 30 Gy at standard fractionation, which is not a tumoricidal dose, although it can provide palliative relief of pain and discomfort in 50 to 70% of patients with metastatic liver disease.[2, 3] In 1987, the Radiation Therapy Oncology Group (RTOG)[4] reported a randomized trial comparing external-beam radiation therapy

(EBRT) plus misonidazole with EBRT alone (21 Gy in seven fractions to whole liver). Of 136 patients, 80% experienced significant pain relief following treatment, although the addition of misonidazole did not improve the therapeutic response.

One method of increasing the dose is hyperfractionation (multiple small doses per day), which could allow a higher total dose without causing significant late effects. The RTOG[5] trial used 1.5 Gy BID, to three dose levels (27 Gy, 30 Gy, and 33 Gy). Median survival at each dose level was approximately 4 months. The risk of radiation-induced lethal damage (RILD) at a total dose of 33 Gy with BID fractionation is similar from that obtained with standard fractionation. Lawrence and colleagues[6] from the University of Michigan, treating patients with liver metastases, used intra-arterial hepatic floxuridine (FUDR) and EBRT (30 Gy in 1.5-Gy BID fractions) to the whole liver, plus a 15- to 30-Gy boost to tumor. They reported a partial response in 48% of patients and stable disease in 45%.

Another method for increasing the radiation dose is three-dimensional conformal radiation therapy. The technique calls for tightly shaped radiation fields that encompass the tumor but minimize the dose to surrounding normal liver tissue. Robertson and colleagues[7] from the University of Michigan treated 22 patients with liver metastases by combining three-dimensional conformal radiation therapy with intra-arterial hepatic FUDR. A total dose of 72.6 Gy (1.5 Gy BID) was prescribed to part of the liver, with no significant radiation hepatitis. Eleven of 22 patients with liver metastases showed an objective response, and the actuarial freedom from hepatic progression was 25% at 1 year.

For 11 patients with hepatocellular cancers treated with the same regimen, the outcome is more encouraging,[8] with 50% freedom from hepatic progression. The median survival was 16 months with an actuarial 4-year survival rate of about 20%, a result approaching the survival rates of treatment by surgical resection.

Radioimmunotherapy has been used in patients with unresectable primary liver tumors. The RTOG[9] reported a randomized trial using EBRT (21 Gy in seven fractions) plus 5-fluorouracil (5-FU) and doxorubicin followed by random administration of either further 5-FU and doxorubicin or iodine 131 antiferritin. Compared with chemotherapy only, radiolabeled antibody and full-dose chemotherapy led to similar rates of partial remission rates (25%) and survival. Median survival rate (6 months) was similar in both groups.

## REFERENCES

1. Okuda K, Ohtuski T, Obata H, et al. Natural history of hepatocellular carcinoma and prognosis in relation to treatment. Cancer 1985;56:918–28.
2. Lawrence TS, Ten Haken RK, Kessler ML, et al. The use of 3-D dose volume analysis to predict radiation hepatitis. Int J Radiat Oncol Biol Phys 1992;23:781–8.
3. Borgelt BB, Gelber R, Brady LW, et al. The palliation of hepatic metastases: results of the RTOG pilot study. Int J Radiat Oncol Biol Phys 1981;7:587–91.
4. Leibel SA, Pajak TF, Massullo V, et al. A comparison of misonidazole sensitized radiation therapy to radiation therapy alone for the palliation of hepatic metastases: results of a RTOG randomized prospective protocol. Int J Radiat Oncol Biol Phys 1987;13:1057–64.
5. Stillwagon GB, Order SE, Guse C, et al. Prognostic factors in unresectable hepatocellular cancer: RTOG study 8301. Int J Radiat Oncol Biol Phys 1991;20:65–71.
6. Lawrence TS, Dworzanin LM, Walker-Andrews SC, et al. Treatment of cancers involving the liver and porta hepatis with external beam irradiation and intraarterial hepatic fluorodeoxyuridine. Int J Radiat Oncol Biol Phys 1991;20:555–61.
7. Robertson JM, Lawrence TS, Walker S, et al. The treatment of colorectal liver metastases with conformal radiation therapy and regional chemotherapy. Int J Radiat Oncol Biol Phys 1995;32:445–50.
8. Robertson JM, Lawrence TS, Andrews JC, et al. Long term results of hepatic artery fluorodeoxyuridine and conformal radiation therapy for primary hepatobiliary cancers. Int J Radiat Oncol Biol Phys 1997;37:325–30.
9. Order S, Pajak T, Leibel S, et al. A randomized prospective trial comparing full dose chemotherapy to 131I antiferritin: an RTOG study. Int J Radiat Oncol Biol Phys 1991;20:953–63.

# CHEMOTHERAPY

● Charles M. Haskell

The role of chemotherapy in the management of primary hepatic cancer is controversial. At present, there is no program or protocol of treatment that can be recommended as *standard* or *established* therapy for this group of patients. Patients with hepatic cancer should be encouraged to participate in clinical trials designed to answer important questions about management.

This section summarizes the chemotherapy of hepatocellular carcinoma in adult patients, including the use of single-agent chemotherapy (see Table 46–6)[1] and combination chemotherapy by systemic administration for patients with advanced disease (see Table 46–7),[1–3] regional infusion chemotherapy (see Table 46–8),[1, 4, 5] transcatheter arterial chemoembolization (TACE) therapy (see Table 46–9),[6–17] and randomized studies comparing TACE with other routes of chemotherapy administration (see Table 46–10).[18–21] Adjuvant

chemotherapy after hepatic resection is summarized in Table 46-11,[22–28] and adjuvant therapy after liver transplantation is summarized in Table 46–12.[29–32] Childhood hepatoblastomas,[33] primary hepatic sarcomas,[34] cholangiocarcinomas, and other primary hepatic neoplasms are not considered here. The reader who is interested in a more detailed discussion of specific drug regimens or contemporary clinical trials involving chemotherapy in the past is referred to a review of this topic by Nerenstone and colleagues.[35]

## SYSTEMIC CHEMOTHERAPY

Table 46–6 summarizes the response rates achieved with single-agent chemotherapy in patients with hepatocellular

*Table 46–6.* Systemic Single-Agent Chemotherapy for Hepatocellular Carcinoma*

| Drug | Patients (No. of CR + PR/Total) | Response Rate (%) |
|---|---|---|
| Doxorubicin | 92/468 | 20 |
| Cyproterone acetate | 5/25 | 20 |
| Ifosfamide | 3/28 | 11 |
| Cisplatin | 10/103 | 10 |
| Mitoxantrone | 18/187 | 9.6 |
| 5-Fluorouracil | 9/105 | 9 |
| Vinblastine | 2/25 | 8 |
| Etoposide | 3/42 | 7 |
| Fludarabine | 0/16 | 0 |
| Trimetrexate | 0/20 | 0 |
| Tamoxifen | 0/30 | 0 |
| Epirubicin | 0/14 | 0 |

*The drugs listed are limited to commercially available agents tested in at least 10 patients. Response rates are based on the number of complete and partial responses reported by the authors of the respective studies. Response rates should not be considered the sole proof of efficacy in the absence of other evidence of benefit.

CR, complete response; PR, partial response.

carcinoma. Patients with advanced hepatoma who respond to chemotherapy appear to live longer than those who do not respond or those who are treated with placebo but this longer survival could be totally unrelated to drug therapy. The median duration of survival in responding patients is approximately 7 to 9 months, and occasional patients survive 2 years or more. Most patients, however, fail to respond to systemic chemotherapy and die a few months after diagnosis. Even the most active single agent, doxorubicin, has a response rate of only 20% (see Table 46–6). This response rate is too low to have any meaningful impact on the survival of entire groups of patients, and many authorities consider such therapy to be excessively toxic for the rare benefit observed.[36] This rarity is demonstrated by a randomized clinical trial from Hong Kong comparing doxorubicin chemotherapy with supportive care alone.[37] There was no difference in overall survival between the two groups of patients.

There has been some interest in the use of tamoxifen in patients with advanced hepatocellular carcinoma, largely based on a randomized trial from Padua that found a significant prolongation of survival in a small group of patients receiving tamoxifen.[38] This group, however, found no actual responses with tamoxifen, and a trial from the Mayo Clinic observed no responses with tamoxifen (see Table 46–6). A randomized trial of tamoxifen versus best supportive care for 496 patients with advanced hepatocellular carcinoma showed no difference in survival between the two groups.[39] It is fair to conclude that tamoxifen is not an effective treatment for these patients.

Numerous combination chemotherapy regimens have been tried in patients with hepatocellular carcinoma (Table 46–7). Several regimens, most of which contain 5-FU or floxuridine, appear to give higher response rates than doxorubicin used as a single agent. None of these regimens can be considered standard therapy or clearly superior to any of the others. These trials illustrate one important point, however. Several suggest that treatment may have major benefit for occasional patients, even though results in the aggregate are unimpressive. For example, Leung and coworkers[3] ob-

tained an overall response rate of only 26% in their study of 5-FU, doxorubicin, cisplatin, and interferon, but 9 of the 50 patients underwent surgical resection after showing a partial response to treatment. Four of these 9 patients had no viable tumor in the resection specimen and appeared to enjoy good postoperative survival. The authors concluded that persistent radiologic lesions may still represent complete pathologic resolution of active disease, with benefit to the patient.

## REGIONAL INFUSION CHEMOTHERAPY

The basic principle of arterial infusion therapy is to administer cytotoxic drugs to a region containing localized tumor through the artery supplying that area. This approach greatly increases the drug concentration in the area of the tumor, compared with administration of the same amount of drug systemically. The blood supply of the liver, roughly 80 to 90%, is derived mainly from the portal vein, whereas the blood supply of the tumor is almost exclusively from the hepatic artery.[40–45] Hepatic artery infusion affords a high concentration of drug in the tumor, estimated to be 5 to 20 times greater than that in the surrounding normal hepatic tissue. This concentration may be graphically shown by the capillary phase of a hepatic artery angiogram, in which tumor stain clearly differentiates the tumor from the surrounding hepatic parenchyma, and by a portogram, in which the tumor is visualized as a nonstaining defect within the opacified normal liver parenchyma. These findings suggest that attempting to deliver antitumor drugs by portal vein catheterization is much less logical than using the hepatic arterial inflow.

Table 46–8 provides an overview of studies of hepatic artery infusion in patients with hepatocellular carcinoma. All

*Table 46–7.* Systemic Combination Chemotherapy for Hepatocellular Carcinoma*

| Combination | Patients (No. of CR + PR/Total) | Response Rate (%) |
|---|---|---|
| 5-FU + mitomycin[1] | 8/19 | 42 |
| Epirubicin + etoposide[2] | 14/36 | 39 |
| 5-FU + doxorubicin + teniposide[1] | 7/24 | 29 |
| 5-FU + teniposide + amsacrine[1] | 6/23 | 26 |
| 5-FU + doxorubicin + cisplatin + interferon alfa[3] | 13/50 | 26 |
| 5-FU + carmustine[1] | 8/23 | 24 |
| Doxorubicin + verapamil[1] | 5/21 | 24 |
| Methotrexate + cyclophosphamide ± vincristine ± 5-FU[1] | 14/60 | 23 |
| Mitoxantrone + interferon-β[1] | 9/38 | 23 |
| 5-FU + methotrexate + prednisone[1] | 2/11 | 18 |
| 5-FU + streptozocin[1] | 3/18 | 17 |
| Doxorubicin + tamoxifen[1] | 4/30 | 16 |
| 5-FU + doxorubicin[1] | 5/38 | 13 |
| 5-FU + semustine[1] | 2/36 | 6 |
| 5-FU + cytarabine[1] | 1/16 | 6 |
| Doxorubicin + interferon alfa[1] | 1/31 | 3 |

*Studies are limited to those testing at least 15 patients. Response rates are approximations and should not be considered proof of efficacy for any individual regimen without other evidence of benefit.

CR, complete response; PR, partial response; 5-FU, 5-fluorouracil.

*Table 46–8.* **Hepatic Artery Infusion Chemotherapy for Hepatocellular Carcinoma***

| Drugs | Patients (No. of CR + PR/Total) | Response Rate (%) |
|---|---|---|
| *Commercially Available Single Agents* | | |
| Floxuridine[1] | 26/46 | 57 |
| Doxorubicin[1] | 8/19 | 42 |
| Cisplatin[1] | 4/10 | 40 |
| Mitomycin[1] | 9/25 | 36 |
| Mitoxantrone[1] | 6/23 | 26 |
| 5-FU[1] | 15/83 | 18 |
| Epirubicin[1] | 8/53 | 15 |
| Methotrexate[1] | 1/2 | — |
| *Combinations of Agents* | | |
| 5-FU + floxuridine[1] | 10/18 | 56 |
| Methotrexate + 5-FU + cisplatin + interferon alfa-2b[4] | 7/15 | 47 |
| 5-FU (CI) + mitoxantrone + cisplatin[5] | 9/27 | 33 |
| 5-FU + doxorubicin + semustine[1] | 3/20 | 15 |
| 5-FU + epirubicin[1] | 2/10 | — |
| 5-FU + doxorubicin (Infusaid pump)[1] | 1/5 | — |
| 5-FU + methotrexate + yttrium 90[1] | 2/3 | — |
| 5-FU + methotrexate[1] | 0/1 | — |

*Response rates are approximations and should not be considered proof of efficacy for any individual regimen without other evidence of benefit.

CR, complete response; PR, partial response; 5-FU, 5-fluorouracil; CI, continuous infusion.

these patients were treated with hepatic artery catheters placed at the time of laparotomy or by the percutaneous Seldinger technique. Results vary greatly from center to center, which can be ascribed, at least in part, to a lack of uniformity in defining what constitutes an objective response. For example, the objective response rate of seven patients who were treated at the University of California Los Angeles (UCLA) was only 14%; however, all but one patient had substantial subjective improvement, and survival appeared to be prolonged. Some of these patients may have been considered objective responders to treatment had they been analyzed in the past at other centers. The combined overall response rate for fluoropyrimidine therapy with either 5-FU or floxuridine in this literature series is 32%, which is superior to the 9% response rate reported in Table 46–5 for 5-FU given systemically. The approximate median survival of all patients treated with 5-FU or floxuridine by the hepatic artery route is 8.5 months, which is superior to the 3-month median seen with systemic 5-FU administration. Finally, the hepatic artery route is occasionally associated with long survival times and is rarely associated with the complete eradication of visible tumor.[46, 47] In a review of patients with unresectable hepatoma who were treated with hepatic artery infusion of 5-FU at UCLA, the median survival in 13 patients was 14 months (range, 3 to 28 months).[1]

Detractors of this form of therapy point out that the impact on median survival in this exceedingly lethal disease, in which survival in the untreated patient is usually measured in weeks, is not impressive. There is a paucity of controlled clinical trials directly comparing systemic administration of chemotherapy with administration by the hepatic arterial route. In one such trial involving doxorubicin, there was no

significant difference in survival times between the two routes of administration (7 months vs. 6.5 months).[48] Adherents of this form of therapy point out that certain patients may have spectacular responses, which warrant its application in every instance possible, and that even those whose survival is not prolonged as dramatically have enough improvement in symptoms to warrant infusion therapy.

Reed and associates[49] have attempted to address these findings in an extensive evaluation of the impact of this type of infusional therapy on patient lifestyle and well-being. They concluded that the patient with some limitation of activity is the most likely to have a perceptible benefit from this form of treatment. They addressed a number of questions. (1) Is the therapy adaptable to the patient's lifestyle? They believed that once patients had adapted to the necessity of wearing an external device, their lifestyle became satisfactory. (2) Is there threatening local (liver) toxicity? Reed and associates[49] noted only limited toxicity that could be attributed to the infusion itself. (3) Are there systemic symptoms? Their experience was that symptoms were minimal. The experience at UCLA generally supports these conclusions.[1]

Because of the poor results with systemic therapy reported in the literature, and in light of this review of the literature, it is reasonable to recommend initiation of chemotherapy with a continuous hepatic artery infusion of 5-FU or floxuridine for patients with unresectable hepatoma that has not spread beyond the liver. The drug is delivered through a catheter placed in the hepatic artery percutaneously by the Seldinger technique.

5-FU is started at a dose of 12 to 14 mg/kg/day. The infusion is administered in the hospital or outpatient environment continuously for 6 to 7 days. If serum markers, such as AFP, are significantly reduced in 2 to 3 weeks or if there is a regression of the size of the tumor, indicating efficacy of the intra-arterial therapy, the patient may benefit from continuous, long-term hepatic artery chemoinfusion.

**Infusaid Pump.** The Infusaid pump (Infusaport Implantable Drug Delivery System, Shiley Infusaid Inc, Norwood, MD, or Portacath Implantable Drug Delivery System, Pharmacia Inc, Piscataway, NJ). It has been widely used in the management of metastatic liver involvement by colorectal cancer, but there is relatively little published experience with this device in patients with hepatocellular carcinoma. The published experience at UCLA with implanting and treating hepatoma with these pumps has been limited to 12 cases, but results have been encouraging.[1] As the use of these devices grows, it is possible that hepatic artery infusion with floxuridine for hepatoma patients will become more prevalent because this technique has the tremendous advantage of being self-contained within the body.

**Infusion by External Pump.** An alternative to the Infusaid pump is the use of totally implantable drug delivery systems, which consist of vascular access ports connected to polymeric silicone (Silastic) catheters. The catheters can be placed in the hepatic artery through the gastroduodenal artery at laparotomy. These are then tunneled subcutaneously and attached to the port, which also is anchored subcutaneously, usually in the upper anterior rib cage. Simple percutaneous needle puncture into the port, usually a round polymeric silicone window in a small metal casing, allows infusion of chemotherapeutic agents. These agents are then pumped in by a small, external, battery-powered chemoinfusion pump

*Table 46–9.* **Transcatheter Arterial Chemoembolization Therapy for Hepatocellular Carcinoma**

| Reference | Drugs | Patients (No.) | Response Rate (%)* | Median Survival | 1-Year Survival (%) | 3-Year Survival (%) | 5-Year Survival (%) |
|---|---|---|---|---|---|---|---|
| Yamada et al (1990)[6] | Mitomycin C and doxorubicin in gelatin | 793 | 75 | | 51 | 12 | |
| Bismuth et al (1992)[7] | Doxorubicin in ethiodized oil and gelatin | 291 | 29 | | | | |
| Hsieh et al (1992)[8] | Various agents in iodized oil and absorbable gelatin sponge | 100 | 24 | | 57 | 21 | |
| Venook et al (1992)[9] | Doxorubicin, mitomycin, and cisplatin in absorbable gelatin sponge and contrast medium | 51 | | Median survival 207 days | | | |
| Tanaka et al (1992)[10] | TACE alone vs. TACE followed by local alcohol injection | 21 | 10 vs. 45 p < 0.05 | | 68 vs. 100 | 0 vs. 85 p < 0.01 | |
| Monden et al (1992)[11] | Doxorubicin, Lipiodol, and absorbable gelatin sponge vs. resection alone | 173 vs. 140 | | | 65 vs. 87 | 30 vs. 66 | 16 vs. 47 |
| Colleoni et al (1998)[12] | 5-FU, leucovorin, and carboplatin by HAI × 3 courses → TACE with mitoxantrone + ethiodized oil + gelatin sponge Q 28 days × 3 | 28 | 43 | 16.6 mo | | | |
| Okusaka et al (1998)[13] | Zinostatin stimalamer–Lipiodol | 30 | 40 | | | | |
| Ikeda et al (1997)[14] | TACE alone vs. TACE followed by oral 5'-deoxy-5-fluorouridine | 20 vs. 20 | 70 vs. 60 | | 75 vs. 85 NSD | 65 vs. 50 NSD | |
| Bhattacharya et al (1995)[15] | Epirubicin-Lipiodol vs [131]I-Lipiodol | 17 vs. 11 | | | 25 vs. 25 | | |
| Ikeda et al (1995)[16] | TACE alone vs. TACE followed by oral tegafur and uracil | 20 vs. 20 | 60 vs. 50 | 28.2 vs. 22.7 mo | 82 | 61 | |
| Raoul et al (1999)[17] | Preoperative intra-arterial injections of Lipiodol radiolabeled with [131]I | 34 | 50 | | | | |

*Combined complete plus partial response rates. Response rates are approximations and should not be considered the sole proof of efficacy for any individual drug or regimen. None of these trials was randomized, but some compared results in otherwise comparable groups of patients.

TACE, transcatheter arterial chemoembolization; 5-FU, 5-fluorouracil; HAI, hepatic artery infusion; NSD, no sign of disease.

*Table 46–10.*  **Randomized Studies Comparing Chemotherapy Routes of Administration in Advanced Hepatocellular Carcinoma**

| Reference | Patients (No.) | Treatment | Comment |
|---|---|---|---|
| Minoyama et al[18] (1995) | 97 | TACE with Lipiodol and 4'epidoxorubicin or acurarubicin | Response rate 39%; 3-yr survival rate 21% |
| | 17 | HAI chemotherapy without Lipiodol | Response rate 18%; Lipiodol treatment "better" |
| Bayraktar et al[19] (1996) | 28* | TACE with Lipiodol and mitomycin C + absorbable gelatin sponge | Mean survival 13 mo ($p < 0.005$) |
| | 15* | Systemic doxorubicin + mitomycin C | Mean survival 7.2 mo |
| | 14* | No chemotherapy | Mean survival 6.9 mos |
| Biselli et al[20] (1997) | 38† | TACE (Lipiodol) vs. HAI chemotherapy | OS better with TACE ($p < 0.05$) |
| Okuda et al[21] (1999) | 73 | HAI cisplatin + 5-FU vs. TACE with Lipiodol | HAI gave best results (statistically significant): 71% response rate and 45.7% survival rate at 5 yr |

\*All patients had cirrhosis.
†All patients elderly.
TACE, transcatheter arterial embolization; HAI, hepatic artery infusion; OS, overall survival.

that the patient carries in a pouch, achieving continual intra-arterial chemoinfusions. An advantage of this approach is that a variety of chemotherapeutic agents and combinations, other than floxuridine or 5-FU, can be used. This approach requires a dedicated, well-trained clinical support team for patient selection and education, pump management, and troubleshooting.

A third alternative is simply hooking up an external chemoinfusion pump to a conventional percutaneous venous catheter for continuous intravenous chemotherapy. The dosages of chemotherapy must be low when this method is used to avoid toxicity, and experience is limited.

**Chemoembolization and Chemotherapy with Hepatic Artery Ligation.**  Numerous investigators have studied either

hepatic artery ligation[50] or dearterialization of the liver by the injection of various materials, combined with various forms of chemotherapy. As discussed previously in the section on surgery, dearterialization by surgical means is rarely employed at this time. There is considerable research interest in chemoembolization, however, which is variably known as TACE or TAE. Examples of materials injected into the hepatic artery include Lipiodol,[51, 52] absorbable gelatin sponge,[53–58] and combined Lipiodol–absorbable gelatin sponge.[59, 60] In most cases, the embolization agent is given with a chemotherapeutic drug, most commonly mitomycin or doxorubicin. Preliminary results with this approach to chemotherapy are summarized in Table 46–9. The results are at least comparable to those seen with intra-arterial

*Table 46–11.*  **Randomized Trials of Adjuvant Chemotherapy for Hepatocellular Carcinoma**

| Reference | Patients (No.) | Treatment | 1-Year Survival (%) | 3-Year Survival (%) | 5-Year Survival (%) | Statistics |
|---|---|---|---|---|---|---|
| Asahara et al[22] (1999) | 67 | Resection alone | | 69.2 | 38.1 | |
| | 68 | Resection + hepatic arterial infusion chemotherapy with doxorubicin-Lipiodol | | 79.1 | 54.5 | $p = 0.086$ |
| Lai et al[23] (1998) | 36 | Resection alone | 69 | 48 | | $p = 0.04$ |
| | 30 | Resection + epirubicin IV + transarterial iodized oil with cisplatin | 50 | 18 | | |
| Ono et al[24] (1997) | 27 | Resection alone | | | | |
| | 29 | Resection + epirubicin (HAI) → epirubicin IV × 3 mo + oral HCFU | | | | NSD at 5 yr |
| Kohno et al[25] (1996) | 40 | Resection + adjuvant PO UFT | 82 | 50 | 49 | |
| | 48 | Resection + adjuvant PO UFT + epirubicin by hepatic artery bolus injection | 90 | 48 | 35 | $p = 0.22$ |
| Nakashima et al[26] (1996) | 48 | Resection alone | 67.2 | 32 | | |
| | 26 | Resection + HAI with cisplatin or a combination of 5-FU + doxorubicin + mitomycin C | 90.3 | 71.3 | | $p < 0.05$ |
| Yamamoto et al[27] (1996) | (67) | Resection alone | | | | |
| | | Resection + oral HCFU | | | | |
| Lygidakis et al[28] (1995) | 20 | Resection alone | | | | |
| | 20 | Resection with preoperative and postoperative local-regional chemotherapy-immunotherapy | | | | NA |

IV, intravenous; HAI, hepatic artery infusion; HCFU, carmofur, 1-hexylcarbamoyl-5-fluorouracil; UFT, tegafur; 5-FU, 5-fluorouracil; NSD, no sign of disease; NA, not available.

*Table 46–12.* Combined-Modality Therapy with Orthotopic Liver Transplantation in Patients with Hepatocellular Carcinoma

| Center | Treatment Added to Hepatectomy with OLT | Patients (No.) | Survival |
|---|---|---|---|
| University of Paris (1994)[29] | HA chemoembolization + RT → OLT → mitoxantrone IV | 9 | 5 patients alive 25–45 mo after OLT |
| Baylor University (1993)[30] | Neoadjuvant chemotherapy → OLT with intraoperative and postoperative doxorubicin | 20 | 9 patients alive NED; 3-yr actuarial survival, 59% |
| UCLA (1995)[31] | OLT → fluorouracil + doxorubicin + cisplatin × 6 mo | 25 | 4-yr actuarial survival, 46% |
| New Jersey (1995)[32] | Neoadjuvant chemotherapy → OLT | 27 | |

OLT, orthotopic liver transplantation; HA, hepatic artery; RT, radiation therapy; IV, intravenous; NED, no evidence of disease.

chemotherapy, although they are probably not as good as those seen with surgical resection in eligible patients.

Relatively few studies have attempted to compare directly the results of TACE with other routes of chemotherapy administration. Table 46–10 summarizes the results of four studies involving a diverse collection of treatments. None of these trials establishes TACE or TAE as being superior to the administration of these drugs by the hepatic arterial route.

## ADJUVANT CHEMOTHERAPY

**Chemotherapy with Hepatic Resection.** There is limited experience with adjuvant chemotherapy for hepatocellular carcinoma. Table 46–11 summarizes the results of adjuvant chemotherapy in seven randomized trials involving a variety of different groups of patients. Several of the trials involve the use of relatively ineffective or nontoxic regimens, whereas others use fairly aggressive treatment. The largest trial is that of Asahara and colleagues.[22] This group compared resection alone with resection followed by hepatic arterial infusion chemotherapy with doxorubicin and lipiodol. The 5-year survival of the group treated with adjvuant therapy was better than that of the resection-alone group (54.5% vs. 38.1%, $p = 0.086$). These results support the continued investigation of this promising approach to management.

**Adjuvant Chemotherapy and Liver Transplantation.** There is limited experience with the aggressive management of hepatocellular carcinoma with transplantation and aggressive chemotherapy (Table 46–12). The longest follow-up of this approach is from UCLA, where the 3-year actuarial survival rate has been reported to be 46%. This rate is impressive compared with the historical experience at UCLA, in which survival for patients matched for extent of disease was only 5.8% at 3 years.[31] Further experience with this combined-modality approach for eligible patients appears warranted.

## IMMUNOTHERAPY

The intriguing relationship between HBV antigens and hepatocellular carcinoma has led to numerous immunologic investigations in patients with this disease. The most important benefit of immunotherapy is in the prevention of chronic hepatitis in individuals exposed to HBV during the perinatal period, as discussed earlier in this chapter. Attempts to treat established hepatitis with interferon are also under way but with uncertain results in terms of the prevention of hepa-

toma. Established hepatocellular carcinoma has occasionally been treated with interferon as well. In one randomized study, interferon therapy was superior to systemic doxorubicin chemotherapy in terms of rates of tumor regression and overall side effects.[61] In other studies, however, interferon therapy has been ineffective when used alone.[62] In another, a variety of biologic response modifiers were used after chemotherapy with 5-FU in the hope of maintaining responses achieved with 5-FU. The results were unimpressive, with no significant benefit identified.[63] Another approach has been the combined use of interleukin-2 with the pineal hormone melatonin.[64] In this provocative study, more than a third of the patients responded to treatment, and the toxicity was minimal. Finally, there have been a number of studies of immunotherapy combined with chemotherapy. Examples include doxorubicin plus the streptococcal agent OK-432,[65] recombinant leukocyte A interferon given with doxorubicin,[66] intra-arterial immunochemotherapy (with interleukin-2, OK-432, doxorubicin, cyclophosphamide, and famotidine),[67] the use of combined transarterial immunotherapy-chemotherapy studies using interferon-γ and interleukin-2,[68] and several studies using lymphokine-activated killer cells.[69-71] Despite some intriguing results, immunotherapy plays little role in the contemporary management of hepatocellular cancer. This approach to treatment remains investigational at this time.

## REFERENCES

1. Haskell CM, Lavey RS, Ramming KP. Liver. In: Haskell CM, ed. Cancer Treatment. 4th ed. Philadelphia: WB Saunders, 1995:512–25.
2. Bobbio-Pallavicini E, Porta C, Moroni M, et al. Epirubicin and etoposide combination chemotherapy to treat hepatocellular carcinoma patients: a phase II study. Eur J Cancer 1997;33:1784–8.
3. Leung TW, Patt YZ, Lau WY, et al. Complete pathological remission is possible with systemic combination chemotherapy for inoperable hepatocellular carcinoma. Clin Cancer Res 1999;5:1676–81.
4. Urabe T, Kaneko S, Matsushita E, et al. Clinical pilot study of intrahepatic arterial chemotherapy with methotrexate, 5-fluorouracil, cisplatin and subcutaneous interferon-alpha-2b for patients with locally advanced hepatocellular carcinoma. Oncology 1998;55:39–47.
5. Okada S, Okusaka T, Ueno H, et al. Phase II trial of cisplatin, mitoxantrone and continuous-infusion 5-fluorouracil (5-FU) (FMP therapy) for hepatocellular carcinoma (HCC). Proc ASCO 1999;18:248a.abstract.
6. Yamada R, Kishi K, Sonomura T, et al. Transcatheter arterial embolization in unresectable hepatocellular carcinoma. Cardiovasc Intervent Radiol 1990;13:135–9.
7. Bismuth H, Morino M, Sherlock D, et al. Primary treatment of hepatocellular carcinoma by arterial chemoembolization. Am J Surg 1992;163:387–94.
8. Hsieh MY, Chang WY, Wang LY, et al. Treatment of hepatocellular carcinoma by transcatheter arterial chemoembolization and analysis of prognostic factors. Cancer Chemother Pharmacol 1992;31:Suppl:S82–5.

9. Venook AP, Stagg RJ, Lewis BJ, et al. Chemoembolization for hepatocellular carcinoma. J Clin Oncol 1990;8:1108–14.
10. Tanaka K, Nakamura S, Numata K, et al. Hepatocellular carcinoma: treatment with percutaneous ethanol injection and transcatheter arterial embolization. Radiology 1992;185:457–60.
11. Monden M, Sakon M, Gotoh M, et al. Selection of therapeutic modalities for hepatocellular carcinoma in patients with multiple hepatic lesions. Cancer Chemother Pharmacol 1992;31:Suppl:S38–44.
12. Colleoni M, Vicario G, Manente P, et al. Activity and tolerability of courses of intra-arterial chemotherapy followed by chemoembolization in unresectable hepatocellular carcinoma. Tumori 1998;84:673–6.
13. Okusaka T, Okada S, Ishii H, et al. Transarterial chemotherapy with zinostatin stimalamer for hepatocellular carcinoma. Oncology 1998;55:276–83.
14. Ikeda K, Saitoh S, Suzuki Y, et al. A prospective randomized administration of 5′-deoxy-5-fluorouridine as adjuvant chemotherapy for hepatocellular carcinoma treated with transcatheter arterial chemoembolization. Am J Clin Oncol 1997;20:202–8.
15. Bhattacharya S, Novell JR, Dusheiko GM, et al. Epirubicin-lipiodol chemotherapy versus 131iodine-lipiodol radiotherapy in the treatment of unresectable hepatocellular carcinoma. Cancer 1995;76:2202–10.
16. Ikeda K, Saitoh S, Koida I, et al. A prospective randomized evaluation of a compound of tegafur and uracil as an adjuvant chemotherapy for hepatocellular carcinoma treated with transcatheter arterial chemoembolization. Am J Clin Oncol 1995;18:204–10.
17. Raoul JL, Messner M, Boucher E, et al. Preoperative treatment of hepatocellular carcinoma with radioactive lipiodol. Proc ASCO 1999;18:243a.abstract.
18. Minoyama A, Yoshikawa M, Ebara M, et al. Study of repeated arterial infusion chemotherapy with a subcutaneously implanted reservoir for advanced hepatocellular carcinoma. J Gastroenterol 1995;30:356-66.
19. Bayraktar Y, Balkanci F, Kayhan B, et al. A comparison of chemoembolization with conventional chemotherapy and symptomatic treatment in cirrhotic patients with hepatocellular carcinoma. Hepatogastroenterology 1996;43:681–7.
20. Biselli M, Forti P, Mucci F, et al. Chemoembolization versus chemotherapy in elderly patients with unresectable hepatocellular carcinoma and contrast uptake as prognostic factor. J Gerontol Series A Biol Sci Med Sci 1997;52:M305–9.
21. Okuda K, Tanaka M, Shibata J, et al. Hepatic arterial infusion chemotherapy with continuous low dose administration of cisplatin and 5-fluorouracil for multiple recurrence of hepatocellular carcinoma after surgical treatment. Oncol Rep 1999;6:587–91.
22. Asahara T, Itamoto T, Katayama K, et al. Adjuvant hepatic arterial infusion chemotherapy after radical hepatectomy for hepatocellular carcinoma—results of long-term follow-up. Hepatogastroenterology 1999;46:1042–8.
23. Lai EC, Lo CM, Fan ST, et al. Postoperative adjuvant chemotherapy after curative resection of hepatocellular carcinoma: a randomized controlled trial. Arch Surg 1998;133:183–8.
24. Ono T, Nagasue N, Kohno H, et al. Adjuvant chemotherapy with epirubicin and carmofur after radical resection of hepatocellular carcinoma: a prospective randomized study. Semin Oncol 1997;24:2 Suppl 6:S6-18–25.
25. Kohno H, Nagasue N, Hayashi T, et al. Postoperative adjuvant chemotherapy after radical hepatic resection for hepatocellular carcinoma (HCC). Hepatogastroenterology 1996;43:1405–9.
26. Nakashima K, Kitano S, Kim YI, et al. Postoperative adjuvant arterial infusion chemotherapy for patients with hepatocellular carcinoma. Hepatogastroenterology 1996;43:1410-4.
27. Yamamoto M, Arii S, Sugahara K, Tobe T. Adjuvant oral chemotherapy to prevent recurrence after curative resection for hepatocellular carcinoma. Br J Surg 1996;83:336–40.
28. Lygidakis NJ, Pothoulakis J, Konstantinidou AE, Spanos H. Hepatocellular carcinoma: surgical resection versus surgical resection combined with pre- and post-operative locoregional immunotherapy-chemotherapy: a prospective randomized study. Anticancer Res 1995;15:543–50.
29. Cherqui D, Piedbois P, Pierga JY, et al. Multimodal adjuvant treatment and liver transplantation for advanced hepatocellular carcinoma: a pilot study. Cancer 1994;73:2721–6.
30. Stone MJ, Klintmalm GB, Polter D, et al. Neoadjuvant chemotherapy and liver transplantation for hepatocellular carcinoma: a pilot study in 20 patients. Gastroenterology 1993;104:196–202.
31. Olthoff KM, Rosove MH, Shackleton CR, et al. Adjuvant chemotherapy improves survival after liver transplantation for hepatocellular carcinoma [erratum appears in Ann Surg 1996;224:686]. Ann Surg 1995;221:735–41.
32. Holman M, Harrison D, Stewart A, et al. Neoadjuvant chemotherapy and orthotopic liver transplantation for hepatocellular carcinoma. N Engl J Med 1995;92:519–22.
33. Holton CP, Burrington JD, Hatch EI. A multiple chemotherapeutic approach to the management of hepatoblastoma: a preliminary report. Cancer 1975;35:1083–7.
34. Tanner AR, Bolton PM, Powell LW. Primary sarcoma of the liver: report of a case with excellent response to hepatic artery ligation and infusion chemotherapy. Gastroenterology 1978;74:121–3.
35. Nerenstone SR, Ihde DC, Friedman MA. Clinical trials in primary hepatocellular carcinoma: current status and future directions. Cancer Treat Rev 1988;15:1–31.
36. Nagahama H, Okada S, Okusaka T, et al. Predictive factors for tumor response to systemic chemotherapy in patients with hepatocellular carcinoma. Jpn J Clin Oncol 1997;27:321–4.
37. Lai C-L, Wu PC, Chan GC, et al. Doxorubicin versus no antitumor therapy in inoperable hepatocellular carcinoma: a prospective randomized trial. Cancer 1988;62:479–83.
38. Farinati F, De Maria N, Fornasiero A, et al. Prospective controlled trial with antiestrogen drug tamoxifen in patients with unresectable hepatocellular carcinoma. Dig Dis Sci 1992;37:659–62.
39. CLIP Group (Cancer of the Liver Italian Programme). Tamoxifen in treatment of hepatocellular carcinoma: a randomised controlled trial. Lancet 1998;352:17–20.
40. Bierman HR, Byron RL, Kelley KH, Grady A. Studies of the blood supply of tumors in man: III. vascular patterns of the liver by hepatic arteriography in vivo. J Natl Cancer Inst 1951;12:107–17.
41. Breedis C, Young G. The blood supply of neoplasms in the liver. Am J Pathol 1954;30:969–985.
42. Healey JE Jr. Vascular patterns in human metastatic liver tumors. Surg Gynecol Obstet 1965;120:1187–93.
43. Almersjö O, Bengmark S, Engevik L, et al. Hepatic artery ligation as pretreatment for liver resection of metastatic cancer. Rev Surg 1966;23:377–80.
44. Segall HN. An experimental anatomical investigation of the blood and bile channels of the liver. Surg Gynecol Obstet 1923;37:152–78.
45. Wright RD. The blood supply of newly developed epithelial tissue in the liver. J Pathol Bacteriol 1937;45:405–14.
46. Davis HL Jr, Ramirez G, Ansfield FJ. Adenocarcinomas of stomach, pancreas, liver, and biliary tracts: survival of 328 patients treated with fluoropyrimidine therapy. Cancer 1974;33:193–7.
47. Anderson JM, Patrick RS, Short DW, Mackey WA. Disappearance of hepatic cancer after intra-arterial fluorouracil. Br Med J 1972;3:454–5.
48. Tzoracoleftherakis EE, Spiliotis JD, Kyriakopoulou T, Kakkos SK. Intra-arterial versus systemic chemotherapy for non-operable hepatocellular carcinoma. Hepatogastroenterology 1999;46:1122–5.
49. Reed ML, Vaitkevicius VK, Al-Sarraf M, et al. The practicality of chronic hepatic artery infusion therapy of primary and metastatic hepatic malignancies: ten-year results of 124 patients in a prospective protocol. Cancer 1981;47:402–9.
50. Al-Jurf AS, Jochimsen PR, Shirazi SS, et al. Hepatic artery ligation and chemotherapeutic infusion in the treatment of hepatic malignancy. J Surg Oncol 1984;27:119–23.
51. Okayasu I, Hatakeyama S, Yoshida T, et al. Selective and persistent deposition and gradual drainage of iodized oil, Lipiodol in the hepatocellular carcinoma after injection into the feeding hepatic artery. Am J Clin Pathol 1988;90:536–44.
52. Takayasu K, Shima Y, Muramatsu Y, et al. Hepatocellular carcinoma: treatment with intraarterial iodized oil with and without chemotherapeutic agents. Radiology 1987;163:345–51.
53. Hsu HC, Wei TC, Tsang YM, et al. Histologic assessment of resected hepatocellular carcinoma after transcatheter hepatic arterial embolization. Cancer 1986;57:1184–91.
54. Furui S, Otomo K, Itai Y, Iio M. Hepatocellular carcinoma treated by transcatheter arterial embolization: progress evaluated by computed tomography. Radiology 1984;150:773–8.
55. Takayasu K, Moriyama N, Muramatsu Y, et al. Hepatic arterial embolization for hepatocellular carcinoma: comparison of CT scans and resected specimens. Radiology 1984;150:661–5.
56. Nakao N, Miura K, Takahashi H, et al. Hepatocellular carcinoma: combined hepatic, arterial, and portal venous embolization. Radiology 1986;161:303–7.
57. Sato Y, Fujiwara K, Ogata I, et al. Transcatheter arterial embolization for hepatocellular carcinoma: benefits and limitations for unresectable

cases with liver cirrhosis evaluated by comparison with other conservative treatments. Cancer 1985;55:2822–5.

58. Sakurai M, Okamura J, Kuroda C. Transcatheter chemo-embolization effective for treating hepatocellular carcinoma: a histopathologic study. Cancer 1984;54:387–92.

59. Shimamura Y, Gunvèn P, Takenaka Y, et al. Combined peripheral and central chemoembolization of liver tumors: experience with lipiodol-doxorubicin and gelatin sponge (L-TAE). Cancer 1988;61:238–42.

60. Sasaki Y, Imaoka S, Kasugai H, et al. A new approach to chemoembolization therapy for hepatoma using ethiodized oil, cisplatin, and gelatin sponge. Cancer 1987;60:1194–203.

61. Lai C-L, Wu PC, Lok AS, et al. Recombinant alpha 2 interferon is superior to doxorubicin for inoperable hepatocellular carcinoma: a prospective randomised trial. Br J Cancer 1989;60:928–33.

62. GITSG. A prospective trial of recombinant human interferon alpha 2B in previously untreated patients with hepatocellular carcinoma. The Gastrointestinal Tumor Study Group. Cancer 1990;66:135–9.

63. Suto T, Fukuda S, Moriya N, et al. Clinical study of biological response modifiers as maintenance therapy for hepatocellular carcinoma. Cancer Chemother Pharmacol 1994;33:Suppl:S145–8.

64. Aldeghi R, Lissoni P, Barni S, et al. Low-dose interleukin-2 subcutaneous immunotherapy in association with the pineal hormone melatonin as a first-line therapy in locally advanced or metastatic hepatocellular carcinoma. Eur J Cancer 1994;30A:167–70.

65. Imaoka S, Sasaki Y, Ishikawa O. Immunochemotherapy in human hepatocellular carcinoma using the streptococcal agent OK-432. J Clin Oncol 1986;4:1645–51.

66. Creagan ET, Long HJ, Frytak S, Moertel CG. Recombinant leukocyte A interferon with doxorubicin: a phase I study in advanced solid neoplasms and implications for hepatocellular carcinoma. Cancer 1988;61:19–22.

67. Oka M, Hazama S, Yoshino S, et al. Intraarterial combined immuno-chemotherapy for unresectable hepatocellular carcinoma: preliminary results. Cancer Immunol Immunother 1994;38:194–200.

68. Lygidakis NJ, Kosmidis P, Ziras N, et al. Combined transarterial targeting locoregional immunotherapy-chemotherapy for patients with unresectable hepatocellular carcinoma: a new alternative for an old problem. J Interferon Cytokine Res 1995;15:467–72.

69. Okuno K, Takagi H, Nakamura T, et al. Treatment for unresectable hepatoma via selective hepatic arterial infusion of lymphokine-activated killer cells generated from autologous spleen cells. Cancer 1986;58:1001–6.

70. Hsieh KH, Shu SY, Lee CS, et al. Lysis of primary hepatic tumours by lymphokine activated killer cells. Gut 1987;28:117–24.

71. Ishikawa T, Imawari M, Moriyama T. Immunotherapy of hepatocellular carcinoma with autologous lymphokine-activated killer cells and/or recombinant interleukin-2. J Cancer Res Clin Oncol 1988;114:283–90.

·······································

# TREATMENT BY STAGE OF DISEASE

• Charles M. Haskell

Ideally, hepatocellular carcinoma should be prevented by measures that reduce the risk of acquiring hepatis. Lacking prevention, one should try to treat the disease when it is a small, early lesion. Although prospective randomized trials have not proved the value of screening for this disease, anecdotal experience and limited trials suggest that this is rational in high-risk populations. Subsequent treatment varies with the size and number of lesions, underlying liver function, and the expertise and experience of the physicians involved in management. My current approach to treatment of established hepatocellular carcinoma is summarized in Figure 46–2.

## STAGES I THROUGH IIIA

Patients with potentially resectable primary hepatic cancer should be offered surgical exploration and possible resection

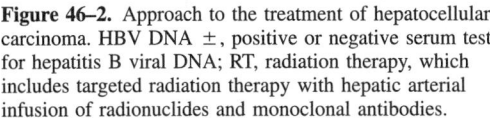
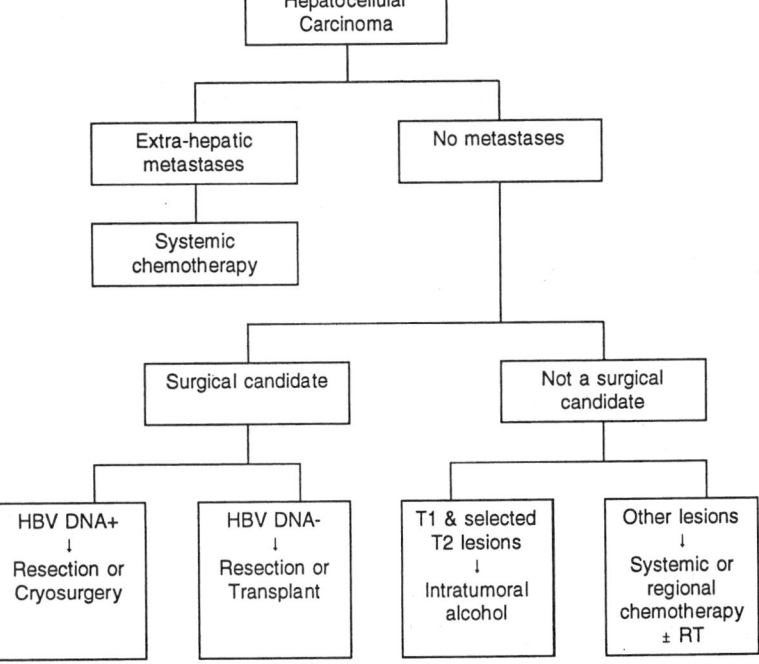

**Figure 46–2.** Approach to the treatment of hepatocellular carcinoma. HBV DNA ±, positive or negative serum test for hepatitis B viral DNA; RT, radiation therapy, which includes targeted radiation therapy with hepatic arterial infusion of radionuclides and monoclonal antibodies.

of the tumor unless there are compelling contraindications to surgery, such as the presence of obvious extrahepatic tumor, extensive hepatic involvement, or medical contraindications to surgery. Cirrhosis of the liver alone is not an absolute contraindication to surgery. Indeed, the only hope of cure for these patients is with partial hepatectomy or liver transplantation.

Patients who undergo exploratory surgery and are found to have inoperable disease, but who have one to three nodules smaller than 3 cm and no evidence of extrahepatic tumor, are candidates for intraoperative injection of 10 to 20 ml of sterile alcohol into the tumor. Percutaneous injection under ultrasonographic guidance can be repeated three times weekly for up to 12 treatments. Alternatively, hepatic artery infusion therapy can be initiated, either with chemotherapy or a radionuclide, or a combination of the two. Patients with focal rather than diffuse hepatic involvement are the best candidates for chemotherapy plus partial liver irradiation. Patients with disease confined to the liver, but in a fashion that precludes localized resection, may also be considered for orthotopic liver transplantation if they have no evidence of hepatitis, preferably combined with chemotherapy.

### STAGES IIIB AND IV

Patients with extrahepatic tumor at the time of laparotomy, and patients who do not undergo exploratory surgery because of obviously unresectable disease, are usually treated with chemotherapy using 5-FU as a single agent. Choosing between systemic and hepatic artery infusion of a fluoropyrimidine depends on the general condition of the patient and the expertise of the treatment team. Some centers use lipiodol-targeted chemotherapy or TAE for these patients instead. Patients who strongly desire continued chemotherapy after initial treatment failure may be considered for other single agents given systemically or by the intra-arterial route.

### SUGGESTIONS FOR ADDITIONAL READING

Di Bisceglie AM (moderator, NIH conference). Hepatocellular carcinoma. Ann Intern Med 1988;108:390–401. *This is a good review of the epidemiology, etiology, diagnosis, and surgical treatment of hepatocellular carcinoma.*

Dusheiko GM, Hobbs KEF, Dick R, Burroughs AK. Treatment of small hepatocellular carcinomas. Lancet 1992;340:285–8. *This article provides a European perspective on the management of small, screen-detected lesions.*

Venook AP. Treatment of hepatocellular carcinoma: too many options? J Clin Oncol 1994;12:1323–34. *This extensive review concludes that prevention is the ideal approach to hepatocellular carcinoma. Surgical cure is rarely possible, whereas other therapeutic maneuvers are difficult to assess because of the paucity of randomized clinical trials.*

Farmer DB, Rosove MH, Shaked A, Busuttil RW. Current treatment modalities for hepatocellular carcinoma. Ann Surg 1994;219:236–47. *This review emphasizes the primacy of surgical resection in treatment of curative intent.*

Leung TW, Patt YZ, Lau WY, et al. Complete pathological remission is possible with systemic combination chemotherapy for inoperable hepatocellular carcinoma. Clin Cancer Res 1999;5:1676–81. *This study shows that pathologic complete remissions are possible in patients with hepatocellular carcinoma using multiagent chemotherapy.*

Asahara T, Itamoto T, Katayama K, et al. Adjuvant hepatic arterial infusion chemotherapy after radical hepatectomy for hepatocellular carcinoma—results of long-term follow-up. Hepatogastroenterology 1999;46:1042–8. *Long-term survival after radical hepatic resections was better in patients treated with adjuvant therapy than in patients treated with surgery alone.*

# CHAPTER 47

# GALLBLADDER

......................................

# NATURAL HISTORY, DIAGNOSIS, AND STAGING

• Charles M. Haskell

### EPIDEMIOLOGY AND ETIOLOGY

**Incidence and Mortality.**[1] The annual incidence of gallbladder cancer in the United States is 1 case per 100,000 population. The annual mortality rate is 0.6 deaths per 100,000, and the overall 5-year survival rate is 13.7%. The disease is more common in women than in men, with annual incidence figures of 1.2 and 0.7 cases per 100,000, respectively. The frequency of gallbladder carcinoma in autopsy series has ranged from 0.2 to 0.8%.[2] Overall this is a rare cancer, composing only 1.4% of all gastrointestinal neoplasms.

**Epidemiology and Risk Factors.** The cause of gallbladder cancer is unknown, but it usually occurs in the presence of gallstones. Indeed, the frequency of gallbladder cancer is directly proportional to the frequency of gallstones in different populations. Several examples serve to illustrate this point. Both gallstones and gallbladder cancer are extremely rare in the Bantu of Africa, whereas both are common in the Native American population. In autopsy studies[3, 4] and one cohort study,[5] for example, gallbladder cancer constituted 8.5 to 30% of all cancers detected in Native Americans. The incidence of gallbladder cancer is influenced by the period of exposure to gallstones[6] and to the size of gallstones. Specifically, Diehl[7] has reported a 10-fold increase in the risk of gallbladder cancer in individuals with gallstones, but only in those with stones 3 cm or larger. Other causes of gallbladder disease may also be associated with gallbladder cancer. For example, chronic typhoid and paratyphoid carriers have a marked increase in their risk of the disease (relative risk 167, confidence interval 54 to 389).[8] Other predisposing factors include gallbladder polyps greater than 1 cm in diameter, calcification of the gallbladder (porcelein gallbladder), and a rare anatomic condition known as *anomalous pancreaticobiliary ductal junction.*[9] Anomalous pancreaticobiliary ductal junction is found mostly among Asians, and it is sometimes associated with a choledochal cyst. Patients with this condition are candidates for prophylactic cholecystectomy with cyst excision.[10]

It must be emphasized that gallbladder cancer remains a rare disease, even in individuals with cholelithiasis. Despite the clear association of gallstones with carcinoma of the gallbladder, the incidence of gallbladder cancer is relatively low in the total population of patients with cholelithiasis (0.66% in one series).[11]

Further details of the cause and epidemiology of gallbladder cancer have been reviewed by Piehler and Crichlow[2] and by Diehl.[12] Studies of oncogene products and growth factors in gallbladder cancer are just beginning to be reported.[13]

## PATHOLOGY

Histologically, cancer of the gallbladder is almost always a form of adenocarcinoma. There is some evidence that this tumor may arise from precursor lesions that include hyperplasia, atypical hyperplasia, and carcinoma in situ.[14, 15]

The Surveillance, Epidemiology, and End Results (SEER) reporting program of the National Cancer Institute recorded 2599 cases of gallbladder cancer between 1977 and 1986. Of the 2399 cases in which histologic type was recorded, 82% were adenocarcinoma, 6% were papillary adenocarcinoma, 5% were mucinous adenocarcinoma, 4% were adenosquamous carcinoma, 2% were squamous carcinoma, and 1% were oat cell carcinoma.[16]

Metastasis occurs primarily through submucosal lymphatics into the regional lymphatics, including the cystic duct nodes, pericholedochal nodes, and superior pancreaticoduodenal nodes. Direct extension is common, and distant metastases, particularly in the abdomen, are not infrequent.[17]

## CLINICAL FEATURES AND DIAGNOSIS

After reviewing 6222 instances of carcinoma of the gallbladder reported in the English language literature since 1960, Piehler and Crichlow[2] identified five ways in which most patients with this disease present. In their review, 43% of patients presented to the physician with findings suggestive of chronic cholecystitis, 34% presented with symptoms of malignant tumors of the biliary tract (jaundice, weight loss, anorexia, persistent aching right upper quadrant pain), 29% presented with symptoms of malignancy outside the biliary tract, 16% presented with symptoms of acute cholecystitis, and the remainder presented with symptoms suggestive of a benign manifestation of disease outside the biliary tree.

Patients presenting with symptoms suggesting gallbladder disease of almost any type should initially be studied by ultrasonography.[18, 19] This study has largely supplanted oral

cholecystography in evaluating patients with potential cholelithiasis, and it is capable of detecting early gallbladder cancer in some patients. For example, Koga and colleagues[20] were able to perform curative resections on four of five patients with early carcinoma of the gallbladder detected by ultrasonography. It should be emphasized, however, that the vast majority of cases of gallbladder cancer are not diagnosed preoperatively, despite the presence of symptoms suggestive of a malignant process involving the hepatobiliary system. In the review by Piehler and Crichlow,[2] for example, only 8.6% of patients were correctly diagnosed preoperatively. Newer imaging procedures, such as magnetic resonance imaging (MRI), may prove more sensitive and accurate in the early diagnosis and staging of this malignancy.[21] Whether MRI will prove to be cost effective has not been determined.

Tumor markers, such as carcinoembryonic antigen (CEA) and CA 19-9 measured in serum, are of little value in the diagnosis and staging of gallbladder cancer. Measurements of CEA and CEA-related substances in bile were more useful in one study,[22] but these findings must be confirmed independently. Rare cases of elevated levels of alpha-fetoprotein in patients with gallbladder cancer and no evidence of hepatic metastases have been reported, so this can represent a type of false-positive reaction in patients with germ cell and hepatocellular neoplasms.[23, 24]

## STAGING

A TNM staging system for gallbladder cancer has been developed jointly by the American Joint Committee on Cancer and the International Union Against Cancer.[25] The current version of this system is presented in Table 47–1 for reference purposes.

## PROGNOSIS

The overall 5-year survival rate in the United States for patients with gallbladder cancer diagnosed between 1989 and 1995 in the SEER database was 13.7%.[1] Prognosis is strongly affected by the TNM stage of disease. Median survival was 19 months for stage I, 7 months for stage II, 4 months for stage III, 2 months for stage IV, and 4 months for all cases combined. Within stage I, patients without vascular invasion had a 31% 5-year survival rate, compared with 13% among those with vascular invasion. Histologic grade also correlates with prognosis, but to a lesser extent than does stage.[16] There is some evidence in the SEER database that papillary adenocarcinoma of the gallbladder may be a more favorable histologic presentation than other histologic types, with a median survival of 20 months and a 2-year survival of 47%. Patients with well-differentiated neoplasms live an average of 13 months longer than those with poorly differentiated lesions.[26]

There is some evidence that the prognosis of patients with gallbladder cancer may be improving in Japan,[27, 28] but not in the United States and Europe.[29] Surgeons from Japan ascribe at least some of the improvement to their use of radical surgical resections, including the removal of lymph nodes. Radical surgery may be especially important in pa-

*Table 47–1.*  **TNM Staging for Primary Neoplasms of the Gallbladder**

*Primary Tumor (T)*

TX  Primary tumor cannot be assessed
T0  No evidence of primary tumor
Tis  Carcinoma in situ
T1  Tumor invades lamina propria or muscle layer
   T1a  Tumor invades lamina propria
   T1b  Tumor invades muscle layer
T2  Tumor invades perimuscular connective tissue; no extension beyond serosa or into liver
T3  Tumor perforates the serosa (visceral peritoneum) or directly invades one adjacent organ, or both (extension 2 cm or less into liver)
T4  Tumor extends more than 2 cm into liver, and/or into two or more adjacent organs (stomach, duodenum, colon, pancreas, omentum, extrahepatic bile ducts, any involvement of liver)

*Regional Lymph Nodes (N)*

NX  Regional lymph nodes cannot be assessed
N0  No regional lymph node metastasis
N1  Metastasis in cystic duct, pericholedochal, and/or hilar lymph nodes (i.e., in the hepatoduodenal ligament)
N2  Metastasis in peripancreatic (head only), periduodenal, periportal, celiac, and/or superior mesenteric lymph nodes

*Distant Metastasis (M)*

MX  Distant metastasis cannot be assessed
M0  No distant metastasis
M1  Distant metastasis

*Stage Grouping*

| Stage 0 | Tis | N0 | M0 |
|---|---|---|---|
| Stage I | T1 | N0 | M0 |
| Stage II | T2 | N0 | M0 |
| Stage III | T1 | N1 | M0 |
|  | T2 | N1 | M0 |
|  | T3 | N0 | M0 |
|  | T3 | N1 | M0 |
| Stage IVA | T4 | N0 | M0 |
|  | T4 | N1 | M0 |
| Stage IVB | Any T | N2 | M0 |
|  | Any T | Any N | M1 |

Used with the permission of the American Joint Committee on Cancer (AJCC®), Chicago, Illinois. The original source for this material is the AJCC® Cancer Staging Manual, 5th ed (1997) published by Lippincott-Raven Publishers, Philadelphia, Pennsylvania.

tients with subserosal invasion, especially in the presence of positive surgical margins.[30]

# REFERENCES

1. SEER Cancer Statistics Review 1973–1996. (See website: http://www-seer.ims.nci.nih.gov.)
2. Piehler JM, Crichlow RW. Primary carcinoma of the gallbladder. Surg Gynecol Obstet 1978;147:929–42.
3. Black WC, Key CR, Carmany TB, Herman D. Carcinoma of the gallbladder in a population of southwestern American Indians. Cancer 1977;39:1267–79.
4. Reichenbach DD: Autopsy incidence of diseases among southwestern American Indians. Arch Pathol 1967;84:81–6.
5. Grimaldi CH, Nelson RG, Pettitt DJ, et al. Increased mortality with gallstone disease: results of a 20-year population-based survey in Pima Indians. Ann Intern Med 1993;118:185–90.
6. Lowenfels AB, Lindström CG, Conway MJ, Hastings PR. Gallstones and risk of gallbladder cancer. J Natl Cancer Inst 1985;75:77–80.
7. Diehl AK. Gallstone size and the risk of gallbladder cancer. JAMA 1983;250:2323–6.
8. Caygill CPJ, Hill MJ, Braddick M, Sharp JC. Cancer mortality in chronic typhoid and paratyphoid carriers. Lancet 1994;343:83–4.
9. De Groen PC, Gores GJ, LaRusso NF, et al. Biliary tract cancers (medical progress). N Engl J Med 1999;341:1368–78.
10. Chijiiwa K, Kimura H, Tanaka M. Malignant potential of the gallbladder in patients with anomalous pancreaticobiliary ductal junction: the difference in risk between patients with and without choledochal cyst. Int Surg 1995;80:61–4.
11. Gerst PH. Primary carcinoma of the gallbladder—a thirty-year summary. Ann Surg 1961;153:369–72.
12. Diehl AK. Epidemiology of gallbladder cancer: a synthesis of recent data. J Natl Cancer Inst 1980;65:1209–14.
13. Yukawa M, Fujimori T, Hirayama D, et al. Expression of oncogene products and growth factors in early gallbladder cancer, advanced gallbladder cancer, and chronic cholecystitis. Hum Pathol 1993;24:37–40.
14. Albores-Saavedra J, Alcántra-Vazquez A, Cruz-Ortiz H, Herrera-Goepfert R. The precursor lesions of invasive gallbladder carcinoma: hyperplasia, atypical hyperplasia, and carcinoma in situ. Cancer 1980;45:919–27.
15. Yamaguchi K, Enjoji M. Carcinoma of the gallbladder: a clinicopathology of 103 patients and a newly proposed staging. Cancer 1988;62:1425–32.
16. Henson DE, Albores-Saavedra J, Corle D. Carcinoma of the gallbladder: histologic types, stage of disease, grade, and survival rates. Cancer 1992;70:1493–7.
17. Warren KW, Hardy KJ, O'Rourke MG. Primary neoplasia of the gallbladder. Surg Gynecol Obstet 1968;126:1036–40.
18. Marton KI, Doubilet P. How to image the gallbladder in suspected cholecystitis. Ann Intern Med 1988;109:722–9.
19. Health and Policy Committee, American College of Physicians. How to study the gallbladder. Ann Intern Med 1988;109:752–4.
20. Koga A, Yamauchi S, Izumi Y, Hamanaka N. Ultrasonographic detection of early and curable carcinoma of the gallbladder. Br J Surg 1985;72:728–30.
21. Sagoh T, Itoh K, Togashi K, et al. Gallbladder carcinoma: evaluation with MR imaging. Radiology 1990;174:131–6.
22. Uchino R, Kanemitsu K, Obayashi H, et al. Carcinoembryonic antigen (CEA) and CEA-related substances in the bile of patients with biliary diseases. Am J Surg 1994;167:306–8.
23. Brown JA, Roberts CS. Elevated serum alpha-fetoprotein levels in primary gallbladder carcinoma without hepatic involvement. Cancer 1992;70:1838–40.
24. Watanabe M, Hori Y, Nojima T, et al. Alpha-fetoprotein–producing carcinoma of the gallbladder. Dig Dis Sci 1993;38:561–4.
25. Fleming ID, Cooper JS, Henson DE, et al, eds. AJCC Cancer Staging Manual. 5th ed. Philadelphia: Lippincott-Raven, 1997:97–100.
26. White K, Kraybill WG, Lopez MJ. Primary carcinoma of the gallbladder: TNM staging and prognosis. J Surg Oncol 1988;39:251–5.
27. Ouchi K, Suzuki M, Saijo S, et al. Do recent advances in diagnosis and operative management improve the outcome of gallbladder carcinoma? Surgery 1993;113:324–9.
28. Shirai Y, Yoshida K, Tsukada K, et al. Radical surgery for gallbladder carcinoma: long-term results. Ann Surg 1992;216:565–8.
29. Cubertafond P, Gainant A, Cucchiaro G. Surgical treatment of 724 carcinomas of the gallbladder: results of the French Surgical Association Survey. Ann Surg 1994;219:275–80.
30. Yamaguchi K, Tsuneyoshi M. Subclinical gallbladder carcinoma. Am J Surg 1992;163:382–6.

# TREATMENT

• Charles M. Haskell • Luu M. Tran • Kenneth P. Ramming

## SURGERY

Surgery is the mainstay of therapy for carcinoma of the gallbladder, despite its bleak prognosis. At present, it offers the only potential for cure. In patients with local invasion, partial hepatectomy should be performed if possible. Regional lymphadenectomy is also indicated in most patients with grossly apparent tumor, and reoperation for the purpose of performing a more extensive local dissection with wedge resection of the liver and regional node dissection should be considered if not carried out initially, even in patients with presumably curative local resections.[1]

Cancer of the gallbladder is so strongly linked to cholelithiasis that the advisability of elective cholecystectomy to prevent this virulent cancer is frequently discussed. Indeed, after the analysis of 15 cases, Blalock[2] advocated prophylactic cholecystectomy in good-risk surgical patients. Moreover, an increasing number of cholecystectomies in the United States and parts of western Europe associated with a declining incidence of gallbladder cancer in these areas has suggested a rationale for such prophylactic surgery on an epidemiologic basis.[3] Nevertheless, the tremendous number of patients with benign gallbladder disease in clinical and autopsy series would lead one away from this conclusion. Because carcinoma of the gallbladder occurs in only about 0.66% of patients with cholelithiasis, prophylactic surgery would be without benefit in more than 99% of patients with asymptomatic stones. However, patients with symptomatic gallstones are candidates for cholecystectomy, as recommended by the American College of Physicians.[4]

The choice of a specific operation for patients with known or suspected gallbladder cancer is different from the choice for a patient with uncomplicated gallstones. The latter patient is likely to choose a laparoscopic procedure, if available, because of the lower morbidity and shorter hospital stay.[5] Laparoscopic surgery is contraindicated in the patient with known carcinoma because of the need for a node dissection in most of these patients and the risk of parietal seeding after the procedure.[6]

## RADIATION THERAPY

Gallbladder carcinoma is usually advanced by the time of diagnosis, with only 20 to 30% of tumors being resectable.[7] In addition, there is a high risk of microscopic residual disease after complete gross resection. In a report from North and colleagues,[8] only 36 of 109 patients undergoing surgery had complete resection (median survival 67 months), whereas 44 had residual disease, with a median survival rate of only 9 months. With the likelihood of locally advanced disease, adjuvant radiation therapy (RT) with or without chemotherapy has been used in several small series.[9–15]

Only retrospective studies are available to support the use of RT, as the rarity of this lesion precludes any meaningful

randomized trial. Vaittinen[9] obtained a median survival of 63 months in 7 patients treated with postoperative RT, compared with 29 months for the 24 patients treated with surgery alone. Nadler and McSherry[10] from Beth Israel Medical Center reviewed 56 cases with gallbladder carcinoma. Although no definite protocols were used, there was a suggestion of improved survival with adjuvant RT or chemotherapy. At Washington University in St. Louis,[5] adjuvant RT was given after cholecystectomy to three patients with gallbladder cancers. Of these, two survived 22+ and 27+ months, respectively, whereas the third died of local disease at 5 months.

Flickinger and colleagues[12] evaluated the role of primary RT in the treatment of 8 patients with gallbladder carcinoma and 55 patients with extrahepatic bile duct tumors. The median survival was 3 and 9 months, respectively. The only long-term survivors were patients treated with liver transplantation and irradiation (22% survival at 4 years). At Washington University in St. Louis,[16] 96 patients were given RT for biliary tract cancers and showed a dose response, namely, an RT dose greater than 40 Gy improved survival more than a dose of less than 40 Gy ($p = 0.003$). There was no survival difference between gallbladder primary cancers and tumors elsewhere in the biliary tract. Todoroki and colleagues[17] used intraoperative RT (IORT) (20 to 30 Gy) with and without external-beam RT in 17 patients with stage IV gallbladder cancers. The 3-year survival rate was 10% for resection plus IORT, but 0% for resection alone.

Adjuvant RT seems to improve survival rates for gallbladder and extrahepatic bile duct tumors.

## CHEMOTHERAPY

Chemotherapy is of unproved value in the treatment of this disease. Little is known about its use, and most reports of chemotherapy for gallbladder cancer combine results with those seen with extrahepatic biliary cancer, as discussed in Chapter 48.

## SUMMARY OF TREATMENT

Surgical therapy is the mainstay of treatment for cancer of the gallbladder. Stage 0 and stage I gallbladder cancers that are found unexpectedly during laparoscopic surgery may be treated effectively with this procedure, but most patients with gallbladder cancer require more radical procedures than can be accomplished by the laparoscopic route. Extended, or radical, cholecystectomy is preferred for patients with stages II, III, and IV gallbladder cancers. Adjacent liver tissue and regional lymph nodes are removed during such extended procedures.

Adjuvant RT is a reasonable, but unproved, treatment for patients with subserosal involvement, positive surgical margins, or positive lymph nodes following radical resection. Patients with locally advanced disease are candidates for primary RT. Chemotherapy plays no significant role in management.

## SUGGESTIONS FOR ADDITIONAL READING

Marton KI, Doubilet P. How to image the gallbladder in suspected cholecystitis. Ann Intern Med 1988;109:722–29. *The importance of ultrasonography in the diagnosis of gallbladder disease is discussed in this review, as well as in a companion position paper from the American College of Physicians.*

De Groen PC, Gores GJ, LaRusso NF, et al. Biliary tract cancers (medical progress). N Engl J Med 1999;341:1368–78. *An excellent review of all biliary tract cancers, including gallbladder cancer.*

## REFERENCES

1. Piehler JM, Crichlow RW. Primary carcinoma of the gallbladder. Surg Gynecol Obstet 1978;147:929–42.
2. Blalock JB Jr. An analysis of 15 cases of gallbladder carcinoma. Am Surg 1978;44:286–9.
3. Diehl AK, Beral V. Cholecystectomy and changing mortality from gallbladder cancer. Lancet 1981;2:187–9.
4. Ransohoff DF, Gracie WA. Treatment of gallstones. Pt 1. Ann Intern Med 1993;119:606–19.
5. Southern Surgeons Club: A prospective analysis of 1518 laparoscopic cholecystectomies. N Engl J Med 1991;324:1073–8 and 325:1517–8.
6. Pezet D, Fondrinier E, Rotman N, et al. Parietal seeding of carcinoma of the gallbladder after laparoscopic cholecystectomy. Br J Surg 1992;79:230.
7. Adson MA, Farnell MB. Hepatobiliary cancer—surgical considerations. Mayo Clin Proc 1981;56:686–99.
8. North JH Jr, Pack MS, Hong C, Rivera DE. Prognostic factors for adenocarcinoma of the gallbladder: an analysis of 162 cases. Am Surg 1998;64:437–40.
9. Vaittinen E. Carcinoma of the gall-bladder: a study of 390 cases diagnosed in Finland 1953–1967. Ann Chir Gynaecol 1970;168:Suppl:1–81.
10. Nadler LH, McSherry CK. Carcinoma of the gallbladder: review of the literature and report on 56 cases at the Beth Israel Medical Center. Mt Sinai J Med 1992;59:47–52.
11. Fields JN, Emami B. Carcinoma of the extrahepatic biliary system: results of primary and adjuvant radiotherapy. Int J Radiat Oncol Biol Phys 1987;13:331–8.
12. Flickinger JC, Epstein AH, Iwatsuki S, et al. Radiation therapy for primary carcinoma of the extrahepatic biliary system: an analysis of 63 cases. Cancer 199;68:289–94.
13. Mahe M, Stampfli C, Romestaing P, et al. Primary carcinoma of the gallbladder: potential for external radiation therapy. Radiother Oncol 1994;33:204–8.
14. Bosset J, Mantion G, Gillet M, et al. Primary carcinoma of the gallbladder: adjuvant postoperative external irradiation. Cancer 1989;64:1843–7.
15. Buskirk SJ, Gunderson LL, Adson MA, et al. Analysis of failure following curative irradiation of gallbladder and extrahepatic bile duct carcinoma. Int J Radiat Oncol Biol Phys 1984;10:2013–23.
16. Kraybill W, Lee H, Picus J, et al. Multidisciplinary treatment of biliary tract cancers. J Surg Oncol 1994;55:239–45.
17. Todoroki T, Iwasaki Y, Orii K, et al. Resection combined with intraoperative radiation therapy (IORT) for stage IV (TNM) gallbladder carcinoma. World J Surg 1991;15:357–66.

# CHAPTER 48

## BILE DUCT CARCINOMAS

## NATURAL HISTORY, DIAGNOSIS, AND STAGING

• Charles M. Haskell

In the eighth and ninth revisions of the International Classification of Disease, intrahepatic biliary cancer has been classified with cancer of the liver, whereas the extrahepatic biliary system has been subclassified into three groups: gallbladder cancer, extrahepatic biliary cancer, and cancer of the ampulla of Vater. These distinctions have proved useful in identifying the unique characteristics of carcinomas of the gallbladder and ampulla of Vater. However, arbitrary distinctions between the intrahepatic and extrahepatic biliary system make less sense because these tumors share important histologic and epidemiologic features.

Tumors of the bile ducts are commonly known as *cholangiocarcinomas*. The term *cholangiocarcinoma* was initially intended for primary tumors of the intrahepatic biliary system[1]; however, the term has more recently been extended to include both the intrahepatic and extrahepatic biliary systems.[2] Perihilar tumors at the bifurcation of the hepatic duct have also been called *Klatskin's tumors* based on Klatskin's

description of this entity in 1965.[3] More recently, perihilar bile duct tumors have been further classified by Bismuth and colleagues into four types.[4] Type I includes tumors below the confluence of the left and right hepatic ducts. Type II includes tumors reaching the confluence. Type III includes tumors that occlude the common hepatic duct and either the right (IIIa) or left (IIIb) hepatic ducts. Type IV includes tumors that are multicentric or involve the confluence and both the right and left hepatic ducts. These distinctions and anatomic relationships are demonstrated in Figure 48–1.

This section reviews the natural history and treatment of intrahepatic and extrahepatic cholangiocarcinomas, exclusive of cancer of the gallbladder and ampulla of Vater. Unusual tumors, such as sarcomas and lymphomas, are not discussed.

### EPIDEMIOLOGY AND ETIOLOGY

**Incidence and Mortality Rates.** The annual incidence of bile duct cancer in the United States is 1.7 cases per

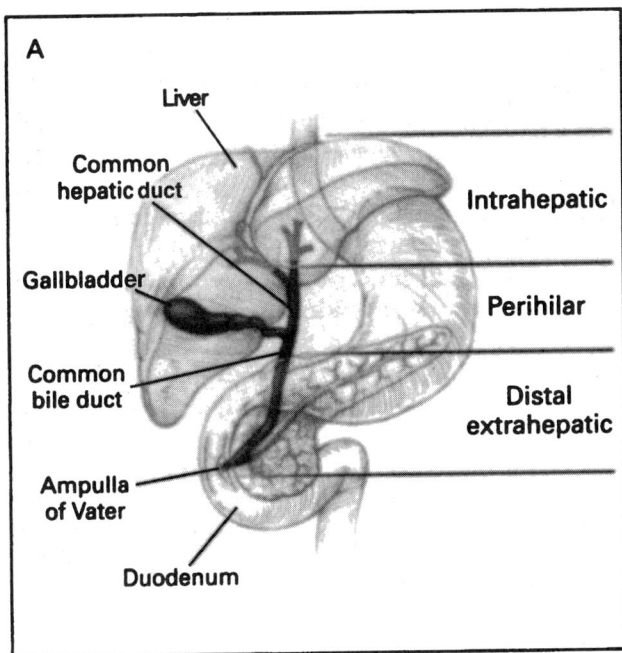

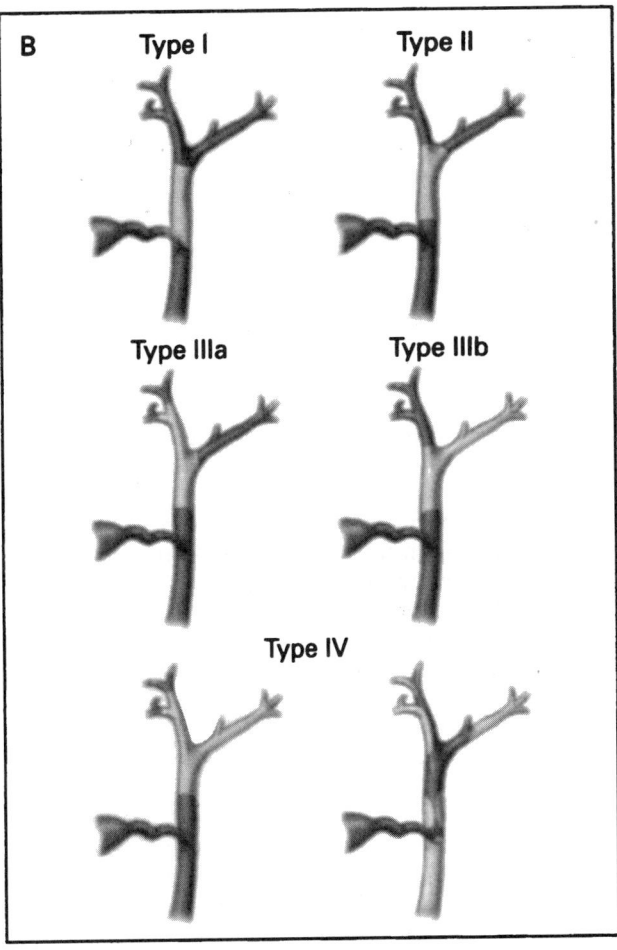

**Figure 48–1.** Classification of cancers of the human biliary tract. *A,* The overall classification of biliary tract cancers. *B,* The Bismuth classification of perihilar cholangiocarcinomas. Light areas represent tumor, whereas the darker areas are the normal biliary tree. (From De Groen PC, Gores GJ, LaRusso NF, et al. Medical Progress: biliary tract cancers. N Engl J Med 1999;341:1369.)

100,000, of which 35% are intrahepatic and 75% are extrahepatic in location.[5] The extrahepatic sites include those in the perihilar area, the distal extrahepatic area, and the ampulla of Vater (which is discussed separately in Chapter 49). The annual mortality rates in the United States for intrahepatic and extrahepatic bile duct cancers are 0.6 and 0.5 deaths per 100,000 population, respectively. The 5-year survival rates for these two groups are 2.8% for intrahepatic tumors and 17% for extrahepatic bile duct cancers. The frequency of bile duct neoplasms increases with advancing age. Most patients with bile duct cancers are in the sixth, seventh, or eighth decade of life.[6] Bile duct cancer is more common in men than in women. The comparative incidence rates for intrahepatic bile duct cancer are 0.8 and 0.5 per 100,000 for men and women, respectively, whereas the comparable figures for men and women for extrahepatic bile duct cancer are 1.3 and 0.9 cases per 100,000 population, respectively.

**Risk Factors.** Although the cause of bile duct carcinoma remains unknown, many authors have speculated about the importance of gallstones as a possible causative factor. However, the association of gallstones with bile duct cancer is less strong than it is with carcinoma of the gallbladder. For example, Jones[7] reported gallstones coexisting with gallbladder carcinoma in 65 to 88% of patients in the series he reviewed, whereas Stewart and associates[8] reported only a 20% incidence of gallstones in patients with bile duct carcinoma. In the 416 cases of bile duct cancer collected by

Sako and colleagues,[9] 161, or 39%, had stones either in the gallbladder or in the bile ducts. Of 103 patients reported by Ross and associates,[10] 30% were known to have had gallstones. Support for a relationship between gallstones and bile duct cancer comes from a Swedish study that found that the risk of biliary cancer significantly decreased beyond 10 years of cholecystectomy.[11]

Bile duct carcinoma has been associated with a history of primary sclerosing cholangitis, with a lifetime risk of about 10% for such patients.[12, 13] Bile duct carcinoma has also been associated with ulcerative colitis[14]; infection with *Clonorchis sinensis*[15]; congenital anomalies such as polycystic disease or congenital hepatic fibrosis, which may slow the flow of bile[16]; and the conversion of environmental agents commonly detoxified in the liver—such as bile acids and deoxycholic acid—to form carcinogens.[16] Although it has not been confirmed, it seems likely that an inflammatory reaction in the duct wall, when combined with the presence of bile, may create an appropriate environment for the development of a malignant tumor.

**Molecular Pathogenesis.** Little is known about the molecular pathogenesis of biliary cancer. Limited studies suggest that the pathogenesis of these tumors is similar to that of other gastrointestinal malignancies. Numerous studies have found mutations of the K-*ras* oncogene in patients with biliary cancer.[17, 18] Other oncogene mutations have been reported for *c-myc*, *c-neu*, Her-2/*neu*, and *c-met*. Mutations in the tumor-suppressor genes p53 and *bcl*-2 have also been reported. Further studies are needed to clarify the importance of these findings.

## PATHOLOGY

Cholangiocarcinomas of the bile ducts can be divided into three types: (1) local or nodular, (2) diffuse, and (3) papillary. Local tumors are approximately 2 cm in diameter and usually consist of an annular, constricting, grayish white lesion. The duct is generally distended above the tumor and collapsed distal to it. Diffuse growths produce extensive thickening of the entire duct, with resultant constriction of the lumen. The duct is often converted to a firm, rigid tube that can easily be confused with sclerosing cholangitis or a benign stricture.[16] A single, prominent tumor mass may not be present.

Depending on its primary site and size, any tumor of this type may extend from the hilus into the liver parenchyma. The diffuse tumor, without a specific tumor nodule but generalized, dense, fibrotic thickening of the duct wall, may be particularly confusing and can make a biopsy of the tumor difficult.[19] The papillary tumor that projects into the lumen of the duct is usually readily identified when the thickened duct is opened. Such a tumor frequently involves multiple areas of the duct mucosa and may be extensive. Rarely, combined hepatocellular-cholangiocarcinomas can occur as well.[20]

On histologic examination, tumors of the bile ducts are almost always found to be various types of adenocarcinoma, which are broadly classified here as *cholangiocarcinomas.* The histologic subtype generally correlates with the gross characteristics of the tumor, ranging from poorly differentiated to well differentiated. The diffusely fibrotic tumor shows a dense sclerotic fibrotic adenocarcinoma, and the grossly nodular tumor is identifiable as papillary adenocarcinoma.

## CLINICAL FEATURES AND DIAGNOSIS

The principal signs and symptoms are those of obstructive jaundice, but unfortunately there are no unique clinical features that specifically identify a malignant bile duct tumor. Sako and coworkers[9] described jaundice in 90% of their patients, usually occurring within 4 months before admission and becoming progressively more severe. Occasionally, patients develop mild postprandial epigastric discomfort, which occurs approximately 2 months before the onset of jaundice. Pain is present in about one third of patients and is the second most noticed symptom. Severe, persistent pruritus is often the most distressing symptom for the patient. The combination of anorexia and weight loss generally appears as the disease progresses. Other signs and symptoms include clay-colored stools, weakness, fever, diarrhea, and chills.

Laboratory studies generally reveal elevated alkaline phosphatase and serum bilirubin levels, anemia, and leukocytosis. Abdominal ultrasonography often discloses dilated bile ducts, and it is usually best to perform this test as the first step in pursuing a radiologic diagnosis.[21, 22] When the obstruction is at or above the common hepatic duct, or when a mass is seen, the sonographic findings can be considered highly suggestive of carcinoma. Sonography may also provide information about the resectability of the lesion, although the sensitivity of sonography for this purpose is only about 19%.[22]

In most cases, computed tomographic scanning is performed to help localize the obstructive lesion and to further evaluate the status of the liver and other intra-abdominal organs for signs of metastatic disease. Magnetic resonance cholangiopancreatography is also a useful test for defining the vascular architecture and the anatomy of the hepatobiliary tree. In many cases, the views of the vasculature are adequate to replace angiography as a preoperative test to rule out vascular invasion or encasement by tumor.

The next diagnostic test to be used for patients with obstructive jaundice is cholangiography. In the face of a markedly elevated serum bilirubin level, the usual oral and intravenous cholangiograms are of no value, so percutaneous transhepatic cholangiography is performed to determine the intrabiliary extent of the disease and to establish the diagnosis.[23] At the University of California, Los Angeles, this test has been successful in demonstrating the intrahepatic biliary system in 100% of patients whose ducts were obstructed and in 60% of patients with nonobstructed intrahepatic biliary systems.[24] The methodology of this procedure has been well described.[23, 25, 26]

Endoscopic retrograde choledochopancreatography is a diagnostic technique that assists in establishing a definitive diagnosis in certain cases of obstructive jaundice. It is possible for skilled endoscopists to cannulate the papilla of Vater and visualize radiographically the bile ducts or the pancreatic duct in 75 to 95% of cases. In a series of 146 patients, duodenoscopy was successfully performed in 144 patients, the papilla of Vater was located in 140 patients, and the ampulla was cannulated in 114 patients. The definitive diagnosis was established in 109 patients, and useful information was obtained in an additional 11 patients.[27] We feel that the use of endoscopic retrograde choledochopancreatography is indicated when the cause of jaundice cannot be determined. If cannulation of the papilla is unsuccessful and the ductal system cannot be adequately visualized, percutaneous transhepatic cholangiography is performed.[28]

Biliary tumors metastasize to the liver and to regional lymph nodes in the hepatoduodenal ligament. Kuwayti and colleagues[29] reported metastases or direct spread in 71.4% of their 63 cases. Extension or metastases to the liver, lymph nodes, pancreas, gastrohepatic lymph, or mediastinum occurred in about 50% of the cases reported by Stewart and coworkers.[8] Frequent invasion of the regional nerve plexus has also been noted. Because of the high frequency of hepatic or regional nodal involvement by this tumor, an abdominal computed tomographic scan is usually indicated before operative intervention to help rule out hepatic involvement. The sensitivity of a computed tomographic scan in detecting unresectable tumor has been reported to be about 44%, with a specificity of 78%.[22] Similarly, in another series,[30] computed tomographic–diagnosed liver metastases and a tumor mass in 53 and 23% of patients, respectively.

The value of tumor markers in the diagnosis of this disease is uncertain, except in certain high-risk settings. For patients with primary sclerosing cholangitis with a high risk of developing cholangiocarcinoma, the CA 19-9 test appears to be useful in screening and early diagnosis. A serum CA

*Table 48–1.* **TNM Staging for Primary Neoplasms of the Extrahepatic Bile Ducts**

*Primary Tumor (T)*

| | |
|---|---|
| TX | Primary tumor cannot be assessed |
| T0 | No evidence of primary tumor |
| Tis | Carcinoma in situ |
| T1 | Tumor invades subepithelial connective tissue or fibromuscular layer |
| T1a | Tumor invades subepithelial connective tissue |
| T1b | Tumor invades fibromuscular layer |
| T2 | Tumor invades perifibromuscular connective tissue |
| T3 | Tumor invades adjacent structures: liver, pancreas, duodenum, gallbladder, colon, stomach |

*Regional Lymph Nodes (N)*

| | |
|---|---|
| NX | Regional lymph nodes cannot be assessed |
| N0 | No regional lymph node metastasis |
| N1 | Metastasis in cystic duct, pericholedochal and/or hilar lymph nodes (i.e., in the hepatoduodenal ligament) |
| N2 | Metastasis in peripancreatic (head only), periduodenal, periportal, celiac, and/or superior mesenteric and/or posterior pancreaticoduodenal lymph nodes |

*Distant Metastasis (M)*

| | |
|---|---|
| MX | Distant metastasis cannot be assessed |
| M0 | No distant metastasis |
| M1 | Distant metastasis |

*Stage Grouping*

| | | | |
|---|---|---|---|
| Stage 0 | Tis | N0 | M0 |
| Stage I | T1 | N0 | M0 |
| Stage II | T2 | N0 | M0 |
| Stage III | T1 | N1 | M0 |
| | T1 | N2 | M0 |
| | T2 | N1 | M0 |
| | T2 | N2 | M0 |
| Stage IVA | T3 | Any N | M0 |
| Stage IVB | Any T | Any N | M1 |

Used with the permission of the American Joint Committee on Cancer (AJCC®), Chicago, Illinois. The original source for this material is the AJCC® Cancer Staging Manual, 5th edition (1997) published by Lippincott-Raven Publishers, Philadelphia, Pennsylvania.

19-9 level greater than 100 U/ml (normal < 40 U/ml) has been reported to have a sensitivity of 89% and a specificity of 86% for the detection of cholangiocarcinoma in such patients.[31] The CA 19-9 test is also useful in following patients after definitive treatment of cholangiocarcinoma.

Other tumor markers are of uncertain or no value in the management of cholangiocarcinoma. One study has suggested that serum *N*-acetyl-β-hexosaminidase is more useful in differentiating between malignant and benign extrahepatic biliary obstruction than is carcinoembryonic antigen.[32] There has been no confirmation of this finding as yet, however, so the value of this or any other test in making this differentiation is uncertain.

## STAGING AND PROGNOSIS

The TNM staging system for intrahepatic bile duct tumors is given in Table 46–1 in the chapter on hepatocellular carcinoma. The TNM staging system for extrahepatic biliary tumors is given in Table 48–1.[33]

The 5-year survival rate for resectable carcinomas of the common bile duct is about 20%, but most patients have unresectable disease.[34] The median survival time for patients with unresectable disease is poor; in a series from the Mayo Clinic it was 5 months.[35] A more detailed assessment of prognosis is given in the following section on surgery.

## REFERENCES

1. Albores-Saavedra J, Henson DE, Sobin LH. Histological typing of tumours of the gallbladder and extrahepatic bile ducts. 2nd ed. Berlin: Springer-Verlag, 1991.
2. De Groen PC, Gores GJ, LaRusso NF, et al. Biliary tract cancers (medical progress). N Engl J Med 1999;341:1368–78.
3. Klatskin G. Adenocarcinoma of the hepatic duct at its bifurcation within the porta hepatis: an unusual tumor with distinctive clinical and pathological features. Am J Med 1965;38:241–56.
4. Bismuth H, Nakache R, Diamond T. Management strategies in resection for hilar cholangiocarcinoma. Ann Surg 1992;215:31–8.
5. SEER Cancer Statistics Review 1973–1996. (See http://www-seer.ims.-nci.nih.gov.)
6. Doll R. Cancer incidence in five continents. New York: Springer-Verlag, 1966.
7. Jones CJ. Carcinoma of the gallbladder—a clinical and pathologic analysis of fifty cases. Ann Surg 1950;132:110–20.
8. Stewart HL, Lieberber MM, Morgan DR. Carcinoma of the extrahepatic bile ducts. Arch Surg 1940;41:662–713.
9. Sako S, Seitzinger GL, Garside E. Carcinoma of the extrahepatic ducts—a review of the literature and report of 6 cases. Surgery 1957;41:416–37.
10. Ross AP, Braasch JW, Warren KW. Carcinoma of the proximal bile ducts. Surg Gynecol Obstet 1973;136:923–8.
11. Ekbom A, Hsieh CC, Yuen J, et al: Risk of extrahepatic bile duct cancer after cholecystectomy. Lancet 1993;342:1262–5.
12. Kornfeld D, Ekbom A, Ihre T. Survival and risk of cholangiocarcinoma in patients with primary sclerosing cholangitis: a population-based study. Scand J Gastroenterol 1997;32:1042–5.
13. Broome U, Olsson R, Loof L, et al. Natural history and prognostic factors in 305 Swedish patients with primary sclerosing cholangitis. Gut 1996;38:610–5.
14. Roberts-Thompson IC, Strickland RG, Mackay IR. Bile duct carcinoma in chronic ulcerative colitis. Aust N Z J Med 1973;3:264–7.
15. Belamaric J. Intrahepatic bile duct carcinoma and *C. sinensis* infection in Hong Kong. Cancer 1973;31:468–73.
16. Gallagher PJ, Millis RR, Mitchinson MJ. Congenital dilatation of the intrahepatic bile ducts with cholangiocarcinoma. J Clin Pathol 1972;25:804–8.
17. Imai M, Hoshi T, Ogawa K. K-*ras* codon 12 mutations in biliary tract tumors detected by polymerase chain reaction denaturing gradient gel electrophoresis. Cancer 1994;73:2727–33.
18. Tada M, Omata M, Ohto M. High incidence of *ras* gene mutation in intrahepatic cholangiocarcinoma. Cancer 1992;69:1115–8.
19. Altemeier WA, Gall EA, Zinniger MM, Hoxworth PI. Sclerosing carcinoma of the major intrahepatic bile ducts. Arch Surg 1957;75:450–60.
20. Goodman ZD, Ishak KG, Langloss JM, et al. Combined hepatocellular-cholangiocarcinoma: a histologic and immunohistochemical study. Cancer 1985;55:124–35.
21. Richter JM, Silverstein MD, Schapiro R. Suspected obstructive jaundice: a decision analysis of diagnostic strategies. Ann Intern Med 1983;99:46–51.
22. Nesbit GM, Johnson CD, James EM, et al. Cholangiocarcinoma: diagnosis and evaluation of resectability by CT and sonography as procedures complementary to cholangiography. AJR Am J Roentgenol 1988;151:933–8.
23. Mueller PR, vanSonnenberg E, Simeone JF. Fine-needle transhepatic cholangiography: indications and usefulness. Ann Intern Med 1982;97:567–72.
24. Longmire WP Jr. Tumors of the extrahepatic biliary radicals. Curr Probl Cancer 1976;1:1–45.
25. Okuda K, Tanikawa K, Emura T, et al. Nonsurgical, percutaneous transhepatic cholangiography—diagnostic significance in medical problems of the liver. Am J Dig Dis 1974;19:21–36.
26. Redeker AG, Karvountzis GG, Richman RH, Horisawa M. Percutane-

ous transhepatic cholangiography: an improved technique. JAMA 1975;231:386–7.

27. Blumgart LH. Endoscopy of the upper gastrointestinal tract. In: Longmire WP Jr, ed. Advances in Surgery. Vol 9. Chicago, Year Book Medical, 1975:97–138.

28. Takagi K, Ikeda S, Nakagawa Y, et al. Retrograde pancreatography and cholangiography by fiber duodenoscope. Gastroenterology 1970;59:445–52.

29. Kuwayti K, Baggenstoss AH, Stauffer MH, Priestley JT. Carcinoma of the major intrahepatic and the extrahepatic bile ducts exclusive of the papilla of Vater. Surg Gynecol Obstet 1957;104:357–66.

30. Mittal B, Deutsch M, Iwatsuki S. Primary cancers of extrahepatic biliary passages. Int J Radiat Oncol Biol Phys 1985;11:849–54.

31. Nichols JC, Gores GJ, LaRusso NF, et al. Diagnostic role of serum CA 19-9 for cholangiocarcinoma in patients with primary sclerosing cholangitis. Mayo Clin Proc 1993;68:874–9.

32. Scapa E, Thomas P, Loewenstein MS, Zamcheck N. Serum beta-*N*-acetyl hexosaminidase (beta-NAH) as a discriminant between malignant and benign extrahepatic biliary obstruction: comparison with carcinoembryonic antigen (CEA). Eur J Cancer Clin Oncol 1985;21:1037–42.

33. Fleming ID, Cooper JS, Henson DE, et al. AJCC Cancer Staging Manual. 5th ed. Philadelphia: Lippincott-Raven, 1997:101–6.

34. Bismuth H, Malt RA. Current concepts in cancer: carcinoma of the biliary tract. N Engl J Med 1979;301:704–6.

35. Moertel CG. Advanced gastrointestinal cancer. New York, Harper & Row, 1969:5.

# SURGERY

● Kenneth P. Ramming

The hope for cure and significant palliation of bile duct cancer has traditionally rested in the hands of the surgeon. At the time of surgery, the first problem is to locate the site of obstruction and identify the true nature of the lesion.

The bile duct is conventionally divided into three general areas: (1) the upper region, including the left and right hepatic ducts, the confluence, and the common hepatic duct; (2) the common duct from the region of the cystic duct to the pancreas; and (3) the intrapancreatic portion of the common duct not included in the papilla of Vater. When the tumor has been visualized and the biopsy specimen procured, the extent of the tumor must be assessed. Endoscopic examination at the time of surgery using choledochoscopy, as reported by Tompkins and colleagues,[1] may demonstrate widely scattered multicentric intraductal tumor growths in patients whose disease otherwise might be considered resectable.

Less than 20% of upper lesions are resectable. The most frequently performed procedure is dilation at the site of obstruction and intubation of the ducts above and below the tumor, usually with a T-tube. Terblanche and associates[2] reported their experience with 21 cases of carcinoma in the upper-third region and describe their adaptation of the U-tube technique for the palliation of malignant biliary obstruction. With the aid of a dilator, one end of the U-tube is passed through the tumor into the right or left hepatic ductal system and is forced through the liver parenchyma, the surface of the liver, and a stab wound in the anterior abdominal wall. The common bile duct is tailored around the middle of the tube, and then the other end of the tube is also brought to the outside through the abdominal wall.

A modification of this technique is the J-tube, in which one end is forced through the liver parenchyma and the right flank, and the other end lies internally in the duodenum in an attempt to facilitate internal biliary drainage.

Tumors of the middle region of the ductal system are treated, when possible, by excision and duct-enteric biliary bypass. Partial hepatic resection and cholangiojejunostomy might also be necessary.

Tumors that are located in the intrapancreatic portion of the common ducts are generally grouped with the periampullary tumors. When possible, these tumors are resected by pancreaticoduodenectomy. An excellent illustrated review of surgery of the hepatic ducts has been assembled by Longmire,[3] including significant contributions of other surgeons in this field.[4–9] More recent reviews of this topic are also available.[10]

Andersson and coworkers[11] have reported a series of 76 patients with cancer of the extrahepatic bile ducts. In lesions located above the ampulla of Vater, survival time was 6.8 months after palliative bypass, as compared with a median of 23 months after resection. Iwasaki and colleagues[12] operated on 14 patients with carcinoma of the extrahepatic biliary system and performed curative resection on 9 of them; 6 of these patients were still alive after a follow-up of 5 to 25 months.

As an alternative to surgical decompression of the biliary tree in patients with obvious unresectable or metastatic disease, several groups have explored the use of nonsurgical decompression.[13–16] These new and still-evolving techniques include endoscopic papillotomy, biliary stenting, balloon dilation, endoprosthesis insertion, and various T-tube manipulations.[16] Palliation in patients with biliary tract neoplasms may be accomplished with minimal morbidity and with an expected duration of about 8 to 12 months.[15] This evolving area deserves careful consideration by those involved in the primary management of these patients. Indeed, increasing numbers of authorities are advocating nonsurgical management of most of these patients.[17] An innovative extension of this approach to therapy has been the use of a laser via percutaneous transhepatic choledochoscopy.[18]

## REFERENCES

1. Tompkins RK, Johnson J, Storm FK, Longmire WP Jr. Operative endoscopy in the management of biliary tract neoplasms. Am J Surg 1976;132:174–82.

2. Terblanche J, Saunders SJ, Louw JH. Prolonged palliation in carcinoma of the man hepatic duct junction. Surgery 1972;71:720–31.

3. Longmire WP Jr. Tumors of the extrahepatic biliary radicals. Curr Probl Cancer 1976;1:1–45.

4. Altemeier WA, Gall EA, Zinniger MM, Hoxworth PI. Sclerosing carcinoma of the major intrahepatic bile ducts. Arch Surg 1957;75:450–60.

5. Molnar W, Stockum AE. Relief of obstructive jaundice through percuta-

neous transhepatic catheter—a new therapeutic method. Am J Roent-genol Radium Ther Nucl Med 1974;122:356–67.

6. Whelton MJ, Petrelli M, George P, et al. Carcinoma at the junction of the main hepatic ducts. Q J Med 1969;38:211–30.

7. Warren KW, Mountain JC, Lloyd-Jones W. Malignant tumours of the bile ducts. Br J Surg 1972;59:501–5.

8. Ingis DA, Farmer RG. Adenocarcinoma of the bile ducts: relationship of anatomic location to clinical features. Am J Dig Dis 1975;20:253–61.

9. Longmire WP Jr, McArthur MS, Bastounis EA, Hiatt J. Carcinoma of the extrahepatic biliary tract. Ann Surg 1973;178:333–45.

10. Ottow RT, August DA, Sugarbaker PH. Treatment of proximal biliary tract carcinoma: an overview of techniques and results. Surgery 1985;97:251–62.

11. Andersson A, Bergdahl L, van der Linden W. Malignant tumors of the extrahepatic bile ducts. Surgery 1977;81:198–202.

12. Iwasaki Y, Ohto M, Todoroki T, et al. Treatment of carcinoma of the biliary system. Surg Gynecol Obstet 1977;144:219–24.

13. Pereiras RV Jr, Rheingold OJ, Huston D, et al. Relief of malignant obstructive jaundice by percutaneous insertion of a permanent prosthe-sis in the biliary tree. Ann Intern Med 1978;89(Pt 1):589–93.

14. Huguet C, Nordlinger B, Ibanez L, et al. Palliative treatment of carci-noma of the hepatic duct junction: intra-hepatic derivation or trans-tumoral intubation? Nouv Presse Med 1982;11:1467–70. author's trans-lation.

15. MacCarty RL. Nonsurgical management of obstructive jaundice in the patient with advanced cancer. JAMA 1980;244:1976–8.

16. Kozarek RA, Sanowski RA. Nonsurgical management of extrahepatic obstructive jaundice. Ann Intern Med 1982;96:743–5.

17. Summerfield JA. Biliary obstruction is best managed by endoscopists. Gut 1988;29:741–5.

18. Kubota Y, Seki T, Nakano T, et al. A case of bile duct cancer treated by laser via percutaneous transhepatic choledochoscopy. Hepatogas-troenterology 1988;35:213–4.

······································

# RADIATION THERAPY

• Luu M. Tran

Surgery remains the primary treatment for bile duct carci-noma. However, at the time of diagnosis, more than 80% of the tumors are unresectable because of their proximity to major blood vessels and also frequently because of liver or lymph node invasion.[1] Only 20% of patients are eligible for curative resection, and mortality rates with this treatment are high. Because achieving complete resection with negative surgical margins is unusual, and with local recurrence rates being as high as 50 to 80%, radiation therapy (RT) has been used in the past as an adjuvant treatment following curative resection or else as primary treatment for unresectable tu-mors.[2, 3]

With these conventional techniques, RT has played only a minor role in the management of hepatobiliary cancer, mainly because of the liver's low tolerance to ionizing radia-tion. The dose is usually not greater than 30 Gy if the whole liver is irradiated using a standard fractionation scheme. This dosage is not effective in preventing recurrent disease following resection and has been used mainly for palliation of painful metastatic liver lesions. To safely augment the action of radiation to the hepatic lesions, newer modalities have been used such as (1) concurrent fluoropyrimidine-based chemotherapy as radiation sensitizer, (2) altered frac-tionation with multiple small-dose daily fractions, and (3) three-dimensional conformal treatment (3D-CRT) to focal hepatic tumors.

## RADIATION TECHNIQUES

The radiation field should encompass the tumor bed as well as the regional lymphatic drainage, such as the porta hepatis and celiac axis. Field borders are defined by CT scan, surgi-cal clips placed at laparotomy, and angiographic and endo-scopic retrograde cholangiopancreatography (ERCP) films. Patients should be treated with multiple and shrinking-field techniques using high-energy photons. When available, 3D-CRT should be used to minimize the dose to the liver, kidneys, small bowel, and spinal cord. The tumor volume is generally treated with a dose ranging from 50 to 54 Gy at 1.8 Gy a day, 5 days per week.

## ADJUVANT RADIATION THERAPY

High local-regional recurrence rates following an apparently curative resection have prompted widespread efforts to de-velop an effective treatment for cholangiocarcinoma.

Given the rarity of the tumor, randomized comparisons between surgery and RT are not practical. Since the 1980s, there have been several conflicting reports regarding the use of adjuvant RT following resection.[4–11] The European Organization for Research and Treatment of Cancer (EORTC)[5] reported the results of 55 patients with biliary tract carcinoma treated either with surgery alone (17 pa-tients) or with postoperative radiation because of residual disease (38 patients). The median survival of the adjuvant group was better than the surgery-alone group (19 months vs. 8 months, respectively). The overall 3-year survival rate was 31% in the irradiated group as compared with 10% in the surgery-alone group ($p = 0.0005$). In patients having residual disease after resection, Schoenthaler and colleagues[9] reported a median survival of 21 months with adjuvant radiation and 11 months without radiation ($p = 0.01$). Con-versely, Pitt and associates[6] from Johns Hopkins showed no survival advantage when postoperative RT was added after curative resection in 50 patients with localized perihilar cholangiocarcinoma.

The use of fluorouracil-based chemotherapy combined with RT has been limited. Willett and colleagues[7] from Massachusetts General Hospital reported a slight improve-ment in survival and local control in the adjuvant radia-tion–5-fluorouracil (5-FU) group over the surgery-alone group for patients with ampullary cancer. However, Schoen-thaler and colleagues[9] and Flickinger and associates[11] re-ported no survival advantage with the addition of chemother-apy. More recently, the University of St. Louis[12] has launched a phase II trial of continuous infusion of 5-FU with 3D-CRT in the adjuvant treatment of 34 patients with pancreatic, ampullary, and biliary cancers. The treatment was well tolerated, and 31 patients were able to complete all planned treatment. To date, it appears that adding chemotherapy to radiation has no survival benefit in the adjuvant setting.

## PRIMARY RADIATION WITH OR WITHOUT CHEMOTHERAPY

Several studies since the late 1980s have supported the usefulness of RT in the management of unresectable biliary duct carcinoma.[13–17] Conventional radiation techniques with external-beam RT (EBRT) have rarely permitted long-term survival, and median survival has ranged from 10 to 16 months. However, RT can provide temporary palliation and occasionally long-term survival in unresectable biliary duct tumors.

Based on the encouraging results of combined chemoradiation in treating other gastrointestinal tract tumors, several institutions have used this approach in the management of locally unresectable or recurrent cancers of the bile duct. Minsky and associates[14] from Memorial Sloan-Kettering hospital reported on 12 patients with extrahepatic biliary carcinoma treated with combined-modality therapy. All received 50 Gy to the tumor bed and nodal area followed by a 1.5 Gy boost with brachytherapy in 10 patients. Chemotherapy with 5-FU and mitomycin C was given concurrently with RT and followed by maintenance treatment. The median survival was 10 months, and the overall 4-year actuarial survival was 36%. The local recurrence was 50%.

Other studies support the combined-modality approach. Weiss and colleagues[18] from Fox Chase Cancer Center observed a survival benefit in patients with gross disease treated with RT plus 5-FU compared with RT alone. McMasters and colleagues[19] reported a study with 91 patients. The median survival was 11 months for 51 patients with unresectable disease and 22 months for the 40 resected cases. For the latter, 9 patients received preoperative chemoradiation therapy and achieved 100% negative surgical margins, as opposed to 54% for those without neoadjuvant treatment.

Encouraging results have been reported by investigators from the University of Michigan,[20] who used intra-arterial hepatic infusion of fluorodeoxyuridine (FdUrd) and 3D-CRT in 11 patients with cholangiocarcinoma and 11 patients with hepatoma. RT consisted of CRT (1.5 to 1.65 Gy per fraction, twice a day) for a total dose of 48 to 66 Gy directly to the tumors and given concurrently with hepatic infusion chemotherapy. Although only 11 patients were able to be evaluated, 10 had objective responses, and the overall freedom from hepatic progression at 2 years was about 50%. As in their earlier reports,[21] the investigators did not see late hepatic complications. These findings of the efficacy of combined modalities are encouraging in view of the overwhelmingly dismal outcome of the disease when using conventional techniques.

Intraluminal transcatheter brachytherapy has been used for bile duct carcinoma, usually in combination with EBRT.[16, 17, 22, 23] Historically, the efficacy of this approach was shown through low dose rate treatment via percutaneous transhepatic drainage tube or ERCP. Montemaggi and co-workers[24] reported an experience of 12 Italian patients (5 had extrahepatic duct carcinoma and 7 had pancreatic head carcinoma) that resulted in 14 months' median survival for bile duct cancer patients. Alden and Mohiuddin[23] from Thomas Jefferson University Hospital reported the treatment results of 24 patients treated with a combined approach: EBRT (46 Gy), brachytherapy implant (25 Gy at 1 cm) and 5-FU, doxorubicin, and mitomycin C. Patients treated with a radiation dose to greater than 55 Gy attained a 2-year survival of 48% as compared with 17% for the no-radiation group. High-dose-rate brachytherapy has gained popularity, prompting physicians to use this new technology to deal with biliary tract tumors. At New York Hospital,[25] a median survival rate of 19 months was reported. This method avoids patient hospitalization and theoretically can minimize normal tissue damage by tailoring the dose distribution tightly around the tumor using a sophisticated treatment planning system (similar to the rationale behind 3D-CRT).

Another method of increasing the radiation dose is to use "altered" fractionation with multiple small-dose fractions per day (as opposed to the conventional fractionation scheme of once-a-day treatment with 1.8 to 2.0 Gy per fraction). Stillwagon and associates[26] reported a Radiation Therapy Oncology Group (RTOG) trial of 194 patients with hepatocellular cancers, the majority (135) with extrahepatic metastasis. All patients were treated with either 21 Gy in 3-Gy fractions once a day or 24 Gy in 1.2-Gy fractions twice a day. The RT was combined with intravenous 5-FU and doxorubicin, followed a month later by radiolabeled antibody. Median survival was only 5 months and response rate was only 21%. Hyperfractionation did not demonstrate a significant improvement over the standard once-a-day treatment.

Robertson and colleagues[20] reported the results of six cases of diffuse hepatocellular carcinoma treated with 1.5 Gy per fraction twice a day to a total of 36 Gy to the whole liver, using conformal treatment technique and concomitant intra-arterial hepatic infusion FdUrd. There was only one objective response. Severe or moderately acute toxicity occurred in 5 of 6 patients. Results, however, were more encouraging for the 11 patients with focal hepatocellular carcinoma for whom the radiation field was restricted to the involved portion of the liver. They further updated the results of 3D-CRT,[20] in which ultrahigh doses ($\geq 70$ Gy) were delivered to the hepatic tumors precisely. There was no significant toxicity, and the median survival of patients with primary hepatobiliary cancer was 19 months, similar to results for those treated with surgical resection. These findings suggested that 3D-CRT and hepatic infusion FdUrd could produce a high, durable response rate.

The anatomic relation of the liver to critical structures such as the pancreas, kidneys, spinal cord, and liver prohibits the delivery of a tumoricidal dose of radiation. This limitation has prompted the use of different techniques, such as intraoperative electron-beam irradiation (IORT). IORT combined with RT has produced good palliation with occasional long-term survival in several series.[27–33] The investigators from Japan[27, 28, 30, 31] demonstrated the potential of IORT in bile duct carcinoma. Using single doses of 25 to 40 Gy IORT, 16 (27%) of 59 patients with unresectable cholangiocarcinoma were reported to be alive, the longest for 18 months.

Todoroki and colleagues[28] observed a 1-year survival of 63% in 11 patients with advanced cholangiocarcinoma treated with an IORT dose of 25 to 30 Gy. Eight of 11 patients who initially presented with complete obstruction achieved recanalization of the bile duct. In the United States, the RTOG[32] conducted a phase I/II trial of EBRT with IORT in the treatment of cholangiocarcinoma. Local recurrence was seen in only 1 of 8 patients with a median follow-up of 10.5 months. Buskirk and colleagues from the Mayo Clinic[33] observed local failure in 9 of 17 patients with advanced tumors treated by EBRT alone (45 to 60 Gy) with and without 5-FU, 3 of 10 patients treated with iridium 192 interstitial implant boost, and 2 of 6 patients who received IORT boost with curative intent.

In summary, patients with cholangiocarcinomas usually present with locally advanced disease, and surgical resection is rarely curative. RT, either as an adjuvant treatment or as primary therapy, may play a role in the management of this lethal disease.

# REFERENCES

1. Langer JC, Langer B, Taylor BR, et al. Carcinoma of the extrahepatic bile ducts: results of an aggressive approach. Surgery 1985;98:752–9.
2. Kopelson G, Galdabini J, Warshaw AL, Gunderson LL. Patterns of failure after curative surgery for extra-hepatic biliary tract carcinoma: implications for adjuvant therapy. Int J Radiat Oncol Biol Phys 1981;7:413–7.
3. Cameron JL, Pitt HA, Zinner MJ, et al. Management of proximal cholangiocarcinomas by surgical resection and radiotherapy. Am J Surg 1990;159:91–7 and 97–8.
4. Vaittinen E. Carcinoma of the gall bladder: a study of 390 cases diagnosed in Finland, 1953–1967. Ann Chir Gynaecol 1970;168:1–81.
5. Gonzalez Gonzalez D, Gerard JP, Maners AW, et al. Results of radiation therapy in carcinoma of the proximal bile duct (Klatskin tumor). Semin Liver Dis 1990;10:131–41.
6. Pitt HA, Nakeeb A, Abrams RA, et al. Perihilar cholangiocarcinoma: postoperative radiotherapy does not improve survival. Ann Surg 1995;221:788–97.
7. Willett CG, Warshaw AL, Convery K, Compton CC. Patterns of failure after pancreaticoduodenectomy for ampullary carcinoma. Surg Gynecol Obstet 1993;176:33–8.
8. Verbeek PC, Van Leeuwen DJ, Van Der Heyde MN, Gonzalez Gonzalez D. Does additive radiotherapy after hilar resection improve survival of cholangiocarcinoma? An analysis in sixty-four patients. Ann Chir 1991;45:350–4.
9. Schoenthaler R, Castro JR, Halberg FE, Phillips TL. Definitive postoperative irradiation of bile duct carcinoma with charged particles and/or photons. Int J Radiat Oncol Biol Phys 1993;27:75–82.
10. Schoenthaler R, Phillips T, Castro J, et al. Carcinoma of the extrahepatic bile ducts: the University of California at San Francisco experience. Ann Surg 1994;219:267–74.
11. Flickinger JC, Epstein AH, Iwatsuki S, et al. Radiation therapy for primary carcinoma of the extrahepatic biliary system: an analysis of 63 cases. Cancer 1991;68:289–94.
12. Picus J, Myerson R, Drebin J, et al. A phase II trial of continuous infusion (CI) 5-FU with 3D-CRT in the adjuvant treatment of pancreatic, ampullary, and biliary cancers. Proc ASCO 1998;17:266a.
13. Kopelson G, Harisiadis L, Tretter P, Chang CH. The role of radiation therapy in cancer of the extrahepatic biliary system: an analysis of 13 patients and a review of the literature of the effectiveness of surgery, chemotherapy, and radiotherapy. Int J Radiat Oncol Biol Phys 1977;2:883–94.
14. Minsky BD, Wessan MF, Armstrong JG, et al. Combined-modality therapy of extrahepatic biliary system cancer. Int J Radiat Oncol Biol Phys 1990;18:1157–63.
15. Mittal B, Duetsch M, Iwatsuki S. Primary cancers of extrahepatic biliary passages. Int J Radiat Oncol Biol Phys 1985;11:849–54.
16. Fields JN, Emami B. Carcinoma of the extrahepatic biliary system: results of primary and adjuvant radiotherapy. Int J Radiat Oncol Biol Phys 1987;13:331–8.
17. Fogel TD, Weissberg JB. The role of radiation therapy in carcinoma of the extrahepatic bile ducts. Int J Radiat Biol Oncol Phys 1984;10:2251–8.
18. Weiss M, Whittington R, Schulz D, et al. Carcinoma of the extrahepatic biliary system: results of primary therapy. Int J Radiat Oncol Biol Phys 1992;24:Suppl 1:213.
19. McMasters KM, Tuttle TM, Leach SD, et al. Neoadjuvant chemoradiation for extrahepatic cholangiocarcinoma. Am J Surg 1997;174:605–8.
20. Robertson JM, Lawrence T, Andrew J, et al. Long-term results of hepatic artery fluorodeoxyuridine and conformal radiation therapy for primary hepatobiliary cancers. In J Radiat Oncol Biol Phys 1997;37:325–30.
21. Robertson J, Lawrence T, Dworzanin L, et al. The treatment of primary hepatobiliary cancers with conformal radiation therapy and regional chemotherapy. J Clin Oncol 1993;11:1286–93.
22. Herskovic AM, Engler MJ, Noell KT. Radical radiotherapy for bile duct carcinoma. Endocuriether Hypertherm Oncol 1985;1:119.
23. Alden ME, Mohiuddin M. The impact of radiation dose in combined external beam and intraluminal Ir-192 brachytherapy for bile duct cancer. Int J Radiat Oncol Biol Phys 1994;28:945–51.
24. Montemaggi P, Costamagna G, Dobelbower R, et al. Intraluminal brachytherapy in the treatment of pancreas and bile duct carcinoma. Int J Radiat Oncol Biol Phys 1995;32:437–43.
25. Merimsky O, Nori D, Rogers D, et al. Conformal high dose rate percutaneous transhepatic intraluminal cholangio-irradiation for unresectable cholangiocarcinoma. Endocuriether Hyperther Oncol 1995;11:115.
26. Stillwagon GB, Order S, Guse C, et al. Prognostic factors in unresectable hepatocellular cancer: Radiation Oncology Group Study 83-01. Int J Radiat Oncol Biol Phys 1991;20:65–71.
27. Abe M, Takahashi M. Intraoperative radiotherapy: the Japanese experience. Int J Radiat Oncol Biol Phys 1981;7:863–8.
28. Todoroki T, Iwasaki Y, Okamua T, et al. Intraoperative radiotherapy for advanced carcinoma of the biliary system. Cancer 1980;46:2179–84.
29. Busse PM, Stone MD, Sheldon TA, et al. Intraoperative radiation therapy for biliary tract carcinoma: results of a 5-year experience. Surgery 1989;105:724–33.
30. Iwasaki Y, Todoroki T, Fukao K, et al. The role of intraoperative radiation therapy in the treatment of bile duct cancer. World J Surg 1988;12:91–8.
31. Abe M, Takahashi M, Yabumoto E, et al. Clinical experience with intraoperative radiotherapy of locally advanced cancers. Cancer 1980;45:40–8.
32. Wolkov HB, Graves GM, Won M, et al. Intraoperative radiation therapy of extrahepatic biliary carcinoma: a report of RTOG-8506. Am J Clin Oncol 1992;15:323–7.
33. Buskirk SJ, Gunderson LL, Adson MA, et al. Analysis of failure following curative irradiation of gallbladder and extrahepatic bile duct carcinoma. Int J Radiat Oncol Biol Phys 1984;10:2013–23.

·······································

# CHEMOTHERAPY

• Charles M. Haskell

## SINGLE-AGENT CHEMOTHERAPY

Although the majority of cytotoxic agents have not received an adequate trial in this group of tumors, the published experience thus far leaves little room for optimism. The response rates achieved with the commercially available chemotherapeutic agents are summarized in Table 48–2.[1-13] Mitomycin appears to be the most active single agent available for this group of tumors, but long-term survival is unlikely with single-agent therapy.

## COMBINATION CHEMOTHERAPY

The results achieved with combination chemotherapy appear in Table 48–3.[3, 6, 14–23] The most active combination appears to be mitomycin plus 5-fluorouracil given by hepatic artery infusion, with a response rate that exceeds 50%.[14, 18] The doses used in the largest study of this combination were 5-FU 1200 mg/m²/day given as a continuous infusion for 4 days, plus mitomycin C, 6 mg/m² by intra-arterial bolus on days 1 and 4 of each course. Courses are repeated every 4 weeks. Some of the responses with this treatment have been durable, including one patient who was free of disease for more than 5 years after the use of this combination.[14]

An alternative regimen for patients without vascular access to the hepatic artery involves intermittent courses of 5-FU (400 mg/m²) and leucovorin (20 mg/m²) given as intravenous boluses daily × 4 days with carboplatin (300 mg/m²) intravenously on day 1 only. Sanz-Altamira and colleagues[15] reported a 21% response rate with this regimen, with one patient having a complete response to therapy. An additional 29% of patients had stable disease for a median duration of 4 months.

There is some suggestion that neoadjuvant or preoperative

**Table 48–3.** Combination Chemotherapy for Carcinoma of the Gallbladder and Extrahepatic Biliary System

| Drugs | Patients* | Response Rate (%)† |
|---|---|---|
| 5-FU + mitomycin by HAI | 8/12 | 67 |
| 5-FU + doxorubicin (Adriamycin) + mitomycin (FAM) | 4/14 | 29 |
| 5-FU + leucovorin + carboplatin | 3/14 | 21 |
| Fluorouracil (5-FU) + semustine | 3/31 | 10 |
| 5-FU + streptozocin | 2/26 | 8 |
| 5-FU + dacarbazine + vincristine + carmustine | 2/2 | |
| Carmustine + mitomycin | 1/2 | |
| Cisplatin + 5-FU + epirubicin by HAI and oral UFT | 1/1 | |
| 5-FU + doxorubicin + cisplatin by HAI | 1/1 | |
| Preoperative HAI cisplatin + 5-FU + doxorubicin + mitomycin | 1/1 | |
| Carmustine + vincristine | 0/3 | |
| 5-FU + mitomycin + cytarabine | 0/5 | |

*Number of complete and partial responses per total number of patients treated.
†Response rates are only approximations of efficacy and are given solely for drugs tested in at least 15 patients.
5-FU, 5-fluorouracil; HAI, hepatic artery infusion; UFT, tegafur.

therapy may be useful, with case reports of long-term survival in patients so treated.[20] The experience with this approach is inadequate for it to be considered standard therapy, but it deserves further study. Combined-modality therapy (chemotherapy plus RT) is discussed in the previous section.

## REFERENCES

1. Crooke ST, Bradner WT. Mitomycin C: a review. Cancer Treat Rev 1976;3:121–39.
2. Moore GE, Bross ID, Ausmans R, et al. Effects of 5-fluorouracil (NSC-19893) in 389 patients with cancer. Eastern Clinical Drug Evaluation Program. Cancer Chemother Rep 1968;52:641–53.
3. Moertel CG. Extrahepatic bile ducts. In: Holland JF, Frei E, eds. Cancer medicine. Philadelphia: Lea & Febiger, 1974:1551–6.
4. Davis HL Jr, Ramirez G, Ansfield FJ. Adenocarcinomas of stomach, pancreas, liver, and biliary tracts: survival of 328 patients treated with fluoropyrimidine therapy. Cancer 1974;33:193–7.
5. Bateman JR, Pugh RP, Cassidy FR, et al. 5-Fluorouracil given once weekly: comparison of intravenous and oral administration. Cancer 1971;28:907–13.
6. Falkson G, MacIntyre JM, Moertel CG. Eastern Cooperative Oncology Group experience with chemotherapy for inoperable gallbladder and bile duct cancer. Cancer 1984;54:965–9.
7. Wittes RE, Adrianza ME, Parsons R, et al. Compilation of phase II results with single antineoplastic agents. Cancer Treat Symp 1985;4:396 and 399.
8. Middleman E, Luce J, Frei E III. Clinical trials with Adriamycin. Cancer 1971;28:844–50.
9. Frytak S, Moertel CG, Schutt AJ, et al. Adriamycin (NSC-123127) therapy for advanced gastrointestinal cancer. Cancer Chemother Rep 1975;59:405–9.
10. Adolphson CC, Carpenter JT Jr. Response to doxorubicin and mitomy-

**Table 48–2.** Single-Agent Chemotherapy for Carcinoma of the Gallbladder and Extrahepatic Biliary System

| Drug | Patients* | Response Rate (%)† |
|---|---|---|
| Mitomycin | 7/15 | 47 |
| 5-Fluorouracil | 6/92 | 7 |
| Streptozocin | 1/22 | 5 |
| Carmustine | 2/4 | |
| Doxorubicin | 1/4 | |
| Dacarbazine | 1/3 | |
| Cyclophosphamide | 1/1 | |
| Cisplatin | 0/3 | |
| Altretamine | 0/3 | |
| Etoposide | 0/1 | |
| Lomustine | 0/4 | |

*Number of complete and partial responses per total number of patients treated.
†Response rates are only approximations of efficacy and are given solely for drugs tested in at least 15 patients.

cin in cholangiocarcinoma: a case report. Cancer Treat Rep 1982;66:209–10.

11. Moertel CG, Reitemeier RJ, Hahn RG, Schutt AJ. 5-(3,3-dimethyl-1-triazeno) imidazole-4-carboxamide (NSC-45388) in patients with gastrointestinal carcinoma. Cancer Chemother Rep 1970;54:471–3.

12. Schutt AJ, Hahn RG, Reitemeier RJ, Moertel CG. A phase 2 study of intermittent high-dose cyclophosphamide therapy of advanced gastrointestinal cancer. Cancer Res 1973;33:2218–20.

13. Moertel CG, Schutt AJ, Reitemeier RJ, Hahn RG. Therapy for gastrointestinal cancer with the nitrosoureas alone and in drug combination. Cancer Treat Rep 1976;60:729–32.

14. Shirai Y, Ohtani T, Tsukada K, Hatakeyama K. Lymph node recurrence of gallbladder carcinoma successfully managed by systemic chemotherapy with 5-fluorouracil and mitomycin C: report of a 5-year survivor. Eur J Surg Oncol 1997;23:457–8.

15. Sanz-Altamira PM, Ferrante K, Jenkins RL, et al. A phase II trial of 5-fluorouracil, leucovorin, and carboplatin in patients with unresectable biliary tree carcinoma. Cancer 1998;82:2321–5.

16. Yokoyama M, Takahashi S, Tateoka H, et al. A case of recurrent gallbladder cancer with marked response to arterial infusion chemotherapy and transarterial embolization. Gan To Kagaku Ryoho 1997;24:9.

17. Lai DT, Storey DW, Waugh R, Stephens FO. Induction chemotherapy via hepatic artery for gallbladder carcinoma. Eur J Surg Oncol 1995;21:690–1.

18. Smith GW, Bukowski RM, Hewlett JS, Groppe CW. Hepatic artery infusion of 5-fluorouracil and mitomycin C in cholangiocarcinoma and gallbladder carcinoma. Cancer 1984;54:1513–6.

19. Harvey JH, Smith FP, Schein PS. 5-Fluorouracil, mitomycin, and doxorubicin (FAM) in carcinoma of the biliary tract. J Clin Oncol 1984;2:1245–8.

20. Kawabata Y, Yano S, Ohishi T, et al. A case of advanced gallbladder cancer responding to neoadjuvant intra-arterial chemotherapy. Gan To Kagaku Ryoho 1999;26:3.

21. Eden EB van, Falkson G, Dyk JJ van, et al. 5-Fluorouracil (5-Fu; NSC-19893), 5-(3,3-dimethyl-1-triazeno) imidazole-4-carboxamide (NSC-45388), vincristine (NSC-67574), and 1,3-bis(2-chloroethyl)-2-nitrosourea (BCNU; NSC-409962) given concomitantly in the treatment of solid tumors in man. Cancer Chemother Rep 1972;56:107–47.

22. Stolinsky DC, Pugh RP, Bohannon RA, et al. Clinical trial of BCNU (NSC-409962) combined with vincristine (NSC-67574) in disseminated gastrointestinal cancer and other neoplasms. Cancer Chemother Rep 1974;58:947–50.

23. De Jager RL, Magill GB, Golbey RB, Krakoff IH. Combination chemotherapy with mitomycin C, 5-fluorouracil, and cytosine arabinoside in gastrointestinal cancer. Cancer Treat Rep 1976;60:1373–5.

......................................

# SUMMARY OF TREATMENT

- Charles M. Haskell

## GENERAL APPROACH TO THE PATIENT

**Cancer Screening.** High-risk groups of patients, such as those with a history of primary sclerosing cholangitis, intraductal stones, cystic diseases of the biliary system, or familial adenomatosis polyposis, should be considered for cancer screening and possible prophylaxis.[1] This may include periodic follow-up by endoscopic retrograde cholangiography or annual measurement of the serum CA 19-9 level, or both.[2]

**Clinical Staging and Presurgical Assessment.** Surgery is the mainstay of therapy for localized neoplasms of the hepatobiliary tree.[3] For patients with a good performance status, reasonable cardiopulmonary function, and no evidence of cirrhosis, surgical resection should be considered if at all possible. The patient should be clinically staged, as discussed previously, and treatment chosen based on the extent of disease, including the presence or absence of the following: distant metastases, extensive regional lymphadenopathy, regional vascular encasement by tumor, or invasion of adjacent organ systems. Other factors to consider in the preoperative phase of evaluation are the nutritional status of the patient, the presence or absence of sepsis, and the extent of biliary cholestasis.

## TREATMENT BY STAGE OF DISEASE

**Stages 0 to III.** The extent of the surgical resection depends on the precise location of the tumor.[4] Localized intrahepatic cholangiocarcinoma is usually managed by hepatic resection alone. Surgical resection for perihilar lesions depends on the specific region involved, as discussed in the section on surgery. Patients with tumors below the confluence of the left and right hepatic ducts (Bismuth type I) or involving the confluence of these ducts (Bismuth type II) are commonly treated with en bloc resection of the extrahepatic bile ducts and gallbladder, regional lymphadenectomy, and Roux-en-Y hepaticojejunostomy. Patients with tumors occluding the common hepatic duct and either the right or the left hepatic duct (Bismuth types IIIa and IIIb, respectively) are treated with the previously described resection plus hepatic lobectomy. In some cases, caudate lobe resection may also be used for patients with type II cholangiocarcinoa. For distal extrahepatic tumors, pancreatoduodenectomy alone is the preferred surgical procedure.

Postoperative surgical-pathologic staging should be performed to complete treatment planning. The goal is to obtain at least a 5-mm proximal surgical margin. If the patient has positive surgical margins, RT should be considered.[1] In this setting, it appears reasonable to combine external-beam irradiation with continuous infusion 5-FU and transcatheter brachytherapy.[5]

**Stage IVA.** Primary RT covering the entire biliary tree may prolong survival in patients who are not candidates for resection or who experience recurrence. Some patients may be treated by endoscopic[6] or percutaneous bypass of unresectable obstructions, although these procedures can be complicated by acute cholangitis.[7] Unresectable lesions should be considered for treatment with external-beam irradiation and transcatheter brachytherapy, either alone or in combination with chemotherapy. For patients with hepatic artery access, the intra-arterial administration of 5-FU and mitomycin appears to be effective in palliating more than half the patients so treated.

**Stage IVB.** Supportive care and comfort measures are indicated, in some cases supplemented by biliary stenting or drainage for the control of symptoms. Systemic chemotherapy given alone in any of several drug combinations may be useful in patients with advanced disease, although the benefit is likely to be short-lived.

## SUGGESTIONS FOR ADDITIONAL READING

De Groen PC, Gores GJ, LaRusso NF, Gunderson LL, Nagorney DM. Medical Progress: biliary tract cancers. N Engl J Med 1999;341:1368–1378.

Brugge WR, Dam J van. Medical Progress: pancreatic and biliary endoscopy. N Engl J Med 1999;341:1808–1816.

## REFERENCES

1. De Groen PC, Barry JA, Schaller WJ. Applying World Wide Web technology to the study of patients with rare diseases. Ann Intern Med 1998;129:107–13.

2. Johlin FC, Voigt M, Wu YM. Surveillance cytology (SC) in the detection of asymptomatic progression to cholangiocarcinoma (CCC) in patients with primary sclerosing cholangitis. Hepatology 1998;28:Suppl:393A. abstract.

3. Tompkins RK, Saunders K, Roslyn JJ, Longmire WP Jr. Changing patterns in diagnosis and management of bile duct cancer. Ann Surg 1990;211:614–20.

4. De Groen PC, Gores GJ, LaRusso NF, et al. Medical Progress: biliary tract cancers. N Engl J Med 1999;341:1368–78.

5. Foo ML, Gunderson LL, Bender CE, Buskirk SJ. External radiation therapy and transcatheter iridium in the treatment of extrahepatic bile duct carcinoma. Int J Radiat Oncol Biol Phys 1997;39:929–35.

6. Summerfield JA. Biliary obstruction is best managed by endoscopists. Gut 1988;29:741–5.

7. Lai ECS, Lo C-M, Choi T-K, et al. Urgent biliary decompression after endoscopic retrograde cholangiopancreatography. Am J Surg 1989;157:121–5.

# CHAPTER 49

# AMPULLA OF VATER

• CHARLES M. HASKELL • LUU M. TRAN • KENNETH P. RAMMING

## Natural History, Diagnosis, and Staging

### EPIDEMIOLOGY AND ETIOLOGY

**Incidence.** Carcinoma of the ampulla of Vater is an extremely rare neoplasm of the duodenum, with close anatomic proximity to both biliary and pancreatic ducts (see Fig. 48–1). It constitutes about 0.01% of all solid tumors and is found in about 0.2% of postmortem examinations.[1]

**Risk Factors.** It has been presumed that this tumor occurs as a sporadic, acquired disease of unknown cause in most patients. However, rare examples of hereditary ampullary carcinoma have been reported. In some cases, this has been part of Gardner's syndrome, with the presumed neoplastic transformation of a duodenal polyp.[2] Periampullary carcinoma has been reported in three siblings who had no evidence of Gardner's syndrome or familial polyposis coli.[3] In patients with familial adenomatous polyposis, about 5 to 10% die of upper gastrointestinal cancer, usually from tumors of periampullary origin.[4]

**Molecular Pathogenesis.** The molecular lesions associated with carcinomas of the ampulla of Vater are similar to those reported elsewhere in the biliary system and gut. Among the abnormalities reported are the following: mutations of K-*ras,* somatic mutations of the APC gene, microsatellite instability, transforming growth factor-β1 receptor gene mutations, hMSH2 and hMLH1 allele losses, mutations of p53, abnormalities of p21/Waf1 protein expression, mutations of the human MUT S homologue 6 gene, and allelic losses at chromosome 5 that are similar to early events in gastric carcinogenesis.[5–15] The most important of these changes involve K-*ras* and the APC gene. Changes in K-*ras* correlate well with tumors arising from biliary duct tissue, whereas abnormalities of APC correlate with morphologic changes consistent with a more intestinal site of origin. These observations support common mechanisms of molecular pathogenesis among tumors of the digestive system, with variations based on precise location and the associated forms of genetic predisposition.

### PATHOLOGY

It is likely that most cases of ampullary carcinoma arise from pre-existing mucosal lesions, such as an adenoma, or from areas of dysplasia.[16–18] These lesions can demonstrate a wide range of differentiation. Thanks to the increasing use of endoscopy, it has become easier to study the histologic spectrum of ampullary tumors. Blackman and Nash[19] reported a series of 35 patients studied by endoscopic biopsy in which there were 11 benign adenomas (31%) and 24 malignant adenocarcinomas (69%). Of the 11 adenomas, 5 had focal areas of hyperplasia. The malignant lesions were subclassified histologically as follows: intestinal-type carcinomas (resembling colonic carcinoma) in 10 patients, anaplastic carcinomas (resembling diffuse gastric carcinoma) in 7 patients, adenocarcinoma in situ in 2 patients, and unoriented, cytologically malignant epithelium in 5 patients. In essentially all the adenocarcinomas diagnosed by this method, there was strong cytoplasmic staining for carcinoembryonic antigen (CEA) by immunohistochemistry. In extremely rare cases, neuroendocrine tumors may also develop in this location.[20]

The spread of ampullary carcinoma is by local infiltration into the walls of the adjacent common ducts, the second portion of the duodenum, and the head of the pancreas. With more extensive local spread, the portal and splenic veins may be involved, and secondary thrombosis of these vessels may occur. Local nodal metastases are demonstrable in about one patient in four at the time of surgical diagnosis. The nodal groups involved, in decreasing order of frequency, are the posterior pancreaticoduodenal node group, the inferior pancreaticoduodenal artery group, and the para-aortic area.[21] Knowledge of this pattern of spread can be useful in planning lymph node dissections for patients undergoing radical resections.

## CLINICAL FEATURES AND DIAGNOSIS

Symptoms of periampullary carcinoma are similar to those seen with obstructive lesions in other parts of the extrahepatic biliary duct, especially the lower common duct. Obstructive jaundice and pain are the most common symptoms, followed by constitutional findings such as weight loss, nausea, and chills. Anemia is frequent.

Diagnosis of this lesion is similar to the diagnostic workup outlined in the chapters on the pancreas (Chapter 45) and the biliary ducts (Chapter 48). Ultrasonography of the biliary system is usually the first step in diagnosis for patients presenting with symptoms of biliary obstruction. The study is useful in identifying the presence or absence of cholelithiasis, and it may provide some tentative localization of a site of obstruction. However, the presence of biliary stones does not necessarily rule out a malignancy, so further resolution of areas of obstruction is usually needed. Magnetic resonance cholangiopancreatography (MRCP) is an excellent next step in providing anatomic resolution of the hepatobiliary tree. Flexible endoscopy, with examination of the duodenum and ampulla, and transhepatic percutaneous cholangiography are additional procedures that may be needed for diagnosis, depending on the findings of standard ultrasonography and the MRCP. Standard CT scan of the abdomen is usually performed to rule out intra-abdominal metastases.

Endoscopic retrograde cholangiopancreatography (ERCP) and biopsy are commonly employed to make a presurgical diagnosis in patients with tumors of the ampulla. In one large series,[22] ERCP supported a diagnosis of cancer in about 90% of cases later confirmed by surgery. The negative predictive values were poor, however, with values of 33% for endoscopic appearance and 50% for endoscopic biopsy. Indeed, some authors have concluded that endoscopic biopsy, even when performed with endoscopic ultrasonography (EUS), is not accurate enough to ensure that an ampullary tumor is benign preoperatively.[23]

EUS is emerging as another useful staging modality, although it is not widely available. In its simplest form, EUS has an accuracy rate of 72 to 74% in predicting the T stage of disease.[24, 25] When used to predict resectability, it is 86 to 100% accurate, depending on the series. When EUS is performed in the presence of a stent placed during an earlier endoscopic procedure, however, the accuracy of staging is decreased.[26] This may underestimate the need for a Whipple resection because of tumor understaging. Another approach to EUS involves the use of sonography performed during ERCP. In a study directly comparing staging by intraductal ultrasonography, standard endoscopic ultrasonography, and CT, intraductal sonography was clearly superior.[27] Intraductal ultrasonography had a sensitivity and specificity of 100%, and the rates of tumor visualization were significantly improved (100% vs. 49.3% vs. 29.6%, respectively).

In some clinics, diagnostic laparoscopy is performed to rule out metastatic disease prior to exploratory laparotomy

for pancreatic and periampullary malignancies. However, modern CT scans of the abdomen have rendered this procedure largely irrelevant. In one series of 180 patients undergoing laparotomy for periampullary or pancreatic cancer, only 10% had metastases in the face of a negative CT scan.[28] Some of these patients needed laparotomy for palliation, so the actual number of patients spared an unnecessary laparotomy by preoperative laparoscopy was small.

Both the CEA and the CA 19-9 tests provide abnormal results in patients with tumors of the ampulla of Vater.[29] Of the two, the CA 19-9 test is more useful in management because elevations of this tumor marker may be useful in diagnosis and in assessing prognosis, and it appears to be more useful than CEA in following the postoperative course of disease. Further discussion of this marker can be found in the chapter on bile duct tumors (Chapter 48).

## STAGING AND PROGNOSIS

The international TNM staging system for carcinomas of the ampulla of Vater is presented in Table 49–1. The course of this disease is often indolent, with the survival time of unresectable disease often being greater than 1 year after diagnosis.[30, 31]

Prognosis is considered in the section on surgical treatment.

**Table 49–1.** TNM Staging for Primary Neoplasms of the Ampulla of Vater

*Primary Tumor (T)*

| | |
|---|---|
| TX | Primary tumor cannot be assessed |
| T0 | No evidence of primary tumor |
| Tis | Carcinoma in situ |
| T1 | Tumor limited to the ampulla of Vater or sphincter of Oddi |
| T2 | Tumor invades duodenal wall |
| T3 | Tumor invades 2 cm or less into the pancreas |
| T4 | Tumor invades more than 2 cm into pancreas and/or into other adjacent organs |

*Regional Lymph Nodes (N)*

| | |
|---|---|
| NX | Regional lymph nodes cannot be assessed |
| N0 | No regional lymph node metastasis |
| N1 | Regional lymph node metastasis |

*Distant Metastasis (M)*

| | |
|---|---|
| MX | Distant metastasis cannot be assessed |
| M0 | No distant metastasis |
| M1 | Distant metastasis |

*Stage Grouping*

| | | | |
|---|---|---|---|
| Stage 0 | Tis | N0 | M0 |
| Stage I | T1 | N0 | M0 |
| Stage II | T2 | N0 | M0 |
| | T3 | N0 | M0 |
| Stage III | T1 | N1 | M0 |
| | T2 | N1 | M0 |
| | T3 | N1 | M0 |
| Stage IV | T4 | Any N | M0 |
| | Any T | Any N | M1 |

Used with the permission of the American Joint Committee on Cancer (AJCC®), Chicago, Illinois. The original source for this material is the AJCC® Cancer Staging Manual, 5th edition (1997) Lippincott-Raven Publishers, Philadelphia, Pennsylvania.

# Treatment

## SURGERY

Because of the usual low grade of malignancy and early symptoms caused by relatively small lesions in this critical anatomic region, the results of surgery for carcinomas of the ampulla of Vater are much better than those for other malignancies in this area. Nevertheless, there is some controversy about what constitutes optimal surgery for patients with this disease. Crile and associates[32, 33] and Shapiro[34] have recommended that the most appropriate management of these patients is by local excision. More recently, Knox and Kingston[35] reported a 50% actuarial survival rate for local excision of this disease compared with a 25% actuarial survival rate for a Whipple procedure. On the surface, this would suggest that more limited surgery is optimal for this tumor. However, this study has been criticized for methodologic reasons,[36] and most other surgeons consider pancreaticoduodenectomy to be the treatment of choice.[37–45] There are generally fewer technical problems when this procedure is performed for carcinomas of the ampulla of Vater than when it is performed for carcinomas of the duodenum or pancreas. When performed in appropriate patients with carcinoma of the ampulla of Vater, the procedure has a mortality rate of about 4%, and the 5-year survival rate is about 30 to 35%.[45]

Patients who undergo exploratory surgery to determine if pancreaticoduodenectomy is possible and who are found to have unresectable disease should have a prophylactic retrocolic gastrojejunostomy as a measure to prevent subsequent gastric outlet obstruction. This recommendation is based on a randomized trial demonstrating a significant decrease in late gastric outlet obstruction without an increased incidence of postoperative complications or extended length of stay.[46]

## RADIATION THERAPY

A report of 10 patients treated with pancreaticoduodenectomy at Massachusetts General Hospital found disease recurrence in 7 of these patients; 3 patients had distant failure, 3 patients had local-regional failure, and 1 patient had both distant and local failure. The position of this tumor allows larger surgical margins and consequently better local control than is possible for gallbladder or more proximal bile duct tumors.[47] Because local failure is less predominant than for other biliary tumors, the rationale for postoperative radiation for grossly resected tumors is less clear. Radiation therapy has been used occasionally both as primary and as adjuvant therapy, but there are too few case reports to evaluate the value of radiation therapy for ampullary tumors. Whether radiation therapy is contemplated for adjuvant or definitive treatment, a reasonable dose is 45 to 50 Gy to the extrahepatic biliary tract and draining lymphatics through opposing anterior-posterior fields with an external-beam or intracavitary boost.

## CHEMOTHERAPY

There is little experience with chemotherapy for patients with this rare tumor. Hoffman and coworkers[48] described their limited experience with preoperative chemotherapy, and Abrams and associates[49] studied the use of postoperative adjuvant therapy. Neither group provided compelling evidence in support of either preoperative or postoperative radiation therapy, chemotherapy, or chemoradiotherapy. We consider the use of adjuvant therapy to be of unproved benefit for patients with carcinomas of the ampulla of Vater.

## SUMMARY OF TREATMENT

The expanded availability of biliary endoscopy has changed the approach to tumors of the periampullary region. Although tumors of this region are rare, lesions of this area are being identified by endoscopy at earlier stages than in the past. Consequently, local resections are more commonly considered for these patients at present.[50] For invasive cancer in this region, however, we continue to favor extended surgery as the cornerstone of management. The addition of adjuvant chemotherapy or radiation therapy, or both, is of unproved benefit in the management of this group of patients.

## SUGGESTIONS FOR ADDITIONAL READING

Kimchi NA, Mindrul V, Broide E, Scapa E. The contribution of endoscopy and biopsy to the diagnosis of periampullary tumors. Endoscopy 1998;30:538–43.

Matory YL, Gaynor J, Brennan M. Carcinoma of the ampulla of Vater. Surg Gynecol Obstet 1993;177:366–70. *This article is a review of 69 patients treated at the Memorial Sloan-Kettering Cancer Center in New York. The median survival in patients treated with resection was 51 months.*

Yeo CJ, Cameron JL. Adenocarcinoma of the ampulla of Vater: a 28-year experience. Ann Surg 1997;225:590–9. *The authors summarize the management of 120 patients with adenocarcinoma of the ampulla of Vater treated at Johns Hopkins University between 1969 and 1996. Resection rates increased from 62% in the 1970s to 82% in the 1980s and 1990s. The overall mortality rate for the procedure was 3.8%, with no deaths in the most recent 45 consecutive patients. Five-year survival for resected patients was 38%.*

## REFERENCES

1. Blumgart LH, Kennedy A. Carcinoma of the ampulla of Vater and duodenum. Br J Surg 1973;60:33–40.
2. Guyton DP, Schreiber H. Intestinal polyposis and periampullary carcinoma—changing concepts. J Surg Oncol 1985;29:158–9.
3. Austin JC, Organ CH Jr, Williams GR, Pitha JV. Vaterian cancer in siblings. Ann Surg 1988;207:655–61.
4. Wallace MH, Phillips RK. Preventative strategies for periampullary tumours in FAP. Ann Oncol 1999;10:Suppl 4:201–3.
5. Howe JR, Klimstra DS, Cordon-Cardo C, et al. K-*ras* mutation in adenomas and carcinomas of the ampulla of vater. Clin Cancer Res 1997;3:129–33.
6. Nagai M, Kawarada Y, Watanabe M, et al. Analysis of microsatellite instability, TGF-beta type II receptor gene mutations, and hMSH2 and hMLH1 allele losses in pancreaticobiliary maljunction–associated biliary tract tumors. Anticancer Res 1999;19:1765–8.
7. Sato T, Konishi K, Kimura H, et al. Adenoma and tiny carcinoma in adenoma of the papilla of Vater—p53 and PCNA. Hepatogastroenterology 1999;46:1959–62.
8. Matsubayashi H, Watanabe H, Yamaguchi T, et al. Differences in mucus and K-*ras* mutation in relation to phenotypes of tumors of the papilla of Vater. Cancer 1999;86:596–607.
9. Zhao B, Kimura W, Futakawa N, et al. p53 and p21/Waf1 protein

expression and K-*ras* codon 12 mutation in carcinoma of the papilla of Vater. Am J Gastroenterol 1999;94:2128–34.

10. Ebert MP, Hoffmann J, Schneider-Stock R, et al. Analysis of K-*ras* gene mutations in rare pancreatic and ampullary tumours. Eur J Gastroenterol Hepatol 1998;10:1025–9.

11. Imai Y, Inoue T, Ishikawa T. Mutations of the human MUT S homologue 6 gene in ampullary carcinoma and gastric cancer. Int J Cancer 1998;78:576–80.

12. Achille A, Baron A, Zamboni G, et al. Chromosome 5 allelic losses are early events in tumours of the papilla of Vater and occur at sites similar to those of gastric cancer. Br J Cancer 1998;78:1653–60.

13. Imai Y, Oda H, Tsurutani N, et al. Frequent somatic mutations of the APC and p53 genes in sporadic ampullary carcinomas. Jpn J Cancer Res 1997;88:846–54.

14. Achille A, Scupoli MT, Magalini AR, et al. APC gene mutations and allelic losses in sporadic ampullary tumours: evidence of genetic difference from tumours associated with familial adenomatous polyposis. Int J Cancer 1996;68:305–12.

15. Chung CH, Wilentz RE, Polak MM, et al. Clinical significance of K-ras oncogene activation in ampullary neoplasms. J Clin Pathol 1996;49:460–4.

16. Baczako K, Büchler M, Beger HG, et al. Morphogenesis and possible precursor lesions of invasive carcinoma of the papilla of Vater: epithelial dysplasia and adenoma. Hum Pathol 1985;16:305–10.

17. Büchler M, Rampf W, Baczako K, et al: Clinical aspects and fine structure of papillary cancer. With special reference to morphological carcinogenesis. Dtsch Med Wochenschr 1984;109:1629–34.

18. Stolte M, Pscherer C. Adenoma-carcinoma sequence in the papilla of Vater. Scand J Gastroenterol 1996;131:366–71.

19. Blackman E, Nash SV. Diagnosis of duodenal and ampullary epithelial neoplasms by endoscopic biopsy: a clinicopathologic and immunohistochemical study. Hum Pathol 1985;16:901–10.

20. Büchler M, Malfertheiner P, Baczako K, et al. A metastatic endocrine-neurogenic tumor of the ampulla of Vater with multiple endocrine immunoreaction—malignant paraganglioma? Digestion 1985;31:54–9.

21. Kayahara M, Nagakawa T, Ohta T, et al. Surgical strategy for carcinoma of the papilla of Vater on the basis of lymphatic spread and mode of recurrence. Surgery 1997;121:611–7.

22. Kimchi NA, Mindrul V, Broide E, Scapa E. The contribution of endoscopy and biopsy to the diagnosis of periampullary tumors. Endoscopy 1998;30:538–43.

23. Sauvanet A, Chapuis O, Hammel P, et al. Are endoscopic procedures able to predict the benignity of ampullary tumors? Am J Surg 1997;174;355–8.

24. Kubo H, Chijiiwa Y, Akahoshi K, et al. Preoperative staging of ampullary tumours by endoscopic ultrasound. Br J Radiol 1999;72:443–7.

25. Buscail L, Pagáes P, Berthâelemy P, et al. Role of EUS in the management of pancreatic and ampullary carcinoma: a prospective study assessing resectability and prognosis. Gastrointest Endosc 1999;50:34–40.

26. Cannon ME, Carpenter SL, Elta GH, et al. EUS compared with CT, magnetic resonance imaging, and angiography and the influence of biliary stenting on staging accuracy of ampullary neoplasms. Gastrointest Endosc 1999;50:27–33.

27. Menzel J, Hoepffner N, Sulkowski U, et al. Polypoid tumors of the major duodenal papilla: preoperative staging with intraductal US, EUS, and CT—a prospective, histopathologically controlled study. Part 1. Gastrointest Endosc 1999;49:349–57.

28. Friess H, Kleeff J, Silva JC, et al. The role of diagnostic laparoscopy in pancreatic and periampullary malignancies. J Am Coll Surg 1998;186:675–82.

29. Kau SY, Shyr YM, Su CH, et al. Diagnostic and prognostic values of CA 19-9 and CEA in periampullary cancers. J Am Coll Surg 199;188:415–20.

30. Crile G Jr, Isbister WH, Hawk WA. Carcinoma of the ampulla of Vater and the terminal bile and pancreatic ducts. Surg Gynecol Obstet 1970;131:1052–4.

31. Warren KW, Cattell RB, Blackburn JP, Nora PF. A long-term appraisal of pancreaticoduodenal resection for peri-ampullary carcinoma. Ann Surg 1962;155:653–62.

32. Crile G Jr. The advantages of bypass operations over radical pancreaticoduodenectomy in the treatment of pancreatic carcinoma. Surg Gynecol Obstet 1970;130:1049–53.

33. Crile G Jr, Isbister WH, Hawk WA. Carcinoma of the ampulla of Vater and the terminal bile and pancreatic ducts. Surg Gynecol Obstet 1970;131:1052–4.

34. Shapiro TM. Adenocarcinoma of the pancreas: a statistical analysis of biliary bypass vs Whipple resection in good risk patients. Ann Surg 1975;182:715–21.

35. Knox RA, Kingston RD. Management of periampullary carcinoma. Br J Surg 1988;75:291–2.

36. Neoptolemos JP, Talbot IC. Ampullary carcinoma. Br J Surg 1988;75:829–30.

37. Kopelson G, Harisiadis L, Tretter P, Chang CH. The role of radiation therapy in cancer of the extra-hepatic biliary system: an analysis of thirteen patients and a review of the literature of the effectiveness of surgery, chemotherapy and radiotherapy. Int J Radiat Oncol Biol Phys 1977;2:883–94.

38. Fish JC, Cleveland BR. Pancreaticoduodenectomy for peri-ampullary carcinoma—analysis of 38 cases. Ann Surg 1964;159:469–76.

39. Wise L, Pizzimbono C, Dehner LP. Periampullary cancer. A clinicopathologic study of sixty-two patients. Am J Surg 1976;131:141–8.

40. Akwari OE, van Heerden JA, Adson MA, Baggenstoss AH. Radical pancreaticoduodenectomy for cancer of the papilla of Vater. Arch Surg 1977;112:451–6.

41. Stephenson LW, Blackstone EH, Aldrete JA. Radical resection for periampullary carcinomas: results in 53 patients. Arch Surg 1977;112:245–9.

42. Barton RM, Copeland EM III. Carcinoma of the ampulla of Vater. Surg Gynecol Obstet 1983;156:297–301.

43. Walsh DB, Eckhauser FE, Cronenwett JL, et al. Adenocarcinoma of the ampulla of Vater. Diagnosis and treatment. Ann Surg 1982;195:152–7.

44. Kellum JM, Clark J, Miller HH. Pancreaticoduodenectomy for resectable malignant periampullary tumors. Surg Gynecol Obstet 1983;157:362–6.

45. Jones BA, Langer B, Taylor BR, Girotti M. Periampullary tumors: which ones should be resected? Am J Surg 1985;149:46–52.

46. Lillemoe KD, Cameron JL, Hardacre JM, et al. Is prophylactic gastrojejunostomy indicated for unresectable periampullary cancer? A prospective randomized trial. Ann Surg 1999;230:322–8.

47. Kopelson G, Galdabini J, Warshaw AL, Gunderson LL. Patterns of failure after curative surgery for extra-hepatic biliary tract carcinoma: implications for adjuvant therapy. Int J Radiat Oncol Biol Phys 1981;7:413–7.

48. Hoffman JP, Cooper HS, Young NA, Pendurthi TK. Preoperative chemotherapy or chemoradiotherapy for the treatment of adenocarcinoma of the pancreas and ampulla of Vater. J Hepatobiliary Pancreatic Surg 1998;5:251–4.

49. Abrams RA, Grochow LB, Chakravarthy A, et al. Intensified adjuvant theapy for pancreatic and periampullary adenocarcinoma: survival results and observations regarding patterns of failure, radiotherapy dose and CA19-9 levels. Int J Radiat Oncol Biol Phys 1999;44:10.

50. Treitschke F, Beger HG. Local resection of benign periampullary tumors. Ann Oncol 1999;10:Suppl 4:212–4.

# CHAPTER 50

# PROSTATE

• SUNAI LEEWANSANGTONG • E. DAVID CRAWFORD

The management of prostate cancer in the United States is currently among the most controversial and confusing issues facing urologists and oncologists. Mass screening of the population for prostate cancer is now feasible, yet experts argue whether this is scientifically or economically rational. In every stage of the disease, proven competing treatment modalities exist, with each side trying to prove that its modality is superior to any other. Respected specialists, many of whom have dedicated their academic careers to the research and treatment of this disease, assert that perhaps no treatment is required for most patients with prostate cancer, whereas other equally dedicated and respected physicians hold that early aggressive treatment of most clinically detectable tumors yields the greatest rewards for the patient and is more cost-effective in the long run. At present, neither of these camps has been able to amass a majority of followers to their side, and they likely never will.

Implicit in the understanding of the natural history of prostate cancer is the fact that it presents in a variety of ways; progresses at variable rates; metastasizes in some, but not, all patients; and has the ability to kill, simply *bother*, or spare its host. In the absence of a reliable early prognostic indicator, the treating physician must weigh the available data in each case, present a wealth of information on tumor biology and modes of treatment to the patient, then tailor therapy based on his or her feelings and the feelings of the patient. The management of prostate cancer was not always so controversial. In the early 1980s, the treatment paradigm by stage was fairly uniform. Patients with small volumes of occult cancer diagnosed unexpectedly by transurethral resection of the prostate were usually observed, whereas patients with larger volumes were treated by external-beam radiation therapy (EBRT). Patients with palpable tumors thought to be confined to the prostate gland or locally extensive were also treated with radiation therapy if they had no evidence for skeletal metastases. A few patients who fulfilled strict preoperative criteria were offered a chance for cure with radical prostatectomy, although it was presumed that this was a high-morbidity procedure, with a 100% chance of impotence and a fair chance of urinary incontinence. A few centers investigated the use of implantable radioactive seeds in efforts to curb the morbidity of external radiation yet provide local control of the disease. Patients with metastatic disease were offered the choice of palliative hormonal blockade with orchiectomy or diethylstilbestrol (DES), usually initiated not at the first sign of metastasis but when the patient became symptomatic from the disease. A series of chemotherapeutic protocols closed in the early 1980s, with the finding that prostate cancer was resistant to all currently available drugs and combinations.

Several landmark studies (reported from 1981 to 1983) brought into question the aforementioned management

schema. An elegant study of the periprostatic anatomy disclosed the location of the important neurovascular bundles responsible for producing and maintaining erections of the penis.[1] A novel surgical procedure was then devised, which was shown to preserve potency reliably in most men and to reduce greatly blood loss and associated surgical morbidity.[2] With 10-year follow-up showing that radiation therapy did not always cure or control prostate cancer, physicians and patients began looking toward surgery again as a rational modality. A re-evaluation of the results of the Veterans Administration Cooperative Urological Research Group (VACURG) study on metastatic prostate cancer prompted a retraction, stating that delayed hormonal ablation may not yield the same cancer-specific survival as early hormonal ablation.[3] With the development of a safe, effective means of *medical castration* came the ability to offer a reasonable alternative to orchiectomy or DES.[4] Finally, the development of a new serum marker for prostate cancer, prostate-specific antigen (PSA), ushered in an era of earlier detection of *silent, nonpalpable* prostate cancers and earlier detection of treatment failure or escape from hormonal control.[5]

In North America, several social factors have a bearing on the aforementioned scientific advances. Improved cardiac care, better antihypertensive and anti-infective medicines, and a purported healthier lifestyle have resulted in longer life for most American men. A man in his late 60s now expects to live an active, independent life into his 80s. The popular media now centers much attention on health issues, with the benefit of a much wiser and well-informed, health-conscious U.S. citizen. Conversely, this omnipresent public scrutiny, when coupled with escalating health care inflation in the United States, which spends 14% of its gross domestic product on health care, has brought about demands that state-of-the-art care continue to be delivered quickly and effectively, yet inexpensively.

All these issues have a direct impact on the present-day management of prostate cancer. Although the management paradigm of the early 1980s may have been simple and comfortable, present-day management strategies attempt to fine-tune diagnostic and treatment efforts to optimize survival in American men and minimize treatment-associated morbidity while working within the constraints of modern society. To this end, current recommendations regarding the management of prostate cancer present an evolving science.

## Natural History, Diagnosis, and Staging

### INCIDENCE AND EPIDEMIOLOGY

In the 1990s, prostate cancer incidence exceeded lung cancer incidence for the first time, making prostate cancer the most commonly diagnosed (noncutaneous) neoplasm in North American men. A total of 179,300 new cases of prostate cancer were estimated to be diagnosed in the United States in 1999, and mortality resulting from the malignancy was expected to exceed 37,000.[6] Between 1987 and 1992, the prostate cancer incidence steadily increased to 84%, but it declined to 46% between 1992 and 1994. The incidence was expected to continue to decline through 1999. Prostate cancer–specific mortality began to decline by 0.5% per year between 1990 and 1994. Aggressive prostate cancer screening programs, heightened public awareness of prostatic diseases, and the rise of a healthier aged population since the late 1980s are all major contributors to this changing incidence.

Calculating the prevalence of prostate cancer is problematic. Several autopsy studies of patients dying with no known history of prostate cancer have shown that occult prostate cancer is a frequent occurrence.[7, 8] Beginning at age 50, the prevalence of histologically confirmed prostate cancer rises throughout each decade until age 80, when it plateaus. It has previously been assumed that younger men in their 30s and 40s were generally free of prostatic cancer risk. Nevertheless, an elegantly performed autopsy study of 159 boys and men 10 to 49 years old dying of trauma disclosed that 25 to 30% of men in their 30s and 36% of men in their 40s harbored histologically documented prostate cancer.[9] If more than one third of all American men older than age 30 harbor prostate cancer, the prevalence of the disease is astounding. Most men with histologically detectable prostate cancer do not develop clinically detectable prostate cancer and die with, rather than of, prostate cancer.

Autopsy studies in other developed countries have shown a prevalence of prostate cancer similar to that of the United States, but incidence and cancer mortality rates vary tremendously.[10] Between 1992 and 1995, an age-adjusted death rate of prostate cancer in the United States was 17.3 per 100,000 men compared with 4.2 per 100,000 men in Japan.[6] Insofar as the prevalence of histologic prostate cancer is similar between these two groups, a genetic or environmental factor must be responsible for the differing natural histories of prostate cancer in the United States and Japan. Japanese immigrants and their first-generation offspring tend to approach the prostate cancer incidence of American men, arguing against a genetic basis for the discrepancies between the two countries. It is presumed that certain environmental factors, such as diet and activity level, are likely responsible for the higher rate of clinically relevant prostate cancer in the United States.

Within the United States, black Americans have a significantly higher incidence (180/100,000 vs. 134/100,000) and mortality rate (53/100,000 vs. 24/100,000) of prostate cancer than white Americans.[11] Correcting for geographic, socioeconomic, and age factors does not alter the doubled prostate cancer death rate experienced by black men in the United States.[12] Autopsy studies confirm that the prevalence of histologically detectable prostate cancer is similar between the two groups, indicating that genetic or environmental factors may select worse variants of prostate cancer in black Americans than in white Americans.[9, 13, 14] In a nationwide, ongoing prostate cancer screening program, the stage of the cancer at presentation in black American men is consistently worse than in the white American cohort.

Although a wealth of epidemiologic information on prostate cancer exists, no clear or consistent causative factor has yet emerged as the primary culprit for the high incidence of prostate cancer in the United States. The high-fat, high-cholesterol, and low-fiber diet consumed by Americans is suspected as a prime candidate, but compelling data are lacking to support this hypothesis. High prostate cancer rates cross all occupational and socioeconomic levels in the United States and affect rural and urban dwellers alike. The rates are equally high in celibate men and sexually active men. Despite the inability of epidemiologic studies to shed light on the pathogenic basis of prostate cancer, elegant research using genetic linkage analysis techniques in families with clusters of prostate cancer cases found that the genetic region where prostatic neoplasia occurs is localized to chromosome 1 band q24 (*HPC1* gene), with 34% of the families being linked to this locus.[15] Although this information may pertain primarily to the hereditary form of prostate cancer and not to the predominant sporadic form, it is hoped that this landmark discovery opens the door to understanding the preliminary steps in the evolution of prostatic cancer.

## PATHOLOGY AND CLASSIFICATION

### Acinar Adenocarcinoma

The prostate is a gland derived embryologically from ingrowth of the primitive urogenital sinus (endoderm) into the mesenchyme. Through mesenchymal and endodermal inductive events, the portion of the urogenital sinus forming the prostate gland arborizes into a highly branched complex gland composed of ducts and acini in a fibromuscular stroma. In young men without benign prostatic hypertrophy (BPH), most of the glandular volume is located in the peripheral zone of the prostate (peripherally located in relation to the urethra), whereas a significant mass of prostatic epithelium resides in the central zone. The transitional zone is the periurethral zone, which is prone to development of BPH. In nonpathologic conditions, the periurethral zone comprises a small percentage of the total prostatic glandular mass. Using axial whole-mount pathologic sectioning, these three zones can be reliably distinguished from one another.

Approximately 95% of all prostatic cancers are adenocarcinomas. Roughly 4% of all prostate malignancies arise from the transitional epithelium of the urethra or ducts as transitional cell carcinoma. Primary carcinoid tumors of the prostate and primary small cell carcinoma of the prostate are rare, as are a wide variety of sarcomas. Primary rhabdomyosarcoma of the prostate occurs in the pediatric population with known frequency, whereas the most common adult sarcoma of the prostate is the leiomyosarcoma.

Most prostatic adenocarcinomas are believed to arise in the peripheral zone, where roughly 70% of the prostatic mass is located. About 10% of carcinomas arise in the central zone, and about 20% of carcinomas arise in the transition zone. Although the central zone cancers are generally larger and presumed to be clinically significant, the transition zone cancers usually detected during transurethral resection of the prostate for BPH are frequently small in volume and often pose no threat to their host.[16] Immunohistochemical staining techniques are invaluable in the differential diagnosis of metastases suspected to be prostatic in origin. Immunoperoxidase staining of specimens with PSA and prostate-specific acid phosphatase (PSAP) reliably diagnose prostatic tissue or metastases.[17] Nevertheless, a few pitfalls in the performance and evaluation of these marker stains bear mention. Poorly differentiated prostatic tumors without glandular formation occasionally fail to stain positive for PSA or PSAP, indicating that both techniques should be used together routinely. Additionally, these high-grade tumors may take up stain only focally, indicating the need for an adequate volume of the biopsy specimen before making a negative diagnosis. Weak focal staining of biopsy tissue must be interpreted with caution because renal cell and breast carcinoma have stained positive for PSAP, as have adenocarcinomas of the bladder or intestine.[18, 19]

### Variant Forms of Adenocarcinoma

**Mucinous Adenocarcinoma.** Mucinous adenocarcinoma is a rare pathologic entity, constituting less than 1% of all prostatic adenocarcinomas. Although most prostatic adenocarcinomas stain positive for mucin and secrete mucosubstances, mucinous adenocarcinoma of the prostate is precisely defined by the presence of lakes of extracellular mucin in at least 25% of the resected tumor. The tumor continues to stain positive for PSA and PSAP. The tumor behaves aggressively, frequently metastasizing to bone and showing resistance to hormonal deprivation therapies.[20] This type of adenocarcinoma is also found in young patients.[21]

**Primary Signet-Ring Cell Carcinoma.** Primary signet-ring cell carcinoma of the prostate is extremely rare. Its appearance results from the presence of intracytoplasmic lumens or from vacuoles. This cell type is negative for neutral and acid mucins but immunoreactive for PSA and PSAP.[22]

**Adenocarcinoma with Endometrioid Features.** Adenocarcinoma with endometrioid features is also a rare pathologic diagnosis, with only 10 cases occurring in one study of 2600 cases of primary prostate cancer.[20] Histologically, the tumor demonstrates a tall pseudostratified columnar epithelium with amphophilic cytoplasm arranged in papillary or complex glandular configurations, often with slit-like lumina. All 10 cases stained positive for PSA and PSAP, indicating a prostatic origin for the tumor and refuting the concept of an endometrial carcinoma arising in a müllerian rest in the prostate. Although most adenocarcinomas with endometrioid features arise in the ductal region of the prostate, they are often associated with concomitant acinar adenocarcinomas elsewhere in the gland.

**Ductal Adenocarcinoma.** Ductal adenocarcinoma denotes primary tumors originating in the primary or peripheral ducts of the prostate. Approximately 0.5% of prostate carcinomas arise in the ductal structures. The histologic characteristics are as described previously for adenocarcinoma with endometrial features, which is a form of ductal carcinoma. In general, these tumors follow an aggressive course, metastasizing early and showing less responsiveness to hormonal blockade.[23] A study showed, however, that the tumor responded well to orthodox microacinar carcinoma therapy, and the longest survival was 12 years.[24]

**Endocrine Paracrine.** Amine precursor uptake and decarboxylation cells are located throughout the prostate, and they are capable of undergoing malignant degeneration, as demonstrated by the presence of carcinoid and oat cell tumors of the prostate.[25] Evidence is mounting that most prostatic adenocarcinomas show some degree of neuroendocrine differentiation focally. These foci stain positive with silver stains and show dendritic processes and neurosecretory granules on electron microscopy. Early evidence points toward a relative hormone resistance for this component of an adenocarcinoma, with a possible poorer prognosis. Because serotonin and various peptides may have a role in this tumor component, specific subtypes of neoplastic cells with neuroendocrine differentiation based on serotonin and peptide profiles should be analyzed for innovative treatment.[26]

### Histologic Grading

In the 1960s and 1970s, VACURG amassed an abundance of data on nearly 5000 prostate cancer patients. Among the many valuable contributions of these studies was the development of a standardized grading system for prostate cancer based primarily on the glandular architecture of the tumor.[27] Nine recurring unique histologic patterns were identified but not ranked in severity. Rather, survival data were accrued independently and compared with the assigned histologic pattern. Certain patterns followed a less lethal course, whereas other patterns followed a rapidly fatal course. Most cases followed an intermediate course, but subtle pattern discrimination permitted further subclassification. The nine patterns were distilled into five grades, with grade 1 being least aggressive and grade 5 most aggressive. Roughly half of the cases showed two separate, unique patterns. The ultimate grading system incorporated the two predominant patterns in any tumor and summed their grades. When assigning a Gleason summation score of 2 to 10 to the tumors in the VACURG study, cancer-specific mortality rose steadily and reliably from scores 2 through 10. The grading system was schematized through a simple drawing and soon adopted (not without considerable debate) throughout the United States.[28] Other grading systems, including some that take into account the degree of nuclear pleomorphism in the tumor, have been used.[29, 30] None has shown clear superiority over the Gleason system in terms of interobserver reproducibility or prognostic reliability. For these reasons, the Gleason system has become the favored approach to grading prostatic adenocarcinomas. Its performance as a prognostic indicator is discussed later.

### Prostatic Intraepithelial Neoplasia

Premalignant changes in the ductal and acinar epithelium are now referred to as *prostatic intraepithelial neoplasia* (PIN). In the past, terms such as *atypical glandular hyperplasia*, *cytologic atypia*, and *intraductal dysplasia* were used to describe abnormalities in the acinar and ductal architecture, cytology, and nuclear morphology. By convention, these terms have been discarded in favor of the designation PIN.

The histologic criteria for diagnosing PIN include crowding and stratification of the luminal epithelial cells of the prostatic acini and ducts, with a definable basal cell layer partially or wholly intact.[31] Invasive prostatic adenocarcinoma lacks a definable basal cell layer. Using ordinary hematoxylin and eosin staining techniques, the basal cell layer of prostatic acini is not reliably seen. In borderline cases of PIN versus invasive carcinoma, anticytokeratin antibody stains, which selectively stain basal cells, may be used to rule out the presence of invasive carcinoma.[31, 32]

The grading of PIN has been divided into low-grade PIN and high-grade PIN. Cytologic criteria for PIN include nuclear pleomorphism, hyperchromasia (in high-grade PIN), and prominent nucleoli (in high-grade PIN) in the luminal epithelial cells.[33, 34] Low-grade PIN is defined by crowding and stratification of the luminal epithelial cells with nuclear pleomorphism. High-grade PIN shows the same crowding and stratification, sometimes with cribriform architecture. The basal cell layer is often disrupted in high-grade PIN. The nuclei in high-grade PIN are pleomorphic or frankly enlarged, often with large, prominent nucleoli. Hyperchromasia is always apparent in high-grade PIN.

PIN fulfills the histologic criteria for a premalignant lesion because of its frequent association with invasive prostatic carcinoma. PIN has been seen in 80 to 100% of prostates with invasive prostate cancer.[31, 33] It is seen much less frequently in normal prostates removed at autopsy.[33] The prevalence of PIN was 65 to 85% in 40- to 70-year-old black men compared with 35 to 60% in white men in the same age range.[34] High-grade PIN prevalence was also higher in young black men.[35] PIN is usually seen in proximity to an invasive lesion.[31] It arises most frequently in the peripheral zone, the zone where most invasive carcinomas are found.[36] It rarely arises in the transitional zone. Several studies showed a high incidence (47 to 57%) of carcinoma in the rebiopsy specimens after a previous biopsy of high-grade PIN. Some investigators suggested a rebiopsy in men with a previous high-grade PIN but not in men with low-grade PIN.[34, 37]

At present, the prognostic value of prostatic biopsy specimens containing PIN alone is indeterminable. Forty percent of noncancerous prostates harbor PIN. Using PIN in the absence of frank carcinoma on biopsy as a threshold criterion for initiating therapy is unwise.

## CLINICAL FEATURES

Men with prostate cancer present in a variety of ways, from an asymptomatic nodule detected on digital rectal examination (DRE) to hemiplegia from spinal cord compression by metastatic deposits. Because of the widespread use of serum PSA measurements for early detection of prostate cancer, an increasing percentage of men now present with asymptomatic disease. When patients present with a prostate nodule and symptoms of lower urinary tract obstruction, the obstructive voiding symptoms are more likely due to concomitant BPH (in the periurethral portion of the gland) than to the carcinoma (arising most frequently in the peripheral zone of the gland). Carcinoma of the prostate may grow large enough to obstruct the urethra partially and cause urinary difficulties. In this scenario, the cancer is usually advanced, with the likelihood of cure slim.

The symptom complex of obstructive urinary complaints combined with axial or long bone pain occurs frequently in men diagnosed with prostate cancer. Technetium 99m bone scintigraphy in this setting usually detects multiple foci of increased uptake in symptomatic and asymptomatic bone sites. If the metastases to the vertebrae are extensive or involve the epidural space, absent rectal sphincter tone, urinary or fecal incontinence, or lower extremity weakness may be present, indicating spinal cord or radicular impingement by tumor—a true oncologic emergency. Less frequent presenting scenarios include bilateral lower extremity edema from lymphatic obstruction by metastases, priapism from locally advanced or metastatic tumor obstructing the penile venous drainage, uremia and hydronephrosis from bilateral ureteral obstruction by a large primary tumor, and life-threatening disseminated intravascular coagulation from extensive myelogenous metastatic deposits or production of anticoagulating substances by the tumor.

It is generally believed that men presenting with symptomatic prostate cancer are usually incurable at diagnosis. This observation has prompted efforts to detect more prostate cancer cases in the asymptomatic stages, when cure may be possible. Screening for prostate cancer using serum PSA measurement or DRE, or both, has become one of the key issues in urologic oncology today.

## Screening for Prostate Cancer

Screening for prostate cancer is the most controversial issue facing American urologists today. Arguments against routine screening center around a purported prohibitive cost of screening, lack of complete knowledge of the natural history of untreated prostate cancer, and fears that early detection efforts would diagnose a preponderance of *clinically insignificant, autopsy incidence* prostatic cancers. The presumption is that many patients who participate in screening programs will be treated unnecessarily for prostate cancer that would not have presented a mortal threat. Proponents of screening contend that properly conducted screening is cost-effective, that low-morbidity treatment for early detected tumors is available, and that screening efforts as currently practiced do not detect *clinically insignificant* tumors.

Several early screening studies that used DRE alone for the early detection of prostate cancer have been published and reviewed.[38] The average cancer detection rate for DRE alone is 1.8%, with the average positive predictive value for DRE calculated at 32%. Although approximately 70% of prostate cancers detected by screening DRE are believed to be clinically confined to the prostate, approximately 50% end up being pathologically outside the gland.[39, 40] DRE is subjective and subject to error. Its efficiency for screening is lower than PSA.[39, 41] At present, DRE has not been used alone in most screening trials. Some screening trials eliminated DRE as a screening test.[42]

Transrectal ultrasonography (TRU) has been used widely in early trials for prostate cancer. These trials do not represent true screening studies in that most studies were performed at urologic referral centers, often in patients with urologic symptoms. The cancer detection rate for TRU varies from 2.6 to 12.4%, with sensitivities varying from 90 to 100% and specificities varying from 65 to 94%.[43, 44] TRU is highly user dependent with a significant learning curve. Although it is believed that TRU does not detect low-volume, clinically insignificant tumors, only about two thirds of classic hypoechogenic foci in the prostate prove to be prostate cancers. Abnormal findings on TRU are neither sufficiently sensitive nor sufficiently specific to be used for screening. At present, some screening studies have not used TRU as a screening method. TRU has been used for biopsy when PSA or DRE is abnormal.

PSA is a serine protease produced by prostatic epithelial cells that is normally secreted in minute amounts into the serum. It has been shown to be an effective tumor marker in following cases of prostate cancer.[5] Efforts have centered around its utility as a screening tool in the early detection of prostate cancer. In general, a PSA less than 4 ng/ml is infrequently associated with prostate cancer, whereas a PSA greater than 10 ng/ml is highly suspicious for cancer. Difficulties arise in the evaluation of patients with values between 4 and 10 because benign conditions predominate in this range of PSA. Several investigators have tried to index the serum PSA level by prostatic weight (PSA density).[45, 46] By dividing the PSA value by the volume of the prostate gland as measured by TRU, it was hoped that the benign glandular hyperplastic contribution to the PSA elevation would be factored out. It appears, however, that the PSA density is neither more sensitive nor more specific than random PSA measurements alone in detecting prostate cancer.[47]

One screening trial has used serum PSA without DRE (n = 1249), with a cancer detection rate of 2.6% when the upper limit of normal for PSA is defined as 4 ng/ml (Hybritech assay).[48] In a follow-up study by the same group of investigators, 701 men (of the previous 1249 men) without an abnormal PSA from the previous year returned for a repeat PSA check, with a resulting second-year cancer detection rate of 2%.[49] In both years of the study, men with a PSA between 4.1 and 10 ng/ml who submitted to biopsy had a 23 to 26% rate of prostate cancer detected. Using the 2-year screening criteria, 75 to 88% of patients with a serum PSA up to 10 ng/ml had organ-confined or specimen-confined tumors when patients were subjected to radical prostatectomy. Overall, 67% of patients in the screening trial electing to undergo radical prostatectomy were cured based on pathologic criteria. Another screening trial (n = 1653) yielded similar results.[50] Using an upper limit of normal of 3.9 ng/ml, a cancer detection rate of 2.2% was obtained. Of patients with a PSA between 4 and 9.9 ng/ml who submitted to biopsy, a 22% rate of prostate cancer was obtained. Of the men in the study with PSA values less than 10 who underwent radical prostatectomy, 59 to 79% had disease confined by the prostatic capsule (presumed surgical cure).

Routine serum PSA measurements are an imperfect means of screening for prostate cancer. The sensitivity and specificity, using an upper limit of normal of 4 ng/ml, are less than 90%, the standard percentage desired for screening efficacy. A single serum value of PSA represents a *snapshot* in assessing the average patient's risk of developing clinically significant prostate cancer. The efforts have centered around longitudinal evaluation of serum PSA values in hopes of improving on the roughly 80% sensitivity and 60% specificity of PSA in a screening setting.[49, 51] A unique study was reported that used archival frozen serum collected over a 25-year span to determine the rate of change of serum PSA over time (PSA velocity) in men with and without prostate diseases.[51] The investigators found that men who ultimately developed prostate cancer experienced an annual rate of rise of serum PSA of 0.75 ng/ml/yr or greater. The slope of the

curve for the rate of change of PSA in men with BPH only was much lower. The rate of change in PSA levels distinguished men with cancer from men with BPH at a specificity of 90%. Finally, the rate change for PSA was operative at PSA levels less than 4 ng/ml. An annual change from 2 ng/ml to 4 ng/ml would be highly predictive for cancer. Others have shown that an annual increase of serum PSA levels by 20% or greater may be indicative of carcinoma.[49] Age-specific reference range (ASRR) has been used for increasing sensitivity and specificity of PSA. The theory is that a PSA level increases with age among men without prostate cancer or men with BPH. Several investigators recommended ASRR levels.[52–54] There are some limitations for using ASRR, however. ASRR increases the specificity in older men and the sensitivity in younger men. Nonetheless, it enhances a higher rate of missed diagnosis for prostate cancer in older patients.[55] Data suggested that men of different races should have different ASRR levels.[56] Free PSA is another effort to increase the specificity of PSA. PSA in serum is composed of a free PSA and complexed PSA compounds that bind to α1-antichymotrypsin or other proteins. Data suggested that the ratio of free PSA and total PSA (complexed plus free) is different between men with and those without prostate cancer; the lower the ratio, the higher the risk of prostate cancer.[57] Free PSA improves the specificity in men with a PSA between 4.1 and 10 ng/ml.

Serum PSA measurement is minimally invasive, simple to perform, and readily available in all parts of the United States. It provides an objective means of determining a man's prostate cancer risk. It does not appear to detect clinically insignificant prostate cancers.[48, 58] In our experience, more than 50% of prostate cancers detected by modest elevations of PSA in the presence of a palpably normal gland show extracapsular carcinoma after radical prostatectomy and extensive pathologic scrutiny (unpublished results). The cost of detecting a single case of prostate cancer using routine screening with PSA has been estimated to be $2000, which compares favorably with the estimated $14,000 using routine mammography for breast cancer screening. Serum PSA values are not altered significantly by routine DRE so that serum may be obtained before or after examination.[59]

The aforementioned study also sought to define the best method for screening by comparing the predictive value of DRE, TRU, and PSA in predicting for a positive biopsy specimen for carcinoma.[50] Multivariate logistic regression analysis was used to compare the value of each study by itself and in combination with each other. PSA is more accurate than DRE or TRU when the three studies are used alone. In the two large screenings (n = 31,953 and 6630), the combination of PSA and DRE had the highest predictive values (46.6 to 48.5%) for positive biopsy when compared with those of PSA alone (31.6 to 32%) or DRE alone (21 to 25.5%). It also showed the highest cancer detection rates (4.7 to 5.8%) when compared with those of PSA alone (3.6 to 4.6%) or DRE alone (3 to 3.2%).[41, 60] This combination also detected 88% of the cancers in high-risk families.[58] In the early 1990s, the American Cancer Society recommended all men between the ages of 50 and 70 with a 10-year life expectancy undergo annual prostate cancer screening with DRE and PSA. Some investigators recommend that DRE not be omitted because 18 to 30% of prostate cancer patients in selected surgical series have a normal PSA.[60, 61] Black men and men with a positive family history for prostate cancer should be screened beginning at age 40 or 45 because these two groups tend to develop prostate cancer at a younger age. The necessity of annual screening in men who have initial normal PSA (<4 ng/ml) was questioned. One longitudinal study (n = 6804) suggested that men with an initial PSA of 0 to 1 ng/ml and 1.1 to 2 ng/ml would be at low risk to develop a PSA value greater than 4 ng/ml (0.9% and 4.1%) and prostate cancer (0.34% and 0.97%) within the next 3 years. In contrast, approximately 34% of men with an initial PSA between 2.1 and 4 ng/ml would develop a PSA value greater than 4 ng/ml, and approximately 6% of these men would develop prostate cancer within the next 3 years.[62] Another study (n = 827) showed similar results.[63] Because most screened men have a PSA value less than 2 ng/ml at initial screening, elimination of annual PSA screening in these groups for the next 3 years may have significant cost savings.

## DIAGNOSIS AND STAGING

The diagnosis and staging of prostate cancer are fairly simple when compared with most other malignancies. Most patients referred to urologists have a suspicious prostate gland on DRE or a suspicious elevation of serum PSA, or both. Biopsy of the prostate is fairly straightforward in this setting. Most urologists have access to TRU; biopsy needle insertion is usually guided into the gland with TRU. Biopsy specimens of all hypoechoic regions in the gland are obtained. Additionally, systematic biopsies of the peripheral zone are recommended because of the nonspecific nature of hypoechoic lesions in the prostate. By preparing patients for biopsy with a Fleet Enema and a prophylactic oral quinolone antibiotic, the rate of iatrogenic urinary tract infection or urosepsis is greatly diminished.

Many European centers and a few centers in the United States continue to use fine-needle aspiration of the prostate to diagnose cancer.[64] Before the advent of the automated core biopsy gun, most patients were admitted to the hospital for prostate biopsy, and they experienced considerable discomfort from the procedure. Fine-needle aspiration offered the advantage of less pain to the patient and could usually be performed on an outpatient basis. By means of TRU and the automated core biopsy gun, most men can undergo transrectal biopsy of the prostate safely and comfortably in an outpatient setting. An experienced cytopathologist is not required, and a Gleason grade and preliminary volume measurement can be assigned to the core biopsy specimen.

Many men are diagnosed with prostate cancer after pathologic review of a prostatic specimen (transurethral resection or open enucleation) removed for presumed benign prostatic hyperplasia. Historically, 10% of men subjected to transurethral resection of the prostate or prostatic enucleation were found to harbor carcinoma in the specimen. It is possible, however, that in the future fewer men will be diagnosed in this manner as more men select nonsurgical treatment for obstructive voiding and are screened for carcinoma with PSA and DRE.

Clinical staging of prostatic carcinoma entails defining the extent of the primary lesion in the prostate and documenting the presence or absence of distant metastases. Despite the introduction of sophisticated imaging modalities into daily practice, there has been little improvement in the ability to document extracapsular prostatic tumor extension. Although technetium 99m bone scintigraphy has shown reliability in ascertaining the presence or absence of osseous metastases, reliable studies to assess the status of the pelvic lymph nodes are lacking. The serum tumor markers PSA and PSAP have utility in staging for prostate cancer, although their reliability is situation dependent. The increased use of radical prostatectomy combined with more careful pathologic staging with the whole-mount technique continues to show the fairly dismal performance of all clinical staging modalities.

### Staging of the Prostate Primary

The three most commonly used clinical staging classification systems are outlined in Table 50–1. Although the Jewett-Whitmore system has been favored in the United States for several decades, the TNM systems are slowly gaining favor because of the more complete description of disease extent (local-regional and metastases). Some controversy centers around the classification of the *PSA-detected tumor*, which does not readily fit into stage A or B (T1 or T2) categories. Longer follow-up with *PSA-detected tumors (T1c)* should disclose whether they behave more like stage A or stage B disease.

**Digital Rectal Examination.** DRE is marginally successful in ensuring that a prostatic nodule is confined to the prostate.[65] Overall, 40% of clinical stage T2 nodules are confined to the organ when careful step sectioning of the radical prostatectomy specimen is carried out. Approximately 50% of clinical stage T2 nodules end up pathologic stage T3 tumors. Using the whole-mount approach (step section approach) to pathologic review detects an additional 20% of tumors that extend outside the prostate capsule.[65] Whether this intense scrutiny of the resected prostate translates into poorer overall survival for patients with minimal extracapsular disease is yet to be proved.

**Transrectal Ultrasonography.** TRU is roughly equal to DRE in detecting extraprostatic extension of tumor. Overall accuracy in correctly diagnosing pathologic stage T2 or T3 disease with TRU is 60%, with a wide variation among institutions.[66, 67] Involvement of the seminal vesicles with tumor is accurately diagnosed 38 to 77% of the time.[66, 68] The sensitivity of TRU in detecting involvement of the periprostatic fat and neurovascular bundles is approximately 66%.[69] The main limitation with TRU is its inability to resolve low-volume or microscopic local extension or isoechoic tumor, whereas it is often capable of verifying large-volume extraprostatic disease. It was supposed that color Doppler TRU might improve the efficiency of detection of isoechoic tumors. Color Doppler TRU, however, appears to offer little advantage over the conventional gray scale imaging.[70]

**Magnetic Resonance Imaging and Computed Tomography.** The periprostatic tissues and seminal vesicles are not well visualized by computed tomography (CT), and clinical staging of localized disease is unrewarding with CT. Overall accuracy in staging the primary lesion is about 65%.[71] Data

*Table 50–1.* **Clinical Staging Systems for Prostate Cancer**

| | Jewett-Whitmore | UICC/AJCC | OSCC |
|---|---|---|---|
| **Nonpalpable Lesion** | | | |
| <3 foci, WD | $A_1$ | T1a | |
| <5% surgical specimen | | | $TA_1$ |
| >3 foci, or MD/PD | $A_2$ | T1b | |
| >5% specimen, or PD | | | $TA_2$ |
| PSA-detected tumor | | T1c | $TA_{psa}$ |
| **Palpable Lesion, Organ Confined** | | | |
| <1.5 cm, one lobe, palpably normal on 3 sides of nodule | $B_1$ | T2a | $TB_1$ |
| >1.5 cm | $B_2$ | T2b | $TB_2$ |
| Both lobes involved | $B_2$ | T2b | $TB_3$ |
| **Palpable Lesion, Non–Organ Confined** | | | |
| Lateral or apical extension | $C_1$ | T3 | |
| Unilateral extension, may include seminal vesicle | $C_2$ | T3 | $TC_1$ |
| Lateral and SV extension | $C_3$ | T3 | |
| Bilateral extension, may include seminal vesicles | | | $TC_2$ |
| Extension into contiguous organs (bladder, rectum, or pelvic side wall) | | T4 | $TC_3$ |
| **Lymph Node Status** | | | |
| Localized disease, elevated enzymatic acid phosphatase | $D_0$ | | $(M_1)$ |
| No regional adenopathy | | N0 | $N_0$ |
| Pelvic lymphadenopathy | $D_1$ | | |
| <2 cm, ≤5 nodes | | N1 | |
| microscopic, biopsy proven | | | $N_1$ |
| macroscopic, 2–5 cm | | | $N_2$ |
| or >5 nodes | | N2 | |
| Bulky adenopathy | | N3 | |
| Para-aortic adenopathy | $D_2$ | | $N_3$ |
| **Disseminated Disease** | | | |
| No evidence of metastasis | | M0 | $M_0$ |
| Osseous metastases | $D_2$ | M1 | $M_{2bone}$ |
| Visceral metastases | $D_2$ | M1 | $M_{2vis}$ |

UICC, Union Internationale Contre Cancer; AJCC, American Joint Committee on Cancer; WD, well differentiated; MD, moderately differentiated; PD, poorly differentiated; SV, seminal vesicle.

showed 11 to 55% sensitivity and 73 to 100% specificity for detecting the extraprostatic spread by CT.[72]

Magnetic resonance imaging (MRI) offers several advantages over CT (and TRU) in staging prostatic carcinoma. Ionizing radiation is avoided. Soft tissue resolution is superior with MRI when using T1-weighted and T2-weighted sequences. The peripheral zone of the gland is distinct from the transitional zone with MRI, and cancers on T1-weighted images show up with characteristically lower signal intensity, permitting diagnosis of extraprostatic disease. Imaging in two or more orthogonal planes is possible with MRI and has been shown to increase local staging accuracy with conventional body coil MRI by 20%.[71] Data showed 13 to 93% sensitivity and 57 to 100% specificity for detecting extraprostatic spread by MRI.[72]

Conventional body coil MRI is being supplanted by endorectal M coil imaging as an investigational tool for staging

prostate cancer. The accuracies of endorectal M coil imaging were approximately 68% for overall staging, 64 to 74% for staging extraprostatic disease, and 77 to 91% for depicting seminal vesicle invasion by carcinoma.[73, 74] Whether MRI improved on DRE in staging the primary lesion was not addressed. Overall accuracy is diminished by the appreciable false-negative rate resulting from the inability of MRI to resolve microscopic extension of tumor.

### Staging of Pelvic Lymph Nodes

Surgical staging of the pelvic lymph nodes remains the gold standard in diagnosing locally metastatic prostatic carcinoma. The incidence of lymph node metastases increases with increasing clinical stage. In the *PSA era*, the incidence of positive lymph nodes in each clinical stage has declined when compared with the *pre-PSA era*. Data showed 3.3 to 5% of lymph node metastases in clinical stage T1 (A2), 5.3 to 17% in clinical stage T2 (B), and 48% in clinical stage T3 (C).[75, 76] It is probable that most prostate cancers are currently being diagnosed at a lower tumor volume than previously, diminishing the likelihood of pelvic metastatic disease.

Laparoscopic pelvic lymphadenectomy has proved to be a useful, minimally invasive method of staging for prostate cancer in a highly select group of patients.[77, 78] The statistical models were developed by using clinical stage, PSA, and Gleason score to estimate the risk of pelvic lymph node metastases.[79, 80] Men with a serum PSA greater than 40 ng/ml, a Gleason sum of 8 or greater, or clinical stage T2b or T3 disease are considered suitable candidates, with the likelihood for metastases with these criteria being about 40 to 50%. Patients with clinical stage T1 or T2a carcinoma, PSA less than 20, and a Gleason sum of 6 or less have a low incidence of pelvic lymph node metastases and should not be considered for this procedure. In the hands of an experienced laparoscopist, the technique is safe, and the lymph node yield is roughly equivalent to an open approach. Hospital stay averages 23 hours, and the convalescence at home is considerably shortened (<1 week).

Axial imaging with CT or MRI is rarely rewarding in the staging of most cases of prostate cancer. The sensitivities were 30 to 60% in most series, with the specificities roughly at 80 to 90%.[72] False-negative results are usually due to the inability of CT or MRI to detect microscopic foci of metastatic disease, whereas false-positive results are due to reactive hyperplasia or other benign conditions. The only useful scenarios for obtaining these studies in previously untreated individuals are in the presence of high PSA levels (>100 ng/ml) or large volumes of poorly differentiated carcinoma on biopsy, where macroscopic metastases are more likely. Identification of pelvic or periaortic adenopathy with aspiration of suspicious nodes through computed tomographic guidance could save the patient exploration.

### Staging for Metastases

**Bone Scintigraphy.** Whole-body bone scans with technetium 99m have been a mainstay in the staging of prostatic carcinoma since the 1980s. Active areas of bone remodeling or activity incorporate the tracer and show high levels of radioactivity on the scintigram. The characteristic bone lesion with metastatic prostate cancer is an osteoblastic lesion, with extremely increased uptake of radiopharmaceutical in the normal bone surrounding the metastasis. The sensitivity for detection of bone lesions is superior to that of plain radiographs, and the specificity is superior to that of serum acid phosphatase levels.[81] Degenerative changes, Paget's disease, and fractures may cause diagnostic confusion, but correlation with site-specific plain radiographs usually reliably differentiates osteoblastic metastases from degenerative or healing changes in the bone.

False-negative results can occur with bone scans. The extreme case is the *superscan*, in which extensive, increased, symmetric uptake is seen. There is usually no isolated *hot spot*. In this scenario, extensive osseous metastases take up most of the tracer, leaving no tracer imaged in the kidneys. The absence of radiotracer in soft tissues, especially the kidneys, confirms the superscan and indicates widespread bone metastases. In cases of equivocal bone scans when site-specific radiographs fail to differentiate metastasis from benign bone disease, MRI of suspected bone lesions reliably confirms metastasis.

A bone scan is relatively expensive, and investigators have attempted to determine the utility of staging bone scintigraphy in men with prostate cancer and low PSA values. In the largest reported series, 852 men with newly diagnosed, untreated prostate cancer and PSA less than 20 ng/ml were evaluated with standard bone scintigraphy.[82] In the range of PSA values from 0 to 10 ng/ml, 3 of 561 (0.5%) men had an abnormal bone scan; in the range of PSA values from 10 to 20 ng/ml, 4 of 285 (1.4%) men had an abnormal scan. The authors concluded that in men with PSA less than 10.1 ng/ml and no bone pain, staging bone scan could be avoided. In 1994, the annual savings of eliminating unnecessary bone and computed tomographic scanning in patients with PSA values of less than 10.1 ng/ml were $114.6 million.[83] Men with poorly differentiated tumors and persistent bone pain should be evaluated by bone scan, however, regardless of PSA level.

**Serum Tumor Markers.** Serum acid phosphatase measurement is among the oldest tumor markers in medicine. It is a glycoprotein found in high concentrations in the epithelium of benign and malignant prostatic tissue. Disruption of the prostatic epithelium, as in metastatic carcinoma, allows the enzyme to enter the bloodstream in minute concentrations. Its primary application is as an immunohistochemical stain to confirm prostatic carcinoma and as a staging tool to document occult metastatic disease.

Several studies have documented the usefulness of serum enzymatic acid phosphatase (EAP) to detect occult metastatic disease.[84, 85] When serum EAP levels are persistently elevated (two or three occasions), metastases to the pelvic lymph nodes are diagnosed 60 to 100% of the time. Some investigators believe that serum EAP offers no unique information over PSA, DRE, Gleason grade, and bone scan.[86] Nevertheless, in cases of large, palpable tumors (T2b or T3) of higher grade, serum EAP is a cost-effective method of assessing pelvic lymph node metastases. Sensitivity for detecting lymphatic metastasis is poor (18% in one study), but specificity is good (>95%). In contrast to PSA, DRE can spuriously elevate serum EAP considerably. Drawing blood

for EAP should be avoided within 1 to 2 weeks of any prostatic manipulation.

Serum PSA values have modest utility in staging prostate cancer. The serum PSA level is roughly correlated with the volume of intracapsular carcinoma in radical prostatectomy specimens at a rate of 3.5 ng/ml/g cancer.[87] As the clinical stage of prostate cancer increases, the serum PSA level increases linearly.[88] As stated previously, at serum levels less than 10 ng/ml, bone metastases as detected by bone scan are rare, and most tumors are confined to the prostatic capsule.[82, 89] At a preoperative level of PSA of 50 ng/ml or greater, seminal vesicle invasion and pelvic lymphadenopathy predominate.[89] PSA levels between 10 and 50 ng/ml are somewhat unpredictable, although at the lower levels organ-confined disease is more likely, and at the higher levels stage T3 disease is most frequent. Levels greater than 100 ng/ml are usually associated with disseminated disease.

Currently the reverse transcriptase polymerase chain reaction of PSA mRNA has been used to detect a metastatic prostate cancer cell in peripheral blood. It was reported that reverse transcriptase polymerase chain reaction of bone marrow samples could detect 19 of 24 patients who had micrometastases that were undetected by conventional methods, such as PSA or bone scintigraphy.[90] The detection rate of prostate cancer cells in patients with metastases was high (88%), and the false-positive rate was low.[91] This procedure has also demonstrated the release of cancer cells into the circulation after TURP.[92] Reverse transcriptase polymerase chain reaction may improve the accuracy of staging metastatic disease and provide the best prognostic indicator. Because of the variation among laboratories, some investigators suggest that clinical decisions not depend on the reverse transcriptase polymerase chain reaction results only.[93]

### Summary of Staging

Careful pathologic staging using the whole-mount (axial step sectioning) technique has shown the significant clinical understaging errors that pervade the management of prostate cancer today. Microscopic capsular perforation, pathologic stage pT3, is a frequent occurrence even in clinical stage T1b and T1c tumors—a jump of two stage categories. The resolution power of all present-day imaging modalities is inadequate to predict this miniscule volume of tumor spread preoperatively. It remains to be seen if the pathologic documentation of such small volumes of extracapsular tumor is succeeded by clinically relevant tumor progression.

Men with prostate cancer and a serum PSA level of less than 10 ng/ml (Hybritech assay) likely do not require further staging work-up if DRE reveals organ-confined disease and the Gleason grade is 7 or less. A DRE that reveals clinical stage T3 disease is usually adequate to ensure extraprostatic disease, although some physicians prefer radiologic confirmation, and endorectal MRI seems to be the modality of choice for detecting periprostatic or seminal vesicle extension. A persistently elevated EAP is strong evidence for metastatic disease, but a normal value does not rule out lymphadenopathy. Laparoscopic lymphadenectomy may play a role in staging these patients because radiation therapy, the most commonly chosen treatment for this stage, should not be used in the presence of metastatic disease.

Most patients presenting with untreated prostate cancer fall into the category of T2b or small T3 disease on DRE, with PSA levels of 15 to 30 ng/ml, and moderately differentiated tumors. Bone scan is recommended in this scenario; CT or MRI is usually unrewarding. The prebiopsy TRU may be helpful in detecting extraprostatic disease, although ultrasonography is relatively insensitive at this task, and therapeutic decisions are not usually based on findings at TRU. The ultimate dilemma is whether or not small volumes of extraprostatic disease almost guaranteed to occur in this case that are managed by surgery or radiation become clinically significant over a 10- to 15-year period.

## PROGNOSTIC INDICATORS

A reliable prognostic indicator would answer many of the unsolved questions surrounding the management of prostate cancer. None of the currently available methods of predicting tumor behavior is universally trusted to guide treatment decisions in all cases of prostate cancer. Prognostication in prostate cancer currently involves weighing the biologic data of tumor grade, stage, suspected volume, and behavior with clinical data such as PSA levels and trends against the individual's age and general health status. Errors in measurement and interpretation abound in all these parameters, leaving the clinician confounded in assigning a risk to the individual patient's tumor. When these uncertainties are combined with the variable performance of present therapeutic modalities, potentially inconsistent results follow. A reliable indicator of prostatic tumor behavior is sorely needed if we are to improve on the present state of the science.

As presented earlier, the Gleason grading system has shown considerable reliability in predicting patient survival.[3, 27] Patients with scores of 2 to 4 have a generally indolent course, whereas those with scores of 8 to 10 suffer from a rapid, aggressive course. In large series of prostate cancer cases, however, two thirds of tumors are graded 5 to 7. The course of an individual in this intermediate grade, although intermediate in relation to the aforementioned subsets, is often unpredictable.

Gleason score is an independent predictor of the presence of lymphatic metastases. The average incidence for grades 2 to 4 is about 10%; for grades 5 to 7, about 33%; and for grades 8 to 10, about 60%.[65, 93] The Gleason sum has also been correlated with the incidence of extracapsular and seminal vesicle extension.[94]

The Gleason system is often criticized for its subjectivity. Nevertheless, if allowances are made for an intraobserver variance of +1 for the interpretation of biopsy material, the Gleason grading system is highly reproducible (85%).[95] Problems occur when attention is directed toward the histologic architecture. The result is often omission of subtle grade 4 tumors, which upgrades the tumor score considerably (usually to a sum of 7). The phenomenon of undergrading biopsy material usually by 1 point when compared with final pathologic grade should always be remembered. Undergrading is believed to be due to systematic bias on the part of the pathologist, who is often reluctant to give credence to a small focus of grade 4 or 5 cancer in a thin biopsy specimen. Sampling error is not suspected to be responsible.

The Gleason grading system has enjoyed widespread support since the 1970s. It proposes to qualify and quantify the rate at which the tumor may progress and not simply document the extent of tumor involvement. It has its greatest usefulness in predicting outcome when it is combined with other prognostic parameters.

*Clinical stage* at presentation has an impact on ultimate survival. Similar to grade, the extreme ends of the staging classifications have fairly predictable outcomes. Most men with stage T1 cancer do not die of their disease, but most men with metastatic stage die of the disease. A patient with a classic T2a nodule can expect a favorable outcome with treatment. Most patients who present with palpable prostate cancer fall into the category of T2b or T3 disease, and the prognosis for these stages is uncertain.

Stage T1a ($A_1$) prostate cancer carries an excellent long-term prognosis. Although in one study 16% of men with T1a disease showed signs of cancer progression when followed for 8 years, nearly half of the men died of other causes, and none died of prostate cancer.[96] Most studies show a progression rate in T1a carcinoma of 10% or less.[97] In surgical series in which stage T1a was managed aggressively, no patients had pelvic lymph node metastases, and 90 to 100% of patients had residual carcinoma in the prostate specimen.[93, 96, 98] Frequently the residual carcinoma is small ($<1$ cm$^3$) and focal, although diffuse, higher-grade tumors may be present 10 to 30% of the time.[96, 98] Repeat transurethral resection of the prostate discloses residual tumor 18 to 37% of the time, but few patients are reclassified as stage T1b ($A_2$) by this method.[99, 100] The relatively indolent nature of stage T1a disease predicts a good prognosis for most with this stage of disease. Young, healthy men may require aggressive management in efforts to avoid the 16% progression rate previously quoted.

Stage T1b ($A_2$) disease carries a much poorer prognosis than T1a and T2a carcinoma. Stage T1b tumors are usually diffuse and of higher volume than small stage T2a nodules, with a greater propensity to lymphatic metastases. Approximately 15% of clinical stage T2a tumors have metastasized to the regional lymphatics at presentation, whereas 30% of clinical stage T1b tumors have disseminated.[93, 101] The natural history of untreated stage T1b carcinoma is tumor progression in 25 to 35% and osseous metastases in 18% at 5 to 10 years.[102–104] With untreated T2a disease, most patients have local progression at a mean interval of 5 years after diagnosis, with 25% requiring transurethral resection of the prostate for symptomatic voiding difficulties.[105] Osseous metastases arise in 20% of these patients during follow-up. The diffuse or higher grade variant of occult prostatic carcinoma behaves more aggressively than the focal variant, confirming the need for the division of stage T1 (A) into T1a ($A_1$) and T1b ($A_2$) categories.

The division of stage T2 (B) prostate cancer into T2a ($B_1$) and T2b ($B_2$) categories in the early 1970s was probably the earliest recognition that tumor volume was prognostically important.[106] In one series, 80% of clinically staged T2a nodules contained tumor volumes of 4 cc or less, whereas T2b nodules and T2c (tumor involves both lobes) contained 2 to 40 cc of tumor, with extraprostatic extension diagnosed frequently.[107] The distinction between T2b and T3 disease clinically is often not clear because of the low sensitivity of DRE. What is clear is that the likelihood for pathologic upstaging to stage T3 in clinically staged T2b nodules is high.[65, 107] Most patients presenting with clinically localized disease fall into this category, and better prognostic indicators are definitely needed.

Although 15% of patients with clinical T2a nodules have pelvic lymph node metastases on surgical staging, 40% of T2b and 50% of T3 tumors are upstaged to N1–N3 ($D_1$) after pelvic lymphadenectomy.[65] Most surgical staging series with pelvic lymphadenectomy were performed before the widespread use of serum PSA as a screening device. The incidence of positive lymph nodes appears to be declining, possibly as a result of earlier detection of cancer; even stage T3 disease may be picked up earlier now. The pathologic manifestation of increased clinical stage is often a greater tumor volume. Whether volume is an independent prognostic indicator is contentious because tumor grade, anatomic location, and ploidy may be ultimately more important in a given tumor's natural course. Low-volume tumors located at the apex are a frequent source of pathologic extraprostatic disease so that volume is not always the primary predictor for tumor behavior. Nevertheless, larger-volume tumors show a propensity for capsular penetration and local dissemination. Palpably large tumors should be highly respected by the treating physician because they may be predictive for extracapsular prostate cancer. As presented earlier, no preoperative study is able to predict reliably cancer volume or extraprostatic disease any better than DRE. Serum PSA is showing promise in this area, but its ultimate reliability in predicting extraprostatic disease is yet to be defined.

Metastatic disease is prognostically important. Nearly all men who present at this stage die of prostate cancer. Patients with M1 ($D_2$) disease can expect a median 30-month survival, whereas those presenting with N1 3M0 disease can expect to live 5 years and sometimes 10 years before succumbing to cancer.[108, 109] Within stage M1 disease, prognosis is altered by the patient's performance status, serum testosterone level, and presence of bone pain and number of osseous metastases on bone scintigraphy.[108, 110] Patients with a good performance status (Eastern Cooperative Oncology Group 0-2), serum testosterone greater than 8.6 nmol/L, and two or fewer metastases in the axial skeleton tend to live longer than patients with poor performance status, lower testosterone levels, and large volumes of osseous metastases at presentation.[108, 110]

*Pretreatment serum PSA* has been an important predictor of the results of definitive treatments for clinically localized prostate cancer. Data suggested that 3- to 5-year rates of biochemical failure stratified by pretreatment PSA less than 4 ng/ml, 4 to 10 ng/ml, 10 to 20 ng/ml, and greater than 20 ng/ml are approximately 8%, 17 to 26%, 45 to 55%, and 55 to 80% for radical prostatectomy series and 0 to 31%, 10 to 56%, 11 to 73%, and 20 to 87% for radiotherapy series.[111] There were variations of the outcomes as well as the definitions of biochemical failure among those series, however. The value of pretreatment PSA for prediction of prostate cancer is still unclear. The combination of pretreatment PSA with other prognostic factors could improve the prognostic accuracy.

The measurement of the DNA content of tumor cells (*ploidy*) using flow cytometric techniques is anticipated as a potential breakthrough in predicting the behavior of prostate cancer. Ploidy analysis shows value in predicting progression of stage T1 cancers and in predicting survival in metastatic cancer.[112] Tumors with a large aneuploid peak on flow cytometry are less likely to respond to hormonal ablation in metastatic cases.[113] Many studies that attempt to define the predictive capacity of flow cytometry fail to stratify by treatment, Gleason grade, and PSA. The value of this technique is still unclear.

*Molecular biomarkers* have also been anticipated as a prognostic factor. p53 presented approximately 3 to 12% in patients with clinically localized disease. p53 was found in 66% of patients with locally advanced disease or metastatic disease.[114] Ki-67 and *bcl-2* have been significantly correlated to PSA recurrence after radical prostatectomy.[115, 116] Many investigators have combined the prognostic variables (e.g., stage, pretreatment PSA, Gleason score, tumor volume, DNA ploidy, p53, *bcl-2*, and Ki-67) into a biostatistical model for predicting the risk of recurrence.[117] Some investigators, however, indicated that p53, Ki-67, and DNA ploidy are not as reliable predictors of survival as stage or Gleason score.[118] The value of these molecular biomarkers for survival prediction is still unresolved.

Currently, many investigators use *neovascularity* as a novel prognostic marker. The essential requirement for tumor progression is the neovascularity. Microvessel density was correlated to the pathologic stage of radical prostatectomy specimens.[119] It showed a 44% sensitivity, 100% specificity, and 100% positive predictive value for organ-confined disease.

Other prognostic indicators are currently being developed or are under evaluation, including analysis of nuclear roundness, nucleolar morphology, neuroendocrine differentiation, androgen receptor status, serum tissue polypeptide antigen levels, and free PSA levels. Although it is hoped that one or more of these markers may show merit as a predictor of tumor behavior, the ultimate key to identifying tumor behavior likely resides in the tumor's genome, and study at the molecular level may yield the greatest rewards.

## Treatment

### OBSERVATION

A large, prospective trial on conservative management of localized prostate cancer in Sweden has generated considerable discussion in the international urologic and oncologic communities.[102] More than 200 men with clinically localized prostate cancer were followed for a mean of 10 years (range, 81 to 165 months). The mean age at presentation was 72 years, and most men had well-differentiated (grade 1–3), occult T1 disease (stage A). One third of the men showed progression of disease or metastasis, requiring transurethral resection of the prostate for relief of local progression causing urinary obstruction or hormonal ablation for disseminated disease. Only 9% of the men have died of prostate cancer, and 47% have died of other causes. This landmark study shows that highly selected, older men with well-differentiated, low-volume prostate cancer frequently die of competing co-morbidities and can be carefully watched and treated for symptomatic progression.

A smaller American series on delayed therapy for localized prostatic carcinoma has been reviewed, with the finding that 61% of patients ultimately require some form of treatment for prostate cancer—usually transurethral resection of the prostate for voiding difficulties (roughly one third) or androgen ablation for metastasis (roughly one fourth).[105] In this series of 75 men with mostly well to moderately differentiated stage T2 tumors at diagnosis, 11 have died of prostate cancer and 18 have died of other causes (7 lost to follow-up). At a median follow-up of about 10 years, median actuarial survival for patients with stage T2a lesions was 216 months; T2b lesions, 138 months; and T2c lesions, 197 months.

The subjects in both of these series represent a highly selected group of men with prostate cancer so that extrapolation to the average American man with prostate cancer is perilous. A meta-analysis of conservative management (observation and delayed hormonal therapy) of clinically localized prostate cancer (n = 828) showed that 10-year disease-specific survival was 87% for men with low-grade and moderate-grade prostate cancer and 34% for those with poorly differentiated prostate cancer.[120] Another study indicated that 65- to 75-year-old men with low-grade localized prostate cancer had a similar risk of dying from prostate cancer compared with the general population within 10 years.[121]

Observation appears to be appropriate for older men with an average life expectancy of 10 years or less and low risk of progression. As discussed later, these results were compared with series using radiation therapy and radical prostatectomy at time of diagnosis.

## RADICAL PROSTATECTOMY

Radical prostatectomy may be carried out through an abdominal or perineal approach. Each approach has its proponents, although neither the abdominal nor the perineal approach is necessarily superior to the other. Neither approach requires peritoneal disruption so that the risk of intra-abdominal adhesions and small bowel obstruction is avoided. The perineal incision does not violate the abdominal fascia and may be less painful to the patient, but staging lymphadenectomy is not possible through the perineal approach (requiring laparotomy or laparoscopy if lymph node status is desired). Most contemporary urologists are not trained in perineal prostatectomy, although the procedure is enjoying a renaissance. Many experienced urologists can carry out open staging lymphadenectomy and radical retropubic prostatectomy in about 2 hours, and nearly all urology residents entering practice today are trained in the retropubic procedure.

Radical prostatectomy is indicated in men with clinically localized adenocarcinoma of the prostate who have a 10-year life expectancy. Some controversy surrounds the use of the procedure in men older than age 70, even if 10 years or more of quality life is predicted. This concern is logical because many men with moderately differentiated stage B carcinoma live 10 years with expectant management (see previous discussion). Radical prostatectomy is not without attendant morbidity, and the mortality rate is about 1%. Even the most physically fit man in his 70s may be well served to select an alternative approach to radical prostatectomy.

The anatomic radical retropubic prostatectomy (potency

sparing) is a proven technique that does not increase the likelihood of positive surgical margins.[122] The overall incidence of positive surgical margins (stage pT3a or pT3b) is 10%, and this is equal to the overall incidence of seminal vesicle involvement (stage pT3c), indicating that these patients have extensive disease as the source for their tumor extensions and are not due to attempts to preserve the neurovascular bundles for potency. Local control with anatomic radical prostatectomy is excellent, with less than 5% local recurrence in clinical stages T1a and T2a disease and less than 8% local recurrence in clinical stage T1b and T2b disease at 5 years. These data compare favorably with reported series that make no attempt to preserve the neurovascular structures. Local recurrence at 5 years in patients with pathologically advanced disease (T3) is 8%. The key feature in preserving local control is early intraoperative identification of potentially advanced nodules and sacrifice of the neurovascular bundle on that side.[122, 123]

Complications from radical prostatectomy have been well defined.[122] Postoperative deep venous thrombosis and pulmonary embolism occur at a rate of 1 to 12% and 1 to 5%. Early postoperative ambulation is the key to avoiding these complications. Systemic anticoagulation has been attempted with minidose heparin subcutaneously or oral warfarin, with no demonstrable advantage over simple attention to early ambulation. The incidence of lymphocele collection with these anticoagulants may be increased. Patients with a known history of hypercoagulability should receive early postoperative anticoagulation.

Anastomotic stricture at the site of bladder neck reconstruction occurs in 3 to 12% of cases. Bladder neck contracture is usually easily remedied with dilatation in the office on one or two occasions. Rarely, endoscopically directed surgical incision is required to ensure an adequate lumen. Urinary incontinence severe enough to require wearing a protective pad occurs in 6% of men.[124, 125] Rarely does a patient require placement of an artificial urinary sphincter. One study showed that more than 50% of men undergoing radical prostatectomy have a component of detrusor instability (*spasticity*) before and after prostatectomy, indicating that the bladder and not the sphincter may be the cause for postprostatectomy incontinence.[126] Another study implicated a functionally shortened urethra as the likely cause.[127] Although stress urinary incontinence requiring wearing a protective pad occurs in less than 10% of men, total incontinence occurs rarely.

Before the landmark work by Walsh and Donker[1] that identified the course of the neurovascular structures responsible for erections, impotence was a nearly universal sequela of radical prostatectomy. With careful attention to the anatomic boundaries of radical prostatectomy, potency can be preserved in 63 to 68% of men.[124, 128] Independent variables related to potency preservation with prostatectomy include age, status of the neurovascular bundles, and pathologic stage.[128] Patients younger than age 50 can expect a 90% chance of return of erections postoperatively, whereas men older than age 70 can expect about a 20% chance of recovery of potency. Men between ages 50 and 70 can expect a 60 to 80% chance of recovery of potency if both neurovascular bundles are preserved, with the chances decreased to 40 to 60% if one neurovascular bundle is widely excised. With increasing pathologic stage, the likelihood for return of potency diminishes probably as a result of tumor invasion of the ipsilateral neurovascular bundle. The return of potency is often delayed 6 to 18 months postoperatively.[128] Implantation of an inflatable penile prosthesis should be deferred for an appropriate time until it is certain that natural erections will not return. Testing of men with postprostatectomy impotence using vasoactive intracavernosal therapy (papaverine) indicates that a vascular cause is as important as a neurogenic cause.[129]

Radical prostatectomy cures most patients with pathologic organ-confined disease. The serum PSA level after radical prostatectomy should decline to undetectable levels (PSA <0.2 ng/ml) within 3 weeks after surgery and should stay undetectable indefinitely.[5] Data suggested that 10-year likelihood of PSA progression-free rates after radical prostatectomy were approximately 71 to 90% in stage T1 or T2, 58 to 82% in stage T3a, 21 to 43% in stage T3b, and 0% in N1.[130] Outcomes in terms of cancer-specific survival are also excellent. Ten-year survival data with the anatomic radical prostatectomy have disclosed a 92 to 97% cancer-specific survival at 10 years and 86 to 94% survival at 15 years.[131] The calculated mean 10-year cancer-specific survival for radical prostatectomy was 93%. The incidence of poorly differentiated tumors in the studies reviewed was 16.6%. The mean number of deaths resulting from prostate cancer was approximately equal to the mean number of deaths resulting from other causes.

Examination of the entire prostate specimen using a 4-mm step section technique has led to the frequent detection of small foci of extraprostatic cancer. Small foci of cancer with a Gleason score of less than 7 do not ordinarily progress to local or distant failure.[132] Larger volumes of extracapsular cancer, high-grade (Gleason 8, 9, 10) extracapsular cancer, and positive surgical margins are all risk factors for local recurrence. The management of patients with positive surgical margins (pT3A or pT3b) or seminal vesicle invasion (pT3c) is unclear. One retrospective report indicated that adjuvant radiotherapy (45 Gy) conferred a survival advantage when compared with historical controls receiving no adjuvant EBRT.[133] Disease-specific 10-year actuarial survival was 78% with adjuvant therapy. Postoperative radiation therapy was least helpful to patients with poorly differentiated tumors (Gleason 8, 9, 10) or seminal vesicle invasion. Another retrospective report (n = 1035) of adjuvant EBRT or hormonal ablation compared with no immediate adjuvant therapy indicated that cause-specific survivals of pathologic stage T3 were 98%, 81%, and 66% at 5, 10, and 15 years.[134] Both adjuvant treatments appeared to have a similar efficacy and significantly decreased local and systemic progression but did not improve cause-specific survival.

Slowly rising PSA levels in patients with previously undetectable PSA levels indicate local recurrence or occult metastatic disease. The management of patients with this predicament is an evolving art. Adjuvant EBRT returns the serum PSA to undetectable levels, only to have them rise again later. TRU-guided biopsy of the urethrovesical anastomotic site should be performed to verify locally recurrent disease before instituting EBRT.[135] At present, adjuvant EBRT improves the local control rate but appears to have little impact on the later development of metastatic disease or death from prostate cancer.[134]

**Neoadjuvant Hormonal Ablation.** Despite the development of strategies for diagnosis and staging of prostate cancer, only 40 to 60% of patients with clinically localized prostate cancer have a pathologic organ-confined specimen after radical prostatectomy. The challenge of neoadjuvant hormonal ablation is to improve the proportion of pathologic organ-confined cancer and to prolong the survival. The available data suggest that neoadjuvant hormonal ablation can significantly improve organ-confined cancer rates (74 to 78% vs. 47 to 49% in control group) and positive margin rates (8 to 10% vs. 33% in control group) in clinically localized prostate cancer (T2).[136, 137] These studies do not have sufficient power to assess the survival end point, however.[136, 138] Even though neoadjuvant hormonal ablation could improve organ-confined and positive margin rates in stage T2, it failed to show these benefits in clinical stage T3.[138]

## RADIATION THERAPY

Tumoricidal doses of radiation may be delivered to the prostate in two ways. Radioactive seeds (e.g., iodine 125, gold 198, iridium 192) may be implanted into the gland, with localized cell death determined by the energy of the radiation source, its radius of penetration, and the natural decay of the isotope. In the 1950s, with the development of reliable sources of photonic energy from cobalt 60 and linear accelerators, megavoltage EBRT assumed pre-eminence as the nonsurgical method for curing prostate cancer. For nearly 30 years, EBRT was the most frequently chosen modality for management of localized or locally advanced prostatic carcinoma.

EBRT for prostate cancer is delivered in fractionated doses of approximately 20 cGy per setting for 32 to 35 visits. The prostatic region receives all 64 to 70 Gy, whereas the entire pelvis, including the first echelon lymph nodes, receives only 50 Gy during the regimen. Technologic developments of MRI or CT with conventional radiographs and computer planning software have improved the ability to localize tumors and spare adjacent organs. A method of EBRT called *three-dimensional conformal radiotherapy* has been shown to deliver high doses with decreased toxicity.[139]

The EBRT results of 30 years of treatment in 1031 men from Stanford University were reported for crude and cancer-specific survival, freedom from relapse, and clinical local control. Most patients were clinically staged T1–T3, with the lymph node status unknown in most of them. Most patients did receive irradiation to the first echelon pelvic lymph nodes, with many also receiving doses to the para-aortic nodes. The use of early or delayed adjuvant hormonal ablation is not addressed in the review. Overall survival depended on clinical stage. Patients with stage T1 cancer enjoyed a life span equal to that of a well-matched cohort without prostate cancer. Median actuarial crude survival for stage T2 disease was 12 to 14 years. Patients with stage T3 disease did poorly, with fewer than half surviving 7 years. It is likely that many patients with stage T3 disease had occult lymphatic metastases, and radiation treatments were doomed to fail in these men. In a subset analysis of 142 men with surgical staging, the 60 men with lymphatic metastases treated with extended radiotherapy did considerably worse than the 80 men who had no lymphatic disease.

Cancer-specific survival also depended on clinical stage.

More than 80% of patients with stage T1 cancer had actuarial disease-specific survival of greater than 20 years. Median cancer-specific survival for stage T2 disease was 14 to 20 years. Cancer-specific survival for stage T3 disease was nearly the same as crude survival in that stage. Failure of local control as defined by growth of tumor on DRE at 10 years was 15 to 25% for stage T2 disease. In a review of international results with EBRT, 10-year disease-specific survival of 62% was calculated for EBRT.[131] A report of long-term outcomes of more than 1000 patients with EBRT from Stanford University indicated that the 15-year survival of stage T1 and T2a cases with proven negative lymph nodes was 53%, whereas 15-year survivals of stage T3 and T4 cases were 18% and 15%.[140, 141]

Morbidity from EBRT of the prostate encompasses collateral damage to the nearby pelvic organs and failure of local control and its attendant morbidity. A review of the delayed complications resulting from radiation by a combined urologic and radiation oncology service provides a fair appraisal of the safety of EBRT.[142] Radiation cystitis, usually only troublesome but sometimes debilitating, occurs in 1 to 5% of patients treated with definitive EBRT. Urethral stricture and bladder neck contracture occur 11% of the time. Transurethral resection of the prostate, before EBRT or after definitive radiation, was the key risk factor in the development of stricture. As a result of the nonpliability of healed, radiated tissue, incision or dilatation of these strictures can precipitate severe stress incontinence or even total (continuous) incontinence. Overall, 4.7% of men treated with definitive EBRT experience significant incontinence. Radiation proctitis occurs in 10% of men, with rectourethral fistula formation requiring colostomy occurring in 2.4%. Anal stenosis occurs infrequently but is not amenable to surgical correction because of the density of the cicatrix, poorly vascularized local tissue, and relative rectosigmoid fixation by EBRT. Erectile difficulties and impotence occur in 20 to 40% of men treated with EBRT. The onset may be delayed 18 months, however. Complications resulting from local progression after EBRT include fistula formation, ureteral obstruction requiring urinary diversion, and bladder outlet obstruction requiring repeated transurethral resection of the prostate.

**Hormonal Ablation Combined with External-Beam Radiation Therapy.** The rationale for addition of EBRT to hormonal ablation in prostate cancer patients is to improve local control and probably prolong survival. This is an alternative treatment to avoid a higher radiation dose by reducing tumor before definitive radiation therapy and to treat disease outside the radiated field.[143] One randomized trial compared EBRT plus 3 years of goserelin acetate with EBRT alone in 401 patients with locally advanced disease.[144] With median follow-up of 45 months, a significant benefit of combined therapies in terms of overall survival at 5 years was demonstrated (79% vs. 48% in control group).

**Brachytherapy.** The history of prostatic brachytherapy spans 80 years, but the technique fell out of favor because of significant local failure rates, increased local morbidity, the need for surgical access, unsure dosimetry resulting from placement errors, and the increased popularity of EBRT and radical prostatectomy. An updated technique using currently available TRU or CT guidance of isotope implantation through the perineum has been able to implant accurately throughout the gland.[145]

The most popular sources for prostatic brachytherapy include palladium 103, gold 198, iridium 192, and iodine 125. Gold 198 has the highest energy level (412 kV) and shortest half-life (2.7 days) of the permanently implantable isotopes, whereas iridium 192 (340 kV, half-life 70 days) requires temporary implantation because of its high energy and longer half-life. The range of doses obtainable with brachytherapy nearly doubles that of EBRT, with approximately 90 to 160 Gy possible by these techniques.

The results with modern brachytherapy have been mixed. The early results of brachytherapy were likely poor because of technical difficulty replacing seeds accurately throughout the prostate gland uniformly.[145] Local control as shown by negative biopsy rates is disappointing.[146] Patients treated with gold 198 implants and EBRT had local failure rates of 40 to 60% for stages T2 and T3 disease. These rates were nearly identical for patients treated with iodine 125 alone. An analysis of stage T2a cases with brachytherapy from the New York Hospital–Queens showed that clinical and biochemical rates of freedom from relapse at 5 years were 79% and 64%.[147] Another report of stage T1–T2 patients treated with iodine 125 and palladium 103 showed that freedom from PSA failure at 4 years was 75%, 74%, and 34% for patients with PSA values of 10 ng/ml, 10.1 to 20 ng/ml, and greater than 20 ng/ml. Patients with Gleason scores of 2 to 6 had 85% negative 2-year biopsies versus 62% for those with a score of 7 or more.[148] Neoadjuvant hormonal ablation has been used for reduction of prostatic volume. It is also used for high-risk features (PSA >10 ng/ml, stage T2b, or Gleason score of 7) to improve outcomes.[148]

An attempt using modern brachytherapy to improve results in stage T2b–T3 tumors was the combination of conformal boost brachytherapy (iridium 192) and EBRT. Preliminary data showed that biochemical control in the brachytherapy boost treatment group was 85% compared with 52% in the EBRT-alone treatment group at 3-year follow-up.[149]

The results of brachytherapy appear to be as effective as EBRT for patients with early stage and low risk features.[145] These were not randomized data, however. A variety of techniques among institutions might affect these results. Long-term (10 to 15 years) outcomes of brachytherapy have not been presented. The value of brachytherapy for prostate cancer needs further follow-up and requires a randomized study for comparison with surgery or EBRT.

## HORMONAL ABLATION

The demonstration of the androgen sensitivity of human prostatic tissue and prostate cancer by Huggins and Hodges[150] was met with overwhelming enthusiasm because it was believed that a simple cure for systemic cancer had been discovered. With experience, the limitations of androgen ablation were readily apparent. Orchiectomy or oral DES were not able to cure disseminated prostate cancer, but long-term local control and significant palliation of metastatic disease were realized.[151] Fifty years after Huggins and Hodges' preliminary report, the demonstration of the

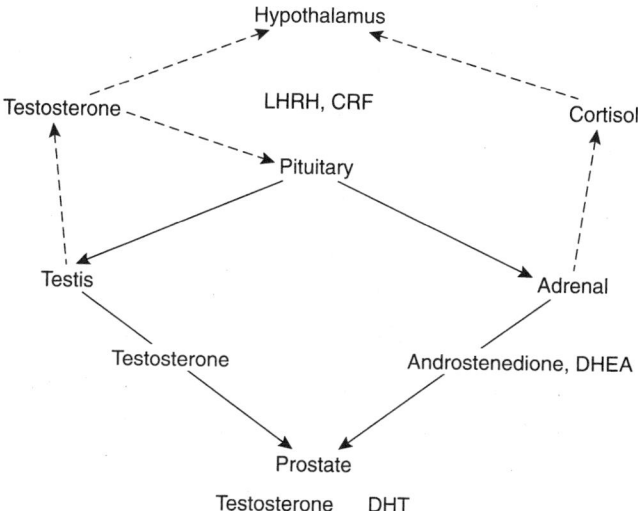

**Figure 50–1.** Endocrine axis in hormone regulation of prostate growth. LHRH, luteinizing hormone–releasing hormone; CRF, cortisol-releasing factor; LH, luteinizing hormone; FSH, follicle-stimulating hormone; ACTH, adrenocorticotropic hormone; DHT, dihydrotestosterone. (Redrawn from Mayer FJ, Crawford ED. Update on combined androgen blockade for metastatic prostate cancer. Adv Urol 1994;7:94.)

androgen sensitivity of human prostate cancer remains the most significant discovery in its treatment.

The endocrine axis responsible for androgen production and control is well characterized (Fig. 50–1). Central control of endocrine function is contained within the hypothalamus, which releases luteinizing hormone–releasing hormone (LHRH) into the anterior pituitary portal circulation in pulsa-tile fashion. The anterior pituitary responds with production and secretion of LH, which is transported systemically and stimulates the interstitial cells of Leydig (testes) to produce and secrete testosterone. In androgen-sensitive cells, testosterone is converted to the more potent androgen dihydrotestosterone by the enzyme 5α-reductase. Dihydrotestosterone is internalized in the nucleus and causes transcription of novel mRNA, with the ultimate translation of key proteins necessary in the maintenance of androgen-responsive cells. Testosterone is capable of negative feedback inhibition at the central level.

The hypothalamic-pituitary-adrenal axis also plays a significant role in androgen physiology. Cortisol-releasing factor stimulates adrenocorticotropic hormone (ACTH) secretion by the anterior pituitary gland. The zona reticularis responds to ACTH stimulation with release of the adrenal androgens dehydroepiandrosterone and androstenedione (along with cortisol). The relatively weak adrenal androgens compose less than 10% of the normal circulating androgen pool. Nevertheless, their importance in the maintenance of metastatic prostate cancer is becoming increasingly evident.

Medical therapies are available to block the above-mentioned endocrine axes at each level (Table 50–2). On the testicular side, the potent LHRH agonists leuprolide (Lupron, depot Lupron) and goserelin (Zoladex) cause pituitary desensitization by altering the normal pulsatile reception of LHRH by the pituitary gland. LH release is greatly diminished, and Leydig cell production of testosterone is diminished to *castration* levels (<50 ng/ml).

Finasteride (Proscar) is a competitive inhibitor of the 5α-reductase enzyme, blocking the conversion of testosterone to dihydrotestosterone.[152] Serum levels of testosterone remain

*Table 50–2.* **Agents Used in Androgen Blockade**

| Class | Mechanism of Action | Comments |
|---|---|---|
| *LHRH Analogues*<br><br>Leuprolide, goserelin | Pituitary desensitization ( ↓ LH, ↓ testosterone synthesis) | Transient flare of symptoms due to initial surge of LH secretion |
| *Steroidal Antiandrogens*<br><br>Megestrol acetate, cyproterone acetate | Primary: competitive inhibition of androgens at the receptor level<br>Secondary: progestational effect overrides the negative feedback of testosterone at the hypothalamus | Require administration of DES 0.1 mg/day to ensure continued pituitary suppression |
| *Nonsteroidal Antiandrogens*<br><br>Flutamide | Competitive inhibitor of androgen binding at the target cell level | Short half-life, weak affinity for androgen receptor |
| Nilutamide | Same as flutamide | Reversible interstitial lung disease in 1–3% of patients; bothersome side effect of impaired adaptation to darkness |
| Bicalutamide (Casodex) | Same as flutamide | Once-daily dosing; greater affinity for androgen receptor than flutamide (4×); 10× more potent than flutamide |
| *Other Agents*<br><br>Aminoglutethimide | Inhibitor of adrenal steroidogenesis by blocking P450-mediated hydroxylation | Requires the administration of hydrocortisone to suppress ACTH levels |
| Ketoconazole | Inhibitor of P450 enzymes in testes and adrenals | Castration levels achieved in <24 hr (useful with impending spinal cord compression) |

LHRH, luteinizing hormone–releasing hormone; LH, luteinizing hormone; DES, diethylstilbestrol; ACTH, adrenocorticotropic hormone.
From Mayer FJ, Crawford ED. Update on combined androgen blockade for metastatic prostate cancer. Adv Urol 1994;7:96.

normal or elevated, but intracellular levels of dihydrotestosterone are considerably lowered. The utility of finasteride in treating prostate carcinoma remains to be elucidated.

The nonsteroidal antiandrogens (flutamide [Eulexin], nilutamide [Anandron], bicalutamide [Casodex]) are a group of drugs capable of competitively binding with testosterone and the adrenal androgens for intracytoplasmic and intranuclear receptors.[153, 154] They have generally negligible stimulatory capability, so they have become a valuable means of blocking the function of testicular and adrenal androgens. Concerns over incomplete blockade of testosterone have limited their utility as monotherapeutic means of androgen blockade. The steroidal antiandrogens cyproterone acetate and megestrol acetate (Megace) have peripheral antiandrogenic function and central inhibitory function at the pituitary level.[155, 156] Use of the steroidal antiandrogens requires coadministration of *minidose* DES (0.1 mg/day) to obviate pituitary escape from antiandrogen control.

Potent inhibitors of adrenal steroidogenesis have been used to treat patients relapsing from hormonal blockade and, infrequently, as first-line therapies for metastatic prostate cancer. Aminoglutethimide was originally marketed as an anticonvulsant but was withdrawn from that indication when several patients developed clinical adrenal insufficiency. It blocks several steps in cytochrome P450–mediated hydroxylation of adrenal steroid precursors. Its physiologic function may be overcome by endogenous ACTH, so the drug must be administered with physiologic doses of hydrocortisone (aminoglutethimide 250 mg three times per day with hydrocortisone 40 mg twice a day).[157] The antifungal ketoconazole, when used at supratherapeutic doses (400 mg three times per day), can also inhibit cytochrome P450–mediated steroidogenesis in the testes and adrenals. It is most effective in managing the patient with impending spinal cord compression resulting from metastases because its use is associated with castration levels of serum testosterone within hours of administration.[158]

The LHRH analogues have shown efficacy equal to DES and bilateral orchiectomy in treating patients with metastatic prostate cancer.[159, 160] Overall, about 60 to 80% of men with metastatic prostate cancer treated with monotherapy (DES, LHRH analogue, orchiectomy, and antiandrogens) experience a subjective and objective response or disease stabilization for a mean duration of 20 to 24 months. Once the hormone-refractory state is achieved, mean duration of survival is 6 to 9 months, with few therapies providing significant response. The antiparasitic agent suramin has shown antineoplastic properties in vitro, including blocking the activity of epidermal growth factor and fibroblast growth factor, and has shown promise in clinical trials for treating hormone-refractory prostate cancer.[161]

The unfavorable cardiovascular profile of DES at doses of 3 mg/day or greater has tempered enthusiasm for its use.[151, 159] DES appears to be a cost-effective means of achieving castration levels of serum testosterone until the cost of hospitalization and treatment of thromboembolic complications are considered. In many studies, a 20 to 25% rate of severe, often fatal cardiovascular and thromboembolic side effects has consistently been shown. Employing DES at 1 mg/day greatly diminished these side effects and was as effective as DES at 5 mg/day or orchiectomy.[3, 162] Orchiectomy is generally well tolerated, with the principal side effects of decreased libido, impotence, gynecomastia, and vasomotor hot flashes. Gynecomastia may be prevented with a short course of EBRT (800 cGy) to the breasts before orchiectomy. The LHRH analogues are well tolerated, with most patients experiencing vasomotor hot flashes (about 60%), impotence, testicular shrinkage, and decreased libido and some patients experiencing peripheral edema (about 10%) and gynecomastia.

The results of the VACURG 1 study indicated that patients originally receiving placebo, then going on to orchiectomy or DES at the first signs of progression, had survival similar to patients receiving orchiectomy or DES at enrollment.[151] It was then inferred that delayed endocrine ablation was preferable to early endocrine ablation. For the next 20 years, most patients with metastatic prostate cancer were managed by delayed hormonal ablation. When cancer-specific survivals were later calculated, however, a benefit of early androgen ablation was seen.[3] Currently, it is generally agreed that symptomatic metastatic disease should be promptly treated by hormonal therapy. The controversy of immediate versus deferred treatment has remained for asymptomatic patients. Data showed that patients with good performance status and few osseous metastases (low-volume disease) have a superior survival if endocrine blockade is initiated at diagnosis.[108] Many studies have shown that early hormonal treatment had delayed progression in surgically proven stage N1–N3 M0 patients.[67, 163] A randomized study of patients with locally advanced or asymptomatic metastatic disease indicated that immediate hormonal ablation had a significant advantage in subjective responses (pain), the prolongation of time to progression, and overall survival compared with the deferred group.[164] Immediate hormonal treatment appears to improve quality of life and prevent complications from advanced metastasis, such as bladder outlet obstruction, uremia, or spinal cord compression.

**Combined Androgen Blockade.** The contribution of the adrenal glands to the maintenance of prostate cancer was suspected in the 1940s, when Huggins and Scott[165] treated several men with hormone-refractory prostate cancer by bilateral adrenalectomy. Survival with this approach was short because of the lack of effective adrenal hormone replacement therapy. *Medical* adrenalectomy was later attempted with cortisol, aminoglutethimide, and ketoconazole, among other agents. Responses to secondary hormonal ablation were variable but enough to keep several endocrinologists and urologists interested in the concept of total androgen ablation. Basic research revealed that although the adrenal androgens account for only 5 to 10% of the circulating androgen pool, they are responsible for 20% of the total intraprostatic dihydrotestosterone.[166] Additionally, 50% of the intraprostatic dihydrotestosterone remains after orchiectomy or medical castration.[167] These basic research findings coupled with the responses seen with medical adrenalectomy became the foundation for the clinical trials in the early 1980s of combined androgen blockade: eliminate testicular androgen by surgical or medical castration combined with an antiandrogen.

The first report of combined androgen blockade was met with considerable enthusiasm.[168] Markedly superior survival with LHRH agonist and antiandrogen therapy was shown in comparison to monotherapy. The study was criticized because of the addition of patients with stage T3 disease and

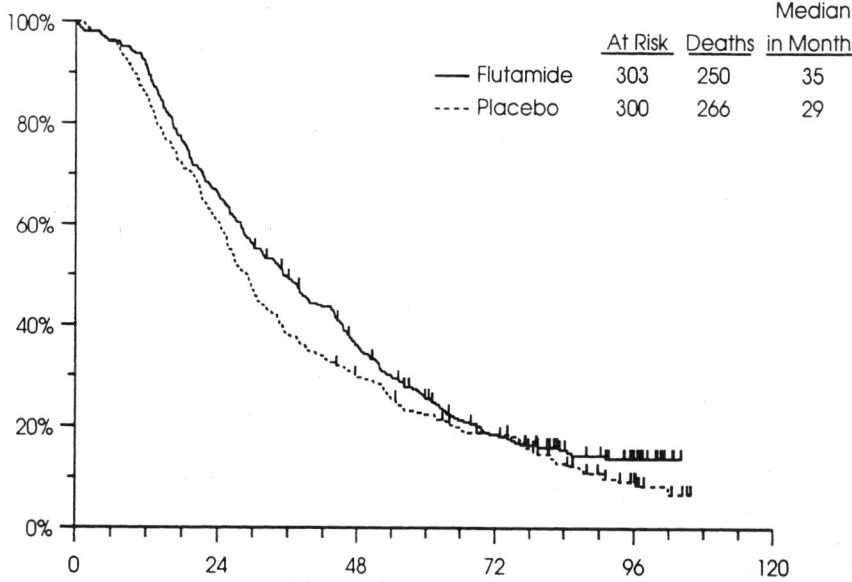

**Figure 50–2.** National Cancer Institute Intergroup Protocol 0036. Leuprolide with flutamide or placebo: overall survival, February 1994.

because of lack of a control arm. The first study to document clearly the benefits of combined androgen blockade was the National Cancer Institute Intergroup Study (0036) of 603 men with newly diagnosed metastatic prostate cancer.[108] Patients receiving leuprolide and flutamide (250 mg PO three times per day) enjoyed longer disease-free intervals and survival when compared with their cohort receiving leuprolide and placebo. Overall a 7-month increased survival was seen in men receiving flutamide (Fig. 50–2). In men with good performance status and minimal osseous metastases, survival was prolonged by 19 months when compared with equally matched subjects not receiving flutamide (Fig. 50–3). Men with poor performance status and widely disseminated disease did not benefit from the addition of flutamide. Flutamide was well tolerated, with 15% of patients experiencing mild or moderate diarrhea. Several other studies have con-

firmed the benefit of adding early adrenal androgen blockade to medical or surgical castration.[169, 170]

Several other studies failed to show survival advantages.[171–174] The results of a large randomized study (n = 1371) failed to show a significant survival benefit of orchiectomy plus 750 mg/day of flutamide compared with orchiectomy alone (33 months vs. 30 months) in patients with metastatic disease.[175] It also failed to show a significant survival benefit in men with good performance status and minimal metastases. Some investigators argued that an insufficient statistical power for showing a survival benefit might be due to an insufficient number of patients, or it may be too early to evaluate survival differences in some trials.

At present, the controversy of an advantage of combined androgen blockade as a first-line therapy for newly diagnosed metastatic disease remains unresolved. Even though

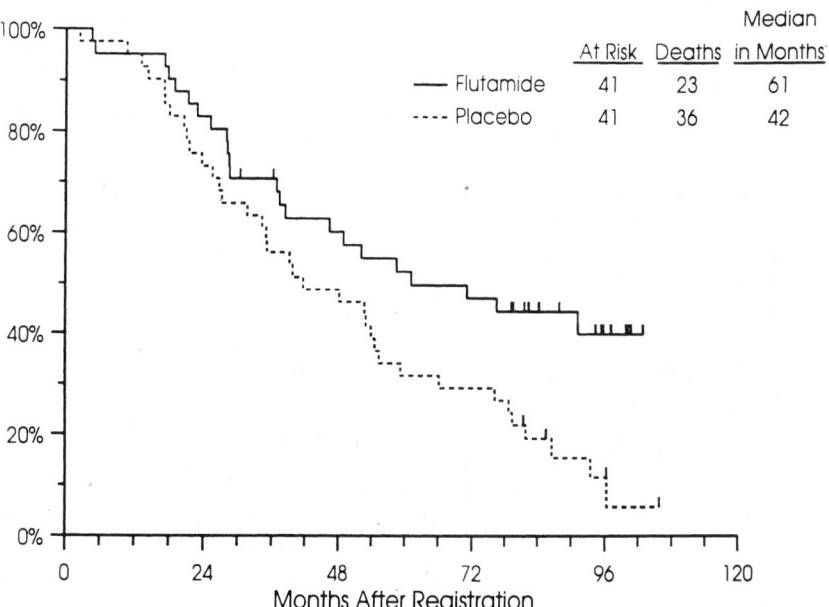

**Figure 50–3.** National Cancer Institute Intergroup Protocol 0036. Leuprolide with flutamide or placebo: overall survival, February 1994, good-prognosis subset.

some studies failed to show a statistically significant difference in terms of survival, most studies showed a benefit of combined androgen blockade in terms of subjective or objective response rates.

**Intermittent Androgen Ablation Therapy.** Most prostatic cancers develop an androgen-independent state during antiandrogen therapy. It has been proposed that intermittent androgen administration may mitigate the development of resistance to antiandrogen therapy.[176] This concept may improve quality of life, reduce side effects and cost of treatment, and probably delay time to development of hormone resistance and tumor progression. One study of 47 patients with two cycles of intermittent combined androgen blockade showed that serum testosterone levels returned to normal range within 8 weeks after stopping treatment.[177] The mean and median times to progression were similar to the expected results of continuous androgen ablation. In nontreatment periods, libido and potency returned in patients who reported normal sexual function before therapy. It remains unclear whether intermittent hormonal therapy alters survival.

**Antiandrogen Withdrawal Syndrome.** In 1993, data showed paradoxical responses, such as a decrease of PSA, symptoms, or objective signs, on withdrawal of flutamide in approximately 40% of patients with progression on LHRH analogue plus flutamide treatment.[178] Many investigators hypothesized that the androgen receptor mechanism probably mutates and recognizes the antiandrogen as a stimulator.[179] The current recommendation for management in patients whose disease progresses after combined androgen blockade therapy is withdrawal of antiandrogens.

## CHEMOTHERAPY AND PALLIATIVE THERAPY

The use of cytotoxic chemotherapy in hormone-refractory prostate cancer has been assiduously reviewed.[180–182] The relatively chemoresistant nature of prostate cancer has been borne out in years of studies with single-agent and multidrug combinations. No single agent has shown superiority over its counterparts, and no drug combination seems particularly effective. Overall, about 10 to 30% of patients experience an objective response or disease stabilization. The median survival using these treatments is 9 months. The low efficacy of cytotoxic chemotherapy might be from a low fraction of actively dividing cells or inherent resistance of tumor cells.

Trials with chemotherapy in prostate cancer are hindered by the lack of radiographic bidimensional disease measurements in most cases because of the proclivity for prostate cancer to metastasize to the bones. Although gross objective data may be obtained when bone scans are radically changed during therapy, standard bone scintigraphy is incapable of providing the measurable disease parameters that are important in evaluating response to chemotherapeutic agents. Serum PSA and PSAP are often used as objective criteria for response, although in widely metastatic disease, PSA is an unreliable measure of tumor volume. Finally, most studies include *disease stabilization* in their response data. If these trials were controlled, disease stabilization might imply a benefit of therapy; nevertheless, most chemotherapeutic trials are nonrandomized and uncontrolled, and disease stabilization may represent nothing more than the natural history of untreated cancer.

Adjuvant chemotherapy has been tried with early endocrine therapy in the hope of capturing the hormone-refractory clones at a lower volume and earlier stage of dedifferentiation.[183] No benefit was seen with the earlier initiation of cytotoxic chemotherapy when compared with hormonal ablation alone. The drug-resistant, slow-growing nature of most prostate cancers makes them particularly resistant to standard chemotherapy. The antiparasitic agent suramin generally yielded 20 to 40% objective response rates and greater than 1-year median survival in metastatic prostate cancer.[181] Data also showed the clinical limitations of suramin, however, including neurotoxicity and adrenal insufficiency. The management of hormone-refractory prostate cancer should be centered around limiting toxicity and providing optimal palliative care for men with a life expectancy of months.

Significant palliation of bone metastases in men with hormone-refractory prostate cancer is possible with EBRT to the metastases or with hemibody irradiation.[184, 185] Patients with solitary, painful osseous metastases treated with 20 to 40 Gy of EBRT experience complete relief 60% of the time and partial relief 80% of the time. Half the patients with multiple painful lesions treated with 30 Gy had complete relief of pain, with most patients experiencing partial relief of bone pain.[184] Complete relief of bone pain in patients treated with hemibody irradiation ranges from 20 to 80%, depending on the extent of disease,[185] and the symptomatic relief of bone pain in patients treated with hemibody irradiation usually persists until death.

Strontium 89 has been used for the palliative treatment of symptomatic osseous metastases. Strontium 89 is a beta-particle emitter with a half-life of 50 days. It is handled as a calcium imitator, with uptake and retention into areas of active bone metabolism. It is *washed out* of healthy bone within 14 days of administration but is retained in the metastatic sites. The approximate absorbed dose locally in the bone lesion varies from 2 to 20 Gy.[186] In randomized trials, the addition of strontium 89 to local field EBRT reduced the rate of progression of painful bone metastases and diminished the likelihood for new lesions to arise.[187] At present, approximately 80% of patients with painful bone lesions resulting from hormone-refractory prostate cancer respond to strontium 89.[188] Currently the bisphosphonate clodronate has also been used for bone pain of metastatic prostate cancer.[189] Clodronate relieves bone pain within 3 days after intravenous administration. It is one of the most cost-effective palliative treatments for metastatic prostate cancer.

## CRYOSURGICAL ABLATION

Freezing the prostate gland was attempted in the 1960s and abandoned because of high associated morbidity and the widespread acceptance of radiation therapy in that era. At that time, the procedure was performed without careful intraoperative imaging, leading to unsure placement of the freezing device, which had obvious implications for success in eradicating cancer and limiting unwarranted freezing of the bladder and rectum. With the advent of modern TRU and the development of safer cryogenic delivery systems, TRU-guided cryoablation of the prostate has re-emerged as an exciting investigative technique for the treatment of clinically localized adenocarcinoma of the prostate.

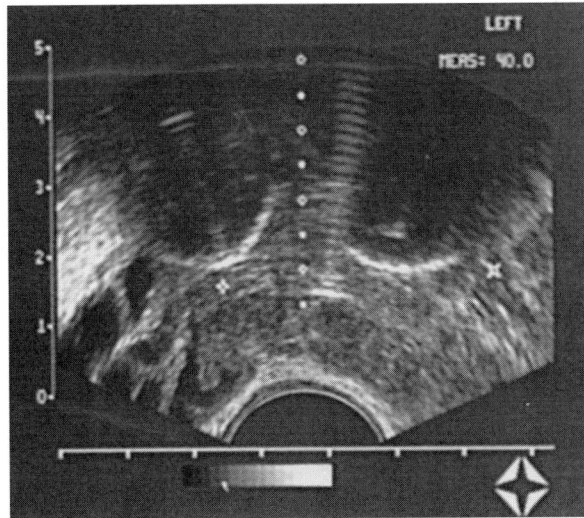

**Figure 50–4.** Transverse ultrasonographic image after placement of five probes within the prostate, showing the upper probes freezing with an anechoic ice ball forming around both superior probes.

Suitable candidates are treated in the operating room under regional or general anesthesia and discharged either the day of the procedure or the following day. The prostate is imaged intraoperatively with real-time TRU. Five stainless steel probes are placed in the prostate gland with ultrasonographic guidance through five small puncture sites in the perineal skin, qualifying the procedure as a minimally invasive technique. The stainless steel probes circulate supercooled liquid nitrogen throughout their steel core; the liquid is not allowed to escape into the tissue. Freezing of the prostate and periprostatic tissue is followed ultrasonographically throughout the procedure (Figs. 50–4 and 50–5). The mass of tissue frozen shows up on the ultrasonogram as an anechoic region termed the *ice ball.* The urethra is protected with a warming catheter. The anterior rectal wall cools but should not be frozen. Close monitoring of the advancement of the ice ball toward the rectal wall and DRE ensure that undue cooling of the anterior rectal wall does not occur.

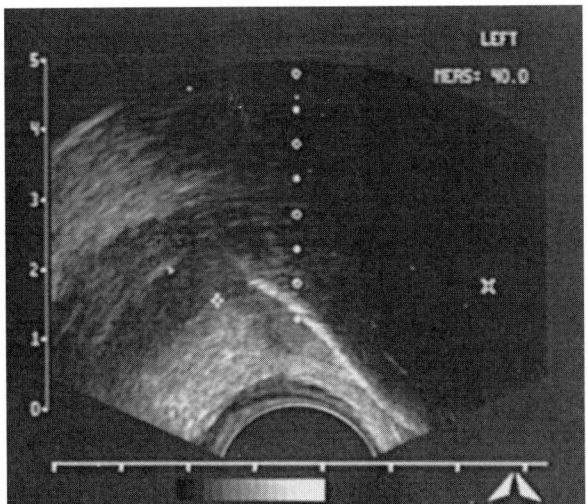

**Figure 50–5.** Transverse view showing the extent of prostatic freezing.

Preliminary results with cryoablation are encouraging.[190] The therapy appears to be well tolerated, with rectal and bladder complications rarely encountered (<5%). Data suggest that cryotherapy results in a postprocedural undetectable PSA rate of 48% and a 23% rate of positive biopsy of residual tissue.[191] The interest in cryotherapy as a primary therapy has declined because of failures and lack of third-party insurance coverage for the procedure.

## SUMMARY OF TREATMENT

In working through a patient's treatment options, it is usually helpful first to categorize the man according to clinical stage. The Gleason grade, patient age, comorbidity, and other factors (e.g., ploidy, personal beliefs) enter into the decision of which treatment is selected. Additionally, the known clinical staging errors in stages T2 and T3 disease must be respected, and the patient's risk for occult disseminated disease must be estimated. Using these simple parameters and a careful patient education regimen on the natural history of prostate cancer, the physician and patient can usually select the best treatment for each individual case.

### Stage T1a

As presented previously, most men with clinical stage T1a disease can be managed on an observation protocol, with frequent clinical examination and PSA measurements. Local progression and dissemination of cancer are rare. The younger man (40 to 60 years) with this stage of disease should strongly consider definitive therapy—either EBRT or radical prostatectomy.

### Stage T1b and T2a

The results of EBRT in this stage are good, as is the cure rate with radical prostatectomy. Classically, about 25 to 30% of men with stage T1b prostate cancer had evidence of pelvic lymph node metastases when subjected to surgical staging, and the results of EBRT with known pelvic lymphadenopathy are poor. Patients with elevations of serum enzymatic acid phosphatase, Gleason 9 or 10 tumors, or PSA greater than 40 ng/ml should be considered for surgical staging before EBRT. In certain instances, when a patient is a poor surgical risk and has a contraindication for EBRT, hormonal ablation is a reasonable approach.

### Stage T1c (Prostate-Specific Antigen–Detected Tumor)

Patients with stage T1c clinically localized disease are best served by some form of definitive therapy. It is a widely held belief that most men with PSA-detected tumors have clinically significant tumors (on tumor volume and pathologic staging criteria) that can be life threatening. There is insufficient information in this new stage classification to recommend either EBRT or surgery definitively.

### Stage T2b and T3

Although the results with EBRT in clinical stage T2b disease are fairly good, the cancer-specific survival with EBRT in clinical stage T3 disease is fairly poor, possibly similar to the natural history of untreated stage T3 disease. With palpably bulky stage T3 disease, the risk for pelvic lymph node metastases is 40 to 50%, so radiation in this scenario should be combined with a period of hormonal ablation for prolongation of disease progression and survival.

With careful pathologic staging after radical prostatectomy, we now know that most clinical stage T2b tumors have escaped the confines of the prostatic capsule. The experience with pathologic stage T3 (no seminal vesicle invasion) disease managed by radical prostatectomy at the Johns Hopkins Hospital indicates that patients with a Gleason grade 6 or less with low-volume pathologic stage T3 disease have excellent 10-year cancer-specific survival with clinically nondetectable disease, as evidenced by serum PSA values less than 0.2 ng/ml.

Patients with bulky stage T3 disease on DRE should not undergo radical prostatectomy because of the high rate of seminal vesicle invasion and pelvic lymph node metastases. An investigative approach includes using LHRH analogue and flutamide in a neoadjuvant protocol before radical prostatectomy (if staging laparoscopic lymph node dissection reveals no metastases). If the prostate gland and the cancerous nodule shrink considerably, radical prostatectomy may be attempted. Preliminary results show that 90% of patients continue to have prostate cancer outside the capsule. The survival results in these patients determine if this is a rational approach. Early hormonal ablation is also a rational approach to the management of patients with stage T3 disease, although it has not been proved superior to observation or the previously mentioned therapies.

### Stages N1–3M0 and M1

Most of the literature supports the initiation of combined androgen blockade, instituted at diagnosis, in metastatic prostate cancer. There is no medical advantage of orchiectomy over LHRH analogue. In some centers, patients with low-volume, microscopic pelvic lymph node metastases (N1 M0) are subjected to radical prostatectomy with early orchiectomy. The results of these trials are controversial because they are never compared with a concomitant control arm or an arm receiving orchiectomy alone.

Patients who fail to respond to hormonal ablation or who relapse after a period of remission should be considered for treatment with investigative agents because the results with standard chemotherapy are dismal. Palliation with long-acting narcotics and the early institution of strontium 89 for symptomatic osseous metastases can preserve a reasonable quality of life for most patients dying of disseminated prostate cancer.

### SUGGESTIONS FOR ADDITIONAL READING

Braddock CH 3rd, Edwards KA, Hasenberg NM, et al. Informed decision making in outpatient practice: time to get back to basics. JAMA 1999;282:2313–20. *This article reviews the principles of patient education for shared decision-making using PSA counseling as an example.*

Screening for prostate cancer. American College of Physicians. Ann Intern Med 1997;126:480–4. *This article provides the practice guidelines for PSA counseling of the American College of Physicians.*

Cox JD, Gallagher MJ, Hammond EH, et al. Consensus statements on radiation therapy of prostate cancer: guidelines for prostate re-biopsy after radiation and for radiation therapy with rising prostate-specific antigen levels after radical prostatectomy. American Society for Therapeutic Radiology and Oncology Consensus Panel. J Clin Oncol 1999;17:1155–63. *Based on the data presented, the panel estimated the prostate rebiopsy negative rates after radiation therapy to range from 62 to 80% for patients with T1–2 tumors and that rebiopsy was not necessary as standard follow-up.*

Oh WK, Pantoff PW. Treatment of locally advanced prostate cancer: is chemotherapy the next step? J Clin Oncol 1999;17:3664–75.

Lichtenstein P, Holm NV, Pia KV, et al. Environmental and heritable factors in the causation of cancer. Analyses of cohorts of twins from Sweden, Denmark, and Finland. N Engl J Med 2000;343:78–85. *Heritable factors were observed to be important in 42% of patients with prostate cancer. This high frequency may explain why it has been difficult to identify environmental risk factors for this disease.*

### REFERENCES

1. Walsh PC, Donker PJ. Impotence following radical prostatectomy: insight into etiology and prevention. J Urol 1982;128:492–7.
2. Eggleston JC, Walsh PC. Radical prostatectomy with preservation of sexual function: pathological findings in the first 100 cases. J Urol 1985;134:1146–8.
3. Byar DP, Corle DK. Hormone therapy for prostate cancer: results of the Veterans Administration Cooperative Urological Research Group studies. NCI Monogr 1988;7:165–70.
4. Leuprolide Study Group. Leuprolide versus diethylstilbestrol for metastatic prostate cancer. N Engl J Med 1984;311:1281–6.
5. Stamey TA, Yang N, Hay AR, et al. Prostate-specific antigen as a serum marker for adenocarcinoma of the prostate. N Engl J Med 1987;317:909–16.
6. Landis SH, Murray T, Bolden S, Wingo PA. Cancer statistics, 1998. CA Cancer J Clin 1999;49:8–31.
7. Scardino PT. Early detection of prostate cancer. Urol Clin North Am 1989;16:635–55.
8. Silvestri F, Bussani R, Pavletic N, Bassan F. Neoplastic and borderline lesions of the prostate: autopsy study and epidemiological data. Pathol Res Pract 1995;191:908–16.
9. Sakr WA, Haas GP, Cassin BF, et al. The frequency of carcinoma and intraepithelial neoplasia of the prostate in young male patients. J Urol 1993;150:379–85.
10. Breslow N, Chan CW, Dhom G, et al. Latent carcinoma of prostate of autopsy in seven areas. Int J Cancer 1977;20:680–8.
11. Parker SL, Davis KJ, Wingo PA, et al. Cancer statistics by race and ethnicity. CA Cancer J Clin 1998;48:31–48.
12. Ernster VL, Winkelstein W Jr, Selvin S, et al. Race, socioeconomic status, and prostatic cancer. Cancer Treat Rep 1977;61:187–91.
13. McNeal JE, Bostwick DG, Kindrachuk RA, et al. Patterns of progression in prostate cancer. Lancet 1986;1:60–3.
14. Guileyardo JM, Johnson WD, Welsh RA, et al. Prevalence of latent prostate carcinoma in two U.S. populations. J Natl Cancer Inst 1980;65:311–6.
15. Gronberg H, Xu J, Smith JR, et al. Early age at diagnosis in families providing evidence of linkage to the hereditary prostate cancer locus (HPC1) on chromosome 1. Cancer Res 1997;57:4707–9.
16. McNeal JE, Redwine EA, Freiha FS, Stamey TA. Zonal distribution of prostatic adenocarcinoma: correlation with histologic pattern and direction of spread. Am J Surg Pathol 1988;12:897–906.
17. Ellis DW, Leffers S, Davies JS, Ng AB. Multiple immunoperoxidase markers in benign hyperplasia and adenocarcinoma of the prostate. Am J Clin Pathol 1984;81:279–84.
18. Epstein JI, Kuhajda FP, Lieberman PH. Prostate-specific acid phosphatase immunoreactivity in adenocarcinomas of the urinary bladder. Hum Pathol 1986;17:939–42.
19. Sobin LH, Hjermstad BM, Sesterhenn IA, Helwig EB. Prostatic acid phosphatase activity in carcinoid tumors. Cancer 1986;58:136–8.
20. Epstein JI, Lieberman PH. Mucinous adenocarcinoma of the prostate gland. Am J Surg Pathol 1985;9:299–308.
21. Jadeja NA, Dogra PN, Gupta NP. Carcinoma of the prostate in young patients: a report of two cases. Urol Int 1994;52:48–51.
22. Ro JY, el-Naggar A, Ayala AG, et al. Signet-ring-cell carcinoma of the prostate: electron-microscopic and immunohistochemical studies of eight cases. Am J Surg Pathol 1988;12:453–60.

23. Epstein JI, Woodruff JM. Adenocarcinoma of the prostate with endometrioid features: a light microscopic and immunohistochemical study of ten cases. Cancer 1986;57:111–9.

24. Millar EK, Sharma NK, Lessells AM. Ductal (endometrioid) adenocarcinoma of the prostate: a clinicopathological study of 16 cases. Histopathology 1996;29:11–9.

25. Cohen RJ, Glezerson G, Taylor LF, et al. The neuroendocrine cell population of the human prostate gland. J Urol 1993;150:365–8.

26. Di Sant'Agnese PA, Cockett AT. The prostatic endocrine-paracrine (neuroendocrine) regulatory system and neuroendocrine differentiation in prostatic carcinoma: a review and future directions in basic research. J Urol 1994;152:1927–31.

27. Gleason DF. Histologic grading and clinical staging of prostatic carcinoma. In: Tannenbaum M, ed. Urologic pathology: the prostate. Philadelphia: Lea & Febiger, 1977:171–97.

28. Murphy GP, Whitmore WF Jr. A report of the workshops on the current status of the histologic grading of prostate cancer. Cancer 1979;44:1490–4.

29. Brawn PN, Ayala AG, Von Eschenbach AC, et al. Histologic grading study of prostate adenocarcinoma: the development of a new system and comparison with other methods—a preliminary study. Cancer 1982;49:525–32.

30. Gaeta JF, Asirwatham JE, Miller G, Murphy GP. Histologic grading of primary prostatic cancer: a new approach to an old problem. J Urol 1980;123:689–93.

31. Bostwick DG, Brawer MK. Prostatic intra-epithelial neoplasia and early invasion in prostate cancer. Cancer 1987;59:788–94.

32. Nagle RB, Ahmann FR, McDaniel KM, et al. Cytokeratin characterization of human prostatic carcinoma and its derived cell lines. Cancer Res 1987;47:281–6.

33. McNeal JE, Bostwick DG. Intraductal dysplasia: a premalignant lesion of the prostate. Hum Pathol 1986;17:64–71.

34. Lipski BA, Garcia RL, Brawer MK. Prostatic intraepithelial neoplasia: significance and management. Semin Urol Oncol 1996;14:149–55.

35. Sakr WA, Grignon DJ, Haas GP, et al. Age and racial distribution of prostatic intraepithelial neoplasia. Eur Urol 1996;30:138–44.

36. Troncoso P, Babaian RJ, Ro JY, et al. Prostatic intraepithelial neoplasia and invasive prostatic adenocarcinoma in cystoprostatectomy specimens. Urology 1989;34:6 Suppl:52–6.

37. Shepherd D, Keetch DW, Humphrey PA, et al. Repeat biopsy strategy in men with isolated prostatic intraepithelial neoplasia on prostate needle biopsy. J Urol 1996;156:460–3.

38. Gerber GS, Chodak GW. Digital rectal examination in the early detection of prostate cancer. Urol Clin North Am 1990;17:739–44.

39. Chodak GW, Keller P, Schoenberg HW. Assessment of screening for prostate cancer using the digital rectal examination. J Urol 1989;141:1136–8.

40. Mueller EJ, Crain TW, Thompson IM, Rodriguez FR. An evaluation of serial digital rectal examinations in screening for prostate cancer. J Urol 1988;140:1445–7.

41. Crawford ED, DeAntoni EP, Etzioni R, et al. Serum prostate-specific antigen and digital rectal examination for early detection of prostate cancer in a national community-based program: The Prostate Cancer Education Council. Urology 1996;47:863–9.

42. Nijs HG, Tordoir DM, Schuurman JH, et al. Randomised trial of prostate cancer screening in The Netherlands: assessment of acceptance and motives for attendance. J Med Screen 1997;4:102–6.

43. Cooner WH, Mosley BR, Rutherford CL Jr, et al. Clinical application of transrectal ultrasonography and prostate specific antigen in the search for prostate cancer. J Urol 1988;139:758–61.

44. Lee F, Littrup PJ, Torp-Pedersen ST, et al. Prostate cancer: comparison of transrectal US and digital rectal examination for screening. Radiology 1988;168:389–94.

45. Littrup PJ, Kane RA, Williams CR, et al. Determination of prostate volume with transrectal US for cancer screening: Part I. comparison with prostate-specific antigen assays. Radiology 1991;178:537–42.

46. Benson MC, Whang IS, Olsson CA, et al. The use of prostate specific antigen density to enhance the predictive value of intermediate levels of serum prostate specific antigen. J Urol 1992;147:817–21.

47. Brawer MK, Aramburu EA, Chen GL, et al. The inability of prostate specific antigen index to enhance the predictive value of prostate specific antigen in the diagnosis of prostatic carcinoma. J Urol 1993;150:369–73.

48. Brawer MK, Chetner MP, Beatie J, et al. Screening for prostatic carcinoma with prostate specific antigen. J Urol 1992;147:841–5.

49. Brawer MK, Beatie J, Wener MH, et al. Screening for prostatic carcinoma with prostate specific antigen: results of the second year. J Urol 1993;150:106–9.

50. Catalona WJ, Smith DS, Ratliff TL, et al. Measurement of prostate-specific antigen in serum as a screening test for prostate cancer. N Engl J Med 1991;324:1156–61.

51. Carter HB, Pearson JD, Metter EJ, et al. Longitudinal evaluation of prostate-specific antigen levels in men with and without prostate disease. JAMA 1992;267:2215–20.

52. Oesterling JE, Jacobsen SJ, Chute CG, et al. Serum prostate-specific antigen in a community-based population of healthy men: establishment of age-specific reference ranges. JAMA 1993;270:860–4.

53. Dalkin BL, Ahmann FR, Kopp JB. Prostate specific antigen levels in men older than 50 years without clinical evidence of prostatic carcinoma. J Urol 1993;150:1837–9.

54. DeAntoni EP, Crawford ED, Oesterling JE, et al. Age- and race-specific reference ranges for prostate-specific antigen from a large community-based study. Urology 1996;48:234–9.

55. Jacobson JO. Can screening for early-stage prostate cancer be rationalized? Hematol Oncol Clin North Am 1996;10:549–64.

56. Oesterling JE, Kumamoto Y, Tsukamoto T, et al. Serum prostate-specific antigen in a community-based population of healthy Japanese men: lower values than for similarly aged white men. Br J Urol 1995;75:347–53.

57. Catalona WJ, Smith DS, Wolfert RL, et al. Evaluation of percentage of free serum prostate-specific antigen to improve specificity of prostate cancer screening. JAMA 1995;274:1214–20.

58. McWhorter WP, Hernandez AD, Meikle AW, et al. A screening study of prostate cancer in high risk families. J Urol 1992;148:826–8.

59. Crawford ED, Schutz MJ, Clejan S, et al. The effect of digital rectal examination on prostate-specific antigen levels. JAMA 1992;267:2227–8.

60. Catalona WJ, Richie JP, Ahmann FR, et al. Comparison of digital rectal examination and serum prostate specific antigen in the early detection of prostate cancer: results of a multicenter clinical trial of 6,630 men. J Urol 1994;151:1283–90.

61. Walsh PC. Why make an early diagnosis of prostate cancer? J Urol 1992;147:853–4.

62. Leewansangtong S, Crawford ED, Stuart GG, et al. Longitudinal follow up from Prostate Cancer Awareness Week (PCAW): screening interval. J Urol 1998;159:5 Suppl:177.abstract.

63. Harris CH, Dalkin BL, Martin E, et al. Prospective longitudinal evaluation of men with initial prostate-specific antigen level of 4 ng/ml or less. J Urol 1997;157:1740–3.

64. Honig SC, Stilmant MM, Klavans MS, et al. The role of fine-needle aspiration biopsy of the prostate in staging adenocarcinoma. Cancer 1992;69:2978–82.

65. Donohue RE, Miller GJ. Adenocarcinoma of the prostate: biopsy to whole mount: Denver VA experience. Urol Clin North Am 1991;18:449–52.

66. Andriole GL, Coplen DE, Mikkelsen DJ, Catalona WJ. Sonographic and pathological staging of patients with clinically localized prostate cancer. J Urol 1989;142:1259–61.

67. Rifkin MD, Zerhouni EA, Gatsonis CA, et al. Comparison of magnetic resonance imaging and ultrasonography in staging early prostate cancer: results of a multi-institutional cooperative trial. N Engl J Med 1990;323:621–6.

68. Salo JO, Kivisaari L, Rannikko S, Lehtonen T. Computerized tomography and transrectal ultrasound in the assessment of local extension of prostatic cancer before radical retropubic prostatectomy. J Urol 1987;137:435–8.

69. Hamper UM, Sheth S, Savader BL. Positional hypoechoic pseudolesions on transrectal sonography of the prostate. AJR Am J Roentgenol 1990;155:1138–9.

70. Clements R. The changing role of transrectal ultrasound in the diagnosis of prostate cancer. Clin Radiol 1996;51:671–6.

71. Hricak H, Dooms GC, Jeffrey RB, et al. Prostatic carcinoma: staging by clinical assessment, CT, and MR imaging. Radiology 1987;162:331–6.

72. Rees MA, Resnick MI, Oesterling JE. Use of prostate-specific antigen, Gleason score, and digital rectal examination in staging patients with newly diagnosed prostate cancer. Urol Clin North Am 1997;24:379–88.

73. Chelsky MJ, Schnall MD, Seidmon EJ, Pollack HM. Use of endorectal surface coil magnetic resonance imaging for local staging of prostate cancer. J Urol 1993;150:391–5.

74. Perrotti M, Kaufman RP Jr, Jennings TA, et al. Endo-rectal coil magnetic resonance imaging in clinically localized prostate cancer: is it accurate? J Urol 1996;156:106–9.

75. Sands ME, Zagars GK, Pollack A, von Eschenbach AC. Serum prostate-specific antigen, clinical stage, pathologic grade, and the incidence of nodal metastases in prostate cancer. Urology 1994;44:215–20.

76. Petros JA, Catalona WJ. Lower incidence of unsuspected lymph node metastases in 521 consecutive patients with clinically localized prostate cancer. J Urol 1992;147:1574–5.

77. Kerbl K, Clayman RV, Petros JA, et al. Staging pelvic lymphadenectomy for prostate cancer: a comparison of laparoscopic and open techniques. J Urol 1993;150:396–9.

78. Schuessler WW, Pharand D, Vancaillie TG. Laparoscopic standard pelvic node dissection for carcinoma of the prostate: is it accurate? J Urol 1993;150:898–901.

79. Bluestein DL, Bostwick DG, Bergstralh EJ, Oesterling JE. Eliminating the need for bilateral pelvic lymphadenectomy in select patients with prostate cancer. J Urol 1994;151:1315–20.

80. Partin AW, Walsh PC. The use of prostate specific antigen, clinical stage and Gleason score to predict pathological stage in men with localized prostate cancer. J Urol 1994;152:172–3.

81. Schaffer DL, Pendergrass HP. Comparison of enzyme, clinical, radiographic, and radionuclide methods of detecting bone metastases from carcinoma of the prostate. Radiology 1976;121:431–4.

82. Oesterling JE, Martin SK, Bergstralh EJ, Lowe FC. The use of prostate-specific antigen in staging patients with newly diagnosed prostate cancer. JAMA 1993;269:57–60.

83. Perez CA. Carcinoma of the prostate: a model for management under impending health care system reform: 1994 RSNA annual oration in radiation oncology. Radiology 1995;196:309–22.

84. Whitesel JA, Donohue RE, Mani JH, et al. Acid phosphatase: its influence on the management of carcinoma of the prostate. J Urol 1984;131:70–2.

85. McDowell GC 2d, Johnson JW, Tenney DM, Johnson DE. Pelvic lymphadenectomy for staging clinically localized prostate cancer: indications, complications, and results in 217 cases. Urology 1990;35:476–82.

86. Lowe FC, Trauzzi SJ. Prostatic acid phosphatase in 1993: its limited clinical utility. Urol Clin North Am 1993;20:589–95.

87. Stamey TA, Kabalin JN, McNeal JE, et al. Prostate specific antigen in the diagnosis and treatment of adenocarcinoma of the prostate. II: radical prostatectomy treated patients. J Urol 1989;141:1076–83.

88. Stamey TA, Kabalin JN. Prostate specific antigen in the diagnosis and treatment of adenocarcinoma of the prostate. I: untreated patients. J Urol 1989;141:1070–5.

89. Lange PH. Prostate-specific antigen for staging prior to surgery and for early detection of recurrence after surgery. Urol Clin North Am 1990;17:813–7.

90. Wood DP Jr, Banks ER, Humphreys S, et al. Identification of bone marrow micrometastases in patients with prostate cancer. Cancer 1994;74:2533–40.

91. Olsson CA, de Vries GM, Buttyan R, Katz AE. Reverse transcriptase-polymerase chain reaction assays for prostate cancer. Urol Clin North Am 1997;24:367–78.

92. Heung YM, Walsh K, Sriprasad S, et al: The detection of prostate cells by the reverse transcription-polymerase chain reaction in the circulation of patients undergoing transurethral resection of the prostate. Bju Int 2000;85:65–9.

93. Verkaik NS, Schröder FH, Romijn JC. Clinical usefulness of RT-PCR detection of hematogenous prostate cancer spread. Urol Res 1997;25:373–84.

94. Oesterling JE, Brendler CB, Epstein JI, Kimball AW Jr, Walsh PC. Correlation of clinical stage, serum prostatic acid phosphatase and preoperative Gleason grade with final pathological stage in 275 patients with clinically localized adenocarcinoma of the prostate. J Urol 1987;138:92–8.

95. Gleason DF. Histologic grading of prostate cancer: a perspective. Hum Pathol 1992;23:273–9.

96. Epstein JI, Oesterling JE, Walsh PC. The volume and anatomical location of residual tumor in radical prostatectomy specimens removed for stage A1 prostate cancer. J Urol 1988;139:975–9.

97. Zhang G, Wasserman NF, Sidi AA, et al. Long-term followup results after expectant management of stage A1 prostatic cancer. J Urol 1991;146:99–103.

98. Greene DR, Egawa S, Neerhut G, et al. The distribution of residual cancer in radical prostatectomy specimens in stage A prostate cancer. J Urol 1991;145:324–9.

99. Parfitt HE Jr, Smith JA Jr, Gliedman JB, Middleton RG. Accuracy of staging in A1 carcinoma of the prostate. Cancer 1983;51:2346–50.

100. McMillen SM, Wettlaufer JN. The role of repeat transurethral biopsy in stage A carcinoma of the prostate. J Urol 1976;116:759–60.

101. Donohue RE, Mani JH, Whitesel JA, et al. Pelvic lymph node dissection: guide to patient management in clinically locally confined adenocarcinoma of prostate. Urology 1982;20:559–65.

102. Johansson JE, Adami HO, Andersson SO, et al. High 10-year survival rate in patients with early, untreated prostatic cancer. JAMA 1992;267:2191–6.

103. Blute ML, Zincke H, Farrow GM. Long-term followup of young patients with stage A adenocarcinoma of the prostate. J Urol 1986;136:840–3.

104. Epstein JI, Paull G, Eggleston JC, Walsh PC. Prognosis of untreated stage A1 prostatic carcinoma: a study of 94 cases with extended followup. J Urol 1986;136:837–9.

105. Whitmore WF Jr. Natural history of low-stage prostatic cancer and the impact of early detection. Urol Clin North Am 1990;17:689–97.

106. Jewett HJ, Eggleston JC, Yawn DH. Radical prostatectomy in the management of carcinoma of the prostate: probable causes of some therapeutic failures. J Urol 1972;107:1034–40.

107. Stamey TA, McNeal JE, Freiha FS, Redwine E. Morphometric and clinical studies on 68 consecutive radical prostatectomies. J Urol 1988;139:1235–41.

108. Crawford ED, Eisenberger MA, McLeod DG, et al. A controlled trial of leuprolide with and without flutamide in prostatic carcinoma. N Engl J Med 1989;321:419–24.

109. Kramolowsky EV. The value of testosterone deprivation in stage D1 carcinoma of the prostate. J Urol 1988;139:1242–4.

110. Chodak GW, Vogelzang NJ, Caplan RJ, et al. Independent prognostic factors in patients with metastatic (stage D2) prostate cancer: The Zoladex Study Group. JAMA 1991;265:618–21.

111. Vicini FA, Horwitz EM, Gonzalez J, Martinez AA. Treatment options for localized prostate cancer based on pretreatment serum prostate specific antigen levels. J Urol 1997;158:319–25.

112. Benson MC, Ring K, Giella J. Flow cytometry in carcinoma of the prostate. Urol Clin North Am 1990;17:885–91.

113. Winkler HZ, Rainwater LM, Myers RP, et al. Stage D1 prostatic adenocarcinoma: significance of nuclear DNA ploidy patterns studied by flow cytometry. Mayo Clin Proc 1988;63:103–12.

114. Corless CL. Evaluating early-stage prostate cancer: what pretreatment criteria best guide therapeutic decision making? Hematol Oncol Clin North Am 1996;10:565–79.

115. Bauer JJ, Sesterhenn IA, Mostofi FK, et al. Elevated levels of apoptosis regulator proteins p53 and bcl-2 are independent prognostic biomarkers in surgically treated clinically localized prostate cancer. J Urol 1996;156:1511–6.

116. Bettencourt MC, Bauer JJ, Sesterhenn IA, et al. Ki-67 expression is a prognostic marker of prostate cancer recurrence after radical prostatectomy. J Urol 1996;156:1064–8.

117. Bauer JJ, Connelly RR, Sesterhenn IA, et al. Biostatistical modeling using traditional variables and genetic biomarkers for predicting the risk of prostate carcinoma recurrence after radical prostatectomy. Cancer 1997;79:952–62.

118. Uzoaru I, Rubenstein M, Mirochnik Y, et al. An evaluation of the markers p53 and Ki-67 for their predictive value in prostate cancer. J Surg Oncol 1998;67:33–7.

119. Siegal JA, Yu E, Brawer MK. Topography of neovascularity in human prostate carcinoma. Cancer 1995;75:2545–51.

120. Chodak GW, Thisted RA, Gerber GS, et al. Results of conservative management of clinically localized prostate cancer. N Engl J Med 1994;330:242–8.

121. Albertsen PC, Fryback DG, Storer BE, et al. Long-term survival among men with conservatively treated localized prostate cancer. JAMA 1995;274:626–31.

122. Walsh PC. Anatomic radical prostatectomy. In: Walsh PC, Retik AB, Vaughan ED Jr, Wain AJ, eds. Campbell's urology. 7th ed. Vol III. Philadelphia: WB Saunders, 1998:2565–88.

123. Catalona WJ. Patient selection for, results of, and impact on tumor resection of potency-sparing radical prostatectomy. Urol Clin North Am 1990;17:819–26.

124. Catalona WJ, Basler JW. Return of erections and urinary continence following nerve sparing radical retropubic prostatectomy. J Urol 1993;150:905–7.

125. Steiner MS, Morton RA, Walsh PC. Impact of anatomical radical prostatectomy on urinary continence. J Urol 1991;145:512–5.

126. Constantinou CE, Freiha FS. Impact of radical prostatectomy on the characteristics of bladder and urethra. J Urol 1992;148:1215–20.

127. Presti JC Jr, Schmidt RA, Narayan PA, et al. Pathophysiology of urinary incontinence after radical prostatectomy. J Urol 1990;143:975–8.

128. Quinlan DM, Leonard MP, Brendler CB, et al. Use of the Benchekroun hydraulic valve as a catheterizable continence mechanism. J Urol 1991;145:1151–5.

129. Bahnson RR, Ratliff TL. Inhibition of mouse bladder tumor proliferation by alpha difluoromethylornithine and interferon in vitro and in vivo. J Urol 1988;139:1367–71.

130. Nadler RB, Andriole GL. Who is best benefited by radical prostatectomy? Hematol Oncol Clin North Am 1996;10:581–93.

131. Adolfsson J, Steineck G, Whitmore WF Jr. Recent results of management of palpable clinically localized prostate cancer. Cancer 1993;72:310–22.

132. Epstein JI, Carmichael MJ, Pizov G, Walsh PC. Influence of capsular penetration on progression following radical prostatectomy: a study of 196 cases with long-term followup. J Urol 1993;150:135–41.

133. Freeman JA, Lieskovsky G, Cook DW, et al. Radical retropubic prostatectomy and postoperative adjuvant radiation for pathological stage C (PcN0) prostate cancer from 1976 to 1989: intermediate findings. J Urol 1993;149:1029–34.

134. Andriole GL. Adjuvant therapy for prostate cancer patients at high risk of recurrence following radical prostatectomy. Eur Urol 1997;32:Suppl 3:65–9.

135. Foster LS, Jajodia P, Fournier G Jr, et al. The value of prostate specific antigen and transrectal ultrasound guided biopsy in detecting prostatic fossa recurrences following radical prostatectomy. J Urol 1993;149:1024–8.

136. Fair WR, Cookson MS, Stroumbakis N, et al. The indications, rationale, and results of neoadjuvant androgen deprivation in the treatment of prostatic cancer: Memorial Sloan-Kettering Cancer Center results. Urology 1997;49:3A Suppl:46–55.

137. Labrie F, Cusan L, Gomez JL, et al. Neoadjuvant hormonal therapy: the Canadian experience. Urology 1997;49:3A Suppl:56–64.

138. Witjes WP, Schulman CC, Debruyne FM. Preliminary results of a prospective randomized study comparing radical prostatectomy versus radical prostatectomy associated with neoadjuvant hormonal combination therapy in T2–3 N0 M0 prostatic carcinoma: The European Study Group on Neoadjuvant Treatment of Prostate Cancer. Urology 1997;49:3A Suppl:65–9.

139. Fukunaga-Johnson N, Sandler HM, McLaughlin PW, et al. Results of 3D conformal radiotherapy in the treatment of localized prostate cancer. Int J Radiat Oncol Biol Phys 1997;38:311–7.

140. Bagshaw MA, Cox RS, Hancock SL. Control of prostate cancer with radiotherapy: long-term results. J Urol 1994;152:1781–5.

141. Bagshaw MA, Kaplan ID, Cox RC. Prostate cancer: radiation therapy for localized disease. Cancer 1993;71:3 Suppl:939–52.

142. Schellhammer PF, Kuban DA, el-Mahdi AM. Treatment of clinical local failure after radiation therapy for prostate carcinoma. J Urol 1993;150:1851–5.

143. Zietman AL, Prince EA, Nakfoor BM, Shipley WU. Neoadjuvant androgen suppression with radiation in the management of locally advanced adenocarcinoma of the prostate: experimental and clinical results. Urology 1997;49:3A Suppl:74–83.

144. Bolla M, Gonzalez D, Warde P, et al. Improved survival in patients with locally advanced prostate cancer treated with radiotherapy and goserelin. N Engl J Med 1997;337:295–300.

145. Grimm PD, Blasko JC, Ragde H, et al. Does brachytherapy have a role in the treatment of prostate cancer? Hematol Oncol Clin North Am 1996;10:653–73.

146. Porter AT, Forman JD. Prostate brachytherapy: an overview. Cancer 1993;71:3 Suppl:953–8.

147. Nori D, Moni J. Current issues in techniques of prostate brachytherapy. Semin Surg Oncol 1997;13:444–53.

148. Stock RG, Stone NN. The effect of prognostic factors on therapeutic outcome following transperineal prostate brachytherapy. Semin Surg Oncol 1997;13:454–60.

149. Stromgerg JS, Martinez AA, Horwitz EM, et al. Conformal high dose rate iridium-192 boost brachytherapy in locally advanced prostate cancer: superior prostate-specific antigen response compared with external beam treatment. Cancer J Sci Am 1997;3:346–52.

150. Huggins C, Hodges CV. Studies of prostatic cancer. 1: the effects of castrations, of estrogen and of androgen injections on serum phosphatases in metastatic carcinoma of prostate. Cancer Res 1941;1:293–307.

151. Veterans' Administrative Co-operative Urological Research Group. Treatment and survival of patients with cancer of the prostate. Surg Gynecol Obstet 1967;124:1011–7.

152. Gormley GJ. Role of 5 alpha-reductase inhibitors in the treatment of advanced prostatic carcinoma. Urol Clin North Am 1991;18:93–8.

153. Crawford ED, Nabors WL. Total androgen ablation: American experience. Urol Clin North Am 1991;18:55–63.

154. Kennealey GT, Furr BJ. Use of the nonsteroidal anti-androgen Casodex in advanced prostatic carcinoma. Urol Clin North Am 1991;18:99–110.

155. Geller J. Megestrol acetate plus low-dose estrogen in the management of advanced prostatic carcinoma. Urol Clin North Am 1991;18:83–91.

156. Goldenberg SL, Bruchovsky N. Use of cyproterone acetate in prostate cancer. Urol Clin North Am 1991;18:111–22.

157. Crawford ED, Ahmann FR, Davis MA, Levasseur YJ. Aminoglutethimide in metastatic adenocarcinoma of the prostate. Prog Clin Biol Res 1987;243A:283–9.

158. Pont A, Williams PL, Azhar S, et al. Ketoconazole blocks testosterone synthesis. Arch Intern Med 1982;142:2137–40.

159. Leuprolide Study Group. Leuprolide versus diethylstilbestrol for metastatic prostate cancer. N Engl J Med 1984;311:1281–6.

160. Peeling WB. Phase III studies to compare goserelin (Zoladex) with orchiectomy and with diethylstilbestrol in treatment of prostatic carcinoma. Urology 1989;33:Suppl:45–52.

161. LaRocca RV, Cooper MR, Uhrich M, et al. Use of suramin in treatment of prostatic carcinoma refractory to conventional hormonal manipulation. Urol Clin North Am 1991;18:123–9.

162. Byar DP. Proceedings: The Veterans Administration Cooperative Urological Research Group's studies of cancer of the prostate. Cancer 1973;32:1126–30.

163. Denis L, Murphy GP. Overview of phase III trials on combined androgen treatment in patients with metastatic prostate cancer. Cancer 1993;72:12 Suppl:3888–95.

164. The Medical Research Council Prostate Cancer Working Party Investigators Group. Immediate versus deferred treatment for advanced prostatic cancer: initial results of the Medical Research Council trial. Br J Urol 1997;79:235–46.

165. Huggins C, Scott WW. Bilateral adrenalectomy in prostatic cancer. Ann Surg 1945;122:1031–41.

166. Harper ME, Pike A, Peeling WB, Griffiths K. Steroidals of adrenal origin metabolized by human prostatic tissue both in vivo and in vitro. J Endocrinol 1974;60:117–25.

167. Labrie F, Luthy I, Veilleux R, et al. New concepts on the androgen sensitivity of prostate cancer. Prog Clin Biol Res 1987;243A:145–72.

168. Labrie F, Dupont A, Belanger A, et al. New approach in the treatment of prostate cancer: complete instead of partial withdrawal of androgens. Prostate 1983;4:579–94.

169. Denis LJ, Carnelro de Moura JL, Bono A, et al. Goserelin acetate and flutamide versus bilateral orchiectomy: a phase III EORTC trial (30853): EORTC GU Group and EORTC Data Center. Urology 1993;42:119–30.

170. Dijkman GA, Janknegt RA, De Reijke TM, Debruyne FM. Long-term efficacy and safety of nilutamide plus castration in advanced prostate cancer, and the significance of early prostate specific antigen normalization: International Anandron Study Group. J Urol 1997;158:160–3.

171. Beland G, Elhilali M, Fradet Y, et al. Total androgen ablation: Canadian experience. Urol Clin North Am 1991;18:75–82.

172. Iversen P, Rasmussen F, Klarskov P, Christensen IJ. Long-term results of Danish Prostatic Cancer Group trial 86: goserelin acetate plus flutamide versus orchiectomy in advanced prostate cancer. Cancer 1993;72:3851–4.

173. Tyrrell CJ, Altwein JE, Klippel F, et al. Multicenter randomized trial comparing Zoladex with Zoladex plus flutamide in the treatment of advanced prostate cancer: survival update. Cancer 1993;72:3878–9.

174. Prostate Cancer Trialists' Collaborative Group. Maximum androgen blockade in advanced prostate cancer: an overview of 22 randomized trials with 3283 deaths in 5710 patients. Lancet 1995;346:265–9.

175. Crawford ED, Eisenberger MA, McLeod DG, et al. Comparison of bilateral orchiectomy with or without flutamide for the treatment of patients with stage D2 adenocarcinoma of the prostate: results of NCI intergroup study 0105 (SWOG and ECOG). J Urol 1997;157:336. abstract.

176. Bruchovsky N, Rennie PS, Coldman AJ, et al. Effects of androgen withdrawal on the stem cell composition of the Shionogi carcinoma. Cancer Res 1990;50:2275–82.

177. Goldenberg SL, Bruchovsky N, Gleave ME, et al. Intermittent androgen suppression in the treatment of prostate cancer: a preliminary report. Urology 1995;45:839–45.

178. Kelly WK, Scher HI. Prostate specific antigen decline after antiandrogen withdrawal: the flutamide withdrawal syndrome. J Urol 1993;149:607–9.

179. Veldscholte J, Berrevoets CA, Brinkmann AO, et al. Anti-androgens and the mutated androgen receptor of LNCaP cells: differential effects on binding affinity, heat-shock protein interaction, and transcription activation. Biochemistry 1992;31:2393–9.

180. Yagoda A, Petrylak D. Cytotoxic chemotherapy for advanced hormone-resistant prostate cancer. Cancer 1993;71:3 Suppl:1098–109.

181. Mani S, Vogelzang NJ. Is "off-protocol" chemotherapy for androgen-independent carcinoma of prostate warranted? Hematol Oncol Clin North Am 1996;10:749–68.

182. Theyer G, Hamilton G. Role of multidrug resistance in tumors of the genitourinary tract. Urology 1994;44:942–50.

183. Murphy GP, Beckley S, Brady MF, et al. Treatment of newly diagnosed metastatic prostate cancer patients with chemotherapy agents in combination with hormones versus hormones alone. Cancer 1983;51:1264–72.

184. Tong D, Gillick L, Hendrickson FR. The palliation of symptomatic osseous metastases: final results of the Study by the Radiation Therapy Oncology Group. Cancer 1982;50:893–9.

185. Poulter CA, Cosmatos D, Rubin P, et al. A report of RTOG 8206: a phase III study of whether the addition of single dose hemibody irradiation to standard fractionated local field irradiation is more effective than local field irradiation alone in the treatment of symptomatic osseous metastases. Int J Radiat Oncol Biol Phys 1992;23:207–14.

186. Breen SL, Powe JE, Porter AT. Dose estimation in strontium-89 radiotherapy of metastatic prostatic carcinoma. J Nucl Med 1992;33:1316–23.

187. Porter AT, McEwan AJ, Powe JE, et al. Results of a randomized phase-III trial to evaluate the efficacy of strontium-89 adjuvant to local field external beam irradiation in the management of endocrine resistant metastatic prostate cancer. Int J Radiat Oncol Biol Phys 1993;25:805–13.

188. Soffen EM, Greenberg A, Baumann J, Corn BW. The role of strontium-89 systemic radiotherapy in the management of osseous metastases from prostate cancer. Tech Urol 1997;3:76–80.

189. Adami S. Bisphosphonates in prostate carcinoma. Cancer 1997;80:8 Suppl:1674–9.

190. Onik GM, Cohen JK, Reyes GD, et al. Transrectal ultrasound-guided percutaneous radical cryosurgical ablation of the prostate. Cancer 1993;72:1291–9.

191. Carroll PR, Presti JC Jr, Small E, Roach M 3rd. Focal therapy for prostate cancer 1996: maximizing outcome. Urology 1997;49:3A Suppl:84–94.

# CHAPTER 51

# BLADDER, RENAL PELVIS, AND URETERS

• SUNAI LEEWANSANGTONG • E. DAVID CRAWFORD

## Bladder

### NATURAL HISTORY

#### Etiology and Epidemiology

Transitional cell carcinoma (TCC) of the bladder is the second most common urologic malignancy. It exhibits the entire spectrum of biologic aggressiveness from benign superficial papilloma to invasive high-grade carcinoma. Most bladder cancers are TCCs. These tumors behave as a *field change*, and the entire urothelium from the renal pelvis to the urethra is at risk.

In 1999, it was estimated that approximately 54,200 new cases of bladder cancer would be diagnosed in the United States—39,100 in men and 15,100 in women.[1] With bladder cancer being 2.6 times more common in men than in women, it was estimated that 8100 men and 4000 women would die from this disease in 1999.[1] Approximately 80% of the estimated 54,200 new cases would be classified as superficial (no invasion of muscularis propria) at diagnosis. Of these, only 10 to 15% would eventually progress to invasive disease.[2] In men, bladder cancer is the fourth most common cancer (6%) after prostate, lung, and colorectal. In women, it is the 10th most common type of cancer.[1] The varying incidence of this disease in men and women is not entirely explained by lifestyle differences, such as cigarette smoking or occupational exposure.[3] The incidence of bladder cancer has been increasing since the 1980s, but mortality from the disease has been decreasing in both men and women. Statistically, this disease is diagnosed more frequently in whites than in African Americans.[4] This increased risk is limited to patients with noninvasive tumors, and some investigators believe that some superficial tumors that are diagnosed in whites may go undiagnosed in African Americans.[5]

There are significant differences in the incidence of bladder cancer among various nationalities. The reported incidence of bladder cancer is higher in the United States and England than in Japan and Finland.[6] In Hawaii, the incidence is more than double in Americans than Japanese.[7] A higher incidence has also been reported in Jewish individuals.[8] It is believed that these differences are probably related to environmental and hereditary influences.

Carcinogenesis is probably initiated by carcinogens that begin malignant transformation by altering the genome. Subsequently, promoters stimulate expression of the altered genome.[9] Exposure to aromatic amines and related compounds or a significant history of cigarette smoking has been reported in more than 50% of all bladder cancer cases.[10] It is estimated that occupational exposure accounts for one fourth to one third of all bladder cancer cases in the United States.[10] The latency period can be 40 to 50 years, but heavy exposure to the carcinogen may hasten the development.

**Chemical Carcinogens.** Several aromatic amines have been linked to bladder cancer in humans, including 2-naphthylamine, benzidine, and 4-aminobiphenyl.[11, 12] Occupational exposure to aromatic amines was related to 25% of bladder cancer patients in some industrialized countries.[11] Exposure to these chemicals and an increased risk of bladder cancer have been identified in workers in leather, rubber, paint, and dyestuff industries; auto workers; metal machinists; dry cleaners; paper manufacturers; rope and twine makers; laboratory workers; dental technicians; barbers and beauticians; physicians; and plumbers.[13–16] Identifying a specific causative agent in an occupational setting has been difficult, however, largely because workers are exposed to numerous related compounds.

An understanding of the metabolic processes that lead to cancer may help identify individuals at increased risk. Aromatic amines are detoxified by acetylation in the liver. In humans, a genetic polymorphism exists. Lower and associates[17] suggested that individuals who were slow acetylators were more susceptible to develop bladder cancer than fast acetylators. Cartwright and coworkers[18] showed a 17-fold increase in bladder cancer among slow acetylators. Other investigators have not confirmed this observation.[19]

**Tobacco.** Epidemiologic studies have shown an association between smoking and bladder cancer since the 1960s. Smokers have a sevenfold increased risk for bladder cancer compared with nonsmokers. Nearly all studies have observed steadily higher risks with increasing amounts smoked.[6] Former cigarette smokers have an incidence of bladder cancer somewhere between that of smokers and nonsmokers.[20] It is estimated that cigarette smoking accounts for 25 to 60% of all bladder cancer cases in industrialized, developed countries.[6] Cigarette smoking is the single most important cause of bladder cancer. Epidemiologic studies examining cigar, pipe, and chewing tobacco have not clearly shown an increased risk for bladder cancer. The exact chemicals in cigarette smoke that cause bladder cancer have not been determined, but several of the aromatic amines, including 4-aminobiphenyl and *o*-toluidine, are present in cigarette smoke. Smokers of air-cured cigarettes, which are rich in arylamines, are three times more likely to develop bladder cancer than those who smoke flue-cured cigarettes.[21]

**Caffeine.** Controversy exists about the association between caffeine-containing beverages and bladder cancer. Epidemiologic studies have varied greatly, with some indicating no increased risk and others showing a slightly increased risk of bladder cancer. The association is complicated because coffee drinking, the use of artificial sweeteners, and cigarette smoking are often coexistent. At this time, there is no strong evidence that caffeine increases the risk of bladder cancer in humans.[22]

**Chronic Cystitis.** Chronic irritation of bladder mucosa by long-term catheters, calculi, or chronic urinary infection is associated with an increased risk of squamous metaplasia and the development of squamous cell carcinoma (SCC).[23] Similarly, chronic irritation of bladder mucosa by infestation by the *Schistosoma haematobium* ova is also associated with an increased risk of SCC. In the Middle East and parts of Africa, where schistosomiasis is endemic, SCC of the bladder (bilharzial bladder cancer) is the most common type of bladder cancer (75%).[24]

Other agents or processes have been associated with an increased risk of bladder cancer. Consumption of large quantities of phenacetin has been correlated with an increased risk of TCC of the bladder and renal pelvis. Piper and colleagues[25] reported a 6.5-fold increase in regular use of phenacetin-containing analgesics in a group of women, age 20 to 49 years, who were diagnosed with bladder cancer.

**Tryptophan Metabolites.** Tryptophan metabolites have been shown to have carcinogenic potential in experimental animals.[26] In humans, studies have found increased urinary tryptophan metabolite levels in bladder cancer patients.[27] High levels of urinary tryptophan have been reported to correlate with tumor recurrence.[28] Some studies, however, suggested that endogenous tryptophan metabolites do not contribute significantly to the development of bladder cancer.[29] The relationship of tryptophan metabolites to bladder carcinogenesis has not been completely resolved.

**Other Causes.** Large doses of saccharin have been shown to be bladder carcinogens in rodents.[30] These studies are controversial, however, because of the extremely high dose of sweeteners given and the fact that cancer occurred only in animals exposed in utero or during the neonatal period.[31] The mechanism of carcinogenesis in rodents appears to be related to the formation of silicate-containing crystals or precipitate, which are cytotoxic to the urothelium. Subsequently, these crystals lead to a chronic proliferative state and, ultimately, the formation of tumors. The conditions necessary for the development of silicate-containing crystals in human urine are unlikely to be met.[22] A meta-analysis of all case-control studies indicated that saccharin is not related to bladder cancer in humans.[32]

Cyclophosphamide therapy has been shown to increase the risk of developing bladder cancer ninefold.[33] Studies showed that the risk of bladder cancer increased 3.2-fold when compared with a control group.[34] Most of these tumors are muscle infiltrating at the time of diagnosis.[35] Finally, arsenic has been indicated as a bladder carcinogen in some countries.[24]

## Pathology and Prognostic Indicators

In the United States, TCC accounts for 90 to 95% of all tumors of the bladder, SCC accounts for 5 to 10%, and adenocarcinoma accounts for approximately 1 to 2%.[36] Squamous cell and adenocarcinomatous elements are often found in association with transitional cell tumors, especially in high-grade tumors. In a large series by Melicow,[36] 70% of bladder tumors were found on the posterior and lateral walls near the ureteral orifices, 20% on the trigone and bladder neck, and 10% on the dome of the bladder (Fig. 51–1). Most bladder tumors occur between the ages of 50 and 80 years. As previously stated, TCC of the bladder encompasses a spectrum of disease, ranging from low-grade superficial papillary tumors to high-grade muscle-invasive disease. Approximately 75 to 80% of TCCs of the bladder present as low-grade tumors confined to the superficial mucosa of the bladder. The risk of recurrence in these patients is about 75%, but only 10 to 15% go on to develop invasive disease.

Bladder cancer is generally divided into superficial and invasive disease because the natural history and treatment of the two forms are different. The term *superficial bladder tumor* is traditionally used to identify a tumor that has not invaded the muscularis. The critical factor with regard to biologic potential, however, is the distinction between tumors that are confined to the mucosa versus those that have penetrated the basement membrane and extended into the lamina propria.[37] Mucosally confined tumors (Ta) and low-

## USUAL *SITES* & *SHAPES* OF BLADDER NEOPLASMS

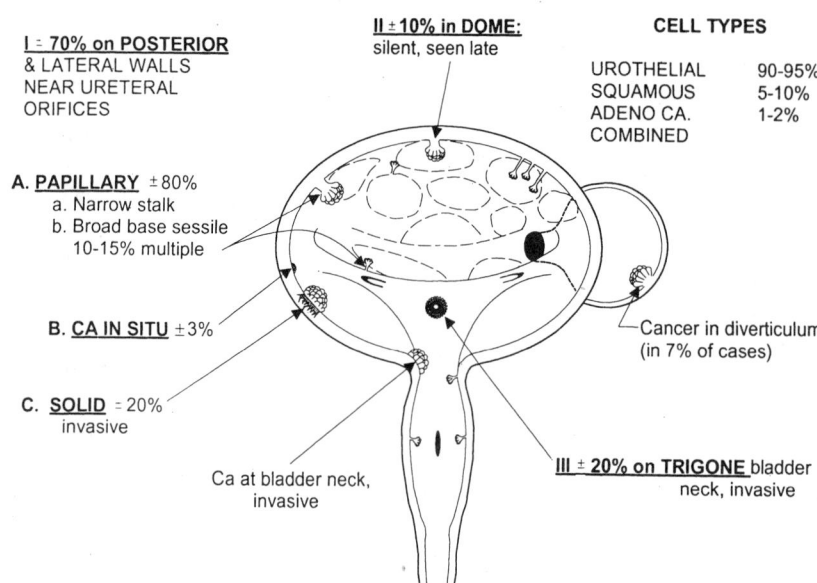

**I = 70% on POSTERIOR**
& LATERAL WALLS
NEAR URETERAL
ORIFICES

**II ± 10% in DOME:**
silent, seen late

**CELL TYPES**

| | |
|---|---|
| UROTHELIAL | 90-95% |
| SQUAMOUS | 5-10% |
| ADENO CA. | 1-2% |
| COMBINED | |

**A. PAPILLARY** ±80%
  a. Narrow stalk
  b. Broad base sessile
  10-15% multiple

**B. CA IN SITU** ±3%

**C. SOLID** = 20%
  invasive

Cancer in diverticulum
(in 7% of cases)

Ca at bladder neck,
invasive

**III ± 20% on TRIGONE** bladder
neck, invasive

**Figure 51–1.** Composite diagram displays gamut of vesical neoplasms from the point of view of site, shape, and cell contents. The relative incidence of each is indicated. (From Melicow MM. Tumors of the bladder: a multifaceted problem. J Urol 1974;112:467.)

grade or moderate-grade tumors are likely to recur but rarely to invade the muscularis.[38] Patients with lamina propria infiltration (T1) eventually have muscle-invasive disease in 25 to 30% of cases.[37, 38] High-grade Ta or any T1 lesions should warrant an aggressive approach, such as adjuvant intravesical therapy.[38]

Carcinoma in situ (CIS), initially described in 1952 by Melicow,[39] was thought to represent the earliest stage of bladder cancer. Subsequent reports documented the development of infiltrative disease in 75% of patients with diffuse CIS.[40] Others have suggested that CIS has limited biologic capacity to invade and metastasize. This suggestion is supported by clinical observations documenting conservative management of patients with the disease for extended periods without the development of invasive cancer.[41] The usual presentation of CIS is with diffuse urothelial involvement in association with one or more bladder tumors. Of bladder tumors, 30 to 70% are associated with CIS, and a higher incidence occurs in association with high-grade tumors. Primary CIS is rarely seen without associated bladder tumors, representing only about 3% of all bladder cancers.[42] No theory of CIS explains all of the clinical observations. When associated with irritative voiding symptoms or when presenting in patients with other papillary tumors, however, CIS is significantly worse in regard to muscle invasion or metastases.[42] When low-grade, low-stage tumors are found to have an associated CIS or severe dysplasia, the probability of subsequent invasion increases dramatically.[43] Another important prognostic factor with CIS is the extent of involvement of the urothelium. Patients with diffuse involvement have a more rapidly progressive course.[43]

Invasive tumors are described as tumors that have invaded the muscularis propria, the perivesical fibroadipose tissue, or adjacent structures. Muscle invasion (T2–T3) of any degree is the usual indication for radical therapy, such as cystectomy with pelvic lymphadenectomy, definitive radiotherapy, neoadjuvant or adjuvant chemotherapy, or combinations of

these. Individual cases of lamina propria invasion associated with high-grade tumors, diffuse CIS, or involvement of the prostatic urethra and cases refractory to conservative management may eventually require radical therapy.

Most patients with invasive bladder cancer have invasive disease at the time of initial presentation. About 50% of patients with muscle-invasive disease already have occult distant metastases at the time of diagnosis; despite radical therapy, 50% of patients who present with muscle-infiltrative cancer develop metastases within 2 years of their initial diagnosis.[44] The most common site of metastases in bladder cancer is the pelvic lymph nodes, occurring in about 78% of patients with metastases.[45] The common sites of vascular metastases from bladder cancer are liver, 38%; lung, 36%; bone, 27%; adrenal, 21%; and intestine, 13%. Any other organ may be involved.[46]

The most clinically useful prognostic parameters for recurrence and subsequent progression in the patient with superficial tumors are grade, stage, lymphatic invasion, tumor size, CIS, papillary or solid tumor configuration, multifocality, and frequency of tumor recurrence. The most important parameters among these are grade, stage, and presence of CIS.[47] Patients with grade III tumors had a 70% incidence of recurrence at 1 year, in contrast to 30% recurrence in patients with grade I tumors and 38% in patients with grade II tumors.[48] Of patients with T1 lesions, 70% had a recurrence within a 3-year period compared with 48% of the patients with stage Ta lesions.[48] Multiplicity of disease has been associated with the likelihood of tumor recurrence rather than disease progression. In patients who initially presented with multiple tumors, the likelihood of recurrence was 90%; the recurrence rate was only 65% in patients with single tumors.[37] The grade of disease correlates with the likelihood of progression. In a National Bladder Cancer Group study, only 2% of grade I tumors, 11% of grade II tumors, and 45% of grade III tumors progressed.[2] A variety of laboratory parameters have also been evaluated in an attempt to predict the biologic potential of bladder tumors. Thompson-Friedenreich (T) antigen expression, lack of ABH blood group antigen, and the presence of epidermal growth factor receptors all portend a worse prognosis for recurrence and progression.[49, 50] Flow cytometry measurement of DNA contents is a useful adjunct to urine cytology.[51, 52] Although aneuploidy is accurate in patients with high-grade tumors or CIS, low-grade tumors, which are usually diploid, often present false-negative results.[51] Quantitative fluorescent image analysis seems to be more sensitive for detecting low-grade tumors.[52] Currently, genetic abnormality is associated with bladder cancer. Loss of pRB gene function is related to high-grade, invasive, or poor prognostic disease.[53] Nuclear accumulation of p53 correlates with poorer prognosis in superficial, invasive, and metastatic disease.[54, 55] There are many requests for standardization of the methodology to assess p53 immunopositivity. At present, the utility of genetic abnormality remains unresolved for clinical management.

## Clinical Presentation

The most common presentation of bladder cancer is painless gross or microscopic hematuria. Bladder irritability, including frequency, urgency, and dysuria, is the second most common presentation; it is present in approximately 20% of patients. These symptoms are more common among patients with CIS or invasive bladder cancer and may be the only presenting symptoms of CIS. Because urinary tract infection and interstitial cystitis can produce similar symptoms, it is important to consider CIS in any patient with a history of chronic irritating voiding symptoms regardless of whether hematuria is present.[40] Because most patients initially present with superficial disease, the physical examination is likely to be completely normal in these patients. Patients with invasive disease may have flank pain from ureteral obstruction, a bladder mass or induration, or lower extremity edema. Occasionally, patients present with symptoms of advanced disease, such as weight loss and abdominal or bone pain.

## Diagnosis

In a patient with hematuria, the diagnostic work-up includes intravenous pyelography, cystoscopy and biopsy, and cytology. Pyelography allows visualization of the upper tracts to help exclude a nonvesical source of the hematuria and to determine whether there is evidence of ureteral obstruction associated with the bladder lesion. Ureteral obstruction is associated with muscle invasion in 92% of patients with TCC of the bladder.[56] Pyelography should be performed before cystoscopy because if an upper tract filling defect is present, retrograde pyelography and selective cytology can be performed to characterize the lesion further. The diagnosis of bladder cancer is established with cystoscopy and biopsy of the lesion. Careful attention should be paid to the remainder of the bladder mucosa and urethra. The mucosa must be evaluated for areas of erythema or irregularity, which may represent CIS. A bimanual examination under anesthesia is also important for staging (see discussion under staging). Exfoliative cytology is an important adjunct in the diagnosis and follow-up of bladder cancer. The limitations of microscopic cytology are that well-differentiated tumors are more

cohesive and not readily shed into the urine. Microscopic cytology is more sensitive in patients with high-grade disease or CIS. Urinary cytology is more than 90% accurate in diagnosing multifocal CIS of the bladder in symptomatic patients.[57] The accuracy of cytologic examination of the urine in the detection of bladder tumors varies considerably and depends greatly on the method of specimen collection, the promptness of fixation, and the skill of the cytologist. Cytology is not a cost-effective means of screening for bladder cancer unless high-risk populations are evaluated.[58] The major role of urine cytology is in the detection of occult urothelial tumors, the screening of high-risk individuals, and the follow-up of urothelial malignancies.

Several novel methods have been used to diagnose or monitor bladder cancer, such as the BTA test (a latex agglutination assay for qualitative detection), NMP22 (nuclear matrix protein), fibrin degradation products, and bladder wash karyometric image analysis.[59–62] These methods may help to detect clinically occult bladder cancer and to increase the interval of cystoscopy.[63] No method or combination of methods has 100% sensitivity and specificity. Selection for clinical use should be based on the desired objective and the performance characteristics of each method.[63]

## Staging and Prognosis

After the cystoscopic diagnosis of a bladder tumor has been made, the patient should be scheduled for transurethral resection of the bladder tumor and for bladder and urethral biopsies under anesthesia. Bladder and urethral *mapping* should be performed to exclude the presence of CIS, which may alter the treatment plan. Mapping should be performed with the cold-cup biopsy forceps so as not to distort mucosal histology. In addition to excretory urography, preoperative staging evaluation should include chest radiograph, serum creatinine, and liver function studies. Some investigators have reported that if serum alkaline phosphatase is elevated, patients should undergo a technetium 99m bone scan to exclude widely metastatic disease.[64] It is our belief, and that of others, that because of the relatively low cost and morbidity of a bone scan, along with its potential impact on treatment, a bone scan should be used routinely in the systemic staging evaluation of muscle-invasive bladder cancer.[65] If the tumor appears invasive (solid rather than papillary) or if it is large (>5 cm), a computed tomographic scan of the abdomen and pelvis should be performed. Although computed tomography (CT) and magnetic resonance imaging (MRI) have limited usefulness in the definition of superficial bladder cancer, CT can determine the presence of bladder wall thickening and aid in the staging of invasive bladder cancer. Loss of the perivesical fat plane on CT or loss of a low-intensity line surrounding the bladder on MRI, especially when using T1-weighted images, suggests but does not confirm extramural tumor extension.[66] Gadolinium–diethylenetriaminepentaacetic acid (DTPA)–enhanced MRI for bladder tumor staging showed improved sensitivity and specificity in detecting muscle invasion (96.2% and 83.3%) relative to transurethral ultrasonography (88.0% and 66.7%) and CT (96.0% and 58.3%).[67] Gadolinium-DTPA also improved the accuracy of dynamic enhanced MRI in superficial bladder cancer.[68] In addition to assessing the extent of the primary tumor, CT provides information about the presence of pelvic and para-aortic lymphadenopathy and the possible presence of liver or adrenal metastases. CT, however, can detect only lymph nodes that are grossly enlarged (>1 cm) and liver metastases that are larger than 2 cm in diameter.[69] If CT or MRI is to be performed, it should be done before local therapy because transurethral resection or radiation therapy may cause perturbation of tissue planes that frequently makes interpretation of CT or MRI invalid for prediction of depth of tumor infiltration. Lymphangiography, which was once used to identify nodal metastases, has been replaced by CT. Liver scans for identifying liver metastases have been supplanted by CT or MRI.

Once the patient is anesthetized, bimanual examination is performed before tumor resection and repeated after the endoscopic resection is completed. The presence of a mass should be noted, along with any evidence of induration or fixation to adjacent structures. The disappearance of a movable mass after resection is most consistent with superficial disease. If the mass is fixed, indurated, or persists after resection, muscle-invasive disease should be suspected. Bimanual examination cannot differentiate benign and malignant bladder fixation in patients with previous radiation therapy or pelvic inflammatory disease. If any of the studies in the metastatic evaluation suggest the presence of metastases, histologic confirmation should be sought by the least invasive means possible, usually fine-needle aspiration biopsy. The primary transurethral resection of the tumor is the most important test for judging the depth of penetration of the tumor. Histologic specimens must be carefully interpreted to distinguish smooth muscle fibers in the lamina propria from those of the detrusor muscle. After the primary tumor is biopsied or resected, the patient is staged.

## Staging System

A staging system for bladder cancer has evolved from observations of the clinical course of different tumors in associa-tion with their depth of penetration through the bladder wall at their initial presentation. The prognosis of bladder cancer depends on the stage and grade of the tumor. In 1946, Jewett and Strong[70] demonstrated the relationship of bladder carcinoma dissemination to the extent of local invasion. This system (later modified by Marshall and colleagues[71]) is used by most urologists in the United States. The shortcoming of this system is the inclusion of CIS in stage 0. It became apparent that the Jewett-Strong-Marshall staging system must be expanded to accommodate additional tumor characteristics. In an attempt to establish an international method of invasion classification, the International Union Against Cancer and the American Joint Committee on Cancer Staging proposed the TNM system.[72] The advantage of this system is that it tends to provide uniformity of staging among all nations. Also, there is separate classification for clinical and pathologic staging. An important advantage is that CIS, originally grouped in stage 0 by the Marshall classification, is separated as a distinct entity (TIS) in the TNM system.[71] A distinction was made between papillary tumors without lamina propria invasion (Ta) and those that had invaded the lamina propria (T1). A comparison of the TNM and Jewett-Strong-Marshall staging systems is shown in Figure 51–2. The clinical significance of separating B1 and B2 or T2 from T3a disease is unclear. The distinction is not supported by differences in survival.[73] The presence of muscle invasion by the tumor appears to be the best predictor of biologic potential of a particular tumor. On this basis, treatment of bladder neoplasms falls broadly into two categories distinguished by the presence or absence of tumor invasion into the muscularis propria.

Several large series have shown that clinical stage often does not correlate with pathologic stage. Approximately 50 to 60% of patients are understaged or overstaged with initial clinical staging. In a review of four large series in the literature, 35% of patients were clinically understaged, and

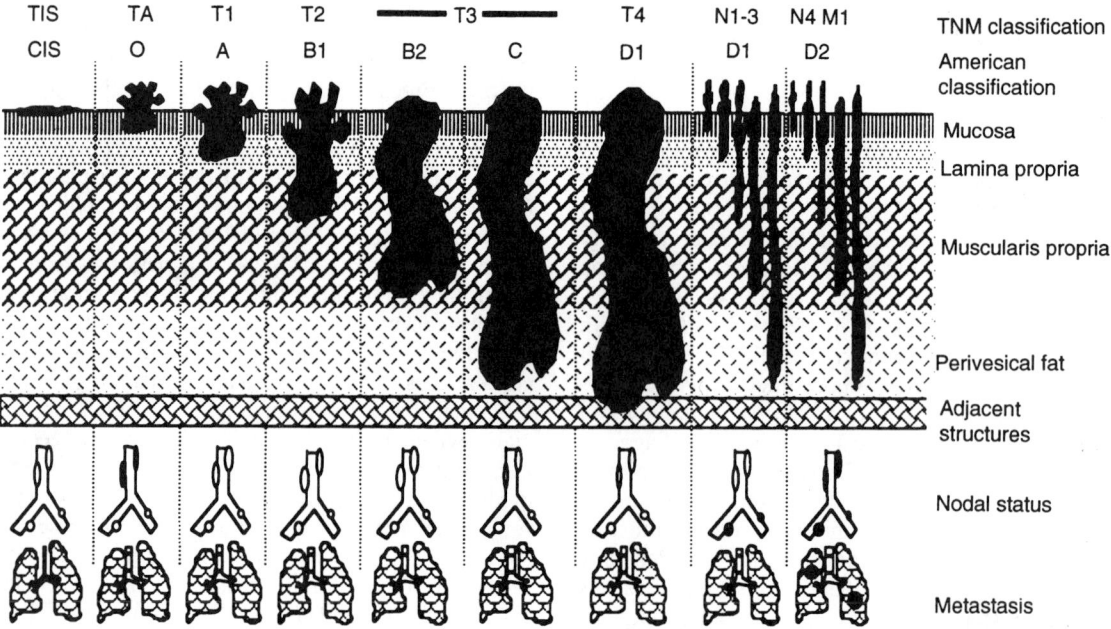

**Figure 51–2.** TNM staging classification for bladder neoplasms. The American Classification (Jewett-Strong-Marshall) is shown for comparison. Tumors T1 (A) or less are considered superficial; tumors T2 (B1) or greater are considered invasive. (From See WA. Staging of advanced bladder cancer. Urol Clin North Am 1992;19:663.)

23% were clinically overstaged.[74] Transurethral resection cannot assess the depth of tumor invasion accurately in all cases.

## MANAGEMENT OF SUPERFICIAL BLADDER CANCER (STAGES Ta AND T1)

**Transurethral Resection.** Most patients with superficial bladder cancer can be adequately treated with transurethral resection or fulguration of the tumor. The overall survival rates of patients with superficial bladder cancer treated with transurethral resection alone are excellent. Five-year survival is approximately 70 to 80%.[75, 76] With superficial bladder cancer, however, recurrence is the rule. About 71% of patients develop tumor recurrences following endoscopic resection, and half of those experience recurrence within 1 year after the original tumor resection.[76] In the study by Althausen and associates,[43] 85% of patients had recurrence of low-grade, low-stage tumors during an 8-year follow-up. As previously stated, the probability of tumor recurrence is directly related to the stage (Ta or T1), histologic grading (grade 1, 2, or 3), size of the tumor, multiplicity of the tumors, and presence of CIS. Recurrence is treated with repeat transurethral resection or fulguration.

A dire prognostic factor is the recurrence of tumors to a higher grade or stage. Approximately 10 to 15% of patients with superficial bladder cancer subsequently develop more aggressive lesions and ultimately require aggressive therapy.[2, 43] T1 tumors have a significantly higher rate of progression than do Ta tumors. Of T1 grade 3 tumors, 48% go on to muscle invasion. Patients with T1 tumors should be considered as having potentially aggressive tumors, especially if they are high grade.[77]

Resectoscope excision of bladder tumors with a *hot loop* is the usual method, but excision with a cold-cup forceps is often suitable. The superficial portion of the tumor is usually resected first and sent to the pathologist as a separate specimen. The deep portion, along with some underlying bladder muscle, is then resected and sent for histologic examination. After the tumor has been completely resected, the base of the resection site is fulgurated. This approach usually produces complete removal of the tumor and provides valuable diagnostic information about the grade and depth of infiltration of the tumor. In patients with a history of low-grade superficial recurrences, it is acceptable to treat these tumors with simple fulguration. This method does not provide tissue for histologic tumor staging or grading, however. In patients with extensive broad-based sessile tumors, which are almost certain to require cystectomy, complete tumor resection is not always necessary, particularly if the tumor is in an area that is difficult to reach with the resectoscope. Attempts at complete resection may result in bladder perforation with dissemination of tumor cells. In such cases, it may be more prudent to begin resecting at the margin of the tumor and progress toward the center, resecting enough tissue to establish the tumor grade and depth of penetration. If this approach is used, frozen sections should document muscle invasion. Tumors encroaching on the ureteral orifices should be resected without regard to the orifice. The orifice should not be fulgurated after the tumor is resected, however. A ureteral stent may be left in place for several days to prevent

obstruction of the orifice by scarring.[78] Tumors arising in bladder diverticula should be biopsied rather than resected. These tumors are best treated definitively with partial or total cystectomy. Transurethral resection should not be attempted because of the high risk of bladder perforation.[78] As previously mentioned, cold-cup biopsy specimens should be taken from areas adjacent to the tumor as well as from the trigone, lateral walls, dome, and, in men, prostatic urethra.

**Adjuvant Therapies.** A variety of treatments have been used as adjuvant therapy in patients with superficial bladder cancer to prevent recurrence and progression, including intravesical chemotherapy and immunotherapy, systemic chemotherapy, photoradiation therapy, laser therapy, and external-beam radiotherapy. Either adjuvant intravesical chemotherapy or immunotherapy is indicated for patients who are at high risk for recurrence or progression. Patients with recurrent tumors, multiple or high-grade tumors, tumors that have invaded the lamina propria, or tumors associated with CIS are candidates to receive adjuvant intravesical therapy. Commonly used therapies are intravesical chemotherapy, including thiotepa, mitomycin C, doxorubicin (Adriamycin), or ethoglucid (Epodyl), and intravesical immunotherapy, including Bacille Calmette-Guérin (BCG) or interferon.

Thiotepa was introduced in 1961 and was the first and most widely used modern intravesical chemotherapeutic agent.[79] The usual protocol is 30 to 60 mg in 30 to 60 ml of saline weekly for 6 to 8 weeks followed by monthly treatments for 1 year. The standard contact time is 1 to 2 hours, based mainly on patient convenience. Thiotepa has been used as a therapeutic as well as a prophylactic agent. When used as definitive therapy, approximately one third of patients show a complete response. After transurethral resection, thiotepa has been shown to reduce recurrence rates to 47% at 2 years compared with 73% in patients not receiving prophylaxis.[80] In this study, 16% of patients receiving thiotepa prophylaxis had tumor progression, 8% developed muscle-invasive disease, and 3% developed distant metastases. In a randomized study, thiotepa failed to reduce recurrence rate and time to first recurrence when compared with no-treatment controls.[81] Therapy is usually delayed about 2 weeks until surgical resection sites have healed. Thiotepa is readily absorbed through the urothelium because of its relatively low molecular weight (189 d) and causes myelosuppression in 15 to 20% of patients.[82] Additional toxicities, such as chemical cystitis or bladder contracture, occur infrequently. Because of the potential for myelosuppression, careful monitoring of the white blood cell and platelet count is mandatory.

Mitomycin C is an antibiotic chemotherapeutic agent that acts by inhibition of DNA synthesis. Because of its higher molecular weight (334 d), it has minimal intravesical absorption, and systemic side effects are uncommon. Its major toxic effects are chemical cystitis and skin rashes that occur from contact of the drug with the skin of the hands and genitalia. Mitomycin C is usually administered in a dose of 40 mg intravesically weekly for 8 weeks followed by monthly maintenance therapy for 1 year. In a combined series of 128 patients, complete tumor responses occurred in 66% of patients and partial responses in another 26%.[83] Mitomycin C appears to have activity in patients in whom thiotepa has failed. In a series by DeFuria and associates,[84]

8 of 9 patients responded to mitomycin C after failure with thiotepa. Soloway[85] reported that 8% of complete responders, 23% of partial responders, and 19% of nonresponders developed muscle-invasive cancer, and 7% died of metastatic bladder cancer. A randomized study by the Southwestern Oncology Group (SWOG) and the Eastern Cooperative Oncology Group (ECOG) showed that 20 mg of mitomycin C given in weekly installations for 6 weeks and then monthly for 1 year in patients with recurrent superficial tumors or CIS was significantly less effective in preventing tumor recurrences than BCG (54% for mitomycin C vs. 39% for BCG).[86] The relatively high cost of mitomycin C compared with the other intravesical agents has also limited its widespread use.

Doxorubicin is another antibiotic chemotherapeutic agent. It shows efficacy equivalent to thiotepa, with a 31% recurrence rate compared with 71% in patients treated with transurethral resection alone.[87] Dosages range from 50 to 90 mg given on widely varying treatment schedules. As with thiotepa, progression to muscle-invasive disease is reported in 16% of patients.[87] The primary side effect is severe cystitis, which occurs in 10 to 25% of patients and can progress to permanent bladder contracture in a few patients. Systemic toxicity is minimal because of doxorubicin's high molecular weight (580 d).

Other intravesical agents have been used for the treatment of superficial bladder cancer, including ethoglucid, which has been used in Europe and Japan with efficacy similar to that of thiotepa.[88] Although thiotepa, mitomycin C, and doxorubicin all eradicate some tumors and decrease recurrence rates, they have minimal impact on the incidence of muscle-invasive recurrences or ultimate cancer death rates. A review of 22 randomized studies of intravesical chemotherapy for superficial bladder cancer showed that maintenance chemotherapy failed to demonstrate a long-term benefit in the incidence of recurrent tumors.[89]

**Intravesical Bacille Calmette-Guérin Therapy.** BCG is an attenuated strain of *Mycobacterium bovis* that has stimulatory effects on immune responses. BCG has been administered intravesically to treat superficial bladder cancer and is generally believed to be the most effective intravesical agent for this purpose.[90] In 1976, Morales and associates[91] introduced intravesical BCG therapy combined with intradermal inoculation as prophylaxis against tumor recurrence in patients with superficial bladder cancer. Subsequently, intradermal inoculation was shown to be unnecessary.[92] BCG is commonly given in three clinical settings: (1) prophylaxis in patients after transurethral resection, in whom there is a high probability of tumor recurrence; (2) treatment of patients with residual papillary TCC other than CIS; and (3) treatment of patients with CIS.[78]

Several strains of BCG have been used, including Pasteur, Armand Frappier, Tice, Connaught, Glaxo, Tokyo, Dutch, and Moreau. All are derived from the original strain developed at the Pasteur Institute. Studies have shown that the effectiveness of BCG may vary considerably from strain to strain and even from lot to lot within the same strain.[93] The Glaxo strain has been reported to be ineffective.[94]

Prospective, randomized trials have shown that BCG is effective against tumor recurrence.[86, 95, 96] Rodrigues Netto and Lemos[97] conducted a randomized trial comparing BCG with thiotepa for prophylaxis. The recurrence rates with BCG were less than 10% compared with 40% for thiotepa. Coplen and associates[98] reported muscle-invasive progression in only 4.1% of 72 patients (55 treated for prophylaxis, 17 for residual tumor) treated with BCG with a mean follow-up of 48 months. Several combined series showed that using BCG for prophylaxis, tumor recurrence rates ranged from 0 to 41%, with most being around 20%, whereas patients not receiving BCG treatments (no treatment, thiotepa, doxorubicin, or mitomycin C) had recurrence rates of 40 to 80%.[78] BCG has also been used to treat residual unresectable tumors, although BCG should not be considered a substitute for the resection of resectable tumors. Overall, when used for this purpose, several series showed a complete response rate of 58%.[78] Herr[99] calculated the net reduction in tumor recurrences between those treated with resection alone and those who received adjuvant therapy, finding a benefit of 42% for those receiving BCG, whereas the net benefit for patients receiving mitomycin C was 12%; for doxorubicin, it was 10%; and for thiotepa, it was 8%. Herr concluded that BCG in the high-risk patient with superficial bladder cancer delayed the disease progression, prolonged the period of bladder preservation, and increased survival. The ten-year progression-free rate was 61.9% for patients treated with BCG compared with 37% for control patients, and the 10-year survival rate for patients treated with BCG was 75%.[96]

Although an optimal treatment schedule has not been established, an induction phase is necessary for the development of an inflammatory and immunologic response within the bladder epithelium and lamina propria. Protocols for prophylaxis with BCG vary widely. All include an induction period of 6-week instillations followed by either some combination of maintenance instillation or no additional therapy. Lamm and associates[100] reported on the results of the SWOG study that compared recurrence rates in patients receiving a single 6-week course of therapy with those continuing with maintenance therapy at 3 months, 6 months, and every 6 months for a period of 3 years. The data indicated that maintenance therapy significantly reduced tumor recurrence and improved survival.

Most investigators recommend waiting 2 weeks following tumor resection before starting BCG therapy. Early administration of BCG may be associated with a greater risk of severe complications. Bladder irritability is the most common side effect of BCG therapy but is expected as a consequence of the immune stimulation and inflammatory reaction that are thought to be essential components of the mechanism of action of BCG. Granulomatous prostatitis commonly occurred following BCG treatment, but only 6% of those patients required treatment.[101] BCG has no direct toxic effect on malignant cells but rather stimulates a generalized immune response that results in tumor destruction. Cystitis typically occurs after the third BCG instillation and may increase in severity with subsequent treatments. The symptoms are frequently associated with mild temperature elevations and malaise. Symptomatic treatment with antipyretics and anticholinergics is recommended. In a review of complications in 2602 patients treated with BCG, symptoms severe enough to require antituberculous therapy occurred in 5% of patients. BCG sepsis was reported in 0.4% of patients, and death occurred in 7 patients.[102] Patients having fever persisting more than 48 hours or greater than 38.5° C for more than 12 hours should be treated with isoniazid 300 mg/day.

Patients that are acutely ill from BCG sepsis should be treated with antituberculous agents plus cycloserine or prednisolone. In Lamm's review, the 7 patients who died either had a traumatic catheterization before instillation therapy or were treated too early after transurethral resection or biopsy. Lamm and associates[102] report that no patient who has been treated with antituberculous agents plus cycloserine or prednisolone has died.

Interferons have been used for superficial bladder cancer because of their antiproliferative, antiangiogenic, and immunostimulator properties.[103] The recurrence rate for 9 million IU of intravesical interferon alfa-2b for 8 weeks in patients with stage Ta and T1 was 45%.[104] A randomized study of stage T1 patients who received 54 million IU interferon alfa-2a weekly for 8 weeks followed by monthly for 9 months versus BCG showed that BCG had a higher efficacy for prophylaxis of the recurrence (69.4% recurrent rate for interferon vs. 39.3% for BCG).[105] Tolerability of interferon was good. The main side effect was flu-like symptoms. No serious side effect was seen.[104, 105]

External-beam radiation therapy has generally proved ineffective in treating patients with superficial bladder cancer. It does not prevent the occurrence of new tumors and may be associated with considerable morbidity, particularly radiation cystitis.[106]

Total or partial cystectomy is rarely required for patients with superficial bladder cancer except for those with severe symptomatic, diffuse, unresectable papillary tumors; CIS that does not respond to intravesical therapy; persistent involvement of prostatic urethra; or persistence of tumors in a nonfunctioning bladder.[107, 108] Because 52% of patients with T1 grade 3 disease do not experience progression, initial cystectomy can represent an overtreatment. When these patients are well selected, intravesical therapy can improve survival and quality of life significantly. The persistent or recurrent T1 grade 3 cancer may be considered for cystectomy.[77]

Photodynamic therapy using hematoporphyrin derivative is based on the selective uptake of porphyrins by neoplastic and dysplastic tissues. If these tissues are irradiated with light of an appropriate wavelength, tumor cells containing porphyrins are killed by the formation of oxygen singlets. Clinical trials have shown some successes against superficial tumors and CIS, but recurrence was common.[109] Adverse effects include generalized cutaneous photosensitivity and bladder contractures in about one fifth of patients. Hematoporphyrin derivative is considered investigational at this time.

Laser fulguration of superficial bladder tumors with the neodymium:yttrium-aluminum-garnet (Nd:YAG) laser has been used with good local control, but its proper role in the treatment of bladder cancer remains unclear. There are no proven definitive therapeutic advantages over standard electrocautery resection. Laser treatment of muscle-invasive tumors has also been used in selected high-risk patients who are either too ill for or refuse cystectomy. In these patients, if the tumors are not too large, the Nd:YAG laser may achieve adequate local control.[110] Laser therapy is theoretically attractive because it can be performed through a small cystoscope using local anesthesia without bleeding or obturator nerve stimulation. The main disadvantage is that the tumor tissue is destroyed by the laser and is not available for histologic examination.

Transurethral resection of superficial bladder carcinoma is the primary modality for treating existing lesions. The incidence of recurrence and progression depends on the initial stage, grade, multiplicity, size of tumor, nuclear ploidy, and presence of CIS. Adjuvant chemotherapy and immunotherapy have been useful in treating tumors with a high likelihood of recurrence or progression.

The traditional follow-up program recommended for patients with superficial bladder cancer includes serial cystoscopies and urine cytology every 3 months for 2 years, every 6 months for 2 years, and then yearly for life. Some investigators believe that patients with low-grade tumors do not need cystoscopy as frequently.[111] Similarly, investigators differ on recommendations for routine monitoring, such as excretory urography (intravenous pyelography), of the upper tracts. A study showed that with median follow-up of 30 months, 16 of 680 patients with bladder cancer subsequently developed upper tract carcinoma. Of 16 patients, 7 presented with gross hematuria and 3 with abdominal pain and fever. This study suggested that routine intravenous pyelography of the upper tract is not indicated during follow-up of patients with bladder cancer.[112] Others, however, suggested that regular intravenous pyelography monitoring should be performed in patients with multiple and recurrent tumors or with tumors involving the ureteral orifice.[113]

## TREATMENT OF CARCINOMA IN SITU

CIS, as described previously, is a high-grade and aggressive manifestation of TCC of the bladder that has a highly variable course. The treatment of CIS has undergone dramatic changes since this malignancy was first recognized. Although cystectomy was once recommended as the initial treatment of choice, other treatments are now available. Treatment of CIS has been revolutionized by the success of BCG. Response data available from 18 series, including 709 patients, show an average complete response rate of 70% (Table 51–1).[114] A SWOG study of 131 patients with CIS randomized treatments between 6-week courses of BCG and doxorubicin. Of the patients treated with BCG, 70% had a complete response, and the median duration of the response was 39 months. Of the patients treated with BCG, 45% were disease free for 5 years compared with 18% of those treated with doxorubicin ($p < 0.001$) (Table 51–2).[115] In another randomized SWOG study, the rate of complete response with BCG was increased by 25% at 6 months with an additional 3-week course of BCG at 3 months. With this regimen, an overall complete response rate of 82% was obtained in 72 patients. In patients with a complete response, maintenance BCG immunotherapy consisting of 3-week treatments at the sixth month followed by treatment every 6 months for 3 years resulted in improving long-term complete response rates from 65% to nearly 90%. With this regimen, the estimated 5-year disease-free rate increased to more than 75%.[114, 116] Because of the response of CIS to BCG therapy, Lamm[114] has stated that radical cystectomy is no longer the generally recommended initial approach. Of patients treated with BCG, 70% can expect a complete response by 3 months, and 82% can expect to have a complete response

*Table 51–1.* Responses to Bacillus Calmette-Guérin in Carcinoma In Situ

| Source | No. Patients | Complete Response (No. [%]) |
|---|---|---|
| Morales | 7 | 5 (71) |
| Herr | 47 | 34 (72) |
| Lamm | 14 | 11 (79) |
| Brosman | 33 | 27 (82) |
| Kelly et al | 12 | 8 (67) |
| Staiano-Colco | 22 | 12 (55) |
| Schellhammer et al | 6 | 6 (100) |
| deKernion et al | 19 | 13 (68) |
| Soloway and Perry | 9 | 5 (56) |
| Kavoussi et al | 59 | 23 (39) |
| Rintala et al | 10 | 4 (40) |
| Brosman | 40 | 28 (70) |
| Steg et al | 30 | 23 (77) |
| Pagano | 27 | 21 (78) |
| Prescott et al | 16 | 14 (88) |
| Reitsma | 153 | 107 (70) |
| SWOG 8216 (1991) | 64 | 45 (70) |
| SWOG 8507 (1991) | | |
| 6 weekly | 78 | 55 (70) |
| 6 + 3 | 72 | 59 (82) |
| Total | 718 | 500 (70) |

SWOG, Southwestern Oncology Group.
From Lamm DL. Carcinoma in situ. Urol Clin North Am 1992; 19:499.

by 6 months with additional 3-week treatments at 3 months. These results are associated with an excellent long-term disease-free survival rate. In patients who fail to respond to an additional trial of BCG immunotherapy or other chemotherapeutic agent, salvage radical cystectomy can be performed. Some investigators have pointed out that although the response rates to intravesical BCG for patients with CIS are favorable, treatment is not successful in all patients. Some have a progression to invasive or metastatic disease.[117] The concern is that because some patients require repeated courses of intravesical therapy before a beneficial effect can be obtained, the tumor may become invasive and metastasize during attempts at conservative therapy. Although it is recommended that patients be offered the option of radical cystectomy, there is no evidence to confirm that cystectomy provides superior survival or quality of life compared with an initial trial of BCG followed by salvage cystectomy if necessary. If progression occurs at any time, the patient is encouraged to undergo cystectomy. Many patients would be

spared radical cystectomy by the use of this approach, but randomized trials are necessary to determine long-term results and survival.

CIS has been treated with intravesical chemotherapeutic agents with somewhat poor results. Response data from 26 studies show complete response with thiotepa in only 38%, with doxorubicin in 48%, and with mitomycin in 53% of patients (Table 51–3).[114] The largest experience with doxorubicin is with SWOG, in which a complete response was seen in only 23 of 67 patients (34%).[115] Most studies of intravesical mitomycin C for CIS have small numbers of patients, with overall results only slightly better than those for doxorubicin.[114] At this time, BCG is the intravesical therapy of choice for patients with CIS.

Patients who continue to demonstrate positive urine cytology results with an endoscopically normal-appearing bladder and mucosal biopsy specimens without evidence of tumor after intravesical BCG therapy are a difficult treatment dilemma. In a series of 18 patients with positive urine cytologic findings but without overt tumor, 11 (61%) had progression to muscle-invasive disease during a follow-up interval of 19 months.[118] Prostatic urethral involvement and ureteral involvement by CIS are known to produce positive cytologic results in the absence of definable bladder pathology. A transurethral resection of the prostate is indicated in these patients to exclude the prostatic urethra as a source of abnormal cells. To exclude ureteral or upper tract involvement, saline barbotage specimens should be collected separately from each ureter. Bilateral retrograde ureteropyelograms should be performed to define the ureters and renal pelvis. If these measures fail to detect the source of the abnormal cells, ureteroscopy with biopsy of the ureteral mucosa and renal pelvis may be necessary to detect CIS. Treatment of these patients should be initiated only when the source of positive cytologic findings has been identified.

Patients in whom BCG immunotherapy fails without evidence of progression may yet be candidates for other forms of treatment, including interferon alfa-2b, bropirimine, keyhole-limpet hemocyanin, or photodynamic therapy.[119, 120] These methods are currently under investigation, and early results are encouraging.[119]

Patients with CIS involving the prostatic urethra may respond to intravesical BCG after transurethral resection of the prostate. Tumor invasion into the prostatic stroma or extensive involvement is best managed by radical cystoprostatectomy.[121]

External-beam radiation has no proven role in the management of CIS. Generally, poor results have been reported.[41]

*Table 51–2.* Results of Treatment with Bacillus Calmette-Guérin or Doxorubicin in Patients with Carcinoma In Situ

| Treatment | No. Patients | Complete Response* (No. [%]) | 95% CI | Median Time to Complete Response (mo) | No. with Treatment Failure† | Median Time to Treatment Failure† (mo) |
|---|---|---|---|---|---|---|
| DOX | 67 | 23 (34) | 23–47 | 3.4 | 15 | 10.2 |
| BCG | 64 | 45 (70) | 58–81 | 2.9 | 19 | 16.5 |

*A complete response was defined as the complete disappearance of disease documented by a normal cystoscopic examination, normal findings on examination of a random biopsy specimen, and normal findings on cytologic analysis of urine. The difference between the groups in the probability of complete response was significant ($p < 0.001$ by two-tailed Fisher's exact test).
†Only data for patients with a complete response were analyzed.
CI, confidence interval; DOX, doxorubicin; BCG, bacillus Calmette-Guérin.
From Lamm DL. A randomized trial of intravesical doxorubicin and immunotherapy with BCG for TCC of the bladder. N Engl J Med 1991;325:1205.

*Table 51–3.* **Chemotherapy Responses in Carcinoma In Situ**

| Source | No. Patients | Complete Response (No. [%]) |
|---|---|---|
| Thiotepa | | |
| Koontz et al | 20 | 11 (55) |
| Proul | 40 | 16 (40) |
| Stanisic et al | 24 | 6 (25) |
| Prout et al | 5 | 1 (20) |
| Subtotal | 89 | 34 (38) |
| Doxorubicin | | |
| Edsmyr and Anderson | 8 | 7 (88) |
| Edsmyr et al | 30 | 20 (67) |
| Duchek and Pavone-Macaluso | 9 | 4 (44) |
| Jakse et al | 15 | 10 (67) |
| Glashan | 55 | 35 (64) |
| Ek et al | 22 | 2 (9) |
| Stanisic et al | 6 | 0 |
| Lamm et al | 67 | 23 (34) |
| Subtotal | 212 | 101 (48) |
| Mitomycin C | | |
| Flüchter et al | 6 | 6 (100) |
| Harrison et al | 6 | 4 (67) |
| Issel et al | 14 | 4 (29) |
| Bouffioux | 5 | 3 (60) |
| Powell | 5 | 3 (60) |
| Soloway | 12 | 5 (42) |
| Koontz et al | 20 | 9 (45) |
| Jauhiainen et al | 11 | 9 (82) |
| Cant et al | 12 | 5 (42) |
| Lucero and Wise | 5 | 4 (80) |
| Hetherington et al | 4 | 4 (100) |
| Stricker et al | 19 | 15 (79) |
| Stanisic et al | 7 | 0 |
| Soloway | 21 | 7 (33) |
| Subtotal | 147 | 78 (53) |
| Chemotherapy total response | 448 | 213 (48) |

From Lamm DL. Carcinoma in situ. Urol Clin North Am 1992; 19:499.

## TREATMENT OF MUSCLE-INVASIVE BLADDER CANCER

Once the diagnosis of muscle invasion (T2–T3) has been established, metastatic disease should be excluded (see under staging). If there is no evidence of metastatic disease, aggressive therapy should be planned. Therapy for muscle-invasive bladder cancer can be divided into bladder preservation and bladder reconstruction. The advantages of bladder preservation include the ability to micturate in a normal fashion and the preservation of potency. These considerations, however, should not preclude the possibility of potentially curative surgery. Radical cystectomy remains the standard by which other modes of therapy are judged. The optimal therapy is yet to be determined.

Transurethral resection is seldom adequate therapy for muscle-invasive bladder cancers. The true depth of the tumor is difficult to assess during the procedure, and in many instances the extent of resection is inadequate to remove the entire microscopic extension of the tumor. Exceptions to this rule are patients with small tumors that have only superficial muscle invasion. Henry and associates[122] reported that 5-year survival rates in patients with stage B1 and B2 bladder tumors treated with transurethral resection alone were better than rates in those treated with preoperative radiation therapy

followed by radical cystectomy, radical cystectomy alone, or definitive radiation therapy alone. Patients treated with transurethral resection generally had smaller tumors than patients in the other groups, however. Herr[123] also reported that appropriately selected patients with muscle-invasive bladder cancer had excellent survival results; 30 of 45 patients (60%) retained their bladder at a mean follow-up of 5 years following transurethral resection. Despite local recurrences, these patients usually were treated by transurethral resections and intravesical BCG. Solsona and colleagues[124] had similar results. Other investigators, however, have reported results that are significantly inferior when compared with results of more radical surgical procedures. These results are generally characterized by a high local failure or recurrence rate.[125] They suggest that resection may play a detrimental role by causing tumor dissemination. Transurethral resection should probably be reserved for patients with small, low-grade tumors with only superficial muscle invasion and for patients who are medically unfit for cystectomy.

Partial or segmental cystectomy is another therapeutic option for selected patients with muscle-invasive bladder cancer. In properly chosen patients, results are comparable to radical cystectomy. A series of partial cystectomy was reviewed by Sweeney and associates.[126] They found that the 5-year survival of patients treated with partial cystectomy was similar to those treated with radical cystectomy. The rates of tumor recurrence were 38 to 78%, with many of them eventually requiring radical cystectomy.[126] A study of combined partial cystectomy and chemotherapy (MVAC [methotrexate, vinblastine, Adriamycin, cisplatin]) in selected invasive bladder cancer patients found that 65% survived more than 5 years. Of those who survived, 54% had a disease-free, normally functioning bladder.[127] These results are no better than partial cystectomy alone, however. The indications for partial cystectomy include patients with a low-grade, unifocal, invasive tumor without evidence of prior tumor, more than 2 cm from the bladder neck, and with no evidence of CIS.[78] Other indications include a tumor in a vesical diverticulum and tumors not amenable to transurethral resection because of size or location.[128] It is also desirable to achieve a 2-cm margin of resection around the tumor.[78] Using these strict selection criteria, few patients are truly candidates for partial cystectomy. Implantation of tumor cells into the surgical wound is a potential complication of this procedure. Wound implantation has been reported in 10 to 20% of patients undergoing partial cystectomy.[129] Wound implantation of tumor cells can be prevented by the preoperative administration of 10 to 12 Gy to the bladder.[130] This dose of radiation is well tolerated and does not interfere with bladder function.

In the United States, radical cystectomy is now the accepted method of treatment for muscle-invasive bladder cancer. The indications for the operation are fairly standard, and the most controversial issues are the role of adjuvant preoperative radiation therapy and the value of pelvic lymphadenectomy. It is difficult to compare radical cystectomy results with results in which radiation therapy or chemotherapy is used alone or in a neoadjuvant or adjuvant setting. Difficulty in comparing these studies is based on differences in patient selection, differences in periods covered, differences in clinical versus pathologic staging, and differences in comparing retrospective with prospective data. Overall survival rates for surgical series indicated 5-year survival rates of 65 to 82% for P2 and P3a disease and 37 to 61% for P3b disease.[78] Some believe this improvement in survival is due to stage migration based on improved preoperative staging and earlier detection rather than a change in the natural history of the disease or an improvement in therapy.[131]

Radical cystectomy in men is usually called a *radical cystoprostatectomy*. This procedure includes a pelvic lymphadenectomy with wide excision of the bladder and prostate along with the bladder pedicles and perivesical fat. Preoperative evaluation of prostatic involvement by bladder TCC is essential for considering urethrectomy. The most common sites of TCC involvement of the prostatic urethra, duct, or stroma in the prostate are at the 5 and 7 o'clock positions adjacent to the verumontanum.[132] Transurethral resection biopsy or needle biopsy should be performed before radical cystectomy.[133] If there is tumor involvement of the prostatic urethra, duct, or stroma, a total urethrectomy should be performed.[78] In women, the standard operation for invasive bladder cancer is wide excision of the bladder and urethra with the uterus and adnexa and the anterior wall of the vagina (anterior pelvic exenteration).[78] The distal ureters should be evaluated by frozen section to ensure that there is no evidence of residual cancer.

The role of pelvic lymphadenectomy is controversial. The incidence of pelvic nodal metastasis in patients undergoing radical cystectomy ranges from 15 to 24% and is related to the depth of the primary tumor's invasion: 6 to 31% for stage P2–P3a; 27 to 59% for stage P3b; and 45 to 60% for stage P4.[134–138] Pelvic lymphadenectomy has been shown to have a therapeutic benefit in a select group of patients— those with only one or two positive lymph nodes. This procedure has not been shown to increase morbidity.[139–141] The least controversial benefit of pelvic lymphadenectomy is in the accurate staging information that is obtained, which becomes more important with regard to adjuvant therapy.[139] If grossly suspicious lymphadenopathy is found to be positive for metastasis on frozen section, cystectomy is usually not performed. The technique of radical cystectomy depends on the preference of the surgeon. For a detailed description of the technique, see the review by Elmajizn and Skinner.[142]

A variety of urinary diversions can be used in patients undergoing cystectomy for invasive bladder cancer. The first type is the ileal conduit, which remains the gold standard because of its low morbidity and because it is extremely well tolerated from a physiologic standpoint. The second type is some form of a continent catheterizable reservoir. These reservoirs can be constructed entirely of ileum, from portions of small and large bowel, entirely of large intestine, or from portions of stomach. The advantage of this type of diversion is that it does not require an external appliance for storing urine. Finally, male patients can be offered an orthotopic or neobladder. With this type of procedure, the neobladder is anastomosed directly to the urethra, and the patient voids using the Valsalva maneuver (Credé voiding). In the past, this type of diversion was not available to women facing cystectomy for TCC because total urethrectomy was recommended for this disease in all female patients. At present, an orthotopic neobladder has become the preferred diversion after cystectomy in most women.[143] The significant risk factors for urethral involvement are bladder neck inva-

sion for all clinical stages and vaginal or cervical invasion for stage T3b or T4.[144] Women who are candidates for orthotopic reconstruction should undergo biopsies of the bladder neck and urethra as part of the preoperative evaluation. Intraoperative frozen sections of the urethra and vaginal margin should be obtained.[144] The various options now available give the patient a more socially acceptable alternative to the standard ileal conduit. Continent reservoirs and diversions must all provide a low-pressure, high-compliance reservoir with adequate capacity that offers the patient continence and ease of emptying. For a detailed description of urinary diversion, see Marayan and Gajendran.[145]

Historically, operative mortality rates for radical cystectomy and urinary diversion were about 10 to 20%, with major postoperative complications ranging substantially higher.[146] More recent series report a mortality rate of only 1 to 2% and an early complication rate of 25 to 30%. The most common complications include wound infection, urine leak, small bowel obstruction, rectal fistula, and medical complications.[147] Impotence following radical cystectomy has been a major disadvantage with the procedure. Walsh and Mostwin[148] described a potency-preserving technique for radical cystectomy and reported a potency rate of 65% compared with 10% in previous series.

In an attempt to decrease pelvic recurrence and increase survival rates, combining radical cystectomy with preoperative radiation therapy was considered. In the 1960s and 1970s, preoperative radiation became standard treatment for muscle-invasive bladder cancer, with 5-year survival rates ranging from 45 to 50%.[149] Significant controversy continues to surround the issue of planned preoperative radiation for invasive bladder cancer. By necessity, the results of all preoperative radiation series are based on clinically staged disease, whereas the surgical series use clinical or pathologic staging, or both. Clinical staging is inaccurate, with pathologic upstaging documented in 35 to 60% of patients.[150] Several prospectively randomized clinical trials have led most urologists to abandon preoperative radiation therapy as standard practice.

The first randomized trial of preoperative radiation therapy, performed by the National Cooperative Bladder Cancer Group in 1976, failed to show a statistically significant difference in the 5-year survival rate of patients treated with integrated therapy.[151] Radiotherapy did not increase the operative morbidity or mortality. This study randomized 233 patients with muscle invasion and no evidence of distant metastases to receive 45 Gy over a 4- to 6-week period followed by radical cystectomy or surgery alone. The weaknesses of this study included a high patient dropout rate, lack of uniformity in treatment delivery, and inconsistencies in reporting pathology and long-term patient follow-up. If all the patients were considered, however, the 5-year survival rates were not significantly different between the two groups. Patients who had surgery alone had a 5-year survival rate of 20% compared with a 23% survival rate for those who also received preoperative radiotherapy.

In another series by Skinner and Lieskovsky,[152] 197 patients were randomized to receive a course of high-dose radiotherapy (16 Gy) over 4 days followed by immediate cystectomy (100 patients) or surgery alone (97 patients). The authors reported no significant difference in 5-year survival, and pelvic recurrence rates were similar: 9% in the group receiving preoperative radiotherapy and 7% in those undergoing surgery alone. The 5-year disease-free survival rates for the patients treated with cystectomy alone were 75% for patients with pathologic stage P2 disease, 44% for P3a and P3b disease, and 36% for P4 disease and positive pelvic nodes. There was a slight difference in the incidence of superficial wound infection and prolonged ileus or small bowel obstruction favoring the nonirradiated group, although this did not reach statistical significance. SWOG reported another randomized clinical trial to help answer this question.[153] They compared 20 Gy of preoperative radiation followed by radical cystectomy within 1 week versus cystectomy alone. The study showed no significant difference in the overall survival between the two groups. Analysis of the available data suggests that preoperative irradiation is not an effective addition to radical surgery alone for the treatment of muscle-invasive bladder cancer. There is a small group of patients who originally responded to this treatment and subsequently proved to be long-term survivors; however, these patients may constitute a subgroup of patients with less aggressive tumors who would have done well with or without preoperative radiation therapy.

Opponents of preoperative radiation therapy cite the potential delay in performing the cystectomy. In patients whose tumors are less radiosensitive, this delay could potentially allow dissemination of a tumor that might have been cured by early cystectomy. Also, although not confirmed in all studies, patients who received preoperative irradiation had a tendency for an increased incidence of wound infections and bowel complications.[152, 154] Because of potential delay in definitive treatment, the potential morbidity, and the lack of supporting data, preoperative radiation therapy for invasive bladder cancer has largely been abandoned by most urologists.

As previously stated, regionally advanced bladder cancer is usually managed surgically in the United States. In Great Britain, primary radiation is the standard treatment, with salvage cystectomy used for local failure.[155] Proponents of radiation therapy cite excessive morbidity and mortality associated with surgery, together with a loss of potency in men and the need for an external appliance. With improved surgical techniques, the development of the potency-sparing radical cystectomy and continent urinary diversions, the latter is less of a concern. Studies have presented convincing data that external-beam radiation alone is not adequate to achieve sustained local control of invasive bladder cancer. Evaluation of several trials of primary radiation alone in patients with clinical stage T2 disease revealed an overall 5-year survival of about 40%. Patients with T3a tumors had a 5-year survival of approximately 35%. For patients with T3b disease, 5-year survival was approximately 20%, with a local recurrence rate of 50 to 70%. For T4 disease, 5-year survival was approximately 10%.[78, 150]

In Great Britain, Blandy and associates[155] advocated a protocol of definitive radiation therapy followed by salvage cystectomy at the first indication of failure. Of patients who have incomplete responses to radiation therapy, however, only 8 to 15% are candidates for salvage cystectomy. In patients treated with salvage cystectomy, the overall 5-year survival rate is approximately 38%, depending on the pathologic findings in the cystectomy specimen. If no residual tumor is found, the 5-year survival is approximately 70%; if

deeply infiltrating tumor is present, the 5-year survival is only 25%.[155] Preoperative assessment of the local tumor extent after definitive radiotherapy is much more difficult than staging primary untreated bladder carcinoma secondary to the dense desmoplastic radiation fibrosis, which fills the pelvis, encases the pelvic vessels, and distorts the lymphatics.[156] In a randomized prospective trial of patients with clinical stage T3 tumors, the M.D. Anderson Cancer Center group reported only a 16% 5-year survival for radiation alone compared with a 48% survival in the group receiving radical cystectomy plus preoperative radiation.[157] A randomized multicenter study of preoperative radiation and cystectomy versus radical radiation and early salvage cystectomy for residual tumors was carried out in 183 patients with stages T2, T3, and T4 by the Danish Vesical Cancer Group.[158] The results showed a trend toward a higher survival rate following treatment with preoperative radiation and cystectomy compared with radical radiation followed by salvage cystectomy in case of residual tumors, but a statistical significance could not be shown. Salvage cystectomy has a mortality rate of 8 to 22%.[155, 156] The controversy of definitive radiation followed by salvage cystectomy versus definitive radical cystectomy alone in invasive bladder cancer remains unresolved. In the United States, definitive radiation therapy is no longer considered an equal alternative as far as tumor-free survival is concerned. It should be reserved for patients who are a poor surgical risk or wish to retain the bladder for overriding personal reasons.

## TREATMENT OF METASTATIC BLADDER CANCER

Approximately 50% of patients with high-grade bladder cancer and deep muscle invasion die of disseminated disease within 2 years of presentation. There is a need for effective systemic therapy as a component of initial local treatment to increase the chance for cure. TCC has shown some response to systemic chemotherapy. Two of the most active commercially available agents are methotrexate and cisplatin, with response rates (complete plus partial response) of 28 to 45% (Table 51–4).[159] Vincristine and doxorubicin are also active but less so than cisplatin and methotrexate. In general, the responses to single agents are incomplete and last a median of 3 to 4 months, with essentially no complete remissions.[159]

A wide variety of combination chemotherapy regimens have been evaluated in clinical trials. One of the principles of developing effective combination chemotherapy programs is to combine agents that have shown independent tumor activity. Because cisplatin and methotrexate are considered the most active single agents, they form the backbone for most currently used combinations for advanced TCC (Table 51–5). Using this approach, an increase in overall and complete response proportions was observed with DDP/MTX (cisplatin and methotrexate), CMV (cisplatin, methotrexate, vinblastine), MVAC, and CISCA (cisplatin, cyclophosphamide, doxorubicin).[160–163] The results with the four-drug regimen MVAC, designed at Memorial Sloan-Kettering Cancer Center in 1983, show three distinct patterns of response: complete clinical and pathologic responses in 25% of patients, partial remission in 48%, and no response in 27%. Within the subgroup of partial responders, 12% were able to undergo surgery to resect residual disease, similar to the

*Table 51–4.* **Results of Single-Agent Trials**

| | No. CR + PR/ Total | % CR + PR | 95% CI (%) |
|---|---|---|---|
| Cisplatin | | | |
| Single institution | 70/206 | 34 | 28–40 |
| Randomized trials | 55/316 | 17 | 13–22 |
| Neoadjuvant | 75/184 | 40 | 34–48 |
| Overall | 200/706 | 28 | 26–32 |
| Carboplatin | 21/186 | 15 | 11–19 |
| Iproplatin (CHIP) | 7/39 | 18 | 6–30 |
| Methotrexate | | | |
| Low dose | 68/236 | 29 | 23–35 |
| High dose | 16/57 | 45 | 37–50 |
| Doxorubicin | 47/274 | 17 | 13–22 |
| Vinblastine | 6/38 | 16 | 4–28 |
| Cyclophosphamide | 30/98 | 31 | 22–40 |
| 5-Fluorouracil | 22/141 | 17 | 11–25 |
| Mitomycin C | 5/42 | 13 | 2–22 |
| Gallium nitrate | 9/29 | 29 | 13–45 |

CR, complete remission; PR, partial remission; CI, confidence interval.
Modified from Scher H, Norton L. Chemotherapy for urothelial tract tumors: breaking the deadlock. Semin Surg Oncol 1992;8:518.

approach used in testicular tumors. These patients were placed in a complete response to chemotherapy and surgery category, for an overall complete response proportion of 36%.[162] With a follow-up of 6 years, the median survival for MVAC-treated patients is 39.2 months for those with advanced nodal disease and 12 months for those presenting with metastases.[164] MVAC has been shown to be superior to single-agent cisplatin and the three-drug regimen CISCA in randomized trials. The definitive trial comparing MVAC and cisplatin included 246 evaluable patients, with complete response proportions of 13% versus 3% and overall response proportions of 39% versus 11.6% ($p = 0.0001$). Similarly, the progression-free survival (10.0 months vs. 4.3 months) and overall survival (12.5 months vs. 8.2 months) ($p = 0.0002$) were significantly greater for the combined-therapy arm.[165] With long-term follow-up evaluation, survival in the MVAC arm has continued to be superior to cisplatin ($p = 0.00015$).[166] Another randomized trial of MVAC and CISCA also showed an advantage for MVAC, with a higher overall response proportion (65% vs. 46%) and longer median survival (18.4 months vs. 9.3 months) for the four-drug regimen ($p = 0.0003$). The MVAC regimen, however, is associated with substantial toxicity, including leukopenia, culture-nega-

tive fever at the time of granulocytopenia, sepsis, mucositis, and renal failure.[165] The patient with metastatic TCC treated with MVAC therapy has a 25% chance, at best, of having a complete response to chemotherapy alone and a 33% chance of having a complete response to chemotherapy with the assistance of a salvage operation. Two thirds of the patients with a complete response relapse within 2 years.[162] Only 17% of patients can expect to remain tumor-free 3 years from the initiation of MVAC chemotherapy. The long-term data showed that only 3.7% are alive and continuously disease free at 6 years.[166] This low durable response rate is achieved at a relatively high price in terms of toxicity to patients who require frequent hospitalizations for granulocytopenic sepsis. At present, however, MVAC combination chemotherapy shows a higher level of response rate, duration of remission, and overall survival when compared with single-agent cisplatin or other combination regimens.

In an attempt to improve results with MVAC, investigators have used recombinant granulocyte colony–stimulating factor to allow escalation of the dose by reducing the side effects. Both mucositis and myelosuppression were ameliorated with the administration of granulocyte colony–stimulating factor.[167] A study at M.D. Anderson Cancer Center used recombinant human granulocyte-macrophage colony-stimulating factor (rhGM-CSF) plus escalated doses of MVAC as salvage for patients whose disease had progressed on MVAC with or without CISCA.[168] Complete and overall response rates of 23% and 40% were observed. Subsequent randomized studies, however, showed that rhGM-CSF could not result in an increased dose intensity of escalated MVAC to decrease side effects.[169] Other studies also indicated that the escalated MVAC with rhGM-CSF had no benefit regarding complete response or survival.[170]

MVAC has become the standard treatment for metastatic bladder cancer. The disappointing long-term results, such as a high relapse rate or a poor prognosis, in patients with complete response including substantial toxicity have prompted the development of novel agents or regimens.[171] Antifolates, taxanes, ifosfamide, gemcitabine, and gallium nitrate have been investigated. Reports of the combination of these agents suggested that response rates were equivalent to those of MVAC but with less toxicity.[172] Further randomized studies need to be conducted to improve the outlook for metastatic bladder cancer.

As noted previously, even after the most skilled surgery and radiation therapy, the incidence of recurrence or persis-

*Table 51–5.* **Results of Combination Programs**

| | | | Response Proportions | | |
|---|---|---|---|---|---|
| Agents* | No. Evaluable Trials | No. Patients | COMPLETE NO. (%) | OVERALL NO. (%) | 95% CI (%) |
| DDP/MTX | 9 | 293 | 41 (14) | 135 (46) | 39–53 |
| CMV | 4 | 157 | 35 (22) | 82 (52) | 43–59 |
| CAP | 10 | 293 | 65 (22) | 166 (57) | 49–64 |
| M-VAC | 12 | 526 | 106 (20) | 281 (53) | 48–58 |

*See text for explanation of abbreviations.
CI, confidence interval.
Modified from Scher HI. Chemotherapy for invasive bladder cancer: neoadjuvant versus adjuvant. Semin Oncol 1990;17:555–565. Copyright © John Wiley & Sons. Reprinted by permission of John Wiley & Sons, Inc.

tence of invasive tumor is greater than 50%. The 5-year survival rate for patients with invasive bladder cancer is approximately 30% after definitive therapy, and only a small percentage have recurrence in the pelvis. It appears that most patients succumb to micrometastatic disease that is present at the time of definitive treatment. Adjuvant chemotherapy has been used in the perioperative management of bladder cancer in an attempt to improve survival after definitive regional management. The principal advantage of adjuvant therapy is that treatment is recommended on the basis of the pathologic findings at surgery. The criteria on which to base the recommendation to offer treatment have not been standardized. Many physicians have chosen to offer treatment when nodal or extravesical tumor extension is documented or when the pathologic specimen shows evidence of vascular or lymphatic invasion.

Several trials using adjuvant chemotherapy have been reported, but most are limited by small numbers of patients and nonrandomization. In a randomized prospective trial, Skinner and coworkers[173] randomized 91 patients to either adjuvant CISCA chemotherapy or observation after radical cystectomy and meticulous pelvic lymph node dissection. The results showed a significant delay in time to progression, with 70% of the chemotherapy group versus 46% of the observation group free of disease at 3 years ($p = 0.001$). Median survival time was 4.3 years, compared with 2.4 years in the observation group ($p = 0.0062$). The number of involved lymph nodes was noted by the authors to be the most important prognostic feature, although no benefit was noted with two or more involved lymph nodes. Protocol violations, however, reduced the significance of the study and the power of the observations. In the chemotherapy arm, 25% of patients randomized to receive chemotherapy did not receive it, and only 48% of the patients completed the planned four cycles. In a randomized trial, 83 patients with stages pT3–pT4a or pN1–pN2 who received MVAC or MVEC (epirubicin replaced doxorubicin) were compared with a group of patients who were observed after surgery.[174] A significant benefit was found in progression-free survival with a follow-up of more than 3 years (58% for adjuvant therapy group vs. 13% for control group, $p = 0.0005$). Freiha and associates[175] conducted a randomized trial of radical cystectomy plus CMV versus radical cystectomy alone. Although a significant advantage for adjuvant chemotherapy was shown in terms of time to metastasis, no difference in survival was observed. At present, the adjuvant chemotherapy could delay time to progression in randomized studies, but this may not translate to a survival benefit. Some randomized studies show an advantage of adjuvant chemotherapy, particularly those who have a single positive lymph node. The small number of patients in each arm in those studies may reduce the power of the study. A large, well-designed, randomized study is needed to determine clearly an advantage of adjuvant chemotherapy after radical cystectomy in high-risk patients.

## NEOADJUVANT CHEMOTHERAPY FOR LOCALLY ADVANCED BLADDER CANCER

Initiation of chemotherapy before definitive regional surgery or radiation has been called *neoadjuvant chemotherapy.*[176]

There are several theoretical advantages to neoadjuvant chemotherapy. First, it allows in vivo assessment of chemosensitivity by observing the response of a marker lesion in the bladder. The response of micrometastases is presumed to be similar to that of the primary lesion. Second, neoadjuvant chemotherapy may produce some downstaging and allow previously unresectable tumor to become resectable. Third, chemotherapy may be carried out in a setting free from postoperative catabolic effects. Fourth, higher dose intensity is possible, and it can be carried out without delay. Finally, an initial response from the primary lesion may be a good prognostic indicator. The disadvantages of neoadjuvant chemotherapy include the fact that not all patients need systemic therapy. Another problem is the reliance on clinical staging to assess response, which is extremely inaccurate.[177] Waiting for a response or the false interpretation of a response can delay definitive treatment. Adjuvant therapy is administered based on pathologic criteria such as nodal metastases or extravesical tumor extension. This timing of chemotherapy may reduce the number of patients unnecessarily exposed to cytotoxic drugs.

The literature available on neoadjuvant therapy is fraught with many problems, including differences in case selection, tumor stage, methods used for staging and restaging, and the criteria of response. Chemotherapy doses and schedules may vary considerably. Scher[178] reviewed 17 published trials comprising 383 patients who received neoadjuvant chemotherapy in an investigative setting. These were mostly nonrandomized studies with fewer than 50 patients per trial. Complete response at cystectomy was reported in 22 to 43% of patients.[178] Herr and colleagues[179] reported 10-year outcomes of 111 patients with stage T2–T3 N0 M0 who responded to MVAC followed by bladder-sparing surgery. They found that 54% achieved a complete clinical response (T0) on transurethral resection, and of 43 patients who had bladder-sparing surgery, 74% were alive and 58% had an intact functional bladder. They suggested that most patients with invasive bladder cancer who achieve T0 status after neoadjuvant MVAC therapy preserve their bladders for 10 years with bladder-sparing surgery.

To assess the true impact of neoadjuvant chemotherapy, randomized trials must be completed with adequate follow-up to observe differences in survival. A randomized study of neoadjuvant cisplatin and doxorubicin in 325 patients undergoing radical cystectomy with stage T1 G3 T2–T4 NX M0 was conducted by The Nordic Cooperative Bladder Cancer Study Group.[180] The corresponding cancer-specific survival rate was 64% for the chemotherapy group and 54% for the control group. No difference was observed for patients with stages T1–T2, but a 15% significant difference ($p = 0.03$) was observed in the overall survival for patients with stages T3–T4. This study showed the benefit of neoadjuvant chemotherapy for patients with locally advanced disease. Another randomized study of CMV neoadjuvant chemotherapy followed by cystectomy or radiation versus cystectomy or radiation alone has been reported by the Medical Research Council/European Organization for Research and Treatment of Cancer. This study indicated that the 2-year disease-free survival rates showed a slight advantage in favor of the CMV arm (51% vs. 45%, $p = 0.06$). Among patients who underwent cystectomy, 33% had no tumor in the pathologic specimens after CMV versus 12%

with no CMV.[181] The chemotherapy regimens in those studies were not the MVAC regimen, which has been the most powerful regimen. Currently, randomized trials of neoadjuvant chemotherapy using MVAC chemotherapy versus no neoadjuvant chemotherapy by SWOG/U.S. Intergroup are complete. It is hoped that the results will help resolve the issue of the value of neoadjuvant MVAC chemotherapy in the treatment of invasive bladder cancer.

Attempts have been made to increase the therapeutic index of chemotherapy by giving intra-arterial infusions. Although preliminary data show that intra-arterial administration of neoadjuvant chemotherapy has demonstrated some activity against TCC of the bladder, it remains to be proved that this mode of therapy increases the efficacy of chemotherapeutic agents.[182, 183] Theoretically the intra-arterial route may result in a higher concentration of the drug delivered to the tumor site and higher local peak concentrations. Perhaps the effective dose might be lowered, decreasing the systemic side effects. The total dose of drugs can be no more than the systemic doses of the regimens used for the treatment of advanced disease if excessive systemic toxicity is to be avoided. For that reason, it is unlikely that the value of this therapy is any greater than when the dose is given systemically in terms of its adjunctive effect on micrometastatic disease. This method cannot be considered routine at present, and further studies are needed to define the role of this route of administration.

In patients with chemotherapy-refractory metastatic urothelial tumors, investigators have found that interferon alfa combined with 5-fluorouracil and gallium nitrate have tumoricidal activity.[172, 184] Gallium nitrate appears to have a limited therapeutic role, however, because its nephrotoxicity makes it difficult to combine with cisplatin-based therapy.

Combination chemotherapy and radiation therapy has been used in patients who were deemed medically unfit for or who refused surgery. This combination is based on laboratory and clinical studies that suggest that cisplatin, by acting as a radiation sensitizer, has synergism with radiation therapy.[185, 186] Results of combined treatment, transurethral resection of bladder tumor (TURBT) followed by concurrent chemotherapy and radiation therapy, in patients with stages T2–T3a showed that individually each local monotherapy of radiation, TURBT, or multidrug chemotherapy achieved a local response rate of 20 to 40%. When these rates were combined, clinically completed response rates were 65 to 80%. The overall survival rate was approximately 50%.[187] Side effects are common, however, with approximately 40% of patients experiencing significant stomatitis, myelosuppression, or renal dysfunction.[186]

The management of invasive and metastatic bladder cancer remains one of the most controversial problems facing urologists. Adjuvant, neoadjuvant, and concurrent chemotherapy for invasive bladder cancer, although offering exciting prospects for the improvement of cure rates, remains investigational. Based on current understanding of the biology of muscle-invasive bladder cancer and the data available regarding its treatment, radical cystectomy with bilateral pelvic lymph node dissection remains the standard of care. The true efficacy of neoadjuvant and adjuvant chemotherapy awaits the results of prospective randomized trials with adequate long-term follow-up.

## SYMPTOMATIC THERAPY FOR ADVANCED BLADDER CANCER

Treatment of the patient with advanced bladder cancer must be directed not only at control of tumor growth and dissemination but also at control of debilitating symptoms. Appropriate use of symptomatic therapy may improve the quality of life to a greater extent than more definitive therapeutic methods.

Hemorrhage from radiation cystitis or uncontrolled tumor can be treated with a 1% alum solution.[188] The solution can be instilled with continuous bladder irrigation without the need for anesthesia and is generally well tolerated. Formalin solutions of 1 to 10% have also been used to control bladder hemorrhage.[189] Formalin solution is exceedingly irritating to the bladder and requires general or regional anesthesia for intravesical instillation. Because a 10% formalin solution may cause fibrosis and obstruction of the ureteral orifices, formalin instillation should begin with a 1% solution and be repeated with a 4% solution, if necessary.[78] Before instillation of formalin, a cystogram should be performed to exclude vesicoureteral reflux. If reflux is present, Fogarty catheters should be passed up both ureters and the patient tilted in the head-up position to protect the upper tracts from the toxic effects of formalin.[190] Helmstein[191] described treatment of intractable bladder hemorrhage by hydrostatic pressure, but this is not advisable because of the risk of bladder rupture. Transurethral resection and fulguration to debulk local bladder tumor may improve the patient's voiding symptoms and help control bleeding, but typically the tumor is widespread and difficult to resect completely. In addition, hemorrhage is frequently diffuse and may be difficult to control. In rare instances, life-threatening hemorrhage can result from hemorrhagic cystitis or uncontrolled bladder tumors. If fulguration, laser treatment, or intravesical alum or formalin instillations fail to control the hemorrhage, it may be necessary to perform transfemoral percutaneous hypogastric artery embolization.[192] If hypogastric embolization or ligation fails to control the hemorrhage, palliative cystectomy may be required as a last resort.

Radiotherapy is often effective in relieving pain from osseous metastases. Pain relief is usually prompt. External-beam radiation therapy has not been effective in palliating pelvic pain, dysuria, and hematuria in patients with inoperable TCC of the bladder.[193] External-beam radiation can increase the symptoms of bladder urgency, pain, and hematuria in addition to causing problems with diarrhea and proctitis.

Urinary diversion is seldom beneficial. Local pain usually indicates invasion of pelvic nerves or bones and is rarely alleviated by diversion. Urinary diversion may allow tamponade of the bladder to stop bleeding and removes the irritation of the urine from the bladder. Diversion to prolong survival in patients with obstructed ureters and impending uremic death is seldom warranted because the average survival of such patients is about 3 months, during which time pain is often severe and difficult to control.[194] It is difficult to divert the urine completely with nephrostomy tubes, and many patients find these tubes uncomfortable. All patients with metastatic disease who are suffering from severe local bladder symptoms should first be treated with more conservative measures to control symptoms before resorting to major surgical intervention.

## SUGGESTIONS FOR ADDITIONAL READING

La Vecchia C, Airoldi L. Human bladder cancer: epidemiological, pathological and mechanistic aspects. IARC Sci Pub 1999;147:139–57.

Sternberg CN. A critical review of the management of bladder cancer. Crit Rev Oncol/Hematol 1999;31:193–207.

van der Meijden AP. Bladder cancer. BMJ 1998;317:1366–9.

Kamat AM, Lamm DL. Intravesical therapy for bladder cancer. Urology 2000;55:161–8.

Sengeløv L, von der Maase H. Radiotherapy in bladder cancer. Radiother Oncol 1999;52:1–14.

## REFERENCES

1. Landis SH, Murray T, Bolden S, Wingo PA. Cancer statistics, 1999. CA Cancer J Clin 1999;49:8–31.
2. Heney NM, Ahmed S, Flanagan MJ, et al. Superficial bladder cancer: progression and recurrence. J Urol 1983;130:1083–6.
3. Hartge P, Harvey EB, Linehan WM, et al. Unexplained excess risk of bladder cancer in men. J Natl Cancer Inst 1990;82:1636–40.
4. Cancer statistics review: 1973–1989. Bethesda, Maryland: National Cancer Institute, 1992.
5. Schairer C, Hartge P, Hoover RN, Silverman DT. Racial differences in bladder cancer risk: a case-control study. Am J Epidemiol 1988;128:1027–37.
6. Morrison AS, Buring JE, Verhoek WG, et al. An international study of smoking and bladder cancer. J Urol 1984;131:650–4.
7. Waterhouse J. Cancer incidence in five continents. Vol 4. Lyon: International Agency for Research in Cancer of the World Health Organization, 1982.
8. Sullivan JW. Epidemiologic survey of bladder cancer in greater New Orleans. J Urol 1982;128:281–3.
9. Cohen SM. Urinary bladder carcinogenesis: initiation-promotion. Semin Oncol 1979;6:157–60.
10. Cole P, Hoover R, Friedell GH. Occupation and cancer of the lower urinary tract. Cancer 1972;29:1250–60.
11. Vineis P, Pirastu R. Aromatic amines and cancer. Cancer Causes Control 1997;8:346–55.
12. Landi MT, Zocchetti C, Bernucci I, et al. Cytochrome P4501A2: enzyme induction and genetic control in determining 4-aminobiphenyl-hemoglobin adduct levels. Cancer Epidemiol Biomarkers Prev 1996;5:693–8.
13. Malker HS, McLaughlin JK, Silverman DT, et al. Occupational risks for bladder cancer among men in Sweden. Cancer Res 1987;47:6763–6.
14. Morrison AS. Advances in the etiology of urothelial cancer. Urol Clin North Am 1984;11:557–66.
15. Silverman DT, Levin LI, Hoover RN. Occupational risks of bladder cancer in the United States. II: nonwhite men. J Natl Cancer Inst 1989;81:1480–3.
16. Silverman DT, Levin LI, Hoover RN, Hartge P. Occupational risks of bladder cancer in the United States. I: white men. J Natl Cancer Inst 1989;81:1472–80.
17. Lower GM Jr, Nilsson T, Nelson CE, et al. N-acetyltransferase phenotype and risk in urinary bladder cancer: approaches in molecular epidemiology: preliminary results in Sweden and Denmark. Environ Health Perspect 1979;29:71–9.
18. Cartwright RA, Glashan RW, Rogers HJ, et al. Role of N-acetyltransferase phenotypes in bladder carcinogenesis: a pharmacogenetic epidemiological approach to bladder cancer. Lancet 1982;2:842–5.
19. Horai Y, Fujita K, Ishizaki T. Genetically determined N-acetylation and oxidation capacities in Japanese patients with non-occupational urinary bladder cancer. Eur J Clin Pharmacol 1989;37:581–7.
20. Augustine A, Hebert JR, Kabat GC, Wynder EL. Bladder cancer in relation to cigarette smoking. Cancer Res 1988;48:4405–8.
21. Bartsch H, Malaveille C, Friesen M, et al. Black (air-cured) and blond (flue-cured) tobacco cancer risk. IV: molecular dosimetry studies implicate aromatic amines as bladder carcinogens. Eur J Cancer 1993;29A:1199–207.
22. Cohen SM, Johansson SL. Epidemiology and etiology of bladder cancer. Urol Clin North Am 1992;19:421–8.
23. Locke JR, Hill DE, Walzer Y. Incidence of squamous cell carcinoma in patients with long-term catheter drainage. J Urol 1985;133:1034–5.
24. Johansson SL, Cohen SM. Epidemiology and etiology of bladder cancer. Semin Surg Oncol 1997;13:291–8.
25. Piper JM, Tonascia J, Matanoski GM. Heavy phenacetin use and bladder cancer in women aged 20 to 49 years. N Engl J Med 1985;313:292–5.
26. Lawrie CA, Renwick AG, Sims J. The urinary excretion of bacterial amino-acid metabolites by rats fed saccharin in the diet. Food Chem Toxicol 1985;23:445–50.
27. Wolf H. Studies on the role of tryptophan metabolites in the genesis of bladder cancer. Acta Chem Scand 1973;433:Suppl:154–68.
28. Teulings FA, Peters HA, Hop WC, et al. A new aspect of the urinary excretion of tryptophan metabolites in patients with cancer of the bladder. Int J Cancer 1978;21:140–6.
29. Renwick AG, Thakrar A, Lawrie CA, George CF. Microbial amino acid metabolites and bladder cancer: no evidence of promoting activity in man. Hum Toxicol 1988;7:267–72.
30. Hicks RM, Wakefield JS, Chowaniec J. Co-carcinogenic action of saccharin in the chemical induction of bladder cancer. Nature 1973;243:347–9. letter.
31. Sontag JM. Experimental identification of genitourinary carcinogens. Urol Clin North Am 1980;7:803–1422.
32. Elcock M, Morgan RW. Update on artificial sweeteners and bladder cancer. Regul Toxicol Pharmacol 1993;17:35–43.
33. O'Keane JC. Carcinoma of the urinary bladder after treatment with cyclophosphamide. N Engl J Med 1988;319:871. letter.
34. Kaldor JM, Day NE, Kittelmann B, et al. Bladder tumours following chemotherapy and radiotherapy for ovarian cancer: a case-control study. Int J Cancer 1995;63:1–6.
35. Durkee C, Benson R Jr. Bladder cancer following administration of cyclophosphamide. Urology 1980;16:145–8.
36. Melicow MM. Tumors of the bladder: a multifaceted problem. J Urol 1974;112:467–78.
37. Smith G, Elton RA, Beynon LL, et al. Prognostic significance of biopsy results of normal-looking mucosa in cases of superficial bladder cancer. Br J Urol 1983;55:665–9.
38. Foresman WH, Messing EM. Bladder cancer: natural history, tumor markers, and early detection strategies. Semin Surg Oncol 1997;13:299–306.
39. Melicow MM. Histological study of vesical urothelium intervening between gross neoplasm in total cystectomy. J Urol 1952;68:261–79.
40. Utz DC, Hanash KA, Farrow GM. The plight of the patient with carcinoma in situ of the bladder. J Urol 1970;103:160–4.
41. Riddle PR, Chisholm GD, Trott PA, Pugh RC. Flat carcinoma in situ of bladder. Br J Urol 1975;47:829–33.
42. Prot GR Jr, Griffin PP, Daly JJ, Heney NM. Carcinoma in situ of the urinary bladder with and without associated vesical neoplasms. Cancer 1983;52:524–32.
43. Althausen AF, Prout GR Jr, Daly JJ. Non-invasive papillary carcinoma of the bladder associated with carcinoma in situ. J Urol 1976;116:575–80.
44. Whitmore WF Jr. Management of invasive bladder neoplasms. Semin Urol 1983;1:34–41.
45. Smith JA Jr, Whitmore WF Jr. Salvage cystectomy for bladder cancer after failure of definitive irradiation. J Urol 1981;125:643–5.
46. Babaian RJ, Johnson DE, Llamas L, Ayala AG. Metastases from transitional cell carcinoma of urinary bladder. Urology 1980;16:142–4.
47. Thrasher JB, Frazier HA, Robertson JE, et al. Clinical variables which serve as predictors of cancer-specific survival among patients treated with radical cystectomy for transitional cell carcinoma of the bladder and prostate. Cancer 1994;73:1708–15.
48. Carbin BE, Ekman P, Gustafson H, et al. Grading of human urothelial carcinoma based on nuclear atypia and mitotic frequency. I: histological description. J Urol 1991;145:968–71.
49. Coon JS, Weinstein RS, Summers JL. Blood group precursor T-antigen expression in human urinary bladder carcinoma. Am J Clin Pathol 1982;77:692–9.
50. Neal DE, Sharples L, Smith K, et al. The epidermal growth factor receptor and the prognosis of bladder cancer. Cancer 1990;65:1619–25.
51. Badalament RA, O'Toole RV, Keyhani-Rofagha S, et al. Flow cytometric analysis of primary and metastatic bladder cancer. J Urol 1990;143:912–6.
52. Parry WL, Hemstreet GP 3d. Cancer detection by quantitative fluorescence image analysis. J Urol 1988;139:270–4.
53. Aprikian AG, Sarkis AS, Reuter VE, et al. Biological markers of

prognosis in transitional cell carcinoma of the bladder: current concepts. Semin Urol 1993;11:137–44.

54. Sarkis AS, Bajorin DF, Reuter VE, et al. Prognostic value of p53 nuclear overexpression in patients with invasive bladder cancer treated with neoadjuvant MVAC. J Clin Oncol 1995;13:1384–90.

55. Lowe SW, Ruley HE, Jacks T, Housman DE. p53-dependent apoptosis modulates the cytotoxicity of anticancer agents. Cell 1993;74:957–67.

56. Hatch TR, Barry JM. The value of excretory urography in staging bladder cancer. J Urol 1986;135:49.

57. Murphy WM, Emerson LD, Chandler RW, et al. Flow cytometry versus urinary cytology in the evaluation of patients with bladder cancer. J Urol 1986;136:815–9.

58. Gamarra MC, Zein T. Cytologic spectrum of bladder cancer. Urology 1984;23:3 Suppl:23–6.

59. Miyanaga N, Akaza H, Kameyama S, et al. Significance of the BTA test in bladder cancer: a multicenter trial. BTA Study Group Japan. Int J Urol 1997;4:557–60.

60. Miyanaga N, Akaza H, Ishikawa S, et al. Clinical evaluation of nuclear matrix protein 22 (NMP22) in urine as a novel marker for urothelial cancer. Eur Urol 1997;31:163–8.

61. Johnston B, Morales A, Emerson L, Lundie M. Rapid detection of bladder cancer: a comparative study of point of care tests. J Urol 1997;158:2098-101.

62. Van der Poel HG, Van Balken MR, Schamhart DH, et al. Bladder wash cytology, quantitative cytology, and the qualitative BTA test in patients with superficial bladder cancer. Urology 1998;51:44–50.

63. Grossman HB. New methods for detection of bladder cancer. Semin Urol Oncol 1998;16:17–22.

64. Brismar J, Gustafson T. Bone scintigraphy in staging of bladder carcinoma. Acta Radiol 1988;29:251–2.

65. See WA, Fuller JR. Staging of advanced bladder cancer: current concepts and pitfalls. Urol Clin North Am 1992;19:663–83.

66. Bryan PJ, Butler HE, LiPuma JP, et al. CT and MR imaging in staging bladder neoplasms. J Comput Assist Tomogr 1987;11:96–101.

67. Tachibana M, Baba S, Deguchi N, et al. Efficacy of gadolinium-diethylenetriaminepentaacetic acid-enhanced magnetic resonance imaging for differentiation between superficial and muscle-invasive tumor of the bladder: a comparative study with computerized tomography and transurethral ultrasonography. J Urol 1991;145:1169–73.

68. Scattoni V, Da Pozzo LF, Colombo R, et al. Dynamic gadolinium-enhanced magnetic resonance imaging in staging of superficial bladder cancer. J Urol 1996;155:1594–9.

69. Voges GE, Tauschke E, Stockle M, et al. Computerized tomography: an unreliable method for accurate staging of bladder tumors in patients who are candidates for radical cystectomy. J Urol 1989;142:972–4.

70. Jewett HJ, Strong GH. Infiltrating carcinoma of the bladder: relation of depth of penetration of the bladder wall to incidence of local extension and metastases. J Urol 1946;366–72.

71. Marshall VF, Holden J, Ma KT. Survival of patients with bladder carcinoma treated by simple segmental resection. Cancer 1956;9:568–71.

72. Hermanek P. UICC-TMN classification of malignant tumors. 4th ed. Heidelberg: Springer-Verlag, 1987.

73. Lieskovsky G. Diagnosis and staging of bladder cancer. In: Skinner DG, Lieskovsky G, eds. Diagnosis and management of genitourinary cancer. Philadelphia: WB Saunders, 1988:264.

74. Bosl GL. American Society of Clinical Oncology educational handbook. Chicago: Society of Clinical Oncology, 1991.

75. Malmstrom PU, Busch C, Norlen BJ. Recurrence, progression and survival in bladder cancer: a retrospective analysis of 232 patients with greater than or equal to 5-year follow-up. Scand J Urol Nephrol 1987;21:185–95.

76. Prout GR Jr, Barton BA, Griffin PP, Friedell GH. Treated history of noninvasive grade 1 transitional cell carcinoma. The National Bladder Cancer Group. J Urol 1992;148:1413–9.

77. Pham HT, Soloway MS. High-risk superficial bladder cancer: intravesical therapy for T1 G3 transitional cell carcinoma of the urinary bladder. Semin Urol Oncol 1997;15:147–53.

78. Messing EM, Catalona WJ. Urothelial tumors of the urinary tract. In: Walsh PC, Retik AB, Vaughan ED Jr, Wein AJ, eds. Campbell's urology. 7th ed. Vol III. Philadelphia: WB Saunders, 1998:2327.

79. Jones HC, Swinney J. Thiothepa in the treatment of the bladder. Lancet 1961;2:615–8.

80. Prout GR Jr, Koontz WW Jr, Coombs LJ, et al. Long-term fate of 90 patients with superficial bladder cancer randomly assigned to receive or not to receive thiotepa. J Urol 1983;130:677–80.

81. Medical Research Council Working Party on Urologic Cancer. The effect of intravesical thiotepa on tumour recurrence after endoscopic treatment of newly diagnosed superficial bladder cancer: a further report with long-term follow-up of a Medical Research Council randomized trial. Br J Urol 1994;73:632–8.

82. Hollister D Jr, Coleman M. Hematologic effects of intravesicular thiotepa therapy for bladder carcinoma. JAMA 1980;244:2065–7.

83. Richie JP. Intravesical chemotherapy: treatment selection, techniques, and results. Urol Clin North Am 1992;19:521–7.

84. DeFuria MD, Bracken RB, Johnson DE, et al. Phase I–II study of mitomycin C topical therapy for low-grade, low stage transitional cell carcinoma of the bladder: an interim report. Cancer Treat Rep 1980;64:225–30.

85. Soloway MS. Intravesical and systemic chemotherapy in the management of superficial bladder cancer. Urol Clin North Am 1984;11:623–35.

86. Lamm DL, Blumenstein BA, Crawford ED, et al. Randomized intergroup comparison of bacillus Calmette-Guerin immunotherapy and mitomycin C chemotherapy prophylaxis in superficial transitional cell carcinoma of the bladder. Urol Oncol 1995;1:119–24.

87. Garnick MB, Schade D, Israel M, et al. Intravesical doxorubicin for prophylaxis in the management of recurrent superficial bladder carcinoma. J Urol 1984;131:43–6.

88. Riddle PR, Wallace DM. Intracavitary chemotherapy for multiple noninvasive bladder tumours. Br J Urol 1971;43:181–4.

89. Lamm DL, Riggs DR, Traynelis CL, Nseyo UO. Apparent failure of current intravesical chemotherapy prophylaxis to influence the long-term course of superficial transitional cell carcinoma of the bladder. J Urol 1995;153:1444–50.

90. Catalona WJ, Ratliff TL. Bacillus Calmette-Guerin and superficial bladder cancer: clinical experience and mechanism of action. Surg Ann 1990;22:363–78.

91. Morales A, Eidinger D, Bruce AW. Intracavitary bacillus Calmette-Guerin in the treatment of superficial bladder tumors. J Urol 1976;116:180–3.

92. Brosman S. Immunotherapy in bladder cancer. In: Pavone-Macaluso M, ed. Bladder tumors and other topics in urologic oncology. New York: Plenum Press, 1980:165.

93. Kelley DR, Ratliff TL, Catalona WJ, et al. Intravesical bacillus Calmette-Guerin therapy for superficial bladder cancer: effect of bacillus Calmette-Guerin viability on treatment results. J Urol 1985;134:48–53.

94. Morales A. Long-term results and complications of intracavitary bacillus Calmette-Guerin therapy for bladder cancer. J Urol 1984;132:457–9.

95. Lamm DL, Thor DE, Harris SC, et al. Bacillus Calmette-Guerin immunotherapy of superficial bladder cancer. J Urol 1980;124:38–40.

96. Herr HW, Schwalb DM, Zhang ZF, et al. Intravesical bacillus Calmette-Guerin therapy prevents tumor progression and death from superficial bladder cancer: ten-year follow-up of a prospective randomized trial. J Clin Oncol 1995;13:1404–8.

97. Rodrigues Netto N Jr, Lemos GC. A comparison of treatment methods for the prophylaxis of recurrent superficial bladder tumors. J Urol 1983;129:33–4.

98. Coplen DE, Marcus MD, Myers JA, et al. Long-term followup of patients treated with 1 or 2, 6-week courses of intravesical bacillus Calmette-Guerin: analysis of possible predictors of response free of tumor. J Urol 1990;144:652–7.

99. Herr HW. Transurethral resection and intravesical therapy of superficial bladder tumors. Urol Clin North Am 1991;18:525–8.

100. Lamm DL, Crawford ED, Blumenstein B, et al. Maintenance BCG immunotherapy of superficial bladder cancer: a randomized prospective Southwest Oncology Group Study. J Urol 1992;147:274A. abstract.

101. Lamm DL, Stogdill VD, Stogdill BJ, Crispen RG. Complications of bacillus Calmette-Guerin immunotherapy in 1,278 patients with bladder cancer. J Urol 1986;135:272–4.

102. Lamm DL, van der Meijden PM, Morales A, et al. Incidence and treatment of complications of bacillus Calmette-Guerin intravesical therapy in superficial bladder cancer. J Urol 1992;147:596–600.

103. Williams RD. Intravesical interferon alfa in the treatment of superficial bladder cancer. Semin Oncol 1988;15:5 Suppl:10–3.

104. Mohanty NK, Gulati P, Saxena S. Role of interferon-alpha-2b in the prevention of superficial carcinoma of the bladder recurrence. Urol Int 1997;59:194–6.

105. Jimenez-Cruz JF, Vera-Donoso CD, Leiva O, et al. Intravesical immu-

noprophylaxis in recurrent superficial bladder cancer (stage T1): multicenter trial comparing bacille Calmette-Guerin and interferon-alpha. Urology 1997;50:529–35.

106. Goffinet DR, Schneider MJ, Glatstein EJ, et al. Bladder cancer: results of radiation therapy in 384 patients. Radiology 1975;117:149–53.

107. Matthews PN, Madden M, Bidgood KA, Fisher C. The clinicopathological features of metastatic superficial papillary bladder cancer. J Urol 1984;132:904–6.

108. Hudson MA. When intravesical measures fail: indications for cystectomy in superficial disease. Urol Clin North Am 1992;19:601–9.

109. Chang SC, Bown SG. Photodynamic therapy: applications in bladder cancer and other malignancies. J Formos Med Assoc 1997;96:853–63.

110. Beisland HO, Sander S. Neodymium-YAG laser irradiation of stage T2 muscle-invasive bladder cancer: long-term results. Br J Urol 1990;65:24–6.

111. Kent DL, Shachter R, Sox HC Jr, et al. Efficient scheduling of cystoscopies in monitoring for recurrent bladder cancer. Med Decis Making 1989;9:26–37.

112. Holmang S, Hedelin H, Anderstrom C, et al. Long term followup of a bladder carcinoma cohort: routine followup urography is not necessary. J Urol 1998;160:45–58.

113. Oldbring J, Glifberg I, Mikulowski P, Hellsten S. Carcinoma of the renal pelvis and ureter following bladder carcinoma: frequency, risk factors and clinicopathological findings. J Urol 1989;141:1311–3.

114. Lamm DL. Long-term results of intravesical therapy for superficial bladder cancer. Urol Clin North Am 1992;19:573–80.

115. Lamm DL, Blumenstein BA, Crawford ED, et al. A randomized trial of intravesical doxorubicin and immunotherapy with bacille Calmette-Guerin for transitional-cell carcinoma of the bladder. N Engl J Med 1991;325:1205–9.

116. Lamm DL. BCG immunotherapy for transitional-cell carcinoma in situ of the bladder. Oncology 1995;9:947–65.

117. Badalament RA, Ortolano V, Burgers JK. Recurrent or aggressive bladder cancer: indications for adjuvant intravesical therapy. Urol Clin North Am 1992;19:485–98.

118. Daly JJ. Carcinoma-in-situ of the urothelium. Urol Clin North Am 1976;3:87–105.

119. Nseyo UO, Lamm DL. Immunotherapy of bladder cancer. Semin Surg Oncol 1997;13:342–9.

120. Erton M, Ilker Y, Akdas K. Carcinoma in situ and treatment options. Int Urol Nephrol 1996;28:33–42.

121. Montie JE, Wood DP Jr, Mendendorp SV, et al. The significance and management of transitional cell carcinoma of the prostate. Semin Urol 1990;8:262–8.

122. Henry K, Miller J, Mori M, et al. Comparison of transurethral resection to radical therapies for stage B bladder tumors. J Urol 1988;140:964–7.

123. Herr HW. Conservative management of muscle-infiltrating bladder cancer: prospective experience. J Urol 1987;138:1162–3.

124. Solsona E, Iborra I, Ricos JV, et al. Feasibility of transurethral resection for muscle-infiltrating carcinoma of the bladder: prospective study. J Urol 1992;147:1513–5.

125. Barnes RW, Dick AL, Hadley HL, Johnston OL. Survival following transurethral resection of bladder carcinoma. Cancer Res 1977; 37:2895–7.

126. Sweeney P, Kursh ED, Resnick MI. Partial cystectomy. Urol Clin North Am 1992;19:701–11.

127. Herr HW, Scher HI. Neoadjuvant chemotherapy and partial cystectomy for invasive bladder cancer. J Clin Oncol 1994;12:975–80.

128. Novick AC, Stewart BH. Partial cystectomy in the treatment of primary and secondary carcinoma of the bladder. J Urol 1976;116:570–4.

129. Magri J. Partial cystectomy: a review of 104 cases. Br J Urol 1962;34:74–87.

130. van der Werf-Messing B. Carcinoma of the bladder treated by suprapubic radium implants: the value of additional external irradiation. Eur J Cancer 1969;5:277–85.

131. Feinstein AR, Sosin DM, Wells CK. The Will Rogers phenomenon: stage migration and new diagnostic techniques as a source of misleading statistics for survival in cancer. N Engl J Med 1985;312:1604–8.

132. Sakamoto N, Tsuneyoshi M, Naito S, Kumazawa J. An adequate sampling of the prostate to identify prostatic involvement by urothelial carcinoma in bladder cancer patients. J Urol 1993;149:318–21.

133. Wood DP Jr, Montie JE, Pontes JE, Levin HS. Identification of transitional cell carcinoma of the prostate in bladder cancer patients: a prospective study. J Urol 1989;142:83–5.

134. Lerner SP, Skinner E, Skinner DG. Radical cystectomy in regionally advanced bladder cancer. Urol Clin North Am 1992;19:713–23.

135. Prout GR Jr, Griffin PP, Shipley WU. Bladder carcinoma as a systemic disease. Cancer 1979;43:2532–9.

136. Giuliani L, Giberti C, Martorana G, et al. Results of radical cystectomy for primary bladder cancer: retrospective study of more than 200 cases. Urology 1985;26:243–8.

137. Wishnow KI, Johnson DE, Ro JY, et al. Incidence, extent and location of unsuspected pelvic lymph node metastasis in patients undergoing radical cystectomy for bladder cancer. J Urol 1987;137:408–10.

138. Soloway MS, Lopez AE, Patel J, Lu Y. Results of radical cystectomy for transitional cell carcinoma of the bladder and the effect of chemotherapy. Cancer 1994;73:1926–31.

139. Skinner DG. Management of invasive bladder cancer: a meticulous pelvic node dissection can make a difference. J Urol 1982;128:34–6.

140. Lerner SP, Skinner DG, Lieskovsky G, et al. The rationale for en bloc pelvic lymph node dissection for bladder cancer patients with nodal metastases: long-term results. J Urol 1993;149:758–65.

141. Vieweg J, Whitmore WF Jr, Herr HW, et al. The role of pelvic lymphadenectomy and radical cystectomy for lymph node positive bladder cancer: the Memorial Sloan-Kettering Cancer Center experience. Cancer 1994;73:3020–8.

142. Elmajizn DA, Skinner DG. The technique of radical cystectomy: a standard anatomic approach. In: Crawford ED, Das S, eds. Current genitourinary cancer surgery. 2nd ed. Baltimore: Williams & Wilkins, 1997:361.

143. Montie JE, Park JM. Orthotopic diversion in women. Semin Urol Oncol 1997;15:184–8.

144. Chen ME, Pisters LL, Malpica A, et al. Risk of urethral, vaginal and cervical involvement in patients undergoing radical cystectomy for bladder cancer: results of a contemporary cystectomy series from M.D. Anderson Cancer Center. J Urol 1997;157:2120–3.

145. Marayan P, Gajendran V. Continent diversion to the urethra. In: Crawford ED, Das S, eds. Current genitourinary cancer surgery. 2nd ed. Baltimore: Williams & Wilkins, 1997:426.

146. Whitmore WK Jr, Marchall VF. Radical total cystectomy for cancer of the bladder: 230 consecutive cases five years later. J Urol 1962;87:853–68.

147. Skinner DG, Crawford ED, Kaufman JJ. Complications of radical cystectomy for carcinoma of the bladder. J Urol 1980;123:640–3.

148. Walsh PC, Mostwin JL. Radical prostatectomy and cystoprostatectomy with preservation of potency: results using a new nerve-sparing technique. Br J Urol 1984;56:694–7.

149. Parsons JT, Million RR. Planned preoperative irradiation in the management of clinical stage B2-C (T3) bladder carcinoma. Int J Radiat Oncol Biol Phys 1988;14:797–810.

150. Wesson MF. Radiation therapy in regionally advanced bladder cancer. Urol Clin North Am 1992;19:725–34.

151. Prout GR Jr. Technique for radical cystectomy. Urol Clin North Am 1976;3:177–93.

152. Skinner DG, Lieskovsky G. Contemporary cystectomy with pelvic node dissection compared to preoperative radiation therapy plus cystectomy in management of invasive bladder cancer. J Urol 1984;131:1069–72.

153. Smith JA Jr, Crawford ED, Paradelo JC, et al. Treatment of advanced bladder cancer with combined preoperative irradiation and radical cystectomy versus radical cystectomy alone: a phase III intergroup study. J Urol 1997;157:805–8.

154. Prout GR Jr, Slack NH, Bross ID. Preoperative irradiation as an adjuvant in the surgical management of invasive bladder carcinoma. J Urol 1971;105:223–31.

155. Blandy JP, England HR, Evans SJ, et al. T3 bladder cancer—the case for salvage cystectomy. Br J Urol 1980;52:506–10.

156. Crawford ED, Skinner DG. Salvage cystectomy after irradiation failure. J Urol 1980;123:32–4.

157. Miller LS. Bladder cancer: superiority of preoperative irradiation and cystectomy in clinical stages B2 and C. Cancer 1977;39:2 Suppl:973–80.

158. Sell A, Jakobsen A, Nerstrom B, et al. Treatment of advanced bladder cancer category T2 T3 and T4a: a randomized multicenter study of preoperative irradiation and cystectomy versus radical irradiation and early salvage cystectomy for residual tumor: DAVECA protocol 8201: Danish Vesical Cancer Group. Scand J Urol Nephrol 1991;138:Suppl:193–201.

159. Scher HI. Systemic chemotherapy in regionally advanced bladder

cancer: theoretical considerations and results. Urol Clin North Am 1992;19:747–59.

160. Stoter G, Splinter TA, Child JA, et al. Combination chemotherapy with cisplatin and methotrexate in advanced transitional cell cancer of the bladder. J Urol 1987;137:663–7.

161. Harker WG, Meyers FJ, Freiha FS, et al. Cisplatin, methotrexate, and vinblastine (CMV): an effective chemotherapy regimen for metastatic transitional cell carcinoma of the urinary tract. A Northern California Oncology Group study. J Clin Oncol 1985;3:1463–70.

162. Sternberg CN, Yagoda A, Scher HI, et al. Methotrexate, vinblastine, doxorubicin, and cisplatin for advanced transitional cell carcinoma of the urothelium: efficacy and patterns of response and relapse. Cancer 1989;64:2448–58.

163. Logothetis CJ, Dexeus FH, Chong C, et al. Cisplatin, cyclophosphamide and doxorubicin chemotherapy for unresectable urothelial tumors: the M.D. Anderson experience. J Urol 1989;141:33–7.

164. Arap W, Scher HI. The value of cytotoxic chemotherapy in locally invasive and metastatic bladder cancer. In: Williams G, ed. Urological cancer: a consensus. London: Edward Arnold Publishers, 1991:185.

165. Loehrer PJ Sr, Einhorn LH, Elson PJ, et al. A randomized comparison of cisplatin alone or in combination with methotrexate, vinblastine, and doxorubicin in patients with metastatic urothelial carcinoma: a cooperative group study. J Clin Oncol 1992;10:1066–73.

166. Saxman SB, Propert KJ, Einhorn LH, et al. Long-term follow-up of a phase III intergroup study of cisplatin alone or in combination with methotrexate, vinblastine, and doxorubicin in patients with metastatic urothelial carcinoma: a cooperative group study. J Clin Oncol 1997;15:2564–9.

167. Gabrilove JL, Jakubowski A, Scher H, et al. Effect of granulocyte colony-stimulating factor on neutropenia and associated morbidity due to chemotherapy for transitional-cell carcinoma of the urothelium. N Engl J Med 1988;318:1414–22.

168. Logothetis CJ, Dexeus FH, Sella A, et al. Escalated therapy for refractory urothelial tumors: methotrexate-vinblastine-doxorubicin-cisplatin plus unglycosylated recombinant human granulocyte-macrophage colony-stimulating factor. J Natl Cancer Inst 1990;82:667–72.

169. Logothetis CJ, Finn LD, Smith T, et al. Escalated MVAC with or without recombinant human granulocyte-macrophage colony-stimulating factor for the initial treatment of advanced malignant urothelial tumors: results of a randomized trial. J Clin Oncol 1995;13:2272–7.

170. Loehrer PJ Sr, Elson P, Dreicer R, et al. Escalated dosages of methotrexate, vinblastine, doxorubicin, and cisplatin plus recombinant human granulocyte colony-stimulating factor in advanced urothelial carcinoma: an Eastern Cooperative Oncology Group trial. J Clin Oncol 1994;12:483–8.

171. Igawa M, Urakami S, Shiina H, et al. Long-term results with M-VAC for advanced urothelial cancer: high relapse rate and low survival in patients with a complete response. Br J Urol 1995;76:321–4.

172. Fagbemi SO, Stadler WM. New chemotherapy regimens for advanced bladder cancer. Semin Urol Oncol 1998;16:23–9.

173. Skinner DG, Daniels JR, Russell CA, et al. The role of adjuvant chemotherapy following cystectomy for invasive bladder cancer: a prospective comparative trial. J Urol 1991;145:459–67.

174. Stockle M, Meyenburg W, Wellek S, et al. Adjuvant polychemotherapy of nonorgan-confined bladder cancer after radical cystectomy revisited: long-term results of a controlled prospective study and further clinical experience. J Urol 1995;153:47–52.

175. Freiha F, Reese J, Torti FM. A randomized trial of radical cystectomy versus radical cystectomy plus cisplatin, vinblastine and methotrexate chemotherapy for muscle invasive bladder cancer. J Urol 1996;155:495–500.

176. Raghavan D, Pearson B, Duval P, et al. Initial intravenous cis-platinum therapy: improved management for invasive high risk bladder cancer. J Urol 1985;133:399–402.

177. Herr HW, Whitmore WF Jr, Morse MJ, et al. Neoadjuvant chemotherapy in invasive bladder cancer: the evolving role of surgery. J Urol 1990;144:1083–8.

178. Scher HI. Chemotherapy for invasive bladder cancer: neoadjuvant versus adjuvant. Semin Oncol 1990;17:555–65, 1990.

179. Herr HW, Bajorin DF, Scher HI. Neoadjuvant chemotherapy and bladder-sparing surgery for invasive bladder cancer: ten-year outcome. J Clin Oncol 1998;16:1298–301.

180. Malmstrom PU, Rintala E, Wahlqvist R, et al. Five-year followup of a prospective trial of radical cystectomy and neoadjuvant chemotherapy: Nordic Cystectomy Trial I: The Nordic Cooperative Bladder Cancer Study Group. J Urol 1996;155:1903–6.

181. Hall RR. Neoadjuvant CMV chemotherapy and cystectomy or radiotherapy in muscle invasive bladder cancer: first analysis of MRC/EORTC trial. Proc ASCO 1996;15:244. abstract.

182. Jacobs SC, Menashe DS, Mewissen MW, Lipchik EO. Intraarterial cisplatin infusion in the management of transitional cell carcinoma of the bladder. Cancer 1989;64:388–91.

183. Galetti TP, Pontes JE, Montie J, et al. Neoadjuvant intra-arterial chemotherapy in the treatment of advanced transitional cell carcinoma of the bladder: results and followup. J Urol 1989;142:1211–5.

184. Logothetis CJ, Hossan E, Sella A, et al. Fluorouracil and recombinant human interferon alfa-2a in the treatment of metastatic chemotherapy-refractory urothelial tumors. J Natl Cancer Inst 1991;83:285–8.

185. Shipley WU, Prout GR Jr, Einstein AB, et al. Treatment of invasive bladder cancer by cisplatin and radiation in patients unsuited for surgery. JAMA 1987;258:931–5.

186. Prout GR Jr, Shipley WU, Kaufman DS, et al. Preliminary results in invasive bladder cancer with transurethral resection, neoadjuvant chemotherapy and combined pelvic irradiation plus cisplatin chemotherapy. J Urol 1990;144:1128–36.

187. Shipley WU, Zietman AL, Kaufman DS, et al. Invasive bladder cancer: treatment strategies using transurethral surgery, chemotherapy and radiation therapy with selection for bladder conservation. Int J Radiat Oncol Biol Phys 1997;39:937–43.

188. Ostroff EB, Chenault OW Jr. Alum irrigation for the control of massive bladder hemorrhage. J Urol 1982;128:929–30.

189. Brown RB. Further experiences with intravesical formalin administration in advanced carcinoma of the bladder. Br J Urol 1970;42:738–9.

190. Fall M, Pettersson S. Ureteral complications after intravesical formalin instillation. J Urol 1979;122:160–2.

191. Helmstein K. Treatment of bladder carcinoma by a hydrostatic pressure technique: report on 43 cases. Br J Urol 1972;44:434–50.

192. Carmignani G, Belgrano E, Puppo P, et al. Transcatheter embolization of the hypogastric arteries in cases of bladder hemorrhage from advanced pelvic cancers: followup in 9 cases. J Urol 1980;124:196–200.

193. Culp DA. Palliative treatment of the patient with disseminated carcinoma of the bladder. Semin Oncol 1979;6:249–53.

194. Yonemoto RH, Chez RA, Byron RL, Getzoft PL. Evaluation of ileal conduit as a palliative procedure. Surg Gynecol Obstet 1965;121:70–8.

# Renal Pelvis and Ureteral Cancer

## NATURAL HISTORY

### Etiology and Epidemiology

Carcinomas of the renal pelvis and ureter are rare malignancies that account for only 2 to 4% of all urothelial tumors.[1] The incidence and mortality statistics in the United States for renal pelvic tumors are limited because they are grouped with renal cell carcinoma.[2] In a review of the American Cancer Society statistics, renal pelvic TCC accounted for 15% of renal tumors.[3] In 1998, the estimated number of new cases for all renal tumors was approximately 29,900.[4] The estimated number for new renal pelvic TCC was approximately 4500. Ureteral tumors are even more uncommon, occurring with one quarter the incidence of renal pelvic tumors, and account for less than 1% of all genitourinary malignant tumors.[5] There has been a 30-fold increase in the number of cases reported since 1934, principally reflecting improvements in available diagnostic techniques and higher survival rates of patients with bladder cancer, who have a greater chance than the general population of developing ureteral carcinoma.[6] Because they are classified separately, epidemiologic data are more readily available for ureteral malignancy. The peak incidence in white men is 10 cases per 100,000 per year. Ureteral tumors are at least twice as common in men as in women and twice as common among whites as blacks.[2] Upper tract urothelial tumors rarely occur before age 40, and the peak incidence is in the 50s and 60s. The mean age of occurrence is 67 years.[3] There is an equal distribution for anatomic site. The distal ureter is reported as the primary site in 73% of patients, the midureter in 24%, and the proximal ureter in only 3%.[7] Bilateral involvement (synchronous or metachronous) occurs in 2 to 5% of sporadic upper tract transitional carcinomas.[8] Upper tract tumors occur in 2 to 4% of patients with bladder cancer.[9] Although performing routine excretory urography for follow-up of the upper tracts in bladder cancer patients is not uniformly recommended, particular attention should be paid to patients with multiple, high-grade, or recurrent tumors and with tumors involving the ureteral orifices. Approximately 30 to 75% of patients with upper tract urothelial tumors have synchronous or metachronous bladder tumors.[10] Tumors of the urothelium represent a diffuse multifocal neoplastic diathesis, and careful monitoring of the remaining urothelial lining by excretory urography, endoscopy, and cytology is mandatory. Exposure to the environmental substances that have been associated with the development of bladder cancer has also been linked to the development of renal pelvic and ureteral carcinoma.

**Occupational Factors.** Occupational carcinogens that are linked with bladder cancer are also associated with the development of renal pelvic and ureteral cancers, including the aromatic amines 2-naphthylamine, benzidine, and 4-aminobiphenyl.[11, 12] These agents are found in the dye, textile, printing, plastic, and rubber industries. Higher levels of exposure to such carcinogens are necessary in the upper tract because of the decreased time of exposure compared with the bladder.

**Tobacco.** Cigarette smoking is a major risk factor for carcinoma of the renal pelvis and ureter. The relative risk was 2.6 in a Denmark study.[13] A strong dose-effect relationship was observed; the heaviest smokers for more than 45 years had an almost eightfold increased risk.[14]

**Phenacetin.** Phenacetin abuse is well documented to be associated with TCC of the upper tracts. Of patients, 22% with renal pelvic tumors and 11% with ureteral tumors gave a history of phenacetin abuse.[15] The risk increases from 3.6-fold to 20-fold when phenacetin abuse occurs with renal papillary necrosis.[16] The lower risk to the bladder may be secondary to the degradation of the aniline-like byproducts of phenacetin when exposed to urine.

**Chronic Inflammation.** Chronic inflammation, infection, and stones may lead to urothelial dysplasia and subsequent tumor formation.[17] Cyclophosphamide metabolites, including acrolein, also increase the risk of upper tract malignancies.[18] Tumors induced by this agent are usually high grade and more aggressive.[19]

**Balkan Nephropathy.** In the Balkan countries of Romania, Greece, Yugoslavia, and Bulgaria, there is an endemic nephropathy that is associated with a 100-fold to 200-fold increased incidence of TCC of the upper tract. TCC associated with Balkan nephropathy has a 10% incidence of bilaterality and behaves in a more indolent fashion than the sporadic form of the disease.[20] Patients more commonly die from intervening renal failure, not from metastatic TCC. Adopting conservative treatment policies for these patients has provided the impetus for using conservative treatment of upper tract urothelial cancers in other clinical settings.

## Pathology

Almost all histologic types of tumor can be found in the renal pelvis and ureter. TCC is the most common and accounts for more than 90% of upper tract urothelial tumors.[7] SCC, which is usually associated with chronic infection and stone disease, accounts for approximately 7% of upper tract tumors.[7] Adenocarcinoma of the renal pelvis or ureter is extremely rare and accounts for less than 1% of upper tract tumors. As with SCC, adenocarcinoma is associated with chronic inflammation and calculi.[21] The upper tract TCC spreads by direct invasion to renal parenchyma or surrounding tissue, mucosal extension, mucosal seeding, or invasion to vascular or lymphatic systems.[22] The most common sites of lymphatic metastases are paracaval and para-aortic as well as the ipsilateral common iliac and pelvic lymph nodes.[23] Similar to renal cell carcinoma, vascular invasions of renal pelvic TCC may include renal veins and vena cava.[22]

Other unusual tumor types, including leiomyosarcoma and carcinosarcoma, rarely occur in the upper urinary tract.[24, 25] Benign polyps can radiographically mimic neoplasms but are more commonly located in the proximal ureter.[26] Inverted papillomas are found in the upper tracts as well as the bladder. Classically, these tumors behave in a benign manner but occasionally undergo malignant transformation.[27] Metastatic tumors to the ureter are most frequently of breast, colorectal, cervical, prostatic, or bladder origin.[28]

## Clinical Presentation

The most common presenting symptom of upper urinary tract neoplasms is gross painless hematuria, which occurs in approximately 80% of patients.[1] Hematuria throughout urination suggests bleeding from the upper urinary tract. Flank pain occurs in approximately one third of patients and is usually dull because of gradual obstruction and distention of the collecting system. Acute flank pain can be secondary to the passage of blood clots. Ten to 15% of patients are asymptomatic, and the tumor is diagnosed as an incidental finding on imaging studies obtained for other reasons.[29] Bladder irritation is seen in 5 to 10% of patients, and constitutional symptoms are seen in approximately 5% of patients. Physical findings are usually absent, but a flank mass secondary to associated hydronephrosis may be present.

## Diagnosis

**Imaging Studies.** A radiolucent filling defect on intravenous urography or retrograde ureteral pyelography is the most common radiologic finding in upper tract urothelial tumors. The filling defect is characteristically irregular and in continuity with the wall of the collecting system (Fig. 51–3).[8] The differential diagnosis includes malignant lesions, a radiolucent calculus, blood clots, fungus ball, benign tumors such as papillomas, inflammatory processes such as ureteritis cystica, sloughed papillae, artifacts, external compression of the collecting system by a crossing vessel, or overlying intestinal gas. In the kidney, the tumor can produce incomplete filling or nonfilling of a renal infundibulum or calyx. Tumors cause obstruction or nonvisualization of the

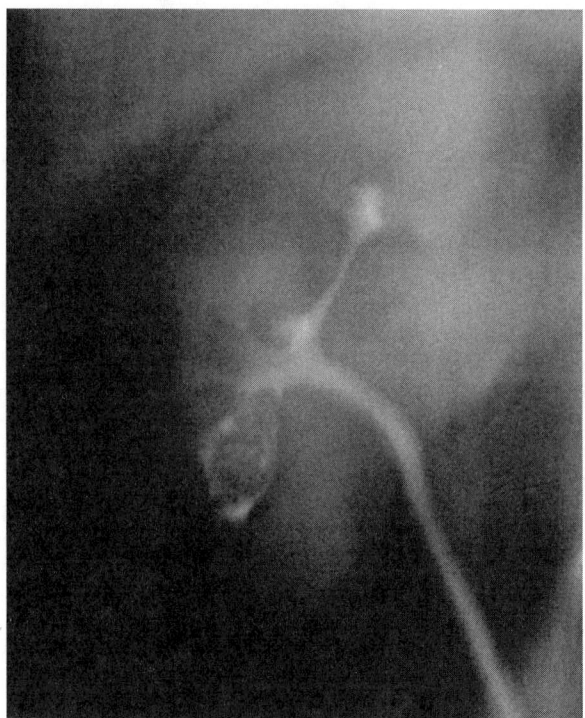

**Figure 51–3.** Filling defect in the renal pelvis.

collecting system in 10 to 30% of cases.[7] This clinical presentation is generally associated with an advanced lesion.[30] It is extremely important to study the contralateral upper urinary tract carefully for subtle filling defects because its status may alter the treatment plan. Retrograde ureteropyelography is useful in the diagnosis of upper tract lesions and is essential when the excretory urogram is inconclusive. Antegrade percutaneous pyelography can be used in special circumstances when a patient has a nonvisualizing kidney and it is not possible to perform a retrograde study; however, it is not advisable because of the risk of seeding tumor cells along the needle tract. In these situations, CT may reveal a soft tissue mass within the collecting system and would render an antegrade pyelogram unnecessary. CT can be useful in the diagnosis and staging of upper tract urothelial tumors. It is helpful in determining the local extent of the primary tumor as well as in evaluating metastases by showing extension into the renal parenchyma or periureteral soft tissues, venous involvement, lymph node involvement, or liver metastases. In some instances, because of its increased sensitivity, CT may delineate a collecting system tumor better than excretory urography would.[31] Ultrasonography can be useful in differentiating radiolucent filling defects caused by nonopaque renal calculi from neoplasms. Other tests in the metastatic evaluation include chest radiography or CT, bone scan, and liver function tests.

**Urine Cytology.** Routine voided or catheterized urinary cytologic studies are of limited value because of the high incidence of false-positive and false-negative results. Positive results from cytologic studies increase as tumor anaplasia increases, varying from 11% for grade I lesions to 83% for grade IV lesions.[32] Even if the voided cytologic finding is positive in a patient with an upper tract filling defect, one cannot be certain of the origin of the malignant cells.

Cystoscopy is a mandatory component of complete evaluation of the upper urinary tracts because of the significant association with bladder tumors. Ureteral catheterization with saline barbotage and brush biopsies can increase diagnostic accuracy of urine cytology to 89%.[33]

**Ureteroscopy.** With the development of the rigid and flexible ureteroscope, ureteroscopy has become a valuable tool in the diagnosis of upper tract urothelial tumors. Ureteropyeloscopy can increase the diagnostic accuracy over the standard diagnostic regimen. The accuracy was 86% for renal pelvic tumors and 90% for ureteral tumors in one study.[34] The major complications of ureteroscopy include a risk of ureteral perforation with extravasation, denudation of mucosa facilitating implantation, or pyelovenous-lymphatic migration of tumor cells.[35, 36] Diagnostic ureteroscopy should be reserved for patients in whom the diagnosis remains in doubt after using conventional diagnostic techniques and for patients in whom treatment would be influenced by the results of the ureteroscopy.

### Staging and Prognosis

Tumor stage and grade are clinically the most useful prognostic variables for upper tract urothelial tumors. The tumor stage is the more important predictor of prognosis than the grade. Huben and associates[37] reported that the median survival for low-grade tumors was 67 months; for high-grade tumors, median survival was only 14 months. The median survival for low-stage tumors was 91 months and for high-stage tumors only 13 months.

The difficulty in establishing the diagnosis as well as the limited accuracy of the available staging procedures has precluded the development of a useful clinical staging system. Instead, classification of renal pelvic and ureteral tumors is based on pathologic findings. After studying 70 patients with renal pelvic tumors, Grabstald and associates[38] proposed a classification based on tumor stage and grade. The most commonly applied form is a modification of this system proposed by Batata and Grabstald[1] and is similar to the Jewett-Marshall-Strong system for bladder cancer (Fig. 51–4). The American Joint Committee on Cancer developed a TNM system for tumors of the ureter and renal pelvis.[39] Table 51–6 displays both systems as well as the estimated 5-year survival rates by stage.

TCC is graded from I to III—highly differentiated to poorly differentiated. The 5-year survival for patients with grade I TCC of the renal pelvis approaches 100%; for grade II, it is 60 to 70%; and for grade III, it is approximately 5%.[38] Representative 5-year survival rates for carcinoma of the ureter are 95% for stage A, 82% for stage B, 29% for stage C, and 0% for stage D.[40] Das and associates[41] reported that there are no significant differences in survival by stage between patients with carcinoma of the renal pelvis and ureter. Data according to the TNM staging system suggested that stage T3 renal pelvic TCC had a better prognosis than stage T3 ureteral TCC because of the renal parenchymal barrier against further invasion.[42] Renal pelvic TCC tumors that minimally invaded the collecting duct or the renal parenchyma had a better prognosis than did those with extensive parenchymal extension.[43] The presence and degree of renal parenchymal involvement may be valuable for staging or prognostic indicators.

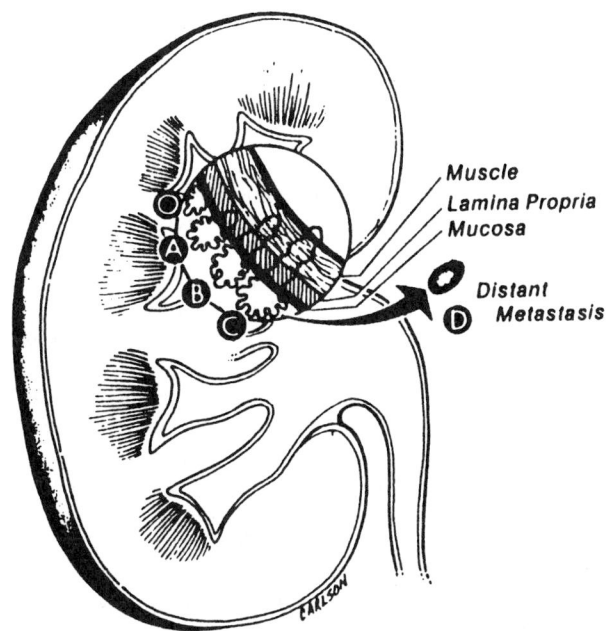

**Figure 51–4.** Staging system modified from Batata and associates, based on the extent of penetration applied to carcinoma of the renal pelvis. (From Babaian RJ, Johnson DE. Carcinoma of the renal pelvis. Cancer Bull 1979;31:21. Copyright Medical Arts Publishing Foundation, Houston, Texas.)

Flow DNA analysis correlates with malignant potential of upper tract urothelial tumors. High-grade tumors are found to be almost uniformly aneuploid, whereas low-grade tumors are less commonly aneuploid. Tumor cell ploidy correlates to grade, stage, and clinical outcome. For high-grade, high-stage tumors, ploidy provides no additional information; however, for low-grade, low-stage tumors, an aneuploid pattern identifies a subgroup of patients who have significantly

poorer survival rates.[44] Al-Abadi and Nagel[45] suggested that DNA ploidy affords no additional prognostic information to grades I and III tumors; however, it does give additional information in grade II tumors. They subclassified grade II tumors as aneuploid (biologically aggressive) and diploid or tetraploid (biologically less aggressive). Studies measuring S-phase fraction of renal pelvis and ureteral tumors revealed that all low-grade tumors have an S-phase fraction less than 10%. The average S-phase fraction for noninvasive tumors was 9.7% and for invasive tumors was 20.9%. The S-phase fraction also appeared to correlate with the biologic potential of the tumor.[46] Although p53 mutations have been shown to correlate with the risk of recurrence and survival, the prognostic value of p53 abnormalities for the upper tract tumors has not been shown to be a good independent prognostic variable.[47, 48]

## TREATMENT

### Surgical Therapy

The accepted treatment for renal pelvic or ureteral tumors is nephroureterectomy with excision of a cuff of bladder and bladder mucosa. Batata and associates[23] reported the 5-year survival outcomes: 91% for stage Tis, Ta, or T1; 43% for stage T2; 23% for stage T3, T4, N1, or N2; and 0% for stage N3 or M1. The high recurrence rate in ureteral stumps following incomplete nephroureterectomy (64%), the low contralateral recurrence rate, and the need for prolonged surveillance of the ipsilateral ureter have all been used to justify this procedure.[49] For most renal pelvic tumors, a radical nephroureterectomy, with removal of the entire ureter including a cuff of bladder, should be performed when there is a normal contralateral kidney. Certain circumstances necessitate a more conservative renal-sparing approach to the treatment of upper tract tumors. Conservative parenchyma-

*Table 51–6.* **Staging Systems and Survival**

| Modified Jewett System | | 5-Year Survival (%) | AJCC TNM System | |
|---|---|---|---|---|
| STAGE | DESCRIPTION | | STAGE | DESCRIPTION |
| | | | TX | Primary tumor cannot be assessed |
| | | | T0 | No evidence of primary tumor |
| | | | Tis | Carcinoma in situ |
| 0 | Confined to mucosa | 100 | Ta | Papillary noninvasive carcinoma |
| A | Involvement through lamina propria | 80–95 | T1 | Tumor invades subepithelial connective tissue |
| B | Into muscular wall | 40–80 | T2 | Tumor invades muscularis |
| C | Periureteral spread | 15–33 | T3 | Tumor invades beyond muscularis into periureteric or peripelvic fat or renal parenchyma |
| D | Metastatic disease | 0 | T4 | Tumor invades adjacent organs or through kidney into perinephric fat |
| | | | NX | Regional lymph nodes cannot be assessed |
| | | | N0 | No regional lymph node metastases |
| | | | N1 | Metastasis in a single lymph node, ≤2 cm in greatest dimension |
| | | | N2 | Metastasis in a single lymph node, >2 cm but not >5 cm in greatest dimension, or multiple lymph nodes, none >5 cm in greatest dimension |
| | | | N3 | Metastasis in a lymph node >5 cm in greatest dimension |
| | | | MX | Presence of distant metastasis cannot be assessed |
| | | | M0 | No distant metastasis |
| | | | M1 | Distant metastasis |

From Crawford ED, Das S. Current genitourinary cancer surgery. Malvern, PA: Lea & Febiger, 1990:106.

sparing procedures for tumors of the upper urinary tract were advocated in 1945 by Vest.[50] In patients with a solitary kidney, bilateral lesions, compromised renal function, or endemic Balkan nephropathy or in patients who are a poor surgical risk, conservative therapy is essential. The preferred treatment is local excision of a renal pelvic tumor, with or without partial nephrectomy. In the case of a ureteral tumor, local excision or ureterectomy is the treatment of choice. The proponents of radical nephroureterectomy with removal of a cuff of bladder emphasize the difficulty in determining the grade and stage of the tumor preoperatively. Advocates of conservative surgical therapy for renal pelvic or ureteral tumors note the poor prognosis associated with advanced lesions, regardless of the form of surgical therapy, and the higher morbidity and mortality rates occurring with more radical procedures. Although nephroureterectomy has traditionally been considered the treatment of choice for upper tract urothelial tumors, experiences with more conservative treatment methods have appeared more frequently in the literature. Mufti and colleagues[51] reported no difference in the 5-year survival rates of patients with low-grade, low-stage upper tract lesions when treated with radical or conservative surgery. When urothelium was left behind after conservative resection, however, there was a 22% recurrence rate on the ipsilateral side. Data suggested that the recurrence rates following conservative surgery of renal pelvic tumors were greater than those following conservative surgery of ureteral tumors.[52] Recurrence was highly associated with multifocality, and in 58 patients treated conservatively, only 3% developed recurrence if the original tumor was solitary versus 50% recurrence if the original tumor was multifocal. Besides multifocality, tumor grade has also been used as an indication for conservative surgery. The 5-year survival rates were 88% and 75% for grade I tumors treated with radical and conservative surgery. For grade II tumors, the 2-year survival rate was 90% for patients treated with radical surgery, whereas 46% of patients treated with conservative surgery survived more than 2 years. The ipsilateral recurrence rate was 28% in patients with grade II tumors treated with conservative surgery.[53, 54] The recommendation for conservative resection is a single, well-differentiated, noninvasive tumor of the upper tract.

For patients with apparent solitary tumors of the lower third of the ureter, especially low-grade tumors, distal ureterectomy and ureteral reimplantation with either a psoas hitch or a Boari flap is an excellent option. Distal ureterectomy for low-grade, low-stage ureteral carcinoma has excellent long-term survival rates. Several series have reported 100% 5-year survival for distal ureterectomy in grade I, stage I TCC of the distal ureter.[1, 7, 10, 40] Mufti and colleagues[51] have suggested that survival and recurrence of upper tract tumors do not depend on their site (renal pelvis, upper or lower ureter) but on their original grade and stage and whether they are single or multifocal. In general, patients with low-grade, low-stage tumors do well with either conservative or radical surgery. Patients with intermediate-grade tumors do better with radical surgery, and patients with high-grade, high-stage tumors do equally poorly with either conservative or radical surgery. Distal ureterectomy is appealing for several other reasons. Approximately 70% of all ureteral tumors are in the distal third of the ureter. Distal ureterectomy and ureteral reimplantation directly into the bladder (ureteroneo-

cystotomy) has a lower rate of morbidity and mortality than does radical nephroureterectomy.[55, 56] Additionally, although most series report only a 2% recurrence rate in the contralateral ureter, some have noted synchronous or metachronous cancer in 10% of patients.[56] This clinical occurrence makes conservative treatment a more attractive approach. For distal ureteral tumors, regardless of tumor grade or stage, distal ureterectomy, including a cuff of bladder with ureteral reimplantation using a psoas hitch or Boari flap, if necessary, is the preferred treatment. It is important to obtain a negative proximal ureteral margin; otherwise a total nephroureterectomy is required. Using this approach, Heney and associates[40] found 5-year survival to be virtually identical, stage for stage and grade for grade, when comparing nephroureterectomy and segmental resection for distal ureteral tumors. Other renal-sparing methods of treating ureteral carcinoma include segmental ureterectomy and ileal interposition, cutaneous ureterostomy, and autotransplantation. Although these procedures may occasionally be effective in certain situations, they have largely fallen out of favor because of significant morbidity and poor results. If conservative therapy is planned, thorough evaluation of the entire urothelium is mandatory. Retrograde pyelography to exclude secondary ureteral or renal pelvic lesions is essential. Brush biopsy, barbotage cytology, or ureteroscopy should be used to provide a better idea of stage and grade. The contralateral ureter and renal pelvis must be carefully evaluated to exclude bilateral tumors.

In patients with Balkan nephropathy, renal-sparing surgery plays a more pronounced role. In a series from the Balkan region, patients died more frequently from renal failure than from metastatic disease.[56]

In general, treatment guidelines for upper tract urothelial tumors are as follows. Most renal pelvic tumors should be treated with radical nephroureterectomy with excision of a cuff of bladder. Upper ureteral and midureteral tumors can be treated with segmental resection if they are low grade and solitary but should be treated with nephroureterectomy if they are high grade and multifocal. Distal ureteral tumors should be treated by distal ureterectomy and ureteroneocystostomy.

**Technique.** Nephroureterectomy can be carried out by a one-incision or two-incision approach. The one-incision technique involves a flank incision that is extended to a paramedian incision down to the symphysis pubis. This incision allows adequate exposure for removing the distal ureter and bladder cuff. With the two-incision approach, a flank incision is used to expose the kidney and proximal ureter, and then a paramedian or Pfannenstiel (transverse lower abdominal) incision is used to remove the distal ureter. Regardless of the incision used, the bladder should be opened and the ureter removed intravesically with a 1-cm cuff around the ureteral orifice. The ureter should not be removed by an extravesical approach. A report of nine cases of *complete nephroureterectomy* performed by tenting up of the ureter resulted in a retained ureteral orifice and intramural ureter as determined by cystoscopy and retrograde ureterogram in all nine patients. Recurrence was subsequently found in two of the nine ureteral stumps.[57] Some authors recommend the instillation of an intravesical chemotherapeutic agent before the procedure to reduce the incidence of spillage and implantation of viable tumor cells.[58]

The value of lymphadenectomy in the treatment of this disease is undetermined. Although it allows for more accurate staging, its therapeutic benefit has not been proved. Babaian and Johnson[7] suggested that the increase in operative time and potential morbidity outweighs the possible benefits of the procedure. Most of the data suggest that if lymph node metastases are present, the patient has widely metastatic disease and would not benefit from a regional lymphadenectomy.[40]

## Endoscopic Treatment

Although conservative therapy has come to play a role in the treatment of upper urinary tract tumors, conservative surgery is still not without the complications of an open surgical procedure. The advent of refined endoscopic instruments and techniques has provided less invasive complementary methods of evaluating and treating upper tract tumors. The principles of endoscopic treatment for upper tract urothelial tumors are the same as for the endoscopic treatment of bladder tumors. The main differences relate to the technical difficulty in gaining access to the urothelium in the upper tract. Advances in ureteroscopic technology allow access to the entire ureter and renal pelvis in most patients. Percutaneous nephroscopy permits access to the renal pelvis. Other considerations in the endoscopic management of upper tract tumors include the comparative thinness of the ureteral wall, making it susceptible to perforation and extravasation of tumor cells. Additionally, the narrow ureteral lumen is susceptible to obstruction from post-treatment scarring and fibrosis. Endoscopic resection of tumor can be accomplished in several ways. A cold-cup biopsy forceps, the standard resectoscope, and the Nd:YAG laser have all been used. Ureteral tumors can usually be treated ureteroscopically. Renal pelvic tumors are more commonly approached percutaneously, especially if they are larger than 1 cm. Overall, ureteral tumors appear to be more amenable to endoscopic treatment than renal pelvic tumors. Schilling and associates[59] reported 16 ureteral tumors in 13 patients treated with Nd:YAG laser phototherapy in the lower ureter with follow-up from 3 to 31 months. They identified no local tumor recurrences and only one new tumor recurrence distal to the original tumor site. Carson[60] reported no recurrence in 8 patients followed 6 to 40 months after ureteroscopic resection of ureteral tumors with the Nd:YAG laser. High recurrence rates of the upper tract tumors treated by endoscopic surgery were demonstrated by several other investigators. Blute and associates[61] indicated a recurrence in 1 of 5 renal pelvic tumors and 2 of 13 ureteral tumors treated by ureteroscopic surgery. Grossman and coworkers[62] found 5 of 8 patients in their series needed further management. Orihuela and Smith[63] reported on a series of 12 patients who underwent percutaneous resection of renal pelvic tumors followed by supplemental therapy consisting of Nd:YAG laser irradiation of the tumor bed and the intrarenal administration of BCG immunotherapy. Recurrence was noted in 6 of 12 patients and was confined to patients with multifocal, high-grade, sessile tumors. Recurrence was unlikely in patients with single, well-localized, low-grade, small, papillary tumors. Stoller and colleagues[64] reported high recurrence rates with endoscopic surgery. With a mean follow-up of 25 months in 20 patients, 44% of patients with renal pelvic tumors and 80% of patients with ureteral tumors experienced recurrence.

Several authors have reported experience with topical instillation therapy in upper tract tumors. In Orihuela and Smith's series[63] of 12 patients, BCG administration appeared to be safe and relatively effective. At 22 months' follow-up, recurrence was seen in 80% of patients who did not receive BCG and in only 16.6% of those who received it. Delivery of topical agents to the renal pelvis is also accomplished with the reflux caused by a double J stent.[65] The potential complications of this method are scarring or obstruction of the collecting system, systemic absorption, and sepsis.[66] At present, the indications and success rate of topical therapy of upper tract TCC are not clear.

Concern has been raised over the potential for retroperitoneal seeding by perforation or of seeding along the nephrostomy tract. Several investigators have reported no retroperitoneal or nephrostomy tract recurrence in patients undergoing percutaneous endosurgery for upper tract TCC.[63, 67] Most patients in these series, however, have been followed for a relatively brief period, usually less than 2 years. Longer follow-up is necessary to determine if there is minimal risk. Some investigators used iridium 192 wire brachytherapy in the nephrostomy tract to avoid retroperitoneal seeding of tumors.[68]

The use of endoscopic surgery for the treatment of upper tract tumors in patients with bilaterally functioning kidneys remains extremely controversial. All series reported in the literature had a small number of patients and were not randomized studies. The long-term results are still unclear. For low-grade tumors of the ureter, recurrence rates and the need for open surgery are low. Additionally, the endoscopic staging of ureteral tumors appears to be fairly accurate. The same does not apply to renal pelvic tumors. Understaging occurs in approximately 60% of the cases, and recurrence rates are much higher.[69] At this time, endoscopic treatment of upper tract tumors should be limited to patients with a solitary kidney and a low-grade, apparently low-stage tumor confined to a single, small focus or to those who are poor candidates to undergo standard surgical procedures. For most patients with TCC of the upper urinary tract, nephroureterectomy or distal ureterectomy, depending on the location of the tumor, remain the treatments of choice.[70]

Careful follow-up after conservative therapy is essential because of high recurrence rates. Urine cytologic studies from the bladder and the affected ureter should be performed every 3 months for 1 year, every 6 months for 2 years, and then once a year for life. Excretory urography should be obtained every 6 months for 2 years and then as necessary. If cytologic findings become positive and no lesions can be identified on radiologic studies, ureteroscopy should be performed. Because of the high incidence of bladder tumors in patients with upper tract TCC, cystoscopy should be performed every 3 months for a year, every 6 months for 2 years, and then every year for life. Recurrence in the urinary tract after conservative resection occurs in 38 to 46% of patients.[63] These recurrent tumors are of a higher grade in approximately 25% of patients.[71] If recurrence is detected in the remaining upper tract, total nephroureterectomy is a reasonable treatment plan, if this is feasible.

## Radiation Therapy

Radiation therapy has been used postoperatively in patients at risk for residual disease or for those at increased risk for local recurrence. A review evaluating postoperative radiation therapy in 26 patients concluded that local control was statistically improved from 34 to 88%. Adjuvant radiation therapy had no impact on distant disease that occurred in approximately 50% of patients regardless of therapy.[72] Similar results were reported by Brookland and Richter.[73] In contrast, another study showed no benefit of adjuvant radiation therapy in invasive TCC of the upper tract.[74] They indicated that with a mean follow-up of 45 months, local tumors relapsed, there was nodal recurrence, and metastases occurred in 4%, 15%, and 54% of patients. To solve this controversy, a prospective randomized study should be conducted. The role of radiation therapy for the upper tract tumors is still ill-defined. Radiation therapy has been effective for palliation of painful osseous metastases from TCC.[29]

## Chemotherapy

Because cisplatin-based chemotherapy has shown some improvement in survival in patients with TCC of the bladder, one might expect similar results in patients with TCC of the renal pelvis and ureter. No randomized prospective trials have been reported, however. Das and associates[41] reported that a group of patients with metastatic upper tract tumors treated with cisplatin-based chemotherapy alone or with radiation had a median survival of 21.5 and 22.2 months. This survival compared favorably with the median survival of 6.4 months in a group of historical controls who did not receive chemotherapy. Five-year survival was no different, however. In another series of 41 patients with TCC who were treated with MVAC (10 patients with renal pelvic or ureteral tumors), the results have been disappointing, with durable complete responses being reported in 5% of the patients. There was a 41% incidence of neutropenic sepsis and a 2% mortality.[75] Cisplatin-based chemotherapy and adjuvant chemotherapy for upper tract TCC have shown some favorable effects but are not without significant side effects. Prospective randomized trials are needed to evaluate the efficacy of chemotherapy for advanced-stage upper tract TCC.

## SUGGESTIONS FOR ADDITIONAL READING

Hall MC, Womack S, Sagalowsky AI, et al. Prognostic factors, recurrence, and survival in transitional cell carcinoma of the upper urinary tract: a 30-year experience in 252 patients. Urology 1998;52:594–601.

Ozsahin M, Zouhair A, Villáa S, et al. Prognostic factors in urothelial renal pelvis and ureter tumours: a multicentre Rare Cancer Network study. Eur J Cancer 1999;35:738–43.

Scher H, Bahnson R, Cohen S, et al. NCCN urothelial cancer practice guidelines. National Comprehensive Cancer Network. Oncology 1998;12(7A):225–71.

## REFERENCES

1. Batata M, Grabstald H. Upper urinary tract urothelial tumors. Urol Clin North Am 1976;3:79–86.
2. 1987 Annual Cancer Statistics Review: including cancer trend: 1950-1985. NIH Publication No. 88-2789. Bethesda, Md.: U.S. Dept. of Health and Human Services, National Cancer Institute, 1987.
3. Guinan P, Vogelzang NJ, Randazzo R, et al. Renal pelvic cancer: a review of 611 patients treated in Illinois 1975–1985: Cancer Incidence and End Results Committee. Urology 1992;40:393–9.
4. Landis SH, Murray T, Bolden S, Wingo PA. Cancer statistics, 1998. CA Cancer J Clin 1998;48:6–29.
5. Huben RP, Mounzer AM, Murphy GP. Tumor grade and stage as prognostic variables in upper tract urothelial tumors. Cancer 1988;62:2016–20.
6. Babaian RJ. Primary carcinoma of the upper urothelium: an overview. In: Crawford ED, ed. Current genitourinary cancer surgery. Philadelphia: Lea & Febiger, 1990:93.
7. Babaian RJ, Johnson DE. Primary carcinoma of the ureter. J Urol 1980;123:357–9.
8. Murphy DM, Zincke H, Furlow WL. Management of high grade transitional cell cancer of the upper urinary tract. J Urol 1981;125:25–9.
9. Shinka T, Uekado Y, Aoshi H, et al. Occurrence of uroepithelial tumors of the upper urinary tract after the initial diagnosis of bladder cancer. J Urol 1988;140:745–8.
10. Anderstrom C, Johansson SL, Pettersson S, Wahlqvist L. Carcinoma of the ureter: a clinicopathologic study of 49 cases. J Urol 1989;142:2 Pt 1:280–3.
11. Vineis P, Pirastu R. Aromatic amines and cancer. Cancer Causes Control 1997;8:346–55.
12. Bartsch H, Malaveille C, Friesen M, et al. Black (air-cured) and blond (flue-cured) tobacco cancer risk. IV: molecular dosimetry studies implicate aromatic amines as bladder carcinogens. Eur J Cancer 1993;29A:1199–207.
13. Ross RK, Paganini-Hill A, Landolph J, et al. Analgesics, cigarette smoking, and other risk factors for cancer of the renal pelvis and ureter. Cancer Res 1989;49:1045–8.
14. McLaughlin JK, Silverman DT, Hsing AW, et al. Cigarette smoking and cancers of the renal pelvis and ureter. Cancer Res 1992;52:254–7.
15. Steffens J, Nagel R. Tumours of the renal pelvis and ureter: observations in 170 patients. Br J Urol 1988;61:277–83.
16. McCredie M, Stewart JH, Carter JJ, et al. Phenacetin and papillary necrosis: independent risk factors for renal pelvic cancer. Kidney Int 1986;30:81–4.
17. Schiff HI, Finkel M, Schapira HE. Transitional cell carcinoma of the ureter associated with cyclophosphamide therapy for benign disease: a case report. J Urol 1982;128:1023–4.
18. Cohen SM, Garland EM, St. John M, et al. Acrolein initiates rat urinary bladder carcinogenesis. Cancer Res 1992;52:3577–81.
19. Brenner DW, Schellhammer PF. Upper tract urothelial malignancy after cyclophosphamide therapy: a case report and literature review. J Urol 1987;137:1226–7.
20. Radovanovic Z, Krajinovic S, Jankovic S, et al. Family history of cancer among cases of upper urothelial tumours in a Balkan nephropathy area. J Cancer Res Clin Oncol 1985;110:181–3.
21. Stein A, Sova Y, Lurie M, Lurie A. Adenocarcinoma of the renal pelvis: report of two cases, one with simultaneous transitional cell carcinoma of the bladder. Urol Int 1988;43:299–301.
22. Jitsukawa S, Nakamura K, Nakayama M, et al. Transitional cell carcinoma of kidney extending into renal vein and inferior vena cava. Urology 1985;25:310–2.
23. Batata MA, Whitmore WF, Hilaris BS, et al. Primary carcinoma of the ureter: a prognostic study. Cancer 1975;35:1626–32.
24. Madgar I, Goldwasser B, Czerniak A, Many M. Leiomyosarcoma of the ureter. Eur Urol 1988;14:487–9.
25. Fleming S. Carcinosarcoma (mixed mesodermal tumor) of the ureter. J Urol 1987;138:1234–5.
26. Fiorelli C, Durval A, Di Cello V, et al. Ureteral intussusception by a fibroepithelial polyp. J Urol 1981;126:110–2.
27. Stower MJ, MacIver AG, Gingell JC, Clarke E. Inverted papilloma of the ureter with malignant change. Br J Urol 1990;65:13–6.
28. Richie JP, Withers G, Ehrlich RM. Ureteral obstruction secondary to metastatic tumors. Surg Gynecol Obstet 1979;148:355–7.
29. Messing EM, Catalona WJ. Urothelial tumors of the urinary tract. In: Walsh PC, Retik AB, Vaughan ED Jr, Wein AJ, eds. Campbell's urology. 7th ed. Vol III. Philadelphia: WB Saunders, 1998:2327.
30. Bloom NA, Vidone RA, Lytton B. Primary carcinoma of the ureter: a report of 102 new cases. J Urol 1970;103:590–8.
31. Kenney PJ, Panicek DM, Witanowski LS. Computed tomography of ureteral disruption. J Comput Assist Tomogr 1987;11:480–4.

32. Zincke H, Aguilo JJ, Farrow GM, et al. Significance of urinary cytology in the early detection of transitional cell cancer of the upper urinary tract. J Urol 1976;116:781–3.

33. Sheline M, Amendola MA, Pollack HM, et al. Fluoroscopically guided retrograde brush biopsy in the diagnosis of transitional cell carcinoma of the upper urinary tract: results in 45 patients. AJR Am J Roentgenol 1989;153:313–6.

34. Blute ML, Segura JW, Patterson DE, et al. Impact of endourology on diagnosis and management of upper urinary tract urothelial cancer. J Urol 1989;141:1298–301.

35. Lim DJ, Shattuck MC, Cook WA. Pyelovenous lymphatic migration of transitional cell carcinoma following flexible ureterorenoscopy. J Urol 1993;149:109–11.

36. Huang A, Low RK, deVere White R. Nephrostomy tract tumor seeding following percutaneous manipulation of a ureteral carcinoma. J Urol 1995;153:1041–2.

37. Huben RP, Mounzer AM, Murphy GP. Tumor grade and stage as prognostic variables in upper tract urothelial tumors. Cancer 1988;62:2016–20.

38. Grabstald H, Whitmore WF, Melamed MR. Renal pelvic tumors. JAMA 1971;218:845–54.

39. American Joint Committee on Cancer. Renal pelvis and ureter. In: Manual for staging of cancer. 3rd ed. Philadelphia: JB Lippincott, 1988:205.

40. Heney NM, Nocks BN, Daly JJ, et al. Prognostic factors in carcinoma of the ureter. J Urol 1981;125:632–6.

41. Das AK, Carson CC, Bolick D, Paulson DF. Primary carcinoma of the upper urinary tract: effect of primary and secondary therapy on survival. Cancer 1990;66:1919–23.

42. Guinan P, Vogelzang NJ, Randazzo R, et al. Renal pelvic cancer: a review of 611 patients treated in Illinois 1975–1985: Cancer Incidence and End Results Committee. Urology 1992;40:393–9.

43. Fujimoto H, Tobisu K, Sakamoto M, et al. Intraductal tumor involvement and renal parenchymal invasion of transitional cell carcinoma in the renal pelvis. J Urol 1995;153:57–60.

44. Blute ML, Tsushima K, Farrow GM, et al. Transitional cell carcinoma of the renal pelvis: nuclear deoxyribonucleic acid ploidy studied by flow cytometry. J Urol 1988;140:944–9.

45. Al-Abadi H, Nagel R. Transitional cell carcinoma of the renal pelvis and ureter: prognostic relevance of nuclear deoxyribonucleic acid ploidy studied by slide cytometry: an 8-year survival time study. J Urol 1992;148:31–7.

46. Nemoto R, Hattori K, Sasaki A, et al. Estimations of the S phase fraction in situ in transitional cell carcinoma of the renal pelvis and ureter with bromodeoxyuridine labelling. Br J Urol 1989;64:339–44.

47. Gardiner RA, Walsh MD, Allen V, et al. Immunohistological expression of p53 in primary pT1 transitional cell bladder cancer in relation to tumour progression. Br J Urol 1994;73:526–32.

48. Terrell RB, Cheville JC, See WA, Cohen MB. Histopathological features and p53 nuclear protein staining as predictors of survival and tumor recurrence in patients with transitional cell carcinoma of the renal pelvis. J Urol 1995;154:1342–7.

49. Kakizoe T, Fujita J, Murase T, et al. Transitional cell carcinoma of the bladder in patients with renal pelvic and ureteral cancer. J Urol 1980;124:17–9.

50. Vest SA. Conservative surgery in certain benign tumors of the ureter. J Urol 1945;53:97–121.

51. Mufti GR, Gove JR, Badenoch DF, et al. Transitional cell carcinoma of the renal pelvis and ureter. Br J Urol 1989;63:135–40.

52. Zincke H, Neves RJ. Feasibility of conservative surgery for transitional cell cancer of the upper urinary tract. Urol Clin North Am 1984;11:717–24.

53. Murphy DM, Zincke H, Furlow WL. Management of high grade transitional cell cancer of the upper urinary tract. J Urol 1981;125:25–9.

54. Murphy DM, Zincke H, Furlow WL. Primary grade 1 transitional cell carcinoma of the renal pelvis and ureter. J Urol 1980;123:629–31.

55. Zungri E. Bone biopsy in solitary lesions on bone scan in genitourinary malignancy. Eur Urol 1990;17:293–5.

56. Petkovic SD. Epidemiology and treatment of renal pelvic and ureteral tumors. J Urol 1975;114:858–65.

57. Strong DW, Pearse HD. Recurrent urothelial tumors following surgery for transitional cell carcinoma of the upper urinary tract. Cancer 1976;38:2173–83.

58. Donohue RE. Radical nephroureterectomy for carcinoma of the renal pelvis and ureter. In: Crawford ED, ed. Current genitourinary cancer surgery. Philadelphia: Lea & Febiger, 1990:102.

59. Schilling A, Bowering R, Keiditsch E. Use of the neodymium-YAG laser in the treatment of ureteral tumors and urethral condylomata acuminata: clinical experience. Eur Urol 1986;12:Suppl 1:30–3.

60. Carson CC 3d. Endoscopic treatment of upper and lower urinary tract lesions using lasers. Semin Urol 1991;9:185–91.

61. Blute ML, Segura JW, Patterson DE, et al. Impact of endourology on diagnosis and management of upper urinary tract urothelial cancer. J Urol 1989;141:1298–301.

62. Grossman HB, Schwartz SL, Konnak JW. Ureteroscopic treatment of urothelial carcinoma of the ureter and renal pelvis. J Urol 1992;148:275–7.

63. Orihuela E, Smith AD. Percutaneous treatment of transitional cell carcinoma of the upper urinary tract. Urol Clin North Am 1988;15:425–31.

64. Stoller ML, Gentle DL, McDonald MW, et al. Endoscopic management of upper tract urothelial tumors. Tech Urol 1997;3:152–7.

65. Mazeman E, Gilliot P. Renal-sparing conservative treatment of the upper urinary tract tumors. Prog Clin Biol Res 1991;370:25–36.

66. Ramsey JC, Soloway MS. Instillation of bacillus Calmette-Guerin into the renal pelvis of a solitary kidney for the treatment of transitional cell carcinoma. J Urol 1990;143:1220–2.

67. Kulp DA, Bagley DH. Does flexible ureteropyeloscopy promote local recurrence of transitional cell carcinoma? J Endourol 1994;8:111–3.

68. Shepherd SF, Patel A, Bidmead AM, et al. Nephrostomy track brachytherapy following percutaneous resection of transitional cell carcinoma of the renal pelvis. Clin Oncol (R Coll Radiol) 1995;7:385–7.

69. Clayman RV, McDougal EM, Nakada SY. Endourology of the upper tract: percutaneous renal and ureteral procedure. In: Walsh PC, Retik AB, Vaughan ED Jr, Wein AJ, eds. Campbell's urology. 7th ed. Vol III. Philadelphia: WB Saunders, 1998:2789.

70. Gerber GS, Lyon ES. Endourological management of upper tract urothelial tumors. J Urol 1993;150:2–7.

71. Mazeman E. Tumours of the upper urinary tract calyces, renal pelvis and ureter. Eur Urol 1976;2:120–6.

72. Cozad SC, Smalley SR, Austenfeld M, et al. Adjuvant radiotherapy in high stage transitional cell carcinoma of the renal pelvis and ureter. Int J Radiat Oncol Biol Phys 1992;24:743–5.

73. Brookland RK, Richter MP. The postoperative irradiation of transitional cell carcinoma of the renal pelvis and ureter. J Urol 1985;133:952–5.

74. Maulard-Durdux C, Dufour B, Hennequin C, et al. Postoperative radiation therapy in 26 patients with invasive transitional cell carcinoma of the upper urinary tract: no impact on survival? J Urol 1996;155:115–7.

75. Tannock I, Gospodarowicz M, Connolly J, Jewett M. M-VAC (methotrexate, vinblastine, doxorubicin and cisplatin) chemotherapy for transitional cell carcinoma: the Princess Margaret Hospital experience. J Urol 1989;142:289–92.

# CHAPTER 52

# URETHRA AND PENIS

• MITCHELL K. RAUCH • JEAN B. DEKERNION

## URETHRAL CANCER

Urethral carcinoma is a rare disease, accounting for less than 1% of all malignancies. Despite the greater length and complexity of the male urethra, urethral cancer remains the only shared genitourinary neoplasm that occurs more frequently in women than in men.[1] The anatomy, pathology, and clinical course of urethral cancer differ between men and women, and these aspects are discussed separately. Also, the management of the anterior urethra in men following radical cystoprostatectomy for invasive transitional cell carcinoma (TCC) is addressed.

As an overview, both male and female urethral cancers are apt to invade surrounding adjacent soft tissues. Also, they tend to metastasize to regional lymph nodes and distant organs early in their clinical course. Therefore, the majority of patients present with advanced disease. These features account for the poor prognosis of urethral tumors despite early, aggressive surgical therapy. In addition, adjuvant therapies such as radiation and chemotherapy are limited in their efficacy.

## Carcinoma of the Female Urethra

### NATURAL HISTORY

#### Epidemiology and Etiology

Urethral cancer was first described in the early 1830s, but through 1996 only about 1500 cases had been reported in the literature. Eighty percent of the reported cases were in women in the sixth and seventh decades, with an age distribution of 29 to 80 years.[2-4] This cancer appears to be more common in white women (85% of cases) than in black women (12% of cases), although a predilection for blacks is seen with adenocarcinoma of the urethra.

The cause of urethral carcinoma in women is still unknown. There are weak associations between urethral cancers and both urethral caruncles and urethral diverticula; however, no data to support a cause-and-effect relationship exist. One series reported a less than 1% incidence of a positive history for urethral caruncle in women with urethral carcinoma.[5] It is possible that early urethral cancers may have been mistaken for caruncles and that only after the lesion failed to respond to therapy was the correct diagnosis made. Also, both adenocarcinomas and TCCs have been reported to occur in urethral diverticula, probably secondary to infection, urinary stasis, and chronic irritation. However, despite the common incidence of urethral diverticula, reported cases of cancer are rare. In any event, a biopsy should be performed with urethral lesions that do not respond to conservative therapy or lesions that enlarge or bleed to rule out urethral carcinoma.[6]

## Anatomy

The female urethra is an epithelial-lined tube that is approximately 4 to 6 cm long. The external urinary meatus lies anterior to the vaginal introitus and just 2 cm inferior to the clitoris. The urethra is arbitrarily divided into an anterior segment (distal third) and a posterior segment (proximal two-thirds) (Fig. 52–1). Urinary continence is maintained by the posterior segment. Surgical excision of the distal third of the urethra does not result in incontinence. This arbitrary division not only reflects continence but also dictates the differences in treatment and prognosis associated with the tumor's location.

The lymphatic channels that drain the female urethra follow two courses. The distal urethra drains into the superficial inguinal nodes, whereas the proximal urethra drains into the deep pelvic nodes,[7] consisting of the external iliac nodes, obturator nodes, or presacral nodes.

## Pathology

The distal two thirds of the female urethra is lined with a stratified squamous epithelium that becomes continuous with the epithelium of the vulva at the urethral meatus. The proximal third of the female urethra is lined with transitional epithelium that merges internally with the lining of the bladder. Beneath the mucosa is the submucosal connective tissue, consisting of elastic fibers, spongy venous sinuses, and the periurethral Skene's glands. These glands usually empty into the urethra at the meatus, but they may extend along the entire urethral length. They are lined with pseudostratified and stratified columnar epithelium.

The pathologic distribution of female urethral carcinomas has been reviewed. The majority of reported cases are squamous cell carcinomas (53%), followed by TCC (14%), adenocarcinomas (14%), undifferentiated carcinoma (2.5%), malignant melanoma (2.3%), and mixed carcinomas, that is,

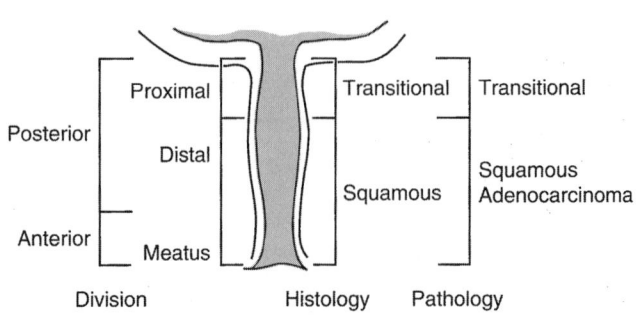

**Figure 52–1.** Division, histology, and pathology of the female urethra. (From Droller MJ, Nyberg L. Urethral carcinoma. AUA Update Series. Vol 2. Lesson 19, 1983.)

squamous cell carcinoma with either adenocarcinoma or TCC (2%). Uncommon primary urethral cancers are clear cell adenocarcinomas and cloacogenic carcinoma.[8] Squamous cell carcinomas may involve the entire female urethra or may be localized to the distal third. Adenocarcinomas of the female urethra tend to arise from the proximal urethra or periurethral glands. They tend to be locally aggressive and highly metastatic.[9, 10]

The natural history of untreated female urethral cancer involves the local extension to adjacent organs (urethral vaginal septum, vagina, bladder neck, or vulva) and metastatic spread to regional lymph nodes. Large, locally advanced meatal lesions may mimic a fungating, primary vulvar carcinoma. Clinical evidence of inguinal lymphadenopathy occurs in 35 to 50% of patients and may be secondary to an inflammatory process of the urethra. However, pathologically proven metastases occur in only 12.5 to 35% of patients.[1, 11, 12] Urethral cancers tend to metastasize to the lung, liver, bone, and brain. Adenocarcinomas of the urethra tend to be more aggressive and are more frequently associated with distant spread.[1]

## Clinical Features and Diagnosis

Most women are symptomatic before seeking medical attention. The most common symptoms are urethral spotting or bleeding. Some patients may present with dysuria, frequency, dyspareunia, or obstructive voiding. A urethral or periurethral neoplasm should be included in the differential diagnosis of urinary retention in women. Other benign urethral conditions that may share the symptoms of a urethral cancer include a caruncle, polyp, prolapse, hemangioma, fibroma, diverticulum, or urethral vaginal fistula.

On physical examination, a meatal mass is commonly seen because the majority of carcinomas originate in the distal urethra or involve the entire urethra. As previously mentioned, a urethral cancer may be discovered as an incidental finding during the evaluation of a urethral caruncle or diverticulum. Adenocarcinomas often present with a bloody discharge and a palpable, soft urethral mass. Urinalysis may contain white and red blood cells, and the urine cytologic findings may be positive.

Urethral tumors are diagnosed by cystourethroscopy and biopsy. At this time, a careful bimanual examination under anesthesia helps evaluate the extent and fixation of the tumor as well as assesses inguinal and pelvic lymphadenopathy. Radiologic tests to help evaluate both local and distant spread include intravenous pyelography, computed tomography (CT) scan, magnetic resonance imaging (MRI), bone scanning, and chest radiography.

## Staging

The TNM classification, introduced by the American Joint Committee on Cancer, provides an exact differentiation of primary tumor invasion, lymph node involvement, and metastasis (Table 52–1). Although the TNM staging system is desirable, the staging, treatment, and prognosis are simplified by anatomically dividing the urethra into anterior or posterior sections or the entire segment.

*Table 52–1.* **International TNM Staging for Both the Male and the Female Urethra**

### Definition of TNM

*Primary Tumor (T) (Male and Female)*

| | |
|---|---|
| TX | Primary tumor cannot be assessed |
| T0 | No evidence of primary tumor |
| Ta | Noninvasive papillary, polypoid, or verrucous carcinoma |
| Tis | Carcinoma *in situ* |
| T1 | Tumor invades subepithelial connective tissue |
| T2 | Tumor invades any of the following: corpus spongiosum, prostate, periurethral muscle |
| T3 | Tumor invades any of the following: corpus cavernosum, beyond prostatic capsule, anterior vagina, bladder neck |
| T4 | Tumor invades other adjacent organs |

*Transitional Cell Carcinoma of the Prostate*

| | | |
|---|---|---|
| Tis | pu | Carcinoma *in situ*, involvement of the prostatic urethra |
| Tis | pd | Carcinoma *in situ*, involvement of the prostatic ducts |
| T1 | | Tumor invades subepithelial connective tissue |
| T2 | | Tumor invades any of the following: prostatic stroma, corpus spongiosum, periurethral muscle |
| T3 | | Tumor invades any of the following: corpus cavernosum, beyond prostatic capsule, bladder neck (extraprostatic extension) |
| T4 | | Tumor invades other adjacent organs (invasion of the bladder) |

*Regional Lymph Nodes (N)*

| | |
|---|---|
| NX | Regional lymph nodes cannot be assessed |
| N0 | No regional lymph node metastasis |
| N1 | Metastasis in a single lymph node, 2 cm or less in greatest dimension |
| N2 | Metastasis in a single node more than 2 cm in greatest dimension, or in multiple lymph nodes |

*Distant Metastasis (M)*

| | |
|---|---|
| MX | Distant metastasis cannot be assessed |
| M0 | No distant metastasis |
| M1 | Distant metastasis |

*Stage Grouping*

| | | | |
|---|---|---|---|
| Stage 0a | Ta | N0 | M0 |
| Stage Ois | Tis | N0 | M0 |
| | Tis pu | N0 | M0 |
| | Tis pd | N0 | M0 |
| Stage I | T1 | N0 | M0 |
| Stage II | T2 | N0 | M0 |
| Stage III | T1 | N1 | M0 |
| | T2 | N1 | M0 |
| | T3 | N0 | M0 |
| | T3 | N1 | M0 |
| Stage IV | T4 | N0 | M0 |
| | T4 | N1 | M0 |
| | Any T | N2 | M0 |
| | Any T | Any N | M1 |

*Histopathologic Grade (G)*

| | |
|---|---|
| GX | Grade cannot be assessed |
| G1 | Well differentiated |
| G2 | Moderately differentiated |
| G3–G4 | Poorly differentiated or undifferentiated |

Used with the permission of the American Joint Committee on Cancer (AJCC®), Chicago, Illinois. The original source for this material is the AJCC® Cancer Staging Manual, 5th edition (1997) published by Lippincott-Raven Publishers, Philadelphia, Pennsylvania.

## Prognosis

The most important features of urethral cancer that relate to survival include anatomic location, size of tumor, and clinical stage. Since the average delay in diagnosing urethral cancer after the appearance of symptoms is 5 months,[11] many patients present with advanced disease. Accordingly, urethral carcinoma has a poor prognosis. At the time of diagnosis, 84% of patients already have muscular invasion or regional lymph node involvement.[13] Larger primary tumors are associated with a poorer survival, and a 3-cm diameter has been suggested as a threshold for a poor prognosis. Patients with tumors less than 2 cm have a 60% 5-year survival rate, whereas patients whose tumors are greater than 5 cm have a 13% 5-year survival.[13–15] With respect to location, it has been shown that distal urethral carcinomas have a better prognosis than proximally located tumors (14 to 40% vs. 0 to 17% 5-year surviva).[8] However, the overall 5-year survival rate for all urethral cancers is still poor and ranges from 12 to 32%. Local recurrence rates may approach 50%, and it is the failure to achieve local disease control that results in morbidity and mortality.[13]

## TREATMENT

Because of the rarity of urethral cancer, no single institution has a large enough series to examine various treatment protocols prospectively. Accordingly, there appears to be a lack of uniformity when treating urethral tumors. Nevertheless, the majority of therapy involves surgical resection. Radiation therapy may also be used for patients with regionally advanced disease, although absolute indications for its use are uncertain. Similarly, for TCCs of the urethra, platinum-based chemotherapy may be effective. However, squamous cell carcinomas and adenocarcinomas are less responsive. More precise recommendations based on the stage of the disease are discussed in the following sections.

### Stages 0a, 0is, and I

Urethral tumors involving the distal third of the urethra and limited to the mucosa (stage Tis and stage Ta) or involving the submucosa (T1) are rare. Yet, they have been successfully managed with either a thorough transurethral resection or a local excision. Laser ablation may also be acceptable for low-grade superficial lesions.[16] The 5-year survival rate for appropriately treated patients should be 90% or better.[4] Unfortunately, tumors in these early stages are rare, and a careful work-up to avoid understaging is indicated.

### Stage II

Tumors of the anterior third of the urethra that infiltrate the urethral muscularis (T2) may be managed by a partial urethrectomy if an adequate margin can be obtained. As much as two thirds of the anterior urethra may be excised without stress or total incontinence resulting from the surgery. Neoplasms involving the proximal urethra or the entire urethra have a much worse prognosis and should be managed more aggressively. These tumors are almost always at least a clinical stage T2, and in more than 50% of cases there is nodal involvement. For localized tumors without inguinal or pelvic lymph node metastases, the treatment of choice is anterior pelvic exenteration and urinary diversion. En bloc resection of the inferior aspect of the pubic symphysis and adjacent urogenital diaphragms may improve local control. Inguinal lymph node dissection should not be performed in

the absence of palpable disease in the groin. Overall, the results have been poor. Five-year survival rates range from 10 to 17%, and local tumor recurrence rates exceed 60%. In an effort to decrease local recurrence, an integrated approach using external-beam radiation therapy with or without interstitial brachytherapy before or after radical surgery has been suggested.[1, 13, 16–18] Several studies have recommended combined modality approaches of preoperative irradiation and chemotherapy (M-VAC [methotrexate, vinblastine, doxorubicin {Adriamycin}, cisplatin] or combined mitomycin-C and 5-fluorouracil) followed by radical cystourethrectomy. Long-term results are still unavailable.

### Stages III and IV

Inguinal lymphadenopathy is a relatively frequent finding, and because 60 to 80% of clinically palpable groin nodes harbor tumor, excisional biopsy of suspicious nodes is mandatory.[1, 8] Prophylactic inguinal lymph node dissection has no survival benefit over a therapeutic dissection and, because of its added morbidity, has been discouraged. Palliative systemic chemotherapy as an adjunct to surgery and radiation may be considered, yet it is seldom curative.

## Carcinoma of the Male Urethra

### NATURAL HISTORY

#### Epidemiology and Etiology

Approximately 600 cases of primary carcinoma of the male urethra have been reported since Thiaudierre described the first case in a young man in 1834. Because the incidence of male urethral tumors is low, no single institution has sufficient experience to outline a definitive treatment plan. No racial or geographic predisposition has been identified to date.

As in females, 70 to 80% of the reported cases of urethral cancer in males are identified during the sixth and seventh decades of life. The exact cause of male urethral tumors is unknown. However, the frequent history or associated finding of chronic urethral irritation has been observed. A past history of urethral stricture, venereal disease, or urethritis is common in most men with urethral tumors. Kaplan and colleagues, in a classic review of 232 patients, noted a history of venereal disease, stricture, or significant trauma in 79% of men with urethral cancer.[19] The association between urethral strictures and urethral cancer is further strengthened by the finding that the bulbomembranous urethra is the most frequent location for both disease processes.[6] Others, however, have argued that urethral cancers may merely be misdiagnosed as urethral strictures and that the symptoms possibly derive from an early, unrecognized urethral carcinoma.[20] In contrast to TCC of the bladder and the upper urinary tracts, in which causative agents such as aromatic amines, cigarette smoking, and analgesic abuse have been identified, there are no known agents responsible for TCC of the urethra.[21] However, Schellhammer and Whitmore have shown an association of TCC of the urethra with concomitant or previous TCCs of the bladder.[22]

## Anatomy

The male urethra is an epithelial-lined tubular structure with an average length of 21 cm that courses from the bladder to the external urinary meatus. The male urethra is divided into four segments: prostatic, membranous, bulbous, and penile (Fig. 52–2). By an anatomic convention, the posterior urethra comprises the prostatic and membranous portions, whereas the more distal segments make up the anterior urethra. However, when considering urethral carcinomas, previous authors have included the bulbous urethra with the posterior segment because of the differences in treatment and prognosis with tumors in this segment compared with those in the anterior, or penile, portion. Therefore, in this discussion, bulbourethral tumors are considered posterior urethral lesions.[6]

The lymphatic drainage of the male urethra is well characterized. The lymphatic channels from the anterior urethra parallel those from the glans penis and corpus spongiosum and drain into the deep inguinal nodes. Lymphatic channels from the posterior urethra (prostatic, membranous, and bulbous urethra) drain into the pelvic lymph node chain, consisting of the external iliac nodes, internal iliac nodes, obturator nodes, or presacral nodes.

## Pathology

The most frequent histologic type is squamous cell carcinoma, accounting for about 78% of all urethral cancers. TCCs account for 15% of all urethral tumors and most often occur in the prostatic urethra. Adenocarcinomas, most frequently found in the membranous urethra, are thought to arise in Cowper's glands and account for 7% of all cases.[19]

The natural history of untreated male urethral cancer is similar to that of female urethral cancer. Male urethral cancers spread by direct extension to adjacent structures (corpora cavernosa, corpus spongiosum, urogenital diaphragm, rectum, prostate, or bladder neck) and then to regional lymph nodes. Similarly, the lung, liver, and bone are the most common sites for distant metastatic spread. However, some series have shown that metastatic disease secondary to hematogenous spread is uncommon and is found in only 12 to 14% of patients. The most frequent cause of death from male urethral carcinoma is infection secondary to local ulceration and subsequent sepsis.[19] Conversely, TCCs of the male urethra are highly aggressive tumors that spread by both hematogenous and lymphatic routes.[6]

## Clinical Features and Diagnosis

Urethral carcinoma in the male is usually a localized destructive lesion. It often results in a delayed diagnosis, and its symptoms are vague and mimic those of a urethral stricture. Men with urethral cancer may present with dysuria, obstructive voiding, hematuria, urinary retention, overflow incontinence, urethral bleeding or discharge, hematospermia, or priapism. The association of these symptoms with a urethral mass is highly suspicious for urethral carcinoma. Urethral carcinoma has also been found in conjunction with urethral abscesses and urethrocutaneous fistulas.

The index of suspicion must be high when treating men with recurrent urethral stricture disease whose strictures require either more frequent dilations or bleed excessively following dilations. Transurethral biopsy of suspicious lesions is usually adequate; however, occasionally repeated deep biopsies must be performed in areas where there is an abscess or phlegmon. A bimanual examination under anesthesia may help delineate local invasion. Also, careful palpation of the inguinal region is critical because, unlike penile cancer, inguinal lymphadenopathy is usually suggestive of metastatic disease rather than infection.[6] Retrograde urethrography is the most helpful radiographic study to diagnose urethral carcinoma. In one series, 60% of patients had suspicious retrograde urethrograms showing long, irregular strictures with extravasation, fistula formation, obstruction, or intraluminal filling defects.[23] Ultrasonography of the urethra may also help in the diagnosis and staging of this tumor, along with assessment of local tumor extension. Lymphadenopathy and distant metastasis may be evaluated by CT, MRI, and chest radiography. Urinary cytologic findings may be positive for urethral cancer in greater than 81% of cases.[19, 23]

## Staging

The TNM staging classification is based on depth of invasion of the primary tumor and the presence or absence of regional lymph node involvement and distant metastasis (Table 52–2).

## Prognosis

Neither histology nor tumor grade has a significant impact on survival. Instead, the stage and location of the tumor are the most important factors affecting prognosis. Anterior urethral carcinomas tend to present early with symptoms and, accordingly, tend to be detected at lower stages. Posterior tumors tend to be more difficult to detect, and in one study, 86% of patients with posterior cancers presented with either stage III or stage IV lesions.[23] Five-year survival rates

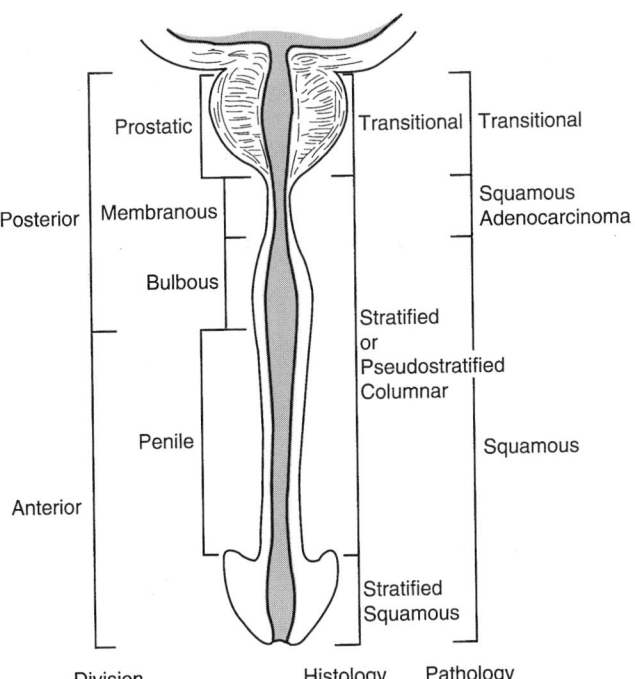

**Figure 52–2.** Division, histology, and pathology of the male urethra. (From Droller MJ, Nyberg L. Urethral carcinoma. AUA Update Series. Vol 2. Lesson 19, 1989.)

*Table 52–2.* **International TNM Staging System for the Penis**

| Definition of TNM | |
| --- | --- |

*Primary Tumor (T)*

| | |
| --- | --- |
| TX | Primary tumor cannot be assessed |
| T0 | No evidence of primary tumor |
| Tis | Carcinoma in situ |
| Ta | Noninvasive verrucous carcinoma |
| T1 | Tumor invades subepithelial connective tissue |
| T2 | Tumor invades corpus spongiosum or cavernosum |
| T3 | Tumor invades urethra or prostate |
| T4 | Tumor invades other adjacent structures |

*Primary Lymph Nodes (N)*

| | |
| --- | --- |
| NX | Regional lymph nodes cannot be assessed |
| N0 | No regional lymph node metastasis |
| N1 | Metastasis in a single superficial, inguinal lymph node |
| N2 | Metastasis in multiple or bilateral superficial inguinal lymph nodes |
| N3 | Metastasis in deep inguinal or pelvic lymph node(s), unilateral or bilateral |

*Distant Metastasis (M)*

| | |
| --- | --- |
| MX | Distant metastasis cannot be assessed |
| M0 | No distant metastasis |
| M1 | Distant metastasis |

*Histopathologic Grade (G)*

| | |
| --- | --- |
| GX | Grade cannot be assessed |
| G1 | Well differentiated |
| G2 | Moderately well differentiated |
| G3-4 | Poorly differentiated or undifferentiated |

*Stage Grouping*

| | | | |
| --- | --- | --- | --- |
| Stage 0 | Tis | N0 | M0 |
| | Ta | N0 | M0 |
| Stage I | T1 | N0 | M0 |
| Stage II | T1 | N1 | M0 |
| | T2 | N0 | M0 |
| | T2 | N1 | M0 |
| Stage III | T1 | N2 | M0 |
| | T2 | N2 | M0 |
| | T3 | N0 | M0 |
| | T3 | N1 | M0 |
| | T3 | N2 | M0 |
| Stage IV | T4 | Any N | M0 |
| | Any T | N3 | M0 |
| | Any T | Any N | M1 |

Used with the permission of the American Joint Committee on Cancer (AJCC®), Chicago, Illinois. The original source for this material is the AJCC® Cancer Staging Manual, 5th edition (1997) published by Lippincott-Raven Publishers, Philadelphia, Pennsylvania.

for stage I and stage II tumors have been reported to be as high as 86%, whereas the 5-year survival rate for stage III and stage IV tumors is only 19%.[3] Unfortunately, invasive cancers represent the majority of cases.

## TREATMENT

Treatment of urethral neoplasms depends on the location (anterior vs. posterior urethra) of the lesion and its extent of involvement. The primary mode of therapy for carcinoma of the male urethra is surgical excision, and its extent depends on the location and stage of the tumor.

### Stages 0a, 0is, and I

The rare low-grade, superficial tumor can be managed with transurethral resection, fulguration, or segmental urethral resection with end-to-end anastomosis.

### Stage II

Adequate treatment of anterior urethral tumors can be achieved with a partial penectomy provided that a 2-cm tumor-free margin proximal to the lesion is obtained. If a partial penectomy would result in a penile stump too short to allow the patient to direct his urinary stream, total penectomy with permanent perineal urethrostomy is indicated. Occasionally, superficially invasive bulbourethral carcinomas can be treated with urethrectomy, partial corporectomy, and perineal urethroplasty, thus sparing the penis.

### Stage III

More advanced carcinomas of the proximal urethra may require radical cystoprostatectomy, pelvic lymph node dissection, and total emasculation.[1, 13, 19] Even with extensive local excision, it may be difficult to obtain adequate surgical margins, and local recurrence has been reported in 40 to 60% of men with invasive tumors.[3, 23] Accordingly, a more radical approach with en bloc pelvic exenteration and inferior rami or pubic bone resection has been advocated.[13, 24, 25] Radiation and chemotherapy have been used mainly for palliative therapy for surgically unresectable tumors or as adjuncts to surgical therapy.[19, 25, 26] Platinum-based chemotherapy has some activity against TCCs of the prostatic urethra; however, other histologic types tend to be unresponsive to chemotherapy. In 1996, two patients with locally advanced squamous cell carcionmas of the proximal deep urethra were treated with a modified Nigro chemoradiation protocol. The initial treatment was by suprapubic cystotomy urinary diversion followed by external beam radiation. Chemotherapy consisted of mitomycin and 5-fluorouracil.[27] Prophylactic inguinal lymph node dissection does not increase survival when compared with therapeutic inguinal lymph node dissection and thus is probably advisable only in patients with palpable lymphadenopathy.

### Stage IV

Metastatic urethral carcinomas have a grave prognosis and are managed similarly to advanced bladder cancer. Currently, patients with squamous cell carcinoma are treated with a regimen of cisplatin, bleomycin, and methotrexate. Those with metastatic TCC receive M-VAC.

## Transitional Cell Carcinoma of the Prostate

The management of patients with primary TCC of the prostate has been reviewed.[28] For patients with superficial or superficially invasive TCC of the prostate, transurethral resection is curative in 50% of cases.[1] Recurrences are common, and in cases of carcinoma in situ, a course of intravesical bacille Calmette-Guérin is given. However, tumors that invade the prostatic stoma are often aggressive, and a radical cystoprostatectomy is recommended.

## Management of the Urethra in Men with Transitional Cell Carcinoma of the Bladder

TCC is a potentially multifocal lesion, and the entire urothelium is at risk in patients with bladder cancer. Several studies have shown that between 4 and 10% of patients develop urethral tumors after undergoing only a radical cystoprostatectomy for TCC.[22, 23, 29] Prophylactic urethrectomy at the time of radical cystoprostatectomy provides the greatest assurance of eliminating the potential for tumor formation in the remnant urethra. However, a urethrectomy adds time and morbidity to an already lengthy operation and seems to be indicated only in patients with overt carcinoma or carcinoma in situ of the prostatic urethra or invasion of the prostate gland. Neobladder reconstruction to the urethra is currently the procedure of choice after cystectomy in most men and is a compelling reason to preserve the urethra whenever possible. In patients with a low risk of urethral involvement by tumor, a conservative approach is indicated and, accordingly, these patients must be followed closely with yearly physical examination of the urethra and urethral washings for cytologic studies. Urethrectomy is then indicated if the urethral wash reveals positive cytologic findings or if a bloody urethral discharge develops.[29]

## Penile Cancer

### NATURAL HISTORY

#### Epidemiology

Carcinoma of the penis, which is uncommon in the developed nations of North America and Europe, constitutes less than 1% of all malignancies in the U.S. male population. However, it accounts for up to 14% of adult male cancers in India, Central Africa, China, and Southeast Asia.[30] In Paraguay, penile cancer is the most common genitourinary tumor (45 to 76% of all genitourinary tumors); in Uganda, where circumcision usually is not performed, penile cancer is the most common male cancer.[30, 31] In Israel, where a ritual neonatal circumcision is commonly performed, penile cancer is exceedingly rare, with an incidence of 0.1 per 100,000 males.[32] Also, the importance of geographic factors when considering the incidence of penile cancer is emphasized by realizing that the incidence among the Chinese living in the continental United States or in Hawaii is lower than that for Chinese living in Asia. Some studies have shown an increased incidence of penile cancer in the black population.[33] Penile cancer is most commonly diagnosed during the sixth and seventh decades of life, and there is an increasing incidence of penile cancer with increasing age.[34]

#### Etiology

The cause of penile cancer is unknown. However, several risk factors are associated with its development.

The presence of a foreskin seems to be the greatest risk factor for the development of penile cancer. This is supported by the fact that Jews, who are routinely circumcised in infancy, and Muslims, who are circumcised between the ages of 4 and 9, rarely develop penile cancer.[35] However, there are case reports of penile carcinoma developing in men who underwent an incomplete circumcision where only a portion of the foreskin was excised.[36] Likewise, men who undergo circumcision later in adolescence or during adulthood for indications such as phimosis or chronic balanoposthitis are not protected against penile cancers. Further evidence for the protective effects of neonatal circumcision is derived from studies examining populations with a high incidence of penile cancer. For example, among Ugandan tribes practicing circumcision, the rate of penile cancer is significantly lower than among those tribes not practicing that ritual.[37] In conclusion, circumcision at birth seems to be an effective prophylactic measure against penile cancer.

Phimosis, which is considered by some to be a risk factor for penile cancer, is the most common coexisting anatomic abnormality found in men with penile cancer. As many as 69% of patients with penile cancer relate a pre-existing history of phimosis alone or with balanoposthitis.[38] Pathologic studies that have examined the foreskins of men with phimosis have shown that epithelial atypia, a putative precursor of malignancy, was noted in 35% of specimens, compared with 0% of specimens obtained in patients without phimosis.[39] Also, different configurations of the phimotic foreskin have been studied with respect to penile cancer, and it appears that a closed preputial cavity prohibits effective penile hygiene and hence may predispose to penile cancer.

Some evidence suggests that penile cancer occurs more commonly in men of lower socioeconomic levels. However, a large population-based Danish study refuted such a relationship, and therefore no definitive conclusions can be drawn. Similarly, even though a history of venereal disease has been reported in up to 22% of patients with penile cancer, causality cannot be proved, and confounding variables such as poor penile hygiene and low circumcision rates may be responsible.[38] Even though penile cancer has been reported to develop in the scarred penile skin after a mutilating circumcision,[36] no definite relationship between penile trauma and penile cancer has been established.[38]

A possible association between viral infections and penile cancer has sparked considerable interest. There is evidence that wives whose husbands have penile cancer have an increased risk of developing cervical cancer. Both these conditions have been related to a herpesvirus infection.[40, 41] Also, data have suggested, but not yet proved, a causative role for the human papillomavirus (HPV) in penile cancer. DNA analysis of squamous cell carcinomas in Brazilian men demonstrated HPV 16 or HPV 18 sequences in 50% of tumors.[42, 43]

#### Anatomical Considerations

Penile cancer usually begins as a small lesion that gradually enlarges to involve the glans, shaft, and corpora. Penetration and subsequent invasion of Buck's fascia and the tunica albuginea permit entrance into the vascular corpora and the potential for vascular dissemination. However, hematogenous spread is rare, and lymphatic metastases are more common. Lymphatics from the prepuce decussate at the base of the penis and drain to the superficial and deep inguinal nodes. The decussation of these lymphatic channels accounts for positive contralateral lymph nodes. The lymphatics of the glans, corpora, and urethra drain into the deep inguinal and external iliac nodes.[44]

Enlarged regional lymph node metastases eventually result in skin necrosis, chronic infection, sepsis, and hemorrhage secondary to erosion into the femoral vessels. Distant metastases usually occur late in the disease and tend to involve the lung, liver, bone, or brain.[45]

## Pathology

By convention, penile tumors have been divided into benign lesions, premalignant (or precancerous) lesions, carcinoma in situ, noninvasive carcinomas, and invasive carcinomas. Metastatic tumors to the penis are rare, with the majority of these lesions originating from the bladder, prostate, or rectum.[46-48]

**Benign Lesions.** Briefly, benign penile lesions include condylomata acuminata, molluscum contagiosum, hirsutoid papillomas, sebaceous cysts, and nevi. These lesions are mentioned only for completeness; discussion of them is beyond the scope of this chapter.

**Premalignant Lesions.** Leukoplakia, giant condyloma acuminatum (Buschke-Löwenstein tumors), and balanitis xerotica obliterans have been termed *premalignant lesions* because of their malignant potential or their close pathologic relationship to squamous cell carcinomas of the penis.

Leukoplakia, which is a rare condition that is associated with chronic irritation, inflammation, and diabetes, appears as sharply defined white cutaneous plaques that tend to involve the meatus. It is often found adjacent to areas of frank squamous carcinoma, but this should not imply that all squamous tumors originate as leukoplakia.[38] Treatment consists of surgical excision, careful histologic examination for invasive cancer, and meticulous follow-up. Balanitis xerotica obliterans is a chronic inflammatory process that occurs in both circumcised and uncircumcised males. Its exact relationship to penile cancer is poorly understood, but the development of overt malignancy in association with this condition has been reported.[49] Balanitis xerotica obliterans may involve the glans, inner prepuce, urethral meatus, or fossa navicularis, and treatment consists of either excision or topical therapy with testosterone or steroid cream.[50]

**Carcinoma in Situ.** Erythroplasia of Queyrat, Bowen's disease, and bowenoid papulosis constitute the three pathologic forms of squamous cell carcinoma in situ of the penis. Erythroplasia of Queyrat occurs mainly on the glans or prepuce and appears as distinct velvety red plaques with ill-defined margins that often ulcerate and are associated with pain and discharge. It is almost never found in circumcised men; progression to invasive carcinoma has been documented.[51] Erythroplasia of Queyrat is clinically and pathologically similar to Bowen's disease. However, Bowen's disease, which is an intraepithelial carcinoma that is similar to Bowen's disease in other areas such as the vulva, generally appears dryer and is often crusted and less painful than erythroplasia of Queyrat. Although Bowen's disease was believed to be associated with other visceral malignancies, case-control studies have not confirmed this. Bowenoid papulosis is histologically identical to erythroplasia of Queyrat and Bowen's disease, but clinically it is more benign. It occurs on the penile shaft of circumcised men age 20 to 40 years and appears as multiple pigmented papules.[52] These lesions range in size from 0.2 to 3 cm in diameter and are associated with HPV 16 infections.[53]

**Noninvasive Carcinoma.** Buschke-Löwenstein tumors (giant condyloma acuminatum, verrucous carcinoma) may be histologically benign despite their large size and malignant appearance. These papillary lesions can develop into large, necrotic, exophytic lesions that may erode into the urethra, fistulize, and eventually destroy the penis. There is controversy regarding its benign or malignant potential, and histologically its appearance is indistinguishable from usual, benign condyloma. However, cases of malignant degeneration with carcinomatous degeneration have been reported.[54] These tumors should be regarded as malignant, and an excision with either a partial or a total penectomy should be performed. Podophyllin, radiation therapy, and 5-fluorouracil have not proved effective.

**Invasive Squamous Cell Carcinoma.** Invasive squamous cell carcinoma of the penis commonly arises on the glans or prepuce, may be predominantly exophytic or diffuse, and frequently ulcerates. It is usually well to moderately well differentiated, and these cells usually invade adjacent tissue.[55] As previously mentioned, Buck's fascia acts as a barrier to the corpora cavernosa. However, once the tumor has invaded the corpora, hematogenous dissemination occurs. Primarily, penile cancers spread to the lymph nodes in a prescribed pattern, first involving the superficial inguinal nodes and then the deep inguinal nodes and finally the pelvic nodes.

## Clinical Features and Diagnosis

Men with penile cancer tend to delay seeking medical care and, on average, present to their physicians 10 months (range, 3 to 26 months) after noting a penile lesion. This delay is attributable to ignorance about disease, personal neglect, denial, embarrassment, and fear of emasculation.[30] Although some studies show no difference in survival rates between patients who present early and those who present later,[33] others show poorer survival rates in men who delay presentation. The tumor is often nontender, and the diagnosis is made by physical examination and biopsy. Careful examination of the inguinal area for lymphadenopathy is extremely important. The differential diagnosis of penile masses includes lymphogranuloma venereum, granuloma inguinale, herpes, syphilis, chancroid, condyloma acuminatum, and traumatic ulceration. Radiologic procedures used to stage penile cancer and assess potential metastatic sites include a chest radiograph; CT of the chest, abdomen, and pelvis; a bone scan; and ultrasonography.

Palpable inguinal lymphadenopathy is associated with benign inflammation in approximately 40 to 50% of patients. This inflammatory reaction tends to subside after excision of the penile mass followed by a course of antibiotics.[30, 56, 57] However, clinically negative inguinal nodes are associated with micrometastasis in 20% of patients.[30] Survival is related to nodal status and, hence, the most accurate evaluation of the inguinal lymph nodes is inguinal dissection. Unfortunately, this procedure is associated with a 30 to 50% morbidity rate and a 3% mortality rate.[58] Some urologists, therefore, advocate either fine-needle aspiration of the inguinal nodes[59] or a limited inguinal dissection directed at a sentinel lymph node located medial to the epigastric-saphenous junction in association with the superficial epigastric vein.[60] However, negative biopsy results with these approaches do not prove the absence of cancer spread, and these patients must be followed closely. Some studies have also suggested relying on the stage of the primary tumor to predict lymph node metastasis. This approach is too simplistic, however, and often leads to understaging of the inguinal lymph nodes.[44]

### Staging

The first staging system for penile cancer was introduced by Jackson.[61] In this staging system, stage I lesions are limited to the glans and prepuce; stage II lesions involve the penile shaft; stage III lesions are operable tumors metastasizing to the inguinal lymph nodes, but without distant metastasis; and stage IV lesions include cases with inoperable inguinal nodes or distant spread (Fig. 52–3). More recently, a TNM staging system has been used, which allows a more precise differentiation among local extension, histologic grade, lymph node involvement, and distant spread (see Table 52–2).

### Prognosis

The 5-year survival rate for patients after surgery for stage I and stage II disease is greater than 70% and 50%, respec-

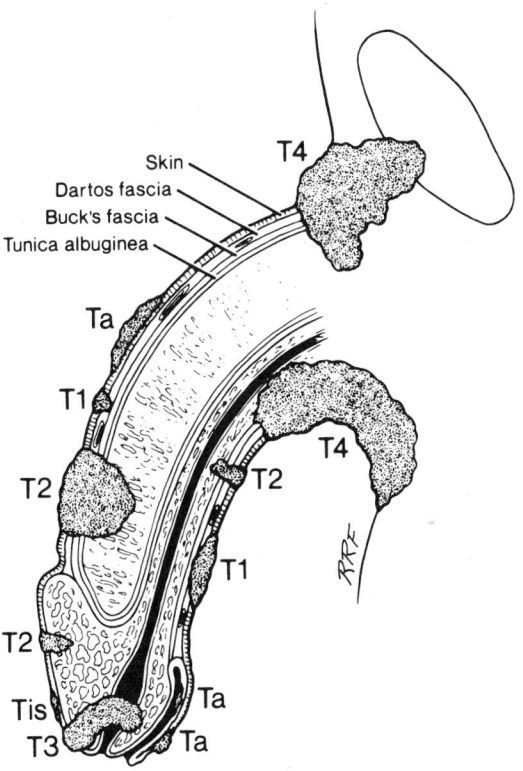

**Figure 52–3.** Because treatment decisions for inguinal node dissections are currently based on the characteristics of the primary lesion, a careful assessment of the depth of invasion of the primary lesion is required. The diagram illustrates the importance of invasion in assigning tumor (T) stage. (From Schellhammer PF, et al: Tumors of the penis. In: Walsh PC, Retik AB, Stamey TA, Vaughan ED, eds. Campbell's urology. 6th ed. Philadelphia: WB Saunders, 1992:1277.)

tively.[30] However, survival is dependent on nodal status and, accordingly, only 27 to 50% of men with stage III tumors survive 5 years. Men with stage IV tumors tend to do poorly, with a 0% 5-year survival rate.[8]

## TREATMENT

The management of the primary penile lesion in penile carcinoma is surgery, and the urologist must achieve adequate tumor control with a 2-cm margin while attempting to maintain a masculine body image and preserve both sexual function and the ability to urinate while standing. Therefore, surgical options include local excision of the tumor, circumcision, partial penectomy, or total penectomy with perineal urethrostomy.

### Stage 0 and Stage I

Carcinoma in situ of the penis is best managed by local excision with intraoperative frozen sections obtained on the margins. Using Mohs' micrographic surgery, selective lesions can be excised, and normal penile tissue can be preserved. Alternatively, superficial squamous cell carcinomas can be managed with topical chemotherapy (5-fluorouracil). However, this therapy is recommended only for reliable patients who can be expected to follow the dosing schedules and attend follow-up visits rigorously.[62] Preliminary results with the neodymium:yttrium-aluminum-garnet (Nd:YAG) hand-held laser have shown that localized penile lesions (Tis, T1, T2) can be excised safely with cosmetically pleasing long-term results.[63, 64] For superficial tumors localized to the foreskin, circumcision alone is a sufficient form of treatment provided that an adequate tumor-free margin can be obtained. No recurrences have been observed at the University of California, Los Angeles,[30] but the recurrence rate in these cases can be as high as 50%.[65]

### Stage II and Stage III

Invasive lesions of the glans and the shaft without lymph node metastasis are treated with partial penectomy with a 2-cm tumor-free margin proximal to the cancer. If the size and location of the tumor prohibit an adequate tumor-free margin, or the remaining stump prohibits voiding while standing, a total penectomy with a perineal urethrostomy is performed. Advocates of a partial penectomy maintain that some degree of sexual capability is maintained and that the patient is able to direct his urinary stream. Any form of penectomy is obviously a psychologically traumatic event, and counseling and support should be offered to all such patients.[38]

The timing and role of inguinal lymphadenectomy remain controversial in the management of penile carcinoma. Lymphadenectomy is curative when lymphatic metastases are limited to the groin, and it is the status and management of these lymph nodes that have the most significant impact on patient survival.[66] However, as previously stated, inguinal lymphadenectomy is associated with significant morbidity, including skin flap necrosis and lower extremity edema. Because of this morbidity, some urologists perform groin dissections only on patients with palpable inguinal lymph nodes and no clinical evidence of distant metastases.[30] Others, however, invoke the observation that 20% of clinically normal groins harbor histologic evidence of tumor, and thus they believe that a lymphadenectomy should be an integral part of the primary treatment of stage II and stage III penile cancers.[58] A modified lymphadenectomy, which spares the saphenous vein and reduces the extent of the dissection, has been suggested as a means to decrease morbidity and render this potentially therapeutic procedure more palatable.[67, 68]

Patients observed with surveillance therapy instead of groin lymphadenectomy must be closely supervised at monthly intervals during the first 3 years because most inguinal metastases occur within this period.[33, 69] Unreliable patients or patients too obese to allow an adequate physical examination of the groin are not suitable candidates for these surveillance options.

In summary, recommended guidelines for inguinal lymphadenectomy are as follows: For men with stage I penile cancers and no palpable adenopathy, an observation program can be used. If adenopathy is detected subsequently, a staged, bilateral inguinal lymphadenectomy is performed. In patients with stage II penile cancer and no palpable adenopathy, a staged, bilateral inguinal lymphadenectomy is appropriate. In patients with stage I or stage II tumors who have palpable adenopathy, a 3-week course of oral antibiotics is appropriate after the primary lesion is excised. Once the inflammation has subsided, clinically positive groins should undergo a staged, bilateral lymphadenectomy.[44] Patients with metastatic disease to the pelvic lymph nodes are seldom cured by surgery. Accordingly, pelvic lymph node dissections are performed only in men with clinically positive inguinal nodes, and if these pelvic nodes are negative, inguinal lymph node dissections are then undertaken.[70]

Survival rates following radiotherapy are comparable to those in surgically treated patients. However, radiation is associated with local recurrence rates ranging from 35 to 62%, and a salvage penectomy is then required. Penile amputation is also sometimes necessary secondary to radiation injury or necrosis following biopsy of the irradiated penis.[45] Adjuvant radiotherapy has been used, but its efficacy is unknown.[71]

## Stage IV

In patients with advanced unresectable inguinal metastases, radiation therapy may result in significant palliation and may postpone local complications. Chemotherapy has been used for metastatic penile cancer, and responses have been noted with bleomycin, 5-fluorouracil, cisplatin, and methotrexate.[72, 73] However, a cooperative Southwest Oncology Group study using cisplatin alone reported only a 15% response rate with a response duration of 1 to 3 months.[74] After a regimen of cisplatin, methotrexate, and bleomycin, large squamous cell carcinomas metastatic to the inguinal lymph nodes completely regressed in several patients as proved by postchemotherapy surgical resections. Combined modality programs using chemotherapy plus surgery or radiotherapy have been used with encouraging results in the treatment of squamous cell carcinoma of the larynx and anus. Similar strategies may be helpful in specific clinical situations.

## SUGGESTIONS FOR ADDITIONAL READING

Crawford ED, Das S, eds. Penile, urethral, and scrotal cancer. Urol Clin North Am 1992;19.

Krieg R, Hoffman R. Current management of unusual genitourinary cancers. Part 1: Penile cancer. Part 2: Urethral cancer. Oncology 1999;13:1347–52 and 1511–7, 1520; discussion 1523–4.

Maden C, Sherman KJ, Beckmann AM, et al. History of circumcision, medical conditions, and sexual activity and risk of penile cancer. J Natl Cancer Inst 1993; 85:19–24. *This article describes a large epidemiologic study in the Pacific Northwest supporting the importance of noncircumcision as a risk factor for penile cancer.*

## REFERENCES

1. Grabstald H. Proceedings: Tumors of the urethra in men and women. Cancer 1973;32:1236–55.
2. Levine RL. Urethral cancer. Cancer 1980;45:Suppl:1965–72.
3. Ray B: In: Javadpour N, ed. Principles and management of urologic cancer. Baltimore, Williams & Wilkins, 1979:445.
4. Hopkins SC. Tumors of the urethra and penis. In: Walsh PC, Retik AB, Vaughn ED, Wein AJ, eds. Campbell's urology. 5th ed. Vol. 2. Philadelphia: WB Saunders, 1986: 1441.
5. McCrea LE. Urethral pathology. Urol Surv 1952;2:85.
6. Palmer TE. Urethral carcinoma. In: Gillenwater JY, ed. Adult and pediatric urology. Vol. 1. Chicago, Year Book Medical, 1987:1315.
7. Carroll PR, Dixon CM. Surgical anatomy of the male and female urethra. Urol Clin North Am 1992;19:339–46.
8. Peterson RO. Urethra. In: Peterson RO, ed. Urologic pathology. Philadelphia: JB Lippincott, 1986:417.
9. Herr H. In Walsh PC, Retik AB, Stamey TA, Vaughan ED, eds. Campbell's urology, 6th ed, Vol 3. Philadelphia: WB Saunders, 1992:3073.
10. Mostofi FK, Davis CJ Jr, Sesterhenn IA. Carcinoma of the male and female urethra. Urol Clin North Am 1992;19:347–58.
11. Sullivan J, Grabstald H. Management of carcinoma of the urethra. In: Skinner DG, deKernion JB, eds. Genitourinary Cancer. Philadelphia: WB Saunders, 1978:419.
12. Desai S, Libertino JA, Zinman L. Primary carcinoma of the female urethra. J Urol 1973;110:693–5.
13. Bracken RB, Johnson DE, Miller LS, et al. Primary carcinoma of the female urethra. J Urol 1976;116:188–92.
14. Akaza H, Homma Y, Koiso K. Clinical evaluation of urethral tumors based on a simple classification system. Eur Urol 1988;14:107–10.
15. Rogers RE, Burns B. Carcinoma of the female urethra. Obstet Gynecol 1969;33:54–7.
16. Grabstald H, Hilaris B, Henschke U, Whitmore WF. Cancer of the female urethra. JAMA 1966;197:835–42.
17. Sailer SL, Shipley WU, Wang CC. Carcinoma of the female urethra: a review of results with radiation therapy. J Urol 1988;140:1–5.
18. Johnson DE. In: Genitourinary tumors: fundamental principles and surgical techniques. Johnson DE, Boileau MA, eds. New York: Grune & Stratton, 1982:267.
19. Kaplan GW, Bulkey GJ, Grayhack JT. Carcinoma of the male urethra. J Urol 1967;98:365–71.
20. Mandler JI, Pool TL. Primary carcinoma of the male urethra. J Urol 1966;96:67–72.
21. Droller MJ. Bladder cancer. Curr Probl Surg 1981;18:205–79.
22. Schellhammer PF, Whitmore WF Jr. Transitional cell carcinoma of the urethra in men having cystectomy for bladder cancer. J Urol 1976;115:56–60.
23. Ray B, Canto AR, Whitmore WF Jr. Experience with primary carcinoma of the male urethra. J Urol 1977;117:591–4.
24. Klein FA, Whitmore WF, Herr HW, et al. Inferior pubic rami resection with en bloc radical excision for invasive proximal urethral carcinoma. Cancer 1983;51:1238–42.
25. Raghavaiah N: Radiotherapy in the treatment of carcinoma of the male urethra. Cancer 1978;41:1313.
26. Bracken RB. Exenterative surgery for posterior urethral cancer. Urology 1982;19:248–51.
27. Oberfield RA, Zinman LN, Leibenhaut M, et al. Management of invasive squamous cell carcinoma of the bulbomembranous male urethra with coordinated chemo-radiotherapy and genital preservation. Br J Urol 1996;78:573–8.
28. Matzkin H, Soloway MS, Hardeman S. Transitional cell carcinoma of the prostate. J Urol 1991;146:1207–12.
29. Ahlering TE, Lieskovsky G, Skinner DG. Indications for urethrectomy

in men undergoing single stage radical cystectomy for bladder cancer. J Urol 1984;131:657–9.

30. deKernion JB. In: Skinner DG, deKernion JB, eds. Genitourinary cancer. Philadelphia: WB Saunders, 1978:494.
31. Dodge OG, Owor R, Templeton AC. Tumors of the male genitalia. Recent Results Cancer Res 1973;41:132–44.
32. Persky L. Epidemiology of cancer of the penis. Recent Results Cancer Res 1977;60:97–109.
33. Johnson DE, Fuerst DE, Ayala AG. Carcinoma of the penis: experience with 153 cases. Urology 1973;1:404–8.
34. Hall NEL. In: Schottenfeld D, ed. Cancer epidemiology and prevention. Philadelphia: WB Saunders, 1982:964.
35. Leiter E, Lefkovitis AM. Circumcision and penile carcinoma. NY State J Med 1975;75:1520–2.
36. Bissada NK, Morcos RR, el Senoussi M. Post-circumcision carcinoma of the penis, clinical aspects. Urology 1986;135:283–5.
37. Schmauz R, Jain DK. Geographical variation of carcinoma of the penis in Uganda. Br J Cancer 1971;25:25–32.
38. Hanash KA, Furlow WL, Utz DC, Harrison EG Jr. Carcinoma of the penis: a clinicopathologic study. J Urol 1970;104:291–7.
39. Reddy CRRM, Devendranath V, Pratap S. Carcinoma of penis—role of phimosis. Urology 1984;24:85–8.
40. Goldberg HM, Pell-Ilderton R, Daw E, Saleh N. Concurrent squamous cell carcinoma of the cervix and penis in a married couple. Br J Obstet Gynecol 1979;86:585–6.
41. Graham S, Priore R, Graham M, et al. Genital cancer in wives of penile cancer patients. Cancer 1979;44:1870–4.
42. Villa LL, Lopes A. Human papillomavirus DNA sequences in penile carcinomas in Brazil. Int J Cancer 1986;37:853–5.
43. McCance DJ, Kalache A, Ashdown K, et al. Human papillomavirus types 16 and 18 in carcinomas of the penis from Brazil. Int J Cancer 1986;37:55–9.
44. Thompson IM. AUA Update Series. 1990;9:1.
45. Schellhammer PE. In: Walsh PC, Retik AB, Stamey TA, Vaughan ED, eds. Campbell's Urology. 6th ed, Vol. 2. Philadelphia: WB Saunders, 1992:1264.
46. Bachrach P, Dahlen CP. Metastatic tumors to the penis. Urology 1973;1:359–62.
47. Tuttle JP, Rous SN, Kinzel RC. Bladder epithelial neoplasms metastatic to glans penis. Urology 1976;8:80–1.
48. Weitzner S. Secondary carcinoma in the penis: report of three cases and literature review. Am Surg 1971;37:563–7.
49. Weigand DA. Lichen sclerosus et atrophicus, multiple dysplastic keratoses, and squamous cell carcinoma of the glans penis. J Dermatol Surg Oncol 1980;6:45–50.
50. Rheinschild GW, Olsen BS. Balanitis xerotica obliterans. J Urol 1970;104:860–3.
51. Rege PR, Evans AT. Erythroplasia of Queyrat. J Urol 1974;111:784–5.
52. Kossow AS, Cotelingam JD, MacFarland F. Bowenoid papulosis of the penis. J Urol 1981;125:124–6.
53. Gross G, Hagedorn M, Ikenberg H, et al. Bowenoid papulosis: presence of human papillomavirus (HPV) structural antigens and of HPV 16 related DNA sequences. Arch Dermatol 1985;121:858–63.
54. Gritsch HA, Randazzo RF, Layfield LJ, deKernion JB. Invasive giant condylomata acuminata: a case report. J Urol 1989;141:950–2.
55. Mostofi FK. Tumors of the male genital system. Washington, D.C.: Armed Forces Institute of Pathology, 1973:277.
56. Catalona WJ. Role of lymphadenectomy in carcinoma of the penis. Urol Clin North Am 1980;7:785–92.
57. Mukamel E, de Kernion JB. Early versus delayed lymph node dissection versus no lymph node dissection in carcinoma of the penis. Urol Clin North Am 1987;14:707–11.
58. McDougal WS, Kirchner FK, Edwards RH, Killion LT. Treatment of carcinoma of the penis: the case for primary lymphadenectomy. J Urol 1986;136:38–41.
59. Scappini P, Piscioli F, Pusiol T, et al. Penile cancer: aspiration biopsy cytology for staging. Cancer 1986;58:1526–33.
60. Cabanas RM. An approach for the treatment of penile carcinoma. Cancer 1977;39:456–66.
61. Jackson SM. The treatment of carcinoma of the penis. Br J Surg 1966;53:33–5.
62. Johnson DE. Neoplastic lesions of the penis. In: deKernion JB, ed. Genitourinary cancer management. Philadelphia: Lea & Febiger, 1987:219.
63. Horenblas S, van Tinteren H, Delemarre JF, et al. Squamous cell carcinoma of the penis—treatment of the primary tumor. J Urol 1992;147:1533–8.
64. Hofstetter A. In: Dixon JA, ed. Surgical applications of lasers. Chicago: Year Book Medical, 1983:146.
65. Narayama AS, Olney LE, Loening SA, et al. Carcinoma of the penis: analysis of 219 cases. Cancer 1982;49:2185–91.
66. Fossa SD, Hall KS, Johannessen NB, et al. Cancer of the penis: experience at the Norwegian Radium Hospital 1974–1985. Eur Urol 1987;13:372–7.
67. Catalona WJ. Modified inguinal lymphadenectomy for carcinoma of the penis with preservation of saphenous veins: technique and preliminary results. J Urol 1988;140:306–10.
68. Catalona WJ. In: Urologic survey. New Scotland: LTI Medica, 1988.
69. Derrick FC, Lynch KM, Kretkowski RC, Yarbrough WJ. Epidermoid carcinoma of the penis: computer analysis of 87 cases. J Urol 1973;110:303–5.
70. Mukamel E. AUA Update Series 1990;9:10.
71. Potter R, Muller RP, Luttke G. Treatment results of surgical and radiologic therapy of penile cancer. Strahlenther Onkol 1988; 164:260–5.
72. Yagoda A, Mukherji B, Young C, et al. Bleomycin, an antitumor antibiotic: clinical experience in 272 patients. Ann Intern Med 1972;77:861–70.
73. Dexeus FH, Logothetis CJ, Sella A, et al. Combination chemotherapy with methotrexate, bleomycin and cisplatin for advanced squamous cell carcinoma of the male genital tract. J Urol 1991;146:1284–7.
74. Gagliano RG, Blumenstein BA, Crawford ED, et al. cis-Diaminedichloroplatinum in the treatment of advanced epidermoid carcinoma of the penis: a Southwest Oncology Group study. J Urol 1989;141:66–7.

# CHAPTER **53**

# KIDNEY

• BARBARA J. GITLITZ • DAVID M. J. HOFFMAN •
• ROBERT A. FIGLIN • ARIE S. BELLDEGRUN •

## Natural History, Diagnosis, and Staging

### EPIDEMIOLOGY

Renal cell carcinoma is the most common malignancy of the kidney and accounts for approximately 2% of all cancers worldwide.[1] Renal cell carcinoma (RCC) is a cancer of adults, primarily of those in the fifth to eighth decades of life, but it may occasionally occur in the period between infancy and young adulthood.[1] Worldwide mortality from kidney cancer is projected to be greater than 100,000 in the year 2000.[2] The highest incidence rates are found in North

America and Scandinavia. It is estimated that there will be approximately 31,200 new cases of cancer of the kidney and renal pelvis in the United States in the year 2000, accounting for about 11,900 U.S. cancer deaths.[3] An analysis of the National Cancer Institute's Surveillance, Epidemiology, and End Results (SEER) program data shows that the incidence of RCC in the United States appears to be rising, and is not simply explained by the increased detection of incidental tumors.[4] Between 1975 and 1995, the age-adjusted incidence rates increased annually by 2.3% among white men, 3.1% for white women, 3.9% among African American men, and 4.3% for African American women. Incidence rates for men are twice those for women. In both sexes, however, incidence rates among African Americans have exceeded those of whites. Asians in the United States have incidence rates approximately half those of other major racial groups.[5]

The origin of the tumor is the proximal convoluted tubule, but the stimulus for neoplastic transformation has not been determined. Environmental factors, pre-existing medical conditions, and occupational factors have been found to be associated with the development of kidney cancer. There is an increased incidence of kidney cancer in both male and female cigarette smokers.[6–8] There is a positive correlation between RCC and obesity[9] and RCC and hypertension.[10] An increased incidence of renal cell carcinoma has been observed in uremic dialysis patients with acquired multicystic kidney disease.[11] Other diseases, such as von Hippel-Lindau (VHL) syndrome,[12] polycystic kidney disease,[13] and lymphoproliferative disorders,[14] have been shown to predispose to the development of renal adenocarcinoma. A less conclusive correlation exists between RCC and diuretics[15] and RCC and phenacetin-containing analgesics (no longer available in the United States).[16] Hormonal agents have not been proved to play a clear role in renal cell etiology, even though diethylstilbestrol (DES) causes typical RCC in adult Syrian hamsters.[17] No epidemiologic study has conclusively related exposure or chosen occupation to RCC. Reports of increased risk, however, include asbestos workers,[18] as well as workers exposed to solvents (dry cleaners), polycyclic aromatic hydrocarbons (coke-oven workers), petroleum products (gas station attendants), and lead and cadmium.[19]

## MOLECULAR GENETICS

RCC occurs in both familial and sporadic forms. Similar to other familially inherited malignancies, such as retinoblastoma, the hereditary form of kidney cancer tends to be multifocal and bilateral, and to occur early in life. To date, four forms of familial RCC have been described: hereditary nonpapillary RCC, VHL disease, hereditary papillary RCC, and hereditary renal oncocytoma. In 1979, Cohen and coworkers performed the initial studies to demonstrate a gene associated with inherited nonpapillary renal cell carcinoma.[20] In this study, karyotypic analysis of a kindred including 10 members with kidney cancer revealed a constitutional translocation of chromosome 3 to chromosome 8[t(3;8) (p14;q24)]. Ninety percent of family members possessing this constitutional translocation developed kidney cancer by age 60, and no individual without the translocation developed kidney cancer. In 1989, a second kindred with inheritable kidney cancer was reported;[21] this family possessed

another constitutional translocation involving 3p—[t(3;6) (p13;q25.1)]. A third kindred has been described with a translocation of chromosome 3 to chromosome 11 as seen in karyotypic analysis of tumor cells only.[22] In all three kindreds, the breakpoint in 3p was in the same 3p13-p14 region first described by Cohen and associates.[20] The only clinical manifestations in affected members of these kindreds was kidney cancer.

A second type of hereditary kidney cancer is that associated with VHL disease, a familial cancer syndrome with autosomal dominant inheritance and variable penetrance. Investigators have consistently demonstrated loss of DNA sequences on the short arm of chromosome 3 in tumors from patients with sporadic kidney cancer, suggesting the presence of a tumor-suppressor gene at this location associated with the development of kidney cancer.[23] Tumors from patients with VHL disease were evaluated for this loss of DNA from chromosome 3p by analysis of restriction fragment length polymorphisms (RFLPs) using polymorphic probes on chromosome 3p. DNA analysis was performed on 17 tumors, along with normal tissue removed from seven affected patients. Loss of chromosome 3p alleles was detected in 11 of 11 renal tumors from the patients with VHL disease.[24] The genotypes of the parents of the patients with VHL disease were determined to show that in each instance it was the wild-type allele (from the unaffected parent) that was deleted in the tumor, leaving the abnormal copy in the affected patient. These results are consistent with the hypothesis of an inherited disease gene present on chromosome 3 that is involved in the emergence of kidney cancer in patients with VHL disease. Thus far, the VHL gene has been localized to an interval between *raf1*, a proto-oncogene that maps to 3p25, and an anonymous marker, D3S18, located telomeric to c-*raf1* at 3p26.[25]

Another form of inherited kidney cancer has been described. Hereditary papillary renal carcinoma (HPRC) was reported in the early 1990s, which led to the identification of the responsible gene, termed c-*met*. The c-*met* gene is a proto-oncogene that, when mutated or damaged, leads to activation of function and subsequent tumorigenesis.[26]

## SPORADIC KIDNEY CANCER

Cytogenetic studies of nonfamilial-associated RCC have demonstrated consistent chromosome 3p deletions. The most commonly observed changes in sporadic cases are losses that include at least the terminal part of 3p (73.4%).[27] Studies have demonstrated loss of heterozygosity (LOH) on 3p loci in tumors from 51 of 58 evaluable patients (88%).[28] No correlation was seen between LOH and disease stage or histologic type. Analysis of the genotype of these tumors identified boundaries that also contain the VHL gene (the location of which has been more precisely narrowed), suggesting that a tumor-suppressor gene in this region is involved in the initiation of sporadic RCC. Abnormalities at other tumor-suppressor gene loci may also be involved in the generation of RCC. Besides chromosome 3, chromosomes 5, 6, 7, and 14 and the sex chromosomes have demonstrated nonrandom aberrations associated with RCC.[29] These findings have led to the introduction of a molecular genetic classification of kidney cancer.

Specific regions that harbor tumor-suppressor capacity appear to be lost preferentially, likely via the processes of translocation and nondisjunction. Examples of putative tumor-suppressor genes lost in RCC include MSH2 (associated with chromophobe subtype RCC), VHL gene, APC, MCC, BRCA1 and 2, Rb1, TP53, and DCC. Each of these genes and their protein products can lead to malignant tumor growth through multiple complex (and incompletely understood) mechanisms. The protein product of the VHL gene regulates both RNA polymerase II transcription and vascular endothelial growth factor (VEGF) mRNA expression, affecting the key angiogenesis factor in RCC.[29]

Work has been directed at the relationship between tumorigenesis and apoptosis. The *bcl*-2 proto-oncogene that regulates apoptosis was found to be overexpressed in a majority of renal cell cancers examined in a study by Huang and coworkers. *Bcl*-2 is critical for normal kidney development and has been found to be overexpressed in chemotherapy-resistant tissues, which may explain in part the resistance of kidney cancer to conventional cytotoxic therapy.[30]

Histopathologic examination of kidneys obtained from radical nephrectomy has demonstrated a significant percentage of additional satellite lesions not detected by standard radiographic studies. Investigators have demonstrated similar LOH patterns from both primary and satellite tumors, indicating likely intrarenal metastases. LOH was detected at chromosome arms 3p, 6q, 8p, 9p, 9q, and 14q. These results have implications for the risk of recurrence with the use of nephron-sparing surgery.[31]

## CLASSIFICATION

RCCs historically have been classified according to cell type (clear cell, granular, spindle, or oncocytic) and histologic growth pattern (acinar, papillary, or sarcomatoid).

The Mainz classification of renal cell tumors is based on both histopathology and cytogenetics and is becoming widely used. Five types of renal cancer are distinguished in this classification:[32-34] clear cell, chromophilic (papillary), chromophobic, oncocytic, and collecting duct (Bellini's duct) tumors. Clear cell tumors make up the majority (75 to 85%), have their origin in the proximal tubule, and are characterized by a deletion of the short arm of chromosome 3. Chromophilic carcinomas account for less than 15% of kidney cancers, have their origin in the proximal tubule, are frequently multifocal and bilateral, and often present as small (<3 cm) lesions.[35] They are not associated with 3p deletions, but often demonstrate monosomy Y, trisomy 7, and trisomy 17.[36] These tumors present at a lower stage and have a more favorable prognosis. Chromophobic tumors are uncommon (<4% of renal cancers), are of cortical collecting duct origin, and are associated with an excellent prognosis.[37] They are not associated with 3p abnormalities but with a hypodiploid number of chromosomes. Renal oncocytomas are also uncommon and are generally benign. Collecting duct tumors are rare, arise from the medullary collecting duct, and are clinically aggressive. They are not associated with any reproducible chromosomal abnormalities.[38]

## CLINICAL FEATURES

Called "the internist's tumor," renal cancer can present with a multitude of varied signs and symptoms. However, many patients fail to have symptoms, thus delaying diagnosis. The major presenting symptoms of RCC in a review of 2366 cases were hematuria (56%), pain (38%), presence of a palpable flank or abdominal mass (36%), and stigmata of local extension or metastatic disease, including weight loss (27%) and fever (11%).[39] The classic triad of symptoms ascribed to renal carcinoma—hematuria, abdominal mass, and flank pain—is found in about 19% of patients and usually indicates far-advanced disease. Vague constitutional symptoms such as fever, night sweats, malaise, and weight loss are frequent and nonspecific. Sudden onset of a varicocele (often left-sided because of testicular vein obstruction)[39] may be the only presenting complaint. Asymptomatic renal carcinomas may be incidental findings on routine physical examination or abdominal computed tomography (CT) performed for other indications.

One to 3% of kidney tumors are bilateral. Twenty-five to 30 percent of patients have metastatic disease at initial presentation.[40] Most frequent sites of distant spread include lung (50 to 60%), bone (30 to 40%), liver (30 to 40%), and brain (5%).[41] Despite its predilection for these organs, renal cancer is notorious for unusual sites of metastasis that involve virtually any organ, including thyroid, pancreas, striated muscle, orbit, skin and subcutaneous tissue, and reproductive tract.

Paraneoplastic syndromes are sometimes associated with renal carcinoma and may be the predominant finding at disease presentation. The finding of a paraneoplastic syndrome does not imply metastatic disease and is not a contraindication to resection of an otherwise localized tumor. Hypercalcemia is the most common of the paraneoplastic syndromes, affecting approximately 20% of patients with RCC.[42] In the absence of bone metastases, the hypercalcemia is mediated by parathyroid hormone–related peptide and other humoral factors such as osteoclast-activating factor, transforming growth factor-α, and tumor necrosis factor.[42] Hypercalcemia associated with bone metastases is not a true paraneoplastic syndrome because it is a direct result of osteolytic bone disease. In approximately 3% of patients, the primary renal carcinoma produces an erythropoietin-like substance by an unknown mechanism, resulting in erythrocytosis.[43] Tumor production of erythropoietin may identify a subset of individuals with RCC that is responsive to immunotherapy with interleukin-2 and alfa-interferon.[44] In 15 to 40% of patients, hypertension is present, and renin production by the tumor has been documented.[45] Another nonhumoral cause of hypertension in these patients is renal artery compression. Fever and anemia are common in RCC patients and are likely mediated by cytokines secreted by the tumor.[43] Other paraneoplastic syndromes observed in RCC include hyperglycemia[46] and amyloidosis.[47]

A recognized syndrome of hepatic dysfunction in the absence of liver metastases (Stauffer's syndrome)[48] has been reported to occur in up to 20% of patients with renal carcinoma. This idiopathic syndrome is characterized by hepatosplenomegaly, fever, elevated alkaline phosphatase levels, prolonged partial thromboplastin time, and elevated serum haptoglobin levels. The cause of Stauffer's syndrome remains unclear, with hepatic biopsies showing a nonspecific hepatitis in the absence of biliary obstruction. Interleukin-6 production by the primary tumor has been implicated.[49] After nephrectomy, liver function may return to normal and the associated hepatomegaly may disappear, but most patients with this syndrome die within 5 years.

## DIAGNOSIS

There are multiple imaging techniques available to help stage RCC. They include CT, magnetic resonance imaging (MRI), ultrasonography, renal angiography (RA), digital subtraction angiography, inferior venacavography, and positron emission tomography (PET). The choice of which modality to use depends on physician preference, patient risk factors, particular strengths of each technique, and availability of resources. The best overall imaging approach should determine stage and extent of disease with accuracy and identify extension into local structures and areas of distant spread.[50]

CT is currently the most widely used study for the evaluation of renal masses. An intravenous contrast bolus is required, and 5-mm sections through the mass should be obtained. Diagnostic difficulties occur with complex cystic lesions that contain thick walls, thick internal septations, large areas of calcification, soft tissue components, or internal hemorrhage. Bosniak described four categories (I to IV) of such cystic lesions with an intent to convey the possibility of malignancy based on their complexity.[51] Further evaluation with ultrasonography may allow characterization of simple cysts with internal hemorrhage as benign; however, complex cysts can be further evaluated by percutaneous cyst puncture under ultrasonographic or computed tomographic guidance, with assay of the cyst fluid for fat, blood, and cells.

CT can identify with excellent accuracy size and location of RCCs greater than 2 cm in diameter. CT is approximately 78% accurate in the detection of tumor extension into the renal vein and approximately 96% accurate in the inferior vena cava (IVC). In identifying lymphadenopathy in the setting of kidney cancer, CT has a sensitivity of approximately 83% and a specificity of 88%. Adjacent organ invasion is identified with a sensitivity of 60% and a specificity approaching 100%.[52]

CT is not without limitations. It cannot detect microscopic invasion of perinephric fat, cannot distinguish between tumor infiltration and inflammatory changes, and is insensitive relative to MRI in distinguishing small collateral vasculature from lymphangitic spread of tumor.[50] Suboptimal technique, avascular masses, questionable extension into liver, and IVC thrombus all pose problems for CT technology.[53] Patients with renal insufficiency and allergy to intravenous contrast are incompletely evaluated with CT.

The technique currently indicated in the majority of cases requiring additional radiographic evaluation is MRI. Unlike CT, which is limited to transaxial planar images, MRI may be performed in sagittal, coronal, or oblique projections. This ability to produce orthogonal images can be helpful in studying the IVC for tumor thrombus. The intrinsic soft tissue contrast of MRI better distinguishes tissues of similar density and direct extension of tumor to adjacent organs, when compared with CT. Intravascular contrast is not required to evaluate vascular structures, and flowing blood can be distinguished from soft tissue masses. Small (<3 cm) lesions may be better studied by MRI.[54]

Disadvantages of MRI include limited availability, unpredictable image quality, longer imaging time, and more restrictive patient requirements. MRI may be reserved for patients with known contraindications to iodinated contrast or suboptimal computed tomographic scans, or when CT findings are equivocal.[55] Overall MRI accuracy in staging RCC is reported to fall between 82% and 96%.[56, 57] Others have reported overall accuracy rates up to 96%.[56, 57] Because of the availability of resources, its overall staging accuracy, lack of expense, noninvasiveness, low associated morbidity, and proven experience, CT remains the first choice in the initial evaluation of patients with known or suspected RCC.[53]

In the past, angiography was considered a mandatory preoperative test before partial nephrectomy and in patients with bilateral tumors in whom the conservation of functioning renal tissue in one or both kidneys was the therapeutic goal. Today, CT and MRI are excellent techniques for preoperative planning for partial nephrectomy. CT- and MRI-derived angiography can outline the vasculature supply to the tumor and the normal parenchyma. Traditional angiography soon may be replaced by MR angiography for this evaluation.

Percutaneous biopsy of renal masses remains controversial owing to risks of hemorrhage, perforation of adjacent viscera, and seeding of the needle tract with tumor cells. This problem has never been reported in association with the use of the thin-walled 20-gauge needle. Percutaneous needle aspiration should be limited to patients in whom a complex cyst is diagnosed by CT or ultrasonography, or both, and in whom mitigating circumstances make angiography or surgery unduly hazardous.

PET has demonstrated limited evaluation thus far for RCC imaging. This technique has been assessed in a study to detect histologically confirmed RCC, confirming 20 of 26 cases.[58] Because of PET reliance on functional properties of viable tumor, small studies have shown encouraging results for the detection of recurrence or progression of disease,[59] and for assessing response to interleukin-2–based therapy,[60] especially when there is a remaining radiographic abnormality (viable tumor vs. necrotic remnant?). Further study is warranted to establish the role of PET in patients with renal cell carcinoma.

## STAGING

As with any malignancy, staging must be based on factors that influence survival. Renal vein involvement has long been thought to be associated with a poor prognosis, but contemporary studies fail to show such a correlation, perhaps owing to the emphasis in recent years on complete excision of the renal veins and the preoperative identification of renal vein involvement. If properly managed, extension of tumor into the renal veins and IVC alone, excluding nodal or perinephric fat involvement, does not compromise survival significantly.[61, 62] The size of the primary tumor is only loosely correlated with survival and is not a major factor in staging.

The staging factors that have been shown to influence prognosis include invasion through the renal capsule, regional lymph node involvement, and distant dissemination. The presence of tumor in the lymph nodes draining the renal parenchyma is a dire prognostic sign and is associated with a 5-year survival rate of less than 20%.[63] Tumor invasion through the renal capsule into the perinephric fat was a greater detriment to survival before the widespread adoption of radical nephrectomy with excision of Gerota's fascia. Even after radical excision of Gerota's fascia with the kidney, the extension of tumor into the perinephric fat decreases the 5-year survival rate to about 50%.[64] When tumor extends to contiguous organs, a patient rarely survives 5 years, even after surgical excision.

Two systems are used to stage renal cell carcinoma. Historically, physicians used Robson's[65] modification of the system of Flocks and Kadesky, which is summarized in Table 53–1. The shortcomings of the system become obvious when it is noted that the survival rate of patients with stage II (or B) tumor is less than that of patients with stage III (or C) disease, indicating an inappropriate assignment of prognostic factors. The grouping of renal vein, vena cava, and lymph node involvement into stage III causes the survival rate to be higher because simple renal vein extension in the absence of nodal metastases is not as dire a prognostic factor. The TNM system is preferred by most investigators because it separates venous involvement from nodal invasion, and thus more explicitly defines the anatomic extent of disease (Table 53–2).[66] A new cutoff point of 7 cm now separates T1 and T2 tumors. Tumors extending into the renal capsule are grouped with those extending into the vein in the T3 category, but they are separated by subclasses (T3a, T3b, T3c). The best way to combine subgroups into meaningful stage groupings, however, is still a matter of controversy.

## PROGNOSIS

The natural history of RCC is more unpredictable than that of most tumors and has been a subject of interest for many decades. The tumor is the second most common neoplasm to undergo spontaneous regression following resection of the primary lesion. Numerous cases of spontaneous regression of RCC have been reported in the literature, and many more have been anecdotally described.[67, 68] Many patients did not have histologic documentation of the metastatic foci, and regression as reported cannot be equated with long-term cure.

Histopathology has prognostic implications. Sarcomatoid

**Table 53–1. Stage Classification of Renal Cell Carcinoma**

| Tumor Status | Robson[65] |
| --- | --- |
| No primary | — |
| Small primary, minimal distortion | A |
| Large tumor, renal distortion | A |
| Involving perinephric tissues | B |
| Involving renal vein | C |
| Involving renal vein and infradiaphragmatic vena cava | C |
| Invading adjacent structures | D |
| Involving superior vena cava | C |
| No nodes involved | A,B |
| Single, ipsilateral node involved | C |
| Involvement of multiple regional nodes | C |
| Fixed regional nodes | C |
| Involved juxtaregional nodes | C |
| Distant metastases | D |

**Table 53–2. International TNM Classification of Renal/Kidney Carcinomas**

**Definitions**

PRIMARY TUMOR (T)

| | |
| --- | --- |
| TX | Primary tumor cannot be assessed |
| T0 | No evidence of primary tumor |
| T1 | Tumor 7 cm or less in greatest dimension limited to the kidney |
| T2 | Tumor more than 7 cm in greatest dimension limited to the kidney |
| T3 | Tumor extends into major veins or invades adrenal gland or perinephric tissues but not beyond Gerota's fascia |
| T3a | Tumor invades adrenal gland or perinephric tissues but not beyond Gerota's fascia |
| T3b | Tumor grossly extends into renal vein(s) or vena cava below diaphragm |
| T3c | Tumor grossly extends into vena cava above diaphragm |
| T4 | Tumor invades beyond Gerota's fascia |

REGIONAL LYMPH NODES (N)*

| | |
| --- | --- |
| NX | Regional lymph nodes cannot be assessed |
| N0 | No regional lymph node metastasis |
| N1 | Metastasis in a single regional lymph node |
| N2 | Metastasis in more than one regional lymph node |

DISTANT METASTASIS (M)

| | |
| --- | --- |
| MX | Distant metastasis cannot be assessed |
| M0 | No distant metastasis |
| M1 | Distant metastasis |

STAGE GROUPING

| | | | |
| --- | --- | --- | --- |
| I | T1 | N0 | M0 |
| II | T2 | N0 | M0 |
| III | T1 | N1 | M0 |
| | T2 | N1 | M0 |
| | T3a | N0 | M0 |
| | T3a | N1 | M0 |
| | T3b | N0 | M0 |
| | T3b | N1 | M0 |
| | T3c | N0 | M0 |
| | T3c | N1 | M0 |
| IV | T4 | Any N | M0 |
| | Any T | N2 | M0 |
| | Any T | Any N | M1 |

*Laterality does not affect the N classification.

Used with the permission of the American Joint Committee on Cancer (AJCC®), Chicago, Illinois. The original source for this material is the AJCC® Cancer Staging Manual, 5th edition (1998) published by Lippincott-Raven Publishers, Philadelphia, Pennsylvania.

changes (associated with either clear cell or chromophilic variants) have a poor prognosis.[69] There is a suggestion that patients with chromophobe tumors have improved prognosis, but this is mostly related to the high proportion of lower stage presentations.[70] Histologic grading of tumor is an important prognostic factor, but it can be variable and may factor out when considered with tumor stage.[71] Molecular prognostic factors such as proliferation markers, karyometric analysis, oncogene expression, and adhesion molecules are a clear area of interest and research. None of these markers has been validated in large prospective studies, and some have conflicting prognostic value.[72]

Survival appears to be mainly dependent on the extent to which tumor has invaded and spread locally and on the presence or absence of distant metastases. Once metastatic disease develops, prognosis is dismal, with 5-year survival rates of 5 to 10%. Maldazys and deKernion[73] examined prognostic factors in 181 cases of metastatic RCC; good performance status, a disease-free interval between nephrectomy and the discovery of metastatic disease (especially if it was longer than 24 months), and the presence of only lung metastases were associated with improved survival.

The Eastern Cooperative Oncology Group (ECOG) examined 610 patients with recurrent or metastatic RCC looking for prognostic variables of potential importance for stratification in clinical trials.[74] Patients were entered into ECOG phase II protocols for advanced RCC between 1975 and 1984. Multivariate analysis identified performance status, the time from initial diagnosis, the number of metastatic sites, a history of recent weight loss, and prior cytotoxic chemotherapy as important factors for survival. The authors then separated patients into five prognostic subgroups, defined according to ECOG performance status *plus* the number of additional significant risk factors per patient (Table 53–3). The median survival for each of the five risk groups ranged from 12.8 to 2.1 months, respectively (Fig. 53–1). Fossa and colleagues[75] performed a similar analysis on a group of 295 patients with metastatic RCC treated with either chemotherapy or interferon alfa, as did Motzer and associates[76] in a group of 670 patients.

An international consensus workshop considered a wide range of prognostic factors for RCC and divided them into categories 1 through 3. Those factors in category 1 were considered well supported in the literature and were used regularly to manage patients.[69] They mainly included patient-related factors, such as performance status, and tumor-related factors, such as TNM stage, number, and sites of metastases.

## Treatment

### SURGERY

**Primary Renal Carcinoma.** The mainstay of treatment of primary renal carcinoma is surgical excision. Radical nephrectomy has become the standard of care and includes the en bloc excision of Gerota's fascia and its contents,

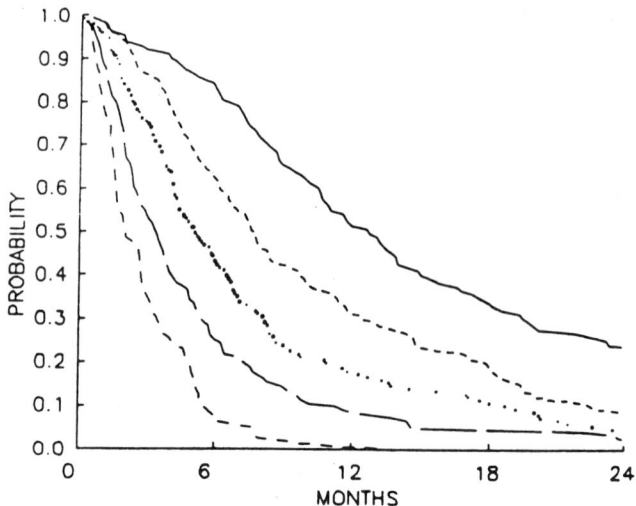

**Figure 53–1.** Survival by risk group. Kaplan-Meier estimates of the survivor function are plotted for each risk group. Risk group 1 (n = 113), —; risk group 2 (n = 141), ---; risk group 3 (n = 151), . . . . .; risk group 4 (n = 123), ---; risk group 5 (n = 82), ----. (From Elson PJ, Witte RS, Trump DL. Prognostic factors for survival in patients with recurrent or metastatic renal cell carcinoma. Cancer Res 1988;48:7310.)

including the kidney, perinephric fat, and adrenal gland.[77] As with many cancer surgeries, the goal is to excise all tumor with wide margins. There has not been a randomized trial proving the merits of radical nephrectomy over simple nephrectomy. Only large, single-institutional case series exist that document patient outcomes outside of studies.[78, 79] Invasion of perinephric fat has been shown to be an important determinant of survival, and this can be expected to be seriously compromised if microscopic or gross tumor is left in Gerota's fascia after a simple nephrectomy. Similarly, although the importance of renal vein invasion has been debated, failure to remove gross tumor from the renal vein results in a poorer prognosis. Therefore, the importance of the radical nephrectomy is obvious for stage T3 and higher stage tumors. Since the early 1990s, however, there has been increasing controversy over the surgical management of the primary tumor. The factors fueling this controversy include the increasing numbers of lower stage, incidentally discovered renal masses; advances in imaging technology that allow improved preoperative staging; improved surgical technique; and advanced options for treating metastatic disease. The surgical questions raised include the role of nephron-sparing surgery, adrenal-sparing radical nephrectomy, and lymph node dissection with radical nephrectomy; the management of tumor extending into the IVC; and the purpose of surgery in the setting of metastatic disease.

The rising incidence of renal cell carcinoma is the result of an increased number of patients with localized tumors, suggesting a migration toward treatment at earlier stages as a result of earlier detection.[4] This is explained in part by the widespread use of noninvasive imaging modalities such as CT and MRI.[80] The literature, for the most part, supports the idea that incidentally discovered tumors are of lower histologic grade and lower pathologic stage and are associated with improved survival.[81] A review of 663 patients with RCC undergoing treatment at UCLA supported a significantly improved survival, lower histologic grade, and earlier

*Table 53–3.* **Risk Groups**

| Effective No. of Risk Factors* | Group | Risk N | Survival Rate (%) 3 MOS | Survival Rate (%) 12 MOS | Median Survival (mo) |
|---|---|---|---|---|---|
| 0,1 | 1 | 113 | 92 | 52 | 12.8 |
| 2 | 2 | 141 | 87 | 31 | 7.7 |
| 3 | 3 | 151 | 76 | 18 | 5.3 |
| 4 | 4 | 123 | 54 | 9 | 3.4 |
| ≥5 | 5 | 82 | 35 | 1 | 2.1 |

*The effective number of risk factors is equal to the sum of the ECOG performance status plus the sum of the values of the four indicator variables included in this model, or this sum minus 1 for those patients scoring 1 on all three of the following: metastatic sites, recent weight loss, and prior chemotherapy. The four indicator variables and score values are as follows: metastatic sites (score of 0 for 0 to 1 sites and score of 1 for 2 or more sites); time from diagnosis (score of 0 for >1 yr, score of 1 for ≤1 yr); prior cytotoxic chemotherapy (score of 0 for no, 1 for yes); and weight loss in prior 6 months (score of 0 for no, 1 for yes).

From Elson PJ, et al. Cancer Res 1988;48:7310.

clinical stage in patients presenting with true incidentally discovered tumor versus a symptomatic presentation.[82] Considering the improvement in preoperative staging, the increasing numbers of incidentally discovered tumors, and the advancements in operative techniques, perhaps radical nephrectomy is not the optimal treatment choice for some patients.

In the past, nephron-sparing surgery was reserved for patients with a functional or anatomic impairment of the contralateral kidney. Currently, appropriately located tumors (inferior or superior pole) of less than 4 cm can be treated with nephron-sparing surgery with excellent long-term survival, even in the face of a normal contralateral kidney.[83] This 4-cm cutoff is based on studies that demonstrate a higher risk of local recurrence for larger tumors.[84] Some authors suggest a cutoff of 2 cm or less for nephron-sparing surgery,[85] again owing to the risk of local recurrence and the multifocal presentation of larger tumors. The incidence of ipsilateral satellite tumors has been reported to be up to 20% in large tumors, decreasing to less than 5% for tumors less than 4 cm.[86] Opponents of nephron-sparing surgery cite the higher risk of bleeding and operative complications associated with this more complex procedure when compared with radical nephrectomy. In addition, the life expectancy of an individual with one kidney is similar to that of an individual with two kidneys, and is associated with a low lifetime risk of developing contralateral RCC. Studies are available in the literature, however, showing no significant difference in survival or local recurrence between selected patients who underwent radical and those who had partial nephrectomy.[87–89]

With the advent of spiral, high-resolution CT, it is possible to assess the status of the primary renal tumor and ipsilateral adrenal gland before surgery. Ipsilateral adrenal involvement has an incidence of about 4% and is associated with a poor prognosis because it usually manifests with lymph node involvement and higher stage primary tumors.[90, 91] It has been estimated that adrenalectomy contributes to cure in less than 0.5% of patients.[92] The incidence of adrenal involvement in the presence of a radiographically normal adrenal gland is less than 5%.[93] Currently, many surgeons advocate ipsilateral adrenalectomy for lesions identified by preoperative staging or during operative exploration and for large upper pole tumors.[91]

Regional node involvement is unquestionably an important prognostic factor because it indicates dissemination, which significantly decreases 5-year survival.[94] Multiple authors have suggested a therapeutic benefit to lymphadenectomy during the radical nephrectomy.[95, 96] Several characteristics of renal carcinoma argue against a therapeutic role for lymphadenectomy. First, the tumor metastasizes through the bloodstream with the same frequency with which it progresses through the lymphatic system, and most patients with positive lymph nodes eventually have bloodborne metastases. Second, the lymphatic drainage of the renal tumor is variable and may occur anywhere in the retroperitoneum. Third, many patients without metastasis to regional lymph nodes develop disseminated disease. The procedure is a valuable method of staging, however, and has become more important as adjuvant clinical treatment trials are instituted.

Extension of RCC into the renal vein and vena cava occurs in about 10% of patients.[97] Many of these patients already have evidence of metastatic disease. However, in the absence of metastases or bulky regional disease, or both, patients should be considered for curative resection. Once venous involvement is associated with local extension of tumor and involvement of regional lymph nodes, the prognosis is poor. The survival of patients with extension into the vena cava alone appears to be dependent on the superior extent of the tumor thrombus, and patients with infradiaphragmatic extension seem to have a prognosis similar to that of patients with low-stage tumors.[98, 99] Extensive surgery for vena cava tumor thrombus, which often involves thoracotomy, cardiopulmonary bypass, and extraction of tumor thrombus from the right atrium, is appropriate only in patients with tumor localized to the kidney without regional or distant, metastases. At experienced centers, this procedure carries a 5 to 10% operative mortality rate, but about 50% of these patients survive 5 years.[100]

**Nephrectomy in Patients with Metastasis.** There are several defensible reasons to excise the primary RCC in the presence of metastatic disease. Palliative nephrectomy for severe symptoms—such as local pain, hemorrhage, and endocrinopathy—appears to be justified in the patient who has a reasonable expectation of living at least 6 months. Nephrectomy in the setting of metastatic disease solely for the purpose of inducing spontaneous remission is never justified. Angioinfarction is another option in patients with intractable pain or hematuria from inoperable local disease.

Patients occasionally present with a limited number of metastases (either synchronously or metachronously) that are treatable by surgery or definitive radiotherapy. The 5-year survival rate after complete excision of solitary metastases is between 25% and 50%, depending on factors such as location and, most important, time from nephrectomy to recurrence.[73, 101]

Another potential indication for palliative nephrectomy is in conjunction with an approved clinical protocol of systemic therapy. Retrospective reviews suggest higher response rates in patients undergoing cytoreductive nephrectomy before cytokine therapy (IL-2 or interferon alfa).[102–104] It has been suggested that resection of residual masses, metastatic or primary, can improve survival after the response to IL-2–based immunotherapy for metastatic RCC.[105] Several patients have had a complete response after resection of residual disease with a favorable response to IL-2–based therapy;[106] ongoing reported survival is 58+ months.[107] Furthermore, the Southwest Oncology Group has completed a randomized trial in 246 patients comparing cytoreduction nephrectomy plus interferon alfa 2b therapy and interferon alfa 2b therapy alone.[107a] The median survival with nephrectomy was 12.5 months compared with 8.1 months without nephrectomy ($p = 0.033$). The results of this study provide strong support for the use of cytoreduction nephrectomy in patients who are eligible for clinical trials of immunotherapy.

Having patients undergo nephrectomy to prepare for adoptive immunotherapy brings forth another controversy in the management of metastatic RCC. Some institutions have reported that up to 40% of patients with metastatic RCC who undergo nephrectomy fail to receive planned systemic immunotherapy because of perioperative morbidity or mortality or because of deterioration of the patient's condition due to progressive disease.[108, 109] In our experience, 89% of 62 patients received planned systemic therapy (tumor-infiltrating lymphocytes (TILs/IL-2) after radical nephrectomy, despite the fact that some of these patients had to undergo complicated operations, including resection of caval thrombus, partial hepatectomy, and splenectomy.[110, 111] Other single-institution experiences support our favorable outcome.[112, 113] It should be noted, however, that in these series, patients are carefully selected for this "aggressive" approach on the basis of parameters such as performance status and lack of brain metastases. Given the results of the randomized study described previously, removing the primary tumor before providing planned systemic immunotherapy can be considered in select patients, especially when they are part of an investigational trial. At UCLA, we consider this "aggressive" approach in select patients with metastatic disease, even when complicated surgeries are involved (vena cava thrombectomy),[114] and histologies (sarcomatoid variants) are unfavorable.[115]

## RADIATION THERAPY

Radiation therapy has been used for RCC in two major areas: (1) as a treatment for metastatic foci, and (2) as an adjuvant to surgical therapy. The role of preoperative radiation therapy can be considered controversial, although it is not a widely used practice. The randomized study conducted by van der Werf-Messing[116] compared results with 30 Gy of preoperative therapy with those when no preoperative radiotherapy was provided. The 5-year survival rate was not improved, although the incidence of recurrence in the renal fossa was significantly diminished. A second randomized trial of preoperative radiation therapy failed to show improvement in overall or disease-free survival.[117] Postoperative radiotherapy similarly has not been shown to affect survival.[118]

An irrefutable role for radiation therapy is in the palliative treatment of metastatic foci. Skeletal metastases usually respond with marked relief of pain and often complete necrosis of the tumor. Complete resolution of abdominal wall and pulmonary metastases after low-dose radiation therapy has been noted. The response rates for use in spinal cord compression have been less successful.[119] Therapy to the renal fossa in patients in whom tumor has been incompletely resected is also ineffective. The radiotherapist should be an important part of the treatment team in patients with metastatic renal cell carcinoma who require palliation.

## HORMONAL THERAPY AND CHEMOTHERAPY

The observation that progestational agents inhibit the growth of diethylstilbestrol (DES)-induced kidney tumors in the golden Syrian hamster model provided the stimulus for clinical trials in humans. Bloom reviewed the literature and reported an objective response rate of approximately 15% in patients with metastatic renal carcinoma.[120] No report has substantiated the role of progestational agents in the treatment of this disease.[121]

Cytotoxic drugs, either alone or in combination, remain the cornerstone of treatment of advanced solid tumors. However, despite the advances made in the treatment of some tumors, RCC remains one of the tumors most refractory to

standard chemotherapy. The search for active cytotoxic drugs for the therapy of advanced RCC continues despite years of discouraging results. A 1993 review by Yagoda[122] of 72 agents evaluated in phase II trials involving more than 3500 patients between 1983 and 1992 demonstrated an objective response rate of only 5.6%, usually of short duration. This review focuses mainly on single-agent therapy but does include results of drug combinations that have been used for RCC. Vinblastine is commonly used as single-agent therapy for RCC, yet weekly intravenous bolus administration yields a response rate of only 7% (complete, plus partial response).[122] Vinblastine used as a continuous infusion showed no improvement in response in the face of increased toxicity. There is interest in the use of floxuridine (FUDR) in the treatment of metastatic RCC. Novel chronobiologic circadian infusion schedules have allowed the administration of higher total FUDR doses with less toxicity than seen with continuous-infusion schedules.[123] A review of many studies using FUDR as a continuous infusion (circadian rhythm and constant rate) shows a response rate of 16% in 284 adequately treated patients.[122] A report from the National Biotherapy Study Group of a phase II trial of continuous-infusion FUDR in combination with alfa interferon found no response among 18 patients despite considerable toxicity.[124] Chemoresistance has been attributed to high levels of expression of the multidrug resistance 1 gene (MDR1) product, P-glycoprotein, which actively effluxes drug from tumor cells.[125] High levels of MDR1 mRNA that are likely to be functioning as a built-in defense mechanism have been described in normal proximal renal tubule cells. Strong MDR1 gene expression in most renal adenocarcinomas has been confirmed and is associated with drug resistance in these tumors.[126] In addition to p-170, the activity of glutathione and associated enzymes has been found to contribute to the MDR of RCC.[127] The possibility of modulating the chemoresistance of RCC is actively being explored in clinical trials, with preliminary disappointing results.[128] In summary, neither hormonal therapy nor chemotherapy has been established for the standard management of patients with metastatic RCC; they should be reserved for clinical trial assessment.

## IMMUNOTHERAPY

**Interferons.** The interferons have diverse immunomodulatory effects and can also inhibit cell proliferation. In 1983, Quesada[129] and deKernion[130] and their associates, in independent studies, reported on the regression of metastatic RCC with a partially purified human α-interferon (α-INF) preparation. In these studies, human leukocyte INF was administered at a dose of 3 million units (MU) by intramuscular injection on either a daily[129, 131] or a Monday-through-Friday[130] schedule, respectively. Responses occurred in 26% and 16.5% of patients treated, respectively.

After these initial reports, numerous phase II trials with the α-interferons (HuINF-αLe, HuINF-αLy, recombinant interferon alfa-2a, recombinant interferon alfa-2b) were conducted to evaluate their efficacy and toxicity profile in this disease.[132, 133] A reproducible objective response rate (complete responses and partial responses) of 15 to 20% was observed. These responses appear independent of the interferon preparation used. An optimal schedule has yet to be determined. Responses have been observed in trials in which the interferon was administered daily, 5 days a week, three times a week, or cyclically. In randomized studies by Kirkwood[132] using HuINF-αLe, and Quesada[131] using interferon alfa-2a, as well as a review of nonrandomized studies, intermediate dosages ($\geq$10 MU/m$^2$) are required to induce objective responses. In general, responses have been correlated with the following patient factors: previous nephrectomy, good performance status, a long disease-free interval, and lung-predominant disease.

The survival rates of 84 evaluable patients with metastatic renal carcinoma treated with interferon alfa in three consecutive trials at UCLA and their relationship to these favorable prognostic variables have been reported.[134] The overall median survival was 49 weeks, similar to the 44-week median survival reported by deKernion[135] a decade earlier. In retrospect, a subset of patients with favorable prognostic variables (disease-free interval > 1 year, excellent performance status, lung metastases only) had a median survival of 155 weeks.

In 1993, the Memorial Sloan-Kettering Cancer Center reported the results of their single-institution experience with interferon alfa-2a for patients with advanced RCC.[102] A total of 159 patients were treated in three consecutive trials, one of which randomized subjects to treatment that included vinblastine. The overall response rate was 10%, with a median survival duration of 11.4 months. Prognostic factors for survival were similar to those reported in previous trials, although patients with metastases confined to the lung had no significant survival benefit. The addition of vinblastine increased hepatotoxicity and myelosuppression without an increase in efficacy.

Median response duration for patients receiving interferon alfa varies from study to study, although 8- to 10-month responses can be expected. The prognostic findings of these studies suggest that many of the interferon-responsive patients with metastatic renal cancer may have prolonged survival because of their inherent natural history, rendering the evaluation of the interferon effect more difficult. Tumor biology may provide additional factors associated with response to interferon alfa. There is evidence suggesting a correlation between clinical response to interferon alfa and expression of a 160-kd kidney-restricted glycoprotein (gp-160) in renal cancer cell lines both in vitro and in animal xenograft models.[136] Renal cell lines expressing gp-160 are resistant, whereas those that are gp-160–negative are sensitive to the antiproliferative effects of interferon alfa.

Another explanation for tumor sensitivity to interferon alfa is the difference in interferon-regulated gene expression. RCC cell lines sensitive to the antiproliferative effects of interferon alfa show downregulation of epidermal growth factor receptors when exposed to the drug. RCC lines resistant to interferon alfa show no such effect on epidermal growth factor receptors.[137] Perhaps in the future, these findings may help differentiate patients whose tumors are likely to respond to treatment. In most patients, a 3-month course of recombinant interferon alfa is sufficient to judge whether they are going to respond. An optimal dosage schedule and preparation have not been determined, although starting at 3 MU three times a week and increasing to 18 MU 3 to 5 times a week, is a commonly used regimen.

Attempts have been made to modify the toxicity profile of interferon alfa. A trial reported by Creagan and colleagues[138] of recombinant interferon alfa-2a with aspirin (acetylsalicylic acid [ASA]), designed to assess the impact of ASA on the constitutional sequelae associated with interferon alfa therapy, demonstrated an objective response rate of 34%, with a median response duration of 10+ months, which are both higher than what one might expect from the literature at large. Constitutional symptoms were no better with ASA than with historical controls. The possible therapeutic potentiation that resulted from ASA added to interferon alfa was assessed in a randomized prospective trial.[139] The results were disappointing, with an overall response rate of 10% in 176 randomized patients. In a randomized trial, indomethacin had little or no effect on the incidence of major constitutional symptoms.[140] Acetaminophen is effective in both the treatment and prophylaxis of interferon alfa–induced constitutional effects and is the general standard of therapy.

Clinical trials of chemotherapy (ie, vinblastine or FUDR) and interferon alfa have yet to demonstrate superior activity when compared with the experience of single-agent interferon alfa.[102, 141–143] Additionally, many of these studies have suggested an increase in the toxicity profile when compared with either drug administered alone. Trials have explored the possibility of synergy between interferon alfa and the retinoid, 13-*cis* retinoic acid (CRA). Preliminary studies suggested synergy[144, 145] with response rates up to 29%. A randomized trial of interferon alfa with or without CRA failed to show a difference in median survival or time to progression.[146]

Investigations have addressed the role of interferon alfa used as an adjuvant for the treatment of high-risk, surgically resected RCC. Most trials have defined high risk as either lymph node positive, or T3 or T4 tumors. Preliminary reports do not suggest any benefit of this approach in terms of disease-free interval or survival.[147, 148]

Clinical trials of interferon beta and interferon gamma have demonstrated limited single-agent activity in renal carcinoma and, based on nonrandomized phase II trials, these agents are not superior to interferon alfa.[149–152] The optimal dose of interferon gamma is yet to be determined. In an attempt to increase the efficacy of interferon gamma, Aulitzky and coworkers[153] designed a phase I–II trial to determine the "biologically active dose" as opposed to the maximally tolerated dose. This dose and schedule, 100 µg subcutaneously administered once a week, resulted in reproducible augmentation in serum $\beta_2$-microglobulins and neopterin serum levels (used as markers for immunomodulation by interferon gamma) with tolerable side effects. The objective response rate in 20 evaluable metastatic renal cell cancer patients treated with this regimen was 30%; a follow-up trial using low-dose gamma-interferon found objective responses in only 1 of 36 subjects.[154] Gleave and associates performed a trial randomizing patients with metastatic renal cell carcinoma to receive either interferon gamma or placebo.[68] No difference in outcome was observed, emphasizing the importance of phase III trials of immunomodulatory agents.

Interferons alfa and gamma demonstrate synergistic antiproliferative effects in vitro;[155] thus there is interest in combining their use in patients. Although these observations provide a rationale for the combined administration of these agents, the schedule, dose, and sequence have not been optimized. Initial reports have demonstrated activity, but it is too soon to determine any superiority over single-agent interferon alfa.[156, 157] There is a suggestion that interferon alfa and interferon gamma administered sequentially can improve both efficacy and side-effect profiles.[156]

**Interleukin-2.** The discovery of the T-cell growth factor interleukin-2 (IL-2) has revolutionized the field of cancer immunotherapy and has opened up new prospects for the treatment of RCC. IL-2 is a cytokine produced and secreted by activated T lymphocytes. This glycoprotein molecule is involved in virtually all immune responses in which T cells play a role, including antitumor immunity. IL-2 has no demonstrable direct antitumor effect but leads to immunologically mediated tumor destruction.[158] The antineoplastic effect of IL-2 has been documented in tumor-bearing animal models, causing regression of established metastases from selected murine tumors.[159]

Early reports from the National Cancer Institute (NCI) demonstrated objective responses in patients with metastatic RCC.[160] An important issue was the durability of these responses and the impact on survival in responding patients. On the basis of data from seven phase II clinical trials involving a total of 255 patients enrolled at 21 institutions, the U.S. Food and Drug Administration (FDA) in 1992 approved the use of IL-2 for the treatment of metastatic RCC (data presented at the FDA Biological Response Modifiers Advisory Committee hearings). The results of this trial were formally published in 1995, and were updated in 1997.[161, 162] The IL-2 doses used and subsequently recommended were either 600,000 IU/kg or 720,000 IU/kg as a 15-minute infusion bolus every 8 hours for a total of 14 doses over 5 days. After a rest period, the same therapy was administered to complete one course. Objective responses were seen in 37 patients (15%), including 7% complete and 8% partial. All responding patients were ECOG 0 or 1. At the time of publication, median duration of response for all responders was 54 months (range, 3–107 +). Median duration of response for complete responders had not been reached, with a median duration for partial responders being 20 months (range, 3–97 +). The conclusion to this study is that high-dose bolus IL-2 is extremely effective for a subset of patients with metastatic RCC. Another large patient series from Rosenberg and associates[163] demonstrated a 19% response rate in 227 patients with metastatic RCC treated with high-dose IL-2. Median duration of response for complete responders had not been reached (range, 39–134 + months), with 80% of complete responders disease free after 3 years. These combined trials attest to the durability and quality of response to high-dose bolus IL-2 in excellent-performance-status patients.

At UCLA, an unpublished series of 124 patients treated with high-dose bolus IL-2 in a non–intensive care unit (ICU) setting for metastatic RCC produced a response rate of 14.5%. Median duration of response for complete responders was 10 + months (range, 4 to 69 months). Median duration of survival for patients with complete response has not been reached (range, 9 + to 85 + months). There were no toxic deaths. Nine (7.3%) patients required transfer to an ICU.

The use of high-dose IL-2 is associated with significant side effects, the most serious of which are hypotension, pulmonary edema, and renal failure. These major toxicities are dose related and appear to result from increased membrane permeability caused by IL-2, leading to fluid and colloid loss into visceral organs and soft tissue spaces. Other common side effects include third spacing of fluid, tachyarrhythmias, mental status changes, fever, chills, diarrhea, nausea, and vomiting. Most side effects are reversible within 72 hours after discontinuation of therapy. However, during therapy, decreased organ perfusion may lead to rare but irreversible events, such as myocardial infarction, gastrointestinal bleeding or perforation, and death. In the FDA's review of 255 patients receiving high-dose IL-2, the drug-related death rate was 4% (11 of 255 patients). In a large review of 1039 courses of high-dose IL-2 administered to 652 cancer patients at the National Cancer Institute, the death rate reported was 1.5%.[164]

Siegel and Puri have published an excellent review of the toxicities of IL-2 and their proposed mechanisms.[165] There is evidence that both tumor necrosis factor-$\alpha$ (TNF-$\alpha$) and nitrous oxide may be mediators of IL-2 toxicity.[166, 167] There are ongoing trials that are evaluating agents to temper the side effects of IL-2 without diminishing response.[168, 169] Therapy with high-dose IL-2 results in severe yet largely reversible toxicities. In anticipation of these toxicities, patients should be carefully evaluated for co-morbid illnesses, which could augment the risk of treatment morbidity or preclude the use of optimal dose intensity.

Alternative infusion schedules have been scrutinized in an attempt to ameliorate the toxicity of high-dose IL-2, yet sustain efficacy. In 1987, West and colleagues[170] treated a group of patients with advanced cancers with escalating doses of IL-2 by continuous intravenous infusion and lymphokine-activated killer (LAK) cells in a conventional oncology unit setting. Objective responses were seen in 15 of 40 patients, all of whom were in the group receiving $18 \times 10^6$ IU/m²/day for 5-day cycles. A European group used a similar schedule of continuous infusion of IL-2 in a phase II study of patients with metastatic RCC.[171] The overall response rate of 20%, with a 7% complete response rate, was similar to that obtained with high-dose bolus injections of IL-2 administered alone or in combination with LAK cell infusion. Although toxicity was similar to that reported from high-dose bolus regimens, no patient was referred to the ICU. Another phase II trial randomizing patients to high-dose bolus IL-2 versus continuous-infusion high-dose IL-2 (with LAK cell infusion in both arms of the trial) produced similar anticancer activity and toxicity in patients with renal cell cancer.[172]

Although response and toxicity were similar between methods of high-dose infusion, these studies suggested that continuous infusion of IL-2 required less total drug administration than did bolus schedules. Other studies have confirmed that IL-2 can be administered safely over a prolonged period with appropriate dose reductions.[173] The possibility that a decrease in the dose intensity of IL-2 may decrease its efficacy is a theoretical concern for patients with RCC. However, many patients are not eligible for high-dose bolus therapy, mainly because of factors such as concomitant disease and advanced age.

Despite the obvious appeal of minimizing the toxicity and rigors of IL-2 administration by lowering the dose, results of treatment with low-dose IL-2 alone are inconsistent. Thompson and colleagues[174] used a combination of intravenous IL-2 and LAK cells to treat 42 patients with metastatic RCC. The first 20 patients were treated with a high-dose regimen, and the last 22 patients with a lower dose for a longer period. The overall response rate was 33%. Despite decreased toxicity in the low-dose group, the response rates did not differ between the groups. Subcutaneously administered low-dose IL-2 has been used in a phase II outpatient regimen with an overall response rate of 20% (two complete responses and seven partial responses) in 46 evaluable patients.[175] As noted by the authors, this regimen shows efficacy and is tolerable even by patients who would be considered ineligible for bolus IL-2 owing to concomitant disease (seen in about 45% of patients in this study). Conversely, Koretz and coworkers[176] did not observe any objective responses in 20 patients treated with either IL-2 alone or IL-2 plus LAK cells using low-dose IL-2 administered by continuous infusion. At present, there is an ongoing phase III trial at the NCI comparing high-dose bolus IL-2 with reduced-dose bolus IL-2 (72,000 IU/kg vs. an outpatient subcutaneous IL-2 regimen).[177]

Table 53–4 summarizes the major clinical investigations of recombinant IL-2 in metastatic RCC.

**Combination Biologic Therapy.** Combination therapy has become a mainstay of therapy for many solid tumors. Because immune surveillance and tumor destruction is a complex, multistep process that involves many aspects of the immune system, the notion of combination therapy with biologic response modifiers seems valid. IL-2 and interferon alfa have differing mechanisms of action: IL-2 acts as an immunomodulator, whereas interferon alfa displays direct antiproliferative effects. Although both recombinant IL-2 and recombinant interferon alfa produce response rates of 15 to 20% as single agents for metastatic RCC, the use of recombinant IL-2 is associated with significant systemic toxicity, thus limiting the number of patients eligible for therapy. There is experimental evidence of additive benefit when interferon alfa and IL-2 are used in combination in the treatment of metastatic RCC. Murine models have suggested that combined administration of interferon alfa and IL-2 may yield synergistic antitumor effects.[185–187] Interferon alfa may augment the immunogenicity of tumors by enhancing expression of major histocompatibility antigens and tumor antigens, making them more susceptible to IL-2–stimulated T lymphocytes.[188, 189]

Initial trials of combination therapy at the NCI demonstrated an overall response rate of 31%; however, the recombinant IL-2 was given in escalating intravenous (IV) bolus

Table 53–4. Representative Clinical Trials of rIL-2 for the Treatment of Metastatic RCC

| Authors | Year | Patients | Response (%) |
|---|---|---|---|
| West et al[170] | 1987 | 40 | 32 |
| Fisher[178] | 1988 | 35 | 16 |
| Rosenberg et al[164] | 1989 | 54 | 22 |
| Bukowski et al[173] | 1990 | 41 | 12 |
| Rosenberg[159] | 1991 | 60 | 18 |
| Geertsen et al[179] | 1992 | 30 | 20 |
| Weiss et al[172] | 1992 | 94 | 18 |
| Atkins et al[180] | 1993 | 71 | 17 |
| Rosenberg et al[181] | 1994 | 143 | 20 |
| **Total** | | 568 | 20 |

Table 53–5. Representative Clinical Trials of Combination of IL-2 and Interferon-α for the Treatment of Metastatic RCC

| Authors | Year | Patients | Response (%) |
|---|---|---|---|
| Rosenberg et al[190] | 1989 | 35 | 31 |
| Budd et al[191] | 1989 | 12 | 8.3 |
| Lee et al[192] | 1989 | 5 | 0 |
| Atzpodien et al[193] | 1990 | 17 | 36 |
| Bergman et al[194] | 1990 | 10 | 20 |
| Kirchner et al[195] | 1990 | 17 | 29 |
| Mittleman et al[196] | 1990 | 18 | 22 |
| Hirsch et al[197] | 1990 | 15 | 40 |
| Bukowski et al[173] | 1990 | 20 | 15 |
| Sznol et al[198] | 1990 | 7 | 43 |
| Figlin et al[207] | 1992 | 52 | 25 |
| Thomas et al[199] | 1992 | 34 | 6 |
| Spencer et al[200] | 1992 | 22 | 5 |
| Budd et al[201] | 1992 | 21 | 10 |
| Ilson et al[202] | 1992 | 34 | 12 |
| Vogelzang et al[106] | 1993 | 42 | 12 |
| Lipton et al[203] | 1993 | 39 | 33 |
| Atkins et al[180] | 1993 | 28 | 11 |
| Atzpodien et al[204] | 1995 | 152 | 25 |
| **Total** | | 580 | 20 |

doses, similar to single-agent recombinant IL-2 bolus therapy.[190] Since then, trials of combination immunotherapy have emphasized low-dose, outpatient-based regimens with more favorable toxicity profiles. Pooled data from major phase I and II trials (Table 53–5) of combined IL-2/interferon alfa therapy for the treatment of RCC demonstrate an objective response rate of 20% and a complete response rate of 5%. Responses have occurred at all sites of disease and have been observed in patients with bulky tumor burdens.

A phase II study by Atkins and associates[205] randomized patients to high-dose IL-2 alone or high-dose IL-2 in combination with interferon alfa in patients with advanced RCC. The combination of cytokines given on an identical schedule with equivalent intensity was not superior to high-dose IL-2 alone; response rates were 17% for the single-drug arm and 11% for the combination arm.

One of the first trials to demonstrate the efficacy of home therapy with IL-2 plus interferon alfa included 35 patients with advanced cancers refractory to standard therapy.[206] Each cycle consisted of a 2-day IL-2 pulse of 9 million IU/m² given subcutaneously every 12 hours, followed by 6 weeks of IL-2 (1.8 million IU/m² daily for 5 days per week) and interferon alfa-2b (5 million IU/m² three times a week). The main adverse effects of fever, chills, nausea, anorexia, and hypotension were limited to World Health Organization severity grades I and II in 29 of 35 patients, with no grade IV toxicities seen in 52 treatment cycles. This home regimen proved less toxic than IL-2 alone, yet the response rates among patients with RCC were similar to those reported for high-dose intravenous regimens of IL-2.

Since 1988, 52 patients at UCLA with measurable metastatic RCC have undergone therapy with the combination of IL-2 and interferon alfa.[207] Patients received low-dose IL-2 by continuous intravenous infusion (38 patients) or by subcutaneous injection (14 patients) on days 1 through 4, and interferon alfa subcutaneously or intramuscularly on days 1 and 4 of each week. In continuous intravenous infusion patients only, the first 4 days' doses were administered on an inpatient basis. The objective response rate was 25% (8% complete responses and 17% partial responses). The duration of response has been 5 to 54+ months, with a median duration of response of 23 months. The overall median duration of survival is 34+ months, with a range of 18 to 58+ months. There were no treatment-related deaths. These results compare favorably with those achieved with high-dose IL-2 alone (4% complete responses and 11% partial responses), and both elderly and severely ill patients (lower Karnofsky performance status) may be safely treated with the low-dose combination regimen on an outpatient basis.

Table 53–5 is a summary of major phase I and II trials of combination interferon alfa and IL-2 in the treatment of metastatic RCC. These studies provided data on 403 patients treated with varying doses, schedules, and routes of administration. The clinical trials, two of which included LAK cell infusions, had a composite response rate of 22% (89 of 403 evaluable patients). Four studies demonstrated that combination IL-2 and interferon alfa therapy could be safely administered on an outpatient basis. The activity of these regimens appears comparable to that of high-dose IL-2–interferon regimens, with considerably less toxicity. These merged data imply that IL-2 dose intensity may be less important in combination regimens. It should be noted that the majority of studies using combined therapy are nonrandomized phase I and II investigations. The largest study, a randomized phase III trial of 425 patients reported by Negrier and colleagues,[208] compared continuous intravenous recombinant IL-2, interferon alfa, and their combination. The investigators found that combination therapy produced responses in 18.6% of patients, with significant prolongation of event-free survival at 1 year. Further phase III studies are needed to define the role of IL-2 in combination with interferon-alfa and to define the dose-response curve of combination therapy.

**Adoptive Immunotherapy.** The demonstration that tumor cells express antigens that can invoke an immune response has formed the basis of attempts to manipulate the immune system to cause improved tumor surveillance and destruction.

*Autolymphocyte Therapy.* The theoretical basis of autolymphocyte therapy (ALT) relies on the activation of memory T lymphocytes in patients with metastatic cancer. These T lymphocytes presumably have been exposed in vivo to tumor antigens and may have the potential for mediating tumor regression after nonspecific activation.[209] In ALT, antibodies to the invariant CD3 component of the T-cell receptor (TCR) are used to activate memory T cells, which results in clonal T-cell proliferation through an IL-2–dependent autocrine pathway.[210]

Enthusiasm for this therapeutic modality began in 1990 when an initial report of a 90-patient randomized trial of ALT versus high-dose cimetidine alone revealed a 2.5-fold survival advantage in the ALT arm with only mild toxicity.[211] However, enthusiasm waned when a phase III randomized trial comparing ALT with single-agent interferon alfa failed to demonstrate a survival advantage. This led to the cessation of commercially produced ALT. There may be a role for ALT in the adjuvant setting[212] or in combination with chemotherapy.[213]

*Lymphokine-Activated Killer Cells.* LAK cells are pe-

ripherally circulating lymphoid cells activated in vitro by the exposure to pharmacologically high concentrations of IL-2.[214] LAK cells cause a nonclassic cytotoxicity distinct from cytotoxic T lymphocytes (CTLs), which are highly specific against a sensitizing antigen and are class I major histocompatibility complex (MHC)-restricted. In contrast, LAK activity is MHC-nonrestricted—tumor target cells derived from syngeneic, allogeneic, or xenogeneic sources are lysed, regardless of target expression of MHC antigens.[215]

The ability to distinguish between tumor cells and normal cells is a hallmark of LAK activity, although the mechanism remains unknown. On target cell adhesion, a number of calcium-dependent phases of LAK cell lytic function occur.[216] A membrane-associated cytotoxin, M-CTX, also aids in target lysis.[217]

After initial preclinical and animal feasibility studies and promising results in humans in early NCI studies, various institutions conducted phase II trials using LAK plus IL-2 for metastatic RCC, with response rates ranging from 9 to 35%. However, three randomized trials[218–220] failed to show an improvement in response rate with the combination of LAK cells and IL-2 as compared with IL-2 alone.

*Tumor-Infiltrating Lymphocytes.* Infiltrating lymphoid cells found in a solid tumor can be isolated and expanded ex vivo with the use of IL-2, and these appear to mediate the destruction of tumor cells 50 to 100 times more potently than do autolymphocytes or LAK cells.[221] TILs were found effective in the elimination of murine pulmonary metastases in the absence of IL-2, although when administered together with low-dose IL-2, TIL effectiveness was enhanced two- to fivefold.[222]

The specificity of TIL antitumor activity is mediated through tumor antigen–TCR interaction and is thus MHC-restricted. TILs secrete cytokines, such as granulocyte-macrophage colony-stimulating factor (GM-CSF)α-INF, and TNF-α in response to autologous tumor stimulation, providing further evidence for immune recognition of tumor antigen.[223]

Several clinical trials have used TILs in the adoptive immunotherapy of advanced human cancers, often in combination with cytotoxic chemotherapy.[224, 225] These studies established the feasibility of using TIL as a treatment for human cancer. To date, there have been comparatively few patients with metastatic RCC treated with TIL. The two largest studies[226–228] report response rates ranging from 12% in 34 patients to 35% in 55 patients. These results compare favorably with the overall response rate seen with high-dose IL-2 alone and have led to a phase III randomized trial of low-dose IL-2 plus CD8+ selected TILs versus low-dose IL-2 alone.[229] However, in the intent-to-treat analysis, the overall response rate was 10.6% and was unaffected by TIL treatment. Technical shortcomings in the study have left open the question of the benefit of TIL therapy.

*Dendritic Cell Therapy.* Dendritic cells are the primary antigen-presenting cells (APCs) responsible for stimulating T-cell–mediated immune response in situ,[230, 231] including antitumor immunity. Dendritic cells are bone marrow–derived leukocytes that lack cell surface markers typical for B-, T-, or NK-cell or monocyte-macrophage lineage. Dendritic cells can be propagated in large numbers from peripheral blood lymphocytes by exposing them to GM-CSF and IL-4 in vitro or in vivo,[232–234] and they exhibit all the important features of APCs crucial for stimulating CD4 and CD8 T-cell subsets.

Dendritic cells offer new directions for the treatment of cancer. The premise behind this interest is that dendritic cells can be isolated from patients, loaded with tumor antigens, and used to induce a specific antitumor response. Dendritic cell–based phase I human trials have already shown promising results in patients with B-cell lymphoma, melanoma, and prostate cancer.[235–237] Work to prepare an autologous tumor lysate–loaded dendritic cell vaccination for the treatment of RCC is under way.[238]

**Future Prospects.** Recent developments in the field of gene therapy have brought forward the concept of vaccine therapy for treating RCC. The UCLA group completed transfection of a renal cancer cell line with plasmid vectors containing the genes for α-INF and IL-2.[216] These cell lines display stable production of high levels of both interferon and IL-2. The cell line failed to grow in T-cell–depleted mice, which prevented the growth of tumors following injection of nontransfected RCC. We hope to develop the ability to stably transfect fresh tumor from patients with cytokine-expressing vectors and prepare tumor vaccines. Animal tumor vaccine models suggest that this therapy holds promise in patients with RCC, especially in the adjuvant setting in patients at high risk for relapse. Another approach to gene therapy is the transfection of TILs with cytokines. The rationale underlying this approach is that TILs traffic directly to tumor deposits, concentrating at those sites to secrete high levels of cytotoxic cytokines. Having received approval from the Recombinant DNA Advisory Committee of the FDA, investigators at UCLA have begun to enroll patients in a trial with genetically altered TILs to study trafficking patterns in patients with RCC.

Both melanoma and renal carcinoma are considered highly immunogenic tumors; however, unlike melanoma, there has been a dearth of RCC-associated antigens to serve as potential targets for RCC-reactive T lymphocytes. The G250 antigen is expressed in 85% of RCCs but not by neighboring normal tissue, and preclinical experiments have demonstrated that cytotoxic T lymphocytes are able to recognize and lyse cells bearing an HLA-A2.1-restricted epitope encoded by G250.*32 This may lead to the use of G250 as a potential target for anti-RCC immunotherapy.

## SUMMARY OF TREATMENT BY STAGE

**T1–T3 N0 M0.** Radical nephrectomy is the treatment of choice, with removal of caval thrombus as needed. Parenchyma-sparing surgery (with perinephric fat and Gerota's fascia) is reserved for bilateral tumors, solitary kidneys, and the rare small (T1) circumscribed polar lesion.

**T4 N0 M0.** Despite the generally dismal results, the absence of alternatives forces us to advise surgical extirpation whenever feasible. The decision about operability cannot be made reliably on clinical or radiologic grounds.

**N+ M0.** Massive lymphadenopathy surrounding the renal pedicle may render the tumor inoperable. In a patient with good performance status, we recommend IL-2–based therapy followed by adjunctive nephrectomy in responding patients. In patients with small-bulk lymphadenopathy, we

proceed with nephrectomy and lymphadenectomy in operable disease. Postoperative adjuvant therapy is not recommended for T1–T4 N0 and N+ completely resected patients.

**M1.** Palliative nephrectomy to relieve severe symptoms of local pain, hemorrhage, or endocrinopathy is a reasonable undertaking in selected patients expected to live 6 months or longer; it is not indicated solely for the purpose of "inducing" a remission. Radiation therapy directed to focal metastases may provide temporary relief, especially in patients with painful bone metastases. IL-2–based therapy (high-dose bolus, lower dose continuous infusion, with or without interferon alfa) should be considered in all patients with adequate performance status and absence of co-morbid disease. Interferon alfa, interferon gamma, and chemotherapy remain alternatives, but the impact of these treatments on survival remains uncertain. Experimental therapy (cell therapy, vaccine therapy, gene therapy) should remain an option for selected patients in well-performed trials in an attempt to improve response rates and survival in this disease.

## SUGGESTIONS FOR ADDITIONAL READING

Motzer RJ, Russo, P, Nanus DM, Berg WJ. Renal cell carcinoma. Curr Probl Cancer 1997;21:185–232. *A comprehensive review of the subject.*
Motzer RJ. Renal cell carcinoma. Semin Oncol 2000;27: April issue. *The issue consists of 13 articles on the natural history and treatment of renal cell carcinoma.*

## REFERENCES

1. Kosary CL, McLaughlin JK. Kidney and renal pelvis. In: Miller BA, Ries LAG, Hankey BF, et al, eds. SEER cancer statistics review, 1973–1990. Bethesda, Md: National Cancer Institute, 1993. (NIH publication no. 93-2789, XI.1–XI.22.)
2. Pisani P, Parkin DM, Ferlay J. Estimates of the worldwide mortality from eighteen major cancers in 1985: implications for prevention and projections of future burden. Int J Cancer 1993;55:891–903.
3. Greenlee RT, Murray T, Bolden S, et al. Cancer statistics 2000. CA Cancer J Clin from ACS 2000;50(1):7–33.
4. Chow WH, Devesa SS, Warren JL, Fraumeni JF. Rising incidence of renal cell cancer in the United States. JAMA 1999;281:1628–31.
5. Miller BA, ed. Racial/ethnic patterns of cancer in the United States, 1988–1992. Bethesda, Md: National Cancer Institute, 1996;56–60. (NIH publication no. 96–4104.)
6. McLaughlin JK, Lindblad P, Mellemgaard A, et al. International renal-cell cancer study. I. tobacco use. Int J Cancer 1995;60:194–8.
7. Yuan JM, Castelao JE, Gago-Dominquez M, et al. Tobacco use in relation to renal cell carcinoma. Cancer Epidemiol Biomarkers Prev 1998;7:429–33.
8. McLaughlin JK, Hrubec Z, Blot WJ, et al. Smoking and cancer mortality among U.S. veterans: a 26-year follow-up. Int J Cancer 1995;60:190–3.
9. Lindblad P, Wolk A, Bergstrom R, et al. The role of obesity and weight fluctuations in the etiology of renal cell cancer: a population-based case-control study. Cancer Epidemiol Biomarkers Prev 1994;3:631–9.
10. Chow WH, McLaughlin JK, Mandel JS, et al. Risk of renal cell carcinoma in relation to diuretics, antihypertensive drugs, and hypertension. Cancer Epidemiol Biomarkers Prev 1995;4:327–31.
11. Matson MA, Cohen EP. Acquired cystic kidney disease: occurrence, prevalence, and renal cancers. Medicine 1990;69:217–26.
12. Latif F, Tory K, Gnarra J, et al. Identification of the von Hippel-Lindau disease tumor suppressor gene. Science 1993;260:1317–20.

13. Rackley RR, Angermeier KW, Levin H, et al. Renal cell carcinoma arising in a regressed multicystic dysplastic kidney. J Urol 1994;152:1543–5.

14. Nishikubo CY, Kunkel LA, Figlin R, et al. An association between renal cell carcinoma and lymphoid malignancies: a case series of eight patients. Cancer 1996;78:2421–6.

15. Fraser GE, Phillips R, Beeson WL. Hypertension, antihypertensive medication and risk of renal carcinoma in California Seventh-Day Adventists. Int J Epidemiol 1990;19:832–8.

16. McLaughlin JK, Blot WJ, Mehl ES. Relation of analgesic use to renal cancer: population-based findings. Natl Cancer Inst Monogr 1985;69:217–22.

17. Goldfarb S, Pugh TD. Morphology and anatomic localization of renal microneoplasms and proximal tubule dysplasias induced by four different estrogens in the hamster. Cancer Res 1990;50:113–9.

18. Selikoff IJ, Hammond EC, Seidman H, et al. Mortality experience of insulation workers in the United States and Canada, 1943–1976. Ann NY Acad Sci 1979;330:91–116.

19. Mandel JS, McLaughlin JK, Schlehofer B, et al. International renal cell cancer study. IV. occupation. Int J Cancer 1995;61:601–5.

20. Cohen AJ, Li FP, Berg S, et al. Hereditary renal-cell carcinoma associated with a chromosomal translocation. N Engl J Med 1979;301:592–5.

21. Kovacs G, Brusa P, de Riese W. Tissue-specific expression of a constitutional 3;6 translocation: development of multiple bilateral renal-cell carcinomas. Int J Cancer 1989;43:422–7.

22. Pathak S, Strong LC, Ferrell RE, et al. Familial renal cell carcinoma with a 3;11 chromosome translocation limited to tumor cells. Science 1982;217:939–41.

23. Zbar B, Brauch H, Talmadge C, et al. Loss of alleles of loci on the short arm of chromosome 3 in renal cell carcinoma. Nature 1987;327:721–4.

24. Tory K, Brauch H, Linehan M, et al. Specific genetic change in tumors associated with von Hippel-Lindau disease. J Natl Cancer Inst 1989;81:1097–1101.

25. Richards FM, Maher ER, Latif F, et al. Detailed genetic mapping of the von Hippel-Lindau disease tumor suppressor gene. J Med Genet 1993;30:104–7.

26. Linehan WM. Kidney cancer: novel model for cancer genetics and therapy. J Urol 1999;162:292.

27. Mitelman F. Catalog of chromosome aberrations in cancer, 5th ed. New York: Whey-Liss, 1995.

28. Anglard P, Trahan E, Liu S, et al. Molecular and cellular characterization of human renal cell carcinoma cell lines. Cancer Res 1992;52:348–56.

29. Erlandsson R. Molecular genetics of renal cell carcinoma. Cancer Genet Cytogenet 1998;104:1–18.

30. Huang A, Fone PD, Gandour-Edwards R, et al. Immunohistochemical analysis of BCL-2 protein expression in renal cell carcinoma. J Urol 1999;162(2):610–3.

31. Miyake H, Nakamura H, Hara I, et al. Multifocal renal cell carcinoma: evidence for a common clonal origin. Clin Cancer Res 1998;4:2491–4.

32. van den Berg E, van der Hout AH, Oosterhuis JW, et al. Cytogenetic analysis of epithelial renal-cell tumors: relationship with a new histopathological classification. Int J Cancer 1993;55:223–7.

33. Weiss LM, Gelb AB, Medeiros LJ. Adult renal epithelial neoplasms. Am J Clin Pathol 1995;103:624–35.

34. Storkel S, van den Berg E. Morphological classification of renal cancer. World J Urol 1995;13:153–8.

35. Mancilla-Jimenez R, Stanley RJ, Blath RA. Papillary renal cell carcinoma: a clinical, radiologic, and pathologic study of 34 cases. Cancer 1976;38:2469–80.

36. Kovacs G, Fuzesi L, Emanual A, et al. Cytogenetics of papillary renal cell tumors. Genes Chromosomes Cancer 1991;3:249–55.

37. Akhtar M, Kardar H, Linjawi T, et al. Chromophobe cell carcinoma of the kidney: a clinicopathologic study of 21 cases. Am J Surg Pathol 1995;19:1245–56.

38. Fuzesi L, Cober M, Mittermayer C: Collecting duct carcinoma: cytogenetic characterization. Histopathology 1992;21:155–60.

39. Ritchie AWS, Chisholm GD. The natural history of renal carcinoma. Semin Oncol 1983;10:390–400.

40. Waters WB, Richie JP. Aggressive surgical approach to renal cell carcinoma: review of 130 cases. J Urol 1979;122:306–9.

41. Ritchie AWS, Chisholm GD. The natural history of renal carcinoma. Semin Oncol 1983;10:390–400.

42. Muggia FM: Overview of cancer-related hypercalcemia: epidemiology and etiology. Semin Oncol 1990;17:3–9.

43. Laski ME, Vugrin D. Paraneoplastic syndrome in hypernephroma. Semin Nephrol 1987;7:123–30.

44. Janik JE, Sznol M, Urba WJ, et al. Erythropoietin productions: a potential marker for interleukin-2/interferon-responsive tumors. Cancer 1995;72(9):2656–9.

45. Lindop GBM, Fleming S. Renin in renal cell carcinoma—an immunocytochemical study using an antibody to pure human renin. J Clin Pathol 1984;37:27–31.

46. Jobe BA, Bierman MH, Mezzacappa FJ. Hyperglycemia as a paraneoplastic endocrinopathy in renal cell carcinoma: a case report and review of the literature. Nebr Med J 1993;78:348–51.

47. Berger L, Sinkoff MWL. Systemic manifestations of hypernephroma. Am J Med 1957;22:791–6.

48. Stauffer MH. Nephrogenic hepatosplenomegaly. Gastroenterology 1961;40:694. abstract.

49. Tsukamoto T, Kumanoto Y, Miyao N, et al. Interleukin-6 in renal cell carcinoma. J Urol 1992;148:1778–82.

50. Bechtold RE, Zagoria RJ. Imaging approach to staging of renal cell carcinoma. Urol Clin North Am 1997;24:507–22.

51. Bosniak MA. The current radiological approach to renal cysts. Radiology 1986;158:110.

52. Johnson CD, Dunnick NR, Cohan RH, et al. Renal adenocarcinoma: CT staging of 100 tumors. AJR Am J Roentgenol 1987;148:59–63.

53. Benson MA, Haaga JR, Resnick MI. Staging renal carcinoma: What is sufficient? Arch Surg 1989;124:71–3.

54. Semelka RC, Shoenut JP, Kroeker MA, et al. Renal lesions: controlled comparison between CT and 1.5T MR imaging with nonenhanced and gadolinium-enhanced fat suppressed spin-echo and breath-hold FLASH techniques. Radiology 1992;182:425–30.

55. Fein AB, Lee JDT, Balfe DM, et al. Diagnosis and staging of renal cell carcinoma: a comparison of MR imaging and CT. AJR Am J Roentgenol 1987;148:749–853.

56. Hricak J, Thoeni RF, Carroll PR, et al. Detection and staging of renal neoplasms: a reassessment of MR imaging. Radiology 1988;166:643–9.

57. Hricak H, Demas B, Williams R, et al. Magnetic resonance imaging in the diagnosis and staging of renal and perirenal neoplasms. Radiology 1985;154:709–15.

58. Bachor R, Kotzerke J, Gottfried HW, et al. Positron emission tomography in diagnosis of renal cell carcinoma. Urologe A 1996;35:146–50.

59. Hoh CK, Seltzer MA, Franklin J, et al. Positron emission tomography in urological oncology. J Urol 1998;159:347–56.

60. Mankoff DA, Thompson JA, Gold P. Identification of interleukin-2–induced complete response in metastatic renal cell carcinoma by FDG PET despite radiographic evidence suggesting persistent tumor. AJR Am J Roentgenol 1997;169:1049–50. abstract.

61. Golimbu M, Al-Askari S, Tessler A, et al. Aggressive treatment of metastatic renal cancer. J Urol 1986;136:805–7.

62. Hatcher PA, Anderson EE, Paulson DF, et al. Surgical management and prognosis of renal cell carcinoma invading the vena cava. J Urol 1991;145:20–3.

63. Golimbu M, Joshi P, Sperber A, et al. Renal cell carcinoma: survival and prognostic factors. Urology 1986;27:291–301.

64. Thrasher JB, Paulson DF. Prognostic factors in renal cancer. Urol Clin North Am 1993;20:247–62.

65. Robson CJ. Results of radical nephrectomy for renal cell carcinoma. J Urol 1969;101:297–301.

66. Sobin LH, Wittekind C, eds. TNM classification of malignant tumours. International Union Against Cancer (UICC). 5th ed. New York: John Wiley 1997:108–12.

67. Oliver RTD, Mehta A, Barnett MJ. A phase 2 study of surveillance in patients with metastatic renal cell carcinoma and assessment of response of such patients to therapy on progression. Mol Biother 1988;1:13–20.

68. Gleave M, Elhilali M, Frodet Y, et al. Interferon gamma-1b compared with placebo in metastatic renal cell carcinoma. N Engl J Med 1998;338:1265.

69. Oda H, Nakatsuru Y, Ishikawa T, et al. Mutations of the p53 gene and p53 protein overexpression are associated with sarcomatoid transformation in renal cell carcinomas. Cancer Res 1995;55:354–9.

70. Crotty TB, Farrow GM, Michael LM. Chromophobe cell renal carcinoma: clinicopathological feature of 50 cases. J Urol 1995;154:964–7.

71. Bostwick DG, Murphy GP. Diagnosis and prognosis of renal cell

carcinoma: highlights from an international consensus workshop. Semin Urol Oncol 1998;16(1):46–52.

72. Franklin JR, deKernion JB. Kidney tumors—What's new? Curr Opin Urol 1995;5:225–30.

73. Maldazys JD, deKernion JB. Prognostic factors in metastatic renal carcinoma. J Urol 1986;136:376.

74. Elson PJ, Robert SW, Trump DL. Prognostic factors for survival in patients with recurrent or metastatic renal cell carcinoma. Cancer Res 1988;48:7310–3.

75. Fossa SD, Kramar A, Droz JP. Prognostic factors and survival in patients with metastatic renal cell carcinoma treated with chemotherapy or interferon-α. Eur J Cancer 1994;30:1310.

76. Motzer RJ, Mazumdar M, Bacik J, et al. Survival and prognostic stratification of 670 patients with advanced renal cell carcinoma. J Clin Oncol 1999;17:2530–40.

77. Novick AC, Strem SB. Surgery of the kidney. In: Walsh PC, Patik AB, Vaughan ED, et al, eds. Campbell's Urology, 7th ed. Philadelphia: WB Saunders, 1998:2973–3061.

78. Skinner DG, Colvin RB, Vermillion CD, et al. Diagnosis and management of renal cell carcinoma: a clinical and pathologic study of 309 patients. Cancer 1971;28:1165–77.

79. Sullivan LD, Westmore DD, McLoughlin MG. Surgical management of renal cell carcinoma at the Vancouver General Hospital: 20-year review. Can J Surg 1979;22:427–31.

80. Jayson M, Sanders H. Increased incidence of serendipitously discovered renal cell carcinoma. Urology 1998;51:203–5.

81. Konnak JW, Grossmann HB. Renal cell carcinoma as an incidental finding. J Urol 1985;134:1094–6.

82. Tsui KH, Shvarts O, Smith R, et al. Renal cell carcinoma: prognostic significance of incidentally detected tumors. J Urol 2000;163:426–30.

83. Butler BP, Novick AC, Miller DP, et al. Management of small unilateral renal cell carcinomas: radical versus nephron-sparing surgery. Urology 1995;45:34–41.

84. Provet J, Tessler A, Brown J, et al. Partial nephrectomy for renal cell carcinoma: indications, results and implications. J Urol 1991;145:472–6.

85. Wunderlich H, Reichelt O, Schumann S, et al. Nephron sparing surgery for renal cell carcinoma 4 cm or less in diameter: indicated or undertreated? J Urol 1998;159:1465–9.

86. Nissenkorn I, Bernheim J. Multicentricity in renal cell carcinoma. J Urol 1995;153:620–2.

87. Belldegrun A, Tsui KH, deKernion JB, et al. Efficacy of nephron sparing surgery for renal cell carcinoma: analysis based on the new 1997 TNM tumor staging. J Clin Oncol 1999;17:2868–6.

88. Morgan WR, Zincke H. Progression and survival after renal-conserving surgery for renal cell carcinoma: experience in 104 patients and extended follow-up. J Urol 1990;144:852–8.

89. D'Armiento M, Damiano R, Feleppa B, et al. Elective conservative surgery for renal carcinoma versus radical nephrectomy: a prospective study. Br J Urol 1997;79:15–9.

90. Shalev M, Cipolla B, Guille F, et al. Is ipsilateral adrenalectomy a necessary component of radical nephrectomy? J Urol 1995;153:1415–7.

91. Sandock DS, Seftel AD, Resnick MI. Adrenal metastases from renal cell carcinoma: role of ipsilateral adrenalectomy and definition of stage. Urology 1997;49:28.

92. Sagalowsky AI, Kadesky KT, Ewalt DM, et al. Factors influencing adrenal metastasis in renal cell carcinoma. J Urol 1994;151:1181–4.

93. Kletscher BA, Qian J, Bostwick DG, et al. Prospective analysis of the incidence of ipsilateral adrenal metastasis in localized renal cell carcinoma. J Urol 1996;155:1844–6.

94. Wood DP Jr. Role of lymphadenectomy in renal cell carcinoma. Urol Clin North Am 1991;18:421–6.

95. Ditonno P, Traficante A, Battaglia M, et al. Role of lymphadenectomy in renal cell carcinoma. Prog Clin Biol Res 1992;378:169–74.

96. Robson CJ. Radical nephrectomy for renal cell carcinoma. J Urol 1963;89:37–42.

97. Hatcher PA, Anderson EE, Paulson DF, et al. Surgical management and prognosis of renal cell carcinoma invading the vena cava. J Urol 1991;145:20.

98. Cherrie RJ, Goldman DG, Lindner A, et al. Prognostic implications of vena caval extension of renal cell carcinoma. J Urol 1982;128:910–2.

99. Sosa RE, Muecke EC, Vaughan ED, et al. Renal cell carcinoma extending into the inferior vena cava: the prognostic significance of the level of vena cava involvement. J Urol 1984;132:1097–1100.

100. Marshall FF, Dietrick DD, Baumgartner WA, et al. Surgical management of renal cell carcinoma with intracaval neoplastic extension above the hepatic veins. J Urol 1988;139:1166–72.

101. Kavolius JP, Mastorakos DP, Pavlovich C, et al. Resection of metastatic renal cell carcinoma. J Clin Oncol 1998;16:2261–6.

102. Minasian LM, Motzer RJ, Gluck L, et al. Interferon alfa-2a in advanced renal cell carcinoma: treatment results and survival in 159 patients with long-term follow-up. J Clin Oncol 1993;11:1368–75.

103. Belldegrun A, Koo AS, Bochner B, et al. Immunotherapy for advanced renal cell cancer: the role of radical nephrectomy. Eur Urol 1990;18:Suppl 2:42–5.

104. Figlin R, Gitlitz B, Franklin J, et al. Interleukin-2 based immunotherapy for the treatment of metastatic renal cell carcinoma: an analysis of 203 consecutively treated patients. Cancer J Sci Am 1997;3:S92.

105. Sherry RM, Pass HI, Rosenberg SA, Yang JC. Surgical resection of metastatic renal cell carcinoma and melanoma after response to interleukin-2–based immunotherapy. Cancer 1992;69:1850–5.

106. Vogelzang NJ, Lipton A, Figlin RA. Subcutaneous interleukin-2 plus interferon alfa-2a in metastatic renal cancer: an outpatient multicenter trial. J Clin Oncol 1993;11:1809–16.

107. Gitlitz BJ, Pierce W, Moldawer N, et al. Long term follow-up and patterns of relapse in metastatic renal cell carcinoma (RCCa) using an outpatient regimen of low dose interleukin-2 (IL-2) and interferon-alpha (IFN): UCLA Kidney Cancer Program. Proc Am Soc Clin Oncol 1994;13:254.

107a. Flanigan RC, Blumenstein BA, Salmon S, Crawford E. Cytoreduction nephrectomy in metastatic renal cancer: the results of Southwest Oncology Group Trial 8949. Proc Am Soc Clin Oncol 2000;19:2a.

108. Walther MM, Alexander RB, Weiss GH, et al. Cytoreductive surgery prior to interleukin-2–based therapy in patients with metastatic renal cell carcinoma. Urology 1993;42:250–8.

109. Flanigan RC. Role of surgery in patients with metastatic renal cell carcinoma. Semin Urol Oncol 1996;14:227–9.

110. Figlin RA, Pierce WC, Kaboo R, et al. Treatment of metastatic renal cell carcinoma with nephrectomy, interleukin-2 and cytokine-primed or CD8(+) selected tumor infiltrating lymphocytes from primary tumor. J Urol 1997;158:740–5.

111. Franklin JR, Figlin RA, Rauch J, et al. Cytoreductive surgery in the management of metastatic renal cell carcinoma: the UCLA experience. Semin Urol Oncol 1996;14(4):230–6.

112. Wolf JS Jr, Aronson FR, Small EJ, Carroll PR. Nephrectomy for metastatic renal cell carcinoma: a component of systemic treatment regimens. J Surg Oncol 1994;55:7–13.

113. Fallick ML, McDermott DF, LaRock D, et al. Nephrectomy before interleukin-2 therapy for patients with metastatic renal cell carcinoma. J Urol 1997;158:1691–5.

114. Naitoh J, Kaplan A, Dorey F, et al. Metastatic renal cell carcinoma with concurrent inferior vena caval invasion: long-term survival after combination therapy with radical nephrectomy, vena caval thrombectomy and postoperative immunotherapy. J Urol 1999;162:46–50.

115. Cangiano T, Liao J, Naitoh J, et al. Sarcomatoid renal cell carcinoma: biologic behavior, prognosis, and response to combined surgical resection and immunotherapy. J Clin Oncol 1999;17:523–8.

116. van der Werf-Messing B. Carcinoma of the kidney. Cancer 1973;32:1056–62.

117. Juusela H, Malmio K, Alfthan D. Preoperative irradiation in the treatment of renal adenocarcinoma. Scand J Urol Nephrol 1977;45:277–83.

118. Finney R. Radiotherapy in the treatment of hypernephroma: a clinical trial. Br J Urol 1973;45:26.

119. Onufrey V, Mohiuddin M. Radiation therapy in the treatment of metastatic renal cell carcinoma. Int J Radiat Oncol Biol Phys 1985;11:2007–9.

120. Bloom HJG. Medroxyprogesterone acetate (Provera) in the treatment of metastatic renal cancer. Br J Cancer 1971;25:250.

121. Kriegmair M, Oberneder R, Hofstetter A. Interferon alfa and vinblastine versus medroxyprogesterone acetate in the treatment of metastatic renal cell carcinoma. Urology 1995;45:758.

122. Yagoda A, Petrylak D, Thompson S. Cytotoxic chemotherapy for advanced renal cell carcinoma. Urol Clin North Am 1993;20:303.

123. Von Roemeling R, Hrushesky WJ. Circadian patterning of continuous floxuridine infusion reduces toxicity and allows higher dose intensity in patients with widespread cancer. J Clin Oncol 1989;7:1710.

124. Soori GS, Schulof RS, Stark JJ, et al. Continuous-infusion floxuridine and alpha interferon in metastatic renal cancer: a national biotherapy study group phase II study. Cancer Invest 1999;17(6):379–84.

125. Nishiyama K, Shirahama T, Yoshimura A. Expression of the multidrug transporter, P-glycoprotein, in renal and transitional cell carcinomas. Cancer 1993;71:3611–9.

126. Naito S, Sakomoto N, Kotoh S, et al. Expression of P-glycoprotein and multidrug resistance in renal cell carcinoma. Eur J Urol 1993;24:156.

127. Mikisch G, Bier H, Bergler W, et al. P-170 glycoprotein, glutathione and associated enzymes in relation to chemoresistance of primary human renal cell carcinomas. Urol Int 1990;45:170–6.

128. Samuels BL, Hollis DR, Rosner GL, et al. Modulation of vinblastine resistance in metastatic renal cell carcinoma with cyclosporin A or tamoxifen: a Cancer and Leukemia Group B study. Clin Cancer Res 1997;3:1977.

129. Quesada JR, Swanson DA, Trindade A, Gutterman JU. Renal cell carcinoma: antitumor effects of leukocyte interferon. Cancer Res 1983;43:940.

130. deKernion B, Sarna G, Figlin R, et al. The treatment of renal cell carcinoma with human leukocyte alpha-interferon. J Urol 1983; 130:1063.

131. Quesada JR, Rios A, Swanson D: Antitumor activity of recombinant derived interferon-alpha in metastatic renal cell carcinoma. J Clin Oncol 1985;3:1522.

132. Kirkwood JM, Ernstoff MS, Davis CA, et al. A randomized study of low and high doses of leukocyte alpha-interferon in metastatic renal cell carcinoma: the American Cancer Society Collaborative Trial. Cancer Res 1985;45:863.

133. Figlin RA, deKernion JB, Mukamel E, et al. Recombinant interferon alfa-2a in metastatic renal cell carcinoma: assessment of antitumor activity and anti-interferon antibody formation. J Clin Oncol 1988;6:1604.

134. Sarna G, Figlin R, deKernion J. Interferon in renal cell carcinoma. The UCLA experience. Cancer 1987;59:Suppl 3:610–2.

135. deKernion JB, Ramming KP, Smith RB. The natural history of metastatic renal cell carcinoma: a computer analysis. J Urol 1978;120:148–52.

136. Nanus DM, Pfeffer LM, Bander NH, et al. Antiproliferative and antitumor effects of alpha-interferon in renal cell carcinomas: correlation with the expression of a kidney-associated differentiation glycoprotein. Cancer Res 1990;50:4190–4.

137. Eisenkraft BL, Nanus DM, Albino AP, Pfeffer LM. Alpha-interferon down-regulates epidermal growth factor receptors on renal carcinoma cells: relation to cellular responsiveness to the antiproliferative action of alpha-interferon. Cancer Res 1991;51:5881–7.

138. Creagan ET, Buckner JC, Hahn RG, et al. An evaluation of recombinant leucocyte A interferon with aspirin in patients with metastatic renal cell cancer. Cancer 1988;61:1787–91.

139. Cregan ET, Twito DI, Johansson SL, et al. A randomized prospective assessment of recombinant leukocyte A human interferon with or without aspirin in advanced renal adenocarcinoma. J Clin Oncol 1991;9:2104.

140. Miller RL, Steis RG, Clark JW, et al. Randomized trial of recombinant alpha 2b-interferon with or without indomethacin in patients with metastatic malignant melanoma. Cancer Res 1989;49:1871.

141. Neidhart JA, Anderson SA, Harris JE, et al. Vinblastine fails to improve response of renal cancer to interferon alfa-n1: high response rate in patients with pulmonary metastases. J Clin Oncol 1991;9:832–6.

142. Fossa SD, Raabe N, Moe B. Recombinant interferon-alpha with or without vinblastine in metastatic renal carcinoma: results of a randomized phase II study. Br J Urol 1989;64:468–71.

143. Soori GS, Schulof RS, Stark JJ, et al. Continuous-infusion floxuridine and alpha interferon in metastatic renal cancer: a national biotherapy study group phase II study. Cancer Invest 1999;17(6):379–84.

144. Motzer RJ, Schwartz L, Murray Law T, et al. Interferon alfa-2a and 13-cisretinoic acid in renal cell carcinoma: antitumor activity in a phase II trial and interactions in vitro. J Clin Oncol 1995;13:1950.

145. Casali A, Sega FM, Casali M, et al. 13-cis retinoic acid and interferon alfa-2a in the treatment of metastatic renal carcinoma. J Exp Clin Cancer Res 1998;17:227.

146. Motzer RJ, Murphy BA, Mazumdar M, et al. Randomized phase III trial of interferon alfa-2a (IFN) versus IFN plus 13-cis-retinoic acid in patients with advanced renal cell carcinoma (RCC). Proc Am Soc Clin Oncol 1999;18:1271.

147. Trump DL, Elson P, Propert K, et al. Randomized, controlled trial of adjuvant therapy with lymphoblastoid interferon in resected, high-risk renal cell carcinoma. Proc Am Soc Clin Oncol 1996;15:648.

148. Pizzocaro G, Piva L, Costa A, et al. Adjuvant interferon to radical nephrectomy in Robson's stage II and III renal cell cancer, a multicenter randomized study with some biological evaluations. Proc Am Soc Clin Oncol 1997;16:1132.

149. Rinehart JJ, Young D, Laforge J, et al. Phase I/II trial of interferon-beta-serine in patients with renal cell carcinoma: immunologic and biological effects. Cancer Res 1987;47:2481–5.

150. Rinehart JJ, Malspeis L, Young D, Neidhart JA. Phase I/II trial of human recombinant interferon gamma in renal cell carcinoma. J Biol Response Mod 1986;5:300.

151. Quesada JR, Kurzrock R, Sherwin SA, Gutterman JU. Phase II studies of recombinant human interferon gamma in metastatic renal cell carcinoma. J Biol Response Mod 1987;6:20.

152. Garnick MB, Reich SD, Maxwell B. Phase I/II study of recombinant interferon gamma in advanced renal cell carcinoma. J Urol 1988;139:251.

153. Aulitzky W, Gastl G, Aulitzky WE, et al. Successful treatment of metastatic renal cell carcinoma with a biologically active dose of recombinant interferon gamma. J Clin Oncol 1989;7:1875–84.

154. Aulitzky WE, Lerche J, Thews A, et al. Low dose gamma-interferon therapy is ineffective in renal cell carcinoma patients with large tumor burdens. Eur J Cancer 1994;30A:940–5.

155. Czarniecki CW, Fennie CW, Powers DB, Estell DA. Synergistic antiviral and antiproliferative activities of E. coli derived human alpha, beta and gamma interferons. J Virol 1984;49:490.

156. Ernstoff MS, Nair S, Bahnson RR, et al. A phase IA trial of sequential administration of recombinant DNA-produced interferons: combination recombinant interferon gamma and recombinant interferon alfa in patients with metastatic renal cell carcinoma. J Clin Oncol 1990;8:1637–49.

157. Bruntsch U, de Mulder PH, ten Bokkel Huinink WW, et al. Phase II study of recombinant human interferon-gamma in metastatic renal cell carcinoma. J Biol Response Mod 1990;9:335.

158. Rosenberg SA. Immunotherapy of cancer using IL-2. Immunol Today 1988;9:58–67.

159. Rosenberg SA. The immunology and gene therapy of cancer. Cancer Res 1991;51(18s):5074.

160. Rosenberg SA, Lotze MT, Muul LM, et al. Observations on the systemic administration of autologous lymphokine-activated killer cells and recombinant interleukin-2 to patients with metastatic cancer. N Engl J Med 1985;313:1485–92.

161. Fyfe G, Fisher RI, Rosenberg SA, et al. Results of treatment of 255 patients with metastatic renal cell carcinoma who received high-dose recombinant interleukin-2 therapy. J Clin Oncol 1995;13:688–96.

162. Fisher RI, Rosenberg SA, Sznol M, et al. High-dose aldesleukin in renal cell carcinoma: long-term survival update. Cancer J Sci Am 1997;3:S70–2.

163. Rosenberg SA, Yang JC, White DE, Steinberg SM. Durability of complete responses in patients with metastatic cancer treated with high-dose interleukin-2. Identification of the antigens mediating response. Ann Surg 1998;228:307–19.

164. Rosenberg SA, Lotze MT, Yang JC, et al. Experience with the use of high-dose interleukin-2 in the treatment of 652 cancer patients. Ann Surg 1989;210:474.

165. Siegel JP, Puri RK. Interleukin-2 toxicity. J Clin Oncol 1991;9:694–704.

166. Mier JW. Pathogenesis of the interleukin-2–induced vascular leak syndrome. In: Atkins MB, ed. Therapeutic applications of interleukin-2. New York: Marcel Dekker, 1993.

167. Hibbs JB Jr, Westenfelder C, Taintor R, et al. Evidence for cytokine-inducible nitric oxide synthesis from L-arginine in patients receiving interleukin-2 therapy. J Clin Invest 1992;89:867–77.

168. DuBois JS, Trehu EG, Mier JW, et al. Randomized placebo-controlled clinical trial of high-dose interleukin-2 in combination with a soluble p75 tumor necrosis factor receptor immunoglobulin G chimera in patients with advanced melanoma and renal cell carcinoma. J Clin Oncol 1997;15:1052–62.

169. Kemeny MM, Botchkina GI, Ochani M, et al. The tetravalent guanyl-hydrazone CNI-1493 blocks the toxic effects of interleukin-2 without diminishing antitumor efficacy. Proc Natl Acad Sci USA 1998;95:4561–6.

170. West WH, Tauer KW, Vannelli JR. Constant infusion recombinant interleukin-2 in adoptive immunotherapy of advanced cancer. N Engl J Med 1987;316:898–905.

171. Geersten PF, Hermann GG, van der Maase H, Steven K. Treatment of

metastatic renal cell carcinoma by continuous infusion of recombinant interleukin-2: a single center phase II study. J Clin Oncol 1992;10:753.

172. Weiss GR, Margolin KA, Aronson FR, et al. A randomized phase II trial of continuous infusion interleukin-2 or bolus injection of interleukin-2 plus lymphokine-activated killer cells for advanced renal cell carcinoma. J Clin Oncol 1992;10:275–81.

173. Bukowski RM, Murthy S, Sergi S. Phase I trial of continuous infusion recombinant interleukin-2 and intermittent recombinant interferon-alpha 2a: clinical effects. J Biol Response Modif 1990;9:538–45.

174. Thompson JA, Shulman KL, Benyunes MC, et al. Prolonged continuous intravenous infusion of interleukin-2 and lymphokine-activated killer-cell therapy for metastatic renal cell carcinoma. J Clin Oncol 1992;10:960–8.

175. Butler J, Sleijfer DT, van der Graaf WTA, et al. A progress report on the outpatient treatment of patients with advanced renal cell carcinoma using subcutaneous recombinant interleukin-2. Semin Oncol 1993;20:16.

176. Koretz MJ, Lawson DH, York RM, et al. Randomized study of interleukin-2 (IL-2) alone vs IL-2 plus lymphokine-activated killer cells for treatment of melanoma and renal cell cancer. Arch Surg 1991;126:898.

177. Yang JC, Rosenberg SA. An ongoing prospective randomized comparison of interleukin-2 regimens for the treatment of metastatic renal cell cancer. Cancer J Sci Am 1997;3:S79–84.

178. Fisher RI. Metastatic renal cell cancer treated with interleukin-2 and lymphokine-activated killer cells. Ann Intern Med 1988;108:518.

179. Geertsen PF, Hermann GG, van der Maase H, et al. Treatment of metastatic renal cell carcinoma by continuous infusion of recombinant interleukin-2: a single center phase II study. J Clin Oncol 1992;10:753.

180. Atkins MB, Sparano J, Fisher RI, et al. Randomized phase II trial of high-dose interleukin-2 either alone or in combination with interferon alpha-2b in advanced renal cell carcinoma. J Clin Oncol 1993;11:661–70.

181. Rosenberg SA, Yang JC, Topalian SL, et al. Treatment of 283 consecutive patients with metastatic melanoma or renal cell cancer using high dose bolus interleukin-2. JAMA 1994;271:907–13.

182. Nanus DM, Pfeffer LN, Bander NH, et al. Antiproliferative and antitumor effects of alpha-interferon in renal cell carcinoma: correlation with the expression of a kidney-associated differentiation glycoprotein. Cancer Res 1990;50:4190–4.

183. Fidler IJ, Heicappell R, Saiki I, et al. Direct antiproliferative effects of recombinant human interferon-alpha:B/D hybrids on human tumor cell lines. Cancer Res 1987;47:2020–7.

184. Mule JJ, Yang JC, Lafreniere R, et al. Identification of cellular mechanisms operational in vivo during the regression of established pulmonary metastases by the systemic administration of high-dose recombinant interleukin-2. J Immunol 1987;139:285–94.

185. Cameron RB, McIntosh JK, Rosenberg SA. Synergistic antitumor effects of combination immunotherapy with recombinant interleukin-2 and recombinant hybrid alpha-interferon in the treatment of established murine hepatic metastases. Cancer Res 1988;48:5810–7.

186. Rosenberg SA, Schwartz S, Speiss PJ. Combination immunotherapy for cancer: synergistic antitumor interactions of interleukin-2, alpha-interferon, and tumor-infiltrating lymphocytes. J Natl Cancer Inst 1988;80:1393–7.

187. Chikkala NF, Lewis I, Ulchaker J, et al. Interactive effects of alpha-interferon A/D and interleukin-2 on murine lymphokine-activated killer activity: analysis at the effector and precursor level. Cancer Res 1990;50:1176–82.

188. Wan YJ, Orrison BM, Lieberman R, et al. Induction of major histocompatibility class I antigens by interferons in undifferentiated F9 cells. J Cell Physiol 1987;130:276–83.

189. Heron I, Hokland M, Berg K. Enhanced expression of B-2-microglobulin and HLA antigens on human lymphoid cells by interferon. Proc Natl Acad Sci USA 1978;75:6215–9.

190. Rosenberg SA, Lotze MT, Yang JC, et al. Combination therapy with interleukin-2 and alpha-interferon for the treatment of patients with advanced cancer. J Clin Oncol 1989;1863–74.

191. Budd GT, Osgood B, Bama B, et al. Phase I clinical trial of interleukin-2 and interferon: toxicity and immunologic effects. Cancer Res 1989;49:6432–6.

192. Lee KH, Talpaz M, Rothenberg JM, et al. Concomitant administration of recombinant human interferon alpha-2A in cancer patients: a phase I study. Cancer Res 1989;49:1726–32.

193. Atzpodien J, Korfer A, Franks RC, et al. Home therapy with recombinant interleukin-2 and interferon alpha-2b in advanced human malignancies. Lancet 1990;35:1509–12.

194. Bergman L, Wiedmann E, Mitrou PS, et al. Interleukin-2 in combination with interferon-alpha in disseminated malignant melanoma and advanced renal cell carcinoma: a phase I/II study. Oncologie 1990;13:137–40.

195. Kirchner H, Korfer A, Palmer PA, et al. Subcutaneous interleukin-2 and interferon alpha-2b in patients with metastatic renal cell cancer. The German outpatient experience. Mol Biother 1990;2:145–54.

196. Mittleman A, Huberman A, Puccio C, et al. A phase I study of recombinant human interleukin-2 and alpha-interferon-2a in patients with renal cell cancer, colorectal cancer, and malignant melanoma. Cancer 1990;66:664–9.

197. Hirsch M, Lipton A, Harvey H, et al. A phase I study of interleukin-2 and interferon alpha 2a as outpatient therapy for patients with advanced malignancy. J Clin Oncol 1990;8:1657–83.

198. Sznol M, Mier JW, Sparano J, et al. A phase I study of high-dose interleukin-2 in combination with interferon-alpha 2b. J Biol Resp Modif 1990;9:529–37.

199. Thomas H, Batron C, Saini A, et al. Sequential interleukin-2 and alpha-interferon for renal cell carcinoma and melanoma. Eur J Cancer 1992;28A:1047–9.

200. Spencer WF, Lineham WM, Walter MM, et al. Immunotherapy with interleukin-2 and alpha-interferon in patients with metastatic renal cell carcinoma with in situ primary cancers: a pilot study. J Urol 1992;147:24–30.

201. Budd GT, Murthy S, Finke J, et al. Phase I trial of high-dose bolus interleukin-2 and interferon alpha-2a in patients with metastatic malignancy. J Clin Oncol 1992;10:804–9.

202. Ilson DH, Motzer RJ, Kradin RL, et al. A phase II trial of interleukin-2 and interferon-alpha-2a in patients with advanced renal cell carcinoma. J Clin Oncol 1992;10:1124–30.

203. Lipton A, Harvey H, Givant E, et al. Interleukin-2 (IL-2) and interferon alpha-2a outpatient therapy for metastatic renal cell carcinoma. J Immunother 1993;13:122–9.

204. Atzpodien J, Hanninen EL, Kirchner H, et al. Multiinstitutional home-therapy trial of recombinant human interleukin-2 and interferon alpha-2 in progressive metastatic renal cell carcinoma. J Clin Oncol 1995;13:497–501.

205. Atkins MB, Sparano J, Fisher RI, et al. Randomized phase II trial of high-dose interleukin-2 either alone or in combination with interferon alpha-2b in advanced renal cell carcinoma. J Clin Oncol 1993;13:497–501.

206. Atzpodian J, Korfer A, Franks RC, et al. Home therapy with recombinant interleukin-2 and interferon alpha-2b in advanced human malignancies. Lancet 1990;35:1509–12.

207. Figlin RA, Belldegrun A, Moldawer N, et al. Concomitant administration of recombinant human interleukin-2 and recombinant interferon alpha-2a: an active outpatient regimen in metastatic renal cell carcinoma. J Clin Oncol 1992;10:414–21.

208. Negrier S, Escudier B, Lasset C, et al. Recombinant human interleukin-2, recombinant interferon alfa-2a, or both in metastatic renal cell carcinoma. N Engl J Med 1996;338:1272.

209. Gray D, Sprent J. Immunological memory. Curr Top Microbiol Immunol 1990;159:1.

210. Herzberg VL, Smith KA. T cell growth without serum. J Immunol 1987;139:998.

211. Osband ME, Lavin PT, Babayan RK, et al. Effect of autolymphocyte therapy on survival and quality of life in patients with metastatic renal cell carcinoma. Lancet 1990;335:994.

212. Sawczuk IS, Graham SD Jr, Miesowicz F, and the ALT Adjuvant Study Group. Randomized, controlled trial of adjuvant therapy with ex vivo activated T cells (ALT) in T1-3a,b,c or T4N+M0 renal cell carcinoma. Proc Am Soc Clin Oncol 1997;16:326a.

213. Gold JE, Masters TR, Babbit B, et al. Ex vivo activated memory T-lymphocytes as adoptive cellular therapy of human renal cell tumour targets with potentiation by cis-diamminedichloroplatinum (II). Br J Urol 1995;76:115.

214. Grimm EA, Robb J, Roth JA, et al. Lymphokine-activated killer cell phenomenon. III. evidence that IL-2 is sufficient for direct activation of peripheral blood lymphocytes into lymphokine-activated killer cells. J Exp Med 1983;158:1356.

215. Rosenberg SA, Lotze MT. Cancer immunotherapy using interleukin-2–activated lymphocytes. Annu Rev Immunol 1986;4:681.

216. Ortaldo JR, Hiserodt JC. Mechanisms of cytotoxicity by natural killer cells. Curr Opin Immunol 1989;2:39.

217. Hiserodt JC. Some thoughts on the cytolytic activity of natural killer lymphocytes. Cancer Cells 1991;3:530.
218. McCabe M, Stablein D, Hawkins MJ. The Modified Group C experience—phase III randomized trials of IL-2 versus IL-2/LAK in advanced renal cell cancer and advanced melanoma. Proc Am Soc Oncol 1991;10:213. abstract 714.
219. Rosenberg SA, Lotze MT, Yang JC, et al. Prospective randomized trial of high dose interleukin 2 alone or in conjunction with lymphokine-activated killer cells for the treatment of patients with advanced cancers. J Natl Cancer Inst 1993;85:622.
220. Law TM, Motzer RJ, Mazumdar M, et al. Phase III randomized trial of interleukin-2 with or without lymphokine-activated killer cells in the treatment of patients with advanced renal cell carcinoma. Cancer 1995;76:824–32.
221. Rosenberg SA, Speiss PJ, Lafreniere R. A new approach to the adoptive immunotherapy of cancer with tumor-infiltrating lymphocytes. Science 1986;233:1318.
222. Speiss PJ, Yang JC, Rosenberg SA. In vivo antitumor activity of tumor infiltrating lymphocytes expanded in recombinant interleukin 2. J Natl Cancer Inst 1987;79:1067.
223. Schwartzentruber DJ, Topalian SL, Mancini MJ, et al. Specific release of granulocyte-macrophage colony-stimulating factor, tumor necrosis factor-alpha, and interferon gamma by tumor-infiltrating lymphocytes after autologous tumor stimulation. J Immunol 1991;146:3674.
224. Topalian SL, Solomon D, Frederick P, et al. Immunotherapy of patients with advanced cancer using tumor-infiltrating lymphocytes and recombinant interleukin-2: a pilot study. J Clin Oncol 1988;6:839.
225. Kradin RL, Lazarus DS, Dubinett SM, et al. Tumour-infiltrating lymphocytes and interleukin 2 in treatment of advanced cancer. Lancet 1989;1:577.
226. Bukowski RM, Sharfman W, Murthy S, et al. Clinical results and characterization of tumor-infiltrating lymphocytes with or without recombinant interleukin 2 in human metastatic renal cell carcinoma. Cancer Res 1991;51:4199.
227. Bukowski RM, Rayman P, Uzzo R, et al. Signal transduction abnormalities in T lymphocytes from patients with advanced renal cell carcinoma: clinical relevance and effects of cytokine therapy. Clin Cancer Res 1998;4:2337–47.
228. Figlin RA, Pierce WC, Kaboo R, et al. Treatment of metastatic renal cell carcinoma with nephrectomy, interleukin-2 and cytokine-primed or CD8(+) selected tumor infiltrating lymphocytes from primary tumor. J Urol 1997;158:740.
229. Figlin RA, Thompson JA, Bukowski RM, et al. Multicenter, randomized, phase III trial of CD8 + tumor-infiltrating lymphocytes in combination with recombinant interleukin-2 in metastatic renal cell carcinoma. J Clin Oncol 1999;17:2521–9.
230. Kiertcher S, Roth M. Human CD14 + leukocytes acquire the phenotype and function of antigen-presenting dendritic cells when cultured in GM-CSF and IL-4. J Leukoc Biol 1996;59:208.
231. Inaba K, Metlay JP, Crowley MT, et al. Dendritic cells as antigen presenting cells in vivo. Intern Rev Immunol 1990;6:197.
232. Sallusto F, Cella M, Danieli C, et al. Efficient presentation of soluble antigen by cultured human dendritic cells is maintained by GM-CSF plus IL-4 and down regulated by tumor necrosis factor-alpha. J Exp Med 1994;179:1109.
233. Romani N, Gruner S, Brang D. Proliferating dendritic cell progenitors in human blood. J Exp Med 1994;180:83.
234. Gitlitz B, Roth M, Kiertscher S, et al. In-vivo generation of dendritic cells by the combination of interleukin-4 and granulocyte macrophage colony stimulating factor in patients with metastatic cancer—a phase I trial. Proc Am Soc Clin Oncol 1998;17:429A.
235. Hsu FJ, Benike C, Fagnoni F, et al. Vaccination of patients with B-cell lymphoma using autologous antigen-pulsed dendritic cells. Nature Med 1996;2:52.
236. Nestle FO, Alijagic S, Gilliet M, et al. Vaccination of melanoma patients with peptide or tumor lysate-pulsed dendritic cells. Nature Med 1998;4:328.
237. Tjoa BA, Simmons SJ, Bowes VA, et al. Evaluation of phase I/II clinical trials in prostate cancer with dendritic cells and PSMA peptides. Prostate 1998;36:39.
238. Hinkle A, Gitlitz B, Mulders P, et al. Dendritic cell therapy for metastatic renal cell carcinoma—a translation phase I clinical trial. Proc Am Soc Clin Oncol 1998;17:432a.

# CHAPTER 54

# TESTIS

• JOHN D. HAINSWORTH • F. ANTHONY GRECO

Testicular cancer is an uncommon neoplasm, representing approximately 1% of all cancers that afflict males.[1] It is, however, the most common malignancy in men age 15 to 35 years and is now curable in most patients. The development of curative therapy for testicular cancer represents one of the major successes in cancer therapy and provides a model for the successful use of multimodal treatment for solid tumors. At present, more than 80% of patients with testicular cancer can be cured with optimal treatment, and the cure rate approaches 100% for patients with low-stage disease. Major advances in the management of testicular cancer have included the development of sensitive and specific serum tumor markers, highly active combination chemotherapy regimens, and modifications in the approach to surgical treatment.

## Natural History

### EPIDEMIOLOGY AND ETIOLOGY

Approximately 7000 men in the United States developed testicular cancer during 1997,[2] and the incidence appears to be increasing worldwide. Testicular cancer occurs four to five times more frequently in white men versus black men and is less common in Asian men.

Most testicular cancers occur in men between the ages of 20 and 35 years, with a second, smaller incidence peak in men older than 50. In infants and young children, embryonal carcinoma and yolk sac tumors predominate, and seminoma is rarely seen on histologic examination. Pure seminoma is the most common testicular neoplasm in men older than 50 years. Approximately 2 to 3% of testicular cancers are bilateral, occurring either simultaneously or sequentially. Nearly half of the men with bilateral testicular tumors also have a history of cryptorchidism.

The cause of testicular cancer remains unknown, although a strong association between cryptorchidism and testicular cancer has been recognized for more than 100 years. Approximately 10% of patients with testicular tumors have a history of cryptorchidism. Estimates of the relative risk of development of testicular cancer in patients with cryptorchidism have varied, but statistics have indicated that the risk is increased by 10 to 15 times.[3] Early orchiopexy reduces the risk, and only a few cases of testicular cancer have been reported in children who have undergone this procedure before the age of 10 years. The development of testicular cancer after early orchiopexy has been reported, however, and the incidence of testicular cancer in the contralateral, normally descended testis is also increased.[4] It is likely that some patients with cryptorchidism have bilateral dysgenesis and remain at risk for the development of testicular cancer even after orchiopexy.

The association of testicular cancer with other factors such as trauma, torsion of the testis, testicular atrophy, and exposure to various toxins has not been well documented.

## PATHOLOGY AND CLASSIFICATION

Ninety-five percent of all primary testicular tumors arise from germinal elements. Various other rare tumors make up the remaining 5%, including tumors arising from Leydig's and Sertoli's stromal elements. Non-Hodgkin's lymphoma occasionally involves the testis as a primary site, but testicular involvement is much more commonly associated with disseminated disease. Testicular metastases from other solid tumors are rare. The remainder of this chapter focuses on tumors arising from germinal elements.

For the purposes of clinical decision-making, germ cell tumors of the testes can be divided into two groups: pure seminoma and a variety of other germ cell neoplasms referred to collectively as *nonseminomatous germ cell tumors.* Several classification systems for germ cell tumors have been proposed, but the revised international classification[5] (Table 54–1) is used almost exclusively in the United States. The other system used widely is the British, in which the various nonseminomatous tumors are referred to as *malignant teratomas* of various types.

Estimates of the relative incidence of the various histologic subtypes differ somewhat, probably because of differences in the way pathologists identify tumors with mixed histologic aspects. Pure seminoma is the most common: 30 to 40% of all testicular tumors. Various nonseminomatous histologies account for the remainder, including embryonal carcinoma (20 to 25%), teratocarcinoma (25%), benign teratoma (5%), choriocarcinoma (1%), and mixed histologies (10 to 15%).[6] Although detailed review of the histopathologic features of germ cell tumors is beyond the scope of this chapter, several important features are reviewed briefly.

*Table 54–1.* **Classification of Germ Cell Tumors**

Seminoma
  Classic (typical)
  Anaplastic
  Spermatocytic
Teratoma
  Mature
  Immature
  Mature or immature with malignant transformation
Embryonal carcinoma
Choriocarcinoma
Yolk sac tumor (endodermal sinus tumor)
Mixed histologic features
  Mixed nonseminoma elements
  Mixed seminoma/nonseminoma

### Seminoma

*Classic Seminoma.* Classic seminoma accounts for 85% of all seminomas and occurs most frequently in the fourth decade of life. Histologically, classic seminoma is composed of sheets of relatively large cells with clear cytoplasm. Syncytiotrophoblastic elements are seen in 10 to 15%, and their presence is correlated with a higher incidence of serum human chorionic gonadotropin (hCG) elevation.

*Anaplastic Seminoma.* Approximately 10% of seminomas are characterized histologically by a higher mitotic rate and the absence of trophoblastic elements. Survival with these so-called anaplastic seminomas is lower than with classic seminoma (70% vs. 90%).[7] However, survival differences are probably related to the tumor stage at diagnosis, which is higher in patients with anaplastic seminoma. When treatment of similar stages is compared, survival rates with classic seminoma and anaplastic seminoma are identical.[8] Therefore, recommendations for treatment are identical to those for classic seminoma.

*Spermatocytic Seminoma.* This neoplasm accounts for 5 to 10% of all seminomas and has a distinct histologic appearance and biologic features. Histologically, the cells resemble those of different phases of the maturing spermatogonia, and it has been postulated that a spermatocytic seminoma originates from relatively mature spermatogonia compared with classic seminoma.[9] Clinically, this tumor occurs predominantly in men older than 50 years, grows slowly, and rarely metastasizes. Prognosis after radical orchiectomy alone is excellent, and prophylactic radiation therapy is not necessary.

**Nonseminomatous Germ Cell Tumors.** The major subtypes of nonseminomas are discussed separately, with the corresponding British subclassification indicated in parentheses.

*Embryonal Carcinoma (Malignant Teratoma, Undifferentiated).* Embryonal carcinoma has a histologic appearance of malignant epithelioid cells arranged in glands or tubules. The mitotic rate is high, with frequent multinucleated cells, vacuolated cytoplasm, and trophoblastic elements. These tumors can secrete hCG, alpha-fetoprotein (AFP), or both.

*Teratocarcinoma (Malignant Teratoma, Intermediate).* This tumor contains a mixture of histologically mature teratoma elements and frankly malignant-appearing tissue. These components are present in various proportions, and in some cases the malignant areas are difficult to locate. When benign teratoma elements predominate, mature teratoma is more likely to remain after completion of chemotherapy. Teratocarcinomas can secrete either β-hCG or AFP.

*Choriocarcinoma (Malignant Teratoma, Trophoblastic).* Pure choriocarcinomas are rare, and the diagnosis requires the presence of two distinct cell types, syncytiotrophoblasts and cytotrophoblasts. Syncytiotrophoblasts are large, multinucleated cells with large, hyperchromatic nuclei. Cytotrophoblasts are closely packed, intermediate-size uniform cells with a distinct border and a single nucleus. Although pure choriocarcinoma is rare, choriocarcinoma components can be seen in 10 to 15% of nonseminomatous tumors. Pure choriocarcinoma produces only β-hCG.

*Yolk Sac Tumor.* This is a rare form derived from the primitive yolk sac or endodermal sinus elements. Pure yolk sac tumors occur in children, usually in extragonadal areas; in adults, pure yolk sac tumors almost always arise in the mediastinum. As with choriocarcinoma, yolk sac elements are a relatively frequent component in mixed tumors. Pure yolk sac tumors produce only AFP.

## CLINICAL COURSE

Germ cell tumors are rapidly growing neoplasms. Nonseminomatous tumors are more aggressive than pure seminomas; at the time of diagnosis, 60 to 70% have metastasized, compared with approximately 25% of seminomas. The metastatic spread of testicular cancer, unlike many other types of cancer, is predictable, and this has greatly aided in the surgical and radiotherapeutic treatment of these patients. The retroperitoneal lymph nodes are almost always the first sites of metastasis; spread to these nodes occurs via the lymphatics. More specifically, tumors of the right testis spread to the retroperitoneal nodes located medial to the insertion of the spermatic vein into the inferior vena cava, and left-sided testicular tumors spread to the nodes immediately caudal and medial to the insertion of the spermatic vein into the renal vein.[10, 11] Metastatic spread to contralateral retroperitoneal nodes is rare and virtually never occurs in the absence of extensive ipsilateral involvement.[10] Likewise, involvement of the suprahilar lymph nodes is rare unless significant retroperitoneal nodal disease is also present at other sites.

Within the testes, tumors usually remain limited within the tunica albuginea, although spread to the epididymis or along the spermatic cord can occur in 10 to 15% of patients. In these patients, lymph node metastases to the external iliac or obturator nodes are sometimes seen. Metastases to the inguinal lymph nodes are rare and are seen only in the rare tumor that extends to involve the scrotum directly or when a transscrotal incision is made in a patient with an unsuspected testicular cancer.

Hematogenous metastasis is common in nonseminomatous tumors but generally occurs after involvement of the retroperitoneal lymph nodes. The lungs are almost always the first site of hematogenous metastasis. Other metastatic sites, such as liver, bone, and brain, are uncommon in nonseminomatous neoplasms and generally occur only in far-advanced cases. In contrast, seminoma rarely spreads through hematogenous channels, and a predilection for bone involvement has been reported.[12]

## CLINICAL FEATURES

Testicular cancer usually presents as a painless swelling or nodule in one testis, noted incidentally by the patient. A heaviness or dull, aching sensation in the scrotum or lower abdomen is often associated. In approximately 10% of patients, acute testicular pain is the presenting symptom. Unfortunately, the diagnosis is sometimes overlooked for intervals of up to 6 months; these delays can be either patient or physician related and can adversely affect prognosis.[13, 14] Improved patient education and the widespread use of public health techniques such as testicular self-examination may result in earlier diagnosis and improved treatment results.

In 10 to 15% of patients, initial symptoms are related to metastatic disease. Most patients presenting in this way have nonseminomatous tumors. Back pain due to retroperitoneal adenopathy is the most common of these symptoms, but occasional patients present with a neck mass, respiratory symptoms, or gastrointestinal complaints. Approximately 5% of patients develop gynecomastia due to high serum levels of hCG.

## DIAGNOSIS

Most testicular cancers are strongly suspected after routine physical examination. Testicular examination should begin with the normal contralateral testis to provide a baseline for the size, contour, and consistency of the normal testis. Careful palpation of the testis is performed between the thumb and first two fingers of the examining hand. Most tumors are felt as firm areas within the body of the testis. The location and consistency of the mass should enable the differential diagnosis of testicular tumors from other benign scrotal lesions (Fig. 54–1).

High-resolution ultrasonography can aid in the clinical evaluation of scrotal masses. With this technique, intrates-

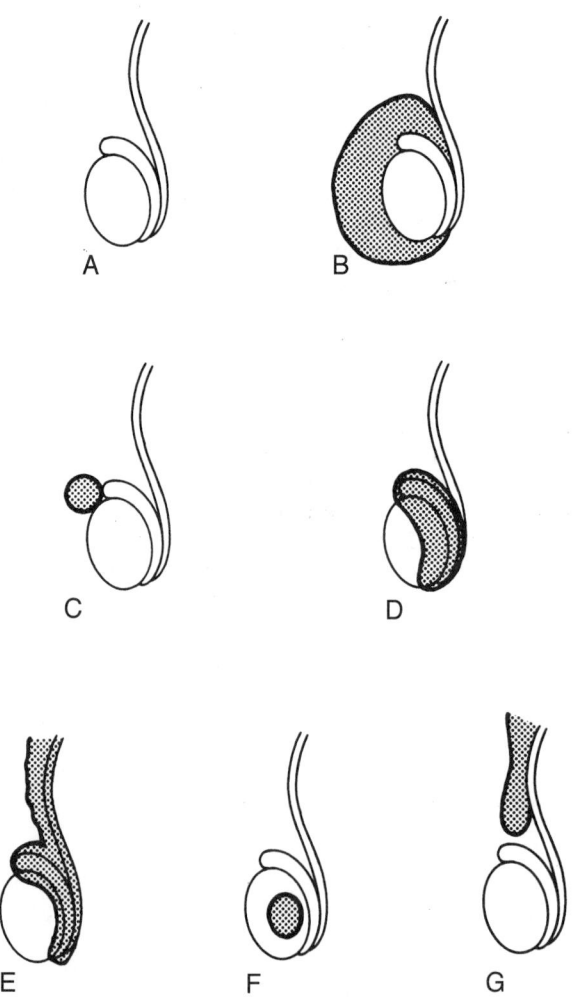

**Figure 54–1.** Differential diagnosis of scrotal lesions. *A,* Normal. *B,* Hydrocele. *C,* Spermatocele. *D,* Epididymitis. *E,* Epididymovasitis (tuberculosis). *F,* Testicular tumor. *G,* Hernia. (From Frank IN, Schwartz SI, eds. Urology. In: Principles of Surgery. 5th ed. New York: McGraw-Hill, 1985:1735.)

ticular and extratesticular masses can be differentiated, as can solid and cystic masses. Ultrasonography can occasionally detect unsuspected small testicular lesions in patients with suspected metastatic germ cell tumors.

In patients with intratesticular masses, testicular cancer must be the provisional diagnosis until proved otherwise. All such masses should initially be explored through an inguinal incision. The blood supply of the spermatic cord at the internal ring should be controlled before the testis is inspected or sampled. If a malignancy is confirmed, the spermatic cord and its tunica should be dissected into the retroperitoneum proximal to the internal ring, ligated, and removed. Transscrotal testicular orchiectomy or biopsy is contraindicated in a patient with suspected testicular cancer because it leaves the inguinal portion of the spermatic cord intact and predisposes the patient to metastases in the scrotal skin, inguinal nodes, and pelvic nodes.

## STAGING

After the diagnosis of testicular cancer, accurate clinical staging is critical to appropriate subsequent management. The predictable patterns of spread, coupled with accurate imaging techniques and sensitive and specific tumor markers, enable accurate clinical staging to be made in most patients.

**Staging Systems.** Several staging systems for germ cell tumors have been proposed, but the revised American Joint Commission on Cancer stage groupings have now been generally accepted (Table 54–2). The three stages defined in this classification are dependent on the size and sites of primary tumor and metastatic disease, as well as levels of serum tumor markers. In general, stage I tumors are confined to the testis, stage II disease is restricted to the retroperitoneal lymph nodes, and stage III disease involves metastases to other nodal sites or visceral locations. The stage at the time of diagnosis differs widely between seminoma and nonseminomatous tumors. Seventy-five percent of patients with pure seminoma have clinical stage I disease at diagnosis, whereas 19% have stage II and only 6% have stage III disease. In contrast, only 20% of patients with nonseminomatous tumors have clinical stage I, whereas 50 to 60% have stage II and 20 to 30% have stage III disease at presentation.

In patients with clinical stage I nonseminoma, several features of the primary tumor are prognostically important. The presence of either lymphatic or vascular invasion or both is associated with a higher incidence of retroperitoneal metastases (about 50%).[15, 16] Invasion through the tunica albuginea into the tunica vaginalis (T2), spermatic cord (T3), or scrotum (T4) is also an adverse prognostic feature.[17] The presence of embryonal carcinoma has also been correlated with a higher incidence of retroperitoneal metastases; however, this feature coexists with vascular invasion and is therefore not independently prognostic. Likewise, the size of the primary tumor within the testis is not an important prognostic factor.[18] These features have not been found to be prognostically important in patients with pure seminoma.

The definition of stage II disease can be based on either clinical or pathologic staging. When clinical staging is used, the transverse diameter of the largest lymph node seen on computerized tomographic scanning has been used to subcategorize the stage II disease (see Table 54–2). The dimensions of retroperitoneal disease dictate treatment in patients with pure seminoma. Pathologic staging in stage II disease is accomplished with retroperitoneal lymph node dissection. The number and size of retroperitoneal lymph nodes are of prognostic importance.[19, 20] When fewer than six nodes are involved with tumor and the largest is less than 2 cm, the recurrence rate is less than 35%. In contrast, more extensive nodal involvement is generally associated with a recurrence rate of 50% or higher.

Within the category of stage III disease, a number of clinical features have been identified as influencing prognosis and are used to determine systemic treatment. Table 54–3 outlines features that separate seminomas and nonseminomatous tumors into good risk, intermediate risk, and poor risk categories.[21] In pure seminoma, pulmonary location of metastases (good risk) versus any other visceral site (intermediate risk) has been the only prognostically important distinction identified. For nonseminomatous tumors, levels of tumor markers, sites of metastases, and primary tumor site (testicular versus extragonadal) all are included in determination of risk category (see Table 54–3). The risk categories defined in this table represent an international consensus derived from several previously defined prognostic classifications.[22–25]

### Staging Evaluation

*Orchiectomy.* The extent of local tumor should be accurately recorded at the time of radical inguinal orchiectomy. Specifically, the pathologist should report whether tumor is confined within the body of the testis (T1), extends beyond the tunica albuginea (T2), involves the epididymis or rete testis (T3), or invades the spermatic cord (T4A) or scrotal wall (T4B). In addition, any lymphatic or vascular invasion should be reported. All of these factors are important in planning treatment for patients with early-stage disease.

*Chest Radiography and Computed Tomography of the Chest.* The standard anteroposterior and lateral chest radiographs provide initial information about the lung parenchyma, but optimal staging also requires computed tomography (CT) of the chest.[26] CT detects lung involvement not suspected on chest radiography in an additional 10% of patients. CT scans should be interpreted cautiously, however, because a substantial proportion of 2- to 5-mm lesions are benign.

*Computed Tomography of the Abdomen.* CT of the abdomen is the most effective means to identify retroperitoneal lymph node involvement. Abnormal lymph nodes as small as 1 to 2 cm can be reliably detected in the upper para-aortic regions. Abnormal computed tomographic findings are therefore accurate in demonstrating metastatic disease. However, the value of abdominal CT in precluding retroperitoneal lymph node involvement is limited. As many as 25 to 30% of patients with normal results on CT scans are found to have retroperitoneal metastases at the time of lymph node dissection.[27] In some of these patients, nodal involvement is minimal and the lymph nodes are not grossly enlarged. In thin patients, retroperitoneal metastases may not be evident on CT even when they are 2 to 3 cm in diameter, owing to the absence of intraperitoneal and retroperitoneal fat planes. The possibility of a false-negative CT scan result becomes important in planning treatment for patients with

*Table 54–2.* **New TNM Staging of Testis Tumors: American Joint Committee on Cancer**

**Primary Tumor (pT)**

| | |
|---|---|
| pTX | Primary tumor cannot be assessed (if no radical orchiectomy has been performed, TX is used) |
| pT0 | No evidence of primary tumor (e.g., histologic scar in testis) |
| pTis | Intratubular germ cell neoplasia (carcinoma in situ) |
| pT1 | Tumor limited to the testis and epididymis without vascular/lymphatic invasion; tumor may invade into the tunica albuginea but not the tunica vaginalis |
| pT2 | Tumor limited to the testis and epididymis with vascular/lymphatic invasion, or tumor extending through the tunica albuginea with involvement of the tunica vaginalis |
| pT3 | Tumor invades the spermatic cord with or without vascular/lymphatic invasion |
| pT4 | Tumor invades the scrotum with or without vascular/lymphatic invasion |

**Regional Lymph Nodes (N)**

*Clinical*

| | |
|---|---|
| NX | Regional lymph nodes cannot be assessed |
| N0 | No regional lymph node metastasis |
| N1 | Lymph node mass 2 cm or less in greatest dimension; or multiple lymph nodes, none more than 2 cm in greatest dimension |
| N2 | Metastasis with a lymph node mass, more than 2 cm but not more than 5 cm in greatest dimension; or multiple lymph nodes, any one mass greater than 2 cm but not more than 5 cm in greatest dimension |
| N3 | Metastasis with a lymph node mass more than 5 cm in greatest dimension |

*Pathologic (pN)*

| | |
|---|---|
| pNX | Regional lymph nodes cannot be assessed |
| pN0 | No regional lymph node metastasis |
| pN1 | Metastasis with a lymph node mass 2 cm or less in greatest dimension and less than or equal to 5 nodes positive, none more than 2 cm in greatest dimension |
| pN2 | Metastasis with a lymph node mass, more than 2 cm but not more than 5 cm in greatest dimension; or more than 5 nodes positive, none more than 5 cm; or evidence of extranodal extension of tumor |
| pN3 | Metastasis with a lymph node mass more than 5 cm in greatest dimension |

**Distant Metastasis (M)**

| | |
|---|---|
| MX | Distant metastasis cannot be assessed |
| M0 | No distant metastasis |
| M1 | Distant metastasis |
| M1a | Nonregional nodal or pulmonary metastasis |
| M1b | Distant metastasis other than to nonregional lymph nodes and lungs |

**Serum Tumor Markers (S)**

| | |
|---|---|
| SX | Marker studies not available or not performed |
| S0 | Marker study levels within normal limits |
| S1 | LDH $<1.5 \times$ N AND |
| hCG | (mIu/ml) $<5000$ AND |
| AFP | (ng/ml) $<1000$ |
| S2 | LDH $1.5–10 \times$ N OR |
| hCG | (mIu/ml) 5000–50,000 OR |
| AFP | (ng/ml) 1000–10,000 |
| S3 | LDH $>10 \times$ N OR |
| hCG | (mIu/ml) $>50,000$ OR |
| AFP | (ng/ml) $>10,000$ |
| N | indicates the upper limit of normal for the LDH assay |

**Stage Grouping**

| | | | | |
|---|---|---|---|---|
| Stage 0 | pTis | N0 | M0 | S0 |
| Stage I | pT1–4 | N0 | M0 | SX |
| Stage IA | pT1 | N0 | M0 | S0 |
| Stage IB | pT2 | N0 | M0 | S0 |
| | pT3 | N0 | M0 | S0 |
| | pT4 | N0 | M0 | S0 |
| Stage IS | Any pT/Tx | N0 | M0 | S1–3 |
| Stage II | Any pT/Tx | N1–3 | M0 | SX |
| Stage IIA | Any pT/Tx | N1 | M0 | S0 |
| | Any pT/Tx | N1 | M0 | S1 |
| Stage IIB | Any pT/Tx | N2 | M0 | S0 |
| | Any pT/Tx | N2 | M0 | S1 |
| Stage IIC | Any pT/Tx | N3 | M0 | S0 |
| | Any pT/Tx | N3 | M0 | S1 |
| Stage III | Any pT/Tx | Any N | M1 | SX |
| Stage IIIA | Any pT/Tx | Any N | M1a | S0 |
| | Any pT/Tx | Any N | M1a | S1 |
| Stage IIIB | Any pT/Tx | N1–3 | M0 | S2 |
| | Any pT/Tx | Any N | M1a | S2 |
| Stage IIIC | Any pT/Tx | N1–3 | M0 | S3 |
| | Any pT/Tx | Any N | M1a | S3 |
| | Any pT/Tx | Any N | M1b | Any S |

clinical stage A; for these patients, observation is a consideration.

***Tumor Markers.*** The staging and management of germ cell tumors have been greatly facilitated by the existence of relatively sensitive and specific tumor markers. By means of radioimmunoassay, minute serum quantities of hCG and AFP can be detected in most patients with nonseminomatous tumors.[17, 28] Measurement of serum lactic dehydrogenase, although much less specific, can provide useful information for the management of advanced seminoma or of nonseminomatous tumors that do not secrete β-hCG or AFP.[29]

hCG is composed of two polypeptide chains (α and β)

and is normally secreted by trophoblastic tissue. In germ cell tumors, syncytiotrophoblastic cells secrete the β subunit of hCG, which can be measured accurately by radioimmunoassay. β-hCG may be secreted by tumors of any nonseminomatous form except the rare pure endodermal sinus tumor. Most patients with high levels have tumors with elements of choriocarcinoma. β-hCG level is elevated in only 10% of patients with pure seminoma at the time of diagnosis and is usually detected only at low levels (<100 ng/ml). High levels of β-hCG in patients with "pure seminoma" should raise suspicion of unrecognized nonseminomatous elements.

AFP is a single-chain glycoprotein normally produced by

*Table 54–3.* **Risk Classification for Advanced Germ Cell Tumors: International Consensus**

| Risk Category | Seminoma | Nonseminoma |
|---|---|---|
| Good risk | Visceral metastases limited to lungs | AFP <1000 ng/ml; hCG <5000 MIU/ml LDH <1.5 × upper limits of normal Visceral metastases limited to lungs |
| Intermediate risk | Nonpulmonary visceral metastases | AFP 1000–10,000 ng/ml hCG 5000–50,000 MIU/ml LDH 1.5–10 × upper limits of normal |
| Poor risk | — | AFP >10,000 ng/ml; hCG >50,000 MIU/ml LDH >10 × upper limits of normal Nonpulmonary visceral metastases Mediastinal primary site |

AFP, alpha-fetoprotein; hCG, human chorionic gonadotropin; LDH, lactate dehydrogenase.

From International Germ Cell Cancer Collaborative Group. International germ cell consensus classification: a prognostic factor–based staging system for metastatic germ cell cancers. J Clin Oncol 1997;15:594–603.

the fetal yolk sac, liver, and gastrointestinal tract. Highest serum concentrations are detected during the 12th to 14th weeks of gestation; levels decline gradually thereafter and are extremely low after 1 year of age. AFP is not present in adult serum except in pathologic states. Elevated AFP levels have been associated with a number of malignancies but are most commonly produced by hepatocellular carcinoma and nonseminomatous germ cell tumors. Tumors of any nonseminomatous variety except pure choriocarcinoma can produce AFP. Pure seminomas *never* produce AFP, however, and any elevation of this marker is indicative of the presence of nonseminomatous elements, even when only seminoma is detected histologically. AFP has a long serum half-life (3 to 4 days); the slow elimination of this substance from the serum must be kept in mind when using serial AFP levels to monitor response to therapy.

Measurement of hCG and AFP provides valuable information for the clinical staging and management of nonseminomatous germ cell neoplasms. Failure of both markers to normalize after orchiectomy indicates the presence of residual tumor. Because one or both markers are elevated in approximately 85% of patients with stage II or III nonseminomatous germ cell tumors, they are extremely valuable in monitoring response to therapy. Persistent elevation of markers after completion of therapy usually indicates persistent viable carcinoma. In addition, detection of rising marker levels in patients who are being monitored after achieving complete remission is often the first indication of relapse and allows early initiation of salvage therapy.

In patients with known testicular cancer, false-positive elevations of hCG and AFP are uncommon. Low-level hCG elevations have been reported in patients who are habitual marijuana users and in patients who are hypogonadal after completion of chemotherapy. In these latter patients, false-positive results are caused by high levels of serum luteinizing hormone (LH), which cross-react with the radioimmuno-

assay for β-hCG. Testosterone replacement in these patients reduces serum LH levels and causes β-hCG determinations to normalize.[30] Elevated serum AFP levels unrelated to testicular cancer are uncommon but can occur in patients with a variety of hepatic disorders. AFP levels are only mildly elevated in nonmalignant conditions and do not rise with sequential determinations.

*Other Staging Procedures.* Routine use of other radiologic staging procedures, including intravenous pyelography, bipedal lymphangiography, gallium scanning, arteriography, and magnetic resonance imaging, provides no useful additional information about most patients. Lymphangiography remains useful for planning treatment for patients with clinical stage I seminoma (discussed later).

## Treatment of Seminoma

Even before the development of effective combination chemotherapy regimens, the treatment of seminoma was gratifying because of the exquisite radiosensitivity of this tumor. Most patients with seminoma present with early-stage disease (stage I or IIA), and radiation therapy cure rates for these stages are high. Even in patients with massive retroperitoneal disease (stages IIB, IIC), radiation therapy is curative in a substantial percentage. With the development of highly effective chemotherapy for patients with advanced-stage or recurrent seminoma, the combined cure rate for all stages is now greater than 90%. In addition, long-term treatment-related sequelae, including infertility, are uncommon.

Before therapy is begun, clinical evaluation of patients with seminoma should be completed as previously described. In addition to standard staging procedures, a bipedal lymphangiogram may be indicated in patients with normal abdominal CT scan results. Lymphangiography can detect abnormal periaortic lymph nodes in 13 to 22% of these patients, permitting greater accuracy of staging.[31, 32] Seminomas differ from nonseminomatous germ cell tumors in that specific histopathologic characteristics of the primary tumor, such as vascular invasion or invasion of the epididymis and spermatic cord, have not been found to be predictive of retroperitoneal node involvement.[33, 34] Serum levels of hCG and AFP should be measured in all patients; patients with elevated AFP levels have nonseminoma and should be treated as such. Patients with modest elevations of β-hCG (<100 ng/ml) should be treated under the standard guidelines for pure seminoma.[35] After careful staging, patients with anaplastic seminoma should also be treated according to standard guidelines for seminoma.[34]

### STAGES I, IIA, AND IIB

After radical orchiectomy, radiation therapy remains the treatment of choice for early-stage seminoma. Numerous large series have documented high cure rates from radiation therapy (Table 54–4).

The radiation therapy field should include the ipsilateral inguinal, iliac, and bilateral para-aortic and caval nodes. Adequate coverage of the renal hilum is most important for left-sided tumors because the testicular lymphatics and the

*Table 54–4.* **Results of Postorchiectomy Radiation Therapy in Early-Stage Seminoma**

| Institution | No. of Patients (STAGE I/IIA) | 5-Year Survival (%) | |
| --- | --- | --- | --- |
| | | STAGE I | STAGE IIA, IIB₁ |
| Royal Marsden Hospital[36] | 232/39 | 97 | 95 |
| M.D. Anderson Cancer Center[33] | 161/37 | 8 | 94 |
| Princess Margaret Hospital[37] | 150/16 | 99 | 94 |
| Massachusetts General Hospital[38] | 135/18 | 98 | 100 |
| Cross Cancer Institute[39] | 147/20 | 98 | 85 |
| Harvard Joint Center[40] | 79/25 | 97 | 96 |
| Johns Hopkins Hospital[31] | 42/16 | 100 | 100 |
| Princess Margaret Hospital[41, 42] | 194/69 | 97 | 94 |
| Total | 1140/240 | 98 | 95 |

testicular vein often drain directly into the renal hilum. The lymphatic drainage on the right side is usually to the lymph nodes at the level of the fourth lumbar vertebra adjacent to the inferior vena cava. For stage I seminoma, a total dose of 3000 cGy is administered using conventional fractionation (150 cGy/day five times a week). For stage IIA or IIB seminoma, a total dose of 3600 cGy is recommended, delivered to the involved nodes with a 5-cm margin. Elective irradiation of the mediastinum is unnecessary in these early-stage cases.[37] Current techniques permit shielding of the contralateral testis so that only approximately 3 cGy is administered during the entire course of treatment. Figure 54–2 shows a standard radiation therapy treatment portal for stage I, IIA, or IIB seminoma of the left testis.

In certain situations, modification of standard radiation therapy technique is required. The ipsilateral internal iliac lymph nodes should be included if the primary tumor invades the epididymis. If a scrotal approach has been made for the orchiectomy, the ipsilateral hemiscrotum needs to be treated. Finally, if the primary tumor demonstrates direct scrotal invasion, the ipsilateral hemiscrotum requires irradiation by a 12- to 15-MeV electron beam field matched to the lower border of the photon field.

Radiation therapy for early-stage seminoma is well tolerated, and most patients have no long-term sequelae. Dyspepsia or ulcer disease has been reported in approximately 5% of patients.[36] Patients usually experience no associated azoospermia or even oligospermia.

The strategy of observation alone for patients with clinical stage I seminoma has been investigated by several centers. Patients were closely monitored with serial markers, chest and abdominal radiographs, and, less frequently, abdominal CT. The recurrence rate with observation alone has been approximately 15%.[41, 43] The salvage rate is high; however, a substantial proportion of these patients have large-volume disease and require chemotherapy at the time of relapse. Median time to recurrence is 12 months, with occasional recurrences as late as 5 years,[41] therefore necessitating prolonged duration of surveillance with abdominal CT. Because radiation therapy produces a high cure rate with minimal toxicity and is less costly than surveillance,[44, 45] radiation

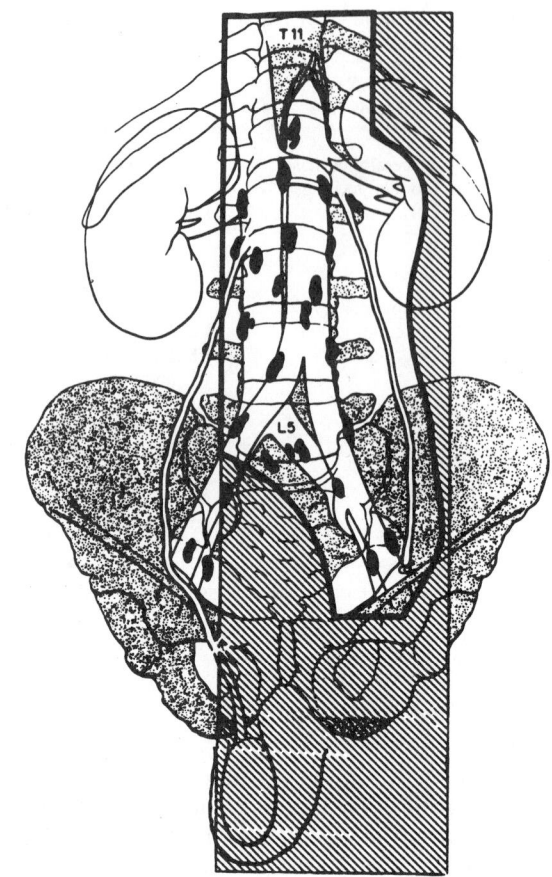

**Figure 54–2.** Contoured anterior and posterior radiation treatment fields for men with clinical stage I or stage IIA left testicular cancer. The diagonally shaded area is an individually made, 8 cm–thick Ostalloy block (shield 2). (Reprinted by permission of the publisher from Reduction of the scatter dose to the testicle outside the radiation treatment fields. Kubo H, Shipley WU, Int J Radiat Oncol Biol Phys 8:1742. Copyright 1982, by Elsevier Science Inc.)

therapy remains the standard treatment for patients with stage I seminoma.

## STAGE IIC (BULKY RETROPERITONEAL ADENOPATHY)

The cure rate from radiation therapy alone decreases markedly when patients have greater than 5 cm adenopathy in the retroperitoneum. In most reported series, long-term survival is approximately 60%.[31, 37–39, 46–48] Most patients who are not cured with radiation therapy suffer relapse at distant sites. Combination chemotherapy for stage IIC seminoma is more effective as a single modality than is radiation therapy, and cure rates of greater than 90% can be expected.[29, 42] Treatment with four courses of cisplatin-based chemotherapy, as described for nonseminomatous germ cell tumors, is therefore the treatment of choice for patients with stage IIC seminoma.

## STAGE III AND RECURRENT SEMINOMA

Patients who have stage III seminoma at presentation or recurrent seminoma after radiation therapy should receive cisplatin-based combination chemotherapy as described for advanced nonseminomatous germ cell tumors. With this approach, more than 90% of patients treated de novo and 80 to 85% of patients treated after radiation are cured.[29, 49] Bleomycin should be used with caution in patients who have received previous mediastinal or pulmonary irradiation. The optimal platinum-based regimen for advanced seminoma is undefined, although most patients are now treated with cisplatin, etoposide, and bleomycin as described for nonseminomatous germ cell tumors. Horwich and colleagues evaluated single-agent carboplatin in patients with stage III seminoma in an effort to reduce the toxicity of therapy.[50] Twenty-seven of 34 patients (80%) remained disease free 12 to 40 months after treatment with single-agent carboplatin. Five of six patients who suffered relapse underwent salvage treatment with cisplatin-containing combination chemotherapy. Because the relapse-free survival following single-agent carboplatin is lower than with combination therapy, the less toxic regimen should be reserved for patients who are unlikely to tolerate standard treatment regimens.

Many patients given chemotherapy for stage IIC or III seminoma have residual radiographic abnormalities after completion of treatment. Some of these patients have residual viable seminoma, but most have only necrotic tumor or fibrosis. Residual benign teratoma has not been observed in these patients. Most patients have residual radiographic abnormalities smaller than 3.0 cm; these patients should be observed without further therapy because the incidence of residual viable seminoma is extremely low.[51, 53] Treatment of the less common patient with a residual abnormality of 3 cm or larger is controversial. In a group of 104 patients described by Puc and associates, 30 (29%) had residual masses 3 cm or larger and 8 of these (27%) had viable seminoma on biopsy.[52] In contrast, Schultz and coworkers reported that eight of nine patients with residual masses 3 cm or larger remained free of progression when monitored without biopsy.[53] Complete retroperitoneal node dissection is extremely difficult after chemotherapy in these patients, owing to severe desmoplastic reaction and obliteration of tissue planes.[54] However, biopsy and resection of residual radiographic abnormalities has been associated with acceptable morbidity, and should be considered so that additional therapy can be administered to patients with residual viable seminoma.

## TREATMENT OF SECOND PRIMARY SEMINOMA

Treatment of a second primary seminoma depends on that administered for the initial tumor. If patients have received previous infradiaphragmatic radiation, a repeat course of this therapy to the necessary dosages can be hazardous. In this situation, observation may be the best policy for patients with clinical stage I seminoma. Those with stage II or III seminoma should receive initial cisplatin-based chemotherapy.

# Treatment of Nonseminoma

Treatment of nonseminomatous germ cell tumors has changed markedly since 1975 and is continuing to evolve.

At present, most of these tumors can be cured, and all should be approached with this intent. The development of highly effective combination chemotherapy is the major therapeutic advance; however, optimal treatment of most patients requires combined modality therapy. Appropriate integration of surgical treatment with systemic chemotherapy is essential for maximizing the cure rate while minimizing the toxicity of therapy. Careful clinical staging is critical for determining the optimal treatment approach.

## STAGE I NONSEMINOMA

The management of clinical stage I nonseminoma is controversial because different treatment approaches have produced similar excellent results. Retroperitoneal lymph node dissection remains the gold standard of therapy; this remains the only accurate staging procedure and is definitive therapy for most patients. However, the alternative approach of active surveillance alone, with intervention only in cases that recur, has also produced excellent results in several large series.[55–63]

**Modified Retroperitoneal Lymph Node Dissection.** When retroperitoneal lymph node dissection is performed in patients with clinical stage I nonseminoma, 20 to 25% are demonstrated to have retroperitoneal lymph node involvement and are therefore upstaged to pathologic stage II. Patients with pathologic stage I nonseminoma have cure rates greater than 95% with retroperitoneal lymph node dissection alone.[64] Approximately 50% of those with pathologic stage II nonseminoma are cured with retroperitoneal lymph node dissection; however, the cure rate is much higher (approximately 80%) in patients with only microscopic lymph node involvement. When retroperitoneal node dissection is complete, almost all subsequent recurrences are pulmonary.

Before 1980, infertility was common after retroperitoneal node dissection, because of either failure of seminal emission or retrograde ejaculation. This complication resulted from disruption of postganglionic sympathetic nerve fibers in the area of the aortic bifurcation. Pioneering work of Narayan and associates in the 1980s, however, demonstrated that fertility could be preserved if the surgical boundaries of retroperitoneal node dissection were modified.[65] The boundaries of right and left retroperitoneal node dissections are diagrammed in Figure 54–3; unilateral dissection below the inferior mesenteric artery and avoidance of the hypogastric plexus over the aortic bifurcation are necessary to preserve fertility. In a large series of patients treated with modified retroperitoneal node dissection, Richie reported preservation of antegrade ejaculatory function in 80 of 85 patients (94%).[66]

**Surveillance.** Because many patients with clinical stage I nonseminoma are cured by radical orchiectomy alone, close surveillance after radical inguinal orchiectomy has been investigated by several centers. Twenty-five to 30% of these patients are destined to experience recurrence without further therapy; therefore, the success of a surveillance approach depends on early detection of recurrence and the availability of curative therapy for such patients. Results of such surveillance studies (Table 54–5) demonstrate that this approach is feasible, with a very low percentage of disease-related fatalities. However, it should be emphasized that

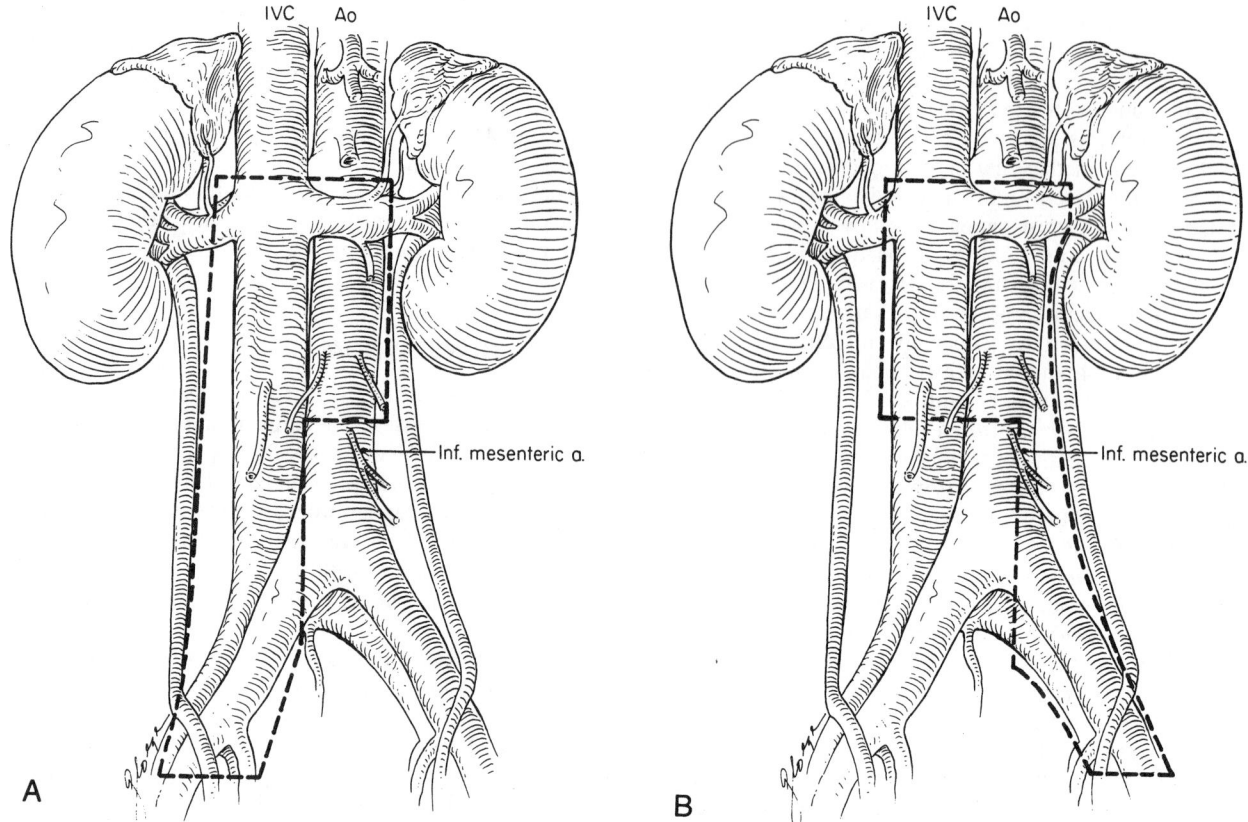

**Figure 54–3.** Anatomic boundaries for modified retroperitoneal lymph node dissection. *A,* Limits of dissection for right-sided tumor. *B,* Limits of dissection for left-sided tumor.

patients in these studies were monitored extremely closely, with physical examination, chest radiography, and tumor markers performed monthly for the first year, every 2 months for the second year, and every 3 to 6 months thereafter. Because most of the recurrences are in the retroperitoneum, abdominal computed tomographic scans are also necessary and should be performed every 2 to 3 months for the first 2 years and at least every 6 months thereafter. Late recurrences have been observed in this group; surveillance is therefore necessary for a minimum of 5 years and possibly 10 years after radical orchiectomy.

The policy of surveillance after radical orchiectomy has

allowed the identification of several prognostic factors in patients with clinical stage I nonseminoma. Adverse prognostic factors include tumor invasion of the epididymis or tunica albuginea (T2 or greater), vascular or lymphatic invasion, or embryonal histology.[15, 66] Patients with one or more of these adverse prognostic factors have a 40% chance of relapse after orchiectomy alone, compared with a 5 to 10% relapse rate in patients with no adverse factors.[15]

**Adjuvant Chemotherapy.** A few reports have documented low recurrence rates when high-risk patients receive two courses of combination chemotherapy following orchiectomy.[67, 68] Although these results are promising, patients are subjected to the temporary toxicity of combination chemotherapy, and this approach cannot be considered standard until more experience is available.

**Choice of Therapy.** Because excellent results can be obtained with several treatment approaches, the choice of treatment must be individualized. Retroperitoneal lymph node dissection is probably the better choice for most patients, because the major treatment-related morbidity (ejaculatory dysfunction) has been minimized by the change in operative technique. Such procedures should ideally be performed only by urologists who are specifically trained and who perform this procedure with some regularity. Patients unable or unwilling to comply with the rigorous follow-up required for adequate surveillance should always be treated with lymph node dissection. Although close follow-up is still necessary after lymph node dissection, recurrence in the retroperitoneum is rare, and frequent abdominal computed

*Table 54–5.* Results of Surveillance for Patients with Clinical Stage I Nonseminoma

| Investigator | Year | No. of Patients | No. of Relapses | No. of Deaths |
|---|---|---|---|---|
| Johnson et al[55] | 1984 | 36 | 12 (33%) | 2 |
| Pizzocaro et al[56] | 1986 | 85 | 23 (27%) | 1 |
| Freedman et al[57] | 1987 | 259 | 70 (27%) | 3 |
| Gelderman et al[58] | 1987 | 54 | 11 (20%) | 0 |
| Rorth et al[59] | 1987 | 79 | 24 (30%) | 2 |
| Raghavan et al[60] | 1988 | 46 | 13 (8%) | 2 |
| Sogani et al[61] | 1988 | 45 | 10 (22%) | 2 |
| Thompson et al[62] | 1988 | 36 | 12 (33%) | 2 |
| Read et al[63] | 1992 | 373 | 100 (27%) | 5 |
| Total | | 1013 | 275 (27%) | 19 (2%) |

tomographic scans thus are unnecessary. Node dissection is probably also advisable for patients with adverse prognostic factors, although these individuals may be at increased risk for systemic recurrence regardless of initial treatment.

Conversely, surveillance is an excellent treatment option for highly motivated patients who wish to avoid retroperitoneal node dissection. Although 20 to 25% of these patients will experience recurrence, treatment with cisplatin-based combination chemotherapy at the time of recurrence is curative in the large majority.

## STAGE II NONSEMINOMA

As in the treatment of stage I seminoma, several treatment alternatives yield excellent results in the management of stage II nonseminoma. Retroperitoneal lymph node dissection was the first curative treatment available; however, results of this procedure are inferior to those achieved in stage I seminoma, and cure is achieved with surgery alone in only 50% of patients with involved retroperitoneal lymph nodes. In addition, the presence of gross metastatic disease in the retroperitoneal lymph nodes often necessitates a more extensive dissection, resulting in ejaculatory dysfunction. Therefore, when retroperitoneal lymph nodes larger than 3 cm are seen on abdominal CT, combination chemotherapy as described for stage III nonseminoma should be the initial treatment. Many patients with bulky retroperitoneal adenopathy require node dissection after completion of chemotherapy (discussed later).

For patients with an area of adenopathy less than 3 cm in diameter on abdominal CT, retroperitoneal lymph node dissection is considered standard therapy. Most of these patients have unilateral adenopathy, and a modified lymph node dissection can be performed.[69] Alternatively, such patients can be treated initially with three courses of combination chemotherapy as described for patients with favorable stage III nonseminoma. Excellent treatment results have been reported with this strategy, although no randomized comparative studies have been performed.[70] However, many patients who receive initial chemotherapy still require subsequent retroperitoneal lymph node dissection. Surgical treatment is necessary for patients who show persistent abnormalities on CT after chemotherapy, as well as for those who have prominent elements of teratocarcinoma in the primary tumor.

After retroperitoneal lymph node dissection, patients with involved retroperitoneal lymph nodes have a substantial risk of recurrence. Again, two reasonable treatment options exist: immediate adjuvant chemotherapy or surveillance in patients whose marker levels normalize. These treatments have been compared in a large randomized study.[20] In this Intergroup trial, 197 patients in complete remission after retroperitoneal lymph node dissection either received two postoperative courses of cisplatin-based combination chemotherapy or were observed and given four courses of chemotherapy at the time of relapse. The surveillance program included physical examination, chest radiography, and testing of serum tumor marker levels monthly during the first year and every 2 months during the second year. As predicted, the relapse rate was much higher in the observation group (49% vs. 2%); however, with early detection of relapse followed by four courses of chemotherapy, long-term disease-free sur-

vival was excellent with either treatment (99% with adjuvant chemotherapy, 97% with initial observation). More recently, excellent results have been reported using two courses of cisplatin and etoposide (omitting bleomycin) in the adjuvant treatment of stage II nonseminoma.[71]

## TREATMENT OF DISSEMINATED (STAGE III) TESTICULAR CANCER

**Initial Combination Chemotherapy.** Testicular cancer was recognized to be an unusual solid tumor as early as the 1960s. A number of chemotherapeutic agents, including dactinomycin, mithramycin, vinblastine, and bleomycin, produced objective response rates of approximately 50%. Approximately 10% of these patients had complete responses, and a small number (approximately 5%) were cured by single-agent therapy. The combination of bleomycin and vinblastine, reported by Samuels and colleagues in 1975, was a marked advance compared with single-agent therapy and produced long-term disease-free survival in approximately 30% of patients.[72] However, the introduction of cisplatin, the most active single agent in this disease, and its successful incorporation into combination regimens began the modern era of combination chemotherapy for advanced testicular cancer.

In 1977, Einhorn and Donohue reported the results of treatment of disseminated testicular cancer with PVB (Platinol [cisplatin], vinblastine, and bleomycin) (Table 54–6).[73] In this study, patients received four courses of chemotherapy

*Table 54–6.* **Selected Cisplatin-Based Combination Chemotherapy Regimens for Treatment of Disseminated Testicular Cancer**

*Historical Regimens*

PVB (original regimen)[73]
  Cisplatin 20 mg/m²/day × 5 days IV over 15–30 min
  Vinblastine 0.2 mg/kg IV bolus days 1 and 2
  Bleomycin 30 units IV bolus weekly
    Four cycles given at 21-day intervals (maintenance vinblastine 0.3 mg/kg IV monthly × 21 mo given in original series)
VAB-6[74]
  Cyclophosphamide 600 mg/m² IV day 1
  Bleomycin 30 units IV bolus day 1
  Bleomycin 20 units/m²/day IV continuous infusion days 1–3
  Dactinomycin 1 mg/m² IV day 1
  Vinblastine 4 mg/m² IV day 1
  Cisplatin 120 mg/m² IV day 4 (saline/mannitol diuresis)
    Three cycles given at 4-wk intervals

*Current Regimens*

PEB[75]
  Cisplatin 20 mg/m²/day × 5 days IV over 15–30 min
  Etoposide 100 mg/m²/day × 5 days IV over 20–30 min
  Bleomycin 30 units IV days 2, 9, and 16
    Three or four courses given at 21-day intervals (number of courses depends on risk factors)
VIP[76]
  Cisplatin 20 mg/m²/day × 5 days IV over 15–30 min
  Ifosfamide 1.2 g/m²/day × 5 days IV over 30–60 min
  Mesna 400 mg/m² IV bolus before therapy, then 1200 mg/m²/day IV continuous infusion
  Etoposide 75 mg/m²/day × 5 days IV (vinblastine 0.11 mg/kg IV push days 1 and 2 substituted for etoposide in VeIP regimen)
    Four cycles given at 21-day intervals

followed by complete restaging (CT of the chest and abdomen, serum tumor markers). Patients in complete remission (normal radiographic results and tumor markers) received maintenance vinblastine monthly for 21 months. Patients with normal serum tumor markers and residual radiographic abnormalities underwent surgical resection 4 to 6 weeks after completion of chemotherapy. Surgical procedures consisted of retroperitoneal lymph node dissection, thoracotomy, median sternotomy, or a combined thoracoabdominal procedure as necessary to resect all radiographic abnormalities. If residual carcinoma was found, patients received two additional courses of cisplatin and vinblastine; patients with no residual tumor received maintenance vinblastine.

With this treatment approach, 33 of 47 patients (70%) achieved a complete remission, and an additional five patients (11%) were rendered disease free after resection of residual teratoma or carcinoma. The relapse rate was low, and 67% of patients had long-term disease-free survival. The major acute chemotherapy-related toxicity was severe myelosuppression, although vinblastine-related gastrointestinal toxicity was also a problem in some patients. Similar results were subsequently reported by Memorial Sloan-Kettering Cancer Center with the VAB-6 regimen (see Table 54–6).[74]

These results represented such a marked improvement over previous therapy that this approach (intensive cisplatin-based chemotherapy followed by surgical resection of residual radiographic abnormalities) has persisted as the model for treatment of advanced testicular cancer. However, refinements have been made in both the chemotherapy regimen and the strategy of surgical resection. Improvements in therapy have been achieved almost exclusively through large, well-conceived randomized trials conducted in cooperative groups in both the United States and Europe. Valid conclusions about treatment efficacy in relatively well treated neoplasms are possible only with such studies, and it is unfortunate that such a logical progression of randomized studies has not taken place in other areas of oncology.

Table 54–7 summarizes the results of the most important randomized trials performed since Einhorn's report of the original PVB regimen. The toxicity of the original PVB regimen was reduced without reducing efficacy by decreasing the vinblastine dose from 0.4 to 0.3 mg/kg[77, 78] and by eliminating maintenance therapy.[79] In the early 1980s, etoposide was found to be an active drug even after cisplatin-containing combination regimens had failed, and curative salvage therapy was achieved with the combination of cisplatin and etoposide.[80] Therefore, etoposide was substituted for vinblastine in the PVB regimen and studied in a randomized setting by the Southeastern Cancer Study Group.[75] In this study containing a total of 244 patients, the 2-year disease-free survival rate was approximately 80% with either treatment. The etoposide-containing regimen was better tolerated, because the vinblastine-related gastrointestinal toxicity and myalgias were eliminated. In addition, retrospective analysis of patients with poor-risk disease showed an advantage of the etoposide-containing combination. On the basis of this study, BEP (bleomycin, etoposide, and Platinol [cisplatin]) replaced PVB as the standard treatment for advanced testicular cancer.

The development of reliable classification systems to separate good-risk and poor-risk patients (see Table 54–3) has allowed subsequent randomized studies to focus on specific patient populations. In general, trials enrolling good-risk patients have attempted to reduce the toxicity of therapy because standard therapy in this group cures more than 90% of cases. Conversely, trials enrolling poor-risk patients have attempted to improve the efficacy of treatment.

The trials recruiting good-risk patients, elaborated in Table 54–7, have allowed further simplification of therapy for these patients. The Southeastern Cancer Study Group found that three courses of BEP were equivalent to four courses in good-risk patients.[81] Elimination of the fourth course of treatment substantially reduces the toxicity of therapy because myelosuppression as well as cumulative bleomycin toxicity is worst during the fourth course. Long-term follow-up has confirmed equivalent survival with only three courses of BEP.[82]

The elimination of bleomycin from the regimen has been investigated by two groups. The Memorial Sloan-Kettering group compared four courses of etoposide and cisplatin with the VAB-6 regimen and found equivalent efficacy and greatly reduced toxicity with the two-drug regimen.[83] A subsequent randomized trial showed that four courses of etoposide and cisplatin were superior to four courses of etoposide and carboplatin.[84] Long-term follow-up of the entire group of patients treated with etoposide-cisplatin in these two sequential Memorial Sloan-Kettering studies showed an 86% disease-free survival.[85] In contrast, the Eastern Cooperative Group found that bleomycin was an important component of treatment when only three courses were given.[86] In this trial, 38% of patients receiving the two-drug regimen had unfavorable treatment outcomes (treatment failure, residual carcinoma at resection, relapse), compared with 17% who received three drugs ($p = 0.004$). Consequently, overall survival was inferior with the two-drug regimen (95% vs. 86%, $p = 0.01$).

The substitution of carboplatin for cisplatin, in an attempt to reduce treatment-related toxicity, has been evaluated in two randomized trials.[84, 87] Both trials showed higher relapse rates and reduced survival among patients receiving carboplatin. Therefore, cisplatin remains an essential component of treatment.

Randomized trials enrolling poor-risk patients have not yet resulted in the identification of a regimen superior to four cycles of BEP. A small randomized trial performed by the National Cancer Institute suggested a benefit from high-dose cisplatin (40 mg/m² daily for 5 days). However, the experimental arm in this trial also included etoposide; this regimen was compared with the standard PVB regimen.[88] It was therefore unclear whether the double-dose cisplatin or the addition of etoposide increased efficacy. The dosage of cisplatin was investigated directly in an Intergroup study.[89] Standard BEP for four cycles was compared with an identical BEP regimen except that the cisplatin dose was doubled in the investigational regimen. No differences in efficacy were observed, and the high-dose cisplatin regimen was much more toxic. More recently, two randomized trials have compared VIP (etoposide, ifosfamide, and cisplatin) with standard BEP, on the basis of the demonstrated efficacy of this regimen in salvage treatment.[76] Both trials showed equivalent efficacy of BEP and VIP, but VIP was associated with greater toxicity.[90, 91]

In summary, selection of appropriate initial chemotherapy

*Table 54–7.* **Important Randomized Trials of Therapy for Disseminated Nonseminomatous Germ Cell Tumors**

| Institution | Year | "Standard" Treatment | Investigational Treatment | Purpose of Study | Results |
|---|---|---|---|---|---|
| Indiana University[77] | 1980 | PVB (vinblastine 0.4 mg/kg) | PVB (vinblastine 0.3 mg/kg) | Reduce myelosuppression | Lower vinblastine dose less toxic, equally effective |
| EORTC[78] | 1986 | PVB (vinblastine 0.4 mg/kg) | PVB (vinblastine 0.3 mg/kg) | Reduce myelosuppression | Lower vinblastine dose less toxic, equally effective |
| SEG[79] | 1987 | PVB (vinblastine 0.3 mg/kg) | PVB without maintenance vinblastine | Reduce toxicity | Maintenance therapy unnecessary |
| SEG[75] | 1987 | PVB × 4 | BEP × 4 | Improve efficacy | BEP less toxic, more effective in poor-risk subgroup |
| *Good Risk Patients* | | | | | |
| SEG[81, 82] | 1989 | BEP × 4 | BEP × 3 | Reduce toxicity | BEP × 3 equally effective, less toxic |
| Memorial Sloan-Kettering[83] | 1988 | VAB-6 × 3 | EP × 4 | Reduce toxicity | EP × 4 equally effective, less toxic |
| ECOG[86] | 1995 | BEP × 3 | EP × 3 | Reduce toxicity | EP × 3 less effective |
| Memorial Sloan-Kettering[84] | 1993 | EP × 4 | Etoposide/carboplatin × 4 | Reduce toxicity | Carboplatin regimen less effective |
| EORTC[87] | 1997 | BEP × 4 | CEB × 4 | Reduce toxicity | Carboplatin regimen less effective |
| *Poor Risk Patients* | | | | | |
| NCI[88] | 1988 | PVB × 4 | PveVB high-dose cisplatin (40 mg/m² × 5) | Improve efficacy | PveVB superior |
| SEG/Intergroup[89] | 1991 | BEP × 4 | BEP × 4 high-dose cisplatin (40 mg/m² × 5) | Improve efficacy | High-dose cisplatin no more efficacious, more toxic than standard BEP |
| EORTC[90] | 1993 | BEP × 4 | VIP × 4 | Improve efficacy | Equal efficacy, VIP more toxic |
| Intergroup[91] | 1998 | BEP × 4 | VIP × 4 | Improve efficacy | Equal efficacy, VIP more toxic |
| EORTC[92] | 1998 | BEP × 4 | BOP/VIP-B | Improve efficacy | Equal efficacy, BOP/VIP more toxic |

PVB, cisplatin, vinblastine, bleomycin; BEP, bleomycin, etoposide, cisplatin; VAB-6, Sloan-Kettering multidrug regimen (see Table 54–6); CEB, carboplatin, etoposide, bleomycin; PveVB, cisplatin, vinblastine, etoposide, bleomycin; VIP, etoposide, ifosfamide, cisplatin; SEG, Southeast Cooperative Oncology Group; EORTC, European Organization for Research and Treatment of Cancer; ECOG, Eastern Cooperative Oncology Group; NCI, National Cancer Institute.

for patients with advanced testicular cancer should follow a careful staging evaluation and should be based on the categorization of the patient as a good or poor risk. Good-risk disease can be treated less intensively while maintaining a cure rate of approximately 90%. At present, three courses of BEP is the best treatment for most patients. Four courses of etoposide and cisplatin produce equivalent results to three courses of BEP and may be preferable for patients with contraindications to bleomycin. Carboplatin is not an equivalent substitute for cisplatin and should be avoided. For patients at poor risk, four courses of BEP probably represent the best available treatment, resulting in a cure rate of approximately 50 to 60%. However, results with early high-dose therapy are promising in poor prognosis patients. Motzer and colleagues have used two courses of high-dose carboplatin, etoposide, and cyclophosphamide in poor risk patients who had poor response after two courses of etoposide-ifosfamide-cisplatin chemotherapy.[93] The 50% disease-free survival achieved in these patients compares favorably with their retrospective results in similar patients treated with standard dose therapy. Randomized trials evaluating high-dose therapy as part of initial treatment are ongoing.

**Surgical Management After Initial Chemotherapy.**
After completion of initial chemotherapy, approximately 30% of patients have normal serum tumor markers but continuing radiographic abnormalities. In the initial PVB series reported by Einhorn and Donohue, such patients underwent radical resection of all radiographic abnormalities 4 to 6 weeks after completion of chemotherapy. The surgical findings were roughly equally divided among necrosis-fibrosis, mature teratoma, and residual carcinoma. Patients with either necrosis-fibrosis or mature teratoma had an excellent prognosis similar to that of patients achieving complete radiographic remission with chemotherapy alone.

In subsequent series, the surgical findings have changed somewhat, for reasons that are unexplained. In more recent large series, only 10 to 20% of patients have residual carcinoma, and more than 50% have either necrotic tumor or fibrosis. Because these patients, now constituting a majority of the group, derive no benefit from surgical resection, the approach adopted has been to delay surgical resection in patients without high risk of residual teratoma or carcinoma. Specifically, these are patients who show no elements of teratocarcinoma in the orchiectomy specimen and who show a greater than 90% radiographic response to chemotherapy. In such patients, serial radiography examinations after completion of chemotherapy often document slow resolution of residual abnormalities. Surgical intervention can be avoided in these patients, although the relapse rate is slightly higher than for those with normal CT findings after chemotherapy.[94, 95] In another small group of patients, tumor markers begin to rise rapidly 2 to 3 months after completion of chemotherapy. Surgical treatment is probably not beneficial in this group either, who instead require salvage chemotherapy.

Although this approach is beneficial for many patients, several points deserve emphasis. First, not all patients are candidates for such a strategy. In particular, patients with teratocarcinoma in the initial orchiectomy specimen have a much higher chance of harboring residual mature teratoma,[96, 97] and resection should be considered without delay in all such individuals. In addition, patients who show stabilization (rather than continued resolution) of residual radiographic abnormalities should undergo resection, even if serum marker levels remain normal. The presence of mature teratoma is more likely in these patients, and the delayed problems of enlarging mature teratoma or late relapse are well recognized.[98–100] As with initial retroperitoneal lymph node dissection, the experience of the urologist who performs such procedures is critical to the outcome. Bilateral retroperitoneal node dissections are usually necessary in these patients; ejaculatory dysfunction is the most frequent complication. Resection of large residual mature teratomas is frequently a complicated and arduous procedure that sometimes requires the combined efforts of urologist, vascular surgeon, and thoracic surgeon.

**Salvage Therapy.** All patients with residual carcinoma after completion of initial therapy require salvage therapy. In general, the duration of initial chemotherapy should be only four courses because patients with incomplete response after this length of therapy are unlikely to have long-term complete response. An exception to this generalization is the group of patients with residual carcinoma completely resected after initial chemotherapy. Without further chemotherapy, the recurrence rate in these patients is greater than 80%. Administration of two additional courses of standard induction chemotherapy (without bleomycin), however, results in a 70% long-term complete remission rate.[101]

In patients who have incomplete response to initial chemotherapy (as evidenced by residual tumor marker elevations) or in those who experience relapse after initial complete response, the chance of cure is relatively poor. However, some patients can still achieve long-term survival with additional chemotherapy. The combination of cisplatin and etoposide after PVB failure was the first regimen found to be curative in approximately 30% of relapsing cases.[80] More recently, the VIP or VeIP (vinblastine substituted for etoposide) combinations (see Table 54–6) have been evaluated, because ifosfamide has substantial activity as a single agent in relapsing patients. Because most patients currently receive etoposide as part of first-line treatment, the VeIP regimen is used most frequently. This regimen, administered for four courses, produces long-term remissions in 15 to 25% of patients.[76, 102] Although only 10% of patients achieving complete remission with first-line chemotherapy experience relapse, the relapse rate after salvage chemotherapy is approximately 50%. Patients with cisplatin resistance (i.e., who show progression while receiving a cisplatin-containing regimen) are much less likely to obtain a complete response. Hematologic toxicity with salvage treatment can be considerable. However, every attempt should be made to administer therapy with full drug doses; the use of cytokines is helpful in these patients.

After salvage chemotherapy, indications for surgical resection are identical to those following first-line therapy. Even if residual carcinoma is present, disease-free survival as high as 40% has been reported if complete resection can be accomplished.[101] Daily use of oral etoposide (50 mg/m² daily for 21 consecutive days, repeated every 28 days for three courses) resulted in a 74% long-term disease-free survival rate in a group of 23 patients in complete remission following salvage therapy.[103] Although no randomized trials have validated this approach, these results compare favorably with retrospective series and suggest a role for this relatively well tolerated maintenance therapy.

*High-Dose Salvage Therapy.* Because salvage therapy with standard dose chemotherapy is curative in only a minority of patients, high-dose therapy has been investigated in this setting. Several of the most active chemotherapeutic agents in the treatment of testicular cancer can be escalated to high doses; these drugs include etoposide, carboplatin, and alkylating agents (cyclophosphamide, ifosfamide). To date, most high-dose regimens have contained etoposide and carboplatin; some have added an alkylating agent as a third drug. At present, published treatment results do not enable the identification of a "best" high-dose regimen.

In early reports of salvage high-dose therapy, most patients had received two or three previous standard-dose regimens and therefore had highly refractory disease. In these patients, who were incurable with standard dose therapy, a complete response rate of 26 to 40% and disease-free survival of 15 to 21% was achieved.[104–106]

High-dose therapy has more recently been incorporated into initial salvage regimens, usually following two courses of vinblastine, ifosfamide, and cisplatin. The incidence of severe treatment-related toxicity is reduced with this approach.[107, 108] Long-term survival of approximately 40% has been reported by several groups using this approach.[109–111] Several prognostic factors can be used to differentiate good-risk from poor-risk patients when high-dose salvage regimens are used. These factors include progressive disease before high-dose chemotherapy, disease refractory to cisplatin, hCG level greater than 1000 ng/ml, and mediastinal nonseminomatous primary tumor.[112] Although no randomized trials have compared standard dose and high-dose therapy as initial salvage treatment, the results with high-dose therapy are very promising, and this approach should be considered when feasible.

## Special Problems in the Treatment of Metastatic Testicular Cancer

### THE TESTIS AS A SANCTUARY SITE

In selected patients with widespread nonseminomatous testicular cancer, initial chemotherapy (rather than orchiectomy) is indicated. Some of these patients have, however, been found to harbor residual active carcinoma in the testis, even at a time when complete remission had been achieved systemically. Greist and associates described 20 patients who underwent delayed orchiectomy after cisplatin-containing combination chemotherapy.[113] These patients were initially thought to have primary retroperitoneal germ cell tumors but subsequently were found to have a primary testicular mass either on physical examination or by testicular ultrasonography. When these patients underwent orchiectomy, three had active carcinoma and six had teratoma remaining in the testis.

Orchiectomy should therefore be performed either before or after therapy in all patients with a known or suspected testicular primary tumor because chemotherapy does not always eradicate carcinoma at this site. If active carcinoma is found, recommendations for further treatment differ; investigators at Indiana University recommended two additional courses of cisplatin-based chemotherapy,[113] whereas others advocated observation alone.[114]

## CENTRAL NERVOUS SYSTEM METASTASES

Metastases to the central nervous system (CNS) are uncommon and occur in less than 5% of patients with advanced testicular cancer. These patients usually have concomitant advanced pulmonary metastases and often have either pure choriocarcinoma or primary mediastinal tumors. When CNS metastases are found at the time of initial diagnosis, the patient should still be approached with curative intent. Whole-brain irradiation should be administered concurrently with cisplatin-based chemotherapy; with this strategy, 30 to 40% of patients achieve long-term survival.[115, 116]

A second group of patients in whom successful salvage therapy is possible are those who experience relapse with an "isolated" CNS metastasis. Surgical resection followed by whole-brain irradiation should be considered if the CNS metastasis is solitary. In addition, two additional courses of chemotherapy are administered. Three of four patients treated in this manner at Indiana University have enjoyed long-term survival.[117]

In patients who develop CNS metastasis at a time when they have progressive, cisplatin-resistant tumor at many other sites, treatment is ineffective and the disease is invariably fatal.

## LATE RELAPSE

Relapse occurring more than 2 years after completion of treatment is unusual, being seen in approximately 3% of patients.[118] Relapse should be distinguished from a second primary testicular cancer, which occurs in approximately 1 to 3% of cured patients. Most late relapses probably arise from residual benign teratoma not removed after completion of initial therapy. Repeat biopsy is important in these patients, because some will have unusual "non–germ cell" histologic features such as sarcoma or neuroendocrine carcinoma. In these patients, re-treatment with germ cell therapy is ineffective, and surgical resection should be considered if the tumor is localized. Patients with germ cell carcinoma at the time of repeat biopsy (or resection if possible) should undergo salvage chemotherapy, although treatment efficacy is markedly reduced in these patients.[118] Patients who are thought to have a second primary testicular cancer should undergo treatment following the same guidelines described for the initial germ cell tumor.

## Late Consequences of Chemotherapy for Testicular Cancer

After successful chemotherapy, 95% of patients return to their pretherapy functional status, and approximately 90% are in full-time employment.[119] Most of the toxicity of therapy is therefore acute, and long-term symptoms are uncommon. Nevertheless, several treatment-related toxicities have been reported.

### INFERTILITY

Infertility is common at the time of initial diagnosis of testicular cancer. In one series, 77% of patients were severely oligospermic and 17% were azoospermic.[120] After completion of cisplatin-based chemotherapy (either PVB or PEB), essentially all patients become azoospermic. After 2 years, however, 50 to 60% of patients who receive three or four courses of treatment have regained a normal sperm count.[120, 121] Patients who receive longer courses of therapy have a higher rate of permanent infertility.[122]

Long-term infertility therefore occurs in approximately 40% of patients after successful treatment and is the most frequent chemotherapy-related toxicity. It is likely that some of these patients (perhaps 10 to 15%) remain infertile because of dysgenetic abnormalities in the contralateral testis rather than as a result of the chemotherapy.

### SECOND MALIGNANCIES

Second malignancies are rare following treatment for testicular cancer. Etoposide causes secondary acute leukemia with a specific cytogenetic abnormality involving chromosome 11 (11q23).[123] This incidence of etoposide-related leukemia is less than 0.5% in patients receiving a cumulative dose of less than 2000 mg/m²,[124, 125] however, and was only 0.8% in a group of patients receiving 3750 to 5300 mg/m².[126] The usual latent period for this treatment-related leukemia is 2 to 4 years.

The risk of other solid tumors increases with time following treatment; in one large group, the observed-to-expected ratio for all solid tumors was 1:54 for 20-year survivors.[127] Most secondary solid tumors (stomach, pancreas, bladder, sarcoma) have been associated with radiotherapy rather than with chemotherapy.[128, 129]

### VASCULAR COMPLICATIONS

Raynaud's phenomenon after treatment of testicular cancer with either PVB or vinblastine and bleomycin was first described in 1981.[130] In the original reported series, 22 of 60 men (37%) developed this complication; its incidence in subsequent studies has been substantially lower (<10%). The pathogenesis is unknown.

Anecdotal reports describe more serious vascular complications. Reported complications have included myocardial infarction and thromboembolic phenomena[131, 132]; however, these reports involved small numbers of patients, and in some cases the vascular events were possibly due to problems other than the chemotherapy.

The incidence of vascular complications has been evaluated in patients with stage II nonseminoma involved in the Intergroup adjuvant study. In this study, patients either were observed without therapy, received two courses of adjuvant chemotherapy, or were treated at the time of relapse with four courses of cisplatin-based combination chemotherapy. The incidence of major vascular complications was not significantly different among the three groups of patients and failed to support a causative role for chemotherapy.[20]

## BLEOMYCIN-RELATED COMPLICATIONS

Bleomycin-related pulmonary toxicity occurs with increasing frequency at cumulative doses exceeding 300 units. Although rare, bleomycin-induced pulmonary fibrosis causes up to 50% of treatment-related fatalities in patients receiving four courses of therapy.[75] Risk factors for this complication include age older than 45 years, previous mediastinal radiation therapy, and pre-existing pulmonary disease. Patients with good-risk metastatic testicular cancer now receive only three courses of treatment and a total bleomycin dose of 270 units; the incidence of pulmonary toxicity in this group is less than 1%.

Although bleomycin pneumonitis typically produces diffuse fibrosis on chest radiography, this complication occasionally shows nodules on the chest film and simulates persistent or progressive testicular cancer.[133] The timing of the appearance of these lesions on chest radiography should make the cause easy to determine.

## Summary

Curative therapy now exists for more than 85% of patients who develop testicular cancer, and all patients should be approached with this intent. Treatment of all patients with stage I or II seminoma or nonseminoma can be accomplished safely and with minimal long-term toxicity. Patients who have stage III nonseminomatous germ cell tumors and who have favorable prognostic features also have a cure rate of approximately 90%, and carefully conducted randomized trials have made it possible to simplify treatment to minimize toxicity. Although cure can be achieved in half of the patients with poor-prognosis stage III nonseminoma, it is this group that remains the major challenge for further therapeutic improvements. Although the earlier use of high-dose therapy will probably result in some additional cures in this patient group, it is likely that major advances will necessitate the identification of new active agents. Several promising new agents, including paclitaxel and gemcitabine, are currently being evaluated in combination regimens.

## SUGGESTIONS FOR ADDITIONAL READING

Bosl GJ, Motzer RJ. Testicular germ-cell cancer. N Engl J Med 1997; 337:242–253. *A concise review of testicular cancer treatment, emphasizing recent changes in management.*

International Germ Cell Cancer Collaborative Group. International germ cell consensus classification: a prognostic factor-based staging system for metastatic germ cell cancers. J Clin Oncol 1997; 15:594–603. *A clinically applicable prognostic system distinguishes good-risk and poor-risk patients and resolves previous inconsistencies among staging systems.*

Beyer J, Kramar A, Mandanas R, et al. High-dose chemotherapy as salvage treatment in germ cell tumors: a multivariate analysis of prognostic factors. J Clin Oncol 1996;14:2638–2645. *Further definition of the role of high-dose salvage therapy.*

## REFERENCES

1. Boring CC, Squires TS, Tong T, Montgomery S. Cancer statistics, 1994. CA Cancer J Clin 1994;44:7.
2. Devesa SS, Blot WJ, Stone BJ, et al. Recent cancer trends in the United States. J Natl Cancer Inst 1995;87:175–82.
3. Farrer JH, Walker AH, Rajfer J. Management of the postpubertal cryptorchid testis: a statistical review. J Urol 1985;134:1071–6.
4. Batata M, Chu F, Hilaris B, et al. Testicular cancer in cryptorchids. Cancer 1982;49:1023.
5. Mostofi FK, Sesterhenn IA. Revised international classification of testicular tumours. In: Jones WG, Harnden P, Appleyard I, eds. Germ cell tumours. III: Advances in the biosciences. Vol. 91. Oxford, England: Pergamon Press, 1994:153–8.
6. Mostofi FK. Proceedings: testicular tumors. Epidemiologic, etiologic, and pathologic features. Cancer 1973;32:1186–201.
7. Bains MS, McCormack PM, Cvitkovic E, et al. Results of combined chemo-surgical therapy for pulmonary metastases from testicular carcinoma. Cancer 1978;41:850–3.
8. Cockburn AG, Vugrin D, Batata M, et al. Poorly differentiated (anaplastic) seminoma of the testis. Cancer 1984;53:1991–4.
9. Muller J, Skakkeback NE, Parkinson MC. The spermatocytic seminoma: views on pathogenesis. Int J Androl 1987;10:147–56.
10. Ray B, Hajdu SI, Whitmore WF Jr. Distribution of retroperitoneal lymph node metastases in testicular germinal tumors. Cancer 1974;33:340–8.
11. Donohue JP, Zachary JM, Maynard BR. Distribution of nodal metastases in nonseminomatous testis cancer. J Urol 1982;128:315–20.
12. Johnson DE, Appelt G, Samuels ML, Luna M. Metastases from testicular carcinoma. Study of 78 autopsied cases. Urology 1976;8:234–9.
13. Bosl GJ, Vogelzang NJ, Goldman A, et al. Impact of delay in diagnosis on clinical stage of testicular cancer. Lancet 1981;2:970.
14. Scher H, Bosl G, Geller N, et al. Impact of symptomatic interval on prognosis of patients with stage III testicular cancer. Urology 1983;21:559.
15. Hoskin P, Dilly S, Easton D, et al. Prognostic factors in stage I nonseminomatous germ cell testicular tumors managed by orchiectomy and surveillance: implications for adjuvant chemotherapy. J Clin Oncol 1986;4:1031.
16. Klepp O, Olsson AM, Henrikson H, et al. Prognostic factors in clinical stage I nonseminomatous germ cell tumors of the testis: multivariate analysis of a prospective multicenter study. Swedish-Norwegian Testicular Cancer Group. J Clin Oncol 1990;8:509.
17. Fung CY, Garnick MB. Clinical stage I carcinoma of the testis: a review. J Clin Oncol 1988;6:734.
18. Raghavan D, Vogelzang NJ, Bosl GJ, et al. Tumor classification and size in germ-cell testicular cancer: influence on the occurrence of metastases. Cancer 1982;50:1591.
19. Richie JP, Kantoff PW. Is adjuvant chemotherapy necessary for patients with stage B1 testicular cancer? J Clin Oncol 1991;9:1393.
20. Williams SD, Stablein DM, Einhorn LH, et al. Immediate adjuvant chemotherapy versus observation with treatment at relapse in pathological stage II testicular cancer. N Engl J Med 1987;317:1433.
21. International Germ Cell Cancer Collaborative Group. International germ cell consensus classification: a prognostic factor–based staging system for metastatic germ cell cancers. J Clin Oncol 1997;15:594–603.
22. Bosl GJ, Geller NL, Cirrincione C, et al. Multivariate analysis of prognostic variables in patients with metastatic testicular cancer. Cancer Res 1983;43:3403.
23. Birch R, Williams S, Cone A, et al. Prognostic factors for favorable outcome in disseminated germ cell tumors. J Clin Oncol 1986;4:400.

24. De Wit R, Stoter G, Sleijfer DT, et al. Four cycles of BEP versus an alternating regimen of PVB and BEP in patients with poor prognostic metastatic testicular nonseminoma: a randomized study of the EORTC Genitourinary Tract Cancer Cooperative Group. Br J Cancer 1995;71:1311.

25. Mead GM. International consensus prognostic classification for metastatic germ cell tumors treated with platinum based chemotherapy: final report of the International Germ Cell Cancer Collaborative Group (IGCCCG). Proc Am Soc Clin Oncol 1995;14:235. abstract.

26. Chang AE, Schaner EG, Conkle DM, et al. Evaluation of computed tomography in the detection of pulmonary metastases: a prospective study. Cancer 1979;43:913.

27. Stomper PC, Kalish LA, Garnick MB, et al. CT and pathologic predictive features of residual mass histologic findings after chemotherapy for nonseminomatous germ cell tumors: can residual malignancy or teratoma be excluded? Radiology 1991;180:711–4.

28. Bosl GJ, Geller NL, Chan EY. Stage migration and the increasing proportion of complete responders in patients with advanced germ cell tumors. Cancer Res 1988;48:3524.

29. Mencel PJ, Motzer RJ, Mazumdar M, et al. Advanced seminoma: treatment results, survival, and prognostic factors in 142 patients. J Clin Oncol 1994;12:120.

30. Catalona WJ, Vaitukaitis JL, Fair WR. Falsely positive specific human chorionic gonadotropin assays in patients with testicular tumors: conversion to negative with testosterone administration. J Urol 1979;122:126.

31. Epstein BE, Order SE, Zinreich ES. Staging, treatment, and results in testicular seminoma. A 12-year report. Cancer 1990;65:405–11.

32. Marks LB, Shipley WU, Walker TG, Waltman AC. Role of lymphangiography in staging testicular seminoma. Urology 1991;38:264–6.

33. Zagars GK, Babian RJ. Stage I testicular seminoma: rationale for postorchidectomy radiation therapy. Int J Radiat Oncol Biol Phys 1987;13:155.

34. Vaeth M, Schultz HP, von der Maase H, et al. Prognostic factors in testicular germ cell tumors. Acta Radiol [Oncol] 1984;23:271.

35. Butcher DN, Gregory WM, Gunter PA, et al. The biological and clinical significance of hCG-containing cells in seminoma. Br J Cancer 1985;51:473.

36. Hamilton C, Horwich A, Easton D, Peckham M. Radiotherapy for stage I seminoma testis: results of treatment and complications. Radiother Oncol 1986;6:115.

37. Thomas G, Rider W, Dembo A, et al. Seminoma of the testis: results of treatment and patterns of failure after radiation therapy. Int J Radiat Oncol Biol Phys 1982;8:165.

38. Dosoretz DE, Shipley WU, Blitzer PH, et al. Megavoltage irradiation for pure testicular seminoma: results and patterns of failure. Cancer 1981;48:2184–90.

39. Willan BD, McGowan DG. Seminoma of the testis: a 22-year experience with radiation therapy. Int J Radiat Oncol Biol Phys 1985;11:1769–75.

40. Lederman GS, Sheldon TA, Chaffey JT, et al. Cardiac disease after mediastinal irradiation for seminoma. Cancer 1987;60:772–6.

41. Warde P, Gospodarowicz MK, Panzarella T, et al. Stage I testicular seminoma: results of adjuvant irradiation and surveillance. J Clin Oncol 1995;13:2255.

42. Warde P, Gospodarowicz M, Panzarella T, et al. Management of stage II seminoma. J Clin Oncol 1998;16:290–4.

43. Horwich A. Surveillance for stage I seminoma of the testis. In: Horwich A, ed. Testicular cancer: investigation and management. London: Chapman & Hall, 1991:109.

44. Sharda NN, Kinsella TJ, Ritter MA. Adjuvant radiation versus observation: a cost analysis of alternate management schemes in early-stage testicular seminoma. J Clin Oncol 1996;14:2933–9.

45. Buchholz TA, Walden TL, Prestidge BR. Cost-effectiveness of post-treatment surveillance after radiation therapy for early stage seminoma. Cancer 1998;82:1126–33.

46. Zagars G, Babaian J. The role of radiation in stage II testicular seminoma. Int J Radiat Oncol Biol Phys 1987;13:163.

47. Gregory C, Peckham M. Results of radiotherapy for stage II testicular seminoma. Radiother Oncol 1986;6:285–92.

48. Ellerbroek N, Tran L, Selch M, et al. Testicular seminoma: a study of 103 cases treated at UCLA. Am J Clin Oncol 1988;11:93.

49. Loehrer PJ, Birch R, Williams SD, et al. Chemotherapy of metastatic seminoma: the Southeastern Cancer Study Group experience. J Clin Oncol 1987;5:1212.

50. Horwich A, Dearnaley DP, Duchesne GM, et al. Simple nontoxic treatment of advanced metastatic seminoma with carboplatin. J Clin Oncol 1989;7:1150–6.

51. Motzer R, Bosl GS, Heelan R, et al. Residual mass: an indication for further therapy in patients with advanced seminoma following systemic chemotherapy. J Clin Oncol 1987;5:1064–71.

52. Puc HS, Heelan R, Mazumdan M, et al. Management of residual mass in advanced seminoma: results and recommendations from the Memorial Sloan-Kettering Cancer Center. J Clin Oncol 1996;14:454–460.

53. Schultz SM, Einhorn LH, Conces DJ Jr, et al. Management of postchemotherapy residual mass in patients with advanced seminoma: Indiana University experience. J Clin Oncol 1989;7:1497–1503.

54. Herr H, Bosl GJ. Residual mass after chemotherapy for seminoma. J Urol 1987:137;1234.

55. Johnson DE, Lo RK, von Eschenback A, et al. Surveillance alone for patients with clinical stage I non-seminomatous germ cell tumors of the testis: preliminary results. J Urol 1984;131:491–3.

56. Pizzocaro G, Zanoni F, Salvioni R, et al. Surveillance or lymph node dissection in clinical stage I non-seminomatous germinal testis cancer? Br J Urol 1985;57:759–62.

57. Freedman LS, Jones WG, Peckham MJ, et al. Histopathology in the prediction of relapse of patients with stage I testicular teratoma treated by orchiectomy alone. Lancet 1987;2:294–8.

58. Gelderman WA, Schraffordt Koops H, Sleijfer DT, et al. Orchidectomy alone in stage I nonseminomatous testicular germ cell tumors. Cancer 1987;59:578–80.

59. Rorth M, Jacobson GK, von der Maase H, et al. Surveillance alone versus radiotherapy after orchiectomy for clinical stage I nonseminomatous testicular cancer. J Clin Oncol 1991;9:1543–8.

60. Raghavan D, Colis B, Levi J, et al. Surveillance for stage I non-seminomatous germ cell tumours of the testis: the optimal protocol has not yet been defined. Br J Urol 1988;61:522–6.

61. Sogani P. Evolution of the management of stage I nonseminomatous germ-cell tumor of the testis. Urol Clin North Am 1991;18:561.

62. Thompson PI, Nixon J, Harvey VJ. Distant relapse in patients with stage I non-seminomatous germ cell tumor of the testis on active surveillance. J Clin Oncol 1988;6:1597–1603.

63. Read G, Stenning S, Cullen M, et al. A Medical Research Council prospective study of surveillance for stage I testicular teratoma. J Clin Oncol 1992;10:1762–71.

64. Oliver RTD, Raja M, Ong J, Gallagher C. Pilot study to evaluate impact of a policy of adjuvant chemotherapy for high risk stage I malignant teratoma on overall relapse rate of stage I cancer patients. J Urol 1992;148:1453.

65. Narayan P, Lange P, Fraley E. Ejaculation and fertility after extended retroperitoneal lymph node dissection for testicular cancer. J Urol 1982;127:685.

66. Richie J. Clinical stage I testicular cancer: the role of modified retroperitoneal lymphadenectomy. J Urol 1990;144:1160.

67. Pont J, Albrecht W, Postner G, et al. Adjuvant chemotherapy for high-risk clinical stage I nonseminomatous testicular germ cell cancer: long term results of a prospective trial. J Clin Oncol 1996;14:441–9.

68. Cullen MH, Stenning SP, Parkinson MC, et al. Short-course adjuvant chemotherapy in high-risk stage I nonseminomatous germ cell tumors of the testis: a Medical Research Council report. J Clin Oncol 1996;14:1106–13.

69. Donohue J, Zachary J, Maynard B. Distribution of nodal metastases in nonseminomatous testis cancer. J Urol 1982;128:315.

70. Logothetis CJ, Swanson DA, Dexeus F, et al. Primary chemotherapy for clinical stage II nonseminomatous germ cell tumors of the testis: a follow-up of 50 patients. J Clin Oncol 1987;5:906–11.

71. Motzer RJ, Sheinfeld J, Mazumdar M, et al. Etoposide and cisplatin adjuvant therapy for patients with pathologic stage II germ cell tumors. J Clin Oncol 1995;13:2700.

72. Samuels ML, Johnson EE, Holoye PY. Continuous intravenous bleomycin therapy with vinblastine in stage III testicular neoplasia. Cancer Chemother Rep 1975;59:563–8.

73. Einhorn LH, Donohue JP. *Cis*-diamminedichloroplatinum, vinblastine, and bleomycin combination chemotherapy in disseminated testicular cancer. Ann Intern Med 1977;87:293–9.

74. Bosl GJ, Gluckman R, Geller NL, et al. VAB-6: an effective chemotherapy regimen for patients with germ-cell tumors. J Clin Oncol 1986;4:1493.

75. Williams SD, Birch R, Einhorn LH, et al. Treatment of disseminated

germ-cell tumors with cisplatin, bleomycin, and either vinblastine or etoposide. N Engl J Med 1987;316:1435.

76. Loehrer PJ, Lauer R, Roth BJ, et al. Salvage therapy in recurrent germ cell cancer: ifosfamide and cisplatin plus either vinblastine or etoposide. Ann Intern Med 1988;109:540.

77. Einhorn LH, Williams SD. Chemotherapy of disseminated testicular cancer. Cancer 1980;46:1339–44.

78. Stoter G, Sleyfer DT, ten Bokkel Huinink WW, et al. High-dose versus low-dose vinblastine in cisplatin-vinblastine-bleomycin combination chemotherapy of nonseminomatous testicular cancer: a randomized study of the EORTC Genitourinary Tract Cancer Cooperative Group. J Clin Oncol 1986;4:1199–206.

79. Einhorn L, Williams S, Troner M, et al. The role of maintenance therapy in disseminated testicular cancer. N Engl J Med 1981; 305:727–9.

80. Hainsworth JD, Williams SD, Einhorn LH, et al. Successful treatment of resistant germinal neoplasms with VP-16 and cisplatin: results of a Southeastern Cancer Study Group trial. J Clin Oncol 1985;3:666–71.

81. Einhorn LH, Williams SD, Loehrer PJ, et al. Evaluation of optimal duration of chemotherapy in favorable-prognosis disseminated germ cell tumors: a Southeastern Cancer Study Group protocol. J Clin Oncol 1989;7:387–91.

82. Saxman SB, Finch D, Gonin R, Einhorn LH. Long-term follow-up of a phase III study of three versus four cycles of bleomycin, etoposide, and cisplatin in favorable prognosis germ-cell tumors: the Indiana University experience. J Clin Oncol 1998;16:702–6.

83. Bosl GJ, Geller NL, Bajorin D, et al. A randomized trial of etoposide-+cisplatin versus vinblastine + bleomycin + cisplatin + cyclophosphamide + dactinomycin in patients with good-prognosis germ cell tumors. J Clin Oncol 1988;6:1231.

84. Bajorin DF, Sarosdy MF, Pfister DG, et al. Randomized trial of etoposide and cisplatin versus etoposide and carboplatin in patients with good-risk germ cell tumors: a multi-institutional study. J Clin Oncol 1993;11:598.

85. Xiao H, Mazumdar M, Bajorin DF, et al. Long-term follow-up of patients with good-risk germ cell tumors treated with etoposide and cisplatin. J Clin Oncol 1997;15:2553–8.

86. Loehrer PJ, Johnson DH, Elson P, et al. Importance of bleomycin in favorable-prognosis disseminated germ cell tumors: an Eastern Cooperative Oncology Group Trial. J Clin Oncol 1995;13:470.

87. Horwich A, Sleijfer DT, Fossa SD, et al. Randomized trial of bleomycin, etoposide, and cisplatin compared with bleomycin, etoposide, and carboplatin in good-prognosis metastatic nonseminomatous germ cell cancer: a Multi-institutional Medical Research Council/European Organization for Research and Treatment of Cancer trial. J Clin Oncol 1997;15:1844–52.

88. Ozols RF, Ihde DC, Linehan WM, et al. A randomized trial of standard chemotherapy versus a high-dose chemotherapy regimen in the treatment of poor prognosis nonseminomatous germ-cell tumors. J Clin Oncol 1988;6:1031.

89. Nichols CR, Williams SD, Loehrer PJ, et al. Randomized study of cisplatin dose intensity in poor-risk germ cell tumors: a Southeastern Oncology Group protocol. J Clin Oncol 1991;9:1163.

90. Stoter G, Sleijfer DT, Schornagel JH, et al. BEP versus VIP in intermediate risk patients with disseminated non-seminomatous testicular cancer. Proc Am Soc Clin Oncol 1993;12:232. abstract.

91. Nichols CR, Catalano PJ, Crawford ED, et al. Randomized comparison of cisplatin and etoposide and either bleomycin or ifosfamide in treatment of advanced disseminated germ tumors: an Eastern Cooperative Oncology Group, Southeast Oncology Group, and Cancer and Leukemia Group B study. J Clin Oncol 1998;16:1287–93.

92. Kaye SB, Mead GM, Fossa S, et al. Intensive induction-sequential chemotherapy with BOP/VIP-B compared with treatment with BEP-EP for poor-prognosis metastatic nonseminomatous germ cell tumor: a randomized Medical Research Council/European Organization for Research and Treatment of Cancer study. J Clin Oncol 1998;16:692–701.

93. Motzer RJ, Mazumdar M, Bajorin DF, et al. High dose carboplatin, etoposide, and cyclophosphamide with autologous bone marrow transplantation in first-line therapy for patients with poor-risk germ cell tumors. J Clin Oncol 1997;15:2546–52.

94. Debono DJ, Heilman DK, Einhorn LH, Donohue JP. Decision analysis for avoiding postchemotherapy surgery in patients with disseminated nonseminomatous germ cell tumors. J Clin Oncol 1971;5:1455–64.

95. Steyerberg EW, Keizer HJ, Fosser SD, et al. Prediction of residual retroperitoneal mass histology after chemotherapy for metastatic non-seminomatous germ cell tumor: multivariate analysis of individual patient data from six study groups. J Clin Oncol 1995;13:1177–87.

96. Gelderman WA, Schraffordt Koops H, Sleijfer DT, et al. Results of adjuvant surgery in patients with stage III and IV nonseminomatous testicular tumors after cisplatin-vinblastine-bleomycin chemotherapy. J Surg Oncol 1988;38:227.

97. Sonneveld DJA, Sliejfer DT, Koops HS, et al. Mature teratoma identified after postchemotherapy surgery in patients with disseminated nonseminomatous testicular germ cell tumors: a plea for an aggressive surgical approach. Cancer 1998;82:1343–51.

98. Lorigan J, Efterhari F, David C, et al. The growing teratoma syndrome: an unusual manifestation of treated nonseminomatous germ cell tumors of the testis. AJR Am J Roentgenol 1988;151:325.

99. Logothetis CJ, Samuels ML, Trindade A, et al. The growing teratoma syndrome. Cancer 1982;50:1629.

100. Baniel J, Foster RS, Gonin R, et al. Late relapse of testicular cancer. J Clin Oncol 1995;13:1170–6.

101. Fox E, Weathers T, Williams S, et al. Outcome analysis for patients with persistent nonteratomatous germ cell tumor in postchemotherapy retroperitoneal lymph node dissections. J Clin Oncol 1993;11:1294.

102. Motzer RJ, Cooper K, Geller NL, et al. The role of ifosfamide plus cisplatin-based chemotherapy as salvage therapy for patients with refractory germ cell tumors. Cancer 1990;66:2476.

103. Cooper MA, Einhorn LH. Maintenance chemotherapy with daily oral etoposide following salvage therapy in patients with germ cell tumors. J Clin Oncol 1995;13:1167–9.

104. Broun ER, Nichols CR, Kneebone P, et al. Long-term outcome of patients with relapsed and refractory germ cell tumors treated with high-dose chemotherapy and autologous bone marrow rescue. Ann Intern Med 1992;117:124.

105. Linkesch W, Greinix HT, Hocker P, et al. Long term follow up of phase I/II trial of ultra-high carboplatin, VP 16, cyclophosphamide with ABMT in refractory or relapsed NSGCT. Proc Am Soc Clin Oncol 1993;12:232. abstract.

106. Motzer R, Mazumdar M, Bosl GJ, et al. High-dose carboplatin, etoposide, and cyclophosphamide for patients with refractory germ cell tumors: treatment results and prognostic factors for survival and toxicity. J Clin Oncol 1996;14:1098.

107. Motzer RJ, Mazumdar M, Gulati SC, et al. Phase II trial of high-dose carboplatin and etoposide with autologous bone marrow transplantation in first-line therapy for patients with poor-risk germ cell tumors. J Natl Cancer Inst 1993;85:1828.

108. Motzer RJ, Gulati SC, Crown JP, et al. High-dose chemotherapy and autologous bone marrow rescue for patients with refractory germ cell tumors: early intervention is better tolerated. Cancer 1992;69:550.

109. Margolin K, Doroshow JH, Ahn C, et al. Treatment of germ cell cancer with two cycles of high-dose ifosfamide, carboplatin, and etoposide with autologous stem-cell support. J Clin Oncol 1996;14:2631–7.

110. Broun ER, Nichols CR, Turns M, et al. Early salvage therapy for germ cell cancer using high dose chemotherapy with autologous bone marrow support. Cancer 1990;73:1716–20.

111. Broun ER, Nichols CR, Gize G, et al. Tandem high dose chemotherapy with autologous bone marrow transplantation for initial relapse of testicular germ cell cancer. Cancer 1997;79:1605–10.

112. Beyer J, Kramar A, Mandanos R, et al. High-dose chemotherapy as salvage treatment in germ cell tumors: a multivariate analysis of prognostic variables. J Clin Oncol 1996;14:2638–45.

113. Greist A, Einhorn LH, Williams SD, et al. Pathologic findings at orchiectomy following chemotherapy for disseminated testicular cancer. J Clin Oncol 1984;2:1025.

114. Chong C, Logothetis CJ, von Eschenback A, et al. Orchiectomy in advanced germ cell cancer following intensive chemotherapy: a comparison of systemic to testicular response. J Urol 1986; 136:1221–3.

115. Rustin GJS, Newlands ES, Bagshawe KD, et al. Successful management of metastatic and primary germ cell tumors in the brain. Cancer 1986;57:2108–13.

116. Bokemeyer C, Nowak P, Haupt A, et al. Treatment of brain metastases in patients with testicular cancer. J Clin Oncol 1997;15:1449–54.

117. Spears WT, Morphis G, Lester G, et al. Brain metastases and testicular tumors; long-term survival. Int J Radiat Oncol Biol Phys 1991;22:17–22.

118. Baniel J, Foster RS, Gonin R, et al. Late relapse of testicular cancer. J Clin Oncol 1995;13:1170–6.

119. Roth BJ, Greist A, Kubilis PS, et al. Cisplatin-based combination chemotherapy for disseminated germ cell tumors: long-term follow-up. J Clin Oncol 1988;6:1239–47.

120. Drasga RE, Einhorn LH, Williams SD, et al. Fertility after chemotherapy for testicular cancer. J Clin Oncol 1983;1:179.

121. Leitner SP, Bosl GJ, Bajorunas D. Gonadal dysfunction in patients treated for metastatic germ-cell tumors. J Clin Oncol 1986;4:1500

122. Lampe H, Horwich A, Norman A, et al. Fertility after chemotherapy for testicular germ cell cancers. J Clin Oncol 1997;15:239–45.

123. DeVore R, Whitlock J, Hainsworth JD, Johnson DH. Therapy-related acute nonlymphocytic leukemia with monocytic morphology and re-arrangement of chromosome 11q. Ann Intern Med 1989;110:740–2.

124. Bajorin DF, Motzer RJ, Rodriquez E, et al. Acute nonlymphocytic leukemia in germ cell tumor patients treated with etoposide-containing chemotherapy. J Natl Cancer Inst 1993;85:60.

125. Nichols CR, Breeden ES, Loehrer PJ. Secondary leukemia associated with a conventional dose of etoposide: review of serial germ cell tumor protocols. J Natl Cancer Inst 1993;85:36.

126. Bokemeyer C, Schmoll H, Kuczyk M, et al. Risk of secondary leukemia following high cumulative doses of etoposide during chemotherapy for testicular cancer. J Natl Cancer Inst 1995;58:58.

127. Travis LB, Curtis RE, Storm H, et al. Risk of second malignant neoplasms among long-term survivors of testicular cancer. J Natl Cancer Inst 1997;89:1429–39.

128. Van Leeuwen F, Stiggelbout A, van den Belt-Dusebout A, et al. Second cancer risk following testicular cancer: a followup study of 1,909 patients. J Clin Oncol 1993;11:415.

129. Jacobsen G, Mellemgaard A, Engelholm S, Moller H. Increased incidence of sarcoma in patients treated for testicular seminoma. Eur J Cancer 1993;29A:664.

130. Vogelzang NJ, Bosl GJ, Johnson K, Kennedy BJ. Raynaud's phenomenon: a common toxicity after combination chemotherapy for testicular cancer. Ann Intern Med 1981;95:288.

131. Doll DC, List AF, Greco FA, et al. Acute vascular ischemic events after cisplatin-based combination chemotherapy for germ cell tumors of the testis. Ann Intern Med 1986;105:48–52.

132. Stoter G, Koopman A, Vendrik C, et al. Ten-year survival and late sequelae in testicular cancer patients treated with cisplatin, vinblastine, and bleomycin. J Clin Oncol 1989;7:1099.

133. Nachman JB, Baum ES, White H, Cruissi FG. Bleomycin-induced pulmonary fibrosis mimicking recurrent metastatic disease in a patient with testicular carcinoma: case report of the CT scan appearance. Cancer 1981;47:236–9.

# PART

# XII

# GYNECOLOGIC NEOPLASMS

• JONATHAN S. BEREK

Gynecologic malignancies will account for more than 77,000 new cases of invasive cancer in women in the United States in 2000. There were more than 36,000 new cases of uterine corpus cancer, more than 23,000 cases of ovarian cancer, and nearly 13,000 cases of invasive cervical cancers. As the cause of cancer death in women, gynecologic cancers rank fourth after respiratory, breast, and gastrointestinal cancers.

The management of gynecologic malignancies involves the use of all cancer therapeutic modalities in a manner that can best control locally invasive as well as metastatic tumors. The subspecialty of gynecologic oncology has evolved to train individuals who can undertake the surgical treatment of these tumors and coordinate the chemotherapy, radiation therapy, and psychosocial counseling necessary for the integrated management of patients with gynecologic malignancy.

# CHAPTER 55

# OVARY AND FALLOPIAN TUBES

## OVARY

• Lee-may Chen • Jonathan S. Berek

Ovarian cancer is the fifth most common cancer in women in the United States, accounting for the most common cause of death among women who develop gynecologic malignancies. In 2000, an estimated 23,100 American women will be diagnosed with ovarian cancer, and 14,000 will succumb to this disease.[1]

Ovarian malignancies fall into the general categories of epithelial tumors, germ cell tumors, sex cord–stromal tumors, and various mixtures of these groups. In addition, the ovary is a site of metastatic carcinomas, such as in breast cancer or Krukenberg's tumors. Approximately 90% of ovarian cancers are derived from coelomic mesothelium and are classified as epithelial ovarian cancers.

## Etiology and Epidemiology

The incidence of ovarian cancer varies in different geographic locations. Western regions, including the United States, Great Britain, and Scandinavia, have rates about three to seven times greater than Japan, where the tumors are relatively rare. Japanese immigrants to the United States experience a significant increase in the incidence of ovarian cancer, approaching that of women born in the United States. There appears to be a racial difference as well in that U.S. whites develop ovarian cancers almost 1.5 times more frequently than do U.S. blacks.[2]

Population-based studies have identified family history as one of the strongest risk factors for the development of ovarian cancer, and the genetics of ovarian cancer is one area of active investigation. Epidemiologic studies have not identified any consistent predisposing factors associated with ovarian cancer, but patient characteristics that have been associated with an increased risk of epithelial ovarian cancer include white race, nulligravity, late age of menopause, a family history of cancer of the ovary or endometrium, and prolonged intervals of ovulation. The Collaborative Ovarian Cancer Group evaluated menstrual characteristics, reproductive characteristics, exogenous hormone use, and prior pelvic surgeries in an analysis of 12 U.S. case-control studies (Table 55–1).[3, 4]

Reproductive factors seem to play a role, including infertility and inability to conceive. The increased prevalence of disease in single women, including nuns, and in nulliparous married women suggests that incessant ovulation, uninterrupted by pregnancy, may predispose women to develop neoplastic changes. Use of fertility drugs to induce ovulation have been implicated in increasing the risk of ovarian cancer,

particularly for borderline tumors.[5, 6] A careful analysis of the various case series demonstrated that infertility treatment did not appear to increase the risk for cancer independently but rather that infertility by itself was an independent risk factor.[7]

Use of oral contraceptives actually decreases the risk of ovarian cancer and endometrial cancer. In a meta-analysis of 20 studies addressing the effects of oral contraceptive pills on ovarian cancer, Hankinson and colleagues found a relative risk of 0.64 associated with any previous use of the pill in both nulliparas and multiparas.[8] Even 3 to 6 months of contraceptive use appears to significantly decrease the relative risk for ovarian cancer.[9] The effects of oral contraceptives appear to remain protective for up to 10 years after cessation of use.

Prior use of postmenopausal hormone replacement has not been shown to alter the risk of epithelial ovarian cancer. There is no association with prior radiation exposure. Unlike cervical cancer, infectious agents, including viruses, have not been associated with this disease. In addition, risk factors associated with the development of endometrial cancer, such as obesity, hypertension, and diabetes, have not been associated with ovarian cancer.

It has been speculated that a causative agent or potentiator could enter the peritoneal cavity through the lower genital tract and spread upward through the uterus and fallopian tubes. Asbestos-contaminated talc was linked to epithelial tumors in one case-control study.[10] Tubal ligation, and to a lesser extent hysterectomy, have been observed to decrease the risk of ovarian cancer by at least one-third.[11] Proposed mechanisms of ovarian cancer protection by tubal ligation include interruption of access to the peritoneal cavity or disruption of ovarian circulation, resulting in less exposure to gonadotropins.

*Table 55–1.* **Risk Factors Associated with Ovarian Cancer**

| Risk Factor | Relative Risk |
| --- | --- |
| Unprotected intercourse >15 yr | 1.6 |
| Infertility with use of fertility drugs | 2.8 |
| Nulligravity | 27 |
| Parity | 0.47 |
| Breast-feeding | 0.81 |
| Oral contraceptive use | 0.66 |
| Tubal ligation | 0.59 |

Adapted from Whittemore AS, Harris R, Intyre J, and the Collaborative Ovarian Cancer Group. Characteristics relating to ovarian cancer risk: collaborative analysis of 12 U.S. case-control studies. II: invasive epithelial ovarian cancers in white women. Am J Epidemiol 1992;136:1184–1203.

## Genetics

The lifetime risk of ovarian carcinoma for women in the United States is about 1.8%.[12] With a positive family history, a woman's risk increases threefold.[13, 14] Most epithelial ovarian cancer is sporadic, with familial or hereditary patterns accounting for less than 15% of all malignancies. Hereditary ovarian cancers generally occur about 10 years earlier than do sporadic lesions. These hereditary cancers have been described in several different syndromes: site-specific ovarian cancer, breast-ovarian cancer, and the Lynch II cancer family syndrome.[15, 16]

Family pedigree analysis of site-specific and breast-ovarian cancers led to the discovery of two genetic susceptibility genes: *BRCA1* and *BRCA2*. The *BRCA1* gene maps to chromosome 17q12–21, and accounts for a significant number of early-onset breast cancers and hereditary ovarian cancers.[17] The *BRCA2* gene maps to chromosome 13q12–13, is associated with male breast cancer, and has a lower penetrance for ovarian cancer than does *BRCA1*.[18, 19] Both are large genes and are predicted to have tumor suppressor functions.[17, 20]

Founder effects of *BRCA1* and *BRCA2* have been identified in several populations, most notably in Ashkenazi Jews in whom up to 2.5% of the population carries one of four genetic mutations: 185delAG, 188del11, and 5382insC mutations in *BRCA1*, and 6174delT mutations in *BRCA2*.[21, 22] Less than 0.5% of the general population carries mutations to *BRCA1* or *BRCA2*. Overall, there are hundreds of mutations identified in *BRCA1* and *BRCA2*, with diverse phenotypes and degrees of penetration. Thus the allelic heterogeneity of these genes confounds our ability to predict the significance of disease for all mutation carriers. The attributable risk of *BRCA1* and *BRCA2* was originally estimated from high-risk families, but with further analysis, the risk of breast cancer in *BRCA1* mutation carriers is 16% by age 70, and the risk of breast cancer is 56%.[23, 24] In addition, there also may be an increased risk for colon cancer, as well as for prostate cancer in male carriers of *BRCA1*.

The use of oral contraceptives has been found to reduce the incidence of ovarian carcinoma in *BRCA1* and *BRCA2* families to a similar degree as that in the general population.[25] Prophylactic oophorectomies have also been recommended after childbearing for mutation carriers, yet they do not completely eliminate the possibility of ovarian cancer.[26, 27]

The Lynch II syndrome describes hereditary nonpolyposis colorectal cancer (HNPCC) associated with other cancers, in particular endometrial, ovarian, urogenital, and other gastrointestinal primaries.[28] Although colorectal cancer is the hallmark disease for HNPCC, endometrial cancer is the second most common malignancy for affected women, and an increased risk of ovarian cancer also exists.[29] Several genes involved with DNA mismatch repair have been associated with HNPCC, including hMSH2, hMLH1, hPMS1, and hPMS2.[30–32]

In all these syndromes, women at risk benefit from a thorough pedigree analysis. A geneticist should evaluate the family pedigree for at least three generations if possible. Decisions about management are best made after careful study and, whenever possible, histologic diagnosis of the family members' ovarian cancer. In 1996, the American Society of Clinical Oncology released a statement regarding

**Table 55–2. Ovarian Cancer Screening Recommendations for Familial Cancer Patients**

| | |
|---|---|
| BRCA1 and BRCA2 | Transvaginal ultrasonography, with color Doppler, every 6–12 mo; begin at age 25–35 |
| HNPCC | Routine surveillance; consider screening if observed in family members |

Data from the Cancer Genetics Study Consortium: Burke W, Daly M, Garber J, et al. Recommendations for follow-up care of individuals with an inherited predisposition to cancer. II: BRCA1 and BRCA2. JAMA 1997;277:997–1003 and Burke W, Petersen G, Lynch P, et al. Recommendations for follow-up care of individuals with an inherited predisposition to cancer. I: hereditary nonpolyposis colon cancer. JAMA 1997;277:915–19.
HNPCC, hereditary nonpolyposis colorectal cancer.

guidelines for indications, the need for appropriate counseling, and informed consent as part of genetic testing for cancer susceptibility.[33]

The management of a woman with a strong family history of epithelial ovarian cancer depends on her age, reproductive plans, and the extent of risk. The plan must be individualized because the value of screening with transvaginal ultrasonography, CA-125 levels, or other procedures has not been clearly established in women at high risk. Current recommendations for screening in high-risk women as outlined by the Cancer Genetics Study Consortium are summarized in Table 55–2.[34, 35]

## Clinical Features and Diagnosis

The diagnosis of an ovarian malignancy is typically made or confirmed at the time of exploratory laparotomy performed for pelvic masses. Symptoms, if present, may not be severe or specific enough to prompt women to seek medical attention. In many cases, malignancy may be unexpected and may already have spread beyond the ovaries at the time of diagnosis. Routine pelvic examination, including cervical and vaginal cytologic evaluation, is of limited value in the early detection of ovarian cancer. Furthermore, no consistently reliable radiologic or serologic screening test is yet available for ovarian neoplasms, prompting the 1994 National Institutes of Health Consensus Conference on Ovarian Cancer to conclude that "there is not evidence available as yet that the current screening modalities of CA-125 and transvaginal ultrasonography can be effectively used for widespread disease screening."[36]

### SCREENING

An ideal screening test is inexpensive, convenient, and has high sensitivity and specificity for detecting early disease. Only detection of early stage disease would affect morbidity or mortality. In contrast to the cervix, colon, or breast, the location of the ovaries in the peritoneal cavity limits their accessibility for direct examination or screening. Screening women in the general population with current technologies has been ineffective for detecting early ovarian cancer. Only 29 cases of ovarian cancer were detected among 36,208 women participating in screening programs; of these cases, only 12 were diagnosed with stage I disease.[37] Focusing on volunteers with a positive family history, 7 cases of ovarian cancer (6 with stage I disease) were detected in more than 3100 patients screened.

Transvaginal ultrasonography has been found to be sensitive in detecting early changes of the ovary associated with tumor growth, but the specificity and positive predictive value limit its use for widespread screening. In a review of prospective ultrasonographic and Doppler screening trials for ovarian cancer, only five cases of stage I invasive epithelial ovarian carcinoma were detected among 11,283 asymptomatic women.[38] To diagnose these five cases, 486 surgical procedures were performed, which averages to 32 surgeries required to diagnose one woman with stage I ovarian cancer. An arbitrary minimal positive predictive value has been set at 10%, suggesting that it would be acceptable to perform 9 surgeries for a false-positive screening test result for each case of ovarian cancer detected.[39]

CA-125 has been found useful in monitoring ovarian cancer, but elevations in CA-125 have been associated with other malignancies, benign conditions such as endometriosis, and even physiologic conditions, including pregnancy and menstruation. CA-125 is elevated in 80 to 85% of ovarian cancer patients, although only 50% have an elevation in stage I disease.[40] If a palpable mass is present, the CA-125 measurement has a positive predictive value of 82% for malignancies.

The specificity of CA-125 may be improved by combining the test with transvaginal ultrasonography or by following the CA-125 levels over time.[39, 41] Using CA-125, followed by abdominal ultrasonography if the CA-125 results were abnormal, Jacobs and colleagues screened 22,000 perimenopausal and postmenopausal women. Forty-one surgeries were performed, which diagnosed 11 cases of ovarian cancer, of which 4 cases were stage I or stage II.[42] On a larger scale, the Prostate, Lung, Colorectal, and Ovary Trial by the National Cancer Institute is in progress to determine whether a 35% decrease in cause-specific mortality can be detected by randomizing 74,000 postmenopausal women with surveillance versus screening with bimanual examination, CA-125 assays, transvaginal ultrasonography, and follow-up for 10 years.[43]

Screening is likely to have the greatest impact in postmenopausal women and ovarian cancer families. At this time, the only recommendations for screening are for women with hereditary cancer syndromes (see Table 55–2).[34, 35] In the future, new markers or technologies may improve the specificity of ovarian cancer screening, but additional study is necessary at this time.

## SYMPTOMS

Most women with epithelial ovarian cancer have vague, nonspecific symptoms.[44, 45] In premenopausal women, menstrual cycles may or may not be regular. If a pelvic mass is compressing the bladder or rectum, she may report urinary frequency or constipation. Occasionally, she may perceive lower abdominal distention or pressure or dyspareunia. Acute symptoms from rupture or torsion are unusual.

In advanced stage disease, patients most often present with symptoms of abdominal distention, bloating, constipation, nausea, anorexia, or early satiety. These symptoms are related to the presence of ascites, omental metastases, or bowel metastases.

## SIGNS

The most important sign is the presence of a pelvic mass on physical examination. A solid, irregular, fixed pelvic mass is highly suggestive of an ovarian malignancy. If a concomitant upper abdominal mass or ascites is present, the diagnosis of ovarian cancer is almost certain. Although the patient usually complains of abdominal symptoms, a pelvic examination should always be performed, lest the presence of a pelvic tumor be missed.

## DIAGNOSIS

The diagnosis of a pelvic mass ultimately requires surgery. The premenopausal patient may undergo a period of observation if the adnexal mass is not clinically suspicious. A cystic mass larger than 8 cm in diameter is likely to be neoplastic. Patients who have solid, fixed, irregularly shaped masses should undergo surgery. Masses that are mobile, cystic, unilateral, and regular in contour may be followed over a period of 2 months. Oral contraceptives may be used to suppress the ovaries hormonally. Lesions that are not neoplastic should regress, as measured by pelvic examination or ultrasonography. If the mass does not regress or increases in size, it must be presumed to be neoplastic and must be removed surgically.

Before the planned exploration, routine hematologic and biochemical assessments should be performed. A preoperative evaluation should include a chest radiograph. Abdominal and pelvic computed tomography (CT) or magnetic resonance imaging (MRI) is not necessary in a patient with a definite pelvic mass but may be helpful in evaluating the urinary tract. Patients with ascites and no pelvic mass should have a computed tomographic or MRI scan with particular attention to the possibility of a liver or pancreatic tumor. The findings rarely preclude laparotomy. Liver-spleen, bone, and brain scans are unnecessary unless symptoms or signs suggest metastases to these sites.

The preoperative evaluation should exclude other primary cancers metastatic to the ovary. Any patient with occult blood in the stool or evidence of intestinal obstruction should be evaluated for a primary colon tumor. A barium enema scan is a more sensitive test than CT. An upper gastrointestinal series is indicated if there are symptoms indicating gastric involvement. Bilateral mammography should be performed in the presence of a breast mass, as breast cancer metastatic to the ovaries can clinically simulate ovarian cancer.

Papanicolau screening of the cervix should be up to date, although its value in the detection of ovarian cancer is limited. Patients who have irregular menses or postmenopausal bleeding should undergo endocervical curettage and endometrial biopsy to exclude the presence of endocervical or endometrial cancer that may be metastatic to the ovary.

## DIFFERENTIAL DIAGNOSIS

Epithelial cancers of the ovary must be differentiated from benign neoplasms and functional cysts. A variety of benign conditions of the reproductive tract can simulate ovarian cancer, such as endometriosis, a pedunculated uterine leiomyoma, and pelvic inflammatory disease. Nongynecologic causes of a pelvic tumor include an inflammatory or neoplastic colon process or metastatic disease. Tumor markers such as CA-125 and carcinoembryonic antigen (CEA) may be useful in distinguishing malignant from benign pelvic masses.[46]

## PATTERNS OF SPREAD

Epithelial ovarian cancers spread primarily by exfoliation of cells into the peritoneal cavity, by lymphatic channels, and by hematogenous spread. The most common and earliest mode of dissemination is by exfoliation of cells that implant along the surfaces of the peritoneal cavity. The cells tend to follow the circulatory path of peritoneal fluid, often moving with the forces of respiration from the pelvis, up the paracolic gutters (especially on the right), along the intestinal mesenteries, and to the right hemidiaphragm. Metastases are typically seen on the posterior cul-de sac, the paracolic gutters, the right diaphragm, the liver capsule, the surfaces of the intestines, and the omentum. The disease seldom invades the intestinal lumen but progressively agglutinates loops of bowel, leading to functional intestinal obstruction, or carcinomatous ileus.

Lymphatic dissemination to the pelvic and para-aortic lymph nodes is common, particularly in clinically advanced disease.[47, 48] Spread through the lymphatic channels of the retroperitoneal lymph nodes and the diaphragm can lead to dissemination of disease into the supraclavicular lymph nodes and pleural space.

Hematogenous dissemination of disease at the time of diagnosis is uncommon, with only 2 to 3% of patients found to have parenchymal involvement of the lungs or liver. Most patients with disease above the diaphragm have a right pleural effusion.[49] Systemic metastases are seen more frequently in patients who have survived for some years. Distant metastases ultimately developed in 38% of patients who originally had intraperitoneal disease.[50] Malignant effusions developed in one quarter of patients with a median survival of 6 months. Significant risk factors for distant metastases were degree of disease involvement at the initial surgery, that is, the presence of ascites, peritoneal carcinomatosis, large metastatic disease, and retroperitoneal lymph nodes.

Death from ovarian cancer usually results from progressive bowel obstruction. Carcinomatosis involving the lumen and mesentery of the small and large intestine often produces an intermittent or incomplete obstruction for a prolonged period, although the tumor does not typically invade the lumen of the intestine.

## Prognostic Factors

The outcome of disease in following treatment can be evaluated in the context of prognostic factors, which can be grouped into pathologic, biologic, and clinical.

## PATHOLOGIC FACTORS

The morphologic and histologic patterns of the lesion are important prognostic variables. In particular, clear cell carcinomas are associated with a worse prognosis than the other histologic types. Histologic grade, determined by the pattern of differentiation and extent of cellular anaplasia, is also of prognostic significance.

## BIOLOGIC FACTORS

Several biologic factors have been correlated with prognosis in epithelial ovarian cancer. Using flow cytometry, Friedlander and colleagues showed that ovarian cancers were commonly aneuploid.[51] Furthermore, this group and others showed that there was a correlation between stage and ploidy.[52–55] Early-stage cancers tend to be diploid, and advanced stage tumors tend to be aneuploid. Multivariate analyses have shown that ploidy is an independent prognostic variable and one of the most significant predictors of survival. The S-phase fraction has also been correlated with prognosis.[56]

More than 60 proto-oncogenes have been identified, and studies have focused on the amplification or expression of these genes and their relationship to the development and progression of ovarian cancer. For example, Slamon and colleagues reported that 30% of epithelial ovarian tumors expressed the HER-2/*neu* oncogene and that this group of patients had a poorer prognosis.[57] Berchuck and colleagues reported a similar incidence, and in their series, patients whose tumors expressed this gene had a poorer median survival: 15.7 months versus 32.8 months.[58] A monoclonal antibody to the HER-2/*neu* receptor has been developed and is called trastuzumab (Herceptin). The Gynecologic Oncology Group is currently studying the response rates of trastuzumab in patients with recurrent ovarian carcinoma.

p53 is a key tumor-suppressor gene involved in transcriptional regulation; mutations appear in many malignancies, including more than 60% of ovarian carcinomas.[59, 60] Kohler and colleagues have identified p53 to be overexpressed in 29% of stage I and stage II ovarian carcinoma patients through immunohistochemistry, with the incidence correlated to the stage, size, and grade of disease.[61] The mutated p53 gene is also the target of an investigational replication-deficient adenovirus containing wild-type p53 being studied in one of the several gene therapy trials at various sites around the United States.

## CLINICAL FACTORS

Ovarian epithelial malignancies are staged according to the 1988 Revised International Federation of Gynecology and Obstetrics (FIGO) system (Table 55–3).[62] A preoperative evaluation should exclude the presence of extraperitoneal metastases. Staging is based on findings at surgical exploration. The importance of thorough surgical staging cannot be overemphasized because subsequent treatments are determined by the stage of disease. A careful search should be undertaken to look for microscopic disease in patients whose exploratory surgery does not reveal macroscopic extraovar-

**Table 55–3. FIGO Staging for Primary Carcinoma of the Ovary**

Stage I. Growth limited to the ovaries

Ia      Growth limited to one ovary. Capsule intact. No tumor on the external surfaces. No ascites containing malignant cells.

Ib      Growth limited to both ovaries. Capsules intact. No tumor on the external surface. No ascites containing malignant cells.

Ic      Either Ia or Ib, but tumor on surface of one or both ovaries, capsule ruptured, ascites containing malignant cells, or positive peritoneal washings.

Stage II. Growth involving one or both ovaries with pelvic extension

IIa      Extension and/or metastasis to the uterus and/or tubes.

IIb      Extension to other pelvic tissues.

IIc      Either IIa or IIb, but tumor on surface of one or both ovaries, capsule ruptured, ascites containing malignant cells, or positive peritoneal washings.

Stage III. Tumor involving one or both ovaries with peritoneal implants outside the pelvis and/or retroperitoneal or inguinal nodes. Superficial liver metastasis equals stage III. Tumor is limited to the true pelvis, but with histologically proven malignant extension to small bowel or omentum.

IIIa      Tumor grossly limited to the true pelvis with negative nodes but with histologically confirmed microscopic seeding of abdominal peritoneal surfaces.

IIIb      Tumor of one or both ovaries with histologically confirmed implants of abdominal peritoneal surfaces; none exceeding 2 cm in diameter. Nodes negative.

IIIc      Abdominal implants >2 cm in diameter and/or positive retroperitoneal or inguinal lymph nodes.

Stage IV. Growth involving one or both ovaries with distant metastasis. If pleural effusion is present, there must be positive cytologic test results to allot a case to stage IV. Parenchymal liver metastasis equals stage IV.

From Pecorelli S, Odicini F, Maisonneuve P, et al. FIGO annual report of the results of treatment in gynaecological cancer: carcinoma of the ovary. J Epidemiol Biostat 1998;3:75–102.

ian disease. Up to one third of patients who have disease clinically confined to the ovary will be upstaged by detection of occult disease through complete surgical staging. In earlier series in which patients did not undergo careful surgical staging, the overall 5-year survival for patients with apparent stage I ovarian cancer was only 60%. With proper staging, 5-year survival rates for stage IA disease is about 90%.[63]

Surgical resection of ovarian tumors should be performed with the tumor intact. A frozen section should be prepared to determine the diagnosis. If the ovarian malignancy appears to be confined to the ovaries or pelvis, a thorough surgical staging should be carried out. Any free fluid in the cul-de-sac should be retrieved and submitted for cytologic evaluation. Washings of the peritoneal cavity should be obtained from the cul-de-sac, paracolic gutters, and hemidiaphragms by instilling and removing 50 to 100 ml of saline. Sending the specimens separately for cytologic analysis maximizes the probability of detecting exfoliated cancer cells.

A systematic exploration of all intra-abdominal surfaces and viscera is performed. Any suspicious area or adhesion should be biopsied. If there is no evidence of disease, multiple intraperitoneal biopsies should be performed, obtaining specimens from the cul-de-sac, both gutters, bladder peritoneum, and bowel mesentery. The diaphragm should be evaluated either by biopsy or by cytologic smear. The omentum should be resected from the transverse colon by performing an infracolic omentectomy. If the gastrocolic ligament pal-

pates normally, it does not need to be resected. The retroperitoneal spaces should be explored to dissect the pelvic and para-aortic lymph nodes. Nodal tissue should be sampled from the external, internal, and common iliac vessels; the obturator fossa; and the para-aortic area. Any enlarged lymph nodes should be resected and submitted separately for histopathologic evaluation.

Occult metastases in apparent stage I or stage II ovarian cancer are not uncommon.[64–68] The importance of careful initial surgical staging is emphasized by the findings of a 1983 cooperative national study in which 100 patients with apparent stage I or stage II disease who were referred for subsequent therapy underwent additional staging surgery.[64] In this series, 29% of patients initially thought to have stage I disease, and 43% of patients thought to have stage II disease, were found to have more advanced disease. One third of patients were upstaged as a result of additional surgery, including one quarter who were upstaged to stage III disease. Histologic grade was a significant predictor of occult metastasis: 16% of patients with grade 1 lesions were upstaged, compared with 34% with grade 2 disease and 46% with grade 3 disease. If a patient is diagnosed with ovarian cancer and has been incompletely staged at her primary surgery, a decision must be made regarding completion of staging and tumor resection versus initiation of chemotherapy with subsequent reassessment.

## Epithelial Carcinomas

The most common neoplasms of the ovary are of "epithelial" origin, accounting for 85 to 90% of cases.[69, 70] The designation of epithelial carcinoma is derived from the fact that the tumor arises embryologically from the coelomic epithelium and adjacent ovarian stroma via neoplastic transformation of surface epithelium. A classification of epithelial ovarian tumors is presented in Table 55–4.[71]

Most epithelial lesions are seen in patients between the ages of 40 and 65. Patients less than 30 years are more likely to have tumors of germ cell origin. After peaking in the fifth and sixth decades of life, the incidence of epithelial ovarian tumors diminishes in the seventh and eighth decades.[63]

### BORDERLINE TUMORS

Tumors of low malignant potential are called *borderline tumors*. These lesions are defined histologically by atypical proliferation and no stromal invasion.[72] The incidence of disease appears to be evenly distributed across the decades. In women less than age 40, one quarter of all nonbenign tumors are borderline; overall, borderline tumors represent approximately 10% of nonbenign ovarian neoplasms (Fig. 55–1).[63]

Molecular and genetic analyses have not demonstrated borderline lesions to be an intermediate step between benign ovarian tumor and carcinoma.[73] No association with hereditary ovarian cancer syndrome has been observed.

The recommended treatment of borderline tumors is surgical resection of the primary tumor with staging. After

**Table 55–4.** Epithelial Ovarian Tumors

| Histologic Type | Cellular Type |
|---|---|
| 1. Serous<br>   Benign<br>   Borderline<br>   Malignant | Endosalpingeal |
| 2. Mucinous<br>   Benign<br>   Borderline<br>   Malignant | Endocervical |
| 3. Endometrioid<br>   Benign<br>   Borderline<br>   Malignant<br>   Epithelial-stromal | Endometrial |
| 4. Clear Cell<br>   Benign<br>   Borderline<br>   Malignant | Müllerian |
| 5. Transitional Cell<br>   Benign Brenner<br>   Borderline Brenner<br>   Malignant Brenner<br>   Non-Brenner Transitional<br>   Cell | Transitional |
| 6. Squamous Cell Tumors | Squamous mixed |
| 6. Mixed Epithelial<br>   Benign<br>   Borderline<br>   Malignant | |
| 7. Undifferentiated | Anaplastic |
| 8. Unclassified | Mesothelioma, and so on |

Adapted from Serov SF, Scully RE, Sobin IH. International Histological Classification of Tumors No. 9: histological typing of ovarian tumours. Geneva: World Health Organization, 1973.

examination of a frozen section and determination that the histologic type is borderline, premenopausal patients who desire to maintain ovarian function may be managed with preservation of the uterus and contralateral ovary. In a study of patients who underwent unilateral ovarian cystectomy for apparent stage I borderline serous tumors, recurrence was noted in 8% of patients 2 to 18 years later, all of whom had curable disease confined to the ovaries.[74] Thus in patients in whom an oophorectomy or cystectomy has been performed and a borderline tumor documented later in the permanent pathologic report, no additional immediate surgery is necessary. The diagnostic accuracy of frozen section in borderline tumors is limited, however, especially with a mucinous histologic type.[75–77] Up to 25% of borderline ovarian tumors at frozen section have been underclassified ovarian malignancies; thus, surgical staging should remain mandatory when frozen section demonstrates a borderline tumor.

There is no evidence that either subsequent chemotherapy or radiation therapy improves survival, but complete staging provides valuable prognostic information. Borderline tumors tend to remain confined to the ovary, with approximately 75% of patients diagnosed with stage I disease.[63] Peritoneal spread of borderline tumors tends to be through surface implantation; although on occasion invasive peritoneal implants are identified in patients in whom the primary ovarian tumor is borderline. The presence of invasive implants is correlated with an adverse prognosis and may be an instance in which cytotoxic chemotherapy may be considered.[78]

Survival for stage I borderline tumors is excellent, approximately 99% at a mean follow-up of 7 years.[73] Because of the indolent nature of borderline tumors, it is perhaps better to consider 10-year survival rather than 5-year survival. In the presence of peritoneal implants (stage III), survival is 96% at 5 years and 77% at 10 years.[78] Progression of disease can lead to intestinal obstruction; treatment of recurrent disease is usually surgical for patients who are candidates.

## PERITONEAL CARCINOMAS

Primary peritoneal carcinoma is a disseminated serous adenocarcinoma of the peritoneum in the presence of normal ovaries. It is histologically indistinguishable from papillary serous ovarian carcinoma but morphologically distinct. Many names have been given to this disease entity, including serous surface papillary carcinoma and extraovarian peritoneal serous papillary carcinoma, reflecting the diagnostic dilemma faced by pathologists in cases of intraperitoneal carcinoma with minimally involved ovaries.[79–83]

Primary peritoneal carcinoma is recognized as a separate clinical entity, distinct from mesotheliomas and primary ovarian carcinomas. In 1993, the Gynecologic Oncology Group established certain criteria to define primary peritoneal carcinoma: ovaries normal in size or enlarged by a benign process, extraovarian involvement greater than ovarian involvement, predominantly serous histology, and surface involvement of less than 5 mm depth and width. Using this clinical definition of primary peritoneal carcinoma based on ovarian size and invasion, 7 to 20% of patients previously identified with primary ovarian carcinoma may be reclassified as having primary peritoneal carcinoma.[81–84] Although it is disputable, it has been suggested that primary peritoneal carcinoma has a worse outcome than its primary ovarian cancer counterpart.[85, 86] Response rates to chemotherapy may be comparable, yet optimal surgical cytoreduction may be more difficult to achieve in the setting of widespread peritoneal disease without a predominant ovarian or pelvic mass.

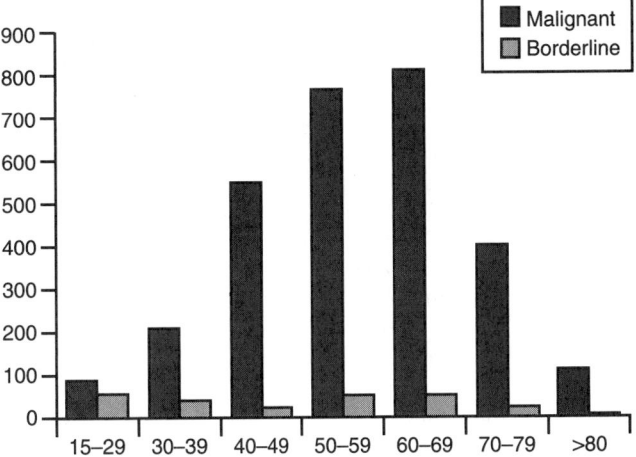

**Figure 55–1.** Distribution of malignant and borderline cases by age groups of patients treated in 1990 to 1992. (Adapted from Pecorelli S, Odicino F, Maisonneuve P, et al. FIGO annual report on the results of treatment in gynaecological cancer. J Epidemiol Biostat 1998;3:75–102.)

The malignant transformation of the peritoneum can produce a condition in which "ovarian cancer" can arise in a patient who has had her ovaries surgically removed many years before. Also, these patients may develop peritoneal carcinomatosis with grossly normal-appearing ovaries. In these cases, the ovaries may be "innocent bystanders" of a diffuse peritoneal process.

## INVASIVE NEOPLASMS

Up to 75% of invasive epithelial ovarian cancers are of the serous histologic type.[87] Less common types are mucinous (9%), endometrioid (10 to 20%), clear cell (6%), transitional cell (1%), and undifferentiated carcinomas (1%).[88–92] Each tumor type has a histologic pattern that reproduces the mucosal features of the lower genital tract. For example, the serous or papillary pattern has an appearance similar to that of the glandular epithelium lining the fallopian tube. Mucinous tumors arise in cells that resemble the endocervical glands, and the endometrioid tumors resemble the endometrium.

Serous carcinomas range from predominantly cystic and papillary to extremely solid and firm tumors. Histologically, the pattern simulates the lining of the fallopian tube. Poorly differentiated forms are grossly indistinguishable from other epithelial tumors. Multiple papillary projections are seen on the surfaces of the tumors. Bilateral tumors exist in about one third of patients with stage I or stage IIA disease, and in as many as two thirds if all stages are included.[88]

Mucinous tumors resemble endocervical epithelium histologically. They tend to remain confined to the ovaries longer than do serous carcinomas and are usually the largest epithelial neoplasms, often 20 cm or more in diameter.[89] The tumors may be multiloculated, with areas of necrosis and hemorrhage. Borderline or malignant tumors may be found in only a small portion of an otherwise benign neoplasm, thus thorough pathologic sampling is necessary. Occasionally, the condition known as pseudomyxoma peritonei is associated with a mucinous carcinoma of the ovary or with a mucinous tumor of the appendix.

Endometrioid tumors closely resemble the components of typical carcinoma of the endometrium. Occasionally these carcinomas arise from foci of endometriosis.[93, 94] The stromal component of an endometrioid tumor may also be malignant, a so-called mixed müllerian tumor or adenosarcoma of the ovary. Endometrioid tumors are bilateral in about 13% of stage I and stage IIA disease but in 30% of all stages.[90]

Clear cell carcinomas of the ovary have also been called mesonephroid carcinomas because of their histologic features that suggest a mesonephric origin. These features include "clear cells," similar to those seen in renal cell carcinomas. These tumors can also arise from endometriosis.[91] Clear cell carcinomas are rarely bilateral.[91]

Brenner's tumors represent 2 to 3% of all ovarian neoplasms, and less than 2% have been reported as borderline or malignant. As many as one half of Brenner's tumors are microscopic, and almost all of these are benign nodules.[92]

## TREATMENT OF LIMITED DISEASE

The primary therapy for stage I epithelial ovarian cancer is surgical staging. In patients who have undergone a thorough staging in which no evidence of spread beyond the ovary has been found, an abdominal hysterectomy with bilateral salpingo-oophorectomy is appropriate. The uterus and contralateral ovary can be preserved in women with stage IA disease who want to preserve fertility.

Patients with stage IA and stage IB, grade 1 disease have an excellent prognosis. In a report by Guthrie and coworkers, the outcome in 656 patients with early-stage epithelial ovarian cancer was studied.[68] No patient who had a properly documented stage I, grade 1 cancer died of the disease. In another series of 194 patients with untreated stage I epithelial ovarian cancer, 5-year survival rates of stage IA, IB, and IC were 94%, 92%, and 84%, respectively.[95] Independent poor prognostic factors included grade, surface disease, and presence of ascites. In a prospective randomized trial carried out by the Gynecologic Oncology Group, observation versus melphalan was studied in patients with stage IA and stage IB, grade 1 disease.[96] There was identical, excellent survival for both groups: 96% survival at 5 years. Furthermore, prolonged exposure to melphalan, an alkylating agent, increased the risk of developing an acute nonlymphocytic leukemia. Without evidence of survival benefit, no adjuvant treatment is recommended for stage IA or stage IB disease, although patients should be followed carefully with periodic pelvic examination and determination of CA-125 titers. Generally, the contralateral ovary and uterus are removed at the completion of childbearing.

In an analysis of factors predictive of relapse in 252 patients from the Princess Margaret Hospital in Toronto, the strongest prognostic factors in stage I ovarian carcinoma are grade, dense adhesions, and large volume (greater than 250 mL) ascites.[97] Neither cyst rupture or capsular penetration was prognostic for relapse in this population. The overall relapse risk of 28% for grade 2 and grade 3 disease was high enough to warrant postoperative treatment, but the best adjuvant therapy is unclear.

In patients whose disease is more poorly differentiated or in whom there are malignant cells in either ascitic fluid or peritoneal washings, additional therapy is indicated. Treatment options for stages IA and IB, grades 2 and 3, and stage IC include chemotherapy and radiation therapy. Some comparisons of these modalities have been made, although most are retrospective and therefore inconclusive.

Chemotherapy for patients with stage IA or IB, grade 2 or 3, and stage IC epithelial ovarian cancer can be either single agent or multiagent. The Gynecologic Oncology Group studied melphalan versus intraperitoneal phosphorus 32 ($^{32}$P) in patients with early-stage disease with unfavorable prognostic features and found similar 5-year survival rates: 81% for melphalan and 78% with $^{32}$P.[98] The impact of treatment on survival cannot be definitively established because an untreated group was not included in the study, yet neither treatment is markedly different from the overall 5-year survival in historical controls.

Cisplatin, carboplatin, and paclitaxel are single agents active against epithelial ovarian cancer, and these agents may be preferable to melphalan in patients with early-stage disease. Cisplatin and cyclophosphamide, with or without doxorubicin, have been used to treat patients with stage I disease, but there are no data comparing the use of combination cisplatin chemotherapy with either single-agent chemotherapy or radiation therapy. The Gynecologic Oncology

Group has completed accrual for a trial in early-stage ovarian cancer, randomizing 3 versus 6 cycles of paclitaxel and carboplatin, but it is still too soon to evaluate survival data on this cohort. Another clinical trial currently under way in the Gynecologic Oncology Group for early-stage ovarian cancer patients is a randomized trial between 3 cycles of paclitaxel and carboplatin versus 3 cycles of paclitaxel and carboplatin plus 12 cycles of weekly paclitaxel.

Radiation therapy may use intraperitoneal radiocolloids or whole-abdomen radiation therapy. In one series of patients treated with $^{32}$P, 5-year survival was 85%.[99] In another series of patients with stage I disease treated with whole-abdomen radiation, the 5-year survival was only 78%.[100] Either modality of radiation produces results similar to those of single-agent chemotherapy but has a higher rate of delayed bowel complications.

Until better data are available, appropriate treatment options for stage IA or IB, grades 2 and 3, and stage IC disease include platinum-based chemotherapy, paclitaxel-based che-motherapy, or intraperitoneal $^{32}$P. Since no form of adjuvant therapy has been shown to improve survival, an option of no treatment can also be considered. Treatment with paclitaxel and carboplatin for three to four cycles seems desirable in young patients.

## TREATMENT OF ADVANCED STAGE DISEASE

The treatment for all advanced-stage tumors is approached in a similar manner, with modifications made for the overall status and general health of the patient, as well as the extent of residual disease present at the time of initiation of treatment (Fig. 55–2).[101]

The patient should undergo initial exploratory surgery with removal of as much diseased tissue as possible. The operation to remove the primary tumor is referred to as *debulking* or *cytoreductive surgery*. Most patients subsequently receive combination chemotherapy for an empirical

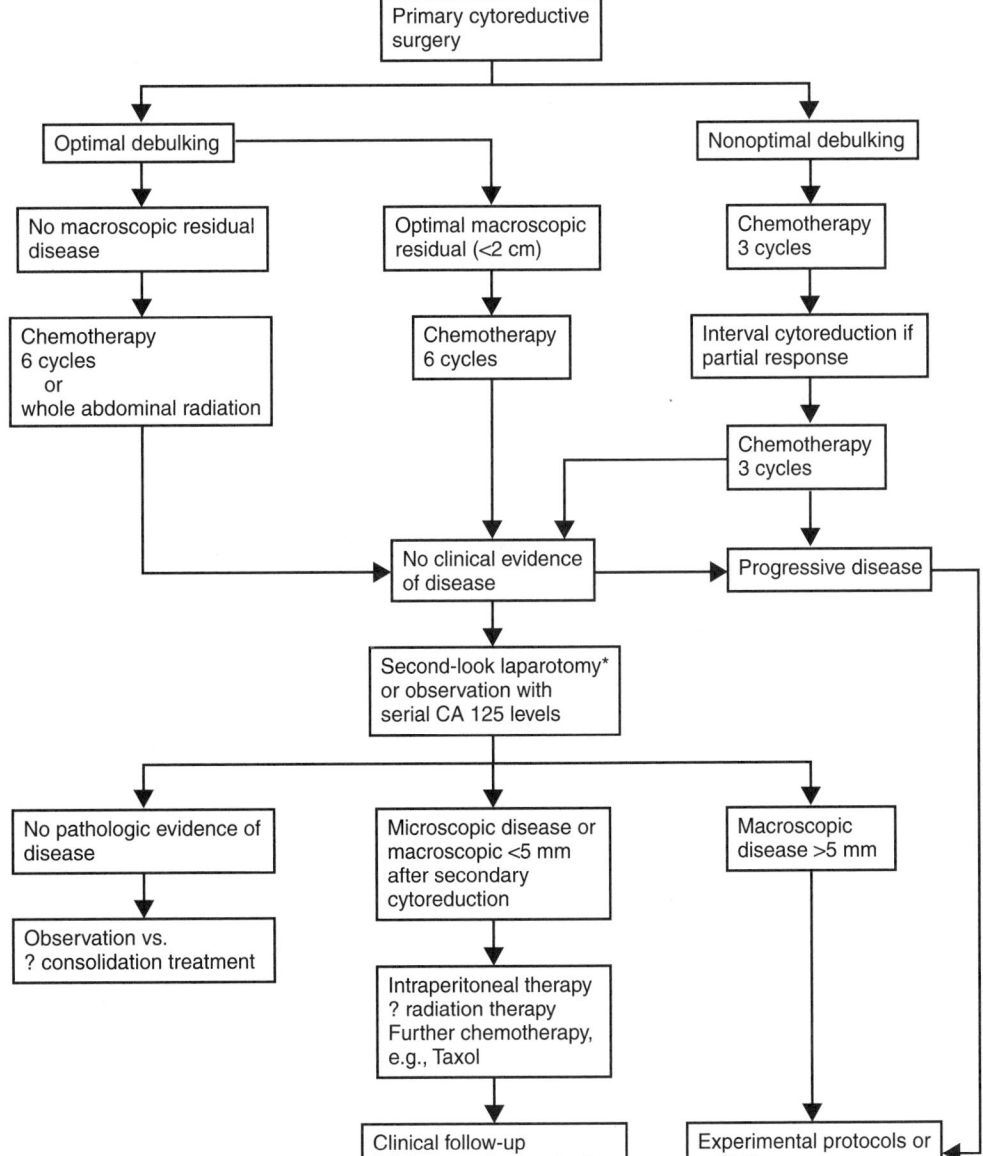

**Figure 55–2.** Treatment scheme for patients with advanced stage ovarian cancer. (Adapted from Berek JS, Hacker NF. Practical gynecologic oncology. 3rd ed. Philadelphia: Lippincott Williams & Wilkins, 2000.)

number of cycles. In patients whose disease is not clinically apparent at the completion of chemotherapy, a reassessment or "second-look" surgery may be performed to determine whether or not a complete response to therapy has occurred. In patients with persistent disease at second-look surgery, a second-line therapy may be recommended. The types of second-line therapy available are extensive but are limited in effectiveness. Immunotherapy and hormonal therapy also may be appropriate in selected circumstances.

## Cytoreductive Surgery

Patients with advanced-stage epithelial ovarian cancer documented at initial exploratory laparotomy should undergo cytoreductive surgery to remove as much tumor and metastatic disease as possible to facilitate the effectiveness of subsequent therapies.[102, 103] Compared with other solid tumors, ovarian carcinoma is relatively chemosensitive; thus reducing tumor volume improves effectiveness of the chemotherapy. The operation typically includes a total abdominal hysterectomy and bilateral salpingo-oophorectomy, along with a complete omentectomy and resection of metastatic lesions on the peritoneal surfaces or from the intestines. The pelvic tumor often directly involves the rectosigmoid colon, the terminal ileum, and the cecum. Some have questioned the ability of cytoreductive surgery to improve the overall outcome of patients with ovarian cancer. There is concern regarding the morbidity associated with these operations; however, the data available suggest that cytoreductive surgery has an acceptable morbidity and is generally beneficial.

The rationale for cytoreductive surgery relates to three general theoretical considerations:

1. Physiologic benefits of tumor mass excision
2. Decreased number of tumor cells and resistant clones, increased growth fraction, and improved tissue perfusion, all increasing the likelihood of response to chemotherapy or radiotherapy
3. Enhanced immunologic competence of the patient

The removal of bulky tumor masses also reduces the volume of ascites. Often, ascites disappears after removal of the primary tumor and a large omental "cake." Removal of the omental cake often alleviates the nausea and early satiety that many patients experience. Removal of intestinal metastases restores adequate intestinal function and may lead to an improvement in the overall nutritional status of the patient, which can facilitate the patient's ability to tolerate subsequent chemotherapy.

The larger the initial tumor burden, the longer the necessary exposure to the drug; therefore, the chance of development of drug resistance is higher. Because the spontaneous mutation rate of tumors is an inherent property of malignancy, the likelihood of phenotypic drug resistance developing also increases with the size of the tumor.[104] This means that the chance of a clone of cells developing that is resistant to a specific agent is related to both the tumor size and its mutation frequency. One of the inherent problems with cytoreductive surgery is that phenotypic drug resistance may have already developed before surgical intervention.

Larger tumor masses tend to be composed of a higher proportion of cells that are either nondividing, or in the $G_0$ resting phase of the cell cycle, making them essentially resistant to chemotherapy. A low growth fraction is characteristic of bulky tumor masses, and cytoreductive surgery can reduce the masses to smaller residual disease with a relatively higher growth fraction. These smaller masses will be inherently more susceptible to cytotoxic therapy. The fractional cell kill hypothesis of Skipper indicates that a constant proportion of the remaining cancer cells are destroyed with each treatment.[105] This theory suggests that a given dose of a drug will kill a constant fraction of cells as long as the growth fraction and phenotype are the same. Therefore, a treatment that reduces a population of tumor cells from $10^9$ to $10^4$ cells also would reduce a population of $10^5$ cells to a single cell ($10^0$). If the absolute number of cells that must be destroyed is lower at the initiation of treatment (i.e., a lower tumor burden), fewer cycles of therapy are necessary to eradicate the cancer provided that the cells are not inherently resistant to the treatment.

If the tumor is large and bulky, it tends to contain areas that are poorly vascularized and necrotic. These areas are exposed to inadequate concentrations of the chemotherapeutic drugs and thus are unable to yield maximal antitumor response. Similarly, these areas are poorly oxygenated so that radiation therapy will be less effective. Thus, the surgical removal of these bulky tumors maximizes the effectiveness of treatment.

Larger tumor masses appear to be more immunosuppressive than smaller tumors. In addition to the nonspecific immunocompromise that occurs with large tumors, bulky tumors may be less amenable to control by host defense mechanisms. The normal mechanism of recognition of abnormal antigens may be overwhelmed and abrogated by the relatively large number of cancer cells. Excess tumor antigen can block the function of cytotoxic lymphocytes.[106]

The principal goal of cytoreductive surgery is the removal of all the primary cancer and its metastases. If resection of all metastases is not feasible, the goal is to reduce the tumor burden by resection of all individual tumors to an optimal status. The concept of *optimal* cytoreduction was initially proposed by Griffiths, who found that the survival of patients whose metastatic disease was resected to less than 1.5 cm in maximal dimension was significantly longer than the survival of those whose lesions were larger.[102] The patients with optimal cytoreduction subsequently had a higher response rate to chemotherapy and longer disease-free intervals.

Results of optimal cytoreduction can be improved by taking the goal to minimal residual disease. Hacker and colleagues showed that patients whose largest residual lesions were 5 mm or less had a median survival of 40 months after surgery, compared with a median survival of 18 months for patients whose tumors were less than 1.5 cm (Fig. 55–3).[103]

A survey by the American College of Surgeons found that the surgery for women diagnosed with ovarian cancer was performed by a gynecologic oncologist in only 24.6% of cases, whereas a gynecologist was the physician in charge in 47% of cases.[107] An analysis of the retrospective data available suggests that cytoreductive surgery is feasible in 70 to 90% of patients when performed by gynecologic oncologists, who are specially trained in ovarian cancer surgery.[108, 109] Median survival and progression-free survival of patients undergoing cytoreductive surgery are inversely related to the extent of residual disease at the completion of

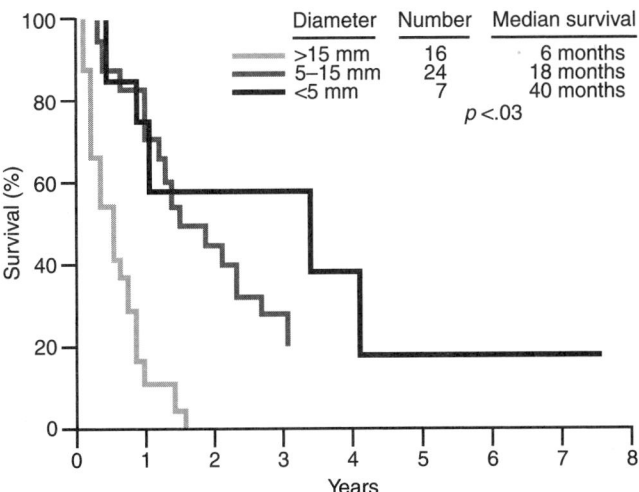

**Figure 55–3.** Survival versus diameter of largest residual disease. (Adapted from Hacker NF, Berek JS, Lagasse LD, et al. Reprinted with permission from the American College of Obstetricians and Gynecologists, 1983, 61, pp. 413–20.)

the laparotomy.[110] The feasibility of optimal cytoreduction does seem to depend on prior experience; therefore, it is important for training programs to continue to teach the skills of cytoreduction techniques. Major morbidity is in the range of 10%.

Intestinal resection in these patients does not appear to increase the overall morbidity of the operation.[108, 111] Diaphragm resection, splenectomy, and other upper abdominal procedures may also be indicated if the patient can be left with minimal residual disease.[112, 113] Performing pelvic and para-aortic lymphadenectomy in patients with no residual intraperitoneal disease has also been reported to improve survival; however, this has not been confirmed in a prospective clinical trial.[114–116]

The resectability of the metastatic tumor is often determined by the size of nodules and the location of disease. Patients whose metastatic disease is very large (i.e. >10 cm before cytoreductive surgery) had a shorter survival than those with smaller metastatic disease.[108] Extensive upper abdominal disease—particularly in the parenchyma of the liver, the porta hepatis, or the lesser omentum, or that involving the base of the small bowel mesentery—may preclude adequate surgical excision of metastatic disease. Such patients may be candidates for interval cytoreduction if they respond well to primary chemotherapy.

In the past, patients with stage IV disease were considered to have a poor prognosis and were not always considered candidates for aggressive cytoreductive surgery. Several studies have focused on the feasibility, morbidity, and effect on survival of primary surgical cytoreduction in stage IV ovarian cancer.[117–120] Optimal tumor cytoreduction to less than 2 cm disease was feasible in 30 to 45% of patients. Patients who underwent optimal cytoreduction enjoyed a median survival of 38 months, compared with 11 months for patients who were left with suboptimal disease. Furthermore, Bristow and colleagues were able to demonstrate that even in the face of unresectable liver lesions, optimal cytoreduction of all extrahepatic disease still provided a survival advantage: median survival 25 months versus 8.5 months.[120]

Thus, the mere presence of intrahepatic or extraperitoneal metastatic ovarian cancer should not by itself be a contraindication for surgical exploration.

Neoadjuvant chemotherapy in ovarian cancer involves the administration of chemotherapy for several cycles prior to attempting surgical resection of disease.[121, 122] Stage IV disease is one area in which neoadjuvant chemotherapy has been proposed as more effective management. Other scenarios for neoadjuvant chemotherapy include patients with malignant ascites but no pelvic mass or patients with malignant ascites but an unresectable pelvic mass. Patient selection for cytoreductive surgery versus neoadjuvant chemotherapy depends greatly on the performance status of the patient along with any comorbidities for surgery. CT imaging criteria have been proposed for prediction of surgical resectability; however, these criteria have never been tested in a prospective fashion.[123, 124] Neoadjuvant chemotherapy followed by interval cytoreductive surgery is of benefit for patients who are unable to undergo primary cytoreductive surgery; however, survival appears to be somewhat compromised, probably related to a larger number of chemoresistant clones at the start of treatment.[121]

### First-Line Chemotherapy

Systemic chemotherapy is the standard treatment for metastatic epithelial ovarian cancer. For many years, an oral single-agent alkylating agent regimen was used, but the introduction of cisplatin in the late 1970s revolutionized the therapeutic approach for most patients. Cisplatin-based chemotherapy was the most frequently used regimen in the 1980s. Paclitaxel became available in the early 1990s, and with the introduction of carboplatin as a less toxic platinum agent, paclitaxel and carboplatin have now become a standard in first-line therapy.

**Single-Agent Therapy.** The use of single-agent chemotherapy in first-line therapy for metastatic ovarian cancer is generally reserved for patients whose overall physical condition precludes the use of more toxic therapy. In elderly or debilitated patients and in those who refuse intravenous chemotherapy, the use of an oral agent is simple and appealing.

The standard dose for the alkylating agent melphalan is 0.2 mg/kg/day given for 5 consecutive days every 4 weeks. In three separate Gynecologic Oncology Group studies treating stage III ovarian cancer (with suboptimal cytoreduction), 193 patients were treated with this regimen. Of these patients, 62 (33%) had a clinical response, with a 16% complete response and a 17% partial response rate.[96] However, the median duration of response was only 7 months, and the median survival was 12 months.

Other active drugs that have been used as single agents include cisplatin, carboplatin, paclitaxel, ifosfamide, doxorubicin, hexamethylmelamine, and 5-fluorouracil.[125, 126] Cisplatin, carboplatin, and paclitaxel appear to be more active than alkylating agents and produce sufficiently high response rates to justify their use in primary therapy. The individual activities and their complementary toxicities serve as the rationale for their incorporation into combination regimens.

**Combination Chemotherapy.** Various combination chemotherapy regimens have been tested in the treatment of advanced epithelial ovarian cancer. A summary of the most common regimens is presented in Table 55–5. Combination chemotherapy has been shown to be superior to single-agent therapy in most patients with advanced epithelial ovarian cancer.[127]

After cisplatin became available for the treatment of ovarian cancer, it was soon recognized to be an active single agent against the disease. Concurrently, it was tested in a variety of combinations with other cytotoxic drugs. One such regimen, CHAP (cyclophosphamide, hexamethylmelamine, doxorubicin [Adriamycin], and cisplatin [Platinol]), was shown to be active and generally tolerable.[128] A prospective randomized study comparing CHAP with Hexa-CAF (hexamethylmelamine, cyclophosphamide, doxorubicin [Adriamycin], and 5-fluorouracil) showed a surgically documented complete response rate of 40% for the CHAP regimen, compared with 19% for the Hexa-CAF regimen.[129] The median survivals were 26 months and 19 months, respectively, suggesting that the cisplatin-based combination was superior. Because of the toxicity of hexamethylmelamine, particularly the depression that some patients developed, hexamethylmelamine was often omitted from the CHAP regimen. In a meta-analysis of patients with advanced-stage ovarian cancer treated with chemotherapy, patients treated with cisplatin-containing combination chemotherapy were compared with those treated without cisplatin. The cisplatin group appeared to have a survival advantage between 2 and 5 years, but these survival differences seemed to disappear by 8 years.[127]

The PAC regimen (cisplatin, doxorubicin [Adriamycin], and cyclophosphamide) has been extensively used for advanced ovarian cancer. Ehrlich and colleagues reported on 56 patients treated with the PAC regimen every 3 weeks for 12 cycles.[130] The median survival of patients with suboptimal residual disease was 23 months, compared with 45 months with optimal residual disease. Most studies using the PAC or PC (cisplatin and cyclophosphamide) regimen report response rates and survival similar to those produced by CHAP.[131, 132]

Because of the cardiotoxicity of doxorubicin, it would be desirable to omit the drug if overall response rates were not significantly changed. A large prospective randomized Dutch study of CHAP versus PC showed that the response rates and median survivals were almost identical.[133] Because the toxicity of PC was significantly less than that of the four-drug treatment, the authors concluded that PC should be considered the treatment of choice.

Several trials have compared PAC and PC.[134–137] No study showed a significant difference in survival between treatment arms. The Gynecologic Oncology Group's randomized prospective comparison of equitoxic doses of PAC and PC showed no benefit to the inclusion of doxorubicin in the combination. A meta-analysis of the combined data of four randomized trials showed a 7% survival advantage at 6 years for patients treated with the doxorubicin-containing regimen. At 8 years, the survival curves appear to converge.

With a two-drug regimen of PC, higher doses of each drug can be used. This is particularly important for cisplatin, for which there is a theoretical dose-response curve; that is, the higher the dose, the greater the theoretical probability of response. Evidence to support the correlation of dose intensity of cisplatin (less than doses used in stem cell transplant) has never been demonstrated clinically. The issue of dose intensification of cisplatin was examined in a prospective trial conducted by the Gynecologic Oncology Group.[138] In this study, 243 patients with suboptimally debulked ovarian cancer were randomized to receive either 50 mg/m$^2$ or 100 mg/m$^2$ cisplatin and 500 mg/m$^2$ cyclophosphamide. There was no difference in response rates, and overall survivals were the same; however, there was a higher toxicity associated with the high-dose regimen. In contrast, a Scottish group reported that patients who received 100 mg/m$^2$ cisplatin and 750 mg/m$^2$ cyclophosphamide had a significantly longer median survival compared with those receiving 50 mg/m$^2$ and the same dose of cyclophosphamide.[139] In their interim analysis, the study was stopped early because the overall median survival was significantly different: 114 weeks in the high-dose group and 69 weeks in the standard dose group. Yet when these patients were followed for long-term survival, even though survival rates at 4 years were still significantly better for the high-dose intensity group, the differences were much less than at 2 years.[140] Thus, a dose effect may exist, but it may only delay recurrence without affecting long-term survival.

The second-generation platinum analogue carboplatin was introduced and developed to have less toxicity than its parent compound cisplatin. In toxicity and early efficacy trials, carboplatin was shown to have lower toxicity.[141–144] Fewer gastrointestinal side effects and less nausea and vomiting were observed than with cisplatin, as well as less nephrotoxicity, neurotoxicity, and ototoxicity. Initial studies showed carboplatin and cisplatin to have a 4:1 equivalency ratio.[142] An approximate dose of 350 to 450 mg/m$^2$ carboplatin can be used initially in patients with a normal serum creatinine level and then adjusted to toxicity. The dose is calculated by using the area under the curve (AUC) and the glomerular filtration rate via the Calvert formula. The target AUC is 6 to 7 for untreated patients with ovarian cancer. Thrombocytopenia is the usual dose-limiting toxicity.

Prospective randomized trials of carboplatin plus cyclophosphamide versus cisplatin plus cyclophosphamide have

*Table 55–5.* **Chemotherapeutic Regimens for Advanced Ovarian Cancer***

| Regimen Drugs | Dose and Schedule |
|---|---|
| **TC** | |
| Paclitaxel | 175 mg/m$^2$ over 3 hr |
| Carboplatin | AUC 5–6 |
| **TP** | |
| Paclitaxel | 135 mg/m$^2$ over 24 hr or 175 mg/m$^2$ over 3 hr |
| Cisplatin | 75 mg/m$^2$ |
| **CC** | |
| Carboplatin | AUC 5–6 |
| Cyclophosphamide | 600 mg/m$^2$ |
| **PC** | |
| Cisplatin | 75 mg/m$^2$ |
| Cyclophosphamide | 750 mg/m$^2$ |
| **PAC** | |
| Cisplatin | 50 mg/m$^2$ |
| Adriamycin | 50 mg/m$^2$ |
| Cyclophosphamide | 500 mg/m$^2$ |

*All regimens given every 3 to 4 weeks.
AUC, area under the curve.

been carried out in patients with suboptimally debulked stage III or IV disease.[143, 144] The carboplatin and cisplatin groups were shown to have equivalent survival with lower toxicity. Median survival was 20 months versus 17.4 months in the Southwest Oncology Group trial, and 27.5 months versus 25 months in the National Cancer Institute of Canada trial. Although the gastrointestinal toxicities of cisplatin can be effectively ameliorated by the use of potent antiemetics, older patients and those with significant medical problems tolerate cisplatin less well, and carboplatin should be the preferred platinum agent.

Paclitaxel (Taxol) is the most recent introduction of a remarkably active agent, and the most active agent since cisplatin was developed. In phase II trials, response rates of 36% were seen in patients with heavily pretreated recurrent disease.[145] This is a higher rate than was seen for cisplatin when it was first tested. In a pair of contemporary randomized trials, the Gynecologic Oncology Group studied the role of paclitaxel in first-line therapy. One study was a comparison between paclitaxel and cyclophosphamide, in combination with cisplatin in optimally debulked stage III disease, and the second was a three-arm comparison of paclitaxel versus cisplatin versus paclitaxel plus cisplatin in suboptimally debulked stage III and stage IV disease.

Paclitaxel alone as a first-line agent had a lower response rate than either cisplatin alone or cisplatin and paclitaxel in combination.[146] There was not a significant difference in survival between cisplatin alone and the cisplatin-paclitaxel combination; however, the combined regimen produced fewer toxicities than did cisplatin alone. The results of the study are confounded by the allowance for crossovers in treatment; similar survival results may be indicative of the results of treating with paclitaxel and cisplatin in series rather than studying the merits of each individual agent.

More patients demonstrated a clinical response to the cisplatin-paclitaxel combination in comparison to the cisplatin-cyclophosphamide combination: 73% versus 60%.[147] Both progression-free survival (18 months vs. 13 months) and overall survival (38 months vs. 24 months) were significantly longer in the cisplatin-paclitaxel group, establishing a platinum-taxane combination as the standard of care for first-line chemotherapy in epithelial ovarian cancer (Fig. 55–4).

The Gynecologic Oncology Group has been studying the combination of cisplatin-paclitaxel versus carboplatin-paclitaxel in optimally debulked stage III disease.[148] Paclitaxel has been studied as a 3-hour infusion to simplify its administration with carboplatin in an outpatient setting. When paclitaxel was administered over 3 hours followed by cisplatin, a high degree of neurotoxicity developed; thus, paclitaxel is still administered for 24 hours prior to cisplatin.[149] Preliminary results of the study confirm the clinical suspicions of many that carboplatin is equally efficacious in first-line therapy, but with a much lower toxicity profile.

Prolonging paclitaxel infusion may also improve tumor response; thus, the Gynecologic Oncology Group is also studying long infusion (96 hours) of paclitaxel versus standard infusion (24 hours) of paclitaxel in combination with cisplatin.

Based on the current data available, chemotherapy with carboplatin and paclitaxel is the combination of choice in patients with advanced disease. It is our preference to use

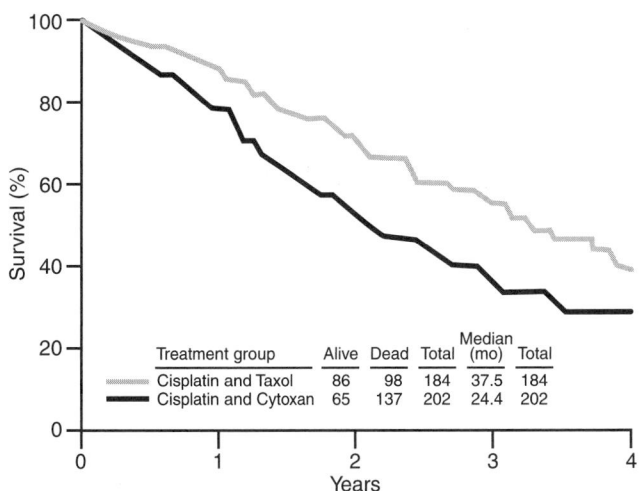

**Figure 55–4.** Survival according to cisplatin-paclitaxel versus cisplatin-cyclophosphamide combination chemotherapy. (Adapted from McGuire WP, Hoskins WJ, Brady MF, et al. Cyclophosphamide and cisplatin compared with paclitaxel and cisplatin in patients with stage III and stage IV ovarian cancer. N Engl J Med 1996;334:1–6.)

paclitaxel at 175 mg/m$^2$ over a 3-hour infusion, followed by carboplatin at an AUC of 5 to 6. The roles of topotecan and doxorubicin in combination chemotherapy regimens remain controversial, and their toxicities may be significant.

Intraperitoneal chemotherapy has been gaining popularity again as well. Following the principles of dose intensity, the theoretical benefit of intraperitoneal chemotherapy is to provide high levels of drug to the tumor on the peritoneal surfaces while minimizing systemic effects. In a Southwest Oncology Group trial, intraperitoneal cisplatin combined with intravenous cyclophosphamide was found to have improved survival (49 months vs. 41 months) with far less ototoxicity and neurotoxicity.[150] The effects of paclitaxel on survival are unknown in combination with intraperitoneal cisplatin, but the Gynecologic Oncology Group is also studying the role of intraperitoneal cisplatin, intravenous paclitaxel, and intraperitoneal paclitaxel versus standard paclitaxel and cisplatin chemotherapy in optimally debulked stage III ovarian carcinoma. Intraperitoneal chemotherapy probably plays a role in patients with minimal residual peritoneal disease, but the exact role of intraperitoneal chemotherapy in all ovarian cancer patients remains to be determined.

High-dose chemotherapy with stem cell rescue has also been studied with interest in many solid tumors, including ovarian cancer.[151, 152] At standard doses of cisplatin or carboplatin, escalating dose intensity has not resulted in improved outcome. Escalating doses even higher may theoretically improve outcome, but in a series from Loyola University, median progression-free survival was only 7 months and overall survival 13 months.[152] Patients who were platinum sensitive and had less than 1 cm greatest residual disease had a better outcome of 19 months progression-free survival and 30 months overall survival. The value of high-dose chemotherapy seems limited.

### Radiation Therapy

For selected patients with metastatic ovarian cancer, an alternative to combination chemotherapy is whole-abdomen radiation therapy. Although this approach is not commonly used in the United States, it is standard treatment in some institutions in Canada for patients with no residual macroscopic disease in the upper abdomen.[100]

Historically, radiation therapy in the cure of epithelial ovarian cancer was confined to use in patients with stage II disease, but the studies on which this idea was based usually were not randomized and varied considerably in the radiation dosages and techniques used. Before 1975, radiation techniques did not cover the entire peritoneum, although now it is clearly recognized that the predominant route of spread in ovarian cancer is intraperitoneal.

Recognizing the peritoneal route of spread of ovarian cancer, investigators at the M. D. Anderson Hospital developed an abdominal radiation technique using a moving strip of radiation.[153] This therapy was shown to be less effective, with greater amounts of residual disease after surgery.

The strongest evidence for the effectiveness of whole-abdomen irradiation in ovarian cancer comes from a study at the Princess Margaret Hospital undertaken from 1971 to 1975.[154] Patients with stages IB, II, and III disease were randomized after stratification by major prognostic factors to receive either pelvic irradiation alone, pelvic irradiation plus chlorambucil for 2 years, or pelvic plus whole-abdomen irradiation using the moving strip technique. The radiation field included the entire peritoneal cavity from above the diaphragm.[155] The dose of radiation was within liver tolerance, and no liver shielding was employed. Conclusions drawn from this study were that upper abdominal irradiation reduced the risk of upper abdominal relapse and improved survival over that achieved with pelvic radiation therapy. The greatest survival benefit was seen in patients with small or no macroscopic lesions.

Because the moving strip technique is cumbersome, a randomized study was undertaken to compare it with open-field whole-abdomen and pelvic irradiation.[156] After stratification by stage, grade, pathologic subtype, and completeness of pelvic surgery, 166 patients were randomized and 105 eligible patients were treated off study with one of the two techniques. The latter group was used in the toxicity analysis only. No significant differences in the 5-year survival rates or relapse-free rates were observed between the open-field technique and the moving strip technique. Acute toxicity was similar for both techniques, although thrombocytopenia was more common with the moving strip technique. Major late complications were also more frequent in the moving strip technique, with 6% of patients requiring bowel surgery compared with only 1% of those treated with the open-field technique. No treatment-related deaths were observed in either group. The open-field technique is now the standard and recommended form of whole-abdomen radiation.

In whole-abdomen radiation therapy, the treatment portal should encompass the entire peritoneal cavity. The superior margins are 1 to 1.5 cm above the domes of the diaphragm, and the lateral margins are 3 to 4 cm beyond the peritoneal reflection. The kidneys should be shielded from the posterior to limit the renal dose to 18 to 20 Gy. The maximal dose over the liver should not exceed 30 Gy. Because of the tolerance of the whole abdomen and the organs therein, it is unsafe to irradiate the entire peritoneal cavity with doses normally used for smaller radical treatments. It is better to treat all the tumor volume with a lower dose than to leave part of the abdomen untreated. Daily fractions sizes of 1 to 1.2 Gy are used because this small daily fraction size decreases the risk of acute nausea, late radiation enteritis, and hepatitis. The boost dose to the pelvis should be applied before or after the abdominal port is established and usually consists of 20 to 22.5 Gy in 1.8- to 2.25-Gy fractions, to a total pelvic dose of 45 to 50 Gy. A boost is not routinely given to the para-aortic lymph nodes or medial domes of the diaphragm because of the possibility of an increased risk of complications.

The use of postoperative whole-abdomen radiation should be limited to patients most likely to benefit from the treatment, that is, patients whose metastatic disease is microscopic or completely resected. The treatment has not been studied in direct comparison to combination chemotherapy. A retrospective review of patients treated with whole-abdomen radiation has identified subgroups of these patients.[157] Patients with stage I grade 1 tumors or borderline malignancies have a high probability of being cured by surgery alone, and radiation therapy is not recommended. Similarly, patients with stage III and stage IV disease and gross residual disease remaining after surgery are best managed with chemotherapeutic approaches. The remaining group of patients are those with stage I grades 2 and 3, or stage II or III lesions with no residual macroscopic disease or small residual disease confined to the true pelvis. Those with grade 2 serous tumors who have only microscopic residual disease are most likely to benefit from whole-abdomen radiation therapy. For those with macroscopic disease, radiation therapy does not produce satisfactory cure rates.[157]

Significant side effects from open-field abdominal radiation are seen in 60% of patients and include symptoms of anorexia, nausea, or vomiting. All patients develop general fatigue. Ten percent develop significant thrombocytopenia or neutropenia. After chemotherapy, about one third of patients have significant myelotoxicity. Radiologic evidence of evidence of basal pneumonitis develops in 15% of patients and it is symptomatic in 1%. The condition is self-limiting and resolves spontaneously. Transient biochemical evidence of liver damage with raised serum alkaline phosphatase levels is seen in 40%, but symptomatic hepatitis is not seen after the open-field technique. About 3% of patients develop episodes of bowel obstruction, about two thirds of which may need surgical correction. The frequency of bowel complications increases if higher total doses or larger fraction sizes are employed. Factors that may add to the risk of bowel obstruction are the extent and number of previous abdominal operations and possibly prior combination chemotherapy.[157]

A trial of three cycles of high dose cisplatin and cyclophosphamide chemotherapy followed by whole-abdomen radiation therapy to consolidate the initial response has been reported.[158] This approach showed no apparent benefit to sequential chemotherapy and radiation therapy in patients with optimal disease.

## ASSESSMENT OF TREATMENT

Many patients who have optimal cytoreductive surgery and subsequent chemotherapy for epithelial ovarian cancer have no evidence of disease at the completion of treatment. Tumor markers and radiologic assessments have proved too insensitive to exclude the presence of subclinical disease accurately. Therefore, a common technique employed in the evaluation of these cancers has been the "second-look" operation. Either laparotomy or laparoscopy has been employed in this circumstance.

The ideal follow-up schedule for patients with disease in remission has also not been standardized. Clinical practice typically involved follow-up visits every 3 months for the first year, every 3 or 4 months for the second year, every 6 months for the following 3 years, and annually thereafter.[159] Serial serum CA-125 levels may detect subclinical disease. CT may or may not detect subclinical disease. Other surveillance modalities include positron emission tomography and intraperitoneal washings through an intraperitoneal port.[160–162] The presumed advantage of early detection of disease recurrence is to be able to reinitiate therapy before the tumor burden becomes more advanced or unmanageable.

## Tumor Markers

Tumor markers are not reliable enough to predict accurately which patients with epithelial lesions have had their tumors completely eradicated. Epithelial carcinomas, unlike germ cell malignancies, do not secrete β-human chorionic gonadotropin (β-hCG), AFP, or other hormonal substances that can be measured by an radioimmunoassay. CEA may be elevated in patients with ovarian cancer, but it is too nonspecific and insensitive to have much use in the management of patients with ovarian cancer.

CA-125 is a surface glycoprotein associated with müllerian epithelial tissues. The CA-125 antigen can serve as a tumor marker for some epithelial ovarian cancers. Although as much as 80% of epithelial cancers are associated with a measurable CA-125 titer in the serum, the levels frequently become undetectable after the initial resection of tumor or early in the course of chemotherapy.

The levels of CA-125 have been correlated with the findings at second-look operations. Positive titers are useful in predicting the presence of disease, and negative titers are an insensitive determinant of the absence of disease. In a prospective study, the predictive value of a positive test result was shown to be 100%, that is, if the CA-125 titer was greater than 35 IU/ml, disease was always detectable in patients at second-look operation.[163] The predictive value of a negative test result was only 56%, that is, if the level was less than 35 IU/ml, disease was still present in 44% of patients at the time of second-look operation. Therefore, CA-125 is not sensitive enough to exclude subclinical disease in many patients.

Serum CA-125 levels can be used during chemotherapy to follow patients whose titer was positive at the initiation of therapy.[164] The rate of change in levels generally correlates with response. Patients with persistently elevated levels of CA-125 after 3 months of treatment most likely have resistant tumors. Persistently elevated or rising titers with treatment usually indicate treatment failure and suggest that continuation of the current regimen is unlikely to be of value.

## Radiologic Assessment

In patients with stage I to stage III epithelial ovarian cancer, radiologic tests have generally been of limited value in assessing the response to therapy in patients with subclinical disease. Ascites can readily be detected, but even large omental metastases can be missed on CT.[165] If liver enzymes are abnormal, the liver can be evaluated with CT or ultrasonography, but extensive liver metastases can be present before they appear on imaging studies. A positive computed tomographic scan and fine-needle aspiration cytology can confirm the presence of disease, which could obviate the need for surgery in some cases, but the false-negative rate of CT is about 45%.

## Second-Look Procedures

A second-look operation is performed in a patient who has no clinical evidence of disease after a prescribed course of chemotherapy to determine the response to therapy. It permits the discontinuation of treatment when there is no pathologic evidence of disease, thereby minimizing the toxicity of treatment. Second-look operations are usually laparotomies, but the laparoscope is also used for this purpose.

The technique of the second-look laparotomy is essentially identical to that of the staging laparotomy. After multiple specimens are obtained for cytologic study, biopsy specimens of the peritoneal surfaces should be obtained, particularly from areas of previously documented tumor. These are the most important areas to biopsy because they are most likely to give a positive result. Any adhesions or surface irregularities should be sampled. A pelvic and para-aortic lymph node dissection below the level of the inferior mesenteric artery should be performed in patients whose nodal tissues have not previously been removed, which is the case for most patients with stage III disease.

Approximately 50 to 60% of patients with advanced-stage disease and a complete clinical response have occult disease detected at second-look operation.[166] About 30% of patients without evidence of macroscopic disease are found to have microscopic metastases.[167] In many patients with microscopic disease, residual disease is detected in only the occasional biopsy or cytologic specimen. Therefore, if a second-look operation is to be performed, a large number of specimens (20 to 30) should be obtained to minimize the false-negative rate of the operation.[168, 169] In selected patients in whom gross residual tumor is discovered at the second-look operation, resection of isolated masses may be performed. The removal of all gross persistent disease might facilitate a response to salvage therapies and also permits the collection of tissue for in vitro analysis.[170, 171] In a series from the Memorial Sloan-Kettering Cancer Center, cytoreduction at the time of second-look operation resulted in a group of patients whose disease was reduced to microscopic proportions. These patients had a 5-year survival of 51%, comparable to the 5-year survival of 62% in patients found to have microscopic disease at second-look operation and much better than the 10% survival of patients left with gross disease. These results were confirmed by a Gynecologic Oncology Group study in which the risk of death was lower among patients whose disease was debulked to a lower disease category.[172] Whether this benefit of cytoreductive surgery at second-look operation reflects tumor biology allowing surgical cytoreduction or direct effect from the cytoreduction itself is unclear.

Second-look laparotomies have not been shown to influence patient survival. Because second-line therapies in patients with persistent disease have not yet demonstrated a clear improvement in overall survival, second-look surgeries are recommended only in a research setting.[164]

The findings at second-look operation do correlate with subsequent outcome and survival.[167, 168, 173, 174] Patients who have no histologic evidence of disease have a significantly longer survival compared with those who have microscopic or macroscopic disease documented at laparotomy.[168, 175] About 50 to 75% of patients with negative results on second-look surgery remain free of disease at 5 years, whereas the median survival of patients with any disease is 12 to 18 months. Patients who remain disease free at 5 years have excellent long-term survival rates. In a 10-year follow-up of patients with negative findings at second-look surgery, only 16% (3 of 19 patients) with at least 5 years of disease-free follow-up had recurrence in the next 60 months.

The extent of residual disease documented at the second-look operation also correlates with patient survival.[167] Patients with microscopic disease have a 5-year survival of 40 to 50% and a median survival of more than 36 months, compared with 12 months for patients with any evidence of macroscopic disease. Clearly it is not possible to sample every potential site of disease, but failure to find disease at a second-look operation is not tantamount to a cure. In addition, disease can become clinically apparent in sites that are occult, such as the liver parenchyma or spleen. Most recurrences after a negative second-look operation are in patients with poorly differentiated cancers.

Variables associated with the outcome of the second-look laparotomy include initial stage, tumor grade, size of the largest metastatic disease site prior to treatment, size of the residual disease, and type of chemotherapy.[176] Unfortunately, there is no single variable or combination of variables that is sufficiently predictive to obviate a planned second-look surgery.[108]

Patients whose tumors are initially stage I or stage II have negative second-look laparotomy rates of 85 to 95% and 60 to 80%, respectively, whereas the rate for patients with stage III or stage IV disease is 30 to 45%.[167, 168, 173, 174, 177] The majority of patients with early-stage disease who have evidence of persistent disease at second-look surgery have more poorly differentiated tumors. The likelihood of negative findings on second-look operation in patients of all stages is about 80% for those with grade 1 tumors, 60 to 70% with grade 2 disease, and only 20% for those with grade 3 disease.[178]

The probability of a negative result on a second-look procedure is higher in patients whose tumor burden prior to initiation of chemotherapy is smaller. Patients whose disease is microscopic or less than 5 mm at the start of therapy have a much higher likelihood of a complete pathologic remission than do patients with more extensive disease.[167] Patients with extensive metastatic tumors also have a lower likelihood of negative findings on second-look operation, regardless of the extent of tumor reduction.

The likelihood of a negative second-look laparotomy is higher in patients who have been treated with a cisplatin-containing regimen compared with those treated with doxorubicin and cyclophosphamide or melphalan alone.[167] In patients with advanced-stage disease, the negative second-look rate is about 35 to 50% with cisplatin-containing regimens,

compared with only about 15 to 25% in patients treated with regimens not including cisplatin.

The second-look laparotomy has helped to define the number of cycles of chemotherapy necessary to achieve a complete response. Six to 9 cycles of cisplatin-containing chemotherapy produce about the same rate of negative second-look laparotomy in patients with advanced-stage disease as do 10 to 12 cycles.[167] These data suggest that epithelial carcinomas that are sensitive to chemotherapy are likely to respond early in the course of treatment. Additional treatment beyond 6 to 9 cycles does not appear to increase the probability of achieving a complete pathologic remission and will only increase treatment toxicity.

The laparoscope has been used for second-look assessment as well.[179–181] The advantage of the procedure is that it is a less invasive operation; the disadvantage is that the visibility is relatively limited by the frequent presence of intraperitoneal adhesions. Also, even in patients in whom visibility is good, the operation requires the technical expertise to be able to evaluate the retroperitoneum. Adhesions under the diaphragm and in the pelvic cul-de-sac are frequently a problem, as they limit the visibility in areas that are frequent sites of metastatic disease.

Open laparoscopy is frequently used. This technique allows the placement of the laparoscope after a cutdown to the fascia of the rectus abdominis in order to enter the peritoneum under direct vision, thus avoiding blind insertion, which can be associated with intestinal injury. Alternatively, a left upper quadrant entry can be used, making the incision just off the 12th rib in the midclavicular line.[180]

The sensitivity of the laparoscopic technique has been determined by performing a laparotomy immediately after negative laparoscopic findings.[182, 183] In one series, 35% of those who had a negative result on laparoscopy had evidence of disease at laparotomy. The false-negative rate of second-look laparoscopy depends on the thoroughness of the laparoscopic evaluation however. Despite obtaining fewer biopsy specimens with laparoscopy, Casey and associates found that this did not hinder the ability to detect disease.[180] Furthermore, laparoscopy was advantageous in minimizing operative time and days of hospitalization.[181] Another strategy is to use the laparoscope immediately prior to a planned laparotomy; if gross disease is detected and resection of tumor is not planned, a laparotomy might be omitted.

## TREATMENT OF RECURRENT OR PERSISTENT DISEASE

### Secondary Cytoreduction

Patients with persistent or recurrent pelvic and abdominal tumors after primary therapy for ovarian cancer occasionally are candidates for surgical excision of their disease. This operation has been referred to as secondary cytoreductive surgery.[170] Tumor resection under these circumstances should be restricted to carefully selected patients for whom resection has a reasonable chance of either prolonging life or significantly palliating symptoms because most patients with persistent or progressive disease after primary therapy do not benefit.

Candidates for secondary cytoreduction should be in good

general medical condition. A suitable patient would be one who has no evidence of ascites, has had a response to prior therapy, and has had a reasonably long disease-free interval from the time of primary diagnosis (at least 9 to 12 months). If the patient has received prior platinum-based therapy, secondary cytoreduction is justified if there has been a long disease-free interval because such patients are likely to respond again to the primary chemotherapy.[184–186]

The goal of secondary cytoreduction is to remove all gross residual tumor or to reduce the metastatic tumor burden to microscopic disease. The results of secondary chemotherapy indicate that volume of residual disease after secondary cytoreduction is still predictive of survival outcome. Janicke and coworkers found a significant difference in survival for 30 patients undergoing secondary cytoreduction.[187] Median survival after complete resection was 29 months, compared with 9 months in patients with disease that was resected to less than 2 cm. A disease-free interval of greater than 12 months before secondary cytoreduction was also associated with a prolongation of median survival by more than 20 months. Similarly, Vaccarello and colleagues reported 57 patients with a median progression-free interval of 33 months after a pathologic complete response to primary cytoreduction and platinum-based chemotherapy.[188] Patients who underwent optimal debulking had a median survival of 41 months. Patients who had suboptimal debulking had a median survival of 23 months, and patients who did not undergo re-exploration had a median survival of 9 months. Again, multivariate analysis confirmed that degree of surgical cytoreduction was the most significant variable affecting survival.

## Second-Line Chemotherapy

If disease persists at the time of second-look laparotomy, or if clinically evident disease develops during primary therapy, patients usually are switched to an alternative treatment, often second-line chemotherapy. The response rates for second-line chemotherapy have been less than 10 to 30% for most drugs tested via the oral or intravenous route.[189] Second-line therapy has not been shown to prolong survival; however, many more agents are now available for use as single agents and in combination.

Depending on prior therapy, persistent disease can be treated with cisplatin, carboplatin, or paclitaxel. In addition, topotecan, gemcitabine, liposomal doxorubicin, vinorelbine, ifosfamide, and hexamethylmelamine have all been shown to have activity in recurrent or persistent disease.

Patients who have responded to platinum-paclitaxel in the past can have a second response to retreatment with the same agents if an appropriate progression-free interval has elapsed. Weekly paclitaxel also appears to have activity in patients previously treated with cisplatin and paclitaxel.[190] Paclitaxel administered at doses of 60 mg/m$^2$ on a weekly basis is well tolerated, with partial response rates of up to 30%.

Topotecan, a topoisomerase I inhibitor, appears to have significant tumor activity against ovarian cancer.[191–194] Response rates seem dependent on prior platinum sensitivity. In a European phase II study, response rates of 26.7% were seen in cisplatin-sensitive patients, 17.8% in cisplatin-resistant patients, and only 5.9% in cisplatin-refractory patients.[192] Neutropenia and thrombocytopenia are significant toxicities associated with topotecan, and growth factor support should be strongly considered for patients who have received prior chemotherapy. Topotecan is also being studied in first-line therapy in combination with paclitaxel and cisplatin.[195] Preliminary toxicity data appear acceptable with the use of granulocyte colony–stimulating factor support.

Gemcitabine is a fluorine-substituted pyrimidine antimetabolite. In patients previously treated with platinum and paclitaxel, Shapiro and colleagues observed an overall response rate of 13% and a median progression-free interval of 7 months.[196] Gemcitabine is well tolerated on a weekly schedule, even in heavily pretreated patients. Uncomplicated neutropenia is the main hematologic toxicity.

Liposomal doxorubicin is a preparation of doxorubicin in a hydrophilic polymer capsule that lessens macrophage uptake and possibly increases tumor localization of the drug. In a platinum-refractory population, Muggia and associates reported an overall response rate of 26%, with a median duration of 5.7 months.[197] Minimal toxicity was observed, the most significant of which was hand-foot syndrome or stomatitis.

Vinorelbine is a vinca alkaloid analogue that inhibits assembly of microtubules. Administered weekly, vinorelbine has been shown to have a 21% response rate in phase II trials.[198] Again, side effects were manageable, including neutropenia, anemia, and worsening of neuropathy.

New strategies in therapy will include combining cytotoxic chemotherapy with agents such as trastuzumab (Herceptin) or gene therapy to approach the tumor targets in a multimodal fashion. Chemoprotectants such as amifostine and growth factors such as granulocyte colony–stimulating factor will also be able to allow continued treatment to the tumor while minimizing toxicity to the patients.[199]

## Biologic Response Modifiers

The interferons have been studied in ovarian cancer patients with minimal residual disease. In one series of 11 patients with less than 5 mm residual disease, the intraperitoneal administration of recombinant interferon alfa augmented peritoneal natural killer cell cytotoxicity and resulted in a surgically documented complete response in 4 patients (36%).[200] Unfortunately these response rates are only temporary. The typical circumstance in which intraperitoneal cytokines has been used is in a research setting after small residual disease has been found at second-look surgery, and these cases have not shown significant improvement with interferon alfa.[201]

Studies using adoptive immunotherapy with lymphokine-activated killer cells, and the concomitant administration of interleukin-2, are in progress for ovarian cancer. In 22 patients treated with intraperitoneal interleukin-2 and lymphokine-activated killer cell therapy, six responses were seen.[202] A major problem encountered with this approach has been excessive regional toxicity, especially peritoneal fibrosis.

## Radiation Therapy

Whole-abdomen radiation therapy given as a second-line treatment has been shown to be potentially effective in carefully selected patients with microscopic disease, but it is associated with relatively high morbidity. In one study, the 3-year survival of patients with minimal residual disease was 58%, but as many as 30% of patients treated with this approach developed intestinal obstruction necessitating exploratory surgery.[203] With current radiation techniques and appropriate fractionation, this risk should be minimized to less than 5%. In a series from Stanford University, 5-year survival of patients with residual disease less than 1.5 cm was 53% but no patients with disease greater than 1.5 cm survived 5 years.[204] Seven percent of patients in this series had late intestinal complications.

Localized radiation can also be administered to patients in fields such as the pelvis, chest, or brain for palliation of symptoms such as vaginal bleeding or pain.[205] Palliative response rates are about 80%, with a median duration of palliation of 4 months, reflecting palliation until death in 90% of cases.

### Hormonal Therapy

The role of progestins in the primary management of patients with epithelial cancer has been investigated by Berqvist and colleagues.[206] Four patients with previously untreated advanced ovarian cancer were given intramuscular medroxyprogesterone acetate. Three patients with mucinous carcinoma had objective responses, the fourth patient, with a serous carcinoma, had rapidly progressive disease.

Rendina and associates reported a series of 41 patients with endometrioid ovarian cancers in whom high-dose intramuscular medroxyprogesterone acetate was used as primary therapy.[207] Estrogen receptor (ER) and progesterone receptor (PR) status appeared to correlate with the histologic grade. Only 5 of 38 well-differentiated tumors were ER and PR negative, whereas 3 of 5 poorly differentiated tumors were PR negative. Seventeen patients could be evaluated for response: three patients had a complete response, one had a partial response, eight had stable disease, and six had progression of disease. Responses to progestin therapy were seen only in patients whose cancers expressed ER or ER plus PR. The results of this study support the concept that endometrioid ovarian cancers are hormonally sensitive tumors, and responses to progestin therapy may be correlated with the receptor content of the primary cancer.

There is no evidence that hormonal therapy alone is appropriate primary therapy for advanced ovarian cancer. Even in combination with multiagent chemotherapy, there are no good data to suggest that the use of medroxyprogesterone acetate or tamoxifen improves the effects of cytotoxic chemotherapy.[208, 209]

The progestational agent most commonly used for the management of recurrent ovarian cancer is medroxyprogesterone acetate, administered in both oral and intramuscular forms. Few responses (3 to 8%) have been observed, but no toxicity has been reported. Geisler used high-dose oral megestrol acetate, 800 mg daily for 1 month, then 400 mg daily thereafter, in the management of recurrent ovarian cancer.[210] Ten of 31 patients (32%) had an objective remission. Six patients had a complete response lasting 5 to 36 months (mean 16.5 months), and 4 patients had a partial response, with a progression-free interval ranging from 4 to 10 months.

Oral tamoxifen has been studied in recurrent epithelial ovarian cancer patients as well. One series from the Gynecologic Oncology Group using tamoxifen 20 mg twice daily in 77 patients demonstrated an objective response rate of 13% (five complete responders and five partial responders).[211] The median progression-free survival time in this series was only 4.4 months, but others have confirmed that many patients can have stabilization of disease even when they have failed to respond to standard cytotoxic chemotherapy.[212] Because the response to second-line cytotoxic chemotherapy is poor, tamoxifen may be a suitable alternative for these patients.

### Prognosis

The prognosis for patients with epithelial ovarian cancer relates to patient age, tumor stage, tumor grade, extent of residual disease, second-look status, and patient performance status.

In all stages of disease, patients younger than 50 years have a 5-year survival of 50 to 60%, compared with 35 to 40% 5-year survival for patients older than 50 years.[63] The 5-year survival for carefully and properly staged patients with stage I tumors is 80 to 90%, depending on the tumor grade. The 5-year survival for stage II and stage IIIA tumors is about 40 to 60% compared with about 25% for stage III and 10% for stage IV disease.

Patients with microscopic residual disease at the start of treatment have a 5-year survival of about 40 to 75%, compared with about 30 to 40% for those with optimally debulked disease, and only 5% for patients with suboptimally debulked disease.[170, 175] Patients without any evidence of disease at second-look laparotomy have a 5-year survival of 50 to 75%, compared with 40 to 50% for those with microscopic disease, and only about 5% for patients with macroscopic disease.

## Nonepithelial Ovarian Neoplasms

Nonepithelial malignancies of the ovary account for up to 20% of all ovarian cancers.[213–215] These include malignancies of germ cell origin (Table 55–6), sex cord–stromal cell origin, metastatic carcinomas to the ovary, and a variety of rare ovarian carcinomas such as sarcomas and lipoid cell tumors.

### GERM CELL MALIGNANCIES

Ranking behind epithelial tumors, germ cell tumors constitute the second largest group of primary ovarian neoplasms. Germ cell tumors are derived from the primordial germ cells of the ovary. During embryonic development, germ cells migrate from the caudal part of the yolk sac, along the dorsal mesentery of the hindgut, before being incorporated into the sex cords of the developing gonads. Although germ cell tumors can arise in extragonadal sites such as the mediastinum and the retroperitoneum, most arise from undifferentiated germ cells in the gonads. In men, germ cell tumors represent more than 95% of testicular cancer cases, and the incidence is also about 10 times greater than that in malignant germ cell tumors in women. Experience in the treatment

*Table 55–6.* World Health Organization Classification of Ovarian Germ Cell Tumors

Dysgerminoma
Yolk sac tumor (endodermal sinus tumor)
Embryonal carcinoma
Polyembryoma
Choriocarcinoma
Teratoma
  Immature
  Mature
    Solid
    Cystic (dermoid)
  Monodermal and highly specialized
    Struma ovarii
    Carcinoid
    Strumal carcinoid
    Others
Mixed forms

Adapted from Serov SF, Scully RE, Sobin IH. International histological classification of tumors No. 9: histological typing of ovarian tumours. Geneva: World Health Organization, 1973.

of testicular tumors has contributed significantly to the advances in the management of ovarian germ cell tumors.

## Classification

The histology of ovarian germ cell tumors follows a classification system developed by the World Health Organization (see Table 55–6).[71] Dysgerminomas are primitive germ cell neoplasms that are incapable of further differentiation. Embryonal carcinomas are composed of undifferentiated cells and are the progenitor lesions of more differentiated germ cell tumors. The tumors that have undergone extraembryonic differentiation recapitulate trophoblastic tissue and yolk sac histology in ovarian choriocarcinoma and endodermal sinus tumors, whereas tumors that have undergone embryonic differentiation recapitulate ectoderm, mesoderm, and endoderm in immature teratomas.

Several tumor markers are secreted by germ cell malignancies and can be clinically useful in the diagnosis and monitoring of patients. Embryonal carcinomas secrete AFP and hCG. Endodermal sinus tumors secrete AFP and choriocarcinomas secrete hCG. Immature teratomas have lost the ability to secrete these tumor markers. Lactate dehydrogenase is commonly produced by dysgerminomas and may be useful for monitoring disease. Placental alkaline phosphatase and $\alpha_1$-antitrypsin can also be detected in association with some germ cell tumors. Based on the patterns of expression between these tumor markers, a classification system of germ cell tumors can be diagrammed (Fig. 55–5).[216]

## Epidemiology

Although 20 to 25% of all benign and malignant ovarian neoplasms are germ cell tumors, only about 3% of these tumors are malignant.[215] Germ cell malignancies account for less than 5% of ovarian cancers in Western countries. In other societies where epithelial ovarian cancers are much less common, germ cell malignancies represent 15 to 20% of ovarian cancers.

In the first two decades of life, approximately two thirds of ovarian tumors are of germ cell origin, of which one third are malignant, accounting for two thirds of ovarian malignancies in this age group.[215] Germ cell tumors are also seen in the third decade of life but thereafter become rare.

## Clinical Features

In contrast to the relatively slow-growing epithelial ovarian tumors, germ cell malignancies grow rapidly and often present with subacute pelvic pain related to capsular distention, hemorrhage, or necrosis. The rapidly enlarging pelvic mass may produce pressure on the bladder or rectum, and menstrual irregularities may also occur in menarchal patients. Some young patients may misinterpret the early symptoms of a neoplasm as those of pregnancy, and this can lead to a delay in the diagnosis. Acute symptoms associated with torsion or rupture of the adnexa can develop. These symptoms may be confused with acute appendicitis. In more advanced cases, ascites may develop, and the patient can present with abdominal distention.

Patients with a palpable adnexal mass should be evaluated according to its characteristics of size, cystic versus solid nature, mobility, and smoothness of the surface (Fig. 55–6).[217] If the lesions are principally solid or a combination of solid and cystic, as might be noted on an ultrasonographic evaluation, a neoplasm is probable and a malignancy must be excluded. The physical examination should search for signs of ascites, pleural effusion, and organomegaly.

Some premenarchal patients may require examination under anesthesia. Adnexal masses 2 cm or larger in premenarchal females or 8 cm or larger in postmenarchal females usually require surgical exploration. In young patients, blood tests should include serum hCG and AFP titers, a complete blood count, and liver function tests. A chest radiograph is important to evaluate for pulmonary or mediastinal metasta-

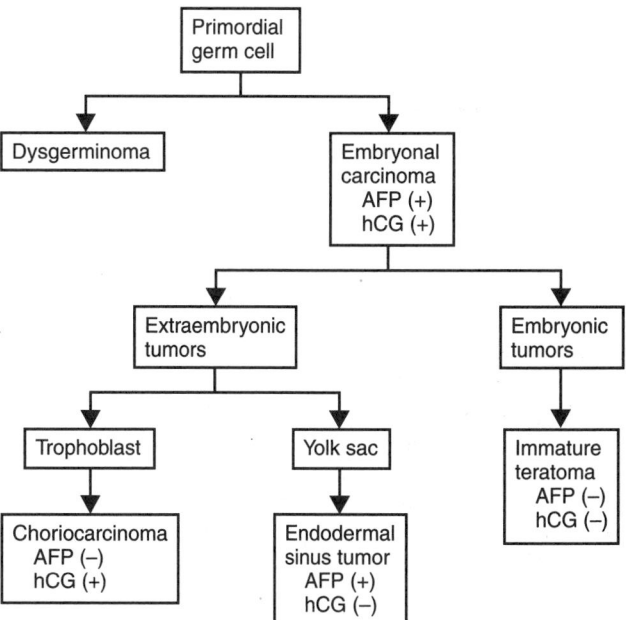

**Figure 55–5.** Relationship of pure malignant germ cell tumors and their secreted marker substances. (Adapted from Berek JS, Hacker NF. Practical gynecological oncology. 3rd ed. Philadelphia: Lippincott Williams & Wilkins, 2000:523–551.)

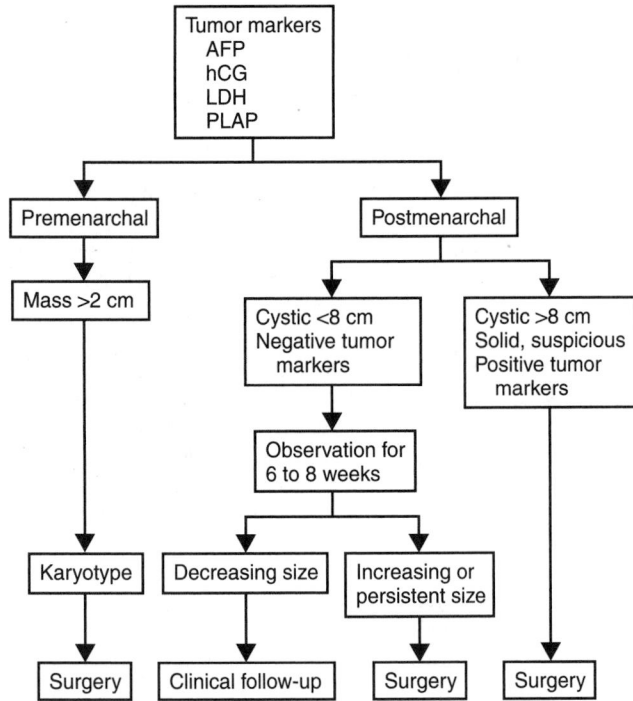

**Figure 55–6.** Evaluation of a pelvic mass in a young female patient. (Adapted from Bristow RE, Berek JS. Surgical management of dysgerminoma. Contemp Ob/Gyn 1998;43:98.)

ses. A karyotype should be obtained preoperatively in premenarchal females because of the propensity of these tumors to arise in dysgenetic gonads. Preoperative CT or MRI may document the presence and extent of retroperitoneal lymphadenopathy or liver metastases, but because these patients require surgical exploration, a more extensive and time-consuming evaluation is unnecessary. Germ cell tumors can grow rapidly; therefore, expediting surgery and moving on to chemotherapy is essential.

## Dysgerminomas

Dysgerminomas are the most common malignant germ cell tumor, composing up to 50% of all ovarian cancers of germ cell origin.[215] They account for 1% of all ovarian cancers but 5 to 10% of ovarian cancer in patients younger than age 20 and 20 to 30% of ovarian malignancies diagnosed in pregnancy. The mean age of dysgerminoma occurrence is 20 to 23 years.[218, 219]

Approximately 5% of dysgerminomas are diagnosed in phenotypic females with abnormal gonads. Most often dysgerminomas are associated with pure gonadal dysgenesis (46XY, bilateral streak gonads) or mixed gonadal dysgenesis (45X/46XY, unilateral streak gonad, contralateral testis), but they can also be associated with androgen insensitivity (46XY, testicular feminization).[215] A premenarchal patient with a pelvic mass should have the karyotype determined.

In most patients with gonadal dysgenesis, dysgerminomas arise in gonadoblastomas, which are benign ovarian tumors composed of germ cells and sex cord stroma. If gonadoblastomas are left in situ in patients with gonadal dysgenesis, more than 50% develop into ovarian malignancies.[220]

Not only are dysgerminomas diagnosed at a younger age,

they also present in an earlier stage. About 75% of patients present with stage I disease, with bilaterality noted in 10 to 15% of these patients.[221, 222] In fact, dysgerminoma is the only germ cell malignancy that has this significant rate of bilaterality, with other germ cell tumors being bilateral rarely. Microscopic disease can be present in 5 to 10% of patients whose contralateral ovary has been preserved.[215] This figure includes patients not treated with additional therapy. Given the chemosensitive nature of dysgerminoma, combination chemotherapy after conservative surgery would likely treat microscopic residual disease.

In the 25% of patients who present with metastatic disease, the tumor most commonly spreads via the lymphatics. It can also spread hematogenously, or by direct extension through the ovarian capsule, with exfoliation and dissemination of cells throughout the peritoneal surfaces. Metastases to the contralateral ovary may occur without other evidence of spread. Bony metastases are rare, and when this occurs lesions are seen principally in the lower vertebrae. Metastases to the lungs, liver, brain, and mediastinum are seen most often in longstanding or recurrent disease.

**Treatment.** An algorithm for the management of ovarian dysgerminoma is presented in Figure 55–7.[216] The treatment of patients with early dysgerminoma is primarily surgical, including the resection of the primary lesion and proper surgical staging. Chemotherapy or radiation therapy, or both, are administered to patients with metastatic disease. Because the patients affected by this disease are young, special consideration must be given to the preservation of fertility.

*Surgery.* The minimal operation for ovarian dysgerminoma is a unilateral oophorectomy. If there is desire to preserve fertility, the contralateral ovary, fallopian tube, and uterus should be left in situ, even in the presence of metastatic disease, because of the sensitivity of the tumor to chemotherapy. In patients with advanced disease whose fertility need not be preserved, it may be appropriate to perform a total abdominal hysterectomy and bilateral salpingo-oophorectomy. In patients whose karyotype analysis reveals a Y chromosome, both ovaries should be removed, although the uterus may be left in situ for possible future embryo transfer.

In patients in whom the neoplasm appears on inspection to be confined to the ovary, a careful staging operation should be undertaken to determine the presence of any occult metastatic disease. All peritoneal surfaces should be inspected and palpated and any suspicious lesions biopsied. Unilateral pelvic lymphadenectomy, along with careful palpation and sampling of enlarged para-aortic nodes, is particularly important to staging. These tumors often metastasize to the para-aortic nodes around the renal vessels. Dysgerminoma is the only germ cell tumor that tends to be bilateral, and not all bilateral lesions have ovarian enlargement. A Tru-Cut biopsy or excisional biopsy of any suspicious lesion is desirable. If a small contralateral tumor is found, it may be possible to resect it and preserve some normal ovary. Bivalving the contralateral ovary has been recommended in the past, but this probably increases the risk of subsequent infertility. A conservative surgical approach does not appear to increase the risk of recurrence.[223]

Although there are less specific data looking at the role of cytoreduction in germ cell tumors, the principles of debulking tumor to minimal residual disease to allow a better response to chemotherapy still apply. In a Gynecologic On-

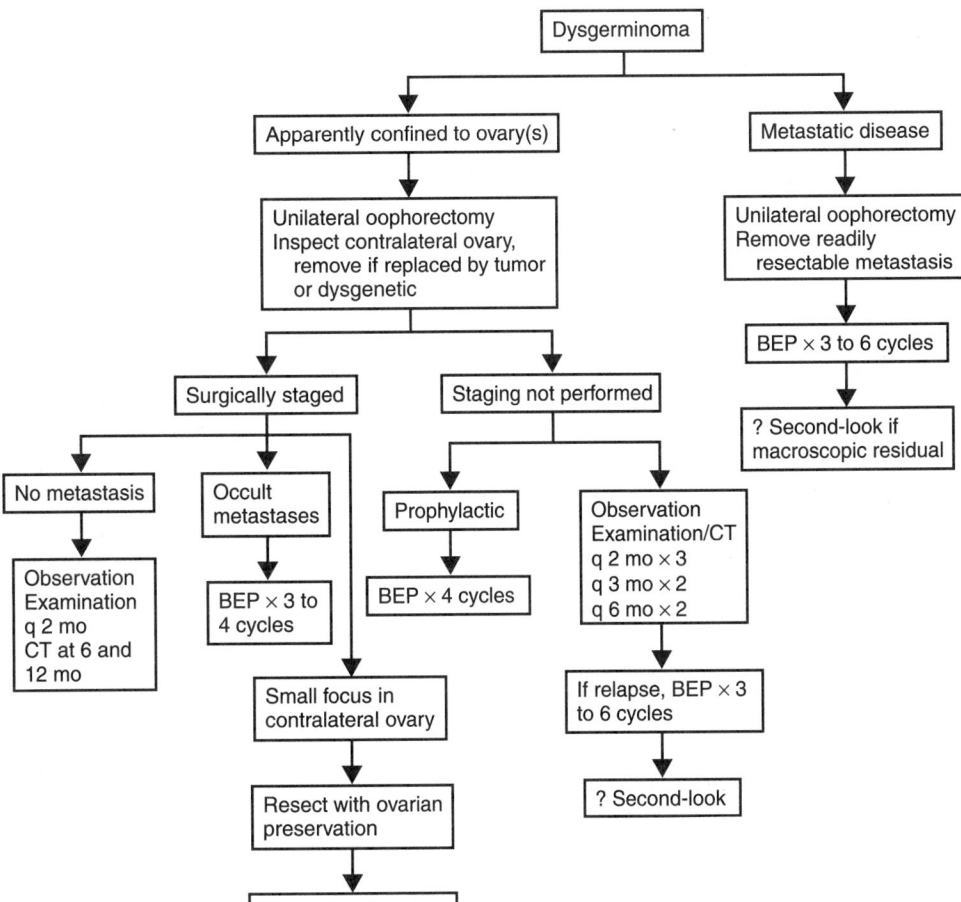

**Figure 55–7.** Algorithm for the management of ovarian dysgerminoma. (Adapted from Berek JS, Hacker NF. Practical gynecologic oncology. 3rd ed. Lippincott Williams & Wilkins, 2000.)

cology Group study, patients with malignant germ cell tumors treated with VAC (vincristine, dactinomycin [Adriamycin], and cyclophosphamide) were more likely to respond to chemotherapy when their disease was completely resected.[224] Although there were no pure dysgerminomas in the group, 15 of 22 (68%) patients with incompletely resected disease did not respond to VAC, whereas only 15 of 54 (28%) patients with completely resected disease did not respond. With improved response rates to newer chemotherapeutic agents, the degree of aggressiveness that should be taken, for example in the presence of high retroperitoneal lymph nodes, is debatable.

Many patients with dysgerminoma have a tumor that is apparently confined to one ovary and are referred after unilateral salpingo-oophorectomy without surgical staging. The options for such patients are a second laparotomy for surgical staging, regular pelvic and abdominal surveillance with CT, and adjuvant chemotherapy. As these are rapidly growing tumors, our preference is to perform regular computed tomographic surveillance. Tumor markers (hCG and AFP) should also be monitored in case there are occult mixed germ cell elements present.

PREGNANCY. Because dysgerminomas tend to occur in young patients, they may coexist with pregnancy. When a stage IA tumor is found, the tumor can be removed intact and the pregnancy continued. In patients with more advanced disease, continuation of the pregnancy will depend on gestational age. Chemotherapy can be given in the second and

third trimesters in the same dosages as given for the nonpregnant patient without apparent detriment to the fetus.

*Chemotherapy.* For many decades, radiation therapy was the traditional postoperative treatment. To achieve equal survival rates while preserving fertility and ovarian function, chemotherapy was used and there have been numerous reports of successful control of metastatic dysgerminomas with systemic chemotherapy, and this should now be considered the treatment of choice.

The most frequently used chemotherapeutic regimen for germ cell tumors is BEP (bleomycin, etoposide, and cisplatin), although PVB (cisplatin [Platinol], vinblastine, and bleomycin) and VAC remain as older alternatives (Table 55–7).[224–231]

The Gynecologic Oncology Group included dysgerminomas in two cisplatin-based chemotherapy trials using PVB and BEP followed by VAC consolidation.[230] Of 20 assessable patients, 19 of 20 were free of disease with a median follow-up of 26 months (range 6 to 68 months). Fourteen of these patients had a second-look operation, all of which produced negative findings. VAC consolidation is probably unnecessary in this group of patients.

Another study at the M. D. Anderson Cancer Center used BEP in 14 patients with residual disease, and all were disease free with long follow-up.[228] These results suggest that patients with advanced-stage, incompletely resected dysgerminoma still have an excellent prognosis when treated with cisplatin-based combination chemotherapy. The optimal regi-

*Table 55–7.* **Combination Intravenous Chemotherapy for Germ Cell Tumors of the Ovary Studied by the Gynecologic Oncology Group**

| Regimen Drugs | Dose and Schedule |
| --- | --- |
| BEP | |
| Bleomycin | 30 units weekly (400 units maximal total dose) |
| Etoposide | 100 mg/m$^2$ × 5 days, every 3 wk |
| Cisplatin | 20 mg/m$^2$ × 5 days, every 3 wk |
| PVB | |
| Cisplatin | 20 mg/m$^2$ × 5 days, every 3 wk |
| Vinblastine | 12 mg/m$^2$ every 3 wk |
| Bleomycin | 20 units/m$^2$ (30 units maximum) every wk |
| VAC | |
| Vincristine | 1.5 mg/m$^2$ (2 mg maximum) every 4 wk |
| Dactinomycin | 0.3 mg/m$^2$ × 5 days every 4 wk |
| Cyclophosphamide | 150 mg/m$^2$ × 5 days every 4 wk |

men is yet unknown, but three to four cycles of BEP seem sufficient.

There appears to be no need to perform a second-look laparotomy in dysgerminoma patients with all macroscopic disease resected at the primary operation.[232] In patients with macroscopic residual disease at the start of chemotherapy, a second-look operation may be able to identify persistent disease. Because effective second-line therapy is available, early identification of persistent disease may improve the prognosis.

*Radiation.* Dysgerminomas are sensitive to radiation therapy, and doses of 25 to 35 Gy may be curative even for gross metastatic disease.[232] However, loss of fertility is a problem with radiation therapy, so it should rarely be used as first-line treatment. For recurrence, however, radiation is effective for disease control.

**Prognosis and Recurrence.** In patients whose initial disease is stage IA, unilateral oophorectomy also results in 5-year disease-free survivals of greater than 95%.[218, 219, 222, 232] Lesions larger than 10 cm in diameter have been suggested to have a higher risk of recurrence, although not all series confirm this association. A microscopic pattern of high mitotic activity also does not seem to be associated with a worse prognosis and should not be a deterrent to conservative therapy.[215]

Most recurrences occur within the first year after initial treatment, the most common sites being the peritoneal cavity and retroperitoneal lymph nodes. These patients should be treated with radiation or chemotherapy, depending on their primary treatment. Patients with recurrent disease who have had no therapy other than surgery should be treated with chemotherapy. If prior chemotherapy with BEP has been given, VAC or PVB may be considered. Alternatively, ifosfamide-based (ifosfamide, cisplatin, and etoposide or vinblastine) regimens have been shown to have activity with durable responses.[233] From the testicular cancer literature, other alternatives to platinum-resistant tumors include high-dose chemotherapy regimens or phase II drugs.[234]

## Immature Teratomas

Immature teratomas contain elements resembling tissues derived from the embryo. Immature teratoma elements may occur in combination with other germ cell tumors as mixed germ cell tumors. The pure immature teratoma accounts for less than 1% of all ovarian cancers but is the second most common germ cell malignancy.[235] These tumors account for 10 to 20% of ovarian cancer in patients younger than 20 years. About 50% of pure immature teratomas of the ovary occur between the ages of 10 and 20 years, and they rarely occur in postmenopausal women. The mean age of immature teratoma occurrence in 17 to 21 years.[236–238]

Immature teratomas are differentiated from their benign mature counterparts through the presence of primitive neuroectodermal tissue. The histologic grade is based on a grading system classifying the quantity and degree of differentiation of the immature tissue.[237] Grade 1 refers to rare foci of immature neural tissue, occupying less than one low-power field in any slide. Grade 2 tumors have moderate quantities of immature neural tissue, occupying two to three low-power fields. Grade 3 tumors have four or more low-power fields on any slide containing fetal neuroepithelium.

The preoperative evaluation and differential diagnosis are the same as for patients with other germ cell tumors. Some of these lesions contain calcifications similar to mature teratomas; these calcifications can be detected by a radiograph of the abdomen or by ultrasonography. The clinical presentation is typically with an abdominal or pelvic mass and may be accompanied by pain. Tumor markers are generally absent unless a mixed germ cell tumor is present.

About two thirds of patients present with stage I disease, although bilaterality is seen in less than 10% of cases.[237–239] Metastatic disease is more likely to be in the form of peritoneal implants and less commonly as lymph node metastases. Preoperative rupture or tumor spill may increase the risk of subsequent peritoneal implants.[240, 241] Hematogenous metastases to the lungs, liver, or brain are uncommon. When present, they are usually seen with late or recurrent disease and most often in tumors that are poorly differentiated.

### Treatment

*Surgery.* In a premenopausal patient whose lesion appears confined to a single ovary, unilateral oophorectomy and surgical staging should be performed. In postmenopausal patients or patients whose childbearing is complete, a total abdominal hysterectomy and bilateral salpingo-oophorectomy may be performed.

Contralateral involvement is rare, and routine resection or wedge resection of the contralateral ovary is unnecessary. An enlarged contralateral ovary may contain a benign cyst or a mature cystic teratoma, which may be managed with an ovarian cystectomy. Any lesions of the peritoneal surfaces should be sampled and submitted for histologic evaluation.

Maximal tumor resection should still be the goal of surgery for this type of ovarian cancer. Patients whose tumors have been incompletely resected prior to treatment have a significantly lower probability of 5-year survival than those whose lesions have been completely resected.

*Chemotherapy.* Patients with stage IA grade 1 tumors have an excellent prognosis, and no adjuvant therapy is required. In patients whose tumors are stage IA grade 2 or 3, or of higher stage, adjuvant chemotherapy should be used.[236, 242]

The most frequently used combination chemotherapeutic regimen in the past has been VAC. The newer approach has been to incorporate cisplatin into the primary treatment of these tumors; thus, BEP is now the most commonly used chemotherapeutic combination (see Table 55–7).

The Gynecologic Oncology Group reported on a series of 76 patients with advanced-stage malignant germ cell tumors, 28 of which had histologic features of immature teratoma. These patients were treated with VAC.[224] Five of 28 (18%) patients had progression or recurrence; 1 of 20 of these patients had completely resected disease at primary surgery compared with 4 of 8 recurrences in patients with incompletely resected disease.

Because of its success in the treatment of testicular tumors and its activity in patients in whom VAC fails, PVB was introduced as a preferable first-line regimen.[225] The Gynecologic Oncology Group studied 97 patients with advanced-stage or recurrent germ cell malignancies, 26 of which had immature teratoma histology. Forty-two of 89 patients (47%, excluding dysgerminomas) ultimately had recurrence, but many were successfully treated with second- or third-line therapy for a 71% 2-year survival.

Vinblastine's side effects include neuromuscular toxicity. In a randomized clinical trial among men with disseminated germ cell tumors, BEP was found to be superior to PVB, with better efficacy and fewer neurologic and gastrointestinal toxicities. Three courses of adjuvant BEP were given in a Gynecologic Oncology Group prospective study of patients with surgically resected nondysgerminomatous germ cell malignancies. Forty-two patients with immature teratoma were in this group; only one patient had relapsed after a median follow-up of 38 months. Overall toxicity was acceptable, although two patients subsequently developed secondary hematologic malignancies. In view of these results, BEP is the preferred treatment regimen for patients with completely resected disease and for patients with gross residual disease, replacing VAC.

The use of bleomycin appears to be important in this group of patients. In a randomized study of three cycles of etoposide plus cisplatin with or without bleomycin (EP vs. BEP) in 166 patients with germ cell tumors of the testes, the BEP regimen had a relapse-free survival of 84% compared with 69% for the EP regimen.[233] In addition, cisplatin may be slightly better than carboplatin in the setting of metastatic germ cell tumors.[243]

The need for a second-look operation in germ cell malignancies has been questioned. It seems not to be justified in patients who have received chemotherapy in an adjuvant setting because chemotherapy in these patients is so effective. In a series of 53 patients with malignant nondysgerminomatous germ cell tumors undergoing second-look laparotomy at M. D. Anderson Cancer Center, only 1 patient was found to have persistent disease. With a median follow-up of 113 months (range 10 to 184 months), 50 of 53 patients were without evidence of disease. One patient had recurrence of disease and died, and 2 others died of leukemia.[244] We continue to prefer second-look surgery in patients with macroscopic residual disease at the start of chemotherapy because there are no reliable tumor markers for this disease, and such patients are at higher risk of relapse.

If a second-look operation is performed, careful sampling of any peritoneal lesions should be performed, and the retroperitoneal lymph nodes should be evaluated carefully. In as many as one quarter of patients, chemotherapeutic retroconversion, or the presence of mature implants after chemother-

apy for a higher grade tumor, may be observed.[244, 245] These implants may represent the differentiation of more primitive disease, or the nonmalignant component of the teratoma that is not chemosensitive. In either case, these mature implants do not confer worse prognosis. If only mature elements are found, chemotherapy should be discontinued. If persistent immature elements are documented, an alternative chemotherapeutic regimen should be used.

***Radiation.*** Radiation therapy is generally not used in the primary treatment of patients with immature teratomas. There is also no evidence that the combination of chemotherapy and radiation has a higher rate of disease control than does chemotherapy alone. Radiation should be reserved for patients with localized persistent disease after chemotherapy.

**Prognosis.** The most important prognostic feature of the immature teratoma is the grade of the lesion.[235, 237] In addition, the stage of disease and the extent of tumor at the initiation of treatment also have an impact on the curability of the lesion. Prior to current state-of-the-art chemotherapy, 5-year survival of patients with grades 1, 2, and 3 tumors was 81%, 60%, and 30%, respectively. With platinum-based combination chemotherapy, the 5-year survival is 90 to 95% for stage I disease and 75% for advanced stage disease. Recurrences are uncommon after the first 2 years of follow-up.[224, 229] Platinum-refractory disease may respond to other chemotherapeutic regimens including VAC, ifosfamide, or EMA-CO (etoposide, methotrexate, dactinomycin, cyclophosphamide, and vincristine). Furthermore, secondary cytoreductive surgery followed by additional chemotherapy may play a role in chemorefractory immature teratomas.[246]

### Endodermal Sinus Tumor

Endodermal sinus tumors have also been referred to as *yolk sac tumors* because they are derived from the primitive yolk sac. These lesions are the third most frequent malignant germ cell tumor of the ovary. About one third of patients are premenarchal at the time of initial presentation. Endodermal sinus tumors are most common in patients in the second and third decades. The mean age of endodermal sinus tumor occurrence is age 19.[247] The most common presenting symptom is abdominal pain, occurring in 80% of patients, whereas an asymptomatic pelvic mass is present in 10% of patients. The tumors tend to be solid and large, with a median size of 15 cm.[215]

Bilaterality is not seen in these lesions, and the other ovary is involved with metastatic disease only when there are other metastases in the peritoneal cavity. About 50% of patients have stage I disease.[232]

Most endodermal sinus tumors secrete AFP; rarely they may elaborate detectable $\alpha_1$-antitrypsin. There is a good correlation between the extent of disease and the level of AFP.[248] The serum level of AFP is useful in monitoring the patient's response to treatment.

### Treatment

***Surgery.*** The treatment of endodermal sinus tumor is surgical exploration, unilateral salpingo-oophorectomy, and a frozen section for diagnosis. The addition of hysterectomy and contralateral oophorectomy does not alter outcome. Any gross metastases should be removed if possible, but extensive surgical staging is not necessary because all patients with endodermal sinus tumor require chemotherapy.

*Chemotherapy.* All patients with endodermal sinus tumors are treated with either adjuvant or therapeutic chemotherapy. Prior to the routine use of combination chemotherapy, the 2-year survival for this disease was only 25%. After the introduction of VAC, this rate improved to 50 to 60%, indicating the chemosensitivity of the majority of these tumors.[224] Furthermore, with conservative surgery and adjuvant chemotherapy, fertility can be preserved as with other germ cell tumors.

PVB has been more effective in the treatment of endodermal sinus tumor, particularly in the treatment of measurable or incompletely resected tumors. In the Gynecologic Oncology Group series, 16 of 29 (55%) patients with endodermal sinus tumor had disease-free survival with a median follow-up of 37 months.[229] Using BEP in optimally resected disease, 24 of 25 (96%) of patients were clinically disease free with a median follow-up of 38 months.[231] Therefore, cisplatin-containing combination chemotherapy, preferably BEP, should be used as primary therapy for endodermal sinus tumor. The optimal number of treatment cycles has not been established; the Gynecologic Oncology Group protocols have used three to four cycles every 3 to 4 weeks. Our policy has been to give three to four cycles for patients with stage I and completely resected disease, and two further cycles after negative tumor marker status for patients with macroscopic residual disease prior to chemotherapy.

The value of a second-look procedure has yet to be established in patients with endodermal sinus tumor.[244] It appears reasonable to omit the operation in patients with pure lesions that are low stage and with normalization of AFP levels. There have been reported cases where the AFP level has returned to normal despite persistent measurable disease; some of these cases have been mixed germ cell tumors. In patients whose AFP titers do not return to normal, persistent disease can be assumed and alternative chemotherapy offered.

### Embryonal Carcinoma

Embryonal carcinoma of the ovary is an extremely rare tumor that is distinguished by large primitive cells resembling the embryonic germ disk.[215] The patients are very young; about half the patients are prepubertal, with the median age of occurrence at age 12. The presentation is usually an adnexal mass, but embryonal carcinomas may secrete estrogens, and patients may exhibit signs or symptoms of precocious pseudopuberty or irregular bleeding. The tumors are typically large and unilateral. About 60% of patients have disease confined to the ovary. These lesions frequently secrete AFP and hCG, which are useful markers for following the response to subsequent therapy.[233]

The treatment of embryonal carcinomas is the same as that for endodermal sinus tumors. Unilateral oophorectomy should be followed by BEP combination chemotherapy.[231] Without chemotherapy, the 5-year survival in one series was only 50%. Chemotherapy in other case series has been curative, even with extraovarian spread.[249–251] Radiation treatment does not appear to be useful as primary treatment.

### Choriocarcinoma of the Ovary

Pure nongestational choriocarcinoma of the ovary is an extremely rare tumor. Histologically, it has the same appearance as gestational choriocarcinoma metastatic to the ovaries.[215] The majority of patients are younger than 20 years. Isosexual precocious pseudopuberty has been seen in the presence of high hCG levels. The presence of hCG can be useful in monitoring the patient's response to treatment.

The prognosis for ovarian choriocarcinoma has been poor, with the majority of patients having metastatic disease to organ parenchyma at the time of initial diagnosis.[252] Ovarian choriocarcinomas may be less responsive to chemotherapy than gestational choriocarcinomas. It has been suggested that ovarian choriocarcinomas be treated with BEP, a germ cell regimen, rather than methotrexate or dactinomycin, a gestational trophoblastic disease regimen.[253]

### Polyembryoma

Polyembryoma of the ovary is another extremely rare tumor that is composed of embryoid bodies, recapitulating the structures of early embryonic development.[215] The lesion tends to present in young premenarchal girls, with signs and symptoms of a pelvic mass and pseudopuberty. AFP and hCG titers may be elevated. Anecdotally, combination chemotherapy has been reported to be effective. One patient with stage IA disease was treated successfully by surgery alone.[254] Recurrent or metastatic disease in two cases consisted of mature teratomatous elements.[255, 256]

### Mixed Germ Cell Tumors

Mixed germ cell malignancies of the ovary contain two or more elements of pure germ cell tumors. The most common component of a mixed germ cell tumor is dysgerminoma, occurring in 80%, followed by endodermal sinus tumor in 70%, immature teratoma in 53%, choriocarcinoma in 20%, and embryonal carcinoma in 20%.[257] The most frequent combination is dysgerminoma and endodermal sinus tumor. The mixed lesions may secrete AFP, hCG, both, or neither, depending on the components of the tumor.

These lesions should be treated with BEP chemotherapy. A serum marker that is initially positive and regresses may reflect regression of only a particular component of a mixed lesion. Therefore, in these patients, a second-look operation may be considered to determine a more precise response to therapy if there was macroscopic disease present at initiation of chemotherapy.

The most important prognostic features of these tumors are the size of the primary tumor and the relative amount of its most malignant component. In stage IA lesions smaller than 10 cm, survival is 100%.[257] Tumors composed of less than one-third endodermal sinus tumor, choriocarcinoma, or grade 3 immature teratoma also have an excellent prognosis, but the prognosis is less favorable when these components represent the majority of the mixed lesions.

## SEX CORD–STROMAL TUMORS

Sex cord–stromal tumors of the ovary account for about 8% of all primary ovarian neoplasms.[258] The tumors in this group are derived from the sex cords and the ovarian mesenchyme or stroma. Various combinations of elements may be present, including "female" elements of granulosa and theca cells,

*Table 55–8.* **Sex Cord–Stromal Tumors**

Granulosa-stromal cell tumors
  Granulosa cell tumor
  Thecoma-fibroma group
    Thecoma
    Fibroma
    Unclassified
Androblastomas: Sertoli-Leydig cell tumors
  Well-differentiated
    Sertoli's cell tumor
    Sertoli-Leydig cell tumor
    Leydig's cell tumor
  Moderately differentiated
  Poorly differentiated (sarcomatoid)
  Retiform
Sex cord tumor with annular tubules
Gynadroblastoma
Steroid cell tumors
  Stromal luteoma
  Leydig's cell tumor; Hilus' cell tumor
Unclassified

Adapted from Serov SF, Scully RE, Sobin IH. International histological classification of tumors No. 9: Histological typing of ovarian tumours. Geneva: World Health Organization, 1973.

and "male" elements of Sertoli's cells and Leydig's cells. The classification of these tumors is also based on these elements (Table 55–8).[71]

## Granulosa–Stromal Cell Tumors

Granulosa cell tumors, thecomas, and fibromas are included in the granulosa-stromal cell tumors. Granulosa cell tumors are considered of low malignant potential. In the rare instance that thecomas and fibromas have morphologic features of malignancy, they may be referred to as *fibrosarcomas.*

Granulosa cell tumors, which may be estrogen secreting, are seen in women of all ages. Approximately 5% of granulosa cell tumors occur in prepubertal girls; the remainder are distributed equally among premenopausal, perimenopausal, and postmenopausal women.[259] Adult versus juvenile histologic type refers to the patterns of growth, and the adult type accounts for 95% of granulosa cell tumors. Bilaterality occurs less than 5% of the time.[258]

Granulosa cell tumors are the most common functional ovarian neoplasms. Prepubertal lesions are associated with sexual pseudoprecocity due to estrogen production in three quarters of cases. In the reproductive age group, patients may have menstrual irregularities or secondary amenorrhea, and in postmenopausal women, abnormal uterine bleeding may be the presenting symptom.[259, 260] Because of the endogenous estrogen effect, endometrial hyperplasia is also frequently present. Approximately 25 to 50% of granulosa cell tumors are associated with endometrial hyperplasia, whereas 5 to 10% are associated with a low-grade endometrial carcinoma.[259, 261]

A mass is usually present. Between 80 and 90% of granulosa cell tumors are confined to the ovary. Advanced metastatic disease with ascites is present in about 10% of cases. Granulosa cell tumors tend to be hemorrhagic; occasionally they may rupture and produce a hemoperitoneum.

The tumors may also spread hematogenously, and patients can develop metastases in the lungs, liver, and brain years after initial diagnosis. Although granulosa cell tumors usually present with stage I disease, this may be somewhat reflective of incomplete staging because 5 to 10% of patients with stage I disease have recurrences 5 to 30 years later.[258, 262] Ten-year survival is approximately 90%, whereas 20-year survival is approximately 75%. Recurrent disease can progress more rapidly.

Serum inhibin may be a valuable tumor marker, particularly in postmenopausal women. Elevated serum inhibin levels have been correlated with preoperative diagnosis and recurrence.[263, 264]

**Treatment.** The treatment of granulosa cell tumors depends on the age of the patient and the extent of disease. For most patients, surgery alone is sufficient therapy, with radiation and chemotherapy reserved for the treatment of advanced, recurrent, or metastatic disease.[259, 260]

*Surgery.* Because granulosa cell tumors are bilateral in only about 2% of patients, performing a unilateral salpingo-oophorectomy is appropriate therapy for stage IA tumors in children or in women desiring future fertility.[262] At the time of surgery, if a granulosa cell tumor is identified by frozen section, a staging operation should be performed, including an assessment of the contralateral ovary. If the opposite ovary appears enlarged, it should be biopsied. In perimenopausal and postmenopausal women for whom ovarian function is no longer significant, a hysterectomy and bilateral salpingo-oophorectomy should be performed. In premenopausal women in whom the uterus is left in situ, an endometrial sampling of the uterus should be performed to evaluate for the possibility of a coexistent endometrial neoplasm.

*Radiation.* The use of radiation therapy has been described in both adjuvant and recurrent settings for granulosa cell tumor; however, its effects on improving survival are unproved.[260] Because of relatively low recurrence rates after primary resection, the data are inconclusive about the independent effects of radiation when considering factors of stage, residual disease, and field of radiation. Disease response has been observed with radiation in metastatic or recurrent disease, and this may be considered when tumor cannot be suitably debulked.

*Chemotherapy.* Patients with stage I disease usually do well with surgical treatment alone, but patients with advanced-stage disease are candidates for adjuvant treatment. Several different combinations of chemotherapeutic agents have been used in metastatic and recurrent disease, yet there has been no consistently effective regimen in these patients. Cisplatin-based combination therapy appears most effective. A combination of bleomycin, etoposide, and cisplatin in a 5-day regimen for four cycles was studied by the Gynecologic Oncology Group for primary and recurrent stromal malignancies of the ovary.[265] Forty-eight of 57 patients were enrolled with granulosa cell tumor. For primary disease, 6 of 15 patients had second-look surgery; 4 of these 6 patients were without pathologic evidence of disease. Of patients with recurrent disease, 9 of 24 evaluable patients demonstrated response (5 complete responders); thus, BEP is also recommended as an active regimen for ovarian stromal malignancies. Intraperitoneal chemotherapy may also be considered for this slow-growing surface disease. The use of hormonal agents such as progestins or anti-estrogens has been suggested, but there are no data available to suggest effectiveness.[262]

**Prognosis.** Granulosa cell tumors have a prolonged natural history and a tendency for late relapse, reflecting their low-grade biology. Ten-year survival of approximately 90% has been reported, with 20-year survival around 75%.[259, 262] Most histologic types have the same prognosis, but the juvenile form tends to recur earlier than the adult form.[258] The presence of residual disease at surgery is probably the most important predictor of progression-free survival, but DNA ploidy appears to be an independent prognostic factor as well.[266]

### Sertoli–Leydig Cell Tumors

Sertoli-Leydig cell tumors are composed of Sertoli's cells, as well as Leydig's cells and other cells of stromal derivation in variable proportions. The mean age of occurrence is 25 years, with 75% of lesions seen in women younger than age 40.[258] Sertoli-Leydig cell tumors behave mostly in a low-grade malignant fashion, although occasionally a poorly differentiated tumor may behave more aggressively.

The tumors typically produce androgens, and clinical virilization is seen in up to two thirds of cases. Signs of virilization include oligomenorrhea or amenorrhea, breast atrophy, acne, hirsutism, clitoromegaly, deepening voice, and male pattern hair loss. Plasma androgen and androstenedione may be elevated with slightly elevated dihydroepiandrostenedione.[258] Rarely, Sertoli-Leydig tumors can produce an estrogen effect, resulting in isosexual precocity and irregular bleeding. Patients without hormonal symptoms present with the usual abdominal symptoms.

**Treatment.** These low-grade lesions are bilateral in less than 1% of cases. The usual treatment for women of reproductive age is unilateral salpingo-oophorectomy and evaluation of the contralateral ovary. Older women should undergo hysterectomy and bilateral salpingo-oophorectomy.

There are insufficient data to document the utility of radiation or chemotherapy in patients with persistent disease.[258] Seven of 57 patients in the Gynecologic Oncology Group trial using BEP in stromal tumors had Sertoli-Leydig cell tumors.[265]

**Prognosis.** These tumors behave in a slow-growing, indolent, fashion. Recurrences are typically early, about two-thirds within 1 year after primary treatment. The 5-year survival is 70 to 90%.

## SARCOMAS

Malignant mixed mesodermal sarcomas of the ovary are rare tumors, and pure sarcomas are even more uncommon. Most lesions are heterologous, and tend to occur in postmenopausal women. The presentation is similar to that of most ovarian malignancies. The lesions are biologically aggressive, and the majority of patients present with metastatic disease.

**Treatment.** The diagnosis of carcinosarcomas of the ovary is usually made at surgery. Optimal cytoreduction appears to contribute to improved outcome in ovarian sarcomas as well as in epithelial ovarian cancers.[267] Platinum-based chemotherapy has also been shown to have activity and appears to give a survival advantage over other chemo-

therapy combinations.[267–269] Median survival has been described at about 18 to 24 months.

## STEROID CELL TUMORS

Steroid cell tumors, or lipoid tumors, are thought to arise in the adrenal cortical rests that reside in the vicinity of the ovary. Stromal luteomas and Leydig's cell tumors may be associated with virilization and occasionally with obesity, hypertension, and glucose intolerance. Rare cases of estrogen secretion and isosexual precocity have been reported. Bilaterality has been noted in only 5% of cases, and extraovarian spread at the time of diagnosis is seen in about 20% of cases.[270]

**Treatment.** Management of steroid cell tumors is by surgical extirpation of the primary lesion. The majority of these tumors have a benign or low-grade behavior. Malignant behavior has been correlated with tumor size greater than 7 cm, two or more mitotic figures per high-power field, necrosis, hemorrhage, and nuclear atypia.[271] There are insufficient data regarding radiation or chemotherapy for this disease.

# Metastatic Tumors

About 5 to 6% of ovarian tumors are metastatic from other organs, most frequently from the female genital tract, the breast, or the gastrointestinal tract. The metastases may occur from direct extension of another pelvic neoplasm, intraperitoneal dissemination, lymphatic spread, or hematogenous spread.

## GYNECOLOGIC METASTASES

Cancers of the genital tract can spread by direct extension to the ovaries, such as in the instance of tubal carcinomas. Under some circumstances, it is difficult to know if the tumor originates in the tube or in the ovary when both are involved. Adenocarcinoma of the endometrium can also spread and become directly implanted on the surface of the ovaries, but two synchronous tumors probably occur with greater frequency. In most cases, there is an endometrioid carcinoma of the ovary associated with an endometrioid carcinoma of the endometrium that is histologically indistinguishable. Cervical cancer of squamous histology rarely spreads to the ovary, but adenocarcinomas can metastasize to the ovaries in about 2% of cases.[272]

## BREAST METASTASES

The frequency of breast cancer metastasizing to the ovaries varies according to the method of determination, but the phenomenon is common. In autopsy series of women who died of metastatic breast cancer, the ovaries were involved in 24% of cases; in 80% of these cases, involvement was bilateral.[273] Similarly, when oophorectomy is performed to palliate advanced breast cancer, 20 to 30% of cases reveal ovarian involvement.[274] In early-stage breast cancer, the incidence of involvement is considerably lower. In most cases, ovarian involvement is occult, or a pelvic mass is discovered after other metastatic disease becomes apparent.

## GASTROINTESTINAL TRACT METASTASES

The Krukenberg tumor, which can account for 30 to 40% of cancers metastatic to the ovaries, arises in the ovarian stroma and has characteristic mucin-filled, signet ring cells.[275] The primary tumor is frequently from the stomach but may also be from the colon, breast, or biliary tract. Krukenberg's tumors are usually bilateral and usually are not discovered until the primary disease is advanced; therefore, prognosis is poor. In some cases, a primary tumor is not found.

In other cases of metastasis from the gastrointestinal tract to the ovary, the tumor does not have the classic histologic appearance of a Krukenberg tumor. Most of these metastases are from the colon and, less commonly, the small intestine. Patients with advanced colorectal cancer may often develop metastases to the ovaries during the course of their disease, and oophorectomy may be indicated in these women to prevent recurrence.

Furthermore, in women with an adnexal tumor and gastrointestinal symptoms, a primary gastrointestinal carcinoma must be considered. CT is helpful, but a barium enema or colonoscopy is more sensitive if the level of suspicion is high.

## CARCINOID METASTASES

Metastatic carcinoid tumors represent less than 2% of metastases to the ovary.[276] Conversely, only 2% of primary carcinoids have ovarian metastases, and only 40% of these patients have carcinoid syndrome at the time of discovery of the metastatic carcinoid. In perimenopausal and postmenopausal women who undergo exploratory surgery for an intestinal carcinoid, it is reasonable to remove the ovaries to prevent subsequent metastases. The discovery of an ovarian carcinoid should prompt a careful search for an intestinal primary.

## LYMPHOMATOUS METASTASES

Lymphomas and leukemias can involve the ovary in a bilateral fashion. About 5% of patients with Hodgkin's disease develop lymphomatous involvement of the ovaries, but this occurs typically with advanced stage disease.[277] With Burkitt's lymphoma, ovarian involvement is common.[278] The ovaries may be the only site of abdominal or pelvic involvement, and in these circumstances, surgical exploration may be indicated. Removal of the large ovarian mass may improve patient comfort and facilitate response to subsequent radiation or chemotherapy. If an intraoperative frozen section of the ovary reveals lymphoma, extensive surgical staging is not necessary, although enlarged lymph nodes should be biopsied. In Hodgkin's disease, a more extensive evaluation may be necessary. Treatment involves that of the lymphoma in general (i.e., CHOP chemotherapy).

# FALLOPIAN TUBES

• Jonathan S. Berek • Lee-may Chen

Carcinoma of the fallopian tubes accounts for 0.3% of all cancers of the female genital tract.[264, 265] In histology and behavior, fallopian tube carcinoma is similar to ovarian cancer; thus, the evaluation and treatment are essentially the same. The fallopian tubes are frequently involved secondarily from other primary sites, most often the ovaries, endometrium, gastrointestinal tract, or breast. They may also be involved in primary peritoneal carcinomas. Almost all cancers are of epithelial origin, most frequently of serous histologic type. Rare sarcomas have also been reported.

## Clinical Features

Tubal cancers are seen most frequently in the fifth and sixth decades of life, with a mean age of 55 to 60 years. There are no known predisposing factors, and preoperative diagnosis is made in only about 5% of cases.[265]

The classic triad of symptoms and signs associated with fallopian tube cancer is (1) a prominent watery vaginal discharge (hydrops tubae profluens), (2) pelvic pain, and (3) a pelvic mass. However, this triad is noted in less than 15% of patients.

Vaginal discharge or bleeding is the most common symptom reported by patients with tubal carcinoma. Abdominal or pelvic pressure and pain are also noted in many patients and may be associated with distention of the fallopian tube by tumor. The presentation may be rather vague and nonspecific. In perimenopausal and postmenopausal women with an unusual, unexplained, or persistent vaginal discharge, the possibility of an occult tubal cancer should be considered. Fallopian tube cancer is often found incidentally in asymptomatic women at the time of abdominal hysterectomy and bilateral salpingo-oophorectomy.

On examination, a pelvic mass is present in about 60% of patients, and ascites may be present if advanced disease exists. Abnormal or adenocarcinoma cells may be seen in cytologic specimens obtained from the cervix in 10% of patients, and these patients have negative results on dilation and curettage.

Tubal cancers spread in much the same manner as epithelial ovarian malignancies, principally by the transcoelomic exfoliation of cells that implant throughout the peritoneal

*Table 55–9.* **FIGO Staging for Carcinoma of the Fallopian Tube (1991)**

**Stage I. Growth limited to the fallopian tube**
Ia   Growth limited to one tube, with extension into the submucosa and/or muscularis, but not penetrating the serosal surface; no ascites.
Ib   Growth limited to both tubes with extension into the submucosa and/or muscularis but not penetrating the serosal surface; no ascites.
Ic   Either Ia or Ib, but with tumor extension through or onto the tubal serosa, or with ascites present containing malignant cells, or with positive peritoneal washings.

**Stage II. Growth involving one or both fallopian tubes with pelvic extension.**
IIa   Extension and/or metastasis to the uterus and/or ovaries.
IIb   Extension to other pelvic tissues.
IIc   Either IIa or IIb, but with ascites present containing malignant cells or with positive peritoneal washings.

**Stage III. Tumor involves one or both fallopian tubes, with peritoneal implants outside the pelvis and/or retroperitoneal or inguinal nodes. Superficial liver metastasis equals stage III. Tumor is limited to the true pelvis, but with histologically proven malignant extension to small bowel or omentum.**
IIIa   Tumor grossly limited to the true pelvis with negative nodes but with histologically confirmed microscopic seeding of abdominal peritoneal surfaces.
IIIb   Tumor of one or both ovaries with histologically confirmed implants of abdominal peritoneal surfaces; none exceeding 2 cm in diameter. Nodes negative.
IIIc   Abdominal implants >2 cm in diameter and/or positive retroperitoneal or inguinal lymph nodes.

**Stage IV. Growth involving one or both fallopian tubes with distant metastasis. If pleural effusion is present, there must be positive cytologic test results to allot a case to stage IV. Parenchymal liver metastasis equals stage IV.**

From Pecorelli S, Odicino F, Maisonneuve P, et al. FIGO annual report of the results of treatment in gynaecological cancer: carcinoma of the ovary. J Epidemiol Biostat 1998;3:75–102.

cavity. Bilaterality is present in only about 3% of cases.[280] About 80% of patients with advanced disease have metastases confined to the peritoneal cavity at the time of diagnosis.[281]

The fallopian tube is also richly permeated with lymphatic channels, and spread to the para-aortic and pelvic lymph nodes is common. Metastases to the para-aortic lymph nodes have been documented in at least 33% of patients with all stages of disease.[282]

The International Federation of Gynecology and Obstetrics (FIGO) staging system for tubal cancer is adopted from the ovarian staging system (Table 55–9).[283] Using this surgical staging system, 37% of patients have stage I disease, 20% have stage II, 31% have stage III, and 10% have stage IV.[283] A somewhat lower incidence of advanced disease is seen in these patients than in patients with epithelial ovarian carcinoma, presumably because symptoms occur earlier.

## Treatment

The treatment for this disease is similar to that for epithelial ovarian cancer.[281, 282, 284] Exploratory surgery is necessary to remove the primary tumor, stage the disease, and resect metastases. After surgery, the most frequently used treatment is combination chemotherapy, although radiation is also used in selected cases.

Patients with a tubal carcinoma should undergo total abdominal hysterectomy and bilateral salpingo-oophorectomy. If there is no gross tumor spread, a staging operation is performed. The retroperitoneal lymph nodes should be adequately evaluated, peritoneal cytology and biopsy specimens obtained, and an infracolic omentectomy performed.

In patients with metastatic disease, an effort should be made to remove as much tumor bulk as possible. The role of cytoreductive surgery in this disease is unclear, but extrapolating from the experience with epithelial ovarian cancer, significant benefit might be expected.

For patients with unstaged disease in whom an occult fallopian tube carcinoma is discovered postoperatively, treatment options include staging laparoscopy or proceeding with chemotherapy in grade 2 to 3 disease.

It appears justifiable to use the same protocols as for epithelial ovarian cancer in patients with epithelial tubal cancers. Data on well-staged lesions are scarce. Therefore, it is unclear whether or not patients with disease confined to the fallopian tube, that is, stage IA grade 1 or 2, benefit from additional therapy.

Although the majority of patients with tubal cancers were treated with radiation in the past, its role in the management of disease remains unclear because patients have not been treated in any consistent manner, and the small numbers preclude any meaningful conclusions.

The overall 5-year survival for patients with epithelial tubal carcinomas is about 40%. This number is higher than that for ovarian cancer, reflecting the somewhat higher proportion of patients with early-stage disease. The outlook is clearly related to the stage of disease. The 5-year survival for patients with stage I disease is about 84%, with stage II disease it is 52%, and for stage III or IV disease it is 15 to 35%.[283]

## SUGGESTIONS FOR ADDITIONAL READING

Chuaqui RF, Cole KA, Emmert-Buck MR, Merino MJ. Histopathology and molecular biology of ovarian epithelial tumors. Ann Diagn Pathol 1998;2:195–207.

Berchuck A. Biomarkers in the ovary. J Cell Biochem 1995;23:Suppl:223–6.

Outwater EK, Dunton CJ. Imaging of the ovary and adnexa: clinical issues and applications of MR imaging. Radiology 1995;194:1–18.

Ronnett BM, Shmookler BM, Sugarbaker PH, Kurman RJ. Pseudomyxoma peritonei: new concepts in diagnosis, origin, nomenclature, and relationship to mucinous borderline (low malignant potential) tumors of the ovary. Anat Pathol 1997;2:197–226.

Tropé C, Kaern J. Management of borderline tumors of the ovary: state of the art. Semin Oncol 1998;25:372–80.

Piura B, Rabinovich A, Yanai-Inbar I, et al. Primary sarcoma of the ovary: report of five cases and review of the literature. Eur J Gynaecol Oncol 1998;19:257–61.

Talerman A. Germ cell tumors of the ovary. Curr Opin Obstet Gynecol 1997;9:44–7.

## REFERENCES

1. Greenlee RT, Murray T, Bolden S, Wingo PA. Cancer statistics, 2000. CA Cancer J Clin 2000;50:7–33.
2. Scully RE, Young RH, Clement PB. General features of ovarian

tumors. In: Tumors of the ovary, maldeveloped gonads, fallopian tube, and broad ligament. Washington, D. C.: Armed Forces Institute of Pathology 1998;27–50.

3. Whittemore AS, Harris R, Intyre J, and the Collaborative Ovarian Cancer Group: Characteristics relating to ovarian cancer risk: collaborative analysis of 12 U. S. case-control studies. II: Invasive epithelial ovarian cancers in white women. Am J Epidemiol 1992;136:1184–1203.

4. Whittemore AS, Harris R, Intyre J, and the Collaborative Ovarian Cancer Group: Characteristics relating to ovarian cancer risk: collaborative analysis of 12 U. S. case-control studies: the pathogenesis of epithelial ovarian cancer. Am J Epidemiol 1992;136:1212–20.

5. Rossing MA, Daling JR, Weiss NS, et al. Ovarian tumors in a cohort of infertile women. N Engl J Med 1994;331:771–6.

6. Shushan A, Paltiel O, Iscovich J, et al. Human menopausal gonadotropin and the risk of epithelial ovarian cancer. Fert Steril 1996;65:13–8.

7. Bristow RE, Karlan BY. Ovulation induction, infertility, and ovarian cancer risk. Fert Steril 1996;66:499–507.

8. Hankinson SE, Colditz GA, Hunter DJ, et al. A quantitative assessment of oral contraceptive use and risk of ovarian cancer. Obstet Gynecol 1992;80:708–14.

9. The Cancer and Steroid Hormone Study of the Centers for Disease Control and the National Institute of Child Health and Human Development. The reduction in risk of ovarian cancer associated with oral contraceptive use. N Engl J Med 1987;316:650–5.

10. Cramer DW, Welch WR, Scully RE, Wojciechowski CA. Ovarian cancer and talc. Cancer 1982;50:372–6.

11. Hankinson SE, Hunter DJ, Colditz GA, et al. Tubal ligation, hysterectomy, and risk of ovarian cancer. JAMA 1993;270:2813–6.

12. Hartge P, Whittemore AS, Intyre J, et al. Rates and risks of ovarian cancer in subgroups of white women in the United States. Obstet Gynecol 1994;84:760–4.

13. Schildkraut, JM, Thompson WD. Familial ovarian cancer: a population-based case-control study. Am J Epidemiol 1988;128:456–66.

14. Kerlikowske K, Brown JS, Grady DG. Should women with familial ovarian cancer undergo prophylactic oophorectomy? Obstet Gynecol 1992;80:700–7.

15. Lynch HT, Albano W, Black L, et al. Familial excess of cancer of the ovary and other anatomic sites. JAMA 1982;245:261–4.

16. Lynch HT, Watson P, Bewtra C, et al. Hereditary ovarian cancer. Cancer 1991;67:1460–6.

17. Miki Y, Swensen J, Shattuck-Eidens D, et al. A strong candidate for the 17q-linked breast and ovarian cancer susceptibility gene BRCA1. Science 1994;266:66–71.

18. Wooster R, Bignall G, Lancaster J, et al. Identification of the breast cancer susceptibility gene BRCA2. Nature 1995;378:789–92.

19. Couch FJ, Farid LM, DeShano ML, et al. BRCA2 germline mutations in male breast cancer cases and breast cancer families. Nat Genet 1996;13:123–5.

20. Tavtigaian SV, Simard J, Rommens J, et al. The complete BRCA2 gene and mutations in chromosome 13q-linked kindreds. Nat Genet 1996;12:333–7.

21. Struewing JP, Abeliovich D, Peretz T, et al. The carrier frequency of the BRCA1 185delAG mutation is approximately 1 percent in Ashkenazi Jewish individuals. Nat Genet 1995;11:198–200.

22. Abeliovich D, Kaduri L, Lere I, et al. The founder mutations 185delAG and 5832insC in BRCA1 and 6174detT in BRCA2 appear in 60% of ovarian cancer and 30% of early-onset breast cancer patients among Ashkenazi women. Am J Hum Genet 1997;60:505–14.

23. Easton DF, Ford D, Bishop DT, and the Breast Cancer Linkage Consortium. Breast and ovarian cancer incidence in BRCA1-mutations carriers. Am J Hum Genet 1995;56:265–71.

24. Struewing JP, Hartge P, Wacholder S, et al. The risk of cancer associated with specific mutations of BRCA1 and BRCA2 among Ashkenazi Jews. N Engl J Med 1997;336:1401–08.

25. Narod SA, Risch H, Moslehi R, et al. Oral contraceptive use and the risk of hereditary ovarian cancer. N Engl J Med 1998;424–8.

26. Tobacman JK, Tucker MA, Kase R, et al. Intra-abdominal carcinomatosis after prophylactic oophorectomy in ovarian cancer prone families. Lancet 1982;2:795–7.

27. Struewing JP, Watson P, Easton DF, et al. Prophlactic oophorectomy in inherited breast/ovarian cancer families. J Natl Cancer Inst 1995;17:33–5.

28. Watson P, Lynch HT. Extracolonic cancer in hereditary nonpolyposis colorectal cancer. Cancer 1993;71:677–85.

29. Aarnio M, Mecklin J-P, Aaltonen LA, et al. Lifetime risk of different cancers in hereditary non-polyposis colorectal cancer (HNPCC) syndrome. Int J Cancer 1995;64:430–5.

30. Fishel R, Lescoe MK, Rao MR, et al. The human mutator gene homologue MSH2 and its association with hereditary nonpolyposis colon cancer. Cell 1993;75:1027–38.

31. Bronner CE, Baker SM, Morrison PT, et al. Mutation in the DNA mismatch repair gene homologue hMLH1 is associated with hereditary nonpolyposis colon cancer. Nature 1994;368:258–61.

32. Nicolaides NC, Papadopoulos N, Liu B, et al. Mutations of two PMS homologues in hereditary nonpolyposis colon cancer. Nature 1994;371:75–80.

33. American Society of Clinical Oncology. Genetic testing for cancer susceptibility. J Clin Oncol 1996;14:1730–6.

34. Burke W, Daly M, Garber J, et al. Recommendations for follow-up care of individuals with an inherited predisposition to cancer. II: BRCA1 and BRCA2. JAMA 1997;277:997–1003.

35. Burke W, Petersen G, Lynch P, et al. Recommendations for follow-up care of individuals with an inherited predisposition to cancer. I: Hereditary nonpolyposis colon cancer. JAMA 1997;277:915–9.

36. National Institutes of Health Consensus Development Conference Statement. Ovarian cancer: screening, treatment, and follow-up. Gynecol Oncol 1994;55:S4–14.

37. Westhoff C. Current status of screening for ovarian cancer. Gynecol Oncol 1994;55:S34–37.

38. Karlan BY, Platt LD. The current status of ultrasound and color Doppler imaging in screening for ovarian cancer. Gynecol Oncol 1994;55:S28–33.

39. Jacobs I, Bridges J, Reynolds C, et al. Multimodal approach to screening for ovarian cancer. Lancet 1988;1:269–71.

40. Jacobs I, Bast RC. The CA125 tumor-associated antigen: a review of the literature. Hum Reprod 1989;4:1–12.

41. Skates SJ, Xu F, Yu Y, et al. Toward an optimal algorithm for ovarian cancer screening with longitudinal tumor markers. Cancer 1995;76:2004–10.

42. Jacobs I, Davies AP, Bridges J, et al. Prevalence screening for ovarian cancer in postmenopausal women by CA125 measurement and ultrasonography. Br Med J 1993;306:1030–4.

43. Kramer BS, Gohagan J, Prorok PC, Smart C. A National Cancer Institute sponsored screening trial for prostate, lung, colorectal, and ovarian cancers. Cancer 1993;71:589–93.

44. Smith EM, Anderson B. The effects of symptoms and delay in seeking diagnosis of stage of disease at diagnosis among women with cancers of the ovary. Cancer 1985;56:2727–32.

45. Flam F, Einhorn N, Sjovall K. Symptomatology of ovarian cancer. Eur J Obstet Gynecol Reprod Biol 1988;27:53–7.

46. Malkasian GD, Knapp RC, Lavin PT, et al. Preoperative evaluation of serum CA125 levels in premenopausal and postmenopausal patients with pelvic masses: discrimination of benign from malignant disease. Am J Obstet Gynecol 1988;159:341–6.

47. Burghardt E, Pickel H, Lahousen M, Stettner H. Pelvic lymphadenectomy in operative treatment of ovarian cancer. Am J Obstet Gynecol 1986;155:315–9.

48. Chen SS, Lee L. Incidence of paraaortic and pelvic lymph node metastasis in epithelial ovarian cancer. Gynecol Oncol 1983;16:95–100.

49. Julian CG, Goss J, Blanchard K, Woodruff JD. Biologic behavior of primary ovarian malignancy. Gynecol Oncol 1974;44:873–84.

50. Dauplat J, Hacker NF, Nieberg RK, Berek JS. Distant metastasis in epithelial ovarian carcinoma. Cancer 1987;60:1561–6.

51. Friedlander ML, Hedley DW, Swanson C, et al. Prediction of long term survivals by flow cytometric analysis of cellular DNA content in patients with advanced ovarian cancer. J Clin Oncol 1988;6:282–90.

52. Murray K, Hopwood L, Volk D, et al. Cytofluorometric analysis of the DNA content in ovarian cancer and its relation to patient survival. Cancer 1989;63:2456–60.

53. Volm M, Bruggeman A, Gunther M, et al. Prognostic relevance of ploidy, proliferation and resistance predictive tests in ovarian carcinoma. Cancer Res 1985;45:5180–5.

54. Blumenfeld D, Braly PS, Ben-Ezra J, et al. Tumor DNA content as a prognostic feature in advanced epithelial ovarian carcinoma. Gynecol Oncol 1987;27:389–402.

55. Khoo SK, Hurst T, Kearsley J, et al. Prognostic significance of tumour ploidy in patients with advanced ovarian carcinoma. Gynecol Oncol 1990;39:284–8.

56. Kallioniemi OP, Punnonen R, Mattila J, et al. Prognostic significance of DNA index, multiploidy and S-phase fraction in ovarian cancer. Cancer 1988;61:334–9.
57. Slamon DJ, Godolphin W, Jones LA, et al. Studies of the HER-2/neu protooncogene in human breast and ovarian cancer. Science 1989;244:707–12.
58. Berchuck A, Kamel A, Whitaker R, et al. Overexpression of HER-2/neu is associated with poor survival in advanced epithelial ovarian cancer. Cancer Res 1990;50:4087–91.
59. Teneriello MG, Ebina M, Linnoila RI, et al. p53 and Ki-ras gene mutations in epithelial ovarian neoplasms. Cancer Res 1993;53:3103–8.
60. Herod JJO, Eliopouslos AG, Warwick J, et al. The prognostic significance of Bcl-2 and p53 expression in ovarian cancer. Cancer Res 1996;56:2178–84.
61. Kohler MF, Kerns BM, Humphrey PA, et al. Mutation and overexpression of p53 in early stage epithelial ovarian cancer. Obstet Gynecol 1993;81:643–50.
62. Peterson F, ed. FIGO annual report on the results of treatment in gynecological cancer. Int J Gynecol Obstet 1991;36:Suppl:1.
63. Pecorelli S, Odicino F, Maisonneuve P, et al. FIGO annual report of the results of treatment in gynaecological cancer: carcinoma of the ovary. J Epidemiol Biostat 1998;3:75–102.
64. Young RC, Decker DG, Wharton JT, et al: Staging laparotomy in early ovarian cancer. JAMA 1983;250:3072–6.
65. Buchsbaum HJ, Lifshitz S. Staging and surgical evaluation of ovarian cancer. Semin Oncol 1984;11:227–37.
66. Piver MS, Barlow JJ, Lele SB, et al. Intraperitoneal chromic phosphate in peritoneoscopically confirmed stage I ovarian adenocarcinoma. Am J Obstet Gynecol 1982;144:836–40.
67. Knapp RC, Friedman EA. Aortic lymph node metastasies in early ovarian cancer. Am J Obstet Gynecol 1974;119:1013–7.
68. Guthrie D, Davy MLJ, Phillips PR. Study of 656 patients with "early" ovarian cancer. Gynecol Oncol 1984;17:363–9.
69. Katsube Y, Berg JW, Silverberg SG. Epidemiologic pathology ovarian tumors. Int J Gynecol Pathol 1982;1:3–16.
70. Koonings PP, Campbell AC, Mishell DR, Grimes DA. Relative frequency of primary ovarian neoplasms: A 10 year review. Obstet Gynecol 1989;74:921–6.
71. Serov SF, Scully RE, Sobin IH. International histological classification of tumors no. 9: histological typing of ovarian tumours. Geneva: World Health Organization, 1973.
72. Russell P. Surface epithelial-stromal tumors of the ovary. In: Kurman RJ, ed. Blaustein's pathology of the female genital tract. 4th ed. New York: Springer Verlag 1994;705–82.
73. Trimble CL, Trimble EL. Management of epithelial ovarian tumors of low malignant potential. Gynecol Oncol 1994;55:S52–61.
74. Lim-Tan SK, Cajigas HE, Scully RE. Ovarian cystectomy for serous borderline tumors: a follow-up study of 35 cases. Obstet Gynecol 1988;72:775–81.
75. Robinson WR, Curtin JP, Morrow CP. Operative staging and conservative surgery in the management of low malignant ovarian tumors. Int J Gynecol Cancer 1992;2:113–8.
76. Menzin AW, Rubin SC, Noumoff JS, LiVolsi VA. The accuracy of a frozen section diagnosis of borderline ovarian malignancy. Gynecol Oncol 1995;59:183–5.
77. Holschneider CH, Nieberg RK, Puniyasavatsut M, et al. Rapid frozen section diagnosis of ovarian neoplasms: inaccuracy in cases of borderline tumors. J Gynecol Tech 1996;2:191–5.
78. Bell DA, Weinstock MA, Scully RE. Peritoneal implants of ovarian serous borderline tumors. Histologic features and prognosis. Cancer 1988;62:2212–2.
79. Swerdlow M. Mesothelioma of the pelvic peritoneum resembling papillary cystadenocarcinoma of the ovary: case report. Am J Obstet Gynecol 1959;77:197–200.
80. Gooneratne S, Sassone M, Blaustein A, Talerman A. Serous surface papillary carcinoma of the ovary: a clinicopathologic study of 16 cases. Int J Gynecol Pathol 1982;1:258–69.
81. Dalrymple JC, Bannatyne P, Russell P, et al. Extraovarian peritoneal serous papillary carcinoma: a clinicopathologic study of 31 cases. Cancer 1989;64:110–5.
82. Lele SB, Piver MS, Matharu J, Tsukada Y. Peritoneal papillary carcinoma. Gynecol Oncol 1988;31:315–20.
83. Fromm G-L, Gershenson DM, Silva EG. Papillary serous carcinoma of the peritoneum. Obstet Gynecol 1990;75;89–95.
84. Mills SE, Andersen WA, Fechner RE, Austin MB. Serous surface papillary carcinoma: a clinicopathologic study of 10 cases and comparison with stage III-IV ovarian serous carcinoma. Am J Surg Pathol 1988;12:827–34.
85. Killackey MA, Davis AR. Papillary serous carcinoma of the peritoneal surface: matched-case comparison with papillary serous ovarian carcinoma. Gynecol Oncol 1993;51:171–4.
86. Bloss JD, Liao S, Buller RE, et al. Extraovarian peritoneal serous papillary carcinoma: a case-control retrospective comparison to papillary adenocarcinoma of the ovary. Gynecol Oncol 1993;50:347–51.
87. Ben-Barush G, Sivan E, Moran O, et al. Primary peritoneal serous papillary carcinoma: a study of 25 cases and comparison with stage III-IV ovarian papillary serous carcinoma. Gynecol Oncol 1996;60:393–6.
88. Scully RE, Young RH, Clement PB. Surface epithelial-stromal tumors and serous tumors. In: Tumors of the ovary, maldeveloped gonads, fallopian tube, and broad ligament. Washington, D. C.: Armed Forces Institute of Pathology, 1998;51–80.
89. Scully RE, Young RH, Clement PB. Mucinous tumors and pseudomyxoma peritonei. In: Tumors of the ovary, maldeveloped gonads, fallopian tube, and broad ligament. Washington, D. C.: Armed Forces Institute of Pathology, 1998;81–106.
90. Scully RE, Young RH, Clement PB. Endometrioid tumors. In: Tumors of the ovary, maldeveloped gonads, fallopian tube, and broad ligament. Washington, D. C.: Armed Forces Institute of Pathology, 1998;107–32.
91. Scully RE, Young RH, Clement PB. Clear cell tumors. In: Tumors of the ovary, maldeveloped gonads, fallopian tube, and broad ligament. Washington, D. C.: Armed Forces Institute of Pathology, 1998;141–52.
92. Scully RE, Young RH, Clement PB. Transitional and squamous cell tumors. In: Tumors of the ovary, maldeveloped gonads, fallopian tube, and broad ligament. Washington, D. C.: Armed Forces Institute of Pathology, 1998;153–64.
93. Heaps JM, Nieberg RK, Berek JS. Malignant neoplasms arising in endometriosis. Obstet Gynecol 1990;75:1023–8.
94. McMeekin DS, Burger RA, Manetta A, et al. Endometrioid adenocarcinoma of the ovary and its relationship to endometriosis. Gynecol Oncol 1995;59:81–6.
95. Ahmed FY, Wiltshaw E, A'Hern PR, et al. Natural history and prognosis of untreated stage IA epithelial ovarian carcinoma. J Clin Oncol 1996;14:2968–75.
96. Hreshchyshyn MM, Park RC, Blessing JA, et al. The role of adjuvant therapy in stage I ovarian cancer. Am J Obstet Gynecol 1980;138:139–45.
97. Dembo AJ, Davy M, Stenwig SF, et al. Prognostic factors in patients with stage I epithelial ovarian cancer. Obstet Gynecol 1990;75:263–73.
98. Young RC, Walton LA, Ellenberg SS, et al. Adjuvant therapy in stage I and II epithelial ovarian cancer: results of two prospective randomized trials. N Engl J Med 1990;322:1021–7.
99. Piver MS, Barlow JJ, Lele SB. Incidence of subclinical metastasis in stage I and II ovarian carcinoma. Obstet Gynecol 1978;52:100–4.
100. Dembo AJ, Bush RS, Beale FA, et al. The Princess Margaret Hospital study of ovarian cancer: stage I, II, and asymptomatic III presentations. Cancer Treat Rep 1979;63:249–54.
101. Berek JS. Epithelial ovarian cancer. In: Berek JS, Hacker NF, eds. Practical gynecologic oncology, 2nd ed. Baltimore: Williams & Wilkins 1994:327–75.
102. Griffiths CT. Surgical resection of tumor bulk in the primary treatment of ovarian carcinoma. Natl Cancer Inst Monogr 1975;42:101–4.
103. Hacker NF, Berek JS, Lagasse LD, et al. Primary cytoreductive surgery for epithelial ovarian cancer. Obstet Gynecol 1983;61:413–20.
104. Goldie JH, Coldman AJ. A mathematical model for relating the drug sensitivity of tumors to their spontaneous mutation rate. Cancer Treat Rep 1979;63:1727–33.
105. Skipper HE. Adjuvant chemotherapy. Cancer 1978;41:936–40.
106. Bookman M, Berek JS. Biologic and immunologic therapy of ovarian cancer. Hematol Oncol Clin North Am 1992;6:941–65.
107. Averette HE, Hoskins W, Nguyen HN, et al. National survey of ovarian carcinoma. I: a patient care evaluation study of the American College of Surgeons. Cancer 1993;71:1629–38.
108. Heintz APM, Hacker NF, Berek JS, et al. Cytoreductive surgery in ovarian carcinoma: feasibility and morbidity. Obstet Gynecol 1986;67:783–8.
109. Chen SS, Bochner R. Assessment of morbidity and mortality in primary cytoreductive surgery for advanced ovarian carcinoma. Gynecol Oncol 1985;20:190–5.

110. Eisenkop SM, Friedman RL, Wang H. Complete cytoreductive surgery is feasible and maximizes survival in patients with advanced epithelial ovarian cancer: a prospective study. Gynecol Oncol 1998;69:103–8.

111. Berek JS, Hacker NF, Lagasse LD. Rectosigmoid colectomy and reanastamosis to facilitate resection of primary and recurrent gynecologic cancer. Obstet Gynecol 1984;64:715–20.

112. Montz FJ, Schlaerth JB, Berek JS. Resection of diaphragmatic peritoneum and muscle: role in cytoreductive surgery for ovarian cancer. Gynecol Oncol 1989;35:338–40.

113. Scarabelli C, Gallo A, Campagnutta E, Carbone A. Splenectomy during primary and secondary cytoreductive surgery for epithelial ovarian carcinoma. Int J Gynecol Cancer 1998;8:215–21.

114. Spirtos NM, Gross GM, Freddo JL, Ballon SC. Cytoreductive surgery in advanced epithelial cancer of the ovary: the impact of aortic and pelvic lymphadenectomy. Gynecol Oncol 1995;56:345–52.

115. Di Re F, Baiocchi G, Fontanelli R, et al. Systematic pelvic and paraaortic lymphadenectomy for advanced ovarian cancer: prognostic significance of node metastases. Gynecol Oncol 1996;62:360–5.

116. Scarabelli C, Gallo A, Visentin MC, et al. Systematic pelvic and para-aortic lymphadenectomy in advanced ovarian cancer patients with no residual intraperitoneal disease. Int J Gynecol Cancer 1997;7:18–26.

117. Curtin JP, Malik R, Venkatraman ES, et al. Stage IV ovarian cancer: impact of surgical debulking. Gynecol Oncol 1997;64:9–12.

118. Liu PC, Benjamin I, Morgan MA, et al. Effect of surgical debulking on survival in stage IV ovarian cancer. Gynecol Oncol 1997;64:4–8.

119. Munkarah AR, Hallum AV, Morris M, et al. Prognostic significance of residual disease in patients with stage IV epithelial ovarian cancer. Gynecol Oncol 1997;64:13–17.

120. Bristow RE, Montz FJ, Lagasse LD, et al. Survival impact of surgical cytoreduction in stage IV epithelial ovarian cancer. Gynecol Oncol 1999;72:278–87.

121. Schwartz PE, Rutherford TJ, Chambers JT, et al. Neoadjuvant chemotherapy for advanced ovarian cancer: long-term survival. Gynecol Oncol 1999;72:93–9.

122. Vergote I, De Wever I, Tjalma W, et al. Neoadjuvant chemotherapy or primary debulking surgery in advanced ovarian carcinoma: a retrospective analysis of 285 patients. Gynecol Oncol 1998;71:431–6.

123. Nelson BE, Rosenfield AT, Schwartz PE. Preoperative abdominopelvic computed tomographic prediction of optimal cytoreduction in epithelial ovarian carcinoma. J Clin Oncol 1993;11:166–72.

124. Meyer JI, Kennedy AW, Friedman R, et al. Ovarian carcinoma: value of CT in predicting success of debulking surgery. AJR Am J Roentgenol 1995;165:875–8.

125. Thigpen JT. Single agent chemotherapy in the management of ovarian carcinoma. In: Alberts DS, Surwit EA, eds. Ovarian cancer. Boston: Martinus Nijhoff, 1985:115–46.

126. Lambert HE, Berry RJ. High dose cisplatin compared with high dose cyclophosphamide in the management of advanced epithelial ovarian cancer (FIGO stages III and IV): report from the North Thames Cooperative Group. Br Med J 1985;290:889–93.

127. Advanced Ovarian Cancer Trialists Group: Chemotherapy in advanced ovarian cancer: an overview of randomized clinical trials. Br Med J 1991;303:884–93.

128. Greco FA, Julian CG, Richardson RL. Advanced ovarian cancer: brief intensive combination chemotherapy and second-look laparotomy. Obstet Gynecol 1981;58:199–205.

129. Neijt JP, van der Burg ME, Vriesendorp R, et al. Randomized trial comparing two combination chemotherapy regimens (Hexa-CAF vs. CHAP-5) in advanced ovarian carcinoma. Cancer 1984;2:594–600.

130. Ehrlich EC, Einhorn L, Williams SD, et al. Chemotherapy for stage III-IV epithelial ovarian cancer with cis-dichorodiamineplatinum (II), Adriamycin, and cyclophosphamide: a preliminary report. Cancer Treat Rep 1979;63:281–8.

131. Ozols RF. Chemotherapy for advanced epithelial ovarian cancer. Hematol Oncol Clin North Am 1992;6:879–94.

132. Neijt JP, ten Bokkel Huinink WW, van der Burg MET, et al. Randomized trial comparing two combination chemotherapy regimens (CHAP-5 versus CP) in advanced ovarian carcinoma: a randomized trial of the Netherlands Joint Study Group for Ovarian Cancer. J Clin Oncol 1987;5:1157–68.

133. Edmonson JH, McCormack GW, Weiand HS. Late emerging survival differences in a comparative study of HCAP versus CP in stage III-IV ovarian carcinoma. In: Salmon S, ed. Adjuvant therapy of cancer. Philadelphia: WB Saunders, 1990:512–21.

134. Omura F, Bundy B, Berek JS, et al. Randomized trial of cyclophosphamide plus cisplatin with or without doxorubicin in ovarian carcinoma: a Gynecologic Oncology Group Study. J Clin Oncol 1989;7:457–65.

135. Bertelsen K, Jakobsen A, Andersen JE, et al. A randomized study of cyclophosphamide and cisplatin with or without doxorubicin in advanced ovarian cancer. Gynecol Oncol 1987;28:161–9.

136. Conte PF, Brazzone M, Chiara S, et al. A randomized trial comparing cisplatin plus cyclophosphamide versus cisplatin, doxorubicin and cyclophosphamide in advanced ovarian cancer. J Clin Oncol 1986;4:965–71.

137. Gruppo Interegionale Cooperativo Oncologia Gincologia: Randomized comparison of cisplatin with cyclophosphamide/cisplatin with cyclophosphamide/doxorubicin/cisplatin in advanced ovarian cancer. Lancet 1987;2:353–9.

138. McGuire WP, Hoskins WJ, Homesley HD, et al. Assessment of dose-intensive therapy in suboptimally debulked ovarian cancer: a Gynecologic Oncology Group study. J Clin Oncol 1995;13:1589–99.

139. Kaye SB, Lewis CR, Paul J, et al. Randomised study of two doses of cisplatin with cyclophosphamide in epithelial ovarian cancer. Lancet 1992;340:329.

140. Kaye SB, Paul J, Cassidy J, et al. Mature results of a randomized trial of two doses of cisplatin for the treatment of ovarian cancer. J Clin Oncol 1996;14:2113–9.

141. ten Bokkel Huinink WW, van der Burg MET, van Oosterom AT, et al. Carboplatin in combination therapy for ovarian cancer. Cancer Treat Rev 1988;15:Suppl:9–15.

142. Calvert AH, Newall DR, Gumbrell LA, et al. Carboplatin dosage: prospective evaluation of a simple formula based on renal function. J Clin Oncol 1989;7:1748.

143. Alberts DS, Green S, Hannigan EV, et al. Improved therapeutic index of carboplatin plus cyclophosphamide: final report by the Southwest Oncology Group of a phase III randomized trial in stages III (suboptimal) and IV ovarian cancer. J Clin Oncol 1992;10:706.

144. Swenerton K, Jeffrey J, Stuart G, et al. Cisplatin-cyclophophamide versus carboplatin-cyclophosphamide in advanced ovarian cancer: a randomized phase III study of the National Cancer Institute of Canada Clinical Trials Group. J Clin Oncol 1992;10:718–26.

145. Thigpen T, Vance RB, McGuire WP, et al. The role of paclitaxel in the management of coelomic epithelial carcinoma of the ovary: a review with emphasis on the Gynecologic Oncology Group experience. Semin Oncol 1995;22:Suppl:23–31.

146. Muggia FM, Braly PS, Brady MF, et al. Phase III cisplatin (P) or paclitaxel, versus their combination in suboptimal stage III and IV epithelial ovarian cancer (EOC): Gynecologic Oncology Group (GOG) Study No. 132. Proc Am Soc Clin Oncol 1997;16:A1257.

147. McGuire WP, Hoskins WJ, Brady MF, et al. Cyclophosphamide and cisplatin compared with paclitaxel and cisplatin in patients with stage III and stage IV ovarian cancer. N Engl J Med 1996;334:1–6.

148. Ozols RF, Bundy BN, Fowler J, et al. Randomized phase III study of cisplatin (CIS)/paclitaxel (PAC) versus carboplatin (carbo)/PAC in optimal stage III epithelial ovarian cancer (OC): a Gynecologic Oncology Group Trial (GOG 158). Proc Am Soc Clin Oncol 1999;18:A1373.

149. Connelly E, Markman M, Kennedy A, et al: Paclitaxel delivered as a 3-hr infusion with cisplatin in patients with gynecologic cancers: unexpected incidence of neurotoxicity. Gynecol Oncol 1996;62:166–8.

150. Alberts DS, Liu PY, Hannigan EV, et al. Intraperitoneal cisplatin plus intravenous cyclophosphamide versus intravenous cisplatin plus intravenous cyclophosphamide for stage III ovarian cancer. N Engl J Med 1996;335:1950–5.

151. Legros M, Dauplat J, Fleury J, et al. High dose chemotherapy with hematopoietic rescue in patients with stage III to IV ovarian cancer: long-term results. J Clin Oncol 1997;15:1302–8.

152. Stiff PJ, Boyer R, Kerger C, et al. High-dose chemotherapy with autologous transplantation for persistent/relapsed ovarian cancer: a multivariate analysis of survival of 100 consecutively treated patients. J Clin Oncol 1997;15:1309–17.

153. Declos L, Smith JP. Ovarian cancer, with special regard to types of radiotherapy. Natl Cancer Inst Monogr 1975;42:129.

154. Dembo AJ, Bush RS, Beale FA, et al. Ovarian carcinoma: improved survival following abdominopelvic irradiation in patients with a completed pelvic operation. Am J Obstet Gynecol 1979;134:793–800.

155. Dembo AJ, Van Dyk J, Japp B, et al. Whole abdominal irradiation by a moving strip technique for patients with ovarian cancer. Int J Radiat Oncol Biol Phys 1982;5:1933–42.

156. Dembo AJ, Bush RS, Beale FA, et al. A randomized clinical trial of

moving strip versus open field whole abdominal irradiation in patients with invasive epithelial cancer of ovary. Int J Radiat Oncol Biol Phys 1983;9:Suppl:97.

157. Dembo AJ. Abdominopelvic radiotherapy in ovarian cancer: a 10-year experience. Cancer 1980;55:2285.

158. Rothenberg ML, Ozols RF, Glatstein E, et al. Dose-intensive induction therapy with cyclophosphamide, cisplatin, and consolidative abdominal radiation in advanced stage epithelial cancer. J Clin Oncol 1992;10:727–34.

159. Barnhill D, O'Connor D, Farley J, et al. Clinical surveillance of gynecologic cancer patients. Gynecol Oncol 1992;46:275–80.

160. Karlan BY, Hawkins R, Hoh C, et al. Whole-body positron emission tomography with 2-[18F]-fluoro-2-deoxy-D-glucose can detect recurrent ovarian carcinoma. Gynecol Oncol 1993;51:175–81.

161. Hubner KF, McDonald TW, Niethammer JG, et al. Assessment of primary and metastatic ovarian cancer by positron emission tomography (PET) using 2-[18F] deoxyglucose (2-[18F]FDG). Gynecol Oncol 1993;51:197–204.

162. Fujiwara K, Yamauchi H, Yoshida T, et al. Relationship between peritoneal washing cytology through implantable port system (IPS-cytology) and second-look laparotomy in ovarian cancer patients with unmeasurable residual disease. Gynecol Oncol 1998;70:231–5.

163. Berek JS, Knapp RC, Malkasian GD, et al. CA125 serum levels correlated with second-look operations among ovarian cancer patients. Obstet Gynecol 1986;67:685–9.

164. Lavin PT, Knapp RC, Malkasian GD, et al. CA125 for the monitoring of ovarian carcinoma during primary therapy. Obstet Gynecol 1987;69:223–7.

165. Brenner DE, Shaff MI, Jones HW, et al. Abdominopelvic computed tomography: evaluation in patients undergoing second-look laparotomy for ovarian carcinoma. Obstet Gynecol 1985;65:715–9.

166. Podratz KC, Cliby WA. Second-look surgery in the management of epithelial ovarian carcinoma. Gynecol Oncol 1994;55:S128–133.

167. Berek JS, Hacker NF, Lagasse LD, et al. Second-look laparotomy in stage III epithelial ovarian cancer: clinical variables associated with disease status. Obstet Gynecol 1984;64:207–12.

168. Gershenson DM, Copeland LJ, Wharton JT, et al. Prognosis of surgically determined complete responders in advanced ovarian cancer. Cancer 1985;55:1129–35.

169. Friedman RL, Eisenkop SM, Wang H. Second-look laparotomy for ovarian cancer provides reliable prognostic information and improves survival. Gynecol Oncol 1997;67:88–94.

170. Berek JS, Hacker NF, Lagasse LD, et al. Survival of patients following secondary cytoreductive surgery in ovarian cancer. Obstet Gynecol 1983;61:189–93.

171. Hoskins WJ, Rubin SC, Dulaney E, et al. Influence of secondary cytoreduction at the time of second-look laparotomy on the survival of patients with epithelial ovarian carcinoma. Gynecol Oncol 1989;34:365–71.

172. Williams L, Brunetto VL, Yordan E, et al. Secondary cytoreductive surgery at second-look laparotomy in advanced ovarian cancer: a Gynecologic Oncology Group Study. Gynecol Oncol 1997;66:171–8.

173. Podratz KC, Malkasian GD Jr, Hilton JF, et al. Second-look laparotomy in ovarian cancer: evaluation of pathologic variables. Am J Obstet Gynecol 1985;152:230–8.

174. Cohen CJ, Goldberg JD, Holland JF, et al. Improved therapy with cisplatin regimens for patients with ovarian carcinoma (FIGO stages III and IV) as measured by surgical end-staging (second-look operation). Am J Obstet Gynecol 1983;145:955–67.

175. Rubin SC, Randall TC, Armstrong KA, et al. Ten-year follow-up of ovarian cancer patients after second-look laparotomy with negative findings. Obstet Gynecol 1999;93:21–4.

176. Gadducci A, Sartori E, Maggino T, et al. Analysis of failures after negative second-look in patients with advanced ovarian cancer: An Italian multicenter study. Gynecol Oncol 1998;68:150–5.

177. Rubin SC, Jones WB, Curtin JP. Second-look laparotomy in stage I ovarian cancer following comprehensive surgical staging. Obstet Gynecol 1993;82:139–42.

178. Webb MJ, Snyder JA, Williams TJ, Decker DG. Second-look laparotomy in ovarian cancer. Gynecol Oncol 1982;14:285–93.

179. Berek JS, Griffith CT, Leventhal JM. Laparoscopy for second-look evaluation in ovarian cancer. Obstet Gynecol 1981;58:192–98.

180. Casey AC, Farias-Eisner R, Pisani AL, et al. What is the role of reassessment laparoscopy in the management of gynecologic cancers in 1995? Gynecol Oncol 1996;60:454–61.

181. Abu-Rustum NR, Barakat RR, Siegel PL, et al. Second-look operation for epithelial ovarian cancer: laparoscopy or laparotomy. Obstet Gynecol 1996;88:549–53.

182. Lele S, Piver MS. Interval laparoscopy prior to second-look laparotomy in ovarian cancer. 1986;68:345.

183. Clough KB, Ladonne JM, Nos C, et al. Second-look for ovarian cancer: laparoscopy or laparotomy? A prospective comparative study. Gynecol Oncol 1999;72:411–7.

184. Gershenson DM, Kavanagh JJ, Copeland LJ, et al. Retreatment of patients with recurrent epithelial ovarian cancer with cisplatin-based chemotherapy. Obstet Gynecol 1989;73:798–802.

185. Markman M, Rothman R, Hakes T, et al. Second-line platinum therapy in patients with ovarian cancer previously treated with cisplatin. J Clin Oncol 1991;9:389.

186. Gore ME, Fryatt I, Wiltshaw E, Dawson T. Treatment of relapsed carcinoma of the ovary with cisplatin or carboplatin following initial treatment with these compounds. Gynecol Oncol 1990;36:207–11.

187. Janicke F, Holscher M, Kuhn W, et al. Radical surgery procedure improves survival time in patients with recurrent ovarian cancer. Cancer 1992;70:2129–36.

188. Vaccarello L, Rubin SC, Vlamis V, et al. Cytoreductive surgery in ovarian carcinoma patients with a documented previously complete surgical response. Gynecol Oncol 1995;57:61–5.

189. Ozols RF. Treatment of recurrent ovarian cancer: increasing options—"recurrent" results. J Clin Oncol 1997;15:2177–80.

190. Fennelly D, Aghajanian C, Shapiro F, et al. Phase I and pharmacologic study of paclitaxel administered weekly in patients with relapsed ovarian cancer. J Clin Oncol 1997;15:187–92.

191. Swisher EM, Mutch DG, Rader JS, et al. Topotecan in platinum- and paclitaxel-resistant ovarian cancer. Gynecol Oncol 1997;66:480–6.

192. Creemers GJ, Bolis G, Gore M, et al. Topotecan, an active drug in the second line treatment of epithelial ovarian cancer: results of a large European phase II study. Gynecol Oncol 1996;14:3056–61.

193. ten Bokkel Huinink W, Gore M, Carmichael J, et al. Topotecan versus paclitaxel for the treatment of recurrent epithelial ovarian cancer. J Clin Oncol 1997;15:2183–93.

194. Bookman MA, Malmstrom H, Bolis G, et al. Topotecan for the treatment of advanced epithelial ovarian cancer: an open-label phase II study in patients treated after prior chemotherapy that contained cisplatin or carboplatin and paclitaxel. J Clin Oncol 1998;16:3345–52.

195. Herben VMM, Nannan Panday VR, Ricel DJ, et al. Phase I and pharmacologic study of the combination of paclitaxel, cisplatin, and topotecan administered intravenously every 21 days as first-line therapy in patients with advanced ovarian cancer. J Clin Oncol 1999;17:747–55.

196. Shapiro JD, Millward MJ, Rischin D, et al. Activity of gemcitabine in patients with advanced ovarian cancer: responses seen following platinum and paclitaxel. Gynecol Oncol 1996;63:89–93.

197. Muggia FM, Hainsworth JD, Jeffers S, et al. Phase II study of liposomal doxorubicin in refractory ovarian cancer: Antitumor activity and toxicity modification by liposomal encapsulation. J Clin Oncol 1997;15:987–93.

198. Bajetta E, Di Leo A, Biganzoli L, et al. Phase Ii study of vinorelbine in patients with pretreated advanced ovarian cancer: activity in platinum-resistant disease. J Clin Oncol 1996;14:2546–51.

199. Kemp G, Rose P, Lurain J, et al. Amifostine pretreatment for protection against cyclophosphamide-induced and cisplatin-induced toxicities: results of a randomized control trial in patients with advanced ovarian cancer. J Clin Oncol 14:2101–12.

200. Berek JS, Hacker NF, Lichtenstein A, et al. Intraperitoneal recombinant α-interferon for "Salvage" Immunotherapy in Stage III Epithelial Ovarian cancer: a Gynecologic Oncology Group study. Cancer Res 1985;45:4447.

201. Bruzzone M, Rubagotti A, Gadducci A, et al. Intraperitoneal carboplatin with or without interferon-α in advanced ovarian cancer patients with minimal residual disease at second-look: a prospective randomized trial of 111 patients. Gynecol Oncol 1997;65:499–505.

202. Steis RG, Urba WJ, VanderMolen LA, et al. Intraperitoneal lymphokine-activated killer cell and interleukin-2 therapy for malignancies limited to the peritoneal cavity. J Clin Oncol 1990;8:1618.

203. Hacker NF, Berek JS, Juilliard G, et al. Whole abdominal radiation as salvage therapy for epithelial ovarian cancer. Obstet Gynecol 1985;65:50.

204. Cmelak AJ, Kapp DS. Long-term survival with whole abdominopelvic irradiation in platinum-refractory persistent or recurrent ovarian cancer. Gynecol Oncol 1997;65:453–60.

205. Corn BW, Lanciano RM, Boente M, et al. Recurrent ovarian cancer: effective radiotherapeutic palliation after chemotherapy failure. Cancer 1994;74:2979–83.

206. Berqvist A, Kullander S, Thorell J. A study of estrogen and progesterone cytosol receptor concentration in benign and malignant ovarian tumors and a review of malignant ovarian tumors treated with medroxyprogesterone acetate. Acta Obstet Gynecol Scand 1981;101:Suppl:75.

207. Rendina GM, Donadio C, Giovannini M. Steroid receptors and progestinic therapy in ovarian endometrioid carcinoma. Eur J Gynaecol Oncol 1982;3:241–6.

208. Kahanpaa KV, Karkkainen J, Nieminen U. Multiagent chemotherapy with and without medroxyprogesterone acetate in the treatment of advanced ovarian cancer. Excerpta Med Congr Ser 1982;611:477.

209. Schwartz PE, Chambers JT, Kohorn EI, et al. Tamoxifen in combination with cytotoxic chemotherapy in advanced epithelial ovarian cancer: A prospective randomized trial. Cancer 1989;36:1074–8.

210. Geisler HE. The use of high-dose megestrol acetate in the treatment of ovarian adenocarcinoma. Semin Oncol 1985;12:Suppl:20–2.

211. Markman M, Iseminger KA, Hatch KD, et al. Tamoxifen in platinum-refractory ovarian cancer: A Gynecologic Oncology Group ancillary report. Gynecol Oncol 1996;62:4–6.

212. Schwartz PE, Keating F, MacLusky N, et al. Tamoxifen therapy for advanced ovarian cancer. Obstet Gynecol 1982;59:583–8.

213. Young RH. Metastatic tumors of the ovary. In: Kurman RJ, ed. Blaustein's pathology of the female genital tract. 4th ed. New York: Springer-Verlag 1994:939–74.

214. Young RH, Scully RE. Sex cord-stromal, steroid cell, and other ovarian tumors with endocrine, paraendocrine, and paraneoplastic manifestations. In: Kurman RJ, ed. Blaustein's pathology of the female genital tract. 4th ed. New York: Springer-Verlag 1994:783–847.

215. Scully RE, Young RH, Clement PB. Germ cell tumors: general features and primitive forms. In: Tumors of the ovary, maldeveloped gonads, fallopian tube, and broad ligament. Washington, D. C.: Armed Forces Institute of Pathology, 1998:239–66.

216. Berek JS, Hacker NF. Nonepithelial ovarian and fallopian tube cancers. In: Berek JS, Hacker NF, eds. Practical gynecologic oncology. 2nd ed. Baltimore: Williams & Wilkins, 1994:377–401.

217. Bristow RE, Berek JS. Surgical management of dysgerminoma. Contemp Obstet Gynecol 1998;43:98–119.

218. Bjorkholm E, Lundell M, Gyftodimos A, Silfversward C: Dysgerminoma: the Radiumhemmet series 1927–1984. Cancer 1990;65:38–44.

219. Gordon A, Lipton D, Woodruff JD. Dysgerminoma: a review of 158 cases from the Emil Novak Ovarian Tumor Registry. Obstet Gynecol 1981;58:497–504.

220. Kurman RJ, Norris HJ. Germ cell tumors of the ovary. Hum Pathol 1978;1:291.

221. Asadourian LA, Taylor HB. Dysgerminoma: an analysis of 105 cases. Obstet Gynecol 1969;33:370–9.

222. DePalo G, Pilorri S, Kenda R, et al. Natural history of dysgerminoma. Am J Obstet Gynecol 1982;143:799–807.

223. Casey AC, Bhodauria S, Shapter A, et al. Dysgerminoma: the role of conservative surgery. Gynecol Oncol 1996;63:352–7.

224. Slayton RE, Park RC, Silverberg SG, et al. Vincristine, dactinomycin, and cyclophosphamide in the treatment of malignant germ cell tumors of the ovary: a Gynecologic Oncology Group Study (a final report). Cancer 1985;56:243–8.

225. Taylor MH, Depetrillo AD, Turner AR. Vinbastine, bleomycin, and cisplatin in malignant germ cell tumors of the ovary. Cancer 1985;56:1341–9.

226. Gershenson DM, Wharton JT, Kline RC, et al. Chemotherapeutic complete remission in patients with metastatic ovarian dysgerminoma. Cancer 1986;58:2594–9.

227. Williams SD, Birch R, Einhorn LH, et al. Treatment of disseminated germ-cell tumors with cisplatin, bleomycin, and either vinblastine or etoposide. N Engl J Med 1987;316:1435–40.

228. Gershenson DM, Morris M, Cangir A, et al. Treatment of malignant germ cell tumors of the ovary with bleomycin, etoposide, and cisplatin. J Clin Oncol 1990;8:715–20.

229. Williams SD, Blessing JA, Moore DH, et al. Cisplatin, vinblastine, and bleomycin in advanced and recurrent ovarian germ-cell tumors: a trial of the Gynecologic Oncology Group. Ann Intern Med 1989;111:22–7.

230. Williams SD, Blessing JA, Hatch KD, Homesley HD. Chemotherapy of advanced dysgerminoma: trials of the Gynecologic Oncology Group. J Clin Oncol 1991;9:1950–5.

231. Williams S, Blessing JA, Liao S, et al. Adjuvant therapy of ovarian germ cell tumors with cisplatin, etoposide, and bleomycin: a trial of the Gynecologic Oncology Group. J Clin Oncol 1994;12:701–6.

232. Thomas GM, Dembo AJ, Hacker NF, DePetrillo AD. Current therapy for dysgerminoma of the ovary. Obstet Gynecol 1987;70:268–75.

233. Loehrer PJ, Elson P, Johnson DH, et al. A randomized trial of cisplatin plus etoposide with or without bleomycin in favorable prognosis disseminated germ cell tumors: an ECOG study. Proc Am Soc Clin Oncol 1991;10:540.

234. Gershenson DM. Update on malignant ovarian germ cell tumors. Cancer 1993;71:1581–90.

235. Scully RE, Young RH, Clement PB. Teratomas (excluding monodermal). In: Tumors of the ovary, maldeveloped gonads, fallopian tube, and broad ligament. Washington, D. C.: Armed Forces Institute of Pathology 1998;267–84.

236. Breen JL, Neubecker RD. Malignant teratoma of the ovary: an analysis of 17 cases. Obstet Gynecol 1963;21:669–81.

237. Norris HJ, Zirkin HJ, Benson WL. Immature (malignant) teratoma of the ovary: a clinical and pathologic study of 58 cases. Cancer 1976;37:2359–72.

238. Gershenson DM, Del Junco G, Silva EG, et al. Immature teratoma of the ovary. Obstet Gynecol 1986;68:624–9.

239. Gallion H, van Nagell JR Jr, Donaldson ES, et al. Immature teratoma of the ovary. Am J Obstet Gynecol 1983;146:361–5.

240. Robboy SJ, Scully RE. Ovarian teratoma with glial implants on the peritoneum: an analysis of 12 cases. Hum Pathol 1970;1:643–53.

241. Nogales FF Jr, Favara BE, Major FJ, Silverberg SG. Immature teratoma of the ovary with a neural component ("solid" teratoma): a clinicopathologic study of 20 cases. Hum Pathol 1976;7:625–42.

242. Curry SL, Smith JP, Gallagher HS. Malignant teratoma of the ovary: prognostic factors and treatment. Am J Obstet Gynecol 1978;131:845–9.

243. Bajorin DF, Sarosdy MF, Bosl GJ, et al. A randomized trial of etoposide plus carboplatin versus etoposide plus cisplatin in patients with metastatic germ cell tumors. J Clin Oncol 1993;11:598–606.

244. Gershenson DM, Copeland LJ, DelJunco G, et al. Second-look laparotomy in the management of malignant germ cell tumors of the ovary. Obstet Gynecol 1986;67:789–93.

245. DiSaia DJ, Saltz A, Kagan AR, Morrow CP. Chemotherapeutic retroconversion of immature teratoma of the ovary. Obstet Gynecol 1977;49:346–50.

246. Munkarah A, Gershenson DM, Levenback C, et al. Salvage surgery for chemorefractory ovarian germ cell tumors. 1994;55:217–23.

247. Gershenson DM, Del Junco G, Herson J, Rutledge FN. Endodermal sinus tumor of the ovary: the M. D. Anderson experience. Obstet Gynecol 1983;61:194–202.

248. Talerman A, Haije WG, Baggerman L. Serum alpha-fetoprotein (AFP) in patients with germ cell tumors of the gonads and extragonadal sites: correlation between endodermal sinus (yolk sac) tumor and raised serum AFP. Cancer 1980;46:380–5.

249. Kurman RJ, Norris HJ. Embryonal carcinoma of the ovary: a clinicopathologic entity distinct from endodermal sinus tumor resembling embryonal carcinoma of the adult testis. Cancer 1976;38:2420–33.

250. Nakakuma K, Tashiro S, Uemura K, Takayama K. Alpha-fetoprotein and human chorionic gonadotropin in embryonal carcinoma of the ovary: an 8-year survival case. Cancer 1983;52:1470–2.

251. Ueda G, Abe Y, Yoshida M, Fujiwara T. Embryonal carcinoma of the ovary: a six-year survival. Int J Gynecol Oncol 1990;31:287–92.

252. Gerbie MV, Brewer JI, Tamimi H. Primary choriocarcinoma of the ovary. Obstet Gynecol Surv 1975;46:720–3.

253. Jacobs AJ, Newland JR, Green RK. Pure choriocarcinoma of the ovary. Obstet Gynecol Surv 1982;37:603–9.

254. Chapman DC, Grover R, Schwartz PE. Conservative management of an ovarian polyembryoma. Obstet Gynecol 1994;83:879–92.

255. King ME, Hubbell MJ, Talerman A. Mixed germ cell tumor of the ovary with a prominent polyembryoma component. Int J Gynecol Pathol 1991;10:88–95.

256. Tsukahara Y, Fukuta T, Yamada T, Nakai I. Retroperitoneal giant tumor formed by migrating polyembroma with numerous erythroid bodies from an ovarian mixed germ cell tumor. Gynecol Obstet Invest 1991;31:58–60.

257. Kurman RJ, Norris HJ. Malignant mixed germ cell tumors of the ovary: a clinical and pathological analysis of 30 cases. Obstet Gynecol 1976;48:579–89.

258. Scully RE, Young RH, Clement PB. Sex cord—stromal tumors, granu-

losa cell tumors. In: Tumors of the ovary, maldeveloped gonads, fallopian tube, and broad ligament. Washington, D. C.: Armed Forces Institute of Pathology, 1998:169–88.

259. Fox H, Agrawal K, Langley FA. A clinicopathologic study of 92 cases of granulosa cell tumor of the ovary with special reference to the factors influencing prognosis. Cancer 1975;35:231–41.

260. Segal R, DePetrilo AD, Thomas G. Clinical review of adult granulosa cell tumors of the ovary. Gynecol Oncol 1995;56:338–44.

261. Gusberg SB, Kardon P. Proliferative endometrial response to theca-granulosa cell tumors. Am J Obstet Gynecol 1967;111:633–43.

262. Bjorkholm E, Petterson F. Granulosa-cell and theca-cell tumors: the clinical picture and long term outcome for the Radiumhemmet series. Acta Obstet Gynecol Scand 1980;59:361–5.

263. Lappohn RE, Burger HG, Bouma J, et al. Inhibin as a marker for granulosa-cell tumors. N Engl J Med 1989;321:790–3.

264. Jobling T, Memers P, Healy DL, et al. A prospective study of inhibin in granulosa cell tumor of the ovary. Gynecol Oncol 1994;55:285–9.

265. Homesley HD, Bundy BN, Hurteau JA, Roth LM. Bleomycin, etoposide, and cisplatin combination therapy of ovarian granulosa cell tumors and other stromal malignancies: a Gynecologic Oncology Group study. Gynecol Oncol 1999;72:131–7.

266. Holland DR, LeRiche J, Swenerton KD, et al. Flow cytometric assessment of DNA ploidy is a useful prognostic factor for patients with granulosa cell ovarian tumors. Int J Gynecol Cancer 1991:227.

267. Sood AK, Sorosky JI, Gelder MS, et al. Primary ovarian sarcoma: analysis of prognostic variables and the role of surgical cytoreduction. Cancer 1998;82:1731–7.

268. Bicher A, Levenback C, Silva EG, et al. Ovarian malignant mixed mullerian tumors treated with platinum-based chemotherapy. Obstet Gynecol 1995;85:735–9.

269. Le T, Krepart GV, Lotocki RJ, Heywood MS. Malignant mixed mesodermal ovarian tumor treatment and prognosis: a 20-year experience. Gynecol Oncol 1997;95:237–40.

270. Scully RE, Young RH, Clement PB: Steroid cell tumors. In: Tumors of the ovary, maldeveloped gonads, fallopian tube, and broad ligament. Washington, DC: Armed Forces Institute of Pathology 1998:227–38.

271. Hayes MC, Scully RE. Ovarian steroid cell tumor (not otherwise specified): a clinicopathological analysis of 63 cases. Am J Surg Pathol 1987;11:835–45.

272. Sutton GP, Bundy BN, Delgado G, et al. Ovarian metastases in stage IB carcinoma of the cervix: a Gynecologic Oncology Group study. Am J Obstet Gynecol 1992;166:50–3.

273. Kasilag FB, Rutledge FN: Metastatic breast carcinoma to the ovary. Am J Obstet Gynecol 1957;74:989.

274. Lee YN, Hori JM. Significance of ovarian metastasis in therapeutic oophorectomy for advanced breast cancer. Cancer 1971;27:1374–8.

275. Woodruff JD, Novak ER. The Krukenberg tumor: study of 48 cases from the Emil Novak Ovarian Tumor Registry. Obstet Gynecol 1960;15:351.

276. Robboy SJ, Scully RE, Norris HJ. Carcinoid metastatic to the ovary: a clinicopathologic analysis of 35 cases. Cancer 1974;33:798–811.

277. Freeman C, Berg JW, Cutler SJ. Occurrence and prognosis of extra-nodal lymphomas. Cancer 1972;29:252–60.

278. Arseneau JC, Canellos GP, Banks DM, et al. American Burkitt's lymphoma: a clinicopathologic study of 30 cases. I: clinical factors relating to prolonged survival. Am J Med 1975;58:314–21.

279. Sedlis A. Carcinoma of the fallopian tube. Surg Clin North Am 1978;58:121–9.

280. Scully RE, Young RH, Clement PB. Tumors of the fallopian tube: histologic classification and cancer staging epithelial and mixed epithelial mesenchymal tumors. In: Tumors of the ovary, maldeveloped gonads, fallopian tube, and broad ligament. Washington, D. C.: Armed Forces Institute of Pathology, 1998:461–76.

281. Podratz KC, Podczaski ES, Gaffey TA, et al. Primary carcinoma of the fallopian tube. Am J Obstet Gynecol 1986;254:1319–26.

282. Tamimi HK, Figge DC. Adenocarcinoma of the uterine tube: potential for lymph node metastases. Am J Obstet Gynecol 1981;141:132–7.

283. Pecorelli S, Odicino F, Maisonneuve P, et al. FIGO annual report of the results of treatment in gynaecological cancer: carcinoma of the fallopian tube. J Epidemiol Biostat 1998;3:63–74.

284. Deppe G, Bruckner HW, Cohen CJ. Combination chemotherapy for advanced carcinoma of the fallopian tube. Obstet Gynecol 1980;56:530–2.

# C H A P T E R  56

## CERVIX

• MICHAEL L. BERMAN • DIANE YAMADA

In the United States, cervical cancer is the 10th most common solid malignant neoplasm. With the advent of Papanicolaou's (Pap) smear screening, the diagnosis of carcinoma in situ has become much more common than that of invasive cervical cancer. Overall, the rate of cervical cancer in the United States decreased in the 20-year period between 1973 and 1994 from 14.2 per 100,000 to 7.8 per 100,000. The American Cancer Society (ACS) predicts that in 2000, in the United States, 12,800 new cases of invasive cervical cancer will be diagnosed and 4600 deaths will result from these cancers.[1] In contrast, cervical cancer is the second most common form of cancer in women worldwide. Cervical cancer screening has a critical role in reducing the incidence and mortality of invasive disease. It has been estimated that 90% of invasive cervical cancers can be prevented by modern screening methods.[2] From data accumulated worldwide, the International Federation of Gynecology and Obstetrics (FIGO) reported that the majority of women who developed cervical cancer between 1992 and 1994 had never had a Pap smear.[3]

More than 80% of cervical cancers are epidermoid (squamous cell). The majority of these arise in the transformation zone, where columnar epithelium is being transformed to squamous epithelium. This area of the cervix typically is easily accessible for cytologic screening. Fifteen to 20% are adenocarcinomas arising from the endocervical canal.[3] The natural history and treatment of these two histologic types are sufficiently different to justify separate discussions. The management of cervical cancer diagnosed during pregnancy is also discussed as a separate topic.

# SQUAMOUS CELL CARCINOMA

## Natural History

### ETIOLOGY AND EPIDEMIOLOGY

Epidemiologic studies have demonstrated that cervical squamous cell cancer and its precursors follow a pattern typical of a sexually transmitted disease. Cervical cancer is not found in virginal women but is commonly found in prostitutes.[4, 5] Reported risk factors include early age at first coitus, early childbearing, numerous sexual partners, venereal infection, and sexual intercourse with high-risk males.[6–8]

Human papillomavirus (HPV) has been recognized as a primary agent responsible for cervical cancer and its precursors. The papillomaviruses are double-stranded DNA tumor viruses known to cause squamous proliferation in humans. They are responsible for the common wart, laryngeal papillomas, and condylomas of the genital tract. In 1971, zur Hausen postulated an etiologic relationship between HPV and cervical cancer. In 1977, Meisels and colleagues[9] observed that koilocytosis, the histopathologic feature thought to be pathognomonic for infection of epithelial cells with HPV, was seen commonly in cervical intraepithelial neoplasia (CIN), the precursor lesion to cervical cancer. He theorized, therefore, that HPV could induce malignant transformation of the cervical squamous epithelium.

HPV DNA was isolated, sequenced, and cloned from cervical cancers by Durst and associates[10] and Schwartz and coworkers.[11] HPV RNA transcripts and protein products have also been identified in cervical carcinomas.[12] More than 60 HPV types are identified; each tends to infect a specific tissue type, with an extensive spectrum of HPV-induced disease. Types 6, 11, 16, 18, 31, and 33 are the most common HPV types found in genital lesions. Types 6 and 11, categorized as low-risk types, usually cause benign warts called *condylomata acuminata* and rarely, if ever, cause an invasive cancer. The high-risk types, 16, 18, 31, 35, 39, 45, 51, 52, 56, and 58, are associated with malignant transformation and are found in cervical cancers and high-grade CIN (CIN 3).[13] Types 16, 18, and 33 have been detected in more than 90% of cervical squamous cell cancers using sensitive detection techniques such as polymerase chain reaction (PCR).[14–16]

An extensive number of epidemiologic studies also support HPV as the principal causative agent of cervical neoplasia. In a prospective study of 1000 patients in the Kaiser-Permanente health maintenance system, 76% of the CIN cases could be attributed to HPV infection. When HPV infection was controlled for, the significance of most other risk factors associated with sexual behavior disappeared, suggesting that HPV infection is an independent risk factor for the development of CIN.[17] A prospective study conducted in Finland on a cohort of 18,814 women compared serologic evidence of HPV 16 infection in patients who did and did not develop cervical cancer. The odds ratio for development of cervical cancer with HPV 16 infection was 12.5 (95% confidence interval 2.7–57, $p<0.001$).[18]

Factors other than HPV have also been associated with cervical squamous cell cancer, suggesting that HPV may be only a promoter or co-carcinogen. Some of these factors include pelvic irradiation, immunodeficiency, vitamin A and vitamin C deficiency, oral contraceptive use, and cigarette smoking.[6, 16, 19] Although a specific mutagenic agent in cigarette smoke has not been identified, the majority of studies support a significant association between cigarette smoking and the development of cervical dysplasia. When compared with levels in nonsmokers, significantly elevated levels of nitrosamine 4-(methylnitrosamino)-1-(3-pyridyl)-1-butanone (NNK), a carcinogen found in cigarette smoke, have been found in the cervical mucus of smokers.[20] It has been postulated that byproducts of cigarette smoke may promote the formation of DNA adducts that result in mutagenesis of the cervical epithelium.[21, 22] Smoking cessation itself has been shown to decrease the size of mildly dysplastic lesions.[23]

The importance of a nutritional effect has not been quantified; however, studies to investigate this association have demonstrated that cervicovaginal and plasma beta-carotene levels are significantly lower in patients with CIN and cervical cancer as compared with healthy controls.[24] Attempts to promote regression of mild and moderate cervical dysplasia using oral beta-carotene have met with some success[25]; however, these results are difficult to quantify because mild dysplasia is frequently known to regress without treatment.[26] Furthermore, topical retinoids (Retin-A) have been shown to reverse CIN 2 lesions to normal significantly more often than use of a placebo applied topically. A mechanism by which dietary deficiencies might influence the risk of developing cervical neoplasia has been reported by Butterworth and colleagues,[27] who found that folate deficiency may facilitate the incorporation of the HPV genome into the epithelial cell chromosomal material.

### PATHOGENESIS

The cervix lends itself to intensive investigation because of its accessibility; therefore, the pathogenesis of the disease has been well studied. The cervix consists of two anatomic parts: the portio vaginalis, which projects into the vagina, and the portio supravaginalis, which lies above the vagina and includes the endocervical mucosa. The portio vaginalis, or exocervix, typically is covered by nonkeratinizing squamous epithelium. The endocervical canal, which leads to the uterine cavity, is lined by columnar mucus-secreting epithelium. The transformation zone between the two cell types consists of columnar epithelium undergoing squamous metaplasia. This metaplastic process is accelerated in utero, at puberty, and at the time of first pregnancy, and it declines in the perimenopausal and postmenopausal years. Coppleson[28] has suggested that the periods of most active metaplasia provide the greatest risk for neoplastic transformation when a suitable inciting agent is present. The end result of squamous metaplasia is the slowly progressive movement of the squamocolumnar junction cephalad into the endocervical canal.

Eighty to 85% of cervical carcinomas are of the squamous cell variety and originate in metaplastic squamous epithelium. The initial event, typically preceding the development of cervical cancer by several years, is a viral induction of atypical metaplasia, which can progress to a recognizable cancer precursor, CIN.

There is a correlation between the presence or absence of viral integration into the cellular DNA caused by different HPV types and the potential for malignant transformation. For example, in lesions infected with low-risk HPV types, the viral DNA remains circular and separate from the host genome in a form known as an *episome*. Conversely, lesions infected with the high-risk HPV types typically demonstrate integration of viral DNA into the host genome. This process occurs in 75% of HPV-16–infected cells and nearly all HPV-18–infected cells.[29, 30] It is this integration that ultimately leads to immortalization (prolonged cellular viability) and transformation of the host cells such that they exhibit anchorage-independent growth. HPV-16 and -18 have two open reading frames, E6 and E7, which are transcriptional units capable of encoding for proteins critical for viral replication. The E7 protein provides the high-risk HPV types with their major immortalizing and transforming ability.[31] E7 binds to protein products of the retinoblastoma gene, pRb, thereby releasing transcription factors such as E2F from the inhibitory effects of pRb.[32] The net effect of pRb binding to E7 is uninhibited cell cycle progression in cells infected with HPV-16 and HPV-18. The E6 product has the ability to bind to the protein product of p53, also a known tumor suppressor gene, that helps to regulate cell growth and division.[33] Binding results in rapid degradation of p53 via a ubiquitin-dependent, proteolytic pathway.[34, 35] p53 degradation disrupts one of the cellular regulatory mechanisms that controls unchecked cellular growth.

Although HPV infection appears to play an essential role in cervical carcinogenesis, the entire process is complex and not fully understood. The premalignant changes incited by HPV infection form a continuum rather than separate and distinct pathologic entities. The disorders within that continuum include the dysplasias and carcinoma in situ and have in common a progressive increase in disorderliness of the epithelial maturation process and degree of cytologic pleomorphism. Three subclassifications of CIN are defined as follows: grade 1, mild dysplasia; grade 2, moderate dysplasia; and grade 3, severe dysplasia and carcinoma in situ. The natural history of CIN in an individual patient is variable. CIN can progress to invasive cancer, remain static for indefinite periods, or regress. Spontaneous regression occurs frequently in CIN 1 but is rare in CIN 2 and 3. Severely dysplastic lesions normally can persist indefinitely or can progress to invasive carcinoma.[36] An estimate of the duration of CIN 3 in women whose disease progresses to invasive cancer is 3 to 10 years, based on data obtained from Pap smear screening programs in British Columbia, Canada, and in Barbados, West Indies.[37] The course of HPV infection and CIN presumably reflects the interaction between the host immune system and the virus. This statement is supported by the observation that women who are taking immunosuppressive drugs have increased susceptibility to HPV-associated diseases.[38] For example, patients who undergo kidney transplantation may have flourishing condylomas and can demonstrate unusually rapid progression of premalignant

cervical lesions to invasive cancer during immunosuppressive treatment.[39] Additionally, studies have found an association between human immunodeficiency virus (HIV) infection and the prevalence of HPV. In a large prospective cohort study, high-risk HPV types were detected with higher frequency in HIV-positive women as compared with HIV-negative women at the initial visit. On subsequent visits, a higher percentage of HIV-positive women tested positively for high-risk HPV types and a higher percentage had persistent HPV infection when compared with seronegative women. HPV prevalence was inversely related to CD4$^+$ counts. Although 74% of women with CD4$^+$ counts of greater than 500/mm$^3$ had detectable high-risk HPV types, 95% of HIV-positive women with CD4$^+$ counts of less than 500/mm$^3$ tested positively for HPV.[40] Overall, HIV-infected women have a fivefold greater risk of developing cervical neoplasia when compared with seronegative women.[41] In up to 4% of HIV-infected women, cervical cancer, which was categorized in 1993 as an acquired immunodeficiency syndrome (AIDS)–defining illness, is the initial presenting illness.[42, 43]

The biologic behavior of invasive cervical cancer is often more predictable than that of CIN. Once cancer extends beneath the basement membrane of the squamous epithelium, the most common route of spread is by direct extension to adjacent structures, including the vagina, paracervical and paravaginal soft tissues, bladder, and rectum. Tumor embolization to regional lymph nodes occurs most frequently with large tumor masses, with advanced stage of disease, and possibly with increasing cytologic anaplasia. Metastasis to the external iliac and obturator lymph nodes accounted for more than 40% of metastases in 744 patients with lymphatic spread.[44] An additional 15 to 20% of metastases were to hypogastric lymph nodes. Metastases to the common iliac and para-aortic lymph nodes occurred secondarily after the external iliac and hypogastric areas were involved. Distant metastasis by the hematogenous route has been reported infrequently and is usually associated with extensive pelvic tumors. The most common sites of hematogenous spread are the lungs, liver, and bone.

## PREVENTION

Dramatic decreases in the mortality rate of women with cancer of the cervix in the developed countries of the world have resulted from the most successful cancer screening program effected for any cancer site.[45, 46] Before the widespread use of the Pap smear, cervical cancer was the leading cause of cancer deaths in American women. Because of the Pap smear, the mortality rate has declined by more than 75%, to 2.9 deaths per 100,000 women per year.[47] According to American Cancer Society (ACS) statistics, the 5-year survival rate has increased from 58% in the 1960s to 71% for white women in the period 1986 to 1993.[48] Of concern is that the 5-year survival rate of 57% for African American women remains significantly lower than that of Caucasian women, largely reflecting more advanced disease at the time of diagnosis.[48, 49]

The improved survival has resulted, in part, from advancements in cervical cancer treatment but, in large part, reflects earlier diagnosis of invasive squamous cell carcinoma. Thus, although the major benefit of cervical cancer screening lies in the potential to detect premalignant disease that is curable by various means of local therapy, an additional, less well documented benefit is the detection of invasive cancers at an earlier stage than previously. Despite these advances, however, cervical cancer remains a frequent cause of cancer mortality in countries where routine screening is not prevalent.

The reasons for our failure to identify and treat all high-risk patients before they have invasive disease are numerous: (1) High-risk patients often do not use screening services; (2) precursors to adenocarcinoma of the cervix are not well detected by Pap smears, and therefore the occurrence rate of adenocarcinoma of the cervix has not been reduced by screening practices[50]; (3) the inherent false-negative rate of the Pap test ranges between 10 and 20%[51]; (4) patients do not always obtain follow-up after an abnormal smear is found; and (5) physicians can err either by failing to perform a Pap smear as a part of a general physical examination or by not recognizing that minor cytologic abnormalities can be associated with CIN or invasive cancer, thereby failing to evaluate the patient further.[52] Data from the National Health Interview Survey in 1992 indicated that one half of women age 60 or older had not had a Pap smear in the past 3 years despite having the same number of physician visits as younger patients during that interval. The observation that one fourth of cervical cancer cases and 41% of cancer deaths occurred in this age group emphasizes the importance of continued screening in the postmenopausal patient population.[53]

Efforts must be directed toward better education of women concerning cervical cancer screening and better education of physicians about the shortcomings of cytologic screening. The Pap smear should ideally not be performed within 24 hours of intercourse or during the menses. In addition, whenever topical therapies are being used, patients should have completed intravaginal antibiotic and antifungal preparations more than a week prior to obtaining a Pap smear. The sensitivity of the test can be improved by ensuring adequate sampling of the ectocervix, the squamocolumnar junction, and the endocervical canal. Use of a cytologic brush within the cervical canal instead of a cotton swab minimizes the likelihood of obtaining an unsatisfactory sample by maximizing the number of endocervical or metaplastic cells. Performing the ectocervical smear before the endocervical smear may reduce the number of Pap smears rendered unsatisfactory by blood. The finding of columnar endocervical cells or metaplastic cells on the Pap smear is reassurance that an adequate specimen was obtained.[54]

False-negative Pap results are seen when the underlying process is obscured by intense inflammation or when the transformation zone is not sampled adequately. The transformation zone is more difficult to evaluate in postmenopausal than premenopausal women because of its location high in the endocervical canal with advancing age. Additionally, the test can be less sensitive in detecting invasive cancer because hemorrhage, necrosis, and intense inflammation, which often accompany this diagnosis, can obscure the underlying disease process. False-negative Pap smears have been reported in up to 15% of patients with invasive cancer.[55]

Because of the diagnostic, therapeutic, and survival advantages of detecting carcinoma of the cervix in an in situ rather than an invasive stage, the ACS and the American College of Obstetrician Gynecologists (ACOG) have recommended the following: "All women who are or have been sexually active or who are 18 and older should have an annual Pap test and pelvic examination. After three or more consecutive satisfactory examinations with normal findings, the Pap test may be performed less frequently at the discretion of a woman's physician."

The rationale for these recommendations is severalfold: (1) The per patient cost of annual cytologic screening is not excessive; (2) the identification and successful treatment of preinvasive disease justify an intensive screening program when compared with the morbidity and mortality associated with invasive cancer; (3) the pelvic and breast examinations performed in conjunction with cervical screening should be conducted annually; (4) it is often not possible to identify a low-risk female population because the sexual activity of a woman's partner is also an important factor and is not easily quantified; and (5) the incidence of cervical carcinoma in older women might be increasing. One study found 55% of newly diagnosed cervical cancer patients to be older than 50 years.[56]

## APPROACH TO THE PATIENT WITH AN ABNORMAL PAP SMEAR

Results of the Pap smear examination have traditionally been reported on a numeric scale, class I through class V. This terminology was often varied and confusing. As a result, this scheme was replaced in most centers by the Bethesda system, which was developed at a workshop in 1988 sponsored by the National Cancer Institute.[57] Refinements in this system were recommended during a second workshop held in 1992. The Pap smear report is given in three parts: (1) statement of specimen adequacy; (2) general categorization (normal, benign cellular changes, and epithelial cell abnormalities); and (3) descriptive diagnoses. The descriptive diagnoses are extensive and include the broad categories of infection, reactive and reparative changes, epithelial cell abnormalities (including malignancy), nonepithelial neoplasms, and hormonal evaluation. Changes associated with HPV infection and all levels of CIN are categorized as *squamous intraepithelial lesions* (SIL). *Low-grade SIL* includes biopsy-proven CIN 1 or changes associated with HPV infection, or both. *High-grade SIL* denotes biopsy-proven CIN 2 and CIN 3. *ASCUS* and *AGCUS* are terms to denote the categories of atypical squamous cells of undetermined significance and atypical glandular cells of undetermined significance, respectively. When patients with ASCUS Pap smears undergo biopsy, up to 30% are found to have clinically significant lesions, although the majority (25%) of these are CIN 1.[58] Persistent ASCUS Pap smear results repeated after 3 to 4 months necessitate further evaluation as outlined in the algorithm for the triage of Pap smears shown in Figure 56–1. The rate of significant findings in patients with AGCUS smears ranges from 17 to 38%. Four to 11% of these patients actually have cancer.[59–61]

Approximately 80% of laboratories have adopted the Bethesda system of reporting, but others continue to use the former system.[57, 62] This change in reporting has permitted clinicians to correlate their clinical assessment with the histopathologic assessment of colposcopically directed biopsies.

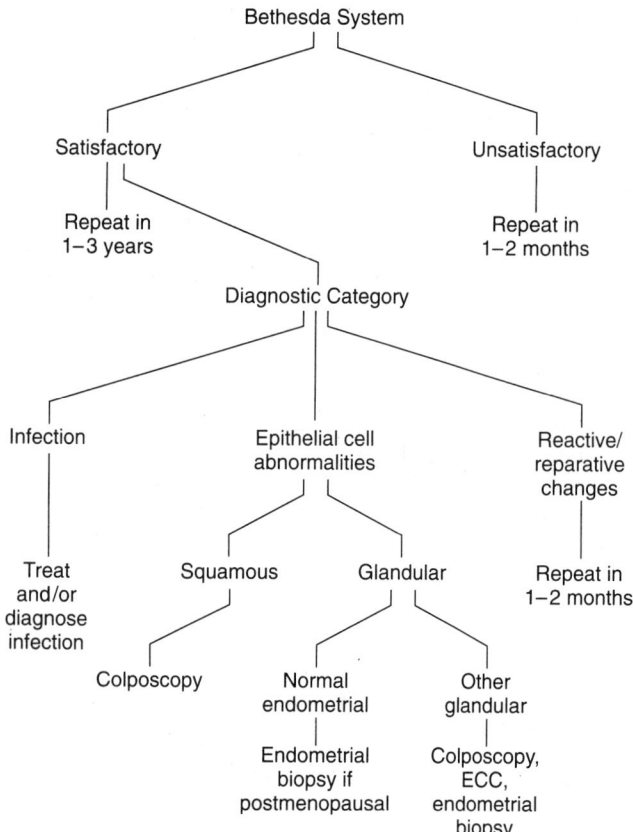

**Figure 56–1.** This algorithm is useful for triaging abnormal Papanicolaou (Pap) smears.

Readers may refer to Kurman and colleagues' guidelines for a comprehensive summary of recommendations for the management of abnormal Pap smears.[63] Colposcopy is the tool used by clinicians to evaluate women with abnormal Pap smear results. The colposcope is a dissecting-type microscope that typically magnifies the cervical area by 7 to 16 times. Three or 5% acetic acid, applied to the cervix, can help identify abnormal areas for directed biopsy.[64] As a general rule, when the examining clinician is able to visualize satisfactorily the entire area of abnormality on the cervix, when no disease is found in the endocervical canal, and when the correlation between the cytologic prediction of disease and the biopsy findings is excellent, treatment can be effected without more extensive biopsy procedures such as conization of the cervix.

Implicit in the evaluation scheme is the need for experience in using the colposcope as a diagnostic tool, an understanding of the natural history of the underlying disease process, and the technical ability to perform the various diagnostic and treatment procedures. In all instances, representative biopsy specimens should be obtained from the abnormal areas on the cervix *in addition* to an endocervical curettage. Examinations must be recorded as either "satisfactory," indicating that the entire transformation zone was visualized with the aid of the colposcope (and, therefore, the entire lesion was visualized), or "unsatisfactory." Satisfactory colposcopy is followed by evaluation of the histologic and cytologic findings and formulation of a treatment plan. Results of the endocervical curettage must be normal, and

the cytologic abnormality must be adequately explained by the biopsy findings to allow treatment by conservative ablative methods.

The most commonly used treatments for CIN are cryotherapy, laser vaporization, and loop electrosurgical excision procedure (LEEP). The goal of these standard treatment approaches is to destroy or excise the lesion and the entire transformation zone to a depth of 6 to 8 mm, including 3 to 5 mm of normal tissue around the periphery of the lesion. Cryotherapy involves freezing the cervix by means of nitrous oxide or other suitable agents.[65] Cryotherapy has efficacy that approaches that of laser vaporization under colposcopic guidance, with a cure rate of 80 to 95% in properly selected patients. Laser vaporization appears to have a higher cure rate than cryotherapy for lesions greater than 3 cm or with 5 mm of extension into the endocervical canal.[66] Follow-up examination after both of these approaches should be performed 3 months after treatment, with a Pap smear and endocervical curettage. If results of both studies are normal, the Pap smear should be repeated at 3-month intervals for 1 year and annually thereafter. This practice promptly identifies treatment failures and recurrences, 90% of which are found within a year.

When the colposcopic examination is unsatisfactory, treatment must include a cervical conization or LEEP. Similarly, dysplastic epithelium found on endocervical curettage or a Pap smear that suggests a degree of CIN greater than that found on cervical biopsy necessitates a cervical conization or LEEP. Because a diagnosis of microinvasive cancer found on a punch biopsy specimen must be viewed as inconclusive for frankly invasive cancer, a conization or LEEP is also required for this finding.

Cervical conization is both a diagnostic and a therapeutic modality and is indicated when the possibility of invasive disease has not been precluded by colposcopic evaluation and directed biopsies. This procedure can be performed using a knife or carbon dioxide laser. When no invasive disease is found in the conization specimen, the cure rate exceeds 90% if the margins of the specimen are negative for CIN; the cure rate drops to 70% if margins are involved with premalignant changes.[67] Patients who have positive cone biopsy margins and who desire future fertility can be monitored conservatively with repeat Pap smears, endocervical curettages, and colposcopically directed biopsies, if indicated, with little risk of progression to invasive cancer.[68, 69] A vaginal or abdominal hysterectomy is indicated for recurrence of high-grade CIN if future childbearing is not desired. Conversely, a cone biopsy can be repeated for endocervical failures and cryotherapy or laser for ectocervical failures, as determined by colposcopy and endocervical curettage, when the patient wishes to avoid hysterectomy. Even after a hysterectomy has been performed, patients remain at risk for vaginal intraepithelial neoplasia and carcinoma; therefore, yearly Pap smear examinations should still be performed.[36]

In many physicians' practices, LEEP has largely replaced conization, cryotherapy, and laser therapy as the usual treatment modality for CIN. It can be performed quickly in the office using local anesthesia, causes minimal discomfort or morbidity, and is much less expensive than conization. As with conizations, more than 90% of patients are cured with this procedure. Similar follow-up as for conization is required. Whether LEEP should be used to replace colposcopically directed cervical biopsies remains controversial. Some practitioners favor this concept because it allows diagnosis and treatment in one step. The major concerns about this approach include (1) the possibility that LEEP might adversely affect cervical function, thereby compromising fertility and increasing premature deliveries, and (2) whether patients with lower grade lesions will be treated overly aggressively.[70, 71] The majority of patients are treated effectively using this approach, which has been proposed as a cost-effective program in underserved areas where resources are limited and follow-up not ensured.[72]

## PRETREATMENT EVALUATION AND STAGING

Cervical cancer is the only gynecologic malignancy that remains clinically staged. The oncology division of FIGO revised the staging system for stage I lesions in 1994 in an effort to have reliable criteria to compare different therapeutic modalities (Table 56–1).[73] Stage IA1 previously was defined as "minimal microscopically evident stromal invasion." The staging revision now specifies a maximum depth of invasion of 3 mm with no more than 7 mm horizontal spread. Lesions with invasion deeper than 3 mm but not greater than 5 mm and no more than 7 mm horizontal spread are defined as stage IA2. In addition, stage IB (lesions confined to the cervix but more extensive than stage IA) has been divided into two subgroups to reflect the difference in prognosis of the bulky stage IB lesions. This subgrouping

distinguishes those lesions greater than 4 cm in diameter (stage IB2) from smaller lesions (stage IB1).

Allowable techniques for patient evaluation include pelvic examination, colposcopy, endocervical curettage, cone biopsy, cystoscopy, proctoscopy, intravenous pyelogram (IVP), barium enema, and radiographic examination of the lungs. Pelvic examination is often performed with the patient under anesthesia and requires thorough inspection and palpation of the vagina and palpation of the parametrial tissues on rectal examination to search for local spread of disease. When qualified examiners disagree about the stage of disease in a particular patient, the lower stage should be assigned. The stage may not be changed at a later date on the basis of new findings. Other diagnostic modalities including imaging techniques or directed lymph nodes biopsies may be used for treatment planning, but the findings cannot affect the clinical stage assigned.

A cost-effective pretreatment staging evaluation is advised, and frequently ordered tests that do not provide useful information should be avoided. Lindell and Anderson[74] reviewed the records of 141 women with cervical cancer to determine how frequently information derived from pretreatment tests changed the stage of disease as determined by pelvic examination alone. One patient whose disease was originally thought to be stage II was found to have lung metastasis on chest radiography. Cystoscopic evaluation revealed mucosal tumor invasion of the bladder in two patients, both of whom were initially thought to have stage III disease. Thus, the final designation of stage differed from

**Table 56–1.** International Federation of Gynecology and Obstetrics Staging of Carcinoma of the Cervix Uteri

| | |
|---|---|
| Stage 0 | Carcinoma in situ, intraepithelial carcimona. |
| Stage I | The carcinoma is strictly confined to the cervix (extension to the corpus should be disregarded). |
| Stage IA | Invasive cancer identified only microscopically. All gross lesions even with superficial invasion are stage 1B cancers. |
| | Invasion is limited to measured stromal invasion with maximal depth of 5.0 mm and no wider than 7.0 mm. |
| Stage IA1 | Measured invasion of stroma no greater than 3.0 mm in depth and no wider than 7.0 mm. |
| Stage IA2 | Measured invasion of stroma greater than 3.0 mm and no greater than 5.0 mm in depth and no wider than 7.0 mm. |
| Stage IB | Clinical lesions confined to the cervix or preclinical lesions greater than 1A. |
| Stage IB1 | Clinical lesions no greater than 4.0 cm in size. |
| Stage IB2 | Clinical lesions greater than 4.0 cm in size. |
| Stage II | The carcinoma extends beyond the cervix but has not extended to the pelvic wall. The carcinoma involves the vagina but not as far as the lower third. |
| Stage IIA | No obvious parametrial involvement. |
| Stage IIB | Obvious parametrial involvement. |
| Stage III | The carcinoma has extended to the pelvic wall. On rectal examination, there is no cancer-free space between the tumor and the pelvic wall. The tumor involves the lower third of the vagina. |
| | All cases with a hydronephrosis or nonfunctioning kidney are included unless they are known to be due to other causes. |
| Stage IIIA | No extension to the pelvic wall. |
| Stage IIIB | Extension to the pelvic wall and/or hydroneophrosis or nonfunctioning kidney. |
| Stage IV | The carcinoma has extended beyond the true pelvis or has clinically involved the mucosa of the bladder or rectum. A bullous edema as such does not permit a case to be allotted to stage IV. |
| Stage IVA | Spread of the growth to adjacent organs. |
| Stage IVB | Spread to distant organs. |

*Notes about the staging:*

The diagnosis of both Stage IA1 and IA2 cases should be based on microscopic examination of removed tissue, preferably a cone, which must include the entire lesion. The depth of invasion should not be more than 5.0 mm taken from the base of the epithelum, either surface or glandular, from which it originates.

The second dimension, the horizonatal spread, must not exceed 7 mm. Vascular space involvement, either venous or lymphatic, should not alter the staging but should be specifically recorded, as it may affect treatment decisions in the future.

Lesions of greater size should be classified as stage 1B.

As a rule, it is impossible to estimate clinically whether a cancer of the cervix has extended to the corpus or not. Extension to the corpus should therefore be disregarded.

A patient with a growth fixed to the pelvic wall by a short and indurated but not nodular parametrium should be allotted to stage IIB. It is impossible, at clinical examination, to decide whether a smooth and indurated parametrium is truly cancerous or only inflammatory. Therefore, the case should be placed in stage III only if the parametrium is nodular on the pelvic wall or if the growth itself extends to the pelvic wall.

From FIGO, Federation Internationale de Gynecologie et d'Obstetrique. Annual report on the results of treatment in gynaecological cancer. J Epidemiol Biostat 1998;3:119.

the extent of disease determined by pelvic examination alone in only 2% of patients. Because of the low yield of cystoscopy, IVP, sigmoidoscopy, and barium enema, patients with disease clinically limited to the cervix may forgo these procedures. With clinical evidence of more advanced disease, however, cystoscopy and IVP are recommended in the pretreatment assessment.

Computed tomography (CT) of the abdomen and pelvis has been advocated as a possible replacement for IVP in patients with advanced disease because it can detect both ureteral obstruction and para-aortic adenopathy. The latter finding might warrant fine-needle aspiration to confirm or refute metastasis to this location. This procedure permits the radiotherapist to select treatment fields in planning radiotherapy. CT appears to be more useful in detecting metastatic cancer in para-aortic lymph nodes than in pelvic lymph nodes. The sensitivity for involved para-aortic lymph nodes ranges from 67 to 71%, in contrast to that for involved pelvic lymph nodes of 25 to 45%.[75, 76] The ability to detect parametrial involvement by CT is poorer than by clinical examination.[77] Magnetic resonance imaging (MRI) has also been used to assess the parametrial and nodal regions in patients with cervical cancer.[78, 79] Overall, CT appears to be superior to MRI for evaluating the para-aortic regions, whereas MRI provides more accurate information about parametrial infiltration. As with CT, the expense of MRI appears to outweigh the benefits when compared with IVP alone and is no more accurate than a careful pelvic examination performed by well-trained gynecologic oncologists and radiotherapists in evaluating the local extent of disease.[80]

Lymphangiography is rarely used because of poor sensitivity and specificity in most series as well as patients' discomfort, excessive cost, and morbidity. In patients with ureteral obstruction, renal scans sometimes prove useful for determining residual renal function. This information can help with the decision to place nephrostomy tubes or provide other means of urinary diversion. Liver-spleen scans have been replaced by CT when liver involvement is suspected on the basis of abnormal liver function test results or clinical evidence of hepatomegaly. In patients who complain of bone pain, appropriate skeletal radiographs and a bone scan should be performed. Other tests can be ordered as judged appropriate by the clinician in order to assess specific patients' complaints that might result from metastatic cancer.

## PROGNOSIS

The most reliable prognostic indicator for patients with carcinoma of the cervix is the clinical stage of disease. According to the latest FIGO statistics derived from 11,945 women treated between 1990 and 1992, patients with stage IA1 and IA2 disease had a 5-year survival in excess of 95%. Women with stage IB disease had a 5-year survival of 80%, stage IIA and IIB 64 to 66%, stage IIIA and IIIB 33 to 39%, stage IVA 17%, and IVB 9%.[3] More advanced stage not only reflects increased tumor burden but also correlates with an increased likelihood of lymph node metastasis.

Clinical staging is inaccurate in a large percentage of cases because lymph node metastases are not detectable by clinical assessment and occult parametrial disease is sometimes discovered only on pathologic assessment of a radical hysterectomy specimen. The subjective nature of the staging process must be understood when reviewing survival data. Errors in staging can be reduced by the use of examination under anesthesia[81] but remain high when compared with findings at operative assessment. This observation has led many investigators to advocate surgical assessment of patients with advanced disease in an attempt to facilitate better treatment selection and improve survival. Nevertheless, after 20 years of clinical experience with operative assessment, the benefit of pretreatment laparotomy in terms of increased survival has not been demonstrated.[82, 83]

Surgical staging does, however, improve our understanding of the disease process and, with advances in radiation and chemotherapy, might lead to survival improvement. The goal of pretreatment operative assessment is to identify disease outside of the planned radiation field. Fine-needle aspiration of para-aortic nodes has proved to be an acceptable alternative to surgical staging when the nodes are enlarged on CT scan.[84] If the para-aortic nodes appear normal on CT, an extraperitoneal lymph node dissection can be helpful for treatment planning in women with locally advanced disease (stage IB2 through IIIB). An extraperitoneal approach to the para-aortic nodes is preferred to transabdominal exploration to avoid adhesion formation because radiation effects on bowel and the resulting complications of bowel obstruction and necrosis are increased when loops of small intestine become fixed in the pelvis.[85] Reports of laparoscopic pelvic and para-aortic lymphadenectomies provide the potential for operative staging at reduced expense and morbidity for this group of patients.

**Lymph Node Involvement.** The presence of lymph nodes with metastases correlates directly with stage of disease, which, in turn, correlates with survival (Table 56–2). By combining data from 31 series, Plentl[44] reported lymph node metastases in 15.4% of 3391 women with stage I disease, 28.6% of 2952 women with stage II disease, and 47% of 217 women with stage III disease. The number of positive pelvic lymph nodes has also been shown to correlate inversely with 5-year survival: 62% with one positive node, 36% for two nodes, 20% for three to four, and 0% for five or greater.[86]

Some patients experience recurrence and die of disease in the absence of lymph node metastases. Many authors have tried to characterize this subset of patients. These patients often have bulky tumors that may be deeply invasive, contain lymphovascular space invasion, have endometrial extension, or involve the surgical margins.[87–89] Boyce and colleagues[90] described 11 of 119 patients with stage I

*Table 56–2.* **Pelvic Node Metatasis with Invasive Carcinoma According to Depth of Stromal Penetration**

| Depth of Invasion (mm)* | No. of Patients | Node Metastasis | |
|---|---|---|---|
| | | NO. OF PATIENTS | (%) |
| 0.1–3.0 | 397 | 1 | 0.2 |
| 3.1–5.0 | 98 | 8 | 8.1 |
| Total 0.1–5.0 | 495 | 9 | 1.8 |

*Stromal invasion from 0.1 to 5.0 mm with and without vascular invasion and confluency.

Adapted from Ferenczy A. In: Kurman R, ed. Blaustein's pathology of the female genital tract. New York: Springer-Verlag, 1978:177.

disease with negative nodes who experienced recurrence following radical hysterectomy. Five of 9 patients with uterine corpus involvement and 3 of 10 with invasion of more than 10 mm combined with lymphovascular invasion experienced recurrence. Burke and colleagues[91] reported 18 patients who suffered recurrence after undergoing radical hysterectomy and pelvic lymphadenectomy in which lymph node metastasis was not found. They found lymphovascular space involvement to be three times as common in the women with recurrence versus those without. On the basis of these observations, adjuvant radiotherapy following surgery for a select group of high-risk patients was studied by the Gynecologic Oncology Group (GOG). In a randomized, prospective study, these patients with risk factors for recurrence had a lower risk of recurrence (27.9% vs. 15.3%) if they received adjuvant pelvic irradiation.[138a]

**Tumor Size.** Although tumor size frequently correlates with the stage of disease, a wide range of tumor sizes is found within each stage. Of 240 patients with stage IB or IIA carcinoma of the cervix, Piver and Chung[92] found lymph node metastases in 21% of 132 patients with tumors up to 3 cm. No significant difference in the risk of lymph node metastases was noted between the two stages studied when corrected for tumor volume. Although stage is an important prognostic factor in cervical cancer, tumor volume within a given stage can influence survival. In addition to the increased risk of regional spread, larger tumor volume increases the risk of central recurrences after radiation therapy. For stage IB tumors, Perez and colleagues[93] determined that the 10-year actuarial pelvic failure rate was 5% for tumors smaller than 2 cm, 15% if the tumor was 2.1 to 5 cm, and 35% for tumors greater than 5 cm. This directly correlated with differences in 10-year disease-free survival that ranged from 90% for stage IB tumors smaller than 2 cm to 47% for those greater than 5 cm.

**Histologic Studies.** Cell type can have prognostic importance, although adenocarcinomas and squamous cell carcinomas have survival probabilities that are similar when corrected for stage. Eighty to 85% of cervical cancers are of the squamous variety and can be categorized into three groups: (1) large cell nonkeratinizing, which is the most common, followed by (2) large cell keratinizing and (3) small cell carcinomas.[94] Whether the large cell nonkeratinizing tumors are associated with a slight survival advantage when compared with large cell keratinizing tumors is debated.[95] The small cell cancers, including small cell undifferentiated tumors, are characterized by the presence of intracellular neuroendocrine secretions and have a particularly dismal outcome.[96] Sheets and colleagues[97] reported the University of California, Irvine, experience with 14 patients with stages IB and IIA. All patients were treated surgically, and nodal metastases were found in 57% of women. All patients had recurrence, and only two were alive with follow-up less than 5 years.

**Endometrial Extension.** Although not included in the FIGO staging system, endometrial extension appears to worsen the prognosis. In a study by Perez and coworkers,[98] the 5-year survival rate fell from 85 to 50% in patients with stage I and from 70 to 45% in patients with stage II if endometrial curettings demonstrated tumor extension to the uterine corpus. When endometrial extension is present, the risk of both lymph node metastasis and central recurrence

after radiation is increased.[99] Positive uterine curettings are often difficult to interpret because they can represent contamination from tumor within the endocervix; therefore, endometrial curettage is not routinely performed in the evaluation of patients with cervical cancer.

**Expression of Molecular Markers and Growth Factors.** With the knowledge of the interaction between the HPV-E6 protein with p53 and the HPV-E7 protein with pRb, the expression of oncogenes is under extensive investigation. Oncogene overexpression may not only play an important role in cervical carcinogenesis but may also be a predictor of a more aggressive phenotype. The detection of certain oncogenes could theoretically be used to determine which patients might benefit from adjuvant radiation therapy or chemotherapy. For example, *bcl-2* is part of a family of genes that control apoptosis. The p53 protein is known to downregulate *bcl-2*. In a group of patients with primary cervical cancer, there was a strong association between loss of *bcl-2* expression and tumor stage. Additionally, there was a correlation between expression of *bcl-2* and overall survival, suggesting that regulation of apoptosis may play a significant role in the behavior of cervical cancer.[100] C-*myc* gene overexpression has also been associated with decreased disease-free survival and higher risk of distant metastases.[101] Likewise, in studies of the c-*erb*2 protein in cervical cancer, positive staining on immunohistochemistry was strongly correlated with poor survival in a group of patients who had stage IB and IIA cervical carcinoma and who were monitored for at least 5 years.[102] Other oncogenes and growth factors being investigated in cervical cancer include Ha-*ras*, epidermal growth factor receptor (EGFR), and transforming growth factor-$\alpha$ (TGF-$\alpha$) and -$\beta$ (TGF-$\beta$).[103–106]

## Treatment

The treatment of patients with cervical cancer is determined primarily by the stage of disease. Preinvasive disease (stage 0) is discussed in the section on treatment of patients with abnormal Pap smears. Microinvasive cancer (stage IA1) can be managed by nonradical surgery in most instances. Early invasive cancer (stages IA, IB, and IIA) can be effectively treated with either radical surgery or radiation therapy. Advanced local disease (stages IIB to IVA) is optimally treated with radiation therapy, and when there is distant disease, chemotherapy can be added. In some patients with a large tumor volume or a poor response to radiation therapy, a combination of radiation and surgery is indicated. Disease recurring after radiation therapy and located centrally in the pelvis can be managed successfully with exenterative surgery. Recurrent disease in the pelvis following surgery is treated with radiation, whereas recurrent disease outside of the pelvis is treated best with chemotherapy.

### STAGES IA1 AND IA2

The FIGO criteria for microinvasive cancer of the cervix adopted in 1994 are listed in Table 56–1. The recurrence rate (1 to 3%) and survival (97%) for patients with stage IA1 and IA2 disease reflect the low incidence of regional or distant spread for stage IA. The distinction between the two stages is made primarily to compare treatment modalities that can be more conservative in patients with less than 3 mm depth of invasion (stage IA1), when the risk of nodal involvement is 0 to 4%.[107] In contrast, the risk of nodal involvement in stage IA2 disease has been reported to range from 2 to 8%.[108, 109]

An excisional cone biopsy is considered adequate therapy for patients with stage IA1 cancers when future childbearing is planned and when long-term follow-up can be ensured.[110–112] The following pathologic criteria should be met: Depth of invasion should not exceed 3 mm, the lesion width should be less than 7 mm, lymphovascular space invasion should not be present, and the epithelial and stromal margins of the cone biopsy specimen should be free of both invasive and preinvasive disease. Follow-up of these patients must be intensive, including Pap smear, colposcopy, and endocervical curettage every 3 months for the first year. Extrafascial hysterectomy via the abdominal approach remains the therapy preferred by most clinicians when childbearing is not contemplated. The abdominal approach allows the surgeon to evaluate the lymph nodes by palpation and to sample any that are suspicious. Because the risk of nodal metastases with stage IA1 disease is so low, a vaginal hysterectomy is also acceptable therapy.

It is recommended that patients with stage IA2 disease undergo a pelvic lymphadenectomy because the risk of regional spread in these cases ranges from 2 to 8%. Whether a radical hysterectomy or a simple hysterectomy should be performed remains controversial. Parametrial disease has only rarely been noted in these patients, so extrafascial hysterectomy may be satisfactory. However, most gynecologic oncologists prefer a modified radical hysterectomy in this group in order to be certain that all of the cervical stroma and medial parametria have been excised.[113] A retrospective review by the GOG focused on patients with stage IA2 disease who had undergone cervical conization followed by radical hysterectomy and pelvic and para-aortic node dissection. Despite the fact that nearly one fourth of the 51 patients had lymphovascular space invasion, none had nodal involvement at surgery or later recurrence.[114] Intracavitary brachytherapy alone may also be used for definitive therapy in these patients; however, the small percentage of women with occult lymph node spread treated in this fashion may experience later recurrence. Accordingly, this approach should be limited only to women who are unable to withstand an operative procedure.

## STAGES IB1 AND IB2

In 1994, FIGO revised the staging system for clinically evident cancers limited to the cervix to reflect the difference in behavior between smaller cervical lesions (≤4 cm, stage IB1) and the larger ones (>4 cm, stage IB2). As expected, many studies have reported higher recurrence rates with larger tumors.[115, 116] Pelvic lymph node metastases occur in 15 to 25% of women with stage IB cancer but appreciably more frequently in stage IB2 than stage IB1. Effective treatment must address these lymph nodes in addition to the cervix, upper vagina, and paracervical and paravaginal tissues. Optimal management can be achieved with radical

hysterectomy and bilateral pelvic lymphadenectomy. Primary radiation therapy can be used with equal cure rates. In many centers, women with early-stage disease who are elderly, who have coexisting medical problems that increase the risk of serious intraoperative or postoperative complications with a radical pelvic operation, and who have primary tumors greater than 5 cm in diameter are treated with radiation, whereas "more favorable" patients undergo surgery. Patients with stage IB2 disease have a poorer 5-year survival (72.8%) when compared with patients with stage IB1 (90.0%), mainly because of the higher risk of regional spread with larger cancers.[117]

**Surgery.** Radical hysterectomy and bilateral pelvic lymphadenectomy include removal of the uterine fundus and cervix with the paracervical and paravaginal tissues at the pelvic side walls in continuity, transection of the ureterosacral ligaments near their sacral attachments, ligation of the uterine vessels at their origin from the hypogastric artery, removal of the upper one third of the vagina with the paracolpos, and excision of pelvic lymph nodes from the common, external, and internal iliac vessels.[118] Extensive dissection of the bladder base and ureters subjects approximately 2 to 3% of patients to the formation of a vesicovaginal or ureterovaginal fistula.[119] Most patients develop transient bladder dysfunction, but the majority recover functionally.[120, 121]

A major advantage of surgery over radiation in the treatment of cervical cancer includes preservation of ovarian function in young women, which obviates the necessity for exogenous estrogen administration and reduces the risk of post-treatment sexual dysfunction. Another possible benefit of ovarian preservation with radical hysterectomy is the potential for oocyte retrieval in those women who might consider surrogate parenting. Ovaries can be preserved because ovarian metastases rarely are seen in early squamous cell carcinoma of the cervix,[122] and these tumors are not stimulated hormonally.[123] The ovaries may be transposed laterally out of the pelvis to avoid the effects of adjuvant pelvic irradiation should it be administered because of poor prognostic factors. Patients should be counseled, however, that even with ovarian transposition, their risk of ovarian failure may be as great as 50% if radiation is required.[124] Surgery will shorten the functional length of the vagina, but lubrication will be maintained. With radiation therapy, the vaginal length, diameter, and lubrication are often affected adversely. Delayed complications of radiation, such as colitis, enteritis, and cystitis, are also avoided with surgery. Because intracavitary radiation cannot be delivered safely to patients with pelvic infections, operative management should be selected for these women. An additional advantage of surgery over radiation is the potential for intraoperative findings to provide important prognostic information that can help identify women at risk for recurrence, for whom adjuvant radiotherapy is indicated.

**Radiation Therapy.** Treatment of patients with stage IB cancer of the cervix by radiation therapy provides effective treatment of the primary tumor and areas at risk for occult metastasis or extension. Treatment consists of teletherapy to the whole pelvis in addition to intracavitary brachytherapy in the uterus, endocervical canal, and vaginal fornices, usually using $^{226}$Ra, $^{137}$Cs, or $^{192}$Ir. Megavoltage linear accelerators used today for teletherapy produce less skin reaction and superior survival results compared with those reported in patients treated with older equipment. A combination of teletherapy and brachytherapy is used. Brachytherapy primarily treats the central portion of the tumor, whereas teletherapy provides a homogeneous radiation dose to the whole pelvis. Standard doses of teletherapy range from 150 to 200 cGy per day, 5 days per week, until 4500 to 5500 cGy is delivered homogeneously to the pelvis. If parametrial disease is still present, limited additional radiation may be delivered with a midline block to protect the bladder and rectosigmoid colon. If para-aortic lymph node metastases are present, 4500 cGy may be delivered to the para-aortic area. At completion of treatment, the central tumor should receive approximately 8000 to 8500 cGy. In bulky tumors, the total dose may reach 9500 cGy. The pelvic side wall should receive 6000 to 6500 cGy. Marcial and Marcial[125] provide an excellent current review of radiotherapy in the treatment of cervical carcinoma.

Intracavitary brachytherapy can deliver large doses of radiation to the primary tumor while sparing nearby structures. This dose-sparing effect occurs because the source of radiation is packed against the tumor and away from the rectum and bladder and because the dose delivered per unit of time varies inversely as the square of the distance from the source of radiation. For example, the bladder and rectum packed 3 cm from a source of intracavitary radium would receive only 11% of the dose of radiation delivered to a tumor located 1 cm from that source. High dose–rate intracavitary radiation is also being used more frequently as an alternative to traditional low dose–rate brachytherapy. With the high dose rates given (50 to 500 cGy/min), the therapy can be administered on an outpatient basis instead of in the required hospital stays with traditional low dose–rate intracavitary brachytherapy.[126]

The sequence of the two radiotherapeutic modalities is often determined by tumor volume and vaginal caliber. When the tumor is less than 1 cm in diameter, the risk of lymph node metastases is small, and therefore intracavitary therapy alone can be curative.[127] Bulky tumors are treated initially with external-beam therapy to the pelvis in order to reduce tumor volume and improve geometry for the placement of implants. Older patients' cancers of less than 3 cm can be treated initially with intracavitary therapy because vaginal narrowing following external therapy might not permit optimal placement of the applicators commonly used for intracavitary therapy, unless the therapist uses an interstitial needle template.[128]

Patients with primary tumors greater than 4 cm are at increased risk for spread to the para-aortic lymph nodes than are those with smaller cancers. The value of prophylactic para-aortic irradiation is controversial, but one prospective trial by the Radiation Therapy Oncology Group (RTOG) with 10 years of follow-up has demonstrated a survival advantage in the group of patients with bulky stage IB, IIA, or IIB cancers who received prophylatic para-aortic plus pelvic irradiation.[129]

Additional situations associated with an increased risk of recurrence after radiation therapy are endometrial extension of tumor, discussed previously, and prolonged interruptions in treatment due to acute radiation reactions or poor patient compliance. For patients with stage IB, Perez and colleagues[130] determined that the pelvic failure rate increased

from 7% in patients with radiation treatment time of 7 weeks or less to 36% if treatment time was prolonged to 9 weeks. Similarly, 10-year survival decreased from 86% with 7 weeks' treatment time to 55% with greater than 9 weeks' total treatment time.

Complications of radiotherapy are often reported to be more frequent and more severe than those seen following radical hysterectomy with bilateral pelvic lymphadenectomy. Perez and associates[131] reported an 8% incidence of severe complications (grade 3) and a 10% incidence of moderate complications in 277 patients with stage IB treated between 1958 and 1977. Subsequent reports have found a 10% major complication rate, including bowel obstruction; rectovaginal, vesicovaginal, and ureterovaginal fistulas; bowel or urinary tract strictures requiring surgical correction; proctitis; cystitis; and vaginal vault necrosis or stenosis.[132] Factors associated with an increased risk of complications following radiotherapy include age younger than 36 years, previous pelvic infections or surgery, central radiation dose greater than 8500 cGy, external irradiation only, high patient volume per radiation oncologist, daily dose greater than 180 cGy, and an extended treatment field.[125] These complications have made surgical therapy more attractive for otherwise healthy women. Surgical complications, excluding transient bladder dysfunction, which is seen frequently, occur in less than 5% of patients and, generally, are more amenable to surgical correction, rarely resulting in long-term disability.

**Radiation Combined with Surgery.** Several clinical situations have been managed with a combination of radiation and surgery. In selected patients with tumors arising within the endocervix, an endophytic pattern of growth can produce concentric expansion of the cervix and lower uterine segment. These so-called barrel-shaped lesions, which often exceed 6 cm in diameter, are usually managed initially with external-beam therapy to the whole pelvis. In many instances, tumor shrinkage is insufficient to permit curative intracavitary placement, and central recurrence can often result in patients' being treated by radiotherapy alone. These patients may be considered for extrafascial hysterectomy 6 to 10 weeks after external-beam therapy and one intracavitary treatment.[133] With lesions greater than 6 cm, a significantly higher survival rate at 10 years' follow-up with combined radiation and surgery versus radiation alone has been reported: 64% versus 45%.[134, 135] The GOG has prospectively addressed the value of extrafascial hysterectomy in lesions exceeding 4 cm after completion of radiation therapy with or without concurrent weekly cisplatin chemotherapy. The authors concluded that the performance of an extrafascial hysterectomy was not a significant benefit in bulky stage IB cancer; however, weekly cisplatin conferred a significant survival benefit.[135a]

Patients at high risk for pelvic recurrences following a radical hysterectomy should be considered for postoperative radiotherapy. Risk factors associated with higher recurrence rates include tumor in or near the surgical margins, parametrial involvement, pelvic lymph node metastases, lymphovascular space involvement, and large tumor volume.[136, 137] Adjuvant radiation in this setting reduces pelvic recurrences, but it was unclear until recently that the combined therapy reduced distant recurrences or increased overall survival.[138] In a prospective randomized clinical trial, the GOG studied the value of adjunctive pelvic radiotherapy in women who had stage IB cancers and who were found on pathologic specimen examination to have poor prognostic factors. The trial closed in 1995 and showed a significant reduction (47%) in both local and distant recurrences in one pelvic radiotherapy arm with acceptable morbidity. Survival data are not yet available.[138a] A subsequent study investigated the role of adjuvant pelvic radiotherapy with or without radiation-sensitizing chemotherapy using concurrent cisplatin and 5 FU in a randomized prospective clinical trial of women with selected high-risk factors. The results of this study again documented a significant survival advantage for patients who received adjuvant chemoradiation compared with those receiving radiation alone.[139a]

**Neoadjuvant Chemotherapy.** Neoadjuvant chemotherapy administered prior to definitive surgery or radiation therapy has been studied in an effort to gain better local-regional control and improve operability. One study demonstrated in a randomized fashion that neoadjuvant chemotherapy can improve survival in bulky stage IB lesions by improving operability.[139] A review of all phase III randomized trials of neoadjuvant therapy, however, failed to demonstrate improved survival with this approach.[140]

## STAGES II AND III

When a cervical tumor extends to the upper vagina and the paracervical soft tissues are clinically uninvolved (stage IIA), treatment can be effected either by radical hysterectomy and pelvic lymphadenectomy or by radiation therapy as described for stage IB. When the tumor extends to paracervical and paravaginal tissues (stage IIB or IIIB) or the distal vagina (stage IIIA), radiation therapy is preferred because adequate margins of resection are difficult to achieve. When lymph node metastases are found by CT-directed fine-needle aspiration or at exploratory laparotomy, radiation treatment is modified, with the dose of radiation to the involved side of the pelvis boosted and the radiation ports extended to include lymphatics one chain above the extent of documented disease.[141] Although the usual pelvic port measures approximately $15 \times 15$ cm and extends to the bottom of the 5th lumbar vertebral body, the port should be extended to the level of the aortic bifurcation (body of the 4th lumbar vertebral body with common iliac metastases or the level of the 12th thoracic vertebra with aortic lymph node metastases).[142]

The value of excising enlarged lymph nodes with metastatic cancer is controversial. One study has shown that the relapse-free survival of 50% in the group that had macroscopically positive but completely resected nodes was the same as in the group that had microscopically positive nodes only. These results would suggest a therapeutic benefit of excising these lymph nodes. By comparison, patients with unresected nodes with gross tumor replacement had a relapse-free rate of 0%.[143, 144]

## STAGE IV

**Radiation and Surgery.** Tumors that extend into the bladder or rectum can be cured infrequently with aggressive radiation therapy, sometimes combined with operation. Gen-

erally, 5000 cGy of external radiation is delivered to the whole pelvis, and if there is good response, 1000 cGy can be given through $10 \times 10$ cm ports and another 1000 cGy through $8 \times 8$ cm ports, for a total dose of 7000 cGy. Pelvic exenteration should then be considered if central disease persists 3 months following completion of therapy. Because radiation therapy alone rarely cures these advanced tumors, a primary exenteration should be considered if disease is not fixed to the lateral pelvic walls. Patients with recurrent disease or tumor fixed to the pelvic sidewall that is not amenable to surgical therapy may elect to have interstitial implantation of [125]I seeds. This treatment can occasionally be successful even in patients with recurrence after radiation therapy.[128]

**Chemotherapy.** Chemotherapy has been used in the treatment of squamous cell carcinomas of the cervix in three clinical situations: (1) as neoadjuvant therapy, (2) as a radiation sensitizer, and (3) as palliative therapy for recurrent or metastatic disease outside of the pelvis. Thus far, neoadjuvant chemotherapy followed by radiotherapy or surgery has not proved effective in improving local control or survival over radiation alone in patients with advanced stage cervical cancer.[145] Cisplatin and 5-fluorouracil are the drugs used most frequently as radiation sensitizers. In 1999, the Radiation Therapy Oncology Group (RTOG), the Southwest Oncology Group (SWOG), and the GOG reported three prospective, randomized trials that evaluated the impact of concurrent cisplatin and 5-FU chemotherapy with radiation in patients with stage IIB to IV disease.[145a–c] One of these trials[145a] treated patients with metastases to the pelvic lymph nodes. In all three trials, patients who received the concurrent chemotherapy had a significant reduction in the risk of death, ranging from approximately 25 to 40%. Based on these three trials, patients who require radiation for treatment of their cervical cancer should also receive concurrent chemotherapy.

For recurrent disease, several agents have clinical activity, with responses seen typically in 15 to 25% of patients (Table 56–3).[146] Agents reported to produce partial responses in this range include cyclophosphamide, 5-fluorouracil, doxorubicin, methotrexate, hexamethylmelamine, mitomycin C, bleomycin, cisplatin, chlorambucil, melphalan, ifosfamide, mitolactol (dibromodulcitol), carboplatin, and vincristine.[147] Of these drugs, cisplatin has been reported by the GOG to have the greatest antitumor activity in advanced squamous carcinoma of the cervix.[146] With a dose of 50 mg/m², 11 of the first 22 patients treated without prior chemotherapy responded. The results were much less favorable in patients who had received prior chemotherapy. The median duration of response for complete responders was 6 months, with a median survival of only 9 months. These figures did not differ significantly from those observed for partial responders. In a review of the literature, the overall objective response rate to cisplatin in the treatment of advanced and recurrent squamous cell carcinoma of the cervix is around 25%.[147, 148] Taxol (paclitaxel) has been studied more recently as a single agent in previously treated cervical cancer patients and has been found to have a 17% overall response rate.[149]

Combination chemotherapy is frequently difficult to administer because of previous pelvic radiotherapy, obstructive uropathy, or general debility. Combinations using myelotoxic

*Table 56–3.* Single-Agent Chemotherapy in Squamous Cell Carcinoma of the Cervix

| Drug | Prior Treatment | Response (%) |
|------|-----------------|--------------|
| **Alkylating agents** | | |
| Cyclophosphamide | Mixed | 38/251 (15) |
| Chlorambucil | Mixed | 11/44 (25) |
| Melphalan | Mixed | 4/20 (20) |
| Ifosfamide | No | 7/46 (15) |
| | Yes | 3/27 (11) |
| | Mixed | 25/84 (29) |
| Mitolactol | No | 16/55 (29) |
| (dibromodulcitol) | No | 7/47 (15) |
| Galactitol | Mixed | 7/36 (19) |
| Semustine | Mixed | 7/94 (7) |
| Lomustine | Mixed | 3/63 (5) |
| Yoshi 864 | Yes | 0/18 (0) |
| **Heavy metal complexes** | | |
| Cisplatin | No | 182/785 (23) |
| | Yes | 8/30 (27) |
| Carboplatin | No | 27/175 (15) |
| Iproplatin | No | 19/177 (11) |
| **Antibiotics** | | |
| Doxorubicin | No | 12/61 (20) |
| | Mixed | 33/205 (16) |
| Mitoxantrone | Yes | 2/26 (8) |
| Esorubicin | Yes | 0/28 (0) |
| Piperazinedione | No | 5/38 (13) |
| Echinomycin | Yes | 2/28 (7) |
| Porfiromycin | No | 17/78 (22) |
| **Antimetabolites** | | |
| 5-Fluorouracil | Mixed | 29/142 (20) |
| Methotrexate | Mixed | 17/96 (18) |
| 6-Mercaptopurine | Mixed | 1/18 (5) |
| Dichloromethotrexate | No | 3/37 (8) |
| Baker's antifol | Mixed | 5/32 (16) |
| **Plant alkaloids** | | |
| Etoposide | Mixed | 0/31 (0) |
| Teniposide | Yes | 3/22 (14) |
| Vincristine | Mixed | 10/55 (18) |
| Vinblastine | Yes | 0/33 (0) |
| | Mixed | 2/20 (10) |
| Vindesine | Mixed | 5/21 (24) |
| Maytansine | Yes | 1/29 (3) |
| **Other agents** | | |
| Hydroxyurea | Mixed | 0/14 (0) |
| Razoxane | Mixed | 5/28 (18) |
| Aminothiadiazole | Yes | 1/21 (5) |
| Amsacrine | Yes | 1/25 (4) |
| PALA | Yes | 0/36 (0) |
| Diaziquone | Yes | 1/26 (4) |
| *N*-methylformamide | Yes | 0/20 (0) |
| Spirogermanium | Yes | 0/18 (0) |
| Hexamethylmelamine | No | 12/64 (19) |

PALA, *N*-(phosphonoacetyl)-L-aspartate.
From Park RC, Thigpen JT. Chemotherapy in advanced and recurrent cervical cancer: a review. CANCER Vol. 71, 1993, p. 1446. Copyright © 1993 American Cancer Society. Reprinted by permission of Wiley-Liss Inc., a subsidiary of John Wiley & Sons, Inc.

and nonmyelotoxic agents have been used over the past several years with variable results. To date, no multidrug regimen produces a response superior to single-agent cisplatin without adding greatly to the toxicity reported with cisplatin alone. Furthermore, no regimen has been associated with improved overall survival. A phase II trial by the GOG using methotrexate, vinblastine, doxorubicin, and cisplatin demonstrated a 66% response rate; however, 50% of the patients experienced grade 3 or 4 neutropenia.[150] The GOG reported on a randomized trial of cisplatin versus cisplatin plus mitolactol versus CIFX (cisplatin plus ifosfamide). The

latter regimen was the most active one, with a 31.1% response rate but with more myelotoxicity and more renal and peripheral neurotoxicity. In addition, the mean time to progression was only 4.6 months.[151]

Brader and colleagues[152] analyzed factors predictive of response to chemotherapy in patients with recurrent cervical cancer. In chemotherapy-naive patients, site of disease recurrence correlated with the probability of response. Patients with recurrence in the previously irradiated field had a 5.3% response rate, as compared with 25.2% for those with recurrence outside the field. Nevertheless, the mean duration of response was only 4.8 months among responders.

**Pelvic Exenteration.** Persistent cervical cancer present at least 3 months after radiation therapy, or recurrent cancer detected after a longer interval, can be managed by pelvic exenteration when disease is confined to the pelvis. The diagnosis typically is suspected if the cervix remains bulky or nodular, if a tumor mass develops following an initial response, if a Pap smear result is abnormal more than 3 months after treatment, or if symptoms such as pain, bleeding, or leg swelling occur. The diagnosis usually can be confirmed by punch biopsy, needle biopsy, curettage of the cervix, or CT-guided fine-needle aspiration. The evaluation of patients with documented or suspected recurrence should include those studies performed in the initial evaluation of patients with untreated carcinoma. As in untreated patients, the pelvic examination is most important because nodular tumor palpated on the lateral pelvic wall is associated with little chance of cure and tumor fixed to the pelvic sidewall at operation is an indication to abandon a contemplated exenteration. Patients are rarely cured if they have leg edema or sciatic pain. Similarly, an IVP documenting ureteral obstruction is associated with a low rate of tumor resectability and of cure. Pelvic exenteration is rarely carried out in patients older than 70 years or in those with impaired pulmonary function, serious cardiac disease, massive obesity, or emotional instability.

Patients with recurrent tumor in the cervix, vagina, or paravaginal soft tissues usually require total pelvic exenteration. Initial steps in the operation include exploration for intraperitoneal spread, repeated biopsies of the lateral pelvic walls, and bilateral pelvic and para-aortic lymphadenectomy. Tumor in any of these areas reflects little chance for cure and, when found, is usually cause to abandon the procedure. If exenteration is performed, the operation involves the removal of the bladder, rectum, vagina, uterus, ovaries, fallopian tubes, and all supporting tissues within the true pelvis. A transverse or sigmoid colon colostomy and urinary diversion are constructed. Less extensive operations occasionally can be used in patients with minimal tumor and include a radical hysterectomy in those with small tumors confined to the cervix or an anterior exenteration in patients with lesions not encroaching on the rectum, uterosacral ligaments, or pararectal areas. Posterior exenteration rarely is performed because it usually is impossible to establish a cancer-free plane between the bladder and the heavily irradiated cervix and because of the high rate of severe bladder dysfunction and urinary tract fistulas that follow this operation.

When the possibility of exenteration is entertained, sophisticated preoperative and postoperative support is required. The physician must prepare the patient emotionally as well as medically. Intraoperative efforts should be directed toward prevention of disability and complications. Early postoperative attention is paid to massive fluid shifts, infection, and bleeding. These patients benefit from total parenteral nutrition because protein sparing facilitates wound healing and convalescence following the ultraradical operation. Although patients rarely die during the intraoperative or early postoperative period, convalescence often takes up to 3 months. This operation is thus undertaken only if there is a reasonable expectation of cure.[153]

The major morbidity and mortality after exenteration result mainly from intestinal complications.[154] Newer techniques used to prevent small intestinal obstruction and fistula include the repair of pelvic floor defects with either a carpet of omentum or a peritoneal graft. Partial closure of the defect in the pelvic floor by anastomosis of sigmoid colon to rectal stump can reduce these bowel complications while permitting subsequent colostomy closure in some patients with tumors that do not extend to the distal rectum. Myocutaneous flaps using the gracilis or rectus abdominis muscle in the construction of a neovagina also fill the anterior pelvis and reduce the rate of small intestine obstruction or fistula formation. Reconstruction of the urinary system traditionally has involved the use of an ileal conduit. Surgical innovations to produce a continent urinary diversion such as the Indiana pouch can eliminate the need for wearing an ostomy appliance for most women undergoing this procedure. If the procedure is completed and the surgical margins are uninvolved, the patient can expect a 40 to 50% chance of cure.

**Cervical Carcinoma Found in Hysterectomy Specimen.** All patients must have a normal Pap smear result or a satisfactory colposcopic examination before a hysterectomy is performed to avoid removal of an invasive cervical cancer by simple hysterectomy. Patients with invasive cervical cancer treated initially by simple hysterectomy can be categorized into four groups.[155] Group I consists of those with stage Ia disease who require no further therapy. Group II includes those with tumor in the surgical specimen with adequate surgical clearance (early stage Ib lesions). These patients can be treated with 5000 cGy whole-pelvis irradiation and can expect an 80% survival.[156] Group III includes patients whose hysterectomy specimen contains microscopic disease extending to the margin of resection. These patients can be treated with whole pelvis irradiation, usually with vaginal apex brachytherapy. Group IV patients have gross residual tumor at the margins of resection and, as expected, have a much poorer survival rate. Treatment for groups II to IV must be started within 6 weeks of hysterectomy because long delays in administering radiotherapy compromise survival even further. Radiotherapy for group IV patients should include both 5000 cGy to the whole pelvis and two vaginal implants. With palpable residual disease following completion of external-beam radiotherapy, interstitial brachytherapy should be considered. Reports of radical parametrectomy, upper vaginectomy, and bilateral pelvic lymphadenectomy in patients in groups II and III indicate excellent cure rates for this approach as well.[157] In one series, 15% of patients were found to have residual disease at the time of re-exploration.[158] Patients treated in this fashion also benefit from the additional prognostic information gained regarding the status of their pelvic lymph nodes.

**Investigation in Progress.** Exciting avenues of new investigation include innovative combinations of conventional modalities such as neoadjuvant chemotherapy preceding surgery or radiation therapy in an effort to minimize tumor volume before administering definitive therapy, adjuvant chemotherapy in conjunction with radiotherapy for bulky and advanced-stage disease, and radiation-sensitizing agents in the management of locally advanced cervical cancers. The greatest impact in cervical cancer research, however, may take place with an emphasis on preventive measures. Work on prophylactic HPV vaccines in several laboratories is currently under way. A number of clinical trials investigating therapeutic vaccines are under way, as well as numerous gene therapy programs targeting the E6 and E7 oncoproteins.

......................................

# ADENOCARCINOMA OF THE CERVIX

## Natural History

The management of adenocarcinoma of the uterine cervix is less well standardized than that of squamous cancers because adenocarcinomas represent only about 15 to 20% of primary cervical lesions.[159] A relative increase in the percentage of adenocarcinomas to squamous cancers is occurring because cervical cancer prevention is largely confined to squamous cell lesions. The earlier detection and treatment of squamous intraepithelial neoplasias has not been accompanied by the frequent detection of a precursor to adenocarcinomas.

### ETIOLOGY

Clear cell adenocarcinoma of the cervix and vagina in women born between 1948 and 1965 has frequently been associated with in utero exposure to the synthetic nonsteroidal estrogen diethylstilbestrol (DES). The Registry for Research on Hormonal Transplacental Carcinogenesis of the University of Chicago identified 519 cases of clear cell carcinoma of the vagina and cervix by June 30, 1985. The mothers of these women were known to have received DES during their pregnancy in 60% of cases, and an unidentified medication or hormone was known to have been taken by another 12%. Ninety-one percent of malignancies have been diagnosed in women between the ages of 15 and 27, with a median age of 19 years. Melnick and colleagues'[160] review of this subject estimates that 1 of every 1000 women exposed in utero to DES will develop clear cell adenocarcinoma. The absence of newer publications on this subject over the past decade suggests that new cases of DES-associated adenocarcinoma are not occurring after these women reach 30 years of age. Recurrent clear cell carcinoma has been detected as long as 20 years after primary therapy; this finding emphasizes the importance of continued follow-up and surveillance.[161] DES-exposed daughters do not appear, however, to have a higher risk of other cancers.[162]

Adenocarcinoma has not traditionally been associated with venereal transmission as reported for squamous cell carcinomas; however, more recent data have demonstrated that many adenocarcinomas also are associated with HPV. In 1986, Smotkin and colleagues[163] reported that HPV DNA could be detected in adenocarcinoma and adenosquamous tumors. This observation has been confirmed by Wilczynski and coworkers[164] at the University of California, Irvine, who detected the presence of HPV-18 in young women with adenocarcinomas. HPV-16 has also been detected in adenocarcinomas, but not as frequently as HPV-18.[165] That HPV was not identified in older women suggests that many causes of this disease may exist.

## ADENOCARCINOMA IN SITU

This precursor to adenocarcinoma was first described in 1952 by Helper and colleagues. The endocervical cells show pleomorphism characteristic of an adenocarcinoma, but they line architecturally normal endocervical glands and do not invade the cervical stroma. In contrast to squamous cell dysplasia, this entity does not necessarily spread contiguously. The diagnosis of adenocarcinoma in situ (AIS) can be made only by LEEP or cervical conization. When diagnosed in this fashion, even when the surgical margins are free of AIS, residual disease sometimes is found in the hysterectomy specimen.[166, 167] The usual recommendation for patients with AIS who do not desire future fertility is hysterectomy. Should the patient desire to maintain fertility, rigorous follow-up with Pap smears and periodic endocervical curettage is required after conization. Hysterectomy should be considered in these women following completion of child bearing.

## PROGNOSIS

Adenocarcinomas may have a slightly poorer prognosis than do squamous cell carcinomas for each stage of disease. For example, the 1998 report by FIGO showed stage I survival to be 78% for adenocarcinoma, compared with 84% for squamous cell carcinoma.[3] As with squamous cell carcinomas, prognosis is related to the presence of lymph node involvement, tumor volume, and stage of disease. The presence of lymphatic space invasion also appears to be an independent high-risk factor. Pelvic radiotherapy may be less likely to cure patients with nodal disease when compared with patients with similar stage of squamous cell carcinomas.[159]

The adenosquamous cell type has a poorer prognosis than adenocarcinoma. Gallup and colleagues[168] reported only a 25% survival of patients with stage IB lesions, some of

**Table 56–4.** Single-Agent Chemotherapy in Adenocarcinoma of the Cervix

| Drug | Prior Treatment | Response (%) |
| --- | --- | --- |
| Cisplatin | No | 4/20 (20) |
| Piperazinedione | Mixed | 2/14 (14) |
| Etoposide | Mixed | 1/19 (5) |
| Galactitol | Mixed | 2/27 (7) |
| Razoxane | Mixed | 1/25 (4) |
| Mitoxantrone | Mixed | 2/25 (8) |
| Diaziquone | Mixed | 2/26 (8) |
| Aminothiadiazole | Mixed | 2/26 (8) |
| Teniposide | Mixed | 1/23 (4) |
| Ifosfamide | Mixed | 3/24 (12) |

From Park RC, Thigpen JT: Chemotherapy in advanced and recurrent cervical cancer: a review. Cancer 1993;71:1448.

whose lesions were smaller than 2 cm. These tumors were of higher grade and had a higher incidence of lymph node metastasis. Patients with stage IB were found to have twice the usual rate of pelvic lymph node metastasis (43%). Recurrences can occur later than with squamous cell cancers, and there might be a higher rate of distant metastasis than with squamous carcinomas.

## Treatment

An analysis of previous reports shows a lack of agreement about the roles of surgery and radiation therapy for invasive lesions. The principal controversy regarding the therapy for stage I disease is whether radical surgery alone or a combination of radiation before surgery is better than radiation alone. Berek and colleagues[169] suggested that surgical removal of the uterus and cervix is important in improving survival. When women with stage I disease were stratified according to the size of the lesion, those who underwent radical hysterectomy or external plus intracavitary radiation therapy followed by simple hysterectomy had a better outcome than others treated with external and intracavitary radiation alone. In addition, about one fifth of the patients who underwent a hysterectomy following radiation had residual disease in the specimen, suggesting that, whenever possible, surgery is indicated for these patients. Combination therapy also appeared beneficial in stage II disease. Thus, the current recommendation for many is surgical removal of the primary tumor, via either radical hysterectomy or limited hysterectomy following radiation therapy. In general, patients with bulkier primary cervical lesions—namely, stage IB2—should receive combination therapy. Patients with more advanced disease (stages III and IV) should be treated in the same manner as those with squamous lesions. As with epidermoid lesions of the cervix, chemotherapy is relatively ineffective (Table 56–4).

...........................

# CERVICAL CANCER IN PREGNANCY

## Carcinoma in Situ

The incidence of carcinoma in situ associated with pregnancy is 1.3 per 1000, or approximately 1 per 770 pregnancies, and the average age of patients is 29.9 years.[170] Prenatal patients should have a routine Pap smear at the first antenatal visit if not done within the past year, and abnormal smears should be followed by colposcopy. The colposcopic appearance of cervical dysplasia tends to be exaggerated during pregnancy; however, colposcopically directed biopsy is a safe, reliable method of diagnosis, reducing the need for conization by 80% or more. A conization is required only if microinvasion is observed on punch biopsy, if the Pap smear suggests that invasive cancer is present, or if it is not possible to visualize the transformation zone adequately and the examination results arouse suspicion of invasive cancer. An endocervical curettage should not be performed during pregnancy because of the risk of hemorrhage and accidental rupture of the fetal membranes.

Carcinoma in situ diagnosed during pregnancy should be managed conservatively once invasive cancer has been precluded. Vaginal delivery is not contraindicated, and definitive treatment should be carried out as in the nonpregnant patient 6 to 8 weeks following delivery. There is a limited place for cesarean hysterectomy in the management of patients with carcinoma in situ who desire sterilization and whose reliability for follow-up may be uncertain; however, the physician must rule out an invasive cancer before considering this approach.

## Invasive Cancer

The incidence of invasive cancer in pregnancy is 0.45 per 1000, or approximately 1 per 2205 pregnancies.[170] Pregnancy complicates an average of 1 in 34 cases of invasive carcinoma of the cervix, and the average age of such patients is 33.8 years. Abnormal vaginal bleeding is the most common symptom and during pregnancy may be attributed to such conditions as threatened abortion or placenta previa. Thus, delayed diagnosis is common during pregnancy, and approximately 50% of cases are not recognized until the postpartum period.

Diagnosis of cervical cancer in pregnancy is usually made by punch biopsy of a gross lesion. Colposcopy is indicated for abnormal cervical cytology, with directed biopsies as necessary. The findings of microinvasion on a punch biopsy specimen or persistently abnormal Pap smear results indicative of invasive disease are indications for cervical conization, which is usually performed between 14 and 20 weeks.[171, 172]

Management of cervical cancer in pregnancy is influenced by the stage of the disease and the gestational age. Invasive cancer less than 3 mm, diagnosed on cone biopsy, may be treated conservatively, and the pregnancy allowed to proceed to term, with colposcopic surveillance every 6 to 8 weeks. At term, definitive treatment may consist of either cesarean hysterectomy or vaginal delivery followed by postpartum extrafascial hysterectomy. If the margins of the conization specimen from which the diagnosis of microinvasive carcinoma was made show evidence of this diagnosis, definitive treatment should be withheld until additional biopsy specimens are taken following delivery to rule out a more extensive process.

In the second trimester, there are no clear guidelines for the management of frankly invasive cancer, and a careful discussion with the patient and her family is necessary to provide sufficient information to permit a rational decision. In general, prior to about 24 weeks' gestation, the patient should be treated without delay; after this time, it may be reasonable to delay therapy for several weeks until fetal viability is achieved, usually around 34 weeks' gestation. Corticosteroid therapy may be used to accelerate lung maturity, and delivery should occur after amniocentesis documents a satisfactory lung status.

For patients with stage IB or early IIA disease, radical hysterectomy and bilateral pelvic lymphadenectomy with preservation of the ovaries provide effective treatment with acceptably low morbidity. Prior to 20 weeks, the operation is usually performed with the fetus in situ, but thereafter the uterus should first be evacuated before hysterectomy.

For more advanced disease, radiation therapy is the treatment of choice. In the first trimester, it is usual to start with external irradiation and anticipate spontaneous abortion. The pregnancy often aborts, before 4000 cGy of external radiation has been given. If this does not occur by the end of the external therapy, uterine curettage should be performed, followed 1 week later by intracavitary therapy. In the second trimester, treatment is the same as in the first trimester until 20 weeks. Thereafter, hysterectomy should be performed before radiation therapy because of the likely delay in spontaneous abortion and the teratogenic risks of the radiation. In the third trimester, delivery by classic cesarean section should be performed prior to beginning radiation therapy.

Invasive adenocarcinomas, even those with minimal invasion, should be treated as frankly invasive cancers.

### PROGNOSIS

The overall prognosis for pregnant women with cervical cancer evaluated as a group is similar to that for nonpregnant women; however, when survival is evaluated by stage of disease, pregnancy seems to have an unfavorable effect on prognosis for more advanced stages. Thus, the favorable overall prognosis for pregnant patients is related to the greater proportion of those with stage I disease, in whom the survival is similar to that of nonpregnant patients.[173] Clinical stage is the most important determinant of prognosis, and gestational age does not influence prognosis when corrected for stage of disease. Vaginal delivery, although not recommended for frankly invasive disease because of the risks of hemorrhage and infection, has not been shown to influence prognosis adversely.

## SUGGESTIONS FOR ADDITIONAL READING

Boone CW, Kelloff GJ, Steele VE. Natural history of intraepithelial neoplasia in humans with implications for cancer chemoprevention strategy. Cancer Res 1992;52:1651–9. *An excellent review.*

Cervical Cancer. NIH Consensus Statement 1996 Apr 1–3;14(1):1–38. *Assessment of current screening, prevention and treatment modalities.*

J Natl Cancer Inst Monogr, 1996, vol 21. *Series of articles discussing cervical cancer topics ranging from HPV vaccines to value of neoadjuvant chemotherapy.*

Koutsky LA, Holmes KK, Critchlow CW, et al. A cohort study of the risk of cervical intraepithelial neoplasia grade 2 or 3 in relation to papillomavirus infection. N Engl J Med 1992;327:1272–8. *A good study supporting an etiologic role for HPV infection.*

Kurman RJ, Henson DE, Herbst AL, et al. Interim guidelines for management of abnormal cervical cytology: the 1992 National Cancer Institute workshop. JAMA 1994;271:23:1866–69. *Provides guidelines for management of abnormal Pap smears.*

Marcial VA, Marcial LV. Radiation therapy of cervical cancer. New developments. Cancer 1993;71:4 Suppl:1438–45.

Park RC, Thigpen JT. Chemotherapy in advanced and recurrent cervical cancer—a review. Cancer 1993;71:Suppl 4:1446–50. *An excellent review.*

Zemlickis D, Lishner M, Degendorfer P, et al. Maternal and fetal outcome after invasive cervical cancer in pregnancy. J Clin Oncol 1991;9:1956–61. *This study suggests that pregnancy leads to an earlier diagnosis of cervical cancer because of regular, pregnancy-associated obstetric examinations. Perspective on the cost-benefit of colposcopy in the evaluation of dyskaryotic cervical smears.*

## REFERENCES

1. Estimated New Cancer Cases and Deaths by Sex for All Sites, United States, 1998, American Cancer Society-Cancer Facts and Figures 1998: Graphical Data. (see http://www.cancer.org/statistics/cff98/graphicaldata.html#aacdrf.) Accessed September 19, 1998.
2. Greenlee RT, Murray T, Bolden S, Wingo PA. Cancer statistics 2000. CA Cancer J Clin 2000;50:7–33.
3. FIGO, Federation Internationale de Gynecologie et d'Obstetrique. Annual report on the results of treatment in gynaecological cancer. J Epidemiol Biostat 1998;3:1:19.
4. Keighley E. Carcinoma of the cervix among prostitutes in a women's prison. Br J Vener Dis 1968;44:254.
5. Taylor RS, Carroll BE, Lloyd JW. Mortality of women in three Catholic religious orders with special references to cancer. Cancer 1959;12:1207.
6. Brinton LA, Tashima KT, Lehman HF, et al. Epidemiology of cervical cancer by cell type. Cancer Res 1987;47:1706–11.
7. Fenoglio CM. Etiologic factors in cervical neoplasia. Semin Oncol 1982;9:349–72.
8. Harris RW, Brinton LA, Cowdell RH, et al. Characteristics of women with dysplasia or carcinoma in situ of the cervix uteri. Br J Cancer 1980;42:359–69.
9. Meisels A, Fortin R, Roy M. Condylomatous lesions of the cervix II. Cytologic, colposcopic and histopathologic study. Acta Cytol 1977;21:379–90.
10. Durst M, Gissmann L, Ikenberg H, zur Hausen H. A papillomavirus DNA from a cervical carcinoma and its prevalence in cancer biopsy samples from different geographic regions. Proc Natl Acad Sci U S A 1983;80:3812–5.
11. Schwartz E, Freeze UK, Gissmann L, et al. Structure and transcription of human papillomavirus sequences in cervical carcinoma cells. Nature 1985;314:111.
12. Smotkin D, Wettstein FO. Transcription of human papillomavirus type 16 early genes in a cervical cancer and a cancer-derived cell line and identification of the E7 protein. Proc Natl Acad Sci U S A 1986;83:4680–4.
13. Koutsky LA, Holmes KK, Critchlow CW, et al. A cohort study of the risk of cervical intraepithelial neoplasia grade 2 or 3 in relation to papillomavirus infection. N Engl J Med 1992;327:1272.
14. Bosch FX, Manos MM, Munoz N, et al. Prevalence of human papillomavirus in cervical cancer: a worldwide perspective, International Biological Study on Cervical Cancer (IBSCC) Study Group. J Natl Cancer Inst 1995;87:796–802.
15. Chichareon S, Herrero R, Munoz N, et al. Risk factors for cervical cancer in Thailand: a case-control study. J Natl Cancer Inst 1998;90:50–6.
16. Ngelangel C, Munoz N, Bosch FX, et al. Causes of cervical cancer in the Philippines: a case-control study. J Natl Cancer Inst 1998;90:43–49.
17. Schiffman MH, Bauer HM, Hoover RN, et al. Epidemiologic evidence showing that human papillomavirus infection causes most cervical intraepithelial neoplasia. J Natl Cancer Inst 1993;85:958–64.
18. Lehtinen M, Dillner J, Knekt P, et al. Serologically diagnosed infection with human papillomavirus type 16 and risk for subsequent development of cervical carcinoma: nested case-control study. Br Med J 1996;312:537–9.
19. Valente PT, Hanjani P. Endocervical neoplasia in long-term users of oral contraceptives: clinical and pathologic observations. Obstet Gynecol 1986;67:695–704.
20. Prookopczyk B, Cox JE, Hoffmann D, Waggoner SE. Identification of tobacco-specific carcinogen in the cervical mucus of smokers and nonsmokers. J Natl Cancer Inst 1997;89:868–73.
21. Ali S, Astley SB, Sheldon TA, et al. Detection and measurement of DNA adducts in the cervix of smokers and non-smokers. Int J Gynaecol Cancer 1994;4:188.
22. Simons AM, Phillips DH, Coleman DV. Damage to DNA in cervical epithelium related to smoking tobacco. Br Med J 1993;306:1444–8.
23. Szarewski A, Jarvis MJ, Sasieni P, et al. Effect of smoking cessation on cervical lesion size. Lancet 1996;347:941–3.
24. Palan PR, Mikhail MS, Basu J, Romney SL. Beta-carotene levels in exfoliated cervicovaginal epithelial cells in cervical intraepithelial neoplasia and cervical cancer. Am J Obstet Gynecol 1992;167:1899–903.
25. Manetta A, Schubert T, Champman J, et al. Beta-carotene treatment of cervical intraepithelial neoplasia: a phase II study. Cancer Epidemiol Biomarkers Prev 1996;5:929–32.
26. Romney SL, Ho GY, Palan PR, et al. Effects of beta-carotene and other factors on outcome of cervical dysplasia and human papillomavirus infection. Gynecol Oncol 1997;65:483–92.
27. Butterworth CE Jr, Hatch KD, Macaluso M, et al. Folate deficiency and cervical dysplasia. JAMA 1992;267:528–33.
28. Coppleson M. Colposcopy. Springfield, Ill.: Charles C Thomas, 1971.
29. Cullen AP, Reid R, Campion M, Lorincz AT. Analysis of the physical state of different human papillomavirus DNAs in intraepithelial and invasive cervical neoplasm. J Virol 1991;65:606–12.
30. Das BC, Sharma JK, Gopalakrishna V, Luthra UK. Analysis by polymerase chain reaction of the physical state of human papillomavirus type 16 in cervical preneoplastic and neoplastic lesions. J Gen Virol 1992;73:2327–36.
31. Phelps WC, Yee CL, Munger K, Howley PM. The human papillomavirus type 16 E7 gene encodes transactivation and transforming functions similar to those of adenovirus E1A. Cell 1988;53:539–47.
32. Chellappan S, Kraus VB, Kroger B, et al. Adenovirus E1A, simian virus 40 tumor antigen, and human papillomavirus E7 protein share the capacity to disrupt the interaction between the transcription factor E2F and the retinoblastoma gene product. Proc Natl Acad Sci U S A 1992;89:4549–53.
33. Werness BA, Levine AJ, Howley PM. Association of human papillomavirus types 16 and 18 E6 proteins with p53. Science 1990;248:76–9.
34. Scheffner M, Werness BA, Huibregtse JM, et al. The E6 oncoprotein encoded by human papillomavirus types 16 and 18 promotes the degradation of p53. Cell 1990;63:1129–36.
35. Scheffner M, Huibregtse JM, Vierstra RD, Howley PM. The HPV-16 and E6-AP complex functions as a ubiquitin-protein ligase in the ubiquitination of p53. Cell 1993;75:495–505.
36. Kolstad P, Klem V. Long-term followup of 1121 cases of carcinoma in situ. Obstet Gynecol 1976;48:125–9.
37. Barron BA, Cahill MC, Richart RM. A statistical model of the natural history of cervical neoplastic disease: the duration of carcinoma in situ. Gynecol Oncol 1978;6:196–205.
38. Krebs HB, Schneider V, Hurt WG, Goplerud DR. Genital condylomas

in immunosuppressed women: a therapeutic challenge. South Med J 1986;79:183–7.

39. Porreco R, Penn I, Droegemueller W, et al. Gynecologic malignancies in immunosuppressed organ homograft recipients. Obstet Gynecol 1975;45:359–64.

40. Sun X, Kuhn L, Ellerbrock TV, Chiasson MA, et al. Human papillomavirus infection in women infected with the human immunodeficiency virus. N Engl J Med 1997;337:1343–9.

41. Mandelblatt JS, Fahs M, Garibaldi K, et al. Association between HIV infection and cervical neoplasia: implications for clinical care of women at risk for both conditions. AIDS 1992;6:173–8.

42. Klevens MR, Fleming PL, Mays MA, Frey R. Characteristics of women with AIDS and invasive cancer. Obstet Gynecol 1996;88:169–73.

43. Maiman M, Fruchter RG, Clark M, et al. Cervical cancer as an AIDS-defining illness. Obstet Gynecol 1997;89:76–80.

44. Plentl AA. Lymphatic system of the female genitalia. Philadelphia: WB Saunders, 1971:85.

45. Walton RJ. Cervical cancer screening programs. Can Med Assoc J 1982;127:953.

46. Parkin DM, Laara E, Muir CS. Estimates of the worldwide frequency of sixteen major cancers in 1980. Int J Cancer 1988;41:184–97.

47. 20-year trends in cancer death rates per 100,000 population 1972–1974 to 1992–1994, American Cancer Society—cancer facts and figures 1998: graphical data. (see http://www.cancer.org/statistics/cff98/graphicaldata.html#aacdrf). Accessed September 19, 1998.

48. Trends in 5-year relative survival rates by race and year of diagnosis, United States, 1960–1993, American Cancer Society—cancer facts and figures 1998: graphical data. (see http://www.cancer.org/statistics/cff98/graphicaldata.html#aacdrf). Accessed September 19, 1998.

49. Mandelblatt J, Andrews H, Kerner J, et al. Determinants of late stage diagnosis of breast and cervical cancer: the impact of age, race, social class, and hospital type. Am J Public Health 1991;81:646–9.

50. Boon ME, de Graaf Guilloud JC, Kok LP, et al. Efficacy of screening for cervical squamous and adenocarcinoma. Cancer 1987;59:862–6.

51. Koss LG. Cervical (Pap) smear. New directions. Cancer 1993;71:1406–12.

52. Koss LG. The Papanicolaou test for cervical cancer detection. A triumph and a tragedy. JAMA 1989;261:737–43.

53. Cervical cancer. NIH Consensus Statement 1996;14:1:1–38.

54. Kivlahan C, Ingram E. Papanicolaou smears without endocervical cells. Are they inadequate? Acta Cytol 1986;30:258–60.

55. Bearman DM, MacMillan JP, Creasman WT. Papanicolaou smear history of patients developing cervical cancer: an assessment of screening protocols. Obstet Gynecol 1987;69:151–5.

56. Anderson GH, Benedet JL, LeRiche JC, et al. Invasive cancer of the cervix in British Columbia: a review of the demography and screening histories of 437 cases seen from 1985–1988. Obstet Gynecol 1992;80:1–4.

57. The 1988 Bethesda System for reporting cervical/vaginal cytological diagnoses. National Cancer Institute workshop. JAMA 1989;262:931–4.

58. Wright TC, Sun XW, Koulos J. Comparison of management algorithms for the evaluation of women with low-grade cytologic abnormalities. Obstet Gynecol 1995;85:202–10.

59. Duska LR, Flynn CF, Chen A, et al. Clinical evaluation of atypical glandular cells of undetermined significance on cervical cytology. Obstet Gynecol 1998;91:278–82.

60. Goff BA, Atanasoff P, Brown E, et al. Endocervical glandular atypia in Papanicolaou smears. Obstet Gynecol 1992;79:101–4.

61. Kennedy AW, Salmieri SS, Wirth SL, et al. Results of the clinical evaluation of atypical glandular cells of undetermined significance (AGCUS) detected on cervical cytology screening. Gynecol Oncol 1996;63:14–8.

62. Kurman RJ, Malkasian GD Jr, Sedlis A, et al. From Papanicolaou to Bethesda: the rationale for a new cervical cytologic classification. Obstet Gynecol 1991;77:779–82.

63. Kurman RJ, Henson DE, Herbst AL, et al. Interim guidelines for management of abnormal cervical cytology. JAMA 1994;271:1866–9.

64. Wright TL, Kurman RJ, Ferenczy A. Precancerous lesions of the cervix. In: Kurman RJ, ed. Blaustein's pathology of the female genital tract. New York: Springer-Verlag, 1987:177.

65. Schantz A, Thormann L. Cyrosurgery for dysplasia of the uterine ectocervix. A randomized study of the efficacy of the single- and double-freeze techniques. Acta Obstet Gynecol Scand 1984;63:417–20.

66. Ferenczy A. Comparison of cryo- and carbon dioxide laser therapy for cervical intraepithelial neoplasia. Obstet Gynecol 1985;66:793–8.

67. Ahlgren M, Ingemarsson I, Lindberg LG, Nordqvist RB. Conization as treatment of carcinoma in situ of the uterine cervix. Obstet Gynecol 1975;46:135–9.

68. Lapaquette TK, Dinh TV, Hannigan EV, et al. Management of patients with positive margins after cervical conization. Obstet Gynecol 1993;82:440–3.

69. Monk A, Pushkin SF, Nelson AL, Gunning JE. Conservative management of options for patients with dysplasia involving endocervical margins of cervical cone biopsy specimens. Am J Obstet Gynecol 1996;174:1695–9.

70. Howe DT, Vincenti AC. Is large loop excision of the transformation zone (LLETZ) more accurate than colposcopically directed punch biopsy in the diagnosis of cervical intraepithelial neoplasia? Br J Obstet Gynecol 1991;98:588–91.

71. Keijser KG, Kenemans P, van der Zanden, et al. Diathermy loop excision in the management of cervical intraepithelial neoplasia: diagnosis and treatment in one procedure. Am J Obstet Gynecol 1992;166:1281–7.

72. Santos C, Galdos R, Alvarez M, et al. One-session management of cervical intraepithelial neoplasia: a solution for developing countries. Gynecol Oncol 1996;61:11–5.

73. Creasman WT. New gynecologic cancer staging. Gynecol Oncol 1995;58:157–8.

74. Lindell LK, Anderson B. Routine pretreatment evaluation of patients with gynecologic cancer. Obstet Gynecol 1987;69:242–6.

75. Matsukuma K, Tsukmoto N, Matsuyama T, et al. Preoperative CT study of lymph nodes in cervical cancer—its correlation with histological findings. Gynecol Oncol 1989;33:168–71.

76. Camilien L, Gordon D, Fruchter RG, et al. Predictive value of computerized tomography in the presurgical evaluation of primary carcinoma of the cervix. Obstet Gynecol 1988;30:209–15.

77. King LA, Talledo OE, Gallup DG, et al. Computed tomography in evaluation of gynecologic malignancies: a retrospective analysis. Am J Obstet Gynecol 1986;155:960–4.

78. Yu KK, Hricak H, Subak LL, et al. Preoperative staging of cervical carcinoma: phased array coil fast spin-echo versus body coil spin-echo T2-weighted MR imaging. AJR AM J Roentgenol 1998;171:707–11.

79. Hricak H, Powell CB, Yu KK, et al. Invasive cervical carcinoma: role of MR imaging in pretreatment work-up—cost minimization and diagnostic efficacy analysis. Radiology 1996;198:403–9.

80. Van Vierzen PB, Massuger LF, Ruys SH, Barentsz JO. Fast dynamic contrast enhanced MR imaging of cervical carcinoma. Clin Radiol 1998;53:183–92.

81. Van Nagell JR Jr, Rodick JW Jr, Lowin DM. The staging of cervical cancer: inevitable discrepancies between clinical staging and pathologic findings. Am J Obstet Gynecol 1971;110:973–8.

82. Jones HW III. In: Ballon SC, ed. Gynecologic oncology: controversies in cancer treatment. Boston: GK Hall Medical Publishers, 1981:167.

83. LaPolla JP, Schlaerth JB, Gaddis, O Morrow CP. The influence of surgical staging on the evaluation and treatment of patients with cervical carcinoma. Gynecol Oncol 1986;24:194–206.

84. Fortier KJ, Clarke-Pearson DL, Creasman WT, Johnston WW. Fine-needle aspiration in gynecology: evaluation of extrapelvic lesions in patients with gynecologic malignancy. Obstet Gynecol 1985;65:67–72.

85. Berman ML, Lagasse LD, Watring WG, et al. The operative evaluation of patients with cervical carcinoma by an extraperitoneal approach. Obstet Gynecol 1977;50:658–64.

86. Tanaka Y, Sawada S, Murata T. Relationship between lymph node metastases and prognosis in patients irradiated postoperatively for carcinoma of the uterine cervix. Acta Radiol 1984;23:455–9.

87. Samlal RAK, van der Valden J, Ten Kate FJW, et al. Surgical pathologic factors that predict recurrence in stage IB and IIA cervical carcinoma patients with negative pelvic lymph nodes. Cancer 1997;80:1234–40.

88. Delgado G, Bundy B, Zaino R, et al. Prospective surgical-pathological study of disease-free interval in patients with stage IB squamous cell carcinoma of the cervix: a Gynecologic Oncology Group study. Gynecol Oncol 1990;38:352–7.

89. Estape RE, Angioli R, Madrigal M, et al. Close vaginal margins as a prognostic factor after radical hysterectomy. Gynecol Oncol 1998;68:229–32.

90. Boyce J, Fruchter RG, Nicastri AG, et al. Prognostic factors in stage I carcinoma of the cervix. Gynecol Oncol 1981;12:154–65.

91. Burke TW, Hoskins WJ, Heller PB, et al. Clinical patterns of tumor recurrence after radical hysterectomy in stage IB cervical carcinoma. Obstet Gynecol 1987;69:382–5.

92. Piver MS, Chung WS. Prognostic significance of cervical lesion size and pelvic node metastases in cervical carcinoma. Obstet Gynecol 1975;46:507–10.

93. Perez CA, Grigsby PW, Chao KS, et al. Tumor size, irradiation dose, and long-term outcome of carcinoma of uterine cervix. Int J Radiat Oncol Biol Phys 1998;41:307–17.

94. Reagan JW, Ng ABP. The cellular manifestations of uterine carcinogenesis. In: Norris HJ, Hertig AT, Abell MR, eds. The uterus. Baltimore: Williams and Wilkins, 1973.

95. Finck FM, Denk M. Cervical carcinoma: relationship between histology and survival following radiation therapy. Obstet Gynecol 1970;35:339–43.

96. Wang PH, Liu YC, Lai CR, et al. Small cell carcinoma of the cervix: analysis of clinical and pathological findings. Eur J Gynaecol Oncol 1998;19:189–92.

97. Sheets EE, Berman ML, Hrountas CK, et al. Surgically treated, early-stage neuroendocrine small-cell cervical carcinoma. Obstet Gynecol 1988;71:10–14.

98. Perez CA, Zivnuska F, Askin F, et al. Prognostic significance of endometrial extension from primary carcinoma of the uterine cervix. Cancer 1975;35:1493–504.

99. Durrance FY, Fletcher GH, Rutledge FN. Analysis of central recurrent disease in stages I and II squamous cell carcinomas of the cervix on intact uterus. Am J Roentgenol Radium Ther Nucl Med 1969;106:831–8.

100. Tjalma W, De Cuyper E, Weyler J, et al. Expression of *bcl*-2 in invasive and in situ carcinoma of the uterine cervix. Am J Obstet Gynecol 1998;178:113–7.

101. Riou GF, Bourhis J, Le MG. The c-*myc* proto-oncogene in invasive carcinomas of the uterine cervix: clinical relevance of overexpression in early stages of the cancer. Anticancer Res 1990;10:1225–31.

102. Hale RJ, Buckley CH, Fox H, et al. Prognostic value of c-*erb*B-2 expression in uterine cervical carcinoma. J Clin Pathol 1992;45:594–6.

103. Kim JW, Kim HS, Kim IK, et al. Transforming growth factor-beta 1 induces apotosis through down-regulation of c-*myc* gene and overexpression of p27Kipl protein in cervical carcinoma. Gynecol Oncol 1998;69:230–6.

104. Van Dam PA, Lowe DG, Watson JV, et al. Multiparameter flow-cytometric quantitation of epidermal growth factor receptor and c-*erb*B-2 oncoprotein in normal and neoplastic tissues of the female genital tract. Gynecol Oncol 1991;42:256–64.

105. Pinion SB, Kennedy JH, Miller RW. Oncogene expression in cervical intraepithelial neoplasia and invasive cancer of the cervix. Lancet 1991;337:819–20.

106. Sagae S, Kuzumaki N, Hisada T, et al. *Ras* oncogene expression and prognosis of invasive squamous cell carcinomas of the uterine cervix. Cancer 1989;63:1577–82.

107. Sevin BU, Nadji M, Averette HE, et al. Microinvasive carcinoma of the cervix. Cancer 1992;63:2121–8.

108. Buckley SL, Tritz DM, Van Le L, et al. Lymph node metastases and prognosis in patients with stage IA2 cervical cancer. Gynecol Oncol 1996;63:4–9.

109. Greer BE, Figge DC, Tamimi HK, et al. Stage IA2 of squamous carcinoma of the cervix: difficult diagnosis and therapeutic dilemma. Am J Obstet Gynecol 1990;162:1406–9.

110. Morris M, Mitchell MF, Silva EG, et al. Cervical conization as definitive therapy for early invasive squamous carcinoma of the cervix. Gynecol Oncol 1993;51:193–6.

111. Tseng CJ, Horng SG, Soong YK, et al. Conservative conization for microinvasive carcinoma of the cervix. Am J Obstet Gynecol 1997;176:1009–10.

112. Roman LD, Felix JC, Muderspach LI, et al. Risk of residual invasive disease in women with microinvasive squamous cancer in a conization specimen. Obstet Gynecol 1997;90:759–64.

113. Van Nagell JR Jr, Greenwell N, Powell DF, et al. Microinvasive carcinoma of the cervix. Am J Obstet Gynecol 1983;145:981–91.

114. Creasman WT, Zaino RJ, Major FJ, et al. Early invasive carcinoma of the cervix (3 to 5 mm invasion): risk factors and prognosis. Am J Obstet Gynecol 1998;178:62–5.

115. Lin HH, Cheng WF, Chan KW, et al. Risk factors for recurrence in patients with stage IB, IIA, and IIB cervical carcinoma after radical hysterectomy and postoperative pelvic irradiation. Obstet Gynecol 1996;88:274–9.

116. Sevin BU, Nadji M, Lampe B, et al. Prognostic factors of early stage cervical cancer treated by radical hysterectomy. Cancer 1995;76:1978–86.

117. Finan MA, DeCesare S, Fiorica JV, et al. Radical hysterectomy for stage IB1 vs IB2 carcinoma of the cervix: does the new staging system predict morbidity and survival? Gynecol Oncol 1996;62:139–47.

118. Parsons L. An atlas of pelvic operations. 2nd ed. Philadelphia: WB Saunders, 1968.

119. Shingleton HM. Cancer of cervix. New York: Churchill Livingstone, 1987.

120. Zanolla R, Monzeglio C, Campo B, et al. Bladder and urethral dysfunction after radical abdominal hysterectomy: rahabilitative treatment. J Surg Oncol 1985;28:190–4.

121. Seski JC, Diokno AC. Bladder dysfunction after radical abdominal hysterectomy. Am J Obstet Gynecol 1977;128:643–51.

122. Tabata M, Ichinoe K, Sakuragi N, et al. Incidence of ovarian metastasis in patients with cancer of the uterine cervix. Gynecol Oncol 1987;28:255–61.

123. Ploch E. Hormonal replacement in patients after cervical cancer treatment. Gynecol Oncol 1987;26:169–77.

124. Feeney DD, Moore DH, Look KY, et al. The fate of the ovaries after radical hysterectomy and ovarian transposition. Gynecol Oncol 1995;56:3–7.

125. Marcial VA, Marcial LV. Radiation therapy of cervical cancer. New developments. Cancer 1993;71:1438–45.

126. Stitt JA. High dose rate intracavitary brachytherapy for gynecologic malignancies. Oncology 1992;6:59–70.

127. Hamberger AD, Fletcher GH, Wharton JT. Results of treatment of early stage I carcinoma of the uterine cervix with intracavitary radium alone. Cancer 1978;41:980–5.

128. Syed AMN. In: Nori D, eds. Radiation therapy of gynecologic cancers. New York: Alan R. Liss, 1987.

129. Rotman M, Pajak TF, Choi K, et al. Prophylactic extended-field irradiation of para-aortic lymph nodes in stage IIB and bulky IB and IIA cervical carcinomas. Ten year treatment results of RTOG 79-20. JAMA 1995;274:387–93.

130. Perez CA, Grigsby PW, Castro-Vita H, Lockett MA. Carcinoma of the uterine cervix. I. Impact of prolongation of treatment time and timing of brachytherapy on outcome of radiation therapy. Int J Radiat Oncol Biol Phys 1995;32:1275–88.

131. Perez CA, Breaux S, Bedwinek JM, et al. Radiation therapy alone in the treatment of carcinoma of the uterine cervix. II. Analysis of complications. Cancer 1984;54:235–46.

132. Hanks GE, Herring DF, Kramer S. Patterns of care outcome studies. Results of the national practice in cancer of the cervix. Cancer 1983;51:959–67.

133. Nelson AJ III, Fletcher GH, Wharton JT. Am J Roentgenol Radium Ther Nucl Med 1975;123:91–9.

134. Thoms WW, Eifel PJ, Smith TL, et al. Bulky endocervical carcinoma: a 23-year experience. Int J Radiat Oncol Biol Phys 1992;23:491–9.

135. Eifel PJ, Thomas WW Jr, Smith TL, et al. The relationship between brachytherapy dose and outcome in patients with bulky endocervical tumors treated with radiation dose. Int J Radiat Oncol Biol Phys 1994;28:113–8.

135a. Keys HM, Bundy BN, Stehman FB, et al. Cisplatin, radiation, and adjuvant hysterectomy compared with radiation and adjuvant hysterectomy for bulky stage IB cervical carcinoma. N Engl J Med 1999;340:1154–61.

136. Delgado G, Bundy BN, Fowler WC Jr, et al. A prospective surgical pathological study of stage I squamous carcinoma of the cervix: a Gynecologic Oncology Group study. Gynecol Oncol 1989;35:314–20.

137. Monk BJ, Cha DS, Walker JL, et al. Extent of disease as an indication for pelvic radiation following radical hysterectomy and bilateral pelvic lymph node dissection in the treatment of stage IB and IIA cervical carcinoma. Gynecol Oncol 1994;54:4–9.

138. Kinney WK, Alvarez RD, Reid GC, et al. Value of adjuvant whole-pelvis irradiation after Wertheim hysterectomy for early-stage squamous carcinoma of the cervix with pelvic nodal metastasis: a matched-control study. Gynecol Oncol 1989;34:258–62.

138a. Sedlis A, Bundy BN, Rotman MZ, et al. A randomized trial of pelvic radiation therapy versus no further therapy in selected patients with stage IB carcinoma of the cervix after radical hysterectomy and pelvic lymphadenectomy: a Gynecologic Oncology Group study. Gynecol Oncol 1999;73:177–83.

139. Sardi JE, Giaroli A, Sananes C, et al. Long-term follow-up of the first randomized trial using neoadjuvant chemotherapy in stage IB squamous carcinoma of the cervix: the final results. Gynecol Oncol 1997;67:61–9.

139a. Peters WA III, Liu PY, Barrett RJ, et al. Cisplatin and 5-fluorouracil plus radiation therapy are superior to radiation therapy as adjunctive in high-risk early-stage carcinoma of the cervix after radical hysterectomy and pelvic lymphadenectomy: report of a phase III intergroup study. (see http://cancertrials.nci.nih.gov/types/cervical/announcement/sumref.html) J Clin Oncol 2000. in press.

140. Shueng PW, Hsu WL, Jen YM, et al. Neoadjuvant chemotherapy followed by radiotherapy should not be a standard approach for locally advanced cervical cancer. Int J Radiat Oncol Biol Phys 1998;40:889–96.

141. Berman ML, Lagasse LD, Ballon SC, et al. Modification of radiation therapy following operative evaluation of patients with cervical carcinoma. Gynecol Oncol 1978;6:328–32.

142. Fletcher GH, Rutledge FN. Extended field technique in the management of the cancers of the uterine cervix. Am J Roentgenol Radium Ther Nucl Med 1972;114:116–22.

143. Potish RA, Downey GO, Adcock LL, et al. The role of surgical debulking in cancer of the uterine cervix. Int J Radiat Oncol Biol Phys 1989;17:979–84.

144. Downey GO, Potish RA, Adcock LL, et al. Pretreatment surgical staging in cervical carcinoma: therapeutic efficacy of pelvic lymph node resection. Am J Obstet Gynecol 1989;160:1055–61.

145. Sundfor K, Trope CG, Hogbewrg T, et al. Radiotherapy and neoadjuvant chemotheapy for cervical carcinoma. A randomized multicenter study of sequential cisplatin and 5-fluorouracil and radiotherapy in advanced cervical carcinoma stage 3B and 4A. Cancer 1996;77:2371–8.

145a. Morris M, Eifel PJ, Lu J, et al. Pelvic radiation with concurrent chemotherapy compared with pelvic and para-aortic radiation for high-risk cervical cancer. N Engl J Med 1999;340:1137–43.

145b. Rose PG, Bundy BN, Watkins EB, et al. Concurrent cisplatin-based radiotherapy and chemotherapy for locally advanced cervical cancer. N Engl J Med 1999;340:1144–53.

145c. Whitney CW, Sause W, Bundy BN, et al. Randomized comparison of fluorouracil plus cisplatin versus hydroxyurea as an adjunct to radiation therapy in stage IIB–IVA carcinoma of the cervix with negative para-aortic lymph nodes: a Gynecologic Oncology Group and Southwest Oncology Group study. J Clin Oncol 1999;17:1339–48.

146. Thigpen T, Shingleton H, Homesley H, et al. *Cis*-platinum in treatment of advanced or recurrent squamous cell carcinoma of the cervix: a phase II study of the Gynecologic Oncology Group. Cancer 1981;48:899–903.

147. Park RC, Thigpen JT. Chemotherapy in advanced and recurrent cervical cancer: a review. Cancer 1993;71:1448.

148. Alberts DS, Garcia D, Mason-Liddil N. Cisplatin in advanced cancer of the cervix: an update. Semin Oncol 1991;18:11–24.

149. McGuire WP, Blessing JA, Moore D, et al. Paclitaxel has moderate activity in squamous cervix cancer: a Gynecologic Oncology Group study. J Clin Oncol 1996;14:792–5.

150. Long HJ III, Cross WG, Wieand HS, et al. Phase II trial of methotrexate, vinblastine, doxorubicin, and cisplatin in advanced/recurrent carcinoma of the uterine cervix and vagina. Gynecol Oncol 1995;57:235–9.

151. Omura GA, Blessing JA, Vaccarello L, et al. Randomized trial of cisplatin versus cisplatin plus mitolactol versus cisplatin plus ifosfamide in advanced squamous carcinoma of the cervix: a Gynecologic Oncology Group study. J Clin Oncol 1997;15:1:165–171.

152. Brader KR, Morris M, Levenback C, et al. Chemotherapy for cervical carcinoma: factors determining response and implications for clinical trial design. J Clin Oncol 1998;16:1879–84.

153. Morley GW. Pelvic exenteration and the treatment of recurrent carcinoma of the cervix. Semin Oncol 1982;9:331–40.

154. Roberts WS, Cavanagh D, Bryson SC, et al. Major morbidity after pelvic exenteration: a seven year experience. Obstet Gynecol 1987;69:617–21.

155. Durrance FY. Radiotherapy following simple hysterectomy in patients with stage I and II carcinoma of the cervix. Am J Roentgenol Radium Ther Nucl Med 1968;102:165–9.

156. Perkins PL, Chu AM, Jose B, et al. Posthysterectomy megavoltage irradiation in the treatment of cervical carcinoma. Gynecol Oncol 1984;17:340–8.

157. Chapman JA, Mannel RS, DiSaia PJ, et al. Surgical treatment of unexpected invasive cervical cancer found at total hysterectomy. Obstet Gynecol 1995;80:931–4.

158. Kinney WK, Egorshin EV, Ballard DJ, Podratz KC. Long term survival and sequelae after surgical management of invasive cervical carcinoma diagnosed at the time of simple hysterectomy. Gynecol Oncol 1992;44:24–7.

159. Brand E, Berek JS, Hacker NF. Controversies in the management of cervical adenocarcinoma. Obstet Gynecol 1988;71:261–9.

160. Melnick S, Cole P, Anderson D, et al. Rates and risks of diethylstilbestrol-related clear cell adenocarcinoma of the vagina and cervix. An update. N Engl J Med 1987;316:514–6.

161. Herbst AL, Anderson D. Clear cell adenocarcinoma of the vagina and cervix secondary to intrauterine exposure to diethylstilbestrol. Semin Surg Oncol 1990;6:343–6.

162. Hatch EE, Palmer JR, Titus-Ernstoff L, et al. Cancer risk in women exposed to diethylstilbestrol in utero. JAMA 1998;280:630–4.

163. Smotkin D, Berek JS, Fu YS, et al. Human papillomavirus deoxyribonucleic acid in adenocarcinoma and adenosquamous carcinoma of the uterine cervix. Obstet Gynecol 1986;68:241–4.

164. Wilczynski SP, Bergen S, Walker J, et al. Human papillomaviruses and cervical cancer: analysis with different viral types. Hum Pathol 1988;19:697–704.

165. Johnson TL, Kim W, Plieth DA, Sarkar FH. Detection of HPV 16/18 DNA in cervical adenocarcinoma using polymerase chain reaction (PCR) methodology. Mod Pathol 1992;5:35–40.

166. Goldstein NS, Mani A. The status and distance of cone biopsy margins as a predictor of excision adequacy for endocervical adenocarcinoma in situ. Am J Clin Pathol 1998;109:727–32.

167. Denehy TR, Gregori CA, Breen JL. Endocervical curettage, cone margins, and residual adenocarcinoma in situ of the cervix. Obstet Gynecol 1997;90:1–6.

168. Gallup DG, Harper RH, Stock RJ. Poor prognosis in patients with adenosquamous cell carcinoma of the cervix. Obstet Gynecol 1985;65:416–22.

169. Berek JS, Castaldo TW, Hacker NF, et al. Adenocarcinoma of the uterine cervix. Cancer 1981;48:2734–41.

170. Hacker NF, Berek JS, Lagasse LD, et al. Carcinoma of the cervix associated with pregnancy. Obstet Gynecol 1982;59:735–46.

171. Choo YC, Chan OLY, Ma HK. Colposcopy in microinvasive carcinoma of the cervix: an enigman of diagnosis. Br J Obstet Gynaecol 1984;92:1156.

172. Hannigan EV, Whitehouse HH, Atkinson WD, Becker SV. Cone biopsy during pregnancy. Obstet Gynecol 1982;60:450–5.

173. Lee RB, Neglia W, Park RC. Cervical carcinoma in pregnancy. Obstet Gynecol 1981;58:584–9.

# CHAPTER 57

# UTERUS

• MICHAEL L. BERMAN • MICHAEL T. McHALE

The endometrium is the most common site of invasive cancer in the female genital tract and the fourth most frequent site of malignancy in women. During 2000, an estimated 36,100 new cases and 6500 deaths will be attributed to endometrial cancer.[1] Although the incidence of endometrial cancer declined slightly during the late 1980s, since the mid-1990s it has remained fairly constant. Although the incidence has remained stable, the number of annual deaths has almost doubled during that period. The cause of this alarming statistic is probably multifactorial; however, it justifies re-evaluating both the pathogenesis and management of this neoplasm.

Characteristically, endometrial cancer is detected early in the course of disease, with at least 75% of new cases confined to the uterus on clinical assessment.[2] The frequency of early cancer detection is high because signs of abnormal genital bleeding are usually seen while the cancer is confined to the uterine corpus. Paradoxically, because survival statistics suggest high curability and because therapeutic measures often involve commonly performed operative procedures, many patients with endometrial cancer are treated without the benefit of careful staging and consultation with physicians who are trained in the management of gynecologic malignancies. Because of a better understanding of the natural history of endometrial cancer and the risk factors that can necessitate modification of therapy, treatment should be initiated only after careful evaluation of the extent of disease and those factors that can place a patient at high risk of failure to respond to standard therapy.[3]

Carcinomas and sarcomas of the uterus are sufficiently different to justify separate discussions in this chapter.

## Carcinomas

### ETIOLOGY AND EPIDEMIOLOGY

Although the definitive cause of adenocarcinoma of the endometrium is unknown, studies suggest that at least two different mechanisms may be related to its pathogenesis.[4] In some individuals, it may develop spontaneously, arising in the presence of an atrophic endometrium, whereas in others it appears to be hormonally derived. Estrogen, either from endogenous sources or administered exogenously, can cause varying degrees of endometrial proliferation known as *simple* and *complex hyperplasia*. Because this finding often precedes or coexists with endometrial cancer, clinicians have long suspected that estrogens can cause this disorder. There appears to be a continuum of endometrial hyperplasias; in the most advanced state, referred to as *complex hyperplasia with atypia,* it is characterized by marked crowding and infolding of glands with severe cytologic atypia. This lesion can be confused with an early carcinoma. It is estimated that 10 to 30% of patients with complex hyperplasia, if untreated, will develop endometrial cancer within 10 years. Furthermore, approximately 20% of women with complex hyperplasia with atypia found on dilation and curettage have a coexisting well-differentiated endometrial cancer elsewhere in the uterine lining. Endometrial hyperplasia without cytologic atypia appears to be reversible in most instances when the source of estrogen is removed or when progestogens are administered cyclically or continuously. However, severely atypical complex hyperplasia is less responsive to hormonal manipulation, especially in postmenopausal women.

Evidence supporting a causal role for exogenous estrogens has been provided by several independent, retrospective, matched-control studies of women with endometrial cancer.[5-9] The risk of cancer developing appears to range from four to eight times that of women not taking exogenous estrogens. Increasing duration and higher doses of estrogen therapy have been associated with an even greater risk of cancer in some studies. Conversely, when daily estrogens are administered with at least 10 days of progestins each month, the increased risk of developing endometrial cancer can be eliminated. In addition to these analyses of risk factors, the observation that the incidence of endometrial cancer in white women paralleled patterns of exogenous estrogen intake in various communities supports the hypothesis that estrogens can cause endometrial cancer.[10] For example, between 1969 and 1973, the California Tumor Registry reported a 60% increase in the incidence of endometrial cancer in the San Francisco Bay Area. Prior to and during that interval, the use of exogenous estrogens in California and throughout the United States increased dramatically with the widespread recognition that estrogens retarded many signs and symptoms of the climacteric in women.[11] Interestingly, with the initial reports linking endometrial cancer to estrogen use, there was a decrease in the numbers of women using estrogens and a reduction in the dosage of estrogens used in many women who continued estrogen therapy. Data from the Kaiser Permanente System in Seattle, Washington, confirmed these trends while demonstrating a concurrent reduction in the incidence of endometrial cancer.[12] This downward trend in endometrial cancer incidence continued until the late 1980s but has remained constant since then. Paradoxically, cigarette smoking is associated with a lower risk of endometrial cancer, inversely related to duration of tobacco use and number of cigarettes smoked.[13]

In addition to the various population trends and retrospective analyses cited, clinicians have recognized for decades that conditions that predispose to hyperestrinism are frequently associated with endometrial cancer (Table 57–1). The risk associated with the various factors can be additive.[14] For example, obesity is a recognized risk factor for endome-

*Table 57–1.* **Conditions Associated with Hyperestrinism and Endometrial Cancer**

| Source and Mechanism of Estrogen Secretion | Condition |
|---|---|
| OVARY | OVARIAN NEOPLASM |
| Increased secretion of $E_1$ | Granulosa-theca cell tumor |
| Increased secretion of A with peripheral conversion to $E_1$ | Sertoli-Leydig cell tumor<br>Hilar cell tumor |
| Increased secretion of A with peripheral conversion to $E_1$ | Stromal hyperplasia (seen with ovarian neoplasm)<br>Mucinous tumors<br>Brenner's tumors<br>Krukenberg's tumors |
| Increased secretion of A with peripheral conversion to $E_1$ | Stromal hyperplasia without ovarian neoplasm (Stein-Leventhal syndrome) |
| ADRENAL | |
| More efficient peripheral conversion of A to $E_1$ | Obesity |
| Exogenous | |
| Direct effect of $E_1$ (which is 35 to 65% of conjugated estrogen) | Oral, vaginal, or injectable estrogens |

$E_1$, estrone; A, androstenedione.

trial cancer and is associated with increased levels of circulating estrogens when compared with those in age-matched thin women. In fact, obesity is one of the best-defined risk factors,[13] with a relative risk (RR) of 2 to 17.7, depending on the parameter chosen (e.g., Quetelet's index vs. weight) and its degree. The increased availability of unopposed peripheral estrogens and the lower concentration of sex hormone–binding globulin in these women can cause endometrial hyperplasia and cancer. Reports that have focused on anthropomorphic measurements in obese women have found that a higher upper body fat localization (android obesity) yields a greater risk for endometrial cancer than do other types of obese body habitus.[15] Diet may be an independent risk factor for endometrial cancer. Goodman and colleagues, in a case-control study, examined the association of diet, body size, and physical activity with the risk of endometrial cancer.[16] Their data suggested that women with a low body mass index and a diet low in plant and animal fats and high in carbohydrates are at a reduced risk for endometrial cancer. Additionally, micronutrients such as beta carotene may have a protective effect against endometrial cancer.[17]

Additional supporting evidence in animal studies includes induction of endometrial cancer with exogenous estrogens and blockage of methylcholanthrene-induced endometrial cancer by ovariectomy in rabbits.[18] Although a causal relationship between estrogens administered exogenously and endometrial cancer was controversial when first reported, the overwhelming body of evidence supports this association.

Clinical trials using tamoxifen in an effort to prevent or treat breast cancers have raised concerns about a possible increased risk of uterine cancer in these women. Tamoxifen exhibits both estrogenic and antiestrogenic properties, depending on the organ, animal, or cell line in question.[19, 20] In the human uterus, tamoxifen primarily exhibits an estrogenic

effect.[19] The Stockholm trial of adjuvant tamoxifen (40 mg daily) in postmenopausal women showed a significant increase (RR 6.4) in the number of new corpus cancers, mainly in women who were treated for more than 2 years.[21] Similarly, the National Surgical Adjuvant Breast and Bowel Project (NSABP) B-14 trial noted an increased risk of endometrial cancer in the tamoxifen-treated patients compared with controls (RR 7.5).[22] Although the risk of endometrial cancer increases following tamoxifen therapy for breast cancer, the net benefit markedly outweighs this risk.

MacDonald and Siiteri[14] postulated the "estrone hypothesis" to explain the association between estrogens and endometrial cancer, suggesting a permissive role of estrone unopposed by progestogens in the development of this malignancy. The constitutional characteristics of obesity, advanced age, and anovulation, which are seen commonly in endometrial cancer patients, are associated with increased extraglandular aromatization of androstenedione from the adrenal gland to estrone. Aromatization appears to occur primarily in adipose tissue and most efficiently in obese, elderly patients, accounting for the increased estrone levels in these individuals. Similarly, young patients with Stein-Leventhal syndrome, who also are at high risk to develop endometrial cancer, secrete increased amounts of androstenedione from the hyperplastic ovarian stroma or, in some instances, from the adrenal gland, providing more substrate to peripheral sites for conversion to estrone.

The pathogenesis for both endometrial hyperplasia and endometrial cancer remains uncertain. However, advances in molecular genetics have shown that the accumulation of genetic alterations may be responsible for the development of neoplasia.[23] Specifically, the identification and role of tumor-suppressor genes in solid tumors have been the focus of many investigations.[24, 25] One of the most common tumor-suppressor genes in human cancer is p53. The gene responsible for this protein is located on the short arm of chromosome 17. It has been hypothesized that this gene may play a role in carcinogenesis when it has been inactivated by a point mutation and loss of heterozygosity.[26, 27] Although p53 expression was first studied in colorectal cancer, it has been extensively examined in gynecologic malignancies, including endometrial cancer. Many investigators have demonstrated the presence of mutant p53 in endometrial cancer and the adverse prognostic impact of such a genetic alteration.[28–31] These studies suggest that alterations in the p53 gene may play an important role in tumorigenesis. Other alterations that have been identified and implicated in the development of endometrial cancer include alterations in the expression of the epidermal growth factor (EGF) receptor, overexpression of the HER-*2/neu* oncoprotein, and point mutations in the *ras* gene family.[32] Although a number of genetic alterations have been identified in patients with endometrial cancer, their roles remain unclear and are the focus of ongoing investigations.

## PATTERNS OF SPREAD

Typically, endometrial cancer disseminates by direct extension to adjacent structures, through the lymphatic system to regional and distant nodes, and infrequently by the hematogenous route to remote sites (Fig. 57–1). Although these

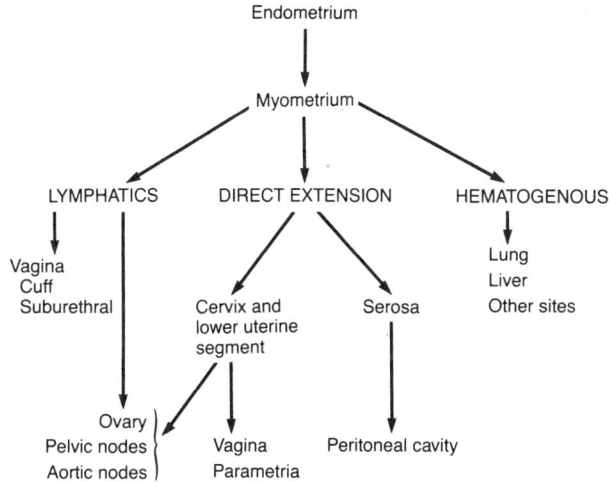

**Figure 57–1.** Patterns of spread of endometrial cancer.

cancers are frequently confined to the endometrium, the initial route of spread appears to be dependent on extension into the underlying myometrium. Most patients with disease outside the uterine corpus who undergo hysterectomy have myometrial penetration extending through at least one half of the thickness of the uterine wall. With increasing depth of myometrial penetration, there is a progressive increase in the incidence of lymph node metastases. In patients with cancer confined to the uterine corpus on clinical assessment, metastases to pelvic lymph nodes are found in up to one third of deeply invasive tumors but in less than 1% of noninvasive tumors.[33, 34] Since most endometrial cancers are confined to the endometrial cavity or are only superficially invasive, the overall risk of lymph node metastases in women with tumors confined to the uterine corpus on clinical assessment is only about 5 to 10%.[35]

Tumors that involve myometrium more extensively can extend to the serosal surface of the uterus. When this occurs, intra-abdominal carcinomatosis can develop by seeding of tumor throughout the peritoneal cavity, with involvement of omentum, liver, diaphragm, and other visceral surfaces in a pattern similar to that commonly seen with epithelial ovarian cancers. Such patients can present with ascites or bowel obstruction. Unusual histologic variants such as the serous papillary carcinoma and clear cell carcinoma of the endometrium metastasize via the peritoneal route much more often than do the other kinds of endometrial cancers. For these two subtypes, peritoneal spread is frequently seen even with more superficially invasive disease.

Lymphatics from the uterus follow the route of the ovarian and uterine blood vessels. Therefore, lymph node metastases can follow the uterine veins to the hypogastric, iliac, aortic, and precaval lymph nodes or can result from direct drainage into the aortic and precaval nodes via the lymphatics accompanying the ovarian vessels. Autopsy data suggest that periaortic nodes are the most frequent sites of metastases, which are often found in the absence of pelvic lymph node involvement.[36] Pelvic and periaortic lymphadenectomies performed in patients undergoing primary operation for cancer confined to the uterine corpus, however, have documented aortic lymph node involvement without positive pelvic lymph nodes in less than 2% of patients.[34] Conversely,

38% of patients with pelvic lymph node metastases also had periaortic metastases. Therefore, the most common route of initial lymphatic spread appears to be the pelvic lymph nodes, with secondary involvement of the periaortic nodes.

Local spread to the cervix reportedly occurs in 5 to 15% of women with endometrial cancer.[2] The biologic behavior of such tumors resembles that of primary cervical carcinoma, with an increased risk of lymph node metastases and extension to the vagina or parametrium. The overall frequency of pelvic lymph node metastases is reported to increase from 8.2% in tumors confined to the uterine fundus to 25.4% in tumors with cervical extension.[37]

The vagina also can be a site of metastases by lymphatic spread or possibly from seeding of the vaginal cuff at the time of hysterectomy. Evaluation of recurrences after hysterectomy in patients who had preoperative intracavitary radium showed the same risk of vaginal metastases in patients with no residual tumor as in those with residual cancer.[38] These data suggest that tumor implantation at operation is an infrequent source of vaginal spread of endometrial cancer and that a more likely origin of these metastases might be paracervical and paravaginal lymphatics. The occurrence of isolated vaginal metastases in the distal vagina also supports this hypothesis.

Involvement of the uterine isthmus or lower uterine segment, as determined by histologic evaluation of hysterectomy specimens, is associated with an increased risk of deep myometrial invasion, anaplasia, lymph node metastases and, hence, poorer survival. In fact, the risk of pelvic lymph node metastases with cervical isthmus tumors is approximately twice that of cancers confined to the corpus (16% vs. 8%).[34]

Ovarian metastases occur in approximately 5% of women with endometrial cancer. The most likely mechanism of ovarian involvement is via the lymphatics in the mesosalpinx and mesovarium. Because primary ovarian neoplasms often coexist with endometrial cancers, they can be confused with metastases from the uterus. Therefore, when cancer is also found in the ovaries, careful histologic evaluation is necessary to distinguish between coexisting and metastatic ovarian tumors. In some instances, this distinction cannot be made. The coexistence of a well-differentiated endometrial cancer and a stage I grade I ovarian endometrioid cancer of similar histologic appearance is associated with a good prognosis.

Involvement of distant sites, including lung, liver, and skeleton, occurs by the hematogenous route and is infrequent. The lungs are the most common sites of distant metastasis and are involved in 2 to 3% of cases, often concurrently with other sites.[39] Although poorly differentiated tumors represent less than 25% of endometrial cancer, 60% of patients with spread to these distant sites have anaplastic cancers.

## NATURAL HISTORY

**Classification.** The relative frequencies of the five histologic types of endometrial cancer in 542 women treated between 1942 and 1971 and reported by Ng and Reagan[40] are shown in Table 57–2. Squamous cell and clear cell tumors of the endometrium are rare and usually aggressive.

In the early 1980s, Hendrickson and colleagues[41] described another histologic subtype of adenocarcinoma whose

*Table 57–2.* **Classification of Endometrial Carcinomas**

| Histologic Type | Relative Frequency (%) |
|---|---|
| Adenocarcinoma | 67.1 |
| Adenoacanthoma | 20.3 |
| Adenosquamous carcinoma | 12.6 |
| Clear cell carcinoma | <1 |
| Squamous carcinoma | <1 |

morphologic appearance is strikingly similar to that of papillary serous carcinomas of the ovary. These "serous papillary carcinomas" of the endometrium accounted for 10% of endometrial cancers in the series of patients reported from Stanford. However, they accounted for 50% of all treatment failures. Biologically, these cancers behave in a pattern similar to that of clear cell cancers, with a tendency for frequent metastasis. Extrauterine spread is found at exploratory laparotomy in more than half of patients believed to have stage I disease prior to surgery.

Confusion exists concerning the interpretation and implications of adenoacanthomas, adenosquamous carcinomas, and adenocarcinomas because the terminology is not used uniformly, and precise criteria for establishing the proper diagnosis are lacking. Adenoacanthoma represents an adenocarcinoma with benign squamous metaplasia; adenosquamous carcinoma contains both malignant glandular and squamous elements, and adenocarcinoma has malignant glandular elements and no squamous components. Adenoacanthomas are usually well differentiated and have the most favorable prognosis, whereas adenosquamous carcinomas are usually anaplastic and, therefore, the most aggressive of the three subtypes.[37]

**Clinical Features and Diagnosis.** Endometrial cancer occurs characteristically in postmenopausal upper middle class obese women, who are often taking estrogen replacement therapy and have a prior menstrual and reproductive history suggestive of prolonged anovulation. Ninety percent of women with endometrial cancer are postmenopausal, and 65% are in the sixth or seventh decade of life.[42] Only 5% of these patients are less than 40 years, and most of these younger women have Stein-Leventhal syndrome and are infertile, massively obese, or diabetic, or show other evidence of endocrinopathy.[43]

Most women with endometrial cancer present initially with complaints of abnormal bleeding characterized as prolonged, excessive, or intermenstrual in the premenopausal woman or as occurring after cessation of menses in the postmenopausal woman. Postmenopausal bleeding is defined as bleeding at least 12 months after cessation of menses. The bleeding patterns associated with endometrial cancer in the postmenopausal woman are indistinguishable from those seen with benign conditions such as vaginal atrophy as well as the premalignant endometrial hyperplasias. Bleeding may be as trivial as a single episode of spotting or severe enough to require transfusion. Although atrophic changes created by a hypoestrogenic state are the most frequent cause of postmenopausal bleeding, up to 20% of these women are found to have cancer and an additional 15 to 25% have endometrial hyperplasia.[44, 45]

Fifteen to 20% of women with endometrial cancer are

asymptomatic, sometimes presenting with an atypical Papanicolaou's (Pap) smear, suggesting an adenocarcinoma. When atypical glandular cells are seen on a Pap smear, the risk that an adenocarcinoma will be found is approximately 20%. The risk increases to approximately 50% in women who are at least 60 years.[46] Even apparently normal endometrial cells in a Pap smear of a postmenopausal woman suggests malignancy. Approximately 10% of postmenopausal women less than 60 years and up to 20% of those who are older with this finding have an adenocarcinoma.[47] The presence of five or more histiocytes per high-power field on cervicovaginal smears of postmenopausal women has also been associated with an increased cytologic sensitivity for endometrial cancer.[48] Five to 10% of patients may present with symptoms of advanced neoplasm, including ascites, bowel obstruction, jaundice, or respiratory embarrassment. Five percent of patients have occult malignancy diagnosed at hysterectomy performed for an apparently unrelated condition.

Endometrial cancer must be considered in any woman beyond 40 years with abnormal uterine bleeding and in younger women with abnormal bleeding associated with infertility or anovulation. With physicians' increasing reliance on vaginal ultrasonography for the screening and diagnosis of a variety of gynecologic conditions, clinicians have noted that marked endometrial thickening in an asymptomatic postmenopausal woman can be the only evidence for a uterine cancer. It has been suggested that endometrial thickness of 10 mm or greater in this population of women warrants endometrial sampling. Endometrial biopsy performed in the office or fractional dilation and curettage of the uterus are the preferred methods for diagnosis in these high-risk patients. Of the office biopsy techniques, sampling by a 3-mm flexible plastic aspirator (e.g., the Pipelle instrument) is preferred because it minimizes patient discomfort and is highly sensitive, with sufficient tissue obtained for diagnosis in 90% of cases and cancer detection approaching 95%.[49] In the symptomatic patient who has insufficient tissue for pathologic evaluation, a dilation and curettage must be considered. Cytologic screening techniques also exist and have varying sensitivities, with 50% accuracy when a specimen is obtained from the exocervix and vaginal pool, 75% with endocervical aspiration, 90% with saline irrigation of the endometrial cavity or the rotating endometrial brush method, and nearly 95% with a jet washer technique.[50] Unlike cytologic techniques used to detect cervical neoplasia, those used to diagnose endometrial neoplasia fail to detect a high percentage of premalignant lesions.

Screening measures for endometrial carcinoma are more costly, complex, and uncomfortable than those used to detect cervical neoplasia, and controlled prospective studies of high-risk populations are needed to evaluate the usefulness of routine screening with these cytologic and biopsy techniques. In patients with a history of abnormal bleeding requiring diagnosis, endocervical curettage also must be performed to rule out a primary endocervical malignancy. When endometrial biopsy and endocervical curettage are either inadequate to rule out a uterine cancer or demonstrate endometrial hyperplasia, a fractional curettage should be performed. When performed in conjunction with hysteroscopy, the diagnostic accuracy of a uterine sampling approaches 100%. Ultrasonography has been used for the screening of both symptomatic and asymptomatic postmenopausal women. Granberg and colleagues[51] evaluated 205 women with postmenopausal bleeding, 18 of whom had endometrial cancer and none with an endometrial stripe less than 8 mm. There was an overlap of the extent of endometrial thickness in women with cancer and those without cancer. Similarly, Bourne and colleagues reported an overlap of endometrial thickness in women with and without endometrial cancer.[52] Other studies have suggested similar findings. Because of the overlap in the endometrial thickness found in women with and without cancer, ultrasonography has not proved to be a cost-effective method of screening for this diagnosis.

**Staging.** The staging of endometrial cancer between July 1974 and 1988 used only clinical criteria and could not be modified by findings at operation. These criteria were replaced in 1988 by surgical criteria based on the recommendations of the Cancer Committee of the International Federation of Gynecology and Obstetrics (FIGO), as shown on Table 57–3.[53] The major impetus for surgical staging resulted from the published work of Sir John Stallworthy and collaborators who reviewed their assessment of disease status in women with endometrial cancer treated by Wertheim's hysterectomy and lymphadenectomy.[54, 55] A critical review of these data led some of the leaders in gynecologic oncology in the United States to develop a surgical staging protocol.[56] This initial pilot study and the expanded Gynecologic Oncology Group (GOG) study noted results similar to the Oxford reports.[34, 57] They found frequent errors in staging based on clinical criteria. Many patients had more extensive disease than expected, and some had less extensive disease than expected preoperatively. These surgical investigations were the catalyst for the 1988 FIGO revisions of endometrial cancer staging from that determined clinically to that discovered at surgery.

The purpose of staging is to provide a common language for study comparisons. This modification of staging criteria permits the evaluation of comparable subgroups of patients with endometrial cancer for treatment response and survival. The older clinical criteria did not permit separation of high-risk from low-risk patients based on important prognostic criteria, including depth of invasion, the extent cervical stromal invasion, and presence of extrauterine spread; the new criteria accomplish this.[58] In a retrospective review of 56 women, whose disease was thought to be limited to the

uterine corpus or uterine cervix, or both, clinical assessment was found to be inaccurate in approximately 40% of the cases as compared with surgical staging.[59]

A pretreatment evaluation typically consists of a medical assessment with a complete blood count; urinalysis; blood urea nitrogen, creatinine, and postprandial blood sugar levels, liver function tests; chest radiograph; and electrocardiogram. An intravenous pyelogram and barium enema are usually performed to rule out coexistent gastrointestinal or urologic disease and to permit future comparison should related symptoms develop. Imaging of the upper abdomen should be considered if liver function test results are abnormal; a lymphangiogram, computed tomographic scan, or magnetic resonance imaging (MRI) can help explain unexpected ureteral obstruction; and bone surveys or scans can be helpful in evaluating occasional patients with pain of uncertain origin. The routine use of computed tomography (CT) and MRI of the pelvis has not been demonstrated to add to the pretreatment evaluation of women with endometrial cancers, and these techniques are not viewed as cost effective for this diagnosis. Reliable information concerning depth of myometrial invasion and cervical extension has been demonstrated with MRI[60]; however, since this information is readily gained by histopathologic assessment of the hysterectomy specimen, the cost of MRI does not justify its use for this purpose. Likewise, the liver and periaortic lymph nodes can often be assessed with MRI or CT, readily demonstrating the presence of adenopathy and hepatic metastasis. Again, since surgery is usually performed, even in women with advanced uterine cancer when feasible to palliate the pelvic tumor, this information rarely results in a change in the initial treatment approach. Transabdominal and vaginal ultrasonography is another means of assessing depth of uterine invasion, although it does not reliably detect extrauterine disease. Although it is less expensive than MRI and CT, the information gained rarely modifies the treatment approach used. Conversely, in the unusual patient with advanced-stage disease in whom primary radiotherapy is planned instead of surgery, abdominal CT or MRI can assist in evaluating the periaortic area and liver more precisely and should be considered prior to planning therapy. Therapeutic decisions should be made after presentation to a tumor board consisting of gynecologic oncologists, radiation therapists, and pathologists.

Patients with stage I disease make up the majority of endometrial cancer cases. The high frequency of stage I is partly the result of public awareness that postmenopausal bleeding is a warning sign of malignancy and partly due to the large fraction of newly diagnosed cases associated with exogenous estrogen intake, which is almost always diagnosed in stage I. Until 1989, patients with stage I disease were subclassified on the basis of both the length of the uterine cavity as measured from the external cervical os and the degree of tumor anaplasia. The purpose of including these two criteria in the staging was to permit the clinician to identify prior to treatment those patients for whom individualization of therapy is most appropriate. In this context, grade of disease has proved more important than uterine size in predicting outcome. Indeed, Malkasian[61] demonstrated that, for each grade of disease, uterine size does not influence the survival probability.

Stage II disease, which implied cervical extension, was

*Table 57–3.* **FIGO Uterine Corpus Cancer Staging***

| Stage | Characteristics |
|-------|-----------------|
| Ia | Tumor limited to endometrium |
| Ib | Invasion of ≤ one half of myometrium |
| Ic | Invasion of > one half of myometrium |
| IIa | Endocervical glandular involvement only |
| IIb | Cervical stromal invasion |
| IIIa | Tumor invades serosa or adnexae, or both, or positive peritoneal cytologic findings |
| IIIb | Vaginal metastases |
| IIIc | Metastases to pelvic or para-aortic lymph nodes, or both |
| IVa | Tumor invasion bladder or bowel mucosa, or both |
| IVb | Distant metastases including intra-abdominal or inguinal lymph node, or both |

*Corpus cancer is surgically staged. Also, each stage is subdivided by histologic differentiation into grades 1, 2, and 3.

From Pecorelli S. Annual report on the results of treatment in gynaecological cancers. J Epidemiol Biostat 1998;3:45.

reported to occur in up to 15% of patients. However, these data were based on the older clinical criteria for staging, and many of these cases were not found to have cervical extension at the time of hysterectomy. This discrepancy resulted because the most common means of evaluating the cervix prior to hysterectomy occurred at the time of fractional curettage of the uterus, when an endocervical curettage specimen was obtained before curettage of the endometrial cavity. Not infrequently, however, malignant glands actually arising in the endometrial cavity were found in the endocervical curettage specimen. There was and continues to be great difficulty in distinguishing these "floaters" from true endocervical extension. The frequency of this diagnostic error has approached 50% of cases reported as stage II disease based on clinical criteria.[62] Primary operative management as suggested by the new staging criteria has helped minimize this source of error in evaluating patients for cervical extension.

**Prognosis.** Prognosis is a function of several interrelated variables, including stage, exogenous estrogen use, depth of myometrial penetration, lymphatic involvement, histologic grade, cell type, uterine size, peritoneal cytologic characteristics, receptor status, and patient age.[32, 42] Unfortunately, it is not possible to assess each of these factors independently to determine their relative importance; nevertheless, it appears that stage is the most important measure of prognosis, as shown in Table 57–4. These data are based on surgical staging of patients treated from 1990 to 1992, with overall survival up to 1997.[63]

The depth of myometrial penetration and tumor grade are the best indicators of risk of extrauterine spread in general and specifically of lymphatic spread. Only 6.4% of 528 patients with cancer confined to the uterine corpus on clinical assessment, who were explored (stage I endometrial cancer) prior to any type of radiotherapy, were found to have pelvic lymph node metastases in a collaborative (GOG) study.[35] Nevertheless, 23.8% of 80 patients in this group with invasion to the outer third of the myometrium had lymph node metastases, as contrasted with 3.2% of 434 patients whose tumors were more superficial. In this study, the grade of tumor was shown to be equally predictive of lymph node metastases. Of 70 patients with grade 3 tumors, 21.4% were found to have pelvic lymph node metastases, as compared with only 4.1% of 440 patients with lower grade tumors. As anticipated from these data, there is a progressive increase in the incidence of deep myometrial invasion with advancing histologic grade. Cheon[64] demonstrated deep myometrial invasion in 12% of 219 patients with grade 1 tumors, 20% of

74 patients with grade 2 tumors, and 46% of 79 patients with grade 3 lesions. Likewise, the GOG study reported 23% outer two-thirds myometrial invasion with grade 1 tumors, as compared with 58% with grade 3 lesions.[34] In this study, both grade and depth of myometrial invasion worked in concert to increase the risk of nodal metastasis. In fact, 34% of women with outer third invasion and grade 3 tumors had pelvic lymph node metastases; 23% of these women also had periaortic metastasis.

The high frequency of nodal spread with deeply invasive or anaplastic tumors is reflected in the reported survival rates. Patients with noninvasive or superficially invasive tumor have an 80 to 85% 5-year relapse-free survival rate, whereas those with deeply invasive tumors have a 60% survival rate.[65] As the tumor becomes less differentiated, the chance of deep myometrial invasion and extrauterine spread increases, and therefore survival decreases. The most recent FIGO review reported 5-year survival statistics of 91.7% for grade 1, 86.7% for grade 2, and 73.6% for grade 3 lesions.[62]

As indicated previously, the cell type can influence the prognosis for these patients. The prognosis appears worse for adenosquamous tumors than for adenoacanthomas or pure adenocarcinomas. The most important factor that determines the prognosis associated with these tumors appears to be the differentiation of malignant glandular elements. Because approximately 75% of adenoacanthomas are well differentiated,[66] they appear to have the best prognosis of the group, with a 71% overall 5-year survival rate and an 84% survival rate in stage I disease. Less than 20% of the adenosquamous tumors are well differentiated, however, and reported 5-year relapse-free survival rates range between 20% and 50%. Overall, adenocarcinomas without squamous elements have a 5-year survival rate of approximately 60%. For a given grade of malignant glandular epithelium, however, the prognosis for a patient with any of these three types of tumor is similar.[66]

Serous papillary carcinomas of the endometrium also have been associated with a poor prognosis. These cancers are considered poorly differentiated, and frequent early recurrences are reported. This subgroup of adenocarcinomas represents less than 10% of the group but might account for nearly half the recurrences. A few small series of patients with this diagnosis have been reported, most of which have confirmed the poor prognosis of this tumor and the frequent patterns of unsuspected intraperitoneal spread. For example, Jeffrey and colleagues[67] reported the understaging of 8 of 15 patients with this diagnosis, only 2 of whom were alive and disease free at 5 years. In a review by Dunton and colleagues,[68] patients with papillary serous adenocarcinomas tended to be 8 to 10 years older than those with other types of adenocarcinoma. Five-year survival rate ranges from only 10 to 50%, with the majority of long-term survivors having stage I tumors without myometrial invasion. Similarly, Goff and associates reported in 50 women with uterine papillary serous carcinoma that 72% had extrauterine disease; half of these women had lymph node metastasis in the absence of myometrial invasion.[69] The rarer tumors of the endometrium, including clear cell or epidermoid carcinoma, have a uniformly poor prognosis, with a 5-year relapse-free rate of approximately 25%.

Peritoneal cytologic findings also have been identified as a factor that can influence prognosis in early-stage endome-

*Table 57–4.* **Carcinoma of the Endometrium: Survival by Surgical Stage**

| Stage | Patients (No.) | 5-Year Survival (%) |
|-------|----------------|---------------------|
| I | 3845 | 87.0 |
| II | 575 | 71.9 |
| III | 694 | 50.8 |
| IV | 167 | 8.8 |

From Pecorelli S, ed. Annual report on the results of treatment in gynecologic cancer. Vol. 23. International Federation of Gynecology and Obstetrics. Milan, Italy: European Institute of Oncology, 1998:45.

trial cancer patients; however, their role as an independent prognostic factor remains controversial.[70] The largest body of data comes from the GOG's extensive clinicopathologic study of clinical stage I carcinoma of the endometrium, which found 12% of 621 patents with positive cytologic findings.[34] In patients with positive cytologic findings, approximately 25% had metastasis to the pelvic lymph nodes, 19% of whom also had metastasis to the para-aortic nodes. In addition, 35% of patients with extrauterine disease (adenexa, nodes, or intraperitoneal disease) had positive washings. The significance of positive cytologic findings remains unclear. Some investigators, such as Kadar and colleagues, found that positive cytologic findings had an adverse survival outcome only in the presence of extrauterine disease.[71] Because the cytologic findings also correlated with other prognostic factors, such as the grade of tumor and the depth of invasion, it is not clear whether peritoneal cytologic findings per se represent an independent prognostic factor. Nevertheless, peritoneal cytologic specimens are obtained easily at operation and should be evaluated even in patients with apparently early disease. The need for adjuvant therapy in the setting of early stage I disease and positive cytologic findings remains to be elucidated.

Age at diagnosis is often overlooked as an important prognostic indicator. Older patients more often present with an advanced stage of disease, more extensive myometrial invasion in early stages, and a poor 5-year survival rate even when corrected for deaths from intercurrent disease.[64] The poor survival rate also results from selective modification of therapy in some patients because of advanced age and coexisting medical conditions. When possible, optimal therapy should not be compromised because of age alone.

Other factors that might influence prognosis include race,[72] status of estrogen and progesterone receptors,[73] DNA content as determined by flow cytometry, vascular invasion,[74] and overexpression of various oncogenes in the cancerous tissues.[75] Although each of these factors has been reported to influence prognosis, in most instances there is considerable overlap with the prognostic factors discussed earlier. For example, the poorer prognosis in black women than in white women partly results because blacks often are not estrogen users and therefore tend to have more poorly differentiated and deeply invasive cancers. In addition, blacks tend to have delays in diagnosis so that advanced-stage disease is present more frequently than in whites. As a second example, the presence of receptors for estrogen (ER +) and progesterone (PR +) has been associated with a better prognosis than that found in women whose tumors are ER and PR negative (ER −, PR −). Yet the receptor status also correlates well with tumor grade and hence depth of myometrial invasion, nodal metastases, and so forth. Despite this observation, there are data that suggest that receptor status might be an independent prognostic variable even after correcting for stage of disease and other prognostic variables.[76] Furthermore, PR status might be a better predictor of prognosis and response to hormonal therapy than ER status.[77]

Some studies suggest that the overexpression of HER-2/neu and C-myc oncogenes may influence prognosis as well in endometrial cancer. For example, Berchuck and colleagues[75] found that overexpression of HER-2/neu was associated with ER cancers, which tended to be of advanced stage and anaplastic. Borst and colleagues[78] made similar observations for the overexpression of both HER-2/neu and C-myc. In addition, as noted previously, there have been extensive investigations regarding both the presence and significance of mutations in the tumor suppressor gene p53. Kohler and associates noted that mutant p53 was overexpressed in 20% of 107 primary endometrial adenocarcinomas, including 9% of stage I to stage II and 40% of stage III and stage IV.[79] In a univariate analysis, overexpression of mutant p53 was associated with multiple poor prognostic factors such as stage, grade, and absence of progesterone receptors. Although several studies have demonstrated the association of p53 with a poor prognosis, it has not been identified as an independent prognostic variable.[80, 81] Furthermore, the relationship of p53 to pathogenesis and prognosis remains unclear.

Overlapping and confounding prognostic variables are also seen when one evaluates the influence of DNA content in endometrial cancer cells as determined by flow cytometry. Tumor aneuploidy has been associated with a poorer prognosis than diploidy; however, the fact that aneuploidy is seen more frequently in more poorly differentiated carcinomas, whereas diploidy is seen more frequently in well-differentiated tumors probably accounts for this observation.

## TREATMENT

The best approach to the management of patients with endometrial cancer should provide satisfactory treatment of the primary tumor, known metastases, and areas at increased risk for metastases. Data that identify and quantify the risk factors cited previously permit the development of rational approaches to the treatment of the various stages and substages of this disease. Unfortunately, many questions concerning optimal treatment remain unanswered because of the difficulty in interpreting data reported in the literature. The magnitude of this problem is great because virtually all studies reported either demonstrate bias in patient selection for the various treatment regimens used or fail to control the factors that influence prognosis within each treatment group.[38]

Prospective, controlled studies have been difficult to carry out. The absence of such studies inevitably has resulted in the systematic inclusion of patients in a treatment group because of age, weight, or other medial conditions, thereby preventing meaningful comparison of data so generated. In addition, there is lack of uniformity within and among studies concerning definitions of stage of disease, determination of tumor grade, means of detecting cervical involvement, and quantification of myometrial invasion. In some reports, extent of disease conforms to the older League of Nations staging, in some reports it conforms to FIGO staging, and in other reports the extent disease does not conform to any standardized staging system. Determination of tumor grade remains subjective, and comparison of histologic grading among studies is often meaningless. Some authors use Broders'[63] grading system (groups I to IV), and others use that recommended by FIGO (grades 1 to 3). Cervical involvement might be evaluated by clinical examination only, cervical punch biopsy, endocervical curettage, cervical conization, or only after evaluating the hysterectomy specimen. Determination of myometrial penetration has been made by dividing the uterine wall in half or in thirds or by otherwise defining superficial, intermediate, and deep invasion. Often unclear is the means of reporting patients lost to follow-up or dying of intercurrent disease. These problems are compounded by the inability to standardize radiation therapy and surgery among studies or even within studies that include patients often spanning the experience of an institution over 2 or 3 decades. Hence, there is a great need for prospective controlled studies designed to minimize the many variables cited.

**Premalignant Disease.** The treatment of premalignant changes in the endometrium (atypical adenomatous hyperplasia) can consist of either operative or medical management. Anovulatory premenopausal women who develop atypical hyperplastic changes in the uterus resulting from unopposed estrogen stimulation are often managed by cyclic progestational therapy. When these women want to bear children, they are best treated with drugs that can initiate ovulation. Perimenopausal and postmenopausal women with these premalignant changes are best managed by hysterectomy. When severely atypical hyperplasia is present in this age group, regression of premalignant changes with proges-

tational therapy is unlikely, and progression to frank carcinoma is a possibility. Conservative medical management in this situation is potentially hazardous, as occult cancers can be found in approximately 20% of hysterectomy specimens in which a recent uterine curettage revealed only atypical adenomatous hyperplasia.

When endometrial hyperplasia either with or without atypia is found on endometrial biopsy, endometrial carcinoma first must be ruled out by curettage of the uterus before specific therapy is begun. If conservative therapy is chosen, an endometrial biopsy should be performed after 3 months of progestational therapy to ensure reversal of the prior findings. Hysterectomy should be carried out if premalignant changes persist.

**Malignant Disease.** The approach to managing patients with endometrial cancer typically employs surgery first, often combined with postoperative radiation therapy when adverse prognostic factors are present (Figs. 57–2 and 57–3). Initial management of patients with suspected stage I disease consists of, at minimum, an abdominal exploration, aspiration of peritoneal fluid for cytologic investigation, and performance of a total abdominal hysterectomy and bilateral

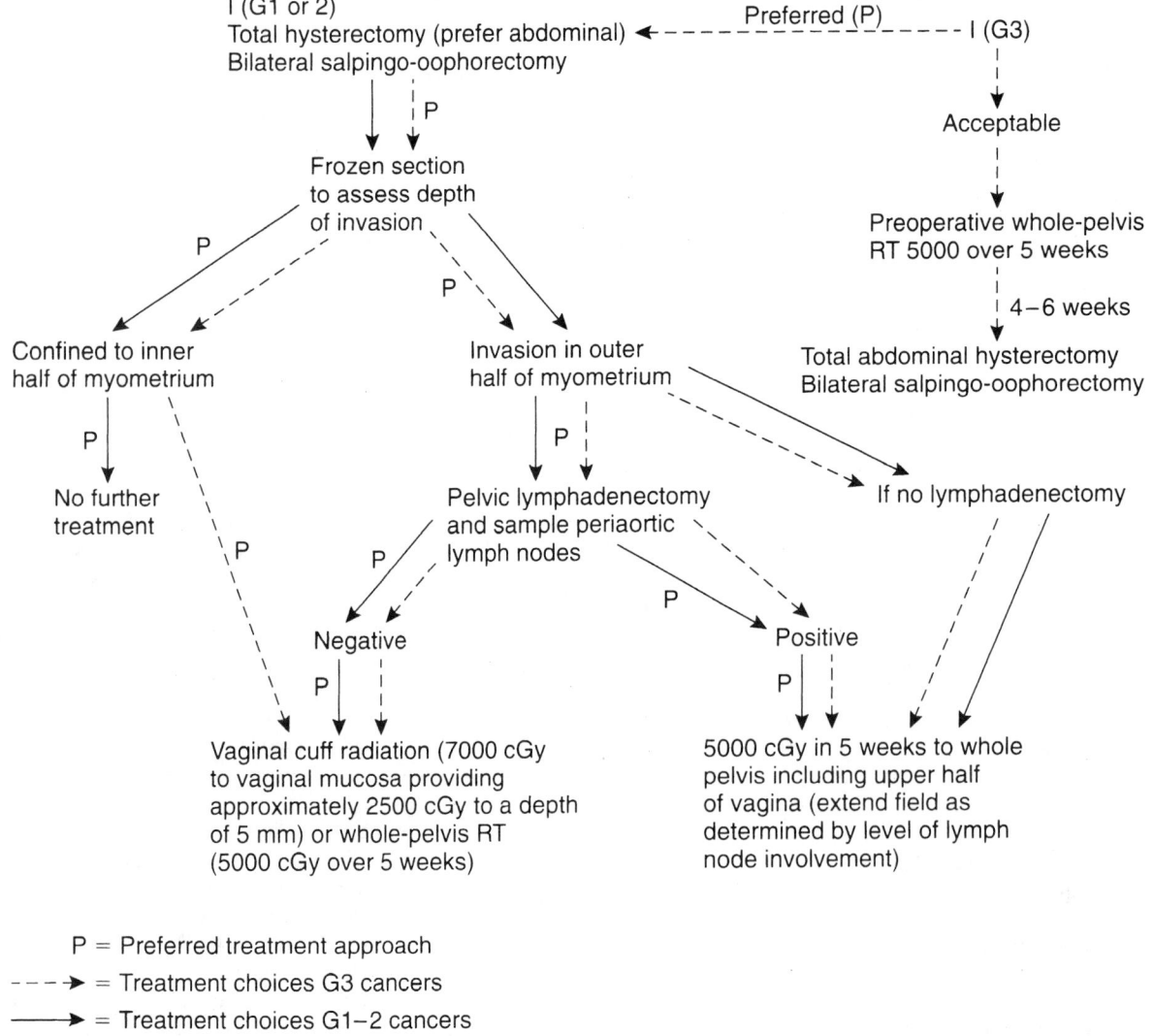

**Figure 57–2.** Treatment of stage I endometrial cancer.

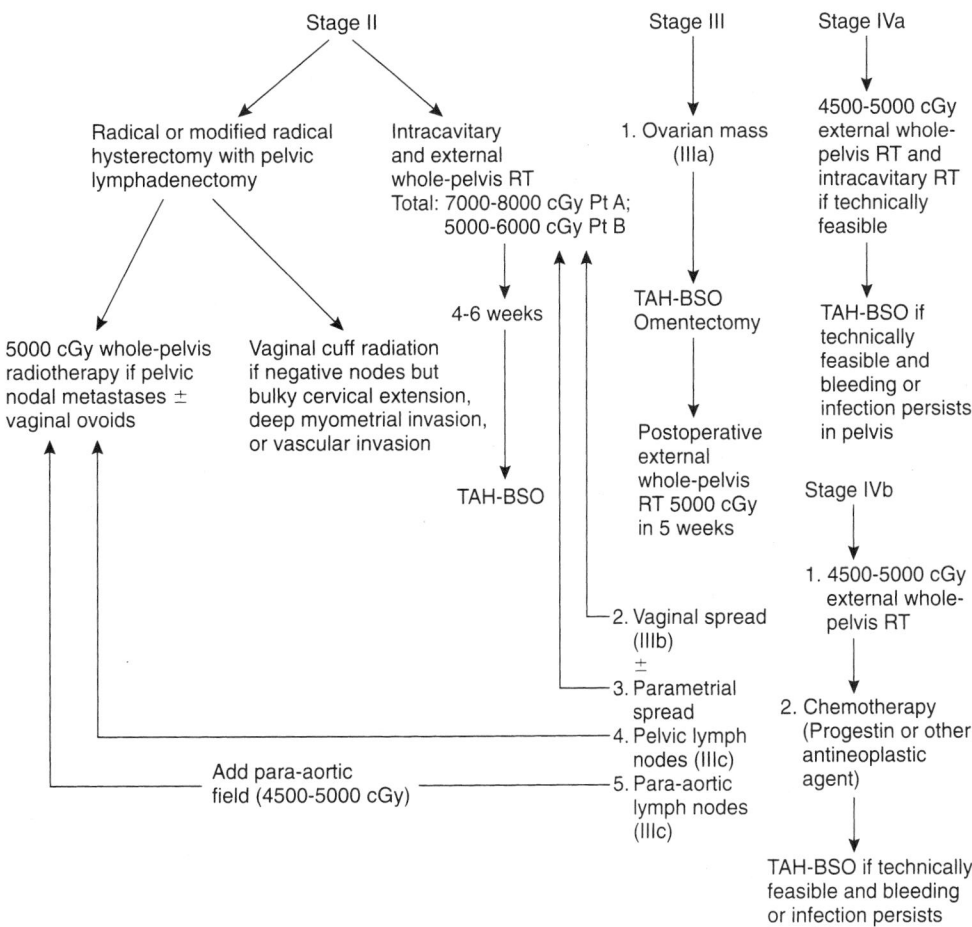

**Figure 57–3.** Treatment of stages II to IV endometrial cancer. TAH-BSO, total abdominal hysterectomy–bilateral salpingo-oophorectomy

salpingo-oophorectomy. Although some investigators have advocated radical hysterectomy with pelvic lymphadenectomy as the treatment of choice,[82] there are no data substantiating improved survival with more extensive resections[3, 83, 84] and no decrease in the risk of subsequent vaginal metastases.[85] Because endometrial cancer rarely spreads to the parametrium without cervical involvement, removal of the parametrium in the absence of clear-cut cervical extension is not warranted.

A vaginal hysterectomy is an acceptable alternative in the occasional patient with suspected stage I carcinoma for whom an abdominal hysterectomy might be attended with excessive morbidity. Morbidly obese patients and those with severe pulmonary or cardiac conditions are managed more safely when the vaginal approach is used, thereby reducing the risk of wound dehiscence, evisceration, pneumonia, and other complications seen more frequently after abdominal surgery.[86] When a vaginal hysterectomy is used, every effort should be made to remove the ovaries also, an approach that can be facilitated by laparoscopic assistance or by performing large unilateral or even bilateral Schuchardt's incisions to improve exposure. Although a vaginal approach precludes abdominal exploration, sampling of lymph nodes and, in some instances, removal of the ovaries, the authors' experience suggests that survival is not compromised in women with stage I, grade 1 or 2 carcinomas.[86] Similarly, Massi and colleagues retrospectively reviewed the survival

of 327 women, clinically thought to have stage I adenocarcinomas, who were treated with vaginal or abdominal hysterectomy.[87] Overall, 180 patients underwent vaginal hysterectomy, and 147 patients had an abdominal hysterectomy. The survival rates were approximately 90% in both groups at 5 and 10 years. In this uncontrolled, retrospective study, route of surgery, histologic tumor type, use of adjuvant radiation and performance of a lymphadenectomy did not have an impact on survival. Accordingly we believe that even with less favorable histologic subtypes, the risks of abdominal surgery in morbidly obese and medically compromised patients outweigh its benefits over the vaginal approach.

Another alternative method of surgically staging patients with presumed stage I disease uses laparoscopy. This approach allows a laparoscopically assisted vaginal hysterectomy, when indicated, and pelvic and periaortic lymph node assessment. Childers and colleagues[88] reported this approach for 59 patients with presumed stage I disease. Eight of these patients required laparotomy for either advanced disease or operative complication. Although this approach provides an alternative to laparotomy that may reduce hospital stay and possibly reduce costs of medical care, its long-term efficacy remains to be proved.

Routine pelvic and periaortic lymphadenectomy or lymph node sampling in women with endometrial cancer has not been demonstrated to improve cure rates for this disease significantly. Nevertheless, women with cancers having poor prognostic features commonly have metastases to pelvic and periaortic lymph nodes. This information gained at the time of surgery markedly influences the decision to use adjuvant radiotherapy. Because this sequence of events often reduces the risk of pelvic recurrence and might also have a favorable impact on survival, in 1988 FIGO adopted a surgical staging system for endometrial cancer that included assessment of the pelvic and para-aortic lymph nodes for metastasis. Although the presence of lymph node metastasis is included in the staging of endometrial cancer (see Table 57–3), lymph node sampling is not required with the evaluation and management of all the patients. Many gynecologic oncologists believe that the indication for lymph node sampling or dissection should reflect the potential for lymphatic involvement. A stage IA, grade 1 endometrial cancer has such a low risk of lymphatic spread that it would not warrant a dissection. However, a moderate- or high-risk lesion may justify sampling the pelvic and periaortic lymph nodes. The lymph node dissection may facilitate postoperative treatment decisions, and provide prognostic information and may be therapeutic. Yokoyama and colleagues[89] noted a poor prognosis in patients with regional lymph nodes containing metaplastic cancer as compared with those without metastasis. This analysis of 63 patients with stages I to III disease found a 22% incidence of pelvic lymph node metastases and a 19% para-aortic incidence of metastases. The survival of patients with periaortic metastasis (usually also associated with pelvic node metastasis) was worse than for those with pelvic node disease alone (44.4% and 80%, respectively). Similarly, Mohan and coworkers[90] suggested that complete lymphadenectomy did not increase morbidity and may modify the use of postoperative radiation.

Although there are no controlled clinical trials demonstrating a clear survival advantage for subsets of women undergoing lymph node sampling or lymphadenectomy, there are data that suggest that such a survival advantage might exist in certain clinical situations. A report by Kilgore and associates[91] clearly documented an improved survival advantage in patients who had multisite lymph node sampling versus those who did not have any sampling. In their comparison of patients who received adjuvant radiation for deep myometrial invasion and grade III lesions, patients with multisite sampling had better survival than did those in whom nodes were not sampled. This strongly suggests a therapeutic benefit for lymphadenectomy for all risk groups. Conversely, others doubt the necessity of both pelvic and para-aortic lymphadenectomy. Belinson and colleagues[92] noted that few patients with early-stage disease have metastases to these nodes, that disease rarely recurs on the pelvic side wall following pelvic radiation whether or not lymph nodes were sampled, and that removal of positive para-aortic lymph nodes rarely results in cure, even when followed by radiotherapy.

Accordingly, the role for lymphadenectomy remains controversial in the management of endometrial cancer. However, in the absence of randomized, prospective trials, the current data provide compelling evidence for lymphadenectomy in the moderate- and high-risk patient. The frequent performance of lymphadenectomy reflects the important prognostic information it provides and the ability to tailor adjuvant radiation therapy based on an accurate assessment of the extent of disease.

The role of adjuvant therapy in patients with cancer confined to the uterus (surgical stage I) also is controversial. Postoperative external-beam radiation traditionally has been given to patients with one or more adverse risk factors, including deep myometrial invasion or high-grade disease; however, there are few supporting data for this approach. Aalders and associates[93] published the only prospective report evaluating adjuvant teletherapy in disease confined to the uterus. This study failed to demonstrate an improved 5-year survival in the group of women treated with radiotherapy. Although the GOG study published by Morrow and coworkers[94] did not randomize stage I patients postoperatively, it also failed to demonstrate a survival advantage in patients who received external-beam radiation over those who did not. Similarly, Irwin and colleagues[95] found no survival advantage for patients who received adjuvant radiotherapy over those who did not in 550 pathologic stage I patients. This study did, however, confirm that adjuvant radiotherapy can reduce the incidence of pelvic recurrence. Additionally, a study by Orr and associates[96] noted that in 310 surgical stage I patients, the risk of pelvic recurrence and survival was not compromised by withholding adjuvant teletherapy. The GOG has completed a controlled clinical trial that will provide additional data regarding the role of adjuvant radiotherapy for this disease.

When lymphadenectomy is not performed, the decision to administer radiation therapy typically is determined by the depth of myometrial penetration and the histologic grade of the tumor. Grade 1 or 2 tumors confined to the endometrium or with inner-half myometrial invasion (stage Ia or Ib) rarely metastasize to lymph nodes or recur in the vagina and can be managed with operation alone. With outer-half myometrial invasion (stage Ic), even tumors with more favorable histologic characteristics frequently metastasize in the pelvis and typically receive whole-pelvis radiotherapy to include the pelvic lymph nodes and the upper half of the vagina. Patients with grade 3 tumors or other unfavorable histologic tumor types, including clear cell, adenosquamous, and serous papillary carcinomas, have a reduced 5-year survival rate and an increased risk of vaginal metastases.[97] All these patients should receive some form of radiotherapy, usually administered to the whole pelvis and encompassing the upper half of the vagina (see Fig. 57–2).

The rationale for combining surgery with radiation lies in the proven ability of the latter to reduce the incidence of vaginal vault recurrences from 15 to approximately 3%.[3, 98] Additionally, radiation therapy can be curative as a single modality in patients who are not candidates for surgery, suggesting that its addition to surgery might be beneficial.

When endometrial cancer extends to the cervix (stage II), treatment traditionally includes the parametria, vagina, and pelvic lymph nodes in addition to the uterus. Two treatment regimens in current use for women with bulky cervical extension include either radical hysterectomy with bilateral pelvic lymphadenectomy or radiation therapy consisting of intracavitary treatment using tandem and ovoids with external whole-pelvis therapy. Most patients with stage II disease have occult cervical extension typically found on histopathologic assessment of the hysterectomy specimen. They are best managed with adjuvant radiotherapy following the initial surgical procedure. Because the risk of pelvic lymph node metastases in stage II disease approaches 30%[37] meticulous attention must be directed to their treatment, whether by surgery or radiotherapy. The treatment approach favored by us is one that depends on the general condition of the patient and the estimated tumor volume within the cervix (stage IIa vs. stage IIb). Patients whose weight, age, and medical condition permit extended surgery can safely undergo either a radical hysterectomy if bulky stage IIb is suspected based on a positive cervical biopsy or a nodular expanded cervix or a modified radical hysterectomy if stage IIa is suspected based on positive endocervical curretage specimens. In both instances, a pelvic lymphadenectomy is performed from the level of the aortic bifurcation superiorly to the distal portion of the external iliac vessels. When nodal metastases or occult parametrial extension is found, approximately 50 Gy whole-pelvis radiotherapy is administered approximately 4 to 6 weeks postoperatively, often in conjunction with brachytherapy. In the absence of these features vaginal vault radiation should be considered without external-beam therapy because the risk of cuff recurrences remains high even after a radical hysterectomy for this disease. In a review of the UCI experience of 70 women with stage II disease treated in this fashion, the actuarial 5-year disease-free survival rate was 65%.[99] One quarter of recurrences were within the pelvis, with the remainder at distant sites. This observation confirms the excellent pelvic control that can be achieved with surgery, usually combined with radiotherapy, and that the majority of failures reflect occult distant metastasis at initial treatment. The authors found that half of the recurrences in this series were from papillary serous cancers and that all the stage II papillary serous cancers recurred. Patients believed to have cervical extension who are not candidates for an extended hysterectomy undergo initial radiotherapy followed by a simple hysterectomy 4 to 6 weeks later (see Fig. 57–3). Preoperative radiotherapy typically consists of 50 Gy external-beam therapy to the whole pelvis without intracavitary therapy when the cervix is not expanded or nodular. When bulky cervical disease is present, intracavitary radiotherapy should be added to the external-beam therapy. If this is not done, the ensuing simple hysterectomy frequently will not encompass the remaining cancer within the cervix.

The treatment of stage III disease when associated with vaginal metastases requires more extensive radiation, and therefore subsequent operation frequently is abandoned. A total of 85 Gy to point A and 60 Gy to point B can be delivered safely, but subsequent operation can cause an unacceptably high risk of gastrointestinal and urologic injuries. Patients who have stage III disease on the basis of ovarian or nodal metastases are managed initially by operation, usually followed by radiation of the whole pelvis. Extended radiation fields are used when nodal metastases are present in the common iliac or periaortic regions. Operation should consist of a total abdominal hysterectomy, bilateral salpingo-oophorectomy, and pelvic and periaortic lymphadenectomy, adding an omentectomy when there is intraperitoneal or adnexal metastasis.

The treatment of stage IV disease is designed primarily for palliation, although a few patients with tumor invading bladder or rectum can be cured with an aggressive approach using surgery combined with radiotherapy. The treatment program we prefer for patients with stage IV cancer is outlined in Figure 57–3. Pelvic exenteration for recurrent

pelvic tumor has only rarely been of value because of the frequent association with occult extrapelvic metastases.[100]

A role for adjuvant chemotherapy in managing patients at high risk for distant metastases cannot be justified at this time. Adjuvant progestational therapy has been used in multiple randomized, prospective trials without a significant decrease in recurrence. The GOG investigated the use of adjuvant doxorubicin in 181 patients with high-risk stage I and stage II disease in a controlled clinical trial. The group of patients treated with cytotoxic chemotherapy fared no better than those who were not treated.[101] Investigators at M.D. Anderson[102] prospectively used cisplatin, doxorubicin, and cyclophosphamide as adjuvant therapy in high-risk patients. Three-year survival was 82% for patients with disease confined to the uterus compared with 46% if there was extrauterine spread. Until more active agents against endometrial cancer are identified, adjuvant chemotherapy will not play an important role in the management of these patients.

**Radiotherapy Alone.** Five-year relapse-free survival rates with radiotherapy alone in patients controlled for stage of disease based on clinical assessment only are significantly lower than those in patients who undergo surgery or a combination of surgery and radiation.[103] In a total of 190 pairs of patients matched stage for stage, there was a significantly higher long-term survival rate for surgery with or without radiation compared with that for radiation alone ($p < 0.01$). The 5- and 10-year relapse-free survival rates in stage I disease were 87% and 76%, respectively, for the group of patients treated with surgery, as compared with 69% and 52% for the irradiated group. Likewise, women treated primarily with radiotherapy do significantly less well than do those who undergo postradiotherapy hysterectomy for this disease.[104] In these series, survival differences were most marked for stages II and III, with survival rates of 82% versus 47% in stage II[105] and 57% versus 18% in stage III.[104] These data suggest that radiatiotherapy alone should be reserved for the patients with significant medical risks and for women with extensive pelvic tumors not amenable to surgery. In contrast to the preceding observations, Fishman and colleagues[106] treated 54 "inoperable" patients with stage I and II disease, based on clinical assessment, with radiotherapy alone. A cohort of 108 operable patients, also staged clinically, was used as a control group. Although a majority of the patients with inoperable disease died of intercurrent disease, the 5-year survival of those that did not die from other causes was 80%. In this small series, the 80% survival was not significantly worse than the survival in the control group. This study supports a role for radiotherapy in the medically inoperable patient.

**Chemotherapy.** Recurrent or metastatic endometrial carcinoma has traditionally been treated with a hormonal agent. Various progestational compounds, including megestrol acetate and 17α-hydroxyprogesterone in a wide range of dosages, have produced objective response rates ranging from 15 to 40%.[107] Other studies have reported response rates of less than 20%.[108] Patients in whom palliation is most likely to be achieved with these compounds characteristically have well-differentiated tumors metastatic to the lung in the absence of other disease and a long disease-free interval after initial treatment. Nearly half these patients show objective improvement, and 5- and 10-year relapse-free survival rates have been reported.[107] Unfortunately, the majority of ad-

*Table 57–5.* **Single-Agent Chemotherapy in Endometrial Carcinoma**

| Drug | No. of Patients Responding/ Patients Treated | Response Rate (%) | Reference |
|---|---|---|---|
| Cisplatin | 11/26 | 42 | 120 |
| Paclitaxel | 10/28 | 36 | 111 |
| Doxorubicin | 86/298 | 29 | 121 |
| Etoposide (VP-16) | 1/29 | 3 | 122 |
| Carboplatin | 7/23 | 30 | 130 |

vanced-stage and recurrent cancers are anaplastic and hence ER − and PR −. Such tumors rarely respond to hormonal therapy and should be considered for first-line cytotoxic chemotherapy.

Patients in whom hormonal treatment fails may be considered for cytotoxic chemotherapy. At least four drugs have demonstrated activity as single agent, namely, cisplatin, doxorubicin, paclitaxel, and carboplatin (Table 57–5). Doxorubicin appears to be the most active, with response rates of 10 to 37% reported, including complete responses in 5 to 20% of patients so treated.[109] Cisplatin and carboplatin apparently have a similar activity, with reported response rates ranging from 4 to 42%.[110] Paclitaxel appears to be a newer promising agent in endometrial cancer treatment. A phase II trial by the GOG, reported by Ball, noted an overall response rate of 36%.[111] There is only modest information on combination chemotherapy for endometrial carcinoma (Table 57–6). Unfortunately, the optimistic results of small preliminary studies generally have not been confirmed when adequate numbers of patients were treated. At present, more work is needed to define the role of both single-agent and combination chemotherapy in endometrial carcinoma; however, there does not appear to be a clear benefit of combination chemotherapy over a single agent in the treatment of women with advanced or recurrent endometrial cancer.

**Follow-Up Assessment.** After completion of any mode of therapy, patients should be followed every 3 months for 2 years because 75% of recurrences take place within that time. Routine follow-up examinations continue every 6 months thereafter and should include an abdominal and pelvic examination with Pap smear. A chest radiograph should be obtained annually for patients with one or more high-risk factors for recurrence. Specific complaints referable to the gastrointestinal tract and urologic or skeletal system should be evaluated. Tumor markers have not proved

*Table 57–6.* **Combination Chemotherapy in Endometrial Carcinoma**

| Drugs | Patients Responding/ Patients Treated | Response Rate (%) | Reference |
|---|---|---|---|
| DOXO + CYC | 8/11 | 73 | 123 |
| DOXO + CYC | 8/26 | 31 | 124 |
| DOXO + CYC + FU + VCR | 10/20 | 50 | 125 |
| DOXO + CYC + FU + Meg | 13/29 | 45 | 126 |

DOXO, doxorubicin (Adriamycin); CYC, cyclophosphamide; FU, 5-fluorouracil; VCR, vincristine; Meg, megestrol acetate.

useful in the subsequent evaluation of endometrial cancer patients. In some instances, carcinoembryonic antigen, CA-125, or CA-19-9 has been elaborated by these tumors. Until more data have been published, the routine use of one or more of these tumor markers in the follow-up of uterine cancer patients does not seem warranted.

## Sarcomas

A group of sarcomas with biologic, histologic, and clinical features distinct from uterine adenocarcinoma can arise from both the endometrial stroma and the myometrium. These tumors account for 2 to 5% of uterine malignancies. Unlike that of adenocarcinomas, the incidence of uterine sarcoma has not increased since the 1970s, suggesting that they are not induced by exogenous estrogen use. Patient age ranges from 30 to 85 years, with an average age of 70. Some investigators suggest that these tumors are more frequent in black women. Although prior pelvic or uterine irradiation has been implicated in the genesis of uterine sarcomas, this has not been substantiated by a review of reported cases. Less than 5% of uterine sarcomas have been preceded by pelvic radiotherapy. When this association is seen, radiotherapy has frequently been administered more than 20 years previously. The triad of obesity, diabetes, and hypertension associated with endometrial adenocarcinoma is also found in women with uterine sarcoma.

### NATURAL HISTORY

**Classification.** Uterine sarcomas can contain both homologous and heterologous elements. Homologous tumors are composed only of those tissues that are indigenous to the uterus (endometrial stroma, smooth muscle, and glandular epithelium), whereas the heterologous types include foreign elements such as cartilage, striated muscle, or bone.[112] Both can exist in pure or mixed form; pure tumors are composed of a single cell type, and mixed tumors contain more than one cell type. Another system classifies the uterine sarcomas on the basis of their origin from the endometrium, myometrium, or nonspecific connective tissue such as blood vessels and nerves (Table 57–7).[113] Sarcomas can occasionally be classified only on the basis of the microscopic appearance of the predominant cell and are designated spindle cell, round cell, or myxoid sarcoma.

Two problems exist in the pathologic interpretation of uterine tumors as sarcomas. The first is to establish malignant potential, and the second is to define the predominant cell type. Efforts to establish definitive criteria of malignancy rely on a determination of the mitotic index.[114] The malignant potential of leiomyosarcomas with more than 10 mitoses per 10 high-power microscopic fields is clear. Tumors with fewer than 5 mitoses per 10 high-power fields are benign. The behavior of tumors with mitotic counts between 5 and 9 per 10 high-power fields is less certain, however, as some may metastasize after operative management, whereas others respond completely to operative removal. Similarly, the virulence of endometrial stromal sarcoma is reflected in the mitotic index. The size of the primary tumor and degree of encapsulation also are of prognostic importance.[115]

**Table 57–7.** Classification of Uterine Sarcomas

Sarcomas
  Homologous
  Pure
    Leiomyosarcoma
    Stroma sarcoma
    Endolymphatic stromal myosis
    Angiosarcoma
    Fibrosarcoma
  Mixed
  Heterologous
  Pure
    Rhabdomyosarcoma
    Chondrosarcoma
    Osteosarcoma
    Liposarcoma
  Mixed
  Malignant mixed müllerian tumors
  Homologous
  Pure—carcinoma with homologous sarcoma
  Mixed
  Heterologous
  Pure—carcinoma with heterologous sarcoma
  Mixed
  Sarcoma, unclassified

Degeneration of a myoma with associated giant cell formation and cellular pleomorphism is often difficult to distinguish from a sarcoma. Retrospective review of tumors diagnosed as leiomyosarcomas reveals that benign cellular myomas can be misdiagnosed as sarcomas.

**Clinical Features and Diagnosis.** The symptoms of patients with uterine sarcomas relate to the tumor's origin from endometrium or myometrium. Sarcomas of endometrial origin often cause abnormal bleeding, whereas abdominal pain and the presence of a pelvic or abdominal mass are less frequent. Nonspecific complaints such as vaginal discharge, weight loss, and dysuria also occur. Sarcomas of myometrial origin frequently present as a painful or asymptomatic pelvic mass. Rapid enlargement of known fibroids in a postmenopausal patient is suggestive of sarcomatous degeneration. Pain is often associated with a rapidly growing tumor and should also arouse suspicion. The incidence of sarcomatous degeneration of a benign leiomyoma is less than 2% and does not warrant hysterectomy in all patients with uterine fibroids.[116]

The early diagnosis of uterine sarcomas is often difficult. Patients who develop postmenopausal bleeding require fractional curettage. On occasion, a poorly differentiated adenocarcinoma with sarcomatoid features is difficult to distinguish from a sarcoma. The diagnosis of tumors that arise from the myometrium is usually made at laparotomy.

**Staging.** No accepted staging system exists for uterine sarcomas, and the FIGO staging of endometrial carcinoma is often applied. Tumors confined to the fundus are designated as stage I. Stages II, III, and IV reflect progressive involvement of the cervix, spread to the pelvic tissues, and distant metastases. Sarcoma spreads by direct extension to involve adjacent tissues, by lymphatic spread to regional and distant lymph nodes, and by the hematogenous pathway to lung, liver, and bone.

**Prognosis.** The prognosis for patients with uterine sarcoma relates to cell type, stage, depth of myometrial penetration, and presence of lymph node metastases. Patients with endometrial stromal sarcoma, a pure homologous tumor, appear to have both higher rates of cure and more frequent control of local disease in the pelvis. Leiomyosarcoma, a pure homologous tumor of myometrial origin, has an unfavorable prognosis because of a tendency to spread early to distant organs. Tumors that contain heterologous elements, such as cartilage and striated muscle, are uniformly associated with a poor prognosis.

Stage correlates both with survival at 2 and 5 years and with control of pelvic disease. It appears, however, that sarcomas are likely to metastasize by the hematogenous pathway and to involve regional and distant lymphatics at an earlier stage than are endometrial adenocarcinomas. Of 28 patients with mixed müllerian tumors, 10 (35.7%) had involvement of pelvic lymph nodes at the time of hysterectomy.[116] Four of these patients also had metastases to aortic lymph nodes. All patients with metastases to pelvic or pelvic and periaortic lymph nodes had invasion of the middle or outer third of the myometrium by the primary tumor.

The survival rate of patients with mixed mesodermal sarcoma is reported to be about 50% for stage I and 10% for stage II, with virtually no survivors among patients with stages III and IV disease. Difficulty in interpreting survival statistics for other cell types relates to the use of different staging systems and small numbers of patients reported. A 2-year survival rate of 50 to 60% has been reported for patients with stage I and stage II leiomyosarcoma, with a 60 to 70% survival rate in stage I and stage II endometrial stromal sarcoma and carcinosarcoma.

## TREATMENT

The overall survival figures reported for many patients with these diseases suggest that no single treatment modality is curative. Total hysterectomy and bilateral salpingo-oophorectomy are adequate to remove the primary tumor in patients with stage I and stage II disease but are often ineffective in the prevention of local recurrence.

The high rate of pelvic lymph node involvement suggests that radiation therapy to the pelvis might be beneficial. It can be administered before or after hysterectomy. Patients with endometrial stromal sarcoma have benefited from pelvic irradiation with improved survival and decreased local and regional recurrence.[117] Patients with leiomyosarcoma have not benefited from pelvic radiotherapy because of a tendency toward distant metastases and relative insensitivity to radiation. Isolated pelvic recurrence is unusual in patients treated by operation and radiatiotherapy. Distant disease accounts for about 50% of recurrences; the other 50% are the result of both regional and distant disease. Ninety percent of patients who develop a recurrence do so within 2 years of diagnosis and initial treatment.

Systemic chemotherapy is a logical adjunct to local therapy for most patients with a sarcoma of the uterus; however, little is known about the value of chemotherapy in treating this group of tumors. The success of doxorubicin in treating soft tissue sarcomas in other sites has led to several studies of its use in patients with pelvic sarcomas.[63, 118] It has been demonstrated to be the most active agent in leiomyosarcomas. Ifosfamide has also demonstrated moderate activity. Multiagent chemotherapy for leiomyosarcoma has failed to

*Table 57–8.* **Chemotherapy in Uterine Sarcoma**

| Drugs | No. of Patients Responding/ Patients Treated | Response Rate (%) | Reference |
|---|---|---|---|
| D | 1/17 | 6 | 127 |
| D + CYC + VCR + DTIC | 1/1 | — | 128 |
| D + VCR + DTIC | 4/6 | — | 129 |
| D* | 13/80 | 16 | 118 |
| | 16/66 | 24 | |
| D* + DTIC | | | 118 |

*Randomized study of D vs. D + DTIC.

D, doxorubicin (Adriamycin); CYC, cyclophosphamide; VCR, vincristine; DTIC, dacarbazine.

demonstrate an improved response in comparison to doxorubicin alone.[119] Currently, ifosfamide and cisplatin appear to be most active in patients with mixed mesodermal tumors. Again, combination therapies do not appear to improve response when compared with ifosfamide alone. These agents have been used in various combinations, but preliminary results are not encouraging (Table 57–8).

At present, studies are ongoing to define the role of chemotherapy in this group of tumors. Given that these cancers are seen infrequently, patients should be encouraged to participate in these studies if at all possible.

## SUGGESTIONS FOR ADDITIONAL READING

Nag S. Modern techniques of radiation therapy for endometrial cancer. Clin Obstet Gynecol 1996;39:728–44.

Creasman WT. Endometrial cancer: incidence, prognostic factors, diagnosis, and treatment. Semin Oncol 1997;S1-24:140–50.

## REFERENCES

1. Greenlee RT, Murray T, Bolden S, Wingo PA. Cancer Statistics, 2000. CA Cancer J Clin 2000;50:7–33.
2. Kottmeir HL. Annual reports of treatment in carcinoma of the uterus, vagina, and ovary. Vol 16. Stockholm, EOS-Tryckerierna, 1976.
3. Gusberg SB. The evolution of modern treatment of corpus cancer. Cancer 1976;38:603–9.
4. Bokhman JV. Two pathogenetic types of endometrial carcinoma. Gynecol Oncol 1983;15:10.
5. McDonald TW, Anneers JF, O'Fallon WM, et al. Exogenous estrogen and endometriod carcinoma: case control and incidence study. Am J Obstet Gynecol 1977;127:572–80.
6. Mack TM, Pike MC, Henderson BE, et al. Estrogens and endometrial cancer in a retirement community. N Engl J Med 1976;294:1262–67.
7. Smith DC, Prentice R, Thompson DJ, Hermann WL. Association of exogenous estrogen and endometrial carcinoma. N Engl J Med 1975;293:1164–7.
8. Ziel HU, Finkle WD. Increased risk of endometrial carcinoma among users of conjugated estrogen. N Engl J Med 1995;293:1167–70.
9. Antunes CF, Stolley PP, Rosenshein MB, et al. Endometrial cancer and estrogen use, report of large case-control study. N Engl J Med 1979;300:9–13.
10. Weiss NS, Szekely DR, Austin DF. Increasing incidence of endometrial cancer in the United States. N Engl J Med 1976;294:1259–62.
11. Greenwald P, Caputo TA, Wolfgang PE. Endometrial cancer after menopausal use of estrogens. Obstet Gynecol 1977;50:239–43.
12. Jick H, Watkins RN, Hunter JR, et al. Replacement estrogens and endometrial cancer. N Engl J Med 1979;300:218–22.
13. Parazzini F, La Vecchia C, Bocciolone L, Franceschi S. The epidemiology of endometrial cancer. Gynecol Oncol 1991;41:1–16.
14. MacDonald PC, Siiteri PK. The relationship between the extraglandular production of estrone and the occurrence of endometrial neoplasia. Gynecol Oncol 1974;2:259–63.
15. Schapira DV. Nutrition and cancer prevention. Prim Care 1992;19:481–91.
16. Goodman MT, Hankin JH, Wilkens LR, et al. Diet, body size, physical activity, and the risk of endometrial cancer. Cancer Res 1997;57:5077–85.
17. Negr E, La Vecchia C, Franceschi S, et al. Intake of selected micronutrients and the risk of endometrial carcinoma. Cancer 1996;77:917–23.
18. Lipsett MB. Estrogen use and cancer risk. JAMA 1977;237:1112–5.
19. Fornander T, Rutqvist LE, Wilking N. Effects of tamoxifen on the female genital tract. Ann NY Acad Sci 1991;622:469–76.
20. Jordan VC, Gottardis MM, Satyaswaroop PG. Tamoxifen-stimulated growth of human endometrial carcinoma. Ann NY Acad Sci 1991;622:439–46.
21. Fornander T, Rutqvist LE, Cedermark B, et al. Adjuvant tamoxifen in early breast cancer: occurrence of new primary cancers. Lancet 1989;1:117–20.
22. Fisher B, Costantino JP, Redmond CK, et al. Endometrial cancer in tamoxifen-treated breast cancer patients: findings from the National Surgical Adjuvant Breast and Bowel Project (NSABP) B-14. J Natl Cancer Inst 1994;86:527–37.
23. Bishop JM. The molecular genetics of cancer. Science 1987;235:305–11.
24. Weinberg RA. Tumor suppressor genes. Science 1991;254:1138–46.
25. Marshall CJ. Tumor suppressor genes. Cell 1991;64:313–26.
26. Levine AJ, Momand J, Finlay CA. The p53 tumour suppressor gene. Nature 1991;351:453–6.
27. Harris CC, Hollstein M. Clinical implications of the p53 tumor-suppressor gene. N Engl J Med 1993;329:1318–27.
28. Kohler MF, Berchuck A, Davidoff AM, et al. Overexpression and mutation of p53 in endometrial carcinoma. Cancer Res 1992;52:1622–7.
29. Khalifa MA, Mannel RS, Haraway SD, et al. Expression of EGFR, HER-2/*neu*, p53, and PCNA in endometrioid, serous papillary, and clear cell endometrial adenocarcinomas. Gynecol Oncol 1994;53:84–9.
30. Kihana T, Hamada K, Inoue Y, et al. Mutation and allelic loss of the p53 gene in endometrial carcinoma: incidence and outcome in 92 surgical patients. Cancer 1995;76:72–8.
31. Geisler JP, Wiemann MC, Zhou Z, et al. p53 as a prognostic indicator in endometrial cancer. Gynecol Oncol 1996;61:245–8.
32. Burke TW, Tortolero-Luna G, Malpica A, et al. Endometrial hyperplasia and endometrial cancer. Obstet Gynecol Clin North Am 1996;23:411–56.
33. Plentl AA. Lymphatic system of female genitalia. Philadelphia: WB Saunders, 1971:123.
34. Creasman WT, Morrow CP, Bundy BN, et al. Surgical pathologic spread patterns of endometrial cancer: a Gynecologic Oncology Group study. Cancer 1987;60:8:Suppl:2035–41.
35. Morrow CP: Gynecological oncology. New York: Springer-Verlag 1987:147.
36. Henriksen E. The lymphatic dissemination in endometrial carcinoma: a study of 188 necropsies. Am J Obstet Gynecol 1975;123:570–6.
37. Berman ML, Ballon SC, Lagasse LD, Watring WG. Prognosis and treatment of endometrial cancer. Am J Obstet Gynecol 1980;136:679–88.
38. Morrow CP, DiSaia PJ, Townsend DE. The role of postoperative irradiation in the management of stage I adenocarcinoma of the endometrium. AJR Am J Roentgenol 127:325–9.
39. Ballon SC, Berman ML, Donaldson RC, et al. Pulmonary metastases of endometrial carcinoma. Gynecol Oncol 1979;7:56–65.
40. Ng AB, Reagan JW. Incidence and prognosis of endometrial carcinoma by histologic grade and extent. Obstet Gynecol 1970;35:437–43.
41. Hendrickson M, Ross J, Eifel P, et al. Uterine papillary serous carcinoma: a highly malignant form of endometriod adenocarcinoma. Am J Surg Pathol 1982;6:93–108.
42. Frick HC, Munnell EW, Richart RM, et al. Carcinoma of the endometrium. Am J Obstet Gynecol 1973;115:663–76.
43. Kempson RL, Pokorny GE. Adenocarcinoma of the endometrium in women aged forty and younger. Cancer 1968;21:650–62.
44. Allen DG, Correy JF, Marsden DE. Abnormal uterine bleeding and cancer of the genital tract. Aust NZ J Obstet Gynaecol 1990;30:81–3.

45. Alberico S, Conoscenti G, Vegliáo P, et al. A clinical and epidemiological study of 245 postmenopausal metrorrhagia patients. Clin Exp Obstet Gynecol 1989;16:113–21.
46. Cherkis RC, Patten SF Jr, Andrews TJ, et al. Significance of normal endometrial cells detected by cervical cytology. Obstet Gynecol 1988;71:242–4.
47. Cherkis RC, Patten SF Jr, Dickinson JC, Dekanich AS. Significance of atypical endometrial cells detected by cervical cytology. Obstet Gynecol 1987;69:786–9.
48. Blumenfeld W, Holly EA, Mansur DL, King EB. Histiocytes and the detection of endometrial adenocarcinoma. Acta Cytol 1985;29:317–22.
49. Chamber JT, Chambers SK. Endometrial sampling: When? Where? Why? With what? Clinical Obstet Gynecol 1992;35:28–39.
50. Cohen CJ, Gusberg SB. Screening for endometrial cancer. Clin Obstet Gynecol 1975;18:27–39.
51. Granberg S, Wiklan, M, Karlsson B, et al. Endometrial thickness as measured by endovaginal ultrasonography for identifying endometrial abnormality. Am J Obstet Gynecol 1991;164:47–52.
52. Bourne TH, Campbell S, Steer CV, et al. Detection of endometrial cancer by transvaginal ultrasonography with color flow imaging and blood flow analysis: a preliminary report. Gynecol Oncol 1991;40:253–9.
53. FIGO News. Int J Gynecol Obstet 1987;28:1987.
54. Lewis BV, Stallworthy JA, Cowdell R. Adenocarcinoma of the body of the uterus. J Obst Gynaecol Br Commonw 1970;77:343–8.
55. Stallworthy JA. Surgery of endometrial cancer in the Bonney tradition. Ann R Coll Surg 1971;48:293–305.
56. Boronow RC. Surgical staging of endometrial cancer: evolution, evaluation, and responsible challenge—a personal perspective. Gynecol Oncol 1997;66:179–89.
57. DiSaia PJ, Creasman WT, Boronow RC, Blessing JA. Risk factors and recurrent patterns in stage I endometrial cancer. Am J Obstet Gynecol 1985;151:1009–15.
58. Homesley HD. Revised 1988 International Federation of Gynecology and Obstetrics staging systems for endometrial and vulvar cancer. Clin Obstet Gynecol 1992;35:89–94.
59. Campbell K, Nuss RC, Benrubi GI. An evaluation of the clinical staging of endometrial cancer. J Reprod Med 1988;33:8–10.
60. Chen SS, Rumancik WM, Spiegel G. Magnetic resonance imaging in stage I endometrial carcinoma. Obstet Gynecol 1990;75:274–7.
61. Malkasian GD Jr. Carcinoma of the endometrium: effect of stage and grade on survival. Cancer 1978;41:996–1001.
62. Berman ML, Afridi MA, Kanbour AI, Ball HG. Risk factors and prognosis in stage II endometrial cancer. Gynecol Oncol 1982;14:49–61.
63. Pecorelli S. Annual report on the results of treatment in gynaecological cancers. J Epidemiol Biostat 1998;3:45.
64. Cheon HK. Prognosis of endometrial carcinoma. Obstet Gynecol 1969;34:680–4.
65. Jones HW III. Treatment of adenocarcinoma of the endometrium. Obstet Gynecol Surv 1975;30:147.
66. Rozier JC, Underwood PB. Use of progestational agents in endometrial adenocarcinoma. Obstet Gynecol 1974;44:60–4.
67. Jeffrey JF, Krepart GV, Lotocki RJ. Papillary serous adenocarcinoma of the endometrium. Obstet Gynecol 1986;67:670–4.
68. Dunton CJ, Balsara G, McFarland M, Hernandez E. Uterine papillary serous carcinoma: a review. Obstet Gynecol Surv 1991;46:97–102.
69. Goff BA, Kato D, Schmidt RA, et al. Uterine papillary serous carcinoma: patterns of metastatic spread. Gynecol Oncol 1994;54:264–8.
70. Turner DA, Gershenson DM, Atkinson N, et al. The prognostic significance of peritoneal cytology for stage I endometrial cancer. Obstet Gynecol 1989;74:775–80.
71. Kadar N, Homesley HD, Malfetano JH. Positive peritoneal cytology is an adverse factor in endometrial carcinoma only if there is other evidence of extrauterine disease. Gynecol Oncol 1992;46:145–9.
72. Cancer among blacks and other minorities: statistical profiles. Washington, D.C.: U.S. Department of Health and Human Services, NIH Publication No. 86–2785, 1986.
73. Soper JT, Christensen CW. Steroid receptors and endometrial cancer. Clin Obstet Gynaecol 1986;13:825–42.
74. Fu YS. Presented at the first meeting of the Gynecologic Cancer Society, Amsterdam, October 4–8, 1987 p 43.
75. Berchuck A, Rodriguez G, Kinney RB, et al. Overexpression of HER-2/neu in endometrial cancer is associated with advanced stage disease. Am J Obstet Gynecol 1991;164:15–21.
76. Creasman WT. Prognostic significance of hormone receptors in endometrial cancer. Cancer 1993;71:1467–70.
77. Kauppila A. Oestrogen and progestin receptors as prognostic indicators in endometrial cancer. A review of the literature. Acta Oncol 1989;28:561–6.
78. Borst MP, Baker VV, Dixon D, et al. Oncogene alterations in endometrial carcinoma. Gynecol Oncol 1990;38:364–6.
79. Kohler MF, Berchuck A, Davidoff AM, et al. Overexpression and mutation of p53 in endometrial carcinoma. Cancer Res 1992;52:1622–7.
80. Reinartz JJ, George E, Leindgen BR, Niethans G. Expression of p53, transforming growth factor alpha, epidermal growth factor receptor, and *cerb*-2 in endometrial carcinoma and correlation with survival and known predictors of survival. Hum Pathol 1994;25:1075–83.
81. Lukes AS, Kohler MF, Pieper MF, et al. Multivariable analysis of DNA ploidy, p53, and HER-2n prognostic factors in endometrial cancer. Cancer 1994;73:2380–5.
82. Lees DH. An evaluation of the treatment in carcinoma of the body of the uterus. J Obstet Gynecol 1969;76:615–23.
83. Rutledge F. The role of radical hysterectomy in adenocarcinoma of the endometrium. Gynecol Oncol 1974;2:3345–7.
84. de Muelenaere GF. The case against Wertheim's hysterectomy in endometrial carcinoma. J Obst Gynaecol 1973;80:728–34.
85. Shanh CA, Green TH. Evaluation of current management of endometrial carcinoma. Obstet Gynecol 39:500–29.
86. Bloss JD, Berman MF, Bloss LP, Buller RE. The use of vaginal hysterectomy for the management of stage I endometrial cancer in the medically compromised patient, Gynecol Oncol 1991;4074–7.
87. Massi G, Savino L, Susini T. Vaginal hysterectomy versus abdominal hysterectomy for the treatment of stage I endometrial adenocarcinoma. Am J Obstet Gynecol 1996;174:1320–6.
88. Childers JM, Brzechffa PR, Hatch KD, Surwit EA. Laparoscopically assisted surgical staging (LASS) of endometrial cancer. Gynecol Oncol 1993;51:33–8.
89. Yokoyama Y, Maruyama H, Sato S, Saito Y. Indispensability of pelvic and paraaortic lymphadenectomy in endometrial cancers. Gynecol Oncol 1997;64:411–7.
90. Mohan DS, Samuels MA, Selim MA, et al. Long-term outcomes of therapeutic pelvic lymphadenectomy for stage I endometrial adenocarcinoma. Gynecol Oncol 98;70:165–171.
91. Kilgore LC, Partridge EE, Alvarez RD, et al. Adenocarcinoma of the endometrium: survival comparisons of patients with and without pelvic nodesampling. Gynecol Oncol 1995;56:29–33.
92. Belinson JL, Lee KR, Badger GJ, et al. Clinical stage I adenocarcinoma of the endometrium—analysis of recurrences and the potential benefit of staging lymphadenectomy. Gynecol Oncol 1992;44:17–23.
93. Aalders J, Abeler V, Kolstad P, Onsrud M. Postoperative external irradiation and prognostic parameters in stage I endometrial carcinoma: clinical and histopathologic study of 540 patients. Obstet Gynecol 1980;56:419–27.
94. Morrow CP, Bundy BN, Kurman RJ, et al. Relationship between surgical-pathological risk factors and outcome in clinical stage I and II carcinoma of the endometrium: a Gynecologic Oncology Group study. Gynecol Oncol 1991;40:55–65.
95. Irwin C, Levin W, Fyles A, et al. The role of adjuvant radiotherapy in carcinoma of the endometrium—results in 550 patients with pathologic stage I disease. Gynecol Oncol 1998;70:247–54.
96. Orr J, Holiman JL, Orr PF. Stage I corpus cancer: is teletherapy necessary? Am J Obstet Gynecol 1997;176:777–8.
97. Beiler DD, Schumtz DA, O'Rourke TL. Carcinoma of the endometrium: radiation and surgery versus surgery alone. Radiology 1972;102:159–64.
98. Graham J. The value of preoperative or postoperative treatment by radium for carcinoma of the uterine body. Surg Gynecol Obstet 1971;132:855–60.
99. Mannel RS, Berman ML, Walker JL, et al. Management of endometrial cancer with suspected cervical involvement. Obstet Gynecol 1990;75:1016–22.
100. Barber HR, Brunschwig A. Treatment and results of recurrent cancer of corpus uteri in patients receiving anterior and total pelvic exenteration 1947–1963. Cancer 1968;22:949–55.
101. Morrow CP, Bundy BN, Homesley HD, et al. Doxorubicin as an adjuvant following surgery and radiation therapy in patients with high-risk endometrial carcinoma, stage I and occult stage II: a Gynecologic Oncology Group study. Gynecol Oncol 1990;36:166–71.

102. Burke TW, Gershenson DM, Morris M, et al. Postoperative adjuvant cisplatin, doxorubicin, and cyclophosphamide (PAC) chemotherapy in women with high-risk endometrial carcinoma. Gynecol Oncol 1994;55:47–50.
103. Bickenbach W, Lochmuller H, Dirlich G, et al. Factor analysis of endometrial carcinoma in relation to treatment. Obstet Gynecol 1967;29:632–6.
104. Ahmad K, Kim YH, Deppe G, et al. Results of treatment in locally advanced carcinoma of the endometrium. Acta Oncol 1990;29:203–9.
105. Backstrom T, Cajander S, Kjellgren O, Persson H. Results of primary radiation treatment of endometrial carcinoma. 20 years' experience of an unselected material from the north of Sweden. Acta Oncol 1989;28:569–75.
106. Fishman DA, Roberts KB, Chambers JT, et al. Radiation therapy as exclusive treatment for medically inoperable patients with stage I and II endometrioid carcinoma with endometrium. Gynecol Oncol 1996;61:189–96.
107. Kohorn EI. Gestagens and endometrial carcinoma. Gynecol Oncol 1976;4:398–411.
108. Moore TD, Phillips PH, Nerenstone SR, Cheson BD. Systemic treatment of advanced and recurrent endometrial carcinoma: current status and future directions. J Clin Oncol 1991;9:1071–88.
109. Thigpen JT, Buchsbaum HJ, Mangan C, Blessing JA. Phase II trial of adriamycin in the treatment of advanced or recurrent endometrial carcinoma: a Gynecologic Oncology Group study. Cancer Treat Rep 1979;63:21–7.
110. Thigpen JT, Blessing JA, Homesley H, et al. Phase II trial of cisplatin as first-line chemotherapy in patients with advanced or recurrent endometrial carcinoma: a Gynecologic Oncology Group study. Gynecol Oncol 1989;33:68–70.
111. Ball H, Blessing JA, Lentz S, Mutch D. A phase II trial of Taxol in advanced and recurrent adenocarcinoma of the endometrium: a Gynecologic Oncology Group study. Gynecol Oncol 1996;62:278–81.
112. Ober WB. NY Acad Sci 1959;75:568.
113. Rutledge F. Gynecology oncology. New York: John Wiley & Sons, 1976:1931.
114. Kempson RL, Bari W. Uterine sarcomas. Classification, diagnosis, and prognosis. Hum Pathol 1970;1:331–49.
115. Norris HJ, Taylor HB. Criteria for histologic diagnosis of leiomyosarcoma. Obstet Gynecol 1972;40:132–4.
116. DiSaia PJ, Morrow CP, Boronow R, et al. Endometrial sarcoma: lymphatic spread pattern. Am J Obstet Gynecol 1978;130:104–5.
117. Gilbert HA, Kagan AR, Lagasse L, et al. The value of radiation therapy in uterine sarcoma. Obstet Gynecol 1975;45:84–8.
118. Omura GA, Major FJ, Blessing JA, et al. A randomized study of adriamycin with and without dimethyl triazenoimidazole carboxamide in advanced uterine sarcomas. Cancer 1983;52:626–32.
119. Sutton G, Blessing JA, Malfetano JH. Ifosfamide and doxorubicin in the treatment of advanced leiomyosarcomas of the uterus: a Gynecologic Oncology Group study. Gynecol Oncol 1996;62:226–9.
120. Seski JC, Edwards CL, Herson J, Rutledge FN. Cisplatin chemotherapy for disseminated endometrial cancer. Obstet Gynecol 1982;59:225–8.
121. Burke TW, Eifel PJ, Muggia FM. Cancer of the uterine body. In: DeVita VT Jr, eds., Cancer—principles and practices of oncology. Philadelphia: JB Lippincott, 1997:1478–99.
122. Slayton RE, Blessing JA, Delgado G. Phase II trial of etoposide in the management of advanced or recurrent endometrial carcinoma: a Gynecologic Oncology Group study. Cancer Treat Rep 1982;66:1669–71.
123. Muggia FM, Chia G, Reed LJ, Romney SL. Doxorubicin-cyclophosphamide: effective chemotherapy for advanced endometrial adenocarcinoma. Am J Obstet Gynecol 1977;128:314–9.
124. Seski JC, Edwards CL, Gershenson DM, Copeland LJ. Doxorubicin and cyclophosphamide chemotherapy for disseminated endometrial cancer. Obstet Gynecol 1981;58:88–91.
125. Kauppila A, Janne O, Kujansuu E, Vihko R. Treatment of advanced endometrial adenocarcinoma with a combined cytotoxic therapy. Predictive value of cytosol estrogen and progestin receptor levels. Cancer 1980;46:2162–7.
126. Deppe G, Jacobs AJ, Bruckner H, Cohen CJ. Chemotherapy of advanced and recurrent endometrial carcinoma with cyclophosphamide, doxorubicin, 5-fluorouracil, and megestrol acetate. Am J Obstet Gynecol 1981;140:313–6.
127. Piver MS, Barlow JJ, Lele SB, Yazigi R. Adriamycin in localized and metastatic uterine sarcomas. J Surg Oncol 1979;12:263–5.
128. Parente JT, Axelrod MR, Levy JL, Chiang CE. Leiomyosarcoma of the uterus with pulmonary metastases: a favorable response to operation and chemotherapy in a patient monitored with serial carcinoembryonic antigen. Am J Obstet Gynecol 1978;131:812–5.
129. Azizi F, Bitran J, Javehari G, Herbst AL. Remission of uterine leiomyosarcomas treated with vincristine, Adriamycin, and dimethyl-triazeno-imidazole carboximide. Am J Obstet Gynecol 1979;133:379–81.
130. Green JB, Green S, Alberts DS, et al. Carboplatin therapy in advanced endometrial cancer. Obstet Gynecol 1990;75:696–700.

# CHAPTER 58

# VULVA

● CHRISTINE H. HOLSCHNEIDER ● JONATHAN S. BEREK

In the early part of the 20th century, vulvar cancer was generally far advanced at the time of diagnosis, and inadequate surgical attempts resulted in 5-year survival rates of less than 25%.[1, 2] Following the surgical principles espoused by the Frenchman Basset,[3] Taussig in the United States and Way in Britain demonstrated 5-year survival rates of about 60% using a radical en bloc resection of the vulva and bilateral regional lymph nodes.[4, 5] Postoperative morbidity with wound breakdown and infection was high and prolonged hospitalization the norm.

Because vulvar cancer is increasingly being diagnosed at an earlier stage and in younger patients, a more individualized and less radical surgical approach to the disease has evolved over the past decades in an effort to decrease morbidity, disfigurement, and interference with body image and sexual function. Such innovations included the radical local excision rather than radical vulvectomy for small and intermediate-size lesions,[6, 7] individualization of the extent of lymphadenectomy,[8–10] and the use of separate groin incisions for the lymph node dissection.[11] For patients with advanced vulvar cancer involving the bladder and rectum, the use of radiation with or without synchronous chemotherapy has decreased the extensiveness of surgery required, allowing for organ preservation in cases in which exenterative procedures historically would have been performed.[12, 13]

## Classification of Epithelial Disorders of the Vulva

In the past, numerous terms were used to denote disorders of epithelial growth and differentiation that produce a variety

*Table 58–1.* International Society for the Study of Vulvar Disease Classification of Vulvar Diseases

| Current Classification | Replaced Former Terms |
| --- | --- |
| Non-neoplastic epithelial disorders of skin and mucosa | Vulvar dystrophies |
| Lichen sclerosus | |
| Squamous hyperplasia | Hyperplastic dystrophy without atypia |
| Other dermatoses (vulvar manifestation of other common dermatoses such as psoriasis, lichen simplex, lichen planus, dermatitis) | |
| Mixed non-neoplastic and neoplastic epithelial disorders | |
| Intraepithelial neoplasia | Hyperplastic dystrophy with atypia |
| Squamous intraepithelial neoplasia | Bowenoid papulosis refers to VIN associated with numerous papules |
| VIN 1 (mild dysplasia) | |
| VIN 2 (moderate dysplasia) | |
| VIN 3 (severe dysplasia, carcinoma in situ) | The following three formerly used terms describe merely variants of VIN 3: erythroplasia of Queyrat, Bowen's disease, and carcinoma in situ simplex |
| Nonsquamous intraepithelial neoplasia | |
| Paget's disease | |
| Noninvasive tumors of melanocytes | |
| Invasive tumors | |

VIN, vulvar intraepithelial neoplasia.
From Committee on Terminology, International Society for the Study of Vulvar Disease: New nomenclature for vulvar disease. Int J Gynecol Pathol 1989;8:83–84.

of gross changes on the vulva. Such terms included *leukoplakia, lichen sclerosus et atrophicus, primary atrophy, sclerotic dermatosis, atrophic and hyperplastic vulvitis, senile vulvitis,* and *kraurosis vulvae*. In 1966, Jeffcoate suggested that these terms did not refer to separate entities because their macroscopic and microscopic appearances were interchangeable. He therefore assigned the generic term *chronic vulvar dystrophy* to the entire group.[14]

In 1976, the International Society for the Study of Vulvar Diseases approved a classification for vulvar dystrophies and atypias.[15] In 1986, this classification was replaced by the currently used classification system of neoplastic and non-neoplastic epithelial disorders of the vulva (Table 58–1).[16]

## Examination of the Vulva

Early-stage disease at diagnosis is the most important prognostic factor in vulvar cancer. Given its location on exposed skin, vulvar cancer and its preinvasive lesions should be amenable to early diagnosis. A gynecologic examination must include a thorough inspection and palpation of the vulva for masses, ulcers, and color changes. Any lesion on the vulva is abnormal and warrants biopsy, with the exception of obviously infectious changes, which then need appropriate work-up, treatment, and biopsy if they persist. Careful palpation of the inguinal region is important.

Diagnostic measures that enhance the suspicion of an

abnormality or that may guide the biopsy to the site of most significant abnormality include colposcopy with acetic acid and staining the vulva with toluidine blue. For colposcopy, cotton balls containing 2 to 5% acetic acid are applied to the vulva and need to be left for several minutes. Intraepithelial neoplasia produces an acetowhite lesion with or without punctations, which should be sampled. Acetic acid precipitates nucleoprotein, which is increased in vulvar intraepithelial neoplasia (VIN) and also in areas of infection or tissue repair. Toluidine blue is a nuclear stain that detects cellular nuclei at the surface of ulcerations, infections, and neoplastic processes. The vulva is painted with 1% toluidine blue, which after 2 minutes is washed off with 1% acetic acid.[17, 18] Abnormal areas retain the blue dye and should be sampled, whereas normal areas remain unstained. False-positive results may be caused by infection or non-neoplastic ulceration, whereas false-negative results may occur in thick hyperkeratotic lesions, as well as ulcerated or abraded lesions, which absorb only a small amount of dye.

Biopsy provides the definitive diagnosis for any vulvar lesion. The area is cleansed with an antiseptic solution and infiltrated with a local anesthetic. The Key dermatologic punch biopsy instrument should be used because it allows for the most accurate orientation of the specimen and evaluation of the thickness of the lesion. Monsel's solution or silver nitrate can be used for hemostasis. Rarely, a suture is needed. If multifocal lesions are found, repeated biopsies may be required. Excisional biopsies should be reserved for cases in which punch biopsy did not yield a satisfactory pathologic specimen, for pigmented lesions, or for select cases with extensive ulceration or induration.

## Noninvasive Lesions of the Vulva

### NON-NEOPLASTIC EPITHELIAL DISORDERS

The association between non-neoplastic epithelial disorders (NNEDs) of the vulva and invasive squamous cell carcinoma has been a matter of debate ever since lichen sclerosus (LS) was first recognized on the vulva. NNEDs are found concurrently with vulvar cancer in 52 to 87% of vulvectomy specimens.[19–22] In the majority of these cases, the diagnosis of NNED has not preceded the detection of cancer, but concomitant NNED was diagnosed on the vulvectomy specimen.[22, 23] However, this association does not prove a causative link. It may merely indicate that NNEDs are the result of local reaction to the same chronic stimulus that contributes to the development of invasive carcinoma. In a review of 3093 cases of symptomatic vulvar LS reported in the literature, Carlson and colleagues found a compiled incidence of vulvar squamous cell carcinoma arising in LS of 4.5%. The reported average duration of LS prior to the diagnosis of carcinoma was 10 years.[24]

**Lichen Sclerosus.** The etiology and pathogenesis of LS, a well-recognized benign epithelial disorder, remain unknown. Proposed theories include reports on the absence of collagenases, increased collagen inhibitor enzyme, and increase in elastase activity.[25] An autoimmune mechanism has been implied, because about 20% of women with LS have other autoimmune disorders.[26] Furthermore, a universally observed increase in the number and activity of certain T cells and Langerhans' cells in LS suggests a possible role of the skin immune system in the pathogenesis of LS.[27] The disorder is characterized histopathologically by epidermal atrophy, with blunting or loss of the rete ridges and concomitant edema of the superficial dermis, giving it an acellular homogeneous appearance. Beneath this zone of hyalinization are underlying inflammatory lymphocytic infiltrates.

LS may be found in all age groups, including prepubertal girls with pruritus. It is most common in postmenopausal white women. Presenting symptoms generally are vulvar pruritus and dyspareunia. LS involves the pudendum and often continues across the perineum and perianal region. The skin is white, sometimes pinkish, thinned, crinkled, and like parchment paper. The skin appears thickened and hyperkeratotic if there is concomitant squamous hyperplasia. Erosions, purpura, and sometimes hemorrhagic areas, fissures, and ulcerations occur with extensive lesions, pruritus, and scratching. A hallmark of LS is the loss of anatomic structural detail with often almost complete disappearance of the labia minora. Shrinkage of the introitus leading to introital stenosis may be found, as well as atrophy of the clitoral structures. Biopsy specimens should be taken to confirm the diagnosis prior to implementing topical therapy. Any other associated disorders should be investigated and treated concomitantly, such as candidiasis or uncontrolled diabetes.

High-potency steroids are the treatment of choice, with greater than 90% subjective and objective response rates.[28–31] Less effective, traditionally used remedies include topical 2% testosterone and 1 to 2% progesterone. Lifetime therapy is generally required to achieve permanent control of the disease. Surgical therapy, such as laser evaporation, wide local excision, or skinning vulvectomy, should be reserved for patients who continue to be severely symptomatic despite many different medical management approaches. Postoperative recurrence rates are as high as 50%.[32]

**Squamous Hyperplasia.** Squamous hyperplasia is seen in about one third of patients with LS. Clinically, the lesions are frequently localized, elevated, and well delineated and have a white or dusky red appearance, depending on the degree of hyperkeratosis. Seen histologically are hyperkeratosis, acanthosis, which causes distortion of the rete pegs, and frequently parakeratosis. Topical steroids are the mainstay of therapy.

## VULVAR INTRAEPITHELIAL NEOPLASIA

The anogenital epithelium is derived from the embryonic cloaca and extends from the cervix to the vagina, vulva, anus, and lower 3 cm of rectal mucosa up to the dentate line. There are similar etiologic factors and clinical presentations for some of the pathologic processes in the lower genital tract, especially the susceptibility to infection with human papillomavirus (HPV) and the potential for preinvasive disease: cervical intraepithelial neoplasia (CIN), vaginal intraepithelial neoplasia (VAIN), VIN, and perianal intraepithelial neoplasia. Therefore, it is not surprising that squamous intraepithelial neoplasia is frequently multicentric, defined as involving several anatomic sites, and multifocal, indicating the presence of several disease foci within the same site. About 10% of patients with CIN 3 have concomi-

tant preinvasive disease at other sites (3% VAIN 3, 7% VIN 2 to 3).[33] Similarly, about 60% of women with VAIN 3 and 60% of those with vulvar VIN 3, are found to have preexisting or synchronous cervical neoplasia.[33–35] Thus, it is important to evaluate all sites potentially involved in the neoplastic process. Although multicentric lesions tend to be associated with the oncogenic HPV types, particularly HPV-16,[36, 37] neoplastic transformation within the stable squamous epithelia of the vulva and vagina is much less common than in the cervix.

**Epidemiology, Etiology, and Malignant Potential.** The incidence of VIN 3 almost doubled over the past two decades, from 1.2 to 2.1 per 100,000 women, with younger patients in the third and fourth decades of life being most commonly affected.[38] This increase is thought to be due to improved surveillance as well as a concomitant rise in HPV infection. Seventy-five percent of cases of VIN 3 affect premenopausal women. Risk factors are similar to those for vulvar cancer, with HPV infection, tobacco use, and immunosuppression being of major importance.[39–41] Although most of the vulvar condylomata acuminata contain the low-risk HPV subtypes 6 and 11, VIN, especially if multifocal or high grade, often contains the oncogenic subtypes 16, 18, and 31. There does not appear to be a racial predisposition to VIN.

The continuum from intraepithelial neoplasia to invasive carcinoma is not as well documented for VIN to vulvar carcinoma as it is for CIN to cervical carcinoma. Although the latency period for progression from preinvasive to invasive disease is about 5 to 10 years in cervical cancer, it appears to be 25 to 30 years in vulvar cancer. The malignant potential of carcinoma in situ of the vulva is still debated. Several studies have focused on the relationship of VIN to vulvar carcinoma. Jones and Rowan found that 88% (seven of eight) women with untreated VIN 3 developed invasive squamous cell carcinoma of the vulva within 8 years.[42] Following initial treatment of VIN 3, 4 to 8% of patients are reported to subsequently develop invasive vulvar carcinoma.[35, 42–44]

**Histopathology.** VIN 3 lesions are subdivided into three types based on their morphologic features, which may occur as pure forms or mixed: warty (condylomatous), basaloid (usual type), and differentiated (simplex type). The warty type is characterized by hyperkeratosis, parakeratosis, and marked proliferation with numerous mitotic figures. Maturation occurs, albeit abnormal. The surface is undulating or spiking, giving it a condylomatous appearance. Surface keratinocytes with koilocytosis, binucleation, or multinucleation are common. The basaloid type has a thickened epithelium with a relatively flat, smooth surface and is composed of atypical immature parabasal type cells with numerous mitotic figures and enlarged hyperchromatic nuclei. The differentiated type is characterized by abnormal cells confined to the parabasal and basal portion of the rete pegs. Mild nuclear atypia may be seen. Keratin pearl formation may be present.[45]

**Clinical Features and Diagnosis.** Approximately half of the patients are asymptomatic. If symptoms exist, pruritus is the most common complaint, although some patients present with an altered appearance of the vulva or a palpable abnormality. Other cases are diagnosed during colposcopy for an abnormal Papanicolaou's (Pap) smear. The minority of patients present with perineal pain or discharge; generally, this is after chronic itching or scratching of the vulva. There is no characteristic clinical appearance, and more than one pattern may be seen in the same patient. About half of the lesions are white and raised,[45] but the color may be red, pink, gray, or brown. Gross warty tumors have been seen in approximately 20% of cases.[44] The distribution of VIN appears to have two distinct forms: Unifocal lesion are predominantly seen in the postmenopausal patient, and their relation to HPV has been less well established. Multifocal lesions are usually HPV associated and tend to occur predominantly in the younger, premenopausal patient. Confluent or multicentric lesions exist in up to two thirds of case.[46] The interlabial grooves, posterior fourchette, and perineum are most frequently affected. More extensive disease is often confluent, involving the labia majora, labia minora, and perianal skin.

**Treatment.** Treatment for VIN must be individualized on the basis of biopsy results, extent of disease, and a patient's symptoms. Management options include wide local excision, skinning vulvectomy, laser ablation, and topical treatment with 5-fluorouracil (5-FU). Local excision of the individual lesion with a 1-cm margin followed by approximation of the defect is the mainstay of therapy because this allows adequate histologic evaluation to exclude invasive foci. For treatment of VIN, removal of the epidermis provides sufficient depth. However, a small amount of underlying dermis should be removed also to allow for exclusion and assessment of invasive disease. An unsuspected underlying invasive squamous cell carcinoma is found in 10 to 22% of patients undergoing surgical excision for VIN 3.[35, 39] This underscores the tremendous additional diagnostic advantage of an excisional treatment over ablative or medical management modalities. VIN recurs in one third of the patients, regardless of whether treatment is by laser, wide local excision, or vulvectomy.[35, 39, 43, 44] In a study by Modesitt and colleagues, margin status correlated significantly with the risk of recurrence, which was 46% for the 39 patients with positive margins and 17% for the 18 patients with negative margins.[39] Additional risk factors for recurrence are grade of VIN and multifocal as well as multicentric disease.[35, 43] For more extensive lesions, skinning vulvectomy, in which the vulvar skin is removed along a relatively avascular plane beneath the epidermis, may be used.[47, 48] Closure can be achieved either primarily or using a split-thickness skin graft. Reported recurrence rates are 27 to 39%.[47, 49]

Conservative therapies aimed at preserving the vulvar anatomy have been attempted, particularly in younger pa-

tients. Topical 5-FU (Efudex) is effective in 40 to 75% of cases.[50, 51] Careful colposcopic examination with biopsies to exclude invasive disease is mandatory prior to 5-FU treatment. The cream causes a chemical desquamation of the lesion, which generally causes a significant amount of burning, pain, inflammation, and edema as well as occasional painful ulcerations. Topical immunotherapy, photodynamic therapy, and the use of chemopreventive agents such as retinyl acetate gel are being investigated. Regardless of the treatment modality used, long-term surveillance of the entire lower genital tract is mandatory.

## PAGET'S DISEASE

**Epidemiology, Etiology, and Malignant Potential.** In 1874, Sir James Paget first described a cutaneous lesion that affects the nipple and areola of the breast and is associated with an underlying ductal carcinoma.[52] The first case of vulvar Paget's disease was reported by Dubreuilh in 1901.[53] Paget's disease of the vulva is a rare intraepithelial lesion accounting for less than 1% of all vulvar neoplasms. It predominantly affects postmenopausal white women at a median age of 60 to 70 years[54, 55] but may occur as early as the fourth decade of life.[56] Although Paget's disease of the breast is universally associated with an underlying malignancy, usually an underlying ductal carcinoma,[57] a vulvar malignancy is found in 20 to 30% of patients with Paget's disease of the vulva. This constitutes an underlying adenocarcinoma of the vulva in about 10% and invasive Paget's disease in an average of 11% of patients (Table 58–2). Most cases of invasion are associated with extensive Paget's disease of the skin.[55] Although an underlying adenocarcinoma may be suspected on clinical examination, the diagnosis of invasion may at times be made only by careful examination of the excised specimen,[58] in particular in cases of invasive Paget's disease.[59] In addition to its link to the risk of a local malignancy, Paget's disease of the vulva may herald synchronous or metachronous invasive cancer in other sites in about 21% of patients (see Table 58–2), such as tumors of the breast, gastrointestinal tract, skin, cervix, endometrium, ovary, bladder, thyroid, or lung.[54, 55, 59–61] When the anal mucosa is involved there is usually an underlying rectal carcinoma.[61] Thus, patients with vulvar Paget's disease should undergo a thorough work-up for malignancy at the time of diagnosis and close cancer surveillance thereafter.[62–64]

The origin of the Paget's cell remains controversial. Electron microscopic studies indicate that it originates from plur-

*Table 58–2.* **Paget's Disease of the Vulva: Underlying Vulvar Adenocarcinoma, Invasive Paget's Disease, Associated Nonvulvar Malignancies, and Recurrent Intraepithelial Paget's Disease**

| Reference | Number | Underlying Vulvar Adenocarcinoma | Invasive Paget's Disease | Associated Nonvulvar Malignancies | Recurrent Intraepithelial Paget's Disease |
|---|---|---|---|---|---|
| Bergen et al[162] | 14 | 0 | 0 | 1 (7%) | 3 (21%) |
| Feuer et al[59] | 19 | 1 (5%) | 2 (11%) | 5 (26%) | 8/17 (47%) |
| Curtin et al[54] | 36 | 5 (14%) | 0 | 9/28 (32%) | 6/28 (21%) |
| Fishman et al[63] | 14 | 2 (14%) | 1 (7%) | 7 (50%) | 5 (36%) |
| Kodama et al[64] | 27 | 9 (33%) | 9 (33%) | 1 (4%) | 4/19 (21%) |
| Fanning et al[55] | 100 | 4 (4%) | 12 (12%) | 20 (20%) | 30/84 (36%) |
| Total | 210 | 21 (10%) | 24 (11%) | 43/202 (21%) | 56/17 (32%) |

ipotent germinative cells in the epidermis.[65, 66] Cells from this layer are the precursors of squamous keratinocytes, sweat gland cells, hair follicles, or other adnexal structures. Some Paget's cells show the ultrastructural characteristics of keratinocytes, whereas others demonstrate the features of glandular cells.[67, 68] This concept of abnormal differentiation from the germinal layer is consistent with the clinical observation of frequently multifocal intraepithelial Paget's disease and explains the typical location of Paget's cells adjacent to the basal layer in both the epidermis and the adnexal structures.[69] Little is understood about the molecular pathogenesis of Paget's disease. Feuer and colleagues found associated koilocytes in 67% of patients with vulvar Paget's disease,[59] but in situ hybridization and polymerase chain reaction DNA studies failed to detect HPV.[70, 71]

**Histopathology.** The disease is characterized by the pathognomonic Paget's cells seen within the epidermis and skin adnexa. Paget cells are large round or oval cells with abundant pale, at times vacuolated cytoplasm and vesicular nuclei. These cells are rich in mucopolysaccharide, a diastase-resistant substance reactive to periodic acid–Schiff staining.[64]

**Clinical Features.** Pruritus, burning, irritation, and tenderness are the most frequent presenting symptoms; they are typically present for prolonged periods.[55, 59] The disease tends to be multifocal. The affected area is usually well demarcated and has a characteristic bright red, erythematous, scaly, eczematoid appearance, with scattered white plaque-like lesions. The disease usually begins in a hair-bearing region of the skin. The disease may initially appear as a localized lesion, but progressive growth results in involvement of the greater part of the vulva with possible extension onto the mons pubis, thighs, and buttocks. Rarely it may extend to involve the mucosa of the rectum, vagina, and urinary tract.[72] These more extensive lesions are usually elevated and have a velvety texture. Persistent weeping is a distressing feature of extensive Paget's disease.

**Treatment.** The mainstay of therapy is surgery. The fact that the extent of histologically demonstrable disease is for greater than that of the visible lesion is clinically relevant to the management of Paget's disease of the vulva.[73] In particular, because a negative resection margin is associated with a 15% recurrence risk and a positive margin with a 35% recurrence risk of Paget's disease, excluding all those cases with initially diagnosed invasion (Table 58–3), a very wide

local excision is required to decrease the likelihood of recurrence. It may be helpful to check the surgical margins with frozen section to assist complete surgical removal of the disease.[54, 61] Although a positive frozen section result may prompt the removal of an additional margin, it is important to recognize that a negative frozen section margin may still have Paget's cells on permanent section in about one third of cases.[54, 62, 63] This may be because of the multifocal nature of the disease, as well as sampling errors. If the disease is extensive, a wide superficial vulvectomy is frequently required. A split-thickness skin graft may be used to cover the defect. A more limited resection aimed at palliation of symptoms may be preferable in the case of a medically unfit patient. An underlying malignancy is not always apparent preoperatively. Thus, the superficial dermis should be removed also, as adnexal structures of the vulvar skin extend as deep as 0.4 cm.[62] Careful sectioning of the underlying apocrine gland–bearing tissue is essential for histologic detection of an occult adenocarcinoma. If any underlying malignancy is present, the treatment should be the same as for other invasive carcinomas of the vulva and usually requires at least a radical wide excision and ipsilateral inguinofemoral lymphadenectomy. The reported recurrence rate for patients with invasive Paget's disease of the vulva is 8% in the largest series to date.[55] The prognosis is largely determined by the initial stage of the disease.[54, 58, 62, 72] Approximately one half of the patients with Paget's disease and an underlying adenocarcinoma are found to have metastatic disease at the time of diagnosis.[55] There are reports of regional lymph node metastases even with minimally invasive Paget's disease.[74]

Intraepithelial Paget's disease of the vulva recurs in about one fourth of cases. The risk correlates with the margin status, as discussed earlier. Nondiploidy is associated with an increased risk of recurrence.[75] The reported median time to recurrence is 3 years. It is not unusual to find recurrences as late as 15 years after diagnosis.[54, 55, 59] Hence, continued postoperative surveillance is warranted. Traditional teaching is that recurrences are generally noninvasive and may thus be treated with minor local excisions or laser therapy if they are detected early. However, there have been case reports of invasive Paget's disease,[59] as well as underlying adenocarcinoma in recurrent Paget's disease.[54, 60] Several reports describe recurrent Paget's disease of the vulva in a split-thickness skin graft even in the absence of underlying malignancy.[76, 77]

*Table 58–3.* **Recurrence of Intraepithelial Paget's Disease in Relation to Margin Status**

| Reference | Recurrence of Intraepithelial Paget's Disease | | | | |
|---|---|---|---|---|---|
| | NEGATIVE MARGIN | | POSITIVE MARGIN | | TOTAL |
| Gunn[73] | 0/1 | | 0/3 | | 0/4 |
| Stacy et al[61] | 0/8 | | 1/2 | (50%) | 1/10 (10%) |
| Bergen et al[62] | 1/8 | (13%) | 2/6 | (33%) | 3/14 (21%) |
| Curtin et al[54] | 3/14 | (21%) | 2/8 | (25%) | 5/22 (23%) |
| Fishman et al[63] | 3/9 | (33%) | 2/5 | (40%) | 5/14 (36%) |
| Kodama et al[64] | 0/10 | | 4/9 | (44%) | 4/19 (21%) |
| Scheistrøen et al[75] | 2/10 | (20%) | 6/15 | (40%) | 8/25 (32%) |
| Total | 9/60 | (15%) | 17/48 | (35%) | 26/108 (24%) |

## Invasive Squamous Cell Vulvar Cancer

### NATURAL HISTORY

Squamous cell carcinoma accounts for about 90% of primary vulvar malignancies,[78] whereas melanoma (5.7%), adenocarcinoma (3.7%), basal cell carcinoma (2%), and sarcoma (1.7%) are much less common.[79] In addition, about 8% of vulvar tumors are metastatic, most commonly from the uterine cervix, followed by endometrium and urinary tract.[80]

**Epidemiology and Etiology.** With 3300 new cases and 900 deaths annually in the United States, vulvar carcinoma is a relatively rare entity,[81] representing about 3 to 5% of all malignancies of the female genital tract. It is generally a disease of postmenopausal women, with 75% of patients older than 50 years at diagnosis. However, 15% of patients develop vulvar cancer before age 40. A second primary malignancy has been reported in up to 27% of cases, predominantly in another region of the lower genital tract, especially the uterine cervix, followed by breast, extragenital skin, and gastrointestinal tract.[82–84]

Squamous cell carcinoma of the vulva is of heterogeneous nature.[85] There appear to be at least two distinct etiologic entities, one that is related to HPV infection (basaloid type) and one that is not (keratinizing type).

The *basaloid* or *warty* histologic type is associated with VIN in more than 80% of cases and tends to occur in the younger patient population. HPV DNA has been found in 55% of patients with VIN, 89% of patients with VIN 3, and in up to 86% of warty or basaloid carcinomas of the vulva.[85, 86] HPV types 16 and 18 are frequently associated with higher grade VIN and are considered to be of greater oncogenic potential. In a population-based study, Madeleine and colleagues found HPV-16–seropositive current smokers to have a 19 times higher risk of developing vulvar cancer than that noted for HPV-16–seronegative nonsmokers.[87] In general, epidemiologic risk factors for the basaloid and warty types are similar to the classic cervical cancer risk factors, such as number of sexual partners, age at coitarche, abnormal Pap smear findings, venereal warts, low socioeconomic status, immunosuppression, and smoking.[85, 88–90] Although these data support the hypothesis that VIN 3 is a precursor for basaloid and warty carcinoma of the vulva, the natural history of VIN remains unclear.

The *keratinizing* type frequently develops in areas adjacent to LS and squamous hyperplasia with or without atypia and tends to occur in older women. HPV DNA is rarely (<10%) detected in these tumors.[85] Alternate, commonly implied etiologic variables are the itch-scratch cycle with hyperplasia and atypical changes in the repaired epithelium.[91] In this context, there has been controversy about the concern that vaginal deodorants, perfumed soaps, and hygiene sprays may contribute to the carcinogenic process insofar as they frequently lead to chronic vulvar irritation and the itch-scratch cycle. Although associated LS and squamous hyperplasia are found in 38 to 83% of patients with keratinizing squamous cell carcinoma,[22, 85, 92] the etiologic role of squamous cell hyperplasia with or without atypia or LS remains controversial. Supportive evidence that some of these lesions could be a precursor for squamous cell carcinomas comes from studies that demonstrate monoclonal expansion of keratinocytes in LS and associated squamous hyperplasia,[93] as well as p53 overexpression and aneuploid DNA content.[24] Some studies in the past found obesity, poor hygiene, hypertension, diabetes mellitus, arteriosclerosis, early menopause, and nulliparity associated with an increased risk for vulvar cancer.[94, 95] Others more recently were unable to confirm any of these as risk factors.[89]

**Signs, Symptoms, and Diagnosis.** Vulvar carcinoma should be amenable to early diagnosis, yet patient and physician delay of the diagnosis is common. In more than 70% of cases, patients report a longstanding history of an intense vulvar pruritus.[84] Other symptoms are a mass, lump, ulcer, bleeding lesion, discharge, or unusual odor. Pain or dysuria tends to develop with midline lesions near the clitoris and

urethra. Pain is also common with bacterial superinfection of the tumor. Only 5% of patients have a presenting complaint of a groin mass or abscess. Nearly 60% of patients do not seek medical care until symptoms persist for more than 10 months. Once medical attention is sought, the diagnosis is frequently delayed for another 3 months. In one fifth of patients it is delayed for more than 12 months during empirical therapy with creams and ointments without a preceding biopsy.[82, 83]

A thorough visual inspection of the vulva should be part of every gynecologic examination. In addition, the vulva, perineum, mons pubis, and inguinal region should be carefully palpated for subcutaneous lesions and lymphadenopathy. Careful determination of the extent of the lesion, its unifocality or multifocality, and involvement of bone, urethra, bladder, vagina, anus, rectum, and lymph nodes is essential. The lesion of a vulvar carcinoma may be clinically inapparent, such as in the presence of VIN or vulvar dystrophies,[39, 96] or in deep induration without an apparent surface lesion. Lesions may be ulcerative, raised, nodular, exophytic, or infiltrative; pigmented, red or white; dry, weeping, or necrotic; tender or painless. Thus, any lesion of the vulva warrants a biopsy. Colposcopy should be performed to include evaluation of the cervix and vagina owing to the high prevalence of multicentric lesions. Needle aspiration biopsies may be helpful for deeply placed indurations.

**Histopathology.** The distribution of vulvar carcinoma is as follows: 60% labia majora and minora, 15% clitoris, and 10% on the perineal body. Approximately 10% of cases are too extensive to determine the site of origin.[97] Squamous carcinoma of the vulva can be divided into three distinct histologic subtypes designated basaloid carcinoma, warty carcinoma, and keratinizing squamous carcinoma.[92] As outlined earlier, basaloid and warty carcinomas of the vulva are generally associated with HPV, whereas the majority of keratinizing squamous carcinomas are not.

**Routes of Spread.** Squamous cell carcinoma of the vulva grows by direct extension to adjacent structures, such as the urethra, bladder, vagina, or anus. It spreads via lymphatic embolization to the regional inguinal and femoral lymph nodes. Lymphatic metastases may occur early in the disease, and 12% of T1 tumors have regional nodal metastases.[10, 82] The typical lymphatic route of spread is via the superficial inguinal nodes, located along the inguinal ligament and saphenous vein below Camper's fascia and above the fascia lata and cribriform fascia.[10] Spread then continues to the deep femoral nodes, which are located along the medial side of the femoral vein within the opening of the fossa ovalis and beneath the cribriform fascia.[98] Cloquet's or Rosenmüller's node is the most cephalad of the deep femoral lymph nodes and lies at the entrance of the femoral canal beneath the inguinal ligament. It is thought of as a sentinel node for metastatic disease to the pelvis. Despite this generally predictable pattern of lymphatic spread, patients with metastases to the deep femoral nodes without involvement of the superficial inguinal nodes have been described by several investigators.[10, 99–101] Corroborative evidence is further provided by Levenback and colleagues, who, in an intraoperative lymphatic mapping study of patients with vulvar cancer, found the sentinel node to be deep to the cribriform fascia in 1 of 21 patients (5%).[102]

The lymphatics of the vulva form a rich network covering

*Table 58–4.* **Incidence of Lymph Node Metastasis in Squamous Cell Carcinoma of the Vulva**

| Reference | Positive Inguinofemoral Nodes | | Positive Pelvic LN/Patients with Pelvic LND | | Positive Pelvic LN with Positive Groin LN | | Positive Pelvic Nodes with Negative Groin LN | |
|---|---|---|---|---|---|---|---|---|
| Rutledge et al[82] | 33/86 | (38%) | 12/72 | (17%) | 12/33 | (36%) | 0/53 | |
| Collins et al[108] | 27/98 | (28%) | 11/98 | (11%) | 7/27 | (26%) | 4/71 | (6%) |
| Morley[109] | 67/180 | (37%) | 6/23 | (26%) | 6/67 | (9%) | 0/113 | |
| Krupp and Blohm[110] | 40/195 | (21%) | 10/195 | (5.1%) | 9/40 | (23%) | 1/155 | (0.6%) |
| Benedet et al[97] | 34/120 | (28%) | 4/51 | (8%) | n.a. | | n.a. | |
| Curry et al[105] | 57/191 | (30%) | 9/52 | (17%) | 9/57 | (16%) | 0/134 | |
| Iversen et al[111] | 90/262 | (34%) | 7/100 | (7%) | 6/90 | (7%) | 1/172 | (0.6%) |
| Hacker et al[9] | 31/113 | (27%) | 6/18 | (33%) | 6/31 | (19%) | 0/82 | |
| Podratz et al[83] | 59/175 | (34%) | 7/114 | (6%) | 7/59 | (12%) | 0/116 | |
| Monaghan and Hammond[112] | 37/134 | (28%) | 3/80 | (4%) | n.a. | | n.a. | |
| Hopkins et al[113] | 61/145 | (42%) | 13/38 | (34%) | 13/61 | (21%) | 0/84 | |
| Keys[103] | 203/588 | (35%) | 15/53 | (28%) | n.a. | | n.a. | |
| Total | 739/2287 | (32%) | 103/894 | (12%) | 75/465 | (16%) | 6/980 | (0.6%) |

LN, lymph nodes; LND, lymph node dissection; n.a., data not available.

its entire surface. The lymphatics from either side anastomose in the midline, and lymphatic drainage from the perineum, clitoris, and anterior labia minora is bilateral. The lymphatic drainage of lesions that are at least 2 cm lateral of the midline is ipsilateral. Contralateral involvement of inguinal lymph nodes without ipsilateral spread is rare in lateral tumors. For patients with unilateral T1 tumors and negative ipsilateral nodes, the risk of contralateral lymph node metastasis is 0.4%.[10] When patients with all stages are considered, this risk increases to 1.7 to 2.8%.[103, 104] If there is metastatic disease in the ipsilateral inguinal nodes, the contralateral and pelvic nodes are at increased risk for metastasis. Although direct lymphatics from the clitoris and Bartholin's gland to the deep pelvic nodes have been described, these channels seem to have minimal clinical significance.[105–107] Lesions involving primarily the vagina may drain directly into the pelvic lymph nodes, whereas perianal lesions can metastasize via the hemorrhoidal lymphatics to the para-aortic lymph nodes.

The overall incidence of inguinofemoral lymph node metastasis is reported to be about 30% (Table 58–4). The incidence of lymph node metastasis is related to lesion size (Table 58–5). For lesions up to 1 cm, the incidence is 5%; it rises to approximately 50% for lesions greater than 4 cm. Laterality of groin node metastasis correlates with the number of lymph nodes involved (Table 58–6). Metastases to pelvic lymph nodes average 16% in patients with positive inguinofemoral nodes (see Table 58–4). Pelvic lymph node involvement is rare in the absence of three or more positive

inguinofemoral nodes; then the risk rises to about 50%.[9, 83, 114] With clinically suspicious groin nodes, the risk of pelvic lymph node involvement is about 33%.[9] Positive pelvic nodes are generally located on the side of the many positive groin nodes.[83]

Hematogenous spread to distant organs, including lung, liver, and bone, is usually a late phenomenon and rarely occurs in the absence of lymphatic metastases. As shown in Table 58–7, only about 4% of patients with less than three positive unilateral groin nodes develop systemic metastases, compared with 66% of patients with three or more positive nodes.

**Staging.** Vulvar carcinoma used to be staged clinically on the basis of tumor size, location, and palpable lymph node status. Clinical assessment of lymph node involvement has been notoriously poor, with false-negative and false-positive rates of approximately 25%.[83, 109] Lymph node metastases, however, are highly significant in terms of survival, and the majority of patients are undergoing primary surgical therapy including lymphadenectomy. Thus, in 1988, the International Federation of Gynecology and Obstetrics (FIGO) abandoned the clinical staging of vulvar cancer in favor of a surgical staging system incorporating the pathologic lymph

*Table 58–5.* **Frequency of Lymph Node Metastases in Relation to Lesion Size in Vulvar Carcinoma**

| Lesion Size (cm) | Number | Positive Nodes | % |
|---|---|---|---|
| <1 | 40 | 2 | 5 |
| 1–2 | 81 | 13 | 16 |
| 2–4 | 33 | 11 | 33.3 |
| >4 | 15 | 8 | 53.3 |

Data from Rutledge F, et al. Am J Obstet Gynecol 1970;106:1117, and Hacker NF, et al. Obstet Gynecol 1983;61:408.

*Table 58–6.* **Correlation of Number of Positive Groin Nodes with Laterality of Groin Node Metastasis**

| Number of Positive Inguinofemoral Nodes | Inguinofemoral Nodes Positive | |
|---|---|---|
| | UNILATERAL | BILATERAL |
| 1 | 40 (52%) | 0 |
| 2 | 23 (30%) | 4 (11%) |
| 3 | 8 (10%) | 11 (31%) |
| 4 | 0 | 9 (25%) |
| 5–6 | 5 (7%) | 4 (11%) |
| 7–9 | 1 (1%) | 5 (14%) |
| ≥10 | 0 | 3 (8%) |
| Total | 77 (100%) | 36 (100%) |

From Homesley H, Bundy BN, Sedlis A, Adcock L. Radiation therapy versus pelvic node resection for carcinoma of the vulva with positive groin nodes. Obstet Gynecol 1986;68:733–740.

*Table 58–7.* **Site of Recurrence in Relation to Number of Positive Unilateral Groin Nodes**

| Nodal Status | Vulva RATIO (%) | Groin RATIO (%) | Pelvis RATIO (%) | Systemic RATIO (%) |
|---|---|---|---|---|
| 1–2 positive | 6/104 (5.8%) | 3/104 (2.9%) | 0/104 (0%) | 4/104 (3.8%) |
| ≥3 positive | 3/9 (33%) | 3/9 (33%) | 4/9 (44%) | 6/9 (66%) |

From Hacker NF, Berek JS, Lagasse LD, et al. Management of regional lymph nodes and their prognostic influence in vulvar disease. Obstet Gynecol 1983;61:408–12. Reprinted with permission from The American College of Obstetricians and Gynecologists.

*Table 58–9.* **Five-Year Survival Versus Surgical International Federation of Gynecology and Obstetrics Staging for Patients with Vulvar Carcinoma Treated Curatively in a Gynecologic Oncology Group**

| Stage | Number | Corrected 5-yr Survival (%) |
|---|---|---|
| I | 148 (26%) | 98% |
| II | 191 (33%) | 85% |
| III | 176 (31%) | 74% |
| IV | 62 (11%) | 31% |
| Total | 577 | 79% |

From Homesley HD, Bundy BN, Sedlis A, et al. Assessment of current FIGO staging of vulvar carcinoma relative to prognostic factors for survival (a GOG study). Am J Obstet Gynecol 1991;164:997–1004.

node status. In 1995, FIGO further modified the stage I grouping to separate T1 lesions invasive to 1 mm or less as stage IA (Table 58–8).[115] Although this surgical staging offers much improvement over the previous clinical staging system, further refinements are still needed. Currently, stage III involves a heterogeneous group of patients including those with a small lesion and distal urethral or vaginal involvement but negative nodes and patients with only one microscopically involved lymph node, all of whom have a good prognosis, as well as those patients with many positive groin nodes, who have a poor prognosis.[116]

**Prognosis and Survival.** The prognosis for patients with early vulvar carcinoma is generally good, with a greater than 90% 5-year survival for patients with stage I and greater than 80% for those with stage II disease. Five-year survival decreases to approximately 70% for stage III and 30% for stage IV disease. Lymph node status is the single most important independent prognostic factor, followed by lesion size.[118] Various other surgicopathologic variables, such as tumor thickness, depth of invasion, histologic grade, and

lymph-vascular space involvement (LVSI), are not independent predictors of survival but rather contribute to lymph node involvement.[117]

***Stage and Lymph Node Status.*** Survival correlates with FIGO stage, as is demonstrated by data from the Gynecologic Oncology Group (GOG) in Table 58–9.[118] Lymph node status is the single most important prognostic factor for survival.[118] Patients with positive nodes have a 5-year survival rate of about 50%, whereas the rate is greater than 90% for those with negative nodes (Table 58–10). Hacker[9] demonstrated in 1983 that if stratified by the number of positive lymph nodes, patients with one microscopic positive node survive almost as long as those with negative nodes, but survival decreases markedly if three or more nodes are positive (Fig. 58–1). The fact that the number of positive nodes is an important prognostic variable has since been confirmed by other investigators.[118, 121] Although some authors find bilaterality of lymph node metastasis per se not to be a risk factor, others note survival to be worse if lymph

*Table 58–8.* **International Federation of Gynecology and Obstetrics Surgical Staging of Vulvar Cancer (FIGO 1995) and TNM Classification of Vulvar Carcinoma**

| FIGO Stage | Comment | TNM Stage | Comment |
|---|---|---|---|
| 0 | Carcinoma in situ | Tis | Carcinoma in situ |
| I | Tumor confined to vulva and/or perineum, ≤2 cm diameter | T1 N0 M0 | T1: Tumor confined to vulva and/or perineum, ≤2 cm diameter |
| IA stromal invasion* ≤1 mm | | | |
| IB stromal invasion >1 mm | | | |
| II | Tumor confined to vulva and/or perineum, >2 cm diameter | T2 N0 M0 | T2: Tumor confined to vulva and/or perineum, >2 cm diameter |
| III | Tumor of any size that invades any of the following: lower urethra, vagina, anus, and/or unilateral regional lymph node metastasis | T3 N0/N1 M0 T1/T2 N1 M0 | T3: Tumor of any size that invades lower urethra, vagina, or anus, and/or (N1) unilateral regional lymph node metastasis |
| IVa | Tumor of any size that invades any of the following: upper urethra, bladder mucosa, rectal mucosa, pelvic bone, and/or bilateral regional lymph node metastasis | T4 any N M0 T1/T2/T3 N2 M0 | T4: Tumor of any size that invades any of the following: upper urethra, bladder mucosa, rectal mucosa, pelvic bone, and/or (N2) bilateral regional lymph node metastasis |
| IVb | Distant metastasis | Any T Any N M1 | M1: Distant metastasis (pelvic lymph node metastasis is M1) |

*The depth of stromal invasion is defined as the measurement of the tumor from the epithelial-stromal junction of the adjacent most superficial dermal papilla to the deepest point of invasion.

Data from Shepherd JH. Staging announcement. FIGO staging of gynecologic cancers; cervical and vulva. Int J Gynecol Cancer 1995;5:319, and Baehrs OH, Henson DE, Hutter RVP, Kennedy BJ, eds. Vulva. In: Manual for staging cancer. 4th ed. American Joint Committee on Cancer. Philadelphia: JB Lippincott, 1992:177–80.

*Table 58–10.* **Five-Year Survival for Patients with Negative Versus Positive Lymph Nodes Treated with Curative Intent**

| Reference | Positive Inguinal Lymph Nodes | | Negative Inguinal Lymph Nodes | |
|---|---|---|---|---|
| | NUMBER | 5-YR SURVIVAL (%) | NUMBER | 5-YR SURVIVAL (%) |
| Rutledge et al[82] | 33 | 39 | 53 | 100 |
| Collins et al[108] | 31 | 19 | n.a. | n.a. |
| Morley[109] | 64 | 39 | 130 | 92 |
| Green[119] | 46 | 61 | 61 | 92 |
| Curry et al[105] | 52 | 42 | n.a. | n.a. |
| Hacker et al[9] | 31 | 66 | 82 | 96 |
| Podratz et al[83] | 59 | 47 | 115 | 90 |
| Monaghan and Hammond[112] | 37 | 24 | 95 | 90 |
| Cavanagh et al[120] | 58 | 38 | 96 | 83 |
| Keys[103] | 203 | 57 | 385 | 91 |
| Total | 614 | 47 | 1017 | 91 |

From Homesley HD, Bundy BN, Sedlis A, et al. Assessment of current FIGO staging of vulvar carcinoma relative to prognostic factors for survival (a GOG study). Am J Obstet Gynecol 1991;164:997–1004.

node metastases are bilateral.[83, 113, 117] Once patients have positive pelvic nodes, survival is as low as 17% (Table 58–11).

***Lesion Size.*** Based on the 588-patient GOG study, Homesley and colleagues found that tumor size, although correlated with lymph node status, was the only other independent predictor for survival in addition to lymph node status (Table 58–12).[118]

***Depth of Invasion.*** Depth of invasion is a major determinant of the risk of lymph node metastasis. Although there is an occasional report of lymph node metastasis with a T1 lesion invasive to 1 mm or less,[122] the risk of lymph node metastasis with less than 1 mm invasion in a T1 lesion is exceedingly small. This risk rises dramatically once the depth of invasion is greater than 1 mm (Table 58–13), underscoring the need for great care in the assessment of depth of invasion.

***Location, Configuration, and Growth Pattern.*** There is controversy about the prognostic significance of tumor location as well as configuration and growth pattern. Clitoral involvement is reported to increase the risk of groin involvement to about 40%.[105, 123] As depth of invasion is a better predictor of lymph node metastasis than tumor thickness, it appears intuitive that infiltrative growth may be more aggressive than exophytic or papillary growth. Evidence suggests that the pattern of invasion may be associated with lymph node status and thus prognosis. Reported rates of lymph node involvement for T1 lesions are 11 to 14% with a broad, pushing front of invasion, versus 29 to 51% with a spray or stellate pattern of invasion.[7, 123]

***Lymph–Vascular Space Involvement.*** The presence of LVSI correlates with the risk for lymph node metastasis and thus survival.[124] Based on GOG data, the risk of inguinofemoral lymph node metastasis with LVSI is almost three times that for negative LVSI (75% vs. 27%).[117]

***Surgical Margin.*** In a University of California, Los Angeles (UCLA), study of squamous cell carcinoma of the vulva, Heaps and colleagues noted that none of the 91 patients with surgical margins greater than 0.8 cm suffered

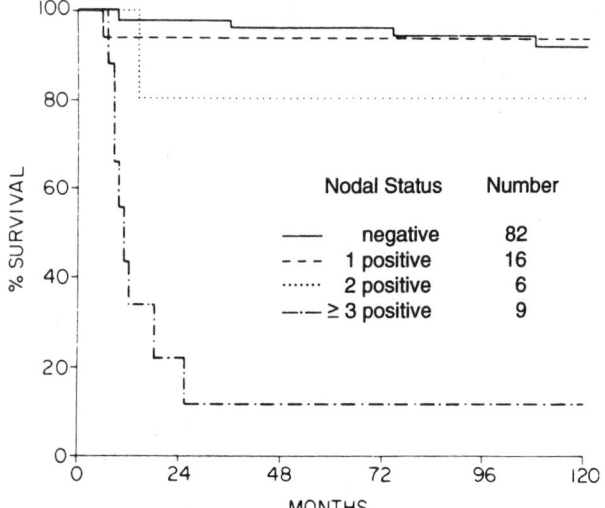

**Figure 58–1.** Corrected survival in relation to inguinofemoral lymph node status. (From Hacker NF, Berek JS, Lagasse LD, et al. Management of regional lymph nodes and their prognostic influence in vulvar cancer. Obstet Gynecol 1983;61:408. Reprinted with permission from the American College of Obstetricians and Gynecologists.)

*Table 58–11.* **Frequency of Pelvic Nodal Involvement in Patients with Positive Inguinofemoral Lymph Nodes in Vulvar Carcinoma and Survival with Positive Pelvic Nodes**

| Reference | 5-Yr Survival with Positive Pelvic Lymph Node | |
|---|---|---|
| | RATIO | % |
| Rutledge et al[82] | 3/12* | 25 |
| Collins et al[108] | 1/11 | 9 |
| Green[119] | 0/2 | 0 |
| Benedet et al[97] | 2/4 | 50 |
| Curry et al[105] | 2/9 | 22.2 |
| Hacker et al[9] | 0/6 | 0 |
| Podratz et al[83] | 1/7 | 14 |
| Cavanagh et al[120] | 2/10 | 20 |
| Homesley et al[114] | 3/15* | 20 |
| Hopkins et al[113] | 1/13 | 8 |
| Total | 15/89 | 17 |

*Two- to 3-yr survival.

*Table 58–12.* Frequency and Relative Survival by Tumor Diameter and Groin Node Status

| Tumor Diameter (cm) | Surgical Groin Node Status | | | | | |
| | NEGATIVE NODES | | | POSITIVE NODES | | |
| | *Number* | *%* | *5-yr Survival* | *Number* | *%* | *5-yr Survival* |
|---|---|---|---|---|---|---|
| ≤2 | 154 | 40 | 98 | 36 | 18 | 79 |
| 2.1–3 | 120 | 32 | 91 | 55 | 28 | 59 |
| 3.1–4 | 37 | 10 | 76 | 44 | 22 | 57 |
| >4 | 70 | 18 | 82 | 64 | 32 | 45 |
| Total | 381 | 100 | | 199 | 100 | |

From Homesley HD, Bundy BN, Sedlis A, et al. Assessment of current FIGO staging of vulvar carcinoma relative to prognostic factors for survival (a GOG study). Am J Obstet Gynecol 1991;164:997–1004.

a local recurrence, compared with 21 of the 44 patients with surgical margins less than 0.8 cm. This led to their conclusion that margin status is the most powerful predictor of local vulvar recurrence.[125] Margin status, however, does not predict survival.[118]

***Grade.*** Histologic grade has been consistently shown to be a predictor of the risk of groin node metastasis.[117] The risk for inguinofemoral lymph node metastasis is 16 to 33% for grade 1, 28 to 48% for grade 2, and 62 to 75% for grade 3 lesions.[126, 127]

***Human Papillomavirus Status.*** Monk and colleagues used polymerase chain reaction to determine the HPV status in 55 vulvar cancers. Ninety-five percent of basaloid, warty, or verrucous tumors were HPV positive, compared with 39% of keratinizing squamous cell carcinomas. In their series, the presence of HPV DNA represented an independent prognostic factor associated with a decreased risk of recurrence and better survival.[128]

## TREATMENT

The failure to control vulvar cancer by limited surgical excision led Basset in 1912 to propose an en bloc dissection of the vulva and regional lymphnodes.[3] Taussig and Way independently demonstrated improved survival with this technique.[2, 4, 5] Radical vulvectomy became the mainstay of treatment for vulvar cancer. Because of the significant physical and psychological morbidity associated with such radical treatment of vulvar cancer, the trend during the past decades

*Table 58–13.* Incidence of Lymph Node Metastasis Versus Depth of Invasion in Patients with T1 Squamous Cell Carcinoma Undergoing Vulvectomy and Inguinal Lymphadenectomy

| Invasion Depth (mm) | No. of Cases | Nodal Metastasis (%) |
|---|---|---|
| <1 | 163 | 0 |
| 1.1–2 | 145 | 11 (7.7) |
| 2.1–3 | 131 | 11 (8.3) |
| 3.1–5 | 101 | 27 (26.7) |
| >5 | 38 | 13 (34.2) |
| Total | 578 | 62 (10.7) |

From Morley GW. Infiltrative carcinoma of the vulva: results of surgical treatment. Am J Obstet Gynecol 1976;124:874–888.

has been to modify this radical surgical approach for patients with early-stage lesions by performing the most conservative surgery possible without jeopardizing the potential for cure. This requires individualization of several aspects of the patient's care: the management of the primary lesion and the management of the lymph nodes, as well as the use of adjuvant or neoadjuvant radiation therapy with or without chemotherapy.

### Management of the Primary Lesion

***Microinvasion—T1A.*** Microinvasive carcinoma of the vulva, first conceptualized by Franklin and Rutledge in 1971,[129] has since been defined by FIGO as a tumor 2 cm or less in diameter with 1 mm or less invasion. Patients with more than one site of invasion are not included in this category. Microinvasive carcinoma carries a clinically insignificant risk of local extension and groin node metastasis. The definition of an adequate excision of this primary lesion is still debated, but a wide, deep excision with a 1- to 2-cm margin into normal surrounding skin appears appropriate.

***Frankly Invasive Carcinoma—T1B.*** Even for more deeply invasive T1 lesions, ample evidence shows that radical local excision provides adequate treatment for the primary tumor in an otherwise normal-appearing vulva. Local recurrence following such treatment is no more common than following radical vulvectomy.[10] This appears to hold true regardless of the depth of invasion. The radical local excision should clear the tumor with a 1- to 2-cm margin and extend down to the level of the inferior fascia of the urogenital diaphragm. Supportive evidence comes from a retrospective review of 135 patients from UCLA with all stages of disease, which revealed that a 1-cm histologically tumor-free surgical margin on the vulva resulted in excellent local control, independent of the primary tumor size and coexisting benign vulvar pathology.[125] However, with an 8-mm or less histologically negative surgical margin, local vulvar recurrences were observed in 21 of 44 (48%) cases. These margin requirements are the same for a radical local excision, radical hemivulvectomy, or radical vulvectomy. In a review of the literature, Hacker and Van der Velden report local recurrences to occur at similar frequencies following radical local excisions and radical vulvectomies performed for early vulvar cancer (Table 58–14).[10] Two large series confirm these findings. Following radical local excision there were 14 invasive vulvar recurrences in a total of 197 patients (7.1%),[101, 130] When detected early, isolated local failure is usually salvageable by additional surgical therapy.[84, 101, 130, 131]

*Table 58–14.* Local Invasive Recurrence After Radical Local Excision and Radical Vulvectomy for T1 Squamous Cell Carcinoma of the Vulva

| | Number | Recurrence | Died of Disease |
|---|---|---|---|
| Radical local excision | 165 | 12 (7.2%) | 1 (0.6%) |
| Radical vulvectomy | 365 | 23 (6.3%) | 2 (0.6%) |

From Hacker NF, Van der Velden J. Conservative management of early vulvar cancer. Cancer 1993;71:1673–7.

In light of the significantly reduced short- and long-term physical and psychological morbidity associated with radical local excision, such conservative surgery is justified and should be attempted whenever possible.

The management of vulvar cancer arising in the presence of VIN or some non-neoplastic vulvar disorder may pose special difficulties. Treatment needs to be individualized on the basis of a patient's age, performance status, and symptoms of concurrent disease. One may choose to perform a radical local excision of the cancer and concurrently a superficial local excision of the VIN or vulvar dystrophy. Alternatively, one can administer steroid treatment for the vulvar dystrophy.

*Midline Lesions.* Radical local excision is most feasible for lateral and perineal vulvar lesions. Midline lesions pose special challenges owing to their proximity to clitoris, urethra, vagina, or anus. For small anterior clitoral or periclitoral lesions, especially in the younger patient, Hacker has suggested that the use of about 5000 cGy external beam radiation therapy followed by biopsies to confirm absence of residual disease may be a feasible alternative to any surgical excision with its associated psychosexual consequences.[132] Even the resection of just a distal portion of the urethra may be associated with compromised continence.[133] For periurethral lesions, as for perineal lesions with close proximity to the anus, consideration should be given to preoperative or postoperative radiation therapy.

*Frankly Invasive Carcinoma—Vulvar Conservation for Early T2 and Early T3 Lesions.* In general, the management of patients with T2 and early T3 lesions consists of radical vulvectomy and bilateral inguinofemoral lymphadenectomy. In the past decade, the indications for conservative surgery for the primary lesion have been extended to selected patients with early T2 and early T3 tumors. Lesions that might be most amenable to this approach are posterior lesions, for which preservation of the mons and clitoris is feasible while allowing for an appropriate surgical margin. The reported experience indicates that radical wide excision is associated with the same outcome as radical vulvectomy.[130, 134, 135] However, studies of long-term survival are still limited. Some validation for this approach comes from UCLA data, which show comparable 5-year survival in patients treated with radical wide excision tailored to the tumor and in those undergoing radical vulvectomy.[136] This is not surprising because the most important predictor of local recurrence is the surgical margin rather than tumor size per se or the extent or type of radical procedure.[125] However, although margin status is a strong predictor of local disease control, it does not predict survival.[118]

Following radical vulvectomy, the defect can usually be closed primarily without tension. If not, a number of options exist: The area may be left open to granulate,[137] or it may be covered with full-thickness skin grafts.[138, 139] Myocutaneous grafts may be developed to cover the defect, such as a gracilis muscle flap or a rectus abdominis muscle flap.[140, 141] Myocutaneous grafts are particularly helpful if the vascular supply to the vulva is compromised owing to prior surgery or radiation therapy.

*Advanced Frankly Invasive Vulvar Carcinoma—Large T3 and T4 Primary Tumors.* To achieve adequate surgical clearance for primary tumors involving the upper urethra, anus, rectum, or rectovaginal septum, pelvic exenteration is needed in addition to radical vulvectomy and bilateral inguinofemoral lymphadenectomy. Such radical procedures carry an extremely high physical and psychological morbidity.[142, 143] Five-year survival rates of about 50% are being reported.[144–146] Surgery alone is rarely curative for patients with fixed or ulcerated groin nodes.

Although radiotherapy alone is associated with low cure rates around 20%,[147] a number of recent small retrospective and prospective studies (Table 58–15) demonstrate that a combined radiosurgical approach offers management advantages for patients with advanced vulvar cancer and may allow for preservation of important structures, such as urethra, anus, and clitoris. Using external beam radiation to shrink the tumor, followed by a more limited resection of the tumor bed and individualized lymph node dissection, 5-year survival rates as high as 76% have been reported.[148] Interestingly, about half of the vulvectomy specimens were without residual tumor.[13, 148] More recent studies suggest that preoperative use of chemoradiation may be associated with even better survival rates than preoperative radiation alone (see Table 58–15). Although initial response rates are excellent, up to 50% local relapse rates have been reported if not combined with surgical excision of the tumor bed.[149] Thus, preoperative chemoradiation followed by surgical excision of the tumor bed should be offered as first-line treatment to these patients who otherwise would require some form of exenterative surgery. Caution is warranted, however, in designing very aggressive management protocols for this largely elderly patient population.

## Management of the Lymph Nodes

*Microinvasion—Stage IA.* The incidence of inguinofemoral lymph node metastasis with a microinvasive squamous cell carcinoma of the vulva is less than 1%, although an occasional patient has a groin recurrence following local excision of a T1 tumor with less than 1 mm stromal invasion.[122] Provided that there are no clinically suspicious inguinal lymph nodes and there is no LVSI, these stage IA lesions do not require lymphadenectomy. In fact, this is the only subgroup of vulvar carcinoma that does not require at least ipsilateral inguinofemoral lymphadenectomy. Great care is required in assessing the depth of invasion, as even 1 to 2 mm of invasion increases the risk of lymph node metastasis from close to zero to almost 8% (see Table 58–13). Recurrence in an undissected groin carries a high mortality (Table 58–16) and is one of the most important causes of preventable death in early vulvar cancer. Thus, all patients with tumors invading more than 1 mm require at least unilateral inguinofemoral lymphadenectomy.

*Frankly Invasive Carcinoma—Separate Groin Incisions.* En bloc dissection of the vulva and inguinofemoral

*Table 58–15.* **Radiation Therapy With or Without Chemotherapy for Patients with Locally Advanced Primary Vulvar Carcinoma**

| Reference | n | Radiation Therapy | Chemotherapy | Response Rate | Recurrent/Persistent Local Disease |
|---|---|---|---|---|---|
| PREOPERATIVE RADIATION THERAPY ± CHEMOTHERAPY | | | | | |
| Hacker et al[13] | 8 | EB ± IC | — | 7 (88%)* | 1/7 (14%) |
| Fairey et al[150] | 7 | EB ± IC | — | 6 (86%)* | 1/6 (17%) |
| Boronow et al[148] | 37 | EB ± IC | — | 34 (81%)* | 5/34 (15%) |
| Rotmensch et al[151] | 16 | EB | — | 11 (63%)* | 4/11 (36%) |
| Berek et al[152] | 12 | EB + IS | 5-FU + CDDP | 11 (92%)* | 0 |
| Levin et al[153] | 6 | EB | 5-FU + Mito | 4 (67%)* | 0 |
| Lupi et al[154] | 24 | EB | 5-FU + Mito | 22 (92%)* | 5/22 (23%) |
| Total | 110 | | | 95 (86%) | 16/80 (20%) |
| CHEMORADIATION ± SURGERY | | | | | |
| Evans et al[155] | 4 | EB ± IS | 5-FU + Mito | 4 (100%) | 2/4 (50%) |
| Russell et al[156] | 18 | EB | 5-FU ± CDDP | 17 (94%) | 1/17 (6%) |
| Scheistrøen and Tropé[157] | 20 | EB | Bleo | 15 (75%) | 10/15 (67%) |
| Wahlen et al[158] | 19 | EB ± IS | 5-FU ± Mito | 17 (89%)† | 5/19 (26%) |
| Eifel et al[159] | 12 | EB | 5-FU + CDDP | 11 (92%) | 6/12 (50%) |
| Cunningham et al[160] | 14 | EB | 5-FU + CDDP | 13 (93%) | 3/12 (25%) |
| Moore et al[161] | 71 | EB | 5-FU + CDDP | 68 (96%) | 22/68 (32%) |
| Total | 158 | | | 145 (92%) | 49/147 (33%) |

*Response rate allowing for organ-preserving surgery.
†Two patients without response to chemoradiation therapy were successfully treated with radical surgery.
EB, external beam radiation therapy; IC, intracavitary radiation therapy; IS, interstitial; Bleo, bleomycin; Mito, mitomycin; 5-FU, 5 fluorouracil; CDDP, cisplatin.

nodes is associated with highly satisfactory survival rates for vulvar cancer, but postoperative morbidity, particularly wound breakdown, is common, frequently prolonging hospitalization. During the past several decades, an increasing number of centers have used separate incisions for the groin dissection rather than the en bloc approach in an attempt to decrease the incidence of wound breakdown (Fig. 58–2*A* and *B*). This technique leaves a skin bridge between the primary tumor and the draining lymph nodes, but examination of the intervening tissue in patients with early nodal metastases has failed to reveal tumor in the connecting lymphatic channels. This is because lymphatic metastasis occurs by embolization rather than by permeation. With advanced involvement of the lymph nodes, retrograde permeation along lymphatic channels may occur,[129] and the separate incision technique may result in skin bridge recurrences unless postoperative radiation therapy is used. In a series of 100 patients in whom separate groin incisions were

*Table 58–16.* **Mortality Rates After Recurrence in an Undissected Groin**

| Reference | Recurrence | Died of Disease |
|---|---|---|
| Rutledge et al[82] | 4 | 3 |
| Magrina et al[162] | 4 | 3 |
| Hoffman et al[163] | 4 | 4 |
| Hacker et al[7] | 3 | 3 |
| Monaghan and Hammond[112] | 4 | 4 |
| Lingard et al[164] | 7 | 7 |
| Stehman et al[101] | 9 | 5 |
| Burke et al[130] | 4 | 3 |
| Total | 39 | 32 (82%) |

used, only two developed metastases in the skin bridge. Both of these patients had clinically suspicious groin lymph nodes and three or more histologically positive nodes.[11] This modification reduces the rate of wound breakdown from 62% to 38%,[164] but its effect on the incidence or severity of lymphedema, one of the most troublesome long-term complications of groin dissection, is less clear.

If a groin node dissection is indicated, it should be a thorough inguinofemoral dissection as GOG data have confirmed. Six patients of 121 with T1 N0–1 tumors suffered groin recurrences after a superficial (inguinal nodes only) groin dissection, even though the inguinal nodes were negative.[110] Comparable failure rates have been reported by Burke and colleagues.[130] Similarly, radiation therapy cannot substitute for groin dissection followed by radiation therapy when indicated, even in patients with clinically negative nodes. The GOG reported a significantly higher incidence of recurrences in groins receiving radiation therapy only.[165] Patients with clinically negative groin nodes were randomized to undergo either groin dissection or groin irradiation in conjunction with radical vulvectomy. The study was closed early because of a significantly higher incidence of recurrences in groins receiving radiation therapy only (19% vs. 0%).

***Frankly Invasive Carcinoma—Lateral Versus Midline Lesions.*** Lateral T1 lesions may undergo ipsilateral inguinofemoral lymphadenectomy. In a review of the literature involving 476 patients, Hacker and Van der Velden found that only 2 (0.4%) lateral T1 lesions had positive contralateral nodes with negative ipsilateral inguinofemoral lymph nodes.[10] Lesions crossing the midline obviously require bilateral inguinofemoral lymphadenectomy. Although there is no clear definition of a "lateral" lesion, it appears that every lesion that is within 2 cm of the midline should be regarded as a "central" lesion and thus requires bilateral groin node

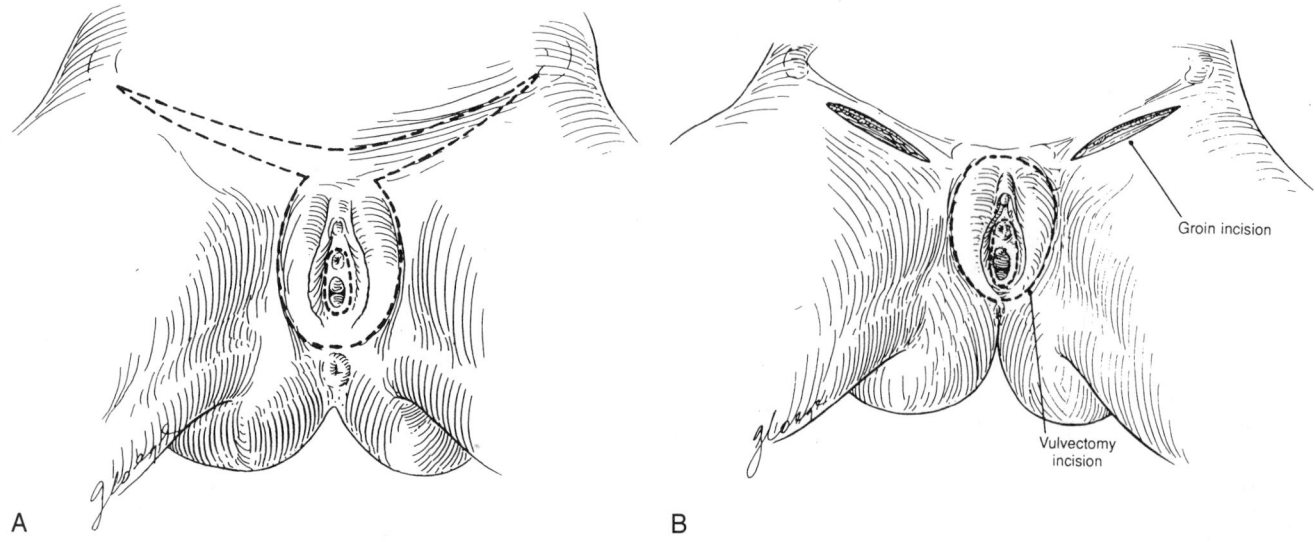

A                                                    B

**Figure 58–2.** *A*, Skin incision for en bloc groin dissection. *B*, Skin incision for groin dissection through separate incisions. (From Hacker NF. Vulvar cancer. In: Berek JS, Hacker NF, eds. Practical gynecologic oncology. 3rd ed. Philadelphia: Lippincott Williams & Wilkins, 2000:553–96.

dissection. Despite evidence that clitoral lymphatics drain directly into pelvic nodes, this has not proved to be of clinical significance.[105–107] Thus, these lesions can be treated following the same principles for lymphadenectomy that apply to all other midline lesions.

*Sentinel Lymph Node Studies.* A complete inguinofemoral lymph node dissection is currently required for all but stage IA lesions. The associated morbidity is high, especially chronic lymphedema. Thus, gynecologic oncologists continue to investigate avenues that might allow for less extensive node dissection while affording the same survival advantage. The use of intraoperative lymphatic mapping techniques is currently being investigated in an attempt to identify the first draining regional lymph node. This technique has been used successfully in patients with other solid tumors, especially breast cancer and melanoma.[166, 167] For these tumors, studies suggest that the isosulfan blue dye and the [99m]Tc-labeled sulfur colloid techniques are suitable. Success rates of 95% with false-negative rates of 0.84% are reported when the two modalities are combined.[168] In patients with vulvar cancer, Levenback and colleagues performed intraoperative lymphatic mapping using isosulfan blue and identified the sentinel node in 18 of 21 (86%) cases. In no case was a nonsentinel node positive if the sentinel node was negative.[102] In another study by DeCesare and coworkers, intraoperative lymphoscintigraphy was used in 10 patients with vulvar cancer. Again, in no case was a nonsentinel node positive if the sentinel node or nodes were negative.[169] These preliminary data suggest that intraoperative lymphatic mapping may be as efficacious in the management of patients with vulvar cancer as it is in other malignancies. The GOG is currently investigating the use of intraoperative lymphatic mapping in patients with vulvar cancer.

*Bulky Groin Nodes and Pelvic Nodes.* Bulky nodes in the groin should be resected, but in anticipation of groin radiation therapy, full groin dissection may be avoided in an attempt to decrease the risk of leg edema. Patients with bulky groin nodes are at increased risk for pelvic lymph

node metastasis. In a review of the UCLA data, Hacker and associates reported that no patient with fewer than three positive groin nodes developed a pelvic recurrence.[11] All patients with positive pelvic nodes had clinically suspicious groin nodes. A similar experience was reported from the M.D. Anderson Hospital by Curry and colleagues.[105] Pelvic recurrences are more frequent after pelvic irradiation than after pelvic lymphadenectomy, possibly because of the failure of external beam radiation therapy to sterilize bulky pelvic lymph nodes.[114] In these cases, preoperative imaging with computed tomography or magnetic resonance imaging may be helpful. If bulky pelvic nodes are shown, they can be resected.

**Complications of Surgical Treatment of Vulvar Cancer.** With use of the separate groin incision technique, the incidence of major wound breakdown or infection in the groin may be reduced from about 53 to 64% to about 14 to 38%.[11, 82, 84, 170] Local care includes cleansing and sharp debridement as necessary, whirlpool, appropriate cultures, and antibiotics. With meticulous care, the wound heals by secondary intention. Seromas occur in about 10 to 20% of cases.[82, 83] The use of suction drains for about 10 days and until the daily output is 30 ml or less may also be helpful for preventing accumulation of blood and lymph and for decreasing infection rates. Lymphocysts, a misnomer because they are unilocular lymph-filled spaces without a distinct epithelial lining, occur in approximately 10% of cases.[171, 172] The accumulation of lymph within the groin produces a cystic mass that becomes painful and frequently secondarily infected. Previous irradiation, metastatic disease to the lymph nodes, ultraradical groin dissection, and heparin use may contribute to the problem.[171, 173, 174] Hemoclips for careful surgical ligation of the afferent and efferent lymphatics, suction drains to obliterate this dead space, and pneumatic compression stockings have been postulated as preventive measures. Once lymphocysts have formed, they require drainage under aseptic conditions, as well as culture and antibiotic treatment if superinfection occurs. Although the use of the separate groin incisions may have reduced chronic lymphedema somewhat, it continues to be one of the most troublesome long-term complications following groin dissection. Reported incidences average around 30% (9 to 69%).[82–84, 170] Associated recurrent lymphangitis and cellulitis are reported in about 10% of patients[83, 170]; these usually respond to oral antibiotics. Physical methods of treatment may reduce edema fluid. Support stockings or elastic bandages are often helpful. In addition, some authors report that the use of 5,6-benzo-alpha-pyrone results in reduction of lymphedema.[175] Urinary tract infections are common following radical vulvar surgery owing to frequent prolonged use of indwelling Foley catheters. Radical vulvectomy that includes removal of a portion of the urethra increases the risk of urinary incontinence. Urinary incontinence with or without associated pelvic relaxation has been reported in 4 to 24% of patients after radical vulvectomy.[133, 170] Rectal incontinence occurs at a significant rate even after partial resection of the external anal sphincter and perianal tissue.[176] Trauma to the femoral nerve from inguinal node dissection causes some degree of anesthesia or paresthesia over the upper anterior surface postoperatively. This is usually self-limited and resolves within months. Less frequent acute complications of radical vulvar surgery and groin dissection are thrombophlebitis, pulmonary embolism, femoral vessel rupture, and osteomyelitis.[82–84, 177] The risk of preoperative death is reported to be around 3%.[79] Introital stenosis, femoral hernia, and rectoperineal fistula are other complications. Long-term treatment complications further include depression, altered body image, and sexual dysfunction.[142, 178] Appropriate preoperative and postoperative information and counseling may help lessen some of the psychological trauma.

**Radiation Therapy With or Without Chemotherapy.** Radiation therapy alone has little place in the primary management of vulvar cancer, but it may be used in conjunction with surgery in a number of situations:

1. For patients with disease involving the rectovaginal septum or upper urethra, preoperative irradiation may cause sufficient shrinkage of the primary tumor to save the patient from primary exenterative surgery and improve disease control. This has been addressed in detail in the discussion of the management of patients with advanced primary disease.

2. Postoperative pelvic and groin irradiation is indicated for patients with two or more occult groin node metastases or one clinically enlarged positive node, as discussed earlier. In 1977, the GOG initiated a prospective trial in which patients with groin nodes were randomized to either ipsilateral pelvic node dissection or bilateral pelvic and groin irradiation. The survival rate for the radiation group (68% at 2 years) was significantly ($p = 0.03$) better than the survival for the pelvic lymphadenectomy group (54% at 2 years). The survival advantage was limited to patients with two or more positive groin nodes or clinically evident groin node metastases. There was a decreased incidence of groin recurrence (5% vs. 24%) with irradiation. Four patients in the radiation group developed pelvic recurrence, compared with one in the pelvic lymphadenectomy group. Thus, although these data do not provide evidence that pelvic irradiation is superior to pelvic lymphadenectomy for the prevention of pelvic recurrences, they do emphasize the value of prophy-

lactic groin irradiation in preventing groin recurrences in patients with clinically suspicious or more than one microscopically positive lymph node.[114] From the foregoing observations it would seem that patients with only one microscopically positive groin node require no further therapy. Patients with two or more positive groin nodes or one large positive groin node are best treated by pelvic and groin irradiation after primary surgery regardless of the type of incision used for the groin dissection.

3. Postoperative radiation therapy may be beneficial in patients with involved or close surgical margins.[179]

4. As suggested by Hacker in 1990, radiation may possibly play a role as primary therapy in women who have small clitoral or periclitoral lesions and in whom surgical resection would have significant psychological consequences.[132]

**Recurrence.** About two thirds of recurrences of vulvar squamous cell carcinoma occur within the first 24 months after initial surgery.[180] Groin recurrences occur significantly sooner (on average, at about 6 months) than vulvar recurrences (at about 3 years).[181] The risk for recurrence of vulvar cancer correlates most closely with the number of positive groin nodes (see Table 58–7). Patients with fewer than three positive groin nodes have a low incidence of recurrence at any site, whereas those with three or more positive nodes have a high incidence of local, regional, and systemic recurrences. Local vulvar recurrences are most likely in patients with primary lesions greater than 4 cm and close (8 mm or less) or positive margins.[125, 182] Once disease has recurred, risk factors for poor outcome are advanced stage, high tumor grade, short disease-free interval, and site of recurrence, with recurrence beyond the vulva being the most important predictor of poor survival.[180, 183] Local recurrences, especially if detected early, are amenable to further surgical excision or radiation therapy, and if this is the only site of recurrence, that patient can usually be saved.[84, 130, 131, 180, 183] Regional or systemic recurrences are difficult problems to manage and are associated with a poor prognosis.[180, 181, 183] Radiation therapy and chemotherapeutic agents that have activity against squamous cell carcinoma are indicated, but response rates are low. Long-term survival is uncommon with regional or distal recurrences.[180–183]

## Adenosquamous Carcinoma

Lever, in 1947, described a distinctive squamous cell carcinoma of the skin composed histologically of both solid areas and gland-like areas.[184] This tumor has a number of synonyms, including adenoid squamous cell carcinoma, pseudoglandular squamous cell carcinoma, and adenoacanthoma of Lever. Most such lesions occur in light-exposed areas, and it has been suggested that they arise from senile keratosis.[185] However, cases have been described as arising from the vulva, where sun exposure would not be a factor.[186, 187] Desquamated cells, many keratinized, may be seen in the glandular lumina, and Lasser and coworkers postulated that the gland-like spaces were areas of acantholysis.[186] Others have suggested that the glandular cells are mucin-producing cells of the skin appendages.[185, 187]

Regardless of their pathogenesis, these tumors of the

vulva seem to be highly aggressive, present at a more advanced stage, and have a higher rate of lymph node metastases than squamous cell carcinoma of the vulva in relation to tumor size.[187] Underwood and colleagues reported an actuarial 5-year survival rate of 6.6% (1 of 18) for patients with adenosquamous carcinoma of the vulva, compared with 77.4% (48 of 77) for patients with squamous cell carcinoma.[187] The counterpart of this tumor elsewhere on the skin behaves in a relatively benign way, suggesting that the vulvar lesion may be a biologically distinct tumor. Treatment should be the same as for squamous cell carcinoma and generally includes radical vulvectomy with bilateral inguinofemoral lymphadenectomy. Postoperative radiation may be indicated.

## Verrucous Carcinoma

Verrucous carcinoma is a variant of squamous cell carcinoma.[188] It was originally described in the oral cavity by Ackerman.[189] Kraus and Perez-Mesa were the first to report its occurrence in the genital tract.[190] Lesions may occur on the cervix, vulva, or vagina. Grossly, the tumors are exophytic, cauliflower-like, or papillary and resemble condylomata acuminata. Microscopically, a tumor with papillary growth is seen, demonstrating hyperkeratosis and parakeratosis. It lacks the central fibrovascular core that is typical of condylomata acuminata and is characterized by the presence of squamous pearls in the deep epithelium that do not exist in condylomata acuminata.[188, 191] The epithelium is well differentiated, cytologic atypia is minimal, and mitoses are seen only occasionally. Invasion occurs across a broad "pushing" front, and unless the base of the lesion is submitted for histologic examination, differentiation from condylomata acuminata or squamous papilloma may be difficult. The gross and microscopic features of verrucous carcinoma are very similar to those of the giant condyloma of Buschke-Löwenstein, and these entities may be successive stages of the same disease process.[191, 192] The cause of these lesions in the female genital tract is unclear, but associated HPV-6 and HPV-11 have been found.[193] Postmenopausal women are typically affected.

Clinically, these tumors are slowly but relentlessly growing lesions that invade adjacent tissues, including bone, causing widespread destruction. Metastases to regional lymph nodes are rare but have been reported.[194] The basic treatment is radical local excision of the primary tumor, although if there are palpably suspicious groin nodes it is difficult to avoid inguinofemoral lymphadenectomy or at least excisional biopsy as well. These enlarged nodes have been reported usually to result from inflammatory hypertrophy.[188] If the nodes contain metastases, radical vulvectomy with bilateral inguinofemoral lymphadenectomy appears indicated. Several small studies failed to demonstrate a significant therapeutic effect of radiation therapy.[188, 190, 194] In addition, several reports indicate that irradiation may induce anaplastic transformation in these lesions and thus should be avoided.[190, 195] Japaze and coworkers reported a corrected 5-year survival of 94% for 17 patients treated with surgery alone, and 42% for 7 patients treated with surgery and radiation. The latter had, however, more advanced disease.[188]

## Bartholin Gland Carcinoma

### NATURAL HISTORY

**Epidemiology and Etiology.** Malignancy of the Bartholin gland was first described by Klob in 1864.[196] Bartholin gland carcinoma is rare, accounting for 2 to 7% of all vulvar malignancies.[107, 197] At an annual incidence of 0.114/100,000, it is five times more common in postmenopausal than in premenopausal (0.025/100,000) women.[198] In a review of the literature, Leuchter and colleagues reported a median age at diagnosis of 57 years, although 38% of the patients were younger than 50 years and the youngest patient described was 14 years old.[107] The cause of Bartholin gland carcinoma is poorly understood. In one small series, HPV has been detected in most squamous cell carcinomas of the Bartholin gland—not, however, in adenocarcinomas.[199]

**Histopathology.** The Bartholin gland is a greater vestibular gland, situated inferior to the bulbocavernosus muscle and superior to the deep perineal muscle. The main duct is lined by stratified squamous epithelium, and this changes to transitional epithelium as the terminal ducts are reached. The gland itself is composed of columnar epithelium. Thus, adenocarcinomas, squamous cell carcinomas, and, rarely, transitional cell carcinomas may arise from the gland. Adenocarcinomas account for about half of the cases; squamous cell carcinomas, close to 40%.[107] Classification of a vulvar carcinoma as arising from the Bartholin gland requires that it fulfill the following criteria:

1. There must be histologic documentation of areas of apparent transition from normal Bartholin epithelium to malignant elements. If that cannot be demonstrated owing to tumor volume, vulvar, vaginal, and rectal epithelium must be carefully sectioned to rule out transition in these areas.
2. Clinical location of the tumor must be in the anatomic region of the Bartholin gland.
3. There may be no evidence of a concurrent primary tumor with similar histologic features elsewhere.[197, 200] Although direct lymphatic channels extend from the Bartholin gland to the pelvic lymph nodes, metastases to the pelvis in the absence of positive inguinal nodes are rare.[107]

**Signs, Symptoms, and Diagnosis.** The most common presenting symptom is a vulvar mass or perineal pain. A history of preceding inflammation of the Bartholin gland may be obtained in up to 10% of patients. Cancer may be mistaken for a benign cyst or abscess, thus delaying diagnosis. Leuchter and colleagues reported that 21 of 90 patients (23%) with Bartholin gland carcinoma initially received an incorrect diagnosis and underwent incision, drainage, and antibiotic therapy before biopsy.[107] Any patient, regardless of age, with a persistent Bartholin gland cyst or abscess unresponsive to standard therapy should be evaluated by biopsy or excision. Because inflammatory disease of the Bartholin gland is uncommon outside the reproductive years and rarely affects postmenopausal women, it may be prudent to obtain histologic evaluation at the time of initial presentation in postmenopausal patients.

**Prognosis and Survival.** Because of the deep location of the gland, cases tend to be more advanced at the time of diagnosis. Less than one third of patients have T1 lesions, and 30 to 50% have lymph node metastases at the time of

*Table 58–17.* Survival of Patients with Bartholin Gland Carcinoma Based on FIGO Stage[107, 197, 201]

| FIGO Stage | No. of Patients | No. of Patients with Recurrence | No. of Patients with NED (Median Follow-up >5 yr) |
|---|---|---|---|
| I | 12 (20%) | 3 (25%) | 11 (92%) |
| II | 15 (25%) | 2 (13%) | 14 (93%) |
| III | 26 (43%) | 8 (31%) | 21 (81%) |
| IV | 7 (12%) | 5 (71%) | 3 (43%) |
| Total | 60 | 18 (30%) | 49 (82%) |

NED, no evidence of disease; FIGO, International Federation of Gynecology and Obstetrics.

diagnosis.[107, 197, 201] Lymph node status is the most important prognostic variable. Patients with stages I and II disease have close to 20% recurrence rates, but more than 90% of patients are reported to be alive and without evidence of disease at a median follow-up of at least 5 years. Prognosis worsens once lymph node metastases are present (Table 58–17).

## TREATMENT

The traditionally recommended treatment is radical vulvectomy and bilateral inguinofemoral lymphadenectomy. Copeland and colleagues at M.D. Anderson Hospital have reported good results with hemivulvectomy or radical local excision for the primary tumor, particularly if postoperative radiation therapy is used locally, which in Copeland's series decreased the likelihood of local recurrence from 27% (6 of 22) to 7% (1 of 14).[197] If the tumor is extensive or fixed to bone, or involves the rectum or anal sphincter, preoperative radiation with or without chemosensitization may decrease the tumor size and extent of surgery needed.

**Adenoid Cystic Carcinoma of Bartholin's Gland.** The adenoid cystic variety, which accounts for 15% of Bartholin's gland carcinomas, takes a more indolent course, is less likely to metastasize to lymph nodes, and carries a somewhat better prognosis.[107, 202] In Copeland and colleagues' review of the literature, 7 of 37 reported cases (19%) were diagnosed during or immediately after pregnancy.[202] Extensive perineural invasion is common and thought to be responsible for the frequent burning and pain associated with and at times preceding the tumor. Local recurrences are common, and metastases, particularly to the lungs, may occur. There is a disparity between progression-free interval and survival curves,[202] reflecting the tendency for late recurrence and the slowly progressive nature of these tumors. For persistent or recurrent disease, radiation therapy with or without chemotherapy may prove to be beneficial.[202–204]

## Malignant Melanoma

### NATURAL HISTORY

**Epidemiology and Etiology.** Malignant melanoma of the vulva is a rare lesion, although it is the second most common vulvar malignancy, accounting for about 4 to 10% of all vulvar cancers.[205] Nearly 5% of all melanomas in women occur on the vulva, which accounts for only 1% of the body's skin surface.[206] Most arise de novo[207] or from preexisting junctional nevi, which may be precursor lesions to melanoma and thus demand excision. Vulvar melanoma occurs predominantly in postmenopausal white women. Vulvar melanoma appears to behave much like other cutaneous melanomas.[208–210]

**Signs, Symptoms, and Diagnosis.** Most patients who develop vulvar melanomas are asymptomatic. A pigmented lesion may be noted on routine examination, or the patient may present with a lesion that may have grown, changed character, or arisen de novo. Some patients present because of itching, bleeding, or a groin mass. Most lesions involve the labia minora or clitoris. There is frequent extension to the urethra or vagina on presentation. Key to improving the outcome in patients with melanoma is early detection. Thus, any pigmented lesion on the vulva requires histologic evaluation. Any nevus on the vulva should be removed, because the majority of nevi on the vulva are junctional and may be precursor lesions to melanoma. Whenever a melanoma is suspected, an excisional biopsy should be performed to allow for pathologic evaluation of the entire lesion.[211] If the lesion is large, an incisional biopsy specimen of sufficient size may be taken from its most significant region. Patients with clinically localized vulvar melanoma beyond the superficial level require careful history and physical examination, chest radiography, and serum lactate dehydrogenase determination.[212] Further testing for metastatic disease may be indicated.

**Histopathology.** There are three basic histologic types. The most common is the superficial spreading melanoma, which tends to remain relatively superficial early in its development. The lentigo maligna melanoma is a flat freckle that sometimes becomes extensive but tends to remain superficial. The third type is nodular melanoma, which is a raised tumor that penetrates deeply and carries an ominous prognosis because it tends to metastasize widely. Amelanotic varieties may occur but are uncommon.

**Routes of Spread.** The pattern of regional metastases resembles that of squamous cell carcinoma of the vulva. However, melanoma tends to spread early not only lymphatically but also hematogenously. The overall incidence of lymph node metastasis in patients with vulvar melanoma is around 20%.[208–210]

**Staging.** The staging is not the same as that for squamous cell carcinoma, because melanomas are usually smaller lesions and tend to metastasize earlier. The prognosis correlates more closely with the depth of tumor penetration. Several staging systems are in use for cutaneous melanoma: The system established by Clark and colleagues depends on the anatomic level of the skin invaded by the melanoma.[213] Survival correlates with the specific subepidermal layer of penetration. The Clark system is less readily applicable to vulvar lesions because of the different skin morphology, as the vulvar skin lacks a well-defined papillary dermis. This makes interpretation at times difficult. Breslow's classification appears to be more adequate for the vulva because it measures in millimeters the tumor thickness to the site of deepest penetration.[214] Chung and colleagues had proposed a modified leveling system for the vulva that retained Clark's definitions for levels I and V but defined levels II, III, and

*Table 58–18.* Microstaging of Vulvar Melanoma

| Level | Extent of Lesion* | | |
|---|---|---|---|
| | CLARK ET AL[213] | CHUNG ET AL[215] | BRESLOW[214] |
| I | Intraepithelial | Intraepithelial | <0.76 mm† |
| II | Into papillary dermis | ≤1 mm from granular layer | 0.76–1.5 mm superficial invasion |
| III | Filling dermal papillae | 1.1–2 mm from granular layer | 1.51–2.25 mm intermediate invasion |
| IV | Into reticular dermis | >2 mm from granular layer | 2.26–3.0 mm intermediate invasion |
| V | Into subcutaneous fat | Into subcutaneous fat | >3.0 mm deep invasion |

*Clark uses level of involvement, Chung uses depth of invasion, and Breslow uses tumor thickness.
†Using Breslow's classification of melanoma, a tumor that is 0.76 mm thick is generally confined to the epidermis and behaves like a carcinoma in situ.

IV using measurements in millimeters.[215] As is evident from Table 58–18, these microstaging systems are not fully comparable. The 1992 American Joint Committee on Cancer (AJCC) melanoma staging combined the Clark and Breslow systems with clinical staging (Table 58–19).

**Prognosis and Survival.** The behavior of melanoma can be unpredictable. Melanomas tend to spread earlier than squamous cell carcinomas, and the overall prognosis is poor. The 5-year survival from several large series reported since 1970 is 32% (Table 58–20), a lower percentage than for vulvar squamous cell carcinoma or cutaneous melanomas in general. This has been largely attributed to an older patient population and a larger proportion of advanced-stage tumors. Prognosis is best predicted by microstaging (Table 58–21). Patients with lesions invading to 1 mm or less have an excellent prognosis, but as depth of invasion increases, prognosis worsens. Chung and colleagues reported corrected 5-year survival rates of 100% for patients with level II lesions (n = 8), 40% with level III and IV lesions (n = 20), and 20% for patients with level V lesions (n = 5). In Chung's series, the 5-year survival rate for patients with positive groin nodes was 13%, and for those with negative nodes, 38%.[215] In addition, tumor volume appears to correlate with prognosis. Patients who have a tumor volume less than 100 mm³ are reported to have an excellent prognosis.[227] In addition to depth of invasion and tumor volume, factors that have an impact on nodal metastasis and survival include a patient's age, AJCC stage, the presence of multifocal or satellite lesions, tumor ulceration, central tumor location, histologic growth pattern, capillary or involvement or LVSI, and aneuploidy.[208–210, 225] The presence of any metastasis confers a very poor prognosis, although long-term survival has been reported in some patients with positive groin nodes.[208, 209]

Survival in patients with lymph nodes metastases appears to decline with the extent and number of nodes involved. Because vulvar melanoma has a propensity for late recurrence, a 5-year survival may not reflect cure.

## TREATMENT

Appropriate treatment of vulvar melanoma continues to be controversial. In part this is because most of the literature on vulvar melanoma consists of small retrospective studies, making it difficult to establish the behavior and treatment of vulvar carcinoma. Most follow a treatment model that combines guidelines for vulvar squamous cell carcinoma and those for cutaneous melanoma in general. These include individualization of management based on microstaging and site of the primary lesion, determination of an appropriate margin of resection, and identification of patients who might benefit from elective regional lymphadenectomy. In line with the trend to more conservative surgery for cutaneous melanoma[229, 230] is a trend toward more conservative management of vulvar melanoma as well.[209, 220, 231] Radical vulvectomy is being performed less frequently, and survival does not appear to be compromised. Current literature on cutaneous melanoma suggests that a 1-cm margin of skin and subcutaneous tissue is adequate for local treatment of a superficial cutaneous melanoma.[232] In a prospective GOG study of 71 patients with vulvar melanoma, the risk of inguinofemoral lymph node metastasis correlates with the Breslow microstage.[210] This GOG study is in keeping with the literature on cutaneous melanoma, which suggests that for superficial lesions (<0.76 mm tumor thickness), the risk for nodal spread is low, that routine regional lymphadenectomy is not

*Table 58–19.* Microstaging Of Vulvar Melanomas

| | Clark's Levels | Chung | Breslow |
|---|---|---|---|
| I | Intraepithelial | Intraepithelial | <0.76 mm |
| II | Into papillary dermis | ≤1 mm from granular layer | 0.76–1.50 mm |
| III | Filling dermal papillae | 1.1–2 mm from granular layer | 1.51–2.25 mm |
| IV | Into reticular dermis | >2 mm from granular layer | 2.26–3.0 mm |
| V | Into subcutaneous fat | Into subcutaneous fat | >3 mm |

*Table 58–20.* Five-Year Survival for Patients with Malignant Melanoma of the Vulva

| Reference | Number | 5-yr Survival (%) |
|---|---|---|
| Yackel et al[217] | 21 | 7 (33) |
| Chung et al[215] | 33 | 10 (30) |
| Karlen et al[218] | 20 | 5 (25) |
| Ariel[219] | 38 | 12 (32) |
| Podratz et al[208] | 48 | 26 (54) |
| Davidson et al[220] | 28 | 7 (25) |
| Bradgate et al[221] | 50 | 15 (30) |
| Total | 238 | 82 (34) |

**Table 58–21.** Prognosis for Patients with Vulvar Melanoma Based on Breslow's Microstaging[209, 222–228]

| Tumor Thickness (mm) | Number | % Died of Disease |
|---|---|---|
| <0.76 | 31 (13%) [19 (8%)] | 7 (23%) [1/19 (5%)]* |
| 0.76–1.5 | 35 (15%) | 6 (17%) |
| 1.51–3.0 | 42 (18%) | 23 (55%) |
| >3.0 | 128 (54%) | 86 (67%) |
| Total | 236 (100%) | 122 (52%) |

*All but one of these seven deaths are reported in one study with an unusually low 5-yr survival of 48% for 12 patients with melanomas of Breslow thickness <0.76 mm.[209]

indicated, and that wide local excision is adequate therapy.[233] For intermediate-thickness (1 to 4 mm) cutaneous melanomas, the excision margin can be safely reduced to 2 cm.[234] Frequent tumor encroachment on midline vulvar structures can make it difficult to obtain adequate margins while avoiding compromise to organ function. Appropriate margin size for involved mucosa remains controversial but should probably at least be equal to the corresponding cutaneous margin. This often requires removal of the clitoris, portions of the distal vagina, or parts of the distal urethra. Careful judgment is required in determining the need for more extensive surgery, such as exenteration, with more extensive organ involvement, especially given the propensity for early lymphatic and hematogenous spread of these tumors. Excision of the underlying layer of the fascia remains controversial. Local management of deep melanomas is less clear owing to the high risk of metastatic disease in these patients. Radical vulvectomy with en bloc bilateral inguinal-femoral lymphadenectomy has traditionally been recommended. However, the trend to individualize and to use less morbid procedures, such as separate groin incisions and radical local excision, often leaves only a few patients who indeed require radical vulvectomy. The value of lymphadenectomy for patients with deeply invasive melanoma is controversial. Patients with cutaneous melanoma thicker than 4 mm have a high risk of both regional and systemic metastases, and they are unlikely to benefit from a regional lymphadenectomy.[233] Site-specific for the vulva is a small amount of data that suggest a possible benefit of elective groin lymphadenectomy and removal of clinically positive nodes.[208, 209] Pelvic lymphadenectomy does not appear to be warranted in patients with lesions confined to the vulva and negative groin nodes. The benefit of pelvic lymphadenectomy for patients with positive groin nodes is probably minimal as well.

If the groin nodes are fixed or ulcerated or the metastatic work-up indicates spread beyond the vulva or groin, palliative wide local excision of the primary and groin lesions should be the only surgical intervention.

**Nonsurgical Treatment.** Vulvar melanoma is less sensitive to radiation and chemotherapy than other cancers. Adjuvant therapy with nonspecific immunostimulants such as bacille Calmette-Guérin or chemotherapeutic agents such as dacarbazine (DTIC) has been tried but without much success. Cancer vaccines are currently under investigation.[235] Treatment with alfa-2b interferon has improved survival for patients with deeply (>4 mm) invasive cutaneous melanoma

and those with lymph node metastases, but patient morbidity is substantial.[236]

**Recurrence.** Recurrent or metastatic disease carries a poor prognosis. Local recurrences are reported in 33% of vulvar melanomas and tend to involve the medial margin of resection, not surprising because central location and mucosal involvement make obtaining an adequate margin difficult. Apparently isolated local or regional recurrences may be amenable to excision. Systemic therapy is of limited palliative benefit.

## Basal Cell Carcinoma

Basal cell carcinomas represent about 2 to 3% of all vulvar cancers, in contrast to their occurrence on sun-exposed skin, where 60 to 65% of all malignancies are basal cell carcinomas.[237] They usually affect postmenopausal white women, two thirds of whom are older than 70 years.[237]

Symptoms are frequently present for a prolonged period and most commonly include irritation, soreness, and pruritus.[237] Basal cell carcinomas typically occur on the anterior vulva, especially the labia majora. They generally are T1 tumors,[237] but giant lesions have been reported.[238] As is typical for basal cell carcinoma elsewhere on the body, they commonly present as the so-called rodent ulcer, a small nodule with a central ulceration and rolled edges. Nodules, plaques, and macules are other morphologic varieties. Diagnosis is made by biopsy. Basal cell carcinomas are locally invasive, although rarely metastasizing.[237, 239, 240] Of the seven well-documented cases of regional lymph node metastases, all had either a deep infiltrating or large (>4 cm) primary tumor.[237]

Radical local excision is adequate treatment, but local disease recurs in about 10 to 20% of cases[237, 241] and may be related to inadequate margins. Regional lymphadenectomy may be indicated in selected cases. About 3 to 5% of basal cell carcinomas contain a malignant squamous component (basosquamous carcinoma). These lesions are more aggressive and should be treated as squamous cell carcinomas.[239] Another variant is the adenoid basal cell carcinoma, which must be differentiated from the more aggressive adenoid cystic carcinoma of the Bartholin's gland or the skin appendages.[239] Basal cell carcinomas are associated with a high incidence of antecedent or concomitant malignancies elsewhere in the body. Benedet and colleagues described 10 patients with other basal cell carcinomas and 10 patients with other primary malignancies in their series of 28 women with vulvar basal cell carcinoma. One of the 28 patients (3.6%) in their series died of metastatic basal cell carcinoma.[237]

## Merkel Cell Carcinoma

Merkel cell tumors, also known as trabecular carcinoma or primary cutaneous neuroendocrine carcinoma, are malignant, small cell, neuroendocrine tumors of the skin. They are thought to be derived from Merkel cells, which are touch-sensitive receptor cells in the basal layer of the epidermis.[242]

At least nine of these tumors have been reported to originate from the vulva.[243] They usually present as a painless sessile mass. These tumors tend to be aggressive, with a high incidence of LVSI and bilateral lymph node metastases, as well as distant metastases. Recommended treatment includes radical local excision with bilateral inguinofemoral lymphadenectomy and adjuvant chemotherapy.[244]

## Vulvar Sarcoma

Vulvar sarcomas represent 1 to 2% of vulvar malignancies. Many histologic types have been reported, including leiomyosarcoma, fibrosarcoma, neurofibrosarcoma, liposarcoma, rhabdomyosarcoma, angiosarcoma, epitheloid sarcoma, malignant fibrous histiocytoma, dermatofibrosarcoma protuberans, malignant schwannoma, and histiocytosis X.

Leiomyosarcomas appear to be the most common variant. Most patients present with an enlarging, often painful mass, usually in the area of the labium majus. Nielsen and colleagues propose that tumors that show at least three of the following four criteria should be considered sarcomas: 5 cm or greater in largest diameter, infiltrative margins, five or more mitotic figures per 10 high-power fields, and moderate to severe cytologic atypia.[245] Treatment must be individualized to the location and extent of disease. Lymphatic metastases are uncommon,[246] and radical wide excision is usually the appropriate local treatment; as with enucleation, the recurrence risk is as great as 70%.[247, 248]

Epithelioid sarcomas may rarely occur on the vulva. Ulbright and colleagues reported that these tumors may mimic a Bartholin's cyst and thus may receive inadequate initial treatment. They tend to behave more aggressively than their extragenital counterparts, with four of five patients dying of metastatic disease in Ulbright's series.[249]

Rhabdomyosarcomas are the most common soft tissue sarcomas in childhood, and 20% involve the pelvis or genitourinary tract.[250] The development of a combined modality treatment approach has made significant improvements in the management of these tumors. Hays and colleagues described nine patients, ages 1 to 19 years, with primary vulvar rhabdomyosarcoma, five of which had embryonal (botryoid) histologic characteristics. Following chemoradiation and wide local excision with or without inguinofemoral lymphadenectomy, eight of nine patients were in long-term remission and one was alive with disease.[251]

Dermatofibrosarcoma protruberans is a rare, cutaneous, low-grade malignancy with a marked tendency for local recurrence but very infrequently metastasizing.[252–254] Few cases are reported to arise in the vulva. They tend to be multinodular, slow growing, and painless. Radical local excision is the recommended treatment.

## Rare Vulvar Malignancies

Apart from those previously mentioned, a number of tumors more commonly seen in other sites of the body may rarely present as an isolated vulvar tumor. These include lymphomas, plasmacytomas, and endodermal sinus (yolk sac) tumors. Treatment for these tumors must be individualized but generally consists of wide local excision and chemotherapy or radiation therapy, depending on the nature of the tumor.

## Metastatic Tumors of the Vulva

About 8% of vulvar tumors are metastatic and originate, in decreasing order of frequency, from cervix, endometrium, kidney, and urethra. Most patients who develop vulvar metastases have an advanced primary tumors at diagnosis. In about one fourth of these patients, the primary lesion and the vulvar metastasis are diagnosed simultaneously.[79]

### REFERENCES

1. Blair-Bell W, Datnow MM. Primary malignant disease of the vulva, with special reference to treatment by operation. J Obset Gynaecol Br Emp 1936;43:755–63.
2. Way S. The anatomy of the lymphatic drainage of the vulva and its influence on the radical operation for carcinoma. Ann R Coll Surg Eng 1948;3:187–209.
3. Basset A. Traitement chirurgical opératoire de l'épithélioma primitif du clitoris. Indications—technique—résultats. Rev Chir 1912;32:546–70.
4. Taussig FJ. Cancer of the vulva. An analysis of 155 cases (1911–40). Am J Obstet Gynecol 1940;40:764–79.
5. Way S. Carcinoma of the vulva. Am J Obstet Gynecol 1960;79:692–7.
6. DiSaia PJ, Creasman WT, Rich WM. An alternate approach to early cancer of the vulva. Am J Obstet Gynecol 1979;133:825–32.
7. Hacker NF, Berek JS, Lagasse LD, et al. Individualization of treatment for stage I squamous cell vulvar carcinoma. Obstet Gynecol 1984;63:155–62.
8. Morris JM. A formula for selective lymphadenectomy. Its application to cancer of the vulva. Obstet Gynecol 1977;50:152–8.
9. Hacker NF, Berek JS, Lagasse LD, et al. Management of regional lymph nodes and their prognostic influence in vulvar cancer. Obstet Gynecol 1983;61:408–12.
10. Hacker NF, Van der Velden J. Conservative management of early vulvar cancer. Cancer 1993;71:1673–7.
11. Hacker NF, Leuchter RS, Berek JS, et al. Radical vulvectomy and bilateral inguinal lymphadenectomy through separate groin incisions. Obstet Gynecol 1981;58:574–9.
12. Boronow RC. Combined therapy as an alternative to exenteration for locally advanced vulvo-vaginal cancer. Rationale and results. Cancer 1982;49:1085–91.
13. Hacker NF, Berek JS, Juillard GJF, Lagasse LD. Preoperative radiation therapy for locally advanced vulvar cancer. Cancer 1984;54:2056–61.
14. Jeffcoate TNA. Chronic vulvar dystrophies. Am J Obstet Gynecol 1966;95:61–74.
15. Gardner HL, Friedrich EG Jr, Kaufmann RH, Woodruff JD. The vulvar dystrophies, atypias, and carcinoma in situ: an invitational symposium. J Reprod Med 1976;17:131–64.
16. Ridley CM, Frankman O, Jones ISC, et al. Announcement. New nomenclature for vulvar disease. Report of the Committee on Terminology, International Society for the Study of Vulvar Disease. Int J Gynecol Pathol 1989;8:83–4.
17. Collins CG, Hansen LH, Theriot E. A clinical stain for use in selecting biopsy sites in patients with vulvar disease. Obstet Gynecol 1966;28:158–63.
18. Joura EA, Zeisler H, Lösch A, et al. Differentiating vulvar intraepithelial neoplasia from nonneoplastic epithelial disorders. The toluidine blue test. J Reprod Med 1998;43:671–4.
19. Leibowitch M, Neill S, Pelisse M, Moyal-Barracco M. The epithelial changes associated with squamous cell carcinoma of the vulva: a review of the clinical, histological, and viral findings in 78 women. Br J Obstet Gynaecol 1990;97:1135–9.
20. Buscema J, Stern J, Woodruff JD. The significance of the histologic alterations adjacent to invasive vulvar carcinoma. Am J Obstet Gynecol 1980;137:902–9.

21. Gómez Rueda N, García A, Vighi S. Epithelial alterations adjacent to invasive squamous carcinoma of the vulva. J Reprod Med 1994;39:526–30.

22. Vilmer C, Cavelier-Balloy B, Nogues C, et al. Analysis of alterations adjacent to invasive vulvar carcinoma and their relationship with the associated carcinoma: a study of 67 cases. Eur J Gynecol Oncol 1998;19:25–31.

23. Kagie MJ. Aspects of malignant progression of vulvar epithelial disorders. Eur J Obstet Gynecol 1998;80:1–3.

24. Carlson JA, Ambros R, Malfetano J, et al. Vulvar lichen sclerosus and squamous cell carcinoma: a cohort, case control, and investigational study with historic perspective; implications for chronic inflammation and sclerosis in the development of neoplasia. Hum Pathol 1998;29:932–48.

25. Godeau G, Frances C, Hornebeck W, et al. Isolation and partial characterization of an elastase-type protease in human vulvar fibroblasts: its possible involvement in vulvar elastic tissue destruction of patients with lichen sclerosus et atrophicus. J Invest Dermatol 1982;78:270–7.

26. Meyrick Thomas RH, McGibbon DH, Ridley CM, Black MM. Anogenital lichen sclerosus in women. J R Soc Med 1996;89:694–8.

27. Carli P, Cattaneo A, Pimpinelli N, et al. Immunohistochemical evidence of skin immune system involvement in vulvar lichen sclerosus et atrophicus. Dermatologica 1991;182:18–22.

28. Dalziel KL, Millard PR, Wojnarowska F. The treatment of vulvar lichen sclerosus with a very potent topical steroid (clobetasol propionate 0.05%) cream. Br J Dermatol 1991;124:461–4.

29. Bracco GL, Carli P, Sonni L, et al. Clinical and histologic effects of topical treatments of vulvar lichen sclerosus. A critical evaluation. J Reprod Med 1993;38:37–40.

30. Dalziel KL, Wojnarowska F. Long-term control of vulval lichen sclerosus after treatment with a potent topical steroid cream. J Reprod Med 1993;38:25–7.

31. Bornstein J, Heifetz S, Kellner Y, et al. Clobatasol dipropionate 0.05% versus testosterone propionate 2% topical application for severe vulvar lichen sclerosus. Am J Obstet Gynecol 1998;178:80–4.

32. Abramov Y, Elchalal U, Abramov D, et al. Surgical treatment of vulvar lichen sclerosus: a review. Obstet Gynecol Surv 1996;51:193–9.

33. Campion MJ. Clinical manifestations and natural history of genital human papilloma virus infection. Obstet Gynecol Clin North Am 1987;14:363–88.

34. Hummer WK, Mussey E, Decker DG, Dockerty MB. Carcinoma in situ of the vagina. Am J Obstet Gynecol 1970;108:1109–16.

35. Hørding U, Junge J, Poulsen H, Lundvall F. Vulvar intraepithelial neoplasia III: a viral disease of undetermined progressive potential. Gynecol Oncol 1995;56:276–9.

36. Ogunbiyi OA, Scholefield JH, Robertson G, et al. Anal human papilloma virus infection and squamous neoplasia in patients with vulvar cancer. Obstet Gynecol 1994;83:212–6.

37. Reid R. Human papillomaviral infection: the key to rational triage of cervical neoplasia. Obstet Gynecol Clin North Am 1987;14:407–29.

38. Sturgeon SR, Brinton LA, Devesa SS, Kurman RJ. In situ and invasive vulvar cancer incidence trends (1973–87). Am J Obstet Gynecol 1992;166:1482–5.

39. Modesitt SC, Waters AB, Walton L, et al. Vulvar intraepithelial neoplasia III: occult cancer and the impact of margin status on recurrence. Obstet Gynecol 1998;92:962–6.

40. Jones RW, Baranyai J, Stables S. Trends in squamous cell carcinoma of the vulva: the influence of vulvar intraepithelial neoplasia. Obstet Gynecol 1997;90:448–52.

41. Wright TC, Koulos JP, Liu P, Sun XW. Invasive vulvar carcinoma in two women infected with human immunodeficiency virus. Gynecol Oncol 1996;60:500–3.

42. Jones RW, Rowan DM. Vulvar intraepithelial neoplasia III: a clinical study of the outcome in 113 cases with relation to the later development of invasive vulvar carcinoma. Obstet Gynecol 1994;84:741–5.

43. Küppers V, Stiller M, Somville T, Bender HG. Risk factors for recurrent VIN. Role of multifocality and grade of disease. J Reprod Med 1997;42:140–44.

44. Buscema J, Woodruff JD, Parmley TH, Genadry R. Carcinoma in situ of the vulva. Obstet Gynecol 1980;55:225–30.

45. Kurman RJ, Norris HJ, Wilkinson EJ, eds. Tumors of the cervix, vagina, and vulva. In: Atlas of tumor pathology. Washington, D.C.: Armed Forces Institute of Pathology, 1992:183–9.

46. Friedrich EG Jr, Wilkinson EG, Fu YS. Carcinoma in situ of the vulva: a continuing challenge. Am J Obstet Gynecol 1980:136:830–43.

47. DiSaia PJ, Rich WM. Surgical approach to multifocal carcinoma in situ of the vulva. Am J Obstet Gynecol 1981;140:136–45.

48. Rutledge F, Sinclair M. Treatment of intraepithelial carcinoma of the vulva by skin excision and graft. Am J Obstet Gynecol 1968;102:806–18.

49. Rettenmaier MA, Berman ML, DiSaia PJ. Skinning vulvectomy for the treatment of multifocal vulvar intraepithelial neoplasia. Obstet Gynecol 1987;69:247–50.

50. Sillman FH, Sedlis A, Boyce JG. A review of lower genital intraepithelial neoplasia and the use of topical 5-fluorouracil. Obstet Gynecol Surv 1985;40:190–220.

51. Krupp PJ. 5-Fluorouracil topical treatment of in situ vulvar cancer. Obstet Gynecol 1978;51:702–6.

52. Paget J. St Bartholomew's Hosp Rep 1874;10:87.

53. Dubreuilh W. Pigmentation of the skin due to demodex folliculorum. Br J Dermatol 1901;13:403.

54. Curtin JP, Rubin SC, Jones WB, et al. Paget's disease of the vulva. Gynecol Oncol 1990;39:374–7.

55. Fanning J, Lambert L, Hale TM, et al. Paget's disease of the vulva: prevalence of associated vulvar adenocarcinoma, invasive Paget's disease, and recurrence after surgical excision. Am J Obstet Gynecol 1999;180:24–7.

56. Helwig EB, Graham JH. Anogenital (extramammary) Paget's disease. Cancer 1963;16:387–403.

57. Navin J. Pathology and fine needle aspiration cytology of the breast. In: Hindle W, ed. Breast disease for gynecologists. Norwalk, Conn.: Appleton & Lange, 1990:183–91.

58. Creasman WT, Gallager HS, Rutledge F. Paget's disease of the vulva. Gynecol Oncol 1975;3:133–48.

59. Feuer GA, Shevchuk M, Calanog A. Vulvar Paget's disease: the need to exclude an invasive lesion. Gynecol Oncol 1990;38:81–9.

60. Hart WR, Millman JB. Progression of intraepithelial Paget's disease of the vulva to invasive carcinoma. Cancer 1977;40:2333–7.

61. Stacy D, Burrell MO, Franklin EW III. Extramammary Paget's disease of the vulva and anus: use of intraoperative frozen-section margins. Am J Obstet Gynecol 1986;155:519–23.

62. Bergen S, DiSaia PJ, Liao SY, Berman ML. Conservative management of extramammary Paget's disease of the vulva. Gynecol Oncol 1989;33:151–6.

63. Fishman DA, Chambers SK, Schwartz PE, et al. Extramammary Paget's disease of the vulva. Gynecol Oncol 1995;56:266–70.

64. Kodama S, Kaneko T, Saito M, et al. A clinicopathologic study of 30 patients with Paget's disease of the vulva. Gynecol Oncol 1995;56:63–70.

65. Fetherston WC, Friedrich EG. The origin and significance of vulvar Paget's disease. Obstet Gynecol 1972;39:735–44.

66. Guarner J, Cohen C, DeRose PB. Histogenesis of extramammary and mammary Paget cells. An immunohistochemical study. Am J Dermatopathol 1989;11:313–8.

67. Koss LG, Brockunier A. Ultrastructural aspects of Paget's disease of the vulva. Arch Pathol 1969;87:592–600.

68. Mazoujian G, Pincus GS, Haagensen DE. Extramammary Paget's disease—evidence for an apocrine origin. Am J Surg Pathol 1984;8:43–50.

69. Friedrich EG, Wilkinson EJ, Steingraeber PH, Lewis JD. Paget's disease of the vulva and carcinoma of the breast. Obstet Gynecol 1975;130–4.

70. Snow SN, Desouky S, Lo JS, Kurtycz D. Failure to detect human papillomavirus DNA in extramammary Paget's disease. Cancer 1992;69:249–51.

71. Takata M, Hatta N, Takehara K. Tumor cells of extramammary Paget's disease do not show either p53 mutation or allelic loss at several selected loci implicated in other cancers. Br J Cancer 1997;76:904–8.

72. Lee RA, Dahlin DC. Paget's disease of the vulva with extension into the urethra, bladder, and ureters: a case report. Am J Obstet Gynecol 1981;140:834–6.

73. Gunn RA, Gallager HS. Vulvar Paget's disease. A topographic study. Cancer 1980;46:590–4.

74. Fine BA, Fowler LJ, Valente PT, Gaudet T. Minimally invasive Paget's disease of the vulva with extensive lymph node metastases. Gynecol Oncol 1995;57:262–5.

75. Scheistrøen M, Tropé C, Kaern J, et al. DNA ploidy and expression of p53 and C-erB-2 in extramammary Paget's disease of the vulva. Gynecol Oncol 1997;64:88–92.

76. Geisler JP, Stowell MJ, Melton ME, et al. Extramammary Paget's

disease of the vulva recurring in a skin graft. Gynecol Oncol 1995;56:446–7.

77. DiSaia PJ, Dorion GE, Cappuccini F, Carpenter PM. A report of two cases of recurrent Paget's disease of the vulva in a split-thickness graft and its possible pathogenesis labeled "retrodissemination." Gynecol Oncol 1995;57:109–112.

78. Rhodes CA, Cummins C, Shafi MI. The management of squamous cell vulval cancer: a population based retrospective study of 411 cases. Br J Obstet Gynaecol 1998;105:200–5.

79. Morrow CP, Curtin JP, eds. Tumors of the vulva. In: Synopsis of gynecologic oncology. 5th ed. New York: Churchill Livingstone, 1998;61–87.

80. Dehner LP. Metastatic and secondary tumors of the vulva. Obstet Gynecol 1973;42:47–57.

81. Landis SH, Murray T, Bolden S, Wingo PA. Cancer statistics 1999. CA Cancer J Clin 1999;49:8–31.

82. Rutledge F, Smith JP, Franklin EW. Carcinoma of the vulva. Am J Obstet Gynecol 1970;106:1117–30.

83. Podratz KC, Symmonds RE, Taylor WF, Williams TJ. Carcinoma of the vulva: analysis of treatment and survival. Obstet Gynecol 1983;61:63–74.

84. Cavanagh D, Fiorica JV, Hoffman MS, et al. Invasive carcinoma of the vulva. Changing trends in surgical management. Am J Obstet Gynecol 1990;163:1007–15.

85. Trimble CL, Hildesheim A, Brinton LA, et al. Heterogeneous etiology of squamous carcinoma of the vulva. Obstet Gynecol 1996;87:59–64.

86. Rusk D, Sutton GP, Look KY, Roman A. Analysis of invasive squamous cell carcinoma of the vulva and vulvar intraepithelial neoplasia for the presence of human papillomavirus DNA. Obstet Gynecol 1991;77:918–22.

87. Madeleine MM, Daling JR, Carter JJ, et al. Cofactors with human papillomavirus in a population-based study of vulvar cancer. J Natl Cancer Inst 1997;89:1516–23.

88. Bloss JD, Liao SY, Wilczynski SP, et al. Clinical and histologic features of vulvar carcinoma analyzed for human papillomavirus status: evidence that squamous cell carcinoma of the vulva has more than one etiology. Hum Pathol 1991;22:711–8.

89. Brinton LA, Nasca PC, Mallin K, et al. Case-control study of cancer of the vulva. Obstet Gynecol 1990;75:859–66.

90. Korn AP, Autry M, DeRemer PA, Tan W. Sensitivity of the Papanicolaou smear in human immunodeficiency virus–infected women. Obstet Gynecol 1994;83:401–4.

91. Zacur H, Genadry R, Woodruff JD. The patient-at-risk for development of vulvar cancer. Gynecol Oncol 1980;9:199–208.

92. Kurman RJ, Toki T, Schiffman MH. Basaloid and warty carcinoma of the vulva. Distinctive types of squamous cell carcinoma frequently associated with human papillomaviruses. Am J Surg Pathol 1993;17:133–45.

93. Tate JE, Mutter GL, Boynton KA, Crum CP. Monoclonal origin of vulvar intraepithelial neoplasia and some vulvar hyperplasias. Am J Pathol 1997;150:315–22.

94. Franklin EW, Rutledge FD. Epidemiology of epidermoid carcinoma of the vulva. Obstet Gynecol 1972;39:165–72.

95. Green TH Jr, Ulfelder H, Meigs JV. Epidermoid carcinoma of the vulva: an analysis of 238 cases. Part I. Am J Obstet Gynecol 1958;75:834–47.

96. Chafe W, Richards A, Morgan L, Wilkinson E. Unrecognized invasive carcinoma in vulvar intraepithelial neoplasia (VIN). Gynecol Oncol 1988;31:154–62.

97. Benedet JL, Turko M, Fairey RN, Boyes DA. Squamous carcinoma of the vulva: results of treatment, 1938–76. Am J Obstet Gynecol 1979;134:201–7.

98. Micheletti L, Borgno G, Barbero M, et al. Deep femoral lymphadenectomy with preservation of the fascia lata. Preliminary report on 42 invasive vulvar carcinomas. J Reprod Med 1990;35:1130–33.

99. Chu J, Tamimi HK, Figge DC. Femoral node metastases with negative superficial inguinal lymph nodes in early vulvar cancer. Am J Obstet Gynecol 1981;140:337–8.

100. Podczaski E, Sexton M, Kaminski P, et al. Recurrent carcinoma of the vulva after conservative treatment for "microinvasive" disease. Gynecol Oncol 1990;39:65–8.

101. Stehman FB, Bundy BN, Dvoretsky PM, Creasman WT. Early stage I carcinoma of the vulva treated with ipsilateral superficial inguinal lymphadenectomy and modified radical hemivulvectomy: a prospective study of the Gynecologic Oncology Group. Obstet Gynecol 1992;79:490–7.

102. Levenback C, Burke TW, Morris M, et al. Potential applications of intraoperative lymphatic mapping in vulvar cancer. Gynecol Oncol 1995;59:216–20.

103. Keys H. Gynecologic Oncology Group randomized trials of combined technique therapy of vulvar cancer. Cancer 1993;71:1691–6.

104. Malfetano JH, Piver MS, Tsukada Y, Reese P. Univariate and multivariate analyses of 5-year survival, recurrence, and inguinal node metastases in stage I and II vulvar carcinoma. J Surg Oncol 1985;30:124–31.

105. Curry SL, Wharton JT, Rutledge F. Positive lymph nodes in vulvar squamous carcinoma. Gynecol Oncol 1980;9:63–7.

106. Piver MS, Xynos FP. Pelvic lymphadenectomy in women with carcinoma of the clitoris. Obstet Gynecol 1977;49:592–5.

107. Leuchter RS, Hacker NF, Voet RL, et al. Primary carcinoma of the Bartholin gland: a report of 14 cases and review of the literature. Obstet Gynecol 1982;60:361–8.

108. Collins CG, Lee FY, Roman-Lopez JJ. Invasive carcinoma of the vulva with lymph node metastasis. Am J Obstet Gynecol 1971;109:446–52.

109. Morley GW. Infiltrative carcinoma of the vulva: results of surgical treatment. Am J Obstet Gynecol 1976;124:874–88.

110. Krupp PJ, Bohm JW. Lymph gland metastases in invasive squamous cell cancer of the vulva. Am J Obstet Gynecol 1978;130:943–52.

111. Iversen T, Aalders JG, Christensen A, Kolstad P. Squamous cell carcinoma of the vulva: a review of 424 patients, 1956–1974. Gynecol Oncol 1980;9:271–9.

112. Monaghan JM, Hammond IG. Pelvic node dissection in the treatment of vulval carcinoma—is it necessary? Br J Obstet Gynaecol 1984;91:270–4.

113. Hopkins MP, Reid CG, Vettrano I, Morley GW. Squamous cell carcinoma of the vulva: prognostic factors influencing survival. Gynecol Oncol 1991;43:113–7.

114. Homesley H, Bundy BN, Sedlis A, Adcock L. Radiation therapy versus pelvic node resection for carcinoma of the vulva with positive groin nodes. Obstet Gynecol 1986;68:733–40.

115. Shepherd JH. Staging announcement. FIGO staging of gynecologic cancers; cervical and vulva. Int J Gynecol Cancer 1995;5:319.

116. Baehrs OH, Henson DE, Hutter RVP, Kennedy BJ, eds. Vulva. In: Manual for staging cancer. 4th ed. American Joint Committee on Cancer. Philadelphia: JB Lippincott, 1992:177–80.

117. Homesley HD, Bundy BN, Sedlis A, et al. Prognostic factors for groin node metastasis in squamous cell carcinoma of the vulva (a GOG study). Gynecol Oncol 1993;49:279–83.

118. Homesley HD, Bundy BN, Sedlis A, et al. Assessment of current FIGO staging of vulvar carcinoma relative to prognostic factors for survival (a GOG study). Am J Obstet Gynecol 1991;164:997–1004.

119. Green TH Jr. Carcinoma of the vulva. A reassessment. Obstet Gynecol 1978;52:462–9.

120. Cavanagh D, Roberts WS, Bryson SCP, et al. Changing trends in the surgical management of invasive carcinoma of the vulva. Surg Gynecol Obstet 1986;162:164–8.

121. Hoffman JS, Kurman NB, Morley GW. Prognostic significance of groin lymph node metastases in squamous carcinoma of the vulva. Obstet Gynecol 1985;66:402–5.

122. Atamdede F, Hoogerland D. Regional lymph node recurrence following local excision for microinvasive vulvar carcinoma. Gynecol Oncol 1989;34:125–8.

123. Boyce J, Fruchter RG, Kasambilides E, et al. Prognostic factors in carcinoma of the vulva. Gynecol Oncol 1985;20:364–77.

124. Iversen T, Abeler V, Aalders J. Individualized treatment of stage I carcinoma of vulva. Obstet Gynecol 1981;57:85–9.

125. Heaps JM, Fu YS, Montz FJ, et al. Surgical-pathologic variables predictive of local recurrences in squamous cell carcinoma of the vulva. Gynecol Oncol 1990;38:309–14.

126. Donaldson ES, Powell DE, Hanson MB, van Nagell JR. Prognostic parameters in invasive vulvar cancer. Gynecol Oncol 1981;11:184–90.

127. Husseinzadeh N, Zaino R, Nahhas WA, Mortel R. The significance of histologic findings in predicting nodal metastases in invasive squamous cell carcinoma of the vulva. Gynecol Oncol 1983;16:105–11.

128. Monk BJ, Burger RA, Lin F, et al. Prognostic significance of human papillomavirus DNA in vulvar carcinoma. Obstet Gynecol 1995;85:709–15.

129. Franklin EW III, Rutledge FD. Prognostic factors in epidermoid carcinoma of the vulva. Obstet Gynecol 1971;37:892–901.

130. Burke TW, Levenback C, Coleman RL, et al. Surgical therapy of T1 and T2 vulvar carcinoma: further experience with radical wide exci-

sion and selective inguinal lymphadenectomy. Gynecol Oncol 1995;57:215–220.

131. Hopkins MP, Reid GC, Morley GW. The surgical management of recurrent squamous cell carcinoma of the vulva. Obstet Gynecol 1990;75:1001–5.

132. Hacker NF. Vulvar cancer. In: Berek JS, Hacker NF, eds. Practical gynecologic oncology. 3rd ed. Philadelphia: Lippincott Williams & Wilkins, 2000:553–96.

133. Reid GC, DeLancey JOL, Hopkins MP, et al. Urinary incontinence following radical vulvectomy. Obstet Gynecol 1990;75:852–8.

134. Burrell MO, Franklin EW III, Campion MJ, et al. The modified radical vulvectomy with groin dissection: an eight-year experience. Am J Obstet Gynecol 1988;159:715–22.

135. Hoffman MS, Roberts WS, Finan MA, et al. A comparative study of radical vulvectomy and modified radical vulvectomy for treatment of invasive squamous cell carcinoma of the vulva. Gynecol Oncol 1992;45:192–7.

136. Farias-Eisner R, Cirisano FD, Grouse D, et al. Conservative and individualized surgery for early squamous carcinoma of the vulva: the treatment of choice for stages I and II (T1–2, N0–1, M0) disease. Gynecol Oncol 1994;53:55–8.

137. Simonsen E, Johnsson JE, Tropé C. Radical vulvectomy with warm-knife and open-wound techniques in vulvar malignancies. Gynecol Oncol 1984;17:22–31.

138. Julian CG, Callison J, Woodruff JD. Plastic management of extensive vulvar defects. Obstet Gynecol 1971;38:193–8.

139. Trelford JD, Deer DA, Ordorica E, et al. Ten-year prospective study in a management change of vulvar carcinoma. Am J Obstet Gynecol 1984;150:288–96.

140. Ballon SC, Donaldson RC, Roberts JA, Lagasse LD. Reconstruction of the vulva using a myocutaneous graft. Gynecol Oncol 1979;7:123–7.

141. Pursell SH, Day TG, Tobin GR. Distally based rectus abdominis flap for reconstruction in radical gynecologic procedures. Gynecol Oncol 1990;37:234–8.

142. Andersen BL, Hacker NF. Psychosexual adjustment after vulvar surgery. Obstet Gynecol 1983;62:457–62.

143. Andersen BL, Hacker NF. Psychosexual adjustment following pelvic exenteration. Obstet Gynecol 1983;61:331–8.

144. Cavanagh D, Shepherd JH. The place of pelvic exenteration in the primary management of advanced carcinoma of the vulva. Gynecol Oncol 1982;13:318–22.

145. Phillips B, Buchsbaum HJ, Lifshitz S. Pelvic exenteration for vulvo-vaginal carcinoma. Am J Obstet Gynecol 1981;141:1038–44.

146. Kaplan AL, Kaufman RH. Management of advanced carcinoma of the vulva. Gynecol Oncol 1975;3:220–32.

147. Bäckström A, Edsmyr F, Wicklund H. Radiotherapy of carcinoma of the vulva. Acta Obstet Gynecol 1972;51:109–15.

148. Boronow RC, Hickman BT, Reagan MT, et al. Combined therapy as an alternative to exenteration for locally advanced vulvovaginal cancer. II. Results, complications, and dosimetric and surgical considerations. Am J Clin Oncol 1987;10:171–81.

149. Thomas G, Dembo A, DePetrillo A, et al. Concurrent radiation and chemotherapy in vulvar carcinoma. Gynecol Oncol 1989;34:263–7.

150. Fairey RN, Mackay PA, Benedet JL, et al. Radiation treatment of carcinoma of the vulva, 1950–80. Am J Obstet Gynecol 1985;151:591–7.

151. Rotmensch J, Rubin SJ, Sutton HG, et al. Preoperative radiotherapy followed by radical vulvectomy with inguinal lymphadenectomy for advanced vulvar carcinomas. Gynecol Oncol 1990;36:181–4.

152. Berek JS, Heaps JM, Fu YS, et al. Concurrent cisplatin and 5-fluorouracil chemotherapy and radiation therapy for advanced-stage squamous carcinoma of the vulva. Gynecol Oncol 1991;42:197–201.

153. Levin W, Goldberg G, Altaras M, et al. The use of concomitant chemotherapy and radiotherapy prior to surgery in advanced stage carcinoma of the vulva. Gynecol Oncol 1986;25:20–5.

154. Lupi G, Raspagliesi F, Zucali R, et al. Combined preoperative chemo-radiotherapy followed by radical surgery in locally advanced vulvar carcinoma. Cancer 1996;77:1472–8.

155. Evans LS, Kersh CR, Constable WC, Taylor PT. Concomitant 5-fluorouracil, mitomycin-C, and radiotherapy for advanced gynecological malignancies. Int J Radiat Oncol Biol Phys 1988;15:901–6.

156. Russell AH, Mesic JB, Scudder SA, et al. Synchronous radiation and cytotoxic chemotherapy for locally advanced or recurrent squamous cancer of the vulva. Gynecol Oncol 1992;47:14–20.

157. Scheistrøen M, Tropé C. Combined bleomycin and irradiation in preoperative treatment of advanced squamous cell carcinoma of the vulva. Acta Oncol 1993;32:657–61.

158. Wahlen SA, Slater JD, Wagner RJ, et al. Concurrent radiation therapy and chemotherapy in the treatment of primary squamous cell carcinoma of the vulva. Cancer 1995;75:2289–94.

159. Eifel PJ, Morris M, Burke TW, et al. Prolonged continuous infusion cisplatin and 5-fluorouracil with radiation for locally advanced carcinoma of the vulva. Gynecol Oncol 1995;59:51–56.

160. Cunningham MJ, Goyer RP, Gibbons SK, et al. Primary radiation, cisplatin, and 5-fluorouracil for advanced squamous carcinoma of the vulva. Gynecol Oncol 1997;66:258–61.

161. Moore DH, Thomas GM, Montana GS, et al. Preoperative chemoradiation for advanced vulvar cancer: a phase II study of the GOG. Int J Radiat Oncol Biol Phys 1998;42:79–85.

162. Magrina JF, Webb MJ, Gaffey TA, Symmonds RE. Stage I squamous cell cancer of the vulva. Am J Obstet Gynecol 1979;134:453–9.

163. Hoffman JS, Kumar NB, Morley GW. Microinvasive squamous carcinoma of the vulva: search for a definition. Obstet Gynecol 1983;61:615–8.

164. Lingard D, Free K, Wright RG, Battistutta D. Invasive squamous cell carcinoma of the vulva: behavior and results in light of changing management regimens. Aust N Z J Obstet Gynaecol 1992;32:137–45.

165. Stehman FB, Bundy BN, Thomas G, et al. Groin dissection versus groin radiation in carcinoma of the vulva: a GOG study. Int J Radiat Oncol Biol Phys 1992;24:389–96.

166. Leong SPL, Steinmetz I, Habib FA, et al. Optimal selective sentinel lymph node dissection in primary malignant melanoma. Arch Surg 1997;132:666–73.

167. Giuliano AE, Jones RC, Brennan M, Statman R. Sentinel lymphadenectomy in breast cancer. J Clin Oncol 1997;15:2345–50.

168. Cox CE, Haddad F, Bass S, et al. Lymphatic mapping in the treatment of breast cancer. Oncology 1998;12:1283–98.

169. DeCesare SL, Fiorica JV, Roberts WS, et al. A pilot study utilizing intraoperative lymphoscintigraphy for identification of the sentinel lymph nodes in vulvar cancer. Gynecol Oncol 1997;66:425–8.

170. Hopkins MP, Reid GC, Morley GW. Radical vulvectomy. The decision for the incision. Cancer 1993;72:799–803.

171. Piver MS, Malfetano JH, Lele SB, Moore RH. Prophylactic anticoagulation as a possible cause of inguinal lymphocyst after radical vulvectomy and inguinal lymphadenectomy. Obstet Gynecol 1983;62:17–21.

172. Daly JW, Pomerance AJ. Groin dissection with prevention of tissue loss and postoperative infection. Obstet Gynecol 1979;53:395–9.

173. Dodd GD, Rutledge F, Wallace S. Postoperative pelvic lymphocysts. Am J Roentgenol 1970;108:312–23.

174. Rutledge F, Dodd GD, Kasilag FB. Lymphocysts: a complication of radical pelvic surgery. Am J Obstet Gynecol 1959;77:1165–75.

175. Casley-Smith JR, Morgan RG, Piller NB. Treatment of lymphedema of the arms and legs with 5,6-benzo-alpha-pyrone. N Engl J Med 1993;329:1158–63.

176. Cavanagh D. Vulvar cancer—continuing evolution in management. Gynecol Oncol 1997;66:362–7.

177. Hoyme UB, Tamimi HK, Eschenbach DA, et al. Osteomyelitis pubis after radical gynecological operations. Obstet Gynecol 1984;63:47S–53S.

178. Thranov I, Klee M. Sexuality among gynecologic cancer patients—a cross-sectional study. Gynecol Oncol 1994;52:14–9.

179. Perez CA, Grigsby PW, Galakatos A, et al. Radiation therapy in management of carcinoma of the vulva with emphasis on conservation therapy. Cancer 1993;71:3707–16.

180. Puira B, Masotina A, Murdoch J, et al. Recurrent squamous cell carcinoma of the vulva: a study of 73 cases. Gynecol Oncol 1993;48:189–95.

181. Stehman FB, Bundy BN, Ball H, Clarke-Pearson DL. Sites of failure and times to failure in carcinoma of the vulva treated conservatively: a GOG study. Am J Obstet Gynecol 1996;174:1128–33.

182. Podratz KC, Symmonds RE, Taylor WF. Carcinoma of the vulva: analysis of treatment failures. Am J Obstet Gynecol 1982;143:340–51.

183. Tilmans AS, Sutton GP, Look KY, et al. Recurrent squamous carcinoma of the vulva. Am J Obstet Gynecol 1992;176:1383–9.

184. Lever WF. Adenoacanthoma of sweat glands. Carcinoma of sweat glands with glandular and epidermal elements; report of four cases. Arch Dermatol Syphilol 1947;56:157–71.

185. Johnson WC, Helwig EB. Adenoid squamous cell carcinoma (adenoacanthoma). A clinicopathologic study of 155 patients. Cancer 1966;19:1639–50.

186. Lasser A, Cornog JL, Morris JM. Adenoid squamous cell carcinoma of the vulva. Cancer 1974;33:224–7.

187. Underwood JW, Adcock LL, Okagaki T. Adenosquamous carcinoma of skin appendages (adenoid squamous cell carcinoma, pseudoglandular squamous cell carcinoma, adenoacanthoma of Lever) of the vulva: a clinical and ultrastructural study. Cancer 1978;42:1851–8.

188. Japaze H, Van Dinh T, Woodruff JD. Verrucous carcinoma of the vulva. Study of 24 cases. Obstet Gynecol 1982;60:462–6.

189. Ackerman LV. Verrucous carcinoma of the oral cavity. Surgery 1948;23:670–8.

190. Kraus FT, Perez-Mesa C. Verrucous carcinoma. Clinical and pathologic study of 105 cases involving oral cavity, larnyx, and genitalia. Cancer 1966;19:26–38.

191. Partridge EE, Murad T, Shingleton HM, et al. Verrucous lesions of the female genitalia. II. Verrucous carcinoma. Am J Obstet Gynecol 1980;137:419–24.

192. Partridge EE, Murad T, Shingleton HM, et al. Verrucous lesions of the female genitalia. I. Giant condyloma. Am J Obstet Gynecol 1980;137:412–8.

193. Kondi-Paphitis A, Deligeorgi-Politi H, Liapis A, Plemenou-Frangou M. Human papillomavirus in verrucous carcinoma of the vulva: an immunopathological study of three cases. Eur J Gynaecol Obstet 1998;19:319–20.

194. Gallouis S. Verrcous carcinoma. Report of three vulvar cases and a review of the literature. Obstet Gynecol 1972;40:502–7.

195. Demian SDE, Bushkin FL, Echevarria RA. Perineural invasion and anaplastic transformation of verrucous carcinoma. Cancer 1973;32:395–401.

196. Klob JM. Pathologische Anatomie der weiblichen Sexualorgane. Vienna, 1864.

197. Copeland LJ, Sneige N, Gershenson DM, et al. Bartholin gland carcinoma. Obstet Gynecol 1986;67:794–801.

198. Visco AG, Del Priore G. Postmenopausal Bartholin gland enlargement: a hospital-based cancer risk assessment. Obstet Gynecol 1996;87:286–90.

199. Felix JC, Cote RJ, Kramer EEW, et al. Carcinomas of Bartholin's gland. Histogenesis and the ethiologic role of human papillomavirus. Am J Pathol 1993;142:925–33.

200. Chamlian DL, Taylor HB. Primary carcinoma of Bartholin's gland. A report of 24 patients. Obstet Gynecol 1972;39:489–94.

201. Wheelock JB, Goplerud DR, Dunn LJ, Oates JF. Primary carcinoma of the Bartholin gland: a report of ten cases. Obstet Gynecol 1984;63:820–4.

202. Copeland LJ, Sneige N, Gershenson DM, et al. Adenoid cystic carcinoma of Bartholin gland. Obstet Gynecol 1986;67:115–20.

203. DePasquale SE, McGuinness TB, Mangan CE, et al. Adenoid cystic carcinoma of Bartholin's gland: a review of the literature and report of a patient. Gynecol Oncol 1996;61:122–5.

204. Rosenberg P, Simonsen E, Risberg B. Adenoid cystic carcinoma of the Bartholin's gland: a report of five new cases treated with surgery and radiotherapy. Gynecol Oncol 1989;34:145–7.

205. Bouma J, Weening JJ, Elders A. Malignant melanoma of the vulva: report of 18 cases. Eur J Obstet Gynecol Reprod Biol 1982;13:237–51.

206. Tasseron EW, van der Esch EP, Hart AAM, et al. A clinicopathological study of 30 melanomas of the vulva. Gynecol Oncol 1992;46:170–5.

207. Dunton CJ, Kautzky M, Hanau C. Malignant melanoma of the vulva: a review. Obstet Gynecol Surv 1995;30:739–46.

208. Podratz KC, Gaffey TA, Symmonds RE, et al. Melanoma of the vulva: an update. Gynecol Oncol 1983;16:153–68.

209. Trimble EL, Lewis JL Jr, Williams LL, et al. Management of vulvar melanoma. Gynecol Oncol 1992;45:254–8.

210. Phillips GL, Bundy BN, Okagaki T, et al. Malignant melanoma of the vulva treated by radical hemivulvectomy. A prospective study of the GOG. Cancer 1994;74:2626–32.

211. Landthaler M, Braun-Falco O, Leitl A, et al. Excisional biopsy as the first therapeutic procedure versus primary wide excision of malignant melanoma. Cancer 1989;64:1612–6.

212. Khansur T, Sanders J, Das SK. Evaluation of staging workup in vulvar melanoma. Arch Surg 1989; 24:847–9.

213. Clark WH, From L, Bernardino EA, Mihm MC. The histogenesis and biological behavior of primary human melanomas of the skin. Cancer Res 1969;29:705–15.

214. Breslow A. Thickness, cross-sectional areas and depth of invasion in the prognosis of cutaneous melanoma. Ann Surg 1970;172:902–8.

215. Chung AF, Woodruff JM, Lewis JL Jr. Malignant melanoma of the vulva: a report of 44 cases. Obstet Gynecol 1975;45:638–46.

216. Baehrs OH, Henson DE, Hutter RVP, Kennedy BJ, eds. Melanoma. In: Manual for staging cancer. 4th ed. American Joint Committee on Cancer. Philadelphia: JB Lippincott, 1992.

217. Yackel DB, Symmonds RE, Kempers RD. Melanoma of the vulva. Obstet Gynecol 1970;35:625–31.

218. Karlen JR, Piver MS, Barlow JJ. Melanoma of the vulva. Obstet Gynecol 1975;45:181–5.

219. Ariel IM. Malignant melanoma of the female genital system: a report of 48 patients and review of the literature. J Surg Oncol 1981;16:371–83.

220. Davidson T, Kissin M, Westbury G. Vulvo-vaginal melanoma—should radical surgery be abandoned? Br J Obstet Gynaecol 1987;94:473–6.

221. Bradgate MG, Rollason TP, McConkey CC, Powell J. Malignant melanoma of the vulva: a clinicopathologic study of 50 women. Br J Obstet Gynaecol 1990;97:124–33.

222. Phillips GL, Twiggs LB, Okagaki T. Vulvar melanoma: a microstaging study. Gynecol Oncol 1982;14:80–8.

223. Jaramillo BA, Ganjei P, Averette HE, et al. Malignant melanoma of the vulva. Obstet Gynecol 1985;66:398–401.

224. Woolcott RJ, Henry RJW, Houghton CRS. Malignant melanoma of the vulva. Australian experience. J Reprod Med 1988;33:699–702.

225. Scheistrøoen M, Tropé C, Kaern J, et al. Malignant melanoma of the vulva. Evaluation of prognostic factors with emphasis on DNA ploidy in 75 patients. Cancer 1995;75:72–80.

226. Piura B, Egan M, Lopes A, Monaghan JM. Malignant melanoma of the vulva: a clinicopathologic study of 18 cases. J Surg Oncol 1992;50:234–40.

227. Beller U, Demopoulos RI, Beckman EM. Vulvovaginal melanoma. A clinicopathologic study. J Reprod Med 1986;31:315–9.

228. Look KY, Roth LM, Sutton GP. Vulvar melanoma reconsidered. Cancer 1993;72:143–6.

229. Aitken DR, Clausen K, Klein JP, James AG. The extent of primary melanoma excision. A re-evaluation—how wide is wide? Ann Surg 1983;198:634–41.

230. Day CL, Mihm MC, Sober AJ, et al. Narrower margins for clinical stage I malignant melanoma; N Engl J Med 1982;306:479–82.

231. Rose PG, Piver MS, Tsukada Y, Lau T. Conservative therapy for melanoma of the vulva. Am J Obstet Gynecol 1988;159:52–5.

232. Veronesi U, Cascinelli N. Narrow excision (1-cm margin): a safe procedure for thin cutaneous melanoma. Arch Surg 1991;126:438–41.

233. Balch CM, Soong SJ, Milton GW, et al. A comparison of prognostic factors and surgical results in 1,786 patients with localized (stage 1) melanoma treated in Alabama, USA, and New South Wales, Australia. Ann Surg 1982;196:677–84.

234. Balch CM, Urist MM, Karakousis CP, et al. Efficacy of 2-cm surgical margins for intermediate-thickness melanomas (1–4 mm): results of a multi-institutional randomized surgical trial. Ann Surg 1993;218:262–9.

235. Wolchok JD, Livingston PO, Houghton AN. Vaccines and other adjuvant therapies for melanoma. Hematol Oncol Clin North Am 1998;12:835–48.

236. Agarwala SS, Kirkwood JM. Adjuvant interferon treatment for melanoma. Hematol Oncol Clin North Am 1998;12:823–33.

237. Benedet JL, Miller DM, Ehlen TG, Bertrand MA. Basal cell carcinoma of the vulva: clinical features and treatment results in 28 patients. Obstet Gynecol 1997;90:765–8.

238. Dudzinski MR, Askin FB, Fowler WC. Giant basal cell carcinoma of the vulva. Obstet Gynecol 1984;63:57S–60S.

239. Hoffman MS, Roberts WS, Ruffolo EH. Basal cell carcinoma of the vulva with inguinal lymph node metastases. Gynecol Oncol 1988;29:113–9.

240. Jimenez HT, Fenoglio CM, Richart RM. Vulvar basal cell carcinoma with metastasis: a case report. Am J Obstet Gynecol 1975;121:285–6.

241. Palladino VS, Duffy JL, Bures GJ. Basal cell carcinoma of the vulva. Cancer 1969;24:460–70.

242. Weissmann A, Camisa C. Friedrich Siegmund Merkel. Part I. The man. Am J Dermatopathol 1982;4:521–6.

243. Scurry J, Brand A, Planner R, et al. Vulvar Merkel cell tumor with glandular and squamous differentiation. Gynecol Oncol 1996;292–7.

244. Cliby W, Soisson AP, Berchuck A, Clarke-Pearson DL. Stage I small cell carcinoma of the vulva treated with vulvectomy, lymphadenectomy, and adjuvant chemotherapy. Cancer 1991;67:2415–17.

245. Nielsen GP, Rosenberg AE, Koerner FC, et al. Smooth-muscle tumors of the vulva. A clinicopathological study of 25 cases and review of the literature. Am J Surg Pathol 1996;20:779–93.
246. Moøller LBK, Nielsen MN, Trolle C. Leiomyosarcoma vulvae: a case report. Acta Obstet Gynecol Scand 1990;69:187–9.
247. Tavassoli FA, Norris HJ. Smooth muscle tumors of the vulva. Obstet Gynecol 1979;53:213–7.
248. Davos I, Abell MR. Soft tissue sarcoma of the vulva. Gynecol Oncol 1976;4:70–86.
249. Ulbright TM, Brokaw SA, Stehman FB, Roth LM. Epitheloid sarcoma of the vulva. Evidence suggesting a more aggressive behavior than extra-genital epitheloid sarcoma. Cancer 1983;52:1462–9.

250. Bell J, Averette H, Davis J, Toledano S. Genital rhabdomyosarcoma: current management and review of the literature. Obstet Gynecol Surv 1986;41:257–63.
251. Hays DM, Shimada H, Raney RB, et al. Clinical staging and treatment results in rhabdomyosarcoma of the female genital tract among children and adolescents. Cancer 1988;61:1893–1903.
252. Barnhill DR, Boling R, Nobles W, et al. Vulvar dermatofibrosarcoma protruberans. Gynecol Oncol 1988;30:149–52.
253. Agress R, Figge DC, Tamimi H, Greer B. Dermatofibrosarcoma protuberans of the vulva. Gynecol Oncol 1983;16:288–91.
254. Bock JE, Andreasson B, Thorn A, Holck S. Dermatofibrosarcoma protuberans of the vulva. Gynecol Oncol 1985;20:129–35.

# CHAPTER 59

# VAGINA

• JOHN C. ELKAS • JONATHAN S. BEREK

Primary cancer of the vagina constitutes 1 to 2% of malignant neoplasms of the female genital tract. Approximately 2100 new cases of vaginal cancer have been estimated to occur in the United States in 2000, with 600 deaths.[1] Vaginal cancer represents one of the most challenging therapeutic problems in gynecologic oncology, and until the late 1930s, the disease was generally considered to be incurable. With improved techniques in radiation therapy and radical surgery, cure of even advanced cases has been well documented. However, although vaginal cancer appears to behave biologically in a fashion similar to cervical cancer,[2] overall cure rates remain generally much lower and morbidity from treatment relatively high. Despite the opportunity today for early diagnosis with routine vaginal examination and Papanicolaou's (Pap) smear, most patients continue to present with disease spread beyond the vagina.

Most vaginal malignancies are metastatic,[3] usually from the cervix or vulva. This is partly related to the International Federation of Gynecology and Obstetrics (FIGO) classification and staging of malignant tumors of the female pelvis, which requires that a tumor that has extended to the portio and reached the area of the external os be regarded as a carcinoma of the cervix, whereas a tumor involving the vulva and vagina is classified as a vulvar carcinoma. Endometrial carcinomas and choriocarcinomas commonly metastasize to the vagina, and tumors from the bladder or rectum may invade the vagina directly. Metastatic tumors are not discussed further in this chapter.

The histologic types of primary vaginal tumors are listed in Table 59–1. Squamous cell carcinomas are the most common, although adenocarcinomas, melanomas, and sarcomas are also seen. The natural history and management of each of these lesions are distinctive, so they are discussed separately in the following sections.

## Squamous Cell Carcinoma

### NATURAL HISTORY

Squamous cell carcinoma is the most common vaginal cancer. The mean age of the patients is approximately 60 years, although the disease is occasionally seen in the third and fourth decades of life. Perez reported that 76% of patients were older than 50 years.[4]

**Etiology.** The cause of squamous cell carcinoma of the vagina is unknown, although interest has focused on the association between human papillomavirus infection and multifocal carcinoma of the lower female genital tract.[5] Vaginal intraepithelial neoplasia (VAIN) has been the subject of increasing attention as a precursor of vaginal cancer, although the true malignant potential of VAIN is not known.[6] Benedet and Saunders reviewed 136 cases of carcinoma in situ of the vagina seen over a 30-year period.[7] Four cases (3%) progressed to invasive vaginal cancer despite various methods of treatment. Lenehan and colleagues reported invasive vaginal cancer following treatment for VAIN in 3 of 59 patients (5%).[6] Chronic local irritation from long-term use of a pessary may be of significance, although pessaries are less commonly used in modern gynecology.[8]

*Table 59–1.* **Primary Vaginal Cancer: Reported Incidence of Histologic Types**

| Histologic Type | Number | % |
|---|---|---|
| Squamous cell | 698 | 83.4 |
| Adenocarcinoma | 74 | 8.9 |
| Sarcoma | 26 | 3.1 |
| Melanoma | 21 | 2.5 |
| Undifferentiated | 8 | 1.0 |
| Small cell | 2 | 0.2 |
| Adenosquamous | 2 | 0.2 |
| Lymphoma | 2 | 0.2 |
| Carcinoid | 1 | 0.1 |
| Total | 834 | 100.0 |

From Berek JS, Hacker NF, eds: Practical gynecologic oncology. Baltimore: Williams & Wilkins, 1994:442. Data from Dunn and Napier, 1966[2]; Rutledge, 1967[8]; Perez et al, 1974[4]; Pride and Buchler, 1977[12]; Ball and Berman, 1982[16]; Benedet et al, 1983[10]; Peters et al, 1985[11]; and Rubin et al, 1985.[9]

Up to 30% of patients with primary vaginal carcinoma have a history of in situ or invasive cervical cancer that was treated at least 5 years earlier.[9-13] In a report from South Carolina, a past history of invasive cervical cancer was present in 20% of cases, and cervical intraepithelial neoplasia was present in 7%. The median interval between the diagnosis of cervical cancer and the diagnosis of vaginal cancer was 14 years, with a range of 5 years 8 months to 28 years.[14] There are three possible mechanisms for this occurrence: (1) occult residual disease, (2) new primary disease arising in an at-risk lower genital tract, and (3) radiation carcinogenicity.

**Screening.** For screening to be cost-effective, the incidence of the disease must be sufficient to justify the cost of screening. In the United States, the age-adjusted incidence rate of vaginal cancer of 0.6 per 100,000 makes routine screening of all patients inappropriate.[15] However, women with a history of cervical intraepithelial or invasive neoplasia are at increased risk and should be carefully monitored with Pap smears.

Up to 59% of patients with vaginal cancer have had a prior hysterectomy.[16] Some authors have suggested that all these patients should be routinely monitored with Pap smears.[17, 18] When vaginal cancer occurs in patients who have had a hysterectomy for benign disease, it is usually more advanced at presentation, presumably because these patients have not been under gynecologic surveillance.[17] However, when age and prior cervical disease are controlled for, there is no increased risk of vaginal cancer in women who have had a hysterectomy for benign disease.[19]

**Symptoms and Signs.** Most patients with vaginal cancer present with painless vaginal bleeding and discharge. The bleeding is usually postmenopausal but may be postcoital. Because the bladder neck is close to the vagina, bladder pain and frequency of micturition occur earlier than with cervical cancer.[7] Posterior tumors may produce tenesmus. About 5% of patients present with pelvic pain because of extension of disease beyond the vagina, and 5 to 10% of patients are asymptomatic, the disease being detected on routine pelvic examination and Pap smear.

Most lesions are situated in the upper third of the vagina, usually on the posterior wall. Macroscopically, the lesions are usually exophytic (fungating, polypoid), but they may be endophytic. Surface ulceration usually occurs late in the course of the disease.

**Diagnosis.** The diagnosis of carcinoma of the vagina is often missed on first examination, particularly if the lesion is small and situated in the lower two thirds of the vagina, where it may be covered by the blades of the speculum. Frick and colleagues reported that at least 10 of 52 cases (19%) in their series had been missed on the initial examination.[20] Definitive diagnosis is usually made by biopsy of a gross lesion, which can often be performed in the office without anesthesia. Particularly in elderly patients or in those with some degree of vaginal stenosis, examination under anesthesia may be desirable to allow adequate biopsy and clinical staging. The latter may require cystoscopy or proctoscopy, depending on the location of the tumor.

In some patients with abnormal Pap smear findings and no gross abnormality, careful vaginal colposcopy and the liberal use of Lugol's iodine to stain the vagina are necessary. This is usually best performed under general anesthesia

to allow wide biopsy of colposcopically abnormal lesions to be taken. For a definite diagnosis of early vaginal carcinoma, it may be necessary to resect the entire vaginal vault and submit it for careful histologic evaluation, as the lesion may be partially buried by closure of the vaginal vault at the time of hysterectomy. Hoffman and colleagues reported 32 patients who underwent upper vaginectomy for VAIN 3.[21] Occult invasive carcinoma was found in nine patients (28%).

**Staging of Vaginal Cancer.** The International Federation of Gynecology and Obstetrics (FIGO) staging for vaginal carcinoma is shown in Table 59–2. The staging is clinical, based on the findings from general physical and pelvic examination, cystoscopy, proctoscopy, and chest and skeletal radiographs if the latter are indicated because of bone pain.

Because it is difficult to determine spread into subvaginal tissues accurately, particularly for anterior or posterior lesions, observer differences are common; this is reflected in the wide range of stage distributions, as well as survival within a given stage, reported in the literature.

Surgical staging for vaginal cancer has been less commonly used than for cervical cancer. However, in selected premenopausal patients, a pretreatment laparotomy may allow better definition of the extent of disease, excision of any grossly enlarged lymph nodes, and cephalad placement of the ovaries into the paracolic gutter beyond the pelvic irradiation field. The distribution by FIGO stage from five contemporary series is shown in Table 59–3. Only about one third of cases present with disease confined to the vagina.

**Patterns of Spread.** Vaginal cancer spreads by the following routes: (1) direct extension to the pelvic soft tissues, pelvic bones, and adjacent organs (bladder and rectum); (2) lymphatic dissemination to the pelvic and later the para-

*Table 59–2.* **International Federation of Gynecology and Obstetrics Staging of Vaginal Cancer**

| | |
|---|---|
| Stage 0 | Carcinoma in situ, intraepithelial carcinoma |
| Stage I | The carcinoma is limited to the vaginal wall |
| Stage II | The carcinoma has involved the subvaginal tissue but has not extended onto the pelvic wall |
| Stage III | The carcinoma has extended onto the pelvic wall |
| Stage IV | The carcinoma has extended beyond the true pelvis or has involved the mucosa of the bladder or rectum |
| Stage IVa | Spread of growth to adjacent organs |
| Stage IVb | Spread to distant organs |

*Table 59–3.* **Primary Vaginal Carcinoma: Distribution by Stage of Disease**

| Stage | Number | % |
|---|---|---|
| I | 226 | 25.8 |
| II | 294 | 33.6 |
| III | 220 | 25.1 |
| IV | 136 | 15.5 |
| Total | 876 | 100.0 |

From Berek JS, Hacker NF, eds: Practical gynecologic oncology. Baltimore: Williams & Wilkins, 1994:445. Data from Pride and Buchler, 1977[12]; Ball and Berman, 1982[16]; Benedet et al, 1983[10]; Peters et al, 1985[11]; Rubin et al, 1985[9]; and Kucera et al, 1985.[24]

*Table 59–4.* **Primary Vaginal Carcinoma: 5-Year Survival**

| Stage | Number | 5-Yr Survival | % |
|---|---|---|---|
| I | 177 | 118 | 66.7 |
| II | 236 | 108 | 45.8 |
| III | 203 | 62 | 30.5 |
| IV | 114 | 20 | 17.5 |
| Overall | 730 | 308 | 42.5 |

From Berek JS, Hacker NF, eds. Practical gynecologic oncology. Baltimo Williams & Wilkins, 1994:447. Data from Pride et al, 1977[11]; Benedet et al, 1983[10]; Kucera et al, 1985[24]; and Rubin et al, 1985.[9]

aortic lymph nodes (lesions in the lower one third of the vagina metastasize directly to the inguinofemoral lymph nodes, with the pelvic nodes being involved secondarily); and (3) hematogenous dissemination to distant organs, including lung, liver, and bone. Hematogenous dissemination is a late phenomenon in vaginal cancer, the disease usually remaining confined to the pelvis for most of its course.

There is little information available on the incidence of lymph node metastases in vaginal cancer because most patients are treated with radiation therapy. Rubin and associates[9] reported that 16 of 38 patients (42%) with all stages of disease had abnormal results on a lymphangiogram, but many of these abnormalities were not confirmed histologically. Al-Kurdi and Monaghan performed lymph node dissections on 35 patients and reported positive pelvic nodes in 10 patients (28%).[22] Positive inguinal nodes were present in 6 of 19 patients (31%) with disease involving the lower vagina.

**Preoperative Evaluation.** Apart from the standard staging investigations, a computed tomographic scan of the pelvis and abdomen may be useful to evaluate the extent of the primary tumor, pelvic and para-aortic lymph nodes, and ureters.

**Prognosis.** The overall 5-year survival rate for vaginal cancer is about 42%, which is about 15% worse than for carcinoma of the cervix or vulva, reflecting the difficulties involved in treating this disease (Table 59–4). Even for patients with stage I disease, the 5-year survival rate is only 67%. Overall survival was markedly higher in younger patients (90% vs. 30% in older patients).[23] Most recurrences occur in the pelvis, so improved radiation therapy, which may include chemoradiation or increasing experience with interstitial techniques, or both, may improve the results.

## TREATMENT

There is no consensus regarding the proper management of primary vaginal cancer, owing in part to the rarity of the disease. Most gynecologic oncology centers in the United States see only two to five new cases per year. Even in some European centers, where referral of oncology cases tends to be more centralized, only about one new case per month can be expected.[24] Therapy must be individualized and varies depending on the stage of disease and site of vaginal involvement, further limiting individual experience.

Anatomic factors and psychological considerations place significant constraints on treatment planning. The close proximity of the vagina to the rectum, bladder, and urethra limits the dose of radiation that can be delivered and restricts the

surgical margins that can be attained unless an exenterative procedure is performed. For most patients, maintenance of a functional vagina is an important factor to be taken into consideration in planning therapy.

**Surgery.** Surgery has a limited role in the treatment of patients with vaginal cancer, but in selected cases, satisfactory results can be achieved.[16, 22] Surgery may be useful in the following circumstances:

1. In patients with stage I disease involving the upper posterior vagina. If the uterus is still in situ, these patients require radical hysterectomy, partial vaginectomy, and bilateral pelvic lymphadenectomy. If the patient has had a hysterectomy, a radical upper vaginectomy can be performed after development of the paravesical and pararectal spaces and dissection of each ureter out to its point of entry into the bladder. In general, the 5-year survival rate for these patients is in the range of 56 to 80%.[22, 25]

2. In young patients requiring radiation therapy. Pretreatment laparotomy in such patients may allow ovarian transposition, surgical staging, and resection of any enlarged lymph nodes.

3. In patients with stage IVa disease, particularly if a rectovaginal or vesicovaginal fistula is present. Primary pelvic exenteration is a suitable treatment option for such patients, provided that they are medically fit. In sexually active patients, vaginal reconstruction should be performed simultaneously, preferably using gracilis myocutaneous grafts.[26]

4. In patients with a central recurrence following radiation therapy. Surgical resection, which frequently necessitates pelvic exenteration, is the only option for this group of patients.

5. A number of reports have described the use of neoadjuvant chemotherapy followed by radical surgery in advanced vaginal carcinoma. Umesaki and colleagues reported an excellent response to irinotecan and cisplatin followed by radical excision.[27] Similarly, Zanetta and coworkers had a 67% response to epirubicin and cisplatin that allowed more than 80% of patients to undergo complete radical excision.[28] As more experience is gained with neoadjuvant chemotherapy, patients with cancers once deemed inoperable may become surgical candidates, and their survival may thus be improved.

**Radiation Therapy.** Radiation therapy is the treatment of choice for all patients except those described earlier and involves an integration of teletherapy and intracavitary-interstitial therapy.[4, 24] Radiation for stage I disease is highly effective, with survival rates of 75 to 95%. In superficial tumors, brachytherapy alone may be used. The recommended dose of 60 to 70 Gy calculated 5 mm beyond the plane of the implant or vaginal mucosa should be given. Deeper stage I tumors should be treated with external beam and brachytherapy delivering 40 to 50 Gy to the pelvic nodes and 70 to 75 Gy to the tumor.

Treatment for stage II and above lesions is usually started with external irradiation to shrink the primary tumor and treat the pelvic lymph nodes. If the lower one third of the vagina is involved, the groin nodes should also be treated or dissected. Intracavitary treatment follows. If the uterus is intact and the lesion involves the upper vagina, an intrauterine tandem and ovoids can be used. If the uterus has been previously removed, a Bloedorn's-type applicator or vaginal cylinder may be used. If the lesion is more deeply invasive (thicker than 0.5 mm), interstitial irradiation, alone or in conjunction with the intracavitary therapy, may be required to improve the dose distribution.

The major determinants of local control are tumor bulk and location; lesions involving the posterior vaginal wall are less likely to be completely treated. Survival rates range between 50 and 85% for stage II disease, between 15 and 30% for stage III, and between 15 and 30% for stage IV disease.[25, 29, 30] Tumor bulk (FIGO stage or tumor volume) also is an important determinant of recurrence. Unfortunately, salvage after relapse is uncommon, and the survival rate after recurrence is only 12%.[29]

Extended-field radiation has rarely been used for patients with vaginal cancer. However, if positive para-aortic nodes are documented following either surgical staging or computed tomographic scanning and fine-needle aspiration cytologic studies, this treatment is appropriate.

Similarly, there is little reported experience with chemoradiation for vaginal cancer. In view of the problem with control of the central tumor, however, consideration should be given to the concurrent use of 5-fluorouracil or cisplatin, or both, with the radiation therapy, as is being done in some centers for other squamous carcinomas.

**Complications of Therapy.** Major complications of therapy are usually reported in 15 to 20% of patients treated for primary vaginal cancer, whether the treatment is by surgery or radiation therapy.[29] The close proximity of the rectum, bladder, and urethra predisposes these structures to injury, and radiation cystitis, rectovaginal or vesicovaginal fistulas, and rectal strictures or ulceration may occur. Radiation necrosis of the vagina occasionally occurs, and radiation-induced fibrosis and subsequent vaginal stenosis are a constant concern. Patients who are sexually active must be encouraged to continue regular intercourse; those who are not sexually active or for whom intercourse is temporarily too painful should be encouraged to use a topical estrogen and a vaginal dilator every second night. Documentation of the adequacy of vaginal function following either surgery or radiation therapy has been inadequate.

## Adenocarcinoma

### NATURAL HISTORY

About 7% of primary vaginal carcinomas are adenocarcinomas, and they affect a younger population of women regardless of whether or not exposure to diethylstilbestrol (DES) in utero has occurred.[31] Adenocarcinomas may arise in areas of vaginal adenosis, particularly in patients exposed to DES in utero, but they probably also arise in wolffian rest elements, periurethral gland,[20] and foci of endometriosis. Secondary tumors from sites such as the colon, endometrium, or ovary should be considered when vaginal adenocarcinoma is diagnosed.

**Diethylstilbestrol Exposure in Utero.** In 1970, Herbst and Scully initially described seven women age 15 to 22 years with clear cell adenocarcinoma of the vagina over a 4-year period.[32] Subsequently, Herbst and colleagues described an association with maternal DES ingestion during pregnancy in six of these seven cases.[33] A Registry for Research on Hormonal Transplacental Carcinogenesis was established by Herbst and Scully in 1971 to investigate the clinical, pathologic, and epidemiologic aspects of clear cell adenocarcinoma of the vagina and cervix occurring in females born after 1940—that is, during the years when DES was used to maintain high-risk pregnancies. As many as 3 million women in the United States may have been exposed to DES in utero. Such high-risk situations included diabetic and twin pregnancies and pregnancies in women with a past history of spontaneous abortion. The use of DES for pregnant patients was discontinued in the United States in 1971.

More than 500 cases of clear cell carcinoma of the vagina or cervix have been reported to the Registry, although only about two thirds of completely investigated cases have a history of prenatal exposure to DES. In all instances, the mother had been treated in the first trimester using some unknown medication, but in 25% of cases there was no indication of maternal hormone ingestion.

These cancers become most frequent after the age of 14 years, and the peak age at diagnosis is 19 years. The oldest reported DES-exposed patient with vaginal clear cell carcinoma was 42 years of age. The estimated risk of clear cell adenocarcinoma in an exposed offspring is 1 in 1000 or less. Approximately 70% of vaginal adenocarcinomas are stage I at diagnosis.

Although DES exposure in utero rarely leads to vaginal adenocarcinoma, vaginal adenosis occurs in about 33% of such patients, and about 25% of exposed females have structural changes of the cervix and vagina. Such changes include a transverse vaginal septum, a cervical collar, a "cockscomb" (a raised ridge, usually on the anterior cervix), and cervical hypoplasia. The occurrence of these abnormalities is related to the dose of medication given and the time of first exposure, the risk being insignificant if administration was begun after the 22nd week of gestation.

Two types of cells have been described in vaginal adenosis and cervical ectropion: the mucinous cell, which resembles the endocervical epithelium, and the tuboendometrial cell. Robboy and colleagues reported foci of atypical tuboendometrial epithelium in 16 of 20 (80%) cases of clear cell adenocarcinoma of the cervix or vagina.[34] The foci were almost immediately adjacent to the tumor, and they suggested that atypical vaginal adenosis and atypical cervical ectropion of the tuboendometrial type may be precursors of clear cell adenocarcinoma. In 1980, Sandberg and Christian reported the appearance of cervicovaginal clear cell adenocarcinoma in only one of a genetically identical (monozygotic) pair of twins simultaneously exposed to DES in utero.[35] Benign teratologic changes were present in both twins. This discordance suggests that factors other than embryonic exposure to DES may be operative in tumorigenesis.

It is recommended that a young woman exposed to DES in utero be initially seen when she begins to menstruate, or at about age 14 years. The most important aspects of the examination are careful inspection and palpation of the entire vagina and cervix and cytologic sampling by direct scraping of the vagina and cervix. Colposcopy is not essential if results of clinical and cytologic evaluation are normal, but staining with half-strength Lugol's iodine delineates areas of adenosis. Although DES-exposed daughters are at an increased risk for clear cell adenocarcinoma of the vagina and cervix, a report by Hatch and colleagues failed to demonstrate an increased risk for other malignancies, although the mean age of their cohort was only 38 years.[36]

**Prognosis.** The overall 5-year survival rate for registry patients, regardless of the mode of therapy, is 78%. Survival correlates well with stage of disease, being 87% for patients with stage I disease, 76% for those with stage II, and 30% for those with stage III.[37]

## TREATMENT

In general, these tumors may be treated in a fashion similar to that for squamous carcinomas, except that in these young patients every effort should be made to preserve vaginal and ovarian function. For early-stage tumors, particularly those involving the upper vagina, radical hysterectomy, pelvic lymphadenectomy, vaginectomy, and replacement of the vagina with a split-thickness skin graft is the standard of care. However, local excision of small primary tumors after negative results of pelvic lymph node dissection is an option for those patients who desire future childbearing. Lymph node dissection prior to conservative surgery is mandatory because up to 16% of patients with stage I disease have positive pelvic nodes.[38] If radiation therapy is used, a pretreatment staging laparotomy to allow pelvic lymphadenectomy and ovarian transposition facilitates an optimal functional outcome and preserves the option of childbearing with assisted reproductive techniques.

## Rare Neoplasms

### VERRUCOUS CARCINOMA

Verrucous carcinomas of the vagina are rare, but their clinical and pathologic features are similar to those of their vulvar counterparts.[39] They are large, warty tumors that are locally aggressive but that have minimal tendency to metastasize. Wide surgical excision of the tumor is the treatment of choice. Regional lymphadenectomy is not required, provided that there is no suspicious adenopathy. Radiation therapy has been implicated in the rapid transformation of such lesions to a more malignant tumor.[40]

### VAGINAL MELANOMA

Malignant melanomas of the vagina are rare, with only some 200 cases reported in the world literature.[41] They presumably arise from melanocytes, which are present in the vagina of 3% of normal women.[42] The average age of the patient is 55 years, but vaginal melanomas have been reported from the third to the ninth decades of life.[43] Clinically, most patients present with vaginal bleeding or discharge. The lesions most commonly arise in the distal vagina, particularly on the anterior wall.[41, 44] They may be nonpigmented and are frequently ulcerated and are therefore easily confused with squamous carcinomas. Most are deeply invasive. Expressed in terms of level of invasion as defined by Chung and coworkers for vulvar melanomas, 13 of 15 vaginal melanomas were at level IV in reports by these investigators.[45, 46] About 60% of cases exhibit spread of melanocytic cells into the adjacent epithelium, and in about 30% of cases the lateral spread is extensive.[24]

Radical surgery has been the mainstay of treatment, and this has often involved anterior, posterior, or total pelvic exenteration, depending on the location of the lesion. Small upper vaginal lesions may be treated by radical hysterectomy, subtotal vaginectomy, and pelvic lymphadenectomy. Small distal vaginal lesions may be amenable to partial vaginectomy, total or partial vulvectomy, and bilateral inguinofemoral lymphadenectomy. If vaginal mucosa is left, frozen sections should be obtained to exclude lateral superficial spread, as the most common site of initial recurrence is the vagina.[46] In line with the management of melanomas in other sites, more conservative operations are now being used (e.g., wide local excision), and Reid and colleagues reported no significant benefit in terms of survival or disease-free interval for radical versus conservative surgery.[41]

Radiation therapy, particularly a combination of external and interstitial, may offer palliation in selected patients and may be combined with local excision for tumor control. Petru and coworkers have shown that primary radiotherapy or adjuvant radiotherapy following local excision yields survival rates similar to those achieved with radical surgery in patients with lesions 3 cm or less in diameter.[47] Chemotherapy for melanoma of the vagina (e.g., with methyl-CCNU or dacarbazine) has not been shown to be effective.

The overall prognosis for patients with vaginal melanoma is poor. Reid and colleagues reviewed the literature and reported that only 14 of 130 patients (10%) survived for 5 years or longer.[41] Six of the 14 patients were treated by radical surgery, 4 with irradiation, and 4 by wide local excision. The overall 5-year survival in many other series is only 10 to 20%.

### VAGINAL SARCOMA

Vaginal sarcomas, such as fibrosarcomas and leiomyosarcomas, are rare tumors. They occasionally result from the treatment of cervical cancer by radiation therapy. They are usually bulky lesions and occur most commonly in the upper vagina. Tavassoli and Norris reported 60 smooth muscle tumors of the vagina, only 5 of which recurred.[48] All the recurrences were seen in tumors greater than 3 cm in diameter, with moderate to marked cytologic atypia and more than five mitoses per 10 high-power fields.

Surgical excision is the mainstay of treatment, and if the lesion is well differentiated and the surgical margins are not involved, as is likely with tumors of low malignant potential, the likelihood of cure is good. For the frankly malignant lesions, lymphatic and hematogenous dissemination is common. The value of adjuvant chemotherapy or pelvic radiation, or both, for such tumors is unknown.

Sarcoma botryoides (embryonal rhabdomyosarcoma) is a highly malignant tumor. Within the female genital tract, sarcoma botryoides is usually found in the vagina during infancy and early childhood, in the cervix during the reproductive years, and in the corpus uteri during the postmenopausal period. Hilgers and colleagues reported a peak incidence for vaginal sarcoma botryoides around 3 years of age, and these lesions may rarely be present at birth.[49]

The term *botryoides* comes from the Greek word *botrys*, which means "grapes," and grossly the tumor usually presents as a polypoid mass extruding from the vagina and resembling a bunch of grapes. Microscopically, the characteristic feature is the presence of cross-striated rhabdomyoblasts (strap cells).

In the past, exenteration was usually performed for these tumors, but more recently, conservative surgery has been used in conjunction with preoperative or postoperative chemotherapy and irradiation without compromising survival.[44, 50] The usual chemotherapy given has been vincristine, actinomycin D, and cyclophosphamide.

## ENDODERMAL SINUS TUMOR (YOLK SAC TUMOR)

These rare germ cell tumors are occasionally found in extragonadal sites such as the vagina. Leverger and colleagues reported 11 such cases from the Institute Gustave-Roussy.[51] The average age of the patients was 10 months, and the presenting symptom was vaginal bleeding. Diagnosis was made by examination and biopsy under anesthesia. All children were cured, with an average follow-up of 3.5 years. Treatment consisted of primary chemotherapy to reduce the tumor volume, followed by either partial colpectomy or radiotherapy, or both.

## SUGGESTIONS FOR ADDITIONAL READING

Hacker NF. Vaginal cancer. In: Berek JS, Hacker NF, eds. Practical gynecologic oncology. 3rd ed. Baltimore: Lippincott Williams & Wilkins, 2000. *This chapter outlines the diagnosis, staging, treatment, and prognosis of vaginal cancer.*

Herbst AL, Anderson S, Hubby MM, et al. Risk factors for the development of diethylstilbestrol-associated clear cell adenocarcinoma: a case-control study. Am J Obstet Gynecol 1986;154:814. *This is review of the Registry experience with clear cell carcinoma of the vagina.*

Eddy GL, Marks RD, Miller MC III, Underweed PB Jr. Primary invasive vaginal carcinoma. Am J Obstet Gynecol 1991;165:292–8. *This article discusses a well-analyzed contemporary series of vaginal cancer from one institution.*

Weinstock MA. Malignant melanoma of the vulva and vagina in the United States: patterns of incidence and population-based estimates of survival. Am J Obstet Gynecol 1994;171:1225. *This is a review of the current epidemiology of melanoma of the lower genital tract.*

## REFERENCES

1. Greenlee RT, Murray T, Bolden S, Wingo PA. Cancer statistics, 2000. CA Cancer J Clin 2000;50:7–33.
2. Dunn LJ, Napier JG. Primary carcinoma of the vagina. Am J Obstet Gynecol 1966;96:1112–6.
3. Gompel C, Silverberg SC. Pathology in gynecology and obstetrics. Philadelphia: JB Lippincott, 1977.
4. Perez CA, Arneson AN, Dehner LP, et al. Radiation therapy in carcinoma of the vagina. Obstet Gynecol 1974;44:862–72.
5. Weed JC, Lozier C, Daniel SJ. Human papilloma virus in multifocal, invasive female genital tract malignancy. Obstet Gynecol 1983;62:832–75.
6. Lenehan PM, Meffe F, Lickrish GM. Vaginal intraepithelial neoplasia: biologic aspects and management. Obstet Gynecol 1986;68:333–7.
7. Benedet JL, Saunders BH. Carcinoma in situ of the vagina. Am J Obstet Gynecol 1984;148:695–700.
8. Rutledge F. Cancer of the vagina. Am J Obstet Gynecol 1967;97:635–55.
9. Rubin SC, Young J, Mikuta JJ. Squamous carcinoma of the vagina: treatment, complications, and long-term follow-up. Gynecol Oncol 1985;20:346–53.
10. Benedet JL, Murphy KJ, Fairey RN, et al. Primary invasive carcinoma of the vagina. Obstet Gynecol 1983;62:715–9.
11. Peters WA, Kumar NB, Morley GW. Carcinoma of the vagina. Cancer 1985;55:892–7.
12. Pride GL, Buchler DA. Carcinoma of vagina 10 or more years following pelvic radiation therapy. Am J Obstet Gynecol 1977;127:513–7.
13. Choo YC, Anderson DG. Neoplasms of the vagina following cervical carcinoma. Gynecol Oncol 1982;14:125–32.
14. Eddy GL, Marks RD, Miller MC, Underwood PB. Primary invasive vaginal carcinoma. Am J Obstet Gynecol 1991;165:292–6.
15. Cramer DW, Cutler SJ. Incidence and histopathology of malignancies of the female genital organs in the United States. Am J Obstet Gynecol 1974;118:443–60.
16. Ball HG, Berman ML. Management of primary vaginal carcinoma. Gynecol Oncol 1982;14:49–61.
17. Stuart GCE, Allen HH, Anderson RJ. Squamous cell carcinoma of the vagina following hysterectomy. Am J Obstet Gynecol 1981;139:311–5.
18. Bell J, Sevin BU, Averette H, et al. Vaginal cancer after hysterectomy for benign disease: value of cytologic screening. Obstet Gynecol 1984;64:699–702.
19. Herman JM, Homesley HD, Dignan MB. Is hysterectomy a risk factor for vaginal cancer? JAMA 1986;256:601–3.
20. Frick HC, Jacox HW, Taylor HC. Primary carcinoma of the vagina. Am J Obstet Gynecol 1968;101:695–703.
21. Hoffman MS, De Ceaare SL, Roberts WS, et al. Upper vaginectomy for in situ and occult superficially invasive carcinoma of the vagina. Am J Obstet Gynecol 1992;166:30–3.
22. Al-Kurdi M, Monaghan JM. Thirty-two years experience in management of primary tumors of the vagina. Br J Obstet Gynaecol 1981;88:1145–50.
23. Creasman WT, Phillips JL, Menck HR. The National Cancer Data Base report on cancer of the vagina. Cancer 1998;83:1033–40.
24. Kucera H, Langer M, Smekal G, et al. Radiotherapy of primary carcinoma of the vagina: management and results of different therapy schemes. Gynecol Oncol 1985;21:87–93.
25. Perez C, Camel H, Galakatos A, et al. Definitive irradiation in carcinoma of the vagina: long-term evaluation of results. Int J Radiat Oncol Biol Phys 1988;15:1283–90.
26. Berek JS, Hacker NF, Lagasse LD. Vaginal reconstruction performed simultaneously with pelvic exenteration. Obstet Gynecol 1984;63:318–23.
27. Umesaki N, Kawamura N, Tsujimura A, et al. Stage II vaginal cancer responding to chemotherapy with irinotecan and cisplatin: a case report. Oncol Rep 1999;6:123–5.
28. Zanetta G, Lissoni A, Gabriele A, et al. Intense neoadjuvant chemotherapy with cisplatin and epirubicin for advanced or bulky cervical and vaginal adenocarcinoma. Gynecol Oncol 1997;64:431–5.
29. Chyle V, Zagars GK, Wheeler JA, et al. Definitive radiotherapy for carcinoma of the vagina: outcome and prognostic factors. Int J Radiat Oncol Biol Phys 1996;35:891–905.
30. Kirkbride P, Fyles A, Rawlings GA, et al. Carcinoma of the vagina—experience at the Princess Margaret Hospital (1974–1989). Gynecol Oncol 1994;56:435–43.
31. Ballon SC, Lagasse LD, Chang NH, et al. Primary adenocarcinoma of the vagina. Surg Gynecol Obstet 1979;149:233–7.
32. Herbst AL, Scully RE. Adenocarcinoma of the vagina in adolescence. Cancer 1970;25:745–57.
33. Herbst AL, Ulfelder H, Poskanzer DC. Adenocarcinoma of the vagina: association of maternal stilbestrol therapy with tumor appearance in young women. N Engl J Med 1971;284:878–81.
34. Robboy SJ, Young RH, Welch WR, et al. Atypical vaginal adenosis and cervical ectropion. Cancer 1984;54:869–75.
35. Sandberg EC, Christian JC. Diethylstilbestrol-exposed monozygotic twins discordant for cervicovaginal clear cell adenocarcinoma. Am J Obstet Gynecol 1980;137:220–8.
36. Hatch EE, Palmer JR, Titus-Ernstoff L, et al. Cancer risk in women exposed to diethylstilbestrol in utero. JAMA 1988;280:630–4.

37. Herbst AL, Cole P, Norusis MJ, et al. Epidemiologic aspects and factors related to survival in 384 Registry cases of clear cell adenocarcinoma of the vagina and cervix. Am J Obstet Gynecol 1979;135:876–86.
38. Herbst AL, Robboy SJ, Scully, RE, et al. Clear-cell adenocarcinoma of the vagina and cervix in girls: analysis of 170 Registry cases. Am J Obstet Gynecol 1974;119:713–24.
39. Isaacs JH. Verrucous carcinoma of the female genital tract. Gynecol Oncol 1976;4:259–69.
40. Gallousis S. Verrucous carcinoma: report of three vulcar cases and review of the literature. Obstet Gynecol 1972;40:502–7.
41. Reid GC, Schmidt RW, Roberts JA, et al. Primary melanoma of the vagina: a clinicopathologic analysis. Obstet Gynecol 1972;40:190–9.
42. Nigogosyam G, De La Pava S, Pickren JW. Melanoblasts in vaginal mucosa. Cancer 1964;17:912–3.
43. Morrow CP, DiSaia PJ. Malignant melanoma of the female genitalia: a clinical analysis. Obstet Gynecol Surv 1976;31:233–71.
44. Dewhurst J: Practical pediatric and adolescent gynecology. New York: Marcel Dekker, 1980.
45. Chung AF, Casey MJ, Flannery JT, et al. Malignant melanoma of the vagina—report of 19 cases. Obstet Gynecol 1980;55:720–7.
46. Chung AF, Woodruff JW, Lewis JL Jr. Malignant melanoma of the vulva: a report of 44 cases. Obstet Gynecol 1975;45:638–46.
47. Petru E, Nagele F, Czerwenka K, et al. Primary malignant melanoma of the vagina: long-term remission following radiation therapy. Gynecol Oncol 1998;70:23–6.
48. Tavassoli FA, Norris HJ. Smooth muscle tumors of the vagina. Obstet Gynecol 1979;53:689–93.
49. Hilgers RD, Malkasian GD, Soule EH. Embryonal rhabdomyosarcoma (botryoid type) of the vagina: a clinicopathologic review. Am J Obstet Gynecol 1970;107:484–502.
50. Mahesh Kumar AP, Wrenn EL, Fleming ID, et al. Combined therapy to prevent complete pelvic exenteration for rhabdomyosarcoma of the vagina or uterus. Cancer 1976;37:118–22.
51. Leverger G, Flamant F, Gerbaulet A, et al. Tumors of the vitelline sac located in the vagina in children. Arch Fr Pediatr 1983;40:85–9.

# CHAPTER 60

# GESTATIONAL TROPHOBLASTIC NEOPLASIA

• ROSS S. BERKOWITZ • DONALD P. GOLDSTEIN

Gestational trophoblastic tumors (GTTs) are rare human tumors that are highly curable even with widespread metastases.[1, 2] The risk of GTT is about 1 in 1200 pregnancies in the United States, but the disease occurs more commonly in Asia and South America. The cause of GTT is not known, and the reason for the increased incidence of the disease in certain geographic areas is unknown. It makes up less than 1% of malignancies in females, but because of its highly curable nature, these patients are best treated in specialized centers.

GTTs are a spectrum of interrelated tumors, including invasive mole, placental site trophoblastic tumor, and choriocarcinoma, that have varying tendencies for local invasion and metastasis. Although GTTs most commonly follow a hydatidiform mole, they may ensue after any gestation, including ectopic or term pregnancy and spontaneous or therapeutic abortion. Important advances have been made in the diagnosis, treatment, and follow-up of patients with GTT since the introduction of chemotherapy. This chapter reviews these advances and discusses the basic principles of management of these patients.

## Molar Pregnancy

### COMPLETE VERSUS PARTIAL MOLAR PREGNANCY

**Pathologic and Chromosomal Features.** Hydatidiform mole may be categorized as either a complete or a partial mole on the basis of gross morphology, histology, and karyotype (Table 60–1).

Complete moles have no identifiable embryonic or fetal tissues. The chorionic villi have generalized swelling and are enveloped by atypical and hyperplastic trophoblast. Complete moles generally have a 46,XX karyotype, and the molar chromosomes are derived entirely from paternal origin.[3] Complete moles usually arise from fertilization of an empty ovum by a haploid sperm that then duplicates its own chromosomes.[4] Although chromosomal DNA in complete moles is entirely paternal in origin, mitochondrial DNA is maternal in origin.[5]

Partial hydatidiform moles are characterized by the following pathologic features: (1) various-sized chorionic villi with focal hydatidiform swelling and cavitation, (2) marked villous scalloping with stromal trophoblastic inclusions, (3) focal trophoblastic hyperplasia, and (4) identifiable fetal or embryonic tissues.[6] Partial moles generally have a triploid karyotype, which results from the fertilization of an apparently normal ovum by two spermatozoa.[7]

**Presenting Signs and Symptoms.** Vaginal bleeding is the most common presenting symptom in patients with complete mole; it occurred in 97% of our patients.[8] The uterine size may be larger than expected for gestational age in about half of the patients with complete mole because the endometrial cavity may be expanded by clot and chorionic tissue. Excessive uterine size is generally associated with markedly ele-

*Table 60–1.* Complete Versus Partial Molar Pregnancy

|  | Complete Mole | Partial Mole |
|---|---|---|
| Fetal or embryonic tissue | Absent | Present |
| Hydatidiform swelling of chorionic villi | Diffuse | Focal |
| Trophoblastic hyperplasia | Diffuse | Focal |
| Scalloping of chorionic villi | Absent | Present |
| Trophoblastic stromal inclusions | Absent | Present |
| Karyotype | 46,XX; 46,XY | Triploid |

vated human chorionic gonadotropin (hCG) blood levels because the uterus is at least partially expanded by hyperplastic trophoblastic tissue. hCG is a regular and predictable secretory product of the trophoblast cell. Elevated levels of hCG may hyperstimulate the ovaries and induce formation of numerous theca-lutein cysts. Toxemia may also develop in patients with complete mole, particularly when the uterus is excessively enlarged and serum hCG levels are high. Complete moles are now being diagnosed earlier in pregnancy, before many of the classic signs and symptoms have developed.

In contrast, patients with partial mole generally do not present with the dramatic clinical features that characterize complete mole. These patients usually present with the signs and symptoms of incomplete or missed abortion, and the diagnosis of partial mole may be considered only after histologic review of the curettage specimens.[9]

## DIAGNOSIS OF HYDATIDIFORM MOLE

**Ultrasonography.** Ultrasonography is a sensitive and reliable technique for diagnosing molar pregnancy. Because of the marked and diffuse swelling of the chorionic villi, complete molar pregnancy produces a characteristic vesicular pattern on ultrasound examination. Ultrasonography may also contribute to the diagnosis of partial mole by demonstrating focal cystic spaces in the placenta.

## NATURAL HISTORY OF MOLAR PREGNANCY

Complete molar pregnancy is well recognized to have a potential for the development of uterine invasion or metastasis. Following molar evacuation, uterine invasion and metastasis occur in 15 and 4% of patients, respectively.[8]

We reviewed 858 patients with complete mole to identify factors that predispose to persistent GTT. At the time of presentation, 41% of the patients had the following signs of marked trophoblastic growth: hCG level greater than 100,000 mIU/ml, uterine size greater than expected for gestational age, and theca-lutein ovarian cysts larger than 6 cm in diameter. After evacuation, 31% of these patients developed uterine invasion and 8.8% developed metastases. The risk for persistent GTT is considerably less for patients who do not present with signs of marked trophoblastic growth. Following molar evacuation, only 3.4% of these patients developed local invasion and 0.6% developed metastases. Therefore, patients with complete moles with markedly elevated hCG values and excessive uterine size are at increased risk of developing postmolar GTT and are categorized as high risk.

Seventeen (5.5%) of our 310 patients with partial mole developed nonmetastatic GTT.[10] Sixteen of these patients were thought to have missed abortion before uterine evacuation. Only one patient presented with theca-lutein cysts, markedly elevated hCG levels, and excessive uterine size. Patients with partial mole who developed persistent tumor did not have clinical characteristics that distinguished them from other patients with partial mole.

## TREATMENT

After diagnosis of a molar pregnancy, the patient is carefully assessed for the presence of associated medical complications, including toxemia and anemia. She is first stabilized, and then a decision must be made about the most appropriate method of evacuation.

If the patient no longer desires to preserve fertility, hysterectomy may be performed. Although hysterectomy eliminates the risks associated with local invasion, it does not prevent metastasis.

Suction curettage is the preferred method of evacuation regardless of uterine size in patients who desire to retain fertility.[11] When suction evacuation is thought to be complete, a sharp curettage should be performed to remove any residual molar tissue.

**Prophylactic Chemotherapy.** The use of prophylactic chemotherapy at the time of molar evacuation remains highly controversial.[12] However, several studies have demonstrated that chemoprophylaxis reduces the risk of postmolar GTT.

Kim and coworkers[13] reported on a prospective randomized study of the use of prophylactic chemotherapy at the time of molar evacuation. Chemoprophylaxis effectively reduced the incidence of postmolar GTT from 47% to 14% in patients with high-risk complete mole. Prophylactic chemotherapy may therefore be particularly useful in the management of high-risk complete mole, especially when hormonal follow-up is unavailable or unreliable.

**Hormonal Follow-up.** After molar evacuation, all patients must be monitored with serial hCG measurements to facilitate the early detection of persistent tumor. Patients are monitored with weekly hCG determinations until values have been nondetectable for 3 weeks and then monthly until they have been nondetectable for 6 months.

Patients are encouraged to use effective contraception during the entire interval of gonadotropin follow-up. If the patient does not desire sterilization, she is confronted with the choice of using either steroidal contraceptives or barrier methods.

The incidence of postmolar GTT has been reported to be increased in patients who used oral contraceptives before gonadotropin remission.[14] However, data from the New England Trophoblastic Disease Center (NETDC) and the Gynecologic Oncology Group indicate that oral contraceptives do not increase the risk of postmolar trophoblastic disease.[15, 16] We therefore believe that oral contraceptives may be safely prescribed after molar evacuation during the entire interval of hCG follow-up.

## Gestational Trophoblastic Tumors

### NATURAL HISTORY

**Nonmetastatic Disease.** Locally invasive GTT develops in 15% of patients following evacuation of a complete mole and infrequently after other pregnancies.[8] These patients may present with irregular vaginal bleeding, theca-lutein cysts, uterine subinvolution or asymmetric enlargement, and elevated hCG levels. Trophoblastic tumor may perforate through the myometrium, producing intraperitoneal bleeding, or erode into uterine vessels, causing vaginal hemorrhage. Bulky necrotic tumor may involve the uterine wall and serve as a nidus for sepsis.

**Metastatic Disease.** Metastatic GTT occurs in 4% of patients after evacuation of a complete mole and infrequently following other gestations.[8] Metastatic GTT is usually associated with the presence of choriocarcinoma. Choriocarcinoma has a tendency for early vascular invasion with widespread dissemination. The most common metastatic sites are as follows: lung, 80%; vagina, 30%; pelvis, 20%; brain, 10%; and liver, 10%. In the absence of pulmonary or vaginal involvement, metastases to the brain, liver, and other sites are rare. Because trophoblastic tumors are highly vascular, metastases are often hemorrhagic. Patients commonly present with signs and symptoms of bleeding from metastases, such as hemoptysis or hepatic rupture.

**Staging System.** An anatomic staging system for GTT has been adopted by the International Federation of Gynecology and Obstetrics (Table 60–2). Stage I is characterized by tumor confined to the uterus. Stage II designates tumor outside the uterus but localized to the vagina or pelvis, or both. Stage III is defined by pulmonary metastases with or without uterine, vaginal, or pelvic involvement. Patients with stage IV have far-advanced disease with involvement of the brain, liver, kidneys, or gastrointestinal tract. Stage IV tumors are generally choriocarcinoma and commonly follow a nonmolar pregnancy.

In addition to anatomic staging, other prognostic variables can be used to predict the likelihood of drug resistance and to assist in selecting appropriate chemotherapy. The World Health Organization has published a prognostic scoring system that reliably predicts the potential for chemotherapy resistance (Table 60–3). When the prognostic score is 8 or greater, the patient is placed in a high-risk category and requires intensive combination chemotherapy to achieve remission. In general, patients with stage I disease have a low-risk score and patients with stage IV disease have a high-risk score. Therefore, the distinction between low and high risk applies mainly to stages II and III GTT.

**Diagnostic Evaluation.** All patients with persistent GTT should undergo a thorough pretreatment evaluation, including a complete history and physical examination; determination of hCG blood levels; hepatic, thyroid, and renal function tests; and determination of baseline levels of peripheral blood and platelet counts. The metastatic work-up should include a chest roentgenogram, ultrasonography of the abdomen and pelvis, computed tomographic (CT) scan of the head, and, in some cases, selective angiography of abdominal and pelvic organs. CT scans have facilitated the early detection of asymptomatic cerebral lesions.[17]

*Table 60–2.* **Staging of Gestational Trophoblast Tumors**

| Stage | Criteria |
|-------|----------|
| I | Confined to uterine corpus |
| II | Metastases to pelvis and vagina |
| III | Metastases to lung |
| IV | Distant metastases |

## TREATMENT

**Stage I.** Table 60–4 reviews the NETDC protocol for the management of stage I disease. The selection of treatment is based primarily on the patient's desire to retain fertility.

If the patient no longer wishes to preserve fertility, hysterectomy with adjuvant single-agent chemotherapy may be performed as primary treatment. Adjuvant chemotherapy is administered for three reasons: (1) to reduce the likelihood of disseminating viable tumor cells at surgery; (2) to maintain the cytotoxic level of chemotherapy in the bloodstream and tissues in case viable tumor cells are disseminated; and (3) to treat any occult metastases that may already be present. Occult pulmonary metastases may be detected by CT scan in about 40% of patients with presumed nonmetastatic disease.[18] Chemotherapy may be safely administered perioperatively without increasing the incidence of surgical complications. Twenty-nine patients were treated by primary hysterectomy and adjuvant chemotherapy at the NETDC, and all had complete remission with no additional therapy.

All patients with nonmetastatic placental-site trophoblastic tumor (PSTT) should be treated with hysterectomy.[19] PSTT is an uncommon variant of choriocarcinoma that is primarily composed of intermediate trophoblastic cells. PSTT is generally resistant to chemotherapy and, owing to the paucity of syncytiotrophoblast, produces low levels of hCG.

Single-agent chemotherapy is the preferred treatment in patients with stage I disease who desire to retain fertility. Primary single-agent chemotherapy was administered to 453 of our patients with stage I GTT, and 416 patients (91.8%) had complete remission. In the remaining 37 patients, remission was subsequently attained with either combination chemotherapy or surgical intervention.

All patients with stages I, II, and III GTT are monitored with weekly hCG values until these have been nondetectable for 3 weeks and are then monitored with monthly values until nondetectable for 12 months. Patients are encouraged to use effective contraception during the entire interval of hCG follow-up.

**Stage II.** The NETDC protocol for the management of stage II disease is outlined in Table 60–5. Although low-risk patients are treated with primary single-agent chemotherapy, high-risk patients are managed with primary combination chemotherapy. Between July 1965 and December 1996, 27 patients with stage II disease were treated at the NETDC, and all had remission. Single-agent chemotherapy induced complete remission in 16 (84.2%) of 19 low-risk patients. In contrast, remission was attained in only two of eight high-risk patients with single-agent treatment.

Vaginal metastases may bleed profusely because they may be highly vascular and friable. Bleeding may be controlled by packing the hemorrhagic lesion or performing wide local excision. Infrequently, hypogastric artery ligation or angiographic embolization may be required to control hemorrhage from vaginal lesions.

**Stage III.** The NETDC protocol for the treatment of stage III disease is reviewed in Table 60–5. Low-risk patients are treated with primary single-agent chemotherapy, and high-risk patients are treated with combination-drug treatment. One hundred thirty-five patients with stage III disease were treated at the NETDC between July 1965 and December

*Table 60–3.* Scoring System Based on Prognostic Factors

| | Score* | | | |
|---|---|---|---|---|
| | 0 | 1 | 2 | 4 |
| Age (yr) | <39 | >39 | | |
| Antecedent pregnancy | H. mole | Abortion | Term | |
| Interval between end of antecedent pregnancy and start of chemotherapy (mo) | <4 | 4–6 | 7–12 | >12 |
| hCG in blood (IU/L) | $<10^3$ | $10^3$–$10^4$ | $10^4$–$10^5$ | $>10^5$ |
| ABO groups | | O or A | B or AB | |
| Largest tumor, including uterine (cm) | <3 | 3–5 | >5 | |
| Site of metastases | | Spleen Kidney | GI tract Liver | Brain |
| Number of metastases | | 1–3 | 4–8 | >8 |
| Prior chemotherapy | | | 1 drug | ≥2 drugs |

*The total score for a patient is obtained by adding the individual scores for each prognostic factor. Total score: <4 = low risk; 5–7 = middle risk; ≥8 = high risk.
H., hydatidiform; hCG, human chorionic gonadotropin; GI, gastrointestinal.
From Bagshawe KD. Treatment of high-risk choriocarcinoma. J Reprod Med 1984;29:813.

1996, and complete remission was achieved in 134 (99%). Gonadotropin remission was induced with single-agent chemotherapy in 72 (80.9%) of 89 patients with low-risk disease and in 13 (28.3%) of 46 patients with high-risk disease. All patients who were resistant to single-agent treatment later had remission with combination chemotherapy.

Thoracotomy has a limited role in the management of stage III GTT. Thoracotomy may be performed if the diagnosis is seriously in question. Furthermore, if a patient has an isolated viable pulmonary nodule despite intensive chemotherapy, thoracotomy may be undertaken to excise the resistant focus. It is important to emphasize that fibrotic nodules may persist indefinitely on chest roentgenogram after complete gonadotropin remission is achieved.

Hysterectomy may be required in patients with metastatic GTT to control uterine hemorrhage or sepsis. Furthermore, in patients with bulky uterine tumor, hysterectomy may substantially reduce the tumor burden and thereby limit the need for multiple courses of chemotherapy.[20]

**Stage IV.** Table 60–6 outlines the NETDC protocol for the management of stage IV disease. These patients are at greatest risk of developing rapidly progressive and resistant tumors despite intensive therapy.

All patients with stage IV disease should be treated with primary intensive combination chemotherapy and the selective use of radiation therapy and surgery.[21] Before 1975, only six (30%) of our 20 patients with stage IV disease had complete remission, but after 1975, 14 (77.8%) of our 18 patients with stage IV tumors had gonadotropin remission. This improvement in survival has resulted from aggressive multimodal treatment.

The management of hepatic metastases is particularly problematic and challenging. Hepatic resection may be required to control acute bleeding and hepatic rupture or to excise resistant tumor.

If cerebral metastases are detected, whole-brain irradiation is promptly instituted at our center. The occurrence of cerebral hemorrhage may be reduced by the use of combination chemotherapy and brain irradiation. Brain irradiation may be both hemostatic and tumoricidal. Yordan and associates[22] reported that deaths due to central nervous system involvement occurred in 11 (44%) of 25 patients treated

*Table 60–4.* Protocol for Treatment of Stage I Gestational Trophoblastic Neoplasia

| | |
|---|---|
| Initial | MTX-FA; if resistant, switch to Act-D, or hysterectomy with adjuvant chemotherapy |
| Resistant | Combination chemotherapy or hysterectomy with adjuvant chemotherapy; local uterine resection |
| Follow-up hCG | Weekly until normal for 3 wk, then monthly until normal for 12 mo |
| Contraception | 12 consecutive mo of normal hCG titers |

MTX, methotrexate; FA, folinic acid; Act-D, actinomycin D; hCG, human chorionic gonadotropin.
Modified from Berek JS, Hacker NF. Practical gynecologic oncology. 3rd ed. Baltimore: Lippincott–Williams & Wilkins, 2000:615–38. Adapted from Goldstein DP, Berkowitz RS, eds. Gestational trophoblastic neoplasms: clinical principles of diagnosis and management. Philadelphia: WB Saunders, 1982.

*Table 60–5.* Protocol for Treatment of Stage II and Stage III Gestational Trophoblastic Neoplasms

| | |
|---|---|
| *Low Risk* * | |
| Initial | MTX-FA; if resistant, switch to Act-D |
| Resistant to both single agents | Combination chemotherapy |
| *High Risk* * | |
| Initial | EMA-CO combination chemotherapy |
| Resistant | PVB |
| *Follow-up hCG* | Weekly until normal for 3 wk, then monthly until normal for 12 mo |
| *Contraception* | Until there have been 12 consecutive mo of normal hCG titers |

*Local resection optional.
MTX, methotrexate; FA, folinic acid; Act-D, actinomycin D; EMA-CO, etoposide, methotrexate, actinomycin D, cyclophosphamide, vincristine (Oncovin); PVB, vinblastine, bleomycin, cisplatin (Platinol); hCG, human chorionic gonadotropin.
Modified from Berek JS, Hacker NF. Practical gynecologic oncology. 3rd ed. Philadelphia: Lippincott–Williams & Wilkins, 2000:615–38. Adapted from Goldstein DP, Berkowitz RS, eds. Gestational trophoblastic neoplasms: clinical principles of diagnosis and management. Philadelphia: WB Saunders, 1982.

**Table 60–6.** Protocol for Treatment of Stage IV Gestational Trophoblastic Neoplasms

| | |
|---|---|
| *Initial* | EMA-CO combination chemotherapy |
| Brain | Whole-head irradiation (3000 cGy) |
| | Craniotomy to manage complications |
| Liver | Resection to manage complications |
| *Resistant** | PVB |
| | Hepatic arterial infusion |
| *Follow-up hCG* | Weekly until normal for 3 wk, then monthly until normal for 24 mo |
| *Contraception* | Until there have been 24 consecutive mo of normal hCG titers |

*Local resection optional.

EMA-CO, etoposide, methotrexate, actinomycin D, cyclophosphamide, vincristine (Oncovin); PVB, vinblastine, bleomycin, cisplatin (Platinol); hCG, human chorionic gonadotropin.

Modified from Berek JS, Hacker NF: Practical gynecologic oncology. 3rd ed. Philadelphia: Lippincott–Williams & Wilkins, 2000:615–38. Adapted from Goldstein DP, Berkowitz RS, eds. Gestational trophoblastic neoplasms: Clinical principles of diagnosis and management. Philadelphia: WB Saunders, 1982.

with chemotherapy alone but in none of 18 patients treated with brain irradiation and chemotherapy.

Rustin and colleagues,[17] however, have reported excellent remission rates in patients with cerebral metastases treated with chemotherapy alone. Eighty-seven percent of their patients with cerebral lesions had sustained remission with intensive combination chemotherapy, including high-dose intravenous and intrathecal methotrexate. Excellent cure rates can therefore be attained in patients with cerebral metastases with intensive chemotherapy alone.

Craniotomy should be performed to manage life-threatening cerebral complications with the hope that the patient will ultimately be cured with chemotherapy. Craniotomy may be necessary to provide acute decompression or to control bleeding. Infrequently, cerebral metastases that are resistant to chemotherapy may be resectable. Fortunately, patients who have cerebral metastases and who attain remission generally have no residual neurologic deficits.

Patients with stage IV disease are monitored with weekly hCG determinations until levels have been nondetectable for 3 weeks, and they are then monitored with monthly determinations until levels have been nondetectable for 24 months. These patients require prolonged gonadotropin follow-up because they have an increased risk of late recurrence.

## Chemotherapy

**Single-Agent Chemotherapy.** Single-agent chemotherapy with various regimens of either actinomycin D or methotrexate has induced comparable and excellent remission rates in both nonmetastatic and metastatic GTT. Investigators have modified the protocols for administering methotrexate and actinomycin D to limit systemic toxicity and length of hospitalization. Bagshawe and Wilde[23] first reported using folinic acid with methotrexate to minimize systemic toxicity. Schlaerth and coworkers[24] have administered single-dose actinomycin D and observed excellent remission rates with limited hospitalization.

Methotrexate–folinic acid has been the preferred single-

agent regimen in the treatment of GTT at the NETDC since 1974.[25] This involves the intramuscular administration of methotrexate in a dosage of 1 mg/kg every other day for four doses, provided that the platelet count is greater than 100,000/ml and the granulocyte count is greater than 1500/ml. Twenty-four hours after each dose of methotrexate, folinic acid (leucovorin) is administered in a dose of 0.1 mg/kg intramuscularly.

Between September 1974 and September 1985, 185 patients with GTT were treated with primary methotrexate–folinic acid at the NETDC. Complete remission was induced in 162 patients (87.6%), and 132 (81.5%) of these patients required only one course of chemotherapy. Methotrexate–folinic acid induced remission in 147 (90.2%) of 163 patients with stage I GTT and in 15 (68.2%) of 22 patients with low-risk stage II and III GTT. Thrombocytopenia, granulocytopenia, and hepatotoxicity occurred in only 11 (5.9%), three (1.6%), and 26 (14.1%) patients, respectively. No patient required platelet transfusions or developed sepsis from myelosuppression. Methotrexate–folinic acid not only induces an excellent remission rate with minimal toxicity but also effectively limits chemotherapy exposure.

*Administration.* The hCG level is measured weekly after each course of chemotherapy, and the hCG regression curve serves as the primary basis for determining the need for further treatment. After the first treatment, further chemotherapy is withheld as long as the hCG level is falling progressively. Additionally, single-agent chemotherapy is not administered at any predetermined or fixed time interval. A second course of chemotherapy is administered under the following conditions: (1) The hCG level remains at a plateau for more than 3 consecutive weeks or re-elevates, and (2) the hCG level does not decline by one log within 18 days after completion of the first treatment.

If a second course of methotrexate–folinic acid is needed, the dosage of methotrexate is unchanged if the patient's response to the first treatment was adequate. An adequate response is defined as a fall in the hCG level by one log following a course of chemotherapy. When the response to the first treatment is inadequate, the dosage of methotrexate is increased to 2 mg/kg in four divided doses. If the response to two courses of methotrexate–folinic acid is inadequate, the patient is considered to be resistant to methotrexate, and actinomycin D is promptly substituted.

**Combination Chemotherapy.** Modified triple therapy with methotrexate–folinic acid, actinomycin D, and cyclophosphamide was the preferred combination-drug regimen at the NETDC in the past.[26] However, primary triple therapy is inadequate as an initial treatment in patients with metastatic disease and a high-risk score.[27] Triple therapy induced remission in only 5 (45%) of 11 patients with metastatic GTT and a high-risk score. Similarly, Dubuc-Lissoir and colleagues[28] observed that primary triple therapy induced remission in only 11 (50%) of 22 patients with metastatic GTT and a high-risk score.

Etoposide (VP-16) has been demonstrated to be an effective antitumor agent in GTT. Primary oral etoposide induced complete sustained remission in 56 (93.3%) of 60 patients with nonmetastatic or low-risk metastatic GTT.[29] Bagshawe[30] reported an 83% remission rate in patients with a high-risk score using a combination-drug regimen that includes etoposide. This regimen (EMA-CO) includes etoposide,

*Table 60–7.* **EMA-CO Regimen for Patients with Gestational Trophoblastic Neoplasms**

| Regimen* | |
| --- | --- |
| **Course I (EMA)** | |
| Day 1 | VP-16, 100 mg/m² IV infusion in 200 ml of saline over 30 min |
| | Actinomycin D, 0.5 mg IV push |
| | Methotrexate, 100 mg/m² IV push, followed by a 200 mg/m² IV infusion over 12 h |
| Day 2 | VP-16, 100 mg/m² IV infusion in 200 ml of saline over 30 min |
| | Actinomycin D, 0.5 mg IV push |
| | Folinic acid, 15 mg IM or PO every 12 hr for 4 doses beginning 24 hr after start of methotrexate |
| **Course 2 (CO)** | |
| Day 8 | Vincristine, 1.0 mg/m² IV push |
| | Cytoxan, 600 mg/m² IV in saline |

*This regimen consists of two courses: course 1 is given on days 1 and 2; course 2 is given on day 8. Course 1 might require overnight hospital stay; course 2 does not. These courses can usually be given on days 1 and 2, 8, 15 and 16, 22, etc., and the intervals should not be extended without cause.

EMA-CO, etoposide (VP-16), methotrexate, actinomycin D, cyclophosphamide (Cytoxan), vincristine (Oncovin).

From Bagshawe KD. Treatment of high-risk choriocarcinoma. J Reprod Med 1984;29:813.

methotrexate, actinomycin D, cyclophosphamide, and vincristine (Oncovin) and is our preferred initial treatment for patients with a high-risk score (Table 60–7). Bolis and co-workers[31] and Schink and colleagues[32] have confirmed that primary EMA-CO induced complete remission in 13 (81%) of 16 patients and all 5 patients in their respective studies, with metastatic GTT and a high-risk score. If patients experience resistance to EMA-CO, remission may still be achieved by substituting etoposide and cisplatin (EMA-EP) for cyclophosphamide and vincristine on day 8.[33]

Following the success of PVB (cisplatin [Platinol], vinblastine, and bleomycin) in testicular tumors, PVB has been used as second-line therapy in GTT. We administered PVB as salvage in seven patients who were resistant to triple therapy or the modified Bagshawe regimen, and four of these patients had remission.[34] Despite advances in primary treatment, we continue to need effective second-line therapies for patients with resistant disease.

Patients who require combination chemotherapy must be treated intensively to achieve remission. We administer combination chemotherapy as frequently as toxicity permits until the patient has three consecutive nondetectable weekly hCG levels. After nondetectable hCG levels have been attained, additional courses of chemotherapy are administered to reduce the risk of relapse.

**Subsequent Pregnancies.** Patients who achieve remission with chemotherapy for persistent GTT should be reassured that they can anticipate a normal reproductive outcome in the future.[35, 36] Patients at the NETDC who received chemotherapy for persistent GTT had 410 later conceptions between June 1, 1965, and December 31, 1992. Those pregnancies resulted in 287 term live births (69.9%), seven stillbirths (2.4%), 17 premature deliveries (4.2%), and four ectopic gestations (1.0%). First- and second-trimester sponta-

neous abortions occurred in 65 (15.9%) and seven (1.7%) of the pregnancies, respectively. Major and minor congenital anomalies were detected at birth in only 7 (2.2%) of 311 term or premature infants.

## SUGGESTION FOR ADDITIONAL READING

Berkowitz RS, Goldstein DP. Chorionic tumors. N Engl J Med 1996;335;23:1740–8.

## REFERENCES

1. Goldstein DP, Berkowitz RS. Gestational trophoblastic neoplasms: clinical principles of diagnosis and management. Philadelphia: WB Saunders, 1982:1–310.
2. Bagshawe KD. Risk and prognostic factors in trophoblastic neoplasia. Cancer 1976;38:3:1373–85.
3. Kajii T, Ohama K. Androgenetic origin of hydatidiform mole. Nature 1977;268:5621:633–4.
4. Yamashita K, Wake N, Araki T, et al. Human lymphocyte antigen expression in hydatidiform mole: androgenesis following fertilization by a haploid sperm. Am J Obstet Gynecol 1979;135:597–600.
5. Azuma C, Saji F, Tokugawa Y, et al. Application of gene amplification by polymerase chain reaction to genetic analysis of molar mitochondrial DNA: the detection of anuclear empty ovum as the cause of complete mole. Gynecol Oncol 1991;40:1:29–33.
6. Szulman AE, Surti U. The syndromes of hydatidiform mole. 11. Morphologic evolution of the complete and partial mole. Am J Obstet Gynecol 1978;132:1:20–7.
7. Lawler SD, Fisher RA, Dent J. A prospective genetic study of complete and partial hydatidiform moles. Am J Obstet Gynecol 1991;164:5 part 1:1270–7.
8. Berkowitz RS, Goldstein DP. Chorionic tumors. N Engl J Med 1996;335:23:1740–8.
9. Berkowitz RS, Goldstein DP, Bernstein MR. Natural history of partial molar pregnancy. Obstet Gynecol 1986;66:677–81.
10. Lage JM, Berkowitz RS, Rice LW, et al. Flow cytometric analysis of DNA content in partial hydatidiform moles with persistent gestational trophoblastic tumor. Obstet Gynecol 1991;77:1:111–5.
11. Berkowitz RS, Goldstein DP. Presentation and management of molar pregnancy. In: Hancock BW, Newlands ES, Berkowitz RS, eds. Gestational trophoblastic disease. London: Chapman and Hall, 1997:127–142.
12. Goldstein DP, Berkowitz RS. Prophylactic chemotherapy of complete molar pregnancy. Semin Oncol 1995;22:2:157–60.
13. Kim DS, Moon H, Kim KT, et al. Effects of prophylactic chemotherapy for persistent trophoblastic disease in patients with complete hydatidiform mole. Obstet Gynecol 1986;67:5:690–4.
14. Stone M, Dent J, Kardana A, Bagshawe KD. Relationship of oral contraception to development of trophoblastic tumour after evacuation of a hydatidiform mole. Br J Obstet Gynaecol 1976;83:913–6.
15. Berkowitz RS, Goldstein DP, Marean AR, Bernstein M. Oral contraceptives and post-molar trophoblastic disease. Obstet Gynecol 1981;58:4:474–7.
16. Curry SL, Schlaerth JB, Kohorn EL, et al. Hormonal contraception and trophoblastic sequelae after hydatidiform mole (a Gynecologic Oncology Group study). Am J Obstet Gynecol 1989;160:4:805–9; discussion 809–11.
17. Rustin GJS, Newlands ES, Begert RHJ, et al. Weekly alternating etoposide, methotrexate, actinomycin D/vincristine and cyclophosphamide chemotherapy for the treatment of CNS metastases of choriocarcinoma. J Clin Oncol 1989;7:900–3.
18. Mutch DG, Soper JT, Baker ME, et al. Role of computed axial tomography of the chest in staging patients with nonmetastatic gestational trophoblastic disease. Obstet Gynecol 1986;68:3:348–52.
19. Finkler NJ, Berkowitz RS, Driscoll SG, et al. Clinical experience with placental site trophoblastic tumors at the New England Trophoblastic Disease Center. Obstet Gynecol 1988;71:854–7.
20. Soper JT. Surgical therapy for gestational trophoblastic disease. J Reprod Med 1994;39:3:168–74.
21. Lurain JR. Management of high-risk gestational trophoblastic disease. J Reprod Med 1998;43:1:44–52.

22. Yordan EL Jr, Schlaerth J, Gaddis O, Morrow CP. Radiation therapy in the management of gestational choriocarcinoma metastatic to the central nervous system. Obstet Gynecol 1987;69:627–630.

23. Bagshawe KD, Wilde CE. Infusion therapy for pelvic trophoblastic tumours. J Obstet Gynaecol Br Commonw 1964;71:565–70.

24. Schlaerth JB, Morrow CP, Nalick RH, Gaddis O Jr. Single-dose actinomycin D in the treatment of postmolar trophoblastic disease. Gynecol Oncol 1984;19:1:53–6.

25. Berkowitz RS, Goldstein DP, Bernstein MR. Ten years experience with methotrexate and folinic acid as primary therapy for gestational trophoblastic disease. Gynecol Oncol 1986;23:111–8.

26. Berkowitz RS, Goldstein DP, Bernstein MR. Modified triple chemotherapy in the management of high-risk metastatic gestational trophoblastic tumors. Gynecol Oncol 1984;19:2:173–81.

27. DuBeshter B, Berkowitz RS, Goldstein DP, et al. Metastatic gestational trophoblastic disease: experience at the New England Trophoblastic Disease Center, 1965–1985. Obstet Gynecol 1987;69:390–5.

28. Dubuc-Lissoir J, Sweizig S, Schlaerth JB, Morrow CP. Metastatic gestational trophoblastic disease: a comparison of prognostic classification systems. Gynecol Oncol 1992;45:1:40–5.

29. Wong LC, Choo YC, Ma HK. Primary oral etoposide therapy in gestational trophoblastic disease: an update. Cancer 1986;58:14–17.

30. Bagshawe KD. Treatment of high-risk choriocarcinoma. J Reprod Med 1984;29:813–20.

31. Bolis G, Bonazzi C, Landoni R, et al. EMA/CO regimen in high-risk gestational trophoblastic tumor (GTT). Gynecol Oncol 1988;31:439–444.

32. Schink JL, Singh DK, Rademaker AW, et al. Etoposide, methotrexate, actinomycin D, cyclophosphamide, and vincristine for the treatment of metastatic, high-risk gestational trophoblastic disease. Obstet Gynecol 1992;80:817–20.

33. Newlands ES, Bagshawe KD, Begent RH, et al. Results with the EMA/CO (etoposide, methotrexate, actinomycin D, cyclophosphamide, vincristine) regimen in high-risk gestational trophoblastic tumours, 1979 to 1989. Br J Obstet Gynaecol 1991;98:6:550–7.

34. DuBeshter B, Berkowitz RS, Goldstein DP, Bernstein M. Vinblastine, cisplatin and bleomycin as salvage therapy for refractory high-risk metastatic gestational trophoblastic disease. J Reprod Med 1989;34:3:189–92.

35. Song H-Z, Wu P-C, Wang Y, et al. Pregnancy outcomes after successful chemotherapy for choriocarcinoma and invasive mole: long-term follow-up. Am J Obstet Gynecol 1988;158:538–45.

36. Berkowitz RS, Im SS, Bernstein MR, Goldstein DP. Gestational trophoblastic disease. Subsequent pregnancy outcome, including repeat molar pregnancy. J Reprod Med 1998;43:1:81–6.

# XIII

# HEAD AND NECK CANCER

• CHARLES M. HASKELL

Neoplasms of the head and neck account for about 4% of all cancer in the United States. Tobacco smoking and heavy alcohol use are important risk factors for the development of cancer of the head and neck, with the possible exception of salivary gland tumors, and smoking cessation and moderation in the use of alcohol are important forms of prevention. Investigational approaches to the prevention of head and neck cancer using various retinoids and other agents are discussed in Chapter 4.

As with most other carcinomas, early diagnosis is the key to management. Prompt referral to a specialist in head and neck surgery is essential for diagnosis. Subsequent management is the responsibility of surgeons and radiation therapists working closely together in order to integrate appropriately a plan of treatment suitable for each anatomic region of the head and neck. The medical oncologist plays only a peripheral role in the treatment of most of these patients, although emerging data support the combined use of chemotherapy and radiation therapy in preserving the quality of life by retaining the larynx in patients with advanced laryngeal carcinoma. This model of combined-modality therapy is under intense investigation and in the future may become the standard of care for several sites in the head and neck. It is hoped that the medical oncologist and general internist will also play an increasing role in cancer prevention and surveillance.

Because of the pivotal role of the surgeon and radiation therapist in the management of head and neck tumors, the chapters in this section are oriented toward the roles of surgery and radiation therapy in each of several distinct anatomic regions. The role of chemotherapy for this entire group of neoplasms is discussed separately in Chapter 66.

# CHAPTER 61

# ORAL CAVITY AND OROPHARYNX

• THOMAS C. CALCATERRA • GUY J. F. JUILLARD •
• KEITH E. BLACKWELL •

Cancers of the oral cavity and oropharynx account for approximately 3% of all cancers in the United States and are responsible for nearly 8000 deaths annually. As with other head and neck cancers, cases in men predominate, although the ratio of afflicted men to women is decreasing owing to the increasing number of women who smoke tobacco.

Many different etiologic factors have been proposed in oral cancer, and some seem definite. Sun exposure is undoubtedly an important etiologic factor in lip cancer, with the lower lip at greater risk. Cancer of the floor of the mouth is seen far more frequently in people who use snuff than in the general population.[1] Similarly, the habitual pipe smoker is prone to cancer of the buccal mucosa. Cigar smoking, which has become increasingly prevalent during the past decade, is also associated with an increased risk of carcinomas of the oral cavity.[2] Excessive smoking and alcohol consumption are certainly related to oral cavity and oropharyngeal cancers, but it is difficult to assess which of these habits is more oncogenic because they usually occur together.[3]

Two epidemiologic studies have suggested that nonsmoking women who use mouthwash may have an increased risk of oral cancer.[4, 5] A third case-control study involving 866 patients and 1249 controls found the risk of oral cancer to be increased 60% for women and 40% for men who used alcohol-containing mouthwash.[6] However, a comprehensive review of the literature found that a definite etiologic relationship between the use of mouthwash and the development of oral cancers has not been well established.[7]

Some oral cavity cancers, particularly those of the buccal mucosa, arise from an area of leukoplakia; fortunately, however, the condition does not usually degenerate into a malignant tumor. Nevertheless, it is important to correct abrading surfaces on dentures or teeth that give rise to leukoplakia or superficial ulceration. In cases of cancer of the tongue, an association with tertiary syphilis was noted when syphilis was prevalent. More recent evidence suggests a possible role for human papillomavirus, which is detected in 59% of oral carcinomas.[8]

The rather high incidence of second and third primary cancers in the oral cavity is of particular importance. Occasionally, multiple primary cancers occur in individuals who do not smoke or drink—usually older women with atrophic oral mucosa that is possibly related to deficiencies of iron and riboflavin.[3] Likewise, it has been postulated that alcoholism leads to similar vitamin and mineral deficiencies.

## Natural History

### CLASSIFICATION AND PATHOLOGY

Squamous cell (epidermoid) cancer is the most common type of cancer (90%) arising in the oral cavity and oropharynx.

In general, cancers originating in the oral cavity are well differentiated, particularly in the lip and buccal mucosa. Those arising in the oropharynx tend to be less well differentiated and have a greater propensity for early metastasis. Oral cavity cancers, which may develop from an area of hyperkeratosis, tend to be exophytic and well differentiated. Some of these tumors become bulky and develop a warty appearance, and they are termed *verrucous cancer*. They are characterized by a papillary architecture, a lack of cellular atypia, and relatively late invasion of the underlying musculatures.

The next most prevalent of the other types of cancers that are seen in the oral cavity and oropharynx is that originating in the numerous nests of salivary gland tissue omnipresent throughout the entire mucosal lining.[9] The usual site for salivary gland tumors is the palate and, less frequently, the floor of the mouth and base of the tongue.[10] These tumors vary in their malignant potential and invasiveness, but in general, they grow slowly and have a tendency to recur locally if not widely resected when first treated. Of particular concern is adenoid cystic carcinoma, which has a remarkable proclivity for distant extension via the perineural lymphatics, resulting in a high incidence of local recurrence and lung metastasis.

Lymphomas are likely to be found in the portion of the oropharynx that contains Waldeyer's ring of lymphoid tissue. Care must be taken during biopsy to avoid a crush artifact of the cells, which makes precise diagnosis difficult.

Melanomas are rarely seen in the oral cavity and oropharynx; however, they may appear as nonpigmented tumors, and diagnosis may be difficult. Immunohistochemical stains for S–100 and HMB–45 play an important role in distinguishing mucosal melanomas from the more common neoplasms of the oral cavity.[11]

## DIAGNOSIS

Although the patient may be aware of symptoms related to an oral cavity or oropharyngeal cancer, the diagnosis is often delayed for several weeks or months. The patient typically attributes the symptoms to a slowly resolving "fever blister" or "tonsillitis" and fails to seek medical attention. Likewise, the first physician consulted generally carries out a therapeutic trial of antibiotics or gargles that further delays diagnosis. It is therefore important to refer patients with any persistent throat pain or nonhealing ulcer to a physician who is capable of performing a thorough head and neck examination and biopsy of any suspicious lesion.

The examination of the oral cavity and oropharynx requires good illumination, which is best provided by a head mirror or head light, and is facilitated by suction, local anesthesia, and various-sized mirrors or fiberoptic telescopes for systematic inspection of the anatomic regions of the oral cavity and oropharynx. Manual palpation is extremely important in examination of the tongue and the floor of the mouth to detect indurated tissue that cannot be seen. The use of intravital staining has assisted in the identification of oral cavity cancer,[12] but a biopsy of sufficient depth to ascertain submucosal extension must also be performed to confirm the presence of cancer. Stage II and larger tumors are often evaluated by magnetic resonance imaging or computed tomographic scanning, or both. The magnetic resonance imaging scan is most often used because of its capacity to define soft tissue planes and anatomic abnormalities. When osseous definition is sought, the computed tomographic scan is usually selected. After completion of the evaluation, detailed drawings or photographs of the cancer should be prepared as a baseline for treatment planning and follow-up.

## STAGING

The oral cavity is divided into several anatomic regions, each of which gives rise to tumors with similar biologic characteristics and prognostic factors. These regions are the lips, alveolar ridges, buccal mucosa, retromolar trigones, floor of the mouth, hard palate, and anterior two thirds of the tongue. The oropharynx is divided from the oral cavity superiorly by the junction of the hard and soft palates, laterally by the anterior tonsillar pillars, and inferiorly by the circumvallate papillae of the tongue. The regions of the oropharynx are the soft palate and uvula, base of the tongue (pharyngeal or posterior third), tonsils, and pharyngeal wall. The classification of the primary tumor is determined by its size (Table 61–1).[13] The recommended tumor (T) designation varies from one anatomic region of the head and neck to another, but the classification of the node (N) and metastasis (M) categories is applicable to all of the areas of the head and neck. Grading of the tumor using Broders' system is recommended for all tumors of the head and neck, although it is not a formal part of the TNM staging system for tumors of this region. Except for salivary gland tumors (Chapter 64), TNM stage groupings are similar throughout the head and neck region. Tables 61–1 and 61–2 provide the TNM staging systems for the tumor types covered in this chapter.

## Clinical Features and Treatment

### ORAL CAVITY

**Lip.** Carcinoma of the lip accounts for 30% of all cancers of the oral cavity, and the vast majority are squamous cell carcinomas. Patients with lip cancer usually present with a nonhealing sore of the lower lip that repeatedly forms a dry crust that bleeds on removal. The tumor may then develop into a bulky exophytic growth or, less commonly, an ulcerative indurated lesion. Associated keratotic lesions may appear on the remaining area of the lip. Almost 95% of such cancers occur on the lower lip, and these are characteristi-

cally more differentiated than upper lip cancers. The incidence of metastasis ranges from 10 to 15% and is greater with tumors of increased size, long durations, and less differentiation. For midline cancers of the lower lip, the most frequent site of cervical metastasis is the submental nodes; for lateral cancers, it is the submandibular nodes. The metastatic incidence of upper lip cancers approaches 50% and usually involves the upper deep jugular lymph node chain.

Lip cancers of stages T1 and T2 can be managed with equal success by irradiation or surgery.[14] When irradiation is the selected method, it is usually delivered by external beam, up to 6000 cGy over 5 to 6 weeks, or by radioactive implant that delivers 6000 to 7000 cGy over 5 or 6 days.

Large lesions are best treated surgically if there is soft tissue destruction or jaw involvement. Surgery usually consists of a V incision for small lesions or a W excision with primary closure for larger cancers involving an area no larger than one third of the lip. A local transposed flap of the opposite lip (Abbé's flap or Estlander's flap) is often used for lesions that involve between one third to two thirds of the lip. For advanced lip cancers that encompass up to two thirds of the lip, a rotational flap from the upper lip (Karadandlzic flap), which preserves the neurovascular supply to the orbicularis oris muscle, is used. Total lip reconstruction is carried out most effectively using a microvascular free flap from the forearm. A radical neck dissection is performed for palpable cervical metastasis, and it is often necessary to remove the periosteum or a cortical margin of the mandible to secure adequate tumor clearance. Postoperative radiation is often used when the lymph nodes are involved.

The 5-year control rate for lower lip cancers is related to the size of the tumor, but on average, it approaches 90% when there is no cervical metastasis. When cervical metastasis is present, however, the favorable prognosis is reduced almost by half. Upper lip cancers have a less favorable prognosis, with a 5-year control rate in the range of 50 to 60%.

**Buccal Mucosa.** Buccal cancers are relatively rare, accounting for only 5% of oral carcinomas. Tumors of the buccal mucosa, often arising in or associated with leukoplakia,[15] are more frequently exophytic than ulcerative and sometimes appear as warty outgrowths (verrucous cancer). These tumors may reach a rather large size before becoming symptomatic, particularly when they are exophytic. The ulcerative lesions are likely to present earlier with pain. When there is extension to the posterior buccal surface, trismus may be present owing to the invasion of the pterygoid muscles. This cancer is seen in an older age group, more so than those cancers located in all other regions of the oral cavity; the mean age of those afflicted with these tumors is in the seventh decade.

Radiation and surgery are equally effective for treatment of early lesions. For small lesions, peroral cone irradiation or radioactive implants are particularly effective. If surgery is performed, the buccal defect is usually repaired with a skin graft. Larger tumors may necessitate the resection of a portion of the mandible or maxillary alveolus. When the tumor extends through the cheek muscles close to skin, the skin must be excised, after which it is either closed primarily or repaired with a rotational neck flap. More extensive resec-

*Table 61–1.* **The International TNM Staging System for Cancer of the Lip and Oral Cavity**

**Definition of TNM**

*Primary Tumor (T)*

Lip and oral cavity

| | |
|---|---|
| TX | Primary tumor cannot be assessed |
| T0 | No evidence of primary tumor |
| Tis | Carcinoma in situ |
| T1 | Tumor 2 cm or less in greatest dimension |
| T2 | Tumor more than 2 cm but not more than 4 cm in greatest dimension |
| T3 | Tumor more than 4 cm in greatest dimension |
| T4 (lip) | Tumor invades adjacent structures (e.g., through cortical bone, tongue, skin of neck) |
| T4 (oral cavity) | Tumor invades adjacent structures (e.g., through cortical bone, into deep [extrinsic] muscle of tongue, maxillary sinus, skin) |

*Regional Lymph Nodes (N)*

| | |
|---|---|
| NX | Regional lymph nodes cannot be assessed |
| N0 | No regional lymph node metastasis |
| N1 | Metastasis in a single ipsilateral lymph node, 3 cm or less in greatest dimension |
| N2 | Metastasis in a single ipsilateral lymph node, more than 3 cm but not more than 6 cm in greatest dimension; or in multiple ipsilateral lymph nodes, none more than 6 cm in greatest dimension; or in bilateral or contralateral lymph nodes, none more than 6 cm in greatest dimension |
| N2a | Metastasis in single ipsilateral lymph node more than 3 cm but not more than 6 cm in greatest dimension |
| N2b | Metastasis in multiple ipsilateral lymph nodes, none more than 6 cm in greatest dimension |
| N2c | Metastasis in bilateral or contralateral lymph nodes, none more than 6 cm in greatest dimension |
| N3 | Metastasis in a lymph node more than 6 cm in greatest dimension |

*Distant Metastasis (M)*

| | |
|---|---|
| MX | Presence of distant metastasis cannot be assessed |
| M0 | No distant metastasis |
| M1 | Distant metastasis |

*Stage Grouping*

| | | | |
|---|---|---|---|
| Stage 0 | Tis | N0 | M0 |
| Stage I | T1 | N0 | M0 |
| Stage II | T2 | N0 | M0 |
| Stage III | T3 | N0 | M0 |
| | T1 | N1 | M0 |
| | T2 | N1 | M0 |
| | T3 | N1 | M0 |
| Stage IV | T4 | N0 | M0 |
| | T4 | N1 | M0 |
| | Any T | N2 | M0 |
| | Any T | N3 | M0 |
| | Any T | Any N | M1 |

*Histopathologic Grade (G)*

| | |
|---|---|
| GX | Grade cannot be assessed |
| G1 | Well differentiated |
| G2 | Moderately differentiated |
| G3 | Poorly differentiated |
| G4 | Undifferentiated |

From Beahrs OH, Henson DE, Hutter RVP, Kennedy BJ. Manual for staging of cancer. 4th ed. Philadelphia: JB Lippincott, 1992:29. Reproduced by permission of the American Joint Committee on Cancer and the publisher.

tions may require reconstruction using pedicled regional flaps or microvascular free flaps.

Metastasis to the submandibular and upper deep cervical nodes tends to occur when the tumor is advanced. The overall 5-year survival rate ranges between 40% and 50%.

**Alveolus, Retromolar Trigine, and Hard Palate.** Alveolar ridge, retromolar trigone, and hard palate tumors are discussed together because cancers in this region demonstrate close adherence to bone, an important consideration in selection of the optimal form of treatment. Inasmuch as pain is not typical during the early stages, these tumors are often confused with a dental infection or epulis. Indeed, the patient may undergo tooth extraction or modification of a denture because of persistent irritation. These tumors are generally well differentiated and may be exophytic or ulcerative. Al-

though squamous cell cancer clearly predominates in tumors of the alveolus and retromolar trigone, at least half of the hard palate cancers are of salivary gland origin. Because of the tumor's proximity to bone, bone involvement is present in most instances, although it may not be confirmed by radiographic studies.

The treatment for these tumors is almost always surgical, unless the patient refuses or has a poor medical status that would substantially increase operative risk.[16] The surgery removes the tumor en bloc, requiring at least a marginal mandibulectomy or partial maxillary alveolectomy. Defects arising after marginal mandibulectomy may be repaired with a split-thickness skin graft or fasciocutaneous free flap. Segmental defects of the anterior mandibular arch are almost always reconstructed with a vascularized bone-containing

*Table 61-2.* The International TNM Staging System for Cancer of the Oropharynx

**Definition of TNM**

*Primary Tumor (T)*

| | |
|---|---|
| TX | Primary tumor cannot be assessed |
| T0 | No evidence of primary tumor |
| Tis | Carcinoma in situ |

*Oropharynx*

| | |
|---|---|
| T1 | Tumor 2 cm or less in greatest dimension |
| T2 | Tumor more than 2 cm but not more than 4 cm in greatest dimension |
| T3 | Tumor more than 4 cm in greatest dimension |
| T4 | Tumor invades adjacent structures (e.g., through cortical bone, soft tissues of neck, deep [extrinsic] muscle of tongue) |

*Regional Lymph Nodes (N)*

| | |
|---|---|
| NX | Regional lymph nodes cannot be assessed |
| N0 | No regional lymph node metastasis |
| N1 | Metastasis in a single ipsilateral lymph node, 3 cm or less in greatest dimension |
| N2 | Metastasis in a single ipsilateral lymph node, more than 3 cm but not more than 6 cm in greatest dimension; or in multiple ipsilateral lymph nodes, none more than 6 cm in greatest dimension; or in bilateral or contralateral lymph nodes, none more than 6 cm in greatest dimension |
| N2a | Metastasis in a single ipsilateral lymph node more than 3 cm but not more than 6 cm in greatest dimension |
| N2b | Metastasis in multiple ispilateral lymph nodes, none more than 6 cm in greatest dimension |
| N2c | Metastasis in bilateral or contralateral lymph nodes, none more than 6 cm in greatest dimension |
| N3 | Metastasis in a lymph node more than 6 cm in greatest dimension |

*Distant Metastasis (M)*

| | |
|---|---|
| MX | Presence of distant metastasis cannot be assessed |
| M0 | No distant metastasis |
| M1 | Distant metastasis |

*Stage Grouping*

| | | | |
|---|---|---|---|
| Stage 0 | Tis | N0 | M0 |
| Stage I | T1 | N0 | M0 |
| Stage II | T2 | N0 | M0 |
| Stage III | T3 | N0 | M0 |
| | T1 | N1 | M0 |
| | T2 | N1 | M0 |
| | T3 | N1 | M0 |
| Stage IV | T4 | N0 | M0 |
| | T4 | N1 | M0 |
| | Any T | N2 | M0 |
| | Any T | N3 | M0 |
| | Any T | Any N | M1 |

*Histopathologic Grade (G)*

| | |
|---|---|
| GX | Grade cannot be assessed |
| G1 | Well differentiated |
| G2 | Moderately differentiated |
| G3 | Poorly differentiated |
| G4 | Undifferentiated |

From Beahrs OH, Henson DE, Hutter RVP, Kennedy BJ. Manual for staging of cancer. 4th ed. Philadelphia: JB Lippincott, 1992:34–5. Reproduced by permission of the American Joint Committee on Cancer and the publisher.

free flap, to prevent oral incompetence. Defects of the maxillary alveolus or hard palate must be obturated with a prosthesis that is worn like a denture to permit normal swallowing and speech. The management of involved cervical lymph nodes requires a neck dissection, and if there is substantial likelihood of metastatic disease in the neck despite negative clinical findings, prophylactic neck dissection or postoperative irradiation should be carried out. The 5-year control rate is related to stage but on average is about 50%.

**Floor of Mouth and Anterior Tongue.** The sites for the majority of intraoral cancers[17] (excluding the lips) are the tongue and floor of the mouth, with the tongue being twice as likely to be afflicted. The area usually involved on the tongue is the middle third of the lateral border; the remainder of the lateral borders and the ventral surface give rise to tumors less commonly. Cancers of the tip of the tongue and dorsal surface are rare. The extent of tongue tumors tends to be underestimated because of their iceberg pattern of growth. It is far more reliable to palpate the underlying induration than to measure the visible portion. Tongue cancers occasionally appear to be superficial, like a patchy desquamation or aphthae.

Floor of mouth cancers account for 10 to 15% of all oral carcinomas. Most cancers of the floor of the mouth arise in the anterior half, in areas of leukoplakia or erythroplasia; this is not characteristic of tongue cancers. Histologically, such tumors tend to be moderately well differentiated, although some can be well differentiated and superficial. Both exophytic and infiltrative growth patterns are seen—the latter more frequently in the tongue.

The symptoms of tongue and floor of the mouth tumors can be negligible during the early stages, often no more than a slight local irritation. As the tumor enlarges, particularly if it is ulcerative, frank pain develops and may radiate to the ear if it is in the posterior half of the oral cavity. If there is direct invasion of the lingual nerve, the pain becomes severe. When there is an open ulcer, the patient or his or her family will notice a foul mouth odor. Deep infiltration into the tongue muscles eventually produces abnormalities in speech and an inability to protrude the tongue. If the submandibular gland duct is invaded, the gland becomes swollen, particularly during eating. A patient occasionally presents with a neck mass, and in such instances the primary site is likely to be a poorly differentiated tumor in the posterior area of the oral cavity.

Diagnosis must include a biopsy of a viable portion of the tumor, with avoidance of any necrotic tissue from the center of an ulcer crater. The evaluation must include a careful search for metastatic neck disease because at least 40% of all tongue cancers present with metastases to the cervical lymph nodes and an additional 20% of patients develop this during the subsequent year.[18] Lymph nodes involved by anterior lesions are likely to be those in the submental and submandibular regions; metastases of posteriorly located cancers first become manifested in the deep cervical chain at the hyoid level. These tumors are prone to occur with other primary tumors in the oral cavity, particularly when they arise in areas of leukoplakia and erythroplasia.

Treatment varies among institutions, probably because the results of surgery and radiation are comparable. Both modalities used alone are reasonably effective with small tumors; however, each is ineffective in advanced disease, especially when there is cervical metastasis. The treatment should be carefully individualized. For patients who have small lesions and who cannot afford speech impairment, radiation is the treatment of choice.[19] Conversely, in chronic alcoholics and heavy smokers, radiation is often poorly tolerated, and therefore wide surgical excision is preferred for treatment of small lesions.[20] The choice of surgery is even more valid if the development of future oral cancers is anticipated, because radiation can usually be administered only once and may later be required for a lesion that cannot be effectively excised.

When tumors are larger than 4 cm or if there is cervical metastasis, combined therapy is recommended. Radiation may be administered by external beam, intraoral cone, or interstitial implantation. The radiation therapist delivers external-beam irradiation in doses compatible with adequate wound healing and minimal surgical morbidity and then completes tumoricidal radiation with interstitial implantation. The latter technique is particularly effective when the tumor mass is not lying adjacent to the mandible.[21] Surgical excision ranges from a simple monobloc excision[22] and primary closure to a composite resection that may include the mandible, most or all of the tongue, and the oropharynx. Obviously, surgery of this magnitude often interferes with speech and hinders swallowing. With these large lesions, it is usually necessary to repair the substantial surgical defect with a pedicled regional flap or a microvascular free flap. The pectoralis myocutaneous flap provides ample skin and muscle to reconstruct large defects of the oral cavity.[23, 24] Because they offer an improved aesthetic and functional outcome, free flaps are preferred for reconstruction of defects

in patients who are suitable medical candidates for tolerating a lengthy surgery, particularly when the resection includes critical areas of the tongue or a segmental resection of the anterior mandible.[25, 26]

In most instances of oral cavity cancers, the neck also has to be treated. Irradiation appears to be equally as effective in eliminating microscopic metastatic disease as radical neck dissection. However, its effectiveness diminishes rapidly when there is palpable metastatic disease, especially if the lymph nodes exceed 3 cm; radical neck dissection is used when the cervical nodes are larger than 3 cm. Radiation may occasionally be used for the primary tumor, with surgery reserved to treat the cervical metastasis after radiation.

The prognosis varies considerably, depending on the size of the primary tumor and the presence of regional metastasis. For small (<2 cm), well-differentiated tumors of the tongue and floor of the mouth without evidence of metastasis, the 5-year survival rate reaches 85%; however, for larger tumors (>4 cm) with cervical metastasis, this rate is only about 25%.

## OROPHARYNX

Several anatomic regions in the oropharynx have been grouped together because oropharyngeal tumors are biologically similar and are treated similarly. The anatomic regions composing the oropharynx are the base of the tongue, tonsillar pillars, tonsils, soft palate and uvula, and lateral and posterior pharyngeal walls extending from the tip of the epiglottis to the soft palate.

The most common tumor in the oropharynx arises from the tonsil; the base of the tongue and the soft palate are next in frequency. It is unusual, however, to find any of these tumors confined to a single anatomic site when first discovered because they grow rather large before becoming obviously symptomatic. This paucity of symptoms when the tumor is small is probably related to a less refined sensory nerve distribution than is found in the oral cavity. Moreover, it is difficult for the patient to visualize or palpate these sites and thus discover the tumor.

Oropharyngeal tumors are generally less well differentiated histologically than those in the oral cavity, ranging from moderately well differentiated to anaplastic. They are more likely to be ulcerative and infiltrating than exophytic in gross configuration. The anterior part of the oropharynx sometimes gives rise to well-differentiated tumors, as is seen occasionally with tumors arising from the anterior tonsillar pillar.

On the whole, the metastatic propensity to regional nodes is significantly higher in the oropharynx than in the oral cavity. In most regions, the metastatic rate exceeds 50%; in the base of the tongue it reaches about 75%. Metastases from small cancers of the tonsil or base of the tongue are frequent. The upper deep jugular nodes, such as the jugulodigastric, typically are the first to become clinically manifest. Bilateral cervical metastases can occur, particularly from tumors of the base of the tongue and the pharyngeal walls. Metastasis to the retropharyngeal nodes portends a poor prognosis.

As the tumor enlarges and ulcerates, the patient experiences pharyngeal pain that may sometimes alter in intensity. In fact, when first evaluated, these tumors are usually considered to be tonsillitis or protracted pharyngitis, and consequently, the patient is given one or more trials of antibiotic therapy. Another common presenting symptom is otalgia. This pain is referred by the glossopharyngeal and vagus nerves, which have sensory branches to the ear and the oropharynx. The development of an asymptomatic neck mass is another frequent mode of presentation. Even a thorough examination sometimes fails to reveal the oropharyngeal tumor; random biopsy specimens ultimately disclose its site. As the tumor enlarges, it may extend into the retromandibular space, causing trismus; extension into the base of the tongue can involve the hypoglossal nerve, paralyzing the tongue. When there is an underlying mass without mucosal ulceration, lymphoma or a tumor of minor salivary gland or mesenchymal origin must be suspected.

The treatment of oropharyngeal tumors requires close cooperation between the surgeon and the radiation therapist. For smaller tumors, radiation therapy is often the initial treatment of choice. It is usually delivered by external radiation and is occasionally supplemented by intraoral cone irradiation or, more frequently, by interstitial radiation.

Cervical metastases of less than N2 stage at presentation can be controlled by irradiation alone with a high likelihood of success. Clinically undetectable occult metastases can be controlled by radiation doses that produce few sequelae (i.e., 45 to 50 Gy in 4.5 to 6 weeks), whereas larger masses require higher doses (i.e., 55 to 65 Gy in 5.5 to 7 weeks) for control. It has been documented that there is poor correlation between the rate of gross reduction of oropharyngeal epidermoid carcinomas and ultimate control by radiation therapy.[27] It is our preference to treat patients with early-stage primary tumors (stages T1 and T2) that present with palpable cervical metastases using initial radiation therapy. Radiation therapy is carried to a tumoricidal dose range of 65 to 70 Gy to the primary tumor site and to the regional lymph nodes. Patients with residual disease at the primary site or in the neck after the completion of radiation therapy undergo salvage surgery. For patients who achieve a complete clinical response after radiation therapy, the stage of the neck disease at presentation determines the need for an elective node dissection. A postirradiation therapy modified radical neck dissection is recommended for all patients who present with stage N2 or greater regional disease, even if there has been complete clinical regression of the cervical lymphadenopathy. We realize that this treatment philosophy is controversial, but we have demonstrated a 40% incidence of microscopic residual disease in the lymph nodes in this situation.[28]

Inasmuch as advanced oropharyngeal tumors (stages T3 and T4) are not likely to be cured by either surgery or irradiation alone, planned combinations of these two modes of therapy are required to maximize the chances for cure.[29] Our current preferred mode of treatment is composite resection of the oropharyngeal tumor and radical neck dissection followed by tumoricidal irradiation. Improvements in reconstructive surgery have allowed us to recommend planned combined therapy to many patients who have advanced oropharyngeal primaries and who previously might have been considered poor candidates for surgical therapy.

Patients with unresectable stage IV cancers are candidates for radiation therapy. A number of clinical trials have been established for these patients using varying doses and combinations of chemotherapy.[30] Drug therapy may be used before (induction) radiation therapy or during (concurrent) radiation therapy. Current evidence suggests that there may be an improved response to concurrent chemotherapy and radiation therapy compared with sequential chemotherapy and radiation therapy.[31] However, patients undergoing concurrent therapy experience more severe toxicity. Radiation therapy protocols include hyperfractionation schedules and brachytherapy. It is yet to be determined that these investigative treatment modalities are superior to conventional radiation therapy.

## SUGGESTIONS FOR ADDITIONAL READING

Blot WJ, Devesa SS, McLaughlin JK, Fraumeni JF Jr. Oral and pharyngeal cancers. Cancer Surv 1994;19–20:23–42. *This article provides a good general review of the subject.*
Blott WJ, McLaughlin JK, Winn DM, et al. Smoking and drinking in relation to oral and pharyngeal cancer. Cancer Res 1988;48:3282–7. *A case-control study involving 2382 individuals suggests that smoking tobacco and drinking alcohol combine to account for approximately three fourths of all oral and pharyngeal cancers in the United States.*
McLaughlin JK, Gridley G, Block G, et al. Dietary factors in oral and pharyngeal cancer. J Natl Cancer Inst 1988;80:1237–43. *This case-control study found an inverse relationship between fruit intake and the risk of oral and pharyngeal cancer. Dietary factors other than alcohol appeared to have no impact on the frequency of the disease in this population. This study suggests that eating a diet high in fruit may provide some degree of protection against oral cancer.*
La Vecchia C, Tavani A, Franceschi S, Levi F, Corrao G, Negri E. Epidemiology and prevention of oral cancer. Oral Oncol 1997;33:302–12. *Descriptive epidemiology of oral and pharyngeal cancer over the last four decades is reviewed. The relative contribution of tobacco exposure, alcohol exposure, dietary factors, and human papillomavirus in the development of oral cancer is discussed.*
Mashberg A, Samit AM. Early detection, diagnosis, and management of oral and oropharyngeal cancer. CA Cancer J Clin 1989;39:67–88. *This article provides a good, short review.*

## REFERENCES

1. Winn DM, Blot WJ, Shy CM, et al. Snuff dipping and oral cancer among women in the southern United States. N Engl J Med 1981;304:745–9.
2. Cigar smoking among teenagers—United States, Massachusetts, and New York, 1996. MMWR Morb Mortal Wkly Rep 1997;46:433–40.
3. Wynder EL. Etiological aspects of squamous cancers of the head and neck. JAMA 1971;215:452–3.
4. Blot WJ, Winn DM, Fraumeni JF Jr. Oral cancer and mouthwash. J Natl Cancer Inst 1983;70:251–3.
5. Wynder EL, Kabat G, Rosenberg S, Levenstein M. Oral cancer and mouthwash use. J Natl Cancer Inst 1983;70:255–260.
6. Winn DM, Blot WJ, McLaughlin JK, et al. Mouthwash use and oral conditions in the risk of oral and pharyngeal cancer. Cancer Res 1991;51:3044–7.
7. Elmore JG, Horwitz RI. Oral cancer and mouthwash use: evaluation of the epidemiologic evidence. Otolaryngol Head Neck Surg 1995;113:253–61.
8. McKaig RG, Baric RS, Olshan AF. Human papillomavirus and head and neck cancer: epidemiology and molecular biology. Head Neck 1998;20:250–65.
9. Shumrick DA. Treatment of malignant tumors of minor salivary glands. Arch Otolaryngol 1968;88:74–9.
10. Kessler DJ, Mickel RA, Calcaterra TC. Malignant salivary gland tumors of the base of the tongue. Arch Otolaryngol 1985;111:664–6.
11. Regauer S, Anderhuber W, Richtig E, et al. Primary mucosal melanomas of the nasal cavity and paranasal sinuses: a clinicopathological analysis of 14 cases. APMIS 1998;106:403–10.
12. Strong MS, Vaughan CW, Incze JS. Toluidine blue in the management of carcinoma of the oral cavity. Arch Otolaryngol 1968;87:527–31.
13. Beahrs OH, Henson DE, Hutter RVP, Kennedy BJ. American Joint Committee on Cancer. Manual for staging of cancer, 4th ed. Philadelphia: JB Lippincott, 1992.

14. Bailey BJ. Management of carcinoma of the lip. Laryngoscope 1977;87:250–60.
15. O'Brien PH, Catlin D. Cancer of the cheek (mucosa). Cancer 1965;18:1392–8.
16. Cady B, Catlin D. Epidermoid cancer of the gum: a 20-year survey. Cancer 1969;23:551–69.
17. Skolnik EM, Saberman MN. Cancer of the tongue. Otolaryngol Clin North Am 1969;2:603–15.
18. Frazell EL. A review of the treatment of cancer of the mobile portion of the tongue. Cancer 1971;28:1178–81.
19. Som ML. Carcinoma of the mobile portion of the tongue: follow-up of previous study. Arch Otolaryngol 1968;87:511–4.
20. Dubner S, Spiro RH. Median mandibulotomy: a critical assessment. Head Neck 1991;13:389–93.
21. Wendt CD, Peters LJ, Delclos L, et al. Primary radiotherapy in the treatment of stage I and II oral tongue cancers: importance of the proportion of therapy delivered with interstitial therapy. Int J Radiat Oncol Biol Phys 1990;18:1287–92.
22. Moloy PJ, Rappaport I, Turnbull FM, et al. Horizontal versus vertical block resection for early floor of mouth carcinoma. Am J Otolaryngol 1989;10:153–60.
23. Cuono CB, Ariyan S. Immediate reconstruction of a composite mandibular defect with a regional osteomusculocutaneous flap. Plast Reconstr Surg 1980;65:477–84.
24. Biller HF, Baek SM, Lawson W, et al. Pectoralis major myocutaneous island flap in head and neck surgery: analysis of complications in 42 cases. Arch Otolaryngol 1981;107:23–6.
25. Urken ML, Weinberg H, Vickery C, et al. Oromandibular reconstruction using microvascular composite free flaps. Report of 71 cases and a new classification scheme for bony, soft-tissue, and neurologic defects. Arch Otolaryngol Head Neck Surg 1991;117:733–44.
26. Urken ML, Buchbinder D, Weinberg H, et al. Functional evaluation following microvascular oromandibular reconstruction of the oral cancer patient: a comparative study of reconstructed and nonreconstructed patients. Laryngoscope 1991;101:935.
27. Goffinet DR, Fee WE Jr, Wells J, et al. [192]Ir pharyngoepiglottic fold interstitial implants. The key to successful treatment of base tongue carcinoma by radiation therapy. Cancer 1985;55:941.
28. Wang S, Wang MB, Calcaterra TC. Radiation therapy followed by neck dissection for small head and neck cancers with advanced cervical metastases. Ann Otol Rhinol Laryngol 1999;108:128–31.
29. Weber RS, Gidley P, Morrison WH, et al. Treatment selection for carcinoma of the base of the tongue. Am J Surg 1990;160:415–9.
30. Merlano M, Corvo R, Margarino G, et al. Combined chemotherapy and radiation therapy in advanced inoperable squamous cell carcinoma of the head and neck. The final report of a randomized trial. Cancer 1991;67:915–21.
31. El-Sayed S, Nelson N. Adjuvant and adjunctive chemotherapy in the management of squamous cell carcinoma of the head and neck: a meta-analysis of respected and randomized trials. J Clin Oncol 1996;14:838–47.

# CHAPTER 62

# NASAL CAVITY AND PARANASAL SINUSES

• THOMAS C. CALCATERRA • GUY J. F. JUILLARD •
• KEITH E. BLACKWELL •

Cancers of the nasal cavity and paranasal sinuses are described in the same chapter because of their anatomic proximity, similar biologic characteristics, and common methods of treatment. They constitute about 5% of all tumors arising from the respiratory tract and approximately 0.5% of all malignancies.[1] As with most head and neck cancers, the peak incidence occurs in the sixth and seventh decades of life, and there is a slight male predominance. The association with tobacco smoking is not as strong as in other carcinomas of the respiratory tract. There appears to be a causal relationship between adenocarcinoma of the nasal cavity or sinuses and certain airborne compounds used in the furniture industry[2] and in the repair or manufacture of footwear.[3] Exposure to nickel refinery fumes has also been implicated,[4] as well as human papillomavirus.[5, 6]

## Natural History

### CLASSIFICATION AND PATHOLOGY

No widely accepted classification of nasal and sinus malignancies exists, inasmuch as such tumors are rarely confined to one anatomic area when first diagnosed. Nasal cavity tumors can sometimes be identified as arising from the septum or lateral nasal wall. Localized tumors of the maxillary sinus have been arbitrarily divided into two groups by Ohngren's line, which is a theoretical plane passing between the medial canthus of the eye and the angle of the mandible.[7] Tumors occurring below this plane, called *infrastructure tumors*, have a more favorable prognosis, whereas those that develop above this plane, called *suprastructure tumors*, have a less favorable outlook owing to their proximity to the orbit and cranium.

The type of tumor generally found in the nasal cavity and paranasal sinuses is squamous cell carcinoma, which represents about 80% of the total. These malignancies are typically intermediate in differentiation, tending to metastasize late to the cervical lymph node network, particularly when they originate in the sinuses. Distant metastases are rare until late in the course of the disease.

A variety of other kinds of malignant tumors may arise in the nasal fossa and paranasal sinuses. Esthesioneuroblastoma (olfactory neuroblastoma) occurs in the upper portion of the nasal cavity and usually presents as polypoid masses that may be confused with lymphomas or undifferentiated carcinomas.[8] Malignant melanomas are found in the nasal cavity and less often in the sinuses. Some melanomas may exhibit a rather unusual indolent course, with only a slight tendency to metastasize,[9] whereas others behave in an aggressive fashion.[10] The entire spectrum of salivary gland tumors may likewise develop in this region inasmuch as nests of salivary gland cells are found throughout the upper respiratory tract. Other rare malignancies that occur in this region include sinonasal undifferentiated carcinoma and neuroendocrine carcinoma.[11, 12] With the advent of immunocytochemical phenotyping of lymphocytes, many of the "lethal midline syndromes" that affect the nose and paranasal sinuses, including lethal midline granuloma, polymorphic reticulosis, and lymphomatoid granulomatosis, are now recognized to be lymphomas.[13] The biologic growth behavior generally corresponds to the degree of histologic differentiation of the specific tumor.

## CLINICAL FEATURES

Tumors of the nasal fossa are typically heralded by unilateral nasal airway obstruction and rhinorrhea, which the patient attributes to an infection or allergy. Occasionally, however, epistaxis or blood streaking of nasal mucus arouses suspicion of the presence of tumor. As the tumor enlarges, the patient may experience facial pain owing to blocked sinus ostia and epiphora or dacryocystitis secondary to invasion of the lacrimal drainage system.

Among paranasal sinus tumors, those occurring in the maxillary sinus predominate. Unfortunately, these usually attain a large size before becoming symptomatic. If the drainage of the sinus is impaired, concomitant sinusitis is likely to develop. The patient may experience pain or looseness of the upper molar teeth with progressive tumor growth, followed later by distortion of the palate. Fullness over the cheek, particularly when accompanied by numbness over the distribution of the intraorbital nerve, strongly suggests a maxillary sinus cancer. Because the orbit is surrounded on three sides by paranasal sinuses (maxillary, ethmoid, and frontal), orbital symptoms are frequently associated with paranasal sinus cancers. The earliest sign is simple displacement of the orbital contents away from the involved sinus, such as upward displacement by a maxillary sinus tumor and lateral displacement by an ethmoid tumor. If the cancer invades the orbital contents, proptosis, limited ocular motor function, and ultimate blindness can develop. Posterior extension of maxillary sinus tumors is often manifested by trismus as the pterygoid muscles are invaded. Likewise, posterior and superior extension of ethmoid sinus cancers to the cavernous sinus results in a number of cranial nerve dysfunctions (first through sixth cranial nerves). Frontal sinus cancers are uncommon, typically invading the anterior cranial fossa before diagnosis.[14] Primary sphenoid sinus cancers, which occur least frequently, become manifested by affecting the neurovascular structures that surround the sinus.[15]

Because of the paucity of early symptoms, cancers in the nasal fossa and paranasal sinuses often reach advanced stages before diagnosis. Both the patient and the clinician often assume the problem to be an inflammatory one, but when prompt resolution of the presumed infection fails to occur, the presence of cancer must be considered. Suspicious-appearing tissue in the nasal fossa can be seen through the nares, particularly with adequate topical vasoconstriction of the nasal mucosa. The development of flexible and rigid fiberoptic nasal telescopes has greatly facilitated the examination of the nasal fossa and paranasal sinus ostia. Persistent sinus symptoms refractory to medical management are usually assessed by a limited or full computed tomographic scan. The radiographic signs of cancer may be difficult to differentiate from those of inflammation, but suspicion is raised by bone erosion, patchy bone sclerosis, and a unilateral discrete soft tissue mass as well as enlargement of the osseous foramina. A magnetic resonance imaging (MRI) scan is often helpful in determining the presence and extent of any intracranial tumor extension.[16] MRI is also useful in distinguishing a tumor mass from postobstructive inflammatory changes that are frequently seen in adjacent paranasal sinuses.[17]

Diagnosis requires histologic confirmation by biopsy; a biopsy of tumors extending to or arising in the nasal fossa can readily be performed through the nares with topical anesthesia. Maxillary sinus puncture with lavage for cytologic study is another method of diagnosis. If transnasal biopsy is not feasible or productive, it is necessary to obtain representative tissue by direct sinusotomy of the involved sinus, using various approaches such as endoscopic sinus surgery, the Caldwell-Luc operation, external ethmoidectomy, or frontal sinusotomy.

## STAGING

The TNM classification for cancer of the maxillary sinus developed by the American Joint Committee on Cancer and the International Union Against Cancer is given in Table 62–1.[18]

## PROGNOSIS

The 5-year survival rates for patients with tumors of the nasal fossa and paranasal sinuses are difficult to summarize because staging is obscure and tumor types vary widely. Tumors arising close to the cranial fossa, such as frontal and sphenoid sinus cancers, have an unfavorable prognosis; indeed, prolonged survival is rare. Tumors involving or extending to the ethmoid sinus and orbit have an intermediate prognosis; with aggressive combined-modality therapy, the 5-year survival rate ranges between 30 and 40%. Tumors that are confined to the nasal fossa and maxillary sinus cavity have the best prognosis, however, with the 5-year survival rate ranging between 45 and 55%.

## TREATMENT

No consensus exists about the optimal treatment of cancers arising in the nasal cavity or paranasal sinuses. The use of surgery or radiation therapy alone has been based on the preference of the involved physician.

For cancers limited to the nasal fossa, either method can be highly successful, with the choice based on tumor type, location, and extent and desire for anatomic preservation.[19]

During the past two decades, increased emphasis has been placed on combining both treatment modalities for carcinomas arising in the paranasal sinuses.

Before a specific treatment plan can be selected, the anatomic extent of the tumor must be ascertained to determine the feasibility of surgical resectability or the volume of tissue to be irradiated, or both. Computed tomographic and MRI scans are helpful in determining the limits of

*Table 62–1.* **The International TNM Staging System for Cancer of the Maxillary Sinus**

*Definition of TNM*

*Primary Tumor (T)*

| | |
|---|---|
| TX | Primary tumor cannot be assessed |
| T0 | No evidence of primary tumor |
| Tis | Carcinoma in situ |
| T1 | Tumor limited to the antral mucosa with no erosion or destruction of bone |
| T2 | Tumor with erosion or destruction of the infrastructure,* including the hard palate and/or the middle nasal meatus |
| T3 | Tumor invades any of the following: skin of cheek, posterior wall of maxillary sinus, floor or medial wall of orbit, anterior ethmoid sinus |
| T4 | Tumor invades orbital contents and/or any of the following: cribriform plate, posterior ethmoid or sphenoid sinuses, nasopharynx, soft palate, pterygomaxillary or temporal fossae, or base of skull |

*Regional Lymph Nodes (N)*

| | |
|---|---|
| NX | Regional lymph nodes cannot be assessed |
| N0 | No regional lymph node metastasis |
| N1 | Metastasis in a single ipsilateral lymph node, 3 cm or less in greatest dimension |
| N2 | Metastasis in a single ipsilateral lymph node, more than 3 cm but not more than 6 cm in greatest dimension, or in multiple ipsilateral lymph nodes, none more than 6 cm in greatest dimension, or in bilateral or contralateral lymph nodes, none more than 6 cm in greatest dimension |
| N2a | Metastasis in a single ipsilateral lymph node more than 3 cm but not more than 6 cm in greatest dimension |
| N2b | Metastasis in multiple ipsilateral lymph nodes, none more than 6 cm in greatest dimension |
| N2c | Metastasis in bilateral or contralateral lymph nodes, none more than 6 cm in greatest dimension |
| N3 | Metastasis in a lymph node more than 6 cm in greatest dimension |

*Distant Metastasis (M)*

| | |
|---|---|
| MX | Distant metastases cannot be assessed |
| M0 | No distant metastasis |
| M1 | Distant metastasis |

*Stage Grouping*

| | | | |
|---|---|---|---|
| Stage 0 | Tis | N0 | M0 |
| Stage I | T1 | N0 | M0 |
| Stage II | T2 | N0 | M0 |
| Stage III | T3 | N0 | M0 |
| | T1 | N1 | M0 |
| | T2 | N1 | M0 |
| | T3 | N1 | M0 |
| Stage IV | T4 | N0 | M0 |
| | T4 | N1 | M0 |
| Stage IVB | Any T | N2 | M0 |
| | Any T | N3 | M0 |
| Stage IVC | Any T | Any N | M1 |

*Ohngren's line, a theoretical plane joining the medial canthus of the eye with the angle of the mandible, is used to divide the maxillary antrum into the anteroinferior portion (the infrastructure) and the superoposterior portion (the suprastructure).

From Beahrs OH, Henson DE, Hutter RVP, Kennedy BJ, eds. Manual for staging of cancer. 4th ed. Philadelphia: JB Lippincott, 1992:45–6. Reproduced by permission of the American Joint Committee on Cancer and the publisher.

these tumors. For high-grade malignancies, surgery is not considered worthwhile if there is evidence of extension across the dura of the anterior or middle cranial fossa or if there is substantial involvement of the pterygoid muscles. With more indolent neoplasms, there may be a role for surgical therapy with intracranial or infratemporal fossa extension using modern skull base techniques, although this subject remains controversial.[20]

The degree of histologic differentiation and the type of tumor modify the approach to treatment. All lymphomas and many poorly differentiated carcinomas are treated with irradiation or chemotherapy, or both. Adenocarcinomas, salivary gland carcinomas, and melanomas are usually treated first by surgery when there is a likelihood that the tumor can be completely encompassed. In most of these instances, postoperative irradiation is also used. Esthesioneuroblastoma is treated effectively by surgery, with some authors also advocating chemotherapy and radiation therapy.

Various treatment plans are followed for epidermoid carcinomas, which compose the majority of these cancers. Some authors favor preoperative irradiation followed immediately by surgery;[21–23] although this planned combined therapy maximizes the cure rate, it unnecessarily sacrifices the sinus or possibly the eye in instances in which irradiation has achieved a cure. At the University of California, Los Angeles, Medical Center, a modification of planned combined irradiation is often used, consisting of surgical removal of the alveolar ridge and hard palate beneath the involved maxillary sinus 6 to 8 weeks after full-dose irradiation. Several biopsy specimens of the maxillary and ethmoid sinuses are then examined by frozen section. If tumor is encountered, a total or extended maxillectomy is immediately performed. In contrast, if no tumor is found, the defect is obdurated as part of a denture. This palatal opening can then be used for future inspection of the sinus cavity to determine whether there are any signs of recurrence. If physicians elect observation of the patient after full-dose irradiation, it is important to re-evaluate this area thoroughly at frequent intervals for at least 3 years. Periodic fiberoptic nasal endoscopy as well as computed tomographic and MRI scans is useful to monitor for recurrence when no surgical cavity is present to make direct examination possible.

The type of surgery chosen for nasal and sinus tumors is predicated on the anatomic extent of the tumor. For tumors occupying the nasal fossa, a lateral rhinotomy and medial maxillectomy allowing an en bloc resection of the septum and lateral nasal wall are often used.[24] Tumors that are confined to the maxillary sinus are treated by maxillectomy, which may or may not involve the removal of the sinus roof (orbital floor). Tumors arising in or extending to the ethmoid sinus usually require the removal of the orbital contents. However, tumors are usually considered inoperable if there is erosion of the pterygoid plates or evidence on computed tomographic scan of involvement of the anterior cranial fossa, sphenoid sinus, or cavernous sinus. In the latter instances, computed tomographic scanning demonstrates that the cribriform plate is absent, that the crista galli is tilted, or that the lateral wall of the sphenoid sinus and foramen rotundum is eroded. In selected instances, tumors that erode the anterior skull base but do not penetrate the dura may be amenable to a combined intracranial and extracranial resection.[25]

The technique of radiation therapy varies according to the type and extent of the tumor. If the tumor is located in the lower aspect of the maxillary sinus, the eye can be shielded to avoid late radiation complications. If postoperative radiation is used, the treatment volume is selected after the surgical specimen has been analyzed to determine the anatomic margins that are at greatest risk for recurrence.

Close cooperation with a maxillofacial prosthodontist is mandatory for maximal rehabilitation of these patients. Indeed, all surgically treated patients who undergo resection of the palate require some type of obturator to seal the sinus and nasal fossa from the oral cavity. Although it is sometimes necessary to resect the nose or cheek, a prosthesis can be worn to fill the defect and provide an acceptable facial appearance.[26] Alternatively, the midface can be surgically reconstructed using autogenous tissues, although several staged procedures are usually required to achieve a satisfactory outcome, and tumor surveillance through an open cavity is not possible after surgical reconstruction.[27, 28]

The treatment of patients with advanced nasal and paranasal sinus cancer is difficult. In many instances, palliation becomes the therapeutic goal. Chemotherapy has assumed an increasingly effective role for patients who suffer from recurrent disease, and it is also being evaluated as an adjunctive modality immediately following initial therapy (see Chapter 66). Others have reported a potential beneficial role for induction chemotherapy, particularly for the treatment of esthesioneuroblastoma.[29] Palliation in recurrent disease can also be accomplished by cryotherapy or local endocavity radiation.

## SUGGESTIONS FOR ADDITIONAL READING

Fukuda K, Shibata A. A case-control study of past history of nasal diseases and maxillary sinus cancer in Hokkaido, Japan. Cancer Res 1988;48:1651–2. *This study identified chronic sinusitis, nasal polyps, a history of cigarette smoking, and an occupational history of being a carpenter, joiner, furniture maker, or other woodworker as statistically significant risk factors for nasal and maxillary sinus cancer for men, whereas no single item was a significant risk factor for women.*

Jacob HE. Chemotherapy for cranial base tumors. J Neurooncol 1994;20:327–35. *This article includes a review of the literature on the use of chemotherapy for esthesioneuroblastoma and salivary gland cancers of the paranasal sinuses. The author concludes that progress in this field has suffered from a lack of multi-institutional protocols to treat these rare cancers.*

Moore C, Greenberg RA, Kane L. Feasibility study of a head and neck (upper aero-digestive tract) cancer examination. J Natl Cancer Inst 1987;79:409–15. *This study suggests that an adequate screening examination of the head and neck area can be accomplished in about 10 minutes, including the use of a fiberoptic pharyngoscope. The authors recommend that this approach to screening be taught to dentists and then studied for its cost and benefit in a controlled clinical trial. This study provides a good review of the pertinent issues in performing screening examinations for cancer of the head and neck area.*

Mosesson RE, Som PM. The radiographic evaluation of sinonasal tumors: an overview. Otolaryngol Clin North Am 1995;28:1097–115. *This article provides a good overview of the role of radiology in the evaluation and treatment of sinonasal tumors.*

Osguthorpe JD. Sinus neoplasia. Arch Otolaryngol Head Neck Surg 1994;120:19–25. *This article includes an overview of the epidemiology, histology, and evaluation of nasal and sinus neoplasms as well as a discussion of surgical advances in facial translocation, skull base dissection, and defect reconstruction. Radiation therapy and chemotherapy are also discussed.*

## REFERENCES

1. Cutler SJ. NCI Monogr 1975;41:1.
2. Acheson ED, Cowdell RH, Hadfield E, MacBeth RG. Nasal cancer in woodworkers in the furniture industry. Br Med J 1968;5605:2:587–96.
3. Lancet 1983;1:856. editorial.
4. Mastromatteo E. Nickel: a review of its occupational health aspects. J Occup Med 1967;9:127–36.
5. Wu TC, Trujillo JM, Kashima HK, Mounts P. Association of human papillomavirus with nasal neoplasia. Lancet 1993;341:522–4.
6. Furuta Y, Takasu T, Asai T, et al. Detection of human papillomavirus DNA in carcinomas of the nasal cavities and paranasal sinuses by polymerase chain reaction. Cancer 1992;69:353–7.
7. Rubin P. Cancer of the head and neck: nose, paranasal sinuses. JAMA 1972;219:336–8.
8. Dulgerov P, Calcaterra T. Esthesioneuroblastoma: the UCLA experience 1970–1990. Laryngoscope 1992;102:843–9.
9. Trapp TK, Fu YS, Calcaterra TC. Melanoma of the nasal and paranasal sinus mucosa. Arch Otolaryngol 1987;113:1086–9.
10. Crawford RI, Tron VA, Ma R, Rivers JK. Sinonasal malignant melanoma—a clinicopathologic analysis of 18 cases. Melanoma Res 1995;5:261–5.
11. Houston GD. Sinonasal undifferentiated carcinoma: report of two cases and review of the literature. Oral Surg Oral Med Oral Pathol Oral Radiol Endod 1998;85:185–8.
12. Chaudhry MR, Akhtar S, Kim DS. Neuroendocrine carcinoma of the ethmoid sinus. Eur Arch Otorhinolaryngol 1994;251:461–3.
13. Cleary KR, Batsakis JG. Sinonasal lymphomas. Ann Otol Rhinol Laryngol 1994;103:911–4.
14. Brownson RJ, Ogura JH. Primary carcinoma of the frontal sinus. Laryngoscope 1971;81:71–89.
15. Van Wart C, Dedo HH, McCoy EG. Carcinoma of the sphenoid sinus. Ann Otol Rhinol Laryngol 1973;82:318–22.
16. Som PM, Shapiro MD, Biller HF, et al. Sinonasal tumors and inflammatory tissues: differentiation with MR imaging. Radiology 1988;167:803–8.
17. Allbery SM, Chaljub G, Cho NL, et al. MR imaging of nasal masses. Radiographics 1995;15:1311–27.
18. Beahrs OH, Henson DE, Hutter RVP, Kennedy BJ, eds. American Joint Committee on Cancer: manual for staging of cancer. 4th ed. Philadelphia: JB Lippincott, 1992.

19. Mendenhall NP, Parsons JT, Cassisi NJ, Million RR. Carcinoma of the nasal vestibule treated with radiation therapy. Laryngoscope 1987;97:626–32.
20. Osguthorpe JD, Patel S. Craniofacial approaches to sinus malignancy. Otolaryngol Clin North Am 1995;28:1239–57.
21. Gallagher TM, Boles R. Carcinoma of the maxillary antrum. Laryngoscope 1970;80:924–32.
22. Schechter GL, Ogura JH. Maxillary sinus malignancy. Laryngoscope 1972;82:796–806.
23. Lewis JS, Castro EB. Cancer of the nasal cavity and paranasal sinuses. J Laryngol Otol 1972;86:255–62.
24. Sessions RB, Larson DL. En bloc ethmoidectomy and medial maxillectomy. Arch Otolaryngol 1977;103:195–202.
25. Sundaresan N, Shah JP. Craniofacial resection for anterior skull base tumors. Head Neck Surg 1988;10:219–24.
26. Beumer J, Calcaterra TC. Prosthetic rehabilitation of large midfacial defects. Laryngoscope 1976;86:280–5.
27. Urken ML, Catalano PJ, Post K, et al. Free tissue transfer for skull base reconstruction: analysis of complications and a classification scheme for defining skull base defects. Arch Otolaryngol Head Neck Surg 1993;119:1318.
28. Hoasjoe DK, Stucker FJ, Aarstad RF. Aesthetic and anatomic considerations for nasal reconstruction. Facial Plast Surg 1994;10:317–21.
29. Polin RS, Sheehan JP, Chenelle AG, et al. The role of preoperative adjuvant treatment in the management of esthesioneuroblastoma: the University of Virginia experience. Neurosurgery 1998;42:1029–37.

# CHAPTER 63

# NASOPHARYNX

• THOMAS C. CALCATERRA • GUY J. F. JUILLARD •
• KEITH E. BLACKWELL

The incidence of nasopharyngeal cancer varies according to race. In the United States' predominantly white population, cancers in this site account for approximately 0.25 to 0.5% of all malignant tumors.[1] The incidence is much higher in Asian populations, particularly in parts of southern China, where this tumor has been reported to constitute 50% of all malignancies.[2] This percentage prevails even when these people emigrate to other parts of the world.[3] Nasopharyngeal tumors occur at an earlier age than do most other head and neck cancers and are not uncommon in the pediatric age group.[4] The occurrence predominates in males in all series, with a ratio of about 2:1.

Isolated reports of nasopharyngeal cancer afflicting the same family have suggested a genetic origin.[5] No specific carcinogens have been proved, but wood[6] and formaldehyde[7] exposure, as well as the inhalation of smoke or eating salted fish,[8] has been associated with the disease. In whites in the United States, cigarette smoking and heavy alcohol use are also implicated.[9] Increased titers of antibody to the Epstein-Barr virus have been demonstrated in patients with nasopharyngeal cancer, suggesting a possible viral etiologic agent.[10, 11] The World Health Organization sponsored a study to test the value of measuring antibodies to Epstein-Barr virus as a test for occult disease, and preliminary results suggested that this may be feasible.[12] This approach has been updated to include screening that can detect recombinant Epstein-Barr virus proteins in serum.[13] The epidemiology of nasopharyngeal carcinoma has been reviewed for the reader interested in more details.[14]

## Natural History

### CLASSIFICATION

The nasopharynx, which is part of the respiratory tract, is situated behind the nasal fossa and below the middle cranial fossa. Its roof principally composes the floor of the sphenoid sinus, and its posterior wall is formed by the basiocciput. Most tumors of the nasopharynx are believed to arise in Rosenmüller's fossa, which is immediately superior to the eustachian tube orifices on the lateral walls. A rich lymphatic system freely communicates with the lymph nodes of the parapharyngeal space and the upper cervical region.

The nasopharyngeal mucosa serves a respiratory function and consists of ciliated pseudocolumnar epithelium and stratified squamous epithelium. The carcinomas arising here are chiefly squamous epithelium (epithelial) in origin, although histologically some may be diffusely infiltrated with lymphocytes (lymphoepitheliomas), which should not be confused with tumors of lymphocytic origin. The differentiation of nasopharyngeal tumors ranges from moderate to anaplastic. Other tumors arising in the nasopharynx include salivary gland cancers, lymphomas, sarcomas, and melanomas.

## CLINICAL FEATURES AND DIAGNOSIS

Nasopharyngeal cancer develops insidiously. Initial nasal stuffiness and excessive nasal mucus discharge are nearly always disregarded. Later, halitosis, blood-streaked mucus, and poorly localized headache signify enlargement of the tumor. Profuse epistaxis is not typical of this tumor.

The first clinical indication of nasopharyngeal cancer frequently may be noted elsewhere, such as fullness in the ear and hearing loss, signifying tumor involvement of the eustachian tube, or gradual, painless enlargement of an upper cervical lymph node, indicating metastasis. Severe pain at the base of the skull, diplopia, and other cranial nerve symptoms point to intracranial extension of the tumor.

Almost 50% of patients have palpable cervical metastasis at the time of diagnosis. The enlarged cervical node characteristically grows beneath the upper portion of the sternocleidomastoid muscle or within the posterior cervical triangle. Although nodal involvement is usually unilateral, there is a significant incidence of bilateral metastasis. At times, the nasopharyngeal tumor may not be readily visible despite repeated examinations of the nasopharynx. When a nasopharyngeal cancer is suspected, such as an occult cervical metastasis, random biopsy specimens of the nasopharynx should be obtained. Any adult with unilateral serous otitis media should also undergo a careful nasopharyngeal examination.

Nasopharyngeal cancers tend to gain access to the cranial cavity via the foramen lacerum. The sixth cranial nerve is usually the first to be affected; the third, fourth, and fifth cranial nerves become involved later, and there may be proptosis of the ipsilateral eye. Horner's syndrome develops when the sympathetic nerve fibers around the carotid artery become involved. Distant metastases are likely to occur, particularly to the lung, liver, or bone.

Nasopharyngeal cancer can usually be diagnosed readily, under local anesthesia, by transnasal or transoral biopsy. Fine-needle aspiration biopsy specimens may also be useful in patients without obvious lesions when combined with DNA amplification of the Epstein-Barr virus genome using the polymerase chain reaction.[15] Examination is greatly facilitated by a fiberoptic telescope placed through the mouth or nose.[16] Biopsies can then be performed under direct vision. The diagnostic work-up, including computed tomographic scanning of the skull base, seeks evidence of bone erosion as well as an enlargement of the jugular foramen or foramen ovale. If there is any indication of intracranial extension, magnetic resonance imaging is also performed.

## STAGING

The TNM staging system of the American Joint Committee on Cancer and the International Union Against Cancer is given in Table 63–1. A critical staging factor in this system is whether or not there is evidence of intracranial extension by the primary tumor.

## PROGNOSIS

The prognosis of nasopharyngeal cancer is determined by the extent of the primary lesion, the presence of metastases, and the tumor histology. Tumors with intracranial extension

*Table 63–1.* **The International TNM Staging System for Cancer of the Nasopharynx**

| *Definition of TNM* | | | |
| --- | --- | --- | --- |
| *Primary Tumor (T)* | | | |
| TX | Primary tumor cannot be assessed | | |
| T0 | No evidence of primary tumor | | |
| Tis | Carcinoma in situ | | |
| *Nasopharynx* | | | |
| T1 | Tumor limited to one subsite of nasopharynx (posterosuperior wall or lateral wall) | | |
| T2 | Tumor invades more than one subsite of nasopharynx | | |
| T3 | Tumor invades nasal cavity and/or oropharynx | | |
| T4 | Tumor invades skull and cranial nerve(s) | | |
| *Regional Lymph Nodes (N)* | | | |
| NX | Regional lymph nodes cannot be assessed | | |
| N0 | No regional lymph node metastasis | | |
| N1 | Metastasis in a single ipsilateral lymph node 3 cm or less in greatest dimension | | |
| N2 | Metastasis in a single ipsilateral lymph node more than 3 cm but not more than 6 cm in greatest dimension, or in several ipsilateral lymph nodes, none more than 6 cm in greatest dimension, or in bilateral or contralateral lymph nodes, none more than 6 cm in greatest dimension | | |
| N2a | Metastasis in a single ipsilateral lymph node more than 3 cm but not more than 6 cm in greatest dimension | | |
| N2b | Metastasis in multiple ipsilateral lymph nodes, none more than 6 cm in greatest dimension | | |
| N2c | Metastasis in bilateral or contralateral lymph nodes, none more than 6 cm in greatest dimension | | |
| N3 | Metastasis in a lymph node more than 6 cm in greatest dimension | | |
| *Distant Metastasis (M)* | | | |
| MX | Presence of distant metastases cannot be assessed | | |
| M0 | No distant metastasis | | |
| M1 | Distant metastasis | | |
| *Stage Grouping* | | | |
| Stage 0 | Tis | N0 | M0 |
| Stage I | T1 | N0 | M0 |
| Stage II | T2 | N0 | M0 |
| Stage III | T3 | N0 | M0 |
| | T1 | N1 | M0 |
| | T2 | N1 | M0 |
| | T3 | N1 | M0 |
| Stage IV | T4 | N0 | M0 |
| | T4 | N1 | M0 |
| | Any T | N2 | M0 |
| | Any T | N3 | M0 |
| | Any T | Any N | M1 |

From Beahrs OH, Henson DE, Hutter RVP, Kennedy BJ, eds. Manual for staging of cancer. 4th ed. Philadelphia: JB Lippincott, 1992:34–5. Reproduced by permission of the American Joint Committee on Cancer and the publisher.

and skull erosion have the worst prognosis; the 5-year survival rate is generally less than 15%. Cervical metastasis, which is frequent with this cancer, also worsens the prognosis. In a series of 966 patients from Taiwan,[17] the overall actuarial and relapse-free survival rates were 43% and 33% at 5 years and 36% and 22% at 10 years, respectively. None of the patients presenting with distant metastases survived more than 4 years. As discussed in the next section, preliminary evidence suggests that combined chemotherapy and radiation therapy might provide improved survival compared with radiation therapy alone.

## Treatment

Irradiation to include the nasopharyngeal primary tumor, the retropharyngeal lymph nodes, and the bilateral cervical lymph nodes has been the traditional treatment of choice for nasopharyngeal carcinoma.[18] The treatment fields include the entire nasopharynx, the posterior nasal cavity, the posterior ethmoid sinus, the sphenoid sinus, the basiocciput, the cavernous sinus, and the pterygoid fossa. Dosages to the primary site and cervical metastases may reach 6500 to 7000 cGy in 6.5 to 8 weeks, whereas 4500 to 5000 cGy in 5 weeks may be used for subclinical cervical metastases. If a palpable mass in the neck persists for 2 or 3 months after irradiation, with no evidence of tumor in the nasopharynx, a radical neck dissection may be indicated.

Evidence suggests that there is a survival advantage of concurrent chemotherapy and radiation therapy when compared with radiation therapy alone for the treatment of advanced nasopharyngeal cancer.[19] A randomized phase III trial carried out by the Southwest Oncology Group documented a 76% 3-year survival rate for patients treated with concurrent radiation therapy and cisplatin followed by three courses of postirradiation cisplatin and fluorouracil. This 3-year survival was statistically improved (p<0.001) when compared with a 46% 3-year survival achieved by patients treated by radiation therapy alone. Pending further validation of these data, it is currently our practice to treat patients with advanced nasopharyngeal carcinoma and with an acceptable performance status using combined chemotherapy and radiation therapy.

Recurrent or residual disease is difficult to manage.[20] A second course of irradiation can be attempted, although the 5-year survival rate is less than 10%, and complications of repeated irradiation can be severe. A brief initial disease-free interval between completion of primary radiotherapy and diagnosis of local failures and advanced T stage and N stage at the time of re-treatment are significant prognosticators predicting poor survival after repeated irradiation.[21] Limited success has been achieved in cases of recurrence using cryotherapy or intracavitary radiation therapy.[22]

In a few centers, surgical salvage of recurrent nasopharyngeal cancer after radiation therapy has been attempted.[23–25] The operative approaches include an anterior approach using a maxillary swing or maxillectomy, a lateral approach through the infratemporal fossa, or transcervical approach using a mandibulotomy. Although short-term results appeared promising, most patients eventually succumbed to their disease. Patients with limited midline recurrences that do not have intracranial extension appear to be the best candidates for surgical salvage after radiation therapy.

## SEQUELAE OF TREATMENT

Because a large volume of normal tissue is irradiated to a high dose, sequelae are frequent and may result in serious, persistent morbidity. Mucosal dryness of varying severity follows irradiation of the parotid gland. Dental problems, related to xerostomia or direct irradiation of the teeth and supporting bone, or both, may develop. Hearing loss and otitis media may follow changes in the auditory tube. Infrequent trismus is due to changes in the pterygoid muscles. The epithelial lining of the external ear canals may become fragile and susceptible to infection. Irradiation of parts of the hypothalamus and temporal lobes of the brain and the pituitary gland rarely produces clinically detectable sequelae. Very rarely, radiation myelopathy of the cervical spinal cord and brain stem has been reported.

## SUGGESTIONS FOR ADDITIONAL READING

Wang DC, Cai WM, Hu YH, Gu XZ. Long-term survival of 1035 cases of nasopharyngeal carcinoma. Cancer 1988;61:2338–41. *The 5-year survival rate for the entire group was 20%, but it was 35% for patients with histologically confirmed, nonmetastatic cancer that was treated with at least 40 Gy.*

Gasparini M, Lombardi F, Rottoli L, et al. Combined radiotherapy and chemotherapy in stage T3 and T4 nasopharyngeal carcinoma in children. J Clin Oncol 1988;6:491–4. *The actuarial 3-year relapse-free survival rate was 75% in 12 children treated with aggressive combined-modality therapy. The analogous survival rate from the authors' historical series was 8%. This study suggests but does not prove that combined therapy is superior to radiation therapy alone.*

Clark JR, Norris CM Jr, Dreyfuss AI, et al. Nasopharyngeal carcinoma: the Dana Farber Cancer Institute experience with 24 patients treated with induction chemotherapy and radiotherapy. Ann Otol Rhinol Laryngol 1987;96:608–14. *Induction chemotherapy resulted in a complete response rate of 29% and a partial response rate of 46%. The 2-year failure-free survival rate for all patients was 57%. The authors conclude that induction chemotherapy for patients with nasopharyngeal carcinoma is an investigational tool of considerable promise.*

Chan AT, Teo PM, Leung TW, Johnson PJ. The role of chemotherapy in the management of nasopharyngeal carcinoma. Cancer 1998;82:1003–12. *The authors perform a review of retrospective and prospective clinical series to assess the role of chemotherapy to treat nasopharyngeal carcinoma. They conclude that nasopharyngeal carcinoma is a chemosensitive tumor, and there is a likely role for chemotherapy to treat local-regional disease and distant metastases.*

Fandi A, Cvitkovic E. Biology and treatment of nasopharyngeal cancer. Curr Opin Oncol 1995;7:255–63. *A brief overview that discusses the epidemiology, pathology, evaluation, and treatment of nasopharyngeal carcinoma.*

## REFERENCES

1. Schnohr P. Survival rates of nasopharyngeal cancer in California: a review of 516 cases from 1942 through 1965. Cancer 1970;25:1099–106.
2. Martin H, Quan S. The racial incidence (Chinese) of nasopharyngeal cancer. Ann Otol Rhinol Laryngol 1951;60:168–74.
3. Laing D. Nasopharyngeal carcinoma. Otolaryngol Clin North Am 1969;2:703–25.
4. Snow JB Jr. Carcinoma of the nasopharynx in children. Ann Otol Rhinol Laryngol 1975;84:817–26.

4. Snow JB Jr. Carcinoma of the nasopharynx in children. Ann Otol Rhinol Laryngol 1975;84:817–26.
5. Hara HJ. Cancer of the nasopharynx: review of the literature and report of 72 cases. Laryngoscope 1969;79:1315–29.
6. Elwood JM. Wood exposure and smoking: association with cancer of the nasal cavity and paranasal sinuses in British Columbia. Can Med Assoc J 1981;124:1573–7.
7. Halperin WE, Goodman M, Stayner L, et al. Nasal cancer in a worker exposed to formaldehyde. JAMA 1983;249:510–2.
8. Armstrong RW, Armstrong MJ, Yu MC, Henderson BE. Salted fish and inhalants as risk factors for nasopharyngeal carcinoma in Malaysian Chinese. Cancer Res 1983;43:2967–70.
9. Nam JM, McLaughlin JK, Blot WJ. Cigarette smoking, alcohol, and nasopharyngeal carcinoma: a case-control study among U.S. whites. J Natl Cancer Inst 1992;84:619–22.
10. Hsu MM, Chiou JF, McCabe BF. Anti-Epstein Barr virus antibody in nasopharyngeal carcinoma. Ann Otol Rhinol Laryngol 1974;83:19–25.
11. Luka J, Deeb ZE, Hartmann DP, et al. Detection of antigens associated with Epstein-Barr virus replication in extracts from biopsy specimens of nasopharyngeal carcinomas. J Natl Cancer Inst 1988;80:1164–7.
12. Pearson GR, Weiland LH, Neel HB, et al. Application of Epstein-Barr virus (EBV) serology to the diagnosis of North American nasopharyngeal carcinoma. Cancer 1983;51:260–8.
13. Littler E, Baylis SA, Zeng Y, et al. Diagnosis of nasopharyngeal carcinoma by means of recombinant Epstein-Barr virus proteins. Lancet 1991;337:685–9.
14. Ablashi DV, Levine PH, Prasad U, Pearson GR. Fourth international symposium on nasopharyngeal carcinoma application of field and laboratory studies to the control of NPC. Cancer Res 1983;43:2375–8.
15. Feinmesser R, Miyazaki I, Cheung R, et al. Diagnosis of nasopharyngeal carcinoma by DNA amplification of tissue obtained by fine-needle aspiration. N Engl J Med 1992;326:17–21.
16. Ward PH, Berci G, Calcaterra TC. Advances in endoscopic examination of the respiratory system. Ann Otol Rhinol Laryngol 1974;83:754–60.
17. Hsu MM, Tu SM. Nasopharyngeal carcinoma in Taiwan. Clinical manifestations and results of therapy. Cancer 1983;52:362–8.
18. Schabinger PR, Reddy S, Hendrickson FR, et al. Carcinoma of the nasopharynx: survival and patterns of recurrence. Int J Radiat Oncol Biol Phys 1985;11:2081–4.
19. Al-Sarraf M, LeBlanc M, Giri PG, et al. Chemoradiotherapy versus radiotherapy in patients with advanced nasopharyngeal cancer: phase III randomized Intergroup study. J Clin Oncol 1998;16:1310–7.
20. Vikram B, Strong EW, Shah JP, et al. Intraoperative radiotherapy in patients with recurrent head and neck cancer. Am J Surg 1985;150:485–7.
21. Teo PM, Kwan WH, Chan AT, et al. How successful is high-dose (> or = 60 Gy) reirradiation using mainly external beams in salvaging local failures of nasopharyngeal carcinoma? Int J Radiat Oncol Biol Phys 1998;40:897–913.
22. Tsao SY. Intracavitary radiotherapy for nasopharyngeal carcinoma—palliation or cure? Ann Acad Med Singapore 1994;23:221–5.
23. Wei WI, Lam KH, Sham JS. New approach to the nasopharynx: the maxillary swing approach. Head Neck 1991;13:200–7.
24. Fee WE, Roberson JB, Goffinet DR. Long-term survival after surgical resection for recurrent nasopharyngeal cancer after radiotherapy failure. Arch Otolaryngol Head Neck Surg 1991;117:1233–6.
25. Morton RP, Liavaag PG, McLean M, Freeman JL. Transcervico-man-

# C H A P T E R  **64**

# SALIVARY GLANDS

• THOMAS C. CALCATERRA • KEITH E. BLACKWELL

Nests of salivary gland cells are normally found throughout the entire upper aerodigestive tract, making it possible for salivary gland tumors to arise anywhere in this anatomic area. The incidence of these tumors is low, representing less than 3% of all human tumors; the overall incidence in the general population is about 1.5 per 100,000.[1]

In a comparison of several large series, no sex predilection could be consistently identified, except for cases of Warthin's tumor, which developed about five times more frequently in men. As a general rule, benign salivary gland tumors occur in younger patients, whereas patients afflicted by malignant tumors are older. The cause of salivary gland tumors is unknown, although one study implicated dental radiographs for parotid gland tumors.[2]

## Natural History

### CLASSIFICATION AND PATHOLOGY

Salivary gland tumors are composed of a complex array of tumor types, varying in growth behavior from indolent to aggressive. Many of the tumors are difficult to classify into specific subgroups, and some overlap histologically.

Acceptable classifications of salivary gland tumors are based on the specific salivary gland cell that is presumed to

have given origin to the neoplasm.[3] The prototype of a salivary gland unit consists of serous or mucous acini that drain to a duct that is divided sequentially into three different portions lined by morphologically different epithelial cells, which are termed *intercalated, striated,* and *excretory.* Myoepithelial cells are located around the periphery of the acini and the intercalated portion of the duct, functioning as contractile cells to force secretions from the acini and intercalated portion of the duct. The intercalated cells are undifferentiated, whereas the striated duct cells are well differentiated.

Using these cell types as progenitors of salivary gland neoplasms, one hypothesis currently favored is that the excretory duct cells give rise to the squamous cell and mucoepidermoid carcinomas.[3] The striated duct cells produce oncocytic tumors, and the intercalated duct cells generate adenoid cystic carcinomas. The acinar cells give rise to the acinic cell carcinomas, mixed tumors, and monomorphic adenomas. Another hypothesis of origin, which is not based on the dedifferentiation of already highly specialized cells such as the acinar and striated duct cells, is the "bicellular theory of origin," which postulates that all salivary gland neoplasms arise from two undifferentiated cell types, the excretory duct cell and the intercalated duct cell.[4]

Salivary gland tumors, which are also classified by anatomic site of origin, are divided into two groups—those of major salivary gland origin and those from the minor salivary glands. The major salivary glands are the parotid, submandibular, and sublingual; the minor salivary glands are distributed as small nests throughout the upper aerodigestive tract. About 75% of salivary gland tumors occur in the parotid gland, 10% occur in the submandibular gland, and 1% occur in the sublingual gland. The remainder develop in the minor glands, the most common site being the palate.[5]

The relative incidence of malignant tumors increases as the size of the originating salivary gland decreases, that is, the frequency of malignancy in parotid gland tumors is about 20%, in submandibular gland tumors it is about 40 to 50%, and in lesser salivary gland tumors it is about 50 to 60%. Fortunately, more than 75% of these tumors arise in the parotid gland, thereby accounting for the fact that the majority of salivary gland tumors are benign.

## DIAGNOSIS

The typical presenting complaint of patients with salivary tumors is a painless mass of variable duration. Although tumors can appear in any portion of the parotid gland, they usually occur in the posterior half. The lump is often considered to be an enlarged lymph node, and therefore antibiotic therapy is generally started. If unattended, salivary gland tumors, particularly the benign ones, can reach substantial proportions before causing difficulties.

Although partial or complete facial paralysis has been reported in benign tumors, this feature almost always heralds a malignancy.[6] Other features suggestive of malignancy are hardness and fixation of the tumor to underlying bone or overlying skin. Although pain is not highly diagnostic of malignancy, it raises suspicion because of possible sensory nerve involvement. Cervical lymph node enlargement suggests malignancy because of the likelihood of regional node metastasis. However, regional node metastasis is uncommon in most parotid gland malignancies, occurring with an appreciable frequency in only patients with high grade mucoepidermoid carcinoma or squamous cell carcinoma, malignant mixed tumor, and adenocarcinoma. When regional metastasis does occur, it is usually late in the course of the disease. The presence of facial paralysis as well as regional node metastasis portends a very unfavorable prognosis despite aggressive therapy.

All patients who are found to have a mass in the region of the major salivary glands should undergo a thorough head and neck examination. When masses occur in the region of the parotid gland, the face and scalp should be carefully inspected for skin lesions, such as melanoma, squamous cell carcinoma, and Merkel's cell carcinoma, because these types of facial skin cancer tend to metastasize first to the periparotid lymph nodes. The posterior and lateral pharyngeal walls should be inspected and palpated because the retropharyngeal space may harbor a primary tumor presenting laterally in the parotid gland area, mimicking a parotid gland tumor. Conversely, a tumor of the deep lobe of the parotid gland may extend medially, appearing as a pharyngeal mass. If the mass is located in the region of the submandibular gland, particular attention should be directed toward the oral cavity because this area may be the site of a primary cancer that has metastasized. The submandibular gland duct must be

carefully palpated bimanually to determine the presence of stones. The fixation of the tumor to the mandible should be assessed, and a determination of the integrity of the lingual and hypoglossal nerve function must be made.

Magnetic resonance imaging plays an increasingly important role in the diagnostic evaluation of salivary gland tumors, particularly of the parotid gland.[7] This imaging method can usually provide precise anatomic information regarding the location of the tumor within the parotid gland and demonstrate the proximity to the facial nerve, stylomastoid foramen, skull base, and parapharyngeal space. Enlarged cervical lymph nodes are readily apparent by this study.

Occasionally, sialography is helpful when a diagnosis of parotitis is being considered, as the appearance of stones or ectasia of the ductal system suggests inflammatory disease.[8]

The definitive diagnosis is usually accomplished by surgical excision; the complete excision of the tumor with an ample margin of normal salivary gland tissue also becomes part of the treatment. The surgeon may wish to identify the tumor type by frozen section examination, or interpretation may await permanent sections. Either method of tumor diagnosis may dictate surgical therapy beyond excisional biopsy.

Cytologic examination of parotid masses by fine-needle aspiration has been shown to be a reliable diagnostic tool in the hands of an experienced cytologist.[9] This diagnostic information is extremely beneficial if the tumor is unresectable or if the clinician strongly suspects metastatic tumor or a lymphoma. In addition, if surgery is planned, knowledge of the tumor type helps the surgeon prepare the patient for the scope of the operation.

## STAGING

The TNM staging system for salivary gland tumors of the American Joint Committee on Cancer and the International Union Against Cancer is presented in Table 64–1.[10]

# Treatment

The successful treatment of salivary gland tumors requires especially close multidisciplinary communication among the surgeon, the pathologist, and the radiotherapist. Only since the 1980s has the biologic aggressiveness of each type of salivary gland tumor been characterized, thereby enabling the development of a rational treatment plan for the various kinds of tumors.

The initial treatment for all primary salivary gland neoplasms is surgical, with the use of wide excision whenever possible. In most instances, the extent of surgical resection is dictated by the tumor type. The various surgical options must be agreed on with the patient in advance so that the surgeon is not limited by lack of consent to perform an appropriate operation.

The first step in surgical therapy is careful exposure of the salivary gland harboring the tumor. This is followed by wide excision of the tumor mass, sparing any vital structure adjacent to the tumor unless it has clearly been infiltrated by tumor. Frozen section examination is then carried out to determine the tumor type. If the pathologist is certain that

*Table 64–1.* **The International TNM Staging System for Cancer of the Salivary Glands**

**Definition of TNM**

*Primary Tumor (T)*

| | |
|---|---|
| TX | Primary tumor cannot be assessed |
| T0 | No evidence of primary tumor |
| T1 | Tumor 2 cm or less in greatest dimension |
| T2 | Tumor more than 2 cm but not more than 4 cm in greatest dimension |
| T3 | Tumor more than 4 cm but not more than 6 cm in greatest dimension |
| T4 | Tumor more than 6 cm in greatest dimension |
| | Note: All categories are subdivided: (a) no local extension; (b) local extension. Local extension is clinical or macroscopic evidence of invasion of skin, soft tissues, bone, or nerve. Microscopic evidence alone is not local extension for classification purposes |

*Regional Lymph Nodes (N)*

| | |
|---|---|
| NX | Regional lymph nodes cannot be assessed |
| N0 | No regional lymph node metastasis |
| N1 | Metastasis in a single ipsilateral lymph node 3 cm or less in greatest dimension |
| N2 | Metastasis in a single ipsilateral lymph node, more than 3 cm but not more than 6 cm in greatest dimension; or, in multiple ipsilateral lymph nodes, none more than 6 cm in greatest dimension; or, in bilateral or contralateral lymph nodes, none more than 6 cm in greatest dimension |
| N2a | Metastasis in single ipsilateral lymph node more than 3 cm but not more than 6 cm in greatest dimension |
| N2b | Metastasis in multiple ipsilateral lymph nodes, none more than 6 cm in greatest dimension |
| N2c | Metastasis in bilateral or contralateral lymph nodes, none more than 6 cm in greatest dimension |
| N3 | Metastasis in a lymph node more than 6 cm in greatest dimension |

*Distant Metastasis (M)*

| | |
|---|---|
| MX | Presence of distant metastases cannot be assessed |
| M0 | No distant metastasis |
| M1 | Distant metastasis |

*Stage Grouping*

| | | | |
|---|---|---|---|
| Stage I | T1a | N0 | M0 |
| | T2a | N0 | M0 |
| Stage II | T1b | N0 | M0 |
| | T2b | N0 | M0 |
| | T3a | N0 | M0 |
| Stage III | T3b | N0 | M0 |
| | T4a | N0 | M0 |
| | Any T | N1 | M0 (except T4b) |
| Stage IV | T4b | Any N | M0 |
| | Any T | N2 | M0 |
| | Any T | N3 | M0 |
| | Any T | Any N | M1 |

From Beahrs OH, Henson DE, Hutter RVP, Kennedy BJ, eds. Manual for staging of cancer. 4th ed. Philadelphia: JB Lippincott, 1992:49–50. Reproduced by permission of the American Joint Committee on Cancer and the publisher.

the tumor is benign or of low-grade malignancy, the excisional biopsy will suffice as adequate therapy. However, if it proves to be of a higher grade of malignancy, it is often necessary to resect a broader margin of the adjacent tissue and follow with radiation therapy.[11]

With parotid gland malignancies, some authors advocate wide resection with ample margins, which may involve sacrifice of the entire facial nerve, the ascending ramus of the mandible, and even the temporal bone. Likewise, if there is possible involvement of the skin, a wide excision can be performed and the defect resurfaced with an advancement neck-chest flap. However, a therapeutic benefit of this aggressive approach has not been demonstrated definitively in the literature, so many surgeons now advocate preservation of vital adjacent structures such as the facial nerve unless they are actually invaded by the cancer. In this instance, postoperative radiation therapy is often used to treat close resection margins. The upper cervical node should be routinely examined and, if frozen section reveals malignancy, a radical neck dissection should be performed. Prophylactic neck dissections are not routinely performed for all parotid gland malignancies because of the low frequency of regional metastasis; however, they are frequently a part of a submandibular gland malignancy resection because of a higher incidence of associated nodal metastasis. Elective lymph node dissection has also been advocated for high-grade mucoepidermoid carcinoma, malignant mixed tumors, adenocarcinoma, squamous cell carcinomas, and facial skin cancers that have metastasized to periparotid lymph nodes.

When the facial nerve or one of its segments has been sacrificed, it has proved worthwhile to replace the nerve using a cable nerve graft, which provides a conduit for subsequent motor fiber regeneration and achieves satisfactory facial function in approximately 9 to 12 months. Suitable donor sensory nerves for facial nerve cable grafting include the great auricular nerve, the supraclavicular sensory plexus of nerves, the sural nerve of the leg, and the antebrachial cutaneous nerve of the forearm. If the orbicularis oculis muscle is paralyzed, the cornea must be preserved by measures such as the frequent application of wetting solutions, eyelid taping, and protective coverings. Lagophthalmos can be prevented by placing a gold weight implant into the paralyzed upper eyelid.

The role of radiation has become clearer in recent years. Certainly it can provide effective palliation for the patient who has an unresectable tumor or metastasis to a salivary gland; however, there is growing evidence that many of the malignant tumors can be eradicated if the tumor mass is grossly removed or at least reduced.[14] In our institution, postoperative tumoricidal irradiation is advised if there is concern about the adequacy of a surgical margin or if the tumor is poorly differentiated.[12]

The palliative use of chemotherapy in patients with salivary gland tumors is discussed in Chapter 66.

## Clinical Features and Treatment of Specific Neoplasms

### BENIGN TUMORS

**Mixed Tumor (Pleomorphic Adenoma).** This most common salivary gland tumor, constituting at least 75% of all benign tumors, is characterized by slow growth, and it usually appears in the superficial lobe of the parotid gland. The tumor may remain quiescent for several months or years and then undergo a period of slow growth. Pain is not a frequent symptom, although a vague pressure sensation may be experienced.

On examination, the mixed tumor is usually solitary, well circumscribed, sometimes lobulated, and usually mobile. Gross examination shows an encapsulated and multilobulated tumor of variable size. Close inspection of the external surface frequently reveals small excrescences jutting out from the capsule. On cut section, the tumor surface is variable, depending on the cellular make-up.

Although the microscopic appearance is diverse, both epithelial and mesenchymal elements must be present for diagnosis. The mesenchymal element may consist of myxoid, fibroid, or chondroid cellular structures that make up the stroma. The ratio of epithelial cells to mesenchymal stroma may vary considerably and probably does not influence the prognosis.[13]

Mixed tumors are best treated by a wide surgical excision. When they are treated by simple enucleation, the recurrence rate may be as high as 50%. Today, the favored treatment for mixed tumors of the parotid gland is superficial lobectomy. Although there is no anatomic division of the parotid gland into lobes, this operation is designed to remove all the parotid gland tissue lateral to the facial nerve. This constitutes the majority of the gland, which is the most likely site for these tumors. The operation requires exposure and careful dissection of the facial nerve and usually affords ample margins of normal parotid gland tissue around the tumor. This approach prevents any tumor spillage and completely encompasses the excrescences or pseudopods that may be on the outer limits of the tumors.

The same principle applies to the surgical management of mixed tumors that are located in the deep lobe of the parotid gland or submandibular gland. Again, a cuff of normal tissue is preserved around the tumor capsule, the only exception being when the tumor lies directly adjacent to a vital structure, such as the facial nerve. In such circumstances, it is reasonable to dissect the tumor carefully from the epineurium. The use of these surgical techniques should keep the recurrence rate at less than 2%; however, in the event of recurrence, repeated surgical excision is often successful. The sacrifice of the facial nerve should be considered only if there is evidence of intracranial extension or for recurrent tumor that presents with facial nerve paralysis. Radiation therapy as the sole therapeutic modality has had limited effectiveness in the treatment of recurrent tumor,[14] although there may be a role for radiation to treat microscopic residual disease after surgical re-excision.[15, 16]

**Warthin's Tumor (Papillary Cystadenoma Lymphomatosum).** Warthin's tumor is almost exclusively confined to the parotid gland, representing between 5% and 10% of all parotid gland tumors. Almost without exception, it is benign and unlikely to recur after adequate removal. This tumor develops at least five times more frequently in males than in females, usually in the fifth or sixth decade of life. It has the highest incidence of bilateral occurrence of all salivary gland tumors (in the range of 5 to 10%).

Warthin's tumor is unique in that it characteristically arises in the inferior pole of the parotid gland and occasionally originates in the lymph nodes adjacent to that part of the gland. The genesis of this tumor remains controversial; indeed, in the opinion of some authors, it is not a true tumor but is similar to an autoimmune disorder such as Hashimoto's thyroiditis.[17] The most commonly accepted theory is that it arises from heterotopic salivary duct tissue in paraparotid lymphoid tissue.[18] The tumor is usually soft or even cystic to palpation, ranging in size from 1 to 6 cm. It tends to be unilocular, encapsulated, and filled with gray or tan fluid. Microscopically, there is a characteristic appearance of intracystic papillary fronds lined by a double layer of cells: an inner layer of cuboidal, darkly staining cells and an outer layer of tall, columnar, nonciliated cells.

The tumor is best treated surgically by wide excision, usually requiring exposure of the facial nerve, and resection of that portion of the superficial lobe that harbors the tumor. The tumor does not shell out well, and there is always the risk of spillage and implantation of tumor cells if this approach is attempted. In the aged or severely ill patient, needle biopsy and observation are reasonable measures because this type of tumor grows slowly and there is essentially no risk of metastasis.

**Monomorphic Adenomas.** A number of other benign tumors of the salivary glands are generally classified together under the term *monomorphic adenomas*, representing 2% or 3% of all salivary gland neoplasms. Included in this group are the oncocytomas, consisting of large polygonal eosinophilic cells with granular cytoplasm. Some authors believe that these lesions may simply represent aggregate hyperplasia of mature cells, inasmuch as they may be multicentric.[19] Oncocytomas are solid and encapsulated, and they tend to grow slowly. Recurrence is uncommon, and malignant degeneration is rare.

Other types of monomorphic adenomas have been described that are characterized by a uniform epithelial pattern throughout the tumor without a myxomatous stroma that distinguishes them from mixed tumors. They are generally found among an older age group and follow a benign course. The basal cell adenoma, the sebaceous adenoma, and the clear cell adenoma are included in this category. The basal cell adenoma consists of uniform strands or islands of spindle cells resembling a basal cell carcinoma of the skin. The most difficult aspect of the diagnosis is to differentiate them from adenoid cystic carcinomas. Sebaceous adenomas are composed of lipid-containing cells that are believed to represent ectopic sebaceous glands in a matrix of lymphoid tissue, not unlike Warthin's tumor. The clear cell adenoma, which is a rare tumor, consists of glycogen-rich cells that resemble those of its counterpart commonly seen in the kidney.

## MALIGNANT TUMORS

**Mucoepidermoid Tumor.** Mucoepidermoid tumors are the most common malignant tumors of the parotid gland, composing approximately one third of all salivary gland malignancies.[20, 21] The second most common site for this tumor is the palate. Although these tumors may develop in patients of any age, the peak incidence is in the fifth decade. The clinical presentation varies according to the histologic grade of the tumor, which may range from well differentiated (low grade) to poorly differentiated (high grade), and the symptoms range from a slow-growing, painless lump to a rapidly expanding mass that causes trismus and facial paralysis. These variations in differentiation and clinical behavior led to the opinion that the better differentiated tumors are benign; however, there have been enough accounts of differentiated tumors infiltrating locally and metastasizing that all grades of this tumor must be considered to be malignant.

The tumors are usually circumscribed but poorly encapsulated and thus may adhere to surrounding structures. Microscopically, the tumor includes both squamous cells and mucin-secreting cells that are believed to arise from the ductal epithelium. In the well-differentiated tumor, multiple cystic spaces are filled with mucin and lined by attenuated squamous cells and mucin-secreting goblet cells. The poorly differentiated tumors mainly show squamous elements without discrete cyst formation and with only a few acinar or mucinous cells.

Not surprisingly, the prognosis varies according to the histologic differentiation. The recurrence rate in patients with well-differentiated tumors is as low as 10 to 15%, whereas for those with poorly differentiated tumors it is about 75%. Initially, the treatment is almost invariably surgical, with an attempt to resect the tumor with a wide margin of normal tissue. A radical neck dissection is considered important by some clinicians for poorly differentiated tumors, particularly when these tumors arise in the submandibular gland.

**Adenoid Cystic Carcinoma.** This tumor composes about 4 to 8% of salivary gland tumors, occurring most frequently in the submandibular, sublingual, and minor salivary glands, but it has been reported in virtually every part of the upper aerodigestive tract.[22–24] Like other salivary gland tumors, it initially presents as an asymptomatic mass, but because of its proclivity to involve nerves, the symptoms of pain and numbness or motor paralysis frequently follow. It is typically slow growing, and survival can be protracted despite the presence of tumor. Distant metastases, particularly to the lung, may be noted many years after the primary tumor is discovered and are seen more commonly than are regional lymph node metastases.

Adenoid cystic carcinomas vary considerably in size, tending to be poorly encapsulated and often exhibiting infiltrative growth into adjacent soft tissue and bone. The microscopic features of this neoplasm are characteristic in that the cells are uniform in size, with darkly stained nuclei arranged in solid cords, a cribriform pattern, or a tubular pattern. Tumors that exhibit the cribriform or tubular architecture are characterized by slow growth and prolonged survival, whereas the solid type of tumor can behave more aggressively. The tendency for this tumor to invade along perineural spaces is well known; such perineural extension can sometimes be noted by concentric enlargement of the osseous foramina of the skull, usually indicating its unresectability.[25]

The majority of patients with adenoid cystic carcinoma survive for 5 years, but this does not mean they are cured. In most series, there is a progressive decline in survival after 5 years; in some, it decreases to as low as 12% at 15 years.[22]

The analysis of successfully managed patients seems to support aggressive therapy at the time the tumor is discovered, which consists of wide surgical excision that may necessitate the sacrifice of all or part of the facial nerve, as well as resection of part of the mandible, temporal bone, or maxilla. Postoperative irradiation may be useful, particularly when the surgical margins are not ample.[26, 27]

**Acinic Cell Tumor.** This tumor represents 1 to 2% of all salivary gland tumors and about 10% of parotid gland malignancies. It was originally considered to be benign, but long-term series have shown that there is a 25% incidence of local recurrence and a 10% incidence of distant metastases.[28, 29]

Acinic cell tumors are characterized by gradual, painless growth and are often present for several years before receiving medical attention. They typically develop as an isolated mass in the superficial lobe of the parotid gland. The histologic configuration appears benign, inasmuch as the predominant granular cells show minimal pleomorphism. The cell cytoplasm ranges from darkly basophilic granules to almost clear cells.

As with other slow-growing salivary gland malignancies, the 5-year survival rate is about 90%, but it continues to diminish significantly with increasing years. Superficial parotidectomy—with total excision of the portion of the parotid gland that contains the tumor—is the preferred treatment for this entity.

**Malignant Mixed Tumor (Carcinoma Arising in Pleomorphic Adenoma).** Most authorities agree that this type of carcinoma arises from a benign mixed tumor, an opinion based on numerous examples of apparent transition to malignancy within the tumor.[30] It is the epithelial element alone that undergoes this transition. This opinion is supported clinically by the frequent history of suddenly accelerated growth of a dormant mass that had existed for several years. Likewise, a mixed tumor may have been removed several years earlier, followed by a rapidly growing recurrence showing malignant histologic features different from those of the original tumor. It has been estimated that between 2% and 5% of all mixed tumors undergo this transition, generally in the parotid gland, in which it represents about 7% of the malignancies.

The prognosis in the first 5 years is less favorable than that for most other salivary gland malignancies; the 5-year survival rate is about 50%. Metastasis occurs in about half of patients, frequently to distant sites such as the lung and the central nervous system.

**Miscellaneous Primary Carcinomas.** A number of other malignancies of the salivary glands are seen infrequently, but they seem to have distinguishable characteristics that enable separate classification. Most are clinically malignant, demonstrating rapid growth and frequent recurrence and ending in the death of the patient. Included in this group of tumors are epidermoid carcinoma, undifferentiated carcinoma, and adenocarcinoma.

These tumors tend to occur in older patients, and rapid growth, hardness, fixation to skin, pain, and facial paralysis indicate malignancy. Grossly, they often infiltrate the salivary gland tissue and adjacent structures, even replacing the entire gland. Thus, the invasion of lymphatics and blood vessels is often apparent microscopically.

The prognosis for these tumors is bleak; regardless of the type of therapy used, the 5-year survival rate is about 25%. The prognosis is even poorer with anaplastic tumors.

## SUGGESTIONS FOR ADDITIONAL READING

Spiro RH. Management of malignant tumors of the salivary glands. Oncology 1998;12:671–80. *This article provides a good review of the contemporary roles of surgery, radiation therapy, and chemotherapy for the management of salivary gland cancers. The author draws on his considerable career experience in treating salivary neoplasms at Memorial Sloan-Kettering Hospital (also see reference 20).*

Bissett RJ, Fitzpatrick PJ. Malignant submandibular gland tumors—a review of 91 patients. Am J Clin Oncol 1988;11:46–51. *The 5-year local-regional control rate was 30% when surgery was combined with radiation therapy. These results suggest that radiation therapy may also play a role in the management of these tumors.*

Ellis ER, Million RR, Mendenhall WM, et al. The use of radiation therapy in the management of minor salivary gland tumors. Int J Radiat Oncol Biol Phys 1988;15:613–7. *In this series of 52 patients, early-stage disease was managed equally well by radiation alone and by combined radiation therapy and surgery; however, combined therapy was clearly superior for patients with advanced tumors.*

Armstrong JG, Harrison LB, Spiro RH, et al. Malignant tumors of major salivary gland origin: a matched-pair analysis of the role of combined surgery and postoperative radiotherapy. Arch Otolaryngol Head Neck Surg 1990;116:290–3. *The results suggest that postoperative radiotherapy significantly improves outcome for patients with advanced disease.*

Armstrong JG, Harrison LB, Thaler HT, et al. The indications for elective treatment of the neck in cancer of the major salivary glands. Cancer 1992;69:615–9. *Routine elective treatment of the neck is not indicated for most patients, with the possible exception of patients with high-grade tumors and those that are T4.*

## REFERENCES

1. Dorn HF. Public Health Monograph No. 56. Washington, D.C.: U.S. Government Printing Office, 1959.
2. Preston-Martin S, Thomas DC, White SC, Cohen D. Prior exposure to medical and dental x-rays related to tumors of the parotid gland. J Natl Cancer Inst 1988;80:943–9.
3. Regezi JA, Batsakis JG. Histogenesis of salivary gland neoplasms. Otolaryngol Clin North Am 1977;10:297–307.
4. Eversole LR. Histogenic classification of salivary tumors. Arch Pathol 1971;92:433–43.
5. Eneroth CM. Salivary gland tumors in the parotid gland, submandibular gland, and the palate region. Cancer 1971;27:1415–8.
6. Eneroth CM. Facial nerve paralysis: a criterion of malignancy in parotid tumors. Arch Otolaryngol 1972;95:300–4.
7. Vogl TJ, Dresel SH, Spath M, et al. Parotid gland: plain and gadolinium-enhanced MR imaging. Radiology 1990:177:667–674.
8. Calcaterra TC, Hemenway WG, Hansen GC, Hanafee WN. The value of sialography in the diagnosis of parotid tumors. A clinicopathological correlation. Arch Otolaryngol 1977;103:727–9.
9. Layfield LJ, Tan P, Glasgow BJ. Fine-needle aspiration of salivary gland lesions. Comparison with frozen sections and histologic findings. Arch Pathol Lab Med 1987;111:346–53.
10. Beahrs OH, Henson DE, Huller RVP, Kennedy BJ, eds. Manual for staging of cancer. 4th ed. Philadelphia: JB Lippincott, 1992.
11. Reddy SP, Marks JE. Treatment of locally advanced, high-grade, malignant tumors of major salivary glands. Laryngoscope 1988;98:450–4.
12. Tran L, Sadeghi A, Hanson D, et al. Major salivary gland tumors: treatment results and prognostic factors. Laryngoscope 1986;96:1139–44.
13. Batsakis JG. Tumors of the major salivary glands. In: Batsakis JG, ed. Tumors of the Head and Neck—Clinical and Pathological Considerations. Baltimore: Williams & Wilkins, 1974:21–37.
14. Fayos JV. The role of radiotherapy in salivary gland neoplasms. Otolaryngol Clin North Am 1977;10:431–5.
15. Samson MJ, Metson R, Wang CC, Montgomery WW. Preservation of the facial nerve in the management of recurrent pleomorphic adenoma. Laryngoscope 1991;101:1060–2.
16. Dawson AK. Radiation therapy in recurrent pleomorphic adenoma of the parotid. Int J Radiat Oncol Biol Phys 1989;16:819–21.
17. Allegra SR. Warthin's tumor: a hypersensitivity disease? Hum Pathol 1971;2:403–20.
18. Thompson AS, Bryant HC. Histogenesis of papillary cystadenoma lymphamatosum (Warthin's tumor) of the parotid salivary gland. Am J Pathol 1950;26:807–49.
19. Cohen MA, Batsakis JG. Oncocytic tumors (oncocytomas) of minor salivary glamds. Arch Otolaryngol 1968;88:71–3.
20. Spiro RH. Salivary neoplasms: overview of a 35-year experience with 2,807 patients. Head Neck 1986;8:177–84.
21. Auclair PL, Goode RK, Ellis GL. Mucoepidermoid carcinoma of intraoral salivary glands: evaluation and application of grading criteria in 143 cases. Cancer 1992;69:2021–30.
22. Eibling DE, Johnson JT, McCoy JP, et al. Flow cytometric evaluation of adenoid cystic carcinoma: correlation with histologic subtype and survival. Am J Surg 1991;162:367–72.
23. Conley J, Dingman DL. Adenoid cystic carcinoma in the head and neck. Arch Otolaryngol 1974;100:81–90.
24. Eby LS, Johnson DS, Baker HW. Adenoid cystic carcinoma of the head and neck. Cancer 1972;29:1160–8.
25. Calcaterra TC, Cherney EF, Hanafee WF. Normal variations in size and neoplastic changes of skull foramina. Laryngoscope 1973;83:1385–97.
26. Frankenthaler RA, Luna MA, Lee SS, et al. Prognostic variables in parotid gland cancer. Arch Otolaryngol Head Neck Surg 1991;117:1251–6.
27. Barnett TA, Kapp DS, Goffinet DR. Adenoid cystic carcinoma of the salivary glands. Management of recurrent, advanced, or persistent disease with hyperthermia and radiation therapy. Cancer 1990;65:2648–56.
28. Batsakis JG, Luna MA, el-Naggar AK. Histopathologic grading of salivary gland neoplasms. II: Acinic cell carcinomas. Ann Otol Rhinol Laryngol 1990;99:929–33.
29. Tortoledo ME, Luna MA, Batsakis JG. Carcinomas ex pleomorphic adenoma and malignant mixed tumors: histomorphologic indexes. Arch Otolaryngol Head Neck Surg 1984;110:172–6.
30. Gerughty RM, Scofield HH, Brown FM, Hennigar GR. Malignant mixed tumors of salivary gland origin. Cancer 1969;24:471–86.

# CHAPTER 65

# LARYNX AND HYPOPHARYNX

• THOMAS C. CALCATERRA • GUY J. F. JUILLARD
• KEITH E. BLACKWELL

Laryngopharyngeal cancer constitutes about 1% of all cancers diagnosed annually in the United States.[1] The American Cancer Society has estimated that each year there are about 12,500 new cases of laryngeal cancer, resulting in 3800 deaths. The annual incidence of hypopharyngeal carcinoma in the United States is approximately 4000 cases per year.[2]

Shumrick[3] reported an increasing incidence of laryngeal cancer that appears to be centered in the industrialized areas of the world.

The onset of laryngeal cancer is highest between the ages of 60 and 65. The age-adjusted incidence of this tumor is approximately 8.1 per 100,000 for men and 0.9 per 100,000

for women,[4] with no significant difference in incidence between whites and blacks. This higher incidence in males is
the case for tumors in all areas of the laryngopharynx, except
for the postcricoid region, in which there is an almost total
reversal of rates, with females predominating.

Epidemiologic studies of laryngeal cancer have established a strong association of the disease with smoking
tobacco and heavy alcohol use.[5–7] The *U.S. Surgeon General's Report on Smoking and Health* reported a strong correlation with heavy smoking. Dysplastic changes in the laryngeal
epithelium can be demonstrated in almost all heavy smokers,
and the degree of these histologic changes seems to develop
in proportion to the amount of exposure to tobacco smoke.[8]
Moderate synergy between alcohol and cigarette smoking
has been reported in epidemiologic studies.[9] Asbestos exposure has increased the risk of laryngeal carcinoma in cigarette smokers in some reports[10, 11] but not all.[7]

Hyperkeratotic lesions of the vocal cords, such as leukoplakia, are considered premalignant, and it has been estimated that about 5% of patients with these lesions develop
invasive carcinoma.[12] Such lesions are found in patients who
abuse the larynx by excessive, loud talking. The atrophic
and chronic inflammatory changes of the pharyngeal mucous
membranes observed in the Plummer-Vinson syndrome have
been associated with cancer in the postcricoid region of
the pharynx.

There has been a correlation between laryngeal cancer
and several viruses. In one series, 95% of laryngeal cancer
patients showed evidence of serum antibodies to herpes
simplex virus–determined proteins, whereas in a comparable
control group, only 5% of individuals were seropositive.[13]
Epstein-Barr virus has been associated with some cases of
supraglottic laryngeal cancer.[14] Human papillomavirus type
16 has been implicated in the cause of laryngeal cancer in
one study.[15]

## Natural History

### ANATOMIC CLASSIFICATION

Cancers of the larynx and hypopharynx are classified according to anatomic sites or compartments that relate to the
tumors' biologic behavior and prognosis. Anatomically, the
larynx can be divided into three regions: supraglottic, glottic,
and subglottic (Fig. 65–1). The supraglottis is composed of
the lingual and laryngeal surfaces of the epiglottis, false
vocal cords, arytenoid cartilages, aryepiglottic folds, and
ventricle. The glottis includes the true vocal cords, extending
to the inferior limit of the vocal muscle, which is about 5
mm below the free margin of the cord, and including the
anterior and posterior commissures. The subglottis is the
region extending from the lower boundary of the glottis to
the lower margin of the cricoid cartilage.

The hypopharynx extends from a transverse plane through
the hyoid bone, corresponding to the pharyngoepiglottic
folds, to a transverse plane through the lower border of the
cricoid cartilage. It is arbitrarily subdivided into four areas:
the paired piriform sinuses, the posterior pharyngeal wall,
and the postcricoid region. The majority of hypopharyngeal
cancers arise in the piriform sinus, with less than 20% of

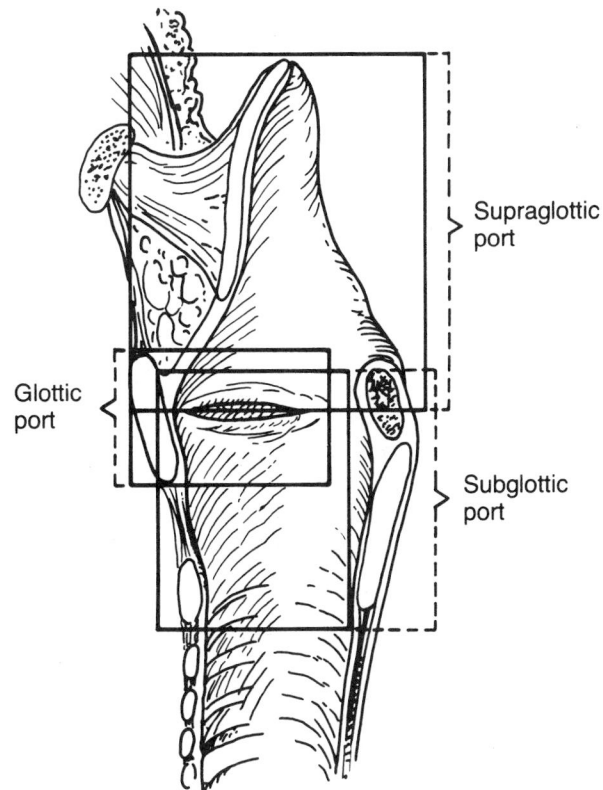

**Figure 65–1.** Schematic illustration of the three divisions of the larynx
used for classification of laryngeal cancer.

such tumors occurring in the postcricoid region or posterior
pharyngeal wall.[2, 16, 17]

Archer and coworkers[18] have proposed an alternative way
of classifying laryngeal cancer based on four anatomic regions that are easily identified by computed tomography
(CT). This classification system has not been widely used,
however.

### PATHOLOGY

Squamous cell carcinoma is found in more than 95% of
laryngeal and hypopharyngeal cancers. Tumors arising from
the vocal cords and intrinsic portions of the larynx tend to
be the best differentiated, whereas those occurring in the
hypopharynx are less well differentiated. In general, the
better differentiated cancers are likely to be exophytic with
well-defined margins, whereas poorly differentiated tumors
are usually ulcerative and indistinctly circumscribed with a
proclivity for submucosal extension.

Carcinoma in situ characteristically arises from the epithelium of the vocal cords and is usually accompanied by
adjacent areas of hyperkeratosis with dysplastic changes.[19]
Moreover, carcinoma in situ may be grossly indistinguishable from hyperkeratotic lesions, appearing as white, gray,
or red patches on the vocal cords. Verrucous carcinomas
are warty exophytic lesions, appearing microscopically like
hyperkeratosis with deep rete pegs; however, they invade
the local tissues with continual slow growth and may expand
enough to destroy underlying cartilage.

Sarcomas and minor salivary gland tumors compose most of the remainder of the primary tumors of the larynx. The sarcomas include fibrosarcoma, chondrosarcoma, rhabdomyosarcoma, and hemangiosarcoma. Occasionally, a squamous cell carcinoma has similar microscopic features and is called a *sarcoma, spindle cell carcinoma,* or *pseudosarcoma.* Cancers that originate in the minor salivary gland, including adenocarcinoma, adenoid cystic carcinoma, and mucoepidermoid carcinoma, comprise less than 1% of all laryngeal cancers.[20] Rarely, primary anaplastic small cell carcinomas may occur as well.[21]

Regional cervical metastasis relates to the anatomic site of the tumor and its differentiation. Highly differentiated tumors, such as verrucous cancers, never metastasize. As the degree of differentiation of the tumor decreases, the rate of metastasis increases. Because of a paucity of lymphatics in the region of the vocal cords, tumors of the glottic larynx have a much lower rate of metastasis than do those occurring in the supraglottic larynx, subglottic larynx, or hypopharynx. Cancers that are confined to the glottis have a low metastatic rate, whereas the rate of metastasis in the inferior hypopharyngeal cancers may reach 80%. There may be a long interval between recognition of the primary tumor in the larynx and pharynx and the recognition of metastasis. The most frequent sites for distant metastasis are the mediastinum and the lung, with the liver, bone, and brain being affected less often.

## SYMPTOMS

Hoarseness is the foremost symptom of laryngeal cancer. The degree of hoarseness depends on the amount of interference with vocal cord function. Since the quality of the voice can be affected by small irregularities of the vocal cord margin, glottic cancers become symptomatic early. The more distant the tumor is from the vocal cords, the larger it will grow before it becomes symptomatic. Supraglottic cancers may cause hoarseness by fixation of the arytenoid cartilages, but typically the voice remains remarkably clear. Because invasion of the recurrent nerve paralyzes the vocal cords, infraglottic tumors tend to produce hoarseness. Characteristically, dyspnea and stridor are later symptoms of glottic and infraglottic tumors. These airway obstructions are caused by the sheer bulk of the tumor, which blocks the airway lumen, and are usually associated with the fixation of one or both vocal cords.

Pain is more characteristic of hypopharyngeal and supraglottic cancers because of their tendencies toward ulcerative growth patterns. Often the patient first feels pain in the ear on the side of the tumor. This referred pain arc is transmitted by the vagus nerve, which has a sensory branch to the tympanic membrane as well as a sensory distribution to the hypopharynx and supraglottic portion of the larynx. The intensity of the pain ranges from slight irritation to severe lancinating pain on swallowing.

Dysphagia may stem from the simple mechanical interference with food transit caused by lesions in the postcricoid region or inferior hypopharynx. Generally, however, difficulty in swallowing is related to mild aspiration because the sphincteric actions of the larynx during swallowing are compromised by the tumor. Significant hemoptysis is uncommon with such tumors, although saliva may be streaked with blood, particularly in cases of large ulcerative tumors.

The occurrence of an asymptomatic metastatic neck mass is typical of a piriform sinus cancer. As with all neck masses of possible metastatic origin, it is imperative, whenever possible, to identify the primary cancer and include it in the initial treatment plan.

## PHYSICAL EXAMINATION

Inspection and palpation of the larynx are highly important measures, inasmuch as irregularity or tenderness of the laryngeal cartilage suggests cartilage invasion or possible perichondritis. The larynx normally produces crepitus on lateral motion across the cervical spine. The absence of this crepitus suggests a tumor near the cricoid cartilage or metastatic involvement of the retropharyngeal lymph nodes. Complete palpation of the neck should be carried out to determine the presence of metastatic adenopathy. Laryngeal and hypopharyngeal metastases can occur in the anterior cervical triangle opposite the hyoid bone. Another group of nodes that may be involved, particularly for intrinsic laryngeal tumors, are those located over the cricothyroid membrane and anterior trachea.

The examination of the endolarynx is accomplished indirectly with a mirror. The visible hypopharynx, the base of the tongue, and the larynx are scanned systematically, with attention directed toward the mobility of the vocal cords, the visible portion of the subglottic space, the symmetry of the arytenoid cartilages, and the cricopharyngeal inlet. To permit adequate examination in a patient with a hyperactive gag response, a local anesthetic spray, such as 2% lidocaine, may be necessary. Inspection of the larynx, particularly the region of the anterior commissure, may be facilitated by use of a narrow-rod lens system that can be adapted for still and video photography.[22]

Another method of examining the larynx in an outpatient setting, particularly in a patient with an active gag reflex, is transnasal fiberoptic laryngoscopy. Although this visualization instrument does not have the magnification and bright illumination of the rod lens system, it almost always provides a comfortable view of the larynx and is easily adaptable to video documentation.

Prior to biopsy of a laryngeal or hypopharyngeal tumor, it is often advisable to perform CT or magnetic resonance imaging (MRI).[23] These techniques provide a permanent record of the extent of the tumor, which is pertinent information for use in the radiation therapy plan. CT is most helpful in assessing the submucosal extent of disease. One can often detect depth of laryngeal muscle invasion as well as involvement of laryngeal cartilage by tumor. Another valuable result of CT is assessment of deep cervical lymph nodes that may be enlarged by metastatic disease but, because of insufficient size or inaccessible location, cannot be examined manually. CT and MRI have contributed significantly to allow more precise anatomic delineation of laryngopharyngeal tumors, which is essential in partial organ surgery.

Direct laryngoscopy is usually employed to obtain tissue for diagnosis and then to corroborate the findings of indirect and radiographic studies. This examination may be performed with either local or general anesthesia. Local anesthesia is accomplished by the topical application of a 4% cocaine solution to the base of the tongue, piriform fossa, and laryngeal vestibule. This is usually supplemented by regional blockade of the glossopharyngeal and superior laryngeal nerves by direct injection of 2% lidocaine.[24] General anesthesia is used more commonly and is indicated whenever maximal relaxation of the laryngeal muscles is required, such as when vocal cord stripping or other endoscopic procedures are indicated, for example, esophagoscopy. When general anesthesia is used, a small endotracheal tube (5.5 to 6.5F) is placed in the posterior commissure for ventilation. The narrowness and flexibility of the tube permit a thorough examination of the entire aerodigestive tract.

Microscopic examination of biopsy tissue is mandatory before any therapeutic measures are undertaken because many lesions of the larynx and pharynx can simulate cancer. Granulomatous infections of the larynx, such as tuberculosis, coccidioidomycosis, and blastomycosis, may grossly resemble cancer, although these infections have a predilection to involve the posterior commissure. Whenever an infection is suspected, the biopsy tissue should be submitted for culture and special staining as well as for routine staining. Papillomas may be solitary and begin de novo in the adult; however, because of their characteristic microscopic appearance, they are rarely difficult to differentiate from cancer. A biopsy should be performed for chronic traumatic lesions of the vocal cords, such as contact ulcers, vocal nodules, and polyps, particularly if the lesion does not respond to voice rest and if the patient is a smoker.

Biopsy specimens should be generous and should include the submucosa. A small superficial biopsy specimen of an exophytic well-differentiated cancer is insufficient for diagnosis by the pathologist. Indeed, to determine histologic invasion, penetration through the basement membrane must be seen. Sometimes this is not evident despite obtaining numerous deep biopsy specimens of a verrucous carcinoma, and the diagnosis must be made on the basis of the tumor's gross appearance and growth pattern.

Detection of residual cancer in the irradiated larynx and pharynx can be difficult, inasmuch as only small nests of tumor may remain after irradiation. The possibility of this situation increases when there is persistent asymmetric edema or ulceration several months after irradiation.[25] In many instances, multiple, sequential biopsies are necessary to document the presence of residual cancer. Sometimes the postirradiation course is indicative of persistent tumor even if biopsy confirmation is lacking.

## STAGING

The TNM staging system for these tumors is shown in Tables 65–1 and 65–2. Table 65–1 provides the details of the tumor definition for the tumors in this anatomic region and Table 65–2 summarizes the node and metastatic classification and the recommended stage groups.[26]

# Treatment

The treatment of carcinoma of the larynx and hypopharynx has long been controversial, but there is little doubt that radiation therapy and surgery must be closely integrated.

*Table 65–1.* **Classification of Laryngeal and Hypopharyngeal Carcinomas Definition of TNM**

*Primary Tumor (T)*

| | |
|---|---|
| TX | Primary tumor cannot be assessed |
| T0 | No evidence of primary tumor |
| Tis | Carcinoma in situ |

*Supraglottis*

| | |
|---|---|
| T1 | Tumor limited to one subsite of the supraglottis with normal vocal cord mobility* |
| T2 | Tumor invades more than one subsite of supraglottis or glottis, with normal vocal cord mobility |
| T3 | Tumor limited to the larynx with vocal cord fixation and/or invades the postcricoid area, medial wall of the pyriform sinus, or pre-epiglottic tissues |
| T4 | Tumor invades through the thyroid cartilage and/or extends to other tissues beyond the larynx (e.g., to the oropharynx or soft tissues of the neck) |

*Glottis*

| | |
|---|---|
| T1 | Tumor limited to the vocal cord(s) (may involve anterior or posterior commissures) with normal mobility |
| T1a | Tumor limited to one vocal cord |
| T1b | Tumor involves both vocal cords |
| T2 | Tumor extends to the supraglottis and/or subglottis, and/or with impaired vocal cord mobility |
| T3 | Tumor limited to the larynx with vocal cord fixation |
| T4 | Tumor invades through the thyroid cartilage and/or extends to other tissues beyond the larynx (e.g., to the oropharynx or soft tissues of the neck) |

*Subglottis*

| | |
|---|---|
| T1 | Tumor limited to the subglottis |
| T2 | Tumor extends to vocal cord(s) with normal or impaired mobility |
| T3 | Tumor limited to the larynx with vocal cord fixation |
| T4 | Tumor invades through the cricoid or thyroid cartilage and/or extends to other tissues beyond the larynx (e.g., to the oropharynx or soft tissues of the neck) |

*Hypopharynx*

| | |
|---|---|
| T1 | Tumor limited to one subsite of hypopharynx* |
| T2 | Tumor invades more than one subsite of hypopharynx or an adjacent site, without fixation of hemilarynx |
| T3 | Tumor invades more than one subsite of hypopharynx or an adjacent site, with fixation of hemilarynx |
| T4 | Tumor invades adjacent structures (e.g., cartilage or soft tissues of neck) |

*Defined by the anatomic boundaries described in the text.
From Beahrs OH, Henson DE, Hutter RVP, Kennedy BJ, eds. Manual for staging of cancer. 4th ed. Philadelphia: JB Lippincott, 1992:34, 40. Reproduced by permission of the American Joint Committee on Cancer and the publisher.

Irradiation may be used (1) as a primary curative modality, either alone or in combination with chemotherapy; (2) as a planned part of combined therapy before or after surgery; or (3) for palliation. Surgery may also be used to achieve any of these three therapeutic goals. Chemotherapy is increasingly used as an adjunct to radiation therapy to conserve the larynx, as discussed in Chapter 66.

The selection of a specific type of therapy is best evaluated in concert by a surgeon, radiation therapist, and medical oncologist. Considerations must include the patient's age, occupational and social needs for precise vocalization, ease of laryngeal and hypopharyngeal evaluation, personal habits (such as smoking and the degree of alcohol consumption),

*Table 65–2.* **Node (N) and Metastasis (M) Classification and Stage Grouping for Carcinomas of the Larynx and Hypopharynx**

*Regional Lymph Nodes (N)*

| | |
|---|---|
| NX | Regional lymph nodes cannot be assessed |
| N0 | No regional lymph node metastasis |
| N1 | Metastasis in a single ipsilateral lymph node, 3 cm or less in greatest dimension |
| N2 | Metastasis in a single ipsilateral lymph node, more than 3 cm but not more than 6 cm in greatest dimension; or, in multiple ipsilateral lymph nodes, none more than 6 cm in greatest dimension; or, in bilateral or contralateral lymph nodes, none more than 6 cm in greatest dimension |
| N2a | Metastasis in a single ipsilateral lymph node more than 3 cm but not more than 6 cm in greatest dimension |
| N2b | Metastasis in multiple ipsilateral lymph nodes, none more than 6 cm in greatest dimension |
| N2c | Metastasis in bilateral or contralateral lymph nodes, none more than 6 cm in greatest dimension |
| N3 | Metastasis in a lymph node more than 6 cm in greatest dimension |

*Distant Metastasis (M)*

| | |
|---|---|
| MX | Presence of distant metastasis cannot be assessed |
| M0 | No distant metastasis |
| M1 | Distant metastasis |

*Stage Grouping*

| | | | |
|---|---|---|---|
| Stage 0 | Tis | N0 | M0 |
| Stage I | T1 | N0 | M0 |
| Stage II | T2 | N0 | M0 |
| Stage III | T3 | N0 | M0 |
| | T1 | N1 | M0 |
| | T2 | N1 | M0 |
| | T3 | N1 | M0 |
| Stage IV | T4 | N0 | M0 |
| | T4 | N1 | M0 |
| | Any T | N2 | M0 |
| | Any T | N3 | M0 |
| | Any T | Any N | M1 |

From Beahrs OH, Henson DE, Hutter RVP, Kennedy BJ, eds. Manual for staging of cancer. 4th ed. Philadelphia: JB Lippincott, 1992:34–5, 41. Reproduced by permission of the American Joint Committee on Cancer and the publisher.

general health, family support, and a number of other factors. Ideally, the treatment decision is discussed in an open forum by physicians who have a special interest in head and neck cancer. A synopsis of the treatment options is then presented to the patient, who should participate in the final decision regarding treatment.

## GLOTTIC CANCER

Tumors of the glottis tend to be well differentiated and slow growing, usually arising in the anterior half of the membranous vocal cord. They can extend anteriorly to the anterior commissure and involve the opposite vocal cord, or they can extend posteriorly to involve the vocal process and arytenoid cartilages. Extension to the anterior commissure is accompanied by an increased frequency of laryngeal cartilage involvement, whereas posterior extension can cause invasion of the cricoid lamina. The progressive growth of a vocal cord cancer inevitably invades the vocal and thyroarytenoid muscles and then limits the mobility of the vocal cord. Fixation of the cord results from substantial invasion of these glottic muscles, from the tumor bulk extending to

the thyroid lamina, and from tumor involvement of the recurrent nerve.[27] Tumor extending more than 1 cm below the glottis often accompanies the invasion of the cricothyroid membrane and the body of the cricoid cartilage.

The lymphatics of the glottis are sparse, and T1 cancers have an extremely low incidence of metastasis (2%). T2 and T3 cancers, which extend to the arytenoid cartilage and subglottic regions, have a metastatic rate of up to 13%, and the node most frequently involved is the Delphian node, which overlies the cricothyroid membrane.

Considerable difference of opinion remains regarding the treatment of carcinoma in situ or microinvasive cancer of the vocal cords. Decortication (stripping) of the vocal cord under the operative microscope and close observation to detect any evidence of recurrence are measures that incur the least morbidity.[28, 29] Radiation therapy is also effective in eradicating this tumor. Doyle and colleagues[30] advise complete stripping of the vocal cord, followed 1 month later by biopsy. If there is any evidence of cancer in the biopsy specimen, irradiation is begun. Miller[31] favors immediate cordectomy via laryngofissure, whereas DeSanto[32] performs a cordectomy via suspension microlaryngoscopy. Small cordal cancers have also been effectively managed by endoscopic carbon dioxide laser excision.[33]

Radiation therapy is almost universally considered the primary treatment modality for invasive T1 and selected T2 cancers of the vocal cord. Small treatment volumes are used to minimize injury to the larynx. Doses of approximately 65 Gy are delivered in 6.5 to 8 weeks. Cure rates with irradiation for these glottic tumors are approximately 90%, with partial laryngectomy being reserved for treatment failures.

With extension to the anterior commissure or arytenoid cartilages, the prognosis worsens for both surgery and irradiation. Some clinicians favor surgery for these lesions,[34, 35] whereas others prefer primary radiation therapy,[36] particularly when the cords remain fully mobile. Patients who have extensive T2 or T3 lesions with cordal fixation are generally considered to be surgical candidates to be treated by either vertical hemilaryngectomy (Fig. 65–2) or total laryngectomy. The extent of partial laryngectomy is tailored to the anatomic involvement by the tumor. Whenever a partial laryngectomy is planned, permission for total laryngectomy must be obtained before surgery is performed. The vertical hemilaryngectomy may include resection of the arytenoid cartilages or the anterior third of the opposite vocal cord, or both. Confirmation of tumor-free margins is determined at the time of surgery by frozen section examination prior to reconstruction and closure.

The goals of glottic reconstruction are (1) to provide a competent sphincter to prevent aspiration, (2) to construct a tissue ledge for phonation (pseudocord) that will ensure a smooth surface for approximation by the opposite vocal cord, and (3) to provide an adequate channel for respiration. Various reconstructive procedures have been described for reconstituting the function of the glottis.[37] Aspiration can generally be prevented by using tissue bulk in place of a resected arytenoid cartilage, and an adequate airway can be maintained by temporarily placing a keel in the anterior aspect of the larynx when the anterior portion of the opposite vocal cord has been resected. Indeed, if both arytenoid cartilages are preserved, at least the anterior half of both vocal cords can be resected for an extensive cancer of the

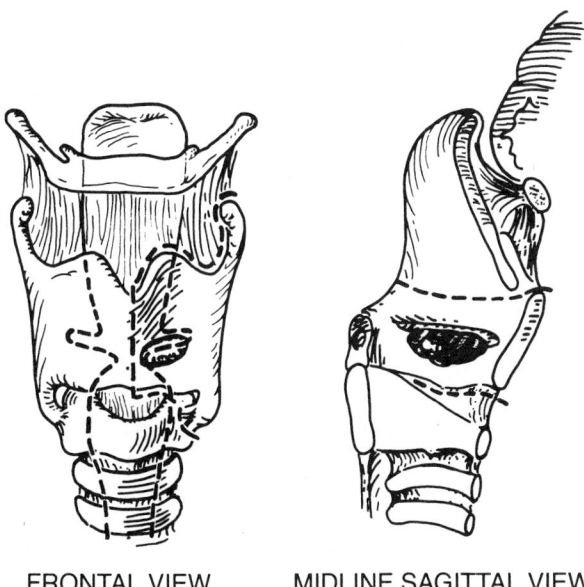

**FRONTAL VIEW**
Cartilage incisions
outlined

**MIDLINE SAGITTAL VIEW**
Mucosal incisions
outlined

**Figure 65–2.** Dotted lines indicate portion of larynx usually excised by horizontal supraglottic laryngectomy. (After Shumrick DA. Supraglottic laryngectomy: its place in the treatment of laryngeal cancer. Arch Otolaryngol 1969;89:629–35.)

anterior commissure.[38] It is important to emphasize that none of the various modifications of vertical hemilaryngectomy provides the same vocal quality as irradiation. However, in most instances, the voice is intelligible despite varying degrees of hoarseness.

When a glottic cancer involves the ventricle (transglottic) or extends below the level of the cricoid cartilage, total laryngectomy is necessary. Because transglottic tumors usually involve laryngeal cartilage, partial laryngeal surgery is inadequate for tumor removal. Resection of a substantial portion of the cricoid cartilage to attempt partial laryngectomy usually results in permanent subglottic stenosis that is inadequate for respiration. Because the incidence of cervical metastasis ranges from 30 to 50%, treatment of the neck is required—usually radical neck dissection that spares the spinal accessory nerve if it is completely free of tumor. In addition, the ipsilateral thyroid lobe is commonly removed because of possible tumor involvement. Postoperative irradiation is employed if the cancer extends outside the confines of the intrinsic larynx or if several nodes in the radical neck dissection contain metastatic tumor.

## SUPRAGLOTTIC CANCER

Supraglottic tumors tend to be exophytic and bulky, sometimes obscuring or hanging down over the vocal cords.[39] Often they invade the pre-epiglottic space, although there definitely appears to be a compartmentalization or barrier to downward involvement of the glottis. When the tumor extends outside the larynx and involves the vallecula, epiglottis, tongue base, or piriform sinus, it behaves more like a hypopharyngeal cancer.

The treatment of supraglottic cancer is usually surgical,

although primary radiation therapy of T1 epiglottic tumors and tumors of the aryepiglottic fold above the level of the hyoid bone (suprahyoid) has been successful.[40] The operation that is generally performed for these cancers is the supraglottic laryngectomy,[41] which is designed to spare the vocal cords by placing the inferior plane of the resection through the laryngeal ventricle just above the vocal cords (Fig. 65–3). This operation may be modified to resect tumors in different parts of the laryngeal vestibule and hypopharynx. The false vocal cords, epiglottis, and entire pre-epiglottic space are typically included in the resection. The resultant defect is closed with a perichondral flap from the thyroid cartilage. Because the incidence of cervical metastasis exceeds 30%, bilateral modified neck dissections are usually performed concomitantly, sparing the spinal accessory nerves and internal jugular veins whenever possible. The patient's primary postoperative handicap—a tendency toward aspiration because only the glottis remains to protect the airway—can be minimized by suspending the laryngeal remnant to the suprahyoid muscles, well under the base of the tongue, to serve as a ledge to cover the laryngeal inlet.[42]

Supracricoid laryngectomy is a voice conservation surgery that is appropriate for select supraglottic and transglottic cancers that would not otherwise be amenable to partial laryngectomy.[43] The indications for this procedure are carcinomas of the supraglottis that involve the glottis and anterior commissure, invade the ventricle, present with a marked limitation of true vocal cord mobility, or invade the thyroid cartilage. This surgery allows resection of the whole thyroid cartilage and paraglottic space, as well as the epiglottis and the whole pre-epiglottic space. The cricoid cartilage, the hyoid bone, and at least one arytenoid cartilage are spared, and the resulting defect is repaired by pexy of the cricoid cartilage to the hyoid bone.

Preoperative or postoperative radiation therapy is frequently used in patients with supraglottic carcinoma. Postop-

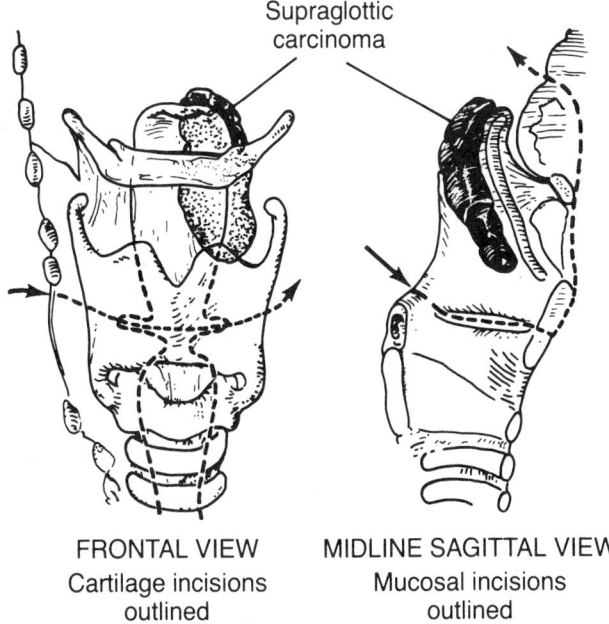

**FRONTAL VIEW**
Cartilage incisions
outlined

**MIDLINE SAGITTAL VIEW**
Mucosal incisions
outlined

**Figure 65–3.** Dotted lines indicate portion of the larynx typically excised by vertical hemilaryngectomy.

erative radiation is particularly valuable in treating close margins or patients with regional metastases. Supraglottic laryngectomy after full-dose irradiation is hazardous because of the high incidence of wound dehiscence and carotid artery rupture resulting from impaired wound healing induced by radiation. Therefore, total laryngectomy is usually necessary for supraglottic cancers that recur after previous radiation therapy.

The prognosis for supraglottic cancers varies according to the site, size, gross configuration, and histologic type. Patients with small (<2 cm) tumors involving the free border of the epiglottis (suprahyoid) have a 5-year survival rate that exceeds 80%.[44] Infiltrative and less well differentiated tumors (particularly those extending to the thyroid cartilage, base of tongue, and piriform sinuses) have a worse prognosis, with 5-year survival rates being in the range of 35 to 50%.

## SUBGLOTTIC CANCER

Subglottic tumors constitute 5 to 10% of all laryngeal cancers.[45] They can grow to a large size before becoming symptomatic, inasmuch as stridor is usually the patient's presenting complaint. There is a relatively high incidence of paratracheal node metastasis (60%).

The treatment of subglottic cancer is total laryngectomy followed by radiation. It is particularly important that the trachea be transected well below the tumor because the mucosal lymphatics spread downward. The surgical resection may be extended to the sixth tracheal ring, including amputation of the manubrium so that the tracheal stoma can be exteriorized without tension.[46]

Both the cervical node dissection and postoperative radiation are directed toward the paratracheal lymphatics, which are the primary source of recurrent disease. In selected low subglottic cancers and recurrent tumors at the stoma, mediastinal resection has been attempted with some success, although the prognosis remains poor.[47]

## HYPOPHARYNGEAL CANCER

Hypopharyngeal tumors usually arise in the piriform sinuses (tending to be large when first discovered), or they may be heralded by a metastatic neck mass.[48] The lymphatics of the piriform sinus are profuse, and therefore the incidence of cervical metastasis, including contralateral metastasis, is high.

Since small lesions are almost never identified, radiation therapy is used as an adjunctive modality; likewise, surgery is rarely used alone as treatment. The choice of surgery varies with the anatomic extent of the tumor. When the tumor is confined to the lateral or anterior wall of the piriform sinus, the glottis can be preserved, with resection of almost all the piriform sinus in selected instances.[49] Since there is a tendency for submucosal extension, surgical margins around the visible tumor must be at least 2 cm in diameter. When the tumor involves the medial wall of the piriform sinus and the arytenoid cartilage, extends to the piriform sinus apex, or invades the posterior wall of the pharynx, a total laryngectomy is usually necessary. Almost

all surgery for piriform sinus cancers involves an ipsilateral cervical node dissection, including removal of nodes in the retropharyngeal area.

Radiation is usually used postoperatively. Such therapy is preferable because it can be planned according to the findings of the surgical specimen. If any surgical margins of the specimen are close to the tumor, irradiation can be boosted to the appropriate area. Moreover, the incidence of wound healing complications is lower with postoperative irradiation.

The prognosis for piriform sinus cancers is generally unfavorable, and the only improved survival statistics have been demonstrated with combined therapy.[50] The analysis of failures typically shows that distant metastasis or recurrent neck disease developed.

Hypopharyngeal tumors, which may also occur in the region of the cricoid cartilage and esophageal inlet, likewise have a poor prognosis because of an early tendency to spread into the mediastinum via retropharyngeal lymphatics or submucosal extension. Radiation therapy is often used, but if it is used alone, the percentage of 5-year survivors is low (5 to 10%). Because the circumference of the pharynx is narrow at the cricoid level, surgical therapy often necessitates resection of most or all the pharynx in addition to laryngectomy.

When there is insufficient tissue to reconstitute the pharyngeal lumen, it is either reconstructed with regional skin flaps or immediately replaced with a free flap or transposed part of the gastrointestinal tract, such as the stomach or large intestine. Reconstruction of the pharynx after subtotal laryngopharyngectomy can be accomplished in a single-stage operation using a pectoralis myocutaneous flap. This flap may be used in conjunction with a dermal graft.[51] The immediate replacement of the pharynx and esophagus at the time of resection using a gastric pull-up or colon interposition flap can be a formidable operation that incurs significant morbidity and mortality, but when successful, it has the advantage of rapidly re-establishing the ability to swallow.[52] Jejunal free flaps and radial forearm free flaps, which use microvascular anastomoses, have also been performed successfully to reconstruct circumferential defects of the hypopharynx, with a lower incidence of perioperative morbidity and mortality when compared with pedicled visceral flaps.[53–55] With these types of extensive surgery, it is beneficial to use postoperative radiation rather than preoperative radiation to maximize healing.

The posterior pharyngeal wall extends from the level of the soft palate to the arytenoid cartilages. Cancers in this region are difficult to cure even if they do not grow large.[50] They tend to spread along the prevertebral fascia and sometimes manifest "skip" areas. Bilateral cervical node metastasis, as well as retropharyngeal node involvement, is particularly common. Surgery combined with radiation is the treatment of choice for these cancers and is usually performed without sacrificing the larynx. The defect may be repaired with a radial forearm free flap.[54] Postoperative radiation should be used to control any surgically untreated neck at risk to harbor occult metastases and to sterilize the region adjacent to the primary tumor. The 5-year prognosis for these tumors, even with combined therapy, is about 5 to 25%.

## ORGAN PRESERVATION PROTOCOLS

Since the early 1990s, there have been increasing efforts to avoid total laryngectomy for patients with advanced laryngeal and hypopharyngeal cancers. Induction or concurrent chemotherapy in conjunction with radiation therapy has been tried, as has hyperfractionation radiation therapy. The largest randomized study to date was reported by Wolf and Hong in patients with operable stage III and stage IV laryngeal cancer.[56] This study showed nearly equal survival rates for induction chemotherapy plus radiation therapy with surgical salvage of treatment failures, when compared with total laryngectomy followed by radiation therapy as the primary treatment. Overall, 64% of patients enrolled in the chemoradiation arm of the study retained their larynges for the duration of the follow-up period. In a follow-up study of organ preservation in patients with stage II to stage IV hypopharyngeal cancer, overall survival was again shown to be similar when comparing chemoradiation with combined surgery and radiation therapy, although the rate of laryngeal preservation was somewhat lower (42%) in the chemoradiation group.[57] This approach to management is discussed further in Chapter 66.

## SUGGESTIONS FOR ADDITIONAL READING

Maciejewski B. Regression rate of metastatic neck lymph nodes after radiation treatment as a prognostic factor for local control. Radiother Oncol 1987;8:301–8. *Complete regression at the end of treatment correlated strongly with local control.*

Stalpers LJA, Verbeek ALM, van Daal WAJ. Results of radiotherapy and surgery for glottic carcinoma. Cancer Treat Rev 1987;14:131–41. *This article provides a detailed review.*

The Department of Veterans Affairs Laryngeal Cancer Study Group: Induction chemotherapy plus radiation compared with surgery plus radiation in patients with advanced laryngeal cancer. N Engl J Med 1991;324:1685. *This randomized study involving 332 patients demonstrated equivalent survival but improved quality of life using chemotherapy plus radiation.*

## REFERENCES

1. Boring CC, Squires TS, Tong T. Cancer statistics, 1993. CA Cancer J Clin 1994;43:7–26.
2. Mansfield EL, Cote DN. Hypopharyngeal carcinoma. J La State Med Soc 1995;147:489–92.
3. Shumrick DA. Supraglottic laryngectomy: its place in the treatment of laryngeal cancer. Arch Otolaryngol 1969;89:629–35.
4. Silverberg E, Lubera JA. Cancer statistics, 1989. CA Cancer J Clin 1989;39:3–20.
5. Lowry WS. Alcoholism in cancer of the head and neck. Laryngoscope 1975;85:1275–80.
6. Tuyns AJ, Esteve J, Raymond L, et al. Cancer of the larynx/hypopharynx, tobacco and alcohol: IARC international case-control study in Turin and Varese (Italy), Zaragoza and Navarra (Spain), Geneva (Switzerland) and Calvados (France). Int J Cancer 1988;41:483–91.
7. Muscat JE, Wynder EL. Tobacco, alcohol, asbestos, and occupational risk factors for laryngeal cancer. Cancer 1992;69:2244–51.
8. Auerbach O, Hammond EC, Garfinkel L. Histologic changes in the larynx in relation to smoking habits. Cancer 1970;25:92–104.
9. Flanders WD, Rothman KJ. Interaction of alcohol and tobacco in laryngeal cancer. Am J Epidemiol 1982;115:371–9.
10. Burch JD, Howe GR, Miller AB, Semenciw R. Tobacco, alcohol, asbestos, and nickel in the etiology of cancer of the larynx: a case-control study. J Natl Cancer Inst 1981;67:1219–24.
11. Brown LM, Mason TJ, Pickle LW, et al. Occupational risk factors for laryngeal cancer on the Texas Gulf Coast. Cancer Res 1988;48:1960–4.
12. Blackwell KE, Calcaterra TC, Fu YS. Laryngeal dysplasia: epidemiology and treatment outcome. Ann Otol Rhinol Laryngol 1995;104:596–602.
13. Sheinin R. Viruses: causative agents of cancer. Laryngoscope 1975;85:468–86.
14. Kiaris H, Ergazaki M, Segas J, Spandidos DA. Detection of Epstein-Barr virus genome in squamous cell carcinomas of the larynx. Int J Biol Markers 1995;10:211–5.
15. Brandsma JL, Steinberg BM, Abramson AL, Winkler B. Presence of human papillomavirus type 16 related sequences in verrucous carcinoma of the larynx. Cancer Res 1986;46:2185–88.
16. Malan JF, Sellars SL, Kranold D. A critical review of hypopharyngeal carcinomas—1975–1985. S Afr J Surg 1993;31:74–8.
17. Elias MM, Hilgers FJ, Keus RB, et al. Carcinoma of the pyriform sinus: a retrospective analysis of treatment results over a 20-year period. Clin Otolaryngol 1995;20:249–53.
18. Archer CR, Yeager VL, Herbold DR. Improved diagnostic accuracy in the TNM staging of laryngeal cancer using a new definition of regions based on computed tomography. J Comput Assist Tomogr 1983;7:610–7.
19. Blackwell KE, Fu YS, Calcaterra TC. Laryngeal dysplasia: a clinicopathologic study. Cancer 1995;75:457–63.
20. Alavi S, Namazie A, Calcaterra TC, Blackwell KE. Glandular carcinoma of the larynx: the UCLA experience. Ann Otol Rhinol Laryngol 1999;108:485–9.
21. Gnepp DR, Ferlito A, Hyams V. Primary anaplastic small cell (oat cell) carcinoma of the larynx: review of the literature and report of 18 cases. Cancer 1983;51:1731–45.
22. Berci G, Calcaterra T, Ward PH. Advances in endoscopic techniques for examination of the larynx and nasopharynx. Can J Otolaryngol 1975;4:768–92.
23. Williams DW. Imaging of laryngeal cancer. Otolaryngol Clin North Am 1997;30:35–58.
24. Calcaterra TC, House J. Local anesthesia for suspension microlaryngoscopy. Ann Otol Rhinol Laryngol 1976;85:71–3.
25. Calcaterra TC, Stern F, Ward PH. Dilemma of delayed radiation injury of the larynx. Ann Otol Rhinol Laryngol 1972;81:501–7.
26. Beahrs OH, Henson DE, Hutter RVP, Kennedy BJ, eds. Manual for staging of cancer. 4th ed. Philadelphia: JB Lippincott, 1992.
27. Kessler DJ, Trapp TK, Calcaterra TC. The treatment of T3 glottic carcinoma with vertical partial laryngectomy. Arch Otolaryngol Head Neck Surg 1987;113:1196–9.
28. Bauer WC, McGavran MH. Carcinoma in situ and evaluation of epithelial changes in laryngopharyngeal biopsies. JAMA 1972;221:72–5.
29. Altmann F, Ginsberg I, Stout AP. Intraepithelial carcinoma (cancer in situ) of the larynx. Arch Otolaryngol 1952;56:121–33.
30. Doyle PJ, Flores A, Douglas GS. Carcinoma in situ of the larynx. Laryngoscope 1977;87:310–6.
31. Miller AH. Carcinoma in situ of the larynx—clinical appearance and treatment. Can J Otol Rhinol Laryngol 1974;3:567–72.
32. DeSanto LW. Selection of treatment for in situ and early invasive carcinoma of the glottis. Can J Otol Rhinol Laryngol 1974;3:552–6.
33. Eckel HE, Thumfart WF. Laser surgery for the treatment of larynx carcinomas: indications, techniques, and preliminary results. Ann Otol Rhinol Laryngol 1992;101:113–8.
34. Kirchner JA, Som ML. The anterior commissure technique of partial laryngectomy: clinical and laboratory observations. Laryngoscope 1975;85:1308–17.
35. Wang MB, Lavey RS, Calcaterra TC. Efficacy and morbidity of partial laryngectomy and postoperative radiation therapy. Laryngoscope 1990;100:1146–51.
36. Wang CC. Factors influencing the success of radiation therapy for T2 and T3 glottic carcinomas. Importance of cord mobility and sex. Am J Clin Oncol 1986;9:517–20.
37. Strasnick B. Regional flaps for reconstruction following conservation laryngeal surgery. Facial Plast Surg 1989;6:251–64.
38. Reino AJ, Lee HY, Lawson W, et al. Management of bilateral glottic tumors. Arch Otolaryngol Head Neck Surg 1997;123:465–73.
39. Kirchner JA, Som ML. Clinical and histological observations on supraglottic cancer. Ann Otol Rhinol Laryngol 1971;80:638–45.
40. Fletcher GH, Jessie RH, Lindberg RD, Koons CR. The place of radiotherapy in the management of the squamous cell carcinoma of the supraglottic larynx. Am J Roentgenol Radium Ther Nuclear Med 1970;108:19–26.
41. Calcaterra TC. Supraglottic laryngectomy with preservation of laryngeal function. Am Surg 1971;37:393–6.
42. Calcaterra TC. Laryngeal suspension after supraglottic laryngectomy. Arch Otolaryngol 1971;94:306–9.
43. Laccourreye H, Laccourreye O, Weinstein G, et al. Supracricoid laryngectomy with cricohyoidopexy: a partial laryngeal procedure for se-

lected supraglottic and transglottic carcinomas. Laryngoscope 1990;100:735–41.

44. Burstein FD, Calcaterra TC. Supraglottic laryngectomy: series report and analysis of results. Laryngoscope 1985;95:833–6.

45. Harrison DFN. The pathology and management of subglottic cancer. Ann Otol Rhinol Laryngol 1971;80:6–12.

46. Harris HH, Butler E. Surgical limits in cancer of the subglottic larynx. Arch Otolaryngol 1968;87:490–3.

47. Hosal IN, Onerci M, Turan E. Peristomal recurrence. Am J Otolaryngol 1993;14:206–8.

48. Kirchner JA. Pyriform sinus cancer: a clinical and laboratory study. Ann Otol Rhinol Laryngol 1975;84:793–803.

49. Ogura JH, Jurema AA, Watson RK. Partial laryngopharyngectomy and neck dissection for pyriform sinus cancer. Laryngoscope 1960;70:1399–1417.

50. Briant TDR, Bryce DP, Smith TJ. Carcinoma of the hypopharynx—a five year follow-up. J Otolaryngol 1977;6:353–62.

51. Fabian R. Pectoralis major myocutaneous flap reconstruction of the laryngopharynx and cervical esophagus. Laryngoscope 1988;98:1227–31.

52. Silver CE. Reconstruction after pharyngolaryngectomy-esophagectomy. Am J Surg 1976;132;428–34.

53. Coleman JJ, Searles JM, Hester TR, et al. Ten years experience with the free jejunal autograft. Am J Surg 1987;154:394–8.

54. Harii K, Ebihara S, Ono I, et al. Pharyngoesophageal reconstruction using a fabricated forearm free flap. Plast Reconstr Surg 1985;75:463–74.

55. Surkin MI, Lawson W, Biller HF. Analysis of the methods of pharyngoesophageal reconstruction. Head Neck 6:953–70, 1984.

56. Wolf GT, Hong WK. Induction chemotherapy for organ preservation in advanced laryngeal cancer: is there a role? Head Neck 1995;17:279–83.

57. Lefebvre JL, Chevalier C, Luboinski B, et al. Larynx preservation in pyriform sinus cancer: preliminary results of a European Organization for Research and Treatment of Cancer phase III trial: EORTC Head and Neck Cancer Cooperative Group. J Natl Cancer Inst 1996;88:890–9.

# CHAPTER 66

# CHEMOTHERAPY OF HEAD AND NECK CANCER

• MAURA L. GILLISON • ARLENE A. FORASTIERE

Squamous cell carcinomas of the oral cavity, pharynx, and larynx constitute most of the approximately 45,000 new cases of head and neck cancer diagnosed annually in the United States. Data from the Cancer Statistics branch of the National Cancer Institute indicate that there was no significant change in the relative 5-year survival of patients over the period from 1960 to 1993 (Table 66–1).[1] Despite improvements in surgery and radiotherapy techniques, the aggressive use of these local therapies has not altered survival rates.

Surgery or radiation therapy has been the standard of care for patients with head and neck squamous cell carcinoma (HNSCC). Local therapy with surgery or radiation has achieved cure rates of approximately 80% in patients with stage I disease and 60% in patients with stage II disease. Most head and neck cancer patients, however, present with locally advanced, stage III or IV disease. Treatment of this patient population with local surgery, or radiotherapy, or both is associated with poor long-term survival because of local recurrence and development of distant metastasis. Multimodality therapy, coordinated by a multidisciplinary team of medical oncologists, radiation oncologists, and head and neck surgeons, has evolved in an attempt to improve local disease control and decrease the incidence of distant metastases.

The role of chemotherapy in the treatment of HNSCC is being increasingly defined. Prior to the 1990s, this role was limited to the palliative care of patients with advanced or recurrent disease. Since the identification of effective combination regimens in this patient population, medical oncologists have had greater involvement in the care of patients with earlier stage disease. Cisplatin and 5-fluorouracil (5-FU) combination chemotherapy, currently the most frequently used and efficacious regimen, has been incorporated into the initial curative treatment of newly diagnosed patients with the goal of improving survival and preserving organ function. In the 1990s, neoadjuvant chemotherapy followed by radiation therapy was shown to preserve organ function successfully in patients with cancer of the larynx and hypopharynx. Concurrent chemoradiotherapy has improved local control and survival for patients with locally advanced nasopharyngeal cancer. At other sites in the head and neck, concurrent chemoradiotherapy has shown promise in the treatment of patients with local-regional, advanced disease and as adjuvant therapy for the postsurgical patient at high risk for recurrence.

*Table 66–1.* **Survival Trends by Site**

| | 5-Year Relative Survival by Year of Diagnosis | | | | |
|---|---|---|---|---|---|
| | 1960–1963 | 1970–1973 | 1974–1976 | 1980–1982 | 1986–1993 |
| *Oral Cavity and Pharynx* | | | | | |
| White | 45 | 43 | 55 | 54 | 55 |
| Black | NA | NA | 36 | 32 | 34 |
| *Larynx* | | | | | |
| White | 53 | 62 | 66 | 69 | 69 |
| Black | NA | NA | 59 | 59 | 54 |

NA, data not available.
Modified from Landis S, Murray T, Bolden S, Wingo P. Cancer statistics, 1998. CA Cancer J Clin 1998;48:6.

## Systemic Therapy for Locally Recurrent, Persistent, or Metastatic Disease

### SINGLE-AGENT CHEMOTHERAPY

Palliation of symptoms and prolongation of survival are the treatment goals when chemotherapy is used for recurrent

*Table 66–2.* **Single Agents with Activity in Recurrent Head and Neck Squamous Cell Carcinoma**

| Agent | No. Patients | Response Rate (%) | Reference |
|---|---|---|---|
| Methotrexate | 988 | 31 | 2 |
| Weekly | 312 | 34 | 2,3 |
| Monthly | 107 | 29 | 3 |
| Cisplatin | 288 | 28 | 2 |
| Carboplatin | 169 | 22 | 2 |
| Bleomycin | 347 | 21 | 2 |
| 5-Fluorouracil | 118 | 15 | 2 |
| Ifosfamide | 99 | 26 | 4–6 |
| Paclitaxel | 33 | 40 | 7 |
| Docetaxel | 66 | 32 | 9 |
| Gemcitabine | 54 | 13 | 8 |

disease in which previous attempts at cure have failed. The agents with clearly demonstrated activity against HNSCC are listed in Table 66–2.[2–9] In general, the expected response rate for a single agent is in the 15 to 30% range. Tumor regression is usually brief in duration (i.e., 2 to 3 months), and responses are almost always partial. There is little impact on survival, which averages 6 months for this population.

Cisplatin, a platinum analogue that forms covalent bonds with DNA, remains the most useful single agent for head and neck cancer. The in vitro synergism of cisplatin with 5-FU and its radiosensitizing properties are important to its activity.[10] As a single agent in total doses ranging from 80 to 120 mg/m² every 3 to 4 weeks, the cumulative response rate is 28%.[2] Cisplatin may be administered as a single intravenous bolus every 3 to 4 weeks, weekly, or on 5 successive days. There is a pharmacokinetic advantage to a 5-day continuous infusion schedule versus 5-day intravenous bolus therapy. This schedule results in a doubling of tumor exposure to the non–protein-bound, active form of cisplatin.[11] Trials have not been performed, however, to determine whether this observed pharmacokinetic difference provides a therapeutic advantage. Most often, cisplatin is administered as a 100 mg/m² intravenous bolus every 3 weeks. Tumor regression is rapid and may be observed within 1 week of treatment. Peripheral neuropathy and ototoxicity are seen after cumulative doses of 400 mg/m² and affect nearly all patients to varying degrees after doses of 600 mg/m².

Because of cisplatin's treatment-limiting neurotoxicity, the analogue carboplatin was developed. Data pooled from phase II trials show carboplatin to have a response rate of 22%.[2] It appears to be less active than cisplatin, although no direct single-agent comparative study has been published. The major toxic effects are myelosuppression, leukopenia, and thrombocytopenia; the drug is administered every 4 weeks to allow marrow recovery. Doses of 400 mg/m² can be administered safely to patients with a creatinine clearance of at least 60 ml/min. Otherwise, the dose should be adjusted using formulas by Egorin and colleagues[12] or Calvert and colleagues,[13] which are based on the pharmacokinetics of carboplatin and account for altered drug elimination when renal function is impaired.

Methotrexate, a classic antifolate, has been used in various dosages and schedules. Weekly dosing appears superior to monthly loading.[14] Randomized trials comparing moder-

ate-dose or high-dose regimens with weekly dosing show higher overall response rates with high-dose regimens but no difference in complete response rates and survival.[15–17] Weekly intravenous dosing starting with 40 mg/m², with escalation by 5 to 10 mg/m²/wk to toxicity or response, is the recommended schedule.

Bleomycin, an antitumor antibiotic, may be administered by intravenous bolus or intramuscular injection once or twice a week or by continuous infusion. Because the drug is cell cycle phase specific, the continuous-infusion schedule may be more effective.[18] Bleomycin does not cause myelosuppression and was therefore an attractive agent for use in combination regimens, primarily in the late 1970s and early 1980s. Cumulative pulmonary toxicity proved treatment limiting.

5-FU, a thymidylate synthase inhibitor, has had limited testing as a single agent. Most data come from broad phase II trials using intermittent bolus dosing.[14, 19] A 15% response rate was reported in 75 assessable patients treated with a total dose of 4 g/m² given by continuous intravenous infusion over 96 hours.[20] 5-FU is most useful in combination with cisplatin and is rarely used as a single agent.

Ifosfamide, an alkylating agent, has undergone testing in patients with HNSCC. Response rates ranging from 6 to 43% have been reported in phase II studies.[4–6] Response appears to depend on the extent of previous treatment. The average dose of ifosfamide used together with the uroprotective agent mesna is 5 g/m².

The taxoids paclitaxel and docetaxel are the most active new agents for HNSCC since the discovery of cisplatin in 1968. Originally isolated from the bark of the Pacific yew *Taxus brevifolia*, paclitaxel affects cells in the $G_2/M$ phase by promoting microtubule assembly.[21] Phase II trials of single-agent paclitaxel have been completed. The Eastern Cooperative Oncology Group (ECOG) evaluated a 250-mg/m² dose administered as a 24-hour continuous infusion every 21 days.[7] In 33 patients with recurrent or metastatic squamous cancers, a 40% complete and partial response rate was observed. A trial of 175 mg/m² administered as a 3-hour infusion resulted in a 20% response rate in the same population of patients.[22] The most commonly observed toxicities include neutropenia, alopecia, and neuropathy. Paclitaxel is also a cell cycle–selective radiosensitizer and has been evaluated in combination with radiotherapy in many phase I and II trials. Continuous infusion (6.5 mg/m²/day), weekly (30 mg/m²/wk), and every-3-week (100 mg/m²) paclitaxel regimens have shown promise in this setting.[23]

Docetaxel, a more potent antimicrotubule agent in vitro than paclitaxel, has shown activity in HNSCC in two phase II trials. The European Organization for Research and Treatment of Cancer (EORTC) reported a trial of docetaxel 100 mg/m² administered every 21 days and observed an overall response in 12 of 37 (32%; 95% confidence interval [CI], 17 to 47) patients with advanced or recurrent HNSCC.[9] A response rate of 42% (95% CI; 24 to 60) with a median duration of response of 5 months was reported by other investigators using the same docetaxel regimen.[24] Other cytotoxic agents that are less well studied but have reported activity include doxorubicin (Adriamycin), vinblastine, cyclophosphamide, hydroxyurea,[2] and the newer agents vinorelbine and gemcitabine.[23]

## COMBINATION CHEMOTHERAPY

Combination regimens have been tested in patients with recurrent, persistent, or metastatic disease, with the goal of achieving higher overall response rates, more durable responses, and prolonged survival when compared with single-agent therapy. Many cisplatin-containing and non–cisplatin-containing regimens have shown promising activity in phase II trials. In 1984, the combination of cisplatin 100 mg/m$^2$ on day 1 and continuous-infusion 5-FU 1000 mg/m$^2$/day for 4 days administered every 21 days was reported to result in an overall response rate of 70% and a complete response rate of 27%.[25] At least a dozen phase II studies using this regimen have been published, and the cumulative response rate was 50%, with a range of 11 to 79%.[26] Several other chemotherapeutic agents have been added to this regimen and produced high response rates. These regimens include cisplatin, 5-FU, and leucovorin (56% overall response, 6% complete response);[27] cisplatin, 5-FU, and bleomycin (50% overall response, 5% complete response);[28] and cisplatin, 5-FU, bleomycin, and methotrexate (63% overall response, 7% complete response).[29]

Large, prospective randomized trials are needed to validate previous, preliminary observations of efficacy in single-institution trials. Randomized trials of promising combination regimens, including cisplatin plus 5-FU, compared with single agents are compiled in Table 66–3.[20, 30–39] Three large multicenter trials have reported statistically significant improvements in overall response rates for cisplatin plus 5-FU when compared with single agents.[20, 36, 38] All three studies reported similar overall response rates of approximately 32% and 6% complete response to the cisplatin plus 5-FU regimen. In one study, 249 patients with recurrent HNSCC were randomized to single-agent cisplatin, or 5-FU, or the combination. Response rates were 17%, 13%, and 32%, respectively.[20] Clavel and colleagues[38] reported an improved response rate when cisplatin plus 5-FU was compared to cisplatin alone. In another three-arm study randomizing 277 HNSCC patients, cisplatin plus 5-FU, but not carboplatin plus 5-FU, improved response rates over single-agent methotrexate (32% vs. 10%; $p<0.001$).[36]

Browman and Cronin[40] performed a meta-analysis of 15 trials comparing single-agent therapy with combination chemotherapy for recurrent or advanced HNSCC. Combination chemotherapy produced a statistically significant increase in response rates when compared with single-agent chemotherapy, and cisplatin plus 5-FU was more efficacious than other combinations. Improved response rates did not result in significant improvements in survival over single-agent therapy in this meta-analysis.[40] The addition of other agents to the cisplatin plus 5-FU regimen was associated with greater toxicity and did not improve complete response rates or survival.[40] The cisplatin plus 5-FU regimen is currently the standard of care.

New agents for the treatment of HNSCC are needed. Given the high response rates observed with single-agent paclitaxel, the combination of cisplatin plus paclitaxel has been evaluated in phase II trials and found to have activity.[41] A randomized trial in patients with advanced or recurrent disease compared high-dose (200 mg/m$^2$) versus low-dose (135 mg/m$^2$) paclitaxel administered as a 24-hour infusion in combination with cisplatin (75 mg/m$^2$ bolus infusion).[39] An identical overall response rate of 35% was observed in both arms of the study. The 24-hour infusion schedule was associated with significant morbidity and mortality because of complications from neutropenia. A 3-hour infusion of paclitaxel 175 mg/m$^2$ and cisplatin 75 mg/m$^2$ is currently being compared with cisplatin plus 5-FU in a randomized trial by ECOG.

The lower response rates observed in randomized trials when compared with small, single-institution studies can largely be explained by patient selection. The most important prognostic factor for response and survival is performance status.[2, 20, 42, 43] Patients with a high tumor burden or bulky disease in previously irradiated sites and patients who have undergone chemotherapy previously are also less likely to respond and have a shortened survival. Even if these patients do show some tumor regression in response to aggressive multiagent therapy, it is likely to be a transient partial response. Although complete response occurs infrequently, studies suggest that patients may benefit from a durable response with prolonged survival.[44–46]

Only one randomized trial has addressed whether chemotherapy improves survival over supportive care alone.[37] A total of 116 patients with advanced or recurrent HNSCC were randomized to receive best supportive care, single agents bleomycin or cisplatin alone, or the combination of bleomycin and cisplatin. The two cisplatin-containing arms

*Table 66–3.* **Randomized Trials of Combination Regimens in Recurrent Head and Neck Squamous Cell Cancer**

| Chemotherapy Regimen | Patients (n) | % Response (% CR) | Median Survival (mo) | Reference |
|---|---|---|---|---|
| P vs. P/MTX/B | 57 | 11 (3) vs. 11 (0) | NR | 30 |
| P vs. P/MTX/L | 79 | 18 (8) vs. 33 (15) | 6.3 vs. 6.9 | 31 |
| MTX vs. P/VCR/B | 51 | 33 (8) vs. 41 (11) | 5.6 vs. 4.0 | 32 |
| MTX vs. MTX/P/B | 163 | 35 (8) vs. 48 (16) | 5.6 vs. 5.6 | 33 |
| MTX vs. P/VBL/B | 190 | 16 (0) vs. 22 (10) | 7.2 vs. 6.8 | 34 |
| SC vs. B vs. P vs. PB | 116 | NA vs. 14 (0) vs. 24 (3) vs. 13 (6) | 2.1 vs. 2.8 vs. 4.2 vs. 4.0* | 37 |
| MTX vs. C/MTX | 40 | 25 (5) vs. 25 (0) | 6.0 vs. 6.0 | 35 |
| MTX vs. C/5-FU vs. P/5-FU | 261 | 10 (2) vs. 21 (2) vs. 32 (6)* | 5.6 vs. 5.0 vs. 6.6 | 36 |
| P vs. 5-FU vs. P/5-FU | 245 | 17 (4) vs. 13 (2) vs. 32 (6)* | 5.0 vs. 6.1 vs. 5.5 | 20 |
| P/MTX/B/VCR vs. P/5-FU vs. P | 382 | 34 (10) vs. 31 (3) vs. 15 (2)* | 7.0 vs. 7.0 vs. 7.0 | 38 |
| PT(high)/P vs. PT(low)/P | 197 | 32 (8) vs. 32 (8) | 7.5 vs. 6.9 | 39 |

*Significant difference.

CR, Complete response; P, cisplatin; MTX, methotrexate; B, bleomycin; L, leucovorin; VCR, vincristine; VBL, vinblastine; SC, supportive care; 5-FU, 5-fluorouracil; PT (high), high-dose paclitaxel; PT (low), low-dose paclitaxel; NA, not available; NR, not reported.

resulted in a small but statistically significant improvement in median survival compared with supportive care alone (4 and 4.2 months vs. 2.1 months). No quality of life measures were performed in this trial to assess the impact of therapy on goals of palliative care, such as pain control or performance status.

A number of single-agent and combination regimens have activity against HNSCC. Some cisplatin-containing combination regimens result in higher overall response rates but are associated with more toxicity and no increase in survival compared with single agents. When considering the treatment of patients with advanced or recurrent HNSCC, the performance status of the patient must be considered, and the goals of palliative care must be carefully weighed against the possible adverse effects of chemotherapy.

## BIOLOGIC THERAPY

Cellular immune defects have long been recognized in head and neck cancer patients.[47, 48] Clinical trials of interferons generally have been disappointing, showing low response rates and poor survival.[49–51] Studies combining cisplatin and 5-FU with interferon or interleukin-2 (IL-2) have not shown enhanced response rates or increased duration of survival. The rationale for studies with IL-2 alone or IL-2 combined with interferon is based on the cell-surface expression of IL-2 receptors in several HNSCC cell lines. Although growth can be inhibited by IL-2 in model systems, clinical trials have reported significant toxicity but no clear benefit.[52] Intralesional or peritumoral injections of low-dose IL-2 have yielded more promising results.[50, 53] In one study, local and systemic activation of antitumor effector cells was documented in response to local administration of IL-2.[54] Monoclonal antibodies directed against antigens expressed on the surface of tumor cells have shown efficacy in the therapy of low-grade lymphomas[55] and breast cancer.[56] Epidermal growth factor receptor is a rational target for such therapy in patients with head and neck cancers because overexpression occurs in most tumors,[57] and levels correlate with risk of local recurrence and survival.[58] Monoclonal antibodies against epidermal growth factor receptor inhibit growth of epidermal growth factor receptor–expressing tumors in animal models, and pilot studies in humans have confirmed localization of antibody to the surface of tumor cells.[59–61] Further efficacy trials are planned. Biologic therapies are a promising focus of clinical and basic research but as yet have no defined role in the management of head and neck cancer.

## Chemotherapy in the Primary Management of Head and Neck Cancer

Pilot studies with cisplatin-based chemotherapy in the 1970s showed that rapid tumor regression occurred in a high percentage of newly diagnosed patients given chemotherapy before surgery or radiation. This observation, coupled with poor long-term survival rates, led to the incorporation of chemotherapy into combined-modality primary curative treatment programs. Patients with the worst prognosis (large primary tumors or regional node involvement, or both, and

stages III and IV disease) were targeted for these investigational therapies. Approximately two thirds of head and neck cancer patients fall into this staging category. Patients whose disease can be completely resected have an approximately 40% 5-year survival rate, whereas less than 20% of patients with unresectable disease survive for 5 years.[62] The causes of death are complications of local-regional disease (50 to 60%), distant metastases (20%), second primary tumors (2 to 6%), and non–cancer-related causes (15%).[63–65] To improve survival, treatments must be designed that increase local-regional control and decrease distant metastases. Three strategies have been under investigation: (1) induction or neoadjuvant chemotherapy, (2) adjuvant chemotherapy, and (3) concomitant administration of radiation and chemotherapy.

## INDUCTION (NEOADJUVANT) CHEMOTHERAPY

The rationale for induction chemotherapy is that reduction in tumor size may improve local control achievable with subsequent definitive surgery or radiotherapy, or both. The use of systemic therapy may affect micrometastatic disease and reduce the incidence of distant metastases, leading to improved survival. Initial multidrug regimens tested as induction chemotherapy in the late 1970s and early 1980s used cisplatin and infusional bleomycin with or without a vinca alkaloid or methotrexate.[62, 66–68] Complete response rates occurred in 20 to 30%, and the overall response rates were approximately 70% in chemotherapy-naive patients. In the 1980s, the cisplatin and infusional 5-FU regimen was developed.[25] Approximately 85% of previously untreated patients had complete response rates of 40 to 50% (Table 66–4).[69–81] About two thirds of clinical complete responses were pathologically confirmed. Interest in a possibly less toxic regimen led to trials with carboplatin and 5-FU. Overall and complete response rates are lower than those reported for the parent drug, cisplatin. A randomized trial of induction cisplatin and 5-FU versus carboplatin and 5-FU in stage IV M0 HNSCC showed significant differences in response rate (92% vs. 76%, $p<0.05$), disease-free survival (47% vs. 24%, $p=0.02$), and 5-year survival (45% vs. 24%, $p=0.03$), indicating that cisplatin and 5-FU is superior.[82]

To intensify cisplatin and 5-FU therapy, investigators added leucovorin, a reduced folate, creating the PFL regimen. Moderate to severe gastrointestinal toxicity and leukopenia necessitating dose reduction were common. Although some studies report complete responses in 50 to 60% of patients,[78, 79] improvements in survival that might justify the added toxicity have not occurred. Another intensive regimen, a combination of PFL plus interferon alfa, has shown promising activity in phase II trials.[83]

Many randomized trials directly comparing induction chemotherapy followed by surgery or radiotherapy with standard local treatment have been published. Many studies were poorly designed, used inferior chemotherapy regimens, or enrolled too few patients.[84] Several randomized trials have examined the addition of three to five cycles of neoadjuvant cisplatin 100 mg/m² intravenous bolus and continuous-infusion 5-FU 1 g/m²/day for 96 to 120 hours to definitive local therapy alone.[85–91] One large multicenter randomized trial has shown a positive result for unresectable stage III or IV patients: Patients with inoperable disease who received four

*Table 66–4.* **Platinum-Based Induction Chemotherapy Regimens**

| Regimen | Cycles (n) | Patients (n) | % CPR + PR (range) | % CR (range) | Reference |
|---|---|---|---|---|---|
| Cisplatin 80–120 mg/m² + 5-FU 800–1000 mg/m²/day × 5 days every 21–28 days | 2–4 | 373 | 85 (73–94) | 35 (19–54) | 69–75 |
| Carboplatin 300–400 mg/m² + 5-FU 1000 mg/m²/day × 4–5 days every 21–28 days | 2–3 | 287 | 79 (53–87) | 28 (13–41) | 76–77 |
| Cisplatin 100–120 mg/m² + 5-FU 400–800 mg/m²/day × 5 days + leucovorin 100–500 mg/m²/day × 5 days every 21–28 days | 2–3 | 151 | 83 (80–95) | 43 (24–65) | 78–81 |

CR, complete response; PR, partial response; 5-FU, 5-fluorouracil.

cycles of cisplatin and 5-FU followed by full-course radiotherapy had an increase in complete response rate, a decrease in distant metastases, and an improved overall survival (24% vs. 10% at 3 years, $p = 0.04$) compared with radiotherapy alone.[89] However, this difference may be explained in part by the poor overall survival in the radiotherapy-alone arm compared with other reports in the literature and has not been reproduced in other trials. Other chemotherapy regimens have been similarly unsuccessful in improving survival. A change in the pattern of failure was observed in several trials, in which patients receiving induction chemotherapy had a reduced incidence of distant metastases.[89, 92–94]

Induction chemotherapy is feasible; it results in high response rates without an increase in complications from subsequent radiotherapy or surgery. Although unsuccessful in improving survival in HNSCC, induction chemotherapy can be used to select patients for organ preservation therapy (see next section).

## INDUCTION CHEMOTHERAPY FOR ORGAN PRESERVATION

Total laryngectomy, the traditional surgical management of advanced cancers of the larynx and hypopharynx (T3 and T4 tumors), can significantly affect a patient's quality of life by causing impairment of swallowing function and a complete loss of voice. Neoadjuvant chemotherapy trials showed that a complete response to chemotherapy predicted a favorable response to subsequent radiotherapy and that patients who achieved a complete response had a survival advantage.[44–46] This advantage encouraged the study of neoadjuvant chemotherapy in patients with operable stage III and IV laryngeal cancer, with the goal of identifying patients who were candidates for organ-preserving, primary radiotherapy.[95]

In 1985, the Veterans Administration Cooperative Studies Program mounted a large national study that randomized 332 patients with stage III or IV laryngeal cancer to either induction chemotherapy (three cycles of cisplatin and 5-FU) followed by radiotherapy or standard laryngectomy and postoperative radiotherapy.[93, 96] Approximately 80% of patients in the neoadjuvant chemotherapy arm achieved a complete response or partial response after two or three cycles of chemotherapy and were eligible for treatment with primary radiotherapy. At a median follow-up of 98 months, there was no significant difference in survival between the two treatment groups (35%). At 4 years, 31% of 161 patients initially randomized to induction chemotherapy had successful laryngeal preservation, and this group also had a lower rate of distant metastases. Sixty-two percent of patients in the chemotherapy arm who survived to 4 years after randomization had a preserved larynx. Although 38% of patients in the chemotherapy arm required salvage laryngectomy, their survival was not different from that of patients initially randomized to surgery. The presence of a T4 tumor increased the risk of failure with induction chemotherapy and the need for salvage surgery.

The EORTC performed a prospective, randomized phase III trial comparing induction chemotherapy and radiation with conventional surgery followed by radiotherapy in patients with operable stage II, III, or IV (T2–T4 N0–N2b) piriform sinus tumors.[92] In contrast to the Veterans Administration trial, only patients who achieved a complete response after two or three cycles of cisplatin 100 mg/m² and 5-FU 1000 mg/m²/day for 120 hours were eligible for radiation therapy. Although patients in the induction chemotherapy arm had a significant reduction in the rate of distant metastases, no difference in survival was observed between the two arms of the study. At a median follow-up of 51 months, 35% of patients in the induction chemotherapy arm were projected to have a preserved larynx at 5 years. The results of these trials, although not showing improvement in survival, have established a role for induction chemotherapy as an alternative treatment for patients with advanced laryngeal or hypopharyngeal cancer who desire preservation of natural speech.

Many investigators are evaluating similar nonsurgical approaches to preserve function of the larynx and other critical sites in the oral cavity and pharynx.[97] Also, functional outcomes of larynx preservation strategies are being evaluated.[98] The Head and Neck Intergroup is conducting a follow-up trial to the Veterans Administration study for stages III and IV resectable laryngeal cancer. Three nonsurgical therapies are being compared: (1) induction cisplatin and 5-FU followed by radiotherapy (control arm), (2) concurrent cisplatin 100 mg/m² every 3 weeks for three doses during radiotherapy, and (3) standard fractionation radiotherapy.[99] Because the Veterans Administration and the EORTC trials did not include radiation therapy–alone arms, this study should clarify the role of induction chemotherapy.[100]

## ADJUVANT CHEMOTHERAPY

Patients with advanced-stage HNSCC are at high risk for death resulting from local-regional failure or distant metastases: 40 to 60% of deaths are due to persistent or recurrent local disease, and 20 to 30% are due to distant metastases. Factors known to increase the risk of local-regional recurrence and distant metastases after surgical resection include positive or close (<5 mm) surgical margins, multiple positive nodes (≥N2), nodal extracapsular spread of disease, and perineural, lymphatic, or vascular invasion.[101, 102] Traditional adjuvant chemotherapy administered after patients have been rendered disease-free by surgery and radiotherapy has been tested in small feasibility trials, with promising results.[46, 103–106]

Several single-agent and combination regimens using methotrexate, bleomycin, 5-FU, and cisplatin have been evaluated in randomized trials, but none has resulted in a survival advantage. The Head and Neck Intergroup conducted a large prospective randomized trial in which patients with negative margins of resection were randomized to immediate postoperative radiotherapy or the experimental arm, consisting of three cycles of cisplatin and 5-FU followed by radiotherapy.[107] This trial showed no significant difference in survival or disease-free survival. An analysis of pattern of failure, however, showed a decrease in distant metastases in the chemotherapy-treated group. A high-risk group of patients (with extracapsular nodal extension, close surgical margins, or carcinoma in situ at the margin of resection) was identified in whom improvement in survival and local-regional control approached statistical significance.[107]

Cisplatin plus 5-FU chemotherapy administered before or after definitive local therapy can decrease distant metastases. Because of a lack of survival advantage, however, there is currently no role for adjuvant chemotherapy in the routine care of patients. Patients at high risk for recurrence and metastases as a result of pathologic features should be encouraged to participate in ongoing trials of adjuvant combined-modality therapy.

## Concomitant Chemoradiation in the Primary Management of Head and Neck Cancer

Attempts to clarify the role of concurrent chemotherapy and radiation in the management of patients with head and neck cancer continue to challenge medical oncologists as well as radiation oncologists and surgeons. Because of poor local control in patients with advanced local-regional disease treated with radiotherapy alone, cytotoxic agents have been administered simultaneously with radiotherapy to potentiate radiation cell kill.[108] Combined-modality regimens studied to date include single-agent and multiagent chemotherapy administered simultaneously with standard fractionated, accelerated, or hyperfractionated radiotherapy or alternated with split-course radiotherapy. Several studies of concurrent chemoradiotherapy have shown improvements in survival, disease-free survival, or local control over radiotherapy alone. In two separate meta-analyses of randomized controlled trials comparing concurrent chemoradiotherapy with radiotherapy, concurrent chemotherapy and radiation therapy significantly reduced the risk of death from head and neck cancer.[109, 110] Concurrent therapy, however, also significantly increases the toxicity of treatment, particularly high-grade mucositis, often resulting in delays in therapy and need for gastrostomy placement.[110]

## UNRESECTABLE, LOCAL-REGIONAL DISEASE (M0)

Several randomized controlled trials of radiotherapy with or without concomitant single-agent bleomycin,[111, 112] mitomycin C,[113] or 5-FU[114] have shown improvements in disease-free or overall survival with the addition of chemotherapy (Table 66–5).[111–121] Cisplatin has been shown to act as an effective radiosensitizer.[10] Weekly low-dose cisplatin (10 to 30 mg/m$^2$)[122] and intermittent high-dose therapy (100 mg/m$^2$ every 3 weeks)[123] with simultaneous standard fractionation radiotherapy have been studied in safety and efficacy trials. One randomized trial in patients with stage III or IV unresectable disease compared weekly cisplatin (20 mg/m$^2$) plus radiotherapy with standard treatment with radiotherapy alone.[124] Chemotherapy-treated patients had a higher complete response rate, 73% versus 59%, but there was no difference in overall survival, possibly owing to the low total dose of cisplatin (120 to 140 mg/m$^2$) given during the 6 to 8 weeks of radiotherapy. The Radiation Therapy Oncology Group evaluated a high intermittent dosing schedule, cisplatin 100 mg/m$^2$ every 3 weeks, in a similar group of patients with locally advanced disease.[123] A 71% complete

*Table 66–5.* **Randomized Trials of Radiotherapy Versus Concomitant Chemoradiotherapy**

| Chemotherapy | Patients (n) | Follow-up (yr) | % OS Control vs. Chemotherapy | % DFS Control vs. Chemotherapy | Reference |
|---|---|---|---|---|---|
| 5-FU | 136 | 5 | 13 vs. 32* | NA | 114 |
| Bleomycin | 157 | 5 | 24 vs. 66* | NA | 111 |
| Bleomycin | 100 | 3 | 24 vs. 43 | 15 vs. 31* | 112 |
| Mitomycin C | 117 | 5 | 40 vs. 48 | 49 vs. 75 | 113 |
| Cisplatin | 83 | 5 | 13 vs. 36* | 23 vs. 45* | 115 |
| Methotrexate | 313 | 5 | 28 vs. 43 | NA | 121 |
| Cisplatin + 5-FU | 157 | 5 | 10 vs. 24* | 9 vs. 21* | 116 |
| Cisplatin + 5-FU + LV | 270 | 3 | 24 vs. 48* | NA | 117 |
| Cisplatin + 5-FU | 110 | 3 | 34 vs. 55 | 44 vs. 70* | 118 |
| Cisplatin + 5-FU | 100 | 4 | 55 vs. 52 | 51 vs. 62* | 119 |
| Carboplatin + 5-FU | 226 | 3 | 31 vs. 51* | 19 vs. 42* | 120 |

*Significant difference.
OS, overall survival; DFS, disease-free survival; 5-FU, 5-fluorouracil; LV, leucovorin.

response rate occurred, and local-regional control and survival estimated at 4 years were superior to the data seen in a historical control group treated with radiotherapy alone.

Combination chemotherapy and concomitant radiotherapy has been explored in a number of phase I and phase II feasibility trials in patients with locally advanced resectable and unresectable disease. Cisplatin plus infusional 5-FU, cisplatin together with 5-FU and leucovorin, and 5-FU plus hydroxyurea are the three most studied regimens.[119, 125–128] Mucositis (often severe) and myelosuppression were common even with split-course radiotherapy and protracted treatment. Several randomized trials of radiation therapy with or without concurrent chemotherapy have been performed (see Table 66–5). The application of these trials to the routine clinical care of patients is confounded by a number of issues. Several trials were performed exclusively in or included patients with resectable disease and did not include a control arm of standard treatment (surgical resection followed by radiation). A randomized trial comparing accelerated fractionation radiotherapy with or without three cycles of concurrent cisplatin, 5-FU, and leucovorin in unresectable disease alone showed improved local control and overall survival (24% vs. 48%, $p<0.001$) at 3 years.[117] By contrast, randomized trials including patients with resectable disease have shown improvements in local control only with the addition of concurrent cisplatin and 5-FU to standard fractionation[129] and accelerated hyperfractionation irradiation.[118]

Alternating chemotherapy with radiation therapy has shown superior tumor cell kill when compared with sequential therapy in vitro and in vivo.[130] In addition, alternating therapy may avoid the severe mucosal toxicity commonly observed with simultaneous therapy.[116, 131] One randomized trial of alternating courses of cisplatin plus 5-FU and radiotherapy compared with radiotherapy alone in patients with locally advanced unresectable disease showed improved progression-free and overall survival for the chemotherapy-treated patients at 5 years (see Table 66–5).[116] Improvements in local control and disease-free survival have been shown with concurrent or alternating chemoradiotherapy when compared with sequential chemotherapy and radiotherapy in several randomized trials.[132] A National Cancer Institute–sponsored, randomized, controlled trial for stage III and stage IV locally advanced unresectable squamous cancers of the oral cavity, oropharynx, hypopharynx, and larynx has completed accrual.[99] The three-arm trial compared (1) neoadjuvent cisplatin 100 mg/m² every 3 weeks for three doses followed by radiotherapy; (2) concurrent cisplatin, infusional 5-FU, and radiotherapy; and (3) standard fractionation radiotherapy (control arm). Arm 2 (concurrent cisplatin, infusional 5-FU, and radiotherapy), significantly improved survival compared with radiotherapy alone and should now be the standard of care.

## POSTOPERATIVE, HIGH-RISK DISEASE

Improvement in local-regional control with concurrent therapy may be more feasible in patients with earlier stage disease (i.e., resected stages III and IV). Postsurgical patients at high risk for recurrence because of extracapsular spread of nodal disease were randomized to standard fractionation radiotherapy with or without weekly cisplatin (50-mg fixed

dose).[115, 133] Five-year survival was improved in the chemotherapy arm (36% vs. 13%, $p<0.01$, with a median survival of 40 months vs. 22 months).[115] The Head and Neck Intergroup is currently conducting a randomized trial of three cycles of adjuvant concurrent cisplatin 100 mg/m² and radiation versus standard fractionation radiation alone.

## CHEMOPREVENTION

Chemoprevention is the use of pharmacologic agents to reverse a premalignant condition or to inhibit events in the multistep process of carcinogenesis.[134] Head and neck cancer patients are particularly prone to develop more than one upper aerodigestive tract tumor because of exposure of the epithelial surface to the carcinogenic effects of excessive alcohol and tobacco. This process is known as *field cancerization*.[135–137] Second primary tumors occur in head and neck cancer patients at a constant rate of 3 to 4% per year.[138, 139] Individuals with stage I or stage II cancers treated for cure are at great risk for another cancer, particularly if they continue to smoke and drink.

Retinoids, the synthetic and natural analogues of vitamin A, and carotenoids can affect epithelial growth and differentiation through binding of nuclear retinoid receptors.[140] The major limitation of the retinoids in clinical use (i.e., vitamin A [retinol], β-all-*trans*-retinoic acid [tretinoin], and 13-*cis*-retinoic acid [isotretinoin]) is acute toxicity: dryness of mucous membranes, skin desquamation, hypertriglyceridemia, and bone tenderness. Chronically, hepatotoxicity and bone remodeling may occur.[134] These compounds are also highly teratogenic and should not be taken by premenopausal women.

The efficacy of retinoids in the treatment of dysplastic leukoplakia and erythroplakia and the prevention of second head and neck primaries has been evaluated in randomized clinical trials.[141] A series of randomized, placebo-controlled trials have shown that 13-*cis*-retinoic acid can cause histologic and clinical reversal of dysplastic leukoplakic lesions.[141] A small randomized trial using 12 months of high-dose 13-*cis*-retinoic acid 50 to 100 mg/m²/day to prevent second malignant tumors in patients with a previous HNSCC showed a significant difference in the incidence of second tumors at 32 months (4% vs. 24%) and 54 months (14% vs. 31%).[142, 143] Benefits of therapy began to dissipate thereafter, however. A trial of 24 months of therapy with another retinoid, etretinate, versus placebo failed to show benefit to therapy.[144] A large multicenter, double-blind, placebo-controlled trial of 36 months of low-dose 13-*cis*-retinoic acid 30 mg/day in patients with treated stage I or stage II HNSCC was completed in 1999. Because of the toxicity of these compounds and the uncertainty of the optimal dose and length of treatment, *cis*-retinoic acid cannot be recommended for routine use until results are reported.

# Cancer of the Nasopharynx

Cancer involving the nasopharynx is uncommon in the United States, making up only 2% of all head and neck cancers. A World Health Organization pathologic classification divides nasopharyngeal tumors into three types: type 1, keratinizing; type 2, nonkeratinizing; and type 3, often termed *undifferentiated, transitional cell,* or *lymphoepithelioma.* All are variants of squamous cell (or epidermoid) carcinoma,[145] and the therapeutic management is the same.

For many reasons, nasopharyngeal carcinomas are often set apart from other tumors of the head and neck.[146] Nasopharyngeal tumors are more likely to present and recur at distant sites when compared with other head and neck tumors. Because of anatomic location, nasopharyngeal primaries cannot be resected with adequate surgical margins, and radiotherapy is the standard treatment for all stages of local-regional disease. Nasopharyngeal tumors, particularly the lymphoepithelioma variant, are highly radiosensitive tumors: Treatment of stage I and stage II disease with external-beam radiotherapy results in 5-year survival rates of 90% and 80%, respectively. In contrast, treatment of patients with N2 or N3 disease is associated with a 30 to 40% 5-year survival with radiotherapy alone.

Chemotherapy has an established role in the palliation of locally recurrent, persistent, or metastatic nasopharyngeal carcinoma and should follow the same guidelines as outlined for squamous cell cancers of other sites in the head and neck. Many trials have been conducted evaluating induction, adjuvant, and concomitant chemoradiation treatment for newly diagnosed patients with regional node involvement.[62] A randomized trial of radiation therapy with or without three cycles of induction BEP (bleomycin, epirubicin, and cisplatin) showed a significant improvement in disease-free survival and reduction of metastases but not overall survival in the chemotherapy arm.[147] Two cycles of cisplatin 100 mg/$m^2$ and 5-FU 1000 mg/$m^2$/day for 72 hours before radiotherapy followed by four cycles after radiotherapy did not significantly improve response rate, disease-free survival, or overall survival when compared with radiation therapy alone.[148]

Concomitant chemoradiotherapy appears to be the most promising treatment for stage III and stage IV nasopharyngeal carcinoma. An Intergroup trial randomized 193 patients to radiotherapy or concomitant chemoradiotherapy with three cycles of cisplatin 100 mg/$m^2$ followed by three cycles of adjuvant cisplatin 80 mg/$m^2$ and 5-FU 1000 mg/$m^2$/day for 96 hours.[149, 150] At a median follow-up of 3.5 years, 147 patients were evaluable for survival analysis. Patients in the chemoradiotherapy arm had significant improvement in progression-free survival (75% vs. 26%, $p < 0.001$) and overall survival (83% vs. 45%, $p < 0.001$) when compared with patients in the radiotherapy-only arm. The importance of the adjuvant therapy to the success of this regimen remains unclear. The highly positive results of this trial have now established this concurrent chemoradiotherapy regimen as the standard of care in the United States for treatment of patients with stage III and stage IV squamous cell carcinoma of the nasopharynx.[151]

## Salivary Gland Cancers

Cancers originating in the salivary glands represent 3% of malignant tumors in the head and neck. The most common on histologic examination are adenoid cystic carcinoma, adenocarcinoma, and mucoepidermoid carcinoma.[152] Survival rates vary widely, depending on histologic type and grade. All types have the potential for distant dissemination to any organ.

Chemotherapy has been used mainly to treat recurrent disease. Because these cancers are infrequent, trials evaluating any chemotherapy agent or combination have covered only small numbers of patients. Essentially, all cytotoxic agents with reported activity in HNSCC have been tried in salivary gland cancers. Cisplatin, 5-FU, doxorubicin, and cyclophosphamide, used singly or in combination, have shown activity. A phase II trial of paclitaxel did not show activity in salivary gland primaries, however (Pinto H, personal communication, 1999). Response rates are in the 20 to 30% range; however, the small number of patients in each study precludes firm conclusions as to the true level of efficacy.[153] Treatment with these agents or investigational drugs is recommended for adenocarcinoma and high-grade mucoepidermoid carcinoma. Metastatic adenoid cystic carcinoma, typically lung metastases, may progress slowly. These patients should be observed only, with chemotherapy held in reserve until the disease shows evidence of more rapid progression.

## Specific Treatment Recommendations

### SQUAMOUS CELL CARCINOMA OF THE ORAL CAVITY, OROPHARYNX, HYPOPHARYNX, LARYNX, AND PARANASAL SINUSES

**Stage I and Stage II Disease.** In general, early-stage cancers (T1–T2 N0) can be treated effectively for cure with single-modality surgery or radiotherapy. The selection of treatment depends on the site, institutional expertise, and patient preference. Early laryngeal cancer is usually treated with radiotherapy, with surgery reserved for salvage of locally recurrent disease. Patients treated with surgical resection who have pathologic features indicating a high risk for recurrence (close or positive margins; multiple positive nodes; extracapsular spread; or perineural, lymphatic, or vascular invasion) should receive adjuvant radiation.

**Stage III and Stage IV (M0) Disease.** Large primary tumors (T3–T4) or regional node involvement, or both, are further classified as resectable (meaning that there is a high likelihood of complete removal of the tumor with negative margins of resection) or unresectable.

*Unresectable Disease.* The standard treatment of unresectable disease in the United States is radiotherapy and concurrent chemotherapy. Because of the two large multicenter positive European trials[89, 116] and the poor results in these patient groups treated with radiotherapy alone (median survival, 12 months), the following treatment options are suggested:

Good to excellent performance status and nutritional status, good renal function (creatinine clearance ≥60 ml/min), compliance expected:
Enroll in an approved protocol evaluating combined-modality treatment.
If no protocol is available, concurrent chemotherapy and standard fractionation radiotherapy with cisplatin 75 or 100 mg/$m^2$ every 3 weeks may be used provided that a multidisciplinary team

experienced in the management of toxicity is administering treatment.

Poor performance status or poor nutrition, poor renal function (creatinine clearance <60 ml/min), or poor expected compliance:

Treat with full-course standard fractionation radiotherapy.

***Resectable Disease.*** For all sites except the supraglottic and glottic larynx and piriform sinus, patients should be treated with surgery and postoperative radiotherapy or enrolled in an approved combined-modality protocol. Patients with larynx and piriform sinus cancer should be offered the option of nonsurgical therapy to preserve their larynx. The options for nonsurgical treatment depend on the patient's suitability for intensive combined-modality treatment.

Good to excellent performance status and nutritional status, good renal function (creatinine clearance ≥60 ml/min), compliance expected:

Enroll in the Head and Neck Intergroup larynx preservation trial through one of the major cooperative groups, or enroll in an approved protocol evaluating sequential or concomitant chemoradiation.

If no protocol is available, use the published Veterans Administration Cooperative Studies Program regimen:[93] cisplatin 100 mg/m² day 1 and 5-FU 1000 mg/m²/24 hours continuous intravenous infusion for 120 hours every 21 days for two cycles. If the response of the primary tumor is at least partial (≥50% disease regression) and there is no progression of neck disease, administer a third cycle of chemotherapy followed by full-course radiotherapy. If response is inadequate after two cycles, the patient should undergo immediate surgery and postoperative radiotherapy.

Poor performance status or poor nutrition, poor renal function, poor compliance expected. These patients are not candidates for organ preservation by induction chemotherapy, and surgery should be recommended. Full-course radiotherapy alone for organ preservation should be reserved as an option for patients with T3 N0 M0 disease, which is the standard of care for this TNM stage in Canada and Great Britain but not accepted standard treatment in the United States.

**Locally Recurrent, Persistent, or Metastatic Disease.** Patients who are not candidates for further salvage surgery or radiation offering the possibility of cure can be considered for palliative chemotherapy. Because none of the currently available chemotherapeutic agents used alone or in combination has led to survival prolongation, patients should be given the opportunity to participate in investigational treatment protocols that evaluate new agents. The decision to treat with established drugs should be guided by known prognostic factors. Patients with a good performance status (ECOG 0 or 1) and no previous chemotherapy should be offered cisplatin plus 5-FU chemotherapy because of its significantly higher response rate compared with single agents and the possibility that they may achieve a complete response and survival benefit. Patients with an ECOG performance status of 2 should receive either supportive care or single-agent therapy (e.g., weekly methotrexate). Patients with an ECOG performance status of 3 should receive best supportive care because they are unlikely to tolerate chemotherapy.

## SQUAMOUS CELL CARCINOMA OF THE NASOPHARYNX

**Stages I and II Disease.** Patients with T1–2bN0–1 tumors should be treated with definitive radiotherapy to the nasopharynx.

**Stages III and IV (M0) Disease.** Patients with advanced local disease should receive concurrent chemoradiotherapy with cisplatin 100 mg/m² as an intravenous bolus on days 1, 22, and 43 during standard fractionation full-course radiotherapy (≥70 Gy). After completion of radiotherapy, three courses of adjuvant cisplatin 80 mg/m² on day 1 and 5-FU 1000 mg/m²/day on days 1 through 4 as a continuous infusion should be administered.[150]

**Stage IV (M1).** Patients should be treated with platinum-based combination chemotherapy as indicated previously.

## SUGGESTIONS FOR ADDITIONAL READING

Fu KK. Combined-modality therapy for head and neck cancer. Oncology 1997;85:1781–90. *This is a comprehensive review (62 references) of induction chemotherapy, adjuvant chemotherapy, and concomitant chemoradiation.*

Vokes EE, Weichselbaum RR, Lippman SM, et al. Head and neck cancer. N Engl J Med 1993;328:184. *This superb review (150 references) emphasizes natural history, epidemiology, biology, diagnosis, and staging. Treatment of metastatic or recurrent disease and chemoprevention are presented in addition to brief summaries of combined-modality therapies.*

Forastiere AA, Panel Chairman: NCCN Practice Guidelines for Head and Neck Cancer. Oncology 1998;12:39–147. *A panel of experts from the National Comprehensive Cancer Network provides guidelines for the current management of squamous cell carcinoma of the head and neck. Guidelines for work-up and clinical staging, in addition to treatment, are provided.*

## REFERENCES

1. Landis S, Murray T, Bolden S, Wingo P. Cancer statistics, 1998. CA Cancer J Clin 1998;48:6–29.
2. Al-Sarraf M. Head and neck cancer: chemotherapy concepts. Semin Oncol 1988;15:70–85.
3. Hong W, Bromer R. Chemotherapy in head and neck cancer. N Engl J Med 1983;308:75–9.
4. Buesa J, Fernandez R, Esteban E, et al. Phase II trial of ifosfamide in recurrent and metastatic head and neck cancer. Ann Oncol 1991;2:151–2.
5. Cervellino J, Araujo C, Pirisi C, et al. Ifosfamide and mesna for the treatment of advanced squamous cell head and neck cancer: a GET-LAC study. Oncology 1991;48:89–92.
6. Verweij J, Alexieva-Figusch J, de Boer M, et al. Ifosfamide in advanced head and neck cancer: a phase II study of the Rotterdam Cooperative Head and Neck Cancer Study Group. Eur J Cancer Clin Oncol 1988;24:795–6.
7. Forastiere A, Shank D, Neuberg D, et al. Final report of a phase II evaluation of paclitaxel in patients with advanced squamous cell carcinoma of the head and neck. Cancer 1998;82:2270–4.
8. Catimel G, Vermorken JB, Clavel M, et al. A phase II study of Gemcitabine (LY 188011) in patients with advanced squamous cell carcinoma of the head and neck. EORTC Early Clinical Trials Group. Ann Oncol 1994;5:543–7.

9. Catimel G, Verweij J, Mattijssen V, et al. Docetaxel (Taxotere): an active drug for the treatment of patients with advanced squamous cell carcinoma of the head and neck. EORTC Early Clinical Trials Group. Ann Oncol 1994;5:533–7.
10. Fu K, Phillips T. Biologic rationale of combined radiotherapy and chemotherapy. Hematol Oncol Clin North Am 1991;5:737–51.
11. Forastiere A, Belliveau J, Goren M, et al. Pharmacokinetic and toxicity evaluation of five-day continuous infusion versus intermittent bolus cis-diamminedichloroplatinum (II) in head and neck cancer patients. Cancer Res 1988;48:3869–74.
12. Egorin M, Van Echo D, Tipping S, et al. Pharmacokinetics and dosage reduction of cis-diammine (1, 1-cyclobutanedicarboxylato) platinum in patients with impaired renal function. Cancer Res 1984;44:5432–8.
13. Calvert A, Newell D, Gumbrell L, et al. Carboplatin dosage: prospective evaluation of a simple formula based on renal function. J Clin Oncol 1989;7:1748–56.
14. Goldsmith M, Carter S. The integration of chemotherapy into a combined modality approach to cancer therapy: V. squamous cell cancer of the head and neck. Cancer Treat Rev 1975;2:137–58.
15. DeConti R, Schoenfeld D. A randomized prospective comparison of intermittent methotrexate, methotrexate with leukovorin, and a methotrexate combination in head and neck cancer. Cancer 1981;48:1061–72.
16. Kirkwood J, Canellos G, Ervin T, et al. Increased therapeutic index using moderate dose methotrexate and leucovorin twice weekly vs. weekly high dose methotrexate-leukovorin in patients with advanced squamous carcinoma of the head and neck: a safe new effective regimen. Cancer 1981;47:2414–21.
17. Taylor S, McGuire W, Hauck W, et al. A randomized comparison of high-dose infusion methotrexate versus standard-dose weekly therapy in head and neck squamous cancer. J Clin Oncol 1984;2:1006–11.
18. Krakoff I, Cvitkovic E, Currie V, et al. Clinical pharmacologic and therapeutic studies of bleomycin given by continuous infusion. Cancer 1977;40:2027–37.
19. Carter S. The chemotherapy of head and neck cancer. Semin Oncol 1977;4:413–24.
20. Jacobs C, Lyman G, Velez-Garcia E, et al. A phase III randomized study comparing cisplatin and fluorouracil as single agents and in combination for advanced squamous cell of the head and neck. J Clin Oncol 1992;10:257–63.
21. Schiff P, Fant J, Horwitz S. Promotion of microtubule assembly in vitro by taxol. Nature 1979;277:665–7.
22. Gebbia V, Testa A, Cannata G, Gebbia N. Single agent paclitaxel in advanced squamous cell head and neck carcinoma. Eur J Cancer 1996;32A:901–2. letter.
23. Schrijvers D, Vermorken JB. Update on the taxoids and other new agents in head and neck cancer therapy. Curr Opin Oncol 1998;10:233–41.
24. Dreyfuss AI, Clark JR, Norris CM, et al. Docetaxel: an active drug for squamous cell carcinoma of the head and neck. J Clin Oncol 1996;14:1672–8.
25. Kish J, Weaver A, Jacobs J, et al. Cisplatin and 5-fluorouracil infusion in patients with recurrent and disseminated epidermoid cancer of the head and neck. Cancer 1984;53:1819–24.
26. Urba SG, Forastiere AA. Systemic therapy of head and neck cancer: most effective agents, areas of promise. Oncology (Huntingt) 1989;3:79–88.
27. Vokes E, Choi K, Schilsky R, et al. Cisplatin, fluorouracil, and high-dose leucovorin for recurrent or metastatic head and neck cancer. J Clin Oncol 1988;6:618–26.
28. Guthrie T, Brubaker L, Porubsky E, et al. Circadian cisplatin, bleomycin and 5-fluorouracil in advanced squamous cell carcinoma of the head and neck. Proc ASCO 1990;9:178.
29. Amrein P. Cisplatin and 5-fluorouracil vs. the same plus bleomycin and methotrexate in recurrent squamous cell carcinoma of the head and neck. Proc ASCO 1990;9:175.
30. Davis S, Kessler W. Randomized comparison of cis-diamminedichloroplatinum versus cis-diamminedichloroplatinum, methotrexate, and bleomycin in recurrent squamous cell carcinoma of the head and neck. Cancer Chemother Pharmacol 1979;3:57–9.
31. Jacobs C, Meyers F, Hendrickson C, et al. A randomized phase III study of ciplatin with or without methotrexate for recurrent squamous cell carcinoma of the head and neck: a Northern California Oncology Group study. Cancer 1983;52:1563–9.
32. Drelichman A, Cummings G, Al-Sarraf M. A randomized trial of the combination of cis-platinum, oncovin and bleomycin (COB) versus methotrexate in patients with advanced squamous cell carcinoma of the head and neck. Cancer 1983;52:399–403.
33. Vogl S, Schoenfeld D, Kaplan B, et al. A randomized prospective comparison of methotrexate with a combination of methotrexate, bleomycin, and cisplatin in head and neck cancer. Cancer 1985;56:432–42.
34. Williams S, Velex-Garcia E, Essessee I, et al. Chemotherapy for head and neck cancer: comparison of cisplatin + vinblastine + bleomycin versus methotrexate. Cancer 1986;57:18–23.
35. Eisenberger M, Krasnov S, Ellenberg S, et al. A comparison of carboplatin plus methorexate versus methotrexate alone in patients with recurrent and metastatic head and neck cancer. J Clin Oncol 1989;7:1341–5.
36. Forastiere A, Metch B, Schuller D, et al. Randomized comparison of cisplatin plus fluorouracil and carboplatin plus fluorouracil versus methotrexate in advanced squamous-cell carcinoma of the head and neck: a Southwest Oncology Group study. J Clin Oncol 1992;10:1245–51.
37. Morton RP, Rugman F, Dorman EB, et al. Cisplatinum and bleomycin for advanced or recurrent squamous cell carcinoma of the head and neck: a randomised factorial phase III controlled trial. Cancer Chemother Pharmacol 1985;15:283–9.
38. Clavel M, Vermorken JB, Cognetti F, et al. Randomized comparison of cisplatin, methotrexate, bleomycin and vincristine (CABO) versus cisplatin and 5-fluorouracil (CF) versus cisplatin (C) in recurrent or metastatic squamous cell carcinoma of the head and neck: a phase III study of the EORTC Head and Neck Cancer Cooperative Group. Ann Oncol 1994;5:521–6.
39. Forastiere A, Leong T, Murphy E, et al. A phase III trial of high-dose paclitaxel + cisplatin + G-CSF versus low-dose paclitaxel + cisplatin in patients with advanced squamous cell carcinoma of the head and neck (HNSCC): an Eastern Cooperative Oncology Group trial. Proc ASCO 1997;16:384a.
40. Browman GP, Cronin L. Standard chemotherapy in squamous cell head and neck cancer: what we have learned from randomized trials. Semin Oncol 1994;21:311–9.
41. Hitt R, Paz-Ares L, Hidalgo M, et al. Phase I/II study of paclitaxel/cisplatin as first-line therapy for locally advanced head and neck cancer. Semin Oncol 1997;24:S19–20–4.
42. Recondo G, Armand J, Tellez-Bernal E, et al. Recurrent and/or metastatic head and neck squamous cell carcinoma: a clinical, univariate and multivariate analysis of response and survival with cisplatin-based chemotherapy. Laryngoscope 1991;101:494–501.
43. Stell P. Survival times in end-stage head and neck cancer. Eur J Surg Oncol 1989;15:407–10.
44. Perry DJ, Weltz MD, Brown AW Jr, et al. Vinblastine, bleomycin and cisplatin for recurrent or metastatic squamous cell carcinoma of the head and neck. Cancer 1982;50:2257–60.
45. Chiuten D, Vogl SE, Kaplan BH, Greenwald E. Effective outpatient combination chemotherapy for advanced cancer of the head and neck. Surg Gynecol Obstet 1980;151:659–62.
46. Ervin TJ, Clark JR, Weichselbaum RR, et al. An analysis of induction and adjuvant chemotherapy in the multidisciplinary treatment of squamous-cell carcinoma of the head and neck. J Clin Oncol 1987;5:10–20.
47. Katz AE. Advances in the immunology of head and neck cancer. Otolaryngol Clin North Am 1980;13:431–6.
48. Newbill ET, Johns ME. Immunology of head and neck cancers. Crit Rev Clin Lab Sci 1983;19:1–25.
49. Vlock DR, Johnson J, Myers E, et al. Preliminary trial of nonrecombinant interferon alpha in recurrent squamous cell carcinoma of the head and neck. Head Neck 1991;13:15–21.
50. Vlock DR, Snyderman CH, Johnson JT, et al. Phase Ib trial of the effect of peritumoral and intranodal injections of interleukin-2 in patients with advanced squamous cell carcinoma of the head and neck: an Eastern Cooperative Oncology Group trial. J Immunother 1994;15:134–9.
51. Dimery IW, Jacobs C, Tseng A Jr, et al. Recombinant interferon-gamma in the treatment of recurrent nasopharyngeal carcinoma. J Biol Response Mod 1989;8:221–6.
52. Urba SG, Forastiere AA, Wolf GT, Amrein PC. Intensive recombinant interleukin-2 and alpha-interferon therapy in patients with advanced head and neck squamous carcinoma. Cancer 1993;71:2326–31.
53. Cortesina G, De Stefani A, Giovarelli M, et al. Treatment of recurrent squamous cell carcinoma of the head and neck with low doses of interleukin-2 injected perilymphatically. Cancer 1988;62:2482–5.

54. Whiteside TL, Letessier E, Hirabayashi H, et al. Evidence for local and systemic activation of immune cells by peritumoral injections of interleukin 2 in patients with advanced squamous cell carcinoma of the head and neck. Cancer Res 1993;53:5654–62.

55. McLaughlin P, Grillo-Lopez AJ, Link BK, et al. Rituximab chimeric anti-CD20 monoclonal antibody therapy for relapsed indolent lymphoma: half of patients respond to a four-dose treatment program. J Clin Oncol 1998;16:2825–33.

56. Cobleigh M, Vogel C, Tripathy D, et al. Efficacy and safety of Herceptin as a single agent in 222 women with Her2 overexpression who relapsed following chemotherapy for metastatic breast cancer. Proc ASCO 1998;17:97a.

57. Salomon DS, Brandt R, Ciardiello F, Normanno N. Epidermal growth factor-related peptides and their receptors in human malignancies. Crit Rev Oncol Hematol 1995;19:183–232.

58. Dassonville O, Formento JL, Francoual M, et al. Expression of epidermal growth factor receptor and survival in upper aerodigestive tract cancer. J Clin Oncol 1993;11:1873–8.

59. Modjtahedi H, Eccles S, Sandle J, et al. Differentiation or immune destruction: two pathways for therapy of squamous cell carcinomas with antibodies to the epidermal growth factor receptor. Cancer Res 1994;54:1695–701.

60. Modjtahedi H, Hickish T, Nicolson M, et al. Phase I trial and tumour localisation of the anti-EGFR monoclonal antibody ICR62 in head and neck or lung cancer. Br J Cancer 1996;73:228–35.

61. Modjtahedi H, Affleck K, Stubberfield C, Dean C. EGFR blockade by tyrosine kinase inhibitor or monoclonal antibody inhibits growth, directs terminal differentiation and induces apoptosis in the human squamous cell carcinoma HN5. Int J Oncol 1998;13:335–42.

62. Dimery IW, Hong WK. Overview of combined modality therapies for head and neck cancer. J Natl Cancer Inst 1993;85:95–111.

63. Tupchong L, Scott CB, Blitzer PH, et al. Randomized study of preoperative versus postoperative radiation therapy in advanced head and neck carcinoma: long-term follow-up of RTOG study 73–03. Int J Radiat Oncol Biol Phys 1991;20:21–8.

64. Marcial VA. Ninth annual del Regato lecture: optimal multidisciplinary management of head and neck cancer. Int J Radiat Oncol Biol Phys 1987;13:393–401.

65. Fazekas J, Pajak TF, Wasserman T, et al. Failure of misonidazole-sensitized radiotherapy to impact upon outcome among stage III–IV squamous cancers of the head and neck. Int J Radiat Oncol Biol Phys 1987;13:1155–60.

66. Randolph VL, Vallejo A, Spiro RH, et al. Combination therapy of advanced head and neck cancer: induction of remissions with diamminedichloroplatinum (II), bleomycin and radiation therapy. Cancer 1978;41:460–7.

67. Hong WK, Shapshay SM, Bhutani R, et al. Induction chemotherapy in advanced squamous head and neck carcinoma with high-dose cisplatinum and bleomycin infusion. Cancer 1979;44:19–25.

68. Glick JH, Marcial V, Richter M, Velez-Garcia E. The adjuvant treatment of inoperable stage III and IV epidermoid carcinoma of the head and neck with platinum and bleomycin infusions prior to definitive radiotherapy: an RTOG pilot study. Cancer 1980;46:1919–24.

69. Amrein PC, Weitzman SA. Treatment of squamous-cell carcinoma of the head and neck with cisplatin and 5-fluorouracil. J Clin Oncol 1985;3:1632–9.

70. Kish J, Drelichman A, Jacobs J, et al. Clinical trial of cisplatin and 5-FU infusion as initial treatment for advanced squamous cell carcinoma of the head and neck. Cancer Treat Rep 1982;66:471–4.

71. Weaver A, Flemming S, Kish J, et al. Cis-platinum and 5-fluorouracil as induction therapy for advanced head and neck cancer. Am J Surg 1982;144:445–8.

72. Thyss A, Schneider M, Santini J, et al. Induction chemotherapy with cis-platinum and 5-fluorouracil for squamous cell carcinoma of the head and neck. Br J Cancer 1986;54:755–60.

73. Jacobs JR, Pajak TF, Kinzie J, et al. Induction chemotherapy in advanced head and neck cancer: a Radiation Therapy Oncology Group Study. Arch Otolaryngol Head Neck Surg 1987;113:193–7.

74. Jacobs C, Goffinet DR, Goffinet L, et al. Chemotherapy as a substitute for surgery in the treatment of advanced resectable head and neck cancer: a report from the Northern California Oncology Group. Cancer 1987;60:1178–83.

75. Clark JR, Fallon BG, Dreyfuss AI, et al. Chemotherapeutic strategies in the multidisciplinary treatment of head and neck cancer. Semin Oncol 1988;15:35–44.

76. Volling P, Schroder M, Rauschning W, et al. Carboplatin: the better platinum in head and neck cancer? Arch Otolaryngol Head Neck Surg 1989;115:695–8.

77. Gregoire V, Beauduin M, Humblet Y, et al. A phase I–II trial of induction chemotherapy with carboplatin and fluorouracil in locally advanced head and neck squamous cell carcinoma: a report from the UCL-Oncology Group, Belgium. J Clin Oncol 1991;9:1385–92.

78. Dreyfuss AI, Clark JR, Wright JE, et al. Continuous infusion high-dose leucovorin with 5-fluorouracil and cisplatin for untreated stage IV carcinoma of the head and neck. Ann Intern Med 1990;112:167–72.

79. Vokes EE, Schilsky RL, Weichselbaum RR, et al. Induction chemotherapy with cisplatin, fluorouracil, and high-dose leucovorin for locally advanced head and neck cancer: a clinical and pharmacologic analysis. J Clin Oncol 1990;8:241–7.

80. Loeffler TM, Lindemann J, Luckhaupt H, et al. Chemotherapy of advanced and relapsed squamous cell cancer of the head and neck with split-dose cisplatinum (DDP), 5-fluorouracil (Fura) and leucovorin (CF). Adv Exp Med Biol 1988;244:267–73.

81. Pfister DG, Bajorin D, Motzer R, et al. Cisplatin, fluorouracil, and leucovorin: increased toxicity without improved response in squamous cell head and neck cancer. Arch Otolaryngol Head Neck Surg 1994;120:89–95.

82. De Andres L, Brunet J, Lopez-Pousa A, et al. Randomized trial of neoadjuvant cisplatin and fluorouracil versus carboplatin and fluorouracil in patients with stage IV-M0 head and neck cancer. J Clin Oncol 1995;13:1493–500.

83. Vokes EE, Ratain MJ, Mick R, et al. Cisplatin, fluorouracil, and leucovorin augmented by interferon alfa-2b in head and neck cancer: a clinical and pharmacologic analysis [published erratum appears in J Clin Oncol 1994;12:643]. J Clin Oncol 1993;11:360–8.

84. Forastiere AA. Randomized trials of induction chemotherapy: a critical review. Hematol Oncol Clin North Am 1991;5:725–36.

85. DiBlasio B, Barbieri W, Bozzetti A, et al. A prospective randomized trial in resectable head and neck carcinoma: locoregional treatment with and without neoadjuvant chemotherapy. Proc ASCO 1994;13:279.

86. Hasegawa Y, Matsura H, Fukushima M, et al. A randomized trial of neoadjuvant chemotherapy with cisplatin and 5-FU in advanced head and neck cancer. Proc ASCO 1994;13:286.

87. Toohill RJ, Anderson T, Byhardt RW, et al. Cisplatin and fluorouracil as neoadjuvant therapy in head and neck cancer: a preliminary report. Arch Otolaryngol Head Neck Surg 1987;113:758–61.

88. Martin M, Malaurie E, Langlet P, et al. A randomized prospective study of CDDP and 5-FU as neoadjuvant chemotherapy in head and neck cancer: a final report. Proc ASCO 1995;14:294.

89. Paccagnella A, Orlando A, Marchiori C, et al. Phase III trial of initial chemotherapy in stage III or IV head and neck cancers: a study by the Gruppo di Studio sui Tumori della Testa e del Collo. J Natl Cancer Inst 1994;86:265–72.

90. Dalley D, Beller E, Aroney R, et al. The value of chemotherapy (CT) prior to definitive local therapy (DLT) in patients with locally advanced squamous cell carcinoma (SCC) of the head and neck (HN). Proc ASCO 1995;14:297.

91. Domenge C, Coche-Dequeant B, Wibault P. Randomized trial of neoadjuvant chemotherapy before radiotherapy in oropharyngeal carcinoma. 4th International Conference on Head and Neck Cancer, Toronto, Canada, 1996. abstract.

92. Lefebvre JL, Chevalier D, Luboinski B, et al. Larynx preservation in pyriform sinus cancer: preliminary results of a European Organization for Research and Treatment of Cancer phase III trial. EORTC Head and Neck Cancer Cooperative Group. J Natl Cancer Inst 1996;88:890–9.

93. Induction chemotherapy plus radiation compared with surgery plus radiation in patients with advanced laryngeal cancer. The Department of Veterans Affairs Laryngeal Cancer Study Group. N Engl J Med 1991;324:1685–90.

94. Schuller DE, Metch B, Stein DW, et al. Preoperative chemotherapy in advanced resectable head and neck cancer: final report of the Southwest Oncology Group. Laryngoscope 1988;98:1205–11.

95. Demard F, Chauvel P, Santini J, et al. Response to chemotherapy as justification for modification of the therapeutic strategy for pharyngo-laryngeal carcinomas. Head Neck 1990;12:225–31.

96. Wolf G, Hong W, Fisher S. Neoadjuvant chemotherapy for organ preservation: current status. 4th International Conference on Head and Neck Cancer, Toronto, Canada, 1996.

97. Carew JF, Shah JP. Advances in multimodality therapy for laryngeal cancer. CA Cancer J Clin 1998;48:211–28.

98. Hillman RE, Walsh MJ, Wolf GT, et al. Functional outcomes following treatment for advanced laryngeal cancer: Part I. voice preservation in advanced laryngeal cancer. Part II. laryngectomy rehabilitation: the state of the art in the VA System. Research Speech-Language Pathologists. Department of Veterans Affairs Laryngeal Cancer Study Group. Ann Otol Rhinol Laryngol 1998;172:Suppl:1–27.

99. Forastiere AA. Cisplatin and radiotherapy in the management of locally advanced head and neck cancer. Int J Radiat Oncol Biol Phys 1993;27:465–70.

100. Forastiere A. Larynx preservation trials: a critical appraisal. Semin Radiat Oncol 1998;8:1–9.

101. Peters L, Goepfert H, Ang K, et al. Evaluation of the dose for postoperative radiation therapy of head and neck cancer: first report of a prospective randomized trial. Int J Radiat Oncol Biol Phys 1993;26:3–11.

102. Cooper J, Pajak T, Forastiere A, et al. Post-operative, concurrent radiochemotherapy for advanced resectable head and neck cancer: a rationale for future investigation based on the RTOG experience. Laryngoscope 1998;21:588–94.

103. Johnson JT, Myers EN, Schramm VL Jr, et al. Adjuvant chemotherapy for high-risk squamous-cell carcinoma of the head and neck. J Clin Oncol 1987;5:456–8.

104. Jacobs JR, Pajak TF, al-Sarraf M, et al. Chemotherapy following surgery for head and neck cancer. A Radiation Therapy Oncology Group Study. Am J Clin Oncol 1989;12:185–9.

105. Vokes EE, Moran WJ, Mick R, et al. Neoadjuvant and adjuvant methotrexate, cisplatin, and fluorouracil in multimodal therapy of head and neck cancer. J Clin Oncol 1989;7:838–45.

106. Jacobs C, Makuch R. Efficacy of adjuvant chemotherapy for patients with resectable head and neck cancer: a subset analysis of the Head and Neck Contracts Program. J Clin Oncol 1990;8:838–47.

107. Laramore GE, Scott CB, al-Sarraf M, et al. Adjuvant chemotherapy for resectable squamous cell carcinomas of the head and neck: report on Intergroup Study 0034. Int J Radiat Oncol Biol Phys 1992;23:705–13.

108. Vokes EE, Weichselbaum RR. Concomitant chemoradiotherapy: rationale and clinical experience in patients with solid tumors [published erratum appears in J Clin Oncol 1990;8:1447]. J Clin Oncol 1990;8:911–34.

109. Bourhis J, Pignon J, Designe L, et al. Meta-analysis of chemotherapy in head and neck cancer (MACH-NC): (1) loco-regional treatment vs same treatment + chemotherapy (CT). Proc ASCO 1998;17:386a.

110. El-Sayed S, Nelson N. Adjuvant and adjunctive chemotherapy in the management of squamous cell carcinoma of the head and neck region: a meta-analysis of prospective and randomized trials. J Clin Oncol 1996;14:838–47.

111. Shanta V, Krishnamurthi S. Combined bleomycin and radiotherapy in oral cancer. Clin Radiol 1980;31:617–20.

112. Fu KK, Phillips TL, Silverberg IJ, et al. Combined radiotherapy and chemotherapy with bleomycin and methotrexate for advanced inoperable head and neck cancer: update of a Northern California Oncology Group randomized trial. J Clin Oncol 1987;5:1410–8.

113. Weissberg JB, Son YH, Papac RJ, et al. Randomized clinical trial of mitomycin C as an adjunct to radiotherapy in head and neck cancer. Int J Radiat Oncol Biol Phys 1989;17:3–9.

114. Lo TC, Wiley AL Jr, Ansfield FJ, et al. Combined radiation therapy and 5-fluorouracil for advanced squamous cell carcinoma of the oral cavity and oropharynx: a randomized study. AJR Am J Roentgenol 1976;126:229–35.

115. Bachaud JM, Cohen-Jonathan E, Alzieu C, et al. Combined postoperative radiotherapy and weekly cisplatin infusion for locally advanced head and neck carcinoma: final report of a randomized trial. Int J Radiat Oncol Biol Phys 1996;36:999–1004.

116. Merlano M, Benasso M, Corvo R, et al. Five-year update of a randomized trial of alternating radiotherapy and chemotherapy compared with radiotherapy alone in treatment of unresectable squamous cell carcinoma of the head and neck. J Natl Cancer Inst 1996;88:583–9.

117. Wendt TG, Grabenbauer GG, Rodel CM, et al. Simultaneous radiochemotherapy versus radiotherapy alone in advanced head and neck cancer: a randomized multicenter study. J Clin Oncol 1998;16:1318–24.

118. Brizel DM, Albers ME, Fisher SR, et al. Hyperfractionated irradiation with or without concurrent chemotherapy for locally advanced head and neck cancer. N Engl J Med 1998;338:1798–804.

119. Adelstein DJ, Kalish LA, Adams GL, et al. Concurrent radiation therapy and chemotherapy for locally unresectable squamous cell head and neck cancer: an Eastern Cooperative Oncology Group pilot study. J Clin Oncol 1993;11:2136–42.

120. Calais G, Alfonsi M, Bardet E, et al. Randomized study comparing radiation alone versus RT with concomitant chemotherapy in stages III and IV oropharynx carcinoma: preliminary results of the 94.01 study from the French Group of Radiation Oncology for Head and Neck Cancer. Proc ASCO 1998;17:385a.

121. Gupta NK, Pointon RC, Wilkinson PM. A randomised clinical trial to contrast radiotherapy with radiotherapy and methotrexate given synchronously in head and neck cancer. Clin Radiol 1987;38:575–81.

122. Haselow R, Adams G, Oken M, et al. Cisplatinum with radiation therapy for locally advanced unresectable head and neck cancer. Proc ASCO 1983;2:160.

123. Marcial VA, Pajak TF, Mohiuddin M, et al. Concomitant cisplatin chemotherapy and radiotherapy in advanced mucosal squamous cell carcinoma of the head and neck: long-term results of the Radiation Therapy Oncology Group study 81–17. Cancer 1990;66:1861–8.

124. Haselow R, Warshaw M, Oken M. Radiation alone versus radiation with weekly low dose cisplatin in unresectable cancer of the head and neck. In: Fee W, Geopfert H, Johns M, eds. Head and neck cancer. Vol. 2. Philadelphia: BC Decker, 1990:279.

125. Taylor SGT, Murthy AK, Caldarelli DD, et al. Combined simultaneous cisplatin/fluorouracil chemotherapy and split course radiation in head and neck cancer. J Clin Oncol 1989;7:846–56.

126. Adelstein DJ, Sharan VM, Damm C, et al. Concurrent radiation therapy, 5-fluorouracil, and cisplatin for stage II, III, and IV, node-negative, squamous cell head and neck cancer: results and surgical implications. Cancer 1992;70:2685–90.

127. Wendt TG, Hartenstein RC, Wustrow TP, Lissner J. Cisplatin, fluorouracil with leucovorin calcium enhancement, and synchronous accelerated radiotherapy in the management of locally advanced head and neck cancer: a phase II study. J Clin Oncol 1989;7:471–6.

128. Vokes EE, Panje WR, Schilsky RL, et al. Hydroxyurea, fluorouracil, and concomitant radiotherapy in poor-prognosis head and neck cancer: a phase I–II study. J Clin Oncol 1989;7:761–8.

129. Adelstein DJ, Saxton JP, Lavertu P, et al. A phase III randomized trial comparing concurrent chemotherapy and radiotherapy with radiotherapy alone in resectable stage III and IV squamous cell head and neck cancer: preliminary results. Head Neck 1997;19:567–75.

130. Looney W, Hopkins H, Tubiana M. Experimental and clinical studies alternating chemotherapy and radiotherapy. Cancer Metastasis Rev 1989;8:53–79.

131. Merlano M, Vitale V, Rosso R, et al. Treatment of advanced squamous-cell carcinoma of the head and neck with alternating chemotherapy and radiotherapy. N Engl J Med 1992;327:1115–21.

132. Fu KK. Combined-modality therapy for head and neck cancer. Oncology (Huntingt) 1997;11:1781–90.

133. Bachaud JM, David JM, Boussin G, Daly N. Combined postoperative radiotherapy and weekly cisplatin infusion for locally advanced squamous cell carcinoma of the head and neck: preliminary report of a randomized trial. Int J Radiat Oncol Biol Phys 1991;20:243–6.

134. Heyne KE, Lippman SM, Hong WK. Chemoprevention in head and neck cancer. Hematol Oncol Clin North Am 1991;5:783–95.

135. Califano J, van der Riet P, Westra W, et al. Genetic progression model for head and neck cancer: implications for field cancerization. Cancer Res 1996;56:2488–92.

136. Papadimitrakopoulou VA, Shin DM, Hong WK. Molecular and cellular biomarkers for field cancerization and multistep process in head and neck tumorigenesis. Cancer Metastasis Rev 1996;15:53–76.

137. Strong MS, Incze J, Vaughan CW. Field cancerization in the aerodigestive tract—its etiology, manifestation, and significance. J Otolaryngol 1984;13:1–6.

138. Cooper JS, Pajak TF, Rubin P, et al. Second malignancies in patients who have head and neck cancer: incidence, effect on survival and implications based on the RTOG experience. Int J Radiat Oncol Biol Phys 1989;17:449–56.

139. Licciardello JT, Spitz MR, Hong WK. Multiple primary cancer in patients with cancer of the head and neck: second cancer of the head and neck, esophagus, and lung. Int J Radiat Oncol Biol Phys 1989;17:467–76.

140. Boone CW, Kelloff GJ, Malone WE. Identification of candidate cancer chemopreventive agents and their evaluation in animal models and human clinical trials: a review. Cancer Res 1990;50:2–9.

141. Khuri FR, Lippman SM, Spitz MR, et al. Molecular epidemiology and retinoid chemoprevention of head and neck cancer. J Natl Cancer Inst 1997;89:199–211.

142. Hong WK, Lippman SM, Itri LM, et al. Prevention of second primary tumors with isotretinoin in squamous-cell carcinoma of the head and neck. N Engl J Med 1990;323:795–801.

143. Hong WK, Lippman SM, Wolf GT. Recent advances in head and neck cancer—larynx preservation and cancer chemoprevention: the Seventeenth Annual Richard and Hinda Rosenthal Foundation Award Lecture. Cancer Res 1993;53:5113–20.

144. Bolla M, Laplanche A, Lefur R, et al. Prevention of second primary tumours with a second generation retinoid in squamous cell carcinoma of oral cavity and oropharynx: long term follow-up. Eur J Cancer 1996;32A:375–6. letter.

145. Vokes EE, Weichselbaum RR, Lippman SM, Hong WK. Head and neck cancer. N Engl J Med 1993;328:184–94.

146. Chan AT, Teo PM, Johnson PJ. Controversies in the management of locoregionally advanced nasopharyngeal carcinoma. Curr Opin Oncol 1998;10:219–25.

147. El Gueddari B. Final results of the VUMCA I randomized trial comparing neoadjuvent chemotherapy (CT) (BEC) plus radiotherapy (RT) alone in undifferentiated nasopharyngeal carcinoma (UNCT). Proc ASCO 1998;17:385a.

148. Chan AT, Teo PM, Leung TW, et al. A prospective randomized study of chemotherapy adjunctive to definitive radiotherapy in advanced nasopharyngeal carcinoma. Int J Radiat Oncol Biol Phys 1995;33:569–77.

149. Al-Sarraf M, LeBlanc M, Giri PG, et al. Chemoradiotherapy versus radiotherapy in patients with advanced nasopharyngeal cancer: phase III randomized Intergroup study 0099. J Clin Oncol 1998;16:1310–7.

150. Al-Sarraf M, LeBlanc M, Giri P, et al. Chemo-radiotherapy vs radiotherapy in patients with advanced nasopharyngeal cancer. Intergroup 0099 phase III study: progress report. Proc ASCO 1998;17:385a.

151. NCCN practice guidelines for head and neck cancer. Oncology (Huntingt) 1998;12:39–147.

152. Spiro RH. Management of malignant tumors of the salivary glands. Oncology (Huntingt) 1998;12:671–80.

153. Suen JY, Johns ME. Chemotherapy for salivary gland cancer. Laryngoscope 1982;92:235–9.

# ENDOCRINE AND NEUROENDOCRINE NEOPLASMS

# CHAPTER 67

# MULTIPLE ENDOCRINE NEOPLASIA

• JOSEPH R. PISEGNA • MARK P. SAWICKI

The endocrine, central nervous, and gastrointestinal systems work closely as a network to fine-tune the amount of hormones released in the body. Neoplastic disease originating from common ancestral cells may involve any of these systems. Patients with neoplastic disease may develop multiple tumors in endocrine, neuroendocrine, or gastroenteropancreatic tissues that follow three specific genetic patterns. Based on the clinical syndrome and prior to the cloning of the affected gene, these three patterns of disease were classified as multiple endocrine neoplasia (MEN). Although the patterns share similarities with regard to the neoplastic cell type, they vary with respect to the clinical syndromes. The three major patterns of disease are called *multiple endocrine neoplasia type 1* (MEN 1), *multiple endocrine neoplasia type 2A* (MEN 2A), and *multiple endocrine neoplasia type 2B* (MEN 2B) (Table 67–1). The recent developments in cloning the genes for MEN 1 and MEN 2 have led to the development of specific genetic tests for these conditions as well as a better understanding of the pattern of gene mutations occurring among affected families.

As shown in Table 67–1, the tumors involved in the MEN syndromes occur within endocrine, gastrointestinal, or neural tissues in a manner that determines their phenotypic expression. This pattern of expression suggests that an ancestral cell that is common among the systems becomes dysregulated, further suggesting a relationship among the nervous, endocrine, and gastrointestinal systems. The cells that link these systems are probably the endocrine and endocrine-like cells that originate from neural tissue, most likely the neural crest during embryologic development.[1] The most common characteristic of these tissues gave rise to the acronym APUD (amine precursor uptake and decarboxylation). Histologically, these tumors are characterized by monotonous sheets of cells that consist of small, compact nuclei that are uniform in appearance and contain electron-dense granules that have either biologically active amines or peptides (see Chapter 71). These granules contain chromogranins (A and C), neuron-specific enolase, and synaptophysins in varying concentrations. The concept of a common ancestral cell that gives rise to the development of neuroendocrine tumors has been accepted by many clinicians[2–4] but resisted by others because of controversy over the neural crest origin of gastroenteropancreatic cells and concern about the biologic relevance of the hypothesis.[5, 6] The identification of genetic abnormalities occurring in these disorders, however, makes the earlier speculation more attractive.

MEN 1, MEN 2A, and MEN 2B are inherited in an autosomal dominant manner, with differing degrees of penetrance. Similarly, the age at which the symptoms develop may vary among members of the same family.[7] There may also be variability in the malignant potential of tumors within a given family.[8] The variable expression and behavior of these tumors, as well as their multicentricity, make their treatment difficult. The diagnosis and treatment of the individual tumors that compose the MEN syndromes are described later in this chapter. The first part of this chapter focuses on the MEN 1 syndrome and the second part includes both forms of the MEN 2 syndrome. Both parts expand the understanding of the unique genetic abnormalities, pathogenesis, diagnosis, and treatment of the syndromes.

## Multiple Endocrine Neoplasia Type 1

### MEN 1 GENETICS

As shown in Table 67–1 the first of the syndromes, MEN 1, is an inherited syndrome characterized by tumors of the parathyroid, pancreas, duodenum, and anterior pituitary and, less commonly, the lung, stomach, thymus, and adrenal gland. The search for the gene that predisposes individuals to MEN 1 was initiated by several groups in the 1980s. In 1988, the MEN 1 gene locus was assigned to 11q13 by genetic linkage analysis.[9] Loss of heterozygosity overlapping the putative gene locus identified in MEN 1 and sporadic tumors suggested that the MEN 1 gene functioned as a tumor-suppressor gene.[10–13] The gene responsible for the syndrome was later identified as containing inactivating mutations associated with the phenotypic expression of MEN 1.[14] The MEN 1 gene contains 10 exons and encodes a ubiquitously expressed 2.8-kb transcript. The predicted 610–amino acid protein product, termed *MENIN*, is unlike any previously known protein. Studies using immunofluorescence, Western blots, and epitope tags with green fluorescent protein indicate that MENIN is a nuclear protein.[15] There are a few mutation hot spots, but there does not appear to

*Table 67–1.* **Clinical Syndromes of Multiple Endocrine Neoplasia (MEN)**

| Syndrome | MEN 1 | MEN 2A | MEN 2B |
|---|---|---|---|
| Pituitary adenoma | X | | |
| Pancreatic islet cell tumor | X | | |
| Zollinger-Ellison syndrome | X | | |
| Parathyroid adenoma | X | X | |
| Parathyroid hyperplasia | X | X | |
| Medullary carcinoma of the thyroid | | X | X |
| Pheochromocytoma | | X | X |
| Neurofibroma | | | X |
| Mucoid neuroma | | | X |
| Ganglioneuromatosis | | | X |

be a correlation between MEN 1 phenotype and gene mutation.[16] The precise role of MENIN in the nucleus is not understood at present.

Now that the gene locus is well described, it is possible to determine the patterns of inheritance observed in MEN 1. For example, familial clustering of MEN 1 was studied in four kindreds from the Burin peninsula/Fortune Bay area of Newfoundland, where affected patients are known to develop prolactinomas, carcinoids, and parathyroid tumors but not pancreatic tumors (referred to as *MEN 1 Burin*). A nonsense mutation in the MEN 1 gene was found to be responsible for the disease in the affected members in all four of the MEN 1/Burin families, providing evidence for the existence of a common founder.[17] Mutation of the MENIN gene is identified in the majority of MEN 1 families. In a large study, germline MEN 1 mutations were identified in 47 of 50 probands with familial MEN 1, in 7 of 8 cases with sporadic MEN 1, and in 1 of 3 cases with atypical sporadic MEN 1.[16] On detailed analysis, it is apparent that most of the MEN 1 germline mutations occur in regions of CpG/CpNpG, short DNA repeats, or single nucleotide repeat motifs that can account for recurring germline mutations in 50% of the mutations in North American MEN 1 families.[18] It is likely that to facilitate the diagnosis and prediction of MEN 1 in patients and their relatives, strategies will be developed to screen for MENIN gene mutations by single-strand conformational polymorphism (SSCP) analysis.[19]

Consistent with Knudson's hypothesis and the tumor suppressor gene paradigm, somatic MEN 1 mutations were also found in pancreatic endocrine tumors, pituitary tumors, carcinoid tumors, and parathyroid tumors not associated with MEN 1.[20–25] It is unknown why some MEN 1 patients and some sporadic tumors do not have MENIN mutations, but it has been suggested that there may be a second tumor-suppressor gene locus neighboring the MENIN gene at 11q13.[26]

By determining the genetic abnormality occurring in patients with MEN 1, using SSCP analysis, an estimation of the age-related penetrance of the disease can be determined. This is important because it provides an estimate of the most likely age at the time of diagnosis. In one study of 63 unrelated MEN 1 families, mutations within the 2790-bp coding region of the MEN 1 gene identified 47 mutations with an age-related penetrance of 7, 52, 87, 98, 99, and 100% at 10, 20, 30, 40, 50, and 60 years of age, respectively.[16] In another study of 84 families with either MEN 1 or MEN 1–related inherited endocrine tumors germline mutations were identified in 87% of the MEN 1 families. In that study, gene carriers were identified by genetic analysis (167 affected and 53 unaffected), and age-related penetrance was estimated to be greater than 95% at age 30 years or more.[27]

## NATURAL HISTORY AND DIAGNOSIS

Although MEN 1 has a high penetrance, there is significant heterogeneity in expression. MEN 1 patients usually (80 to 90% of cases) have asymptomatic primary hyperparathyroidism or complications of hypercalcemia at the time of initial diagnosis.[28–31] Development of tumors at other sites is variable even within families. Only a minority of patients have clinically important tumors at more than two sites, with the pancreas being the most common second site. Clinically significant disease is usually diagnosed during the third or fourth decade of life. The clinical findings include, in descending order of frequency, nephrolithiasis, peptic ulcer disease, hypoglycemia, headache, visual field loss, hypopituitarism, acromegaly, galactorrhea, amenorrhea, Cushing's syndrome, and complications related to the development of islet cell tumors of the pancreas (described in Chapter 69). Prospective biochemical screening programs detect asymptomatic affected individuals at a much earlier age.[32, 33] Biochemical screening should begin at age 10 and be performed annually. This screening should include ionized serum calcium and peptide hormone levels. A reasonable peptide screening panel includes serum prolactin, insulin-like growth factor I (IGF-I), parathyroid hormone (PTH), gastrin, insulin, glucagon, and pancreatic polypeptide. Since the MEN 1 gene has been identified, prenatal testing is now feasible. Once routine genetic testing is available, all at-risk family members should be offered screening and genetic counseling to determine who should be followed by biochemical screening.

Virtually every patient with MEN 1 develops evidence of primary hyperparathyroidism.[28, 34–36] Approximately one third of these patients are asymptomatic at the time of diagnosis.[28] The diagnosis should be confirmed by the measurement of elevated ionized calcium levels on at least two occasions and elevated intact PTH levels. The parathyroid glands may contain multiple adenomas or areas of hyperplasia, and years may pass before a pancreatic islet cell tumor or a pituitary adenoma becomes evident. Even with familial clustering there are differences in disease expression. In one study, two patterns of hyperparathyroidism were found.[37] One group had solitary or double adenomas, and recurrence after resection was uncommon, whereas the other group had hyperplasia, and persistent or recurrent disease was common.

Pancreatic endocrine tumors are identified in approximately 60% of MEN 1 patients.[35, 38, 39] The most common functional tumor is a gastrinoma; less commonly an insulinoma is found. The Zollinger-Ellison syndrome (ZES) occurs in approximately one third of patients with MEN 1, although the relationship between the timing for the development of the two diseases may be unrelated because a diagnosis of MEN 1 frequently precedes the development of ZES. The diagnosis of ZES is based on an elevated fasting serum gastrin level and may be confirmed by a positive secretin stimulation test. In many cases, the severity of the ZES can be decreased by parathyroidectomy, which serves to reduce the level of hypercalcemia and thus reduce gastric acid secretion.[40] The majority of gastrinomas are occult (<1 cm), multiple, and found within the gastrinoma triangle.[39, 41, 42] Tumor is frequently found within lymph nodes, but hepatic metastases are infrequent in most series (Table 67–2). Consequently, there is a high metastatic rate reported for these tumors, but the clinical significance of tumor within lymph nodes may be questionable. Moreover, patients with hepatic metastases have a relatively good prognosis because of the slow progression of the disease. Because of the unique tumor biology of gastrinomas, the management of MEN 1 associated with ZES is controversial. Some have advocated aggressive surgical management, whereas others suggest that surgical resection does not result in cure.[29, 38, 39, 42, 43] In one series of 10 patients with MEN 1 who underwent surgical

*Table 67–2.* **Metastases in MEN 1 Patients**

| Institution | Tumor in Lymph Nodes No. (%) | Hepatic Metastases No. (%) | Reference |
|---|---|---|---|
| NIH | 13/18 (73) | 3/18 (17) | 75 |
| University of Tasmania | 7/32 (22) | 4/32 (13) | 42 |
| Bichat-Claude Bernard | 7/45 (16) | 14/45 (31) | 38 |
| University of Michigan | 14/34 (41) | 1/34 (3) | 39 |
| Vrije Universiteit Brussel | 7/18 (39) | 1/18 (6) | 41 |

resection of gastrinoma, only 1 patient (10%) had a short-term cure that lasted only 3 months. In contrast, another study of 40 MEN 1 patients with functional syndromes treated with surgery reported that 68% of the 34 patients with ZES remained eugastrinemic for as long as 19 years.[39] The differences between these studies in part reflect differing operative strategy and varied tumor biology. Multicenter trials combined with genetic tumor analysis may help identify the best operative candidates.

Pituitary tumors are clinically evident in as much as 65% of MEN 1 patients.[44–46] They may be the presenting endocrinopathy in young patients.[28] Usually they are prolactin-producing or, less commonly, growth hormone–producing microadenomas. Cushing's disease is less common in most series. Larger tumors may produce symptoms because of mass effect, for example, visual field loss or hypopituitarism. Diagnosis of these tumors is usually by measurement of elevated serum prolactin or growth hormone levels. Magnetic resonance imaging (MRI) or computed tomography (CT) may demonstrate the tumor, but many microadenomas are too small to image. These tumors behave in similar fashion to that noted for their more common sporadic counterparts and therefore are treated in a comparable fashion.

Adrenal tumors are found in as many as one third of patients.[47, 48] Usually they are benign cortical adenomas, cortical or nodular hyperplasia, and rarely malignant tumors. Most of these tumors are nonfunctional and are identified incidentally during imaging studies of the pancreas. Most patients who have adrenal tumors also have pancreatic endocrine tumors.[48] Although most of these tumors are hormonally silent, diagnostic tests should be performed to identify potentially functional tumors. Serum potassium and cortisol levels and 24-hour urinary catecholamine levels should be measured. Dexamethasone suppression tests may be performed if clinically warranted.

Carcinoid tumors particularly involving the duodenum are seen in some cases of MEN 1 and occur more frequently when both ZES and MEN 1 are present.[49, 50] Gastric, bronchial, and thymic carcinoids may also be found.[35, 51, 52] Duodenal carcinoids usually do not metastasize and may be managed endoscopically.[53] Bronchial carcinoids are usually benign and occur most often in women. Thymic carcinoids tend to occur in men who are heavy smokers and can be particularly aggressive.[28, 54] These tumors are generally diagnosed by CT.

As in the gastrointestinal tract, specific dermatologic disturbances have been identified in MEN 1. These tumors include multiple angiofibromas, collagenomas, and lipomas. In a study from the group at the National Institutes of Health, skin biopsies from five patients with MEN 1 identified allelic deletion of the MEN 1 gene, suggesting that a loss of function mutation of the MEN 1 gene may provide a basis for the development of these skin disorders in patients with MEN 1.[55] One patient with malignant carcinoid diagnosed as rosacea was reported and was later found to have an additional functioning parathyroid tumor.[56] The percentage of patients with MEN 1 who develop skin lesions and the number of clinical manifestations are unknown. For example, there has been one case report of a patient with diffuse petechiae, severe thrombocytopenia, hemolytic anemia, and MEN 1 that suggested an association of thrombotic thrombocytopenia purpura with MEN 1. This observation raises the question of a genetic linkage or hormonal interaction, or both, between the two disorders.[57] The association of MEN 1 syndrome with other neoplastic proliferations, such as pulmonary lymphangioleiomyoma and malignant lymphoma, has also been reported.[58, 59]

## DIAGNOSTIC IMAGING STUDIES

Radiologically identifiable pancreatic endocrine tumors are a frequent requirement for exploration in patients with MEN 1 and pose the most significant challenge to accurately imaged tumors. Delay in identifying the site of tumor involvement may lead to a 30 to 50% incidence of metastases. Based on results obtained from 25 MEN 1 patients, conventional pancreatic imaging was shown to be insensitive and nonspecific for recognizing even substantial pancreatic tumors associated with MEN 1.[60] With regard to imaging studies, the value of [$^{111}$In]-somatostatin receptor scintigraphy (SRS) has been shown to have a higher sensitivity than conventional diagnostic modalities for detecting pancreatic tumors. In one study of 48 patients (37 with carcinoid and pancreatic endocrine tumors and medullary carcinoma of the thyroid and 11 with neuroendocrine syndromes) 35 of 48 patients had positive SRS results. In 88% of the patients with positive conventional imaging, the SRS was also positive. In 50% of the patients with negative conventional imaging studies, the SRS was positive, indicating that SRS is both sensitive and specific for the diagnosis of these tumors.[61] In another study, MRI was compared with other imaging modalities for the diagnosis of pancreatic or extrapancreatic tumors in patients with ZES. MRI had an overall sensitivity of 83% compared with angiography (61%), CT (56%), and ultrasonography (50%).[62] Although MEN 1 patients were not included in this study, the results are consistent with more recent data in patients with both MEN 1 and ZES (unpublished data). Endoscopic ultrasonography is particularly useful for identifying pancreatic and duodenal tumors.[63] With the development of endoscopic ultrasonography (EUS) as a sensitive imaging modality in the detection of primary neuroendocrine tumors of the duodenum and pancreas, the current recommendations are that patients undergo imaging with a combination of EUS, SRS, CT, and MRI. By combining these imaging modalities, tumors can be detected in more than 80% of cases (see Chapter 69).

## MEDICAL AND SURGICAL MANAGEMENT

**Surgical Management of MEN 1.** Surgical management of MEN 1 patients is challenging because not only is the disease rare but different centers have reported varied experience with the medical and surgical management of these patients. A few centers have published large collective experiences with the surgical management of these patients. The surgical strategy adopted by these centers often reflects their local experience. For example, in some centers the primary determinant of MEN 1–associated mortality was metastatic pancreatic endocrine tumors, whereas in another it was metastatic thymic carcinoids. The natural history for the disease in these different kindreds dictates the aggressiveness needed for surgical extirpation of tumors. Thus, the surgical management of MEN 1 patients must consider that there are varied presentations and biologic behaviors for these inherited tumors. It is therefore best to consider each patient individually, primarily within the context of the natural history of the disease within that particular family and secondarily in relation to the regional experience.

**Parathyroid Hyperplasia.** The vast majority of MEN 1 patients have primary hyperparathyroidism at the time of diagnosis. If left untreated, many of these patients develop renal failure; therefore, subtotal parathyroidectomy is recommended for all MEN 1 patients with primary hyperparathyroidism. Some authors have recommended selective parathyroid surgery for patients with symptoms or calcium levels greater than 11 mg/dl.[29] It is best to perform parathyroidectomy prior to surgery for gastrinoma, as the patient's peptic ulcer disease will be more easily controlled this way. Preoperative imaging is generally unnecessary unless the patient is being surgically treated for recurrent hyperparathyroidism. Most patients have four-gland hyperplasia. The two surgical options are subtotal three-gland resection and total parathyroidectomy with autotransplantation.[64] The former operation is preferred by many because of the lower incidence of permanent hypoparathyroidism. In both approaches, the cervical thymus should be removed because this is the most common location for a supernumerary parathyroid gland as well as a frequent cause for persistent postoperative hyperparathyroidism. Less extensive resection may rarely be necessary for selected patients who truly have only one- or two-gland involvement. The initial surgical success rate is greater than 90% in patients with subtotal resection.[65] The recurrence rate after operation is much higher than that for MEN 2A and sporadic disease. Patients may have recurrence as late as 20 years after operation, and it may be as high as 68% with long-term follow-up.[65, 66] These patients rarely develop parathyroid carcinoma. Annual screening of serum ionized calcium levels is sufficient to detect recurrent disease.

**Pancreatic Endocrine Tumors.** The biologic behavior of MEN 1 pancreatic endocrine tumors is extremely varied, and their surgical management is different from that for their sporadic counterparts. Deaths from pituitary tumor or malignant endocrine tumors within the thorax are just as common or more common than deaths from pancreatic malignant neoplasms in some series.[54] This has resulted in considerable controversy regarding the aggressiveness of operation and several surgical strategies for the management of these patients. Most of the MEN 1 pancreatic tumors are asymptom-

atic. Usually multiple small asymptomatic tumors are found throughout the pancreas, and they are often benign.[67] In some families, however, pancreatic endocrine tumors do not occur in any members (MEN 1 Burin). Symptomatic tumors include gastrinomas and insulinomas and less commonly glucagonomas, VIPomas, and somatostatinomas. Because the malignant potential of these tumors is unclear, and there is no good multicenter controlled analysis of these tumors in MEN 1 patients, we regard any macroscopic tumor as potentially malignant.

Gastrinomas are present in up to 30% of MEN 1 patients.[64] Usually these tumors are multicentric and found within the duodenum and pancreatic head. For this reason, endoscopic ultrasonography is helpful in preoperative localization. Helical CT with pancreatic phase imaging and Octreoscan are also helpful in identifying tumors preoperatively. The latter imaging studies are also sensitive in identifying extensive hepatic metastases, which has a significant impact on the operative strategy for these patients. Transhepatic venous sampling can regionalize gastrinomas, but we have not advocated this study because of the associated co-morbidity. None of the imaging modalities is as sensitive as operative exploration by an experienced surgeon. Resection of all gastrinoma tumors identified, including duodenal, pancreatic, and lymph node tumors, can result in eugastrinemia in as many as two thirds of patients.

Insulinomas are present in 10% of MEN 1 patients. These tumors are found frequently within the pancreatic tail, but unlike their sporadic counterparts, they are usually multiple. In contrast to gastrinomas, these tumors are rarely ectopic and usually are not metastatic. Preoperative imaging can be helpful, but like gastrinomas the offending tumor may not be visualized. Octreoscan in particular is significantly less sensitive for insulinomas than for gastrinomas. Hyperinsulinemia resulting from an insulinoma in MEN 1 is a rare, but potentially curable, tumor because the majority are benign. In one surgical series, distal subtotal pancreatectomy with enucleation of pancreatic insulinomas that were detected intraoperatively resulted in the immediate cure of two patients, suggesting that distal subtotal pancreatectomy and enucleation is the treatment of choice for the management of insulinoma occurring in the setting of MEN 1.[68] Some groups have advocated total pancreatectomy for patients with MEN 1 if the pancreatic tumor has caused high morbidity and mortality within the family, especially if several tumors are present in the pancreas.[69] In general, the management of MEN 1 pancreatic endocrine tumors can be categorized as follows:

1. *Abnormal serum hormone levels but no demonstrable tumor.* This group of patients frequently has elevated pancreatic polypeptide or gastrin levels. Extensive imaging in these patients does not reveal any identifiable tumor. These patients should not be operated on unless their hormone-related symptoms cannot be controlled medically. They should be followed with annual imaging studies.

2. *Asymptomatic patient with macroscopic pancreatic tumor.* Most patients with MEN 1 are found to have multiple small nonfunctional pancreatic tumors. Some of these are occult, whereas others grow to a large size and metastasize. It is controversial whether to remove all these tumors. In general, the growth rate of these tumors is slow, and partial

pancreatectomy will ultimately be followed by additional tumors developing in the pancreatic remnant. It is unknown how many of these tumors will progress to malignancy, and current radiologic and biopsy techniques cannot distinguish benign from malignant tumors. The propensity of tumors to become malignant may vary among kindreds. Some kindreds may have uniform malignant potential, whereas others may not. If this information is known, aggressive surgical intervention may be warranted. In general, tumors larger than 2 cm should be considered malignant, and these patients should undergo surgery.

3. *Symptomatic hormone syndrome and macroscopic tumor.* These patients undergo exploratory surgery if they have demonstrable tumor. Most of these patients have gastrinomas and less commonly insulinomas. Other functional tumors are uncommon. The majority of gastrinomas in these patients are in the duodenal wall and adjacent tissues. Since these individuals have multifocal gastrinomas at the same time they have multiple non-gastrinomas, it can be challenging to resect all gastrinomas. Some groups have had success with transhepatic venous gastrin sampling to localize occult tumors and achieve eugastrinemia.[39, 70, 71] Other groups only resect large gastrinomas (>3 cm) clearly identified by imaging and verified by transhepatic venous sampling.[29, 72] Others consider gastrinomas hopelessly incurable and treat them medically.[38, 73] The frequency of hepatic metastases in these patients varies. In general, the prognosis for MEN 1–associated gastrinomas is better than that for sporadic gastrinomas.[74, 75] Many of these gastrinomas may be small compared with the other nongastrinoma pancreatic tumors in the same patient. Surgical resection of MEN 1 gastrinomas is frequently unsuccessful for permanently normalizing serum gastrin levels, but gastrin levels may be sufficiently lowered to assist in control of the peptic ulcer disease. In some series, pancreatic but not duodenal gastrinoma was a high risk factor for the development of hepatic metastases. Advanced age and tumor size are also risk factors. Usually the hepatic metastases are present at the time of diagnosis or operation.

Insulinomas are more straightforward in MEN 1 than are gastrinomas.[39] They are less common, less malignant, almost always found within the pancreas, and frequently multiple. Transhepatic venous sampling can be helpful in defining the location of the tumor. Surgical exploration is frequently successful but requires a distal pancreatectomy.[76]

4. *Hepatic metastases.* Patients with metastatic tumor may live for many years and may fare better than their counterparts with sporadic tumors.[38] Metachronous hepatic metastases are less common in most series. Limited hepatic involvement may be resectable or amenable to cryotherapy. Hepatic transplantation probably has a limited role in these patients.

**Pituitary Tumors.** As many as 65% of MEN 1 patients have clinically important pituitary tumors. These patients frequently have prolactinomas or growth hormone–secreting tumors. Other functional tumors are less frequent. Annual screening with serum prolactin α subunit and IGF-I and imaging every 3 years will identify most clinically relevant disease. Patients with prolactinomas frequently respond to the dopamine agonist bromocriptine. Growth hormone–secreting tumors may respond to octreotide. There is no effective drug therapy for the nonfunctional tumors. Patients

who do not respond should be considered for surgery. Other tumors should be treated surgically.

**Adrenal Tumors.** Adrenal abnormalities occur in one third of MEN 1 patients. Most are cortical adenomas or hyperplasia and of no clinical consequence. They generally do not require surgical intervention. Carcinomas are rare. Tumor size should be followed by annual imaging studies. Tumors larger than 4 cm should be surgically removed.

**Thymic Tumors.** In some families, thymic carcinoids are a significant cause of death. These tumors are usually diagnosed late and are highly malignant. Cervical thymectomy should be performed at the time of parathyroidectomy to minimize the risk of this tumor's developing. CT should be performed to screen for these tumors.

**Chemotherapy, Biotherapy and Radiotherapy.** Surgery is the cornerstone of therapy for neuroendocrine tumors. Adjuvant chemotherapy is generally not indicated but may be effective in patients with metastatic disease.[77] Fortunately, a minority of MEN 1 patients develop metastatic disease, and it usually arises from pancreatic endocrine tumors, although in one series thymic carcinoids significantly contributed to tumor-related deaths.[54] Metastatic pancreatic endocrine tumors may benefit from tumor debulking to assist in control of disease symptoms related to hormone production. Proton pump inhibitors are effective in controlling acid secretion in patients with ZES, and diazoxide may be effective in patients with uncontrolled hyperinsulinemia. Cytotoxic chemotherapy is generally ineffective for controlling tumor growth, but streptozotocin and 5-fluorouracil may be effective in a small percentage of patients. Biotherapy with somatostatin analogues and interferon-α is modestly effective in alleviating hormone-related symptoms and may inhibit tumor growth in a smaller percentage. Unfortunately, progress in the development of effective chemotherapy regimens has been hampered by the lack of multicenter controlled trials. External-beam radiation therapy is not helpful, but ongoing trials using [111]In-DTPA (diethylenetriamine pentaacetic acid)-octreotide and 90Y DOTA (1,4,7,10-tetra-azacyclododecane-N,N′,N″,N‴-tetra-acetic acid)-octreotide may prove effective.

## PROGNOSIS

The lethality of endocrine tumors associated with the MEN 1 syndrome has been controversial. In one study to determine the cause and age of death in 59 MEN 1 patients, 27 died directly of MEN 1–specific illness and 32 from non–MEN 1 causes. The causes of death in the MEN 1 patients included islet cell tumor (n = 12), ulcer disease (n = 6), hypercalcemia-uremia (n = 3), carcinoid tumor (n = 6), and nonendocrine malignancies (n = 9). In general, death in MEN 1–affected individuals occurred in younger patients with a median age of 47 years, and pancreatic islet cell tumors were the most common cause of death in these patients.[69]

## Multiple Endocrine Neoplasia Type 2

### MEN 2 GENETICS

MEN 2, like MEN 1, is an autosomal dominant inherited disease.[78, 79] In contrast to the tumor-suppressor gene mechanism responsible for MEN 1, the development of tumors in patients with MEN 2 occurs from mutations in a proto-oncogene. This proto-oncogene, called *ret*, encodes a receptor tyrosine kinase that may have a role in the development of neural crest cells and thereby may provide an understanding of the development of tumor cells originating embryologically from the neural crest. *ret* ligands include glial cell line–derived neurotrophic factor and neurturin, which compose a family of transforming growth factor-β–related neurotrophic factors, which have trophic influences on neuronal cells. Germline mutations in one of eight distinct codons contained in *ret* give rise to the three types of MEN 2, namely, MEN 2A (60%), MEN 2B (5%), and familial medullary thyroid carcinoma (FMTC) (35%). Because of the limited spectrum of mutations found within the majority of MEN 2 patients, genetic testing is feasible. It is important that detection of the *ret* proto-oncogene mutation be carried out early in the course of the disease, prior to the development of clinical or biochemical evidence of disease. Early diagnosis and treatment are essential to ensure a good prognosis for patients with this disease.

Optimally, a combination of genetic and biochemical testing should be performed in the evaluation of at-risk MEN 2 patients. In one study, the authors concluded that biochemical tests can be replaced by direct DNA mutation analysis as the first-line screening in identifying gene carriers of MEN 2A.[80] The discovery of specific mutations in the *ret* proto-oncogene can now reliably predict MEN 2A, MEN 2B, and FMTC, permitting genetic screening of at-risk individuals. The availability of polymorphic DNA probes permits the use of restriction fragment-length polymorphisms (RFLPs) to identify carriers of the gene rapidly if mutations cannot be identified within the RET gene.[81, 82] It should be stated that undergoing genetic testing may lead to anxiety and depression in these patients but also relief, even in the face of a positive test outcome.[83] Therefore, every effort should be made to counsel patients appropriately both before and after genetic testing. Prenatal screening for *ret* mutations by genetic analysis of the DNA isolated from the chorionic villi can also be performed during routine amniocentesis and the information used to counsel at-risk patients.[84, 85]

## MEN 2A NATURAL HISTORY AND DIAGNOSIS

MEN 2A (Sipple's syndrome) is an autosomal dominant inherited disease characterized by medullary thyroid cancer, pheochromocytoma, and hyperparathyroidism.[86] This syndrome usually presents as a mass in the neck in a middle-aged person and proves to be a bilateral medullary carcinoma of the thyroid.[87, 88] Unilateral or bilateral pheochromocytomas and mild hypercalcemia from parathyroid hyperplasia are also frequently present. It has approximately 70 to 90% penetrance and a variable age of onset. Although there is high penetrance, the expressivity of these multiple endocrine problems varies. In a study of 44 families with MEN 2A, only 41% of cases were clinically manifested by the age of 70. However, 93% of genetic carriers could be identified by age 31 using standard biochemical diagnostic tests.

Genetic carriers of MEN 2 can be identified with 95% accuracy using genetic screening, and these patients are candidates for attempts at early diagnosis. A consensus state-

ment from Europe calls for measurement of basal and pentagastrin- and calcium-stimulated serum levels of calcitonin by radioimmunoassay starting at the age of 3 and continuing annually until age 35. Annual screening for pheochromocytoma, by measuring the urinary excretion of catecholamines, and for hyperparathyroidism, using serum calcium determinations, is also indicated.[89] Because MEN 2 frequently affects women during the childbearing years, significant attention has focused on their obstetric management. The diagnosis of MEN 2A preceding pregnancy may be associated with a normal obstetric outcome in the absence of hypertension associated with pheochromocytoma.[90]

Medullary thyroid carcinomas (MTCs) occur sporadically (75 to 95%) and as part of MEN 2. The prognosis in patients with MEN 2A is in part determined by the development of the very malignant MTC. This is generally the first tumor identified in these patients and is a nearly constant feature. MTC associated with MEN 2A is generally considered less virulent than MEN 2B, although this perspective has been challenged. Unlike sporadic MTC, MEN 2–associated MTC is invariably bilateral, multicentric, and preceded by C-cell hyperplasia. Because the concentration of C cells is highest within the upper poles of the thyroid, these tumors tend to occur in the superior portions of the gland. Fine-needle aspiration biopsy of MTC shows a characteristic amyloid staining that is valuable for diagnosis. These tumors produce large amounts of calcitonin, and immunohistochemistry for this peptide confirms the diagnosis. These tumors metastasize early, usually to the central lymph nodes of the neck and then to distant sites. Although the tumors can spread early, the risk of metastases increases with the size of the tumor. Ten-year survival is 10 to 30% if metastases are present at the time of diagnosis, compared with 80% if they are absent.[91]

Although genetic testing for MTC does not completely replace the predictive value of routine serum calcitonin measurements, small elevations of serum calcitonin may lead to a false-positive diagnosis of MTC. Therefore, DNA testing in addition to measuring the serum calcitonin yields the optimal diagnosis of MEN 2A.[92] One European study suggests that in addition to serum calcitonin, serum chromogranin A is predictive of advanced disease.[93] The use of specific immunologic stains, such as those against pancreatic polypeptide, have been proposed to differentiate familial and sporadic forms of MTC; however, additional studies have yet to be performed to characterize its specificity.[94]

Like MCT, pheochromocytomas occur sporadically or less commonly as part of MEN 2. The most common clinical feature in patients with the sporadic form is hypertension, whereas one study reported that in MEN 2A, only 35% of patients develop hypertension. Furthermore, that study reported that all the pheochromocytomas identified with the MEN 2A syndrome occurred bilaterally, compared with none of the sporadic pheochromocytomas.[95]

The risk for pheochromocytoma and hyperparathyroidism in patients with MEN 2A is clearly associated with the presence of the *ret* mutation at codon 634.[96] In another study, the position of the RET mutation was reported to be related to the disease phenotype, with codon 634 mutations predictive of families predisposed to pheochromocytoma. The authors of this report suggest that in addition to performing 24-hour urinary epinephrine excretion and diagnostic imaging studies, a determination of this point mutation should be obtained in all patients, including those with tumors that appear to be "sporadic."[97] In another study of 29 tumors obtained from "sporadic" cases, 3 tumors (10%) were found to have a mutation in one of the three exons, indicating that somatic mutations in the *ret* proto-oncogene may contribute to tumorigenesis in a small percentage of sporadic pheochromocytomas.[98]

In one study, the prevalence of pheochromocytoma was 40% and that of hyperparathyroidism was 35%.[99] The highest diagnostic and treatment priority for these patients is the pheochromocytomas. The elaboration of catecholamines by this tumor places the patient at risk of sudden death during anesthesia resulting from the rapid and high levels of secreted catecholamines. These tumors primarily produce epinephrine. Cardiovascular events are a significant cause of death in these patients. Therefore, it is essential to rule out the possibility of pheochromocytoma in any patient with MCT, either with or without primary hyperparathyroidism. Screening should begin at age 5 with 24-hour urinary metanephrine levels. Unlike MEN 2B, pheochromocytomas typically present unilaterally in MEN 2A. A combination of imaging studies such as CT, MRI, and scanning with $^{131}$I-metaiodobenzylguanidine ($^{131}$I-MIBG), now makes it possible to localize these tumors accurately.[100]

Hyperparathyroidism is clinically relevant in 15 to 25% of patients with MEN 2A. The patients typically have four-gland hyperplasia with elevated calcium and PTH levels. Similar to MEN 1, imaging with sestamibi scan usually is not helpful in these patients.

It has been reported that MEN 2A is occasionally associated with Hirschsprung's disease, indicating that both syndromes may be linked to germline mutations in the *ret* proto-oncogene. Using genomic DNA isolated from affected individuals and molecular techniques it has been observed that Hirschsprung's disease is associated with a RET exon 10 mutation and occurs more commonly than originally understood.[101] In approximately 25% of patients with Hirschsprung's disease, germline mutations occur in the RET gene.[102]

## MEN 2B NATURAL HISTORY AND DIAGNOSIS

MEN 2B is an autosomal dominant genetic variant of MEN 2 in which MCT and pheochromocytomas are associated not with parathyroid disease but rather with multiple mucosal neuromas or neurofibromas, intestinal ganglioneuromatosis, characteristic facies, and a marfanoid habitus.[103, 104] This variant is usually diagnosed in childhood because of the mucosal neuromatosis and characteristic facies. MEN 2B resembles MEN 2A in that both disorders are inherited in an autosomal dominant fashion and include MCT and pheochromocytoma. The two disorders differ in that only patients with MEN 2B develop neuromas of the mucous membranes.[105] MEN 2B is considered to be a more malignant variant of the MEN 2 syndrome because the pheochromocytomas tend to be bilateral and frequently result in malignant hypertension.[100] In addition, these patients may present with mucosal neuromas, ganglioneuromas of the intestinal tract, and skeletal and ophthalmic abnormalities. On presentation, the patients may provide a history of hyper-

tension and diarrhea or constipation, or both. On physical examination they have the typical nodules of neuromas on the tongue, lips, cheeks, and eyelids and a broadened nasal bridge. There are also typical facial radiographic features that are consistent with this disorder.[106] In addition to the oral and facial abnormalities associated with this syndrome, diffuse ganglioneuromatosis of the alimentary tract is also a characteristic finding in MEN 2. A case of severe diverticulitis has been reported to be associated with MEN 2B, suggesting that other gastrointestinal syndromes may also be associated with this syndrome.[107]

## MEDICAL AND SURGICAL MANAGEMENT OF MEN 2

Of the two subtypes of MEN 2, MEN 2B is the more lethal. Since the development of genetic testing for MEN 2, the role of prophylactic surgery has been addressed and defined.

**Parathyroid Neoplasia.** Management of the parathyroid disease requires the identification and resection of all enlarged glands for cure, but routine subtotal resection need not be performed because this condition occurs in less than 20% of patients, it is readily cured, and recurrence is uncommon.[108, 109] Some authorities have advocated a more aggressive approach, including total parathyroidectomy with autotransplantation.[65]

**Pheochromocytoma.** Pheochromocytomas develop in approximately 50% of MEN 2 patients.[110] Adrenal disease in these patients is frequently bilateral (70%). Ectopic tumors are uncommon. The pathologic features include medullary hyperplasia, pheochromocytoma, and malignant pheochromocytoma, although the latter is uncommon in most series. Most of the patients have adrenal medullary hyperplasia. In the absence of overt symptoms or biochemical abnormalities, this tumor should be not be surgically treated. Pheochromocytoma is the initial presenting tumor in less than 10% of patients. Patients are usually symptomatic at the time of diagnosis. Any MEN 2 patient with a pheochromocytoma should be referred for operation. CT and MIBG studies may reveal unilateral disease or bilateral disease. For patients with unilateral disease, prophylactic resection of the normal or minimally diseased contralateral adrenal gland is controversial. Follow-up of patients with unilateral adrenals remaining should include annual physical examinations and 24-hour urinary catecholamine measurements. After unilateral adrenalectomy, the opposite adrenal develops a pheochromocytoma in 50% of patients over a 5-year period. Patients who have had bilateral adrenalectomy do not have recurrent disease but are at significant risk for addisonian crisis.

**Medullary Thyroid Cancer.** Nearly all patients with MEN 2A and MEN 2B develop MTC. This is the primary determinant for survival in these patients. Multifocal MTCs arise from hyperplasia of thyroid C cells. Early lymph node metastases are common, and distant metastases portend a poor prognosis. MTC in MEN 2B is particularly virulent.[111] Some advocate the use of prophylactic thyroidectomy in affected family members, with close attention to baseline calcitonin levels.[91] The more recent trend is to offer genetic testing and early prophylactic thyroidectomy to prevent the development of MTC.[112, 113] In one study, a 10-year-old boy diagnosed with MEN 2 by DNA testing had normal calcitonin levels but had metastatic MTC at the time of operation.[112] In another study, RET mutations were detected in suspected family members, leading to early thyroidectomy to prevent the development of medullary thyroid carcinoma.[114] In another study, RET mutations at exons 10, 11, and 16 were assessed in tumor DNA extracted from 13 fresh frozen MTCs and a RET mutation was detected in every tumor, including a novel mutation, a 6-bp deletion preceding the cysteine-634, in a sporadic case of MTC.[115] For these reasons, operation at an early age (as early as 5 years) prior to the development of clinically detectable disease based on genetic testing has been advocated. Total thyroidectomy, central lymph node dissection, and parathyroid autotransplantation should be performed in all patients. Preoperative imaging generally is not helpful, but evaluation for the presence of pheochromocytoma is essential. There is no effective radiation therapy, chemotherapy, or hormonal therapy. After thyroidectomy, the patient should receive thyroid replacement. Follow-up with annual basal and stimulated serum calcitonin levels helps identify tumor recurrences.

## PROGNOSIS

The prognosis for MEN 2 is largely determined by the stage of MTC at the time of diagnosis. Since even small MTCs can metastasize at an early age, aggressive surgical management of these patients is warranted. Still, a significant number of patients have complications related to their pheochromocytomas. The relatively high lethality of this disease supports early and thorough genetic and biochemical screening of these patients.

## SUGGESTIONS FOR ADDITIONAL READING

Moley JF, Lairmore TC, Phay JE. Hereditary endocrinopathies. Curr Probl Surg 1999;36:653–762.

Marx S, Spiegel AM, Skarulis MC, et al. Multiple endocrine neoplasia type 1: clinical and genetic topics. Ann Intern Med 1998;129:484–94.

Heshmati HM, Hofbauer LC. Multiple endocrine neoplasia type 2: recent progress in diagnosis and management. Eur J Endocrinol 1997;137:572–8.

Eng C. RET proto-oncogene in the development of human cancer. J Clin Oncol 1999;17:380–93.

## REFERENCES

1. Pearse AG. The cytochemistry and ultrastructure of polypeptide hormone-producing cells of the APUD series and the embryologic, physiologic and pathologic implications of the concept. J Histochem Cytochem 1969;17:303–13.
2. Pearse AG. Islet cell precursors are neurones. Nature 1982;295:96–7.
3. Jager RM, Polk HCJ. Carcinoid apudomas. Curr Probl Cancer 1977;1:1–53.
4. Teitelman G, Joh TH, Reis DJ. Transformation of catecholaminergic precursors into glucagon (A) cells in mouse embryonic pancreas. Proc Natl Acad Sci USA 1981;78:5225–9.
5. Skrabanek P. APUD concept: hypothesis or tautology? Med Hypotheses 1980;6:437–40.
6. Stevens RE, Moore GE. Inadequacy of APUD concept in explaining production of peptide hormones by tumours. Lancet 1983;1:118–9.
7. Hershon KS, Kelly WA, Shaw CM, et al. Prolactinomas as part of the multiple endocrine neoplastic syndrome type 1. Am J Med 1983;74:713–20.
8. Emmertsen K, Elbrond O, Nielsen HE, et al. Familial medullary thyroid carcinoma in multiple endocrine neoplasia (MEN) IIa: diagnosis and problems in treatment. Eur J Cancer Clin Oncol 1982;18:645–50.
9. Larsson C, Skogseid B, Oberg K, et al. Multiple endocrine neoplasia type 1 gene maps to chromosome 11 and is lost in insulinoma. Nature 1988;332:85–7.
10. Thakker RV, Bouloux P, Wooding C, et al. Association of parathyroid tumors in multiple endocrine neoplasia type 1 with loss of alleles on chromosome 11. N Engl J Med 1989;321:218–24.
11. Bystrom C, Larsson C, Blomberg C, et al. Localization of the MEN1 gene to a small region within chromosome 11q13 by deletion mapping in tumors. Proc Natl Acad Sci USA 1990;87:1968–72.
12. Bale AE, Norton JA, Wong EL, et al. Allelic loss on chromosome 11 in hereditary and sporadic tumors related to familial multiple endocrine neoplasia type 1. Cancer Res 1991;51:1154–7.
13. Sawicki MP, Wan YJY, Johnson CL, et al. Loss of heterozygosity on chromosome 11 in sporadic gastrinomas. Hum Genet 1992;89:445–9.
14. Chandrasekharappa SC, Guru SC, Manickam P, et al. Positional cloning of the gene for multiple endocrine neoplasia-type 1. Science 1997;276:404–7.
15. Guru SC, Goldsmith PK, Burns AL, et al. Menin, the product of the MEN1 gene, is a nuclear protein. Proc Natl Acad Sci USA 1998;95:1630–4.
16. Bassett JHD, Forbes SA, Pannett AAJ, et al. Characterization of mutations in patients with multiple endocrine neoplasia type 1. Am J Hum Genet 1998;62:232–44.
17. Olufemi SE, Green JS, Manickam P, et al. Common ancestral mutation in the MEN1 gene is likely responsible for the prolactinoma variant of MEN1 (MEN1Burin) in four kindreds from Newfoundland. Hum Mutat 1998;11:264–9.
18. Agarwal SK, Debelenko LV, Kester MB, et al. Analysis of recurrent germline mutations in the MEN1 gene encountered in apparently unrelated families. Hum Mutat 1998;12:75–82.
19. Karges W, Ludwig L, Kessler H, et al. Menin mutations in the diagnosis and prediction of multiple endocrine neoplasia type 1. Langenbecks Arch Surg 1998;383:183–6.
20. Marx SJ, Agarwal SK, Kester MB, et al. Germline and somatic mutation of the gene for multiple endocrine neoplasia type 1 (MEN1). J Intern Med 1998;243:447–53.
21. Wang EH, Ebrahimi SA, Wu AY, et al. Mutation of the MENIN gene in sporadic pancreatic endocrine tumors. Cancer Res 1998;58:4417–20.
22. Heppner C, Kester MB, Agarwal SK, et al. Somatic mutation of the MEN1 gene in parathyroid tumours. Nature Genet 1997;16:375–378.
23. Zhuang Z, Vortmeyer AO, Pack S, et al. Somatic mutations of the MEN1 tumor suppressor gene in sporadic gastrinomas and insulinomas. Cancer Res 1997;57:4682–4686.
24. Zhuang Z, Ezzat SZ, Vortmeyer AO, et al. Mutations of the MEN1 tumor suppressor gene in pituitary tumors. Cancer Res 1997;57:5446–5451.
25. Debelenko LV, Brambilla E, Agarwal SK, et al. Identification of MEN1 gene mutations in sporadic carcinoid tumors of the lung. Hum Mol Genet 1997;6:2285–2290.
26. Chakrabarti R, Srivatsan ES, Wood TF, et al. Deletion mapping of endocrine tumors localizes a second tumor suppressor gene on chromosome band 11q13. Genes Chromosomes.Cancer 1998;22:130–137.
27. Giraud S, Zhang CX, Serova-Sinilnikova O., Wautot V. Germline mutation analysis in patients with MEN1 and related disorders. Am J Hum Genet 1998;63:455–67.
28. Shepherd JJ. The natural history of multiple endocrine neoplasia type 1. Highly uncommon or highly unrecognized? Arch Surg 1991;126:935–52.
29. Chanson P, Cadiot G, Murat A. Management of patients and subjects at risk for multiple endocrine neoplasia type 1: MEN 1. GENEM 1. Groupe d'Etude des neoplasies endocriniennes multiples de type 1. Horm Res 1997;47:211–20.
30. Wermer P. Genetic aspects of adenomatosis of endocrine glands. Am J Med 1954;16:363–71.
31. Oberg K, Walinder O, Bostrom H, et al. Peptide hormone markers in screening for endocrine tumors in multiple endocrine adenomatosis type I. Am J Med 1982;73:619–30.

32. Skogseid B, Oberg K. Experience with multiple endocrine neoplasia type 1 screening. J Intern Med 1995;238:255–61.
33. Oberg K, Skogseid B. The ultimate biochemical diagnosis of endocrine pancreatic tumours in MEN-1. J Intern Med 1998;243:471–6.
34. Ballard HS, Frame B, Hartsock RJ. Familial multiple endocrine adenoma–peptic ulcer complex. Medicine 1964;43:481–516.
35. Burgess JR, Greenaway TM, Shepherd JJ. Expression of the MEN-1 gene in a large kindred with multiple endocrine neoplasia type 1. J Intern Med 1998;243:465–70.
36. Marx SJ, Vinik AI, Santen RJ, et al. Multiple endocrine neoplasia type I: assessment of laboratory tests to screen for the gene in a large kindred. Medicine (Baltimore) 1986;65:226–41.
37. Kraimps JL, Duh QY, Demeure M, Clark OH. Hyperparathyroidism in multiple endocrine neoplasia syndrome. Surgery 1992;112:1080–6.
38. Mignon M, Ruszniewski P, Podevin P, et al. Current approach to the management of gastrinoma and insulinoma in adults with multiple endocrine neoplasia type I. World J Surg 1993;17:489–97.
39. Thompson NW. Current concepts in the surgical management of multiple endocrine neoplasia type 1 pancreatic-duodenal disease: results in the treatment of 40 patients with Zollinger-Ellison syndrome, hypoglycaemia or both. J Intern Med 1998;243:495–500.
40. Norton JA, Cornelius MJ, Doppman JL, et al. Effect of parathyroidectomy in patients with hyperparathyroidism, Zollinger-Ellison syndrome, and multiple endocrine neoplasia type I: a prospective study. Surgery 1987;102:958–66.
41. Pipeleers-Marichal M, Donow C, Heitz PU, Kloppel G. Pathologic aspects of gastrinomas in patients with Zollinger-Ellison syndrome with and without multiple endocrine neoplasia type I. World J Surg 1993;17:481–8.
42. Shepherd JJ, Challis DR, Davies PF, et al. Multiple endocrine neoplasm, type 1. Gastrinomas, pancreatic neoplasms, microcarcinoids, the Zollinger-Ellison syndrome, lymph nodes, and hepatic metastases. Arch Surg 1993;128:1133–42.
43. Sugg SL, Norton JA, Fraker DL, et al. A prospective study of intraoperative methods to diagnose and resect duodenal gastrinomas. Ann Surg 1993;218:138–144.
44. Skogseid B, Eriksson B, Lundqvist G, et al. Multiple endocrine neoplasia type 1: a 10-year prospective screening study in four kindreds. J Clin Endocrinol Metab 1991;73:281–287.
45. Burgess JR, Shepherd JJ, Parameswaran V, et al. Spectrum of pituitary disease in multiple endocrine neoplasia type 1 (MEN 1): clinical, biochemical, and radiological features of pituitary disease in a large MEN 1 kindred. J Clin Endocrinol Metab 1996;81:2642–2646.
46. Capella C, Riva C, Leutner M, La Rosa S. Pituitary lesions in multiple endocrine neoplasia syndrome (MENS) type 1. Pathol Res Pract 1995;191:345–347.
47. Skogseid B, Larsson C, Lindgren PG, et al. Clinical and genetic features of adrenocortical lesions in multiple endocrine neoplasia type 1. J Clin Endocrinol Metab 1992;75:76–81.
48. Burgess JR, Harle RA, Tucker P, et al. Adrenal lesions in a large kindred with multiple endocrine neoplasia type 1. Arch Surg 1996;131:699–702.
49. Yazawa K, Kuroda T, Watanabe H, et al. Multiple carcinoids of the duodenum accompanied by type I familial multiple endocrine neoplasia. Surg Today 1998;28:636–9.
50. Debelenko LV, Emmert-Buck MR, Zhuang Z, et al. The multiple endocrine neoplasia type I gene locus is involved in the pathogenesis of type II gastric carcinoids. Gastroenterology 1997;113:773–81.
51. Duh QY, Hybarger CP, Geist R, et al. Carcinoids associated with multiple endocrine neoplasia syndromes. Am J Surg 1987;154:142–8.
52. Teh BT, McArdle J, Chan SP, et al. Clinicopathologic studies of thymic carcinoids in multiple endocrine neoplasia type 1. Medicine 1997;76:21–9.
53. Akerstrom G. Management of carcinoid tumors of the stomach, duodenum, and pancreas. World J Surg 1996;20:173–82.
54. Wilkinson S, Teh BT, Davey KR, et al. Cause of death in multiple endocrine neoplasia type 1. Arch Surg 1993;128:683–90.
55. Pack S, Turner ML, Zhuang Z, et al. Cutaneous tumors in patients with multiple endocrine neoplasia type 1 show allelic deletion of the MEN1 gene. J Invest Dermatol 1998;110:438–40.
56. Creamer JD, Whittaker SJ, Griffiths WA. Multiple endocrine neoplasia type 1 presenting as rosacea. Clin Exp Dermatol 1996;21:170–1.
57. Kouides PA, Phatak PD, Cramer SF. Fatal thrombotic thrombocytopenic purpura (TTP) presenting concurrently with metastatic multiple endocrine neoplasia (MEN) type I. Hematopathol Mol Hematol 1996;10:161–70.
58. Carnevale V, Romagnoli E, Remotti D, et al. Pulmonary lymphangioleiomyoma in a patient with multiple endocrine neoplasia type I. J Endocrinol Invest 1997;20:282–5.
59. Toshimori H, Okamoto M, Nakatsuru K, et al. Multiple endocrine neoplasia type 1 associated with malignant lymphoma and other complications. Intern Med 1996;35:849–54.
60. Skogseid B, Oberg K, Akerstrom G, et al. Limited tumor involvement found at multiple endocrine neoplasia type I pancreatic exploration: can it be predicted by preoperative tumor localization? World J Surg 1998;22:673–7.
61. Shi W, Johnston CF, Buchanan KD, et al. Localization of neuroendocrine tumours with [$^{111}$In]DTPA-octreotide scintigraphy (Octreoscan): a comparative study with CT and MR imaging. Q J Med 1998;91:295–301.
62. Pisegna JR, Doppman JL, Norton JA, et al. Prospective comparative study of ability of MR imaging and other imaging modalities to localize tumors in patients with Zollinger-Ellison syndrome. Dig Dis Sci 1993;38:1318–28.
63. Cadiot G, Lebtahi R, Sarda L, et al. Preoperative detection of duodenal gastrinomas and peripancreatic lymph nodes by somatostatin receptor scintigraphy. Groupe d'Etude du Syndrome de Zollinger-Ellison. Gastroenterology 1996;111:845–54.
64. Thompson NW. The surgical management of hyperparathyroidism and endocrine disease of the pancreas in the multiple endocrine neoplasia type 1 patient. J Intern Med 1995;238:269–80.
65. O'Riordain DS, O'Brien T, Grant CS, et al. Surgical management of primary hyperparathyroidism in multiple endocrine neoplasia types 1 and 2. Surgery 1993;114:1031–7.
66. Burgess JR, David R, Parameswaran V, et al. The outcome of subtotal parathyroidectomy for the treatment of hyperparathyroidism in multiple endocrine neoplasia type 1. Arch Surg 1998;133:126–9.
67. Skogseid B, Oberg K, Eriksson B, et al. Surgery for asymptomatic pancreatic lesion in multiple endocrine neoplasia type I. World J Surg 1996;20:872–6.
68. Lo CY, Lam KY, Fan ST. Surgical strategy for insulinomas in multiple endocrine neoplasia type I. Am J Surg 1998;175:305–7.
69. Doherty GM, Olson JA, Frisella MM, et al. Lethality of multiple endocrine neoplasia type I. World J Surg 1998;22:581–6.
70. Thompson NW, Pasieka J, Fukuuchi A. Duodenal gastrinomas, duodenotomy, and duodenal exploration in the surgical management of Zollinger-Ellison syndrome. World J Surg 1993;17:455–62.
71. Thompson NW, Bondeson AG, Bondeson L, Vinik A. The surgical treatment of gastrinoma in MEN I syndrome patients. Surgery 1989;106:1081–5.
72. Fraker DL, Norton JA. The role of surgery in the management of islet cell tumors. Gastroenterol Clin North Am 1989;18:805–30.
73. Mignon M, Cadiot G. Diagnostic and therapeutic criteria in patients with Zollinger-Ellison syndrome and multiple endocrine neoplasia type 1. J Intern Med 1998;243:489–94.
74. Melvin WS, Johnson JA, Sparks J, et al. Long-term prognosis of Zollinger-Ellison syndrome in multiple endocrine neoplasia. Surgery 1993;114:1183–8.
75. Weber HC, Venzon DJ, Lin JT, et al. Determinants of metastatic rate and survival in patients with Zollinger-Ellison syndrome: a prospective long-term study. Gastroenterology 1995;108:1637–49.
76. Demeure MJ, Klonoff DC, Karam JH, et al. Insulinomas associated with multiple endocrine neoplasia type I: the need for a different surgical approach. Surgery 1991;110:998–1004.
77. Oberg K. Advances in chemotherapy and biotherapy of endocrine tumors. Curr Opin Oncol 1998;10:58–65.
78. Ponder BA. The gene causing multiple endocrine neoplasia type 2 MEN 2. Ann Med 1994;26:199–203.
79. Mulligan LM, Ponder BA. Genetic basis of endocrine disease: multiple endocrine neoplasia type 2. J Clin Endocrinol Metab 1995;80:1989–95.
80. Oriola J, Hernandez C, Simo R, et al. Genetic analysis of seven Mediterranean families with multiple endocrine neoplasia type 2A. Clin Endocrinol (Oxf) 1996;44:207–12.
81. Marsh DJ, Robinson BG, Andrew S, et al. A rapid screening method for the detection of mutations in the RET proto-oncogene in multiple endocrine neoplasia type 2A and familial medullary thyroid carcinoma families. Genomics 1994;23:477–9.
82. Sobol H, Narod SA, Nakamura Y, et al. Screening for multiple endocrine neoplasia type 2a with DNA-polymorphism analysis. N Engl J Med 1989;321:996–1001.

83. Grosfeld FJ, Lips CJ, Ten Kroode HF, et al. Psychosocial consequences of DNA analysis for MEN type 2. Oncology 1996;10:141–6.

84. Libroia A, Verga U, Vecchi G, et al. Seventeen-year-long follow-up of a family affected by type 2A multiple endocrine neoplasia (MEN 2A). J Endocrinol Invest 1998;21:87–92.

85. Mathew CG, Easton DF, Nakamura Y, Ponder BA. Presymptomatic screening for multiple endocrine neoplasia type 2A with linked DNA markers. The MEN 2A International Collaborative Group. Lancet 1991;337:7–11.

86. Sipple JH. The association of pheochromocytoma with carcinoma of the thyroid. Am J Med 1961;31:163–6.

87. Keiser HR, Beaven MA, Doppman J, et al. Sipple's syndrome: medullary thyroid carcinoma, pheochromocytoma, and parathyroid disease: studies in a large family. NIH conference. Ann Intern Med 1973;78:561–79.

88. Wells SAJ, Ontjes DA. Multiple endocrine neoplasia type II. Annu Rev Med 1976;27:263–8.

89. Calmettes C, Ponder BA, Fischer JA, Raue F. Early diagnosis of the multiple endocrine neoplasia type 2 syndrome: consensus statement. European Community Concerted Action: Medullary Thyroid Carcinoma. Eur J Clin Invest 1992;22:755–60.

90. Wax JR, Eggleston MKJ, Teague KE. Pregnancy complicated by multiple endocrine neoplasia type IIA (Sipple's syndrome). Am J Obstet Gynecol 1997;177:461–2.

91. Conte-Devolx B, Schuffenecker I, Niccoli P, et al. Multiple endocrine neoplasia type 2: management of patients and subjects at risk. French Study Group on Calcitonin-Secreting Tumors GETC. Horm Res 1997;47:221–6.

92. Decker RA, Peacock ML, Borst MJ, et al. Progress in genetic screening of multiple endocrine neoplasia type 2A: is calcitonin testing obsolete? Surgery 1995;118:257–63.

93. Blind E, Schmidt-Gayk H, Sinn HP, et al. Chromogranin A as tumor marker in medullary thyroid carcinoma. Thyroid 1992;2:5–10.

94. O'Hare MM, Shaw C, Johnston CF, et al. Pancreatic polypeptide immunoreactivity in medullary carcinoma of the thyroid: identification and characterisation by radioimmunoassay, immunocytochemistry and high performance liquid chromatography. Regul Pept 1986;14:169–80.

95. Pomares FJ, Canas R, Rodriguez JM, et al. Differences between sporadic and multiple endocrine neoplasia type 2A phaeochromocytoma. Clin Endocrinol (Oxf) 1998;48:195–200.

96. Schuffenecker I, Virally-Monod M, Brohet R, et al. Risk and penetrance of primary hyperparathyroidism in multiple endocrine neoplasia type 2A families with mutations at codon 634 of the RET proto-oncogene. Groupe d'Etude des Tumeurs à Calcitonine. J Clin Endocrinol Metab 1998;83:487–91.

97. Frank-Raue K, Kratt T, Heoppner W, et al. Diagnosis and management of pheochromocytomas in patients with multiple endocrine neoplasia type 2—relevance of specific mutations in the RET proto-oncogene. Eur J Endocrinol 1996;135:222–5.

98. Lindor NM, Honchel R, Khosla S, Thibodeau SN. Mutations in the RET protooncogene in sporadic pheochromocytomas. J Clin Endocrinol Metab 1995;80:627–9.

99. Howe JR, Norton JA, Wells SAJ. Prevalence of pheochromocytoma and hyperparathyroidism in multiple endocrine neoplasia type 2A: results of long-term follow-up. Surgery 1993;114:1070–7.

100. Jansson S, Tisell LE, Fjalling M, et al. Early diagnosis of and surgical strategy for adrenal medullary disease in MEN II gene carriers. Surgery 1988;103:11–8.

101. Decker RA, Peacock ML. Occurrence of MEN 2a in familial Hirschsprung's disease: a new indication for genetic testing of the RET proto-oncogene. J Pediatr Surg 1998;33:207–14.

102. Eng C, Mulligan LM. Mutations of the RET proto-oncogene in the multiple endocrine neoplasia type 2 syndromes, related sporadic tumours, and Hirschsprung disease. Hum Mutat 1997;9:97–109.

103. Williams ED, Pollock DJ. Multiple mucosal neuromata with endocrine tumours: a syndrome allied to von Recklinghausen's disease. J Pathol Bacteriol 1966;91:71–80.

104. Carney JA, Go VL, Sizemore GW, Hayles AB. Alimentary-tract ganglioneuromatosis. A major component of the syndrome of multiple endocrine neoplasia, type 2b. N Engl J Med 1976;295:1287–91.

105. Norum RA, Lafreniere RG, O'Neal LW, et al. Linkage of the multiple endocrine neoplasia type 2B gene (MEN2B) to chromosome 10 markers linked to MEN2A. Genomics 1990;8:313–7.

106. Schenberg ME, Zajac JD, Lim-Tio S, et al. Multiple endocrine neoplasia syndrome—type 2b. Case report and review. Int J Oral Maxillofac Surg 1992;21:110–4.

107. Eyer SD, Snover DC, Delaney JP. Diverticulitis in the multiple endocrine neoplasia type II B syndrome. Am J Gastroenterol 1988;83:183–6.

108. Kraimps JL, Denizot A, Carnaille B, et al. Primary hyperparathyroidism in multiple endocrine neoplasia type IIa: retrospective French multicentric study. Groupe d'Etude des Tumeurs à Calcitonine (GETC), French Calcitonin Tumors Study Group, French Association of Endocrine Surgeons. World J Surg 1996;20:808–12.

109. Decker RA, Geiger JD, Cox CE, et al. Prophylactic surgery for multiple endocrine neoplasia type IIa after genetic diagnosis: is parathyroid transplantation indicated? World J Surg 1996;20:814–20.

110. Lairmore TC, Ball DW, Baylin SB, Wells SAJ. Management of pheochromocytomas in patients with multiple endocrine neoplasia type 2 syndromes. Ann Surg 1993;217:595–601.

111. O'Riordain DS, O'Brien T, Weaver AL, et al. Medullary thyroid carcinoma in multiple endocrine neoplasia types 2A and 2B. Surgery 1994;116:1017–23.

112. Lairmore TC, Frisella MM, Wells SJ. Genetic testing and early thyroidectomy for inherited medullary thyroid carcinoma. Ann Med 1996;28:401–6.

113. Lips CJ, Landsvater RM, Hoppener JW, et al. Clinical screening as compared with DNA analysis in families with multiple endocrine neoplasia type 2A. N Engl J Med 1994;331:828–35.

114. Gelston AL, Delisle MB, Patel YC. Multiple endocrine adenomatosis type I. Occurrence in an octogenarian with high levels of circulating pancreatic polypeptide. JAMA 1982;247:665–6.

115. Jhiang SM, Fithian L, Weghorst CM, et al. RET mutation screening in MEN2 patients and discovery of a novel mutation in a sporadic medullary thyroid carcinoma. Thyroid 1996;6:115–21.

# CHAPTER 68

# THYROID GLAND

• JEROME M. HERSHMAN • WILLIAM H. BLAHD • H. EARL GORDON

## Natural History

### ETIOLOGY

Radiation to the thyroid may induce benign and malignant thyroid neoplasms. After radiation, benign neoplasms of the thyroid are severalfold more frequent than carcinoma. In Chicago, head and neck radiation was associated with a 6% incidence of subsequent thyroid carcinoma.[1] The incidence of thyroid cancer is proportional to the dose of radiation from 0.1 to 3 Gy with a flattening at 10 Gy.[2, 3] Thyroid carcinoma has resulted from radiation given to the thymic region of infants, the tonsils and adenoids of children, and the face of adolescents with acne, and the scalp in children with tinea capitis. The latent period between the radiation and the recognition of a thyroid neoplasm has most commonly been 20 to 35 years, with a peak at 25 to 29 years,[2] but thyroid tumors have been found as soon as 5 years and as long as 50 years after the radiation treatment. There is a trend for decreased risk with increasing age.

After the Chernobyl nuclear reactor accident in 1986, a great increase in thyroid cancer was found in children.[4] The greatest frequency has been in children less than 5 years at the time of the accident, including children exposed in utero. The mean latency period from exposure was about 7 years and was shorter in the youngest children. The cancer has been attributed to iodine radioisotopes released by the damaged reactor.

There is also an increased risk of thyroid cancer after radiation of the neck with 25 to 40 Gy for Hodgkin's disease.[5] However, hypothyroidism has been the main thyroid problem in patients receiving more than 40 Gy to the thyroid for treatment of Hodgkin's disease or cancer of the larynx. About one fifth to two thirds of these patients develop hypothyroidism.[5, 6] Nearly all the radiation-related thyroid cancers have been of the papillary type. The Chernobyl data reiterate the lesson learned from study of external radiation, namely, that the younger the child, the greater the risk of radiation-related thyroid cancer.

Thyroid carcinoma is approximately three times more common in women than in men, as are most thyroid diseases.

The cellular *myc* proto-oncogene is expressed in human thyroid follicular adenomas and papillary carcinomas.[7] Thyrotropin increases expression of this oncogene in human thyroid neoplasms and expression of the *ras* and *fos* proto-oncogenes in cultured rat thyroid cells. Mutations of *ras* oncogenes are equally prevalent in benign and malignant thyroid tumors, suggesting that these mutations are early lesions in thyroid cell neoplasia.[8]

Activation of the *ret* oncogene is found in one fifth of papillary thyroid carcinomas in adults and about two thirds of those in children, with a higher frequency in children irradiated by the Chernobyl fallout.[9, 10] The *ret* oncogene is also highly expressed in medullary carcinoma in patients with multiple endocrine neoplasia.[11] Mutational inactivation of the p53 tumor-suppressor gene is prevalent in anaplastic thyroid carcinoma.[12] p53 gene mutations have been found in 18% of radiation-related papillary thyroid cancers[13] and in 61% of the tall cell variant of papillary carcinoma, which may be responsible for the worse prognosis of this variant.[14]

Other growth factors—including epidermal growth factor, insulin-like growth factor, basic fibroblast growth factor, tumor necrosis factor-α, transforming growth factor-β, and Met/hepatocyte growth factor—may play important roles in thyroid cell growth, neoplasia, and metastases.[15–17]

### EPIDEMIOLOGY

The estimated number of new cases of thyroid cancer in the United States in 1998 was 17,200.[18] Thyroid cancer makes up about 1.4% of all new cancers. The relationship between endemic goiter and thyroid carcinoma has been carefully studied. In an endemic goiter region of Colombia, thyroid carcinoma was found in 1% of autopsy specimens and was responsible for death in 0.6%.[19] The incidence of thyroid carcinoma in this region was fivefold greater than that in the state of New York. In Switzerland, the use of iodized salt reduced both the incidence of endemic goiter and the death rate from thyroid carcinoma.[20] However, the decline in the incidence of goiter in the United States has not been associated with a reduction in the incidence of thyroid carcinoma. In Austria, there has been a shift in the ratio of the forms of differentiated thyroid carcinoma with the use of iodized salt: The incidence of follicular carcinoma declined and that of papillary carcinoma increased.[21]

### Heredity

Medullary thyroid carcinoma, a tumor of the calcitonin-secreting cells, is a component of multiple endocrine neoplasia, type 2 (MEN 2) as are bilateral pheochromocytoma and parathyroid hyperplasia. Patients with MEN, type 2b (MEN 2b) have multiple mucosal neuromas and a marfanoid habitus. Although medullary carcinoma is a hereditary disorder and follows a pattern of autosomal dominant inheritance, most cases are sporadic rather than familial.[22] There is a familial form of papillary thyroid carcinoma.[23]

### Effect of Thyroid-Stimulating Hormone on Thyroid Tumors

The anterior pituitary hormone thyroid-stimulating hormone (TSH, thyrotropin) stimulates many biosynthetic processes within the thyroid gland and promotes its growth. The removal of thyrotropin causes involution of the thyroid.

Papillary and follicular thyroid carcinomas generally possess a lower level of normal biosynthetic activity. In scans performed with radioiodine, these tumors usually do not concentrate radioiodine to the same extent that adjacent normal thyroid tissue does, giving rise to the term *cold nodule*. This information has often been misinterpreted by inference that hypofunctioning tumors (in relation to the concentration of radioiodine) are not affected by thyrotropin. However, several studies have shown that benign and malignant (differentiated) thyroid tumors have receptors for thyrotropin and that this hormone increases adenylcyclase activity, the cyclic adenosine monophosphate concentration, and the oxidation of glucose by the tumors.[24] Growth of the tumor is probably dependent on these processes and is therefore influenced by thyrotropin. Anaplastic thyroid carcinoma lacks the receptor for thyrotropin.[24] The membrane transport protein that is responsible for uptake of iodide, called the sodium-iodide symporter, is present in papillary thyroid carcinomas, but its expression is probably reduced and tends to decrease in metastases.[25]

## CLASSIFICATION

Table 68-1 shows the histopathologic classification and frequency of the different forms of thyroid carcinoma. The differentiated thyroid cancers, papillary and follicular, compose 80% of thyroid cancers.

## CLINICAL FEATURES

Thyroid cancer usually presents as a discrete mass in the thyroid. The onset is insidious, and the tumor is often discovered on routine physical examination. Sometimes rapid growth of the tumor may call it to the attention of the patient. Significant enlargement within a period of a few weeks to a few months suggests a cancer or hemorrhage into a thyroid cyst.

The consistency of malignant tumors varies from firm or even stony to that of normal thyroid tissue. The lack of movement of the thyroid nodule with swallowing, and fixation of the tumor to adjacent structures indicates malignancy. Thyroid carcinoma may metastasize to local lymph nodes, to the contralateral thyroid lobe, and to adjacent cervical structures. In some patients there is cervical lymphadenopathy due to metastases, without a palpable nodule in the

*Table 68-1.* **Histopathologic Classification of Thyroid Cancer**

| Type | Frequency (%) |
| --- | --- |
| Papillary (with or without follicular foci) | 62 |
| Follicular (note extent of invasion of tumor capsule) | 18 |
| Medullary | 6 |
| Undifferentiated (anaplastic) | 10 |
| Lymphoma | 4 |

Modified from Van Herle AJ, Uller RP: Thyroid cancer: classification, clinical features, diagnosis, and therapy. In: Hershman JM, Bray GA, eds. The thyroid: physiology and treatment of disease. Oxford: Pergamon Press, 1979:505.

thyroid. Distant metastases occur most often in lung and bone.

Lateral displacement of the trachea and esophagus is more often due to a large multinodular goiter than to a carcinoma. Vocal cord palsy is indicative of a cancer involving the homolateral recurrent laryngeal nerve, although a large benign goiter may also compress this nerve.

## DIAGNOSIS

A battery of special diagnostic tests is often used to determine the cause of a thyroid nodule. Thyroid scans with radioiodine show the ability of the nodule to concentrate radioiodine in comparison with the rest of the gland. If the nodule concentrates nearly all the radioiodine and is hyperfunctional ("hot"), the lesion is almost certainly not a carcinoma. Thyroid scans have limited utility for making the diagnosis of thyroid carcinoma. Although nearly all thyroid cancers appear as hypofunctional ("cold") areas if they are large enough, benign processes such as cysts, inflammation, colloid goiter, or adenomas are usually "cold" on the scan as well.

Ultrasonography is useful in differentiating cystic nodules from solid lesions. Thyroid cysts are nearly always benign, but solid or mixed solid and cystic lesions may be malignant. In middle-aged and older individuals, neck ultrasonograms reveal thyroid nodules, usually less than 1.5 cm, in one fourth to two thirds of the population. If these "incidentalomas" are smaller than 1 cm, they do not require evaluation or follow-up.

Fine-needle aspiration biopsy is a safe procedure, and cytologic study of the aspirated cells has been found useful. This technique has become the principal method for evaluating patients with thyroid nodules and has been recommended as the initial diagnostic approach, based on its sensitivity, specificity, and cost effectiveness.[26] The cytologic examination can diagnose colloid goiter, lymphocytic thyroiditis, papillary carcinoma, follicular lesions, medullary carcinoma, and undifferentiated carcinoma. Unfortunately, cytologic studies cannot distinguish between follicular adenoma and follicular carcinoma. The sensitivity and specificity of fine-needle aspiration generally exceed 90%, and the overall diagnostic accuracy is 95%.[26] The incidence of false-positive diagnoses of carcinoma is about 3%; the false-positive group increases greatly if all suspicious lesions are considered indicative of carcinoma.[26] False-negative results occur in about 5% of cases.[26] The aspiration of fluid permits the diagnosis of thyroid cysts, and the resulting decompression provides therapy for the cyst.

Ultrasonography may disclose psammoma bodies in papillary carcinoma that appear as punctate calcifications. Large, irregular calcifications usually represent calcified degenerative areas in a multinodular goiter or carcinoma.

Several blood tests may be helpful. Measurements of serum thyroxine and triiodothyronine concentrations are generally normal; elevated levels indicate that the thyroid nodule is hyperfunctioning and exclude malignancy. Low levels of circulating thyroid hormones and elevated serum thyrotropin concentrations indicate hypothyroidism and suggest that the thyroid enlargement results from compensatory hypertrophy. The measurement of antithyroid antibodies (antiperoxidase or antithyroglobulin antibodies) yields diagnostic titers in about 90% of patients with nodular goiter caused by chronic lymphocytic thyroiditis. Serum thyroglobulin concentrations are elevated in a large proportion of patients with nodular goiter, regardless of the cause, so this test is not useful in distinguishing benign processes from thyroid carcinoma.

Serum calcitonin levels are elevated in patients with medullary thyroid carcinoma. Screening of patients with nodular thyroid disease by measurement of serum calcitonin preoperatively has uncovered a prevalence of medullary carcinoma of 0.4 to 1.4%; however, most of these tumors were only a few millimeters.[27, 28] To screen for medullary thyroid carcinoma in family members of patients with MEN 2, analysis of *ret* oncogene mutations in DNA is more sensitive and specific than measurement of calcitonin after pentagastrin stimulation.[29]

## STAGING AND PROGNOSIS

Table 68–2 presents the staging of thyroid cancer by the TNM classification. This system compares favorably with staging by other classifications.[30] In spite of the varied manifestations of thyroid cancer, the rate of growth, the mode of spread, and the response to therapy are reasonably predictable for each of the four subgroups. Because of the slow growth of the differentiated types, survival statistics usually reflect a composite of various therapeutic approaches that have evolved over the years. An analysis of 700 patients with differentiated (papillary and follicular) thyroid carcinoma by the TNM classification showed recurrence rates of 15%, 22%, 46%, and 67% in stages 1 to 4, respectively, and death rates of 2%, 16%, 30%, and 61% in stages 1 to 4, respectively.[31]

**Papillary Adenocarcinoma.** The mode of extension of this thyroid tumor is primarily by way of the lymphatics, with positive lymph node involvement in approximately 40 to 50% of patients.[32] In contrast to malignancy arising in almost all other organs, the presence of lymph node metastases does not necessarily have an adverse effect on the outcome of the disease.[33] Although some studies suggest that lymph node involvement may actually exert a protective effect on the patient, others do not support this finding.[34, 35]

It is generally recognized that the prognosis is poorer in patients older than age 40.[34] The presence of lesions 5 cm or larger and extrathyroidal extension of the cancer are additional factors that usually have an adverse effect on the outcome.[34] In contrast, small papillary lesions ($\leq$1.5 cm) are almost invariably curable.

**Follicular Carcinoma.** There is a propensity for vascular invasion in follicular carcinoma. Although the overall 10-year survival rate is reported at 72 to 88%, it decreases to 34 to 44% in selected patients who demonstrate a moderate to marked degree of invasion.[34] Spread to regional lymph nodes is uncommon compared with papillary lesions. Distant metastases, when present, are most frequently found in the lung and bone. The Hürthle cell (oncocytic) variant has a worse prognosis.

**Medullary Carcinoma.** This lesion is much more aggressive than the differentiated neoplasms. The overall 5-year survival rate is 69% at 10 years and 65% at 15 years after diagnosis.[22] Survival tends to be better in patients with the familial form of the disease. In patients without cervical lymph node metastases, the survival closely approximates the rates for normal individuals of comparable age. Regional lymph node spread is common, but unlike the papillary type, distant metastases may occur in the lung, liver, and elsewhere. Cellular heterogeneity with few calcitonin-containing cells indicates a more virulent neoplasm and a grave prognosis.[36]

**Anaplastic Carcinoma.** These neoplasms are highly lethal regardless of treatment. Most patients will die of their disease within 6 to 12 months of diagnosis.[37]

**Lymphoma.** Primary lymphoma of the thyroid gland (usually non-Hodgkin's type) is being reported with increasing frequency[38] (see Chapter 94). There is nearly always coexistent Hashimoto's thyroiditis. The disorder presents as a rapidly growing thyroid mass. Open surgical biopsy is necessary to confirm the diagnosis. Treatment with chemotherapy and radiation has resulted in an 8-year survival rate of nearly 100%.[39]

# Treatment

## SURGERY

Surgical therapy is the definitive treatment for thyroid cancer. When patients with a suspicious lesion are evaluated by the diagnostic methods previously described, the course of action will be clarified in the majority of cases.

Surgery is indicated (1) if a fine-needle aspirate indicates malignancy and (2) if the aspirate reveals a follicular neoplasm that is suggestive of a follicular carcinoma. Histologic examination of the entire nodule is required to establish the diagnosis. If the fine-needle biopsy result is benign or nondiagnostic, neck exploration may still be indicated. This will depend on a thorough evaluation of symptoms, physical findings and other risk factors, such as the age of the patient and the size of the nodule.

Although there is general agreement that surgical excision is the only primary treatment for thyroid carcinoma, the extent of resection remains controversial. This applies not only to the amount of thyroid gland that should be resected but also to the management of regional lymph nodes. The lack of consensus in surgical management is due to the unique characteristics of thyroid carcinoma compared with most neoplasms arising in other sites. First, the relatively low incidence of thyroid carcinoma makes it difficult for any individual or medical center to accumulate a broad experience. Second, the slow rate in most thyroid cancers dictates that follow-up must be measured over a time span of 20 to 30 years. Consequently, there are no prospective randomized studies that compare the merits of one therapeutic modality with another. Therefore, our decisions must depend on retrospective studies.

The major factors that dictate the extent of the operative procedure are (1) the size and distribution of the carcinoma within the thyroid gland, (2) the presence or absence of metastases, (3) extension of the cancer beyond the capsule of the thyroid gland, and (4) the histologic type of the neoplasm. Because the biologic behavior of the tumor is influenced so greatly by the pathologic classification, it is useful to consider the surgical approach on the basis of the predominant cell type.

*Table 68–2.* **Staging of Thyroid Cancer Using the TNM Classification**

**Definition of TNM**

*Primary Tumor (T)*

Note: All categories may be subdivided: (a) solitary tumor, (b) multifocal (the largest determines the classification).

TX   Primary tumor cannot be assessed
T0   No evidence of primary tumor
T1   Tumor 1 cm or less in greatest dimension limited to the thyroid
T2   Tumor more than 1 cm but not more than 4 cm in greatest dimension limited to the thyroid
T3   Tumor more than 4 cm in greatest dimension limited to the thyroid
T4   Tumor of any size extending beyond the thyroid capsule

*Regional Lymph Nodes (N)*

Regional lymph nodes are the cervical and upper mediastinal lymph nodes

NX   Regional lymph nodes cannot be assessed
N0   No regional lymph node metastasis
N1   Regional lymph node metastasis
  N1a   Metastasis in ipsilateral cervical lymph node(s)
  N1b   Metastasis in bilateral, midline, or contralateral cervical or mediastinal lymph nodes

*Distant Metastasis (M)*

MX   Presence of distant metastasis cannot be assessed
M0   No distant metastasis
M1   Distant metastasis

*Stage Grouping*

Separate stage groupings are recommended for papillary, follicular, medullary, or undifferentiated (anaplastic).

*Papillary or Follicular*

|           | *UNDER 45 YEARS*   | *45 YEARS AND OLDER* |
|-----------|--------------------|----------------------|
| Stage I   | Any T, Any N, M0   | T1, N0, M0           |
| Stage II  | Any T, Any N, M1   | T2, N0, M0           |
|           |                    | T3, N0, M0           |
| Stage III |                    | T4, N0, M0           |
|           |                    | Any T, N1, M0        |
| Stage IV  |                    | Any T, Any N, M1     |

*Medullary*

| Stage I   | T1    | N0    | M0 |
|-----------|-------|-------|----|
| Stage II  | T2    | N0    | M0 |
|           | T3    | N0    | M0 |
|           | T4    | N0    | M0 |
| Stage III | Any T | N1    | M0 |
| Stage IV  | Any T | Any N | M1 |

*Undifferentiated (anaplastic)*

All cases are stage IV.

| Stage IV | Any T | Any N | Any M |
|----------|-------|-------|-------|

*Histopathologic Type*

There are four major histopathologic types:

Papillary carcinoma (including those with follicular foci)
Follicular carcinoma
Medullary carcinoma
Undifferentiated (anaplastic) carcinoma

Used with the permission of the American Joint Committee on Cancer (AJCC®), Chicago, Illinois. The original source for this material is the AJCC® Cancer Staging Manual, 5th edition (1997) published by Lippincott-Raven Publishers, Philadelphia, Pennsylvania.

**Well-Differentiated Adenocarcinoma (Papillary and Follicular).** Although there are some basic behavioral differences between these two cell types, there are enough similarities to justify considering them as one group. In the approach to a single suspicious nodule, a total lobectomy on the affected side is most frequently the biopsy procedure of choice. Exceptions would be those few small lesions that can be removed easily with a wide margin of normal tissue. Incisional biopsy or enucleation should never be performed.

After the diagnosis of carcinoma has been established, a

decision must be made with regard to the extent of thyroid tissue to be removed. This remains one of the most controversial aspects in the surgical management of this disease. Those who favor a total thyroidectomy base their decision on the high incidence of multicentric foci of carcinoma, with a reported incidence of 20 to 80% with bilateral involvement in one third of cases.[40, 41] Clark and Duh[42] recommend a total thyroidectomy for most patients with a lesion bigger than 1 cm. In a study of the impact of therapy on 698 patients with stage II or III differentiated thyroid carcinoma, Mazzaferri and Jhiang found that 30-year recurrence rates were greater following subtotal thyroidectomy compared with total thyroidectomy (40% and 26%, respectively).[35] Other experts also favor total thyroidectomy[40, 43, 44] except for the small circumscribed lesions for which a lobectomy would likely be curative.

In contrast, a number of surgeons favor a more conservative approach for intrathyroidal cancer.[45–48] Vickery and colleagues[45] reviewed the experience in 237 patients with papillary carcinoma at Massachusetts General Hospital. Subtotal thyroidectomies were performed in 176 patients; 131 of these procedures were lobectomies. They concluded that the patients treated with a subtotal resection had an outcome comparable to 61 patients undergoing total thyroidectomy. The proponents of the conservative approach support their view with two principal arguments. The first relates to the recognized risk of permanent hypoparathyroidism and recurrent laryngeal nerve injury associated with total thyroidectomy. Second, although acknowledging the frequency of multicentricity and the potential risk of local recurrence with the more limited procedures, they argue that these factors have little bearing on the eventual outcome of the disease.

A reasonable compromise is to perform a near-total thyroidectomy, preserving 2 to 3 grams of thyroid tissue posteriorly on the side of least involvement of carcinoma.[40, 44, 49] In experienced hands, this procedure can be carried out with low morbidity if one carefully identifies and preserves the recurrent nerve and parathyroid glands. The remnant of thyroid tissue preserved can be ablated postoperatively with radioactive iodine. The total elimination of all thyroid tissue carries the additional benefit of enabling one to identify and treat recurrences and metastases with radioactive iodine. This approach, combining the use of radioiodine (I131) with surgery, has proved to be a highly effective means of controlling the disease.

Despite the recognized risk of total thyroidectomy, this procedure must be used in patients with extensive bilateral carcinoma. When there is extrathyroidal extension of cancer, resection of adjacent tissues may also be required. A total (or near-total) resection must be performed in all patients with follicular carcinoma showing vascular and capsular invasion.

With regard to the management of the regional lymph nodes, there is now general agreement that prophylactic neck dissections have no value in the treatment of thyroid cancer. The presence of metastatic cancer, confirmed at the time of operation, is the indication for the removal of cervical lymph nodes in this disease. The thyroid is unique in that the routes of lymphatic drainage are accessible for examination at the time the primary tumor is removed. The extent of lymph node dissection to be performed will depend on the magnitude and extent of node involvement.

Although there are divergent views with regard to the extent of regional lymph node dissection, most surgeons have joined the trend toward a more conservative resection that is limited to the extent of clinical node involvement. Consequently, the standard radical neck dissection should be performed only in occasional patients in whom the metastatic disease in the lateral neck cannot be removed with a lesser resection. Even fairly extensive involvement of lateral cervical nodes can be adequately removed in most patients with a modified type of neck dissection, resulting in the preservation of the sternocleidomastoid muscle, the spinal accessory nerve and, usually, the internal jugular vein as well.

If the presence of positive node involvement is confined to the anterior neck in the region of the thyroid, it is reasonable to limit the dissection to this area. An en bloc anatomic anterior or central neck dissection can be readily accomplished through the conventional neck incision. Care must be taken to encompass the lymphatic tissue along the recurrent nerves.

With papillary carcinoma, cervical lymph node involvement and distant metastases are much more common in children younger than 17 years than in adults. This observation was reported by Zimmerman and colleagues[50] in their long-term follow-up of 1039 patients treated at the Mayo Clinic. Despite being more aggressive at initial evaluation, thyroid carcinoma was much less lethal in children than in adults.

**Medullary Carcinoma.** Special considerations apply to the management of medullary thyroid carcinoma (MTC) because of the more aggressive nature of the neoplasm, the propensity for metastases, and the possible association with other endocrine disorders.[51–53] Pheochromocytomas also occur in 20 to 40% of patients within this category.[51, 52] Approximately 75% of patients with MTC fall within the sporadic category, with the peak incidence occurring in the fifth and sixth decades of life. The neoplasm in this group is almost always confined to one lobe of the thyroid, in contrast to the familial groups, in which bilateral involvement is present in the majority of cases.[52, 53] The prognosis is usually better than in those with the MEN 2b syndrome.

All patients with MTC require a total thyroidectomy, along with a central lymph node dissection.[42, 51–54] The latter should extend from the hyoid to the sternal notch and laterally to the jugular veins. Patients with MEN 2a who have associated hyperplasia of the parathyroid glands require at least a subtotal parathyroidectomy. Lairmore and Wells[51] and Dunn and Farndon[53] advocate a total removal of all four parathyroid glands with autotransplantation of parathyroid tissue. Patients with involvement of lateral cervical nodes require a lateral modified radical neck dissection. A conventional radical neck dissection would not be indicated unless there is extension of the tumor to the sternocleidomastoid muscle or internal jugular veins. Clark and Duh[42] advocate a more aggressive approach because nodal metastases are present in more than 50% of patients. They recommend that an ipsilateral modified neck dissection be performed in all patients in whom the primary lesion is 3 cm or larger.

In view of the association of pheochromocytomas with MEN 2a and MEN 2b, a thorough evaluation of this possibility must first be carried out. Any coexistent pheochromocytomas should be removed prior to cervical exploration to avoid hypertensive crises during the neck operation.

Basal and stimulated calcitonin levels detect residual or recurrent disease following operation.[55] Several reports have stressed the value of selective venous samplings of calcitonin to evaluate the extent of the disease and the site of metastatic lesions.[51, 53] Frank-Raue and colleagues have demonstrated a marked improvement in survival by identifying the exact locations of metastatic lesions by selective venous samplings and removing them by microdissection.[56]

Family members at risk for developing MTC should be screened in early childhood. If the *ret* oncogene mutation is found, a prophylactic thyroidectomy performed prior to the development of clinical features may be curative.[52]

**Hürthle Cell Carcinoma.** Hürthle cell neoplasms are uncommon and occur more frequently in women and in individuals older than 50 years. In the series from the Johns Hopkins Hospital, the incidence of carcinoma was 35%, and it was 65% in tumors larger than 4 cm.[57]

In a large series reported by Grant from the Mayo Clinic, he emphasizes the many similarities that exist between Hürthle cell carcinoma and follicular carcinoma.[49] A definitive diagnosis cannot be made by fine-needle aspiration and may be difficult on frozen section as well. The diagnostic criteria for both neoplasms is based on the finding of capsular and vascular invasion. When metastasis occurs, it is by the hematogenous route and is infrequent to lymph nodes. There is general agreement that a total or near-total thyroidectomy should be performed on all patients with Hürthle cell carcinoma.

**Anaplastic Carcinoma.** These tumors grow rapidly and are uniformly fatal. Because of local invasion of midline structures, local removal by total thyroidectomy is recommended but is frequently impossible. External irradiation may provide some degree of palliation. Nilsson and colleagues reported eight patients (10%) who survived more than 2 years with combinations of chemotherapy, radiation therapy, and surgery.[58]

## RADIOIODINE THERAPY

Although the majority of thyroid adenocarcinomas can be removed surgically, there is often uncertainty as to the completeness of the surgical resection and concern about the presence of local or distant metastases. Radioiodine ($^{131}$I) has been used as adjunctive therapy in the management of thyroid adenocarcinoma for more than 45 years. There is mounting evidence that indicates increased survival and decreased tumor recurrence in patients who have received radioiodine therapy.[35, 43, 59]

The efficacy of radioiodine therapy, with rare exceptions, is directly related to tumor uptake and retention. Under appropriate conditions, radioiodine uptake has been attained in 50 to 80% of adenocarcinomas of the thyroid. Efficient uptake and response to radioiodine is observed in tumors that are of the differentiated cell type, such as papillary or follicular, whereas anaplastic carcinomas and medullary carcinomas do not concentrate radioiodine. Effective tumor uptake is approximately 0.5% of the radioiodine dose per gram with a biologic half-life of approximately 4 days. From the administration of 5.6 gigabecquerel (GBq; equivalent to 150 mCi) of $^{131}$I, a tumor may receive as much as 250 Gy or five times the absorbed dose that can be delivered by a

course of external radiation therapy. Moreover, this dose will be delivered to every functional metastasis regardless of its size or location in the body, and tumor tissue will receive several hundred times the radiation exposure received by the rest of the body.

**Radioiodine Ablation of Postsurgical Thyroid Tissue.** It is necessary to ablate with radioiodine any residual thyroid tissue that has not been removed surgically because the complete ablation of all normal thyroid tissue usually ensures therapeutically effective radioiodine uptake in remaining tumor deposits and tumor metastases. Ablation of small thyroid remnants after near-total thyroidectomy may be accomplished by the administration of 1.1 to 3.7 GBq (30 to 100 mCi) of $^{131}$I.[30] Ablation of thyroid remnants is usually carried out 1 to 3 months after thyroidectomy. The first scan after surgery is performed preferably with 0.5 mCi $^{123}$I because scan doses of $^{123}$I do not prevent uptake of subsequent therapeutic doses of $^{131}$I, whereas this may happen with large scan doses of $^{131}$I (see further on). In a report of 49 patients, successful ablation was achieved in 84% when the dose administered was proportional to the radioiodine uptake in the neck measured 48 hours after a scanning dose of 2 mCi.[60] Approximately 6 to 12 months after ablation, whole-body radioiodine imaging is performed to assess the completeness of ablation. Subsequent management is based on the results of the imaging procedure.

The ablation of small thyroid remnants after near-total thyroidectomy is controversial, particularly in patients with limited disease and no evidence of nodal metastases. However, there are a number of arguments that suggest the value of ablative therapy, including the possible elimination of residual microscopic foci of cancer in thyroid remnants and the removal of residual thyroid tissue as a source of thyroglobulin complicating post-therapy management. DeGroot and colleagues[59] reported that radioiodine ablation of postsurgical remnants decreases the risk of recurrence and death in patients older than age 45 who have tumors larger than 1 cm.

Controversy with respect to ablation of postsurgical thyroid remnants is most apparent in patients with differentiated thyroid cancer in the 20- to 40-year age group when there is no evidence of extraglandular involvement and tumors are smaller than 1 cm. Although these individuals ordinarily have a good prognosis without complementary radioiodine therapy, over a 20-year period there may be a 5 to 10% recurrence rate and a death rate of 1 to 2%.[59] To determine the risk to this subgroup from a single ablative dose of radioiodine, the radiobiologic consequences were evaluated in terms of lifetime cancer and genetic risks (Table 68–3). It would appear from these data that the radiobiologic effects of a single 3.7-GBq (100 mCi) $^{131}$I ablation dose are insignificant with respect to carcinogenesis and mutagenesis.

**Radioiodine Therapy of Cancer.** The objective of treating thyroid cancer with radioiodine is to destroy all functioning thyroid cancer tissue. The following indications should be considered in evaluating patients with well-differentiated thyroid cancer for possible radioiodine treatment: inoperable primary cancer, residual postoperative cancer in the cervical region, metastases to cervical or mediastinal lymph nodes, distant metastases, and recurrent cancer.

Before radioiodine therapy is given, the ability of residual or metastatic thyroid cancer to concentrate radioiodine is

*Table 68–3.* **Fatal Cancer and Genetic Risks: 3.7 GBq (100 mCi) $^{131}$I Dose**

|  | Breast | Leukemia | Genetic |
| --- | --- | --- | --- |
| Expected incidence in population (%) | 4.04 | 0.01 | 10.60 |
| Expected excess incidence after 100 mCi $^{131}$I dose (%) | 0.08 | 0.03 | 0.28 |

Data from Boring CC, Squires TS, Tong T. Cancer statistics, 1992. CA Cancer J Clin 1992;42:19–38; Beir V. Health effects of exposure to low levels of ionizing radiation. Washington, DC: National Research Council, 1990, and Blahd W. Management of thyroid cancer. Compr Ther 1993;19:197–202.

evaluated by radioiodine imaging procedures. If levothyroxine (T$_4$) has been administered, it must be discontinued for 4 to 6 weeks. Studies have shown that withdrawing triiodothyronine (T$_3$) replacement for 2 weeks is as good as withdrawing it for 4 weeks in attaining radioiodine uptake in functional metastases. T$_3$ is cleared from the body much more rapidly than is T$_4$. The shorter period of withdrawal minimizes the period of hypothyroidism. Accordingly, patients are switched from suppression therapy with T$_4$ to a corresponding dose of T$_3$ for 4 weeks to allow metabolic disposal of the T$_4$. This is followed by 2 weeks of T$_3$ withdrawal. Serum thyrotropin concentration also is measured before radioiodine imaging is begun. Optimally, serum thyrotropin levels should exceed 30 mU/L. Measurement of serum thyrotropin may help identify the rare individual who does not respond to the brief period of T$_3$ withdrawal.

**Exogenous Thyrotropin.** Bovine thyrotropin has been withdrawn from use because of concern that the bovine protein could be contaminated with the agent causing Jacob-Creutzfeldt disease. Fortunately, recombinant human thyrotropin is now available. It is given to increase the accumulation of radioiodine in thyroid cancer metastases.[61] In a second phase III trial, scans after two injections of 0.9 mg human thyrotropin were as effective as withdrawal of thyroid hormone for detection of thyroid remnants and cancer on radioiodine scans. The main advantage of human thyrotropin used in this way is that patients do not have symptomatic hypothyroidism.[61]

**Iodine Contamination.** Patients undergoing radioiodine ablation or treatment, or whole-body imaging with radioiodine, must avoid contamination with iodine-containing medications and radiographic contrast media. In addition, it is probably helpful to restrict dietary iodine to 50 μg/day or less for 2 weeks before the radioiodine therapy through a low-iodine diet.[62]

**Radioiodine Dosimetry.** Once adequate tumor uptake has been ensured by radioiodine imaging studies, therapeutic doses of radioiodine are administered. Most therapists use an empirical dose of radioiodine that varies from 3.7 to 7.4 GBq (100 to 200 mCi) depending on the location and extent of metastatic tumor distribution. This dose range has been found to be without significant complications in most patients.

Several studies have reported that performing dosimetric calculations for specific cases may result in predictably better success rates while at the same time limiting higher radioiodine exposure to those individuals who require larger thera-

peutic doses.[63, 64] Maxon and colleagues[63] suggest that a uniformly good response should be possible with a minimal tumor dose of 80 to 100 Gy if dosimetry is based on estimation of the mass of postsurgical residual cancer tissue, the percent uptake in cancerous lesions, and the effective half-life of radioiodine in the lesions. It is worthwhile to perform scans 10 to 14 days after the therapeutic dose because these scans may reveal sites of uptake that are not detected on diagnostic scans.[65] In general, radioiodine therapy doses are given at intervals of 6 to 12 months until there is no demonstrable evidence of functioning tumor tissue on radioiodine imaging.

**Complications.** In accordance with radiation therapy principles, the maximal amount of $^{131}$I that can be safely administered should be given. The limiting factor is the possibility of complications from the damaging effects of radioiodine on normal or vital tissues. Whole-body irradiation from usual therapeutic doses of radioiodine is estimated to be 0.2 to 0.4 Gy. Generally, complications are minor and rarely interfere with therapeutic endeavors.[64] Rarely transient radiation thyroiditis may occur, persisting for 2 to 3 weeks. Occasionally, swelling of the parotid or submaxillary salivary glands may be observed shortly after therapy, which usually persists for several days but sometimes for longer periods.

Bone marrow depression is uncommon with the usual dosage regimens, except when bone metastases are present. Pulmonary fibrosis has been reported in patients with pulmonary metastases after repeated administration of large therapeutic doses. Some cases of leukemia have been reported after large total cumulative radioiodine doses. However, no case of leukemia was found in a study of 846 patients treated with an average dose of 7.2 GBq $^{131}$I.[66] The transformation of previously differentiated tumors to rapidly growing anaplastic cancers may occur in a small percentage of patients. Since this is known to occur spontaneously in untreated thyroid carcinomas, there appears to be no evidence to implicate radiation as the cause of tumor transformation. Table 68–3 gives additional information on the genetic risks of radioiodine therapy.

**Follow-up Treatment and Management**

*Radioiodine Imaging.* Following total thyroid cancer ablation, radioiodine imaging with test doses of 74 to 111 MBq (2 to 3 mCi) of $^{131}$I is performed at regular intervals. Diagnostic doses in excess of 2 mCi may "stun" the thyroid tissue and reduce the uptake of subsequent therapeutic doses.[67] If there is tumor recurrence by scan, the patient is re-treated. If there is demonstrable persistent or progressive disease with undetectable uptake of radioiodine, suppressive doses of T$_4$ are resumed, and the patient is evaluated for treatment with external radiation therapy or chemotherapy.

Long-term follow-up is important. The recurrence of tumor after radioiodine ablation of all functioning tumor tissue has been observed in more than half of patients who have tumor metastases and in one fourth of patients who did not have metastases. Recurrences have been observed as late as 30 years after the initial treatment despite negative interval diagnostic studies.[68] In view of the possibility of late recurrence, all patients in whom total radioiodine ablation has been attained should be followed by means of diagnostic imaging studies at 1- to 3-year intervals for a minimum of 10 years to ensure that they remain free of recurrent tumor.

In most instances, recurrence occurs at the same site and responds to treatment with radioiodine.

*Serum Thyroglobulin.* Although whole-body imaging with radioiodine has been considered to be the "gold standard" for detecting recurrent disease, it is a formidable procedure requiring withdrawal of thyroid hormone and periods of symptomatic hypothyroidism, unless scans are performed after administration of human thyrotropin. Several reports suggest that the determination of serum thyroglobulin may be as sensitive in the detection of recurrent thyroid cancer as whole-body imaging, and that it may supplement or even replace routine whole-body imaging in the management and follow-up of patients who appear to be in remission.[69, 70]

Thyroglobulin is a large glycoprotein molecule found in normal thyroid gland follicular tissue. The normal thyroid gland secretes small amounts of thyroglobulin that may be detected in low concentration in the blood of normal individuals by sensitive immunoassays. Most differentiated thyroid carcinomas also secrete thyroglobulin, including the Hürthle cell variant of follicular carcinoma that often does not concentrate radioiodine. Medullary and anaplastic carcinomas do not secrete thyroglobulin. Patients with differentiated thyroid carcinomas may have elevated serum thyroglobulin preoperatively; however, similar elevations are often found in patients with benign thyroid neoplasms and in patients with goiter of other causes. Consequently, serum thyroglobulin is of little help in the preoperative evaluation of thyroid cancer, but it is a useful marker for metastatic disease in patients who have had total thyroid gland removal.

Serial monitoring of thyroglobulin in patients who have had total thyroid gland removal will detect residual tumor tissue or metastases or the recurrence of tumor.[71] Because autoantibodies to thyroglobulin interfere with the measurement, antibody determination is performed routinely with each measurement of thyroglobulin.[72] Elevated levels of thyroglobulin in a patient receiving thyroid hormone suppression therapy is a clear indication for a radioiodine body scan. Low levels generally exclude the presence of residual or recurrent thyroid carcinoma. Borderline serum thyroglobulin concentrations should be evaluated after withdrawal of $T_4$ or after the administration of recombinant human thyrotropin. Elevated thyroglobulin levels under these circumstances are indicative of the presence of recurrent tumor or metastases. Patients with bone and lung metastases have the highest thyroglobulin concentrations, and those with metastases to the lymph nodes the lowest concentrations. Elevated thyroglobulin levels have been observed when radioiodine body scans were negative, but generally there is good correlation between abnormal scans and elevated thyroglobulin concentrations. In some patients with elevated thyroglobulin levels and normal results on [131]I scanning, a repeat [131]I scan using a therapeutic dose of radioiodine will disclose unsuspected areas of metastatic tumor. Rarely, the [131]I scan is positive, and the serum thyroglobulin determination is negative. In general, the measurement of serum thyroglobulin complements radioiodine body imaging in the management of cancer patients.

*New Imaging Agents.* When thyroglobulin is elevated despite a negative radioiodine scan, a total body thallium-201 ([201]Tl) scan may be useful in detecting tumor that has lost its radioiodine concentrating ability. [201]Tl acts as a potassium analogue. It concentrates primarily in myocardium and skeletal muscles but also concentrates in tumor tissues. [201]Tl scintigraphy is simple to perform. It does not require that the patient discontinue thyroid hormone replacement, and it can be completed in one visit. In studies comparing [201]Tl with radioiodine imaging and serum thyroglobulin determinations, [201]Tl imaging had the greatest sensitivity (94%), whereas radioiodine had the highest specificity (99%).[73] However, [201]Tl scans are not recommended as the sole imaging test in follow-up studies of thyroid cancer. In medullary carcinoma that is radioiodine negative, [201]Tl may be of value in the localization of calcitonin-producing metastases.

There have been several reports of the use of technetium-99m–labeled methoxyisobutylnitrile (Sestamibi) or tetrofosmin as an alternative imaging agents in the follow-up of differentiated thyroid carcinoma and also recurrent medullary and Hürthle cell carcinoma.[74, 75] These agents are taken up by mitochondria in metabolically active tissues. These scans have been useful for detecting recurrent disease in the neck as well as metastases, and are probably more sensitive than [201]Tl scans. They can be performed without discontinuing thyroxine suppression therapy.

Metastases from differentiated thyroid cancers have been demonstrated by positron emission tomography (PET) using fluorine-18–labeled fluorodeoxyglucose in patients whose metastases failed to accumulate radioiodine.[76, 77] PET scans are positive in carcinomas that do not accumulate radioiodine.

Follow-up of patients may also include ultrasonography for recurrent local disease in the neck, computed tomography, or magnetic resonance imaging. Currently in the post–radioiodine therapy follow-up and management of thyroid cancer, there are several excellent alternative imaging modalities that, when used in conjunction with radioiodine imaging and thyroglobulin determinations, provide a high probability for the detection of recurrent or metastatic disease.

**Results of Radioiodine Therapy.** Although the therapeutic efficacy of radioiodine in the management of differentiated thyroid cancer has never been documented by randomized studies, there are a number of reports that establish its utility. DeGroot and coworkers[59] at the University of Chicago analyzed the course of papillary carcinoma in 269 patients. The average follow-up period was 12 years. The majority of patients underwent either total or near-total thyroidectomy, which was followed by radioiodine thyroid ablation in more than half the patients. Using this approach, there was a 25% recurrence rate. Only 8.2% of the patients died of cancer during the follow-up period, which extended in some instances to 38 years.

The largest radioiodine therapy series comprising 1599 patients with differentiated thyroid cancer was reported by Samaan and colleagues[43] at the University of Texas M.D. Anderson Cancer Center. The median follow-up for these patients was 11 years, with a maximal follow-up of 43 years. Sixty-six percent of the patients had total thyroidectomy, 7% received external radiation therapy, and 46% had radioactive iodine therapy. The overall recurrence rate was 23%, and 11% of the patients died. The authors state that radioiodine therapy was the most important prognostic indicator of increased "disease-free interval" and that it significantly increased survival. No benefit was obtained from external radiation therapy. Mazzaferri and Jhiang[35] reported the analysis of 1355 patients with papillary or follicular thyroid carcinoma who had a median follow-up of 16 years. Patients treated with total or near-total thyroidectomy and radioiodine had significantly fewer recurrences, especially when the postsurgical thyroid remnant was ablated by radioiodine. After a follow-up of 30 years, no patient who had radioiodine ablation had died of carcinoma.

The results of radioiodine therapy have been much less rewarding in patients with surgically unresectable tumor or gross residual disease in the neck and in patients with skeletal involvement. Brown and colleagues[78] observed neither objective improvement nor survival times exceeding 5 years in patients who received radioiodine therapy for bone metastases.

Accordingly, in some patients, limited or no therapeutic benefit is obtained with radioiodine therapy, whereas in others large and disseminated tumor masses disappear, and no evidence of recurrence of tumor tissue can be demonstrated. In view of this variability in response, it is important that radioiodine therapy be used judiciously in the appropriate clinical situation and for the histologic type of tumor that can be expected to be clinically responsive. In this regard, radioiodine is of little or no value in the treatment of medullary carcinoma. Metaiodobenzylguanidine labeled with [131]I has been used with only limited therapeutic success, although meaningful pain palliation has been achieved.[79]

## EXTERNAL RADIATION THERAPY

Conventional radiation therapy may be detrimental to the success of radioiodine therapy in thyroid adenocarcinomas and should not precede therapeutic efforts with radioiodine. External radiation therapy in the management of thyroid cancer has been reserved for anaplastic carcinoma and lymphoma and differentiated cancer that does not concentrate radioiodine. Therapy is best given with high-energy electrons. Beneficial results with 35 to 70 Gy have been reported in the treatment of local recurrence in some differentiated thyroid cancers that did not take up radioiodine. Tubiana and colleagues reported 97 patients treated with external radiation therapy after incomplete surgical excision. The incidence of local recurrence at 15 years was 11% in the irradiated group and 23% in those treated with surgery alone, even though the irradiated patients had larger and more extensive tumors.[68] In older patients with invasive papillary carcinoma (stage pT4) and positive lymph nodes, 50 to 60 Gy external radiation significantly reduced the 10-year recurrence rate.[80]

## CHEMOTHERAPY

**Thyroid Hormone.** There have been no trials of treatment with thyroid hormone as primary therapy. Instead, it is used after surgical therapy and radioiodine. In most instances, the administration of thyroid hormone is regarded as an adjuvant to prevent the recurrence of the tumor. The use of thyroid hormone to suppress thyrotropin secretion after resection of differentiated thyroid cancer has been practiced for many years. As noted previously, thyrotropin is an important growth factor for thyroid follicular cells, and in

a few cases metastatic thyroid carcinoma has diminished markedly after treatment with thyroid hormone. Several studies have demonstrated that the recurrence rate of differentiated thyroid carcinoma was significantly reduced by administration of thyroid hormone.[33, 35]

Suppression of pituitary thyrotropin secretion may be achieved with thyroid hormone in doses that are only slightly greater than those of customary replacement. The preparation of choice is sodium levothyroxine (thyroxine) because the serum concentrations of thyroxine and triiodothyronine are more stable in patients treated with thyroxine. About 2 to 6 hours after administration of desiccated thyroid or triiodothyronine, there are large supraphysiologic peaks of serum T3 concentration, which fall to lower levels over the next 24 hours, thus making therapy with these preparations less physiologic. With the use of ultrasensitive immunometric assays for serum thyrotropin concentration, subnormal levels can be measured with confidence.[81] The therapeutic dose of thyroxine should be adjusted to maintain a subnormal serum thyrotropin level, preferably a level of less than 0.1 mU/L (normal 0.4 to 4 mU/L), without causing symptoms of hyperthyroidism. This may require daily thyroxine doses of 2.5 µg/kg, which are 50 to 75 g greater than the usual daily replacement dose.[82] The dose should be adjusted for each patient. Relapse-free survival is longer in patients maintained with constantly suppressed thyrotropin than in those with nonsuppressed thyroptropin.[83, 84]

Excessive doses of thyroxine, desiccated thyroid, or triiodothyronine have been advocated in the past. Such doses should be avoided, however, because they may produce disturbing symptoms of thyrotoxicosis and may exert deleterious effects on the heart and cause demineralization of bone if continued chronically. In men and young women, suppressive doses of thyroxine do not cause osteopenia, but this may occur in postmenopausal women. It can be prevented with replacement estrogen therapy and calcium supplements of 1 g daily.

**Cytotoxic Agents.** Doxorubicin and bleomycin are active single agents in thyroid cancer.[85–88] Twenty-three other single agents and 25 drug combinations have been tested for activity, but the results are inconclusive because of the small number of patients treated.[87] Two cooperative groups have been studying combination chemotherapy for thyroid carcinoma,[87] and results from the Eastern Cooperative Oncology Group have been published.[89] In this randomized study, a small number of patients with advanced, aggressive disease enjoyed prolonged disease-free survival off chemotherapy following the intravenous use of cisplatin 40 mg/m2 and doxorubicin 60 mg/m2, given every 3 weeks. This combination was more toxic than doxorubicin used alone, but there were no deaths from toxicity, and the combined response rate in 84 patients was 26%. However, cisplatin plus doxorubicin was ineffective in a study performed by the Southeastern Cancer Study Group.[90] In a summary of the literature on treatment with doxorubicin,[91] its use was recommended for differentiated carcinoma or MTC only after exhaustion of all conventional therapies, but it should be used in conjunction with conventional therapy for anaplastic (undifferentiated thyroid carcinoma). In 33 patients with anaplastic thyroid carcinoma treated with external radiation, doxorubicin 20 mg/wk for 3 weeks, followed by surgery and doxorubicin for 2 more weeks, the median survival was only 4 months, but in 4 patients survival with no evidence of disease exceeded 2 years.[92] A patient with medullary carcinoma responded to the combination of dacarbazine and 5-fluorouracil.[93]

We recommend that eligible patients be treated as part of an experimental protocol if possible. If not, patients with metastatic undifferentiated thyroid carcinoma or aggressive differentiated carcinoma that is refractory to radiation therapy may be treated with doxorubicin, as described in Chapter 9.

## SUGGESTIONS FOR ADDITIONAL READING

Schlumberger MJ. Papillary and follicular thyroid carcinoma. N Engl J Med 1998;338:297–306.

Gharib H, Goellner JR. Fine-needle aspiration biopsy of the thyroid: an appraisal. Ann Intern Med 1993;118:282–9. *This is an excellent review of this important diagnostic test.*

Dulgeroff AJ, Hershman JM. Medical therapy for differentiated thyroid carcinoma. Endocr Rev 1994;15:500–15.

Samaan NA, Schultz PN, Hickey RC, et al. The results of various modalities of treatment of well differentiated thyroid carcinomas: a retrospective review of 1599 patients. J Clin Endocrinol Metab 1992;75:714. *This is the largest study of the treatment of thyroid cancer.*

## REFERENCES

1. Favus M, Schneider A, Stachura M, et al. Thyroid malignancy as a late consequence of head and neck irradiation: clinical-pathological correlation of 1056 patients. N Engl J Med 1976;294:1019–25.
2. Schneider AB, Ron E, Lubin J, et al. Dose-response relationships for radiation-induced thyroid cancer and thyroid nodules: evidence for the prolonged effects of radiation on the thyroid. J Clin Endocrinol Metab 1993; 77:362–9.
3. Ron E, Lubin JH, Shore RE, et al. Thyroid cancer after exposure to external radiation: a pooled analysis of seven studies. Radiation Research 1995; 141:259–77.
4. Pacini F, Vorontsova T, Demidchik EP, et al. Post-Chernobyl thyroid carcinoma in Belarus children and adolescents: comparison with naturally occurring thyroid carcinoma in Italy and France. J Clin Endocrinol Metab 1997;82:3563–9.
5. Hancock SL, Cox RS, McDougall IR. Thyroid diseases after treatment of Hodgkin's disease. New Engl J Med 1991;325:599–605.
6. Vrabec DP, Heffron TJ. Hypothyroidism following treatment for head and neck cancer. Ann Otol Rhinol Laryngol 1981;90:449–53.
7. Yamashita S, Ong J, Fagin JA, Melmed S. Expression of the *myc* cellular proto-oncogene in human thyroid tissue. J Clin Endocrinol Metab 1986; 63:1170–3.
8. Fagin JA. Genetic basis of endocrine disease 3: Molecular defects in thyroid gland neoplasia. J Clin Endocrinol Metab 1992;75:1398–1400.
9. Santoro M, Carlomagno F, Hay ID, et al. Ret oncogene activation in human thyroid neoplasms is restricted to the papillary cancer subtype. J Clin Invest 1992;89:1517–22.
10. Nikiforov YE, Rowland JM, Bove KE, et al. Distinct patter of ret oncogene rearrangements in morphological variants of radiation-induced and sporadic thyroid papillary carcinomas in children. Cancer Res 1997;57:1690–94.
11. Itoh F, Ishizaka Y, Tahira T, et al. Identification and analysis of the ret proto-oncogene promoter region in neuroblastoma cell lines and medullary thyroid carcinomas from MEN2A patients. Oncogene 1992;7:1201–6.
12. Fagin JA, Matsuo K, Karmakar A, et al. High prevalence of mutations of the p53 gene in poorly differentiated human thyroid carcinomas. J Clin Invest 1993;91:179–84.
13. Fogelfeld L, Bauer TK, Schneider AB, et al. p53 gene mutations in radiation-induced thyroid cancer. J Clin Endocrinol Metab 1996;81:3039–44.
14. Ruter A, Dreifus J, Jones, et al. Overexpression of p53 in tall cell variants of papillary thyroid carcinoma. Surgery 1996;12:1046–50.
15. Pang XP, Hershman JM. Differential effects of growth factors on [3H]thymidine incorporation and [125I]iodine uptake in FRTL-5 rat thyroid cells. Proc Soc Exp Biol Med 1990;194:240–4.
16. Pang XP, Park M, Hershman J. Transforming growth factor-β blocks protein kinase-A-mediated iodide transport and protein kinase-c-mediated DNA synthesis in FRTL-5 rat thyroid cells. Endocrinology 1992;131:45–50.
17. Belfiore A, Gangemi P, Costantino A, et al. Negative/low expression of the Met/hepatocyte growth factor receptor identifies papillary thyroid carcinomas with high risk of distant metastases. J Clin Endocrinol Metab 1997;82:2322–88.
18. Landis SH, Taylor M, Bolden S, et al. Cancer statistics, 1998. CA 1998;48:6–29.
19. Wahner HW, Cuello C, Correa P, et al. Thyroid carcinoma in an endemic goiter area, Cali, Colombia. Am J Med 1966;40:58–66.
20. Van Herle AJ, Uller RP. Thyroid cancer: Classification, clinical features, diagnosis, and therapy. In: Hershman JM, ed. The thyroid. Physiology and treatment of disease. Oxford: Pergamon Press, 1979:505–31.
21. Bacher-Stier C, Riccabona G, Totsch M, et al. Incidence and clinical characteristics of thyroid carcinoma after iodine prophylaxis in an endemic goiter country. Thyroid 1997;7:733–41.
22. Bergholm U, Bergstrom R, Ekbom A. Long term follow-up of patients with medullary carcinoma of the thyroid. Cancer 1997;79:132–8.
23. Loh KC. Familial nonmedullary thyroid carcinoma: a meta-review of case series. Thyroid 1997;7:107–13.
24. Clark OH, Gerene PL, Goretzki P, et al. Characterization of the thyrotropin receptor-adenylate cyclase system in neoplastic human thyroid tissue. J Clin Endocrinol Metab 1983;57:140.
25. Arturi F, Russo D, Schlumberger M, et al. Iodide symporter gene expression in human thyroid tumors. J Clin Endocrinol Metab 1998;83:2493–6.
26. Gharib H, Goellner JR. Fine-needle aspiration biopsy of the thyroid: an appraisal. Ann Intern Med 1993;118:282–9.
27. Pacini F, Fontanelli M, Fugazzola L, et al. Routine measurement of serum calcitonin in nodular thyroid diseases allows the preoperative diagnosis of unsuspected sporadic medullary thyroid carcinoma. J Clin Endocrinol Metab 1994;78:826–9.
28. Niccoli P, Wion-Barbot N, Caron P, et al. Interest of routine measurement of serum calcitonin: study in a large series of thyroidectomized patients. The French Medullary Study Group. J Clin Endocrinol Metab 1997;82:338–41.
29. Marsh DJ, Learoyd DL, Robinson BG. Medullary thyroid carcinoma: recent advances and management update. Thyroid 1995;5:407–24.
30. Dulgeroff AJ, Hershman JM. Medical therapy for differentiated thyroid carcinoma. Endocr Rev 1994;15:500–15.
31. Loh KC, Greenspan FS, Gee L, et al. Pathological tumor-node-metastasis (pTNM) staging for papillary and follicular thyroid carcinomas: a retrospective analysis of 700 patients. J Clin Endocrinol Metab 1997;82:3533–62.
32. Mazzaferri EL, Young RL, Oertel JE, et al. Papillary thyroid carcinoma: the impact of therapy in 576 patients. Medicine 1977;56:171–96.
33. Samaan NA, Maheshwari YK, Nader S, et al. Impact of therapy for differentiated carcinoma of the thyroid: an analysis of 706 cases. J Clin Endocrinol Metab 1983;56:1131–8.
34. Simpson WJ, McKinney SE, Carruthers JS, et al. Papillary and follicular thyroid cancer: prognostic factors in 1,578 patients. Am J Med 1987;83:479–88.
35. Mazzaferri EL, Jhiang SM. Long-term impact of initial surgical and medical therapy on papillary and follicular thyroid cancer. Am J Med 1994;97:418–28.
36. Lippman SM, Mendelsohn G, Trum DL, et al. The prognostic and biological significance of cellular heterogeneity in medullary thyroid carcinoma: a study of calcitonin, L-dopa decarboxylase, and histaminase. J Clin Endocrinol Metab 1982;54:233–40.
37. Ain KB. Anaplastic thyroid carcinoma: behavior, biology and therapeutic approaches. Thyroid 1998;8:715–26.
38. Hamburger JI, Miller JM, Kini SR. Lymphoma of the thyroid. Ann Intern Med 1983;99:685–93.
39. Matsuzuka F, Miyauchi A, Katayama S, et al. Clinical aspects of primary thyroid lymphoma: diagnosis and treatment based on our experience of 119 cases. Thyroid 1993;3:93–9
40. Schlumberger MJ. Papillary and follicular thyroid carcinoma. N Engl J Med 1998;338:297–306.
41. Patwardham N, Cataldo T, Braverman LE. Surgical management of the patient with papillary cancer. Surg Clin North Am 1995;75:449–64.

42. Clark OH, Duh Q. Thyroid cancer. Med Clin North Am 1991;75:211–34.

43. Samaan NA, Schultz PN, Hickey RC, et al. The results of various modalities of treatment of well differentiated thyroid carcinoma: a retrospective review of 1599 patients. J Clin Endocrinol Metab 1992;75:714–20.

44. Gagel RF, Goepfert H, Callender DL. Changing concepts in the pathogenesis and management of thyroid carcinoma. CA Cancer J Clin 1996;46:261–83.

45. Vickery AL, Chliu-an W, Walker AM. Treatment of intrathyroidal papillary carcinoma of the thyroid. Cancer 1987;60:2587–95.

46. Wanebo H, Coburn M, Teates D, et al. Total thyroidectomy does enhance disease control or survival even in high-risk patients with differentiated thyroid cancer. Ann Surg 1998;227:912–21.

47. Sanders LE, Cady B. Differentiated thyroid cancer: reexamination of risk groups and outcome of treatment. Arch Surg 1998;133:419–25.

48. Cady B. Papillary carcinoma of the thyroid. Semin Surg Oncol 1991;7:81–6.

49. Grant CS. Operative and postoperative management of the patient with follicular and Hürthle cell carcinoma: do they differ? Surg Clin North Am 1995;75:395–403.

50. Zimmerman D, Hay ID, Gough IR, et al. Papillary thyroid carcinoma in children and adults. Long-term follow-up of 1039 patients conservatively treated at one institution during three decades. Surgery 1988:104:1157–66.

51. Lairmore TC, Wells SA. Medullary carcinoma of the thyroid: current diagnosis and management. Semin Surg Oncol 1992;7:92–9.

52. Robbins J. Thyroid cancer: a lethal neoplasm. Ann Intern Med 1991;115:133–47.

53. Dunn JM, Farndon JR. Medullary thyroid carcinoma. Br J Surg 1993;80:6–9.

54. Moley JF. Medullary thyroid cancer. Surg Clin North Am 1995;75:405–20.

55. Gharib H, Mc Conahey WM, Tigs RD, et al. Medullary thyroid carcinoma: clinicopathologic features and long-term follow-up of 65 patients treated during 1946 through 1970. Mayo Clin Proc 1992;67:934–40.

56. Frank-Raue F, Raue R, Buhr HJ, et al. Localization of occult persisting medullary thyroid carcinoma before mircrosurgical reoperation: high sensitivity of selective venous catheterization. Thyroid 1992;2:113–7.

57. Chen H, Nicol TL, Zeiger MA, et al. Hürthle cell neoplasms of the thyroid: are there factors predictive of malignancy? Ann Surg 1998;227:542–6.

58. Nilsson O, Lindeberg J, Zedenius J, et al. Anaplastic giant cell carcinoma of the thyroid gland: treatment and survival over a 25-year period. World J Surg 1998;22:725–30.

59. DeGroot LJ, Kaplan EL, McCormick M, Straus FH. Natural history, treatment, and course of papillary thyroid carcinoma. J Clin Endocrinol Metab 1990;71:414–24.

60. Hodgson DC, Brierley JD, Tsang RW, et al. Prescribing [131]iodine based on neck uptake produces effective thyroid ablation and reduced hospital stay. Radio Oncol 1998;47:325–30.

61. Haugen BR, Pacini F, Reiners C, et al. A comparison of recombinant human thyrotropin and thyroid hormone withdrawal for the detection of thyroid remnant or cancer. J Clin Endocrinol Metab 1999;84:3877–85.

62. Lakshmanan M, Schaffer A, Robbins J, et al. A simplified low iodine diet in I-131 scanning and therapy of thyroid cancer. Clin Nucl Med 1988;13:866–8.

63. Maxon HR, Englaro EE, Thomas SR. Radioiodine-131 therapy for well-differentiated thyroid cancer—a quantitative radiation dosimetric approach: outcome and validation in 85 patients. J Nucl Med 1992;33:1132–6.

64. Bushnell DL, Boles MA, Kaufman GE, et al. Complications, sequelae and dosimetry of iodine-131 therapy for thyroid carcinoma. J Nucl Med 1992;33:2214–21.

65. Sherman SI, Tielens ET, Sostre S, et al. Clinical utility of posttreatment radioiodine scans in the management of patients with thyroid carcinoma. J Clin Endocrinol Metab 1994;78:629–34.

66. de Vathaire F, Schlumberger M, Delisle MJ, et al. Leukaemias and cancers following iodine-131 administration for thyroid cancer. Br J Cancer 1997;75:734–9.

67. Park HM, Perkins OW, Edmondson JW, et al. Influence of diagnostic radioiodines on the uptake of ablative dose of iodine-131. Thyroid 1994;4:49–54.

68. Tubiana M, Haddad E, Schlumberger M, et al. External radiotherapy in thyroid cancers. Cancer 1985;55:2062–71.

69. Ashcraft MW, Van Herle AJ. The comparative value of serum thyroglobulin measurements and iodine 131 total body scans in the follow-up study of patients with treated differentiated thyroid cancer. Am J Med 1981;71:806–14.

70. Blahd WH. Serum thyroglobulin in the management of thyroid cancer. J Nucl Med 1990;31:1771–3.

71. Schlumberger M, Baudin E. Serum thyroglobulin determination in the follow-up of patients with differentiated thyroid carcinoma. Eur J Endocrinol 1998;138:249–52.

72. Spencer CA, Takeuchi M, Kazarosyan M, et al. Serum thyroglobulin autoantibodies: prevalence, influence on serum thyroglobulin measurement, and prognostic significance in patients with differentiated thyroid carcinoma. J Clin Endocrinol Metab 1998;83:1121–7.

73. Hofenagel CA, Delprat CC, Marcuse HR, de Vijlder JJ. Role of thallium-201 total body scintigraphy in follow-up of thyroid carcinoma. J Nucl Med 1986;27:1854–7.

74. Alam MS, Kasagi K, Misaki T, et al. Diagnostic value of technetium-99m methoxyisobutyl isonitrile ([99m]Tc-MIBI) scintigraphy in detecting thyroid cancer metastases: a critical evaluation. Thyroid, 1998;8:1091–100.

75. Gallowitsch HJ, Mikosch P, Kresnik E, et al. Thyroglobulin and low-dose iodine-131 and technetium-99m-tetrofosmin whole-body scintigraphy in differentiated thyroid carcinoma. J Nucl Med 1998;39:870–5.

76. Feine U. Fluor-18-deoxyglucose positron emission tomography in differentiated thyroid cancer. Eur J Endocrinol 1998;138:492–6.

77. Grunwald F, Menzel C, Bender H, et al. Comparison of [18]FDG-PET with [131]iodine and [99m]Tc-sestamibi scintigraphy in differentiated thyroid cancer. Thyroid 1997;7:327–35.

78. Brown AP, Greening WP, McCready VR, et al. Radioiodine treatment of metastatic thyroid carcinoma: the Royal Marsden Hospital experience. Br J Radiol 1984;57:323–7.

79. Hoefnagel CA, Delprat CC, Valdes Olmos RA. Role of [131I]metaiodobenzylguanidine therapy in medullary thyroid carcinoma. J Nucl Biol Med 1991;35:334–6.

80. Farahati J, Reiners C, Stuschke M, et al. Differentiated thyroid cancer. Impact of adjuvant external radiotherapy in patients with perithyroidal tumor infiltration (stage pT4). Cancer 1996;77:172–80.

81. Ross DS, Daniels GH, Gouveia D. The use and limitations of a chemiluminescent thyrotropin assay as a single thyroid function test in an out-patient endocrine clinic. J Clin Endocrinol Metab 1990;71:764–9.

82. Burmeister LA, Goumaz MO, Mariash CN, Oppenheimer JH. Levo-thyroxine dose requirements for thyrotropin suppression in the treatment of differentiated thyroid cancer. J Clin Endocrinol Metab 1992;75:344–50.

83. Pujol P, Daures JP, Nsakala N, et al. Degree of thyrotropin suppression as a prognostic determinant in differentiated thyroid cancer. J Clin Endocrinol Metab 1996;81:4318–23.

84. Cooper DS, Specker B, Ho M, et al. Thyrotropin suppression and disease progression in patients with differentiated thyroid cancer: results from the National Thyroid Cancer Treatment Cooperative Registry. Thyroid 1998;8:737–44.

85. Gottlieb JA, Hill CS Jr. Chemotherapy of thyroid cancer with Adriamycin: experience with 30 patients. N Engl J Med 1974;290:193–7.

86. Shimaoka K. Adjunctive management of thyroid cancer: chemotherapy. J Surg Oncol 1987;15:283–6.

87. Poster DS, Bruno S, Penta J, et al. Current status of chemotherapy in the treatment of advanced carcinoma of the thyroid gland. Cancer Clin Trials 1981;4:301–7.

88. Benker G, Reinwein D. Results of chemotherapy in thyroid cancer. Dtsch Med Wochenschr 1983;108:403–6.

89. Shimaoka K, Schoenfeld DA, DeWys WD, et al. A randomized trial of doxorubicin versus doxorubicin plus cisplatin in patients with advanced thyroid carcinoma. Cancer 1985;56:2155–60.

90. Williams SD, Birch R, Einhorn LH. Phase II evaluation of doxorubicin plus cisplatin in advanced thryoid cancer: a Southeastern Cancer Study Group Trial. Cancer Treat Rep 1986;70:405–7.

91. Ahuja S, Ernst H. Chemotherapy of thyroid carcinoma. J Endocrinol Invest 1987;10:303–10.

92. Tennvall J, Lundell G, Hallquist A, et al. Combined doxorubicin, hyperfractionated radiotherapy, and surgery in anaplastic thyroid carcinoma. Cancer 1994;74:1348–54.

93. Petursson SR. Metastatic medullary thyroid carcinoma: complete response to combination chemotherapy with dacarbazine and 5-fluorouracil. Cancer 1988;62:1899–1903.

# CHAPTER 69

# NEUROENDOCRINE PANCREAS

• JOSEPH R. PISEGNA • MARK P. SAWICKI

## Natural History, Diagnosis, and Staging

Pancreatic neuroendocrine tumors, although rare, pose a significant challenge to the clinician because they produce unique clinical syndromes. Their diagnosis, which is difficult and often delayed, requires a high index of suspicion and confirmation with biochemical tests. In this section, the epidemiology, pathology, and clinical syndromes for the major functional groups of tumors are discussed for alpha cells (glucagonomas), beta cells (insulinomas), and delta cells (Zollinger-Ellison syndrome [ZES] tumors or gastrinomas); *pancreatic cholera* or diarrheogenic tumors and somatostatinomas are also discussed. The latter part of the chapter focuses on localization modalities and treatment strategies. Because most neuroendocrine tumors of the pancreas have similar biologic characteristics, the approach to diagnosis and treatment can be applied to all classes of neuroendocrine tumors of the pancreas.

## EPIDEMIOLOGY AND PATHOLOGY

In general, pancreatic neuroendocrine tumors are rare and account for less than 1% of malignant tumors and have a prevalence of approximately 10 persons per 1 million.[1] Insulinomas are the most prevalent of the islet cell tumors, and most (approximately 90%) are benign. In contrast, gastrinomas are the next most common islet cell tumors, and most of these are malignant (65%). In one series of 53 patients (age range, 14 to 17 years; mean, 48 years; median, 60 years), autopsies revealed an incidence rate of 0.11%, with most being insulinomas (62%) and the remaining being gastrinomas (6%) and glucagonomas (4%). The annual incidence of functional neuroendocrine tumors of the pancreas is approximately 0.2 per 100,000 population.[2]

Neuroendocrine tumors are a heterogeneous group of tumors characterized by combinations of argentaffin cells possessing granules that stain positive for chromogranins, synaptophysins, or neurotensin.[3, 4] Although most primary neuroendocrine tumors of the pancreas secrete either one or a combination of neuroamines, neuropeptides, or other biologically active peptides, others are not associated with the secretion of a particular hormone and are classified as silent. The pancreatic neuroendocrine tumors are thought to arise from a common ancestral cell belonging to the amine precursor uptake and decarboxylation cell. Histologically, monotonous sheets of cells containing small, compact nuclei that are uniform in appearance characterize these tumors. By electron microscopy, the cells contain electron-dense granules with biologically active amines or peptides. These granules contain chromogranins (A and C), neuron-specific enolase, and synaptophysins in varying concentrations.

Specific immunohistochemical stains are usually positive for the detection of one or more of these products and are routinely used for the definitive pathologic identification of neuroendocrine tumors. In one series, immunohistochemical stains showed evidence of multihormone production in 18% of cases, with all tumors having stained for at least one of the following six markers: neuron-specific enolase, chromogranin, synaptophysin, insulin, glucagon, or somatostatin. The authors of this study concluded that of the three markers, chromogranin, neuron-specific enolase, and synaptophysin were predictive as initial screening if used in combination and led to the detection of 92% of the tumors in their series.[3]

Many other nonendocrine tumors may also stain positive with these immunohistochemical stains, including certain colorectal adenocarcinomas.[5] Adenocarcinomas of the colon and rectum, which have a strong affinity for chromogranin staining, have a greater likelihood for malignant potential.[6, 7] Most pancreatic islet cell tumors stain positive for multiple peptide hormones, and the staining patterns are not necessarily predictive of the serum expression of these hormones.[8] It is also possible that some islet cell tumors possess granules and secrete yet unidentified hormones. In one case, an islet cell tumor metastatic to the liver was shown to possess granules containing the recently identified peptide, pituitary adenylate cyclase activating polypeptide, a close peptide relative to vasoactive intestinal polypeptide (VIP) (Pisegna JR, unpublished report, 1999). Controversy exists over the significance of the expression and release of human chorionic gonadotropin. It has been proposed that elevated serum elevations of β-human chorionic gonadotropin are associated with increased malignancy; however, this association has not been consistently established.

In general, the serum level of a particular peptide hormone, as determined by radioimmunoassay, has no predictive value for assessing the malignant potential of pancreatic neuroendocrine tumors. The size of a neuroendocrine tumor does not correlate with the level of hormone production or the severity of the clinical syndrome. For example, the serum gastrin levels associated with gastrinomas are not associated with the level of gastric acid secretion or tumor bulk. One reason for this dissociation is that even though a particular neuroendocrine tumor may produce sufficient quantities of a hormone to lead to a clinical syndrome, the patient may remain asymptomatic because of receptor desensitization on the target tissue. The excess hormone secretion by the tumor has no biologic significance. Although the size of neuroendocrine tumors bears little relation to the levels of a particular hormone secreted into the circulation, their size may increase the risk for metastatic spread of the tumor as well as the morbidity and mortality of the patients.

Although neuroendocrine tumors of the pancreas are

grouped together by common histologic features, their distribution may be a consequence of embryologic development from the ventral (cluster 1) or dorsal (cluster 2) pancreatic buds. In this series, cluster 1 tumors (gastrinomas, pancreatic polypeptide–secreting tumors, and somatostatinomas) occurred to the right of the superior mesenteric artery in 75% of cases, whereas cluster 2 tumors (insulinomas, glucagonomas) occurred to the left of the superior mesenteric artery in 75% of cases.[8] A special case can be made for the association of pancreatic neuroendocrine tumors arising in the setting of multiple endocrine neoplasia, type 1 (MEN 1). Functional pancreatic neuroendocrine tumors arise in approximately one third of patients with the hereditary MEN 1 syndrome. The clinical features of MEN 1 are covered in more detail in Chapter 67.

## ALPHA CELL TUMORS (GLUCAGONOMAS)

Glucagonomas are tumors involving functioning pancreatic alpha cells. Tumors of the alpha cells are rare, with fewer than 200 cases reported so far. Classically the *glucagonoma syndrome* is characterized by a distinctive rash; weight loss; stomatitis; glossitis; mild diabetes; hypoaminoacidemia; a normochromic, normocytic anemia; and a susceptibility to deep vein thrombosis and neuropsychiatric disturbances. Glucagonomas are more common in women than in men and have a peak incidence in patients age 50 to 60. These tumors are usually larger than 5 cm in diameter, and more than 50% are malignant, in contrast to the low prevalence of malignancy for insulinomas (see later). Although earlier reports suggest that these tumors were more commonly located in the body and tail of the pancreas, more recent reports indicate that location in the head of the pancreas is common.[9, 10] The evolving description of glucagonomas may parallel that of insulinomas, which were originally reported to be much more common in the body and tail but are now considered to occur with equal frequency throughout the pancreas.

The characteristic rash in glucagonoma is necrolytic migratory erythema, first described by Wilkinson.[11] The cardinal features of the rash are erosions and crusting, which tend to be seen on the buttocks, groin, central parts of the face, and distal aspects of the lower extremities. Marked erythema with plaques, pustules, and bullae is usually present. Fungal and bacterial superinfections as well as sparse scalp hair and thin, friable nails are common. The factors associated with the development of this skin rash have not been determined. It has been postulated that the rash may be associated with the development of hypoaminoaciduria, which is related to the elevated use of amino acids for gluconeogenesis because of elevated glucagon levels. In one patient with a glucagonoma, an increased clearance of infused amino acids suggested that the effects of glucagon may be specifically mediated by renal mechanisms.[12] Therapies with zinc hydration, which may improve the hypoaminoacidemia, have been reported to improve this rash.[13, 14] A high-protein diet has brought serum amino acid levels to normal without an improvement in the rash,[15] whereas the rash has responded favorably to intravenous infusion of amino acids.[16] Another report documents that zinc levels were normal in a patient with glucagonoma but without a

skin rash.[17] The response to local and oral zinc supplementation as well as omega-3 fatty acids, which are known largely to reverse the signs of zinc deficiency, suggests that zinc deficiency is important in the genesis of the rash associated with glucagonomas.[18] The fact that the rash may subsequently reappear, however, suggests that zinc deficiency is not the sole explanation. The rash has responded dramatically when glucagon concentrations were lowered by treatment with a long-acting somatostatin analogue in the presence of continued hypoaminoacidemia and lowered zinc levels.[13] In another case, a patient with necrolytic migratory erythema and a high plasma glucagon concentration showed significant improvement in the skin rash following treatment with the somatostatin analogue octreotide (Sandostatin) 400 µg/day.[19] This sequence points toward an important effect of glucagon itself (or some other unidentified tumor product) on the genesis of the rash.

Hyperglucagonemia is directly responsible for the mild diabetes through stimulation of hepatic glucose production by enhanced glycogenolysis and gluconeogenesis. It is common for patients to be euglycemic despite excessive plasma glucagon levels, and the levels of glucagon do not generally correlate with the degree of diabetes but are probably best correlated to the particular patient's insulin stores.[13, 20–23] As with patients harboring insulinomas who have an increased percentage of proinsulin, the plasma from patients with glucagonomas contains greater than normal amounts of a high-molecular-weight molecule reacting with the glucagon antibody. This molecule is probably preproglucagon, which is pancreatic glucagon with C-terminal and N-terminal extensions. There is failure of the normal cleavage of the prohormones of insulin (insulinomas) and glucagon (glucagonomas) in these islet cell tumors. Preproglucagon has been identified as enteroglucagon, which may be produced in the cells in the intestine and is a putative growth factor for gut mucosa. This would explain the association of glucagonomas with mucosal thickening and villous hypertrophy throughout the small intestine.[24–26] Despite its actions as an incretin, the direct actions of glucagon on catabolism probably account for the weight loss associated with the syndrome. These actions are supported by the reversal of weight loss following the administration of the somatostatin analogue octreotide.[27] In addition to the known clinical associations with glucagonomas, there is one case in the literature of an association of glucagonoma and calculous pancreatitis. Because of the general rarity of glucagonomas, it can be concluded that the association between glucagonoma and calculous pancreatitis is merely coincidental or etiologically related.[28]

In general, the diagnosis of glucagonoma should be considered in any patient presenting with dermatitis that is not responsive to topical therapy and is associated with an elevated serum glucose level and weight loss. Frequently the diagnosis is first suspected on dermatologic grounds.[29, 30] A definitive diagnosis is made by finding a high plasma glucagon concentration in the absence of any other cause, such as renal failure or severe stress. The diagnosis can be confirmed by immunocytochemistry of the isolated tumor using a glucagon antibody. Elevated fasting plasma levels of pancreatic glucagon, often in excess of 1000 pg/ml (normal <150 pg/ml) is observed. An elevation of glucagon greater than 1000 pg/ml is virtually pathognomonic for the diagnosis of glucagonoma. There are no specific provocative studies to confirm an elevated glucagon level. Because glucagonomas can be part of MEN 1 syndrome, further appropriate endocrine testing in these patients is important (Chapter 67). Similarly, the presence of dermatitis, hyperglycemia, and weight loss should raise the level of suspicion for a glucagon-secreting tumor in a patient with MEN 1 syndrome.

## BETA CELL TUMORS (INSULINOMAS)

Insulinomas are tumors involving functioning pancreatic beta cells.[1] Insulinomas that secrete excessive amounts of insulin may clinically manifest as a hormone syndrome with hypoglycemia.[31] Insulinomas occur more often in women than in men and are usually diagnosed in patients in their 30s or 40s.[32-37] Pancreatic islet cell tumors of the pancreas are rare in children, but there is at least one report of an insulinoma occurring in a child.[38] Approximately 80% of patients with insulinomas have single benign adenomas, 10% have malignant tumors, and 10% have multiple benign tumors that are frequently part of MEN 1 syndrome. Most insulinomas are small (usually <2 cm in diameter) and are located with equal frequency in the head, body, and tail of the pancreas. These patients present with symptoms of hypoglycemia during fasting conditions, such as occurs before breakfast. Because the blood glucose may drift down slowly as fasting ensues, the symptoms of hypoglycemia (tachycardia, nervousness, weakness, circumoral and extremity tingling, sweating, and tremor) that are due to sympathetic nervous system activity may be absent or minimal. These patients may present with the more confusing symptoms of depressed central nervous system function (headache, transient neurologic syndromes, visual difficulties, mental confusion, personality changes, and convulsions). Weight gain is common because chronic hyperinsulinemia and hypoglycemia lead to excessive caloric intake and lipogenesis. Dogs provide a useful model to investigate insulinomas because they have been described frequently and have similar signs of neuroglycopenia with increased concentrations of plasma catecholamines.[39, 40] A correlation between hyperinsulinemia and essential hypertension does not appear to occur.[41] Although rare, insulinomas can occur in the setting of non–insulin-dependent or insulin-dependent diabetes mellitus.[42] The incidence of insulinomas occurring in the setting of pregnancy is unknown. There was one case of an insulinoma found during the first trimester of pregnancy that manifested as repeat hypoglycemic episodes, and this diagnosis should be considered in cases of postpartum hypoglycemia.[43]

To prove that an endocrine gland is overactive and functioning autonomously, one must show that it cannot be suppressed normally. In the normal state, fasting inhibits the release of insulin. The key to diagnosing an insulinoma is to document an inappropriately high insulin level for the resulting glucose concentration that occurs during fasting conditions. Although glucose concentrations may drop to 30 to 35 mg/dl in normal patients (especially in women) after a 3-day fast, insulin levels decrease proportionally more.[44] There are several ways to relate glucose and insulin concentrations during fasting,[45] such as the simple insulin (units/ml)/glucose (mg/dl) ratio.[46] In normal subjects, this ratio remains less

than 0.3 as fasting continues, whereas in patients with inappropriate insulin secretion, the ratio almost invariably rises to more than 0.3.[47] To perform this study in a patient suspected of having an insulinoma, the patient undergoes an overnight fast, and serum glucose and insulin levels are obtained every 4 to 6 hours for 72 hours or until symptoms of hypoglycemia occur. The test should be terminated if the serum glucose level falls to less than 40 mg/dl or if symptoms of hypoglycemia develop. It is recommended that these studies be performed in a hospital setting. Symptomatic hypoglycemia takes place within 24 hours of the start of the fast in two thirds of the patients with insulinomas and within 48 hours in 95%. The remaining 5% of patients require the full 3 days of fasting. The test is considered positive if serum insulin remains stable or increases in the setting of hypoglycemia or if the insulin/glucose ratio is greater that 0.3. High insulin concentrations are not necessary to make the diagnosis. A value of 25 to 40 units/ml at a time when glucose concentration has fallen to less than 40 mg/dl is considered positive. Although provocative testing with tolbutamide, leucine, glucagon, and calcium is sometimes used, false-positive and false-negative results are common. We no longer use these tests. An oral glucose tolerance test is generally not helpful because serum glucose levels may remain unchanged, rise to within normal limits, or rise to abnormally high levels.

The measurement of proinsulin is helpful in diagnosing insulinomas. The beta islet cells of the pancreas synthesize proinsulin. Proinsulin is composed of two amino acid chains that are connected by a 33 amino acid–connecting peptide, termed *C-peptide*. Both insulin and the C-peptide are secreted in similar amounts. In normal individuals, the percentage of proinsulin in the fasting plasma is less than 20% of the total immunoreactive insulin, whereas this level is increased to 25 to 75% among patients with an insulinoma.[48-50] Aggressive insulinomas are more often associated with the highest levels of proinsulin (50 to 75%).[49] Antibodies that are able to distinguish between insulin and proinsulin have facilitated the measurement of proinsulin concentrations directly rather than as a proportion of total immunoreactive insulin levels. Patients with insulinoma have increased amounts of circulating proinsulin and either a normal or elevated level of C-peptide[51] that can be measured in blood or urine. The major advantage of measuring C-peptide levels is the ability to distinguish endogenous insulin levels in the presence of exogenous administration of insulin.[52] In patients suspected of surreptitiously using insulin, the proinsulin level is normal, and C-peptide levels are decreased. It is probably wise to measure fasting levels because these are the values usually reported by the laboratory, and a small amount of proinsulin may be secreted following a meal.[53] In one series, the diagnosis of insulinoma was established by a glucose level of 40 mg/dl with a serum insulin level of 6 μU/ml, a C-peptide level greater than 200 pmol/L, and negative screen for sulfonylurea.[54]

Once a biochemical diagnosis of insulinoma is established, preoperative localization of the tumor is required because insulinomas are frequently small (<2 cm).[55-57] Despite the small size of insulinomas, 90% are solitary, and nearly 100% are intrapancreatic. Considering that approximately 95% of insulinomas can be successfully removed at surgery by an experienced surgeon after careful palpation and sometimes guided by intraoperative ultrasonography, it seems prudent (and cost-effective) to reserve the invasive localizing procedure to patients who have had an unsuccessful exploration.

## DELTA CELL TUMORS (GASTRINOMA AND ZOLLINGER-ELLISON SYNDROME)

ZES is caused by excessive gastric acid secretion resulting from a gastrin-producing delta cell tumor (gastrinoma).[58, 59] In 1955, Zollinger and Ellison published their landmark article that characterized the gastrinoma syndrome and presented a hypothesis for the pancreatic endocrine origin of the gastric hypersecretion and ulcer disease. Classically the gastric acid hypersecretion associated with the tumor results in multiple duodenal postbulbar ulcerations. Nearly 50% of patients with ZES, however, have esophagitis, which may be more difficult to treat than the peptic ulcer disease.[60] Gastrinomas are estimated to occur in 0.1 to 3 individuals per 1 million in the United States.[61] Gastrinomas occur with nearly equal frequency in the duodenum and pancreas, and both are equally malignant.[62] ZES is associated with MEN 1 in approximately one third of patients.[58, 63, 64] A family history of endocrinopathy and the presence of other tumors, especially in the parathyroids and pituitary, characterize the co-occurrence of ZES with MEN 1 syndrome. It is important to recognize the diagnosis of MEN 1 occurring in the setting of ZES because the management is different (discussed in Chapter 67). Patients with ZES without MEN 1 (sporadic gastrinomas) frequently have multiple tumors. The tumors are difficult to find and in about one third of cases are not located at the time of surgery.[62, 65, 66] Because in the past,

many of these undiscoverable tumors were duodenal gastrinomas, the use of operative endoscopic transillumination of the bowel wall has markedly improved the ability to detect these tumors.[62, 67]

The diagnosis of ZES is suspected in patients with severe gastroduodenal ulcer symptoms; however, diarrhea and abdominal pain are more consistent symptoms. These symptoms occur when large amounts of acid enter the duodenum, destroy pancreatic lipase, and damage the small bowel mucosa, resulting in a malabsorption syndrome. Generally the physical examination is normal in most patients and is not useful in making the diagnosis of ZES. The diagnosis is made when the fasting serum gastrin (>100 pg/ml) is found in the absence of achlorhydria (Fig. 69–1). Patients with gastrinoma usually have levels greater than 500 pg/ml, and a level greater than 900 pg/ml is almost always diagnostic of ZES. In patients without ZES taking proton-pump inhibitors, such as omeprazole or lansoprazole, elevations in serum gastrin are common and occur in the setting of reduced acid secretion; however, serum gastrin is generally less than 200 pg/ml. Lipemic serum can falsely elevate the gastrin level to a clearly diagnostic value.[68] Renal insufficiency can also lead to an elevated serum gastrin level, resulting from a reduction in the renal clearance of gastrin.[69] Exogenous administration of gastrin in humans[70] and rodents[71] is associated with an increase in renal excretion of sodium that is mediated, at least in part, by the gastrin receptor, cholecystokinin type B (CCKB), which has been cloned in both species.[72, 73]

In nearly 50% of patients with gastrinoma, an equivocal serum gastrin concentration is observed, and provocative testing is required in these patients to establish the correct diagnosis.[74] In patients with borderline elevated gastrin val-

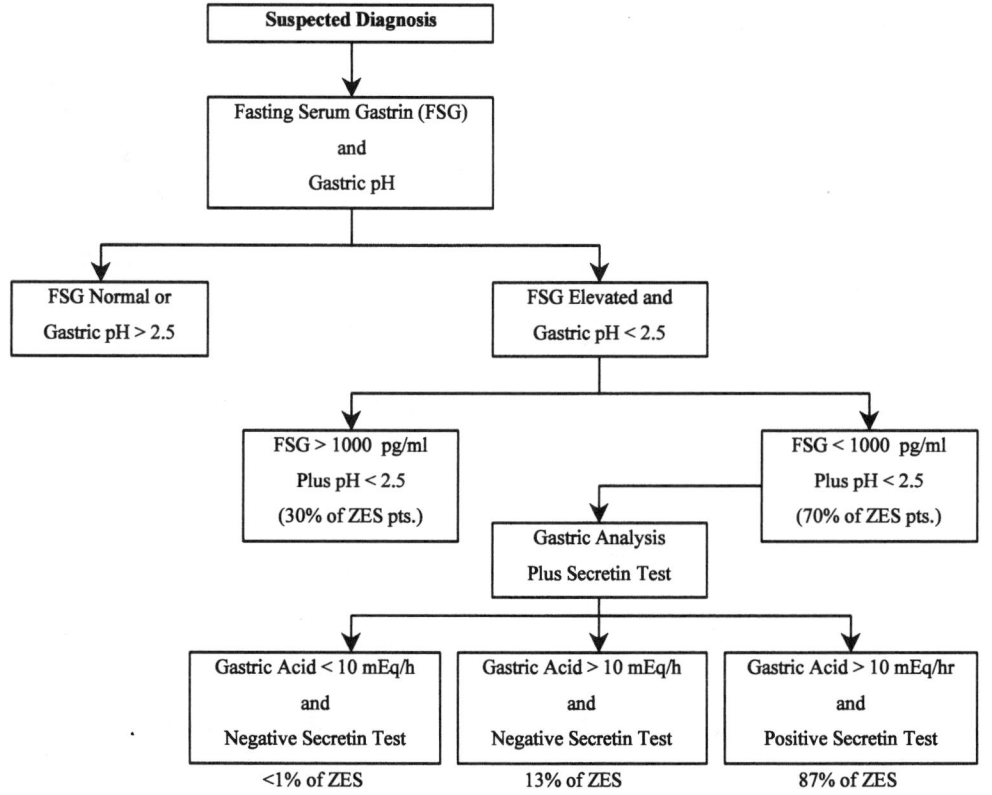

**Figure 69–1.** Algorithm for the diagnosis of Zollinger-Ellison syndrome (ZES).

ues (e.g., 200 to 500 pg/ml) in whom ZES is suspected, a secretin provocative test (see Fig. 69–1) is sensitive and specific for the diagnosis of ZES .[75] This test is performed by measuring serum gastrin at baseline and following the administration of secretin (2 units/kg intravenously as a bolus). A rise in the gastrin level of greater than 200 pg/ml within 15 minutes is diagnostic of gastrinoma in 87 to 93% of patients with ZES.[75] Alternatively, calcium provocative testing can be performed in equivocal cases, although this test is less sensitive than the secretin infusion test.[76] In patients in whom the diagnosis of the ZES is suspected but cannot be definitively proved, testing for *Helicobacter pylori* may be helpful. In patients with duodenal (but not gastric) ulcers, a negative test for the organism increases the pretest probability from 10 to 20% to a post-test range of 61 to 78%.[77] The prevalence of *H. pylori* in patients with ZES is lower than that in the general population and is not an independent risk factor for the genesis of peptic ulcerations in ZES patients.[78] In patients with ZES, there are frequently multiple hormone elevations, such as adrenocorticotropic hormone (ACTH), that carry a risk of the development of Cushing's syndrome and a more ominous prognosis.[79] Cushing's syndrome occurs in approximately 20% of patients with MEN 1 syndrome and is caused by the overproduction of ACTH by the pituitary gland.[80] The occurrence of Cushing's syndrome in sporadic ZES generally carries a worse prognosis and occurs in advanced disease with metastases.[81] In contrast to MEN 1 syndrome, the syndrome in sporadic ZES occurs because of the ectopic production of ACTH.

Once the diagnosis of ZES has been established, the determination and control of gastric acid secretion is the next most important step in its management.[81] With gastrinomas, severe peptic ulcer disease and upper gastrointestinal hemorrhage are a greater threat than the growth of metastatic tumor. Therapy has been directed mostly toward control of acid hypersecretion. Gastric analysis is not only an objective measure of the adequacy of medical management of ZES but also can be used in the diagnostic work-up of ZES. The presence of gastric acid hypersecretion is determined with the use of gastric analysis and the titration of four 15-minute acid collections using 0.1N sodium hydroxide. Basal acid output (BAO) is less than 10 mEq/hr in normal subjects and is increased in the presence of hypergastrinemia. Using the gastrin analogue, pentagastrin, the maximal acid output (MAO) can be determined. Because patients with ZES have BAO that are nearly as high as MAO, it is logical that the BAO/MAO ratio should be nearly 1.0.[82–84] Although BAO and MAO parallel the course of ZES, following curative gastrinoma resection, as defined by having a normal serum gastrin and a negative secretin infusion test, BAO and MAO may remain elevated in nearly 50% of patients.[85] One reason for this continued elevation is the expansion of parietal cell mass as a consequence of long-term hypergastrinemia. Following curative gastrinoma resection, the major indices that predict cure are the fasting serum gastrin and the secretin infusion test. Even following curative gastrinoma resection, patients require long-term gastric analysis to assess the adequacy of gastric antisecretory medication.[85] Prevention of peptic ulcerations is attainable with a reduction in gastric acid secretion to less than 10 mEq/hr. Ideally, BAO should be maintained at less than 5 mEq/hr for uncomplicated ZES and at less than 1 to 2 mEq/hr for complicated ZES, such as

that occurring in association with MEN 1, gastroesophageal reflux disease, or postgastrectomy.[86]

Initial treatment previously consisted of H2-receptor antagonists, but currently the newer proton-pump inhibitors are used.[87, 88] Although useful, H2-receptor antagonists have a lower efficacy and shorter duration of action and consequently require high doses for the adequate control of gastric acid secretion. The median dose of ranitidine required to control gastric acid secretion fully is 1.2 g/day, with 6 g/day required in difficult to control cases. Despite the high doses required, H2-receptor antagonists continue to be safe, including use during pregnancy.[89] Acid secretion can be controlled acutely in patients unable to take oral medications in 70% of patients with an infusion of ranitidine 1 mg/kg/hr; 4 mg/kg/hr controls gastric acid hypersecretion in all patients with ZES.[90]

The advent of the substituted benzimidazoles, which block the final step in gastric acid production by the gastric parietal cell, has heralded improved outcomes in patients with ZES [91, 92] and have replaced H2-receptor antagonists as the first-line agents for the control of gastric acid secretion in patients with ZES.[93] Omeprazole, the first of the proton-pump inhibitors, is effective in the control of gastric acid secretion in 99% of patients with ZES, with a dose range of 10 to 180 mg/24 hr.[91] The initial oral dosage of omeprazole should be 60 mg/day, with subsequent dose adjustments based on gastric acid analysis. Proton-pump inhibitors in a dosage of 60 mg/day control acid output in most patients, and 60 mg every 12 hours controls gastric acid secretion in all ZES patients.[90] Often, doses can then be reduced slowly and progressively. MEN 1 patients with difficult to control gastric acid secretion may have these difficulties related to hypercalcemia secondary to hyperparathyroidism.[90] The dose of omeprazole in ZES patients can be safely reduced to 20 mg once or twice daily in most patients.[92] Omeprazole and another substituted benzimidzole, lansoprazole,[94] are equally efficacious in the management of gastric acid hypersecretion in ZES patients.[95] Other substituted benzimidazoles, pantoprazole and rabeprazole, have been under investigation for the management of gastric acid hypersecretion in ZES. Pantoprazole is being studied for oral and intravenous administration for ZES when oral therapy is not feasible (i.e., during surgery or chemotherapy). In early studies, intravenous pantoprazole was found efficacious for rapid and prolonged acid suppression.[96] An intravenous proton-pump inhibitor has the advantage over the oral formulation because it can be used in situations in which oral feeding is not feasible, such as during the perioperative period, during acute upper gastrointestinal hemorrhage, or during the administration of chemotherapy, when patients frequently have nausea and vomiting.

In early studies involving proton-pump inhibitors, concern was raised over the development of gastric carcinoid tumors in rodents. Gastrin stimulates not only the release of histamine from enterochromaffin-like (ECL) cells, but also the growth of the ECL cells, and long-term hypergastrinemia may lead to the transformation of ECL cells to carcinoids.[97] Argyrophil carcinoid tumor has been reported in sporadic ZES, suggesting that the chronic hypergastrinemia associated with this syndrome may lead to fundic carcinoid development in nongenetically predisposed individuals.[98] In a more comprehensive study of patients with ZES taking high doses of proton-pump inhibitors for a prolonged period, however, no changes indicative of malignant transformation were observed in successive gastric biopsy samples, suggesting that the use of proton-pump inhibitors is safe.[99, 100] The trophic effect of gastrin on ECL cells appears to be increased in women and in patients with MEN 1 syndrome, suggesting that genetic traits are important determinants for the promotion of gastric carcinoids.[101] Suppression of hypergastrinemia, by antrectomy or with somatostatin analogues, may result in regression of ECL-cell hyperplasia and ECL-cell carcinoid.[102] These gastric carcinoids occurring in the setting of ZES and MEN 1 require surveillance by endoscopy and, in cases in which there is significant growth, should be resected endoscopically or surgically.[103] Hypergastrinemia also has been proposed to be important in the genesis of colon adenocarcinomas; however, the mechanisms involved in this association are unclear.[104]

Once gastric acid hypersecretion is safely under control, the next most important objective is to localize and treat the gastrinoma tumor (Fig. 69–2). The localization of islet cell tumors has undergone significant improvement with advanced radiologic imaging studies (discussed in more detail later). The first aim is to attempt to cure the disease through surgical resection. When this is not possible, the second goal is to reduce the metastatic spread of the gastrinoma. To address the first of these aims, management depends on whether the patient presents with the sporadic or the hereditary form of ZES (MEN 1). In patients with the sporadic form of ZES and without liver metastases, it is currently possible to localize and remove surgically the endocrine tumors, and this process has been improved by refinements in modern medical imaging, which are discussed later in this chapter. Once localized and resected, the cure of gastrinoma

in even the most sophisticated surgical center is 60% at 5 years. The percentage of patients who develop liver metastases depends on whether surgical resection is performed. Metastases develop in greater than 20% of patients who have not undergone surgery, compared with less than 5% in patients who have had surgery performed for cure (Fig. 69–3). In patients with ZES and MEN 1, surgical cure is not generally possible, and surgical resection is recommended in selected patients. Surgical resection in these cases involves a pancreatoduodenectomy.[105] In one case, a duodenal wall gastrinoma was cured endoscopically; however, the procedure may be associated with perforation because of the submucosal localization.[106] One explanation for the normalization in serum gastrin resulting from total gastrectomy may be due to the excision of occult duodenal wall gastrinomas.[107] In select cases, surgical intervention is aimed at reducing the gastric acid secretion rather than attempting a surgical cure.[108] Islet cell tumors of the pancreas also have been reported to result in pancreatic duct stricture that can be diagnosed by endoscopic retrograde cholangiopancreatography, and surgical intervention should be directed at palliation or correction of the stricture.[109, 110] Disseminated malignancy can occur and mainly involves spread to the liver, lymph nodes, and bone. With the improved control of gastric acid hypersecretion, metastatic spread is now the principal determinant of early death.[111]

## DIARRHEOGENIC TUMORS OF THE PANCREAS (VIPOMA)

Most cases of pancreatic cholera (also called *watery diarrhea, hypokalemia achlorhydria syndrome*) are caused by an

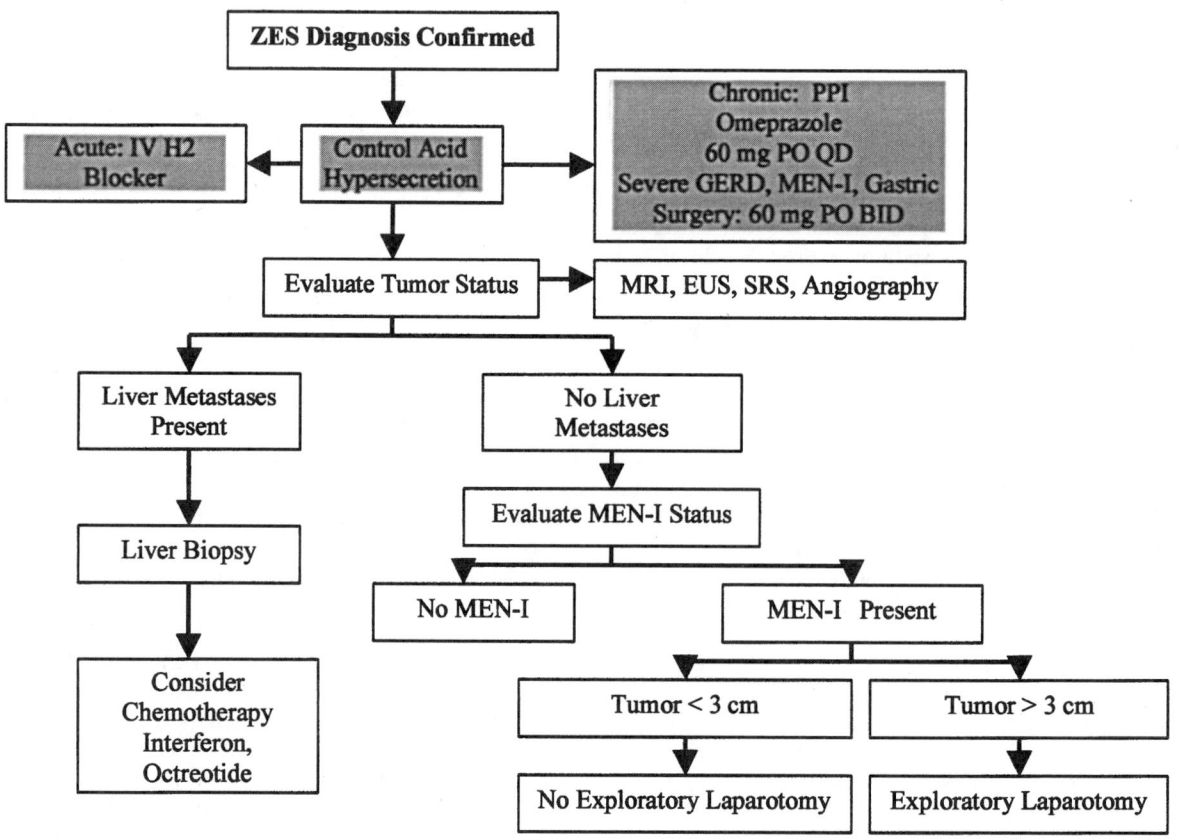

**Figure 69–2.** Protocol for the evaluation of ZES.

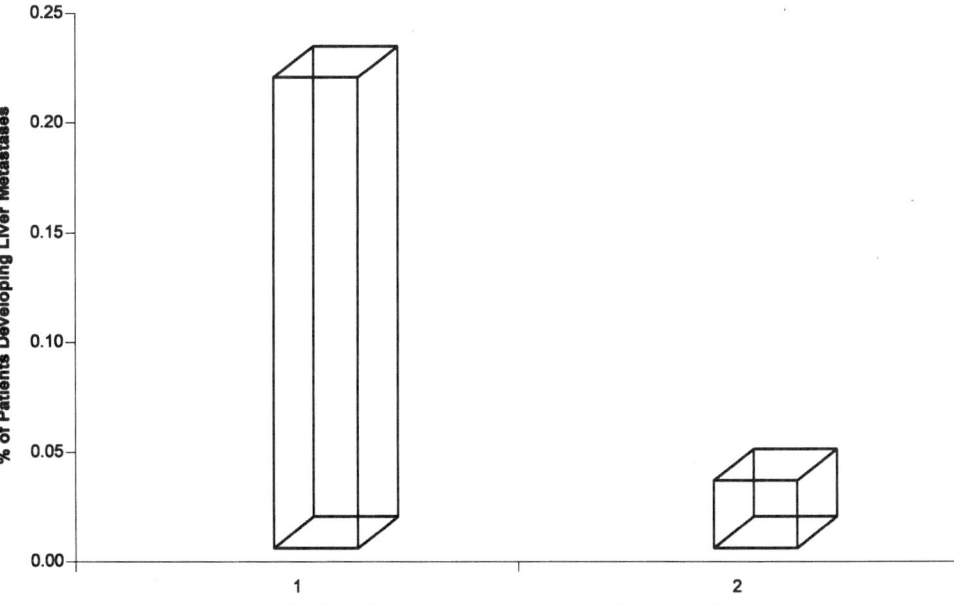

**Figure 69–3.** Percentage of patients with ZES who develop liver metastases.

islet cell tumor of the pancreas that secretes VIP or peptide histidine isoleucine.[112] Classically, this syndrome is characterized by profuse watery diarrhea, massive gastrointestinal losses of potassium, a low serum potassium level, and extreme weakness. Gastric acid secretion is usually low or absent, even after stimulation with pentagastrin, as a result of the inhibitory effects of VIP on gastric acid secretion. Stool volume averages about 5 L/day during acute episodes and contains more than 300 mEq of potassium (20 times normal). Severe metabolic acidosis may result from loss of bicarbonate in the stool. Many patients are also hypercalcemic, possibly from secretion by the tumor of parathyroid hormone–related protein. Abnormal glucose tolerance may result from decreased insulin secretion secondary to hypokalemia. The diagnosis of VIPoma should be considered in patients with severe diarrhea associated with hypokalemia and should be studied carefully for other causes before the diagnosis of this syndrome is entertained seriously. Chronic laxative abuse is a frequent explanation, and an elevated osmolar gap in the 24-hour stool collection is generally observed. Patients with VIPoma should be distinguished from patients with pseudopancreatic cholera syndrome; excluding laxative abuse and a reliable VIP radioimmunoassay are generally needed for differential diagnosis.[117] In normal conditions, the serum VIP level is generally less than 170 pg/ml in the fasting state. The use of a reliable laboratory for the determination of serum VIP levels is critical because in contrast to gastrin, VIP can easily degrade. It is recommended that the serum be fractionated by centrifugation shortly after collection and that the serum component be kept frozen until analysis to avoid false-negative values. Levels greater than 900 pg/ml are commonly observed.[113, 114] Similar to glucagonomas and insulinomas, tumor processing of VIP is impaired, and pre-proVIP levels can be detected in the circulation.[115]

Preoperative staging with endoscopic ultrasonography, spiral computed tomography (CT), and angiography should be used in an attempt to localize VIPomas. Approximately 80%

of VIPomas are solitary, are located in the body or tail, and can be readily resected. About half the lesions are malignant, and three fourths of these malignancies have metastasized by the time of exploration. In children, however, most tumors secreting VIP are ganglioneuromas rather than islet cell lesions. Approximately 200 cases of VIPomas have been described.[113, 116] In cases of metastatic spread, the symptoms can generally be controlled with the subcutaneous administration of octreotide.

## SOMATOSTATINOMAS

Somatostatinomas are delta cell tumors that arise in the pancreas in most cases, although they may also occur in the intestine.[117–121] The syndrome results from secretion of somatostatin by an islet cell tumor of the pancreas, which, in most cases, is malignant and accompanied by hepatic metastases. In many cases, the tumor is identified unexpectedly at the time of surgery for other conditions. In most cases because of the excessive production of somatostatin, the presenting features include diabetes mellitus, cholelithiasis, diarrhea, and steatorrhea. Most cases of pancreatic somatostatinomas are symptomatic, whereas most intestinal somatostatinomas are silent.[122] The syndrome results from the overproduction of somatostatin, a tetradecapeptide that has protean effects on the gastrointestinal system. Somatostatin is a potent inhibitor of gastric acid secretion and is normally released from the gastric delta cells. Consequently, patients with somatostatinomas frequently have decreased gastric acid secretion.[123] Somatostatin is also a potent inhibitor of pancreatic acinar function and reduces the release of pancreatic enzymes by cholecystokinin. Consequently, patients frequently have pancreatic steatorrhea and a reduction in the intestinal absorption of lipids and vitamins such as vitamin $B_{12}$ and folate.[124] Somatostatin is a potent inhibitor of intestinal and gallbladder smooth muscle contraction and leads to the development of gallstones and abnormal gastrointestinal motility. In one series, however, 23 cases of pancreatic somatostatinoma were reviewed, and there were no cases of cholelithiasis, suggesting that gallstones are less frequently encountered than originally thought.[121] The effect of octreotide on gastrointestinal hormone secretion is one of the reasons that the somatostatin analogue has utility in the management of excessive hormone secretion in conditions such as gastrinoma, glucagonoma, insulinoma, and carcinoid tumors.[125-131] Serum levels of calcitonin and IgM may be elevated. Recognizing the clinical syndrome and measuring increased concentrations of somatostatin in the serum may establish the diagnosis. Although there is no specific provocative test for somatostatinomas, tolbutamide and arginine may stimulate an increase in somatostatin levels of the serum.[91, 132, 133] In most cases, however, the somatostatin syndrome has been unsuspected until histologic evidence of metastatic islet cell carcinoma has been obtained. Only about 30 patients with this rare syndrome have been reported in the literature thus far.[124, 134-137] Duodenal somatostatinomas with carcinoid tumors,[138-140] von Hippel–Lindau disease, and von Recklinghausen's disease or neurofibromatosis[138, 139, 141, 142] have been described.

## PANCREATIC POLYPEPTIDE-SECRETING TUMORS OF THE PANCREAS

Pancreatic polypeptide-secreting tumors of the pancreas (PPomas) are broadly classified along with nonfunctional pancreatic islet cell tumors because PPomas are not associated with a clinical syndrome. The presentation is typically that of a patient being evaluated for cachexia, weight loss, and hepatomegaly with CT or magnetic resonance imaging (MRI) evidence of multiple hepatic metastases. Pathologically, these tumors resemble other islet cell tumors. The diagnosis of PPoma is confirmed by the presence of elevated serum levels of pancreatic polypeptide by radioimmunoassay.[143-145] It is unclear why patients with elevated serum pancreatic polypeptide levels fail to have symptoms, but presumably the hormone released is not biologically active. The role of pancreatic polypeptide in the gastrointestinal tract has been investigated by several groups to determine its physiologic function. Patients with PPoma generally present in their 40s or 50s, and it is not unusual for patients 70 years old to have these tumors.[143, 144, 146] Most of these patients have widely metastatic disease (70 to 90% of cases).[143-145] The primary tumor is almost invariably situated in the pancreas and is large (7.5 cm) at the time of imaging.[143-145] In solitary lesions of the pancreas, surgical resection is indicated. There are few data in the literature regarding the long-term cure rate following pancreatic resection in these cases. Response to octreotide therapy in patients with widely metastatic disease has not been well characterized. The existence of islet cell tumors that secrete other hormonal markers also has not been well characterized. Many patients with metastatic islet cell tumors may present with hypercalcemia. Similar to small cell tumors of the lung, this hypercalcemia is thought to be due to the tumor release of parathyroid hormone or a parathyroid hormone–releasing hormone. There is one case of an islet cell tumor of the pancreas that stained positively with pancreatic polypeptide and a novel biologically inactive hormone called *pituitary adenylate acti-*

*vating polypeptide* (Pisegna JR, unpublished data, 1999). It is likely that other biologically active peptides exist that have not yet been isolated.

## GROWTH HORMONE–RELEASING FACTOR TUMORS OF THE PANCREAS AND NEUROTENSINOMAS

Growth hormone–releasing factor tumors (GRFomas) generally are rare, occur predominantly in the pancreas, and secrete excessive amounts of growth hormone–releasing factor, leading to a syndrome characterized by acromegaly. The first case was identified in 1982.[147, 148] The tumors are generally large, and most are benign. There is an association between GRFomas and patients with ZES and MEN 1 syndrome. GRFomas should be considered in the differential diagnosis of acromegaly, especially when associated with ZES and MEN 1. The diagnosis is established by measuring the serum levels of growth hormone–releasing factor by radioimmunoassay.

Neurotensinomas are rare and are difficult to identify because their symptom complex results from excessive VIP secretion, making the clinical diagnosis difficult. These patients present with edema, hypotension, cyanosis, and flushing.[123]

## PANCREATIC ISLET CELL TUMOR LOCALIZATION

Advances in imaging studies have greatly increased the yield for the detection of primary and metastatic islet cell tumors.[149] Following the diagnosis and confirmation of islet cell tumor disease by the identification of elevated peptide hormones and the control of symptoms, the next most important aspect of management is the identification of the primary tumor. These generally occur in the pancreas, duodenum, or peripancreatic soft tissues. It is also important to exclude the presence of metastatic disease, generally in the liver or bone. Because the cure of these tumors depends on the resection of primary disease, proper identification of the primary tumor provides guidance to the surgeon and reduces intraoperative time for exploration. The preoperative diagnosis of metastatic tumor is important because in cases of widely metastatic disease, surgery for curative resection is generally not recommended and may guide management directed more at palliative ablative cryotherapy or hepatic transplantation if indicated.

Percutaneous ultrasonography, CT, angiography, and MRI have been studied and shown to be important for the preoperative staging of disease (Fig. 69–4). Improvements in abdominal imaging have increased the diagnostic yield for the detection of tumors. In one study, MRI short tau inversion-recovery (STIR) (Fig. 69–4B) was shown to be the most sensitive study for the evaluation of hepatic metastases, compared with CT (Fig. 69–4A), ultrasonography, or angiography.[150] Endoscopic ultrasonography (EUS), (Fig. 69–4D), which is performed more routinely now, also has been shown to be sensitive for the detection of primary pancreatic and duodenal gastrinomas. The Octreoscan (somatostatin receptor scintigraphy) was shown to be sensitive for the detection of primary islet cell tumors of the pancreas and nearly as

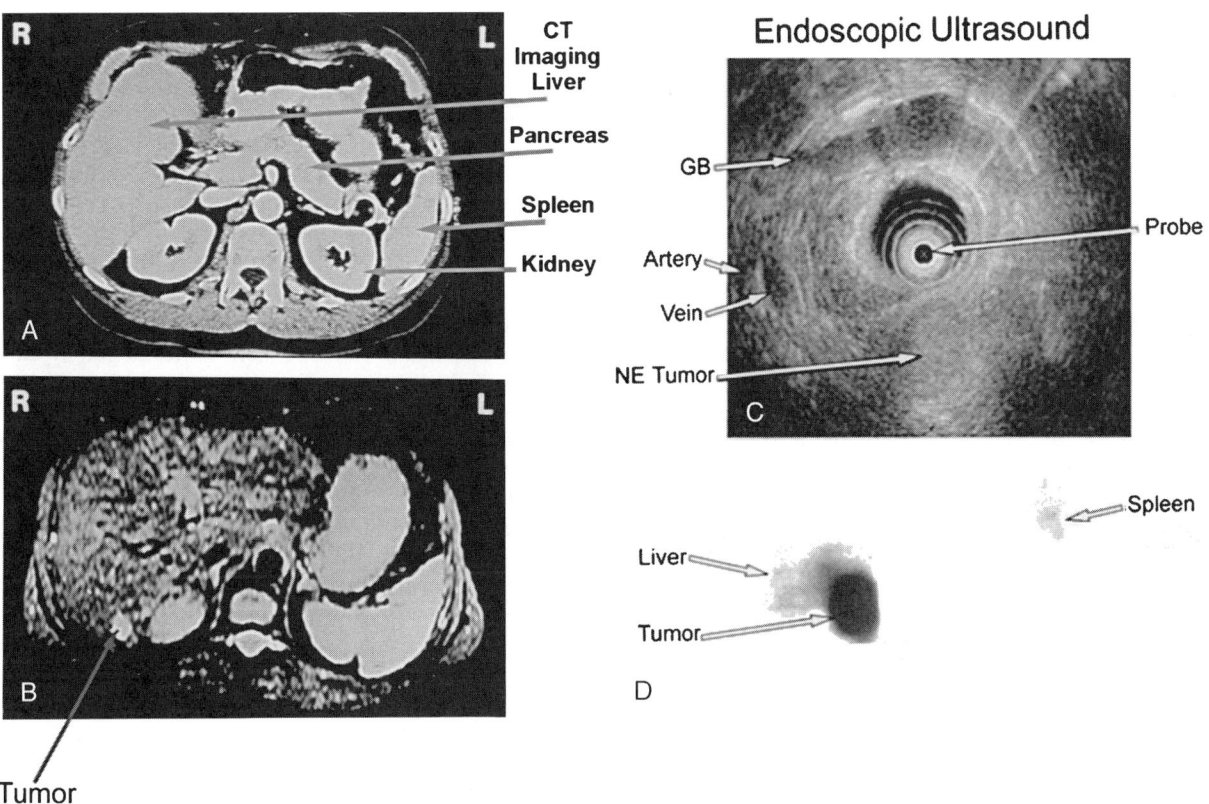

**Figure 69–4.** Imaging modalities for the localization of islet cell tumors. *A,* CT scans of the abdomen. *B,* MRI of the abdomen. *C,* Endoscopic ultrasonography. *D,* Octreoscan (somatostatin receptor scintigraphy).

sensitive for the detection of hepatic metastases. Endoscopic localization of tumors is possible in rare cases; endoscopic extirpation of tumor carries a high risk for perforation because most of these tumors are submucosal. It is preferable in these cases to perform fine-needle aspiration for cytologic evaluation.[151] Spiral CT is now recommended over standard CT of the abdomen and is nearly as sensitive as MRI in the diagnosis of hepatic metastases (unpublished observations). Positron emission tomography (PET) is also increasingly used in the preoperative imaging of islet cell tumors; however, no large study has yet been performed to determine its sensitivity for detecting tumors of the pancreas or liver. In general, islet cell tumors of the pancreas are hypervascular, and when they occur in the liver, they must be distinguished from hemangiomas, which also are hypervascular. In these cases and especially given the common occurrence of hemangiomas, the Octreoscan may be useful because only islet cell tumors are positive. In other cases, an increase in tumor size with serial imaging can establish the diagnosis of islet cell tumor.[152] Of the entire group of islet cell tumors that involve the pancreas, insulinomas, given their small size, can be difficult to diagnose without the use of specialized imaging studies. The modalities available for localization previously included selective arteriography,[55–57] ultrasonography, rapid computed tomographic scanning with contrast,[56, 57, 153] and transhepatic selective venous sampling.[154–158] The sensitivity for the first three approaches is approximately 50 to 75%.[154–157] There is no doubt that transhepatic selective venous sampling is more accurate in the preoperative localization of insulinomas.[154–158] Using this approach, veins draining various parts of the pancreas are catheterized by a

transhepatic approach, and samples are collected for measurement of insulin concentration.[159] By assessing the gradients of insulin sampled from these tributaries, it is possible to identify more accurately the location of an insulinoma. The use of another invasive procedure for localization, selective intra-arterial injection of calcium with measurement of hepatic vein insulin levels, reportedly has an increased sensitivity for localizing insulinomas.[160–162] A twofold rise of hepatic vein insulin concentrations within 30 to 60 seconds of the calcium injection is considered sufficiently sensitive for localization. Generally, injection is as follows: gastroduodenal, superior head and neck, superior mesenteric, inferior head and uncinate process, splenic, body and tail, hepatic, and liver metastases. In addition to these invasive radiologic studies, somatostatin receptor scintigraphy, intraoperative ultrasonography (IOUS), and EUS are emerging as useful imaging approaches to localizing islet cell tumors of the pancreas. One report documents a case of insulinoma that was localized using a laparoscopic ultrasonographic probe.[163] The intravenous administration of [111In]DTPA-D-Phe-octreotide followed by whole-body gamma camera scintigraphy localizes islet cell tumors with a sensitivity of 75%, specificity of 100%, positive predictive value of 63%, and overall accuracy of 82% in 28 patients studied for 12 months.[164] Another technique for the localization of insulinomas is IOUS. At least one series recommends the use of IOUS as the definitive imaging study for localizing insulinomas.[165] IOUS is as sensitive as the other invasive procedures in localizing tumors. Moreover, it not only is more cost-effective but also gives the surgeon anatomic information regarding the location of pancreatic ducts, which is helpful in deciding between simple enucleation or pancreatic resection.[166] Finally, the development of EUS has resulted in the successful preoperative localization of 100% of insulinomas located in the head and body of the pancreas but (as might be expected) in only 40% of tumors located in the tail in a small number of patients.[167] By EUS, insulinomas may appear round, homogeneous, and slightly hypoechoic, compared with the pancreatic parenchyma.[168, 169]

Of the remaining islet cell tumors of the pancreas, gastrinomas have been the most studied of the tumors with respect to the diagnostic sensitivity and specificity of the localization studies. The ability to localize and resect gastrinomas has been greatly facilitated by the use of advanced imaging studies, as with the long-acting somatostatin analogue octreotide, which is frequently used as a tracer to localize tumors.[164, 170] Ultrasonography, CT, MRI, EUS, and intraoperative duodenal transillumination and sonography have greatly increased the yield for identification of islet cell tumors.[62, 150, 171, 172] With these improved imaging studies, duodenal wall gastrinomas are more frequently detected and now account for nearly half the total cases.[62] In some cases, the use of portal venous sampling and angiography with stimulation can lead to a sensitivity for detecting tumors that approaches 70 to 80% in selected series.[173–175]

## Surgical Management

### INSULINOMA

With insulinomas, surgery should be undertaken promptly because the tumor may be malignant, and with repeated attacks of hypoglycemia, permanent cerebral damage may occur. Because these tumors are interesting, many physicians are tempted to explore every possibility in their efforts to diagnose and localize these tumors. Because of the rarity of these tumors and the rapid advancement of imaging techniques, however, determining which tests are necessary for preoperative evaluation remains controversial. In most series, these techniques are not as sensitive as intraoperative palpation combined with intraoperative ultrasonography.[176–179] Most lesions are not seen on computed tomographic scans because they are too small. CT should be performed, however, to evaluate the patient for metastatic disease.[180] In experienced hands, this may be the only preoperative imaging test necessary. EUS appears to be sensitive (85%) and may be the optimal modality if the expertise is available.[181, 182] Other imaging modalities are useful in selected patients or when an initial operative exploration has failed to identify the tumor, which occurs in less than 10% of patients.

Selective angiography shows the tumor in about 50% of cases.[176, 183] This technique may be particularly helpful in centers where the surgical experience is limited and conventional imaging modalities fail to identify the tumor. Percutaneous transhepatic venous catheterization allows sampling of blood draining from the pancreas at multiple sites along the splenic and portal veins.[184] Insulin is measured in the samples, and the point at which the insulin concentration rises sharply indicates the location of the tumor. This technique can regionalize the location of the tumor and facilitate precise intraoperative localization.[185, 186] Calcium angiography, in which calcium gluconate is injected into specific pancreatic arteries and hepatic venous blood is collected for insulin assay, may be even more sensitive.[187–189]

Some authorities discontinue diazoxide for 1 week or more before operation because of the association of diazoxide with hypotension on induction of anesthesia. Others, however, consider this risk to be minimal and of less importance than the risk of hypoglycemia for that added period. At surgery, the entire pancreas must be fully mobilized and carefully palpated to find the tumor. Intraoperative ultrasonography is useful.[190] Many tumors may be small, soft, and difficult to palpate. Intraoperative ultrasonography can help to identify these tumors. The tumor should be enucleated if it is superficial. If it is deeply situated near the pancreatic duct, it should be removed as part of a partial pancreatectomy. Tumors in the head of the gland can nearly always be enucleated, so a pancreaticoduodenectomy is not often indicated.[191] If the tumor cannot be found and the results of venous sampling studies suggest its location, that portion of the pancreas should be resected. A Whipple resection may be appropriate if these studies indicate that the tumor is in the head of the gland. Insulinoma can be successfully treated by an experienced surgeon in more than 90% of patients.[192]

If the tumor cannot be localized at operation, blind pancreatic resection is controversial. If no localizing information is available, the distal half of the pancreas is removed, and a pathologist slices the specimen up into thin sections to look for the tumor. If it is found, the operation is concluded. If not, more is removed until an 80% distal pancreatectomy has been performed. Because the tumors are evenly distributed, this confers an 80% probability of cure.[193] For islet cell hyperplasia, nesidioblastosis, or multiple benign adenomas, distal subtotal pancreatectomy is indicated to decrease insulin levels sufficiently so that medical management can be more effective. For malignant insulinomas, resection of the primary tumor and debulking of metastases are warranted if the procedures are technically feasible and safe.

### GASTRINOMA

The ability to control gastric acid secretion adequately in patients with ZES has shifted the emphasis of surgery from gastric resection to identification and resection of the tumors for cure. The current recommendations for the management of patients with ZES are shown in Table 69–1. There has been a major change in understanding of the biology of these tumors in the 1990s, and consequently the ability to cure these patients has improved. With aggressive surgical management, 50 to 80% of patients can be cured.[194–196]

Surgical management should be directed at complete tumor resection to effect cure of the syndrome and to prevent the development of metastasis.[194, 196–198] All patients with the sporadic form of ZES should undergo a surgical resection aimed at cure, even if the primary tumor is not identified by imaging studies. In patients with MEN 1, the role of surgery is less clear-cut. In one series of 10 patients with MEN 1 and ZES who underwent surgical resection, only 1 patient was cured immediately postoperatively; however, that person suffered a recurrence at 3 months (Norton J, unpublished data, 1992). Because patients with gastrinoma and MEN 1 syndrome have multiple small pancreatic tumors that cannot

**Table 69–1.** Current Recommendations for the Management of Zollinger-Ellison Syndrome

MRI and SRS are the first-line imaging studies for evaluating the presence of gastrinoma metastatic to the liver

SRS, EUS, and selective angiography are the most sensitive studies for the preoperative localization of gastrinomas

Surgical exploration, intraoperative ultrasonography, and duodenal transillumination are indicated in all patients who are operative candidates

In patients with MEN 1, surgical exploration should be considered in patients with primary tumors >3 cm without evidence of metastatic disease

Medical therapy for metastatic gastrinoma has not been clearly established. The use of combination chemotherapy and interferon and octreotide are currently under investigation

MRI, magnetic resonance imaging; SRS, somatostatin receptor scintigraphy; EUS, endoscopic ultrasound; MEN 1, multiple endocrine neoplasia type 1.

be completely resected, some physicians agree that operation is not necessary.[63, 199, 200] If these patients also have hyperparathyroidism, parathyroidectomy should be performed promptly because it may dramatically improve the acid peptic disease.

Computed tomographic scans usually show pancreatic tumors if they are greater than 3 cm in diameter and are helpful to identify hepatic metastases. Octreoscan is now generally available and is the most sensitive test for identifying gastrinomas.[201] Octreoscan identifies 80% of tumors and is particularly useful in patients with tumors located at unexpected sites, such as the heart or lungs.[202, 203] Smaller tumors may also be localized with MRI.[204] To localize duodenal tumors, selective arterial secretin injection studies have a greater than 90% positive predictability rate and may be more sensitive than portal venous sampling.[205, 206]

At operation, a thorough exploration of the abdomen should be performed with initial emphasis placed on the gastrinoma triangle.[207] Greater than 80% of the tumors are found in the *gastrinoma triangle*, which includes the area of the common bile duct, the duodenum, and the head and neck of the pancreas.[208, 209] Distant sites, such as the lung, heart, ovaries, kidney, and mesentery, have been found to contain gastrinomas.[209–211] If the tumor is found in the pancreas at operation, it should be enucleated, if possible. Pancreaticoduodenectomy is usually not needed. Ultrasonography may be useful to detect small lesions deep within the gland but not those in extrapancreatic sites. Intraoperative endoscopy to transilluminate the duodenal wall and duodenotomy may help in locating a duodenal tumor.[67, 212] These are often small and occur in more than 50% of cases. Resection of duodenal tumors or lymph nodes, or both, that contain gastrinoma appears to have cured some patients, with serum gastrin concentrations returning to normal.[208, 213–220] In about 15% of patients, however, the tumor is never identified. Liver resection is appropriate in the rare patient with a primary liver gastrinoma and patients with limited metastases.[221] Total gastrectomy should be performed in patients whose ulcer disease is refractory to medical therapy and who are unable to undergo resection of the tumor.

## NONFUNCTIONAL GLUCAGONOMAS AND DIARRHEOGENIC TUMORS

Most nonfunctional glucagonomas and diarrheogenic tumors are malignant and have metastasized by the time of diagno-

sis. Preoperative localization is rarely a problem because the tumors are often large and evident on CT. At operation, the tumor should be resected, and if metastases are present, they should be debulked. Even if all the tumor cannot be resected, subtotal resection may result in considerable palliation. With widespread hepatic metastases, placement of a hepatic artery catheter is indicated for postoperative therapy (see later discussion). The characteristic rash of glucagonoma usually improves within several days and clears rapidly, even with debulking.

## POSTOPERATIVE FOLLOW-UP

Follow-up of a patient with pancreatic neuroendocrine tumor depends on the type of tumor. In general, these are slowly growing tumors, and annual follow-up is usually sufficient. Every patient should have their serum tumor markers reevaluated immediately after surgery. A patient who had a successful resection of a benign insulinoma does not need long-term follow-up past 5 years, unless the patient subsequently develops symptoms. Malignant insulinomas need close follow-up to treat ongoing or developing metastases. Gastrinomas are more difficult to predict. These patients need lifelong follow-up with annual fasting serum gastrin levels. Secretin testing and octreotide scanning should be performed on anyone who has evidence of recurrence. Nonfunctional tumors should be followed for at least 5 years annually by serial CT and serum markers, if they were initially elevated.

## Nonsurgical Management of Metastatic Islet Cell Tumors

### RADIATION THERAPY

The treatment of metastatic deposits with radiation has not been associated with significant relief of symptoms. Because most metastatic lesions are in the liver, treatment with high-voltage radiation carries with it the risk of hepatic decompensation or failure. In one case, a patient with unresectable, locally advanced endocrine pancreatic carcinoma (measuring $5 \times 5 \times 6$ cm) was completely cured by external-beam radiation therapy (40 Gy). The authors concluded from the complete response observed in this case report and an additional four cases in the literature that external-beam radiation therapy should be considered in locally unresectable endocrine pancreatic carcinomas.[222] Bone metastases involving the central skeleton, as observed in more advanced cases of metastatic gastrinoma, are associated with a poor prognosis. In these patients, radiotherapy results in good symptom control in about 50% of the cases.[223]

### CHEMOTHERAPY AND HORMONE THERAPY

In general, chemotherapy is not highly efficacious for use in islet cell tumors; experience with single and combination agents yields less than a 29% response rate. Hormonal agents, such as octreotide and interferon alfa, when used as monotherapy, yield better response rates. Combination agents, as investigated by ongoing clinical studies, may offer significant promise.

**Glucagonoma.** The relative rarity of this lesion precludes any large experience with chemotherapy. Since an initial successful case report by Kessinger and colleagues[224] on the use of dacarbazine, a series of reports has confirmed a useful role for this drug in patients with symptomatic glucagonoma.[225–229] Dacarbazine is the drug of choice for symptomatic glucagonoma; its use is discussed in Chapter 10. Other drugs and drug combinations have not been nearly as useful as dacarbazine.[21] A few patients have responded to streptozocin, a glucosamine nitrosourea isolated from *Streptomyces achromogenes*.[24, 230] One patient, whose treatment with 5-fluorouracil (5-FU), streptozocin, and dacarbazine failed, responded to lomustine.[231] The combination of streptozocin plus 5-FU is not effective for glucagonomas.[24]

The markedly elevated glucagon levels and consequent clinical syndrome seen in these patients have improved with the long-acting somatostatin analogue octreotide.[230, 232, 233] This improvement is accompanied by a prompt improvement in the rash but no effect on tumor size. The use of octreotide is discussed in Chapter 10.

**Insulinoma.** In cases in which surgical resection does not lead to cure and hyperinsulinemia and hypoglycemia persist, diazoxide (Proglycem) is usually used to treat the hypoglycemia. This preparation should not be confused with intravenous diazoxide (Hyperstat), which is administered as a bolus to lower dangerously high blood pressure. Diazoxide is a nondiuretic benzothiadiazide that causes hyperglycemia in normal individuals and animals. Diazoxide is known to inhibit insulin secretion by the beta cell directly[234]; to stimulate epinephrine production by the adrenal medulla, which may further block insulin secretion[235] and inhibit peripheral glucose utilization[236, 237]; and to block hepatic glucose production directly.[238] The usual dose is 100 mg orally three or four times daily. Side effects may include nausea, sodium retention (for which a diuretic is added), tachycardia (due to epinephrine secretion), eosinophilia, granulocytopenia, neutropenia, thrombocytopenia, lymphocytosis, and hyperuricemia. Approximately half the patients respond to diazoxide.[239] Because oral diazoxide may be ineffective in many cases, other agents have been tried for the treatment of hypoglycemia. These include phenytoin (Dilantin),[240–242] chlorpromazine,[243] propranolol, the calcium channel blocker verapamil,[244] and octreotide.[232, 245] Diazoxide does not affect tumor growth.

Streptozocin localizes to and destroys normal and neoplastic beta cells. This intravenously administered agent is the most active chemotherapeutic agent in patients with metastatic insulinoma.[246] Streptozocin causes objective tumor regression and amelioration of hypoglycemia. L-Asparaginase[247] and doxorubicin (Adriamycin)[248, 249] have occasionally been effective in patients who are unresponsive to streptozocin. These agents are discussed further in Chapter 10. In view of the toxicity of streptozocin and these other agents, the use of chemotherapy is limited to patients with metastatic and unresectable tumors. Combination chemotherapy appears to be even more effective than single-agent therapy for insulinomas. Adding 5-FU to streptozocin markedly improved the response rate to 50% in one study.[230] A subsequent randomized study has shown that the combination of streptozocin and doxorubicin is even more effective than the combination of 5-FU and streptozocin.[250] The median survival was 2.2 years with streptozocin plus doxorubicin, compared with 1.4 years with streptozocin plus 5-FU ($p = 0.004$).[228] For patients with active heart disease, the combination of 5-FU plus streptozocin should be used instead of the doxorubicin-containing combination. Patients with hepatic metastases as the dominant site of disease may benefit from chemoembolization therapy, as reviewed in Chapter 104 and in an excellent review from the Mayo Clinic.[251]

**Gastrinoma.** The role of chemotherapy and hormonal therapy has been extensively studied in patients with metastatic gastrinoma tumors and serves as a model to determine potential efficacies for other noninsulinoma islet cell tumors of the pancreas. Chemotherapy has been reserved primarily for patients with ZES with enlarging liver metastases. These patients may be candidates for transcatheter arterial embolization through the hepatic artery, as discussed in Chapter 104. Streptozocin, 5-FU, doxorubicin, and tubercidin, as well as combinations of these agents, have been used in patients with ZES and metastatic gastrinoma.[144, 252–255] One study indicated that the combination of streptozocin and 5-FU was more effective than streptozocin alone.[230] At the National Institutes of Health, a combination of streptozocin, 5-FU, and doxorubicin had been used previously for patients with metastatic gastrinoma; however, because of the lack of tumor response, the toxicity associated with these agents, and the short-lasting response, these agents are no longer routinely used.[256, 257] In patients with ZES, the amount of tumor burden might not correlate with the degree of gastric acid suppression. Reduction in acid output may not accompany a decrease in tumor size, and adequate pharmacologic control of gastric hypersecretion must be maintained unless the patient has had a total gastrectomy.

Studies have been performed by our group as well as others to investigate the efficacy of hormonal therapies for the management of metastatic gastrinomas. In one study, alfa-interferon was shown to reduce tumor growth in 40% of patients treated with doses of 5 million units daily for at least 6 months.[256] In European studies, alfa-interferon had little to no effect on the progression of metastatic gastrinomas. Octreotide has been used in other studies and shown to have minimal results when used alone. Studies are under way to investigate the response to combination therapy with octreotide and alfa-interferon. The combination of these two agents is currently under study at UCLA (unpublished). The use of high-dose indium-radiolabeled analogues of somatostatin to target and irradiate metastatic islet cell tumors locally is also an area of investigation.

**VIPomas.** Streptozocin has produced remissions in several cases, but nephrotoxicity may limit its effectiveness in VIPomas. Selective arterial administration is preferred when renal function is impaired. Treatment with long-acting somatostatin analogues (Sandostatin LAR) decreases VIP levels, controls diarrhea, and may even reduce tumor size and should be used as initial therapy. The effect persists indefinitely in most patients, but for a few patients the response is only transient. If severe diarrhea continues, therapy with corticosteroids or indomethacin may be of benefit. The use of octreotide acetate is discussed in Chapter 10. The addition of alfa-interferon to this regimen, for possible tumor remission, needs to be explored further.

**Somatostatinoma.** A variety of agents have been used, including streptozocin, dacarbazine, and 5-FU. In general, these agents are ineffective in the treatment of somatostatinomas.

## SUGGESTIONS FOR ADDITIONAL READING

Richardson P, Hawkey CJ, Stack WA. Proton pump inhibitors: pharmacology and rationale for use in gastrointestinal disorders. Drugs 1998;56:307–35.

Norton JA. Gastrinoma: advances in localization and treatment. Surg Oncol Clin North Am 1998;7:845–61.

Jensen RT. Management of the Zollinger-Ellison syndrome in patients with multiple endocrine neoplasia type 1. J Intern Med 1998;243:477–88.

Stabile BE. Islet cell tumors. Gastroenterologist 1997;5:213–32.

Yu F, Venzon DJ, Serrano J, et al. Prospective study of the clinical course, prognostic factors, causes of death, and survival in patients with long-standing Zollinger-Ellison syndrome. J Clin Oncol 1999;17:615–30.

Fishbeyn VA, Norton JA, Benya RV, et al. Assessment and prediction of long-term cure in patients with the Zollinger-Ellison syndrome: the best approach. Ann Intern Med 1993;119:199–206.

Moertel CG, Johnson CM, McKusick MA, et al. The management of patients with advanced carcinoid tumors and islet cell carcinomas. Ann Intern Med 1994;120:302–9.

## REFERENCES

1. Boden G. Insulinoma and glucagonoma. Semin Oncol 1987;14:253–62.
2. SEER Cancer Statistics Review 1973-1996. (See http://www-seer.ims.nci.nih.gov.)
3. O'Connor DT, Deftos LJ. Secretion of chromogranin A by peptide-producing endocrine neoplasms. N Engl J Med 1986;314:1145–51.
4. Del Valle J, Yamada T. Zollinger-Ellison syndrome. In: Yamada T, ed. Textbook of gastroenterology. Philadelphia: JB Lippincott, 1991.
5. Lew EA, Lewin KJ, Zarchy T, Pisegna JR. Adenocarcinoma of the colon with neuroendocrine features and secretory diarrhea. Am J Gastroenterol 1999;94:1692–4.
6. Saclarides TJ, Szekuga D, Staren ED. Neuroendocrine cancers of the colon and rectum: results of a ten-year experience. Dis Col Rectum 1994;37:635–42.
7. Gaffey MJ, Mills SE, Lack EE. Neuroendocrine carcinoma of the colon and rectum: a clinicopathologic, ultrastructural, and immunohistochemical study of 24 cases. Am J Surg Pathol 1990;14:1010–23.
8. Howard TJ, Stabile BE, Zinner MJ, et al. Anatomic distribution of pancreatic endocrine tumors. Am J Surg 1990;159:258–64.
9. Wawrukiewicz AS, Rösch J, Keller FS, Lieberman DA. Glucagonoma and its angiographic diagnosis. Cardiovasc Intervent Radiol 1982;5:318–24.
10. Breatnach ES, Han SY, Rahatzad MT, Stanley RJ. CT evaluation of glucagonomas. J Comput Assist Tomogr 1985;9:25–9.
11. Wilkinson DS. Necrolytic migratory erythema with carcinoma of the pancreas. Trans St John's Hosp Dermatol Soc 1973;59:244–50.
12. Almdal TP, Heindorff H, Bardram L, Vilstrup H. Increased amino acid clearance and urea synthsis in a patient with glucagonoma. Gut 1990;31:946–8.
13. Holst JJ. Glucagon-producing tumors. In: Cohen S, Soloway D, eds. Hormone producing tumors of the gastrointestinal tract. New York: Churchill Livingstone, 1978:57.
14. Marynick SP, Fagadau WR, Duncan LA. Malignant glucagonoma syndrome: response to chemotherapy. Ann Intern Med 1980;93:453.
15. Abraira C, DeBartolo M, Katzen R, Lawrence AM. Disappearance of glucagonoma rash after surgical resection, but not during dietary normalization of serum amino acids. Am J Clin Nutr 1984;39:351–5.
16. Shepherd ME, Raimer SS, Tyring SK, Smith EB. Treatment of necrolytic migratory erythema in glucagonoma. J Am Acad Dermatol 1991;25:925–8.
17. Parr JH, Ramsay ID, Keeling PW, et al. Glucagonoma without cutaneous manifestations. Postgrad Med J 1985;61:737–8.
18. Altimari AF, Bhoopalam N, O'Dorsio T, et al. Use of a somatostatin analog (SMS 201–995) in the glucagonoma syndrome. Surgery 1986;100:989–96.
19. Rosenbaum A, Flourie B, Chagnon S, et al. Octreotide (SMS 201–995) in the treatment of metastatic glucagonoma: report of one case and review of the literature. Digestion 1989;42:116–20.
20. Maton PN, Gardner JD, Jensen RT. Use of long-acting somatostatin analog SMS 201–995 in patients with pancreatic islet cell tumors. Dig Dis Sci 1989;34:28S–39S.
21. Leichter SB. Clinical and metabolic aspects of glucagonoma. Medicine 1980;59:100–13.
22. Service FJ. Insulinoma and other islet-cell tumors. Cancer Treat Res 1997;89:335–46.
23. Holst JJ, Helland S, Ingemannson S, et al. Functional studies in patient with the glucagonoma syndrome. Diabetologia 1979;17:151–6.
24. Stacpoole PW. The glucagonoma syndrome: clinical features, diagnosis, and treatment. Endocr Rev 1981;2:347–61.
25. Jones B, Fishman EK, Bayless TM, Siegelman SS. Villous hypertrophy of the small bowel in a patient with glucagonoma. J Comput Assist Tomogr 1983;7:334–7.
26. Stevens FM, Flanagan RW, O'Gorman D, Buchanan KD. Glucagonoma syndrome demonstrating giant duodenal villi. Gut 1984;25:784–91.
27. Boden G, Ryan IG, Eisenschmid BL, et al. Treatment of inoperable glucagonoma with the long-acting somatostatin analogue SMS 201–995. N Engl J Med 1986;314:1686–9.
28. Mao C, Pour PM, Howard JM. Glucagonoma associated with calculous pancreatitis. HPB Surg 1996;9:77–81.
29. Kasper CS. Necrolytic migratory erythema: unresolved problems in diagnosis and pathogenesis: a case report and literature review. Cutis 1992;49:120–2,125–8.
30. Rappaport KD, White JW Jr. 45-year-old man with dermatitis and weight loss. Mayo Clin Proc 1995;70:785–8.
31. Mozell E, Stenzel P, Woltering EA, et al. Functional endocrine tumors of the pancreas: clinical presentation, diagnosis, and treatment. Curr Probl Surg 1990;27:301–86.
32. Galbut DL, Markowitz AM. Insulinoma: diagnosis, surgical management and long-term follow-up: review of 41 cases. Am J Surg 1980;139:682–90.
33. Gierchsky KE, Halse J, Mathisen W, et al. Endocrine tumors of the pancreas. Scand J Gastroenterol 1980;15:129–35.
34. Glickman MH, Hart MJ, White TT. Insulinoma in Seattle: 39 cases in 30 years. Am J Surg 1980;140:119–25.
35. Le Quesne LP, Nabarro JD, Kurtz A, Zweig S. The management of insulin tumours of the pancreas. Br J Surg 1979;66:373–8.
36. Service FJ, Dale AJ, Elveback LR, Jiang NS. Insulinoma: clinical and diagnostic features of 60 consecutive cases. Mayo Clin Proc 1976;51:417–29.
37. van Heerden JA, Edis AJ, Service FJ. The surgical aspects of insulinomas. Ann Surg 1979;189:677–82.
38. Jaksic T, Yaman M, Thorner P, et al. A 20-year review of pediatric pancreatic tumors. J Pediatr Surg 1992;27:1315–7.
39. Meleo K. Management of insuloma patients with refractory hypoglycemia. Probl Vet Med 1990;2:602–9.
40. Eckersley GN, Fockema A, Williams JH, et al. An insulinoma causing hypoglycaemia and seizures in a dog: case report and literature review. J S Afr Vet Assoc 1987;58:187–92.
41. Sawicki PT, Baba T, Berger M, Starke A. Normal blood pressure in patients with insulinoma despite hyperinsulinemia and insulin resistance. J Am Soc Nephrol 1992;3:4 Suppl:S64–8.
42. Svartberg J, Stridsberg M, Wilander E, et al. Tumour-induced hypoglycaemia in a patient with insulin-dependent diabetes mellitus. J Intern Med 1996;239:181–5.
43. Garner PR, Tsang R. Insulinoma complicating pregnancy presenting with hypoglycemic coma after delivery: a case report and review of the literature. Obstet Gynecol 1989;73:5 Pt 2:847–9.
44. Merimee TJ, Tyson JE. Stabilization of plasma glucose during fasting: normal variations in two separate studies. N Engl J Med 1974;291:1275–8.
45. Davidson MB. Hypoglycemia in adults. In: Lavin N, ed. Manual of endocrinology and metabolism. 2nd ed. Boston: Little, Brown, 1994:459.
46. Fajans SS, Vinik AI. Insulin-producing islet cell tumors. Endocrinol Metab Clin North Am 1989;18:45–74.
47. Merimee TJ. Hypoglycemia in man: pathologic and physiologic variants. Diabetes 1977;26:161.

48. Gutman RA, Lazarus NR, Penhos JC, et al. Circulating proinsulin-like material in patients with functioning insulinomas. N Engl J Med 1971;284:1003–8.

49. Sherman BM, Pek S, Fajans SS, et al. Plasma proinsulin in patients with functioning pancreatic islet cell tumors. J Clin Endocrinol Metab 1972;35:271–80.

50. Cohen RM, Given BD, Licinio-Paixao J, et al. Proinsulin radioimmunoassay in the evaluation of insulinomas and familial hyperproinsulinemia. Metabolism 1986;35:1137–46.

51. Grunberger G, Weiner JL, Silverman R, et al. Factitious hypoglycemia due to surreptitious administration of insulin: diagnosis, treatment, and long-term follow-up. Ann Intern Med 1988;108:252–7.

52. Rendell M. The expanding clinical use of C-peptide radioimmunoassay. Acta Diabetol 1983;20:105–13.

53. Bonser AM, Garcia-Webb P. C-peptide measurement and its clinical usefulness: a review. Ann Clin Biochem 1981;18:Pt 4:200–6.

54. Grant CS. Gastrointestinal endocrine tumours: insulinoma. Baillieres Clin Gastroenterol 1996;10:645–71.

55. Gray RK, Rösch J, Grollman JH Jr. Arteriography in the diagnosis of islet-cell tumors. Radiology 1970;97:39–44.

56. Stark DD, Moss AA, Goldberg HI, Deveney CW. CT of pancreatic islet cell tumors. Radiology 1984;150:491–4.

57. Rossi P, Baert A, Passariello R, et al. CT functioning tumors of the pancreas. AJR Am J Roentgenol 1985;144:57–60.

58. Vinayek R, Frucht H, Chiang HC, et al. Zollinger-Ellison syndrome: recent advances in the management of the gastrinoma. Gastroenterol Clin North Am 1990;19:197–217.

59. Berg CL, Wolfe MM. Zollinger-Ellison syndrome. Med Clin North Am 1991;75:903–21.

60. Day JP, Richter JE. Medical and surgical conditions predisposing to gastroesophageal reflux disease. Gastroenterol Clin North Am 1990;19:587–607.

61. Hirschowitz BI. Zollinger-Ellison syndrome: pathogenesis, diagnosis, and management. Am J Gastroenterol 1997;92:4 Suppl:44S–8S.

62. Sugg SL, Norton JA, Fraker DL, et al. A prospective study of intraoperative methods to diagnose and resect duodenal gastrinomas. Ann Surg 1993;218:138–44.

63. van Heerden JA, Smith SL, Miller LJ. Management of the Zollinger-Ellison syndrome in patients with multiple endocrine neoplasia type I. Surgery 1986;100:971–7.

64. Fishbeyn VA, Norton JA, Benya RV, et al. Assessment and prediction of long-term cure in patients with the Zollinger-Ellison syndrome: the best approach. Ann Intern Med 1993;119:199–206.

65. Thompson JC, Lewis BG, Wiener I, Townsend CM Jr. The role of surgery in the Zollinger-Ellison syndrome. Ann Surg 1983;197:594–607.

66. Vinik AI, Thompson N. Controversies in the management of Zollinger-Ellison syndrome. Ann Intern Med 1986;105:956–9.

67. Frucht H, Norton JA, London JF, et al. Detection of duodenal gastrinomas by operative endoscopic transillumination: a prospective study. Gastroenterology 1990;99:1622–7.

68. Romeo DP, Weesner RE, Giannella RA. Misdiagnosis of the Zollinger-Ellison syndrome due to hyperlipidemia. Gastroenterology 1990;99:1511–3.

69. Schjönsby H, Willassen Y. Renal extraction of endogenous gastrin in patients with normal renal function. Scand J Gastroenterol 1977;12:205–7.

70. Pisegna JR, Lew E, Tarasova N, et al. The cholecystokinin type B receptor (CCKBR) in the human kidney mediates gastrin-stimulated urinary sodium excretion. Gastroenterology 1998;114:G4797.

71. Pisegna JR, Tarasova NI, Kopp JA, et al. Meal-stimulated gastrointestinal hormonal control of renal function. Unpublished data, 1999.

72. Pisegna JR, de Weerth A, Huppi K, Wank SA. Molecular cloning of the human brain and gastric cholecystokinin receptor: structure, functional expression and chromosomal localization. Biochem Biophys Res Commun 1992;189:296–303.

73. Wank SA, Pisegna JR, de Weerth A. Brain and gastrointestinal cholecystokinin receptor family: structure and functional expression. Proc Natl Acad Sci U S A 1992;89:8691–5.

74. Wolfe MM, Jensen RT. Zollinger-Ellison syndrome: current concepts in diagnosis and management. N Engl J Med 1987;317:1200–9.

75. Bloom SR, Long RG, Bryant MG, et al. Clinical, biochemical and pathological studies on 62 VIPomas. Gastroenterology 1980;78:5 Pt 2:1143.

76. Vezzadini C, Poggioli R, Casoni I, Vezzadini P. Use of calcium

77. Sonnenberg A, Townsend WF. Testing for *Helicobacter pylori* in the diagnosis of Zollinger-Ellison syndrome. Am J Gastroenterol 1991;86:606–8.

78. Weber HC, Venzon DJ, Jensen RT, Metz DC. Studies on the interrelation between Zollinger-Ellison syndrome, *Helicobacter pylori,* and proton pump inhibitor therapy. Gastroenterology 1997;112:84–91.

79. Lyons DF, Eisen BR, Clark MR, et al. Concurrent Cushing's and Zollinger-Ellison syndromes in a patient with islet cell carcinoma: case report and review of the literature. Am J Med 1984;76:729–33.

80. Maton PN, Gardner JD, Jensen RT. Cushing's syndrome in patients with the Zollinger-Ellison syndrome. N Engl J Med 1986;315:1–5.

81. Fass R, Rosen HR, Walsh JH. Zollinger-Ellison syndrome: diagnosis and management. Hosp Pract 1995;30:73–6.

82. Arps H, Dietel M, Schulz A, et al. Pancreatic endocrine carcinoma with ectopic PTH-production and paraneoplastic hypercalcaemia. Virchows Arch A Pathol Anat Histopathol 1986;408:497–503.

83. Fajans SS, Floyd JC Jr. Fasting hypoglycemia in adults. N Engl J Med 1976;294:766–72.

84. Domschke S, Domschke W, Bloom SR, et al. Vasoactive intestinal peptide in man: pharmacokinetics, metabolic and circulatory effects. Gut 1978;19:1049–53.

85. Pisegna JR, Norton JA, Slimak GG, et al. Effects of curative gastrinoma resection on gastric secretory function and antisecretory drug requirement in the Zollinger-Ellison syndrome. Gastroenterology 1992;102:767–78.

86. Hirschowitz BI. Zollinger-Ellison syndrome: pathogenesis, diagnosis, and management. Am J Gastroenterol 1997;92:Suppl:44S–8S.

87. Richardson CT, Peters MN, Feldman M, et al. Treatment of Zollinger-Ellison syndrome with exploratory laparotomy, proximal gastric vagotomy, and H2-receptor antagonists: a prospective study. Gastroenterology 1985;89:357–67.

88. McArthur KE, Collen MJ, Maton PN. Omeprazole: effective, convenient therapy for Zollinger-Ellison syndrome. Gastroenterology 1985;88:939–44.

89. Stewart CA, Termanini B, Sutliff VE, et al. Management of the Zollinger-Ellison syndrome in pregnancy. Am J Obstet Gynecol 1997;176:Pt I:224–33.

90. Maton PN. Zollinger-Ellison syndrome: recognition and management of acid hypersecretion. Drugs 1996;52:33–44.

91. Frucht H, Maton PN, Jensen RT. Use of omeprazole in patients with Zollinger-Ellison syndrome. Dig Dis Sci 1991;36:394–404.

92. Metz DC, Pisegna JR, Fishbeyn VA, et al. Currently used doses of omeprazole in Zollinger-Ellison syndrome are too high. Gastroenterology 1992;103:1498–508.

93. Maton PN. Role of acid suppressants in patients with Zollinger-Ellison syndrome. Aliment Pharmacol Ther 1991;5:Suppl 1:25–35.

94. Garnett WR. Lansoprazole: a proton pump inhibitor. Ann Pharmacother 1996;30:1425–36.

95. Metz DC, Pisegna JR, Ringham GL, et al. Prospective study of efficacy and safety of lansoprazole in Zollinger-Ellison syndrome. Dig Dis Sci 1993;38:245–56.

96. Metz DC, Lew E, Forsmark CE, et al. Intravenous (IV) pantoprazole (PANTO) rapidly and effectively controls acid output (AO) in patients with Zollinger-Ellison syndrome (ZES). Gastroenterology 1998;114:G0926.

97. Waldum HL, Brenna E, Kleveland PM, Mignon, M. Gastrin—physiological and pathophysiological role: clinical consequences. Dig Dis 1995;13:25–38.

98. Cadiot G, Vissuzaine C, Potet F, et al. Fundic argyrophil carcinoid tumor in a patient with sporadic-type Zollinger-Ellison syndrome. Dig Dis Sci 1995;40:1275–8.

99. Helander HF, Rutgersson K, Helander KG, et al. Stereologic investigations of human gastric mucosa: II. oxyntic mucosa from patients with Zollinger-Ellison syndrome. Scand J Gastroenterol 1992;27:875–83.

100. Sölvell L. The clinical safety of omeprazole. Digestion 1990;47:Suppl 1:59–63.

101. Solcia E, Capella C, Fiocca R, et al. Gastric argyrophil carcinoidosis in patients with Zollinger-Ellison syndrome due to type 1 multiple endocrine neoplasia: a newly recognized association. Am J Surg Pathol 1990;14:503–13.

102. Bordi C, D'Adda T, Azzoni C, et al. Hypergastrinemia and gastric enterochromaffin-like cells. Am J Surg Pathol 1995;19:Suppl 1:S8–19.

103. Gilligan CJ, Lawton GP, Tang LH, et al. Gastric carcinoid tumors: the

biology and therapy of an enigmatic and controversial lesion. Am J Gastroenterol 1995;90:338–52.

104. Joshi SN, Gardner JD. Gastrin and colon cancer: a unifying hypothesis. Dig Dis 1996;14:334–44.

105. Delcore R, Friesen SR. Role of pancreatoduodenectomy in the management of primary duodenal wall gastrinomas in patients with Zollinger-Ellison syndrome. Surgery 1992;112:1016–22.

106. Straus E, Raufman JP, Samuel S, et al. Endoscopic cure of the Zollinger-Ellison syndrome. Gastrointest Endosc 1992;38:709–11.

107. Delcore R, Friesen SR. Zollinger-Ellison syndrome: a new look at regression of gastrinomas. Arch Surg 1991;126:556–8.

108. Jensen RT. Should the 1996 citation for Zollinger-Ellison syndrome read: "Acid-reducing surgery in, aggressive resection out"? Am J Gastroenterol 1996;91:1067–70.

109. Heller SJ, Ferrari AP, Carr-Locke DL, et al. Pancreatic duct stricture caused by islet cell tumors. Am J Gastroenterol 1996;91:147–9.

110. Rothmund M, Stinner B, Arnold R. Endocrine pancreatic carcinoma. Eur J Surg Oncol 1991;17:191–9.

111. Mignon M, Cadiot G, Marmuse JP, Lewin MJ. Is gastrinoma a medical disease? Yale J Biol Med 1996;69:289–300.

112. O'Dorisio TM, Mekhjian HS, Gaginella TS. Medical therapy of VIPomas. Endocrinol Metab Clin North Am 1989;18:545–56.

113. Alberti KG, Oxbury JM, Higgins G. Factitious hypoglycaemia: chlorpropamide self-administration by a non-diabetic. Br Med J 1972;1:87–8.

114. O'Dorisio TM, Mekhjian HS. VIPoma syndrome. In: Cohen S, Soloway RD, eds. Hormone producing tumors of the pancreas. New York: Churchill Livingstone, 1985:101.

115. Rønnov-Jensen D, Gether U, Fahrenkrug J. PreproVIP-derived peptides in tissue and plasma from patients with VIP-producing tumours. Eur J Clin Invest 1991;21:154–60.

116. Smale BF. Surgical disease of the pancreas. In: Howard JM, ed. Surgical disease of the pancreas. Philadelphia: Lea & Febiger, 1987:860.

117. Boden G, Shimoyama R. Somatostatinoma. In: Cohen S, Soloway RD, eds. Hormone-producing tumors of the gastrointestinal tract. New York: Churchill Livingstone, 1985:85.

118. Reber HA. In: Howard JM, ed. Surgical disease of the pancreas. Philadelphia: Lea & Febiger, 1987:865.

119. Krejs GJ, Orci L, Conlon JM, et al. Somatostatinoma syndrome: biochemical, morphologic and clinical features. N Engl J Med 1979;301:285–92.

120. Lowry SF, Burt ME, Brennan MF. Glucose turnover and gluconeogenesis in a patient with somatostatinoma. Surgery 1981;89:309–13.

121. Konomi K, Chijiiwa K, Katsuta T, Yamaguchi K. Pancreatic somatostatinoma: a case report and review of the literature. J Surg Oncol 1990;43:259–65.

122. Vinik AI, Moattari AR. Treatment of endocrine tumors of the pancreas. Endocrinol Metab Clin North Am 1989;18:483–518.

123. Vinik AI, Strodel WE, Eckhauser FE, et al. Somatostatinomas, PPomas, neurotensinomas. Semin Oncol 1987;14:263–81.

124. Galmiche JP, Chayvialle JA, Dubois PM, et al. Calcitonin-producing pancreatic somatostatinoma. Gastroenterology 1980;78:1577–83.

125. Walsh JH. Gastrointestinal hormones. In: Johnson LR, ed. Physiology of the gastrointestinal tract. New York: Raven Press, 1987:1981.

126. Boden G, Sivitz MC, Owen OE, et al. Somatostatin suppresses secretin and pancreatic exocrine secretion. Science 1975;190:163–5.

127. Koerker DJ, Ruch W, Chideckel E, et al. Somatostatin: hypothalamic inhibitor of the endocrine pancreas. Science 1974;184:482–4.

128. Bloom SR, Mortimer CH, Thorner MO, et al. Inhibition of gastrin and gastric-acid secretion by growth-hormone release-inhibiting hormone. Lancet 1974;2:1106–9.

129. Schlegel W, Raptis S, Harvey RF, et al. Inhibition of cholecystokinin-pancreozymin release by somatostatin. Lancet 1977;2:166–8.

130. Ormsbee HS 3rd, Koehler SL, Telford GL. Somatostatin inhibits motilin-induced interdigestive contractile activity in the dog. Am J Dig Dis 1978;23:781–8.

131. Reichlin S. Somatostatin. N Engl J Med 1983;309:1495–501.

132. Samols E, Weir GC, Ramseur R, et al. Modulation of pancreatic somatostatin by adrenergic and cholinergic agonism and by hyper- and hypoglycemic sulfonamides. Metabolism 1978;27:1219–21.

133. Boden G, Baile CA, McLauglin CL, Matschinsky FM. Effects of starvation and obesity on somatostatin, insulin, and glucagon release from an isolated perfused organ system. Am J Physiol 1981;241:E215–20.

134. Schusdziarra V, Grube D, Seifert H, et al. Somatostatinoma syndrome: clinical, morphological and metabolic features and therapeutic aspects. Klin Wochenshr 1983;61:681–9.

135. Pipeleers D, Somers G, Gepts W, et al. Plasma pancreatic hormone levels in a case of somatostatinoma: diagnostic and therapeutic implications. J Clin Endocrinol Metab 1979;49:572–9.

136. Axelrod L, Bush MA, Hirsch HJ, Loo SW. Malignant somatostatinoma: clinical features and metabolic studies. J Clin Endocrinol Metab 1981;52:886–96.

137. Wright J, Abolfathi A, Penman E, Marks V. Pancreatic somatostatinoma presenting with hypoglycaemia. Clin Endocrinol 1980; 12:603–8.

138. Swinburn BA, Yeong ML, Lane MR, et al. Neurofibromatosis associated with somatostatinoma: a report of two patients. Clin Endocrinol 1988;28:353–9.

139. Ohtsuki Y, Sonobe H, Mizobuchi T, et al. Duodenal carcinoid (somatostatinoma) combined with von Recklinghausen's disease: a case report and review of the literature. Acta Pathol Jpn 1989;39:141–6.

140. Soga J, Suzuki T, Yoshikawa K, et al. Carcinoid somatostatinoma of the duodenum. Eur J Cancer 1990;26:1107–8.

141. Hagen EC, Houben GM, Nikkels RE, et al. Exocrine pancreatic insufficiency and pancreatic fibrosis due to duodenal somatostatinoma in a patient with neurofibromatosis. Pancreas 1992;7:98–104.

142. Maki M, Kaneko Y, Ohta Y, et al. Somatostatinoma of the pancreas associated with von Hippel-Lindau disease. Intern Med 1995;34:661–5.

143. Kent RB, van Heerden JA, Weiland LH. Nonfunctioning islet cell tumors. Ann Surg 1981;193:185–90.

144. Eckhauser FE, Cheung PS, Vinik A, et al. Nonfunctioning malignant neuroendocrine tumors of the pancreas. Surgery 1986;100:978–88.

145. Eriksson B, Oberg K, Skogseid B. Neuroendocrine pancreatic tumors: clinical findings in a prospective study of 84 patients. Acta Oncol 1989;28:373–7.

146. Grama D, Eriksson B, Mårtensson H, et al. Clinical characteristics, treatment and survival in patients with pancreatic tumors causing hormonal syndromes. World J Surg 1992;16:632–9.

147. Rivier J, Spress J, Thorner M, Vale W. Characterization of a growth hormone-releasing factor from a human pancreatic islet tumour. Nature 1982;300:276–8.

148. Thorner MO, Perryman RL, Cronin MJ, et al. Somatotroph hyperplasia: successful treatment of acromegaly by removal of a pancreatic islet tumor secreting a growth hormone-releasing factor. J Clin Invest 1982;70:965–77.

149. Keogan MT, Baker ME. Computed tomography and magnetic resonance imaging in the assessment of pancreatic disease. Gastrointest Endosc Clin N Am 1995;5:31–59.

150. Pisegna JR, Doppman JL, Norton JA, et al. Prospective comparative study of ability of MR imaging and other imaging modalities to localize tumors in patients with Zollinger-Ellison syndrome. Dig Dis Sci 1993;38:1318–28.

151. Benya RV, Metz DA, Hijazi YM, et al. Fine needle aspiration cytology of submucosal nodules in patients with Zollinger-Ellison syndrome. Am J Gastroenterol 1993;88:258–65.

152. Termanini B, Gibril F, Doppman JL, et al. Distinguishing small hepatic hemangiomas from vascular liver metastases in gastrinoma: use of a somatostatin-receptor scintigraphic agent. Radiology 1997;202:151–8.

153. Günther RW, Klose KJ, Rückert K, et al. Islet-cell tumors: detection of small lesions with computed tomography and ultrasound. Radiology 1983;148:485–8.

154. Pedrazzoli S, Feltrin G, Dodi G, et al. Usefulness of transhepatic portal catheterization in the treatment of insulinomas. Br J Surg 1980;67:557–61.

155. Rayfield EJ, Goldberg IJ, Giegerich EW, et al. Transportal blood sampling for preoperative localization of insulinomas. Mt Sinai J Med 1983;50:258–62.

156. Kinoshita Y, Nonaka H, Suzuki S, et al. Accurate localization of insulinoma using percutaneous transhepatic portal venous sampling—usefulness of simultaneous measurement of plasma insulin and glucagon levels. Clin Endocrinol 1985;23:587–93.

157. Doherty GM, Doppman JL, Shawker TH, et al. Results of a prospective strategy to diagnose, localize, and resect insulinomas. Surgery 1991;110:989–96.

158. Vinik AI, Delbridge L, Moattari R, et al. Transhepatic portal vein catheterization for localization of insulinomas: a ten-year experience. Surgery 1991;109:1–11.

159. Pereiras R Jr. Percutaneous transhepatic portography. J Lab Res Methods Biol Med 1983;7:391–403.
160. Doppman JL, Miller DL, Chang R, et al. Insulinomas: localization with selective intra-arterial injection of calcium. Radiology 1991;178:237–41.
161. Brightbill TC, Templeton EO, Sperling D, Mooney LP. Insulinoma: detection by intraoperative ultrasonography. J Clin Ultrasound 1992;20:615-7.
162. Kung AW, Chan FL, Tam SC, Lam KS. Case report: localization of occult insulinoma by intra-arterial stimulation with calcium and venous sampling technique. Clin Radiol 1992;46:55–6.
163. Sussman LA, Christie R, Whittle DE. Laparoscopic excision of distal pancreas including insulinoma. Aust N Z J Surg 1996;66:414–6.
164. Modlin IM, Cornelius E, Lawton GP. Use of an isotopic somatostatin receptor probe to image gut endocrine tumors. Arch Surg 1995;130:367–73.
165. Owens LV, Huth JF, Cance WG. Insulinoma: pitfalls in preoperative localization. Eur J Surg Oncol 1995;21:326–8.
166. van Heerden JA, Grant CS, Czako PF, et al. Occult functioning insulinomas: which localizing studies are indicated? Surgery 1992;112:1010–4.
167. Palazzo L, Roseau G, Salmeron M. Endoscopic ultrasonography in the preoperative localization of pancreatic endocrine tumors. Endoscopy 1992;24:Suppl 1:350–3.
168. Scott BA, Gatenby RA. Imaging advances in the diagnosis of endocrine neoplasia. Curr Opin Oncol 1998;10:37–42.
169. Knobel B, Rosman P, Czerniak A. Endoscopic ultrasonography for the preoperative localization of insulinoma—a new, useful modality: case report and review of the literature. Isr J Med Sci 1995;31:365–7.
170. Perry RR, Vinik AI. Endocrine tumors of the gastrointestinal tract. Annu Rev Med 1996;47:57–68.
171. Gorman B, Reading CC. Imaging of gastrointestinal neuroendocrine tumors. Semin Ultrasound CT MR 1995;16:331-41.
172. Meko JB, Norton JA. Management of patients with Zollinger-Ellison syndrome. Annu Rev Med 1995;46:395–411.
173. Cherner JA, Doppman JL, Norton JA, et al. Selective venous sampling for gastrin to localize gastrinomas: a prospective assessment. Ann Intern Med 1986;105:841–7.
174. Maton PN, Miller DL, Doppman JL, et al. Role of selective angiography in the management of patients with Zollinger-Ellison syndrome. Gastroenterology 1987;92:913–8.
175. Roche A, Raisonnier A, Gillon-Asavouret MC. Pancreatic venous sampling and arteriography in localizing insulinomas and gastrinomas: procedure and results in 55 cases. Radiology 1982;145:621–7.
176. Grant CS. Surgical aspects of hyperinsulinemic hypoglycemia. Endocrinol Metab Clin North Am 1999;28:533–54.
177. Norton JA. Intraoperative methods to stage and localize pancreatic and duodenal tumors. Ann Oncol 1999;10:Suppl 4:182–4.
178. Huai JC, Zhang W, Niu HO, et al. Localization and surgical treatment of pancreatic insulinomas guided by intraoperative ultrasound. Am J Surg 1998;175:18–21.
179. Correnti S, Liverani A, Antonini G, et al. Intraoperative ultrasonography for pancreatic insulinomas. Hepatogastroenterology 1996;43:207–11.
180. King CM, Reznek RH, Dacie JE, Wass JA. Imaging islet cell tumours. Clin Radiol 1994;49:295–303.
181. Rösch T, Lightdale CJ, Botet JF, et al. Localization of pancreatic endocrine tumors by endoscopic ultrasonography. N Engl J Med 1992;326:1721–6.
182. Schumacher B, Lubke HJ, Frieling T, et al. Prospective study on the detection of insulinomas by endoscopic ultrasonography. Endoscopy 1996;28:273–6.
183. Boukhman MP, Karam JM, Shaver J, et al. Localization of insulinomas. Arch Surg 1999;134:818–22.
184. Vinik AI, Delbridge L, Moattari R, et al. Transhepatic portal vein catheterization for localization of insulinomas: a ten-year experience. Surgery 1991;109:1–11.
185. Pasieka JL, McLeod MK, Thompson NW, Burney RE. Surgical approach to insulinomas: assessing the need for preoperative localization. Arch Surg 1992;127:442–7.
186. Doherty GM, Doppman JL, Shawker TH, et al. Results of a prospective strategy to diagnose, localize, and resect insulinomas. Surgery 1991;110:989–96.
187. Doppman JL, Miller DL, Chang R, et al. Intraarterial calcium stimulation test for detection of insulinomas. World J Surg 1993;17:439–43.
188. Pereira PL, Roche AJ, Maier GW, et al. Insulinoma and islet cell hyperplasia: value of the calcium intraarterial stimulation test when findings of other preoperative studies are negative. Radiology 1998;206:703–9.
189. Doppman JL, Chang R, Fraker DL, et al. Localization of insulinomas to regions of the pancreas by intra-arterial stimulation with calcium. Ann Intern Med 1995;123:269–73.
190. Zeiger MA, Shawker TH, Norton JA. Use of intraoperative ultrasonography to localize islet cell tumors. World J Surg 1993;17:448–54.
191. Phan GQ, Yeo CJ, Cameron JL, et al. Pancreaticoduodenectomy for selected periampullary neuroendocrine tumors: fifty patients. Surgery 1997;122:989–96.
192. Norton JA. Intra-operative procedures to localize endocrine tumors of the pancreas and duodenum. Ital J Gastroenterol Hepatol 1999;31:Suppl 2:S195–7.
193. Rothmund M, Angelini L, Brunt LM, et al. Surgery for benign insulinoma: an international review. World J Surg 1990;14:393–8.
194. Norton JA, Fraker DL, Alexander HR, et al. Surgery to cure the Zollinger-Ellison syndrome. N Engl J Med 1999;341:635–44.
195. Norton JA, Doppman JL, Jensen RT. Curative resection in Zollinger-Ellison syndrome: results of a 10-year prospective study. Ann Surg 1992;215:8–18.
196. Howard TJ, Zinner MJ, Stabile BE, Passaro E Jr. Gastrinoma excision for cure: a prospective analysis. Ann Surg 1990;211:9–14.
197. Townsend CM Jr, Thompson JC. Surgical management of tumors that produce gastrointestinal hormones. Annu Rev Med 1985;36:111–24.
198. Stabile BE, Passaro E Jr. Benign and malignant gastrinoma. Am J Surg 1985;149:144–50.
199. Sheppard BC, Norton JA, Doppman JL, et al. Management of islet cell tumors in patients with multiple endocrine neoplasia: a prospective study. Surgery 1989;106:1108–17.
200. Thompson NW. Surgical treatment of the endocrine pancreas and Zollinger-Ellison syndrome in the MEN 1 syndrome. Henry Ford Hosp Med J 1992;40:195–8.
201. Alexander HR, Fraker DL, Norton JA, et al. Prospective study of somatostatin receptor scintigraphy and its effect on operative outcome in patients with Zollinger-Ellison syndrome. Ann Surg 1998;228:228–38.
202. Gibril F, Curtis LT, Termanini B, et al. Primary cardiac gastrinoma causing Zollinger-Ellison syndrome. Gastroenterology 1997;112:567–74.
203. Corleto VD, Scopinaro F, Angeletti S, et al. Somatostatin receptor localization of pancreatic endocrine tumors. World J Surg 1996;20:241–4.
204. Semelka RC, Cumming MJ, Shoenut JP, et al. Islet cell tumors: comparison of dynamic contrast-enhanced CT and MR imaging with dynamic gadolinium enhancement and fat suppression. Radiology 1993;186:799–802.
205. Thom AK, Norton JA, Doppman JL, et al. Prospective study of the use of intraarterial secretin injection and portal venous sampling to localize duodenal gastrinomas. Surgery 1992;112:1002–8.
206. Imamura M, Takahashi K. Use of selective arterial secretin injection test to guide surgery in patients with Zollinger-Ellison syndrome. World J Surg 1993;17:433–8.
207. Stabile BE, Morrow DJ, Passaro E Jr. The gastrinoma triangle: operative implications. Am J Surg 1984;147:25–31.
208. Howard TJ, Sawicki MP, Stabile BE, et al. Biologic behavior of sporadic gastrinoma located to the right and left of the superior mesenteric artery. Am J Surg 1993;165:101–5.
209. Howard TJ, Stabile BE, Zinner MJ, et al. Anatomic distribution of pancreatic endocrine tumors. Am J Surg 1990;159:258–64.
210. Sawicki MP, Howard TJ, Dalton M, et al. The dichotomous distribution of gastrinomas. Arch Surg 1990;125:1584–7.
211. Bhagavan BS, Slavin RE, Goldberg J, Rao RN. Ectopic gastrinoma and Zollinger-Ellison syndrome. Hum Pathol 1986;17:584–92.
212. Sugg SL, Norton JA, Fraker DL, et al. A prospective study of intraoperative methods to diagnose and resect duodenal gastrinomas. Ann Surg 1993;218:138–44.
213. Thompson NW, Pasieka J, Fukuuchi A. Duodenal gastrinomas, duodenotomy, and duodenal exploration in the surgical management of Zollinger-Ellison syndrome. World J Surg 1993;17:455–62.
214. Norton JA, Doppman JL, Jensen RT. Curative resection in Zollinger-Ellison syndrome: results of a 10-year prospective study. Ann Surg 1992;215:8–18.
215. Weber HC, Venzon DJ, Lin JT, et al. Determinants of metastatic rate

and survival in patients with Zollinger-Ellison syndrome: a prospective long-term study. Gastroenterology 1995;108:1637–49.

216. Arnold WS, Fraker DL, Alexander HR, et al. Apparent lymph node primary gastrinoma. Surgery 1994;116:1123–9.

217. Delcore R Jr, Cheung LY, Friesen SR. Outcome of lymph node involvement in patients with the Zollinger-Ellison syndrome. Ann Surg 1988;208:291–8.

218. Kitagawa M, Hayakawa T, Kondo T, et al. Gastrinoma in a mesenteric lymph node. Am J Gastroenterol 1989;84:660–2.

219. MacGillivray DC, Rushin JM, Zeiger MA, Shakir KM. The significance of gastrinomas found in peripancreatic lymph nodes. Surgery 1991;109:558–62.

220. Perrier ND, Batts KP, Thompson GB, et al. An immunohistochemical survey for neuroendocrine cells in regional pancreatic lymph nodes: a plausible explanation for primary nodal gastrinomas? Mayo Clinic Pancreatic Surgery Group. Surgery 1995;118:957–65.

221. Norton JA, Doherty GM, Fraker DL, et al. Surgical treatment of localized gastrinoma within the liver: a prospective study. Surgery 1998;124:1145–52.

222. Tennvall J, Ljungberg O, Ahrén B, et al. Radiotherapy for unresectable endocrine pancreatic carcinomas. Eur J Surg Oncol 1992;18:73–6.

223. Tennvall J, Ljungberg O, Ahrén B, et al. Radiotherapy for unresectable endocrine pancreatic carcinomas. Eur J Surg Oncol 1992;18:73–6.

224. Kessinger A, Lemon HM, Foley JF. The glucagonoma syndrome and its management. J Surg Oncol 1977;9:419–24.

225. Marynick SP, Fagadau WR, Duncan LA. Malignant glucagonoma syndrome: response to chemotherapy. Ann Intern Med 1980;93:453–4.

226. Awrich AE, Peetz M, Fletcher WS. Dimethyltriazenoimidazole carboxamide therapy of islet cell carcinoma of the pancreas. J Surg Oncol 1981;17:321–6.

227. Strauss GM, Weitzman SA, Aoki TT. Dimethyltriazenoimidazole carboxamide therapy of malignant glucagonoma. Ann Intern Med 1979;90:57–8.

228. Duncan LA, Marynick SP. Glucagonoma and dacarbazine. Ann Intern Med 1982;97:930.

229. Altimari AF, Badrinath K, Reisel HJ, Prinz RA. DTIC therapy in patients with malignant intra-abdominal neuroendocrine tumors. Surgery 1987;102:1009–17.

230. Moertel CG, Hanley JA, Johnson LA. Streptozocin alone compared with streptozocin plus fluorouracil in the treatment of advanced islet-cell carcinoma. N Engl J Med 1980;303:1189–94.

231. Khandekar JD, Sriratana P. Response of glucagonoma syndrome to lomustine. Cancer Treat Rep 1986;70:433–4.

232. Kvols LK, Buck M, Moertel CG, et al. Treatment of metastatic islet cell carcinoma with a somatostatin analogue (SMS 201–995). Ann Intern Med 1987;107:162–8.

233. Wood SM, Kraenzlin ME, Adrian TE, Bloom SR. Treatment of patients with pancreatic endocrine tumours using a new long-acting somatostatin analogue symptomatic and peptide responses. Gut 1985;26:438–44.

234. Loubatières A, Mariani MM, Alric R. The action of diazoxide on insulin secretion, medullo-adrenal secretion, and the liberation of catecholamines. Ann N Y Acad Sci 1968;150:226–41.

235. Porte D Jr, Graber AL, Kuzuya T, Williams RH. The effect of epinephrine on immunoreactive insulin levels in man. J Clin Invest 1966;45:228–36.

236. Daniel WF, Arthur HR. Hypoglycemia, insulinoma, and other hormone-secreting tumors of the pancreas. In: Braunwald E, ed. Harrison's principles of internal medicine. New York: McGraw-Hill, 1987:1804.

237. Abramson EA, Arky RA. Role of beta-adrenergic receptors in counter-regulation to insulin-induced hypoglycemia. Diabetes 1968;17:141–6.

238. Altszuler N, Moraru E, Hampshire J. On the mechanism of diazoxide-induced hyperglycemia. Diabetes 1977;26:931–5.

239. Stefanini P, Carboni M, Patrassi N. Problems of the management of insulinomas: review of 132 cases treated with medical measures. Acta Diabetol 1974;11:71–7.

240. Knopp RH, Scheinin JC, Freinkel N. Diphenylhydantoin and an insulin-secreting islet adenoma. Arch Intern Med 1972;130:904-8.

241. Brodows RG, Campbell RG. Control of refractory fasting hypoglycemia in a patient with suspected insulinoma with diphenylhydantoin. J Clin Endocrinol Metab 1974;38:159–62.

242. Hofeldt FD, Dippe SE, Levin SR, et al. Effects of diphenylhydantoin upon glucose-induced insulin secretion in three patients with insulinoma. Diabetes 1974;23:192–8.

243. Federspil G, Casara D, Stauffacher W. Chlorpromazine in the treatment of endogenous organic hyperinsulinism. Diabetologia 1974;10:189–91.

244. Ulbrecht JS, Schmeltz R, Aarons JH, Greene DA. Insulinoma in a 94-year-old woman: long-term therapy with verapamil. Diabetes Care 1986;9:186–8.

245. Osei K, O'Dorisio TM. Malignant insulinoma: effects of a somatostatin analog (compound 201–995) on serum glucose, growth, and gastro-entero-pancreatic hormones. Ann Intern Med 1985;103:223–5.

246. Broder LE, Carter SK. Pancreatic islet cell carcinoma: II. results of therapy with streptozotocin in 52 patients. Ann Intern Med 1973;79:108–18.

247. Sadoff L. Control of hypoglycemia with L-asparaginase in a patient with islet cell cancer. J Clin Endocrinol Metab 1973;36:334–7.

248. Eastman RC, Come SE, Strewler GJ, et al. Adriamycin therapy for advanced insulinoma. J Clin Endocrinol Metab 1977;44:142–8.

249. Moertel CG, Lavin PT, Hahn RG. Phase II trial of doxorubicin therapy for advanced islet cell carcinoma. Cancer Treat Rep 1982;66:1567–9.

250. Moertel CG, Lefkopoulo M, Lipsitz S, et al. Streptozocin-doxorubicin, streptozocin-fluorouracil or chlorozotocin in the treatment of advanced islet-cell carcinoma. N Engl J Med 1992;326:519–23.

251. Moertel CG, Johnson CM, McKusick MA, et al. The management of patients with advanced carcinoid tumors and islet cell carcinomas. Ann Intern Med 1994;120:302–9.

252. Thompson NW, Eckhauser FE. Malignant islet-cell tumors of the pancreas. World J Surg 1984;8:940–51.

253. Geelhoed GW, Bass BL, Mertz SL, Becker KL. Somatostatin analog: effects on hypergastrinemia and hypercalcitoninemia. Surgery 1986;100:962–70.

254. Mignon M, Ruszniewski P, Haffar S, et al. Current approach to the management of tumoral process in patients with gastrinoma. World J Surg 1986;10:703–10.

255. Howard JM, Ghent CN, Carey LS, et al. Diagnostic efficacy of hepatic computed tomography in the detection of body iron overload. Gastroenterology 1983;84:209–15.

256. Pisegna JR, Slimak GG, Doppman JL, et al. An evaluation of human recombinant alpha interferon in patients with metastatic gastrinoma. Gastroenterology 1993;105:1179–83.

257. von Schrenck T, Howard JM, Doppman JL. Prospective study of chemotherapy in patients with metastatic gastrinoma. Gastroenterology 1988;94:1326–34.

# CHAPTER 70

# ADRENAL GLAND

• CHARLES M. HASKELL • MARK P. SAWICKI

Benign nodules of the adrenal gland are extremely common, with a prevalence of 3% in autopsy studies of individuals who died after age 50.[1] However, malignant tumors of the adrenal gland are rare lesions that afflict about two persons per million.[2, 3] Thus, most of what is known about malignant tumors of the adrenal gland comes from small series and case reports. This section draws especially from the published experience of the Mayo Clinic,[4] Memorial Sloan-Kettering Cancer Center,[5, 6] the M.D. Anderson Hospital,[7] and the Cleveland Clinic.[8] The two major malignant neoplasms of this organ are adrenocortical carcinomas and pheochromocytomas. Each will be discussed separately.

## Adrenocortical Carcinoma

### NATURAL HISTORY, DIAGNOSIS, AND STAGING

#### Epidemiology and Etiology

The cause of sporadic cases of adrenocortical carcinoma is unknown, but numerous observations support a multistep process of carcinogenesis similar to that reported for tumors arising in other sites. Genes (and chromosomes) implicated in carcinogenesis in the adrenal cortex in one review include *IGF-II* on chromosome 11p15.5, *p57* (*KIP2*) on chromosome 11p15, *p53* on chromosome 17p13, and an unidentified gene on chromosome 9q34.[1] Changes in the expression of certain transcription factors (GATA-4 and GATA-6) have been reported,[9] as has inactivation of the p16 tumor-suppressor gene on chromosome 9p21.[10] The importance of these various abnormalities and the most frequent sequence of events have yet to be defined. It is likely that the sequence of events may differ between children and adults. Specifically, one study suggests that the pattern of molecular changes in childhood adrenocortical tumors is most consistent with an embryonal origin for children but not for adults.[11]

Adrenal cortical neoplasms may arise as part of several familial cancer syndromes. One is the Beckwith-Wiedemann syndrome in children, which is a growth disorder characterized by macroglossia, gigantism, and omphalocele.[12, 13] Another is Li-Fraumeni syndrome, which includes familial susceptibility to several tumors, including sarcomas, breast cancer, lung cancer, and adrenocortical carcinoma.[14, 15] Other examples include multiple endocrine neoplasia, type 1; familial congenital adrenal hyperplasia; the Carnery complex; and the McCune-Albright syndrome.[1] These associations all fit the models of carcinogenesis discussed in Chapter 2.

#### Pathology

Adrenocortical carcinomas can be large when discovered. In one series, the average tumor weighed 736 g, and the largest weighed 1 kg.[16] The large size of these lesions underlines the insidious nature of their growth and development. They are frequently encapsulated, lobulated, soft, or cystic masses that are friable. The cut surface of the tumor usually shows extensive areas of necrosis and hemorrhage.[7]

The histology of these neoplasms varies considerably, but certain neuroendocrine markers can be useful in diagnosis. Immunohistochemistry can identify intermediate filament proteins, and vimentin is present in all patients with adequate handling of tissue.[17] Indeed, the absence of vimentin in an adrenal tumor suggests that the tumor is not an adrenocortical carcinoma provided that the tissue has been appropriately processed for immunohistochemistry. In some tumors, polygonal cells resembling normal cells of the adrenal cortex are found, whereas in others the cells are extremely anaplastic and show marked nuclear and cellular pleomorphism. The number of mitotic figures per high-powered microscopic field also varies greatly from patient to patient.

In many cases it is difficult to distinguish between benign and malignant tumors. Capsular or vascular invasion and the presence of metastatic disease are unambiguous indications of adrenocortical carcinoma, as opposed to a benign adrenal tumor. A variety of other histologic features are of some use in distinguishing between benign and malignant lesions; tumor weight and mitotic activity appear to be the most useful of these.[18] The number of mitoses is probably especially important. Weiss and colleagues[19] found a worse prognosis for patients with more than 20 mitoses per 50 high-powered microscopic fields compared with a smaller number of mitoses. They proposed that tumors be designated as low or high grade based on this number of mitoses.

DNA content, as assessed by flow cytometry, has been reported as a guide to the degree of malignancy.[20–23] Unfortunately, not all studies agree about how aneuploidy influences outcome. Usually, aneuploidy confers a worse prognosis; in one series, however, aneuploidy was associated with longer survival.[24] Medeiros and Weiss from the National Cancer Institute have concluded that DNA ploidy is of minimal value in the diagnosis and management of adrenocortical carcinoma.[25] Other markers that have been proposed to assist differential diagnosis include assessments of MiB-1–positive nuclei per 1000 tumor cells and the expression of p53.[26] Further study is needed to place these newer tumor markers in diagnostic perspective.

#### Classification

Adrenocortical tumors are functional or nonfunctional, depending on the endocrine status of the patient. There are no histologic features that separate functional from nonfunctional adrenal tumors.[7]

**Functional Tumors.** Adrenocortical carcinomas are considered functional if there is excessive cortisol production that lacks both diurnal variation and suppression by dexamethasone. Patients with this type of tumor usually have the clinical signs of Cushing's syndrome. From the reverse perspective, approximately 10% of Cushing's syndrome is caused by a malignant adrenal tumor. Excessive production of other hormones, such as aldosterone, testosterone, or estradiol, may be associated with Conn's syndrome, virilization syndromes, or feminization syndromes, respectively.[27] Because of their endocrinologic manifestations, the functioning tumors tend to be smaller at the time of surgical exploration.

**Nonfunctional Tumors.** Tumors in this class are usually large at discovery, have not produced any clinical endocrine syndrome, and do not contain unusually high amounts of hormones.

## Clinical Features

In a review of 1891 cases from the literature, adrenocortical carcinoma was more common in women (58.6%) than in men (41.4%).[28] The age distribution was bimodal, with peaks in the first and fifth decades. Adrenocortical carcinomas in children were more likely to be functional (about 84%), whereas they were more likely to be nonfunctional in older patients (84%). Most of the tumors were too advanced at diagnosis for surgical cure (68%).

Other studies confirm that adrenocortical carcinomas are lethal tumors with highly variable survival rates, which vary from a low of 8% at 1 year to a high of 44% at 5 years.[8, 29, 30] Metastases to lung, liver, lymph nodes, or bone, or combinations of these sites, are commonly found at initial presentation (Table 70–1). There is no clear predilection for these tumors to involve one side with more frequency than the other; bilateral carcinomas occur in about 4% of cases.[7]

The major presenting symptoms in most patients with adrenocortical carcinoma are abdominal pain, weakness, and weight loss. In most series, physical signs of an abdominal mass, distant lymphadenopathy, hepatomegaly, and leg edema are common at the time of presentation. In addition, patients with functioning tumors that are producing excess cortisol will show the cardinal features of Cushing's syndrome (central obesity, cutaneous striae, osteoporosis, hypertension, diabetes, plethora, and hirsutism). Clitoral hypertrophy, deepening of the voice, receding hair at the temples, and acne may be the result of excessive androgen production. Breast enlargement in men and children and precocious puberty in girls are signs of excessive estrogen production. Primary aldosteronism due to adrenocortical carcinoma is rare, but when it occurs, potassium depletion, edema, and hypertension are present.

## Diagnosis

For patients with suspected excess production of corticosteroids, either of two screening tests can be recommended. One is the measurement of plasma cortisol level in both the morning and evening, and the other is the 24-hour urinary level of free cortisol. A value greater than 100 μg in a 24-hour urine collection is considered abnormal.[7] In establishing a diagnosis of Cushing's syndrome, the traditional approach has been to perform both a low-dose and a high-dose dexamethasone suppression test.[31] The low-dose suppression test involves giving 1 mg of dexamethasone at 11 PM, followed the next morning by a serum cortisol determination, which should be less than 5 μg/dl. A value greater than 10 μg/dl is highly suspicious for Cushing's syndrome. The next step is to try to differentiate pituitary-dependent adrenocorticotropic hormone (ACTH) hypersecretion from the ectopic ACTH syndrome and primary glucocorticoid-secreting adrenal tumors. This usually involves a high-dose dexamethasone suppression test in which the patient takes 2 mg dexamethasone every 6 hours for 48 hours, with simultaneous collection of urine for 3 days. In this test, urinary cortisol levels are reduced by at least 50% in patients with pituitary-dependent Cushing's syndrome but not in patients with the ectopic ACTH syndrome or an adrenal tumor. The sensitivity and specificity of this test can be increased by measuring the suppression of both the free cortisol and 17-hydroxysteroid levels in urine.[32] The specificity is reportedly 100% if the urine free cortisol is decreased more than 90% and the 17-hydroxysteroid excretion is decreased by more than 64%. Tyrrell and colleagues recommend an alternative to this form of high-dose dexamethasone suppression test.[33] It involves obtaining a plasma cortisol level between 0700 and 0800 hours on the day of the test, oral ingestion of 8 mg of dexamethasone at 2300 hours on that same day, and a repeat plasma cortisol determination between 0700 and 0800 hours on the following morning. There should be at least a 50% or greater reduction in the plasma cortisol level after dexamethasone administration compared with the baseline value.

Using the low-dose and high-dose dexamethasone suppression tests and the clinical findings of the individual patient, one can often distinguish between an adrenal source of excessive cortisol and either a pituitary or ectopic source of ACTH overproduction. If the diagnosis remains obscure, the next step is to measure the plasma ACTH level. It should be low in patients with an adrenal source of cortisol excess. Another test that may be useful in some patients is the corticotropin-releasing hormone (CRH) test.[34, 35] In patients with Cushing's disease (from a pituitary tumor) there is a normal or exaggerated ACTH and cortisol response to CRH administration, whereas patients with ectopic ACTH secretion and non–ACTH-dependent causes of excess cortisol production fail to respond to CRH.[34, 36] Another test is the overnight metyrapone test, as described by Sindler and colleagues.[37] Only rarely must one measure urinary 17-hydroxycorticosteroids, 17-ketosteroids, testosterone, and estradiol.[38]

Once an adrenal tumor is suspected, a computed tomo-

*Table 70–1.* Sites of Metastases at the Time of Diagnosis of Adrenocortical Cancer

| Organ | Cases (%) |
|---|---|
| Lungs | 60 |
| Liver | 53 |
| Lymph nodes | 47 |
| Abdomen | 43 |
| Bones | 33 |
| Kidneys | 20 |
| Brain | 10 |

Modified from Hajjar RA, Hill CS Jr, Samaan NA. Adrenal cortical carcinoma: a study of 32 patients. Cancer 1975;35:549–54.

graphic scan of the retroperitoneal area is the most reliable way to establish the presence of a suprarenal mass.[39] Alternatively, magnetic resonance imaging (MRI) can also visualize this area of the abdomen.[40] Preliminary results suggest that MRI can distinguish benign from malignant adrenal lesions.[41] Confirmation of the ability of MRI to make this distinction is needed. Adrenal scintigraphy with [131]I-6-β-iodomethylnorcholesterol (NP-59) may also provide useful information about adrenal masses discovered by computed tomography (CT) or MRI. This is especially true of nonfunctional adrenal masses found as an incidental finding by CT or MRI. Adrenal scintigraphy with NP-59 is usually positive in patients with adrenal adenomas or hyperplasia, whereas there is little or no imaging of adrenal masses due to metastatic malignancy, adrenal cysts, or adrenocortical carcinomas.[42, 43] In rare cases, direct biopsy with computed tomographic guidance may provide the diagnosis.[44]

Patients with suspected adrenocortical carcinoma should be screened for metastatic disease before surgical exploration. CT and MRI are frequently inaccurate in diagnosing liver involvement by tumor, but these studies are more accurate in assessing other areas of the abdomen. Other preoperative staging studies should include a chest radiograph, a biochemical screening panel, and a bone scan. One study suggests that PET may be a useful staging procedure for these patients.[45]

Adrenal masses found incidentally by abdominal CT are an increasing problem. Most of these lesions are benign adrenal adenomas. They are present as an incidental finding in as many as 3% of all autopsies.[1] Copeland has studied the differential diagnosis of incidental adrenal masses found by CT.[46] He makes the point that lesions smaller than 6 cm are almost never nonfunctional adrenocortical carcinomas. However, subsequent studies have shown that CT frequently underestimates the size of adrenal masses, especially when they are small.[47] Hopefully, refinements in the metaiodobenzylguanidine (MIBG) scan or a related technique may prove useful in distinguishing between small carcinomas and the more common benign forms of adrenal enlargement.

### Staging

The American Joint Committee on Cancer and the International Union Against Cancer have not adopted any staging system for this disease. The simplest unofficial system classifies these tumors as local, regional, or metastatic in extent. Macfarlane[48] developed a variant of this simple system that Sullivan and coworkers[49] later modified (Table 70–2). Bradley[50] devised an alternative pathologic staging system for adrenocortical tumors that added tumor grade and the completeness of tumor resection as important prognostic variables. Until a standard staging system is adopted, the system given in Table 70–2 can be used.

### Prognosis

The most important prognostic factors are the stage of disease (see Table 70–2), the number of mitoses per 50 high-powered microscopic fields (≥20), and possibly the degree of aneuploidy found by flow cytometry. A series from the Cleveland Clinic illustrates the importance of stage.[8] In this series of 82 patients, the 5-year survival rate for 40 patients

*Table 70–2.* **Staging System for Carcinoma of the Adrenal Cortex**

*TNM Designations*

| | |
|---|---|
| T1 | Tumor <5 cm, no invasion |
| T2 | Tumor >5 cm, no invasion |
| T3 | Tumor any size, locally invading but not involving adjacent organs |
| T4 | Tumor any size, locally invading adjacent organs |
| N0 | No positive regional nodes |
| N1 | Positive regional nodes |
| M0 | No distant metastasis |
| M1 | Distant metastasis present |

*Stage Groupings*

| | |
|---|---|
| I | T1 N0 M0 |
| II | T2 N0 M0 |
| III | T1 or T2 N1 M0; T3 N0 M0 |
| IV | Any T any N M1; T3 N1; T4 |

From Macfarlane DA. Cancer of the adrenal cortex: the natural history, prognosis, and treatment in a study of 55 cases. Ann R Coll Surg Engl 1958;23:155 as modified by Sullivan M, Boileau M, Hodges CV. Adrenal cortical carcinoma. J Urol 1978;120:660.

with localized disease was 44%, for 9 patients with regional disease it was 12%, and for 33 patients with metastatic disease it was 6%. A series of 156 patients from France provides similar 5-year survival results, as follows: overall, 34%; curative surgery group, 42%; local disease only, 53%; regional disease, 24%. The median survival for patients treated palliatively was 6 months.[51] Only rare patients with extensive regional or metastatic disease have been cured by a combination of surgical excision and chemotherapy.[52] A single case of spontaneous regression of adrenocortical carcinoma in a newborn has been reported.[53]

## TREATMENT

### Surgery

Complete surgical resection, if at all possible, is the treatment of choice for malignant adrenal tumors.[54] The operative approach should be an aggressive one that attempts to remove all visible tumor and metastases as completely as possible. This point cannot be overemphasized because the majority of patients present with advanced disease (stage III to stage IV). If the regional lymph nodes are enlarged, they should be removed with the tumor. Tumors with intracaval extension of tumor thrombus can be excised with cardiac bypass techniques in selected patients.[55] Reports of prolonged survival and reduced symptoms in patients who have had repeated excisions of metastatic deposits should encourage the surgeon to take an aggressive approach.[56] In a series of 20 untreated patients, the average survival time was only 2.7 months from the time of diagnosis.[57] In contrast, multiple surgical series have shown that complete surgical resection increases survival.[54, 56, 58]

There are four basic surgical approaches to adrenal tumors: anterior, posterior, flank, and thoracoabdominal.[59] Although the posterior or flank approaches are generally recommended for many adrenal cortical tumors because of their lower morbidity, there is general agreement that these approaches are contraindicated for patients with adrenocortical carcinomas. Laparoscopic surgery has been used for patients with benign tumors, but this treatment technique is inappropriate for patients with adrenocortical carcinoma.[60] A transabdominal approach allows thorough exploration of the abdomen and adequate exposure. With extremely large tumors (>10 cm), a thoracoabdominal approach provides the optimal exposure.

One should control endocrine problems (such as hypertension, diabetes, edema) as much as possible before surgery. Postoperatively, corticosteroids should be prescribed if all adrenal tissue has been removed. Follow-up of patients with functional tumors should include periodic reassessment of steroid levels. This is a good guide to possible recurrence or progression of the disease process.

Recurrent disease after "curative" resection is common. Surgical therapy is of occasional palliative value in patients with recurrent disease. In a study of 45 patients with recurrence, the mean survival time was more than doubled in patients who underwent reoperation.[56] Local recurrences should be aggressively resected. Limited pulmonary and hepatic metastases should be considered for palliative resection. There are several reports of prolonged survival after multiple thoracotomies to resect metastatic adrenocortical carcinoma to the lung.[61–63]

## Radiation Therapy

Radiation therapy has been reported to be of some benefit as an adjunct to surgery for patients with stage III disease,[64] but most centers consider radiation therapy of limited value in primary management. It may have a limited palliative role in patients with symptomatic metastases. For example, one group reported that palliative doses of irradiation delivered over 2 to 3 weeks resulted in relief of pain from metastases, healing of osseous lesions, and relief of localized intestinal obstruction.[65] Occasionally, radiation therapy provides prolonged local control of unresectable lesions.

## Chemotherapy

**Treatment of Advanced Disease.** Table 70–3 lists chemotherapeutic agents that have been studied for the treatment of patients with advanced or metastatic adrenocortical carcinomas.[66–84] The most active single agent is probably mitotane, but cisplatin is also active based on limited studies of the drug used alone and more extensive studies using cisplatin-based regimens of combination chemotherapy. Patients with unresectable or metastatic adrenocortical carcinoma, of both the functional and nonfunctional types, should be given a trial treatment with mitotane.[2, 52, 85–87] Chapter 10 summarizes the pharmacology and clinical use of this drug. It is useful in about one fourth of such cases but only rarely with apparent cure[52] or prolonged remission.[88, 89] In one case,[89] a patient remained in remission for 12 years while receiving a total of 13 kg of mitotane. Mitotane has also been used to treat Cushing's syndrome and the ectopic ACTH syndrome[90]; however, mitotane is rarely recommended for these problems because surgical treatment is generally superior.

There is a growing experience with combination chemotherapy for patients with advanced adrenocortical carcinoma. Cisplatin and etoposide appear to be an active combination, and the addition of mitotane and doxorubicin appears to further increase the efficacy of the combination. There is speculation that this may relate to the fact that resistance to cisplatin, etoposide, and doxorubicin is mediated through P-glycoprotein, and mitotane appears to inhibit this mechanism of multiple drug resistance. The role of P-glycoprotein in adrenocortical cancer has been studied in the hope that overexpression of the multiple drug resistance phenotype

*Table 70–3.* **Chemotherapy for Adrenocortical Carcinomas**

| Drugs | Patients (No. CR + PR/total) | Response Rate (%) |
|---|---|---|
| *Single-Agent Chemotherapy* | | |
| Cisplatin[69–71] | 10/18 | 56 |
| Mitotane[64–68] | 25/106 | 24 |
| Doxorubicin | | |
| First line (before mitotane)[67] | 3/16 | 19 |
| Second line (after mitotane)[67] | 0/15 | 0 |
| Ketoconazole[72] | 1/1 | |
| Carmustine[73] | 0/2 | |
| Methotrexate[73] | 0/1 | |
| Vinblastine[73] | 0/1 | |
| Altretamine[69] | 0/1 | |
| Streptozocin[69] | 0/1 | |
| *Combination Chemotherapy* | | |
| Mitotane + cisplatin + doxorubicin + etoposide[80] | 15/28 | 54 |
| Cisplatin + etoposide[77, 81, 82] | 9/21 | 43 |
| Mitotane + cisplatin[74] | 11/37 | 30 |
| Fluorouracil + doxorubicin + cisplatin[75] | 3/13 | 23 |
| Cyclophosphamide + doxorubicin + cisplatin (CAP)[76] | 2/11 | 18 |
| Mitotane + streptozocin[78] | 2/3 | |
| Cisplatin + etoposide + bleomycin[66] | 2/4 | |
| Cisplatin + etoposide + cyclophosphamide + vincristine[79] | 1/1 | |

CR + PR, the number of complete plus partial responses.

may explain the refractory nature of adrenocortical cancer to chemotherapy. In one study, P-glycoprotein was found in all patients enrolled.[91] In another study, 53% of the patients expressed P-glycoprotein. Paradoxically, three patients with high levels of P-glycoprotein had complete responses to mitotane, whereas another three patients with P-glycoprotein–negative tumors failed to respond.[92] These unexpected results deserve further study.

The role of combination chemotherapy for this rare disease remains incompletely defined, but it appears reasonable to offer cisplatin-based combination chemotherapy (with or without mitotane) to motivated patients with a good performance status and reasonable hematopoietic, renal, and cardiac function.

Symptomatic patients with functional tumors that fail to respond to mitotane or combination chemotherapy may be considered for therapy with aminoglutethimide (see Chapter 10) or metyrapone.[93, 94] However, these agents do nothing for the underlying disease, and metyrapone treatment may precipitate hypertension and hypokalemia. Octreotide acetate has been reported effective in the treatment of ectopic Cushing's syndrome.[95] This drug deserves further evaluation in patients with adrenocortical carcinoma.

**Adjuvant Therapy.** Mitotane has been used as an adjuvant therapy after surgical resection, with variable results. Some groups have reported anecdotal experiences suggesting benefit, whereas others consider the drug ineffective as adjuvant therapy.[96] Resolution of this controversy can only come from an appropriately controlled clinical trial, although such a trial is unlikely given the rare occurrence of this tumor type.

## SUMMARY OF TREATMENT FOR ADRENOCORTICAL CARCINOMA

The mainstay of treatment is surgical excision of the tumor. This may be useful for the primary tumor and in many cases for local recurrence. The roles of adjunctive radiation therapy or chemotherapy, or both, are difficult to assess. Adjunctive therapy is not recommended for patients with stages I, II, and III disease (as defined in Table 70–2). However, the poor survival rate of patients with resected stage IV disease justifies consideration of adjunctive mitotane therapy in highly motivated patients with good performance status and baseline organ function.[2, 50, 97] Patients with advanced, unresectable disease may be offered palliative therapy with mitotane or cisplatin-based chemotherapy, or a combination of the two.

## Pheochromocytoma

### NATURAL HISTORY, DIAGNOSIS, AND STAGING

Pheochromocytoma is a neoplasm of chromaffin cells that may arise as a unilateral or bilateral tumor within the adrenal medullary tissue or as nonmalignant tumors scattered in the adrenal glands and other catechol-secreting tissues throughout the body.[98] The term *paraganglioma* is sometimes used to describe pheochromocytomas when they arise outside the adrenal gland.

### Epidemiology and Etiology

Pheochromocytomas are rare neoplasms with an approximate incidence of 2 to 3 cases/million per year in the United States and Scandinavia.[99] Autopsy studies suggest that about one third of pheochromocytomas are not diagnosed during the life of the patient. The incidence of malignant pheochromocytoma is uncertain, with estimates varying between 5% and 46%, with a likely average figure of about 13%.[99] Surveillance, Epidemiology, and End Results data suggest an overall incidence of malignant pheochromocytoma of about 0.04 cases per 100,000 population.

There is an association of pheochromocytoma with other endocrine tumors, most notably those seen in multiple endocrine neoplasia, type 2 (MEN 2), including medullary carcinoma of the thyroid, hyperplasia of the parathyroid glands, and bilateral adrenal medullary pheochromocytomas (see Chapter 67). A variant of this syndrome (MEN 2b) replaces parathyroid disease with a marfanoid habitus, a characteristic facies, and mucosal neuromas of the lip and intestines. There is also an association of pheochromocytoma with nonendocrine familial syndromes, including von Hippel-Lindau disease, which is known to have an abnormal gene on chromosome 3,[100, 101] and more rarely in neurofibromatosis and von Recklinghausen's disease.[102]

Ninety percent of pheochromocytomas are sporadic and unrelated to familial syndromes. The approximate distribution of some important forms of pheochromocytoma can be described by the "rough rule of 10s."[99] Specifically, about 10% of pheochromocytomas occur in children, 10% are associated with familial syndromes, about 10% of sporadic cases are bilateral, about 10% are extra-adrenal, and 10% are malignant.

The cause of pheochromocytomas is unknown. Deletion mapping of chromosome 1p and chromosome 22q suggests that inactivation of multiple tumor-suppressor genes may be required in the pathogenesis of this tumor.[103]

### Classification

Ten percent of pheochromocytomas are malignant and eventually recur in ectopic, nonchromaffin tissue. As with other endocrine tumors, the behavior of the tumor is more important in defining malignancy than is histologic appearance alone. Proof of malignancy usually rests on definitive evidence of spread to liver, lung, bone, or other nonsympathetic chain areas. The differentiation between multicentric primary sites and metastatic sites can be a problem. Two ancillary procedures have been studied for their potential in distinguishing between benign and malignant forms of pheochromocytoma. Flow cytometric analysis of DNA for the presence of aneuploidy or tetraploidy has been studied in Taiwan[104] and at the Mayo Clinic.[105] Both studies suggest that the presence of aneuploidy or tetraploidy is associated with a poor prognosis. Another approach is the measurement of serum levels of neuron-specific enolase (NSE). In a study from France, all the patients with benign pheochromocytomas had normal levels of NSE, whereas half the patients with malignant pheochromocytomas had elevated levels.[106]

Eighty percent of pheochromocytomas occur in adults, with the remainder occurring in children. In children, approximately 20 to 40% are either bilateral or multiple. The malignant potential of pheochromocytomas in children is unclear. In a series of 19 patients with MEN 2 reported at the Mayo Clinic,[107] 4 had metastatic pheochromocytoma, which is roughly twice the expected number.

## Clinical Features

The symptoms and signs of pheochromocytoma result from the release of excessive amounts of catecholamines (epinephrine or norepinephrine, or both). This causes hypertension in most patients, which can be either paroxysmal (72%) or sustained (47%).[108] A wide variety of other clinical manifestations can be induced as well, as illustrated by Table 70–4.[109]

Rarely, patients will present with atypical or milder symptoms, which include headache, nervousness, palpitations, nausea, weakness, anorexia, flushing, dizziness, and shortness of breath. A single case has also been reported of a pheochromocytoma presenting as fever of unknown origin without hypertension.[110] These attacks may occur infrequently, making immediate diagnosis difficult or even impossible. Between attacks blood pressure can be normal, and patients are frequently classified as "functional." Individuals presenting with such a constellation of symptoms require careful testing, sometimes repeatedly over long periods, to exclude the presence of a catechol-producing tumor. Rarely, a diagnosis of factitious pheochromocytoma should be considered.[111] Another rare presentation (3 of 27 patients treated in one series) was characterized by multiple organ system

*Table 70–4.* **Symptoms and Signs of Pheochromocytoma**

| Finding | Approximate Percentage | |
|---|---|---|
| | ADULT | CHILD |
| *Symptoms* | | |
| Persistent hypertension | 65 | 92 |
| Paroxysmal hypertension | 30 | 8 |
| Headache | 80 | 81 |
| Sweating | 70 | 68 |
| Palpitations, nervousness | 60 | 34 |
| Pallor of face | 40 | 27 |
| Tremor | 40 | 0 |
| Nausea | 30 | 56 |
| Weakness, fatigue | 25 | 27 |
| Weight loss | 15 | 44 |
| Abdominal or chest pain | 15 | 35 |
| Dyspnea | 15 | 16 |
| Visual changes | 10 | 44 |
| Constipation | 5 | 8 |
| Raynaud's phenomenon | 5 | 0 |
| Convulsions | 3 | 23 |
| Polydipsia, polyuria | | 25 |
| Puffy, red, cyanotic hands | | 11 |
| *Signs* | | |
| Fasting blood glucose >120 mg/dl | 40 | 40 |
| Glycosuria | 10 | 3 |
| Eyeground changes | 30 | 70 |

From Hume DM. In: Astwood EB, Cassidy CE, eds. Clinical endocrinology. Vol. 2. New York: Grune & Stratton, 1968:519.

failure, high fever, encephalopathy, and vascular lability. Successful treatment required prompt diagnosis, vigorous medical preparation, and emergency adrenalectomy if the patient's condition continued to deteriorate.[112]

Physical examination of pheochromocytoma patients is most often normal but may show physiologic findings related to the excess catechols or to the presence of an abdominal mass. Most patients are thin. When sustained catechol release is present, they may appear tremulous, with excessive sweating. Tachypnea and tachycardia are also frequently present. Evidence of associated findings (such as café au lait spots in neurofibromatosis; retinal manifestations, i.e., cherry red spots with von Hippel-Lindau or Sturge-Weber disease; and retinal vascular abnormalities seen in patients with long-standing sustained hypertension) can be helpful clues. Objectively, attacks are accompanied by diagnostic elevations in urine and blood catecholamine levels.

Abdominal palpation, especially if vigorous and in the vicinity of a pheochromocytoma, frequently precipitates a hypertensive attack. This can be hazardous and because biochemical testing is readily available, abdominal massage should be avoided. Attacks can be precipitated by a variety of stimuli such as exercise; emotional trauma; physical trauma; increases in intra-abdominal pressure caused by micturition, sneezing, and coughing; and the ingestion of alcohol. Most important is the recognition of paroxysmal attacks during anesthetic induction, any operative procedure, or bodily stress. After an attack, patients frequently feel extremely weak.

A family history of thyroid tumors or hyperparathyroidism in any patient with episodic hypertension or a firm diagnosis of pheochromocytoma, or both, are absolute indications to search for the existence of the more general MEN syndrome that is associated with a pheochromocytoma. Investigation of the entire kindred by means of pentagastrin or calcium infusions should be carried out, looking for diagnostic elevations of calcitonin. Assays of catecholamines in serum or urine require investigation as well if MEN 2 is diagnosed in the index case.

## Laboratory Diagnosis

In the routine evaluation of patients with sustained hypertension, a single determination of vanillylmandelic acid (VMA) and metanephrine levels from a 24-hour urine specimen is sufficient to exclude the diagnosis of pheochromocytoma in greater than 95% of patients. The combination of urinary metanephrines and VMA had a sensitivity of 98% in detecting the disease in patients seen at the Mayo Clinic between 1980 and 1992.[108]

Catecholamine levels should be assayed when urinary determinations of VMA and metanephrines give inconclusive results and the suspicion of pheochromocytoma is high, that is, there is sustained hypertension with paroxysmal symptoms. Pharmacologic testing of patients suspected of having pheochromocytomas has been greatly facilitated by the development of analytic methods for the determination of plasma catecholamines. The overwhelming majority of patients with catechol-secreting tumors have baseline elevations in norepinephrine and some, albeit lesser, elevations of epinephrine. In rare cases, suppression of catecholamines with clonidine may be required to establish a biochemical diagnosis of pheochromocytoma.[113]

The finding of increased norepinephrine and epinephrine levels in a 2-hour timed urine specimen begun at the onset of an attack can help make a diagnosis when a patient has paroxysmal attacks that suggest a pheochromocytoma. With few exceptions, patients whose hypertension is caused by a pheochromocytoma have abnormally high levels of norepinephrine or epinephrine, or both, immediately following an attack.

Patients with pheochromocytomas seldom have increased urinary excretion of dopa, dopamine, and homovanillic acid (HVA). Previously, it was thought that abnormally high levels of dopamine or HVA, or both, occurred exclusively with malignant pheochromocytomas. However, patients with benign tumors have been described as having high dopamine or HVA excretion.[114] Chromogranin A is also elevated in patients with pheochromocytoma.[115]

The preoperative demonstration of pheochromocytoma has improved remarkably since the advent of ultrasonography, CT, and MRI.[40] Adrenal tumors as small as 2 cm in diameter are routinely visualized by the use of a combination of these techniques. The Mayo Clinic has reported the positive and negative predictive values for localization of tumors by CT as 95% and 100%, respectively.[108]

Pheochromocytomas tend to be vascular tumors, and 90% of cases can be visualized easily by selective aortography; however, arteriography may precipitate a hypertensive crisis and should be avoided. Scintigraphic localization has been achieved by MIBG.[116] Tumor masses of 0.4 to 63 g with predominant norepinephrine or epinephrine, or both, have been equivalently visualized. Venous catheterization of the superior and inferior vena cava is a useful aid to tumor localization in extra-adrenal tumors, which tend to produce exclusively noradrenaline. The procedure should be considered when strong evidence exists for a norepinephrine-producing pheochromocytoma and attempts to visualize the tumor within the adrenal or abdominal cavity by noninvasive methods fail to uncover a mass. In selective venous sampling, the primary diagnostic feature is an increase in the measured plasma catechols at the approximate level that coincides with the venous drainage from the tumor.

### Staging

There is no established staging system for pheochromocytomas.

### Prognosis

In a review at the Mayo Clinic of 110 patients treated by primary resection between 1980 and 1992, the perioperative mortality rate was less than 1%.[108] With routine alpha and β-blockade, there were no complications associated with intraoperative hypertension. Perioperative morbidity was 16%, and more than 90% of patients were restored to a condition of normotension. An earlier review from the Mayo Clinic of 138 surgically treated patients reported the overall recurrence rate for benign and malignant tumors resected to be 9.8% and the 5-year survival rate for patients with malignant tumors to be 44%.[117]

### TREATMENT

The successful treatment of pheochromocytoma requires a team approach. Multiple specialists may be required, including internists, endocrinologists, medical oncologists, anesthesiologists, radiologists, and surgeons. Each specialist has a critical role in the management of the patient with this disease, ranging from the initial accurate diagnosis and localization of the tumor to the surgeon and anesthesiologist, whose combined efforts can minimize perioperative morbidity and mortality. This is especially true when patients have other complicating medical conditions, such as pregnancy.[118]

### Surgery

Surgical resection is the mainstay of treatment, and it should be prompt and aggressive. The general philosophy is to gently "steal the tumor away from the patient." For this reason, excellent exposure is required, and this is best achieved by an anterior approach.[119] Early control and ligation of the adrenal vein, if possible, along with minimal manipulation of the tumor, requires an anterior approach. Exposure of the right adrenal gland is achieved by extensive kocherization of the duodenum and downward traction of the kidney with superior retraction of the right lobe of the liver. The left adrenal gland can be approached by entry into the lesser sac and superior or inferior mobilization of the pancreas. Alternatively, the left adrenal may be approached by medial rotation of the spleen and pancreas.

A growing experience with laparoscopic transabdominal adrenalectomy suggests this is a safe procedure in experienced hands.[60] This approach is amenable for small (<8 cm) benign tumors. There is no difference in the frequency of intraoperative hypertensive episodes or blood loss when compared with the traditional anterior approach.[120] The intraoperative blood pressure management is identical to that for the open technique. Patients undergoing laparoscopy in general have less pain, a shorter hospitalization, and require less recuperation time. Bilateral and unilateral tumors can be removed by this approach. However, patients whose tumors cannot be visualized preoperatively should be explored through an open anterior approach. In addition, the open approach should be used in patients with malignant tumors or tumors with local extension. The laparoscopic retroperitoneal approach is not recommended.

Before the planned surgical extirpation of the tumor, patients should have a symptom-free period, during which blood volume, myocardial stress, and the emotional consequences of longstanding catechol excess can be controlled. This can be accomplished through pharmacologic control with α-blockers and, at times, β-blockers, which allows smoother intraoperative and postoperative periods.[121] β-Blockers should never precede α-blockade, because this may precipitate general vasoconstriction from the unopposed α-adrenergic activity.

In the usual case, treatment is begun with the α-blocker phenoxybenzamine.[122] Therapy is initiated at 10 mg twice daily, with a gradual increase in dosage to approximately 30 to 160 mg daily, depending on the patient's symptomatic response. In well-blocked individuals, almost all the catechol-mediated symptoms and signs are controlled by the use of this agent. The principal reported toxicity has been mild and transient sedation. If significant tachycardia continues after initiation of therapy with phenoxybenzamine, β-blockers (such as propranolol) may be used to control the tachycardia after correction of hypovolemia. As an alternative, prazosin may be used instead of phenoxybenzamine. The duration of α-blockade prior to surgery should be 7 to 10 days. β-Blockade can be initiated 3 days prior to surgery.

The anesthesia management of these patients during surgery is aimed at providing blockage of hypertension during manipulation of the tumor and its excision and the reversal of these effects to prevent hypotension after the tumor has been removed. The initial steps can be managed with phenoxybenzamine and propranolol, and the latter step with norepinephrine and fluids, if necessary. Surgical morbidity and mortality have been greatly reduced by appropriate preoperative preparation of the patient.[123] Prior to the era of pharmacologic blocking, the operative mortality rate was in the range of 20%. Swan-Ganz catheter monitoring may be necessary in selected patients with significant cardiac disease.

Some controversy exists in the literature regarding the continued use of α- and β-blockers during the intraoperative period. Although some anesthesiologists and surgeons favor the continued use of phenoxybenzamine and propranolol during the intraoperative period, there are some anesthesiologists who feel that the drug should be discontinued prior to the planned operative procedure and that the patient's blood pressure should be controlled intraoperatively with a nitroprusside drip. This latter method has been reported to be useful in intraoperative localization of the catechol-secreting tumor, since gentle palpation of the operative site can result in blood pressure elevations because of catechol release. These hypertensive episodes can easily be controlled with nitroprusside. In the postoperative period, patients whose therapy with α- and β-blockers was discontinued 3 to 5 days before the operation have been noted to have less prolonged anesthetic effects and shorter mean postoperative hospitalization times.

In the case of metastatic disease, an attempt should be made to remove all possible sites of tumor deposits. This type of "debulking" may enable the patient to survive longer, with subsequent more effective chemotherapy of lesions that are not resectable. An anterior transabdominal approach is preferred because of the need to explore the entire abdomen for possible extra-adrenal sites of tumor. Recurrences should be aggressively treated surgically because patient survival up to 20 years has been reported after the removal of such lesions. In patients who are found to have Sipple's syndrome or MEN 2, the pheochromocytomas should be excised first, and later attention should be given to the thyroid and parathyroid tumors.

### Radiation Therapy

Some authors feel that external-beam radiation therapy is useful in the palliation of metastatic disease,[124] especially for the management of painful bone metastases.

About 60% of patients concentrate MIBG, and there has been interest in the use of [131]I-labeled MIBG for treatment.[125–128] Early studies of radiolabeled MIBG found a composite response rate of 40% in 30 patients, but none of these responses was complete or durable. In a review of 116 reported patients, Loh and colleagues found that 76% of patients had symptomatic improvement, 30% had objective regression of tumor, 45% had hormonal responses, and 5 patients had complete tumor and hormonal responses lasting from 16 to 58+ months.[128] The authors concluded that [131]I-MIBG may be useful in the palliation of selected patients with malignant pheochromocytoma.

### Medical Management of Malignant Pheochromocytoma

Medical management of malignant pheochromocytoma is reserved for cases in which the tumor has metastasized or cannot be located at surgery or when medical contraindications preclude an exploratory laparotomy. Metastatic pheochromocytoma tends to be a slow-growing tumor, and both the morbidity and mortality rates of this disease can be directly related to the cardiovascular complications produced by the prolonged elevated catechol secretion. Long-term symptomatic palliation can be obtained in some patients with the chronic oral administration of phenoxybenzamine in divided doses of 30 to 100 mg daily. Direct inhibition of catechol synthesis in patients with pheochromocytoma has been achieved with the experimental agent α-methylparatyrosine.

Relatively little is known about the value of single-agent cytotoxic chemotherapy in the treatment of malignant pheochromocytoma. Anecdotal experience with streptozocin suggests it may lower catecholamine levels, but there is no convincing evidence of prolonged survival.[129, 130]

There is only limited information available about the use of combination chemotherapy in patients with malignant pheochromocytoma.[99] The only useful regimen tested to date is the combination of cyclophosphamide, vincristine, and dacarbazine. Keiser and coworkers[131] initially studied three patients with cyclophosphamide, vincristine, and dacarbazine, with promising results. A subsequent, larger study by Averbuch and colleagues[132] of the U.S. National Cancer Institute extended these results in 14 patients. These investigators treated 14 patients with cyclophosphamide (750 mg/m² intravenously on day 1), vincristine (1.4 mg/m² intravenously on day 1), and dacarbazine (600 mg/m² intravenously on days 1 and 2) every 21 days. Complete and partial responses were seen in 79% of the patients, with a median duration of 22 months. All the patients who responded had objectively improved performance status and blood pressure. The toxic side effects were tolerable, including the expected hematologic, neurologic, and gastrointestinal effects of these three drugs (see Chapter 10). Additional anecdotal evidence of a palliative benefit from this regimen in one of two patients has been published from Europe.[133] One of two patients was also reported to respond in a study from Japan.[134]

There has been one report of combined [131]I-MIBG and multiagent chemotherapy.[135] Further experience with this combination is needed before it can be recommended for general use.

### SUMMARY OF TREATMENT FOR PHEOCHROMOCYTOMA

The successful treatment of pheochromocytoma requires broad access to the expertise of endocrinologists, medical oncologists, diagnostic radiologists, anesthesiologists, and surgeons. Management depends on making an accurate diagnosis, preoperative control of hypertension with phenoxybenzamine, careful intraoperative management of blood pressure by the anesthesiologist, and an aggressive surgical resection through an anterior approach. Patients with persistent hypertension may require continued antihypertensive therapy, and some patients may benefit from repeated resection of metastatic disease. External-beam radiation therapy and chemotherapy are not useful in the adjuvant setting but may be of modest palliative benefit in patients with metastatic disease and symptoms other than hypertension. Highly motivated patients with a good performance status and normal organ function may benefit from the palliative use of $^{131}$I-MIBG or combination chemotherapy (cyclophosphamide, vincristine, and dacarbazine).

## SUGGESTIONS FOR ADDITIONAL READING

Luton J-P, Cerdas S, Billaud L, et al. Clinical features of adrenocortical carcinoma, prognostic factors, and the effect of mitotane therapy. N Engl J Med 1990;322:1195–1201.

Bornstein SR, Stratakis CA, Chrousos GP. Adrenocortical tumors: recent advances in basic concepts and clinical management. Ann Intern Med 1999;130:759–71.

Schulick RD, Brennan MF. Adrenocortical carcinoma. World J Urol 1999;17:26–34.

Cryer PE. Pheochromocytoma. West J Med 1992;156:399–407.

Orchard T, Grant CS, van Heerden JA, et al. Pheochromocytoma—continuing evolution of surgical therapy. Surgery 1993;114:1153–9.

Lairmore TC, Ball DW, Baylin SB, Wells SA. Management of pheochromocytomas in patients with multiple endocrine neoplasia type-2 syndromes. Ann Surg 1993;217:595–603.

Manger WM, Gifford RW Jr, eds. Clinical and experimental pheochromocytoma. 2nd ed. Cambridge, Mass: Blackwell Science, 1996:570.

## REFERENCES

1. Bornstein SR, Stratakis CA, Chrousos GP. Adrenocortical tumors: recent advances in basic concepts and clinical management. Ann Intern Med 1999;130:759–71.
2. Hutter AM Jr, Kayhoe DE. Adrenal cortical carcinoma: clinical features of 138 patients. Am J Med 1966;41:572–80.
3. Hutter AM Jr, Kayhoe DE. Adrenal cortical carcinoma: results of treatment with *o,p'DDD* in 138 patients. Am J Med 1966;41:581–92.
4. Henley DJ, van Heerden JA, Grant CS, et al. Adrenal cortical carcinoma—a continuing challenge. Surgery 1983;94:926–31.
5. Brennan MF. Adrenocortical carcinoma. CA Cancer J Clin 1987;37:348–65.
6. Cohn K, Gottesman L, Brennan M. Adrenocortical carcinoma. Surgery 1986;100:1170–7.
7. Samaan NA, Hickey RC. Adrenal cortical carcinoma. Semin Oncol 1987;14:292–6.
8. Bodie B, Novick AC, Pontes JE, et al. The Cleveland Clinic experience with adrenal cortical carcinoma. J Urol 1989;141:257–60.
9. Kiiveri S, Siltanen S, Rahman N, et al. Reciprocal changes in the expression of transcription factors GATA-4 and GATA-6 accompany adrenocortical tumorigenesis in mice and humans. Mol Med 1999;5:490–501.
10. Pilon C, Pistorello M, Moscon A, et al. Inactivation of the p16 tumor suppressor gene in adrenocortical tumors. J Clin Endocrinol Metab 1999;84:2776–9.
11. James LA, Kelsey AM, Birch JM, Varley JM. Highly consistent genetic alterations in childhood adrenocortical tumours detected by comparative genomic hybridization. Br J Cancer 1999;81:300–4.
12. Müller S, Gadner H, Weber B, et al. Wilms' tumor and adrenocortical carcinoma with hemihypertrophy and hamartomas. Eur J Pediatr 1978;127:219–26.
13. Hayward NK, Little MH, Mortimer RH, et al. Generation of homozygosity at the c-Ha-ras-1 locus on chromosome 11p in an adrenal adenoma from an adult with Wiedemann-Beckwith syndrome. Cancer Genet Cytogenet 1988;30:127–32.
14. Li FP, Fraumeni JF Jr. Prospective study of a family cancer syndrome. JAMA 1982;247:2692–4.
15. Lynch HT, Katz DA, Bogard PJ, Lynch JF. The sarcoma, breast cancer, lung cancer, and adrenocortical carcinoma syndrome revisited: childhood cancer. Am J Dis Child 1985;139:134–6.
16. Kay S. Hyperplasia and neoplasia of the adrenal gland. Pathol Annu 1976;11:103–39.
17. Miettinen M. Neuroendocrine differentiation in adrenocortical carcinoma: new immunohistochemical findings supported by electron microscopy. Lab Invest 1992;66:169–74.
18. van Slooten H, Schaberg A, Smeenk D, Moolenaar AJ. Morphologic characteristics of benign and malignant adrenocortical tumors. Cancer 1985;55:766–73.
19. Weiss LM, Medeiros LJ, Vickery AL Jr. Pathologic features of prognostic significance in adrenocortical carcinoma. Am J Surg Pathol 1989;13:202–6.
20. Bowlby LS, DeBault LE, Abraham SR. Flow cytometric analysis of adrenal cortical tumor DNA. Relationship between cellular DNA and histopathologic classification. Cancer 1986;58:1499–505.
21. Hosaka Y, Rainwater LM, Grant CS, et al. Adrenocortical carcinoma: nuclear deoxyribonucleic acid ploidy studied by flow cytometry. Surgery 1987;102:1027–34.
22. Taylor SR, Roederer M, Murphy RF. Flow cytometric DNA analysis of adrenocortical tumors in children. Cancer 1987;59:2059–63.
23. Amberson JB, Vaughan ED Jr, Gray GF, Naus GJ. Flow cytometric analysis of nuclear DNA from adrenocortical neoplasms: a retrospective study using paraffin-embedded tissue. Cancer 1987;59:2091–5.
24. Haak HR, Cornelisse CJ, Hermans J, et al. Nuclear DNA content and morphological characteristics in the prognosis of adrenocortical carcinoma. Br J Cancer 1993;68:151–5.
25. Medeiros LJ, Weiss LM. New developments in the pathologic diagnosis of adrenal cortical neoplasms: a review. Am J Clin Pathol 1992;97:73–83.
26. Vargas MP, Vargas HI, Kleiner DE, Merino MJ. Adrenocortical neoplasms: role of prognostic markers MIB-1, p53, and RB. Am J Surg Pathol 1997;21:556–62.
27. Tang CK, Gray GF. Adrenocortical neoplasms: prognosis and morphology. Urology 1975;5:691–5.
28. Wooten MD, King DK. Adrenal cortical carcinoma: epidemiology and treatment with mitotane and a review of the literature. Cancer 1993;72:3145–55.
29. Hajjar RA, Hickey RC, Samaan NA. Adrenal cortical carcinoma: a study of 32 patients. Cancer 1975;35:549–54.
30. Nader S, Hickey RC, Sellin RV, Samaan NA. Adrenal cortical carcinoma: a study of 77 cases. Cancer 1983;52:707–11.
31. Ashcraft MW, Van Herle AJ, Vener SL, Geffner DL. Serum cortisol levels in Cushing's syndrome after low- and high-dose dexamethasone suppression. Ann Intern Med 1982;97:21–6.
32. Flack MR, Oldfield EH, Cutler GB Jr, et al. Urine free cortisol in the high-dose dexamethasone suppression test for the differential diagnosis of the Cushing syndrome. Ann Intern Med 1992;116:211–7.
33. Tyrrell JB, Findling JW, Aron DC, et al. An overnight high-dose dexamethasone suppression test for rapid differential diagnosis of Cushing's syndrome. Ann Intern Med 1986;104:180–6.
34. Nieman LK, Loriaux DL. Corticotropin-releasing hormone: clinical applications. Annu Rev Med 1989;40:331–9.
35. Yanovski JA, Cutler GB Jr, Chrousos GP, Nieman LK. Corticotropin-releasing hormone stimulation following low-dose dexamethasone administration: a new test to distinguish Cushing's syndrome from pseudo-Cushing's states. JAMA 1993;269:2232–8.
36. Nieman LK, Chrousos GP, Oldfield EH, et al. The ovine corticotropin-releasing hormone stimulation test and the dexamethasone suppression test in the differential diagnosis of Cushing's syndrome. Ann Intern Med 1986;105:862–7.
37. Sindler BH, Griffing GT, Melby JC. The superiority of the metyrapone test versus the high-dose dexamethasone test in the differential diagnosis of Cushing's syndrome. Am J Med 1983;74:657–62.
38. Richie JP, Gittes RF. Carcinoma of the adrenal cortex. Cancer 1980;45:Suppl:1957–64.
39. Abrams HL, Siegelman SS, Adams DF, et al. Computed tomography versus ultrasound of the adrenal gland: a prospective study. Radiology 1982;143:121–8.

40. Doppman JL, Reinig JW, Dwyer AJ, et al. Differentiation of adrenal masses by magnetic resonance imaging. Surgery 1987;102:1018–26.
41. Mitchell DG, Crovello M, Matteucci T, et al. Benign adrenocortical masses: diagnosis with chemical shift MR imaging. Radiology 1992;185:345–51.
42. Fig LM, Gross MD, Shapiro B, et al. Adrenal localization in the adrenocorticotropic hormone–independent Cushing syndrome. Ann Intern Med 1988;109:547–53.
43. Gross MD, Shapiro B, Bouffard JA, et al. Distinguishing benign from malignant euadrenal masses. Ann Intern Med 1988;109:613–8.
44. Bernardino ME, Walther MM, Phillips VM, et al. CT-guided adrenal biopsy: accuracy, safety, and indications. AJR Am J Roentgenol 1985;144:67–9.
45. Schumacher T, Brink I, Moser E, Nitzsche EU. Imaging of an adrenal cortex carcinoma and its metastasis with FDG-PET. German. Nuklearmedizin 1999;38:124–6.
46. Copeland PM. The incidentally discovered adrenal mass. Ann Intern Med 1983;98:940–5.
47. Cerfolio RJ, Vaughan ED Jr, Brennan TG Jr, Hirvela ER. Accuracy of computed tomography in predicting adrenal tumor size. Surg Gynecol Obstet 1993;176:307–9.
48. Macfarlane DA. Cancer of the adrenal cortex—the natural history, prognosis and treatment in a study of 55 cases. Ann R Coll Surg Engl 1958;23:155–86.
49. Sullivan M, Boileau M, Hodges CV. Adrenal cortical carcinoma. J Urol 1978;120:660–5.
50. Bradley EL III. Primary and adjunctive therapy in carcinoma of the adrenal cortex. Surg Gynecol Obstet 1975;141:507–16.
51. Icard P, Chapuis Y, Andreassian B, et al. Adrenocortical carcinoma in surgically treated patients: a retrospective study on 156 cases by the French Association of Endocrine Surgery. Surgery 1992;112:972–9.
52. Ostuni JA, Roginsky MS. Metastatic adrenal cortical carcinoma: documented cure with combined chemotherapy. Arch Intern Med 1975;135:1257–8.
53. Saracco S, Abramowsky C, Taylor S, et al. Spontaneously regressing adrenocortical carcinoma in a newborn: a case report with DNA ploidy analysis. Cancer 1988;62:507–11.
54. Harrison L, Gaudin P, Brennan M. Pathologic features of prognostic significance for adrenocortical carcinoma after curative resection. Arch Surg 1999;134:181–5.
55. Hedican S, Marshall F. Adrenocortical carcinoma with intracaval extension. J Urol 1997;158:2056–61.
56. Pommier R, Brennan M. An eleven year experience with adrenocortical carcinoma. Surgery 1992;112:963–71.
57. Mac Farlane D. Cancer of the adrenal cortex: the natural history, prognosis, and treatment in a study of fifty-five cases. Ann R Coll Surg Engl 1958;23:155–86.
58. Icard P, Chapius Y, Andreassian B, et al. Adrenocortical carcinoma in surgically treated patients: a retrospective study on 156 cases by the French Association of Endocrine Surgery. Surgery 1992;112:972–80.
59. Prinz R, Falimirski M. Operative approaches to the adrenal gland. In: Clark OH, Duy QY, eds. Textbook of Endocrine Surgery. Philadelphia: WB Saunders, 1997:529–34.
60. Barresi R, Prinz R. Laparoscopic adrenalectomy. Arch Surg 1999;134:212–7.
61. Appelqvist P, Kostiainen S. Multiple thoracotomy combined with chemotherapy in metastatic adrenal cortical carcinoma: a case report and review of the literature. J Surg Oncol 1983;24:1–4.
62. Potter D, Strott C, Javadpour N, Roth JA. Prolonged survival following six pulmonary resections for metastatic adrenal cortical carcinoma: a case report. J Surg Oncol 1984;25:273–7.
63. Kwauk S, Burt M. Pulmonary metastases from adrenal cortical carcinoma: results of resection. J Surg Oncol 1993;53:243–6.
64. Markoe AM, Serber W, Micaily B, Brady LW. Radiation therapy for adjunctive treatment of adrenal cortical carcinoma. Am J Clin Oncol 1991;14:170–4.
65. Percarpio B, Knowlton AH. Radiation therapy of adrenal cortical carcinoma. Acta Radiol: Ther Phys Biol 1976;15:288–92.
66. van Slooten H, Moolenaar AJ, van Seters AP, Smeenk D. The treatment of adrenocortical carcinoma with o,p'-DDD: prognostic implications of serum level monitoring. Eur J Cancer Clin Oncol 1984;20:47–53.
67. Boven E, Vermorken JB, van Slooten H, Pinedo HM. Complete response of metastasized adrenal cortical carcinoma with o,p'-DDD: case report and literature review. Cancer 1984;53:26–9.
68. Hesketh PJ, McCaffrey RP, Finkel HE, et al. Cisplatin-based treatment of adrenocortical carcinoma. Cancer Treat Rep 1987;71:222–4.
69. Decker RA, Elson P, Hogan TF, et al. Eastern Cooperative Oncology Group study 1879: mitotane and adriamycin in patients with advanced adrenocortical carcinoma. Surgery 1991;110:1006–13.
70. Luton JP, Cerdas S, Billaud L, et al. Clinical features of adrenocortical carcinoma, prognostic factors, and the effect of mitotane therapy. N Engl J Med 1990;322:1195–201.
71. Wittes RE, Adrianza ME, Parsons R, et al. Compilation of phase II results with single antineoplastic agents. Cancer Treat Symp 1985;4:122–9.
72. Tattersall MH, Lander H, Bain B, et al. Cis-platinum treatment of metastatic adrenal carcinoma. Med J Aust 1980;1:419–21.
73. Grapski RT, Lopez JA, Krikorian JG, Melby JC. Cisplatin chemotherapy of adrenocortical carcinoma. Proc ASCO 1983;2:232.
74. Contreras P, Rojas A, Biagini L, et al. Regression of metastatic adrenal carcinoma during palliative ketoconazole treatment. Lancet 1985;2:151–2.
75. Haq MM, Legha SS, Samaan NA, et al. Cytotoxic chemotherapy in adrenal cortical carcinoma. Cancer Treat Rep 1980;64:909–13.
76. Bukowski RM, Wolfe M, Levine HS, et al. Phase II trial of mitotane and cisplatin in patients with adrenal carcinoma: a Southwest Oncology Group study. J Clin Oncol 1993;11:161–5.
77. Schlumberger M, Brugieres L, Gicquel C, et al. 5-Fluorouracil, doxorubicin, and cisplatin as treatment for adrenal cortical carcinoma. Cancer 1991;67:2997–3000.
78. van Slooten H, van Oosterom AT. CAP (cyclophosphamide, doxorubicin, and cisplatin) regimen in adrenal cortical carcinoma. Cancer Treat Rep 1983;67:377–9.
79. Johnson DH, Greco FA. Treatment of metastatic adrenal cortical carcinoma with cisplatin and etoposide (VP-16). Cancer 1986;58:2198–202.
80. Eriksson B, Oberg K, Curstedt T, et al. Treatment of hormone-producing adrenocortical cancer with o,p'DDD and streptozocin. Cancer 1987;59:1398–403.
81. Crock PA, Clark AC. Combination chemotherapy for adrenal carcinoma: response in a 5½-year-old male. Med Pediatr Oncol 1989;17:62–5.
82. Berruti A, Terzolo M, Pia A, et al. Mitotane associated with etoposide, doxorubicin, and cisplatin in the treatment of advanced adrenocortical carcinoma: Italian Group for the Study of Adrenal Cancer. Cancer 1998;83:2194–200.
83. Zidan J, Shpendler M, Robinson E. Treatment of metastatic adrenal cortical carcinoma with etoposide (VP-16) and cisplatin after failure with o,p'DDD: clinical case reports. Am J Clin Oncol 1996;19:229–31.
84. Bonacci R, Gigliotti A, Baudin E, et al. Cytotoxic therapy with etoposide and cisplatin in advanced adrenocortical carcinoma: Reseau Comete INSERM. Br J Cancer 1998;78:546–9.
85. Becker D, Schumacher OP. o,p'DDD therapy in invasive adrenocortical carcinoma. Ann Intern Med 1975;82:677–9.
86. Lubitz JA, Freeman L, Okun R. Mitotane use in inoperable adrenal cortical carcinoma. JAMA 1973;223:1109–12.
87. Molnar GD, Mattox UR, Bahn RC. Clinical and therapeutic observations in adrenal cancer: a report on 7 patients treated with o,p'-DDD. Cancer 1963;16:259–68.
88. McKiernan P, Doyle DA, Duffy GJ, et al. o,p'-DDD and adrenal carcinoma. Ir J Med Sci 1978;147:437–40.
89. Jarabak J, Rice K. Metastatic adrenal cortical carcinoma: prolonged regression with mitotane therapy. JAMA 1981;246:1706–7.
90. Temple TE Jr, Jones DJ Jr, Liddle GW, Dexter RN. Treatment of Cushing's disease: correction of hypercortisolism by o,p'DDD without induction of aldosterone deficiency. N Engl J Med 1969;281:801–5.
91. Flynn SD, Murren JR, Kirby WM, et al. P-glycoprotein expression and multidrug resistance in adrenocortical carcinoma. Surgery 1992;112:981–6.
92. Haak HR, van Seters AP, Moolenaar AJ, Fleuren GJ. Expression of P-glycoprotein in relation to clinical manifestation, treatment and prognosis of adrenocortical cancer. Eur J Cancer 1993;29A:1036–8.
93. Melby JC, Cyr MS, Dale SL. Reduction of adrenal-steroid production by an inhibitor of cholesterol biosynthesis. N Engl J Med 1961;264:583–7.
94. Fukushima DK, Gallagher TF, Greenberg W, Pearson OH. Studies with an adrenal inhibitor in adrenal carcinoma. J Clin Endocrinol 1960;20:1234–45.

95. De Rosa G, Testa A, Liberale I, et al. Successful treatment of ectopic Cushing's syndrome with the long-acting somatostatin analog octreotide. Exp Clin Endocrinol 1993;101:319–25.

96. Vassilopoulou-Sellin R, Guinee VF, Klein MJ, et al. Impact of adjuvant mitotane on the clinical course of patients with adrenocortical cancer. Cancer 1993;71:3119–23.

97. Schteingart DE, Motazedi A, Noonan RA, Thompson NW. Treatment of adrenal carcinomas. Arch Surg 1982;117:1142–6.

98. Scott HW Jr. In: Sabiston DC, ed. Davis-Christopher: Textbook of Surgery. 11th ed. Philadelphia: WB Saunders, 1977.

99. Wu L-T, Chahinian AP, Baylin SB, et al. Neoplasms of the neuroendocrine system. In: Holland JF, Frei E, Bast RC Jr, et al, eds. Cancer Medicine. 4th ed. 1997:1581–90.

100. Tisherman SE, Tisherman BG, Tisherman SA, et al. Three-decade investigation of familial pheochromocytoma: an allele of von Hippel-Lindau disease? Arch Intern Med 1993;153:2550–6.

101. Gautier JF, Schlumberger M, Fonseca E, et al. Familial pheochromocytoma and Van Hippel-Lindau disease. Presse Med 1990;19:1494–6.

102. Nakagawara A, Ikeda K, Tsuneyoshi M. Malignant pheochromocytoma with ganglioneuroblastomatous elements in a patient with von Recklinghausen's disease. Cancer 1985;55:2794–8.

103. Shin E, Fujita S, Takami K, et al. Deletion mapping of chromosome 1p and 22q in pheochromocytoma. Jpn J Cancer Res 1993;84:402–8.

104. Pang LC, Tsao KC. Flow cytometric DNA analysis for the determination of malignant potential in adrenal and extra-adrenal pheochromocytomas or paragangliomas. Arch Pathol Lab Med 1993;117:1142–7.

105. Nativ O, Grant CS, Sheps SG, et al. The clinical significance of nuclear DNA ploidy pattern in 184 patients with pheochromocytoma. Cancer 1992;69:2683–7.

106. Grouzmann E, Gicquel C, Plouin PF, et al. Neuropeptide Y and neuron-specific enolase levels in benign and malignant pheochromocytomas. Cancer 1990;66:1833–5.

107. Carney JA, Sizemore GW, Sheps SG. Adrenal medullary disease in multiple endocrine neoplasia, type 2: pheochromocytoma and its precursors. Am J Clin Pathol 1976;66:279–90.

108. Orchard T, Grant CS, van Heerden JA, Weaver A. Pheochromocytoma—continuing evolution of surgical therapy. Surgery 1993;114:1153–8.

109. Hume DM. In: Astwood EB, ed. Clinical endocrinology. Vol. 2. New York: Grune & Stratton, 1968:519.

110. Dawson J, Harding LK. Phaeochromocytoma presenting as pyrexia of undetermined origin: diagnosis using gallium-67. Br Med J 1982;284:1164.

111. Portioli I, Valcavi R. Factitious phaeochromocytoma: a case for Sherlock Holmes. Br Med J (Clin Res Ed) 1981;283:1660–1.

112. Newell KA, Prinz RA, Pickleman J, et al. Pheochromocytoma multisystem crisis: a surgical emergency. Arch Surg 1988;123:956–9.

113. Sjoberg RJ, Simcic KJ, Kidd GS. The clonidine suppression test for pheochromocytoma: a review of its utility and pitfalls. Arch Intern Med 1992;152:1193–7.

114. Voorhess ML. Neuroblastoma-pheochromocytoma: products and pathogenesis. Ann NY Acad Sci 1974;230:187–94.

115. Hsiao RJ, Neumann HP, Parmer RJ, et al. Chromogranin A in familial pheochromocytoma: diagnostic screening value, prediction of tumor mass, and post-resection kinetics indicating two-compartment distribution. Am J Med 1990;88:607–13.

116. Sisson JC, Frager MS, Valk TW, et al. Scintigraphic localization of pheochromocytoma. N Engl J Med 1981;305:12–7.

117. Remine WH, Chong GC, Van Heerden JA, et al. Current management of pheochromocytoma. Ann Surg 1974;179:740–8.

118. Freier DT, Thompson NW. Pheochromocytoma and pregnancy: the epitome of high risk. Surgery 1993;114:1148–52.

119. Grant C. Pheochromocytoma. In: Clark OH, Duy QY, eds. Textbook of endocrine surgery. Philadelphia: WB Saunders, 1997:513–22.

120. Fernandez-Cruz L, Taura P, Saenz A, et al. Laparoscopic approach to pheochromocytoma: hemodynamic changes and catecholamine secretion. World J Surg 1996;20:762–8.

121. Craco R, Eckaldt J, Wiswell J. Pheochromocytoma treatment with alpha and beta adrenergic agents. JAMA 1977;202:807–10.

122. Russell W, Metcalfe I, Tonkin A, Frewin D. The preoperative management of pheochromocytoma. Anesth Intensive Care 1998;26:196–200.

123. Samaan N, Hickey R, Shutts P. Diagnosis, localization, and management of pheochromocytoma. Cancer 1988;62:2451–60.

124. James RE, Baker HL Jr, Scanlon PW. The roentgenologic aspects of metastatic pheochromocytoma. Am J Roentgenol Radium Ther Nucl Med 1972;115:783–93.

125. McEwan AJ, Shapiro B, Sisson JC, et al. Radio-iodobenzylguanidine for the scintigraphic location and therapy of adrenergic tumors. Semin Nucl Med 1985;15:132–53.

126. Krempf M, Lumbroso J, Mornex R, et al. Use of m-[131I]iodobenzylguanidine in the treatment of malignant pheochromocytoma. J Clin Endocrinol Metab 1991;72:455–61.

127. Feldman JM, Frankel N, Coleman RE. Platelet uptake of the pheochromocytoma-scanning agent 131I-meta-iodobenzylguanadine. Metabolism 1984;33:397–9.

128. Loh KC, Fitzgerald PA, Matthay KK, et al. The treatment of malignant pheochromocytoma with iodine-131 metaiodobenzylguanidine (131I-MIBG): a comprehensive review of 116 reported patients. J Endocrinol Invest 1997;20:648–58.

129. Feldman JM. Treatment of metastatic pheochromocytoma with streptozocin. Arch Intern Med 1983;143:1799–800.

130. Gross DJ, Schlank E, Ipp E. Streptozotocin therapy for malignant pheochromocytoma. Arch Intern Med 1985;145:367–8.

131. Keiser HR, Goldstein DS, Wade JL, et al. Treatment of malignant pheochromocytoma with combination chemotherapy. Hypertension 1985;7(3 Pt 2):I18–24.

132. Averbuch SD, Steakley CS, Young RC, et al. Malignant pheochromocytoma: effective treatment with a combination of cyclophosphamide, vincristine, and dacarbazine. Ann Intern Med 1988;109:267–73.

133. Senan S, Reed N, Connell J. Palliation of malignant phaeochromocytoma with combination chemotherapy. Eur J Cancer 1992;28A:1006–7.

134. Noshiro T, Honma H, Shimizu K, et al. Two cases of malignant pheochromocytoma treated with cyclophosphamide, vincristine and dacarbazine in a combined chemotherapy. Endocr J 1996;43:279–84.

135. Sisson JC, Shapiro B, Shulkin BL, et al. Treatment of malignant pheochromocytomas with 131-I metaiodobenzylguanidine and chemotherapy. Am J Clin Oncol 1999;22:364–70.

# CHAPTER 71

# CARCINOID TUMORS

• LARRY K. KVOLS • ARVIND CHAUDHRY

Carcinoid tumors are rare tumors with an approximate incidence of one to two per 100,000 population.[1] These tumors have a natural history that is unlike any other malignant disease, and histologically they present a monotony of innocuous-appearing cells with rare mitotic figures, leading to the misnomer of *carcinoid*. Patients may present with a mix of tumor-related symptoms and signs with unusual endocrine syndromes that have fascinated physicians for decades. Although it had been known for 60 years that carcinoid tumors develop in enterochromaffin cells, it was the work of Pearse

*Table 71–1.* Sites of Carcinoid Tumors

|  | Surgical Patients (%) (4000 cases) | Necropsy (%) (201 cases) |
|---|---|---|
| Appendix | 45 | 3 |
| Small bowel | 30 | 76 |
| Rectum | 15 | 1.5 |
| Bronchus | 5 | 9 |
| Colon | 5 | 6 |
| Stomach | 3 | 2.5 |
| Ovary | 1 | 0 |
| Other | 0 | 2 |

Data from Peskin GW. Small bowel tumors including carcinoid. In: Hardy J, ed. Rhoad's textbook of surgery. Philadelphia: JB Lippincott, 1977:1167 and Berge T, Jinell F. Carcinoid tumors: frequency in a defined population during a 12-year period. Acta Pathol Microbiol Scand 1976;84:322.

in the late 1960's that provided the unifying concept of the APUD or *a*mine *p*recursor *u*ptake and *d*ecarboxylation system. This term, although rarely used today, provided a histogenetic explanation for carcinoid tumors occurring in diverse sites such as the lung,[2, 3] biliary tree, pancreas,[4] stomach, duodenum,[5, 6] small intestine, colon, rectum, ovary,[7] cervix,[8] testis,[9, 10] thymus,[11] kidney,[12] and larynx (Table 71–1).[13] The APUD concept also provided a new way to approach the rare occurrence of carcinoid tumors in some of the multiple endocrine neoplasia (MEN) syndromes, (MEN 1 and MEN 2),[14] as well as its association with the ectopic production of various peptides (adrenocorticotropic hormone, growth hormone, insulin, gastrin, calcitonin, β-melanocyte–stimulating hormone, antidiuretic hormone, human chorionic gonadotropin [hCG], and vasoactive intestinal peptide).[4, 5, 14–16]

Many of the clinical and diagnostic considerations in

carcinoid tumors relate to the synthesis of serotonin and other biologically active materials. Serotonin synthesis and metabolism play a key role in understanding this disease. The schematic representation shown in Figure 71–1 emphasizes the shunting of tryptophan away from its usual metabolic pathway to form niacin and protein. Some gastric and bronchial carcinoids lack aromatic L-amino acid decarboxylase and release large amounts of 5-hydroxytryptophan (5-HTP) into the blood. Metabolites in the urine then include 5-HTP, 5-hydroxytryptamine (5-HT or serotonin), and less 5-hydroxyindoleacetic acid (5-HIAA) than is expected. The detailed biochemical, endocrinologic, and biologic characteristics of the carcinoid tumors are beyond the scope of this section and are reviewed extensively in other sources.[17–20]

## Natural History, Diagnosis, and Staging

### CLASSIFICATION AND PATHOLOGY

Because of the difference in the histologic appearance of carcinoid tumors occurring in different parts of the gut, as well as differences in histochemistry and frequency of association with various other clinical syndromes, Williams and Sandler have classified carcinoid tumors as being of foregut, midgut, and hindgut derivation. Table 71–2 lists some of the characteristics of carcinoid tumors that are derived from different embryonic divisions of the gut. Carcinoids are also frequently classified broadly as gastric, bronchial, or intestinal, the latter of which includes carcinoid tumors arising from the small intestine, appendix, and rectum.

**Bronchial Carcinoids.** Since the 1990s, bronchial carci-

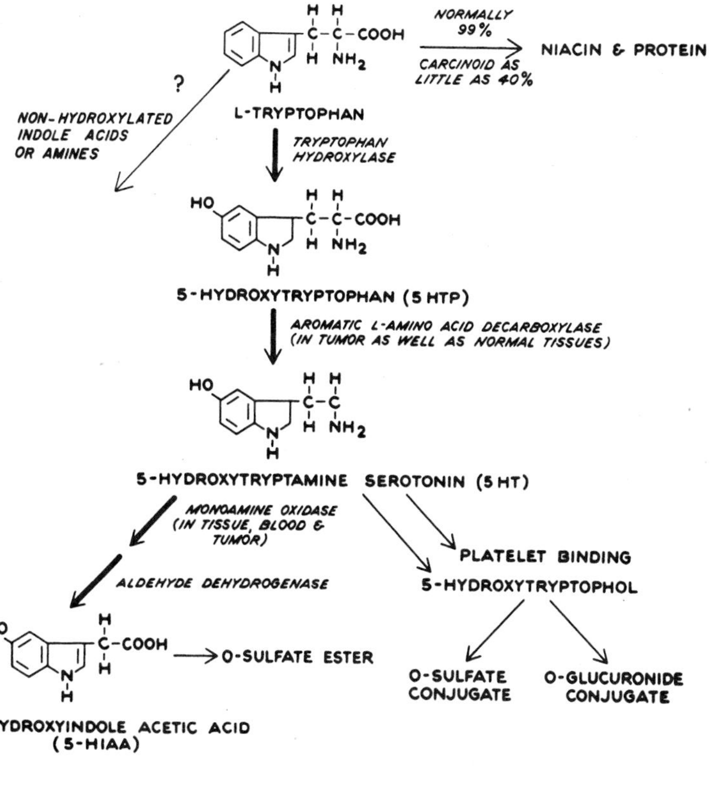

**Figure 71–1.** Metabolism of tryptophan in a patient with carcinoid syndrome. Heavy arrows indicate the shunting of tryptophan away from its usual metabolic pathway to form niacin and protein. Heavy arrows leading from serotonin show the major metabolites of serotonin excreted in the urine (see text for further discussion). (From Melmon KL. The endocrinologic manifestations of the carcinoid tumor. In: Williams RH, ed. Textbook of Endocrinology. 6th ed. Philadelphia: WB Saunders, 1981.)

*Table 71–2.* **Characteristics of Carcinoid Tumors Derived from Different Embryonic Divisions of the Gut**

| Characteristic | Foregut | Midgut | Hindgut |
|---|---|---|---|
| Histologic structure | Trabecular pattern | Characteristic solid nests | Atypical; tendency to trabecular |
| Argentaffin and diazo reactions | Usually negative | Positive | Often negative |
| Tumor 5-HT | Low | High | Not detected |
| 5-HTP secretion | Frequent | Rare | Not detected |
| Urinary 5-HIAA | Normal | High | Normal |
| Metastases into bone (usually osteoblastic) and skin | Common | Unusual | Common |

5-HT, 5-hydroxytryptamine; 5-HTP, 5-hydroxy-L-tryptophan; 5-HIAA, 5-hydroxyindole acetic acid.
Data from Melmon KL. The endocrinologic manifestations of the carcinoid tumor. In: Williams RH, ed. Textbook of endocrinology. 6th ed. Philadelphia: WB Saunders, 1981 and Williams ED, Sandler M. The classification of carcinoid tumours. Lancet 1963;1:238.

noids have been recognized more frequently and account for about 30% of all carcinoid tumors. The classification of bronchial carcinoid tumors is the subject of considerable debate.[21] Lung neuroendocrine tumors have been classified into four categories: the typical carcinoid (Kulchitsky cell carcinoma [KCC] I), atypical carcinoid (KCC II), intermediate small cell neuroendocrine carcinomas, and small cell neuroendocrine carcinomas (KCC III).[21-23] The different categories have different prognoses, varying from excellent for typical carcinoids to poor for small cell neuroendocrine carcinomas.[21-23]

**Gastric Carcinoids.** Gastric carcinoids are most uncommon and make up part of the neoplastic evolution that ranges from argentaffin cell hyperplasia to "carcinoid tumorlets," small benign-behaving tumors, and larger metastasizing cancer. This usually multicentric display is most frequently observed in pernicious anemia. It has been presumed that increased levels of gastrin play a trophic role in inducing these hyperplastic and neoplastic phenomena. The presence of hypergastrinemia, typical histologic features, no serosal involvement, and a size less than 2 cm are favorable prognostic signs.

**Intestinal Carcinoids.** More than 95% of all gastrointestinal carcinoids originate in only three sites: the appendix, rectum, and small intestine (Table 71–3).

*Carcinoids of the Appendix.* These are relatively common neoplasms. The overall prevalence was 0.32% among 34,505 patients who underwent appendectomy.[24] Because most of these tumors were found incidentally, the observed prevalence probably approaches the prevalence of the general population. Because only a small proportion of the

*Table 71–3.* **Metastatic Behavior of and Syndrome Production by Carcinoid Tumors**

| Site | Metastasizing (%) | With Syndrome (%) |
|---|---|---|
| Colon | 60 | 5 |
| Small bowel | 30 | 7 |
| Bronchus | 30 | 15 |
| Stomach | 25 | 5 |
| Rectum | 15 | 0 |
| Ovary | 5 | 50 |
| Appendix | 1 | Rare |

Data from Melmon KL. The endocrinologic manifestations of the carcinoid tumor. In: Williams RH, ed. Textbook of endocrinology. 5th ed. Philadelphia: WB Saunders, 1974:1084, Grahame-Smith DG. Carcinoid syndrome. London, William Heinemann Medical Books, 1972, and Jager RM. Carcinoid apudomas. Curr Probl Cancer 1977;1:1.

general population undergoes appendectomy, it can be assumed that most patients with carcinoid tumors of this vestigial organ bear them comfortably without treatment, and these neoplasms have no influence on life expectancy. Most appendiceal carcinoids are less than 1 cm in diameter and rarely ever metastasize. Simple appendectomy without further follow-up is justified in all patients with appendiceal carcinoids 1 cm or less in diameter and probably in all patients with tumors of less than 2 cm diameter, irrespective of the degree of local invasion. Only carcinoids of 2 cm or more in largest dimension should prompt consideration of a more radical operation. The presence of vascular invasion and involvement of the mesoappendix in a younger patient are factors that may favor more radical surgery for tumors greater than 2 cm.

*Carcinoids of the Rectum.* For reasons that are unclear, 99% of rectal carcinoids occur in a small zone between 4 and 13 cm above the dentate line. In contrast to carcinoids of the small intestine, multicentricity of these neoplasms within the rectum is rare (2%). On hematoxylin staining, they are indistinguishable from other carcinoids, but they do not take up silver and histochemically they usually do not show evidence of serotonin production. This may explain the fact that however widely they metastasize, they usually do not give rise to the carcinoid syndrome. Eighty percent of rectal carcinoids are smaller than 1 cm, and only 5% are larger than 2 cm in diameter. Size as a prognostic factor for metastases is similar to that for appendiceal carcinoids, and patients with carcinoids 2 cm or larger should have a full-scale cancer operation.

*Carcinoids of the Small Bowel.* The small intestine is the most common location for carcinoids of clinical significance. An annual incidence rate of 0.28 per 100,000 population in 1987 was reported by the Surveillance Epidemiology and End Results (SEER, Division of Cancer Prevention and Control, National Cancer Institute, 1987). Translated nationally, this means that approximately 600 new cases occur yearly. The frequency of intestinal carcinoids increases exponentially moving caudad from the duodenum. Forty percent of carcinoids of the small intestine are located within 2 feet of the ileocecal valve. Carcinoids of the colon are rare. Another unusual feature of small bowel carcinoids is a remarkable tendency to multicentricity. Twenty-five percent of patients had more than one lesion.

The most common clinical presentation for small bowel carcinoids is periodic abdominal pain. Because of its small size and deep mucosal site of origin, the primary small bowel carcinoid can present as intussusception. When the carcinoid invades the mesentery, it stimulates an intense fibroblastic reaction that may present as partial or complete small bowel obstruction. This has been shown to be related to the paracrine action of growth factors like β-fibroblast growth factor, transforming growth factor-β, platelet-derived growth factor, and epidermal growth factor.[25] A classic picture is a fully active patient with large masses in a grossly enlarged liver; there are minimal symptoms and normal or near-normal results on liver function tests. After the liver, the most common site of distant metastases is bone. The duration of symptoms before diagnosis varies from 2 to 20 years. Half the symptomatic patients are found at initial surgery to have unresectable disease. Five-year survival for incurable abdominal disease is estimated to be 50%; for those with hepatic metastases, the 5 year survival is 30%, with the median survival no longer than 3 years.

Histologically, carcinoid tumors are composed of monotonous sheets of small, round cells with uniform nuclei and cytoplasms.[20] Characteristically, carcinoid tumors either take up and reduce silver (argentaffin reaction) or take it up but do not reduce it (argyrophilic reaction).[26] Immunohistochemical localization of chromogranin, synaptophysin, and neuron-specific enolase are also used.[27] The chromogranins (A, B, and C) are a family of acidic polypeptides that are the major component of the secretory granules of many neuroendocrine cell types.[28] There is usually a close correspondence between neuroendocrine cells sharing chromogranin A immunoreactivity and an argyrophilic reaction, which may be partially explained by the fact that pure chromogranin is argyrophilic.[28] In addition to the general histologic neuroendocrine tumor markers, specific markers that identify serotonin, such as the argentaffin reaction of Masson or antibodies to serotonin, may be useful in identification of a tumor as carcinoid.

Foregut tumors (bronchus, stomach, duodenum, and pancreas) are argentaffin negative and tend to have low serotonin content. These tumors may metastasize to bone. In contrast, midgut carcinoids (jejunum, ileum, and ascending colon) are argentaffin positive and have a high serotonin content and rarely metastasize to bone. Hindgut tumors (transverse colon, descending colon, and rectum) are argentaffin negative, rarely contain serotonin, and may metastasize to bone. The argentaffin reaction is highly specific for serotonin-containing carcinoid tumors. Mitotic figures are rare; most of these tumors are diploid on flow cytometry, although aneuploidy is not unusual.[29, 30] However, unlike many other tumors, aneuploidy has an uncertain prognostic importance. Evaluation of the biologic behavior of these tumors with

antibody (Ki-67) against proliferating nuclear antigen may represent a viable option.[31] Immunohistochemical stains for L-dopa decarboxylase and chromogranin A are especially useful in diagnosis. When examined by electron microscopy or by special stains, carcinoid cells contain a variety of neuroendocrine marker substances that include neuron-specific enolase, Leu-7 antigen, and S-100 protein. There are at least five histologic patterns of growth, and they differ in prognosis. The median survivals found with these five subtypes in a study by the Eastern Cooperative Oncology Group[32] were as follows: insular (2.9 years), trabecular (2.5 years), glandular (0.9 years), undifferentiated (0.5 years), and mixed (1.4 to 4 years, depending on the mixture seen).

## CLINICAL FEATURES

**Malignant Carcinoid Syndrome.** Table 71–4 summarizes the major patterns of the carcinoid syndrome; the "classic syndrome" is that for tumors arising in the ileum.[17–19] Serotonin is well established as the cause of diarrhea in these patients, and it is also the putative cause of fibrotic changes in the heart and elsewhere. A wide variety of substances may contribute to other features and include substance P,[33] dopamine, tachykinins,[34, 35] and even growth hormone–releasing factor.[36]

Flushing may be the most bothersome component of the carcinoid syndrome for some patients. It is important to distinguish the flushing attacks from other possible causes of flushing, which include the idiopathic flushing syndrome,[37] postmenopausal state, chlorpropamide-alcohol flush, panic attacks, medullary thyroid carcinoma, systemic mastocytosis, and autonomic epilepsy. The flushing with carcinoid syndrome is usually associated with visible facial redness and is sometimes associated with wheezing, abdominal pain, and elevation of urinary 5-HIAA.

Diarrhea in the typical patient is usually mild and responsive to diphenoxylate or loperamide. Only rarely does diarrhea have a steatorrheic element and, again, this may be related more to mechanical problems of tumor or surgery than to the syndrome per se. Uncommonly, diarrhea may be exceedingly profuse, associated with life-threatening fluid and electrolyte losses.

The occurrence and severity of the syndrome is directly related to tumor bulk in an area that drains into the systemic circulation. This almost always implies distant metastases; the exceptions are carcinoids developing in teratomas of the ovary or testis. The most dramatic manifestation of the

*Table 71–4.* **Carcinoid Syndromes by Anatomic Site**

| Syndrome | Bronchus | Stomach | Ileum |
|---|---|---|---|
| Flush | Severe, prolonged with facial edema | Blotchy, often continuous | Episodic (3–10 min, worse after eating, exertion, alcohol) |
| Diarrhea | Infrequent | Less severe | Severe |
| Bronchoconstriction | Infrequent | Frequent | Sporadic, asthma-like attacks, may be severe |
| Cardiac lesions | Left side | Infrequent | Right side |
| Miscellaneous | Sudden death | Hypotension, peptic ulcers | |

Data from Melmon KL. The endocrinologic manifestations of the carcinoid tumor. In: Williams RH, ed. Textbook of endocrinology. 5th ed. Philadelphia: WB Saunders, 1974:1084, Grahame-Smith DG. Carcinoid syndrome. London: William Heinemann Medical Books, 1972, and Jager RM. Carcinoid apudomas. Curr Probl Cancer 1977;1:1.

malignant carcinoid syndrome is the carcinoid crisis, which is generally observed in patients with foregut carcinoids or greatly elevated 5-HIAA levels. This condition may occur spontaneously or may be precipitated by physically stressful conditions, particularly the induction of anesthesia. It is characterized by an intense generalized flush that may persist for hours or days and may be observed after a course of chemotherapy. It is also associated with severe exacerbation of diarrhea, tachyarrhythmias, and severe hypotension and previously was often a terminal event. Carcinoid crises may be prevented with octreotide.

**Carcinoid Heart Disease.** Carcinoid heart disease is more common than was previously recognized because of advances in echocardiography and Doppler techniques. It is common in patients with a long history of carcinoid syndrome and is usually associated with higher 5-HIAA levels. The pathologic features of carcinoid heart disease are distinctive and restricted to the endocardium and subendocardium, leaving the deeper architecture of the valve preserved. From a clinical standpoint, carcinoid heart disease presents with the characteristic murmurs of the respective valves involved, and the most common functional impairment is due to right-sided heart failure.[38] The associated hepatomegaly, ascites, and edema may produce a confusing clinical picture when mixed with abdominal malignant disease and hepatic metastases. Occasionally, when symptoms are severe, valve surgery may result in dramatic improvement of symptoms.[39]

## DIAGNOSIS

Patients presenting with carcinoid syndrome usually have the diagnosis confirmed by measurement of the 24-hour urinary excretion of 5-HIAA.[17–19] A value in excess of 9 mg/24 hr in a person without malabsorption or a value in excess of 30 mg/24 hr in the case of malabsorption may be considered confirmatory. Certain foods or drugs may give a false-positive result (bananas, walnuts, avocados, pineapples, reserpine, and glyceryl guaiacolate–containing cough syrups). Phenothiazines may give a false-negative result. Patients with gastric or, rarely, bronchial carcinoids may not have diagnostic elevations of 5-HIAA because of the lack of L-amino acid decarboxylase.[17] In these patients, confirmation of the diagnosis may require a search for 5-HT and 5-HTP in the urine by paper chromatography. In patients with symptomatic carcinoid tumors, there is a delay in diagnosis varying from 1 to 2 years in different studies. Attempts are being made to identify specific and sensitive serum markers for carcinoid tumors that may allow earlier diagnosis. In one study, urinary 5-HIAA had a sensitivity of 73% and a specificity of 100%; plasma substance P had a sensitivity of 32% and a specificity of 85%; and plasma neurotensin had a sensitivity of 41% and a specificity of 60%.[40] Other substances that have been tested include plasma neuropeptide K, plasma pancreatic polypeptide concentration, α-hCG, β-hCG, and chromogranin A, B, and C. Using specific radioimmunoassays in a study of 44 patients with carcinoid tumors, 100% had elevated plasma chromogranin A levels, 86% had elevated chromogranin B levels, and 5% had elevated chromogranin C levels.[41] These studies are not specific for carcinoid tumors because increased levels occur with high frequency in patients with endocrine pancreatic tumors and certain other neuroendocrine tumors.

Diagnosis ultimately depends on the histologic examination of tissue. Silver stains are generally required to confirm the diagnosis, but results with immunoperoxidase techniques using antibodies to a variety of neuroendocrine substances have simplified the process.

**Localization.** Unlike most other tumors, carcinoid tumors metastasize to the liver without causing functional liver abnormalities. Thus, liver function tests are of little value in screening,[42] and most patients with suspected abdominal carcinoid tumors benefit from a preoperative computed tomographic scan of the abdomen.[43, 44] A number of techniques, including gastrointestinal endoscopy, imaging studies (ultrasonography, computed tomography, magnetic resonance imaging, and angiography), endoscopic ultrasonography, selective venous sampling for various hormones, and various forms of radionuclide scanning have been used to determine the location of the primary tumor as well as the extent of tumor spread. The main problem is localizing small bowel carcinoids, which may be small and can be missed by barium studies. Carcinoid tumors possess high-affinity receptors for the hormone somatostatin in 88% of cases.[45] Five subtypes (numbered SSTR-1 to SSTR-5) of somatostatin receptors have been described.[46] An advance in localizing carcinoid tumors is the development of [111]In-DTPA-D-Phe1 octreotide scintigraphy (Octreoscan). Octreotide binds with high affinity to SSTR-2 and with a slightly less affinity to SSTR-3 and SSTR-5. Limited data show carcinoid tumors express SSTR-2, with SSTR-5 being less frequently expressed. This has been used as an adjunct in the diagnosis and staging of patients with carcinoid tumors.[47] In one series, known tumor sites were visualized in 32 of 37 patients (86%) in whom histologically proven sites were still present. To visualize hepatic metastases, it is critical that single-photon emission computed tomography be performed. Previously unsuspected extrahepatic localization or sites were found in 20 of 37 patients. Octreoscan imaging may be potentially useful before aggressive cytoreductive surgery to be certain that all sites of metastatic disease have been identified. As a consequence of the ability of Octreoscan to demonstrate somatostatin receptor–positive tumors, it can be used to select patients who are likely to respond favorably to octreotide treatment.

Another test that appears useful for selected patients is the [131]I-metaiodobenzylguanidine scan ([131]I-MIBG)[43, 44], which is concentrated by a sodium-dependent neuronal pump in pheochromocytomas; it is also concentrated by carcinoid tumors. The overall sensitivity is reported as 55 to 70%, with a specificity of 95%. However, octreotide scanning is reported to be more sensitive (96% vs. 70%).[45]

## STAGING AND PROGNOSIS

There is no established staging system for carcinoid tumors. As discussed earlier, size has been established as an important predictor for metastatic disease in carcinoid tumors arising from the appendix and rectum.[48, 49] Additional prognostic factors include histologic subtype, location (Table 71–5), and several other factors reported by Greenberg and associates.[50] Prognosis for gastrointestinal carcinoid tumors

*Table 71–5.* **Five-Year Survival Rates (%) in Patients with Carcinoid Tumors**

| Site | Stage | | | |
| | Local | Regional Lymph Nodes | Distant Metastasis | Overall |
| --- | --- | --- | --- | --- |
| Appendix | 99 | 99 | 27 | 99 |
| Bronchus | 96 | 71 | 11 | 87 |
| Rectum | 92 | 44 | 7 | 83 |
| Small bowel | 75 | 59 | 19 | 54 |
| Stomach | 93 | 23 | 0 | 52 |
| Colon | 77 | 65 | 17 | 52 |

From Godwin JD II. Carcinoid tumors: an analysis of 2837 cases. Cancer 1975;36:560.

was adversely affected by increasing age, advanced stage of disease, location within the large intestine, and occurrence of another malignancy. It should be noted that the prognosis for individual patients is unpredictable. In fact, highly variable survival data have been reported by different groups. This may, at least in part, be related to the lack of a widely accepted TNM system for staging.

## Treatment

### SURGERY

Surgical removal of all neoplastic tissue is the preferred therapy for primary tumors.[19] Surgical resection of metastatic disease was also the preferred palliative treatment for recurrence until the introduction of octreotide acetate, which now dominates palliative management.[51] The extent of the surgical resection is dependent on the location of the tumor, its size, its anticipated stage, and the general condition of the patient. More specific guidelines for selected sites are presented in the following sections.

**Appendix.** Small appendiceal carcinoids (<2 cm) are managed by appendectomy unless the lesion is adjacent to the cecal wall or involves lymph nodes. A rare larger lesion or one that involves the cecum or lymph nodes requires right hemicolectomy with removal of regional nodes, unless the patient is elderly or has a high operative risk.[52] Regional lymph node involvement is uncommon, although it may occur with lesions as small as 1 cm.[53]

**Small Bowel.** Since about one third of these carcinoids metastasize, en bloc resection is indicated, including the lymph nodes draining the tumor plus at least 10 cm of the bowel on either side of the lesion. If the tumor is within 5 cm of the ileocecal valve, a right hemicolectomy may be necessary.[19] If the small bowel carcinoid is too extensive for curative resection, one should still resect as much of the tumor as possible to reduce tumor bulk or perform intestinal diversion if there is any obstruction. Every attempt should be made to remove all visible tumor; if this is not feasible, a subtotal resection should be attempted.[1] In every case, however, one must remember the tendency of this tumor to cause fibrosis and to be associated with malabsorption. There is some evidence that this may be the result of mesenteric angiopathy.[54] Whatever the cause, the mesenteric vasculature must be protected and the amount of small bowel resected kept to the minimum necessary to accomplish the debulking

procedure. The anastomoses should be hand sewn because multiple anastomoses with a stapling device in the small bowel can result in prolonged and intractable ileus.

**Rectum.** Carcinoid tumors in this location are extremely rare and almost always benign.[55] For reasons that are not clear, 99% of rectal carcinoids occur in a small zone between 4 and 13 cm above the dentate line. More than 80% of the tumors are smaller than 1 cm; they virtually never metastasize and may be treated with local fulguration. Tumors that are 1 to 2 cm are in the "gray zone," where there is some room for clinical judgment based on patient age, operative risk, and the necessity for and acceptability of a permanent colostomy. A reasonable approach would seem to be wide local excision, proceeding to more radical surgery only if there is deep invasion. Rectal ultrasonography may be useful in identifying regional nodal metastases. If the tumor is 2 cm or larger, a full-scale cancer operation should be performed.[20]

**Bronchial Carcinoids.** Various parenchyma-saving procedures have been tried in patients with bronchial carcinoids. However, it now appears that such procedures are inadequate.[56, 57] We therefore recommend that the minimal surgical procedure be a lobotomy.

**Liver Metastases.** Metastatic involvement of the liver is not a contraindication to the palliative resection of symptomatic primary and metastatic carcinoid tumors in patients whose tumors are refractory to octreotide. If hepatic metastases are limited to a single lobe of the liver, partial hepatectomy should be performed.[19, 58–61] If hepatic metastases are bilateral, enucleation of these lesions may be performed, if feasible.[19] One report suggests that hepatic transplantation may be a reasonable treatment in highly selected patients.[62] If multiple liver metastases preclude partial hepatectomy or enucleation and if the patient demonstrates progressive deterioration with liver-dominant disease, interruption of hepatic arterial blood flow may be considered provided that the portal vein is patent. This has been accomplished by a variety of techniques, including the following: hepatic artery ligation alone;[61, 63–66] hepatic artery ligation around a catheter with the subsequent infusion of cytotoxic drugs;[66] use of embolic fragments of gelatin or absorbable gelatin sponge (Gelfoam),[66–68] polyvinyl alcohol foam (Ivalon) particles,[68, 69] or lyophilized dura mater;[70] and a Swan-Ganz balloon tip catheter.[71] Although none of these reports involves large numbers of patients, all report some degree of success. Of these approaches we concur with Melia and colleagues[66] and the Mayo Clinic group[72] that hepatic artery obliteration by an embolization technique appears to be the safest and simplest choice. The role of systemic chemotherapy or regional infusion chemotherapy for hepatic metastasis is discussed in a subsequent section.

**Cardiac Disease.** Endocardial plaques may accompany the carcinoid syndrome and result in cardiac failure. These plaques specifically involve the mural and valvular endocardium on the right side of the heart.[73] Indeed, as many as one third of patients with the carcinoid syndrome ultimately develop evidence of tricuspid or pulmonary valve disease.[74] Cardiac surgery may be useful in selected patients in whom the metastatic disease and the carcinoid syndrome are reasonably controlled and right-sided congestive heart failure is dominating the clinical picture.[75]

**Anesthesia Considerations.** Patients with the carcinoid syndrome may tolerate anesthesia poorly.[6, 76–79] Bronchospasm and hypotension are the usual problems encountered, but on rare occasion hypertensive crises may be seen. In general, the major problems can be ascribed to either serotonin or kallikrein-bradykinin. Careful preoperative assessment and treatment is mandatory, and the anesthetist must be prepared for the potential intraoperative problems that may occur. One of the keys to successful anesthetic management of patients with carcinoid is good communication between oncologist, surgeon, and anesthetist. The suggested management for such patients includes preoperative hydration and premedication with an antiserotonin agent such as cyproheptadine and in severe cases with an antibradykinin agent (phenothiazine). Glucocorticoids may also be given. Every effort should be made to avoid factors that precipitate a carcinoid crisis, such as prolonged attempts at intubation and manually stimulating the tumor. For example, aggressive scrubbing of the abdominal wall in a patient with hepatomegaly may precipitate release of vasoactive substances.

The intraoperative management of the carcinoid syndrome has been dramatically simplified by the availability of the somatostatin analogue octreotide. Previously untreated patients with metastatic carcinoid and the carcinoid syndrome should be premedicated with octreotide at a dose of 150 to 500 μg given subcutaneously at least three times daily for 3 to 7 days before surgery if time allows. In an emergency situation, 500 to 1000 μg may be given intravenously just before surgery and repeated intraoperatively as necessary. This drug should be available in the operating room for all patients with the carcinoid syndrome who are undergoing surgery.

## RADIATION THERAPY

Several reports suggest that radiation therapy can play a modest palliative role in the management of selected patients with inoperable carcinoid tumors.[80, 81] In the past, one study suggested that whole abdomen radiation therapy may be useful in some patients,[82] but the subsequent experience at the same institution failed to support the use of this modality.[83] At present, the main indication for the use of radiation therapy is in the palliative treatment of painful bone metastases.[19]

## CHEMOTHERAPY

Cytotoxic chemotherapy plays only a minimal role in the management of metastatic carcinoid, and it should be

avoided in the early stages of the disease.[84] The indolent course of the tumor in many patients, the exacerbation of symptoms that may result from treatment, and the marginal evidence for a life-prolonging effect of chemotherapy all support this recommendation. However, systemic chemotherapy is sometimes justifiable in patients with progressive, symptomatic tumors that have failed more conservative symptomatic treatment. This is particularly true of rare variants of malignant carcinoids that behave in a particularly aggressive fashion such as the anaplastic neuroendocrine tumors.[85] Systemic chemotherapy may also be indicated after hepatic artery occlusion, as discussed further on. Several end points in the literature are used to claim success of a particular agent in single-institution, nonrandomized trials. End points include relief of diarrhea, wheezing, and flushing; reduction of blood or urine levels of biochemical markers to less than 50%; and reduction of tumor mass.

**Single-Agent Chemotherapy.** The results obtained to date with single-agent chemotherapy are summarized in Table 71–6. The highest response rate (CR + PR) shown in this table is for melphalan (28%), but there is a wide consensus that melphalan is not useful in this disease when administered alone. Similarly, streptozocin, doxorubicin, and 5-fluorouracil all yield response rates of at least 20%, but they are nearly always short in duration. Indeed, only rarely has single-agent chemotherapy been associated with long-lasting responses. An example of such a rare event was reported by van Hazel and colleagues, in which one patient enjoyed more than an 8-year response to intermittent dactinomycin therapy.[86]

**Combination Chemotherapy.** The response rates achieved to date with combination chemotherapy are superior to those seen with single-agent therapy but only marginally superior for most combinations that are given without hepatic artery occlusion before the chemotherapy (Table 71–7). The combination of 5-fluorouracil plus streptozocin was one of the treatment arms in a randomized multi-institutional trial performed by investigators in the Eastern Cooperative Oncology Group.[87] This randomized trial compared 5-fluorouracil plus streptozocin with cyclophosphamide plus streptozocin in more than 80 patients. The objective response rates were 33% and 26%, respectively, but this was not a

*Table 71–6.* **Single-Agent Systemic Therapy for Carcinoid Tumors**

| Drug | No. of Patients (CR + PR/Total) | Response Rate (%) |
|---|---|---|
| Melphalan[112] | 5/18 | 28 |
| Streptozocin[113] | 7/31 | 23 |
| Doxorubicin[88, 113, 114] | 26/125 | 21 |
| 5-Fluorouracil[87, 113, 115] | 10/49 | 20 |
| Dactinomycin[116] | 4/22 | 18 |
| Cyclophosphamide[87, 113, 115, 117] | 4/25 | 16 |
| Dacarbazine[11, 116, 118] | 11/73 | 15 |
| Tamoxifen[112, 119, 120, 121] | 2/14 | 14 |
| Etoposide[122] | 2/17 | 12 |
| Cisplatin[123, 124] | 1/16 | 6 |
| Interferon alfa[95] | 16/111 | 15 |
| Octreotide[106] | 4/25 | 16 |

CR + PR, Number of complete plus partial responses as defined by a 50% or greater reduction in the sum of the products of measurements of the greater and lesser diameters of all measurable lesions.

*Table 71–7.* Combination Therapy for Carcinoid Tumors

| Drug Combination | No. of Patients (CR + PR/Total) | Response Rate (%) |
|---|---|---|
| Doxo + FU + dacarbazine + streptozocin[72] | 21/28 | 75* |
| Doxo + FU + cyclophosphamide + streptozocin[125] | 20/56 | 36 |
| Doxo + FU + cyclophosphamide[126] | 5/17 | 29 |
| Cyclophosphamide + streptozocin[87] | 12/47 | 26 |
| FU + streptozocin[87, 126, 127] | 42/180 | 23 |
| Cyclophosphamide + methotrexate[128, 129] | 6/27 | 22 |
| Doxo + streptozocin (q wk)[130] | 2/9 | — |

*Chemotherapy given after chemoembolization or hepatic artery ligation, as described in the text.
CR + PR, Number of complete plus partial responses as defined in Table 71–6; FU, 5-fluorouracil; Doxo, doxorubicin (Adriamycin).

statistically significant difference. The Eastern Cooperative Oncology Group then proceeded with another randomized study that compared streptozocin and 5-fluorouracil with monthly doxorubicin.[88] The streptozotocin was given every 10 weeks instead of every 5 weeks in an attempt to reduce the incidence of nausea and vomiting. The response rate in both arms was 23%. The median survival in most chemotherapy trials in patients with metastatic carcinoid tumors ranged between 8 and 12 months.

**Hepatic Artery Infusion Chemotherapy.** The role of chemotherapy by hepatic artery infusion is controversial.[18, 89] We currently avoid this technique because of the prolonged hospitalization that often results and because of the complications of the procedure. Moreover, the available data suggest that tumor shrinkage is no more likely with this approach than it is with single-agent therapy or combination chemotherapy (Table 71–8).

**Hepatic Arterial Devascularization Followed by Chemotherapy.** A growing body of evidence suggests that this is the optimal approach to treatment for patients with liver-dominant metastatic disease, as reviewed by Moertel and colleagues.[72]

The combination most favored by these authors is the combination of 5-fluorouracil plus doxorubicin alternating with dacarbazine plus streptozocin.[72] This regimen was associated with a 75% regression rate in patients treated first with hepatic artery occlusion, and survival was better than in patients treated solely with hepatic artery occlusion. Significant nausea is the rule with this regimen, and the drug has caused the exacerbation of the carcinoid syndrome in some patients. The spectrum of toxicity is wide, given the

diverse list of toxic side effects possible with each of the individual agents. The protocol developed at the Mayo Clinic is as follows:[72] Patients with an indication for laparotomy, such as symptoms of intermittent small bowel obstruction, may undergo hepatic artery ligation, but most others are treated by hepatic artery catheterization followed by embolization with absorbable gelatin sponge or polyvinyl alcohol, or both. Octreotide is used to prevent an exacerbation of the symptoms from carcinoid syndrome induced by embolization. Subsequently, after full recovery from embolization, chemotherapy is initiated (usually 3 or 4 weeks after embolization). The regimen includes doxorubicin 60 mg/m$^2$ intravenous bolus on day 1 and dacarbazine at a daily dose of 250 mg/m$^2$ intravenous bolus on days 1 to 5. Four weeks later, streptozocin is given in a dose of 500 mg/m$^2$, and fluorouracil is given at 400 mg/m$^2$, both by intravenous injection daily for 5 days. At 8 weeks, the cycle is repeated, but the interval between the cycles of doxorubicin plus dacarbazine and 5-fluorouracil plus streptozocin is increased to 5 weeks. Chemotherapy is continued until the patient has stabilized at a maximal tumor regression. Doxorubicin is limited to a total dose of 400 mg/m$^2$, and streptozocin is discontinued if the serum creatinine level reaches 2 mg/dl or greater.

Preliminary studies from other institutions also suggest that chemoembolization in which cytotoxic agents are injected concomitantly with the embolic material is effective in some patients.[90–92] Chemoembolization appears to be reasonably well tolerated, and studies are needed to compare this approach to bland embolization followed by chemotherapy.

*Table 71–8.* Hepatic Artery Infusion Chemotherapy for the Treatment of Carcinoid Tumors Metastatic to Liver

| Drug/Study | No. of Patients (CR + PR/Total) | Response Rate (%) |
|---|---|---|
| 5-Fluorouracil | | |
| Reed[131] | 1/1 | — |
| Melia[132] | 2/15* | 13 |
| Farndon[133] | 0/2 | — |
| Murray-Lyon[134] | 2/2† | — |
| Overall | 5/20 | 25 |

*Three patients received fluorouracil by portal vein infusion.
†With ligation of hepatic artery.
CR + PR, Number of complete plus partial responses, as defined in Table 71–6.

## BIOLOGIC RESPONSE MODIFIERS

One of the exciting prospects for improving the treatment of carcinoid tumors lies with biologic response modifiers. Two major groups of agents have been evaluated: the interferons and analogues of somatostatin.

**Interferons.** Human leukocyte interferon and recombinant interferon alfa have both been used in the management of this disease.[93–105] In an initial study from Scandinavia,[94] 36 patients with metastatic carcinoid were treated with interferon at doses of 3 to 6 million units/day. Seventeen of 36 patients had an objective response with greater than 50% reduction of urinary 5-HIAA. Four of these 17 patients had a significant tumor response (11%) with two complete remissions. Subsequently, in a large prospective study 111 patients were treated with interferon[95] and achieved an objective tumor response of 15%. Fifty-three of these patients had received prior chemotherapy with 5-fluorouracil and streptozocin. Survival of patients treated with interferon alone was more than 80 months, and in patients who received chemotherapy followed by interferon, survival was 64 months. This was significantly better than the 8 to 12 month survival in historical controls who received chemotherapy alone. These results could be influenced by patient selection and need to be confirmed by randomized studies. Interferon treatment was associated with side effects that included flu-like syndrome (89%), fatigue (70%), weight loss (57%), cytopenias (31%), liver function abnormalities (31%), and clinical thyroid disease in 76% of patients with thyroid antibodies. The toxicity of the interferons appears tolerable, but the optimal dose and preparation of interferon remains undefined, and some reports have been pessimistic.[105] More recent efforts to use interferons in combination with octreotide suggest that this combination may be superior to the use of interferon alone.[106]

**Somatostatin Analogues.** An important advance in the palliative management of the carcinoid syndrome has been achieved with the availability of octreotide, an analogue of natural somatostatin. In the initial experience using octreotide in 53 patients with metastatic carcinoid and carcinoid syndrome, 25 patients were treated at a dose of 150 μg subcutaneously three times daily. Flushing and diarrhea associated with the syndrome were promptly relieved in 22 patients. Eighteen of 25 (72%) patients had a greater than 50% reduction of urinary 5-HIAA after therapy.[107] Subsequently, 28 patients were treated with a higher dose of 500 μg three times daily.[109] All patients had a decrease in urinary 5-HIAA and 18 of 28 patients had a greater than 50% reduction. Although octreotide reduces the size of carcinoid tumors in only 5 to 11% of cases, the drug can dramatically improve the symptoms of the carcinoid syndrome.[107–110] One study suggested that a good response to octreotide may be predicted by measuring the level of somatostatin receptors in malignant neuroendocrine tissue.[111] Currently, however, the same information can be obtained by performing an octreoscan because avid uptake on the scan is highly predictive of a favorable response to octreotide.

## SUMMARY OF TREATMENT

**Management of the Tumor.** Surgical resection is the mainstay of management for carcinoid tumors. The most common site of metastatic disease is the liver, which may benefit from surgical resection if the disease is limited. Radiofrequency ablation can be used to destroy tumors up to 4 cm in diameter by sound waves. It may be used as an adjunct to surgical resection or in lieu of surgery in some cases. More extensive disease in the liver may respond to hepatic artery embolization or hepatic artery ligation followed by systemic chemotherapy (doxorubicin plus dacarbazine plus streptozocin plus fluorouracil) as described by Moertel and associates.[72] Progressive disease with symptoms related to tumor mass may be treated with interferon or experimental chemotherapy. Occasionally patients with carcinoid heart disease may benefit from tricuspid valve replacement and pulmonary valvectomy.

**Management of the Carcinoid Syndrome.** Patients with highly symptomatic carcinoid tumors should be carefully assessed for pharmacologic control of the various forms of the carcinoid syndrome and should be given nutritional supplementation, including niacin. Flushing can be treated by avoiding precipitating factors, such as certain foods or alcohol. Diarrhea can be treated with nonprescription antidiarrheal agents or in severe cases tincture of opium. Wheezing can be treated with bronchodilators. If these symptomatic measures fail to control the symptoms of the carcinoid syndrome, the patient should be treated with octreotide, which is the gold standard for the management of hormone-related clinical symptoms. The usual starting dose is 150 μg administered subcutaneously three times daily. If symptom control is only partial at this dosage level, larger doses can be tried (from 250 to 500 μg TID). A microencapsulated long-acting release (LAR) formulation of octreotide has been developed for once-monthly intramuscular dosing. A multicenter study demonstrated that once steady-state concentrations are achieved, octreotide LAR given at 4-week intervals controls the symptoms of carcinoid syndrome at least as well as three daily shots. This has the potential for improving the patient's quality of life. Octreotide should also be administered prophylactically at times of stress that might induce symptoms, such as before and after surgery or chemotherapy. Further clinical trials are needed to identify more effective agents. Radioactive somatostatin analogues are in phase I testing, and angiogenesis inhibitors will be evaluated in the near future. Some of the newer chemotherapy agents are being tested in phase II studies.

## SUGGESTIONS FOR ADDITIONAL READING

Moertel CG. An odyssey in the land of small tumors. J Clin Oncol 1987;5:1503–22. *This review is based on Dr. Moertel's Karnofsky Memorial Lecture delivered to the American Society of Clinical Oncology in May 1987.*

Grahame-Smith DG. What is the cause of the carcinoid flush? Gut 1987;28:1413–6. *This article presents a brief discussion of the various kinds of carcinoid flush and their putative causes.*

Gorden P, Comi RJ, Maton PN, Go VLW. Somatostatin and somatostatin analogue (SMS 201–995) in treatment of hormone-secreting tumors of the pituitary and gastrointestinal tract and non-neoplastic diseases of the gut. Ann Intern Med 1989;110:35–50. *This article discusses an NIH conference summarizing the biology of somatostatin and the use of octreotide acetate. The authors state that 90% of patients with flushing due to the carcinoid syndrome respond to this therapy.*

Moertel CG, Johnson CM, McKusick MA, et al. The management of patients with advanced carcinoid tumors and islet cell carcinomas. Ann Intern Med 1994;120:302–9. *This review emphasizes embolization followed by chemotherapy for liver-dominant disease.*

Kulke MH, Mayer RJ. Carcinoid tumors. N Engl J Med 1999;340:858–68. *This is an excellent review of the subject.*

## REFERENCES

1. Richardson CT, Walsh JH. The value of a histamine H2-receptor antagonist in the management of patients with the Zollinger-Ellison syndrome. N Engl J Med 1976;294:133–5.
2. Salyer DC, Salyer WR, Eggleston JC. Bronchial carcinoid tumors. Cancer 1975;36:1522–37.
3. Godwin JD II, Brown CC. Comparative epidemiology of carcinoid and oat-cell tumors of the lung. Cancer 1977;40:1671–3.
4. Gordon DL, Lo MC, Schwartz MA. Carcinoid of the pancreas. Am J Med 1971;51:412–5.

5. Hirata Y, Sakamoto N, Yamamoto H, et al. Gastric carcinoid with ectopic production of ACTH and beta-MSH. Cancer 1976;37:377–85.

6. Friesen SR, Hermreck AS, Mantz FA Jr. Glucagon, gastrin, and carcinoid tumors of the duodenum, pancreas, and stomach: polypeptide "apudomas" of the foregut. Am J Surg 1974;127:90–101.

7. Chatterjee K, Heather JC. Carcinoid heart disease from primary ovarian carcinoid tumors: a case report and review of the literature. Am J Med 1968;45:643–8.

8. Albores-Saavedra J, Larraza O, Poucell S, Rodriguez Martinez HA. Carcinoid of the uterine cervix: additional observations on a new tumor entity. Cancer 1976;38:2328–42.

9. Berdjis C, Mostofi FK. Carcinoid tumors of the testis. J Urol 1977:118:777–82.

10. Sullivan JL, Packer JT, Bryant M. Primary malignant carcinoid of the testis. Arch Pathol Lab Med 1981;105:515–7.

11. Salyer WR, Salyer DC, Eggleston JC. Carcinoid tumors of the thymus. Cancer 1976;37:958–73.

12. Kojiro M, Ohishi H, Isobe H. Carcinoid tumor occurring in cystic teratoma of the kidney: a case report. Cancer 1976;8:1636–40.

13. Goldman NC, Hood CI, Singleton GT. Carcinoid of the larynx. Arch Otolaryngol 1969;90:64–7.

14. Berg B, Biorklund A, Grimelius L, et al. A new pattern of multiple endocrine adenomatosis: chemodectoma, bronchial carcinoid, GH-producing pituitary adenoma, and hyperplasia of the parathyroid glands, and antral and duodenal gastrin cells. Acta Med Scand 1976;200:321–6.

15. Oberg K, Wide L. hCG and hCG subunits as tumor markers in patients with endocrine pancreatic tumors and carcinoids. Acta Endocrinol (Copenh) 1981;98:256–60.

16. Feldman JM, Plonk JW, Bivens CH, et al. Growth hormone and prolactin secretion in the carcinoid syndrome. Am J Med Sci 1975;269:333–47.

17. Melmon KL. The endocrinologic manifestations of the carcinoid tumor. In: Williams RH, ed. Textbook of Endocrinology. 5th ed. Philadelphia: WB Saunders, 1974:1084.

18. Grahame-Smith DG. The carcinoid syndrome. London: William Heinemann Medical Books, 1972.

19. Jager RM, Polk HC Jr. Carcinoid apudomas. Curr Probl Cancer 1977;1:1–53.

20. Moertel CG. Karnofsky memorial lecture: an odyssey in the land of small tumors. J Clin Oncol 1987;5:1502–22.

21. Dusmet M, McKneally MF. Bronchial and thymic carcinoid tumors: a review. Digestion 1994;55:70.

22. Bonato M, Cerati M, Pagani A, et al. Differential diagnostic patterns of lung neuroendocrine tumors. Virchows Arch (Pathol Anat) 1992;420:201–11.

23. Hasleton PS. Histopathology and prognostic factors in bronchial carcinoid tumors. Thorax 1994;49:Suppl:S56–62.

24. Moertel CG, Dockerty MB, Judd ES. Carcinoid tumors of the vermiform appendix. Cancer 1968;21:270–8.

25. Chaudhry A, Funa K, Oberg K. Expression of growth factor peptides and their receptors in neuroendocrine tumors of the digestive system. Acta Oncol 1993;32:107–14.

26. Creutzfeld W. Historical background and natural history of carcinoids. Digestion 1994;55:Suppl 3:3–10.

27. Wilander E. Diagnostic pathology of gastrointestinal and pancreatic neuroendocrine tumours. Acta Oncol 1989;28:363–9.

28. Wilander E, Scheibenpflug L, Eriksson B, Oberg K. Diagnostic criteria of classical carcinoids. Acta Oncol 1991;30:469–75.

29. Kujari H, Joensuu H, Klemi P, et al. A flow cytometric analysis of 23 carcinoid tumors. Cancer 1988;61:2517–20.

30. Tsushima K, Nagorney DM, Weiland LH, Lieber MM. The relationship of flow cytometric DNA analysis and clinicopathology in small-intestinal carcinoids. Surgery 1989;105:366–73.

31. Chaudhry A, Oberg K, Wilander E. A study of biological behavior based on the expression of a proliferating antigen in neuroendocrine tumors of the digestive system. Tumor Biol 1992;13:27–30.

32. Johnson LA, Lavin P, Moertel CG, et al. Carcinoids: the association of histologic growth pattern and survival. Cancer 1983;51:882–9.

33. Strodel WE, Vinik AI, Jaffe BM, et al. Substance P in the localization of a carcinoid tumor. J Surg Oncol 1984;27:106–11.

34. Norheim I, Wilander E, Oberg K, et al. Tachykinin production by carcinoid tumours in culture. Eur J Cancer Clin Oncol 1987;23:689–95.

35. Bishop AE, Hamid QA, Adams C, et al. Expression of tachykinins by ileal and lung carcinoid tumors assessed by combined in situ hybridization, immunocytochemistry, and radioimmunoassay. Cancer 1989;63:1129–37.

36. Berger G, Trouillas J, Bloch B, et al. Multihormonal carcinoid tumor of the pancreas: secreting growth hormone-releasing factor as a cause of acromegaly. Cancer 1984;54:2097–108.

37. Aldrich LB, Moattari AR, Vinik AI. Distinguishing features of idiopathic flushing and carcinoid syndrome. Arch Intern Med 1988;148:2614–8.

38. Pellika PA, Tajik AJ, Khandheria BK, et al. Carcinoid heart disease: clinical and echocardiographic spectrum in 74 patients. Circulation 1993;1987:1188–96.

39. Connolly HM. Outcome of cardiac surgery for carcinoid heart disease. J Am Coll Cardiol 1995;25:410–6.

40. Feldmann JM, Odorisio TM. The role of neuropeptides and serotonin in the diagnosis of carcinoid tumors. Am J Med 1986;81:41–8.

41. Stridsberg M, Oberg K, Li Q, Engstrom U, Lundqvist G. Measurement of chromogranin A, chromogranin B, (secretogranin I), chromogranin C (secretogranin II) and pancreastatin in plasma and urine from patients with carcinoid tumors and endocrine pancreatic tumors. J Endocrinol 1995;144:49–59.

42. Moinuddin M, Dean P, Vander Zwaag R, Dragutsky M. The limitation of liver function tests in metastatic carcinoid tumors. Cancer 1987;59:1304–6.

43. Bomanji J, Levison DA, Zuzarte J, Britton KE. Imaging of carcinoid tumors with iodine-123 metaiodobenzylguanidine. J Nucl Med 1987;28:1907–10.

44. Jodrell DI, Irvine AT, McCready VR, et al. The use of $^{131}$I-MIBG in the imaging of metastatic carcinoid tumours. Br J Cancer 1988;58:663–4.

45. Krenning EP. Somatostatin receptor scintigraphy with [$^{111}$In-DTPA-D-Phe1]-and [$^{123}$I I-Tyr3]-octreotide: the Rotterdam experience with more than 1000 patients. Eur J Nucl Med 1993;20:716–31.

46. Reubi JC. Expression of somatostatin receptors in normal, inflamed, and neoplastic human gastrointestinal tissues. Ann NY Acad Sci 1994;733:122–37.

47. Krenning EP, Kwekkeboom DJ, Pauwels S, et al. Somatostatin receptor scintigraphy. In: Freeman LM, ed. Nuclear Medicine Annual 1995. New York: Raven Press.

48. Thompson GB, van Heerden JA, Martin JK Jr, et al. Carcinoid tumors of the gastrointestinal tract: presentation, management, and prognosis. Surgery 1985;98:1054–63.

49. Sauven P, Ridge JA, Quan SH, Sigurdson ER. Anorectal carcinoid tumors: is aggressive surgery warranted? Ann Surg 1990;211:67–71.

50. Greenberg RS, Baumgarten DA, Clark WS, et al. Prognostic factors for gastrointestinal and bronchopulmonary carcinoid tumors. Cancer 1987;60:2476–83.

51. Ahlman H, Schersten T, Tisell LE. Surgical treatment of patients with the carcinoid syndrome. Acta Oncol 1989;28:403–7.

52. Moertel CG, Weiland LH, Nagorney DM, Dockerty MB. Carcinoid tumor of the appendix: treatment and prognosis. N Engl J Med 1987;317:1699–1701.

53. Syracuse DC, Perzin KH, Price JB, et al. Carcinoid tumors of the appendix: mesoappendiceal extension and nodal metastases. Ann Surg 1979;190:58–63.

54. Eckhauser FE, Argenta LC, Strodel WE, et al. Mesenteric angiopathy, intestinal gangrene, and midgut carcinoids. Surgery 1981;90:720–8.

55. Burke M, Shepherd N, Mann CV. Carcinoid tumours of the rectum and anus. Br J Surg 1987;74:358–61.

56. Blondal T, Grimelius L, Nou E, et al. Argyrophil carcinoid tumors of the lung: incidence, clinical study, and follow-up of 46 patients. Chest 1980;78:840–4.

57. Aberg T, Blondal T, Nou E, Malmaeus J. The choice of operation for bronchial carcinoids. Ann Thorac Surg 1981;32: 19–22.

58. Zeegen R, Rothwell-Jackson R, Sandler M. Massive hepatic resection for the carcinoid syndrome. Gut 1969;10: 617–22.

59. Gillett DJ, Smith RC. Treatment of the carcinoid syndrome by hemihepatectomy and radical excision of the primary lesion. Am J Surg 1974;128:95–9.

60. Battersby C, Egerton WS. A carcinoid saga. Aust N Z J Surg 1974;44:32–84.

61. Que FG, Nagorney DM, Batts KP, et al. Hepatic resection for metastatic neuroendocrine carcinomas. Am J Surg 1995;169:36–43.

62. Le Treut YP, Delpero JR, Dousset B, et al. Results of liver transplantation in the treatment of metastatic neuroendocrine tumors: a 31-case French multicentric report. Ann Surg 1997;225:355–64.

63. McDermott WV Jr, Hensle TW. Metastatic carcinoid to the liver treated by hepatic dearterialization. Ann Surg 1974;180:305–8.

64. Jugdutt BI, Watanabe M, Turner FW. Hepatic artery ligation in treatment of carcinoid syndrome. Can Med Assoc J 1975;112:325–7.

65. Khoury GA, Divine T, Bolt DE. Complete liver dearterialization and the carcinoid syndrome. Br J Surg 1979;66:253–6.

66. Melia WM, Nunnerley HB, Johnson PJ, Williams R. Use of arterial devascularization and cytotoxic drugs in 30 patients with the carcinoid syndrome. Br J Cancer 1982;46:331–9.

67. Allison DJ, Modlin IM, Jenkins WJ. Treatment of carcinoid liver metastases by hepatic-artery embolization. Lancet 1977;2:1323–5.

68. Mitty HA, Warner RR, Newman LH, et al. Control of carcinoid syndrome with hepatic artery embolization. Radiology 1985;155:623–6.

69. Carrasco CH, Chuang VP, Wallace S. Apudomas metastatic to the liver: treatment by hepatic artery embolization. Radiology 1983;149:79–83.

70. Odurny A, Birch SJ. Hepatic arterial embolization in patients with metastatic carcinoid tumours. Clin Radiol 1985;36:597–602.

71. Helmer RE III, Morettin LB, Costanzi JJ. Hepatic artery occlusion with perfusion in the treatment of carcinoid syndrome. Oncology 1981;38:361–4.

72. Moertel CG, Johnson CM, McKusick MA, et al. The management of patients with advanced carcinoid tumors and islet cell carcinomas. Ann Intern Med 1994;120:302–9.

73. Ross EM, Roberts WC. The carcinoid syndrome: comparison of 21 necropsy subjects with carcinoid heart disease to 15 necropsy subjects without carcinoid heart disease. Am J Med 1985;79:339–54.

74. Pellikka PA, Tajik AJ, Khandheria MK, et al. Carcinoid heart disease: clinical and echocardiographic spectrum in 74 patients. Circulation 1993;87:1188–96.

75. Connolly HM, Nishimura RA, Smith HC, et al. Outcome of cardiac surgery for carcinoid heart disease. J Am Coll Cardiol 1995;25:410–6.

76. Marsh HM, Martin JK, Kvols LK, et al. Carcinoid crisis during anesthesia: successful treatment with a somatostatin analogue. Anesthesiology 1987;66:89–91.

77. Vaughn DJ, Brunner MD. Anaesthesia for patients with carcinoid syndrome. Int Anaesthesiol Clin 1997;35:120–42.

78. Murphy DM, Lockhart CH, Burrington JD. Anaesthetic considerations in bronchial adenoma. Can Anaesth Soc J 1975;22:710–4.

79. Desmonts JM. In: Conseiller C, eds. Anaesthesia and postoperative care in uncommon diseases, post graduate course. XIIth International Meeting of Anesthesiology and Resuscitation, 1980. New York: Elsevier North-Holland, 1981:159.

80. Samlowski WE, Eyre HJ, Sause WT. Evaluation of the response of unresectable carcinoid tumors to radiotherapy. Int J Radiat Oncol Biol Phys 1986;12:301–5.

81. Abrams RA, King D, Wilson JF. Objective response of malignant carcinoid to radiation therapy. Int J Radiat Oncol Biol Phys 1987;13:869–73.

82. Gaitan-Gaitan A, Rider WD, Bush RS. Carcinoid tumor-cure by irradiation. Int J Radiat Oncol Biol Phys 1975;1:9–13.

83. Keane TJ, Rider WD, Harwood AR, et al. Whole abdominal radiation in the management of metastatic gastrointestinal carcinoid tumor. Int J Radiat Oncol Biol Phys 1981;7:1519–21.

84. Moertel CG. Treatment of the carcinoid tumor and the malignant carcinoid syndrome. J Clin Oncol 1983;1:727–40. Review.

85. Moertel CG, Kvols LK, O'Connell MJ, Rubin J. Treatment of neuroendocrine carcinomas with combined etoposide and cisplatin; evidence of major therapeutic activity in the anaplastic variants of these neoplasms. Cancer 68:227–32, 1991.

86. van Hazel GA, Rubin J, Moertel CG. Treatment of metastatic carcinoid tumor with dactinomycin or dacarbazine. Cancer Treat Rep 1983;67:583–5.

87. Moertel CG, Hanley JA. Combination chemotherapy trials in metastatic carcinoid tumor and the malignant carcinoid syndrome. Cancer Clin Trials 1979;2:327–34.

88. Engstrom PF, Lavin PT, Moertel CG, et al. Streptozocin plus fluorouracil versus doxorubicin therapy for metastatic carcinoid tumor. J Clin Oncol 1984;2:1255–9.

89. Hill GJ. Carcinoid tumors: pharmacological therapy. Oncology 1971;25:329–43.

90. Ruszniewski P, Rougier P, Roche A, et al. Hepatic arterial chemoembolization in patients with liver metastases of endocrine tumors. A prospective phase II study in 24 patients. Cancer 1993;71:2624–30.

91. Wangberg B, Geterud K, Nilsson O, et al. Embolization therapy in the midgut carcinoid syndrome: just tumor ischemia? Acta Oncol 1993;32:251–6.

92. Hajarizadeh H, Ivancev K, Mueller CR, et al. Effective palliative treatment of metastatic carcinoid tumors with intra-arterial chemotherapy/chemoembolization combined with octreotide acetate. Am J Surg 1992;163:479–3.

93. Oberg K, Funa K, Alm G. Effects of leukocyte interferon on clinical symptoms and hormone levels in patients with mid-gut carcinoid tumors and carcinoid syndrome. N Engl J Med 1983;309:129–33.

94. Oberg K, Norheim I, Lind E, et al. Treatment of malignant carcinoid tumors with human leukocyte interferon: long-term results. Cancer Treat Rep 1986;70:1297–1304.

95. Oberg K, Eriksson B. The role of interferons in the management of carcinoid tumors. Acta Oncol 1991;30:519–22.

96. Biesma B, Willemse PH, Mulder NH, et al. Recombinant interferon alpha-2b in patients with metastatic apudomas: effect on tumours and tumor markers. Br J Cancer 1992;66:850–5.

97. Basser RL, Lieschke GJ, Sheridan WP, et al. Recombinant alpha-2b interferon in patients with malignant carcinoid tumor. Aust N Z J Med 1991;21:875–8.

98. Joensuu H, Kumpulainen E, Grohn P. Treatment of metastatic carcinoid tumor with recombinant interferon alfa. Eur J Cancer 1992;28A:1650–3.

99. Schober C, Schmoll E, Schmoll HJ, et al. Antitumor effect and symptomatic control with interferon alpha 2b in patients with endocrine active tumours. Eur J Cancer 1992;28A:1664–6.

100. Di Bartolomeo M, Bajetta E, Zilembo N, et al. Treatment of carcinoid syndrome with recombinant interferon alpha-2a. Acta Oncol 1993;32:235–8.

101. Ahren B, Engman K, Lindblom A. Tolerance to long-term treatment of malignant midgut carcinoid with a highly purified human leukocyte alpha-interferon. Anticancer Res 1992;12:881–4.

102. Ahren B, Engman K, Lindblom A. Treatment of malignant midgut carcinoid with a highly purified human leukocyte alpha interferon. Anticancer Res 1992;12:129–33.

103. Smith DB, Scarffe JH, Wagstaff J, Johnston RJ. Phase II trial of rDNA alfa 2b interferon in patients with malignant carcinoid tumor. Cancer Treat Rep 1987;71:1265–6.

104. Oberg K, Alm G, Magnusson A, et al. Treatment of malignant carcinoid tumors with recombinant interferon alfa-2b: development of neutralizing interferon antibodies and possible loss of antitumor activity. J Natl Cancer Inst 1989;81:531–5.

105. Välimäki M, Jarvinen H, Salmela P, et al. Is the treatment of metastatic carcinoid tumor with interferon not as successful as suggested? Cancer 1991;67:547–49.

106. Janson ET, Oberg K. Long-term management of the carcinoid syndrome: treatment with octreotide alone and in combination with alpha-interferon. Acta Oncol 1993;32:225–9.

107. Kvols LK, Moertel CG, O'Connell MJ, et al. Treatment of the malignant carcinoid syndrome. Evaluation of a long-acting somatostatin analogue. N Engl J Med 1986;315:663–6.

108. Souquet J-C, Sassolas G, Forichon J, et al. Clinical and hormonal effects of a long-acting somatostatin analogue in pancreatic endocrine tumors and in carcinoid syndrome. Cancer 1987;59:1654–60.

109. Kvols LK, Moertel CG, Schutt AJ, Rubin J. Treatment of malignant carcinoid syndrome with a long acting somatostatin analogue (SMS 201–995): preliminary evidence that more is not better. Proc Am Soc Clin Oncol 1987;6:95.

110. Balks HJ, Conlon JM, Creutzfeldt W, Stockmann F. Effect of a long-acting somatostatin analogue (octreotide) on circulating tachykinins and the pentagastrin-induced carcinoid flush. Eur J Clin Pharmacol 1989;36:133–7.

111. Kvols LK, Reubi JC, Horisberger U, et al. The presence of somatostatin receptors in malignant neuroendocrine tumor tissue predicts responsiveness to octreotide. Yale J Biol Med 1992;65:505–18.

112. Lotito CA, Mengel CE. Effect of melphalan in the malignant carcinoid syndrome. Arch Intern Med 1969;124:36–8.

113. Moertel CG. Treatment of the carcinoid tumor and the malignant carcinoid syndrome. J Clin Oncol 1983;1:727–40.

114. Solomon A, Sonada T, Patterson FK. Response of metastatic malignant carcinoid tumor to Adriamycin (NSC-123127). Cancer Treat Rep 1976;60:273–6.

115. Legha SS, Valdivieso M, Nelson RS, et al. Chemotherapy for metastatic carcinoid tumors: experiences with 32 patients and a review of the literature. Cancer Treat Rep 1977;61:1699–1703.

116. van Hazel GA, Rubin J, Moertel CG. Treatment of metastatic carcinoid tumor with dactinomycin or dacarbazine. Cancer Treat Rep 1983;67:583–5.
117. Melia WM, Nunnerley HB, Johnson PJ, Williams R. Use of arterial devascularization and cytotoxic drugs in 30 patients with the carcinoid syndrome. Br J Cancer 1982;46:331–9.
118. Kessinger A, Foley JF, Lemon HM. Use of DTIC in the malignant carcinoid syndrome. Cancer Treat Rep 1977;61:101–2.
119. Haskell CM. In: Haskell CM, ed. Cancer Treatment. 2nd ed. Philadelphia: WB Saunders, 1985:591.
120. Stathopoulos GP, Karvountzis GG, Yiotis J. Tamoxifen in carcinoid syndrome. N Engl J Med 1981;305:52.
121. Myers CF, Ershler WB, Tannenbaum MA, Barth R. Tamoxifen and carcinoid tumor. Ann Intern Med 1982;96:383.
122. Kelsen D, Fiore J, Heelan R, et al. Phase II trial of etoposide in APUD tumors. Cancer Treat Rep 1987;71:305–7.
123. Moertel CG, Rubin J, O'Connell MJ. Phase II study of cisplatin therapy in patients with metastatic carcinoid tumor and the malignant carcinoid syndrome. Cancer Treat Rep 1986;70:1459–60.
124. Pratt CB, Hayes A, Green AA, et al. Pharmacokinetic evaluation of cisplatin in children with malignant solid tumors: a phase II study. Cancer Treat Rep 1981;65:1021–6.
125. Bukowski RM, Johnson KG, Peterson RF, et al. A phase II trial of combination chemotherapy in patients with metastatic carcinoid tumors: a Southwest Oncology Group Study. Cancer 1987;60:2891–5.
126. Chernicoff D, Bukowski RM, Groppe CW Jr, Hewlett JS. Combination chemotherapy for islet cell carcinoma and metastatic carcinoid tumors with 5-fluorouracil and streptozotocin. Cancer Treat Rep 1979;63:795–6.
127. Oberg K, Norheim I, Lundqvist G, Wide L. Cytotoxic treatment in patients with malignant carcinoid tumors: response to streptozocin—alone or in combination with 5-FU. Acta Oncol 1987;26:429–32.
128. Mengel CE. In: Holland JF, eds. Cancer medicine. Philadelphia: Lea & Febiger, 1982:1818.
129. Moertel CG, O'Connell MJ, Reitemeier RJ, Rubin J. Evaluation of combined cyclophosphamide and methotrexate therapy in the treatment of metastatic carcinoid tumor and the malignant carcinoid syndrome. Cancer Treat Rep 1984;68:665–7.
130. Frame J, Kelsen D, Kemeny N, et al. A phase II trial of streptozotocin and Adriamycin in advanced APUD tumors. Am J Clin Oncol 1988;11:490–5.
131. Reed ML. Treatment of disseminated carcinoid tumors including hepatic-artery catheterization. N Engl J Med 1963;269:1005–10.
132. Melia WM, Nunnerley HB, Johnson PJ, Williams R. Use of arterial devascularization and cytotoxic drugs in 30 patients with the carcinoid syndrome. Br J Cancer 1982;46:331–9.
133. Farndon JR. The carcinoid syndrome: methods of treatment and recent experience with hepatic artery ligation and infusion. Clin Oncol 1977;3:365–75.
134. Murray-Lyon IM, Parsons VA, Blendis LM, et al. Treatment of secondary hepatic tumours by ligation of hepatic artery and infusion of cytotoxic drugs. Lancet 1970;2:172–5.

# XV

# PRIMARY NEOPLASMS OF THE NERVOUS SYSTEM

# CHAPTER 72

# BRAIN

• TIMOTHY CLOUGHESY • MICHAEL T. SELCH • LINDA LIAU

In the United States, 35,000 primary brain tumors are diagnosed every year. Brain tumor is second only to stroke as a cause of neurologic death and causes 2.5% of all cancer deaths. Astrocytoma is the most common primary brain tumor (50%). In children, brain tumor is second only to leukemia as a cause of death. In the age group 15 to 34 years, brain tumor is the third most common cause of death.

Metastatic brain tumors are more prevalent than primary brain tumors. Autopsy series show that approximately 25 to 30% of patients with systemic cancer have involvement of the nervous system. This percentage translates to approximately 125,000 patients a year in the United States. Brain metastasis most commonly occurs in the setting of systemic relapse in patients with advanced disease. In 15% of cases, the primary cancer is heralded by neurologic symptoms. Metastatic brain tumors are reported to be solitary in 50% of patients.

The development of computed tomography (CT) and magnetic resonance imaging (MRI) techniques has resulted in earlier and more accurate diagnosis. Functional tests, magnetic resonance spectroscopy, thallium-201 spectroscopy, and positron emission tomography (PET) are useful in determining the grade of astrocytic tumors. They may separate tumor recurrence from radiation necrosis and help in obtaining the best site for stereotactic brain biopsy.

Despite significant progress in making a rapid and accurate diagnosis, the prognosis for malignant tumors remains poor. Because many different tumors can be identified in the brain and its coverings, a definitive pathologic diagnosis is strongly recommended prior to treatment.

Research efforts are expanding in molecular biology, and a phase III trial of *gene therapy* has completed enrollment. Changes in the sequence of treatment and new therapies are being studied. Antiangiogenesis agents, signal transduction inhibitors, anti-invasion agents, immunotoxins, immunotherapy, new chemotherapeutic agents, novel radiation sensitizers, advances in radiosurgery, interstial delivery methods, thermoablative techniques, and real-time MRI neurosurgical approaches are being studied for the treatment of primary and metastatic central nervous system (CNS) cancer.

## Natural History

### EPIDEMIOLOGY

At present, there are no known epidemiologic factors clearly related to gliomas or other types of CNS neoplasms. Incidence figures differ depending on the population studied. In one study, the average annual incidence rate for all primary brain tumors was estimated at 12.6 per 100,000 population,[1]

of which approximately 28% were gliomas. These figures, based on an analysis of the Rochester, Minnesota, population, represent combined autopsy and clinical statistics and are higher than in some other studies.[2] The finding of meningiomas, the most common type of previously undiagnosed brain tumor encountered at postmortem examination, probably explains the higher overall incidence rate of tumors and a lower relative percentage of gliomas in that study.[2, 3] Several surveys have described the preponderance of tumors of the astrocytoma series among males and of meningiomas among females.[1, 2] The higher incidence of gliomas in males seems to apply equally to adult and pediatric age groups in a ratio of 3:2. Incidence curves for gliomas show a peak between ages 6 and 10 and again between ages 45 and 64 years, after which the incidence declines.[4] Well-differentiated astrocytomas appear to be more common in a younger age group, whereas malignant astrocytomas and glioblastomas occur more frequently in older patients.[2] The incidence of gliomas is higher among North American whites, whereas meningiomas, pituitary adenomas, and nerve sheath tumors are more common among blacks.[5] The frequency with which the various tumors are encountered is given in Tables 72–1 and 72–2.

The epidemiology of metastatic lesions relates to the primary tumor type. The incidence rate for metastatic tumors to the nervous system is estimated at 11.1 per 100,000 population, with such tumors representing 41% of CNS neoplasms in a combined clinical and autopsy survey.[1, 6]

### Etiology

To date, the cause of most spontaneously occurring CNS tumors remains unknown. Radiation exposure has been cited as a possible etiologic factor in some tumors. Meningiomas, astrocytomas, and sarcomas have been reported in patients who have received radiation treatment for unrelated problems, for example, pituitary tumors. Studies of children irradiated for tinea capitis[7] and of atomic bomb survivors[8] suggest that children may be particularly sensitive to the effects of radiation with respect to CNS neoplasia. Underlying endocrine influences may be important because it appears that in both males and females the incidence decreases coincident with decreasing sex hormone levels.[4]

Neurofibromatosis consists of two distinct inherited disorders, the genes for which are located on separate chromosomes.[9] Neurofibromatosis type I (NF I) is characterized by multiple brown skin macules (café au lait spots), iris hamartomas (Lisch nodules), and multiple skin neurofibromas. It is also associated with optic gliomas, spinal and peripheral nerve neurofibromas, and bone abnormalities. Schwann's cell tumors may occur on any nerve in patients with NF I, but bilateral acoustic neuromas almost never

**Table 72–1.** Frequency of Intracranial Gliomas (All Ages)

| Type | % |
|---|---|
| Glioblastomas | 55.0 |
| Astrocytomas | 20.5 |
| Ependymomas | 6.0 |
| Medulloblastomas | 6.0 |
| Oligodendrogliomas | 5.0 |
| Choroid plexus papillomas | 2.0 |
| Colloid cysts | 2.0 |

From Koos WT, Miller MH. Intracranial tumors of infants and children. St. Louis: CV Mosby, 1971.

develop. In contrast, the hallmark of NF II is bilateral acoustic neuromas. Bilateral acoustic neuromas are inherited in an autosomal dominant pattern with greater than 95% penetrance so that any offspring of an affected parent has a 50% risk of developing these tumors.

Genetically, NF I and NF II are inherited as autosomal dominant disorders. The gene responsible for NF I is located on the long arm of chromasome 17 and has spontaneous mutations in 30% of cases. Its gene product, neurofibromin, is thought to play a tumor-suppressor role, suppressing the p21-*ras* oncogene pathway. NF II has been traced to a deletion within the q12 arm of chromosome 22. Spontaneous mutations occur in 50% of cases. Schwannomin, the gene product, is thought to be involved in cytoplasm and cell membrane, playing a role in cellular movement, division, growth, and communication. It has been suggested that growth factors play a role in the development of neurofibromas.

Tuberous sclerosis, another disorder with a genetic predisposition, is associated with mental retardation, acneiform facies, and intraventricular giant cell astrocytomas. Patients with Rendu-Osler-Weber syndrome are reported to develop cerebellar hemangioblastomas; Turcot's syndrome, a familial polyposis of the colon, is associated with malignant gliomas of the CNS.

Patients with meningiomas have often been found to have abnormalities of chromosome 22, usually in the form of translocations and dislocations. Attempts are being made to define different glioblastoma multiformes by genetic pathways.

Immunosuppression, in transplant recipients and patients with acquired immunodeficiency syndrome (AIDS), has been shown to increase markedly the risk of primary lymphoma of the brain. CNS lymphoma is also increased in patients with Sjögren's syndrome and immunoglobulin A deficiency.

**Table 72–2.** Frequency of Brain Tumors in Infancy and Childhood

| Type | % |
|---|---|
| Spongioblastomas, including cerebellar astrocytomas | 21.7 |
| Medulloblastomas | 18.9 |
| Astrocytomas | 10.1 |
| Ependymomas | 8.7 |
| Glioblastomas | 4.6 |

From Koos WT, Miller MH. Intracranial tumors of infants and children. St. Louis: CV Mosby, 1971.

Patients with CNS lymphomas also have a high incidence of infection with Epstein-Barr virus. DNA from tumor tissue but not from normal brain tissue was shown to contain the Epstein-Barr virus genome.

At present, there is little evidence that viral infections play a role in the other human CNS tumors. A human polyoma JC virus injected into primates has produced tumors compatible with human astrocytomas after an 18-month incubation period. Murine astrocytomas can be produced by purified avian sarcoma virus, and Rous sarcoma virus has produced a malignant astrocytoma in dogs.

Environmental carcinogens have not been proved to induce human brain tumors. Ethylnitrosoureas and methylnitrosoureas and anthracene derivatives induce glial tumors in the offspring of maternal rats treated with these agents. Vinyl chloride and rubber industry work have been implicated by a few clinical studies as risk factors in humans.

## MOLECULAR BIOLOGY

Information on the molecular basis of how oncogenes and tumor-suppressor genes determine the behavior of malignant cells is increasing at a rapid pace. The number of new oncogenes being reported in the literature is growing along with the definition of downstream events and the molecular pathways exploited. Tumor-suppressor genes and oncogenes associated with gliomas are listed in Table 72–3. Many of these oncogenes encode for growth factors or growth factor receptors. For example, the *erb*B oncogene expressed in some gliomas codes for the epidermal growth factor (EGF) receptor on the malignant cell's membrane, whereas the c-*sis* oncogene makes platelet-derived growth factor (PDGF). Many of the growth factor receptors that are encoded for by oncogenes are nonfunctional. The biologic behavior of cancer cells is probably determined by their particular combination of oncogenes. An understanding of the molecular biology of cancer not only gives insight into the development of cancer, but also yields new possibilities for therapeutic intervention. Readers interested in details on the genetic changes involving all tumors of the CNS are referred to the book edited by Kleihues and Cavenee.[10]

**Table 72–3.** Oncogenes and Tumor-Suppressor Genes in Brain Tumors

| Growth Factors | Tumor-Suppressor Genes |
|---|---|
| EGF-R | p53 |
| PDGF/PDGF-R | PTEN |
| FGF-2/FGF-R | mdm2-2 |
| IGFI/IGF-IR | NF1 |
| C-*eRB*-B2 | Rb |
| Hepatocyte growth factor | p16-cdkn2 |
| | APC |

| *Other Proto-Oncogenes* | |
|---|---|
| TGF-B | |
| *myc* | |
| *ras* | |
| *ros* | |
| *gli* | |

# BIOLOGY

**Primary Tumors.** The biology of primary tumors of the brain and spinal cord cannot be discussed without reference to their histologic classification. In a broad sense, neuroepithelial tumors derived from the three major glial cell types range from those made up of well-differentiated cells to highly anaplastic tumors in which the basic cell type is difficult to recognize. Astrocytomas, oligodendrogliomas, and ependymomas all exist in such a range of tumor variants.

The mitotic index of glioblastomas is surprisingly low, and kinetic studies have shown that more than 50% of the tumor cell population is in the nonproliferative ($G_0$) phase.[11] The picture is further complicated by the fact that glial tumors are often not homogeneous with respect to the degree of cell differentiation or the predominant cell type. This lack of homogeneity is reflected in the growth kinetics of the tumors.[12] The degree of malignancy of primary CNS tumors, however, is never less than that of the most anaplastic portion of the tumor. This is an important consideration when the physician is asked to make a statement regarding tumor prognosis on the basis of a needle biopsy specimen because this limited technique could introduce a sampling error.

Glial tumors grow primarily by contiguity, infiltrating the surrounding brain or cord parenchyma as they extend. Highly anaplastic tumors may grow so rapidly that excessive demands are placed on the regional blood and oxygen supply, resulting in regional tissue necrosis within the tumor. Glioblastomas may use a variety of molecular approaches to stimulate proliferation of neoplastic vessels within the neoplasm. Hemorrhage into tumors has been considered to occur more frequently than is seen clinically. Significant hemorrhage is encountered particularly in association with glioblastoma, oligodendrogliomas, and pituitary adenomas as well as with metastatic melanomas, choriocarcinomas, hypernephroma, and lung cancer.

In addition to growth by direct contiguous extension, primary tumors may extend within the CNS by implanting beneath the leptomeninges or the ependyma and by forming perineuronal and perivascular aggregates of the tumor cells beyond the margins of the main tumor mass. These formations, known as Scherer's secondary structures, are seen only in association with primary CNS tumors and may be indicative of early anaplasia.[13, 14] Tumor cells also seem capable of growing along heavily myelinated structures, such as the corpus callosum, expanding into another mass beyond the restrictive confines of the myelinated structure. This growth gives rise to the characteristic appearance of so-called butterfly lesions of the cerebral hemispheres. Approximately 2.5% of gliomas show evidence of multicentric origin.

All primary CNS tumors, but most commonly medulloblastomas, pineal cell tumors, germinomas, and fourth ventricle ependymomas as well as papillomas of the choroid plexus, appear capable of shedding cells into the cerebrospinal fluid (CSF), which can then be detected by cytologic examination. Retinoblastomas (see Chapter 77) share this property. Perhaps only the histologically most benign tumors do not seed into the CSF in this manner. Secondary tumor implants within the spinal subarachnoid space are, however, rare except for the group of tumors just listed.[15, 16] Metastasis

of primary malignant brain tumors outside the CNS is even more uncommon, although sporadic reports of such cases have appeared in the literature.[17–19]

As is the case with tumors of other organ systems, the presence of a primary brain tumor is accompanied by changes in the host's immune system. Careful studies of patients with malignant gliomas have shown that there is a decreased number of circulating lymphocytes, particularly T cells; decreased blastogenesis of lymphocytes; and depressed skin-test reactivity to common antigens.[20–23] A glioma-associated antigen has been postulated on the basis of some investigations,[24] whereas other studies point to the presence of a meningioma-associated antigen.[25, 26] There is some evidence for the presence of glioma-specific antibodies or antigen-antibody complexes, and the possibility exists that there are circulating blocking factors that impair the cytotoxic response to the tumor, such as transforming growth factor-$\beta$ (TGF-$\beta$).[27]

**Metastatic Tumors.** Metastatic tumors to the brain may arise from any primary neoplasm capable of hematogenous dissemination. The frequency with which different primary tumors are represented in one series is indicated in Table 72–4. Metastatic tumors probably appear with equal frequency among men and women. Surveys fail to substantiate that one hemisphere is more likely to be involved than the other.[28]

Certain primary neoplasms, in particular, carcinoma of the breast and lymphomas, tend to give rise to diffuse leptomeningeal carcinomatosis.[29] Dural invasion also is most common for metastatic tumors arising from the breast. Solitary brain metastases originate most commonly from the breast or hypernephroma primaries.

Although metastatic carcinomas may be in contact with the subarachnoid space or the ventricular system, allowing tumor cells to be recovered in the CSF, most such freely floating cells in the CSF rarely, if ever, give rise to subarachnoid implants over the spinal cord or cauda equina.[16] Sarcomatous tumors, by contrast, may give rise to such meningeal

*Table 72–4.* **Source of Metastatic Tumors to the Brain**

| Tumor | Neurology Statistics 456 PATIENTS (%) | Neurosurgery Statistics 2037 PATIENTS (%) | Autopsy Statistics 1067 CASES (%) |
|---|---|---|---|
| Lung | 40.0 | 36.0 | 34.0 |
| Breast | 21.0 | 14.0 | 22.0 |
| Hypernephroma | 7.5 | 8.0 | 6.0 |
| Melanoma | 4.5 | 5.0 | 5.5 |
| Gastrointestinal tract | 9.0 | 6.0 | 8.5 |
| Thyroid | 1.0 | 2.0 | 2.0 |
| Female genitalia | 4.0 | 3.0 | 4.5 |
| Male genitalia | 1.0 | 0.5 | 1.0 |
| Prostate | 1.0 | 0.5 | 2.0 |
| Face | 1.5 | 2.0 | 2.0 |
| Other carcinomas | 2.0 | 2.0 | 5.0 |
| Sarcomas | 2.0 | 1.0 | 3.0 |
| Unknown primary | 5.5 | 20.0 | 4.5 |

From Penzholz H. Metastatic diseases of the central nervous system caused by malignant tumors: a clinical study on the basis of 158 individual cases of a neurosurgical clinic. Acta Neurochir (Wien) 1968;Suppl 16:1–205.

metastases. The subject of metastatic tumors to the brain has been analyzed in detail.[27]

## CLASSIFICATION

Table 72–5 gives the classification of primary tumors of the CNS as recommended by the World Health Organization for universal adoption.[30]

## CLINICAL FEATURES

In time, all tumors may be expected to produce symptoms by one or more of the following mechanisms: (1) increased intracranial pressure, which may be due to the tumor mass, peritumoral edema, and obstruction of CSF pathways; (2) local biochemical changes, which may act to depolarize neurons within or adjacent to the tumor, triggering seizure activity; (3) local destruction of brain tissue, resulting in neurologic deficits; (4) stretching, distortion, or compression of surrounding neural structures (cranial nerves), which are themselves not infiltrated by tumors; (5) remote effects on other organ systems resulting from the alteration of neuroendocrine function or elaboration of active substances by the tumor; and (6) stretching of the dura and stretching or distortion of the basal arteries composing the circle of Willis, giving rise to headache.

Intracranial pressure may be elevated as a result of the

*Table 72–5.* **WHO Histologic Typing of Central Nervous System Tumors**

| | |
|---|---|
| *1* | *Tumors of Neuroepithelial Tissue* |
| 1.1 | *Astrocytic tumors* |
| 1.1.1 | Astrocytoma |
| 1.1.1.1 | Variants: Fibrillary |
| 1.1.1.2 | Protoplasmic |
| 1.1.1.3 | Gemistocytic |
| 1.1.2 | Anaplastic (malignant) astrocytoma |
| 1.1.3 | Glioblastoma |
| 1.1.3.1 | Variants: Giant cell glioblastoma |
| 1.1.3.2 | Gliosarcoma |
| 1.1.4 | Pilocytic astrocytoma |
| 1.1.5 | Pleomorphic xanthoastrocytoma |
| 1.1.6 | Subependymal giant cell astrocytoma (tuberous sclerosis) |
| 1.2 | *Oligodendroglial tumors* |
| 1.2.1 | Oligodendroglioma |
| 1.2.2. | Anaplastic (malignant) oligodendroglioma |
| 1.3 | *Ependymal tumors* |
| 1.3.1 | Ependymoma |
| 1.3.1.1 | Variants: Cellular |
| 1.3.1.2 | Papillary |
| 1.3.1.3 | Clear cell |
| 1.3.2 | Anaplastic (malignant) ependymoma |
| 1.3.3 | Myxopapillary ependymoma |
| 1.3.4 | Subependymoma |
| 1.4 | *Mixed gliomas* |
| 1.4.1 | Oligoastrocytoma |
| 1.4.2 | Anaplastic (malignant) oligoastrocytoma |
| 1.4.3 | Others |
| 1.5 | *Choroid plexus tumors* |
| 1.5.1 | Choroid plexus papilloma |
| 1.5.2 | Choroid plexus carcinoma |
| 1.6 | *Neuroepithelial tumors of uncertain origin* |
| 1.6.1 | Astroblastoma |
| 1.6.2 | Polar spongioblastoma |
| 1.6.3 | Gliomatosis cerebri |
| 1.7 | *Neuronal and mixed neuronal-glial tumors* |
| 1.7.1 | Gangliocytoma |
| 1.7.2 | Dysplastic gangliocytoma of cerebellum (Lhermitte-Duclos) |
| 1.7.3 | Desmoplastic infantile ganglioglioma |
| 1.7.4 | Dysembryoplastic neuroepithelial tumor |
| 1.7.5 | Ganglioglioma |
| 1.7.6 | Anaplastic (malignant) ganglioglioma |
| 1.7.7 | Central neurocytoma |
| 1.7.8 | Paraganglioma of the filum terminale |
| 1.7.9 | Olfactory neuroblastoma (esthesioneuroblastoma) |
| 1.7.9.1 | Variant: Olfactory neuroepithelioma |
| 1.8 | *Pineal parenchymal tumors* |
| 1.8.1 | Pineocytoma |
| 1.8.2 | Pineoblastoma |
| 1.8.3 | Mixed/transitional pineal tumors |
| 1.9 | *Embryonal tumors* |
| 1.9.1 | Medulloepithelioma |
| 1.9.2 | Neuroblastoma |
| 1.9.2.1 | Variant: Ganglioneuroblastoma |
| 1.9.3 | Ependymoblastoma |
| 1.9.4 | Primitive neuroectodermal tumors |
| 1.9.4.1 | Medulloblastoma |
| 1.9.4.1.1 | Variants: Desmoplastic medulloblastoma |
| 1.9.4.1.2 | Medullomyoblastoma |
| 1.9.4.1.3 | Melanotic medulloblastoma |
| *2* | *Tumors of Cranial and Spinal Nerves* |
| 2.1 | *Schwannoma* (neurilemoma, neurinoma) |
| 2.1.1 | Variants: Cellular |
| 2.1.2 | Plexiform |
| 2.1.3 | Melanotic |
| 2.2 | *Neurofibroma* |
| 2.2.1 | Circumscribed (solitary) |
| 2.2.2 | Plexiform |
| 2.3 | *Malignant peripheral nerve sheath tumor (MPNST) (neurogenic sarcoma, anaplastic neurofibroma, malignant schwannoma)* |
| 2.3.1 | Variants: Epithelioid |
| 2.3.2 | MPNST with divergent mesenchymal and/or epithelial differentiation |
| 2.3.3 | Melanotic |
| *3* | *Tumors of the Meninges* |
| 3.1 | *Tumors of meningothelial cells* |
| 3.1.1 | Meningioma |
| 3.1.1.1 | Variants: Meningothelial |
| 3.1.1.2 | Fibrous (fibroblastic) |
| 3.1.1.3 | Transitional (mixed) |
| 3.1.1.4 | Psammomatous |
| 3.1.1.5 | Angiomatous |
| 3.1.1.6 | Microcystic |
| 3.1.1.7 | Secretory |
| 3.1.1.8 | Clear cell |
| 3.1.1.9 | Chordoid |
| 3.1.1.10 | Lymphoplasmacyte-rich |
| 3.1.1.11 | Metaplastic |
| 3.1.2 | Atypical meningioma |
| 3.1.3 | Papillary meningioma |
| 3.1.4 | Anaplastic (malignant) meningioma |
| 3.1.3. | Papillary meningioma |
| 3.1.4 | Anaplastic (malignant) meningioma |
| 3.2 | *Mesenchymal, nonmeningothelial tumors* *Benign neoplasms* |
| 3.2.1 | Osteocartilaginous tumors |
| 3.2.2 | Lipoma |
| 3.2.3 | Fibrous histiocytoma |
| 3.2.4 | Others |

*Table continued on following page*

*Table 72–5.* **WHO Histologic Typing of Central Nervous System Tumors** *Continued*

|       | *Malignant neoplasms*                        |       |                                                      |
|-------|----------------------------------------------|-------|------------------------------------------------------|
| 3.2.5 | Hemangiopericytoma                           | 6     | *Cysts and Tumor-like Lesions*                       |
| 3.2.6 | Chondrosarcoma                               | 6.1   | Rathke's cleft cyst                                  |
| 3.2.6.1 | Variant: Mesenchymal chondrosarcoma        | 6.2   | Epidermoid cyst                                      |
| 3.2.7 | Malignant fibrous histiocytoma               | 6.3   | Dermoid cyst                                         |
| 3.2.8 | Rhabdomyosarcoma                             | 6.4   | Colloid cyst of the third ventricle                  |
| 3.2.9 | Meningeal sarcomatosis                       | 6.5   | Enterogenous cyst                                    |
| 3.2.10 | Others                                      | 6.6   | Neuroglial cyst                                      |
|       |                                              | 6.7   | Granular cell tumor (choristoma, pituicytoma)        |
| 3.3   | *Primary melanocytic lesions*                | 6.8   | Hypothalamic neuronal hamartoma                      |
| 3.3.1 | Diffuse melanosis                            | 6.9   | Nasal glial heterotopia                              |
| 3.3.2 | Melanocytoma                                 | 6.10  | Plasma cell granuloma                                |
| 3.3.3 | Malignant melanoma                           |       |                                                      |
| 3.3.3.1 | Variant: Meningeal melanomatosis           | 7     | *Tumors of the Sellar Region*                        |
|       |                                              | 7.1   | Pituitary adenoma                                    |
| 3.4   | *Tumors of uncertain histogenesis*           | 7.2   | Pituitary carcinoma                                  |
| 3.4.1 | Hemangioblastoma (capillary hemangioblastoma) | 7.3  | Craniopharyngioma                                    |
|       |                                              | 7.3.1 | Variants: Adamantinomatous                           |
| 4     | *Lymphomas and Hematopoietic Neoplasms*      | 7.3.2 | Papillary                                            |
| 4.1   | Malignant lymphomas                          | 8     | *Local Extensions From Regional Tumors*              |
| 4.2   | Plasmacytoma                                 |       |                                                      |
| 4.3   | Granulocytic sarcoma                         | 8.1   | Paraganglioma (chemodectoma)                         |
| 4.4   | Others                                       | 8.2   | Chordoma                                             |
|       |                                              | 8.3   | Chondroma, chondrosarcoma                            |
| 5     | *Germ Cell Tumors*                           | 8.4   | Carcinoma                                            |
| 5.1   | Germinoma                                    | 9     | *Metastatic Tumors*                                  |
| 5.2   | Embryonal carcinoma                          |       |                                                      |
| 5.3   | Yolk sac tumor (endodermal sinus tumor)      | 10    | *Unclassified Tumors*                                |
| 5.4   | Choriocarcinoma                              |       |                                                      |
| 5.5   | Teratoma                                     |       |                                                      |
| 5.5.1 | Immature                                     |       |                                                      |
| 5.5.2 | Mature                                       |       |                                                      |
| 5.5.3 | Teratoma with malignant transformation       |       |                                                      |
| 5.6   | Mixed germ cell tumors                       |       |                                                      |

From Kleihues P, Burger PC, Scheithauer BW. Histological typing of tumors of the central nervous system. World Health Organization, International Histological Classification of Tumors. Berlin: Springer-Verlag, 1993.

tumor mass itself, but sometimes the mass effect of peritumoral edema may be as great as, or greater than, that of the tumor nodule. Cerebral edema is a major contributing factor to the increased intracranial pressure. The magnitude of peritumoral edema is particularly great in more rapidly growing neoplasms and in the case of metastatic tumors. Intracranial pressure may also be elevated because the tumor and surrounding edema obstruct the ventricular system. This obstruction most commonly occurs at or near the interventricular foramen, at the third ventricle and the aqueduct of Sylvius, or near the outlet foramina of the fourth ventricle. Increased intracranial pressure gives rise to rather nonspecific symptoms and signs, including headache, nausea and vomiting, obscuration of vision, papilledema, and in young children spreading of cranial sutures.

The irritative action that tumor or edema may exert on the involved brain can lead to seizures, which may be focal or generalized. Rarely a prolonged state of seizure activity—status epilepticus—may develop, which could have a fatal outcome if it is not or cannot be treated adequately.

Local destruction of brain tissue may also be the result of tumor or peritumoral edema, or both, and can cause the loss of neural function appropriate to the area of brain involved. The resulting clinical picture can be quite variable and may include disturbances of motor, speed, sensory, visual, or intellectual function or personality changes. Cranial nerves often are stretched or distorted by tumor so as to interfere in their function. The clinical picture resulting from such cranial nerve deficit can be of localizing value, although stretching of the most frequently involved nerve—the abducens (VI)—is nonspecific and often does not aid the anatomic localization of the tumor. Intracranial tumors may also exhibit remote effects if they impinge on or involve neuroendocrine structures, such as the hypothalamus or pituitary gland.

## MECHANISMS OF DEATH

The most common cause of death from brain tumors is a herniation syndrome resulting from increased mass effect. In the case of cerebral hemisphere lesions, medial temporal lobe herniation commonly results in the medial displacement of the uncus of the temporal lobe, producing compression and stretching of the brain stem. Posterior fossa tumors may compress the lower brain stem directly or produce herniation of the cerebellar tonsils with medullary compression. In all these situations, coma and respiratory arrest ensue. Not infrequently the compressive effect on the brain stem is somewhat more gradual, and the patient first becomes comatose. During this time, there is a great risk of aspiration and pneumonia. Some patients die as a result of uncontrolled seizure activity. In the setting of hospice care, it is not uncommon for a patient to die of dehydration after the patient is no longer able to swallow or from a pulmonary embolism.

# DIAGNOSIS

The evaluation of a patient with a suspected solitary intracerebral lesion should begin with a careful history and general physical examination. Gradual rather than abrupt onset and a relentless progression of neurologic symptoms and signs suggest a neoplastic rather than a vascular lesion. Rapid progression of clinical abnormalities may suggest obstructive hydrocephalus, brain edema or intratumoral hemorrhage with brain herniation, seizures with Todd's paralysis, and the presence of a more malignant lesion or neoplastic involvement with considerable associated perifocal edema or hemorrhage into the tumor.

The first neurodiagnostic procedure performed is frequently a CT scan or MRI. A CT scan with bone windows is useful for some skull base tumors. MRI gives greater anatomic detail than CT scanning and is now considered the imaging modality of choice for parenchymal lesions of the brain and spinal cord. The ability to provide detailed images in the sagittal and coronal planes is also an advantage of MRI over CT scanning. Magnetic resonance angiography can show the relationship of major vessels to the tumor.

Although newer generation CT and MRI scanners continue to improve resolution and to shorten the time required for image analysis, neither CT scanning nor MRI specifically images tumor tissue. These techniques provide information about the mass effect produced by tumors: changes in tumor density, water content, or areas of blood-brain barrier breakdown visible after the administration of iodinated or ferromagnetic contrast agents. The inability to image tumor tissue specifically remains a major problem for neuro-oncologists and neurosurgeons because primary brain tumors frequently extend beyond what is considered the tumor's outermost border on CT scans or MRI studies.

Other imaging modalities, such as thallium-201 single-photon emission computed tomography (SPECT), and fludeoxyglucose (FDG)-PET, may be helpful in confirming the imaging diagnosis of more malignant types of tumors but do not provide significant uptake in the setting of low-grade tumors or in tumors without breaching of the blood-brain barrier, as is the case for thalium-201 SPECT. Magnetic resonance spectroscopy gives additional information, especially with regard to the cellularity of a given tumor once the diagnosis has been made. These modalities may be useful to the surgeon when selecting sites for biopsy so as to avoid sampling error.

A diagnostic lumbar puncture can be undertaken safely if there is no evidence of a mass lesion with increased intracranial pressure or mass shift. In most instances, it is best to obtain a CT scan or MRI first and to perform the lumbar puncture only if it is thought that it will yield additional critical information. Examination of the CSF may show an increase in the overall number of cells, and tumor cells may be present. The routine cell count may record tumor cells simply as *mononuclear* cells. A specific cytologic examination should be undertaken and may be a helpful diagnostic study. This is particularly true in situations in which the diagnosis of meningeal carcinomatosis or a nodular metastasis in contact with CSF is under consideration. CSF protein levels are commonly elevated in the presence of an intracranial tumor, and glucose values may be low. Various tumor markers have been identified in CSF.[31–34]

# STAGING

Although a TNM staging classification has been published by the American Joint Committee on Cancer, it is not widely employed and is not discussed further in this chapter.

# PROGNOSIS

**Primary Central Nervous System Tumors.** Factors affecting the prognosis of patients with primary brain tumors include age of patient, histologic grade (ranging from well differentiated to very poorly differentiated), performance status, and whether a gross total imaging resection can be safely achieved. Although all these factors are significant with respect to prognosis, the variety of primary tumors and the differences in their biologic behavior make it difficult to apply these factors rigidly to all tumors to formulate a prognosis. It is necessary to elaborate to some degree on the criteria listed. For instance, even the most differentiated cerebral glioma, if not totally resectable, as is true of most, may ultimately lead to the death of the host by virtue of its mass effect. Juvenile cerebellar astrocytomas form an exceptional group, however, and cures of this type of tumor are not uncommon.[35] Proximity to the brain stem, CSF obstruction, and seeding must be emphasized in considering the prognosis of a patient with medulloblastoma.

In addition to the prognostic factors just presented, one must consider the following in approaching the question of tumor prognosis: (1) cystic versus solid nature of the tumor; (2) vascularity of the tumor; (3) limitations on resectability imposed by lateralization of the tumor, (i.e., speech-dominant hemisphere) or localization of the tumor within the deep structures of the brain precluding resection (i.e., basal ganglia or thalamus); (4) radiosensitivity of the tumor—medulloblastomas (which are often difficult to resect totally), pineal tumors, and ependymomas are among the most sensitive to x-ray therapy; (5) quality of survival, reflecting many aspects of function, including motor and intellectual function—rough quantitation using Karnofsky ratings (see Chapter 8) has proved useful in assessing these factors; (6) obstruction of CSF pathways necessitating a shunting procedure; and (7) dissemination of the tumor within the subarachnoid space or, rarely, outside the CNS.

**Metastatic Tumors Involving the Central Nervous System.** The prognosis for survival of patients with metastatic lesions involving the CNS requires consideration of some factors different from those that apply to primary tumors. Key considerations are the nature of the tumor of origin, how well it is controlled, and how extensively it has spread. Factors that apply specifically to CNS involvement include (1) the number and size of metastatic foci and how they affect cerebral mass dynamics; (2) the extent of peritumoral edema and its responsiveness to pharmacologic agents, that is, corticosteroids, as well as the patient's ability to tolerate such therapy; (3) resectability of a solitary tumor focus and the possibility of local recurrence at the site of the metastatic tumor resection; and (4) radiosensitivity of the (primary) tumor and availability of unexplored routes of chemotherapy or endocrine manipulation.

# Principles of Treatment

## PERITUMORAL EDEMA AND STEROIDS

Before discussing specific modalities of brain tumor therapy, some measures that may be useful as adjuncts to operative and nonoperative therapy are noted. From a practical point of view, corticosteroids are employed most commonly for the treatment of increased intracranial pressure and for the reduction of cerebral edema that surrounds brain tumors.

Peritumoral edema (PTE) is an area surrounding the tumor that contains an increase in a plasma ultrafiltrate in the extracellular space. PTE occurs as a result of the tumor or tumor growth. Most typically the edema is present immediately surrounding the tumor, but also it can be seen distant to the tumor seeming to follow white matter tracts. PTE is typically classified as vasogenic because the underlying abnormality is an abnormal blood-tumor barrier accounting for the accumulation of water and protein into the interstitial space. A cytotoxic component may also play a role because malignant gliomas frequently undergo necrosis from ischemia by simply outgrowing its blood supply.

**Corticosteroids.** Corticosteroid effect on brain tumors and PTE has been postulated to have multiple mechanisms, including (1) vascular permeability, (2) cytotoxic effect, (3) decreased rate of tumor formation, and (4) decreased CSF formation. Typically a favorable response was detected within 24 to 48 hours with the maximum response by 1 week. A study of patients with clinically significant PTE showed that 4 mg of dexamethasone was as effective as 8 or 16 mg in divided daily doses and produced fewer side effects when measuring Karnofsky performance status. The corticosteroid-associated side effects increase in number after more than 3 weeks of drug use. After a therapeutic response is obtained, one should taper corticosteroids to the lowest effective dose to avoid such adverse effects as steroid diabetes, gastrointestinal hemorrhages, proximal myopathy, and psychiatric disturbances.

A typical starting dosage of dexamethasone is 16 mg/day in divided doses. If there is a good response within 48 hours, that dosage should be continued until the disappearance of alarming neurologic signs. The dosage should then be tapered down to the lowest possible effective dose. If there is no significant response, efficacy can be attained by doubling the dose and redoubling every 48 hours up to a dosage of 100 mg/day. Responses can be seen at these higher levels.

**Osmotic Dehydration.** Mannitol is thought to have three possible mechanisms of action: (1) osmotic effect, (2) improvement of rheologic aspects, and (3) diuretic effect. The osmotic effect pulls free water out of the extracellular space and into the vasculature, decreasing PTE. The rheologic effects allow for increased blood cell deformity and better oxygen delivery to tissue as well as diluting hemoglobin and fibrinogen, which lowers the viscosity of blood. This lower viscosity allows for less blood volume, lowering intracranial pressure, that can meet the same nutritional needs. Mannitol is also a diuretic, which causes an eventual negative fluid balance and dehydration of the brain, if urine fluid loss is not replenished. Mannitol can also have a *rebound* effect. In brain tumors, the blood-brain barrier is not intact in certain regions. Over time, mannitol can accumulate in the extracellular space, causing an osmotic gradient that draws water

into the extracellular space. A second possible cause of rebound may be related to dehydration and lowering of systemic blood pressure, which, in turn, may critically lower cerebral perfusion pressure. This decrease in cerebral perfusion pressure leads to vasodilatation, which increases the blood volume in the intracranial cavity and increases intracranial pressure. In general, mannitol should not be considered as a form of definitive treatment of PTE, but it is readily effective in patients with critically elevated intracranial pressure and should be instituted while other measures are ongoing to lower intracranial pressure and mass effect. A typical dose of mannitol is 0.25 to 1.0 g/kg every 6 to 12 hours. The goals for osmolality are 310 to 320 mOsm and two thirds of the diuresed volume should be replaced.

**Diuretics.** Diuretics such as furosemide have been used as an adjunct to the treatment of PTE. Furosemide has an additive effect with dexamethasone when measuring water content by CT scanning. Its main mechanism of action in lowering intracranial pressure is most likely secondary to its dehydration effects. A decrease in CSF production rate could lead to an increased clearance of the interstitial fluid toward the ventricle or other CSF spaces. Acetazolamide can be considered effective by a similar mechanism. Acetazolamide is not traditionally used in the setting of PTE. A typical dose of furosemide is 10 to 20 mg every 6 to 12 hours.

**Summary.** PTE is successfully treated with corticosteroids; however, the side effects are at times intolerable. These side effects have led to an attempt to find other agents that might be as effective in the definitive treatment of PTE. Traditional measures for treatment of critically increased intracranial pressure should always be employed. At present, corticosteroids provide for most of the symptomatic treatment of PTE. The development of other agents to treat PTE would help decrease much of the morbidity associated with the present approaches.

**Clinical Conditions of Concern in Patients with Peritumoral Edema**

*Fluid and Electrolyte Balance.* Fluid balance is important in patients with PTE. Overhydration can lead to an increase in interstitial fluid accumulation, especially in the setting of hypo-osmolality, such as hyponatremia. Identification of the cause of hyponatremia is vital, and appropriate correction helps prevent clinical deterioration. Hydration during chemotherapy treatment can accentuate PTE, causing clinical deterioration during treatment.

*Hypertension.* Hypertension can exacerbate PTE. An increase in blood pressure increases the hydrostatic pressure in the capillary bed, especially when the pressures are greater than the upper limits of autoregulation. This increase in hydrostatic pressure can lead to an increase in the formation rate of PTE because the blood-tumor barrier capillary bed has increased permeability. Clinicians must always remember that adequate cerebral perfusion pressure is imperative to prevent ischemia in the setting of increased intracranial pressure, but excessive hypertension can cause clinical deterioration.

*Seizures.* Patients with significant PTE and increased intracranial pressure can show local changes in cerebral blood flow. Seizures create tremendous metabolic needs, which result in increased blood flow to meet these metabolic needs. This increased blood flow can increase intracranial pressure from baseline and might cause ischemia, which is manifested as a prolonged or permanent neurologic deficit, which might be pathophysiologically different from the short-lived (24 to 48 hours) Todd's phenomenon that occurs in partial epilepsies. Adequate control of seizures is imperative in patients with PTE and increased intracranial pressure.

## ANTICONVULSANTS

Of patients, 70% with primary parenchymal tumors and 40% with metastatic brain tumors develop seizures. Anticonvulsants are commonly used in these patients. Anticonvulsants can cause significant side effects, and seizures can cause devastating sequelae; physicians should strongly consider which patients are appropriate for use of anticonvulsants. Patients who present with seizures should have anticonvulsants initiated. Often, simple focal seizures in the setting of mass effect can lead to permanent neurologic deficits postictally. In the most extreme setting, a generalized tonic-clonic seizure can lead to cerebral herniation in a patient with significant mass effect. Complete control of seizure activity is optimal for best patient care. Treatment with anticonvulsants does not come without risk, however: Phenytoin frequently causes a rash and neurocognitive effects; carbamazepine causes a drug rash, neutropenia, and hyponatremia; valproic acid causes weight gain, tremor, and hair loss and has been associated with platelet and bleeding disorders; and phenobarbital causes sedation. Anticonvulsants that induce hepatic enzymes (phenytoin, carbamazepine, and phenobarbital) can interact with some chemotherapy agents, leading to significant underdosing of the cancer treatment. We tend to treat all patients with primary brain tumors and metastatic brain tumors with significant mass effect or a predilection toward hemorrhage (melanoma, renal cell carcinoma, choriocarcinoma). Any patient who develops a seizure should be treated. We typically start with phenytoin, carbamazepine, or valproic acid. Monotherapy is always preferred, and when necessary, levels should be pushed to the upper limit of the therapeutic range. A variety of new anticonvulsants are on the market, and these should be used typically as *add-on* agents if monotherapy is unsuccessful. Blood levels of these drugs should be checked in 10 to 14 days to ascertain that therapeutic levels have been reached, then every month after that. The reader is referred to standard textbooks of pharmacology for details of drug administration and therapeutic drug levels.

## SURGERY

Total elimination of primary intraparenchymatous tumors by surgery alone is extremely rare. It is more appropriate to speak of an *imaging complete resection*. In dealing with tumors of the brain, the goals of surgery include (1) establishing a histologic diagnosis and (2) reducing intracranial pressure by removing as much tumor as safely possible. Cytoreduction may also decrease the immunosuppressive effects of gliomas and allow time for the patient to benefit from radiation therapy and chemotherapy, extending life expectancy.

The reader is referred to additional texts for the technical aspects of brain tumor surgery, which are beyond the scope of this chapter.[36–38] Surgery performed in patients with increased intracranial pressure requires special precautions before operation, during the induction and maintenance of anesthesia, and with respect to the surgical procedure itself.[39] Modern surgical image-guided systems, functional mapping (functional MRI, optical imaging, and electrophysiology), and operative MRI suites are particularly useful for maximum tumor resection, especially near eloquent brain locations.

The planning of surgical therapy depends on the individual tumor. The factors discussed under prognosis are weighed before, and to some extent during, the course of the operation to determine the procedure best suited for a particular case.[36] A variety of surgical procedures can be carried out. The details of surgery differ according to the histology and anatomic site of the different tumors and are discussed in the next section.

## RADIATION THERAPY AND CHEMOTHERAPY

The details of radiation therapy and chemotherapy differ according to the histology and anatomic site of the respective tumors. These topics are discussed in the next section.

## IMMUNOTHERAPY

Immunotherapy of brain tumors is undergoing intensive evaluation at this time. Past attempts have been unsuccessful to date.

## Treatment of Specific Tumors

### ANAPLASTIC ASTROCYTOMA AND GLIOBLASTOMA

Neoplasms of anaplastic astroglial cells are termed *malignant astrocytomas*. These astrocytic tumors, in contrast to their low-grade counterparts, display many of the classic microscopic features of malignancy—necrosis, neovascularity, nuclear pleomorphism, bizarre mitoses, and invasiveness—although distant hematogenous metastases are rarely a feature of their natural history. This group of tumors has for decades been recognized as heterogeneous because of its highly variegated gross morphology, microscopic appearance, and radiographic picture. In a review of Brain Tumor Cooperative Group (BTCG) cases, Giangaspero and Burger[40] noted that 70% of malignant astrocytomas contained more than one malignant cell type. The heterogeneity of malignant gliomas has been extended to the subcellular level.[41–44] Malignant astrocytomas are composed of subpopulations of neoplastic cells with divergent kinetics, antigenicity, biochemistry, radiochemosensitivity, and neoplastic potential. The therapeutic resistance displayed by this group of lesions is perhaps due to a failure to target appropriately each of the discrete tumor cell populations present with the unique therapies to which it is most sensitive.

Malignant astrocytomas generally present at an older age, as compared with low-grade astrocytomas. In Scanlon and

Taylor's[45] review of the Mayo Clinic series, the mean age of presentation for patients with malignant astrocytomas was 49.5 years. Patients with this type of tumor tend to be symptomatic for a shorter period of time; however, they are generally more profoundly impaired than those with benign astrocytomas in similar locations.

Although malignant astrocytomas are often considered a uniform group from a therapeutic standpoint, there appears to be value in subclassifying these gliomas into prognostically unique categories based on microscopic appearance. Subclassification schemes based on embryologic maturation of astroglia, cellular anaplasia of the neoplastic glial cells, and histologic features of the neoplasm have all been used enthusiastically. The prognostic usefulness of these various schemes remains controversial. According to Sheline,[46] no matter which classification scheme is used, some patients with this diagnosis do relatively well for a time, whereas others survive for an astonishingly short period. The histologic subclassification scheme proposed by Russell[13] and Rubinstein[14] correlates most accurately with prognosis. This system separates malignant astrocytomas into two prognostically unique subgroups, based on the presence or absence of coagulative necrosis. Tumors without areas of necrosis are termed *astrocytoma with anaplastic features (AAF)*; necrotic tumors are termed *glioblastoma multiforme (GBM)*. The prognostic utility of this subclassification scheme was shown by Nelson and coworkers,[47] who reported on 503 patients with malignant glioma entered in an Eastern Cooperative Oncology Group (ECOG)/Radiation Therapy Oncology Group (RTOG) trial of radiation therapy with and without chemotherapy. It was discovered that of these patients, 91 (18%) had AAF, and 412 (82%) had GBM. The respective median and 18-month survival rates for AAF and GBM were 28 months versus 8 months and 62% versus 15%. The same authors then applied the subclassification scheme of Kernohan and Sayre[88] to this group of patients. This grading system is based on cellular anaplasia and is used widely for malignant astrocytomas. In this system, the malignant glioma with a lesser degree of anaplasia is termed *grade 3,* whereas the GBM is termed *grade 4.* When Nelson and coworkers[47] used this system, a poor correlation with survival was noted.

According to most authors, the presence or absence of necrosis is the most important feature differentiating patients harboring malignant glioma who have potential long-term survival from those with extremely rapid demise. Burger and coworkers,[48] reviewing three BTCG trials and employing the Russell and Rubinstein system, collected 175 AAF patients and 1265 GBM patients. The respective median and 2-year survival rates were 22 months versus 10 months and 40% versus 10%. The GBM patients were significantly older than the AAF patients (56 years vs. 46 years) but when corrected for age, the prognostic significance of GBM versus AAF was maintained.

Donahue and associates[49] showed by multivariate analysis that the presence of an oligodendroglial component was a significant prognostic variable for anaplastic astrocytomas (AAs) treated in a RTOG trial of altered fractionation. The median survival times for those with and without any oligodendroglial component were 7 and 3 years. In this same RTOG experience, an oligodendroglial component conferred a favorable prognosis for GBM patients, but the magnitude of improvement was far less than for AAF patients.

Gliosarcoma is a bimorphic nervous system tumor composed of high-grade glial cells and sarcomatous elements.[50] The latter may be malignant fibrous histiocytoma, osteosarcoma, chondrosarcoma, or rhabdomyosarcoma. Galanis and colleagues[50] showed the survival of patients with gliosarcoma was equivalent to that of patients with GBM in a series of 18 Mayo Clinic patients. No patient developed extraneural relapse.

Lesion size, as determined on a contrast-enhanced CT scan, was not found to correlate with prognosis by Reeves and Marks[51] in a series of 56 such tumors not otherwise subclassified. With a cutoff of 300 mm$^2$, there was no significant difference in median survival time between small and large lesions. Known prognostic factors, such as age, extent of resection, radiation dose, and performance status, were found to be equally distributed among small and large tumors. The lack of correlation between lesion size and prognosis was true whether treatment had consisted of surgery plus irradiation or of surgery, irradiation, and chemotherapy.

## Surgery

In considering surgery for malignant high-grade astrocytomas, it should be remembered that the following three factors affect longevity: (1) age, (2) histologic grade, and (3) performance status (i.e., Karnofsky score) at presentation. For AA and GBM, cytoreductive surgery followed by external-beam radiation (of approximately 6000 cGy to the tumor) has been the standard against which other treatments are compared.[52] Some neurosurgeons challenge this view, however, and argue that surgery may be justified to reduce mass effect but not simply for reducing tumor burden.[53, 54] Overall, one must consider that malignant astrocytomas cannot be cured with surgery, and so the goal of treatment should be to prolong quality survival. This goal can usually be accomplished with imaging complete tumor resection for lobar gliomas in noneloquent areas. If the tumor is confined to the pole of a lobe, a lobectomy carried out through healthy tissue can be considered. Maximal surgical resection for young patients (<65 years old) in good neurologic condition is justified. In this group, it is generally accepted that the more complete the surgical resection, the more effective the adjuvant therapy (e.g., chemotherapy or immunotherapy) and the longer the duration of quality survival.[55]

In elderly patients with poor Karnofsky scores, the benefit conferred by surgery is modest. In a study of patients older than 65 years of age with malignant astrocytomas, median survival was 17 weeks after biopsy and postoperative radiation versus 30 weeks after surgery and radiation.[56] In older patients in poor medical or neurologic condition, stereotactic biopsy (instead of open surgery) may be indicated, especially for tumors located in eloquent or inaccessible areas of the brain. The diagnostic yield of biopsy is highest when targets within the low-density necrotic center and the enhancing rim are chosen.[57] In a study of 91 cases of malignant gliomas within *critical locations* (i.e., deep, midline, or eloquent brain tissue), it was found that cytoreductive surgery did not improve survival significantly in the few patients that underwent resection, and the authors argued that biopsy followed by radiation therapy may be the appropriate treatment for these deep nonlobar malignant astrocytomas.[58]

*Table 72–6.* **Radiation Therapy for Anaplastic Astrocytoma**

| Author* | Therapy | Survival (%) | | |
|---|---|---|---|---|
| | | 1 YEAR | 3 YEAR | 5 YEAR |
| Uihlein[66] | S | — | 7 | 3 |
| | S + RT | — | 27 | 16 |
| Stage[65] | S | 12 | 8 | 0 |
| | S + RT | 54 | 31 | 10 |
| Sheline[395] | S | — | — | 22 |
| Kramer[405] | S + RT | — | — | 19 |
| Marsa[396] | S + RT | 60 | 31 | 26 |
| Garcia[391] | S | — | — | 30 |
| | S | — | — | 50 |
| Boyages[68] | S + RT | 50 | 19 | 19 |

*Only the first author is given.
S, surgery; RT, radiation therapy.

Greater than 90% of recurrent gliomas recur at or near the original tumor margins.[59] Reoperation for recurrent gliomas extends survival by an additional 36 weeks in patients with GBM and 88 weeks in patients with AA. The duration of high-quality survival (i.e., Karnofsky performance score >70), however, was extended only 10 weeks for GBM and 83 weeks for AA. Morbidity was 5 to 18% higher with reoperations, with infection, wound dehiscence, or both three times more likely than primary operations.[60, 61] In selecting surgery for tumor recurrence, all these factors need to be taken into account.

### Radiation Therapy

External-beam radiation therapy, administered postoperatively, has become the standard of management for patients with malignant glioma. A multitude of retrospective reviews clearly shows the improvement in quantity and quality of survival following radiation therapy of malignant astrocytomas. Employing modern irradiation techniques for AAs, 15 to 30% 5-year survival rates can be achieved; such figures are rarely achieved with surgery alone (Table 72–6). Radiation therapy for GBM, although virtually never achieving long-term tumor control, can significantly improve short-term end points, such as median survival. Following external-beam irradiation to adequate dose, median survival for GBM patients is 10 to 14 months (Table 72–7).

Three randomized trials support the use of radiation ther-

*Table 72–7.* **Radiation Therapy for Glioblastoma**

| Author* | Therapy | Survival (%) | | |
|---|---|---|---|---|
| | | 6 MONTHS | 1 YEAR | 2 YEAR |
| Taveras[406] | S | 14 | 5 | 0 |
| | S + RT | 60 | 30 | 8 |
| Uihlein[66] | S | 30 | 15 | 8 |
| | S + RT | 70 | 41 | 6 |
| Marsa[396] | S + RT | 70 | 31 | 8 |
| Rutten[407] | S + RT | 82 | 32 | 18 |
| Boyages[68] | S + RT | 70 | 17 | 0 |

*Only the first author is given.
S, surgery; RT, radiation therapy.

apy for these tumors. Walker and associates[62, 63] have published the results of a BTCG study of 222 evaluable patients with malignant astrocytoma (90% glioblastoma, 10% AA). The patients were well stratified for potential prognostic factors. Randomized treatment arms included *supportive care* only, carmustine (BCNU) (80 mg/m²/day for 3 days, every 6 to 8 weeks), radiotherapy (50 to 60 Gy to the whole brain in 6 to 7 weeks), or radiotherapy plus BCNU. Median survival times were 14 weeks for supportive care, 18.5 weeks for BCNU, 36 weeks for radiotherapy, and 34.5 weeks for combined radiotherapy and BCNU. There was an improvement, however, with the last quartile of patients regarding survival who had received chemotherapy in addition to radiation therapy. Patients in the treatment arms including radiotherapy had a significantly ($p = 0.001$) better median survival than those not receiving radiotherapy.

Kristiansen and coworkers[64] have reported the results of a three-armed randomized trial performed by the Scandinavian Glioma Study Group (SGSG) involving 118 patients with malignant astrocytomas. Following partial resection, patients were randomized to external-beam radiotherapy (45 Gy to the whole brain in 5 weeks), radiotherapy plus bleomycin (180 mg total dose), or no therapy other than supportive care. Median survival times were 10.8 months in the two groups receiving radiation therapy versus 5.2 months in the group having operative intervention only. One-year survivals were 33% in the radiotherapy groups versus 8% in the surgery-only group.

The results of the randomized trials by the BTCG and SGSG confirm that radiation therapy confers a definite, albeit transitory, benefit to patients with this type of tumor. Despite some negative opinions in the literature, radiation therapy is a valuable adjunct in the treatment of these difficult tumors and is included in treatment programs by all cooperative groups.

The proper dose of photon radiation for control of malignant astrocytomas remains in dispute. Analysis of older literature is complicated by the use of doses that are clearly inadequate by modern standards.[65, 66] Uihlein and colleagues[66] showed longer survival for patients who received more than 35 Gy, compared with those receiving lesser doses. The bulk of doses employed by these groups is now considered inadequate for patients with volumes of tumor commonly encountered with malignant astrocytoma. The trend has been to deliver tumor doses in excess of 50 Gy. Most authors now recommend 60 Gy. The tumor dose is determined by the tolerance of surrounding normal brain parenchyma, rather than by any strict relationship between the number of viable tumor clonogens present and the theoretical dose necessary for acceptable probability of tumor control.

Whether, in fact, a dose-response relationship exists for this tumor type remains in controversy. The British Medical Research Council reported significantly better results with 60 Gy in 30 factions compared with 45 Gy in 20 fractions.[67] Median and overall survivals with the higher dose were 12 months and 18% compared with 9 months and 11% with the lower dose. The BTCG has shown a statistically significant improvement in median survival time of glioblastoma patients when external-beam doses were increased from 50 to 60 Gy.[63] Median survival times following doses of 50, 55, and 60 Gy were 28 weeks, 36 weeks, and 42 weeks. Radiation dose was not a randomized variable in the BTCG study. Boyages and Tiver[68] have reported evidence for improved survival for grade 3 malignant astrocytomas receiving greater than conventional doses of radiation. In a nonrandom series, the 2-year survival rates with less than 60 Gy, 60 Gy, and more than 60 Gy were 13%, 28%, and 33%. These reports remain among the few in the literature that support a dose response within the *conventional* range for malignant astrocytoma. Most authors reviewing patients treated with modern diagnostic and therapeutic approaches cannot show such a dose response.

Several authors recommend shorter-course radiotherapy for malignant glioma patients with poor prognosis. Bauman and associates[69] showed equivalent survival for patients 65 years or older and with poor Karnofsky performance scores receiving 30 Gy in 10 fractions compared with standard radiotherapy. For elderly patients with good Karnofsky performance scores, however, prognosis following short-course radiotherapy was inferior to the standard approach. In a randomized trial of conventional and hypofractionated therapy, Glinski[70] found equivalent survival for AAF patients. Results for the GBM patients were superior with hypofractionated radiotherapy.

That the size of an external-beam portal for irradiation of a malignant astrocytoma must be considerably larger than the grossly evident tumor is not in dispute. Malignant gliomas are microscopically infiltrative for a distance unappreciated even by MRI but clearly shown by necropsy. Scherer[70a] has convincingly shown perineuronal and perivascular satellitosis, so-called secondary tumor deposits, several centimeters from the main compact tumor mass and its surrounding infiltrative margin. These relatively distant tumor foci could potentially be missed with a restricted radiation portal. Concannon and colleagues[70b] stressed that the poor portal delineation in the kilovoltage era was a direct result of the employment of inaccurate diagnostic tests, such as isotope brain scans, pneumoencephalograms, and angiograms. These studies yielded poor tumor localization (defined as >20% of the lesion outside the indicated volume) in 48% of cases. Others have reported similar high levels of inaccuracy of neuroradiologic definition of malignant astrocytoma in the pre-CT, pre-MRI era.[71] Because of these accumulating data, whole-brain irradiation was previously advocated for malignant gliomas.

Hochberg and Pruitt[72] have cogently questioned the assumptions on which radiotherapists have argued for whole-brain irradiation. Of 35 patients (16 received radiation therapy, 19 did not) who had a CT scan within 2 months of death, the microscopic margin of tumor as determined at necropsy was within 2 cm of the margin depicted on contrast-enhanced CT scan in 29 patients. Of the six patients in whom tumor was more extensive on necropsy than on CT scan, two had spinal subarachoid disease, and two had lesions that failed to take up contrast. The contrast-enhanced CT scan is highly accurate in predicting microscopic tumor margins.

The second group studied by Hochberg and Pruitt[72] involved 42 patients scanned serially following irradiation until tumor recurrence. Twenty-eight patients also underwent necropsy. In 80% of these patients, the recurrence was within the primary site or within 2 cm of the margin of the primary site. In 20%, tumor recurrence was the 2-cm limit; four patients had recurrence in parenchyma more than 2 cm from the original primary lesion without simultaneous local recurrence, and four patients had neuraxial seeding. The third group consisted of 131 untreated patients subjected to necropsy. In this natural history group, 3% displayed multicentric malignant astrocytoma, a finding similar to that of other reports.[73–75] The authors concluded from these series are that there is little justification for routine whole-brain irradiation in the management of malignant astrocytoma since the advent of modern neuroradiology.

De Schryver and colleagues[75a] have reported 64% 1-year and 43% 2-year survival rates, using well-designed partial-brain portals. Because no controlled study has incriminated remote brain failure to be as clinically significant a problem as in-field recurrence, there is no a priori reason to expect whole-brain irradiation to yield survival rates superior to irradiation of carefully planned, limited-volume fields.

The volume of brain to be irradiated in these patients must be individualized on the basis of modern neuroradiologic studies. Well-designed, partial-brain portals appear appropriate for patients harboring a ring-enhancing lesion. Whole-brain irradiation for all or a portion of therapy may prove superior for certain high-risk patients with lesions near a ventricle, poorly defined thalamic lesions, butterfly gliomas, lesions that display irregular enhancement on CT scan in any site, and the rare multicentric astrocytoma. The use of MRI refines further the interface between the normal brain parenchyma and the infiltrating edge of a malignant glioma.[76–78]

Malignant gliomas are only moderately sensitive to radiotherapy. Investigators in Ontario documented imaging response in 22 of 63 cases, but only 3 were complete.[75] Barker and colleagues[79] at the University of California San Francisco (UCSF) reported at least 25% reduction in contrast-enhancing tumor area in 43% of patients. Tumor area was stable or increased in the remainder. In both series, the first follow-up imaging study was done immediately after the conclusion of radiotherapy. In the Ontario trial, 20 of 22 responses were noted at the first follow-up image. The incidence of protracted radiation response was uncommon, in contradistinction to conventional concepts. The prognostic significance of tumor response remains uncertain. Barker and colleagues[79] cautioned that postoperative, preradiotherapy imaging to assess residual disease and, by extension, provide a standard for judging potential post-treatment response, should be carried out before postoperative day 4. Postoperative scans performed after that time could be confounded by spurious contrast enhancement resulting from inflammation that would tend to dissipate over the time course of radiotherapy and result in a false judgment of response.

## Chemotherapy

**Glioblastoma Multiforme.** GBM has had poor responses to chemotherapy, A meta-analysis showed benefit in 10% of patients with GBM.[80] A BTCG study[62, 63] showed a benefit in the last quartile of patients who received chemotherapy and radiation versus those with radiation alone. Careful review of the histopathology could not *weed out* the more chemoresponsive tumors.[81] We believe there are patients who can benefit from chemotherapy. Some GBM are differentially responsive to chemotherapy: One GBM may respond to one type of alkylating agent, whereas another responds to a topoisomerase inhibitor. Only a small percentage of patients respond to chemotherapy, and so consideration must be given to the timing and choice of chemotherapy. Modestly effective chemotherapies alone or in combination for GBM include nitrosourea-based chemotherapies, cisplatin, procarbazine, vincristine, camptothecin-11 (CPT-11), carboplatin, temozolomide, and etoposide.

### Adjuvant Therapy

NEOADJUVANT. Some studies have touted positive results with neoadjuvant use of chemotherapy.[82, 83] To date, however, no regimen has been shown to provide an improvement in quality of life, progression-free survival, or survival. Neoadjuvant therapy should be limited to the investigational arena.

ADJUVANT. The role of adjuvant chemotherapy following radiation therapy is unclear. Patients who are younger (<45 years of age), with better performance status (Karnofsky performance score >80) and with smaller tumor volumes may be more likely to show benefit. One has to consider that radiation may hold the tumor stable for some time (3 to 12 months). If this situation occurs, the true determination of efficacy of the adjuvant chemotherapy would be difficult to measure. If only 10% of patients benefit from adjuvant chemotherapy, 90% suffer only the side effects of treatment, and possibly prolonged treatment, in the adjuvant setting.

### Recurrent or Progressive Disease.

Response to treatment in the setting of recurrent or progressive disease is easy to monitor. The likelihood of responding to chemotherapy is small, but occasionally there are rather dramatic responses that are durable. The above-mentioned chemotherapies should be considered alone or in combination. One should strongly consider the use of investigational therapies or clinical trials in the recurrent setting for all gliomas. Most recurrent malignant high-grade astrocytomas have a median time to tumor progression of 8 to 10 weeks for GBM and 12 to 18 weeks for AAF. Median survival for GBM and AAF in the recurrent setting is 20 weeks and 30 to 40 weeks.

### Method of Delivery.

Intra-arterial and intralesional therapies have been studied by investigators. To date, investigators have not yet been able to show any improvement in response or survival as compared with patients treated with systemic chemotherapies. There has been increased toxicity with many of these delivery methods, however. High-dose chemotherapy with stem cell rescue or autologous bone marrow transplant has yet to show superior results when compared with *normal-dose* treatment in any treatment setting with malignant high-grade astrocytoma.[84]

### Biologic Agents.

High-dose tamoxifen,[85] *cis*-retinoic acid,[86] all-*trans*-retinoic acid, interferon beta,[87] and thalidomide have all shown efficacy in phase II studies of recurrent malignant gliomas. A number of ongoing clinical trials are looking at signal transduction inhibitors, antiangiogenesis agents, inhibitors of drug resistance, and anti-invasion agents, which may show benefits alone or in combination with chemotherapy or radiation therapy.

### Anaplastic Astrocytomas.

AAs are more chemoresponsive than GBM. The same chemotherapy agents considered for use in GBM should be considered with this tumor. Adjuvant treatment with PCV (procarbazine, CCNU, vincristine) has been traditionally used, but an analysis comparing PCV with BCNU alone showed no clear benefit to the

combination therapy. Any of the *effective* chemotherapy regimens could be considered in the adjuvant setting. Chemotherapy is also a strong treatment consideration with recurrent AAs. The chemotherapy agents mentioned previously should be strongly considered and used in combination or alone. The use of investigational approaches or clinical trials should be always a strong consideration.

## LOW-GRADE ASTROCYTOMAS

Low-grade astrocytomas are neoplasms composed of relatively well-differentiated astroglial cells. They may assume a diffuse, infiltrative growth pattern or a more circumscribed, piloid morphology. These tumors have traditionally been graded pathologically using the schemes of Kernohan,[88] Russell[13] and Rubinstein,[14] or Daumas-Duport and colleagues.[76] Whether there is a true, independent prognostic difference between grade 1 and 2 tumors remains debatable, but most authors conclude that a real difference exists.[45, 89]

Patients with low-grade astrocytic gliomas are generally symptomatic for a longer period than those with malignant astrocytoma. Low-grade tumors also present at a younger age than the malignant varieties. In Scanlon and Taylor's[45] review of the Mayo Clinic experience, the mean age of patient presentation was 27 years. This series, however, shows the tendency of some authors to lump all CNS sites and all age groups together when analyzing low-grade astrocytic gliomas. As a result, some series include not only patients with cerebral hemispheric tumors, but also those with optic, cerebellar, and brain stem gliomas. Other series eliminate tumors in one or more of these disparate sites when considering the natural history, treatment options, and therapy outcomes.

When only adult patients with hemispheric tumors are considered, the median age has been reported to be 49 years.[68] Because of their vastly different prognoses, optic gliomas, cerebellar gliomas, and brain stem gliomas are dealt with separately in this chapter. The data cited on low-grade astrocytic gliomas in this section, however, reflect the mixed populations available in the literature. Therapeutic outcomes and potential prognostic parameters should be considered with this proviso in mind.

### Surgery

The surgical indications for low-grade astrocytomas are not definitively elucidated. It has been argued that no well-designed study has shown that surgery for supratentorial low-grade gliomas has any benefit. The argument is that these tumors are slowly growing and that there is no harm in waiting until progression on imaging or malignant degeneration is documented before initiating aggressive treatment.[90] Although this view has been challenged, a definitive well-controlled, randomized study has yet to be performed. Despite the fact that surgery is not curative for most infiltrating gliomas, surgery is considered the treatment of choice in the following situations of low-grade astrocytomas: (1) childhood cerebellar and supratentorial pilocytic astrocytomas, (2) large tumors with significant mass effect, (3) tumors obstructing CSF flow, and (4) lesions causing intractable seizures.[91] Because the natural history of pilocytic low-grade astrocytomas is slow growth, the treatment of choice is surgical excision of the maximal amount of tumor that can be removed safely without producing a neurologic deficit. In some, invasion of the brain stem, cranial nerves, or major blood vessels may limit surgical resection. In tumors composed of a nodule with a *true cyst,* excision of the nodule is sufficient because the cyst wall is non-neoplastic and need not be removed. Some tumors have a so-called false cyst that enhances on CT scan or MRI, which usually contains tumor and should be removed. Because of the high long-term survival rate (5, 10, and 20 years) and the relatively high complication rate of radiation therapy over this long time interval,[92] it is recommended these patients do not undergo radiation therapy postoperatively. Instead, patients with pilocytic astrocytomas should be followed with serial MRI studies and reoperated on if there is recurrence. Radiation therapy is indicated only for recurrent tumor that is not resectable or for recurrence that has degenerated to more malignant histology.

## Radiation Therapy

After complete resection of a low-grade astrocytic glioma, there is no accepted role for adjuvant radiotherapy.[89, 93–96] Leibel and associates[35] showed 100% 5- and 10-year survival after complete resection alone. In Fazekas and colleagues,[97] retrospective series, the 5-year survival after *complete resection* was 90%, but there was progressive tumor relapse and patient death, culminating in a 25% 10-year survival. Despite the overall poor survival, Fazekas and colleagues showed no improvement with the use of postoperative irradiation after complete resection. This finding was most likely due to a maldistribution of tumor sites and patient ages between the groups treated with and without radiotherapy. Others have shown frequent tumor relapse many years after complete resection alone for low-grade gliomas.[89, 93–96] There is no apparent impact of radiotherapy in these series of completely resected patients. These series imply there may be a substantial relapse rate following total removal of an ordinary astrocytoma. Several authors recommend postoperative radiotherapy in the setting of complete resection.[68, 93] The series mentioned previously, however, fail to employ postoperative imaging studies to evaluate the completeness of resection. Until the relapse pattern of astrocytomas following documented total resection is elucidated, most authors do not advocate irradiation in the setting of macroscopic complete tumor removal.[98–100]

The role of radiotherapy following incomplete resection of low-grade astrocytomas remains controversial because of the slow growth rate of these tumors, their long natural history, and the belief that they are radioresistant (Table 72–8). Leibel and coworkers[35] showed 5-, 10-, and 20-year survivals of 46%, 35%, and 23% respectively with a combined approach versus 19%, 11%, and 0% with incomplete resection alone. The survival advantage was seen in grade 1 and 2, in adults and children, and in all sites. Five-year survival rates of 40 to 64% and median survivals of 4 to 8 years have been reported for patients irradiated after less than complete resection.[93, 94, 98, 99, 101–105] Ten-year survival rates following combined therapy vary from 25 to 37%.[98, 106] Several authors report that radiotherapy following incomplete resection significantly affects only short-term

*Table 72–8.* **Radiation Therapy for Low-Grade Astrocytomas**

| Author* | Therapy | Survival (%) | | |
|---|---|---|---|---|
| | | 1 YEAR | 5 YEAR | 10 YEAR |
| Levy[408] | Cr or Pr | 81 | 26 | — |
| | Pr + RT | 82 | 36 | — |
| Bouchard[394] | Pr + RT | 62 | 49 | 35 |
| Stage[65] | Pr | 50 | 20 | — |
| | Pr + RT | 80 | 40 | — |
| Leibel[35] | Cr | 100 | 100 | 100 |
| | Pr | 51 | 19 | 11 |
| | Pr + RT | 80 | 46 | 35 |
| Fazekas[97] | Cr | 95 | 90 | 25 |
| | Pr | 43 | 13 | — |
| | Pr + RT | 85 | 41 | 28 |
| Rutten[407] | Pr + RT | 90 | 44 | — |

*Only the first author is given.
Cr, complete resection; Pr, partial resection; RT, radiation therapy.

survival.[99, 107] Finally, several authors report no survival impact of radiotherapy at any time period.[95, 96] These series imply radiotherapy delays, but does not prevent, ultimate reappearance of low-grade ordinary astrocytoma. Until the results of randomized trials are available, postoperative radiotherapy should be reserved for patients with subtotal resections at greatest risk for relapse or those with unrelenting symptoms. Rogers and coworkers[108] reported benefit of radiotherapy for patients with low-grade astrocytomas and medically intractable seizures.

Multiple authors report no significant dose-response relationship for low-grade astrocytomas. The European Organization for Research and Treatment of Cancer (EORTC) randomized 379 adults with low-grade gliomas to 45 or 59.4 Gy following resection and reported equivalent 5-year relapse-free and overall survival rates.[104] Several authors report a nonsignificant trend favoring doses greater than 50 Gy.[93, 98, 107] There has been no documented relationship between field size and survival for the low-grade astrocytomas.[93, 98, 109]

The post-treatment functional class of low-grade astrocytoma patients is unchanged for 2 years according to North and coworkers.[110] After that interval, however, a significant decline in functional class was observed. This decline is most pronounced in the pediatric age group, in which only 11% of patients remained in the best performance classes. There were no long-term cognitive defects in adults, but 50% of children were cognitively impaired. These authors could find no statistically significant association of radiotherapy with later cognitive deficits.

The radiographic response of low-grade glial neoplasms is typically modest.[111] Fisher and coworkers[111] reported the results of serial imaging in 19 patients receiving a median of 54 Gy following incomplete resection. Ten of 19 showed some response, and 4 showed a complete response. Mean volume reduction for the entire group was 30%. The mean time to maximum response was 14 months. Maximum response was achieved in five patients at the first follow-up scan done at a median of 3.3 months after radiotherapy. In the remaining five, maximum response required 7 months to 5 years. There was no apparent correlation between the eventual local control rate and the imaging response rate.

## Chemotherapy

The role of chemotherapy of low-grade astrocytoma is usually limited to the recurrent setting. The same agents listed for GBM should be considered. Some authors strongly favor the use of carboplatin alone[112] or in combination with vincristine[113] or etoposide in this setting.

## OLIGODENDROGLIOMAS

Oligodendrogliomas are common brain tumors, constituting 5 to 10% of gliomas when mixed tumors are included. They occur twice as often in males. Patients commonly have a prior history of neurologic symptoms, including seizure and focal signs. Calcifications are noted in half the cases on CT scan. There is a predilection for the frontal lobe. There is a risk of intratumoral hemorrhage, meningeal spread, and distant metastasis. Anaplastic oligodendrogliomas and mixed oligoastrocytomas with a high-grade astrocytic component are malignant tumors with a poor prognosis.

In contrast to the case with astrocytic gliomas, the standard grading systems do not appear to correlate with prognosis. Histopathologic grading schemes that significantly correlate with median and 5-year survivals have been proposed by Smith and colleagues[114] from the Armed Forces Institute of Pathology and by Burger and Green[115] from Duke University. In the former study, pleomorphism was the most significant correlate of prognosis, whereas in the latter series, tumor necrosis was the most significant determinant. Shaw and coworkers[116] showed that the Kernohan and the St. Anne/Mayo systems separated mixed oligodendroglial tumors into prognostically meaningful high and low grades. The former system proved to be a better discriminator. The distribution of purported histologic determinants of survival among nonrandomly assigned treatment groups must be accounted for when analyzing results of therapy for this tumor. Chromosomal analysis has been evaluated in helping define prognostic groups. Cairncross and coworkers[117] have shown loss of chromosome 1p and 19q are highly statistically significant determinants of not only chemoresponsiveness, but also survival.

## Surgery

Surgery is the principal treatment of choice for oligodendrogliomas. It has been shown that aggressive resection of these tumors leads to longer survival and results in fewer complications than *partial debulking* operations.[118] Whenever possible, a gross total resection should be attempted. This type of tumor usually appears as a pinkish or reddish friable mass. There may be a well-circumscribed plane of demarcation between tumor and what appears to be normal brain. This plane allows oligodendrogliomas to be removed more completely than their astrocytic counterparts, which may account for its better prognosis following surgery. As a group, regardless of histologic grade, median survival for surgically treated oligodendrogliomas is 35 months postoperatively, and mean survival is 52 months following surgery.[119] In one study, patients with oligodendrogliomas in the frontal lobes were found to survive longer (37 months postoperatively) than those with temporal lobe tumors (28 months

postoperatively).[119] This finding is probably due to the increased ease of radical surgical resection of frontal lobe tumors versus those in other locations.

## Radiation Therapy

There is no established role for irradiation following complete removal of an oligodendroglioma.[120] Postoperative irradiation remains controversial following subtotal resection of an oligodendroglioma. Reedy and coworkers[121] from the Cleveland Clinic reported identical 5-year survivals with or without addition of postoperative irradiation in a series of 48 patients. In that retrospective review, radiotherapy doses varied from 22 to 65 Gy, and a higher proportion of surgery-only patients had complete resection compared with those undergoing radiation postoperatively. Other series showing no benefit to adjunctive radiotherapy can be similarly criticized.[122, 123]

There are sufficient data in the literature showing improved survival with radiation therapy to justify its use (Table 72–9). Sheline[124] reported 5- and 10-year survival rates of 31% and 25% with incomplete resection alone versus 85% and 55% with the combined approach. In a meta-analysis of 425 patients from the literature, Shimizu and colleagues[398] reported a significant survival advantage when irradiation followed subtotal resection. The 5-year survival rates with and without radiotherapy were 56% and 42% ($p < 0.01$).

The best results of adjunctive irradiation have been reported following doses of 50 to 55 Gy in standard fractionation to a limited volume.[98, 125] Packer and colleagues[126] described three pediatric patients with *malignant* posterior fossa oligodendroglioma who received local-field irradiation. All three patients had extension of disease outside these fields (two spinal seeding, one subfrontal meninges) without evidence of local failure. A fourth patient with a similar tumor was free of disease 2 years after elective craniospinal axis irradiation. Radiotherapy of the neuraxis should be considered strongly for the rare high-grade, posterior fossa oligodendroglioma.

## Chemotherapy

The role of chemotherapy is usually limited to anaplastic oligodendrogliomas, anaplastic mixed gliomas, recurrent or

*Table 72–9.* **Radiation Therapy for Oligodendroglioma**

| Author* | Therapy | Survival (%) 5 YEAR | 10 YEAR |
|---|---|---|---|
| Bailey[131] | S | 37 | — |
| Richmond[393] | S + RT | 53 | — |
| Bouchard[394] | S + RT | 56 | 33 |
| Sheline[395] | S | 31 | 55 |
| | S + RT | 85 | 35 |
| Marsa[396] | S + RT | 74 | 35 |
| Chin[397] | S | 82 | — |
| | S + RT | 100 | — |
| Shimizu[398] | S | 42 | — |
| | S + RT | 56 | — |

*Only the first author is given.
S, surgery; RT, radiation therapy.

aggressive oligodendrogliomas, or recurrent or aggressive mixed gliomas.[127–130] This tumor type is the one setting with gliomas in which chemotherapy responsiveness is common. Typically, PCV is used and, with anaplastic tumors, often in the neoadjuvant setting. Some investigators are pursuing treatment with high-dose chemotherapy in anaplastic tumors, showing a response after one or two cycles of PCV. The advent of chromosomal determination of response may allow for a more individually tailored treatment in these patients.[117]

## MEDULLOBLASTOMAS

Medulloblastomas were described by Bailey and Cushing in 1925.[131] They are posterior fossa lesions seen primarily in children, in whom they account for 20% of CNS tumors. Medulloblastomas are of uncertain histogenesis. In their classic form, they arise from the roof of the fourth ventricle and project into the cerebellar vermis. Extensive disease involving the cerebellar hemispheres, the brain stem, or both is possible, but subarachnoid seeding remains the most notorious feature of this tumor's natural history. The true risk of seeding is uncertain because virtually all patients receive craniospinal irradiation for this tumor. In Cushing's original series, there was one survivor among 61 cases treated by surgery with or without local-field irradiation. In the series by McFarland and coworkers[132] of 420 collected cases, the risk of late CSF seeding appeared to be 33%. Some of McFarland's patients received craniospinal-axis irradiation, so this cannot be considered a natural history series. When meningeal disease does become apparent, either because of uncontrolled CSF tumor that was present but unsuspected at diagnosis or because of late seeding associated with a posterior fossa recurrence, it involves the spinal subarachnoid space in 95% of cases and the cerebral meninges in 5%.[132]

Metastatic disease outside the CNS was formerly an extraordinarily rare event. According to Kleinman and associates,[133] the risk of distant metastases may approach 5% today. Whether extra-CNS metastases are in any way related to ventricular shunting remains a highly controversial question.[133–136] It appears that if extra-CNS metastases occur, they do so sooner than in nonshunted patients (mean, 1.3 vs. 2.0 years).[133] According to Berry and associates,[135] membrane (Millipore) filters do not prevent systemic metastases in shunted patients. The increasing number of reports of systemic metastases of medulloblastoma may be a manifestation of the improving prospects for long-term survival in this formerly fatal malignancy.

MRI studies of the spinal axis must be included in the diagnostic evaluation of patients with medulloblastoma, and currently MRI is used in place of myelograms.[74, 137] In a series of 38 patients, Deutsch and coworkers[74] demonstrated 12 positive myelograms. In this series as well as others, CSF cytology was a poor predictor of imaging findings. CSF analysis complements, but does not replace, myelography in these patients. Deutsch and coworkers[74] recommended that myelography (now MRI) be performed 2 to 3 weeks after posterior fossa surgery, so as to avoid any confusion with contamination of the subarachnoid space by surgical manipulation of the tumor.

## Surgery

The treatment of choice for medulloblastoma is surgical resection of as much tumor as possible without causing neurologic deficit, followed by craniospinal radiation therapy. Because this type of tumor has a high propensity to recur and seed in the subarachnoid space, postoperative radiation is necessary, and the details of radiotherapy are discussed subsequently. Medulloblastomas usually arise in the vermis of the cerebellum, and invasion into the floor of the fourth ventricle and brain stem often limits complete excision. It is generally believed that leaving a small residual tumor on the brain stem is preferable to removing every last remnant attached to the brain stem, which is likely to cause significant neurologic deficit and promote seeding of tumor cells. The location of these tumors near the roof of the fourth ventricle also predisposes patients with medulloblastomas to early obstructive hydrocephalus. It has been estimated that 30 to 40% of children required permanent ventriculoperitoneal shunting of CSF following posterior fossa resection of tumor. The risk of shunt-related seeding into the peritoneum has been shown to be 10 to 20%.[138, 139] In the past, tumor filters were frequently used in attempts to minimize seeding, but these filters were associated with a higher incidence of shunt obstruction. Endoscopic third ventriculostomy may be considered for patients with obstructive hydrocephalus secondary to tumors in the posterior fossa.[140]

## Radiation Therapy

After maximal safe resection of tumor, appropriate therapy includes irradiation of the entire neuraxis. As shown by several retrospective reviews, there is no place for irradiation of limited volumes of the CNS in the management of medulloblastoma.[141, 142] Landberg and colleagues[141] showed that 5-year survival for these patients was related to irradiation technique. After irradiation of the posterior fossa only, 5% of the patients were alive, whereas 25% were alive for a similar period following radiation therapy to the posterior fossa and spinal axis, and 53% were alive following craniospinal-axis irradiation. With routine craniospinal irradiation, 5-year survival rates of 28 to 47% were achieved in older series covering primarily the kilovoltage era. More recent reports are more encouraging; having employed megavoltage and a clearer understanding of dose response, these reports show overall 5-year survival rates greater than 50% (Table 72–10).

The technical difficulties of craniospinal irradiation are well known. Lateral whole-brain fields with separate posterior spinal fields and moving junctions are generally used. Tokars and associates[143] described excellent results with a single *hockey-stick* field. They reported a 73% 5-year survival rate in patients treated with this technique versus a 17% historical survival rate with the conventional approach. Tokars and associates[143] believed that improved results were due to the avoidance of junctional hot or cold spots that occur with gapped fields. The posterior fossa dose was higher with the hockey-stick approach, however, than in the historical control patients. This increased dose, rather than the change in technique, may have been responsible for the improved cure rate.

The width of the posterior spinal field should rarely

*Table 72–10.* **Survival of Patients with Medulloblastoma Following Radiation Therapy**

| Author* | 5-Year Survival (%) |
|---|---|
| Cumberlin[399] | 63 |
| Brown[400] | 50 |
| Smith[142] | 59 |
| Tokars[143] | 73 |
| Berry[135] | 64 |
| Chin[401] | 80 |
| Silverman[134] | 85 |
| Kopelson[158] | 56 |
| Miralbell[154] | 57 |
| Khafaga[156] | 57 |

*Only the first author is given.

exceed 5 cm when linear accelerator photons are used. The CSF extends laterally to the intervertebral foramina.[144] According to Jenkin,[144] the distance between the lateral margins of the posterior vertebral body pedicles is at least equal to the distance between the foramina. The maximal interpedicular separation is approximately 4 cm at the fifth lumbar segment. According to Halperin,[145] the sacral end of the spinal field need not be widened to include the sacroiliac joints (*spade*). The CSF surrounds the lumbar and sacral nerve roots within the dural sac but only to the level of the neural foramina.[144, 145] In children, the foraminal separation at the second sacral segment is approximately 5 cm. The caudal end of the neuraxis field should be widened only an additional 1.2 to 1.8 cm to irradiate sacral nerve roots adequately. It is not appropriate to set the inferior border of the spinal field arbitrarily at the second sacral body. The caudal end of the dural sac is variable using gadolinium-enhanced sagittal MRI.[146] The termination is determined by the convergence of the anterior and posterior dural walls. This point varies from the first through the fifth sacral segments. Involvement of the leptomeninges by spinal seeding may contribute to further caudal extension of the convergence point.

The traditional approach to comprehensive neuraxis radiotherapy for medulloblastoma also involves a boost of the entire posterior fossa. Establishing the boundaries of the posterior fossa for boost field planning proved difficult in the pre-MRI era. Solit and Goldwein[147] have clearly shown that the most accurate method for defining the extent of the posterior fossa involves use of sagittal MRI at the time of simulation. In the absence of MRI, however, Drayer and coworkers[148] have described a method to determine the apex of the tentorium using bone landmarks seen on a standard lateral skull simulator film. This method predicted the location of the apex to within 10 mm in most patients.

Local control and survival of patients following radiation therapy are strongly related to posterior fossa dose. The best-documented results have occurred after a dose of 50 to 55 Gy to the posterior fossa. When both optimal fields and posterior fossa doses of 50 Gy or greater are used, many authors report 5-year survival rates of 75% or higher (see Table 72–10). When doses to the posterior fossa are less than 50 Gy, 5-year survival rates of 25 to 40% are commonly reported. Allen and associates[149] showed an apparent improvement in local control following hyperfractionation and chemotherapy. Twenty-three patients with Chang stage T3/

T4 or M-positive medulloblastomas received 72 Gy to the posterior fossa. Fourteen of 15 T3/T4 tumors remained free of relapse for a median of 75 months. This aggressive approach proved less effective for patients who were M positive at diagnosis.

The appropriate dose for the uninvolved brain and spine remains controversial. Tumor recurrence in initially uninvolved areas may be the result of seeding from a concomitant posterior fossa recurrence or a geographic miss of the primary tumor, as opposed to an indication that the applied prophylactic dose was too low to control occult subarachnoid disease. With regard to the spinal prophylactic dose, advocates of either more than 30 Gy or less than 30 Gy can be found. Brand and colleagues[150] have published the results of a nonrandom trial. Patients were separated into low-risk and high-risk groups on the basis of age, stage, and extent of resection. In both groups, there were no significant differences in spinal control or survival when doses of 25 Gy or more than 30 Gy were used for spinal prophylaxis. Solitary spinal recurrence was extremely rare. Tumors that did occur were virtually always associated with local recurrence in the posterior fossa, and this latter phenomenon was unrelated to spinal dose. The Children's Cancer Study Group performed a randomized trial of 35 Gy versus 24 Gy neuraxis dose for low-risk patients.[151] The trial was stopped because of an unacceptable rate of neuraxis relapses in the low-dose group. Similar discouraging results were reported from a randomized Society Internationale Oncologie pediatric trial of 25 Gy versus 35 Gy for low-risk patients.[144] These data imply that reduced neuraxis dose should be employed in the setting of a clinical trial.

Generally, doses to the uninvolved portions of the brain are 35 Gy or more. Jereb and coworkers[152] have called attention to recurrence in the cribriform plate area, possibly resulting from a relative underdosage in this region as a consequence of eye shielding. Jereb and coworkers[152] recommend an electron-beam boost to the anterior cribriform plate region to prevent such recurrence. Proper eye shielding and an appreciation of the penumbra inherent in many radiotherapy units may also prevent recurrence in this region without the need to resort to an electron boost. Miralbell and associates[153] found a significant relationship between subfrontal and subtemporal failure and the adequacy of the whole-brain field used during neuraxis therapy. The authors found no relation between supratentorial control and adequacy of the whole-brain field around the cerebral convexity. This latter finding implies that supratentorial relapse may be related to the effects of gravity and that the entire supratentorium may not require elective radiotherapy. Miralbell and colleagues[154] have published a proton-beam plan for medulloblastoma that effectively irradiates the entire ventricular system and subfrontal and subtemporal area but avoids the remainder of the cortex. Clinical efficacy of this unique approach remains to be established.

The posterior fossa remains the most common site of recurrence. At least two thirds of treatment failures have a component of local recurrence, and approximately 25% have a component of spinal seeding. Isolated spinal recurrence or relapse in portions of the brain outside the posterior fossa are rare. Most recurrence, in any site, occurs within a time frame predicted by Collins' rule: that is, within a period of time equal to the life span of the child at the time of diagnosis plus 9 months.[155] According to Raimondi and Tomita,[136] only patients less than 2 years old at diagnosis obey Collins' rule.

Despite the foregoing, there remains little evidence that the entire posterior fossa requires the full boost dose. It is uncertain whether local relapse reflects relapse within the tumor bed or elsewhere in the posterior fossa. Khafaga and associates[156] reported poorer control following boost with less than a 2-cm margin around the bed compared with all larger volumes. In the review of technique by Miralbell and colleagues[153] previously cited, there was no statistically significant relationship between local control and the adequacy of posterior fossa fields. Should the boost dose be delivered to the entire posterior fossa, Fukunaga-Johnson and colleagues[156a] advocate that conformal techniques be used. This method permits irradiation of the entire posterior fossa with significant cochlear dose reduction compared with standard parallel opposed fields. Cochlear dose reduction by conformal radiotherapy is achieved, however, at the cost of modest dose increase to the pituitary and mandible.

The influence on prognosis of the extent of resection is difficult to separate from confounding variables, such as tumor size and posterior fossa dose. According to Silverman and colleagues[134] and Mealey and Hall,[157] when only patients receiving optimal radiation fields and dose are considered, there are no prognostic differences between total resection, subtotal resection, and biopsy only. Extent of surgery may not be an independent prognostic factor in the data from Kopelson and colleagues.[158] For T1 and T2 lesions, there was no prognostic significance to degree (total resection equaled partial resection; virtually none had biopsy only), and T3 and T4 tumors rarely had any surgery other than biopsy. In Kopelson's overall patient group, those who had radical surgery did better than those with biopsy only.[158] Packer and associates[159] report similar data from the University of Pennsylvania. Patients who underwent gross total removal had a 70% 5-year survival rate versus a 36% survival for those with less than gross total removal.

Prognosis for adults appears to be the same as for pediatric patients.[158] This situation may be due to the higher incidence of the desmoplastic variant in adults.[160, 161] In a large review of adult patients, Carrie and colleagues[160] from the Institut Gustave Roussy reported 46 of 156 patients available for histologic review had the desmoplastic variant. In this series, the 10-year survival and relapse-free survival rates were 51% and 48%. Multivariate analysis revealed significantly shorter survival associated with classic cell type, brain stem invasion, fourth ventricular involvement, and spinal dose less than 30 Gy. In all adult series, the posterior fossa remains the most common site of relapse, occasionally 8 years after treatment.[160]

## Chemotherapy

Recurrent medulloblastoma is responsive to various agents, and this observation stimulated randomized and nonrandomized adjuvant trials.[157, 162–164] The Pediatric Oncology Group (POG) evaluated MOPP (mechlorethamine, vincristine [Oncovin], procarbazine, prednisone) in 71 patients. No significant difference in relapse-free survival was noted with chemotherapy.[165] Overall survival was superior with MOPP if results were corrected for age. Subgroup analysis revealed

that MOPP significantly improved the relapse-free and overall survival of patients older than 5 years. The Childrens Cancer Group (CCG) evaluated CCNU, vincristine, and prednisone in 179 patients.[166] No significant difference in relapse-free or overall survival rates was found. Subgroup analysis revealed significant benefit to chemotherapy only for T3/T4/M+ patients. Five-year overall rates were 61% and 19%. Relapse-free rates were 46% and 0%. The SIOP evaluated CCNU and vincristine in 285 patients.[167] No significant survival differences were found. Subgroups benefiting from chemotherapy were patients with brain stem invasion, patients with residual tumor, and patients younger than 2 years old. Packer and colleagues[168] employed CCNU, vincristine, and cisplatin for high-risk patients. They reported 87% 5-year survival, which was significantly better than that of historical controls treated by radiotherapy alone.

Chemotherapy has been administered before radiotherapy to delay or defer irradiation of infants and to decrease tumor burden of those with residual disease. In a POG trial, Duffner and colleagues[169] used vincristine, cyclophosphamide, cisplatin, and etoposide in 198 infants. Patients younger than 24 months old received 2 years of therapy, whereas patients 24 to 36 months old received 1 year of therapy. Radiotherapy was to be delivered to patients at 4 years of age or at progression during chemotherapy. The overall progression-free survival rates for the older and younger infants were 41% and 39%. Respective overall survival rates were 75% and 53%. Survival rate was particularly encouraging for patients who were M negative and completely resected or showing complete response to chemotherapy. There were 13 patients free of disease after chemotherapy who never were irradiated. Eleven remain free of relapse a median of 1 year after treatment. Geyer and coworkers[170] reported a similar CCG trial in 96 patients. Patients younger than 18 months old received *8 in 1.* Although the protocol specified posterior fossa radiotherapy after two cycles of treatment or craniospinal therapy 1 year after diagnosis, few patients were ever irradiated. Results were considerably poorer than in the POG trial. The 3-year progression-free survival rate was 25% and 30% percent in those M negative and totally resected. The median time to relapse was 6 months, implying failure during chemotherapy administration.

These two trials leave the question of deferred radiotherapy unanswered. In the POG trial and in the St. Jude's Hospital experience, long-term relapse-free survival is possible in patients with an incomplete response, but not progressive disease, following a full course of chemotherapy and who then receive neuraxis radiotherapy.[171, 172] The results of radiotherapy delivered to those with progression during chemotherapy appear less encouraging, particularly in those who then show less than complete response to neuraxis irradiation.

Chemotherapy may permit lowering the craniospinal dose of radiotherapy. Preradiation chemotherapy has resulted in clearing of the CSF of malignant cells. Goldwein and associates[173] delivered 1800 cGy to the neuraxis and standard 50 to 55 Gy to the posterior fossa plus vincristine and CCNU and cisplatin to good-risk patients. Three of 10 patients experienced recurrence in the spine. Halberg and colleagues[174] used 25 Gy to the neuraxis and 54 Gy to the primary site plus procarbazine and hydroxyurea for high-risk patients. They reported 56% 5-year relapse-free survival without significantly higher spine relapse than historical controls. Bouffet and associates[175] stressed that elimination of neuraxis radiotherapy may be unwise even for patients responding to preradiation chemotherapy. In their report of the French M4 trial, 9 of 13 relapses involved the supratentorium when patients received preradiotherapy drugs and irradiation of the posterior fossa and spine only. Gentet and coworkers[176] reported the results of the successor trial to the French M4. Patients older than 3 years received 27 Gy whole brain, 30 to 36 Gy to the spine, and 50 to 55 Gy to the posterior fossa. Patients younger than 3 received the same doses except 20 Gy to the whole brain. Chemotherapy consisted of *8 in 1*. The 5-year, relapse-free survival rates for good-risk and poor-risk patients were 74% and 57%. Many patients received whole-brain doses greater than protocol specifications. Univariate analysis revealed whole-brain doses greater than or less than 30 Gy were not associated with tumor relapse rates.

# EPENDYMOMAS

Ependymomas are glial tumors, described by Bailey in 1926, that arise from ependymal cells lining the ventricles, central spinal canal, conus medullaris, and filum terminale.[101] Cranial ependymomas may originate in the supratentorium, where they often have a more prominent parenchymal than intraventricular component, or the infratentorium, where they arise from the midline of the fourth ventricle. In this latter location, involvement of the upper cervical spinal cord is common.[177] Cranial ependymomas are seen predominantly in children and young adults at an average age of 23 years for unselected patients. The relative frequency of supratentorial and infratentorial ependymomas is controversial, but generally the latter site predominates in all age groups. This predominance is especially true in the pediatric age group, in which ependymoma is the third most common infratentorial tumor, following cerebellar astrocytoma and medulloblastoma.[178]

Ependymomas grow slowly, and the duration of symptoms can be correspondingly long.[179] Histologic subtyping (cellular, epithelial, myxopapillary, anaplastic) appears to be of limited therapeutic or prognostic usefulness for cranial ependymomas.[180] Histologic grading according to the systems of Kernohan or Rubinstein has been difficult to apply to ependymomas. Patients with low-grade ependymomas fare significantly better than those with high-grade lesions according to many authors. Mork and Loken[178] found no impact of grade on survival until after 4 years. Survival beyond that point was significantly better for low-grade tumors. Kovalic and associates[181] confirmed the prognostic value of grade in a multivariate analysis of 31 patients. The 10-year relapse-free survivals were 55% for low-grade ependymomas and 26% for high-grade tumors. Many other authors, however, report that grade does not predict reliably the biologic behavior of ependymoma.[182–184]

The reported incidence of both grades of cranial ependymoma by site is controversial. In unselected patients, there is generally an equal incidence of high-grade and low-grade ependymomas.[181, 185] There is a greater frequency of benign ependymoma in infratentorial tumors, whereas high-grade lesions predominate in the supratentorium.[183, 186] Ross and Rubinstein[185] stressed that the ependymoblastoma must be separated from otherwise malignant ependymoma when analyzing patients. The ependymoblastoma is now considered to be a primitive neuroectodermal tumor with ependymal differentiation and is more properly considered with the medulloblastoma. The ependymoblastoma presents in the supratentorium of patients younger than 5 years old, and median survival is generally 12 to 20 months.[187, 188] The reader is cautioned that many literature series examining the relationship of grade and prognosis of ependymomas fail to exclude ependymoblastoma from the group of otherwise *malignant* ependymoma.

Before treatment, CSF examination and spinal imaging are recommended. In four series, positive cytologic findings were reported in 6 of 93 examinations.[181, 183, 189] CSF dissemination at diagnosis appears uncommon in children younger than 3 years old. In a POG evaluation of 43 children, CSF was positive in 2, and none showed imaging evidence of subarachnoid involvement.

The influence of primary site on prognosis is more controversial and, in part, reflects the grade distribution of the patients studied (Table 72–11). Better outcome has been reported for infratentorial ependymomas by many authors.[183, 190, 191] Kovalic and associates[181] reported a 10-year relapse-free survival of 48% for infratentorial tumors compared with 0% for supratentorial disease ($p = 0.0025$ univariate). In that series, all supratentorial tumors were high grade, and when the authors used multivariate analysis, no significance was found for tumor site. McLaughlin and colleagues[190] reported that site was the only significant prognostic factor in their multivariate analysis. The 10-year overall survival rates for supratentorial and infratentorial lesions were 20% and 45%.[190] Several other groups report superior prognosis for supratentorial ependymomas[192] or no influence of location.[184]

Data from Princess Margaret Hospital and the Christie Hospital indicate that the prognosis for adults is superior to that of children.[193, 194] Chin and coworkers[195] from Kentucky reported a 17% 5-year survival for adults compared with 50% for children. Most authors have found that younger children, variously defined, have poorer prognosis than older children. Kovalic and associates[181] employed multivariate analysis and showed no relationship between patient age and prognosis.

## Surgery

After the diagnosis of an intracranial mass that is believed to be consistent with ependymoma, the initial therapy of

*Table 72–11.* **Influence of Site on Survival with Ependymoma**

| Author* | Supratentorial (%) | Infratentorial (%) |
|---|---|---|
| Phillps[402] | 42 (80)† | 69 (90)† |
| Kricheff[403] | 22 | 45 |
| Kim[198] | 46 | 33 |
| Marks[404] | 32 | 57 |
| Chin[195] | 37 | 47 |
| McLaughlin[190] | 20 | 45 |

*Only the first author is given.
†Numbers in parentheses represent percent of patients finishing course of radiation, as discussed in text.

choice should be surgery, with the goal of maximal possible resection of the tumor without causing neurologic deficit. When invasion of the brain stem (for infratentorial tumors) or eloquent cortex (for supratentorial tumors) is extensive, total excision is often not possible, and good surgical judgment should be exercised. Operative mortality for these lesions was estimated to be 20 to 50%.[178] In more recent series with modern microneurosurgical techniques, mortality rates are reported to be 0 to 2% for supratentorial ependymomas and 5 to 8% for infratentorial lesions.[192, 196] After surgery, a lumbar puncture, myelogram, or spinal MRI scan should be performed to look for *drop metastases*.

## Radiation Therapy

Postoperative irradiation, although performed in a nonrandomized fashion, has been shown to improve survival in many series (Table 72–12). Regardless of grade, site, age, dose, or volume, overall 5-year survival rates of 37 to 79% have been reported when radiotherapy was part of the therapeutic approach. Among 35 irradiated children with infratentorial ependymoma in Toronto, 5-year survival was 87% with total resection compared with 30% with lesser resection (*p*<0.01).[189] At Children's Hospital of Philadelphia, 5-year progression-free survival was 60% for patients with total or near-total resection compared with 21% for patients with lesser removal (*p*<0.01).[192] No prognostic significance of resection in irradiated patients was reported by others.[183, 190, 197] This discrepancy may be due to the method of analyzing degree of resection. Investigators at the Children's Hospital of Boston used postoperative imaging to judge the degree of resection. The 5-year progression-free survival was 75% in patients without residual tumor on imaging compared with 0% for patients with residual tumor. In that same series, however, surgical assessment of the degree of resection did not correlate with prognosis.

Many authors report better survival following doses greater than 45 Gy.[183, 198, 199] Although a dose effect is commonly reported, it is not a universal finding.[197] Wallner and associates[200] from UCSF stated that a dose effect exists—local control and survival being clearly inferior when less than 45 Gy is administered—but it is uncertain whether doses approaching 55 Gy yield substantially better results than doses between 45 and 50 Gy. Finally, in multivariate

*Table 72–12.* **Survival with Cranial Ependymoma Following Radiation Therapy and Surgery**

| Author* | 5-Year Survival (%) |
|---|---|
| Kim[198] | 37 |
| Chin[195] | 37 |
| Mørk[178] | 40 |
| Kricheff[403] | 41 |
| Salazar[179] | 45 |
| Bloom[163] | 47 |
| Phillips[402] | 56 |
| Bouchard[394] | 60 |
| Marsa[396] | 79 |
| Garrett[193] | 43 |
| Pierre-Kahn[243a] | 51 |
| Shaw[93] | 61 |

*Only the first author is given.

analyses, Kovalic and coworkers[181] found 10-year relapse-free survivals of 49% with at least 50 Gy and 31% with lower doses (*p*=0.05).

The appropriate volume of CNS to irradiate is the most controversial aspect of management because of the uncertain risk of spinal seeding. The risk of leptomeningeal recurrence, previously reported to be 66%, has been shown to be low for ependymomas.[184, 191] Vanuytsel and Brada[200a] reviewed the literature and reported an overall rate of seeding of 7% for all types of ependymoma. The development of seeding was not influenced by use of elective craniospinal-axis irradiation. The rates for high-grade ependymomas with and without craniospinal-axis irradiation were 9% and 7%. The rates for low-grade tumors were 9% and 2%. Overall, seeding was reported for 1.7% of supratentorial lesions and 9.7% of infratentorial lesions. Local recurrence was a factor in spinal relapse. The authors found 3% spinal relapse when the primary tumor was controlled and 10% when local recurrence was documented. No difference in spinal seeding with or without craniospinal-axis irradiation was noted for patients with local control or local failure. Many authors report that isolated spinal relapse is a rare event, and most such relapses occur in the setting of local failure. These data imply that there is no role for elective craniospinal-axis irradiation in any primary ependymoma. Elective craniospinal-axis irradiation was previously recommended for all high-grade ependymomas. Many series have shown no significant advantage to elective craniospinal-axis irradiation for any grade of ependymoma. Goldwein and colleagues[183] continue to advise craniospinal-axis irradiation for all high-grade infratentorial tumors and high-grade supratentorial tumors with ventricular impingement. These authors published the results of treatment for 17 children with anaplastic ependymomas.[201] Two-year survival rates were 40% with local fields and 52% with craniospinal-axis irradiation. All authors recommend craniospinal-axis irradiation for patients with evidence of leptomeningeal dissemination at diagnosis of ependymoblastoma. There is little evidence that local control following partial brain irradiation is significantly inferior to whole-brain treatment.[191, 197]

Median time to relapse following radiotherapy varies from 16 to 40 months in the literature. Isolated local failure accounts for most relapses after radiotherapy. Goldwein and coworkers[183] documented that recurrent ependymoma may be more or less differentiated than the initial tumor. Distant metastases are uncommon but reported for ependymomas. Newton and coworkers[202] reported an incidence of 6% at Memorial Sloan-Kettering and reviewed the literature. The mean age of patients experiencing recurrence outside the CNS was 15 years, and the mean interval to metastases was 29 months. Malignant ependymoma and ependymoblastoma were most likely to metastasize.

## Chemotherapy

There have been few data regarding chemotherapy in ependymoma. The studies have shown limited efficacy in patients with ependymoma. Use of chemotherapy has been limited to recurrent ependymoma or anaplastic ependymoma. Agents used that have shown limited efficacy include carboplatin, cisplatin, etoposide, and vincristine.

## PINEAL TUMORS

Pineal body tumors are rare brain lesions seen primarily in males during the first two decades of life. They account for 8% of pediatric CNS malignancies. They are notoriously common in Japan. Histologically, primary pineal tumors fall into one of three categories: germinal, parenchymal, and glial. Germinal neoplasms consist of germinomas, which histologically resemble testicular seminoma or ovarian dysgerminoma, or other germ cell tumors, including teratoma, teratocarcinoma, embryomal carcinoma, choriocarcinoma, endodermal sinus tumor, and yolk sac tumor. Germinomas account for approximately 50% of all pineal germ cell neoplasms.[203] True germinomas have previously been termed *pinealomas, pineal dysgerminomas,* and *atypical teratomas.* Glial tumors are composed of the various grades of astrocytomas and arise from the quadrigeminal plate, secondarily involving the pineal gland. Tumors of the pineal parenchyma (neuroectoderm) consist of well-differentiated pineocytomas and poorly differentiated pineoblastomas.

Pineal tumors may spread by any one of four major routes. Contiguous spread to the floor and walls of the third ventricle, quadrigeminal plate, aqueduct, pituitary gland, hypothalamus, and cerebellum has been documented.[204] This situation is especially true for germinomas, and because they constitute most pineal tumors, the overall risk of brain invasion is high.[205] Cerebellar involvement is particularly ominous.[206] Spinal and cerebral subarachnoid seeding are possible from any tumor that potentially invades the ventricular surface. The incidence of such dissemination is controversial because of the histologic variability and uncertainty inherent in treatment of these tumors as well as the lack of analysis of cumulative risk. In six series, CSF cytology was positive at diagnosis in only 16 of 100 germinoma patients evaluated by lumbar puncture or imaging.[207–211] In a review of the UCSF experience with confirmed or suspected germ cell tumors of all histologies, spinal MRI was negative for metastatic disease in 30 of 31 evaluable patients. In the same report, myelography was negative in 35 of 36 cases.[212]

Pineoblastomas represent another histologic type capable of seeding. In this regard, they are thought to resemble medulloblastomas and primitive neuroectodermal tumors. Pineocytomas have generally been considered low-grade malignancies unlikely to seed. Data from the University of Pennsylvania challenge this assumption. The authors describe several cases of these tumors in children that recurred locally and in the spine, despite craniospinal-axis irradiation.

Pineal tumors classically produce paralysis of upward gaze (Parinaud's syndrome) resulting from pressure on the corpora quadrigemina of the midbrain. Posterior extension can lead to obstructive hydrocephalus or hypothalamic dysfunction. The suprasellar germinoma, or *ectopic pinealoma,* is a variant of a true pineal germinoma in which the pineal body is normal, but germinoma tissue involves the pituitary infundibulum. This tumor produces a triad of diabetes insipidus, homonymous hemianopsia, and pituitary insufficiency. The double midline tumor is another unusual entity, involving pineal and suprasellar areas. Most double midline lesions prove to be germinomas if biopsy is performed. There is an association of an autosomal dominant bilateral retinoblastoma with a subsequent pineoblastoma (trilateral retinoblastoma). Histologically, these two entities may be difficult to

separate. Because the pineal lesions arise years after treatment of the retinal tumors, many considered the former a metastasis of the latter. The pineal tumor is now recognized as a true second malignancy.[213–215] Also reported are a malignant germ cell tumor arising years after removal of a benign teratoma[216] and a suprasellar germinoma associated with a hypothalamic glioma.[217]

MRI has proved to be the best available diagnostic tool and may aid in establishing histologic diagnosis.[218–220] Attention has been given to identifying serum and CSF markers for pineal tumors. Alpha-fetoprotein and β-human chorionic gonadotrophin elevations in serum and CSF have been reported for patients with nongerminoma germ cell tumors.[221] Modest elevation of β-human chorionic gonadotrophin less than 100 has been reported for nongerminoma or pure germinoma.[222, 223] Elevation of melatonin and hydroxyindole-O-methyl transferase have been reported with pineal parenchymal tumors.

Modern microsurgical approaches have made surgical removal, when indicated, a safe procedure. Biopsy verification of tumor is now advocated by most neurosurgeons and radiation oncologists. Reliance on the *radiation biopsy* has fallen into disfavor. Nongerminoma histology has been documented at relapse following irradiation for presumed germinoma or germinoma proved by biopsy.[211, 224]

### Surgery

The optimal management strategy for pineal region tumors has yet to be determined. The indications for open surgical resection, stereotactic biopsy, and *trial radiation therapy* (without tissue diagnosis) are still controversial. It is generally agreed that germinomas are radiosensitive and best treated with radiation therapy. In the past, if a pineal region tumor had the classic imaging characteristics of a germinoma on MRI, some advocated no surgery and giving a test dose of radiation. If the tumor responded, radiation therapy could be continued without surgical diagnosis of a presumed germinoma.[225] Others argued that a tissue diagnosis by stereotactic biopsy was necessary before exposing patients with benign or radioresistant tumors to needless radiation.[226] As modern neurosurgical navigation techniques have improved, the risks of surgical biopsy have correspondingly decreased, and most neurosurgeons and neuro-oncologists discourage radiation treatment of pineal region tumors without tissue diagnosis. A report found the mortality and morbidity rate of stereotactic biopsies in this area to be 1.3% and 7%. Another shortcoming of stereotactic biopsy is that it may fail to disclose the histologic heterogeneity of some pineal tumors.[227]

There is still controversy regarding the role of stereotactic biopsy versus open resection for pineal tumors. Some believe that because the pineal region has numerous large vessels (e.g., vein of Galen, basal veins of Rosenthal, internal cerebral veins), a closed biopsy may be riskier than an open operation.[228] Because the diagnostic rate of stereotactic biopsies is only about 94%,[226] some neurosurgeons argue that most pineal tumors should be considered for open resection as the initial form of management.[228] Surgery is the treatment of choice for radioresistant tumors (e.g., malignant nongerminomas) and is potentially curative for benign tumors in this region (e.g., pinealomas, teratomas, and pilocytic astrocytomas). For patients presenting acutely with obstructive hydrocephalus, one may re-establish obstructed CSF pathways by removing the offending element of tumor that compresses the third ventricle or the aqueduct of Sylvius. A significant number of patients with pineal region tumors can avoid permanent ventricular shunting after open surgical resection of lesions, which would prevent the possible shunt-induced seeding of tumor cells.[139] Despite certain advantages, however, open surgery is still reportedly associated with a 5 to 10% morbidity rate, even in the best neurosurgical hands. Postoperative complications include Parinaud's syndrome, new visual field deficits, epidural fluid collections, infection, and cerebellar ataxia.[226, 227]

### Radiation Therapy

Individual centers generally report 5-year relapse-free survival rates of 85 to 100% for verified germinomas.[229, 230] Several groups report inferior results in patients irradiated on a presumptive diagnosis of germinoma,[212, 231] although others report equivalent results.[222] Patients with nongerminoma germ cell tumors have reported 5-year relapse-free survival rates following irradiation of 6 to 60%. At the Mayo Clinic, survival of nongerminoma germ cell tumors was related to the use of CT scanning and histology and the degree of resection.[232] There was no impact of radiotherapy on survival for patients with mature or immature teratomas. For all other histologies, survival was significantly better following adjunctive radiotherapy than resection alone. Survival rates for patients with pineal glial tumors depends on tumor differentiation. Pineoblastoma was previously associated with poor survival.[233] More recent reports are more encouraging.[234, 235] The survival of patients with pineocytoma is uncertain because of the rarity of the disease.[233] Pineocytomas with prominent glial or neuronal differentiation may behave as benign lesions. It is likely that varying amounts of such differentiation account for the divergent results reported for pineocytomas.

The minimal effective dose for CNS germinomas has not been established reliably. Although histologic complete response of germinomas has been documented following doses of 16 Gy,[236] there is little indication that the radiosensitivity of CNS germinomas equals that of testicular seminomas. Most series, although not randomized, report the highest rates of survival and local control with doses greater than 50 Gy.[229, 230, 237] Current UCSF recommendations are tumor doses of 50 Gy for germinoma and 55 to 60 Gy for nongerminomas.[212] Schild and associates[234] reported higher local relapse for pineal parenchymal lesions receiving less than 50 Gy compared with higher doses.

Appropriate field size for cranial radiotherapy is undefined for pineal region tumors. Many series published before the routine use of CT scanning suggested inferior results with local fields.[210, 232] Salazar and colleagues[204] reported 10-year survival rates of 70% for germinoma patients receiving whole-brain irradiation compared with 50% following irradiation of the ventricular system or a local field. One of 12 patients recurred locally following whole-brain treatment, whereas 6 of 10 did so with smaller fields. Whole-brain irradiation, treatment of the ventricular system, and local fields have all been advised. The UCSF group advocates 24 Gy to the entire ventricular system followed by boosts of 26

Gy for germinoma and 30 to 36 Gy for nongerminomas. According to Bradfield and Perez,[229] when field size is adequate to prevent marginal failure, tumor size is not prognostic.

The risk of spinal relapse and the role of prophylactic craniospinal-axis irradiation for pineal region tumors are contentious. Lindstadt and coworkers[237a] reviewed the literature and reported an average rate of spinal recurrence of 8% (range, 0 to 25%) for verified germinoma patients receiving craniospinal-axis irradiation. The average for verified patients not receiving craniospinal-axis irradiation was 23% (range, 0 to 55%). The average rates for unverified germinomas with and without craniospinal-axis irradiation were 11% (range, 0 to 25%) and 9% (range; 0 to 33%). In the experience at UCSF, 1 of 31 verified or presumed germinomas relapsed in the spine following partial brain treatment. Craniospinal-axis irradiation does not prevent leptomeningeal seeding reliably because spine relapse frequently occurs in association with local tumor recurrence.

Many authors continue to advise elective craniospinal-axis irradiation.[209] Dearnaley and colleagues[238] reported that the average rate of isolated spine failure in the literature was 7% without craniospinal-axis irradiation compared with none of 74 patients with craniospinal-axis irradiation from the literature. The salvage rate of patients with spinal relapse is admittedly low, and this constitutes a prime argument for elective craniospinal-axis irradiation.

Nongerminoma germ cell tumors are uncommon, and the risk of spinal seeding is undetermined. Craniospinal-axis irradiation has been advocated for all nongerminomas[231] or for endodermal sinus tumors.[209] At UCSF, 44 patients with various confirmed or suspected germ cell tumors and negative evaluations of the spine underwent radiotherapy that excluded the neuraxis. Isolated spinal relapse was noted in 2%, whereas five others relapsed in the meninges at the time of local failure.[212] Malignant teratoma may be at particular risk for spinal seeding.[232]

Craniospinal-axis irradiation is recommended for patients with malignant CSF cytology, those with radiographic evidence of leptomeningeal or ventricular seeding, and those with gross spillage during resection. Craniospinal-axis irradiation is generally recommended for patients with double midline tumors.

### Chemotherapy

Both germinoma germ cell tumors and nongerminoma germ cell tumors of the CNS are sensitive to chemotherapy. Agents used include carboplatin, etoposide, and bleomycin and cyclophosphamide in combination or alone. Greater than 50% of the patients studied showed a complete response when chemotherapy was given in the neoadjuvant setting.[239, 240] We do not advocate use of chemotherapy in the neoadjuvant or adjuvant setting outside of a clinical trial at this time, but chemotherapy can provide a benefit in the recurrent setting.

## BRAIN STEM

Brain stem tumors are seen primarily in children and young adults. Pontomedullary tumors are especially predominant in the pediatric population, in which they account for 15% of CNS tumors. In a review of the McGill University experience, 50% of all brain stem tumors occurred in patients younger than 15 years old. Tumors in this region frequently involve more than one brain stem structure.[241]

Antemortem specimens are often unavailable from these sites. When pathologic material was available, from biopsy or necropsy, astrocytic gliomas accounted for most tumors.[242, 243] Pierre-Kahn and colleagues[243a] reported a series of 75 children undergoing resection of brain stem tumors, predominantly exophytic and surface lesions. Pure glial tumors were noted in 69 patients (58 astrocytomas and 11 oligodendrogliomas), whereas the remainder included ganglioglioma, primitive neuroectodermal tumor, and ependymoma. The grade distribution of these astrocytomas is debatable. In some series, brain stem gliomas, especially pontine, are primarily high grade[244]; in other series, low-grade tumors prevail, or an equal distribution of grades is reported.[245] Autopsy information accounted for a substantial amount of pathologic diagnoses in these historical series, histologic information is derived from a selected group of patients. According to Panitch and Berg,[246] the symptomatic duration is inversely related to grade of a brain stem tumor.

Although technically feasible and relatively nonmorbid, histologic confirmation of malignancy may not be necessary for brain stem tumors. Modern neuroimaging has attained remarkable specificity, sensitivity, and predictive value.[247, 248] Although rare benign processes are occasionally reported from necropsy following empirical irradiation, patients undergoing irradiation following a radiographic diagnosis of glioma have a survival identical to those undergoing irradiation after biopsy confirmation of tumor.[249] MRI is superior to CT scanning for evaluating brain stem gliomas.[247, 250] In the experience of Packer and colleagues,[248] MRI showed more extensive disease than CT scanning in 50% of cases. Histopathologic evidence of tumor corresponds most closely to the signal abnormality seen with long TR/TE imaging sequences.[241] Albright and associates[251] and Stroink and coworkers[252] believe the precontrast CT tumor density is prognostic for brain stem gliomas. Patients with an intrinsic, hypodense lesion have an inferior survival following irradiation compared with patients with isodense or hyperdense lesions. The degree and pattern of CT enhancement appear unrelated to tumor grade or prognosis for brain stem patients.

## Surgery

Surgery for brain stem and midbrain gliomas is usually not recommended. It has been argued that even biopsies should not be performed for diffuse infiltrating brain stem lesions because diagnosis can likely be made based on MRI, and surgical biopsy does not change treatment or outcome.[253] The one exception when surgery may be indicated for brain stem or midbrain tumors is the surgical resection of lesions with an exophytic component.[254] These tumors may protrude into the ventricles and tend to be lower grade. The surgical goals of operating on exophytic brain stem or midbrain tumors are (1) to enhance survival by subtotal removal of the exophytic component[255] or (2) to establish a diagnosis because radiographic differentiation of exophytic brain stem gliomas from other tumors (e.g., medulloblastoma, ependymoma, dermoids) may be difficult.[253]

## Radiotherapy

Primary irradiation is the therapeutic modality of choice for midbrain or brain stem gliomas. Survival of irradiated patients is superior to those receiving no specific therapy. Panitch and Berg[246] showed an average survival time of 15 months without radiation versus 47 months with radiotherapy. Symptomatic stabilization or improvement is reported in 60 to 80% of irradiated patients.[256] The 5-year survival for brain stem gliomas following radiotherapy varies from 15 to 38%. Medullary tumors appear to do better than pontine tumors. Thalamic or midbrain tumors yield 40 to 72% 5-year survival. Quality of life following irradiation is reportedly good, even for patients younger than 3 years old.[257, 258]

No randomized trials have been undertaken to determine the optimal dose for these tumors. The earlier data from the orthovoltage era are not useful for decision-making because of necessarily low doses and poor survival. Modern literature supports tumor doses of 50 to 55 Gy, but there is no clear dose-response relationship using higher doses.[242, 243, 251] Kim and associates[258a] reported 20% 5-year survival with doses greater than 50 Gy versus no survival with lesser doses. Hibi and coworkers[259] reported significant improvement in radiographic response rate as tumor dose increased from less than 45 Gy to greater than 65 Gy. Survival, however, decreased with tumor doses greater than 55 Gy, possibly as a result of neurotoxicity.

Field size for brain stem gliomas should include the neuroimaging tumor volume plus a judicious margin of uninvolved parenchyma. Gliomas in this region spread contiguously, and the extent of spread is grade related. Pontine lesions may extend cephalocaudal into the diencephalon and medulla as well as posteriorly into the cerebellum. Mantravadi and coworkers[260] reported that the cerebellum was involved in 9 of 17 patients with pontine gliomas at autopsy. Medullary lesions may involve the cervical cord. The pattern of relapse of brain stem gliomas following modern radiotherapeutic management is overwhelmingly within the portal or at its margins. In the combined Washington University and Duke University experience, in-field recurrence was noted in 91 of 96 relapsing patients.[243, 261]

Survival following primary radiotherapy appears to be related to histologic grade.[262] Albright and colleagues[251] reported 65% 2-year survival for low-grade gliomas compared with 14% for anaplastic gliomas. Age is a significant prognostic factor. Bloom and coworkers[262a] reported that older children fare better than younger patients. Kim and associates[258a] found superior survival at 10 years for children younger than age 15 with brain stem tumors. Neurologic response to irradiation, measured 1 month after therapy, may be prognostic. Kim and associates[258a] showed a 50% survival among *responders* versus no 5-year survivors among *nonresponders*. The significance of specific symptoms remains controversial. Albright and colleagues[263] have established the significance of cranial nerve palsy at diagnosis. Five-year survival among patients without palsy was 38% compared with 0% for those with a cranial nerve deficit. Eifel and coworkers[242] at the Joint Center for Radiation Therapy published data supporting the influence of sex on prognosis. They reported that the survival rates for males and females with thalamic tumors were 92% and 46%. Survival rates for infratentorial brain stem gliomas according to gender were 40% and 20%. The morphologic growth pattern may have prognostic value. Albright and colleagues[263] reported a 50% survival rate for exophytic lesions compared with 13% for intrinsic brain stem tumors. Hoffman and coworkers[255] reported no tumor deaths among 10 exophytic lesions, including 6 managed with subtotal resection alone.

Efforts to improve radiotherapy results have centered on altered fractionation. Various centers and cooperative groups have used hyperfractionation and escalated tumor doses to 78 Gy. Despite this aggressive approach, reported survivals are no better than historical results with conventional radiotherapy. Investigators at UCSF reported 2-year survival of 62% for thalamic and midbrain tumors and 16% for pontomedullary lesions following hyperfractionated radiotherapy.[264] Two-year survival for focal tumors was 70% compared with 5% for diffuse intrinsic lesions. Packer and associates[265] also commented that the inclusion of favorable subsets of patients—low-grade gliomas, adults, focal intrinsic lesions, diencephalic tumors—may produce an apparent advantage in altered fractionation trials. The role of altered fractionation remains undefined for brain stem gliomas. A randomized POG trial showed no survival differences between 70.2 Gy by hyperfractionation versus 54 Gy by conventional techniques.[266] Investigators in the United Kingdom reported no benefit to an accelerated fractionation approach of 1.8 Gy twice per day to 48.6 to 50.4 Gy.9.[267]

### Chemotherapy

Brain stem gliomas are rarely responsive to chemotherapy. Agents thought to show some efficacy are those listed in the section on malignant gliomas.

## OPTIC GLIOMAS

Tumors originating in the optic nerve or chiasm are rare lesions, seen predominantly in the pediatric population.[268–270] The rarity of this tumor and the difficulty in examining young patients often lead to delays in diagnosis exceeding 1 year.[270, 271] von Recklinghausen's disease occurs in 20 to 50% of these patients but carries no prognostic significance.[272–274] Bilateral optic glioma may be more common with von Recklinghausen's disease.[269, 275]

The most common tumor in this area is a low-grade astrocytic glioma.[276, 277] Malignant optic gliomas occur rarely in adults. Although Hoyt and Baghdassarian[278] suggested that these lesions may represent benign congenital hamartoma, cell culture studies as well as clinical progression of untreated cases suggest the neoplastic nature of this entity.[279–281]

There is no accepted staging system for optic tumors, although most authors subdivide lesions into those confined to an optic nerve, those with chiasmal involvement, and those with hypothalamic involvement. The former situation is encountered rarely: Hoyt and Baghdassarian[278] documented 19%; Montgomery and colleagues,[282] 31%; and Danoff and colleagues,[268] 0%. In virtually all series, chiasmal lesions with or without posterior extension to the hypothalamus and third ventricle prevail.

### Surgery

Optic gliomas involving a single optic nerve, causing proptosis and vision loss, should be treated by a transcranial excision of the nerve from the globe all the way back to the optic chiasm. A transorbital approach alone is not appropriate because tumor should not be left on the optic nerve stump. Tumors involving the chiasm are generally not treated surgically except for biopsy or CSF shunting to reduce intracranial pressure. Rarely, surgery is sometimes indicated to remove the exophytic component of an optic tumor to try to improve vision.

### Radiation Therapy

Surgical removal is advocated for patients already blind from localized optic nerve tumor. Long-term local control approaches 100% if the proximal resection margin is free of tumor.[186, 271, 272, 280, 281] Partial resection alone has been reported to be successful; in the UCSF experience, five of six patients were free of progression from 4 to 13 years.[283] Radiation therapy with surgical salvage is recommended when useful vision remains. Several centers report local control of optic nerve gliomas following radiotherapy, although few patients have been treated. Investigators at Washington University reported 100% actuarial 15-year freedom from progression for five patients.[186] Most authors recommend adjuvant irradiation should the proximal nerve margin disclose histologic evidence of tumor.[284, 285] Gaini and associates[271] controlled all five patients with resected optic gliomas showing tumor infiltration of the intracanalicular portion. Adjuvant irradiation may be withheld in very young patients, although clinicians must recognize that any subsequent relapse is likely to involve the chiasm.

Posterior tumors, accounting for most optic lesions, are more aggressive than their anterior counterparts. Surgical resection is associated with serious morbidity and is advisable only for the rare exophytic tumor.[286, 287] Primary radiotherapy has been shown to be effective for chiasmal gliomas.[288] Flickinger and coworkers[272] and Kovalic and colleagues[186] have documented 15-year freedom-from-progression rates of 75% and 87%. Danoff and associates[268] reported 5- and 10-year survival rates of 100% and 90% for anterior tumors compared with 71% and 66% for tumors involving hypothalamus or third ventricle. Gaini and coworkers[271] reported no relapses among eight patients with anterior chiasmal tumors followed 5 to 30 years. This report is to be compared with relapse in 12 of 18 irradiated posterior tumors. Despite the undeniable success of radiotherapy, many observers recommend surveillance of pediatric patients with anterior chiasmal gliomas. Jenkin and colleagues[289] reported a 10-year relapse-free survival rate of 86% for irradiated anterior gliomas compared with 75% for selected untreated patients. In Jenkin's experience, all patients with anterior chiasmal tumors were alive at 10 years regardless of initial management.[289] Observation is rarely recommended for posterior gliomas.[290–292] Rodriguez and associates[291] reported that the median time to progression for patients with irradiated posterior gliomas was 70 months compared with 30 months for untreated patients ($p<0.01$). Alvord and Lofton[279] reported progressive disease in 50% of patients with hypothalamic extension and 75% with hydrocephalus. Salvage therapy generally failed in these patients, and their survival rates were low, in contrast to the successful salvage of patients with more anterior gliomas. The Princess Margaret Hospital now recommends surveillance of stringently selected posterior glioms.[289] The 10-year progression-free survival rate for 13 observed patients was 52% compared with 75% for 18 irradiated patients. Tao and coworkers[274] irradiated 29 patients with optic chiasmal gliomas showing either clinical or radiographic progression. The 15-year overall and progression-free survivals were 85% and 82%. The apparent success of deferred radiotherapy implies that there may be a role for surveillance of selected pediatric patients with either anterior or posterior chiasmal gliomas. Radiotherapy in this setting could be withheld until the tumor enlarges on two successive imaging studies or there are two successive declines in visual acuity. Patients eligible for surveillance are those with minimal visual or hypothalamic dysfunction and documented evidence of a nonprogressive clinical course. Surveillance requires much of the clinician and the parents. According to Iraci and colleagues,[293] "the line of therapeutic abstention demands considerable powers of decision and perserveration." Borit and Richardson[290] found no histologic differences between stable optic gliomas and tumors that progressed during surveillance.

Most authors recommend 50 Gy in standard fractions to a local field for tumors in this area. Montgomery and associates[282] reported 100% disease-free survival following at least 50 Gy compared with 40% with lesser doses. In a UCSF review, local progression was noted in 56% of chiasmal gliomas receiving less than 50 Gy compared with 22% with higher doses.[283] Flickinger and coworkers[272] at Pittsburgh found a statistically significant association between dose and local control of chiasmal gliomas. In their nonrandom, retrospective series, the highest local control was achieved with doses of at least 1385 roentgen equivalent tumor (ret). The pattern of relapse for irradiated optic apparatus gliomas is overwhelmingly local.[270, 274] Flickinger and coworkers[272] found no significant impact of field size on progression-free survival. An effort should be made to exclude the retinae from treatment portals for chiasmal tumors. Optic chiasm tumors have been reported to invade the globe, but this is so unusual as to mitigate against routine ocular irradiation.[294]

The response of visual dysfunction to radiotherapy is controversial. Several centers report virtually no visual improvement following treatment. Many authors, however, note frequent amelioration of visual complaints. Visual decrement following radiotherapy is extremely unusual, provided that the dose fraction size was 1.8 to 2.0 Gy. Horwich and associates[276] caution that late visual decrement indicates tumor recurrence and not radiation-induced damage. Late endocrine failure has been linked to irradiation but can also be present before irradiation in 20% of patients.[272, 295]

## Chemotherapy

Some investigators have advocated using chemotherapy before radiation, especially in patients younger than 5 years old. In one series, carboplatin and vincristine were used with newly diagnosed disease.[113] More than half showed an objective shrinkage of tumor, and more than 90% had either clinical improvements or disease stabilization during treatment. This type of treatment may delay the need for radiation

therapy in the very young or may provide a salvage treatment in those with recurrent disease.

## MENINGIOMAS

### Surgery

The primary treatment modality recommended for symptomatic meningiomas is gross total surgical excision. Incidental meningiomas without symptoms may be managed expectantly with serial MRI studies because many meningiomas tend to grow slowly, and some *burn out* and stop growing. The recurrence rate is related to tumor location and the ability to resect the tumor and its dural attachment. The Simpson grading system for meningiomas[296] measures the extent of surgical tumor removal and is the most important factor in the prognostication of recurrence. In a 1980 study, gross total tumor removal was associated with an 11 to 15% recurrence rate, whereas incomplete removal had a 29% recurrence.[297] In a more recent retrospective series of 135 meningiomas at UCSF, recurrence rate was 4% after gross total excision and 32 to 60% after partial resection.[298] Five-year recurrence rates after partial resections have been reported to be 37 to 85%, whereas the overall 20-year recurrence rate has been estimated to be 19 to 50% in different surgical series.[299–301]

The role of radiotherapy following incomplete resection of benign meningiomas remains controversial. Condra and colleagues[302] reported a 15-year local control rate of 87% following subtotal resection and postoperative radiotherapy, a result equivalent to that of patients undergoing total resection. By comparison, local control following incomplete resection alone was 30%. In the UCSF experience, 84 patients underwent incomplete resection with an average follow-up of 78 months.[298] The local progression rate for patients receiving immediate irradiation was 32% compared with 60% for patients managed by partial excision alone ($p < 0.05$). Sixteen patients received radiotherapy at the time of tumor progression, and a subsequent progression was noted in 40%. Carella and associates[303] from New York University also reported superior results with immediate compared with deferred irradiation. They reported that 41 of 43 patients were alive following immediate radiotherapy compared with 8 of 14 when radiation therapy was used as part of salvage therapy. In a literature review, Salazar[304] claimed that the average recurrence rate was 18% following immediate radiotherapy and 43% following salvage surgery plus deferred radiotherapy.

Several groups report no significant disadvantage to deferred radiation therapy. Miralbell and coworkers[304a] reported 8-year progression-free survival rates of 88% following immediate irradiation and 78% when irradiation was delivered to relapsing patients. Eight-year progression-free survival rates were 48% when no radiotherapy was delivered after the initial incomplete resection. Most authors report that the time interval to subsequent relapse is lengthened when radiotherapy is administered to patients with recurrent meningioma.[305] Authors claiming no local control advantage or lengthening of recurrence-free interval have irradiated only a small number of patients or provide no technical details of irradiation.[306]

Virtually all authors recommend immediate postoperative radiotherapy for malignant meningiomas and hemangiopericytoma and hemangioblastoma regardless of degree of resection. In the UCSF experience with 23 partially resected malignant tumors, 5-year relapse-free survival following radiotherapy was 48%. King and coworkers[305] documented significant prolongation of recurrence-free interval for angioblastic and sarcomatous meningiomas. Mean interval to relapse for patients with angioblastic tumors was 72 months following radiotherapy compared with 39 months without radiotherapy. The values for meningeal sarcomas were 83 and 10 months. Guthrie and colleagues[307] reported the largest experience with hemangiopericytoma. Five-year recurrence rates were 36% for irradiated patients compared with 90% without radiotherapy. Median intervals to recurrence were 58 and 29 months. Because 80% of irradiated patients eventually experienced recurrence by 15 years, these data imply that postoperative radiotherapy does not ensure permanent eradication of hemangiopericytoma. Bastin and Mehta[308] reviewed the literature on meningeal hemangiopericytoma. Mean survivals for patients managed with surgery or surgery plus radiotherapy were 65 and 96 months.

All authors recommend restricted volume radiotherapy for meningiomas. Goldsmith and associates[309] recommended 1- to 2-cm margins around the postoperative tumor volume for benign meningiomas and 3 cm around the preoperative volume for malignant tumors. Marginal recurrence following partial brain radiotherapy has been observed only for a large skull base meningioma with extracranial extension.[309] Virtually all relapses following radiotherapy occur within the treatment volume. The UCSF experience was updated by Goldsmith and associates.[309] Postoperative radiotherapy was routinely used for 117 subtotally resected benign patients. The 5- and 10-year progression-free survivals were 89% and 77%. The 5-year progression-free survivals in the CT and MRI era compared with earlier periods were 98% and 77%. Eng and associates[310] have outlined a sophisticated three-field conformal radiotherapy technique for optic sheath meningioma. This approach results in significantly less chiasm and pituitary dose compared with conventional field arrangements.

Stereotactic cerebral irradiation, or radiosurgery, has proved effective for meningiomas. The unique capabilities of radiosurgery make this approach valuable for selected meningiomas in close proximity to critical normal structures. Kondziolka and associates[311] irradiated 50 meningiomas using the multisource gamma knife. The tumors were located in the parasellar, petrous, or cavernous sinus regions. The 2-year actuarial local control rate was 96%.

The evidence for a dose-response relationship for meningiomas is controversial. The UCSF group reported a significant impact of dose for benign and malignant tumors.[309] The 5-year progression-free survivals for benign meningiomas receiving 52 Gy or less compared with higher doses were 65% and 93%. Progression-free survival for malignant tumors receiving 53 Gy or less compared with greater than 53 Gy were 17% and 63%. Several investigators reported no significant local progression differences over the range 50 to 65 Gy.[303, 312] Goldsmith and coworkers[313] have reviewed all published cases of radiation optic neuropathy. Two of the 42 cases in the literature were a result of radiotherapy for meningiomas. The authors developed an isotoxicity model

for neuropathy based on total dose and number of fractions. They documented a low risk of neuropathy with a scheme of 54 Gy in 30 fractions. Based on the foregoing and in the absence of randomized trials, most authors recommend 50 to 55 Gy for residual benign meningioma and 55 to 60 Gy for malignant tumors.

The clinical response of irradiated meningiomas is often surprisingly rapid. Smith and associates[314, 315] as well as others[316, 317] have documented gratifying improvement in visual acuity and visual fields following primary radiotherapy for optic sheath meningiomas. Five of the 50 patients irradiated by the Pittsburgh radiosurgery group responded clinically 6 to 36 months following large single-fraction treatment.[311]

Despite clinical response of meningiomas to ionizing radiation, their radiographic resolution is imperceptibly slow. In series using CT scanning, minimal tumor shrinkage was noted, even for patients showing symptomatic improvement and followed for many years.[318] Loss of central contrast enhancement on CT occurs rarely after conventional radiotherapy for meningiomas. Radiographic response appears more often following radiosurgery. The Pittsburgh group reported that 54% of patients followed at least 12 months showed a decrease in tumor size. Loss of central contrast enhancement occurred 3 months after radiosurgery and was associated with later tumor shrinkage.[311]

Vascular meningeal tumors may respond sufficiently to preoperative radiotherapy to permit resection. Wara and associates[318a] reported that the tumors of 8 of 12 preoperatively treated patients became resectable 6 months after irradiation. Others have reported that the hemangiopericytoma may be the most responsive meningeal tumor to preoperative irradiation.[297, 319]

### Chemotherapy

Mifepristone (RU486), an antiprogesterone, is being studied for use in recurrent meningioma.[320] Hydroxyurea at a dosage of 1000 to 1500 mg/day (approximately 20 mg/kg/day) has been shown to cause objective tumor shrinkage in recurrent meningomas (benign and malignant variants).[321] Other chemotherapies have shown activity in recurrent meningiomas in isolated cases (combinations of doxorubicin [Adriamycin] and dacarbazine or ifosfamide and mesna).[322]

### LYMPHOMA

Primary central nervous system lymphoma (PCNSL) is a non-Hodgkin's lymphoma that arises in the absence of apparent systemic lymphoma. The tumor is typically of B-cell origin and large cell morphology.[323] PCNSL accounts for 1% of primary intracranial neoplasms. It is the most common brain tumor seen in AIDS (see Chapter 101).[324] Increased risk accompanies congenital and acquired immunosuppression, as in transplant recipients, and chronic granulomatous, inflammatory, and vasculitic disease. The incidence in the apparently immunocompetent population has increased threefold since the 1980s.[325] In immunosuppressed patients, the Epstein-Barr virus genome can be identified in more than 90% of cases by in situ hybridization or polymerase chain reaction; it is generally not seen in immunocompetent patients.

The tumor is seen in a supratentorial location three times more commonly than below the tentorium. There is a predilection for involvement of the periventricular region, corpus callosum, thalamus, and basal ganglia. One third to one half of the patients have multiple deposits. The vitreous and retina of the eye can be involved in 15 to 20% of patients and may precede brain infiltration.[326] The meninges are involved in 25% of newly diagnosed cases and may herald the disease in 7% of patients.

In the immunosuppressed population, an infectious cause for the mass must be excluded. If toxoplasmosis is a consideration, a therapeutic trial of antibiotics is provided, and thereafter the brain imaging studies are repeated. If there is no response, a CT-guided stereotactic brain biopsy is performed.

When the tumor presents as a solitary mass, it cannot be separated from other causes by cranial imaging studies. Because this tumor may be responsive to corticosteroid treatment, it is important to proceed with the diagnostic evaluation, including brain biopsy, before use of these agents if clinically feasible.

The staging of patients with PCNSL should include the following:

1. Slit-lamp examination of the vitreous
2. Cell surface marker study of the vitreous fluid or vitrectomy if clinically indicated (or both)
3. Polymerase chain reaction and cell surface marker studies of the CSF if feasible
4. Serologic testing for syphilis and human immunodeficiency virus type 1 (HIV-1) antibodies

Routine evaluation for systemic lymphoma is not required.

### Surgery

Surgical resection, whether partial or gross total, does not alter the prognosis of patients with PCNSL. The only role for surgery in this tumor type is for diagnostic biopsy. Stereotactic image–guided techniques are the preferred surgical procedures for these tumors, which are often deep.[327]

### Radiation Therapy

Radiation therapy is the mainstay of therapy for intracranial lymphoma. The best results have been reported with whole-brain irradiation with or without a tumor boost.[325, 326] There is little indication of a dose response greater than 50 to 60 Gy for the large cell varieties.[328, 329] Although PCNSL is radioresponsive, relapse is the rule, and long-term survival is uncommon.[328] The pattern of relapse is predominantly local following whole-brain radiotherapy. Efforts to restrict the field of radiotherapy result in relapse in parenchyma initially uninvolved with lymphoma.[325] Isolated relapse in the meninges and spinal cord is unusual, and routine neuraxis irradiation is not indicated. Prognosis is related most strongly to initial performance status, gender, and age.[328, 329] The disease is more aggressive in immunocompromised than immunocompetent individuals.[330, 331] Radiation is the treatment of choice for vitreal or retinal lymphoma. The entire

orbit to the inferior orbital ridge is included in the field, to a total dose of 40 to 50 Gy.

### Chemotherapy

The most appropriate regimen of chemotherapy, if any, is not defined. DeAngelis and colleagues[332, 333] have used neoadjuvant methotrexate, whole-brain radiation therapy, intrathecal methotrexate, and two cycles of high-dose cytarabine. This group reported a median relapse-free survival of 40 months following this approach.[333] Other regimens, such as CHOP (cyclophosphamide, hydroxydauriomycin, Oncovin, prednisone), are also under investigation.[334]

## METASTASES

Approximately 25% of cancer patients develop brain metastases, most often from lung, breast, gastrointestinal, melanoma, and kidney primaries. Immediate management involves the administration of dexamethasone to decrease peritumoral edema. The response to this drug, however, has been shown to be dose dependent in a linear fashion. Renaudin and colleagues[335] showed initial antiedema requirements of 96 mg of dexamethasone per day in some patients.

### Surgery

Surgical treatment of metastatic brain tumors may be considered when there is a solitary brain lesion if (1) the primary disease is quiescent, (2) the lesion is surgically accessible without causing additional neurologic deficit, (3) the lesion has significant mass effect causing symptoms of life-threatening herniation, (4) the primary tumor is known to be relatively radioresistant, and (5) the primary diagnosis is unknown. Surgical resection of brain metastases in the face of uncontrolled systemic cancer or significant neurologic deficit is usually not warranted.[336]

The survival rate for patients with multiple brain metastases is generally much worse than those with solitary lesions.[337] Multiple metastases are usually treated with radiation therapy without surgery. In one study, it was shown that if total excision of all metastatic lesions is possible, patients with multiple brain metastases have a survival similar to those with single lesions following surgical removal.[338] If total resection of all lesions is not possible (i.e., if part of one or more tumors must be left behind), however, there is no improvement in survival afforded by the addition of surgery, and radiation therapy alone is the recommended treatment of choice. The indications for surgery for multiple brain metastases are (1) palliative treatment to reduce mass effect if one particular lesion is clearly causing symptoms or is immediately life-threatening, (2) multiple lesions that are all accessible and amenable to total removal, and (3) diagnosis of unknown primary cancer.[225]

Stereotactic procedures should be considered for the following: (1) lesions that are not appropriate for open surgery (e.g., deep lesions or multiple small tumors) or (2) patients who are poor candidates for long surgical procedures. When open surgical resection is justified, most operative brain metastases present near the surface of the brain. For those that are not visible on the surface, intraoperative ultrasound or image-guided navigational techniques should be used to localize the lesion. In contrast to primary glial tumors, brain metastases usually have a well-defined border. A plane of separation between tumor and normal brain can usually be identified during surgery, often allowing gross total removal of metastatic brain tumors.

Some authors have advocated stereotactic radiosurgery as the definitive noninvasive treatment for brain metastases. Although there has not yet been a well-controlled, prospectively randomized study to compare open surgery with stereotactic radiosurgery, one retrospective study suggests that stereotactic radiosurgery may be comparable to surgery.[339] Another study, however, found median survival to be 7.5 months with stereotactic radiosurgery and 16.4 months with open surgery, suggesting that surgical resection may be advantageous over stereotactic radiosurgery for control of cerebral metastases.[340] Radiographic local control rate has been estimated at 88% following radiosurgery,[341] whereas advocates of open surgery cite complete local control following gross total resection. The advantages of stereotactic radiosurgery are that it is noninvasive and there is no risk of intraoperative hemorrhage, infection, or mechanical spread of tumor cells.

Surgical removal of solitary brain metastases has been reported with encouraging results, especially in those with suitably situated lesions occurring after a prolonged period of primary tumor control.[286, 342, 343] In patients with a solitary metastasis, Patchell and coworkers[344] showed a significant survival and local control advantage to resection and whole-brain radiotherapy versus radiotherapy alone in a randomized trial. The role of adjuvant radiotherapy following resection is controversial. Nonrandomized series demonstrate a significant benefit to postoperative treatment[345] or no discernible advantage. Patchell and associates[346] also showed a significant reduction in intracranial relapse rate with the addition of adjuvant radiotherapy following resection of a single lesion in a randomized trial.

## Radiation Therapy

Whole-brain radiation alone is the major form of treatment for patients not eligible for resection. Early investigators arbitrarily selected doses of 30 to 40 Gy in 3 to 4 weeks. The largest experience with primary irradiation of brain metastases is that of the RTOG, which randomized more than 2000 patients to a variety of regimens (20 Gy over 1 week, 30 Gy over 2 weeks, 40 Gy over 3 weeks, 40 Gy over 4 weeks) to answer questions regarding maximal palliative benefit with minimal patient time and expense. Reports from initial RTOG trials showed no significant impact of dose and time parameters on palliation, survival, or incidence of CNS death.[347–350] Subsequent trials by this group showed no benefit from the addition of misonidazole or 5-bromo-2-deoxy-uridine to radiotherapy.[351, 352]

Analysis of the RTOG trials has served to identify patient and radiographic characteristics influencing prognosis of those with metastases. These features include age, performance status, control of the primary lesion, presence of extracranial disease, and number of lesions. Median survival following radiotherapy for patients with a maximum of favorable features is 7 months versus 2 months with few or no favorable features.[353, 354] Even among patients with the

most favorable prognosis, however, there is no impact of dose and time factors in the RTOG experience. A CT study documented the ineffectiveness of radiotherapy for metastases larger than 1.5 cm in diameter.

The impact of dose escalation beyond the RTOG standards is uncertain. There are retrospective and randomized prospective data evaluating 1000 cGy in a single dose for brain metastases.[355–357] Response rate, median survival, time to progression, and complications appear similar to those with fractionated schedules. Investigators at the Royal Marsden Hospital showed no survival benefit to a 15-Gy tumor boost following whole-brain irradiation.[358] The RTOG employed accelerated fractionation and showed a nearly significant survival advantage for patients with a solitary lesion receiving 54 to 70 Gy compared with lower doses.[359, 360] Nieder and associates[361] documented significantly higher radiographic response rate following 40 to 60 Gy compared with lower doses, although survivals were not similarly affected.

There is increasing experience with stereotactic radiotherapy for brain metastases. Crude local control rates following this innovative therapy approach 90%, although actuarial rates are typically 60 to 70%.[339, 362] In view of these relatively high control rates, the role of whole-brain radiotherapy has been called into question. Nonrandom trials document superior results following combined treatment versus radiosurgery alone.[341, 363]

## GLOMUS JUGULARE TUMORS

Chemoreceptors are specialized neurosensory tissues located in the carotid body, aortic body, vagus nerve, glomus tympanicum, auricular and tympanic nerves, and jugular bulb region of the jugular vein.[364] Tumors of the chemoreceptors have been generically called *chemodectomas, paragangliomas,* or *receptomas.* A chemodectoma of the jugular bulb has been called a *glomus jugulare tumor.* All chemodectomas, regardless of site, are tumors composed of nests of epithelioid cells and nerve fibers in a high vascular stroma.[365–367] These lesions are histologically benign, but the glomus jugulare tumors are malignant by nature of their critical location and capability for local invasion. According to Tidwell and Montague,[364] local invasiveness appears proportional to the tumor vascularity. Glomus jugulare tumors do not secrete catechols,[368] but Tidwell and Montague[364] report that an occasional patient presents with a pheochromocytoma-like syndrome.

Patients with these tumors tend to be women in their 30s or 40s.[288, 369–372] Familial cases and bilaterality have been reported. A long prediagnostic course is typical. Throughout the literature, a delay in therapy of 1 to 5 years is common. Typical signs and symptoms include deafness, tinnitus, vertigo, otorrhea, bleeding, otalgia, facial palsy, ear canal mass, and deficits of cranial nerves IX to XII. Glomus jugulare tumors are capable of petrous bone destruction. They may also rarely present with dysphagia and a pulsatile pharyngeal mass.

There is no agreed-on staging system for chemodectomas in this region. Approximately 50% of tumors arise from glomic tissue of the tympanicum, tympanic nerve, or auditory nerve. The other 50% are true lesions of the jugular bulb. McCabe and colleagues[373] have proposed that these tumors be subdivided into lesions of the tympanic membrane, lesions of the tympanomastoid, and lesions of the petrous bone. For true glomus jugulare tumors, most authors agree that patients with intracranial extent fare worse than patients with disease confined to the jugular bulb. Cummings and colleagues,[368] however, have stated that the presence or absence of cranial nerve deficits did not correlate with eventual tumor control by radiotherapy.

## Surgery

Surgery is generally recommended for chemodectomas of the tympanic membrane and tympanomastoid regions. Postoperative radiation therapy may be employed when the completeness of resection is in question. Surgery for true glomus jugulare tumors is difficult because of the proximity of the seventh and eighth cranial nerves as well as the risk of bleeding. Even if achieved, *complete resection* is no guarantee of permanent eradication of tumor. When all degrees of resection are included, recurrence rates for petrous tumors are high. In the experience of Newman and colleagues,[367] 11 of 14 patients had recurrence, all within 3 to 5 years of surgery. In the experience of Hatfield and associates,[366] 8 of 16 tumors recurred, all within 4 years of surgery.

## Radiation Therapy

The role of radiation therapy for glomus jugulare tumors remains controversial, owing mainly to the failure of these tumors to regress completely following treatment. The *no evidence of disease* concept is useless with this unusual neoplasm because the regression rate is extraordinarily slow following irradiation. Far better end points are freedom from progression and freedom from symptoms. When analyzed in this fashion, primary radiotherapy yields control rates of 80 to 100%.[374–377] Springate and associates[378] reviewed the literature and reported 195 patients treated with primary radiotherapy. The average mean follow-up period was 7 to 10 years, and the overall local control rate was 93%. Dawes and coworkers[379] reported an actuarial 20-year progression-free survival rate of 77% following radiotherapy. Virtually all authors agree that chemodectomas are best irradiated to doses of 40 to 50 Gy. In a literature review, Kim and associates[371] reported 25% of patients receiving less than 40 Gy experienced recurrence compared with 1.4% of those receiving more than 40 Gy.

In most radiotherapy series, there is an impressive, if delayed, palliation of symptoms despite persistence of tumor mass. Tinnitus, pain, vertigo, and aural discharge respond well in most patients. Auditory deficits respond partially in 50% of patients.[377] Deficits of other cranial nerves only rarely improve.[377] The glomus jugulare tumor shows relative radioresistance to modern treatment. Mumber and Greven[377] reported imaging evidence of tumor decrease in 30% and stabilization in the remainder of irradiated patients with a median of 11 years' follow-up. The tumor cells respond, albeit slowly, but there is minimal response of tumor vascularity. Maruyama and colleagues[365] performed angiography before irradiation and 3 years following treatment. No vascular response was detected in three patients despite reduction of tumor mass and alleviation of symptoms in all patients.

Complications following irradiation of temporal bone chemodectomas are rare. The overall incidences of brain necrosis, bone necrosis, or new cranial neuropathy are each less than 2%.[378, 380] Wang and colleagues[381] reported a significant dose effect for radiotherapy complications. In their experience, serious late morbidity occurred only with doses greater than 64 Gy. Springate and coworkers[378] reported a single in-field second malignancy occurring in 379 irradiated patients. Mumber and coworkers[377] added an occipital bone osteosacoma, bringing the world experience with radiation-associated malignancies to 0.54% of all treated patients. Hawthorne and colleagues[382] found that salvage surgery of patients failing radiotherapy was not more morbid than primary resection of glomus jugulare tumors.

## CEREBELLAR ASTROCYTOMAS

Cerebellar neoplasms of the astrocytic series form a special subgroup of gliomas. Their grade distribution, resectability, and natural history are in contrast to those of cerebral hemispheric gliomas. These tumor occur most commonly in childhood and account for the most frequent pediatric brain tumors.[383, 384] In several series, the average patient age varied from 6.5 to 9 years.[384, 385]

Cerebellar astrocytomas are true proliferative neoplasms, although generally of low grade.[384] These tumors have correspondingly indolent growth rate. Two histologic varieties have been described.[386] The more common form is the classic juvenile pilocytic astrocytoma. This tumor, accounting for 75% of all cerebellar astrocytomas, is of low grade, is well circumscribed, and predominates in childhood.[387] A less common form is the diffuse cerebellar astrocytoma. This variant, accounting for 25% of lesions, is more often of high grade, is infiltrative, and is seen in adult patients. Either histologic variant can present as a cystic or solid tumor.[386, 387]

In the past, cystic cerebellar astrocytomas were believed to have a good prognosis, whereas solid tumors were thought to do poorly. According to Gjerris and Klinken,[386] this difference in prognosis may be due not to inherent differences in the natural history of cystic and solid cerebellar astrocytomas but rather to the distribution of piloid and diffuse histologic features among these tumors. Cystic varieties are predominately piloid, whereas solid tumors more often have a diffuse histologic pattern and a natural course resembling that of cerebral astrocytomas. According to many authors, there is no significant correlation of survival with the gross appearance of a cerebellar astrocytoma.[386–388] Gjerris and Klinken,[386] however, reported that tumor histology was prognostic. Twenty-five-year survival for juvenile piloid tumors was 94% compared with 38% for diffuse lesions ($p < 0.001$). Diffuse solid tumors showed the poorest survival rate in that series. In a multivariate analysis, Hayostek and associates[389] concurred that histologic subtype was the most significant predictor of survival.

## Surgery

Approximately 50 to 75% of piloid cerebellar astrocytomas are amenable to complete surgical resection. The prognosis in this setting is excellent, with many authors reporting 80% or greater 5- and 10-year survival rates with prolonged follow-up of radically resected patients.[390–392] Gjerris and Klinken[386] have shown 100% 10-year survival for 29 completely resected juvenile pilocytic cerebellar astrocytomas, whether cystic (23 of 23) or solid (6 of 6). The same authors reported 40% 10-year survival for 10 completely resected diffuse tumors. Diffuse cystic tumors appeared to do better than diffuse solid tumors, but patient numbers in these subcategories are small. Ilgren and Stiller[182] reported 25-year disease-free and overall survival rates of 95% in a series of 50 completely resected patients. There is no apparent need for radiotherapy following gross total resection confirmed by imaging. Contrast enhancement in the resection cavity occurs frequently several months after surgery. This occurrence has not been associated with tumor relapse.[392]

## Radiation Therapy

The role of radiotherapy following subtotal resection of cerebellar astrocytoma remains controversial. There are numerous examples of long-term progression-free survival in this setting without adjunctive irradiation. Many authors report no benefit following irradiation. Ilgren and Stiller[182] reported the 20-year relapse-free rate was 33% with radiotherapy versus 27% following subtotal resection alone. Garcia and coworkers[391] reported 20-year actuarial survival rates were 70% with radiotherapy compared with 65% without radiotherapy.

Several groups advocate postoperative radiotherapy for all subtotally resected cerebellar astrocytomas. Dose-response analysis has rarely been reported for cerebellar astrocytomas. Wallner and coworkers[392] reviewed the UCSF experience with piloid astrocytomas in any site. Local control was superior at greater than 46 Gy, but a limited patient population prevented formal dose-response analysis. There were no survival differences at greater than or less than 45 Gy in the Mayo series.[389] All authors recommend irradiating a restricted volume when treating low-grade lesions. Leptomeningeal dissemination is unusual even if a cerebellar astrocytoma involves the vermis.

At present, complete resection, if accompanied by minimal morbidity, is the treatment of choice for these tumors. This approach is often possible for piloid tumors, which are usually cystic, and no further therapy is indicated if resection is truly complete. For the incompletely resected piloid tumors, a policy of watchful waiting with surgical salvage of recurrent disease appears worthwhile, although immediate postoperative irradiation yields greater disease-free survival. Diffuse cerebellar astrocytomas, similar to standard low-grade cerebral astrocytomas, are generally not amenable to complete resection. These tumors should be treated similar to partially resected grade 1 and 2 tumors elsewhere in the CNS, with limited-volume radiation therapy.

## Chemotherapy

Patients with pilocytic astrocytomas, similar to those with optic gliomas, may benefit from the use of chemotherapy in the very young patient or in patients with recurrent disease.[113] The agents to consider in this setting include carboplatin, vincristine, nitrosourea-based chemotherapies, and etoposide.

## SUGGESTIONS FOR ADDITIONAL READING

Rasheed BK, Wiltshire RN, Bigner SH, Bigner DD. Molecular pathogenesis of malignant gliomas. Curr Opin Oncol 1999;11:162–7.

Avgeropoulos NG, Batchelor TT. New treatment strategies for malignant gliomas. Oncologist 1999;4:209–24.

Brandes AA, Vastola F, Monfardini S. Reoperation in recurrent high-grade gliomas: literature review of prognostic factors and outcome. Am J Clin Oncol 1999;22:387–90.

Shafman TD, Loeffler JS. Novel radiation technologies for malignant gliomas. Curr Opin Oncol 1999;11:147–51.

Burton E, Prados M. New chemotherapy options for the treatment of malignant gliomas. Curr Opin Oncol 1999;11:157–61.

Cokgor I, Friedman HS, Friedman AH. Chemotherapy for adults with malignant glioma. Cancer Invest 1999;17:264–72.

Davey P. Brain metastases. Curr Probl Cancer 1999;23:59–98.

## REFERENCES

1. Percy AK, Elveback LR, Okazaki H, Kurland LT. Neoplasms of the central nervous system: epidemiologic considerations. Neurology 1972;22:40–8.
2. Schoenberg BS, Christine BW, Whisnant JP. The descriptive epidemiology of primary intracranial neoplasms: the Connecticut experience. Am J Epidemiol 1976;104:499–510.
3. Choi NW, Schuman LM, Gullen WH. Epidemiology of primary central nervous system neoplasms: II. case-control study. Am J Epidemiol 1970;91:467–85.
4. Hopewell JW, Edwards DN, Wiernik G. Sex dependence of human intracranial gliomata. Br J Cancer 1976;34:666–70.
5. Fan KJ, Kovi J, Earle KM. The ethnic distribution of primary central nervous system tumors: AFIP, 1958 to 1970. J Neuropathol Exp Neurol 1977;36:41–9.
6. Barker DJ, Weller RO, Garfield JS. Epidemiology of primary tumours of the brain and spinal cord: a regional survey in southern England. J Neurol Neurosurg Psychiatry 1976;39:290–6.
7. Ron E, Modan B, Boice JD Jr, et al. Tumors of the brain and nervous system after radiotherapy in childhood. N Engl J Med 1988;319:1033–9.
8. Jablon S, Tachikawa K, Belsky JL, Steer A. Cancer in Japanese exposed as children to atomic bombs. Lancet 1971;1:927–32.
9. Martuza RL, Eldridge R. Neurofibromatosis 2 (bilateral acoustic neurofibromatosis). N Engl J Med 1988;318:684–8.
10. Kleihues P, Cavenee WK. Pathology and genetics of tumors of the nervous system. Lyon, France: International Agency for Research, 1998.
11. Hoshino T, Barker M, Wilson CB, et al. Cell kinetics of human gliomas. J Neurosurg 1972;37:15–26.
12. Hoshino T, Townsend JJ, Muraoka I, Wilson CB. An autoradiographic study of human gliomas: growth kinetics of anaplastic astrocytoma and glioblastoma multiforme. Brain 1980;103:967–84.
13. Russell DS. Pathology of tumors of the nervous system. Baltimore: Williams & Wilkins, 1977.
14. Rubinstein LJ. Tumors of the central nervous system. Washington, D.C.: Armed Forces Institute of Pathology, 1972.
15. Bryan P. CSF seeding of intra-cranial tumours: a study of 96 cases. Clin Radiol 1974;25:355–60.
16. Batzdorf U, Gold V. Dispersion of central nervous system tumors: correlation between clinical aspects and tissue culture studies. J Neurosurg 1974;41:691–8.
17. Smith DR, Hardman JM, Earle KM. Metastasizing neuroectodermal tumors of the central nervous system. J Neurosurg 1969;31:50–8.
18. Anzil AP. Glioblastoma multiforme with extracranial metastases in the absence of previous craniotomy: case report. J Neurosurg 1970;33:88–94.
19. Komatsu K, Hiratsuka H, Takahashi S, et al. Widespread extracranial metastases of glioblastoma multiforme: report of case and clinicopathological review of cases in literature. Bull Tokyo Med Dent Univ 1972;19:29–49.
20. Brooks WH, Roszman TL, Mahaley MS, Woosley RE. Immunobiology of primary intracranial tumours: II. analysis of lymphocyte subpopulations in patients with primary brain tumours. Clin Exp Immunol 1977;29:61–6.

21. Young HF, Sakalas R, Kaplan AM. Inhibition of cell-mediated immunity in patients with brain tumors. Surg Neurol 1976;5:19–23.
22. Mahaley MS Jr, Brooks WH, Roszman TL, et al. Immunobiology of primary intracranial tumors: Part 1. studies of the cellular and humoral general immune competence of brain-tumor patients. J Neurosurg 1977;46:467–76.
23. Woosley RE, Mahaley MS Jr, Mahaley JL, et al. Immunobiology of primary intracranial tumors: Part 3. microcytotoxicity assays of specific immune responses of brain tumor patients. J Neurosurg 1977;47:871–85.
24. Trouillas P. Immunology and immunotherapy of cerebral tumors: current status. Rev Neurol (Paris) 1973;128:23–38.
25. Catalano LW Jr, Harter DH, Hsu KC. Common antigen in meningioma-derived cell cultures. Science 1972;175:180–2.
26. Winters WD, Rich JR. Human meningioma antigens. Int J Cancer 1975;15:815–22.
27. Apuzzo ML, Sheikh KM. Tumor immunology: a neurosurgical perspective: I. general concepts of tumor immunology. Bull Los Angeles Neurol Soc 1976;41:168–75.
28. Penzholz H. Metastatic diseases of the central nervous system caused by malignant tumors: a clinical study on the basis of 158 individual cases of a neurosurgical clinic. Acta Neurochir (Wien) 1968:Suppl 16:1–205.
29. Olson ME, Chernik NL, Posner JB. Infiltration of the leptomeninges by systemic cancer: a clinical and pathologic study. Arch Neurol 1974;30:122–37.
30. Kleihues P, Burger PC, Scheithauer BW. The new WHO classification of brain tumours. Brain Pathol 1993;3:255–68.
31. Marton LJ, Edwards MS, Levin VA, et al. Predictive value of cerebrospinal fluid polyamines in medulloblastoma. Cancer Res 1979; 39:993–7.
32. Fulton DS, Levin VA, Lubich WP, et al. Cerebrospinal fluid polyamines in patients with glioblastoma multiforme and anaplastic astrocytoma. Cancer Res 1980;40:3293–6.
33. Marton LJ, Edwards MS, Levin VA, et al. CSF polyamines: a new and important means of monitoring patients with medulloblastoma. Cancer 1981;47:757–60.
34. Wasserstrom WR, Schwartz MK, Fleisher M, Posner JB. Cerebrospinal fluid biochemical markers in central nervous system tumors: a review. Ann Clin Lab Sci 1981;11:239–51.
35. Leibel SA, Sheline GE, Wara WM, et al. The role of radiation therapy in the treatment of astrocytomas. Cancer 1975;35:1551–7.
36. Rhoton A. General and micro-operative techniques. In: Youmans JR, ed. Neurological surgery. Vol. 4. Philadelphia: WB Saunders, 1996:724.
37. Salcman M. Supratentorial gliomas: clinical features and surgical therapy. In: Wilkins R, Rengachary S, eds. Neurosurgery. Vol. I. New York: McGraw-Hill, 1996:777.
38. Wilkins R. Principles of neurosurgical operative technique. In: Wilkins R, Rengachary S, eds. Neurosurgery. Vol. I. New York: McGraw-Hill, 1996:517.
39. Becker DP, Young HF, Vries JK, Sakalas R. Monitoring in patients with brain tumors. Clin Neurosurg 1975;22:364–88.
40. Giangaspero F, Burger PC. Correlations between cytologic composition and biologic behavior in the glioblastoma multiforme: a postmortem study of 50 cases. Cancer 1983;52:2320–33.
41. Salcman M. Survival in glioblastoma: historical perspective. Neurosurgery 1980;7:435–9.
42. Salcman M, Kaplan RS, Samaras GM, et al. Aggressive multimodality therapy based on a multicompartmental model of glioblastoma. Surgery 1982;92:250–9.
43. Bigner DD. Biology of gliomas: potential clinical implications of glioma cellular heterogeneity. Neurosurgery 1981;9:320–6.
44. Bigner DD, Bigner SH, Ponten J, et al. Heterogeneity of genotypic and phenotypic characteristics of fifteen permanent cell lines derived from human gliomas. J Neuropathol Exp Neurol 1981;40:201–29.
45. Scanlon PW, Taylor WF. Radiotherapy of intracranial astrocytomas: analysis of 417 cases treated from 1960 through 1969. Neurosurgery 1979;5:301–8.
46. Sheline GE. Radiation therapy of tumors of the central nervous system in childhood. Cancer 1975;35:957–64.
47. Nelson JS, Tsukada Y, Schoenfeld D, et al. Necrosis as a prognostic criterion in malignant supratentorial, astrocytic gliomas. Cancer 1983;52:550–4.
48. Burger PC, Vogel FS, Green SB, Strike TA. Glioblastoma multiforme and anaplastic astrocytoma: pathologic criteria and prognostic implications. Cancer 1985;56:1106–11.
49. Donahue B, Scott CB, Nelson JS, et al. Influence of an oligodendroglial component on the survival of patients with anaplastic astrocytomas: a report of Radiation Therapy Oncology Group 83–02. A prospective study of short-course radiotherapy in poor prognosis glioblastoma multiforme. Int J Radiat Oncol Biol Phys 1997;38:911–4.
50. Galanis E, Buckner JC, Dinapoli RP, et al. Clinical outcome of gliosarcoma compared with glioblastoma multiforme: North Central Cancer Treatment Group results. J Neurosurg 1998;89:425–30.
51. Reeves GI, Marks JE. Prognostic significance of lesion size for glioblastoma multiforme. Radiology 1979;132:469–71.
52. Leibel S, Sheline G. Radiation therapy for neoplasms of the brain. J Neurosurg 1987;66:1–22.
53. Apuzzo M. Survival after stereotactic biopsy of of malignant gliomas. Neurosurgery 1988;22:472–3.
54. Quigley M, Maroon J. The relationship between survival and the extent of resection in patients with supratentorial malignant gliomas. Neurosurgery 1991;29:385–9.
55. Kornblith P. The role of cytotoxic chemotherapy in the treatment of malignant brain tumors. Surg Neurol 1995;44:551–2.
56. Kelly P, Hunt C. The limited value of cytoreductive surgery in elderly patients with malignant gliomas. Neurosurgery 1994;33:62–7.
57. Greene G, Hitchon P, Schelper R, et al. Diagnostic yield in CT-guided stereotactic biopsy of gliomas. J Neurosurg 1989;71:494–7.
58. Coffey R, Lunsford L, Taylor F. Survival after stereotactic biopsy of malignant gliomas. Neurosurgery 1988;22:465–73.
59. Choucair A, Levin V, Gutin P, et al. Development of multiple lesions during radiation therapy and chemotherapy. J Neurosurg 1986; 65:654–8.
60. Ammirati M, Galicich J, Arbit E, et al. Reoperation in the treatment of recurrent intracranial malignant gliomas. Neurosurgery 1987;21: 607–14.
61. Harsh G, Levin V, Gutin P, et al. Reoperation for recurrent glioblastoma and anaplastic astrocytoma. Neurosurgery 1987;21:615–21.
62. Walker MD, Alexander E Jr, Hunt WE, et al. Evaluation of BCNU and/or radiotherapy in the treatment of anaplastic gliomas: a cooperative clinical trial. J Neurosurg 1978;49:333–43.
63. Walker MD, Strike TA, Sheline GE. An analysis of dose-effect relationship in the radiotherapy of malignant gliomas. Int J Radiat Oncol Biol Phys 1979;5:1725–31.
64. Kristiansen K, Hagen S, Kollevold T, et al. Combined modality therapy of operated astrocytomas grade III and IV: confirmation of the value of postoperative irradiation and lack of potentiation of bleomycin on survival time: a prospective multicenter trial of the Scandinavian Glioblastoma Study Group. Cancer 1981;47:649–52.
65. Stage WS, Stein JJ. Treatment of malignant astrocytomas. Am J Roentgenol Radium Ther Nucl Med 1974;120:7–18.
66. Uihlein A, Colby MY Jr, Layton DD, et al. Comparison of surgery and surgery plus irradiation in the treatment of supratentorial gliomas. Acta Radiol Ther Phys Biol 1966;5:67–78.
67. Bleehen NM, Stenning SP. A Medical Research Council trial of two radiotherapy doses in the treatment of grades 3 and 4 astrocytoma. The Medical Research Council Brain Tumour Working Party. Br J Cancer 1991;64:769–74.
68. Boyages J, Tiver KW. Cerebral hemisphere astrocytoma: treatment results. Radiother Oncol 1987;8:209–16.
69. Bauman GS, Gaspar LE, Fisher BJ, et al. A prospective study of short-course radiotherapy in poor prognosis glioblastoma multiforme. Int J Radiat Oncol Biol Phys 1994;29:835–9.
70. Glinski B. Postoperative hypofractionated radiotherapy versus conventionally fractionated radiotherapy in malignant gliomas: a preliminary report on a randomized trial. J Neurooncol 1993;16:167–72.
70a. Scherer HJ. A critical review: the pathology of cranial glioma. J Neurol Psychiatry 1940;3:147.
70b. Concannon JP, Kramer S, Berry R. The extent of intracranial gliomatas at autopsy and its relationship to techniques used in radiation therapy of brain tumors. Am J Roentgenol Radium Ther Nucl Med 1960;84:99–107.
71. Salazar OM, Rubin P. The spread of glioblastoma multiforme as a determining factor in the radiation treated volume. Int J Radiat Oncol Biol Phys 1976;1:627–37.
72. Hochberg FH, Pruitt A. Assumptions in the radiotherapy of glioblastoma. Neurology 1980;30:907–11.
73. Kaplan WD, Takvorian T, Morris JH, et al. Thallium-201 brain tumor imaging: a comparative study with pathologic correlation. J Nucl Med 1987;28:47–52.

74. Deutsch M, Laurent JP, Cohen ME. Myelography for staging medulloblastoma. Cancer 1985;56:1763–6.

75. Gaspar LE, Fisher BJ, MacDonald DR, et al. Malignant glioma timing of response to radiation therapy: radiation response and survival time in patients with glioblastoma multiforme. Int J Radiat Oncol Biol Phys 1993;25:877–9.

75a. de Schryver A, Greitz T, Forsby N, Brun A. Localized shaped field radiotherapy of malignant glioblastoma multiforme. Int J Radiat Oncol Biol Phys 1976;1:713–16.

76. Daumas-Duport C, Scheithauer BW, Kelly PJ. A histologic and cytologic method for the spatial definition of gliomas. Mayo Clin Proc 1987;62:435–49.

77. Kelly PJ, Daumas-Duport C, Scheithauer BW, et al. Stereotactic histologic correlations of computed tomography– and magnetic resonance imaging–defined abnormalities in patients with glial neoplasms. Mayo Clin Proc 1987;62:450–9.

78. Burger PC. The anatomy of astrocytomas. Mayo Clin Proc 1987; 62:527–9.

79. Barker FG 2nd, Prados MD, Chang SM, et al. Radiation response and survival time in patients with glioblastoma multiforme. J Neurosurg 1996;84:442–8.

80. Fine HA, Dear KB, Loeffler JS, et al. Meta-analysis of radiation therapy with and without adjuvant chemotherapy for malignant gliomas in adults. Cancer 1993;71:2585–97.

81. DeAngelis LM, Burger PC, Green SB, Cairncross JG. Malignant glioma: who benefits from adjuvant chemotherapy? Ann Neurol 1998;44:691–5.

82. Grossman SA, Wharam M, Sheidler V, et al. Phase II study of continuous infusion carmustine and cisplatin followed by cranial irradiation in adults with newly diagnosed high-grade astrocytoma. J Clin Oncol 1997;15:2596–603.

83. Gruber ML, Glass J, Choudhri H, Nirenberg A. Carboplatin chemotherapy before irradiation in newly diagnosed glioblastoma multiforme. Am J Clin Oncol 1998;21:338–40.

84. Petersdorf SH, Livingston RB. High dose chemotherapy for the treatment of malignant brain tumors. J Neurooncol 1994;20:155–63.

85. Couldwell WT, Hinton DR, Surnock AA, et al. Treatment of recurrent malignant gliomas with chronic oral high-dose tamoxifen. Clin Cancer Res 1996;2:619–22.

86. Yung WK, Kyritsis AP, Gleason MJ, Levin VA. Treatment of recurrent malignant gliomas with high-dose 13-cis-retinoic acid. Clin Cancer Res 1996;2:1931–5.

87. Yung WK, Prados M, Levin VA, et al. Intravenous recombinant interferon beta in patients with recurrent malignant gliomas: a phase I/II study. J Clin Oncol 1991;9:1945–9.

88. Kernohan JW, Sayre GP. Tumors of the central nervous system. Washington, D.C.: Armed Forces Institute of Pathology, 1952.

89. Laws ER Jr, Taylor WF, Clifton MB, Okazaki H. Neurosurgical management of low-grade astrocytoma of the cerebral hemispheres. J Neurosurg 1984;61:665–73.

90. Cairncross J, Laperriere N. Low-grade glioma: to treat or not to treat? Arch Neurol 1989;46:1238–9.

91. Greenberg M. Handbook of neurosurgery. Vol. I. Lakeland, Fla.: Greenberg Graphics, 1997:248.

92. Radcliffe J, Packer R, Atkins T, et al. Three- and four-year cognitive outcome in children with noncortical brain tumors treated with whole-brain radiotherapy. Ann Neurol 1992;32:551–4.

93. Shaw EG, Daumas-Duport C, Scheithauer BW, et al. Radiation therapy in the management of low-grade supratentorial astrocytomas. J Neurosurg 1989;70:853–61.

94. McCormack BM, Miller DC, Budzilovich GN, et al. Treatment and survival of low-grade astrocytoma in adults—1977–1988. Neurosurgery 1992;31:636–42.

95. Piepmeier JM. Observations on the current treatment of low-grade astrocytic tumors of the cerebral hemispheres. J Neurosurg 1987; 67:177–81.

96. Soffietti R, Chio A, Giordana MT, et al. Prognostic factors in well-differentiated cerebral astrocytomas in the adult. Neurosurgery 1989;24:686–92.

97. Fazekas JT, Garcia DM, Fulling KH, Marks JE. Treatment of grades I and II brain astrocytomas: the value of radiation therapy in addition to surgery for astrocytomas of the adult cerebrum. Int J Radiat Oncol Biol Phys 1977;2:661–6.

98. Whitton AC, Bloom HJ. Low grade glioma of the cerebral hemispheres in adults: a retrospective analysis of 88 cases. Int J Radiat Oncol Biol Phys 1990;18:783–6.

99. Weir B, Grace M. The relative significance of factors affecting postoperative survival in astrocytomas, grades one and two. Can J Neurol Sci 1976;3:47–50.

100. Hirsch JF, Sainte Rose C, Pierre-Kahn A, et al. Benign astrocytic and oligodendrocytic tumors of the cerebral hemispheres in children: postoperative radiotherapy of supratentorial low-grade gliomas. J Neurosurg 1989;70:568–72.

101. Walker MD, Hurwitz BS. BCNU (1,3-bis(2-chloroethyl)-1-nitrosourea; NSC-409962) in the treatment of malignant brain tumors preliminary report. Cancer Chemother Rep 1970;54:263–71.

102. Trojanowski T, Peszynski J, Turowski K, et al. Quality of survival of patients with brain gliomas treated with postoperative CCNU and radiation therapy. J Neurosurg 1989;70:18–23.

103. Janny P, Cure H, Mohr M, et al. Low grade supratentorial astrocytomas: management and prognostic factors: survival after stereotactic biopsy and irradiation of cerebral nonanaplastic, nonpilocytic astrocytoma. J Neurosurg 1995;82:523–9.

104. Karim AB, Maat B, Hatlevoll R, et al. A randomized trial on dose-response in radiation therapy of low-grade cerebral glioma. European Organization for Research and Treatment of Cancer (EORTC) Study 22844. Int J Radiat Oncol Biol Phys 1996;36:549–56.

105. Lunsford LD, Somaza S, Kondziolka D, Flickinger JC. Survival after stereotactic biopsy and irradiation of cerebral nonanaplastic, nonpilocytic astrocytoma. J Neurosurg 1995;82:523–9.

106. Shibamoto Y, Kitakabu Y, Takahashi M, et al. Supratentorial low-grade astrocytoma: correlation of computed tomography findings with effect of radiation therapy and prognostic variables. Cancer 1993;72:190–5.

107. Young RC, Walker MD, Canellos GP, et al. Initial clinical trials with methyl-CCNU 1-(2-chloroethyl)-3-(4-methyl cyclohexyl)-1-nitrosourea (MeCCNU). Cancer 1973;31:1164–9.

108. Rogers LR, Morris HH, Lupica K. Effect of cranial irradiation on seizure frequency in adults with low-grade astrocytoma and medically intractable epilepsy. Neurology 1993;43:1599–601.

109. Levin VA, Crafts DC, Norman DM, et al. Criteria for evaluating patients undergoing chemotherapy for malignant brain tumors. J Neurosurg 1977;47:329–35.

110. North CA, North RB, Epstein JA, et al. Low-grade cerebral astrocytomas: survival and quality of life after radiation therapy: patterns of tumor progression after radiotherapy for low-grade gliomas: analysis from the computed tomography/magnetic resonance imaging era. Cancer 1990;66:6–14.

111. Fisher BJ, Bauman GS, Leighton CE, et al: Low-grade gliomas in children: tumor volume response to radiation. J Neurosurg 1998; 88:969–74.

112. Friedman HS, Lovell S, Rasheed K, Friedman AH. Treatment of adults with progressive oligodendroglioma with carboplatin (CBDCA): preliminary results. Writing Committee for The Brain Tumor Center at Duke. Med Pediatr Oncol 1998;31:16–8.

113. Packer RJ, Ater J, Allen J, et al. Carboplatin and vincristine chemotherapy for children with newly diagnosed progressive low-grade gliomas. J Neurosurg 1997;86:747–54.

114. Smith MT, Ludwig CL, Godfrey AD, et al. Grading of oligodendrogliomas: role of radiation therapy in the treatment of cerebral oligodendroglioma: an analysis of 57 cases and a literature review. Cancer 1983;52:2107–14.

115. Burger PC, Green SB. Patient age, histologic features, and length of survival in patients with glioblastoma multiforme. Cancer 1987; 59:1617–25.

116. Shaw EG, Scheithauer BW, O'Fallon JR, et al. Oligodendrogliomas: the Mayo Clinic experience. J Neurosurg 1992;76:428–34.

117. Cairncross JG, Ueki K, Zlatescu MC, et al. Specific genetic predictors of chemotherapeutic response and survival in patients with anaplastic oligodendrogliomas. J Natl Cancer Inst 1998;90:1473–9.

118. Ciric I, Ammirati M, Vick N, et al. Supratentorial gliomas: surgical considerations and immediate post-operative results. Neurosurgery 1987;21:21–6.

119. Mork S, Lindegaard K, Halvorsen T, et al. Oligodendroglioma: incidence and biological behavior in a defined population. J Neurosurg 1985;63:881–9.

120. Lindegaard KF, Mork SJ, Eide GE, et al. Statistical analysis of clinicopathological features, radiotherapy, and survival in 170 cases of oligodendroglioma. J Neurosurg 1987;67:224–30.

121. Reedy DP, Bay JW, Hahn JF. Role of radiation therapy in the treatment of cerebral oligodendroglioma: an analysis of 57 cases and a literature review. Neurosurgery 1983;13:499–503.

122. Bullard DE, Rawlings CEd, Phillips B, et al. Oligodendroglioma: an analysis of the value of radiation therapy. Cancer 1987;60:2179–88.
123. Dohrmann GJ, Farwell JR, Flannery JT. Oligodendrogliomas in children. Surg Neurol 1978;10:21–5.
124. Sheline GE. The importance of distinguishing tumor grade in malignant gliomas: treatment and prognosis. Int J Radiat Oncol Biol Phys 1976;1:781–6.
125. Shaw EG, Evans RG, Scheithauer BW, et al. Postoperative radiotherapy of intracranial ependymoma in pediatric and adult patients: the definition of the ependymoblastoma. Int J Radiat Oncol Biol Phys 1987;13:1457–62.
126. Packer RJ, Sutton LN, Rorke LB, et al. Oligodendroglioma of the posterior fossa in childhood. Cancer 1985;56:195–9.
127. Cairncross JG, Macdonald DR, Glass J, et al. Successful chemotherapy for recurrent malignant oligodendroglioma: the treatment of oligodendrogliomas and mixed oligodendroglioma-astrocytomas with PCV chemotherapy. Ann Neurol 1988;23:360–4.
128. Cairncross G, Macdonald D, Ludwin S, et al. Chemotherapy for anaplastic oligodendroglioma. National Cancer Institute of Canada Clinical Trials Group. J Clin Oncol 1994;12:2013–21.
129. Glass J, Hochberg FH, Gruber ML, et al. The treatment of oligodendrogliomas and mixed oligodendroglioma-astrocytomas with PCV chemotherapy. J Neurosurg 1992;76:741–5.
130. Macdonald DR, Gaspar LE, Cairncross JG. Successful chemotherapy for newly diagnosed aggressive oligodendroglioma. Ann Neurol 1990;27:573–4.
131. Bailey P. A classification of the tumors of the glioma group on histogenic basis with a correlated study of prognosis. Philadelphia: JB Lippincott, 1926.
132. McFarland DR, Horwitz H, Saenger EL, Bahr GK. Medulloblastoma—a review of prognosis and survival. Br J Radiol 1969;42:198–214.
133. Kleinman GM, Hochberg FH, Richardson EP Jr. Systemic metastases from medulloblastoma: report of two cases and review of the literature. Cancer 1981;48:2296–309.
134. Silverman CL, Simpson JR, Berry MP, et al. Cerebellar medulloblastoma: the importance of posterior fossa dose to survival and patterns of failure. Int J Radiat Oncol Biol Phys 1982;8:1869–76.
135. Berry MP, Jenkin RD, Keen CW, et al. Radiation treatment for medulloblastoma: a 21-year review. J Neurosurg 1981;55:43–51.
136. Raimondi AJ, Tomita T. Medulloblastoma in childhood. Acta Neurochir (Wien) 1979;50:127–38.
137. Deutsch M, Reigel DH. Myelography and cytology in the treatment of medulloblastoma. Int J Radiat Oncol Biol Phys 1981;7:721–5.
138. Laurent J, Cheek W. Brain tumors in children. J Pediatr Neurosci 1985;1:15–32.
139. Berger M, Baumeister B, Geyer J, et al. The risks of metastases from shunting in children with primary central nervous system tumors. J Neurosurg 1991;74:872–7.
140. Bergsneider M, Frazee J. Ventricular endoscopy. In: DeSalles A, Lufkin R, eds. Minimally invasive therapy of the brain. New York: Thieme, 1997:254.
141. Landberg TG, Lindgren ML, Cavallin-Stahl EK, et al. Improvements in the radiotherapy of medulloblastoma, 1946–1975. Cancer 1980;45:670–8.
142. Smith CE, Long DM, Jones TK Jr, Levitt SH. Medulloblastoma: an analysis of time-dose relationships and recurrence patterns. Cancer 1973;32:722–8.
143. Tokars RP, Sutton HG, Griem ML. Cerebellar medulloblastoma: results of a new method of radiation treatment. Cancer 1979;43:129–36.
144. Jenkin D. The radiation treatment of medulloblastoma. J Neurooncol 1996;29:45–54.
145. Halperin EC. Concerning the inferior portion of the spinal radiotherapy field for malignancies that disseminate via the cerebrospinal fluid. Int J Radiat Oncol Biol Phys 1993;26:357–62.
146. Dunbar SF, Barnes PD, Tarbell NJ. Radiologic determination of the caudal border of the spinal field in cranial spinal irradiation. Int J Radiat Oncol Biol Phys 1993;26:669–73.
147. Solit DB, Goldwein JW. Posterior fossa: analysis of a popular technique for estimating the location in children with medulloblastoma. Radiology 1995;195:697–8.
148. Drayer JA, Marks LB, Bentel G, Halperin EC. Defining the superior border of posterior fossa radiation treatment fields. Int J Radiat Oncol Biol Phys 1998;41:625–9.
149. Allen JC, Donahue B, DaRosso R, Nirenberg A. Hyperfractionated craniospinal radiotherapy and adjuvant chemotherapy for children with newly diagnosed medulloblastoma and other primitive neuroectodermal tumors. Int J Radiat Oncol Biol Phys 1996;36:1155–61.
150. Brand WN, Schneider PA, Tokars RP. Long-term results of a pilot study of low dose cranial-spinal irradiation for cerebellar medulloblastoma. Int J Radiat Oncol Biol Phys 1987;13:1641–5.
151. Deutsch M, Thomas PR, Krischer J, et al. Results of a prospective randomized trial comparing standard dose neuraxis irradiation (3,600 cGy/20) with reduced neuraxis irradiation (2,340 cGy/13) in patients with low-stage medulloblastoma. A Combined Children's Cancer Group–Pediatric Oncology Group Study. Pediatr Neurosurg 1996;24:167–77.
152. Jereb B, Reid A, Ahuja RK, et al. Patterns of failure in patients with medulloblastoma: period of risk for recurrence in medulloblastoma. Cancer 1982;50:2941–7.
153. Miralbell R, Bleher A, Huguenin P, et al. Pediatric medulloblastoma: radiation treatment technique and patterns of failure. Int J Radiat Oncol Biol Phys 1997;37:523–9.
154. Miralbell R, Lomax A, Russo M. Potential role of proton therapy in the treatment of pediatric medulloblastoma/primitive neuro-ectodermal tumors: spinal theca irradiation. Int J Radiat Oncol Biol Phys 1997;38:805–11.
155. Quest DO, Brisman R, Antunes JL, Housepian EM. Period of risk for recurrence in medulloblastoma. J Neurosurg 1978;48:159–63.
156. Khafaga Y, Kandil AE, Jamshed A, et al. Treatment results for 149 medulloblastoma patients from one institution. Int J Radiat Oncol Biol Phys 1996;35:501–6.
156a. Fukunaga-Johnson N, Sandler HM, Marsh R, Martel MK. The use of 3D conformal radiotherapy (3D CRT) to spare the cochlea in patients with medulloblastoma. Int J Radiat Oncol Biol Phys 1998;41:77–82.
157. Mealey J Jr, Hall PV. Medulloblastoma in children: survival and treatment. J Neurosurg 1977;46:56–64.
158. Kopelson G, Linggood RM, Kleinman GM. Medulloblastoma: the identification of prognostic subgroups and implications for multimodality management. Cancer 1983;51:312–9.
159. Packer RJ, Sutton LN, Rorke LB, et al. Prognostic importance of cellular differentiation in medulloblastoma of childhood. J Neurosurg 1984;61:296–301.
160. Carrie C, Lasset C, Alapetite C, et al. Multivariate analysis of prognostic factors in adult patients with medulloblastoma: retrospective study of 156 patients. Cancer 1994;74:2352–60.
161. Prados MD, Warnick RE, Wara WM, et al. Medulloblastoma in adults: nitrogen mustard, vincristine, procarbazine, and prednisone as adjuvant chemotherapy in the treatment of medulloblastoma. A Pediatric Oncology Group study. Int J Radiat Oncol Biol Phys 1995;32:1145–52.
162. Shapiro WR, Park TS, Hoffman HJ, et al. Chemotherapy of primary malignant brain tumors in children: experience at the Hospital for Sick Children, Toronto, 1950–1980. Cancer 1975;35:965–72.
163. Bloom HJ. Combined modality therapy for intracranial tumors. Cancer 1975;35:111–20.
164. Park TS, Hoffman HJ, Hendrick EB, et al. Medulloblastoma: clinical presentation and management. J Neurosurg 1983;58:543–52.
165. Krischer JP, Ragab AH, Kun L, et al. Nitrogen mustard, vincristine, procarbazine, and prednisone as adjuvant chemotherapy in the treatment of medulloblastoma. A Pediatric Oncology Group study. J Neurosurg 1991;74:905–9.
166. Evans AE, Jenkin RD, Sposto R, et al. The treatment of medulloblastoma: results of a prospective randomized trial of radiation therapy with and without CCNU, vincristine, and prednisone. J Neurosurg 1990;72:572–82.
167. Tait DM, Thornton-Jones H, Bloom HJ, et al. Adjuvant chemotherapy for medulloblastoma: the first multi-centre control trial of the International Society of Paediatric Oncology (SIOP I). Eur J Cancer 1990;26:464–9.
168. Packer RJ, Sutton LN, Goldwein JW, et al. Improved survival with the use of adjuvant chemotherapy in the treatment of medulloblastoma. J Neurosurg 1991;74:433–40.
169. Duffner PK, Horowitz ME, Krischer JP, et al. Postoperative chemotherapy and delayed radiation in children less than three years of age with malignant brain tumors. N Engl J Med 1993;328:1725–31.
170. Geyer JR, Zeltzer PM, Boyett JM, et al. Survival of infants with primitive neuroectodermal tumors or malignant ependymomas of the CNS treated with eight drugs in 1 day: a report from the Children's Cancer Group. J Clin Oncol 1994;12:1607–15.

171. Gajjar A, Mulhern RK, Heideman RL, et al. Medulloblastoma in very young children: outcome of definitive craniospinal irradiation following incomplete response to chemotherapy. J Clin Oncol 1994;12:1212–6.

172. Hartsell WF, Gajjar A, Heideman RL, et al. Patterns of failure in children with medulloblastoma: effects of preirradiation chemotherapy. Int J Radiat Oncol Biol Phys 1997;39:15–24.

173. Goldwein JW, Radcliffe J, Packer RJ, et al. Results of a pilot study of low-dose craniospinal radiation therapy plus chemotherapy for children younger than 5 years with primitive neuroectodermal tumors. Cancer 1993;71:2647–52.

174. Halberg FE, Wara WM, Fippin LF, et al. Low-dose craniospinal radiation therapy for medulloblastoma. Int J Radiat Oncol Biol Phys 1991;20:651–4.

175. Bouffet E, Bernard JL, Frappaz D, et al. M4 protocol for cerebellar medulloblastoma: supratentorial radiotherapy may not be avoided. Int J Radiat Oncol Biol Phys 1992;24:79–85.

176. Gentet JC, Bouffet E, Doz F, et al. Preirradiation chemotherapy including "eight drugs in 1 day" regimen and high-dose methotrexate in childhood medulloblastoma: results of the M7 French Cooperative Study. J Neurosurg 1995;82:608–14.

177. Shapiro WR. Chemotherapy of primary malignant brain tumors in children. Cancer 1975;35:965–72.

178. Mork SJ, Loken AC. Ependymoma: a follow-up study of 101 cases. Cancer 1977;40:907–15.

179. Salazar OM, Rubin P, Bassano D, Marcial VA. Improved survival of patients with intracranial ependymomas by irradiation: dose selection and field extension. Cancer 1975;35:1563–73.

180. Barone BM, Elvidge AR. Ependymomas: a clinical survey. J Neurosurg 1970;33:428–38.

181. Kovalic JJ, Flaris N, Grigsby PW, et al. Intracranial ependymoma long term outcome, patterns of failure. J Neurooncol 1993;15:125–31.

182. Ilgren EB, Stiller CA. Cerebellar astrocytomas: therapeutic management. Acta Neurochir (Wien) 1986;81:11–26.

183. Goldwein JW, Glauser TA, Packer RJ, et al. Recurrent intracranial ependymomas in children: survival, patterns of failure, and prognostic factors. Cancer 1990;66:557–63.

184. Robertson PL, Zeltzer PM, Boyett JM, et al. Survival and prognostic factors following radiation therapy and chemotherapy for ependymomas in children: a report of the Children's Cancer Group. J Neurosurg 1998;88:695–703.

185. Ross GW, Rubinstein LJ. Lack of histopathological correlation of malignant ependymomas with postoperative survival. J Neurosurg 1989;70:31–6.

186. Kovalic JJ, Grigsby PW, Shepard MJ, et al. Radiation therapy for gliomas of the optic nerve and chiasm. Int J Radiat Oncol Biol Phys 1990;18:927–32.

187. Mork SJ, Rubinstein LJ, Wada C, et al. Ependymoblastoma: a reappraisal of a rare embryonal tumor. Cancer 1985;55:1536–42.

188. Wada C, Kurata A, Hirose R, et al. Primary leptomeningeal ependymoblastoma: case report. J Neurosurg 1986;64:968–73.

189. Nazar GB, Hoffman HJ, Becker LE, et al. Infratentorial ependymomas in childhood: prognostic factors and treatment. J Neurosurg 1990;72:408–17.

190. McLaughlin MP, Marcus RB Jr, Buatti JM, et al. Ependymoma: results, prognostic factors and treatment recommendations. Int J Radiat Oncol Biol Phys 1998;40:845–50.

191. Merchant TE, Haida T, Wang MH, et al. Anaplastic ependymoma: treatment of pediatric patients with or without craniospinal radiation therapy. J Neurosurg 1997;86:943–9.

192. Sutton LN, Goldwein J, Perilongo G, et al. Prognostic factors in childhood ependymomas. Pediatr Neurosurg 1990;16:57–65.

193. Garrett PG, Simpson WJ. Ependymomas: results of radiation treatment. Int J Radiat Oncol Biol Phys 1983;9:1121–4.

194. Bloom HJ. Intracranial tumors: response and resistance to therapeutic endeavors, 1970–1980. Int J Radiat Oncol Biol Phys 1982;8:1083–113.

195. Chin HW, Maruyama Y, Markesbery W, et al. Intracranial ependymoma: results of radiotherapy at the University of Kentucky. Cancer 1982;49:2276–80.

196. Ikezaki K, Matsushima T, Inoue T, et al. Correlation of microanatomical localization with postoperative survival in posterior fossa ependymomas. Neurosurgery 1993;32:38–44.

197. Carrie C, Mottolese C, Bouffet E, et al. Non-metastatic childhood ependymomas. Radiother Oncol 1995;36:101–6.

198. Kim YH, Fayos JV, Garrett PG, Simpson WJ. Intracranial ependymomas: results of radiation treatment. Radiology 1977;124:805–8.

199. Salazar OM. A better understanding of CNS seeding and a brighter outlook for postoperatively irradiated patients with ependymomas. Int J Radiat Oncol Biol Phys 1983;9:1231–4.

200. Wallner KE, Wara WM, Sheline GE, Davis RL. Intracranial ependymomas: results of treatment with partial or whole brain irradiation without spinal irradiation. Int J Radiat Oncol Biol Phys 1986;12:1937–41.

200a. Vanuytsel L, Braada M. The role of prophylactic spinal irradiation in localized intracranial ependymoma. Int J Radiat Oncol Biol Phys 1991;21:825–30.

201. Goldwein JW, Corn BW, Finlay JL, et al. Is craniospinal irradiation required to cure children with malignant (anaplastic) intracranial ependymomas? Cancer 1991;67:2766–71.

202. Newton HB, Henson J, Walker RW. Extraneural metastases in ependymoma. J Neurooncol 1992;14:135–42.

203. Jennings MT, Gelman R, Hochberg F, et al. Intracranial germ-cell tumors: natural history and pathogenesis. J Neurosurg 1985;63:155–67.

204. Salazar OM, Castro-Vita H, Bakos RS, et al. Radiation therapy for tumors of the pineal region. Int J Radiat Oncol Biol Phys 1979;5:491–9.

205. Griffin BR, Griffin TW, Tong DY, et al. Pineal region tumors: results of radiation therapy and indications for elective spinal irradiation. Int J Radiat Oncol Biol Phys 1981;7:605–8.

206. Smith NJ, El-Mahdi AM, Constable WC. Results of irradiation of tumors in the region of the pineal body. Acta Radiol Ther Phys Biol 1976;15:17–22.

207. Dattoli MJ, Newall J. Radiation therapy for intracranial germinoma: the case for limited volume treatment. Int J Radiat Oncol Biol Phys 1990;19:429–33.

208. Legido A, Packer RJ, Sutton LN, et al. Suprasellar germinomas in childhood: a reappraisal. Cancer 1989;63:340–4.

209. Linggood RM, Chapman PH. Pineal tumors. J Neurooncol 1992;12:85–91.

210. Haddock MG, Schild SE, Scheithauer BW, Schomberg PJ. Radiation therapy for histologically confirmed primary central nervous system germinoma. Int J Radiat Oncol Biol Phys 1997;38:915–23.

211. Hardenbergh PH, Golden J, Billet A, et al. Intracranial germinoma: the case for lower dose radiation therapy. Int J Radiat Oncol Biol Phys 1997;39:419–26.

212. Wolden SL, Wara WM, Larson DA, et al. Radiation therapy for primary intracranial germ-cell tumors. Int J Radiat Oncol Biol Phys 1995;32:943–9.

213. Meadows A. Trilateral retinoblastoma. Med Pediatr Oncol 1986;14:323–6.

214. Bader JL, Miller RW, Meadows AT, et al. Trilateral retinoblastoma. Lancet 1980;2:582–3.

215. Blach LE, McCormick B, Abramson DH, Ellsworth RM. Trilateral retinoblastoma incidence and outcome: a decade of experience. Int J Radiat Oncol Biol Phys 1994;29:729–33.

216. Czirjak S, Pasztor E, Slowik F, et al. Third ventricle germinoma after total removal of intrasellar teratoma: case report. J Neurosurg 1992;77:643–7.

217. Shuangshoti S. Combined occurrence of third ventricular germinoma and hypothalamic mixed glioma. J Surg Oncol 1986;31:148–52.

218. Takeuchi J, Handa H, Otsuka S, Takebe Y. Neuroradiological aspects of suprasella germinoma. Neuroradiology 1979;17:153–9.

219. Dupont MG, Gerard JM, Flament-Durand J, et al. Pathognomonic aspect of germinoma on CT scan. Neuroradiology 1977;14:209–11.

220. Kleefield J, Solis OJ, Davis KR, et al. Computed tomography of tumors of the pineal region. Comput Tomogr 1977;1:257–65.

221. Takeuchi J, Handa H, Oda Y, Uchida Y. Alpha-fetoprotein in intracranial malignant teratoma. Surg Neurol 1979;12:400–4.

222. Shirato H, Nishio M, Sawamura Y, et al. Analysis of long-term treatment of intracranial germinoma. Int J Radiat Oncol Biol Phys 1997;37:511–5.

223. Shibamoto Y, Takahashi M, Sasai K. Prognosis of intracranial germinoma with syncytiotrophoblastic giant cells treated by radiation therapy. Int J Radiat Oncol Biol Phys 1997;37:505–10.

224. Chapman PH, Linggood RM. The management of pineal area tumors: a recent reappraisal. Cancer 1980;46:1253–7.

225. Posner J. Diagnosis and treatment of metastases to the brain. Clin Bull 1974;4:47–57.

226. Regis J, Bouillot P, Rouby-Volot F, et al. Pineal region tumors and

the role of stereotactic biopsy: review of the mortality, morbidity, and diagnostic rates in 370 cases. Neurosurgery 1996;39:907–14.

227. Schneider J, Chandrasoma P, Nedzi L, Apuzzo M. Neoplasms of the pineal and third ventricular region. In: Youmans J, ed. Neurological surgery. Vol. 4. Philadelphia: WB Saunders, 1997:2715.

228. Kelly P. Pineal region tumors and the role of stereotactic biopsy. Neurosurgery 1996;32:320–1.

229. Bradfield JS, Perez CA. Pineal tumors and ectopic pinealomas: analysis of treatment and failures. Radiology 1972;103:399–406.

230. Wara WM, Fellows CF, Sheline GE, et al. Radiation therapy for pineal tumors and suprasellar germinomas. Radiology 1977;124:221–3.

231. Hoffman HJ, Otsubo H, Hendrick EB, et al. Intracranial germ-cell tumors in children. J Neurosurg 1991;74:545–51.

232. Schild SE, Haddock MG, Scheithauer BW, et al. Nongerminomatous germ cell tumors of the brain. Int J Radiat Oncol Biol Phys 1996;36:557–63.

233. Borit A, Blackwood W, Mair WG, et al. The separation of pineocytoma from pineoblastoma. Cancer 1980;45:1408–18.

234. Schild SE, Scheithauer BW, Schomberg PJ, et al. Pineal parenchymal tumors: clinical, pathologic, and therapeutic aspects. Cancer 1993;72:870–80.

235. Jakacki RI, Zeltzer PM, Boyett JM, et al. Survival and prognostic factors following radiation and/or chemotherapy for primitive neuroectodermal tumors of the pineal region in infants and children: a report of the Children's Cancer Group. J Clin Oncol 1995;13:1377–83.

236. Aydin F, Ghatak NR, Radie-Keane K, et al. The short-term effect of low-dose radiation on intracranial germinoma: a pathologic study. Cancer 1992;69:2322–6.

237. Sung DI, Harisliadis L, Chang CH. Midline pineal tumors and suprasellar germinomas: highly curable by irradiation. Radiology 1978;128:745–51.

237a. Linstedt D, Wara WM, Edwards MS, et al. Radiotherapy of primary intracranial germinomas: the case against routine craniospinal irradiation. Int J Radiat Oncol Biol Phys 1988;15:291–7.

238. Dearnaley DP, A'Hern RP, Whittaker S, Bloom HJ. Pineal and CNS germ cell tumors: Royal Marsden Hospital experience 1962–1987. Int J Radiat Oncol Biol Phys 1990;18:773–81.

239. Balmaceda C, Heller G, Rosenblum M, et al. Chemotherapy without irradiation—a novel approach for newly diagnosed CNS germ cell tumors: results of an international cooperative trial. The First International Central Nervous System Germ Cell Tumor Study. J Clin Oncol 1996;14:2908–15.

240. Allen JC, DaRosso RC, Donahue B, Nirenberg A. A phase II trial of preirradiation carboplatin in newly diagnosed germinoma of the central nervous system. Cancer 1994;74:940–4.

241. Barkovich AJ, Krischer J, Kun LE, et al. Brain stem gliomas: a classification system based on magnetic resonance imaging. Cancer 1987;60:2901–6.

242. Eifel PJ, Cassady JR, Belli JA. Radiation therapy of tumors of the brainstem and midbrain in children: experience of the Joint Center for Radiation Therapy and Children's Hospital Medical Center (1971–1981). Int J Radiat Oncol Biol Phys 1987;13:847–52.

243. Grigsby PW, Thomas PR, Schwartz HG, Fineberg B. Irradiation of primary thalamic and brainstem tumors in a pediatric population: a 33-year experience. Cancer 1987;60:2901–6.

243a. Pierre-Kahn A, Hirsch JF, Vinchon M, et al. Surgical management of brain-stem tumors in children: results and statistical analysis of 75 cases. J Neurosurg 1993;79:845–52.

244. Greenberger JS, Cassady JR, Levene MB, et al. Radiation therapy of thalamic, midbrain and brain stem gliomas. Radiology 1977;122:463–8.

245. Whyte TR, Colby MY Jr, Layton DD Jr. Radiation therapy of brainstem tumors. Radiology 1969;93:413–6.

246. Panitch HS, Berg BO. Brain stem tumors of childhood and adolescence. Am J Dis Child 1970;119:465–72.

247. Bilaniuk LT, Zimmerman RA, Littman P, et al. Computed tomography of brain stem gliomas in children. Radiology 1980;134:89–95.

248. Packer RJ, Zimmerman RA, Luerssen TG, et al. Brainstem gliomas of childhood: magnetic resonance imaging. Neurology 1985;35:397–401.

249. Guiney MJ, Smith JG, Hughes P, et al. Contemporary management of adult and pediatric brain stem gliomas. Int J Radiat Oncol Biol Phys 1993;25:235–41.

250. Epstein FJ, Farmer JP. Brain-stem glioma growth patterns. J Neurosurg 1993;78:408–12.

251. Albright AL, Guthkelch AN, Packer RJ, et al. Prognostic factors in pediatric brain-stem gliomas. J Neurosurg 1986;65:751–5.

252. Stroink AR, Hoffman HJ, Hendrick EB, Humphreys RP. Diagnosis and management of pediatric brain-stem gliomas. J Neurosurg 1986;65:745–50.

253. Albright A, Packer R, Zimmerman R, et al. Magnetic resonance scans should replace biopsies for the diagnosis of diffuse brainstem gliomas: a report from the Children's Cancer Group. Neurosurgery 1993;33:1026–30.

254. Pollack I, Hoffman H, Humphreys R, et al. The long-term outcome after surgical treatment of dorsally exophytic brainstem gliomas. J Neurosurg 1993;78:859–63.

255. Hoffman HJ, Becker L, Craven MA. A clinically and pathologically distinct group of benign brain stem gliomas. Neurosurgery 1980;7:243–8.

256. Urtasun RC. $^{60}$Co radiation treatment of pontine gliomas. Radiology 1972;104:385–7.

257. Skowronska-Gardas A. Radiotherapy of midbrain and brainstem tumours in children. Radiother Oncol 1991;21:240–4.

258. Freeman CR, Krischer J, Sanford RA, et al. Hyperfractionated radiation therapy in brain stem tumors: results of treatment at the 7020 cGy dose level of Pediatric Oncology Group study #8495. Cancer 1991;68:474–81.

258a. Kim TH, Chin HW, Pollan S, et al. Radiotherapy of primary brain stem tumors. Int J Radiat Oncol Biol Phys 1980;6:51–7.

259. Hibi T, Shitara N, Genka S, et al. Radiotherapy for pediatric brain stem glioma: radiation dose, response, and survival. Neurosurgery 1992;31:643–50.

260. Mantravadi RV, Phatak R, Bellur S, et al. Brain stem gliomas: an autopsy study of 25 cases. Cancer 1982;49:1294–6.

261. Halperin EC, Wehn SM, Scott JW, et al. Selection of a management strategy for pediatric brainstem tumors. Med Pediatr Oncol 1989;17:117–26.

262. Littman P, Jarrett P, Bilaniuk LT, et al. Pediatric brain stem gliomas. Cancer 1980;45:2787–92.

262a. Bloom HJ, Glees J, Bell J, et al. The treatment and long-term prognosis of children with intracranial tumors: a study of 610 cases, 1950–1981. Int J Radiat Oncol Biol Phys 1990;18:723–45.

263. Albright AL, Price RA, Guthkelch AN, et al. Brain stem gliomas of children: a clinicopathological study. Cancer 1983;52:2313–9.

264. Prados MD, Wara WM, Edwards MS, et al. The treatment of brain stem and thalamic gliomas with 78 Gy of hyperfractionated radiation therapy. Int J Radiat Oncol Biol Phys 1995;32:85–91.

265. Packer RJ, Boyett JM, Zimmerman RA, et al. Outcome of children with brain stem gliomas after treatment with 7800 cGy of hyperfractionated radiotherapy. A Childrens Cancer Group Phase I/II Trial. Cancer 1994;74:1827–34.

266. Freeman CR, Farmer JP. Pediatric brain stem gliomas: a review. Int J Radiat Oncol Biol Phys 1998;40:265–71.

267. Lewis J, Lucraft H, Gholkar A. UKCCSG study of accelerated radiotherapy for pediatric brain stem gliomas. United Kingdom Childhood Cancer Study Group. Int J Radiat Oncol Biol Phys 1997;38:925–9.

268. Danoff BF, Kramer S, Thompson N. The radiotherapeutic management of optic nerve gliomas in children. Int J Radiat Oncol Biol Phys 1980;6:45–50.

269. Tenny RT, Laws ER Jr, Younge BR, Rush JA. The neurosurgical management of optic glioma: results in 104 patients. J Neurosurg 1982;57:452–8.

270. Weiss L, Sagerman RH, King GA, et al. Controversy in the management of optic nerve glioma. Cancer 1987;59:1000–4.

271. Gaini SM, Tomei G, Arienta C, et al. Optic nerve and chiasm gliomas in children. J Neurosurg Sci 1982;26:33–9.

272. Flickinger JC, Torres C, Deutsch M. Management of low-grade gliomas of the optic nerve and chiasm. Cancer 1988;61:635–42.

273. Safneck JR, Napier LB, Halliday WC. Malignant astrocytoma of the optic nerve in a child. Can J Neurol Sci 1992;19:498–503.

274. Tao ML, Barnes PD, Billett AL, et al. Childhood optic chiasm gliomas: radiographic response following radiotherapy and long-term clinical outcome. Int J Radiat Oncol Biol Phys 1997;39:579–87.

275. Housepian EM, Chi TL. Neurofibromatosis and optic pathways gliomas. J Neurooncol 1993;15:51–5.

276. Horwich A, Bloom HJ, Packer RJ, et al. Optic gliomas: radiation therapy and prognosis. Int J Radiat Oncol Biol Phys 1985;11:1067–79.

277. Packer RJ, Savino PJ, Bilaniuk LT, et al. Chiasmatic gliomas of childhood: a reappraisal of natural history and effectiveness of cranial irradiation. Childs Brain 1983;10:393–403.

278. Hoyt WF, Baghdassarian SA. Optic glioma of childhood: natural history and rationale for conservative management. Br J Ophthalmol 1969;53:793–8.

279. Alvord EC Jr, Lofton S. Gliomas of the optic nerve or chiasm: outcome by patients' age, tumor site, and treatment. J Neurosurg 1988;68:85–98.

280. Dutton JJ. Optic nerve gliomas and meningiomas. Neurol Clin 1991;9:163–77.

281. Rush JA, Younge BR, Campbell RJ, MacCarty CS. Optic glioma: long-term follow-up of 85 histopathologically verified cases. Ophthalmology 1982;89:1213–9.

282. Montgomery AB, Griffin T, Parker RG, et al. Optic nerve glioma: the role of radiation therapy. Cancer 1977;40:2079–80.

283. Wong JY, Uhl V, Wara WM, Sheline GE. Optic gliomas: a reanalysis of the University of California, San Francisco experience. Cancer 1987;60:1847–55.

284. Heiskanen O, Raitta C, Torsti R. The management and prognosis of gliomas of the optic pathways in children. Acta Neurochir (Wien) 1978;43:193–9.

285. DeSousa AL, Kalsbeck JE, Mealey J Jr, et al. Optic chiasmatic glioma in children. Am J Ophthal 1979;87:376–81.

286. Dosoretz DE, Blitzer PH, Wang CC, et al. Management of glioma of the optic nerve and/or chiasm: an analysis of 20 cases. Cancer 1980;45:1467–71.

287. Wisoff JH, Abbott R, Epstein F. Surgical management of exophytic chiasmatic-hypothalamic tumors of childhood. J Neurosurg 1990;73:661–7.

288. Arthur K. Radiotherapy in chemodectoma of the glomus jugulare. Clin Radiol 1977;28:415–7.

289. Jenkin D, Angyalfi S, Becker L, et al. Optic glioma in children: surveillance, resection, or irradiation? Int J Radiat Oncol Biol Phys 1993;25:215–25.

290. Borit A, Richardson EP Jr. The biological and clinical behaviour of pilocytic astrocytomas of the optic pathways. Brain 1982;105:161–87.

291. Rodriquez LA, Edwards MS, Levin VA. Management of hypothalamic gliomas in children: an analysis of 33 cases. Neurosurgery 1990;26:242–6.

292. Capo H, Kupersmith MJ. Efficacy and complications of radiotherapy of anterior visual pathway tumors. Neurol Clin 1991;9:179–203.

293. Iraci G, Gerosa M, Tomazzoli L, et al. Gliomas of the optic nerve and chiasm: a clinical review. Childs Brain 1981;8:326–49.

294. de Keizer RJ, de Wolff-Rouendaal D, Bots GT, et al. Optic glioma with intraocular tumor and seeding in a child with neurofibromatosis. Am J Ophthalmol 1989;108:717–25.

295. Pierce SM, Barnes PD, Loeffler JS, et al. Definitive radiation therapy in the management of symptomatic patients with optic glioma: survival and long-term effects. Cancer 1990;65:45–52.

296. Simpson D. The recurrence of intracranial meningiomas after surgical treatment. J Neurol Neurosurg Psychiatry 1957;20:22–39.

297. Yamashita J, Handa H, Iwaki K, et al. Recurrence of intracranial meningiomas, with special reference to radiotherapy. Surg Neurol 1980;14:33–40.

298. Barbaro NM, Gutin PH, Wilson CB, et al. Radiation therapy in the treatment of partially resected meningiomas. Neurosurgery 1987;20:525–8.

299. Jaaskelainen J. Seemingly complete removal of histologically benign intracranial meningioma: late recurrence. Surg Neurol 1986;26:461–9.

300. Adegbite A, Khan M, Paine K, et al. Recurrence of intracranial meningiomas after surgical treatment. J Neurosurg 1983;58:51–6.

301. Mirimanoff R, Dosoretz D, Lingood R, et al. Meningioma: analysis of recurrence and progression following neurosurgical resection. J Neurosurg 1985;62:18–24.

302. Condra KS, Buatti JM, Mendenhall WM, et al. Benign meningiomas: primary treatment selection affects survival. Int J Radiat Oncol Biol Phys 1997;39:427–36.

303. Carella RJ, Ransohoff J, Newall J. Role of radiation therapy in the management of meningioma. Neurosurgery 1982;10:332–9.

304. Salazar OM. Ensuring local control in meningiomas. Int J Radiat Oncol Biol Phys 1988;15:501–4.

304a. Miralbell R, Linggood RM, de la Monte S, et al. The role of radiotherapy in the treatment of subtotally resected benign meningiomas. J Neurooncol 1992;13:157–64.

305. King DL, Chang CH, Pool JL. Radiotherapy in the management of meningiomas. Acta Radiol Ther Phys Biol 1966;5:26–33.

306. Jaaskelainen J, Haltia M, Servo A. Atypical and anaplastic meningiomas: radiology, surgery, radiotherapy, and outcome. Surg Neurol 1986;25:233–42.

307. Guthrie BL, Ebersold MJ, Scheithauer BW, Shaw EG. Meningeal hemangiopericytoma: histopathological features, treatment, and long-term follow-up of 44 cases. Neurosurgery 1989;25:514–22.

308. Bastin KT, Mehta MP. Meningeal hemangiopericytoma: defining the role for radiation therapy. J Neurooncol 1992;14:277–87.

309. Goldsmith BJ, Wara WM, Wilson CB, Larson DA. Postoperative irradiation for subtotally resected meningiomas: a retrospective analysis of 140 patients treated from 1967 to 1990. J Neurosurg 1994;80:195–201.

310. Eng TY, Albright NW, Kuwahara G, et al. Precision radiation therapy for optic nerve sheath meningiomas. Int J Radiat Oncol Biol Phys 1992;22:1093–8.

311. Kondziolka D, Lunsford LD, Coffey RJ, Flickinger JC. Stereotactic radiosurgery of meningiomas. J Neurosurg 1991;74:552–9.

312. Taylor BW Jr, Marcus RB Jr, Friedman WA, et al. The meningioma controversy: postoperative radiation therapy. Int J Radiat Oncol Biol Phys 1988;15:299–304.

313. Goldsmith BJ, Rosenthal SA, Wara WM, Larson DA. Optic neuropathy after irradiation of meningioma. Radiology 1992;185:71–6.

314. Smith JL, Vuksanovic MM, Yates BM, Bienfang DC. Radiation therapy for primary optic nerve meningiomas. J Clin Neuroophthalmol 1981;1:85–99.

315. Smith JL, McCrary JAD, Ray BS, Vuksanovic MM. Managing menacing meningioma. J Clin Neuroophthalmol 1983;3:169–79.

316. Ito M, Ishizawa A, Miyaoka M, et al. Intraorbital meningiomas: surgical management and role of radiation therapy. Surg Neurol 1988;29:448–53.

317. Sibony PA, Krauss HR, Kennerdell JS, et al. Optic nerve sheath meningiomas: clinical manifestations. Ophthalmology 1984;91:1313–26.

318. Maire JP, Caudry M, Guerin J, et al. Fractionated radiation therapy in the treatment of intracranial meningiomas: local control, functional efficacy, and tolerance in 91 patients. Int J Radiat Biol Phys 1995;33:315–21.

318a. Wara WM, Sheline GE, Newman H, et al. Radiation therapy of meningiomas. Am J Roentgenol Radium Ther Nucl Med 1975;123:453–8.

319. Jaaskelainen J, Servo A, Haltia M, et al. Intracranial hemangiopericytoma: radiology, surgery, radiotherapy, and outcome in 21 patients. Surg Neurol 1985;23:227–36.

320. Grunberg SM. Role of antiprogestational therapy for meningiomas. Hum Reprod 1994;9:Suppl 1:202–7.

321. Schrell UM, Rittig MG, Anders M, et al. Hydroxyurea for treatment of unresectable and recurrent meningiomas: II. decrease in the size of meningiomas in patients treated with hydroxyurea. J Neurosurg 1997;86:840–4.

322. Kyritsis AP. Chemotherapy for meningiomas. J Neurooncol 1996;29:269–72.

323. Tomlinson FH, Kurtin PJ, Suman VJ, et al. Primary intracerebral malignant lymphoma: a clinicopathological study of 89 patients. J Neurosurg 1995;82:558–66.

324. Rosenblum ML, Levy RM, Bredesen DE, et al. Primary central nervous system lymphomas in patients with AIDS. Ann Neurol 1988;23:Suppl:S13–6.

325. Selch MT, Shimizu KT, De Salles AF, et al. Primary central nervous system lymphoma: results at the University of California at Los Angeles and review of the literature. Am J Clin Oncol 1994;17:286–93.

326. Peterson K, Gordon KB, Heinemann MH, DeAngelis LM. The clinical spectrum of ocular lymphoma. Cancer 1993;72:843–9.

327. O'Neill B, Kelly P, Earle J, et al. Computer-assisted stereotactic biopsy for the diagnosis of primary central nervous system lymphoma. Neurology 1987;37:1160–4.

328. Nelson DF, Martz KL, Bonner H, et al. Non-Hodgkin's lymphoma of the brain: can high dose, large volume radiation therapy improve survival? Report on a prospective trial by the Radiation Therapy Oncology Group (RTOG): RTOG 8315. Int J Radiat Oncol Biol Phys 1992;23:9–17.

329. Corry J, Smith JG, Wirth A, et al. Primary central nervous system lymphoma: age and performance status are more important than treatment modality. Int J Radiat Oncol Biol Phys 1998;41:615–20.

330. Corn BW, Donahue BR, Rosenstock JG, et al. Performance status and age as independent predictors of survival among AIDS patients with primary CNS lymphoma: a multivariate analysis of a multi-institutional experience. Cancer J Sci Am 1997;3:52–6.

331. Fine HA, Mayer RJ. Primary central nervous system lymphoma. Ann Intern Med 1993;119:1093–104.

332. DeAngelis LM, Yahalom J, Thaler HT, Kher U. Combined modality therapy for primary CNS lymphoma. J Clin Oncol 1992;10:635–43.

333. Abrey LE, DeAngelis LM, Yahalom J. Long-term survival in primary CNS lymphoma. J Clin Oncol 1998;16:859–63.

334. O'Neill BP, O'Fallon JR, Earle JD, et al. Primary central nervous system non-Hodgkin's lymphoma: survival advantages with combined initial therapy? Int J Radiat Oncol Biol Phys 1995;33:663–73.

335. Renaudin J, Fewer D, Wilson CB, et al. Dose dependency of decadron in patients with partially excised brain tumors. J Neurosurg 1973; 39:302–5.

336. Smalley S, Laws E, O'Fallon J, et al. Resection for solitary brain metastasis: role of adjuvant radiation and prognostic variables in 229 patients. J Neurosurg 1992;77:531–40.

337. DeAngelis L, Mandell L, Thaler H, et al. The role of postoperative radiotherapy after resection of single brain metastases. Neurosurgery 1989;24:798–804.

338. Bindal R, Sawaya R, Leavens M, et al. Surgical treatment of multiple brain metastases. J Neurosurg 1993;79:210–6.

339. Alexander E 3rd, Moriarty TM, Davis RB, et al. Stereotactic radiosurgery for the definitive, noninvasive treatment of brain metastases. J Natl Cancer Inst 1995;87:34–40.

340. Bindal A, Bindal R, Hess K, et al. Surgery versus radiosurgery in the treatment of brain metastasis. J Neurosurg 1996;84:748–54.

341. Fuller BG, Kaplan ID, Adler J, et al. Stereotaxic radiosurgery for brain metastases: the importance of adjuvant whole brain irradiation. Int J Radiat Oncol Biol Phys 1992;23:413–8.

342. Galicich JH, Sundaresan N, Arbit E, et al. Surgical treatment of single brain metastasis: factors associated with survival. Cancer 1980; 45:381–6.

343. Winston KR, Walsh JW, Fischer EG. Results of operative treatment of intracranial metastatic tumors. Cancer 1980;45:2639–45.

344. Patchell RA, Tibbs PA, Walsh JW, et al. A randomized trial of surgery in the treatment of single metastases to the brain. N Engl J Med 1990;322:494–500.

345. Smalley SR, Schray MF, Laws ER Jr, O'Fallon JR. Adjuvant radiation therapy after surgical resection of solitary brain metastasis: association with pattern of failure and survival. Int J Radiat Oncol Biol Phys 1987;13:1611–6.

346. Patchell RA, Tibbs PA, Regine WF, et al. Postoperative radiotherapy in the treatment of single metastases to the brain: a randomized trial. JAMA 1998;280:1485–9.

347. Hendrickson FR. Palliation of cerebral metastases. Int J Radiat Oncol Biol Phys 1977;2:1223–4.

348. Borgelt B, Gelber R, Kramer S, et al. The palliation of brain metastases: final results of the first two studies by the Radiation Therapy Oncology Group. Int J Radiat Oncol Biol Phys 1980;6:1–9.

349. Kurtz JM, Gelber R, Brady LW, et al. The palliation of brain metastases in a favorable patient population: a randomized clinical trial by the Radiation Therapy Oncology Group. Int J Radiat Oncol Biol Phys 1981;7:891–5.

350. Gelber RD, Larson M, Borgelt BB, et al. Equivalence of radiation schedules for the palliative treatment of brain metastases in patients with favorable prognosis. Cancer 1981;48:1749–53.

351. Phillips TL, Scott CB, Leibel SA, et al. Results of a randomized comparison of radiotherapy and bromodeoxyuridine with radiotherapy alone for brain metastases: report of RTOG trial 89–05. Int J Radiat Oncol Biol Phys 1995;33:339–48.

352. Komarnicky LT, Phillips TL, Martz K, et al. A randomized phase III protocol for the evaluation of misonidazole combined with radiation in the treatment of patients with brain metastases (RTOG-7916). Int J Radiat Oncol Biol Phys 1991;20:53–8.

353. Swift PS, Phillips T, Martz K, et al. CT characteristics of patients with brain metastases treated in RTOG study 79–16. Int J Radiat Oncol Biol Phys 1993;25:209–14.

354. Gaspar L, Scott C, Rotman M, et al. Recursive partitioning analysis (RPA) of prognostic factors in three Radiation Therapy Oncology Group (RTOG) brain metastases trials. Int J Radiat Oncol Biol Phys 1997;37:745–51.

355. Hindo WA, DeTrana FAD, Lee MS, Hendrickson FR. Large dose increment irradiation in treatment of cerebral metastases. Cancer 1970;26:138–41.

356. Shehata WM, Hendrickson FR, Hindo WA. Rapid fractionation technique and re-treatment of cerebral metastases by irradiation. Cancer 1974;34:257–61.

357. Harwood AR, Simson WJ. Radiation therapy of cerebral metastases: a randomized prospective clinical trial. Int J Radiat Oncol Biol Phys 1977;2:1091–4.

358. Hoskin PJ, Crow J, Ford HT. The influence of extent and local management on the outcome of radiotherapy for brain metastases. Int J Radiat Oncol Biol Phys 1990;19:111–5.

359. Epstein BE, Scott CB, Sause WT, et al. Improved survival duration in patients with unresected solitary brain metastasis using accelerated hyperfractionated radiation therapy at total doses of 54.4 gray and greater: results of Radiation Therapy Oncology Group 85–28. Cancer 1993;71:1362–7.

360. Sause WT, Scott C, Krisch R, et al. Phase I/II trial of accelerated fractionation in brain metastases RTOG 85–28. Int J Radiat Oncol Biol Phys 1993;26:653–7.

361. Nieder C, Berberich W, Nestle U, et al. Relation between local result and total dose of radiotherapy for brain metastases. Int J Radiat Oncol Biol Phys 1995;33:349–55.

362. Flickinger JC, Kondziolka D, Lunsford LD, et al. A multi-institutional experience with stereotactic radiosurgery for solitary brain metastasis. Int J Radiat Oncol Biol Phys 1994;28:797–802.

363. Pirzkall A, Debus J, Lohr F, et al. Radiosurgery alone or in combination with whole-brain radiotherapy for brain metastases. J Clin Oncol 1998;16:3563–9.

364. Tidwell TJ, Montague ED. Chemodectomas involving the temporal bone. Radiology 1975;116:147–9.

365. Maruyama Y, Gold LH, Kieffer SA. Clinical and angiographic evaluation of radiotherapeutic response of glomus jugulare tumors. Radiology 1971;101:397–9.

366. Hatfield PM, James AE, Schulz MD. Chemodectomas of the glomus jugulare. Cancer 1972;30:1164–8.

367. Newman H, Rowe JF Jr, Phillips TL. Radiation therapy of the glomus jugulare tumor. Am J Roentgenol Radium Ther Nucl Med 1973; 118:663–9.

368. Cummings BJ, Beale FA, Garrett PG, et al. The treatment of glomus tumors in the temporal bone by megavoltage radiation. Cancer 1984;53:2635–40.

369. Gibbin KP, Henk JM. Glomus jugulare tumours in South Wales—a twenty-year review. Clin Radiol 1978;29:607–9.

370. Simko TG, Griffin TW, Gerdes AJ, et al. The role of radiation therapy in the treatment of glomus jugulare tumors. Cancer 1978;42:104–6.

371. Kim JA, Elkon D, Lim ML, et al. Optimum dose of radiotherapy for chemodectomas of the middle ear. Int J Radiat Oncol Biol Phys 1980;6:815–9.

372. Reddy EK, Mansfield CM, Hartman GV. Chemodectoma of glomus jugulare. Cancer 1983;52:337–40.

373. McCabe BF, Fletcher M, Galanis E, et al. Selection of therapy of glomus jugulare tumors: clinical outcome of gliosarcoma compared with glioblastoma multiforme: North Central Cancer Treatment Group results. Arch Otolaryngol 1969;89:156–9.

374. Pryzant RM, Chou JL, Easley JD. Twenty year experience with radiation therapy for temporal bone chemodectomas. Int J Radiat Oncol Biol Phys 1989;17:1303–7.

375. Larner JM, Hahn SS, Spaulding CA, Constable WC. Glomus jugulare tumors: long-term control by radiation therapy. Cancer 1992;69:1813–7.

376. Powell S, Peters N, Harmer C. Chemodectoma of the head and neck: results of treatment in 84 patients. Int J Radiat Oncol Biol Phys 1992;22:919–24.

377. Mumber MP, Greven KM. Control of advanced chemodectomas of the head and neck with irradiation. Am J Clin Oncol 1995;18:389–91.

378. Springate SC, Haraf D, Weichselbaum RR. Temporal bone chemodectomas comparing surgery and radiation therapy. Oncology (Huntingt) 1991;5:131–7.

379. Dawes PJ, Filippou M, Welch AR, Dawes JD. The management of glomus jugulare tumours. Clin Otolaryngol 1987;12:15–24.

380. Boyle JO, Shimm DS, Coulthard SW, et al. Radiation therapy for paragangliomas of the temporal bone. Laryngoscope 1990;100:896–901.

381. Wang ML, Hussey DH, Doornbos JF, et al: Chemodectoma of the temporal bone: a comparison of surgical and radiotherapeutic results. Int J Radiat Oncol Biol Phys 1988;14:643–8.

382. Hawthorne MR, Makek MS, Harris JP, Fisch U. The histopathological and clinical features of irradiated and nonirradiated temporal paragangliomas. Laryngoscope 1988;98:325–31.

383. Bloom H: Clinical management. In: Bloom H, ed. Cancer in children. New York: Springer-Verlag, 1975:93.

384. Farwell JR, Dohrmann GJ, Flannery JT, Wang CC. Central nervous system tumors in children. Cancer 1977;40:3123–32.

385. Geissinger JD. Astrocytomas of the cerebellum in children: long-term study. Arch Neurol 1971;24:125–35.
386. Gjerris F, Klinken L. Long-term prognosis in children with benign cerebellar astrocytoma. J Neurosurg 1978;49:179.
387. Szenasy J, Slowik F. Prognosis of benign cerebellar astrocytomas in children. Childs Brain 1983;10:39–47.
388. Garcia DM, Latifi HR, Simpson JR, Picker S. Astrocytomas of the cerebellum in children. J Neurosurg 1989;71:661–4.
389. Hayostek CJ, Shaw EG, Scheithauer B, et al. Astrocytomas of the cerebellum: A comparative clinicopathologic study of pilocytic and diffuse astrocytomas. Cancer 1993;72:856–69.
390. Larson DA, Wara WM, Edwards MS. Management of childhood cerebellar astrocytoma. Int J Radiat Oncol Biol Phys 1990;18:971–3.
391. Garcia DM, Marks JE, Latifi HR, Kliefoth AB. Childhood cerebellar astrocytomas: is there a role for postoperative irradiation? Int J Radiat Oncol Biol Phys 1990;18:815–8.
392. Wallner KE, Gonzales MF, Edwards MS, et al. Treatment results of juvenile pilocytic astrocytoma. J Neurosurg 1988;69:171–6.
393. Richmond J. Cancer. In: Raven R, ed. Cancer. Vol. 5. London: Butterworth & Co., 1959:375.
394. Bouchard J. Radiation therapy of tumors and disease of the nervous system. Philadelphia: Lea & Febiger, 1966.
395. Sheline GE, Boldrey E, Karlsberg P, Phillips T. Therapeutic considerations in tumors affecting the central nervous system: oligodendrogliomas. Radiology 1964;82:84–9.
396. Marsa GW, Goffinet DR, Rubinstein LJ, Bagshaw MA. Megavoltage irradiation in the treatment of gliomas of the brain and spinal cord. Cancer 1975;36:1681–9.
397. Chin HW, Hazel JJ, Kim TH, Webster JH. Oligodendrogliomas: I. a clinical study of cerebral oligodendrogliomas. Cancer 1980;45:1458–66.
398. Shimizu KT. Management of oligodendroglioma. Radiology 1993;186:569–72.
399. Cumberlin RL, Luk KH, Wara WM, et al. Medulloblastoma: treatment results and effect on normal tissues. Cancer 1979;43:1014–20.
400. Brown RC, Gunderson L, Plenk HP. Medulloblastoma: a review of the LDS hospital experience. Cancer 1977;40:56–60.
401. Chin HW, Maruyama Y: Results of radiation treatment of cerebellar medulloblastoma. Int J Radiat Oncol Biol Phys 1981;7:737–42.
402. Phillips TL. Sheline GE, Boldrey E: Therapeutic considerations in tumors affecting the central nervous system: ependymomas. Am J Roentgenol Radium Ther Nucl Med 1964; 83:88–105.
403. Kricheff II, Becker M, Schneck SA, Taveras JM: Intracranial ependymomas: a study of survival in 65 cases treated by surgery and irradiation. Am J Roentgenol Radium Ther Nucl Med 1964;91:167–75.
404. Marks JE, Adler SJ. A comparative study of ependymomas by site of origin. Int J Radiat Oncol Biol Phys 1982;8:37–43.
405. Kramer S. Radiation therapy in the management of malignant gliomas. In: Seventh national cancer conference proceedings. Philadelphia: JB Lippincott, 1973:823.
406. Taveras JM, Thompson HG, Pool JL: Should we treat glioblastoma multiforme? A study of survival in 425 cases. Am J Roentgenol Radium Ther Nucl Med 1962;87:473–9.
407. Rutten EHJM, Kazem I, Sloof JL, Walder AMD. Postoperative radiation therapy in the management of brain astrocytoma—retrospective study of 142 patients. Int J Radiat Oncol Biol Phys 1981;7:191–5.
408. Levy LF, Elvidge AR. Astrocytoma of the brain and spinal cord: a review of 176 cases, 1940–1949. J Neurosurg 1956;13:413–43.

# CHAPTER 73

# SPINAL CORD

......................................

# NATURAL HISTORY, DIAGNOSIS, AND STAGING

• Ulrich Batzdorf • Charles M. Haskell

## EPIDEMIOLOGY AND ETIOLOGY

Spinal cord tumors, both primary and metastatic, are less common than cerebral tumors in a ratio of 1:7 to 1:10, depending on the nature of the hospital population studied.[1] The epidemiology of spinal cord tumors has not been studied separately from that of other central nervous system (CNS) tumors.[2] Considerations applicable to metastatic tumors are those that relate to individual tumor type. An association of primary spinal tumors, often multiple, with central von Recklinghausen's disease and von Hippel-Lindau disease is recognized.

Nothing is known about the etiology of these tumors, and the same considerations that were cited with respect to the etiology of primary brain tumors in Chapter 72 probably apply. Molecular biologic studies of primary spinal cord neoplasms have been reported only rarely and the results have been inconclusive.[3]

The original primary site of metastatic tumors has been analyzed in various series.[4] Findings depend to a considerable extent on the nature of the hospital population studied and the particular areas of interest within the field of oncology that are emphasized.

## BIOLOGY

Extramedullary intradural tumors are most commonly either benign neurilemomas (schwannomas) or meningiomas. Primary intraspinal tumors, corresponding to the tumor categories in Table 73–1, are frequently of a less malignant nature than corresponding tumors of the brain. Thus, ependymo-

**Table 73–1.** Frequency of Primary Intraspinal Tumors in a Series of 1322 Cases at Mayo Clinic

| Tumor | Percent |
|---|---|
| Schwannomas | 29.0 |
| Meningiomas | 25.5 |
| Gliomas, including extramedullary | 22.0 |
| Sarcomas | 11.9 |
| Vascular tumors | 6.2 |
| Chordomas | 4.0 |
| Epidermoid and other tumors | 1.4 |

From Slooff JL, et al, eds. Primary intramedullary tumors of the spinal cord and filum terminale. Philadelphia: WB Saunders, 1964.

*Table 73–2.* Frequency of Primary Intraspinal Intramedullary Gliomas

| Tumor | Percent |
|---|---|
| Ependymomas | 63.0 |
| Astrocytomas (grades 1 and 2) | 24.4 |
| Glioblastomas (astrocytomas grades 3 and 4) | 7.5 |
| Oligodendrogliomas | 3.0 |
| Other tumors | 2.0 |

From Rubenstein LI. Tumors of the central nervous system. Washington, DC: Armed Forces Institute of Pathology, 1972:3.

mas, both those occurring in the cord and those that arise in the filum terminale, are generally well differentiated. These tumors expand the cord as they grow and, like extramedullary tumors, may ultimately block the circulation of cerebrospinal fluid (CSF), compartmentalizing the fluid below the level of the tumor. Because of selective resorption of water from the CSF, there is a progressive increase in protein concentration of fluid below the level of the tumor, which reaches high levels if there is a complete subarachnoid block. In addition, these tumors may generate cysts, which frequently contain yellowish fluid with high protein content.

Spinal cord tumors produce neurologic symptoms by compression of myelinated tracts and anterior horn cells, and possibly by vascular mechanisms.[5] Occlusion and thrombosis of extradural veins may occur. Astrocytomas, particularly the rare malignant tumors of this type, may also cause destruction of spinal cord tissue.

## CLASSIFICATION

Spinal tumors are commonly classified by both location and histologic nature (Tables 73–1 to 73–3). Extramedullary tumors displace rather than invade neural tissue. However, extradural metastatic tumors usually spare the dura mater, which appears to act as a barrier to tumor extension.

Histologically, spinal cord tumors represent several of the tumor categories listed in the classification of CNS tumors (Table 73–4). Most common among these are neurilemomas (schwannomas), meningiomas, and gliomas, but many other varieties of tumors are also encountered in small numbers. Metastatic tumors of the spine also may be classified with respect to their anatomic location (Tables 73–4 and 73–5). Strict separation of these categories is not always possible, however.

*Table 73–3.* Classification of Spinal Tumors

| By Levels | By Location |
|---|---|
| Cord | Extramedullary 71% |
| Cervical | Extradural |
| Thoracic | Intradural |
| Lumbar | |
| Cauda equina | Intramedullary 29% |
| Lumbar sacral | |

From Greenwood J. Spinal cord tumors. In: Youmans JR, ed. Neurological surgery. Philadelphia: WB Saunders, 1973:1516.

*Table 73–4.* Metastatic Spinal Tumors with Potential Neurologic Complications

Metastases to vertebrae
  Osteoblastic
  Osteolytic with or without vertebral collapse
Epidural metastases
  By extension from vertebrae
  By extension from paravertebral tumor
  Hematogenous
Subarachnoid ("meningeal") dissemination
Intramedullary nodular foci

It is not uncommon for tumors involving the vertebral bodies to extend into the epidural space, at which point they may form a carpet that compresses or constricts the spinal cord. Another form of metastatic tumor to be considered is that developing from the seeding of primary brain tumors. The most common examples of such tumors are seen in relation to medulloblastomas, retinoblastomas, pineal gland tumors, and ependymomas. The multifocal nature of these secondary deposits creates special problems with respect to their therapy.

## CLINICAL FEATURES AND DIAGNOSIS

The clinical manifestations of spinal cord tumors include local spinal pain, which usually precedes progressive neurologic deficit. Pain may be relatively diffuse over the involved area of the spine, but it often has a radicular component as well when one or more nerve roots are compressed, stretched, or infiltrated by the tumor. Radicular pain is encountered in the extremities or may be perceived as a band-like pain in dermatomal distribution over the trunk. Neurologic manifestations include motor and sensory deficits, as well as loss of sphincter control. Sphincter problems are more commonly encountered as an early sign when the tumor is intramedullary. Acute urine retention in a patient known to have cancer should always arouse the suspicion of spinal cord compression or cauda equina involvement.

The diagnosis of spinal cord tumors is made both by clinical examination and by radiologic and imaging techniques. The clinical examination should place special emphasis on motor and reflex evaluation of the extremities, on the

*Table 73–5.* Primary Sites of Metastatic Spinal Tumors

| Origin | Cases (No.) | Percent |
|---|---|---|
| Carcinomas | | |
|   Breast | 15 | 19.2 |
|   Lung | 14 | 17.9 |
|   Prostate | 7 | 9.0 |
|   Colon and rectum | 6 | 7.7 |
|   Kidney | 5 | 6.4 |
|   Unknown | 11 | 14.1 |
| Sarcoma | 6 | 7.7 |
| Melanoma | 4 | 5.2 |
| Others | 10 | 12.8 |
| Total | 78 | 100.0 |

From Vieth RG, Odom GL. Neurosurgery 1965;23:501.

assessment of sensory level, and on evaluating the intactness of sacral cutaneous reflexes and sphincter tone. In children, scoliosis may herald the presence of a cord tumor.

Motor weakness may develop asymmetrically, although with severe cord compression, the deficit tends to become symmetric. Unsteadiness is occasionally seen before weakness. Deep tendon reflexes are usually hyperactive, plantar responses become extensor responses, and superficial abdominal reflexes disappear. Patients with diffuse meningeal involvement of the cauda equina or of individual nerve roots often show loss of deep tendon reflexes in association with pain and weakness. Sensory deficit tends to ascend, reaching a "level" as cord involvement becomes more complete.

Slowly growing spinal tumors may produce erosive changes of the vertebral spine, which often are apparent on plain roentgenograms or on tomographic views of the spine as a scalloping distortion of the vertebral body outline, thinning of a pedicle, enlargement of a nerve root foramen, or scoliosis. More rapidly growing metastatic lesions of the spine may show partial or complete collapse of vertebral bodies, sometimes with angulation of the spine, which may, in turn, result in spinal cord compression. Osteolytic and osteoblastic changes are seen in less advanced situations. Tomography is also helpful in more clearly demonstrating paravertebral soft tissue masses, which may accompany a variety of spinal tumors, including schwannomas, neuroblastomas, and metastatic lesions.

Isotope scanning is a helpful diagnostic tool for the early identification of vertebral metastases because it is often capable of identifying the lesions long before they would be detected on roentgenography.[6, 7]

Magnetic resonance imaging (MRI) is, in many instances, the first study to be performed in patients undergoing evaluation of spinal tumor, both primary and metastatic. It is, of course, noninvasive and therefore does not disturb spinal fluid dynamics, as does myelography, which requires lumbar puncture. Contrast myelography is, however, still useful in clarifying and demonstrating the precise level of spinal involvement in diagnostically difficult cases. Water-soluble contrast material is now universally used and has the advantage of not requiring removal at the conclusion of the radiologic examination. This is a consideration of particular importance when a total myelographic block is demonstrated because precipitous changes in the CSF pressure would hazard impaction of the tumor against the spinal cord. Computed tomography (CT), in conjunction with metrizamide myelography, is a particularly useful tool.

Because of refinements in MRI techniques and the complete safety associated with this modality, a surgical decision and plan can now be made in most patients without myelography. MRI and myelography distinguish cord tumors from non-neoplastic conditions, such as transverse myelitis and radiation myelitis. The latter, in particular, may merit consideration in cancer patients whose neurologic deficit would correlate with an irradiated segment of cord. Edelson and associates[8] also cite the rare occurrence of spinal epidural hematomas in patients with depressed platelet counts. Such lesions may closely mimic metastatic tumor, both clinically and on myelography. The MRI study should encompass the entire spinal cord because lesions may be multifocal, especially those that are metastatic from distant sites.[9]

CSF protein is often elevated in the presence of an intraspinal tumor. When a complete subarachnoid block exists, the protein level may reach several grams per deciliter. CSF cytology may be helpful in patients suspected of having a metastatic spinal cord lesion, but who do not have a demonstrable tumor mass.

## STAGING

The *AJCC Cancer Staging Manual*[10] does not provide a staging guide for spinal tumors.

## PROGNOSIS

The prognosis of spinal tumors must be considered from two points of view: (1) with respect to restoration or preservation of neural function and (2) with regard to local tumor control and survival. The time course over which cord compression develops is most important with respect to the prognosis for recovery or stabilization of neurologic function. Impaired spinal cord function due to a compressive lesion shows a surprising potential for recovery after surgery if the tumor was growing slowly. Examples of this are encountered with meningiomas, neurilemomas (schwannomas), and some intraparenchymatous tumors. By contrast, recovery of neurologic function following decompressive surgery for a metastatic spinal tumor is often disappointing; the loss of neurologic function due to such lesions often develops precipitously over the course of a few days or even hours. The prognosis for recovery is inversely proportional to the severity of the deficit at the time of therapy and the duration of neurologic symptoms.[5]

Total tumor removal is generally possible in most spinal neurilemomas and meningiomas. Recurrences may develop, however, from residual tumor foci if total removal was not or could not be accomplished. Primary intraparenchymatous tumors may or may not lend themselves to total removal by surgery. Total removal is often possible for intraspinal ependymomas but is rarely accomplished in astrocytomas.[5, 11] Ependymomas may recur, although usually after a long period, if initial removal was not total. Primary malignant gliomas of the spinal cord have a poor prognosis for survival; most patients live less than 2 years after combined surgery and radiation therapy.[12]

Metastatic spinal tumors are practically never totally resectable. There is, of course, also a great likelihood that other metastatic foci are present elsewhere in the body so that palliation rather than cure becomes the primary aim of therapy. The importance of palliation cannot be overemphasized for these patients, who may live with the consequences of cord compression for many months or even years after diagnosis. This is especially true for patients with breast cancer or prostate cancer. The earliest possible diagnosis of cord compression should be attempted in such patients to minimize the dreaded complications of intractable pain and paralysis.[13, 14] Death from spinal cord tumors usually occurs by one of two mechanisms: High cervical cord tumors (at or above the C4 level) may produce respiratory embarrassment, whereas tumors located more distally often lead to chronic urinary tract disease.

## REFERENCES

1. Sloof JL. Primary intramedullary tumors of the spinal cord and filum terminale. Philadelphia: WB Saunders, 1964.

2. Barker DJ, Weller RO, Garfield JS. Epidemiology of primary tumours of the brain and spinal cord: a regional survey in southern England. J Neurol Neurosurg Psychiatry 1976;39:290–6.
3. Prayson RA. Cyclin D1 and MIB-1 immunohistochemistry in ependymomas: a study of 41 cases. Am J Clin Pathol 1998;110:629–34.
4. Vieth RG, Odom GL. Extradural spinal metastases and their neurosurgical treatment. J Neurosurg 1965;23:501–8.
5. Connolly ES: Spinal cord tumors in adults. In: Youmans JR, ed. Neurological surgery. 2nd ed. Philadelphia: WB Saunders, 1982:3196.
6. Kagan AR, Gilbert HA. The detection of occult metastases with imaging studies. Int J Radiat Oncol Biol Phys 1976:529–33.
7. Yeh SD. Bone scans in the early detection of cancer. Clin Bull 1975:11–9.
8. Edelson RN, Chernik NL, Posner JB. Spinal subdural hematomas complicating lumbar puncture. Arch Neurol 1974;31:134–7.
9. Cook AM, Lau TN, Tomlinson MJ, et al. Magnetic resonance imaging of the whole spine in suspected malignant spinal cord compression: impact on management. Clin Oncol (Royal College Radiologists) 1998;10:39–43.
10. Fleming ID, Cooper JS, Henson DE, et al, eds. AJCC cancer staging manual. 5th ed. Philadelphia: Lippincott-Raven, 1997:281–3.
11. McCormick PC, Stein BM. Intramedullary tumors in adults. Neurosurg Clin North Am 1990:609–30.
12. Mortara R, Parker JC Jr, Brooks WH. Glioblastoma multiforme of the spinal cord. Surg Neurol 1974:115–9.
13. Solberg A, Bremnes RM. Metastatic spinal cord compression: diagnostic delay, treatment, and outcome. Anticancer Res 1999;19(1B):677–84.
14. Abrahm JL. Management of pain and spinal cord compression in patients with advanced cancer. ACP-ASIM end-of-life care consensus panel. American College of Physicians–American Society of Internal Medicine. Ann Intern Med 1999;131:37–46.

......................................

# SURGICAL TREATMENT

• Ulrich Batzdorf

## PRIMARY SPINAL CORD TUMORS

The initial treatment of primary spinal tumors is always surgical. Advances in surgical technique, in particular, the use of bipolar coagulation and microsurgery, have made the removal of primary tumors safer for the patient and have permitted more complete resection of these lesions. Astrocytomas and ependymomas often have a considerable longitudinal extent within the spinal cord, requiring meticulous intraspinal surgery.[1-4] Astrocytomas are more difficult to remove because they are less clearly demarcated from surrounding cord tissue than are ependymomas. The favorable results after resection of even extensive astrocytomas in children reflect the advances in microsurgical technique.[5] Malignant glial tumors of the cord are rare, and their diffuse intraspinal growth prevents extensive removal.[1, 6] Ependymomas are highly radiosensitive, but the advisability of routine postoperative irradiation is controversial at this time.[1, 7, 8] Radiation treatment is clearly justified, however, for patients with only partially resectable ependymomas. Hemangioblastomas of the spinal cord should be totally excised and do not require radiation therapy.[9]

Notable differences exist in the incidence of primary spinal cord tumors among pediatric and adult populations. Astrocytomas of the spinal cord are more common in children, representing approximately 59% of intramedullary tumors. Ependymomas, which make up approximately 50% of intramedullary tumors in adults, account for approximately 28% of these tumors in children.[10] It has also been observed that malignant spinal cord tumors, such as glioblastomas, are more common in children than in adults.[11] Conversely, tumors such as schwannomas, meningiomas, and hemangioblastomas are rare in children. A major concern is the development of postoperative spinal deformity in children who undergo laminectomy for spinal cord tumor removal. In one report, this late development occurred in 40% of patients.[11, 12]

Refinements in microsurgical technique have permitted more complete tumor resection. The general experience is that the relapse rate, even for anaplastic cord tumors, is much reduced when a complete tumor resection can be performed.[13] Ependymomas are often more sharply demarcated from surrounding cord tissue than are astrocytomas.[11] This may account for the somewhat better disease-free periods associated with ependymomas, as a group. In one series of 23 patients, only one patient had evidence of tumor recurrence with a mean follow-up of 5 years.[14-16] Although there may be an increase in neurologic deficits postoperatively, the majority of patients either return to their preoperative neurologic status or improve.[15] In general, the postoperative deficit correlates best with the extent of preoperative neurologic loss.[15, 17]

Ependymomas of the filum terminale constitute a special subgroup of ependymomas, both histologically and with respect to prognosis. These tumors often are discrete and compress only the surrounding nerve roots of the cauda equina, but in some instances the tumor infiltrates between the nerve roots, making total surgical removal almost impossible.[18, 19] A literature survey indicated that radiation therapy was given to 41% of patients with filum ependymomas, with 50% of these patients showing improvement.[18]

The correlation between extent of tumor resection and long-term outcome is much less clear in patients with spinal cord astrocytomas. Even patients with histologically lower grade astrocytomas (grades 1 and 2) showed a 36% mortality at 38 months, and an equal percentage remained stable during this follow-up period; all seven patients with higher grade astrocytomas (grades 3 and 4) died of their tumor.[14] Another study of 21 spinal cord astrocytomas treated by biopsy, or by subtotal or total removal followed by radiation therapy showed a 5-year survival of 57% and 5-year recurrence-free survival of 44%.[20] Fifteen of 17 adult patients with intramedullary astrocytomas remained free of clinical evidence of tumor recurrence at 50 months following surgery; radiation therapy in these low-grade tumors following previous surgical attempts did not prevent tumor growth.[21]

## METASTATIC TUMORS

Initial treatment of metastatic tumors of the spinal cord is also often surgical, although the specific circumstances must be considered carefully before any treatment is planned.[22] A distinction must be made between metastatic foci associated with neurologic impairment and those that are totally asymptomatic, having been diagnosed only by routine scanning or other imaging techniques, or manifested by pain.[23] When there is no neurologic involvement, or when spinal and root pain is the major symptom, irradiation or chemotherapy, or both, may be preferred forms of therapy. Pain due to metastatic spinal involvement may respond to bracing, particularly when further adjunctive therapy, such as radiation therapy or endocrine-directed treatments, can then be implemented. Occasionally, pain can be managed only with spinal stabilization procedures, which are appropriate for patients with a reasonably long life expectancy.[24] MRI is the diagnostic modality of choice for the initial evaluation of these patients; contrast-enhanced MRI has all but eliminated the need for myelography. The presence of metallic implants, pacemakers, and metal artifacts is now the most common indication for myelography in such patients.

The physician must distinguish whether cord involvement is the result of vertebral collapse, with bone protruding into the spinal canal; a vascular occlusive phenomenon produced by tumor; or epidural tumor, which is the most common form of spinal involvement. Vertebral collapse produces mechanical bony compression of the cord that cannot be expected to improve with treatment other than mechanical decompression. However, the hazards of further distortion of the spine after removal of ligamentous support and posterior laminectomy must be carefully considered. Occasionally, such patients become candidates for a spinal stabilization procedure, using methyl methacrylate or instrumentation techniques.[24–27]

Spinal epidural metastases are the most common form of spinal metastatic disease. The treatment plan must take into consideration the extent of neurologic impairment and the nature of the primary neoplasm. Patients who have little neurologic impairment have a better immediate prognosis. Those who are already paraplegic have a poor prognosis for significant recovery irrespective of the treatment employed. The longer the neurologic deficit has been present, the worse the prognosis for recovery. However, Barron and colleagues[28] pointed out that surgical results were better, even in paraplegic patients, if the condition was gradual in onset; they further noted that patients with spastic paraplegia did better than those with flaccid paraplegia. Therefore, early recognition of metastatic involvement of the spine becomes of paramount importance, as does establishment of the presence of cord compression. Active therapy should be initiated as soon as there is evidence of neurologic impairment. The progression of neurologic deficit is often rapid, and hours may make a significant difference in the outcome of therapy.

Most neurosurgeons prefer the certainty of immediate surgical spinal cord decompression once the diagnosis of epidural compression is made. This is particularly true when spinal cord dysfunction is partial, that is, when there is much to be gained by preventing further progression. Decompressive laminectomy for metastatic disease in the face of total paraplegia, particularly if present for many hours, is probably futile. Surgical decompression of metastatic disease should be followed by radiation therapy. Posner,[29] in a small nonrandomized series of patients, showed that the results of surgical therapy followed by radiation therapy alone were comparable. Although he did take into account the radiosensitivity of the tumor, it is difficult to tell whether or not sufficient consideration was given to the rate of progression of neurologic symptoms prior to therapy in his comparison study. As was mentioned previously, neurologic deficit may progress rapidly, and existing deficit frequently is not reversible.

The suggestion by Posner[29] that surgical decompression is indicated if the patient deteriorates over a 48- to 72-hour period of radiation therapy is therefore fraught with considerable danger. Any evidence of deterioration while the patient is undergoing radiation therapy should be considered an indication for immediate decompressive surgery. This implies that patients who are treated nonoperatively must be followed extremely closely by a competent examiner.[30] A randomized study by Young and King[31] suggests that the presence or absence of a myelographic block correlates better with outcome than the treatment modality employed for metastatic cord tumors. MRI allows localization of the metastatic tumor to be made. Laminectomy generally relieves only those tumors that are dorsal or dorsolateral to the spinal cord; more extensive procedures are required to remove or decompress anteriorly located metastases.

The benefits of surgery for metastatic disease result from both tumor removal and bony decompression. Patients with solitary spinal metastases of slowly growing tumors occasionally may be candidates for radical tumor excision involving resection of portions of the spinal column and subsequent stabilization.[24, 27] Pain relief may be gratifying after decompression or stabilization procedures.[28]

## REFERENCES

1. Connolly ES. Spinal cord tumors in adults. In: Youmans JR, ed. Neurological surgery. 2nd ed. Philadelphia: WB Saunders, 1982:3196.
2. Stein BM. Surgery of intramedullary spinal cord tumors. Clin Neurosurg 1979;26:529–42.
3. McCormick PC, Stein BM. Intramedullary tumors in adults. Neurosurg Clin North Am 1990;609–30.
4. Epstein FJ, Farmer JP, Freed D. Adult intramedullary astrocytomas of the spinal cord. J Neurosurg 1992;77:355–9.
5. Epstein FJ, Farmer JP. Pediatric spinal cord tumor surgery. Neurosurg Clin North Am 1990;1:569–90.
6. Sloof JL. Primary intramedullary tumors of the spinal cord and filum terminale. Philadelphia: WB Saunders, 1964.
7. Bouchard J. Radiation therapy of tumors and diseases of the nervous system. Philadelphia: Lea & Febiger, 1966.
8. Scott M. Infiltrating ependymomas of the cauda equina. Treatment by conservative surgery plus radiotherapy. J Neurosurg 1974;41:446–8.
9. Murota T, Symon L. Surgical management of hemangioblastoma of the spinal cord: a report of 18 cases. Neurosurgery 1989;25:699–707.
10. Epstein F, Epstein N. Intramedullary tumors of the spinal cord. In: Section of Pediatric Neurosurgery of the American Association of Neurological Surgeons, ed. Pediatric neurosurgery. New York: Grune & Stratton; London: Academic Press, 1982:529–40.
11. Steinbok P, Cochrane DD, Poskitt K. Intramedullary spinal cord tumors in children. Neurosurg Clin North Am 1992;3:931–45.
12. Reimer R, Onofrio BM. Astrocytomas of the spinal cord in children and adolescents. J Neurosurg 1985;63:669–75.
13. Przybylski GJ, Albright AL, Martinez AJ. Spinal cord astrocytomas: long-term results comparing treatments in children. Childs Nerv Syst 1997;13:375–82.
14. Cooper PR. Outcome after operative treatment of intramedullary spinal cord tumors in adults: intermediate and long-term results in 51 patients. Neurosurgery 1989;25:855–59.
15. Epstein FJ, Farmer J-P, Freed D. Adult intramedullary spinal cord ependymomas: the result of surgery in 38 patients. J Neurosurg 1993;79:204–9.
16. McCormick PC, Torres R, Post KD, et al. Intramedullary ependymoma of the spinal cord. J Neurosurg 1990;72:523–32.

17. Constantini S, Houten J, Miller DC, et al. Intramedullary spinal cord tumors in children under the age of 3 years. J Neurosurg 1996; 85:1036–43.
18. Celli P, Cervoni L, Cantore G. Ependymoma of the filum terminale: treatment and prognostic factors in a series of 28 cases. Acta Neurochir 1993;124:99–103.
19. Schweitzer JS, Batzdorf U. Ependymoma of the cauda equina region: diagnosis, treatment and outcome in 15 patients. Neurosurgery 1992;30:202–7.
20. Sandler HM, Papadopoulos SM, Thornton AF, et al. Spinal cord astrocytomas: results of therapy. Neurosurgery 1992;30:490–3.
21. Epstein FJ, Farmer J-P, Freed D. Adult intramedullary astrocytomas of the spinal cord. J Neurosurg 1992;77:355–9.
22. Constans JP, de Divitiis E, Donzelli R, et al. Spinal metastases with neurological manifestations. Review of 600 cases. J Neurosurg 1983;59:111–8.
23. Vieth RG, Odom GL. Extradural spinal metastases and their neurosurgical treatment. J Neurosurg 1965;23:501–8.
24. Sundaresan N, Galicich JH, Bains MS, et al. Vertebral body resection in the treatment of cancer involving the spine. Cancer 1984;53:1393.
25. Scoville WB, Palmer AH, Samra K, Chong G. The use of acrylic plastic for vertebral replacement or fixation in metastatic disease of the spine. Technical note. J Neurosurg 1967;27:274–9.
26. Hoppenstein R. Immediate spinal stabilization using an acrylic prosthesis (preliminary report). Bull Hosp Jt Dis 1972;33:66–75.
27. Kirkpatrick DB, Dawson E, Haskell CM, Batzdorf U. Metastatic carcinoid presenting as a spinal tumor. Surg Neurol 1975;283–7.
28. Barron KD, Hirano A, Araki S, Terry RD. Experience with metastatic neoplasms involving the spinal cord. Neurology 1959;91–106.
29. Posner JB. Management of central nervous system metastases. Semin Oncol 1977;481–91.
30. Cobb CA 3d, Leavens ME, Eckles N. Indications for nonoperative treatment of spinal cord compression due to breast cancer. J Neurosurg 1977;47:653–8.
31. Young RF, Post EM, King GA. Treatment of spinal epidural metastases. Randomized prospective comparison of laminectomy and radiotherapy. J Neurosurg 1980;53:741–8.

# RADIATION THERAPY

• Michael Selch

Tumors of the spine may be divided into extradural and intradural lesions. The latter are further subdivided into extramedullary and intramedullary growths. Primary tumors of the spine are rare, with an annual incidence in the United States of approximately 2000 cases. Primary extradural lesions account for 10% of this total and are represented by chordomas, chondrosarcomas, and so forth. Extradural spinal tumors are more commonly secondary, metastatic epidural lesions. Primary intradural-extramedullary tumors account for 65% of the total incidence. These tumors are commonly benign (meningioma, schwannoma, paraganglioma).[1, 2] Malignant intradural-extramedullary lesions are unusual, but chondrosarcoma and hemangioendothelioma have been reported.[3, 4] Secondary carcinomatous meningitis or metastatic deposits from an intracranial tumor such as medulloblastoma may also occur. Primary intradural-intramedullary tumors represent 25% of the total incidence and are commonly referred to as spinal cord tumors. These lesions are virtually always malignant and are most frequently ependymomas or astrocytomas.[5] Tumors of the cauda equina and filum terminale, although technically intradural-extramedullary lesions, are conventionally included with tumors of the true spinal cord. Primary hemangioblastomas, oligodendrogliomas, and lymphomas, as well as secondary systemic metastases, are infrequently reported in an intramedullary location.[6–8] Benign entities such as infarct, infection, vascular anomaly, sinus histiocytosis, and lipoma arise rarely within the spinal cord but may mimic malignancy.[9–18] This section examines the role of radiation therapy in the treatment of patients with intramedullary malignancies.

## EPENDYMOMA

These tumors represent less than 2% of central nervous system malignancies. There is a slight male preponderance.[19–34] Spinal ependymomas typically present in young adults. Reported median age varies from 27 to 43 years.[19, 20, 22, 24–29, 35] Children are rarely affected.[30, 31] The adult/pediatric

ratio is 10:1, according to DiMarco and colleagues.[23] Overall, ependymoma accounts for more spinal cord tumors than astrocytoma.[24, 25, 34] If the extramedullary conus-filum tumors are excluded, however, the incidence of intramedullary ependymoma and astrocytoma is approximately equal.[25] Extramedullary-intradural ependymoma of the thoracic cord has been reported.[36] Histologic variants encountered in spinal cord ependymomas include cellular, epithelial, myxopapillary, anaplastic, and mixed types.[19, 20] In a review of 59 spinal cord ependymomas, Waldron and associates from Toronto noted 32 were cellular, 16 were myxopapillary, 4 were anaplastic, and the histologic subtype was unspecified in 7 patients.[34] Virtually all spinal cord ependymomas are of low grade.[19, 20, 22–24, 28, 29, 32] In the Toronto experience, 32 patients had well-differentiated ependymoma, 20 tumors had intermediate differentiation, 4 were poorly differentiated, and 3 were unspecified.[34] Intramedullary ependymal cysts are rare but may mimic malignancy.[37] Primary anaplastic spinal cord ependymoma is so unusual that this finding should stimulate a search for an underlying intracranial tumor of similar histology.[21, 38] The majority of spinal ependymomas arise in the distal cord, especially the filum terminale and conus medullaris.[24, 32, 33, 39, 40] Tumors of the distal cord are almost exclusively myxopapillary; intramedullary lesions are generally cellular.[19, 20, 29, 32, 41] Ependymomas affect a mean of four to seven cord segments.[20, 22, 28] They are typically solitary, but multifocality has been reported in 14%.[22, 25, 42] Cystic degeneration was previously believed to be uncommon for spinal ependymomas. Reviews, however, indicate that rostral-caudal cyst formation is as common for ependymomas as for spinal astrocytomas.[26, 28] McCormick and coworkers reported cysts associated with spinal ependymomas in 19 of 23 cases. In no case, moreover, were tumor cells found in either cyst walls or fluid.[28] Contrast enhancement of the cyst wall using T1-weighted MRI suggests malignancy of the cyst lining.[5] Extraneural metastases are rarely reported following management of spinal ependymoma.[43] In contradistinction is the known distant metastatic potential of the myxopapillary sacrococcygeal ependymoma.

This unusual extraspinal tumor, thought to arise from heterotopic ependymal rests or the coccygeal medullary vestige, histologically resembles a spinal ependymoma but must be clinically separated from it.[44] Although it is slow growing and apparently indolent, a metastatic potential as high as 17% has been reported for the retrosacral variety.[19, 45, 46, 47] Median symptom duration of spinal ependymoma patients varies from 18 to 73 months.[20, 26, 29, 33, 35, 48] Delay in diagnosis due to the protean nature of symptoms is particularly common for low-grade caudal tumors.[33, 49]

## Treatment Using Surgical Resection

Resection should be attempted in spinal ependymomas. Ependymomas are often smoothly encapsulated, displacing the spinal cord rather than infiltrating neural tissue.[19, 26, 28] Reported rates of intact, gross total resection vary from 25 to 88%.[19, 26, 27, 30, 32, 33, 34, 42, 50-52] Ependymomas of the filum terminale are more amenable to complete resection than are intramedullary lesions.[19, 24] Guidetti and colleagues totally resected 9 of 10 filum-caudal tumors compared with 27 of 38 true cord lesions.[51] Sonneland and colleagues advocated radical resection for encapsulated ependymomas limited to the filum and free of nerve root attachment.[19] McCormick and coworkers and Epstein and colleagues, however, believe that the majority of intramedullary ependymomas are totally resectable because of recent advances in microsurgery.[28, 50] Developing a plane of dissection may prove difficult for the rare high-grade ependymoma.[53]

Recurrence of low-grade spinal cord ependymoma is unlikely following intact, gross total resection.[42, 48, 50, 52, 53] Epstein and associates reported no relapses in a series of 33 completely resected intramedullary ependymomas.[50] In a collection of small series, there were four recurrences in a group of 55 complete resections.[19, 24, 27, 30, 33] Surgical series do not advocate adjunctive irradiation following intact, gross total removal provided high-quality MRI follow-up is available. Guidetti and colleagues reported equivalent 10-year survival with or without irradiation following total resection.[51] Spinal ependymoma patients who were irradiated following "total resection" appeared to have a higher local relapse rate than patients who were not irradiated. In combined series, six relapses were identified in 22 irradiated patients.[19, 20, 22, 39, 49, 54] These substantial recurrence rates and the nonrandom use of radiotherapy imply selection bias. Dissections in these patients may have been performed piecemeal or otherwise compromised. These patients are more properly included with those whose tumors were subtotally resected.

No significant deterioration of neurologic function occurs following a competently performed complete resection of spinal ependymoma.[26, 27] Cooper reported stable or improved lower extremity symptoms in 21 of 29 patients.[26] Stable or improved upper extremity complaints were noted in 13 of 15 patients. McCormick and associates reported transient worsening in 20 of 23 completely resected intramedullary tumor patients.[28] In only 3 patients, however, were the new deficits permanent. In general, postoperative neurologic status is better predicted by the magnitude of preoperative deficits than by the extent of surgery.[26, 50, 53, 55]

The recurrence rate following subtotal resection alone appears unacceptable, although few patients have been subjected to this approach. Twenty-seven such patients have

been reported and 17 have recurrence of disease.[19, 22, 23, 26, 28, 32, 42] Local progression is also common after near-total removal. Cooper reported relapse in 4 of 21 patients undergoing at least near-total resection.[26] Three of those relapses occurred in patients in whom the resection was judged to be 99% complete.

## Radiation Therapy

Multiple retrospective reviews document encouraging survival rates following irradiation of spinal ependymoma patients undergoing subtotal resection or decompressive laminectomy.[19-26, 28, 29, 31, 33, 34, 39, 42, 52-57] In a series of 21 ependymomas, Lindstadt and colleagues reported 5-, 10-, and 15-year overall survival rates of 93%, 93% and 46%, respectively.[25] Corresponding progression-free survival rates were 81%, 58%, and 29%. Shaw and associates reported 5- and 10-year survival rates of 95% in a series of 22 irradiated patients.[20] Corresponding progression-free rates were 81% and 71%, respectively. Garrett and Simpson from Toronto treated 41 patients and reported an 83% 5-year survival rate.[21] This experience was updated by Waldron and colleagues.[34] The authors routinely irradiated 59 patients, 16 after gross total resection. The 5-year relapse-free survival rates following biopsy and partial resection compared with total resection were 84% and 81%, respectively. The results with gross incomplete resection and radiotherapy were similar to those with gross total resection in a series of 34 ependymomas from the Netherlands.[52] The respective 10-year survival rates after gross total resection, partial resection plus radiotherapy, and biopsy plus radiotherapy were 93%, 90%, and 100%, respectively. Respective local relapse rates were 12%, 38%, and 0%. In the literature, the local control rate of irradiated spinal cord ependymomas varies from 75% to 100% with a minimum 5-year follow-up.[19, 21, 25, 34, 39, 42, 58] Although local relapse has been noted as long as 16 years after radiotherapy, the median interval varies from 17 to 48 months.[20, 34, 56] Spinal cord symptoms are palliated by radiotherapy.[32, 55] In the series of Kopelson and coworkers, 45 neurologic deficits were present before irradiation. Thirty-four were totally alleviated, and 8 were improved after irradiation.[54] Although irradiation should be administered routinely following all but uncomplicated total resections, previous radiotherapy renders subsequent operations more hazardous.[22, 28]

Most authors recommend radiotherapy to a volume encompassing the tumor plus a margin varying from 2 to 6 cm for low-grade tumors.[22-25, 34, 39, 42, 52, 57, 59] Clovis and colleagues advocated a margin of at least two vertebral bodies.[32] Coverage of the entire thecal sac must be provided for caudal lesions.[34] Failure to electively irradiate this entire compartment resulted in recurrence in 2 of 6 patients, according to Wen and colleagues.[29] No relapses were reported in 7 patients receiving thecal sac treatment. There is no role for routine neuraxis irradiation of low-grade ependymoma. Following conventional treatment, virtually all recurrences are reported to be within the local radiotherapy field.[19-21, 25, 39, 40, 56, 57, 60] Neuraxis seeding has been reported in 5.8 to 7% of patients with spinal ependymomas.[19, 24, 57] DiMarco and coworkers reviewed the literature and identified CSF seeding in 14 of 300 patients.[23] High-grade ependymomas occurred in 4 of the 14 patients. Elective neuraxis irradiation should be considered for the high-grade ependymoma and in patients with multifocal presentations.[20, 21, 23, 25, 32, 59] In the Toronto experience reviewed by Waldron and colleagues, relapses out of the radiotherapy field were noted following limited-volume treatment of intermediate/high-grade tumors.[34] Although the volume of irradiation was not a significant predictor of relapse-free survival, the authors recommended neuraxis radiotherapy for all anaplastic ependymomas. Local recurrence and failure within the brain have, however, been reported despite neuraxis irradiation.[24, 34] Hulshof and coworkers used local fields for three high-grade ependymomas and four with multifocal lesions.[42] Two patients with high-grade tumors were alive without relapse at 2 and 10 years. The third relapsed at a distant site. All 4 with multifocal tumors were alive with a mean follow-up of 80 months; one patient had residual disease.

A dose-response relationship has not been demonstrated for spinal ependymomas. Lindstadt and associates reported no difference in survival or control rates over the range 45.6 to 52.9 Gy.[25] Waldron and colleagues reported 5-year relapse-free survival of 89% following less than 50 Gy compared with 82% after 50 Gy or more. The difference was not significant by univariate analysis. Shaw and colleagues reported a 35% local recurrence rate following doses of 50 Gy or less compared with 20% local relapse above 50 Gy, but the difference was not significantly different.[20] DiMarco and colleagues reported inferior control with less than 45 Gy, but that observation was based on only three patients.[23] Dose-effect analysis has been hampered by the narrow range of applied doses and the relative sparsity of recurrences.[24, 42, 54] Most authors recommend total doses between 40 and 45 Gy for caudal ependymomas[40, 56] and 45 to 50 Gy for lesions of the true cord.[29, 34, 39, 52, 56, 57] Shaw and colleagues advocate 55 Gy delivered by shrinking field technique.[20]

Age and gender are not prognostic for patients with spinal ependymomas.[20, 34, 40, 42] There is no difference in survival of irradiated patients following biopsy alone compared with subtotal resection.[20, 40, 42, 60] Extensive debulking, however, may positively influence palliation.[51] Most authors report no prognostic significance of tumor location.[7, 20, 42, 60] Garcia reported 5-year survival rates of 100% and 60% for ependymomas of the cauda equina and true cord, respectively.[40] This difference, which was lost at the 10-year follow-up, was ascribed to a preponderance of myxopapillary tumors in the cauda equina. Others have reported a favorable prognosis for myxopapillary ependymomas,[56, 59] but histologic subtype does not appear to influence prognosis significantly.[19, 22] Tumor grade may be more predictive of prognosis than histology. Waldron and colleagues reported 97% 5-year relapse-free survival for well-differentiated ependymoma compared with 63% for intermediate to high-grade tumors ($p = 0.001$, univariate).[34] Whitaker and coworkers reported that survival was significantly better for grade 1 ependymomas than for higher grades. In their multivariate analysis, tumor grade was the only factor that significantly influenced survival.[24]

Although salvage therapy of recurrent spinal ependymoma is viewed with general pessimism,[24] several groups have documented encouraging survival following judicious reirradiation and reoperation.[20, 25, 32, 34, 42]

## ASTROCYTOMA

Astrocytomas present in children and young adults. Reported median age varies from 5 to 40 years.[22, 25, 52, 61, 62] Spinal cord astrocytomas are more common than ependymomas in childhood. The gender distribution of spinal cord astrocytomas is controversial. In a large series of 79 patients from the Mayo Clinic, the overall male/female ratio was 1.3:1.[62] The preponderance of astrocytomas arise in the rostral spinal cord.[42, 62–64] The incidence of cervicomedullary and thoracic lesions is approximately equal.[61, 62, 63, 65] The filum terminale and cauda equina are rarely involved.[25, 65] Multifocal intramedullary tumors are rarely reported.[42, 59, 66] Spinal astrocytomas are typically low-grade tumors; frequently, they resemble the piloid cerebellar variant.[19, 42, 49, 51, 62, 65, 67–69] In the Mayo Clinic series, for instance, 43 patients had pilocytic astrocytomas; 25 were diffuse fibrillary tumors, and 11 were not histologically specified.[62] Investigators at New York University, however, found no piloid lesions among 27 children younger than 3 years.[70] Intramedullary, high-grade astrocytomas are unusual.[42, 52, 62, 64, 70, 71] Cohen and colleagues reported 19 high-grade astrocytomas in a series of 170 total cases.[61] Oligodendrogliomas and mixed gliomas have been reported.[62, 64, 68] Dedifferentiation of low-grade to high-grade astrocytoma occurs rarely.[50, 61, 72] Like ependymoma, the astrocytoma frequently involves multiple cord segments.[63] According to Minehan and colleagues, piloid tumors, unlike fibrillary lesions, are more likely to involve more than four vertebral levels.[62] Extensive tumor is possible in the very young because of an underappreciation of symptoms. Constantini and coworkers reported that tumor involved an average of seven vertebral levels in their series of patients younger than 3 years.[70] Cystic degeneration, which is often extensive, has been reported in 38 to 50% of patients.[26, 50, 70] Epstein and colleagues reported holocord involvement by tumor and cyst in 14 of 19 pediatric patients.[50] Median symptom duration averages 2 years for low-grade tumors and 5 weeks for the high-grade type.[61, 63, 71, 72]

Spinal cord astrocytomas are infiltrative neoplasms.[26, 73] A cleavage plane is difficult to develop, and most authors believe a gross total resection is precluded. Guidetti and associates completely resected two of 53 spinal astrocytomas.[51] Cooper reported local recurrence in 5 of 12 spinal astrocytoma patients undergoing at least 99% resections.[26] Epstein and colleagues, in contrast, advocate gross total resection while admitting residual tumor cells are likely. They believe these cells remain dormant and reported freedom from recurrence in 17 of 19 adult patients with completely resected low-grade astrocytomas (mean follow-up, 50 months).[50] Five of 6 patients with high-grade tumors had local recurrence within 23 months. This same group reported freedom from recurrence in all 19 pediatric patients with resected astrocytomas (14 holocord tumor, 5 focal tumor).[50]

Despite the difficulty of achieving gross total resection, the role of adjunctive radiotherapy for spinal astrocytomas remains surprisingly controversial. Guidetti and coworkers reported no survival differences following nonrandom irradiation of subtotally resected patients.[51] Several groups advocate withholding radiotherapy until clinical or imaging evidence of progression occurs.[49, 50] Constantini and associates, in particular, cautioned against irradiating young children.[70] In their series, gross total resection was accomplished in 19 of 27 patients. Adjunctive radiotherapy was delivered to 2 of 3 patients with high-grade tumors. The 5-year relapse-free survival rate was 76% and the median time to relapse was 94 months. The authors consider radiotherapy deleterious to bone growth and nervous system function and a possible cause of tumor dedifferentiation. Others have reported occasional second malignancies following spinal cord irradiation.[64] Postoperative irradiation, nevertheless, must be considered the standard of care. Lindstadt and colleagues reported 5- and 15-year survival rates of 91% and 74%, respectively, following irradiation of 15 patients.[25] Relapse-free survival rates at 5 and 15 years were 66% and 53%, respectively. 5- and 10-year survival rates in the large Mayo Clinic series were 55% and 50%, respectively.[62] In the literature, 5-year survival varies from 50 to 90%.[39, 40, 42, 52, 60, 63, 71] Local control rates vary from 50 to 75%.[25, 39, 54, 65, 71]

Radiotherapy volume follows the guidelines for ependymoma.[39, 40] Elective thecal sac irradiation does not appear necessary. Following local treatment of low-grade tumor, virtually all recurrences are within the radiotherapy field.[39, 59, 60, 65] Leptomeningeal dissemination is rarely reported following therapy of low-grade tumor.[72] Neuraxis seeding is reported almost exclusively with high-grade astrocytomas or dedifferentiated low-grade tumors.[42, 52, 72, 74–77] Local relapse often accompanies or antedates dissemination. Cohen and colleagues reported clinical or necropsy evidence of neuraxis dissemination in 11 of 19 high-grade tumors.[61] Mixed oligoastrocytoma may also be a risk factor for seeding.[59] In view of the apparent risk of dissemination, neuraxis radiotherapy should be reserved for patients with high-grade spinal cord astrocytomas or the rare patient with leptomeningeal deposits at diagnosis.

A dose-response relationship could not be established by Linstadt and coworkers over the range 45 to 52 Gy.[25] Minehan and associates noted no significant difference in relapse-free survival between those receiving greater or less than 50 Gy.[62] Virtually all authors recommend 45 to 50 Gy.[39, 59, 62, 63, 65, 71] Radiation cordectomy has been advocated for patients with poor motor function as a result of their tumor.[52] Hyperfractionation remains of unproved benefit for spinal astrocytomas. In an animal model, the predicted sparing effect of hyperfractionation on spinal cord tolerance was confirmed by Niewald and coworkers.[78]

Tumor grade is the most significant factor for prognosis in astrocytomas. Kopelson and Linggood reported a 5-year survival rate of 89% for low-grade lesions compared with no survival for high-grade tumors.[59] Minehan and associates reported 81% 10-year survival for piloid astrocytomas compared with 15% for diffuse fibrillary tumors.[62] In the latter subgroup, survival was 25% for low-grade tumors compared with 0% for high-grade lesions. Many others confirm the dismal long-term outlook for high-grade lesions.[25, 26, 52, 62, 63, 65, 71] Degree of surgical resection prior to irradiation was not found to be a prognostic indicator by several groups.[49, 54, 61, 62] Hulshof and coworkers reported fewer relapses following radiation therapy and partial resection compared with biopsy and radiotherapy but could not attach statistical significance.[42] Attempted resection may facilitate neuraxis dissemination of high-grade tumors.[61]

The role of chemotherapy is under investigation. Allen and associates described their experience with aggressive "8-in-1" chemotherapy plus irradiation for pediatric patients with high-grade spinal cord astrocytoma.[75] Thirteen patients were treated as part of a Children's Cancer Study Group protocol. Six patients had leptomeningeal seeding detected by MRI at diagnosis. Five-year progression-free and overall survival rates were 46% and 54%, respectively. Seven patients had recurrence, three in the primary site and four in

the primary plus the leptomeninges. In two of the latter patients, disseminated tumor was not present at diagnosis. Radiotherapy was withheld from three patients owing to young age, and all had disease progression within 9 months. The study implies that aggressive chemotherapy and radiotherapy may yield results superior to those with radiotherapy alone for high-grade lesions. Chemotherapy alone does not appear capable of preventing tumor growth.

## HEMANGIOBLASTOMA

Hemangioblastomas are vascular tumors that represent less than 5% of spinal tumors. Approximately 60% are intramedullary and 30% are associated with von Hippel-Lindau disease.[79] The vast majority are located in the thoracic or cervical cord, and cyst formation is common. Intramedullary hemorrhage of hemangioblastoma may result in profound spinal cord damage.[80] The primary treatment is surgery and some reports have stated that radiation therapy plays no role.[81, 82] Richardson and colleagues, however, report 5-year progression-free survival of a patient with an extensive hemangioblastoma managed with myelotomy and 46.5 Gy.[6]

## LYMPHOMA

There are ten reported cases of intramedullary non-Hodgkin's lymphoma.[83–86] Intermediate- and high-grade morphology are more common than low-grade lymphoma. Irradiation has been the mainstay of treatment. The incidence of neuraxis dissemination implies that craniospinal irradiation may have a greater role in spinal lymphoma than primary brain lymphoma.[84] Dose recommendations follow the guidelines for brain lesions (see Chapter 72). Extraneural dissemination is uncommon but has been reported by McDonald and colleagues.[86] The prognosis appears as dismal as its cranial counterpart.

## METASTATIC CANCER

Intramedullary involvement by systemic malignancy occurs much less frequently than epidural or intradural-extramedullary dissemination. Grem and associates reviewed the available literature.[7] Approximately 100 cases have been reported. Intramedullary involvement is discovered at necropsy in less than 1% of cases. Lung cancer is most frequently reported. Small cell and non–small cell carcinoma are equally represented.[7, 8] Solitary intramedullary metastasis is uncommon. Approximately two thirds of patients have concurrent disease elsewhere in the CNS.[7] Surgery is important for establishing diagnosis but does not result in neurologic improvement. Radiotherapy is of definite palliative benefit.[7, 8] If an imaging search reveals no other CNS involvement, the radiotherapeutic guidelines for spinal ependymoma-astrocytoma may be applied to intramedullary metastases.

## OLIGODENDROGLIOMAS

These lesions account for less than 2% of intramedullary tumors. Fortuna and colleagues reviewed the literature in

1980 and reported 38 cases.[87] The mean age was 28 years, and the gender incidence was equal. The filum was rarely involved, but all locations in the true cord were equally represented with a slight thoracic predominance. The tumor usually affects several cord segments, but holocord extent is possible. Patients are symptomatic for several years. Oscillating complaints characterized by a sudden exacerbation are typical. Intratumoral hemorrhage, a feature noted in one third of patients, explains the latter observation. Spinal oligodendrogliomas are primarily low-grade tumors. Unlike their cranial counterparts, calcification is uncommon in spinal lesions. The role of radiotherapy in the management of these rare tumors is uncertain. Fortuna reported that postoperative irradiation appeared to lengthen survival. Five of 11 patients expiring after surgery plus irradiation had a mean survival of 35.5 months. Five of 27 patients who died after surgery alone had a mean survival of 8.4 months. Leptomeningeal dissemination was noted by Fortuna in six of ten necropsy procedures. This finding was most often reported for the gelatinous type of primary tumor, as opposed to the solid type, and suggests a role for extended-field radiotherapy for this variant.

## UNUSUAL TUMORS

Pleomorphic xanthoastrocytoma (PXA) of the spinal cord was reported by Herpers and colleagues.[88] The role of radiation in this uncommon CNS tumor remains undefined. The PXA typically follows an indolent course regardless of the degree of resection or use of adjuvant therapy. Occasionally, the natural history of PXA is unpredictable. The patient described by Herpers and associates relapsed within 8 months of gross total resection.

Neurocytoma of the cord was described by Tatter and associates.[89] This neuronal tumor typically behaves in a benign fashion when located in the brain. The prognostic significance of the usual histologic indicators of malignancy (eg, mitotic figures, necrosis) is uncertain for neurocytoma. They reported a patient who remained free of progression for 10 years following biopsy plus irradiation with a dose of 43.2 Gy. A second patient relapsed locally within 1 year following partial resection plus 50.7 Gy. This tumor initially demonstrated mitotic figures. The authors advocated reserving irradiation for true anaplastic spinal neurocytoma or until progressive disease is documented.

Hamilton and coworkers described intramedullary Langerhans' cell histiocytosis (eg, eosinophilic granuloma, histiocytosis-X).[90] Marked radiographic response of a cervical lesion was noted following a radiation dose of 20 Gy. This radiosensitivity is typical of extracranial Langerhans' cell histiocytosis.

Several Japanese authors reported intramedullary germinomas.[91, 92] Spinal germinoma is radioresponsive, similar to its cranial counterpart. All reported cases received postoperative radiotherapy, either to the entire spine or to a local field. Tumor dose varied from 35 to 40 Gy. The presence of tumor syncytiotrophoblasts may be a predictor of relapse.[92]

## COMPLICATIONS

Myelitis has been rarely reported following radiotherapy provided according to the aforementioned dose recommendations. Lindstadt reported a single case out of 39 irradiated cord tumors.[25] This patient received 50.4 Gy in 28 equal increments. It has been suggested that a spinal cord damaged by surgery or tumor may have an impaired tolerance to irradiation.[93] Kopelson evaluated all 1-year survivors following irradiation of spinal cord tumors and reported no increased incidence of myelitis when standard tolerance doses were used.[56] Myelopathy is more frequent when intrathecal Au 198 is administered.[40, 56] This form of therapy should be avoided in the management of spinal cord tumors. Reirradiation of the spinal cord has traditionally been avoided owing to concerns over myelitis. Mason and coworkers, however, demonstrated in a guinea pig model that recovery of the spinal cord is possible following irradiation. The capacity for the cord to tolerate retreatment appears to depend on the initial dose and passage of sufficient time for recovery.[94]

## REFERENCES

1. Seppälä MT, Haltia MJ, Sankila RJ, et al. Long-term outcome after removal of spinal schwannoma: a clinicopathological study of 187 cases. J Neurosurg 1995;83:621–6.
2. Seppälä MT, Haltia MJ, Sankila RJ, et al. Long-term outcome after removal of spinal neurofibroma. J Neurosurg 1995;82:572–7 & 1995;83:186.
3. Ranjan A, Chacko G, Joseph T, Chandi SM. Intraspinal mesenchymal chondrosarcoma. Case report. J Neurosurg 1994;80:928–30.
4. Mahdavi Z, Grafe MR, Ostrup R, et al. Spindle cell hemangioendothelioma of the spinal cord. J Neurooncol 1996;27:231–4.
5. Tartaglino LM, Flanders AE, Rapoport RJ. Intramedullary causes of myelopathy. Semin Ultrasound CT MR 1994;15:158–88.
6. Richardson RG, Griffin TW, Parker RG. Intramedullary hemangioblastoma of the spinal cord: definitive management with irradiation. Cancer 1980;45:49–50.
7. Grem JL, Burgess J, Trump DL. Clinical features and natural history of intramedullary spinal cord metastasis. Cancer 1985;56:2305–14.
8. Murphy KC, Feld R, Evans WK, et al. Intramedullary spinal cord metastases from small cell carcinoma of the lung. J Clin Oncol 1983;1:99–106.
9. Taxy JB. Paraganglioma of the cauda equina. Report of a rare tumor. Cancer 1983;51:1904–6.
10. Soffer D, Pittaluga S, Caine Y, Feinsod M. Paraganglioma of cauda equina. A report of a case and review of the literature. Cancer 1983;51:1907–10.
11. Herregodts P, Vloeberghs M, Schmedding E, et al. Solitary dorsal intramedullary schwannoma. Case report. J Neurosurg 1991;74:816–20.
12. Preul MC, Leblanc R, Tampieri D, et al. Spinal angiolipomas. Report of three cases. J Neurosurg 1993;78:280–6.
13. Andrews BT, Kwei U, Greco C, Miller RG. Infarct of the conus medullaris simulating a spinal cord tumor: case report. Surg Neurol 1991;35:139–42.
14. Selwa LM, Brunberg JA, Mandell SH, Garofalo EA. Spinal cord schistosomiasis: a pediatric case mimicking intrinsic cord neoplasm. Neurology 1991;41:755–7.
15. Anson JA, Spetzler RF. Surgical resection of intramedullary spinal cord cavernous malformations. J Neurosurg 1993;78:446–51.
16. Osenbach RK. Isolated extranodal sinus histiocytosis presenting as an intramedullary spinal cord tumor with paraplegia. Case report. J Neurosurg 1996;85:692–6.
17. Lee M, Rezai AR, Abbott R, et al. Intramedullary spinal cord lipomas. J Neurosurg 1995;82:394–400.
18. Resnick DK, Comey CH, Welch WC, et al. Isolated toxoplasmosis of the thoracic spinal cord in a patient with acquired immunodeficiency syndrome. Case report. J Neurosurg 1995;82:493–6.
19. Sonneland PR, Scheithauer BW, Onofrio BM. Myxopapillary ependymoma. A clinicopathologic and immunocytochemical study of 77 cases. Cancer 1985;56:883–93.
20. Shaw EG, Evans RG, Scheithauer BW, et al. Radiotherapeutic management of adult intraspinal ependymomas. Int J Radiat Oncol Biol Phys 1986;12:323–7.
21. Garrett PG, Simpson WJ. Ependymomas: results of radiation treatment. Int J Radiat Oncol Biol Phys 1983;9:1121–4.

22. Ross DA, McKeever PE, Sandler HM, Muraszko KM. Myxopapillary ependymoma. Results of nucleolar organizing region staining. Cancer 1993;71:3114–8.

23. DiMarco A, Griso C, Pradella R, et al. Postoperative management of primary spinal cord ependymomas. Acta Oncol 1988;27:371–5.

24. Whitaker SJ, Bessell EM, Ashley SE, et al. Postoperative radiotherapy in the management of spinal cord ependymoma. J Neurosurg 1991;74:720–8.

25. Lindstadt DE, Wara WM, Leibel SA, et al. Postoperative radiotherapy of primary spinal cord tumors. Int J Radiat Oncol Biol Phys 1989;16:1397–403.

26. Cooper PR. Outcome after operative treatment of intramedullary spinal cord tumors in adults: intermediate and long-term results in 51 patients. Neurosurgery 1989;25:855–9.

27. Rawlings CE 3d, Giangaspero F, Burger PC, Bullard DE. Ependymomas: a clinicopathologic study. Surg Neurol 1988;29:271–81.

28. McCormick PC, Torres R, Post KD, Stein BM. Intramedullary ependymoma of the spinal cord. J Neurosurg 1990;72:523–32.

29. Wen BC, Hussey DH, Hitchon PW, et al. The role of radiation therapy in the management of ependymomas of the spinal cord. Int J Radiat Oncol Biol Phys 1991;20:781–6.

30. Chan HS, Becker LE, Hoffman HJ, et al. Myxopapillary ependymoma of the filum terminale and cauda equina in childhood: report of seven cases and review of the literature. Neurosurgery 1984;14:204–10.

31. Boggan JE, Hoff JT, Wara WM, Boldrey EB. Intraspinal tumors in children. West J Med 1980;133:108–14.

32. Clover LL, Hazuka MB, Kinzie JJ. Spinal cord ependymomas treated with surgery and radiation therapy. A review of 11 cases. Am J Clin Oncol 1993;16:350–3.

33. Fearnside MR, Adams CB. Tumours of the cauda equina. J Neurol Neurosurg Psychiatry 1978;41:24–31.

34. Waldron JN, Laperriere NJ, Jaakkimainen L, et al. Spinal cord ependymomas: a retrospective analysis of 59 cases. Int J Radiat Oncol Biol Phys 1993;27:223–9.

35. Sloof JL: Primary intramedullary tumors of the spinal cord and filum terminale. Philadelphia: WB Saunders, 1964.

36. Wolfla CE, Azzarelli B, Shah MV. Primary extramedullary ependymoma of the thoracic spine. Case illustration. J Neurosurg 1997;87:643.

37. Robertson DP, Kirkpatrick JB, Harper RL, Mawad ME. Spinal intramedullary ependymal cyst. Report of three cases. J Neurosurg 1991;75:312–6.

38. Read G. The treatment of ependymoma of the brain or spinal canal by radiotherapy: a report of 79 cases. Clin Radiol 1984;35:163–6.

39. Schwade JG, Wara WM, Sheline GE, et al. Management of primary spinal cord tumors. Int J Radiat Oncol Biol Phys 1978;4:389–93.

40. Garcia DM. Primary spinal cord tumors treated with surgery and postoperative irradiation. Int J Radiat Oncol Biol Phys 1985;11:1933–9.

41. Specht CS, Smith TW, DeGirolami U, Price JM. Myxopapillary ependymoma of the filum terminale. A light and electron microscopic study. Cancer 1986;58:310–7.

42. Hulshof MC, Menten J, Dito JJ, et al. Treatment results in primary intraspinal gliomas. Radiother Oncol 1993;29:294–300.

43. Rubinstein LJ, Logan WJ. Extraneural metastases in ependymoma of the cauda equina. J Neurol Neurosurg Psychiatry 1970;33:763–70.

44. Anderson MS. Myxopapillary ependymomas presenting in the soft tissue over the sacrococcygeal region. Cancer 1966;19:585–90.

45. Lemberger A, Stein M, Doron J, et al. Sacrococcygeal extradural ependymoma. Cancer 1989;64:1156–9.

46. Miralbell R, Louis DN, O'Keeffe D, et al. Metastatic ependymoma of the sacrum. Cancer 1990;65:2353–5.

47. Wolff M, Santiago H, Duby MM. Delayed distant metastasis from a subcutaneous sacrococcygeal ependymoma. Case report, with tissue culture, ultrastructural observations, and review of the literature. Cancer 1972;30:1046–67.

48. Cooper PR, Epstein F. Radical resection of intramedullary spinal cord tumors in adults. Recent experience in 29 patients. J Neurosurg 1985;63:492–9.

49. DeSousa AL, Kalsbeck JE, Mealey J Jr. Intraspinal tumors in children. A review of 81 cases. J Neurosurg 1979;51:437–45.

50. Epstein FJ, Farmer JP, Freed D. Adult intramedullary spinal cord ependymomas: the result of surgery in 38 patients. J Neurosurg 1993;79:204–9.

51. Guidetti B, Mercuri S, Vagnozzi R. Long-term results of the surgical treatment of 129 intramedullary spinal gliomas. J Neurosurg 1981;54:323–30.

52. Shirato H, Kamada T, Hida K, et al. The role of radiotherapy in the management of spinal cord glioma. Int J Radiat Oncol Biol Phys 1995;33:323–8.

53. Fischer G, Mansuy L. Total removal of intramedullary ependymomas: follow-up study of 16 cases. Surg Neurol 1980;14:243–9.

54. Kopelson G, Linggood RM, Kleinman GM, et al. Management of intramedullary spinal cord tumors. Radiology 1980;135:473–9.

55. Scott M. Infiltrating ependymomas of the cauda equina. Treatment by conservative surgery plus radiotherapy. J Neurosurg 1974;41:446–8.

56. Kopelson G. Radiation tolerance of the spinal cord previously damaged by tumor and operation: long term neurological improvement and time-dose-volume relationships after irradiation of intraspinal gliomas. Int J Radiat Oncol Biol Phys 1982;8:925–9.

57. Peschel RE, Kapp DS, Cardinale F, Manuelidis EE. Ependymomas of the spinal cord. Int J Radiat Oncol Biol Phys 1983;9:1093–6.

58. Leibel SA, Sheline GE, Wara WM, et al. The role of radiation therapy in the treatment of astrocytomas. Cancer 1975;35:1551–7.

59. Kopelson G, Linggood RM. Intramedullary spinal cord astrocytoma versus glioblastoma: the prognostic importance of histologic grade. Cancer 1982;50:732–5.

60. Chun HC, Schmidt-Ullrich RK, Wolfson A, et al. External beam radiotherapy for primary spinal cord tumors. J Neurooncol 1990;9:211–7.

61. Cohen AR, Wisoff JH, Allen JC, Epstein F. Malignant astrocytomas of the spinal cord. J Neurosurg 1989;70:50–4.

62. Minehan KJ, Shaw EG, Scheithauer BW, et al. Spinal cord astrocytoma: pathological and treatment considerations. J Neurosurg 1995;83:590–5.

63. Reimer R, Onofrio BM. Astrocytomas of the spinal cord in children and adolescents. J Neurosurg 1985;63:669–75.

64. O'Sullivan C, Jenkin RD, Doherty MA, et al. Spinal cord tumors in children: long-term results of combined surgical and radiation treatment. J Neurosurg 1994;81:507–12.

65. Rossitch E Jr, Zeidman SM, Burger PC, et al. Clinical and pathological analysis of spinal cord astrocytomas in children. Neurosurgery 1990;27:193–6.

66. Roda JM, Gutiérez-Molina M. Multiple intraspinal low-grade astrocytomas mixed with lipoma (astrolipoma). Case report. J Neurosurg 1995;82:891–4.

67. Epstein F, Epstein N. Surgical treatment of spinal cord astrocytomas of childhood. A series of 19 patients. J Neurosurg 1982;57:685–9.

68. Helseth A, Mørk SJ. Primary intraspinal neoplasms in Norway, 1955 to 1986. A population-based survey of 467 patients. J Neurosurg 1989;71:842–5.

69. Epstein FJ, Farmer JP, Freed D. Adult intramedullary astrocytomas of the spinal cord. J Neurosurg 1992;77:355–9.

70. Constantini S, Houten J, Miller DC, et al. Intramedullary spinal cord tumors in children under the age of 3 years. J Neurosurg 1996;85:1036–43.

71. Sandler HM, Papadopoulos SM, Thornton AF Jr, Ross DA. Spinal cord astrocytomas: results of therapy. Neurosurgery 1992;30:490–3.

72. Bell WO, Packer RJ, Seigel KR, et al. Leptomeningeal spread of intramedullary spinal cord tumors. Report of three cases. J Neurosurg 1988;69:295–300.

73. Malis LI. Intramedullary spinal cord tumors. Clin Neurosurg 1978;25:512–39.

74. Tijssen CC, Sluzewski M. Spinal astrocytoma with intracranial metastases. J Neurooncol 1993;18:49–52.

75. Allen JC, Aviner S, Yates AJ, et al. Treatment of high-grade spinal cord astrocytoma of childhood with "8-in-1" chemotherapy and radiotherapy: a pilot study of CCG-945. Children's Cancer Group. J Neurosurg 1998;88:215–20.

76. Claus D, Sieber E, Engelhardt A, et al. Ascending central nervous spreading of a spinal astrocytoma. J Neurooncol 1995;25:245–50.

77. Johnson DL, Schwarz S. Intracranial metastases from malignant spinal-cord astrocytoma. Case report. J Neurosurg 1987;66:621–5.

78. Niewald M, Feldmann U, Feiden W, et al. Multivariate logistic analysis of dose-effect relationship and latency of radiomyelopathy after hyperfractionated and conventionally fractionated radiotherapy in animal experiments. Int J Radiat Oncol Biol Phys 1998;41:681–8.

79. Rawe SE, Van Gilder JC, Rothman SL. Radiographic diagnostic evaluation and surgical treatment of multiple cerebellar, brain stem, and spinal cord hemangioblastomas. Surg Neurol 1978;9:337–41.

80. Yu JS, Short MP, Schumacher J, et al. Intramedullary hemorrhage in spinal cord hemangioblastoma. Report of two cases. J Neurosurg 1994;81:937–40.

81. Browne TR, Adams RD, Roberson GH. Hemangioblastoma of the spinal cord. Review and report of five cases. Arch Neurol 1976;33:435–41.

82. Hurth M. [Intraspinal hemangioblastomas]. Neurochirurgie 1975; 21(Suppl 1):1–136.
83. Mitsumoto H, Breuer AC, Lederman RJ. Malignant lymphoma of the central nervous system: a case of primary spinal intramedullary involvement. Cancer 1980;46:1258–62.
84. Hautzer NW, Aiyesimoju A, Robitaille Y. "Primary" spinal intramedullary lymphomas: a review. Ann Neurol 1983;14:62–6.
85. Slowik F, Mayer A, Afra D, et al. Primary spinal intramedullary malignant lymphoma. A case report. Surg Neurol 1990;33:132–8.
86. McDonald AC, Nicoll JA, Rampling R. Intramedullary non-Hodgkin's lymphoma of the spinal cord: a case report and literature review. J Neurooncol 1995;23:257–63.
87. Fortuna A, Celli P, Palma L. Oligodendrogliomas of the spinal cord. Acta Neurochir 1980;52:305–29.
88. Herpers MJ, Freling G, Beuls EA. Pleomorphic xanthoastrocytoma in the spinal cord. Case report. J Neurosurg 1994;80:564–9.
89. Tatter SB, Borges LF, Louis DN. Central neurocytomas of the cervical spinal cord. Report of two cases. J Neurosurg 1994;81:288–93 & 1995;82:706.
90. Hamilton B, Connolly ES, Mitchell WT, Jr. Isolated intramedullary histiocytosis-X of the cervical spinal cord. Case report. J Neurosurg 1995;83:716–8.
91. Miyauchi A, Matsumoto K, Kohmura E, et al. Primary intramedullary spinal cord germinoma. Case report. J Neurosurg 1996;84:1060–1.
92. Hisa S, Morinaga S, Kobayashi Y, et al. Intramedullary spinal cord germinoma producing HCG and precocious puberty in a boy. Cancer 1985;55:2845–9.
93. Marsa GW, Goffinet DR, Rubinstein LJ, Bagshaw MA. Megavoltage irradiation in the treatment of gliomas of the brain and spinal cord. Cancer 1975;36:1681–9.
94. Mason KA, Withers HR, Chiang CS. Late effects of radiation on the lumbar spinal cord of guinea pigs: re-treatment tolerance. Int J Radiat Oncol Biol Phys 1993;26:643–8.

# TREATMENT WITH CHEMOTHERAPY

• Charles M. Haskell

The experience with chemotherapeutic management of primary spinal cord tumors is extremely limited. Extrapolating from the treatment of brain tumors, one may presume that ependymomas would respond to the nitrosoureas and that spinal glioblastomas may be somewhat responsive. Chemotherapy is a reasonable consideration for patients with multiple intraspinal subarachnoid seedling lesions and for patients with chemotherapy-responsive metastatic neoplasms.[1]

Most patients with spinal neoplasms require treatment with corticosteroids, especially during the course of radiation therapy. High-dose therapy is well established based on the results of a well-designed randomized clinical trial comparing radiation therapy with high-dose dexamethasone (96-mg IV bolus, then 24 mg PO QID × 3 days, then taper over 10 days) versus radiation therapy without dexamethasone.[2] Radiation therapy was successful in 81% of the patients treated with high-dose dexamethasone compared with 63% of those receiving no dexamethasone. Six months after treatment, 59% of the patients treated with dexamethasone were still ambulatory compared with 33% of the patients receiving radiation therapy without dexamethasone.

Although the efficacy of dexamethasone is unquestioned, there is controversy about what constitutes the optimal dose. Because of the potential toxicity of high-dose dexamethasone, many clinicians prefer the use of moderate doses (such as 10-mg IV bolus, then 4 mg IV QID, with tapering over 2 weeks). However, the efficacy of moderate-dose dexamethasone has never been directly compared with high-dose treatment in a randomized clinical trial.[3] Nevertheless, moderate-dose therapy is so widely used and its benefits so widely accepted that it represents a reasonable alternative to high-dose therapy. Nothing short of a randomized comparison of high-dose and moderate-dose dexamethasone therapy will resolve the dilemma of identifying the optimal dose for this agent.

Chemotherapy is indicated for most patients with leptomeningeal involvement and positive findings on cytologic examination of the CSF.[4,5] Intrathecal methotrexate is usually used, as was described in Chapter 10, but the use of intrathecal thiotepa[6] or cytarabine[7] may also be considered. There is no evidence that combination chemotherapy is more effective than single-agent intrathecal chemotherapy for these patients.[8] There is investigational interest in the use of intrathecal chemotherapy with carmustine encapsulated in liposomes.[9] In some patients, methotrexate may be administered via an Ommaya reservoir to improve drug distribution within the CSF.[10] In nearly all patients, the intrathecal chemotherapy is combined with radiation therapy. This approach is primarily palliative, but occasionally, patients enjoy prolonged benefit (>2 years) with therapy.[5,11]

## IMMUNOTHERAPY

There has been no experience with immunotherapy of primary spinal cord tumors. There has been one study of intrathecal radiolabeled monoclonal antibodies for the treatment of leptomeningeal neoplasms, but it is too soon to assess the value of this or other immunotherapeutic techniques in the management of spinal neoplasms.[12]

## REFERENCES

1. Bleyer WA, Byrne TN: Leptomeningeal cancer in leukemia and solid tumors. Curr Probl Cancer 1988;12:181–238.
2. Sorensen S, Helweg-Larsen S, Mouridsen H, et al. Effect of high-dose dexamethasone in carcinomatous metastatic spinal cord compression treated with radiotherapy: A randomised trial. Eur J Cancer 1994;30A:22–7.
3. Loblaw DA, Laperriere NJ. Emergency treatment of malignant extradural spinal cord compression: an evidence-based guideline. J Clin Oncol 1998;16:1613–24.
4. Theodore WH, Gendelman S. Meningeal carcinomatosis. Arch Neurol 1981;38:696–9.
5. Wasserstrom WR, Glass JP, Posner JB. Diagnosis and treatment of leptomeningeal metastases from solid tumors: experience with 90 patients. Cancer 1982;49:759–72.
6. Trump DL, Grossman SA, Thompson G, et al. Treatment of neoplastic meningitis with intraventricular thiotepa and methotrexate. Cancer Treat Rep 1982;66:1549–51.

7. Fulton DS, Levin VA, Gutin PH, et al. Intrathecal cytosine arabinoside for the treatment of meningeal metastases from malignant brain tumors and systemic tumors. Cancer Chemother Pharmacol 1982:285–91.

8. Hitchins RN, Bell DR, Woods RL, Levi JA. A prospective randomized trial of single-agent versus combination chemotherapy in meningeal carcinomatosis. J Clin Oncol 1987:1655–62.

9. Kitamura I, Kochi M, Matsumoto Y, et al. Intrathecal chemotherapy with 1,3-bis(2-chloroethyl)-1-nitrosourea encapsulated into hybrid liposomes for meningeal gliomatosis: an experimental study. Cancer Res 1996;56:3986–92.

10. Grossman SA, Trump DL, Chen DC, et al. Cerebrospinal fluid flow abnormalities in patients with neoplastic meningitis. An evaluation using [111]indium-DTPA ventriculography. Am J Med 1982;73:641–7.

11. Kopelson G, Parkinson D, Rudders RA. Long term survivors with leptomeningeal tumor involvement. Int J Radiat Oncol Biol Phys 1983:119–20.

12. Papanastassiou V, Pizer BL, Chandler CL, et al. Pharmacokinetics and dose estimates following intrathecal administration of [131]I-monoclonal antibodies for the treatment of central nervous system malignancies. Int J Radiat Oncol Biol Phys 1995;31:541–52.

# APPROACH TO THE PATIENT WITH SUSPECTED SPINAL CORD COMPRESSION

• Charles M. Haskell

The goal of management for patients with suspected spinal cord compression is palliation in nearly all cases. Early diagnosis is essential, and it is important to be alert to the possible significance of new-onset back pain in the cancer patient. In the past, algorithms of management for patients with back pain were strongly oriented toward the use of traditional myelography.[1] The advent of MRI has modified this algorithm to include the early use of MRI to rule out spinal cord compression in high-risk patients. An approach to diagnosis that incorporates MRI in such patients is provided in Figure 73–1.[2]

Once the diagnosis of spinal cord compression is estab-

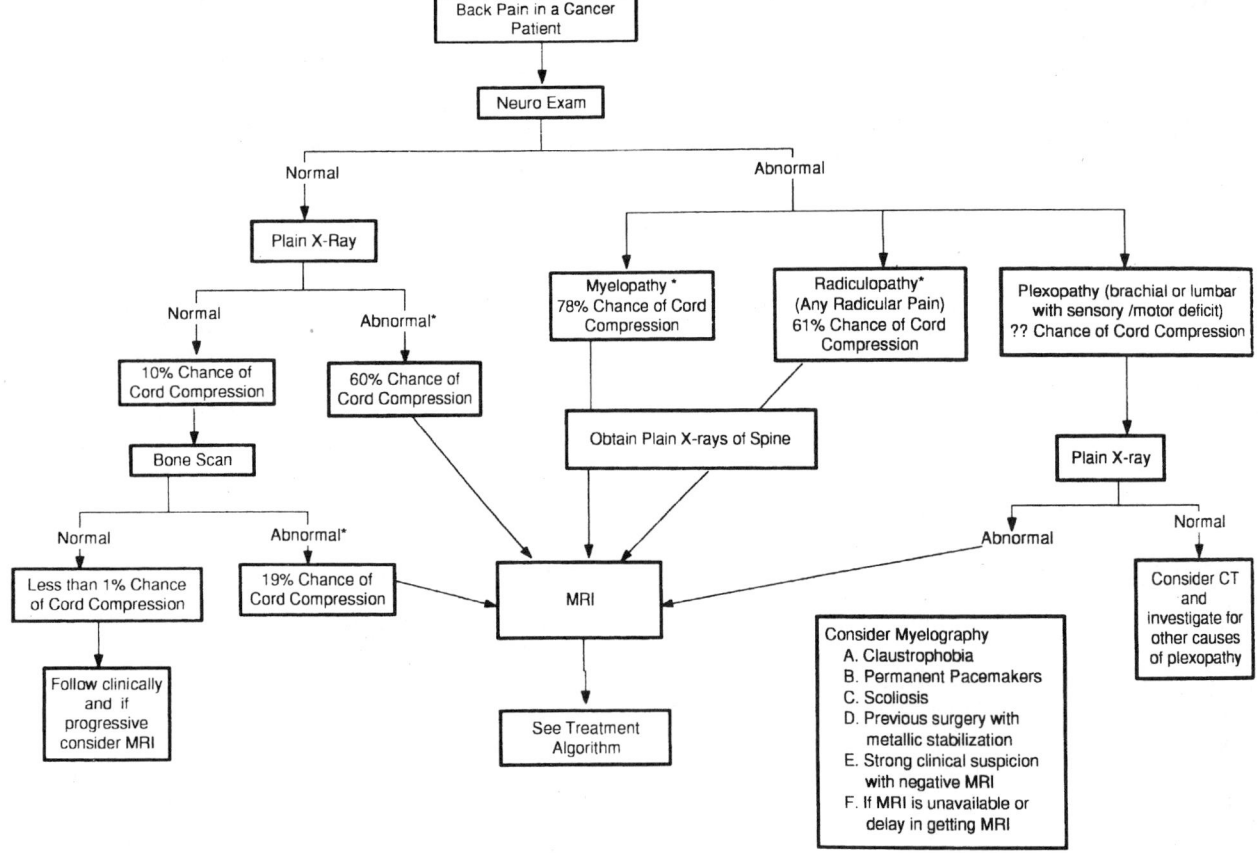

**Figure 73–1.** Algorithm for evaluation of back pain in a patient with cancer. Always consider rebiopsy if the disease-free interval is more than 2 years or if the tumor is solitary. The key reasoning principle is to define anatomically the extent of cord involvement. The goal is to make an early diagnosis to prevent paralysis. Note that all cancer patients with back pain do not need magnetic resonance imaging (MRI) for evaluation, especially with a normal neurologic examination, radiographs, and bone scans. Asterisks indicate start of dexamethasone, 10 mg IV, followed by 4 mg IV or PO every 6 hours whenever there is suspicion of cord compression. From Tummala R. Spinal cord compression. In: Djulbegović B, Sullivan DM, eds. Decision making in oncology—evidence-based management. New York: Churchill Livingstone, 1997:432.

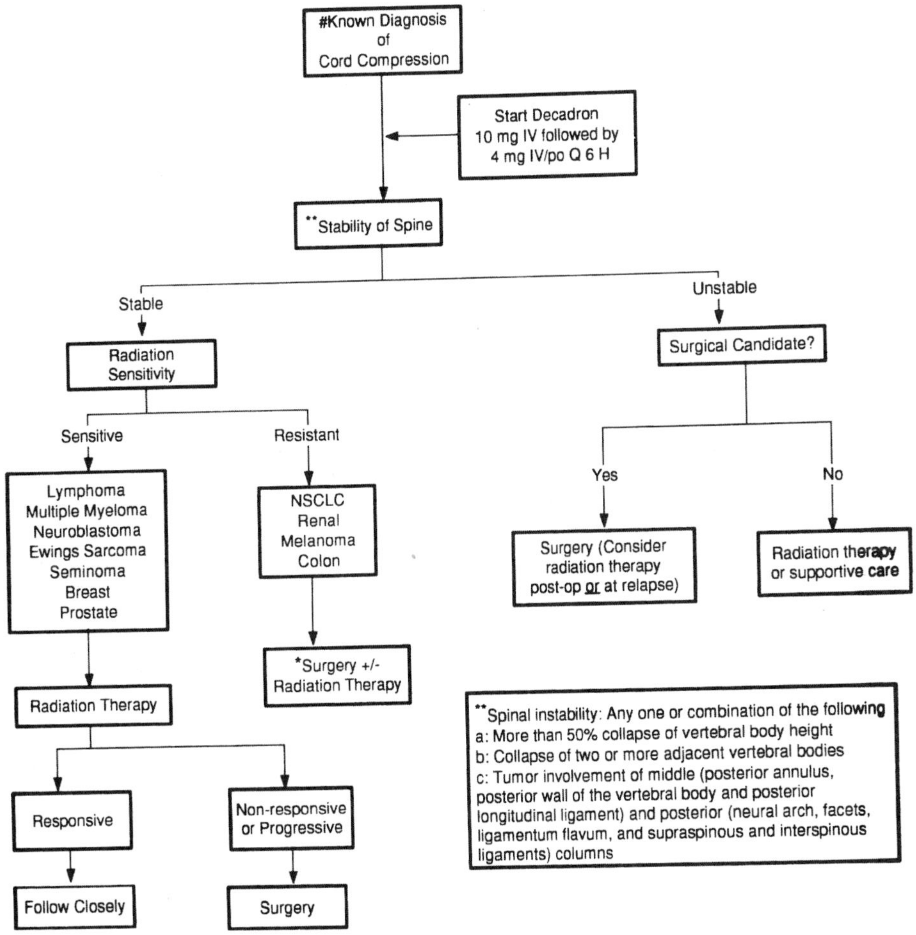

**Figure 73–2.** Algorithm for management of known cord compression in a cancer patient. The key reasoning principle is to determine spinal stability and tumor sensitivity to radiation therapy. The goal is palliation with maintenance or recovery of ambulatory status. Consider chemotherapy in addition to radiation therapy and surgery if the primary tumor is chemosensitive. A single asterisk indicates a need to consider surgery if the expected survival is at least 4 months and the patient is medically stable. A number sign (#) indicates that a specific cancer diagnosis has been made. From Tummala R. Spinal cord compression. In: Djulbegović B, Sullivan DM, eds. Decision making in oncology—evidence-based management. New York: Churchill Livingstone, 1997:434.

lished, prompt treatment is critical to prevent unnecessary morbidity and loss of function.[3–5] No single protocol of management can be recommended because of the relative lack of randomized clinical trials addressing this important concern.[6] An approach to treatment is provided in Figure 73–2.[2] These guidelines are not absolute and may be modified based on the experience and expertise of the treating physicians and institution.

## SUGGESTIONS FOR ADDITIONAL READING

Abrahm JL. Management of pain and spinal cord compression in patients with advanced cancer. ACP-ASIM end-of-life care consensus panel. American College of Physicians–American Society of Internal Medicine. Ann Intern Med 1999;131:37–46.

Byrne TN. Spinal cord compression from epidural metastases. N Engl J Med 1992;614–9.

## REFERENCES

1. Redmond J III, Friedl KE, Cornell P, et al. Clinical usefulness of an algorithm for the early diagnosis of spinal metastatic disease. J Clin Oncol 1988:154–7.
2. Tummala R. Spinal cord compression. In: Djulbegović B, Sullivan DM, eds. Decision making in oncology—evidence-based management. New York: Churchill Livingstone, 1997:431–5.
3. Abrahm JL. Management of pain and spinal cord compression in patients with advanced cancer. ACP-ASIM end-of-life care consensus panel. American College of Physicians–American Society of Internal Medicine. Ann Intern Med 1999;131:37–46.
4. Solberg A, Bremnes RM. Metastatic spinal cord compression: diagnostic delay, treatment, and outcome. Anticancer Res 1999;19(1B):677–84.
5. Husband DJ. Malignant spinal cord compression: prospective study of delays in referral and treatment. BMJ (Clin Res Ed) 1998;317:18–21.
6. Loblaw DA, Laperriere NJ. Emergency treatment of malignant extradural spinal cord compression: an evidence-based guideline. J Clin Oncol 1998;16:1613–24.

# XVI

# MELANOMA AND SKIN CANCER

# CHAPTER 74

# MALIGNANT MELANOMA OF THE SKIN

• ALISTAIR J. COCHRAN • JOHN A. GLASPY •
• ANTONI RIBAS • JAMES E. ECONOMOU •

## Natural History, Diagnosis, and Staging

### EPIDEMIOLOGY AND ETIOLOGY

Melanoma, a malignant neoplasm derived from melanocytes of the skin and other sites, continues to increase in frequency worldwide and is now more common than Hodgkin's disease and primary brain tumors. In the United States, the annual incidence of melanoma has more than doubled from 6 cases per 100,000 population in 1981.[1] Australia reports the highest incidence of melanoma, with 30 new cases annually for every 100,000 persons in Queensland.[2] In the United States and Canada, the rate of increase of melanoma is greater than for any other tumor except lung cancer in women. According to the American Cancer Society, 44,200 new cases of malignant melanoma were expected in the United States during 1999, compared with the 13,600 new cases recorded in 1978.[1, 3] An examination of possible reasons for the increase in melanoma incidence shows two patterns that may reflect a trend. First, the increased incidence of melanoma is proportionally greater in the relatively young than in individuals older than 65 years. Second, the increase preferentially affects certain anatomic sites. There has been a slight increase in the prevalence of melanoma of the head and face, but this is less marked than the increase in incidence on the legs of women and the trunk of men. Data now evolving suggest that the rate of increase of melanoma incidence may be beginning to flatten, although worry persists that continued thinning of the ozone layer or extension of the hole in the ozone layer may lead to a further (and possibly substantial) increase in skin cancer and melanoma.

The increase in melanoma frequency is greatest on body sites where sun exposure has increased because of changes in clothing styles and materials and in recreational habits. Melanoma rarely occurs on *double-covered* areas, such as locations where brassieres or underpants are worn. The sun-protective capacity of clothing is being closely examined, and different fabrics are assigned a solar protection factor (SPF) in the same way that sunscreen preparations have been graded.

Although the exact cause of melanoma is unknown, sunlight— in particular ultraviolet light—has been implicated as a (probably major) factor.[4] In whites, an increase in the incidence and the death rate of melanoma has been correlated with decreasing latitude.[4–6] This increased incidence has been noted particularly in fairer-skinned individuals of celtic extraction. A markedly lower incidence of melanoma has been shown in other races and in more darkly pigmented whites.[4, 5] The role of sunlight in the induction of melanoma is probably complex, and factors such as timing and severity of sunburns may be at least as important as the cumulative dose.[7] For the development of lentigo maligna melanoma (LMM), chronic long-term exposure to the sun, as may occur in individuals occupationally exposed to the sun (farmers, fishermen, and lifeguards), is considered necessary. In the case of nodular melanoma or superficial spreading melanoma, it is suggested that short high-intensity exposure (possibly inducing sunburn) of skin that is not normally exposed to sunlight may lead to malignant transformation of melanocytes. Intensive sunlight exposure in childhood or adolescence, known to lead to an increase in nevocytic nevi, some of which may be melanoma precursors, is probably most hazardous.[8, 9]

The anatomic distribution of primary melanomas differs from that of other sun-induced neoplasms. Basal and squamous cell carcinomas, for example, occur most commonly on the head, neck, forearm, and dorsum of the hand, and their incidence increases with age and cumulative exposure to sunlight. Melanomas are common in regions of the body that have seldom been directly exposed to sunlight and, with the exception of LMM, do not show a progressive increase in frequency with age.

Strategies to reduce melanoma incidence have focused on education of susceptible populations on the avoidance of excessive exposure to sunlight, especially in the vulnerable early years of life. This strategy comprises education of individuals who care for the young, including parents, teachers, and educational administrators, and the development of governmental policy and expenditures to create shade in areas where the population undertakes outdoor work and rest and recreation. Doubt has been cast on the ability of sunscreens to prevent skin cancer, including melanoma.

**Familial Melanoma.** Certain families have a high incidence of melanoma. The incidence of familial melanoma is 5 to 10%, and for a person with a family history of melanoma, the probability of developing the disease is three to four times the expected sporadic incidence in the general population. Multiple primary melanomas are more frequent (11 to 27%) and arise at an earlier age in members of melanoma families.[4, 5]

Some melanoma-prone families are distinguished further by the occurrence of multiple (usually large) moles that are atypical on clinical and histologic examinations. This syndrome has been variously called the *familial atypical multiple mole melanoma syndrome*, the *B-K mole syndrome*, and the *dysplastic nevus syndrome*.[10] The term *dysplastic nevus* is still widely used, although some do not like it because of the difficulty of defining precisely the nature of dysplasia. Attempts to identify and introduce a more acceptable terminology continue but new and better terms, such as *atypical mole*, have not yet achieved universal (or even wide) acceptance.

Affected individuals have multiple (usually) macular moles that are large (>5 mm in diameter) relative to common nevi, have more irregular borders, and show a patchwork of colored areas consisting of brown, black, and reddish pink foci that may be sharply delineated. These moles are most common on the upper torso and arms but are found on the breasts and buttocks, the double-covered areas on which common nevi are extremely rare. In contrast to conventional nevi, which do not usually develop after young adulthood, new dysplastic nevi continue to appear in adults after the period when the acquisition of new common nevi is usual. Microscopically, these are active junction or compound nevi with well-described patterns of melanocytic atypia, dermal fibrosis, telangiectasia, and lymphohistiocytic infiltration. Malignant melanomas arise more frequently in association with dysplastic nevi than with conventional nevi. They are usually of superficial spreading type, arise in younger patients (mean age, 34 years) than sporadic malignant melanoma (mean age, 51 years), and are often multiple. Dysplastic nevus–associated malignant melanomas are often relatively thin, which accords well with the relatively favorable prognosis of patients with such lesions. Although most dysplastic nevi occur in a multiple lesion–family context, similar melanocytic dysplasia may be observed in the epidermis adjacent to ostensibly sporadic melanoma, and it is suggested that in some lesions the melanoma arises from a sporadic dysplastic nevus that may index a forme fruste of the dysplastic nevus syndrome.

The relationship of dysplastic nevi to malignant melanoma is complex. In some melanoma patients with a family history of melanoma and multiple clinically dysplastic nevi, the tumors arise from lesions that are regarded clinically and histologically as dysplastic nevi. In other such patients, melanomas may arise from ostensibly normal skin away from dysplastic nevi. Dysplastic nevi can apparently serve as melanoma precursors and as indicators of susceptibility to the development of cutaneous malignant melanoma.

At a practical level, inquiry for a family history of melanoma is mandatory in all patients, and the presence of multiple large, ugly nevi or of the characteristic histologic findings of melanocytic dysplasia requires consideration of dysplastic nevus syndrome in the differential diagnosis. If the syndrome is identified, the patient should be examined for multiple primary tumors and counseled on the need for follow-up and the desirability of family screening.

The genetic mechanism for the transmission of the tendency to develop melanoma is not known but has been attributed to an autosomal dominant single gene with incomplete penetrance. It has also been suggested that the genetic transmission is polygenic from an undetermined number of alleles at separate loci, perhaps influenced by a cytoplasmic component. No relationship between exposure to airborne or work-related carcinogens has been established. Although the increased cancer risk in most families with the dysplastic nevus syndrome is exclusively for malignant melanoma, kindreds have been described in which a susceptibility to other cancers has been observed. For a complete and balanced account of this difficult and important area, the interested reader is referred to a review by Elder and colleagues.[11]

**Other Etiologic Factors.** The possible role of trauma as a cause of melanoma has been controversial. Some patients give a history of recent trauma, which they associate with the growth of a lesion, but often they are actually reporting trauma secondary to the developed prominence of a growing lesion (traumatic determinism). A high incidence of melanoma of the soles of the feet has been reported in Africans who go barefoot as opposed to those who wear shoes. It has been suggested, however, that the occurrence of melanoma on the soles of the feet of Africans may reflect the distribution of nevi on that site in the members of some tribes.[12] The tendency has been to discount the role of trauma in melanoma development.

A body of evidence is developing that the use of sun lamps or beds, which are artificial sources of ultraviolet radiation, may be associated with an increased risk of melanoma.[13, 14] We know of no good evidence that melanoma incidence is related to exposure to fluorescent light sources, dietary factors, oral contraceptive use, alcohol consumption, or tobacco use.

## CLASSIFICATION

The American Joint Committee on Cancer accepts five different forms of extraocular melanoma occurring in humans (Table 74–1). Of these, LMM, superficial spreading melanoma (SSM), and nodular melanoma (NM) constitute 80 to 85% of the total.[15] For comparison, an update of the 1972 Sydney classification is also included for reference purposes.

**Lentigo Maligna Melanoma.** LMM arises from lentigo maligna (melanotic freckle of Hutchinson or precancerous melanosis of Dubreuilh). LMM constitutes about 10% of all primary cutaneous melanomas and is found most commonly in older patients (median age, 70 years) on chronically sun-exposed areas of the face, neck, and dorsum of the arm and hand. Although classically a disease of the elderly, it can affect much younger individuals in regions of bright sunlight. This lesion has no sex predilection and often appears as a dome-shaped tumor in a large (3- to 4-cm diameter), irregular, tan to dark brown-black lesion with a flat surface.

*Table 74–1.* **Classification of Extraocular Melanoma**

*American Joint Committee on Cancer Classification\**

Lentigo maligna melanoma (Hutchinson's freckle)
Radial spreading (superficial spreading)
Nodular
Acral lentiginous
Unclassified

*Amended Sydney Classification†*

Malignant melanoma, adjacent component of superficial spreading type
Malignant melanoma, adjacent component of lentigo maligna type
Malignant melanoma, adjacent component of acral lentiginous type
Malignant melanoma, adjacent component of mucosal lentiginous type
Malignant melanoma, no adjacent component (nodular melanoma)
Malignant melanoma, unclassified histogenetic type

\*Adapted from Beahrs OH, et al (eds): American Joint Committee on Cancer: manual for staging of cancer. 4th ed. Philadelphia: JP Lippincott, 1992. Melanomas are also identified according to site (mucosal, ocular, vaginal, and urethral). A rare desmoplastic variant also exists (Egbert B, Kempson R, Sagebiel R. Desmoplastic malignant melanoma: a clinicohistopathologic study of 25 cases. Cancer 1988;62:2033–41).

†McGovern VJ, Cochran AJ, Van der Esch EP, et al. The classification of malignant melanoma, its histological reporting and registration: a revision of the 1972 Sydney classification. Pathology 1986;18:12–21.

Areas of hypopigmentation in the lesion, representing regressive phenomena, may be present. The precursor of this lesion, lentigo maligna or Hutchinson's melanotic freckle, may be present for 15 to 20 years before *invasive* melanoma develops. The shape of a patch of lentigo maligna often changes dramatically over time, a phenomenon that is best appreciated when serial photographs from the family album are compared.

**Superficial Spreading Melanoma.** SSM is the most common form of cutaneous melanoma, making up 70% of all melanomas. It has a peak incidence in individuals in their 40s but is common throughout adulthood. SSM is more common in men than in women in the regions of the head, neck, and trunk but is more common in women on the extremities, particularly the lower extremities. It is the melanoma most commonly associated with dysplastic nevus syndrome. The term *superficial* refers to the pattern of early development of the tumor and peripheral growth of the early lesion within the epidermis (radial growth phase). The subsequent vertically invasive stage of the tumor is *not* confined to superficial cutaneous tissues, and the vertically invasive component per se is not distinguishable from the vertically invasive component of other types of melanoma.

SSM tends to be somewhat less irregular in outline than LMM, although it often has notched borders. These lesions are characteristically multicolored, with shades of tan, brown, black, blue, red, and white. Early in their development, they may be barely palpable. These melanomas may have long periods of radial growth, which may persist for 1 to 5 years or longer before invasion occurs.

**Nodular Melanoma.** NM represents 10 to 15% of all cutaneous melanomas. With a median age of onset of 49 years, NM tends to have the earliest occurrence of the three common types. There is no true sex predilection, but it most commonly occurs on the trunk of men. NM lesions are typically dark blue to black but may be amelanotic (when they are notoriously difficult to diagnose). They are characterized by a complete absence of melanocytic anomaly in the adjacent epidermis and are associated with rapid vertical invasion of the dermis. The duration of such lesions before diagnosis is typically a few months to 2 years. The differential features of the common types of melanoma are summarized in Table 74–2.

**Acral Lentiginous Melanoma.** Acral lentiginous melanoma (ALM) occurs in glabrous skin, including the subungual regions, and represents 3 to 5% of melanomas. It occurs with almost equal frequency on the hands and feet, with the most common sites being under the nails of the thumb and the great toe. The tumor is characterized by lentiginous (a proliferation of melanocytes singly and in nests that are largely confined to the basal layer of the epidermis and the skin appendages) proliferation of atypical (sometimes dendritic) melanocytes in the epidermis adjacent to the invasive tumor and by a macroscopically visible macular area of increased pigmentation around the invasive tumor. SSM and NM also occur in glabrous skin.

Although melanomas are uncommon in African Americans, subungual melanomas in this group represent 15 to 20% of the total melanomas. These lesions may have long periods of growth and are frequently misdiagnosed as fungal infections, hematomas, and ingrown nails.[16] Two thirds of these patients have had some form of minor surgical procedure performed before a diagnosis of melanoma was suspected.

**Mucosal Lentiginous Melanoma.** Mucosal lentiginous melanoma is similar in clinical and microscopic appearance to ALM and may occur in a variety of mucosal areas, including the vulva, anus, penis, vagina, oral cavity, and conjunctiva. Such melanomas are more frequent in individuals of African and Asian descent. Although many mucosal melanomas are lentiginous in type, NM and SSM may also develop in these sites.

**Less Common Types of Melanomas.** Congenital nevi are cutaneous hamartomas predominantly composed of neural crest cells, although sometimes incorporating mesenchymal elements. They affect 1 to 2% of neonates; divide readily into small (15 mm), medium (15 to 199 mm), and large (>200 mm) nevi; and are often verrucous and hairy. Microscopically, they are compound nevi (75%) or intradermal (25%) and are composed of variably sized nevocytes with admixed neural crest elements. Some simulate Spitz nevus or blue nevus, and islands of benign cartilage may occur. Melanoma arises uncommonly in congenital nevi (probably around 3% despite some claims for figures as high as 31%). Most frequently, melanoma arises in one of these lesions, especially the large nevi,[17] in the first 5 years of life,

*Table 74–2.* **Differential Clinical Features of the Common Types of Melanoma**

| Type of Melanoma | Common Locations | Median Age (yr) | Sex Predilection | Duration | Identifying Features of Radial Growth Phase* |
|---|---|---|---|---|---|
| Lentigo maligna | Sun-exposed surfaces; head and neck most common | 70 | None | 5–15 yr | Flat. Shades of tan to black. Frequent areas of hypopigmentation |
| Superficial spreading | All body surfaces | 56 | Males: head, neck, trunk Females: lower legs | 1–5 yr | Flat to slightly raised. Irregular margins. Shades of brown, black, pink Areas of hypopigmentation |
| Nodular | All body surfaces | 49 | None overall Males: head, neck, trunk | 1 mo–2 yr | None |
| Acral lentiginous | Volar and subungual areas | 59 | Slight female preponderance | 2 mo–10 yr | Tan to dark-brown macule |
| Mucosal lentiginous | Oral, ocular, and genital mucosa | 56 | Slight male preponderance but varies from area to area | 4–20 yr | Tan to dark-brown macular area |

*The invasive tumors in each melanoma subtype are basically similar, varying from low convex to polypoid in shape and from dark blue-black to light tan or even (amelanotic) reddish pink in color. They are usually hairless and may be ulcerated.

although the lifetime risk for malignant transformation of a congenital nevus is said to be greater than that for common moles. Most tumors arising in congenital nevi are malignant melanomas, but neurogenic sarcomas, liposarcomas, and rhabdomyosarcomas as well as undifferentiated small round cell and spindle cell tumors do occur.

Blue nevi are benign proliferations of melanogenic cells in the dermis related to the congenital sacrococcygeal lesions known as *mongolian spots*, the bluish discolorations of the face known as *nevus of Ota*, and the similar lesions of the deltoid area called *nevus of Ito*. Rarely, malignant melanoma may arise from the epidermis overlying a blue nevus or from the dermal cells of a blue nevus.[17]

## DEVELOPMENTAL BIOLOGY

Clinical and histologic observations indicate that although many malignant melanomas arise in association with pre-existing melanocytic lesions, a few arise from clinically normal skin.[18] Although some antecedent lesions are truly nevocytic, many are the atypical melanocytic proliferations that compose the horizontal or radial growth phase of SSM, LMM, ALM, or mucosal lentiginous type of melanoma. Although malignant melanomas arise in association with common congenital or acquired nevocytic nevi, others are associated with dysplastic nevi.

Most melanomas have two distinctive phases of growth—an initial radial growth (horizontal) phase and a later vertical growth phase. During radial growth, the melanoma spreads out above the basal lamina. This initial phase of radial growth is not associated with metastasis, and in certain types of melanoma, such as SSM, LMM, and ALM, it may last for many years. (The prolonged radial growth phase helped create the controversy over whether all or most melanomas arise from a pre-existing nevocytic lesion.) Eventually the vertical growth phase supervenes, a phase that may give rise to cell populations that can metastasize. It has been suggested that the radial growth phase does not truly end until the melanoma cells evolve to a point at which they can survive and proliferate to form multicelled colonies in the dermis, an event that signals the development of the capacity to metastasize. Melanomas in which there are single melanoma cells present in the upper dermis but no multicelled colonies are to be regarded as being still in the (invasive) radial growth phase and having no capacity to metastasize.[19]

## DIAGNOSIS

Most primary malignant melanomas should be identifiable on inspection, given an adequate history, some experience, and a high level of suspicion. The classic clinical signs of melanoma are alterations in the lesion's color, recent enlargement in height or width, development of nodularity, pruritus, ulceration, and bleeding. These features often apply to a melanoma that has invaded deeply into the dermis and reflect an advanced tumor. More subtle signs, such as irregular or angular borders and variegated color with shades of pink, red, white, and blue, are frequently seen in early melanomas, particularly SSM.[18] The articles of Mihm and

colleagues,[20] Kopf and associates,[21] Clark,[22] and Cochran and colleagues[23] contain excellent descriptions of these changes illustrated with color photographs.

**Biopsy.** The biopsy of a suspicious nevus is the first surgical consideration for melanoma. An excisional biopsy that includes a small amount of subcutaneous tissue is the preferred method because it removes the lesion totally and allows for accurate microstaging. For lesions that are larger than 2 cm or for large lesions on the face, an incisional biopsy may be indicated. Concern that an incisional biopsy through a melanoma might worsen the prognosis has not been validated. An incisional biopsy should be performed through the portion of the lesion that appears most irregular or nodular. The biopsy specimen should include a portion of adjacent normal skin. Shave biopsies, although they may be adequate to make a diagnosis, are not ideal because they often remove any possibilities of accurate microstaging. Biopsy techniques have been well illustrated by Cochran and colleagues.[23]

**Work-Up Before Definitive Therapy.** Once a diagnosis is made, work-up is usually straightforward. A complete physical examination to look for evidence of dysplastic nevus syndrome, in-transit metastases, regional lymph node involvement, other primary melanomas, and distant metastases should be undertaken. Multiple primary melanomas occur in 4 to 5% of all melanoma patients, and most are usually discovered within 1 year of the original diagnosis. The association of multiple primary melanomas and the dysplastic nevus syndrome has been discussed. The biopsy specimen should be identified as primary melanoma; microstaged for measured width of ulceration, Breslow thickness, and the Clark level (see later); and assessed, at a minimum, for mitotic rate, lymphatic and vascular invasion, and completeness of excision.[24] A preoperative chest radiograph, complete blood count, and liver function studies (including lactate dehydrogenase) are usually undertaken. Preoperative liver, brain, and bone scans in patients with stage I disease who do not have clinical or laboratory evidence of metastases are rarely positive and are usually not indicated. In situations in which a surgical approach to the regional lymph nodes is being contemplated, lymphoscintigraphic location of the draining node groups is appropriate and essential for sentinel node biopsy (see later).

## CLINICAL AND PATHOLOGIC STAGING

In the past, melanomas have usually been clinically staged by the system of the International Union Against Cancer or the M.D. Anderson Cancer Center (Table 74–3). Attempts to refine staging continue, and the American Joint Committee on Cancer has produced an interesting schema,[15] which is under revision at the time of this writing.

In 1953, Allen and Spitz[25] first attempted to predict the biologic behavior of melanoma by histologic staging of the primary. Since then, several systems have been devised,[26–28] but the methods of Clark[29] and Breslow[30] are those that have been most widely used. In the Clark system, the primary melanoma is classified according to its microanatomic level of invasion of the dermis (Fig. 74–1). Clark's original observations suggested that progressive invasion through the levels of the dermis was associated with an increasingly poor

*Table 74–3.* **Historically Important Staging Systems for Melanoma**

| UICC* Classification | | M.D. Anderson Classification | | |
|---|---|---|---|---|
| Stage I | Primary with satellites within 5 cm of primary | Stage 0 | Superficial melanoma | |
| Stage II | Involvement of lymph node–draining basin with or without in-transit metastases | Stage I | No metastases–primary only | |
| | | | 1a | Intact primary |
| Stage III | Disseminated melanoma | | 1b | Primary locally excised |
| | | | 1c | Multiple primary melanomas |
| | | Stage II | Local recurrence of metastases All melanotic lesions within 3 cm of primary site | |
| | | Stage III | Regional metastases (>3 cm for primary) | |
| | | | IIIa | In-transit metastases |
| | | | IIIb | Regional lymph nodes |
| | | | IIIab | Intradermal and regional lymph nodes |
| | | Stage IV | Distant metastases | |
| | | | IVa | Cutaneous |
| | | | IVb | Visceral |
| | | | IVc | Lymph nodes |
| | | | IVac | Combinations of above |

*International Union Against Cancer.

prognosis, an observation that has been confirmed repeatedly.

A level I melanoma is equivalent to in situ melanoma and lies in the epidermis above a basal lamina that may or may not be intact. The natural history of level I melanoma is not completely known. In particular, clinicians do not know the proportion of such lesions progressing to invasive melanoma. This lesion is thought to have no metastatic potential, probably because there are neither blood vessels nor lymphatics above the basal lamina. As noted earlier, the concept of melanoma without potential for metastasis has been extended to include tumors in which there are single melanoma cells in the dermis but in which the capacity for local growth into multicelled colonies has not yet developed.

Some pathologists have used terms such as *atypical melanocytic hyperplasia* as synonyms for melanoma in situ. This practice has led to confusion because others used such terms to describe atypical melanocytic lesions that, although possible precursors of melanoma, had not developed fully into melanoma in situ. We strongly recommend that melanoma in situ be so called and that patient apprehension be alleviated by careful explanation of the lack of metastatic potential for such lesions.

Once the melanoma has penetrated the basal lamina into the papillary dermis, it is classified as level II. In the earliest stages of level II invasion, in which there are only single melanoma cells in the papillary dermis, the metastatic potential of the lesion remains zero. Once the tumor cells acquire the capacity to multiply in the dermis and form multicelled colonies, there is an initially small possibility of metastases that progressively increases with further evolution of the melanoma. As the melanoma continues to invade and expand the papillary dermis, it eventually reaches and abuts the papillary-reticular interface, when it is classified as level III. A level IV melanoma invades into the reticular dermis and level V tumors penetrate into the underlying subcutaneous fat. There are practical problems in applying this ostensibly simple system, especially where there is fibrous regression, a pre-existing nevus, or a heavy lymphoid infiltrate in and around the invasive tumor.[31] Some would abandon the Clark technique, but we believe that that would be premature and consider that there are cases in which the Clark level can be assessed accurately in the face of difficulty in evaluating the Breslow thickness.

The simplest and most accurate single predictor of prognosis in primary melanoma is the measurement, with an

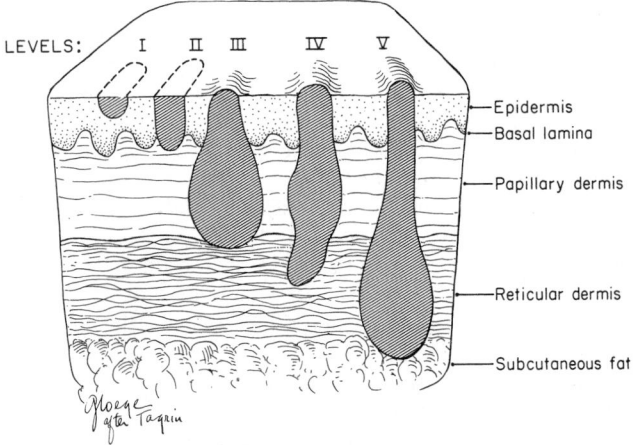

**Figure 74–1.** Diagram of Clark's levels of invasion. (From Grabb WC, ed. Plastic surgery: a concise guide to clinical practice. Boston: Little, Brown, 1968.)

**Table 74–4.** AJCC Staging of Malignant Melanoma

*Primary Tumor (pT)*

pTX     Primary tumor cannot be assessed
pT0     No evidence of primary tumor
pTis     Melanoma in situ (atypical melanocytic hyperplasia, severe melanocytic dysplasia), not an invasive malignant lesion (Clark's Level I)
pT1     Tumor 0.75 mm or less in thickness and invades the papillary dermis (Clark's Level II)
pT2     Tumor more than 0.75 mm but not more than 1.5 mm in thickness and/or invades to papillary-reticular dermal interface (Clark's Level III)
pT3     Tumor more than 1.5 mm but not more than 4 mm in thickness and/or invades the reticular dermis (Clark's Level IV)
    pT3a     Tumor more than 1.5 mm but not more than 3 mm in thickness
    pT3b     Tumor more than 3 mm but not more than 4 mm in thickness
pT4     Tumor more than 4 mm in thickness and/or invades the subcutaneous tissue (Clark's Level V) and/or satellite(s) within 2 cm of the primary tumor
    pT4a     Tumor more than 4 mm in thickness and/or invades the subcutaneous tissue
    pT4b     Satellite(s) within 2 cm of the primary tumor

*Regional Lymph Nodes (N)*

NX     Regional lymph nodes cannot be assessed
N0     No regional lymph node metastasis
N1     Metastasis 3 cm or less in greatest dimension in any regional lymph node(s)
N2     Metastasis more than 3 cm in greatest dimension in any regional lymph node(s) and/or in-transit metastasis*
    N2a     Metastasis more than 3 cm in greatest diameter in any regional lymph node(s)
    N2b     In-transit metastasis*
    N2c     Both (N2a and N2b)

*Distant Metastasis (M)*

MX     Distant metastasis cannot be assessed
M0     No distant metastasis
M1     Distant metastasis
    M1a     Metastasis in skin or subcutaneous tissue or lymph node(s) beyond the regional lymph nodes
    M1b     Visceral metastasis

*Stage Grouping*

| Stage 0 | pTis | N0 | M0 |
|---|---|---|---|
| Stage I | pT1 | N0 | M0 |
| | pT2 | N0 | M0 |
| Stage II | pT3 | N0 | M0 |
| Stage III | pT4 | N0 | M0 |
| | Any pT | N1 | M0 |
| | Any pT | N2 | M0 |
| Stage IV | Any pT | Any N | M1 |

*Note: In-transit metastasis involves skin or subcutaneous tissue >2 cm from the primary tumor but not beyond the regional lymph nodes.

Used with the permission of the American Joint Committee on Cancer (AJCC®), Chicago, Illinois. The original source for this material is the AJCC® Cancer Staging Manual, 5th edition (1997) published by Lippincott-Raven Publishers, Philadelphia, Pennsylvania.

ocular micrometer, of the thickness of the primary tumor from the granular layer of the epidermis or the base of an ulcer to the deepest contiguous melanoma cell. Some pathologists include deep satellites in this measurement. If these are included, that should be indicated in the report. This technique, described by Breslow,[30] has found wide acceptance despite problems of application in melanomas in which tumor cells intermingle with or abut nevi and in melanomas associated with a thick epidermis or multiple

crowded pilosebaceous units. The rule is that the thicker the melanoma, the more likely it is to produce metastases (lesions <0.76 mm rarely produce metastases, whereas those >1.7 mm often metastasize). The accuracy of the Breslow technique is such that subsequent performance of a Clark level assessment adds little to prognostic accuracy in most cases. We continue to report both measures, however, because in the face of technical problems that impede accurate assessment of one parameter, the other is usually more reliable.[31]

For example, consideration of Clark level may compensate for overestimation or underestimation of tumor thickness when the epidermis is notably thick or thin. The capacity of melanoma cells to penetrate the coarse collagen of the reticular dermis may indicate the acquisition of special biologic characteristics. Because of the wide acceptance of the Breslow thickness evaluation and the Clark levels in assessing prognosis, the American Joint Committee on Cancer and the International Union Against Cancer have adopted a new international TNM staging system for melanoma (Table 74–4) that may become the standard of reference for clinical practice and research.

## PROGNOSIS

Many factors have been identified that influence survival, such as age, sex, anatomic location, size, level, thickness, type of primary, and status and number of involved regional lymph nodes.[24] Women with primary melanoma have a better prognosis than men, and premenopausal women survive better than those who are postmenopausal. An age-related decline in prognosis has been reported for men, but it is not as marked as that in women. Male and female patients with melanomas of the extremities survive better than those with melanomas of the head and neck. Patients with truncal melanomas, particularly on the back, have the least favorable survival rate. The use of microstaging of the primary tumor (combining level and tumor thickness) and assessment of the presence or absence of melanoma metastases in the regional lymph nodes are the most important parameters indicating the likelihood of survival.

The Clark levels provide information regarding the probability of regional lymph node metastases and survival (Table 74–5). Cady[32] reported a retrospective study of 176 patients and found overall survival for level II at 6 years to be 86%,

**Table 74–5.** Clark's Levels and 5-Year Survival

| Level | Lymph Node Metastases | No. Patients | 5-Year Survival (%) |
|---|---|---|---|
| II | + | 1 | 100 |
| | − | 18 | 100 |
| III | + | 2 | 100 |
| | − | 44 | 91 |
| IV | + | 11 | 27 |
| | − | 33 | 82 |
| V | + | 3 | 0 |
| | − | 1 | 0 |

From Wanebo JH, et al. Selection of the optimum surgical treatment of stage I melanoma by depth of microinvasion. Ann Surg 1975;182:302–13.

for levels III and IV to be 67%, and for level V to be 11%. Wanebo and colleagues[33] reported 100% survival at 10 years in clinical stage I patients with level II melanoma of an extremity. Patients with level III and level IV melanomas had a 77% and 57% survival rate, but only one of six patients (17%) with level V melanoma was alive at 10 years.

The thickness of the tumor offers prognostic information that is similar to level and, in most cases, is a simpler and probably more accurate index of likely outcome. In several series, the 5-year survival rate for lesions less than 0.5 mm thick was 100%, whereas patients with lesions thicker than 3 mm had a 5-year survival rate less than 30%. Wanebo and colleagues[33] have proposed a rule of thumb, stating that the 5-year mortality rate is approximately 10 times the measured thickness of the primary tumor in millimeters. Tumor thickness has also been claimed to predict survival after lymph node dissection. Other relevant histologic observations are measured width of ulceration, mitotic rate per square millimeter, and presence or absence of lymphatic or blood vascular invasion.[24]

Although level and thickness of the primary tumor are important prognosticators, the tumor status of the regional lymph nodes is also an excellent indicator of ultimate survival; patients without nodal spread of tumor survive markedly better than those with tumor extension to the nodes.[24, 34] We have shown too that there is a direct correlation between the amount of tumor present in the nodes and survival: 47% of patients with three or fewer tumor-positive nodes surviving 5 years after lymphadenectomy compared with 21% of patients with four or more tumor-positive nodes.[35] This finding has been confirmed by numerous other studies.[34] We have also shown that a combination of the number of lymph nodes containing tumor and the relative volume of tumor present (assessed by quantitative morphometry) provides a highly accurate index of the likelihood of survival or of death from melanoma.[36]

Immunohistochemistry permits more detailed microstaging of lymph nodes for metastases. Using antibodies to S-100 protein and melanoma-associated antigens,[37] we have observed that conventional histologic techniques underestimate the number of tumor-containing lymph nodes by 30% in stage II patients[38] and by 15% in stage I patients.[39] Assessment of nodes in this manner increases greatly prognostic accuracy for the individual patient and provides more homogeneous groups of patients for trial stratification. The development of the capacity to identify small numbers of tumor cells (occult tumor cells not readily detectable in hematoxylin and eosin sections) in the regional nodes (and other tissues) of patients with melanoma (and other malignancies[40, 41]) was the basis for the development of the surgical technique of selective lymphadenectomy[42, 43] for the management of clinical stage I patients with high-risk primary melanoma (see later). The study of ploidy and cytogenetic analysis of primary[44, 45] and metastatic[46] melanomas also may yield useful prognostic information.

No discussion of prognosis for patients with melanoma would be complete without noting the highly variable course of the disease in occasional patients. Spontaneous regressions of primary melanoma have been well documented,[47] and rare patients may enjoy prolonged survival despite the presence of substantial metastatic disease. The biologic basis for these unexpectedly long remissions is unclear, but the leading hypothesis relates these remissions to successful control of the disease by host immune factors.

# Treatment

## SURGERY

**Primary Melanoma.** The only effective therapy for primary melanoma at present is surgical resection. Because melanomas are notorious for early lymphatic spread beyond their clinically detectable borders, the treatment of choice is wide excision. The rationale for wide excision is based on the work of Handley,[48] who excised a 5-cm margin of grossly normal tissue around a primary melanoma. Although the original width of wide excision was empirical, Cochran[49, 50] described an increased frequency of melanocytes in areas of skin that appeared clinically normal, and Wong[51] showed melanocytic activation 4 cm away from some primary melanomas. A 5-cm surgical margin for primary cutaneous melanoma has been the traditional recommendation. The argument is that occult foci of melanoma or transformed melanocytes may be present within this circular area of peritumoral skin, which, if not excised, leads to recurrence and metastasis.

The need for such wide margins has been challenged by several clinical trials. A World Health Organization (WHO) randomized study[52] of 612 patients showed that a 1-cm margin was just as effective as a 3-cm margin for primary melanomas no more than 1 mm thick. The optimal margin for melanomas thicker than 1 mm remains unresolved; a Melanoma Intergroup trial is currently comparing 2-cm versus 4-cm margins for melanomas 1 to 4 mm thick.

The following are current recommendations for surgical margins: (1) melanoma in situ, 0.5 to 1 cm; (2) melanomas less than 1 mm thick, 1 cm; and (3) melanomas greater than 1 mm thick, 2 to 3 cm. The surgical margin can also be adjusted by consideration of anatomic site (e.g., face) and other prognostic factors.

Although the depth of excision may include the underlying fascia, a review of recurrence and survival data for patients in whom fascia was not removed has shown no difference.[53] In deciding whether to remove fascia, it is necessary to consider that in some anatomic sites the summary removal of underlying fascia may hinder function, whereas in others this technique may improve skin graft healing.

Because subcutaneous tissue and fascia are nonexistent in the subungual areas, appropriate treatment for melanoma in these locations usually involves amputation at the level of the distal interphalangeal joint. For extensive lesions, amputation of an entire digit may be necessary.

**Regional Lymphadenectomy.** For the patient with clinically suspicious or pathologically proven metastases to regional lymph nodes, regional lymphadenectomy is indicated. A major controversy exists over whether or not early lymph node dissection in patients with clinically negative lymph nodes offers a therapeutic advantage over later dissection of obvious nodal metastases. Some have advised elective lymph node dissection for all patients with clinical stage I melanoma, whereas others prefer to wait, with close and regular surveillance and therapeutic lymphadenectomy as soon as there is any suggestion of nodal metastases. Neither approach is ideal. Several long-term studies of elective node dissection conducted at single institutions[54–57] have indicated therapeutic benefit for patients with primary melanomas of an intermediate Clark level or Breslow thickness. Survival after elective dissection of nodes that contain clinically occult metastases is substantially better than after therapeutic dissection for clinically detectable disease.[35, 58–62] Despite these reports of therapeutic benefit from elective dissection, the results of two randomized clinical trials of this approach in clinical stage I melanoma have failed to show a statistically significant overall survival advantage for the patients receiving elective dissections,[63–65] but even in these studies there is some suggestion of benefit for patients with intermediate-level melanomas.

A prospective multi-institutional randomized trial was conducted by the Intergroup Melanoma Surgical Program in which 740 stage I and II melanoma patients underwent immediate lymph node dissection or observation. The overall 5-year survival between these two groups was not significantly different. A subset analysis suggested that younger patients (<60 years) undergoing immediate surgery enjoyed improved survival.[66]

A method is needed to identify, within the total population of stage I patients, those who have or are likely to have occult nodal metastases. Such a technique would permit limitation of the application of elective node dissection to those few individuals most likely to benefit and avoid unnecessary surgery, with its attendant morbidity, for patients who are truly stage I. For this purpose, we have developed the technique of selective lymphadenectomy based on lymphatic mapping.[67, 68] The technique is based on animal studies that showed the regularity of lymphatic drainage patterns from cutaneous sites. Blue dye injected intradermally into young cats entered the lymphatics within minutes and subsequently passed to a regional node. Dye injected at a given site reliably reached a predictable lymph node in almost all animals.

A prospective study was next performed in 223 patients with clinical stage I melanoma.[42] Blue dye was injected intradermally into the area around a primary tumor or prior local excision site. The technique cannot be used after wide local excision because of disruption of the lymphatic. The skin over the regional nodes was then reflected to allow identification of blue-colored lymphatic channels and lymph nodes. The first node to take up the dye is the *sentinel* lymph node. This node was removed for intraoperative evaluation by immediate histologic evaluation and rapid immunohistochemical staining for S-100 protein, HMB45, and NKIC3 (monoclonal antibodies with relative specificity for melanoma). In the initial stages of the study, the remaining nonsentinel lymph nodes were dissected and examined with routine hematoxylin and eosin sections[42] and immunohistochemistry.

At least one sentinel node was identified in 194 of 237 (82%) lymphadenectomy specimens. The frequency of success increased as the operating surgeons gained experience with the technique. Micrometastases were found in at least one sentinel lymph node in 40 (21%) of these specimens. Twenty-three of the micrometastases were diagnosed by hematoxylin and eosin frozen section and confirmed by rapid immunohistochemistry, whereas 17 were negative on hematoxylin and eosin frozen section and detected in sections stained by immunohistochemistry. Thicker primary melanomas were more often associated with micrometastases. The incidence of micrometastasis was 9.8% in lesions less than 1.5 mm thick and 36.9% in lesions greater than 1.5 mm thick ($p <.001$).[67]

Micrometastases were found exclusively in nonsentinel lymph nodes in only two cases. These results occurred early in the study, before it was realized that the dye passes quickly from the sentinel node to nonsentinel nodes higher in the chain. Additional dye injections during operative manipulations prevented this problem in subsequent cases. In all other cases in which nonblue, nonsentinel nodes contained tumor, tumor was also present in a blue sentinel lymph node.

Our data show that early metastasis in cutaneous melanoma is limited to identifiable sentinel nodes that can be selectively removed at surgery and evaluated for the presence of tumor. Elective dissection can now be applied selectively to those patients most likely to benefit from such an approach. This approach offers a practical alternative to the "wait and see" tactic that dooms some patients to metastasis and death and to the broad use of elective dissection with its associated morbidity. If the sentinel node does not contain tumor at intraoperative evaluation, the morbidity of complete lymphadenectomy can be avoided (for about 80% of patients). Clinical stage I patients with micrometastases have a better chance of long-term survival (approximately 80% 5-year survival rate) if the nodes are removed before metastases grow to a clinically detectable size (15 to 25% 5-year survival rate).[69, 70]

Technical refinement of lymphatic mapping includes the use of technetium 99m sulfide colloid-based lymphoscintigraphy. This approach allows the precise intraoperative localization of the radioactive sentinel node with a hand-held gamma detector. This measure improves the success rate in identifying these nodes and removing them through a minimally invasive surgical procedure.[71]

**Palliative Surgery.** Surgery is not generally indicated for the treatment of disseminated melanoma, but there are occasional, highly selective indications in which surgery can offer relief of symptoms and improvement in quality of life. Melanoma frequently metastasizes to the gastrointestinal tract and produces bleeding, obstruction, or intussusception. Patients with nonterminal disease having significant gastrointestinal symptoms may often be symptomatically palliated by resection of the metastatic lesions.

Melanoma of an extremity may produce massive local subcutaneous and intracutaneous metastases with little or no evidence of distant dissemination. Such patients may benefit from a regional hyperthermic perfusion. Amputations are now not usual for such disease but may be indicated in selected instances.

A single melanoma metastasis to the lung without evidence of other pulmonary or visceral involvement is uncommon. An occasional patient may be found with a pulmonary metastasis and no other evidence of disease on careful metastatic work-up. If the tumor doubling time is greater than 40 days, consideration should be given to surgical resection.[72] Cahan[73] reported 19 patients who had excision of melanoma metastases to the lung. Of 12 patients who had resection of a solitary metastasis, 4 were alive at 5-year follow-up. In a review of our own experience, we found 25% of patients with resected pulmonary metastases alive at 5 years.[74]

*Solitary* brain metastases are infrequent. In such cases, neurosurgical resection followed by whole-brain irradiation has occasionally prolonged survival for several years. Because there are occasional long-term survivors from radiation therapy alone, it is difficult to decide what role neurosurgical decompression plays in this group of patients. Patients with superficial solitary lesions in noncritical areas of the brain seem to be the best candidates for surgical resection.

## RADIATION THERAPY

The most important roles for radiation therapy in the management of melanoma are in the treatment of brain metastases and following therapeutic lymph node dissection for bulky disease.

## CHEMOTHERAPY

**Treatment of Advanced Disease.** The results of chemotherapy for metastatic melanoma have been disappointing. In general, the disease is refractory to single-agent and multiagent chemotherapy. The responses reported in most therapeutic protocols are in tumors in nonvisceral sites. Liver metastases rarely respond to any type of treatment. One exception to this observation may be in younger patients with metastatic melanoma. Despite the fact that the disease is rare in patients younger than 20 years old, it may be much more responsive to multiagent chemotherapy than is the case in older patients, and long-term complete remissions have been reported.[75]

Dacarbazine (DTIC) has had the most extensive clinical trials of any single agent, with a reported response rate of 22% based on 978 reported cases (Table 74–6). Long-term sustained complete responses occur in 1 to 2% of cases, and relapse is rare in patients who remain in complete remission for 2 years.[75]

**Table 74–6.** Single-Agent Chemotherapy for Melanoma*

| Agent | Patients (No.) | Response Rate (%) |
|---|---|---|
| Teniposide[75] | 25 | 28 |
| Procarbazine[75] | 28 | 25 |
| Dacarbazine[75] | 978 | 22 |
| Carmustine[75–77] | 122 | 18 |
| Cisplatin[75–78] | 110 | 15 |
| Paclitaxel[75, 76] | 34 | 15 |
| Carboplatin | 58 | 14 |
| Lomustine[75–80, 82, 83, 175] | 257 | 12 |
| Estramustine[75] | 26 | 12 |
| Ifosfamide[76, 77] | 34 | 6 |
| Mitomycin[75] | 26 | 8 |
| Tamoxifen[75–80, 82, 176–178] | 203 | 6 |

*Response rates are based on the number of patients with a complete or partial response (50%) divided by the number of evaluable patients treated. Investigational agents and commercially available agents with response rates approximating 0% are not listed.

**Table 74–7.** Combination Chemotherapy Regimens with Dacarbazine for Melanoma*

| Drugs Added to Dacarbazine | Patients (No.) | Response Rate (%) |
|---|---|---|
| Cisplatin, carmustine, tamoxifen[95, 96] | 40 | 53 |
| Lomustine, bleomycin, vindesine[179] | 20 | 45 |
| Cyclophosphamide[180] | 43 | 42 |
| Cisplatin, vinblastine[181] | 59 | 41 |
| Cisplatin, vinblastine, bleomycin, mitolactol[182] | 20 | 35 |
| Cyclophosphamide, vincristine, BCG[183] | 50 | 34 |
| Lomustine, bleomycin, vincristine[184, 185] | 118 | 33 |
| Cisplatin[186, 189] | 82 | 28 |
| Carmustine, hydroxyurea, levamisole[190] | 104 | 25 |
| Carmustine, hydroxyurea[190] | 73 | 24 |
| Cisplatin, vindesine[191] | 105 | 24 |
| Dactinomycin[190, 192] | 103 | 22 |
| Lomustine[191] | 38 | 18 |
| Carmustine, vincristine, dactinomycin[192] | 30 | 17 |
| Vindesine[193] | 46 | 17 |
| Vinblastine, bleomycin, cisplatin, dibromodulcitol[194] | 22 | 17 |
| Cisplatin, procarbazine[187] | 13 | 15 |
| Carmustine, vincristine, bleomycin[195] | 14 | 7 |

*Response rates are based on the number of patients with a complete or partial response (50%) divided by the number of evaluable patients treated. Investigational agents and commercially available agents with response rates approximating 0% are not listed.

BCG, bacille Calmette-Guérin.

DTIC has been given by several different dosage schedules,[76–80] including a single-dose regimen.[75] Currently, DTIC is considered to be the single agent of choice in the treatment of melanoma. Guidelines for its use are given in Chapter 10.

The nitrosoureas are the next most active single agents. Many patients have been treated with commercially available and investigational nitrosoureas, with a response rate of 12 to 18% (see Table 74–6). Very high dose carmustine (BCNU), given without autologous bone marrow transplantation, produced a response rate of 22% in 18 evaluable patients, and all responses were partial.[75] The nitrosoureas are no better than DTIC as single-agent chemotherapy for metastatic melanoma, even at very high doses.

Other single agents that have undergone adequate clinical trials are cisplatin and several investigational agents (see Table 74–6). Several small trials have suggested a possible therapeutic benefit from the following drugs: teniposide, procarbazine, idarubicin, carboplatin, and ifosfamide. Many contemporary reports indicate a lack of activity for such drugs as mitoxantrone, AZQ, bruceantin (NSC-165, 563), esorubicin, doxifluridine, streptozocin, high-dose methotrexate with folinic acid rescue, epirubicin, L-alanosine (NSC-153, 353), spirogermanium, and bisantrene.

Several observations suggest that melanomas may be influenced by hormones. Lesions rarely appear before puberty, women have a better prognosis than men,[81] and melanoma may progress rapidly during pregnancy in some patients. These observations have prompted a search for hormone receptors on melanoma cells. Estrogen and progesterone receptors have been found in some melanomas.[75–80, 82, 83] Estrogen receptors were found in 118 of 427 patients (28%). Treatment with tamoxifen has been disappointing (see Table 74–6), however. The tumor cells of some patients who responded to tamoxifen had no detectable hormone receptors. The significance of the presence of hormone receptors on

*Table 74-8.* Combination Chemotherapy for Melanoma not Including Dacarbazine

| Drugs | Patients (No.) | Response Rate (%) |
|---|---|---|
| Cisplatin + WR-2721[196] | 36 | 53 |
| Cisplatin + lomustine + bleomycin[197] | 25 | 48 |
| Bleomycin + vinblastine[198] | 9 | 44 |
| Cisplatin + vindesine + PALA disodium[199] | 21 | 43 |
| Nimustine + peplomycin + vincristine[200] | 30 | 43 |
| Lomustine + bleomycin + vincristine[201] | 49 | 35 |
| Lomustine + procarbazine + vincristine + cyclophosphamide[202] | 12 | 33 |
| Lomustine + procarbazine + vincristine[203–206] | 152 | 32 |
| Cisplatin + vindesine + etoposide[207] | 16 | 31 |
| Cisplatin + vinblastine + bleomycin[208–211] | 120 | 22 |
| Lomustine + benznidazole[212] | 18 | 22 |
| Cisplatin + vindesine[213] | 61 | 21 |
| Carmustine + mitolactol[214] | 20 | 20 |
| Cisplatin + vindesine + lomustine[207] | 15 | 20 |
| Carmustine + 6-thioguanine[215] | 35 | 17 |
| Cisplatin + cytarabine[216] | 25 | 16 |

*Response rates are based on the number of patients with a complete or partial response (50%) divided by the number of evaluable patients treated. Investigational agents and commercially available agents with response rates approximating 0% are not listed.

melanoma cells remains unknown, and the role of hormonal manipulation in the management of melanoma is uncertain.

**Combination Chemotherapy.** Many combination chemotherapy regimens have been tried in phase II and phase III clinical trials in patients with metastatic melanoma in attempts to improve response rates. These studies can be divided into those that include DTIC (the most active single agent) (Table 74–7) and those that do not (Table 74–8). Marked variations in response rates are seen with similar regimens reported by different investigators owing to the small number of patients in each study as well as the tumor burden heterogeneity of patient groups. Most of the studies without DTIC include one of the other active agents, such as the nitrosoureas or cisplatin.

Despite some studies in which higher response rates were observed than those reported for DTIC, no multiagent combination is currently significantly more efficacious. Several randomized clinical trials comparing combination chemo-

therapy versus DTIC alone have shown that there is no statistically significant improvement in response rate or survival for combination chemotherapy (Table 74–9).[84–94] In addition, combination chemotherapy is usually more toxic. Despite the fact that large numbers of patients have been entered into many phase II and phase III treatment protocols in metastatic melanoma, the search for newer and better drugs is ongoing.

Tamoxifen has been included in some chemotherapeutic regimens with apparent improvement in response rates. Del Prete and colleagues[95] reported a 55% response rate in 20 patients (four complete responses, seven partial responses) with a combination of DTIC, BCNU, cisplatin, and tamoxifen. A subsequent trial omitting tamoxifen yielded a response rate of only 10%.[96] Other studies have confirmed that tamoxifen may provide a favorable contribution in combined regimens despite its ineffectiveness as a single agent.[97] Tamoxifen appears to enhance the antiproliferative effects of

*Table 74-9.* Selected Randomized Phase III Clinical Trials of Chemotherapy in Metastatic Melanoma

| Study | Treatment | Patients (No.) | Response Rate (%) | Comments |
|---|---|---|---|---|
| Italian Oncology (Cocconi et al[89]) | Dacarbazine vs. dacarbazine + tamoxifen | 52 / 60 | 12 / 28 | Improved RR and survival in women only on dacarbazine + tamoxifen |
| South Africa (Falkson et al[90]) | Dacarbazine vs. dacarbazine + IFN | 31 / 30 | 20 / 53 | Improved RR and survival for dacarbazine + IFN |
| Canadian Oncology Group (Rusthoven et al[91]) | CDB vs. CDB + tamoxifen | 100 / 104 | 21 / 30 | No benefit for addition of tamoxifen to CDB |
| NCCTG–Mayo Clinic (Creagan et al[92]) | CDB vs. CDB + tamoxifen | 92 / 92 | 33 / 27 | No benefit for addition of tamoxifen to CDB |
| ECOG 3690 (Falkson et al[93]) | Dacarbazine vs. dacarbazine + IFN vs. dacarbazine + tamoxifen vs. dacarbazine + IFN + tamoxifen | 69 / 68 / 66 / 68 | 15 / 21 / 18 / 19 | No benefit for addition of IFN and/or tamoxifen to dacarbazine |
| ECOG 91–140 (Chapman et al[94]) | Dacarbazine vs. CBCT | | | Preliminary results: no significant difference in survival between the two arms |

RR, response rate; IFN, interferon; CDB, cisplatin, dacarbazine, carmustine; CBCT, dacarbazine, cisplatin, carmustine, and tamoxifen.
From Atkins MB, Gollob JA. Chemotherapy and cytokine-based immunotherapy for high-risk and metastatic melanoma. Adv Oncol 1999; 15:22–9.

cisplatin in vitro.[98] Nevertheless, as shown in Table 74–9, tamoxifen has not enhanced the cytotoxic effects of other drugs in appropriately controlled, phase III randomized clinical trials.

**Adjuvant Chemotherapy.** Patients with metastases to regional lymph nodes are at high risk for developing systemic metastases and eventually dying of melanoma. In an effort to benefit these patients, postoperative adjuvant trials have been initiated. Although DTIC is still considered the drug of choice in treating disseminated melanoma, adjuvant trials in patients with stage II melanoma have shown no improvement in survival with DTIC alone,[99, 100] DTIC plus immunotherapy,[101, 102] or DTIC plus cyclophosphamide,[103] as compared with surgery alone.

**Regional Perfusion.** Chemotherapeutic regional perfusion was first reported in 1958 for control of locally recurrent disease.[104] The status of this strategy has been reviewed by Fraker.[105] The technique involves isolating the blood supply to a limb and inserting arterial and venous catheters. A tourniquet is applied, and the limb is perfused by means of a cardiac bypass pump and an oxygenator. Melphalan is the drug that has been used most commonly, and it is infused with or without heat. Results from a study comparing heated and unheated melphalan implied longer survival in the heated melphalan group,[106] a result confirmed by others who showed improved results from heat when the perfused agent was nitrogen mustard[107] or melphalan with or without dactinomycin.[108] Other drugs found to be useful in isolated perfusion for malignant melanoma of the limbs include cisplatin,[109, 110] DTIC,[111, 112] and combination chemotherapy with cisplatin and DTIC.[113] Radiation therapy has also been combined with intra-arterial infusion therapy using DTIC, with apparent improvement of local-regional control. An excellent review by Muchmore and colleagues[114] provides extensive information on this technique.

In patients with stage I disease, the risk of local-regional failure is highest if the primary tumor is Clark's level IV or V. Retrospective analysis of such patients treated with isolated limb perfusion indicates that some patients may benefit.[115] Hyperthermic limb perfusion has been most efficacious in the treatment of recurrent melanoma of the extremity. Patients have been treated with a wide variety of chemotherapeutic agents and different surgical techniques; regardless of the agents and techniques used, survival has been reported to be improved over that of patients with limb recurrences treated with surgery alone. A randomized trial of patients with stages I, II, and III melanoma reported benefit for perfusion-treated patients, regardless of stage.[116] Trials of regional perfusion, combining tumor necrosis factor (TNF)-α, interferon (IFN) alfa, and melphalan, have shown dramatic responses.[117]

Hyperthermic regional perfusion has local, regional, and systemic side effects and complications.[118, 119] Its definitive role in the treatment of patients with melanoma is not yet entirely clear, and this technique is usually appropriately performed only in the setting of a clinical trial.

**High-Dose Chemotherapy with Autologous Bone Marrow Transplantation.** Several groups are pursuing the use of extremely high doses of chemotherapy followed by an autologous bone marrow transplant.[120–123] These studies have generally shown higher response rates than seen with standard dose therapy, but there has been no appreciable impact on long-term survival. This approach to treatment remains investigational at this time.

## IMMUNOTHERAPY

Among the best-characterized human tumor antigens are those of melanoma. Putative tumor-specific antigens include MAGE 1 and MAGE 2,[124] which have been molecularly cloned, as well as ganglioside antigens such as GM2 and GD3[125] and less well characterized protein antigens.

Early immunotherapeutic efforts were made by Morton and coworkers[126] using direct intralesional injections of bacille Calmette-Guérin (BCG). This treatment resulted in greater than 90% of cutaneous melanoma nodules regressing. These seminal investigations provided the clinical foundation for subsequent immunotherapeutic efforts.

Active immunization of patients with allogeneic or autologous melanoma in combination with immunologic adjuvants such as BCG has, in the past, yielded low and inconsistent response rates in patients with measurable disease. Subsequent results, however, have been more consistent.[127, 128] Correlations have been made between therapeutic responses and the induction of cytotoxic T-cell precursors, and the generation of cellular or humoral immune responses may provide an intermediate end point for analysis of these experimental regimens.[129] Some retrospective clinical trials have suggested efficacy of whole-cell vaccines in an adjuvant setting, but these require confirmatory prospective randomized trials.

Passive immunotherapy employs tumor-directed antibodies in an attempt to induce antibody-dependent cellular cytotoxicity. A number of monoclonal antibodies have been described[130] and are being used in clinical trials.[131] Monoclonal antibody R24 directed against ganglioside GD3 has been used in combination with colony-stimulating factors or prepared as an immunotoxin by coupling it to toxins such as ricin.[132–134] A number of minor responses have been described from these phase I clinical trials of passive immunotherapy. This modality should be considered investigational. The use of tumor-specific antibody in generating an ADCC response is well founded from in vitro animal data. The use of colony-stimulating factors such as granulocyte-macrophage colony-stimulating factor (GM-CSF) and granulocyte colony–stimulating factor (G-CSF) may augment the number and activity of effector cells and their potential to interact with antibody-coated tumor cells.

The last 10 years have ushered in the field of biologic therapy of cancer using recombinant cytokines. For melanoma, the interferons have been the best-studied biologic agents. Interferons can modulate effector cell function; upregulate expression of major histocompatibility class antigens and tumor antigens; and, through a variety of mechanisms, enhance immune-mediated killing of tumor cells.[135, 136] The overall response rate of melanoma patients to IFN alfa-2 is approximately 15%, with less than a third of these being complete.[137–139] Lower response rates to IFN alfa-2 have been reported.[140] Intralesional injections of IFN show an increased response but without any improvement systemically.[141] IFN alfa-2 is currently being tested in an adjuvant setting in many cooperative trials (Table 74–10).[142–147] Early results supported the use of IFN, but a true survival benefit for the

*Table 74–10.* **Adjuvant Interferon-Alfa Trials in Malignant Melanoma**

| Study | Treatment | Stage of Disease | Results |
|---|---|---|---|
| ECOG 1684 (Kirkwood et al[142]) | Observation vs. HD IFN induction × 4 wk, then SC maintenance | IIB and III | IFN significantly better for relapse-free and overall survival in node-positive patients |
| NCCTG (Creagan et al[143]) | Observation vs. HD IFN IM twice a week × 12 wk | II and III | No overall difference; trend favoring IFN in node-positive patients |
| WHO (Cascinelli[144]) | Observation vs. LD IFN-alfa-2a SC twice a week × 3 yr | III | No difference in disease-free or overall survival |
| French (Grob et al[145]) | Observation vs. LD IFN-alfa-2a SC twice a week × 3 yr | II | 25% reduction in risk of relapse in IFN arm; no overall survival benefit |
| Austrian (Pehamberger et al[146]) | Observation vs. LD IFN twice a week × 18 mo | II | Relapse-free survival benefit in IFN arm at 3 years; no overall survival benefit |
| ECOG 1690 (Kirkwood et al[147]) | Observation vs. LD IFN × 2 yr vs. HD IFN as in 1684 | IIB and III | Relapse-free survival benefit but no overall survival benefit in HD IFN arm only |

HD, high dose; IFN, interferon; SC, subcutaneously; IM, intramuscularly
From Atkins MB, Gollob JA: Chemotherapy and cytokine-based immunotherapy for high-risk and metastatic melanoma. Adv Oncol 1999; 15:22–9.

use of IFN in the adjuvant setting has been difficult to prove unequivocally.

Interleukin-2 (IL-2) has been studied extensively in the treatment of human melanoma. This cytokine is produced by activated T cells and is a potent activation signal for a variety of cells, including T cells, B cells, natural killer cells, and monocytes. The administration of IL-2 as a single agent at the maximal tolerable dosages yields objective response rates of 16 to 22%.[148, 149] The complete response rate is, however, less than 5%.

The adoptive transfer of lymphokine-activated killer cells does not appear to increase the response rate above that which can be achieved with IL-2 alone.[150] An alternative source of lymphocytes for ex vivo expansion and adoptive transfer is the leukocytes found within tumor deposits—tumor-infiltrating lymphocytes (TILs).[151] This labor-intensive and costly treatment appears to yield response rates of the order of 35%[152–154] but does not seem to increase the number of complete responses. The precise mechanism of the clinical response to TILs is under study.[155]

TNF is an immunoregulatory cytokine produced by macrophages and other cells with a broad range of effector functions. TNF can induce the elaboration of other cytokines, may induce expression of cell surface antigens, and may have direct cytotoxic effects on target cells.[156] Clinical trials using TNF in melanoma have been disappointing, characterized by considerable toxicity and low response rates.[157] TNF has been used as an agent for treatment of in-transit melanoma of the extremity using intra-arterial isolated perfusion therapy.[117] The combination of TNF, IFN, and melphalan has yielded response rates of nearly 90% in this specialized clinical setting. Many other biologic agents are on the hori-

zon for employment in melanoma clinical trials, including IL-1, IL-4, and IL-6. It is hoped that combinations of biologic and chemotherapeutic agents will have higher therapeutic indices.

## GENE THERAPY OF MELANOMA

The lack of effective treatment for advanced disease and the well-documented reports of occasional spontaneous remissions (thought to be immune mediated) in patients with malignant melanoma have made this disease a common target for experimental gene therapy protocols. Of the 193 human cancer gene therapy trials approved so far by the U.S. Office of Biotechnology Activities, Recombinant DNA Advisory Committee (RAC), 51 were approved targeting patients with melanoma.

Initial trials used gene transfer techniques to answer biologic questions. These were gene-marking studies, in which a gene (most frequently a gene conferring resistance to growth in a tissue culture medium containing the antibiotics neomycin and hygromycin) would be introduced into cells to allow their tracking after being reinfused into humans. Two trials conducted in patients with melanoma (Table 74–11) studied the in vivo biology of TIL. The original hypothesis was that TIL would have the capacity to home to tumor deposits. These studies revealed that even though gene-marked TILs were recovered from melanoma lesions,[158] the ability of TILs to localize in tumor lesions was not enhanced compared with marked lymphocytes obtained from peripheral blood.[159]

The initiation of an immune response requires two immu-

*Table 74–11.* **Gene Marking Studies**

| Author | Gene | Purpose | Vector | Target Cell | Gene Transfer | Clinical Phase |
|---|---|---|---|---|---|---|
| Rosenberg[158] | Neo | Gene marking of TIL | Retrovirus | TIL | In vitro | I |
| Economou[159] | Neo | Gene marking of TIL and PBMC | Retrovirus | TIL | In vitro | I |
| Yee[217] | Hygro | Gene marking of tyrosinase-specific CTL | Retrovirus | CTL | In vitro | I |

Neo, neomycin resistance gene; hygro, hygromycin phosphotransferase; TIL, tumor-infiltrating lymphocytes; PBMC, peripheral blood mononuclear cell; CTL, cytotoxic T lymphocytes.

*Table 74–12.* Tumor Vaccines

| Investigator | Gene | Purpose | Vector | Target Cell | Gene Transfer | Clinical Phase |
|---|---|---|---|---|---|---|
| Lotze | IL-2 | Autologous tumor vaccine | Retrovirus | Autologous tumor cells | In vitro | I |
| Rosenberg | TNF | Autologous tumor vaccine | Retrovirus | Autologous tumor cells | In vitro | I |
| Rosenberg | IL-2 | Autologous tumor vaccine | Retrovirus | Autologous tumor cells | In vitro | I |
| Gansbacher | IL-2 | Allogeneic tumor vaccine | Retrovirus | Allogeneic tumor cells | In vitro | I |
| Lotze | IL-4 | Autologous tumor vaccine | Retrovirus | Autologous tumor cells | In vitro | I |
| Seigler | IFN-γ | Autologous tumor vaccine | Retrovirus | Autologous tumor cells | In vitro | I |
| Das Gupta | IL-2 | Allogeneic tumor vaccine | Retrovirus | Allogeneic tumor cells | In vitro | I |
| Economou | IL-2 | Allogeneic tumor vaccine | Retrovirus | Allogeneic tumor cells | In vitro | I |
| Lotze | IL-12 | Intratumoral autologous fibroblasts | Retrovirus | Autologous fibroblasts | In vitro | I |
| Dranoff | GM-CSF | Autologous tumor vaccine | Retrovirus | Autologous tumor cells | In vitro | I |
| Economou | IL-7 | Allogeneic tumor vaccine | Retrovirus | Allogeneic tumor cells | In vitro | I |
| Mahvi | GM-CSF | Autologous tumor vaccine | Gene gun | Autologous tumor cells | In vitro | I |
| Das Gupta | IL-2 | Allogeneic tumor vaccine | Retrovirus | Allogeneic tumor cells | In vitro | I |
| Park | IL-12 | Intratumoral autologous fibroblasts | Retrovirus | Autologous fibroblasts | In vitro | I |
| Dranoff | GM-CSF | Autologous tumor vaccine | Adenovirus | Autologous tumor cells | In vitro | I |
| Lotze | IL-12 | Intratumoral autologous fibroblasts | Retrovirus | Autologous fibroblasts | In vitro | II |
| Suzuki | GM-CSF | Autologous tumor vaccine | Adenovirus | Autologous tumor cells | In vitro | I |

IL, interleukin; TNF, tumor necrosis factor; IFN: interferon; GM-CSF: granulocyte-macrophage colony-stimulating factor.

nologic signals. Signal 1 corresponds to an antigen bound to the major histocompatibility complex (MHC), whereas signal 2 is mediated by the costimulatory molecules B7.1 and B7.2.[160] The production of activating cytokines potentiates further the immune response and leads to the activation and proliferation of cytotoxic T lymphocytes. Tumor cells express signal 1 (antigen/MHC) without signal 2 (costimulation), which leads to an anergic immune response and tumor escape from the immune system. In an attempt to make the tumor cells more immunogenic and optimal antigen presenters to the immune system, genes of costimulatory molecules (B7.1) and cytokines (IL-2, IL-4, IL-7, IL-12, IFN, GM-CSF) were introduced into autologous tumor cells in what has been known as *tumor vaccines* (Table 74–12). The major practical limitation of this approach is the requirement of establishing in vitro tumor cell lines from melanoma cells obtained from each patient, which later have to be stably transfected with the immune stimulatory gene and selected in vitro, a process that may take more than a month. To circumvent this problem, several investigators gene-modified patient's skin fibroblasts, which are more easily cultured in vitro than tumor cells, and delivered them admixed with autologous tumor cells or directly injected intralesionally (see Table 74–12). This stratagem would provide the immune-stimulatory cytokines in a paracrine (local) fashion at the site of tumor antigens in the melanoma lesion. The growing knowledge describing the specific recognition of certain allogeneic melanoma cell lines by lymphocytes isolated from different patients led to the hypothesis that shared melanoma antigens existed. A previously established tumor cell line stably transfected with an immunostimulatory gene might provide the adequate signal 1 (antigen/MHC) for initiating an antitumor immune response. The genes introduced into these allogeneic tumor vaccines were similar to the ones used in the more labor-intensive autologous tumor vaccine strategies (see Table 74–12).

The immune system tries to protect the *self* and reject the *nonself*. This distinction is based on the recognition of an autologous MHC subtype. A foreign MHC subtype stimulates a vigorous immune response. By antigen spreading, the immune response to the foreign MHC molecule may potentiate a response to melanoma antigens that previously were unrecognized by the immune system. To exploit this possibility, the gene coding for the human MHC subtype HLA-B7 has been introduced into allogeneic melanoma cell lines or directly into melanoma lesions in vivo (Table 74–13). This approach has consistently generated objective response rates of 10 to 25% in several clinical trials in patients with melanoma and is currently in phase III trials to determine its benefits over DTIC chemotherapy. Another strategy of direct intratumoral injection of a gene is the direct injection of a plasmid coding the gene for IL-2 coated with liposomes to allow fusion of the DNA-liposome complex directly to the tumor cells. Conceptually, this approach is similar to the autologous tumor vaccine approach but circumvents many of its problems and makes it more widely applicable (see Table 74–13).

An unexpected finding from preclinical studies of tumor vaccine approaches has been that the cells of the tumor vaccines do not directly stimulate an immune response. Studies in chimeric mouse models have established that there is a requirement for antigen processing by host antigen-presenting cells (APC) for the tumor vaccine strategies to stimulate an immune response. The common theme would be that the immune stimulatory genes would attract host APC, which would take up and process tumor antigens at the tumor vaccine site, present them on their surface together with costimulatory molecules and cytokines (signal 1 plus signal 2), and then initiate an antitumor immune response.[161] The understanding of this mechanism of immune stimulation together with the recognition and full characterization of melanoma-associated antigens (MAGE, MART-1/Melan-A, gp100, tyrosinase, tyrosinase-related protein)[162, 163] has led to the strategies known as *genetic immunization* (Table 74–14). These strategies attempt to immunize patients with the gene coding for a melanoma antigen to stimulate an antitumor immune response, with special emphasis on effective means to target these melanoma antigens for presentation by host APC.

Initial studies did not involve gene transfer techniques

*Table 74–13.* Allogeneic Major Histocompatibility Complex and In Vivo Intratumoral Gene Delivery

| Investigator | Gene | Purpose | Vector | Target Cell | Gene Transfer | Clinical Phase |
|---|---|---|---|---|---|---|
| Nabel | HLA-B7 | In vivo transfer | Cationic lipid DNA complex | Intratumoral injection | In vivo | I |
| Sznol | HLA-B7 | Allogeneic MHC tumor vaccine | Cationic lipid DNA complex | Autologous tumor cells | In vivo | I |
| Hersch | HLA-B7 | In vivo transfer | Cationic lipid DNA complex | Intratumoral injection | In vivo | I |
| Hersch | IL-2 | In vivo transfer | Cationic lipid DNA complex | Intratumoral injection | In vivo | I |
| Chang | HLA-B7 | In vivo transfer | Cationic lipid DNA complex | Intratumoral injection | In vivo | I |
| Hersch | HLA-B7 | In vivo transfer | Cationic lipid DNA complex | Intratumoral injection | In vivo | II |
| Hersch | Il-2 | In vivo transfer | Cationic lipid DNA complex | Intratumoral injection | In vivo | II |
| Conry | IL-12 | In vivo transfer | Canarypox virus | Intratumoral injection | In vivo | I |
| Conry | HLA-B7 | In vivo transfer | Canarypox virus | Intratumoral injection | In vivo | I |
| Gonzalez | HLA-B7 + IL-2 | In vivo transfer | Cationic lipid DNA complex | Intratumoral injection | In vivo | I |
| Dreim | HLA-B7 | In vivo transfer | Cationic lipid DNA complex | Intratumoral injection | In vivo | II |
| Thompson | HLA-B7 | In vivo transfer | Cationic lipid DNA complex | Intratumoral injection | In vivo | III |
| Walsh | IL-2 + SEB | In vivo transfer | Cationic lipid DNA complex | Intratumoral injection | In vivo | I |
| Schuchter | B7.1 | In vivo transfer | Adenovirus | Intratumoral injection | In vivo | I |
| Rosenblatt | IFN-γ | In vivo transfer | Adenovirus | Intratumoral injection | In vivo | I |
| Hersch | HLA-B7 + IL-2 | In vivo transfer | Cationic lipid DNA complex | Intratumoral injection | In vivo | I |

HLA, human leukocyte antigen; IL, interleukin; MHC, major histocompatibility complex; IFN, interferon; SEB, *Staphylococcus* endotoxin B.

but have shown that immunization with melanoma tumor antigens leads to clinical responses. An antigenic epitope derived from the gp100 melanoma antigen was administered emulsified in the immunologic adjuvant incomplete Freund's adjuvant, which had the role of attracting host APC, together with systemic recombinant IL-2. This treatment led to an objective response rate of 42% in patients with advanced melanoma with the HLA-A2.1 subtype.[164] In another clinical trial, patients with melanoma were immunized with dendritic cells (the most powerful APC known)[165] pulsed with peptides derived from the melanoma antigens MAGE, MART-1/Melan-A, gp100, and tyrosinase, also leading to objective responses in patients with HLA-A1 or HLA-A2.1 subtypes.[166] Expression of the full DNA sequence of the tumor antigen has several potential advantages over these peptide-based strategies, including more durable presentation of the stimulatory antigen to the immune system; the isolation of the peptide sequence presented by each MHC subtype would not be required (these peptide sequences are known only for the most common HLA subtypes, which make them suitable for treating less than 50% of whites with melanoma); the potential for MHC class I and class II epitope presentation; and the simultaneous presentation of multiple antigen-derived epitopes, reducing the potential risk of escape of mutant tumor cells. Studies in which replication-defective viral vectors expressing genes from melanoma tumor antigens were directly injected into patients have failed to show that this strategy can effectively generate antigen-specific responses.[167] Other strategies, better suited for targeting the melanoma tumor antigen to expression on APC, include the intramuscular or intradermal delivery (by gene gun) of naked DNA plasmids or the gene modification of the patient's cultured dendritic cells (see Table 74–14). The most effective vectors to gene-modify dendritic cells are replication-incompetent viral vectors (adenovirus, retrovirus) as opposed to a variety of physical strategies.[168] When gene-modified dendritic cells have been tested in preclinical models of genetic immunization, encouraging levels of antigen-specific immune responses have been generated.[169–173]

Several gene therapy protocols have expanded on the work with TILs and activated lymphocytes (Table 74–15). Assuming that TILs would target specifically to tumor de-

*Table 74–14.* Genetic Immunotherapy

| Investigator | Gene | Purpose | Vector | Target Cell | Gene Transfer | Clinical Phase |
|---|---|---|---|---|---|---|
| Rosenberg | MART-1 | Genetic immunization | Adenovirus | SC immunization | In vitro | I |
| Rosenberg | gp100 | Genetic immunization | Adenovirus | SC or IM immunization | In vitro | I |
| Rosenberg | MART-1 | Genetic immunization | Fowlpox virus | IM immunization | In vitro | I |
| Rosenberg | gp100 | Genetic immunization | Fowlpox virus | IM immunization | In vitro | I |
| Rosenberg | MART-1 | Genetic immunization | Vaccinia virus | IM immunization | In vitro | I |
| Rosenberg | gp100 | Genetic immunization | Naked DNA | IM immunization | In vitro | I |
| Economou | MART-1 | Genetic immunization | Adenovirus | Dendritic cells | In vitro | I |
| Conry | MART-1 | Genetic immunization | Naked DNA | IM immunization | In vitro | I |
| Haluska | MART-1 + gp100 | Genetic immunization | Adenovirus | Dendritic cells | In vitro | I |
| Albertini | gp100 + GM-CSF | Genetic immunization | Gene gun | SC immunization | In vitro | I |
| Rosenberg | gp100 | Genetic immunization | Fowlpox virus | IM or IV immunization | In vitro | I |
| Topalian | Tyrosinase | Genetic immunization | Fowlpox virus | IM immunization | In vitro | I |

GM = CSF, granulocyte-macrophage colony-stimulating factor; SC, subcutaneously; IM, intramuscularly; IV, intravenous.

*Table 74–15.* **Adoptive Transfer**

| Investigator | Gene | Purpose | Vector | Target Cell | Gene Transfer | Clinical Phase |
|---|---|---|---|---|---|---|
| Rosenberg | TNF | Transduction of TIL | Retrovirus | TIL | In vitro | I |
| Chang | GM-CSF | Adoptive immunotherapy | Retrovirus | Autologous tumor cells used to stimulate CTL | In vitro | I |
| Chang | HLA-B7 | Adoptive immunotherapy | Cationic lipid DNA complex | Intratumoral injection to stimulate TIL | In vitro | I |

TNF, tumor necrosis factor; GM-CSF, granulocyte-macrophage colony-stimulating factor; TIL, tumor-infiltrating lymphocytes; CTL, cytotoxic T lymphocytes.

posits, the gene for TNF-α was introduced into these lymphocytes to allow localized high levels of TNF-α expression in melanoma lesions. It has been difficult to show convincingly, however, that these TILs selectively localize in melanoma lesions. Other strategies have used gene transfer techniques to stimulate lymphocytes, which are expanded in vitro in media containing IL-2 and reinfused into patients (adoptive transfer strategies).

Most of these clinical approaches are still in phase I clinical testing, trying to show the feasibility of the treatment protocol and define the safety, toxicity, and optimal dosing for further clinical development. In general, gene therapy approaches have proven to be safe, and surrogate markers of activity in patients with advanced cancers (detection of specific immune responses) encourage further clinical development. Other areas of research in gene therapy for melanoma include the use of specifically targeted replication-defective viral vectors, intended to deliver a toxic gene directly into the tumor cell by virtue of targeting a specific surface marker present on melanoma cells but not normal cells. This targeting can be achieved by modifying the cell surface receptor-binding site for viral vectors. Also, tumor-specific promoters have been used to express certain genes selectively in tumor cells as opposed to normal cells. Other strategies include the use of cytolytic replication-selective virus, in which viral replication is allowed only in tumor cells and not in normal tissues. These cytolytic viruses can exploit tumor characteristics for selective viral replication (lack of functional p53 or retinoblastoma genes), have tumor-specific promoters guiding viral replication, or use viruses that target and replicate only in cells containing melanoma surface molecules. For immune-based approaches, a strategy has focused on genetically modifying lymphocytes instead of modifying tumor antigen presentation. Lymphocytes recognize tumor antigens by the T-cell receptor, and several T-cell receptors specific for melanoma antigens have been cloned. The introduction of the gene for a melanoma-specific T-cell receptor into cytotoxic T lymphocytes, followed by ex vivo activation with IL-2 and expansion, may create large numbers of antigen-specific T cells for adoptive transfer into patients.

## SUMMARY OF TREATMENT BY STAGE

Surgical excision is the cornerstone of treatment for melanoma. Other modalities may also be required for the individual patient, and the best integration of these modalities is often controversial. Figures 74–2 and 74–3 illustrate our general approach to this disease as a function of stage.

The search for improved cytotoxic and immunostimulative agents is continuing, but at this time few promising advances have been made. It is easy to speculate that when better agents are available, treatment results will improve. For now, however, the best hope for improving survival results in this disease is through earlier diagnosis. Education is a key means currently available that would be highly effective and could be implemented with relatively little cost. Cutaneous melanoma, in contrast to visceral solid tumors, can be detected at early stages. On the basis of the assumption that early-level and early-depth melanomas metastasize infrequently and are associated with a good prognosis, one would predict that a public health and community education program could be highly successful, especially when coupled with a physician education program about the biology of melanoma and the most effective treatment methods. Because the warning signs of melanoma may be extremely subtle, it is recommended that all nevi brought to the attention of a physician warrant biopsy and a pathologic review by an experienced pathologist.

Australia, which has the highest incidence of melanoma of any country in the world, is a model test of this thesis. It would appear that in Australia either melanoma is biologically less malignant or, more likely, public and physician

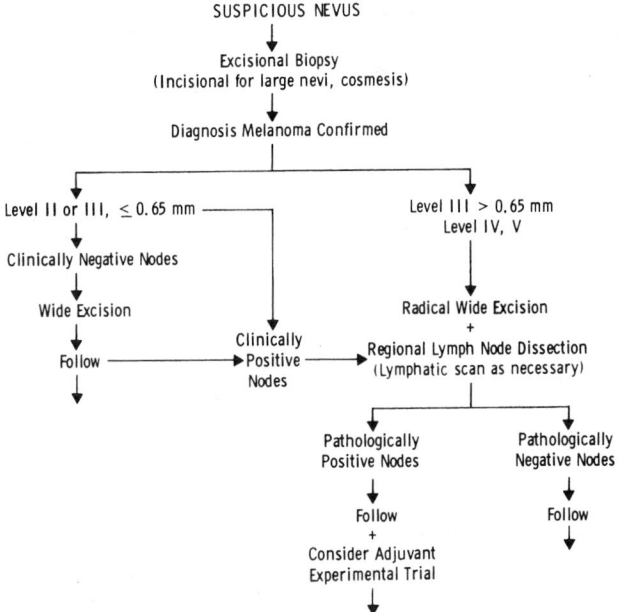

**Figure 74–2.** Management of stage I and stage II melanomas. See text for a discussion of the role of the sentinel node in management.

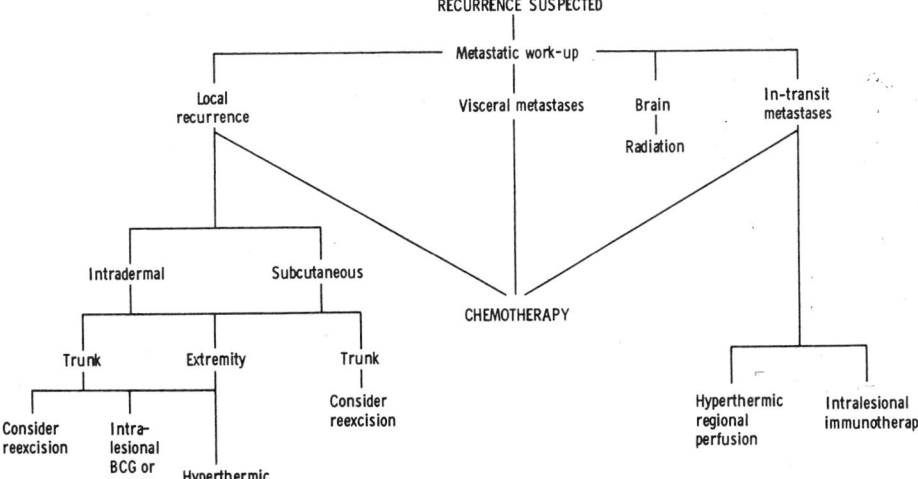

**Figure 74–3.** Management of stage III melanomas. BCG, bacillus Calmette-Guérin; DNCB, dinitrochlorobenzene.

awareness have reduced the mortality.[174] A carefully planned public health and education program could offer the greatest impact on melanoma statistics in the United States.

## SUGGESTIONS FOR ADDITIONAL READING

Cochran AJ, Bailly C, Paul E, Remotti F. Melanocytic tumors: a guide to diagnosis. Philadelphia: Lippincott-Raven, 1997.

Slominski A, Wortsman J, Nickoloff B, et al. Molecular pathology of malignant melanoma. Am J Clin Pathol 1998;110:788–94.

Lang PG Jr. Malignant melanoma. Med Clin North Am 1998;82:1325–58.

Kroon BB, Nieweg OE, Hoekstra HJ, Lejeune FJ. Principles and guidelines for surgeons: management of cutaneous malignant melanoma. European Society of Surgical Oncology Brussels. Eur J Surg Oncol 1997;23:550–8.

Cooper JS. The evolution of the role of radiation therapy in the management of mucocutaneous malignant melanoma. Hematol Oncol Clin North Am 1998;12:849–62.

Hersh EM, Stopeck AT. Advances in the biological therapy and gene therapy of malignant disease. Clin Cancer Res 1997;3:12 Pt 2:2623–9.

Dickler MN, Coit DG, Meyers ML. Adjuvant therapy of malignant melanoma. Surg Oncol Clin North Am 1997;6:793–812.

Toma S, Ugolini D, Palumbo R. Tamoxifen in the treatment of metastatic malignant melanoma: still a controversy? Int J Oncol 1999;15:321–37.

Abbott KL, Harman GS. Combination chemotherapy for disseminated malignant melanoma. Anticancer Drugs 1995;6:489–97

Durán García E, Santolaya R, Requena T. Treatment of malignant melanoma. Ann Pharmacother 1999;33:730–8.

Meisenberg B. High-dose chemotherapy and autologous stem cell support for patients with malignant melanoma. Bone Marrow Transplant 1996;17:903–6.

Atkins MB, Gollob JA. Chemotherapy and cytokine-based immunotherapy for high-risk and metastatic melanoma. Adv Oncol 1999;15:22–9.

## REFERENCES

1. Young JL Jr, Percy CL, Asire AJ, et al. Cancer incidence and mortality in the United States, 1973–77. Monogr Natl Cancer Inst 1981;57:1–187.
2. Cancer incidence in five continents. IARC Publication No. 88. Lyon: IARC, 1987.
3. Landis SH, Murray T, Bolden S, Wingo PA. Cancer statistics, 1999. CA Cancer J Clin 1999;49:8–31.
4. Longstreth J. Cutaneous malignant melanoma and ultraviolet radiation: a review. Cancer Metastasis Rev 1988;7:321–33.
5. Beardmore GL. In: McCarthy WH, ed. Melanoma and skin cancer:

6. Elwood JM, Lee JA, Walter SD, et al. Relationship of melanoma and other skin cancer mortality to latitude and ultraviolet radiation in the United States and Canada. Int J Epidemiol 1974;3:325–32.
7. Armstrong BK. Epidemiology of malignant melanoma: intermittent or total accumulated exposure to the sun? J Dermatol Surg Oncol 1988;14:835–49.
8. Osterlind A, Tucker MA, Stone BJ, Jensen OM. The Danish case-control study of cutaneous malignant melanoma: II. importance of UV-light exposure. Int J Cancer 1988;42:319–24.
9. Zanetti R, Franceschi S, Rosso S, et al. Cutaneous melanoma and sunburns in childhood in a southern European population. Eur J Cancer 1992;28A:1172–6.
10. Clark WH Jr, Reimer RR, Greene M, et al. Origin of familial malignant melanomas from heritable melanocytic lesions: 'the B-K mole syndrome.' Arch Dermatol 1978;114:732–8.
11. Elder DE, Clark WH Jr, Elenitsas R, et al. The early and intermediate precursor lesions of tumor progression in the melanocytic system: common acquired nevi and atypical (dysplastic) nevi. Semin Diagn Pathol 1993;10:18–35.
12. Lewis MG. Malignant melanoma in Uganda. (The relationship between pigmentation and malignant melanoma on the soles of the feet.) Br J Cancer 1967;21:483–95.
13. Autier P, Joarlette M, Lejeune F, et al. Cutaneous malignant melanoma and exposure to sun beds: a descriptive study in Belgium. Melanoma Res 1991;1:69–74.
14. Swerdlow AJ, English JS, MacKie RM, et al. Fluorescent lights, ultraviolet lamps, and risk of cutaneous melanoma [published erratum appears in Br Med J 1988;297:1172]. Br Med J 1988;297:647–50.
15. Fleming ID, Cooper JS, Henson DE, et al, eds. AJCC cancer staging manual. 5th ed. Philadelphia: Lippincott-Raven, 1997:163–7.
16. Pack GT, Oropeza R. Subungual melanoma. Surg Gynecol Obstet 1967;124:571–82.
17. Cochran AJ, Bailly C, Paul E, Dolbeau D. Nevi, other than dysplastic and Spitz nevi. Semin Diagn Pathol 1993;10:3–17.
18. Barnhill RL, Mihm MC Jr. The histopathology of cutaneous malignant melanoma. Semin Diagn Pathol 1993;10:47–75.
19. Clark WH Jr, Elder DE, Guerry D 4th, et al. Model predicting survival in stage I melanoma based on tumor progression [see comments]. J Natl Cancer Inst 1989;81:1893–904.
20. Mihm MC Jr, Fitzpatrick TB, Brown MM, et al. Early detection of primary cutaneous malignant melanoma: a color atlas. N Engl J Med 1973;289:989–96.
21. Kopf AW, Bart RS, Rodriguez-sains RS: Malignant melanoma: a review. J Dermatol Surg Oncol 1977;3:41–125.
22. Clark WH Jr, ed. Human malignant melanoma. New York: Grune & Stratton, 1979:33.
23. Cochran AJ, Bailly C, Paul E, Remotti F. Melanocytic tumors: a guide to diagnosis. Philadelphia: Lippincott-Raven, 1997.
24. Cochran AJ. In: Nathanson L, ed. Current research and clinical man-

agement of melanoma. Philadelphia: Kluwer Academic Publishers, 1993:69–102.

25. Allen AC, Spitz S. Malignant melanoma: a clinicopathologic analysis of the critera for diagnosis and prognosis. Cancer 1953;6:1–45.

26. Cochran AJ. Method of assessing prognosis in patients with malignant melanoma. Lancet 1968;2:1062–4.

27. Mackie RM, Spilg WG, Thomas CE, Cochran AJ. Cell-mediated immunity in patients with malignant melanoma. Br J Dermatol 1972;87:523–8.

28. Schmoeckel C, Nejad KK, Braun-Falco O. [Prognostic index in malignant melanoma: a better method to determine metastasis risk]. Pathologe 1980;1:71–8.

29. Clark WH Jr. A classification of malignant melanoma in man correlated with histogenesis and biologic behavior. In: Montagna W, ed. Advances in biology of the skin: the pigmentary system. Vol. 8. London: Pergamon Press, 1967:621.

30. Breslow A. Thickness, cross-sectional areas and depth of invasion in the prognosis of cutaneous melanoma. Ann Surg 1970;172:902–8.

31. Prade M, Sancho-Garnier H, Cesarini JP, Cochran A. Difficulties encountered in the application of Clark classification and the Breslow thickness measurement in cutaneous malignant melanoma. Int J Cancer 1980;26:159–63.

32. Cady B. "Prophylactic" lymph node dissection in melanoma: does it help? J Clin Oncol 1988;6:2–4. editorial.

33. Wanebo HJ, Fortner JG, Woodruff J, et al. Selection of the optimum surgical treatment of stage I melanoma by depth of microinvasion: use of the combined microstage technique (Clark-Breslow). Ann Surg 1975;182:302–15.

34. Robert ME, Wen DR, Cochran AJ. Pathological evaluation of the regional lymph nodes in malignant melanoma. Semin Diagn Pathol 1993;10:102–15.

35. Callery C, Cochran AJ, Roe DJ. Factors prognostic for survival in patients with malignant melanoma spread to the regional lymph nodes. Ann Surg 1982;196:69–75.

36. Cochran AJ, Lana AM, Wen DR. Histomorphometry in the assessment of prognosis in stage II malignant melanoma. Am J Surg Pathol 1989;3:600–4.

37. Ruiter DJ, Bröcker EB. Immunohistochemistry in the evaluation of melanocytic tumors. Semin Diagn Pathol 1993;10:76–91.

38. Cochran AJ, Wen DR, Herschman HR. Occult melanoma in lymph nodes detected by antiserum to S-100 protein. Int J Cancer 1984;34:159–63.

39. Cochran AJ, Wen DR, Morton DL. Occult tumor cells in the lymph nodes of patients with pathological stage I malignant melanoma: an immunohistological study [see comments]. Am J Surg Pathol 1988;12:612–8.

40. Chen ZL, Wen DR, Coulson WF, et al. Occult metastases in the axillary lymph nodes of patients with breast cancer node negative by clinical and histologic examination and conventional histology. Dis Markers 1991;9:239–48.

41. Chen ZL, Perez S, Holmes EC, et al. Frequency and distribution of occult micrometastases in lymph nodes of patients with non-small-cell lung carcinoma. J Natl Cancer Inst 1993;85:493–8.

42. Morton DL, Wen DR, Wong JH, et al. Technical details of intraoperative lymphatic mapping for early stage melanoma. Arch Surg 1992;127:392–9.

43. Morton DL, Wen D-R, Foshag LJ, Cochran AJ. Use of intraoperative lymphatic mapping and selective lymphadenectomy to identify candidates for adjuvant therapy of melanoma. In: Salmon SE, ed. Adjuvant therapy of cancer VII. Philadelphia: JB Lippincott, 1993:393–97.

44. Kheir SM, Bines SD, Vonroenn JH, et al. Prognostic significance of DNA aneuploidy in stage I cutaneous melanoma. Ann Surg 1988;207:455–61.

45. Silver HK, Karim KA, Le Riche J, et al. Nuclear DNA, serum sialic acid and measured depth in malignant melanoma for predicting disease recurrence and survival. Int J Cancer 1989;44:31–4.

46. Zeng QS, Fu YS, Cochran AJ. Nuclear DNA measurements of metastatic melanoma by a computerized digital imaging system. Hum Pathol 1990;21:1112–6.

47. Giuliano AE, Cochran AJ, Morton DL. Melanoma from unknown primary site and amelanotic melanoma. Semin Oncol 1982;9:442–7.

48. Handley WS. The pathology of melanotic growths in relation to their operative environment. Lancet 1907;1:996–1003.

49. Cochran AJ. Malignant melanoma: a review of experience in Glasgow, Scotland. Cancer 1969;23:1190–9.

50. Cochran AJ. Studies of the melanocytes of the epidermis adjacent to tumors. J Invest Dermatol 1971;57:38–43.

51. Wong CK. A study of melanocytes in the normal skin surrounding malignant melanomata. Dermatologica 1970;141:215–25.

52. Veronesi U, Cascinelli N. Narrow excision (1-cm margin): a safe procedure for thin cutaneous melanoma. Arch Surg 1991;126:438–41.

53. Kenady DE, Brown BW, McBride CM. Excision of underlying fascia with a primary malignant melanoma: effect on recurrence and survival rates. Surgery 1982;92:615–8.

54. Balch CM, Murad TM, Soong SJ, et al. Tumor thickness as a guide to surgical management of clinical stage I melanoma patients. Cancer 1979;43:883–8.

55. Balch CM, Soong SJ, Milton GW, et al. A comparison of prognostic factors and surgical results in 1,786 patients with localized (stage I) melanoma treated in Alabama, USA, and New South Wales, Australia. Ann Surg 1982;196:677–84.

56. Milton GW, Shaw HM, McCarthy WH, et al. Prophylactic lymph node dissection in clinical stage I cutaneous malignant melanoma: results of surgical treatment in 1319 patients. Br J Surg 1982;69:108–11.

57. Reintgen DS, Cox EB, McCarty KS Jr, et al. Efficacy of elective lymph node dissection in patients with intermediate thickness primary melanoma. Ann Surg 1983;198:379–85.

58. Das Gupta TK. Results of treatment of 269 patients with primary cutaneous melanoma: a five-year prospective study. Ann Surg 1977;186:201–9.

59. Balch CM, Soong SJ, Murad TM, et al. A multifactorial analysis of melanoma: III. prognostic factors in melanoma patients with lymph node metastases (stage II). Ann Surg 1981;193:377–88.

60. Cohen MH, Ketcham AS, Felix EL, et al. Prognostic factors in patients undergoing lymphadenectomy for malignant melanoma. Ann Surg 1977;186:635–42.

61. McNeer G, Das Gupta T. Prognosis in malignant melanoma. Surgery 1964;56:512–8.

62. Roses DF, Provet JA, Harris MN, et al. Prognosis of patients with pathologic stage II cutaneous malignant melanoma. Ann Surg 1985;201:103–7.

63. Sim FH, Taylor WF, Ivins JC, et al. A prospective randomized study of the efficacy of routine elective lymphadenectomy in management of malignant melanoma: preliminary results. Cancer 1978;41:948–56.

64. Veronesi U, Adamus J, Bandiera DC, et al. Inefficacy of immediate node dissection in stage 1 melanoma of the limbs. N Engl J Med 1977;297:627–30.

65. Veronesi U, Adamus J, Bandiera DC, et al. Delayed regional lymph node dissection in stage I melanoma of the skin of the lower extremities. Cancer 1982;49:2420–30.

66. Balch CM, Soong S-J, Bartolucci AA, et al. Efficacy of an elective regional lymph node dissection of 1 to 4 mm thick melanoma for patients 60 years of age and younger. Ann Surg 1996;224:255–66.

67. Cochran AJ, Wen DR, Morton DL. Management of the regional lymph nodes in patients with cutaneous malignant melanoma. World J Surg 1992;16:214–21.

68. Morton DL, Wen DR, Foshag LJ, et al. Intraoperative lymphatic mapping and selective cervical lymphadenectomy for early-stage melanomas of the head and neck. J Clin Oncol 1993;11:1751–6.

69. Day CL Jr, Mihm MC Jr, Lew RA, et al. Prognostic factors for patients with clinical stage I melanoma of intermediate thickness (1.51–3.39 mm): a conceptual model for tumor growth and metastasis. Ann Surg 1982;195:35–43.

70. Cochran AJ. Histology and prognosis in malignant melanoma. J Pathol 1969;97:459–68.

71. O'Brien CJ, Uren RF, Thompson JF, et al. Prediction of potential metastatic sites in cutaneous head and neck melanoma using lymphoscintigraphy. Am J Surg 1995;170:461–6.

72. Morton DL, Joseph WL, Ketcham AS, et al. Surgical resection and adjunctive immunotherapy for selected patients with multiple pulmonary metastases. Ann Surg 1973;178:360–6.

73. Cahan WG. Excision of melanoma metastases to lung: problems in diagnosis and management. Ann Surg 1973;178:703–9.

74. Wong JH, Cagle LA, Morton DL. Surgical treatment of lymph nodes with metastatic melanoma from unknown primary site. Arch Surg 1987;122:1380–3.

75. Hayes FA, Green AA. Malignant melanoma in childhood: clinical course and response to chemotherapy. J Clin Oncol 1984;2:1229–34.

76. Hill GJ II, Krementz ET, Hill HZ. Dimethyl triazeno imidazole car-

boxamide and combination therapy for melanoma: IV. Late results after complete response to chemotherapy (Central Oncology Group protocols 7130, 7131, and 7131A). Cancer 1984;53:1299–305.

77. Wagner DE, Ramirez G, Weiss AJ, Hill G Jr. Combination phase 1-II study of imidazole carboxamide (NCS45388). Oncology 1972;26:310–6.
78. Luce JK. Chemotherapy of malignant melanoma. Cancer 1972;30:1604–15.
79. Nathanson L, Wolter J, Horton J, et al. Characteristics of prognosis and response to an imidazole carboxamide in malignant melanoma. Clin Pharmacol Ther 1971;12:955–62.
80. Costanza ME, Nathanson L, Lenhard R, et al. Therapy of malignant melanoma with an imidazole carboxamide and bis-chloroethyl nitrosourea. Cancer 1972;30:1457–61.
81. Cochran AJ. Malignant melanoma: a review of experience in Glasgow, Scotland. Cancer 1969;23:1190–9.
82. Costanzi JJ. DTIC (NSC-45388) studies in the Southwest Oncology Group. Cancer Treat Rep 1976;60:189–92.
83. Costanza ME, Nathanson L, Schoenfeld D, et al. Results with methyl-CCNU and DTIC in metastatic melanoma. Cancer 1977;40:1010–5.
84. Coates AS, Bishop J, Mann GJ, Raghavan D. Chemotherapy in metastatic melanoma: phase II studies of amsacrine, mitoxantrone and bisantrene. Eur J Cancer Clin Oncol 1986;22:97–100.
85. Chauvergne J, Bui NB, Cappelaere P, et al. [Chemotherapy in advanced malignant melanoma: results of a controlled trial comparing a combination of dacarbazine (DTIC) and detorubicin with dacarbazine alone.] Semaine des Hopitaux 1982;58:2697–701.
86. Luikart SD, Kennealey GT, Kirkwood JM. Randomized phase III trial of vinblastine, bleomycin, and cis-dichlorodiammine-platinum versus dacarbazine in malignant melanoma. J Clin Oncol 1984;2:164–8.
87. Lopez M, Perno CF, Di Lauro L, et al. Controlled study of DTIC versus DTIC plus epirubicin in metastatic malignant melanoma. Invest New Drugs 1984;2:319–22.
88. Hill GJ 2d, Metter GE, Krementz ET, et al. DTIC and combination therapy for melanoma: II. Escalating schedules of DTIC with BCNU, CCNU, and vincristine. Cancer Treat Rep 1979;63:1989–92.
89. Cocconi G, Bella M, Calabresi F, et al. Treatment of metastatic malignant melanoma with dacarbazine plus tamoxifen. N Engl J Med 1992;327:516–23.
90. Falkson CI, Falkson G, Falkson HC. Improved results with the addition of interferon alfa-2b to dacarbazine in the treatment of patients with metastatic malignant melanoma. J Clin Oncol 1991;9:1403–8.
91. Rusthoven JJ, Quirt IC, Iscoe NA, et al. Randomized, double-blind, placebo-controlled trial comparing the response rates of carmustine, dacarbazine, and cisplatin with and without tamoxifen in patients with metastatic melanoma. National Cancer Institute of Canada Clinical Trials Group. J Clin Oncol 1996;14:2083–90.
92. Creagan ET, Suman VJ, Dalton RJ, et al. Phase III clinical trial of the combination of cisplatin, dacarbazine, and carmustine with or without tamoxifen in patients with advanced malignant melanoma. J Clin Oncol 1999;17:1884–90.
93. Falkson CI, Ibrahim J, Kirkwood JM, et al. Phase III trial of dacarbazine versus dacarbazine with interferon alfa-2b versus dacarbazine with tamoxifen versus dacarbazine with interferon alfa-2b and tamoxifen in patients with metastatic malignant melanoma: an Eastern Cooperative Oncology Group study. J Clin Oncol 1998;16:1743–51.
94. Chapman PB, Einhorn LH, Meyers ML, et al. Phase III multicenter randomized trial of the Darmouth regimen versus dacarbazine in patients with metastatic melanoma. J Clin Oncol 1999;17:2745–51.
95. Del Prete SA, Maurer LH, O'Donnell J, et al. Combination chemotherapy with cisplatin, carmustine, dacarbazine, and tamoxifen in metastatic melanoma. Cancer Treat Rep 1984;68:1403-5.
96. McClay EF, Mastrangelo MJ, Bellet RE, Berd D. Combination chemotherapy and hormonal therapy in the treatment of malignant melanoma. Cancer Treat Rep 1987;71:465–9.
97. McClay EF, Mastrangelo MJ, Sprandio JD, et al. The importance of tamoxifen to a cisplatin-containing regimen in the treatment of metastatic melanoma. Cancer 1989;63:1292–5.
98. Hofmann J, Doppler W, Jakob A, et al. Enhancement of the antiproliferative effect of cis-diamminedichloroplatinum (II) and nitrogen mustard by inhibitors of protein kinase C. Int J Cancer 1988;42:382–8.
99. Veronesi U, Adamus J, Aubert C, et al. A randomized trial of adjuvant chemotherapy and immunotherapy in cutaneous melanoma. N Engl J Med 1982;307:913–6.
100. Hill GJ 2d, Moss SE, Golomb FM, et al. DTIC and combination therapy for melanoma: III. DTIC (NSC 45388) Surgical Adjuvant Study COG PROTOCOL 7040. Cancer 1981;47:2556–62.
101. Knost JA, Reynolds V, Greco FA, Oldham RK. Adjuvant chemoimmunotherapy stage I/II malignant melanoma. J Surg Oncol 1982;19:165–70.
102. Abdi EA, Hanson J, McPherson TA. Adjuvant chemoimmunotherapy after regional lymphadenectomy for malignant melanoma. Am J Clin Oncol 1987;10:117–22.
103. Balch CM, Murray D, Presant C, Bartolucci AA. Ineffectiveness of adjuvant chemotherapy using DTIC and cyclophosphamide in patients with resectable metastatic melanoma. Surgery 1984;95:454–9.
104. Creech O Jr, Krementz ET, Ryan RF, Winblad JN. Chemotherapy of cancer: regional perfusion utilizing an extracorporeal circuit. Ann Surg 1958;148:616–32.
105. Fraker DL. Hyperthermic regional perfusion for melanoma and sarcoma of the limbs. Curr Probl Surg 1999;36:843–907.
106. Stehlin JS, Giovanella BC, de Ipolyi PD, et al. Results of hyperthermic perfusion for melanoma of the extremities. Surg Gynecol Obstet 1975;140:339–48.
107. Shiu MH, Knapper WH, Fortner JG, et al. Regional isolated limb perfusion of melanoma in transit metastases using mechlorethamine (nitrogen mustard). J Clin Oncol 1986;4:1819–26.
108. Martijn H, Oldhoff J, Schraffordt Koops H. Regional perfusion in the treatment of patients with a locally metastasized malignant melanoma of the limbs. Eur J Cancer 1981;17:471–6.
109. Calvo DB 3d, Patt YZ, Wallace S, et al. Phase I–II trial of percutaneous intra-arterial cis-diamminedichloroplatinum (II) for regionally confined malignancy. Cancer 1980;45:1278–83.
110. Klein ES, Ben-Ari GY. Isolation perfusion with cisplatin for malignant melanoma of the limbs. Cancer 1987;59:1068–71.
111. Ariyan S, Mitchell MS, Kirkwood JM. Regional isolated perfusion of high risk melanoma of the extremities with imidazole carboxamide. Surg Gynecol Obstet 1984;158:238–42.
112. Gundersen S, Hager B, Tausjø J. Radiation in combination with intra-arterial infusion therapy with dacarbazine for metastatic malignant melanoma localized to a lower extremity. Cancer Treat Rep 1986;70:1015–7.
113. Aigner K, Hild P, Henneking K, et al. Regional perfusion with cisplatinum and dacarbazine. Recent Results Cancer Res 1983;86:239–45.
114. Muchmore JH, Carter RD, Krementz ET. Regional perfusion for malignant melanoma and soft tissue sarcoma: a review. Cancer Invest 1985;3:129–43.
115. Baas PC, Hoekstra HJ, Schraffordt Koops H, et al. Hyperthermic isolated regional perfusion in the treatment of extremity melanoma in children and adolescents. Cancer 1989;63:199–203.
116. Ghussen F, Krüger I, Groth W, Stützer H. [Randomized melanoma study of perfusion of the extremities: results of treatment 2 1/2 years after premature discontinuation.] Chirurg 1986;57:619–23.
117. Lienard D, Ewalenko P, Delmotte JJ, et al. High-dose recombinant tumor necrosis factor alpha in combination with interferon gamma and melphalan in isolation perfusion of the limbs for melanoma and sarcoma. J Clin Oncol 1992;10:52–60.
118. Didolkar MS, Fitzpatrick JL, Jackson AJ, Johnston GS. Toxicity and complications of vascular isolation and hyperthermic perfusion with imidazole carboxamide (DTIC) in melanoma. Cancer 1986;57:1961–6.
119. van Geel AN, van Wijk J, Wieberdink J. Functional morbidity after regional isolated perfusion of the limb for melanoma. Cancer 1989;63:1092–6.
120. Lazarus HM, Herzig RH, Wolff SN, et al. Treatment of metastatic malignant melanoma with intensive melphalan and autologous bone marrow transplantation. Cancer Treat Rep 1985;69:473–7.
121. Tchekmedyian NS, Tait N, Van Echo D, Aisner J. High-dose chemotherapy without autologous bone marrow transplantation in melanoma. J Clin Oncol 1986;4:1811–8.
122. Wolff SN, Herzig RH, Fay JW, et al. High-dose thiotepa with autologous bone marrow transplantation for metastatic malignant melanoma: results of phase I and II studies of the North American Bone Marrow Transplantation Group. J Clin Oncol 1989;7:245–9.
123. Ciobanu N, Dutcher J, Gucalp R, et al. High dose chemotherapy with autologous bone marrow transplantation (ABMT) for malignant melanoma after failure of interleukin-2 (IL2) and lymphokine activated killer (LAK) cells. Proc ASCO 1989;8:281.
124. van der Bruggen P, Traversari C, Chomez P, et al. A gene encoding an antigen recognized by cytolytic T lymphocytes on a human melanoma. Science 1991;254:1643–7.

125. Morton DL, Ravindranath MH, Irie RF. Tumor gangliosides as targets for active specific immunotherapy of melanoma in man. Prog Brain Res 1994;101:251–75.

126. Morton DL, Eilber FR, Holmes EC, et al. BCG immunotherapy of malignant melanoma: summary of a seven-year experience. Ann Surg 1974;180:635–43.

127. Morton DL, Foshag LJ, Hoon DS, et al. Prolongation of survival in metastatic melanoma after active specific immunotherapy with a new polyvalent melanoma vaccine [published erratum appears in Ann Surg 1993;217:309]. Ann Surg 1992;216:463–82.

128. Mitchell MS, Kan-Mitchell J, Kempf RA, et al. Active specific immunotherapy for melanoma: phase I trial of allogeneic lysates and a novel adjuvant. Cancer Res 1988;48:5883–93.

129. Bystryn JC. Immunogenicity and clinical activity of a polyvalent melanoma antigen vaccine prepared from shed antigens. Ann N Y Acad Sci 1993;690:190–203.

130. Hellström I, Brown JP, Hellström KE. Workshop on monoclonal antibodies to human melanoma-associated antigens: findings of the Seattle group. Hybridoma 1982;1:399–402.

131. Jost LM. Immunotherapy of melanoma. In: Lejeune FJ, ed. Malignant melanoma: medical and surgical management. New York: McGraw-Hill, 1994:303.

132. Dippold WG, Bernhard H, Dienes HP, et al: Immunotherapy in patients with advanced malignant melanoma using monoclonal anti-melanoma antibody ricin A immunotoxin. Eur J Cancer Clin Oncol 1988;24:S65–8.

133. Vadhan-Raj S, Cordon-Cardo C, Carswell E, et al. Phase I trial of a mouse monoclonal antibody against GD3 ganglioside in patients with melanoma: induction of inflammatory responses at tumor sites. J Clin Oncol 1988;6:1636–48.

134. Spitler LE, del Rio M, Khentigan A, et al. Therapy of patients with malignant melanoma using a monoclonal antimelanoma antibody-ricin A chain immunotoxin. Cancer Res 1987;47:1717–23.

135. Stewart T. The interferon system. New York: Academic Press, 1979.

136. Lengyel P. Biochemistry of interferons and their actions. Ann Rev Biochem 1982;51:251–82.

137. Sertoli MR, Bernengo MG, Ardizzoni A, et al. Phase II trial of recombinant alfa-2b interferon in the treatment of metastatic skin melanoma. Oncology 1989;46:96–8.

138. Robinson WA, Mughal TI, Thomas MR, et al. Treatment of metastatic malignant melanoma with recombinant interferon alfa 2. Immunobiology 1986;172:275–82.

139. Dorval T, Palangie T, Jouve M, et al. Clinical phase II trial of recombinant DNA interferon (interferon alfa 2b) in patients with metastatic malignant melanoma. Cancer 1986;58:215–8.

140. Kirkwood JM, Ernstoff MS, Davis CA, et al. Comparison of intramuscular and intravenous recombinant alfa-2 interferon in melanoma and other cancers. Ann Intern Med 1985;103:32–6.

141. von Wussow P, Block B, Hartmann F, Deicher H. Intralesional interferon-alfa therapy in advanced malignant melanoma. Cancer 1988;61:1071–4.

142. Kirkwood JM, Strawderman MH, Ernstoff MS, et al. Interferon alfa-2b adjuvant therapy of high-risk resected cutaneous melanoma: the Eastern Cooperative Oncology Group trial EST 1684. J Clin Oncol 1996;14:7–17.

143. Creagan ET, Dalton RJ, Ahmann DL, et al. Randomized, surgical adjuvant clinical trial of recombinant interferon alfa-2a in selected patients with malignant melanoma. J Clin Oncol 1995;13:2776–83.

144. Cascinelli N. Evaluation of efficacy of adjuant rIFN-2-alfa in melanoma patients with regional node metastases. Proc ASCO 1995;14:410.

145. Grob JJ, Dreno B, Delaunay M, et al. Long-term results of adjuvant therapy with low dose IFN-alfa2A in resected primary melanoma thicker than 1.5 mm without clinically detectable node metastases. Proc ASCO 1998;17:514a.abstract.

146. Pehamberger H, Soyer HP, Steiner A, et al. Adjuvant interferon alfa-2a treatment in resected primary stage II cutaneous melanoma. Austrian Malignant Melanoma Cooperative Group. J Clin Oncol 1998;16:1425–9.

147. Kirkwood JM, Ibrahim J, Sondak V, et al. Preliminary analysis of the E1690/S9111/C9190 intergroup postoperative adjuvant trial of high- and low-dose IFNa2b (HDI and LDI) in high-risk primary or lymph node metastatic melanoma. Proc ASCO 1999;18:437A.abstract 2072.

148. Lotze MT, Chang AE, Seipp CA, et al. High-dose recombinant interleukin 2 in the treatment of patients with disseminated cancer: responses, treatment-related morbidity, and histologic findings. JAMA 1986;256:3117–24.

149. Parkinson DR, Abrams JS, Wiernik PH, et al. Interleukin-2 therapy in patients with metastatic malignant melanoma: a phase II study. J Clin Oncol 1990;8:1650–6.

150. Rosenberg SA, Lotze MT, Yang JC, et al. Prospective randomized trial of high-dose interleukin-2 alone or in conjunction with lymphokine-activated killer cells for the treatment of patients with advanced cancer [published erratum appears in J Natl Cancer Inst 1993; 85:1091]. J Natl Cancer Inst 1993;85:622–32.

151. Spiess PJ, Yang JC, Rosenberg SA: In vivo antitumor activity of tumor-infiltrating lymphocytes expanded in recombinant interleukin-2. J Natl Cancer Inst 1987;79:1067–75.

152. Kradin RL, Kurnick JT, Lazarus DS, et al. Tumour-infiltrating lymphocytes and interleukin-2 in treatment of advanced cancer. Lancet 1989;1:577–80.

153. Sondel PM, Sosman JA, Hank JA, et al. Tumor-infiltrating lymphocytes and interleukin-2 in melanomas. N Engl J Med 1989;320:1418–9. letter.

154. Dillman RO, Oldham RK, Barth NM, et al. Continuous interleukin-2 and tumor-infiltrating lymphocytes as treatment of advanced melanoma: a national biotherapy study group trial. Cancer 1991;68:1–8.

155. Aebersold P, Hyatt C, Johnson S, et al. Lysis of autologous melanoma cells by tumor-infiltrating lymphocytes: association with clinical response. J Natl Cancer Inst 1991;83:932–7.

156. Ruggiero V, Latham K, Baglioni C. Cytostatic and cytotoxic activity of tumor necrosis factor on human cancer cells. J Immunol 1987;138:2711–7.

157. Quan WD Jr, Mitchell MS. Immunology and immunotherapy of melanoma. Cancer Treat Res 1993;65:257–77.

158. Rosenberg SA, Aebersold P, Cornetta K, et al. Gene transfer into humans—immunotherapy of patients with advanced melanoma, using tumor-infiltrating lymphocytes modified by retroviral gene transduction. N Engl J Med 1990;323:570–8.

159. Economou JS, Belldegrun AS, Glaspy J, et al. In vivo trafficking of adoptively transferred interleukin-2 expanded tumor-infiltrating lymphocytes and peripheral blood lymphocytes: results of a double gene marking trial. J Clin Invest 1996;97:515–21.

160. Bretscher P, Cohn M. A theory of self-nonself discrimination. Science 1970;169:1042–9.

161. Huang AY, Golumbek P, Ahmadzadeh M, et al. Role of bone marrow-derived cells in presenting MHC class I-restricted tumor antigens. Science 1994;264:961–5.

162. Boon T, van der Bruggen P. Human tumor antigens recognized by T lymphocytes. J Exp Med 1996;183:725–9.

163. Rosenberg SA, Kawakami Y, Robbins PF, Wang R. Identification of the genes encoding cancer antigens: implications for cancer immunotherapy. Adv Cancer Res 1996;70:145–77.

164. Rosenberg SA, Yang JC, Schwartzentruber DJ, et al. Immunologic and therapeutic evaluation of a synthetic peptide vaccine for the treatment of patients with metastatic melanoma. Nat Med 1998;4:321–7.

165. Banchereau J, Steinman RM. Dendritic cells and the control of immunity. Nature 1998;392:245–52.

166. Nestle FO, Alijagic S, Gilliet M, et al. Vaccination of melanoma patients with peptide- or tumor lysate-pulsed dendritic cells. Nat Med 1998;4:328–32.

167. Rosenberg SA, Zhai Y, Yang JC, et al. Immunizing patients with metastatic melanoma using recombinant adenoviruses encoding MART-1 or gp100 melanoma antigens. J Natl Cancer Inst 1998;90:1894–900.

168. Arthur JF, Butterfield LH, Roth MD, et al. A comparison of gene transfer methods in human dendritic cells. Cancer Gene Ther 1997;4:17–25.

169. Brossart P, Goldrath AW, Butz EA, et al. Virus-mediated delivery of antigenic epitopes into dendritic cells as a means to induce CTL. J Immunol 1997;158:3270–6.

170. Ribas A, Butterfield LH, McBride WH, et al. Genetic immunization for the melanoma antigen MART-1/Melan-A using recombinant adenovirus-transduced murine dendritic cells. Cancer Res 1997;57:2865–9.

171. Specht JM, Wang G, Do MT, et al. Dendritic cells retrovirally transduced with a model antigen gene are therapeutically effective against established pulmonary metastases. J Exp Med 1997;186:1213–21.

172. Song W, Kong HL, Carpenter H, et al. Dendritic cells genetically

modified with an adenovirus vector encoding the cDNA for a model antigen induce protective and therapeutic antitumor immunity. J Exp Med 1997;186:1247–56.

173. Butterfield LH, Jilani SM, Chakraborty NG, et al. Generation of melanoma-specific cytotoxic T lymphocytes by dendritic cells transduced with a MART-1 adenovirus. J Immunol 1998;161:5607–13.

174. Balch CM Soong SJ, Milton GW, et al. Changing trends in cutaneous melanoma over a quarter century in Alabama, USA, and New South Wales, Australia. Cancer 1983;52:1748–53.

175. Pritchard KI, Quirt IC, Cowan DH, et al. DTIC therapy in metastatic malignant melanoma: a simplified dose schedule. Cancer Treat Rep 1980;64:1123–6.

176. Karakousis CP, Lopez RE, Bhakoo HS, et al. Estrogen and progesterone receptors and tamoxifen in malignant melanoma. Cancer Treat Rep 1980;64:819–27.

177. Wagstaff J, Thatcher N, Rankin E, Crowther D. Tamoxifen in the treatment of metastatic malignant melanoma. Cancer Treat Rep 1982;66:1771.

178. Leichman CG, Samson MK, Baker LH. Phase II trial of tamoxifen in malignant melanoma. Cancer Treat Rep 1982;66:1447.

179. Young DW, Lever RS, English JS, MacKie RM. The use of BELD combination chemotherapy (bleomycin, vindesine, CCNU, and DTIC) in advanced malignant melanoma. Cancer 1985;55:1879–81.

180. Rudolf Z, Plesnicar S. Chemotherapy of disseminated malignant melanoma with imidazol carboxamide (DTIC) and cyclophosphamide: preliminary results. Anticancer Res 1982;2:37–9.

181. Carey RW, Anderson JR, Green M, et al. Treatment of metastatic malignant melanoma with vinblastine, dacarbazine, and cisplatin: a report from the Cancer and Leukemia Group B. Cancer Treat Rep 1986;70:329–31.

182. Richman SP, Woodcock TM, Kubota TT, et al. Phase II trial of vinblastine, bleomycin, and cisplatin (VBP) followed by dacarbazine and mitolactol in metastatic melanoma. Cancer Treat Rep 1984; 68:1395–6.

183. Byrne MG, Reynolds PM. Phase II study of cyclophosphamide, vincristine and D.T.I.C. +/− B.C.G. in the treatment of malignant melanoma. Aust N Z J Med 1982;12:260–6.

184. Seigler HF, Lucas VS Jr, Pickett NJ, Huang AT. DTIC, CCNU, bleomycin and vincristine (BOLD) in metastatic melanoma. Cancer 1980;46:2346–8.

185. York RM, Foltz AT. Bleomycin, vincristine, lomustine, and DTIC chemotherapy for metastatic melanoma. Cancer 1986;61:2183–6.

186. Goodnight JE Jr, Moseley HS, Eilber FR, et al. Cis-dichlorodiammine-platinum (II) alone and combined with DTIC for treatment of disseminated malignant melanoma. Cancer Treat Rep 1979;63:2005–7.

187. Karakousis CP, Getaz EP, Bjornsson S, et al: cis-Dichlorodiammine-platinum (II) and DTIC in malignant melanoma. Cancer Treat Rep 1979;63:2009–10.

188. Oratz R, Speyer JL, Green M, et al. Treatment of metastatic malignant melanoma with dacarbazine and cisplatin. Cancer Treat Rep 1987;71:877–8.

189. Fletcher WS, Green S, Fletcher JR, et al. Evaluation of cis-platinum and DTIC combination chemotherapy in disseminated melanoma: a Southwest Oncology Group study. Am J Clin Oncol 1988;11:589–93.

190. Costanzi JJ, Fletcher WS, Balcerzak SP, et al. Combination chemotherapy plus levamisole in the treatment of disseminated malignant melanoma: a Southwest Oncology Group study. Cancer 1984;53:833–6.

191. Verschraegen CF, Kleeberg UR, Mulder J, et al. Combination of cisplatin, vindesine, and dacarbazine in advanced malignant melanoma: a phase II study of the EORTC Malignant Melanoma Cooperative Group. Cancer 1988;62:1061–5.

192. Creagan ET, Schutt AJ, Long HJ, Green SJ. Phase II study: the combination DTIC, BCNU, actinomycin D, and vincristine in disseminated malignant melanoma. Med Pediatr Oncol 1987;14:86–7.

193. Vorobiof DA, Sarli R, Falkson G. Combination chemotherapy with dacarbazine and vindesine in the treatment of metastatic malignant melanoma. Cancer Treat Rep 1986;70:927–8.

194. Gentile PS, Epremian BE, Seeger J, et al. A phase II trial of vinblastine, bleomycin, and cisplatin induction followed by dacarbazine and dibromodulcitol maintenance in the treatment of metastatic melanoma: a follow-up study of twenty-two patients. Am J Clin Oncol 1988;11:666–8.

195. Cohen SM, Ohnuma T, Cheung T, Holland JF. Bleomycin, carmustine, vincristine, and dacarbazine in patients with metastatic malignant melanoma. Cancer Treat Rep 1983;67:947–8.

196. Glover D, Glick JH, Weiler C, et al. WR-2721 and high-dose cisplatin: an active combination in the treatment of metastatic melanoma. J Clin Oncol 1987;5:574–8.

197. Cohen SM, Ohnuma T, Ambinder EP, Holland JF. Lomustine, bleomycin, and cisplatin in patients with metastatic malignant melanoma. Cancer Treat Rep 1986;70:688–9.

198. Nathanson L, Wittenberg BK. Pilot study of vinblastine and bleomycin combination in the treatment of metastatic melanoma. Cancer Treat Rep 1980;64:133–7.

199. Voigt H, Kleeberg UR. PALA, vindesine, and cisplatin combination chemotherapy in advanced malignant melanoma: a pilot study. Cancer 1984;53:2058–62.

200. Ikeda S, Tajima K, Miyasato H, et al. New combination chemotherapy for malignant melanoma—PAV (peplomycin, ACNU, VCR) therapy. Gan To Kagaku Ryoho 1983;10:2198–204.

201. Abele R, Bernheim J, Cumps E, et al. Re-evaluation of the combination of CCNU, vincristine, and bleomycin in the treatment of malignant disseminated melanoma. Cancer Treat Rep 1981;65:505–6.

202. Green MR, Dillman RO, Horton C. Procarbazine, vincristine, CCNU, and cyclophosphamide (POCC) in the treatment of metastatic malignant melanoma. Cancer Treat Rep 1980;64:139–42.

203. Carmo-Pereira J, Costa FO, Pimentel P, Henriques E. Combination cytotoxic chemotherapy with CCNU, procarbazine, and vincristine in disseminated cutaneous malignant melanoma: 3 years' follow-up. Cancer Treat Rep 1980;64:143–5.

204. Carmo-Periera J, Costa FO, Henriques E. Combination cytotoxic chemotherapy with procarbazine, vincristine, and lomustine (POC) in disseminated malignant melanoma: 8 years' follow-up. Cancer Treat Rep 1984;68:1211–4.

205. Shelley W, Quirt I, Bodurtha A, et al. Lomustine, vincristine, and procarbazine in the treatment of metastatic malignant melanoma. Cancer Treat Rep 1985;69:941–4.

206. Repetto L, Grimaldi A, Ardizzoni A, et al. Metastatic malignant melanoma treated with procarbazine, vincristine, and lomustine (POC). Chemioterapia 1987;6:63–5.

207. Bajetta E, Buzzoni R, Viviani S, et al. Prospective randomized trial in advanced malignant melanoma with cis-platinum, vindesine, and etoposide vs. cis-platinum, vindesine, and lomustine. Am J Clin Oncol 1985;8:401–5.

208. Johnson DH, Presant C, Einhorn L, et al. Cisplatin, vinblastine, and bleomycin in the treatment of metastatic melanoma: a phase II study of the Southeastern Cancer Study Group. Cancer Treat Rep 1985;69:821–4.

209. Nathanson L, Kaufman SD, Carey RW. Vinblastine, infusion, bleomycin, and cis-dichlorodiammine-platinum chemotherapy in metastatic melanoma. Cancer 1981;48:1290–4.

210. York RM, Lawson DH, McKay J. Treatment of metastatic malignant melanoma with vinblastine, bleomycin by infusion, and cisplatin. Cancer 1983;52:2220–2.

211. Creagan ET, Ahmann DL, Schutt AJ, Green SJ. Phase II study of the combination of vinblastine, bleomycin, and cisplatin in advanced malignant melanoma. Cancer Treat Rep 1982;66:567–9.

212. Bleehen NM, Roberts JT, Newman HF. A phase II study of CCNU with benznidazole for metastatic malignant melanoma. Int J Radiat Oncol Biol Phys 1986;12:1401–3.

213. Mulder JH, Dodion P, Cavalli F, et al. Cisplatin and vindesine combination chemotherapy in advanced malignant melanoma: an EORTC phase II study. Eur J Cancer Clin Oncol 1982;18:1297–301.

214. Clamon G, Sinkey C, Jochimsen P. Phase II study of dibromodulcitol and BCNU in metastatic malignant melanoma. Am J Clin Oncol 1985;8:244–6.

215. Morton RF, Creagan ET, Veeder MH, et al. Phase II study of the combination of carmustine and 6-thioguanine in advanced malignant melanoma. Cancer Treat Rep 1987;71:429–30.

216. Bajetta E, Verusio C, Bonfante V, Bonadonna G. Cytarabine and cisplatin in advanced malignant melanoma. Cancer Treat Rep 1986;70:1441–2.

217. Yee C, Gilbert MJ, Riddell SR, et al. Isolation of tyrosinase-specific CD8+ and D4+ T cell clones from the peripheral blood of melanoma patients following in vitro stimulation with recombinant vaccinia virus. J Immunol 1996;157:4079–86.

# CHAPTER 75

# MALIGNANT MELANOMA OF THE EYE

● ROBERT E. ENGSTROM, JR. ● HECTOR L. SULIT
● BRADLEY R. STRAATSMA

Uveal melanoma is the most frequent primary, life-threatening, intraocular tumor encountered by ophthalmologists in adults. The overall incidence of intraocular melanoma in the United States and Europe is about 5 to 7.5/million per year. This figure increases sharply after the age of 50 to about 21/million per year. It is overwhelmingly a disease that afflicts white individuals, who account for 97% of all patients with uveal melanoma. In the Collaborative Ocular Melanoma Study (COMS) enucleation specimens confirmed uveal melanoma in other ethnic populations in the following frequency: Hispanic, 2.1%; African American, 0.5%; Asian or Pacific Islanders, 0.3%; and Native Americans, 0.2%.[1] The median patient age at diagnosis is 60 years.

Ocular malignant melanoma may arise from any of the different structures of the eye that contain stromal melanocytes. The most common location is in the uveal tissue, which is composed of the choroid, ciliary body, and iris, in descending order of frequency of involvement. Primary melanoma of the ocular adnexa, conjunctiva, and orbit is rare.

## Classification of Uveal Melanoma

In 1931, Callender published a classification system for uveal melanoma based on cellular characteristics and prognosis following enucleation.[2] The Callender classification was subsequently modified by McLean and associates[3] at the Armed Forces Institute of Pathology (AFIP) to consist of spindle cell nevus, spindle cell malignant melanoma, mixed cell melanoma, and epithelioid cell melanoma. This modification resulted in a more precise classification of melanoma cells and improved the accuracy of predicting clinical outcomes. Technologic advances have led to a description of other features of uveal melanoma that may have prognostic significance including nucleolar area,[4] nucleolar organizer regions,[5] tumor vascular patterns,[6] and tumor vascular density.[7] Preoperative angiographic[8] and ultrasonographic assessment[9, 10] may provide clinically useful information in identifying patients at higher risk of developing metastatic disease based on the in vivo identification of microvascular anomalies.

## Diagnostic Studies for Uveal Melanoma

### ANGIOGRAPHY

Both fluorescein and indocyanine green (ICG) angiography are useful in establishing an accurate diagnosis of uveal melanoma. By defining the vascular patterns of a suspicious lesion, fluorescein angiography helps differentiate a benign from a malignant chorioretinal mass. Malignant melanoma typically exhibits a double circulation with early hyperfluorescent mottling and punctate areas of dye leakage in the late phases of the study. Metastatic carcinoma to the choroid can also present with similar angiographic features. ICG angiography allows visualization through the retinal pigment epithelium (which blocks fluorescein transmission) highlighting the deeper choroidal vascular components of choroidal melanoma. Lesions that receive their vascular supply directly from the choroid (such as choroidal melanoma and choroidal hemangioma) demonstrate early hyperfluorescence with late staining. A characteristic surrounding halo of hypofluorescence can be seen in the middle to late stages of the ICG angiogram and is suggestive of choroidal melanoma. This angiographic appearance may represent a vascular "steal" phenomenon from adjacent choroidal vessels.[11] High-resolution confocal ICG angiography with scanning laser ophthalmoscopy may provide even more detailed information of the internal vascular characteristics of choroidal melanoma that may prove to be of prognostic significance.[8]

### ULTRASONOGRAPHY

Diagnostic A and B scan ultrasonography further enhances diagnostic accuracy by demonstrating the internal acoustic properties of the mass. The A scan shows choroidal melanoma as an elevated area with a sharp anterior border and low internal spike motions in a linear graphic display. The B scan gives a two-dimensional picture of the echo patterns of the tissue encountered. Choroidal melanoma is characterized by internal hollowing, choroidal excavation, and orbital shadowing. Dynamic internal characteristics of the tumor during B scan ultrasonography allow subjective assessment of tumor vascularity. Ultrasonography is less reliable when the tumor height is less than 2 mm. Ultrasonographic biomicroscopy uses a high-frequency probe that limits the depth of tissue penetration but provides enhanced resolution of anterior ocular structures. Ultrasonographic biomicroscopy is particularly valuable in establishing the anterior extent of ciliary body or anterior choroidal melanoma[12] or the posterior extent of iris melanoma. Newer generations of three-dimensional ultrasonography may allow for in vivo quantitative volumetric assessment of tumor growth, for internal vascular characteristics that may be prognostically important (such as scatterers indicative of vascular loops or networks),[9, 10] and for monitoring tumor shrinkage after treatment. Newer imaging techniques using optical coherence tomography and scanning laser topographic imaging may also prove useful in monitoring for subtle growth of tumors located in and around the macula and optic nerve head.

## RADIOGRAPHIC IMAGING

Neuroimaging, including computed tomography (CT)[13, 14] and high-resolution orbital magnetic resonance imaging (MRI),[15, 16] may allow preoperative detection of transscleral tumor extension and may also be useful in the diagnosis of patients with visually dense media opacities that preclude direct visualization of the tumor by ophthalmoscopy or angiography. If ultrasonography suggests possible extrascleral extension of the tumor, CT or MRI may provide enhanced orbital detection of tumor spread that would be important from a surgical treatment perspective. With thin sectioning or high-resolution scans using surface coils, both CT and MRI can detect lesions as small as 2 mm in height. The differential radiographic appearance of melanoma compared with the water-rich vitreous or orbital fat can be useful in establishing the diagnosis of uveal melanoma in difficult cases. Ultrasonography is generally more reliable, and less expensive, for establishing the diagnosis of intraocular tumors. CT or MRI of the abdomen is recommended for preoperative metastatic evaluation.

## Risk Factors for Ocular Melanoma

The biologic and histopathologic characteristics of ocular melanoma differ significantly from those of cutaneous melanoma, suggesting that these two conditions should be considered different diseases.[17] A number of risk factors, including genetic predisposition, race, iris color, exposure to sunlight, history of atypical cutaneous nevi, and occupational exposure, have been investigated. Although these studies are informative, they are not definitive.

### GENETICS

In a series of articles assessing the familial risk for uveal melanoma, Singh and colleagues found that first-degree relatives of a proband patient with uveal melanoma had a 21-fold increased likelihood of developing uveal melanoma compared with the general population.[18] Familial uveal melanoma occurs in up to 0.6% of patients diagnosed with uveal melanoma, and two thirds of these patients have an affected first-degree relative.[19] Furthermore, although exceptionally rare (occurring in only 8 cases of 4500 reviewed), bilateral primary uveal melanoma occurs more frequently than would be expected on the basis of chance alone, suggesting a genetic predisposition in these individuals.[20] Cases of bilateral uveal melanoma were not related to familial cases but did demonstrate a greater association with ocular melanocytosis.

Cytogenetic abnormalities of uveal melanoma characterized by monosomy 3 and trisomy 8q have been shown to increase the rate of developing metastatic disease, suggesting that chromosomal aberrations may contribute to the lethality

of uveal melanoma.[21, 22] Although present in up to 50% of all cancers, alteration of p53 (a tumor-suppressor gene) is uncommon in uveal melanoma.[23] Furthermore, although mutations in the p16 gene are present in up to one half of patients with familial predisposition to cutaneous melanoma, this mutation has not been associated with uveal melanoma, suggesting that different genetic mechanisms are responsible for these two forms of melanoma.[17]

### ULTRAVIOLET IRRADIATION AND EYE COLOR

Sunlight exposure is a recognized and accepted risk factor for the development of cutaneous melanoma; however, its role in the development of uveal melanoma remains controversial. Tucker and colleagues in 1985 described a case-control study of 444 patients with uveal melanoma and found a 2.7 increased relative risk for the development of uveal melanoma for persons born in the southern United States.[24] They also found that individuals with blue irises were 1.7 times more likely to develop uveal melanoma than brown-eyed individuals. Similar findings have been described by Holly and associates, who found an association between uveal melanoma and blue irises, as well as exposure to intense ultraviolet light resulting in sunburn or following accidental exposure to welding burns or snowblindness.[25] The findings of Tucker and colleagues have been questioned on the basis of statistical bias,[26] and other investigators have failed to identify an increased risk of sunlight exposure to uveal melanoma.[27, 28]

### DYSPLASTIC NEVI

Controversy exists regarding the relationship between dysplastic nevi and uveal melanoma. Dysplastic nevi have been associated with an increased likelihood of ocular nevi (conjunctival, iris, and choroid), as well as uveal melanoma.[29, 30] This association, however, has not been universally observed.[31]

### OCCUPATIONAL RISKS

Case-control studies have been performed that appear to link occupations in agriculture or farming with an increased risk for the development of uveal melanoma.[32] Other individuals with intense exposure to ultraviolet light (see preceding discussion), welding, and asbestos, as well as those involved with chemical use may also be at increased risk for melanoma.[33, 34] The actual number of cases of uveal melanoma associated with occupational exposures that present each year is unknown.

## Clinical Features and Diagnosis

### EYELID MELANOMA

Malignant neoplasms of the eyelid are composed almost exclusively of basal cell and squamous cell carcinomas.

Malignant melanoma of the eyelid occurs at an annual rate of only 0.6 per million white patients.[35] Malignant melanoma of the eyelid skin exhibits a similar clinical appearance and biologic behavior to cutaneous melanoma elsewhere. An alteration in pigmentation or growth in a previously stable pigmented lesion may indicate malignant development. The diagnosis is based on clinical appearance, and suspicious lesions should be either followed closely or excised for histopathologic confirmation.

## CONJUNCTIVAL MELANOMA

Conjunctival nevus is the most common conjunctival melanocytic lesion. These benign lesions may demonstrate rapid cystoid degeneration, suggesting malignant transformation. Conjunctival melanoma is suggested by an absence of cystoid degenerative changes or the presence of dense vascularization, pigmentation, or growth. Conjunctival melanoma may present as a single nodular lesion or as diffuse, multifocal disease. Treatment and prognosis depend strongly on tumor location, discrete or diffuse distribution, and the degree of underlying scleral invasion.

## IRIS MELANOMA

Iris melanoma accounts for between 3% and 10% of patients with ocular melanoma. The inferior iris is involved in up to 80% of patients, suggesting a possible causative relationship to ultraviolet radiation exposure.[24] It may present as a localized or diffuse pigmented lesion associated with distortion of the pupil (corectopia), eversion of the pupillary margin (ectropion uveae), neovascularization, infiltration into the chamber angle structures, elevation of intraocular pressure, and sector cataract formation where the mass contacts the lens.

Unlike melanoma of the eyelid, conjunctiva, ciliary body, or choroid, iris melanoma is biologically more benign and can remain stable over a long period of follow-up. Clinical features suggestive of iris melanoma include a basal diameter greater than 3 mm, pigment dispersion, prominent tumor vascularity, elevated intraocular pressure, and tumor-related symptoms.[36] Excision of iris lesions with these characteristics revealed a diagnostic accuracy for melanoma of 89%. Of pigmented iris lesions not possessing these features on initial presentation, only 6% demonstrated growth within 5 years. Lesions with larger basal diameters at presentation were most likely to show future growth.

## CILIARY BODY MELANOMA

Malignant melanoma in the ciliary body may first become clinically apparent from its extension into the iris root, choroid, or episclera. The lens may be displaced, resulting in irregular lenticular astigmatism and blurred vision. Blurred vision may also result from regional dysfunction of the infiltrated ciliary body with associated localized impairment of accommodation. Unexplained blurred vision with increasing astigmatic refractive error should prompt a dilated fundus examination. Ciliary body melanomas may present

at a more advanced stage because of the clinically silent nature of lesions arising from this anatomic location within the eye. Tumor exudation from a ciliary body melanoma typically drains through the normal anterior segment structures rather than producing a visually symptomatic retinal detachment, which can delay diagnosis. Sectorial cataract may develop through physical contact of the lens with the ciliary body mass.

## CHOROIDAL MELANOCYTIC LESIONS

**Choroidal Nevus.** Because of its importance in the differential diagnosis of choroidal melanoma, it is valuable to highlight the seminal clinical features of choroidal nevus. This lesion is present in 3% of eyes in clinical series and in up to 6.5% of eyes in autopsy series.[37] Although progenitor cells likely exist at birth, choroidal nevi are uncommon until the onset of puberty.[38] Assuming that all cases of choroidal melanoma arise from choroidal nevi, it has been estimated that only 1 in 5000 individuals with choroidal nevi will develop choroidal melanoma over a 10-year period.[39] Appropriate follow-up includes fundus photography to establish baseline appearance, with annual assessment thereafter. More suspicious nevi (larger basal size or height, associated yellow or orange pigment, drusen, or associated collection of subretinal fluid) should be followed every 6 months to monitor for growth.[40]

**Choroidal Melanoma.** Malignant melanoma of the choroid usually appears as a dome- or mushroom-shaped, grayish brown choroidal mass. Exudative retinal detachment adjacent to or remote from the tumor is a hallmark finding. Lipofuscin granules, representing degenerated retinal pigment epithelium and neurosensory retina, appear as fleck-shaped orange pigmentation on the tumor surface. Lipofuscin may not always be detectable on clinical examination.

Melanoma of both the ciliary body and choroid are best visualized clinically by indirect ophthalmoscopy and contact lens biomicroscopy. Transscleral transillumination facilitates the differentiation of potentially degenerative cystic or hemorrhagic lesions from vascularized malignant lesions. Most choroidal melanomas are diagnosed accurately by clinical appearance combined with adjunctive diagnostic testing. Choroidal melanoma located posterior to the equator of the globe usually causes visual symptoms early in development. Melanoma of the anterior choroid or ciliary body may be clinically silent, allowing larger growth prior to detection. The fellow eye should be thoroughly examined to ascertain its functional status and to look for clues (such as degenerative disease) that may suggest the nature of the suspicious lesion in the involved eye.

A clinical subset of choroidal melanoma includes diffuse choroidal melanoma.[41] This variant composes only 3% of cases of choroidal melanoma and is characterized by predominantly marginal expansion rather than vertical growth. There is also a tendency for these lesions to occur around the optic nerve head. Recognition of this variant is important because delay in diagnosis and treatment can adversely affect prognosis. Careful monitoring of all lesion borders through serial fundus photography is essential in assessing growth.

If the diagnosis of uveal melanoma remains clinically indeterminate, fine-needle aspiration biopsy (FNAB) may be used successfully to arrive at the correct diagnosis with minimal reported ocular morbidity.[42–44] Routine FNAB during surgical plaque placement can provide prognostic information by permitting cellular classification of the tumor,[45] and it resulted in a change in surgical treatment in 9% of patients at one center.[43]

Transretinal biopsies are performed following a limited pars plana vitrectomy overlying the tumor, followed by penetration of the choroidal mass with a 25- to 30-gauge needle under direct visualization and high aspiration. Transscleral biopsies are performed after defining the tumor margins by transpupillary transillumination. A partial-thickness scleral flap is constructed in an area corresponding to the central aspect of the tumor. Both biopsy approaches use repeated core aspirations by performing a piston-like movement of the embedded needle tip within the tumor under high aspiration. Vacuum aspiration is allowed to equilibrate completely prior to needle removal to avoid aspiration of irrigation fluid (transretinal route) or air (transscleral route) into the needle hub. Intraocular pressure should be increased to minimize bleeding by either route, and the scleral flap overlying the biopsy site is sutured closed to avoid tumor seeding. Plaque placement is then performed overlying the base of the tumor in standard fashion. The expertise of a cytopathologist familiar with ocular tissue and tumor cell morphology is essential to accurate FNAB diagnosis.

Lesions simulating choroidal melanoma include age-related extramacular disciform degeneration with or without intralesional or subretinal hemorrhage, choroidal nevus, metastatic tumors to the choroid, discrete choroidal hemangioma, or localized pigmentary abnormalities of the retinal pigment epithelium including chorioretinal inflammatory disease or congenital hypertrophy of the retinal pigment epithelium.[46]

## Diagnostic Assessment Following Ocular Diagnosis

A general medical evaluation is mandatory whenever a malignant intraocular tumor is suspected. The discovery of an extraocular metastasis or a primary site elsewhere, together with other general health problems, would certainly influence treatment decisions. Uveal melanoma spreads preferentially to the liver. The medical work-up should include a careful history and physical examination; complete blood count; liver enzyme testing, including gamma-glutamyl-transpeptidase[47]; urinalysis; and chest radiography. Patients with large choroidal melanomas, tumors that involve the ciliary body, or abnormal liver enzymes should also be evaluated with radiographic or ultrasonographic imaging of the liver to detect possible metastatic disease. Metastatic uveal melanoma is detected in up to 2.5% of patients during the initial surveillance following a clinical diagnosis of ocular melanoma without other known systemic dissemination.[48]

## Treatment of Ocular Melanoma

### EYELID MELANOMA

For melanoma of the eyelid skin, wide local excision, possibly combined with contiguous resection of lymphatics and regional lymph nodes, is recommended.[49] It is estimated that about 30% of patients with malignant melanoma of the skin and the conjunctiva have metastasis to the regional lymphatics.

### CONJUNCTIVAL MELANOMA

Malignant melanoma of the conjunctiva is rare. Treatment has consisted of surgical excision ranging from local excision to orbital exenteration. The treatment is strongly dependent on the location and distribution of suspicious tumor sites. Favorable locations include the limbal and bulbar conjunctiva; unfavorable locations include the palpebral conjunctiva, fornices, caruncle, and plica semilunares.[50]

Techniques of surgical excision include removal of the entire mass with a margin of normal-appearing tissue. If the lesion is located at the limbus, or if it extends onto the cornea, a corneal epitheliectomy combined with a partial lamellar scleroconjunctivectomy followed by supplemental cryotherapy should be used.[51] Wide local excisions with supplemental cryotherapy are necessary for conjunctival melanoma located away from the corneoscleral limbus.

Lommatzsch treated 66 patients with conjunctival melanoma using a strontium 90–yttrium 90 beta-ray applicator.[52] A daily dose of 10 Gy, up to a total of 150 to 200 Gy, was given, with 77% of patients showing tumor regression or no growth during a 3- to 10-year follow-up period.

If regional spread of conjunctival melanoma is detected within parotid gland lymph nodes, a radical en bloc dissection of the orbital contents, parotid gland, and regional lymphatics is recommended.[53]

### IRIS MELANOMA

Suspected iris melanoma is usually managed by clinical observation. If growth or change in the lesion is documented, iridectomy with removal of the involved iris is usually performed. There is a risk of disseminating tumor cells into the extrabulbar tissues during excision, so utmost care should be taken throughout the procedure to avoid direct instrument disruption of the mass. The prognosis of iris melanoma is much better than that of choroidal melanoma with a 3% metastatic risk.[54] If iris melanoma extends into the anterior chamber angle structures, en bloc excision with partial-thickness corneoscleral resection and iridocyclectomy, or full-thickness excision followed by tectonic grafting, is required.[55] Brachytherapy with iodine 125 ($^{125}$I) or palladium 103 ($^{103}$Pd) has also been shown to be successful when placed over the corneoscleral junction to treat iris and ciliary body lesions.[56] The cornea demonstrates great resiliency in recovering from this local irradiation insult, but iris neovascularization may occur with neovascular glaucoma, and cataract is also common.

### CILIARY BODY MELANOMA

Ciliary body melanoma that involves fewer than 3 clock hours may be managed by local resection or radiation therapy, but the relative advantages of these treatment modalities are unclear when outcomes are analyzed.[57] Ciliary body tumors that involve more than 4 clock hours are usually better treated by enucleation because of the attendant high complication rate associated with any of the conservative management approaches. Local resection of ciliary body melanomas, with or without the iris or choroid, may be an en bloc or full-thickness procedure with corneal or scleral graft or partial-thickness, lamellar excision.[58] Histopathologic data demonstrate the presence of microscopic tumor spread within the sclera in up to two thirds of eyes and may explain the high rate of local recurrence following resection techniques.[59] Wide surgical margins in these globe-sparing procedures may result in substantial visual morbidity.

## CHOROIDAL MELANOMA

In the clinical setting, management decisions applied to uveal melanoma are influenced by a variety of factors. Among these are the tumor size and anatomic location within the eye; the condition of the fellow eye; the patient's medical history and current health, age, and personal treatment preferences; and the treatment modalities and expertise available at the treatment medical center. Tumor size is the strongest single factor affecting treatment recommendations.

The preoperative diagnostic accuracy of choroidal melanoma has improved over the past two decades. Historically, about 20% of eyes enucleated for suspected choroidal malignant melanoma were found to contain benign simulating lesions. This error has been reduced to less than 1% in most centers because of increased clinical experience, routine use of multiple examination techniques, and the preoperative use of contemporary diagnostic studies.[1, 60]

Histopathologic analysis of the 1527 eyes enucleated in both the medium and large tumor trials of the COMS has been reported.[1] Tumor invasion of the sclera was present in 55% of eyes (preoperative extrascleral extension was an exclusion criterion for the COMS), retinal invasion was seen in 49%, and malignant cells in the vitreous were present in 25% of eyes.

**Small Choroidal Melanoma.** Small choroidal melanoma is defined as melanoma measuring less than 10 mm in basal diameter and less than 2.5 mm in elevation. Simulating lesions are an important consideration when deciding whether a patient with a presumed small choroidal melanoma should be treated. It is generally believed that a brief period of observation does not significantly affect patient survival, as the size of the majority of these tumors remains stable over 5 years. Approximately one third of small choroidal melanomas demonstrate growth after 5 years of follow-up.[61] Identification of features predictive of growth, and of subsequent development of metastatic disease, is helpful in selecting appropriate patients for early treatment. Because growth of small choroidal melanoma has been associated with a sixfold increase in metastatic risk, it is important to recognize these clinical features. Prognostic features for potential growth include greater initial tumor thickness, presence of retinal detachment or subretinal fluid, presence of orange pigment over the tumor surface, and visual symptoms associated with the tumor.[62] Clinical features suggestive of a stable lesion include presence of drusen, adjacent or overlying retinal pigment epithelial atrophy, and presence of intra-

retinal pigment migration. Angiography is important in the assessment of small melanocytic lesions of the choroid because ultrasonography of small lesions is less reliable.

Once a diagnosis of primary malignant uveal melanoma is made, small, active melanomas can be treated by either radiation or enucleation. Various alternative treatments designed to offer better vision preservation have been suggested for the treatment of small choroidal melanoma, including laser photocoagulation (transpupillary thermotherapy [TTT]), radiation using lower energy radioisotopes ($^{103}$Pd), and adjunctive microwave thermal treatment, which allows lower radiation dosages to be effective. These experimental techniques are discussed later in this chapter.

**Medium Choroidal Melanoma.** These melanomas are defined as having a basal diameter of up to 16 mm and a height between 2.5 and 10 mm. The best treatment for medium-sized choroidal melanomas that also provides the longest metastatic-free survival remains unknown.[63, 64] Enucleation was the accepted standard treatment until radiotherapy was recognized as an alternative that allowed preservation of the eye while achieving local tumor control. Long-term patient survival is the primary goal by which the success of any treatment for uveal melanoma should be measured. If the globe is preserved, long-term visual retention is the secondary goal that is used as a gauge of treatment success. No study has demonstrated in a prospective, randomized manner any survival advantage of enucleation over radiation therapy in the treatment of choroidal melanoma.

The COMS is a prospective, randomized study designed to evaluate patients with medium-sized choroidal melanoma treated by either enucleation or $^{125}$I brachytherapy. Recruitment into this trial was completed in July 1998, and meaningful results should become available as adequate numbers of patients complete at least 5 years of follow-up.

## ENUCLEATION

Until the results of controlled trials are known, controversy will continue regarding the advantages or disadvantages of enucleation and radiation therapy for melanoma. A survival benefit from early enucleation has been suggested by many investigators,[65–67] Conversely, it has also been suggested that enucleation does not improve survival and may in fact even contribute to an increase in the mortality rate observed during the 3-year period after surgery.[68, 69] This perceived enhanced mortality following enucleation was attributed to either tumor cell dispersion encountered during surgical manipulation or an alteration in the host immune state, allowing cellular proliferation. This "Zimmerman hypothesis" was subsequently challenged on the basis of statistical bias, with analysis of the same data set revealing an increased death rate from metastatic disease in years 2 to 5 rather than in the first year after surgery as was suggested by Zimmerman and colleagues.[69] These findings were similar to those observed in the natural history of other forms of cancer and did not support a deleterious effect of enucleation surgery on survival.

Tumor cells may be released into the bloodstream in greater numbers during the handling of the globe undergoing enucleation. Various modifications of the surgical technique for enucleation have been developed to minimize globe manipulation and hence possible tumor cell dissemination. One group of investigators developed a "no-touch" technique of enucleation, whereby the globe is frozen with liquid nitrogen running through silicon tubing applied around the eye before excision.[71]

Current enucleation technique usually uses replacement of orbital volume with porous integrated orbital implants. These implants become vascularized from the orbital tissue and provide improved motility when integrated with the extraocular muscles. Complications following placement of integrated orbital implants occur in less than 1% of patients and consist primarily of anterior exposure of the implant or infection.[72]

## RADIATION THERAPY

Radiation therapy for choroidal melanoma offers a globe-sparing alternative to enucleation. A comprehensive review of the history and indications of radiotherapy for the treatment of choroidal melanoma has been published.[73] Radiation can be administered via placement of an ophthalmic plaque (brachytherapy) containing a radioactive isotope of [125]I, [103]Pd, or ruthenium-106 ([106]Ru) sutured to the scleral surface immediately external to the base of the intraocular tumor. Because the source of radiation is placed immediately adjacent to the tumor, deleterious effects of radiation on normal ocular structures are minimized but not eliminated. Teletherapy is an alternative route of radiation delivery using either charged-particle (external beam) proton or helium ions.[74–76] Choroidal melanoma cells are resistant to conventional external-beam radiation therapy at dosages that do not destroy the associated ocular structures within the radiation zone.

The radioisotope [125]I has shown theoretical and biologic advantages over the other radioactive sources used previously.[77, 78] It is a low-energy, gamma-emitting isotope that can be shielded easily with thin metal plaques and has its energies directed toward the tumor, with minimal exposure of adjacent normal tissues and personnel handling the material. Despite the fact that the energy level is lower than that of cobalt 60, [125]I is more effective in killing tumor cells because of its higher relative biologic efficiency. The recommended apical tumor dose is 100 Gy. The main problem with this artificial isotope is the difficulty in dosimetry because of the low energy emitted.

Radiation with proton and helium ion charged particles (external beam) is delivered to the tumor externally through air from a cyclotron. These particles have a "Bragg peak" of ionization so that radiation energy is maximized at the end of the beam range. The Bragg peak, which has very well defined lateral and distal margins, can be focused precisely to a localized area by modulating the beam at its energy source. When the radiation is delivered uniformly to the tumor, the normal tissues laterally at a distance of 3 mm are spared. However, because of the cylindrical radiation field necessary for treatment, and because the radiation field must pass through the anterior structures of the eye for tumors of the posterior globe, up to 70% of the dose delivered to the tumor will also be absorbed by the lids, cornea, and lens.[73] As lesions treated approach the anterior segment of the eye, the shift in the targeted zone results in even greater radiation dosages being delivered to these otherwise normal structures.

All the reported forms of radiotherapy for ocular melanoma are effective in controlling local tumor growth. Rates of local control of the tumor are dependent on the radiation dose, dose rate, tumor location, and length of follow-up. Rates also vary among centers using the same isotope for treatment. Pooling of data from reports with comparable dose delivery (84 Gy) and follow-up reveal an average local tumor control rate of 93%, a secondary enucleation rate of 16%, and a retained visual acuity equal to or better than 20/200 in at least 45% of patients.[73]

Resolution of the exudative retinal detachment within the first 6 months after treatment is usually the first evidence of a successful tumor response. Tumor thickness gradually decreases, but only a few tumors totally regress. A rapid decrease in tumor height after treatment may actually indicate a poor prognosis, as this may reflect a biologically more active tumor with a greater risk for metastatic spread.[79] The absence of continued tumor growth is generally accepted as local tumor control. One or 2 years after treatment, a dark, charcoal-like, shrunken mass is usually seen in place of the original lesion in successfully treated cases. Radiation response is monitored every few months by indirect ophthalmoscopy, biomicroscopy, and ultrasonography.

Ocular complications following radiation therapy are common. The type of ocular complication is affected by the route of radiation delivery. Anterior segment structures are often affected by external-beam radiotherapy, resulting in cataract, neovascular glaucoma, keratopathy, dry eye problems due to damage to the main and accessory lacrimal glands, eyelid erythema, growth abnormality or loss of eyelashes, and punctal occlusions. Ninety percent of patients with large tumors and associated retinal detachment not amenable to plaque therapy who underwent proton-beam radiotherapy developed iris neovascularization within 4 years of treatment.[80] One third of these patients eventually required enucleation to manage ocular pain. Delivery of external radiotherapy through two ports may allow reduced anterior segment absorption, thereby decreasing some of the morbidity unique to this treatment approach.[81]

Radioactive plaque complications such as severe radiation retinopathy, papillitis, and maculopathy occur more commonly when the tumor is located posterior to the equator of the globe. Anterior lesions treated with plaque have a higher rate of cataract formation and anterior segment complications, including neovascular glaucoma that may require secondary enucleation in up to a third of patients.

## Prognostic Features of Uveal Melanoma

Investigators have scrutinized the various clinical and histopathologic features that may influence the prognosis of ciliary body and choroidal malignant melanoma.[82] The size of the tumor is the single most important prognostic factor, with larger tumors having a worse prognosis. Larger tumors are also less likely to be composed of predominantly spindle cells when compared with medium-sized tumors and are more likely to involve the anterior choroid and ciliary body.

Melanoma features that have been suggested as important in the development of metastatic disease include the number of epithelioid cells per high-power field greater than 2, the lower inverse standard deviation of nucleolar areas,[83] and the tumor's anterior border location beyond the equator. Cytomorphometric analysis has also found prognostic significance in the standard deviation of nuclear area and mean of the largest 10 nucleoli as they correlate with the modified Callender classification.[84]

In 1993, Folberg and colleagues[6] suggested that histopathologic features of choroidal melanoma consisting of microvascular networks and parallel vessels with cross-linking possessed independent prognostic significance for metastatic death from uveal melanoma. These features are unique to uveal melanoma and have not been found in benign melanocytic nevi.[85] The prognostic value of this microvascular classification of uveal melanoma has been expanded to include quantification of tumor area[86] and microvessel density.[7] These risk factors have not been supported in histopathologic studies from patients enrolled in prospective, randomized trials and therefore should be interpreted with caution.

Growth of uveal melanoma through the eye wall (extrascleral extension) portends a poor prognosis.[87] Although more common in larger choroidal melanomas, extrascleral extension has also been reported in patients with small tumors.[88] Ultrasonographic "pseudoextension" of uveal melanoma may occur in up to 9% of patients and is more common in lesions adjacent to the optic nerve or extraocular muscles.[89] Patients who demonstrate possible extrascleral extension by ultrasonography should be evaluated by orbital MRI to further confirm this finding.[90, 91]

If extrascleral extension is confirmed during surgery, gross debulking of any orbital tumor is recommended. Postoperative external beam radiotherapy can be considered, but orbital exenteration has not demonstrated a survival advantage.[92] The prognostic significance of the Callender classification system applies only to choroidal and ciliary body melanoma without extrascleral extension.

# Mortality from Ocular Melanoma

## CONJUNCTIVAL MELANOMA

The mortality rates from conjunctival malignant melanoma depend on tumor location. Tumors located in an unfavorable location (anywhere except in an epibulbar location) have a 2.2-fold increased mortality. Mixed cell tumors also have a 3-fold increased mortality when compared with spindle cell conjunctival melanoma, and multifocal tumors demonstrate a 5-fold increased mortality compared with single tumors. Tumor thickness is only prognostically important if location, cell type, and number of lesions are also unfavorable. Overall, the 5-year survival rate is between 83 and 86%,[50, 93] with 10-year survival rates decreasing to between 69% and 73%.

## IRIS MELANOMA

Most melanocytic iris tumors are benign and do not enlarge appreciably during long periods of follow-up. Clinical features predictive of iris melanoma and possible growth were outlined previously. Mortality from metastatic iris melanoma is low, probably because of early detection and the predomi-

nance of spindle cell composition. Metastatic disease from iris melanoma is estimated at 3% and occurred most commonly when tumor excision was incomplete or the tumor was inadvertently transected during removal.[54] The mean time to development of metastatic disease following histologic diagnosis has been reported at 6.5 years, but 5- and 10-year survival rates cannot be accurately determined because of the infrequent nature of this condition.

## CHOROIDAL MELANOMA

An estimate of postenucleation 5-year mortality rates by tumor size was made by pooled analysis of design-comparable publications between 1966 and 1988.[94] The combined weighted mortality estimates were 16% for small tumors, 32% for medium tumors, and 53% for large tumors. Subsequent data from prospective, randomized trials have demonstrated a 5-year all-cause mortality of 6% in patients with small choroidal melanoma.[95] Patients with large choroidal melanoma were found to have a 5-year all-cause mortality of 43% following enucleation alone. Patients who received pre-enucleation radiation therapy had significantly lower mitotic activity within their tumors and a 5-year all-cause mortality of 38%, which was not statistically significant compared with enucleation alone.[96] Prospective survival data for patients with medium-sized choroidal melanoma has yet to be reported.

Failure of local control of tumor growth occurs infrequently. In one study, continued tumor growth was seen in 10% of eyes following radiotherapy after an actuarialized 5-year period.[97] The location of continued growth was categorized as marginal in 41% of eyes (indicating a probable edge miss during treatment) or vertical in 59% of eyes (indicating tumor radioresistance). Intraoperative localization of radioactive plaque placement has identified that 14% of plaques placed by conventional clinical techniques did not fully cover all tumor margins and required intraoperative repositioning.[98] All tumors requiring plaque repositioning had one margin within the posterior pole or were immediately adjacent to the optic nerve.

Intraocular tumor recurrence may increase the risk of subsequent metastasis.[99] Enucleation for tumor regrowth was associated with decreased survival when compared with patients with complete local tumor control.[100] A frequent cause of enucleation is intractable pain in blind eyes that develop neovascular glaucoma. Enucleation in this population (ocular complications from radiation therapy with a clinically inactive tumor) did not increase the risk of subsequent development of metastatic disease.

About 85 to 90% of patients treated by irradiation retain their eyes more than 5 years. However, retention of vision of 20/200 or better is a function of the length of time of observation after treatment, the size of the tumor, radiation dosage, and the location of the tumor in relation to the macula and optic disk.[101, 102]

The outcomes of either brachytherapy or teletherapy for treatment of ocular melanoma appear to be comparable in terms of mortality rate, retention of vision, and ocular complications.[73, 101] Furthermore, available data following treatment by enucleation or radiotherapy do not suggest whether either may provide a greater survival advantage.[103–105] As noted previously, prospective data have been reported addressing the survival of patients with untreated small choroidal melanoma as well as in patients with large melanoma who received enucleation with or without pre-enucleation radiation. Until survival results are known from the prospective COMS medium tumor trial, the absence of a survival advantage attributed to either radiotherapy or enucleation in the management of medium-sized tumors will remain unknown.

## Treatment of Metastatic Uveal Melanoma

As the orbit is devoid of lymphatic drainage, uveal melanoma spreads hematogenously in a preferential manner to the liver. Patients who develop metastasis from uveal melanoma have a median interval time to death of 18 weeks.[106] Isolated hepatic metastases are usually managed by surgical excision,[107, 108] or if more diffuse hepatic involvement exists, by intrahepatic chemoembolization with cisplatin-based regimens. The 23-year experience from the M.D. Anderson Cancer Center for metastatic uveal melanoma reveals a 36% response rate by this technique compared with less than 1% when conventional systemic chemotherapy is used.[109] Data from the Eastern Cooperative Oncology Group, which used strict definitions for complete and partial responses, found that none of the 51 patients with metastatic uveal melanoma demonstrated any response to therapy, compared with a 13% response rate in patients with metastatic cutaneous melanoma.[106] A comprehensive review of treatments for metastatic uveal and cutaneous melanoma has been published that further illustrates the exceptionally poor prognosis for both of these cancers, but particularly that for uveal melanoma.[110]

## Alternative Treatment Modalities for Uveal Melanoma

### TRANSPUPILLARY THERMOTHERAPY

In 1995, Oosterhuis and coworkers reported using the transpupil delivery of long-duration (1-minute exposures) and large beam diameter (1.5 to 4.5 mm) diode laser energy (810 nm) for the treatment of patients with choroidal melanoma (TTT).[111] Six of the 12 patients reported had insufficient response to previous brachytherapy with [106]Ru. A reduction in tumor height was observed in 11 of 12 patients, but follow-up intervals were limited. Their experience with 50 patients was subsequently reported with similar treatment reponses, but the mean follow-up period remained short at 20.5 months.[112] In the largest study to date, Shields and colleagues reported a treatment success rate of decreased mean tumor height from 2.8 to 1.4 mm in 94% of 100 treated patients.[113] Visual outcomes were generally favorable, but the mean follow-up period was limited at only 14 months.

TTT is limited to patients with small or small-medium choroidal melanoma with clear ocular media. The maximal penetration of thermal necrosis following TTT has been shown to be 4 mm.[114] Visual loss is expected in lesions located within the macula or adjacent to the optic nerve because of thermal injury to the retina. Adjunctive use of TTT with lower dose brachytherapy may minimize some of the combined morbidity inherent with each of these treatment modalities. Incomplete or inadequate treatment can result in retention of viable tumor cells even if treatment is combined with brachytherapy.[115] Because the primary goal of any treatment for uveal melanoma is patient survival, until long-term prospective data are reported, the appropriate use of this treatment will remain uncertain.

### HYPERTHERMIA

Hyperthermia has been used as a radiation sensitizer and may allow for significant dose reduction during brachytherapy and potentially minimize the retinal and ocular morbidity associated with radiation therapy. Finger reported on the treatment of 48 patients whose tumors were heated using microwave technology to an apical temperature of 42° C for 45 minutes. Radiation dose reduction was performed in 38 patients. With a mean follow-up of 5 years, local treatment failures and secondary ocular complications were comparable to those in patients treated with radiation alone, but preservation of visual acuity was better in patients treated with adjunctive hyperthermia.[116] Tumor hyperthermia has also been achieved ultrasonographically[117] and by application of ferromagnetic energy.[118]

### PHOTODYNAMIC THERAPY

Hematoporphyrin derivatives have been used to photosensitize tumors prior to application of light energy. These compounds are activated by light energy in the near infrared spectrum to create oxygen radicals within the tumor vasculature. In a rabbit choroidal melanoma model, treatment with photodynamic therapy (PDT) resulted in tumor regression in 12 of 20 animals.[119] In a similar study using the benzoporphyrin derivative, verteporfin, all animals treated with PDT showed arrest of tumor growth with histologic necrosis. None of the animals treated with light alone or verteporfin without PDT showed alterations in tumor histopathology.[120]

PDT in the treatment of humans with uveal melanoma has been reported.[121] Cessation of tumor growth was reported in 76% of patients after 1 year, in 62% of patients after 2 years, and in only 38% of patients after 3 years of follow-up as estimated by Kaplan-Meier estimates. Although these rates compare less favorably with those reported after radiotherapy, the utility of PDT as an adjunctive treatment remains to be determined.

### TRANSSCLERAL RESECTION

Surgical excision of choroidal and ciliary body melanomas is technically possible, with the goal of therapy being preservation of the globe and the potential of retaining some vision. Of 34 patients undergoing this procedure with an average of just more than 5 years of follow-up, 11 patients ultimately required enucleation for intraocular complications or local tumor recurrence (five eyes); metastatic disease was reported in only 2 patients.[58] Median final visual acuity was counting fingers. Shields and colleagues retrospectively reviewed their experience in 95 patients who underwent partial lamellar sclerouvectomy for ciliary body and choroidal tumors over a 16-year period.[122] Intraocular complications were frequent, but preoperative visual acuity was preserved in one quarter of patients after 5 years of follow-up. This approach was recommended only for selected tumors that had basal diameters less than 12 mm, did not involve the pars plicata of the ciliary body, and did not extend more than 4 mm posterior to the equator of the globe. Given the development of newer treatment techniques, and the efficacy of established radiotherapy treatment modalities that also allow some preservation of vision (particularly for lesions located in the anterior choroid treated by plaque radiotherapy), the use of local tumor resection is probably best reserved for the management of iris and ciliary body melanoma.

## SUGGESTIONS FOR ADDITIONAL READING

Houlston RS, Damato BE. Genetic predisposition to ocular melanoma. Eye 1999;13:Pt 1:43–6.

Cather JC, Cather JC, Soparker CN, Nelson BR. Ocular melanoma. Cutis 1999;63:285–92.

Grin JM, Grant-Kels JM, Grin CM, et al. Ocular melanomas and melanocytic lesions of the eye. J Am Acad Dermatol 1998;38:5 Pt 1:716–30.

## REFERENCES

1. The Collaborative Ocular Melanoma Study Group: Histopathologic characteristics of uveal melanomas in eyes enucleated from the Collaborative Ocular Melanoma Study: COMS report no. 6. Am J Ophthalmol 1998;125:745–66.
2. Callender GR. Malignant melanotic tumors of the eye: a study of histologic types in 111 cases. Trans Am Acad Ophthalmol Otolaryngol 1931;36:131–42.
3. McLean IW, Foster WK, Zimmerman LE, Gamel JW. Modifications of Callender's classification of uveal melanoma at the Armed Forces Institute of Pathology. Am J Ophthalmol 1983;96:502–9.
4. Gamel JW, McLean IW. Computerized histopathologic assessment of malignant potential. II: A practical method for predicting survival following enucleation for uveal melanoma. Cancer 1983;52:1032–8.
5. Marcus DM, Minkovitz JB, Wardwell SD, et al. The value of nucleolar organizer regions in uveal melanoma. Am J Ophthalmol 1990;110:527–34.
6. Folberg R, Rummelt V, Parys-Van Ginderdeuren R, et al. The prognostic value of tumor blood vessel morphotogy in primary uveal melanoma. Ophthalmology 1993;100:1389–98.
7. Foss AJ, Alexander AA, Jefferies LW, et al. Microvessel count predicts survival in uveal melanoma. Cancer Res 1996;56:2900–3.
8. Mueller AJ, Bartsch D, Folbret R, et al. Imaging the microvasculature of choroidal melanomas with confocal indocyanine green scanning laser ophthalmoscopy. Arch Ophthalmol 1998:116:31–9.
9. Coleman DJ, Rondeau MJ, Silverman RH, et al. Correlation of microcirculation architecture with ultrasound backscatter parameters of uveal melanoma. Eur J Ophthalmol 1995;5:96–106.
10. Silverman RH, Folberg R, Boldt HC, et al. Correlation of ultrasound parameter imaging with microcirculatory patterns in uveal melanomas. Ultrasound Med Biol 1997;23:573–81.
11. Shields CL, Shields JA, DePotter P. Patterns of indocyanine green videoangiography of choroidal tumors. Br J Ophthalmol 1995;79:237–45.
12. Maberly DA, Pavlin CJ, McGowan HD, et al. Ultrasound biomicroscopic imaging of the anterior aspect of peripheral choroidal melanomas. Am J Ophthalmol 1997;123:506–14.
13. Augsburger JJ, Peyster RG, Markoe AM, et al. Computed tomography of posterior uveal melanomas. Arch Ophthalmol 1987;105:1512–6.
14. Peyster RG, Augsburger JJ, Shields JA, et al. Choroidal melanoma: comparison of CT, funduscopy and US. Radiology 1985;156:675–80.
15. Chambers RB, Davidorf FH, McAdoo JF, Chakeres DW. Magnetic resonance imaging of uveal melanomas. Arch Ophthalmol 1987;105:917–21.
16. Mafee MF, Peyman GA, Peace JH, et al. Magnetic resonance imaging in the evaluation and differentiation of uveal melanoma. Ophthalmology 1987;94:341–8.
17. Albert DM. The ocular melanoma story. LIII Edward Jackson Memorial Lecture: part II. Am J Ophthalmol 1997;123:729–41.
18. Singh AD, Wang MX, Donoso LA, et al. Familial uveal melanoma. III: Is the occurrence of familial uveal melanoma coincidental? Arch Ophthalmol 1996;114:1101–4.
19. Singh AD, Shields CL, DePotter P, et al. Familial uveal melanoma. Clinical observations on 56 patients. Arch Ophthalmol 1996;114:392–9.
20. Singh AD, Shields CL, Shields JA, DePotter P. Bilateral primary uveal melanoma. Bad luck or bad genes? Ophthalmology 1996;103:256–62.
21. Prescher G, Bornfeld N, Hirche H, et al. Prognostic implications of monosomy 3 in uveal melanoma. Lancet 1996;347:1222–5.
22. Sisley K, Rennie IG, Parsons MA, et al. Abnormalities of chromosomes 3 and 8 in posterior uveal melanoma correlate with prognosis. Genes Chrom Cancer 1997;19:22–8.
23. Kishore K, Ghazvini S, Char DH, et al. p53 gene and cell cycling in uveal melanoma. Am J Ophthalmol 1996;121:561–7.
24. Tucker MA, Shields JA, Hartge P, et al. Sunlight exposure as risk factor for intraocular malignant melanoma. N Engl J Med 1985;313:789–92.
25. Holly EA, Aston DA, Char DH, et al. Uveal melanoma in relation to ultraviolet light exposure and host factors. Cancer Res 1990;50:5773–7.
26. Egan KM, Seddon JM, Glynn RJ, et al. Epidemiologic aspects of uveal melanoma. Surv Ophthalmol 1988;32:239–51.
27. Scotto J, Fraumeni JF, Lee JAH. Melanomas of the eye and other noncutaneous sites: epidemiologic aspects. J Natl Cancer Inst 1976;56:489–91.
28. Dolin PJ, Foss AJ, Hungerford JL. Uveal melanoma: is solar ultraviolet radiation a risk factor? Ophthalmol Epidemiol 1994;1:27–30.
29. van Hees CL, de Boer A, Jager MJ, et al. Are atypical nevi a risk factor for uveal melanoma? A case-control study. J Invest Derm 1994;103:202–5.
30. Hammer H, Olah J, Toth-Molnar E. Dysplastic nevi are a risk factor for uveal melanoma. Eur J Ophthalmol 1996;6:472–4.
31. Taylor MR, Guerry D, Bondi EE, et al. Lack of association between intraocular melanoma and cutaneous dysplastic nevi. Am J Ophthalmol 1984;98:478–82.
32. Ajana UA, Seddon JM, Hsieh C, et al. Occupation and risk of uveal melanaoma. An exploratory study. Cancer 1992;70:2891–900.
33. Holly EA, Aston DA, Ahn DK, Smith AH. Intraocular melanoma linked to occupations and chemical exposures. Epidemiology 1996;7:55–61.
34. Albert DM, Puliafito CA, Fulton AB, et al. Increased incidence of choroidal malignant melanoma occurring in a single population of chemical workers. Am J Ophthalmol 1980;89:323–37.
35. Margo CE, Mulla ZD. Malignant tumors of the eyelid: a population-based study of non-basal cell and non-squamous cell malignant neoplasms. Arch Ophthalmol 1998;116:195–8.
36. Harbour JW, Augsburger JJ, Eagle RC. Initial management and follow-up of melanocytic iris tumors. Ophthalmology 1995;102:1987–93.
37. Hale PN, Allen RA, Straatsma BR. Benign melanomas (nevi) of the choroid and ciliary body. Arch Ophthalmol 1965;74:532–8.
38. Gass JDM. Problems in the differential diagnosis of choroidal nevi and malignant melanomas. Trans Am Acad Ophthalmol Otol 1977;83:OP19–46.
39. Ganley JP, Comstock GW. Benign nevi and malignant melanomas of the choroid. Am J Ophthalmol 1973;76:19–25.
40. Augsburger JJ, Schroeder RP, Territo C, et al. Clinical parameters predictive of enlargement of melanocytic choroidal lesions. Br J Ophthalmol 1989;73:911–7.
41. Shields CL, Shields JA, DePotter P, et al. Diffuse choroidal melanoma: clinical features predictive of metastasis. Arch Ophthalmol 1996;114:956–63.
42. Augsburger JJ, Shields JA. Fine needle aspiration biopsy of solid

intraocular tumors: indications, instrumentation and techniques. Ophthalmic Surg 1984;15:34–40.

43. Char DH, Miller T. Accuracy of presumed uveal melanoma diagnosis before alternative therapy. Br J Ophthalmol 1995;79:692–6.

44. Glasgow BJ, Brown HH, Zargoza AM, Foos RY. Quantitation of tumor seeding from fine needle aspiration of ocular melanomas. Am J Ophthalmol 1988;105:538–46.

45. Char DH, Kroll SM, Miller T, et al. Irradiated uveal melanomas: cytopathologic correlation with prognosis. Am J Ophth 1996;122:509–13.

46. Shields JA, Augsburger JJ, Brown GC, Stephens RF. The differential diagnosis of posterior uveal melanoma. Ophthalmology 1980;87:518–22.

47. Munjal D, Chawla PL, Lokich JJ, Zamcheck N. Carcinoembryonic antigen and phosphohexose isomerase, gamma-glutamyl traspeptidase and lactate dehydrogenase levels in patients with and without liver metastases. Cancer 1976;37:1800–7.

48. Wagoner MD, Albert DM. The incidence of metastases from untreated ciliary body and choroidal melanoma. Arch Ophthalmol 1982;100:939–40.

49. Reese AB. Pigmented tumors. In: Reese AB, ed. Tumors of the eye. 3rd ed. Hagerstown: Harper & Row, 1976:173–262.

50. Paridaens ADA, Minassian DC, McCartney ACE, Hungerford JL. Prognostic factors in primary malignant melanoma of the conjunctiva: a clinicopathological study of 256 cases. Br J Ophthalmol 1994;78:252–9.

51. Shields JA, Shields CL, DePotter P. Surgical management of conjunctival tumors: the 1994 Lynn B. McMahan lecture. Arch Ophthalmol 1997;115:808–15.

52. Lommatzsch PK. Beta irradiation of conjunctival melanomas. Trans Ophthalmol Soc UK 1977;97:378–80.

53. Travis LW, Rice DH, McClatchey KD, Wallace SW. Malignant melanoma of conjunctiva metastatic to parotid gland: reports of cases and discussion of surgical management. Laryngoscope 1977;87:2000–7.

54. Geisse LJ, Robertson DM. Iris melanomas. Am J Ophthalmol 1985;99:638–48.

55. Naumann GO, Rummelt V. Block excision of tumors of the anterior uvea: report on 68 consecutive patients. Ophthalmology 1996;103:2017–27.

56. Shields CL, Shields JA, DePotter P, et al. Treatment of non-resectable malignant iris tumours with custom designed plaque radiotherapy. Br J Ophthalmol 1995;79:306–12.

57. Char DH. Radiation therapy for uveal melanomas involving the ciliary body. Trans Ophthalmol Soc UK 1986;105:252–6.

58. Peyman GA, Juarez CP, Diamond JG, Raichand M. Ten years experience with eye wall resection for uveal malignant melanomas. Ophthalmology 1984;91:1720–5.

59. Damato BE, Paul J, Foulds WS. Predictive factors of visual outcome after local resection of choroidal melanoma. Br J Ophthalmol 1993;77:616–23.

60. The Collaborative Ocular Melanoma Study Group: Accuracy of diagnosis of choroidal melanomas in the Collaborative Ocular Melanoma Study Group: COMS report no. 1. Arch Ophthalmol 1990;108:1268–1273.

61. The Collaborative Ocular Melanoma Study Group: Factors predictive of growth and treatment of small choroidal melanoma: COMS report no. 5. Arch Ophthalmol 1997;115:1537–44.

62. Shields CL, Shields JA, Kiratli H, et al. Risk factors for growth and metastasis of small choroidal melanocytic lesions. Ophthalmology 1995;102:1351–61.

63. Fine SL. No one knows the preferred management for choroidal melanoma. Am J Ophthalmol 1996;122:106–8.

64. Schachat AP. Management of uveal melanoma: a continuing dilemma: Collaborative Ocular Melanoma Study Group. Cancer 1994;74:3073–5.

65. Paul EV, Parnell L, Fraker M. Prognosis of malignant melanomas of the choroid and ciliary body. Int Ophthalmol Clin 1962;2:387–402.

66. Shammas HF, Blodi FC. Prognostic factors in choroidal and ciliary body melanomas. Arch Ophthalmol 1977;95:63–9.

67. Burns RP, Fraunfeld FT, Klass AM. A laboratory evaluation of enucleation in treatment of intraocular malignant melanoma. Arch Ophthalmol 1962;67:490–500.

68. Raivio I. Uveal melanoma in Finland: an epidemiological, histological and prognostic study. Acta Ophthalmol (Kbh) 1977;133:Suppl:1–64.

69. Zimmerman LE, McLean IW, Foster WD. Does enucleation of the eye containing a malignant melanoma prevent or accelerate the dissemination of tumour cells? Br J Ophthalmol 1978;62:420–5.

70. Seigel D, Myers M, Ferris F, Steinhorn SC. Survival rates after enucleation of eyes with malignant melanoma. Am J Ophthalmol 1979;87:761–5.

71. Fraunfelder FT, Boozman FW, Wilson RS, Thomas AH. No-touch technique for intraocular malignant melanomas. Arch Ophthalmol 1977;95:1616–20.

72. Shields CL, Shields JA, DePotter P, Singh AD. Problems with the hydroxyapatite orbital implant: experience with 250 consecutive cases. Br J Ophthalmol 1994;78:702–6.

73. Finger PT. Radiation therapy for choroidal melanoma. Surv Ophthalmol 1997;42:215–32.

74. Gragoudas ES, Seddon JM, Egan K, et al. Long-term results of proton beam irradiated uveal melanomas. Ophthalmology 1987;94:349–53.

75. Wilkes SR, Gragoudas ES. Regression patterns of uveal melanomas after proton beam irradiation. Ophthalmology 1982;89:840–4.

76. Char DH, Saunders W, Castro JR, et al. Helium ion therapy for choroidal melanoma. Ophthalmology 1983;90:1219–25.

77. Packer S, Rotman M, Salanitro P. Iodine-125 irradiation of choroidal melanoma: clinical experience. Ophthalmology 1984;91:1700–08.

78. Earle J, Kline RW, Robertson DM. Selection of iodine 125 for the Collaborative Ocular Melanoma Study. Arch Ophthalmol 1987;105:763–4.

79. Augsburger JJ, Gamel JW, Shields JA, et al. Post-irradiation regression of choroidal melanomas as a risk factor for death from metastatic disease. Ophthalmology 1987;94:1173–7.

80. Foss AJ, Whelehan I, Hungerford JL, et al. Predictive factors for the development of rubeosis following proton beam radiotherapy for uveal melanoma. Br J Ophthalmol 1997;81:748–54.

81. Daftari IK, Char DH, Verhey LJ, et al. Anterior segment sparing to reduce charged particle radiotherapy complications in uveal melanoma. Int J Radiat Oncol Biol Phys 1997;39:997–1010.

82. Mooy CM, DeJong PTVM. Prognostic parameters in uveal melanoma: a review. Surv Ophthalmol 1996;41:215–28.

83. Donoso LA, Augsburger JJ, Shields JA, et al. Metastatic uveal melanoma: correlation between survival time and cytomorphometry of primary tumors. Arch Ophthalmol 1986;104:76–8.

84. Coleman K, Baak JP, van Diest PJ, Mullaney J. Prognostic value of morphometric features and the Callender classification in uveal melanomas. Ophthalmology 1996;103:1634–41.

85. Rummelt V, Folberg R, Rummelt C, et al. Microcirculation architecture of melanocytic nevi and malignant melanomas of the ciliary body and choroid: a comparative histopathologic and ultrastructural study. Ophthalmology 1994;101:718–27.

86. Mehaffey MG, Folberg R, Meyer M, et al. Relative importance of quantifying area and vascular patterns in uveal melanomas. Am J Ophthalmol 1997;123:798–809.

87. Pach JM, Robertson DM, Taney BS, et al. Prognostic factors in choroidal and ciliary body melanomas with extrascleral extension. Am J Ophthalmol 1986;101:325–31.

88. Duffin RM, Straatsma BR, Foos RY, Kerman BM. Small malignant melanoma of the choroid with extraocular extension. Arch Ophthalmol 1981;99:1827–30.

89. Murphy ML, Mieler WF, Williams DF, Lewandowski MF. Echographic pseudoextension of uveal melanomas. Graefes Arch Clin Exp Ophthalmol 1995;233:399–406.

90. Hosten N, Bornfeld N, Wassmuth R, et al. Uveal melanoma: detection of extraocular growth with MR imaging and US. Radiology 1997;202:61–7.

91. De Potter P, Flanders AE, Shields JA, et al. The role of fat-suppression technique and gadopentetate dimeglumine in magnetic resonance imaging evaluation of intraocular tumors and simulating lesions. Arch Ophthalmol 1994;112:340–8.

92. Kersten RC, Tse DT, Anderson RL, Blodi FC. The role of orbital exenteration in choroidal melanoma with extrascleral extension. Ophthalmology 1985;92:436–43.

93. Norregaard JC, Gerner N, Jensen OA, Prause JU. Malignant melanoma of the conjunctiva occurrence and survival following surgery and radiotherapy in a Danish population. Graefes Arch Clin Exp Ophthalmol 1996;234:569–72.

94. Diener-West M, Hawkins BS, Markowitz JA, Schachat AP. A review of mortality from choroidal melanoma. II: A meta-analysis of 5-year mortality rates following enucleation, 1966 through 1988. Arch Ophthalmol 1992;110:245–50.

95. The Collaborative Ocular Melanoma Study Group: Mortality in patients with small choroidal melanoma: COMS report no. 4. Arch Ophthalmol 1997;115:886–93.

96. The Collaborative Ocular Melanoma Study Group: The Collaborative Ocular Melanoma Study (COMS) randomized trial of pre-enucleation radiation of large choroidal melanoma. II: Initial mortality findings: COMS report no. 10. Am J Ophthalmol 1998;125:779–96.

97. Harbour JW, Char DH, Kroll S, et al. Metastatic risk for distinct patterns of postirradiation local recurrence of posterior uveal melanoma. Ophthalmology 1997;104:1785–92.

98. Harbour JW, Murray TG, Frazier-Byrne S, et al. Intraoperative echographic localization of iodine 125 episcleral radioactive plaques for posterior uveal melanoma. Retina 1996;16:129–34.

99. Gragoudas ES, Egan KM, Seddon JM, et al. Intraocular recurrence of uveal melanoma after proton beam irradiation. Ophthalmology 1992;99:760–6.

100. Egan KM, Ryan LM, Gragoudas ES. Survival implications of enucleation after definitive radiotherapy for choroidal melanoma: an example of regression on time-dependent covariates. Arch Ophthalmol 1998;116:366–70.

101. Char DH, Kroll S, Quivey JM, Castro J. Long-term visual outcome of radiated uveal melanomas in eyes eligible for randomization to enucleation versus brachytherapy. Br J Ophthalmol 1996;80:117–24.

102. Packer S, Stoller S, Lesser ML, et al. Long-term results of iodine 125 irradiation of uveal melanoma. Ophthalmology 1992;99:767–74.

103. Straatsma BR, Fine SL, Earle JD, et al. Enucleation versus plaque irradiation for choroidal melanoma. Ophthalmology 1988;95:1000–4.

104. Augsburger JJ, Correa ZM, Freire J, Brady LW. Long-term survival in choroidal and ciliary body melanoma after enucleation versus plaque radiation therapy. Ophthalmology 1998;105:1670–8.

105. Seddon JM, Gragoudas ES, Albert DM, et al. Comparison of survival rates for patients with uveal melanoma after treatment with proton beam irradiation or enucleation. Am J Ophthalmol 1985;99:282–90.

106. Albert DM, Ryan LM, Borden EC. Metastatic ocular and cutaneous melanoma: a comparison of patient characteristics and prognosis. Arch Ophthalmol 1996;114:107–8.

107. Gunduz K, Shields JA, Shields CL, et al. Surgical removal of solitary hepatic metastasis from choroidal melanoma. Am J Ophthalmol 1998;125:407–9.

108. Salmon RJ, Levy C, Plancher C, et al. Treatment of liver metastases from uveal melanoma by combined surgery-chemotherapy. Eur J Surg Oncol 1998;24:P127–30.

109. Bedikian AY, Legha SS, Mavligit G, et al. Treatment of uveal melanoma metastatic to the liver: a review of the M.D. Anderson Cancer Center experience and prognostic factors. Cancer 1995;76:1665–70.

110. Albert DM, Niffenegger AR, Willson JKV. Treatment of metastatic uveal melanoma: review and recommendations. Surv Ophthalmol 1992;36:429–38.

111. Oosterhuis JA, Journee-de Korver HG, Kakebeeke-Kemme HM, Bleeker JC. Transpupillary thermotherapy in choroidal melanomas. Arch Ophthalmol 1995;113:315–21.

112. Oosterhuis JA, Journee-de Korver HG, Keunen JEE. Transpupillary thermotherapy: results in 50 patients with choroidal melanoma. Arch Ophthalmol 1998;116:157–62.

113. Shields CL, Shields JA, Cater J, et al. Transpupillary thermotherapy for choroidal melanoma: tumor control and visual results in 100 consecutive cases. Ophthalmology 1998;105:581–90.

114. Journee-de Korver JG, Oosterhuis JA, deWolff-Rouendaal D, Kemme H. Histopathological findings in human choroidal melanomas after transpupillary thermotherapy. Br J Ophthalmol 1997;81:234–9.

115. Diaz CE, Capone A, Grossniklaus HE. Clinicopathologic findings in recurrent choroidal melanoma after transpupillary thermotherapy. Ophthalmology 1998;105:1419–24.

116. Finger PT. Microwave thermoradiotherapy for uveal melanoma: results of a 10-year study. Ophthalmology 1997;104:1794–1803.

117. Coleman DJ, Silverman AH, Ursea A, et al. Ultrasonically induced hyperthermia for adjunctive treatment of intraocular malignant melanoma. Retina 1997;17:109–17.

118. Murray TG, Steeves AA, Gentry L, et al. Ferromagnetic hyperthermia: functional and histopathologic effects on normal rabbit ocular tissue. Int J Hypertherm 1997;13:423–36.

119. Gonzales VH, Hu LK, Theodossiadis PG, et al. Photodynamic therapy of pigmented choroidal melanomas. Invest Ophthalmol Vis Sci 1995;36:871–8.

120. Kim AY, Hu LK, Foster BS, et al. Photodynamic therapy of pigmented choroidal melanomas of greater than 3-mm thickness. Ophthalmology 1996;103:2029–36.

121. Favilla I, Favilla ML, Gosbell AD, et al. Photodynamic therapy: a 5-year study of its effectiveness in the treatment of posterior uveal melanoma, and evaluation of haematoporphyrin uptake and photocytotoxicity of melanoma cells in tissue culture. Melanoma Res 1995;5:355–64.

122. Shields JA, Shields CL, Shah P, Sivalingam V. Partial lamellar sclerouvectomy for ciliary body and choroidal tumors. Ophthalmology 1991;98:971–83.

# CHAPTER 76

# SKIN CANCER

• WILLIAM V. R. SHELLOW

About 1 million individuals develop nonmelanoma skin cancer in the United States annually, representing about one third of all cancers. The overwhelming majority of these are either basal cell carcinoma (BCC) or squamous cell carcinoma (SCC). Nonmelanoma skin cancer is nearly always limited to the skin and is generally diagnosed and treated by dermatologists. These tumors almost never pose a serious threat to the patient's life, but they can cause serious morbidity and occasional mortality if they are long neglected or improperly treated.

This chapter is limited to a brief consideration of carcinomas of the skin, excluding lesions on the eyelids, vulva, penis, and anus. Comments on epidemiology and etiology relate almost entirely to SCC and BCC because other nonmelanoma skin carcinomas are rare. Melanoma, cutaneous T-cell lymphoma, and Kaposi's sarcoma are discussed elsewhere in this book.

## Natural History

### EPIDEMIOLOGY

The incidence of BCC and SCC is highest in individuals with fair skin, light eyes, and light hair; in those who have been exposed to the most sunlight; and in those who tend to sunburn easily.[1] It is highest in whites, much lower in Asians, and lower still in blacks. Among white populations, BCC is much more common than SCC; in dark-skinned races, SCC predominates.

The probability of developing multiple primary BCCs and SCCs is high. The chance of developing a second primary has been estimated to be almost 50% in men and more than 30% in women, with an incidence rate 140 times that of first primaries. About 80% of patients with x-ray–induced tumors develop multiple lesions. Therefore, individuals who have had one primary skin cancer should be followed carefully for the probable development of a new primary tumor in the future.[2]

## ETIOLOGY

The cause of skin cancer is multifactorial. Ionizing radiation, chemical carcinogens, burns, scars, ulcerations, discoid lupus erythematosus, and predisposing genetic disorders (xeroderma pigmentosum and the basal cell nevus syndrome in particular) may all have a contributing causal role. The most important cause by far, however, is actinic damage from solar ultraviolet radiation. Mechanisms include damage to DNA and its repair system, as well as alterations to the immune system. Sun exposure may serve as both an initiating factor and a promoting factor in multistage carcinogenesis in the skin.

SCC and BCC are uncommon sequelae to radiation therapy given to treat malignant disease. In patients so treated who develop chronic radiation dermatitis, less than 5% are ultimately expected to develop cutaneous malignancies in these areas. However, such tumors are much more common in those who develop chronic radiation dermatitis after irradiation for benign conditions. This has been found to occur in 20 to 40% of patients treated for acne, hirsutism, psoriasis, hemangioma, or benign ulcers, or those exposed accidentally.[3, 4] It usually takes longer than 15 years for these tumors to develop. The predominant radiation-induced tumor on the face is BCC; elsewhere, it is SCC.

BCC and SCC are being discovered with increasing frequency in patients who are immunosuppressed for various reasons, including acquired immunodeficiency syndrome, renal and other organ transplantation, and methotrexate therapy for psoriasis. In renal transplant patients, the risk of developing SCC was increased more than 253 times, and the risk of developing BCC was increased 10 times.[5] Patients with lymphocytic lymphoma or leukemia also have a particularly high rate of metastatic SCC.

## CLASSIFICATION

Classifications of precancerous and frankly malignant forms of nonmelanoma skin cancer are presented in Tables 76–1 and 76–2.

Actinic keratoses (solar keratoses, senile keratoses) biologically may be considered carcinoma in situ. They are hyperkeratotic lesions arising on sun-exposed skin that frequently shows other effects of actinic damage. No accurate figures exist for the incidence of malignant transformation to SCC, but the risk of malignant transformation is probably less than 1%. Clinically, actinic keratoses are well-circumscribed macules with rough, scaly surfaces that may be thickened. They are often shades of red and brown, but they may also be the same color as the surrounding skin, or gray

*Table 76–1.* **Classification of Precancerous and Related Lesions**

Actinic keratoses
  Idiopathic
    Keratosis senilis
    Disseminated actinic porokeratosis
    Lichen planus–like keratosis
  Chemically induced
    Arsenical keratoses
      Palmoplantar keratoses
      Bowenoid lesions
    Tar and pitch keratoses
Bowen's disease
Erythroplasia of Queyrat
Cutaneous horns
Intraepidermal carcinoma
  Jadassohn type
  Borst type
  Paget type

From Pinkus H. In: Fitzpatrick TB, et al, eds. Dermatology in general medicine, 2nd ed. New York: McGraw-Hill, 1979:401.

or black. They are usually several millimeters in diameter but vary from a pinpoint to several centimeters in size. Crusting, thickening, and ulceration are signs that should raise suspicion of frank malignant transformation.

The clinical and histologic features of BCC and SCC are summarized in Table 76–3.

## DIAGNOSIS

Dermatologists become adept at clinically diagnosing skin cancers, but even experienced dermatologists make errors when diagnosing BCC. Therefore, if there is any doubt as to the diagnosis, a small biopsy specimen should be taken before definitive treatment is instituted.

## STAGING AND PROGNOSIS

The American Joint Committee on Cancer (AJCC) staging system for nonmelanoma skin cancers (excluding lesions of the eyelid, vulva, and penis) is given in Table 76–4.

**Basal Cell Carcinoma.** The AJCC staging system is rarely used for BCC because the lesion almost never metastasizes. Of the millions of cases known to have occurred in the past, only about 200 cases of metastatic disease have been reported. Most of the morbidity of aggressive cases

*Table 76–2.* **Classification of Cutaneous Neoplasms**

Basal cell carcinoma (BCC)
  Noduloulcerative BCC
  Superficial BCC
  Pigmented BCC
  Morpheaform (sclerosing) BCC
Squamous cell carcinoma (SCC) (including)
  Bowen's disease
  Keratoacanthoma
Other
  Apocrine carcinoma
  Eccrine carcinoma
  Sebaceous carcinoma
  Merkel cell tumor
  Extramammary Paget's disease

*Table 76–3.* Differential Clinical and Histologic Features of Basal Cell Carcinoma (BCC) and Squamous Cell Carcinoma (SCC)

| Clinical Type | Clinical Characteristics | Histologic Type | Histologic Characteristics |
|---|---|---|---|
| Noduloulcerative BCC | Usually on head and neck. Rolled pearly or translucent border. Telangiectasis on surface. | Solid | Masses of basophilic cells. Large nuclei and little cytoplasm. Peripheral palisading and retraction connected to epidermis. Lack of intercellular bridges. |
| | Most common type. | Keratotic | Features of solid type. Masses of keratin: "horn cysts." |
| | | Cystic | Features of solid type. Cystic spaces in tumor. |
| | | Adenoid | Features of solid type. Tubular gland–like structures. |
| Superficial BCC | Usually on trunk or extremities. Tends to be multiple. May be large. Erythematous macule with slight scaling on surface. Mimics many benign conditions. | Superficial | Buds of small groups of basophilic cells from the epidermis into the superficial dermis. |
| Pigmented BCC | Features of above types. Black or brown pigmentation. May suggest melanoma. Usually in brown-eyed individuals. | Pigmented | Features of above types. Melanin deposition. |
| Morpheaform BCC (sclerosing) | Usually on head. Fibrotic, ivory appearance. Borders difficult to define. Telangiectasis. | Morpheaform | Fine strands of basophilic cells embedded in dense fibrous stroma. |
| SCC | May occur anywhere, but usually on damaged skin. Nonhealing ulcerations with indurated border. | SCC | Masses of cells invading into the dermis that vary from well differentiated to anaplastic. |

comes from destruction of local structures, such as the eye, ear, and nose. When BCC causes death, it is usually from intracranial extension of a locally aggressive tumor rather than from distant metastases.

**Squamous Cell Carcinoma.** The AJCC staging system

*Table 76–4.* American Joint Committee on Cancer (AJCC) Staging of Skin Cancer*

**Primary Tumor (T)†**
TX Primary tumor cannot be assessed
T0 No evidence of primary tumor
Tis Carcinoma in situ
T1 Tumor 2 cm or less in greatest dimension
T2 Tumor more than 2 cm but not more than 5 cm in greatest dimension
T3 Tumor more than 5 cm in greatest dimension
T4 Tumor invades deep extradermal structures (eg, cartilage, skeletal muscle, or bone)
**Regional Lymph Nodes (N)**
NX Regional lymph nodes cannot be assessed
N0 No regional lymph node metastasis
N1 Regional lymph node metastasis
**Distant Metastasis (M)**
MX Presence of distant metastasis cannot be assessed
M0 No distant metastasis
M1 Distant metastasis
**STAGE GROUPING**

| Stage 0 | Tis | N0 | M0 |
|---|---|---|---|
| Stage I | T1 | N0 | M0 |
| Stage II | T2 | N0 | M0 |
| | T3 | N0 | M0 |
| Stage III | T4 | N0 | M0 |
| | Any T | N1 | M0 |
| Stage IV | Any T | Any N | M1 |

*Excluding lesions of the eyelid, vulva, and penis.
†In the case of multiple simultaneous tumors, the tumor with the highest T category will be classified, and the number of separate tumors will be indicated in parentheses (eg, T2[5]).
Used with the permission of the American Joint Committee on Cancer (AJCC®), Chicago, Illinois. The original source for this material is the AJCC® Cancer Staging Handbook, 5th edition (1998) published by Lippincott-Raven Publishers, Philadelphia, Pennsylvania.

for skin cancer is rarely used by clinicians treating SCC, despite the fact that SCC is known to be capable of extensive local invasion, lymphatic spread and, occasionally, distant metastases. The risk of metastatic involvement by SCC has variably been estimated to be as low as 2% for patients without known risk factors for dissemination, and as high as 15 to 35% in patients with various predisposing conditions such as immunosuppression.

The grade of the lesion may have prognostic importance. The most widely used system of grading is that of Broders, which defines four grades based on the percentage of cells that appear to be differentiating. The degree of atypicality of the cells, the depth of penetration of the tumor, and the presence or absence of perineural invasion also serve as prognostic factors.

**Other Nonmelanoma Skin Carcinomas.** The AJCC staging system is applicable to the other forms of carcinoma discussed in this chapter.

## Treatment of Actinic Keratoses

Because actinic keratoses result from exposure to sunlight, they are theoretically preventable. Prophylactic measures instituted early in life, including avoidance of sun exposure and the use of protective measures such as sunscreens and opaque clothing by fair-skinned individuals, would prevent these lesions. Once a patient has developed lesions, sun protection must be stressed in the hope of preventing further ultraviolet damage to the skin.

Actinic keratoses rarely exhibit malignant biologic behavior. Because these lesions are noninvasive and contained entirely within the epidermis, the use of treatment methods that limit destruction to the epidermis should eradicate the lesions, leaving minimal or no scarring. A wide variety of treatments may be effective, including cryosurgery with liquid nitrogen, curettage (with or without electrodesiccation), and topical therapy with 5-fluorouracil (either alone or with adjuncts such as high-potency topical steroids or topical tretinoin [Retin-A]). Alternative approaches include chemical peeling with trichloroacetic acid or phenol, dermabrasion, and laser resurfacing.

Radiation therapy is not indicated for the treatment of actinic keratoses. Surgical procedures that use excision of the full thickness of the skin and closure with sutures are rarely necessary for actinic keratosis. An exception to this tenet occurs when there is concern that the lesion may actually be an SCC and it is small enough and located in an area where excisional biopsy will give an excellent cosmetic result.

# Treatment of Basal Cell and Squamous Cell Carcinomas

Conventional means of treating both BCC and SCC include curettage and electrodesiccation, surgical excision, Mohs' micrographic surgery, cryosurgery, and radiation. In certain select circumstances, chemotherapy and immunotherapy may be appropriate. The most important goal of treatment is the cure of disease. The preservation of cosmesis and function is an important secondary consideration. When failure of treatment occurs, it is usually because of an inappropriate and excessive attempt to preserve cosmesis at the expense of obtaining a cure.

For the vast majority of BCCs and SCCs, any of five generally accepted modalities is likely to produce a cure when performed by someone who is expert in its use. Mohs' micrographic surgery is indicated for tumors that are thought to be difficult to treat and cure. Certain tumors may be particularly difficult to treat because of anatomic location (eg, nasal, periorbital, and auricular areas), histologic type (eg, morpheaform BCC), subclinical extension, or the fact that they are recurrent tumors. It is particularly important to cure these more difficult lesions because failure to do so may result in loss of vital structures or even death.

The cure rates among studies, and even with different modalities within the same study, are not truly comparable. Patients are not randomized before a particular modality is chosen. For example, cases treated by Mohs' micrographic surgery techniques are specially selected for their challenging nature. Techniques may vary from one study to the next, and even within a particular study in which multiple physicians are involved. Some of the studies are derived from the experience with difficult cases selected for referral, whereas others are generated from private practices. It is striking that with expert therapy and a variety of modalities, the cure rates typically exceed 90%; therefore, any physician using any of the available treatment modalities should expect a high probability of curing the cutaneous malignancy.

BCCs and SCCs that recur are much more difficult to cure. Whichever method is selected, patients must be followed closely over many years for signs of recurrent tumors and for development of new primaries, although recurrences usually appear within the first 3 years.

## CURETTAGE AND ELECTRODESICCATION

Curettage and electrodesiccation can be used for either BCC or SCC, although it is more commonly employed for BCC. This method takes advantage of the difference in feel of the mushy neoplastic tissue compared with the firmer normal cutis. Normal skin is minimally damaged when firmly scraped with a sharp curette, whereas most epidermal tumors are easily removed with this instrument.

A small shave biopsy to confirm the presence of a malignancy should be taken before any treatment is begun.

After infiltration of the lesion with a local anesthetic, the bulk of the tumor is curetted and may be sent for histologic verification of diagnosis. Information as to clearance of tumor is not available from such a specimen. Subsequently, the base and edges of the resulting cavity are vigorously scraped with a smaller curette, with exploration for any extensions of tumor. The base and edges are then electrodesiccated. Generally, this procedure is repeated at least once.[6] The resulting eschar-covered wound heals in 2 to 6 weeks, depending on the size and location, eventually leaving a flat, white scar.

In general, cosmetic results are surprisingly good with curettage and electrodesiccation. Occasionally, a hypertrophic scar may result from this procedure, but it usually resolves spontaneously. If it fails to resolve within 3 months, corticosteroid injections into the scar generally produce satisfactory flattening. Rarely, a true keloid may develop, the therapy of which is variably successful.

Curettage and electrodesiccation can be superior to non-Mohs' excisional surgery or radiation in the treatment of large superficial lesions of BCC.[7] The superficial nature of such lesions allows their removal in entirety by this method, with an excellent cosmetic result. Scalpel surgery and closure require either long scars or the use of flaps or grafts and may represent overtreatment for large superficial BCC. Radiation therapy tends to leave cosmetically unacceptable scars on the trunk and extremities.

The morpheaform type of BCC is not suitable for treatment with curettage and electrodesiccation because the dense sclerotic stroma does not allow differentiation of the tumor from the surrounding cutis by feel with a curette. Recurrent tumors that contain dense fibrotic scar are also more difficult to treat with this method; therefore, it should not be used. If a punch biopsy is used to verify malignancy in such cases, the curette will penetrate into the tract made by the punch, and end up in the subcutaneous fat. If curettage and electrodesiccation are contemplated from the outset, a shave biopsy is the diagnostic approach of choice. In addition, lesions that penetrate into fat, cartilage, or bone pose problems for removal of the entire tumor with a curette. Lesions that penetrate deeply into the nasolabial fold or the forehead and large lesions involving the eyelid or the nasovestibular area are more difficult to treat with this method. Such tumors require Mohs' micrographic surgery by which the extensions of the cancer can be traced out.

When BCC and SCC reappear following curettage and electrodesiccation, they tend to recur in the margin because of the lack of aggressiveness of technique, or because the lesions were morpheaform. When recurrences are seen, they tend to be superficial and to appear within 2 years of initial treatment. However, they may involve a broader area than is clinically apparent, so serious consideration should be given to removal of the previous scar, in addition to the area of clinically recurrent tumor. Conventional wisdom dictates that a different technique be used to treat a recurrent lesion than was used initially.

Cure rates using curettage and electrodesiccation for both BCC and SCC are greater than 90% in some series.[8]

## SURGERY

In general, surgical techniques for the treatment of BCCs and SCCs involve excision of the lesion, including a margin of at least 4 mm beyond what is clinically felt to be the extent of the tumor.[9, 10] For large tumors, margins of 5 to 10 mm are recommended.[11] Another rule of thumb for SCCs is that the surgical margins should be about 6 mm beyond the lesion. These borders may be checked for clearance with frozen sections if there are particular doubts, and the excised specimen can be marked so that if permanent sections show that the tumor has not been cleared, the physician will know where the residual tumor lies. The incision includes the full thickness of the skin down to the subcutaneous fat. Wounds are usually closed in layers by suturing, although large lesions may be allowed to heal by secondary intention (granulation), often with good cosmetic results. Larger lesions may be closed with a wide variety of local and distant flaps or grafts. It is important, however, not to hide residual tumor beneath skin flaps or full-thickness grafts.

If the pathologic specimen shows extension of SCC to the margins of the excision, a repeat procedure should be performed to eliminate the residual tumor. Tumors that already have been recurrent, that are of morpheaform histology, or that have been incompletely excised at both lateral and deep margins have a particularly high rate of recurrence and should nearly always receive further treatment (most desirably with Mohs' micrographic surgery) rather than being subjected to a "wait and see" approach. Lesions covered by full-thickness grafts or by flaps may recur as deep nodules and may remain hidden for a long time. Therefore, in these types of wound repair, one must be assured that the tumor has been cleared by an adequate margin, and if it becomes known that inadequate margins have been taken, early retreatment is likely to be tissue sparing.

The surgical removal of BCC and SCC has several advantages. All except the largest and most invasive lesions may be treated using local anesthesia on an outpatient basis. Healing is generally rapid, the rate of infection is low, cosmetic results are usually good to excellent, all histologic types may be treated, and the specimen may be checked for clearance of tumor at the margins, giving further assurance that the patient has been adequately treated. Frozen sections may be obtained at the time of operation, but their accuracy in cutaneous lesions is not as high as in other areas, and they are not available to most dermatologists.

### Mohs' Micrographic Surgery

Micrographic surgery is a technique pioneered by Frederick Mohs in the 1930s that involves carefully controlled microscopic monitoring in the excision of skin cancer. It originally referred only to a method of fixing the tissue chemically in situ with zinc chloride paste, followed by surgical removal, with microscopic examination of the lesion. This is now referred to as the "fixed-tissue technique" in contrast to the more recently developed "fresh-tissue technique,"[12] in which the tissues are not chemically treated in situ but rather are examined in a special manner as frozen sections. In both techniques, the sine qua non is the careful mapping of the horizontal sections of tissue, which are meticulously examined for residual tumor. This preserves normal tissue while ensuring that the entire tumor is removed because the excision is carried out in stages until tumor-free planes are achieved.[13] The advantage of Mohs' surgery over conventional frozen sections is that the entire surface of the tumor, including both lateral and deep margins, is completely examined. Therefore, microscopic finger-like extensions of tumor that would be missed if only random "bread-loafed" sections of the tumor were examined, as with standard frozen sections, may be discovered and treated.[14]

The vast majority of procedures are now done using the fresh-tissue technique. However, the fixed-tissue technique may be a better choice for treatment of very large BCCs and SCCs, especially those that invade bone or cartilage or the meninges or brain, or for deeply invasive SCC of the erectile tissue of the penis.

Mohs' surgery offers the advantage of relative assurance that the entire tumor has been removed, coupled with minimal sacrifice of normal tissue. This makes it an ideal therapy for lesions located near functionally or cosmetically critical structures. Although series using either of the two types of Mohs' micrographic surgery generally have selected the most difficult BCCs and SCCs, the highest cure rates of any method of skin cancer treatment are consistently associated with this technique.

Large, deeply infiltrating lesions; tumors involving the periorbital region, fingers, or penis; and those spreading along perichondrial or periosteal planes are particularly suitable for this treatment modality. Tumors in which it is difficult to determine borders clinically, such as morpheaform, micronodular, and infiltrative BCCs, also lend themselves well to Mohs' surgery.

One of the most important indications for using micrographic surgery is treatment of recurrent tumors.[15] Rather than a difference in cure rate of just a few percentage points, the cure rate for recurrent lesions treated by Mohs' surgery is markedly superior to that of other modalities. In various series, cure rates in treating recurrent BCC range from 41 to 88% for curettage and desiccation, from 60 to 95% for excisional surgery, and from 73 to 89% for radiation. These are compared with cure rates of 95 to 97% for Mohs' micrographic surgery.[9]

Mohs has written of his own results, which included patients with some of the most difficult to treat and far-advanced BCCs and SCCs who were referred to him from all over the world. His cure rates are impressive. For almost 8000 such primary BCCs, he attained a cure rate of 99.8% with the fixed-tissue technique after a follow-up of at least 5 years. For nearly 1400 recurrent BCCs, his 5-year follow-up figures showed a 96.8% cure rate; for all BCCs, it was 99.3 percent. For SCCs followed for at least 5 years, many of which were far advanced at the time of treatment, his figure was 94.4% without recurrence. These cure rates have been corroborated by others.[16, 17]

The relative disadvantages of Mohs' surgery include the relatively few physicians who are expert in its use and the increased time and expense of the procedure. It offers only a slight advantage in the management and cure rates of routine BCC and SCC. For BCCs and SCCs that are recurrent, morpheaform, extensive, or infiltrating; that involve vital areas; or that are otherwise difficult to treat, Mohs' surgery is the treatment of choice.

### Cryosurgery

Cryosurgery involves the destruction of tumor by the use of liquid nitrogen to induce cold temperatures. To accomplish this, it is necessary to attain a temperature of at least $-25°$ C in the entire tumor. The alterations produced within cells, tissues, and blood vessels by this rapid change in temperature result in irreversible destruction of the cells. The cold temperature forms an ice ball in the tissue; the cells that survive later die of anoxemia produced by vascular thrombosis that occurs when the small vessels are frozen. These effects are enhanced by application of a double freeze-thaw cycle.[18, 19] Some investigators suggest that temperatures as low as $-50°$ C should be attained because cellular electrolytes are crystallized by the time this temperature has been reached, and therefore cell death is ensured. The details of cryosurgery have been provided in previous editions of this book and in textbooks of dermatology.

BCCs and SCCs on the face that are treated with cryosurgery usually heal within 1 month, but healing may take considerably longer in other locations, especially the lower aspect of the legs. Hypopigmentation is common after this technique has been used.

Lesions that have indistinct borders are less suitable for cryosurgical treatment because there is no way to ensure that the entire tumor is being treated adequately unless a large surrounding area of normal skin is also treated. Cryosurgery is not the preferred method for morpheaform BCC. For other tumors with indistinct borders, a combined technique of curettage, to delineate the extent of the tumor, followed by cryosurgery has been used with success. This combined technique is particularly helpful for treatment of invasive BCCs that, with curettage, have been found to extend into underlying cartilage.

Serious complications of cryosurgery are exceedingly rare. Cryosurgery should be avoided in areas where large nerves are located because this technique can cause severe, but generally reversible, neuropathy.

### RADIATION THERAPY

BCC and SCC are moderately radiosensitive tumors. Cure rates can be comparable to those with other standard modalities, although follow-up data of longer than 5 years are sparse. Radiotherapy is currently used less frequently in treating BCC or SCC than are most of the other standard modalities, largely because it requires special skills, expensive equipment, and multiple patient visits.

Numerous effective radiation treatment regimens exist for BCC and SCC. They range mainly from 45 to 55 Gy with x-rays of varying penetration, generally given as 15 to 20 treatments over 3 to 4 weeks, although some physicians use lesser or greater fractions.[20–22]

Four reasons have been offered to explain why radiation therapy may fail to cure BCC and SCC: underestimation of the marginal extension of the tumor ("geographic miss"), inadequate dosage reaching the depth of the tumor, inadequate treatment schedule, and lack of radiosensitivity of the tumor. Of these, geographic miss is thought to be the main reason for treatment failure.

Electron-beam therapy has been used successfully on occasion in the treatment of particularly large BCC and SCC. Other cases of far-advanced BCC and SCC that defied treatment by any other method have been managed with complex radiation therapy techniques, such as the telecobalt apparatus.

Usually, young patients with BCC or SCC are better treated with modalities other than radiation because altered skin color, atrophy, and telangiectases may develop many years after radiation therapy in the treated areas. Patients with blond hair and blue eyes are more susceptible to these changes. The delayed development of skin cancer is usually not a problem for individuals who are elderly at the time of treatment.

Radiation is a particularly useful treatment for lesions at sites in which destruction of tissue is undesirable for functional or cosmetic reasons. It may be useful for either BCC or SCC involving the eyelids, the alae nasi, the tip of the nose, or the ear. Larger lesions may do well with radiation. Lesions on the trunk and lower extremities are responsive to radiation but often heal with poor cosmetic results. There may even be residual nonmalignant ulcerations after several years.

Radiation therapy is relatively contraindicated in two groups of tumors. Most authorities question the efficacy of radiation therapy for the treatment of morpheaform BCC because cosmesis appears to be inferior to that of other methods of treatment and the cure rates have been unpredictable. Radiation therapists also question the role of radiation therapy in the treatment of skin cancer that develops in areas of previous irradiation.

### TOPICAL CHEMOTHERAPY

A variety of topical chemotherapeutic agents have been administered experimentally in the treatment of skin cancer, but the current approval for such use is limited to 5% 5-fluorouracil (5-FU) exclusively for the histologic category of superficial BCC. This is based on a 93% cure rate in 113 lesions that were proven histologically to be of this type.[23] This method results in no systemic toxicity, little or no scarring, and rapid healing. However, whenever practical, conventional means of treatment are still recommended for these lesions because cure rates are close to 100% for superficial BCCs treated with other modalities. 5-FU definitely should not be used as therapy for recurrent lesions.

### Alternative Therapies

#### IMMUNOTHERAPY

In the mid-1960s, it was noted that the induction of a cutaneous delayed hypersensitivity reaction resulted in the elimination of multiple superficial BCCs. Agents capable of inducing such a reaction include dinitrochlorobenzene (DNCB),[24] mechlorethamine, purified protein derivative to tuberculin, squaric acid dibutyl ester, diphencyprone, and bacille Calmette-Guérin. Use of such agents for the treatment of skin cancer is generally referred to as immunotherapy, although the precise mechanism of antineoplastic action is incompletely defined.

In general, superficial BCCs are more sensitive to these agents than is normal skin. It is therefore possible to use a weaker strength for treating tumors than the lowest concentration that causes an inflammatory response in normal skin, as determined by patch testing. The medication can then be applied to the entire affected area rather than to just the visible tumor without causing a marked reaction, except in the clinically apparent tumor and in microscopic foci of involvement by malignant and premalignant cells. Therefore, small lesions may be recognized and treated earlier in their course than would ordinarily be possible. Such reactions of allergic contact dermatitis have been used, with cure rates generally between 60 and 90% for BCC.

Patients who have xeroderma pigmentosum, the nevoid basal cell carcinoma syndrome, chronic arsenic exposure, extensive chronic radiation dermatitis, or long-term exposure to excessive actinic radiation may have large numbers of skin cancers. The substantial area of the body surface involved may make treatment by surgical excision, curettage and electrodesiccation, cryosurgery, or radiation therapy a difficult and disfiguring undertaking. It is in patients with multiple skin cancers that topical immunotherapy has its biggest role.

Immunotherapy can also be used prophylactically for patients who develop a vast number of cutaneous neoplasms. Studies in three xeroderma pigmentosum patients, in whom one side was treated with conventional therapy and the other side with intermittent courses of DNCB in an attempt to prevent new tumors, showed 177 new tumors on the control sides of the three patients and only 10 new tumors on the sides receiving DNCB immunoprophylaxis over the course of 1 year. Patients with other conditions resulting in multiple epidermal neoplasms have also demonstrated remarkably reduced rates of new tumor formation with immunotherapy.

Combinations of two or more agents, such as a cell-mediated immune response stimulator and a chemotherapeutic agent, such as 5-FU, may be more effective than single-agent therapy. A delayed hypersensitivity reaction can be elicited by a combination of two antigens in concentrations that fail to elicit the reaction when either is given alone. The selective response on application to the tumor may be the result of the adjuvant effect of an additional antigenic agent added to weak tumor antigens, resulting in a delayed hypersensitivity reaction.

Numerous small studies testing the injection of interferon into BCC have shown it to be a fairly effective treatment. Nevertheless, this treatment is not widely used, most likely owing to the expense of the drug and its side effects.

## LASER SURGERY

Although not standard therapy at this time, a variety of laser-based techniques have been used to treat skin cancer.

Examples of lasers tested in the past include the ruby laser, the argon laser, and the neodymium:yttrium-aluminum-garnet (Nd:YAG) laser. The carbon dioxide laser, for example, can be used for either vaporization or cutting of tissues, depending on how the beam is focused. Laser surgery tends to be a fast procedure, but some studies have shown a high recurrence rate after laser therapy for skin cancer. Further study is needed to place this technique into perspective for the treatment of skin cancer.[25]

Another form of laser treatment for skin cancers currently under investigation is called *photodynamic therapy*. It involves the use of porphyrin derivatives as photosensitizers either by injection or topically, followed by the use of a tunable dye laser as the activating light source. Topical δ-amino levulinic acid has been applied to skin tumors. This precursor is converted to a porphyrin; it then reacts with visible light to destroy superficial tumors. A report shows poor long-term cure rates for superficial BCC and SCC treated with this modality.[26]

## SYSTEMIC CHEMOTHERAPY

Systemic chemotherapy plays no role in localized skin cancer, and metastatic disease occurs so rarely that systematic testing of drugs in this setting is precluded. There is no clearly indicated treatment for metastatic BCC, although small series suggest that cisplatin may be useful, either alone or in combination with doxorubicin.[27]

## RETINOIDS

Synthetic retinoids offer some potential in the treatment of skin malignancies.[28] They inhibit chemical carcinogenesis and the proliferation of malignant cell lines, and they have been shown to suppress malignant transformation in vitro. They also inhibit tumor promotion and the induction of ornithine decarboxylase by phorbol esters. They may also interfere with tumor initiation.

Although both isotretinoin and etretinate have induced remission in both BCC and SCC when taken systemically, cure rates are 10% or less.[29] Studies are currently under way to determine if topical tretinoin can prevent the formation of new skin cancers.

## SUMMARY OF TREATMENT FOR SQUAMOUS CELL CARCINOMA AND BASAL CELL CARCINOMA

The vast majority of BCCs and SCCs are curable with surgical excision, curettage and electrodesiccation, radiation therapy, cryosurgery, Mohs' micrographic surgery, or laser surgery (Table 76–5). However, these lesions should not be regarded too lightly because they are capable of producing significant morbidity and occasional mortality if they are long neglected or improperly treated. When a particularly aggressive tumor is encountered, the mode of therapy should be tailored to the characteristics of both the particular patient and the lesions.

*Table 76–5.* Treatment Method Options

| Premalignant or Malignant Lesion | Preferred Method(s) | Alternatives |
|---|---|---|
| Actinic keratosis | Cryosurgery | Electrosurgery |
| | 5-Fluorouracil | Curettage and electrodesiccation (C&ED) |
| Basal cell carcinoma | Curettage and electrodesiccation | Radiation therapy |
| | Excision (shave or ellipse) | Cryosurgery |
| | Mohs' surgery (depending on the tumor variety, size, and location) | Immunotherapy (superficial types) |
| Squamous cell carcinoma (SCC) | Curettage and electrodesiccation | Cryosurgery |
| | Excision (shave or ellipse) | Radiation therapy |
| | Mohs' surgery (depending on the tumor size and location) | |
| Bowen's disease (Intraepidermal SCC) | Curettage and electrodesiccation | Cryosurgery |
| | Excision (shave or ellipse) | |

## Treatment of Rare Skin Tumors

### APOCRINE CARCINOMA

Apocrine carcinoma is an extremely rare tumor that usually arises in the axilla, but it can also arise from apocrine glands in the vulva, external auditory meatus, and eyelid. These lesions can invade locally and metastasize to distant sites. Staging is by the AJCC tumor-node-metastasis (TNM) system, as was described previously.

Treatment is usually limited to surgical excision, but radiation therapy is sometimes useful for locally advanced lesions. The role of chemotherapy in patients with advanced-stage disease is unclear.

### ECCRINE CARCINOMA

This rare tumor has no characteristic site of development. Histologically, it is a form of adenocarcinoma, and it may mimic a metastatic adenocarcinoma from some other site. These lesions are usually locally destructive and they tend to recur after surgical excision. They may metastasize to regional and distant lymph node sites. The role of combined-modality therapy is uncertain.

### SEBACEOUS CARCINOMA

Although uncommon, sebaceous carcinoma accounts for up to 5% of all cutaneous neoplasms. It usually develops clinically as a slowly growing, hard, yellow nodule arising in glands of the eyelid. It may also arise in many other sites, including the face, scalp, or even more distant sites. These lesions are capable of local invasion and distant metastasis and are generally treated by surgical excision. The possible role of combined-modality therapy is uncertain.

### MERKEL CELL TUMORS

Merkel cells are neuroendocrine cells of the skin. Neoplasms of these cells behave like neuroendocrine tumors arising elsewhere, such as small cell carcinoma of the lung. They have a propensity to metastasize widely, and they frequently recur after local therapy. Central nervous system involvement is not unusual with this neoplasm.

Most patients with Merkel cell neoplasms should be treated with combined-modality therapy.[30] Limited lesions may be treated surgically with adjunctive radiation therapy; more advanced disease should benefit from chemotherapy. Active regimens of chemotherapy include all those being used for small cell lung cancer.

### EXTRAMAMMARY PAGET'S DISEASE

Extramammary Paget's disease is a rare epidermal neoplasm that arises mainly in the elderly. It may occur in apocrine gland areas, such as the axilla, vulva, scrotum, or perianal areas. It may also result from direct extension of an adenocarcinoma from a contiguous organ.

Surgical excision is the usual treatment, although radiation therapy is an acceptable alternative for many patients. Chemotherapy is rarely used.

### SUGGESTIONS FOR ADDITIONAL READING

Tai PTH, Yu E, Winquist E, et al. Chemotherapy in neuroendocrine/Merkel cell carcinoma of the skin: case series and review of 204 cases. J Clin Oncol 2000;18:2493–99.

Preston DS, Stern RS. Nonmelanoma cancers of the skin. N Engl J Med 1992;327:1649–62. review article. *A superb review that includes excellent pictures of lesions.*

Moy RL, Taheri DP, Ostad A, eds. Practical management of skin cancer. Philadelphia: Lippincott–Williams & Wilkins, 1998. *A succinct reference with 225 color photographs and a practical discussion of all treatment modalities for skin cancer, including recommendations for various types.*

### REFERENCES

1. Zaynoun S, Lina AA, Shabib J, et al. The relationship of sun exposure and solar elastosis to basal cell carcinoma. J Am Acad Dermatol 1985; 12:522–5.
2. Karagas MR, Stukel TA, Greenberg R, et al. Risk of subsequent basal cell carcinoma and squamous cell carcinoma of the skin among patients with prior skin cancer. JAMA 1992;267:3305–10.
3. Burns FJ. Cancer risk associated with therapeutic irradiation of the skin. Arch Dermatol 1989;21:475–8.
4. Martin H, Strong E, Spiro RH. Radiation-induced skin cancer of the head and neck. Cancer 1970;25:61–71.
5. Hartevelt MM, Blavnick JN, Kootte AM, et al. Incidence of skin cancer after renal transplantation in the Netherlands. Transplantation 1990;49:506–9.

6. Spiller WF, Spiller RF. Treatment of basal cell epithelioma by curettage and electrodesiccation. J Am Acad Dermatol 1984;11:808–14.

7. Kopf AW, Bart RS, Schrager D, et al. Curettage-electrodesiccation of basal cell carcinomas. Arch Dermatol 1977;113:439–43.

8. Salasche SJ. Status of curettage and desiccation in the treatment of primary basal cell carcinoma. J Am Acad Dermatol 1984;10:285.

9. Rowe DE, Carroll RJ, Day CL Jr. Long term recurrence rates in previously untreated (primary) basal cell carcinoma: implications for patient follow-up. J Dermatol Surg Oncol 1989;15:315–27.

10. Wolf DJ, Zitelli JA. Surgical margins for basal cell carcinoma. Arch Dermatol 1987;123:340–4.

11. Brodland DG, Zitelli JA. Surgical margins for excision of primary cutaneous squamous cell carcinoma. J Am Acad Dermatol 1992; 27:241–8.

12. Tromovitch TA, Stegman SJ. Microscopically controlled excision of skin tumors. Arch Dermatol 1974;110:231–2.

13. Swanson NA. Mohs' surgery: technique, indications, applications and the future. Arch Dermatol 1983;119:761–73.

14. Davidson TM, Nahum AM, Astarita RW. Microscopic controlled excisions for epidermoid carcinoma of the head and neck. Otolaryngol Head Neck Surg 1981;89:244–51.

15. Silverman ML, Kopf AW, Bart RS, et al. Recurrence rates of treated basal cell carcinomas. J Dermatol Surg Oncol 1992;18:471–6.

16. Robins P, Menn H. Chemosurgery in the treatment of skin cancer. Hosp Pract 1970;5:40–50.

17. Tromovitch TA, Stegman SJ. Microscopic controlled excision of cutaneous tumors: chemosurgery, fresh tissue technique. Cancer 1978;41:653–8.

18. Zacarian SA. Cryosurgery of skin cancer: fundamentals of technique and application. Cutis 1975;16:449–60.

19. Torre D. Cryosurgery instrumentation and depth dose monitoring. Clinics in Dermatology: Advances in cryosurgery. Vol. 8. New York: Elsevier, 1990:48.

20. Mendenhal WM, Parson JT, Mendenhall NP, et al. T2-T4 carcinoma of the skin of the head and neck, treated with radical irradiation. Int J Radiat Oncol Biol Phys 1987;13:975–81.

21. Farina AT, Leider M, Newall J, et al. Modern radiotherapy for malignant epitheliomas. Arch Dermatol 1977;113:650–4.

22. Lovett RD, Perez CA, Shapiro SJ, et al. External irradiation of epithelial skin cancer. Int J Radiat Oncol Biol Phys 1990;19:235–42.

23. Klein E. Tumors of skin. IX. Local cytostatic therapy of cutaneous and mucosal premalignant and malignant lesion. NY State J Med 1968;68:886–9.

24. Levis WR, Kraemer KH, Klinger WG, et al. Topical immunotherapy of basal cell carcinomas with dinitrochlorobenzene. Cancer Res 1973; 33:3036–42.

25. Adams EL, Price NM. Treatment of basal cell carcinomas with the CO2 laser. J Dermatol Surg Oncol 1989;15:803–6.

26. Fink-Puches R, Soyer HP, Hofer A, et al. Long-term follow-up and histological changes of superficial nonmelanoma skin cancers treated with topical delta-aminolevulinic acid photodynamic therapy. Arch Dermatol 1998;134:821–6.

27. Pfeiffer P, Hansen O, Rose C. Systemic cytotoxic therapy of basal cell carcinoma: a review of the literature. Eur J Cancer 1990;26:73–7.

28. Lippman SM, Parkinson DR, Itri LM, et al. 13-*cis*-retinoic acid and interferon: effective combination therapy for advanced squamous cell carcinoma of the skin. J Natl Cancer Inst 1992;84:235–41.

29. Hughes BR, Marks R, Pearse AD, Gaskell SA. Clinical response and tissue effects of etretinate treatment of patients with solar keratosis and basal cell carcinoma. J Am Acad Dermatol 1988;18:522–9.

30. Yiengpruksawan A, Coit DG, Thaler HT, et al. Merkel cell carcinoma: Prognosis and management. Arch Surg 1991;126:1514–9.

# XVII

# PEDIATRIC NEOPLASMS

# CHAPTER 77

# RETINOBLASTOMA

• MARCIO H. MALOGOLOWKIN • DAVID M. TISHLER • MAY LIN TAO

## Natural History

Retinoblastoma is a rare malignant neoplasm of the embryonic retina. It is the most common malignancy of the eye in children and one of the most common causes of childhood blindness. With early diagnosis and modern therapeutic approaches, the survival rate currently exceeds 90% in most industrialized countries. Retinoblastoma has played a critical role in the development of modern concepts of molecular carcinogenesis, and it provided an early example of the potential therapeutic value of combined-modality therapy.

The treatment of retinoblastoma is oriented toward saving vision, as well as life, to the greatest extent possible. Consequently, treatment usually involves both surgery and radiation therapy. The role of chemotherapy to reduce the size of retinoblastoma tumors followed by local therapy (thereby decreasing the need for radiotherapy and enucleation) is currently under investigation.

## EPIDEMIOLOGY

Retinoblastoma accounts for about 1% of all cancer-related deaths between birth and age 15.[1] Although this cancer is usually recognized within the first 2 years of life, it has been reported in both newborns and adults.[2]

The reported incidence is about 1 per 20,000 live births,[3, 4] but there is evidence that the frequency of tumor occurrence may be increasing.[4-7] For example, Tarkkanen and Tuovinen[6] reported a progressive change in the frequency of tumor recognition in Finland, increasing from 1 per 82,000 live births in 1919 to 1 per 16,000 live births in 1964. This apparent increase in the incidence of retinoblastoma is partially accounted for by better diagnosis and reporting. However, there is an actual increase in this genetically transmitted cancer due to the growing number of survivors who are producing more offspring.

Although it has been stated that there is no racial predilection,[8] a high incidence of retinoblastoma has been reported in several countries (Haiti, Nigeria, Jamaica) where the population is predominantly of African origin.[9, 10] There is no sex predilection.[8] Pendergrass and Davis,[11] in a large population-based survey in the United States, reported no difference in incidence between blacks and whites, but other nonwhites had rates greater than four times those of the white population.

## GENETICS

The Rb-1 gene is a tumor-suppressor gene. When it is absent or inactivated, retinoblastoma develops. The gene has been localized to chromosome 13, band q14, and since its discovery, numerous deletions have been described. According to Knudson's two-hit theory, tumorigenesis occurs as the result of two separate mutational events leading to inactivation or loss of the Rb-1 gene.[12] In hereditary cases, the first hit or mutation is present in the germline, whereas in nonhereditary cases, it occurs in somatic retinal cells. The second hit invariably occurs in somatic cells and initiates tumor formation. Most Rb-1 germline mutations are minute deletional defects, duplications, or point mutations that are detectable only by molecular analysis.

The Rb-1 gene product has been identified, and it appears to be a cell cycle regulator that also inhibits expression of genes involved in control of cell proliferation. The absence of normal Rb-1 thus leads to oncogenesis via promotion of uncontrolled cellular growth.[13]

Retinoblastoma is a model disease for revealing the association between genetics and cancer because it can occur in both hereditary and sporadic forms.[14] Although a positive family history may be documented in approximately 10% of retinoblastoma patients, about 40% of patients actually have hereditary disease. Inheritance is autosomal dominant with approximately 90% penetration. These patients have disease that is usually bilateral and multifocal, and they have an increased risk of secondary nonocular tumors. In contrast, nonhereditary disease occurs in about 60% of patients; in those cases, the tumors are primarily unilateral and unifocal, and there is no increased incidence of secondary malignancy. Fifteen percent of patients with unilateral retinoblastoma may have hereditary disease. Genetic counseling, supported by the use of Rb-1 DNA sequencing, can assist in the identification of patients with germline disease, thus allowing early detection and improved prognosis.[15]

Rb-1 gene mutations have been identified in other human tumors. Osteosarcomas, both with and without a history of retinoblastoma, have been identified with aberrant alterations of 13q14, a finding that is suggestive of shared tumorigenesis.[16] Rb-1 abnormalities have also been described in other soft tissue sarcomas,[17] breast carcinoma,[18] and small cell carcinoma of the lung.[19]

## PATHOLOGY

Retinoblastoma probably develops from neuroblastic tissue that forms the retinal photoreceptors.[20] The tumor may originate in the inner retinal layers and grow into the vitreous (endophytic), or it may originate in the outer retinal layers and extend into the subretinal space with the consequent detachment of the retina (exophytic). This growth pattern apparently has no prognostic significance, except that the endophytic type may be easier to diagnose. Rarely, tumor may thicken the retina without formation of a mass and consequently present clinically as "uveitis."[21] The basic retinoblastoma cells are either small and round or polygonal, with a relatively large nucleus and sparse cytoplasm.

Most retinoblastomas are structured as rosettes, which are composed of columnar cells in a circular arrangement around a lumen containing a hyaluronidase-resistant acid mucopolysaccharide.[22] Fleurettes, which are flower-like arrangements of cell processes in retinoblastoma cells with photoreceptor differentiation, can be identified occasionally.[20] The clinical significance of these structures is uncertain, for Ellsworth[3] has found no relationship to prognosis, whereas Tsukahara[23] and Ts'o and coworkers[20] have claimed a correlation with reduced tumor-related mortality but greater resistance to radiation.

## CLINICAL FEATURES AND DIAGNOSIS

The frequencies of presenting symptoms and signs, as recorded by Ellsworth,[24] are white or "cat's-eye" reflex, 56%; strabismus, 20% (esotropia, 11%; exotropia, 9%); red, painful eye with glaucoma, 7%; poor vision, 5%; incidental finding on routine examination, 3%; unilateral mydriasis, 2%; heterochromia iridis, 1%; hyphema, 1%; "strange expression," 0.5%; nystagmus, 0.5%; white spots on iris, 0.5%; and others, for example, failure to eat and thrive, 0.5%. These findings, most often leukokoria or strabismus, or both, usually are noted by the parent, family doctor, or pediatrician and are referred to the ophthalmologist for definitive diagnosis.

Multiple tumors can be identified in 75% of the eyes examined by indirect ophthalmoscopy with scleral depression.[3] Eighty percent of these tumors originate anterior to the equator of the globe. The mean number per patient is 4.7, and multiple tumors are now thought to signify a germinal mutation.

Two characteristic findings of retinoblastoma are vitreous seeding and flocculent calcification, which are documented in about 75% of patients by roentgenographic or ultrasonic examination or computed tomography (CT). Although the findings in most patients are characteristic of retinoblastoma, other conditions must be differentiated, including infection, retinal hemorrhage and detachment, and vascular malformation. Good differential diagnosis requires examination by personnel who are experienced in the recognition and treatment of retinoblastoma, a disease that is rare in the usual medical practice.

Some researchers report that elevated urinary excretion of vanillylmandelic acid and homovanillic acid before treatment, followed by decreased post-treatment levels, can be a diagnostic aid,[25] but this has not been confirmed by others.[26] Lactic dehydrogenase (LDH), a ubiquitous intracellular enzyme, was first reported as elevated in specimens from paracentesis of the anterior chamber of patients with retinoblastoma by Dias and colleagues in 1971.[27] An elevation two to three times the control value is highly suggestive of retinoblastoma and may be detected before the disease is clinically apparent. Ellsworth[3] reported an 8% incidence of false-negative tests and an occasional false-positive result. The validity of the aqueous/blood ratio of LDH has been questioned, and some authors suggest that total aqueous

LDH is a better index of the presence or absence of retinoblastoma.[28] Aqueous LDH activity has been found to correlate with the presence of tumor in the anterior chamber, but it is not a good indicator of other clinical or histopathologic characteristics of retinoblastoma.[29] Elevated carcinoembryonic antigen and alpha-fetoprotein levels, which drop after therapy, have been reported.[30] Extrascleral extension of tumor, as well as calcification, may be detected by CT.[31] Ultrasonography may be helpful in defining tumor when the visual examination is obstructed by cataract or vitreous opacity, or the tumor growth pattern is primarily endophytic. The pattern must be distinguished from vitreous hemorrhage. Retinoblastoma cells have been detected in the aspirate of the anterior chamber of patients presenting with hypopyon or uveitis.[32]

## STAGING AND PROGNOSIS

Reese and collaborators[33] and Ellsworth[3] developed a staging system that correlates the extent and anatomic location of retinoblastoma with preservation of useful vision following treatment (Table 77–1). This staging system forms the basis for our subsequent discussion of treatment. An alternative staging scheme, with specific treatment recommendations for each stage, has also been proposed by Howarth and colleagues,[34] and the American Joint Committee on Cancer and the International Union Against Cancer have developed a tumor-node-metastasis (TNM) staging scheme for retinoblastoma.[35] Neither of these latter systems will be discussed further because we have not used them personally and the published data on their prognostic value are scant.

Certain features of the enucleation specimen have prognostic correlation. When tumor extends to the cut end of the optic nerve (10 to 12 mm posterior to the lamina cribrosa sclerae), the mortality rate may be as high as 60%, whereas mortality decreases to about 40% if tumor extends beyond the lamina cribrosa sclerae but not to the end of the cut optic nerve, and to about 15% if tumor does not extend beyond the lamina cribrosa sclerae.[36] Much higher survival rates have been reported, however, in cases of extension of the tumor beyond the lamina cribrosa that have no involve-

---

*Table 77–1.* **Staging System for Retinoblastoma**

**Group I (very favorable)**
Solitary tumor, smaller than 4 disk diameters, at or behind equator
Multiple tumors, none larger than 4 disk diameters, all at or behind equator
**Group II (favorable)**
Solitary tumor, 4 to 10 disk diameters in size, at or behind equator
Multiple tumors, 4 to 10 disk diameters in size, all behind equator
**Group III (doubtful)**
Any lesion anterior to equator
Solitary tumor larger than 10 disk diameters, behind equator
**Group IV (unfavorable)**
Multiple tumors, some larger than 10 disk diameters
Any lesion extending anterior to ora serrata
**Group V (very unfavorable)**
Massive tumors involving over one half of retina
Vitreous seeding

From Reese AB, et al. Arch Ophthalmol 1955;53:505; and Ellsworth RM. The practical management of retinoblastoma. Trans Am Ophthalmol Soc 1969;67:462–532. Copyright 1955, American Medical Association.

ment of the sclera, iris, or resection line of the optic nerve.[37] The involvement of the choroid has been reported in approximately two thirds of all enucleated eyes[38] and is compatible with high survival rates when the sclera, iris, ciliary body, and resection site of the optic nerve are not involved.[37] The spread of tumor through or beyond the sclera is a dire prognostic sign. Distant metastases, most frequently to the central nervous system (CNS), skull, long bones, lung, and lymph nodes, are not compatible with survival by current treatment methods. A rare long-term survivor of metastatic disease has been reported, however, after aggressive radiation, chemotherapy, and surgical management.[39]

There has been some controversy about the necessary extent of staging procedures before surgical therapy in patients with retinoblastoma. In some studies, patients have been subjected to lumbar puncture and bone marrow aspirations preoperatively, while others have questioned the need for these studies. Pratt and colleagues[40] performed lumber punctures and bone marrow aspirations in 114 or more patients as part of a large study. They rarely found cerebrospinal fluid (CSF) or bone marrow involvement unless patients had symptoms, signs, or histologic evidence of tumor dissemination preoperatively. Both procedures were recommended, however, for patients with such findings or, if after enucleation, there was evidence of extraglobar extension.

Successful treatment of retinoblastoma is measured not only by patient survival—the primary concern, of course—but also by preservation of useful vision, which is usually defined as visual acuity ranging from 20/20 to 20/200. Tumor-related deaths are secondary to intracranial spread or hematogenous metastases, or both, and usually occur within 5 years of diagnosis. However, 10 to 15% of these patients may die with metastatic tumor more than 10 years following diagnosis.[3]

# Treatment

## INITIAL THERAPY

**Overview.** Classically, the primary treatment modalities for retinoblastoma have been enucleation external beam irradiation, or a combination of these. Secondary or adjuvant modes of treatment have included photocoagulation, cryotherapy, radioactive plaques, laser hyperthermia, and chemotherapy. Because retinoblastoma is usually a localized disease, the chance of cure is excellent (overall, approximately 90% 5-year survival) and cure should be the primary goal of treatment. Given this relatively favorable situation, however, every effort should be made to preserve the vision of an affected, but still sighted eye.

In general, children with unilateral disease have locally advanced tumors that typically present with a leukokoria ("cat's-eye" reflex) or strabismus resulting from a tumor in the macular area. Because these children have little hope of vision, they are often treated by enucleation. In bilateral disease, the traditional approach has been to enucleate the eye with more advanced disease and treat the remaining eye with external-beam irradiation if there is potentially viable retina remaining. However, enucleation of the eye that is more severely affected is indicated only if that eye is blind;

otherwise, an effort should be made to preserve both eyes. The use of chemotherapy to reduce tumor size, followed by local therapy, has been the subject of multiple small clinical trials; however, further investigation is required to confirm the value of this approach for the treatment of intraocular retinoblastoma.

**Enucleation.** Enucleation for the treatment of retinoblastoma involves severing the rectus muscles, placing anterior traction on the globe, and cutting the optic nerve near its exit from the socket with an attempt to secure a long segment (≥10 mm) of nerve. Postoperative external-beam radiation is added if there is significant tumor involvement of the optic nerve or sclera, if tumor is at the cut end of the nerve, or if there is gross residual disease. Enucleation is indicated when one or, in unfortunate instances, both eyes are blind, or when there is a local recurrence of tumor that cannot be controlled by other, more conservative means. Orbital growth may be reduced after enucleation, particularly if the child is younger than 3 years at the time of surgery. Prostheses can be fitted after surgery, which may result in more symmetric orbital development.

**Local Therapies.** Cryotherapy, photocoagulation, laser hyperthermia, and radioactive plaques have traditionally been used for unifocal or limited disease.[41] In the past, local therapy was avoided for patients with either bilateral disease or multifocal disease, or who were otherwise at high risk for developing multifocal disease; however, in the modern era, local therapy is being used in these situations in conjunction with chemotherapy, as will be discussed later. In general, these modalities cannot be used if the tumor is too proximal to either the optic disk or the macula. In select cases, these local therapies may be used for small-tumor recurrence after previous external-beam irradiation.

There is a renewed interest in local therapies, particularly the application of radioactive plaques (ie, cobalt 60, iodine 125, iridium 192, ruthenium 109). Radioactive plaque therapy is suitable for tumors of 15 mm basal diameter or smaller that are located more than 3 mm from the optic disk or fovea, with only limited vitreous seeding over the tumor apex. The advantage is that ocular and regional complications associated with external-beam irradiation can be avoided. Before the operative procedure is begun, the tumor's anatomy and location are mapped out by ultrasonography and physical examination, with later confirmation by an examination performed with the patient under anesthesia. The surgeon opens the conjunctiva around the periphery of the limbus, and the eye is rotated to locate the tumor, usually by either transillumination or ultrasonography. The plaque is sutured to the sclera, the eye is rotated back, and the conjunctiva is closed. The plaque is in place for approximately 3 to 5 days, during which the patient is generally hospitalized. When plaques are used as a single modality for treatment of a small primary tumor or for recurrent tumors after other treatment, the typical dose prescribed to the tumor apex is 35 to 40 Gy. However, with the increasing use of chemotherapy as primary treatment for localized disease, the occurrence of retinitis has led to dose reduction.

**External-Beam Radiotherapy.** External-beam irradiation typically is used when retinoblastoma is multifocal, too large for local therapies, complicated by vitreous seeding, or close to the macula or optic nerve with some vision intact. These situations are, in fact, common. Hilgartner first reported the successful treatment of retinoblastoma by x-rays in 1903.[42] The Reese-Ellsworth staging system can predict the probability of success of irradiation.[3] Larger tumors are harder to control with irradiation. The advantage of external-beam irradiation over local therapies is that the whole retina can be treated, as it is felt that these patients have a field defect.

Patient immobilization is critical to striking the balance between precise localization and treatment of the retina, and minimization of irradiation of normal tissue. Given the young age of these patients, daily anesthesia is generally required for treatment. A radiation oncologist must choose from a number of treatment techniques, which differ in the trade-off between treatment of the entire retinal surface and sparing of the lens, contralateral eye, and other structures such as the frontal lobes. For anteriorly located tumors with increased risk of cataract formation, particular attention must be paid to adequate coverage, or treatment failure may result in this location. The typical modern-era dose is 40 to 45 Gy in daily fractions of 1.8 to 2 Gy per day, 5 days per week. In earlier times, when anesthesia techniques were less sophisticated, patients were treated four times a week in 2.5-Gy fractions with resultant increase in late effects (ie, chorioretinitis).[43, 44] Today, proton treatment and fractionated stereotactic radiation therapy[45] are only two of the innovative methods used to minimize irradiation of normal tissue and to reduce late effects.

If both eyes have the possibility for sight, bilateral irradiation or chemotherapy followed by local therapy may be advised. However, if later follow-up examination under anesthesia shows no evidence of tumor response to treatment, the eye should be enucleated.

**Chemotherapy.** Chemotherapy use has been limited to the treatment of patients with extraocular disease who develop regional or distant metastases because the overall survival rate for patients with retinoblastoma treated with surgery or radiotherapy has been greater than 90%.

Chemotherapeutic agents previously used for the treatment of patients with retinoblastoma have included vincristine, cyclophosphamide, doxorubicin, ifosfamide, and cisplatin.[46] Although these agents have been reported to induce tumor reduction, they have limited efficacy for the treatment of intraocular disease and are associated with significant toxicities. Studies by both the Children's Cancer Group and the Pediatric Oncology Group, as well as the St. Jude Children's Research Center, have sought to determine the efficacy of adjuvant chemotherapy in retinoblastoma.[34, 47, 48] These studies indicate that the combination of vincristine and cyclophosphamide, with or without doxorubicin (Adriamycin), is tolerable and is associated with manageable morbidity. However, neither study has clearly established the added efficacy of these agents as adjuvants to primary therapy.

Conversely, the benefit of adjuvant chemotherapy for patients with extraocular disease has been well documented.[49–53] Zelter and colleagues[49] from Argentina reported their experience with combined-modality therapy in 72 patients in whom the treatment approach was determined by St. Jude staging.[47] Patients with extraocular extension beyond the sclera, the cut end of the optic nerve, or both (stage III) were treated with vincristine, cyclophosphamide, and doxorubicin; those at greatest risk of CNS spread were also

treated with triple intrathecal chemotherapy. Furher intensification using CECA (cisplatin, etoposide, cyclophosphamide, and doxorubicin [Adriamycin]) was used for the small number of patients with bloodborne metastases (stage IV). At a median follow-up of 63 months for patients with unilateral disease and 81 months for patients with bilateral disease, 46% survival was seen in patients with stage III disease. All patients with stage IV disease experienced progression. Toxicity results were acceptable. In another study from Argentina, Schvartzman and colleagues[50] reported on 116 patients treated in a single institution with a combined-modality approach. Twenty-nine patients with stage II disease (orbital or postlaminar invasion) received vincristine, cyclophosphamide, and doxorubicin for 57 weeks with or without orbital radiotherapy and intrathecal chemotherapy for those with extension beyond the cut end of the optic nerve. Patients with CNS disease (stage III) or hematogenous metastasis (stage IV) also received cisplatin and etoposide with cranial or craniospinal radiotherapy. After a median follow-up time of 39 months (12 to 84 months), the overall survival for stage II patients was 85%, and only 25% for those with more advanced stages of disease.

Despite the overall improvement in survival rate of patients with retinoblastoma, patients with CNS involvement or hematogenous metastases continue to have a poor outcome. Several studies have shown that intensive multiagent therapy can be successful in prolonging the survival of these patients.[52, 54] In one report, Grabowski and coworkers included five patients with hematogenous spread.[54] At a mean follow-up of 48 months, three of the five patients were alive with no evidence of disease. Their combined-modality approach included surgical decompression of calvarial lesions, whole-brain radiation therapy (18 to 24 Gy) for those with documented CSF or CNS disease, and systemic chemotherapy with vincristine, cyclophosphamide, and doxorubicin, as well as intrathecal or intra–Ommaya reservoir chemotherapy with methotrexate and cytarabine.

Encouraging reports suggest that increasing the chemotherapy dose intensity may improve survival in extraocular retinoblastoma, as several centers have used high-dose chemoradiotherapy and rescue with autologous bone marrow transplantation to treat small numbers of patients with extraocular disease successfully.[55–57]

The reduced efficacy of chemotherapy for intraocular retinoblastoma may be a result of the poor intraocular penetration of systemic drugs, and the frequent expression of the MDR-1 P-glycoprotein in these tumors. Reports have demonstrated that the use of cyclosporine in combination with chemotherapy (vincristine, teniposide, and carboplatin) can block P-glycoprotein function and reverse multidrug resistance.[58, 59] Chan and colleagues reported on the treatment of 22 patients with cyclosporine, vincristine, teniposide, and carboplatin followed by local therapy.[58] When compared with 19 historical control patients treated with various combinations of chemotherapy regimens without cyclosporine, radiation, and similar local therapy, the study patients showed significantly better long-term responses, and their vision was saved without radiation treatment or enucleation. At a median follow-up of 2.4 years, the relapse-free survival rates were 76% and 37% ($p = 0.032$) for study patients and historical control patients, respectively.

In an attempt to preserve vision by eliminating the need

for enucleation and radiotherapy, and to reduce the risk of late effects, including the development of second malignant neoplasms, many trials have explored the use of chemoreduction plus sequential aggressive local therapy for the treatment of intraocular retinoblastoma.[59-63] Preliminary reports of these trials have demonstrated the usefulness of chemotherapy in reducing intraocular retinoblastoma, while allowing the effective use of local therapy; elimination of both radiation therapy and enucleation for some patients with retinoblastoma has been achieved. Greenwald and Strauss treated six patients (11 eyes, 33 tumors) with six to seven cycles of intravenous carboplatin and etoposide followed by local therapy with cryotherapy or laser.[61] At 12 to 40 months of follow-up, 8 eyes had been preserved, including 5 eyes with large tumors and all 4 eyes with vitreous seeding. Shields and associates treated intraocular tumors in 32 patients (130 tumors, 52 eyes) with chemoreduction using vincristine, etoposide, and carboplatin followed by adjuvant local therapy.[60] At a mean follow-up of 17 months (range, 13 to 27 months), the authors were able to avoid enucleation or external-beam radiation in 42% of these patients. Murphree and coworkers reviewed the outcomes of patients treated with systemic carboplatin; followed by continuous diode laser hyperthermia (thermochemotherapy) or systemic chemotherapy with vincristine, etoposide, and carboplatin; then sequential aggressive local therapy (chemotherapy/ SALT).[63] Success was defined as eradication of tumor without enucleation or external-beam radiation. Successful results were seen in 26 of 38 eyes treated with thermochemotherapy and in 10 of 35 eyes treated with chemotherapy/ SALT. However, in contrast to other reports, less successful results were achieved in eyes with diffuse vitreous seeding or extensive subretinal seeding; enucleation and external-beam radiation could not be avoided in these patients.

The development of collaborative multi-institutional research will help to further define the role and efficacy of chemoreduction treatment of intraocular retinoblastoma, both in salvaging eyes and in reducing long-term complications such as second malignant neoplasms. Patients with retinoblastoma should be referred to centers involved in these collaborative research efforts so they may be offered the best therapeutic options and expertise; such referrals will also further our knowledge of such a rare tumor. Novel approaches such as subconjunctival chemotherapy and gene therapy are starting to be evaluated in the treatment of patients with retinoblastoma.

## LATE EFFECTS OF THERAPY

The late effects of treatment of retinoblastoma are related to treatment modality (surgery, radiotherapy, and chemotherapy) and host susceptibility (age at diagnosis, hereditary vs. nonhereditary disease). As with all investigations of incidence and severity of late effects, time from treatment is an important co-variable; thus, studies could be expected to elucidate new findings as a patient cohort ages. Retinoblastoma, as a treatable and curable disease, presents a unique opportunity for researchers to investigate the long-term effects of specific cancer therapies. Follow-up of such patients can provide us with valuable information as we attempt to "detoxify" treatment in this population.

**Radiation Therapy.** The effects of external-beam radiotherapy have been well characterized. Although megavoltage has supplanted orthovoltage as the radiation modality (with lower bone doses and equal dose delivery to bone and soft tissues), significant late complications have been observed frequently. Imhof and colleagues[64] evaluated 68 patients with bilateral or unilateral disease (120 orbits) who had been treated at age 2 weeks to 53 months (mean, 11 months) with radiation (45 Gy in 15 fractions at three fractions weekly) with or without enucleation and who were 1 to 10 years from therapy (mean, 8 years). They found that irradiation caused significant orbital and midfacial growth retardation when growth was compared with that of nonirradiated orbits, and that patients younger than 6 months at the time of treatment sustained more growth impairment than did older children. Although they reported that enucleation had no additive effect on growth retardation beyond that of radiation therapy, other studies have shown reduced orbital growth after enucleation alone. They concluded that radiation is exceptionally deleterious to the very young patient and that investigation of other forms of treatment that would enable postponement or deletion of radiation was warranted. Pradhan and associates[65] retrospectively examined 120 patients (192 eyes) who had received external-beam orbital radiotherapy (approximately 42 Gy) with and without chemotherapy (vincristine, doxorubicin, and cyclophosphamide). These patients were treated at a mean age of 31 months, and they were subsequently evaluated at a follow-up mean of 48 months from treatment. Complications occurred in approximately 50% of patients and included cataracts, retinopathy, vitreous hemorrhage, glaucoma, optic neuropathy, keratopathy, and dry eye. Half of all patients retained vision in the treated eye. Hypofractionation of radiation therapy (using a high dose per fraction, >2.5 Gy, as was done in an earlier era) appears to contribute to a higher risk of retinopathy.[44] Late effects of treatment in 99 patients with bilateral retinoblastoma were evaluated by Messmer and coworkers.[66] Patients were treated with a variety of modalities, including photo- or cryocoagulation, radiation therapy, enucleation, or all of these. The median follow-up was 15 years. Useful vision was documented in 81 of 96 preserved eyes. Tumor site (central location) and presence of cataract were factors responsible for poor visual acuity. Complications of photocoagulation included iridic atrophy and localized traction retinal detachment. Midfacial hypoplasia and radiation dermatosis were common complications, which occurred more frequently after orthovoltage than after megavoltage radiotherapy.

**Chemotherapy.** Late effects of chemotherapeutic drugs are well documented.[67] Agents that have been previously used to treat retinoblastoma (vincristine, cyclophosphamide, and doxorubicin) have predictable dose- and age-related short- and long-term toxicities. Current combination therapy using carboplatin, etoposide-teniposide, vincristine, and cyclosporine, has been infrequently studied for late effects, and young age at treatment remains a risk factor of concern for long-term complications of treatment. The topoisomerase inhibitors etoposide and teniposide have been associated with secondary leukemias, and close follow-up of young children treated with these agents is warranted.[68] Unknown at this time is whether the mutagenic and genotoxic effects of chemotherapeutic drugs are of increased concern in a patient population already predisposed to second malignancies (see later). Follow-up data of very young patients treated with chemotherapy for retinoblastoma will be enlightening; findings should guide the planning of future therapy protocols.

**Second Malignant Neoplasms.** The elevated incidence of secondary cancers in survivors of retinoblastoma highlights the association of Rb-1 gene abnormalities with subsequent nonocular tumor.[69] Bone and soft tissue sarcomas, specifically osteosarcomas, occur in retinoblastoma patients at a rate approximately 500 times greater than that expected in the general population. Two thirds of secondary osteosarcomas occur within the radiation field, and one third occur outside the field or in nonirradiated patients. Retinoblastoma patients are repeatedly overrepresented in reported series of secondary bone sarcomas, and the Late Effects Study Group, a consortium of 13 pediatric oncology institutions, has reported that 30% of secondary osteosarcomas occur in patients with retinoblastoma. The mean interval to these second malignant neoplasms is about 11 years for sarcomas occurring in the treated radiation field, and 13.5 years for those occurring outside the irradiated area.[70]

In a large cohort incidence study of more than 1600 patients, Wong and coworkers reported a 51% cumulative occurrence of secondary malignancy at 50 years after diagnosis for hereditary retinoblastoma, compared with 5% for nonhereditary cases.[71] The cumulative probability of death from a second cancer was 26% at 40 years after bilateral retinoblastoma, and 1.5% for unilateral disease.[72] Radiotherapy further influenced the risk of development of secondary malignancy; at 50 years, the cumulative incidence of secondary malignancy was 58% in irradiated hereditary retinoblastoma versus 27% in nonirradiated inherited disease.[72] The risk of secondary malignancy was further influenced by escalation of the radiation dose, as well as enlargement of the field of radiation.[73] Roarty and associates demonstrated that the 30-year incidence of secondary malignancy was 29% within the radiation field and 8% outside the field.[74] This latter incidence corresponds to the 6% rate of second cancers for those patients who did not receive radiation therapy.

In summary, genetic predisposition has a substantial impact on the risk of subsequent cancers in patients with retinoblastoma; this risk is increased by radiation. Reduction or elimination of radiation may decrease therapy-associated second malignancies. Given the increased survival of patients with retinoblastoma, it is of paramount importance that patients at risk of developing a second tumor be carefully surveyed.

## SUGGESTIONS FOR ADDITIONAL READING

Herwig S, Strauss M. The retinoblastoma protein: a master regulator of cell cycle, differentiation and apoptosis. Eur J Biochem 1997;246:581–601.

Knudson AG. Hereditary cancer: two hits revisited. J Cancer Res Clin Oncol 1996;122:135–40.

Shields CL, Shields JA. Recent developments in the management of retinoblastoma. J Pediatr Ophthalmol Strabismus 1999;36:8–18.

Fontanesi J, Pratt CB, Hustu HO, et al. Use of irradiation for therapy of retinoblastoma in children more than 1 year old: the St. Jude Children's Research Hospital experience and review of literature. Med Pediatr Oncol 1995;24:321–6.

Bhisitkul RB, Mukai S. Emerging chemotherapeutic strategies in the man-

agement of intraocular retinoblastoma. Int Ophthalmol Clin 1997;37:201–14.

Moll AC, Imhof SM, Bouter LM, Tan KE. Second primary tumors in patients with retinoblastoma. A review of the literature. Ophthalmic Genet 1997;18:27–34.

## REFERENCES

1. Miller RW. Fifty-two forms of childhood cancer: United States mortality experience, 1960–1966. J Pediatr 1969;75:685–9.
2. Bedford MA. Treatment of retinoblastoma. Adv Ophthalmol 1975;31:2–32.
3. Ellsworth RM. The practical management of retinoblastoma. Trans Am Ophthalmol Soc 1969;67:462–534.
4. Franchise J. In: Boniuk M, ed. Ocular and adnexal tumors. St. Louis: CV Mosby, 1964:123.
5. Schappert-Kimmijser J, Hemmes GD, Nijland R. The heredity of retinoblastoma. Ophthalmologica 1966;151:197–213.
6. Tarkkanen A, Tuovinen E. Retinoblastoma in Finland 1912–1964. Acta Ophthalmol 1971;49:293–300.
7. Barry G, Mullaney J. Retinoblastoma in the Republic of Ireland (1955–70). Trans Ophthalmol Soc UK 1971;91:839–55.
8. Ellsworth R. Tumors of the retina. In: Tasman W, ed. Retinal diseases in children. New York: Harper & Row, 1971.
9. Kodilinye HC. Retinoblastoma in Nigeria: problems of treatment. Am J Ophthalmol 1967;63:469–81.
10. Bras G, Cole H, Ashmeade-Dyer A, Watler DC. Report on 141 childhood malignancies observed in Jamaica. J Natl Cancer Inst 1969;43:417–21.
11. Pendergrass TW, Davis S. Incidence of retinoblastoma in the United States. Arch Ophthalmol 1980;98:1204–10.
12. Knudson AG Jr, Hethcote HW, Brown BW. Mutation and childhood cancer: a probabilistic model for the incidence of retinoblastoma. Proc Natl Acad Sci USA 1975;72:5116–20.
13. Zhang K, Wang MX, Munier F, et al. Molecular genetics of retinoblastoma. Int Ophthalmol Clin 1993;33:53–65.
14. Knudson AG Jr. Mutation and cancer: statistical study of retinoblastoma. Proc Natl Acad Sci USA 1971;68:820–3.
15. Yandell DW, Campbell TA, Dayton SH, et al. Oncogenic point mutations in the human retinoblastoma gene: their application to genetic counseling. N Engl J Med 1989;321:1689–95.
16. Hansen MF, Koufos A, Gallie, et al. Osteosarcoma and retinoblastoma: a shared chromosomal mechanism revealing recessive predisposition. Proc Natl Acad Sci USA 1985;82:6216–20.
17. Weichselbaum RR, Beckett M, Diamond A. Some retinoblastomas, osteosarcomas, and soft tissue sarcomas may share a common etiology. Proc Natl Acad Sci USA 1988;85:2106–9.
18. Lee EY, To H, Shew JY, et al. Inactivation of the retinoblastoma susceptibility gene in human breast cancers. Science 1988;241:218–21.
19. Yokota J, Wada M, Shimosato Y, et al. Loss of heterozygosity on chromosomes 3, 13, and 17 in small-cell carcinoma and on chromosome 3 in adenocarcinoma of the lung. Proc Natl Acad Sci USA 1987; 84:9252–6.
20. Ts'o MO, Fine BS, Zimmerman LE. The nature of retinoblastoma. II. Photoreceptor differentiation: an electron microscopic study. Am J Ophthalmol 1970;69:350–9.
21. Howard GM, Ellsworth RM. Differential diagnosis of retinoblastoma. Am J Ophthalmol 1965;60:618–27.
22. Zimmerman LE. Applications of histochemical methods for the demonstration of acid mucopolysaccharides to ophthalmic pathology. Trans Am Acad Ophthalmol Otolaryngol 1958;62:697–701.
23. Tsukahara I. A histopathological study on the prognosis and radiosensitivity of retinoblastoma. Arch Ophthalmol 1960;63:1005–8.
24. Ellsworth RM. Orbital retinoblastoma. Trans Am Ophthalmol Soc 1974;72:79–88.
25. Brown DH. The clinicopathology of retinoblastoma. Am J Ophthalmol 1966;61:508–14.
26. Renelt P, Trieschmann W. Vanilmandelic acid urinary excretion in the diagnosis of retinoblastoma. Albrecht von Graefes Arch Klin Exp Ophthalmol 1973;188:281–3.
27. Dias PL, Shanmuganathan SS, Rajaratnam M. Lactic dehydrogenase activity of aqueous humour in retinoblastoma. Br J Ophthalmol 1971;55:130–2.
28. Abramson DH, Piro PA, Ellsworth RM, et al. Lactate dehydrogenase

levels and isozyme patterns. Measurements in the aqueous humor and serum of retinoblastoma patients. Arch Ophthalmol 1979;97:870–1.

29. Piro PA Jr, Abramson DH, Ellsworth RM, Kitchin D. Aqueous humor lactate dehydrogenase in retinoblastoma patients. Clinicopathologic correlations. Arch Ophthalmol 1978;96:1823–5.

30. Michelson JB, Felberg NT, Shields JA. Fetal antigens in retinoblastoma. Cancer 1976;37:719–23.

31. Goldberg L, Danziger A. Computed tomographic scanning in the management of retinoblastoma. Am J Ophthalmol 1977;84:380–2.

32. Hogan MJ, Wood IS, Godfrey WA. Aqueous humor cytology in uveitis. Arch Ophthalmol 1973;89:217–20.

33. Reese AB, Hyman GA, Merriam GR Jr, et al. Treatment of retinoblastoma by radiation and triethylenemelamine. Arch Ophthalmol 1955;53:505–13.

34. Howarth C, Meyer D, Hustu HO, et al. Stage-related combined modality treatment of retinoblastoma. Results of a prospective study. Cancer 1980;45:851–8.

35. Beahrs OH, eds. Manual for staging of cancer, 4th ed. Philadelphia: JB Lippincott, 1992:235.

36. Ellsworth RM. Retinoblastoma. Mod Probl Ophthalmol 1977; 18:94–100.

37. Stannard C, Lipper S, Sealy R, Sevel D. Retinoblastoma: correlation of invasion of the optic nerve and choroid with prognosis and metastases. Br J Ophthalmol 1979;63:560–70.

38. Redler LD, Ellsworth RM. Prognostic importance of choroidal invasion in retinobastoma. Arch Ophthalmol 1973;90:294–6.

39. Judisch GF, Apple DJ, Fratkin JD. Retinoblastoma. A survivor 12 years after treatment for metastatic disease. Arch Ophthalmol 1980;98:711–3.

40. Pratt CB, Meyer D, Chenaille P, Crom DB. The use of bone marrow aspirations and lumbar punctures at the time of diagnosis of retinoblastoma. J Clin Oncol 1989;7:140–3.

41. Halperin EC. In: Halperin EC, Constine LS, Tarbell NJ, Kun LE, eds. Pediatric radiation oncology, 2nd ed. New York: Raven Press, 1994:140.

42. Hilgartner HL. Report of case of double glioma treated with x-ray. Tex Med J 1903;18:322–3.

43. Thompson RW, Small RC, Stein JJ. Treatment of retinoblastoma. Am J Roentgenol Radium Ther Nucl Med 1972;114:16–23.

44. Coucke PA, Schmid C, Balmer A, et al. Hypofractionation in retinoblastoma: an increased risk of retinopathy. Radiother Oncol 1993;28:157–61.

45. Loeffler JS. In: DeSalles AAF, Goetsch SJ, eds. Stereotactic surgery and radiosurgery. Madison, Medical Physics Publishing, 1993:307.

46. White L. Chemotherapy in retinoblastoma: current status and future directions. Am J Pediatr Hematol/Oncol 1991 (Summer);13:189–201.

47. Wolff JA, Boesel CP, Dyment PG, et al. Treatment of retinoblastoma. Excerpta Med Int Congr Ser 1981;570:364–8.

48. Höpping W, Schmitt G. The treatment of retinoblastoma. Mod Probl Ophthalmol 1977;18:106–12.

49. Zelter M, Damel A, Gonzalez G, Schwartz L. A prospective study on the treatment of retinoblastoma in 72 patients. Cancer 1991;68:1685–90.

50. Schvartzman E, Chantada G, Fandiäno A, et al. Results of a stage-based protocol for the treatment of retinoblastoma. J Clin Oncol 1996;14:1532–6.

51. Doz F, Khelfaoui F, Mosseri V, et al. The role of chemotherapy in orbital involvement of retinoblastoma. The experience of a single institution with 33 patients. Cancer 1994;74:722–32.

52. Pratt CB, Fontanesi J, Chenaille P, et al. Chemotherapy for extraocular retinoblastoma. Pediatr Hematol Oncol 1994;11:301–9.

53. Advani SH, Rao SR, Iyer RS, et al. Pilot study of sequential combination chemotherapy in advanced and recurrent retinoblastoma. Med Pediatr Oncol 1994;22:125–8.

54. Grabowski EF, McCormick B, Ellsworth RE, et al. Extraocular retinoblastoma: first sustained remissions with aggressive multi-modality therapy. Proc ASCO 1988;7:258.

55. Saleh RA, Gross S, Cassano W, Gee A. Metastatic retinoblastoma successfully treated with immunomagnetic purged autologous bone marrow transplantation. Cancer 1988;62:2301–3.

56. Saarinen UM, Sariola H, Hovi L. Recurrent disseminated retinoblastoma treated by high-dose chemotherapy, total body irradiation, and autologous bone marrow rescue. Am J Pediatr Hematol/Oncol 1991;13:315–9.

57. Namouni F, Doz F, Tanguy ML, et al. High-dose chemotherapy with carboplatin, etoposide and cyclophosphamide followed by a haematopoietic stem cell rescue in patients with high-risk retinoblastoma: a SFOP and SFGM study. Eur J Cancer 1997;33:2368–75.

58. Charm HSL, DeBoer G, Thiessen JJ, et al. Combining cyclosporin with chemotherapy controls intraocular retinoblastoma without requiring radiation. Clin Cancer Res 1996;2:1499–508.

59. Gallie BL, Budning A, DeBoer G, et al. Chemotherapy with focal therapy can cure intraocular retinoblastoma without radiotherapy. Arch Ophthalmol 1996;114:1321–8.

60. Shields CL, Shields JA, Needle M, et al. Combined chemoreduction and adjuvant treatment for intraocular retinoblastoma. Ophthalmology 1997;104:2101–11.

61. Greenwald MJ, Strauss LC. Treatment of intraocular retinoblastoma with carboplatin and etoposide chemotherapy. Ophthalmology 1996;103:19897-97.

62. Shields CL, De Potter P, Himelstein BP, et al. Chemoreduction in the initial management of intraocular retinoblastoma. Arch Ophthalmol 1996;114:1330–8.

63. Murphree AL, Villabianca JG, Deegan WF 3rd, et al. Chemotherapy plus local treatment in the management of intraocular retinoblastoma. Arch Ophthalmol 1996;114:1348–56.

64. Imhof SM, Mourits MP, Hofman P, et al. Quantification of orbital and mid-facial growth retardation after megavoltage external beam irradiation in children with retinoblastoma. Ophthalmology 1996; 103:263–8.

65. Pradhan DG, Sandridge AL, Mullaney P, et al. Radiation therapy for retinoblastoma: a retrospective review of 120 patients. Int J Radiat Oncol Biol Phys 1997;39:3–13.

66. Messmer EP, Fritze H, Mohr C, et al. Long-term treatment effects in patients with bilateral retinoblastoma: ocular and midfacial findings. Graefes Arch Clin Exp Ophthalmol 1991;229:309–14.

67. Grossi M. Management and long-term complications of pediatric cancer. Pediatr Clin North Am 1998;45:1637–58.

68. van Leeuwen FE, Chorus AM, van den Belt-Dusebout AW, et al. Leukemia risk following Hodgkin's disease: relation to cumulative dose of alkylating agents, treatment with teniposide combinations, number of episodes of chemotherapy, and bone marrow damage. J Clin Oncol 1994;12:1063–73.

69. Meadows AT, Baum E, Fossati-Bellani F, et al. Second malignant neoplasms in children: an update from the Late Effects Study Group. J Clin Oncol 1985;3:532–8.

70. Newton WA Jr, Meadows AT, Shimada H, et al. Bone sarcomas as second malignant neoplasms following childhood cancer. Cancer 1991;67:193–201.

71. Wong FL, Boice JD Jr, Abramson DH, et al. Cancer incidence after retinoblastoma. Radiation dose and sarcoma risk. JAMA 1997;278:1262–7.

72. Eng C, Li FP, Abramson DH, et al. Mortality from second tumors among long-term survivors of retinoblastoma. J Natl Cancer Inst 1993;85:1121–8.

73. Abramson DH, Ellsworth RM, Kitchin FD, Tung G. Second nonocular tumors in retinoblastoma survivors. Are they radiation induced? Ophthalmology 1984;91:1351–5.

74. Roarty JD, McLean IW, Zimmerman LE. Incidence of second neoplasms in patients with bilateral retinoblastoma. Ophthalmology 1988;95:1583–7.

# CHAPTER 78

# WILMS' TUMOR

• MARCIO H. MALOGOLOWKIN • MAY LIN TAO • NANCY KLIPFEL •
• SUNITA M. BHUTA • JAMES B. ATKINSON •

## Natural History

The survival rate of children with Wilms' tumor (WT) has risen from approximately 20% to greater than 90% since the late 1960s.[1] This success has been the result of the methodical multidisciplinary efforts of pediatric oncologists, surgeons, pathologists, and radiation oncologists through clinical trials conducted by the National Wilms' Tumor Study Group (NWTS) and the International Society of Pediatric Oncology (SIOP).

Since the late 1960s, these successive clinical trials have continued to improve survival, refine therapy, and decrease the acute and long-term morbidity associated with the treatment of children with WT. These trials have also served as a major source for the investigation of the epidemiology and biology of this tumor.

### EPIDEMIOLOGY

Approximately 1 in 10,000 children younger than 15 years of age worldwide develops WT. Each year in the United States, 460 new cases are diagnosed, which represents 5 to 6% of all childhood cancers diagnosed per year in the United States.[2] Worldwide, the incidence rates are about the same for boys and girls. In the United States, however, there is a slightly higher incidence among girls as well as for blacks when compared with whites.[3] More than 75% of the cases occur in children younger than 5 years of age, with a peak incidence around 3 years of age.[4] An increased frequency of this malignancy has been reported in patients with congenital sporadic aniridia,[5] hemihypertrophy or focal gigantism,[6] neurofibromatosis,[7] anomalies of the genitourinary system, mental retardation, and microcephaly. Genetic syndromes that predispose children to the development of WT include WAGR syndrome (WT, aniridia, genitourinary malformations, and mental retardation), Drash's syndrome (intersexual disorders, nephropathy, and WT), and Beckwith-Wiedemann syndrome (macroglossia, organomegaly, omphalocele, and hemihypertrophy). The incidence of WT in WAGR, Drash's, and Beckwith-Wiedemann syndromes has been reported to be greater than 30%, greater than 90%, and less than 5%.[8] Familial cases are rare; however, linear transmission[9] and the occasional concurrence of WT in siblings and identical twins[10] probably reflect an inherited predisposition that may become more apparent as more patients survive to reproductive age.[11]

### GENETICS

WT parallels retinoblastoma in several ways: both malignancies occur in the very young, arise from embryonal cells, can develop unilaterally or bilaterally, and can occur in hereditary and nonhereditary (sporadic) forms. Based on epidemiologic observations, Knudson and Strong[12] have proposed a *two-hit* hypothesis as an etiologic explanation for these tumors. According to this hypothesis, two mutational genetic events are needed to produce a tumor. The first event may be constitutional (occurs in all cells and is transmitted from an affected parent), or it may be somatic. Subsequently the function of the complementary normal gene is lost by one of several mechanisms, leading to tumor formation. In hereditary cases, the first mutation occurs in a germ cell before conception so that all cells in the offspring carry the first mutation. In the nonhereditary cases, both mutations occur after conception. The isolation of the retinoblastoma gene located at 13q14 provided the first molecular confirmation of the two-hit hypothesis.[13]

Several molecular findings have pointed to the existence of a similar tumor-suppressor gene, which when inactivated or lost leads to development of a WT. The deletion of a small portion of the short arm of chromosome 11 has been reported in familial cases of WT associated with other congenital anomalies.[14, 15] A candidate gene (WT1) for the WAGR syndrome has been localized to chromosome 11p13.[16] This gene encodes a zinc-finger protein that functions as a repressor of transcription. In vitro studies have shown that this protein inhibits synthesis of platelet-derived growth factor.[17] A second locus, associated with the Beckwith-Wiedemann syndrome, localizes to chromosome 11p15 and reflects paternal uniparental disomy, resulting in increased expression of insulin-like growth factor II.[18] A third WT locus has been identified on chromosome 16q,[19] but deletion of these genes is not necessary for the appearance of WT.[20, 21] The cause of WT has not been defined completely,[22] but loss of heterozygosity at specific tumor-suppressor loci has been a recurrent observation.

### CLINICAL FEATURES AND DIAGNOSIS

The most common initial manifestation of WT is a large, asymptomatic, unilateral upper abdominal mass, generally discovered incidentally by a parent or physician. The tumor is solid, discrete, nontender, and usually fixed to the posterior abdomen. Other malignant tumors found in the same location include neuroblastoma, rhabdomyosarcoma, and hepatic tumors. Because WTs may be cystic or contain necrotic tissue, cystic lesions of the kidney must be considered in the differential diagnosis. Benign cystic abdominal masses in children include multicystic or hydronephrotic kidneys and mesenteric, choledochal, and duplication cysts.

WTs usually enlarge rapidly shortly before detection. Although they are believed to be embryonal in origin, they apparently remain dormant until their doubling rate increases sharply before detection. The presence of hypertension (owing to the secretion of renin by the tumor),[23] erythrocytosis (owing to the secretion of erythropoietin by the tumor),[24] and vague symptoms of abdominal pain, fever, and weight loss should arouse diagnostic suspicion. Excessive palpation of the mass should be avoided because it may dislodge malignant cells or cause hemorrhage.

Readily available diagnostic studies establish the diagnosis of WT in most patients. Routine urinalysis results are frequently normal, but 15 to 20% of patients have hematuria, especially older children. Chest radiographs should be part of the initial diagnostic work-up. Approximately 10% of patients, particularly older ones, have radiographic evidence of pulmonary metastases at the time of diagnosis.[25]

General baseline laboratory studies are usually normal preoperatively but may be extremely helpful for following the patient through the postoperative period and subsequent therapeutic course. The initial work-up should include a complete blood count, serum creatinine and electrolyte levels, and liver function tests. Serum renin and erythropoietin levels may be elevated. In contrast to neuroblastoma, urinary catecholamine metabolites, especially vanillylmandelic acid and homovanillic acid, are not significantly elevated. Bone marrow aspiration and bone surveys (or bone scans) for metastatic disease are not usually performed unless the possibility of neuroblastoma is considered likely or unless the diagnosis of clear cell sarcoma is made. Clear cell sarcomas have a unique predilection for metastasis to bone[26] and brain.[27] Patients with tumors of this histologic type require bone scan and computed tomography (CT) or magnetic resonance imaging (MRI) of the brain for reliable staging.

Plain abdominal films usually show displacement of bowel gas shadows away from the tumor. In contrast to neuroblastoma, calcification of a WT is unusual. Abdominal ultrasonography examination is helpful to rule out a renal cyst (Fig. 78–1).[28] Real-time ultrasonography or MRI should be performed to screen for tumor extension into the renal vein or vena cava (Fig. 78–2).[29] CT or MRI also can determine the relationship of the mass to other abdominal organs

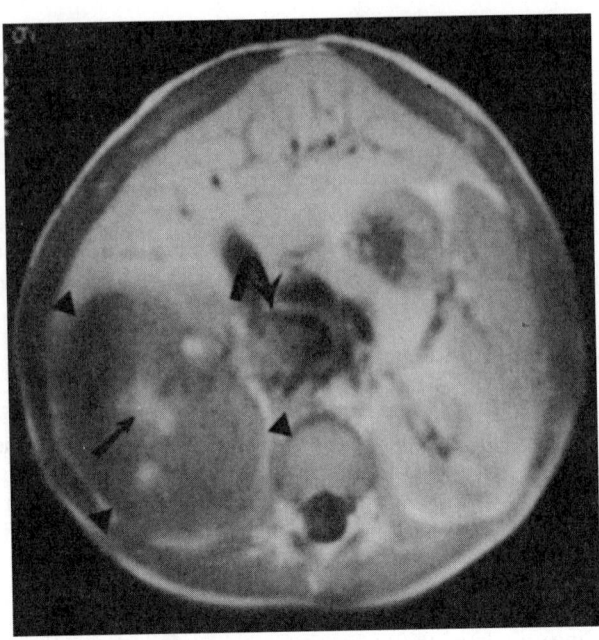

**Figure 78–2.** Axial SE (500/18) magnetic resonance image demonstrates a mass of medium-signal intensity *(arrowheads)*. Inside the mass are areas of high-signal intensity due to hemorrhage *(arrow)*. A tumor thrombus is seen extending into and expanding the inferior vena cava *(curved arrow)*. (Courtesy of R. B. Dietrich.)

as well as the status of the contralateral kidney.[29–31] Clear visualization of the contralateral kidney to rule out bilateral tumor or another abnormality is essential before excisional surgery is attempted.

Intravenous pyelography (IVP) is rarely useful in early diagnosis or the screening of high-risk patients.[32] IVP may be used when imaging with ultrasonography, CT, or MRI is equivocal, and it may be more useful than CT with contrast media in planning radiation therapy fields. IVP typically shows distortion of the kidney and splaying of the calices. When the tumor is extensive, the involved kidney may not show any excretory function. Selective renal arteriography is not performed unless some unusual feature of the tumor requires clarification.

NWTS-4 (1987–1994) advised against the use of computed tomographic scans of the chest to diagnose the presence of metastatic disease that cannot be confirmed by chest radiography because of the risk of a false-positive interpretation and the increased toxicity of therapy in patients treated for stage IV disease. For patients classified as stage IV because of chest computed tomographic scan alone, NWTS-4 recommended confirmation by open lung biopsy.[33]

## STAGING

Early studies of the NWTS used a staging classification based on the extent of disease at diagnosis.[25] The original classification correlated well with prognosis except that patients with regional node involvement did poorly, and patients with limited tumor spillage during surgery did somewhat better than expected. The staging system was changed in 1978 (Table 78–1). The validity of the modifications was confirmed in a subsequent study,[34] yet the American Joint

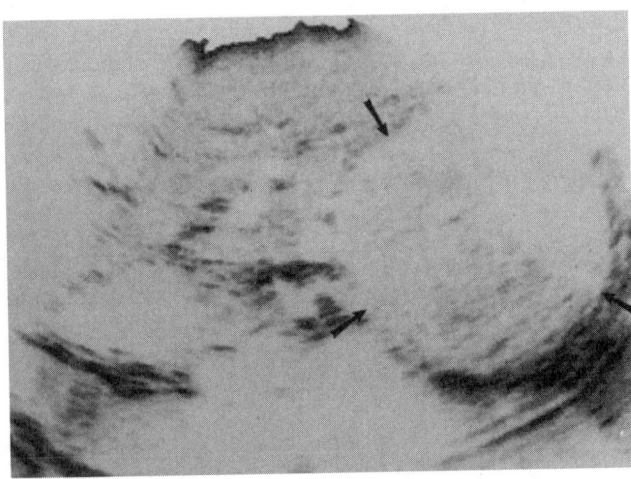

**Figure 78–1.** Transverse abdominal ultrasonography demonstrates a large homogeneous solid mass replacing the kidney *(arrows)*. (Courtesy of R. B. Dietrich.)

***Table 78–1.* Staging of Wilms' Tumor (1978)**

*Stage I*

Tumor limited to kidney and completely excised. Renal capsule intact and tumor not ruptured during removal. No residual tumor beyond margins of resection

*Stage II*

Tumor extends beyond kidney but is completely excised. There is regional extension of tumor by penetration through renal capsule into perirenal soft tissues. Vessels outside kidney may be involved, tumor may have been biopsied, or local spillage of tumor confined to ipsilateral flank may have occurred. No residual tumor at or beyond margins of resection

*Stage III*

Tumor not completely resected, but residual nonhematogenous tumor is confined to abdomen. One or more of the following may occur: regional node involvement, diffuse peritoneal contamination by tumor, penetration of peritoneal surface by tumor, peritoneal implants present, gross or microscopic extension of tumor beyond surgical margins, tumor unresectable because of infiltration into vital structures

*Stage IV*

Hematogenous metastases present

*Stage V*

Bilateral renal involvement

Committee on Cancer[35] has developed another staging system. The two staging systems are similar except for the manner of classifying bilateral disease.

## PATHOLOGY

Gross examination of a WT reveals a large, soft, pale gray nodular mass that markedly distorts the renal contours. Gross cysts, hemorrhage, and necrosis are common. There is usually a sharply defined tumor-kidney junction. A pseudocapsule composed of compressed renal parenchyma and fibrous tissue often surrounds the tumor. Microscopically, WT is classically described as a triphasic *embryonic tumor* composed of blastema, stroma, and epithelium. It is now recognized, however, that biphasic and monophasic variants exist. The metanephric blastemic elements consist of undifferentiated small round cells. The stromal components predominantly consist of fibrous or myxoid tissue but can also contain smooth muscle, striated muscle, adipose tissue, cartilage, bone, squamous or glandular epithelium, melanocytes, or neuroglial tissue.[36]

Beckwith and Palmer,[37] on the basis of their extensive review of WT through the NWTS, separated WT into favorable and unfavorable histologies. The favorable tumors (80% of the total) show the usual triphasic pattern as described previously (Fig. 78–3A). The unfavorable tumors are further divided into the anaplastic and sarcomatous variants. The unfavorable morphology is characterized by anaplasia, which is defined as pleomorphic cells with hyperchromatic nuclei at least three times the size of normal nuclei and atypical, multipolar mitotic figures (see Fig. 78–3C). Focal anaplasia is defined as one or a few sharply localized regions located within the primary tumor, without anaplasia elsewhere (extratumoral or extrarenal).[38] Focal anaplasia does not alter the

prognosis from favorable histology stage I tumors. Diffuse anaplasia includes the following: anaplasia outside the primary tumor, in multiple sites, at the margin, outside the parenchyma, in vessels, in metastatic lesions, in a biopsy sample, or in an incomplete sample. In stage IV cases, 8 of 8 children with focal anaplasia were long-term relapse-free survivors, and 22 of 23 cases with primary lesion diffuse anaplasia died of the tumor. Anaplasia appears to correlate with resistance to therapy rather than increased tumor aggressiveness.[38]

Nephrogenic rests (embryonic renal tissue) are present in 30 to 40% of WT cases[39] but are seen in less than 1% of neonatal autopsies. These rests have the potential to regress completely, become hyperplastic, become neoplastic, and evolve into WT. Intralobar rests are located within the inner portions of the cortex and medulla, whereas perilobar rests are at the periphery of the renal lobe (subcapsular). The presence of multiple or diffuse nephrogenic rests is termed *nephroblastomatosis* and increases the risk of bilateral WT. Nephroblastomatosis shows some of the same genetic changes as WT as well as others (del 4q and 4p).[40]

The genetics of WT are complex (beyond the two-hit model) and are subject to paternal isodisomy and genomic imprinting.[41] Many have normal karyotypes, but molecular analysis reveals the genetic changes. In addition to the *WT1* (11p13) deletions and *WT2* (11p15) mutations, the following have been identified: losses in 1p, 7p, 11p, 16q, 17p; gains in 1q, 7q, 10q, 12q; and trisomies 8 and 18.[40] No correlation has been established between chromosomal composition and histology or tumor stage. Poorer prognosis has been associated with loss of heterozygosity at 1p and 16q, however.[40, 42, 43] Mutation of p53 (<10% of WT cases) is associated with anaplasia and diminished survival.[42] The prognostic significance of DNA ploidy is uncertain.[42] NWTS-5 has as one of its main objectives determination of the prognostic significance of the loss of heterozygosity of chromosomes 16q and 1p as well as of the increased DNA content. The confirmation of the association of these markers with poor outcome may lead to the development of more intensified therapy for these patients.

Two other primary renal neoplasms—clear cell sarcoma of the kidney (CCSK) and malignant rhabdoid tumor of the kidney (RTK)—are now recognized as distinct from WT and have poor prognosis. Clear cell sarcomas are rare (about 4% of primary renal tumors) and are composed of nests and cords of spindle-shaped cells with a branching vascular network and fibrous bands. These cells have bland nuclei with finely dispersed chromatin, rare mitotic figures, and clear, vacuolated, or eosinophilic cytoplasm with indistinct cell borders (see Fig. 78–3B). Malignant rhabdoid tumors (about 2% of primary renal tumors) are composed of loose sheets of polygonal cells with abundant glassy eosinophilic cytoplasm, large eccentric nuclei with prominent nucleoli, and mitotic figures (see Fig. 78–3D). The characteristic feature that is essential for diagnosis is the presence of large, oval, cytoplasmic hyaline inclusions that, by electron microscopy, are shown to be composed of whorled, intermediate-type cytofilaments.[44]

## Treatment

The principal modalities of treatment for WT are surgery, radiation therapy, and chemotherapy. These are nearly al-

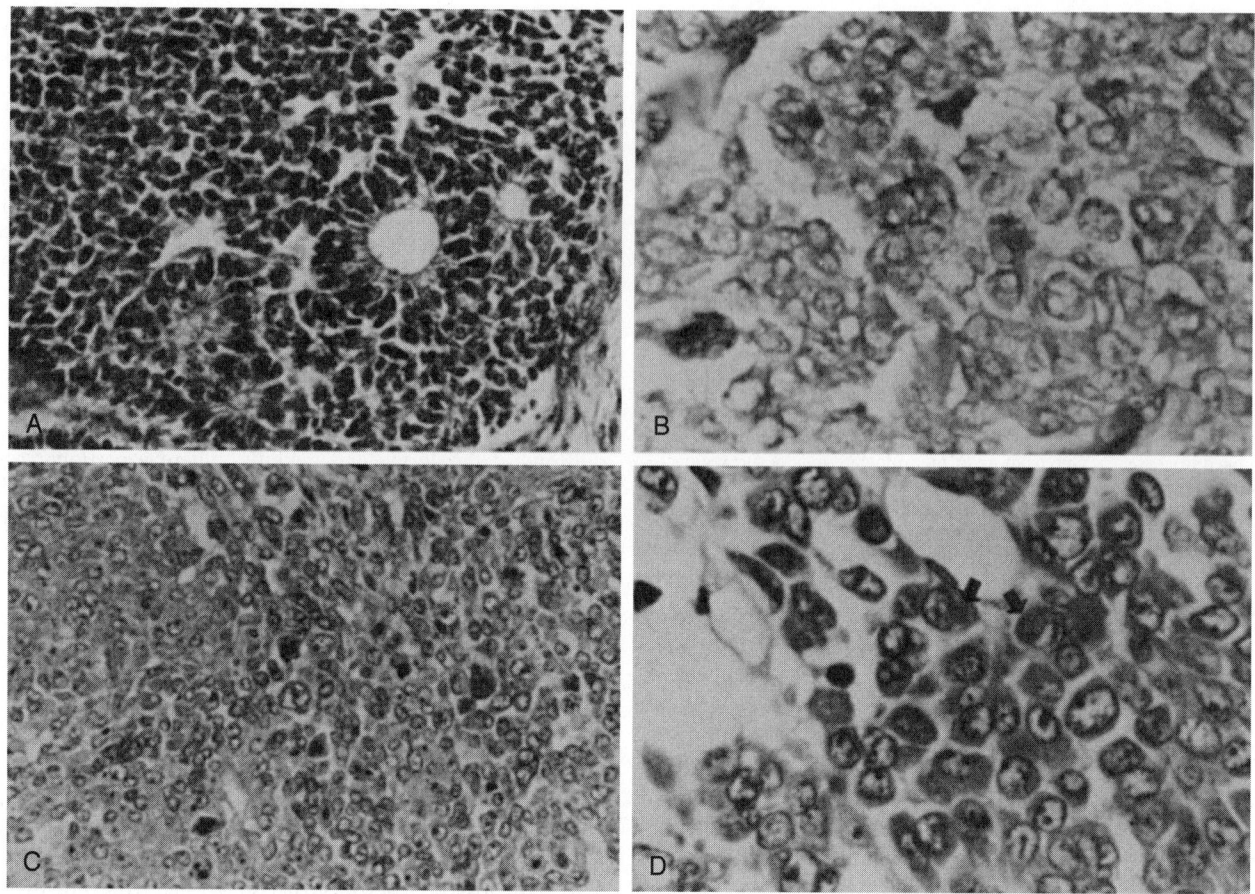

**Figure 78–3.** *A,* Favorable-histology Wilms' tumor with a blastemic pattern and central tubular differentiation. (H & E × 200) *B,* Clear cell sarcoma pattern with large neoplastic cells containing prominent vesicular nuclei surrounded by pale, indistinct cytoplasm. (H & E × 400) *C,* Anaplastic Wilms' tumor characterized by polygonal cells showing marked variation in nuclear sizes and shape. Occasional giant cells are present as well as mitotic figures, including atypical forms. (H & E × 200) *D,* Malignant rhabdoid tumor composed of loosely cohesive polygonal cells with eosinophilic cytoplasm. Occasional cells contain intracytoplasmic inclusions *(arrows).* (H & E × 400)

ways used in combination, rarely alone. The coordinated efforts of surgeons, pediatric oncologists, and radiation therapists are essential to obtain an optimal outcome for patients with WT.

## SURGERY

The child with possible WT may be referred to the surgeon early in the diagnosis, and it is essential that the surgeon be familiar with the differential diagnosis and initial management. Once the diagnosis is made, the surgeon becomes a critical part of the team because surgery is an important part of the multimodality therapy required for cure.

Surgical therapy, usually including initial excision of the tumor, is the mainstay of treatment in most patients. The staging of patients is a critical step leading to recommendations for additional treatment with radiation and chemotherapy after surgery. The surgeon should assist the oncologist and radiation therapist in determining accurately the stage of the patient.

It is essential that the surgeon plan to obtain adequate tissue samples and observations at the time of treatment. As noted elsewhere in this chapter, the histologic examination of tumors allows for them to be separated into favorable and unfavorable histology. In patients whose tumors have been resected, the surgeon should be certain the tissue is promptly preserved for subsequent examination. In cases in which the tumor is not to be removed initially, it is important that adequate tissue samples be obtained before any chemotherapy or radiation. This sampling may require either a large-bore needle biopsy or, preferably, an open biopsy performed by the surgeon. In the case of bilateral tumors, it is best to obtain tissue samples from both tumors because the two sides may differ in terms of their prognostic grouping as a favorable or unfavorable tumor.

The surgeon should observe the regional lymph nodes carefully for evidence of disease. Lymph node samples should be obtained at the time of biopsy or excision to confirm the presence or absence of disease. Children in this age group may frequently have large nodes in the mesentery and periaortic region that do not contain metastatic disease.

The surgeon may be required to evaluate potential metastatic disease in the lung. This evaluation may be accomplished by a limited thoracotomy or by thoracoscopy, if single-lung ventilation can be achieved, given the size of the patient. This technique is usually difficult in children weighing less than 20 kg.

The initial operative approach to these patients should be planned after the completion of studies outlined previously.

The surgeon should have knowledge as to the location of the tumor, status of the contralateral kidney, and any evidence of intravascular extension of the tumor and metastatic disease before beginning the operation. Children should be anesthetized in a warm environment. It is essential that adequate monitoring and vascular access be established at the beginning of the operation. Children with advanced-stage disease benefit from initial placement of a Hickman catheter or implanted port to be used during the surgery and for subsequent care. This placement is not required in stage I and II patients, in whom a simple percutaneous access is sufficient. Arterial monitoring and temperature monitoring are needed.

Most surgeons prefer a transperitoneal approach to the tumor, a technique that allows convenient access if the tumor is adherent to the colon, liver, or other organs. A retroperitoneal approach may be used if the tumor is small. The planned operation is uncomplicated. The approach most commonly used is a chevron upper abdominal incision with potential for extension either in the vertical midline or thoracic extension into the chest. It is critical that adequate exposure be obtained to allow for the safe removal of the tumor without rupture or injury to adjacent vascular structures or other organs.

The initial exploration of the abdomen should readily identify the primary tumor and assess the involvement of any vital structures. If resection is possible, this should be accomplished in almost all cases of unilateral disease. Although initial biopsy and delayed excision of the primary tumor has been advocated, this approach may lead to conversion to an unresectable tumor at a later time for patients that respond poorly to chemotherapy. This has been reported to be the case in 8% of patients so treated. Judgment must be used in weighing the risk of initial resection against the benefit of early tumor removal.

Once a decision has been reached to proceed with resection, the rest of the abdomen should be explored. The liver should be carefully palpated for any evidence of metastatic disease. The contralateral kidney is exposed and Gerota's fascia opened. Both surfaces of the contralateral kidney should be examined for any evidence of disease. Mobilization of the kidney can proceed, using gentle techniques to avoid rupture of the tumor. If rupture should occur, every effort should be made to keep the tumor spill localized and the defect in the tumor sutured. Adhesion of the tumor to the colon, mesentery, liver, spleen, pancreas, diaphragm, aorta, or vena cava is commonly encountered. As the dissection progresses, the surgeon should determine if these adhesions can be divided successfully or if resection of contiguous organs is required. In most cases, the simple separation of these attachments should be feasible. Care should be exercised in identifying the aorta, superior mesenteric vessels, vena cava, and contralateral renal vein. Because of the large size of the tumor mass, these structures can be distorted and injured inadvertently in the course of the operation. The ureter should be preserved until resection is ensured. Care should be exercised not to injure the ureter or the contralateral kidney.

Division of the renal vein and artery requires special attention. The vessels should be isolated and clearly identified before division. Any evidence of tumor extension into the renal vein can usually be handled by control of the infrahepatic vena cava. Extension of tumor beyond the he-

patic vena cava has been handled in the past with use of cardiopulmonary bypass. With the availability of effective chemotherapy, these patients should probably have an initial biopsy and delayed surgery. Most of the extensive intravascular disease resolves. These patients are also likely to have disseminated disease and require systemic therapy in any case.

Lymph node sampling is important to prognosis and guiding subsequent therapy. The surgeon should obtain samples of the nodes from the involved renal hilum, ipsilateral and contralateral periaortic, and vena caval node samples. A therapeutic lymph node dissection is not required.

In selected cases of unilateral disease and in almost all cases of bilateral tumors, it may be prudent to delay surgical resection of the primary tumor until after the initiation of chemotherapy. Criteria for delay in patients with unilateral disease may include patients diagnosed and biopsied when presenting with an acute abdomen and patients with significant hemorrhage or other acute presentation. Operative findings may also suggest it is unsafe to proceed with initial surgical resection because of invasion of the aorta, superior mesenteric vessels, or other vital structures. Tumors with sarcomatous elements may be extremely vascular and difficult to resect before chemotherapy.

Patients may present with bilateral tumors either synchronously or at a later time. This presentation is rare, involving 4 to 8% of patients with WTs. The strategy for successful management without incurring end-stage renal failure is complex. Patients presenting with bilateral tumors should have a complete evaluation and metastatic work-up. The usual recommendation is that both kidneys should undergo biopsy to confirm the histology and to direct therapy toward the most unfavorable histology found. A delay that averages 60 days allows for delivery of sufficient chemotherapy to achieve a response. Frequently, the tumor that may have been the largest proves to be the kidney, which can be spared. Preservation of renal function requires a minimum of 20% of the original renal mass. In patients eventually requiring bilateral nephrectomy, the consideration for transplantation should be delayed a minimum of 3 years beyond completion of treatment.

Common sites of metastasis for WT include local and regional lymph nodes; direct extension to the liver, pancreas, or spleen; and vascular spread to the lungs. Surgical therapy in the early phases of treatment is primarily to confirm the presence of disease in these sites by biopsy when required. Later in the course of treatment, direct surgical excision may be indicated as therapy in resistant cases. Surgery may also have a role in patients with local or distant recurrence to establish the diagnosis or to provide local tumor control. In most cases, the metastatic disease can be resolved with chemotherapy and radiation.

Intraoperative complications are usually related to excessive bleeding or injury to vital structures as a result of distortion of the anatomy by the large tumor mass. The best treatment for these complications is prevention. Early assessment of the vascularity of the tumor and the potential for safe resection should be performed. It is essential that all vital structures be identified before division of any large vessels in the course of tumor resection.

Postoperative complications include those that would be expected with any large retroperitoneal operation. Postoperative bleeding, small bowel obstruction, small bowel intussusception, and wound healing complications should be encountered in less than 3% of patients. Patients with bilateral disease are at significant risk for the long-term complication of end-stage renal failure requiring dialysis and transplantation.

## RADIOTHERAPY

In 1950, Gross and Neuhauser[45] first showed the benefits of routine postoperative radiation to the renal fossa in patients with WT, yielding a 47% long-term disease-free survival rate. Although this was an era before chemotherapy, the inherent radioresponsiveness of WT was acknowledged. Since then, the NWTS and the SIOP trials have defined the interrelationship between adjuvant radiation therapy and chemotherapy, progressively limiting the indications for and the intensity of irradiation without apparent deleterious effect on survival rates.

The NWTS-1 (1969–1973) showed that flank irradiation for children younger than 2 years of age did not improve the 90% disease-free survival rate achieved with postoperative dactinomycin alone.[46] Subsequently, the results of NWTS-2 (1974–1978) and NWTS-3 (1979–1986) showed that radiation therapy could be eliminated when vincristine was added to dactinomycin in all favorable histology stage I and stage II patients.[47, 48] Also in NWTS-3, improved results were seen for stage III patients with either two drugs (vincristine and dactinomycin) plus 20-Gy flank irradiation or three drugs (vincristine, dactinomycin, and doxorubicin [Adriamycin]) plus 10 Gy compared with only two drugs with 10-Gy irradiation.[48] These results suggested that doxorubicin could compensate for a lower radiation dose. Overall the results of NWTS-3 showed that 62% of patients (stage I or stage II favorable histology) needed neither radiation therapy nor the cardiotoxic doxorubicin. NWTS-4 (1987–1994) was designed to reduce toxicity and costs, primarily with regard to chemotherapy.[49] Patients with abdominal stage III favorable histology or any stage patient with clear cell sarcoma histology received radiation (10.8 Gy) to the abdomen. For those with anaplastic histology, radiation continued to be age-adjusted, ranging from 12.6 Gy for infants to 37.8 Gy for those older than 40 months.

NWTS-5, which opened in 1995, has no randomizations. All patients with abdominal stage III favorable histology, stage II through IV anaplastic histology, and stage I through IV CCSK or rhabdoid histology receive 10.8 Gy to the flank with the option for an additional 10.8-Gy boost if there is greater than 3-cm residual disease. Age-adjusted dosing for anaplastic histology has been eliminated because there was no apparent dose-response relationship in NWTS-3; however, these conclusions may not be valid because the numbers in the analysis were small, and prior dosing was based on age and not assigned randomly.

The SIOP studies have primarily used a preoperative approach with flank radiotherapy or combination chemotherapy, or both, as a means to decrease the number of patients whose tumors rupture at time of nephrectomy. The first SIOP study showed that prenephrectomy radiotherapy diminished the risk of intraoperative tumor rupture from 33% (20 of 60) to 4% (3 of 72).[61] A subsequent randomized trial (SIOP-5)

showed almost no difference in the frequency of tumor rupture between the use of preoperative radiotherapy with dactinomycin (9% [7 of 76]) versus preoperative chemotherapy with vincristine and dactinomycin (6% [5 of 88]).[50] In SIOP-6, patients with stage II and negative nodes after preoperative chemotherapy and surgery had an increased incidence of abdominal relapse if they were not irradiated, suggesting that downstaging may be misleading.[51] In the United States, preoperative therapy is rarely carried out except in select patients in whom serious technical difficulties with excision are anticipated or when there is a high risk for surgical complications, such as when there is intracaval extension.

If given, radiation therapy should begin in the immediate postoperative period. Delayed initiation of treatment beyond 10 days following surgery has been related to increased abdominal recurrence. Most relapses related to delayed start of therapy have been in patients with unfavorable histologies.[52] Local-regional irradiation treatment fields should be designed to encompass the tumor bed, as defined by preoperative imaging surgical clips and a 1-cm margin. To avoid late scoliosis (secondary to differential growth resulting from inhomogeneous dosing across the vertebral bodies) and to treat para-aortic lymph nodes adequately, the entire width of the vertebral bodies is treated, while avoiding the remaining kidney. The lateral field is placed at the properitoneal line to include the abdominal cavity but spare subcutaneous tissue, if possible. Whole-abdomen irradiation is given when there is diffuse peritoneal seeding, gross spillage at surgery, or preoperative intraperitoneal rupture. Femoral heads are blocked, and dose to more than one third of the remaining kidney is restricted to a maximum of 14.4 Gy.

The importance of regional irradiation in ultimate disease control is most evident in the failure to achieve secondary survival following abdominal relapse, particularly if prior radiation therapy was given. With appropriate radiation as part of the frontline therapy for favorable histology WT, the frequency of abdominal relapse should be low, 0 to 4%.[52] Reported survival after local recurrence is historically poor, 0 to 20%.[53, 54]

Although local-regional failure after integrated multimodality therapy carries an ominous prognosis, children who have pulmonary metastasis may be successfully approached with the addition of bilateral lung irradiation to 12 Gy, with the option for a boost of 7.5 Gy or excision for residual foci. In the United Kingdom Children's Cancer Study Group Trial 1, the management of stage IV favorable histology patients included bilateral pulmonary irradiation only if there was no evidence of tumor on chest radiography at 12 weeks, in contrast to NWTS recommendations. Their 6-year survival rate of 65% was significantly worse than the NWTS 4-year survival rate of 82% for patients with stage IV favorable histology.[55] Controversy remains about the need for pulmonary irradiation if disease is detected by computed tomographic scan only and not seen on chest radiograph.[56] NWTS-5 allows the physician to choose treatment or not. Radiation is also recommended for other metastatic sites, the recommended doses being 30.6 Gy to whole brain for cerebral metastases, as seen in CCSK and rhabdoid; 30.6 Gy to bone metastases, as usually seen with CCSK; and 19.8 Gy for diffuse or unresectable liver metastases with the option for boost.

## CHEMOTHERAPY

Results of the first three NWTS trials[25, 57, 58] showed that postoperative abdominal radiotherapy was not necessary for patients with stage I favorable histology or anaplastic histology or for those with stage II favorable histology when treated with postnephrectomy chemotherapy with vincristine and dactinomycin. The results of these three trials also demonstrated that the addition of doxorubicin to the combination of vincristine and dactinomycin increased relapse-free survival rate for those with stage III or IV favorable histology WT. In addition, the trial results showed that abdominal radiotherapy could be decreased to 10 Gy for stage III favorable histology patients receiving a three-drug regimen with vincristine, dactinomycin, and doxorubicin.

The NWTS-3 suggested that the addition of cyclophosphamide to the combination of vincristine, dactinomycin, and doxorubicin for patients with stages II to IV anaplastic histology WT who received abdominal radiotherapy improved the outcome.[58] This suggestion was confirmed further by additional patient accrual in the NWTS-4.[59] All patients with CCSK entered in the NWTS-3 received abdominal radiation and were randomized to the same three-drug versus four-drug regimens; however, the addition of cyclophosphamide did not improve their prognosis.[60] Patients with RTK have responded poorly to all treatments evaluated by the NWTS, and their 4-year survival rate has continued to be less than 25%.[58]

The administration of preoperative flank radiotherapy, combination chemotherapy, or both, as tested by consecutive SIOP studies, was shown to be effective in reducing the incidence of tumor rupture during surgery.[61, 62] The use of preoperative therapy must be balanced against the risks involved in administering radiotherapy or chemotherapy without a tissue diagnosis. These include the modification of tumor histology by treatment and the loss of staging information. The current NWTS recommendation for patients given preoperative chemotherapy is that they be considered stage III and receive doxorubicin, with the attendant late risk of cardiomyopathy.[63] Unless the tumor is clearly too large to approach surgically, preoperative therapy is discouraged.

The NWTS-4 attempted to diminish discomfort, inconvenience, and cost by consolidating the use of dactinomycin from the traditional 5-day course (standard) to a single large dose (pulse intensive).[65] A total of 1687 previously untreated children with stages I to II favorable histology, stage I anaplastic histology WT (low-risk group), stages II to IV favorable histology WT, or stages I to IV CCSK (high-risk group) were randomized to receive standard or pulse-intensive treatment regimens. The NWTS-4 was also designed to compare the efficacy of short versus long courses of therapy. Patients were randomized after completion of 6 months of chemotherapy to discontinue (short) or to continue (long) for 9 additional months of treatment with their previously assigned regimens.

There was no difference in the 2-year relapse-free survival rates between the standard versus the pulse-intensive regimens. The 2-year relapse-free survival rates for low-risk patients treated with standard and pulse-intensive regimens were 91.3% and 91.4%. For the high-risk patients treated with standard and pulse-intensive regimens, the 2-year relapse-free survival rates were 87.3% and 90%.[64] The pulse-

intensive regimen permitted administration of chemotherapy at a higher dose intensity, with less severe hematologic toxicity and the requirement of fewer physician and hospital encounters.[65] No statistical difference was noted for low-risk or high-risk patients treated with the short-term or long-term treatment regimens.[66]

Overall, the outcome of children with WT has continued to improve. The 2-year relapse-free survival and overall survival rates after a median follow-up of 4.8 years for the children entered in the NWTS-4 are presented in Table 78-2.[64]

Patients who present with bilateral WT (stage V) account for approximately 6% of all cases. Survival of these patients entered in the NWTS trials is greater than 70% at 10 years after diagnosis.[67] Their risk of developing renal failure was 9.9% on NWTS-3 and 3.8% on NWTS-4, however.[68] This risk has led to the recommendation that these patients be submitted to bilateral renal biopsies with staging of each kidney followed by chemotherapy to shrink the tumor and facilitate renal-sparing procedures.

Although the overall relapse rate for children with WT has decreased to less than 15%, the long-term survival rate for patients with recurrent disease remains less than 30% at best.[54, 69, 70] Factors associated with a favorable outcome after relapse include initial stage I or II, treatment with vincristine and dactinomycin only, no prior radiotherapy, favorable histology, and relapse more than 6 months after initial diagnosis. All other patients have a poor outcome and a high risk of treatment failure. The poor outcome of these patients with recurrent WT has led to the investigation of the role of ifosfamide, etoposide, and platinum agents as single agents or in combination for the treatment of these patients.[71-76] These studies have shown response rates greater than 40%; however, the results are transitory, and the outcome has continued to be poor. Malogolowkin (unpublished data, 1999) treated 26 patients with high-risk recurrent WT with carboplatin and etoposide alternating with ifosfamide and doxorubicin. The 3-year disease-free survival rate was 58% with acceptable toxicity. High-dose chemotherapy followed by autologous stem cell rescue has been used for the treatment of patients with high-risk recurrent WT.[77-79] Pein and colleagues[79] reported for the French Society of Pediatric Oncology on 29 patients with high-risk recurrent WT who received treatment with high-dose chemotherapy followed by autologous stem cell rescue. Despite high treatment-related toxicity, the disease-free survival and overall survival rates at 3 years were $50 \pm 17\%$ and $60 \pm 18\%$, respectively.

*Table 78-2.* **Two-Year Relapse-Free Survival and Overall Survival Rates for Patients Entered in the Fourth National Wilms' Tumor Study Group**

| Stage/Histology | Relapse-Free Survival (%) | Overall Survival (%) |
|---|---|---|
| I/FH | 93.7 | 99.2 |
| I/Ana | 90.6 | 89.4 |
| II/FH | 87.8 | 97.3 |
| III/FH | 93.2 | 98.8 |
| IV/FH | 80.9 | 90.1 |
| I-IV/CCSK | 84.6 | 98.1 |

FH, favorable histology; Ana, anaplasia; CCSK, clear cell sarcoma of kidney.

## LONG-TERM SEQUELAE OF TREATMENT

Improvements in the relapse-free survival of patients with WT have raised concerns about the late effects of successful cancer therapy in children.[80] Scoliosis, kyphosis, and soft tissue underdevelopment have been seen after the use of radiotherapy for patients with WT. In a NWTS late-effects study, scoliosis was seen in 61% of irradiated patients versus 9% of nonirradiated patients.[81] Abdominal irradiation may also produce decreased sitting height and a less apparent decreased standing height.[82] Abdominal irradiation may also affect outcome of pregnancy related to abnormal uterine or pelvic development. One study examined children who were treated at seven different centers from 1931 through 1979, with doses to the abdomen as high as 40 Gy.[83] Among the 114 pregnancies in women who had received abdominal radiotherapy for WT, an adverse outcome occurred in 34 (30%). There were 17 perinatal deaths (5 in premature low-birth-weight infants) and 17 other low-birth-weight infants. Compared with white women in the United States, the irradiated women had an increased perinatal mortality rate (relative risk, 7.9) and an excess of low-birth-weight infants (relative risk, 4.0). In contrast, an adverse outcome was found in 2 (3%) of the 77 pregnancies in nonirradiated female patients with WT and wives of male patients.

Interactions with dactinomycin and doxorubicin may magnify potential complications, such as Budd-Chiari syndrome, pneumonitis, and nephritis. In a study in NWTS-2 patients, the combination of radiation therapy and chemotherapy resulted in a hepatotoxicity rate of 6.2%.[47] In the same study, pneumonitis was identified in approximately 10% of patients receiving 14-Gy whole-lung irradiation along with dactinomycin and vincristine.

Congestive heart failure is a known complication of therapy with anthracyclines, and its effects can be manifest 4 to 20 years after completion of therapy.[63] Analysis of the patients treated on the first three NWTS trials revealed eight cases of congestive heart failure not related to renal failure or pulmonary hypertension.[84] The cumulative frequency of congestive heart failure was 1.7% at 15 years after diagnosis among children treated with doxorubicin. The onset of symptoms was 1.3 to 11.7 years after diagnosis of WT. The percentage increased to 5.4% of those whose treatment included whole-lung irradiation, compared with 1% of those whose treatment did not.

Children with WT are at greater risk for impaired renal function resulting from radiotherapy to the remaining nephrons and the use of potentially nephrotoxic chemotherapeutic agents. There is also a theoretical risk as a result of hyperfiltration of the remaining nephrons following removal of a critical mass of renal tissue. Of the 5823 children registered to the NWTS between October 1969 and July 1993, 55 were found to have renal failure. Of these, 39 had bilateral tumors, 15 had unilateral tumors, and 1 had a WT in a solitary kidney. The incidence of renal failure in bilateral and unilateral tumors was 9% and 0.3%. The most common causes of renal failure were bilateral nephrectomy (24 patients), Drash's syndrome (12 patients), radiation nephritis (6 patients), and progressive tumor in the remaining kidney (5 patients). These findings support the use of parenchymal-sparing procedures for children with bilateral WT but not for those with unilateral WT and a normal contralateral kidney.[68]

Childhood cancer survivors have an increased risk of developing a second malignant neoplasm. Breslow and colleagues[85] analyzed 5278 evaluable patients entered in the NWTS trials to determine the incidence and factors associated with an increased risk of developing a second malignant neoplasm. A total of 43 second malignant neoplasms were observed, whereas only 5.1 cases were expected. Fifteen years after the diagnosis of WT, the cumulative incidence of a second malignant neoplasm was 1.6% and increasing steadily. Previous treatment with abdominal radiation therapy, prior treatment with doxorubicin, and treatment for relapse increased the relative risk of developing a second malignant neoplasm. Advances in molecular biology may assist in the future in the identification of patients at high risk for developing a second malignant neoplasm.

## SUGGESTIONS FOR ADDITIONAL READING

Huff V. Wilms' tumor genetics. Am J Med Genet 1998;79:260–7.

Green DM, D'Angio GJ, Beckwith JB, et al. Wilms' tumor. CA Cancer J Clin 1996;46:46–63.

Tawil A, Cox JN, Roth AD, et al. Wilms' tumor in the adult—report of a case and review of the literature. Pathol Res Pract 1999;195:105–11.

Egeler RM, Wolff JE, Anderson RA, Coppes MJ. Long-term complications and post-treatment follow-up of patients with Wilms' tumor. Semin Urol Oncol 1999;17:55–61.

## REFERENCES

1. Jones PG. Tumors of infancy and childhood. Oxford: Blackwell Scientific Publications, 1976:491.
2. D'Angio GJ. In: Pizzo PA, Poplack DG, eds. Principles and practice of pediatric oncology. 3rd ed. Philadelphia: JB Lippincott, 1997.
3. Breslow N, Olshan A, Beckwith JB, Green DM. Epidemiology of Wilms' tumor. Med Pediatr Oncol 1993;21:172-81.
4. Breslow N, Beckwith JB, Ciol M, Sharples K. Age distribution of Wilms' tumor: report from the National Wilms' Tumor Study. Cancer Res 1988;48:1653–7.
5. Fraumeni JF Jr, Glass AG. Wilms' tumor and congenital aniridia. JAMA 1968;206:825–8.
6. Fraumeni JF Jr, Geiser CF, Manning MD. Wilms' tumor and congenital hemihypertrophy: report of five new cases and review of literature. Pediatrics 1967;40:886–99.
7. Stay EJ, Vawter G. The relationship between nephroblastoma and neurofibromatosis (von Recklinghausen's disease). Cancer 1977;39:2550–5.
8. Coppes MJ, Haber DA, Grundy PE. Genetic events in the development of Wilms' tumor. N Engl J Med 1994;331:586–90.
9. Brown WT, Puranik SR, Altman DH, Hardin HC Jr. Wilms' tumor in three successive generations. Surgery 1972;72:756–61.
10. Knudson AG Jr. The genetics of childhood cancer. Cancer 1975;35:Suppl:1022–6.
11. Matsunaga E. Genetics of Wilms' tumor. Hum Genet 1981;57:231.
12. Knudson AG Jr, Strong LC. Mutation and cancer: a model for Wilms' tumor of the kidney. J Natl Cancer Inst 1972;48:313–24.
13. Friend SH, Bernards R, Rogelj S, et al. A human DNA segment with properties of the gene that predisposes to retinoblastoma and osteosarcoma. Nature 1986;323:643–6.
14. Riccardi VM, Sujansky E, Smith AC, Francke U. Chromosomal imbalance in the aniridia-Wilms' tumor association: 11p interstitial deletion. Pediatrics 1978;61:604–10.
15. Yunis JJ, Ramsay NK. Familial occurrence of the aniridia-Wilms' tumor syndrome with deletion 11p13–14.1. J Pediatr 1980;96:1027–30.
16. Call KM, Glaser T, Ito CY, et al. Isolation and characterization of a zinc finger polypeptide gene at the human chromosome 11 Wilms' tumor locus. Cell 1990;60:509–20.
17. Gashler AL, Bonthron DT, Madden SL, et al. Human platelet-derived growth factor A chain is transcriptionally repressed by the Wilms' tumor suppressor WT1. Proc Natl Acad Sci U S A 1992;89:10984–8.

18. Ogawa O, Eccles MR, Szeto J, et al. Relaxation of insulin-like growth factor II gene imprinting implicated in Wilms' tumour. Nature 1993;362:749–51.

19. Maw MA, Grundy PE, Millow LJ, et al. A third Wilms' tumor locus on chromosome 16q. Cancer Res 1992;52:3094–8.

20. de Martinville B, Francke U. The c-Ha-ras1, insulin and beta-globin loci map outside the deletion associated with aniridia-Wilms' tumour. Nature 1983;305:641–3.

21. Huerre C, Despoisse S, Gilgenkrantz S, et al. c-Ha-ras1 is not deleted in aniridia-Wilms' tumour association. Nature 1983;305:638–41.

22. Breslow NE, Beckwith JB. Epidemiological features of Wilms' tumor: results of the National Wilms' Tumor Study. J Natl Cancer Inst 1982;68:429–36.

23. Mitchell JD, Baxter TJ, Blair-West JR, McCredie DA. Renin levels in nephroblastoma (Wilms' tumour): report of a renin-secreting tumour. Arch Dis Child 1970;45:376–84.

24. Shalet MF, Holder TM, Walters TR. Erythropoietin-producing Wilms' tumor. J Pediatr 1967;70:615–7.

25. D'Angio GJ, Evans AE, Breslow N, et al. The treatment of Wilms' tumor: results of the national Wilms' tumor study. Cancer 1976;38:633–46.

26. Haas JE, Bonadio JF, Beckwith JB. Clear cell sarcoma of the kidney with emphasis on ultrastructural studies. Cancer 1984;54:2978–87.

27. Bonnin JM, Rubinstein LJ, Palmer NF, Beckwith JB. The association of embryonal tumors originating in the kidney and in the brain: a report of seven cases. Cancer 1984;54:2137–46.

28. Ehrlich RM, Bloomberg SD, Gyepes MT, et al. Wilms tumor, misdiagnosed preoperatively: a review of 19 National Wilms Tumor Study I cases. J Urol 1979;122:790–2.

29. Cohen MD, Siddiqui A, Weetman R, et al. A rational approach to the radiologic evaluation of children with Wilms' tumor. Cancer 1982;50:887–92.

30. Kangarloo H, Dietrich RB, Ehrlich RM, et al. Magnetic resonance imaging of Wilms tumor. Urology 1986;28:203–7.

31. Dietrich RB, Kangarloo H. Kidneys in infants and children: evaluation with MR. Radiology 1986;159:215–21.

32. Palmer N, Evans AE. The association of aniridia and Wilms' tumor: methods of surveillance and diagnosis. Med Pediatr Oncol 1983;11:73–5.

33. Green DM, Fernbach DJ, Norkool P, et al. The treatment of Wilms' tumor patients with pulmonary metastases detected only with computed tomography: a report from the National Wilms' Tumor Study. J Clin Oncol 1991;9:1776–81.

34. Farewell VT, D'Angio GJ, Breslow N, Norkool P. Retrospective validation of a new staging system for Wilms' tumor. Cancer Clin Trials 1981;4:167–71.

35. Beahrs OH, ed. American Joint Committee on Cancer: manual for staging of cancer. 4th ed. Philadelphia: JB Lippincott, 1992.

36. Fernandes ET, Parham DM, Ribeiro RC, et al. Teratoid Wilms' tumor: the St. Jude experience. J Pediatr Surg 1988;23:1131–4.

37. Beckwith JB, Palmer NF. Histopathology and prognosis of Wilms tumors: results from the First National Wilms' Tumor Study. Cancer 1978;41:1937–48.

38. Faria P, Beckwith JB, Mishra K, et al. Focal versus diffuse anaplasia in Wilms tumor—new definitions with prognostic significance: a report from the National Wilms Tumor Study Group. Am J Surg Pathol 1996;20:909–20.

39. Beckwith JB, Kiviat NB, Bonadio JF. Nephrogenic rests, nephroblastomatosis, and the pathogenesis of Wilms' tumor. Pediatr Pathol 1990;10:1–36.

40. Steenman M, Redeker B, de Meulemeester M, et al. Comparative genomic hybridization analysis of Wilms tumors. Cytogenet Cell Genet 1997;77:296–303.

41. Miozzo M, Perotti D, Minoletti F, et al. Mapping of a putative tumor suppressor locus to proximal 7p in Wilms tumors. Genomics 1996;37:310–5.

42. Wiener JS, Coppes MJ, Ritchey ML. Current concepts in the biology and management of Wilms tumor. J Urol 1998;159:1316–25.

43. Grundy PE, Telzerow PE, Breslow N, et al. Loss of heterozygosity for chromosomes 16q and 1p in Wilms' tumors predicts an adverse outcome. Cancer Res 1994;54:2331–3.

44. Haas JE, Palmer NF, Weinberg AG, Beckwith JB. Ultrastructure of malignant rhabdoid tumor of the kidney: a distinctive renal tumor of children. Hum Pathol 1981;12:646–57.

45. Gross RE, Neuhauser EBD. Treatment of mixed tumors of the kidney in childhood. Pediatrics 1950;6:843.

46. D'Angio GJ, Evans AE, Breslow N, et al. The treatment of Wilms' tumor: results of the national Wilms' tumor study. Cancer 1976;38:633–46.

47. D'Angio GJ, Evans A, Breslow N, et al. The treatment of Wilms' tumor: results of the Second National Wilms' Tumor Study. Cancer 1981;47:2302.

48. D'Angio GJ, Breslow N, Beckwith JB, et al. Treatment of Wilms' tumor: results of the Third National Wilms' Tumor Study. Cancer 1989;64:349–60.

49. Green DM, Breslow NE, Evans I, et al. The effect of chemotherapy dose intensity on the hematological toxicity of the treatment for Wilms' tumor: a report from the National Wilms' Tumor Study. Am J Pediatr Hematol Oncol 1994;16:207–12.

50. Lemerle J, Voute PA, Tournade MF, et al. Effectiveness of preoperative chemotherapy in Wilms' tumor: results of an International Society of Paediatric Oncology (SIOP) clinical trial. J Clin Oncol 1983;1:604–9.

51. Jereb B, Burgers JM, Tournade MF, et al. Radiotherapy in the SIOP (International Society of Pediatric Oncology) nephroblastoma studies: a review. Med Pediatr Oncol 1994;22:221–7.

52. Thomas PR, Tefft M, Farewell VT, et al. Abdominal relapses in irradiated second National Wilms' Tumor Study patients. J Clin Oncol 1984;2:1098–101.

53. D'Angio GJ, Tefft M, Breslow N, Meyer JA. Radiation therapy of Wilms' tumor: results according to dose, field, post-operative timing and histology. Int J Radiat Oncol Biol Phys 1978;4:769–80.

54. Grundy P, Breslow N, Green DM, et al. Prognostic factors for children with recurrent Wilms' tumor: results from the Second and Third National Wilms' Tumor Study. J Clin Oncol 1989;7:638–47.

55. Pritchard J, Imeson J, Barnes J, et al. Results of the United Kingdom Children's Cancer Study Group first Wilms' Tumor Study. J Clin Oncol 1995;13:124–33.

56. Green DM, Fernbach DJ, Norkool P, et al. The treatment of Wilms' tumor patients with pulmonary metastases detected only with computed tomography: a report from the National Wilms' Tumor Study. J Clin Oncol 1991;9:1776–81.

57. D'Angio GJ, Evans A, Breslow N, et al. The treatment of Wilms' tumor: results of the Second National Wilms' Tumor Study. Cancer 1981;47:2302–11.

58. D'Angio GJ, Breslow N, Beckwith JB, et al. Treatment of Wilms' tumor: results of the Third National Wilms' Tumor Study. Cancer 1989;64:349–60.

59. Green DM, Beckwith JB, Breslow NE, et al. Treatment of children with stages II to IV anaplastic Wilms' tumor: a report from the National Wilms' Tumor Study Group. J Clin Oncol 1994;12:2126–31.

60. Green DM, Breslow NE, Beckwith JB, et al. Treatment of children with clear-cell sarcoma of the kidney: a report from the National Wilms' Tumor Study Group. J Clin Oncol 1994;12:2132–7.

61. Lemerle J, Voute PA, Tournade MF, et al. Preoperative versus postoperative radiotherapy, single versus multiple courses of actinomycin D, in the treatment of Wilms' tumor: preliminary results of a controlled clinical trial conducted by the International Society of Paediatric Oncology (S.I.O.P.). Cancer 1976;38:647–54.

62. Lemerle J, Voute PA, Tournade MF, et al. Effectiveness of preoperative chemotherapy in Wilms' tumor: results of an International Society of Paediatric Oncology (SIOP) clinical trial. J Clin Oncol 1983;1:604–9.

63. Steinherz LJ, Steinherz PG, Tan CT, et al. Cardiac toxicity 4 to 20 years after completing anthracycline therapy. JAMA 1991;266:1672–7.

64. Green DM, Breslow NE, Beckwith JB, et al. Comparison between single-dose and divided-dose administration of dactinomycin and doxorubicin for patients with Wilms' tumor: a report from the National Wilms' Tumor Study Group. J Clin Oncol 1998;16:237–45.

65. Green DM, Breslow NE, Evans I, et al. The effect of chemotherapy dose intensity on the hematological toxicity of the treatment for Wilms' tumor: a report from the National Wilms' Tumor Study. Am J Pediatr Hematol Oncol 1994;16:207–12.

66. Green DM, Breslow NE, Beckwith JB, et al. Effect of duration of treatment on treatment outcome and cost of treatment for Wilms' tumor: a report from the National Wilms' Tumor Study Group. J Clin Oncol 1998;16:3744–51.

67. Montgomery BT, Kelalis PP, Blute ML, et al. Extended followup of bilateral Wilms tumor: results of the National Wilms Tumor Study. J Urol 1991;146:Pt 2:514–8.

68. Ritchey ML, Green DM, Thomas PR, et al. Renal failure in Wilms' tumor patients: a report from the National Wilms' Tumor Study Group. Med Pediatr Oncol 1996;26:75–80.

69. Groot-Loonen JJ, Pinkerton CR, Morris-Jones PH, Pritchard J. How curable is relapsed Wilms' tumour? The United Kingdom Children's Cancer Study Group. Arch Dis Child 1990;65:968–70.
70. Pinkerton CR, Groot-Loonen JJ, Morris-Jones PH, Pritchard J. Response rates in relapsed Wilms' tumor: a need for new effective agents. Cancer 1991;67:567–71.
71. Tournade MF, Lemerle J, Brunat-Mentigny M, et al. Ifosfamide is an active drug in Wilms' tumor: a phase II study conducted by the French Society of Pediatric Oncology. J Clin Oncol 1988;6:793–6.
72. Pein F, Pinkerton R, Tournade MF, et al. Etoposide in relapsed or refractory Wilms' tumor: a phase II study by the French Society of Pediatric Oncology and the United Kingdom Children's Cancer Study Group. J Clin Oncol 1993;11:1478–81.
73. de Camargo B, Melaragno R, Saba e Silva N, et al. Phase II study of carboplatin as a single drug for relapsed Wilms' tumor: experience of the Brazilian Wilms' Tumor Study Group. Med Pediatr Oncol 1994;22:258–60.
74. Douglass EC, Williams JA, Sackey K, Casper R. Efficacy of combination cisplatin (DDP) and VP-16 in the treatment of recurrent and advanced Wilms' tumor (WT). Proc ASCO 1986;5:201.
75. Loh W, Ortega JA, Wolff J, Baranko P. Cisplatin/VP 16 for the retrieval of Wilms' tumor relapsing on chemotherapy. Proc ASCO 1987;6:222.
76. Miser J, Krailo M, Hammond GD. The combination of ifosfamide (IFOS), etoposide (VP16), and mesna (M): a very active regimen in the treatment of recurrent Wilms' tumor (WT). Proc ASCO 1993; 12:417.
77. Warkentin PI, Brochstein JA, Strandjord SE, et al. High dose therapy followed by autologous stem cell rescue for recurrent Wilms' tumor (WT). Proc ASCO 1993;12:414.
78. Kletzel M, Becton DL, Berry DH. Single institution experience with high-dose cyclophosphamide, continuous infusion vincristine, escalating doses of VP-16-213, and total body irradiation with unpurged bone marrow rescue in children with neuroblastoma. Med Pediatr Oncol 1992;20:64–7.
79. Pein F, Michon J, Valteau-Couanet D, et al. High-dose melphalan, etoposide, and carboplatin followed by autologous stem-cell rescue in pediatric high-risk recurrent Wilms' tumor: a French Society of Pediatric Oncology study. J Clin Oncol 1998;16:3295–301.
80. Meadows AT, Baum E, Fossati-Bellani F, et al. Second malignant neoplasms in children: an update from the Late Effects Study Group. J Clin Oncol 1985;3:532–8.
81. Evans AE, Norkool P, Evans I, et al. Late effects of treatment for Wilms' tumor: a report from the National Wilms' Tumor Study Group. Cancer 1991;67:331–6.
82. Wallace WH, Shalet SM, Morris-Jones PH, et al. Effect of abdominal irradiation on growth in boys treated for a Wilms' tumor. Med Pediatr Oncol 1990;18:441–6.
83. Li FP, Gimbrere K, Gelber RD, et al. Outcome of pregnancy in survivors of Wilms' tumor. JAMA 1987;257:216–9.
84. Green DM, Breslow J, Beckwith J, et al. A comparison between single dose and divided dose administration of dactinomycin and doxorubicin: a report from the National Wilms' Tumor Study Group. Proc ASCO 1996;15:457.
85. Breslow NE, Takashima JR, Whitton JA, et al. Second malignant neoplasms following treatment for Wilm's tumor: a report from the National Wilms' Tumor Study Group. J Clin Oncol 1995;13:1851–9.

# CHAPTER 79

# NEUROBLASTOMA

• C. PATRICK REYNOLDS • ROBERT C. SEEGER

Neuroblastoma is a tumor of the peripheral nervous system that accounts for 8% of childhood cancers.[1] The spectrum of clinical behavior manifested by this tumor ranges from spontaneous regression with no therapy to rapidly progressive disease in spite of combination chemotherapy.[2–5] According to a variety of clinical and laboratory prognostic factors, low-, intermediate-, and high-risk groups of patients can be defined at diagnosis based on expected outcome after conventional therapy. Classifying neuroblastoma patients into risk groups is important to avoid overtreating or undertreating a given patient.

The clinical diversity of neuroblastomas is associated with molecular genetic and other biologic differences. For example, patients who are cured by surgery alone have localized tumors that lack genomic amplification of the *MYCN* proto-oncogene, do not grow in vitro, and usually are histologically differentiated. By contrast, conventional treatment is rarely successful for patients whose metastatic neuroblastomas exhibit amplification of the *MYCN* proto-oncogene, and are poorly differentiated.

Forty percent of children with neuroblastoma have low- or intermediate-risk tumors, and they nearly all become long-term, disease-free survivors following conventional therapy, which includes surgery, local irradiation, and chemotherapy. However, 60% have high-risk tumors, and these patients infrequently become long-term survivors after conventional therapy. A phase III study has shown improved event-free survival for high-risk neuroblastoma patients treated with aggressive chemoradiotherapy followed by the differentiating agent 13-cis-retinoic acid. However, as tumor recurrence remains a significant problem for high-risk neuroblastoma, more effective therapeutic approaches must be developed and tested in prospective randomized trials.

This chapter reviews the clinical features of neuroblastoma and the various clinical and laboratory methods used for diagnostic and prognostic assessment of the patient. We then discuss currently available therapeutic approaches based on the prognosis of the patient and briefly review new approaches to therapy being tested in clinical trials.

## Natural History, Diagnosis, and Staging

### CLINICAL FEATURES

Neuroblastoma is predominantly a disease of early childhood. About one half of neuroblastoma patients are diagnosed within the first 2 years of life.[4,6] Approximately 50% of infants and 70% of older neuroblastoma patients have disseminated disease at diagnosis.[7] Presenting symptoms in such patients are often manifestations of widespread tumor, such as weight loss, bone pain, pallor, and easy bruising. These vague symptoms can result in delays in the correct diagnosis. Less common is the incidental discovery of a mass. Occasionally, the presenting symptom is due to neurologic defects resulting from extension of paraspinal tumors into the epidural space,[8] Horner's syndrome from a mediastinal tumor, or a paraneoplastic syndrome related to the tumor, such as opsoclonus-myoclonus[9] or vasoactive intestinal peptide–induced watery diarrhea.[10]

The primary tumor can arise at any point where there is tissue of the sympathetic nervous system; the majority of primary tumors arise in the adrenal glands (Fig. 79–1).[4] The most common site of metastatic disease is the bone marrow, followed by the bone, liver, and lymph nodes. Although the older literature contains reports of neuroblastomas arising in nonsympathetic peripheral nerves, such tumors are now considered to be distinct from neuroblastoma.[11, 12]

## INITIAL EVALUATION

The extent of disease should be determined by evaluating the primary site, potential sites of metastatic disease, and the degree of elevation of tumor markers. Tests should include a chest radiograph; computed tomography (CT) or magnetic resonance imaging (MRI) of the chest, abdomen, and pelvis; a skeletal survey or $^{99m}$Tc-diphosphonate bone scan; or both, and a $^{131}$I-metaiodobenzylguanidine (MIBG) scan.[13–16] Bilateral iliac crest bone marrow aspirates and biopsies should be performed, as this increases the probability of detecting tumor in the marrow.[17] Analysis of urine for catecholamine metabolites[5, 18] (vanillylmandelic acid [VMA] and homovanillic acid [HVA]) can aid in the diagnosis and in monitoring tumor response; measurement of serum ferritin[19] aids in assessing the patient's risk group (see the section Serum Markers).

Surgery, whether for complete or partial resection of the primary tumor or for biopsy, is necessary in patients with local (stage 1 and 2) or regional (stage 3) disease. This provides tumor tissue for diagnosis and prognostication, and it also allows examination and biopsy of regional lymph nodes. Patients with disseminated disease (stages 4 and 4-S) who have demonstrable tumor cells in bone marrow and elevated urine HVA or VMA, or both, do not require surgery to establish a diagnosis. However, patients with stage 4 or 4-S disease who are diagnosed in the first year of life must be tested for *MYCN* gene amplification, which can be carried out on tumor tissue or bone marrow having >10% tumor cells. Biopsy or excision of primary or metastatic tumor is also strongly recommended for stage 4 patients older than 1

year at diagnosis because prognostic and biologic information obtained from tumor tissue may guide future therapies. If urine HVA and VMA are normal in a patient with disseminated disease, tumor tissue must be obtained to establish the diagnosis. In addition to tissue submitted for histopathology, tumor tissue should be used to prepare nonfixed touch preparations for *MYCN* analysis by fluorescence in situ hybridization (FISH); fresh tissue in culture medium should be submitted for ploidy and cell culture; and as much tissue as possible should be frozen immediately, without fixation, for future diagnostic and prognostic studies. Such frozen material is not only invaluable for research but can also be used as needed for diagnostic immunohistochemistry or confirmatory analysis of various prognostic markers. Because laboratory investigations of biologic, diagnostic, prognostic, and therapeutic questions are dependent on both frozen and cultured viable tumor tissue, every effort should be made to plan for full utilization of tissue before surgery is undertaken.

## DIAGNOSIS

Establishing a diagnosis of neuroblastoma is often routine but can occasionally be difficult.[20] Histopathologic examination of primary or metastatic tumor is usually diagnostic. However, undifferentiated neuroblastomas can be confused with primitive neuroectodermal tumor (PNET), peripheral neuroepithelioma, Ewing's sarcoma, rhabdomyosarcoma, lymphoma, and even leukemia.[20, 21] A number of diagnostic markers exist that are valuable in resolving diagnostic dilemmas. Before the current battery of diagnostic tests was available, it was common to consider any extracranial small, round cell tumor of neural origin to be a neuroblastoma. However, clinical and biologic studies now assist in distinguishing neuroblastoma from related neural tumors, including peripheral PNET and esthesioneuroblastoma.[11, 12, 22–26] For most of these tumors, the clinical presentation of the patient aids in distinguishing them from neuroblastoma; we have summarized the clinical features of these tumors in Table 79–1.

**Catecholamines.** Catecholamine metabolites are abnormally elevated in the urine of nearly all patients with neuroblastoma.[5, 18] A diagnosis of neuroblastoma can be established by demonstrating that the tumor is catecholamine positive and that it is a small, round cell tumor (the latter can be determined with primary or metastatic tumor, or with a marrow aspirate and biopsy). However, every effort to obtain tumor tissue should be made to ensure the potential

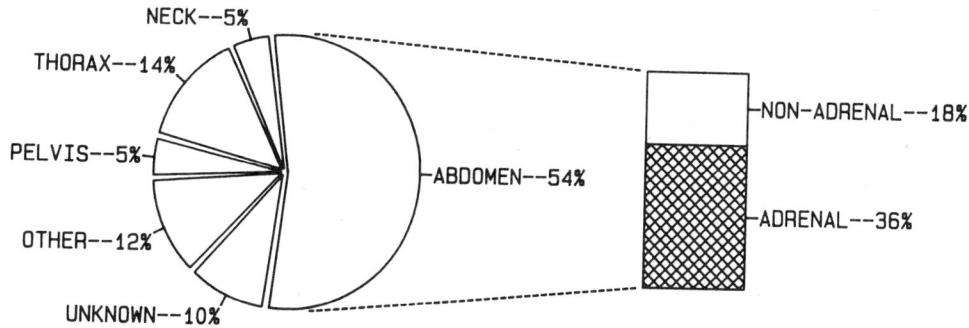

**Figure 79–1.** Sites of origin for primary neuroblastoma. (Data from Jaffe N. Neuroblastoma: review of the literature and an examination of factors contributing to its enigmatic character. Cancer Treat Rev 1976;3:61 and Hayes FA. In: Pizzo PA, eds. Principles and practice of pediatric oncology. Philadelphia: JB Lippincott, 1989:607.)

NECK--5%
THORAX--14%
PELVIS--5%
OTHER--12%
UNKNOWN--10%
ABDOMEN--54%
NON-ADRENAL--18%
ADRENAL--36%

*Table 79–1.* Comparison of Neuroblastoma and Related Neural Tumors

| Tumor | Site or Origin | Histopathology | Ultrastructure | Catecholamines | Cytogenetics | *MYCN* Amplification | Other Markers |
|---|---|---|---|---|---|---|---|
| Neuroblastoma | Sites of sympathetic nervous system | Small, round tumor with neurofibrillary stroma, occasionally with pseudorosettes and/or ganglion cells | Neural, including neurosecretory granules | Most are positive | 1pdel, double minutes, and homogeneously staining regions | Present in 30% | Most HLA class I negative; NSE + TH positive |
| PNET | Thorax, chest wall, pelvis, extremities | Primitive small, round cell tumor | Neural, including neurosecretory granules | All negative | Many have t(11;22) | All negative | HLA class I positive NSE positive TH negative |
| Esthesioneuroblastoma | Olfactory nerve | Primitive small, round cell tumor | Neural, including neurosecretory granules | Most are negative | Some have t(11;22) | Negative in all studied | HLA class I positive |

PNET, primitive neuroectodermal tumor; NSE, neuron-specific enolase; TH, tyrosine hydroxylase.

for laboratory tests useful in assessing prognosis. In addition to being a diagnostic marker, urine catecholamine metabolites are useful for detecting increases or decreases in tumor burden. It should be noted that although a catecholamine-negative tumor can still be a neuroblastoma, PNETs have been found to be uniformly catecholamine-negative.[22] The usual method for establishing that a tumor is catecholaminergic is measurement of catecholamine metabolites in the patient's urine (primarily VMA and HVA).[5, 18] As is shown in Table 79–2, nearly 85% of patients show elevated VMA or HVA in urine.[27–41]

Many neuroblastomas appear to produce only dopamine (which forms HVA); others produce primarily norepinephrine (which forms VMA). Because of this, one can increase to approximately 95% the proportion of neuroblastoma patients detected by measuring metabolites from both pathways. Urine studies do not require timed specimens if urine creatinine is measured so that the VMA and HVA can be expressed in relationship to the creatine level (to correct for urine dilution concentration).

Although qualitative "spot" tests for urine VMA are available, they have a high incidence of false-positive and false-negative results; therefore, the use of quantitative methods is preferred.[5, 18] The spot tests, as well as quantitative tests, have been used to screen for neuroblastoma.[42, 43] An alternative to urinary catecholamine metabolites is the direct measurement of catecholamines in tumor tissue. This can be accomplished using glyoxylic acid to induce catecholamine fluorescence[44]; catecholamine-positive tumor cells can be readily identified in touch preparations from tumor tissue or in smears made from bone marrow aspirates. Because of the high sensitivity of the catecholamine fluorescence method, it has been found to be positive occasionally when urine VMA and HVA levels were not elevated.[20, 44] Similarly, detection in tumor tissue of tyrosine hydroxylase RNA (the rate-limiting enzyme in catecholamine synthesis) is a highly specific and sensitive diagnostic marker for neuroblastoma, even for tumors that fail to show catecholamine excretion in urine or catecholamine positivity in tissue by glyoxylic acid.[45]

*Table 79–2.* **Frequency of Elevated Catecholamine Metabolites in the Urine at Diagnosis**

| VMA | HVA | Reference |
|---|---|---|
| 10/17 | — | 27 |
| 21/21 | 9/17 | 28 |
| 58/75 | 32/43 | 29 |
| 11/12 | 13/14 | 30 |
| 10/13 | — | 31 |
| 74/87 | 27/46 | 32 |
| 19/29 | 21/29 | 33 |
| 35/37 | 34/37 | 34 |
| 33/38 | — | 35 |
| 12/16 | — | 36 |
| 13/16 | 9/14 | 37 |
| 13/16 | 12/12 | 38 |
| 16/18 | — | 39 |
| 48/54 | 48/54 | 40 |
| 246/288 | 237/260 | 41 |
| 619/737 | 442/526 | Elevated levels/total |
| **84.0%** | **84.0%** | **% with elevated levels** |

VMA, vanillylmandelic acid; HVA, homovanillic acid.

**Histopathology.** The histologic appearance of neuroblastoma varies widely, depending on the degree of differentiation.[20, 21, 46] In its most undifferentiated form, neuroblastoma is a small, round cell tumor composed of sheets of round cells with scant cytoplasm and little stroma. More differentiated tumors have evidence of neurofibrillary stroma and occasionally show pseudorosette formation. The most differentiated malignant form of the tumor, ganglioneuroblastoma, contains undifferentiated cell clusters mixed with ganglion cells embedded in a neurofibrillary stroma. A benign tumor that resembles sympathetic ganglion tissue is known as a *ganglioneuroma.* These tumors have been shown to result from maturation of malignant neuroblastoma.[47, 48]

If ganglion cells or pseudorosettes can be demonstrated in a tumor that is otherwise consistent with neuroblastoma, light microscopy is diagnostic. In the absence of such features, it is unwise to rely on light microscopy alone. Ultrastructural evidence of neural origin, such as neuronal processes and especially dense-core neurosecretory granules, is valuable in distinguishing neuroblastoma from Ewing's sarcoma, rhabdomyosarcoma, and lymphoma.[21, 44] However, ultrastructure does not distinguish between neuroblastoma and PNET, or other tumors of neural origin.[11, 22]

Observation of tumor cells in short-term culture can be useful in establishing a diagnosis. In neuroblastoma, such cultures almost always display a distinct morphology in which clumps of round cells extend long processes (neurites). The typical morphology of neuroblastoma is not seen in any of the other small, round cell tumors.[20, 44, 49] Although one can see short neural processes in cultures of a PNET, long processes and especially formation of bundles by multiple parallel neurites are seen only in neuroblastoma.

A variety of chromosomal abnormalities have been associated with neuroblastoma (including chromosome 1p deletions, double minute chromosomes, and homogeneously staining regions), but none is diagnostic for neuroblastoma.[50, 51] Cytogenetics occasionally can be helpful in excluding neuroblastoma if an 11;22 translocation is observed (indicating a diagnosis of peripheral primitive neuroectodermal tumor or Ewing's sarcoma),[52, 53] and detection of the EWS/FLI-1 transcript by reverse transcriptase polymerase chain reaction (RT-PCR) can also be used to identify tumors with the characteristic 11;22 translocation.[24]

Antisera to neuron-specific enolase (NSE) have been used by a number of laboratories to demonstrate the neural origin of tumors. Although NSE is detectable in both neuroblastoma and PNET, it is not seen in Ewing's sarcoma and lymphoma.[54] However, caution must be used in interpreting data using this test, as there is a great variability in reactivity depending on the source of the antiserum, and a positive reaction of anti-NSE with rhabdomyosarcomas has been reported.[54, 55] Monoclonal antibodies against NSE have been reported, which may eliminate some of the false-positive reactions seen with antisera to NSE.[56, 57] Monoclonal antibodies to neurofilament proteins have also been used to establish the neural origin of tumors. The higher specificity and reproducibility of monoclonal antibodies should theoretically make the antineurofilament antibodies excellent markers,[58] but such antibodies are not routinely used for diagnostic purposes.

Monoclonal antibodies to cell surface antigens have been studied for their potential to distinguish the various small, round cell tumors. Most of these studies have examined small panels of cell lines or small numbers of tumors and have not established a definitive role for various anti–cell surface antibodies.[59–62] Use of an antibody that recognizes the human leukocyte antigen (HLA) class I antigen (W6/32) and an antineuroblastoma antibody (such as HSAN 1.2)[60, 62] in combination can be useful, as most neuroblastomas (unlike Ewing's sarcoma, rhabdomyosarcoma, PNET, or lymphoma) show weak or negative HLA class I expression.

Another approach to distinguishing neuroblastoma from similar tumors has been to determine the pattern of gene expression by Northern analysis or by RT-PCR.[22, 45] This approach may enable definition of patterns of expression that are diagnostic for a given disease; as greater numbers of pathology laboratories become facile at doing such molecular studies, this approach may become routine.

## IDENTIFICATION OF RISK GROUPS

Analysis of prognostic factors is necessary for providing appropriate therapy and for interpreting the results of clinical trials. As we review in this section, evaluation of a number of prognostic factors is required for optimal prediction of clinical outcome and for assigning patients to risk groups. Although the biologic basis of aggressive tumor behavior (and especially the lack of aggressive behavior) is only partially understood, there now exist a variety of clinical parameters and laboratory tests that contribute to prognostic assessment.

**Stage.** As with most solid tumors, the degree of tumor spread plays a major role in determining clinical outcome. Nearly all neuroblastoma patients with localized disease have an excellent outcome, whereas most patients with extensive metastases have high-risk disease.[63–66] However, there are notable exceptions, such as infants with metastatic stage 4-S disease (who usually have a very good prognosis),[67–69] or patients with localized tumors that have amplication of the *MYCN* oncogene (who usually have high-risk disease).[64, 70] Such exceptions require that the stage of a patient be considered together with other prognostic indicators, especially the age of the patient,[4] the genomic amplification of *MYCN*,[64] and the histopathology.[46] It is also important to remember that all staging systems are based on methods for detecting disease that were available at the time the staging system was developed. As more sensitive methods for detecting tumor spread become available, staging must still be conducted using "routine" methods, but detection of occult disease provides additional prognostic information.

Four major staging systems have been developed for neuroblastoma. The oldest of these, developed by Evans and colleagues and used by the Children's Cancer Group (CCG), identifies five stages of disease—four that are dependent on degree of tumor spread, and one "special" stage that pertains to infants with a constellation of clinical features associated with a favorable prognosis.[71] A second staging system, which was developed at St. Jude Children's Research Hospital and is used by the Pediatric Oncology Group (POG), is based on a combination of tumor spread (including "surgical-pathologic" staging) and degree of tumor resection.[72] A third system is based on the Tumor Node Metastasis (TNM)

system of the International Union Against Cancer (UICC).[19] The existence of these three systems and the various modifications of them used by several groups have created problems in comparing the results of therapy among various centers. This problem was addressed in two international conferences; the result was a new International Neuroblastoma Staging System (INSS) that is being adopted worldwide.[19, 73] The CCG, POG, and consensus staging systems are shown in Table 79–3, and the INSS is illustrated in Figure 79–2.

**Sensitive Detection of Occult Disease.** Methods that enhance the sensitivity of detecting metastatic disease can be used to improve diagnostic evaluation, may allow more accurate staging of patients, and will likely be useful for monitoring disease activity. However, use of such new methods for clinical decisions must proceed with caution until substantial experience is acquired. One of the more commonly available new methods for detecting neuroblastoma employs the radiolabeled catecholamine analogue $^{131}$I-MIBG, which is accumulated in the tumor tissue via the neuroblastoma catecholamine uptake system.[16, 74–76] Initial studies suggest that MIBG scans are more sensitive than other radiologic techniques for detecting small areas of tumor involvement. Radiolabeled monoclonal antibodies that bind to neuroblastoma have also been used for imaging studies,[77, 78] but such reagents are not optimal for the repeated scanning needed to monitor disease activity because they can induce anti–mouse antibody responses.

Monoclonal antibodies to neuroblastoma have also been used to develop highly sensitive methods for detecting bone marrow metastasis. Although detection of tumor in a routine smear from a bone marrow aspirate can often require as much as 5% tumor cells, use of anti–neuroblastoma antibodies (with immunofluorescence or immunoperoxidase staining) can allow detection of one tumor cell per $10^3$ to $10^5$, depending on the antibodies and methods used.[79–85] A study using an immunoperoxidase method with a sensitivity of one in $10^5$ has shown that some stage 2 and stage 3 patients have subclinical marrow involvement and that the quantity of tumor cells detected has prognostic significance.[79] Sensitive detection and quantitation of marrow tumor content may also prove useful in determining response to therapy and could identify a subset of patients with persistent tumor in the marrow during induction who are at high risk for disease progression.[86] Studies using RT-PCR to detect tumor in marrow (due to expression of mRNA for tyrosine hydroxylase or the neuronal gene PGP 9.5) have shown that detection of one tumor cell per $10^6$ marrow or blood cells is possible.[87–89] The clinical significance of detecting such small numbers of tumor cells remains to be determined in clinical trials. Identification of a neuroblastoma cell in bone marrow by immunocytology is shown in Figure 79–3.

**Surgical Staging.** Although the original staging system for neuroblastoma described by Evans and associates[71] did not use lymph node involvement as a criterion for staging, some studies have suggested an influence of microscopic lymph node involvement on prognosis, especially in patients with localized disease.[72] These observations are reflected in the international staging system (see Table 79–2). It should be noted that lymph node sampling must be done at diagnosis rather than after chemotherapy, and some centers recom-

**Table 79–3. Staging Systems for Defining the Extent of Disease at Diagnosis**

**Evans/CCG Staging System**[71]

| | |
|---|---|
| Stage I | Tumor confined to the organ or structure of origin. |
| Stage II | Tumor extending in continuity beyond the organ or structure of origin but not crossing the midline. Regional lymph nodes on the homolateral side may be involved. |
| Stage III | Tumors extending in continuity beyond the midline. Regional lymph nodes bilaterally may be involved. |
| Stage IV | Remote disease involving bone, parenchymatous organs, soft tissues or distant lymph node groups, or bone marrow. |
| Stage IV-S | Patients who would otherwise be stage I or II but who have remote disease confined to one or more of the following sites: liver, skin, or bone marrow (without evidence of bone metastases). |

**St. Jude/POG Staging System**[72]

| | |
|---|---|
| Stage A | Complete gross excision of primary tumor, margins histologically negative. Intracavitary lymph nodes not intimately adhered to and removed with resected tumor are histologically free of tumor. If primary is in abdomen (including pelvis), liver is histologically free of tumor. |
| Stage B | Incomplete gross resection of primary tumor. Lymph nodes and liver histologically free of tumors, as in stage A. |
| Stage C | Complete or incomplete gross resection of primary tumor. Intracavitary nodes histologically positive for tumor. Liver histologically free of tumor. |
| Stage D | Disseminated disease beyond intracavitary nodes (ie, bone marrow, bone, liver, skin, or lymph nodes beyond cavity containing primary tumor). |

**International Staging System (INSS)**[19,73]

| | |
|---|---|
| Stage 1 | Localized tumor with complete gross excision, with or without microscopic residual disease; representative ipsilateral and contralateral lymph nodes negative for tumor microscopically (nodes attached to and removed with the primary tumor may be positive). |
| Stage 2A | Localized tumor with incomplete gross excision; representative ipsilateral nonadherent lymph nodes negative for tumor microscopically. |
| Stage 2B | Localized tumor with or without complete gross excision, with ipsilateral nonadherent lymph nodes positive for tumor. Enlarged contralateral lymph nodes must be negative microscopically. |
| Stage 3 | Unresectable unilateral tumor infiltrating across the midline,* with or without regional lymph node involvement; or localized unilateral tumor with contralateral regional lymph node involvement; or midline tumor with bilateral extension by infiltration (unresectable) or by lymph node involvement. |
| Stage 4 | Any primary tumor with dissemination to distant lymph nodes, bone, bone marrow, liver, skin, and/or other organs (except as defined in stage 4-S). |
| Stage 4-S | Localized primary tumor (as defined for stage 1, 2A, or 2B), with dissemination limited to liver, skin, and/or bone marrow.† (This stage is limited to infants younger than 1 yr of age.) |

*The midline is defined as the vertebral column. Tumors originating on one side and crossing the midline must infiltrate to or beyond the opposite side of the vertebral column.

†Marrow involvement in stage 4-S should be minimal (<10% of total nucleated cells). More extensive marrow involvement should be considered stage 4. If MIBG scan is done, it must be negative in the marrow for stage 4-S.

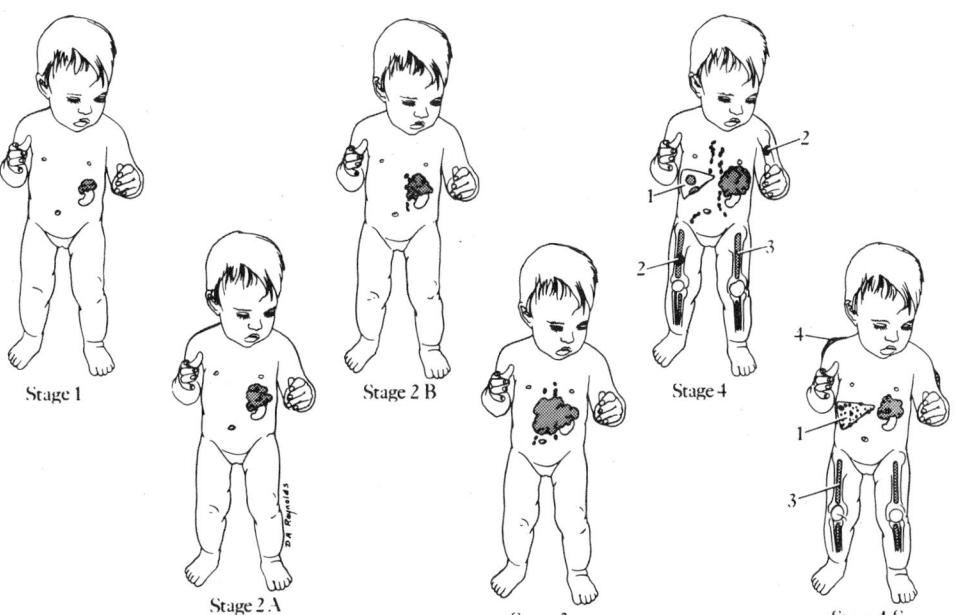

**Figure 79–2.** Depiction of the International Neuroblastoma Staging System (INSS) summarized in Table 79–3. Numbers point to sites of metastatic disease: 1 = liver, 2 = bone, 3 = bone marrow, 4 = skin.

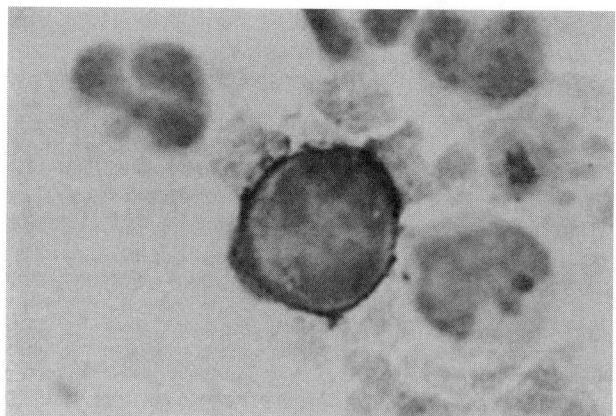

**Figure 79–3.** Neuroblastoma cell in bone marrow identified by immunocytology.

mend needle biopsy of the liver to exclude microscopic disease.

The ability to completely resect primary tumors can also have prognostic significance in some patients. Although incomplete resection does not seem to influence survival in patients with stage 2 disease,[66] patients with resectable stage 3 tumors (either at diagnosis or after chemotherapy) do significantly better than those in whom complete resection cannot be performed.[90] It is unclear whether the latter result reflects the inherent biology of the tumors studied, or if it indicates that surgical removal of mass disease contributes to successful combination therapy. It is important to note that the extent of resection is a major determinant of stage in the INSS system. Because INSS stage for local or regional tumors depends on the extent of resection, it will be important to develop standard surgical guidelines if this criterion is to be reliable and reproducible.

**Age.** The age of the patient at diagnosis is an important prognostic variable. Patients who are younger than 1 year of age (infants) at diagnosis do significantly better than older patients. Although the age of the patient does not seem to affect the prognosis of low-stage patients, infants with widespread disease (and tumors lacking *MYCN* amplification) do not have as poor a prognosis as older patients with stage 4 disease.[63, 64] Also, some reports indicate that children who are older than 6 years of age at diagnosis have less aggressive disease than do those between 1 and 6 years; nevertheless, the group of patients older than 6 years of age at diagnosis is not usually distinguished for the purpose of assigning therapy.[91]

**Histopathology.** A variety of histopathologic classification schemes have been used as prognostic indicators. The majority of these focus on the degree of differentiation of the tumor, usually dividing the tumor into various grades based on the degree of differentiation.[92–94] The most widely accepted classification scheme identifies patients with a "favorable" or "unfavorable" prognosis, based on histopathology and age, as described by Shimada and coworkers.[46] The Shimada classification divides tumors into stroma-rich and stroma-poor groups, with the stroma-rich group considered favorable (>90% survival) unless nodular elements of immature cells are present (18% survival). Stroma-poor tumors are generally classified as unfavorable (<5% survival); how-

ever, if the patient is younger than 18 months and has a low mitotic-karyorrhexis index or is 18 to 60 months, has a low mitotic-karyorrhexis index, and at least 5% of cells show evidence of differentiation, good survival (84%) is predicted. This latter scheme is unusual in that age is used in conjunction with the histopathology. Subsequent studies have confirmed the value of the Shimada classification in predicting survival. It is used by most investigators worldwide in conjunction with other prognostic factors to stratify therapy.[95–98]

**Serum Markers.** Ferritin produced by neuroblastoma cells can lead to elevations of serum ferritin to above-normal values. Hann and colleagues have shown that in stage 3 patients, elevated ferritin (above 142 ng/ml) is associated with poor survival (12%); in contrast, a normal ferritin level predicted a better survival rate (64%).[99] Elevated levels were also associated with poorer outcome in stage 4 patients (8% survival) than were normal levels (21% survival). Although the serum ferritin level at diagnosis is of prognostic value, serial determinations during therapy must be interpreted with caution as blood transfusions can result in elevated ferritin levels.[100]

High levels of NSE in serum (>100 ng/ml) are seen primarily in patients with stage 3 and stage 4 disease. High levels of serum NSE are associated with a worse prognosis in stage 3 patients and in stage 4 infants.[101] High serum levels at diagnosis of chromogranin A,[102] ganglioside GD2,[103] and lactate dehydrogenase[104, 105] all have been reported to indicate a worse prognosis compared with low or normal levels of these markers.

**Tumor Cell DNA Content.** Using flow cytometry, the distribution of DNA content in a tumor specimen can be compared with the DNA content of normal cells. Look and colleagues found that 77% of infants with neuroblastoma had tumor cells with hyperdiploid DNA content and that clinical outcome for these patients was superior to that of infants whose tumors had diploid DNA content.[106] Subsequent studies have confirmed the favorable clinical outcome associated with a hyperdiploid DNA content[107] and have also showed that a high number of cells in $S/G_2/M$ phases of the cell cycle (as determined by DNA content) was associated with a poor outcome.[108] In the latter study, substitution of cell cycle determination by flow cytometry for the mitotic-karyorrhexis index in the Shimada classification appeared to improve the accuracy of the latter in predicting clinical outcome. Although DNA ploidy analysis identifies infants with a poor outcome, it does not appear to provide valuable prognostic information for children older than 2 years at diagnosis.[109]

***MYCN* Oncogene Amplification.** Genomic amplification of the *MYCN* oncogene is seen in about 30% of patients with neuroblastoma and is most commonly found in patients with widespread disease.[110] Study of a large number of untreated primary tumors at diagnosis demonstrated a highly significant relationship between *MYCN* gene amplification and early progression of disease.[64] This relationship was independent of the stage of disease and age at diagnosis; for example, even infants with stage 2 disease had a poor prognosis if *MYCN* was amplified. Subsequent studies have confirmed that *MYCN* gene amplification is predictive of a poor prognosis.[70, 98, 107, 111–116] Because *MYCN* amplification is seen at diagnosis in primary tumors,[64] and nonamplified tumors have not been observed to develop amplification later in the course of the disease,[115] it is likely that amplification plays a role in the tumorigenesis of those tumors with amplified *MYCN*. The latter concept is supported by a close correlation of *MYCN* gene amplification with loss of genetic material from chromosome 1p.[117]

Although most studies of the prognostic significance of *MYCN* have measured amplification of the gene, some investigators have studied the relationship of MYCN expression to clinical outcome. High levels of MYCN RNA expression have been seen in virtually all tumors with gene amplification.[114, 116, 118] However, overexpression of MYCN RNA has also been observed in tumors without amplification, and some of these tumors did not behave aggressively.[116] This suggests that MYCN expression without gene amplification may not be sufficient for causing aggressive tumor behavior. An antiserum to the MYCN protein has also been used to study MYCN expression.[118, 119] Overexpression of *MYCN* has also been observed in nonamplified tumors by immunohistology, but the pattern of staining is uniform and distinct from that seen in tumors with genomic amplification. The pattern of MYCN immunostaining allows identification of tumors with *MYCN* gene amplification owing to their unique "starry sky" pattern of staining.[118] *MYCN* amplification can also be detected rapidly using PCR,[120] or by fluorescent in situ hybridization (FISH).[121–123] FISH is currently the most widely used approach in assessing tumors for *MYCN* amplification.

**Gene Expression.** Elevated or reduced levels of expression for several different genes have been associated with clinical behavior in neuroblastoma. Aggressive neuroblastomas do not express the high-affinity nerve growth factor receptor (TrkA), whether or not they show *MYCN* amplification.[124, 125] Expression of the multidrug resistance gene product, P-glycoprotein, has been studied by several different investigators, some showing that it correlates with poor outcome in neuroblastoma, and others showing that it does not.[126, 127] Other genes in which expression has been reported to be associated with outcome or stage include nm23,[128] c-*src*,[139, 130] *ras*,[131] proliferating cell nuclear antigen (PCNA),[132] Hsp27,[133] the multidrug resistance protein (MRP),[134] and telomerase activity[135, 136] or expression of the telomerase RNA component.[136, 137] Whether or not these markers identify subgroups of patients who are independent of other risk factors will require further prospective study using multivariate analysis.

**Tumor Growth In Vitro and in Xenografts.** The ability of neuroblastoma cells to proliferate in tissue culture and form continuous cell lines has been associated with aggressive tumor behavior in the patient and poor clinical outcome.[138] Although the biologic basis of this phenomenon may be attributed to *MYCN* amplification in some cases, there are examples in which tumor cells from aggressive tumors that lack *MYCN* amplification have formed cell lines.[139] Similarly, the ability of neuroblastomas to form xenografts in athymic (nude) mice has also been associated with poor outcome.[140]

# Treatment

## THERAPY BASED ON RISK GROUPS

Evaluating combinations of prognostic factors is essential for accurate prognostication in neuroblastoma.[65] Based on

the strong influence of age, stage, histopathology, and *MYCN* gene amplification on clinical outcome, it is possible to identify three groups of patients with a high degree of accuracy: those with low-, intermediate-, and high-risk disease.[64, 98] The characteristics of these groups are shown in Table 79–4. Accurate prognostication for patients who have mixed prognostic indicators can be difficult. Decisions about therapy for such patients should be made based on the summation of as many prognostic factors as one has available. Because the effect of a new therapy on the outcome of a given risk group is unknown, it is essential that as many prognostic factors as possible be evaluated for all patients entered into clinical trials. This will facilitate comparison of outcome for defined risk groups in different studies.

This section reviews the current therapies for each of the three major risk groups (low, intermediate, and high). For simplicity, we have used the INSS staging system for categorization of risk groups. It should be noted that some caution must be used for risk groups in which INSS staging has changed from the Evans staging system because the outcome data used to develop these risk groups are principally from patients staged by the Evans system. For example, completely resected large tumors can be an INSS 1, and would have been an Evans stage III. For any patients in whom INSS staging would be significantly different than older staging systems, particular attention must be addressed to all prognostic features of the patient when decisions about therapy are made.

**Low-Risk Patients.** Patients in this risk group have stage 1, stage 2, or stage 4-S tumors without amplification of *MYCN* or other high-risk factors. These patients have a high

---

*Table 79–4.* **Risk Groups Based on Prognostic Markers**

**Low Risk (Survival >80 to 100% with Surgery Alone)**

*All stage 1*

*Stage 2:*
Without amplification of *MYCN*

*Stage 4-S:*
Without amplification of *MYCN*
Without telomerase expression
With hyperdiploid DNA content

**Intermediate Risk (Survival >80% with Surgery, Conventional Chemotherapy, Local Irradiation)**

*Stage 3:*
Without amplication of *MYCN*
With favorable histopathology (Shimada)
Without elevated serum ferritin or neuron-specific enolase
With no or few occult tumor cells in marrow by immunocytology

*Stage 4, diagnosed younger than 1 year of age:*
Without amplification of *MYCN*
With favorable histopathology
Without elevated serum ferritin or neuron-specific enolase
With no or few occult tumor cells in marrow by immunocytology

**High Risk (Survival <10 to 15% with Conventional Chemotherapy, Surgery, Local Irradiation)**

*Stage 4, diagnosed at one year of age or older*

*Any clinical stage or age:*
With *MYCN* amplification
With unfavorable histopathology

likelihood of disease-free survival when treated with surgery alone (see Table 79–4). Stage 1 patients have a greater than 95% probability of survival after surgery alone; the probability of survival for stage 2 patients is greater than 85%, even if resection is incomplete.[66, 141] The addition of chemotherapy or local irradiation, or both, to surgery does not improve outcome for stage 2 patients, even if tumor remains after surgery.[66] However, chemotherapy is effective for stage 2 tumors that cause cord compression, thus removing the long-term complications of laminectomy and radiotherapy.[142, 143] Some, but not all, studies indicate that localized tumors with positive ipsilateral regional lymph nodes (now classified as INSS stage 2B) have a poorer outcome than those without lymph node involvement and may require chemotherapy after surgery.[72, 144–146] Because the prognostic significance of INSS stage 2B is not yet clear, it is acceptable to treat these patients with surgery and close observation if biologic and histopathologic prognostic factors are favorable.

Most stage 4-S patients have a favorable prognosis (greater than 80% survival if the tumors lack high-risk biologic features), and many of these tumors spontaneously regress with minimal or no chemotherapy.[67–69, 147, 148] Deaths in this group usually occur in patients diagnosed before 2 months of age and result from respiratory embarrassment or coagulopathy, or both, due to extensive liver metastases or complications of therapy. A retrospective review of 44 stage 4-S patients showed no positive effects from chemotherapy or irradiation for patients diagnosed from 3 to 12 months of age.[68] Thus, supportive care only is generally recommended, unless hepatic metastases are causing significant clinical problems: In such patients, local irradiation to the liver (4.5 Gy, "cross table") can provide significant benefit.[67, 149] In this procedure, the entire liver does not need to be treated, and the vertebral column, kidneys, and ovaries should be avoided if possible. "Mild" chemotherapy consisting of one or two agents (eg, cyclophosphamide alone or with doxorubicin or vincristine) has also been effective in treating liver involvement; however, systemic toxicity can be severe.[67]

Some 4-S tumors grow progressively, particularly those with diploid tumor DNA content, amplification of *MYCN*, or telomerase expression; this underscores the importance of analyzing primary or metastatic tumor tissue for prognostic markers.[111, 113, 135–137, 148, 150, 151] Current data suggest that intensive, combined-modality therapy is appropriate for stage 4-S patients with *MYCN*-amplified tumors, but effective regimens have not yet been defined in a prospective study.

**Intermediate-Risk Patients.** Patients with no high-risk factors, who have stage 3 disease diagnosed at any age or stage 4 disease diagnosed before 1 year of age, are included in this group. They have a greater than 80% likelihood of disease-free survival after therapy with conventional chemotherapy, surgery and, if necessary, local irradiation.

Approximately 50% of patients with Evans stage III disease are in this group. Most studies indicate that their likelihood of long-term, disease-free survival is greater than 80%. Their tumors have a favorable histologic pattern and lack *MYCN* gene amplification; their serum tumor markers (ferritin, neuron-specific enolase, lactate dehydrogenase, ganglioside $G_{D2}$, and chromogranin A) are normal or nearly so; and they have no or few occult tumor cells in their marrow (<6 per $10^5$ normal cells) as shown by immunocytology.[46, 64, 79, 95, 99, 103, 104, 152] Under INSS staging, a completely resected

tumor that formerly would have been a stage III neuroblastoma would be classified as a stage 1. Some protocols now mandate that such patients with no adverse risk factors not receive chemotherapy, but it should be noted that the usual practice in the past was to treat such patients, and a number of regimens have been investigated.[64, 90, 99] Current studies use the most active drugs (eg, cyclophosphamide, doxorubicin, etoposide, cisplatin; Table 79–5) for a relatively short period (22–38 weeks, depending on response). Nearly half of Evans stage III tumors can be completely resected at diagnosis or after chemotherapy and local irradiation, and tumor resectability confers a positive prognosis.[90] It is not clear whether the favorable prognosis associated with complete resection reflects inherent tumor biology or a therapeutic effect of surgery. Postoperative irradiation is usually given to residual tumor unless the patient was diagnosed before 1 year of age.[90, 153]

Patients with stage 4 disease diagnosed before 1 year of age who do not have high-risk factors have a greater than 80% probability of survival when treated with conventional multimodal therapy.[46, 64, 99, 101, 154] These tumors have a favorable histologic pattern, a hyperdiploid DNA content, and no *MYCN* gene amplification; serum ferritin and neuron-specific enolase are normal or nearly so.[46, 64, 99, 101, 106] A number of chemotherapy regimens have been reported (see Table 79–5) and, as with stage 3 disease, current regimens use surgery together with the most active drugs (eg, cyclophosphamide, doxorubicin, etoposide, and cisplatin) for a relatively short period (22–38 weeks, depending on response).[154–156]

Until recently, all patients with stage 4 disease who were diagnosed during the first year of life were treated similarly but in a prospective study, this approach was not successful for infants with high-risk factors.[154] Therefore, it is critical to identify patients who are at high risk and to treat them as such from the time of diagnosis. Analyses of *MYCN* and of histopathology are currently used by the cooperative group in the United States to identify high-risk stage 4 infants.[157]

**High-Risk Patients.** All patients diagnosed after 1 year of age with metastatic disease[19, 73] and all patients (regardless of age or stage) whose tumors show *MYCN* genomic amplification fall into this group.[64, 70, 111–116] Patients with stage 3 tumors that have unfavorable histopathologic features also have high-risk disease.[46, 95–97] Based on a CCG prospective randomized trial[158] (see later), most investigators treat high-risk patients with multiagent induction chemotherapy, attain local control with surgery and radiation, achieve consolidation using intensive myeloablative therapy, and finally, provide postconsolidation therapy of minimal residual disease using the differentiating agent 13-cis-retinoic acid. Although outcome for high-risk patients treated with the preceding multimodality approach has improved over that with previous therapies, disease-free survival from time of diagnosis for high-risk patients (especially for those with stage 4 disease diagnosed after 1 year of age) is still far from satisfactory. It is therefore important to enter high-risk neuroblastoma patients in clinical trials whenever possible so that newer and more effective therapies can be identified. Ideally, such trials will incorporate elements of therapy already proved effective (induction chemotherapy, myeloablative therapy, and 13-cis-retinoic acid therapy of minimal residual disease).

*Table 79–5.* Chemotherapy Regimens Used for Neuroblastoma

| Chemotherapy | Number of Patients | Response (%) CR + PR | Estimated 2-Year Survival (%) | Reference |
|---|---|---|---|---|
| ctx/vcr/dtic | 60 | 80 | 23 | 195 |
| ctx/vcr/dtic/dox | 44 | 82 | 18 | 195 |
| ctx/vcr/F3T/pap | 21 | 80 | 46 | 196 |
| ctx/vcr/dox | 46 | 69 | 19 | 197 |
| ctx/vcr | 23 | 57 | 22 | 197 |
| ctx/dox | 68 | 71 | 23 | 155 |
| vcr/dox/HN2 | 14 | NA | 25 | 3 |
| ctx/vcr/dtic/dox/cddp/HN2 | 20 | NA | 46 | 3 |
| ctx/vcr/cddp/tenip ± dox | 42 | 74 | 38 | 198 |
| ctx/vcr/dox/Fu/araC/hydr (high dose) | 33 | 88 | NA | 199 |
| ctx/vcr/dox/Fu/araC/hydr (mod. dose) | 14 | 57 | NA | 199 |
| ctx/vcr/dox/cddp/tenip | 35 | 96 | NA | 200 |
| cddp/etop | 17 | 70 | NA | 201 |
| ctx/dtic/dox/cddp/tenip | 28 | NA | 25 | 202 |
| ctx/dox/cddp/etop | 74 | 76 | 34 | 189 |
| cddp/etop/ifos/vcr/dox | 51 | 55 | NA | 203 |
| dox/cddp/etop/ifos | 40 | 43 | NA | 204 |
| ctx/dox/vcr/etop/cddp | 24 | 87 | NA | 205 |

These studies include predominantly stage IV patients diagnosed after 1 year of age; however, some include stage IV patients diagnosed in the first year of life and some stage III patients.

AraC, cytarabine; cddp, cisplatin; ctx, cyclophosphamide; dox, doxorubicin; dtic, dacarbazine; etop, etoposide; F3T, trifluoro-methyl-2-deoxyuridine; Fu, fluorouracil; HN2, mechlorethamine; hydr, hydroxyurea; ifos, ifosfamide; pap, papaverine; tenip, teniposide; vcr, vincristine; NA, not available; CR, complete response; PR, partial response.

## STANDARD TREATMENT MODALITIES

**Surgery.** Resection or partial resection of the primary tumor continues to be the major therapy for patients with localized disease. The use of chemotherapy as an adjuvant to surgery in stage 2 patients has been tested and was found not to improve clinical outcome.[159] Similarly, an analysis of the effect of radiotherapy on the outcome of stage 2 patients after surgery indicates that surgery alone is adequate, even if all of the tumor is not removed.[66] By contrast, patients with stage 3 tumors who have residual disease after surgery do poorly compared with those stage 3 patients in whom the tumor can be completely resected.[90] Because of the difficulty in removing many stage 4 and some stage 3 tumors, it has become common practice to delay attempts at definitive surgical removal of the primary tumor until after several courses of chemotherapy.[160–162] However, for apparent stage 3 patients, biopsy and exploration of the primary site still must be carried out at diagnosis to obtain tumor tissue for diagnosis, to examine regional lymph nodes, and to obtain tumor tissue for prognostic studies. In addition, if the INSS staging system is used, surgery is necessary to determine stage, which relates to the extent of resection.

Whenever possible, surgery should be performed for patients with stage 4 disease. This is particularly important for patients diagnosed before 1 year of age because evaluation of *MYCN* provides prognostic information. Although the benefit of removing residual tumor in stage 4 patients after chemotherapy has not been proved in clinical trials, most centers advocate the practice to remove mass disease in which hypoxic and poorly perfused tumor cells can survive intensive consolidation therapy.

If surgical removal of primary paraspinous tumors is undertaken at diagnosis, care should be taken to rule out extradural extension of the tumor. When the paraspinal portion of such "dumbbell" tumors is removed, substantial expansion can be induced in the extradural portion of the tumor, leading to acute neurologic problems.[163] In the past, it was common to treat or prevent cord compression from such tumors with laminectomy or radiotherapy. However, data indicate that using chemotherapy alone in such cases can avoid the long-term complications of laminectomy or radiotherapy without increasing the risk of neurologic impairment.[143]

**Radiotherapy.** Both clinical experience and studies of human tumors in nude mice have shown neuroblastoma to be a radiosensitive tumor.[164–170] However, because there are potentially serious late complications from primary radiation therapy (eg, scoliosis, renal failure), surgical resection should be the local therapy of choice for patients with surgically approachable disease. Also, primary radiotherapy should be avoided for patients who may undergo intensive chemoradiotherapy and autologous bone marrow transplantation (BMT) because the patient's own marrow or peripheral blood stem cells (PBSCs) must be spared from radiation until they are harvested and cryopreserved and because excess initial local radiation can compromise subsequent delivery of local and total body irradiation.

Patients with surgically unresectable neuroblastoma have been managed with induction chemotherapy followed by a delayed second operation.[63, 160, 162] Reported clinical complete response rates vary, but microscopic residual tumor is found in 20 to 50% so it is appropriate to deliver radiation therapy to unresected mass disease before proceeding with systemic consolidation therapy.

The role of adjuvant radiotherapy in localized neuroblastoma is controversial owing to the lack of randomized trials. Early studies suggested a role for radiotherapy in localized neuroblastoma with inoperable tumors. Although favorable survival in nonrandom studies of patients undergoing minimal surgery plus postoperative external-beam radiotherapy has been reported,[166, 167] and primary irradiation has demonstrated curative potential for mediastinal neuro-blastoma,[171] several nonrandomized studies suggest that adjuvant radiotherapy does not improve survival in stage I or II neuroblastoma.[171-174] A retrospective analysis of 150 stage II patients showed that survival for those 75 patients receiving surgery alone (even with incomplete resection) was not distinguishable from that for the 66 patients who received radiotherapy after surgery.[66] This indicates that stage II patients should not receive adjuvant radiotherapy, regardless of the degree of residual disease left following surgery, unless neurologic complications secondary to spinal cord compression occur. The exception to this would be stage II tumors with *MYCN* amplification,[64] which are aggressive and should be treated with myeloablative therapy, in addition to local radiotherapy.[175]

Stage III abdominal tumors can be completely resected, either at diagnosis or after chemotherapy or radiation therapy, in nearly one half of cases. Postoperative irradiation of residual tumor, in conjunction with chemotherapy, is used routinely and radiotherapy in this group of patients appears to improve survival over incomplete surgery alone.[144] However, in stage III patients younger than 1 year of age with residual disease, irradiation generally is withheld in favor of chemotherapy.[176]

In stage IV disease, the role of primary site radiotherapy remains undefined. Although there is evidence that local radiation therapy of stage D (IV) tumors decreases local recurrence, it has not improved survival when used with conventional chemotherapy.[144] This suggests that unresectable local tumor often can be effectively treated with radiation; thus, it is generally agreed, though not proved, that local irradiation to residual tumor contributes to the success of intensive consolidation therapy. A myeloablative chemoradiotherapy trial included dose-escalated carboplatin and etoposide over previously used levels by omitting total-body irradiation and giving local radiation (1.5 Gy BID for 7 days for a total dose of 21 Gy) to the site and margins of the primary tumor at the time of surgical resection.[177] The local irradiation likely played a role in the markedly diminished relapse rate in the primary tumor site that was observed in this study. As mentioned earlier, radiation therapy must be used with caution in patients expected to undergo myeloablative therapy so that the ability to harvest adequate hematopoietic stem cells is preserved. Owing to concerns about hepatotoxicity, many investigators opt to deliver local radiation to patients after completion of myeloablative chemotherapy.

The dose of local irradiation needed to control neuroblastoma has not been established by randomized clinical trials. Uncontrolled data appear to support a dose-response relationship, with doses of 25 Gy or more yielding superior results.[167] Most physicians now recommend tailoring the dose to patient age. For children younger than 1 year of age, doses of 9 to 15 Gy are recommended; for patients 1 to 2 years of age, 15 to 25 Gy is recommended.[168, 169] In one study, a higher local recurrence rate in older patients was associated with radiation doses lower than 17 Gy.[170] This suggests that for those older than 2 years of age, doses approaching 25 Gy should be given.

The volume of residual disease may affect the dose of radiation necessary for tumor control, but this has not been determined in clinical trials. Field determination depends on tumor location, surrounding vital structures, and tumor margins marked during surgery with radiopaque clips. Tumors adjacent to, or invading, the spine should be treated with fields that include the entire width of the spine and adjacent soft tissues, to minimize the risk of kyphosis and scoliosis.[170]

In stage IV-S neuroblastoma with significant hepatic enlargement, 450 Gy to the liver can have a dramatic benefit in decreasing respiratory compromise.[178] However, because of the long-term potential complications of radiotherapy and the excellent prognosis of stage IV-S patients, radiotherapy should be avoided whenever possible.

Because of the poor prognosis of advanced neuroblastoma, several innovative radiotherapeutic techniques have been tested for patients with stage IV disease. Segmental total-body irradiation, fractionated low-dose total-body irradiation, and sequential hemibody irradiation have been used with chemotherapy.[179-181] None of these techniques has proved superior to conventional chemotherapy. Some investigators have also explored intraoperative radiotherapy as a means to improve local tumor control because of its ability to deliver higher radiation doses while sparing normal tissues.[165, 182, 183] Myeloablative chemoradiotherapy supported by autologous hematopoietic stem cell transplantation (ASCT), in which 10 to 12.5 Gy total-body irradiation (TBI) is part of the pre-ASCT therapy,[175, 184-187] improves outcome for high-risk patients; however, whether or not TBI is necessary for optimal results has not been determined (see later, Myeloablative Therapy Without TBI).

**Chemotherapy.** As with radiotherapy, stage I or II patients whose tumors lack *MYCN* amplification have an excellent prognosis and do not require adjuvant chemotherapy, even if surgical resection is not complete.[64, 66, 188] Although the prognosis for infants with stage IV-S tumors is excellent, such patients can develop respiratory problems due to tumor expansion prior to spontaneous regression.[67] In such cases, chemotherapy has been successful in shrinking the tumor, but most centers use "mild" regimens of one or two agents.

Aggressive multiagent chemotherapy is used for high-risk patients, but past experience has shown that the chances of long-term survival for such patients treated with chemotherapy are not high.[3, 64] The probability of long-term survival can be improved for many high-risk patients by using consolidation with myeloablative chemoradiotherapy and autologous hematopoietic stem cell transplantation (AHSCT).[175, 184-187, 189] Currently, initial chemotherapy is used for cytoreductive purposes, and harvest of hematopoietic stem cells and surgery occur between courses of induction chemotherapy. The success of an induction chemotherapy regimen is measured by its ability to reduce tumor burden and prevent progressive disease and to facilitate surgical resection, as well as the ability of the patient to tolerate subsequent intensive consolidation. Use of multiagent regimens is also appropriate for stage III patients who may not undergo consolidation but require aggressive cytoreductive chemotherapy before undergoing delayed surgery.[90] Multiagent chemotherapy has also been used in place of laminectomy or radiotherapy to minimize neurologic sequelae from extradural tumors.[143]

A number of drugs have been shown to be active against neuroblastoma as single agents and in various combinations, including cyclophosphamide, ifosfamide, cisplatin, carboplatin, iproplatin, doxorubicin, teniposide, etoposide, L-phenylalanine mustard, vincristine, dacarbazine, and topotecan.[7, 190–192] In most high-risk patients, an initial response to multiagent chemotherapy is seen, but progressive tumor growth usually occurs subsequently.[64, 175, 193] Although studies have suggested that scheduling drugs so as to recruit tumor into the cell cycle before administration of S-phase–active agents is beneficial,[155, 194] design of recent multiagent chemotherapy regimens has been mostly empirical, or such design has been based on theoretical concerns about tumor cell cycle effects or drug resistance, or both. This has led to a number of complex regimens (see Table 79–5).[3, 155, 189, 195–205] Currently, there are no randomized comparisons to prove that one particular regimen is superior to another, although the more recent multiagent regimens are clearly superior to older two- and three-agent regimens that were less intensive. Based on the response rate reported for one highly aggressive induction regimen,[205] many investigators are currently using that regimen (or variations of it) for induction of neuroblastoma patients with high-risk disease. Further study will be needed to determine if such aggressive induction regimens achieve a true benefit compared with less aggressive regimens in terms of tumor response (and ultimately disease-free survival after completion of myeloablative therapy). Advantages in terms of disease control seen with aggressive induction regimens will also need to be balanced against the risk of inducing secondary leukemias,[206, 207] although early harvest of hematopoietic stem cells during the course of induction chemotherapy could decrease the rate of secondary leukemias after myeloablative therapy.

**Myeloablative Therapy.** The initial good response seen in many neuroblastoma patients who develop recurrent tumor has prompted the study of methods to intensify the dose of therapy delivered to such patients in hopes of increasing the proportion of patients who achieve long-term disease-free survival.[208] Pilot investigations of high-dose chemotherapy and bone marrow transplantation (BMT), with or without total-body irradiation, suggest that such an approach improved the outcome for some poor-prognosis neuroblastoma patients.[175, 177, 184–189, 209–222] The results of representative studies employing myeloablative therapy before disease progression are summarized in Table 79–6. Long-term disease-free survival is improved over nonmyeloablative chemotherapy by treating patients before disease progression

with very intensive multiagent regimens, some of which use total-body irradiation (TBI). Although myeloablative therapy has been successful in some relapsed patients, the prognosis for patients who have developed progressive disease still remains poor with current myeloablative regimens.[177, 187]

***CCG-3891 Phase III Trial.*** A prospective phase III randomized trial (CCG-3891) was undertaken by the Children's Cancer Group (CCG) to determine if myeloablative therapy supported by purged autologous BMT (ABMT) resulted in higher event-free survival (EFS) than did intensive nonmyeloablative consolidation chemotherapy for patients with high-risk neuroblastoma.[158] Patients entering the study received induction chemotherapy with cisplatin, cyclophosphamide, doxorubicin, and etoposide and were randomized at 28 weeks to a single round of myeloablative therapy with melphalan, carboplatin, etoposide, and TBI (190 patients), or to three rounds of intensive, nonmyeloablative chemotherapy using cisplatin, etoposide, doxorubicin, and ifosfamide/mesna (189 patients). During the induction chemotherapy, patients underwent marrow harvest, surgical resection, and radiotherapy to residual disease, as needed. After completion of either myeloablative or nonmyeloablative consolidation therapy, patients were eligible for a second randomization to test the efficacy of 13-cis-retinoic acid against minimal residual disease (see later). As is shown in Figure 79–4A (intent-to-treat analysis),[158] patients randomized to purged ABMT had a significantly better EFS than did patients randomized to nonmyeloablative chemotherapy; also, the 3-year EFS from time of first randomization was 34% ± 4% for ABMT patients, compared with 22% ± 4% for those randomized to consolidation chemotherapy ($p = 0.034$). Total hospital days were equal for both arms of the study at 46 days.

**Autologous Bone Marrow and Peripheral Blood Stem Cell Purging.** The risk of graft-versus-host disease and the lack of suitable marrow donors limit the use of allogeneic BMT to approximately 25% of patients. This has prompted widespread use of autologous BMT; however, because the frequency of bone marrow metastasis in neuroblastoma is high (approximately 75% of stage IV patients at diagnosis),[79] there is a definite risk of infusing tumorigenic cells with the marrow. Indeed, there are several case reports suggesting that recurrent neuroblastoma after autologous BMT (miliary

*Table 79–6.* **Myeloablative Therapy for High-Risk Neuroblastoma Prior to Disease Progression**

| Regimen | Number of Patients | Estimated % Survival | | Follow-up in Months | | References |
|---|---|---|---|---|---|---|
| | | 2 YR | 3 YR | MEDIAN | (RANGE) | |
| L-PAM | 12 | 25 | NA | 33 | (18–35) | 307 |
| L-PAM | 15 | 33 | 33 | 39 | (29–54) | 209 |
| L-PAM/BCNU/tenip | 33 | 51 | 38 | 28 | (8–50) | 195 |
| L-PAM/vcr/TBI | 37 | 44 | NA | 6 | (3–48) | 185 |
| L-PAM/vcr/TBI | 62 | 40 | 25 | 55 | (NA) | 212 |
| L-PAM/tenip/dox/cddp/ | 31 | 56 | 56 | 7 | (1–44) | 187 |
| L-PAM/tenip/dox/cddp/TBI | 45 | 45 | 45 | 29 | (17–44) | 213 |
| L-PAM/etop/cddp/bcnu | 16 | 44 | NA | 39 | (20–46) | 308 |
| L-PAM/etop/carbo/TBI | 67 | NA | 48 | 40 | (28–64) | 189 |
| L-PAM/etop/carbo/TBI | 129 | NA | 43 | 43 | (2–89) | 175 |
| L-PAM/etop/carbo/LI | 77 | NA | 62 | 30 | (4–90) | 177 |

Carbo, carboplatin; BCNU, carmustine; cddp, cisplatin; dox, doxorubicin; etop, etoposide; L-PAM, L-phenylalanine mustard (melphalan); tenip, teniposide; vcr, vincristine; TBI, total body irradiation; LI, local irradiation; NA, not available.

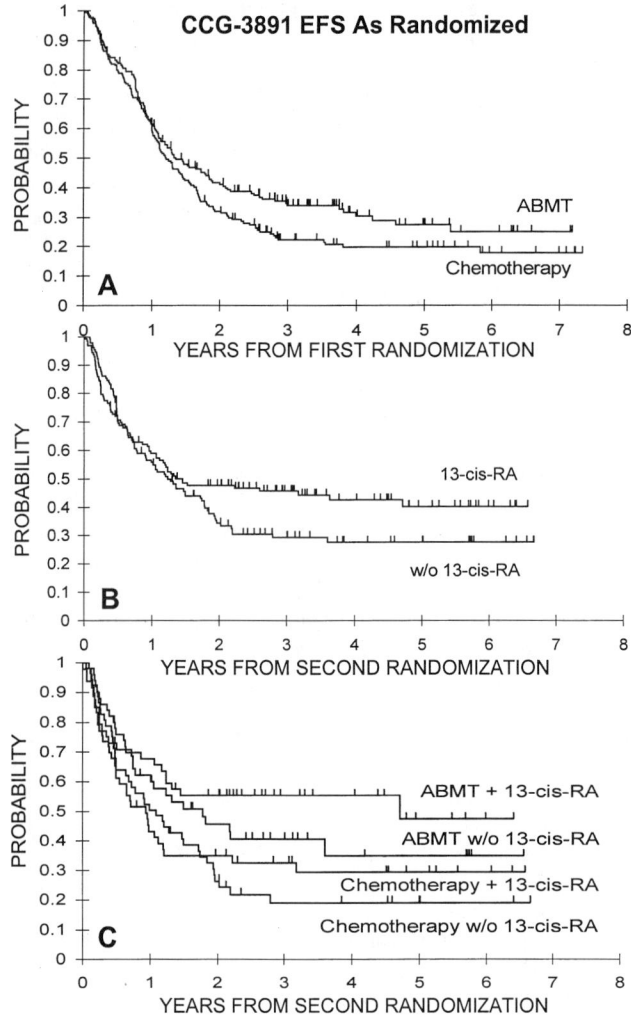

**Figure 79–4.** Summary of event-free survival (EFS) analyses (as randomized) from the CCG-3891 trial.[175] *A,* The primary randomization demonstrated improved EFS for myeloablative therapy supported with purged autologous bone marrow transplantation relative to patients randomized to nonmyeloablative chemotherapy. *B,* Results from the second randomization showed improved EFS for patients randomized to receive 13-cis-retinoic acid given after completion of either myeloablative therapy or consolidation chemotherapy relative to those randomized to no further therapy. *C,* A composite of the four possible treatment groups defined by patients who entered both the first and second randomizations of CCG-3891.

metastases in the lung) resulted from the marrow infusion.[223, 224] Also, a study in which autologous cells were marked with the neomycin-resistance gene demonstrated that neuroblastoma cells in autologous marrow can contribute to relapse.[225]

Several methods for purging tumor cells from bone marrow harvested for autologous transplantation have been developed. The most widely used method employs physical removal of the tumor cells using magnetic microspheres and anti–neuroblastoma monoclonal antibodies.[175, 185, 208, 226, 227] The use of such purging methods, combined with verification of tumor removal with sensitive detection methods,[79, 83, 228–230] should minimize the possibility that tumor recurrence after autologous BMT is due to tumor infused with the marrow. Proving that purging of marrow decreases tumor recurrence

in neuroblastoma in a randomized trial has not been undertaken owing to the high frequency with which neuroblastoma cells are detected in harvested autologous bone marrow. However, a nonrandomized comparison of high-risk neuroblastoma patients who underwent allogeneic BMT versus patients who underwent purged autologous BMT showed an apparent lower relapse rate in the autologous BMT patients, suggesting that autologous marrow purged in the manner used for that study does not contain sufficient tumor cells to cause tumor recurrence in most patients.[231] Studies employing myeloablative therapy have focused on using peripheral blood stem cells (PBSCs) owing to the more rapid rate of engraftment and the lower frequency of tumor contamination seen with PBSCs relative to bone marrow.[89, 232, 233–238] It is currently unknown if the small numbers of tumor cells that may be present in PBSCs can contribute to tumor relapse, but PBSCs can be purged using methods similar to those used for bone marrow. An ongoing Children's Oncology Group (COG) study is comparing, in a randomized phase III trial, unpurged PBSCs to PBSCs purged with immunomagnetic beads.

**Differentiation Therapy with 13-cis-Retinoic Acid.** Anecdotal trials of 13-cis-retinoic acid in neuroblastoma showed responses of mass disease and marrow metastases, including a complete response with a 2-year remission in one patient.[239, 240] Although some responses were seen in neuroblastoma patients with progressive disease in a CCG phase II trial of 13-cis-retinoic acid the overall activity of 13-cis-retinoic acid at a dose of 100 mg/m²/day against progressive disease was disappointing.[241] For 13-cis-retinoic acid to be effective in patients, it was likely that drug levels known to be effective in vitro against neuroblastoma (5 to 10 μM in 2-week pulses) would have to be achieved.[242] A phase I trial showed that an intermittent schedule of 13-cis-retinoic acid (2 weeks of therapy/month) allowed dose escalation to a maximally tolerated dose (MTD) of 160 mg/m²/day in post-BMT patients,[243] with the dose-limiting toxicity being hypercalcemia.[244] Complete responses were seen in the phase I trial in 4 of the 10 patients with measurable disease after myeloablative therapy and bone marrow transplantation; 2 of those 4 patients entered a prolonged remission (>2 years).[243] The latter observation suggested that those patients receiving 13-cis-retinoic acid with no measurable disease could benefit from the drug preventing tumor recurrence.[240]

Because 13-cis-retinoic acid was shown to be tolerable when given soon after ABMT, a second randomization (factorial design) was added to the CCG-3891 study to determine in a prospective fashion if 13-cis-retinoic acid could effectively eradicate minimal residual disease.[175] Patients who completed either myeloablative or nonmyeloablative consolidation therapy were randomized to no further therapy or to receive 13-cis-retinoic acid at 160 mg/m²/day (divided and given BID) for 2 weeks each month over a 6-month period. Patients who had documented active tumor by biopsy at the end of consolidation were nonrandomly assigned to receive 13-cis-retinoic acid. A total of 130 patients were randomized to receive 13-cis-retinoic acid, and 128 patients were randomized to no further therapy. There were 37 patients nonrandomly assigned to 13-cis-retinoic acid for proven residual tumor and 24 patients who refused the second randomization, 4 of whom chose to receive 13-cis-retinoic acid. As shown in Figure 79–4*B,* the 3-year EFS (intent-to-treat analysis) from the time of second randomization for patients randomized to 13-cis-retinoic acid was 46% ± 6%, which was significantly better than the 3-year EFS of 29% ± 5% for those randomized to no further therapy ($p = 0.027$). The effect of 13-cis-retinoic acid was most pronounced in a setting of truly minimal residual disease, as subset analysis showed the most significant effect for 13-cis-retinoic acid in stage IV patients was for those who achieved initial complete remission. The positive benefit of 13-cis-retinoic acid for those patients with minimal residual disease was not seen for children who were nonrandomly assigned to 13-cis-retinoic acid for histologically proven residual disease, as this latter group showed a 3-year EFS of 12% ± 6%.

Toxicity of 13-cis-retinoic acid seen in the CCG-3891 trial[158] was similar to that seen in the phase I trial of post-BMT high-dose, pulse 13-cis-retinoic acid.[243, 244] Toxicities included transaminase elevation (2%), renal effects (2%), gastrointestinal complications (2%), skin disorders (2%), infection (12%), and hypercalcemia (1%). Hematologic toxicities were seen in 9% of patients, but these lessened as time increased from the end of cytotoxic therapy, probably reflecting previous intensive treatment with myelotoxic drugs. Five patients who had undergone ABMT and also received 13-cis-retinoic acid developed hematuria, proteinuria, and hypertension accompanied by creatinine elevation to a maximum of 1.8. Because a syndrome of hypertension, hematuria, and proteinuria has been previously reported following ABMT in patients who were not treated with 13-cis-retinoic acid, it is possible that the renal toxicity seen in those 5 patients was not retinoid related.[158] The most common toxicity with 13-cis-retinoic acid was skin toxicity, which occurred at low grades in most patients, but was rarely severe (only 2% of patients had grade 3 to 4 skin toxicity). Good supportive care, including avoidance of sunlight, use of vitamin E cream for the lips, and application of other moisturizing creams, has been helpful in minimizing skin toxicity.

**Combining Myeloablative Therapy and 13-cis-Retinoic Acid.** Because of the two randomizations in the CCG-3891 study, one can examine the apparent EFS for the four different treatment groups created, although small group size of each of these four treatment groups limits statistical power, and the two different randomization time points preclude a formal analysis (Figure 79–4*C*). Treatment with 13-cis-retinoic acid appeared to be beneficial for patients who received either ABMT or nonmyeloablative chemotherapy. The 3-year EFS from time of second randomization in patients undergoing both randomizations was higher for ABMT and 13-cis-retinoic acid (55% ± 10%), compared with ABMT alone (41% ± 10%; $p = 0.28$). The 3-year EFS for chemotherapy and 13-cis-retinoic acid was 33% ± 7%, compared with chemotherapy alone (19% ± 7%; $p = 0.17$). The EFS curves in Figure 79–4*C* can be shown only from the time of second randomization; therefore, not all patients are included from the first randomization. Thus, one must interpret these curves with caution. However, the significant improvement seen in EFS both for ABMT in the first randomization and for 13-cis-retinoic acid in the second randomization, supports that Figure 79–4*C* shows the highest EFS that can be achieved with ABMT followed by 13-cis-retinoic acid. It is likely that myeloablative therapy was most

effective in reducing disease burden before 13-cis-retinoic acid therapy. The outcome for patients treated with both ABMT and 13-cis-retinoic acid, taken together with the poor survival of patients who had documented active disease at the time they began 13-cis-retinoic acid therapy, emphasizes that the optimal application for 13-cis-retinoic acid is in a setting of minimal residual disease.[158]

## NEW THERAPEUTIC APPROACHES

**Myeloablative Therapy Without Total-Body Irradiation.** Even with the improved survival seen with current myeloablative regimens, more than one half of patients still die from tumor recurrence. One approach to improving outcome would be to develop myeloablative regimens that achieve more effective tumor cell kills with tolerable toxicity. The CCG-3891 study[158] showed that delivering the maximal intensity of therapy in a single setting (using hematopoietic stem cell support) achieved a higher EFS than did multiple courses of submyeloablative therapy. However, CCG-3891 did not define which components of the carboplatin, etoposide, melphalan plus total body irradiation (CEM-TBI) chemoradiotherapy regimen are needed to achieve optimal results. A limited-institution study sought to develop an improved myeloablative regimen (CEM plus local irradiation [CEM-LI]) by eliminating TBI, substituting local radiotherapy to the primary tumor site, and determining if the carboplatin and etoposide could be further dose escalated when given without the TBI.[177] The intent of using local radiotherapy was to decrease the rate of relapse in the site of the primary tumor, which is a site of relapse for 50% of those patients with recurrent tumor after myeloablative therapy.[245] For patients with a glomerluar filtration rate (GFR) of ≥100 ml/min/1.73 m$^2$, the maximally tolerated dose of carboplatin (1700 mg/m$^2$) and etoposide (1350 mg/m$^2$) in the CEM-LI regimen is substantially higher than what was used in CEM-TBI; the relapse rate at the primary tumor site was lower (only 3 of the 20 relapses); and the 3-year EFS for the 77 patients treated with CEM-LI in first response was 62% ± 20%. Because results with CEM-LI were at least as good as those obtained with CEM-TBI, CEM-LI is being used in the current COG phase III study for high-risk neuroblastoma.

**Tandem Autologous Stem Cell Transplantation.** Other investigators have attempted to achieve greater antitumor efficacy by delivering two sequential myeloablative regimens (tandem AHSCT).[246, 247] This approach has been facilitated by the use of PBSCs for hematopoietic reconstitution, as it is often possible to collect enough PBSCs for two infusions. Limited institution studies have shown this approach to be feasible, and tandem-AHSCT may be tested in cooperative group studies in the future.

**Metaiodobenzylguanidine.** In addition to being used for tumor detection, radiolabeled MIBG has been used therapeutically.[75, 248, 249] Although some responses have been observed, one of the limiting factors in using MIBG has been the dose limitation imposed by its hematopoietic toxicity (probably enhanced by tumor uptake of the drug in bone marrow).[248, 250] Pilot studies using AHSCT suggest that higher, and potentially more effective, doses of MIBG can be achieved using AHSCT to overcome myelotoxicity.[251, 252] Because specialized treatment facilities are necessary for therapeutic application of radiopharmaceuticals, at least for the near future, only limited institutions will be using MIBG for therapy.

*Overcoming Drug Resistance.* The poor response to chemotherapy seen in patients who develop recurrent neuroblastoma after therapy (especially relapse after myeloablative therapy) indicates that recurrent tumor cells have acquired resistance to multiple classes of drugs. Indeed, a sustained multidrug resistance phenotype (including resistance to alkylating agents) is seen in neuroblastoma cell lines established at time of relapse after therapy (especially in those established at relapse after myeloablative therapy).[253, 254] Future development of agents that are effective against such drug-resistant tumor cells is necessary to improve outcome for many patients because the degree of drug resistance in tested cell lines cannot be overcome by dose escalation within clinically tolerable levels.[253, 254]

One mechanism by which tumor cells can detoxify alkylating agents and platinum chemotherapy is by conjugation of the drugs to glutathione (GSH), a ubiquitous tripeptide used by cells in detoxifiying xenobiotics and free radicals. Depletion of GSH using buthionine sulfoximine (BSO), an inhibitor of the rate-limiting GSH synthetic enzyme (glutamylcysteine synthase), has been shown to be highly toxic to neuroblastoma in vitro, indicating an unusual dependence of neuroblastoma cells on GSH as an antioxidant to handle a high degree of endogenous reactive oxygen species.[255] BSO is strikingly synergistic against neuroblastoma in vitro when combined with melphalan,[256] and a pilot clinical trial demonstrated response in relapsed neuroblastoma to 15 mg/m$^2$ of melphalan given with BSO, including patients relapsing after myeloablative doses of melphalan (210 mg/m$^2$).[257] Because the major toxicity of BSO-melphalan appears to be hematopoietic,[257] an ongoing clinical study is determining the MTD of melphalan given with BSO, together with hematopoietc stem cell support. If tolerable, BSO-melphalan could be used in future myeloablative regimens for high-risk neuroblastoma.

**Immunotherapy.** Neuroblastomas express antigens recognized by monoclonal antibodies. Most preclinical and clinical therapeutic studies with antibodies have targeted disialoganglioside (GD2) because it is strongly expressed on the surface of neuroblastoma cells.[258, 259] Anti-GD2 antibodies have induced responses in patients,[260–263] probably because of complement-dependent cytotoxicity and antibody-dependent cellular cytotoxicity (ADCC).[264–266] Cytokines can enhance ADCC by activating cytotoxic natural killer cells (IL-2) and neutrophils (GM-CSF).[264, 267–273] Phase I studies have tested the combination of IL-2 and murine anti-GD2 antibody 14G2A[274, 275] in patients with recurrent neuroblastoma; also, GM-CSF and the murine/human chimeric anti-GD2 antibody ch 14.18 has been combined following myeloablative therapy and ABMT.[276] Common toxicities in the latter study included neuropathic pain (50%), fever (43%), nausea and vomiting (25%), urticarial eruption (19%), and hypotension (14%). A planned COG phase III randomized study will determine if a chimeric anti-GD2 antibody, given together with alternating courses of GM-CSF and IL-2 after myeloablative therapy and before 13-cis-retinoic acid, improves EFS over myeloablative therapy followed by 13-cis-retinoic acid alone.

Use of radiolabeled antibodies has shown that selective

localization to tumor sites can be achieved[77, 78]; such an approach may be used to deliver radioisotopes selectively to neuroblastoma. However, as with therapy using MIBG, radiotherapy with antibodies requires highly specialized care and facilities, thus limiting widespread use.

Neuroblastomas also express antigens that could be used to generate cytotoxic T lymphocytes (CTLs). Potential immunogens include tumor cells that have been transduced with cytokine genes such as IL-2[277, 278] or IFN-γ,[279] GD2 conjugated to a carrier protein,[280] anti-GD2 anti-idiotype antibodies,[281–283] and MAGE family proteins or peptides.[284] One study found that patients who developed anti-idiotype antibodies against anti-GD2 had a better outcome than those who did not; however, CTLs or antibody responses to the anti-idiotype antibody were not demonstrated.[281]

Immunotherapy probably will be most effective against relatively small numbers of tumor cells such as those persisting after myeloablative therapy supported by AHSCT. Neutrophils increase within 3 weeks after AHSCT, and both granulocyte colony-stimulating factor (G-CSF) and GM-CSF accelerate hematopoietic recovery.[285] Although it has not been extensively studied, neutrophils from patients who have undergone AHSCT are functional in ADCC in vitro.[286] ADCC against tumor cells also can be mediated by natural killer cells, lymphokine-activated killer cells, monocytes and macrophages, or a combination. Neutrophil cytotoxicity, primarily due to membrane damage, likely will not be affected if tumor cells develop resistance to apoptosis. Induction of active immunity within the first few months after AHSCT may be problematic because patients are not fully immunocompetent. However, tumor-pulsed dendritic cells may be capable of inducing CTL in this setting.[287] Another potential barrier to active immunotherapy is that neuroblastoma cells express low levels of antigen-processing and presentation genes, including LMP-2, LMP-7, TAP-1, and MHC class I, which are necessary for presentation of target peptides to CTLs. Effective CTL antitumor immunity against neuroblastoma would require not only restoration of immunocompetence but also upregulation of antigen processing and presentation genes with, for example, IFN-γ.[279]

Antibody-cytokine fusion proteins (immunocytokines) combine the targeting ability of antibodies with the functional activity of cytokines. Because the cytokine is approximately 20% of the fusion protein,[288] large amounts can be delivered to the tumor microenvironment by the antibody. Immunocytokines, depending on their molecular composition, could create a microenvironment that results in (1) complement activation with generation of chemoattractants for neutrophils; (2) complement-dependent cytotoxicity against tumor cells; (3) ADCC against tumor cells mediated by activated neutrophils, natural killer cells, monocytes-macrophages, or a combination; and (4) attraction of dendritic cells that process tumor-associated antigens and then induce antitumor immune responses by T cells or B cells, or both. An anti-GD2/IL-2 immunocytokine eradicated hepatic metastases of neuroblastomas in SCID mice that had been reconstituted with human lymphokine (IL-2)-activated killer cells.[289, 290] In contrast, the combination of monoclonal anti-GD2 antibody and IL-2 at doses equivalent to the immunocytokine only reduced tumor load. In a syngeneic murine model of GD2-expressing melanoma, targeting with an anti-GD2 antibody/IL-2 immunocytokine resulted in generation of CD8$^+$ T lymphocytes that could eradicate tumor as well as prevent tumor growth.[291] Based on these data, phase I studies of a humanized anti-GD2/IL-2 immunocytokine for neuroblastoma are under way in Germany and the United States (Handgretinger R and Sondel P, personal communications, 2000). Neutrophil cytotoxicity is enhanced by mixing GM-CSF with antibody,[268–271, 273] and activation of neutrophil ADCC using a humanized anti-GD2/GM-CSF immunocytokine hu14.18/GM-CSF also mediates effective anti-neuroblastoma ADCC in vitro.[292] Anti-GD2/GM-CSF immunocytokines effectively mediate ADCC against drug-resistant neuroblastoma cell lines, including those derived from tumors that recurred after autologous or allogeneic BMT.[293] If tolerated, these new agents could be effective against tumor cells that persist after myeloablative therapy.

**Fenretinide.** A synthetic retinoid made in the late 1960s, *N*-(4-hydroxyphenyl) retinamide or fenretinide (4-HPR) has been reported to inhibit the growth of neuroblastoma cell lines in vitro with 1 to 10 micromolar concentrations in a dose-dependent manner[294–296]; 4-HPR was also highly active against retinoic acid–resistant and highly alkylator- and etoposide-resistant cell lines established after myeloablative therapy neuroblastoma cell lines at 5- to 10-$\mu$M drug levels.[240, 297] In contrast to 13-cis-retinoic acid and all-*trans*-retinoic acid, 4-HPR does not induce maturational changes but is cytotoxic, causing large increases in tumor cell ceramide and both apoptosis and necrosis.[297] Toxicity of 4-HPR in chemoprevention clinical trials has been minimal and no hematologic toxicity has been reported, with the major clinical toxicity of 4-HPR being decreased night vision due to decreased plasma retinol levels.[298] A phase I trial of fenretinide in pediatric solid tumors (CCG-09709) is currently in progress, having achieved to date dose levels from 350 to 1499 mg/m$^2$/day. Preliminary results[299] showed that peak plasma levels of >5 $\mu$M 4-HPR are being obtained at doses of 800 to 1200 mg/m$^2$/day, thus approaching levels that are highly effective against neuroblastoma in vitro, with dose escalation still under way.

As 4-HPR has been shown to achieve multilog cytotoxicity in neuroblastoma cell lines resistant to 13-cis-retinoic acid,[300] 4-HPR may be effective against 13-cis-retinoic acid–resistant neuroblastomas. Thus, one possible clinical application of fenretinide will be the treatment of high-risk neuroblastoma patients who have been treated with myeloablative therapy and then 13-cis-retinoic acid, who can then be subsequently treated with 4-HPR to eliminate residual tumor cells resistant to prior therapy. Future trials also will likely use 4-HPR in combination with agents that modulate ceramide metabolism so as to increase the antitumor activity of 4-HPR.[301]

**Other New Agents.** There have been a number of laboratory studies of agents showing antineuroblastoma activity, but we have limited our discussion to drugs used in clinical trials. Preclinical work in neuroblastoma has been reported on drugs that have been used in clinical trials for other diseases, and it is likely that such drugs will be tested on neuroblastoma patients in the near future. Potential new approaches include antiangiogenesis agents such as TMP-470,[302] integrin antagonists with antiangiogenic effects,[303] and deferoxamine, an iron-chelating agent that is toxic to neuroblastoma cells.[304–306]

## SUMMARY

Because neuroblastoma is a relatively rare tumor, developing improved therapies will require entry of as many eligible patients as possible into clinical trials. Continued investigation is needed in the areas of biology, risk assessment, and therapy, especially for high-risk patients. Based on the most recently completed large randomized trial for high-risk neuroblastoma, the most effective therapy requires aggressive chemotherapy from the time of diagnosis, intensification with myeloablative therapy, and then 13-cis-retinoic acid. Further improvements in outcome will depend on the development of new approaches that can be tolerated by patients and that will overcome tumor resistance to existing therapies. It is particularly important to develop strategies for eradicating minimal residual disease that persists following intensive myeloablative chemoradiotherapy and subsequent 13-cis-retinoic acid. Potential future therapies for neuroblastoma aimed at minimal residual disease that remains after current modalities include monoclonal antibody combined with cytokines, new retinoids, and immunization strategies, all of which are currently being studied in clinical trials.

## SUGGESTIONS FOR ADDITIONAL READING

Seeger RC, Brodeur GM, Sather H, et al. Association of multiple copies of the N-*myc* oncogene with rapid progression of neuroblastomas. N Engl J Med 1985;313:1111–6.

Kushner BH, Nai-Kong VC. Neuroblastoma. Pediatr Ann 1988;17:269–84. review.

Seeger RC, Atkins J, Reynolds CP. Neuroblastoma. In: Holland J, et al, eds. *Cancer medicine.* 4th ed. Philadelphia: Lea & Febiger, pp 2991–3020, 1996.

Seeger RC, Reynolds CP. Neuroblastoma. In: Forman SJ, Blume KG, Thomas ED, eds. Bone marrow transplantation. 2nd ed. Cambridge: Blackwell Scientific, Publ., 1999:1071–83.

Matthay KK, Villablanca JG, Seeger RC, et al. Treatment of high risk neuroblastoma with intensive chemotherapy, radiotherapy, autologous bone marrow transplantation, and 13-cis-retinoic acid. N Engl J Med 1999;341:1165–73.

Brodeur GM, Sawada T, Tsuchida Y, Voute PA, eds. Neuroblastoma. Amsterdam: Elsevier Science 2000.

## REFERENCES

1. Linet MS, Ries LA, Smith MA, et al. Cancer surveillance series: recent trends in childhood cancer incidence and mortality in the United States. J Natl Cancer Inst 1999;91:1051–58.
2. Grosfeld JL, Schatzlein M, Ballantine TV, et al. Metastatic neuroblastoma: factors influencing survival. J Pediatr Surg 1978;13:59–65.
3. Rosen EM, Cassady JR, Frantz CN, et al. Neuroblastoma: the Joint Center for Radiation Therapy/Dana-Farber Cancer Institute/Children's Hospital experience. J Clin Oncol 1984;2:719–32.
4. Jaffe N. Neuroblastoma: review of the literature and an examination of factors contributing to its enigmatic character. Cancer Treat Rev 1976;3:61–82.
5. Lopez-Ibor B, Schwartz AD. Neuroblastoma. Pediatr Clin North Am 1985;32:755–78. review.
6. Breslow N, McCann B. Statistical estimation of prognosis for children with neuroblastoma. Cancer Res 1971;31:2098–103.
7. Kushner BH, Cheung NK. Neuroblastoma. Pediatr Ann 1988;17:269–84.
8. Traggis DG, Filler RM, Druckman H, et al. Prognosis for children with neuroblastoma presenting with paralysis. J Pediatr Surg 1977;12:419–25.
9. Altman AJ, Baehner RL. Favorable prognosis for survival in children

with coincident opso-myoclonus and neuroblastoma. Cancer 1976; 37:846–52.

10. Kaplan SJ, Holbrook CT, McDaniel HG, et al. Vasoactive intestinal peptide secreting tumors of childhood. Am J Dis Child 1980;134:21–4.

11. Dehner LP. Peripheral and central primitive neuroectodermal tumors. A nosologic concept seeking a consensus. Arch Pathol Lab Med 1986;110:997–1005.

12. Granowetter L. Ewing's sarcoma and extracranial primitive neuroectodermal tumors. Curr Opin Oncol 1996;8:305–10. review.

13. Bomanji J, Conry BG, Britton KE, Reznek RH. Imaging neural crest tumours with 123I-metaiodobenzylguanidine and x-ray computed tomography: a comparative study. Clin Radiol 1988;39:502–6.

14. Claudiani F, Garaventa A, Scopinaro G, et al. Diagnostic and therapeutic use of 131I-metaiodobenzylguanidine in children with neuroblastoma. J Nucl Med Allied Sci 1988;32:1–6.

15. Feine U, Muller-Schauenburg W, Treuner J, Klingebiel T. Metaiodobenzylguanidine (MIBG) labeled with 123I/131I in neuroblastoma diagnosis and follow-up treatment with a review of the diagnostic results of the International Workshop of Pediatric Oncology held in Rome, September 1986. Med Pediatr Oncol 1987;15:181–7.

16. Perel Y, Conway J, Kletzel M, et al. Clinical impact and prognostic value of metaiodobenzylguanidine imaging in children with metastatic neuroblastoma. J Pediatr Hematol Oncol 1999;21:13–8.

17. Franklin IM, Pritchard J. Detection of bone marrow invasion by neuroblastoma is improved by sampling at two sites with both aspirates and trephine biopsies. J Clin Pathol 1983;36:1215–8.

18. Fitzgibbon MC, Tormey WP. Paediatric reference ranges for urinary catecholamines/metabolites and their relevance in neuroblastoma diagnosis. Ann Clin Biochem 1994;31:1–11. review.

19. Brodeur GM, Seeger RC, Barrett A, et al. International criteria for diagnosis, staging, and response to treatment in patients with neuroblastoma. J Clin Oncol 1988;6:1874–81.

20. Reynolds CP, Smith RG, Frenkel EP. The diagnostic dilemma of the "small round cell neoplasm": catecholamine fluorescence and tissue culture morphology as markers for neuroblastoma. Cancer 1981; 48:2088–94.

21. Triche TJ, Askin FB. Neuroblastoma and the differential diagnosis of small-, round-, blue-cell tumors. Hum Pathol 1983;14:569–95.

22. Thiele CJ, McKeon C, Triche TJ, et al. Differential protooncogene expression characterizes histopathologically indistinguishable tumors of the peripheral nervous system. J Clin Invest 1987;80:804–11.

23. Jurgens H, Bier V, Harms D, et al. Malignant peripheral neuroectodermal tumors. A retrospective analysis of 42 patients. Cancer 1988; 61:349–57.

24. May WA, Denny CT. Biology of EWS/FLI and related fusion genes in Ewing's sarcoma and primitive neuroectodermal tumor. Curr Top Microbiol Immunol 1997;220:143–50. review.

25. Triche TJ. Neuroblastoma and other childhood neural tumors: a review. Pediatr Pathol 1990;10:175–93. review.

26. Israel MA, Miser JS, Triche TJ, Kinsella T. Neuroepithelial tumors. In: Pizzo PA, Poplack DG, eds. Principles and practices of pediatric oncology. Philadelphia: JB Lippincott, 1989:623–34.

27. Voorhess ML, Gardner LI. Studies of catecholamine excretion by children with neural tumors. J Clin Endocrinol 1962;22:126–33.

28. von Studnitz W, Kaser H, Sjoerdsma A. Spectrum of catecholamine biochemistry in patients with neuroblastoma. N Engl J Med 1993;269:232–5.

29. Williams CM, Greer M. Homovanillic acid and vanillylmandelic acid in diagnosis of neuroblastoma. J Am Med Assoc 1963;183:840–6.

30. Greer M, Anton AH, Williams CM, et al. Tumors of neural crest origin. Arch Neurol 1965;13:139–48.

31. McKendrick T, Edwards RWH. The execretion of 4-hydroxy-3-methoxy-mandelic acid by children. Arch Dis Child 1965;40:418–25.

32. Kaser H. Catecholamine-producing neural tumors other than pheochromocytoma. Pharmacol Rev 1966;18:659–65.

33. Hinterberger H, Bartholomew RJ. Catecholamines and their acidic metabolites in urine and in tumour tissue in neuroblastoma, ganglioneuroma and phaeochromocytoma. Clin Chim Acta 1969;23:169–75.

34. Gitlow SE, Bertani LM, Rausen A, et al. Diagnosis of neuroblastoma by qualitative and quantitative determination of catecholamine metabolites in urine. Cancer 1970;25:1377–83.

35. Moyano MB, Bergada C, Becu L. Catecholamine excretion in forty children with sympathoblastoma. J Pediatr 1970;77:239–44.

36. Helson L, Fleisher M, Bethune V, et al. Urinary cystathionine, catecholamine, and metabolites in patients with neuroblastoma. Clin Chem 1972;18:613–5.

37. Liebner EJ, Rosenthal IM. Serial catecholamines in the radiation management of children with neuroblastoma. Cancer 1973;32:623–33.

38. Voorhess ML. Neuroblastoma-pheochromocytoma: products and pathogenesis. Ann NY Acad Sci 1974;230:187–94.

39. Bond JV. Clinical significance of catecholamine excretion levels in diagnosis and treatment of neuroblastoma. Arch Dis Child 1975; 50:691–5.

40. Laug WE, Siegel SE, Shaw KN, et al. Initial urinary catecholamine metabolite concentrations and prognosis in neuroblastoma. Pediatrics 1978;62:77–83.

41. LaBrosse EH, Com-Nougue C, Zucker JM, et al. Urinary excretion of 3-methoxy-4-hydroxymandelic acid and 3-methoxy-4-hydroxyphenylacetic acid by 288 patients with neuroblastoma and related neural crest tumors. Cancer Res 1980;40:1995–2001.

42. Sawada T, Sugimoto T, Tanaka T, et al. Number and cure rate of neuroblastoma cases detected by the mass screening program in Japan: future aspects. Med Pediatr Oncol 1987;15:14–7.

43. Tuchman M, Lemieux B, Woods WG. Screening for neuroblastoma in infants: investigate or implement? Pediatrics 1990;86:791–3. editorial.

44. Reynolds CP, German DC, Weinberg AG, Smith RG. Catecholamine fluorescence and tissue culture morphology. Technics in the diagnosis of neuroblastoma. Am J Clin Pathol 1981;75:275–82.

45. Wang YL, Einhorn PA, Triche TJ, et al. Expression of PGP9.5 and tyrosine hydroxylase in childhood small round cell tumors. Clin Cancer Res 2000;6:551–8.

46. Shimada H, Chatten J, Newton WA, Jr, et al. Histopathologic prognostic factors in neuroblastic tumors: definition of subtypes of ganglioneuroblastoma and an age-linked classification of neuroblastomas. J Natl Cancer Inst 1984;73:405–16.

47. McLaughlin JE, Urich H. Maturing neuroblastoma and ganglioneuroblastoma: a study of four cases with long survival. J Pathol 1977;121:19–26.

48. Sitarz AL, Santulli TV, Wigger HJ, Berdon WE. Complete maturation of neuroblastoma with bone metastases in documented stages. J Pediatr Surg 1975;10:533–6.

49. Layfield LJ, Glasgow B, Ostrzega N, Reynolds CP. Fine-needle aspiration cytology and the diagnosis of neoplasms in the pediatric age group. Diagn Cytopathol 1991;7:451–61.

50. Brodeur GM, Green AA, Hayes FA, et al. Cytogenetic features of human neuroblastomas and cell lines. Cancer Res 1981;41:4678–86.

51. Gilbert F, Feder M, Balaban G, et al. Human neuroblastomas and abnormalities of chromosomes 1 and 17. Cancer Res 1984;44:5444–9.

52. Whang-Peng J, Triche TJ, Knutsen T, et al. Chromosome translocation in peripheral neuroepithelioma. N Engl J Med 1984;311:584–5.

53. Whang-Peng J, Triche TJ, Knutsen T, et al. Cytogenetic characterization of selected small round cell tumors of childhood. Cancer Genet Cytogenet 1986;21:185–208.

54. Tsokos M, Linnoila RI, Chandra RS, Triche TJ. Neuron-specific enolase in the diagnosis of neuroblastoma and other small, round-cell tumors in children. Hum Pathol 1984;15:575–84.

55. Triche TJ, Tsokos M, Linnoila RI, et al. NSE in neuroblastoma and other round cell tumors of childhood. Prog Clin Biol Res 1985;175:295–317.

56. Seshi B, Bell CEJ. Preparation and characterization of monoclonal antibodies to human neuron-specific enolase. Hybridoma 1985;4:13–25.

57. Thomas P, Battifora H, Manderino GL, Patrick J. A monoclonal antibody against neuron-specific enolase. Immunohistochemical comparison with a polyclonal antiserum. Am J Clin Pathol 1987;88:146–52.

58. Osborn M, Dirk T, Kaser H, et al. Immunohistochemical localization of neurofilaments and neuron-specific enolase in 29 cases of neuroblastoma. Am J Pathol 1986;122:433–42.

59. Kemshead JT, Coakham HB. The use of monoclonal antibodies for the diagnosis of intracranial malignancies and the small round cell tumours of childhood. J Pathol 1983;141:249–57.

60. Smith RG, Reynolds CP. Monoclonal antibody recognizing a human neuroblastoma–associated antigen. Diagn Clin Immunol 1987;5:209–20.

61. Gibson FM, Kemshead JT. A monoclonal antibody (FMG25) that can differentiate neuroblastoma from other small round-cell tumours of childhood. Int J Cancer 1987;39:554–9.

62. Donner L, Triche TJ, Israel MA, et al. A panel of monoclonal antibodies which discriminate neuroblastoma from Ewing's sarcoma, rhabdomyosarcoma, neuroepithelioma, and hematopoietic malignancies. Prog Clin Biol Res 1985;175:347–66.

63. Grosfeld JL, Ballantine TV, Baehner RL. Experience with "second-look" operations in pediatric solid tumors. J Pediatr Surg 1978; 13:275–80.

64. Seeger RC, Brodeur GM, Sather H, et al. Association of multiple copies of the N-myc oncogene with rapid progression of neuroblastomas. N Engl J Med 1985;313:1111–6.

65. Evans AE, DAngio GJ, Propert K, et al. Prognostic factors in neuroblastoma. Cancer 1987;59:1853–9.

66. Matthay KK, Sather HN, Seeger RC, et al. Excellent outcome of stage II neuroblastoma is independent of residual disease and radiation therapy. J Clin Oncol 1989;7:236–44.

67. Mancini AF, Rosito P, Vitelli A, et al. IV-S neuroblastoma: a cooperative study of 30 children. Med Pediatr Oncol 1984;12:155–61.

68. Nickerson HJ, Nesbit ME, Grosfeld JL, et al. Comparison of stage IV and IV-S neuroblastoma in the first year of life. Med Pediatr Oncol 1985;13:261–8.

69. Evans AE, Baum E, Chard R. Do infants with stage IV-S neuroblastoma need treatment? Arch Dis Child 1981;56:271–4.

70. Nakagawara A, Ikeda K, Tsuda T, et al. Amplification of N-myc oncogene in stage II and IVS neuroblastomas may be a prognostic indicator. J Pediatr Surg 1987;22:415–8.

71. Evans AE, D'Angio GJ, Randolph J. A proposed staging for children with neuroblastoma: Children's Cancer Study Group A. Cancer 1971;27:374–8.

72. Hayes FA, Green A, Hustu HO, Kumar M. Surgicopathologic staging of neuroblastoma: prognostic significance of regional lymph node metastases. J Pediatr 1983;102:59–62.

73. Brodeur GM, Pritchard J, Berthold F, et al. Revisions of the international criteria for neuroblastoma diagnosis, staging, and response to treatment. Prog Clin Biol Res 1993;11:1466–77.

74. Bomanji J, Conry BG, Britton KE, Reznek RH. Imaging neural crest tumors with 123I-metaiodobenzylguanidine and x-ray computed tomography: a comparative study. Clin Radiol 1988;39:502–6.

75. Claudiani F, Garaventa A, Scopinaro G, et al. Diagnostic and therapeutic use of 131I-metaiodobenzylguanidine in children with neuroblastoma. J Nucl Med Allied Sci 1988;32:1–6.

76. Feine U, Mueller Schauenburg W, Treuner J, Klingebiel T. Metaiodobenzylguanidine (MIBG) labeled with 123I/131I in neuroblastoma diagnosis and follow-up treatment with a review of the diagnostic results of the International Workshop of Pediatric Oncology held in Rome, September 1986. Med Pediatr Oncol 1987;15:181–7.

77. Miraldi FD, Nelson AD, Kraly C, et al. Diagnostic imaging of human neuroblastoma with radiolabeled antibody. Radiology 1986; 161:413–8.

78. Cheung NK, Neely JE, Landmeier B, et al. Targeting of ganglioside GD2 monoclonal antibody to neuroblastoma. J Nucl Med 1987; 28:1577–83.

79. Moss TJ, Reynolds CP, Sather HN, et al. Prognostic value of immunocytologic detection of bone marrow metastases in neuroblastoma. N Engl J Med 1991;324:219–26.

80. Evans AE, Griffin GC, Tartaglione M, Kennett RH. A method of detecting neuroblastoma in human bone marrow by means of two monoclonal antibodies PI 153/3 and KE2. Hybridoma 1985;4:289–96.

81. Cheung NK, Von HoffDD, Strandjord SE, Coccia PF. Detection of neuroblastoma cells in bone marrow using GD2 specific monoclonal antibodies. J Clin Oncol 1986;4:363–9.

82. Moss TJ, Seeger RC, Kindler Rohrborn A, et al. Immunohistologic detection and phenotyping of neuroblastoma cells in bone marrow using cytoplasmic neuron specific enolase and cell surface antigens. Prog Clin Biol Res 1985;175:367–78.

83. Reynolds CP, Moss TJ, Seeger RC, et al. Sensitive detection of neuroblastoma cells in bone marrow for monitoring the efficacy of marrow purging procedures. Prog Clin Biol Res 1985;175:425–41.

84. Beck D, Maritaz O, Gross N, et al. Immunocytochemical detection of neuroblastoma cells infiltrating clinical bone marrow samples. Eur J Pediatr 1988;147:609–12.

85. Favrot MC, Frappaz D, Maritaz O, et al. Histological, cytological and immunological analyses are complementary for the detection of neuroblastoma cells in bone marrow. Br J Cancer 1986;54:637–41.

86. Matthay K, Reynolds CP, Stram D, Seeger RC. Quantitative tumor cell content of bone marrow and blood as an early predictor of response in high risk neuroblastoma: A Children's Cancer Group study. Proc Am Soc Clin Oncol 1997;16:512a. abstract.

87. Mattano L Jr, Moss TJ, Emerson SG. Sensitive detection of rare circulating neuroblastoma cells by the reverse transcriptase–polymerase chain reaction. Cancer Res 1992;52:4701–5.

88. Naito H, Kuzumaki N, Uchino J, et al. Detection of tyrosine hydroxylase mRNA and minimal neuroblastoma cells by the reverse transcription–polymerase chain reaction. Eur J Cancer 1991;27:762–5.

89. Miyajima Y, Horibe K, Fukuda M, et al. Sequential detection of tumor cells in the peripheral blood and bone marrow of patients with stage IV neuroblastoma by the reverse transcription–polymerase chain reaction for tyrosine hydroxylase mRNA. Cancer 1996;77:1214–9.

90. Haase GM, Wong KY, deLorimier AA, et al. Improvement in survival after excision of primary tumor in stage III neuroblastoma. J Pediatr Surg 1989;24:194–200.

91. Blatt J, Gula MJ, Orlando SJ, et al. Indolent course of advanced neuroblastoma in children older than 6 years at diagnosis. Cancer 1995;76:890–4.

92. Beckwith CR, Martin RF. Observations on the histopathology of neuroblastomas. J Pediatr Surg 1968;1:106–10.

93. Makinen J. Microscopic patterns as a guide to prognosis of neuroblastoma in childhood. Cancer 1972;29:1637–46.

94. Dehner LP. Classic neuroblastoma: histopathologic grading as a prognostic indicator. The Shimada system and its progenitors. Am J Pediatr Hematol Oncol 1988;10:143–54.

95. Chatten J, Shimada H, Sather HN, et al. Prognostic value of histopathology in advanced neuroblastoma: a report from the Children's Cancer Study Group. Hum Pathol 1988;19:1187–98.

96. Shimada H, Ambros IM, Dehner LP, et al. The International Neuroblastoma Pathology Classification (the Shimada system). Cancer 1999;86:364–72.

97. Shimada H, Ambros IM, Dehner LP, et al. Terminology and morphologic criteria of neuroblastic tumors: recommendations by the International Neuroblastoma Pathology Committee. Cancer 1999;86:349–63.

98. Shimada H, Stram DO, Chatten J, et al. Identification of subsets of neuroblastomas by combined histopathologic and N-myc analysis. J Natl Cancer Inst 1995;87:1470–6.

99. Hann HW, Evans AE, Siegel SE, et al. Prognostic importance of serum ferritin in patients with Stages III and IV neuroblastoma: the Children's Cancer Study Group experience. Cancer Res 1985; 45:2843–8.

100. Imashuku S, Yamanaka H, Morioka Y, Todo S. Serum ferritin in stage IV neuroblastoma. Am J Pediatr Hematol Oncol 1988;10:39–41.

101. Zeltzer PM, Marangos PJ, Parma AM, et al. Raised neuron-specific enolase in serum of children with metastatic neuroblastoma. A report from the Children's Cancer Study Group. Lancet 1983;2:361–3.

102. Wassberg E, Stridsberg M, Christofferson R. Plasma levels of chromogranin A are directly proportional to tumour burden in neuroblastoma. J Endocrinol 1996;151:225–30.

103. Ladisch S, Wu ZL, Feig S, et al. Shedding of GD2 ganglioside by human neuroblastoma. Int J Cancer 1987;39:73–6.

104. Quinn JJ, Altman AJ, Frantz CN. Serum lactic dehydrogenase, an indicator of tumor activity in neuroblastoma. J Pediatr 1980;97:89–91. abstract.

105. Joshi VV, Cantor AB, Brodeur GM, et al. Correlation between morphologic and other prognostic markers of neuroblastoma. A study of histologic grade, DNA index, N-myc gene copy number, and lactic dehydrogenase in patients in the Pediatric Oncology Group. Cancer 1993;71:3173–81.

106. Look AT, Hayes FA, Nitschke R, et al. Cellular DNA content as a predictor of response to chemotherapy in infants with unresectable neuroblastoma. N Engl J Med 1984;311:231–5.

107. Bowman LC, Castleberry RP, Cantor A, et al. Genetic staging of unresectable or metastatic neuroblastoma in infants: a Pediatric Oncology Group study. J Natl Cancer Inst 1997;89:373–80.

108. Gansler T, Chatten J, Varello M, et al. Flow cytometric DNA analysis of neuroblastoma. Correlation with histology and clinical outcome. Cancer 1986;58:2453–8.

109. Look AT, Hayes FA, Shuster JJ, et al. Clinical relevance of tumor cell ploidy and N-myc gene amplification in childhood neuroblastoma: a Pediatric Oncology Group study. J Clin Oncol 1991;9:581–91.

110. Brodeur GM, Seeger RC, Schwab M, et al. Amplification of N-myc in untreated human neuroblastomas correlates with advanced disease stage. Science 1984;224:1121–4.

111. Cohn SL, Herst CV, Maurer HS, Rosen ST. N-myc amplification in an infant with stage IVS neuroblastoma. J Clin Oncol 1987;5:1441–4.

112. Tsuda H, Shimosato Y, Upton MP, et al. Retrospective study on amplification of N-myc and c-myc genes in pediatric solid tumors and its association with prognosis and tumor differentiation. Lab Invest 1988;59:321–7.

113. Tsuda T, Obara M, Hirano H, et al. Analysis of N-myc amplification in relation to disease stage and histologic types in human neuroblastomas. Cancer 1987;60:820–6.

114. Bartram CR, Berthold F. Amplification and expression of the N-myc gene in neuroblastoma. Eur J Pediatr 1987;146:162–5.

115. Brodeur GM, Hayes FA, Green AA, et al. Consistent N-myc copy number in simultaneous or consecutive neuroblastoma samples from sixty individual patients. Cancer Res 1987;47:4248–53.

116. Nisen PD, Waber PG, Rich MA, et al. N-myc oncogene RNA expression in neuroblastoma. J Natl Cancer Inst 1988;80:1633–7.

117. Fong CT, Dracopoli NC, White PS, et al. Loss of heterozygosity for the short arm of chromosome 1 in human neuroblastomas: correlation with N-myc amplification. Proc Natl Acad Sci USA 1989;86:3753–7.

118. Seeger RC, Wada R, Brodeur GM, et al. Expression of N-myc by neuroblastomas with one or multiple copies of the oncogene. Prog Clin Biol Res 1988;271:41–9.

119. Slamon DJ, Boone TC, Seeger RC, et al. Identification and characterization of the protein encoded by the human N-myc oncogene. Science 1986;232:768–72.

120. Crabbe DC, Peters J, Seeger RC. Rapid detection of MYCN gene amplification in neuroblastomas using the polymerase chain reaction. Diagn Mol Pathol 1992;1:229–34.

121. Leong PK, Thorner P, Yeger H, et al. Detection of MYCN gene amplification and deletions of chromosome 1p in neuroblastoma by in situ hybridization using routine histologic sections. Lab Invest 1993;69:43–50.

122. Shapiro DN, Valentine MB, Rowe ST, et al. Detection of N-mycn gene amplification by fluorescence in situ hybridization. Diagnostic utility for neuroblastoma. Am J Pathol 1993;142:1339–46.

123. Taylor CP, McGuckin AG, Bown NP, et al. Rapid detection of prognostic genetic factors in neuroblastoma using fluorescence in situ hybridisation on tumour imprints and bone marrow smears. United Kingdom Children's Cancer Study Group. Br J Cancer 1994;69:445–51.

124. Nakagawara A, Arima Nakagawara M, Scavarda NJ, et al. Association between high levels of expression of the TRK gene and favorable outcome in human neuroblastoma. N Engl J Med 1993;328:847–54.

125. Suzuki T, Bogenmann E, Shimada H, et al. Lack of high-affinity nerve growth factor receptors in aggressive neuroblastomas. J Natl Cancer Inst 1993;85:377–84.

126. Chan HS, DeBoer G, Thorner PS, et al. Multidrug resistance. Clinical opportunities in diagnosis and circumvention. Hematol Oncol Clin North Am 1994;8:383–410.

127. Dhooge CR, De Moerloose BM, Benoit YC, et al. Expression of the MDR1 gene product P-glycoprotein in childhood neuroblastoma. Cancer 1997;80:1250–7.

128. Leone A, Seeger RC, Hong CM, et al. Evidence for nm23 RNA overexpression, DNA amplification and mutation in aggressive childhood neuroblastomas. Oncogene 1993;8:855–65.

129. Bjelfman C, Hedborg F, Johansson I, et al. Expression of the neuronal form of pp60c-src in neuroblastoma in relation to clinical stage and prognosis. Cancer Res 1990;50:6908–14.

130. Matsunaga T, Takahashi H, Ohnuma N, et al. Expression of N-myc and c-src protooncogenes correlating to the undifferentiated phenotype and prognosis of primary neuroblastomas. Cancer Res 1991;51:3148–52.

131. Nakada K, Fujioka T, Kitagawa H, et al. Expressions of N-myc and ras oncogene products in neuroblastoma and their correlations with prognosis. Jpn J Clin Oncol 1993;23:149–55.

132. Keim DR, Hailat N, Kuick R, et al. PCNA levels in neuroblastoma are increased in tumors with an amplified N-myc gene and in metastatic stage tumors. Clin Exp Metastasis 1993;11:83–90.

133. Ungar DR, Hailat N, Strahler JR, et al. Hsp27 expression in neuroblastoma: correlation with disease stage. J Natl Cancer Inst 1994;86:780–4.

134. Norris MD, Bordow SB, Marshall GM, et al. Expression of the gene for multidrug-resistance-associated protein and outcome in patients with neuroblastoma. N Engl J Med 1996;334:231–8.

135. Hiyama E, Hiyama K, Yokoyama T, et al. Correlating telomerase activity levels with human neuroblastoma outcomes. Nature Med 1995;1:249–55.

136. Hiyama E, Reynolds CP. Telomerase as a biological and prognostic marker in neuroblastoma. In: Brodeur GM, Sawada T, Tsuchida Y, Voute PA, eds. Neuroblastoma. Amsterdam: Elsevier Science BV, 2000:159–74.

137. Reynolds CP, Zuo JJ, Kim NW, et al. Telomerase expression in primary neuroblastomas. Eur J Cancer 1997;33A:1929–31.

138. Reynolds CP, Frenkel EP, Smith RG. Growth characteristics of neuroblastoma in vitro correlate with patient survival. Trans Assoc Am Physicians 1980;93:203–11.

139. Reynolds CP, Tomayko MM, Donner L, et al. Biological classification of cell lines derived from human extracranial neural tumors. Prog Clin Biol Res 1988;271:291–306.

140. George BA, Yanik G, Wells RJ, et al. Growth patterns of human neuroblastoma xenografts and their relationship to treatment outcome. Cancer 1993;72:3331–9.

141. Nitschke R, Smith EI, Shochat S, et al. Localized neuroblastoma treated by surgery: a Pediatric Oncology Group Study. J Clin Oncol 1988;6:1271–9.

142. Hayes FA, Thompson EI, Hvizdala E, et al. Chemotherapy as an alternative to laminectomy and radiation in the management of epidural tumor. J Pediatr 1984;104:221–4.

143. Hayes FA, Green AA, O Connor DM. Chemotherapeutic management of epidural neuroblastoma. Med Pediatr Oncol 1989;17:6–8.

144. Rosen EM, Cassady JR, Kretschmar C, et al. Influence of local-regional lymph node metastases on prognosis in neuroblastoma. Med Pediatr Oncol 1984;12:260–3.

145. Ninane J, Pritchard J, Morris Jones PH, et al. Stage II neuroblastoma. Adverse prognostic significance of lymph node involvement. Arch Dis Child 1982;57:438–42.

146. Evans AE, Albo V, D'Angio GJ, et al. Factors influencing survival of children with non-metastatic neuroblastoma. Cancer 1976;38:661–6.

147. DeBernardi B, Pianca C, Boni L, et al. Disseminated neuroblastoma (stage IV and IV-S) in the first year of life. Outcome related to age and stage. Italian Cooperative Group on Neuroblastoma. Cancer 1992;70:1625–33.

148. Katzenstein HM, Bowman LC, Brodeur GM, et al. Prognostic significance of age, MYCN oncogene amplification, tumor cell ploidy, and histology in 110 infants with stage D(S) neuroblastoma: the pediatric oncology group experience—a pediatric oncology group study. J Clin Oncol 1998;16:2007–17.

149. Suarez A, Hartman O, Vassal G, et al. Treatment of stage IV-S neuroblastoma: a study of 34 cases treated between 1982 and 1987. Med Pediatr Oncol 1991;19:473–7.

150. Wilson PC, Coppes MJ, Solh H, et al. Neuroblastoma stage IV-S: a heterogeneous disease. Med Pediatr Oncol 1991;19:467–72.

151. Garvin J, Bendit I, Nisen PD. N-myc oncogene expression and amplification in metastatic lesions of stage IV-S neuroblastoma. Cancer 1990;65:2572–5.

152. Hsiao RJ, Seeger RC, Yu AL, O Connor DT. Chromogranin A in children with neuroblastoma. Serum concentration parallels disease stage and predicts survival. J Clin Invest 1990;85:1555–9.

153. Castleberry RP, Kun LE, Shuster JJ, et al. Radiotherapy improves the outlook for patients older than 1 year with Pediatric Oncology Group stage C neuroblastoma. J Clin Oncol 1991;9:789–95.

154. Matthay KK, Lukens J, Stram D, et al. Prognosis for stage IV neuroblastoma less than one year at diagnosis: a prospective Children's Cancer Group study. Proc Am Soc Clin Oncol 1995;14:446. abstract.

155. Green AA, Hayes FA, Hustu HO. Sequential cyclophosphamide and doxorubicin for induction of complete remission in children with disseminated neuroblastoma. Cancer 1981;48:2310–7.

156. Kretschmar CS, Frantz CN, Rosen EM, et al. Improved prognosis for infants with stage IV neuroblastoma. J Clin Oncol 1984;2:799–803.

157. DuBois SG, Kalika Y, Lukens JN, et al. Metastatic sites in stage IV and IVS neuroblastoma correlate with age, tumor biology, and survival. J Pediatr Hematol/Oncol 1999;21:181–9.

158. Matthay K, Villablanca JG, Seeger RC, et al. Treatment of high risk neuroblastoma with intensive chemotherapy, radiotherapy, autologous bone marrow transplantation, and 13-cis-retinoic acid. N Engl J Med 1999;341:1165–73.

159. Evans AR, Brand W, de Lorimier A, et al. Results in children with local and regional neuroblastoma managed with and without vincristine, cyclophosphamide, and imidazolecarboxamide. A report from the Children's Cancer Study Group. Am J Clin Oncol 1984;7:3–7.

160. Smith EI, Krous HF, Tunell WP, Hitch DC. The impact of chemotherapy and radiation therapy on secondary operation for neuroblastoma. Ann Surg 1980;191:561–69.

161. Moss TJ, Fonkalsrud EW, Feig SA, et al. Delayed surgery and bone marrow transplantation for widespread neuroblastoma. Ann Surg 1987;206:514–20.

162. Sitarz A, Finklestein J, Grosfeld J, et al. An evaluation of the role of surgery in disseminated neuroblastoma: a report from the Children's Cancer Study Group. J Pediatr Surg 1983;18:147–51.

163. Akwari OE, Payne WS, Onofrio BM, et al. Dumbbell neurogenic tumors of the mediastinum. Diagnosis and management. Mayo Clin Proc 1978;53:353–8.

164. Deacon JM, Wilson PA, Peckham MJ. The radiobiology of human neuroblastoma. Radiother Oncol 1985;3:201–9.

165. Leavey PJ, Odom LF, Poole M, et al. Intra-operative radiation therapy in pediatric neuroblastoma. Med Pediatr Oncol 1997;28:424–8.

166. Wittenborg MH. Roentgen therapy in neuroblastoma. Radiology 1950;54:670–88.

167. Perez CA, Vietti T, Ackerman LV, et al. Tumors of the sympathetic nervous system in children. An appraisal of treatment and results. Radiology 1967;88:750–60.

168. Jacobson GM, Sause WT, OBrien RT. Dose response analysis of pediatric neuroblastoma to megavoltage radiation. Am J Clin Oncol 1984;7:693–7.

169. Jacobson HM, Marcus RB Jr, Thar TL, et al. Pediatric neuroblastoma: postoperative radiation therapy using less than 2000 rad. Int J Radiat Oncol Biol Phys 1983;9:501–5.

170. Halperin EC, Cox EB. Radiation therapy in the management of neuroblastoma: the Duke University Medical Center experience 1967–1984. Int J Radiat Oncol Biol Phys 1986;12:1829–37.

171. Filler RM, Traggis DG, Jaffe N, Vawter GF. Favorable outlook for children with mediastinal neuroblastoma. J Pediatr Surg 1972;7:136–43.

172. DeBernardi B, Rogers D, Carli M, et al. Localized neuroblastoma. Surgical and pathologic staging. Cancer 1987;60:1066–72.

173. Koop CE, Johnson DG. Neuroblastoma: an assessment of therapy in reference to staging. J Pediatr Surg 1971;6:595–600.

174. Zucker JM, Margulis E. Radiochemotherapy of postoperative minimal residual disease in neuroblastoma. Recent Results Cancer Res 1978;68:423–30.

175. Matthay K, Villablanca JG, Seeger RC, et al. Treatment of high risk neuroblastoma with intensive chemotherapy, radiotherapy, autologous bone marrow transplantation, and 13-cis-retinoic acid. N Engl J Med 1999;341:1165–73.

176. Nitschke R, Humphrey GB, Sexauer CL, Smith EI. Neuroblastoma: therapy for infants with good prognosis. Med Pediatr Oncol 1983;11:154–8.

177. Villablanca JG, Matthay KK, Swift P, et al. Phase I trial of carboplatin, etoposide, melpahalan and local irradiation (CEM-LI) with purged autologous bone marrow transplantation (ABMT) for high risk neuroblastoma. Med Pediatr Oncol 1999;33:170.

178. Peschel RE, Chen M, Seashore J. The treatment of massive hepatomegaly in stage IV-S neuroblastoma. Int J Radiat Oncol Biol Phys 1981;7:549–53.

179. Green AA, Hustu HO, Palmer R, Pinkel D. Total-body sequential segmental irradiation and combination chemotherapy for children with disseminated neuroblastoma. Cancer 1976;38:2250–7.

180. Helson L, Jereb B, Vogel R. Sequential hemi-body irradiation (HBI) in treatment of advanced neuroblastoma: a pilot study. Int J Radiat Oncol Biol Phys 1981;7:531–4.

181. Kun LE, Casper JT, Kline RW, Piaskowski VD. Fractionated total body irradiation for metastatic neuroblastoma. Int J Radiat Oncol Biol Phys 1981;7:1599–1602.

182. Haase GM, Meagher DPJ, McNeely LK, et al. Electron beam intraoperative radiation therapy for pediatric neoplasms. Cancer 1994;74:740–7.

183. Aitken DR, Hopkins GA, Archambeau JO, et al. Intraoperative radiotherapy in the treatment of neuroblastoma: report of a pilot study. Ann Surg Oncol 1995;2:343–50.

184. August CS, Serota FT, Koch PA, et al. Treatment of advanced neuroblastoma with supralethal chemotherapy, radiation, and allogeneic or autologous marrow reconstitution. J Clin Oncol 1984;2:609–16.

185. Philip T, Bernard JL, Zucker JM, et al. High-dose chemoradiotherapy with bone marrow transplantation as consolidation treatment in neuroblastoma: an unselected group of stage IV patients over 1 year of age. J Clin Oncol 1987;5:266–71.

186. Pinkerton CR, Philip T, Biron P, et al. High-dose melphalan, vincristine, and total-body irradiation with autologous bone marrow transplantation in children with relapsed neuroblastoma: a phase II study. Med Pediatr Oncol 1987;15:236–40.

187. Seeger RC, Moss TJ, Feig SA, et al. Bone marrow transplantation for poor prognosis neuroblastoma. Prog Clin Biol Res 1988;271:203–13.

188. Evans AE, Albo V, D'Angio GJ, et al. Cyclophosphamide treatment of patients with localized and regional neuroblastoma: a randomized study. Cancer 1976;38:655–60.

189. Stram DO, Matthay KK, O'Leary M, et al. Consolidation chemoradiotherapy and autologous bone marrow transplantation versus continued chemotherapy for metastatic neuroblastoma: a report of two concurrent Children's Cancer Group studies. J Clin Oncol 1996;14:2417–26.

190. Hayes FA, Smith EI. Neuroblastoma. In: Pizzo PA, Poplack DG, eds. Principles and practice of pediatric oncology. Philadelphia: JB Lippincott 1989;607–22.

191. Castleberry RP, Cantor AB, Green AA, et al. Phase II investigational window using carboplatin, iproplatin, ifosfamide, and epirubicin in children with untreated disseminated neuroblastoma: a Pediatric Oncology Group study. J Clin Oncol 1994;12:1616–20.

192. Nitschke R, Parkhurst J, Sullivan J, et al. Topotecan in pediatric patients with recurrent and progressive solid tumors: a Pediatric Oncology Group phase II study. J Pediatr Hematol Oncol 1998;20:315–8.

193. Finklestein JZ, Klemperer MR, Evans AE. Multiagent chemotherapy for children with metastatic neuroblastoma; a report from the Children's Cancer Study Group. Med Pediatr Oncol 1979;6:179.

194. Hayes FA, Green AA, Mauer AM. Correlation of cell kinetic and clinical response to chemotherapy in disseminated neuroblastoma. Cancer Res 1977;37:3766–70.

195. Finklestein JZ, Klemperer MR, Evans A, et al. Multiagent chemotherapy for children with metastatic neuroblastoma: a report from Children's Cancer Study Group. Med Pediatr Oncol 1979;6:179–88.

196. Nitschke R, Cangir A, Crist W, Berry DH. Intensive chemotherapy for metastatic neuroblastoma: a Southwest Oncology Group study. Med Pediatr Oncol 1980;8:281–8.

197. Ninane J, Pritchard J, Malpas JS. Chemotherapy of advanced neuroblastoma: does adriamycin contribute? Arch Dis Child 1981;56:544–8.

198. Shafford EA, Rogers DW, Pritchard J. Advanced neuroblastoma: improved response rate using a multiagent regimen (OPEC) including sequential cisplatin and VM-26. J Clin Oncol 1984;2:742–7.

199. Kushner BH, Helson L. Coordinated use of sequentially escalated cyclophosphamide and cell-cycle-specific chemotherapy (N4SE protocol) for advanced neuroblastoma: experience with 100 patients. J Clin Oncol 1987;5:1746–51.

200. Bernard JL, Philip T, Zucker JM, et al. Sequential cisplatin/VM-26 and vincristine/cyclophosphamide/doxorubicin in metastatic neuroblastoma: an effective alternating non-cross-resistant regimen? J Clin Oncol 1987;5:1952–9.

201. Hartmann O, Pinkerton CR, Philip T, et al. Very-high-dose cisplatin and etoposide in children with untreated advanced neuroblastoma. J Clin Oncol 1988;6:44–50.

202. Ikeda K, Nakagawara A, Yano H, et al. Improved survival rates in children over 1 year of age with stage III or IV neuroblastoma following an intensive chemotherapeutic regimen. J Pediatr Surg 1989;24:189–93.

203. Pinkerton CR, Zucker JM, Hartmann O, et al. Short duration, high dose, alternating chemotherapy in metastatic neuroblastoma. (ENSG 3C induction regimen). The European Neuroblastoma Study Group. Br J Cancer 1990;62:319–23.

204. Campbell LA, Seeger RC, Harris RE, et al. Escalating dose of continuous infusion combination chemotherapy for refractory neuroblastoma. J Clin Oncol 1993;11:623–9.

205. Kushner BH, LaQuaglia MP, Bonilla MA, et al. Highly effective induction therapy for stage 4 neuroblastoma in children over 1 year of age. J Clin Oncol 1994;12:2607–13.

206. Kushner BH, Cheung NK, Kramer K, et al. Neuroblastoma and treatment-related myelodysplasia/leukemia: the Memorial Sloan-Kettering experience and a literature review. J Clin Oncol 1998;16:3880–9. review.

207. Kushner BH, Heller G, Cheung NK, et al. High risk of leukemia after short-term dose-intensive chemotherapy in young patients with solid tumors. J Clin Oncol 1998;16:3016–20.

208. Seeger RC, Reynolds CP. Treatment of high-risk solid tumors of childhood with intensive therapy and autologous bone marrow transplantation. Pediatr Clin North Am 1991;38:393–424.

209. Hartmann O, Kalifa C, Benhamou E, et al. Treatment of advanced neuroblastoma with high-dose melphalan and autologous bone marrow transplantation. Cancer Chemother Pharmacol 1986;16:165–9.

210. Hartmann O, Benhamou E, Beaujean F, et al. Repeated high-dose chemotherapy followed by purged autologous bone marrow transplantation as consolidation therapy in metastatic neuroblastoma. J Clin Oncol 1987;5:1205–11.

211. Graham-Pole J, Pick T, Casper J, et al. Myeolablative treatment for children with metastatic neuroblastoma supported by bone marrow infusions: progress and problems. Autol Bone Marrow Transplant 1989;559.

212. Philip T, Zucker JM, Bernard JL, et al. The LMCE1 unselected group of stage IV neuroblastoma revisited with a median follow up of 59 months after ABMT. Prog Clin Biol Res 1991;366:517–26.

213. Seeger RC, Villablanca JG, Matthay KK, et al. Intensive chemoradiotherapy and autologous bone marrow transplantation for poor prognosis neuroblastoma. Prog Clin Biol Res 1991;366:527–33.

214. Philip T, Chauvin F, Michon J, et al. A pilot study of double ABMT in advanced neuroblastoma (32 patients). In: Dicke KA, Spitzer G, Jagannath S, Evinger-Hodges MJ, eds. Autologous bone marrow transplantation. Houston: University of Texas M.D. Anderson Cancer Center, 1989:799.

215. Evans AE, August CS, Kamani N, et al. Bone marrow transplantation for high risk neuroblastoma at the Children's Hospital of Philadelphia: an update. Med Pediatr Oncol 1994;23:323–7.

216. Ladenstein R, Lasset C, Hartmann O, et al. Impact of megatherapy on survival after relapse from stage 4 neuroblastoma in patients over 1 year of age at diagnosis: a report from the European Group for Bone Marrow Transplantation. J Clin Oncol 1993;11:2330–41.

217. Kremens B, Klingebiel T, Herrmann F, et al. High-dose consolidation with local radiation and bone marrow rescue in patients with advanced neuroblastoma. Med Pediatr Oncol 1994;23:470–5.

218. Ladenstein R, Lasset C, Hartmann O, et al. Comparison of auto-versus allografting as consolidation of primary treatments in advanced neuroblastoma over one year of age at diagnosis: report from the European Group for Bone Marrow Transplantation. Bone Marrow Transplant 1994;14:37–46.

219. Mugishima H, Harada K, Suzuki T, et al. Comprehensive treatment of advanced neuroblastoma involving autologous bone marrow transplant. Acta Paediatr Japn 1995;37:493–9.

220. Kamani N, August CS, Bunin N, et al. A study of thiotepa, etoposide and fractionated total body irradiation as a preparative regimen prior to bone marrow transplantation for poor prognosis patients with neuroblastoma. Bone Marrow Transplant 1996;17:911–6.

221. Hartmann O, Valteau-Couanet D, Benhamou E, et al. Stage IV neuroblastoma in patients over 1 year of age at diagnosis: consolidation of poor responders with combined busulfan, cyclophosphamide and melphalan followed by in vitro mafosfamide-purged autologous bone marrow transplantation. Eur J Cancer 1997;33:2126–9.

222. Garaventa A, Rondelli R, Lanino E, et al. Myeloablative therapy and bone marrow rescue in advanced neuroblastoma. Report from the Italian Bone Marrow Transplant Registry. Italian Association of Pediatric Hematology-Oncology, BMT Group. Bone Marrow Transplant 1996;18:125–30.

223. Glorieux P, Bouffet E, Philip I, et al. Metastatic interstitial pneumonitis after autologous bone marrow transplantation. A consequence of reinjection of malignant cells? Cancer 1986;58:2136–9.

224. Graeve JL, deAlarcon PA, Sato Y, et al. Miliary pulmonary neuroblastoma. A risk of autologous bone marrow transplantation? Cancer 1988;62:2125–7.

225. Rill DR, Santana VM, Roberts WM, et al. Direct demonstration that autologous bone marrow transplantation for solid tumors can return a multiplicity of tumorigenic cells. Blood 1994;84:380–3.

226. Reynolds CP, Moss TJ, Feig SA. Treatment of poor prognosis neuroblastoma with intensive therapy and autologous bone marrow transplantation. In: Dicke KA, Spitzer G, Jagannath S, Evinger-Hodges MJ, eds. Autologous bone marrow transplantation. Houston: University of Texas M.D. Anderson Cancer Center, 1989:575.

227. Treleaven JG, Gibson FM, Ugelstad J, et al. Removal of neuroblastoma cells from bone marrow with monoclonal antibodies conjugated to magnetic microspheres. Lancet 1984;1:70–3.

228. Cheung IY, Barber D, Cheung NK. Detection of microscopic neuroblastoma in marrow by histology, immunocytology, and reverse transcription–PCR of multiple molecular markers. Clin Cancer Res 1998;4:2801–5.

229. Tchirkov A, Kanold J, Giollant M, et al. Molecular monitoring of tumor cell contamination in leukapheresis products from stage IV neuroblastoma patients before and after positive CD34 selection. Med Pediatr Oncol 1998;30:228–32.

230. Lode HN, Handgretinger R, Schuermann U, et al. Detection of neuroblastoma cells in CD34 + selected peripheral stem cells using a combination of tyrosine hydroxylase nested RT-PCR and anti-ganglioside GD2 immunocytochemistry. Eur J Cancer 1997;33:2024–30.

231. Matthay KK, Seeger RC, Reynolds CP, et al. Allogeneic versus autologous purged bone marrow transplantation for neuroblastoma: a report from the Children's Cancer Group. J Clin Oncol 1994; 12:2382–9.

232. Handgretinger R, Greil J, Schurmann U, et al. Positive selection and transplantation of peripheral CD34 + progenitor cells: feasibility and purging efficacy in pediatric patients with neuroblastoma. J Hematother 1997;6:235–42.

233. Cohn SL, Moss TJ, Hoover M, et al. Treatment of poor-risk neuroblastoma patients with high-dose chemotherapy and autologous peripheral stem cell rescue. Bone Marrow Transplant 1997;20:543–51.

234. Kletzel M, Longino R, Rademaker AW, et al. Peripheral blood stem cell transplantation in young children: experience with harvesting, mobilization and engraftment. Pediatr Transplant 1998;2:191–6.

235. Eguchi H, Takaue Y, Kawano Y, et al. Peripheral blood stem cell autografts for the treatment of children over 1 year old with stage IV neuroblastoma: a long-term follow-up. Bone Marrow Transplant 1998;21:1011–4.

236. Kletzel M, Abella EM, Sandler ES, et al. Thiotepa and cyclophosphamide with stem cell rescue for consolidation therapy for children with high-risk neuroblastoma: a phase I/II study of the Pediatric Blood and Marrow Transplant Consortium. J Pediatr Hematol/Oncol 1998;20:49–54.

237. Berger M, Kanold J, Rapatel C, et al. Feasibility of a PB CD34 + cell transplantation procedure using standard leukapheresis products in very small children. Bone Marrow Transplant 1997;20:191–8.

238. Moss TJ, Sanders DG, Lasky LC, Bostrom B. Contamination of peripheral blood stem cell harvests by circulating neuroblastoma cells. Blood 1990;76:1879–83.

239. Reynolds CP, Kane DJ, Einhorn PA, et al. Response of neuroblastoma to retinoic acid in vitro and in vivo. Prog Clin Biol Res 1991;366:203–11.

240. Reynolds CP, Lie SO. Retinoid therapy of neuroblastoma. In: Brodeur GM, Sawada T, Tsuchida Y, Voute PA, eds. Neuroblastoma. Amsterdam: Elsevier Science BV, 2000:519–40.

241. Finklestein JZ, Krailo MD, Lenarsky C, et al. 13-cis-Retinoic acid (NSC 122758) in the treatment of children with metastatic neuroblastoma unresponsive to conventional chemotherapy: report from the Children's Cancer Study Group. Med Pediatr Oncol 1992;20:307–11.

242. Reynolds CP, Schindler PF, Jones DM, et al. Comparison of 13-cis-retinoic acid to trans-retinoic acid using human neuroblastoma cell lines. Prog Clin Biol Res 1994;385:237–44.

243. Villablanca JG, Khan AA, Avramis VI, et al. Phase I trial of 13-cis-retinoic acid in children with neuroblastoma following bone marrow transplantation. J Clin Oncol 1995;13:894–901.

244. Villablanca JG, Khan AA, Avramis VI, Reynolds CP. Hypercalcemia: a dose-limiting toxicity associated with 13-cis-retinoic acid. Am J Pediatr Hematol Oncol 1993;15:410–5.

245. Matthay KK, Atkinson JB, Stram DO, et al. Patterns of relapse after autologous purged bone marrow transplantation for neuroblastoma: a Children's Cancer Group pilot study. J Clin Oncol 1993;11:2226–33.

246. Philip T, Ladenstein R, Zucker JM, et al. Double megatherapy and autologous bone marrow transplantation for advanced neuroblastoma: the LMCE2 study. Br J Cancer 1993;67:119–27.

247. Kawa-Ha K, Yumura-Yagi K, Inoue M, et al. Results of single and double autografts for high-risk neuroblastoma patients. Bone Marrow Transplant 1996;17:957–62.

248. Treuner J, Klingebiel T, Bruchelt G, et al. Treatment of neuroblastoma with metaiodobenzylguanidine: results and side effects. Med Pediatr Oncol 1987;15:199–202.

249. Garaventa A, Bellagamba O, Lo Piccolo MS, et al. 131I-metaiodobenzylguanidine (131I-MIBG) therapy for residual neuroblastoma: a mono-institutional experience with 43 patients. Br J Cancer 1999;81:1371–84.

250. Sisson JC, Hutchinson RJ, Carey JE, et al. Toxicity from treatment of neuroblastoma with 131I-meta-iodobenzylguanidine. Eur J Nucl Med 1988;14:337–40.

251. Matthay KK, DeSantes K, Hasegawa B, et al. Phase I dose escalation of 131I-metaiodobenzylguanidine with autologous bone marrow support in refractory neuroblastoma. J Clin Oncol 1998;16:229–36.

252. Goldberg SS, DeSantes K, Huberty JP, et al. Engraftment after myeloablative doses of 131I-metaiodobenzylguanidine followed by autologous bone marrow transplantation for treatment of refractory neuroblastoma. Med Pediatr Oncol 1998;30:339–46.

253. Keshelava N, Seeger RC, Groshen S, Reynolds CP. Drug resistance

patterns of human neuroblastoma cell lines derived from patients at different phases of therapy. Cancer Res 1998;58:5396–5405.

254. Keshelava N, Groshen S, Reynolds CP. Cross-resistance of topisomerase I and II inhibitors in neuroblastoma cell lines. Cancer Chemother Pharmacol 2000;45:1–8.

255. Anderson CP, Tsai JM, Meek WE, et al. Depletion of glutathione by buthionine sulfoxine is cytotoxic for human neuroblastoma cell lines via apoptosis. Exp Cell Res 1999;246:183–92.

256. Anderson CP, Tsai JM, Chan WW, et al. Buthionine sulfoximine (BSO) is cytotoxic and enhances the activity of melphalan for human neuroblastoma cell lines. Eur J Cancer 1997;33:2016–9.

257. Anderson CP, Seeger RC, Matthay KK, et al. Buthionine sulfoximine (BSO) and melphalan (L-PAM) is active against recurrent neuroblastoma. Med Pediatr Oncol 1999;33:158.

258. Wu ZL, Schwartz E, Seeger RC, Ladisch S. Expression of GD2 ganglioside by untreated primary human neuroblastomas. Cancer Res 1986;46:440–3.

259. Schulz G, Cheresh DA, Varki NM, et al. Detection of ganglioside GD2 in tumor tissues and sera of neuroblastoma patients. Cancer Res 1984;44:5914–20.

260. Cheung NK, Lazarus H, Miraldi FD, et al. Ganglioside GD2 specific monoclonal antibody 3F8: a phase I study in patients with neuroblastoma and malignant melanoma. J Clin Oncol 1987;5:1430–40.

261. Handgretinger R, Baader P, Dopfer R, et al. A phase I study of neuroblastoma with the anti-ganglioside GD2 antibody 14.G2a. Cancer Immunol Immunother 1992;35:199–204.

262. Murray JL, Cunningham JE, Brewer H, et al. Phase I trial of murine monoclonal antibody 14G2a administered by prolonged intravenous infusion in patients with neuroectodermal tumors. J Clin Oncol 1994;12:184–93.

263. Handgretinger R, Anderson K, Lang P, et al. A phase I study of human/mouse chimeric antiganglioside GD2 antibody ch14.18 in patients with neuroblastoma. Eur J Cancer 1995;31A:261–7.

264. Kushner BH, Cheung NK. Clinically effective monoclonal antibody 3F8 mediates nonoxidative lysis of human neuroectodermal tumor cells by polymorphonuclear leukocytes. Cancer Res 1991;51:4865–4870.

265. Barker E, Mueller BM, Handgretinger R, et al. Effect of a chimeric anti-ganglioside GD2 antibody on cell-mediated lysis of human neuroblastoma cells. Cancer Res 1991;51:144–9.

266. Bruchelt G, Handgretinger R, Fierlbeck G, et al. Lysis of neuroblastoma cells by the ADCC-reaction: granulocytes of patients with chronic granulomatous disease are more effective than those of healthy donors. Immunol Lett 1989;22:217–20.

267. Hank JA, Robinson RR, Surfus J, et al. Augmentation of antibody dependent cell mediated cytotoxicity following in vivo therapy with recombinant interleukin 2. Cancer Res 1990;50:5234–9.

268. Kushner BH, Cheung NK. GM-CSF enhances 3F8 monoclonal antibody-dependent cellular cytotoxicity against human melanoma and neuroblastoma. Blood 1989;73:1936–41.

269. Barker E, Reisfeld RA. A mechanism for neutrophil-mediated lysis of human neuroblastoma cells. Cancer Res 1993;53:362–7.

270. Michon J, Moutel S, Barbet J, et al. In vitro killing of neuroblastoma cells by neutrophils derived from granulocyte colony-stimulating factor–treated cancer patients using an anti-disialoganglioside/anti-Fc gamma RI bispecific antibody. Blood 1995;86:1124–30.

271. Baldwin GC, Chung GY, Kaslander C, et al. Colony-stimulating factor enhancement of myeloid effector cell cytotoxicity towards neuroectodermal tumour cells. Br J Haematol 1993;83:545–53.

272. Sondel PM, Hank JA. Combination therapy with interleukin-2 and antitumor monoclonal antibodies. Cancer J Sci Am 1998;3:121–7.

273. Chen RL, Reynolds CP, Seeger RC. Neutrophils are cytotoxic and growth-inhibitin for neuroblastoma cells with an anti-GD2 antibody but, without cytotoxicity, can be growth-stimulating. Cancer Immunol Immunother 2000;48:603–12.

274. Hank JA, Surfus J, Gan J, et al. Treatment of neuroblastoma patients with antiganglioside GD2 antibody plus interleukin-2 induces antibody-dependent cellular cytotoxicity against neuroblastoma detected in vitro. J Immunother 1994;15:29–37.

275. Frost JD, Hank JA, Reaman GH, et al. A phase I/IB trial of murine monoclonal anti-GD2 antibody 14.G2a plus interleukin-2 in children with refractory neuroblastoma: a report of the Children's Cancer Group. Cancer 1997;80:317–33.

276. Ozkaynak MF, Krailo M, Sondel PM, et al. Phase I study of chimeric human/murine anti-GD2 monoclonal antibody (ch14.18) with GM-

277. Katsanis E, Orchard PJ, Bausero MA, et al. Interleukin-2 gene transfer into murine neuroblastoma decreases tumorigenicity and enhances systemic immunity causing regression of preestablished retroperitoneal tumors. J Immunother Emphasis Tumor Immunol 1994;15:81–90.

278. Bowman L, Grossmann M, Rill D, et al. IL-2 adenovector-transduced autologous tumor cells induce antitumor immune responses in patients with neuroblastoma. Blood 1998;92:1941–49.

279. Ucar K, Seeger RC, Challita PM, et al. Sustained cytokine production and immunophenotypic changes in human neuroblastoma cell lines transduced with a human gamma interferon vector. Cancer Gene Ther 1995;2:171–181.

280. Livingston PO. Approaches to augmenting the immunogenicity of melanoma gangliosides: from whole melanoma cells to ganglioside-KLH conjugate vaccines. Immunol Rev 1995;145:147–166.

281. Cheung NK, Cheung IY, Canete A, et al. Antibody response to murine anti-GD2 monoclonal antibodies: correlation with patient survival. Cancer Res 1994;54:2228–2233.

282. Cheung NK, Canete A, Cheung IY, et al. Disialoganglioside GD2 anti-idiotypic monoclonal antibodies. Int J Cancer 1993;54:499–505.

283. Zhao XJ, Cheung NK. GD2 oligosaccharide: target for cytotoxic T lymphocytes. J Exp Med 1995;182:67–74.

284. Corrias MV, Scaruffi P, Occhino M, et al. Expression of MAGE-1, MAGE-3 and MART-1 genes in neuroblastoma. Int J Cancer 1996;69:403–7.

285. Peters WP. The effect of recombinant human colony-stimulating factors on hematopoietic reconstitution following autologous bone marrow transplantation. Semin Hematol 1989;26:18–23.

286. Ericson SG, Guyre CA, Benoit NE, et al. Antibody-dependent cellular cytotoxicity (ADCC) function of peripheral blood polymorphonuclear neutrophils (PMN) after autologous bone marrow transplantation (ABMT). Bone Marrow Transplant 1995;16:787–91.

287. Choi D, Perrin M, Hoffmann S, et al. Dendritic cell-based vaccines in the setting of peripheral blood stem cell transplantation: CD34 + cell–depleted mobilized peripheral blood can serve as a source of potent dendritic cells. Clin Cancer Res 1998;4:2709–16.

288. Gillies SD, Young D, Lo KM, Roberts S. Biological activity and in vivo clearance of antitumor antibody/cytokine fusion proteins. Bioconjug Chem 1993;4:230–5.

289. Sabzevari H, Gillies SD, Mueller BM, et al. A recombinant antibody-interleukin 2 fusion protein suppresses growth of hepatic human neuroblastoma metastases in severe combined immunodeficiency mice. Proc Natl Acad Sci USA 1994;91:9626–30.

290. Pancook JD, Becker JC, Gillies SD, Reisfeld RA. Eradication of established hepatic human neuroblastoma metastases in mice with severe combined immunodeficiency by antibody-targeted interleukin-2. Cancer Immunol Immunother 1996;42:88–92.

291. Becker JC, Varki N, Gillies SD, et al. Long-lived and transferable tumor immunity in mice after targeted interleukin-2 therapy. J Clin Invest 1996;98:2801–4.

292. Batova A, Kamps A, Gillies SD, et al. The Ch14.18-GM-CSF fusion protein is effective at mediating antibody-dependent cellular cytotoxicity and complement-dependent cytotoxicity in vitro. Clin Cancer Res 1999;5:4259–63.

293. Chen RL, Reynolds CP, Keshelava N, et al. Neutrophils and mononuclear cells (MNC) are cytotoxic for chemotherapy-sensitive and -resistant neuroblastoma cell lines with an anti-GD2/GM-CSF fusion protein. Proc Am Assoc Cancer Res 1999;40:355. abstract.

294. Ponzoni M, Bocca P, Chiesa V, et al. Differential effects of N-(4-hydroxyphenyl)retinamide and retinoic acid on neuroblastoma cells: apoptosis versus differentiation. Cancer Res 1995;55:853–61.

295. Di Vinci A, Geido E, Infusini E, Giaretti W. Neuroblastoma cell apoptosis induced by the synthetic retinoid N-(4-hydroxyphenyl)retinamide. Int J Cancer 1994;59:422–6.

296. Mariotti A, Marcora E, Bunone G, et al. N-(4-hydroxyphenyl)retinamide: a potent inducer of apoptosis in human neuroblastoma cells. J Natl Cancer Inst 1994;86:1245–7.

297. Maurer BJ, Metelitsa LS, Seeger RC, et al. N-(4-hydroxyphenyl)retinamide increases ceramide and reactive oxygen species and induces mixed apoptosis/necrosis in neuroblastoma cell lines. J Natl Cancer Inst 1999;91:1138–46.

298. Decensi A, Torrisi R, Polizzi A, et al. Effect of the synthetic retinoid fenretinide on dark adaptation and the ocular surface. J Natl Cancer Inst 1994;86:105–10.

299. Bagniewski PG, Reid JM, Villablanca JG, et al. A phase I pharmacokinetic study of fenretinide (HPR) in children with high-risk solid tumors. Proc Am Assoc Cancer Res 1999;40:92. abstract.

300. Reynolds CP, Melton LJ, Wang YL. N-(4-hydroxyphenyl)retinamide is highly active against retinoic acid resistant neuroblastoma cell lines. Proc Am Assoc Cancer Res 1997;38:25.

301. Maurer BJ, Metelitsa LS, Seeger RC, et al. Fenretinide (4-HPR) induces ceramide in neuroblastoma and 4-HPR cytotoxicity is increased by modulators of ceramide metabolism. Med Pediatr Oncol 1999;33:227.

302. Wassberg E, Pahlman S, Westlin JE, Christofferson R. The angiogenesis inhibitor TNP-470 reduces the growth rate of human neuroblastoma in nude rats. Pediatr Res 1997;41:327–33.

303. Lode HN, Moehler T, Xiang R, et al. Synergy between an antiangiogenic integrin alpha antagonist and an antibody-cytokine fusion protein eradicates spontaneous tumor metastases. Proc Natl Acad Sci USA 1999;96:1591–6.

304. Blatt J, Stitely S. Antineuroblastoma activity of desferoxamine in human cell lines. Cancer Res 1987;47:1749–50.

305. Blatt J, Taylor SR, Stitely S. Mechanism of antineuroblastoma activity of deferoxamine in vitro. J Lab Clin Med 1988;112:433–6.

306. Donfrancesco A, Deb G, Dominici C, et al. Effects of a single course of deferoxamine in neuroblastoma patients. Cancer Res 1990;50:4929–30.

307. Pritchard J, McElwain TJ, Graham-Pole J. High-dose melphalan with autologous marrow for treatment of advanced neuroblastoma. Br J Cancer 1982;45:86–94.

308. Kushner BH, O Reilly RJ, Mandell LR, et al. Myeloablative combination chemotherapy without total body irradiation for neuroblastoma. J Clin Oncol 1991;9:274–9.

# CHAPTER 80

# HISTIOCYTIC DISORDERS

• KENNETH L. McCLAIN

There are relatively few truly malignant diseases of histiocytes when the clinical, cytologic, and molecular biologic characteristics of histiocytic proliferations are examined. However, oncologists and hematologists are the primary caregivers for many patients with these disorders because antineoplastic chemotherapy drugs or radiotherapy, or both, may be the treatment of choice for patients with extensive disease. The confusing terminology and multiple cell types of the histiocytic lineage are at the root of the problem of understanding these disorders. Diseases of these cells can be classified into three broad categories based first on the absence of definitive malignant cell behavior in (1) the Langerhans' cell histiocytosis group derived from the dendritic Langerhans' cell, (2) the hemophagocytic diseases associated with proliferation of benign monocytes, and (3) the truly malignant disorders of the first two. As will be evident from the subsequent discussion, the controversy surrounding these classifications persists. Many experts who treat these diseases have endeavored to streamline the terminology because the historical eponyms associated with the histiocytic proliferations have led to unnecessary confusion.

## Histiocyte Lineage

Both the primary antigen-*processing* macrophages and the antigen-*presenting* dendritic cells are derived from CD34$^+$ hematopoietic stem cells in the bone marrow under the influence of cytokines, including granulocyte-macrophage colony-stimulating factor (GM-CSF), tumor necrosis factor-α (TNF-α), interleukin-4 (IL-4), and others.[1–3] Circulating monocytes that produce tissue-resident macrophages seem to represent one clear path of differentiation because they express little or no CD1a or S-100 on the cell surface, but they do stain for CD11b, CD15A, and CD68. Intracellular enzymes with prominent expression include lysozyme, acid phosphatase, and antitrypsin. Langerhans' and dendritic cells have abundant expression of CD1a and S-100 on the cell surface, but they do not express CD11b, CD15A, and CD68, which are prominently represented on the surface of macrophages. Likewise, the intracellular enzymes characteristic of the macrophages are not expressed in the dendritic or Langerhans' cells.[4] Finally, a unique characteristic of the Langerhans' cells is the pentalaminar Birbeck granule, which is found by electron microscopic examination of normal and most pathologic Langerhans' cells.[5]

If the dendritic or Langerhans' cells and macrophages developed clearly and simply to these definitive cell morphologies, it would be easier to understand the diseases associated with them. However, it appears there is a continuum of cells developing from dendritic cell and macrophage progenitors into *indeterminate cells* (which could be migrating Langerhans' cells); the *mature Langerhans' cells* interact with antigens, then T lymphocytes, and finally become *interdigitating dendritic cells*.[6] Macrophages and perhaps dendritic cell precursors also develop into another variant called the *dermal dendrocyte*.

One may thus divide the histiocytic disorders into categories of (1) clearly malignant diseases, such as monocytic leukemias and solid tumors of dendritic or macrophage type, and (2) histiocytic proliferations that clearly do not meet the criteria of malignancy. In this second category, Favara and coworkers have included dendritic cell–related disorders: Langerhans' cell histiocytosis (LCH), secondary dendritic cell processes, juvenile xanthogranuloma, and dendritic histiocytomas, as contrasted with the macrophage-related disorders, including the various hemophagocytic syndromes, Rosai-Dorfman disease, macrophage-related histiocytomas, and others such as the multicentric reticulohistiocytomas.[6] The category *malignant histiocytosis* has fallen out of favor because true malignancies of dendritic cells are extremely rare, and the majority of cases once believed to be malignant histiocytosis has now been identified as anaplastic large cell lymphomas of either T- or B-lymphoid derivations.[7]

# Langerhans' Cell Histiocytosis

## BIOLOGY

A proliferation of CD1a$^+$, S-100$^+$ Langerhans' cells with their characteristic large, folded nuclei can be found in skin, bone, lymph nodes, spleen, liver, bone marrow, lung, pituitary, and various locations of the brain. Both the age of the patient and the number and dysfunction of organ systems involved are recognized as important prognostic elements for the outcome of therapy. Three groups have confirmed that the pathologic Langerhans' cells represent clonal proliferations.[8–10] Although clonality has been equated with malignancy in lymphoid and other cancers, this is not necessarily the case in histiocytic disorders. Willman and associates clearly showed that patients who had LCH in single bone lesions had the same extent of clonality as did those with diffuse disease.[8] The biology of the disease is clearly different between these two patient groups, so clonality alone does not define a "malignant" behavior of cells. Until recently, there were no cytogenetic data on LCH. Betts and colleagues published the karyotypes from four children with LCH.[11] Three of these patients had single bone lesions and one was an infant with diffuse disease. There were no clonal abnormalities and only one translocation t(2:4)(p21;q33). Additions and deletions of several different chromosomes were found, as was an increase in chromosomal breaks. Because clonal abnormalities were not found, one cannot use these data to support the concept of a malignancy in the classic sense.

In addition to these data, an increased incidence of malignancies has been associated with LCH. Some patients are found to have concurrent LCH and malignancy, and others develop malignancy after the onset of LCH. (See later for more details.) At the very least, this suggests that the chromosome instability noted in the few cases summarized earlier puts patients with LCH at higher risk for malignant transformation in various cell lineages. Until more cytogenetic and molecular data are available, the debate about LCH as a malignancy or a proliferative disease of diverse biologic behavior will go on.

The cytokine milieu of LCH lesions suggests that abnormal regulation of several growth factors for histiocytes could be responsible for the proliferation of Langerhans' cells in these lesions, which are characterized by increased amounts of interleukin-1 (IL-1), interleukin-6 (IL-6), prostaglandin E$_2$, gamma interferon GM-CSF, TNF-$\alpha$, and leukemia inhibitory factor.[10, 12, 13] As yet, there are no molecular defects or viral causes identified that can explain the increased production of these cytokines within the lesions but not in surrounding normal cells.[14]

## CLINICAL PRESENTATION

This is a disease of both children and adults, with an apparent incidence of 2 to 5 per million for children, and occurring perhaps one third as frequently in adults.[15, 16] The most common site of this disease is bone, with the skull being most frequently involved (40%), followed by the femur (13%), ribs (13%), pelvis (12%), vertebra (9%), and mandible (8%).[17] Among children and adults, nearly 80% present with a single painful lesion. Proptosis may be dramatic with orbital involvement and concurrent otitis externa; profuse white material drains from the canal if the mastoid is diseased. When LCH affects the mandible, the teeth may be loose and appear to be floating in a clear space as seen in a plain radiograph. Radiographs of the other bones show lytic lesions with sharp borders that develop sclerosis on healing.[18] Collapse of vertebrae in patients with LCH may cause cord compression.[19]

Skin involvement in children most often presents as a seborrheic rash behind the ears or on the scalp; also, an erythematous, papular rash may develop on the abdomen. Some infants present at birth with a self-healing form of LCH manifested as purplish brown nodular lesions that appear on any part of the body but are most prominent on the trunk and abdomen.[20] Adults and children can have deeply ulcerated lesions in the groin and genital region. Sometimes, extreme hypertrophy of the gingiva occurs, with involvement of the soft and hard palates.

When LCH develops in the lymph nodes, the cervical regions are usually the sole site of disease, but axillary, mediastinal, and abdominal lymphadenopathy can be identified in patients with diffuse disease. Splenic and hepatic enlargement is most often found in children with extensive LCH. Bone marrow involvement is less likely unless several other organs are involved and thrombocytopenia is present.[21]

Pulmonary LCH is found in a variable number of children, depending on whether purely clinical or radiographic criteria are used.[22, 23] Pulmonary disease was found in nearly 40% of children with multisystem disease using clinical or radiologic evidence, or both, but it is rare overall in pediatric cases and it is never the sole lesion.[22] Radiologic findings of pneumothoraces, interstitial infiltrates, nodular infiltrates, honeycombing, and formation of bullae were documented in 8 of 42 patients in another series.[23] The incidence in adults is less well characterized, but it is clearly higher among smokers. Patients present with dyspnea, cough, and chest pain.[24] Older patients and those with markedly decreased pulmonary function at the time of presentation had the worst prognosis. Among the pulmonary function tests, the vital capacity and D$_{LCO}$ (the diffusing capacity of lung for carbon dioxide) were most often abnormal, but the forced expiratory volume in 1 second/forced vital capacity (FEV$_1$/FVC) also held a highly predictive value for a poor outcome.[25]

Central nervous system LCH is identified most often because of pituitary-hypothalamic infiltration that causes diabetes insipidus (DI) and may occur as a presenting symptom, or later after initial bone disease has been treated. Children with periorbital disease and proptosis seem to be at particular risk for DI. This complication of LCH seems to occur equally in adults and children.[26, 27] With more extensive involvement of the hypothalamic-pituitary system, some patients have galactorrhea, hypothyroidism, hypoadrenalism, growth hormone deficiency, and amenorrhea. There has been intensive study of a perplexing group of LCH patients with other brain lesions.[28] The incidence of this complication is not known, but it is clearly higher in patients with multisystem disease involving the temporal, orbital, or other skull bones, and in those with DI or other endocrinopathies. Magnetic resonance imaging defines lesions of the white or gray matter with or without enhancement, as well as extraparenchymal lesions of the dura, arachnoid, or choroid plexus, and atrophic and pituitary lesions. The histopathology of LCH, detailed descriptions of specific brain areas involved, and possible treatment regimens are reviewed by Grois and associates.[29]

## EVALUATION AND TREATMENT

Children and adults with LCH of only one site (especially bone, skin, or pituitary) may be treated with minimal therapy (see later). However, the key initial question is whether the patient has disease that is truly confined to a single site. It is prudent to do a basic staging evaluation so that the extent of disease can be ascertained (Table 80–1).

In rare diseases with variable behavior (such as LCH), there is a tendency for physicians to treat patients with a plethora of therapies. Without an understanding of the natural history of such diseases or an organized approach to standardized treatment regimens, no advancement is made and patients ultimately suffer. Table 80–2 summarizes the options for treatment of the varied forms of LCH. Obviously, disease in single sites such as bone or skin responds to many different therapeutic modalities.[30, 31] Often, the key question is whether treatment with chemotherapy or radiotherapy is warranted at all. For children with disease in more than one organ system and organ dysfunction, the Histiocyte Society

**Table 80–1.** Initial Evaluation of Patients with Langerhans' Cell Histiocytosis

Complete history and physical examination
Complete blood count with differential
Urinalysis and osmolality (after overnight water deprivation)
Electrolyte determination
Liver function tests (AST/ALT, bilirubin, albumin, total protein, may include PT/PTT)
Chest radiograph
Skeletal survey, including skull series
Radionuclide bone scan
CT of head if patient has proptosis or possible mastoid disease
Biopsy of presenting site of disease: If bone lesion or possibly a single lymph node, perform curettage or complete lymph node excision.
**(NOTE: Save frozen tissue for biologic studies—see recommendations for therapy.)**
*Follow-up recommendations:* If laboratory test is abnormal, repeat monthly except urine osmolality, which can be done at 3- to 6-month intervals. Skeletal radiographs of only the involved area may be repeated at 6-month intervals.
*Additional studies as indicated by initial findings:* Bone marrow aspirate and biopsy: if anemia not explained by iron deficiency or "chronic disease," leukopenia, and thrombocytopenia
Pulmonary function tests: if abnormal chest x-ray or pulmonary symptoms
Lung biopsy/bronchoalveolar lavage: for definitive diagnosis of pulmonary LCH (recommended in all patients with suspicious chest radiographs)
Small bowel radiographs and biopsy: chronic diarrhea, failure to thrive
Liver biopsy: abnormal liver function test results
MRI of brain: evidence of DI, suspicion of parenchymal involvement
Panoramic dental radiography of mandible and maxilla: gingival or other oral involvement (*Also, patient should consult an oral surgeon*)
Endocrine evaluation: DI, short stature, galactorrhea, abnormal puberty, abnormal brain MRI
Otolaryngology consultation: otitis externa, mastoid involvement by CT of skull (*Patient should also have an audiogram*)

AST, aspartate transaminase; ALT, alanine transaminase; PT, prothrombin time; PTT, partial thromboplastin time; CT, computed tomography; LCH, Langerhans' cell histiocytosis; MRI, magnetic resonance imaging; DI, diabetes insipidus.

**Table 80–2.** Treatment of Langerhans' Cell Histiocytosis

SINGLE-SITE DISEASE
 Skin: *PUVA* (psoralen and ultraviolet A irradiation)
   *Nitrogen mustard:* Very effective for ulcerated lesions and those not responding to systemic therapy
   *Thalidomide:* Currently used for adults; pediatric trial ongoing
   *No treatment* for infants with purplish brown nodules
 Bone: *Curettage* of lesion ± *injection of steroids* locally during procedure
   *Radiotherapy:* For large skull lesions with incomplete excision, vertebral lesions with cord compression, or neck or femur when bone unstable
   *Indomethacin*[30]: May be sufficient symptomatic treatment of lesions in noncritical areas, which could remit spontaneously
 Lymph node: *Complete excision* may be sufficient therapy for a single node
SINGLE-ORGAN SYSTEM/MULTIPLE SITES
 Patients with multiple bone lesions or lymph nodes are usually included in this group. The current Histiocyte Society recommendations (LCH-II Protocol, Helmut Gadner, Chairperson)[31] are to use a 6-week course of oral prednisone, weekly vinblastine for 6 weeks, and a continuation treatment lasting 18 weeks with daily mercaptopurine, as well as weekly pulses of oral prednisone and intravenous vinblastine every 3 weeks. (Treatment Arm A.) (Contact Histiocyte Society for protocol.)
MULTISYSTEM DISEASE/OLDER THAN 2 YEARS OF AGE
 (Without involvement of the hematopoietic system, liver, lungs, or spleen). Same treatment as for patients with single-organ or multiple-site disease.
MULTISYSTEM DISEASE: ANY AGE WITH INVOLVEMENT OF LIVER, SPLEEN, LUNGS, OR HEMATOPOIETIC SYSTEM
 Patients are randomized between Treatment Arm A given above and Treatment Arm B (Initial treatment: 6 weeks of oral prednisone, intravenous vinblastine, *and* VP-16 weekly).
 Continuation treatment: Continuous oral mercaptopurine for 18 weeks, with pulses of vinblastine and VP-16 every 3 weeks.
RECURRENT OR RESISTANT DISEASE
 A salvage protocol by the Histiocyte Society uses 2-CdA (2-chlorodeoxyadenosine) with or without Ara-C (cytosine arabinoside) because these two agents have been shown to have activity against LCH.[33,34] Other agents such as cyclosporine and interferon have been effective in a limited number of patients, but have not proven the test of time as being clearly superior. Again, registering resistant patients into standardized protocols will help advance the care of these patients more quickly than if they are treated in "random" ways by investigators throughout the world. Additional salvage protocols using new agents are currently under development, and information regarding these can be obtained from the Histiocyte Society.

has available treatment protocols that are designed to advance the understanding of LCH. It is also the goal of the Histiocyte Society to develop standardized treatment strategies for adults—especially those with pulmonary disease. I urge all physicians with LCH patients to register them into Histiocyte Society protocols so that more effective and safe therapies may be devised. Besides the protocols for new patients, there are treatment strategies available for patients with resistant or recurrent LCH. The U.S. Histiocyte Protocol coordinator is Stacey Nicholson, PhD, who can be reached at the University of Oregon Health Science Center, Phone 503–494–1543, FAX 503–494–0714, E-mail: *Nicholss@OHSU.EDU*. Information can also be obtained from Mr. Jeff Toughill of the Histiocytosis Association of America, Phone 609–589–6606, FAX 609–589–6614, E-mail: *histiocyte@aol.com* or from this author, Phone 713–770–4208, FAX 713–770–4107, E-mail: *kmcclain @txccc.org*.

## PROGNOSIS

For patients older than 2 years, with disease at single or multiple bone sites, the chance of disease-free survival is 100%, but up to 12% have recurrences.[31] When soft tissues are involved with or without bone lesions, 96% of patients survived in one study, but 23% had recurrences. Not surprisingly, the children with organ dysfunction (elevated liver function test results, hypoalbuminemia, anemia, leukopenia or thrombocytopenia, or pulmonary dysfunction) had a much worse prognosis. They were reported to have a 62% chance of survival, and recurrences were 42%. However, these results are improved from historical reports in which less than 10% of such patients survived.[32] Therapeutic strategies for patients with resistant disease include treatment with 2-chlorodeoxyadenosine (2-CdA) and cytosine arabinoside, vincristine, and prednisolone and bone marrow transplantation, although the latter has not been very successful.[33–36]

There are no controlled studies of adults with LCH, so one must rely on reported series of patients from single institutions. Malpas and Norton reported deaths in 25% of patients with single-site disease and in 50 to 63% of those with disease at multiple sites.[37] In adults, pulmonary LCH may be fatal in one quarter of patients.[25] The lack of solid data for these patients makes it obvious that controlled trials are needed.

## LATE EFFECTS AND SECONDARY PROBLEMS OF LANGERHANS' CELL HISTIOCYTOSIS

DI usually can be well controlled with DDAVP (1-deamino-8-D-arginine vasopressin). Patients with short stature and other endocrinopathies need additional hormonal support. Chronic orthopedic problems from the effects of LCH or from treatment of the spine and long bones are significant for a few patients. Chronic effects of steroid therapy have been blamed for the obesity and bone problems of some individuals. When VP-16 (etoposide) was initially used in the treatment of LCH, there was a high level of concern that many patients would develop secondary leukemias. There were some cases reported, but these individuals had several grams of VP-16 as opposed to the more moderate doses used in the Histiocyte Society and other trials.[31, 38] There have been few patients with secondary leukemia reported in the trials with moderate doses.[39]

Egeler and associates have documented the relatively high frequency of leukemias, lymphomas, and solid tumors in patients with LCH.[40] A little more than one half of the acute lymphoblastic leukemia cases occurred 6 to 12 months before the onset of LCH. However, a majority of the non-lymphoblastic leukemia cases developed more than 2 years after treatment of LCH. Although these could be secondary to the therapy given for diffuse or polyostotic LCH, the types of leukemia were not characteristic of the epipodophyllotoxin-associated FAB M4 or M5 type with t(11q23). Lymphomas associated with LCH are usually found concurrently, and the LCH is most likely a secondary nodal response to cytokines from the malignant lymphoma cells. The latency of solid tumors is 12 years; many of the malignancies occurred in radiation fields used for treatment of LCH.

# Hemophagocytic Syndromes (Hemophagocytic Lymphohistiocytosis)

Cells of the monocyte-macrophage lineage may be activated to ingest normal hematopoietic cells and cause damage to the liver and central nervous system in children and adults. The eponyms associated with these syndromes have been confusing, especially because the disease may have a familial association or may be secondary to another process. The autosomal recessive familial syndrome is obviously not defined until a second member of a family is affected.[41] Thus the initial case may be thought to be secondary to *infection* (viral, bacterial, fungal, or protozoal) or *malignancy* or associated with *immune deficiency* (Chédiak-Higashi syndrome, autoimmune lymphoproliferative [Purtilo] syndrome, or collagen vascular diseases such as rheumatoid arthritis and lupus). Some patients with leukemia, multiple myeloma, thymoma, carcinoma, or germ cell tumors have also been reported to develop this syndrome before or during treatment for the malignancy.[42] Others present with the hemophagocytic syndrome, but have an occult malignancy such as T- or NK-cell leukemia or a lymphoma. Many of the patients with malignancy-associated hemophagocytic syndromes are also infected with one of the viruses known to trigger the disease.

## BIOLOGY

One immunologic marker of these syndromes is a marked decrease or absence of NK-cell function.[43] This defect persists in familial cases, even when the patient is in remission. However, in patients with infection-associated hemophagocytic syndrome, the NK function may return to normal when signs and symptoms are absent. How the NK defect relates to the pathophysiology of the syndrome is not known, but it may provide an important marker for following the disease and defining patients at risk. Hypercytokinemia of the IL-1 receptor antagonist, a soluble IL-2 receptor, IL-6, gamma interferon, and tumor necrosis factor-$\alpha$ all have been found in patients with hemophagocytic syndromes.[44, 45]

## CLINICAL PRESENTATION

The majority of patients with familial hemophagocytic lymphohistiocytosis (FLH) syndrome present during the first 6 months of life with fever, splenomegaly, and hepatomegaly, sometimes associated with lymph node enlargement, skin rash, and neurologic symptoms.[46] These patients have pancytopenia, hypertriglyceridemia, hyperbilirubinemia, elevated alanine aminotransferase levels, and coagulopathy. Of special note are the markedly elevated levels of ferritin (>10,000 ng/ml) in most patients.[47] Diagnostic criteria for the syndrome have been developed of which the major elements are fever greater than 38.5° C for longer than 7 days, splenomegaly, cytopenias of two or more lineages, hypertriglyceridemia or hypofibrinogenemia, and hemophagocytosis in the bone marrow, spleen, or lymph nodes.[48] Many times, the clinical signs and symptoms clearly point to this syndrome, but histologic evidence of hemophagocytosis is not found in the bone marrow. Repeat aspiration and biopsies are often necessary for confirmation. The presenting symptoms and signs are essentially the same as those for infection-associated or malignancy-associated disease.

## THERAPY

The optimal therapy for the majority of patients with these syndromes is a combination of decadron, VP-16, cyclosporine, and intrathecal methotrexate, which is the current Histiocyte Society protocol (HLH-94).[49] For those with familial disease, a bone marrow transplant is necessary to correct the underlying defect.[50] A variety of therapies have been used for treating patients who have an infection-associated or malignancy-associated hemophagocytic syndrome. Unfortunately, it is not always clear if a young patient has the familial defect; thus, the HLH-94 protocol should be used as initial therapy for all children younger than 10 years. For older children and adults, treatments with cyclosporine, antithymocyte globulin, or high-dose immunoglobulin may be reasonable as initial therapies, but those who do not respond may require the same treatment as patients with familial disease.[51, 52] The use of antiviral agents such as acyclovir is controversial; in my opinion, these are not effective in treating Epstein-Barr virus (EBV)–related hemophagocytic syndrome. In cases of cytomegalovirus-associated disease, ganciclovir may be useful.

## PROGNOSIS

Among children with the familial form of this disease, less than 10% survive with chemotherapy or immunotherapy alone.[46] However, with bone marrow transplant, more than 60% were surviving 5 years after the procedure. Patients with infection-associated and malignancy-associated hemophagocytic syndromes have varying survival rates, depending on their age and underlying disease. The mortality of children younger than 3 years with the infection-associated syndrome is greater than 60%, but it is 38% in those older than age 3.[42] Some patients who are immunosuppressed and develop infection-associated hemophagocytosis respond when the immunosuppressive agents are withdrawn.[53]

## Sinus Histiocytosis with Massive Lymphadenopathy (Rosai-Dorfman Disease)

### CLINICAL PRESENTATION

The pathologic histiocytes of macrophage origin in this disease infiltrate the sinuses of lymph nodes and phagocytose lymphocytes and plasma cells, as well as erythrocytes.[54] Although the histiocytes are S-100 positive, they are CD1a negative unlike the Langerhans' cells, which are positive for both markers. Patients present from infancy to adulthood, most often with dramatically enlarged cervical lymph nodes and fever. Although extranodal involvement is rare initially, nearly half of patients may develop involvement of another site during the course of the disease. Skin, bones, liver,

spleen, and lung may be affected. Laboratory evaluations show leukocytosis, anemia, polyclonal hypergammaglobulinemia, and an increased erythrocyte sedimentation rate. Although EBV has not been found in the nodes, human herpes virus type 6 was identified in several patients.[55, 56]

## THERAPY

Many cases are self-limited and do not require therapy. However, multiorgan involvement or dysfunction and association with immune dysfunction are poor prognostic indicators and indicate the necessity for treatment.[57] A variety of therapies have been used, including steroids, interferon, and chemotherapy, with success in some cases.[58–60]

## Malignant Histiocytic Diseases

There is some debate about the identity of true malignancies of Langerhans' histiocytes because the majority of patients with "histiocytic lymphoma or malignant histiocytosis" reported in the literature probably had one of the variants of large cell lymphoma.[6] After exclusion of those patients with anaplastic large cell lymphomas and other T- or B-lineage large cell lymphomas, the number with true malignancies of histiocytes becomes very small. Favara and colleagues have suggested that such diseases be considered sarcomas of histiocytic or macrophage-related lineage.[6] There are, of course, the monocytic leukemias (FAB M4 and M5). Descriptions of the clinical presentation, biology, and treatment of both large cell lymphomas and monocytic leukemias are presented elsewhere in this book. I will limit my discussion here to the few cases recognized as sarcomas of histiocytic origin.

Favara and coworkers have outlined markers for histiocytic cells that are the most specific, including: macrophage colony–stimulating factor (M-CSF) receptor, lysozyme, Ki-M8, S-100+ large cells, Ki-M4, cathepsin D and E, CD21, and CD35.[6] If a dendritic or histiocytic cell proliferation meets a combination of criteria of "malignant," such as having a clonal cytogenetic abnormality, an aneuploid DNA profile, malignant histo- or cytomorphology, monoclonality, and an aggressive clinical course, it would be fair to classify it as a histiocytic sarcoma.

## CLINICAL PRESENTATION

Males and females of any age are affected equally by the macrophage-related histiocytic sarcomas, with infiltration of liver, spleen, lymph nodes, and skin.[61] Systemic symptoms of fever and wasting may occur. Infiltration of the bone marrow ultimately is found in approximately one quarter of patients.

In the dendritic or Langerhans' cell sarcomas, patients are less likely to have systemic symptoms and rather develop localized involvement of the skin[62] or lymph nodes, or both; however, two patients with multiorgan system involvement have been reported.[63] These authors noted that the aggressive infiltration of heart, pancreas, stomach, and muscle, besides the usual lymphoid tissues, brain, and liver, made the malignant histiocytosis-X a distinct entity from the classic form of Langerhans' cell histiocytosis. Patients with the malignant form did not respond to chemotherapy. However, Levine and associates reported favorable responses of these patients to cyclophosphamide, doxorubicin, vincristine, and prednisone.[64] Others have used a combination of etoposide and cisplatin with ifosfamide or radiation therapy to achieve durable remissions in patients with histiocytic malignancies.[65]

## Conclusion

The histiocytic diseases of children and adults are somewhat less confusing than they were in the past; however, our understanding of the pathophysiology of the various entities is still fragmentary. It is hoped that new insights into the biology of dendritic cells will speed the work of attaining an understanding of LCH. Additional work on the macrophage lineage, perhaps as it relates to control of apoptosis, may bring us closer to an understanding of the hemophagocytic syndromes. Organized protocols for treating many of these rare diseases are available to all investigators who register patients into the studies (see earlier). Only through the use of standardized treatments can we advance our knowledge.

### SUGGESTIONS FOR ADDITIONAL READING

Pritchard J, Beverley PCL, Chu AC, et al, eds. The Proceedings of the Nikolas Symposia on the Histiocytoses 1989–1993. Br J Cancer 1994;70:Suppl XXIII. *Seventeen articles written by experts involved in an annual "think tank" symposium to define new strategies for basic and clinical research of the histiocytic diseases.*

Egeler RM, D'Angio GJ. Langerhans cell histiocytosis. Hematol/Oncol Clin North Am 1998;Vol. 2. *The latest information about Langerhans' cell histiocytosis, hemophagocytic syndromes, and the debate on malignant histiocytosis. This volume best summarizes the state of knowledge on histiocytic diseases of children and adults, with updated views on disease biology, histopathology, and disease classification, as well as clinical presentation, therapeutic trials, and prognostic factors.*

Vassallo R, Ryu JH, Colby TV, et al. Pulmonary Langerhans'-cell histiocytosis. N Engl J Med 2000;342:1969–78. *An excellent review.*

### REFERENCES

1. Reid CD, Fryer PR, Clifford C, et al. Identification of hematopoietic progenitors of macrophages and dendritic Langerhans cells (DL-CFU) in human bone marrow and peripheral blood. Blood 1990;76:1139–49.
2. Caux C, Dezutter-Dambuyant C, Schmitt D, Banchereau J. GM-CSF and TNF-alpha cooperate in the generation of dendritic Langerhans cells. Nature 1992;360:258–61.
3. Palucka KA, Taquet N, Sanchez-Chapuis F, Gluckman JC. Dendritic cells as the terminal stage of monocyte differentiation. J Immunol 1998;160:4587–95.
4. Cline MJ. Histiocytes and histiocytosis. Blood 1994;84:2840–53.
5. Birbeck MS, Breathnach AS, Everall JD. An electron microscopic study of basal melanocyte and high level clear cell (Langerhans cell) in vitiligo. J Invest Dermatol 1961;37:51–64.
6. Favara B, Feller AC, Pauli M, et al. Contemporary classification of histiocytic disorders. Med Pediatr Oncol 1997;29:157–63.
7. Bucsky P, Favara B, Feller AC, et al. Malignant histiocytosis and large cell anaplastic (Ki-1) lymphoma in childhood: guidelines for differential diagnosis—report of the Histiocyte Society. Med Pediatr Oncol 1994;22:200–3.
8. Willman CL, Busque L, Griffith BB, et al. Langerhans'-cell histiocytosis (histiocytosis X)—a clonal proliferative disease. N Engl J Med 1994;331:154–60.
9. Yu RC, Chu C, Buluwela L, Chu AC. Clonal proliferation of Langerhans cells in Langerhans cell histiocytosis. Lancet 1994;343:767–8.
10. Kannorakis G, Abbas A. The role of cytokines in the pathogenesis of Langerhans cell histiocytosis. Br J Cancer 1994;70:Suppl 23: S37–40.
11. Betts DR, Leibundgut KE, Feldges A, et al. Cytogenetic abnormalities in Langerhans cell histiocytosis. Br J Cancer 1998;77:552–5.
12. Arenzana-Seisdedos F, Barbey S, Virelizier JL, et al. Histiocytosis X purified (T6+) cells from bone granuloma produce interleukin-1 and prostaglandin E2 in culture. J Clin Invest 1986;77:326–31.
13. Steiner G, Tschachler E, Tani M, et al. Interleukin 2 receptors on cultured murine epidermal Langerhans cells. J Immunol 1986;137:155–62.
14. McClain K, Jin H, Gresik V, et al. Langerhans cell histiocytosis: lack of a viral etiology. Am J Hematol 1994;47:16–20.
15. Carstensen H, Ornvold K. The epidemiology of Langerhans cell histiocytosis in children in Denmark, 1975–1989. Med Pediatr Oncol 1993;21:387–8.
16. Malpas JS. Langerhans cell histiocytosis in adults. In: Egeler RM, D'Angio GJ, eds. Langerhans cell histiocytosis, hematology/oncology clinics of North America. Philadelphia: WB Saunders, 1998:259–68.
17. Slater JM, Swarm OJ. Eosinophilic granuloma of bone. Med Pediatr Oncol 1980;8:151–64.
18. Alexander JE, Seibert JJ, Berry DH, et al. Prognostic factors for healing of bone lesions in histiocytosis X. Pediatr Radiol 1988;18:326–32.
19. Bollini G, Jouve JL, Gentet JC, et al. Bone lesions in histiocytosis X. J Pediatr Orthop 1991;11:469–77.
20. Hashimoto K, Pritzker MS. Electron microscopic study of reticulohistiocytoma: an unusual case of congenital, self-healing reticulohistiocytosis. Arch Dermatol 1973;107:263–70.
21. McClain K, Ramsay NKC, Robison L, et al. Bone marrow involvement in histiocytosis X. Med Pediatr Oncol 1983;11:167–71.
22. Ha SY, Helms P, Fletcher M, et al. Lung involvement in Langerhans' cell histiocytosis: prevalence, clinical features, and outcome. Pediatrics 1992;89:466–9.
23. Smets A, Mortele K, De Praeter G, et al. Pulmonary and mediastinal lesions in children with Langerhans cell histiocytosis. Pediatr Radiol 1997;27:873–6.
24. Travis WD, Borok Z, Roum JH, et al. Pulmonary Langerhans cell granulomatosis (histiocytosis X). A clinico-pathologic study of 48 cases. Am J Surg Pathol 1993;17:971–86.
25. Delobbe A, Durieu J, Duhamel A, Wallaert B. Determinants of survival in pulmonary Langerhans' cell granulomatosis (histiocytosis X). Eur Respir J 1996;9:2002–6.
26. Kilpatrick SE, Wenger DE, Gilchrist GS, et al. Langerhans cell histiocytosis (histiocytosis X) of bone. Cancer 1995;76:2471–84.
27. Dunger DB, Broadbent V, Yeoman E, et al. The frequency and natural history of diabetes insipidus in children with Langerhans cell histiocytosis. N Engl J Med 1989;321:1157–63.
28. Grois N, Broadbent V, Favara BF, et al. Report of the Histiocyte Society Workshop on "Central Nervous System (CNS) Disease in Langerhans cell histiocytosis (LCH)." Med Pediatr Oncol 1997;29:73–7.
29. Grois NG, Favara BE, Mostbeck GH, Prayer D. Central nervous system disease in Langerhans cell histiocytosis. In: Egeler RM, D'Angio GJ, eds. Langerhans cell histiocytosis, hematology/oncology clinics of North America. Philadelphia, WB Saunders, 1998:287–305.
30. Oliver L, Munn ST, Broadbent V, Pritchard J. Indomethacin—a useful "adjunctive" therapy in Langerhans cell histiocytosis (LCH). abstract. 12th Annual Meeting of the Histiocyte Society, Vienna, Austria, Sept. 28–30, 1996.
31. Gadner H, Heitger A, Grois N, et al. Treatment strategy for disseminated Langerhans cell histiocytosis. Med Pediatr Oncol 1994;23:72–80.
32. Greenberger JS, Crocker AC, Vawter G, et al. Results of treatment of 127 patients with systemic histiocytosis (Lettere-Siwe syndrome, Schuller-Christian syndrome, and multifocal eosinophilic granuloma). Medicine 1981;60:311–38.
33. Saven A, Figueroa ML, Piro LD, Rosenblatt JD. 2-Chlorodeoxy-adenosine to treat refractory histiocytosis X. letter. N Engl J Med 1993;5:734–5.
34. Egeler RM, de Kraker J, Voute PA. Cytosine-arabinoside, vincristine, and prednisolone in the treatment of children with disseminated Langerhans cell histiocytosis with organ dysfunction: experience at a single institution. Med Pediatr Oncol 1993;21:265–70.

35. Stoll M, Freund M, Schmid H, et al. Allogeneic bone marrow transplantation for Langerhans' cell histiocytosis. Cancer 1990;66:284–8.
36. Greinix HT, Storb R, Sanders JE, Petersen FB. Marrow transplantation for treatment of multisystem progressive Langerhans cell histiocytosis. Bone Marrow Transplant 1992;10:39–44.
37. Malpas JS, Norton AJ. Langerhans cell histiocytosis in the adult. Med Pediatr Oncol 1996;27:540–6.
38. Haupt R, Fears TR, Heise A, et al. Risk of secondary leukemia after treatment with etoposide (VP-16) for Langerhans' cell histiocytosis in Italian and Austrian-German populations. Int J Cancer 1997;71:9–13.
39. Stine KC, Saylors RL, Sawer JR, Becton DL. Secondary acute myelogenous leukemia following safe exposure to etoposide. J Clin Oncol 1997;15:1583–6.
40. Egeler RM, Neglia J, Puccetti DM, et al. The association of Langerhans cell histiocytosis with malignant neoplasms. Cancer 1993;71:865–73.
41. Henter J-I, Elinder G. Familial hemophagocytic lymphohistiocytosis. Clinical review based on the findings in seven children. Acta Paediatr Scand 1991;80:269–78.
42. Janka G, Imashuku S, Elinder G, et al. Infection- and malignancy-associated hemophagocytic syndrome. In: Egeler RM, D'Angio GJ, eds. Langerhans cell histiocytosis, hematology/oncology clinics of North America. Philadelphia: WB Saunders, 1998:435–44.
43. Eife R, Janka G, Belohradsky B, et al. Defective natural killer cell function and interferon production in familial hemophagocytic lymphohistiocytosis. Med Pediatr Oncol 1986;14:111–7.
44. Fujiwara F, Hibi S, Imashuku S. Hypercytokinemia in hemophagocytic syndrome. Am J Pediatr Hematol Oncol 1993;15:92–8.
45. Ohga S, Matsuzaki A, Nishizaki M, et al. Inflammatory cytokines in virus-associated hemophagocytic syndrome. Am J Pediatr Hematol/Oncol 1993;15:291–8.
46. Arico M, Janka G, Fischer A, et al. Hemophagocytic lymphohistiocytosis: diagnosis, treatment and prognostic factors. Report of 122 children from the international registry. Leukemia 1996;10:197–203.
47. Esumi N, Ikushima S, Hibi S, et al. High serum ferritin level as a marker of malignant histiocytosis and virus-associated hemophagocytic syndrome. Cancer 1988;61:2071–6.
48. Henter J-I, Elinder G, Ost A. Diagnostic guideline for hemophagocytic lymphohistiocytosis. Semin Oncol 1991;18:29–33.
49. Henter J-I, Arico M, Egeler M, et al. HLH-94. A treatment protocol for hemophagocytic lymphohistiocytosis. Med Pediatr Oncol 1997;28:342–50.
50. Blanche S, Canigilia M, Girault D, et al. Treatment of hemophagocytic lymphohistiocytosis with chemotherapy and bone marrow transplantation: a single-center study of 22 cases. Blood 1991;78:51–4.
51. Chen R-L, Lin K-H, Lin D-T. Immunomodulation treatment for childhood virus–associated haemophagocytic lymphohistiocytosis. Br J Haematol 1995;89:282–91.
52. Stephan JL, Donadieu J, Ledeist F, et al. Treatment of familial hemophagocytic lymphohistiocytosis with antithymocyte globulins, steroids, and cyclosporin A. Blood 1993;82:2319–23.
53. Risdall RJ, McKenna RW, Nesbit ME, et al. Virus-associated hemophagocytic syndrome. Cancer 1979;44:993–1002.
54. Rosai J, Dorfman RF. Sinus histiocytosis with massive lymphadenopathy. A newly recognized benign clinicopathological entity. Arch Pathol 1969;87:63–70.
55. Tsang WY, Yip TT, Chan JK. The Rosai-Dorfman disease histiocytes are not infected by Epstein-Barr virus. Histopathology 1994;25:88–92.
56. Levine PH, Jahan N, Murari P, et al. Detection of human herpesvirus 6 in tissues involved by sinus histiocytosis with massive lymphadenopathy (Rosai-Dorfman disease). J Infect Dis 1992;166:291–5.
57. Rosai J, Dorfman RF. Sinus histiocytosis with massive lymphadenopathy: a pseudolymphomatous benign disorder. Analysis of 34 cases. Cancer 1972;30:1174–9.
58. Sita G, Guffanti A, Colombi M, et al. Rosai-Dorfman syndrome with extranodal localizations and response to glucocorticoids. Haematologica 1996;81:165–7.
59. Palomera L, Domingo JM, Olave T, et al. Sinus histiocytosis with massive lymphadenopathy: complete response to low-dose interferon-alpha. J Clin Oncol 1997;15:2176.
60. Horneff G, Jurgems H, Hort W, et al. Sinus histiocytosis with massive lymphadenopathy (Rosai-Dorfman disease): response to methotrexate and mercaptopurine. Med Pediatr Oncol 1996;27:187–92.
61. Schmidt D. Monocyte/macrophage system and malignancies. Med Pediatr Oncol 1994;23:444–9.
62. Tani M, Ishii N, Kumagai M, et al. Malignant Langerhans cell tumour. Br J Dermatol 1992;126:398–402.
63. Ben-Ezra J, Bailery A, Azumi N, et al. Malignant histiocytosis X. A distinct clinicopathologic entity. Cancer 1991;68:1050–60.
64. Levine EG, Hanson CA, Jaszcz W, Peterson BA. True histiocytic lymphoma. Semin Oncol 1991;18:39–49.
65. Soslow RA, Davis RE, Warnke RA, et al. True histiocytic lymphoma following therapy for lymphoblastic neoplasms. Blood 1996;87:5207–12.

# CHAPTER 81

# OSTEOGENIC SARCOMA

• GERALD ROSEN • CHARLES A. FORSCHER •
• FREDERICK R. EILBER • JEFFREY J. ECKARDT • YAO-SHI FU

Osteogenic sarcoma is a malignant spindle cell sarcoma that produces bone or osteoid. It may also produce cartilage (chondrosarcomatous variety) or an abundant fibrous tissue matrix (fibrosarcomatous or malignant fibrous histiocytomatous matrix). All tumors classified as osteogenic sarcoma produce some degree of bone or tumor osteoid (Fig. 81–1). Osteogenic sarcoma is the most common primary malignant bone tumor found in children and adolescents. It can occur in all age groups, however. Males are affected more than females; the male/female ratio is approximately 1.5:1.0.[1, 2]

Osteogenic sarcoma is usually a primary tumor of bone. It occurs rarely as a secondary tumor after irradiation for other malignancies. It can also occur as a soft tissue tumor. Soft tissue sarcomas, or extraosseous osteogenic sarcomas, are rare in the absence of a history of radiation therapy and are usually found in patients older than age 40. The presumptive diagnosis of an extraosseous osteogenic sarcoma in someone younger than 40 years of age should raise suspicion that a benign condition known as *myositis ossificans* may be present. Myositis ossificans is a post-traumatic soft tissue injury whose reparative process can look malignant if a biopsy specimen of the lesion is obtained within 2 to 3 weeks of the inciting event.

As is the case with other spindle cell sarcomas of bone and soft tissue, osteogenic sarcoma can occur in low-grade and high-grade malignant forms. The former is usually cured by surgery alone. High-grade osteogenic sarcoma has a propensity to metastasize to the lung and other bones. Osteogenic sarcoma occurs in certain distinct clinical settings, and some of them are considered in this chapter.

## Classic Primary Osteogenic Sarcoma

Classic primary osteogenic sarcoma occurs with a peak incidence between the ages of 10 and 20 years. It is almost always of high-grade histologic malignancy, even if not always mirrored by high-grade histologic anaplasia. Its peak incidence in females is 13.5 years and in males is 14.5 years, corresponding to the peak adolescent growth spurt in each sex. It classically involves the medullary cavity of bone, and radiographs frequently show increased density (sclerosis) as a result of the osteoid production in the primary bone lesion. Bone production within a primary osteogenic sarcoma usually takes place in the more mature or central part of the lesion, however, and the malignant spindle cell stroma can extend beyond the classic radiographic appearance of sclerosis within the bone. This intramedullary extension is best detected with a magnetic resonance imaging (MRI) scan of the lesion area (Fig. 81–2).

The most frequent site of involvement is the knee area, with the distal femur representing the most common primary site. The proximal tibia is second in frequency, and the proximal humerus is third. Rarely the tumor occurs in the distal radius and proximal femur. It is said that when one pictures the fetal position, osteogenic sarcoma occurs in the most superior parts of the bone, assuming this fetal position, that is, proximal humerus, distal radius and ulna, distal femur, and proximal tibia.

Most classic osteogenic sarcomas in adolescents are of

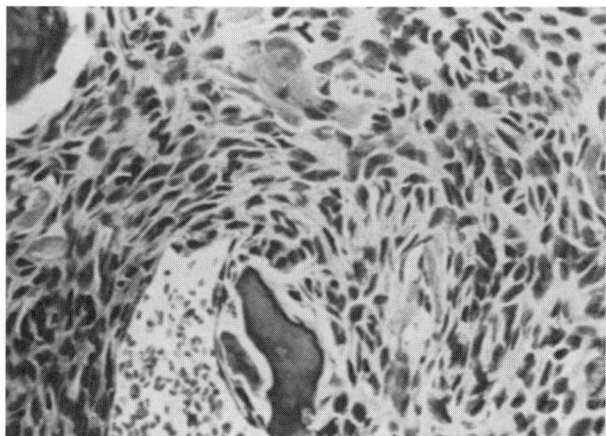

**Figure 81–1.** Bone biopsy demonstrating a malignant spindle cell stroma; note the elongated, large nuclei showing variation in size and shape. This could be either a malignant fibrous histiocytoma primary tumor of bone or an osteogenic sarcoma of bone. The demonstration of tumor osteoid production would be diagnostic of osteogenic sarcoma, however. (×400)

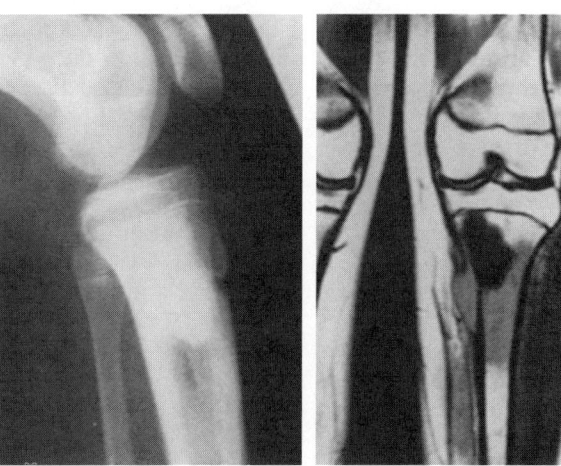

**Figure 81–2.** Osteogenic sarcoma of the proximal tibia. The radiographic appearance is that of a sclerotic lesion in the proximal tibial metaphysis. Magnetic resonance imaging (MRI) demonstrates a sclerotic bone-producing area by the intensely dark area in the proximal tibial metaphysis. However, there is extended marrow fat attenuation demonstrating tumor involvement of the proximal half of the tibia.

high-grade malignancy, but a rare low-grade form (or central osteogenic sarcoma) arising in the medullary canal of bone exists. It represents 1 to 3% of all medullary forms of osteogenic sarcoma. In these tumors, the fibrous tumor resembles a desmoid tumor (fibromatosis) with only a mild to moderate increase in cellularity. The nuclear atypia is mild and subtle, and the mitotic activity is low or absent. Osteoid deposits may be limited in amount or indistinguishable from the woven bone (immature osteoid) seen in fibrous dysplasia. For these reasons, low-grade osteogenic sarcoma is one of the most difficult bone tumors to diagnose, especially in a small, superficial biopsy specimen, which may not be representative of the lesion or does not provide the permeative pattern of marrow infiltration that is usually seen in malignant tumors. It is essential to correlate pathologic and radiologic findings to reach a correct diagnosis in these rare tumors, which often give clinicians and pathologists a difficult diagnostic problem following an incisional biopsy.

A rare malignant form of osteogenic sarcoma that occurs in children younger than age 10 is multifocal sclerosing osteogenic sarcoma. It is usually an osteoblastic lesion that presents with multiple simultaneous primary sites in the metaphyseal ends of most of the bones. In our experience, this type of rare but highly malignant tumor represents approximately 1 to 2% of all primary osteogenic sarcomas in children. It usually presents with an elevated serum alkaline phosphatase, as do approximately 50% of all osteogenic sarcomas, and there is rapid dissemination to the lung and soft tissues. Two such patients in our experience were diagnosed after the discovery of subcutaneous nodules (Fig. 81–3).

Osteogenic sarcoma can occur in various histologic forms. These have been referred to as *osteoblastic, chondroblastic, fibroblastic, telangiectatic, giant cell rich, malignant fibrous histiocytoma (MFH)–like,* and others. These terms refer to the matrix, degree of vascularity, and simulation of other primary bone tumors, such as giant cell tumor and MFH. About 50% of osteogenic sarcomas are of the osteoblastic type, in which most of the tumor matrix is composed of malignant osteoid. Chondroblastic osteogenic sarcoma shows cartilaginous differentiation in most of the matrix. There is osteoid production in all of these histologic subvarieties of osteogenic sarcoma, and production of osteoid in the predominantly chondroblastic tumor leads one to diagnose osteogenic sarcoma rather than chondrosarcoma. The convention of assigning the term *osteogenic sarcoma* to tumors even with minimal osteoid production has been adhered to because these tumors behave with high biologic aggressiveness characteristic of osteogenic sarcoma. Osteogenic sarcoma has a much higher propensity to metastasize than does the pure chondrosarcoma, for example.

The fibrosarcomatous variety of osteogenic sarcoma can resemble a fibrosarcoma histologically, or if malignant giant cells are present, the sarcoma can resemble an MFH of bone, but tumor osteoid production can be detected in parts of the lesion. The differential diagnosis between a primary MFH of bone that sometimes can produce small amounts of osteoid and a true fibrous histiocytic osteogenic sarcoma of bone is still being debated. High-grade MFH and osteogenic sarcomas are treated identically with regard to surgical procedures and chemotherapy.

The telangiectatic osteogenic sarcoma is by definition a purely lytic tumor that is sometimes difficult to differentiate from an aneurysmal bone cyst. One should always be suspicious of an aneurysmal bone cyst that occurs in the younger age group and not rest with that diagnosis until examination of adequate tissue has ruled out the presence of a telangiectatic osteogenic sarcoma. The telangiectatic variety of osteogenic sarcoma tends to grow rapidly and is highly malignant.

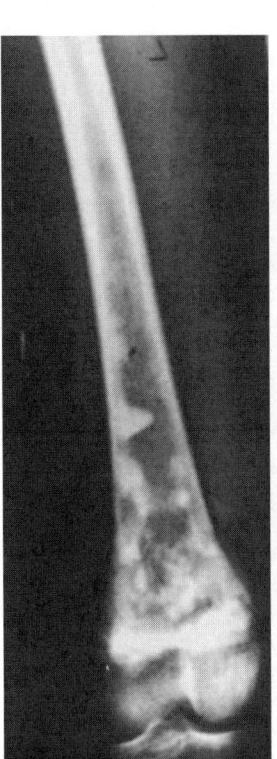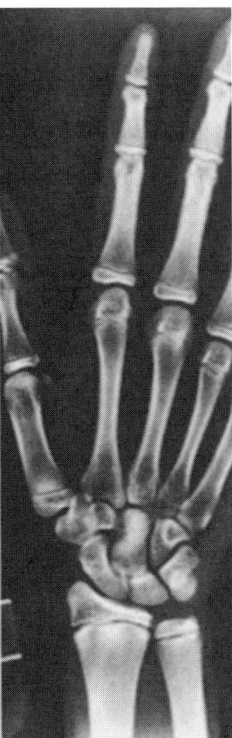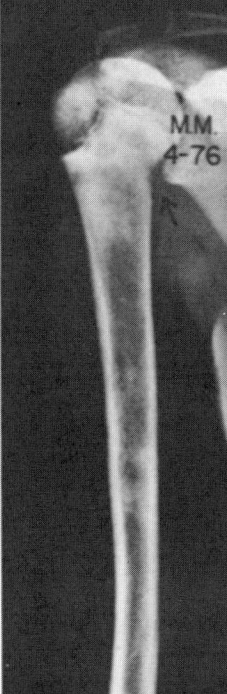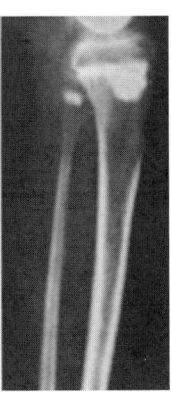

**Figure 81–3.** Multifocal sclerosing osteogenic sarcoma in a 10-year-old girl. Note the multiple sclerotic lesions in the distal femoral epiphyses. At the bottom of the picture (cut off) there is also intense sclerosis of the tibial metaphysis. There are also sclerotic lesions in the center panel in the distal radius and ulna. The humerus also demonstrates multiple sclerotic foci within that bone. The lesions within each individual bone, particularly the femur and humerus, appear to be multifocal within the bone, as well as occurring multifocally throughout multiple bones at the time of diagnosis. Fortunately, this condition is rare because it is uniformly lethal.

Telangiectatic osteogenic sarcoma histologically appears to have large, dilated vascular channels, but the lining of these channels is of malignant spindle cells. In telangiectatic osteogenic sarcoma, malignant or neoplastic osteoid production is typically noted in some of the histologic sections. Telangiectatic osteogenic sarcoma was once thought to have a uniformly lethal outcome because it is a rapidly growing tumor that behaves in a lethal fashion, metastasizing early. With the use of combination chemotherapy, as is used for other forms of osteogenic sarcoma, however, telangiectatic osteogenic sarcoma appears to be just as responsive, and cure rates are as high as in the typical osteoblastic type of osteogenic sarcoma.[3]

Small cell osteogenic sarcoma usually produces a scant amount of osteoid or cartilage. If this element is not identified, malignant lymphoma and Ewing's sarcoma should be excluded by immunohistochemical staining.

## Periosteal Osteogenic Sarcoma

Periosteal osteogenic sarcoma tends to occur in a slightly older age group; it has a peak incidence between the ages of 15 and 25. The tumor arises on the surface of the bone and is somewhat rare. In our experience, the most common site has been the diaphyseal area of the femur and the proximal tibial metaphysis. These lesions produce a characteristic radiographic appearance of arising on the surface of the bone with minimal, although usually some, involvement of the medullary canal. Histologically, these tumors resemble pure chondrosarcomas. Within the predominant chondrosarcomatous matrix, there is tumor osteoid production, however. Frequently, these tumors are mistaken for pure chondrosarcomas. These tumors arise in young adults between the ages of 15 and 25 as a rule, however, and the classic pure chondrosarcoma usually does not arise in patients before the age of 40. The diagnosis of a pure chondrosarcoma in a patient younger than age 40 should always raise suspicion that one may be dealing with a periosteal osteogenic sarcoma, particularly if the lesion is in the femur or tibia, the most common sites for periosteal osteogenic sarcoma. This differential diagnosis is important because most chondrosarcomas seen in the older age group are usually of low to intermediate grade and do not metastasize; they are treated with surgery alone. Periosteal osteogenic sarcoma metastasizes greater than 50% of the time and requires treatment with systemic chemotherapy similar to an osteogenic sarcoma.

Periosteal osteogenic sarcoma should be distinguished from parosteal osteogenic sarcoma (discussed next). The latter is usually a low-grade tumor, whereas periosteal osteogenic sarcoma is usually of high-grade malignancy.[4]

## Parosteal Osteogenic Sarcoma

Parosteal osteogenic sarcoma (or juxtacortical osteogenic sarcoma) is a distinct clinical entity. This tumor also frequently arises on the surface of bone, but in contrast to periosteal osteogenic sarcoma, it rarely involves the medullary canal unless it is far advanced. Although periosteal osteogenic sarcoma is more common in males, parosteal osteogenic sarcoma is slightly more common in females. Parosteal osteogenic sarcoma is most common between the ages of 20 and 30 and has a characteristic radiographic picture of an exophytic bone lesion that commonly occurs on the posterior aspect of the distal femur.[5] Most parosteal osteogenic sarcomas are of low-grade malignancy, containing regularly arranged bone and well-differentiated fibrosarcomatous stroma, and can be cured surgically. Occasionally, in far-advanced or locally recurrent parosteal osteogenic sarcomas, one finds a high-grade malignant stroma, indicating that the tumor is capable of producing metastases.[6]

Because parosteal osteogenic sarcoma is usually of low-grade malignancy, we recommend it be treated with surgery alone followed by careful histologic analysis of the resected specimen. If high-grade osteogenic sarcoma elements are found within the specimen, postoperative adjuvant chemotherapy is recommended.

## Osteogenic Sarcoma of the Jaw

When osteogenic sarcoma arises in the maxilla or mandible, the epidemiology is different from that of classic osteogenic sarcoma arising in the extremity. Jaw primary lesions are most common in the age range of 20 to 40 years and are more common in males than females. The tumor usually arises in the maxilla or mandible, producing pain or swelling around the gums, and is frequently detected during a dental examination. Most osteogenic sarcomas of the jaw are high-grade lesions. Patients with mandibular osteogenic sarcomas have a better outcome than those with maxillary osteogenic sarcoma because the former are predominantly of the chondroblastic type and amenable to segmental resection. Maxillary osteogenic sarcomas tend to be less differentiated and to involve the base of the skull, rendering complete surgical resection difficult at times.

In addition to the risk of local recurrence, distant metastases occur. When one encounters a high-grade osteogenic sarcoma of the maxilla or mandible, the patient should be treated in a multidisciplinary fashion with preoperative chemotherapy followed by surgical resection and then further postoperative chemotherapy, similar to treatment of classic osteogenic sarcoma of the extremity.

It frequently is difficult to obtain permanent local control of jaw tumors. The surgeon usually underestimates the extent of tumor because it sometimes appears to be well localized. We always recommend a hemimaxillectomy or hemimandibulectomy for treatment of these diseases. The most common pitfall in treating osteogenic sarcomas of the jaw is to believe one is dealing with a small localized lesion (the impression one gets from imaging studies) and to perform a segmental resection. Frequently, these lesions recur in the remnants of the mandible and grow into the infratemporal fossa, rendering it completely inoperable, leading to the patient's death, whether the tumor is of high-grade or low-grade malignancy. The reconstruction for a hemimandibulectomy or hemimaxillectomy is functionally and cosmetically good, and these surgical procedures are the procedures of choice for any osteogenic sarcoma of the jaw, no matter how small it may appear to be at diagnosis.[7, 8]

## Osteogenic Sarcoma Arising in Paget's Disease

Osteogenic sarcoma arising in Paget's disease is almost always highly malignant. It arises in longstanding pagetic lesions and is rare in persons younger than age 60. We have seen two patients in their 50s with osteogenic sarcoma arising in Paget's disease, however. The incidence of osteogenic sarcoma in patients with Paget's disease is approximately 1000 times that of the normal population. It can occur in monostotic or polyostotic Paget's disease. Because Paget's disease frequently involves the axial skeleton, osteogenic sarcoma arising in Paget's disease tends to affect the pelvis and proximal femur most commonly. Osteogenic sarcoma arising in solitary Paget's disease of the spine has also been described.

Because osteogenic sarcoma arising in Paget's disease is almost always malignant, treatment with preoperative and postoperative chemotherapy (described later) should be given to all these patients. Because they are usually older with a poor performance status and sometimes impaired renal function, these patients represent a special problem in that their tolerance for chemotherapy is not as great as that of the young adolescent with osteogenic sarcoma. With proper precautions and careful monitoring of renal function (modifications are frequently necessary in chemotherapy), these patients can be treated successfully, however. With modern chemotherapy, the prognosis for Paget's sarcoma has become much better. It will not approach the superior results obtained for the extremity lesions, however, because of the problem of local control with some of the spinal and pelvic primary tumors, which require radical surgical removal for cure of the disease as well.

## Postirradiation Osteogenic Sarcoma

Osteogenic sarcoma occurs in patients cured of other malignancies when radiation therapy has been used. Characteristically the osteogenic sarcoma occurs in the irradiated field; however, in patients who receive large doses of curative radiation therapy, there may be enough irradiation outside the planned radiation field to cause a postirradiation sarcoma in adjacent bone and soft tissue structures. Postirradiation osteogenic sarcomas are more common when higher doses of radiation therapy have been used, and it is hoped that the use of radiation therapy at lower doses combined with chemotherapy in the treatment of certain curable diseases, such as Hodgkin's disease, testicular tumors, primary lymphomas, and brain tumors, will lead to a lower incidence of postirradiation sarcomas. Classically the median time from radiation therapy to the occurrence of a postirradiation sarcoma is 10 to 11 years; we have seen a postirradiation sarcoma 4 years after radiation therapy as well as 25 years after therapy.

Most postirradiation sarcomas are highly malignant and should be treated with preoperative chemotherapy and radical resection. Because most patients receiving radiation therapy for curable diseases, such as Hodgkin's disease or lymphomas, receive axial radiation therapy, complete surgical excision of an axial tumor may not be feasible. The initial surgical resection usually leads to problems with local control, however. Use of preoperative chemotherapy may help to obtain better local control in these high-risk patients. Classically, postirradiation sarcomas occur in the sternum, sternoclavicular joint, and cervical and thoracic spine in patients treated for lymphomas, seminomas, or Hodgkin's disease; the next most common area is the pelvis in patients who are treated for pelvic malignancies. Recurrences of postirradiation sarcomas following treatment frequently have been noted to be multifocal in the irradiated area and may not represent true surgical failures of treatment but rather new primary lesions in the irradiated site.

When postirradiation sarcomas are approached surgically without preoperative chemotherapy, the typical sarcoma around the sternoclavicular joint or in the sternum is usually resected with poor margins. Postoperatively the patient never heals the extensive surgical reconstruction satisfactorily because of tumor regrowth. These patients commonly are found to have malignant pleural effusions and pulmonary metastases before their discharge from the hospital after an initial surgical attempt. It is extremely important to institute systemic chemotherapy in these patients as rapidly as the diagnosis can be made following an incisional biopsy. After a complete response to chemotherapy and shrinkage of the soft tissue mass, it is recommended that complete wide surgical excision be attempted. At that time, the patient is at much less risk for developing postoperative complications resulting from tumor regrowth or metastatic disease, or both.

## Osteogenic Sarcoma and Retinoblastoma

A rare form of osteogenic sarcoma, which sheds some light on the cause of this disease, is osteogenic sarcoma arising in patients with familial or bilateral retinoblastoma. Familial retinoblastoma is a bilateral congenital disease. It is usually treated by enucleation of the more involved eye, with radiation therapy to the other orbit in an effort to preserve sight. In such patients, the incidence of osteogenic sarcoma in the irradiated site (usually the maxilla) is 1000 times that in the normal population. Although this form of osteogenic sarcoma usually occurs in a time frame compatible with a postirradiation osteogenic sarcoma, that is, approximately 10 to 20 years after treatment for retinoblastoma, patients with familial retinoblastoma also have an incidence 500 times that of the normal population of osteogenic sarcomas arising in distant, nonirradiated sites, such as the distal femur.

All patients with bilateral retinoblastoma and approximately 10% of patients with unilateral disease exhibit DNA deletions in region 13q14 on the long arm of chromosome 13. This finding supports the *two-hit* hypothesis proposed by Knudson. Those with the bilateral, hereditary form of the disease have the initial *hit* in the germline, with the second hit in the retinal cell. In the sporadic, unilateral form, both hits occur in the retinal cell. These second hits may be associated with the ability of viral oncogenes to bind the Rb gene, leading to inactivation of the Rb gene product. A detailed discussion of the pathogenesis of retinoblastoma is provided in Chapter 2 and Chapter 77.[9–15]

Osteogenic sarcoma arising in patients with familial retinoblastoma is usually fully malignant. Tumors arising in the maxilla pose a special problem in local control. They are managed best by preoperative chemotherapy as described for classic osteogenic sarcoma, followed by radical surgical removal (hemimaxillectomy). Although this operation sounds radical, it leads to surprisingly good cosmetic results and minimal disfigurement when performed by an experienced head and neck surgeon. With any surgery less than a hemimaxillectomy, local recurrence usually follows. Because there already has been a contralateral enucleation of the eye, removal of the infraorbital ridge (usually the closest margin) is not a functional problem that otherwise would cause double vision.

## Diagnosis and Staging

Most patients who present with osteogenic sarcoma of the extremity complain of pain before soft tissue swelling. This situation is true of any primary tumor of bone because stretching of the periosteum usually causes pain before there is discernible swelling. Diagnostic radiographs are called for in most adolescents who complain of pain in the knee without a significant history of trauma. Soft tissue swelling is a late sign of an osteogenic sarcoma, which usually by then is obvious.

Characteristically the plain radiograph of the involved bone shows a mixed sclerotic or lytic lesion in the affected area. The tumor erodes through the cortex, causing elevation of the periosteum (Codman's triangle), and goes on to produce significant soft tissue swelling. Any time there is periosteal elevation in an apparent bone lesion, this is an indication for a biopsy.

Biopsy material should be obtained by a large-core tissue biopsy or, preferably, an open biopsy. The use of cytologic or fine-needle aspirations for the diagnosis of a malignant bone tumor is not recommended. This approach frequently leads to underdiagnosis or an incorrect diagnosis. The cytologic preparation of some material may make the characteristic spindle cells of a malignant spindle cell tumor become round and smaller so that the cells resemble the small cells of Ewing's sarcoma. Although the diagnosis of malignancy can be made by fine-needle aspiration and cytologic examination, the type of malignancy cannot always be determined with 100% accuracy. In our experience, fine-needle aspiration has led to the erroneous diagnosis of small cell tumor when one is actually dealing with an osteogenic sarcoma.

The treatments for these two distinct classes of malignant bone tumor are entirely different. If a core tissue biopsy or open biopsy is being done, it is important to include the cortex and inner structure of the bone as well as the soft tissue mass in the specimen because frequently the advancing edge of a soft tissue mass is more undifferentiated and does not produce osteoid. Although a specimen from the soft tissue component would lead to the diagnosis of a malignant bone tumor, the diagnosis of osteogenic sarcoma might not be evident.

Modern surgery for osteogenic sarcoma consists of limb-salvage surgery and not amputation. The principles of surgical oncology dictate that the biopsy scar be removed at the time of the definitive resection. It is important to place the biopsy tract in an area where it can be excised totally. Failure to remove a biopsy tract or needle tract might lead to local recurrence following the cessation of therapy. It is always preferable when one suspects a malignant bone tumor to refer the patient for the initial biopsy to the surgeon who would do the definitive surgery.

Once the biopsy has established the diagnosis of osteogenic sarcoma, the work-up to determine the extent of disease should be done as rapidly as possible and should include, in addition to adequate simple radiographs of the primary lesion, a computed tomographic scan to determine the extent of bone destruction. MRI is useful in determining the extent of intramedullary involvement with tumor. We scan from the proximal to the distal joint of the involved bone to facilitate accurate measurement of the tumor and ordering of a custom-made endoprosthesis for the limb-salvage surgery.

A bone scan should be done to rule out other bone metastases. A bone scan may also be helpful in determining intramedullary involvement of bone because osteogenic sarcomas, such as parosteal sarcomas or periosteal sarcomas, that arise on the surface and involve only the cortices can sometimes produce a picture of purely cortical involvement without medullary involvement on the bone scan. The computed tomographic scan is much better in discerning the intramedullary, cortical, and soft tissue extent of tumor, however.

A computed tomographic scan of the chest should be performed to rule out the presence of pulmonary metastases. The presence of small metastases at diagnosis does not preclude a cure. We have seen complete resolution of radiographically distinct large pulmonary metastases that were not detected on computed tomography (CT) performed 2 days after the first high-dose methotrexate treatment. After this patient stopped therapy, he had a recurrence of pulmonary disease in the area where he had this pulmonary metastasis to begin with, which was noted on a posteroanterior chest radiograph that was eventually sent from his referring institution. The patient did not have a thoracotomy to remove residual disease because we thought that the computed tomographic scan was negative and the original chest radiograph was poorly labeled and could have been that of someone else. It is important to obtain the computed tomographic scan of the chest before any treatment.

If the computed tomographic scan of the chest shows the presence of any pulmonary nodules, they should be resected following resection of the primary tumor or at least before stopping all therapy. Even if the nodules disappear completely, the patient should have a thoracotomy. Microscopic small deposits of residual tumor can exist that are likely to recur in the original CT-positive areas if the patient does not have a thoracotomy and removal of the residual disease (which can be readily palpated as a small *grain of sand* by the thoracic surgeon). In an adolescent with a classic osteogenic sarcoma, there is no such thing as an *old calcified granuloma* until that diagnosis is histologically established following the removal of such a lesion from the lung.

About 60% of patients with osteogenic sarcoma, or approximately 100% of patients with predominantly the osteoblastic variety of osteogenic sarcoma, have an elevated serum alkaline phosphatase level at diagnosis. The serum alkaline phosphatase should be determined before the start of treatment so that this value can be used as a tumor marker to help assess the response of the patient's tumor to preoperative chemotherapy. Highly elevated serum alkaline phosphatase levels have been associated with a poor prognosis in the past.[16] This association stands to reason because the abnormally elevated serum alkaline phosphatase is a reflection of tumor mass when the tumor is producing this enzyme. Patients with highly elevated serum alkaline phosphatase levels were noted to have a poor prognosis, as were patients with tumors of large volume.

With modern chemotherapy, the serum alkaline phosphatase, if elevated, can be used as a tumor marker, and a rapid return toward normal of the elevated serum alkaline phosphatase indicates a successful use of preoperative chemotherapy, whereas a lack of quick reduction of the serum alkaline phosphatase may be an indication that the patient's chemotherapy is ineffective, and perhaps alternative therapy should be embarked on. In our experience, an elevated serum alkaline phosphatase that rapidly returns to normal with the institution of chemotherapy leads to a good prognosis rather than a poor one.

Molecular markers, such as level of P-glycoprotein expression or HER-2/*neu* overexpression, are assuming importance as prognostic markers as well. High levels of P-glycoprotein or HER-2/*neu* are associated with poor outcomes. Novel approaches and therapies may be indicated when these markers are elevated. The integration of traditional histologic evaluation with newer molecular techniques is currently under evaluation.[17–24]

Other diagnostic studies that are helpful in evaluating the response to preoperative chemotherapy include radionuclide scanning of the regional area with thallium 201 (²⁰¹Tl) or sestamibi (MIBI), which is labeled with technetium for better resolution; MIBI, similar to ²⁰¹Tl, is now used in most nuclear medicine departments for routine cardiac scans. Both of these agents are metabolites of potassium and are rapidly taken up into cells that have an active potassium pump. This includes the myocardium as well as growing tumors. Both of these agents measure tumor cell turnover and viability rather than reactive osteoid production, which is what is measured by a routine bone scan, and can remain positive

even after tumor cells have been destroyed if the bone is repairing itself. The use of serial ²⁰¹Tl or technetium MIBI scans can predict the effect of preoperative chemotherapy by showing a decrease in uptake after 1 or 2 months of preoperative chemotherapy.[25]

We perform a baseline MIBI scan before the start of treatment and then approximately 1 month after the initiation of preoperative chemotherapy to document decreased uptake, which correlates with a good response to preoperative chemotherapy (Fig. 81–4). It is not acceptable to continue patients on preoperative chemotherapy if they are not responding to treatment because this may lead to tumor progression at the local site and distant metastases while ineffective chemotherapy is being given. This situation happens rarely; however, if one is to use preoperative chemotherapy, it is important for the treating physicians to understand and know the status of the tumor and be sure it is responding at every point during the course of preoperative chemotherapy. If the serum alkaline phosphatase is elevated because of tumor, this serves as an excellent marker as well.

Positron emission tomography is useful as an assessment tool in evaluating the response to preoperative chemotherapy. Decreases in uptake of fludeoxyglucose correlate with the amount of tumor necrosis observed at the time of surgery.[26–29]

## Treatment

### SURGERY

Historically the principal treatment for osteogenic sarcoma consisted of amputation. Because of the rare finding of skip areas of osteogenic sarcoma proximal to distal femur lesions and the usual advanced size that osteogenic sarcomas attained before diagnosis in the past, surgical cure in the few patients who were cured surgically was thought to be obtained at a joint above the location of the original primary tumor. For a lesion in the distal femur, surgery included a hip disarticulation, proximal femur lesions usually required a hemipelvectomy, and proximal humerus lesions were treated with a forequarter amputation. A suspected 25% incidence of *skip metastasis* within the same bone of involvement as the primary tumor perpetuated this radical surgical treatment (*extracompartmental amputation*). The in-

**Figure 81–4.** Serial thallium 201 scans in a patient with osteogenic sarcoma of the tibia. Note the intense uptake prior to therapy. After 2 months (or approximately two thirds of the preoperative chemotherapy regimen), there is marked diminution of thallium uptake. This patient had 100% necrosis when the resected specimen was examined histologically.

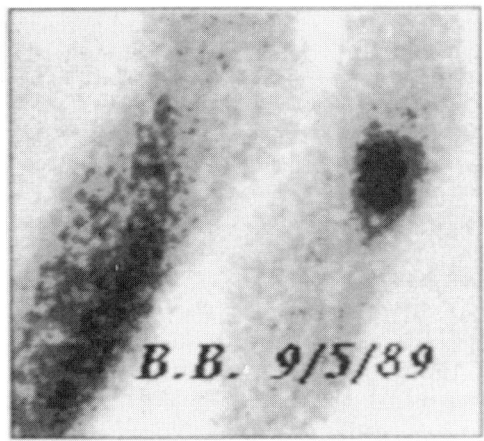
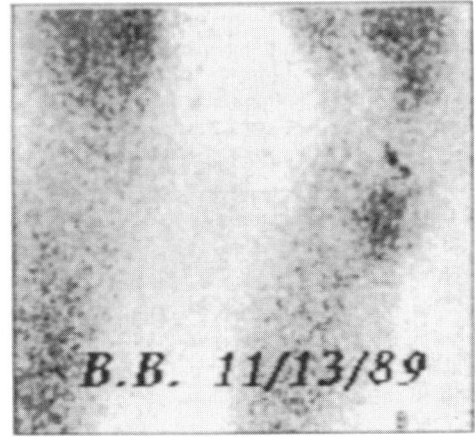

cidence of skip metastases is probably less than 10% (and was only 3.5% in 287 surgical specimens in our experience).

The rare finding of a skip metastasis can now be detected readily with preoperative MRI scans of the involved bone. Rarely, particularly in the unusual form of multifocal sclerosing disease, one can see pretherapy skip metastases on the radiograph or bone scan in addition to the MRI scan. If skip metastases are present, they are dealt with appropriately when planning surgery; however, transmedullary resections or amputations for distal femur lesions have not led to an undue incidence of local recurrences resulting from skip metastases within the bone.

Modern limb-salvage surgery for osteogenic sarcoma was first performed on a routine basis by Marcove[30] when it was decided to embark on this experimental surgery in 1973. At that time, it took approximately 2 to 3 months to have a custom endoprosthesis made to replace the tumorous bone and knee joint for distal femur and proximal tibial lesions. The desire to do limb-salvage surgery led to the era of preoperative chemotherapy.[30]

While an endoprosthesis was being produced, patients underwent aggressive preoperative chemotherapy for osteogenic sarcoma. Limb-salvage surgery was not possible until effective chemotherapy that could control the primary tumor was available because medical opinion before that time was to do an immediate amputation, lest the tumor metastasize while the primary tumor was still in situ.

Today, limb-salvage surgery is the norm for patients with osteogenic sarcoma of the extremity. Although limb function in early limb-salvage surgery patients was not good, it has improved dramatically. The primary reason for early poor function after limb-salvage surgery was the belief that the entire knee joint, including the patella, had to be resected in the treatment of distal femur and proximal tibia lesions. This belief led to sacrifice of the entire extensor mechanism of the lower extremity, and the patient's ambulation was not much better than if he or she had an amputation and an artificial limb.

After examining many operative specimens, it became apparent that few lesions of the distal femur or proximal tibia invaded through the synovial lining of the joint space. This natural barrier to tumor spread permits saving the patella and the extensor mechanism in many patients. Pioneering work by Eckardt and Eilber[31, 32] at the University of California at Los Angeles with this type of intra-articular resection for osteogenic sarcoma has led to excellent function (Figs. 81–5 and 81–6).

Another limitation to limb-salvage surgery has been in children who would have unacceptable leg-length discrepancy should they survive through their adolescent growth spurt to adulthood. This problem has been overcome by the use of the expandable endoprosthesis, that is, one that can be lengthened every 6 months to keep up with the growth of the child. This expandable prosthesis has been used successfully by Lewis in New York, Eckardt in Los Angeles, and Kotz in Vienna.[33]

The Tichoff-Lindberg resection, which involves resection of the proximal humerus, scapula, and clavicle, was first used by Marcove in New York and Salzer in Vienna as limb-salvage surgery for proximal humerus lesions. Although a radical procedure that results in no function of the shoulder joint, it is still a utilitarian operation because hand and forearm function can be preserved in most patients. It is far superior to a forequarter amputation.

With the use of preoperative chemotherapy, many large primary lesions of the proximal humerus can be shrunk to the point at which only the proximal humerus need be resected, and a proximal humeral prosthesis can allow limited shoulder function as well as hand and forearm function and a better cosmetic result (Figs. 81–7 and 81–8).

The functional results of surgery for osteogenic sarcoma have improved dramatically in the last 10 years. This improvement predominantly is due to the interests of orthopedic oncologists who entered the field because of enthusiasm about the high survival rates produced in this disease through the use of chemotherapy. Chemotherapy can now lead to cure for most patients with osteogenic sarcoma; when given preoperatively, it can shrink the primary tumor, define the surgical margins better, and decrease markedly the vascularity of the tumor before resection surgery (see Fig. 81–7).

## CHEMOTHERAPY

The development of effective chemotherapy for the treatment of osteogenic sarcoma was hampered by the fact that patients presenting with metastatic osteogenic sarcoma frequently presented late in their disease and usually had a life expectancy of less than 1 or 2 months following the onset of pulmonary metastases. Nevertheless, early studies showed that some agents, including mitomycin C and doxorubicin (Adriamycin), were somewhat effective in producing remissions in patients with metastatic osteogenic sarcoma. Mitomycin C did not produce consistent responses and produced cumulative, long-term toxicity and the rare catastrophic side effect of hemolytic uremic syndrome. Doxorubicin was the first drug to be shown to be more uniformly successful in the treatment of metastatic osteogenic sarcoma; however, it was noted early on that there was a distinct dose-response curve that existed in the treatment of metastatic osteogenic sarcoma with doxorubicin.[34] When doxorubicin is used as a single agent to treat osteogenic sarcoma, the response rate is significant only when doses of 90 mg/m$^2$ or higher are used.

High-dose methotrexate with leucovorin rescue was first shown to be effective in the treatment of metastatic osteogenic sarcoma in the early 1970s. At that time, doses in the range of 300 to 400 mg/kg (8 to 12 g/m$^2$) were necessary to obtain consistent response rates.

During the phase I and II studies of the drug cisplatin, in which it was used in fractionated doses of 20 mg/m$^2$/day for 5 days, no responses in any patient with sarcoma were noted in our experience. It was not until cisplatin was given in large doses (120 mg/m$^2$), which was facilitated by the use of mannitol diuresis to prevent unacceptable kidney toxicity, that responses were seen in metastatic osteogenic sarcoma with this agent.

The drug ifosfamide has been available in Europe since 1968. It was not until the mid-1980s that it was used in higher dose forms, however, and shown to be effective in the treatment of metastatic osteogenic sarcoma. In many European trials as well as trials in the United States, doses of 6 to 10 g/m$^2$ produced a response rate of 20 to 30% in metastatic osteogenic sarcoma.[35, 36] In our experience, escalation of the dose to 14 g/m$^2$ produced a major response

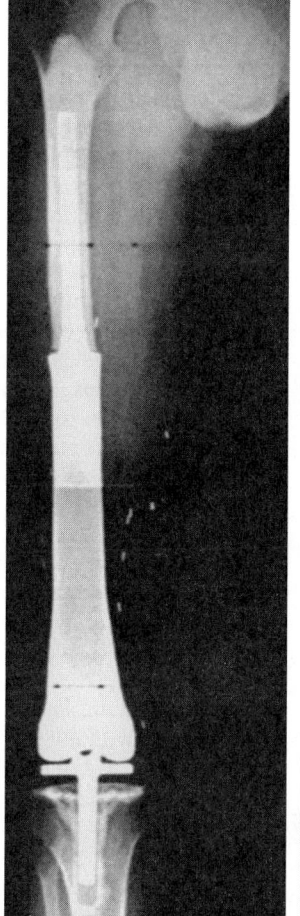

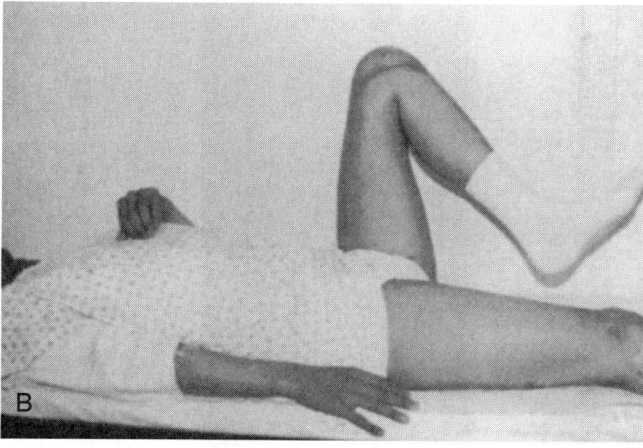

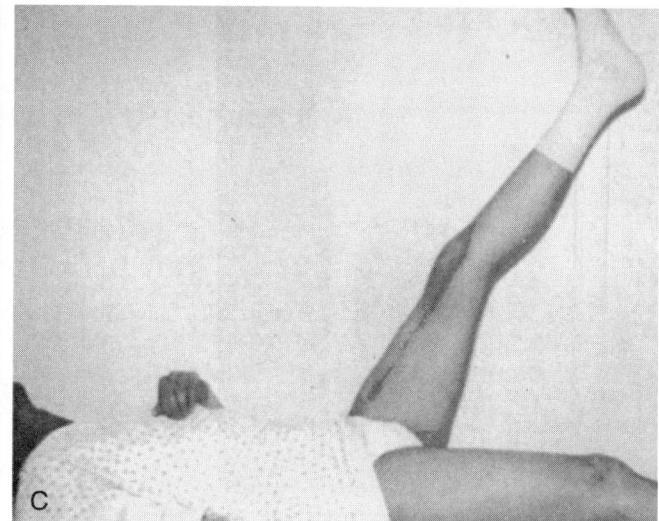

**Figure 81–5.** Endoprosthetic replacement in a patient with osteogenic sarcoma of the distal femur *(A)*. *B,* Note the almost perfect knee joint flexion with the prosthetic replacement. *C,* Total extension of the knee joint. Patients with this type of endoprosthesis have almost normal function. Their only limitation is playing contact sports.

in two thirds of patients (67%) with metastatic osteogenic sarcoma.[37] The drugs effective in the treatment of metastatic osteogenic sarcoma are listed in Table 81–1.

Combination chemotherapy effective in the treatment of metastatic osteogenic sarcoma is summarized in Table 81–2. BCD (bleomycin, cyclophosphamide, and dactinomycin) was first used in the mid-1970s.[38] This combination chemotherapy was put together in an effort to find chemotherapy effective in patients who had exhausted the amount of doxorubicin they could receive but who still suffered from metastatic osteogenic sarcoma. At that time, cyclophosphamide was commonly used in high doses (1200 mg/m²). Cyclophosphamide was combined with bleomycin and dactinomycin, which were the two other antibiotic classes of antineoplastic

agents other than doxorubicin or daunomycin that were available then.

BCD was effective in producing seven major responses in the first 13 patients with metastatic disease to be treated. BCD chemotherapy appeared to be active in the treatment of primary tumors in patients who had no prior treatment, particularly with doxorubicin. The combination of BCD was incorporated with high-dose methotrexate and high-dose doxorubicin, the other two most effective single agents in the treatment of osteogenic sarcoma, in the earliest chemotherapy protocols used for preoperative and postoperative chemotherapy for primary disease.[39]

*Table 81–1.* **Osteosarcoma Single-Agent Chemotherapy**

| Active Single Agents | Dose | Response Rate (%) |
|---|---|---|
| Mitomycin C | 0.5–1.0 mg/kg | 20 |
| Doxorubicin (Adriamycin) | 90 mg/m² | 30 |
| High-dose MTX | 8–12 g/m² | 50 |
| Cisplatin | 120 mg/m² | 20 |
| Ifosfamide | 6–14 g/m² | 20–67 |

MTX, methotrexate.

*Table 81–2.* **Osteosarcoma Combination Chemotherapy**

| Active Combinations | Dose | Response Rate (%) |
|---|---|---|
| Bleomycin | 30–40 mg/m² | up to 55 |
| Cyclophosphamide | 1200 mg/m² | |
| Dactinomycin | 1.2 mg/m² | |
| Doxorubicin (Adriamycin) | 60 mg/m² | 40–60 |
| Cisplatin | 120 mg/m² | |
| Ifosfamide | 18 g/m² | >75 |
| Bleomycin | 40 mg/m² | |
| G-CSF rescue | 480 µg/day | |

G-CSF, granulocyte colony–stimulating factor.

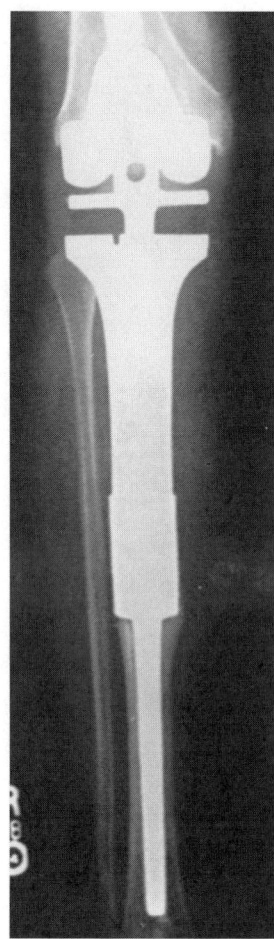

**Figure 81–6.** Proximal tibia and knee joint replacement for osteogenic sarcoma of the tibia.

Cisplatin at a dose of 120 mg/m² produced objective major responses in only 20% of patients with metastatic osteogenic sarcoma. In a series of patients with metastatic osteogenic sarcoma who were recalcitrant to single-agent doxorubicin, we added doxorubicin at the dose of 60 mg/m² to cisplatin at the dose of 120 mg/m² because the two drugs did not have overlapping toxicities at those doses. We were able to show that this combination of doxorubicin and cisplatin produced a response rate of 40%, or roughly twice that of cisplatin alone in patients with metastatic osteogenic sarcoma.[40]

With the introduction of granulocyte colony–stimulating factor (G-CSF), we have been able to escalate the dose of ifosfamide to 18 g/m². This combination of ifosfamide and G-CSF rescue has produced dramatic responses in patients with advanced metastatic disease who had become resistant to all other drugs, including ifosfamide at the dose of 14 g/m² (Fig. 81–9).

## PREOPERATIVE CHEMOTHERAPY FOR PRIMARY OSTEOGENIC SARCOMA

We first started using preoperative chemotherapy before limb-salvage surgery for the treatment of primary osteogenic sarcoma in 1973. Early protocols consisted of high-dose

methotrexate, cyclophosphamide, and doxorubicin. In 1975, after treatment of the first 30 patients, we correlated the histologic effect of the preoperative treatment with survival in patients with osteogenic sarcoma. The resected specimens of patients who underwent preoperative chemotherapy were analyzed extensively by examining 30 to 75 histologic sections from the resected tumors. We found that approximately half of the patients had no evidence of residual osteogenic sarcoma in the resected specimen (Fig. 81–10). Of the 15 patients who had no evidence of active tumor, or what we called a *good response* to preoperative chemotherapy, all 15, or 100% of them, were disease-free survivors.

At that time we defined a good response to chemotherapy as follows: After examining multiple sections from the entire resected specimen, we found the entire specimen to be totally necrotic, or we could identify only isolated foci of viable-appearing tumor cells in one or two of the multiple sections that we examined. There were no confluent, high-power (40 objective) microscopic fields of viable tumor seen in any of the microscopic sections.[41, 42] Various investigators have interpreted our good response as *80%* or *90%* necrosis; 80% or 90% necrosis is not what we would call a good response because if only 10% of the tumor is viable, there would still be numerous microscopic, high-power fields of confluent resistant tumor present after chemotherapy (Table 81–3).

In dealing with numerous pathology laboratories throughout the years, we find it is difficult to have pathologists report the tumor specimen in other than a *percentage of necrosis*. Over the years, we have nominally defined a good response to primary osteosarcoma as *greater than 95% necrosis*; however, in reality, the good response is that defined in Table 81–3. What is really important about the effect of chemotherapy on the primary tumor is not how much tumor necrosis is present but rather how much viable tumor remains. Viable tumor remaining after chemotherapy is an indication of chemotherapy-resistant tumor and represents a threat for systemic metastases.

Early chemotherapy protocols before 1976 produced cure rates only in the vicinity of 50%. Nevertheless, this was a significant advance in the treatment of osteogenic sarcoma, particularly considering that most of those patients were able to undergo limb-salvage surgery rather than amputation.

In our experience in treating metastatic and primary osteogenic sarcoma, the most effective drug in the treatment of this disease is high-dose methotrexate with leucovorin rescue. It was not until approximately 1976, when we understood fully the pharmacokinetics of methotrexate elimination and the guidelines for leucovorin rescue in the exceptional patient who does not excrete methotrexate at a normal rate, that we were able to escalate the dose of high-dose methotrexate safely to its effective dose for children, which is 12 g/m².[43] The first formal regimen to use this dose of high-dose methotrexate also used doxorubicin at a dose of 90 mg/m² and BCD chemotherapy. This protocol, which we called *T-7*, produced a 75% complete response rate in 53 patients who were given preoperative chemotherapy for primary tumors. Of that group of patients, 83% are still disease-free survivors at a minimum follow-up of 15 years at this time.[41]

With the definition of the active combination of cisplatin plus doxorubicin in 1981, we added this combination to the postoperative chemotherapy for patients who did not have a good response to preoperative chemotherapy with the T-7

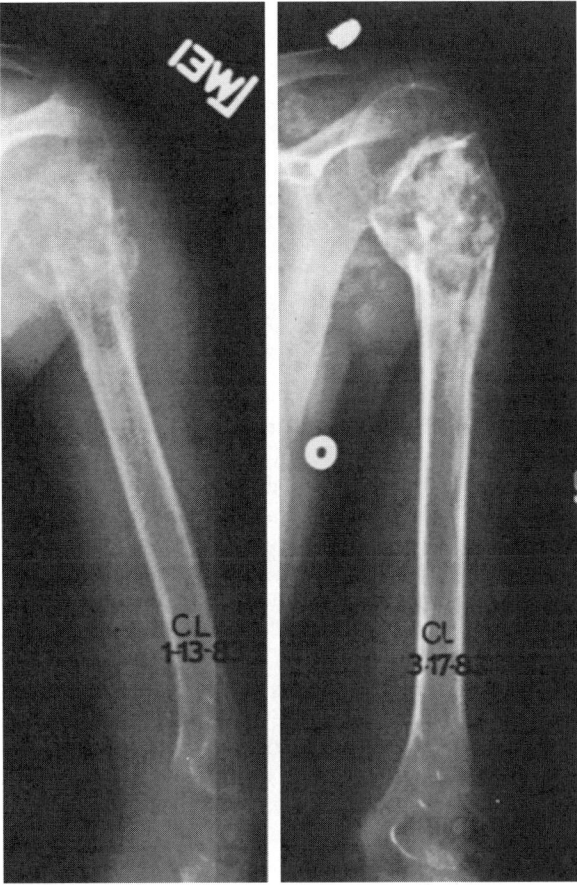

**Figure 81–7.** *Left,* Osteogenic sarcoma of the proximal humerus. There is a destructive, pathologically fractured lesion with a large soft tissue mass obscuring the picture of the shoulder joint. *Right,* After preoperative chemotherapy of only 2 months' duration, there is complete resolution of the soft tissue mass and the bone has gone on to heal. Under these circumstances, it was possible to resect just the proximal humerus, leaving the shoulder joint intact. The cosmetic results are demonstrated in Figure 81–8.

regimen. This treatment regimen became known as the *T-10* regimen.[44] Although the results were as good as those of the T-7 regimen (80% 10-year disease-free survival), we did not increase the survival rate for patients who did not have a good response to preoperative chemotherapy with high-dose methotrexate, BCD, and doxorubicin by the addition of the highly toxic cisplatin combined with doxorubicin. It appeared that patients who responded well to high-dose methotrexate–based chemotherapy continued to do well, and the addition of cisplatin combined with doxorubicin did not increase the survival rate for the few patients who were poor responders to the above-mentioned regimen.

In 1981, we modified the T-10 regimen (the *T-12* regimen) by eliminating postoperative high-dose methotrexate in patients who did not have a good response to preoperative high-dose methotrexate–based chemotherapy. Also, we stopped chemotherapy short in the good responders, with a total of only 15 weeks of chemotherapy consisting of eight high-dose methotrexate treatments and three BCD treatments. The poor responders went on to have a total of six postoperative cisplatin and doxorubicin treatments.[39] In the T-12 regimen, we did not increase the cure rate for the

patients who did not have a good response to preoperative high-dose methotrexate with leucovorin rescue. It appeared we lowered their cure rate by eliminating the high-dose methotrexate, although this was ineffective in producing a complete response in the primary tumor, for the postoperative chemotherapy course. We originally thought that switching directly to cisplatin and doxorubicin without wasting more time with what apparently was ineffective high-dose methotrexate could increase the cure rate, but instead the cure rate decreased to a 5-year disease-free survival of 67% for 81 patients treated on the T-12 regimen. This was an indication that even though high-dose methotrexate did not produce a complete response in approximately half of the patients, it was still useful in prolonging disease-free survival in some of those patients.

The next treatment regimen we embarked on replaced the BCD chemotherapy preoperatively with what appeared to be the more active combination of cisplatin and doxorubicin (T-14). After 2 years, it became apparent that the overall disease-free survival was no better than that produced by the T-12 chemotherapy regimen. The T-14 regimen eliminated high-dose methotrexate in the postoperative treatment of patients who did not have a good response of the primary tumor to preoperative chemotherapy.

With the enthusiasm for the extremely high activity of high-dose ifosfamide in metastatic osteogenic sarcoma, the T-19 chemotherapy regimen incorporated high-dose ifosfamide in the preoperative chemotherapy regimen. In this regimen, high-dose methotrexate, given as the first treatment to patients, was evaluated after only two treatments, and if a response was not apparent on clinical grounds and the thallium scan did not show improvement following two high-dose methotrexate treatments, high-dose methotrexate was dropped altogether from the treatment regimen. This treatment regimen produced two patients who had a complete response of the primary tumor to preoperative chemotherapy without further high-dose methotrexate after the first two doses. Although both of these patients had 100% tumor necrosis in their primary tumor, both developed pulmonary

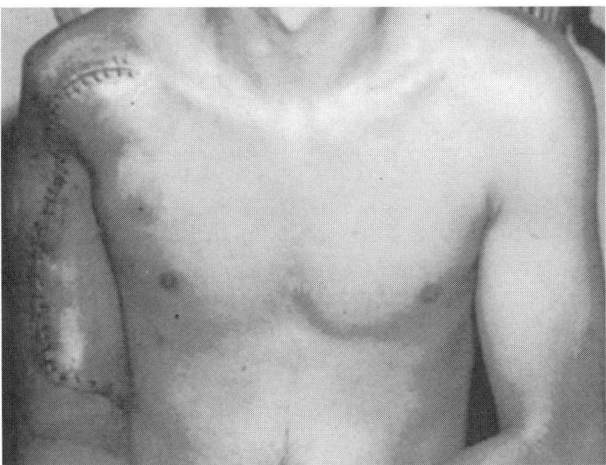

**Figure 81–8.** Postoperative picture of a patient after replacement of the proximal humerus for osteogenic sarcoma. The cosmetic result has gone on to be almost perfect, and although there is limitation in movement around the shoulder joint, the patient can use his right hand for fine motor skills.

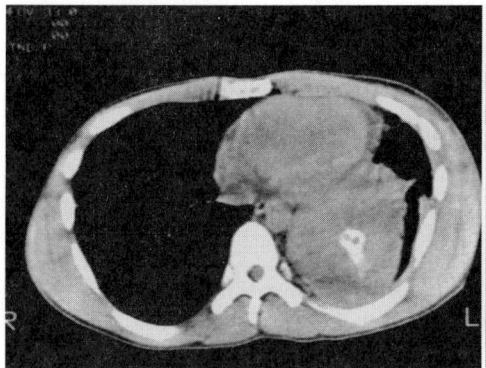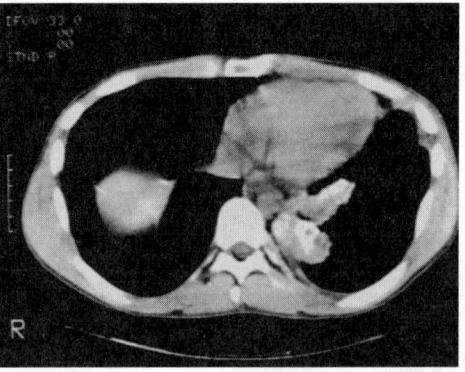

**Figure 81–9.** This patient developed a large, inoperable pulmonary metastasis after treatment with ifosfamide at a dose of 14 g/m². After surgical resection, it was noted that the tumor was totally necrotic. The patient was alive and disease free (without any treatment) 1 year later.

metastases within 6 months of completion of chemotherapy. This phenomenon had not been observed before, that is, a complete response to preoperative chemotherapy and the rapid development of pulmonary metastases.

By this time, it became exceedingly apparent that high-dose methotrexate plays a major role in the treatment of osteogenic sarcoma. All of the survival data that we had generated dealing with the prognosis related to the response of the primary tumor to preoperative chemotherapy were valid for protocols that achieved a good response to preoperative chemotherapy primarily with high-dose methotrexate and leucovorin rescue. This experience has led us to a new treatment regimen for osteogenic sarcoma to be discussed later. First, however, we review the results of treatment with the various aforementioned treatment regimens over 15 years because even though not yet ideal, the improvement in survival has been remarkable, not only in our hands but also in the hands of numerous investigators throughout the world who have adopted these types of treatment regimens for osteogenic sarcoma.

## RESULTS

Since 1976, we have treated 295 patients with preoperative chemotherapy on the T-7, T-10, T-12, T-14, and T-19 chemo-

therapy regimens. Of the entire 295 patients, the 10-year disease-free survival is 73%, with a 69% event-free survival. Approximately 4% of the total number of patients were salvaged with more chemotherapy after relapse. These results are enumerated in Figure 81–11.[39, 41, 44, 45]

Before the use of chemotherapy for the treatment of osteogenic sarcoma, children always had a worse prognosis than adults. Children 10 years old or younger had a disease-free survival of less than 10% following amputation, and adults had disease-free survivals in the range of 20 to 30%, depending on their age and the site of the primary tumor. With earlier chemotherapy protocols that produced disease-free survival rates in the range of 40 to 50%, children still did worse than adults, with disease-free survivals of around 30% versus 60 to 70% for adolescents and adults.

Since the institution of chemotherapy regimens containing 12 g/m² of high-dose methotrexate for children in 1976, our data indicate that this survival trend has been reversed, and younger children do better. In the results reported here, children younger than 11 years old who received high-dose methotrexate at the dose of 12 g/m² had a 10-year disease-free survival of 89%, which is significantly better than that of the older patients. Patients older than age 30 had the worst disease-free survival at 10 years (64%), presumably as a result of lower doses of high-dose methotrexate used for adults (8 g/m²) and the fact that many of the older patients did not have adequate renal function to tolerate the prescribed number of high-dose methotrexate treatments called for in the regimen because of renal complications (Fig. 81–12).

Because of this remarkable finding, it is now our practice to give all patients, regardless of their age, 12 g/m² of high-dose methotrexate. In patients who do not appear to respond to that dose, the dose is escalated somewhat to a range of 15 g/m². Doses higher than 15 g/m² have seldom been effective in our hands; however, it was thought that escalating the dose beyond 12 g/m² might bring the patient above the *threshold* dose for that patient, which appears to be required to make high-dose methotrexate effective in the treatment of individual patients with osteogenic sarcoma.

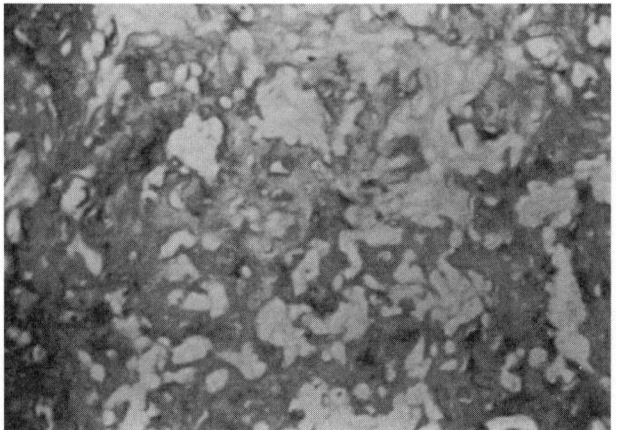

**Figure 81–10.** Representative section from a resected specimen of osteogenic sarcoma after preoperative chemotherapy. Shown in this area, which was representative of the entire specimen, is just dense tumor osteoid. There is a conspicuous lack of tumor cells within the bone lacunae, and no soft tissue tumor mass is present. This bony, hard substance represents totally necrotic osteogenic sarcoma after chemotherapy. (×400)

*Table 81–3.* **Osteosarcoma Therapy: Response of Primary Tumor**

*Good response*
Either totally necrotic or only isolated foci of viable-appearing tumor cells in one or two sections
No confluent areas (high-power fields) of viable tumor
*Note:* 80% or 90% necrosis does not represent a good response

## ENTIRE GROUP
## N=287

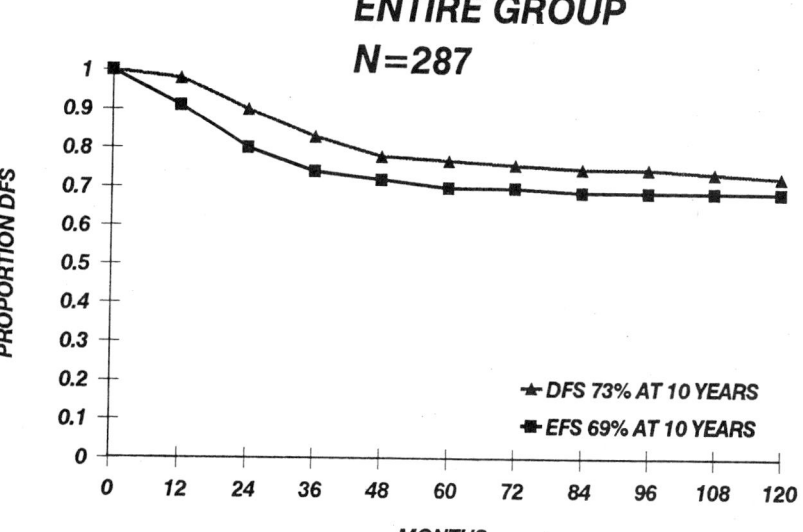

**Figure 81–11.** Survival of patients treated on the T-7, T-10, T-12, T-14, and T-19 chemotherapy regimens. At 10 years' follow-up, almost three-quarters of the patients were surviving free of disease. DFS, disease-free survival; EFS, event-free survival.

Our long-term results of therapy for osteogenic sarcoma continue to point out some important prognostic variables. The response to preoperative chemotherapy remains an important prognostic indicator. In our entire experience in the treatment of 295 patients with preoperative chemotherapy, the 10-year disease-free survival in patients with a good histologic response to preoperative chemotherapy was 92% versus 61% for patients who did not have a complete response (Table 81–4; Fig. 81–13).

The most significant prognostic variable in our patient population was a local recurrence. Even in the face of the most aggressive salvage therapy, including radical amputation and high-dose ifosfamide, as well as high-dose methotrexate and repeat thoracotomies for metastatic disease, all but 2 of the 19 patients who developed local recurrences have died of their disease. This is an extremely important reminder to surgeons who attempt limb-salvage surgery under the questionable circumstances of large tumors. There is still a place for amputation in the modern treatment of

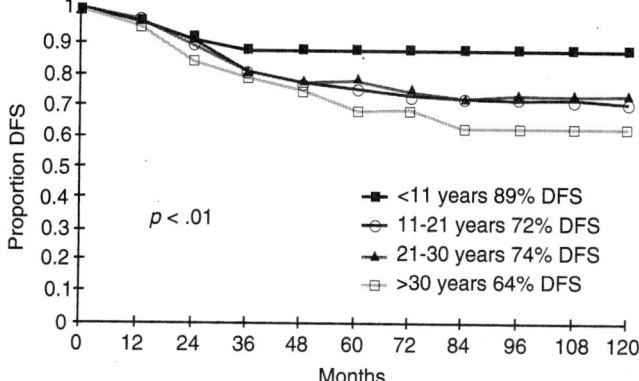

**Figure 81–12.** Survival of patients according to age. The survival of those 10 years or younger is significantly better than that of older adolescent or adult patients. This is attributed to the higher dose of high-dose methotrexate used in this age group (12 g/m²) versus the lower dose (8 g/m²) used in the older patients. Before the use of high-dose methotrexate in these dosages, children age 10 years or less had a worse prognosis than did older adolescents.

some patients with osteogenic sarcoma. The event of a local recurrence of tumor is almost a death warrant for the patient; as indicated in Figure 81–14, a local recurrence has a significant impact on survival ($p<0.00001$).

Our current chemotherapy regimen (T-20) is depicted in Figure 81–15. This treatment protocol uses high-dose methotrexate with leucovorin rescue at the dose of 12 g/m² in all patients. The few patients who do not have a complete response to preoperative chemotherapy repeat the same chemotherapy containing high-dose methotrexate with leucovorin rescue, with the methotrexate dose escalated to 15 g/m². The good responders to preoperative chemotherapy repeat the regimen (see Fig. 81–15). This regimen also incorporates ifosfamide at a dose of 18 g/m², which to date has produced the highest response rate in evaluable metastatic disease in our experience.

Doxorubicin is also used at a dose of 50 mg/m²/day for two doses (100 mg/m²). The combination of cisplatin and doxorubicin is also used; however, all patients receive only two doses of this highly toxic treatment. It is hoped that the addition of high-dose ifosfamide and high-dose single-agent doxorubicin as well as multiple courses of high-dose methotrexate for all patients will increase the cure rate to greater than that seen in the original T-7 chemotherapy regimen, which has produced disease-free survival of 83% at 15 years.

### SUPPORTIVE CARE

Since the 1980s, chemotherapy for osteogenic sarcoma has improved as a result of the availability of good supportive

*Table 81–4.* **Chemotherapy for Osteosarcoma**

| Regimen | CR (%) | DFS (%) |
|---------|--------|---------|
| T-7 | 75 | 83 (15 yr) |
| T-10 | 49 | 80 (12 yr) |
| T-12 | 44 | 67 (5 yr) |
| T-14 | 60 | 71 (4 yr) |
| T-19 | 75 | 75 (2 yr) |

CR, complete response; DFS, disease-free survival (minimum follow-up).

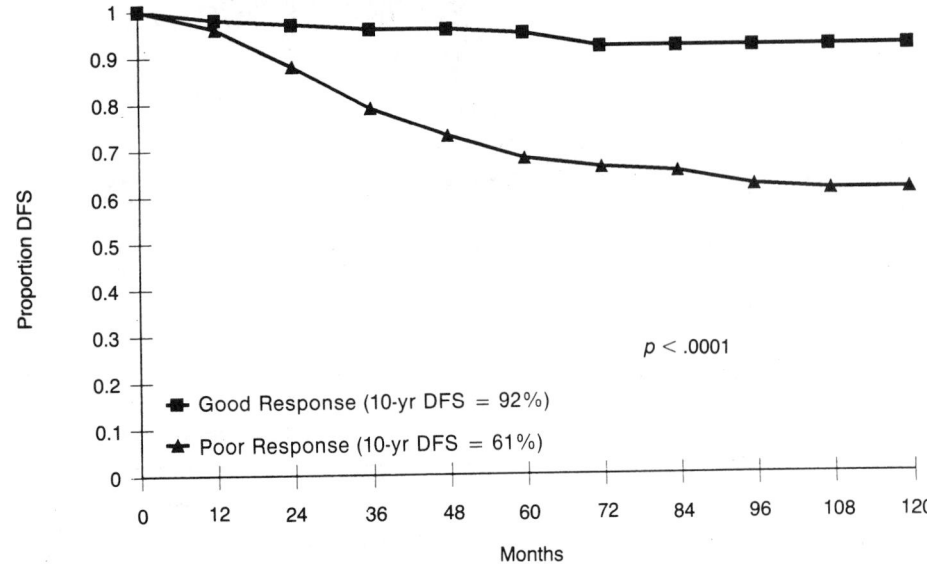

**Figure 81–13.** Survival in osteogenic sarcoma according to the histologic response to preoperative chemotherapy. Patients having a good response to preoperative chemotherapy, nominally defined as greater than 95% necrosis (which actually represents patients whose entire specimen was examined and found to be totally necrotic or contained only microscopic foci of variable tumor cells with no confluent high-power microscopic fields of tumor present), represented approximately 50% of the entire population. Their disease-free survival was 92% at 10 years, compared with 61% for incomplete (or "less than 95% necrosis") responders. The response to preoperative chemotherapy remains a powerful prognostic indicator of survival ($p<0.0001$).

care. Initially the definition of the pharmacokinetics of methotrexate and leucovorin rescue enabled us to increase the dose of high-dose methotrexate to make it effective and still safe in all patients treated. The guidelines for the administration of high-dose methotrexate with leucovorin rescue have been reported extensively by us and others.[43, 46] The use of high-dose ifosfamide at 18 g/m$^2$ and high-dose, single-agent doxorubicin at 100 mg/m$^2$ requires supportive treatment with G-CSF. This drug treatment ameliorates the profound neutropenia found with high-dose ifosfamide and seems to have ameliorated the severe stomatitis that one usually sees at these high doses of doxorubicin because these effects have not been a problem in our patients. G-CSF is administered at the dose of 480 μg/day for 7 days or longer until the patient is no longer neutropenic (if neutropenia does ensue).

All patients are followed meticulously with frequent blood counts, hemoglobin values are maintained at greater than 9.0 g/dl, and platelet transfusions are given when indicated. The need for transfusions as well as intravenous antibiotics for neutropenic fever is minimized in this treatment regimen because of the use of G-CSF. The treatment team must be continuously diligent and aware that this can happen, however, because neutropenic sepsis and the need for transfusions occur in approximately 25 to 30% of patients. The quick onset of these side effects can make a treatment regimen, such as the one depicted in Figure 81–15,

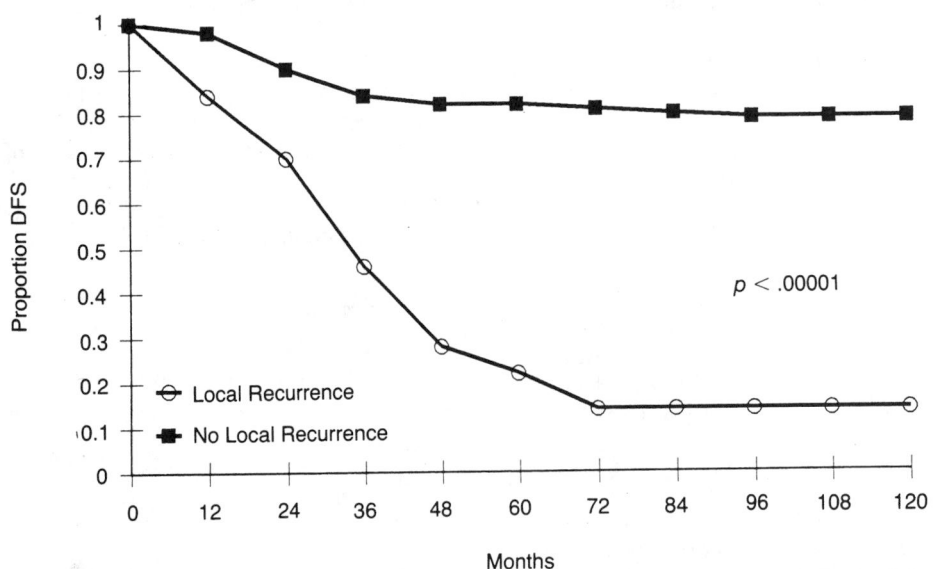

**Figure 81–14.** Osteogenic sarcoma survival by local control. A local recurrence in the primary tumor site is an extremely ominous prognostic indicator. These patients' survival is severely compromised ($p<0.0001$). We are extremely aware of the poor prognosis of patients with local recurrence; whenever a patient presents with metastatic disease, we search carefully for even the smallest of local recurrences. In two such instances, small local recurrences, which were not clinically apparent, were detected by arteriography and thallium 201 scanning. The finding of these local recurrences led to immediate amputations in these two patients, who were the only two survivors of the 19 patients who developed local recurrences in our experience.

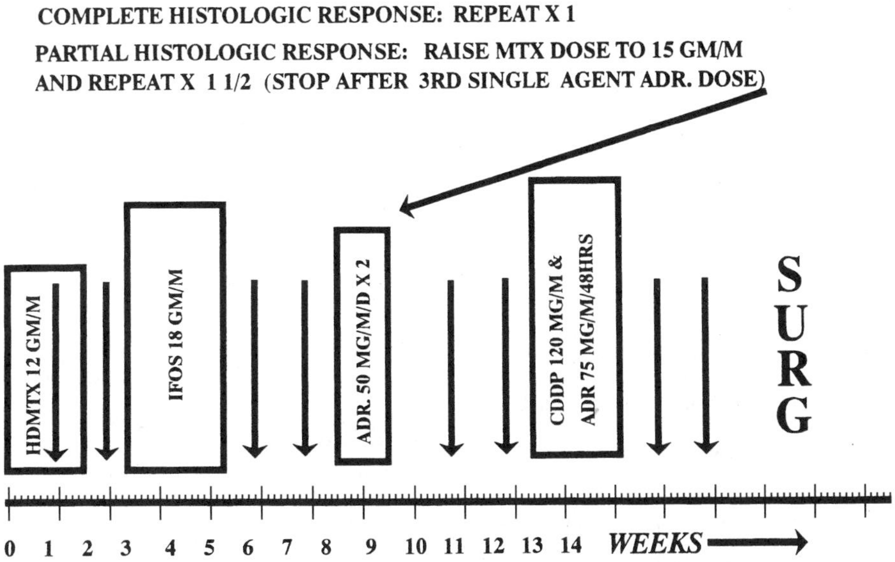

COMPLETE HISTOLOGIC RESPONSE: REPEAT X 1

PARTIAL HISTOLOGIC RESPONSE: RAISE MTX DOSE TO 15 GM/M
AND REPEAT X 1 1/2 (STOP AFTER 3RD SINGLE AGENT ADR. DOSE)

**Figure 81–15.** Our current chemotherapy regimen for the treatment of osteogenic sarcoma reincorporates multiple doses of high-dose methotrexate at a dose of 12 mg/m² for all patients. Ifosfamide (IFOS) at a dose of 18 g/m² is given over a 9-day course, with 2 g/m² given as a 4-hour bolus and then 2 g/m² daily by 24-hour continuous infusion for 8 additional days. Mesna is given at equimolar doses with ifosfamide, and patients also receive supplemental sodium bicarbonate at a dose of 200 mEq/day with 3 or 4 hours of intravenous hydration and supplemental oral potassium as well. Granulocyte colony–stimulating factor (G-CSF) is used for at least 7 days, starting the day after the high-dose ifosfamide. Doxorubicin (Adriamycin [ADR]) is given at a dose of 100 mg/m² divided over 2 consecutive days. The incidence of stomatitis has also been greatly ameliorated through the use of G-CSF after doxorubicin. Supportive care and continual monitoring of the blood counts, as well as of methotrexate (MTX) levels, is necessary in these patients. HDMTX, High-dose methotrexate; CDDP, *cis*-diamminedichloroplatinum.

extremely dangerous to use. We recommend that this chemotherapy regimen be used only in centers in which there is a team of experts containing physicians and nurses who are available 24 hours a day to monitor patients and respond to their needs at any time.

## Conclusions

Osteogenic sarcoma has become a highly treatable and highly curable disease. The treatment of this disease requires special expertise in surgical oncology and chemotherapy. Our extensive experience in treating patients with primary osteogenic sarcoma has elucidated some important conclusions. High-dose methotrexate remains the most important drug in the treatment of osteogenic sarcoma. Survival rates greater than 60% appear to be related to high-dose methotrexate utilization, even in partial responders to preoperative chemotherapy. To achieve survival rates greater than 60%, high-dose methotrexate cannot be replaced by other seemingly more active drugs. Adequate high-dose methotrexate is needed even after a complete response to preoperative chemotherapy. The premature cessation of high-dose methotrexate therapy because the patient has already achieved a complete response of the primary tumor is not an indication that the patient will be guaranteed a cure, as has been shown in the poorer results of our T-12, T-14, and T-19 chemotherapy regimens compared with the T-7 and T-10 regimens.

Several trials have suggested that the use of doxorubicin and cisplatin combinations may produce survival rates equivalent to multiagent chemotherapy, such as the T-10 regimen.[47] Although some patients may be curable with less

aggressive regimens, the goal of therapy should be to treat successfully the largest number of patients possible. The progression-free survival rates with doxorubicin and cisplatin are less than 50%, which is unsatisfactory in this disease. Newer regimens that incorporate ifosfamide and maintain the use of methotrexate produce higher rates of good pathologic responses and improved overall survival rates.[47–50]

Although we have been critical of past treatment protocols because they have failed to increase the cure rate for osteogenic sarcoma higher than that originally attained with the T-7 and T-10 chemotherapy regimens, the results obtained on these treatment regimens for patients with osteogenic sarcoma are truly remarkable. We have increased the relapse-free survival rate to the vicinity of 60% from that of 20% before the days of chemotherapy. Nearly 100% of patients are able to undergo limb-salvage surgery rather than amputation. The quantity and quality of survival for this disease have been truly enhanced.

## SUGGESTIONS FOR ADDITIONAL READING

Weis LD. The success of limb-salvage surgery in the adolescent patient with osteogenic sarcoma. Adolesc Med 1999;10:451–8.

Humphrey GM, Brown I, Squire R, et al. Extraosseous osteogenic sarcoma—a rare pediatric malignancy: case report and review of the literature. J Pediatr Surg 1999;34:1025–8.

La Quaglia MP. Osteosarcoma: specific tumor management and results. Chest Surg Clin North Am 1998;8:77–95.

van der Woude HJ, Bloem JL, Hogendoorn PC. Preoperative evaluation and monitoring chemotherapy in patients with high-grade osteogenic and Ewing's sarcoma: review of current imaging modalities. Skeletal Radiol 1998;27:57–71.

Bramwell VH. The role of chemotherapy in osteogenic sarcoma. Crit Rev Oncol Hematol 1995;20:61–85.

Kay R, Eckardt JJ, Mira J. Osteogenic sarcoma in a retinoblastoma patient. Clin Orthop 1996;323:284–7.

Ward W, Yang R, Eckardt JJ. Endoprosthetic bone reconstruction following malignant tumor resection in skeletally immature patients. Pediatr Orthop Oncol 1996;27:493–501.

# REFERENCES

1. Mirra J. Bone tumors: clinical, radiologic and pathologic correlations. Philadelphia: Lea & Febiger, 1989.
2. Huvos AG. Bone tumors: diagnosis, treatment and prognosis. 2nd ed. Philadelphia: WB Saunders, 1991.
3. Rosen G, Huvos AG, Marcove R, Nirenberg A. Telangiectatic osteogenic sarcoma: improved survival with combination chemotherapy. Clin Orthop 1986;207:164–73.
4. Ritts GD, Pritchard DJ, Unni KK, et al. Periosteal osteosarcoma. Clin Orthop 1987;219:299–307.
5. Schajowicz F, McGuire MH, Santini Araujo E, et al. Osteosarcomas arising on the surfaces of long bones. J Bone Joint Surg Am 1988;70:555–64.
6. Sauer DD, Chase DR. Case report 461: dedifferentiated parosteal osteosarcoma. Skeletal Radiol 1988;17:72–6.
7. Clark JL, Unni KK, Dahlin DC, Devine KD. Osteosarcoma of the jaw. Cancer 1983;51:2311–6.
8. Mark RJ, Sercarz JA, Tran L, et al. Osteogenic sarcoma of the head and neck: The UCLA experience. Arch Otolaryngol Head Neck Surg 1991;117:761–6.
9. Knudson AG Jr. Mutation and cancer: statistical study of retinoblastoma. Proc Natl Acad Sci U S A 1971;68:820–3.
10. Ludlow JW, DeCaprio JA, Huang CM, et al. SV40 large T antigen binds preferentially to an underphosphorylated member of the retinoblastoma susceptibility gene product family. Cell 1989;56:57–65.
11. Whyte P, Buchkovich KJ, Horowitz JM, et al. Association between an oncogene and an anti-oncogene: the adenovirus E1A proteins bind to the retinoblastoma gene product. Nature 1988;334:124–9.
12. DeCaprio JA, Ludlow JW, Figge J, et al. SV40 large tumor antigen forms a specific complex with the product of the retinoblastoma susceptibility gene. Cell 1988;54:275–83.
13. Cance WG, Brennan MF, Dudas ME, et al. Altered expression of the retinoblastoma gene product in human sarcomas. N Engl J Med 1990;323:1457–62.
14. Friend SH, Bernards R, Rogelj S, et al. A human DNA segment with properties of the gene that predisposes to retinoblastoma and osteosarcoma. Nature 1986;323:643–6.
15. Friend SH, Horowitz JM, Gerber MR, et al. Deletions of a DNA sequence in retinoblastomas and mesenchymal tumors: organization of the sequence and its encoded protein. Proc Natl Acad Sci U S A 1987;84:9059–63 and 1988;85:2234.
16. Bacci G, Picci P, Ferrari S, et al. Prognostic significance of serum alkaline phosphatase measurements in patients with osteosarcoma treated with adjuvant or neoadjuvant chemotherapy. Cancer 1993;71:1224–30.
17. Tomar G, Cohen IJ, Kidron D, et al. Prognostic factors in non-metastatic limb osteosarcoma: a 20 year experience of one center. Int J Oncol 1999;15:179–85.
18. Baldini N, Scotlandi K, Serra M, et al. P-glycoprotein expression in osteosarcoma: a basis for risk-adapted adjuvant chemotherapy. J Orthop Res 1999;17:629–32.
19. Kusuzaki K, Hirata M, Takeshita H, et al. Relationship between P-glycoprotein positivity, doxorubicin binding ability and histologic response to chemotherapy in osteosarcoma. Cancer Lett 1999;138:203–4.
20. Baldini N, Scotlandi K, Barbanti-Bradano G, et al. Expression of P-glycoprotein in high-grade osteosarcoma in relation to clinical outcome. N Engl J Med 1995;333:1380–5.
21. Serra M, Maurici D, Scotlandi K, et al. Relationship between P-glycoprotein expression and p53 status in high-grade osteosarcoma. Int J Oncol 1999;14:301–7.
22. Chan HS, Grogan TM, Haddad G, et al. P-Glycoprotein expression: critical determinant in the response to osteosarcoma chemotherapy. J Natl Cancer Inst 1997;89:1706–15.
23. Gorlick R, Huvos AG, Heller G, et al. Expression of HER2/erbB-2 correlates with survival in osteosarcoma. J Clin Oncol 1999;17:2781–8.
24. Bacci G, Ferrari S, Mercuri M, et al. Predictive factors for local recurrence in osteosarcoma: 540 patients with extremity tumors followed for minimum 2.5 years after neoadjuvant chemotherapy. Acta Orthop Scand 1998;69:230–6.
25. Rosen G, Loren GJ, Brien EW, et al. Serial thallium-201 scintigraphy in osteosarcoma: correlation with tumor necrosis after preoperative chemotherapy. Clin Orthop 1993;293:302–6.
26. Schulte M, Brecht-Krauss D, Werner M, et al. Evaluation of neoadjuvant therapy response of osteogenic sarcoma using FDG PET. J Nucl Med 1999;40:1637–43.
27. Shulkin BL, Mitchell DS, Ungar DR, et al. Neoplasms in a pediatric population: 2-[F-18]-fluoro-2-deoxy-D-glucose PET studies. Radiology 1995;194:495–500.
28. Hoh CK, Hawkins RA, Glaspy JA, et al. Cancer detection with whole-body PET using 2-[18F] fluoro-2-deoxy-D-glucose. J Comput Assist Tomogr 1993;17:582–9.
29. Hoh CK, Hawkins RA, Dahlbom M, et al. Whole body skeletal imaging with [18F] fluoride ion and PET. J Comput Assist Tomogr 1993;17:34–41.
30. Marcove RC. New trends in the treatment of osteogenic sarcoma. Orthop Dig 1975;3:11.
31. Eckardt JJ, Matthews JG 2d, Eilber FR. Endoprosthetic reconstruction after bone tumor resections of the proximal tibia. Orthop Clin North Am 1991;22:149–60.
32. Eckardt JJ, Eilber FR, Rosen G, et al. Endoprosthetic replacement for stage IIB osteosarcoma. Clin Orthop 1991;270:202–13.
33. Eckardt JJ, Kabo M, Kelley C, et al. Expandable endoprosthesis reconstruction in skeletally immature patients with tumors. Clin Orthop 2000;373:51–61.
34. Cores EP, Holland JF, Wang JJ, Sinks LF. Doxorubicin in disseminated osteosarcoma. JAMA 1972;221:1132–8.
35. Antman KH, Elias A, Ryan L. Ifosfamide and mesna: response and toxicity at standard- and high-dose schedules. Semin Oncol 1990;17:Suppl 4:68–73.
36. Gasparini M. High-dose ifosfamide alone and in combination for solid malignancies in childhood. Cancer Chemother Pharmacol 1986;18:Suppl 2:S18.
37. Chawla SP, Rosen G, Lowenbraun S. Role of high dose ifosphamide (HDI) in recurrent osteosarcoma. Proc ASCO 1990;9:310.
38. Mosende C, Gutierrez M, Caparros B, Rosen G. Combination chemotherapy with bleomycin, cyclophosphamide and dactinomycin for the treatment of osteogenic sarcoma. Cancer 1977;40:2779–86.
39. Rosen G. Preoperative (neoadjuvant) chemotherapy for osteogenic sarcoma: a ten year experience. Orthopedics 1985;8:659–64.
40. Rosen G. Cisplatinum in metastatic osteogenic sarcoma. In: Prestayko AW, Crooke ST, Carter SK, eds. Cisplatin—current status and new developments. New York: Academic Press, 1980:465.
41. Rosen G, Marcove RC, Caparros B, et al. Primary osteogenic sarcoma: the rationale for preoperative chemotherapy and delayed surgery. Cancer 1979;43:2163–77.
42. Rosen G, Murphy ML, Huvos AG, et al. Chemotherapy, en bloc resection, and prosthetic bone replacement in the treatment of osteogenic sarcoma. Cancer 1976;37:1–11.
43. Rosen G, Nirenberg A. Chemotherapy for osteogenic sarcoma: an investigative method, not a recipe. Cancer Treat Rep 1982;66:1687–97.
44. Rosen G, Caparros B, Huvos AG, et al. Preoperative chemotherapy for osteogenic sarcoma: selection of postoperative adjuvant chemotherapy based on the response of the primary tumor to preoperative chemotherapy. Cancer 1982;49:1221–30.
45. Glasser DB, Lane JM, Huvos A, et al. Survival, prognosis, and therapeutic response in osteogenic sarcoma: the Memorial Hospital experience. Cancer 1992;69:698–708.
46. Grem JL, King SA, Wittes RE, Leyland-Jones B. The role of methotrexate in osteosarcoma. J Natl Cancer Inst 1988;80:626–55.
47. Souhami RL, Craft AW, Van der Eijken JW, et al. Randomised trial of two regimens of chemotherapy in operable osteosarcoma: a study of the European Osteosarcoma Intergroup. Lancet 1997;350:911–7.
48. Bramwell V, Burgers M, Sneath R, et al. A comparison of two short intensive adjuvant chemotherapy regimens in operable osteosarcoma of limbs in children and young adults: the first study of the European Osteosarcoma Intergroup. J Clin Oncol 1992;10:1579–91.
49. Bielack S, Kempf-Bielack B, Schwenzer D, et al. Neoadjuvant therapy for localized osteosarcoma of extremities: results from the Cooperative Osteosarcoma Study Group (COSS) of 925 patients. Klin Pediatr 1999;211:260–70.
50. Philip T, Blay JY, Brunat-Mentigny M, et al. Standards, options and recommendations (SOR) for diagnosis, treatment and follow-up of osteosarcoma. Bull Cancer 1999;86:159–76.

# CHAPTER 82

# EWING'S SARCOMA

• GERALD ROSEN • CHARLES A. FORSCHER •
• FREDERICK R. EILBER • JEFFREY J. ECKARDT • YAO-SHI FU

## Natural History

### OVERVIEW

Ewing's sarcoma of bone is a rare malignancy affecting primarily adolescents. It was originally described by Ewing in 1921.[1] Ewing's sarcoma of bone differs markedly from osteogenic sarcoma (the most common malignant bone tumor seen in adolescents and young adults) in that it is composed of primitive, small round cells rather than the typical spindle cell stroma seen in osteogenic sarcoma and the soft tissue sarcomas of adults. Ewing's sarcoma has a propensity to occur in the diaphysis, or midshaft, of long bones rather than the metaphysis, which is most common for osteogenic sarcoma. Metaphyseal Ewing's sarcomas do occur, however. Ewing's sarcoma also has a propensity to occur in the flat bones of the pelvis as well as the scapula and spine. As noted previously, Ewing's sarcoma is primarily a disease of children and adolescents, rarely occurring in adults older than age 25. In the rare instance when older patients are diagnosed as having Ewing's sarcoma, one has to be certain that the diagnosis is not a primary lymphoma of bone, which becomes more common in adults but also occurs in children and adolescents. Ewing's sarcoma of bone in anyone older than age 21 has a poor prognosis.

Before the use of systemic chemotherapy for the treatment of Ewing's sarcoma, the natural history of the disease was dismal. When the tumor was treated with local therapy alone, good local control appeared to be attainable with megavoltage high-dose radiation therapy to the entire involved bone or radical surgery (amputation). Only approximately 10% of the patients survived with local therapy alone. Within 1 year of treating the primary tumor, approximately 90% of patients developed disseminated bone and pulmonary metastases. Ewing's sarcoma disseminates to the lung and other bones. Involvement of other bones is more common than in osteogenic sarcoma. The most frequent site of metastatic disease is the lung, followed by the skull, pelvis, and other bones. The most common site of primary tumor involvement of Ewing's sarcoma is the femur, followed by the pelvis and other long bones. The flat bones, such as the ribs, vertebral bodies, and scapula, can also be sites of primary disease.[2, 3]

In 1974, we described the first successful use of a four-drug, adjuvant chemotherapy protocol to increase the cure rate in Ewing's sarcoma.[4] In that first small series of patients using four drugs, including doxorubicin (Adriamycin), cyclophosphamide, vincristine, and dactinomycin, we achieved 75% disease-free survival in patients with localized Ewing's sarcoma. This experience heralded the onset of the use of adjuvant or systemic chemotherapy, which produced dramatic improvement in the treatment and prognosis of Ewing's sarcoma.

With most patients surviving disease after adjuvant treatment, it became apparent that the natural history of Ewing's sarcoma treated with radiation therapy included local recurrences after short or prolonged intervals if patients did not die of metastatic pulmonary disease. This observation was made possible only after the dramatic decrease in the occurrence of metastases brought about by the use of adjuvant chemotherapy. In patients who relapsed with metastatic disease after adjuvant chemotherapy, many were noted to harbor local recurrences in the primary, irradiated site.

We had one patient develop a local recurrence of Ewing's sarcoma of the pelvis 14 years after treatment with radiation for the primary tumor. The recurrence was Ewing's sarcoma and not a postirradiation sarcoma, which is usually a spindle cell sarcoma such as osteogenic sarcoma or malignant fibrous histiocytoma. This new understanding of the natural history of Ewing's sarcoma as a result of treatment with chemotherapy has led to important considerations for the treatment of the primary tumor with surgery and radiation therapy.[5]

### DIAGNOSIS

Characteristically, Ewing's sarcoma presents as a painful, diaphyseal lesion in one of the long bones, such as the femur or tibia. It can also present as a soft tissue swelling associated with a painful lesion in a flat bone, such as the pelvis or scapula. The diaphyseal long bone lesion has a characteristic *onionskin* appearance, caused by periosteal new bone being produced as the periosteum is being pushed out of the bone and into the soft tissue. This onionskin appearance can be seen in flat bone lesions as well, but it is not necessarily diagnostic of Ewing's sarcoma (Figs. 82–1 and 82–2). Magnetic resonance imaging (MRI) of the involved bone usually shows extensive marrow involvement as well (Fig. 82–3).

The differential diagnosis of Ewing's sarcoma on histologic examination of a biopsy specimen must exclude any round cell tumor that can arise in bone. The most important differential diagnosis exists between Ewing's sarcoma and primary lymphoma of bone. Ewing's sarcoma tends to be more of a lytic destructive lesion than lymphoma, which tends to have a mixed sclerotic and lytic appearance on radiography or an entirely sclerotic appearance as a result of reactive bone formation secondary to tumor destruction within the bone. Ewing's sarcoma of bone usually has a relatively greater soft tissue mass compared with a primary lymphoma of bone (see Fig. 82–3). Primary lymphomas of bone can develop significant soft tissue masses but usually

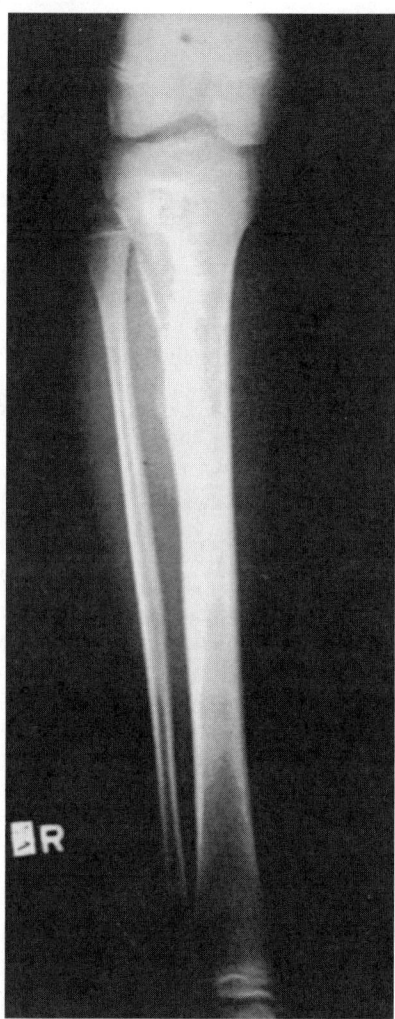

**Figure 82–1.** Radiograph of Ewing's sarcoma of the tibia. There is a discernible lytic lesion in the superior lateral aspect of the tibia. Just below that, periosteal elevation typical of Ewing's sarcoma can be seen. Differential diagnosis includes possible osteomyelitis.

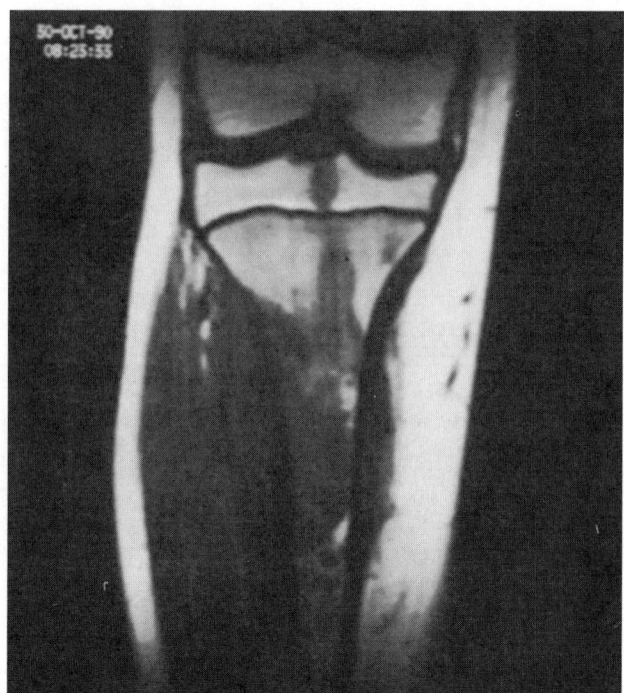

**Figure 82–2.** Ewing's sarcoma of the proximal tibia: magnetic resonance image of the lesion depicted in Figure 82–1. Note the extensive involvement of the medullary canal of the tibia. Medullary involvement of tumor is much better appreciated on MRI than on radiography.

bone lesion includes Ewing's sarcoma of bone, osteomyelitis, or perhaps both.

Histologically, Ewing's sarcoma consists of sheets of small, round cells with small, round nuclei containing *smoky* chromatin and prominent nucleoli. The cells and nuclei are monotonously uniform in shape, and cytoplasmic borders are relatively indistinct (Fig. 82–4). Lymphomas show more hyperchromatism, plumper nuclei, more variation in size and shape, and more distinct cytoplasmic borders. The histo-

do so late in their course. The presenting symptoms of Ewing's sarcoma of bone are usually pain and soft tissue swelling, whereas a lymphoma may present with only pain for a longer period without significant soft tissue swelling. These are only relative differences between the presentation of the two diseases; the clinician must be aware that primary lymphomas of bone do occur in the same age group as do Ewing's sarcomas.

It has been said that fever is part of the clinical picture of Ewing's sarcoma. This may be true, but we believe that fever associated with Ewing's sarcoma may be the result of secondary osteomyelitis. It is well known that Ewing's sarcoma grows rapidly and frequently produces a great deal of necrosis within the tumor. The finding of pus at open biopsy does not rule out the presence of Ewing's sarcoma, and any time the diagnosis of Ewing's sarcoma is suspected and a biopsy is done, one should always take adequate tissue for histologic and microbiologic evaluation if what appears to be pus is encountered. Frequently the *pus* is necrotic Ewing's sarcoma or Ewing's sarcoma that is secondarily infected. The differential diagnosis of periosteal elevation in a painful

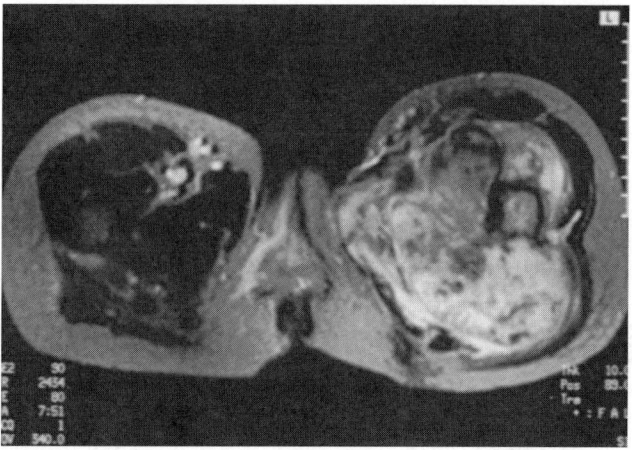

**Figure 82–3.** Ewing's sarcoma of the proximal femur. Note the extensive, large soft tissue mass filling the entire posterior, medial, and portion of the anterolateral compartments of the soft tissues of the proximal thigh on this T2-weighted MRI scan. Ewing's sarcoma characteristically produces much larger soft tissue masses in the primary site than do other small cell sarcomas of bone (e.g., lymphomas of bone).

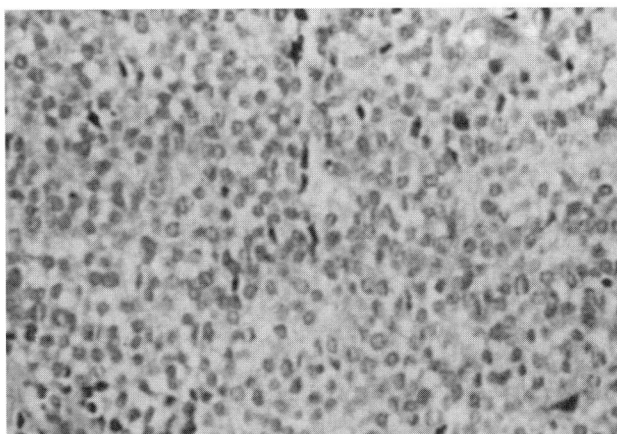

**Figure 82–4.** Histologic high-power microscopic field of a Ewing sarcoma. Note the monotonous array of small, round, slightly vesiculated nuclei with prominent nucleoli. The cytoplasmic borders are typically indistinct.

logic differential diagnosis of Ewing's sarcoma includes all other small round cell tumors.

The diagnosis of Ewing's sarcoma was traditionally made by exclusion and by the presence of glycogen using the periodic acid–Schiff stain.[6] The current use of immunohistochemistry has markedly improved the diagnostic accuracy for Ewing's sarcoma, especially the availability of monoclonal antibody HBA-71 against the cell-surface antigen P-30/32$^{mic2}$. However, lymphoblastic lymphoma, acute lymphoblastic leukemia, and rare sarcomas and carcinomas may react with the HBA-71 monoclonal antibody.[7] Greater than 90% of Ewing's sarcomas react with HBA-71 and antivimentin. Vimentin is a cytoskeletal protein expressed by almost all types of mesenchymal cells. PNET does not express vimentin but expresses neuron-specific enolase, S-100 protein, and neurofilament proteins.

Ewing's sarcoma and PNET have similar reciprocal translocations t(11;22) (q24;12). In view of these two tumors sharing a similar genetic marker and their cytogenetic similarities, their histologic relationship is probably closer than previously realized (however, we have always thought that Ewing's sarcoma and PNET should be treated in the same manner).[8–10] With the demonstration of similar cytogenetic markers, our original suggestion that the treatment of these tumors was similar has now been adopted by most of the oncology community. The most common fusion protein EWS-FLI 1 is produced by this translocation. Its presence can be detected by fluorescent in situ hybridization or reverse transcriptase–polymerase chain reaction. Detection of this protein can aid in rapid confirmation of the diagnosis. A study has suggested that the specific EWS-FLI 1 variant has prognostic significance as well (type 1 has a better prognosis than other types).[11–13]

Most lymphomas are common leukocyte antigen positive, and additional B- and T-lymphocyte markers can distinguish them from Ewing's sarcoma. It is preferable to distinguish a lymphoma from Ewing's sarcoma of bone on the basis of radiographic, clinical, and morphologic appearance, however. In our experience, immunoperoxidase stains applied to bone biopsy specimens may lead to an erroneous diagnosis because decalcification of the bone specimen can often invalidate the accuracy of immunoperoxidase stains.

If properly used, immunoperoxidase stains can distinguish between primary Ewing's sarcoma and metastatic rhabdomyosarcoma. Muscle antigen tests, such as immunoperoxidase stains for myoglobin, myosin, or common muscle antigen, are positive only for patients with rhabdomyosarcoma.

Metastatic neuroblastomas can be distinguished from Ewing's sarcomas by the immunohistochemical expression of neuroendocrine markers such as S-100 protein, chromogranin, and synaptophysin, and nonreactivity with HBA-71 antibody. PNETs are treated in the same way as Ewing's sarcoma. The latter is noted for its total lack of differentiation; it stains positively only for vimentin on immunoperoxidase staining and, as noted previously, it reacts positively with the HBA-71 monoclonal antibody.

The lack of a finding of differentiation markers in small cell sarcomas that arise in soft tissue has led to the classification of a soft tissue tumor called *extraosseous Ewing's sarcoma*. This latter entity is treated in a fashion similar to Ewing's sarcoma of bone, with one important exception. Primary small cell sarcomas of bone, such as Ewing's sarcoma, do not metastasize to regional lymph nodes. Primary small cell sarcomas of soft tissue origin, however, such as embryonal rhabdomyosarcomas, small cell liposarcomas, Merkel cell tumors, and extraosseous Ewing's sarcoma, have at least a 20% incidence of regional node involvement. When one is dealing with extraosseous Ewing's sarcoma, treatment differs in that regional lymph nodes must be biopsied and sometimes given radiation therapy if positive nodes are found or suspected.

## PRETREATMENT WORK-UP

Once the diagnosis of Ewing's sarcoma is established, the patient should undergo additional imaging studies, including a computed tomographic scan of the chest to rule out pulmonary metastases. It is important to do this immediately before starting therapy because Ewing's sarcoma is exquisitely sensitive to chemotherapy, and small pulmonary metastases that exist before the start of treatment can disappear completely within 1 or 2 days of the beginning of treatment. This staging is an important aspect of treatment because if pulmonary metastases are present at the time of diagnosis, they can recur after chemotherapy is finished. The addition of bilateral pulmonary irradiation to patients who have been noted to have small pulmonary metastases before treatment, however, has resulted in cure rates almost as high as those obtained for patients with primary tumor only at the start of treatment.[15]

A bone scan should be done to rule out the presence of other bone metastases. Particular attention should be paid to the skull, which is the most frequent bone site of metastatic disease in Ewing's sarcoma. An entire body scan should be done. We have seen patients referred with bone scans limited to the lesion area or region of the body containing the primary lesion. This type of bone scan is inadequate for staging of Ewing's sarcoma. MRI of the involved extremity should be performed. It shows the extent of marrow involvement within the bone and acts as a guideline for the surgeon, who eventually resects the involved bone as part of the multidisciplinary treatment plan for Ewing's sarcoma.

Bone marrow aspiration should be performed to rule out early bone marrow involvement. Although such involvement is usually a late phenomenon in the natural history of Ewing's sarcoma, it can be found in some patients who have had longstanding, extensive lesions, such as those in the pelvis, which can go undiagnosed for long periods. Early extensive involvement of bone marrow, particularly diffuse involvement, is a more common phenomenon in the lymphomas of children and adolescents than in Ewing's sarcoma.

As noted earlier, extraosseous Ewing's sarcomas have a 20 to 30% chance of metastasizing to regional lymph nodes, and in the work-up for that disease, we perform regional node biopsies before starting treatment. The incidence of regional node involvement in Ewing's sarcoma of bone is extremely low, and in our experience it has never occurred. Regional node dissection or sampling is not indicated in primary Ewing's sarcoma of bone. The presence of regional nodes that are clinically positive should lead one to suspect that the small cell sarcoma is of soft tissue origin and secondarily involves bone or may be a primary lymphoma of bone that does metastasize to regional lymph nodes. In suspected primary Ewing's sarcoma in a small child, in which the incidence of neuroblastoma is higher and the probability of metastatic neuroblastoma is high on the differential diagnosis list, it may be wise to order an intravenous pyelogram or do a computed tomographic scan of the abdomen to look at the adrenal glands and paraspinal structures to detect an undiagnosed primary neuroblastoma.

## Treatment

The use of primary radiation therapy and adjuvant chemotherapy to produce a high survival rate in Ewing's sarcoma had led to the observation that many treatment failures were due to local recurrences. This observation was thought to be particularly true in the bulkier pelvic tumors, but in our experience it was just as true in smaller extremity primaries. The Intergroup Ewing's Sarcoma Study reported a local recurrence rate of approximately 30% in pelvic lesions after radiation therapy alone. This group also reported almost a 30% local recurrence rate in humerus lesions.[16]

These lesions included ones that were documented histologically; however, most of the patients in that study did not have adequate follow-up to determine whether those who relapsed did have a local recurrence. Many patients died at home or under the care of family physicians after they had relapses, and the autopsy rate in this group was not high. It is suspected that the local recurrence rate in pelvic lesions is much higher than 30%. In our experience, axial lesions, including those of the pelvis treated with radiation therapy alone, have a local recurrence rate that approaches 100%. The one patient we treated who was a disease-free survivor after primary radiation therapy to a large, inoperable pelvic lesion relapsed with a local recurrence 14 years after radiation therapy. Histologic biopsy of the recurrence documented it to be Ewing's sarcoma similar to that the patient originally had 14 years earlier.

We initially advocated the use of surgical resection for all patients with Ewing's sarcoma in the mid-1970s, after we observed that survivors who underwent chemotherapy

develop local recurrences.[5] Although there was a great deal of controversy at that time, most of the oncology community has accepted the fact that the use of surgery as well as radiation therapy is extremely important in the management of primary Ewing's sarcoma. We reported a significant increase in the cure rate for patients with pelvic Ewing's sarcomas treated with surgery plus radiation therapy compared with those treated without surgery. Other groups, including the Mayo Clinic and the German-Austrian Cooperative Ewing's Sarcoma Study groups, have also reported much higher cure rates in patients who have had surgical treatment of the primary tumor.

Nevertheless, radiation therapy plays an important role in the treatment of Ewing's sarcoma. As mentioned earlier, radiation can be curative in patients who present with pulmonary metastases when they are given postchemotherapy bilateral pulmonary irradiation in small doses after a complete remission has been obtained. We have given bilateral prophylactic lung irradiation to patients who presented with pulmonary metastases after they had gone into complete remission at the dose rate of 1 Gy/day for 14 doses. This small biologic dose of radiation appears to be effective in preventing once-present pulmonary metastases from returning after chemotherapy is stopped. This effectiveness has also been observed in the European Intergroup Study.[17]

We believe that radiation therapy plays a role in treatment of the primary tumor. We treat the entire involved bone with radiation therapy to a dose of 45 Gy. When possible, we prefer to avoid the growing epiphyseal ends of the bone in young children; however, we obtain a margin of at least several centimeters above and below where the tumor is identified in the medullary cavity on the MRI scan of the primary tumor.

Radiation therapy is particularly important in dealing with rib lesions. Rib lesions have a high propensity to recur in the thoracic cage area and, in particular, produce *dropped* metastases to the diaphragm. Because of these phenomena, patients who have had primary Ewing's sarcomas of the rib have usually had a poor prognosis. Most PNETs arise in the chest wall, and many Ewing's sarcomas of the rib are now classified as PNETs. This tumor also was known for its poor prognosis because of multiple recurrences in the thoracic area. With the judicious use of radiation therapy, as described later, and surgery, primary rib lesions of Ewing's sarcoma or PNET can have cure rates as favorable as those of primary Ewing's tumors of other areas.

In primary rib lesions, concomitant with the use of systemic chemotherapy, we give radiation therapy to a dose of 45 Gy to a large field, including one rib space above the location of the lesion all the way down to and including the diaphragm. The entire chest wall and pleura are irradiated as well as the entire diaphragm. This approach requires sophisticated radiation planning. Sometime electrons can be used for the chest wall with a photon boost to the diaphragm, or photons alone can be used with multiple fields to avoid irradiating the lung and underlying mediastinal structures. With this type of therapy and the surgical resection of the entire involved rib, patients with rib lesions can have a good prognosis or at least one as good as that of those with small primary extremity lesions.

The entire rib must be resected from the costosternal junction to the costovertebral junction because small portions

*Table 82–1.* **Ewing's Sarcoma of Chest or Rib\*: Characteristics**

Recurs after irradiation
Recurs in remaining involved rib
Recurs in pleural spaces and on diaphragm

\*Includes primitive neuroectodermal tumor of soft tissue origin.

of rib left in situ have been known to harbor disease that becomes manifest later on in the patient's life. The theory that the entire marrow cavity of the involved bone is usually microscopically involved with Ewing's sarcoma at the time of diagnosis seems to be particularly true in the case of rib lesions. In our experience, radiation therapy to the entire rib has not prevented recurrences in small pieces of rib that were left behind, even after the lesion area was excised (Tables 82–1 and 82–2).

## SURGERY

Surgical resection of Ewing's sarcoma in all patients is advisable. Since the mid-1980s, all primary Ewing's sarcoma lesions have been subjected to surgical resection as part of combined-modality treatment. Most patients undergo limb-salvage surgery. Preoperative chemotherapy and preoperative radiation therapy usually bring about total regression of the soft tissue component in most tumors. This preoperative therapy makes surgical excision and safe limb-salvage surgery possible, as it does in osteogenic sarcoma. In Ewing's sarcoma, chemotherapy is usually much more effective in eliminating totally all soft tissue components of the tumor, and the addition of 45 Gy of radiation therapy to the entire bone as preoperative therapy ensures temporary sterilization of the bone before resection of the lesion area.

Surgical resection may consist of resection of the diaphysis of the tumor in a long bone with the insertion of an intercalary device, as depicted in Figure 82–5. Lesions that approximate the knee joint can undergo total knee replacement in surgical procedures similar to that used for osteogenic sarcoma of the femur or tibia. A scapula prosthesis that was used in patients with primary lesions of the scapula has also been described. For pelvic lesions, resection of the involved portion of the bone is usually locally curative (Fig. 82–6).

Because many patients with Ewing's sarcoma are skeletally immature, reconstruction of the appendicular skeleton after resection remains challenging because of the continued growth of the contralateral extremity. In this situation, the use of the expandable endoprosthesis, as described by several authors, including Eckardt[18] in our group, has been extremely helpful.

The timing of surgery is important. In the usual extremity lesion, we prefer to give preoperative chemotherapy and

*Table 82–2.* **Ewing's Sarcoma of Chest Wall or Rib\*: Treatment Plan**

Wide surgical resection
Preoperative irradiation of chest wall from one rib superior to the lesion, down to and including the diaphragm
Resection of entire involved rib from vertebral to sternal articulations

\*Includes primitive neuroectodermal tumor of soft tissue origin.

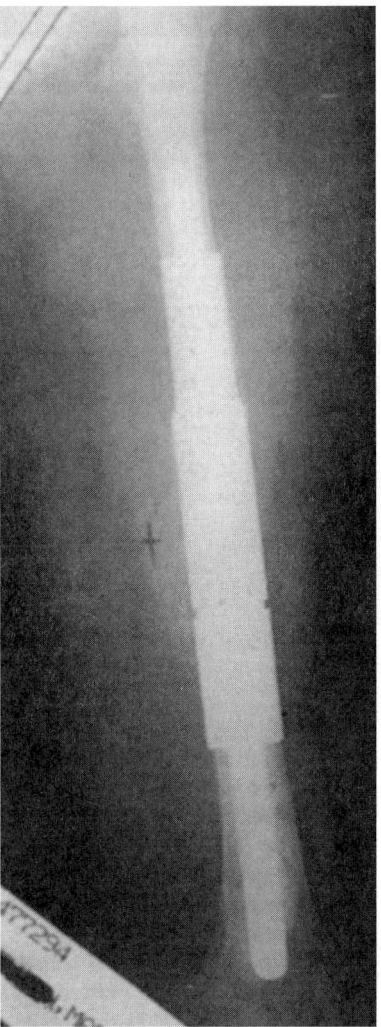

**Figure 82–5.** Endoprosthetic replacement of the femoral diaphysis for Ewing's sarcoma. After preoperative chemotherapy and radiation therapy, this patient underwent resection of the tumor-containing midportion of the femur, with an endoprosthesis placed in the surgical defect to restore complete function of the lower extremity. For patients who have not reached skeletal maturity, such endoprosthetic devices can now be made expandable and can undergo periodic lengthening to adjust for skeletal growth in younger patients.

preoperative radiation therapy for about 3 months. This approach has the advantage of early systemic treatment to arrest and eradicate systemic micrometastatic disease, which is presumed to be present in all patients. Preoperative therapy shrinks the soft tissue mass and sterilizes the operative field, making limb salvage much easier in most patients. After surgical resection, we continue with postoperative chemotherapy for approximately 3 months before the cessation of all therapy in our patients. The timing of surgery has to remain somewhat individualized, however, being based on the patient's primary tumor site and reaction to chemotherapy and radiation therapy.

Rarely, patients do not have adequate shrinkage of the primary tumor. This situation may be particularly true in a few patients with longstanding pelvic lesions who have developed tumors that are resistant to chemotherapy. These patients have only a slight, minor response and then rapidly

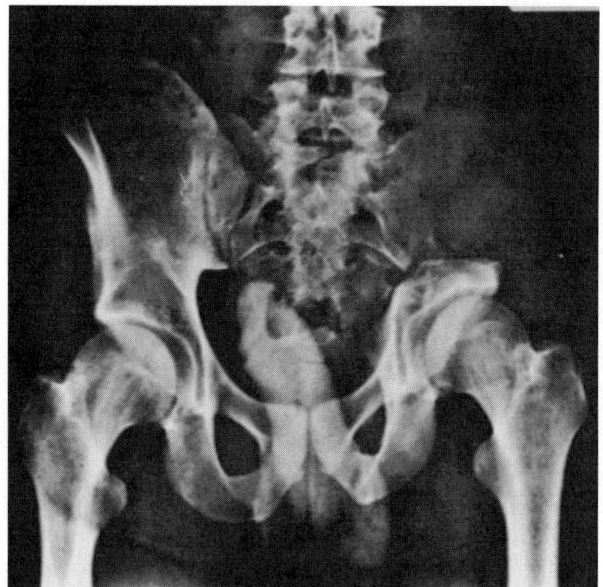

**Figure 82–6.** Surgical resection of the iliac wing in a patient who had a large Ewing sarcoma of the ilium. After preoperative chemotherapy and radiation therapy to the hemipelvis, a resection of the tumor-bearing portion of the ilium was performed. This type of surgery ensures against local recurrence of disease, which in our experience has occurred almost uniformly in patients who do not have surgical resection of the lesion but rather rely on radiation therapy alone for local control. This patient has survived 18 years from the time of his primary treatment. His only disability is a slight extremity shortening due to instability of the upper pelvis, which was corrected by putting a lift in his shoe.

have a regrowth of the tumor. This is an ominous prognostic sign that may make it necessary to proceed to radical surgery (amputation) if progressive tumor growth is documented. In this situation, because the prognosis is so grim, postoperative chemotherapy may be ineffective and the patient may best be referred for some form of experimental therapy.

Patients with lesions in the spine may need to undergo extensive surgery and reconstruction to remove the primary tumor. Surgery consists of a staged procedure in which the spine may be stabilized from behind before an anterior approach to remove the entire vertebral body. This approach frequently involves bone grafting and the insertion of additional hardware at the time of surgery. The postoperative recuperative period for this type of surgery (for the bone graft to heal) can be extensive. For all practical purposes, it is almost impossible to administer postoperative chemotherapy in a timely fashion in such patients. It is our practice in patients with spine lesions to complete the entire 6 months of chemotherapy. If the patient has sustained a complete response in the primary area after preoperative radiation therapy (45 Gy), only at the end of chemotherapy do we perform a surgical resection.

The completion of chemotherapy before surgery in the latter instance usually ensures systemic control of disease, and it allows the patient an indefinite time to recuperate from complicated spinal surgery. All patients need to be individualized on the basis of considerations such as those few given earlier for the timing of multidisciplinary treatment. The general plan for treating most Ewing's tumors is outlined in Figure 82–7.

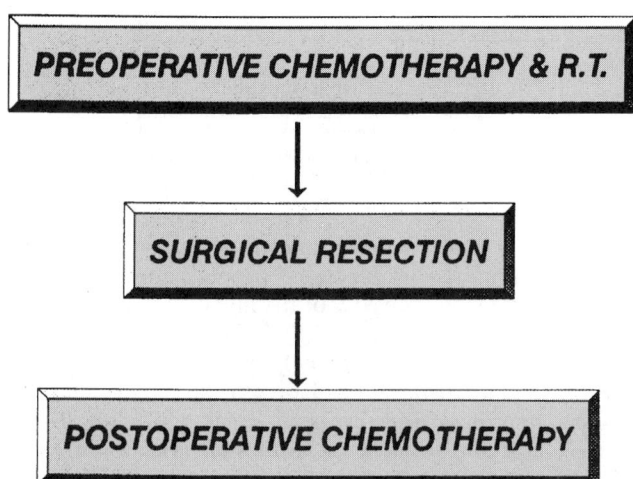

**Figure 82–7.** The treatment strategy for Ewing's sarcoma includes preoperative chemotherapy, as described in the text, and preoperative radiation therapy (R.T.). For preoperative radiation therapy, a dose of approximately 45 Gy should not be exceeded to ensure proper tissue healing after surgical resection. This strategy seems to prevent local recurrences of primary Ewing's sarcoma, which, in the days of modern chemotherapy for the prevention of metastatic disease, was one of the main reasons for failure to cure the patient.

## CHEMOTHERAPY

**Background.** Untreated Ewing's sarcoma is exquisitely sensitive to most chemotherapeutic agents (Table 82–3). In most instances, when Ewing's sarcoma recurs after conventional chemotherapy, the tumor is resistant to further chemotherapy. Ewing's sarcoma shows a rapid acquisition of multidrug resistance after recurrences in most patients. We consider it important to treat Ewing's sarcoma with maximal doses of maximally effective chemotherapy.

The mainstay of chemotherapy for Ewing's sarcoma has been high-dose alkylating agent therapy. It was well known in the mid-1960s that nitrogen mustard, given at the dose of 0.4 mg/kg (twice that used in MOPP [mechlorethamine, Oncovin (vincristine), procarbazine, prednisone] chemotherapy), could shrink a large primary Ewing sarcoma rapidly. The problem with nitrogen mustard was that resistance to further treatment would develop quickly after the patient's relapse. Nitrogen mustard also has cumulative myelosuppressive effects on the bone marrow. Although vincristine and dactinomycin showed minimal but definite activity in the early 1970s in the treatment of Ewing's sarcoma, these agents were only minimally effective, and resistance developed quickly.

The first multidrug chemotherapy regimens used were combinations of dactinomycin, vincristine, and cyclophosphamide. Our first adjuvant chemotherapy protocol for Ewing's sarcoma, reported in 1974, consisted of vincristine,

**Table 82–3.** Ewing's Sarcoma: Effective Drugs

| | |
|---|---|
| Dactinomycin | Doxorubicin (Adriamycin)* |
| Vincristine | Ifosfamide |
| Cyclophosphamide | High-dose ifosfamide* |
| High-dose cyclophosphamide | |

*Most effective agents in recurrent disease.

dactinomycin, cyclophosphamide, and doxorubicin.[4] We gave cyclophosphamide at the then relatively large dose of 1200 mg/m² and included doxorubicin in a protocol that was started in 1970 because of the early recognition of its extraordinary activity in Ewing's sarcoma. The Children's Cancer Study Group and the Intergroup Ewing's Sarcoma Study added doxorubicin to their treatment regimen for Ewing's sarcoma after they reconfirmed its activity in the early 1980s. The problem with all of these supposedly active drug combinations is that when tumor recurs, it is usually resistant to all of these forms of systemic therapy. One possible exception was cyclophosphamide because patients who had relapsed after the above-mentioned chemotherapy usually responded uniformly to cyclophosphamide given at twice the dose given before (2400 mg/m²).

In the past, we have used a multidisciplinary treatment protocol consisting of combination cyclophosphamide, doxorubicin, and low-dose methotrexate, alternating with high-dose cyclophosphamide (1200 mg/m²/day for 2 consecutive days), for the treatment of primary Ewing's sarcoma. This regimen was effective in most patients and led to cure rates of approximately 75 to 80% when surgery was used in addition to radiation therapy for local treatment. These results were no better than those obtained in the early 1970s, however, and it was well recognized that more effective chemotherapy would be desirable. The use of very high dose cyclophosphamide (50 mg/kg × 4 with the addition of other agents, such as busulfan with autologous bone marrow rescue) did not increase the cure rate significantly for high-risk patients in our hands and the hands of other investigators.

We had observed that approximately 10% of our patients, mainly those with extremely bulky tumors, would develop early resistance to chemotherapy during the preoperative chemotherapy phase. These patients were found to have a great deal of viable tumor present at the time of surgical resection, and this was associated with an extremely poor prognosis. These observations have been confirmed by Jurgens and colleagues[19] in the German-Austrian Cooperative Ewing's Sarcoma Study, in which they found a greater than 70% cure rate in patients who had more than 90% tumor necrosis noted at the time of surgical resection versus a cure rate of less than 30% in patients who had more viable tumor present. Others have confirmed this observation, and the histologic response to preoperative chemotherapy is an important predictor of outcome in Ewing's sarcoma.[20–22]

All of the above-mentioned observations led to the conclusion that the problem with Ewing's sarcoma is the development of early resistance. It might be advisable to treat Ewing's sarcoma with maximal-dose chemotherapy with agents that are maximally effective in the treatment of that disease. To that end, we recognized early the futility of continuing chemotherapy for more than 6 months with agents such as vincristine and dactinomycin, which seemed to have little activity, if any at all, in patients who had resistant or recurrent disease.

The emergence of ifosfamide for the treatment of Ewing's sarcoma has offered some new hope for a more active agent for this disease.[19, 23] In 1989, we observed a high response rate of recurrent Ewing's sarcoma treated with high-dose ifosfamide (14 g/m²) in patients who were resistant to cyclophosphamide at equally myelosuppressive high doses. The enthusiasm for ifosfamide chemotherapy was dampened somewhat by a report from the French that chemotherapy for Ewing's sarcoma with ifosfamide is no better, and perhaps more toxic, than conventional chemotherapy.[24] They used ifosfamide at 6 g/m², however, which is a relatively small dose and does not take advantage of the fact that at even twice the dose they used, ifosfamide is not as myelosuppressive as cyclophosphamide as used in the treatment of Ewing's sarcoma. The toxicity observed by the French in their ifosfamide protocol was primarily cardiac in nature. Cardiac toxicity has been observed infrequently with ifosfamide and, generally, in those who have had prior exposure to chest irradiation or anthracyclines, or both. The importance of the early use of ifosfamide alone or with etoposide in Ewing's sarcoma has been found in numerous studies in the United States and Europe. Chemotherapy regimens that have added or included ifosfamide have generally produced better results than those observed with the use of vincristine, actinomycin D, and cytoxan and doxorubicin.[25–30]

With the introduction of granulocyte colony–stimulating factor (G-CSF), we were able to escalate the dose of ifosfamide to 20 g/m², given by a continuous infusion of 2 g/m²/day over 9 days after a 4-hour initial bolus of 2 g/m². At this dose level, we observed continued remissions in patients who had multiple drug–resistant metastatic lesions. Many of these patients had extremely bulky metastatic disease and would respond to this high dose of ifosfamide with good partial or complete remissions that lasted for approximately 3 months. We found that they could then be re-treated every 3 months and have continued remission for as long as they were able to tolerate the drug. In these latter patients who had multiple courses of high-dose ifosfamide, the dose-limiting toxicity was renal in nature.

**Current Practice.** Because of the status quo with adjuvant chemotherapy, the evidence that high-dose ifosfamide was extremely active in the treatment of Ewing's tumor, and the fact that doxorubicin was the next most active agent identified in the treatment of this disease, we elected to embark on a new chemotherapy regimen using the two most active agents in the treatment of Ewing's tumor—high-dose ifosfamide and doxorubicin. We believed that these agents should be administered in their maximally tolerable doses to try to avoid the emergence of drug resistance in patients with Ewing's sarcoma. The availability of G-CSF would make maximally tolerable doses of these agents no more toxic than the older regimens without G-CSF. Also, we could treat patients with large amounts of drug in an effort to attain the rapid regression of disease and avoid drug resistance over a relatively short period without prolonging the patient's toxicity for periods of 1 year (which is what other regimens called for with less effective drugs).

In 1990, we changed our treatment regimen for the treatment of primary Ewing's sarcoma to include high-dose ifosfamide at its maximally tolerable dose (without stem cell or bone marrow support), 20 g/m² given by continuous infusion over 9 days, alternating with doxorubicin at its maximally tolerable dose of 100 mg/m² (50 mg/m²/day for 2 days). Because of the intensity of treatment, we believed that patients could tolerate no more than four doses of each drug. The treatment regimen is outlined in Table 82–4 and has the advantage of administering maximally effective doses of the most active agents to patients with Ewing's sarcoma. After

*Table 82–4.* **Ewing's Sarcoma Chemotherapy (Four Cycles)**

Ifosfamide 20 g/m² (total dose) given over 9 days
G-CSF 480 µg days 10–16

*Alternating with*
Doxorubicin (Adriamycin) 100 mg/m² (total dose) given over 2 days
G-CSF 480 µg days 3–9

G-CSF, granulocyte colony–stimulating factor.

two cycles (or two treatments with each agent), we usually perform surgery on the patient (after concomitant radiation therapy to the lesional area). Postoperatively the patient receives two more cycles of chemotherapy. After a total of four cycles of this chemotherapy, the patient has had a cumulative dose of doxorubicin of 400 mg/m² and a cumulative dose of ifosfamide of 80 g/m², yet the entire chemotherapy regimen takes only 6 months to administer under ideal circumstances.

We have been able to administer this chemotherapy regimen in the outpatient department for all of our patients and have avoided hospitalization. These patients need intensive supportive care, however, which is discussed later. We believe that because there is a dose-response curve that has been shown in multiple studies for ifosfamide and doxorubicin, and because these are the two most active agents in the treatment of this disease, patients would be served best by treatment with this regimen and not wasting valuable time in continuing with less effective drugs, such as dactinomycin or vincristine. It is our hope that this regimen will break the 75 to 80% cure rate barrier that has been standard and constant since the early 1970s, when we first showed the value of adjuvant chemotherapy for the treatment of Ewing's sarcoma. To date, this regimen has produced striking regressions of large, bulky primary tumors in high-risk patients. We believe this is the best available treatment for this disease at this time, but no data are available to indicate that we have achieved a higher cure rate.

**High-Dose Chemotherapy.** For patients who present with multifocal bone disease, patients who present with large pelvic primary tumors, or patients who relapse after initial therapy, high-dose regimens—*megatherapy*—with bone marrow or stem cell support are currently under investigation, with encouraging early results.[31–33] Combinations of radiation and chemotherapy have usually been used (i.e., total-body irradiation and melphalan). It is not clear at this time if any one regimen is superior.

## SUPPORTIVE CARE

Supportive care is important for patients undergoing intensive chemotherapy for Ewing's sarcoma. All patients develop significant neutropenia, thrombocytopenia, and anemia after each treatment course. We routinely follow the patients after each chemotherapy course with a complete blood count and platelet count beginning 1 week from the start of chemotherapy and continuing every other day until they pass through the nadir white count and platelet count. We prophylactically transfuse patients with packed red cells for a hemoglobin less than 9.5 g/dl when we know the white cell count is still falling. With this measure, we have not had any significant

episodes of shock or decreased blood pressure in patients who become febrile while neutropenic. We also transfuse platelets to patients whose platelet count falls to less than 25,000/µl. We perform all of this supportive care as well as the chemotherapy on an outpatient basis. Outpatient treatment is generally better accepted by patients and is significantly better tolerated by adolescents and children, who usually can continue to attend school and live at home with family support during this period of treatment.

Patients who develop fever while neutropenic are given intravenous antibiotics. We currently give 2 g of ceftriaxone (or 50 mg/kg) every 24 hours. Patients are given gentamicin at the dose of 5 to 7 mg/kg/24 hours divided into three equal doses, which is administered automatically through a portable pump that turns on and gives the infusion every 8 hours. We adjust the dose of gentamicin pharmacokinetically based on the peak and trough levels that are measured when the patient comes back the next day for follow-up. Patients are discharged from the outpatient setting only if they are stable and become afebrile while under observation in our outpatient facility within 24 hours.

As curative chemotherapy regimens become more intensive, supportive care and facilities that can handle this treatment on an outpatient basis become extremely important. Intensive regimens such as this one would traditionally be given to hospitalized patients (particularly high-dose ifosfamide). Usually by the end of the 9-day ifosfamide infusion, patients are already neutropenic. If they were to be hospitalized, they would probably remain in the hospital for continued treatment with antibiotics and transfusions and would then be ready for their next treatment by the time of discharge.

It is unacceptable to devise more intensive and, it is hoped, more curative regimens if they require continued hospitalization. Expense is a secondary consideration. Most of these children require the supportive care of family and school life. In addition to providing all the medical supportive care, it is necessary for the teams of social workers to ensure accessibility of treatment to patients as well as to administer to the psychosocial needs of these patients. In a totally supportive treatment setting, such as that described, patients can undergo the most intensive therapy in hopes of attaining a cure for their disease in a relatively short time without totally disrupting the family structure and the educational or vocational needs of the patient. It has been our experience that poor socioeconomic conditions and adverse psychosocial circumstances are the two most important factors leading to the lack of accessibility and the lack of compliance with treatment. These are high-risk factors that need to be addressed with the same diligence as the demanding chemotherapy regimen and complicated timing of multidisciplinary treatment.

## SUGGESTIONS FOR ADDITIONAL READING

de Alava E, Gerald WL. Molecular biology of the Ewing's sarcoma/primitive neuroectodermal tumor family. J Clin Oncol 2000;18:204–13.

Dehner LP. The evolution of the diagnosis and understanding of primitive and embryonic neoplasms in children: living through an epoch. Mod Pathol 1998;11:669–85.

van der Woude HJ, Bloem JL, Hogendoorn PC. Preoperative evaluation and monitoring chemotherapy in patients with high-grade osteogenic and Ewing's sarcoma: review of current imaging modalities. Skeletal Radiol 1998;27:57–71.

Grier HE. The Ewing family of tumors: Ewing's sarcoma and primitive neuroectodermal tumors. Pediatr Clin North Am 1997;44:991–1004.

Maurel J, Rosell R, Lorenzo JC. Poor prognosis Ewing's sarcoma and peripheral primitive neuroectodermal tumours (PNET). Cancer Treat Rev 1996;22:425–36.

Eckardt JJ, Kabo M, Kelley C, et al. Expandable endoprosthesis reconstruction in skeletally immature patients with tumors. Clin Orthop 2000;373:51–61.

Kay R, Eckardt JJ, Mirra J. Osteogenic sarcoma and Ewing's sarcoma in a retinoblastoma patient. Clin Orthop 1996;323:284–7.

Yang R, Eckardt JJ, Eilber F, et al. Surgical indications for Ewing's sarcoma of the pelvis. Cancer 1995;76:1388–97.

# REFERENCES

1. Ewing J. Diffuse endothelioma of bone. Proc N Y Pathol Soc 1921;21:17–24.
2. Dahlin DC, Coventry MB, Scanlon PW. Ewing's sarcoma: a critical analysis of 165 cases. J Bone Joint Surg Am 1961;43:185–92.
3. Boyer CW Jr, Brickner TJ Jr, Perry RH. Ewing's sarcoma: case against surgery. Cancer 1967;20:1602–6.
4. Rosen G, Wollner N, Tan C, et al. Proceedings: disease-free survival in children with Ewing's sarcoma treated with radiation therapy and adjuvant four-drug sequential chemotherapy. Cancer 1974;33:384–93.
5. Rosen G. Primary Ewing's sarcoma: the multidisciplinary lesion. Int J Radiat Oncol Biol Phys 1978;4:527–32.
6. Dehner LP. Primitive neuroectodermal tumor and Ewing's sarcoma. Am J Surg Pathol 1993;17:1–13.
7. Stevenson AJ, Chatten J, Bertoni F, Miettinen M. CD99 ($p^{30/32 \text{ MIC2}}$) neuroectodermal/Ewing's sarcoma antigen as an immunohistochemical marker: review of more than 600 tumors and the literature experience. Appl Immunohistochem 1994;2:231–40.
8. Rettig WJ, Garin-Chesa P, Huvos AG. Ewing's sarcoma: new approaches to histogenesis and molecular plasticity. Lab Invest 1992;66:133–7.
9. May WA, Gishizky ML, Lessnick SL, et al. Ewing sarcoma 11;22 translocation produces a chimeric transcription factor that requires the DNA-binding domain encoded by FLI1 for transformation. Proc Natl Acad Sci U S A 1993;90:5752–6.
10. Taylor C, Patel K, Jones T, et al. Diagnosis of Ewing's sarcoma and peripheral neuroectodermal tumour based on the detection of t(11;22) using fluorescence in situ hybridisation. Br J Cancer 1993;67:128–33.
11. Downing JR, Head DR, Parham DM, et al. Detection of the (11;22)(q24;Q12) translocation of Ewing's sarcoma and peripheral neuroectodermal tumor by reverse transcription polymerase chain reaction. Am J Pathol 1993;143:1294–300.
12. de Alava E, Kawai A, Healey JH, et al. EWS-FLI1 fusion transcript structure is an independent determinant of prognosis in Ewing's sarcoma. J Clin Oncol 1998;16:1248–55.
13. McLean TW, Hertel C, Young ML, et al. Late events in pediatric patients with Ewing's sarcoma/primitive neuroectodermal tumor of bone: the Dana-Farber Cancer Institute/Children's Hospital experience. J Pediatr Hematol Oncol 1999;21:486–93.
14. Hibshoosh H, Lattes R. Immunohistochemical and molecular genetic approaches to soft tissue diagnosis: a primer. Semin Oncol 1997;24:515–25.
15. Wessalowski R, Jurgens H, Bodenstein H, et al. [Results of treatment of primary metastatic Ewing sarcoma: a retrospective analysis of 48 patients]. Klin Padiatr 1988;200:253–60.
16. Evans R, Nesbit M, Askin F, et al. Local recurrence, rate and sites of metastases, and time to relapse as a function of treatment regimen, size of primary and surgical history in 62 patients presenting with non-metastatic Ewing's sarcoma of the pelvic bones. Int J Radiat Oncol Biol Phys 1985;11:129–36.
17. Paulussen M, Ahrens S, Burdach S, et al. Primary metastatic (stage IV) Ewing tumor: survival analysis of 171 patients from the EICESS studies: European Intergroup Cooperative Ewing Sarcoma Studies. Ann Oncol 1998;9:275–81.
18. Eckardt JJ, Eilber FR, Rosen G, et al. Limb salvage versus amputation for malignant tumors other than osteogenic sarcoma. In: Yamamuro T, ed. New developments for limb salvage in musculoskeletal tumors. Kyocera Orthopaedic Symposium. Tokyo: Springer-Verlag, 1989:77–81.
19. Jurgens H, Exner U, Kuhl J, et al. High-dose ifosfamide with mesna uroprotection in Ewing's sarcoma. Cancer Chemother Pharmacol 1989;24:Suppl 1:S40–4.
20. Bacci G, Picci P, Mercuri M, et al. Predictive factors of histological response to primary chemotherapy in Ewing's sarcoma. Acta Oncol 1998;37:671–6.
21. Wunder JS, Paulian G, Huvos AG, et al. The histological response to chemotherapy as a predictor of the oncological outcome of operative treatment of Ewing sarcoma. J Bone Joint Surg Am 1998;80:1020–33.
22. Nilbert M, Saeter G, Elomaa I, et al. Ewing's sarcoma treatment in Scandinavia 1984–1990: ten year results of the Scandinavian Sarcoma Group Protocol SSGIV. Acta Oncol 1998;37:375–8.
23. Meyer WH, Kun L, Marina N, et al. Ifosfamide plus etoposide in newly diagnosed Ewing's sarcoma of bone. J Clin Oncol 1992;10:1737–42.
24. Oberlin O, Habrand JL, Zucker JM, et al. No benefit of ifosfamide in Ewing's sarcoma: a nonrandomized study of the French Society of Pediatric Oncology. J Clin Oncol 1992;10:1407–12.
25. Quezado ZM, Wilson WH, Cunnion RE, et al. High-dose ifosfamide is associated with severe, reversible cardiac dysfunction. Ann Intern Med 1993;118:31–6.
26. Ferrari S, Mercuri M, Rosito P, et al. Ifosfamide and actinomycin-D, added in the induction phase to vincristine, cyclophosphamide and doxorubicin, improve histologic response and prognosis in patients with non metastatic Ewing's sarcoma of the extremity. J Chemother 1998;10:484–91.
27. Craft A, Cotterill S, Malcolm A, et al. Ifosfamide-containing chemotherapy in Ewing's sarcoma: the Second United Kingdom Children's Cancer Study Group and the Medical Research Council Ewing's Tumor Study. J Clin Oncol 1998;16:3628–33.
28. Gururangan S, Marina NM, Luo X, et al. Treatment of children with peripheral primitive neuroectodermal tumor or extraosseous Ewing's tumor with Ewing's-directed therapy. J Pediatr Hematol Oncol 1998;20:55–6.
29. Wexler LH, DeLaney TF, Tsokos M, et al. Ifosfamide and etoposide plus vincristine, doxorubicin, and cyclophosphamide for newly diagnosed Ewing's sarcoma family of tumors. Cancer 1996;78:901–11.
30. Grier H, Krailo M, Link M, et al. Improved outcome in non-metastatic Ewing's sarcoma and PNET of bone with the addition of ifosfamide and etoposide to vincristine, Adriamycin, cyclophosphamide and actinomycin: a Children's Cancer Group and Pediatric Oncology Group Report. Proc ASCO 1994;13:421.
31. Laws HJ, Burdach S, van Kaich B, et al. Multimodality diagnostics and megatherapy in poor prognosis tumor patients: a single center report. Strahlenther Onkol 1999;175:488–94.
32. Pape H, Laws HJ, Burdach S, et al. Radiotherapy and high-dose chemotherapy in advanced Ewing's. Strahlenther Onkol 1999;175:484–7.
33. Astra A, Whelan JS, Calvagna V, et al. High-dose busulphan/melphalan with autologous stem cell rescue in Ewing's sarcoma. Bone Marrow Transplant 1997;20:843–6.

# CHAPTER 83

# SOFT TISSUE SARCOMAS

- CHARLES A. FORSCHER • CARSTEN E. KAMPE
- FREDERICK R. EILBER

Malignant tumors of the soft tissues account for less than 1% of all malignancies diagnosed annually. According to the American Cancer Society, there are about 7800 new cases diagnosed in the United States every year, and 4400 persons die of these tumors annually.[1] Soft tissue sarcomas are unusual primary malignant tumors and are characterized by diversity not only in histologic appearance, but also in biologic behavior and anatomic locations.

Soft tissue sarcomas can occur in any age group. They are more common in older patients, however; about 15% affect persons younger than 15 years old, and about 40% affect persons 55 years old or older.[2] Most childhood tumors are rhabdomyosarcomas or undifferentiated tumors, arising primarily in the head and neck area. The incidence of soft tissue tumors in adults tends to be highest in the extremities; the retroperitoneum is affected less often, and the head and neck is the least affected area.[3] Sex incidence is approximately equal in males and females, and there is no racial predilection.

The cause of soft tissue sarcomas is unknown. This group of tumors has been associated with several genetically transmitted diseases (Table 83–1), including the inherited sarcoma, breast, lung, and adrenocortical carcinoma syndrome described by Li and Fraumeni[4] and by Lynch and colleagues[5] and the Beckwith-Wiedemann syndrome in children.[6, 7] Patients with von Recklinghausen's disease have a 7 to 10% chance of developing neurofibrosarcoma.[8–10] Soft tissue sarcomas are thought to occur with slightly increased frequency in patients with intestinal polyposis, Gardner's syndrome, Werner's syndrome, tuberous sclerosis, and the basal cell nevus syndrome.[11–14]

Much progress has been made in the genetic characterization of sarcomas.[15] Virtually all soft tissue sarcomas contain consistent clonal chromosomal aberrations,[16] many of which have potential use in the diagnosis of sarcomas.[17] Rearrangements or losses of tumor-suppressor genes (e.g., Rb1 and p53) have been shown in several soft tissue sarcomas.[18–20] Evidence is also accumulating of the involvement of oncogenes, particularly K-*ras* and N-*ras*, in the development of embryonal rhabdomyosarcoma.[15] Especially exciting is the discovery of specific chromosomal translocations that are unique to particular classes and subclasses of soft tissue sarcomas. For example, the translocation t(X;18) is almost invariably found in synovial sarcoma.[21–23] Characteristic chromosomal translocations have now been cloned in Ewing's sarcoma,[24] alveolar rhabdomyosarcoma,[25] and myxoid liposarcoma.[26] Specific fusion proteins resulting from these translocations are emerging as diagnostic, prognostic, and potentially therapeutic aids.[27] Each of these translocations involves a DNA transcription factor, which is presumed to modify the expression of other genes that contribute to neoplastic transformation. Most sarcomas are currently thought to represent new mutations. Nevertheless, young patients should be evaluated thoroughly with respect to a family history, the goal being to identify risk to close relatives.

There are also reported cases of malignant soft tissue tumors developing in injured tissues, such as those arising from foreign body implants,[28] from granulating wounds or burn scars,[29] and after radiation injury.[30] These tumors have been reported in patients with chronic lymphedematous extremities, principally those occurring after mastectomy (Stewart-Treves syndrome), as well as in cases of chronic congenital lymphedema.[31, 32] The development of sarcomas in pre-existing lesions is extremely uncommon. Similarly, although there are numerous reports to suggest various associations, there is no proven link between the development of soft tissue sarcomas in humans and a history of trauma, exposure to chemical carcinogens (including Agent Orange[33, 34]), or viral infections. Mesothelioma and Kaposi's sarcoma are exceptions and are discussed in Chapters 38 and 100.

## Natural History

### CLASSIFICATION AND HISTOPATHOLOGY

The terminology for malignant tumors of the soft tissues is complicated and confusing. At present, there are at least 55

*Table 83–1.* **Genetic Predisposition to Sarcoma Development**

| Autosomal Dominant Disorder | Sarcoma Type | Chromosomal Location | Gene |
|---|---|---|---|
| Li-Fraumeni syndrome | Many, especially rhabdomyosarcoma | 17p13 | P53 |
| Gardner's syndrome | Fibromatosis | 15q21–22 | APC |
| Beckwith-Wiedemann syndrome | Rhabdomyosarcoma | 11p15 | Unknown |
| von Recklinghausen's neurofibromatosis | Malignant peripheral nerve sheath tumors | 17q11.2 | NFI |
| Familial retinoblastoma | Many | 13q14 | RBI |

From Cooper CS, Clark J. Molecular biological studies on soft tissue sarcomas. In: Verweij J, Pinedo HM, Suit HD, eds. Multidisciplinary treatment of soft tissue sarcomas. Boston: Kluwer Academic, 1993:38.

different histologic subtypes of soft tissue sarcoma. Commonly recognized types and their frequency are given in Table 83–2. The first universally accepted classification for soft tissue sarcomas was proposed by the World Health Organization in 1969.[35] Since then, several changes have been made, and a histogenic classification based on proliferating cell type is now in common use.[2] By this scheme, each tumor is classified according to the appearance of the tissue it has formed rather than the type of cell from which the tumor arose. Fluctuations in the reported relative frequency of the different types of sarcomas is a reflection of the differences in diagnostic criteria used by pathologists. In older studies, fibrosarcoma was the most frequent sarcoma. Currently, malignant fibrous histiocytoma, liposarcoma, and leiomyosarcoma are the most frequent sarcomas in adult patients.

Separation into histogenetic type, by means of light microscopy, has been useful and reproducible for well-differentiated tumors. As the tumor becomes more undifferentiated, it becomes much more difficult to determine its normal histogenic counterpart, however. In poorly differentiated tumors, applying the histologic criteria of matrix production, cytoplasmic details, and overall architecture to determine the most likely histogenesis has been difficult, and disagreement between reference pathologists is common.[36–39]

Immunohistochemical staining has improved the approach to the classification of soft tissue sarcomas greatly.[40–42] Commonly used, commercially available markers are listed in Table 83–3. Immunohistochemistry has its greatest utility in confirming histologically suspected diagnoses of rhabdomyosarcoma,[43] synovial sarcoma,[44] clear cell sarcoma,[45] and epithelioid sarcoma.[46] Immunohistochemistry can be useful in distinguishing leiomyosarcoma and other types of gastrointestinal stromal tumors.[47–50] It is less often

*Table 83–3.* **Immunohistochemistry: Useful Markers for Sarcoma Typing on Paraffin Sections**

| Markers | Comments |
|---|---|
| Vimentin | Mesenchymal differentiation |
| Cytokeratin, epithelial membrane antigen | Epithelial differentiation (synovial sarcoma, epithelioid sarcoma) |
| Desmin, muscle actin | Muscle differentiation |
| Alpha-smooth muscle actin | Smooth muscle differentiation |
| Myoglobin | Striated muscle differentiation |
| S100 protein | Marker for Schwann cells, chondrocytes, adipocytes, melanocytes |
| HMB45 | Melanotic differentiation |
| Factor VIII R-Ag, CD 34, *Ulex europaeus* | Endothelial differentiation |
| Collagen IV | Marker for basement membranes |

From Coindre JM. In: Verweij J, Pinedo HM, Suit HD, eds. Multidisciplinary treatment of soft tissue sarcomas. Boston: Kluwer Academic, 1993:9.

useful for malignant schwannoma, angiosarcoma, and chondrosarcoma, and no specific markers exist for malignant fibrous histiocytoma, fibrosarcoma, hemangiopericytoma, and alveolar soft part sarcoma. Electron microscopy plays a smaller role in the assessment of soft tissue sarcomas. It can be helpful in identifying diverse cellular constituents, but it often serves merely to confirm the diagnosis suggested by light microscopy.[51]

Histopathologic grade is of greater value to the clinician than the exact histopathologic type because it has a greater ability to predict the biologic behavior of soft tissue sarcomas.[37, 52–54] Consequently, knowledge of the histologic grade is critical to developing proper patient management strategy and often is used to direct the most efficient use of chemotherapy. For example, Elias and colleagues[55] reported that response to palliative chemotherapy in 105 patients with advanced sarcoma was correlated with histologic grade and mitosis rate.

Many grading systems have come into use.[52, 54, 56–59] Of the generally accepted grading criteria for malignancy examined in these grading systems (e.g., nuclear morphology, degree of cellularity, cellular anaplasia, mitotic activity, necrosis, invasion), the two most important parameters for grading soft tissue sarcomas have been the number of mitotic figures and the extent of necrosis.[60–62] As with the assignment of tumor histologic type, the reproducibility of grading between reference pathologists is less than perfect (generally in the range of 60 to 75%),[37, 52] underlining the importance of expert pathologic evaluation in the work-up and planning of treatment of patients with soft tissue sarcomas. Additional shortcomings of current grading systems include the American Joint Committee on Cancer's automatic attribution of some sarcomas (e.g., synovial sarcoma as grade 3). Available data suggest that this practice is unwarranted. For example, a small fraction of patients with synovial sarcoma appear to have true low-grade disease based on a high degree of glandularity and a low mitotic rate.[63, 64] These tumors appear not to metastasize with a frequency warranting aggressive chemotherapy.

It is clear from several histologic studies of soft tissue sarcoma that there is no true tumor capsule, even though

*Table 83–2.* **Frequency of Adult Soft Tissue Sarcoma in Two Large Series**

| Histology | Enjoji et al, 1984 (n = 664), % | Coindre et al, 1993 (n = 711), % |
|---|---|---|
| Malignant fibrous histiocytoma | 30.3 | 30.4 |
| Liposarcoma | 11.1 | 13.7 |
| Leiomyosarcoma | 9.9 | 10.4 |
| Synovial sarcoma | 5.9 | 8.4 |
| Malignant schwannoma | 5.0 | 7.2 |
| Fibrosarcoma | 5.6 | 4.9 |
| Rhabdomyosarcoma | 6.6 | 2.4 |
| Hemangiosarcoma | 3.8 | 3.5 |
| Extraskeletal chondrosarcoma | 3.8 | 1.6 |
| Malignant hemangiopericytoma | 2.6 | NR |
| Malignant mesothelioma | 1.8 | NR |
| Clear cell sarcoma | 2.6 | 0.8 |
| Epithelioid sarcoma | 0.8 | 1.3 |
| Alveolar soft part sarcoma | 1.1 | 0.8 |
| Malignant neuroepithelioma | 0.8 | NR |
| Ewing's sarcoma | 0.3 | 1.3 |
| Extraskeletal osteosarcoma | 0.5 | 0.8 |
| Malignant mesenchymoma | 0.2 | 0.1 |
| Unclassified | 7.4 | 12.4 |

NR, not reported.

Modified from Enjoji M, Hashimoto H. Diagnosis of soft tissue sarcomas. Pathol Res Pract 1984;178:215 and Coindre JM. Pathology and grading of soft tissue sarcomas. In: Verweij J, Pinedo HM, Suit HD, eds. Multidisciplinary treatment of soft tissue sarcomas. Boston: Kluwer Academic 1993:4.

these tumors may appear to be grossly encapsulated. The pseudocapsule consists of compressed normal surrounding cells that have been invaded microscopically by the malignant cells.

## CLINICAL FEATURES

Malignant soft tissue tumors often present as large local masses. The growth is relatively slow in most cases, and the tumors seldom cause early symptoms so that they are often appreciated only when the mass has reached a relatively large size. If contiguous areas, such as nerve or vascular structures, are compressed, the major symptoms are paresthesias, lymphedema, and venous engorgement. Direct invasion of nerve and blood vessels occurs in less than 5% of cases, however, and most of the symptoms can be related to a mass effect with compression of normal structures.

These tumors tend to spread in a three-dimensional fashion, but the greatest microscopic extension appears to occur along fascial planes. Metastases to regional lymph nodes are extremely uncommon, with the exception of rhabdomyosarcoma and synovial cell sarcoma, both of which metastasize to regional lymph nodes in 8 to 10% of cases.[65]

The primary metastatic site is the lung.[66, 67] Approximately 70% of patients who die of soft tissue sarcomas do so because of an uncontrolled primary or metastatic disease confined to the lung. The most common metastatic site for patients with primary retroperitoneal sarcomas is the peritoneal cavity, from peritoneal seeding or from metastasis to the liver. Metastases to the bone and other soft tissue sites and rarely to the central nervous system have been reported.

## DIAGNOSIS

When a patient presents with an ill-defined soft tissue mass and when the tumor is not superficial (in the subcutaneous tissue), additional work-up should be undertaken. Although most patients have a history of antecedent trauma, this usually serves merely to call attention to a pre-existing lesion. Persistence of a soft tissue mass with conservative therapy should alert the physician to an additional soft tissue tumor. Plain radiographs are useful to determine whether there is a primary bone problem. Computed tomography (CT) scanning and magnetic resonance imaging (MRI) have proved to be the most definitive diagnostic modalities in detecting a soft tissue tumor.[68–72] Most of the soft tissue tumor density is different from that of normal muscle, and these tumors appear as a relatively clearly defined, soft tissue tumor mass. Distinction between the tumor and normal muscle is clear, and the separation of a true tumor from a muscle pull or hematoma, the most common clinical differential diagnosis, has been relatively reliable.

Once the diagnostic imaging suggests a definite soft tissue tumor, careful consideration of the type of biopsy incision is mandatory. Fine-needle aspirate or core-needle biopsy often gives a diagnosis of malignancy but seldom gives the exact histogenesis or the grade.[73] Open incisional biopsy, with the direction of incision placed so that it can be incorporated in a subsequent excision, is mandatory. Careful hemostasis and disturbance of as few tissue planes as possible is also advis-

able. Incisional biopsy is the procedure of choice, and excisional biopsies should not be done for these tumors.

## CLINICAL STAGING AND PROGNOSIS

The prognosis for patients with soft tissue sarcomas is based on the histopathology and the local anatomic extent of the disease. The American Joint Committee on Cancer organized a task force to study the problems inherent in soft tissue sarcomas, including their rarity, the difficulty in making an accurate histologic diagnosis, and the lack of a widely accepted system for assessing prognosis. The committee evaluated the end results of surgical therapy in 1215 patients from 13 institutions in whom surgery was the primary treatment.[74] It soon became clear that there was a marked disagreement among the reference pathologists regarding the tissue of origin for many of these tumors. It also became apparent that the tissue of origin was less important in the prognosis than the grade of the tumor (necrosis and number of mitotic figures per high-power field). It was reasonably easy to standardize a reproducible system for assessing the grade of the tumor. A staging system based on the TNM system was developed, with the addition of a G category that represents the tumor grade (Table 83–4).

After these tumors had been classified and the outcome of all cases evaluated, it was possible to stage these sarcomas as clinicopathologic stage I through stage IV. The 5-year survival rate for stage I tumors is 70 to greater than 90%; for stage II, 55 to 70%; for stage III, 20 to 50%; and for stage IV, 4 to 20% (Table 83–5). The even separation in survival curves argues for the usefulness and reproducibility of this clinicopathologic staging system. The system obviates the need for exact histologic classification of tumors and relies on the more objective evaluation of the number of mitoses per high-power field (i.e., the determination of grade).[38, 48] The exceptions are that rhabdomyosarcomas and synovial cell sarcomas are by definition grade 3 tumors.

## Treatment

### SURGERY

Surgery was the first form of treatment applied systematically to soft tissue sarcomas and remains an essential element in the care of patients with these neoplasms. As a local treatment modality, surgery requires a complete and total en bloc excision of the primary tumor. Local excision of gross tumor with a narrow margin or enucleation cannot be classified as complete excision. With local excision, a 90% incidence of local recurrence has been reported.[38, 75, 76] This high local failure rate is related directly to the mistaken impression that these tumors are surrounded by a true anatomic capsule.

**Muscle Group Excision.** Well-differentiated tumors arising in a muscle group or fascial plane can be treated successfully if excision includes the entire soft tissue part from origin to insertion and encompasses the adjacent fascial planes. For example, if the tumor arises in the sartorius muscle of the thigh, an operation that encompasses the

*Table 83–4.* **International TNM Staging Classification for Soft Tissue Sarcomas**

*Histopathologic Grade (G)\**

| | |
|---|---|
| GX | Grade cannot be assessed |
| G1 | Well differentiated |
| G2 | Moderately differentiated |
| G3 | Poorly differentiated |
| G4 | Undifferentiated |

*Definition of TNM*

*Primary Tumor (T)*

| | |
|---|---|
| TX | Primary tumor cannot be assessed |
| T0 | No evidence of primary tumor |
| T1 | Tumor 5 cm or less in greatest dimension |
| T1a | Superficial tumor |
| T1b | Deep tumor |
| T2 | Tumor more than 5 cm in greatest dimension |
| T2a | Superficial tumor |
| T2b | Deep tumor |

*Regional Lymph Nodes (N)*

| | |
|---|---|
| NX | Regional lymph nodes cannot be assessed |
| N0 | No regional lymph node metastasis |
| N1 | Regional lymph node metastasis |

*Distant Metastasis (M)*

| | |
|---|---|
| MX | Presence of distant metastasis cannot be assessed |
| M0 | No distant metastasis |
| M1 | Distant metastasis |

*Stage Grouping*

| | | | | |
|---|---|---|---|---|
| Stage I | | | | |
| A (Low grade, small, superficial and deep) | G1–2 | T1a–1b | N0 | M0 |
| B (Low grade, large, superficial) | G1–2 | T2a | N0 | M0 |
| Stage II | | | | |
| A (Low grade, large, deep) | G1–2 | T2b | N0 | M0 |
| B (High grade, small, superficial, deep) | G3–4 | T1a–1b | N0 | M0 |
| C (High grade, large, superficial) | G3–4 | T2a | N0 | M0 |
| Stage III (High grade, large, deep) | G3–4 | T2b | N0 | M0 |
| Stage IV (any metastasis) | Any G | Any T | N1 | M0 |
| | Any G | Any T | N0 | M1 |

\*Note: Superficial tumor is located exclusively above the superficial fascia without invasion of the fascia; deep tumor is located either exclusively beneath the superficial fascia, or superficial to the fascia with invasion of or through the fascia, or superficial and beneath the fascia. Retroperitoneal, mediastinal, and pelvic sarcomas are classified as deep tumors.

Used with the permission of the American Joint Committee on Cancer (AJCC\*), Chicago, Illinois. The original source for this material is the AJCC\* Cancer Staging Manual, 5th edition (1997) published by Lippincott-Raven Publishers, Philadelphia, Pennsylvania.

The following histological types of tumors are not included: Kaposi's sarcoma, dermatofibrosarcoma, desmoid type of fibrosarcoma grade I and sarcoma arising from the dura mater, brain, parenchymatous organs or hollow viscera.

*Table 83–5.* **Five-Year Survival Rates by Stage**

| Stage | 1954–69\* | 1987† | 1991‡ |
|---|---|---|---|
| I | 75 | 79 | >90 |
| II | 52 | 65 | 70 |
| III | 28 | 45 | 20–50 |
| IV | 7 | 10 | <20 |

\*From a nationwide survey of 2355 patients from 504 hospitals carried out under the auspices of the Commission on Cancer of the American College of Surgeons; Russell W. Cancer 1977;40:1562.

†A retrospective study of 702 sarcomas collected from 13 different institutions: Lawrence W. Ann Surg 1987;205:349.

‡From PDQ, Physician Data Query, 1991.

sartorius completely from origin to insertion plus the adjacent fascial plane is appropriate. Regional lymph node dissection is usually not performed. Most patients with soft tissue sarcomas do not present with tumors in a specified muscle group, however.

**Amputation.** In previous years, amputation was believed to be the procedure of choice for most patients with soft tissue sarcomas. This belief was partially because patients often presented with large tumors, and local excisions were not feasible. Previous experience with local excision and enucleation resulted in a higher local failure rate. The necessity for amputation was based on the fact that these tumors involving an entire anatomic compartment had tumor spread within this compartment. These principles were proved to be of value when surgery was the only treatment method used. When these principles of resection of the entire compartment are adhered to, the local failure rate with surgery alone has been reduced to 25 to 30%.[77] With surgery alone, however, the amputation rate remains high, and amputation is necessary in approximately 50 to 60% of cases. Certain anatomic locations, such as the head and neck, retroperitoneum, and sublocations within the extremity (e.g., the groin and subcutaneous tissue), do not lend themselves well to this principle of compartment resection.

What has become clear over the years, whether surgery is the primary method or whether chemotherapy and radiation are added as adjuvants, is the fact that total excision of the tumor and pathologically confirmed clear margins create the best situation for achieving local tumor control. It is apparent that to achieve this the diagnosis must be known preoperatively so that operations can be planned in an orderly fashion. Also required are large incisions for adequate exposure; exposure of major adjacent structures, such as blood vessels and nerves; and pathologic confirmation of tumor-free margins at the time of surgery.

**Retroperitoneal Sarcomas.** Surgical treatment of retroperitoneal sarcomas often is difficult because of the large size of the tumor by the time diagnosis is made and because of the lack of well-defined compartments and the proximity of adjacent structures. The principles for excision of these tumors in the retroperitoneum are similar to those for tumors in an extremity, however. Complete excision of the tumor is mandatory, and resection of adjacent viscera may be necessary.

**Head and Neck Sarcomas.** Malignant sarcomas of the head and neck, although rare, present additional problems for complete surgical extirpation. As with tumors arising in the retroperitoneum, complete en bloc excision of these tumors with an adequate surgical margin is seldom possible because of the narrow anatomic limits of the spaces in the head and neck and the interrelated fascial planes. The local recurrence rates in the head and neck with surgery alone, even with extensive resections, is 50%.

**Summary of Surgical Principles.** Complete surgical excision of well-differentiated small tumors has been highly successful, with a recurrence rate of less than 10% and an overall survival rate of nearly 80%. Complete surgical excision requires an accurate preoperative diagnosis and a well-planned operation. In patients with larger and higher grade tumors (clinicopathologic stages II and III), the local recurrence rate is much higher with surgery alone, as is the amputation rate. In these higher grade lesions, multimodality therapy appears to give better functional results as well as better overall local tumor control than surgery alone. Regardless of the situation, pathologic confirmation of tumor-free margins is necessary in all surgery for soft tissue sarcomas.

## RADIATION THERAPY

Radiation therapy when used alone is of marginal value in the treatment of soft tissue sarcomas.[78] When used alone as the primary mode of therapy, it results in a local recurrence rate of approximately 80 to 85% and survival rates of less than 10%. Lindberg and colleagues[79] have examined the role of radiation therapy as an adjunct to complete surgical excision for this group of tumors. Patients with primary tumors located distal to the elbow or distal to the knee have been treated by complete excision of all gross tumor and have been given high-dose postoperative radiation therapy in the range of 55 to 65 Gy. With this combination, the local recurrence rate for patients with extremity sarcomas was less than 10%, with a limb-salvage rate of approximately 95%. In contrast, the predicted local recurrence rate with this limited surgical excision was considered to be approximately 60%.

These results appear to be equal to those achieved with muscle group excision and radical amputation, and this has been confirmed in numerous subsequent reports.[80–84] In treating more proximally placed tumors in the thigh or those occurring in the head and neck or trunk, the local control rate was much less, and local recurrence rates were found to be approximately 20 to 35%. This combination therapy has not been as efficacious for tumors located in the retroperitoneum because of the dose limitations in irradiating the abdominal structures. The rationale for the high-dose postoperative radiation therapy to the involved tumor bed was based on the hypothesis that even though the gross tumors were radioresistant, the microscopic residual disease present after local excision was not resistant.[85] More recently, preoperative radiation therapy has been combined with conservative surgery. Preoperative radiation has the theoretical advantage of rendering some marginally resectable lesions resectable.

An additional adjuvant radiation therapy technique has been used by Arbeit and coworkers[86] at Memorial Hospital. Patients had en bloc local excision of soft tissue sarcomas of the extremity, immediately followed by the insertion of plastic catheters into the tumor bed, then afterloading with iridium-192 seeds. The average dose of radiation therapy delivered by this technique was 4500 cGy. Nonrandomized studies using these brachytherapy techniques showed a local recurrence rate of 18%. Additional adjuvant radiation therapy techniques used to date include combined brachytherapy and external-beam radiation,[82] hyperfractionation radiotherapy,[84, 87] intraoperative radiotherapy,[88, 89] fast neutron therapy,[90, 91] and the use of iododeoxyuridine as a radiation sensitizer.[92, 93] Whether or not these methods of therapy are superior to standard postoperative external-beam radiation therapy is currently under investigation.

## CHEMOTHERAPY

Although soft tissue sarcomas have a history of extreme resistance to chemotherapy drugs, several agents have been identified that are effective for these tumors. Doxorubicin (Adriamycin) induces a beneficial response in approximately 30% of patients with disseminated disease.[94] There is a steep dose-response relationship as well as a correlation of dose and survival in patients with metastatic soft tissue sarcoma.[95, 96] Its dose-limiting side effect is cardiotoxicity (as described in Chapter 10). Continuous infusion decreases the risk of cardiotoxicity and the severity of nausea and vomiting, while maintaining equivalent antitumor activity.[97–99] Ifosfamide gives a similar response rate and appears to have a dose-response relationship.[100–103] Ifosfamide is also the most active salvage agent for patients who have failed a doxorubicin-containing regimen. Single-agent dacarbazine (DIC) gives a response rate of 15 to 18% and is particularly active in leiomyosarcoma.[104, 105] Epirubicin is also reported to have a response rate of 18% in pretreated patients.[106] Minor activity has been reported for methotrexate, cytoxan, 5-fluorouracil (5-FU), etoposide, cisplatin, carboplatin, and edatrexate. Combination chemotherapy with CYVADIC (cyclophosphamide, vincristine, doxorubicin [Adriamycin], dacarbazine), originally described by Gottlieb, leads to an approximately 25 to 30% response rate.[107–109] The combinations of doxorubicin and DIC; doxorubicin and ifosfamide; and mesna, doxorubicin, ifosfamide, and DIC (MAID) have shown an even higher response rate—47% in patients with evaluable metastatic disease.[55, 102] Although higher response rates have been observed in many series with combination chemotherapy, there has been no significant improvement in survival. A large, randomized European trial showed no advantage in response rate when ifosfamide was added to doxorubicin, compared with doxorubicin alone.[110–114]

Given the limited efficacy of standard doses of the active drugs in soft tissue sarcomas and their dose-response relationship, efforts have focused on escalating the dose of antineoplastic agents. This dose escalation has, in turn, increased the need to address the problems associated with myelosuppression. One method used to ensure prompt recovery of the bone marrow after high doses of chemotherapy has been the use of autologous bone marrow transplantation.[115–117] Investigators have also attempted to dose-intensify standard chemotherapy regimens using colony-stimulating factor to alleviate myelosuppression.[118–122] One of the highest response rates seen so far is 43%, with an 8% complete response rate in the European Organization for Research in Cancer Therapy (EORTC) cooperative group study using granulocyte-macrophage colony-stimulating factor support with high-dose doxorubicin and ifosfamide in patients with advanced soft tissue sarcomas.[123] The most dramatic results with chemotherapy have been those achieved by vincristine, dactinomycin, and cyclophosphamide in childhood rhabdomyosarcomas; the response rate approaches 90%, even with disseminated disease.[124, 125] For most adult patients with advanced sarcomas, combination chemotherapy continues to provide no advantage over single-agent therapy in terms of palliation or survival.

Additional routes of chemotherapy administration have been studied. Original studies by Haskell and colleagues[126] suggested the intra-arterial route for doxorubicin may be more effective than the systemic route in selected patients because a high concentration of the drug in a local treatment area can be achieved. Eilber and associates[127, 128] described preoperative treatment regimens in patients with large soft tissue sarcomas of the extremity, employing intra-arterial doxorubicin followed by rapid-fraction radiation, followed subsequently by complete surgical excision. The local recurrence rate in this series has been less than 8%, and limb salvage has been greater than 95%. More recently, Eilber and colleagues[129] have shown that intravenous administration of currently active drugs is as effective as and less complicated than the intra-arterial route. Isolated limb perfusion using combinations of hyperthermia, chemotherapy, and biologic agents (i.e., interferon) has shown utility in achieving good local control of advanced extremity sarcomas. In some series, previously unresectable lesions have been rendered resectable. The exact contribution of each agent in these regimens is not clear and is under investigation. The eventual role of these regimens in the therapy of soft tissue sarcoma needs to be defined in controlled trials.[130–135]

## ADJUVANT CHEMOTHERAPY

There have been several reported prospective, randomized trials of adjuvant chemotherapy in the postoperative setting in patients with high-grade sarcomas.[136–154] Table 83–6 shows the various reported adjuvant trials limited to extremity sarcomas and the agents used. These trials are not directly comparable because some included patients with grades 2 and 3 sarcomas, whereas others included only grade 3 lesions. These trials included varying numbers of patients and have different follow-up intervals. The reported results in the single-agent adjuvant trials are overwhelmingly negative, however.[155–159] The only exception is the report from Bologna of an improved disease-free survival in patients with high-grade sarcomas receiving single-agent adjuvant doxorubicin chemotherapy.[145]

The importance of extended follow-up was shown in a 1993 report of the late results of this trial, which showed that 5 of 76 patients developed relapsed disease longer than 5 years from treatment.[146] All the other trials have shown no distinct survival advantage for patients receiving single-agent adjuvant chemotherapy. Of the trials using multiple chemotherapeutic agents,[113, 136, 137, 142, 161, 162] two showed a

significant disease-free survival advantage for patients with tumors confined to the extremity.[137, 162] The National Cancer Institute studies using doxorubicin, cyclophosphamide, and methotrexate initially showed a significant increase in disease-free survival and overall survival for patients with extremity sarcomas at 5-year follow-up. Overall survival advantage lost statistical significance after re-evaluation 2 years later (median follow-up 7.1 years), however. Randomized trials of adjuvant chemotherapy in patients with nonextremity sarcomas have all failed to show any statistically significant benefit. Meta-analyses of adjuvant chemotherapy for advanced soft tissue sarcomas have shown a benefit in recurrence-free survival and local and distant recurrence-free interval, however. There is also a trend toward improved overall survival. In one series, the greatest benefit was seen in patients with extremity sarcomas.[163, 164] Newer regimens that incorporate ifosfamide with doxorubicin or epirubicin appear to be promising in the adjuvant setting as well. An Italian study has shown an overall survival benefit for the use of ifosfamide and epirubicin chemotherapy. Additional studies and longer term follow-up are necessary.[165,166]

Systemic chemotherapy is now being studied for use as a neoadjuvant before surgery. Neoadjuvant chemotherapy has some advantages over treatment limited to the postoperative setting. The presence of evaluable tumor allows the determination of the sensitivity to chemotherapy clinically and pathologically. The degree of sensitivity to preoperative chemotherapy may yield valuable prognostic information and may guide postoperative therapy. The tumor may be downstaged, rendering some tumors more amenable to surgical intervention and rendering some previously unresectable tumors resectable. Drug delivery to the primary tumor may also be enhanced because the tumor's vascular supply has not yet been disturbed by surgery and radiation therapy. Nonrandomized studies include those by Rouessé and coworkers,[165] who reported a 38% response rate in a small group of patients treated with a variety of neoadjuvant chemotherapy schedules; Elias and associates,[166] who reported a response rate of 64% in 22 patients with inoperable primary tumors treated with neoadjuvant chemotherapy; and Pezzi and associates,[167] who obtained a 40% response rate in

*Table 83–6.* **Randomized Studies of Adjuvant Chemotherapy for Extremity Sarcomas**

| Institution | Drugs | N | Observation | | Chemotherapy | | Reference |
|---|---|---|---|---|---|---|---|
| | | | %DFS | %S | %DFS | %S | |
| UCLA | A | 119 | 58 | 75 | 58 | 78 | 152 |
| Bologna | A | 77 | 42 | 68 | 68* | 88* | 145, 146 |
| SSG | A | 155 | NR | NR | NR | NR | 150 |
| DFCI/MGH, ECOG, ISSG | A | 101 | 64 | 67 | 78 | 79 | 151 |
| Mayo | A VCDAd | 48 | 67 | 82 | 86 | 88 | 142, 159 |
| MDA | A VCAd | 46 | 35 | 57 | 55 | 65 | 113 |
| EORTC | A VCDt | 223 | 66 | 74 | 77 | 81 | 136 |
| NCI | A C M | 67 | 54 | 60 | 75* | 83 | 160 |
| Bergonié | A VCDt | 36 | NR | NR | NR* | NR* | 137 |

*Significantly greater than observation group, $p \leq 0.05$.

A, Adriamycin (doxorubicin); Ad, actinomycin D; C, Cytoxan; D, doxorubicin (Adriamycin); Dt, dacarbazine; V, vincristine; M, methotrexate; %DFS, percent disease-free survival; %S, percent surviving; UCLA, University of California, Los Angeles; Bologna, Instituto Ortopedico Rizzoli, Bologna; SSG, Scandinavian Sarcoma Group; DFCI, Dana Farber Cancer Institute; MGH, Massachusetts General Hospital; ECOG, Eastern Cooperative Oncology Group; ISSG, Intergroup Sarcoma Study Group; Mayo, Mayo Clinic; MDA, M.D. Anderson Cancer Center; EORTC, European Organization for Research on Treatment of Cancer Institute; NCI, National Cancer Institute; Bergonié, Fondation Bergonié, Bordeaux; NR, not reported.

Adapted from De Vita VT, Hellman S, Rosenberg SA. Cancer principles and practice of oncology. 4th ed. Philadelphia: JB Lippincott, 1993:1471.

46 patients treated with preoperative doxorubicin-containing chemotherapy regimens.

## SUMMARY OF TREATMENT

Integration of modalities is considered most appropriately as a function of the anatomic region of involvement.

**Extremity Tumors.** Most extremity tumors in children are rhabdomyosarcomas. The most appropriate means of therapy appears to be initiation of chemotherapy with VAC (vincristine, doxorubicin [Adriamycin], cyclophosphamide), complete surgical excision if possible, and postoperative radiation therapy with continuing cycling of chemotherapy.

In adults with extremity tumors, several factors must be taken into consideration. Localized tumors that are small, well circumscribed, well differentiated, and of low grade can be treated adequately by wide surgical excision. Clinicopathologic stage I and stage II tumors do not appear to require local or systemic postoperative adjuvant therapy with radiation or chemotherapy because local recurrence rates are less than 10% and survival rates are high. In patients with grade 2 lesions that are more proximally placed and larger, however, integration of combinations of surgery and radiation therapy (either preoperatively or postoperatively) appears to improve local tumor control.[168] In patients with clinicopathologic stage III or IV tumors or those that are well differentiated but proximally placed, additional therapy before or after surgery appears to be advisable.[169]

Although local recurrence is a major problem, distant metastatic spread is the most important determinant of patient survival. Increased control of metastases requires some form of systemically active therapy. Surgical resection of pulmonary metastases has been performed in selected patients whose primary tumor has been controlled, who lack extrapulmonary disease, and who have adequate cardiopulmonary reserve. Important prognostic factors include tumor histology, number of pulmonary nodules, and disease-free interval. The single most important predictor of survival for metastasectomy is the completeness of resection, however. Median sternotomy is recommended because both lungs can be examined and because approximately 40% of bilateral metastases are missed on conventional computed tomographic scans. Resection of five pulmonary metastases resulted in a prolonged disease-free survival and possible cure for a subset of patients (approximately 20 to 35%).[170–172] Several series have also documented a 25 to 35% 5-year survival rate in selected patients undergoing aggressive repeated metastasectomies.[171–173]

**Head and Neck Tumors.** For patients with head and neck sarcomas, the appropriate method of therapy is yet to be defined. In childhood head and neck sarcomas, primary treatment with VAC chemotherapy combined with radiation after adequate biopsy is the treatment of choice. Radical surgical resection is required infrequently.

In adults with sarcomas of the head and neck, a combination of surgical excision and radiation therapy appears to be essential. Whether there is an advantage to doing this preoperatively or postoperatively is not defined clearly.

**Retroperitoneal Sarcoma.** Complete excision of retroperitoneal sarcomas should be carried out in all cases, regardless of the grade, when technically possible. Once the diagnosis is made, the use of preoperative radiation therapy or combination chemotherapy, or both, has been shown to reduce tumor size in approximately 40% of the cases and to clarify resection margins. This treatment has allowed a much more complete surgical excision of the primary tumor. There are no randomized trials directly comparing preoperative or neoadjuvant therapy in retroperitoneal sarcomas with surgery and postoperative therapy, however.

## PROSPECTS FOR THE FUTURE

Significant progress has been made in understanding of the biology and in the recognition and treatment of soft tissue sarcomas. The availability of computed tomographic scanning and especially refinements in MRI technology have facilitated greatly the delineation and detection of these tumors. The recognition that tumor grade is the dominant prognostic variable has resulted in more common use of the grading system and a more uniform reporting and stratification of end results. Multimodality therapy with surgery, radiation, and chemotherapy has resulted in a marked improvement in local tumor control for patients with high-grade soft tissue sarcomas in the extremities. The combination of modalities has allowed smaller surgical excisions of the primary tumor and a greater incidence of preservation of the extremity and much of its function.

There are currently several methods of performing multimodality therapy, including neoadjuvant therapy and postoperative therapy. The combination of surgery and radiation, either preoperatively or postoperatively, is of proven efficacy for patients with soft tissue sarcoma. Chemotherapy is playing an increasing role in primary tumor therapy. The availability of doxorubicin, DIC, and ifosfamide has added significantly to the clinical armamentarium. Ongoing trials will define better the usefulness of dose-intensified regimens made possible with the use of cytokines and bone marrow transplantation. Combination chemotherapy and radiation are of value in the neoadjuvant setting. Surgical resection of pulmonary metastases is beneficial in a subset of patients and provides a 20 to 25% long-term survival. As a result of advances in surgery, chemotherapy, and radiation and by the successful integration of these modalities, the overall survival and quality of life for patients with soft tissue sarcoma continue to improve. It is also hoped that the wealth of knowledge gained regarding the biology of sarcomas will soon lead to novel and more effective therapies.

## SUGGESTIONS FOR ADDITIONAL READING

Graadt van Roggen JF, Bovée JV, Morreau J, Hogendoorn PC. Diagnostic and prognostic implications of the unfolding molecular biology of bone and soft tissue tumours. J Clin Pathol 1999;52:481–9.

Murray EM, Werner D, Greeff EA, Taylor DA. Postradiation sarcomas: 20 cases and a literature review. Int J Radiat Oncol Biol Phys 1999;45:951–61.

Rougraff B. The diagnosis and management of soft tissue sarcomas of the extremities in the adult. Curr Probl Cancer 1999;23:1–50.

Patel SR, Benjamin RS. New chemotherapeutic strategies for soft tissue sarcomas. Semin Surg Oncol 1999;17:47–51.

## REFERENCES

1. Landis SH, Murray T, Bolden S, Wingo PA. Cancer statistics, 1999. CA Cancer J Clin 1999;49:8–31.

2. Enzinger FM. Soft tissue tumors. 2nd ed. Washington, D.C.: CV Mosby, 1988:2.
3. Torosian MH, Friedrich C, Godbold J, et al. Soft-tissue sarcoma: initial characteristics and prognostic factors in patients with and without metastatic disease. Semin Surg Oncol 1988;4:13–9.
4. Li FP, Fraumeni JF Jr. Prospective study of a family cancer syndrome. JAMA 1982;247:2692–4.
5. Lynch HT, Katz DA, Bogard PJ, Lynch JF. The sarcoma, breast cancer, lung cancer, and adrenocortical carcinoma syndrome revisited: childhood cancer. Am J Dis Child 1985;139:134–6.
6. Muller S, Gadner H, Weber B, et al. Wilms' tumor and adrenocortical carcinoma with hemihypertrophy and hamartomas. Eur J Pediatr 1978;127:219–26.
7. Hayward NK, Little MH, Mortimer RH, et al. Generation of homozygosity at the c-Ha-ras-1 locus on chromosome 11p in an adrenal adenoma from an adult with Wiedemann-Beckwith syndrome. Cancer Genet Cytogenet 1988;30:127–32.
8. Sørensen SA, Mulvihill JJ, Nielsen A. Long-term follow-up of von Recklinghausen neurofibromatosis: survival and malignant neoplasms. N Engl J Med 1986;314:1010–5.
9. Ginsburg DS, Hernandez E, Johnson JW. Sarcoma complicating von Recklinghausen disease in pregnancy. Obstet Gynecol 1981;58:385–7.
10. Verola O, Dallot A, Audebaud G, et al. [Neurogenic sarcoma in Von Recklinghausen's disease: histological, immunohistochemical and ultrastructural study of 6 cases.] Arch Anat Cytol Pathol 1985;33:5–16.
11. Fraumeni JF Jr, Vogel CL, Easton JM. Sarcomas and multiple polyposis in a kindred: a genetic variety of hereditary polyposis? Arch Intern Med 1968;121:57–61.
12. Usui M, Ishii S, Yamawaki S, Hirayama T. The occurrence of soft tissue sarcomas in three siblings with Werner's syndrome. Cancer 1984;54:2580–6.
13. Józwiak S, Górnicki J, Michalowicz R, Gastol P. [A case of renal clear cell sarcoma in a child with tuberous sclerosis.] Wiad Lek 1993;46:846–8.
14. Schweisguth O, Gerard-Marchant R, Lemerle J. [Basal cell nevus syndrome: association with congenital rhabdomyosarcoma.] Arch Fr Pediatr 1968;25:1083–93.
15. Cooper CS, Stratton MR. Soft tissue tumours: the genetic basis of development. Carcinogenesis 1991;12:155–65.
16. Sandberg AA, Turc-Carel C, Gemmill RM. Chromosomes in solid tumors and beyond. Cancer Res 1988;48:1049–59.
17. Fletcher JA, Kozakewich HP, Hoffer FA, et al. Diagnostic relevance of clonal cytogenetic aberrations in malignant soft-tissue tumors. N Engl J Med 1991;324:436–42.
18. Malkin D, Jolly KW, Barbier N, et al. Germline mutations of the p53 tumor-suppressor gene in children and young adults with second malignant neoplasms. N Engl J Med 1992;326:1309–15.
19. Toguchida J, Yamaguchi T, Dayton SH, et al. Prevalence and spectrum of germline mutations of the p53 gene among patients with sarcoma. N Engl J Med 1992;326:1301–8.
20. Brachman DG, Hallahan DE, Beckett MA, et al. p53 gene mutations and abnormal retinoblastoma protein in radiation-induced human sarcomas. Cancer Res 1991;51:23 Pt 1:6393–6.
21. Limon J, Dal Cin P, Sandberg AA. Translocations involving the X chromosome in solid tumors: presentation of two sarcomas with t(X;18)(q13;p11). Cancer Genet Cytogenet 1986;23:87–91.
22. Turc-Carel C, Dal Cin P, Limon J, et al. Translocation X;18 in synovial sarcoma. Cancer Genet Cytogenet 1986;23:93.
23. Smith S, Reeves BR, Wong L, Fisher C. A consistent chromosome translocation in synovial sarcoma. Cancer Genet Cytogenet 1987;26:179–80.
24. Delattre O, Zucman J, Plougastel B, et al. Gene fusion with an ETS DNA-binding domain caused by chromosome translocation in human tumours. Nature 1992;359:162–5.
25. Barr FG, Galili N, Holick J, et al. Rearrangement of the PAX3 paired box gene in the paediatric solid tumour alveolar rhabdomyosarcoma. Nat Genet 1993;3:113–7.
26. Aman P, Ron D, Mandahl N, et al. Rearrangement of the transcription factor gene CHOP in myxoid liposarcomas with t(12;16)(q13;p11). Genes Chromosomes Cancer 1992;5:278–85.
27. Kawai A, Woodruff J, Healey J, et al. SYT gene fusion as a determinant of morphology and prognosis in synovial sarcoma. N Engl J Med 1998;338:153–60.
28. Brand KG. Cancer associated with asbestosis, schistosomiasis, foreign bodies, and scars. In: Becker FF, ed. Cancer 1: a comprehensive treatise, 2nd edition. Etiology: chemical and physical carcinogenesis. New York: Plenum Press, 1975:661–692.
29. Hempelmann LH, Hall WJ, Phillips M, et al. Neoplasms in persons treated with x-rays in infancy: fourth survey in 20 years. J Natl Cancer Inst 1975;55:519–30.
30. Ruka W, Sikorowa L, Iwanowska J, Romeyko M. Induced soft tissue sarcomas following radiation treatment for uterine carcinomas. Eur J Surg Oncol 1991;17:585–93.
31. Stewart FW, Treves N. Lymphangiosarcoma in postmastectomy lymphedema: a report of six cases in elephantiasis chirurgica. Cancer 1948;1:64–81.
32. Francis KC, Lindquist HD. Lymphangiosarcoma of the lower extremity involved with chronic lymphedema. Am J Surg 1970;100:617–619.
33. Greenwald P, Kovasznay B, Collins DN, Therriault G. Sarcomas of soft tissues after Vietnam service. J Natl Cancer Inst 1984;73:1107–9.
34. Kang H, Enzinger FM, Breslin P, et al. Soft tissue sarcoma and military service in Vietnam: a case-control study [published erratum appears in J Natl Cancer Inst 1987 Nov;79(5):1173]. J Natl Cancer Inst 1987;79:693–9.
35. Enzinger FM. Histological classification of soft tissue tumours. Geneva: World Health Organization, 1969.
36. Shiraki M, Enterline HT, Brooks JJ, et al. Pathologic analysis of advanced adult soft tissue sarcomas, bone sarcomas, and mesotheliomas: the Eastern Cooperative Oncology Group (ECOG) experience. Cancer 1989;64:484–90.
37. Coindre JM, Trojani M, Contesso G, et al. Reproducibility of a histopathologic grading system for adult soft tissue sarcoma. Cancer 1986;58:306–9.
38. Presant CA, Russell WO, Alexander RW, Fu YS. Soft-tissue and bone sarcoma histopathology peer review: the frequency of disagreement in diagnosis and the need for second pathology opinions: the Southeastern Cancer Study Group experience. J Clin Oncol 1986;4:1658–61.
39. Alvegard TA, Berg NO. Histopathology peer review of high-grade soft tissue sarcoma: the Scandinavian Sarcoma Group experience. J Clin Oncol 1989;7:1845–51.
40. Roholl PJ, De Jong AS, Ramaekers FC. Application of markers in the diagnosis of soft tissue tumours. Histopathology 1985;9:1019–35.
41. Brooks JJ. Immunohistochemistry in sarcomas. In: Ryan JR, Baker LO, eds. Recent concepts in sarcoma treatment: Proceedings of the International Symposium on Sarcomas, Tarpon Springs, Florida, October 8–10, 1987. Boston: Kluwer Academic, 1988:48–58.
42. Fletcher CD. The use of immunohistochemistry in the diagnosis of soft tissue tumours. Histopathology 1986;10:771–3.
43. Azumi N, Ben-Ezra J, Battifora H. Immunophenotypic diagnosis of leiomyosarcomas and rhabdomyosarcomas with monoclonal antibodies to muscle-specific actin and desmin in formalin-fixed tissue. Mod Pathol 1988;1:469–74.
44. Ordonez NG, Mahfouz SM, Mackay B. Synovial sarcoma: an immunohistochemical and ultrastructural study. Hum Pathol 1990;21:733–49.
45. Kindblom LG, Lodding P, Angervall L. Clear-cell sarcoma of tendons and aponeuroses: an immunohistochemical and electron microscopic analysis indicating neural crest origin. Virchows Arch A Pathol Anat Histopathol 1983;401:109–28.
46. Chase DR, Enzinger FM, Weiss SW, Langloss JM. Keratin in epithelioid sarcoma: an immunohistochemical study. Am J Surg Pathol 1984;8:435–41.
47. Miettinen M, Sarlomo-Rikala M, Lasota J. Gastrointestinal stromal tumors: recent advances in understanding of their biology. Hum Pathol 1999;30:1213–20.
48. Sircar K, Hewlett BR, Huizinga JD, et al. Interstitial cells of Cajal as precursors of gastrointestinal stromal tumors. Am J Surg Pathol 1999;23:377–89.
49. Miettinen M, Sarlomo-Rikala M, Lasota J. Gastrointestinal stromal tumours. Ann Chir Gynaecol 1998;87:278–81.
50. Sarlomo-Rikala M, Kovatich AJ, Barusevicius A, Miettinen M. CD117: a sensitive marker for gastrointestinal stromal tumors that is more specific than CD34. Mod Pathol 1998;11:728–34.
51. Fisher C. The value of electronmicroscopy and immunohistochemistry in the diagnosis of soft tissue sarcomas: a study of 200 cases. Histopathology 1990;16:441–54.
52. Costa J, Wesley RA, Glatstein E, Rosenberg SA. The grading of soft tissue sarcomas: results of a clinicohistopathologic correlation in a series of 163 cases. Cancer 1984;53:530–41.

53. Lack EE, Steinberg SM, White DE, et al. Extremity soft tissue sarcomas: analysis of prognostic variables in 300 cases and evaluation of tumor necrosis as a factor in stratifying higher-grade sarcomas. J Surg Oncol 1989;41:263–73.

54. Trojani M, Contesso G, Coindre JM, et al. Soft-tissue sarcomas of adults: study of pathological prognostic variables and definition of a histopathological grading system. Int J Cancer 1984;33:37–42.

55. Elias A, Ryan L, Sulkes A, et al. Response to mesna, doxorubicin, ifosfamide, and dacarbazine in 108 patients with metastatic or unresectable sarcoma and no prior chemotherapy. J Clin Oncol 1989;7:1208–16.

56. Hadju SI. Pathology of soft tissue tumors. Philadelphia: Lea & Febiger, 1979.

57. Markhede G, Angervall L, Stener B. A multivariate analysis of the prognosis after surgical treatment of malignant soft-tissue tumors. Cancer 1982;49:1721–33.

58. Myhre-Jensen O, Kaae S, Madsen EH, Sneppen O. Histopathological grading in soft-tissue tumours: relation to survival in 261 surgically treated patients. Acta Pathol Microbiol Immunol Scand [A] 1983;91:145–50.

59. Van Unnik JAM, Coindre JM, Contesso G, et al. Grading of soft tissue sarcomas: experience of the EORTC soft tissue and bone sarcoma group. In: Ryan JR, Baker LO, eds. Recent concepts in sarcoma treatment: Proceedings of the International Symposium on Sarcomas, Tarpon Springs, Florida, October 8–10, 1987. Boston: Kluwer Academic, 1988:7–13.

60. Albus-Lutter CE, de Stéfani E, van Unnik JAM. Clinicopathologic relations in soft tissue sarcomas. In: Van Oosterom AT, van Unnik JAM, eds. Management of soft tissue and bone sarcomas. New York: Raven Press, 1986:27.

61. Broders AC, Hargrave R. Meyerding HW. Pathological features of soft tissue fibrosarcoma—with special reference to the grading of its malignancy. Surg Gynecol Obstet 1939;69:267–280.

62. Mandard AM, Chasle J, Mandard JC, et al. The pathologist's role in a multidisciplinary approach for soft part tissue sarcoma: a reappraisal (39 cases). J Surg Oncol 1981;17:69–81.

63. Cagle LA, Mirra JM, Storm FK, et al. Histologic features relating to prognosis in synovial sarcoma. Cancer 1987;59:1810–4.

64. Kampe CE, Rosen G, Eilber F, et al. Synovial sarcoma: a study of intensive chemotherapy in 14 patients with localized disease. Cancer 1993;72:2161–9.

65. Mazeron JJ, Suit HD. Lymph nodes as sites of metastases from sarcomas of soft tissue. Cancer 1987;60:1800–8.

66. Potter DA, Glenn J, Kinsella T, et al. Patterns of recurrence in patients with high-grade soft-tissue sarcomas. J Clin Oncol 1985;3:353–66.

67. Kavanagh J, Yap B, Luna M, Tashima C. Metastatic patterns of adult soft tissue sarcomas. Proc Am Assoc Cancer Res 1980;21:480.

68. Chang AE, Matory YL, Dwyer AJ, et al. Magnetic resonance imaging versus computed tomography in the evaluation of soft tissue tumors of the extremities. Ann Surg 1987;205:340–8.

69. Pettersson H, Gillespy T 3d, Hamlin DJ, et al. Primary musculoskeletal tumors: examination with MR imaging compared with conventional modalities. Radiology 1987;164:237–41.

70. Herrlin K, Ling LB, Pettersson H, et al. Gadolinium-DTPA enhancement of soft tissue tumors in magnetic resonance imaging. Acta Radiol 1990;31:233–6.

71. Shinkwin MA, Lenkinski RE, Daly JM, et al. Integrated magnetic resonance imaging and phosphorus spectroscopy of soft tissue tumors. Cancer 1991;67:1849–58.

72. Dewhirst MW, Sostman HD, Leopold KA, et al. Soft-tissue sarcomas: MR imaging and MR spectroscopy for prognosis and therapy monitoring: work in progress. Radiology 1990;174:3 Pt 1:847–53.

73. Barth RJ Jr, Merino MJ, Solomon D, et al. A prospective study of the value of core needle biopsy and fine needle aspiration in the diagnosis of soft tissue masses. Surgery 1992;112:536–43.

74. Russell WO, Cohen J, Enzinger F, et al. A clinical and pathological staging system for soft tissue sarcomas. Cancer 1977;40:1562–70.

75. Bowden L, Booher RJ. The principles and techniques of resection of soft parts for sarcoma. Surgery 1958;44:963–77.

76. Gerner RE, Moore GE, Pickren JW. Soft tissue sarcomas. Ann Surg 1975;181:803–8.

77. Enneking WF, Spanier SS, Malawer MM. The effect of the anatomic setting on the results of surgical procedures for soft parts sarcoma of the thigh. Cancer 1981;47:1005–22.

78. Tepper JE, Suit HD. Radiation therapy alone for sarcoma of soft tissue. Cancer 1985;56:475–9.

79. Lindberg RD, Martin RG, Romsdahl MM, Barkley HT Jr. Conservative surgery and postoperative radiotherapy in 300 adults with soft-tissue sarcomas. Cancer 1981;47:2391–7.

80. Brant TA, Parsons JT, Marcus RB Jr, et al. Preoperative irradiation for soft tissue sarcomas of the trunk and extremities in adults. Int J Radiat Oncol Biol Phys 1990;19:899–906.

81. Pao WJ, Pilepich MV. Postoperative radiotherapy in the treatment of extremity soft tissue sarcomas. Int J Radiat Oncol Biol Phys 1990;19:907–11.

82. Schray MF, Gunderson LL, Sim FH, et al. Soft tissue sarcoma: integration of brachytherapy, resection, and external irradiation. Cancer 1990;66:451–6.

83. Shiu MH, Hilaris BS, Harrison LB, Brennan MF. Brachytherapy and function-saving resection of soft tissue sarcoma arising in the limb. Int J Radiat Oncol Biol Phys 1991;21:1485–92.

84. Robinson M, Cassoni A, Harmer C, et al. High dose hyperfractionated radiotherapy in the treatment of extremity soft tissue sarcomas. Radiother Oncol 1991;22:118–26.

85. Suit HD, Mankin HJ, Wood WC, et al. Treatment of the patient with stage M0 soft tissue sarcoma. J Clin Oncol 1988;6:854–62.

86. Arbeit JM, Hilaris BS, Brennan MF. Wound complications in the multimodality treatment of extremity and superficial truncal sarcomas. J Clin Oncol 1987;5:480–8.

87. Darendeliler E, Onat H, Inanç ES, et al. Hyperfractionated radiotherapy (H-RT) and concomitant continuous infusion (CCI) epirubicin in locally advanced soft tissue sarcomas (STS). Proc ASCO 1993;12:471.

88. Kinsella TJ, Sindelar WF, Lack E, et al. Preliminary results of a randomized study of adjuvant radiation therapy in resectable adult retroperitoneal soft tissue sarcomas. J Clin Oncol 1988;6:18–25.

89. Willett CG, Suit HD, Tepper JE, et al. Intraoperative electron beam radiation therapy for retroperitoneal soft tissue sarcoma. Cancer 1991;68:278–83.

90. Schmitt G, Mills EE, Levin V, et al. The role of neutrons in the treatment of soft tissue sarcomas. Cancer 1989;64:2064–8.

91. Pelton JG, Del Rowe JD, Bolen JW, et al. Fast neutron radiotherapy for soft tissue sarcomas: University of Washington experience and review of the world's literature. Am J Clin Oncol 1986;9:397–400.

92. Goffman T, Tochner Z, Glatstein E. Primary treatment of large and massive adult sarcomas with iododeoxyuridine and aggressive hyperfractionated irradiation. Cancer 1991;67:572–6.

93. Sussman J, Lawrence T, Robertson J, et al. Short-term continuous infusion of IUDR produces potentially radiosensitizing incorporation in soft tissue sarcomas. Proc ASCO 1993;12:471.

94. Gottlieb JA, Baker LH, Quagliana JM, et al. Chemotherapy of sarcomas with a combination of Adriamycin and dimethyl triazeno imidazole carboxamide. Cancer 1972;30:1632–8.

95. O'Bryan RM, Baker LH, Gottlieb JE, et al. Dose response evaluation of Adriamycin in human neoplasia. Cancer 1977;39:1940–8.

96. Bodey GP, Rodriguez V, Murphy WK, et al. Protected environment—prophylactic antibiotic program for malignant sarcomas: randomized trial during remission induction chemotherapy. Cancer 1981;47:2422–9.

97. Casper E, Magill G, Freidrich C, et al. Prospective randomized trial of adjuvant Adriamycin (A) by bolus (B) vs 72-hour continuous infusion (CI) in patients (pts) with high grade soft tissue sarcoma (HGS). Proc ASCO 1989;8:320.

98. Baker L, Green S, Ryan J, et al. SWOG 8024: combined modality therapy for disseminated soft tissue sarcoma, Phase III. Proc ASCO 1987;6:138.

99. Brennan MF, Friedrich C, Almadrones L, Magill G. Prospective randomized trial examining the cardiac toxicity of adjuvant doxorubicin in high grade extremity sarcomas. In: Salmon S, ed. Adjuvant therapy of cancer. Vol V. Orlando: Grune & Stratton, 1987:745–51.

100. Brain E, Le Cesne A, Le Chevalier T, et al. High dose ifosfamide (HDI) can circumvent resistance to standard dose ifosfamide (SDI) in advanced soft tissue sarcomas (ASTS). Proc ASCO 1993;12:470.

101. Elias AD, Eder JP, Shea T, et al. High-dose ifosfamide with mesna uroprotection: a phase I study. J Clin Oncol 1990;8:170–8.

102. Antman KH, Ryan L, Elias A, et al. Response to ifosfamide and mesna: 124 previously treated patients with metastatic or unresectable sarcoma [published erratum appears in J Clin Oncol 1989 Sep;7(9):1369]. J Clin Oncol 1989;7:126–31.

103. Bramwell VH, Mouridsen HT, Santoro A, et al. Cyclophosphamide versus ifosfamide: final report of a randomized phase II trial in adult soft tissue sarcomas. Eur J Cancer Clin Oncol 1987;23:311–21.

104. Rosen G, Chawla S, Hamburg S, Lowenbraun S. Phase II study of high dose continuous infusion dimethyl triazeno imidazole carboxamide (DTIC) in metastatic leiomyosarcoma (LMS). Proc ASCO 1990;9:313.

105. Buesa JM, Mouridsen HT, van Oosterom AT, et al. High-dose DTIC in advanced soft-tissue sarcomas in the adult: a phase II study of the E.O.R.T.C. Soft Tissue and Bone Sarcoma Group. Ann Oncol 1991;2:307–9.

106. Mouridsen HT, Bastholt L, Somers R, et al. Adriamycin versus epirubicin in advanced soft tissue sarcomas: a randomized phase II/phase III study of the EORTC Soft Tissue and Bone Sarcoma Group. Eur J Cancer Clin Oncol 1987;23:1477–83.

107. Yap BS, Baker LH, Sinkovics JG, et al. Cyclophosphamide, vincristine, Adriamycin, and DTIC (CYVADIC) combination chemotherapy for the treatment of advanced sarcomas. Cancer Treat Rep 1980;64:93–8.

108. Baker LH, Benjamin R, Fine G, et al. Combination chemotherapy in the management of disseminated soft tissue sarcomas—a Southwest Oncology Group (SWOG) study. Proc Am Assoc Cancer Res & Am Soc Clin Oncol 1979;20:378.

109. Pinedo HM, Vendrik CPJ, Bramwell VHC, et al. Re-evaluation of the CYVADIC regimen for metastatic soft tissue sarcoma. Proc Am Assoc Cancer Res & Am Soc Clin Oncol 1979;20:346.

110. Edmonson JH, Ryan L, Blum RH, et al. Randomized comparison of doxorubicin alone vs ifosfamide and doxorubicin or mitomycin, doxorubicin, cisplatin against advanced soft tissue sarcomas. J Clin Oncol 1993;11:1269–75.

111. Antman K, Crowley J, Balcerzak SP, et al. An intergroup phase III randomized study of doxorubicin and dacarbazine with or without ifosfamide and mesna in advanced tissue bone sarcomas. J Clin Oncol 1993;11:1276–85.

112. Santoro A, Tursz T, Mouridsen H, et al. Doxorubicin versus CY-VADIC versus doxorubicin plus ifosfamide in first-line treatment of advanced sarcomas: a study of the EORTC. J Clin Oncol 1995;13:1537–45.

113. Benjamin RS, Terjanian TO, Fenoglio CJ, et al. The importance of combination chemotherapy for adjuvant treatment of high-risk patients with soft-tissue sarcomas of the extremities. In: Salmon SE, ed. Adjuvant therapy of cancer. Vol V. Philadelphia: W.B. Saunders, 1987:735–44.

114. Lindberg RD, Murphy WK, Benjamin RS, et al. Adjuvant chemotherapy in the treatment of primary soft tissue sarcomas: preliminary report. In: Management of bone and soft tissue tumors. Chicago: Year Book Medical Publishers, 1977:343–52.

115. Elias AD, Ayash LJ, Eder JP, et al. A phase I study of high-dose ifosfamide and escalating doses of carboplatin with autologous bone marrow support. J Clin Oncol 1991;9:320–7.

116. Pinkerton CR, Groot-Loonen J, Barrett A, et al. Rapid VAC high dose melphalan regimen, a novel chemotherapy approach in childhood soft tissue sarcomas. Br J Cancer 1991;64:381–5.

117. Pinkerton CR. Megatherapy for soft tissue sarcomas: EBMT experience. Bone Marrow Transplant 1991;7:Suppl 3:120–2.

118. Vadhan-Raj S, Broxmeyer HE, Hittelman WN, et al. Abrogating chemotherapy-induced myelosuppression by recombinant granulocyte-macrophage colony-stimulating factor in patients with sarcoma: protection at the progenitor cell level. J Clin Oncol 1992;10:1266–77.

119. Steward WP, Verweij J, Somers R, et al. High dose chemotherapy (CT) with two schedules of recombinant human granulocyte-macrophage colony-stimulating factor (rhGM-CSF) in the treatment of advanced adult soft tissue sarcomas (STS). Proc ASCO 1991;10:349.

120. Toner GC, Bishop JF, Fennessy A, et al. Escalation of dose intensity of single agent epirubicin with granulocyte-macrophage colony stimulating factor (GM-CSF). Proc ASCO 1992;11:415.

121. Patel SR, Vadhan-Raj S, Trevino C, et al. Phase II study of high dose ifosfamide (HDI) + G-CSF in patients (pts) with malignant bone tumors (BT) and metastatic soft-tissue sarcomas (STS). Proc ASCO 1992;11:413.

122. Chevallier V, Bui NB, Bonichon F, et al. Efficacy of rG-CSF on hematological tolerance to MAID chemotherapy in sarcoma patients and impact on dose intensity. Proc ASCO 1992;11:412.

123. Steward WP, Verweij J, Somers R, et al. Granulocyte-macrophage colony-stimulating factor allows safe escalation of dose-intensity of chemotherapy in metastatic adult soft tissue sarcomas: a study of the European Organization for Research and Treatment of Cancer Soft Tissue and Bone Sarcoma Group. J Clin Oncol 1993;11:15–21.

124. Maurer HM, Moon T, Donaldson M, et al. The intergroup rhabdomyosarcoma study: a preliminary report. Cancer 1977;40:2015–26.

125. Donaldson SS, Castro JR, Wilbur JR, Jesse RH Jr. Rhabdomyosarcoma of head and neck in children: combination treatment by surgery, irradiation, and chemotherapy. Cancer 1973;31:26–35.

126. Haskell CM, Eilber FR, Morton DL. Adriamycin (NSC-123127) by arterial infusion. Cancer Chemother Rep 1975;6:Pt III:187–9.

127. Eilber FR, Morton DL, Eckardt J, et al. Limb salvage for skeletal and soft tissue sarcomas: multidisciplinary preoperative therapy. Cancer 1984;53:2579–84.

128. Eilber FR, Giuliano AE, Hugh J, et al. Limb salvage for high-grade soft tissue sarcomas of the extremity: experience at the University of California, Los Angeles. Cancer Treat Symp 1985;3:49–57.

129. Eilber FR, Giuliano AE, Huth JF, et al. Intravenous vs intraarterial Adriamycin, 2800 r radiation and surgical excision for extremity soft tissue sarcomas: a randomized prospective trial. Proc ASCO 1990;9:309.

130. Eggermont AMM, Schraffordt Koops H, Lienard D, et al. Isolated limb perfusion with high dose tumor necrosis factor-α in combination with IFN-γ and melphalan for irresectable extremity soft tissue sarcomas: a multicenter trial. J Clin Oncol 1996;14:2656–65.

131. Eggermont AMM, Schraffordt Koops H, Klausner J, et al. Isolated limb perfusion with tumor necrosis factor-α and melphalan in 186 patients with locally advanced extremity sarcomas: the cumulative multicenter European experience. Ann Surg 1996;224:756–65.

132. Plaat BE, Molenaar WM, Mastik MF, et al. Hyperthermic isolated limb perfusion with tumor necrosis factor-alpha and melphalan in patients with locally advanced soft tissue sarcomas: treatment response and clinical outcome related to changes in proliferation and apoptosis. Clin Cancer Res 1999;5:1650–7.

133. Lev-Chelouche D, Abu-Abeid S, Kollander Y, et al. Multifocal soft tissue sarcoma: limb salvage following hyperthermic isolated limb perfusion with high-dose tumor necrosis factor and melphalan. J Surg Oncol 1999;70:185–9.

134. Olieman AF, van Ginkel RJ, Molenaar WM, et al. Hyperthermic isolated limb perfusion with tumour necrosis factor-alpha and melphalan as palliative limb-saving treatment in patients with locally advanced soft-tissue sarcomas of the extremities with regional or distant metastases: is it worthwhile? Arch Orthop Trauma Surg 1998;188:70–4.

135. Schraffordt Koops H, Eggermont AM, Lienard D, et al. Hyperthermic isolated limb perfusion with tumour necrosis factor and melphalan as treatment of locally advanced or recurrent soft tissue sarcomas of the extremities. Radiother Oncol 1998;48:1–4.

136. Bramwell V, Rouessé J, Steward W, et al. European experience of adjuvant chemotherapy for soft tissue sarcoma: interim report of a randomized trial of CYVADIC versus control. In: Ryan JR, Baker LO, eds. Recent concepts in sarcoma treatment: Proceedings of the International Symposium on Sarcomas, Tarpon Springs, Florida, October 8–10, 1987. Boston: Kluwer Academic, 1988:156–63.

137. Ravaud A, Bui NB, Coindre J-M, et al. Adjuvant chemotherpy with Cyvadic in high risk soft tissue sarcoma: a randomized prospective trial. In: Salmon SE, ed. Adjuvant therapy of cancer. Vol VI. Philadelphia: WB Saunders, 1990:556–66.

138. Rosenberg SA, Tepper J, Glatstein E, et al. Prospective randomized evaluation of adjuvant chemotherapy in adults with soft tissue sarcomas of the extremities. Cancer 1983;52:424–34.

139. Rosenberg SA. Prospective randomized trials demonstrating the efficacy of adjuvant chemotherapy in adult patients with soft tissue sarcomas. Cancer Treat Rep 1984;68:1067–78.

140. Rosenberg SA, Chang AE, Glatstein E. Adjuvant chemotherapy for treatment of extremity soft tissue sarcomas: review of National Cancer Institute experience. Cancer Treat Symp 1985;3:83–8.

141. Antman K, Suit H, Amato D, et al. Preliminary results of a randomized trial of adjuvant doxorubicin for sarcomas: lack of apparent difference between treatment groups. J Clin Oncol 1984;2:601–8.

142. Edmonson JH, Fleming TR, Ivins JC, et al. Randomized study of systemic chemotherapy following complete excision of nonosseous sarcomas. J Clin Oncol 1984;2:1390–6.

143. Baker LH. Adjuvant therapy for soft tissue sarcomas. In: Ryan JR, Baker LO, eds. Recent concepts in sarcoma treatment: Proceedings of the International Symposium on Sarcomas, Tarpon Springs, Florida, October 8–10, 1987. Boston: Kluwer Academic, 1988:130–35.

144. Antman K, Amato D, Lerner H, et al. Adjuvant doxorubicin for sarcoma: data from the Eastern Cooperative Oncology Group and

Dana-Farber Cancer Institute/Massachusetts General Hospital studies. Cancer Treat Symp 1985;3:109–15.

145. Picci P, Bacci G, Gherlinzoni F, et al. Results of a randomized trial for the treatment of localized soft tissue tumors (STS) of the extremities in adult patients. In: Ryan JR, Baker LO, eds. Recent concepts in sarcoma treatment: Proceedings of the International Symposium on Sarcomas, Tarpon Springs, Florida, October 8–10, 1987. Boston: Kluwer Academic, 1988:144–48.

146. Gherlinzini F, Picci P, Bacci G, et al. Late results of a randomized trial for the treatment of soft tissue sarcomas of the extremities in adult patients. Proc ASCO 1993;12:468.

147. Gherlinzoni F, Bacci G, Picci P, et al. A randomized trial for the treatment of high-grade soft-tissue sarcomas of the extremities: preliminary observations. J Clin Oncol 1986;4:552–8.

148. Eilber FR, Giuliano AE, Hugh JF, Morton DL. Adjuvant Adriamycin in high-grade extremity soft-tissue sarcoma—a randomized prospective trial. Proc ASCO 1986;5:125.

149. Lerner HJ, Amato DA, Savlov ED, et al. Eastern Cooperative Oncology Group: a comparison of adjuvant doxorubicin and observation for patients with localized soft tissue sarcoma. J Clin Oncol 1987;5:613–7.

150. Alvegard TA, Sigurdsson H, Mouridsen H, et al. Adjuvant chemotherapy with doxorubicin in high-grade soft tissue sarcoma: a randomized trial of the Scandinavian Sarcoma Group. J Clin Oncol 1989;7:1504–13.

151. Antman K, Ryan L, Borden E, et al. Pooled results from three randomized adjuvant studies of doxorubicin versus observation in soft tissue sarcoma: 10 year results and review of the literature. In: Salmon SE, ed. Adjuvant therapy of cancer. Vol VI. Philadelphia: WB Saunders, 1990:529–43.

152. Eilber FR, Giuliano AE, Huth JF, Morton DL. Postoperative adjuvant chemotherapy (Adriamycin) in high grade extremity soft tissue sarcoma: a randomized prospective trial. In: Salmon SE, ed. Adjuvant therapy of cancer. Vol V. Orlando: Grune & Stratton, 1987:719–24.

153. Omura GA, Blessing JA, Major F, et al. A randomized clinical trial of adjuvant Adriamycin in uterine sarcomas: a Gynecologic Oncology Group Study. J Clin Oncol 1985;3:1240–5.

154. Wilson RE, Wood WC, Lerner HL, et al. Doxorubicin chemotherapy in the treatment of soft-tissue sarcoma: combined results of two randomized trials. Arch Surg 1986;121:1354–59.

155. Alvegård T, for the Scandinavian Sarcoma Group. Adjuvant chemotherapy with Adriamycin in high grade malignant soft tissue sarcoma—a Scandinavian randomized study. Proc ASCO 1986;5:125.

156. Eilber FR, Giuliano AE, Huth JF, Morton DL. A randomized prospective trial using postoperative adjuvant chemotherapy (Adriamycin) in high-grade extremity soft-tissue sarcoma. Am J Clin Oncol 1988;11:39–45.

157. Antman K, Amato D, Pilepich M, et al. A preliminary analysis of a randomized intergroup (SWOG, ECOG, CALGB, NCOG) trial of adjuvant doxorubicin for soft tissue sarcomas. In: Salmon S, ed. Adjuvant therapy of cancer. Vol V. Orlando: Grune & Stratton, 1987:725–34.

158. Gherlinzoni F, Bacci, G, Picci P, et al. A randomized trial for the treatment of high-grade soft-tissue sarcomas of the extremities: preliminary observations. J Clin Oncol 1986;4:552–8.

159. Bramwell VHC, Rouessé J, Santoro A, et al. European experience of adjuvant chemotherapy for soft tissue sarcoma: preliminary report of randomized trial of cyclophosphamide, vincristine, doxorubicin, and dacarbazine. Cancer Treat Symp 1985;3:99–107.

160. Chang AE, Kinsella T, Glatstein E, et al. Adjuvant chemotherapy for patients with high-grade soft-tissue sarcomas of the extremity. J Clin Oncol 1988;6:1491–500.

161. Sarcoma Meta-Analysis collaboration. Adjuvant chemotherapy for localised resectable soft-tissue sarcoma of adults: meta-analysis of individual data. Lancet 1997;350:1647–53.

162. Zalupski MM, Ryan JR, Hussein ME, et al. Defining the role of adjuvant chemotherapy for patients with soft tissue sarcoma of the extremities. In: Salmon SE, ed. Adjuvant therapy of cancer VII. Philadelphia: JB Lippincott, 1993:385–92.

163. Frustaci S, Gherlinzoni F, De Paoli A, et al. Maintenance of efficacy of adjuvant chemotherapy (CT) in soft tissue sarcoma (STS) of the extremities: up-date of a randomized trial. Proc ASCO 1999;18:546a.

164. Frustaci S, Gherlinzoni F, De Paoli A, et al. Preliminary results of an adjuvant randomized trial on high risk extremity soft tissue sarcomas (STS): the interim analysis. Proc ASCO 1997;16:496a.

165. Rouessé JG, Friedman S, Sevin DM, et al. Preoperative induction chemotherapy in the treatment of locally advanced soft tissue sarcomas. Cancer 1987;60:296–300.

166. Elias A, Ryan L, Sulkes A, et al. Response to mesna, doxorubicin, ifosfamide, and dacarbazine in 108 patients with metastatic or unresectable sarcoma and no prior chemotherapy. J Clin Oncol 1989;7:1208–16.

167. Pezzi CM, Pollock RE, Evans HL, et al. Preoperative chemotherapy for soft-tissue sarcomas of the extremities. Ann Surg 1990;211:476–81.

168. Suit HD, Mankin HJ, Wood WC, Proppe KH. Preoperative, intraoperative, and postoperative radiation in the treatment of primary soft tissue sarcoma. Cancer 1985;55:2659–67.

169. Goodnight JE Jr, Bargar WL, Voegeli T, Blaisdell FW. Limb-sparing surgery for extremity sarcomas after preoperative intraarterial doxorubicin and radiation therapy. Am J Surg 1985;150:109–13.

170. Pastorino U, Valente M, Gasparini M, et al. Lung resection for metastatic sarcomas: total survival from primary treatment. J Surg Oncol 1989;40:275–80.

171. Jablons D, Steinberg SM, Roth J, et al. Metastasectomy for soft tissue sarcoma: further evidence for efficacy and prognostic indicators. J Thorac Cardiovasc Surg 1989;97:695–705.

172. Casson AG, Putnam JB, Natarajan G, et al. Five-year survival after pulmonary metastasectomy for adult soft tissue sarcoma. Cancer 1992;69:662–8.

173. Pogrebniak HW, Roth JA, Steinberg SM, et al. Reoperative pulmonary resection in patients with metastatic soft tissue sarcoma. Ann Thorac Surg 1991;52:197–203.

# PART

# XIX

# MYELOID NEOPLASMS

• CHARLES M. HASKELL

Hematopoiesis involves two major divisions: myelopoiesis and lymphopoiesis. The neoplastic diseases of myelopoiesis are considered in this section; lymphoid neoplasms are considered in Part XX. Myeloid neoplasms constitute about 1% of all new cancer cases seen annually in the United States. The diseases discussed in this part include acute myeloid leukemia (AML), the myeloproliferative and myelodysplastic syndromes, and chronic myelogenous leukemia.

# CHAPTER 84

# ACUTE MYELOID LEUKEMIA

- FRANCIS J. GILES • MICHAEL ANDREEFF • MICHAEL J. KEATING

## Natural History, Diagnosis, and Staging

### EPIDEMIOLOGY

Risk factors for acute leukemia include increasing age, male gender, ethnicity, genetic and hematologic diseases, radiation, and other environmental or occupational exposures.[1] Acute myeloid leukemia (AML) is not considered heritable, although there is an increased incidence of childhood leukemia among identical twins.[1]

Increased rates of AML occur with Down syndrome, Fanconi's anemia, Bloom's syndrome, Bruton-type X-linked agammaglobulinemia, hereditary ataxia-telangiectasia, severe combined immunodeficiency, Wiskott-Aldrich syndrome, Klinefelter's syndrome, Shwachmann-Diamond-Oski syndrome, and Kostmann's syndrome.[1] Myelodysplastic syndromes (MDS), paroxysmal nocturnal hemoglobinuria, aplastic anemia, and myeloproliferative diseases are associated with increased risk for developing AML and are therefore termed *antecedent hematologic disorders* (AHD).[2-4]

The incidence of acute leukemia is increased among survivors of the Hiroshima/Nagasaki explosions, as well as among those exposed to nuclear weapons testing in the western United States during the 1950s. In these cases, acute leukemias increased after a latency of 1 to 2 years, peaked at 5 to 6 years, and remained elevated for more than 20 years.[5] Increased rates of acute leukemia have also been documented among patients treated with therapeutic doses of radiation and radioactive agents (thorium dioxide [Thorotrast] dye, radium, phosphorus 32). The association of acute leukemias with nonionizing radiation exposure (e.g., electromagnetic fields, microwaves), although intriguing, is less well established.[6-8] Occupational exposure is another important risk factor, inasmuch as the incidence of AML has been positively associated with exposure to a variety of chemicals and drugs.[9-11] Hair dyes are associated with increased leukemia rates.[8] Workers in occupations that may expose them to ionizing radiation, metal fumes, or solvents are at increased risk for acute leukemia. Benzene is particularly associated with both aplastic anemia and leukemia.[12, 13] AML is the most common benzene-associated leukemia.[11] Benzene-associated AML may occur 5 to 20 years or more after a significant exposure and is an occupational hazard in several industries (woodworking, leather working, welding, rubber working, petrochemicals).[14-17] Paint, embalming fluid, xylene, ethylene oxide, and herbicides have also been linked to AML.[18-20]

Cytotoxic chemotherapy for a previous malignancy (particularly regimens using alkylating agents and topoisomerase II inhibitors) are factors associated with an increased incidence of AML.[21-23] Other drugs associated with increased AML rates are chloramphenicol, phenylbutazone, chloroquine, methoxypsoralen, lysergic acid diethylamide (LSD), and various analgesics.[24-27] Smoking is associated with an increased risk for leukemia. Several studies suggest that smokers have a higher relative risk of developing AML (1.4 to 1.7) than do nonsmokers; the data also suggest a dose-response effect.[28-30]

### CLASSIFICATION

The French-American-British (FAB) Working Group devised a classification system in 1976 based on morphologic and cytochemical features.[31] Updated classification schema have included immunologic and cytogenetic information that further characterizes AML subtypes (Table 84–1).[32, 33] The reproducibility of the FAB classification is limited and, with some exceptions (M3, M4Eo, M6, L3), the FAB system does not correlate well with therapeutic response or prognosis. A panel of cytochemical stains complements morphologic information and is crucial in establishing the correct diagnosis. The most commonly used stains are myeloperoxidase (MPO), Sudan black B (SBB), nonspecific esterase (NSE), chloroacetate esterase (CAE), acid phosphatase, periodic acid–Schiff (PAS), and terminal deoxynucleotidyl transferase (TdT). The peroxidase reaction detects the presence of MPO in the primary (azurophilic) granules of myeloid and monocytic cells. Auer rods are needle-like, cylindrical collections of primary (MPO$^+$) granules and are prominent in the M2, M3, and M5 AML subtypes.

SBB marks intracellular lipids located in secondary (basophilic) granules of myeloid and monocytic cells, although it is not as sensitive a marker as MPO. Staining for NSE is characteristic of monocytic cells, although weak staining of myeloid cells may be noted. CAE is detected in monocytic cells. PAS and acid phosphatase staining, when used in combination with other cytochemical studies, may help delineate leukemic subtypes. TdT staining is often positive in immature lymphoid phenotypes.

AML is the diagnosis when 3% of leukemic blasts are MPO positive or SBB positive by light microscopy. Some subtypes of AML (e.g., M0, M5, M7) or undifferentiated/biphenotypic leukemias may have less than 3% MPO positive blasts by light microscopy; immunophenotyping, electron microscopy (EM), or other studies can usually identify these cases.

If the blasts are MPO positive or SBB positive, the NSE stain will help further distinguish the M1 through M3 (NSE negative) from the M4 (NSE positive) subtypes. The M5 subtype may be either MPO positive or MPO negative but is always NSE positive. The M6 and M7 subtypes stain for PAS and platelet peroxidase, respectively.

Cell cycle kinetics, as determined with flow cytometry, may provide useful information.[34, 35] A variety of techniques (bromodeoxyuridine [BUdR]/5-iododeoxyuridine [IUdR], acridine orange, proliferating cell nuclear antigen) permits detection of leukemic subpopulations, changes in growth fraction, and proliferation rates. A large number of nonproliferating G0 cells at diagnosis is associated with low complete response (CR) rates, short remission duration, and short survival.[36] This finding provided the basis for the use of growth factors to recruit cells into the cell cycle prior to induction chemotherapy—an approach that has led to generally poor clinical results.[37, 38] Acute promyelocytic leukemia (APL) is characterized by the lowest number of proliferating cells among the AML subtypes.

Immunoglobulin gene rearrangement studies detect abnormalities not only among B-cell acute lymphocytic leukemia (ALL) but also among 10 to 20% of AML patients and 10 to 15% of T-cell ALL patients.[39] Rearrangement of the T-cell receptors α, β, or γ may be seen in T-cell ALL, as well as in a fraction of B-cell ALL and AML patients.[39]

Karyotypic analysis provides the single most important prognostic information in AML.[40-42] Most, but not all, patients with abnormalities of chromosome 5 or 7 have only a 5 to 10% long-term survival, with a considerably superior survival in patients with t(15;17), t(8;21), or inversion of chromosome 16. Techniques such as fluorescent in situ hybridization (FISH) and polymerase chain reaction (PCR) have increased the sensitivity of cytogenetic analysis.[43-45]

### French-American-British Subtypes

M0 undifferentiated acute myeloblastic leukemia composes 2 to 3% of AML cases.[46] The blasts are large and agranular (type I blasts), lack Auer rods, and are without evidence of maturation. The blasts are MPO negative by light microscopy but may be MPO positive by EM. Other myeloid stains are either negative or barely detectable.

M1 acute myeloblastic leukemia composes 20% of AML cases. In this subtype, more than 90% of the myeloid cells in the marrow are myeloblasts (type I or II). Minimal myeloid differentiation is seen (3% promyelocytes), and Auer rods are infrequent. The M1 subtype is frequently associated

*Table 84–1.* **French-American-British (FAB) Classification of Acute Myeloid Leukemia**

| FAB | Description | Percentage |
|-----|-------------|------------|
| M0 | AML without cytologic maturation | 5–7 |
| M1 | AML with minimal maturation | 20 |
| M2 | AML with significant maturation | 30 |
| M3 | Hypergranular promyelocytic leukemia | 10 |
| M4 | Acute myelomonocytic leukemia | 25 |
| M5A | Acute monocytic leukemia (poorly differentiated) | 4 |
| M5B | Acute monocytic leukemia (well differentiated) | 6 |
| M6 | Acute erythroleukemia | 5 |
| M7 | Acute megakaryocytic leukemia | Very rare |

The percentage of AML is greater than 100% because the M0 type was not a formal part of the FAB classification when the percentages were determined. Most of the patients with M0 AML would have been previously diagnosed with acute lymphoblastic leukemia or acute undifferentiated leukemia. Acute mast cell leukemia does not appear in the FAB classification because it is considered too rare to be included.

From Bennett JM. Classification of the acute leukemias: cytochemical and morphologic considerations. In: Wiernik PH, Canellos GP, Kyle RA, Schiffer CA, eds. Neoplastic diseases of the blood. 2nd ed. New York: Churchill Livingstone, 1991:169–181.

with t(9;22), a cytogenetic abnormality found in 3% of AML patients.

M2 acute myeloblastic leukemia with differentiation composes 30% of AML cases. Usually 10% of cells show evidence of differentiation, although less than 20% of these are monocytic. Promyelocytes vary from 3 to 20% of myeloid cells, and occasional myelocytes are seen. Myeloblasts may vary in size or shape, contain at least one nucleolus, and have Auer rods. The pale blue cytoplasm of many M2 blasts may be granular (type II blasts) and may demonstrate basophilia. The t(8;21) abnormality, found in 15 to 18% of M2 patients, is associated with abnormal neutrophil maturation (hypogranular blasts, pseudo–Pelger-Huët anomaly), and eosinophilia.[47-49] Clinically, 25% of these patients have splenomegaly and 20% develop chloromas, including facial chloromas.[49] CR rates and survival are relatively good for this small subgroup.[47] Other subgroups of M2 exhibit erythroid hyperplasia or eosinophilia and cytogenetic abnormalities, including 80% with 9q−, and also −X/−Y.[42]

M3 APL represents approximately 10% of all AML cases.[50-52] M3 is uniquely characterized by the presence of heavily granulated promyelocytes, bilobed nuclei, and multiple Auer rods. Calculations of the percentage of malignant cells include both blasts and promyelocytes (>30% promyelocytes needed for diagnosis). A micro/hypogranular variant of the M3 subtype (M3v) contains fine granules and Auer rods that, although difficult to discern on light microscopy, are more readily found on EM. The M3v variant constitutes 20 to 25% of all M3 cases and resembles the M3 subtype in all other respects.[53] The t(15;17) abnormality, found in virtually all M3 cases, is pathognomonic for the M3 subtype. The PML gene is translocated from chromosome 15 to chromosome 17, thus interrupting the retinoic acid receptor α (RARα) gene located on 17q21. This cytogenetic abnormality results in an abnormal RARα gene. The 106-kd chimeric fusion product, PML-RARα, contains a zinc-finger protein that may interact with RAR binding and functions as a DNA nuclear binding-transcription factor.[54]

M4 acute myelomonocytic leukemia accounts for 25 to 30% of AML cases.[55] In this subtype, myeloid cells compose at least 20% of bone marrow cells, and monocytic cells may compose 20 to 80% of the nonerythroid nucleated blood cells in the marrow. Monocytic cells are usually more abundant in the peripheral blood of M4 patients. If, however, less than 20% of the marrow cells are monocytic, the diagnosis of M4 may be established if there are greater than $5 \times 10^9$/L monocytes in the peripheral blood. This subtype sometimes exhibits Auer rods, increased serum lysozyme levels, gingival hypertrophy, and leukemia cutis. The monocytic cells are NSE positive and CD14+; the myeloid cells are MPO positive or SBB positive. Cytogenetic abnormalities found in (although not unique to) M4 include t(9;11), trisomy 4, and abnormalities of chromosomes 11 (11q23) and 16 (16q22). Acute myelomonocytic leukemia with eosinophilia (M4Eo) is an M4 variant characterized by the presence of greater than 5% abnormal eosinophilic precursors in the bone marrow.[56] The eosinophils in this variant are unusual in that they contain a single unsegmented nucleus and large, basophilic granules and are CAE positive.[16] The M4Eo variant is associated with inversion or deletion of chromosome 16q22 (a karyotype also found in some cases of M2, M4, and M5). Standard-dose chemotherapy in M4Eo results in high CR rates and relatively high survival. CR rates with high-dose cytosine arabinoside (ara-C) among patients with M4Eo and abnormalities of 16q22 are high. Unusual patterns of relapse are observed, particularly with respect to the central nervous system, such as leptomeningeal disease or chloromas, or both.[57]

In M5 acute monocytic leukemias, which represent approximately 10% of AML cases, greater than 80% of the nonerythroid bone marrow elements are monocytic.[58, 59] The M5 subtype is divided into M5a (4% of AML cases) and M5− (6% of AML cases). M5a is present if greater than 80% of the monocytic cells are monoblasts and less than 3% exhibit differentiation. M5a blasts are large, contain one to three large nucleoli, have low nuclear-cytoplasmic ratios with basophilic cytoplasm, and lack Auer rods. The M5− subtype exhibits a mixture of promonocytic and monocytic cells, often with large granules; monoblasts compose less than 80% of the monocytic cells. Auer rods may also be present. Among the cytogenetic abnormalities frequently found in M5 patients are abnormalities of 11q, often involving the 11q23 locus. The t(9;11) abnormality (10% of AML cases) disrupts a region of α interferon genes (chromosome 9), permitting the interferon β1 gene to translocate to the 11q23 locus; the 11q23–24 locus, containing the *c-ets-1* proto-oncogene, is translocated to the 9q22 breakpoint.[60] Patients with t(9;11) are generally young and may present with cutaneous, gingival, or central nervous system leukemic infiltration.[49]

M6 acute erythroleukemia composes 4 to 5% of AML cases and represents 10 to 20% of secondary leukemias.[61] The hematologic appearance of M6 may vary, ranging from anemia (with both myelodysplastic and megaloblastic features) to AML, which morphologically resembles the M1, M2, or M4 subtype. The M6 subtype is diagnosed if 50% of all nucleated bone marrow cells are erythroblasts and the nonerythroid marrow contains 30% blasts. Di Guglielmo's syndrome, in which greater than 70% of bone marrow cells are bizarre, dysplastic erythroblasts, occurs in only 10% of M6 cases. The erythroblasts contain multiple, multilobulated nuclei with megaloblastic features, are strongly PAS positive (block-like patterns may be observed), and demonstrate immunophenotypically the presence of carbonic anhydrase and glycophorin. The myeloblasts, though, are MPO positive and SBB positive and may contain Auer rods.

M7 acute megakaryoblastic leukemia represents approximately 1 to 3% of AML cases.[58, 62] Although blast size and the number of nucleoli may vary, dysplastic changes and a high nuclear-cytoplasmic ratio are usually apparent. The blast cytoplasm is hypogranular, variable in amount, and contains cytoplasmic blebs (platelet budding), which are visible at the periphery. The bone marrow may show evidence of fibrosis, and marrow aspirates may be "dry." Pancytopenia, megakaryoblasts, and micromegakaryocytes are also present. Blasts are MPO negative and SBB negative but may be focally positive for α-naphthyl butyrate esterase. M7 blasts are immunophenotypically positive for CD13, CD33, glycoprotein Ib, and CD41 (glycoprotein IIb/IIIa). Although no cytogenetic abnormalities are specifically associated with the M7 subtype, many cases exhibit abnormalities of chromosomes 5 and 7, as well as +8, +10, t(1;4), and inv(3q). M7 may involve multipotent stem cells.[63] M7 AML has a poor prognosis.

## Immunophenotyping of Acute Myeloid Leukemia

In the normal bone marrow, the antigens designated CD34, CD13, and CD33 appear early in myelomonocytic differentiation.[64] The further differentiation into neutrophil lineage is characterized by the loss of CD34 and acquisition of CD15, accompanied by a decrease of CD33 density and the subsequent acquisition of CD11b. Maturation toward the monocytic lineage is associated with loss of CD34 and acquisition of CD11b, followed by acquisition of CD15 and CD14. Studies of AML by multiparameter flow cytometry revealed heterogeneity in the pattern of antigen expression. Terstappen and coworkers observed four patterns of aberrant antigen expression in AML: (1) expression of nonmyeloid antigens, (2) asynchronous expression of myeloid antigens (i.e., co-expression of CD34 and CD15), (3) overexpression of antigen density of myeloid-associated antigens, and (4) absence of myeloid antigens.[65]

The myeloid-associated monoclonal antibodies (mAbs) are most valuable in cases of poorly differentiated AML, in which the diagnosis is unclear by standard morphologic evaluation by light microscopy. AML-M0 can be diagnosed with certainty only by the reactivity with mAbs against myeloid-associated antigens. The mAbs against CD13, CD14, CD15, CD33, CD34, and human leukocyte antigen (HLA-DR) are most useful for the identification of AML. CD13 and CD33 are present in most cases of AML, whereas CD34 is not lineage restricted. Also, mAbs against MPO have been shown to be more sensitive than the cytochemical test for MPO using light microscopy.[66] Glycophorin A antibody is often useful in confirming the diagnosis of erythroleukemia (AML-M6).[67] Likewise, antibodies against platelet glycoprotein (CD41, CD42, CD61) are valuable in the diagnosis of megakaryoblastic leukemia, AML-M7, but the definitive test is the determination of platelet peroxidase by electron microscopy. The ligand for the stem cell factor c-kit is highly expressed in a subset of AML, and limited expression of c-kit on primitive cells in the normal bone marrow (1 to 3% of bone marrow mononuclear cells) makes this marker more specific for leukemia than other myeloid-associated markers.[68]

Lymphoid antigens are frequently expressed in AML (2 to 60%), depending on the number of mAbs and the methodology used, and are generally of little prognostic significance.[65, 69] B-lineage–associated antigens CD10, CD19, and CD24 are found less frequently in AML. CD56, the natural killer cell–associated antigen, has also been found in AML, most often in the M4 and M5 subgroups.[70]

## Mixed-Lineage Leukemia

Despite the recognition of acute leukemias expressing antigens of more than one lineage (lineage infidelity, lineage promiscuity), no consensus exists regarding their definition, terminology, diagnostic criteria, or biologic implication. The expression of a single aberrant marker such as otherwise typical AML with TdT or ALL with one myeloid-associated antigen does not qualify for classification as "mixed lineage." Different lineage markers appear either on the same blasts or separately on more than one population of blasts. Catovsky and coworkers have proposed a scoring system for this group using various parameters including morphology, cytochemistry, immunophenotype, and gene rearrangement for immunoglobulin and T-cell receptor.[59] Prognosis and optimal treatment for mixed-lineage leukemia remain to be determined. Kantarjian and coworkers found that therapy such as that used in ALL may be successful in AML cases that are morphologically more compatible with lymphoid lineage in a study in which T-cell morphology and membrane markers and MPO positivity by EM were noted.[71]

## MONITORING OF MINIMAL RESIDUAL DISEASE BY IMMUNOPHENOTYPING, FLUORESCENCE-ACTIVATED CELL SORTING, AND FLUORESCENT IN SITU HYBRIDIZATION ANALYSIS

The conventional criteria of CR are based on morphologic evaluation of bone marrow samples. CR is defined as less than 5% of blasts in bone marrow aspirates and normal peripheral blood counts, which reflects the detection limit of cytomorphologic evaluation. Flow cytometric immunophenotyping can improve the detection of minimal residual disease (MRD). The detection limit of leukemic cells by immunologic marker studies varies greatly depending on the antigenic make-up of the blasts and the techniques used. The reported detection limits range from 0.01 to 1%.[72–75] The phenotypic deviation of leukemic cells from normal cells enables one to detect a small number of leukemic cells by multiparameter analysis. In particular, dual staining of leukemic cells with nuclear TdT and surface membrane marker is a sensitive technique for both ALL and AML.

Drach and coworkers and Reading and associates studied the marrow of patients with AML in remission by two-color flow cytometry.[76, 77] In the latter study, all 6 patients with greater than 0.2% of leukemic cells expressing the initial immunophenotype relapsed, whereas 9 of 10 patients with less than 0.2% of these cells remained in remission. These data suggest that the presence of leukemic cells detected by flow cytometry in a "CR" patient indicates probable ultimate failure of therapy. The full spectrum of aberrant antigen expression in non–steady-state hematopoiesis, however, remains to be studied, and the therapeutic decision based on these results must be undertaken cautiously.

An extension of these approaches to MRD assessment is the combination of immunophenotyping with FISH using chromosome-specific and translocation-specific DNA probes. Bone marrow progenitor cells (CD34+) are separated by fluorescence-activated cell sorting (FACS) and analyzed for clonal chromosomal abnormalities by molecular cytogenetics using alpha-satellite probes for centromeric repeat sequences. FISH allows the cytogenetic analysis of dividing and nondividing interphase cells. As few as 1 leukemic cell in 10,000 normal cells is detectable (0.01%). In addition, labeling with BUdR, in combination with FISH, allows assessment of the proliferation of normal and leukemic progenitor cells.[78–80] These specific and sensitive techniques may allow the exact monitoring of MRD far below the level of microscopic detection, with the aim of developing new therapeutic strategies for the eradication or control of residual leukemia cells.

## Treatment of Acute Myeloid Leukemia

The prognosis for newly diagnosed untreated AML is changing rapidly.[81] This section focuses on advances in this field inasmuch as there are few recent developments in the treatment of patients with relapsed or refractory disease. Current treatment strategies for AML are broadly classified into two main phases: remission induction and postremission therapy (consolidation, intensification, and maintenance). Remission is defined as the presence of less than 5% blasts in a normocellular bone marrow, normalization of the peripheral blood counts with a granulocyte count greater than $1 \times 10^9$/L, and a platelet count greater than $100 \times 10^9$/L. Remission duration is determined from the time of documented response until relapse occurs. Survival is measured from the date therapy is started. We review here the different therapeutic strategies and investigational modalities of AML therapy used at the M.D. Anderson Cancer Center (MDACC) during the past three decades (Figs. 84–1 to 84–5).

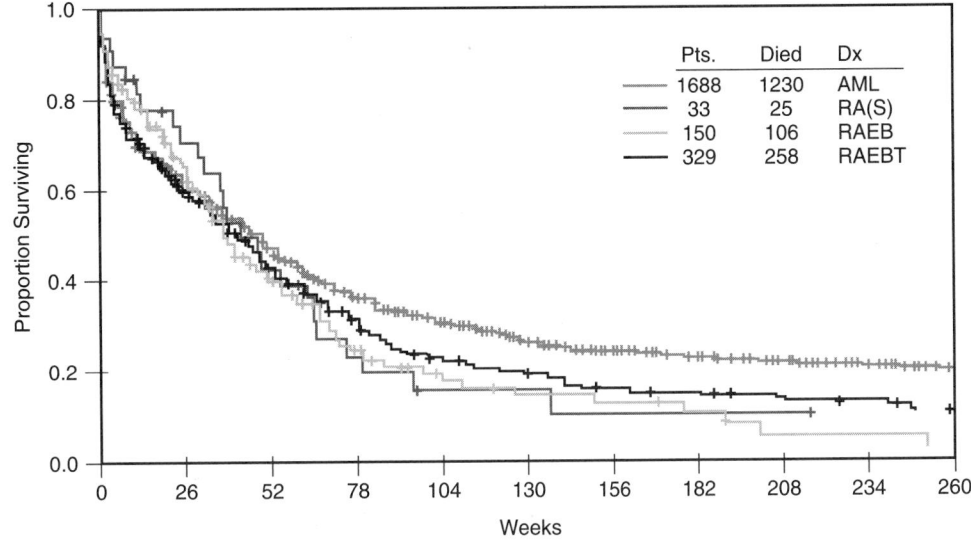

**Figure 84–1.** Survival in acute myeloid leukemia (AML) and myelodysplastic syndrome (MDS) subgroups at the M.D. Anderson Cancer Center.

| Pts. | Died | Dx |
|------|------|------|
| 1688 | 1230 | AML |
| 33 | 25 | RA(S) |
| 150 | 106 | RAEB |
| 329 | 258 | RAEBT |

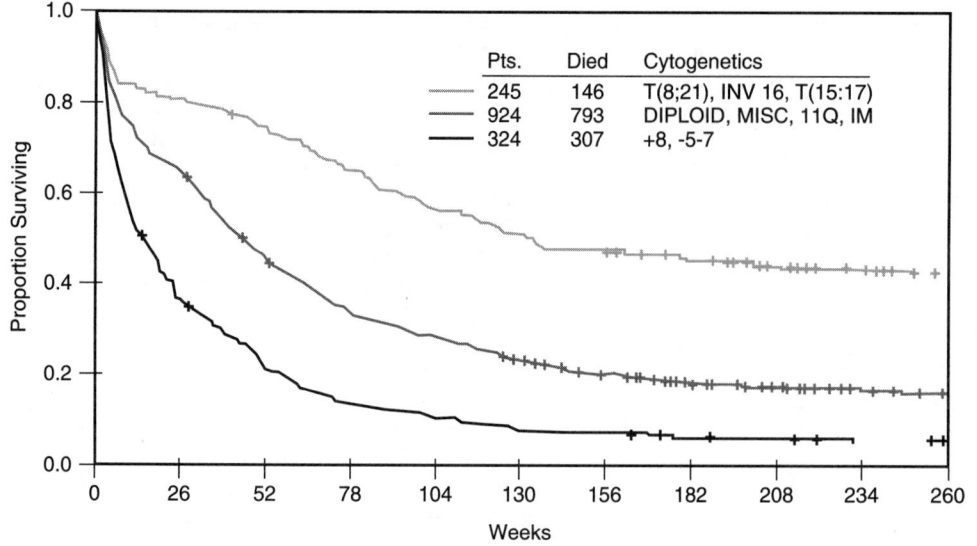

**Figure 84–2.** Survival in AML patients by cytogenetics.

**Figure 84–3.** Survival in AML patients by time periods.

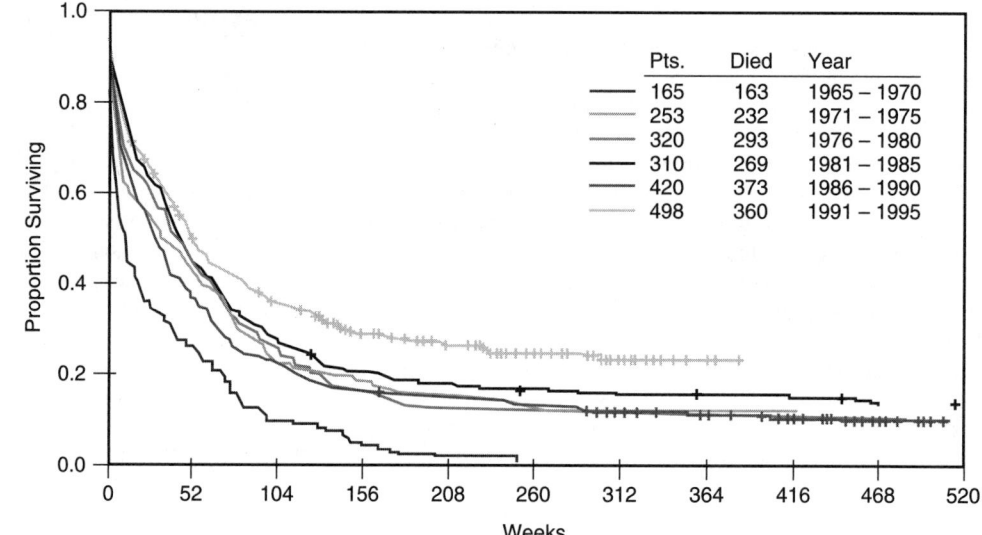

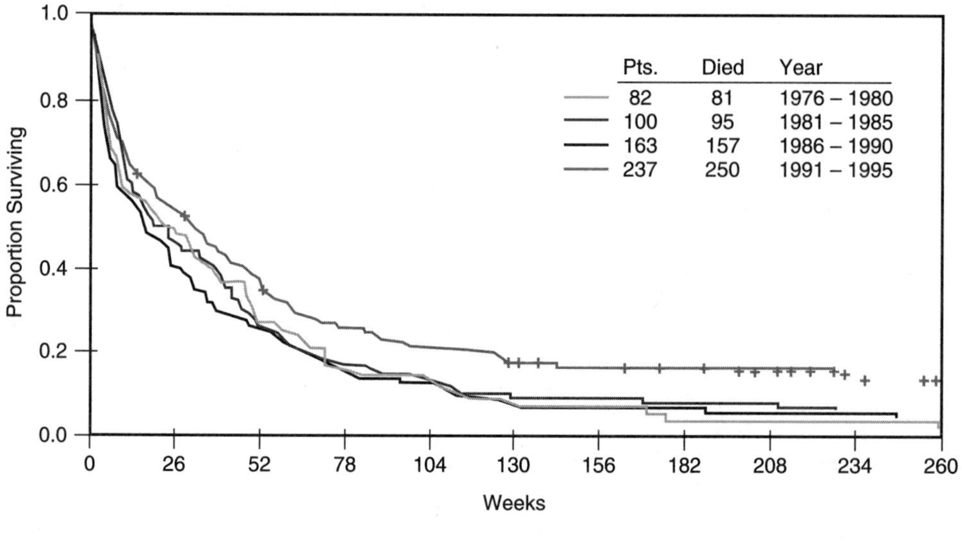

**Figure 84–4.** Survival in AML patients by year group +8, −5/−7, 11Q, MISC.

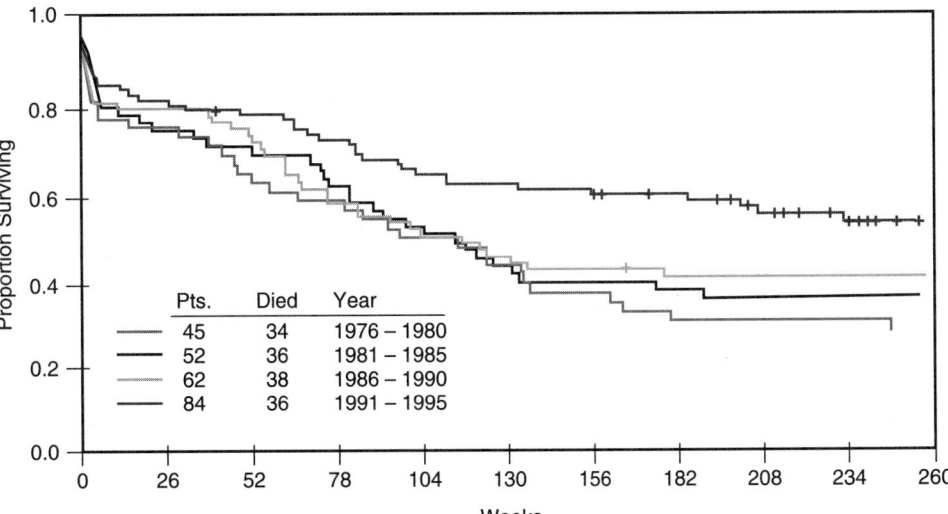

**Figure 84–5.** Survival in AML patients by year group T (8:21), INV 16, T(15;17).

| Pts. | Died | Year |
|------|------|------|
| 45 | 34 | 1976 – 1980 |
| 52 | 36 | 1981 – 1985 |
| 62 | 38 | 1986 – 1990 |
| 84 | 36 | 1991 – 1995 |

## INDUCTION THERAPY

Freireich and associates first demonstrated that achievement of CR, defined by a platelet count less than $1 \times 10^9/L$, a neutrophil count greater than $1 \times 10^9/L$, and a marrow with less than 5% blasts, was essential to subsequent survival in newly diagnosed AML.[82] It is well known, however, that remissions in AML patients who require more than one cycle to achieve CR are brief.[83] The MDACC group has extended these findings by demonstrating that even among patients with AML or MDS who enter CR after one cycle of therapy, there is an inverse association between time to CR and subsequent survival time, with patients who require more than 50 days to enter CR (generally because of slow platelet recovery) having a prognosis closer to patients who never achieve CR than to patients who achieve CR more quickly.[84] This inverse association is independent of factors such as cytogenetics or specific treatment, such as high-dose versus standard-dose ara-C. Of 1101 patients with AML, refractory anemia with excess blasts (RAEB), or refractory anemia with excess blasts in transformation (RAEB-t) treated at the MDACC between 1980 and 1996, 740 (67%) achieved CR; 508 of these 740 (69%) patients had died (80% had disease recurrence before death). The authors estimated time to CR, time from CR to death or residual survival after CR, and residual disease-free survival (DFS) for these patients. There was a strong inverse association between time to CR and both time from CR to death and residual DFS that was independent of cytogenetic status, age, or treatment. The residual survival time of patients who required greater than 50 days to enter CR was closer to the residual survival time of resistant patients than to that of patients known to be in CR within approximately 30 days of the start of treatment. Time to CR is an independent predictor of residual survival and DFS[AU1]. These data have led us to define an "early CR" as one achieved after only one cycle of therapy and within 50 days of the start of that cycle, and to focus on achievement of an early CR as the goal of induction therapy.

Cytoreductive therapy is used to decrease the leukemic burden to a level that will permit restoration of normal hematopoiesis. Remission-induction regimens usually combine ara-C and an anthracycline. CR rates are highly dependent on blast karyotype but, in general, 55 to 75% of all AML patients achieve CR; however, 50 to 70% of these patients relapse and die within 2 years. Relapse beyond 3 years in CR becomes relatively infrequent.[85, 86]

Ara-C remains the most active antileukemic drug and is the backbone of the majority of remission-induction regimens. The dose and schedule of ara-C varies, but doses of 100 to 200 mg/m², administered either as an intermittent bolus or by continuous infusion, demonstrate similar efficacy. The duration of ara-C treatment also varies, although treatment for 7 days is most common. Higher doses of ara-C may be used (1.5 to 3 g/m² every 12 hours for 4 to 6 days), with overall results comparable to standard-dose ara-C plus anthracycline combinations.

The choice among different anthracyclines is controversial. Initially combinations of ara-C and doxorubicin were the standard used for AML induction therapy. Daunorubicin soon replaced doxorubicin because daunorubicin is less toxic and equally active in combination with ara-C. The full role of liposomal preparations such as daunorubicin citrate (DaunoXome) is currently being assessed.[87–89] These latter agents are of particular interest because of their potential to be less susceptible to MDR modulation. Daunorubicin is usually administered in doses of 45 to 60 mg/m² for 3 days, in combination with ara-C. Idarubicin, and to a lesser extent mitoxantrone, have emerged as alternative anthracycline induction agents. Idarubicin is usually administered at doses of 12 mg/m² for 3 days. Three randomized studies comparing idarubicin and daunorubicin in combination with ara-C have found that the idarubicin plus ara-C combination induced higher CR rates, duration, and survival.[90–93] Mitoxantrone is at least as active as idarubicin, and no clearly optimal anthracycline for AML induction has yet been defined.[94–103]

Modifications of remission-induction regimens have added active non–cross-resistant agents (e.g., thioguanine [TG], etoposide)—none of these strategies has been proved to offer significant survival advantages over standard-dose ara-C/anthracycline combinations.[104–107]

Modifications of the "3 + 7" schema have included an extension of ara-C infusion to "3 + 10," with equivalent results in one trial.[106] A comparison of "3 + 10 + 6TG" in the Medical Research Council IX trial demonstrated a higher CR rate as compared with "1 + 5 + 6TG."[108] A Cancer and Leukemia Group B trial comparing "3 + 7" and "2 + 5" showed the former to be a superior induction regimen.[86]

Although the combination of ara-C with an anthracycline (i.e., "3 + 7") is widely used, this is a relatively ineffective regimen. Remission rates may approach 75% in patients with favorable prognoses. Remission rates range from 30 to 50% among poor-risk patients (e.g., those with advanced age, unfavorable cytogenetics, secondary AML, AHD, or poor performance status). In patients with abnormalities of chromosomes 5, 7, and 8, CR rates are on the order of 20 to 30%, although not all these patients have an equally dismal prognosis, as published by Estey and associates.[109] We examined three factors known to be prognostic in AML for their prognostic significance in 400 $-5/-7$ patients treated at MDACC from 1980 to 1998 for AML or MDS. Outcomes were better in $-5/-7$ patients with a simple (rather than complex) karyotype, with greater than 1 normal metaphase (rather than only metaphases containing $-5/-7$), and without an AHD. The 10% of patients with a simple karyotype, greater than one normal metaphase, and no AHD not only had a better outcome than the other $-5/-7$ patients but also had essentially identical outcomes to 669 AML/MDS patients with a normal karyotype treated at MDACC during the same period. Thus all AML patients with $-5/-7$ should not necessarily be regarded as having a highly unfavorable prognosis. These data also highlight the need to refine prognosis within each of the cytogenetic subsets of AML.

Our current front-line regimen for patients with relatively good prognosis cytogenetics is the CAT (cyclophosphamide, ara-C, topotecan) regimen. We and others have documented the activity of topotecan as a single agent and when combined with ara-C in AML and MDS patients.[110-119] The CAT regimen is at least as effective as any prior regimen in this patient cohort and may be less toxic. In a 1998 therapeutic study we looked at the potential benefit of adding retinoic acid (ATRA) (potential to lower concentrations of the antiapoptotic protein bcl-2[120]) or granulocyte colony–stimulating factor (G-CSF), or both, to induction therapy.[121] Accordingly, we randomized 215 patients with newly diagnosed AML (153 patients) or high-risk MDS (RAEB or RAEB-t, 62 patients) to receive fludarabine + ara-C + idarubicin (FAI) alone, FAI + ATRA, FAI + G-CSF, or FAI + ATRA + G-CSF. Eligibility required one of the following: age older than 71 years, a history of abnormal blood counts before MDACC presentation, secondary AML/MDS, failure to respond to one prior course of chemotherapy given outside MDACC, or abnormal renal or hepatic function. For the two treatment arms containing ATRA, ATRA was given 2 days (day 2) before the beginning of, and continued for 3 days after, completion of FAI. For the two treatment arms including G-CSF, G-CSF began on day 1 and continued until neutrophil recovery. Patients with white blood cell counts (WBCs) greater than $50 \times 10^9$/L began ATRA on day 1 and G-CSF on day 2.

Events (death, failure to achieve CR, or relapse from CR) have occurred in 77% of the 215 patients. Reflecting the poor prognosis of the patients entered, the CR rate was only 51%, median event-free survival (EFS) time once in CR was 36 weeks, and median survival time was 28 weeks. A Cox regression analysis indicated that, after accounting for patient prognostic variables, none of the three adjuvant treatment combinations (FAI + ATRA, FAI + G-CSF, FAI + ATRA + G-CSF) affected survival, EFS, or EFS once in CR compared with FAI. Similarly, there were no significant effects of either ATRA ignoring G-CSF, or of G-CSF ignoring ATRA. As previously found, a diagnosis of RAEB or RAEB-t rather than AML was insignificant. There were no indications that the effect of ATRA differed according to cytogenetic group, diagnosis (AML or MDS), or treatment schedule. Logistic regression analysis indicated that, after accounting for prognosis, addition of G-CSF +/− ATRA to FAI improved CR rate versus either FAI or FAI + ATRA, but G-CSF had no effect on the other outcomes. We concluded that the addition of ATRA +/− G-CSF to FAI had no effect on CR rate, survival, EFS, or EFS in CR in poor prognosis, newly diagnosed AML or high-risk MDS.[121]

We had a similarly negative experience with the addition of lisofylline to induction therapy. To determine whether the addition of lisofylline to idarubicin (12 mg/m² daily × 3) and ara-C (1.5 g/m² daily × 4) affected the rates of infection, serious infection, CR, or mortality during remission induction of newly diagnosed AML, RAEB-t, or RAEB, we randomized 70 patients to 3 mg/kg lisofylline or placebo every 6 hours intravenously (IV) to begin 6 hours before the first dose of idarubicin and to continue until recovery of neutrophil and platelet counts or for 28 days, whichever came first.[122] The study was double-blinded and infections were tabulated separately and independently at MDACC and by a three-member outside panel of experts. Logistic regression was used to assess the relative effects of treatment arm, age, performance status, treatment site (laminar air flow room or not), and karyotype on rates of infection and serious infection following the first course of chemotherapy and on CR rates. There was 84% and 87% concordance between the expert panel and MDACC enumerations of infection and serious infections, respectively. Both analyses found no significant differences between the rates of infection or serious infection in the placebo and lisofylline groups. CR, 60-day, and overall mortality rates were similar in the two groups, as were time to neutrophil and blood count recovery and outcome once in CR. Logistic regression analyses supported the preceding conclusions. Severe nausea and vomiting and mucositis were more frequent in the lisofylline group.

Numerous investigators have focused on the escalation of ara-C doses during and after induction therapy. No differences in CR rates were observed between conventional and high-dose regimens (Australian Leukemia Study Group: high-dose ara-C [HDAC] = 3 g/m² every 12 hours for 4 days[104]; Southwest Oncology Group [SWOG]: HDAC = 2 g/m² every 12 hours for 6 days).[123] Remission durations were longer, however, in the HDAC patients in the Australian study. The benefit of HDAC was found to be limited to younger patients, inasmuch as toxicity was increased in patients older than 60 years. The Cancer and Leukemia Group B study randomized patients to HDAC 3 g/m² every 12 hours every other day for six doses, ara-C 400 mg/m² daily for 5 days continuous infusion (CI), and ara-C 100 mg/m² daily for 5 days CI.[124] In this study, 1088 adults with newly diagnosed AML received 3 + 7 daunorubicin/ara-C; 693 achieved CR, 596 were randomized. After a median follow-up of 52 months, the DFS rates in the three treatment groups were significantly different ($p = 0.003$). Relative to the 100-mg group, the hazard ratios were 0.67 for the 3-g group (95% confidence interval, 0.53 to 0.86) and 0.75 for the 400-mg group (95% confidence interval, 0.60 to 0.94). The probability of remaining in CR at 4 years for patients 60 years or younger was 24% in the 100-mg group, 29% in the 400-mg group, and 44% in the 3-g group ($p = 0.002$). In contrast, for patients older than 60 years, the probability of remaining disease-free after 4 years was less than 16% in all groups.

The principal new drugs we have investigated in de novo AML patients have been fludarabine (+ ara-C +/− idarubicin) and topotecan (+ ara-C +/− cyclophosphamide). Early CR rates in patients with adverse karyotypes are shown in Table 84–2. These data combine patients with RAEB or RAEB-t and patients with AML because this distinction is not predictive of response to AML-type therapy, after accounting for factors such as age, cytogenetics, and the like.[125] Overall CR rates remain less than 50%, not to mention the extreme brevity of many of even the early CRs.

**Therapy of Acute Promyelocytic Leukemia.** The therapy of M3 AML is dominated by current attempts to optimize ATRA therapy. Most patients relapse if treated with ATRA alone (median remission duration, 9 months) and require subsequent chemotherapy to achieve and maintain prolonged remission.[126–128] Treatment with ATRA is associated with a transient leukocytosis, which peaks at 3 weeks. ATRA-treated M3 patients are at increased risk of pulmonary leukostasis, particularly during transient leukocytosis.[129] Disseminated intravascular coagulation, which may result from the release of procoagulants from dying or lysed cells, also responds to ATRA treatment. Pseudotumor cerebri can develop and is responsive to acetazolamide. Supportive care during M3-associated disseminated intravascular coagulation is crucial to survival, with aggressive transfusions of platelets, fresh-frozen plasma, and cryoprecipitate as required. We have found liposomal ATRA to be effective in APL and capable of inducing molecular remissions.[130] The induction of reverse transcriptase PCR negativity for the PMR:RAR hybrid mRNA has become a therapeutic end point in APL.[131, 132] No optimal therapy has been defined for patients who fail to achieve or maintain reverse transcriptase PCR negativity following ATRA/anthracycline induction.[133, 134] Data on arsenic trioxide are being explored in this context.[135–138] A particularly difficult issue is the initial therapy of APL patients with a high WBC, who have a very poor prognosis.[132]

## POSTREMISSION THERAPY

Much effort has gone into attempts to define optimal postremission treatment strategies for patients in CR. The benefit of such treatment is well established, but no one approach has clearly emerged as superior. If one chooses intensive chemotherapy as consolidation, HDAC is the current best established regimen. The SWOG conducted a randomized trial comparing HDAC with standard-dose ara-C (SDAC) for CR induction of previously untreated AML and compared these ara-C regimens as consolidation therapy.[123] Patients younger than 65 years with de novo or secondary AML were randomized for induction between SDAC 200 mg/m²/day for 7 days by CI or HDAC at 2 g/m² IV every 12 hours for 12 doses; both groups received daunorubicin at 45 mg/m²/day IV for 3 days. Patients in CR following SDAC were randomized to receive either two additional courses of daunorubicin/SDAC or one course of daunorubicin/HDAC. Patients in CR following HDAC were nonrandomly assigned to receive one additional course of daunorubicin/HDAC. Of patients randomized between SDAC (n = 493) and HDAC (n = 172) induction, 361 achieved CR. The CR rate was slightly poorer with HDAC: 55% versus 58% with SDAC for patients younger than 50 years, and 45% (HDAC) versus 53% (SDAC) for patients age 50 to 64 (age-adjusted one-tailed $p = 0.96$). With a median follow-up time of 51 months, survival was not significantly better with HDAC ($p = 0.41$); the estimated survival rate at 4 years was 32% (HDAC) versus 22% (SDAC) for those younger than 50 years, and 13% (HDAC) versus 11% (SDAC) for those age 50 to 64. However, relapse-free survival was somewhat better following HDAC induction ($p = 0.049$): 33% (HDAC) versus 21% (SDAC) at 4 years for those younger than 50 years, and 21% (HDAC) versus 9% (SDAC) for those age 50 to 64. Induction with HDAC was associated with a significantly increased risk of fatal ($p = 0.0033$) and neurologic ($p < 0.0001$) toxicity. Among patients who achieved CR with SDAC, survival and DFS following consolidation randomization were not significantly better with HDAC compared with SDAC ($p = 0.77$ and 0.46, respectively). Patients who received both HDAC induction and consolidation had the best postremission outcomes; however, the proportion of CR patients who did not go on to protocol consolidation therapy was more than twice as high after HDAC induction compared with SDAC. Induction therapy with daunorubicin/HDAC was associated with greater toxicity than daunorubicin/SDAC, but with no improvement in CR rate or survival. Following CR induction with SDAC, consolidation with HDAC increased toxicity but not survival or DFS. In a nonrandomized comparison, patients who received both

*Table 84–2.* **Early Complete Response Rates in Patients with Adverse Karyotypes**

| Cytogenetic Group | Fludarabine-containing | Topotecan + Ara-C +/− ATRA | Cyclophosphamide + Ara-C + Topotecan +/− ATRA |
|---|---|---|---|
| −5, 5q−, −7, or 7q− (−5/−7) | 69/205 (34%) | 16/30 (53%) | 15/29 (52%) |
| Other abnormal (e.g., +8, del 11q) | 73/166 (44%) | 10/26 (38%) | 13/30 (43%) |
| **Totals** | 142/371 (38%) | 26/56 (46%) | 28/59 (47%) |

ATRA, retinoic acid.

HDAC induction and consolidation had superior survival and DFS compared with those who received SDAC induction with either SDAC or HDAC consolidation.

A major focus of prospective randomized studies in CR patients has been whether allogeneic or autologous stem cell transplantation (SCT) is superior to HDAC as consolidation therapy. In general no evidence that SCT is superior has been convincingly demonstrated. A U.S. multicenter study compared HDAC (single course of 3 g/m² over 3 hours IV every 12 hours for 12 doses) versus allogeneic versus autologous SCT in a cohort of 518 patients in CR from a group of 740 AML patients (70%) age 16 to 55 at time of diagnosis.[139] Patients were induced with idarubicin/ara-C. After complete remission had been achieved, idarubicin (2 days) and ara-C (5 days) were administered. Patients with histocompatible siblings were offered allogeneic SCT, whereas the remaining patients were randomly assigned to receive a single HDAC course or autologous SCT treated with 4-hydroperoxycyclophosphamide. Oral busulfan and IV cyclophosphamide were used as preparative regimens for both allogeneic and autologous SCT. In an intention-to-treat analysis, there was no significant difference in DFS among patients receiving HDAC or either form of SCT. The median follow-up was 4 years. Survival after CR was somewhat better after HDAC than after autologous SCT ($p = 0.05$). There was a slight advantage in terms of overall survival with HDAC compared with allogeneic SCT ($p = 0.04$).

Data from the Medical Research Council AML 10 study suggested some advantage for autologous SCT in certain patient subsets.[140] Following three courses of intensive chemotherapy, bone marrow was harvested from patients (<56 years) in CR who lacked an HLA-matched sibling donor. These patients were then randomized to receive, after one more course of chemotherapy, no further treatment (n = 191) or autologous SCT with cyclophosphamide/TBI conditioning (n = 190). Three hundred eighty-one patients were randomized (38% of those eligible). Of the 190 patients allocated to autologous SCT, 126 received it. On intention-to-treat analysis, the number of relapses was substantially lower in the autologous SCT group than in the group assigned no further treatment (64/190 [37%] versus 101/191 [58%], $p = 0.0007$), resulting in superior DFS at 7 years (53% versus 40%; $p = 0.04$). These benefits were observed in all risk groups and age groups. There were more deaths in CR in the autologous SCT group than in the no-further-treatment group (22 [12%] versus 7 [4%], $p = 0.0008$). In children (<15 years) and patients with good-risk disease, survival from relapse in the no-further-treatment group was 35% and 38% at 2 years, respectively. There was an overall survival advantage in the autologous SCT group at 7 years (57% vs. 45%, $p = 0.2$). Thus the addition of autologous SCT to four courses of intensive chemotherapy substantially reduced the risk of relapse in all risk groups, leading to improvement in long-term survival in this United Kingdom cohort of patients. The authors suggested that considering the relatively effective salvage therapy for children or patients with good-risk disease who relapse from chemotherapy, and the mortality, morbidity, and cost of autologous SCT, this procedure be offered in second remission in these patient groups.[140]

In one of two major French studies addressing this issue, superiority was claimed for the allogeneic SCT approach.[141]

Of a cohort of 204 adult patients with de novo AML, 162 (79.4%) achieved a CR. Of 135 patients who were still in CR after consolidation, 96 patients were younger than 46 years and 36 had an HLA-identical sibling donor and were allocated for allogeneic SCT; the other 60 patients received either autologous SCT or further chemotherapy. The 3-year DFS was higher in allogeneic SCT patients (66.5 ± 16%) than in the other group (42.4 ± 13%) ($p < 0.05$). The actuarial risk of relapse at 3 years was significantly lower for SCT patients (24 ± 15%) than for others (56 ± 13%; $p < 0.009$). However, data from a second French group appears to confirm that an optimal approach has yet to be defined.[142] A Groupe Ouest Est Leucemies Aigues Myeloblastiques randomized study compared allogeneic SCT, autologous SCT, and intensive consolidation chemotherapy in a cohort of 517 patients with de novo AML, age 15 to 50. After achievement of a CR, patients up to the age of 40 who had an HLA-identical sibling were assigned to undergo an allogeneic SCT. All other patients received a first course of HDAC and anthracycline. They were then randomly assigned to receive either a second course of high-dose amsacrine and etoposide or a combination of busulfan and cyclophosphamide followed by an unpurged autologous SCT. Of 367 patients who achieved CR, only 219 (59.5%) actually received the planned intensive postremission treatment (73 allogeneic SCT, 75 autologous SCT, and 71 intensive chemotherapy). With a median follow-up of 62 months, the 4-year DFS of the 367 CR patients was 39.5%. The 4-year overall survival (OS) of the 517 eligible patients was 40.5%. In multivariate analysis, the type of postremission therapy had no significant impact on the outcome. There was no difference in the 4-year DFS and OS between 88 patients for whom an allogeneic SCT was scheduled (44% and 53%, respectively) and 134 patients of the same age category and without an HLA-identical sibling (38% and 53%, respectively). Similarly, there was no difference in the outcome between autologous SCT and intensive chemotherapy. The 4-year DFS was 44% for the 86 patients randomly assigned to autologous SCT and 40% for the 78 patients assigned to intensive chemotherapy. The 4-year OS was similar in the two groups (50% vs. 54.5%). These latter data appear to reflect the overall current literature on the issue of consolidation therapy of CR in AML.

The optimal duration of postremission treatment as it pertains to maintenance therapy is unclear. Maintenance regimens use brief courses of chemotherapy, administered monthly and in low doses, for a period lasting anywhere from 1 to 5 years after achieving or consolidating a clinical remission, or both. No consistent significant advantage for maintenance chemotherapy when compared with induction and consolidation alone has been demonstrated in AML.[93, 101, 106, 143–146]

Two aspects of supportive care in induction therapy of AML are especially worthy of discussion based on current data. The first is the use of recombinant growth factors, specifically G-CSF and granulocyte-macrophage colony-stimulating factor (GM-CSF). In a prospective, randomized, placebo-controlled, U.S. multicenter study conducted by the Eastern Cooperative Oncology Group, recombinant GM-CSF has been shown to improve survival in elderly AML patients by reducing induction chemotherapy–related deaths.[37, 147–149] This reduction in mortality was associated with reductions in fatal sepsis, fungal infections, and metabolic abnormalities, the latter reflecting reduced sepsis or toxic anti-infective agents, or both. A number of similarly designed studies have failed to show a similar reduction in mortality associated with the use of G-CSF.[150–152] A SWOG study involved 234 patients, 55 years or older with de novo or secondary AML, who were randomized to daunorubicin/ara-C plus either placebo or G-CSF. The CR rate was not affected; it was 50% in the placebo and 41% in the G-CSF group. Median OS was also similar—9 months in the placebo and 6 months in the G-CSF arms. There was a significant 15% reduction in the time to neutrophil recovery in the G-CSF patients. G-CSF had no impact on recovery from thrombocytopenia, duration of first hospitalization, incidence of infection, frequency of total documented infections, or number of fatal infections.[150] A report from a Groupe Ouest Est Leucemies Aigues Myeloblastiques study concerned the use of G-CSF as support for high-dose consolidation therapy in CR patients.[151] In this prospective randomized study, G-CSF did significantly reduce the median duration of neutropenia, median duration of hospitalization, median duration of IV antibiotics, and the median duration of antifungal therapy. However, the incidence of microbiologically documented infections, toxic death rate, the 2-year DFS, and the 2-year OS were not affected by G-CSF administration. These differences in impact of GM-CSF and G-CSF are potentially attributable to the former's ability to enhance monocyte replication and function.[153] A large body of data would indicate that GM-CSF may well have an advantage in terms of reducing the incidence of, and reducing the lethality from, invasive fungal and other opportunistic infections. These data are particularly relevant to therapy of AML in elderly patients in whom empirical dose reduction of induction chemotherapy dosage is not useful, toxicity of "full" dose induction is high, and CR rates, EFS, and OS are particularly poor.[154]

A second aspect of supportive care on which the current literature is relatively sparse is the use of therapeutic leukapheresis in hyperleukocytic AML; no data have been published that attempt to define the impact on survival from this procedure. Between 1992 and 1999, we saw 146 patients with newly diagnosed AML (APL excluded) and an initial WBC greater than $50 \times 10^9$/L; 71 of these patients underwent leukapheresis at the discretion of their treating doctors. We compared outcome (early mortality, CR, and OS) rates in the patients who did and those who did not undergo apheresis. After accounting for covariates relevant to these outcomes—including age, performance status, and cytogenetics—there was evidence ($p = 0.006$) that apheresis reduced 2-week mortality rate and a suggestion ($p = 0.06$) that this resulted in a higher CR rate. However, there was no evidence that apheresis lengthened longer term or OS; if anything the suggestion was the converse ($p = 0.06$). This may reflect the fact that the patients chosen to have apheresis had unfavorable prognoses as defined by variables that were not captured in our data set, inasmuch as the alternative explanation—that apheresis per se shortens OS—seems unlikely.

## TREATMENT OF REFRACTORY AND RELAPSED ACUTE MYELOID LEUKEMIA

There is no standard definition of what comprises refractory AML. In terms of suitable candidates for investigational

therapy, there may be decreasing acceptance of the following subgroups: patients who have had multiple relapses, patients in first relapse with an initial CR less than 6 to 12 months, primary resistant patients, patients in first relapse with CR greater than 12 months, patients who fail to get a CR with the first course of therapy, patients who get a CR but take longer than 50 days to do so, and de novo patients with known adverse prognostic features (see Table 84–2). However, MDACC data show clearly that the prognosis in all these subgroups remains dire. One subgroup of particular note is patients who relapse after a relatively brief CR, in whom we have found that although they have a higher second CR rate if given an HDAC-containing regimen rather than phase I agents, OS is equivalent. In patients with an initial CR duration of 12 months or more, an HDAC-containing regimen is associated with both a higher CR and better OS than phase I agents. However, it must be emphasized that an HDAC regimen may well involve a novel combination, that is, a phase II study, and that as most doses of even an active agent in a phase I study are given at inactive doses during the dose-finding portion of the study, comparisons are difficult. These issues are of increasing complexity as the failure of current approaches becomes more evident and the number of investigational agents increases.

Novel agents and approaches that are currently being explored in AML therapy include CMA676,[155, 156] anti-CD33 antibodies,[157–159] anti GM-CSF antibodies,[160, 161] anti-CD45 antibodies,[155] anti-CD52 (Campath-1H) antibodies,[162] anti-TNF antibodies,[163] troxacitabine,[164] tallimustine,[165] homoharringtonine,[166] decitabine,[167] dolastatin,[168] MGI 114,[169] clofarabine,[170] DX-8951f,[171] 9-aminocamptothecin,[172] bryostatin,[173] inhibition of farnesyl transferases,[174] mdr modulation,[175] hypomethylation agents,[176–179] vaccination strategies,[180] antisense therapy,[181] telomerase inhibitors,[182] and antiangiogenic agents.[183]

All these approaches hold potential merit. Inhibition of angiogenesis is of particular interest at present. We have reported that cellular vascular endothelial growth factor (VEGF) levels are elevated in patients with AML with prognostic import.[184] Subsequently, Hussong and coworkers documented increased angiogenesis in diagnostic marrow from AML patients.[185] We have established that plasma VEGF levels are elevated and prognostic in AML, although they are elevated but not prognostic in RAEB and RAEB-t patients. Plasma levels of basic fibroblast growth factor are elevated in patients with both AML and MDS but are not of prognostic significance in either. Thus angiogenesis inhibition may be worthwhile in AML. SU5416 is a synthetic small molecule shown in screening assays to be a potent and selective inhibitor of the tyrosine kinase activity of Flk-1, a receptor tyrosine kinase expressed on the surface of endothelial cells.[186] SU5416 is believed to interfere with the catalytic activity of Flk-1 and, as a putative adenine mimic, may bind to the adenosine triphosphate–binding pocket in the kinase domain. Binding of VEGF to the extracellular domain of Flk-1 activates the tyrosyl-kinase activity in the cytoplasmic portion of the molecule, beginning a signaling cascade leading to cellular proliferation.[187] It is believed that inhibition of this signaling pathway by SU5416 will result in inhibition of endothelial cell proliferation and the sprouting of new vessels. We are investigating the activity of SU5416 in

AML patients in whom front-line CAT therapy has been unsuccessful.

Clearly the most important developments in AML therapy since the last edition of this book have been the enormous increase in knowledge of the pathophysiology of AML and the truly translational research that is developing novel therapeutic approaches based on this knowledge.

## SUGGESTIONS FOR ADDITIONAL READING

Felix CA. Secondary leukemias induced by topoisomerase-targeted drugs. Biochim Biophys Acta 1998;1400:233–55.

McCulloch EA. Toward a leukemia treatment strategy based on the probability of stem cell death: an essay in honor of Dr. Emil J Freireich. Clin Cancer Res 1997;3(12 Pt 2):2676–81.

Waxman S. Differentiation therapy in acute myelogenous leukemia (non-APL). Leukemia 2000;14:491–6.

Keating MJ. Leukemia: a model for drug development. Clin Cancer Res 1997;3(12 Pt 2):2598–604.

Estey EH. Treatment of relapsed and refractory acute myelogenous leukemia. Leukemia 2000;14:476–9.

Anasetti C. Transplantation of hematopoietic stem cells from alternate donors in acute myelogenous leukemia. Leukemia 2000;14:502–4.

## REFERENCES

1. Sandler DP. Epidemiology of acute myelogenous leukemia. Semin Oncol 1987;14:359–64.
2. Schwartz CL, Cohen HJ. Preleukemic syndromes and other syndromes predisposing to leukemia. Pediatr Clin North Am 1988;35:853–71.
3. Tooze JA, Marsh JC, Gordon-Smith EC. Clonal evolution of aplastic anaemia to myelodysplasia/acute myeloid leukaemia and paroxysmal nocturnal haemoglobinuria. Leuk Lymphoma 1999;33:231–41.
4. Hoyle CF, de Bastos M, Wheatley K, et al. AML associated with previous cytotoxic therapy, MDS or myeloproliferative disorders: results from the MRC's 9th AML trial. Br J Haematol 1989;72:45–53.
5. Kato H, Schull WJ. Studies of the mortality of A-bomb survivors. 7. Mortality, 1950–1978: Part I. Cancer mortality. Radiat Res 1982;90:395–432.
6. Fulton JP, Cobb S, Preble L, et al. Electrical wiring configurations and childhood leukemia in Rhode Island. Am J Epidemiol 1980;111:292–6.
7. Modan B. Cancer and leukemia risks after low level radiation—controversy, facts and future. Med Oncol Tumor Pharmacother 1987;4:151–61.
8. Sandler DP. Recent studies in leukemia epidemiology. Curr Opin Oncol 1995;7:12–8.
9. Polednak AP, Stehney AF, Rowland RE. Mortality among women first employed before 1930 in the U.S. radium dial-painting industry. A group ascertained from employment lists. Am J Epidemiol 1978;107:179–95.
10. Hornung RW, Ward E, Morris JA, Rinsky RA. Hematologic effects of benzene: a thirty-five year longitudinal study of rubber workers. Toxicol Ind Health 1989;5:1153–8.
11. Rinsky RA. Benzene and leukemia: an epidemiologic risk assessment. Environ Health Perspect 1989;82:189–91.
12. Crump KS. Risk of benzene-induced leukemia predicted from the Pliofilm cohort. Environ Health Perspect 1996;104:Suppl 6:1437–41.
13. Paxton MB. Leukemia risk associated with benzene exposure in the Pliofilm cohort. Environ Health Perspect 1996;104:Suppl 6:1431–6.
14. Stellman SD, Garfinkel L. Cancer mortality among woodworkers. Am J Ind Med 1984;5:343–57.
15. Silverstein M, Maizlish N, Park R, Mirer F. Mortality among workers exposed to coal tar pitch volatiles and welding emissions: an exercise in epidemiologic triage. Am J Public Health 1985;75:1283–7.
16. Matanoski G, Elliott E, Tao X, et al. Lymphohematopoietic cancers and butadiene and styrene exposure in synthetic rubber manufacture. Ann N Y Acad Sci 1997;837:157–69.
17. Straif K, Weiland SK, Werner B, et al. Workplace risk factors for cancer in the German rubber industry: Part 2. Mortality from non-respiratory cancers. Occup Environ Med 1998;55:325–32.
18. Hayes RB, Blair A, Stewart PA, et al. Mortality of U.S. embalmers and funeral directors. Am J Ind Med 1990;18:641–52.
19. Lynge E, Anttila A, Hemminki K. Organic solvents and cancer. Cancer Causes Control 1997;8:406–19.
20. Bertazzi PA, Pesatori AC, Bernucci I, et al. Dioxin exposure and human leukemias and lymphomas. Lessons from the Seveso accident and studies on industrial workers. Leukemia 1999;13:Suppl 1:S72–4.
21. Smith MA, Rubinstein L, Anderson JR, et al. Secondary leukemia or myelodysplastic syndrome after treatment with epipodophyllotoxins. J Clin Oncol 1999;17:569–77.
22. Levine EG, Bloomfield CD. Leukemias and myelodysplastic syndromes secondary to drug, radiation, and environmental exposure. Semin Oncol 1992;19:47–84.
23. Travis LB, Holowaty EJ, Bergfeldt K, et al. Risk of leukemia after platinum-based chemotherapy for ovarian cancer. N Engl J Med 1999;340:351–7.
24. Kumana CR, Chau RY, Chan TK. Chloramphenicol use and childhood leukaemia. Lancet 1988;1:476–7.
25. Friedman GD. Phenylbutazone, musculoskeletal disease, and leukemia. J Chronic Dis 1982;35:233–43.
26. Adamson RH, Seiber SM. Chemically induced leukemia in humans. Environ Health Perspect 1981;39:93–103.
27. Nagaratnam N, Chetiyawardana AD, Rajiyah S. Aplasia and leukemia following chloroquine therapy. Postgrad Med J 1978;54:108–12.
28. Kane EV, Roman E, Cartwright R, et al. Tobacco and the risk of acute leukaemia in adults. Br J Cancer 1999;81:1228–33.
29. Davico L, Sacerdote C, Ciccone G, et al. Chromosome 8, occupational exposures, smoking, and acute nonlymphocytic leukemias: a population-based study. Cancer Epidemiol Biomarkers Prev 1998;7:1123–5.
30. Zeeb H, Blettner M. Adult leukaemia: what is the role of currently known risk factors? Radiat Environ Biophys 1998;36:217–28.
31. Bennett JM, Catovsky D, Daniel MT, et al. Proposals for the classification of the acute leukaemias. French-American-British (FAB) cooperative group. Br J Haematol 1976;33:451–8.
32. Lee EJ, Pollak A, Leavitt RD, et al. Minimally differentiated acute nonlymphocytic leukemia: a distinct entity. Blood 1987;70:1400–6.
33. Bennett JM, Catovsky D, Daniel MT, et al. Proposal for the recognition of minimally differentiated acute myeloid leukaemia (AML-M0). Br J Haematol 1991;78:325–9.
34. Andreeff M. Cell kinetics of leukemia. Semin Hematol 1986;23:300–14.
35. Toba K, Koike T, Watanabe K, et al. Cell kinetic study of normal human bone marrow hematopoiesis and acute leukemia using 7AAD/PY. Eur J Haematol 2000;64:10–21.
36. Andreeff M, Assing G, Cirrincione C. Prognostic value of DNA/RNA flow cytometry in myeloblastic and lymphoblastic leukemia in adults: RNA content and S-phase predict remission duration and survival in multi-variate analysis. Ann N Y Acad Sci 1986;468:387–406.
37. Rowe JM, Liesveld JL. Hematopoietic growth factors and acute leukemia. Cancer Treat Res 1999;99:195–226.
38. Hoelzer D, Seipelt G. Granulocyte colony-stimulating factor and granulocyte-macrophage colony-stimulating factor in the treatment of myeloid leukemia. Curr Opin Hematol 1995;2:196–203.
39. Hirsch-Ginsberg C, Huh YO, Kagan J, et al. Advances in the diagnosis of acute leukemia. Hematol Oncol Clin North Am 1993;7:1–46.
40. Keating MJ, Cork A, Broach Y, et al. Toward a clinically relevant cytogenetic classification of acute myelogenous leukemia. Leuk Res 1987;11:119–33.
41. Keating MJ, Smith TL, Kantarjian H, et al. Cytogenetic pattern in acute myelogenous leukemia: a major reproducible determinant of outcome. Leukemia 1988;2:403–12.
42. Machnicki JL, Bloomfield CD. Clinical significance of the cytogenetics of acute leukemias. Oncology (Huntingt) 1990;4:23–30; discussion 35–6.
43. Rowley JD. The role of chromosome translocations in leukemogenesis. Semin Hematol 1999;36:59–72.
44. van Dongen JJ, Macintyre EA, Gabert JA, et al. Standardized RT-PCR analysis of fusion gene transcripts from chromosome aberrations in acute leukemia for detection of minimal residual disease. Report of the BIOMED-1 Concerted Action: investigation of minimal residual disease in acute leukemia. Leukemia 1999;13:1901–28.
45. Arkesteijn G, Jumelet E, Hagenbeek A, et al. Reverse chromosome painting for the identification of marker chromosomes and complex translocations in leukemia. Cytometry 1999;35:117–24.

46. Kotylo PK, Seo IS, Smith FO, et al. Flow cytometric immunophenotypic characterization of pediatric and adult minimally differentiated acute myeloid leukemia (AML-M0). Am J Clin Pathol 2000;113:193–200.

47. Swirsky DM, Li YS, Matthews JG, et al. 8;21 translocation in acute granulocytic leukaemia: cytological, cytochemical and clinical features. Br J Haematol 1984;56:199–213.

48. Berger R, Flandrin G, Bernheim A, et al. Cytogenetic studies on 519 consecutive de novo acute nonlymphocytic leukemias. Cancer Genet Cytogenet 1987;29:9–21.

49. Koeffler HP. Syndromes of acute nonlymphocytic leukemia. Ann Intern Med 1987;107:748–58.

50. Slack JL. The biology and treatment of acute progranulocytic leukemia. Curr Opin Oncol 1999;11:9–13.

51. Frankel SR, Powell BL. Current approaches to acute promyelocytic leukemia. Cancer Treat Res 1999;99:125–53.

52. Slack JL, Gallagher RE. The molecular biology of acute promyelocytic leukemia. Cancer Treat Res 1999;99:75–124.

53. Golomb HM, Rowley JD, Vardiman JW, et al. "Microgranular" acute promyelocytic leukemia: a distinct clinical, ultrastructural, and cytogenetic entity. Blood 1980;55:253–9.

54. Tallman MS. Therapy of acute promyelocytic leukemia: all-trans retinoic acid and beyond. Leukemia 1998;12:Suppl 1:S37–40.

55. Dunphy CH. Comprehensive review of adult acute myelogenous leukemia: cytomorphological, enzyme cytochemical, flow cytometric immunophenotypic, and cytogenetic findings. J Clin Lab Anal 1999;13:19–26.

56. Liu PP, Hajra A, Wijmenga C, Collins FS. Molecular pathogenesis of the chromosome 16 inversion in the M4Eo subtype of acute myeloid leukemia. Blood 1995;85:2289–302.

57. Holmes R, Keating MJ, Cork A, et al. A unique pattern of central nervous system leukemia in acute myelomonocytic leukemia associated with inv(16)(p13q22). Blood 1985;65:1071–8.

58. Peterson BA, Levine EG. Uncommon subtypes of acute nonlymphocytic leukemia: clinical features and management of FAB M5, M6 and M7. Semin Oncol 1987;14:425–34.

59. Catovsky D, Matutes E, Buccheri V, et al. A classification of acute leukaemia for the 1990s. Ann Hematol 1991;62:16–21.

60. Oikawa T, Yamada T, Kihara-Negishi F, et al. The role of Ets family transcription factor PU.1 in hematopoietic cell differentiation, proliferation and apoptosis. Cell Death Differ 1999;6:599–608.

61. Goldberg SL, Noel P, Klumpp TR, Dewald GW. The erythroid leukemias: a comparative study of erythroleukemia (FAB M6) and Di Guglielmo disease. Am J Clin Oncol 1998;21:42–7.

62. Garand R, Robillard N. Immunophenotypic characterization of acute leukemias and chronic lymphoproliferative disorders: practical recommendations and classifications. Hematol Cell Ther 1996;38:471–86.

63. Cuneo A, Mecucci C, Kerim S, et al. Multipotent stem cell involvement in megakaryoblastic leukemia: cytologic and cytogenetic evidence in 15 patients. Blood 1989;74:1781–90.

64. Terstappen LW, Loken MR. Myeloid cell differentiation in normal bone marrow and acute myeloid leukemia assessed by multi-dimensional flow cytometry. Anal Cell Pathol 1990;2:229–40.

65. Terstappen LW, Konemann S, Safford M, et al. Flow cytometric characterization of acute myeloid leukemia. Part 1. Significance of light scattering properties. Leukemia 1991;5:315–21.

66. van der Schoot CE, Daams GM, Pinkster J, et al. Monoclonal antibodies against myeloperoxidase are valuable immunological reagents for the diagnosis of acute myeloid leukaemia. Br J Haematol 1990;74:173–8.

67. Kurec AS, Cruz VE, Barrett D, et al. Immunophenotyping of acute leukemias using paraffin-embedded tissue sections. Am J Clin Pathol 1990;93:502–9.

68. Vliagoftis H, Worobec AS, Metcalfe DD. The protooncogene c-kit and c-kit ligand in human disease. J Allergy Clin Immunol 1997;100:435–40.

69. Lauria F, Raspadori D, Ventura MA, et al. The presence of lymphoid-associated antigens in adult acute myeloid leukemia is devoid of prognostic relevance. Stem Cells 1995;13:428–34.

70. Krishnan K, Ross CW, Adams PT, et al. Neural cell-adhesion molecule (CD 56)-positive, t(8;21) acute myeloid leukemia (AML, M-2) and granulocytic sarcoma. Ann Hematol 1994;69:321–3.

71. Kantarjian HM, Hirsch-Ginsberg C, Yee G, et al. Mixed-lineage leukemia revisited: acute lymphocytic leukemia with myeloperoxidase-positive blasts by electron microscopy [see comments]. Blood 1990;76:808–13.

72. Campana D, Yokota S, Coustan-Smith E, et al. The detection of residual acute lymphoblastic leukemia cells with immunologic methods and polymerase chain reaction: a comparative study. Leukemia 1990;4:609–14.

73. Campana D, Coustan-Smith E, Janossy G. The immunologic detection of minimal residual disease in acute leukemia. Blood 1990;76:163–71.

74. Campana D, Coustan-Smith E, Behm FG. The definition of remission in acute leukemia with immunologic techniques. Bone Marrow Transplant 1991;8:429–37.

75. Gore SD, Kastan MB, Goodman SN, Civin CI. Detection of minimal residual T cell acute lymphoblastic leukemia by flow cytometry. J Immunol Methods 1990;132:275–86.

76. Drach J, Drach D, Glassl H, et al. Flow cytometric determination of atypical antigen expression in acute leukemia for the study of minimal residual disease. Cytometry 1992;13:893–901.

77. Reading CL, Estey EH, Huh YO, et al. Expression of unusual immunophenotype combinations in acute myelogenous leukemia. Blood 1993;81:3083–90.

78. San-Miguel JF, Bartram C, Campana D, Andreeff M. Minimal residual disease in hematologic malignancies. Rev Invest Clin 1994;Suppl:147–52.

79. Engel H, Goodacre A, Keyhani A, et al. Minimal residual disease in acute myelogenous leukaemia and myelodysplastic syndromes: a follow-up of patients in clinical remission. Br J Haematol 1997;99:64–75.

80. Engel H, Drach J, Keyhani A, et al. Quantitation of minimal residual disease in acute myelogenous leukemia and myelodysplastic syndromes in complete remission by molecular cytogenetics of progenitor cells. Leukemia 1999;13:568–77.

81. Keating MJ, Estey E, Kantarjian H, et al. Evolution of treatment for acute myelogenous leukemia and myelodysplastic syndrome at M.D. Anderson Cancer Center 1985–1991. Leukemia 1992;6:78–80.

82. Freireich EJ. Four decades of therapy for AML. Leukemia 1998;12:Suppl 1:S54–6.

83. Anderlini P, Ghaddar HM, Smith TL, et al. Factors predicting complete remission and subsequent disease-free survival after a second course of induction therapy in patients with acute myelogenous leukemia resistant to the first. Leukemia 1996;10:964–9.

84. Estey EH, Shen Y, Thall PF. Effect of time to complete remission on subsequent survival and disease-free survival time in AML, RAEB-t, and RAEB. Blood 2000;95:72–7.

85. Kantarjian HM, Keating MJ, Walters RS, et al. The characteristics and outcome of patients with late relapse acute myelogenous leukemia. J Clin Oncol 1988;6:232–8.

86. Schiffer CA, Dodge R, Larson RA. Long-term follow-up of Cancer and Leukemia Group B studies in acute myeloid leukemia. Cancer 1997;80:2210–4.

87. Cortes J, O'Brien S, Estey E, et al. Phase I study of liposomal daunorubicin in patients with acute leukemia. Invest New Drugs 1999;17:81–7.

88. Michieli M, Damiani D, Ermacora A, et al. Liposome-encapsulated daunorubicin for PGP-related multidrug resistance. Br J Haematol 1999;106:92–9.

89. Wang Y, Eksborg S, Lewensohn R, et al. In vitro cellular accumulation and cytotoxicity of liposomal and conventional formulations of daunorubicin and doxorubicin in resistant K562 cells. Anticancer Drugs 1999;10:921–8.

90. Berman E, Wiernik P, Vogler R, et al. Long-term follow-up of three randomized trials comparing idarubicin and daunorubicin as induction therapies for patients with untreated acute myeloid leukemia. Cancer 1997;80:2181–5.

91. Wiernik PH, Banks PL, Case DC Jr, et al. Cytarabine plus idarubicin or daunorubicin as induction and consolidation therapy for previously untreated adult patients with acute myeloid leukemia. Blood 1992;79:313–9.

92. Berman E, Heller G, Santorsa J, et al. Results of a randomized trial comparing idarubicin and cytosine arabinoside with daunorubicin and cytosine arabinoside in adult patients with newly diagnosed acute myelogenous leukemia. Blood 1991;77:1666–74.

93. Vogler WR, Winton EF, Gordon DS, et al. A randomized comparison of postremission therapy in acute myelogenous leukemia: a Southeastern Cancer Study Group trial. Blood 1984;63:1039–45.

94. Wahlin A, Hornsten P, Hedenus M, Malm C. Mitoxantrone and cytarabine versus daunorubicin and cytarabine in previously untreated patients with acute myeloid leukemia. Cancer Chemother Pharmacol 1991;28:480–3.

95. Liu Yin JA, Johnson PR, Davies JM, et al. Mitozantrone and cytosine arabinoside as first-line therapy in elderly patients with acute myeloid leukaemia. Br J Haematol 1991;79:415–20.

96. Sierra J, Granena A, Bosch F, et al. Mitoxantrone and intermediate-dose cytosine arabinoside for poor-risk acute leukemias: response to treatment and factors influencing outcome. Hematol Oncol 1992;10:301–9.

97. Haas R, Ho AD, Del Valle F, et al. Idarubicin/cytosine arabinoside and mitoxantrone/etoposide for the treatment of de novo acute myelogenous leukemia. Semin Oncol 1993;20:20–6.

98. MacCallum PK, Rohatiner AZ, Davis CL, et al. Mitoxantrone and cytosine arabinoside as treatment for acute myeloblastic leukemia in older patients. Ann Hematol 1995;71:35–9.

99. Bow EJ, Sutherland JA, Kilpatrick MG, et al. Therapy of untreated acute myeloid leukemia in the elderly: remission-induction using a non-cytarabine-containing regimen of mitoxantrone plus etoposide. J Clin Oncol 1996;14:1345–52.

100. Feldman EJ, Seiter K, Damon L, et al. A randomized trial of high- vs standard-dose mitoxantrone with cytarabine in elderly patients with acute myeloid leukemia. Leukemia 1997;11:485–9.

101. Lowenberg B, Suciu S, Archimbaud E, et al. Mitoxantrone versus daunorubicin in induction-consolidation chemotherapy—the value of low-dose cytarabine for maintenance of remission, and an assessment of prognostic factors in acute myeloid leukemia in the elderly: final report. European Organization for the Research and Treatment of Cancer and the Dutch-Belgian Hemato-Oncology Cooperative Hovon Group. J Clin Oncol 1998;16:872–81.

102. Kern W, Aul C, Maschmeyer G, et al. Superiority of high-dose over intermediate-dose cytosine arabinoside in the treatment of patients with high-risk acute myeloid leukemia: results of an age-adjusted prospective randomized comparison. Leukemia 1998;12:1049–55.

103. Lambertenghi Deliliers G, Annaloro C, et al. Idarubicin in the therapy of acute myeloid leukemia: final analysis in 57 previously untreated patients. Semin Oncol 1993;20:27–33.

104. Bishop JF, Matthews JP, Young GA, et al. Intensified induction chemotherapy with high dose cytarabine and etoposide for acute myeloid leukemia: a review and updated results of the Australian Leukemia Study Group. Leuk Lymphoma 1998;28:315–27.

105. Bishop JF, Lowenthal RM, Joshua D, et al. Etoposide in acute non-lymphocytic leukemia. Australian Leukemia Study Group. Blood 1990;75:27–32.

106. Preisler H, Davis RB, Kirshner J, et al. Comparison of three remission induction regimens and two postinduction strategies for the treatment of acute nonlymphocytic leukemia: a Cancer and Leukemia Group B study. Blood 1987;69:1441–9.

107. Archimbaud E, Jehn U, Thomas X, et al. Multicenter randomized phase II trial of idarubicin vs mitoxantrone, combined with VP-16 and cytarabine for induction/consolidation therapy, followed by a feasibility study of autologous peripheral blood stem cell transplantation in elderly patients with acute myeloid leukemia. Leukemia 1999;13:843–9.

108. Rees JK. Chemotherapy of acute myeloid leukaemia (AML) in UK: past, present and future. Bone Marrow Transplant 1989;4:Suppl 1:110–3.

109. Estey EH, Pierce S, Keating MJ. Identification of a group of AML/MDS patients with a relatively favorable prognosis who have chromosome 5 and/or 7 abnormalities. Haematologica 2000;85:246–249.

110. Beran M, Kantarjian H. Results of topotecan-based combination therapy in patients with myelodysplastic syndromes and chronic myelomonocytic leukemia. Semin Hematol 1999;36:3–10.

111. Beran M, Estey E, O'Brien S, et al. Topotecan and cytarabine is an active combination regimen in myelodysplastic syndromes and chronic myelomonocytic leukemia. J Clin Oncol 1999;17:2819–30.

112. Vey N, Kantarjian H, Beran M, et al. Combination of topotecan with cytarabine or etoposide in patients with refractory or relapsed acute myeloid leukemia: results of a randomized phase I/II study. Invest New Drugs 1999;17:89–95.

113. Beran M, Estey E, O'Brien SM, et al. Results of topotecan single-agent therapy in patients with myelodysplastic syndromes and chronic myelomonocytic leukemia. Leuk Lymphoma 1998;31:521–31.

114. Beran M, Kantarjian H. Topotecan in the treatment of hematologic malignancies. Semin Hematol 1998;35:26–31.

115. Beran M, Kantarjian H, O'Brien S, et al. Topotecan, a topoisomerase I inhibitor, is active in the treatment of myelodysplastic syndrome and chronic myelomonocytic leukemia. Blood 1996;88:2473–9.

116. Kantarjian HM, Beran M, Ellis A, et al. Phase I study of topotecan, a new topoisomerase I inhibitor, in patients with refractory or relapsed acute leukemia. Blood 1993;81:1146–51.

117. Seiter K, Feldman EJ, Halicka HD, et al. Phase I clinical and laboratory evaluation of topotecan and cytarabine in patients with acute leukemia. J Clin Oncol 1997;15:44–51.

118. Rowinsky EK, Adjei A, Donehower RC, et al. Phase I and pharmacodynamic study of the topoisomerase I-inhibitor topotecan in patients with refractory acute leukemia. J Clin Oncol 1994;12:2193–203.

119. Rowinsky EK, Kaufmann SH, Baker SD, et al. A phase I and pharmacological study of topotecan infused over 30 minutes for five days in patients with refractory acute leukemia. Clin Cancer Res 1996;2:1921–30.

120. Hu ZB, Minden MD, McCulloch EA. Phosphorylation of BCL-2 after exposure of human leukemic cells to retinoic acid. Blood 1998;92:1768–75.

121. Estey EH, Thall PF, Pierce S, et al. Randomized phase II study of fludarabine + cytosine arabinoside + idarubicin +/− all-trans retinoic acid +/− granulocyte colony-stimulating factor in poor prognosis newly diagnosed acute myeloid leukemia and myelodysplastic syndrome. Blood 1999;93:2478–84.

122. Estey EH, Thall PF, Reed P, et al. Treatment of newly diagnosed AML, RAEB-t or RAEB with lisofylline or placebo in addition to chemotherapy. Leukemia 1999;13:850–4.

123. Weick JK, Kopecky KJ, Appelbaum FR, et al. A randomized investigation of high-dose versus standard-dose cytosine arabinoside with daunorubicin in patients with previously untreated acute myeloid leukemia: a Southwest Oncology Group study. Blood 1996;88:2841–51.

124. Mayer RJ, Davis RB, Schiffer CA, et al. Intensive postremission chemotherapy in adults with acute myeloid leukemia. Cancer and Leukemia Group B. N Engl J Med 1994;331:896–903.

125. Estey EH, Keating MJ, Dixon DO, et al. Karyotype is prognostically more important than the FAB system's distinction between myelodysplastic syndrome and acute myelogenous leukemia. Hematol Pathol 1987;1:203–8.

126. Degos L. Is acute promyelocytic leukemia a curable disease? Treatment strategy for a long-term survival. Leukemia 1994;8:S6–8.

127. Fenaux P. Treatment of newly diagnosed APL. The best choice is not ATRA or chemotherapy . . . but a combination of both. European APL Group. Leukemia 1994;8:S59–61; discussion S62.

128. Fenaux P, Chastang C, Degos L. Treatment of newly diagnosed acute promyelocytic leukemia (APL) by a combination of all-trans retinoic acid (ATRA) and chemotherapy. French APL Group. Leukemia 1994;8:S42–7.

129. Fenaux P, Le Deley MC, Castaigne S, et al. Effect of all transretinoic acid in newly diagnosed acute promyelocytic leukemia. Results of a multicenter randomized trial. European APL 91 Group. Blood 1993;82:3241–9.

130. Estey EH, Giles FJ, Kantarjian H, et al. Molecular remissions induced by liposomal-encapsulated all-trans retinoic acid in newly diagnosed acute promyelocytic leukemia. Blood 1999;94:2230–5.

131. Weil SC. Minimal residual disease in acute promyelocytic leukemia. Clin Lab Med 2000;20:105–17, ix.

132. Burnett AK, Grimwade D, Solomon E, et al. Presenting white blood cell count and kinetics of molecular remission predict prognosis in acute promyelocytic leukemia treated with all-trans retinoic acid: result of the Randomized MRC Trial. Blood 1999;93:4131–43.

133. Lo Coco F, Diverio D, Avvisati G, et al. Therapy of molecular relapse in acute promyelocytic leukemia. Blood 1999;94:2225–9.

134. Agis H, Weltermann A, Mitterbauer G, et al. Successful treatment with arsenic trioxide of a patient with ATRA-resistant relapse of acute promyelocytic leukemia. Ann Hematol 1999;78:329–32.

135. Zhang P. The use of arsenic trioxide (As2O3) in the treatment of acute promyelocytic leukemia. J Biol Regul Homeost Agents 1999;13:195–200.

136. Hu J, Shen ZX, Sun GL, et al. Long-term survival and prognostic study in acute promyelocytic leukemia treated with all-trans-retinoic acid, chemotherapy, and As2O3: an experience of 120 patients at a single institution. Int J Hematol 1999;70:248–60.

137. Shen ZX, Chen GQ, Ni JH, et al. Use of arsenic trioxide (As2O3) in the treatment of acute promyelocytic leukemia (APL): II. Clinical efficacy and pharmacokinetics in relapsed patients. Blood 1997;89:3354–60.

138. Chen GQ, Shi XG, Tang W, et al. Use of arsenic trioxide (As2O3) in

the treatment of acute promyelocytic leukemia (APL): I. As2O3 exerts dose-dependent dual effects on APL cells. Blood 1997;89:3345–53.

139. Cassileth PA, Harrington DP, Appelbaum FR, et al. Chemotherapy compared with autologous or allogeneic bone marrow transplantation in the management of acute myeloid leukemia in first remission [see comments]. N Engl J Med 1998;339:1649–56.

140. Burnett AK, Goldstone AH, Stevens RM, et al. Randomised comparison of addition of autologous bone-marrow transplantation to intensive chemotherapy for acute myeloid leukaemia in first remission: results of MRC AML 10 trial. UK Medical Research Council Adult and Children's Leukaemia Working Parties. Lancet 1998;351:700–8.

141. Reiffers J, Stoppa AM, Attal M, et al. Allogeneic vs autologous stem cell transplantation vs chemotherapy in patients with acute myeloid leukemia in first remission: the BGMT 87 study. Leukemia 1996;10:1874–82.

142. Harousseau JL, Cahn JY, Pignon B, et al. Comparison of autologous bone marrow transplantation and intensive chemotherapy as postremission therapy in adult acute myeloid leukemia. The Groupe Ouest Est Leucemies Aigues Myeloblastiques (GOELAM). Blood 1997;90:2978–86.

143. Champlin R, Jacobs A, Gale RP, et al. Prolonged survival in acute myelogenous leukaemia without maintenance chemotherapy. Lancet 1984;1:894–6.

144. Survival in acute myeloblastic leukemia is not prolonged by remission maintenance or early reinduction chemotherapy. The Toronto Leukemia Study Group. Leuk Res 1988;12:195–200.

145. Sauter C, Berchtold W, Fopp M, et al. Acute myelogenous leukaemia: maintenance chemotherapy after early consolidation treatment does not prolong survival. Lancet 1984;1:379–82.

146. Kantarjian HM, Keating MJ, Walters RS, et al. Early intensification and short-term maintenance chemotherapy does not prolong survival in acute myelogenous leukemia. Cancer 1986;58:1603–8.

147. Rowe JM, Andersen JW, Mazza JJ, et al. A randomized placebo-controlled phase III study of granulocyte-macrophage colony-stimulating factor in adult patients (> 55 to 70 years of age) with acute myelogenous leukemia: a study of the Eastern Cooperative Oncology Group (E1490). Blood 1995;86:457–62.

148. Rowe JM. Treatment of acute myeloid leukemia with cytokines: effect on duration of neutropenia and response to infections. Clin Infect Dis 1998;26:1290–4.

149. Bennett CL, Stinson TJ, Tallman MS, et al. Economic analysis of a randomized placebo-controlled phase III study of granulocyte macrophage colony stimulating factor in adult patients (> 55 to 70 years of age) with acute myelogenous leukemia. Eastern Cooperative Oncology Group (E1490). Ann Oncol 1999;10:177–82.

150. Godwin JE, Kopecky KJ, Head DR, et al. A double-blind placebo-controlled trial of granulocyte colony-stimulating factor in elderly patients with previously untreated acute myeloid leukemia: a Southwest Oncology Group study (9031). Blood 1998;91:3607–15.

151. Harousseau JL, Witz B, Lioure B, et al. Granulocyte colony-stimulating factor after intensive consolidation chemotherapy in acute myeloid leukemia: results of a randomized trial of the Groupe Ouest-Est Leucemies Aigues Myeloblastiques. J Clin Oncol 2000;18:780.

152. Heil G, Hoelzer D, Sanz MA, et al. A randomized, double-blind, placebo-controlled, phase III study of filgrastim in remission induction and consolidation therapy for adults with de novo acute myeloid leukemia. The International Acute Myeloid Leukemia Study Group. Blood 1997;90:4710–8.

153. Giles FJ. Monocyte-macrophages, granulocyte-macrophage colony-stimulating factor, and prolonged survival among patients with acute myeloid leukemia and stem cell transplants. Clin Infect Dis 1998;26:1282–9.

154. Hiddemann W, Kern W, Schoch C, et al. Management of acute myeloid leukemia in elderly patients. J Clin Oncol 1999;17:3569–76.

155. Sievers EL. Clinical studies of new "biologic" approaches to therapy of acute myeloid leukemia with monoclonal antibodies and immunoconjugates. Curr Opin Oncol 2000;12:30–5.

156. Appelbaum FR. Antibody-targeted therapy for myeloid leukemia. Semin Hematol 1999;36:2–8.

157. Jurcic JG, DeBlasio T, Dumont L, et al. Molecular remission induction with retinoic acid and anti-CD33 monoclonal antibody HuM195 in acute promyelocytic leukemia. Clin Cancer Res 2000;6:372–80.

158. Kossman SE, Scheinberg DA, Jurcic JG, et al. A phase I trial of humanized monoclonal antibody HuM195 (anti-CD33) with low-dose interleukin 2 in acute myelogenous leukemia. Clin Cancer Res 1999;5:2748–55.

159. Sgouros G, Ballangrud AM, Jurcic JG, et al. Pharmacokinetics and dosimetry of an alpha-particle emitter labeled antibody: 213Bi-HuM195 (anti-CD33) in patients with leukemia. J Nucl Med 1999;40:1935–46.

160. Bouabdallah R, Olive D, Meyer P, et al. Anti-GM-CSF monoclonal antibody therapy for refractory acute leukemia. Leuk Lymphoma 1998;30:539–49.

161. Frankel AE, Hall PD, McLain C, et al. Cell-specific modulation of drug resistance in acute myeloid leukemic blasts by diphtheria fusion toxin, DT388-GMCSF. Bioconjug Chem 1998;9:490–6.

162. Maloney DG. Advances in immunotherapy of hematologic malignancies. Curr Opin Hematol 1998;5:237–43.

163. Barak V, Nisman B, Polliack A. The tumor necrosis factor family correlation with disease activity and response to treatment in hairy cell leukemia. Eur J Haematol 1999;62:71–5.

164. Siu LL, Attardo G, Izbicka E, et al. Activity of (-)-2′-deoxy-3′-oxacytidine (BCH-4556) against human tumor colony-forming units. Ann Oncol 1998;9:885–91.

165. Beran M, Jeha S, O'Brien S, et al. Tallimustine, an effective antileukemic agent in a severe combined immunodeficient mouse model of adult myelogenous leukemia, induces remissions in a phase I study. Clin Cancer Res 1997;3:2377–84.

166. Kantarjian HM, Estey EH, Keating MA. New chemotherapeutic agents in acute myeloid leukemia. Leukemia 1996;10 Suppl 1:S4–6.

167. Kantarjian HM, O'Brien SM, Estey E, et al. Decitabine studies in chronic and acute myelogenous leukemia. Leukemia 1997;11:Suppl 1:S35–6.

168. Poncet J, Hortala L, Busquet M, et al. Synthesis and antiproliferative activity of a cyclic analog of dolastatin 10. Bioorg Med Chem Lett 1998;8:2855–8.

169. Kelner MJ, McMorris TC, Estes L, et al. Anti-leukemic action of the novel agent MGI 114 (HMAF) and synergistic action with topotecan. Leukemia 2000;14:136–41.

170. Keating MJ. Chronic lymphocytic leukemia. Semin Oncol 1999;26:107–14.

171. Vey N, Giles FJ, Kantarjian H, et al. The topoisomerase I inhibitor DX-8951f is active in a severe combined immunodeficient mouse model of human acute myelogenous leukemia. Clin Cancer Res 2000;6:731–6.

172. Vey N, Kantarjian H, Tran H, et al. Phase I and pharmacologic study of 9-aminocamptothecin colloidal dispersion formulation in patients with refractory or relapsed acute leukemia. Ann Oncol 1999;10:577–83.

173. Grant S. Modulation of ara-C induced apoptosis in leukemia by the PKC activator bryostatin 1. Front Biosci 1997;2:d242–52.

174. Beaupre DM, Kurzrock R. RAS and leukemia: from basic mechanisms to gene-directed therapy. J Clin Oncol 1999;17:1071–9.

175. Advani R, Saba HI, Tallman MS, et al. Treatment of refractory and relapsed acute myelogenous leukemia with combination chemotherapy plus the multidrug resistance modulator PSC 833 (Valspodar). Blood 1999;93:787–95.

176. Gattei V, Aldinucci D, Petti MC, et al. In vitro and in vivo effects of 5-aza-2′-deoxycytidine (Decitabine) on clonogenic cells from acute myeloid leukemia patients. Leukemia 1993;7:Suppl 1:42–8.

177. Guo SX, Taki T, Ohnishi H, et al. Hypermethylation of p16 and p15 genes and RB protein expression in acute leukemia. Leuk Res 2000;24:39–46.

178. Melki JR, Vincent PC, Clark SJ. Concurrent DNA hypermethylation of multiple genes in acute myeloid leukemia. Cancer Res 1999;59:3730–40.

179. Issa JP, Baylin SB, Herman JG. DNA methylation changes in hematologic malignancies: biologic and clinical implications. Leukemia 1997;11:Suppl 1:S7–11.

180. Dunussi-Joannopoulos K, Runyon K, et al. Vaccines with interleukin-12–transduced acute myeloid leukemia cells elicit very potent therapeutic and long-lasting protective immunity. Blood 1999;94:4263–73.

181. Cotter FE. Antisense therapy of hematologic malignancies. Semin Hematol 1999;36:9–14.

182. Engelhardt M, Mackenzie K, Drullinsky P, et al. Telomerase activity and telomere length in acute and chronic leukemia, pre– and post–ex vivo culture. Cancer Res 2000;60:610–7.

183. Hatfill SJ, Fester ED, de Beer DP, Bohm L. Induction of morphological differentiation in the human leukemic cell line K562 by exposure to thalidomide metabolites. Leuk Res 1991;15:129–36.

184. Aguayo A, Estey E, Kantarjian H, et al. Cellular vascular endothelial

growth factor is a predictor of outcome in patients with acute myeloid leukemia. Blood 1999;94:3717–21.
185. Hussong JW, Rodgers GM, Shami PJ. Evidence of increased angiogenesis in patients with acute myeloid leukemia. Blood 2000;95:309–13.
186. Fong TA, Shawver LK, Sun L, et al. SU5416 is a potent and selective inhibitor of the vascular endothelial growth factor receptor (Flk-1/

KDR) that inhibits tyrosine kinase catalysis, tumor vascularization, and growth of multiple tumor types. Cancer Res 1999;59:99–106.
187. Bernatchez PN, Soker S, Sirois MG. Vascular endothelial growth factor effect on endothelial cell proliferation, migration, and platelet-activating factor synthesis is Flk-1-dependent. J Biol Chem 1999;274:31047–54.

# CHAPTER 85

# MYELOPROLIFERATIVE AND MYELODYSPLASTIC SYNDROMES

● ROBERT S. NEGRIN ● PETER L. GREENBERG

The myeloproliferative and myelodysplastic syndromes are characterized by abnormal growth and differentiation of one or more hematopoietic cell lineages. All of these diseases have the capacity to undergo transformation to overt leukemia. Among the myeloproliferative disorders (MPDs), four patterns of excessive cellular growth have been described: (1) chronic myelogenous leukemia (CML), (2) polycythemia vera (PV), (3) essential thrombocythemia (ET), and (4) agnogenic myeloid metaplasia (AMM). In 1951, Dameschek[1] proposed that these entities were related and that they be considered MPDs. CML is discussed separately in Chapter 86. Although this framework is useful, there are patients who present with features of MPD but remain unclassifiable. The cause of the MPDs remains unknown. In some instances, a history of exposure to ionizing radiation or carcinogenic chemicals can be elicited. A central feature in these disorders is that they are clonally derived.

## Myeloproliferative Disorders

### POLYCYTHEMIA VERA

PV is a rare disorder with an incidence of approximately 5 to 15 cases per 1 million population per year.[2, 3] PV is characterized by an expansion of the red blood cell (RBC) mass. Most patients with PV also have evidence of myeloproliferation of other cell lines, such as an elevated white blood cell count or platelet count or splenomegaly.[4] The clinical syndrome of PV is related to the increase in RBC mass and resultant hyperviscosity. Complications of this disorder include bleeding or thrombosis, particularly in elderly patients and those with thrombocytosis, as well as the potential for conversion to acute leukemia.[5–7] PV is a chronic condition, with most patients having a protracted clinical course that lasts 10 to 15 years or more. A bone marrow examination typically shows erythroid hyperplasia with normal cytogenetics and enhanced growth of erythroid colonies in vitro without added erythropoietin (EPO).[8–10] After a certain period, patients may enter a spent or myelofibrotic phase of the disease or progress to acute leukemia.[11] Disease appearance is generally sporadic, although familial predisposition has rarely been observed.[12]

**Clinical Features.** Patients with PV may present with a wide range of clinical complaints, including headache, weakness, dizziness, visual disturbances, joint symptoms, and weight loss. Pruritus is often experienced after a warm bath. Patients may present with venous or arterial thromboses.[6, 13] Unusual locations for thrombotic events occur relatively frequently in patients with PV, such as Budd-Chiari syndrome.[14] On physical examination, cyanosis, hepatomegaly, and diastolic hypertension are frequent findings.[7] Approximately 75% of patients also have splenomegaly.

Laboratory evaluation typically reveals an elevated hematocrit and an increased RBC mass. The plasma volume is usually normal or slightly increased. RBC morphology is typically normal except for microcytosis associated with coexisting iron deficiency. Of patients, 60% have a leukocytosis with neutrophilia and basophilia. Most patients have a mild to moderate thrombocytosis with platelet counts typically in the range of 400,000 to 800,000/mm$^3$. In contrast to CML, the leukocyte alkaline phosphatase (LAP) score is elevated in approximately 70% of patients. Hyperuricemia is common and may be complicated by gout.

**Differential Diagnosis.** PV is characterized by an increase in RBC mass. This increase requires documentation with a blood volume study with direct measurement of the RBC mass and the plasma volume.[15] Diagnostic criteria have been established by the Polycythemia Vera Study Group (PVSG) (Table 85–1). In addition to an elevated RBC mass, the presence of splenomegaly is an important finding on physical examination. As discussed previously, PV patients typically have a leukocytosis and thrombocytosis. A bone marrow biopsy usually shows erythroid hyperplasia with low or absent iron stores. Additional laboratory tests include a normal arterial oxygen saturation and elevated serum vitamin B$_{12}$, vitamin B$_{12}$–binding proteins, and LAP score.

The major differential diagnosis of PV includes secondary erythrocytosis or decreased plasma volume. Occasionally, additional tests are required to evaluate patients with PV further. These tests may include in vitro marrow culture to show erythroid colony formation in the absence of exogenous EPO, quantitation of serum EPO levels (low in PV), and analysis of clonality by restriction fragment-length polymorphism.[16]

Patients may be encountered with MPDs who have ele-

**Table 85–1.** Polycythemia Vera Diagnostic Criteria*

*Category A*

1. Total red cell mass
   Male ≥36 ml/kg body weight
   Female ≥32 ml/kg body weight
2. Arterial oxygen saturation >92%
3. Splenomegaly

*Category B*

1. Thrombocytosis (platelets >400,000/mm³)
2. Leukocytosis (white blood cells >12,000/mm³)
3. Increased leukocyte alkaline phosphatase score
4. Serum vitamin $B_{12}$ >900 pg/mL or vitamin $B_{12}$ binding capacity >2200 pg/ml

*Diagnosis of polycythemia vera requires A1 + A2 + A3 or A1 + A2 and any two features from category B.[7]

vated RBC mass yet do not fit the criteria established by the PVSG. This situation occurs particularly when evaluating patients with an isolated pure erythrocytosis who do not have splenomegaly, leukocytosis, or thrombocytosis.[17] Occasionally, patients require careful follow-up with repeated examination until a definitive diagnosis can be made. An alternative schema for the diagnosis of PV has included the measurement of the serum EPO level, which if low in the presence of an elevated hemoglobin level, establishes the diagnosis of PV.[18] For patients with an elevated hemoglobin level, a bone marrow examination and evaluation of erythroid colony growth is then indicated.

PV must also be distinguished from other MPDs, which can have important implications for therapeutic decisions. CML can be distinguished by myeloid abnormalities of blood and marrow and by cytogenetic analysis of the bone marrow in which the characteristic Philadelphia chromosome (9;22 translocation) is observed in approximately 90% of patients or by amplification of chimeric bcr/abl transcripts assayed using the polymerase chain reaction. Measurement of the LAP score may also be useful because it is characteristically low in patients with CML. AMM can occasionally be difficult to distinguish from postpolycythemic myeloid metaplasia. Evaluation of prior blood counts can help distinguish these two entities. PV with marked thrombocytosis can easily be confused with ET, especially in patients with PV who are iron deficient.

**Treatment.** The median survival of patients with untreated PV is approximately 18 months.[5, 19] Dramatic improvement in overall survival has been achieved through a series of therapeutic interventions; however, optimal therapy remains an area of ongoing debate. A series of randomized clinical trials has been conducted by the PVSG that has been instrumental in understanding the treatment of PV. The PVSG closed in 1997.[20]

The mainstay of therapy has been therapeutic phlebotomy, generally to maintain the hematocrit less than 45%. In the first randomized trial of the PVSG, patients received phlebotomy alone or phlebotomy with phosphorus 32 (³²P) or chlorambucil. Although survival was similar in the three groups, patients in the chlorambucil treatment arm had an excess rate of leukemic transformation, greater than 10% at 5 years.[19] There was an early increase in thrombosis in the patients treated with phlebotomy alone. Longer-term follow-

up has revealed an increased proportion of patients who developed myelofibrosis and splenomegaly who were treated with phlebotomy alone.[21] Subsequently the ³²P-treated patients were shown to have increased leukemic transformation after 10 years from the start of treatment, which was dependent on the dose of ³²P received. The median survival of patients treated with ³²P alone was found to be 13.5 years versus 15.2 years, representing a difference of only 10%.[21] The increase in thrombosis was largely in older patients who likely had atherosclerotic disease. The addition of aspirin and dipyridamole to phlebotomy was not beneficial in reducing the risk of thrombosis in the entire cohort of patients.[22] Aspirin has been useful, however, in preventing further thrombotic events in patients with a prior history of thromboses. The addition of hydroxyurea to patients treated with ³²P was evaluated in a randomized study of 461 patients older than age 65 years. In this study, patients were randomized to receive low-dose hydroxyurea (5 to 10 mg/kg/day) after the first ³²P-induced remission or not. This strategy did not control the disease, with 25% of patients having excessive platelet counts and no reduction in the rate of serious vascular events. The treatment was associated with a significantly increased rate of leukemic transformation beyond 8 years.[23] In the entire group, life expectancy was shorter for patients who received ³²P and hydroxyurea (9.3 years) as compared with ³²P alone (10.9 years). The one group that appeared to benefit were patients who had a short remission (<2 years) following ³²P treatment alone.

As a result of the failure of phlebotomy alone and the increased leukemogenic risk of ³²P and chlorambucil, other agents have been explored in the treatment of PV. Hydroxyurea and pipobroman have been studied. Hydroxyurea was used in nonrandomized trials by the PVSG.[24, 25] A randomized study comparing hydroxyurea with pipobroman in 292 PV patients younger than age 65 was reported by the French Polycythemia Study Group. In this study, hydroxyurea was initiated at a dose of 25 mg/kg/day and pipobroman at a dose of 1.2 mg/kg/day with both drugs followed by low-dose maintenance therapy. Drug tolerance was often poor, and hematologic stability, especially with respect to platelet count, was often inadequate. The risk of thromboembolic events was similar in both groups. Survival was no different and was less than in normal age-matched controls. The risk of leukemic progression was also no different between the two groups and was approximately 10% by 13 years.[26] These results suggested that the potential benefits of hydroxyurea and pipobroman were not as great as initially thought, with significant toxicity and less hematologic control. The actuarial risk of leukemic transformation was not different from that of ³²P, and the rate of progression to myelofibrosis was higher with hydroxyurea than with pipobroman. A slightly lower risk of leukemic transformation (5.5%) was reported in a nonrandomized evaluation of pipobroman.[27]

Other approaches have been attempted with promising results in small numbers of patients. The quinazolin derivative anagrelide has been used to treat the thrombocytosis of MPDs.[28] In one study of 577 patients with MPDs, of whom 68 had PV, 93% of patients had a reduction in platelet count of at least 50% at doses of of 0.5 to 1 mg four times daily.[29] Although most patients with PV had no change in their hematocrit while being treated with this drug, some decrease in hematocrit was noted in approximately one third of patients. Adverse reactions are rare but include cardiac toxicities. Longer-term follow-up is required to determine the efficacy of this treatment in reducing thrombotic events.

Interferon alfa has been used to control the erythrocytosis of PV. In several small trials, reductions in hematocrit and platelet counts have been observed.[30, 31] In longer-term treatment of 11 patients, interferon alfa controlled the erythrocytosis without phlebotomy for 12 to 72 months. None of the patients had thrombotic events.[32] These data were updated with continued encouraging results, although the number of patients treated remains relatively small.[33] In a larger study, 36 patients previously treated with phlebotomy or conventional cytostatic agents (or both) were treated with interferon alfa-2a at a dose of $3 \times 10^6$ U subcutaneously three times weekly. Responses were noted in 20 patients with relatively short follow-up. Further evaluation of this agent in randomized trials is warranted.

Patients with pruritus can be a challenging clinical problem. $H_1$ or $H_2$ histamine antagonists may be beneficial alone or in combination. Cholestyramine has also been used in some patients.[34]

Based on these studies, treatment recommendations are presented in Table 85–2. No therapeutic modality has emerged that is optimal, and modifications are required based on the clinical situation.

**Prognosis.** The clinical course of patients with PV is generally indolent and controllable with the measures outlined previously. Leukemic transformation is an ominous event and occurs in a small proportion of patients, particularly those previously treated with high doses of alkylator chemotherapy. Approximately 5 to 15% of patients develop postpolycythemic myeloid metaplasia.[35]

## ESSENTIAL THROMBOCYTHEMIA

ET is characterized by an increase in the number of platelets with a corresponding expansion in the number and size of megakaryocytes in the bone marrow.[36] Patients often have splenomegaly and are prone to bleeding and thrombosis. Similar to the other MPDs, this disorder has been found to be clonal in origin.[37, 38] The incidence of this disorder is unknown; however, estimates of approximately 10 cases per 1 million population have been made. In one population-based study in North America, a sex-adjusted incidence rate of 2.53 cases per 100,000 population annually was observed.[39] The average age at diagnosis is 50 to 60 years in most series, and the disorder occurs with equal frequency in

*Table 85–2.* **Treatment Recommendations for Patients with Polycythemia Vera**

| Patients | Treatment |
|---|---|
| Patients without thrombosis | Phlebotomy to maintain hematocrit <45% |
| Patients with thrombocytosis and previous thrombosis | Phlebotomy plus hematologic suppression with hydroxyurea |
| Persistent thrombocytosis | Antiplatelet agents should be considered: Anagrelide or interferon alfa |
| Elderly patients (>65 yr) and nonresponsive to the above | $^{32}$P 2.3 mCi/m$^2$ IV every 12 wk as needed to suppress thrombocytosis |

IV, intravenously.

men and women. Thrombopoietic levels in the peripheral blood as well as mRNA production in bone marrow stromal cells from patients with ET have been reported to be similar to normal individuals.[40] Most cases are sporadic; however, multiple cases within a family have been reported.[41] In one instance of familial ET, serum thrombopoietin (TPO) levels were significantly elevated in affected family members, which was associated with a one-base deletion in the 5′-untranslated region of the TPO gene.[41a]

**Clinical Features.** Patients with ET may present with a myriad of clinical complaints, or the disorder may be detected by routine blood studies. The major clinical problem associated with this entity is bleeding and thrombosis.[42–44] In one study, the risk of hemorrhage was estimated to be 0.33% per patient at risk per year as compared with the risk of thrombosis of 6.6% per patient at risk per year. Age, a previous thrombotic event, and a long duration of thrombocytosis were all risk factors for thrombosis.[44] Arterial thrombosis was more common than venous thrombosis. The risk of thrombosis does not appear to correlate with the platelet count.[42, 45] In one study, severe clinical complications occurred in 22% of patients with ET who had platelet counts less than 600,000/mm$^3$.[46] Platelets are frequently found to be qualitatively abnormal by standard morphology and by ultrastructural analysis.

In most patients, the physical examination is generally unremarkable except for splenomegaly in approximately 50% and hepatomegaly in 20% of patients.[47] Most patients are otherwise generally asymptomatic.

The hallmark of ET is the elevation in platelet number. To make the diagnosis of ET, a sustained platelet count of greater than 450,000 to 600,000/mm$^3$ is required. Immature myeloid cells and nucleated red blood cells are observed in approximately 25% of patients. Most patients have abnormalities in platelet size with megathrombocytes. Bone marrow examination generally reveals a hypercellular marrow with an excess of megakaryocytes, many of which are large and have abnormal morphology and are found in clusters. Bleeding times are frequently abnormally prolonged.[48] Cytogenetic studies on the bone marrow cells are generally normal. The diagnostic criteria for the diagnosis of ET have been updated.[49]

**Differential Diagnosis.** Primary ET must be distinguished from other secondary causes of thrombocytosis as well as other MPDs. Patients with myelodysplastic syndromes occasionally present with elevated platelet counts, especially those with the 5q– chromosomal abnormality.[50] There are many reasons for secondary thrombocytosis, including chronic inflammation, occult cancer, gastrointestinal bleeding, autoimmune disorders such as rheumatoid arthritis, ankylosing spondylitis, inflammatory bowel disease, and iron deficiency anemia. It is necessary to attempt to exclude secondary causes of thrombocytosis when considering this diagnosis. Platelet counts greater than $1 \times 10^6$/mm$^3$ are rarely due to secondary causes. RBC mass and volume studies are occasionally necessary to rule out PV. Bone marrow cytogenetics are useful to detect the Philadelphia chromosome characteristic of CML. Most patients with ET show spontaneous megakaryocyte or erythroid growth, or both, in vitro, which may be useful in distinguishing this entity from reactive thrombocytosis.[51] This autonomous megakaryocytic growth is not related to a c-mp1 mutation or autocrine stimulation by Mp1.[52]

Occasionally, it is necessary to determine whether clonal hematopoiesis is present to evaluate patients with ET. The finding of clonal hematopoiesis effectively rules out a secondary cause for the thrombocytosis. A significant proportion (50% in one study) of patients with diagnostic criteria of ET may not have clonal hematopoiesis, however. Patients without clonal hematopoiesis had a significantly lower risk of thrombotic complications.[53] This finding could be useful for determining when to initiate treatment.[54] In other cases, careful follow-up is required until the diagnosis is established, or the thrombocytosis resolves.

**Treatment.** The treatment of patients with ET is controversial. Traditionally, treatment has been initiated when platelet counts exceeded $10^6$/mm³. The thrombotic risk of young patients who are asymptomatic may be no different from the general population, and treatment may not be warranted.[44] However, because of the poor correlation between platelet count and thrombosis,[46] relatively benign course of most patients with ET, and leukemogenic potential of myelosuppressive therapy, this recommendation has been reconsidered. The predictive features of major vascular complications were evaluated in one study of 148 patients with ET. Of these patients, 37 had a history of a vascular complication at the time of diagnosis of ET. Patients older than age 60 years, patients with a history of major ischemia, and patients with hypercholesterolemia were at high risk of a major vascular complication.[55]

Patients who develop complications of ET, such as hemorrhage, thrombosis, or neurologic symptoms, warrant treatment. If immediate control of the platelet count is required, platelet pheresis should be instituted. The benefits of this therapy are relatively short-lived, and myelosuppressive therapy is also required. In the initial studies of the PVSG, melphalan was found to be superior to $^{32}$P. Because of the concern of leukemogeneity with alkylating agents, however, other approaches have been investigated.

Hydroxyurea has been widely studied with demonstrated efficacy in reducing the platelet count. An initial dose of 30 mg/kg has been used, with reduction to 15 mg/kg after the first week. The dose is then adjusted to reduce the platelet count while avoiding leukopenia. A randomized trial comparing hydroxyurea with no myelosuppressive therapy was performed in 114 patients with ET. Of these patients, 46% had a history of prior thrombosis. After a median follow-up of 27 months, 2 patients (3.6%) treated with hydroxyurea had a thrombotic episode compared with 14 patients (24%) in the control group ($p = 0.003$).[56] The risk of leukemia with hydroxyurea appears to be less than with alkylating agents; however, concern is still warranted. In one study, 357 patients with ET followed over a 20-year period were evaluated for leukemic risk associated with hydroxyurea therapy. With a median follow-up of 98 months, 17 patients (4.5%) had progressed to acute myelogenous leukemia or myelodysplastic syndromes. Fourteen of those patients had received hydroxyurea at some point in their treatment course.[57]

Encouraging results have been obtained with anagrelide in the treatment of patients with ET. In one study of 335 patients, 94% responded with a reduction of platelets by at least 50% or to an absolute number of less than 600,000/mm³. This reduction has been accomplished with an oral daily dose of 0.5 to 1.0 mg four times daily. Side effects have been limiting in 16% of patients and include nausea, headache, diarrhea, and congestive heart failure.[29] Some patients have been treated for more than 5 years without the need for dosage adjustment. The mechanism of action of anagrelide is not known definitively. The drug is believed to inhibit the maturation of megakaryocytes.[28] Anagrelide was effective in preventing complications in patients with ET. Anagrelide was approved by the U.S. Food and Drug Administration for the treatment of ET in 1997. It should not be used during pregnancy, and caution is advised in patients with heart disease.[58]

Other treatment approaches have been investigated. Interferon alfa has been used to treat small numbers of patients with a response rate of approximately 60%.[59] The role of this agent in the management of patients with ET is not defined. Interferon has been used to treat ET during pregnancy.[60]

The use of platelet antiaggregating drugs is controversial because of the known risk of bleeding in patients with ET. Transient ischemic attacks and erythromelalgia in these patients have been reported to respond to treatment with aspirin with or without dipyridamole.[61, 62] Patients with prior symptomatic events should be treated with antiplatelet agents (e.g., aspirin, ticlopidine) with or without chemotherapy to reduce platelet counts.

**Prognosis.** The clinical course of patients with ET is generally indolent. Ten-year survival is 60 to 80%. The decision to initiate treatment must be made on the basis of the clinical characteristics of the individual patient.[63]

## AGNOGENIC MYELOID METAPLASIA

AMM is characterized by a leukoerythroblastic reaction in the blood, some degree of marrow fibrosis, and hepatic and splenic enlargement. Other names for this disorder include *myelosclerosis* and *idiopathic myelofibrosis*. Similar to the other MPDs, the cause of this disorder is unknown. The hematopoietic cells are clonal in origin, whereas the resultant fibrosis derives from other tissue. AMM may present as the initial disorder, or the other MPDs may evolve into an entity morphologically resembling this disorder. The incidence of this disorder has been estimated to be 1.46 cases per 100,000 population annually with a female/male ratio of 1:6.[64]

**Clinical Features.** Patients with AMM generally present with fatigue associated with anemia. Approximately 20% of patients are asymptomatic at presentation. The most common complaints include fatigue, symptoms related to splenic enlargement, and weight loss.[65] Most patients with AMM are middle-aged to elderly.

On physical examination, splenomegaly is almost always present and may be profound. Hepatomegaly is also a frequent finding. Most patients are anemic with normal RBC indices. Platelet counts may be elevated or suppressed. Most patients have a leukocytosis. The peripheral blood smear is a useful tool in making this diagnosis because of the leukoerythroblastic abnormalities that are frequently present, including myeloid immaturity, nucleated RBCs, poikilocytes, and teardrop RBCs. Myeloblasts are occasionally observed.

Some patients have prolonged prothrombin and activated partial thromboplastin times because of a deficiency of factor

V.[66] Prolonged bleeding times are found in 10 to 20% of patients as a result of the qualitatively abnormal platelets. Bone marrow aspiration is typically difficult because of the presence of fibrosis. Bone marrow biopsy specimens show this fibrosis as well as hypercellularity. Osteosclerosis is also typically present.

A variety of immunologic abnormalities have been reported in patients with AMM, including the presence of antinuclear antibodies, elevated rheumatoid factor titer, positive Coombs' test, and circulating immune complexes.[67, 68] Cytokines have been measured in the serum of AMM patients. TPO levels were found to be elevated as compared with normal controls, and the serum TPO level correlated with the degree of bone marrow fibrosis. Interleukin (IL)-6 levels were also elevated in patients with AMM.[69]

**Differential Diagnosis.** AMM must be differentiated from other causes of marrow fibrosis. Secondary myelofibrosis may result from a variety of causes, including metastatic cancer, especially owing to lymphoma or carcinoma of the stomach, breast, lung, or prostate. Hodgkin's disease can result in marrow fibrosis. Disseminated tuberculosis and histoplasmosis have also been associated with secondary myelofibrosis.[70] Approximately 10% of patients with myelodysplastic syndrome may have marrow fibrosis and be difficult to distinguish from AMM.[71] Hairy cell leukemia can be confused with AMM because of the presence of splenomegaly and marrow fibrosis in this disorder.[72] AMM must also be distinguished from other MPDs, especially PV and CML. Bone marrow cytogenetics and molecular analysis of bcr/abl fusion transcripts are extremely useful in ruling out CML.

Acute myelofibrosis is a distinct entity from AMM. In this disorder, patients generally present acutely with fever and pancytopenia. Splenomegaly is typically not found. Bone marrow biopsy specimens reveal an increase in myeloblasts that often express megakaryocytic markers.[73, 74] This disorder generally runs an aggressive course.

**Treatment.** Patients with AMM generally have a chronic course, and many do not require therapy. Patients who develop constitutional symptoms, such as fever, night sweats, weight loss, progressive splenomegaly, and anemia, often have a more progressive course and require therapy.

The mainstay of treatment in this disorder is supportive care generally with transfusional support. Corticosteroids may be useful for patients with immunologic abnormalities, and folic acid may be needed because of the rapid turnover of hematopoietic cells. Androgenic steroids have been used in anemic patients with responses in approximately 20 to 30%.[75, 76] Because most of these patients have ineffective hematopoiesis, this latter approach is generally not useful.

The splenomegaly that develops in some patients can be a challenging clinical problem. Myelosuppression with busulfan or hydroxyurea may be useful if the suppression in blood counts is tolerated. Splenic irradiation has been used in some patients with occasional benefit but is often complicated by hematologic toxicity. Interferon alfa has been used in small numbers of patients with AMM and has been effective in lowering platelet and white blood cell counts as well as reducing splenomegaly.[77, 78] The role of interferon alfa in treating this disorder remains relatively undefined.

The role of splenectomy in the treatment of patients with AMM has been controversial. Because extramedullary hematopoiesis is common in this disorder, concern has centered on the removal of significant hematopoietic tissue. Because the hematopoietic production is generally ineffective, removal of the spleen has not caused decreased blood counts. In addition, patients with AMM are generally elderly and debilitated, making splenectomy a difficult surgical procedure. Nevertheless, splenectomy may improve the anemia and thrombocytopenia in a significant percentage of patients with AMM.[79] A report suggested that splenectomy may increase the risk of blastic transformation into acute myeloid leukemia in patients with AMM.[80] This concept was challenged[81]; however, additional information on this point is needed, which may provide interesting insights into the mechanism of disease progression. The indications for splenectomy include painful splenomegaly, refractory thrombocytopenia with persisting marrow megakaryocytes, and refractory hemolytic anemia.

Bone marrow transplantation has been performed in selected patients with AMM. Because most patients are elderly, this procedure is not appropriate for most patients with this disorder. Cure of this disease is possible, however, with allogeneic bone marrow transplantation. Following transplantation, the fibrosis in the bone marrow has been reported to reverse.[82, 83] As a result of improved techniques, the upper age limit for transplantation has been extended to 60 years in many centers. Bone marrow transplantation should be considered for selected patients with AMM younger than age 60 who have histocompatible sibling donors. In one study of 12 patients with extensive fibrosis who underwent allogeneic transplantation for AMM with human leukocyte antigen (HLA)–matched sibling donors, the 4-year overall survival and event-free survival were 71% and 59%. In a larger study of 55 AMM patients with a median age of 42 years, the 5-year probability of survival was 47% for the overall group and 54% for patients who received an unmanipulated HLA-matched related transplant. Age and karyotype were important prognostic indicators.[84, 84a]

**Prognosis.** The course of most patients with AMM is generally indolent. Progressive anemia, thrombocytopenia, and splenomegaly generally herald progression of disease, which is often difficult to treat effectively. Because most patients with AMM are elderly, effective supportive care is the mainstay of treatment and can be a challenging clinical task.

# Myelodysplastic Syndromes

## CLINICAL FEATURES

The myelodysplastic syndromes (MDS) describe patients with clonal refractory cytopenias whose marrows show characteristic dysplastic changes in at least two of the three hematopoietic cell lines and have a propensity to undergo transformation into acute myeloid leukemia. The French American and British (FAB) morphologic classification[85] has been relatively useful for determining prognosis in MDS (Table 85–3). MDS patients having refractory anemia with excess of blasts (RAEB, 5 to 20% marrow blasts) and those with RAEB in transformation (RAEB-T, 21 to 30% marrow blasts) have relatively poor prognoses, with median survivals generally 5 to 12 months. In contrast, refractory anemia

*Table 85–3.* Myelodysplastic Syndrome Subtypes FAB Cooperative Group Criteria

| | Bone Marrow Blasts (%) | | Peripheral Blood Blasts (%) | | Auer Rods | Monocytes >1 × 10⁹/L | Ring Sideroblasts >15% of Nucleated Marrow Cells |
|---|---|---|---|---|---|---|---|
| RA | <5 | | ≤1 | | − | − | − |
| RARS | <5 | | ≤1 | | − | − | + |
| RAEB | 5–20 | | <5 | | − | − | ± |
| CMML | ≤20 | | <5 | | − | + | ± |
| RAEB-T | 21–30 | or | ≥5 | or | + | ± | ± |

(RA, <5% blasts) or RA with ringed sideroblasts (RARS, <5% blasts and >15% ringed sideroblasts of the erythroid marrow cells) MDS subtypes have median survivals of approximately 3 to 6 years. The proportion of these individuals who transformed to acute myeloid leukemia varied similarly; in the high-risk RAEB/RAEB-T patients, this incidence was 40 to 50% compared with 5 to 15% in the low-risk RA/RARS group. In a study evaluating time to disease evolution, 25% of patients with RAEB and 55% of patients with RAEB-T underwent transformation to acute myeloid leukemia at 1 year, and 35% and 65% at 2 years.[86] In contrast, for patients with RA, the incidence was 5% and 10% at 1 and 2 years, whereas none of the RARS patients underwent leukemic transformation within 2 years. Chronic myelomonocytic leukemia (CMML) has been categorized as MDS, although it often has characteristics of an MPD. The criteria for CMML include a peripheral monocytosis exceeding 1 × 10³/mm³; increased numbers of monocytic cells in the bone marrow; dysplasia in the erythroid, megakaryocytic, or granulocytic series; fewer than 5% circulating blasts; and fewer than 30% marrow blasts.[87] Within the RAEB and CMML subgroups, an increased proportion of marrow blasts indicates a poorer prognosis.

Primary MDS is predominantly a disease in the elderly, with greater than 80% of the patients being older than 60 years of age.[88, 89] Beyond 70 years of age, the incidence of MDS is approximately 22 to 45 per 10⁵ population, indicating that MDS is as prevalent as the other most common hematologic malignancies of the aged (i.e., chronic lymphocytic leukemia and multiple myeloma).

Secondary MDS (i.e., resulting from prior toxic chemical exposure or chemoradiotherapy) may occur at all ages. This secondary form of MDS is emerging as a significant clinical problem and may cause substantial morbidity and mortality with or without progression to acute myeloid leukemia.[90, 91] The increasing incidence of secondary MDS and acute myeloid leukemia reflects a number of factors, including a longer period of risk resulting from successful treatment of solid tumors, more intensive treatment regimens combining high-dose chemotherapy and irradiation, broader use of adjuvant chemoirradiation in solid tumor therapy, and environmental pollution and exposure to chemicals and carcinogens (particularly organic solvents) in industrialized nations. Generally, these patients have poorer prognoses than those with primary MDS.[90] In secondary MDS, abnormal karyotypes are evident in virtually all patients, the presence of multiple chromosome aberrations is the rule, and chromosomes 5 and 7 are most frequently (85%) involved. Accumulating experience in therapy-related leukemia suggests that chemo-

therapeutic agents may have different leukemogenic potentials that are associated with differing pathophysiologic processes. The classic therapy-related leukemia, involving chromosome 5 and 7 abnormalities and implicating alkylating agents and irradiation, remains the most common form. Two additional forms of therapy-related leukemia have been described: one attributed to exposure to topoisomerase II–active chemotherapeutic agents and involving the chromosome 11q23 locus and the other involving the chromosome 21q22 locus.[91]

## PROGNOSTIC CATEGORIZATION

To determine better the relative efficacy of different treatment approaches, the untreated natural history of these patients has needed improved definition. Although the FAB classification has been relatively effective for categorizing MDS patients since its development in 1982,[85] its prognostic limitations have become apparent, and numerous classification systems have been proposed. To attempt to improve on these disparate systems, a collaborative International MDS Risk Analysis Workshop combined cytogenetic, morphologic, and clinical data from a large group of untreated primary MDS patients. Critical prognostic variables were determined and refined, were weighted according to their prognostic statistical power, and led to the development of the International Prognostic Scoring System (IPSS) for MDS (Table 85–4).[92] In this system, percent marrow blasts (four categories—0 to 5%, 6 to 10%, 11 to 20%, 21 to 30%), specified cytogenetic abnormalities, and number of cytopenias were evaluated in combination, and four risk groups for survival and acute myeloid leukemia evolution were defined: low, intermediate-1, intermediate-2, and high. Cytogenetic risk groups were good (normal, 5q− alone, 20q− alone, −Y alone) and poor risk (chromosome 7 or complex [≥3] abnormalities). Median survivals for these untreated risk groups were 5.7, 3.5, 1.2, and 0.4 years; median times to 25% evolution to acute myeloid leukemia for patients in these groups were 9.4, 3.3, 1.1, and 0.2 years. Age stratification was also an important variable required for evaluation of survival (shortened survival with increased age, partly dependent on comorbid conditions of the elderly). Using these parameters, this system for assessing prognosis in MDS was improved compared with a number of prior methods, including FAB. The various MDS scoring systems and relevant prognostic clinical parameters have been reviewed.[93]

**Table 85–4.** International Prognostic Scoring System for Myelodysplastic Syndromes: Survival and AML Evolution

| Prognostic Variable | Score Value | | | | |
|---|---|---|---|---|---|
| | 0 | 0.5 | 1.0 | 1.5 | 2.0 |
| Marrow blasts (%) | <5 | 5–10 | — | 11–20 | 21–30 |
| Karyotype* | Good | Intermediate | Poor | | |
| Cytopenias | 0/1 | 2/3 | | | |

| Risk Group | Score |
|---|---|
| Low | 0 |
| INT-1 | 0.5–1.0 |
| INT-2 | 1.5–2.0 |
| High | ≥2.5 |

*Good = normal, − Y, del(5q), del(20q); Poor = complex (≥3 abnormalities) or chromosome 7 anomalies; Intermediate = other abnormalities.

Modified from Greenberg P, Cox C, Le Beau MM, et al. International scoring system for evaluating prognosis in myelodysplastic syndromes. Blood 1997; 89:2079–88.

## RISK-BASED TREATMENT

Mortality and morbidity in MDS are related to the morphologic subtype and are due to a variety of causes, including evolution to acute myeloid leukemia, infection, and bleeding complications related to the patients' dominant cytopenias. Because most of these patients are elderly, concomitant nonhematologic diseases associated with an elderly patient population also substantially contribute to their demises.

A variety of treatment approaches have been used in MDS, with supportive care generally being the mainstay of therapy in the community. Patients should be treated as needed with antibiotics for infection and with RBC and platelet transfusions for symptomatic anemia and thrombocytopenic bleeding. Long-term RBC transfusion support may lead to iron overload and hemochromatosis. When it is anticipated that patients will have prolonged transfusion requirements, regular desferrioxamine chelation treatment should be considered.[93a] Because these diseases are characterized by macrocytic anemias, vitamin $B_{12}$ and folate deficiencies need to be excluded. MDS is relatively indolent and predominates in the elderly. A therapeutic challenge has been to provide treatment modalities having adequate support for the patients' dominant cytopenias without causing excessive toxicity. These elderly patients frequently have concomitant medical illnesses that limit therapeutic options markedly. As indicated earlier, patients with abnormal cytogenetics, in vitro marrow myeloid clonal growth patterns, and more deranged clinical and marrow morphologic features have poorer prognoses. These abnormalities generally correlate with the more advanced FAB and IPSS classifications. Because of this variability of prognoses in subgroups of patients with MDS, to analyze the therapeutic efficacy of different treatments, stratification according to these risk categories is necessary.

Categorization of MDS patients into prognostic subgroups appears valuable for appropriately designing and analyzing therapeutic trials—and for selecting therapeutic options. A group of clinicians composing the MDS Panel for Practice Guidelines of the National Comprehensive Cancer Network (NCCN) suggested that therapeutic approaches be based on

three clinical features: (1) the patient's age, (2) performance status, and (3) IPSS-defined risk category.[94] *High-intensity* (defined as requiring hospitalization, e.g., intensive chemotherapy, bone marrow transplantation) as well as *low-intensity* (generally outpatient-type treatments, such as hematopoietic growth factors [HGFs], differentiation-inducing agents, biologic response modifiers, low-intensity chemotherapy) therapies are available to treat MDS patients. Using the NCCN MDS Guidelines approach in the treatment plan for patients 60 years old or younger, with good or excellent performance status in the IPSS intermediate-2 or high risk categories, high-intensity therapies would predominantly be considered. These relatively younger patients in the low or intermediate-1 category would generally be considered for low-intensity therapy. For patients older than age 60 with good performance status, low-intensity therapy would be of prime interest, although selected patients could be candidates for high-intensity therapies. For patients older than age 60 with poor performance status, proposed treatment would predominantly be supportive care or low-intensity therapies.

The results of studies evaluating specific therapeutic approaches are discussed subsequently. Virtually all of these treatments are still experimental; comparative clinical trials using these study designs and stratifications are needed to determine the relative value of each therapeutic modality. Because the relative toxicities and efficacy of many of these treatments are not yet well known, involvement of MDS patients in clinical trials is suggested.

## HIGH-INTENSITY THERAPY

### Induction Chemotherapy

Regarding the use of high-intensity treatment modalities, because a substantial proportion of hematopoietic precursors from patients with advanced MDS have demonstrable overexpression of the multidrug resistance gene *MDR1*,[95] agents that modulate this chemotherapy extrusion pump may prove useful as an adjunct to chemotherapy. Several trials using such multidrug resistance modulators plus standard acute myeloid leukemia–type induction chemotherapy have been performed in patients with high-risk MDS or acute myeloid leukemia post MDS, showing encouraging response rates.[96–98] Studies using these *resistant acute myeloid leukemia* treatment approaches are continuing. Standard chemotherapy in this group of patients has generally not been as effective as in de novo acute myeloid leukemia.[99] A trial using topotecan plus cytosine arabinoside in MDS has had encouraging results[100]; however, the durability of this response has not been established.

### Bone Marrow Transplantation

Although the elderly age of most MDS patients and donor availability issues limit the proportion of MDS patients eligible for bone marrow transplantation, studies using allogeneic marrow transplantation (HLA-matched sibling or unrelated donors) for MDS have been reported.[101–104] A portion (approximately 30 to 40%) of MDS patients have prolonged disease-free survival after bone marrow transplantation (generally younger patients with initially good performance status). Relapse and transplant-related mortality occur in a substantial portion (20 to 35% each) of patients. The relapse rate is higher in patients with advanced MDS and those with poor-risk cytogenetics; mortality and morbidity are higher in those who are more elderly and those receiving transplants from unrelated donors.[101–104] Methods are currently aimed at improving the conditioning and supportive regimens for MDS patients, including the experimental use of nonmyeloablative (*mini*) stem cell transplants.[105] The use of bone marrow transplantation (allogeneic or autologous) is being evaluated in high-risk MDS patients after chemotherapy-induced remission.[106]

## LOW-INTENSITY THERAPY

### Hematopoietic Growth Factors

Defective proliferation of hematopoietic precursors within MDS marrow is related to their decreased responsiveness to or decreased production of HGFs. Because some leukemic cells have enhanced proliferative responses to the colony-stimulating factors (CSFs) in vitro,[107] concern exists regarding the safety of using such agents in responsive neoplastic cells. To evaluate the proliferative versus differentiative responsiveness of hematopoietic precursors in MDS to HGFs and to determine the possible clinical utility of CSF treatment, several laboratories have assessed in vitro proliferative, differentiative, and regenerative responses of marrow cells from these patients to recombinant human granulocyte colony–stimulating factor (G-CSF) and granulocyte-macrophage colony-stimulating factor (GM-CSF).[107] These in vitro findings suggested the possible efficacy of these recombinant human CSFs in this clinical setting and led to therapeutic trials with these agents.[108]

**Granulocyte-Macrophage Colony-Stimulating Factor.** Following the initial phase I–II trials, which showed the efficacy of GM-CSF for short-term improvement of neutrophil counts in most MDS patients, a multicenter study[109] provided information regarding the use of GM-CSF in relatively low-risk MDS patients (i.e., RA patients, RAEB patients with <10% marrow blasts) for periods up to 2 months. Eighty-two patients (50 RA, 32 RAEB) received either of two different, fixed daily dose levels of GM-CSF. Nearly all of the MDS patients treated with GM-CSF responded with increased neutrophil counts. Only 35% of the patients completed 8 weeks of treatment, however, and the drug was discontinued in the others because of progression of disease, local infiltrates, flu-like syndromes, hyperleukocytosis, or bone pain. In 25% of the patients, platelet counts decreased during GM-CSF administration to less than 50% of baseline values, whereas two patients had increases in platelets. Six patients had progressive disease, two of whom with RAEB developed acute leukemia; erythroid responses did not occur. No differences in responses were shown between the two dose levels of GM-CSF used. The impact of GM-CSF on progression of disease could not be addressed because of the small number of patients and short duration of treatment. A preliminary report has indicated similar results of another multi-institutional randomized trial of GM-CSF treatment for periods generally up to 6 months versus observation in 21 patients with MDS, with crossover occurring in patients

with infections.[110] A decrease in infections in the GM-CSF group was reported. These studies showed some of the relative tradeoffs of potential difficulties and benefits of long-term administration of GM-CSF in patients with MDS.

In two studies, patients with low-risk and high-risk subtypes of MDS received GM-CSF plus low-dose cytarabine (Ara-C) for 2 weeks at different schedules for several months.[111, 112] Evaluation of responses indicated that approximately equal thirds of the patients showed clinical improvement, stable disease, or progressive disease or toxic deaths. Adverse events were noted in more than half of the patients, including major hemorrhage and infections, often leading to discontinuation of treatment, with most of the adverse events being due to the low-dose Ara C. The median survival of these patients was similar to that of prior controlled studies using low-dose Ara C alone.[113]

**Granulocyte Colony–Stimulating Factor.** Following initial phase I–II trials that showed a high degree of efficacy for improving neutrophil counts in most MDS patients with G-CSF therapy,[114, 115] a phase III international randomized trial of 102 patients with high-risk MDS (RAEB and RAEB-T), comparing long-term G-CSF administration with observation, was performed to attempt to determine the impact of G-CSF on the natural history of the disease.[116] The G-CSF treatment, which improved neutrophil counts in nearly all patients, was generally well tolerated, with few patients withdrawing from the study because of adverse events. No difference was noted in the incidence of or time to progression to acute myeloid leukemia for RAEB or RAEB-T patients who were in the G-CSF or observation arms of the study. Survival for RAEB-T patients was similar in both groups. For RAEB patients, however, the median survival was shorter in patients receiving G-CSF (10 months vs. 21 months), with an increase in disease-related nonleukemic deaths. The RAEB patients receiving G-CSF showed median survival time similar to previously reported RAEB survival data in the literature, whereas the RAEB patients in the observation group had prolonged survival. Although balanced for most clinical parameters, an increased proportion of RAEB patients receiving G-CSF (29% vs. 14%) were in the poor prognostic risk category, based on the scoring system, which used the proportion of marrow blasts, platelets, and age.[117] Decreased survival in RAEB patients receiving G-CSF was evident only in this high-risk group, compared with that for the high-risk RAEB patients in the observation group. The difference of survival in RAEB patients may be related to the increased number of high-risk patients included in the G-CSF group or the unusually long survival of high-risk patients in the observation group. These disparate therapeutic responses indicate that major biologic differences in MDS are defined by these clinical risk features, stressing the importance of enhancing the precision of these prognostic parameters for the design and analysis of clinical trials. The impact of G-CSF treatment on the incidence of infections is being evaluated in these patients.

**Interleukin-3.** Relatively short-term clinical trials have reported the effects of IL-3 therapy in low-risk MDS patients.[118–120] These studies indicated modest improvements in neutrophils, which, however, were not as prominent as those shown with G-CSF or GM-CSF. Only limited responses occurred in the other cell lines. These data indicate that IL-3 needs to be combined with other hematopoietic cytokines to achieve substantial improvement in the cytopenias in MDS.

**Interleukin-6.** To attempt to improve circulating platelet levels in low-risk MDS, 22 such patients were treated with IL-6.[121] Platelet count responses occurred in eight patients. These responses, however, were noted in only 3 of 11 patients (27%) with less than 20,000 platelets/mm³. Moderate to severe toxicity plus constitutional symptoms occurred without leukocyte improvement, and worsening anemia developed in a substantial portion of these patients. Because of the adverse events, few patients could continue this treatment for several months.

**Erythropoietin.** Serum EPO levels may be suboptimally elevated in MDS patients relative to their degree of anemia.[122] Recombinant human EPO therapy has been instituted to attempt to correct the hypoproductive anemias. Numerous reports have detailed the erythroid responses of MDS patients to this form of treatment.[108] The initial studies using EPO in MDS indicated that approximately 20% of patients responded to EPO. Generally the patients required relatively high doses of EPO ($\geq$150 U/kg/day) for their responses. This limited in vivo responsiveness of MDS marrow cells to EPO is not totally unexpected because the defective erythroid precursors in MDS have shown suboptimal in vitro responses to EPO alone, particularly for erythrocyte burst-forming units growth.[123, 124]

**Erythropoietin Plus Granulocyte Colony–Stimulating Factor.** Hematopoietic cytokines such as G-CSF are synergistic with EPO, enhancing marrow erythrocyte burst-forming units numbers or responsiveness to EPO in vitro in MDS,[124] suggesting their potential to provide more prominent in vivo erythroid responses in combination than with either agent alone. Several studies describing effects of such combination therapy with G-CSF and EPO to treat the anemia of MDS[125–128] have substantiated this thesis. Approximately 40 to 45% of patients receiving this combination treatment (G-CSF 1 μg/kg/day plus EPO 150 to 300 U/kg/day subcutaneously) had substantial erythroid responses (i.e., decreased transfusion requirements and increased hemoglobin levels), and nearly all patients had neutrophil responses. Extension of these trials indicated that erythroid responses persisted for many months in most patients receiving both factors.[127, 128] Erythroid responses were more frequent in patients with less advanced pancytopenia, lower endogenous EPO levels (<200 to 500 mU/mL), less prior RBC transfusion need, and marrow-ringed sideroblasts.[129] Patients with ringed sideroblasts, who respond poorly to EPO alone, showed a response rate of 60% to the combined therapy. On discontinuing G-CSF, approximately half maintained their responses, whereas the remainder required both factors, consistent with the synergistic effects of these two agents for a portion of MDS patients. Responses, if they were to occur, generally occurred within 6 to 8 weeks. If no response occurred within this time frame, the drugs should be discontinued. The relatively high expense of these doses of drugs needs to be compared with the risk of transfusion and the expenses attendant with transfusion therapy.

### Biologic Response Modifiers

Preliminary studies using the phosphothiol drug *amifostine (Ethyol)*, which has antioxidant properties, have shown the ability of this drug to cause trilineage hematopoietic responses in 30 to 40% of MDS patients (generally at doses of 200 to 300 mg/m² three times per week intravenously for 3 weeks each course; two to four courses were administered) in addition to its in vitro hematopoietic stimulatory activity.[130, 131] Clinically relevant responses are somewhat less common. Extended trials are ongoing to determine the relative efficacy of this agent in MDS.

Some MDS patients are believed to have immune-mediated hematopoietic suppression. These are predominantly patients with hypoplastic MDS. A portion of these patients (generally those who are younger with normal cytogenetics, marrow hypoplasia, evidence for a paroxysmal nocturnal hemoglobinuria (PNH) clonal process, and early-stage disease) have responded to anti-immune therapies such as *antithymocyte globulin* and *cyclosporine*.[132–134] The antithymocyte globulin was given at a dose of 40 mg/kg/day intravenously for four doses; serum sickness occurred in virtually all patients, generally controllable by concomitant use of steroids.

Enhanced intramedullary apoptosis of the hematopoietic cells occurs in MDS causing ineffective hematopoiesis and peripheral cytopenias.[135, 136] Some of this apoptosis has been attributed to increased intramedullary elaboration of inhibitory cytokines, such as tumor necrosis factor.[137] Clinical trials are ongoing in MDS using the *tumor necrosis factor receptor fusion protein (Enbrel)* to attempt to decrease such inhibitory effects and their attendant cytopenias.

### Low-Dose Chemotherapy

A phase III randomized clinical trial treating MDS with *5-AZA-2'-deoxycytidine (5-aza)* has been performed by the Cancer and Leukemia Group B (CALGB).[138] These data suggest the potential of 5-aza to decrease the evolution of MDS to acute myeloid leukemia, albeit without differences in survival. The drug can be administered in the outpatient setting (75 mg/m²/day subcutaneously for 5 days monthly for several months) and is considered to be a low-intensity form of therapy. Although cytogenetic data are not available, not permitting strict comparability of risk groups in the two arms of the study, and a crossover design limited outcome analysis, the study results indicate that 5-aza could be considered for selected high-risk and low-risk patients.

New agents attempting to alter the pathophysiologic mechanisms underlying these disorders are being studied. For patients with this chronic, generally indolent disease with substantial comorbidities, methods to evaluate and to improve quality of life as well as objective hematologic parameters are important. Clinical trials in MDS evaluating risk-based therapies should provide results permitting improved approaches to patients with these disorders.

### SUGGESTIONS FOR ADDITIONAL READING

Gilbert HS. Historical perspective on the treatment of essential thrombocythemia and polycythemia vera. Semin Hematol 1999;36:1:Suppl 2:19–22.

Michiels JJ, Barbui T, Finazzi G, et al. Diagnosis and treatment of polycythemia vera and possible future study designs of the PVSG. Leuk Lymphoma 2000;36:239–53.

Karp JE, Sarkodee-Adoo CB. Therapy-related acute leukemia. Clin Lab Med 2000;20:71–81.

Heaney ML, Golde DW. Myelodysplasia. N Engl J Med 1999;340:1649–60.

# REFERENCES

1. Dameshek W. Some speculations on the myeloproliferative syndromes. Blood 1951;6:372. editorial.
2. Modan B. An epidemiological study of polycythemia vera. Blood 1965;26:657.
3. Silverstein MN. Polycythemia, 1935–1969: an epidemiologic survey in Rochester, Minnesota. Mayo Clin Proc 1972;46:751.
4. Berlin N. Diagnosis and classification of polycythemia. Semin Hematol 1985;12:339.
5. Chievitz E. Complications and causes of death in polycythemia vera. Acta Med Scand 1962;172:513.
6. Pearson TC. Vascular occlusive episodes and venous treatment in primary proliferative polycythemia. Lancet 1978;2:1219.
7. Berk PD. Therapeutic recommendations in polycythemia vera based on Polycythemia Vera Study Group protocols. Semin Hematol 1986;23:132.
8. Prchal JF. Bone marrow responses in polycythemia vera. N Engl J Med 1974;290:1382.
9. Golde DW. Polycythemia vera: hormonal modulation of erythropoiesis in vitro. Blood 1977;49:399.
10. Zanjani ED. Erythroid colony formation by polycythemia vera bone marrow in vitro: dependence on erythropoietin. J Clin Invest 1977;59:841.
11. Wasserman LRL. Polycythemia vera—its course and treatment: relation to myeloid metaplasia and leukemia. Bull N Y Acad Med 1954;3:343.
12. Inaba T, Shimazaki C, Hirai H, et al. Familial polycythemia vera in father and daughter. Am J Hematol 1996;51:172.letter.
13. Najean Y. Polycythemia vera in young people: an analysis of 58 cases diagnosed before 40 years. Br J Haematol 1987;67:285.
14. Mitchell MC. Budd-Chiari syndrome: etiology, diagnosis and management. Medicine 1982;61:199.
15. International Committee for Standardization in Haematology. Recommended methods for measurement of red cell and plasma volume. J Nucl Med 1980;21:793.
16. Gilliland G. Determination of clonality in myeloproliferative diseases using polymerase chain reaction. Clin Res 1989;37:801.
17. Najean Y. Pure erythrocytosis: reappraisal of a study of 51 cases. Am J Hematol 1981;10:124.
18. Tefferi A. Diagnosing polycythemia vera: a paradigm shift. Mayo Clin Proc 1999;74:159.
19. Wasserman LR. The management of polycythemia vera. Br J Haematol 1971;21:371.
20. Berlin NI. Prologue: polycythemia vera: the closing of the Wasserman-Polycythemia Vera Study Group era. Semin Hematol 1997;34:1.
21. Najean Y, Rain JD. The very long-term evolution of polycythemia vera: an analysis of 318 patients initially treated by phlebotomy or $^{32}$P between 1969 and 1981. Semin Hematol 1997;34:6.
22. Tantaglis AP. Adverse effects of anti-aggregating platelet therapy in the treatment of polycythemia vera. Semin Hematol 1986;23:172.
23. Najean Y, Rain JD. Treatment of polycythemia vera: use of $^{32}$P alone or in combination with maintenance therapy using hydroxyurea in 461 patients greater than 65 years of age. The French Polycythemia Study Group. Blood 1997;89:2319.
24. Donovan PB. Treatment of polycythemia vera with hydroxyurea. Am J Hematol 1984;17:329.
25. Sharon R. Treatment of polycythemia vera with hydroxyurea. Cancer 1986;57:718.
26. Najean Y, Rain RD. Treatment of polycythemia vera: the use of hydroxyurea and pipobroman in 292 patients under the age of 65 years. Blood 1997;90:3370.
27. Petti MC, Spadea A, Avvisati G, et al. Polycythemia vera treated with pipobroman as single agent: low incidence of secondary leukemia in a cohort of patients observed during 20 years (1971–1991). Leukemia 1998;12:869.
28. Silverstein MN. Anagrelide: a new drug for treating thrombocytosis. N Engl J Med 1988;318:1292.
29. Anagrelide Study Group. Anagrelide, a therapy for thrombocythemic states: experience in 577 patients. Am J Med 1992;92:69.
30. Silver RT. Recombinant interferon-alpha for treatment of polycythemia vera. Lancet 1988;1:403.
31. Talpaz M. Recombinant interferon-alpha therapy of Philadelphia chromosome-negative myeloproliferative disorders with thrombocytosis. Am J Med 1989;86:554.
32. Silver RT. Interferon-a2b: a new treatment for polycythemia vera. Ann Intern Med 1993;119:1091.
33. Foa P, Massaro P, Ribera S, et al. Role of interferon alpha-2a in the treatment of polycythemia vera. Am J Hematol 1995;48:55.
34. Chanarin I. Relief of intractable pruritus in polycythemia rubra vera with cholestyramine. Br J Haematol 1985;29:669.
35. Silverstein MN. The evolution into and treatment of late stage polycythemia vera. Semin Hematol 1986;3:79.
36. Preston EE. Primary thrombocythaemia. Lancet 1982;1:1021.
37. Fialkow PJ. Evidence that essential thrombocythemia is a clonal disorder with origin in a multipotent stem cell. Blood 1981;58:916.
38. Singal U. Essential thrombocythemia: a clonal disorder of hematopoietic stem cell. Am J Hematol 1983;14:193.
39. Mesa RA, Silverstein MN, Jacobsen SJ, et al. Population-based incidence and survival figures in essential thrombocythemia and agnogenic myeloid metaplasia: an Olmsted County Study, 1976–1995. Am J Hematol 1999;61:10.
40. Hirayama Y, Sakamaki S, Matsunaga T, et al. Concentrations of thrombopoietin in bone marrow in normal subjects and in patients with idiopathic thrombocytopenic purpura, aplastic anemia, and essential thrombocythemia correlate with its mRNA expression of bone marrow stromal cells. Blood 1998;92:46.
41. Eystem ME. Familial essential thrombocythemia. Am J Med 1986;80:497.
41a. Kondo T, Okabe M, Sanada M, et al. Familial essential thrombocythemia associated with one-base deletion in the 5'-untranslated region of the thrombopoietin gene. Blood 1998;92:1091.
42. Belluci S. Essential thrombocythemias: clinical, evolutionary and biological data. Cancer 1986;58:2440.
43. Hehlmann R. Essential thrombocythemia: clinical characteristics and cause of 61 cases. Cancer 1988;61:2487.
44. Cartelazzo S. Incidence and risk factors for thrombotic complications in a historical cohort of 100 patients with essential thrombocythemia. J Clin Oncol 1990;8:556.
45. Buss DH. The incidence of thrombotic and hemorrhagic disorders in association with extreme thrombocytosis: an analysis of 129 cases. Am J Hematol 1985;20:36.
46. Regev A, Stark P, Blickstein D, Lahav M. Thrombotic complications in essential thrombocythemia with relatively low platelet counts. Am J Hematol 1997;56:168.
47. Murphy S. Essential thrombocythemia: an interim report from the Polycythemia Vera Study Group. Semin Hematol 1986;23:177.
48. Ginsburg AD. Platelet function in patients with high platelet counts. Ann Intern Med 1985;92:506.
49. Murphy S, Peterson P, Iland H, Laszlo J. Experience of the Polycythemia Vera Study Group with essential thrombocythemia: a final report on diagnostic criteria, survival, and leukemic transition by treatment. Semin Hematol 1997;34:29.
50. Swolin B. On the 5q-deletion, clinical and cytogenetic observations in ten patients and review of the literature. Blood 1981;58:986.
51. Michiels JJ, Juvonen E. Proposal for revised diagnostic criteria of essential thrombocythemia and polycythemia vera by the Thrombocythemia Vera Study Group. Semin Thromb Hemost 1997;23:339.
52. Taksin AL, Couedic JPL, Dusander-Fourt I, et al. Autonomous megakaryocyte growth in essential thrombocythemia and idiopathic myelofibrosis is not related to a c-mp1 mutation or to an autocrine stimulation by Mp1-L. Blood Rev 1997;11:1.
53. Harrison CN, Gale RE, Machin SJ, Linch DC. A large proportion of patients with a diagnosis of essential thrombocythemia do not have a clonal disorder and may be a lower risk of thrombotic complications. Blood 1999;93:417.
54. Nimer SD. Essential thrombocythemia: another heterogeneous disease better understood? Blood 1999;93:415.
55. Besses C, Cervantes F, Pereira A, et al. Major vascular complications in essential thrombocythemia: a study of the predictive factors in a series of 148 patients. Leukemia 1999;13:150.
56. Cortelazzo S, Finazzi G, Ruggeri M, et al. Hydroxyurea for patients with essential thrombocythemia and a high risk of thrombosis. N Engl J Med 1995;332:1132.
57. Sterkers Y, Preudhomme C, Lai JL, et al. Acute myeloid leukemia

and myelodysplastic syndromes following essential thrombocythemia treated with hydroxyurea: high proportion of cases with 17p deletion. Blood 1998;91:616.

58. Silverstein MN, Tefferi A. Treatment of essential thrombocythemia with anagrelide. Semin Hematol 1999;36:23.

59. Lazzarino M. Interferon alpha 2b as treatment for Philadelphia-chromosome negative myeloproliferative disorders with excessive thrombocytosis. Br J Haematol 1989;72:173.

60. Delage R, Demers C, Cantin G, Roy J. Treatment of essential thrombocythemia during pregnancy with interferon-alpha. Obstet Gynecol 1996;87:814.

61. Jabaily J. Neurologic manifestations of essential thrombocythemia. Ann Intern Med 1983;99:513.

62. Michels JI. Erythromelalgia caused by platelet-mediated arteriolar inflammation and thrombocytosis in thrombocythemia. Ann Intern Med 1985;102:466.

63. Barbui T, Finazzi G. Clinical parameters for determining when and when not to treat essential thrombocythemia. Semin Hematol 1999;36:14.

64. Mesa RA, Silverstein MN, Jacobsen SJ, et al. Population-based incidence and survival figures in essential thrombocythemia and agnogenic myeloid metaplasia: an Olmsted County Study, 1976–1995. Am J Hematol 1999;61:10.

65. Varki A. The syndrome of idiopathic myelofibrosis: clinicopathologic review with emphasis on the prognostic variables predicting survival. Medicine 1983;62:353.

66. Silverstein MN. Agnogenic myeloid metaplasia. Acton, Mass.: Publishing Sciences Group, 1985.

67. Gordon BR. Immunologic abnormalities in myelofibrosis with activation of the complement system. Blood 1981;58:904.

68. Rondeau E. Immune disorders in agnogenic myeloid metaplasia: relation to fibrosis. Br J Haematol 1983;53:467.

69. Wang JC, Chen C, Lou LH, Mora M. Blood thrombopoietin, IL-2 and IL-11 in patients with agnogenic myeloid metaplasia. Leukemia 1997;11:1827.

70. Crail HW. Myelofibrosis associated with tuberculosis—a report of four cases. Blood 1948;3:1426.

71. Pagiluca A. Myelofibrosis in primary myelodysplastic syndromes: a clinicopathological study of 10 cases. Br J Haematol 1989;71:499.

72. Golomb HM. Hairy cell leukemia: a clinical review of 71 cases. Ann Intern Med 1978;89:677.

73. Kergsman KL. Acute myelofibrosis: an accelerated variant of agnogenic myeloid metaplasia. Ann Intern Med 1981;74:232.

74. Bearman RM. Acute malignant myelosclerosis. Cancer 1979;43:279.

75. Gardner FH. Androgens and erythropoiesis: III. further evaluation of testosterone treatment of myelofibrosis. N Engl J Med 1966;274:420.

76. Besa EC. Analysis of the androgen response of 23 patients with agnogenic myeloid metaplasia: the value of chromosomal studies in predicting response and survival. Cancer 1982;49:308.

77. Radin AI. Interferon therapy for agnogenic myeloid metaplasia complicated by immune hemolytic anemia. Hematol Pathol 1991;5:83.

78. Parmeggiani L. Alpha interferon in the treatment of symptomatic myelofibrosis with myeloid metaplasia. Eur J Haematol 1987;39:228.

79. Silverstein MN. Splenectomy in myeloid metaplasia. Blood 1979;53:515.

80. Barosi G, Ambrosetti A, Centra A, et al. Splenectomy and risk of blast transformation in myelofibrosis with myeloid metaplasia: Italian Cooperative Study Group on myeloid metaplasia. Blood 1998;91:3630.

81. Porcu P, Neiman RS, Orazi A. Splenectomy in agnogenic myeloid metaplasia. Blood 1999;93:2132. letter.

82. Dolak I. Allogeneic bone marrow transplantation for primary myelofibrosis. Br J Haematol 1989;71:158.

83. Wolf JL. Reversal of acute ("malignant") myelosclerosis by allogeneic bone marrow transplantation. Blood 1982;59:191.

84. Guardiola P, Esperou H, Cazals-Hatem D, et al. Allogeneic bone marrow transplantation for agnogenic myeloid metaplasia. French Society of Bone Marrow Transplantation. Br J Haematol 1997;98:1004.

84a. Guardiola P, Anderson JE, Bandini G, et al. Allogeneic stem cell transplantation for agnogenic myeloid metaplasia: a European Group for Blood and Marrow Transplantation, Societe Francaise de Greffe de Moelle, Gruppo Italiano per il Trapianto del Midollo Osseo, and Fred Hutchinson Cancer Research Center Collaborative Study. Blood 1999;93:2831.

85. Bennett JM, Catovsky D, Daniel MT, et al. FAB Cooperative Group: proposal for the classification of the myelodysplastic syndromes. Br J Haematol 1982;51:189–99.

86. Sanz GF, Sanz MA, Vallespi T, et al. Two regression models and a scoring system for predicting survival and planning treatment in myelodysplastic syndromes: a multivariate analysis of prognostic factors in 370 patients. Blood 1989;74:395–408.

87. Storniolo AM, Moloney WC, Rosenthal DS, et al. Chronic myelomonocytic leukemia. Leukemia 1990;4:766–70.

88. Oscier D. Myelodysplastic syndromes. Ballieres Clin Haematol 1987;1:389.

89. Aul C, Gatterman N, Schneider W. Age-related incidence and other epidemiological aspects of myelodysplastic syndrome. Br J Haematol 1992;82:385.

90. Kantarjian H, Keating M, Walters R, et al. Therapy-related leukemia and myelodysplastic syndrome: clinical, cytogenetic, and prognostic features. J Clin Oncol 1986;4:1743–57.

91. Pedersen-Bjergaard J. Radiotherapy- and chemotherapy-induced myelodysplasia and acute myeloid leukemia: a review. Leuk Res 1992;16:61–5.

92. Greenberg P, Cox C, Le Beau MM, et al. International scoring system for evaluating prognosis in myelodysplastic syndromes. Blood 1997;89:2079–88.

93. Greenberg PL, Sanz GF, Sanz MA. Prognostic scoring systems for risk assessment in myelodysplastic syndromes. Trends Exp Clin Med 1999;9:17–31.

93a. Jensen PD, Heickendorff L, Pedersen B, et al. The effect of iron chelation on haemopoiesis in MDS patients with transfusional iron overload. Br J Haematol 1996;94:288–99.

94. Greenberg PL, Bishop M, Deeg J, et al. NCCN practice guidelines for myelodysplastic syndromes. Oncology 1998;12:53–80.

95. Sonneveld P, et al. Expression of MDR-1 in marrow cells from patients with myelodysplastic syndrome. Leukemia 1993;7:963.

96. List A, Spier C, Greer J, et al. Phase I/II trial of cyclosporine as a chemotherapy resistance modifier in acute leukemia. J Clin Oncol 1993;11:1652–60.

97. Advani R, Saba H, Rowe JM, et al. Treatment of refractory/relapsed AML with chemotherapy plus the multi-drug resistance modulator PSC833 (valspodar). Blood 1999;93:787–95.

98. Wattel E, Solary E, Hecquet B, et al. Quinine improves the results of intensive chemotherapy in myelodysplastic syndromes expressing P glycoprotein: results of a randomized study. Br J Haematol 1998;102:1015–24.

99. Tricot G, De Bock R, Dekker A, et al. The role of aggressive chemotherapy in the treatment of myelodysplastic syndromes. Br J Haematol 1986;63:477.

100. Beran M, Kantarjian H, Keating M, et al. Results of combination chemotherapy with topotecan and high-dose cytosine arabinoside in previously untreated patients with high-risk myelodysplastic syndrome and chronic myelomonocytic leukemia. Blood 1997;90:Suppl 1:583a.

101. Anderson JE, Appelbaum F, Fisher L, et al. Allogeneic bone marrow transplantation for 93 patients with myelodysplastic syndrome. Blood 1993;82:677–81.

102. Anderson JE, Thomas ED. The Seattle experience with bone marrow transplantation for MDS. Leuk Res 1997;21:Suppl 1:S51.

103. Nevill TJ, Fung HC, Shepherd JD, et al. Cytogenetic abnormalities in primary myelodysplastic syndrome are highly predictive of outcome after allogeneic bone marrow transplantation. Blood 1998;92:1910–7.

104. Anderson JE, Anasetti C, Appelbaum FR. Unrelated donor marrow transplantation for myelodysplasia (MDS) and MDS-related acute myeloid leukaemia. Br J Haematol 1996;93:59.

105. Giralt S, Estey E, Albitar M, et al. Engraftment of allogeneic hematopoietic progenitor cells with purine analog-containing chemotherapy: harnessing graft-versus-leukemia without myeloablative therapy. Blood 1997;89:4531–6.

106. Wattel E, Solary E, Leleu X, et al. A prospective study of autologous bone marrow or peripheral blood stem cell transplantation after intensive chemotherapy in myelodysplastic syndromes. Leukemia 1999;13:524–9.

107. Greenberg PL. Biologic and clinical implications of marrow culture studies in the myelodysplastic syndromes. Semin Hematol 1996;33:163–75.

108. Greenberg PL. Treatment of MDS with hemopoietic growth factors. Semin Oncol 1992;19:106–14.

109. Willemze R, van der Lely N, Zwierzina H, et al. A randomized phase

I/II multicenter study of recombinant human GM-CSF therapy for patients with myelodysplastic syndromes and a relatively low risk of acute leukemia. Ann Hematol 1992;64:173–80.

110. Schuster MW, Larson R, Thompson JA, et al. Randomized trial of subcutaneous GM-CSF versus observation in patients with myelodysplastic syndrome. Blood 1990;76:Suppl 1:318a.

111. Economopoulos T, Papageorgiou E, Stathakis N, et al. Treatment of myelodysplastic syndromes with human granulocyte-macrophage colony-stimulating factor (GM-CSF) or GM-CSF combined with low-dose cytosine arabinoside. Eur J Haematol 1992;49:138–42.

112. Gerhartz HH, Marcus R, Delmer A, et al. A randomised Phase II study of low-dose cytosine arabinoside plus GM-CSF in MDS with a high risk of developing leukemia. Leukemia 1994;8:16–23.

113. Miller KB, Kim K, Morrison FS, et al. Evaluation of low dose Ara C vs. supportive care in the treatment of MDS: a Phase III intergroup study. Ann Hematol 1992;65:162.

114. Negrin RS, Haeuber DH, Nagler A, et al. Treatment of myelodysplastic syndromes with recombinant human granulocyte colony stimulating factor. Ann Intern Med 1992;110:976–84.

115. Negrin RS, Nagler A, Kobayashi Y, et al. Maintenance treatment of patients with myelodysplastic syndromes using recombinant human granulocyte colony stimulating factor. Blood 1992;78:36–43.

116. Greenberg P, Taylor K, Larson R, et al. Phase III randomized multicenter trial of G-CSF vs. observation for MDS. Blood 1993;82:Suppl 1:196a.

117. Sanz GF, Sanz MA, Vallespi T, et al. Two regression models and a scoring system for predicting survival and planning treatment in myelodysplastic syndromes: a multivariate analysis of prognostic factors in 370 patients. Blood 1989;74:395–408.

118. Ganser A, Seipelt G, Lindemann A, et al. Effects of recombinant human interleukin-3 in patients with myelodysplastic syndromes. Blood 1990;6:455.

119. Kurzrock R, Talpaz M, Estrov Z, et al. Phase I study of recombinant human interleukin-3 in patients with bone marrow failure. J Clin Oncol 1991;9:1241–50.

120. Ganser A, Ottmann OG, Seipelt G, et al. Effect of long-term treatment with recombinant human interleukin-3 in patients with myelodysplastic syndromes. Leukemia 1993;7:696–701.

121. Gordon MS, Nemunaitis J, Hoffman R, et al. A Phase I trial of recombinant human interleukin-6 in patients with myelodysplastic syndromes and thrombocytopenia. Blood 1995;85:3066–76.

122. Jacobs A, Janowska-Wieczorek A, Caro J, et al. Circulating erythropoietin in patients with myelodysplastic syndromes. Br J Haematol 1989;73:36–9.

123. Merchav S, Nielsen OJ, Rosenbaum H, et al. In vitro studies of erythropoietin-dependent regulation of erythropoiesis in myelodysplastic syndromes. Leukemia 1990;4:771–4.

124. Greenberg PL, Negrin R, Ginzton N. G-CSF synergizes with erythropoietin for enhancing erythroid colony formation in myelodysplastic syndromes. Blood 1991;78:38a.

125. Negrin RS, Stein R, Doherty K, et al. Treatment of the anemias of MDS using recombinant human granulocyte colony-stimulating factor in combination with erythropoietin. Blood 1993;82:737–43.

126. Hellstrom-Lindberg E, Birgegard G, Carlsson M, et al. A combination of G-CSF and erythropoietin may synergistically improve the anaemia in patients with MDS. Leuk Lymph 1993;11:221–8.

127. Negrin RS, Stein R, Doherty K, et al. Maintenance treatment of the anemia of myelodysplastic syndromes with recombinant human G-CSF plus erythropoietin: evidence for in vivo synergy. Blood 1996;87:4076–81.

128. Hellstrom-Lindberg E, Ahlgren T, Begguin Y, et al. Treatment of the anemia of myelodysplastic syndromes with G-CSF plus erythropoietin: results from a randomized Phase II study and long term follow up on 71 patients. Blood 1998;92:68–75.

129. Hellstrom-Lindberg E, Negrin R, Stein R, et al. Erythroid response to treatment with G-CSF plus erythropoietin for the anemia of patients with myelodysplastic syndromes: proposal for a predictive model. Br J Haematol 1997;99:344.

130. List AF, Brasfield F, Heaton R, et al. Stimulation of hematopoiesis by amifostine in patients with myelodysplastic syndrome. Blood 1997;90:3364.

131. List AF, Holmes H, Vempaty H, et al. Phase II study of amifostine in patients with myelodysplastic syndromes: impact on hematopoiesis. Blood 1998;92:Suppl 1:714a.

132. Molldrem J, Caples M, Mavroudis D, et al. Antithymocyte globulin for patients with myelodysplastic syndromes. Br J Haematol 1997;99:699.

133. Dunn DE, Tanawattanacharoen P, Boccuni P, et al. Paroxysmal nocturnal hemoglobinuria cells in patients with bone marrow failure syndromes. Ann Intern Med 1999;131:401.

134. Jonasova A, Neuwirtova R, Cermak J, et al. Promising cyclosporin A therapy for myelodysplastic syndrome. Leuk Res 1997;21:842.

135. Raza A, Mundle S, Iftikhar A, et al. Simultaneous assessment of cell kinetics and programmed cell death in bone marrow biopsies of MDS reveals extensive apoptosis as the probable basis for ineffective hematopoiesis. Am J Hematol 1995;48:143.

136. Rajapaksa R, Ginzton N, Rott L, Greenberg P. Altered oncoprotein expression and apoptosis in myelodysplastic syndrome marrow cells. Blood 1996;88:4275.

137. Gersuk GM, Beckham C, Loken MR. A role for tumour necrosis factor-alpha, Fas and Fas-Ligand in marrow failure associated with myelodysplastic syndrome. Br J Haematol 1998;103:176–88.

138. Silverman L, Demakos E, Peterson B, et al. A randomized controlled trial of subcutaneous azacytidine (AZA C) in patients with the myelodysplastic syndrome (MDS): a study of the CALGB. Proc ASCO 1998;17:14a.

# CHAPTER 86

# CHRONIC MYELOGENOUS LEUKEMIA

• MICHAEL LILL • H. PHILLIP KOEFFLER

## Natural History, Diagnosis, and Staging

### EPIDEMIOLOGY AND ETIOLOGY

Chronic myelogenous (myeloid) leukemia (CML) is an acquired clonal myeloproliferative disorder originating from malignant transformation at a multipotential stem cell level. The age-adjusted incidence of CML in the United States is 1.4 cases per 100,000 per annum. There is a sex bias, with the age-adjusted rate for males being 1.8 per annum and for females 1.1 per annum. No racial difference in incidence occurs. The incidence increases with age. The rate in the population older than age 65 years is 7 per 100,000 per annum versus 0.8 per 100,000 per annum in individuals younger than age 65 years. The incidence peaks in the greater than 85 age group with 12.6 cases per 100,000 per annum. The median age at diagnosis is 49 years. The incidence of CML has been stable since the early 1970s.[1]

The cause of CML is unknown, although an increased incidence has been associated with exposure to ionizing radiation and to benzene. The 5-year survival of patients with CML has increased from 22.4% in 1974 through 1976 to 32% in 1989 through 1994.[1] This increased survival probably reflects earlier diagnosis (i.e., lead-time bias) and improved treatment in younger patients.

## BIOLOGY

CML is characterized clinically by increased proliferation and accumulation of a myeloid cell population with variable functional abnormalities and a triphasic course (chronic, accelerated, and blast phases). The hallmark of this disease is the presence of the abnormal fusion protein, BCR ABL, usually resulting from a reciprocal translocation between chromosomes 9 and 22 (t9;22,Ph[1]). In CML patients, the Philadelphia (Ph[1]) chromosome can be found in metaphases of neutrophil, eosinophil, basophil, erythroblast, platelet, B cell, monocyte, and macrophage precursors. Neither marrow nor skin fibroblasts display Ph[1] during metaphase. T lymphocyte clones derived from patients with CML have been shown to express BCR ABL.

Ph[1] is an abbreviated chromosome 22 (22q−) resulting from an unequal reciprocal translocation (9;22), in which most of the distal end of 22 is exchanged for a small terminal piece of the long arm of chromosome 9 (9q+). Approximately 5% of Ph[1]-positive CML patients show variant cytogenetic changes, of which half are three-way translocations involving chromosomes 9 and 22 and another chromosome.[2] The breakpoints in chromosomes 9 and 22 are at bands q34.1 and q1.21, resulting in a t(9;22) (q34.1;q1.21) that transposes the c-*sis* proto-oncogene from chromosome 22 to chromosome 9 and the cellular Abelson (c-*abl*) proto-oncogene from chromosome 9 to chromosome 22, in proximity to the breakpoint cluster region gene (*bcr*) (Fig. 86–1).[3–8] This latter hybrid *bcr-abl* oncogene produces an abnormal 8.5-kb RNA, in contrast to the normal *abl* transcripts of 6.8 and 7.4 kb.[9] The abnormal mRNA produced by *bcr-abl* encodes for a 210-kd (p210) fusion protein that exhibits tyrosine kinase activity and shows considerable homology to the catalytic subunit of 3′,5′-cyclic adenosine monophosphate (cAMP).[10]

Although usually located in the intron 5′ of exon 2, the breakpoint on chromosome 9 may be variable, ranging over a 200-kb region upstream of the 5′ end of the v-*abl* homologous region.[11] *abl* exons 1a and 1b are sometimes also translocated to chromosome 22, but their transcripts are spliced out of the mature mRNA. In contrast, Ph[1]-positive CML patients and some 50% of Ph[1]-positive acute lymphoblastic leukemia (ALL) and acute nonlymphoblastic leukemia patients have breakpoints on chromosome 22 that cluster in a region about 5.8 kb long, termed the *major breakpoint cluster region* (m-bcr).[12–19] m-bcr encompasses four exons (exons 12 through 15, but usually referred to as exons *b1* through *b4*). The breakpoint on chromosome 22 is located 3′ of the Cλ gene; the lambda chain coding region usually remains on Ph[1] in a 5′ orientation to the translocated c-*abl* gene.[20]

In Ph[1]-positive CML, the breakpoints within m-bcr have been assigned to a 3′ or 5′ location. Depending on whether the hybrid oncogene involves exon 3 or exon 2 of the m-bcr and exon 2 of *abl*, two distinct RNA messages are produced: b3a2 or b2a2. Although the 3′ *bcr* breakpoints often result in b3a2 and 5′ breakpoints in b2a2 messages, some patients with 5′ breakpoints produce a b3a2 message. The hybrid b3a2 mRNA and the protein for which it codes differ in size by 75 bases and 25 amino acids from b2a2 and its product. This spectrum of abnormalities at the DNA and RNA levels has been variably associated with different disease features (e.g., thrombocytosis or distinct prognostic groups), but no conclusive findings have been published to date.[16–20]

The mechanisms conferring a growth advantage on CML cells over normal hematopoietic cells are unknown. A reduced duration of stroma-CML hematopoietic cell interaction has been documented and attributed to abnormalities in the patterns of adherence of CML cells to the stromal matrix.[21] Reduced or abnormal contact with stromal elements in CML may abrogate the normal maturation of cell surface moieties, for example, cytoadhesion molecules (CAM), HLA-DR, required for a normal proliferation-maturation sequence.[22, 23] Interferon alfa has been shown in vitro to reverse some of these adhesion abnormalities.[24, 25] Discordant nuclear/cytoplasmic maturation in CML may also confer a growth advantage over normal hematopoietic cells.[26]

A causal association between Ph[1] and the initiation and perpetuation of CML has been established in many models, including one in which complementary DNA (cDNA) encoding for p210 was introduced into mouse marrow cells, which were reinfused into lethally irradiated mice.[27–29] After 2 to 8 weeks, some mice developed CML-like disorders, including leukocytosis and splenomegaly, monocyte and macrophage extramedullary tumors, and ALL. This spectrum of disorders is similar to the pathogenesis of human CML and suggests that *bcr-abl* rearrangement may be sufficient not only for development of chronic phase CML, but also for its transformation into blast phase disease.

The signaling pathway of p210[BCR-ABL] involved in giving CML cells a growth advantage is still being elucidated. The BCR-ABL fusion protein has several domains that allow multiple protein/protein interactions with adapter proteins, such as growth factor receptor-bound protein 2 (GRB2), the CRK-oncogene-like protein (CRKL), casitas B-lineage lymphoma protein (CBL), and SRC homology 2-containing protein (SHC). These adapter proteins connect the p210[BCR-ABL] to many secondary signaling pathways, including activation of *ras*, PI-3 kinase, JAK-STAT kinases, and focal adhesion kinases.[30] Their activation provides stimulating signals to genes associated with cell proliferation and suppression of the pathways of apoptosis (programmed cell death) by activation of nuclear targets, such as c-*jun*, c-*fos*, cyclin D, *bcl-2*, and c-*myc*.

Activation of these genes may confer on the CML progenitors the capacity to escape partially the normal dependency on growth factors and, in part, to withstand the deleterious effects of cytotoxic drugs and radiation.[31–33] The activation of focal adhesion kinases perhaps results in defective adherence of the immature hematopoietic CML cells to the marrow stromal elements, which may facilitate their release into the blood. Clearly, further investigations are needed to dissect how the BCR-ABL fusion protein provides a growth advantage to the leukemic clone of cells.

About 20% of adults and 5% of children with ALL have Ph[1] in their blast cells.[34] These children are usually older than Ph[1]-negative ALL patients (median, 8 years) and frequently have a higher median white blood cell count, L1 blast cell morphology, and a high incidence of central ner-

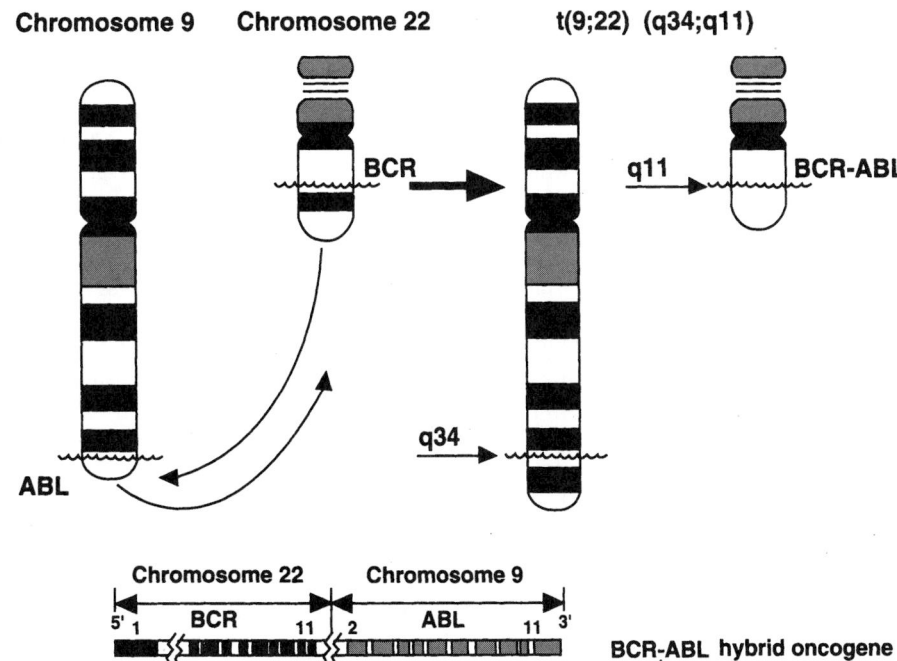

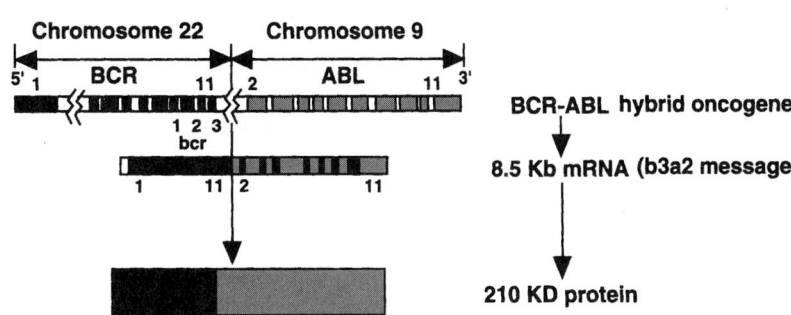

**Figure 86–1.** The Philadelphia chromosome in chronic myelogenous leukemia and associated molecular abnormalities. (From Kantarjian HM, Deisseroth A, Kurzrock R, et al. Chronic myelogenous leukemia: a concise update. Blood 1993;82:694.)

vous system leukemia at diagnosis. Their prognosis is inferior to that of Ph[1]-negative ALL patients. In Ph[1]-positive acute leukemia, 50% of patients have a breakpoint within the m-bcr region, which results in a 7.5-kb mRNA encoding for a 190-kd (p190) protein. Although, in contrast to p190 acute leukemia, chronic phase disease may follow induction therapy in some patients with p210 Ph[1]-positive acute leukemia, the clinical features and prognoses are similar in p210 and p190 acute leukemias.[35]

About 10% of patients with the clinical presentation of CML lack the Ph[1] chromosome. Earlier studies suggested that Ph[1]-negative disease carried a much poorer prognosis.[36] Further studies showed, however, that approximately one third of these individuals have molecular evidence of *bcr* gene rearrangement, and the clinical features and prognosis of these patients are essentially identical to those with Ph[1]-positive disease.[37] Patients with complex translocations resulting in a Ph[1] chromosome have a similar prognosis to patients with the standard t(9;22).[38] In contrast, patients who were Ph[1]-negative and *bcr*-negative were older and had more thrombocytopenia, less basophilia, and an increased monocytosis in blood and marrow. The median survival of Ph[1]-negative, *bcr*-negative patients was significantly less than either Ph[1]-positive, *bcr*-positive patients or Ph[1]-negative, *bcr*-positive patients (25 months vs. 72 months vs. 60 months). These data strongly support the concept that *bcr*-negative disease should be considered a distinct entity. The absence of either Ph[1] or BCR-ABL rearrangement excludes a diagnosis of CML.

CML in children is a rare disorder that behaves similarly to adult Ph[1]-positive CML. Juvenile CML is now known as *juvenile chronic myelomonocytic leukemia* and is Ph[1]-negative. This disease has a peak incidence at age 1 or 2 years. The disease is associated with monosomy 7 and abnormalities in the NF1 gene. Splenomegaly and lymphadenopathy are prominent; myeloid progenitors from these patients can grow spontaneously when their marrow is plated in soft-gel culture, and these patients have a marked elevation of fetal hemoglobin. The response to cytotoxic therapy is poor, and median survival is less than 1 year.

## PATHOLOGY

At diagnosis, circulating erythrocyte burst-forming unit and granulocyte-macrophage colony-forming unit progenitor numbers in CML may be increased 180-fold and 9000-fold.[39, 40] CML marrow hyperplasia of all myeloid stages is caused by progenitor cell expansion, a slower cell cycle, prolonged maturation-division times, and delayed compartmental transit. Circulating neutrophils from CML patients display several striking functional defects. An absent or low leukocyte alkaline phosphatase (LAP) activity is characteristic of CML. With infection, inflammation, secondary malignancy, pregnancy, splenectomy, or peripheral blood remission as a consequence of therapy, the LAP score can rise to normal or high levels. Occasionally, inflammatory or malignant disease can produce a leukemoid reaction, with leukocytosis, immature circulating granulocytes, hyperplasia of the bone marrow, and slight hepatosplenomegaly. Patients with leukemoid reaction are Ph[1]-negative and usually have neither a low LAP score nor an absolute basophilia in the peripheral blood. Low LAP scores are not specific for CML and may be seen in paroxysmal nocturnal hemoglobinuria, congenital hypophosphatasia, and some cases of idiopathic myelofibrosis or acute myeloid leukemia. LAP deficiency in CML represents a quantitative deficiency of enzyme, the pathophysiologic significance of which is unknown.

Other granulocyte abnormalities in CML include subnormal adhesiveness to bone marrow stromal surfaces, delayed emigration to extravascular sites, reduction in phagocytic and bacteriocidal activities, and subnormal lactoferrin and lysozyme content. The CML granulocytes capable of extravascular migration (as determined by the skin window technique) are more active in phagocytosis and show higher LAP activities than do kindred cells trapped in the circulation.[41] Phagocytic activity, release of lactoferrin, adhesion to endothelium, and extravascular migration capability appear to be linked granulocyte properties involving CAM, all of which are depressed in CML. Marrow biopsy in CML reveals hyperproliferation of all stages and classes of myeloid cells impinging on erythroid elements and causing a striking rise in the myeloid/erythroid ratio. Bands plus segmented neutrophils, metamyelocytes, and the combined numbers of myeloblasts, promyelocytes, and myelocytes occur in three equivalent proportions, denoting a marked shift toward myeloid immaturity. Megakaryocytic hyperplasia is common, and dysplastic changes variably affect all cell lines. In 30% of CML patients, Gaucher-like cells may be found in the marrow and spleen, reflecting consumption by mononuclear phagocytes of leukocyte sphingolipids released by leukemic granulocytes. Gaucher's disease results from the absence of sphingolipid hydrolase; in CML, the Gaucher-like cells have active hydrolase but are overwhelmed by the substrate load.

Increased production of uric acid, with hyperuricemia and hyperuricosuria, is common in untreated CML. If cytolytic therapy causes a heavy additional burden of filtered purines, urate nephropathy or urinary tract blockage may ensue. Formation of urate stones is common in CML, and some patients with latent gout may develop overt gouty arthritis or nephropathy. Serum vitamin B12 levels are increased in proportion to the amounts of transcobalamins I and III released during breakdown of CML granulocytes.[42] Serum vitamin B12 levels rise in proportion to the white cell count. Transcobalamin II, the physiologic vitamin B12 carrier, is not increased and may be decreased in CML.

## CLINICAL FEATURES

The diagnosis of CML is made on the basis of the findings of leukocytosis with basophilia and the presence of the *bcr-abl* rearrangement. Usually, routine cytogenetic analysis is used to detect Ph[1]. Fluorescent in situ hybridization can also be used. This technique relies on the fluorescent labeling of a segment of DNA that encompasses the *abl* gene and the labeling, with a different color, of the bcr DNA segment. These segments are hybridized to the chromosomes of the hematopoietic cells of the individual. If the *abl* and bcr are translocated, they can be easily seen on the wrong chromosome. A third technique is polymerase chain reaction (PCR) analysis. Nucleotide primers span the potential sites of rearrangement of the *bcr-abl* genes. These are used with cDNA of the hematopoietic cells of the individual, DNA

polymerase, and additional nucleotides. A visible nucleotide segment (band) is made on gels if bcr and *abl* are fused. In Ph[1]-negative patients with a clinical diagnosis of CML, PCR or Southern blot analysis for bcr rearrangement can identify Ph[1]-negative, bcr-positive CML patients. In the area of patient follow-up, quantitation of bcr rearrangement has not yet been standardized in relation to cytogenetic studies. Southern blots had been used to monitor the effect of therapy in patients with Ph[1]-negative, bcr-positive disease, but it is slow, labor-intensive, and much less sensitive than the PCR technique. PCR techniques can detect residual disease at one CML cell in a population of $10^4$ to $10^5$ *normal cells.*

At diagnosis, the white cell count is typically $170 \times 10^9$/L, the platelet count $500 \times 10^9$/L, and the hemoglobin concentration approximately 12 mg/dl.[43] For many patients, CML is an insidious disorder with a slow pace of early myeloproliferative progression. Elevations of the granulocyte count may go unrecognized for months or years. At this subclinical stage, preleukemic myelodysplastic aberrations are generally demonstrable, including basophilia, leftward shift in blood granulocyte maturity marked by the presence of metamyelocytes and myelocytes, and a profound lowering of the LAP scores.

As the granulocyte count rises to $50 \times 10^9$/L, the spleen becomes palpably enlarged, and hypermetabolic symptoms develop. Common presenting symptoms of chronic phase CML include fatigue (65% of patients), abdominal fullness (35% of patients), and weight loss (20% of patients).[44] Less common but frequent presenting symptoms are diminished exercise tolerance, night sweats, bone pain, and easy bruising.

Splenomegaly is the most common physical finding on initial examination, being detected in 55 to 70% of patients. The magnitude of splenomegaly correlates well with the total body granulocyte mass and the blood granulocyte count. The enlarged spleen is firm and not tender (unless splenic infarction has occurred). The degree of splenomegaly is an indication of the duration of the chronic phase; gross splenomegaly predicts a shorter time to blast crisis. Hepatomegaly is less common (30 to 50% of patients) and much less spectacularly present. Lymphadenopathy is uncommon in chronic phase CML, and its appearance suggests either accelerated or blast phase disease.

Occasionally, initial symptoms are caused by hemorrhage or infection, but these are uncommon in the chronic phase of CML because many neutrophils still function normally, and severe thrombocytopenia is rare. About 30% of CML patients experience focal or diffuse increases in marrow reticulin fibers (reticulin fibrosis) early in the disease, and 20% develop extensive new collagen formation (collagen fibrosis). Minor degrees of marrow fibrosis occur in many CML patients and appear not to imply necessarily a poor prognosis; a rapid rate of development of extensive myelofibrosis is a poor prognostic feature, however. Fibroblasts are not derived from the leukemic clone but represent a secondary reaction to leukemic infiltration.[44] Intravascular plugs of leukemic cells are a serious hazard in CML, particularly in patients younger than 20 years old at diagnosis, 50% of whom present with white cell counts greater than $300 \times 10^9$/L. Leukostasis is also a particular problem in 60% of childhood cases, reflecting the high white cell counts in children with Ph[1]-positive CML. The diverse consequences of severe leukostasis may include central nervous system hemorrhage, headache, dizziness, mental confusion, central or peripheral neuropathy, digital gangrene, cardiorespiratory failure, priapism, and marrow necrosis. Intraocular visible manifestations include papilledema, retinal hemorrhages, and venous engorgement.

Bleeding and thrombosis are uncommon in the chronic phase of CML, but patients with extreme thrombocythemia tend to have thrombotic and hemorrhagic problems, whereas those with marked leukocytosis are prone to thrombotic complications. Disseminated intravascular coagulation may occasionally be seen in the blast phase of the disease.

Blood basophil levels are elevated in almost all patients with Ph$^1$-positive CML (average 4% on white cell differential counts). Eosinophil levels are usually excessive, and monocytosis is common. Rapid rises in basophil counts are predictive of impending blast phase. As CML patients enter blast phase, basophilia may become extreme, and manifestations of hyperhistaminemia, including diarrhea, flushing, urticaria, and bronchospasm, may appear. Persistence of even a 1% basophilia (with or without granules) should prompt a search for CML, polycythemia vera, or myelofibrosis.

Platelet counts in CML have no fixed relationship to other blood cell counts. Platelet levels are subnormal in 10% of patients at diagnosis, and thrombocytopenia is rarely significant in the chronic phase. Levels of platelets are elevated in 50% of patients; in some, thrombocytosis may be extreme, reaching levels of $1000 \times 10^9$/L or more in 10%. Most CML patients have anemia at diagnosis, but generally it is mild, rarely warranting transfusion. Thereafter the hemoglobin concentration shows a crude inverse correlation with the white cell count. Nucleated red cells are found in the blood of all CML patients, and all cell lines show myelodysplastic changes, among which mononuclear megakaryocytes, hypogranular granulocytes, giant metamyelocytes, hyposegmented or hypersegmented neutrophils, and hypogranular or microgranular basophils are common.

Blast phase disease is usually characterized by rising blast counts in the peripheral blood and bone marrow and lack of response to therapy (Table 86–1). During this period, extramedullary myeloblast tumors (chloromas) can develop, especially in bone, lymph nodes, central nervous system, skin, lungs, stomach, and heart.

Many patients go through a period of malaise, fever, increasing splenomegaly, progressive anemia, increasing basophilia, increasing thrombocytosis, and leukocytosis before blast crisis. This phase, known as the *accelerated phase*, may be characterized by all the clinical manifestations of blast crisis without an increase in the percentage of blast cells in the blood and bone marrow.

Meningeal leukemia occurs in more than 5% of patients during the accelerated phase of CML, usually as a prodrome of lymphoid blast transformation. Meningeal leukemia is uncommon in myeloid blast transformation, but central nervous system involvement may be manifest as a localized tumor (granulocyte sarcoma). These myeloid tumors or infiltrates are capable of compressing the spinal cord. CML causes destructive bone lesions during the chronic phase in only 3% of patients, but hypercalcemia and lytic bone lesions may occur in accelerated or blast phase disease.

The two major morphologic subgroups of blast crisis are the myeloblastic and lymphoblastic (usually B) types;

*Table 86–1.* **Blast Phase Criteria***

*Major Criteria*

>30% blasts plus promyelocytes in bone marrow
>20% blasts in bone marrow

*Minor Criteria (Accelerated Phase Characteristics)*

Bone marrow
  Reticulin fibrosis (not present at diagnosis of chronic phase)
  Trilineage dysplasia
    Pseudo-Pelger cells
      *or*
    Megaloblastoid changes
      *or*
    Dysplastic megakaryocytes
  >20% basophils plus eosinophils
Cytogenetic
  Multiple Ph$^1$ or other chromosomal abnormalities in addition to the Ph$^1$
Peripheral blood
  ≥30% blasts plus promyelocytes or ≥15% blasts
  Platelets <100 × 10$^9$/L in the absence of cytoreductive therapy
  Hemoglobin <10.0 g/dl
  WCC >50 × 10$^9$/L refractory to therapy
  Basophils ≥20%
Clinical (signs and symptoms)
Extramedullary leukemia
Fever of undetermined origin >38° C for 7 days
Weight loss >10% of total body weight
>25% increase in spleen size (in the midclavicular line)

*One major or any 3 of the 12 minor criteria are equivalent to blast phase disease.
Ph$^1$, Philadelphia chromosome; WCC, white cell count.

erythroblastic, megakaryocytic, mixed, and undifferentiated forms also occur.[45] In 60% of patients, the blast cells are AML-like. In about 30%, blast cells have a lymphocytic morphology, express the common ALL antigen (CALLA, *CD10*), and contain terminal deoxynucleotidyltransferase (TdT), which is often found in the cells of patients with ALL.

During transition to the accelerated phase, Ph$^1$ appears in 100% of hematopoietic cells; in 80% of patients, additional chromosomal abnormalities develop, resulting in cells with modal chromosome numbers of 47 to 50. In patients with only a single new chromosome change, this involves acquisition of a second Ph$^1$, isochromosome for the long arm of 17, +8, +19, or t(15;17), in descending order of frequency. Isochromosome 17 is almost always associated with a mutation of the p53 tumor-suppressor gene. Chromosomal loss occurs rarely, usually as −7, with an incidence of only 3%.

## PROGNOSIS AND STAGING

For most CML patients, disease progression is divisible into three stages: the chronic phase, in which hematologic progression is generally predictable and uniform; the accelerated phase, marked by the beginning of transformation to an acute leukemia-like illness; and the terminal blast crisis, manifested by blast forms predominating in marrow and blood and, possibly, in most other organs. About 20% of patients have no discernible accelerated phase, and their disease abruptly transforms from chronic to blast phase.

Prognosis has improved in more recent cohorts of CML

patients because of earlier diagnosis, improved therapy, and better supportive care. With routine screening tests, more patients are diagnosed in the asymptomatic phase, often with low tumor loads. Analyses of a cohort of 830 CML patients have shown significant changes in the presenting features of patients seen before 1983 in contrast to those seen since 1983.[46] These include an increase in the percentage of patients with asymptomatic disease (15% vs. 37%, $p<0.01$) and a decrease in the percentage with splenomegaly (76% vs. 54%, $p<0.01$), hepatomegaly (46% vs. 18%, $p<0.01$), white cell count of $100 \times 10^9/L$ (69% vs. 56%, $p<0.01$), and marrow blasts less than 5% (16% vs. 9%, $p<0.01$).

The current median survival in CML is about 50 to 60 months and is highly dependent on therapy. The survival rates are 75 to 85% at 3 years and 50 to 60% at 5 years. Patients treated with hydroxyurea have mortality rates of 5 to 10% during the first year after diagnosis. The mortality rate increases during the second year, and thereafter it is approximately 25% per year.[47] These rates of development of blast crises are significantly lower in patients receiving interferon alfa therapy.

Most treated CML patients are symptom free until accelerated or blast phase develops. The median survival in the blast phase is usually 2 months if the patient does not experience a remission. Approximately 30% of patients in the blast phase have a remission following cytotoxic therapy, and survival in these patients lasts an average of 7 months.

Several staging systems based on multivariate studies of different risk factors and prognosis have been proposed for CML.[48–54] Characteristics associated with a poor prognosis include age of 60 years or more, black race, poor performance status, anemia, high or low platelet count ($<150 \times 10^9/L$ or $>700 \times 10^9/L$), high proportion of blasts and promyelocytes or basophils in the peripheral blood, high proportion of marrow blasts ($\geq5\%$) or marrow basophils ($\geq3\%$), decreased marrow megakaryocytes, and cytogenetic abnormalities in addition to Ph[1]. Prognostic models that categorize CML patients into good (median survival, 5 to 6 years), intermediate (median survival, 3 to 4 years), or poor risk (median survival, 2 years) groups are of major clinical significance.[53]

## Treatment

### CHRONIC PHASE

The introduction of busulfan (1953), hydroxyurea (1972), and interferon alfa (1986) as first-line therapeutic agents in chronic phase CML has proved to mark successive improvements in median survival. Data have clearly shown the superiority of hydroxyurea over busulfan and the superiority of interferon alfa over either agent. Allogeneic bone marrow transplantation (BMT) is curative for most patients who possess a donor but is associated with a high early mortality. The technology of allogeneic BMT is also in a state of flux with the development of unrelated BMT, haploidentical BMT, unrelated cord blood transplantation, nonmyeloablative transplant regimens, and donor leukocyte infusions.

As a result, the appropriate initial treatment strategy for a patient presenting with chronic phase CML remains contro-

versial, with strong institutional biases present in the literature. Busulfan has proved to be superior to irradiation or other drugs such as melphalan, 6-mercaptopurine and chlorambucil, and it provides inexpensive good disease control with moderate toxicity when administered orally.[55] It is associated with skin pigmentation; unpredictably prolonged myelosuppression (10% of patients); and, rarely, organ fibrosis (pulmonary, cardiac, marrow) and an Addison's disease–like syndrome.

Busulfan and hydroxyurea produce hematologic remissions in greater than 80% of patients with chronic phase CML. These agents usually have no effect on the cytogenetic status of the marrow, and persistence of Ph[1]-positive cells in most ($>90\%$) marrow metaphases is the norm. Ph[1] suppression has been observed occasionally when unpredictable prolonged myelosuppression is induced by busulfan therapy. With single-agent hydroxyurea therapy, cytogenetic responses occur in less than 1% of patients and are minor and transient.[44]

The clear superiority of hydroxyurea over busulfan in terms of contribution to prolongation of survival has been established by a prospective randomized study conducted in 409 previously untreated chronic phase CML patients.[44] These patients were entered in the study between July 1983 and January 1991 by the German CML group and randomized to therapy with either busulfan or hydroxyurea.

Of 409 study patients in whom marrow cytogenetics were performed, 90.7% were Ph[1]-positive. The percentage of Ph[1] patients in the low-risk, intermediate-risk, and high-risk groups according to Sokal's prognostic subgrouping was 26%, 38%, and 36%. These subgroupings were highly predictive of survival, with median survivals of 6.5 years, 4.5 years, and 3 years ($p<0.0001$). The median survival of the Ph[1]-positive patients treated with busulfan was 45.4 months; this was in contrast to those treated with hydroxyurea, in whom it was 58.2 months ($p=0.008$). The median survival of all study patients (Ph[1]-positive, Ph[1]-negative, cytogenetic status unknown) treated with busulfan was 43.6 months, in contrast to the equivalent patient group treated with hydroxyurea, in whom it was 56.2 months ($p=0.01$). The median duration of chronic phase (as defined by time to blast phase or resistance to frontline therapy) in all study patients treated with busulfan was 37 months, in contrast to the equivalent group treated with hydroxyurea, in whom it was 47 months ($p=0.04$). The significant survival advantage conferred by hydroxyurea was evident in all Sokal prognostic subgroups.

Sixty-four patients became resistant to frontline therapy (busulfan in 41, hydroxyurea in 23) before developing blast phase disease and were crossed over to therapy with the alternative agent. The median survival from time of crossover of those patients treated with busulfan, having failed hydroxyurea, was 2.45 years; in contrast, those treated with hydroxyurea, having failed busulfan, survived for a median 0.9 years ($p=0.002$). Eleven patients (17%) developed overt blast crisis within 1 month of therapy crossover, and their resistance to frontline therapy was a manifestation of accelerated phase disease. Patients (25%) whose reason for crossover of therapy was the development of peripheral cytopenias or marrow aplasia, or both, were all in the busulfan primary therapy group. Although these are complicating factors, the dates do suggest that busulfan therapy may have a role for patients who become overtly resistant to hydroxyurea. Except for this circumstance or when it is used as a component of conditioning therapy for BMT, busulfan has no current role in the therapy of CML.

Many factors may contribute to the superiority of hydroxyurea over busulfan. Busulfan is known to be leukemogenic in other myeloproliferative disorders (e.g., polycythemia vera), whereas hydroxyurea has little known ability to be leukemogenic. Hydroxyurea can be used to maintain a lower white cell count than busulfan, and this more rigid control may, in turn, reflect less tumor burden. A relevant hypothesis may be that the lower the tumor burden, the less the chance of blast transformation because the number of proliferating malignant cells available for further mutations decreases as the overall tumor bulk decreases. Perhaps the greater the degree of prolonged reduction of white cell count in CML, the better the survival, regardless of the cytostatic agent used. Such a thesis needs to be addressed in future studies.

The initial studies of single-agent recombinant or nonrecombinant interferon alfa therapy of chronic phase CML recorded complete hematologic response (CHR) rates of 70 to 80% and cytogenetic response rates of 30 to 40%.[56–58] Cytogenetic responses are usually categorized as complete if no Ph¹-positive cells are detected in the marrow; major, if they are detectable in 1 to 34% of metaphases; and minor, if they are detectable in 35 to 90% of marrow metaphases. Single-agent interferon alfa studies were followed by attempts to combine it with other biologic agents, intensive combination chemotherapy regimens, hydroxyurea, and low-dose cytosine arabinoside (ara-C).[59–63] The median survival of 313 early chronic phase CML patients treated in a series of single-arm studies with interferon alfa regimens at the M.D. Anderson Cancer Center was 65 months.[47] Many other studies have confirmed that interferon alfa achieves CHRs in 70 to 80% of patients, cytogenetic responses in 30 to 40%, and major cytogenetic responses in 20 to 25%.[64–67]

Differences in the reported rates of CHR and cytogenetic response in various studies may be related to the CML phase in which patients are treated, the patient risk group and pretreatment characteristics, and the dose schedule of interferon alfa (Table 86–2). In early chronic phase CML, interferon alfa at a dose of 5 million U/m² daily, or at the lower maximally tolerated individual dose, was found to be necessary to achieve optimal CHR and cytogenetic response rates.[68] The unique ability of interferon alfa to achieve a 20 to 25% complete cytogenetic remission rate in a non-BMT setting may well explain its positive effect on median survival in CML.

In an analysis of 49 patients achieving cytogenetic responses for periods of 2 to 8 years, 4 had lost their cytogenetic response and reverted to 90% or more Ph¹-positive metaphases.[47] Thirty-four (69%) patients were in ongoing complete cytogenetic remission. Sixteen of the 34 patients had stopped interferon alfa therapy because of toxicities (5 patients) or either patient or physician choice (11 patients). At the time of reporting, 57% of patients were in continuous complete cytogenetic remission either on or off interferon alfa therapy, whereas 80% had a durable major cytogenetic response. Accounting for the time to achieve the maximal cytogenetic response (median time 22 months for complete, 18 months for major, and 12 months for minor), the duration of cytogenetic response was longest in patients achieving a complete cytogenetic response. PCR studies for *bcr-abl* were positive in all M.D. Anderson patients who had complete cytogenetic remissions while on interferon alfa therapy.[69] This level of residual disease may not be clinically relevant because it does not predict consistently for subsequent relapse. Among patients studied after allogeneic BMT, more than 75% have at least one positive PCR result within 12 months post-BMT, and 40 to 50% are positive at 12 months. Only 25% of the latter group go on to develop overt CML relapse.[70–78] Interferon alfa is effective at suppressing cytogenetic and clinical relapse after allogeneic BMT.[79–81]

The clear superiority of interferon alfa over hydroxyurea has been established by a prospective randomized study conducted in 322 previously untreated chronic phase CML patients by the Italian Cooperative Study Group on Chronic Myeloid Leukemia.[48] These patients were randomized to receive interferon alfa 5 million U/m²/day (218 patients) or hydroxyurea (104 patients) as induction and maintenance treatment. At 2 years' follow-up on this study, interferon alfa was associated with a reduction in the rate of development of blast phase disease (27% in the hydroxyurea cohort vs. 19% in the interferon alfa patients). At 4 years, 25% of interferon

*Table 86–2.* **Parameters Associated with Differences in Response to Interferon Alfa in Philadelphia Chromosome–Positive Chronic Myelogenous Leukemia**

| Parameter | Category | CHR (%) | Cytogenetic Response (%) | |
| | | | ANY | MAJOR |
|---|---|---|---|---|
| CML phase (interferon alfa 5 Mu/m² daily) | Early chronic | 60–80 | 40–50 | 20–30 |
| | Late chronic | 50–60 | 10–20 | <10 |
| | Accelerated | 30–40 | <10 | 0 |
| | Blast | 5–10 | <10 | 0 |
| Risk category in early chronic phase | Low | 80–90 | 60 | 40 |
| | Intermediate | 50–60 | 40 | 20–30 |
| | High | 20–60 | 10–20 | 5–10 |
| Dose of interferon alfa | 5 Mu/m² daily | 80 | 50–60 | 40 |
| | 5 Mu/m² Tiw | 70 | 40 | 20 |
| | 2 Mu/m² Tiw | 30–40 | 20 | 5–10 |
| | <2 Mu/m² Tiw | 20–30 | <10 | 0 |

CHR, complete hematologic remission; CML, chronic myelogenous leukemia; Mu, million units; Tiw, subcutaneously 3 times weekly.

alfa–treated patients had major cytogenetic responses compared with none in hydroxyurea-treated patients. Of patients who had a cytogenetic response, 85% were alive at 5 years in contrast to 40% survival among those with no cytogenetic response ($p = 0.0001$). The median survival of the $Ph^1$-positive patients treated with hydroxyurea was 49 months, in contrast to those treated with interferon alfa, in whom it was not reached at 60 months ($p = 0.004$). The superior median survival for the interferon alfa cohort held for the low-risk to intermediate-risk prognostic subgroup (not reached vs. 50 months, $p = 0.004$) and the high-risk group (56 months vs. 38 months, $p = 0.02$).

The French CML Study Group performed a randomized study of interferon alfa alone versus interferon alfa together with ara-C.[63] Patient selection depended, in part, on age and risk factors (Sokal score) and the presence or absence of a matched sibling donor; 745 patients were randomized. The interferon alfa plus ara-C group had more CHRs (66% vs. 55%), more major cytogenetic responses (41% vs. 24%), and more complete cytogenetic responses (15% vs. 9%) than the interferon alfa group. The probability of cytogenetic response was significantly correlated with risk group. In the interferon alfa plus ara-C group, the major cytogenetic response rate at 12 months was 47% for those at low risk, 39% for those at intermediate risk, and 19% for those at high risk. The probability of major cytogenetic response at 24 months increased to 54% in the interferon alfa plus ara-C group and 41% in the interferon alfa group. At 3 years, the estimated survival rates were 85.7% in the interferon alfa plus ara-C group versus 79.1% in the interferon alfa group. All differences were statistically significant and in favor of interferon alfa plus ara-C. Patients who achieved partial or complete cytogenetic responses lived longer than patients with either no response or minor response. The median survival has not yet been reached.

These studies establish the gold standard for interferon alfa–based treatment strategies for CML but do not address the issue of timing or sequencing of interferon alfa–based strategies and allogeneic BMT. Despite clear evidence of its therapeutic advantage, many significant problems may occur with the use of an optimal dose of interferon alfa.[47] Key issues are toxicity and cost. Patients aged 60 years or older tolerate therapy less well than younger patients. Interferon alfa is associated in most individuals with early flu-like side effects (fever, chills, postnasal drip, anorexia, lack of appetite, bone aches). These are not dose limiting, can be managed symptomatically (bedtime administration, acetaminophen), and are minimized by adequate patient education and starting therapy at 50% of the desired dose for the first week. Reducing the initial white cell count counts to less than 20 $10^9$/L with cytotoxic therapy also lessens the leukocytosis-associated side effects (fever, chills, musculoskeletal pains). Tachyphylaxis to the acute adverse effects of interferon alfa usually develops within 1 to 2 weeks.

Delayed adverse effects are dose limiting in 10 to 20% of patients. Adverse effects include persistent fatigue, weight loss, neurotoxicity, depression, insomnia, alopecia, and occasional immune-mediated complications, such as immune-mediated hemolysis or thrombocytopenia, collagen vascular disorders such as rheumatoid arthritis and systemic lupus erythematosus, nephrotic syndromes, and hypothyroidism. Rare cases of cardiac dysfunction (arrhythmias, congestive heart failure) have been reported. Severe autoimmune phenomenon, cardiac dysfunction, refractory depression, or severe neurotoxicity necessitates discontinuation of interferon alfa therapy. Immune-mediated thyroid disease does not require interferon alfa discontinuation and may be managed by standard therapy.[82] Interferon alfa dose reductions are required for grade 3 or 4 toxicity (50% dose reduction after recovery) or a persistent grade 2 toxicity that is not improved by symptomatic support (25% dose reduction).

## BONE MARROW TRANSPLANTATION

The selection of candidates for allogeneic BMT and the timing of the procedure remain controversial. Approximately one third of patients younger than 55 years of age have an appropriately matched sibling donor, and 50% of the remainder have a matched unrelated donor. Transplant-related mortality increases with age. Matched related donor BMT can clearly eradicate $Ph^1$-positive disease and results in long-term survival for 55 to 75% of patients.[83-90] Relapse rates post–matched related donor BMT range from 13 to 20%. Actuarial survival postrelapse has been reported as 36% at 6 years; this rate probably does not reflect current technology. Twelve of 28 patients who had a second allogeneic matched related donor BMT for relapsed CML died from transplant-related toxicity and 5 died from recurrent leukemia. Long-term survival was 25%.[91]

Matched unrelated donor BMT is also curative in CML, with long-term survival rates of 40 to 60%.[92-96] Relapse rates are lower, but transplant-related mortality and morbidity are higher. The development of high-resolution molecular typing is likely to improve donor selection and improve transplant-related mortality, while reducing donor availability. Unrelated cord blood transplant offers the hope of expanding the donor pool by increasing the tolerable degree of human leukocyte antigen (HLA) mismatching; however, it remains to be seen how well adults would engraft with a small dose of cells, and the relative lack of graft-versus-host disease (GVHD) may result in an increased relapse of CML post-transplant.

The risk of relapse after BMT has been closely correlated with immune disparities between recipient and donor—the *graft versus leukemia* effect. The highest risk for relapse is seen with syngeneic BMT and T cell–depleted BMT, next highest with allogeneic matched related donor BMT without GVHD, then allogeneic BMT with GVHD, and lowest with matched unrelated donor BMT. These observations led to studies of augmentation of the immune response in patients with relapsed CML after BMT. Interferon alfa can reverse cytogenetic relapse; however, the treatment of choice currently is donor leukocyte infusion.

Response rates for donor leukocyte infusion are 60 to 73% and were durable in 87 to 89% of patients.[97, 98] Fatal GVHD can occur. The incidence of GVHD is associated with the dose of infused T lymphocytes. Some patients respond to lower doses of T lymphocytes; a dose of $1 \times 10^7$ T lymphocytes/kg is recommended initially.[99] The success of donor leukocyte infusion therapy has led to interest in nonmyeloablative conditioning regimens. This approach remains experimental but has the possibility of reducing substantially transplant-related mortality, particularly in the older population.

A variety of BMT-related variables have an effect on the outcome of transplantation for CML. The busulfan and cytoxan regimen is at least equivalent and may be superior to total-body irradiation and Cytoxan as a conditioning regimen. The addition of a short course of methotrexate to the GVHD prophylactic regimen clearly decreases the relapse rate after BMT. Several articles have suggested that interferon alfa has an adverse effect on the results of allogeneic BMT, and this adverse effect is related to the duration of therapy with interferon alfa. This issue is unresolved.[100–102]

## ACCELERATED AND BLAST PHASES

Although therapies for accelerated and blast phases are discussed together as per most current literature, ample evidence exists that future studies should address these as distinct phases. Patients whose only sign of accelerated phase disease is cytogenetic progression have a better prognosis than patients with overt transition from chronic phase. With the onset of blast phase, resistance to all available chronic phase therapies is evident. The lack of efficacy of regimens used in acute myeloid leukemia is dramatically illustrated by the observation that 70% of blast phase patients relapse after they receive *marrow ablative* therapy as allogeneic BMT conditioning. With current results (15 to 25% disease-free survival in accelerated phase, 5 to 15% in blast phase), all eligible patients with accelerated phase disease should be offered allogeneic BMT. In blast phase, improvements in survival are needed before allogeneic BMT can be recommended.

Of the 30% of patients who have a lymphoblastoid blast transformation, approximately 30 to 50% respond to chemotherapy.[103] At least two or three courses of ALL induction-like therapy should be given to these patients before their disease is judged to be refractory. Approximately 70% of patients who are TdT-positive respond to vincristine and prednisone, whereas less than 10% of TdT-negative patients show improvement. If remission is achieved, the marrow morphology and karyotype revert to the chronic phase of Ph[1]-positive CML. Allogeneic BMT should be offered to these patients, when possible. For patients with lymphoblastoid blast phase disease, oral methotrexate 15 to 20 mg/m[2] twice weekly or oral hydroxyurea 20 to 30 mg/kg as a single daily dose may be effective. Monthly doses of vincristine, with or without prednisone, appear to be essential for prolonged maintenance of remission. Meningeal leukemia is a major problem in blast phase patients who respond to initial therapy. Treatment is with twice-weekly intrathecal injection of ara-C 100 mg or with methotrexate 10 to 15 mg with or without leucovorin rescue 12 to 15 mg/m[2] given orally or parenterally beginning 24 hours after the instillation of intrathecal methotrexate and continuing for 48 hours. Either drug is given until the spinal fluid pleocytosis clears. This treatment is followed by weekly intrathecal maintenance therapy, after which twice monthly, then monthly maintenance therapy is instituted. Cranial irradiation (24 Gy) should be given, especially when cranial nerve deficits are present. The role of prophylactic central nervous system therapy has not been defined. Other extramedullary sites of blast transformation, such as skin, bones, or lymph nodes, are usually radiosensitive and can be controlled with radiotherapy.

Some CML patients have an abrupt onset of blast phase associated with a rapidly rising white cell count. If leukostasis occurs, daily hydroxyurea 50 to 75 mg/kg, cytosine arabinoside 2 to 4 mg/kg every 12 hours, and aggressive leukapheresis may be used. Splenectomy in advanced CML is associated with increased morbidity and mortality without any obvious therapeutic benefit; splenic irradiation, however, may be effective for some patients as a palliative measure. Patients who enter the accelerated or blast phase of CML should, when possible, be offered investigational therapy. For most patients, supportive measures alone are the mainstay of management.

## EXPERIMENTAL THERAPIES

High-dose chemotherapy with autologous stem cell transplantation is under investigation at several centers. Ph[1]-negative cells persist in the marrow during the chronic phase of CML, and selective transplantation of Ph[1]-negative cells using a variety of strategies is desirable. Patients become Ph[1]-negative, but essentially all patients relapse with CML. Transplanted patients appear to be living longer than expected, although this remains to be proved.[104–114]

A variety of therapies are attempting to target *bcr-abl* as a disease-specific marker. These techniques include antisense approaches, ribozymes, specific tyrosine kinase inhibitors, and immune therapies. Preliminary data with tyrosine kinase inhibitors appear particularly encouraging. The development of these novel therapeutic approaches is a source of ongoing excitement in the study of CML.

## TREATMENT SUMMARY

Most centers now use an algorithmic approach to the treatment of CML with an attempt to individualize therapy based on risk factors for disease and therapy.[115, 116] Our current practice is that patients younger than 45 years old with a 6/6 or 5/6 HLA-matched sibling should be offered BMT within the first year after diagnosis. Patients between 45 and 55 years old with a high Sokal score and a matched sibling should also receive BMT within 1 year of diagnosis. Patients older than age 55 should not receive BMT except in the context of a clinical trial. All other patients should receive a trial of interferon alfa and ara-C for at least 12 months. Patients who have not shown a major cytogenetic response after 12 months should receive matched unrelated donor BMT if an appropriate donor is available. Unrelated cord blood transplantation remains experimental, as does autologous stem cell transplantation. Patients who do not have a donor and who have not had a cytogenetic response to interferon alfa and ara-C should be continued on this regimen for at least another 12 months and possibly indefinitely.

## SUGGESTIONS FOR ADDITIONAL READING

Sawyers CL. Chronic myeloid leukemia. N Engl J Med 1999;340:1330–40.
Lee SJ, Anasetti C, Horowitz MM, Antin JH. Initial therapy for chronic

myelogenous leukemia: playing the odds. J Clin Oncol 1998;16:2897–903. editorial.

Faderl S, Talpaz M, Estrov Z, et al. The biology of chronic myeloid leukemia. N Engl J Med 1999;341:164–72.

McGlave PB, De Fabritiis P, Deisseroth A, et al. Autologous transplants for chronic myelogenous leukaemia: results from eight transplant groups. Lancet 1994;343:1486–8.

Kolb HJ, Schattenberg A, Goldman JM, et al. Graft-versus-leukemia effect of donor lymphocyte transfusions in marrow grafted patients. European Group for Blood and Marrow Transplantation Working Party Chronic Leukemia. Blood 1995;86:2041–50.

Delforge M, Boogaerts MA, McGlave PB, et al. BCR/ABL-CD34(+)HLA-DR-progenitor cells in early chronic phase, but not in more advanced phases, of chronic myelogenous leukemia are polyclonal. Blood 1999;93:284–92.

Ringdén O, Remberger M, Runde V, et al. Peripheral blood stem cell transplantation from unrelated donors: a comparison with marrow transplantation. Blood 1999;94:455–64.

Guilhot F, Chastang C, Michallet M, et al. Interferon alfa-2b combined with cytarabine versus interferon alone in chronic myelogenous leukemia. French Chronic Myeloid Leukemia Study Group. N Engl J Med 1997;337:223–9.

# REFERENCES

1. SEER Cancer Statistics Review 1973–1996. (see http://www.seer.ims. nci.nih.gov.)

2. Sandberg AA. Chromosomes and causation of human cancer and leukemia: XL. the Ph1 and other translocations in CML. Cancer 1980;46:2221–6.

3. Heisterkamp N, Groffen J, Stephenson JR, et al. Chromosomal localization of human cellular homologues of two viral oncogenes. Nature 1982;299:747–9.

4. De Kelin A, van Kessel AG, Grosveld G, et al. A cellular oncogene is translocated to the Philadelphia chromosome in chronic myelocytic leukaemia. Nature 1982;300:765–7.

5. Shtivelman E, Lifshitz B, Gale RP, Canaani E. Fused transcript of abl and bcr genes in chronic myelogenous leukaemia. Nature 1985;315:550–4.

6. Heisterkamp N, Stam K, Groffen J, et al. Structural organization of the bcr gene and its role in the Ph¹ translocation. Nature 1985;315:758–61.

7. Kurzrock R, Gutterman JU, Talpaz M. The molecular genetics of Philadelphia chromosome-positive leukemias. N Engl J Med 1988;319:990–8.

8. Prakash O, Yunis JJ. High resolution chromosomes of the t(9;22) positive leukemias. Cancer Genet Cytogenet 1984;11:361–7.

9. Stam K Jr, Heisterkamp N, Grosveld G, et al. Evidence of a new chimeric bcr/c-abl mRNA in patients with chronic myelocytic leukemia and the Philadelphia chromosome. N Engl J Med 1985;313:1429–33.

10. Davis RL, Konopka JB, Witte ON. Activation of the c-abl oncogene by viral transduction or chromosomal translocation generates altered c-abl proteins with similar in vitro kinase properties. Mol Cell Biol 1985;5:204–13.

11. Heisterkamp N, Stephenson JR, Groffen J, et al. Localization of the c-abl oncogene adjacent to a translocation break point in chronic myelocytic leukemia. Nature 1983;306:239–42.

12. Groffen J, Stephenson JR, Heisterkamp N, et al. Philadelphia chromosomal breakpoints are clustered within a limited region, bcr, on chromosome 22. Cell 1984;36:93–9.

13. Teyssier JR, Bartram CR, Deville J, et al. c-abl Oncogene and chromosome 22 "bcr" juxtaposition in chronic myelogenous leukemia. N Engl J Med 1985;312:1393–4.

14. Leibowitz D, Schaefer-Rego K, Popenoe DW, et al. Variable breakpoints on the Philadelphia chromosome in chronic myelogenous leukemia. Blood 1985;66:243–5.

15. Schaefer-Rego K, Dudek H, Popenoe D, et al. CML patients in blast crisis have breakpoints localized to a specific region of the BCR. Blood 1987;70:448–55.

16. Mills KI, MacKenzie ED, Birnie GD. The site of the breakpoint within the bcr is a prognostic factor in Philadelphia-positive CML patients. Blood 1988;72:1237–41.

17. Opalka B, Wandl U, Beer U, et al. Breakpoint localization within the M-bcr and clinical course do not correlate in patients with chronic

myelogenous leukemia undergoing alfa interferon therapy. Leukemia 1991;5:452–6.

18. Mills KI, Benn P, Birnie GD. Does the breakpoint within the major breakpoint cluster region (M-bcr) influence the duration of the chronic phase in chronic myeloid leukemia? An analytical comparison of current literature. Blood 1991;78:1155–61.

19. Inokuchi K, Inoue T, Tojo A, et al. A possible correlation between the type of bcr-abl hybrid messenger RNA and platelet count in Philadelphia-positive chronic myelogenous leukemia. Blood 1991;78:3125–7.

20. Goyns MH, Young BD, van Kessel AG, et al. Regional mapping of the human immunoglobulin lambda light chain to the Philadelphia chromosome in chronic myeloid leukaemia. Leuk Res 1984;8:547–53.

21. Gordon MY, Dowding CR, Riley GP, et al. Altered adhesive interactions with marrow stroma of haematopoietic progenitor cells in chronic myeloid leukaemia. Nature 1987;328:342–4.

22. Schlossman SF, Chess L, Humphreys RE, Strominger JL. Distribution of Ia-like molecules on the surface of normal and leukemic human cells. Proc Natl Acad Sci U S A 1976;73:1288–92.

23. Verfaillie CM, McCarthy JB, McGlave PB. Mechanisms underlying abnormal trafficking of malignant progenitors in chronic myelogenous leukemia: decreased adhesion to stroma and fibronectin but increased adhesion to the basement membrane components laminin and collagen type IV. J Clin Invest 1992;90:1232–41.

24. Dowding C, Guo AP, Osterholz J, et al. Interferon-alpha overrides the deficient adhesion of chronic myeloid leukemia primitive progenitor cells to bone marrow stromal cells. Blood 1991;78:499–505.

25. Upadhyaya G, Guba SC, Sih SA, et al. Interferon-alpha restores the deficient expression of the cytoadhesion molecule lymphocyte function antigen-3 by chronic myelogenous leukemia progenitor cells. J Clin Invest 1991;88:2131–6.

26. Strife A, Lambek C, Wisniewski D, et al. Discordant maturation as the primary biological defect in chronic myeloid leukemia. Cancer Res 1988;48:1035–41 and 3298.

27. McLaughlin J, Chianese E, Witte ON. In vitro transformation of immature hematopoietic cells by the P210 BCR/ABL oncogene product of the Philadelphia chromosome. Proc Natl Acad Sci U S A 1987;84:6558–62.

28. Hariharan IK, Harris AW, Crawford M, et al. A bcr-v-abl oncogene induces lymphomas in transgenic mice. Mol Cell Biol 1989;9:2798–805.

29. Daley GQ, Van Etten RA, Baltimore D. Induction of chronic myelogenous leukemia in mice by the P210bcr/abl gene of the Philadelphia chromosome. Science 1990;247:824–30.

30. Puil L, Liu J, Gish G, et al. Bcr-Abl oncoproteins bind directly to activators of the Ras signalling pathway. EMBO J 1994;13:764–73.

31. Sirard C, Laneuville P, Dick JE. Expression of bcr-abl abrogates factor-dependent growth of human hemaotpoietic M07E cells by an autocrine mechanism. Blood 1994;83:1575–85.

32. McGahon A, Bissonnette R, Schmitt M, et al. BCR-ABL maintains resistance of chronic myelogenous leukemia cells to apoptotic cell death. Blood 1994;83:1179–87.

33. Faderl S, Talpaz M, Estrov Z, et al. The biology of chronic myeloid leukemia. N Engl J Med 1999;341:164–72.

34. Chan LC, Karhi KK, Rayter SI, et al. A novel abl protein expressed in Philadelphia chromosome positive acute lymphoblastic leukaemia. Nature 1987;325:635–7.

35. Secker-Walker LM, Cooke HM, Browett PJ, et al. Variable Philadelphia breakpoints and potential lineage restriction of bcr rearrangement in acute lymphoblastic leukaemia. Blood 1988;72:784–91.

36. Ezdinli EZ, Sokal JE, Crosswhite L, Sandberg AA. Philadelphia-chromosome-positive and -negative chronic myelocytic leukemia. Ann Intern Med 1970;72:175–82.

37. Cortez D, Reuther G, Pendergast AM. The Bcr-Abl tyrosine kinase activates mitogenic signaling pathways and stimulates G1-to-S phase transition in hematopoietic cells. Oncogene 1997;15:2333–42.

38. Wang TY, Raza A, Sait SN, et al. A t(11;21)(13;q22) in Ph-positive chronic myelogenous leukemia. Cancer Genet Cytogenet 1988;31:187–91.

39. Goldman JM, Shiota F, Th'ng KH, et al. Circulating granulocytic and erythroid progenitor cells in chronic granulocytic leukaemia. Br J Haematol 1980;46:7–13.

40. Martin H, Hibbin JA, Dowding C, et al. Purification of haemopoietic progenitor cells from patients with chronic granulocytic leukaemia using percoll density gradients and elutriation. Br J Haematol 1986;63:187–98.

41. Tornyos K. Phagocytic activity of cells of the inflammatory exudate in human leukemia. Cancer Res 1967;27:1756–60.

42. Zittoun J, Zittoun R, Marquet J, Sultan C. The three transcobalamins in myeloproliferative disorders and acute leukaemia. Br J Haematol 1975;31:287–98.

43 Hehlmann R, Heimpel H, Hasford J, et al. Randomized comparison of busulfan and hydroxyurea in chronic myelogenous leukemia: prolongation of survival by hydroxyurea. The German CML Study Group. Blood 1993;82:398–407.

44. Greenberg BR, Wilson FD, Woo L, Jenks HM. Cytogenetics of fibroblastic colonies in Ph1-positive chronic myelogenous leukemia. Blood 1978;51:1039–44.

45. Kantarjian HM, Keating MJ, Talpaz M, et al. Chronic myelogenous leukemia in blast crisis: analysis of 242 patients. Am J Med 1987;83:445–54.

46. Kantarjian HM, Deisseroth A, Kurzrock R, et al. Chronic myelogenous leukemia: a concise update. Blood 1993;82:691–703.

47. Sokal JE, Cox EB, Baccarani M, et al. Prognostic discrimination in "good-risk" chronic granulocytic leukemia. Blood 1984;63:789–99.

48. Tura S, Baccarani M, Corbelli G. Staging of chronic myeloid leukemia. Br J Haematol 1981;47:105–19.

49. Cervantes F, Rozman C. A multivariate analysis of prognostic factors in chronic myeloid leukemia. Blood 1982;60:1298–304.

50. Wareham NJ, Johnso SA, Goldman JM. Relationship of the duration of the chronic phase in chronic granulocytic leukaemia to the need for treatment during the first year after diagnosis. Cancer Chemother Pharmacol 1982;8:205–10.

51. Sokal JE, Baccarani M, Tura S, et al. Prognostic discrimination among younger patients with chronic granulocytic leukemia: relevance to bone marrow transplantation. Blood 1985;66:1352–7.

52. Kantarjian HM, Smith TL, McCredie KB, et al. Chronic myelogenous leukemia: a multivariate analysis of the associations of patient characteristics and therapy with survival. Blood 1985;66:1326–35.

53. Prabhu M, Kochupillai V, Sharma S, et al. Prognostic assessment of various parameters in chronic myeloid leukemia. Cancer 1986;58:1357–60.

54. Sokal JE, Gomez GA, Baccarani M, et al. Prognostic significance of additional cytogenetic abnormalities at diagnosis of Philadelphia chromosome-positive chronic granulocytic leukemia. Blood 1988;72:294–8.

55. Anonymous. Treatment of chronic granulocytic leukemia. Br Med J 1968;1:196–7. editorial.

56. Talpaz M, McCredie KB, Mavligit GM, Gutterman JU. Leukocyte interferon-induced myeloid cytoreduction in chronic myelogenous leukemia. Blood 1983;62:689–92.

57. Talpaz M, Kantarjian HM, McCredie K, et al. Hematologic remission and cytogenetic improvement induced by recombinant human interferon alpha A in chronic myelogenous leukemia. N Engl J Med 1986;314:1065–9.

58. Talpaz M, Kantarjian HM, McCredie KB, et al. Clinical investigation of human alpha interferon in chronic myelogenous leukemia. Blood 1987;69:1280–8.

59. Talpaz M, Kurzrock R, Kantarjian H, et al. A phase II study alternating alpha-2a-interferon and gamma-interferon therapy in patients with chronic myelogenous leukemia. Cancer 1991;68:2125–30.

60. Giles FJ, Aitchison R, Syndercombe-Court D, et al. Recombinant alpha 2B interferon in combination with oral chemotherapy in late chronic phase chronic myeloid leukaemia. Leuk Lymph 1992;7:99–102.

61. Kantarjian HM, Talpaz M, LeMaistre CF, et al. Intensive combination chemotherapy and autologous bone marrow transplantation leads to the reappearance of Philadelphia chromosome-negative cells in chronic myelogenous leukemia. Cancer 1991;67:2959–65.

62. Kantarjian HM, Keating MJ, Estey EH, et al. Treatment of advanced stages of Philadelphia chromosome-positive chronic myelogenous leukemia with interferon-alpha and low-dose cytarabine. J Clin Oncol 1992;10:772–8.

63. Guilhot F, Lamagnère JP, Harousseau JL, et al. Interferon Alfa-2b combined with cytarabine versus interferon alone in chronic myelogenous leukemia. N Engl J Med 1997;337:223–9.

64. Alimena G, Morra E, Lazzarino M, et al. Interferon alpha-2b as therapy for Ph'-positive chronic myelogenous leukemia: a study of 82 patients treated with intermittent or daily administration. Blood 1988;72:642–7.

65. Niederle N, Moritz T, Kloke O, et al. Interferon alfa-2b in acute- and chronic-phase chronic myelogenous leukaemia: initial response and long-term results in 54 patients. Eur J Cancer 1991;27:Suppl 4:7–14.

66. Morra E, Alimena G, Lazzarino M, et al. Evolving modalities of treatment with interferon alfa-2b for Ph1-positive chronic myelogenous leukaemia. Eur J Cancer 1991;27:Suppl 4:14–7.

67. Freund M, von Wussow P, Diedrich H, et al. Recombinant human interferon (IFN) alpha-2b in chronic myelogenous leukaemia: dose dependency of response and frequency of neutralizing anti-interferon antibodies. Br J Haematol 1989;72:350–6.

68. Talpaz M, Kantarjian H, Kurzrock R, et al. Interferon-alpha produces sustained cytogenetic responses in chronic myelogenous leukemia: Philadelphia chromosome-positive patients. Ann Intern Med 1991;114:532–8.

69. Lee MS, Kantarjian H, Talpaz M, et al. Detection of minimal residual disease by polymerase chain reaction in Philadelphia chromosome-positive chronic myelogenous leukemia following interferon therapy. Blood 1992;79:1920–3.

70. Roth M, Antin JH, Bingham EL, Ginsburg D. Detection of Philadelphia chromosome-positive cells by the polymerase chain reaction following bone marrow transplant for chronic myelogenous leukemia. Blood 1989;74:882–5.

71. Morgan GJ, Hughes T, Janssen JW, et al. Polymerase chain reaction for detection of residual leukaemia. Lancet 1989;1:928–9.

72. Lange W, Snyder DS, Castro R, et al. Detection by enzymatic amplification of bcr-abl mRNA in peripheral blood and bone marrow cells of patients with chronic myelogenous leukemia. Blood 1989;73:1735–41.

73. Hughes TP, Morgan GJ, Martiat P, Goldman JM. Detection of residual leukemia after bone marrow transplant for chronic myeloid leukemia: role of polymerase chain reaction in predicting relapse. Blood 1991;77:874–8.

74. Negrin RS, Blume KG. The use of the polymerase chain reaction for the detection of minimal residual malignant disease. Blood 1991;78:225–8.

75. Opalka B, Wandl UB, Becher R, et al. Minimal residual disease in patients with chronic myelogenous leukemia undergoing long-term treatment with recombinant interferon alpha-2b alone or in combination with interferon gamma. Blood 1991;78:2188–93.

76. Delage R, Soiffer RJ, Dear K, Ritz J. Clinical significance of bcr-abl gene rearrangement detected by polymerase chain reaction after allogeneic bone marrow transplantation in chronic myelogenous leukemia. Blood 1991;78:2759–67.

77. Oguma N, Shigeta C, Takauchi K, et al. Molecular elimination of the minimal residual Ph1 clone with IFN alpha in CML. Lancet 1992;339:557–8.

78. Mahon FX, Daheron L, Malinge MC, et al. Polymerase chain reaction detection of residual disease in chronic myeloid leukemia patients in complete cytogenetic remission under interferon with or without chemotherapy. Leukemia 1992;6:1232–4.

79. Klingemann HG, Grigg AP, Wilkie-Boyd K, et al. Treatment with recombinant interferon (alpha-2b) early after bone marrow transplantation in patients at high risk for relapse. Blood 1991;78:3306–11 and 1992;79:3397.

80. Higano CS, Raskind WH, Singer JW. Use of alpha interferon for the treatment of relapse of chronic myelogenous leukemia in chronic phase after allogeneic bone marrow transplantation. Blood 1992;80:1437–42.

81. Higano C, Raskind W, Singer J. Alpha interferon (IFN) treatment of cytogenetic-only relapse of chronic myelogenous leukemia (CML) after marrow transplantation (BMT). Proc ASCO 1993;12:307.

82. Giles FJ, Worman CP, Jewell AP, Goldstone AH. Recombinant alpha-interferons, thyroid irradiation and thyroid disease. Acta Haematol 1991;85:160–3.

83. Thomas ED, Clift RA, Fefer A, et al. Marrow transplantation for the treatment of chronic myelogenous leukemia. Ann Intern Med 1986;104:155–63.

84. Doney K, Buckner CD, Sale GE, et al. Treatment of chronic granulocytic leukemia by chemotherapy, total body irradiation and allogeneic bone marrow transplantation. Exp Hematol 1978;6:738–47.

85. Fefer A, Cheever MA, Thomas ED, et al. Disappearance of Ph1-positive cells in four patients with chronic granulocytic leukemia after chemotherapy, irradiation and marrow transplantation from an identical twin. N Engl J Med 1979;300:333–7.

86. Doney KC, Buckner CD, Thomas ED, et al. Allogeneic bone marrow transplantation for chronic granulocytic leukemia. Exp Hematol 1981;9:966–71.

87. Fefer A, Cheever MA, Greenberg PD, et al. Treatment of chronic

granulocytic leukemia with chemoradiotherapy and transplantation of marrow from identical twins. N Engl J Med 1982;306:63–8.

88. Clift RA, Buckner CD, Thomas ED, et al. Treatment of chronic granulocytic leukaemia in chronic phase by allogeneic marrow transplantation. Lancet 1982;2:621–3.

89. Goldman JM, Baughan AS, McCarthy DM, et al. Marrow transplantation for patients in the chronic phase of chronic granulocytic leukaemia. Lancet 1982;2:623–5.

90. Gale PG, Horowitz MM, Ash RC, et al. Identical-twin bone marrow transplants for leukemia. Ann Intern Med 1994;120:646–52.

91. Radich JP, Sanders JE, Buckner CD, et al. Second allogeneic marrow transplantation for patients with recurrent leukemia after initial transplant with total-body irradiation-containing regimens. J Clin Oncol 1993;11:304–13.

92. Beatty PG, Clift RA, Mickelson EM, et al. Marrow transplantation from related donors other than HLA-identical siblings. N Engl J Med 1985;313:765–71.

93. Beatty PG, Anasetti C, Hansen JA, et al. Marrow transplantation from unrelated donors for treatment of hematologic malignancies: effect of mismatching for one HLA Locus. Blood 1993;81:249–53.

94. Mcglave P, Bartsch G, Anasetti C, et al. Unrelated donor marrow transplantation therapy for chronic myelogenous leukemia: initial experience of the national marrow donor program. Blood 1993;81:543–49.

95. Kernan NA, Bartsch G, Ash RC, et al. Analysis of 462 transplantations from unrelated donors facilitated by the national marrow donor program. N Engl J Med 1993;328:593–601.

96. Hansen JA, Clift RA, Thomas ED, et al. Transplantation of marrow from an unrelated donor to a patient with acute leukemia. N Engl J Med 1980;303:565–7.

97. Collins RH Jr, Shpilberg O, Drobyski WR, et al. Donor leukocyte infusions in 140 patients with relapsed malignancy after allogeneic bone marrow transplantation. J Clin Oncol 1997;15:433–44.

98. Drobyski WR, Keever CA, Roth MS, et al. Salvage immunotherapy using donor leukocyte infusions as treatment for relapsed chronic myelogenous leukemia after allogeneic bone marrow transplantation: efficacy and toxicity of a defined T-cell dose. Blood 1993;82:2310–8.

99. McKinnon S, Papadopoulos EB, Carabasi, MH, et al. Adoptive immunotherapy evaluating escalating doses of donor leukocytes for relapse of chronic myeloid leukemia after bone marrow transplantation: separation of graft-versus-leukemia responses from graft-versus-host disease. Blood 1995;86:1261–8.

100. Morton AJ, Gooley T, Hansen JA, et al. Association between pretransplant interferon-alpha and outcome after unrelated donor marrow transplantation for chronic myelogenous leukemia in chronic phase. Blood 1998;92:394–401.

101. Giralt SA, Kantarjian HM, Talpaz M, et al. Effect of prior interferon alpha therapy on the outcome of allogeneic bone marrow transplantation for chronic myelogenous leukemia. J Clin Oncol 1993;11:1055–61.

102. Beelen DW, Graeven U, Elmaagacli AH, et al. Prolonged administration of interferon-alpha in patients with chronic-phase Philadelphia

chromosome-positive chronic myelogenous leukemia before allogeneic bone marrow transplantation may adversely affect transplant outcome. Blood 1995;85:2981–90.

103. Derderian PM, Kantarjian HM, Talpaz M, et al. Chronic myelogenous leukemia in the lymphoid blastic phase: characteristics, treatment response, and prognosis. Am J Med 1993;94:69–74.

104. Barnett MJ, Eaves CJ, Phillips GL, et al. Autografting with cultured marrow in chronic myeloid leukemia: results of a pilot study. Blood 1994;84:724–32.

105. Talpaz M, Kantarjian H, Liang J, et al. Percentage of Philadelphia chromosome (Ph)-negative and Ph-positive cells found after autologous transplantation for chronic myelogenous leukemia depends on percentage of diploid cells induced by conventional-dose chemotherapy before collection of autologous cells. Blood 1995;85:3257–63.

106. Coulombel L, Kalousek DK, Eaves CJ, et al. Long-term marrow culture reveals chromosomally normal hematopoietic progenitor cells in patients with Philadelphia chromosome-positive chronic myelogenous leukemia. N Engl J Med 1983;308:1493–8.

107. Körbling M, Burke P, Braine H, et al. Successful engraftment of blood derived normal hemopoietic stem cells in chronic myelogenous leukemia. Exp Hematol 1981;9:6684–90.

108. Carlo-Stella C, Mangoni L, Almici C, et al. Autologous transplant for chronic myelogenous leukemia using marrow treated ex vivo with mafosfamide. Bone Marrow Transplant 1994;14:425–32.

109. Reiffers J, Goldman J, Meloni G, et al. Autologous stem cell transplantation in chronic myelogenous leukemia: a retrospective analysis of the European Group for Bone Marrow Transplantation. Bone Marrow Transplant 1994;14:407–10.

110. Kantarjian HM, Talpaz M, Andersson B, et al. High doses of cyclophosphamide, etoposide and total body irradiation followed by autologous stem cell transplantation in the management of patients with chronic myelogenous leukemia. Bone Marrow Transplant 1994;14:57–61.

111. Kantarjian HM, Talpaz M, LeMaistre CF, et al. Intensive combination chemotherapy and autologous bone marrow transplantation leads to the reappearance of Philadelphia chromosome-negative cells in chronic myelogenous leukemia. Cancer 1991;67:2959–65.

112. Kantarjian HM, Talpaz M, Hester J, et al. Collection of peripheral-blood diploid cells from chronic myelogenous leukemia patients early in the recovery phase from myelosuppression induced by intensive-dose chemotherapy. J Clin Oncol 1995;13:553–9.

113. Reiffers J, Trouette R, Marit G, et al. Autologous blood stem cell transplantation for chronic granulocytic leukaemia in transformation: a report of 47 cases. Br J Haematol 1991;77:339–45.

114. McGlave PB, De Fabritiis P, Deisseroth A, et al. Autologous transplants for chronic myelogenous leukaemia: results from eight transplant groups. Lancet 1994;343:1486–8.

115. Sawyers CL. Chronic myeloid leukemia. N Engl J Med 1999; 340:1330–40.

116. Lee SJ, Anasetti C, Horowitz MM, Antin JH. Initial therapy for chronic myelogenous leukemia: playing the odds. J Clin Oncol 1998; 16:2897–903.

# LYMPHOID NEOPLASMS

# CHAPTER 87

# HODGKIN'S LYMPHOMA

• CHRISTOS EMMANOUILIDES • JONATHAN SAID • PETER ROSEN

Hodgkin's lymphoma (HL) is a relatively uncommon hematologic malignancy, accounting for 0.7% of all new cases of cancer in the United States and for 0.3% of cancer-related deaths, with approximately 9000 new cases diagnosed annually. The incidence of HL has been stable, in contrast to the rising incidence of non-Hodgkin's lymphoma. HL is a unique malignancy in many ways: The malignant cells in HL (Reed-Sternberg [RS] cells) constitute the minority of the associated tumor, which consists mostly of a reactive inflammatory infiltrate. There has been controversy regarding the cell of origin of the malignant clone, although somatic mutations of the immunoglobulin heavy chain gene are seen in many and suggest a B-lymphocyte derivation is most likely. For that reason, the term *Hodgkin's lymphoma* has been proposed as more accurate compared with the prior term *Hodgkin's disease*. More importantly, HL is potentially curable with chemotherapy combinations or radiotherapy so that most patients with limited disease and about half of patients with extensive disease can be rendered permanently disease free.

The classification and therapeutic approaches to HL have undergone several changes in the 1990s. Lymphocyte-predominant HL (LPHL) is now considered to be a clinicopathologically distinct lymphoma of B-cell type. LPHL is believed to be separate from the other forms of HL, which are now classified as *classic* HL. Earlier therapeutic approaches to HL favored radiation therapy, whereas combination chemotherapy was reserved for patients considered incurable by radiation treatment. This approach necessitated meticulous assessment of the extent of disease, often including surgical staging. Awareness of long-term sequelae of radiation treatment among survivors and newer chemotherapy combinations have altered thinking, making chemotherapy the main treatment modality and changing the objectives of radiation. Currently, clinical research efforts in the treatment of HL aim at either maintaining the highly successful treatment outcomes for patients with limited-stage disease, while reducing long-term toxicity, or increasing the cure rate of patients who have a relatively adverse prognosis.

## Natural History, Diagnosis, and Staging

### EPIDEMIOLOGY AND ETIOLOGY

The overall annual incidence of HL in the United States is 3 cases per 100,000 population. Incidence peaks occur during early and late adulthood. Childhood HL, although rare in the United States, occurs more commonly in underdeveloped countries. Young adults tend to have the nodular sclerosing form of HL, which often presents with localized disease.

Although the cause of HL is unknown, an infectious agent has long been suspected. Several inconclusive reports indicative of horizontal transmission have appeared in the literature but are usually open to criticism or alternative explanations.[1-4] A hypothetical infectious mechanism, which attempts to explain the epidemiologic differences between the childhood HL that occurs in underdeveloped countries and the young adult form of HL of Western countries, argues that improved living conditions delay exposure to the infectious agent until later in life. Possibly, development of HL is a rare manifestation of a common infection, with increasing penetration as the patient's age of infection increases. Lack of increased incidence among medical personnel or marital partners of patients with HL, however, as well as several negative epidemiologic studies for horizontal transmission contradict this hypothesis.

Multiple lines of evidence suggest a possible role for the Epstein-Barr virus (EBV). In countries of different living standards, the distinct age range of first EBV exposure fits epidemiologically with the age of peak incidence of HL.[5] Occasional dramatic cases of HL have been associated with persistence of EBV infection in some families.[6] An altered antibody response to EBV before the diagnosis of HL has been observed in patients, suggestive of enhanced activation of the virus. EBV genes and EBV clonality have been found in the RS cells of approximately 40% of the studied cases of HL. This phenomenon is intriguing but not clearly understood.[7] Depending on techniques used, variable percentages of EBV positivity in HL have been observed.[8-10] EBV is commonly present in cases of mixed cellularity HL (75%) and in economically developing populations, such as South America.[11, 12] EBV latent membrane protein has potent growth-transforming activity and upregulates the expression of *bcl-2*. It is frequently positive in lymphocyte depletion HL and invariably present in aggressive forms of HL that occur in patients infected with human immunodeficiency virus (HIV).[13] These results should be interpreted with caution, however, because it is hard to distinguish between a bystander or a causative role in the pathogenesis of HL.

There has been much debate regarding the cell of origin of the RS cell. Molecular techniques have identified immunoglobulin gene rearrangements in many cases, but features consistent with dendritic cell lineage have also been observed, suggestive of a possible fusion between a B cell and a dendritic cell as the original malignant event in HL.[14, 15] Nevertheless, although the nature of the RS cell in classic HL remains in question, most studies favor a lymphoid derivation with the existence of B-cell and rare T-cell phenotypes.[16, 17] Sensitive polymerase chain reaction analysis of RS cells have revealed VDJ rearrangements in many, although not all, of the cases of classic HL, suggesting that most RS cells are B cell derived and related to the germinal

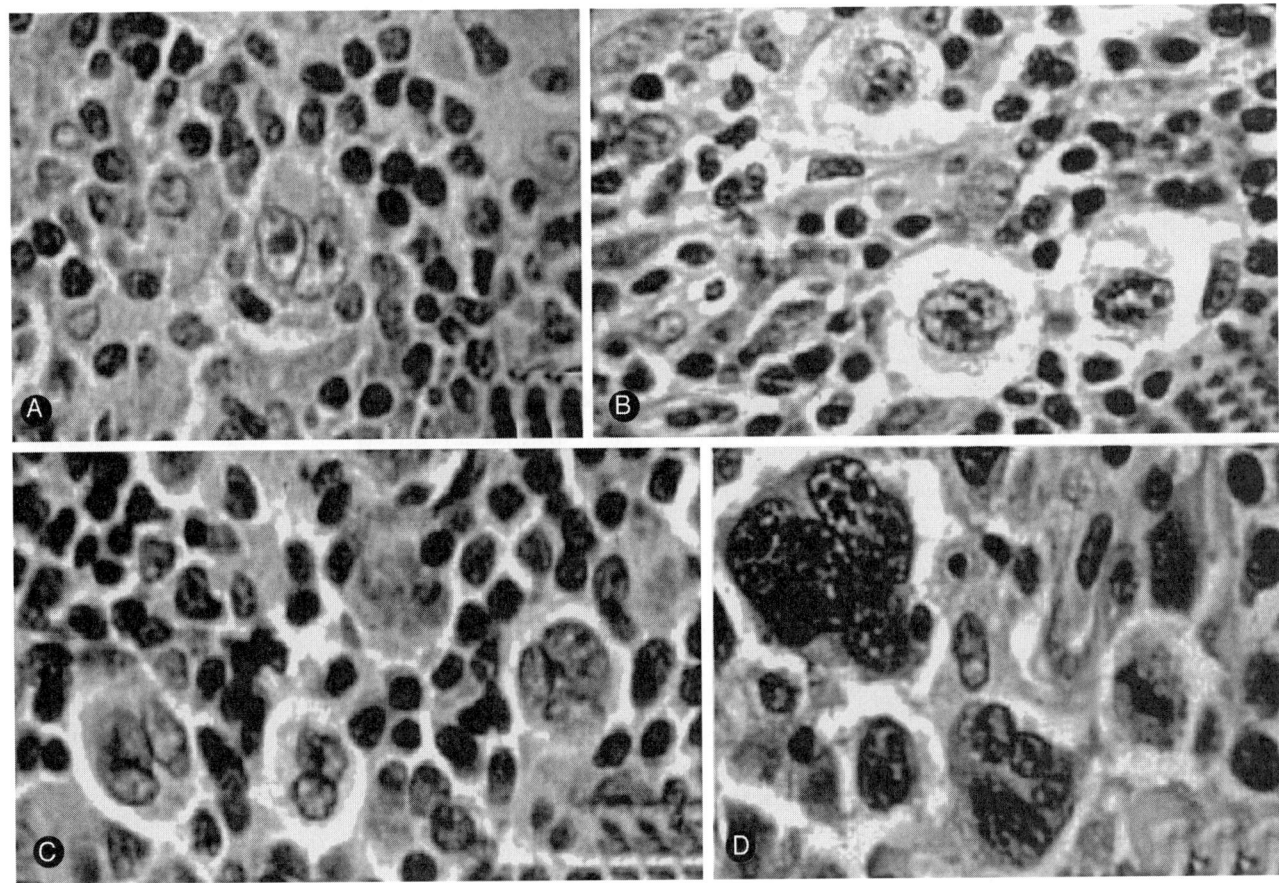

**Figure 87–1.** Reed-Sternberg cells and variants. Diagnostic RS cells are large polypoid cells with two or more vesicular nuclei and large inclusion-like nucleoli *(A)*. Lacunar cells seen in nodular sclerosis *(B)* have abundant pale cytoplasm causing a lacunar artifact in formalin-fixed tissues. "L&H" cells seen in lymphocyte predominance Hodgkin's lymphoma have "popcorn" nuclei and inconspicuous nucleoli *(C)*. Sarcomatoid or reticular variants in lymphocyte depletion include mutlinucleated forms with a more pleomorphic appearance *(D)*.

center or post–germinal center–derived memory B cells.[18] Technical factors may explain observed discrepancies among various investigators.[19]

## CLASSIFICATION (PATHOLOGY)

The diagnosis of HL rests on identifying a diagnostic RS cell in the appropriate cellular background of small lymphocytes, histiocytes, plasma cells, and eosinophils. The classification of HL has undergone modifications with the understanding that LPHL is a separate disease entity from what is currently called *classic* HL (Table 87–1).[20] Diagnostic RS cells are large polyploid cells with two or more vesicular nuclei and usually have large inclusion-like eosinophilic nucleoli. Multinucleated and wreath-like forms are also seen. In addi-

tion to diagnostic cells, there are less diagnostically reliable mononuclear RS or Hodgkin cells and variants (Fig. 87–1). The latter include *L&H* (lymphocyte and histiocyte) *cells* seen in LPHL (see later), lacunar cells seen in nodular sclerosis HL (NSHL), and sarcomatoid or reticular variants in lymphocyte depletion (see later).

Immunohistochemistry has proved useful in characterizing RS cells and differentiating HL from non-Hodgkin's lymphomas, some of which may contain RS-like cells. The characteristic immunophenotype of RS cells is shown in Table 87–2.

### Lymphocyte-Predominant Hodgkin's Lymphoma

Although traditionally classified with HL, there is consensus that LPHL is a clinically and pathologically distinct lymphoma of B-cell type.[21] The distinctive but often subtle

*Table 87–1.* **Classification of Hodgkin's Lymphoma**

| |
|---|
| Lymphocyte predominant Hodgkin's lymphoma |
| Classic Hodgkin's lymphoma |
|     Lymphocyte-rich |
|     Nodular sclerosis |
|     Mixed cellularity |
|     Lymphocyte depletion |

*Table 87–2.* **Immunohistochemistry of Reed-Sternberg Cells**

| | |
|---|---|
| CD15 (Leu M1) | + (approximately 75% of cases) |
| CD30 (Ki1, BerH2) | + |
| CD20 (L26) | ± (approximately 25% of cases positive) |
| CD45 (LCA) | − |

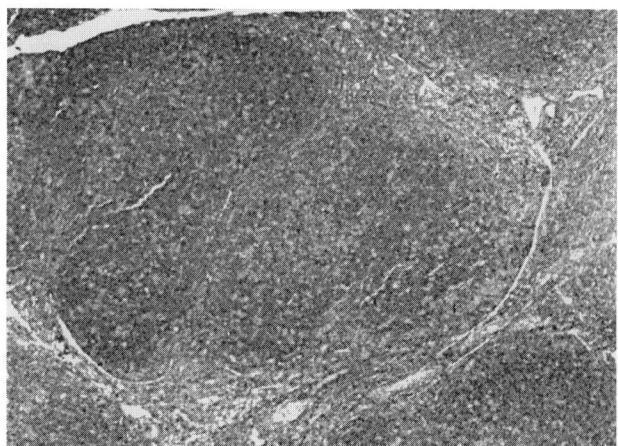

**Figure 87–2.** Nodular lymphocyte predominance Hodgkin's lymphoma. Nodal architecture is effaced by vaguely nodular proliferation. Even in this low-power photomicrograph, the "L&H" cells appear as paler cells within the nodules.

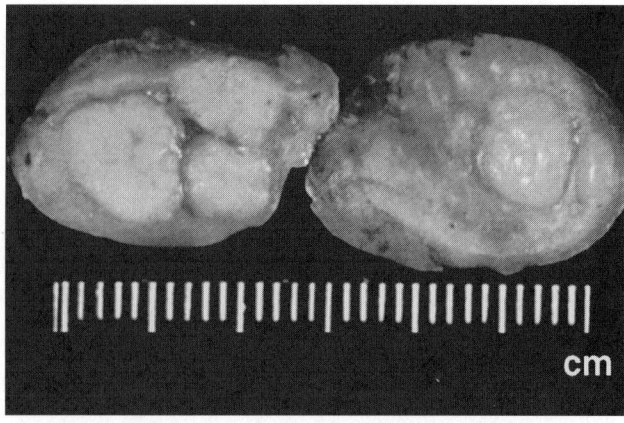

**Figure 87–3.** Nodular sclerosing Hodgkin's lymphoma. The cut surface of this lymph node reveals tumor nodules surrounded by bands of sclerosis.

nodularity of the proliferation as well as the association with progressively transformed germinal centers has suggested a relationship with the lymphoid follicle (Fig. 87–2). The L&H variant RS cells are uniformly of B-cell type, staining for CD45 (leukocyte common antigen), CD20, and epithelial membrane antigen (EMA; in 50% of the cases) and J chain in many cases.[22, 23] They are negative for the characteristic RS cell markers CD15 and CD30. There is a population of distinctly reactive natural killer and T lymphocytes in LPHL that react with CD57 and characteristically surround the L&H cells.[24] Similar to low-grade, B-cell non-Hodgkin's lymphoma, cases of LPHL may have delayed relapses that progress to large B-cell lymphomas over time.[25, 26]

Nodes involved with LPHL may be completely effaced or retain a rim of reactive lymph node. The proliferation may be nodular or nodular and diffuse. It is seldom, if ever, entirely diffuse.[27] The interfollicular pattern that is seen in some cases of classic HL is not usually present in LPHL. The small lymphocytes in the nodules are mostly B-cell type and have regular nuclear outlines or minor nuclear irregularities. L&H cells are large polyploid cells with lobulated nuclei, vesicular chromatin, and inconspicuous

nucleoli. These cells have been appropriately referred to as *popcorn* cells by Lukes,[27a] who pioneered the early classification of HL. They are usually numerous within the nodules.

Some controversies exist regarding LPHL, including the clonal nature of the L&H cell and its progression to large cell lymphoma. Evidence suggests that cases of LPHL with increased L&H cells do not necessarily indicate transformation to large cell lymphoma[26, 28] and have been reported negative for clonal populations with standard polymerase chain reaction techniques.[27] Immunohistochemical studies have shown immunoglobulin light chain restriction in cases of LPHL,[29] however, suggesting a clonal B-cell process.

### Nodular Sclerosing Hodgkin's Lymphoma

In addition to the presence of classic RS cells in the appropriate background, sclerosis and lacunar RS cells are required to diagnose NSHL (Figs. 87–3 and 87–4). Although the amount of sclerosis is variable, minimal criteria include the presence of a thickened capsule with a single sclerotic band. Lacunar cells are large cells with irregular nuclei, vesicular chromatin, and variably prominent nucleoli. In B5 fixed preparations, the cells have abundant clear cytoplasm,

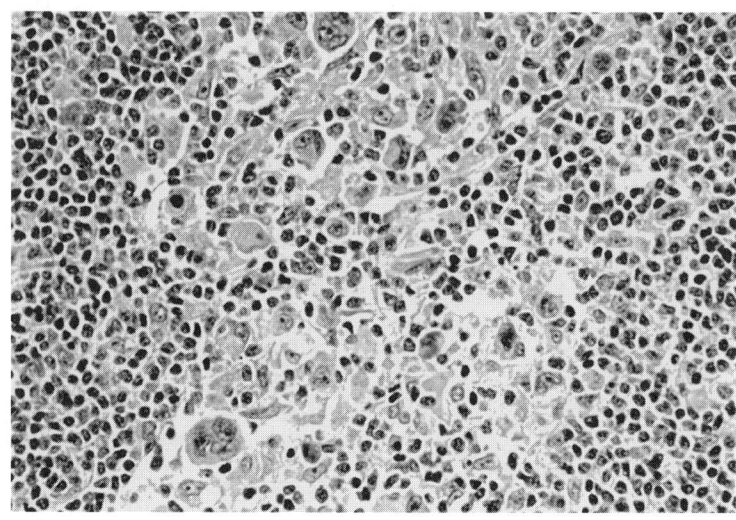

**Figure 87–4.** Nodule from a case of nodular sclerosis showing numerous lacunar Reed-Sternberg variants in a background of predominantly small lymphocytes.

but with formalin fixation, the cytoplasm shrinks, giving the characteristic lacunar artifact.

Attempts have been made to subclassify NSHL into clinically relevant subtypes. Studies of a large series of patients from the British National Lymphoma Investigation (BNLI) and the Netherlands as well as some studies conducted in the United States indicate that cases with large numbers of RS cells (grade 2) had a poorer outcome.[30]

Although NSHL does not usually cause problems in diagnosis, confusion may occur with less common variants. These may include NSHL with minimal or no sclerosis (so-called cellular phase) or where there are large clusters or sheets of lacunar cells (syncytial variant). Particularly in small biopsy or needle cores, sheets of monomorphous lacunar cells can be mistaken for non-Hodgkin's lymphoma, metastatic carcinoma, or other neoplasms.[31] There are increasing clues that NSHL may be related to the germinal follicles. These clues include the nodular pattern, B-cell markers for the RS cells in some cases, and a background meshwork of dendritic cells that stain with CD21.[16, 32] Although the RS cells may be positive for the *bcl-2* protein, they lack the t(14;18) gene rearrangement seen in follicular lymphoma.

### Mixed-Cellularity Hodgkin's Lymphoma

Mixed-cellularity HL (MCHL) is less common than NSHL in the United States but relatively common in developing countries and in patients infected with HIV. EBV is positive in RS cells in a high percentage of cases. MCHL is characterized by diagnostic RS cells, which are often numerous, present in an appropriate background of small lymphocytes, histiocytes, eosinophils, and plasma cells (Fig. 87–5).

### Lymphocyte-Depletion Hodgkin's Lymphoma

The diagnosis of lymphocyte-depletion HL (LDHL) has become problematic, and many previously diagnosed cases turn out to be non-Hodgkin's lymphomas. This diagnostic difficulty is particularly true for CD30 (Ki-1) anaplastic large cell lymphomas (ALCL), some of which may have a

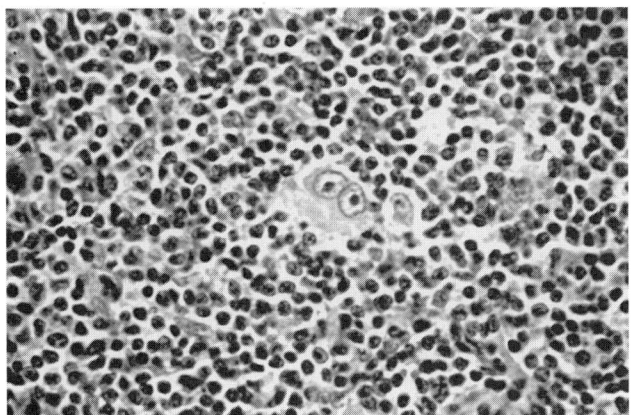

**Figure 87–5.** Mixed cellularity Hodgkin's lymphoma showing a diagnostic Reed-Steinberg cell in a background of small lymphocytes and plasma cells.

*Table 87–3.* **Comparison of Phenotype Between Classic Reed-Sternberg Cells and Anaplastic Large Cell Lymphoma**

| | Antigen | | | | | |
| --- | --- | --- | --- | --- | --- | --- |
| | CD15 | CD45(LCA) | CD30 | CD20 | CD3 | EMA |
| RS cells | + | − | + | +/− | −/+ | − |
| ALCL | − | + | + | −/+ | +/− | + |

RS, Reed-Sternberg; ALCL, anaplastic large cell lymphoma.

Hodgkin's-like appearance.[33] Immunophenotyping and cytogenetics may be helpful in this differentiation. In contrast to RS cells, ALCL cells are positive for the leukocyte common antigen (CD45), usually express one or more T-cell or B-cell markers (frequently T cell), and are negative for CD15 (Leu-M1) (Table 87–3). In some cases of ALCL, the translocation [t(2;5)] is present. This results in the expression of the NPM-ALK fusion protein, which can be detected by immunohistochemistry. These findings are not seen in HL.

Two overlapping variants of LDHL are described: reticular and diffuse fibrosis.[34] The reticular variant contains frequent pleomorphic Hodgkin's cells, many of which in retrospect probably represented cases of non-Hodgkin's lymphomas, particularly ALCL. The diffuse fibrosis variant is rare but should be recognized because of its unusual presentation and clinical course. This entity is characterized by a paucicellular eosinophilic nonbirefringent background, an inflammatory infiltrate, proliferation of fibroblasts or myofibroblasts, and the presence of Hodgkin's and RS cells, which may be sparse. This form of LDHL may be overlooked by the pathologist, particularly because it may present in the liver and bone marrow rather than lymph nodes.[35]

## DIAGNOSIS OF HODGKIN'S LYMPHOMA IN EXTRANODAL SITES

Although staging laparotomies are rarely performed today, routine staging procedures, which include bone marrow and sometimes liver biopsies, are used to assess involvement by HL. In the bone marrow, classic HL infiltrates are often associated with sclerosis, a mixed cellular background, and the presence of Hodgkin's cells. In patients with known HL, diagnosis of bone marrow and liver infiltration requires the presence of Hodgkin's cells or RS variants. The typical multinucleated RS cells are not necessarily required, however.

## DIAGNOSIS OF HODGKIN'S LYMPHOMA IN FINE-NEEDLE ASPIRATES

Fine-needle aspiration is increasingly used for the diagnosis of lymphoma. This technique may be of value in evaluating residual or recurrent disease in patients with known HL. Extreme caution should be taken in the de novo diagnosis of HL. Because RS-like cells occur in non-Hodgkin's lymphomas as well as benign conditions, tissue confirmation should be sought in almost all cases initially diagnosed as HL by fine-needle aspiration.

## EVALUATION AND STAGING

HL typically arises in the lymph nodes of the chest and neck, although in less than 20% of the cases, the disease presents in infradiaphragmatic sites. Extranodal presentations, which are not associated with adjacent primary lymph node involvement, are extremely rare and may suggest an alternative diagnosis. A surgical biopsy is almost always required for the diagnosis of the disease. Because the tumor consists of relatively few malignant cells interspersed among a reactive cellular infiltrate as previously noted, a needle biopsy is frequently nondiagnostic. The histologic subtypes of classic HL appear to have little impact on outcome, although the rare LDHL has an ominous prognosis. HL usually spreads by contiguity from one lymph node chain to adjacent chains and eventually through hematogenous dissemination to extralymphatic tissues.

Clinically, NSHL usually presents in the supraclavicular location or in the anterior mediastinum and often spreads to the cervical nodes, axilla, or upper abdomen. Many patients with NSHL are asymptomatic. Patients with MCHL are often symptomatic with fevers, weight loss, and night sweats. Frequently the retroperitoneum is involved, whereas the mediastinum is often spared. LDHL is rare and presents most often in the elderly with major constitutional symptoms. There is often no peripheral adenopathy, and the diagnosis is frequently made by bone marrow examination or liver biopsy in the presence of fever of unknown origin, cytopenias, and altered hepatic tests. LPHL is frequently found as an isolated high cervical lymph node or in the axilla or groin in an asymptomatic patient. LPHL is typically a disease of young men. NSHL is seen in late adolescence and early adulthood with equal incidence in both sexes. LDHL is mostly a disease of the elderly, whereas MCHL has a broad age range.

The Ann Arbor classification system with the Cotswolds modifications is used for the staging of HL (Table 87–4). This system is based on the fact that HL usually spreads by contiguity to predictable lymph node sites. Four stages are recognized based on the extent of lymphatic involvement or the spread to distant extralymphatic organs. Lack of systemic symptoms is specified as *A*, whereas *B* indicates presence of unexplained weight loss greater than 10%, fevers, or night sweats. *X* denotes the presence of bulky disease, such as a greater than 10 cm nodal mass or mediastinal disease comprising more than a third of the transverse dimension of the diaphragm as seen on a posteroanterior chest radiograph. *E* denotes localized solitary involvement of extralymphatic tissue by limited direct extension from an involved nodal area. An important distinction is whether staging has been assessed by routine physical examination and imaging (clinical staging [CS]) or if it has been supported by a staging laparotomy (surgical or pathologic staging [PS]). Conclusions regarding treatment outcomes derived from surgically staged patients may not necessarily apply to patients who are clinically staged.

The goal of the evaluation and staging of the patient is to obtain information of prognostic value and to define the extent of the disease so that an optimal treatment plan may be applied. Elevated sedimentation rate, anemia, bulky disease, B symptoms, and extranodal involvement are commonly sought in the evaluation of the patient as possible adverse prognostic factors. Routine laboratory tests should include a complete blood count with differential, serum albumin, liver chemistries, creatinine, and erythrocyte sedimentation rate. Computed tomography (CT) of the neck, chest, abdomen, and pelvis are routinely performed. A gallium scan is useful for assessing uptake by large tumor masses, which following treatment result in residual masses because of scar tissue that is no longer gallium avid. This phenomenon is particularly common in the mediastinum. The differentiation of scar from viable tumor is critical in the restaging process. The sensitivity of gallium scanning for this purpose has not been well defined. It has been reported that positron emission tomography scanning using fluorodeoxyglucose may also provide reliable restaging of residual masses.[36, 37] Positron emission tomography scans appear to have a strong negative predictive value greater than 90% but a somewhat weaker positive predictive value. The exact role of this promising technique in the management of HL is currently under clinical investigation.

In the past, bipedal lymphangiography had been commonly used to stage HL. In expert hands, it does appear to add to the assessment of the retroperitoneal lymph nodes. The procedure is infrequently performed even in large academic centers, however, and interpretation of the findings can be problematic. Bone marrow aspirates and biopsies should be performed in patients with B symptoms, significant anemia, or cytopenias and patients with stage III disease or greater, even though the overall incidence of bone marrow involvement in HL is low (<10%), with the exception of HIV-positive patients. Bone scans should be performed in the presence of bone pain, hypercalcemia, or elevation of serum alkaline phosphatase.

Aggressive staging that has historically included laparotomy is probably no longer indicated because a larger proportion of patients receive chemotherapy as part of their treatment. Even when radiation alone is used as treatment of early disease, pathologic staging including laparotomy with splenectomy does not affect survival. Previously, staging laparotomies including splenectomies with intraoperative lymph node and liver biopsies were performed for patients with no or inconclusive clinically apparent disease below the diaphragm. A negative laparotomy would lead to treatment with radiation therapy alone, avoiding the patient's exposure to the relatively toxic MOPP (mustine hydrochloride, vinblastine [Oncovin], procarbazine, prednisone) combination chemotherapy of that time. Given the advent of nonleukemogenic, gonadal-sparing effective regimens (ABVD [doxorubicin (Adriamycin), bleomycin, vinblastine, dacarbazine] and related regimens) as well as the excellent results of combined chemoradiotherapy treatment approaches for early-stage HL, however, staging laparotomies have been largely abandoned because the rationale for their use is obsolete. It is now widely accepted that clinical staging suffices to direct the physician in planning the optimal treatment. The large number of patients that have undergone exploratory laparotomy and splenectomy in the past, however, have contributed to understanding of the mode in

**Table 87–4.** Ann Arbor (AJCC) and Cotswolds Staging Classifications of Hodgkin's Disease

*Ann Arbor/AJCC Stage Grouping\**

| | |
|---|---|
| Stage I | Involvement of single lymph node region (I) or localized involvement of a single extralymphatic organ or site ($I_E$) |
| Stage II | Involvement of two or more lymph node regions on the same side of the diaphragm (II) or localized involvement of a single associated extralymphatic organ or site and its regional lymph node(s) with or without involvement of other lymph node regions on the same side of the diaphragm ($II_E$). *Note:* The number of lymph node regions involved may be indicated by a subscript (e.g., $II_3$) |
| Stage III | Involvement of lymph node regions on both sides of the diaphragm (III), which may also be accompanied by localized involvement of an associated extralymphatic organ or site ($III_E$), by involvement of the spleen ($III_S$), or both ($III_{E+S}$) |
| Stage IV | Disseminated (multifocal) involvement of one or more extralymphatic organs, with or without associated lymph node involvement, or isolated extralymphatic organ involvement with distant (nonregional) nodal involvement |

*Systemic Symptoms*

Each stage is subdivided into A and B categories. B for those with defined systemic symptoms and A for those without. The B designation is given to those patients with (1) unexplained loss of 10% of body weight in the 6 months before admission; (2) unexplained fever with temperatures >38° C, and (3) drenching night sweats. Pruritus alone does not qualify for B classification, nor does a short febrile illness associated with an infection†

*Cotswolds Modifications of the Staging Classification‡*

| | |
|---|---|
| Stage II | Involvement of two or more lymph node regions on the same side of the diaphragm (the mediastinum is considered as a single site, whereas hilar lymph nodes are considered bilaterally). The number of anatomic sites should be indicated by a subscript (e.g., $II_3$) |
| Stage III | Involvement of lymph node regions, or structures on both sides of the diaphragm, is further divided into |
| $III_1$ | With or without involvement of splenic, hilar, celiac, or portal lymph nodes |
| $III_2$ | With involvement of para-aortic, iliac, and/or mesenteric lymph nodes |

*Additional Designation Applicable to any Stage of Disease*

| | |
|---|---|
| A, B, E | Same as for the Ann Arbor/AJCC classification system |
| X | Bulky disease (widening of the mediastinum by more than one third or the presence of a nodal mass with a maximal dimension >10 cm) |
| CS | Clinical stage |
| PS | Pathologic stage |

\* From Beahr OH, et al, eds. American Joint Committee on Cancer: Manual for staging of cancer. 4th ed. Philadelphia: JB Lippincott, 1992:253.

† *Note:* Pruritus as a systemic symptom remains controversial. This symptom is hard to define quantitatively and uniformly, but when it is recurrent, generalized, and otherwise unexplained, and when it ebbs and flows in parallel with disease activity, it may be the equivalent of a B symptom.

‡ From Lister TA, Crowther D, Sutcliffe SB, et al. Report of a committee convened to discuss the evaluation and staging of patients with Hodgkin's disease: Cotswolds Meeting. J Clin Oncol 1989;7:1630–6.

which the disease spreads. It is known that a favorable group of patients that includes women with CS I nonbulky mediastinal disease, patients with CS I LPHL, and patients with unilateral high cervical presentation has less than a 10% chance of being upstaged by laparotomy. It was also found that abdominal CT has poor predictive value in assessing splenic involvement: Half of patients with enlarged or abnormal-appearing spleens have negative histology after splenectomy. About one third of normal-appearing spleens are found to be pathologically involved.[38] Positron emission tomography (PET) is used increasingly for staging and assessment of residual masses and tends to replace gallium scans.

## PROGNOSTIC FACTORS

Most prognostic systems apply to patients with extensive disease because with current treatment, patients with limited HL usually have an excellent disease-free and overall survival. Identification of subgroups of patients with advanced HL who have a relatively reduced chance of disease-free survival may define the target population for attempting intensified treatment. Extensive disease, increased age, and systemic symptoms have been considered adverse prognostic factors intuitively and after retrospective analysis. Several other factors have been shown in different analyses to carry adverse prognostic value, although they have not been always reproducible: anemia, elevated sedimentation rate, and

other markers of a *cytokine release syndrome* suggestive of tumor-related inflammation, such as cytopenia and pruritus.[39-41] Elevation of serum interleukin (IL)-10 has also been proposed as an independent prognostic risk factor.[42] The results of a retrospective analysis of 4695 patients by an international group representing 25 centers have been published.[43] This group included mostly patients with stage III or IV disease, although patients with early-stage disease were included when they were treated with systemic chemotherapy because of bulk or systemic symptoms. Although the usual adverse prognostic factors (previously described) emerged after univariate analysis of the data, the final Cox regression model resulting from multivariate analysis identified seven independent prognostic factors, each conferring a relative risk of 1.29 to 1.49 for relapse (Table 87–5). In this group of patients treated predominantly with full-course doxorubicin-containing chemotherapy, neither bulk nor histology was proved to be an independent factor. Patients with no adverse factors had an 84% freedom from progression (FFP), whereas the presence of each factor depressed the FFP curve plateau by about 8% (Fig. 87–6). This broadly based model is expected to constitute the point of reference for future clinical trials.

## Treatment

Treatment of HL almost always should be planned with curative intent and is directed by the stage of the disease,

*Table 87–5.* Prognostic Factors in Hodgkin's Lymphoma

| Factor | Relative Risk of Relapse |
|---|---|
| Albumin <4 g/dl | 1.49 |
| Hemoglobin <10.5 g/dl | 1.35 |
| Male sex | 1.35 |
| Stage IV disease | 1.26 |
| Age ≥45 yr | 1.39 |
| White cell count >15,000/mm³ | 1.41 |
| Lymphocyte count <600/mm³ or <8% of white cell count | 1.38 |

From Hasenclever D, Diehl V. A prognostic score for advanced Hodgkin's disease. N Engl J Med 1998;339:1506–14.

systemic symptoms, and expected sequelae of the treatment, which depend on the age of the patient, comorbid conditions, and therapeutic modalities used. Long-term treatment-related complications are especially important given the young age of many patients and the likelihood of long-term survival. The first decision to be made is whether a patient requires chemotherapy alone, radiation treatment alone, or a combination of both. Aggressive staging including staging laparotomy is usually unnecessary, unless it has a definite impact on this decision-making.

## HISTORICAL PERSPECTIVE

HL was one of the first non–surgically curable malignancies to be successfully treated first with radiation and subsequently with chemotherapy. In the early days of cancer treatment, single-agent chemotherapy was the accepted standard of care. Consequently, many of the early drugs used to treat cancer were adequately studied in newly diagnosed patients with HL who were not candidates for radiation; procarbazine, vinblastine, mechlorethamine, chlorambucil, vincristine, and cyclophosphamide were reported to produce at least a 60% response rate in untreated HL patients.[44] The responses were usually short-lived and incomplete, however. In the 1960s, the advantages of combination chemotherapy treatment became evident.[45] In the United States, the National Cancer Institute (NCI) developed the four-drug combination MOPP, which proved to be curative for patients with extensive HL (stage III to IV).[46] MOPP and MOPP-like regimens constitute the first generation of alkylating agent–based treatments of HL. In a 20-year follow-up report on MOPP-treated patients,[47] 66% of the complete responders were in remission more than 10 years from the end of the treatment, leading to a 50% disease-specific survival. Approximately 10 years after the advent of MOPP, the ABVD regimen was developed by Bonadonna and Santoro in Milan.[48] ABVD represents a second-generation regimen and has been the basis of the treatment of advanced HL in the 1990s because of its favorable toxicity profile and an improved outcome in multicenter randomized studies. Currently, aggressive, nonmyeloablative regimens have been developed with the help of hematopoietic growth factors. Such regimens appear promising in large phase II studies and have been compared with ABVD. These regimens provide significantly higher dose intensity and may possibly replace ABVD for high-risk subgroups of patients, as discussed subsequently.

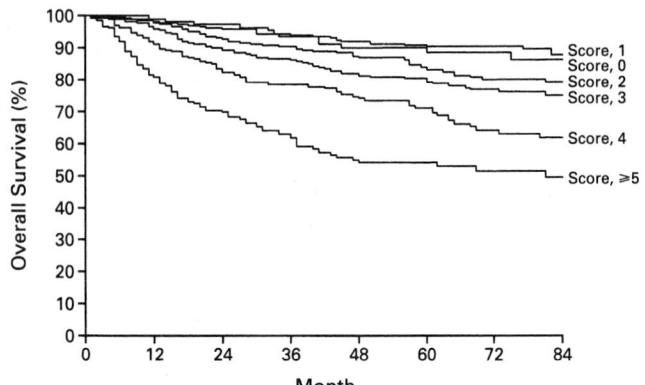

**Figure 87–6.** Use of the prognostic score to predict rates of freedom from progression of disease *(A)* and overall survival *(B)* in 1618 patients with advanced Hodgkin's lymphoma. (The number and percentage of patients with each score were as follows: a score of 0 = 115 patients (7%); 1 = 360 (22%); 2 = 464 (29%); 3 = 378 (23%); 4 = 190 (12%); and 5 or higher = 111 (7%). (From Hasenclever D, Diehl V. A prognostic score for advanced Hodgkin's disease. N Engl J Med 339:1506–14, 1998, copyright © 1998 Massachusetts Medical Society. All rights reserved.)

Several general conclusions can be derived from a multitude of clinical studies and meta-analyses. In most studies directly comparing chemotherapy with radiation therapy, treatment with chemotherapy was equal to or better than radiation monotherapy; this is true even in early-stage disease,[49] the only exception being one trial comparing MOPP with radiation therapy.[50] Consolidative radiation following curative chemotherapy can probably improve disease-free survival, if all disease can be encompassed in the radiation field. It is not clear, however, that overall survival is affected. The one clear exception to this generalization is cases of bulky mediastinal disease, in which radiation therapy appears to influence survival favorably.[51] Successful salvage treatments, which include myeloablative high-dose chemotherapy supported by stem cell transplantation, make the demonstration of the survival benefit of a given primary treatment difficult. Radiation treatment is associated with a significant risk of organ toxicity and, more importantly, of secondary malignancies, which are most likely related to the dose and extent of radiation. Long-term sequelae of chemotherapy include sterility and hematologic malignancies (MOPP) and cardiotoxicity and pulmonary toxicity (ABVD).

## RADIATION THERAPY

Although Senn prematurely claimed a "curative effect" of irradiation for patients with HL in 1903, widespread interest in the curative potential of radiation therapy was not aroused until a report by Peters[52] in 1950. Modern concepts of radiation therapy for HL date to the work of Gilbert,[53] first reported in 1925. His fundamental principle was the destruction of all tumor during the initial course of treatment by extending the irradiated volume from known sites of tumor to suspected sites of involvement within the limits of patients' tolerance. The necessary delivery of large radiation doses to large tissue volumes was not possible with the equipment that was available at the time, however. Nevertheless, with estimated tumor doses that did not exceed 10 Gy, in 1939 Gilbert[54] reported a 5-year survival rate of 34.2% for selected patients treated as planned. The introduction of megavoltage equipment in the 1950s resulted in development of therapeutic techniques that made it possible to deliver *adequate* radiation doses to large tissue volumes with tolerable complications. Soon after the development of the linear accelerator, it became apparent that radiation treatment could cure most patients with stage I to II HL. Principles of radiation monotherapy included the use of extended fields that included prophylactic full doses to areas of inapparent but possible contiguous involvement and the use of parallel opposed anteroposterior portals. These goals required relatively large treatment portals.

According to the *extended field irradiation* principle, patients with high cervical stage I can be treated with a mantle field that involves the cervical, upper mediastinal, supraclavicular, and axillary areas; patients with involvement of the mediastinum usually receive a mantle field as well as an upper abdominal port, including para-aortic nodes and spleen, defined as *subtotal lymphoid irradiation* (STLI) (Fig. 87–7). A large subset of HL patients with pathologic stage I or IIA disease have a 10-year relapse-free survival of about 80%. This low-risk group includes patients with supradi-

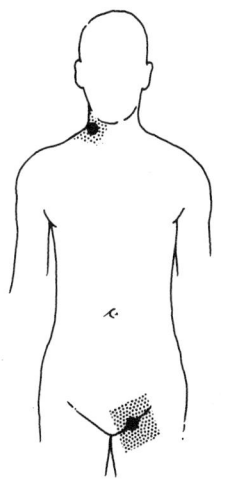 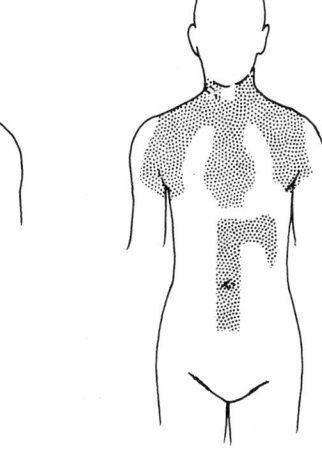

A  Involved field irradiation

B  Subtotal nodal irradiation including mantle and spade fields

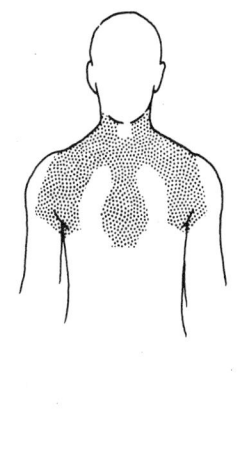 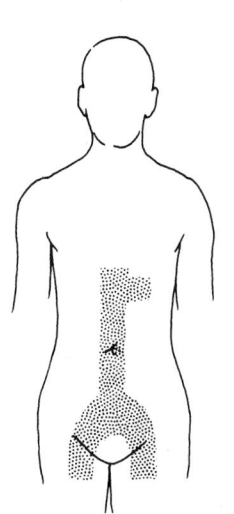

C  Mantle field irradiation

D  Inverted-Y field irradiation

**Figure 87–7.** Common radiation fields in the treatment of Hodgkin's lymphoma.

aphragmatic nonbulky disease who are well served by STLI. The benefit of irradiating areas below the diaphragm for disease that is apparently limited to the area above the diaphragm has been well documented by several trials.[55, 56] Additional fields covering Waldeyer's ring and the preauricular nodes are indicated in the presence of HL in these regions in the upper neck. Patients with early-stage inguinal or femoral disease may be treated with irradiation of pelvic and para-aortic nodes and the spleen (inverted Y field irradiation).

Patients with stage IIIA disease may receive total lymphoid irradiation (TLI), which combines mantle and inverted Y irradiation. If the disease is limited to lymphatic structures above the renal hila after surgical staging (PS III1A), patients have a generally favorable survival similar to PS IIA. The disease-free survival drops to less than 50% in patients with PS III2A, which includes involvement of the lower para-aortic or mesenteric nodes.[57] Currently, radiation monotherapy is not the preferred treatment of CS or PS IIIA disease.

The supradiaphragmatic and subdiaphragmatic fields are not treated concurrently because the large treatment volume produces excessive fatigue, nausea, vomiting, anorexia, and myelosuppression. The region carrying the larger tumor burden is treated first. A break of treatment for 3 to 4 weeks is given after completion of the first region to permit the patient to recover appetite and energy. There is substantial variation in the doses used for the treatment of HL at various institutions. Earlier, higher doses were generally used, whereas currently there is a trend to reduce doses. An influential analysis suggesting a linear increase in control probability with increasing dose up to 44 Gy was published by Kaplan[58] in 1966. His review of data from Stanford showed a 4.4% recurrence rate for involved sites after 35 to 40 Gy, compared with a 1.4% recurrence rate after 44 Gy. A later analysis of published series suggested a plateau in tumor control rate at a dose of approximately 35 Gy.[59] Doses above this level do not decrease further the 4% recurrence rate for previously involved sites, although they do add to the acute and chronic morbidity of treatment. For uninvolved areas or contiguous areas, a smaller radiation dose is sufficient; a dose of 25 to 30 Gy is sufficient to prevent recurrences in uninvolved areas in 99% of patients. When radiation monotherapy is used, it is reasonable to deliver approximately 35 Gy to clinically involved sites, 30 Gy to contiguous clinically negative areas, and 25 Gy to noncontiguous clinically negative areas. When involved field radiation is given as consolidative treatment after a complete response to chemotherapy, 20 Gy may be sufficient. No increase in control rate was found in one randomized trial that compared 40 Gy with 20 Gy. Higher doses are usually given as consolidation therapy to sites of bulky (X) disease, especially with residual mass after chemotherapy.

Long-term complications of radiotherapy are not trivial. The risk for development of solid tumors, especially cancers of the lung and breast, emerges after the first decade following treatment and appears to remain increased for several decades, probably throughout adult life.[60, 61] Using actuarial analyses, approximately one in four long-term survivors develops a malignancy. The risk for secondary malignancies is particularly increased in children and young adults.[62] The development of secondary leukemia is probably less important, unless there is concomitant exposure to MOPP-like regimens. Premature closure of the epiphysis is a concern in children. Tissue damage of the heart, lungs, and thyroid may lead to functional impairment and potentiation of chemotherapy-related toxicity.[63–65] Long-term survivors of HL must be followed rigorously and have periodic physical examinations, with counseling to avoid high-risk behaviors, and women should have annual mammograms beginning within 5 to 10 years after treatment or by age 30.

Practices related to the use of radiation therapy in the treatment of HL were established in the early 1960s and changed dramatically in the 1990s. Because of the significant risk of carcinogenesis, modern treatment strategies for HL tend to employ less intense dosage and limited radiation fields. This trend was made possible by the demonstration of the efficacy of combined-modality chemotherapy and radiation therapy in early and intermediately advanced HL (see later). As a result, radiotherapy monotherapy is now

less commonly prescribed. Most patients receive adjuvant involved field radiation after an abbreviated or a full course of chemotherapy. The only absolute indication for radiation therapy in addition to a full course of chemotherapy is the presence of bulky mediastinal disease as noted earlier. Several studies have shown that consolidation radiotherapy to a total of 20 to 30 Gy can be limited to involved fields without obvious adverse effects on relapse or survival. This consolidation therapy represents a significant reduction in the dosages of radiation that were previously administered. The effect of chemotherapy in reducing tumor size allows for more narrow fields, sparing normal tissues from radiation exposure. Currently, randomized studies are being conducted to define the lowest possible radiation dose that can be given without compromising outcome. Radiation therapy can also be used for emergency situations, such as airway obstruction, spinal cord compression, nerve compression, or ureteral obstruction, although chemotherapy is equally efficacious unless the patient is chemotherapy resistant.

## TREATMENT ACCORDING TO CLINICAL PRESENTATION

The preliminary decision in designing the therapeutic strategy in a newly diagnosed patient with HL is based on the extent of the disease. If the disease is limited enough (very early), radiation monotherapy can be administered. Extensive disease warrants full-course chemotherapy, whereas a combined-modality approach employing abbreviated chemotherapy is preferable in early-stage or intermediate-stage disease. Various presentations can be classified as very early, early, early-intermediate, and extensive as described subsequently (Table 87–6).

### Very Early Disease: Selected Patients with Stage IA (CS)

Selected patients with very limited–stage HL can be treated successfully with radiation therapy only. Analysis of large

**Table 87–6. Outline of Treatment According to Clinical Presentation**

| Presentation | Recommended Treatment |
|---|---|
| Very early disease: IA<br>High solitary cervical<br>Female with stage I nonbulky NSHL mediastinal<br>Lymphocyte predominant cervical or epitrochlear<br>Absence of bulk, anemia, ESR elevation, inflammatory signs | Radiation monotherapy |
| Early stage: IA–IIA<br>Favorable: Absence of bulk, anemia, ESR elevation, inflammatory signs | Combined modality with 2–4 cycles of first line or a lesser regimen and involved field radiation therapy |
| With adverse factors (intermediate) | Combined modality with 4 cycles of first-line regimen and involved field radiation |
| Extensive disease: clinical stage III–IV, Bulky, B symptoms | Full-course chemotherapy plus radiation of bulky site (especially mediastinal) |

NSHL, nodular sclerosis Hodgkin's lymphoma; ESR, erythrocyte sedimentation rate.

series of laparotomy-staged patients from Stanford and the Royal Marsden Hospital as well as experience with LPHL has identified patients who have less than a 10% chance of positive laparotomy.[66–68] These categories include patients who have no suggestive signs of systemic disease (e.g., B symptoms, elevation of sedimentation rate, anemia), have nonbulky disease, and fall into one of the following categories: patients with unilateral high cervical presentation, women with nonbulky anterior mediastinal stage I NSHL, or patients with epitrochlear or cervical LPHL. Such patients can be treated with mantle field irradiation or similar extended field ports (*mini-mantle* may be used for high cervical presentations). Such patients constitute a small minority of all new cases, however. A somewhat broader *very favorable group* comprising all stage IA female patients younger than 40 years old with nonbulky mass and with NSHL or LPHL histology had a 23% relapse rate after mantle field irradiation.[69] The use of strict criteria to define patients who should receive such local or extended field irradiation alone is recommended.

## Early Stage: IA to IIA

**Is There a Role for Laparotomy?** The chance of discovering unsuspected infradiaphragmatic disease in patients with CS I or II HL, who do not fall within the aforementioned strictly defined categories, is approximately 30 to 40%. In the past, patients would undergo staging laparotomy. If they were PS I or II, they would be treated with subtotal lymphoid irradiation, with an expected disease-free survival of about 80%. At least 30% of the patients would be upstaged, whereas 20% would relapse despite negative abdominal staging. Laparotomy is associated with perioperative morbidity and results in delay of treatment. The clinical benefit of performing laparotomy has not been shown in a randomized trial. A European Organization for Research and Treatment of Cancer (EORTC) study randomized patients with favorable stage I or II disease to either staging laparotomy and treatment based on the result of such staging or immediate subtotal nodal irradiation based on clinical staging. At 6 years, FFP was 83% versus 78%, whereas survival was 89% versus 93%. Surgical staging did not appear to improve survival.[70] As noted, these results, along with the advent of nonleukemogenic gonadal-sparing chemotherapy, enable the safe and effective administration of combined-modality treatments in patients with early and intermediate presentations of HL, rendering laparotomy unnecessary.

**Combined-Modality Treatment.** Combined-modality therapy offers the advantage of treating clinically inapparent disease, obviating the need for laparotomy. Chemotherapy makes it possible to avoid extensive radiation fields and to reduce the total dose of radiation to the involved sites. Combined-modality treatment usually includes an abbreviated chemotherapy course and relatively smaller irradiation fields and lower dosages than those required if no chemotherapy were given. Consequently, it is hoped that such brief exposure to chemotherapy and the lesser extent of irradiation will lead to attenuated long-term sequelae of either treatment modality.

It has been known that the radiation field can be reduced when combined-modality treatment is used without compromising cure rates. An early study in pathologically staged HL patients by the Stanford group proved equivalent clinical outcome between subtotal node irradiation and involved field radiation plus six full cycles of MOPP. This study indicated that chemotherapy can be used successfully to limit the extent of the irradiation field.[71]

A related question is whether involved field radiation adds anything to full-course chemotherapy. A meta-analysis of randomized studies comparing a full course of chemotherapy versus full chemotherapy followed by radiation suggests a 10% improvement of disease-free survival. This improvement was limited to the patients with early-stage HL (I to IIIa); no difference in overall survival was noted.[72] Combined-modality treatment for early-stage HL appears to improve tumor control, without necessarily improving survival. Notwithstanding the lack of survival benefit, improvement in freedom from relapse is a legitimate goal, especially in young patients with HL because the long-term sequelae of retreatment may be avoided.

The next logical question is whether less than a full course of chemotherapy may suffice for the combined-modality treatment of early-stage HL. This concept was first validated using four cycles of MOPP chemotherapy and mantle field radiation, with an 89% reported FFP among early-stage and intermediate-stage HL patients.[73] Limiting the dose and the extent of the irradiation field further is expected to reduce the long-term risks of heart and lung damage and secondary malignancies, such as breast and lung cancer.[74, 61]

Because MOPP is a leukemogenic drug combination that also causes infertility in most patients, efforts have been made to evaluate alternative chemotherapy regimens for favorable (no tumor bulk, lack of B symptoms, no elevation of sedimentation rate, no anemia), early CS HL to be used in conjunction with involved field radiation. A combination of vinblastine, bleomycin, and methotrexate with involved field radiation in clinically staged patients has been studied by the Stanford group, with a 20% improvement in 10-year disease-free survival compared with extended subtotal or total nodal irradiation.[75] Similarly the EORTC has compared six cycles EBVP (epirubicin, bleomycin, vinblastine, prednisone) and involved field radiation with STLI in favorable CS I to II patients. The EORTC study showed a superiority in 5-year event-free survival by 9% (90% vs. 81%) for combined-modality therapy, but as is often the case, no difference in overall survival was noted.[76] A brief aggressive 4-week regimen of VAPEC-B (vincristine, doxorubicin, prednisone, etoposide, cyclophosphamide, bleomycin) with involved field radiation has been found superior to irradiation alone in an English study, producing a 3-year disease-free survival of 91% versus 73%.[77] This study can be criticized, however, because it also used limited radiation fields in the control arm. An update on the outcome of clinically staged patients with favorable HL (nonbulky CS I, IIA) treated with VBM (vinblastine, bleomycin, methotrexate) combined with involved field irradiation showed no difference in disease-free survival when compared with studies of extended field radiation.[78]

The VBM regimen was designed to be a less intense regimen used as an adjunct to radiotherapy for early disease; combinations such as VAPEC-B or EBVP seem to be inferior to standard first-line combinations as shown in randomized trials.[79, 80] It remains unclear whether they are preferable to short courses of ABVD when given as the chemotherapy component of a combined-modality regimen for patients with CS I or II without adverse prognostic factors.

It is widely accepted that the traditional first-line regimens (ABVD, MOPP, or related regimens) are preferable as part of a combined-modality treatment for patients with early-stage disease and adverse features (e.g., anemia, increased sedimentation rate, tumor bulk). Good results using 4 months of ABVD alternating with MOPP chemotherapy followed by involved or extended field irradiation in CS I, II, and limited IIIA patients, including patients with adverse factors, have been published with a reported FFP exceeding 80%. In this study, the amount of postchemotherapy radiation administered to patients without bulky disease (20 Gy vs. 40 Gy) did not affect relapses or survival.[81] Four cycles of ABVD used in a combined-modality program had been favorably compared with STLI in a randomized trial by the Milan group, which also showed that the extent of radiation after combined-modality treatment (involved field vs. extended field) did not affect outcome.[82] All patients achieved a complete response, whereas a 94% FFP was reported after a median follow-up of 3 years. These two important studies taken together indicate that patients with I to IIA disease, including those with more adverse clinical presentations, can be treated effectively with an abbreviated course of ABVD-based chemotherapy and involved field radiation. For patients without bulky disease, lower doses of radiation (20 to 30 Gy) may suffice. The use of an effective regimen such as ABVD allows reduction of extent and dose of radiation safely without increase in treatment failure, suggesting at least equivalent survival compared with extended field radiation therapy alone, possibly with fewer long-term radiation effects.

The aforementioned conclusions are supported by a meta-analysis of eight randomized trials comparing extent of radiation field in combined-modality treatments showing that extended field radiation therapy reduced the chance of recurrences but did not affect survival.[83] In the same meta-analysis, when combined-modality treatment was compared with extensive radiation therapy, a trend for better survival was noted in the combined-modality group (reduction of annual odds from dying from HL was 21%, $p = 0.07$). This meta-analysis included studies with different chemotherapy combinations, including regimens inferior to first-line standard treatments.

Available data suggest that for patients with CS IA and IIA HL, combined-modality treatment with an abbreviated course of chemotherapy and involved field irradiation constitutes the therapeutic approach of choice; however, more long-term data regarding outcome and complication rates are needed before a final statement can be made. For patients with adverse factors, a first-line regimen such as ABVD is preferable. Ongoing studies are comparing various chemotherapy regimens to ABVD or the duration of ABVD treatment to try to define the minimum chemotherapy intensity or duration of therapy as well as dose of radiation required without compromising disease-free and overall survival.

### Advanced (Extensive) Hodgkin's Disease

**When Should Full-Course Combination Chemotherapy Be Considered?** Patients with advanced disease require a full course of chemotherapy. This generally implies treatment with six to eight 4-week cycles of treatment with either MOPP-like or ABVD-like regimens or intense combinations of at least equivalent chemotherapy intensity. Such regimens are expected to produce a complete response. It is widely accepted that a minimum of two cycles of treatment is required after complete response is achieved before stopping treatment. For fast responders, six cycles of a conventional regimen are considered sufficient, whereas seven or eight cycles may be given when the response is slower. It is often difficult to assess a complete response in patients with residual masses that may remain stable or disappear slowly because of scarring. Gallium scans or positron emission tomography scans may be useful for this distinction. A lack of complete response, allowing for residual masses, is not a satisfactory outcome, and such individuals should be considered for dose intensification (transplant) or, less often, salvage with radiation therapy. In addition to patients with obvious extensive disease (stage IV) who are treated with full-course combination chemotherapy, the following categories of patients should also be considered as having advanced disease and probably be treated similarly.

*B Disease.* Patients with B symptoms (fever, night sweats, weight loss) even with low CS (I, II) are commonly found to have extensive disease at laparotomy (positive 40 to 50%) and have a high relapse rate if treated with radiation only.[84] Even surgically staged patients with weight loss and fever have a 50% relapse rate when treated with radiation therapy.[85] Patients with B symptoms, especially weight loss and fever, regardless of CS should be considered as having advanced disease and should probably be treated with full-course chemotherapy. The presence of night sweats alone did not seem to confer an adverse prognosis independently in one series. Combined-modality treatment with an abbreviated first-line regimen and involved field radiation may be considered as an alternative to full-dose chemotherapy in selected *early* B cases but with caution.

*Stage IIIA Disease.* Radiation therapy is often insufficient in stage III disease. The utility of chemotherapy even in good prognosis $III_1A$ HL has been documented in a comparative study: TLI produced a 55% FFP, whereas the FFP was 94% in the combined-modality treatment.[86] Chemotherapy alone has produced excellent results in patients with stage IIIA disease with reported FFP at least 90%.[87] Randomized studies have not documented survival advantage by adding radiation to full-course chemotherapy except in the case of bulky mediastinal disease.[88] A published meta-analysis suggested a trend toward increased treatment control by adding radiation to full-course chemotherapy, but it was not statistically significant.[72] Full-course chemotherapy should be the preferred treatment of patients with CS IIIA HD. The role of consolidative radiation is an option of questionable benefit.

*Bulky Mediastinal Disease.* Bulky disease is defined as a nodal mass greater than 10 cm or a mediastinal mass greater than one third of the maximal thoracic diameter. Treatment of patients with a large mediastinal mass with radiation therapy and probably with chemotherapy alone results in relapse in about half of the patients.[89] A randomized trial involving patients with bulky mediastinal disease comparing radiation alone and six courses of chemotherapy followed by involved field radiation showed a significantly improved 10-year freedom from relapse rate for patients treated with combined-modality therapy (81% vs. 45%).[90] For patients with stage IV disease, the benefit of irradiation of the bulky mediastinal mass after a complete course of chemotherapy, although widely practiced, is less well documented. It is believed that a benefit is obtained, although it did not reach statistical significance in a meta-analysis of more than 300 patients.[65] Also the choice of a chemotherapy regimen in patients who are going to have extensive radiation to the mediastinum may be problematic, given the potential cardiac and pulmonary toxicity of ABVD. Results of a treatment program including 65 patients treated with six cycles of alternating MOPP and ABVD followed by mantle irradiation reported an 85% complete response and a projected FFP of 72%.[91] Although the evidence is less compelling, patients with a bulky site other than mediastinum may be treated in a similar manner with radiation to the site of bulk. The benefit of a full course of chemotherapy in patients with bulky disease outside the mediastinum who receive involved field radiation is unclear, unless they have other features of advanced HL.

**Which Is the Preferred Primary Chemotherapy Regimen for Advanced Hodgkin's Lymphoma?** MOPP was the first highly successful combination chemotherapy regimen for HL (Tables 87–7 and 87–8), producing a complete response in 80% of patients and achieving a 50% cure rate in patients with extensive disease.[92] For almost two decades, MOPP remained the mainstay of treatment and was an excellent paradigm of the principle of clinically important synergy achieved by multiagent chemotherapy. In this paradigm, agents with independent activity and nonoverlapping toxicities were chosen to construct a highly effective regimen for a sensitive malignancy. MOPP is given every 4 weeks for six cycles or two cycles beyond maximal clinical response. Although it appears that dose reduction may affect treatment outcome adversely, maintaining the prescribed dose intensity of MOPP has been a difficult task for clinicians. The acute toxicities of MOPP include severe nausea, peripheral neuropathy, and alopecia. The initially recommended dose of vincristine 1.4 mg/m² could not be tolerated by patients outside the NCI because of neuropathy, and a dose cap of 2 mg has been customary. The nausea was reduced by substituting chlorambucil for mechlorethamine (nitrogen mustard), and neurotoxicity was decreased by using vinblastine instead of vincristine (ClVPP [chlorambucil, vinblastine, procarbazine, prednisone]).[93] Several other variations of MOPP have been reported without any significant therapeutic advantage. Despite drug substitutions or modifications, major late morbidity associated with MOPP and related protocols included sterility and an increased incidence of leukemia.

The ABVD regimen was first developed in Milan as a salvage regimen for the treatment of MOPP failures and included drugs considered to be non–cross-resistant with those of MOPP.[48] Because of its efficacy and improved toxicity profile, it was soon tested as first-line treatment. ABVD causes less nausea, gonadal suppression, leukemogenesis, and neurotoxicity. ABVD causes more cardiopulmonary complications, however. The long-term safety of ABVD in young adults is to some extent uncertain, particularly when combined with chest irradiation. ABVD is given every 2 weeks with a cycle defined as two administrations of the drugs. Six cycles or two cycles beyond complete response

***Table 87–7.* Traditional First-Line Chemotherapy Regimens for Hodgkin's Lymphoma**

| Regimen | Dose (mg/m² or U/m²) | Days |
|---|---|---|
| ABVD (28 days) | | |
| Doxorubicin | 25 | 1, 15 |
| Bleomycin | 10 | 1, 15 |
| Vinblastine | 6 | 1, 15 |
| Dacarbazine | 375 | 1, 15 |
| MOPP (28 days) | | |
| Mechlorethamine | 6 | 1, 8 |
| Vincristine | 1.4 | 1, 8 |
| Procarbazine (PO) | 100 | 1–14 |
| Prednisone (PO) | 40 | 1–14 |
| MOPP/ABV (28 days) | | |
| Mechlorethamine | 6 | 1 |
| Vincristine | 1.4 | 1 |
| Procarbazine (PO) | 100 | 1–7 |
| Prednisone (PO) | 40 | 1–14 |
| Doxorubicin | 35 | 8 |
| Bleomycin | 10 | 8 |
| Vinblastine | 6 | 8 |
| COPP (28 days) | | |
| Cyclophosphamide | 650 | 1, 8 |
| Vincristine | 1.4 | 1, 8 |
| Procarbazine (PO) | 100 | 1–14 |
| Prednisone (PO) | 40 | 1–14 |
| Ch1VPP (28 days) | | |
| Chlorambucil (PO total) | 6 | 1–14 |
| Vinblastine (max 10) | 6 | 1, 8 |
| Procarbazine (PO) | 100 | 1–14 |
| Prednisone (PO) | 40 | 1–14 |

*For combined modality treatment of favorable patients:*

| | | |
|---|---|---|
| EBVP (28 days) | | |
| Epirubicin | 70 | 1 |
| Bleomycin | 10 | 1 |
| Vinblastine | 6 | 1 |
| Prednisone (PO) | 40 | 1–5 |
| VBM (28 days) | | |
| Vinblastine | 6 | 1,8 |
| Bleomycin | 10* | 1,8 |
| Methotrexate | 30 | 1,8 |
| (4-week cycle) | | |

* Bleomycin was reduced to 2.5 mg/m² after radiation therapy.

are defined as a full course. When compared directly with MOPP, ABVD produces a better complete response rate and disease-free survival (complete response, 82% vs. 67%; disease-free survival, 61% vs. 50%).[94] Alternating MOPP and ABVD cycles was found to be significantly superior to MOPP alone in at least two large randomized studies in terms of remission rates and overall survival.[95] The MOPP-ABVD alternate regimen was not statistically superior to ABVD, however.[94] Even if the inferior results of MOPP may be due partially to toxicity-related dose reductions, ABVD or related regimens appear to be more tolerable and at least as effective in treating patients with HL. Nonalkylating regimens that do not include bleomycin such as EVA (etoposide, vinblastine, doxorubicin) and others have been reported.[96] Although they have been tested less rigorously, they can be used instead of ABVD if bleomycin-related pulmonary toxicity occurs.

Subsequently a *hybrid* regimen MOPP/ABV was developed in Vancouver, which emphasized increased dose intensity.[97] Despite this possible advantage, direct comparison of the hybrid treatment with alternating MOPP and ABVD by

*Table 87–8.* Salvage Regimens for Hodgkin's Lymphoma

| Regimen | Dose (mg or U/m²) | Days |
|---|---|---|
| EVA (28 days) | | |
| Etoposide | 100 | 1,2,3 |
| Vinblastine | 6 | 1 |
| Doxorubicin | 50 | 1 |
| miniBEAM (28 days) | | |
| BCNU | 60 | 1 |
| Etoposide | 75 | 2–5 |
| Ara-C | 100 BID | 2–5 |
| Melphalan | 30 | 6 |
| VAPEC-B (28 days) | | |
| Vincristine | 1.4 | 8, 22 |
| Doxorubicin | 35 | 1,15 |
| Prednisone (PO) | 50 (total) | Daily for first 6 weeks |
| | 25 (total) | Daily for latter 6 weeks |
| Etoposide | 100 | 15, 16, 17, 18, 19 |
| Cyclophosphamide | 350 | 1 |
| Bleomycin | 10 | 8 |
| Prophylactic cotrimoxazole (for a total of three 4-week cycles) | | |
| CEP (28 days) | | |
| Lomustine (PO) | 80 | 1 |
| Etoposide (PO) | 100 | 1–5 |
| Prednimustine (PO) | 60 | 1–5 |
| DHAP (28 days) | | |
| Dexamethasone (total) | 40 | 1–4 |
| Cisplatin | 100 | 1 (continuous infusion) |
| Ara-C | 2000 q 12 hr × 2 | |
| MINE (28 days) | | |
| Ifosfamide | 1.33 | 1–3 |
| Mitoxantrone | 10 | 1 |
| Etoposide | 65 | 1–3 |

the NCI of Canada group and the Italian group showed no difference in efficacy, with greater toxicity produced by the hybrid.[98, 99] An Intergroup randomized study comparing MOPP and ABV with ABVD was terminated prematurely because of increased mortality in the hybrid arm, whereas no difference in efficacy was apparent.[101] One large American cooperative group study involving 691 patients showed superiority of the hybrid regimen compared with alternating cycles of MOPP and ABVD, with an 8-year survival outcome of 79% versus 71% in favor of the hybrid.[101] Considering all of the above-mentioned studies, it still remains unclear whether the hybrid regimen is superior to ABVD. Its use may be justified, however, in patients with extensive disease and no comorbid conditions who are not concerned about sterility.

Based on the previous discussion, ABVD emerges as the current gold standard combination chemotherapy for patients with extensive HL. Alternating MOPP and ABVD is probably equivalent and can be considered for patients scheduled to receive mediastinal irradiation who have no concerns about maintaining fertility.

Because the dose intensity delivered seems to be an important factor in predicting outcome in patients treated with MOPP or ABVD, several groups have designed dose-intense regimens that deliver more chemotherapy in a shorter time. The Stanford group designed a weekly regimen of seven drugs known as *Stanford V* delivered over 12 weeks (Table 87–9).[102] Consolidative radiation therapy is used. My-

elosuppressive drugs alternate with relatively marrow-sparing agents. In the pilot phase II study, patients with bulky stage II, stage III, and stage IV disease treated according to Stanford V achieved a 93% 6-year actuarial survival, with an 89% FFP.[103, 104] Prompted by these excellent results, the Stanford V regimen is currently being compared with ABVD in a randomized fashion.

A different intense regimen, BEACOPP (bleomycin, etoposide, doxorubicin, cyclophosphamide, vincristine, procarbazine, prednisone), has been developed by the German Hodgkin's Disease Study Group (GHDSG) and has been further tested in a dose-escalated manner. The seven drugs in BEACOPP are given in a 3-week cycle, in contrast to MOPP and ABV, which is given every 4 weeks. Procarbazine is given for 7 days, whereas doxorubicin is given only on day 1, allowing for cycling every 3 weeks, in contrast to MOPP and ABV. In addition, the active agent etoposide is incorporated in this program. In a phase II study, the regimen produced a 97% response rate.[105]

Dose escalation has been performed aided by mandatory use of growth factors. A maximum tolerated BEACOPP dosage was defined that involves increased doses of etoposide, doxorubicin, and cyclophosphamide to 200%, 140%, and 192% of baseline. The preliminary results of a three-arm randomized clinical study comparing COPP (cyclophosphamide, vincristine, procarbazine, prednisone) and ABVD with standard-dose BEACOPP or escalated BEACOPP involving approximately 700 evaluable patients have been reported.[106] The complete response rate for COPP and ABVD was 83% and was inferior to the 92% complete response for the combined BEACOPP arms. Twelve percent of the COPP-ABVD patients had progressive disease, whereas only 6% of the BEACOPP patients had progression.

*Table 87–9.* Dose-Intense Regimens

| Regimen | Dose (mg or U/m²) | Days |
|---|---|---|
| Stanford V (28 days)* | | |
| Doxorubicin | 25 | 1, 15 |
| Vinblastine | 6 | 1,15 |
| Mechlorethamine | 6 | 1, 15 |
| Vincristine | 1.4 | 8, 22 |
| Bleomycin | 5 | 8, 22 |
| Etoposide | 60 | 15 |
| Prednisone | 40 QOD | |
| BEACOPP (21 days) | | |
| Bleomycin | 10 | 8 |
| Etoposide | 100 | 1–3 |
| Doxorubicin | 25 | 1 |
| Cyclophosphamide | 650 | 1 |
| Vincristine | 1.4 | 8 |
| Procarbazine (PO) | 100 | 1–7 |
| Prednisone (PO) | 40 | 1–14 |
| BEACOPP (escalated) | | |
| Bleomycin | 10 | 8 |
| Etoposide | 200 | 1–3 |
| Doxorubicin | 35 | 1 |
| Cyclophosphamide | 1250 | 1 |
| Vincristine | 1.4 | 8 |
| Procarbazine (PO) | 100 | 1–7 |
| Prednisone (PO) | 40 | 1–14 |

*For a total of three 4-week cycles.
QOD, every other day.

The 2-year survival was 89% for the COPP-ABVD arm, 94% for standard BEACOPP, and 96% for escalated BEACOPP. There was no difference in secondary malignancies, although leukemia was observed only in the BEACOPP arms.

Based on these results, enrollment in the COPP-ABVD arm was discontinued. Escalated BEACOPP produced a 95% complete response compared with 88% in standard BEACOPP. Only 2% of the higher dose arm experienced relapse compared with 9% of the standard dose arm. Significantly more cytopenias were noted after escalated BEACOPP, but the incidence of life-threatening events was not increased. Patients with adverse prognostic factors seem to derive more benefit from dose escalation. If these encouraging results are sustained after longer follow-up and can be validated by other groups, this may suggest that moderate dose intensification may benefit certain patients with advanced or high-risk HL. Incorporation of a myeloablative high-dose regimen followed by autologous hematopoietic stem cell transplantation as part of induction treatment of HL has been proposed and is currently being tested in a randomized study in high-risk patients with advanced HL, as defined by the adverse prognostic factors discussed earlier.

For patients with extensive nonbulky disease, the addition of radiotherapy to previously involved sites of disease following chemotherapy has not been proved to have an impact on disease-free or overall survival. In patients with advanced disease, reduction of first-line chemotherapy even if supported by radiation therapy adversely affects long-term survival.[72] As previously noted, patients with bulky mediastinal masses should probably be consolidated with involved field radiation. By inference, patients with extensive disease and a bulky site outside the mediastinum may also receive radiation to the site of bulk, although this practice is not fully supported in the literature.

## TREATMENT OF RELAPSED OR REFRACTORY HODGKIN'S LYMPHOMA

About 30% of patients treated with radiation therapy alone are destined to relapse. Most relapses occur within the first 3 years, but rare relapses beyond the fifth year and up to 20 years have been described.[107] These chemotherapy-naive patients often relapse in previously unirradiated sites and have an excellent chance of successful treatment with front-line chemotherapy regimens.[108] In patients who relapse after traditional first-line chemotherapy, salvage standard-dose chemotherapy (MOPP, ABVD, or equivalent) produces prolonged remission in 10 to 30% of the treated patients.[109] For such patients, adverse prognostic factors include short initial remission (<1 year), older age, extensive disease including organ involvement, and relapse both within and outside radiation ports. Patients with long remissions can be treated with the same or similar regimen as used for induction, or a different first-line regimen can be used (e.g., patients who had received ABVD may be treated with MOPP; patients who had received MOPP may be treated with ABVD). Salvage regimens for patients failing front-line combinations often contain nitrosoureas and etoposide and are given with palliative intent.[110] As noted, patients who relapse in less than 1 year after initial therapy have a particularly poor prognosis.[109, 111] Isolated nonbulky relapses in lymph nodes can be salvaged with radiation alone with an occasional long-term disease-free survival.[112]

Patients failing to achieve a complete response after initial therapy (so-called refractory disease) have a particularly dismal prognosis if treated conventionally and have transient responses to standard-dose front-line or salvage chemotherapy. It is possible that a rare patient with disease limited to one site may be rendered tumor-free by radiation.

### High-Dose Therapy

Because of the disappointing results of conventional salvage treatments seen in relapsed or refractory HL, patients who do not achieve a complete response or have recurrent disease after adequate front-line chemotherapy should be considered for autologous stem cell transplantation. Autologous stem cell transplantation enables the administration of high-dose, myeloablative chemotherapy or chemoradiotherapy (with total-body radiation) with curative intent. When first developed, this procedure involved autologous bone marrow harvesting as a source of hematopoietic precursors; however, the bone marrow has been largely replaced by mobilized peripheral stem cells. The advantages of the latter include more rapid engraftment and easier procurement by performing large-volume leukapheresis. Reece and colleagues[113] reported 30 patients with primary refractory HL who were treated with a dose-intense program supported by autologous stem cells: A 42% actuarial progression-free survival was noted in this group of patients with a poor prognosis. Sixty patients with relapsed HL treated with high-dose chemotherapy and stem cell support were compared with historic matched controls treated with conventional chemotherapy. Event-free survival at 4 years (55% vs. 25%) and overall survival (55% vs. 46%) favored the transplanted patients. The benefit seemed more evident in patients with an adverse prognosis (i.e., refractory disease or relapse within 1 year).[113] Similarly the Stanford group reported a significant improvement in outcome after high-dose treatment with autologous stem cell support in patients with refractory or relapsed HL, who achieved a 53% event-free survival compared with 27% for historic controls.[114] Gianni and colleagues[116] have reported excellent results with a sequential high-dose chemotherapy program, with a 71% event-free survival for relapsed and 31% for refractory patients.

In many other phase II reports, which used different entry criteria and conditioning regimens with varying length of follow-up, 3- to 5-year progression-free survivals of 25 to 64% have been reported.[117–123] In general, a disease-free survival of 20 to 40% for refractory patients and 45 to 65% for relapsing patients can be expected after an autologous stem cell transplant, which compares favorably with historic controls employing standard-dose therapy. Adverse factors emerging from the above-mentioned reports include the number of previous treatments, resistance to chemotherapy, tumor bulk at the time of transplant, systemic symptoms, short duration of initial remission, and extranodal relapses. The prognostic factors differ from study to study, and it is difficult to generalize. It is unknown whether a particular high-dose conditioning regimen or the inclusion of total-body irradiation is superior. Generally, total-body irradiation is avoided in patients who have had mantle field or other extensive prior irradiation. Spot irradiation to bulky or dominant site is often administered, before or after the transplant. At the University of California Los Angeles (UCLA), a total-body irradiation–based conditioning regimen is used when prior radiation history permits. If spot irradiation is needed, it is administered immediately preceding total-body irradiation so that the area of interest receives the scheduled total radiation dose without interruption. Postengraftment irradiation is avoided.

These encouraging data suggest that essentially all refractory or relapsed patients should be considered candidates for a high-dose treatment program, if they maintain satisfactory organ function. Patients intended for such treatments often first receive a salvage cytoreductive regimen designed to reduce tumor bulk and determine chemosensitivity. The value and the optimization of this practice are not entirely clear. Prolonged exposure to salvage chemotherapy may impair the mobilization of stem cells, and the benefits of cytoreduction should be weighed against this risk. Various cytoreductive regimens have been used in preparation for a transplant. Theoretically a preparatory regimen should not contain the drugs used in the high-dose combination to avoid induction of resistance. *Hodgkin's-specific* regimens of substantial efficacy include VAPEC-B,[124] mini-BEAM (BCNU, etoposide, ara-C, melphalan),[125] EVA,[96] and MINE (mitoguazone, ifosfamide, vinorelbine, etoposide)[126]; salvage lymphoma regimens such as DHAP (dexamethasone, cytarabine, cisplatin) and MINE may also be used. The upper age limit for an autologous transplant is unclear. At UCLA, non-total-body irradiation autologous stem cell transplants are performed in selected patients up to the age of 70, with tolerable toxicity.

### Palliative Chemotherapy

Patients who do not qualify for transplant and have remained in remission for more than 1 year can be treated with a first-line regimen, with a possibility of achieving a second durable remission. There is no established curative treatment for multiply relapsed patients who are not transplant candidates. If the performance status allows, one of the salvage combination regimens described earlier can be used. Patients failing standard combination therapy or salvage chemotherapy including autologous transplantation may still respond to single-agent regimens. In an earlier study, oral CCNU at a dose of 100 mg/m² every 6 weeks has been reported to have a 60% response rate.[127] Nitrosoureas have also been used in a variety of third-line combination regimens against HL, such as oral CEP (CCNU, etoposide, prednimustine).[110] Other single agents with defined activity that may be used as palliative agents include vinblastine[128] and oral etoposide.[129] Newer agents with promise include gemcitabine,[130] vinorelbine,[131] and possibly mitoguazone.[132] Such patients are frequently candidates for phase I or II trials.

### TOXICITY ASSOCIATED WITH CHEMOTHERAPY AND RADIATION THERAPY

MOPP and similar agents are mainly associated with secondary myelodysplasia, leukemia, and sterility. Alkylating agent–related myelodysplasia or acute myeloid leukemia is usually characterized by deletions or abnormalities involving the long arms of chromosomes 5 and 7. The cumulative incidence of leukemia is approximately 2% at 20 years, and leukemia commonly occurs within 8 years after treatment.[133] Alkylating agent–related myelodysplasia and acute leukemia have a dire prognosis; allogeneic bone marrow transplantation may be considered for the treatment of eligible young patients. Radiation adds to the risk of MOPP-related myelodysplasia syndrome or acute myeloid leukemia. Multiple chemotherapy exposures or high-dose chemotherapy increase the risk as well.

In males, azoospermia associated with follicle-stimulating hormone elevation but without impotence or hypogonadism is the rule after a full course of MOPP.[134] Irreversible amenorrhea develops in almost all women older than age 25, whereas younger women may have return of their menses.[135] Women who remain fertile may conceive without ill effects on the fetus. Cessation of ovulation by luteinizing hormone–releasing hormone analogues or hormonal supplementation seem to protect male and female rodents from chemotherapy-related infertility, but studies involving humans have been disappointing.[135, 136] Amenorrhea and infertility are also common but rarely reversible complications of autologous transplantation. MOPP-related leukemogenesis and infertility are dose dependent. Permanent infertility has not been associated with ABVD. Sperm banking or egg harvesting and hormone replacement in women should be considered. Of male patients presenting with untreated HL, 70% have some sperm abnormality, and 8% may have azoospermia; there is no clear explanation for this phenomenon.[138]

Doxorubicin, which is a component of ABVD and related regimens, is a well-known cardiotoxic agent. The incidence of cardiotoxicity is related to the cumulative dose and most likely to peak serum levels. The cumulative dose of doxorubicin in ABVD is usually 300 mg/m², which is below the clinically significant cardiotoxic level when given without radiation. Administration of mediastinal radiation increases the chance of cardiomyopathy, pericarditis, or coronary artery disease and the potential for delayed cardiomyopathy at doses of doxorubicin similar to ABVD.[139]

Bleomycin usually causes mild and subclinical reduction of diffusion capacity, which improves slowly after the completion of treatment. Idiosyncratic severe pulmonary toxicity is occasionally seen at cumulative doses of bleomycin greater than 50 mg. In combination with mediastinal radiation, more severe pulmonary toxicity has been reported, which may include pulmonary infiltrates, restrictive defects, and exertional dyspnea.[140] These effects depend, in part, on the total dose of bleomycin and radiation field. Because the pulmonary toxicity of the combination of ABVD and radiation can rarely be fatal, some recommend the use of ABVD alternating with MOPP if a full course of chemotherapy and mediastinal irradiation is anticipated. Rare cases of severe and sometimes fatal hyperpyrexia have been reported with bleomycin in HL.

Other chemotherapy-related toxicities include vinca alkaloid–associated peripheral neuropathy and constipation as well as the known toxicities associated with corticosteroids. The neutropenia, anemia, and thrombocytopenia that accompany chemotherapy for HL are usually readily reversible. The use of neutrophil growth factors should be reserved for patients who are unable to receive the full dose of prescribed chemotherapy in a timely fashion. Erythropoietin may be indicated for symptomatic anemic patients.

Non-Hodgkin's lymphomas can rarely present synchronously with HL. HL survivors are also at increased risk of developing non-Hodgkin's lymphoma.[141, 142] It is unclear if this increased risk is related to a common cause, an immunodeficiency associated with HD, or treatment. Such lymphomas are often extranodal and of aggressive histology.[143] Their management is unclear, and they often have an ominous prognosis, suggesting a role for high-dose myeloablative therapy.

There is a well-described and definite increase in solid tumors in long-term survivors of HL who received radiation therapy.[144–146] Such tumors have a peak incidence during and following the second decade after the treatment. Most, but not all, arise within or near the radiation fields. The most common cancers are lung cancer, especially in smokers; breast cancer; and stomach cancer. Less common malignancies include melanoma, thyroid cancer, head and neck cancers, and sarcomas. The cumulative incidence is 8 to 24% in various studies.[146, 147] The risk seems to be higher for younger patients who receive radiation treatment. In a report from Stanford, the relative risk of developing breast cancer in girls irradiated before the age of 15 was 136; in patients irradiated between the ages of 15 and 24, it was 19. No increased risk was identified for women treated after age 30.[148] Because of the latency of 10 to 20 years for the development of solid tumors, it is still premature to conclude that there will be a lesser impact from currently used limited radiation ports or dosages in terms of secondary malignancies, but this eventuality is eagerly anticipated. The significant risk of developing cancers necessitates careful monitoring of long-term HL survivors, with annual mammograms starting about 10 years after the treatment and frequent physical examinations.

## SPECIAL PRESENTATIONS

### Infradiaphragmatic

Generally the same rules of treatment as in patients with supradiaphragmatic disease apply to patients with infradiaphragmatic disease. If patients present with CS IA peripheral (inguinal or femoral) disease, inverted Y field radiation with or without splenic irradiation may be sufficient, although combined-modality therapy with involved field radiation is increasingly used. For more extensive IIA disease or retroperitoneal IA disease, a combined-modality program is more appropriate. These recommendations are based on earlier experience derived from routine staging laparotomy.[149]

### Childhood Hodgkin's Lymphoma

HL in children is relatively uncommon in the United States but occurs with increased incidence in the Third World. Attention to the toxicity of a selected program is of paramount importance in developing children. Because of the adverse effects of radiation on growing bones and muscles, extensive radiation fields or high dosages should be avoided. Most children or adolescents should probably be treated with a full chemotherapy course, preferably ABVD alternating

with MOPP to avoid sterility and cardiotoxicity. Low-dose adjuvant radiation treatment not exceeding 25 Gy can be considered.[150]

### Pregnancy

Common staging procedures and treatment for HL may have adverse effects on the developing embryo during the first trimester of pregnancy. An abortion should be considered based on the stage and symptomatic state of the mother, rather than delaying treatment until delivery. In later pregnancy, treatment of favorable disease can often be delayed for a few months, until delivery. Staging can be completed during pregnancy by avoiding radiologic tests and using alternative methods, such as ultrasonography or possibly magnetic resonance imaging. During the first trimester, radiation of threatening thoracic disease can be performed safely with appropriate shielding. Chemotherapy can be tolerated well during the third trimester so that first-line treatment can be administered if required by an adverse presentation.

### Human Immunodeficiency Virus

HIV is probably associated with a fivefold to eightfold increased incidence of HL.[151] This increase is significantly smaller compared with the increased risk for non-Hodgkin's lymphoma, which is estimated at 200. It appears that such patients present with more advanced disease, however, with bone marrow involvement and are often relatively difficult to manage because of concomitant morbidity associated with HIV infection.[152] Full treatment should be administered to patients with a good state of health and relatively preserved CD4 counts. Caution should be observed in patients with significant comorbid conditions and poor performance status. The expected benefits of controlling HL should be weighed against the patient's prognosis resulting from immunodeficiency and expected treatment-related complications. Often a carefully designed palliative treatment program is preferable to full treatment for patients with advanced acquired immunodeficiency syndrome.

### Lymphocytic-Predominant Hodgkin's Lymphoma

LPHL is now considered to be an indolent B-cell lymphoma. It is believed that it is a distinct entity with a different epidemiology and natural history. It is more common in young men and in older ages. For older adults, the incidence rises with age, similar to low-grade lymphomas. Bulky disease or involvement of the spleen are uncommon, whereas infradiaphragmatic disease is more common compared with classic HL. The distinct pathologic features have been described earlier. Patients with early disease may have an excellent response to treatment. Patients with advanced disease also achieve remissions but commonly have late relapses. No plateau in disease-free survival is seen for 20 years, reminiscent of the natural history of indolent lymphomas. It is currently unclear how this disease should be treated and whether treatment other than that applied for HL may produce better results. Some patients are being observed expectantly. Given the rarity and long natural history of LPHL, it is unlikely that any alternative treatment will emerge soon; it is therefore reasonable to continue treating patients applying principles used in the treatment of HL.

## Future Directions

As mentioned earlier, dose intensification with or without an autologous transplant early in the treatment of HL with poor prognostic features is currently being explored. When the long-term toxicity of such methods is better defined, and if survival differences are sustained after longer follow-up, such treatment approaches may be accepted as the preferred management for a subgroup of patients with a relatively adverse prognosis. The identification of such a subgroup may be facilitated by the advent of a new, clinically relevant, risk stratification system as noted earlier.

In addition to optimizing chemotherapy-based treatments, alternative approaches have been tested. The use of cytokines, such as interferon alfa, especially as maintenance treatment after dose intensification, has been tested in feasibility trials with inconclusive results so far.[153] Therapeutic strategies have been developed based on the expression of the CD-30 or CD-25 antigen by the RS cells. Anti-CD-25 and anti-CD-30 immunotoxins have been tested with good results in animal HL models.[154–156] An anti-CD-25 ricin-A immunotoxin has been tested in a phase I–II study because the overexpression of CD-25 antigen by RS cells compared with normal lymphocytes is believed to confer substantial differential uptake.[157, 158] Moderate toxicity but also two partial responses were observed in a group of 20 heavily pretreated patients. The use of bispecific anti-CD30 antibodies aimed at bringing in proximity immune effector cells has been tested successfully in the laboratory[159] and tried in patients. Two responses were seen among 15 patients enrolled in a pilot trial, whereas no substantial toxicity was noted.[160] Targeted radioimmunotherapy using a technetium-labeled anti-CD30 antibody has been tested in a phase I feasibility study.[161] A phase I trial of the DAB-IL-2 fusion diphtheria toxin has been reported to have produced a response in one patient.[162] Several other ongoing studies are evaluating immunotherapeutic approaches in the treatment of HL. The available preliminary results suggest a possible role of such treatments, potentially in combination with other modalities.

The high treatment-related toxicity of allogeneic bone marrow or peripheral stem cell transplantation limits application to young patients with refractory disease and suitable donors. The advent of nonmyeloablative but sufficiently immunosuppressive conditioning regimens that enable donor hematopoietic stem cell engraftment with minimal toxicity may widen the candidate patient population for allogeneic transplants.[163] Whether the presumed graft-versus-lymphoma effect would be adequate in suppressing HL remains to be seen.

## REFERENCES

1. Grufferman S, Cole P, Smith PG, et al. Hodgkin's disease in siblings. N Engl J Med 1977;296:248–50.
2. Vianna NJ, Greenwald P, Brady J, et al. Hodgkin's disease cases with features of community outbreak. Ann Intern Med 1972;77:169–80.
3. Schimpff SC, Schimpff CR, Brager DM, et al. Leukaemia and lymphoma patients interlinked by prior social contact. Lancet 1975;1:124–9.
4. Davis S. Case aggregation in young adult Hodgkin's disease: etiologic evidence from a population experience. Cancer 1986;57:1602–12.
5. Mueller N. Epidemiologic studies assessing the role of the Epstein-Barr virus in Hodgkin's disease. Yale J Biol Med 1987;60:321–32.
6. Donhuijsen-Ant R, Abken H, Bornkamm G, et al. Fatal Hodgkin and non-Hodgkin lymphoma associated with persistent Epstein-Barr virus in four brothers. Ann Intern Med 1988;109:946–52.
7. Weiss LM, Chen YY, Liu XF, et al. Epstein-Barr virus and Hodgkin's disease: correlative in situ hybridization and polymerase chain reaction study. Am J Pathol 1991;139:1259–65.
8. Staal SP, Ambinder R, Beschorner WE, et al. A survey of Epstein-Barr virus DNA in lymphoid tissue: frequent detection in Hodgkin's disease. Am J Clin Pathol 1989;91:1–5.
9. Weiss LM, Movahed LA, Warnke RA, et al. Detection of Epstein-Barr viral genomes in Reed-Sternberg cells of Hodgkin's disease. N Engl J Med 1989;320:502–6.
10. Henderson EE, Franks C, Fronko G. Chemical carcinogen Epstein-Barr virus (EBV) synergism: EBV genome amplification and site-specific mutation during transformation. Int J Cancer 1989;43:72–9.
11. Khan G, Norton AJ, Slavin G. Epstein-Barr virus in Hodgkin disease: relation to age and subtype. Cancer 1992;71:3124–9.
12. Ambinder RF, Browning PJ, Lorenzana I, et al. Epstein-Barr virus and childhood Hodgkin's disease in Honduras and the United States. Blood 1993;81:462–7.
13. Pinkus GS, Lones M, Shintaku IP, et al. Immunohistochemical detection of Epstein-Barr virus encoded latent membrane protein in Reed-Sternberg cells and variants of Hodgkin's disease. Mod Pathol 1994;7:454–61.
14. Tamaru J, Hummel M, Zemlin M, et al. Hodgkin's disease with a B-cell phenotype often shows a VDJ rearrangement and somatic mutations in the VH genes. Blood 1994;84:708–15.
15. Sinkovics JG. Discovery of the hybridoma principle in 1968–69 immortalization of the specific antibody producing cell by fusion with a lymphoma cell. J Med 1985;16:509–24.
16. Haluska FG, Brufsky AM, Canellos GP. The cellular biology of the Reed-Sternberg cell. Blood 1994;84:1005–19.
17. Kadin ME, Muramoto L, Said J. Expression of T-cell antigens on Reed-Sternberg cells in a subset of patients with nodular sclerosing and mixed cellularity Hodgkin's disease. Am J Pathol 1988;130:345–53.
18. Brauninger A, Hansman ML, Strickler JG. Identification of common germinal center B-cell precursors in two patients with both Hodgkin's disease and non-Hodgkin's disease. N Engl J Med 1999;340:1239–47.
19. Hummel M, Marafioti T, Stein H. Clonality of Reed-Sternberg cells in Hodgkin's disease. N Engl J Med 1999;340:394–5.
20. Jaffe ES, Harris NL, Diebold J, et al. World Health Organization classification of neoplastic disease of the hematopoietic and lymphoid tissues: a progress report. Am J Clin Pathol 1999;111:Suppl 1:S8–S12.
21. Pinkus GS, Said JW. Hodgkin's disease, lymphocyte predominance type, nodular—a distinct entity? Am J Pathol 1985;118:1–6.
22. Stein H, Hansmann ML, Lennert K, et al. Reed-Sternberg and Hodgkin cells in lymphocyte predominant Hodgkin's disease of nodular subtype contain J chain. Am J Clin Pathol 1986;86:292–7.
23. Pinkus GS, Said JW. Hodgkin's disease, lymphocyte predominance type, nodular—further evidence for a B cell derivation: L & H variants of Reed-Sternberg cells express L26, a pan B cell marker. Am J Pathol 1988;133:211–7.
24. Poppema S. The nature of the lymphocytes surrounding Reed-Sternberg cells in nodular lymphocyte predominance and in other types of Hodgkin's disease. Am J Pathol 1989;135:351–7.
25. Hansmann M-L, Stein H, Fellbaum C, et al. Nodular paragranuloma can transform into high-grade malignant lymphoma of B type. Hum Pathol 1989;20:1969–75.
26. Sundeen JT, Cossman J, Jaffe ES. Lymphocyte predominant Hodgkin's disease with coexistent "large cell lymphoma." Am J Surg Pathol 1988;12:599–606.
27. Hansmann M-L, Stein H, Dallenbach F, et al. Diffuse lymphocyte-predominant Hodgkin's disease (diffuse paragranuloma). Am J Pathol 1991;138:29–36.
27a. Lukes RJ. Criteria for involvement of lymph nodes, bone marrow, spleen and liver in Hodgkin's disease. Cancer Res 1971;1757–67.
28. Greiner TC, Gascoyne RD, Anderson ME, et al. Nodular lymphocyte

predominant-Hodgkin's disease associated with large cell lymphoma: analysis of immunoglobulin gene rearrangements by VJ PCR. Blood 1996;88:657–66.

29. Schmid C, Sargent C, Isaacson PG. L and H cells in nodular lymphocyte predominant Hodgkin's disease show immunoglobulin light-chain restriction. Am J Pathol 1991;139:1281–9.

30. Ferry JA, Linggood RM, Convery KM, et al. Hodgkin disease, nodular sclerosis type. Cancer 1993;71:457–63.

31. Strickler JG, Michie SA, Warnke RA, et al. The "syncytial variant" of nodular sclerosing Hodgkin's disease. Am J Surg Pathol 1986;10:470–7.

32. Delsol G, Meggetto F, Cohen-Knafo E, et al. Relation of follicular dendritic cells to Reed-Sternberg cells of Hodgkin's disease with emphasis on expression of CD21 antigen. Am J Pathol 1993;142:1729–38.

33. Leoncini L, Del Vecchio MT, Kraft R, et al. Hodgkin's disease and CD30-positive anaplastic large cell lymphomas—a spectrum of malignant disorders. Am J Pathol 1990;137:1047–57.

34. Neiman RS, Rosen PJ, Lukes RJ. Lymphocyte-depletion Hodgkin's disease: a clinicopathological entity. N Engl J Med 1973;288:751–5.

35. Kinney MC, Greer JP, Stein RS, et al. Lymphocyte-depletion Hodgkin's disease: histopathologic diagnosis of marrow involvement. Am J Surg Pathol 1986;10:219–26.

36. Bangerter M, Korzerke J, Grieshammer M, et al. Role of whole body FDG-PET in predicting relapse in residual masses after treatment of lymphoma. Blood 1998;92:Suppl 1:242a.

37. Borbenyi Z, Papos M, Tron L, et al. Clinical significance of FDG-PET and MIBI scintigraphy in post-treatment follow-up of residual masses in patients with malignant lymphoma. Blood 1998;92:Suppl 1:242a.

38. Castellino RA, Hoppe RT, Blanck N, et al. Computed tomography, lymphography and staging laparotomy: correlations in initial staging of Hodgkin's disease. AJR Am J Roentgenol 1984;143:37–41.

39. Gisselbrecht C, Ferme C. Prognostic factors in advanced Hodgkin's disease: problems and pitfalls: towards an international prognostic index. Leuk Lymphoma 1995;15:Suppl 1:23–4.

40. Straus DJ. High risk Hodgkin's disease prognostic factors. Leuk Lymphoma 1995;15:41–2.

41. Specht L. Prognostic factors in Hodgkin's disease. Cancer Treat Rev 1991;18:21–53.

42. Sarris AH, Viviani S, Bonfante V, et al. A prognostic model for Hodgkin's disease based on IL-10. Blood 1998;92:Suppl 1:243a.

43. Hasenclever D, Diehl V, Armitage JD, et al. A prognostic score for advanced Hodgkin's disease. N Engl J Med 1998;339:1506–14.

44. Carter SK, Livingston RB. Single agent therapy for Hodgkin's disease. Arch Intern Med 1973;131:377–87.

45. Lacher MJ. Combined vinblastine and chlorambucil therapy for Hodgkin's disease. Ann Intern Med 1965;62:468–76.

46. Frei E III, De Vita VT, Moxley JH, et al. Approaches to improving the chemotherapy of Hodgkin's disease. Cancer Res 1966;26:1284–9.

47. Longo DL, Young RC, Wesley M, et al. Twenty years of MOPP therapy for Hodgkin's disease. J Clin Oncol 1986;4:1295–306.

48. Bonadonna G, Santoro A. ABVD chemotherapy in the treatment of Hodgkin's disease. Cancer Treat Rev 1982;9:21–35.

49. Longo DL, Glatstein E, Duffey PL, et al. Radiation therapy vs. combination chemotherapy in the treatment of early-stage Hodgkin's disease: seven year results of a prospective randomized trial. J Clin Oncol 1991;9:906–17.

50. Biti GP, Cimino G, Cartoni C, et al. Extended field radiotherapy is superior to MOPP chemotherapy for the treatment of pathologic stage I–IIA Hodgkin's disease: a 8 year update of an Italian prospective study. J Clin Oncol 1992;10:378–82.

51. Longo DL, Russo A, Duffey PL, et al. Treatment of advanced stage massive mediastinal disease: the case for combined modality treatment. J Clin Oncol 1991;9:227–35.

52. Peters MV. Study of survival in Hodgkin's disease treated radiologically. AJR Am J Roentgenol 1950;63:299–311.

53. Gilbert R. La Roentgentherapie de la granulomatose maligne. J Radiol Electrol 1925;9:509.

54. Gilbert R. Radiotherapy in Hodgkin's disease; anatomical and clinical foundations; governing principles; results. AJR Am J Roentgenol 1939;41:198–241.

55. Shore T, Nelson N, Weinerman B. A meta-analysis of stages I and II Hodgkin's disease. Cancer 1990;65:1155–60.

56. Rosenberg SA, Kaplan HS. The evolution and summary results of the Stanford randomized clinical trials of the management of Hodgkin's disease: 1962–1984. Int J Radiat Oncol Biol Phys 1985;11:5–22.

57. Desser RK, Golomb HM, Ultman JE, et al. Prognostic classification of Hodgkin's disease in pathologic stage III based on anatomic consideration. Blood 1977;49:883–93.

58. Kaplan HS. Evidence of tumoricidal level in radiotherapy of Hodgkin's disease. Cancer Res 1966;26:1221–4.

59. Fletcher GH. The interplay of radiocurability and tolerance in the irradiation of human cancers. J Radiol Electrol 1975;56:383–400.

60. Mauch PM, Kalish LA, Marcus KC. Second malignancies after treatment for laparotomy staged IA–IIB Hodgkin's disease: long term analysis of risk factors and outcome. Blood 1996;87:3625–32.

61. Van Leeuwen FE, Klokman WJ, Hagenbeek A, et al. Second cancer risk following Hodgkin's disease: a 20-year follow-up study. J Clin Oncol 1994;12:312–25.

62. Wolden SL, Lamborn KR, Cleary SF, et al. Second cancer following pediatric Hodgkin's disease. J Clin Oncol 1998;16:536–44.

63. Constine LS, Schwartz RG, Savage DE, et al. Cardiac function, perfusion and morbidity in irradiated long-term survivors of Hodgkin's disease. Int J Radiat Oncol Biol Phys 1997;39:897–906.

64. Hudson MM, Paquette CA, Lee J, et al. Increased mortality after successful treatment of Hodgkin's disease. J Clin Oncol 1998;16:3592–600.

65. Zinzani PL, Gherlinzoni F, Piovaccari G, et al. Cardiac injury as late toxicity of mediastinal radiation therapy for Hodgkin's disease patients. Haematologica 1996;81:132–7.

66. Leibenhaut MH, Hoppe RT, Efron B, et al. Prognostic indicators of laparotomy findings in clinical stage I–II supradiaphragmatic HD. J Clin Oncol 1989;7:81–91.

67. Brada M, Easton DF, Horwich A, Peckman MJ. Clinical presentation as a predictor of laparotomy findings in supradiaphragmatic stage I and II HD. Radiother Oncol 1986;5:15–22.

68. Russell KJ, Hoppe RT, Colby TV, et al. Lymphocyte predominant HD: clinical presentation and results of treatment. Radiother Oncol 1984;1:197–205.

69. Hagenbeek A, Carde P, Noordijk E, et al. Prognostic factor tailored treatment of early stage Hodgkin's disease: results of a prospective randomized phase III clinical trial in 762 patients (H7 study). Blood 1997;90:Suppl 1:2603a.

70. Carde P, Hagenbeek K, Hayat M, et al. Clinical staging versus laparotomy and combined modality with MOPP versus ABVD in early stage Hodgkin's disease: the H6 twin randomized trials from the European Organization for Research and Treatment of Cancer Lymphoma Cooperative Group. J Clin Oncol 1993;11:2258–72.

71. Rosenberg SA. Laparotomy and splenectomy in Hodgkin's disease: a reappraisal after 20 years. Scand J Med 1985;34:289–92.

72. Loeffler M, Brosteanu O, Hasenclever D, et al. Meta-analysis of chemotherapy versus combined modality treatment trials in Hodgkin's disease. J Clin Oncol 1998;16:818–29.

73. Straus D, Yahalom J, Gaynor J, et al. Four cycles of chemotherapy and regional radiation therapy for clinical early stage and intermediate stage HD. Cancer 1992;69:1052–60.

74. Hancock S, Tucker M, Hoppe R. Factors affecting late mortality from heart disease after treatment of Hodgkin's disease. JAMA 1993;270:1949–55.

75. Horning SJ, Hoppe RT, Hancock SL, et al. Vinblastine, bleomycin and methotrexate: an effective adjuvant in favorable Hodgkin's disease. J Clin Oncol 1988;6:1822–31.

76. Carde P, Noordijk EM, Hagenbeek A, et al. Superiority of EBVP/IF over STNI in favorable clinical stage I–II Hodgkin's disease: the EORTC-GPMC H7F randomized trial. Proc ASCO 1997;16:13a.

77. Radford JA, Cowan RA, Ryder WDJ, et al. Four weeks of neoadjuvant chemotherapy significantly reduces the progression rate in patients treated with limited field radiotherapy for clinical stage IA/IIA Hodgkin's disease: results of a randomized pilot study. Ann Oncol 1996;7:66.abstract.

78. Horning SJ, Hoppe RT, Mason J, et al. Stanford-Kaiser Permanente G1 study for cinical stage I to IIa Hodgkin's disease: subtotal lymphoid irradiation versus vinblastine, methotrexate and bleomycin chemotherapy and regional irradiation. J Clin Oncol 1997;15:1736–44.

79. Radford JA, Rohatiner AZS, Dunlop DJ, et al. A randomized trial comparing weekly VAPEC-B chemotherapy with the ChlVPP/EVA hybrid regimen in previously untreated Hodgkin's disease. Proc ASCO 1997;16:12a.

80. Noordijk EM, Carde P, Mandard AM, et al. Preliminary results of the

EORTC-GPMC controlled clinical trial H7 in early stage Hodgkin's disease. Ann Oncol 1994;5:Suppl 2:107–12.

81. Loeffler M, Diehl V, Pfreundschuh M, et al. Dose-response relationship of complementary radiotherapy following 4 cycles of combination chemotherapy in intermediate stage HD. J Clin Oncol 1997;15:2275–87.

82. Santoro A, Bonfante V, Viviani S, et al. Subtotal nodal vs involved field irradiation after 4 cycles of ABVD in early stage HD. Proc ASCO 1996;15:415a.

83. Specht L, Gray RG, Clarke MJ, et al. Influence of more extensive radiotherapy and adjuvant chemotherapy on long term outcome of early stage Hodgkin's disease: a meta-analysis of 23 randomized trials involving 3,888 patients. J Clin Oncol 1998;16:830–43.

84. Crnkovich MJ, Hoppe RT, Rosenberg SA, et al. Stage IIB Hodgkin's disease: the Stanford experience. J Clin Oncol 1986;4:472–9.

85. Crnkovich MJ, Leopold K, Hoppe RT, et al. Stage I to IIB Hodgkin's disease: the combined experience at Stanford University and the Joint Center for Radiation Therapy. J Clin Oncol 1987;5:1041–9.

86. Marcus KC, Kalish LA, Coleman CN, et al. Improved survival in patients with limited stage IIIA HD treated with combined radiation therapy and chemotherapy. J Clin Oncol 1994;12:2567–72.

87. Lister TA, Dorreen MS, Faux M, et al. The treatment of stage IIIA Hodgkin's disease. J Clin Oncol 1983;1:745–9.

88. Grozea PN, de Persio EJ, Coltman CA, et al. A Southwest Oncology Group Study: chemotherapy versus chemotherapy plus radiotherapy in the treatment of stage III Hodgkin's disease. Recent Results Cancer Res 1982;80:83–91.

89. Mauch P, Gorshein D, Cunningham J, et al. Influence of mediastinal adenopathy on site and frequency of relapse in patients with Hodgkin's disease. Cancer Treat Rep 1982;66:809–17.

90. Hoppe RT, Coleman CN, Cox RS, et al. The management of stage I–II Hodgkin's disease with irradiation alone or combined modality therapy: the Stanford experience. Blood 1982;59:455–65.

91. Longo DL, Russo A, Duffey PL, et al. Treatment of advanced stage massive mediastinal Hodgkin's disease: the case of combined modality treatment. J Clin Oncol 1991;9:227–35.

92. De Vita VT, Serpick AA, Carbone PP. Combination chemotherapy in the treatment of advanced Hodgkin's disease. Ann Intern Med 1970;73:881–95.

93. The International ChlVPP treatment group. ChlVPP therapy for Hodgkin's disease: experience of 960 patients. Ann Oncol 1995;6:167–72.

94. Canellos GP, Anderson JR, Propert KL, et al. Chemotherapy of advanced Hodgkin's disease with MOPP, ABVD, or MOPP alternating with ABVD. N Engl J Med 1992;327:1478–84.

95. Bonadonna G. Chemotherapy strategies to improve control of Hodgkin's disease: the Richard and Hinda Rosenthal Foundation Award Lecture. Cancer Res 1982;42:4309–20.

96. Canellos GP, Petroni GR, Barcos M, et al. Etoposide vinblastine and doxorubicin: an active regimen in the treatment of Hodgkin's disease in relapse following MOPP. J Clin Oncol 1995;13:2005–11.

97. Klimo P, Connors JM. MOPP/ABV hybrid program: combination chemotherapy based on early introduction of seven effective drugs for advanced Hodgkin's disease. J Clin Oncol 1985;3:1174–82.

98. Connors JM, Klimo P, Adams G, et al. Treatment of advanced Hodgkin's disease with chemotherapy: comparison of MOPP/ABV hybrid regimen with alternating courses of MOPP/ABVD. J Clin Oncol 1997;15:1638–45.

99. Viviani S, Bonadonna G, Santoro A, et al. Alternating versus hybrid MOPP and ABVD combinations in advanced Hodgkin's disease: ten year results. J Clin Oncol 1996;5:1421–30.

100. Duggan D, Petroni G, Johnson J, et al. MOPP/ABV vs ABVD for advanced Hodgkin's disease: a preliminary report of CALGB 8952 (with SWOG, ECOG, NCIC). Proc ASCO 1997;16:12a.

101. Glick JH, Young ML, Harrington D, et al. MOPP/ABV hybrid chemotherapy for advanced Hodgkin's disease significantly improves failure-free survival and overall survival: the 8 year results of an intergoup trial. J Clin Oncol 98;16:19–26.

102. Bartlett N, Rosenberg SA, Hoppe RT, et al. Brief chemotherapy: Stanford V and adjuvant radiotherapy for bulky or advanced stage Hodgkin's disease: a preliminary report. J Clin Oncol 1995;13:1080–8.

103. Horning SJ, Hoppe RT, Bartlett NL, et al. Brief chemotherapy: Stanford V and involved field radiotherapy are highly effective for advanced Hodgkin's disease. Proc ASCO 1998;17:16a.

104. Horning SJ, Rosenberg SA, Hoppe RT, et al. Brief chemotherapy (Stanford V) and adjuvant radiotherapy for bulky or advanced Hodgkin's disease: an update. Ann Oncol 1996;7:Suppl 4:105.

105. Diehl V, Sieber M, Ruffer U, et al. BEACOPP: an intensified chemotherapy regimen in advanced Hodgkin's disease. Ann Oncol 1997;8:143–8.

106. Diehl V, Franklin J, Sieber M, et al. Increased efficacy through moderate dose escalation of chemotherapy: interim report from the HD9 randomized trial for advanced Hodgkin's disease. Blood 1998;92:Suppl 1:485a.

107. Herman TS, Hoppe RT, Donaldson SS, et al. Late relapse among patients treated for Hodgkin's disease. Ann Intern Med 1985;102:292–7.

108. Roach M III, Brophy N, Cox R, et al. Prognostic factors for patients relapsing after chemotherapy for early-stage Hodgkin's disease. J Clin Oncol 1990;8:623–9.

109. Longo DL, Duffey PL, Young R, et al. Conventional dose salvage combination chemotherapy in patients relapsing with Hodgkin's disease after combination chemotherapy. J Clin Oncol 1992;10:210–8.

110. Bonadonna G, Viviani S, Valagussa P, et al. Third line salvage chemotherapy in Hodgkin's disease. Semin Oncol 1985;12:Suppl 2:23–5.

111. Santoro A, Bonfante V, Bonadonna G. Salvage chemotherapy with ABVD in MOPP-resistant Hodgkin's disease. Ann Intern Med 1982;96:139–43.

112. Brada M, Eeles R, Ashley S, et al. Salvage radiotherapy in recurrent Hodgkin's disease. Ann Oncol 1992;3:131–5.

113. Reece DE, Barnett MJ, Shepherd JD, et al. High dose cyclophosphamide-carmustine and etoposide with or without cis-platin and autologous transplantation in patients who fail to enter a complete remission after combination chemotherapy. Blood 1995;86:451–6.

114. Lohri A, Barnett M, Fairey RN, et al. Outcome of treatment of first relapse in Hodgkin's disease after primary chemotherapy. Blood 1991;77:2292–8.

115. Yuen AR, Rosenberg SA, Hoppe RT, et al. Comparison between conventional salvage therapy and high dose therapy with autografting for refractory or recurrent Hodgkin's disease. Blood 1997;89:814–22.

116. Gianni AM, Sienna S, Bregni M, et al. High-dose sequential chemoradiotherapy with peripheral blood progenitor cell support for relapsed or refractory Hodgkin's disease: a 6 year update. Ann Oncol 1993;4:889–91.

117. Bierman PJ, Bagin RG, Jargannath S, et al. High dose chemotherapy followed by autologous hematopoietic rescue in Hodgkin's disease: long-term follow-up of 128 patients. Ann Oncol 1993;4:767–73.

118. Reece DE, Connors JM, Spinelli JJ, et al. Intensive therapy with cyclophosphamide, carmustine, etoposide ± cisplatin and autologous marrow transplantation for Hodgkin's disease in first relapse after combination chemotherapy. Blood 1994;83:1193–9.

119. Chopra R, McMillan AK, Lynch DC, et al. The place of high dose BEAM therapy and autologous bone marrow transplantation in poor risk Hodgkin's disease. Blood 1993;81:1137–45.

120. Rapoport AP, Rowe JM, Koides PA, et al. One hundred autotransplants for relapsed or refractory Hodgkin's disease and lymphoma: value of pretransplant status in predicting outcome. J Clin Oncol 1993;11:2351–61.

121. Nademanee A, O'Donnell MR, Snyder DS, et al. High dose chemotherapy with or without total body irradiation followed by autologous bone marrow and/or peripheral stem cell transplantation for patients with relapsed and refractory Hodgkin's disease. Blood 1995;85:1381–90.

122. Horning SJ, Chao NJ, Negrin RS, et al. High dose therapy and autologous hematopoietic progenitor cell transplantation for recurrent or refractory Hodgkin's disease. Blood 1997;89:801–13.

123. Crump M, Smith AM, Brandwein J, et al. High dose etoposide and melphalan and autologous bone marrow transplantation for patients with advanced Hodgkin's disease: importance of disease status at transplant. J Clin Oncol 1993;11:704–11.

124. Radford JA, Crowther D. Treatment of relapsed Hodgkin's disease using a weekly regimen of short duration: results of a pilot study in 20 patients. Ann Oncol 1991;2:505–9.

125. Colwill R, Crump M, Couture F, et al. Mini-BEAM as a salvage therapy for relapsed or refractory Hodgkin's disease before intensive therapy and autologous bone marrow transplantation. J Clin Oncol 1995;13:396–402.

126. Ferme C, Bastion Y, Lepage E, et al. The MINE regimen as intensive salvage chemotherapy for relapsed and refractory Hodgkin's disease. Ann Oncol 1995;6:543–9.

127. Hansen HH, Selawry OS, Pajak TF, et al. The superiority of CCNU in the treatment of advanced Hodgkin's disease. Cancer 1981;47:14–8.

128. Little R, Wittes RE, Longo DL, et al. Vinblastine for recurrent Hodgkin's disease following autologous bone marrow transplant. J Clin Oncol 1998;16:584–8.

129. Taylor RE, McElwain TJ, Barrett A, et al. Etoposide as a salvage agent in relapsed advanced lymphoid malignancies: a phase II study. Cancer Chemother Pharmacol 1982;7:175–7.

130. Tesch H, Santoro A, Fiedler F, et al. Phase II study of gemcitabine in pretreated Hodgkin's disease, results of a multicenter study. Blood 1997;90:Suppl 1:339a.

131. Devizzi L, Santoro A, Bonvante V. Vinorelbine: an active drug for the management of patients with heavily pretreated Hodgkin's disease. Ann Oncol 1994;5:517–20.

132. Williams T, Fay J, Giles F, et al. Palliative mitoguazone therapy for advanced Hodgkin's disease following intensive therapy and autologous bone marrow reconstitution. Proc ASCO 1998;17:24a.

133. Van Leeuwen FE, Chorus AM, van den Belt-Dusebout AW, et al. Leukemia risk following Hodgkin's disease: relation to cumulative dose of alkylating agents, treatment with teniposide combinations, number of episodes of chemotherapy and bone marrow damage. J Clin Oncol 1994;12:1063–73.

134. Viviani S, Santoro A, Ragni G, et al. Gonadal toxicity after combination chemotherapy for Hodgkin's disease: comparative results of MOPP versus ABVD. Eur J Cancer Clin Oncol 1985;21:601–5.

135. Schilsky RL, Sherins RJ, Hubbard SM, et al. Long term follow up of ovarian function in women treated with MOPP chemotherapy for Hodgkin's disease. Am J Med 1981;71:552–6.

136. Waxman JH, Ahmed R, Smith D, et al. Failure to preserve fertility in patients with Hodgkin's disease. Cancer Chemother Pharmacol 1987;19:159–62.

137. Chapman RM, Sutcliffe SB. Protection of ovarian function by oral contraceptives in women receiving chemotherapy for Hodgkin's disease. Blood 1981;58:849–51.

138. Breuer K, Sieber M, Grotenhermen FJ, et al. Male gonadal dysfunction in untreated Hodgkin's disease patients. Blood 1998;92:Suppl 1:86a.

139. Brice P, Tredaniel J, Monsuez JJ, et al. Cardiopulmonary toxicity after 3 courses of ABVD and mediastinal irradiation in favorable HD. Ann Oncol 1991;Suppl 2:73–6.

140. Hirsh A, Vandor Els H, Straus DJ, et al. Effect of ABVD chemotherapy with and without mantle or mediastinal irradiation on pulmonary function and symptoms in early stage Hodgkin's disease. J Clin Oncol 1996;14:1297–305.

141. Armitage JO, Dick FR, Goeken JA, et al. Second lymphoid malignant neoplasms occurring in patients treated for Hodgkin's disease. Arch Intern Med 1983;143:445–50.

142. Krikorian JH, Burke JS, Rosenberg SA, et al. Occurrence of non-Hodgkin's lymphoma after therapy for Hodgkin's disease. N Engl J Med 1979;300:452–8.

143. Zarate-Osorno A, Madeiros LJ, Longo DL, et al. Non-Hodgkin's lymphomas arising in patients successfully treated for Hodgkin's disease: a clinical, histologic and immunophenotypic study of 14 cases. Am J Surg Pathol 1992;16:885–95.

144. Tucker MA, Coleman CN, Cox RS, et al. Risk of second cancers after treatment of Hodgkin's disease. N Engl J Med 1988;318:76–81.

145. Kushner BH, Zauber A, Tan CTC. Second malignancies after childhood Hodgkin's disease: the Memorial Sloan Kettering Cancer Center experience. Cancer 1988;62:1364–70.

146. Cimino G, Papa G, Tura S, et al. Second primary cancers following Hodgkin's disease: updated results of an Italian multicenter study. J Clin Oncol 1991;9:432–7.

147. Meadows AT, Obringer AC, Marrero O, et al. Second malignant neoplasms following childhood Hodgkin's disease: treatment and splenectomy as risk factors. Med Pediatr Oncol 1989;17:477–84.

148. Hancock SL, Tucker MA, Hoppe RT, et al. Breast cancer after treatment of Hodgkin's disease. J Natl Cancer Inst 1993;85:25–31.

149. Krikorian JG, Portlock CS, Mauch PM, et al. Hodgkin's disease presenting below the diaphragm: a review. J Clin Oncol 1986;4:1551–62.

150. Donaldson NN. Hodgkin's disease in children. Semin Oncol 1990;17:736–48.

151. Biggar RJ. Epidemiologic clues to the etiology of cancer in AIDS. 2nd National AIDS Malignancy Conference, Bethesda, Md., 1998.abstract S2.

151a. Biggar RJ, Rabkin CS. The epidemiology of AIDS-related neoplasms. Hematol Oncol Clin North Am 1996;10:997–1010.

152. Prior E, Goldberg AF, Conjalka MS, et al. Hodgkin's disease in homosexual men: an AIDS related phenomenon? Am J Med 1986;81:1085–8.

153. Schenkein DP, Dixon P, Desforges JF, et al. A phase I/II study of cyclophosphamide, carboplatin and etoposide and autologous hematopoietic stem cell transplantation with posttransplant interferon alfa-2b for patients with lymphoma and Hodgkin's disease. J Clin Oncol 1994;12:2423–31.

154. Sforzini S, Bolognesi A, Meazza R, et al. Targeting type 1 ribosome inactivating proteins to CD30 or CD25 hematologic neoplasias by bispecific antibodies. J Hematol 1995;4:429–32.

155. Schnell R, Linnartz C, Katouzi AA, et al. Development of new ricin A chain immunotoxins with potent anti-tumor effects against human Hodgkin's cells in vitro and disseminated Hodgkin tumors in SCID mice using high-affinity monoclonal antibodies directed against the CD30 antigen. Int J Cancer 1995;63:238–44.

156. Terenzi A, Bolognesi A, Pasqualucci L, et al. Anti-CD30 (BERH2) immunotoxins containing the type-1 ribosome inactivating proteins momordin and PAP-S display powerful antitumour activity against CD30+ tumour cells in vitro and in SCID mice. Br J Haematol 1996;92:872–9.

157. Engert A, Diehl V, Schnell R, et al. A phase-I study of an anti-CD25 ricin A-chain immunotoxin (RFT5-SMPT-dgA) in patients with refractory Hodgkin's lymphoma. Blood 1997;89:403–10.

158. Schnell R, Vitetta E, Schindler J, et al. Clinical trials with an anti-CD25 ricin A-chain experimental immunotoxin (RFT5-SMPT-dgA) in Hodgkin lymphoma. Leuk Lymphoma 1998;30:525–37.

159. Hombach A, Jung W, Pohl C, et al. A CD16/CD30 bispecific antibody induces lysis of Hodgkin cells by unstimulated natural killer cells in vitro and in vivo. Int J Cancer 1993;55:830–6.

160. Hartmann F, Renner C, Jung W, et al. Treatment of refractory Hodgkin's disease with an anti-CD16/CD30 bispecific antibody. Blood 1997;89:2042–7.

161. Winkler U, Scheidhaurer K, Stein H, et al. Treatment of patients with relapsed Hodgkin's lymphoma using the radioimmunoconjugate 99mTc-BERH2 (antiCD30): results of a clinical study. Blood 1998;92:Suppl 1:417a.

162. Tepler I, Schwartz G, Parker K, et al. Phase I trial of an interleukin-2 fusion toxin (DAB486IL-2) in hematologic malignancies: complete response in a patient with Hodgkin's disease refractory to chemotherapy. Cancer 1994;73:1276–85.

163. Khouri IF, Keating M, Korbling M, et al. Transplant-lite: induction of graft versus malignancy using fludarabine based nonablative chemotherapy and allogeneic blood progenitor cell transplantation as treatment for lymphoid malignancies. J Clin Oncol 1998;16:2817–24.

# CHAPTER 88

# NATURAL HISTORY, DIAGNOSIS, AND STAGING OF THE NON-HODGKIN'S LYMPHOMAS

• THOMAS M. GROGAN • MARINA A. JARAMILLO •
• THOMAS P. MILLER •

Non-Hodgkin's lymphomas (NHLs) are primary lymphoid malignancies that are characterized by initial sensitivity to treatment with radiotherapy and cytotoxic drugs. The group is heterogeneous with regard to histologic appearance, cellular and molecular biology, and overall clinical course. These diseases interest clinicians in part because of the treatable nature of the disease, at least initially; the potential for cure; and the physician's ability to relieve symptoms predictably. Investigators target these diseases for a disproportionate number of studies because they provide so many suitable clinical paradigms of laboratory phenomena. In view of this enthusiasm for investigation and treatment, one might expect that patient outcome has dramatically improved. That does not seem to be the case as judged by long-term outcome studies and by the recent results of the National High Priority Lymphoma Trial comparing standard combination chemotherapy (CHOP) to newer third-generation chemotherapy programs.[1] Furthermore, these diseases are no longer uncommon.

The estimated number of new cases of NHL in the United States was 56,800 for 1999, and the number of deaths from NHL in 1999 was 25,700.[2] The incidence increased by 50% between 1973 and 1987 from 8.7 diagnoses of lymphoma per 100,000 to 13.1 per 100,000 persons.[3] As a result of this increased incidence and the plateau in therapeutic outcome, mortality rates per 100,000 adjusted for age and standardized to the 1970 census population distribution demonstrated a disturbing trend. There was a 56% increase in mortality rate from 1959 to 1989, whereas the mortality rate due to Hodgkin's disease fell by 66% during those same years.[2]

These trends should not dampen enthusiasm for treating these patients but should encourage vigorous further study of these diseases at the laboratory and clinical level. There will be no progress toward improved outcome if there is no change in understanding and if currently available treatment is viewed as acceptable treatment. Our approach to this introductory chapter on NHLs is to summarize the current state of understanding briefly, to discuss the shortcomings of these models, and to introduce newer concepts. We place particular emphasis on the Revised European-American Lymphoma (REAL) classification scheme because it fully integrates morphology, immunophenotype, and genotype.[4]

## Etiology

Although there are numerous associations linking lymphomas with chemical agents, genetic alterations, and infectious agents (Table 88–1), conclusive proof of cause is elusive because proof entails difficult experiments such as removing

the putative lymphomagenic agent and showing decreased lymphoma incidence.[5, 6] Although strong associations exist with specific agents (human T-cell leukemia/lymphoma virus, type I [HTLV-I], and Epstein-Barr virus [EBV]), the exact sequence of events leading to lymphoma is not yet explained.[6] Nonetheless, some generalities are understood. In particular, it appears that more than one event is necessary for lymphoma to develop, leading to the "two-hit" or "multihit" theory of lymphomagenesis.[7] Endemic Burkitt's lymphoma is an example of the two-hit theory of lymphomagenesis. Burkitt's lymphoma is common in areas of holoendemic malaria. Acute malaria reduces specific T-cell immunosurveillance of EBV, leading to B-cell clonal expansion.[8] In the context of sustained B-cell proliferation, there is a consequent genetic accident: translocation of the c-myc (chromosome 8) proto-oncogene to the immunoglobulin H (IgH) joining region (chromosome 14) (t(8;14)).[8] This translocation, in turn, leads to an immortalized clone because of the c-myc mitogenic factor coming under IgH transcriptional control.[8–10] This well-described sequence comes close to describing the "two-step" hypothesis of lymphoma pathogenesis. Human immunodeficiency virus (HIV-1)–associated lymphoma and body cavity lymphoma are additional examples because both commonly entail two- or even three-hit lymphomagenesis. HIV-1–associated lymphoma typically involves initial HIV-1 infection of T-helper cells, resulting in loss of immunosurveillance and emergence of EBV and human herpesvirus 8 (HHV8) in body cavity lymphoma.[11]

Other causative associations are described further on and include the association of lymphoma with specific chemical agents (herbicides and hair dyes), with immune-altered states (Sjögren's syndrome, HIV infection, after organ transplantation), and with specific viral agents (HTLV-II, HTLV-III, HHV8,[11] hepatitis C [HCV]),[12] and specific bacterial agents (*Helicobacter pylori*,[13] *Mycobacterium tuberculosis*).[14] Al-

**Table 88–1.** Lymphomas with Known Infectious Cause

| Lymphoma Type | Agent |
|---|---|
| Burkitt's Post-transplant Hodgkin's | Epstein-Barr virus (EBV) |
| AIDS-Associated | HIV-1/EBV/HHV8 |
| Japanese T-cell | HIV-III |
| Body cavity | HHV8 |
| Pyothorax-associated | *Mycobacterium tuberculosis* |
| Mucosa-associated | *Helicobacter pylori* |
| Mediterranean | Intestinal pathogen |
| Immunocytoma | Hepatitis C |

HIV-1, human immunodeficiency virus, type 1; HHV8, human herpes virus, type 8; HIV-III, human immunodeficiency virus, type 3; AIDS, acquired immunodeficiency syndrome.

though these agents and conditions seem numerous, they account for only a minority of lymphoma cases. The majority of cases have not been associated with recognizable causative agents.[6]

Immune dysfunctional states are associated with a higher incidence of lymphoma. In particular, post-transplantation patients receiving immunosuppressive agents, especially those receiving anti-OKT3 immunosuppressive therapy, have a higher incidence of NHL.[15] Mediterranean lymphoma is associated with prior gastrointestinal infections and malabsorption.[16] Patients with X-linked lymphoproliferative syndrome have inherited immunodeficiency to EBV and an increased risk of developing NHL.[17] Patients with severe combined immune deficiency develop aggressive lymphomas after thymic or marrow transplantation.[18] There is also an increased incidence of NHL among acquired immunodeficiency syndrome (AIDS) patients. Estimates of the number of AIDS-related lymphomas in 1992 varied from 2900 to 9800.[19] Thus AIDS-related lymphomas account for 8 to 27% of all NHL. In AIDS-related lymphoma, two causative factors are operative: the HIV-1 virus and EVB. HIV-1 destroys T-helper cells, reducing immunosurveillance and allowing escape of EBV. Thus, a viral infection leads to an altered immune state and additional viral assault. HIV-1–infected patients also occasionally develop a peculiar complication known as body cavity lymphoma, which is caused by a second virus: HHV8.[11] Oddly, body cavity lymphoma may also occur independent of HIV-1 in close association with *M. tuberculosis*.[14] Sjögren's syndrome and angioimmunoblastic lymphadenopathy (AILD) are two additional altered immune states that have a high association with lymphoma. Sjögren's syndrome is highly associated with the development of mucosa-associated lymphomas (MALTomas) and angioimmunoblastic lymphadenopathy is highly associated with the development of peripheral T-cell lymphoma.[20–22]

Chemical agents, and in particular herbicides, have been correlated with an increased lymphoma incidence. Herbicide use (phenoxyacetate acid herbicides) has been associated with excess risk of NHLs among farm workers in several studies.[23–25] However, a retrospective cohort study of 5172 workers exposed to dioxin showed no increased risk for NHL.[26] The increased risk of NHLs associated with herbicides seems to apply to both patients and their pets. Households with dogs who developed lymphoma applied 2,4-dichlorophenoxyacetic acid herbicide more frequently to their lawns than did control owners (odds ratio = 1.3).[27] This relative risk rose with the time of exposure to herbicide. Hair dye use has variably been associated with an increased risk of NHL.[28, 29] In particular, Nebraska women who used hair dye had an increased relative risk of developing NHL (relative risk = 1.7).[28] This relative risk increased with prolonged exposure. However, Thun and colleagues reported that women using hair dyes are generally not at increased risk for developing NHLs, although prolonged use (>20 years) of black dyes may be associated with increased risk.[29]

Regarding an infectious cause, there is a growing list of both bacterial and viral agents associated with lymphomagenesis (see Table 88–1). Additional viruses associated with lymphomas include HTLV-1 (HIV-3), which is associated with T-cell neoplasms in both Japan and nonendemic regions.[30] Additionally, a rare form of T-cell hairy cell leukemia is specifically associated with HTLV-II (HIV-2).[31] Most recently, there has been an association made between HCV and a newly defined lymphoma known as an *immunocytoma*. Finally, as mentioned earlier and further detailed later, Burkitt's lymphoma in endemic areas is highly associated with the presence of EBV.[32] Regarding bacteria, there are currently at least two known associations: *M. tuberculosis* and *H. pylori* in MALToma. *H. pylori* is found in 92% of gastric MALTomas. Through antigen stimulation and persistence, *H. pylori* results in clonal evolution from a polyclonal to a oligoclonal to a malignant monoclonal state. Triple-antibiotic therapy may prove curative in 70% of cases.[22]

## Biology

### NORMAL LYMPHOID DEVELOPMENT AND FUNCTION

**B-Cell Development.** Physiologic B-cell development results in an antibody-producing cell.[33, 34] The presentation of foreign antigen by lymph node accessory cells (dendritic reticulum cells) in the germinal centers stimulates production of a unique "idiotypic" antibody relevant to binding and opsonization of the presented antigen. Through a process of clonal evolution over a period of several weeks, the perfect antibody with high affinity is selected.[33, 34] Antibody diversity is generated through a series of gene translocations or rearrangements that result in a unique sequence of juxtaposed VDJ genes (heavy chain) and VJ genes (light chain). The germline DNA contains 1000 V (variable) genes, 10 D (diversity) genes, and 4 different J (joining) genes. These genes combine in a unique combination, much as each railroad train is a unique combination of component box cars. This multiplicity of gene combinations, coupled with ongoing somatic mutations within the germinal center, creates great diversity in the B-cell antibody system, ensuring a high-affinity antibody match to virtually any antigen given enough time.[33, 34]

Ig expression is a complex process that varies greatly with developmental stage[33–37] (Fig. 88–1 and Table 88–2). An early "pre-pre"–B cell has a heavy chain rearrangement but no phenotypic Ig. A "pre-B"–cell has phenotypic cytoplasmic "mu" heavy chains without surface Ig. The subsequent midstage B cell has lost cytoplasmic mu but expresses surface Ig, whereas activated B cells (immunoblasts) variably lose surface Ig and express cytoplasmic Ig. Finally, plasma cells, the paradigm of the B-cell antibody secretion, have no surface Ig, only cytoplasmic Ig[36, 37] (see Fig. 88–1).

There is an additional phenomenon known as *heavy chain switching* whereby midphase surface-Ig–bearing B cells acquire IgD expression in response to initial antigen contact. Subsequent clonal development may lead to a sequence from cytoplasmic IgM to surface IgD, IgG, IgA, and IgE.[33–37] This heavy chain switching phenomenon also has a microanatomic basis with IgD expression in the mantle zone around germinal centers, whereas IgM and IgG are found within germinal centers.[38] The implication is that B cells move around in the developmental process.

Besides heavy chain switching, the characteristic feature of B cells is their capacity to form follicles in the lymph

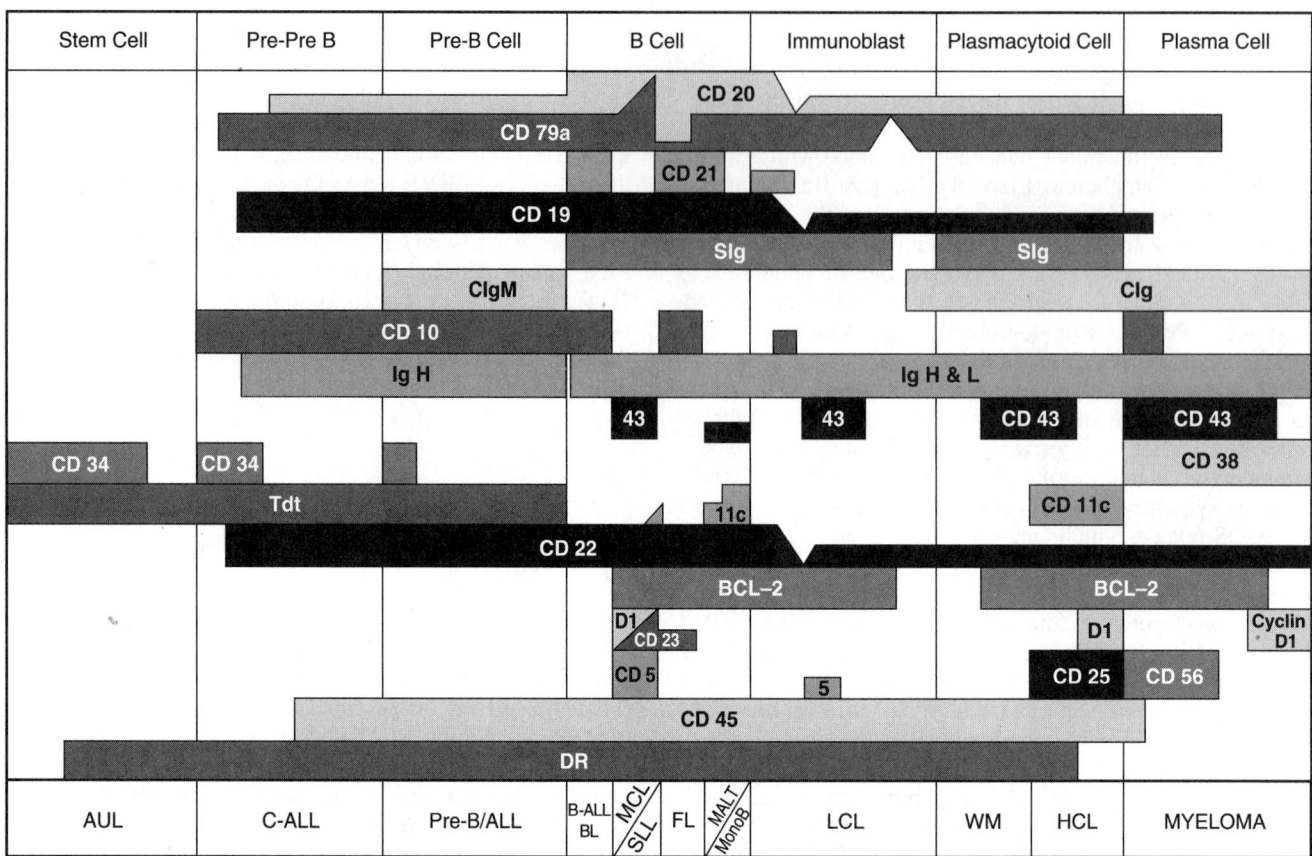

**Figure 88–1.** B-cell phenotypic and genotypic changes. Diagrammatic representation of the range of B-cell antigenic and Ig gene expression in both normal B-cell development (ontogeny) and the B-cell neoplasms derived from each stage of ontogeny. AUL, acute undifferentiated leukemia; C-ALL, common acute lymphoblastic leukemia; pre-B-ALL, pre B-cell acute lymphoblastic leukemia; B-ALL, B-cell acute lymphoblastic leukemia; BL, Burkitt's/Burkitt's-like leukemia-lymphoma; SLL, small lymphocytic lymphoma; LCL, large cell lymphoma; WM, Waldenstom's macroglobulinemia; HCL, hairy cell leukemia; MYELOMA, multiple myeloma; MCL, mantle cell lymphoma; FL, follicular lymphoma; MALT, mucosa-associated lymphomas; Mono-B, monocytoid B-cell lymphoma.

nodes, spleen, bone marrow, and tonsils.[38, 39] They also circulate in the peripheral blood. B cells are thought to traffic or home within these sites. B-cell neoplasms frequently retain and recapitulate this pattern of spread, with neoplastic cells appearing simultaneously in the nodes, marrow, and spleen. In normal tissues, B cells are typically polyclonal or polytypic with cells bearing light chains (lambda, kappa) and heavy chains (gamma, mu, alpha, delta, epsilon) admixed. Kappa-bearing cells usually outnumber lambda-bearing cells by 2:1 or 3:1.[38–40] In neoplastic B-cell lymphomas, there emerges from this polyclonal circumstance a single monotypic clone, as described further on.[36, 37]

When an antigen enters the body for the first time, production of low-affinity IgM antibodies occurs. When the same antigen is presented to the immune system a second time, there is an immediate response, with production of high-affinity IgG antibodies. The process of somatic mutation in the V regions of the Ig genes, which occurs exclusively in the germinal center and results in the random production of antigens with different degrees of affinity by the eliciting antigen, explains this phenomenon.[41] B cells that express antibodies of low affinity are eliminated by apoptosis, whereas the ones producing high-affinity immunoglobulin are preserved and become memory B cells or plasma cells. Thus, B cells can be *subclassified* into three

groups according to their relation with the germinal center, which results in a specific pattern of somatic mutations of the immunoglobulin genes. Cells that have not entered the germinal center and that lack somatic mutations are referred to as *pre–germinal center* B cells or *naive mature* B cells. These cells include the majority of the circulation B cells as well as B cells of primary lymphoid follicles and mantle zones. B cells that have ongoing somatic mutations are called *germinal center* B cells and include centroblasts and centrocytes. Finally, cells that have established somatic mutations in the absence of ongoing mutations are designated *post–germinal center* B cells. Memory B cells of marginal zones and plasma cells compose the latter group.[41]

Besides immunoglobulin, B cells characteristically express pan–B antigens, as shown in Figure 88–1 and Table 88–2. As shown, immature B cells express the nuclear enzyme terminal deoxynucleotidyl transferase (Tdt) and the common acute lymphocytic leukemia antigen (CD10) but not Ig, whereas the midstage B cell expresses surface Ig and no Tdt.[35] The mature plasma cells, the paradigm of B cell, although strongly secreting Ig, paradoxically have no pan–B antigen expression. Note the co-expression of some T-cell–associated antigens, CD5 in certain B-cell subsets, CD25 in hairy cell leukemia, and macrophage-associated antigens, CD11c in hairy cell leukemia[40] (see Fig 88–1).

*Table 88–2.* **Key Human Leukocyte Antigens**

| CD | Other Names | Cell Type | Function |
|---|---|---|---|
| CD1a | T6, Leu 6 | Thy, LC, DC | T-cell response regulation |
| CD2 | T11, Leu 2 | Thy, T, NK | CD58 Rp |
| CD3 | T3, Leu 4 | T, Thy, NK | TCR associated |
| CD4 | T4, Leu 3 | Thy, h/iT, PB-M | MHC class II; HIV Rp |
| CD5 | T1, Leu 1 | Thy, T, B subset | CD72 ligand; B-cell Rp |
| CD7 | Leu 9 | Thy, T subset, NK | Unknown |
| CD8 | T8, Leu 2 | Thy, s/cT, NK sub | MHC class I Rp |
| CD10 | CALLA | Pre-B, GC, Neu, some Epi | Membrane-associated peptidase |
| CD11a | LFA-1α chain | Leu | ICAM ligand |
| CD11b | Mo1, Mac-1α | G, M, NK, T/B subsets | C3bi Rp |
| CD11c | Leu M5, p150/95, CR4 | M, NK, G, T/B subsets, HCL | C3bi Rp; CD18 |
| CD15 | Leu M1, X-hapten | G, M, LC, some Epi, RSC | Unknown |
| CD16 | Leu 11, FcγRIII | NK, G, M | FCγ receptor III |
| CD18 | LFA-1β chain | Leu | β chain to CD11 |
| CD19 | B4, Leu 12 | B, DRC | CD21 ligand; signal transducer |
| CD20 | B1, Leu 16, Leu 26 | B | Ca ion channel |
| CD21 | B2, CR2 | B subset, DRC, MZ | C3d Rp; EBV Rp |
| CD22 | BL-CAM, Leu 14 | B cell, HCL | CD45RO ligand |
| CD23 | BLAST-2, FcεRII | B subset, M, DRC, LC | Fc receptor II |
| CD25 | Tac, IL-2 Rp | Act T/B/M, HCL | IL-2 Rp α chain |
| CD28 | Tp44, T44 | Thy, T subset, PC | B7 (CD80) ligand |
| CD30 | Ki-1, Ber-H2 | Act T/B/NK; RSC, ALCL | CD 153 ligand |
| CD34 | My10, GP105-120 | Progenitors, End | Cell-cell adhesion |
| CD38 | T10 | PC | ADP ribosyl cyclase |
| CD43 | Leukosialin, sialophorin | Leu (except B), PC subset | CD54 ligand |
| CD44 | Pgp-1, H-CAM | Broad expression | Homing receptors |
| CD45 | T200, LCA | Leu | Tyrosine phosphatase |
| CD45RO | UCHL-1 | T, B subset, M | CD22 ligand |
| CD45RA | 4KB5 | B, T subset, M | Unknown |
| CDw49a | VLAα1 | Act T, M | Laminin-1, collagen ligand |
| CDw49b | VLAα2 | PL, Meg, M, Act T, B | Collagen, laminin ligand |
| CDw49c | VLAα3 | B, adhesion cell lines | Collagen, laminin-5, FN ligand |
| CDw49d | VLAα4 | M, B, T, Thy, Eo, NK | CD106, FN ligand |
| CDw49e | VLAα5 | Adherent and nonadherent cells | FN ligand |
| CDw49f | VLAα6 | Plat, Meg, M, End, Epi | Laminin ligand |
| CD54 | ICAM-1 | Broad activation | LFA-1, Mac-1 ligand |
| CD56 | NCAM, NKH1, Leu 19 | NK, T subset, MM, CNS | Isoform of N-CAM |
| CD57 | Leu 7, HNK1 | NK, T/B subsets | Unknown |
| CD58 | LFA3 | Leuk, Ery, End, Epi | CD2 ligand |
| CD72 | Lyb-2 | Pan B, M (spleen, liver) | CD5 ligand |
| CD77 | Gb3, BLA | GC, Burkitt's, FL | CD19 ligand |
| CD80 | B7, BB1 | Act T/B, M | CD28, CD152 ligand |
| CD83 | HB15 | LC, DC | Unknown |
| CD86 | B70, B7-2 | IDC, LC | CD28, CD152 ligand |
| CD99 | E2, MIC2 | hematologic cells, ES | T-cell adhesion, apoptosis |

B, B-cells; PC, plasma cells; T, T-cells; h/iT, helper/inducer T; s/cT, suppressor/cytotoxic T; Thy, thymocytes; GC, germinal center B cells; MZ, mantle cells; G, granulocytes; Leu, leukocytes; Meg, megakaryocytes; M, monocytes/macrophages; NK, natural killer; PL, platelets; Eo, eosinophils; Ery, red blood cells; DC, dendritic cells; IDC, interdigitating dendritic cells; LC, Langerhans cell; End, endothelial cells; Epi, epithelial cells; RSC, Reed-Sternberg cells; ALCL, anaplastic large cell lymphoma; FL, follicular lymphoma; HCL, hairy cell leukemia; MM, multiple myeloma; ES, Ewing's sarcoma; CNS, central nervous system; Rp, receptor; FN, fibronectin; Act, activated.

**T-Cell Development.** Physiologic T-cell development results in effector cells responsible for cell-mediated immunity.[42, 43] These include specifically T-cytotoxic cells, T-suppressor cells, and T-helper cells. Although these cells are embryologically derived from the marrow, maturation occurs in the thymus; hence, the designation T cells. Devoid of immunoglobulin, T cells co-express enzymes and surface molecules relevant to their developmental state (Fig. 88–2).[42, 43] Immature T cells co-express Tdt, CD1a, and simultaneous T-helper/T-cytotoxic antigens CD4 and CD8. In contrast, mature post-thymic T cells lose Tdt and express either T-helper or T-cytotoxic antigens, but not both. In the lymphoid tissues around the body, T cells generally outnumber B cells by 3:1 or 4:1.[38–40] Specifically among T cells, T-helper cells generally outnumber T-suppressor/T-cytotoxic

cells by a factor of 3:1 or 4:1 in a polyclonal configuration. Within specific lymphoid organs, T cells are found in the paracortex of lymph nodes, in the periarteriolar lymphoid sheaths of splenic white pulp, in the marrow, and in the peripheral blood as the dominant lymphoid element.[38–40]

Functionally, T cells may interact with self (e.g., B cells) or with nonself (foreign antigens). Reactivity with B cells is mediated through a variety of molecules, including cell adhesion molecules (CAMs), integrins (e.g., LFA-1), and their ligands (e.g., ICAM)[44] (Fig. 88–3). This process is described in detail later. In addition, reactivity with nonself antigen entails reactivity of the T-cell antigen receptor (TCR), a two-chain heterodimer (alpha and beta TCR chains), with the major histocompatibility complex.[42, 43] The alpha and beta TCR(TCR2) chains are immunoglobulin superfamily mem-

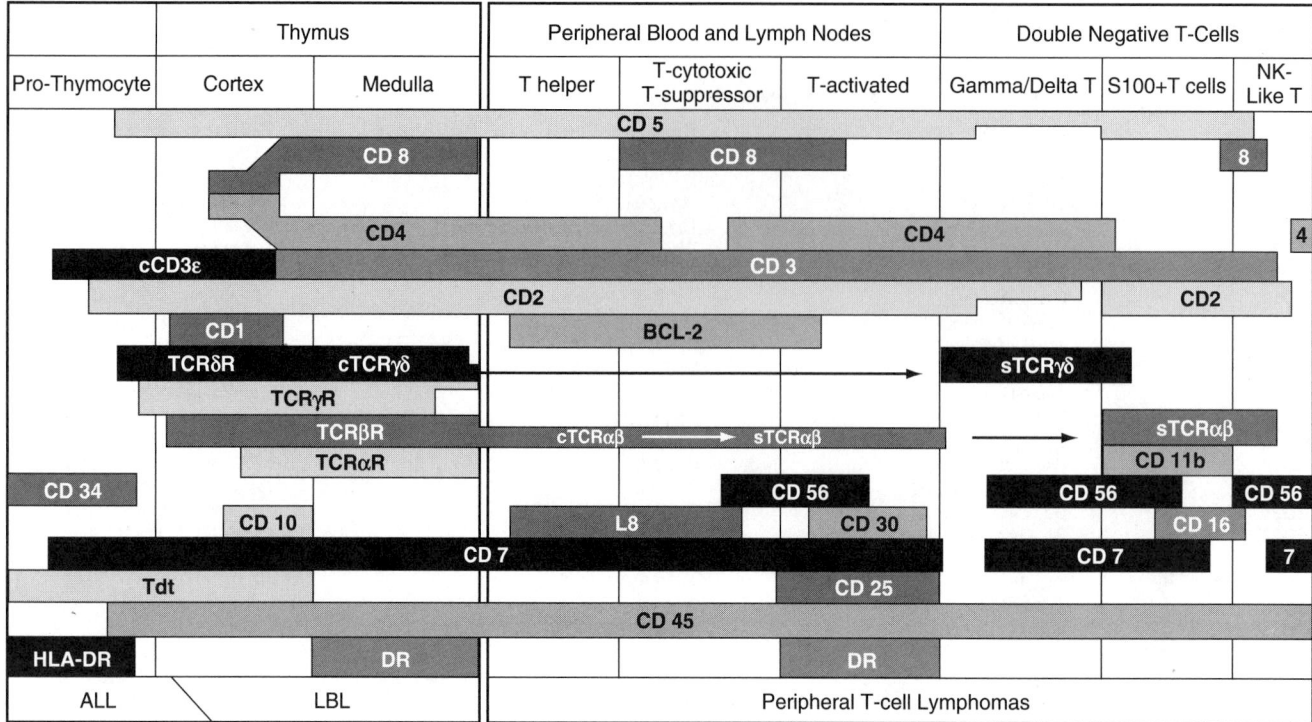

**Figure 88–2.** T-cell phenotypic and genotypic changes. Diagrammatic representation of the range of T-cell antigenic and T antigen receptor (TCR) gene expression in both normal T-cell ontogeny and T-cell neoplasms derived from the developmental phases. See Table 88–1 for descriptions of antibodies. ALL, acute lymphoblastic leukemia; LBL, lymphoblastic lymphoma.

bers that, like B-cell Ig, have hypervariable regions that create diversity relevant to antigen recognition. As with the Ig genes, there is a multiplicity of V, J, and D gene regions, which may be translocated in unique combinations of T-antigen receptor domains. A second T-antigen receptor gene group composed of the gamma and delta genes may give rise to similar diversity among other T-cell subsets.[42, 43] Progenitor T cells in the thymus first undergo gamma and delta gene rearrangement; if no functional gamma/delta receptor is produced, the alpha and beta genes undergo re-

arrangement. The majority of both thymocytes and circulating T cells express TRC alpha/beta, whereas less than 5% express TCR gamma/delta. The latter cells are found in epithelia, including epidermis and intestinal mucosa.

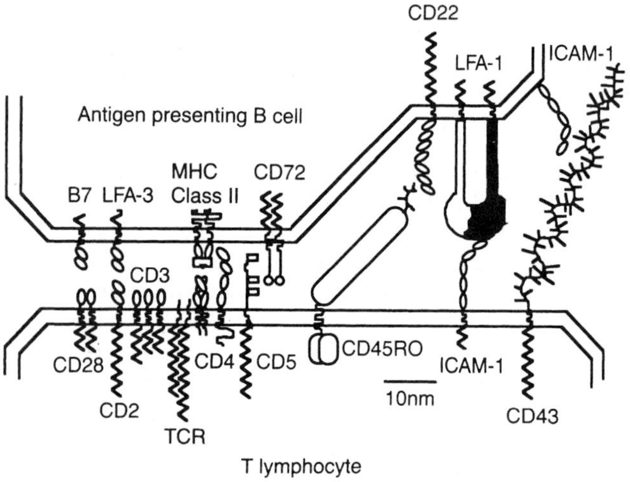

**B-Cell and T-Cell Interactions.** As illustrated in Figure 88–3, a variety of molecules mediate B-cell/T-cell interactions. They include CAMs (e.g., ICAM), integrins (e.g., LFA-1), selectins (e.g., LAM-1), and immunoglobulin superfamily molecules (e.g., CD22).[44–47] Differential expression of these molecules is relevant to cell behavior. A prime example is the LFA-1/ICAM1 interaction illustrated in Figure 88–3.[48] This molecular pairing is a critical factor for (1) B-cell homotypic adhesion, (2) T-cell adhesion for cytotoxic T-lymphocyte (CTL) recognition and T-cell immunosurveillance, and (3) lymphocyte endothelial cell interaction.[44–47] In pathologic circumstances, low expression of both LFA-1 and ICAM-1 may result in (1) loss of B-cell cohesion, aiding tumor dissemination and (2) loss of adhesion relevant to CTL recognition, resulting in lost T-cell immunosurveillance.[49]

T-cell immunosurveillance (see Fig. 88–3) is a complex interaction that is both antigen independent and antigen dependent. In the initial independent phase, LFA-1 is a critical facilitator of T-cell adhesion. The combined LFA-ICAM I ligand interaction is essential for initial CTL recognition. The next step is cross-linking of the T-cell antigen receptor through binding to both foreign antigen and HLA antigens on the opposing cell.[44–47]

Histocompatibility antigens (HLAs) are polymorphic cell surface antigens that serve as recognition structures in cell self-recognition, cell-cell interaction, immunosurveillance, and tumor and foreign antigen rejection.[50, 51] These surface glycoproteins are the products of complex gene arrays found

**Figure 88–3.** Diagrammatic representation of B- and T-cell interactions. See Table 88–2 for descriptions of CD designations. (Adapted from Barclay N. Leucocyte fact book, Chatham, Harcourt Brace Jovanovich: 1993:224.)

on chromosome 6. One family, known as HLA class I, is subdivided into subunits A, B, and C, with both constant and variable regions. The HLA-1 A, B, and C surface antigens are major determinants of graft rejection and serve as self-recognition elements for cytotoxic T cells in foreign body or tumor rejection. A second family, known as HLA class II or Ia (immune-associated gene), is subdivided into DP, DR, and DQ subunits, again with both constant and variable regions. Class II HLA-DP, -DR, and -DQ cell surface antigens function in antigen presentation and in self-recognition by helper T cells, which are also relevant to tumor containment via secondary stimulation of T-cell cytotoxicity.[50, 51]

Besides CAMs and HLA molecules, a third class of molecules known as costimulatory molecules (CSMs) are necessary for effective B- versus T-cell interaction and consequent immunosurveillance.[52] Key CSMs include CD80 and CD86 (see Fig. 88–3), which interact with CD28 on T cells. In particular, after CAM ensure B-cell/T-cell docking and HLA ensures recognition of foreign protein in context of self, the CD80/CD86 CSMs provide the signal for T cells to be activated. Without this costimulation, T-cell immunosurveillance would undergo apoptosis, and an anergic response would prevail.[52]

There are multiple adhesion and recognition molecules that participate in strengthening cell adhesion and lead to effective T-cell surveillance, which serves to eliminate aberrant tumor cells.[52]

**Sessile Versus Mobile Phenotype.** Critical to lymphoid cell development and function is the regulated ability of lymphocytes to either stay put or migrate "home" and invade target organs. Specific phenotypes are now associated with either the sessile or mobile phenotype.[47] Regarding the sessile phenotype, it is thought that the integrin molecules known as the very late activation (VLA) molecules—including VLA-4, VLA-5, and VLA-6—are important for cell attachment of the extracellular matrix (ECM) (see Table 88–2).[53, 54] In particular, it is the beta-1 chain of VLA that mediates interaction with fibronectin (FN) and laminin (LN), giving lymphoid cells an anchoring effect in the ECM.[47] This VLA-FN-LN bond is the putative sessile phenotype that delineates lymphoid cell anchoring at the sites of inflammation and in lymphoid organs. Lymphoid cell mobility also might be affected at the cellular level as VLA-5 associates with the cytoskeletal element talin.[55] Additionally, VLA-5 binding to FN is known to induce collagenase expression, which may affect lymph cell invasiveness.[56]

Regarding collagenases, the expression of human type IV collagenase, a member of the metalloproteinase (MP) family, was found in human lymphoblastic cell lines.[57] This expression correlates with the ability of these lymphoid cells to invade reconstituted basement membrane in vitro and to metastasize in vivo. In this instance, the MP enzyme was thought to be responsible for the degradation of collagen IV in basement membranes.[57]

The activity of tissue MP is held in check by tissue inhibitors of MPs. It is thought that extensive remodeling of the ECM occurs through rapid, localized, transient induction of proteinases and inhibitors under the influence of growth factors, hormones, and cytokines.[58] Loss of control of the extracellular proteolytic balance leads to an excess of degradative enzymes over inhibitory activities and results in ECM destruction and lymphoma invasion in some extranodal sites.[59]

In contrast, the mobile phenotype is associated with lymphoid cell migration, homing, and organ specificity. In particular, the lymphocyte "homing" receptor (LHR, CD44, Hemes 3) is known to play a role in lymphocyte dissemination and trafficking.[60] It is known that the LHR interacts with a complementary receptor on the vascular endothelium (complementary addressins) within the postcapillary venules of the lymph nodes. This interaction facilitates entry of recirculating mature memory cells into and out of the lymph nodes. Thus, circulating peripheral blood T cells and B cells have high-level LHR expression, whereas anchored, sessile germinal center cells express very low level LHR.[61]

Finally, one last molecule—leukocyte adhesion molecule-1 (LAM-1, TQ1, Leu 8), is involved in the binding of human leukocytes to high endothelial venules and may be relevant to lymphoid cell dissemination.[62] In a study by Spertini and colleagues,[62] LAM-1 positivity correlated with the ability of lymphoid cells to migrate through the circulation and disseminate. It was also noted that downmodulation of LAM-1 was increased in the presence of protein kinase C inhibitors.[62] Thus, LAM-1 appears as another player in the sessile versus mobile phenotype.

Ultimately, multifactorial phenotypic analysis is needed to define the complete mobile versus sessile phenotype. As emphasized by Springer in his "area code hypothesis,"[63, 64] the transition from mobile to sessile phenotype may require the correct sequential expression of a specific selectin, integrin, and immunoglobulin-like CAM. Therefore, the analysis of the biologic function of any CAM requires knowledge of its adjacent, tandemly regulated CAM molecules.

**Proliferative Versus Resting Memory Status.** With a given foreign antigen, some lymphoid cells are specifically stimulated to proliferation and activation, whereas immediately adjacent clones are not stimulated. In germinal centers, there is either initial clonal expression and subsequent prolonged survival of high-affinity matched clones or loss or culling out of low-affinity clones. The balance between proliferation and resting status and between clonal expansion and clonal demise is largely regulated by proto-oncogenes, which are protein gene products that control lymphoid cell proliferation, differentiation, and survival.[65]

To date there are three oncogene categories relevant to this process: (1) growth-promoting genes, (2) tumor suppressor genes, and (3) death-sparing survival genes. The first two categories relate directly to cell growth, whereas the third is independent of growth.[65]

The category I growth-promoting genes include nuclear transcription factors like c-*myc* and signal transduction factors like *ras* (a G protein) or *abl* (a tyrosine kinase). A gain of function through greater amplification or promotion of these genes results in increased, unbridled growth. The category II tumor-suppressor oncogenes are the counterbalancing genes that include the retinoblastoma (Rb) genes and the p53 gene family. They both inhibit growth in their wild form. These genes serve as a natural check on unbridled proliferation, unless their functions are lost through mutation or allotypic deletion. In reactive lymphoid tissues, little if any wild-type p53 or c-*myc* is found, suggesting that scant amounts are required for normal physiologic function. In certain lymphomas, p53 exists in abundance, but in mutated form with altered function.[65]

Independent of proliferation, lymphoid cells may be immortalized by an entirely separate means, that is, by avoidance of cell death. In particular, death-sparing or anti-death genes, in the form of a new category of oncogenes, bcl-2 (category III oncogenes), may be responsible.[66] The *bcl-*2 oncogene appears to regulate a phenomenon known as *programmed cell death*, which is a cell "suicide" pathway that naturally restricts cell numbers by self-pruning or culling. In physiologic B-cell clonal expansion, some clones show high affinity to antigen and are immortalized as memory B cells, whereas other B cells show low affinity and are eliminated via programmed cell death.[58] Programmed cell death causes apoptosis. a morphologically distinct cell death with pyknotic nuclei.[66] It is thought that the bcl-2 oncogenic protein expression blocks programmed cell death and apoptosis and thereby spares a cell from sudden demise. Furthermore, as a consequence of bcl-2 expression, the cell is left in G0 arrest, a resting state. Proliferative escape from this resting state is possible only through subsequent activation, consistent with memory B- and T-cell behavior.[66, 67]

## MALIGNANT STATE

**Concept of Malignant Phenotype-Genotype.** Neoplastic lymphoid cells differ from normal lymphoid cells by manifesting a wide array of aberrant changes. These genotypic and phenotypic aberrancies, detailed further on, combine to lead to a single immortalized clone. This singular clone has admixed neoplastic aberrancies and normal lymphoid features.[68] For example, a neoplastic B cell might express a single light chain and heavy chain Ig (monoclonality) but also retain normal LHRs, allowing the neoplastic cell to follow normal homing patterns and to thereby colonize other nodes and extranodal sites (e.g., bone marrow).[40, 68] The collective "malignant" aberrancies of neoplastic lymphoid cells are shown in Table 88–3. The listed malignant properties and their associated molecular or phenotypic markers allow speculation as to the biologic principles at play in lymphoma tumorigenicity. Most commonly, lymphomas present with an amalgam of these "malignant" traits and normal lymphoid traits.[68]

**Monoclonality.** Fundamentally, lymphoma represents a single immortalized clone, and as such it is a paradigm of monoclonality.[33, 34, 42, 43] In neoplastic mid- and late-phase B-cell lymphomas, there is usually light chain and heavy chain Ig restriction, indicating a monoclonal B-cell proliferation.[33, 34] Figure 88–4 demonstrates this light chain and heavy chain restriction in a follicular lymphoma, in contrast with the polyclonal pattern of a reactive lymph node. This figure illustrates the importance of the microanatomic context—that is, the monoclonality is evident within follicles and yet it may be polyclonal in adjacent normal tissues. Thus, monoclonality is defined contextually.[40] Additional genetic evidence of clonality comes from demonstrating clonal rearrangement of Ig heavy chain and light chain genes in B-cell tumors (Fig. 88–5).

Although T-cell lymphomas typically also derive from a single clone, monoclonality may be difficult to judge on a phenotypic basis. Normally, T-helper and T-cytotoxic/Y-suppressor cells are admixed in a 3 to 4:1 ratio.[39, 40] In mature T-cell neoplasia, one subset may be present to the near exclusion of the other, as shown in Figure 88–6. The difficulty is that some reactive T-cell proliferations may also show a remarkable predominance of one subset without being neoplastic.[69] In this circumstance, judgment of T-cell monoclonality is greatly aided by immunoblot assessment of T-antigen receptor genes to establish clonal rearrangements. However, even molecular assay of clonality may prove problematic unless both alpha/beta and gamma/delta assays are performed.[41, 42] Furthermore, phenotypically proven mature T-cell lymphomas without TCR rearrangements have been described.[70] Finally, the issue of clonality is clouded with immature T-cell neoplasms, as tumors with both T subsets and those with neither are described.[71] Nonetheless, in these lymphoblastic lymphomas (LBLs), the unique presence of Tdt and CD1 usually ensure proper lineage identification[71] (Fig. 88–7; see also Fig. 88–2).

In certain etiologic and clinical circumstances, notably HIV-related lymphomas and post-transplantation lymphomas, judgment of monoclonality may be highly ambiguous. In these circumstances, lymphoid tumors that appear morphologically neoplastic have proved to be variously monoclonal, oligoclonal, or polyclonal by genotyping.[72] Some of the latter were self-limiting when immunosuppressive therapy ceased, suggesting that clonality may not always equate precisely with true malignancy.[72]

**Lineage Aberrancies.** Although monoclonality is a powerful indicator of likely lymphoid neoplasia, it is not the sole determinant, as other notable phenotypic aberrancies herald the neoplastic condition. In particular, two lineage-related

*Table 88–3.* **Malignant Properties of Lymphoma**

| Malignant Phenotypes | Markers | Biologic Principles |
|---|---|---|
| High proliferative rate | Ki67, p53, C-*myc* | Loss of growth control |
| Low proliferative rate | *bcl*-2 | Resting status conferred |
| Loss of CAM | LFA-1, CD54, CD22 | Loss of cell cohesion |
| Gain of CAM | CD56 | Extranodal localization |
| Loss of lineage Ag (Pan–B-T) | CD2, CD5, CD22, CD23 | Loss of cell cohesion |
| Loss of HLA | HLA I, HLA II | Loss of immunosurveillance |
| Loss of T-TIL | CD3, CD4, CD8 | Loss of immunosurveillance |
| Drug resistance protein | P-glycoprotein | Gain of efflux pump |
| Homing receptor expression | CD44 | Gain of mobile phenotype |
| Collagenase expression | Collagenase IV | Gain in invasiveness |

## FOLLICULAR LYMPHOMA

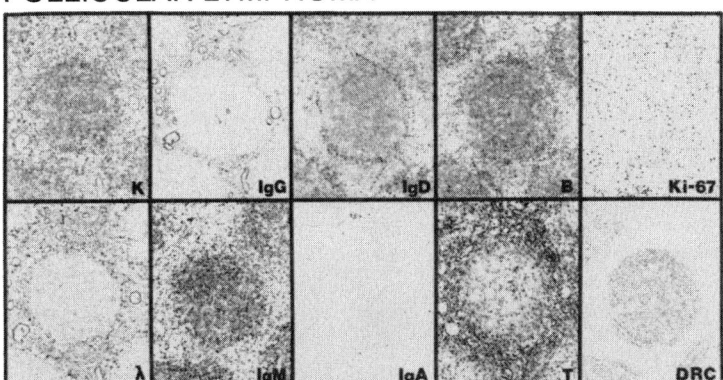

## REACTIVE LYMPH NODE

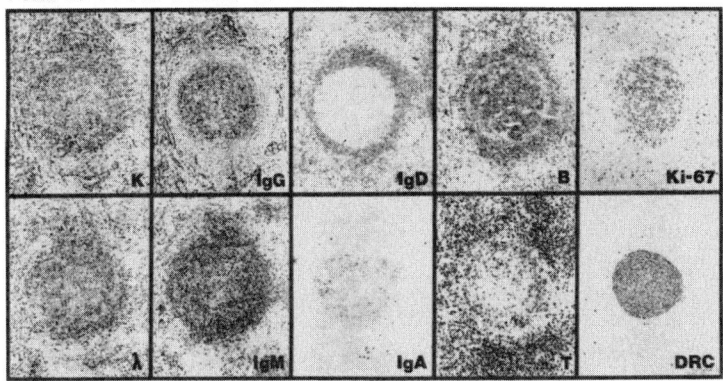

**Figure 88–4.** Comparison of monoclonal follicular lymphoma and polyclonal reactive lymph node tissue section phenotypes. DRC, dendritic reticulum cell (detected with CD21); Ki-67, anti-proliferation antibody directed at nuclear proliferation protein.

phenomena are associated with lymphoid neoplasia: (1) loss of pan–B-cell and pan–T-cell antigens and (2) unusual cross-lineage co-expressions.[73, 74] In the first instance, either B- or T-cell lymphomas may fail to express, or lose expression of, some pan–B-cell or pan-T-cell antigens, indicating a novel, aberrant phenotype that has no normal counterpart.[73, 74] For example, certain mature B-cell lymphomas may fail to express either a heavy chain or light chain Ig, presenting a phenotype with no normal counterpart. The phenomenon of idiosyncratic phenotypes indicates that lymphomas are not invariant mimics of normalcy.[73, 74] Unusual cross-lineage co-expressions include (1) CD5/T antigen co-expression in B-cell small lymphocytic lymphoma (SLL); (2) CD25/T-cell growth factor in hairy cell leukemia, (3) CD11c/histiocytic antigen in B-cell hairy cell leukemias, (4) CD15/myeloid antigen in some NHLs, (5) CD20/pan–B antigen in some T-cell lymphomas, and (6) CD43/pan–T antigen in some B-cell lymphomas.[73] These cross-lineage expressions may have a normal counterpart in the form of a rare (<1%) population. However, in the neoplastic process, the emergence of this rare clone to predominance is heralded by the unexpected cross-lineage pattern of markers.

The phenomenon of lineage antigen loss has been studied with regard to patient outcome. In one study, progressive loss of multiple lineage molecules was related to a progressively worse prognosis.[75] This suggests a series of additional deletional events in lymphoma progression, akin to the allotypic deletional events described in colon cancer progression.[75]

**Oncogenic and Chromosomal Changes.** Malignant transformation of lymphoid cells is commonly triggered by genetic changes, including chromosomal translocations, deletions, gene rearrangements, mutations, and alterations. These alterations frequently involve oncogenes, which (as described earlier) are critical to the control of lymphoid cell proliferation, differentiation, and survival. Fundamentally, lymphoid neoplasia is due to the immortalization of a single lymphoid clone, which gains a survival advantage. This process is aided by altered oncogenes, which may either increase cell proliferation or spare cells from death. Commonly, oncogene alteration may be associated with a chromosomal translocation or genetic mutation. A specific chromosomal change and a specific altered oncogene may, in turn, be associated with a specific morphologic subset of malignant lymphoma, as detailed in Table 88–4.[65]

Category I, category II, and category III oncogene alterations are described in lymphomas. A prime example of a category I alteration is c-*myc* upregulation in Burkitt's lymphoma. In this instance, the t(8;14) chromosomal translocation juxtaposes the c-*myc* oncogene on chromosome 8 with the heavy chain locus (IgH) on chromosome 14, leading to deregulated c-*myc* expression, presumably by bringing c-*myc* under the influence of transcription control elements associated with IgH.[9, 10, 76] The upregulated c-*myc* is a nuclear mitogenic factor leading to loss of proliferative control. Assay with Ki67 (directed at a nuclear proliferation protein) in Burkitt's lymphoma reveals a high proliferative index (>80% Ki67 positivity), representing the highest proliferative rate and shortest median survival of any lymphoma.[77] Some c-*myc* rearrangements occur independent of Burkitt's lymphoma and the t(8;14) translocation. In particular, high-grade gastrointestinal lymphomas may have c-*myc* deregu-

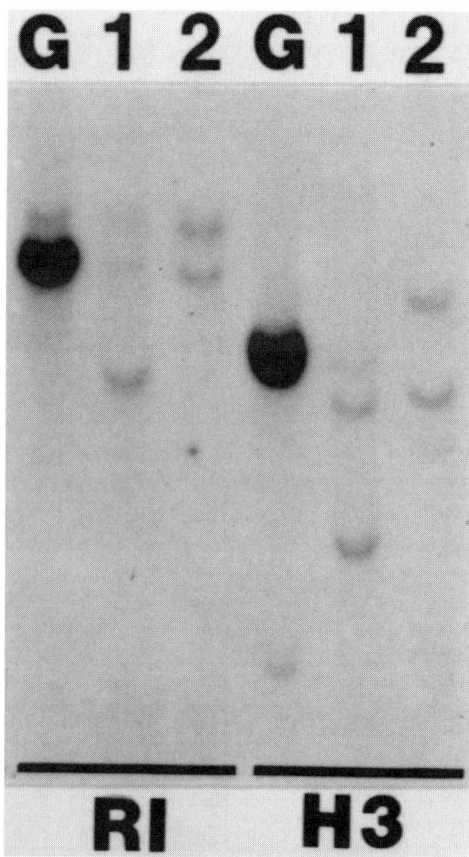

**Figure 88–5.** Southern blot demonstrating clonal, nongermline, bands (rearrangements) in two B-cell lymphomas (1, 2). G, germline band in placental control tissue. R1 and H3, restriction enzyme digestions of DNA.

lated without translocation. In general, c-*myc* upregulation is associated with an extranodal localization.[78] Some low-grade follicular lymphomas may progress to high-grade status, with c-*myc* oncogene increase as the hallmark.[79, 80]

The tumor-suppressor gene p53, a category II oncogene, is prevalent in certain lymphomas.[81, 82] In reactive lymphoid tissues, little if any wild-type p53 is found, suggesting that scant amounts are required for normal physiologic function.[81, 82] In some lymphomas, p53 exists in abundance, but in mutated form with altered function. In particular, altered p53 is readily found in high-grade Burkitt's lymphoma and large cell immunoblastic lymphomas (31% of cases).[81, 82] In these high-grade lymphomas, p53 is in a nonfunctional mutated form incapable of tumor suppression. Although rare among low-grade lymphomas, p53 oncogene expression nonetheless is abundant in the scattered large cells of low-grade lymphomas, suggesting that p53 may play a role in subsequent tumor progression to large cell type.[82] p53 overexpression in follicular lymphoma is a late event heralding clinical progression.[83] Mutated p53 and deregulated c-*myc* are especially common in HIV-associated lymphomas. This association of both a category I and category II oncogene is a reminder that secondary, tandem, add-on genetic change may be a common event in lymphoma progression and tumorigenicity.[82]

Among category III oncogenes, the physiologic role for *bcl*-2 in obviating cell death and arresting proliferation may

persist in pathologic circumstances affecting tumor cell survival and proliferation rate. Among lymphomas, the deregulated *bcl*-2 oncogene is most commonly associated with follicular lymphomas (95% are *bcl*-2 positive).[84–86] The chronic, indolent, ever-relapsing clinical behavior of follicular lymphomas is consistent with the prolonging of cell survival by the *bcl*-2 oncogene. Indeed, the seeming incurability of follicular lymphomas with cycle-specific therapy may reflect the arrest of cells in the G0 resting state.

Among *bcl*-2–positive follicular lymphomas, the majority have the t(14;18)(q32;q21) chromosomal translocation, which juxtaposes the *bcl*-2 proto-oncogenes on chromosome 18 with the immunoglobulin heavy chain locus (IgH) on chromosome 14. This leads to deregulated *bcl*-2 expression, presumably by bringing *bcl*-2 under transcriptional control of the IgH locus. Some follicular lymphomas express *bcl*-2 independent of this translocation, suggesting that other factors may lead to *bcl*-2 upregulation, which may, in turn, be subject to modulation.[84–86]

A variable number of diffuse lymphomas express deregulated *bcl*-2, both related to and unrelated to the t(14;18) translocation.[87–89] In some cases, *bcl*-2 expression (e.g., related to t[14;18]), may be taken as an indicator of derivation from a low-grade predecessor (e.g., follicular small cleaved cell lymphoma).[90] In other instances (without the t[14;18]), it may be a de novo change. This de novo change, found among mature T-cell lymphomas, may explain their lower Ki67 rate relative to B-cell large cell lymphoma (LCL) (see further on). Regarding *bcl*-2–related prognosis, the results are mixed, with some studies finding a prognostic effect and others not finding such an effect.[88–92] Three of these studies found prolonged survival among relapsed NHL patients who were *bcl*-2 positive, suggesting that arrest in low proliferative state may be a factor in relapse and long-term survival after relapse.[88–90] In contrast, one study found poor survival, suggesting that *bcl*-2–positive patients have long-surviving cells that are subject to secondary genetic change, leading to greater tumorigenicity.[92] Regarding "add-on" genetic change, experimental work with mated *bcl*-2 and *myc* transgenic mice demonstrated that *bcl*-2–positive, *myc*-positive tumors were highly lethal.[93] In humans, some *bcl*-2–positive follicular small cleaved cell lymphoma may evolve into a high-grade Burkitt's-like (c-*myc*–positive) lymphoma, which is also particularly lethal.[79, 80] Because *bcl*-2 may block apoptosis commonly associated with c-*myc* mitogenesis, this may be a particularly potent combination. More recent human clinical studies of follicular lymphoma revealed that overexpression of mutated p53 oncogene in the context of preceding *bcl*-2 overexpression heralded progression to more lethality.[83] All this points to the future need for testing relevant gene products from all three categories of oncogenes to establish the level of genetic abnormality and tumorigenicity.

**Loss of Proliferative Control.** Flow cytometric "S" phase and tritiated thymidine labeling have previously shown a high correlation between proliferative rates and lymphoma histologic grade and diagnosis.[94, 95] More recently, tissue section immunostaining with Ki67, a monoclonal antibody directed at a nuclear proliferation antigen, has been used to confirm this association of proliferation to grade.[96, 97] The Ki67 assay allows delineation of relevant microanatomy (e.g., whether proliferative cells are within or outside of

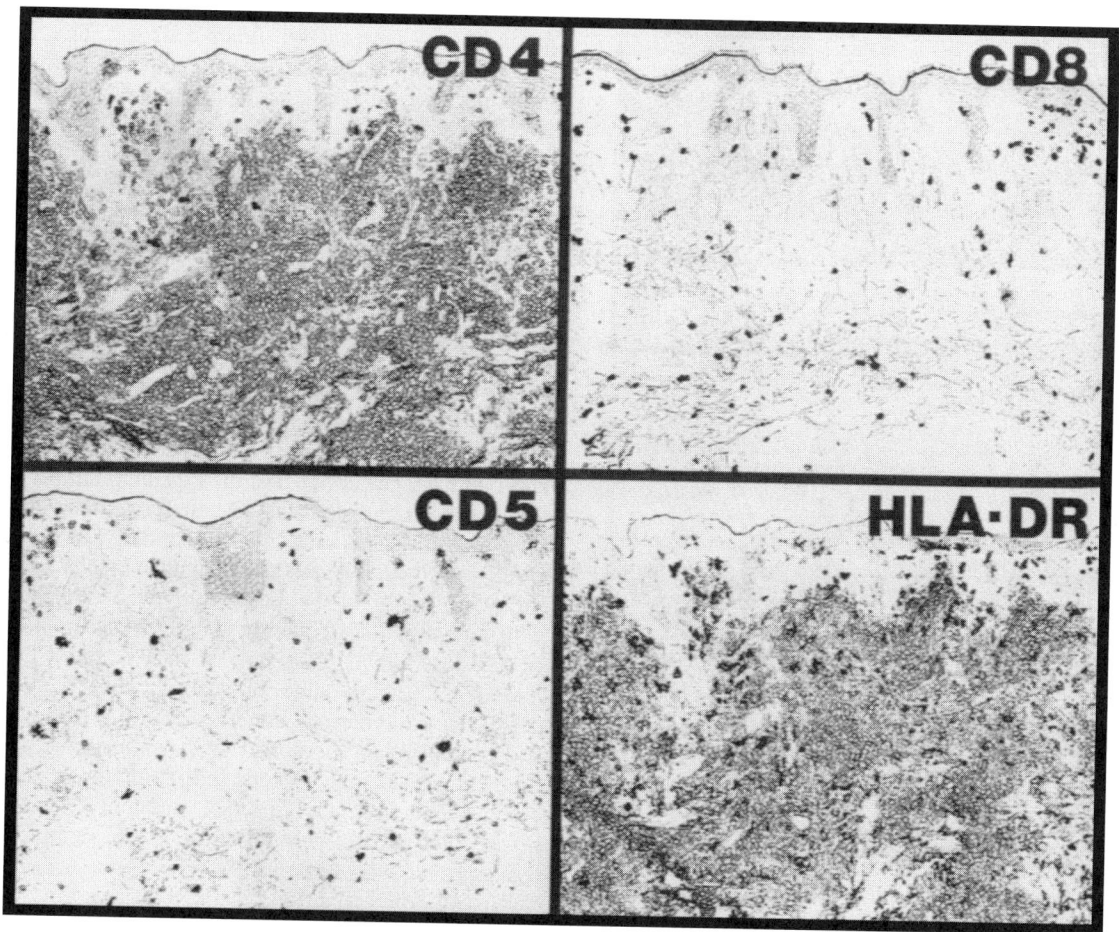

**Figure 88–6.** Peripheral T-cell lymphoma of skin with a novel T-cell phenotype (absent CD5 and CD8), T-helper expression (CD4), and activated status (HLA-DR).

neoplastic follicles) (Fig. 88–8). One Ki67 immunostaining study in particular revealed a sharp delineation among follicular lymphoma subtypes (see Fig. 88–8). Specifically, the follicular small cleaved cell lymphomas had a 5% proliferative rate, compared with 29% for follicular mixed lymphomas and 45% for follicular LCLs.[98] Thus, Ki67 may provide an objective quantitative measure to allow refinement of follicular lymphoma categorization, in contrast with morphologic studies of follicular lymphoma, which could not distinguish reproducibly between the subtypes.[99]

Among low-intermediate grade small cell lymphomas, two separate studies indicate that a proliferative index of greater than 20% or 25% identifies a more aggressive course. Thus, Ki67 may delineate distinctly separate clinical courses within a single morphologic entity.[100, 101]

Among intermediate large cell and high-grade lymphomas, retrospective studies that included small heterogeneous clinical groups have produced conflicting results.[97, 102] However, a more recent Southwest Oncology Group (SWOG) prospective trial of uniformly staged and treated patients revealed that patients with a Ki67 value greater than 80% had a 1-year survival of 18% compared with 82% for a Ki67 value less than 80%. A multifactored analysis revealed that a proliferative rate of greater than 80% is an independent prognostic variable with a relative risk of 16.6.[103]

The poor outcome associated with high proliferation suggests a biologic principle: loss of proliferative control is associated with poor outcome (see Table 88–3). The mechanism underlying this loss of control appears multifactorial, including both oncogenic and immunoregulatory alterations. As discussed earlier, alterations in nuclear mitogenic factors (e.g., C-*myc*, *bcl*-2, p53) or associated memory T cells may lead to proliferative escape of the tumor.[67, 101]

**Altered B-Cell Versus T-Cell Interactions.** As described earlier, normal lymphoid cell interactions, cohesion, and immunosurveillance are highly predicated on expression of surface recognition molecules. In this context, it is not surprising that loss or lack of expression of adhesion-recognition-costimulatory molecules (e.g., HLA, ICAM, LFA-1, CD86) is a broad phenomenon of biologic importance in lymphomas (see Table 88–3). In general, two factors may be at play: loss of lymphoid cell cohesion and loss of the adhesion molecules relevant to immunosurveillance.[47, 52, 101, 104]

Loss of cohesion, as a factor in lymphoma tumorigenicity, fits nicely with the general observation in solid tumors that lack or loss of CAM expression facilitates tumor progression in the metastatic cascade hypothesized by Liotta and colleagues.[105] Three relevant lymphoma examples may be cited: (1) loss of ICAM-1, normally found on mature B cells has been correlated with leukemic behavior in NHL[106]; (2) CD22 loss among B-cell LCL is associated with poor prognosis[743]; and (3) LFA-1–deficient mutants have shown greater invasiveness, suggesting altered or lost adhesiveness.[107]

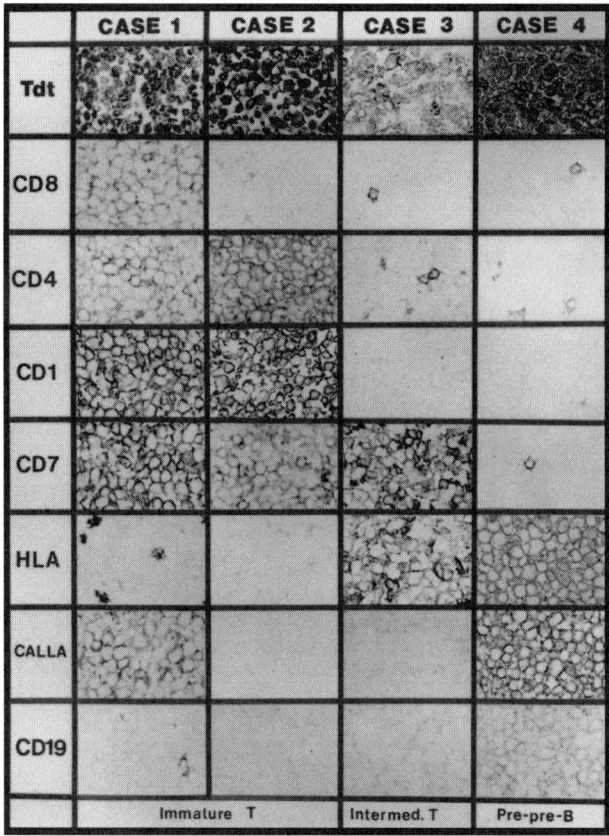

**Figure 88–7.** Comparative immunotypes of lymphoblastic lymphoma. Tdt, terminal deoxynucleotidyl transferase; CALLA, common acute lymphoblastic leukemia antigen.

Regarding loss of T-cell immunosurveillance, several examples may be cited. First, loss of LFA-1, necessary for initial T-cell docking, is more common in higher grade lymphomas, suggesting that LFA-1 loss relates to greater tumorigenicity in lymphoma.[104] More specifically, lymphomas lacking LFA-1 are known as poor stimulators of the CTL response. It is thought that loss of LFA results in loss of T-cell adherence to B cells, thereby obviating immunosurveillance.[104]

Second, because HLA antigens are required in the presen-

tation of new antigens on tumor cells to CTLs, absence of HLA in lymphoma may lead to escape from immunosurveillance because of a lack of tumor immunogenicity. Studies from several groups[108–112] have indeed found that loss of class I or class II antigens predict a poor prognosis; other studies do not.[113, 114] Nonetheless, HLA loss, as with LFA-1, follows an ascending scale of aberrancy with increasing lymphoma grade, again suggesting that HLA loss is an inherent part of increased tumorigenicity in lymphoma.[97]

Third, loss of costimulatory molecules has been associated with a loss of T-cell immunosurveillance with T-cell tumor infiltrating lymphocytes (T-TILs).

The importance of T-cell immunosurveillance in B-cell neoplasia has been underscored in a number of studies.[115–118] In particular, in these studies, lymphoma relapse and patient survival have been related to the type and number of specific T-cell subsets that infiltrate B-cell lymphomas (T-TILs). In one study of B-cell LCL, the finding of CTLs below the 6% level was invariably associated with patient relapse.[118] In a follow-up study to the latter study, the relapsing patients with low T-TILs frequently demonstrated either HLA or LFA-1 loss (85%)[115] or loss of CD80 and CD86.[52] This loss of recognition-adhesion-costimulatory molecule status correlates with loss of immunosurveillance, tumor escape, and prompt relapse. Another study emphasized a decreased frequency of memory T cells in high-grade, relative to low-grade, lymphoma, implying that a memory T-TIL response, rather than naive T-cell response, is active in maintaining less aggressive NHL status.[116–117]

Not all lymphoma tumorigenicity relates to CAM loss. In other instances, a gain of CAM status may affect tumorigenicity. A case in point is the T-cell lymphoma–associated expression of NCAM (CD56-positive lymphoma).[119–121] This oncofetal adhesion molecule, which is highly analogous to carcinoembryonic antigen, is expressed in 25% of peripheral T-cell or NK-like T-cell lymphomas.[119] NCAM studies by both the SWOG repository[119] and Wong and colleagues[120] found that these NCAM-positive lymphomas show a striking predilection for unusual sites of involvement, including the nasopharynx, the central nervous system, skeletal muscle, and the gastrointestinal tract. These anatomic sites naturally express high levels of NCAM, and the known "like-like" homophilic attraction of NCAM molecules could account

*Table 88–4.* **Genotypic Alterations in Lymphoma**

| Oncogene/Gene | Alteration | Protein | Disease |
|---|---|---|---|
| *bcl*-1 | t(11;14) | Cyclin D1 | MCL |
| *bcl*-2 | t(14;18) | Antiapoptosis | FL |
| *bcl*-3 | t(14;19) | NF-κB inhibitor | CLL/SLL |
| c-*myc* | t(8;14); t(2;8); t(8;22) | Mitogenic factor | BL |
| *bcl*-6 | t(3;14) | Zn-finger transcription factor | LBCL |
| API-2 | t(11;18) | Antiapoptosis | MALToma |
| FGFR3 | t(4;14) | Fibroblast growth factor 3 | Myeloma |
| PAX5 | t(9;14) | B-cell differentiation factor | Immunocytoma |
| ALK-1 | t(2;5) | Ki-1 | ALCL |
| TCR (α, β, γ) | rearrangement | — | PTL |
| TCR (δ) | deletion | — | PTL |
| c-*abl* | t(9;22) | p190 bcr-abl | PTL |

ALCL, anaplastic large cell lymphoma; BL, Burkitt's lymphoma; CLL/SLL, chronic lymphocytic leukemia/small lymphocytic lymphoma; FL, follicular lymphoma; LBCL, large cell lymphoma; MALT, mucosa-associated lymphoma; MCL, mantle cell lymphoma; PTL, peripheral T-cell lymphoma

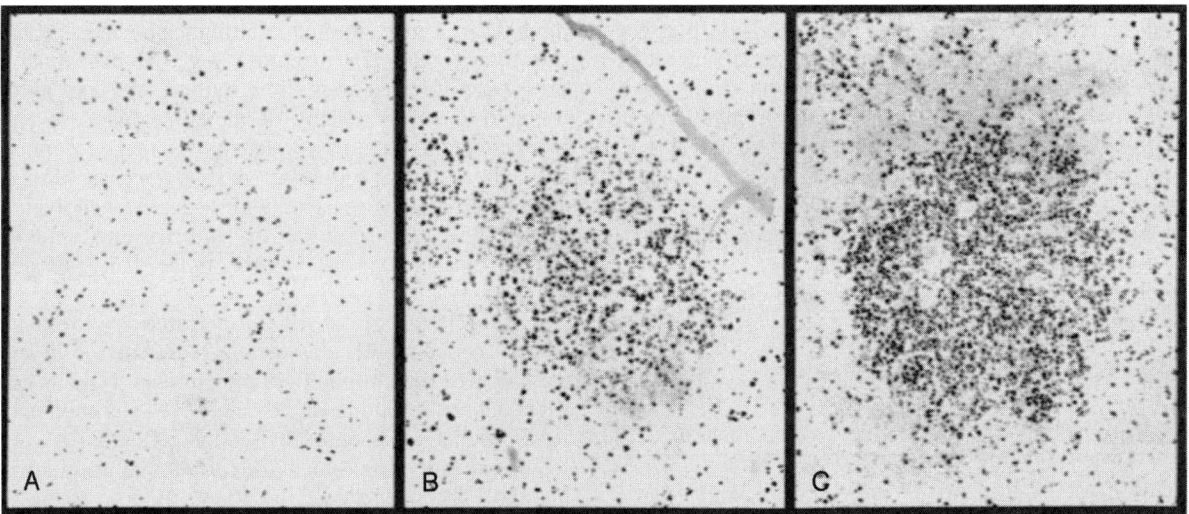

**Figure 88–8.** The range of cell proliferation among follicular lymphomas as revealed by Ki67. *A,* Follicular small cleaved. *B,* Follicular mixed. *C,* Follicular large cell.

for the preferential homing of NCAM-positive lymphomas to these sites.[119, 121]

The observation that NCAM-positive lymphomas with a propensity toward central nervous system invasion have a high α2,8-linked polysialic acid content is intriguing because similar α2,8-linked polysialic acid expression is thought to dictate entry of neuroinvasive bacteria into the meninges.[122] This suggests that glycosylation of surface receptors may sometimes be the pivotal factor in site-specific lymphoma spread.

**Effect of Sessile Versus Mobile Phenotype.** Recent findings suggest that expression of the LHR (CD44, Hermes 3) plays an important role in the dissemination of NHL and that this mechanism of lymphoma spread exerts an unfavorable prognostic influence.[61, 123–125] NHL with a putative derivation from mobile, recirculating, or mature memory T and mature B lymphocytes almost invariably expresses high levels of the LHR, whereas NHLs of sessile derivation (e.g., germinal centers) express lower levels of the LHR. This gives further credence to the notion that a sessile-mobile phenotype may be relevant to lymphoma dissemination.[47, 61]

In a survey by Pals and colleagues, high-level LHR expression occurred in 85% of patients with stage III and stage IV LCL, whereas it occurred in only 12% of patients with stage I and stage II disease.[60] This correlation between LHR expression and disease stage suggesting that there is a "stage-specific" phenotype has been confirmed to varying degrees by others.[124, 125] In any case, the correlation in the Pals study[60] is not absolute because 15% of patients with stage III and stage IV LCL had low-level LHR and 12% of patients with stage I and stage II LCL had high levels. This suggests that molecules other than LHR are relevant to dissemination. Indeed, LFA-1 is also involved in lymphocyte migration through high endothelial venules. In a study of LHR-negative lymphomas, lack of LFA-1β expression correlated with dissemination and poor outcome, whereas LHR-negative LFA-1β–positive lymphomas did not disseminate and had favorable outcome.[123]

Several studies now suggest that LHR staining intensity

is an independent prognostic factor in multivariate analysis of lymphoma. In one study, the actuarial survival rate at 2 years in patients with high levels of CD44 was 47% versus 91% among patients with low CD44 levels.[60] Similarly, poor response to treatment (i.e., lack of remission, relapse, or death from lymphoma) was more common among patients with lymphomas expressing a high level of CD44. In the study by Jalkanen and associates, the actuarial survival rate at 5 years in patients with high LHR was 45% versus 74% in patients with low or no LHR.[123] From a clinical perspective, CD44 not only identifies lymphomas with high metastatic potential and poor prognosis but also identifies and defines a new entity among lymphomas. This new entity is a subgroup characterized by high histologic grade and large S-phase fraction (high proliferative index) with LHR negativity, showing a decreased tendency for dissemination and a generally favorable prognosis.[123, 124] Because morphologic high-grade malignant lymphomas receive aggressive combination chemotherapy with toxicity that might be life threatening, identification of a subgroup with less serious prognosis and a tendency to remain localized may be of therapeutic importance.[123, 124]

**Drug Resistance Phenotype.** P-glycoprotein is a transmembrane protein thought to function as an efflux pump, removing cytotoxic or xenobiotic agents from cells and thereby protecting them from toxic effects.[126] P-glycoprotein expression is described in normal hematopoietic elements (e.g., CD34+ stem cells, CD56+ T cells) and in hematopoietic neoplasms.[127, 128] In patients with lymphomas, detectable levels of P-glycoprotein are uncommon (2%) in untreated patients and frequent (64%) in those with clinically drug-resistant disease.[126] Several reports[129, 130] indicate that the presence of P-glycoprotein in malignant lymphomas is associated with poor response to therapy, although other studies do not find this association.[131] Recent clinical data suggest that patients with P-glycoprotein–positive lymphoma benefit from alternative supplemental therapy with chemosensitizers (e.g., verapamil, quinine, cyclosporine) that may competitively combine with P-glycoprotein and reverse the efflux pump effect.[126] In 18 patients with drug-refractory lymphoma, 72% responded to standard chemotherapy plus the added P-glycoprotein–binding chemosensitizers, suggesting that carefully selected lymphoma patients with clinical evidence of multidrug resistance and detectable P-glycoprotein benefit from this alternative therapy.[126] This suggests that P-glycoprotein is an important object of clinical immunophenotypic assay among patients with lymphoma (see Table 88–2). As described earlier, the high frequency of physiologic P-glycoprotein expression among CD56[+] T cells may explain the relatively poor survival among patients with CD56[+] lymphomas.[118, 119]

## Diagnosis

The integration of morphologic, immunologic, and genetic findings is pivotal to the proper diagnosis of lymphomas as espoused in the REAL classification.[4] Fundamentally, the diagnosis of malignant lymphoma is determined by the precepts of established histologic criteria. Histologic examination determines if the normal tissue architecture is altered and what pattern of lymphoid infiltration is present. It establishes the presence of pleomorphism consistent with hematopoietic neoplasia. It excludes reactive patterns and establishes the histologic category of NHL.[40, 102] Although the histologic diagnosis still remains the "gold standard" on which clinical management is based, phenotyping and genotyping serve as independent exercises to reveal the specific chemistry of the pathologic cells. In short, histology determines whether a pathologic pattern exists and typing determines additional, adjunctive chemical detail of aberrancy. In complex phenotypic and genotypic circumstances, morphology remains critical. For example, the large blastic cells judged to be malignant may be of one phenotype or genotype, whereas the small lymphoid cells judged to be reactive may be of another phenotype or genotype.

As neoplasms of the immune system, lymphomas are best understood biologically by studying their molecular properties, including both phenotypic and genotypic features. NHLs may originate in B cells, T cells, NK cells, or NK-like T cells. Distinction among these subtypes can be made on the basis of phenotypic and molecular features of the tumor cells. The majority of NHLs (80%) are of B-cell origin. The remainder are in large part T-cell tumors. Tumors of NK or NK-like T-cells are uncommon. Tumors of T and B cells show a wide range of phenotypic expression, which can be related to a specific phase of lymphoid ontogeny.[40, 102] Tumor cells are thought to be arrested in a specific stage of lymphoid differentiation and, accordingly, to match the functions and behavior of normal lymphoid counterparts. For example, normal B cells form follicles within lymph nodes; malignant B cells of germinal center origin recapitulate this behavior with nodule formation throughout nodal and extranodal sites. Figures 88–1 and 88–2 show schematic illustrations of the phenotypic and genotypic changes associated with the stepwise differentiation of B cells and T cells and their pathologic counterparts.

The depth of our understanding of lymphoid cells and their tumors has been greatly enhanced by new reagents (e.g., monoclonal antibodies, DNA and RNA probes), new techniques (e.g., tissue section immunohistochemistry, im-

munofluorescence, immunoblotting, polymerase chain reaction [PCR]), and new machines (e.g., cytocentrifuge, epifluorescence microscopes, flow cytometers, and automated immunostainers).[132] Many of these methods use panels of monoclonal antibodies to detect the range of phenotypic antigenic expression. Cluster designation has been used to classify antibodies reactive with a given phenotypic target. Table 88–2 lists some of the more useful antibody and cluster designations among the more than 140 described to date.

**Histopathology.** As demonstrated in the Nebraska study[133] of the REAL classification,[4] the interobserver reproducibility of the morphologic categories of NHL is generally excellent, representing an advance over the previous Working Formulation scheme,[134] although certain REAL subtypes require phenotyping to achieve certainty (Burkitt's-like lymphoma). The imagery of the REAL is now so well established that a well-prepared glass biopsy slide is usually classified readily by light microscopy, and concordance is found readily in expert panels such as the SWOG Pathology Committee.[135] It is the "technically poor slide" that defeats agreement. Quality slides begin with adept gross examination and appropriate tissue preservation (both snap freezing and fixation), followed by proper cutting and staining. Quality slides begin with the pathologist being present in the operating room or outpatient clinic to receive the specimen. This presence may represent the most difficult and most important component of lymphoma diagnosis and classification.

After touch preparations are made, tissue preparation should include (at a minimum) fixation for histologic examination (neutral buffered formalin, 4 to 8 hours, 2-mm thickness) and snap-freezing of tissue for some specialized studies. Some specialized procedures like genotyping, flow cytometry, cytogenetics, tissue section Ig typing, or Southern blotting require fresh tissue. For this reason, the habit of placing lymphoid biopsy specimens entirely into formalin is not acceptable.[40, 102] A pea- to almond-sized portion of tissue may be placed in OCT compound and snap frozen at $-150°C$, either in isopentane quenched in liquid nitrogen or in liquid nitrogen alone, and then stored in an airtight container at $-80°$ C. Sectioning tissue as thin as possible entails use of sharp knives (e.g., disposable blades) to give 3-μm sections.

**Immunophenotypic Studies.** After serial sectioning, tissue section immunohistochemistry may be performed to allow delineation of the combined microanatomic and immunologic topography of the lesion (see Fig. 88–4). This immunoarchitectural analysis allows discrimination between neoplastic cells (e.g., follicular lymphoma cells) and surrounding or admixed host-response cells (e.g., T-TCLs). Alternatively, a portion of the fresh lymphoma sample may be placed in suspension to allow analysis with flow cytometry. This method allows quantitation of markers, sizing of cells, and co-localization of antigens. This mode of analysis accounts for populations of cells, not single-cell analysis or microanatomic detail, which are so frequently of importance in lymphoma diagnosis.

**Genetic Analysis.** Antigen receptor gene analysis (including in particular both Ig and T-cell receptor genes) provides evidence of clonality.[33, 34, 41, 42] Cytogenetic analysis in the form of karyotyping provides further evidence of clonality and may provide evidence of unique marker status (e.g., t(14;18) in follicular lymphoma) (see Table 88–4).

The Ig gene and TCR gene analysis typically involves Southern blot analysis of DNA extracted from fresh or frozen tissue. The DNA cut with restriction enzymes yields a ladder of DNA fragments that are dispersed on agarose gel in an electric field. This is transferred to a nylon membrane and hybridized to a radioactively labeled DNA probe specific for the gene site of interest. If a single clone is present, a single band appears in other than the germline location; otherwise in physiologic lymphoid proliferations, the signal is dispersed to the point of nondetectability except at the germline band, which represents background stromal cells without rearranged genes. Clonal, nongermline bands in a B-cell lymphoma are illustrated in Figure 88–5. In T-cell neoplasia, in which phenotypic demonstration of clonality may be problematic, TCR rearrangement by Southern blotting may be critically definitive (e.g., distinguishing AILD from AILD-like lymphoma).

The PCR method has proved useful in delineating lymphoid genetic aberrancies. In particular, the reverse transcriptase enzyme coupled with primers surrounding the gene target site (e.g., site of *bcl*-2 translocation) and the Taq polymerase enzyme are used to generate, by multiple heat cycles, a greatly amplified portion of relevant genetic material. This may be sequenced to establish genetic specificity or mutated status. It may delineate rare mutational events of diagnostic importance (mutated p53 in follicular lymphoma progression).[83]

**Non-Hodgkin's Lymphomas Versus Hodgkin's Disease.** The distinction between NHL and Hodgkin's disease is crucial in order to optimize management and subsequent outcome. Traditionally, the distinction has been the pathologist's responsibility. However, clinicians can alert their colleagues to clinical presentations that suggest possible mistaken diagnoses. Further histologic study, or use of immunohistochemical technology or molecular analysis, may confirm the clinician's suspicion.

Hodgkin's disease is mistakenly diagnosed in about 13% of patients entered in clinical trials, and most of the errors involve mistaking diffuse mixed or diffuse large cell NHLs for mixed cellularity or lymphocyte-depleted Hodgkin's disease.[136, 137] Most of those pathology errors can be anticipated by recognizing basic differences in clinical presentation between patients with Hodgkin's disease and patients with NHL. Hodgkin's disease is a unique cancer that has a predictable pattern of spread and remains confined to the lymphatic system for long periods. NHLs are hematogenous diseases, with resultant variable organ and nodal spread. Retrospective studies of mistaken diagnoses of Hodgkin's disease have correlated unusual presenting clinical features with a high probability of mistaken diagnoses. These unusual features include unusual extranodal sites of disease involvement (sites other than bone marrow and liver; noncontiguous pattern of spread; and involvement of the inguinal, femoral, or mesenteric nodes). Histologic subtypes associated with a high rate of mistaken diagnoses include lymphocyte-depleted and mixed-cellularity Hodgkin's disease. These histologic subtypes, combined with any of the hallmark clinical features, suggest a high probability of a pathologic error. In a prospective test of these criteria, 17 of 107 patients were identified as having possible errors in diagnosis. Subsequent

expert review identified 15 histologic errors. Eight (53%) of the 15 errors had been anticipated by application of the clinical criteria for mistaken diagnoses. Thus, an understanding of the difference in the initial spread of disease between Hodgkin's disease and NHL can alert the clinician and pathologist to potential errors in diagnosis.[136, 137]

## Classification

Emphasizing the integration of all available morphologic and laboratory data to establish the multiparameter definition of discreet lymphoma entities, the International Lymphoma Study Group has codified and published the classification.[4] By combining morphologic, immunologic, cytogenetic, and molecular biologic features, this classification lists 34 biologically well-defined lymphoma entities (Table 88–5). This classification places the emphasis on the underlying biologic aberrations of the specific lymphoma subtypes. This scheme anticipates development of new treatment strategies targeted toward specific lymphoma aberrations representing phenotype-adapted, etiology-based therapy. A case in point is the MALToma, which, in the gut, may initially be antigen-driven in relation to *H. pylori* and might be cured by triple-antibiotic therapy.[4, 22]

It is in this context of a more precise biologic definition of lymphomas that we review here some features of the new REAL classification. Since the REAL classification, in both full[1] and abbreviated forms, has been published previously,[4] this chapter provides a different focal point. It elaborates on selected non-Hodgkin's entities from the total REAL listing (see Table 88–5).[4] It emphasizes the immunophenotypic (see Figs. 88–1 and 88–2) and microanatomic features (see Figs. 88–4 and 88–6 to 88–8).

### REVISED EUROPEAN-AMERICAN LYMPHOMA CLASSIFICATION OF LYMPHOMAS

#### B-Cell Lymphomas

As shown in Figure 88–1, the immunotypes of the B-cell neoplasms reflect the stages of normal B-cell development. Broadly speaking, there are precursor B-cell neoplasms that derive from B cells before antigen experience and mature or peripheral B-cell neoplasms that derive after antigen or after bone marrow stage development. The category of B-cell lymphomas broadly includes the small lymphoid cell B-cell entities that are typically indolent or low grade and the B-cell lymphoma with a large or blastic cell component that is typically intermediate or high grade.

**Precursor B-Lymphoblastic Leukemia/Lymphoma.** Although the majority of LBLs are of immature T-cell phenotype (as described further on), a minority (15%) are of immature pre–pre-B or pre–B-cell phenotype (see Figs. 88–1 and 88–7).[71, 138–141] These immature B-cell and T-cell LBLs are morphologically indistinguishable. The lymphoblastic cells express the nuclear enzyme Tdt and lack immunoglobulin, although the pre–B-cell forms may express cytoplasmic mu and not surface Ig.[71, 138, 139] A rare pre-B LBL with primary hepatic involvement is described recapitulating em-

**Table 88–5. The Revised European-American Classification of Lymphoid Neoplasms**

B-cell neoplasms
  *Precursor B-cell neoplasm*
    Precursor B-lymphoblastic leukemia/lymphoma
  *Peripheral B-cell neoplasms*
    B-cell chronic lymphocytic leukemia/prolymphocytic leukemia/small
      lymphocytic lymphoma
    Lymphoplasmacytoid lymphoma (immunocytoma)
    Mantle cell lymphoma
    Follicle center lymphoma predominantly follicular (subtype: follicle
      center lymphoma, diffuse small cell)
    Marginal zone B-cell lymphoma
      Extranodal (low-grade B-cell lymphoma of mucosa-associated
        lymphoid tissue type)
      Nodal (± monocytoid B cells)
        Splenic marginal zone B-cell lymphoma (± circulating villous
          lymphocytes)
    Hairy cell leukemia
    Plasmacytoma/myeloma
    Diffuse large B-cell lymphoma (subtype: primary mediastinal large
      B-cell lymphoma)
    Burkitt's lymphoma
    High-grade B-cell lymphoma, Burkitt's-like
T-cell and postulated natural killer (NK) cell neoplasms
  *Precursor T-cell neoplasm*
    Precursor T-lymphoblastic lymphoma/leukemia
  *Peripheral T-cell and postulated NK cell neoplasms*
    T-cell chronic lymphocytic leukemia/prolymphocytic leukemia
    Large granular lymphocyte leukemia
      T-cell type
      Natural killer cell type
    Mycosis fungoides/Sezary's syndrome
    Peripheral T-cell lymphomas, unspecified
    Provisional subtypes: Subcutaneous panniculitic T-cell lymphoma and
      angioimmunoblastic T-cell lymphoma
    Angiocentric lymphoma
    Intestinal T-cell lymphoma (± enteropathy)
    Adult T-cell lymphoma/leukemia, HTLV-1 +
    Anaplastic large cell lymphoma, T-cell and NK-cell types
    Anaplastic large cell lymphoma, Hodgkin's-like
Hodgkin's Disease
  Lymphocyte predominance (nodular ± diffuse)
  Nodular sclerosis
  Mixed cellularity
  Lymphocyte depletion
  Lymphocyte-rich classic Hodgkin's disease
  Unclassifiable (malignant lymphoma, B-cell lymphoma, T-cell
    lymphoma, Hodgkin's disease)

HTLV, human T-cell leukemia/lymphoma.

bryonic pre–B-cell origin in the liver.[140] Some also express CD10 (CALLA) CD34 (proliferative cell nuclear antigen [PCNA]), and other early B-cell antigens (e.g., CD19), further indicative of immaturity. Later B antigens (CD20,22) and universal antigens (e.g., CD45) may be lacking (see Fig. 88–2).

Although precursor acute lymphoblastic lymphoma (ALL) and B-cell lymphoblastic lymphoma (B-LBL) may present with leukemia-like marrow and peripheral blood involvement. B-LBL also has a high incidence of cutaneous and osteolytic bone lesions and may be without the usual mediastinal involvement of T-cell lymphoblastic lymphoma (T-LBL).[138, 141]

**Small Lymphocytic Lymphoma.** This tissue counterpart of chronic lymphocytic leukemia (CLL) is composed of small, round, monotonous lymphoid cells with clumped "tortoise-shell–like" chromatin and inapparent nucleoli

growing in a diffuse pattern.[142, 143] Mitotic figures are rare. Larger prolymphocytes and immunoblasts are clustered in pseudofollicles or proliferation centers.[128, 129] These proliferation centers may falsely suggest a high-grade lesion, but follow-up studies indicate either no effect[144] or a favorable effect[145] on survival.

The immunophenotype is typically (>95%) of B-cell type with a characteristic amalgam of findings: faint monoclonal immunoglobulin expression and general pan–B antigen (CD19, CD20, CD 22, CD23) expression with CD5 pan–T antigen expression.[146–148] Characteristically, CD22 and CD20 expression is weaker than CD19 expression, with the latter sometimes undetectable. Expression of IgD and CD5 in SLL has a high association with eventual lymphocytosis, further blurring the distinction from CLL.[147, 148] The lack of CD5 and IgD in nonleukemic SLL suggests that these molecules are relevant to SLL cell spread and localization.[147, 148] The normal cellular equivalent of SLL is the CD5+ autoantibody–producing B cells at the edge of germinal centers[149] and in primary fetal follicles.[150]

Gene rearrangements generally show rearrangement of the immunoglobulin heavy and light chain genes. T-cell receptor genes are in the germline configuration.

Cytogenetics reveal trisomy 12 (one third of cases)[151] and translocations of chromosomes 11 and 14.[152] Rarely *bcl*-1 rearrangements are reported.[153]

The course of this neoplasm is indolent, reflecting the low proliferative rate and resting cell status. In the 1982 NCI WF study, SLL constituted 3.6% of the 1175 patients with a median age of 60 years and a median survival of 5.8 years.[139] During the course of the disease, patients with SLL may undergo transformation to a higher grade lymphoid malignancy. This progression is usually to a LCL (Richter's syndrome)[154] or to prolymphocytic leukemia-lymphoma (PLL)[155] or rarely to Hodgkin's disease.[156] Richter's syndrome typically presents as a "composite" low- and high-grade lymphoma following 2 to 4 years of SLL or CLL. The median survival from the diagnosis of Richter's syndrome is 4 months.[156] The PLL typically manifests an aggressive clinical course with a high white blood cell count and splenomegaly.[155] These transforming entities typically lose CD5 and increase surface Ig expression.[157] Transition to aggressive disease is also heralded by high mitotic rate[158] (>30/20 high power field) and a high proliferative rate (>20%) as measured by Ki67.[159]

**Immunocytoma (Lymphoplasmacytoid Lymphoma).** This lymphoma is composed of small lymphocytes, plasmacytoid lymphocytes, and plasma cells. Intranuclear (Dutcher's bodies) and intracytoplasmic (Russell's bodies) inclusions are common, as is associated gammopathy due to monoclonal Ig secretion.[4, 160] Many cases represent Waldenström's macroglobulinemia with monoclonal IgM secretion, hyperviscosity syndromes, and widespread involvement of marrow and lymph nodes,[134, 146] although rare patients with isolated nodal involvement of IgG or IgA type are described. Immunocytomas usually lack CD5 and CD10, in contrast with CLL and follicular lymphoma.[4]

There is a newly found association between HCV virus infection and immunocytomas.[12] There is also a newly described molecular lesion in the form of a translocation t(9;14) of the PAX5 gene, which is a B-cell transcription factor.[161] The specificity of both the causative agent and the molecular lesion suggests that some of the newly described discreet categories of the REAL classification like immunocytoma are worthy of separate consideration and of their own names.

Regarding the association with HCV, a strong prevalence of HCV was found in 30% of immunocytomas in an additional study, whereas HCV was a rarity in other lymphomas and was found in only 2.9% of the endemic population.[12] The majority of these HCV-positive lymphomas secrete a cryoprecipitable IgM,K component with rheumatoid factor activity and frequently present with liver or kidney involvement. There are many similarities with essential mixed cryoglobulinemia (EMC), which is of interest given the therapeutic efficacy of interferon alfa in EMC.[162] Currently HCV is thought to cause immunocytoma indirectly: since it not endowed with reverse transcriptase or oncogenes, it may stimulate a polyclonal proliferation from which a neoplastic indolent single clone emerges similar to *H. pylori* in MALT-associated lymphomas.

Regarding the molecular lesion, 50% of immunocytomas have a translocation of t(9;14). Analysis of the 9q13 breakpoint (also found in a heavy chain disease) reveals overexpression (11×) of the PAX5 gene encoding B-cell–specific transcription factors relevant to B-cell proliferation and differentiation.[163] The PAX5 gene is juxtaposed and falls under the transcriptional control of the IgH locus. The PAX5 gene alteration appears to be a distinctive molecular lesion uniquely associated with immunocytoma.

**Follicular Lymphomas.** This heterogeneous group of lymphomas derives from germinal center cells.[164, 165] Expectedly, they are morphologically and immunologically similar to normal germinal center cells. Accordingly, they typically have a nodular or follicular growth pattern, although they eventually spread beyond the follicles to efface the node diffusely.[166] Thus, germinal center–derived lymphomas include not only the follicular lymphomas but also some diffuse LCLs and high-grade entities such as Burkitt's lymphoma.[167]

The archetypal follicular lymphomas show a characteristic histologic appearance: effacement of the node by round, uniformly sized nodules. In particular, the finding of greater than 60 nodules per 40× microscopic field is a strong diagnostic indicator of follicular lymphoma.[168] Previously, the old WF cytologic subdivisions included those with a predominance of small angular lymphoid cells (category B), those with a large cell predominance (category D), and those with admixed large and small cells (category C). The latter category C mixed follicular lymphomas was variously defined as having either 20 to 50% large cells[167] or 5 to 15 large cells/high power field.[169] There appears to be a continuous gradation in the number of large cells. In practice, an individual[169] pathologist may effectively predict outcome in follicular lymphoma by grading the proportion of large cells; yet subdivision agreement is not reproducible among groups of pathologists.[170, 171] For this reason, the REAL classification dropped *subclassification,* leaving two provisional categories based on the prominence of large cells. The finding by SWOG that survival greater than 20 years in follicular lymphoma subtypes is identical (Fig. 88–9) supports the notion that morphologic subtyping of follicular lymphoma is not clinically useful, as recognized by the REAL classification.[172]

Immunologically, follicular lymphomas are B-cell neo-

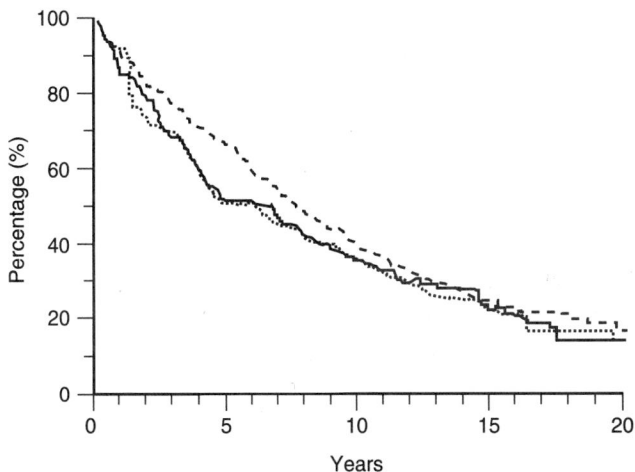

| | At Risk | Deaths | 10 Year Estimate |
|---|---|---|---|
| - - - FSC | 259 | 202 | 40% |
| ········· FM | 77 | 61 | 35% |
| —— FL | 53 | 43 | 37% |

**Figure 88–9.** Follicular lymphoma subtype survival curves (SWOG; overall survival).

plasms with expected monoclonal surface immunoglobulin and pan–B antigen expression[40, 173] (see Fig. 88–4). Similar to normal germinal center cells, follicular lymphoma cells may express CD10; in contrast with other low-grade malignant lymphomas, follicular lymphomas do not express CD5.[173] Follicular lymphoma characteristically preserves the germinal center microanatomic environment of dendritic reticulum cells and T-helper cells.[40, 173] Follicular lymphoma cells retain normal germinal center homing properties (e.g., CD44 expression) and typically show simultaneous marrow, spleen, and liver involvement (stage III to stage IV).[40, 173] In contrast with normal GC, follicular lymphoma nodules constitutively overexpress the bcl-2 protein (see further on), which is a useful diagnostic finding that distinguishes neoplastic from reactive follicles.[174]

With genetic analysis, 70 to 95% of follicular lymphomas have a chromosomal translocation, t(14;18), involving rearrangement of the *bcl*-2 gene, resulting in overexpression of an "antideath" oncogene that immortalizes follicular lymphoma cells in the resting state.[175, 176] This finding is consistent with the known "hypoproliferative" nature of follicular lymphoma and the clinically indolent course.[177]

Clinically, follicular lymphoma characteristically occurs in adults and rarely in children.[178] The course is generally indolent, with poorer prognosis associated with increasing large cell content.[152, 161] Any degree of follicularity in follicular lymphomas, despite associated diffuse growth, indicates a favorable prognosis.[166, 179, 180] In contrast, purely diffuse cases and large cell follicular lymphoma with less than 25% follicularity have a worse prognosis.[166, 181–184] Progression to higher grade lymphoma (e.g., LCL) occurs in 30% of cases and may be heralded by additional tandem genetic changes (e.g., p53 mutation), with consequent loss of suppressor gene effect and loss of proliferative control.[83]

**Marginal Zone B-Cell Lymphoma.** This group of B-cell neoplasms has distinctive histologic and clinical features. It includes (1) extranodal low-grade B-cell lymphoma of mucosa-associated lymphoid tissue MALToma),[4, 185] (2) nodal monocytoid B-cell lymphoma,[185] and (3) splenic marginal zone lymphoma.[186] These entities have sufficient morphologic and immunophenotypic similarities to suggest that they may be related. In particular, they have in common tissue-specific microanatomic homing pattern outside the germinal centers. Histologically, all three specifically involve the lymphoid tissues in a patchy or circular pattern outside the follicular mantle zones in the region known as the marginal zone.[186–193] These entities are considered in more detail.

***Mucosa-Associated B-Cell Lymphoma.*** This low-grade lymphoma typically involves epithelial-lined organs (e.g., the gastrointestinal tract, lung, salivary gland, thymus, breast, orbit, conjunctiva, and skin). Most characteristically, the epithelial surface is directly involved by the neoplastic lymphoid cells forming lymphoepithelial lesions that appear as lacunae of lymphocytes within the mucosa.[13, 17, 185] The adjacent mucosa and submucosa typically shows a lymphocytic infiltrate in the marginal zone of adjacent lymphoid follicles.[13, 17, 185] The lymphoid cells range from small, round (category A WF) to small, cleaved (category E WF) to slightly cleaved (centrocyte-like) cells.[17, 185] Typically, there may be admixed small lymphoid cells with clear cytoplasm known as monocytoid B cells.[13, 17, 185] Plasmacytoid differentiation is common. The various cell components may be stratified in the mucosa, giving a multiphasic appearance.[13, 17, 185] Clinically, this lymphoma remains localized without systemic spread for a considerable time, with relapse frequent at the same site.[185–191] When localized, it may be cured by local therapy;[185–191] when disseminated (30%), it is thought to behave like nodal low-grade B-cell lymphomas.[192] Some studies suggest that proliferation in some MALTomas may be antigen driven[193] and that therapy directed at the antigen may result in regression.[194] Specifically, triple-antibiotic therapy may result in ablation of *H. pylori* and, in turn, gastric lymphoma MALToma.[194] However, SWOG[195] and other studies[196] suggest that systemic involvement may be more frequent than previously reported. These low-grade histologic types may convert to high-grade lesions, and more distant nodes may show involvement in a marginal, monocytoid pattern. Phenotypic studies reveal co-expression of monotypic Ig and pan–B antigens with absent CD5, CD10, or CD23, as found in other lymphocytic lymphomas.[148, 197] The IgH and IgL genes are rearranged,[198] whereas *bcl*-1 and BC-2 genes remain in germline configuration.[199] Trisomy 3 or t(11;18) may be seen.[200] There is a slight female predominance, with most cases being stage I and stage II.[13, 17, 185] Normal follicles may be invaded to cause a follicular colonization pattern.[201] Many patients have a history of autoimmune disease such as Sjögren's syndrome or Hashimoto's thyroiditis.[185] In patients with Sjögren's syndrome, there is an association with MALToma with specific involvement of the myoepithelial sialadenitis lesions by neoplastic MALToma cells.[202] The myoepithelial sialadenitis is considered benign until there is evidence of Ig gene rearrangement, lymphoepithelial islands efface the epithelial islands, the lymphoid cells show cytologic atypia, or distant nodes are involved.[202] Similar criteria apply to the diagnosis of gastric MALToma.[203]

***Monocytoid B-Cell Lymphoma.*** Most monocytoid B-cell lymphomatous infiltrations occur in conjunction with extra-nodal MALTomas, and considerable overlap exists with these two entities.[204] Nonetheless, monocytoid B-cell lymphomas may also occur solely in a nodal disseminated pattern, suggesting an entity separable from MALToma.[205–213] The nodal monocytoid B lymphomas are distinguished from reactive monocytoid infiltrates by their greater pleomorphism, nuclear irregularity, and higher mitotic rate.[213] The monocytoid B lymphoma cells, like the reactive monocytoid cells, occur in sinuses, but the neoplastic form shows a confluent pattern and follicular colonization.[213] There is a high association of composite lymphoma with other low-grade histologic types, suggesting that the monocytoid B-cell population may evolve different morphologic expressions.[207] Like MALToma, it is often associated with Sjögren's syndrome[210] and may be localized, with marrow and peripheral blood involvement uncommon.[211, 212] Phenotypically, it shows a similar phenotype, with notable CD11c positivity in conjunction with monotypic Ig and overexpression of *bcl*-2, unlike *bcl*-2–negative normal monocytoid cells.[207] The clinical course is indolent, and when disseminated it is not curable.[212] Transformation to LCL may occur.[208, 209]

***Splenic Marginal Zone Lymphoma.*** This spleen-borne marginal zone lymphoma is a rare entity found in only 1% of cases (4 in 376) in a SWOG study of indolent lymphoma.[195] Its rarity and newly described status preclude definitive comment, as the entity requires further clarification.[4] However, the following observations have been made to date: (1) characteristically there is splenic involvement at the white pulp margin encircling central germinal centers and mantle zones; (2) secondary red pulp involvement may be extensive, simulating hairy cell leukemia; (3) a range of lymphoid cells are seen, from small lymphoid to monocytoid to those with a villous cytoplasm akin to the previously described splenic lymphoma with villous lymphocytes; (4) patients typically have disseminated disease with peripheral blood and marrow involvement; and (5) the course may be indolent, with splenectomy followed by prolonged remission.[4]

**Mantle Cell Lymphoma.** This lymphoma was initially defined as centrocytic lymphoma by Tolksdorf and colleagues,[214] intermediately differentiated lymphocytic lymphoma by Berard and Dorfman,[215] and mantle zone lymphoma by Weisenburger and colleagues.[216, 217] It is derived from cells of the follicular mantle zone.[216] There are two histologic patterns, including the nodular variant and the diffuse variant. In the American literature, the nodular variant was typically referred to as the mantle zone lymphoma, whereas the diffuse type was typically referred to as the diffuse intermediate differentiated lymphocytic lymphoma.[218] The tumor cells are small, slightly irregular oval to round lymphocytes with moderate chromatin condensation. Larger transformed cells are rare. Rarely, histologic transformation to a lymphoblastic large cell or highly proliferative form may occur.[219] Many cases have scattered epithelial histiocytes, creating a "starry-sky" pattern.[4] The tumor cells express monotypic surface Ig and co-express CD5 with typical absence of CD10, CD11c, and CD23. A prominent disorganized meshwork of follicular dendritic cells (FDCs) is present, in contrast to the tight-knit FDCs of follicular lymphoma. The absence of CD25 is useful in distinguishing mantle cell lymphoma (MCL) from B-CLL; CD5 is useful in distinguishing this tumor from follicular lymphoma or marginal zone lymphoma.[148, 220] There is a chromosomal translocation t(11;14) that involves the *bcl*-1 locus on chromosome 11 and the IgH locus on chromosome 14.[221] This translocation results in overexpression of the *prad*-1 proto-oncogene that encodes the cell cycle cyclin D1, which is not normally expressed in physiologic lymphoid cells.[221] Clinically, the tumor is more prevalent in older males, who usually present with stage III or stage IV disease. Sites involved include lymph nodes, spleen, peripheral blood, marrow, Waldeyer's rings, and the gastrointestinal tract in the form of multifocal lymphomatous polyps.[222] The latter involvement is submucosal in association with polyps, with evident lymphoepithelial lesions as found in MALToma. The disease course is surprisingly aggressive (median survival of 30 months), as the survival curves do not show evidence of a plateau.

MCL, as a small cell lymphocytic entity, is an excellent case in point, demonstrating how classifications evolve over time. A SWOG review found that most MCLs in the WF were category E—diffuse small cleaved cell lymphoma.[195] Previously, WF category E (diffuse small cleaved cell [DSCL]) were called diffuse poorly differentiated lymphocytic lymphomas. Figure 88–10 illustrates the evolution of these entities from the 1975 Rappaport classification diffuse poorly differentiated lymphocytic lymphomas to the 1982 WF category E, which showed more favorable median survival as category I LBLs were lifted out of the general diffuse poorly differentiated lymphocytic lymphoma category. In 1994, the old WF category E was further split by the REAL classification to list MCL separately, showing a foreshortened survival for MCL relative to DSCL.[195] As the three time points (1975, 1982, 1994) show, our classification schemes are evolving to separate more discreet homogenous biologic entities. These discrete biologic entities are most

effectively delineated by entity-specific markers—that is, MCL and cyclin D1 and LBL and Tdt.

### Diffuse Aggressive B-Cell Lymphomas

***Diffuse Large B-Cell Lymphomas.*** Previously, there were two categories of diffuse large cell lymphoma (DLCL) in the WF, which were meant to convey two separate origins: the DLCL derived from follicular center cells (FCCs) and those derived from activated immunoblasts.[134] The FCCs were composed of large noncleaved (centroblastic) and large cleaved (centrocytic) types. The immunoblastic category included four morphologic subtypes: clear cell, polymorphous and epithelioid (of presumed T-cell type), and plasmacytoid (of presumed B-cell type).[134] In practice, this morphologic heterogenicity precluded reproducible subcategorization. Indeed, the WF DLCL categories G and H alone are not reliably separable by pathologists.[223] Furthermore, the survival differences in categories G and H are minimal (e.g., 1.5 years vs. 1.3 years in median survival), leaving the importance of the distinction in question.[134] Finally, some of the subcategories (e.g., DLCL, immunoblastic lymphoma [IBL] with an epithelioid histiocyte component) may be of B-cell lineage, not the expected T-cell type, further bringing into question the sacrosanct nature of these distinctions.[224] Ultimately, the REAL classification, recognizing the difficulty of large cell subcategorization, reduced LCL to one histologic category with phenotype to separate B-cell from T-cell DLCL.[4] The prediction of phenotype of DLCL by cytologic characterizations is only correct between 61 and 80% of the time, so phenotyping has become a gold standard of the REAL classification.[225, 226]

Immunotyping of DLCL reveals that 80% are B cell, 15% are T cell, 4% are null cell, and 1% are biphenotypic.[227, 228] Although DLCLs comprise a great variety of B- and T-cell phenotypes, they have in common expression of various

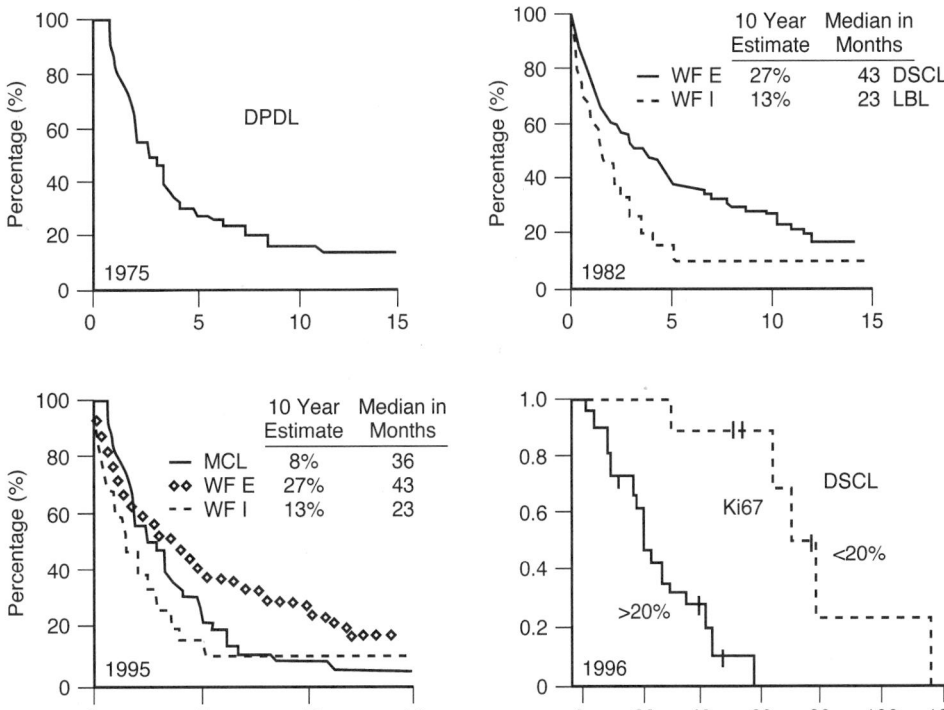

**Figure 88–10.** Survival curves demonstrating evolution of diffuse poorly differentiated lymphocytic lymphoma categorization.

activation antigens (e.g., HLA-DR). DLCLs may present challenges because loss of pan–B antigens and pan–T antigens may accompany their transformed status.[228] The propensity for DLCL to present in extranodal sites has been mentioned. It is emphasized that DLCL may involve any tissue site in the body. In some cases, the extranodal DLCL may be accompanied by compartmentalizing fibrosis, giving a nesting appearance and suggesting carcinoma.[229] DLCL phenotyping may identify prognostic differences, as described further on. Genotyping DLCL reveals a host of cytogenetic abnormalities. In particular, bcl-2 overexpression related to t(14;18) has been described and may indicate an late-relapsing incurable variant of DLCL.[88, 230]

*Burkitt's and Burkitt's-Like Lymphomas.* This high-grade lymphoma is a monomorphic proliferation of intermediate-sized cells with round blastic nuclei and multiple[2–5] basophilic nucleoli.[231] The Burkitt cells have ample "squared-off" cytoplasm, which, in touch preparations, is basophilic and contains vacuoles. There is a high mitotic rate and a starry-sky pattern reflecting ingested apoptotic tumor cells within macrophages.[231] The usual pattern of growth is diffuse, although involved germinal centers suggest follicular derivation.[167] There is a morphologic variation known as Burkitt's-like lymphoma (BLL), a provisional REAL category that shows greater nuclear viability (pleomorphism). BLL typically has nuclei containing one to two eosinophilic nuclei with basophilic vacuolated cytoplasm.[232, 233] The latter appearance is intermediate between Burkitt's and large cell immunoblastic lymphomas. BLL is the most common lymphoma, complicating HIV,[234] treated Hodgkin's disease,[235] and appearing after the immunosuppressive post-transplantation state.[236]

Immunologic findings reflect the likely germinal center origin with pan–B antigen expression, including CD10 and monoclonal immunoglobulin expression (lambda > kappa, M > G).[237, 238] Burkitt's lymphomas typically have absent expression of both LFA-1 (CD18) and ICAM (CD54).[239] The loss of these CAMs relevant to B-cell and T-cell interaction has been shown to result in poor T-cell immunosurveillance of Burkitt's cells and may also account for loss of B-cell cohesion and ready extranodal spread.[104] Occasional Burkitt's-like tumors are described of more immature pre–B-cell (Tdt⁺ CIgM⁺) phenotype.[240] Rare examples of BLL of T-cell phenotype have been described.[241]

Genetic analysis reveals that most cases have a translocation of c-*myc* from chromosome 8 to the Ig heavy chain region on chromosome 14 [t(8;14)] or less often to the light chain focus on 2[t(2;8)] or 22[t(8;22)].[9, 10] In endemic African cases, the breakpoint on chromosome 14 involves the heavy chain joining region, suggesting that the translocation occurs in an early B cell before Ig gene rearrangement is completed.[9, 10] In nonendemic cases, the translocation involves the Ig heavy chain switch region, suggesting events at a later B-cell stage.[9, 10] Burkitt's-like tumors are associated with the same translocation, although the c-*myc* rearrangement is less common and the bcl-2 gene rearrangement t(14;18) is found in 30% of cases, suggesting a different genetic profile from the Burkitt's tumor.[242] In another SWOG study of BLL using fluorescent in situ hybridization assays, BLL demonstrated a high (85%) percentage of t(8;14), suggesting that BLL and Burkitt's lymphoma have in common the distinctive t(8;14) genetic aberration.

On this basis, the conclusion was drawn that BLL, a provisional REAL category, should be considered a morphologic variant of Burkitt's lymphoma.[243]

EBV genomes are present in the tumor cells in 90% of African Burkitt's cases,[244] in 20% of nonendemic Burkitt's lymphoma,[245] and in 40% of cases associated with HIV.[246] It is thought that loss of specific T-cell immunosurveillance of EBV in germinal centers is a pivotal event in pathogenesis.[247] In particular, there is direct evidence that T-cell control of EBV-infected B cells is lost during *Plasmodium falciparum* malaria. This finding may at least partly explain the high incidence of Burkitt's lymphoma in the malarious regions of Uganda.[8]

Endemic African Burkitt's lymphoma is a distinctive clinicopathologic entity, with children (median age 7 years) usually presenting with large extranodal masses involving the jaw and other facial bones, gonads, breast, intestine (distal ileum, cecum, and mesentery), kidney, and other visceral organs.[248, 249] Gonadal and breast involvement may inexplicably be bilateral.[249] Rare cases present in leukemic phase appearing as L3-ALL.[250] More typically, the leukemic phase, along with central nervous system involvement, is a terminal event.[249] Nonendemic Burkitt's lymphoma and Burkitt's-like variants occur more commonly in adults, without jaw or gonadal tumors but with large abdominal masses.[232, 233] In rare instances, BLLs may present in the jaw, as described in one HIV-associated outbreak.[251] The Burkitt's tumor is highly aggressive, reflecting the high proliferative rate (KI67 >95%), with the poorest survival of any WF category (median survival 0.7 years),[134] yet cures are recorded and prognosis in children is said to correlate with disease bulk.[252] In some studies, survival is similar for the Burkitt's lymphoma and BLL subtypes,[253, 254] whereas in others the BLL subgroups fare more poorly.[133, 134]

**The "Lost" B-Cell Entities.** The previous WF classification had an array of intermediate- and high-grade lymphomas. These diffuse lymphomas included small cleaved (category E), mixed cell (category F), large cell (category G), immunoblastic large cell (category H), and small noncleaved (category J). The REAL classification compressed these categories, considering that subsets of large cell are clinically meaningless and that both diffuse small cell and mixed cell are in fact an amalgam of diverse lymphomas with different origins and natural histories and not biologically homogenous.[4]

A review by SWOG finds comparable clinical outcomes among categories E, F, G, and H, suggesting that these categories are indeed rationally considered comparable and may be compressed into one category as in the REAL classification of diffuse large cell B-cell lymphoma.[255]

Among indolent B-cell lymphomas, follicular lymphomas are suggested as a single REAL category, with subsets or grades being provisional. This reflects the broader biologic view that the small, large, and mixed subsets of follicular lymphoma have comparable 20-year survival, as evidenced in a SWOG retrospective review from the 1970s (see Fig. 88–9).[172]

### T-Cell and Natural Killer Cell Lymphomas

**Precursor T-Lymphoblastic Lymphoma/Leukemia.** LBLs of immature T-cell type (morphologically indistinguishable from immature B-LBLs) have blastic nuclei with fine dusky chromatin, inconspicuous nucleoli, and scant cytoplasm. The majority of LBL (85%) (see Figs. 88–1 and 88–7) have an immature T-cell phenotype that mimics the cortex of the thymus.[71, 256–258] As shown in Figures 88–1 and 88–7, this immaturity is manifested by co-expression of T-helper (CD4) and T cytotoxic antigens (CD8), with strong nuclear co-expression of the thymic-derived nuclear enzyme Tdt. The more immature forms co-express CD10 (CALLA) and lack HLA-DR. More mature T-LBLs have a single functional subset (e.g., CD4) and lack CALLA. Rarely, as shown in Figure 88–7 (case 3), even more mature forms occur with faint Tdt and aberrant T antigens (e.g., $CD7^+$, $CD1^-$, $CD4^-$, $CD8^-$). In the latter instance of more mature T-LBLs, the patients nonetheless fit the clinicopathologic profile of LBL with mediastinal presentation in young males, subsequent leukemic involvement, and classic convoluted LBL morphologic features.[71] There is considerable overlap with T-ALL, with peripheral blood and marrow involvement in one third of LBL cases. Sanctuary sites such as the gonads and central nervous system are commonly involved. This similarity to T-ALL (e.g., involvement of sanctuary sites, similar phenotype) prompts treating LBL similar to ALL. Rarely, T-LBL may express natural killer cell antigens ($CD16^+$, $CD57^+$); these patients follow an aggressive course and females predominate in contrast with the usual T-LBL male predominance.[259]

**Peripheral T-Cell Lymphomas.** Peripheral T-cell lymphoma (PTL) is an immunologically defined category of NHL that was not present in older morphologic classifications like the WF but is emphasized in immunologically based classifications like the Kiel classification or the REAL classification.[4] The emergence of PTL as a lymphoma category despite diverse morphologic features and outcome reflects several facts, for example, (1) its immunologic specificity, that is, mature, post-thymic, activated T-cell status with "novel" aberrant pan–T expression and (2) PTL as a broad category has spawned specific entities of etiologic definition (e.g., HIV III–related PTL, clinical distinctiveness (e.g., gluten enteropathy–associated PTL, organ specificity (e.g., hepatosplenic PTL), phenotypic specificity (e.g., NK-like $CD56^+$ PTL), morphologic distinctiveness (e.g., anaplastic lymphoma), and cytogenetic definition (e.g., anaplastic LCL with the t(2;5) translocation.[4] In short, there has emerged under the rubric of PTL a number of distinct clinical, pathologic entities not accounted for in the WF but now tabulated in the REAL scheme.[1] This section focuses on both the broad categorization of PTL[260–288] (Table 88–6) and some of the newly listed REAL PTL provisional entities (see Table 88–5).

*Immunophenotypic Features Of Peripheral T-Cell Lymphomas.* By definition, PTLs are neoplasms of mature T cells that derive from peripheral lymphoid sites outside the thymus, in contrast with a central thymic origin for immature T-cell LBLs.[260–265] As neoplastic cells derived from post-thymic T cells, these cells then expectedly express pan–T cells (e.g., CD2, CD5, CD7), lack immature antigens (e.g., CD1, CD10, CD34), and lack B-cell antigens, as shown in Figure 88–2.

A more useful phenotypic finding of diagnostic import in PTL is the aberrant "idiosyncratic" loss of pan–T antigens

**Table 88–6.** Peripheral T-Cell Lymphoma Variants

| *Working Formulation Category All Diffuse* | *(Percent)* |
|---|---|
| Small cell | ~15 |
| Mixed | ~40 |
| Large cell | ~45 |
| Others | Rare |

*Additional Morphologic Categories*

Clear cell immunoblastic sarcoma (Lukes, Collins)
T-zone lymphoma (Lennert)
Medium-size-cell lymphomas (Japanese)
Hodgkin's-like non-Hodgkin's lymphoma
Plasmacytoid PTL
Anaplastic large cell

*Lymphokine-Related Categories*

Abundant epithelioid histiocytes (Lennert's lymphoma)
PTL with plasmacytosis and gammopathy
PTL with aberrant myelocytopoiesis and eosinophilia
Erythrophagocytic PTL simulating malignant histiocytosis
PTL with hypercalcemia

*Organ-Associated Categories*

CNS: CD56-positive PTL
Cutaneous: low-grade mycosis fungoides
          high grade: mostly large cell
Gut: gluten-sensitive enteropathy-associated
Spleen: PTL simulating hairy cell leukemia
Blood: T-CLL, T-prolymphohistiocytic and large granular cell
    leukemia, Sezary's syndrome

*Vessel-Associated Categories*

Angioimmunoblastic lymphadenopathy–like (AILD-like)
Angiocentric, angiodestructive immunoproliferative lymphoma
Lymphomatoid granulomatosis (pulmonary)
Midline malignant reticulosis (nasal)

*Virus Associated*

Adult T-cell lymphoma/leukemia of Japan and Caribbean
    (HTLV-1 associated)
T-cell hairy cell leukemia (HTLV-II associated)
HIV-associated PTL (HTLV-iII associated)

*Cytogenetic Specific*

Anaplastic large cell (t(2;5))

PTL, peripheral T-cell lymphoma; CNS, central nervous system; HTLV, human T-cell leukemia/lymphoma; HIV, human immunodeficiency virus.

(CD2, CD3, CD5, CD7), as illustrated in Figure 88–6.[265–270] In the majority of PTLs (80%), there is loss of one or more pan–T antigens. This phenotypic loss, which is inconsistent with the expected physiologic phenotype as shown in Figure 88–2, is highly associated with clonal rearrangement of the T-cell antigen receptor genes in PTL and is decidedly not usual in benign inflammatory T-cell proliferations.[260–275] These abnormal PTL phenotypes have no corresponding counterpart in normal T-ontogeny. This suggests that, unlike B-cell neoplasms, PTLs are not as likely to recapitulate normal lymphoid development slavishly. This novel or idiosyncratic phenotype of PTL helps define PTL as a distinct aberrant immunologic entity, and the failure of PTL to fully mimic normalcy can serve a diagnostic purpose.[265–275] The use of pan–T antigen loss to establish neoplasia has some caveats, notably that occasionally a pan–T antigen (e.g., CD7 in cutaneous infiltrates) may be absent in inflammatory conditions.[24] Therefore, the loss of more than one pan–T antigen and (in particular one beyond CD7) is more reliable for diagnosis.

Besides loss of pan–T antigens, another lineage-related phenomenon of PTL serves as a diagnostic aid: unusual cross-lineage co-expression. In particular, CD20 pan–B antigen may be expressed rarely in some PTLs.[275] In this instance, the CD20$^+$ 3$^+$ PTL has a normal counterpart in the form of a rare (<1%) population of normal circulating T cells. However, in the neoplastic process, the emergence of this rare clone to predominance is decidedly pathologic, and the unexpected cross-lineage pattern of markers is the key phenotypic clue.[274]

Besides the common T-helper PTL and less frequent T-cytotoxic PTL, other variants of PTL exist. These include rare cases of aberrant double expression of CD4 and CD8.[266] This CD4$^+$/CD8$^+$ PTL mimics the thymic cortex phenotype except that Tdt is absent and it is, in fact, a mature aberrant PTL phenotype. There are also PTLs with absence of both CD4 and CD8, known as *double-negative* PTL.[260] These include PTL with gamma/delta rearrangements without CD4 and CD8, as shown in Figure 88–1, and S100$^+$ PTL with some natural killer cell (NK)-like antigen co-expressions.[4] Finally, there are double-negative PTLs without S100 and with NK antigens (e.g., CD56), which represent NK-like PTL variants.[4]

Lastly, many PTLs are mature T-cell neoplasms derived from activated T cells and therefore have abundant expression of activation antigens (e.g., HLA-DR), interleukin (IL)-2 receptors (CD25), T-cell activation antigen, and CD30 Ki1 antigen, a nerve growth factor receptor.[4]

**Selected T-Cell Entities.** Among the specified and provisional subtypes of PTL shown in Table 88–5, several entities (five) are selected for further discussion and illustration.[276–288]

*CD30 Ki1–Positive Anaplastic Large Cell Lymphoma.* This neoplasm is composed of anaplastic, large blastic lymphoid cells that express the Ki1 (CD30) antigen.[4] The characteristic features are the large blastic cells with elaborate polylobated "wreath-like" nuclei growing in a sinusoidal, cohesive pattern. This sinusoidal pattern strongly raises the suspicion of possible metastatic carcinoma, seminoma, or melanoma prior to immunotyping.[289–291] The tumor cells of anaplastic large cell lymphoma (ALCL) are typically much larger (two to three times) the usual LCL cells. Lymphohistiocytic and small cell variants have been described. There are two major histologic variants: (1) the classic variant that occurs in a sinusoidal pattern as described earlier and (2) Hodgkin's-like variant, which has morphologic similarity to Hodgkin's disease by virtue of a nodular growth pattern, syncytial growth, large polylobated cells, and surrounding bands of growth, and fibrous sclerosis.[4]

By definition, the tumor cells are CD30$^+$. Additionally, most (70%) are of mature T-cell lineage with variable expression of CD3 and CD4.[289–291] There are several antigens that are highly associated with ALCL and may therefore be considered ALCL-associated antigens: BNH9,[292] EMA,[293] CBF78,[294] and the nucleophosmin-alkaline kinase fusion protein, ALK-1. Occasionally CD30$^+$ ALCLs are of null or B-cell lineage. TCRII gene rearrangements occur in 60% of cases, with 40% being TCRII silent.[290] Cytogenetic studies

reveal that some (12 to 50%) cases have a unique translocation t(2,5)(p23;q35), which results in the fusion of the nucleophosmin gene on 5q35 with a novel anaplastic lymphoma kinase (ALK) gene on chromosome 2p23.[295–298] A higher percentage of t2;5 is observed in pediatric cases.[295–298]

Clinically, two major profiles relevant to outcome are described: systemic and cutaneous ALCL.[299, 300] The latter type typically presents in localized cutaneous form, and it may either regress spontaneously or follow an indolent but nonetheless incurable course. The systemic form is disseminated and has a more aggressive course, although complete cure is possible at the rate (35 to 40%) described in regular LCL. Among the disseminated systemic forms of ALCL, the classic subset matches the clinical profile of a diffuse non-Hodgkin's LCL.[299, 300] In contrast, the Hodgkin's-like variant has shown a high propensity to involve the mediastinum in young girls, once again mimicking Hodgkin's disease.[301] However, phenotyping distinction from Hodgkin's disease is unequivocal, as described further on. Since the large polylobated nuclei of Reed-Sternberg cells in Hodgkin's disease also express CD30, distinction of ALCL from Hodgkin's disease both morphologically and immunologically may be difficult. ALCL differs from Hodgkin's disease by its usual phenotypic profile: CD30$^+$ CD15$^-$ CD45$^+$ pan–T$^+$ or pan–B$^+$, which contrasts with the usual Hodgkin's phenotype: CD30$^+$ 15$^+$ 45$^-$ T$^-$ B$^-$. There are also newly delineated anaplastic-associated antigens (ALK-1, CBF78, BNH9, and EMA), which are characteristically expressed in ALCL and not in Hodgkin's disease.[292–294] Finally the 2,5 translocation is also highly associated with ALCL and not with Hodgkin's disease.

*HIV-III (HTLV-1)–Associated Japanese T-Cell Lymphoma/Leukemia.* A mature T-cell lymphoma/leukemia caused by the human retrovirus variously known as human immunodeficiency virus (HIV-III) or human T-cell leukemia virus 1 (HTLV-1) is endemic in southwestern Japan, the Caribbean, and the southeastern United States.[302–311] Pronounced nuclear pleomorphism with hyperlobated nuclei (flower cells or clover leaf cells) are found in the peripheral blood.[306] The nodes are involved with a heterogeneous mix of small and large lymphoid cells, with some multinucleate cells similar to Reed-Sternberg cells.[302] Common sites of involvement include lymph nodes, skin, liver, spleen, central nervous system, bone marrow, and peripheral blood, with widespread stage IV presentation most frequent.

Typical HTLV-1–associated neoplastic cells have a natural T-helper cell phenotype, with co-expression of CD2, CD3, CD4, and CD5, with absent CD7. The IL-2 receptor (CD25) commonly is highly expressed. The occasional admixed large Reed-Sternberg cells may be CD30-positive or CD15-positive, adding to diagnostic difficulty.[305–308] TCRII genes typically are clonally rearranged. Demonstration of monoclonal or oligoclonal integration of HIV-III (HTLV-1) provirus by Southern blotting provides definitive proof of cause. More recently, PCR has demonstrated proviral sequences in DNA extracted from tissues fixed in formalin and embedded in paraffin.[309, 312]

This entity occurs in adults in the endemic areas of Kyushu, Japan; the Caribbean; and the southern United States. The latter patients are largely but not exclusively blacks.[307, 308] The acute form presents with a high peripheral white blood cell count, hepatosplenomegaly, hypercalcemia, and lytic bone lesions with an aggressive course (survival <1 year).[306] Rarely, it may occur as chronic or smoldering subtypes, frequently with a predominance of cutaneous involvement.

Hypercalcemia and lytic bone lesions are commonly found. Biopsies of lytic bone lesions typically show increased osteoclastic activity with bony resorption and no evidence of local bony involvement by lymphoma/leukemia. The focal osteoclastic activity appears to be an untoward effect of the *tax* gene product of HTLV-1, which induces a parathyroid-like hormone, resulting in osteoclast activity and hypercalcemia.[313]

Cutaneous involvement may be confused with mycosis fungoides–Sézary syndrome. In particular, epidermal clustered lymphoid invasion may occur in the form of Pautrier's microabscesses, greatly mimicking mycosis fungoides.[302–306] HTLV-1–associated disease resembles the d'emblée variant of mycosis fungoides without a chronic premycotic phase. As a differentiating point, the typical acute fulminant course of HTLV-1–associated T-cell lymphoma/leukemia contrasts with the indolent disease course of mycosis fungoides. Ultimately, Southern blot or PCR evidence of HTLV-1 viral sequences allows definitive distinction.[309, 312]

***Subcutaneous Panniculitic Peripheral T-Cell Lymphomas.*** Panniculitic peripheral T-cell lymphomas are lymphomas that involve primarily the subcutaneous tissues, morphologically resembling panniculitis, hence their name.[314–317] The classic case is associated with a hemophagocytic syndrome. These lymphomas primarily involve the subcutaneous tissues, with some infiltration of the deep dermis. Superficial dermal and epidermal involvement are not characteristic but have been described in occasional cases.[314] Lymphoid cells infiltrate between fat cells, forming a "lace-like" pattern that creates the morphologic similarity to panniculitis. Focal aggregates and small sheets of lymphoid cells are also seen. The lymphoid infiltrate may be bland in early lesions, making differentiation from benign panniculitis difficult. More advanced lesions show a mixed infiltrate of small and large cells with irregular nuclear outlines and coarsely clumped chromatin. Most of these infiltrates would be classified as large cell by the REAL classification scheme.[314–317]

Karyorrhexis and frequent mitotic figures are characteristic. Larger lesions show necrosis of connective tissue and fat. Scattered single benign histiocytes, granulomas, and foreign body giant cells may be seen within these areas of necrosis. In cases associated with the hemophagocytic syndrome, erythrophagocytosis by histiocytes is present. Unlike the angiocentric T-cell lymphomas, angiocentricity and angioinvasion are not characteristic.[314–317]

With paraffin section immunohistochemistry, panniculitic PTL stains with the T-cell–associated antigen UCHL1 and may also stain with other T-cell markers such as CD43. Detailed immunophenotypic data are limited in this disease; four of five patient samples tested by Gonzalez and colleagues[314] were CD4+; the remaining case was CD8+. Antigenic aberrancy may be observed.[314] Rearrangement of the T-cell receptor beta chain gene is characteristic of the disease in the few cases tested but may not be identified in every case.[314, 315]

Patients are adults (reported age range 19 to 54 years) who present with subcutaneous nodules 1 to 13 cm in size, classically of the extremities. Most patients develop an asso-

ciated hemophagocytic syndrome, either at the time of diagnosis of panniculitic PTL or subsequently in the disease course. The hemophagocytic syndrome has been attributed to cytokine production by the malignant T cells.[317] The hemophagocytic syndrome is generally florid and is often fatal. Several reports describe patients who initially presented with skin lesions that clinically and morphologically resembled benign panniculitis several years before developing a morphologically recognizable panniculitic PTL in tandem with a hemophagocytic syndrome.[315–317] Whether these represent precursor lesions of PTL is as yet unknown.

The differential diagnosis of panniculitic hemophagocytic syndrome includes viral-associated hemophagocytic syndrome. Patients with the latter disease may have a skin exanthem from a viral illness but do not show the subcutaneous infiltrate seen in panniculitic PTL. Furthermore, they lack the pleomorphism found in panniculitic PTL.

***Enteropathy-Associated T-Cell Lymphoma (Intestinal T-Cell Lymphoma).*** This peripheral T-cell lymphoma is derived from the intraepithelial mucosal T cells of the small bowel and is frequently associated with celiac disease.[318–325]

Enteropathy-associated T-cell lymphoma (EATL) usually involves the small bowel, in particular the jejunum in which more than 70% of the neoplasms are found, and is frequently multifocal.[318, 319] The tumor infiltrates the lamina propria and overlying epithelium and may invade through the muscularis propria, leading to thickening of the bowel wall. Malignant cells invade the epithelium singly and in groups, giving rise to tumor cell collections resembling Pautrier's microabscesses in mycosis fungoides and also resembling the lymphoepithelial lesions of clustered mucosal invasion found in MALTomas.[321] More extensive epithelial involvement leads to extensive mucosal ulceration and associated inflammation. The tumor cells are usually large or immunoblastic, although in a minority of cases, a predominant small cell component is found. Scattered Reed-Sternberg–like cells are frequently found. Admixed plasma cells and eosinophils may be found. In areas grossly uninvolved by neoplasm, there may be a background of celiac disease changes (villous atrophy) and increased numbers of normal-appearing intraepithelial T cells. Microscopic foci of intramucosal tumor may be found within this background of celiac disease distant from the main tumor mass.[318] Background celiac disease changes, however, are not seen in a significant number of cases.

Involved lymph nodes show paracortical infiltration by malignant cells. Generalized disease can involve not only lymph nodes but also other sites, including spleen, liver, and lung.[318, 319]

The neoplastic cells are T cells, with a characteristic CD3+ CD7+ CD4− CD8− or CD8+ phenotype; CD5 and HLA-DR are generally absent.[318] The CD3+ CD7+ CD4− CD8− double-negative phenotype is also found in a proportion of intraepithelial T cells in normal small intestine. It is this same T-cell subset that is expanded in celiac disease.[323] The tumor cells also frequently express HML-1, an antigen expressed by, although not specific for, intestinal intraepithelial T-cells.[72, 74] By paraffin immunohistochemistry, the neoplastic cells stain with CD3 and CD45RO. CD30 is also frequently expressed[320] and may be a useful marker to detect malignant cells in areas in which the neoplastic infiltrate is obscured by acute inflammation from mucosal ulceration. The tumor cells also express p53 and generally show a high proliferative index when stained with MIB1, a marker of proliferating cells.[320] Genotyping shows rearrangement of the T-cell receptor beta chain gene. This rearrangement is also frequently detected in areas of the small bowel unaffected by tumor but involved by celiac disease.[320, 324] and has also been described in small bowel biopsies from a patient with adult-onset celiac disease who lacked histologic evidence of malignant lymphoma, suggesting that the celiac disease lesions may in fact be precursor T-cell lymphoma lesions in some cases.[324]

EATL is a disease of older patients, with a median age of about 60 years. Although controversial, it is generally believed that the disease is strongly associated with celiac disease. Many patients present with celiac disease–type symptoms with months to years of abdominal pain and weight loss. However, a significant number of individuals present with an acute abdominal emergency including perforation or obstruction[318] without antecedent celiac disease symptoms.

The disease is generally aggressive with frequent recurrences. The majority of patients die within 6 months of diagnosis. Survival is better in patients with localized (stage I) disease than in those with advanced disease.[318]

These lymphomas may be mistaken for high-grade MALT-type B-cell lymphomas because of the epitheliotropism (mucosal lymphoepithelial lesions) of the lymphoid cells. Immunohistochemistry reliably differentiates these two entities.

***Hepatosplenic T Gamma/Delta Cell Lymphoma.*** This neoplasm consists of gamma/delta double-negative T cells and is characteristically associated with hepatosplenomegaly but with minimal lymph node involvement.[326–328] In the spleen, there is sinusoidal infiltration of the red pulp by fairly uniform, medium-sized lymphoid cells that have oval or folded, somewhat condensed chromatin and moderate amounts of pale cytoplasm.[326] Splenic involvement may lead to massive splenic enlargement. A similar lymphoid infiltrate is seen in the hepatic sinusoids. Lymph node involvement is likewise characterized by a sinusoidal and interfollicular neoplastic infiltrate, leading to partial or complete nodal effacement.

The neoplastic cells phenotype as CD3$^+$ TCR-1$^+$. Characteristically, they lack both CD4 and CD8 expression and are double negative by typing (see Fig. 88–2). Expression of the other pan T–cell antigens CD2 and CD5 may be weak or absent.[327, 328] Most of the cases described express NCAM CD56.[326–328] In paraffin section immunohistochemistry, the neoplastic infiltrate phenotypes as a T-cell infiltrate (CD3$^+$ UCHL1$^+$ CD43$^+$).

The disease may be aggressive, requiring multiagent chemotherapy. Patients typically present with fever, myalgia, arthralgia, and weight loss. This may lead to a clinical evaluation for fever of unknown origin. Splenomegaly or hepatomegaly may be presenting signs or may develop during the course of the illness. The peripheral blood shows a normal white blood cell count and anemia. There may be either thrombocytopenia or thrombocytosis. Although the white blood cell count is normal, examination of the peripheral smear reveals the presence of atypical lymphocytes; these may account for only a small percentage of cells at initial presentation. The disease sometimes may not respond to multiagent chemotherapy.

Differential diagnosis of the splenic infiltrate includes T-cell lymphoma, hairy cell leukemia, and myeloid leukemia. The differential diagnosis in the lymph nodes would include T-cell lymphoma and a leukemic infiltrate. Immunophenotyping either on fresh or paraffin-fixed tissue is essential to ensure the correct diagnosis. Since helper and CTL antigens are absent, demonstration of the TCR1 gamma/delta framework determinants is essential. Furthermore, an absence of S100 is essential in excluding S100$^+$ PTL, which also may have a sinusoidal hepatosplenic pattern of involvement.

## Staging

The goals of the initial staging evaluation of the patient with NHL have changed since the 1980s. At a time when treatment for NHLs was modeled on Hodgkin's disease, aggressive techniques including surgery were regularly used. Consequently, the Ann Arbor system of staging Hodgkin's disease was extended to patients with NHL.[329] The purpose was to identify patients with visually localized disease so that potentially curative radiation therapy could be prescribed.[330, 331] As our understanding of NHLs has evolved so that it is now considered a hematogenous or systemic disease, and as effective systemic chemotherapy has developed, the need for rigorous staging procedures has lessened.[332]

The systemic nature of NHL is suggested by our current realization that most normal lymphocytes regularly travel through the body. Unless the cell machinery for traveling is lost as part of malignant development, malignant lymphocytes will continue to move throughout the body. The disease is likely systemic from its inception. Clinical evidence for this phenomenon is found in three observations: (1) most patients have visible evidence of systemic disease at diagnosis. Only 5 to 10% of follicular lymphomas and 20% of diffuse histologic types are visually localized at diagnosis after clinical assessment.[333] (2) Laparotomy reveals occult abdominal disease in 20% of patients with clinically localized disease.[334] (3) Initial recurrence at a distant site occurs in 10 to 25% of patients during radiation therapy as initial management[335–337] for visually localized disease. These clinical observations led to trials of initial chemotherapy for localized stages of intermediate- and high-grade histologic types, which resulted in apparent improved outcome based on survival.[338] Moreover, the number of relapses at distant sites was decreased. For example, patients with stage II LCL treated with radiation therapy alone are reported to have 5-year survival rates of 0 to 46%, whereas stage II diffuse LCL patients treated with initial doxorubicin-containing chemotherapy appear to have a 5-year disease-free survival ranging from 64 to 81%.[339] Thus, the development of potentially curative chemotherapy for a disease with a high propensity for systemic spread has obviated much of the need for meticulous staging procedures.

**Ann Arbor System.** The Ann Arbor system is largely based on the expectation of anatomic spread of disease, predictable patterns of disease involvement, and the effectiveness of regionally directed therapy (radiation therapy). The Ann Arbor staging system is summarized in Table 88–7. The stage of disease at diagnosis (Ann Arbor stage I, II, III, or IV) is modified by indicating the presence (B) or absence

*Table 88–7.* Ann Arbor Staging System

*Stage I*

Involvement of a single lymph node region (1) or of a single extralymphatic organ or site ($I_E$)

*Stage II*

Involvement of two or more lymph node regions on the same side of the diaphragm (II) or localized of extralymphatic organ or site and of one or more lymph node regions on the same side of diaphragm ($II_E$). An optional recommendation is that the numbers of node regions involved be indicated by a subscript (i.e., $II_3$)

*Stage III*

Involvement of lymph node regions on both sides of the diaphragm (III), which may also be accompanied by localized involvement of extralymphatic organ or site ($III_E$) or by involvement of the spleen ($III_S$), or both ($III_{SE}$)

*Stage IV*

Diffuse or disseminated involvement of one or more extralymphatic organs or tissues with or without associated lymph node enlargement. The reason for classifying the patient as stage IV should be identified further by defining site by symbols

(A) of specific systemic symptoms known to effect outcome adversely.[340–355] Specific B symptoms include weight loss exceeding 10% of usual weight during the 6 months prior to diagnosis, unexplained fevers with temperatures exceeding 38° C, and night sweats. These specific systemic symptoms are seen in approximately 10% of patients with stage I or stage II disease and in 40% of patients with stage III or stage IV disease.[340, 350] For patients with NHL, staging procedures are usually limited to clinical techniques and include history, physical examination, radiographic studies, isotopic scans, peripheral blood counts, serum chemistry panels, and bone marrow biopsy. Clinical evidence of liver involvement usually includes an enlarged liver and either elevated levels of liver enzymes or an abnormal liver scan. Involvement of the spleen usually requires a palpable spleen or the presence of filling defects on scan.

**Modifications to the Ann Arbor System.** The Ann Arbor system has been modified for the purpose of treatment consideration the reporting of clinical trial results for patients with NHL. One commonly used modification is the subdivision of patients with stage II disease into two groups based on tumor measurements (Table 88–8). Any tumor mass exceeding 10 cm in a single diameter or any mediastinal mass exceeding one third of the maximal chest diameter is defined as *bulky disease*. Patients with stage II nonbulky disease are

classified with all stage I patients as *localized* disease. Patients with stage II bulky disease are classified with all stage III and stage IV patients as having *advanced* disease. This functional division of the Ann Arbor system has been based largely on a report by Fisher and colleagues that demonstrated that stage II patients had a worse outcome than stage III patients.[351]

The definition of bulky disease is also based on retrospective analyses of prognostic factors identifying 10-cm lesions as a poor risk variable and on definitions of bulky mediastinal disease based on observations of treatment outcome in patients with Hodgkin's disease.[352] In an unpublished, updated analysis of a previously reported prospective trial for patients with advanced disease, overall survival for patients with bulky stage II disease was 49% at 5 years compared with 46% for patients with stage III and stage IV disease.[1] That intergroup study of more than 1000 patients convincingly demonstrates that outcome for bulky stage II disease is nearly identical to stage III and stage IV disease.[1] Nevertheless, the predictive model developed by the International NHL Prognostic Factors Project (described further on) found Ann Arbor stage to be one of the important predictors of outcome using the conventional division of stages I and II versus stages III and IV.[340]

The process of staging also serves to identify sites of problematic disease or impending complications of treatment, which is not usually a concern in patients with Hodgkin's disease. Potential problems that may influence the decision to treat or affect the drugs chosen for treatment include hydronephrosis (caused by ureteral obstruction), hyperbilirubinemia (caused by intrahepatic or extrahepatic obstruction), and spinal cord or inferior vena cava obstruction caused by compression.

In summary, staging still has a role in the management of patients with NHLs, albeit less critical than for patients with Hodgkin's disease in which the role of staging is crucial and central to decisions regarding treatment. In general, patients with advanced NHLs require treatment with chemotherapy, whereas radiation therapy combined with less chemotherapy may have a role in the treatment of patients with localized NHLs, as summarized in Table 88–9. In contrast to Hodgkin's disease, in which determination of the correct Ann Arbor stage of disease is critical to treatment planning, the determination of the extent of NHL is only one of several important prognostic variables.

## Prognostic Factors

### PRETREATMENT CLINICAL VARIABLES

There are many pretreatment features in patients with NHLs that correlate with prognosis. These prognostic variables

*Table 88–8.* The Modified Ann Arbor System of Staging for Non-Hodgkin's Lymphoma

| Ann Arbor Stage | Modification | Current Common Use Stage |
|---|---|---|
| I | None | Early or localized |
| II | Nonbulky | |
| II | Bulky | |
| III | None | Advanced |
| IV | None | |

*Table 88–9.* Clinical Stage As Related to Generalized Treatment Approaches for Each Histologic Grade*

| Histologic Type | Clinical Stage | Treatment Approach |
|---|---|---|
| Low grade | Localized | Wide-field radiotherapy |
| | Advanced | Systemic palliative chemotherapy |
| Intermediate or high grade | Localized or advanced | Initial doxorubicin-containing chemotherapy designed for cure |

*Details of treatment are discussed in subsequent chapters.

have largely been identified after retrospective analyses of therapy-based studies or experiences and are therefore limited to data routinely collected and stored as part of the initial staging evaluation. Thus, clinical observations, including patient demographics, number and sites of disease involvement, and presenting symptoms, are commonly analyzed for prognostic importance. Laboratory determinations, including peripheral blood counts and serum enzymes, which are routinely tabulated as part of the pretreatment staging process, are also available for statistical analyses. Details of histologic features based on morphologic review have also been extensively analyzed and were discussed earlier in this chapter. These clinical and laboratory features form the basis of most prognostic index systems because they are easily obtained and universally available. Some of the more commonly used or cited variables are listed in Table 88–10.

**Host Characteristics.** Of the variables listed in Table 88–9 age is probably one of the most important and powerful variables associated with outcome. It has been found to be a significant prognostic indicator in nearly every study in which adequate numbers of patients over the range of ages studied are available for analysis.[340–344, 346–348] Age appears to be a continuous variable, with older patients having a worse prognosis than younger patients (Table 88–11).[346, 348] Survival seems to be adversely affected by older age, whereas complete remission rates may not be influenced.[348]

Although some authors have accounted for the effect of age on survival by censoring deaths due to causes other than lymphoma, the mortality rate of older patients after treatment for lymphoma in most studies exceeds that of the general population after adjustment for age.[346, 355, 356] Age is associated with prognosis regardless of histologic subtype.[346, 347] Poor performance status and the presence of B symptoms are additional clinical characteristics that are often associated with poor outcome (see Table 88–10).[340–349, 357]

**Tumor Characteristics.** Several features associated with disease distribution and tumor burden are frequently found to correlate with poor prognosis, including advanced stage, the number of nodal sites involved, and the number of extranodal sites involved (see Table 88–10).[340–344, 358, 359] In general, these latter parameters probably measure tumor burden. Most studies find significant differences in outcome

when comparing survival for patients with stage I and stage II disease to patients with stage III and stage IV disease.[344, 347, 348, 360] However, there is little difference in survival between patients with stage III disease and patients with stage IV disease.[348, 358] Patients with stage II disease appear to be a heterogeneous group, and outcome varies considerably. Patients with stage II disease that is less than 10 cm in maximal diameter (nonbulky) and is also regionally confined, allowing treatment within a single radiation port, seem to have an excellent prognosis, whereas patients with stage II bulky disease may have a prognosis similar to that of patients with stage III or stage IV disease.[349, 350]

The anatomic distribution of disease can also be expressed as the number of nodal sites of disease or the number of extranodal sites of disease and often correlates with prognosis (see Table 88–10). An increased number of disease sites probably reflects increased tumor burden but may also reflect disease aggressiveness or host competence (as previously discussed in the section Biology). Many specific sites of disease involvement have been associated with poor outcome, including the bone marrow, gastrointestinal tract, mediastinum, liver, and spleen.[340, 348] The analysis of the prognostic significance of involvement of specific extranodal sites of disease is confounded by many factors, including the relative low sensitivity of radiographic techniques for detecting disease in many sites. Thus, the apparent effect of specific disease site involvement on prognosis may in part be a reflection of low-sensitivity detection, allowing lesser tumor masses to go undetected.

**Predictive Models.** To further refine prognostic information, individual clinical variables have been combined to construct models predicting outcome.[359–361] These models have largely been based on retrospective analysis of cooperative group therapeutic trials or single institution experience of several trials conducted over a period of many years. Typically, a series of univariate analyses is used to identify potential prognostic factors to be incorporated into a model for predicting outcome. Frequently, multiple cutpoints for each variable are also analyzed so that outcome differences are maximized. Variables and cutpoints resulting in maximal separation of outcome are incorporated into the model. Usually, the number of poor-risk clinical variables is determined for each patient. Patients are grouped according to the number of poor-risk variables, and outcome is compared among risk groups.

There are many reports of such analyses, and the following three examples are typical. Coiffier and colleagues described a model incorporating serum lactic dehydrogenase (LDH), Ann Arbor stage, individual tumor size, and the number of extranodal sites of disease and retrospectively tested this model on 737 patients treated in a therapeutic trial.[359] Patients were grouped according to the number of adverse risk factors into good, intermediate, and poor prognosis, having complete remission rates of 93%, 83%, and 61%, respectively, and 3-year actuarial survival rates of 88%, 71%, and 41%, respectively.[359] Danieu and associates used 127 patients from consecutive clinical trials and found that serum LDH, the number and location of individual sites of disease, and age combined to give the best separation of survival curves.[361] Patients were grouped into four categories with 4-year actuarial survival varying from 15 (worst group) to 80% (best group). The M.D. Anderson group studied

*Table 88–10.* **Commonly Used Prognostic Variables**

| Variable (Reference) | Usual Comparison (Better vs. Worse) |
|---|---|
| *Age[309–313, 315–317, 346, 348] | ≤60 y vs. >60 years |
| Serum albumin[309, 330] | ≥30 g/L vs. ≤30 g/L |
| Bone marrow[309, 313, 314, 316, 318] | Uninvolved vs. involved |
| *Number of extranodal sites[309, 313, 314, 316, 330] | <2 sites vs. ≥2 sites |
| Gastrointestinal tract[309, 318] | Uninvolved vs. involved |
| Hemoglobin[311, 312, 318] | ≥12 g/dl vs. <12 g/dl |
| *Serum LDH[309, 316, 318, 329, 330, 333] | Normal vs. elevated |
| Number of nodal sites[315, 329] | ≤2 sites vs. >2 sites |
| *Performance status[309, 313, 328] | ECOG 0,1 vs. ECOG 2,3 |
| Sex[310, 312, 318] | Female vs. male |
| *Ann Arbor stage[309, 316, 318, 329, 330, 333] | I, II vs. III, IV |
| Symptoms (B)[309–318] | Absent vs. present |
| Tumor size[309–318] | <10 cm vs. ≥10 cm |

*Variables used in the new International Prognostic Index are indicated with asterisks. LDH, lactate dehydrogenase; ECOG, Eastern Cooperative Oncology Group.

prognostic factors in detail. One of their first proposals incorporated tumor burden based on size and location of disease and serum LDH levels.[358] Three groups of patients were identified having 5-year survival rates ranging from 87% to 20%, whereas Ann Arbor stage did not provide meaningful discrimination among the same group of 105 patients. None of these specific models has been widely used by other groups, even though the principles of incorporating a measure of tumor burden and LDH have been widely used.

**International Prognostic Index.** In an attempt to standardize result reporting and allow improved comparisons among clinical trials, Shipp and colleagues proposed an International Prognostic Index.[340] The index is based on an analysis of pretreatment clinical features and outcome in 3273 patients with intermediate- and high-grade histologic types from 16 cooperative groups and single institutions throughout North America and Europe. Five features were independently associated with survival, including age, number of extranodal sites of disease, serum LDH levels, performance status, and Ann Arbor stage (see Table 88–10; asterisks denote variables used). An International Prognostic Index was established by classifying patients according to the number of risk factors present at the time of diagnosis from this list of five variables. Table 88–12 summarizes the risk categories within the International Prognostic Index and provides corresponding 5-year survival rates for each risk category. The International Prognostic Index has been tested subsequently on a separate group of patients.[1] Patients with stage III or stage IV intermediate- or high-grade lymphomas were entered on SWOG study 8516 (Intergroup study 0067) comparing CHOP (cyclophosphamide, hydroxydaunomycin, Oncovin [vincristine], prednisone) to three third-generation regimens. After categorizing patients according to the International Prognostic Index, outcome based on survival was correctly predicted by the International Prognostic Index risk category as shown in Table 88–12. Thus, the International Prognostic Index appears to have clinical utility. The International Prognostic Index has potential for wide acceptance because it is based on easily obtained and reproducible clinical variables. It will likely provide a benchmark for comparing new therapies, selecting patients with high risk of death for new or experimental therapy, and providing clinicians with reproducible treatment outcome expectations to guide and advise their patients.

## PRETREATMENT LABORATORY VARIABLES

The utility of laboratory-based variables to predict outcome for patients with NHLs has been studied for several decades.

*Table 88–11.* **Effect of Age on Survival***

| Histologic Type | Age (Yr) | Median Survival (Mo) | % Alive at 10 Yr |
|---|---|---|---|
| All low grades (P1) | <40 | 114 | 48 |
| | 40–59 | 85 | 36 |
| | ≥60 | 66 | 26 |
| Diffuse large cell (*) | <55 | 50 | 48 |
| | 55–64 | 24 | 29 |
| | >65 | 16 | 22 |

*Data from Southwest Oncology Group trials of CHOP (cyclophosphamide, doxorubicin, vincristine, and prednisone) chemotherapy. Updated for Survival and Previously published (P1) or not (*).

*Table 88–12.* **The International Prognostic Index Compares Risk to Survival***

| Risk Category | No. of Risk Factors† | 5-Yr Survival Rate | |
|---|---|---|---|
| | | ORIGINAL MODEL (%) | SWOG (%) |
| *8516* | | | |
| Low | 0, 1 | 73 | 55 |
| Low-intermediate | 2 | 50 | 44 |
| High-intermediate | 3 | 43 | 37 |
| High | 4.5 | 26 | 27 |

*The 5-year survival rates of the original model are compared with the 5-year survival rates of the Southwest Oncology Group (SWOG) 8516.[1]
†Based on the International Prognostic Index.[340]

Measurements of serum albumin, β2-microglobulin, and serum LDH levels and peripheral blood counts, including the hemoglobin level, platelet count, and lymphocyte count all have been related to outcome. A prognostic factor index based on laboratory values has potential advantages over currently used systems by providing simple, quantitative, reproducible measurements over a continuous range of possibilities. A laboratory-based system would eliminate the inherent subjectivity of performance status evaluation and radiographic interpretation used to assign Ann Arbor stage. Investigators have focused attention on two serum factors associated with outcome: serum LDH and β2-microglobulin.

**Serum Lactic Dehydrogenase.** The serum LDH level is frequently found to be associated with outcome. LDH is identified in nearly every study of prognostic factors as an important variable (see Table 88–10).[340, 347, 349, 358, 359, 362] In most studies of prognostic factors that fail to identify LDH, serum values of LDH were not available for analysis.[341, 343, 350] Elevated serum levels of LDH were first shown to be associated with lymphoma by Bierman and colleagues in 1957.[363] Ferraris and associates in 1979 and Schneider and coworkers in 1980 related LDH levels to histologic grade (lymphocytic lymphomas versus histiocytic lymphomas) and to overall survival.[364, 365] It is unclear whether the increased LDH is related to a tumor or to a host event. LDH likely measures cellular catabolism (the enzyme is released from injured cells), which can be related to stage (tumor burden), proliferation (growth rate), or the product of tumor burden and proliferation.[366] Thus, it appears that LDH is an important predictor of outcome in patients with lymphoma, but elevated levels of LDH have not been precisely related to a single biologic event.

**Serum β2-Microglobulin.** The serum β2-microglobulin is a low-molecular-weight cell membrane protein associated with the major histocompatibility complex class I antigens.[367] β2-microglobulin is found on the membranes of most nucleated cells and in unbound form in the plasma, where it has no known function and probably reflects cell membrane turnover. A variety of disease states and malignant conditions have been associated with increased serum levels of β2-microglobulin, including NHL.[368] More than 80% of patients with NHLs may have elevated levels of serum β2-microglobulin prior to treatment, and the serum level seems to correlate with tumor cell mass.[369, 370] Elevated levels of serum β2-microglobulin have been found to correlate variously with complete remission rate, relapse rate, relapse-free survival, time to treatment failure, and overall survival in both low-grade and intermediate-grade lymphomas.[369, 371, 372] For example, Litam and colleagues showed that serum levels greater than 3 mg/L provided important prognostic information among 80 patients with low-grade NHL.[371] At 42 months of follow-up, no patients with a β2-microglobulin level 3 mg/L or greater were projected to be in remission as compared with 85% of patients with a β2-microglobulin level less than 3 mg/L.

**Tumor Proliferative Rates.** The growth fraction of lymphoma has previously been studied with a variety of techniques, including assessment of DNA content using flow cytometry and uptake of thymidine using radioactive tritiated labeling.[94, 95] These methods have shown that high proliferative rates in lymphoma biopsies correlate with poor prognosis. Although generally useful, these methods have limitations. In particular, flow cytometry uses a suspension of cells, which results in loss of microanatomic detail, thus obscuring differences between tumor cells and surrounding normal lymphoid tissue. Although radiolabeling may preserve microanatomic features, it is time-consuming and requires special facilities to ensure laboratory safety and thus generally is not available to the practicing oncologist.

Immunohistochemical assessment of proliferating antigens using tissue sections is a more recent development.[96, 97] In this method, the monoclonal antibody Ki67 detects a nuclear antigen found throughout the cell cycle (G1, G2, S, M) but not in resting cells (G0), allowing a quantifiable determination of the growth fraction of lymphoma cells while retaining histologic architecture.[373] The Ki67 antibody applied to frozen tissue sections is comparable to the tritiated thymidine-determined labeling index.[374] The proportion of cells marked by Ki67 has been shown to correlate with histologic grade and outcome in retrospective studies.[96, 97, 374] Ki67 was also found useful in identifying a group of patients with rapidly progressive and fatal disease in a prospective trial of intermediate- and high-grade NHL.[103] A proliferative index of 80% (proportion of Ki67-positive cells) identified a group of patients (18%) who had poor outcome. Overall survival was significantly reduced in these patients with a high proliferative index compared with patients with a low proliferative index ($p = 0.001$). One-year survival estimates were 82% (low proliferative index) versus 18% (high proliferative index). A multivariate regression analysis comparing the effect of the proliferative rate to performance status, age, extranodal sites of disease, stage, and serum LDH level (as defined by the International Prognostic Index) confirmed the independent effect of proliferation on survival. In this study incorporating the proliferative index, stage (tumor burden), and LDH, the relative risk assigned to each factor (relative risk 5.9, 1.3, and 0.8, respectively) suggests that a direct measure of the growth rate is a more powerful prognostic tool than serum LDH levels and largely displaces LDH as a significant variable.

The utility of Ki67-determined proliferative rates has also been tested in patients with lower grades of NHL.[100, 101] The Stanford group found that Ki67 values greater than 20% identified a more aggressive clinical course among patients with diffuse SLLs.[101] The Arizona group showed that within the single histologic group of diffuse small cleaved cell lymphoma, patients with a Ki67 proliferative rate greater

than 20% had a median survival of 20 months compared with 80 months for those with a low index.[100] Thus, the Ki67-determined proliferative index appears to have utility within several histologic subgroups of lymphoma and may prove valuable for selecting patients to receive more aggressive therapy.

## IMMUNOHISTOCHEMICAL VARIABLES

Immunohistochemistry has been used to detect cell surface, cytoplasmic, and nuclear antigens that correlate with prognosis. The clinical utility of these methods has been reviewed in detail.[68, 102] Although the use of immunohistochemistry to define markers of prognostic significance is largely developmental in that most of the published studies are retrospective analyses of patient outcome incorporating heterogeneous clinical features and variable treatment and assay conditions, this area of investigation is of interest inasmuch as the antigens detected may reflect important biologic principles and influence future treatment strategies. Table 88–13 summarizes some of the markers of prognosis detectable with immunohistochemical techniques. Relevant to Table 88–13, Figure 88–11 illustrates several immunophenotypic features that are predictive of poor outcome in a consecutive series of 105 patients with diffuse LCL at the University of Arizona. This figure, a composite of six published papers from the single study, reveals that poor outcome relates to (1) loss or absent HLA-DR antigen, (2) a high proliferative rate with a Ki67 value greater than 60%, (3) presence of T-cell lineage, (4) loss of a pan–B antigen (CD22), and (5) a deficiency of T-TILs (CD8). Finally, as shown in the illustrated model, these immunologic parameters were important independent predictors of outcome among these patients with LCL and have value in identifying patients who will fail current therapy.[360] Recent multi-institutional, prospective studies by SWOG and Groupe d'Etudes des Lymphomes des L'Adulte have confirmed the association of high proliferative rate via Ki67[103] and T-cell phenotype as predictors of poor outcome.[268]

**Cell Lineage.** The prognostic significance of determining B-cell versus T-cell lineage is well established among certain subtypes of lymphoma, specifically LBL.[71] The utility of determining B-cell versus T-cell phenotype among other diffuse intermediate- and high-grade lymphomas is more

*Table 88–13.* **New Laboratory Markers of Prognosis Detectable with Immunohistochemical Techniques**

| Laboratory Variable | Description |
| --- | --- |
| Proliferative rates | High growth rates correlate with shortened survival |
| Lineage (T vs. B) | T-cell phenotype may correlate with shortened relapse-free survival and survival |
| Tumor infiltrating lymphocytes (T-TILs) | Low proportion of T-TILs correlate with shortened survival |
| Neural cell adhesion molecule (NCAM) with | NCAM correlates with disease location |
| Histocompatibility antigens | Low proportion of T-TILs correlates with shortened survival |
| Multiple drug resistance (MDR) | Detectable MDR levels found in treatment-resistant disease |

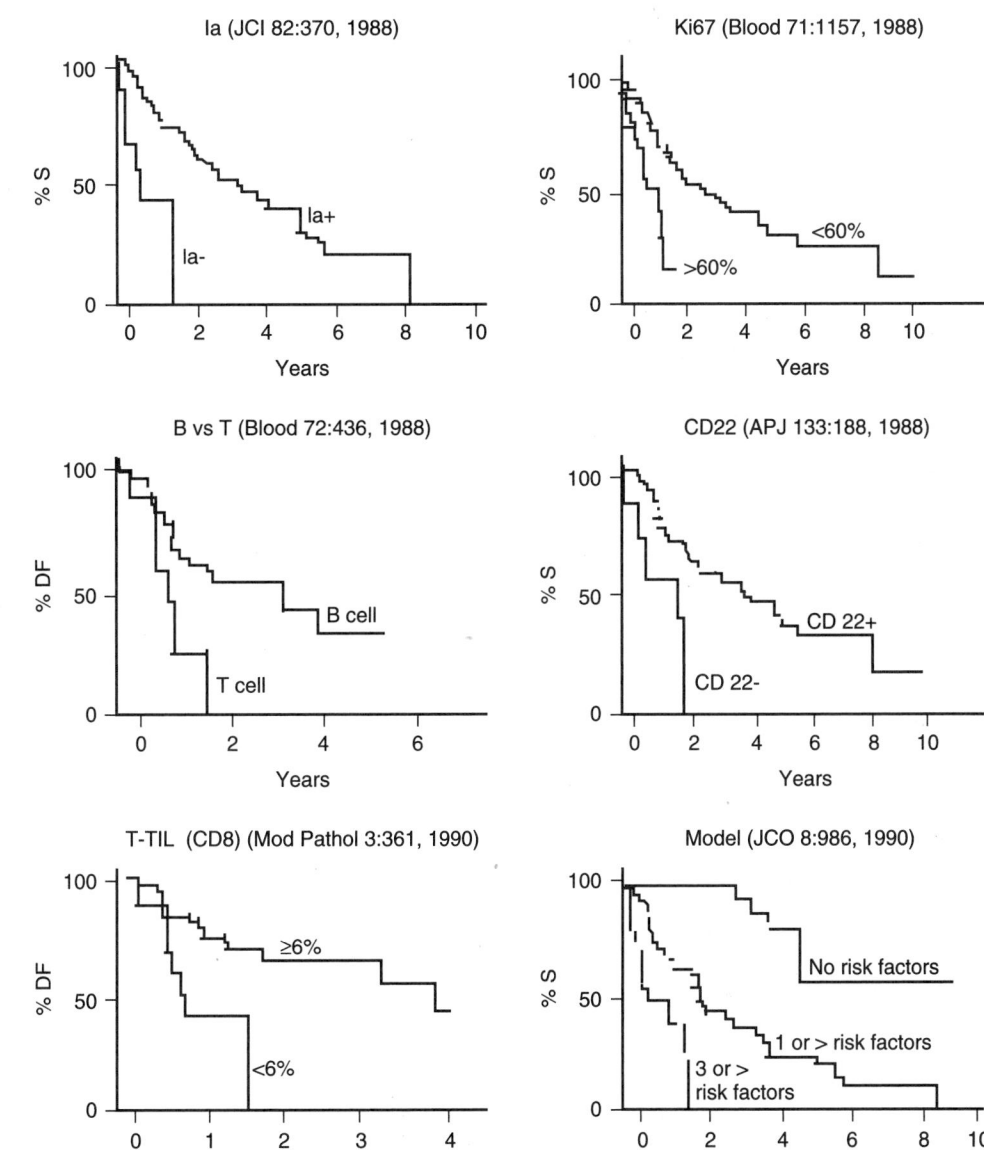

**Figure 88–11.** Laboratory predictors of survival in large cell lymphoma.

controversial, with some studies showing no difference in outcome and others showing a clear survival difference.[265–268]

Studies that focused on a single histologic subtype or used a prospective trial design have shown that patients with T-cell lymphomas have a shortened survival or relapse-free survival compared with patients with B-cell lymphomas.[92, 100, 124, 267, 268] The biologic significance of the association of cell lineage with outcome is currently unknown but may reflect other important cofactors. For example, normal human T-cell lymphocytes have been shown to express higher levels of P-glycoprotein than do normal human B-cell lymphocytes.[375] P-glycoprotein is associated with multidrug resistance (see further on), and increased levels in malignant T-cell lymphocytes may explain higher relapse rates.

**Deficient Tumor-Infiltrating Lymphocyte Response.** The relapse rate and overall survival of lymphoma patients have also been shown to correlate with the type and number of specific T-cell subsets that infiltrate B-cell lymphomas.[101, 115–118] In one study of B-cell diffuse LCL, the finding of low T-cytotoxic cells within the tumor mass (<6% T-cell/tumor cells) was associated with disease relapse.[118] In a separate study of diffuse small cell lymphomas, the proportion of infiltrating host helper T cells predicted overall survival.[101] These studies suggest that the magnitude, subset type, activation state, and memory status of the T-TIL response determined from biopsy specimens from patients with B-cell lymphomas are independent predictors of clinical outcome. Further, the poor outcome associated with low T-TIL response may be improved by upregulating T-TIL with IL-2, resulting in improved immunosurveillance.[117]

**Histocompatibility Antigen Loss.** Deficient T-TIL response may be related to host immunocompetence and tumor HLA status (human leukocyte antigen expression). List and colleagues have shown that low T-TIL in B-cell diffuse LCL correlated with both allograft-associated or HIV-associated lymphoma and loss of HLA determinants in sporadic lymphoma in immunocompetent patients.[115] Loss of HLA determinants has been shown independently to correlate with poor overall survival.[108–112] In one prognostic model, Slymen and associates demonstrated that loss of the HLA-DR antigen was the most important or powerful predictor of poor outcome of all laboratory and clinical features tested.[360] Loss of HLA from malignant B cells may result in a blunted host response, as reflected in those studies of poor outcome associated with loss of T-TIL.

**Neural Cell Adhesion Molecule.** NCAM has been found on the cell surface of some T-cell lymphomas. Two studies have shown a striking predilection of NCAM-positive lymphomas for unusual sites of disease involvement, including the nasopharynx, the central nervous system, skeletal muscle, and the gastrointestinal tract.[119, 120] These anatomic sites are known to be naturally high expressors of NCAM and the like-like or homophilic attraction of NCAM molecules might account for the preferential homing of NCAM-positive lymphomas to these sites.[121] Lymphoma involving either the central nervous system or the nasopharynx is known to portend a poor outcome, and in both clinical correlative trials of NCAM and outcome the median survival of NCAM-positive lymphomas was less than 50% of the median survival of NCAM-negative lymphomas.[119]

**P-Glycoprotein Expression.** Finally, detectable levels of P-glycoprotein have been associated with clinical drug resistance.[129, 130] P-glycoprotein is a transmembrane protein thought to function as an efflux pump removing cytotoxic and xenobiotic agents from cells.[127] P-glycoprotein is found in normal hematopoietic elements and variably in hematopoietic neoplasms.[127, 128, 375] Among newly diagnosed and untreated lymphomas, detectable level of P-glycoprotein is uncommon (2%), but it is frequently found in heavily pretreated patients with clinical evidence of drug resistance (64%).[126] In multiple myeloma it has been shown that the incidence of P-glycoprotein detection is a function of the total dose of prior therapy with either vincristine or doxorubicin.[376] P-glycoprotein has not been related to prognosis in newly diagnosed lymphoma, presumably because the detection methods were not adequately sensitive to detect the low but critical level that affects outcome.[131] As detection methods improve, P-glycoprotein may be shown to correlate with prognosis, and efforts to improve therapy might target this molecule to prevent relapse by overcoming multidrug resistance.

In summary, outcome for patients with NHL can be partially predicted by using any of myriad clinical and laboratory markers of prognosis. Using combinations of clinical features in a prognostic model is a reproducibly effective tool for determining overall survival and projecting median survival. These efforts are best used for comparing treatment programs and for selecting patients for specific treatments. However, prognostic factors based on clinical features do not give insight into the biology of treatment failure, whereas some laboratory-determined features of lymphoma offer prospects for formulating testable hypotheses and designing new treatment strategies. Many prognostic factors have greater utility than clinical staging alone and have largely replaced anatomic staging as important determinants of outcome and treatment.

## Natural History (Clinical Course)

The NHLs are a heterogeneous group of diseases having variable causes, numerous molecular aberrations, distinct morphologic appearances, myriad clinical presentations, and outcomes ranging from death within weeks to cure. Nevertheless, these distinct diseases share some common features worthy of emphasis. This fifth edition of Haskell's *Cancer Treatment* contains a description of many of the histologic subtypes of NHL in detail in a previous section in this chapter (Classification) and discussions of the clinical course for specific histologic types in subsequent chapters. The following discussion primarily serves as an overview to compare and contrast the clinical course of the histologic subtypes.

In the now outmoded WF, the terms *low-grade, favorable,* and *indolent* were often used interchangeably to describe lymphomas having relatively slow growth rates and long median survival durations. In general, these terms described the histologic subtypes of low grade in the WF. The terms *high grade, unfavorable,* and *aggressive* were used to describe lymphomas having relatively rapid growth rates and short median survival times. In general, these terms described the histologic subtypes of the intermediate-grade and high-grade categories of the WF classification system. There are two additional features that distinguish low-grade from intermediate and high-grade histologic types. First, low-grade histologic types have a survival curve characterized by a constant slope over time, indicating a constant risk of death over long periods.[341] Higher grade histologic types, in contrast, have survival curve slopes that change over time and frequently become flat. The point at which the slope becomes flat indicates the proportion of patients cured of lymphoma. Second, treatment does not seem to influence overall survival of patients with low-grade histologic types, whereas doxorubicin-containing treatment has dramatically altered the shape of the survival curve for patients with higher grade histologic types.[1, 341, 377–379] These clinical features are summarized by the stylized survival curves in Figure 88–12.

A primary goal of the initial evaluation of newly diag-

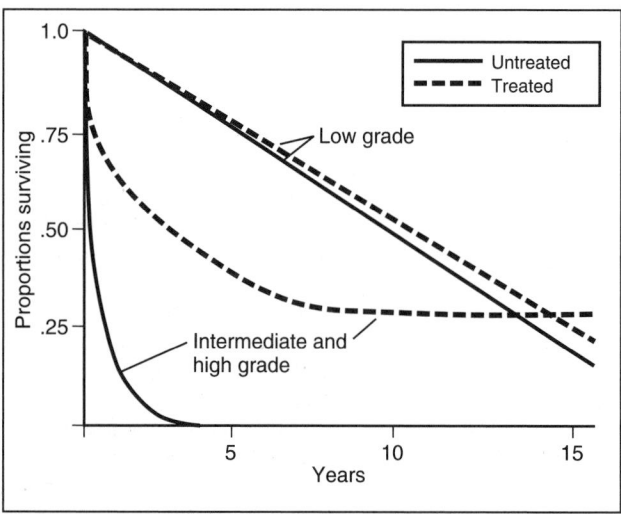

**Figure 88–12.** These stylized survival curves demonstrate the major differences between patients with low-grade histologies of non-Hodgkin's lymphomas and intermediate- and high-grade histologies with regard to medial survival and slope. Note that treatment does not appreciably affect the overall survival of low-grade histologies but dramatically changes the shape of the survival curve for intermediate- and high-grade histologies.

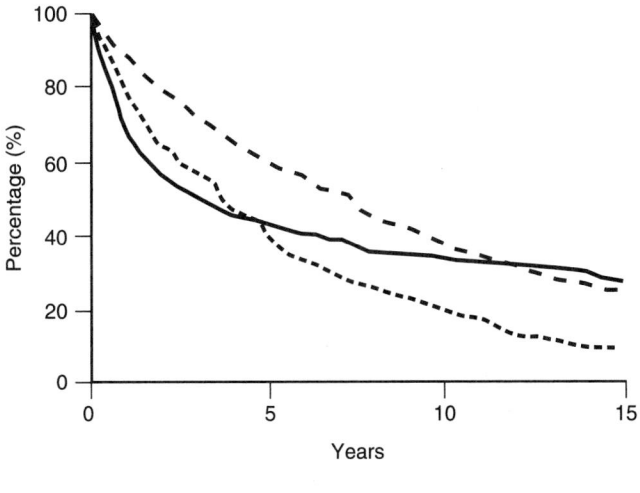

| | At Risk | Deaths | 10 Year Estimate | Median in Months |
|---|---|---|---|---|
| – – Low risk | 533 | 384 | 38% | 86 |
| ···· Intermediate risk | 271 | 227 | 21% | 45 |
| —— High risk | 1364 | 844 | 35% | 39 |

**Figure 88–13.** Southwest Oncology Group (SWOG) survival of Revised European-American Lymphoma (REAL) risk groups.

nosed NHL is to determine whether the patient should receive treatment designed for palliation and relief of symptoms or whether more aggressive combination chemotherapy designed with a potential for cure should be used. The decision has been primarily based on the histologic diagnosis. Patients presenting with a histologic subtype that has been associated with a constant slope of survival over time generally receive treatment designed for palliation. Histologic subtypes previously associated with a potential for cure as evidenced by the flattening of the slope of the survival curve over time are usually treated with initial doxorubicin-containing chemotherapy designed for cure.

There were problems with the WF classification schema, including excessive outcome variability among the low-grade histologic types, nonreproducibility of follicular subtypes based on cytologic assessment, and unnecessary subdivisions within the diffuse large cell categories. The REAL classification system has already been shown to help overcome many of these deficiencies, and although seemingly more detailed and complicated for the practicing clinician, it can be used efficiently to determine prognosis and help select appropriate treatment.[133, 255] (Fig. 88–13)

Within the REAL classification system, follicular lymphomas are lumped into one category and assigned grades (I to III) in an effort to downplay distinctions between histologic subtypes. The WF arbitrarily included follicular LCL in the intermediate-grade histologic group, implying a potential for cure. The distinction had two associated problems. First, even expert hematopathologists could not reliably distinguish histologic subtypes of follicular lymphomas, making outcome analyses based on morphologic assessment an irrelevant exercise.[171, 380–382] Second, long-term analyses of outcome have demonstrated that all patients with follicular lymphomas, regardless of histologic subtype, eventually relapse and die of lymphoma.[378, 383, 384] The inevitable relapse of patients with follicular lymphoma occurs even after they

receive initial treatment with a doxorubicin-containing regimen. Long-term follow-up of patients with follicular lymphomas produces a survival curve that has a constant slope and a median survival in the range of 9 years. The REAL classification recognizes another entity having a constant relapse rate and long median survival, the monocytoid B-cell lymphoma. Patients having either follicular lymphoma or monocytoid B-cell lymphoma have a low histologic risk for early death.

From the practicing clinician's point of view, the most important contribution of the REAL system has been to identify a variety of diffuse small cell diseases that, in general, respond poorly to treatment and have a more aggressive clinical course than the follicular lymphomas. These diseases include MCL, SLL, lymphoplasmacytoid lymphoma, diffuse small-cleaved cell lymphoma, and likely, disseminated MALTomas. Patients with these diseases have a median survival in the range of 3 to 5 years or half that of the lowest histologic risk group. There is no evidence that these patients have an intermediate risk for early death. Finally, there remains the group of patients with lymphomas characterized by high proliferative rates and a potential for cure using aggressive chemotherapy. These lymphomas include the diffuse LCLs, Burkitt's lymphoma and BLL, ALCL, and LBL. These patients have a high risk for early death from lymphoma. Survival curves demonstrate a distinct change in the shape of the curve over time, with a plateau indicating the potential for cure. An analysis of overall survival of more than 2000 patients with advanced-stage disease who were treated with a doxorubicin-containing regimen is provided in Figure 88–13 to demonstrate these concepts.[255]

These clinical and biologic features describe patient groups and reflect average outcome. However, there is wide variability in outcome among individual patients within each histologic subgroup. For example, the proliferative rate determined by the Ki67 monoclonal antibody varied from 0 to 60% in one study of small cell lymphocytic lymphomas.[101] In another study of a single histologic subset (diffuse small cleaved cell) the Ki67-determined proliferative rate varied from less than 10% to greater than 90%.[100] Survival is similarly variable even within a single histologic subgroup. With more than 20 years of follow-up, Dana and associates have shown survival varies from less than 1 year to more than 20 years for patients with WF low-grade NHLs.[341] Thus, there are patients with rapidly growing, rapidly lethal low-grade lymphomas, and there are patients with slower growing, more indolent intermediate-grade lymphomas. The terms *low, intermediate, and high grade* are statistically derived descriptions that obscure the extraordinary tumor heterogeneity and variable clinical course within each category. Clinicians must combine accurate histologic diagnoses with known prognostic factors to modify standard treatment for some patients. The following chapters address these issues in detail as each histologic grade is reviewed.

## REFERENCES

1. Fisher RI, Gaynor ER, Dahlberg S, et al. Comparison of a standard regimen (CHOP) with three intensive chemotherapy regimens for advanced non-Hodgkin's lymphoma. N Engl J Med 1993;328:1002–6.

2. Cancer Statistics, 1999. CA Cancer J Clin 1999;49:8–31.

3. Reynolds T. Non-Hodgkin's lymphoma rate climbed rapidly. J Natl Cancer Inst 1991;83:232–3.

4. Harris NL, Jaffe ES, Stein H, et al. A revised European-American classification of lymphoid neoplasms: a proposal from the International Lymphoma Study Group. Blood 1994;84:1361.

5. Geser A, Brubaker G, Draper CC. Effect of a malaria suppression program on the incidence of African Burkitt's lymphoma. Am J Epidemiol 1989;129:740–52.

6. Buchbinder A, Gallo RC. Lymphoma: etiologic considerations. In: Wiernik PH, Canellos GP, Kyle RA, Schiffer CA, eds. Neoplastic diseases of blood. New York: Churchill Livingstone, 1989:609–19.

7. Salmon SE, Seligmann M. B-cell neoplasia in man. Lancet 1974;2:1230–3.

8. Whittle HC, Brown J, Marsh K, et al. T-cell control of Epstein-Barr virus–infected B cells is lost during *P. falciparum* malaria. Nature 1984;312:449–52.

9. Pelicci PG, Knowles DM 2d, Magrath I, Dalla-Favera R. Chromosomal breakpoints and structural alterations of the c-*myc* locus differ in endemic and sporadic forms of Burkitt lymphoma. Proc Natl Acad Sci 1986;83:2984–8.

10. Neri A, Barriga F, Knowles DM, et al. Different regions of the immunoglobulin heavy-chain locus are involved in chromosomal translocations in distinct pathogenetic forms of Burkitt lymphoma. Proc Natl Acad Sci 1988;85:2748–52.

11. Nador RG, Cesarman E, Chadburn Adawson DB, et al. Primary effusion lymphoma: a distinct clinicopathologic entity associated with the Kaposi sarcoma–associated herpes virus. Blood 1996;88:645–56.

12. Silvestri F, Pipan C, Barillari G, et al. Prevalence of hepatitis C virus infection in patients with lymphoproliferative disorders. Blood 1996;87:4296–301.

13. Isaacson P, Spencer J. Malignant lymphoma of mucosa-associated lymphoid tissue. Histopathology 1987;11:445.

14. Kinoshita T, Ishii K, Taira Y, Naganuma H. Malignant lymphoma arising from chronic tuberculous empyema. Acta Radiol 1997; 38:833–5.

15. Swinnen LJ, Costanzo-Nordin MR, Fisher SG, et al. Increased incidence of lymphoproliferative disorder after immunosuppression with the monoclonal antibody OKT3 in cardiac-transplant recipients. N Engl J Med 1990;323:1723–8.

16. Ramot B. Hulu N. Primary intestinal lymphoma and its relation to alpha heavy chain disease. Br J Cancer 1975;31:343–9.

17. Harrington DS, Weisenburger DD, Purtilo DT. Malignant lymphoma in the X-linked lymphoproliferative syndrome. Cancer 1987;59:1419–29.

18. Shearer WT, Ritz J, Finegold MJ, et al. Epstein-Barr virus–associated B-cell proliferations of diverse clonal origins after bone marrow transplantation in a 12-year-old patient with severe combined immunodeficiency. N Engl J Med 1985;312:1151–9.

19. Gail MH, Pluda JM, Rabkin CS, et al. Projections of the incidence of non-Hodgkin's lymphoma related to acquired immunodeficiency syndrome. J Natl Cancer Inst 1991;83:695–701.

20. Kassan SS, Thomas TL, Moutsopoulos HM, et al. Increased risk of lymphoma in sicca syndrome. Ann Intern Med 1978;89:888–92.

21. Nathwani BN, Rappaport H, Moran EM, et al. Malignant lymphoma arising in angioimmunoblastic lymphadenopathy. Cancer 1978; 41:578–606.

22. Isaacson PG. Lymphomas of mucosa-associated lymphoid tissue (MALT). Histopathology 1990;16:617–9.

23. Wigle DT, Semenciw RM, Wilkins K, et al. Mortality study of Canadian male farm operators: non-Hodgkin's lymphoma mortality and agricultural practices in Saskatchewan. J Natl Cancer Inst 1990;82:572–82.

24. Hoar SK, Blair A, Holmes FF, et al. Agricultural herbicide use and risk of lymphoma and soft-tissue sarcoma. JAMA 1986;256:1141–7.

25. Woods JS, Polissar L, Severson RK, et al. Soft tissue sarcoma and non-Hodgkin's lymphoma in relation to phenoxyherbicide and chlorinated phenol exposure in western Washington. J Natl Cancer Inst 1987;78:899–910.

26. Fingerhut MA, Halperin WE, Marlow DA, Piacitelli LA, et al. Cancer mortality in workers exposed to 2,3,7,8-tetrachlorodibenzo-p-dioxin. N Engl J Med 1991;324:212–8.

27. Hayes HM, Tarone RE, Cantor KP, et al. Case-control study of canine malignant lymphoma: positive association with dog owner's use of 2,4-dichlorophenoxyacetic acid herbicides. J Natl Cancer Inst 1991;83:1226–31.

28. Zahm SH, Weisenburger DD, Babbitt PA, et al. Use of hair coloring products and the risk of lymphoma, multiple myeloma, and chronic lymphocytic leukemia. Am J Public Health 1992;82:990–7.

29. Thun MJ, Altekruse SF, Namboodiri MM, et al. Hair dye use and risk of fatal cancers in U.S. women. J Natl Cancer Inst 1994;86:210–5.

30. Chadburn A, Athan E, Wieczorek R, Knowles DM. Detection and characterization of human T-cell lymphotropic virus type I (HTLV-I) associated T-cell neoplasms in an HTLV-I nonendemic region by polymerase chain reaction. Blood 1991;77:2419–30.

31. Kalyanaraman VS, Sarngadharan MG, Robert-Guroff M, et al. A new subtype of human T-cell leukemia virus (HTLV-II) associated with a T-cell variant of hairy cell leukemia. Science 1982;218:571–3.

32. Goldstein JA, Bernstein RL. Burkitt's lymphoma and the role of Epstein-Barr virus. J Trop Pediatr 1990;36:114–20.

33. Leder P. The genetics of antibody diversity. Sci Am 1982;246:102–15.

34. Tonegawa S. Somatic generation of antibody diversity. Nature 1983;302:575–81.

35. Brack C, Hirama M, Lenhard-Schuller R, Tonegawa S. A complete immunoglobulin gene is created by somatic recombination. Cell 1978;15:1–14.

36. Nadler LM, Ritz J, Griffin JD, et al. Diagnosis and treatment of human leukemias and lymphomas utilizing monoclonal antibodies. Prog Hematol 1981;12;187–225.

37. Foon KA, Nakano GM, Koller CA, et al. Response to 2′-deoxycofor-*myc*in after failure of interferon-alpha in nonsplenectomized patients with hairy cell leukemia. Blood 1986;68:297–300.

38. Grogan TM, Rangel CS, Richter LC, et al. Further delineation of the immunoarchitecture of the human spleen. Lymphology 1984;17:61–8.

39. Stein H, Bonk A, Tolksdorf G, et al. Immunohistologic analysis of the organization of normal lymphoid tissue and non-Hodgkin's lymphomas. J Histochem Cytochem 1980;28:746–60.

40. Grogan T. Immunologic approaches to the classification and management of lymphomas and leukemias. Boston: Kluwer Academic, 1988:36

41. Stein H. Lymphocyte differentiation. In: Mason DY, Harris LH, eds. Human lymphoma: clinical implications of the REAL classification. London: Springer, 1999.

42. Minden MD, Mak TW. The structure of the T cell antigen receptor genes in normal and malignant T cells. Blood 1986;68:327–36.

43. Waldmann TA, Davis MM, Bongiovanni KF, Korsmeyer SJ. Rearrangements of genes for the antigen receptor on T cells as markers of lineage and clonality in human lymphoid neoplasms. N Engl J Med 1985;313:776–83.

44. Dustin ML, Springer TA. Role of lymphocyte adhesion receptors in transient interactions and cell locomotion. Ann Rev Immunol 1991;9:27–66.

45. Makgoba MW, Sanders ME, Ginther Luce GE, Dustin ML, et al. ICAM-1 a ligand for LFA-1-dependent adhesion of B, T and myeloid cells. Nature 1988;331:86–8.

46. Hamann A, Jablonski-Westrich D, Duijvestijn A, et al. Evidence for an accessory role of LFA-1 in lymphocyte-high endothelium interaction during homing. J Immunol 1988;140:693–9.

47. Shimizu Y, van Seventer GA, Horgan KJ, Shaw S. Roles of adhesion molecules in T-cell recognition: fundamental similarities between four integrins on resting human T cells (LFA-1, VLA-4, VLA-5, VLA-6) in expression, binding, and costimulation. Immunol Rev 1990; 114:109–43.

48. Barclay N. Section II: CD54. The leukocyte antigen facts book. Chatham: Academic Press, 1993:224.

49. Albelda SM. Role of integrins and other cell adhesion molecules in tumor progression and metastasis. Lab Invest 1993;68:4–17.

50. Tanaka K, Yoshioka T, Bieberich C, Jay G. Role of the major histocompatibility complex class I antigens in tumor growth and metastasis. Ann Rev Immunol 1988;6:359–80.

51. Hammerling GJ, Klar D, Pulm W, et al. The influence of major histocompatibility complex class I antigens on tumor growth and metastasis. Biochim Biophys Acta 1987;907:245–59.

52. Stopeck AT, Gessner A, Miller T, et al. Loss of B7.2 (CD86) and ICAM-1 (CD54) expression is associated with decreased tumor infiltrating T lymphocytes in diffuse B cell large cell lymphoma. Clin Cancer Res (in press).

53. Buck CA, Horwitz AF. Cell surface receptors for extracellular matrix molecules. Ann Rev Cell Biol 1987;3:179–205.

54. Hemler ME. Adhesive protein receptors on hematopoietic cells. Immunol Today 1988;9:109–13.
55. Horwitz A, Duggan K, Buck C, et al. Interaction of plasma membrane fibronectin receptor with talin—a transmembrane linkage. Nature 1986;320:531–3.
56. Werb Z, Tremble PM, Behrendtsen O, et al. Signal transduction through the fibronectin receptor induces collagenase and stromelysin gene expression. J Cell Biol 1989;109:877–89.
57. Hendrix MJ, Seftor EA, Grogan TM, et al. Expression of type IV collagenase correlates with the invasion of human lymphoblastoid cell lines and pathogenesis in SCID mice. Mol Cell Probe 1992;6:59–65.
58. Matrisian LM. Metalloproteinases and their inhibitors in matrix remodeling. Trends Genet 1990;6:121–5.
59. Pruisinkiewiwicz C, Zhang CL, Kossakowska AE, et al. Interleukin-6 regulation of matrix metalloproteinase (MMP-2 and MMP-9) and tissue inhibitor of metalloproteinase (TIMP-1) expression in malignant non-Hodgkin's lymphomas. Blood 1999;94:2080–9,
60. Pals ST, Horst E, Ossekoppele GJ, et al. Expression of lymphocyte homing receptor as a mechanism of dissemination in non-Hodgkin's lymphoma. Blood 1989;73:885–8.
61. Horst E, Meijer CJ, Radaskiewicz T, et al. Expression of a human homing receptor (CD44) in lymphoid malignancies and related stages of lymphoid development. Leukemia 1990;4:383–9.
62. Spertini O, Freedman AS, Belvin MP, et al. Regulation of leukocyte adhesion molecule-1 (TQ1, Leu-8) expression and shedding by normal and malignant cells. Leukemia 1991;5:300–8.
63. Ezzell C. Sticky situations: picking apart the molecules that glue cells together. Sci News 1992;141:392.
64. Lawrence MB, Springer TA. Leukocytes roll on a selectin at physiologic flow rates: distinction from and prerequisite for adhesion through integrins. Cell 1991;65:859–73.
65. Korsmeyer SJ. *Bcl*-2 initiates a new category of oncogenes: regulators of cell death. Blood 1992;80:879–86.
66. Nunez G, London L, Hockenbery D, et al. Deregulated *Bcl*-2 gene expression selectively prolongs survival of growth factor–deprived hemopoietic cell lines. J Immunol 1990;144:3602–10.
67. Wyllie AH. Apoptosis: cell death in tissue regulation. J Pathol 1987;153:313–6.
68. Grogan TM, Miller TP. Immunobiologic correlates of prognosis in lymphoma. Semins Oncol 1993;20:58–74.
69. Grogan TM, Payne CM, Payne TB, et al. Cutaneous myiasis: immunohistologic and ultrastructural morphometric features of a human botfly lesion. Am J Dermatopathol 1987;9:232–9.
70. Weiss LM, Picker LJ, Grogan TM, et al. Absence of clonal beta and gamma T-cell receptor gene rearrangements in a subset of peripheral T-cell lymphomas. Am J Pathol 1988;130:436–42.
71. Grogan T, Spier C, Wirt DP, et al. Immunologic complexity of lymphoblastic lymphoma. Diagn Immunol 1986;4:81–8.
72. Lippman SM, Volk JR, Spier CM, Grogan TM. Clonal ambiguity of human immunodeficiency virus–associated lymphomas. Similarity to posttransplant lymphomas. Arch Pathol Lab Med 1988;112:128–32.
73. Picker LJ, Weiss LM, Medeiros LJ, et al. Immunophenotypic criteria for the diagnosis of non-Hodgkin's lymphoma. Am J Pathol 1987;128:181–201.
74. Grogan TM, Fielder K, Rangel C, et al. Peripheral T-cell lymphoma: aggressive disease with heterogeneous immunotypes. Am J Clin Pathol 1985;83:279–88.
75. Spier CM, Grogan TM, Lippman SM, et al. The aberrancy of immunophenotype and immunoglobulin status as indicators of prognosis in B cell diffuse large cell lymphoma. Am J Pathol 1988;133:118–26.
76. Klein G. The role of gene dosage and genetic transpositions in carcinogenesis. Nature 1981;294:313–8.
77. Garcia CF, Weiss LM, Warnke RA. Small noncleaved cell lymphoma: an immunophenotypic study of 18 cases and comparison with large cell lymphoma. Hum Pathol 1986;17:454–61.
78. Raghoebier S, Kramer MH, van Krieken JH, et al. Essential differences in oncogene involvement between primary nodal and extranodal large cell lymphoma. Blood 1991;78:2680–5.
79. Mintzer DM, Andreeff M, Filippa DA, et al. Progression of nodular poorly differentiated lymphocytic lymphoma to Burkitt's-like lymphoma. Blood 1984;64:415–21.
80. Weiss LM, Warnke RA. Follicular lymphoma with blastic conversion: a report of two cases with confirmation by immunoperoxidase studies on bone marrow sections. Am J Clin Pathol 1985;83:681–6.
81. Gaidano G, Ballerini P, Gong JZ, et al. p53 mutations in human lymphoid malignancies: association with Burkitt lymphoma and chronic lymphocytic leukemia. Proc Natl Acad Sci U S A 1991;88:5413–7.
82. Said JW, Barrera R, Shintaku IP, et al. Immunohistochemical analysis of p53 expression in malignant lymphomas. Am J Pathol 1992;141:1343–8.
83. Sander CA, Yano T, Clark HM, et al. p53 mutation is associated with progression in follicular lymphomas. Blood 1993;82:1994–2004.
84. Tsujimoto Y, Gorham J, Cossman J, et al. The t(14;18) chromosome translocations involved in B-cell neoplasms result from mistakes in VDJ joining. Science 1985;229:1390–3.
85. Bakhshi A, Jensen JP, Goldman P, et al. Cloning the chromosomal breakpoint of t(14;18) human lymphomas: clustering around JH on chromosome 14 and near a transcriptional unit on 18. Cell 1985;41:899–906.
86. Cleary ML, Sklar J. Nucleotide sequence of a t(14;18) chromosomal breakpoint in follicular lymphoma and demonstration of a breakpoint-cluster region near a transcriptionally active locus on chromosome 18. Proc Natl Acad Sci U S A 1985;82:7439–43.
87. Pezzella F, Tse AG, Cordell JL, et al. Expression of the *bcl*-2 oncogene protein is not specific for the 14;18 chromosomal translocation. Am J Am J Pathol 1990;137:225–32.
88. Miller TP, Levy N, Bailey NP, et al. The *bcl*-2 gene translocation (t14;18) identifies a subgroup of patients with diffuse large cell lymphoma having an indolent clinical course with late relapse. Proc ASCO 1994;13:370.
89. Leith CP, Willman CL, Spier CM, et al. The presence of *bcl*-1 and *bcl*-2 gene rearrangements in diffuse small cleaved-cell lymphoma: a disease with diverse molecular and immunophenotypic findings. Diagn Mol Biol 1994;3:178–83.
90. Offit K, Wong G, Filippa DA, et al. Cytogenetic analysis of 434 consecutively ascertained specimens of non-Hodgkin's lymphoma: clinical correlations. Blood 1991;77:1508–15.
91. Pezzella F, Jones M, Ralfkiaer E, et al. Evaluation of *bcl*-2 protein expression and 14;18 translocation as prognostic markers in follicular lymphoma. Br J Cancer 1992;65:87–9.
92. Yunis JJ, Mayer MG, Arnesen MA, et al. *bcl*-2 and other genomic alterations in the prognosis of large-cell lymphoma. N Engl J Med 1989;320:1047–54.
93. Strasser A, Harris AW, Bath ML, Cory S. Novel primitive lymphoid tumours induced in transgenic mice by cooperation between *myc* and *bcl*-2. Nature 1990;348:331–3.
94. Bauer KD, Merkel DE, Winter JN, et al. Prognostic implications of ploidy and proliferative activity in diffuse large cell lymphomas. Cancer Res 1986;46:3173–8.
95. Del Bino G, Silvestrini R, Costa A, et al. Morphological and clinical significance of cell kinetics in non-Hodgkin's lymphomas. Basic Applied Histochem 1986;30:197–202.
96. Gerdes J, Stein H, Pileri S, et al. Prognostic relevance of tumour-cell growth fraction in malignant non-Hodgkin's lymphomas. Lancet 1987;2:448–9.
97. Grogan TM, Lippman SM, Spier CM, et al. Independent prognostic significance of a nuclear proliferation antigen in diffuse large cell lymphomas as determined by the monoclonal antibody Ki-67. Blood 1988;71:1157–60.
98. Grogan T, Dalton W, Rybski J, et al. Optimization of immunocytochemical P-glycoprotein assessment in multidrug-resistant plasma cell myeloma using three antibodies. Lab Invest 1990;63:815–24.
99. Ellison DJ, Nathwani BN, Metter GE, et al. Mitotic counts in follicular lymphomas. Hum Pathol 1987;18:502–5.
100. Leith CP, Spier CM, Grogan TM, et al. Diffuse small cleaved-cell lymphoma: a heterogeneous disease with distinct immunobiologic subsets. J Clin Oncol 1992;10:1259–65.
101. Medeiros LJ, Picker LJ, Gelb AB, et al. Numbers of host "helper" T cells and proliferating cells predict survival in diffuse small-cell lymphomas. J Clin Oncol 1989 7:1009–17.
102. Grogan TM, Miller TP. New biologic markers in non-Hodgkin's lymphomas. Hematol Oncol Clin North Am 1991;5:925–33.
103. Miller TP, Grogan TM, Dahlberg S, et al. Prognostic significance of the Ki-67–associated proliferative antigen in aggressive non-Hodgkin's lymphomas: a prospective Southwest Oncology Group trial. Blood 1994;83:1460–6.
104. Clayberger C, Wright A, Medeiros LJ, et al. Absence of cell surface

LFA-1 as a mechanism of escape from immunosurveillance. Lancet 1987;2:533–6.

105. Liotta LA, Tryggvason K, Garbisa S, et al. Metastatic potential correlates with enzymatic degradation of basement membrane collagen. Nature 1980;284:67–8.

106. Stauder R, Greil R, Schulz TF, et al. Expression of leucocyte function-associated antigen-1 and 7F7-antigen, an adhesion molecule related to intercellular adhesion molecule-1 (ICAM-1) in non-Hodgkin lymphomas and leukaemias: possible influence on growth pattern and leukaemic behaviour. Clin Exp Immunol 1989;77:234–8.

107. Roossien FF, de Rijk D, Bikker A, Roos E. Involvement of LFA-1 in lymphoma invasion and metastasis demonstrated with LFA-1–deficient mutants. J Cell Biol 1989;108:1979–85.

108. Miller TP, Lippman SM, Spier CM, et al. HLA-DR (Ia) immune phenotype predicts outcome for patients with diffuse large cell lymphoma. J Clin Invest 1988;82:370–2.

109. Rybski JA, Spier CM, Miller TP, et al. Prediction of outcome in diffuse large cell lymphoma by the major histocompatibility complex class II (HLA-DR, DP. DQ) and class I (HLA-A, B, C) phenotype: leukemia and Lymphoma 1991;6:31–8.

110. Hart S, Toghill P, Vaughan-Hudson G. Phenotypic analysis of large cell lymphoma in paraffin section: the relationship to prognosis and natural history. abstract. Third International Conference on Malignant Lymphoma, Lugano, Switzerland, 1987.

111. Kluin PK. Phenotypic analysis of large cell lymphoma in paraffin section: the relationship to prognosis and natural history. abstract. Third International Conference on Malignant Lymphoma, Lugano, Switzerland, 1987.

112. Momburg F, Herrmann B, Moldenhauer G, Moller P. B-cell lymphomas of high-grade malignancy frequently lack HLA-DR, -DP and -DQ antigens and associated invariant chain. Int J Cancer 1987;40:598–603.

113. O'Keane JC, Mack C, Lynch E, et al. Prognostic correlation of HLA-DR expression in large cell lymphoma as determined by LN3 antibody staining. An Eastern Cooperative Oncology Group (ECOG) study. Cancer 1990;66:1147–53.

114. Medeiros LJ, Gelb AB, Wolfson K, et al. Major histocompatibility complex class I and class II antigen expression in diffuse large cell and large cell immunoblastic lymphomas: absence of a correlation between antigen expression and clinical outcome. Am J Pathol 1993;143:1086–97.

115. List AF, Spier CM, Miller TP, Grogan TM. Deficient tumor-infiltrating T-lymphocyte response in malignant lymphoma: relationship to HLA expression and host immunocompetence. Leukemia 1993;7:398–403.

116. Jacob MC, Favre M, Lemarc'Hadour F, et al. CD45RA expression by CD4 T lymphocytes in tumors invaded by B-cell non-Hodgkin's lymphoma (NHL) or Hodgkin's disease (Hodgkin's disease). Am J Hematol 1992;39:45–51.

117. Jacob MC, Piccinni MP, Bonnefoix T, et al. T lymphocytes from invaded lymph nodes in patients with B-cell–derived non-Hodgkin's lymphoma: reactivity toward the malignant clone. Blood 1990;75:1154–62.

118. Lippman SM, Spier CM, Miller TP, et al. Tumor-infiltrating T-lymphocytes in B-cell diffuse large cell lymphoma related to disease course. Mod Pathol 1990;3:361–7.

119. Kern WF, Spier CM, Hanneman EH, et al. Neural cell adhesion molecule-positive peripheral T-cell lymphoma: a rare variant with a propensity for unusual sites of involvement. Blood 1992;79:2432–7.

120. Wong KF, Chan JK, Ng CS, et al. CD56 (NKH1)-positive hematolymphoid malignancies: an aggressive neoplasm featuring frequent cutaneous/mucosal involvement, cytoplasmic azurophilic granules, and angiocentricity. Hum Pathol 1992;23:798–804.

121. Kern WF, Spier CM, Miller TP, Grogan TM. NCAM (CD56)-positive malignant lymphoma. Leuk Lymphoma 1193;12:1–10.

122. Grogan T, Guptil V, Mullen J, et al. Polysialated NCAM as a neurodeterminant in malignant lymphoma.Lab Invest 1994;70:110a.

123. Jalkanen S, Joensuu H, Soderstrom KO, Klemi P. Lymphocyte homing and clinical behavior of non-Hodgkin's lymphoma. J Clin Invest 1991;87:1835–40.

124. Jalkanen S, Joensuu H, Klemi P. Prognostic value of lymphocyte homing receptor and S phase fraction in non-Hodgkin's lymphoma. Blood 1990;75:1549–56.

125. Picker LJ, Medeiros LJ, Weiss LM, et al. Expression of lymphocyte homing receptor antigen in non-Hodgkin's lymphoma. Am J Pathol 1988;130:496–504.

126. Miller TP, Grogan TM, Dalton WS, et al. P-glycoprotein expression in malignant lymphoma and reversal of clinical drug resistance with chemotherapy plus high-dose verapamil. J Clin Oncol 1991;9:17–24.

127. Chaudhary PM, Mechetner EB, Roninson IB. Expression and activity of the multidrug resistance P-glycoprotein in human peripheral blood lymphocytes. Blood 1992;80:2735–9.

128. Drach D, Zhao S, Drach J, et al. Subpopulations of normal peripheral blood and bone marrow cells express a functional multidrug resistant phenotype. Blood 1992;80:2729–34.

129. Dan S, Esumi M, Sawada U, et al. Expression of a multidrug-resistance gene in human malignant lymphoma and related disorders. Leuk Res 1991;15:1139–43.

130. Pileri SA, Sabattini E, Falini B, et al. Immunohistochemical detection of the multidrug transport protein P170 in human normal tissues and malignant lymphomas. Histopathology 1991;19:131–40.

131. Niehans GA, Jaszcz W, Brunetto V, et al. Immunohistochemical identification of P-glycoprotein in previously untreated, diffuse large cell and immunoblastic lymphomas. Cancer Res 1992;52:3768–75.

132. Grogan TM, Rangel C, Rimsza L, et al. Clinical and research applications of rapid, kinetic-mode automated double labelled immunohistochemistry and in situ hybridization. Adv Pathol Lab Med 1995;8:86–96.

133. The Non-Hodgkins Lymphoma Classification Project. A clinical evaluation of the International Lymphoma Study Group classification of non-Hodgkins lymphoma. Blood 1997;89:3909–18.

134. Rosenberg SA. The non-Hodgkin's lymphoma Pathologic Classification Project. NCI sponsored study of classifications of non-Hodgkin's lymphoma: summary and description of a working formulation for clinical usage. Blood 1982;49:2112–35.

135. Grogan TM, Miller TP, Fisher RI. A Southwest Oncology Group perspective on the Revised European American Classification. Hematol Oncol 1997;11:819–46.

136. Braziel RM, Oyama K. Mistaken diagnoses of Hodgkin's disease. Hematol Oncol 1997;11:863–92.

137. Miller TP, Byrne GE, Jones SE. Mistaken clinical and pathologic diagnoses of Hodgkin's disease: a Southwest Oncology Group study. Can Treat Rep 1982;66:645–51.

138. Cossman J, Chused TM, Fisher RI, et al. Diversity of immunological phenotypes of lymphoblastic lymphoma. Cancer Res 1983;43:4486–90.

139. Weiss LM, Bindl JM, Picozzi VJ, et al. Lymphoblastic lymphoma: an immunophenotype study of 26 cases with comparison to T cell acute lymphoblastic leukemia. Blood 1986;67:474.

140. Verdi CJ, Grogan TM, Protell R, et al. Liver biopsy immunotyping to characterize lymphoid malignancies. Hepatology 1986;6:6.

141. Sander C, Medeiros L, Abruzzo L, et al. Lymphoblastic lymphoma presenting in cutaneous sites: a clinicopathologic analysis of six cases. J Am Acad Dermatol 1991;25:1023.

142. Pangalis GA, Nathwani BN, Rappaport H. Malignant lymphoma, well differentiated lymphocytic: its relationship with chronic lymphocytic leukemia and macroglobulinemia of Waldenstrom. Cancer 1977; 39:999–1010.

143. Ben-Ezra J, Burke JS, Swartz WG, et al. Small lymphocytic lymphoma: a clinicopathologic analysis of 268 cases. Blood 1989;73:579–87.

144. Dick FR, Maca RD. The lymph node in chronic lymphocytic leukemia. Cancer 1978;41:283–92.

145. Morrison WH, Hoppe RT, Weiss LM, et al. Small lymphocytic lymphoma. J Clin Oncol 1989;7:598–606.

146. Spier CM, Grogan TM, Fielder K, et al. Immunophenotypes in "well-differentiated" lymphoproliferative disorders, with emphasis on small lymphocytic lymphoma. Hum Pathol 1986;17:1126–36.

147. Harris NL, Bhan AK. B-cell neoplasms of the lymphocytic, lymphoplasmacytoid, and plasma cell types: immunohistologic analysis and clinical correlation. Hum Pathol 1985;16:829–37.

148. Zukerberg LR, Medeiros LJ, Ferry JA, Harris NL. Diffuse low-grade B-cell lymphomas: four clinically distinct subtypes defined by a combination of morphologic and immunophenotypic features. Am J Clin Pathol 1993;100:373–85.

149. Bofill M, Janossy G, Janossa M, et al. Human B cell development. J Immunol 1985;134:1531–8.

150. Antin JH, Emerson SG, Martin P, et al. LEU-1 (CD5) B cells: a major lymphoid subpopulation in human fetal spleen: phenotypic and functional studies. J Immunol 1986;136:505–10.

151. Knuutila S, Elonen E, Teerenhovi L, et al. Trisomy 12 in B cells of patients with B-cell chronic lymphocytic leukemia. N Engl J Med 1986;314:865–9.

152. Levine EG, Arthur DC, Frizzera G, et al. There are differences in cytogenetic abnormalities among histologic subtypes of the non-Hodgkin's lymphomas. Blood 1985;66:1414–22.

153. Athan E, Foitl DR, Knowles DM. *bcl*-1 rearrangement: frequency and clinical significance among B-cell chronic lymphocytic leukemias and non-Hodgkin's lymphomas. Am J Pathol 1991;138:591–9.

154. Richter MN. Generalized reticular cell sarcoma of lymph nodes associated with lymphatic leukemia. Am J Pathol 1928;4:285–92.

155. Melo JV, Catovsky D, Galton DA. The relationship between chronic lymphocytic leukaemia and prolymphocytic leukaemia. I: Clinical and laboratory features of 300 patients and characterization of an intermediate group. Br J Haematol 1985;63:377–87.

156. Brecher M, Banks PM. Hodgkin's disease variant of Richter's syndrome: report of eight cases. Am J Clin Pathol 1990;93:333–9.

157. Harousseau JL, Flandrin G, Tricot G, et al. Malignant lymphoma supervening in chronic lymphocytic leukemia and related disorders: Richter's syndrome: a study of 25 cases. Cancer 1981;48:1302–8.

158. Evans HL, Butler JJ, Youness EL. Malignant lymphoma, small lymphocytic type: a clinicopathologic study of 84 cases with suggested criteria for intermediate lymphocytic lymphoma. Cancer 1978; 41:1440–55.

159. Medeiros LJ, Picker LJ, Gelb AB, et al. Numbers of host "helper" T cells and proliferating cells predict survival in diffuse small-cell lymphomas. J Clin Oncol 1989;7:1009–17.

160. Harris NL, Bhan AK. B-cell neoplasms of the lymphocytic, lymphoplasmacytoid, and plasma cell types: immunohistologic analysis and clinical correlation. Hum Pathol 1985;16:829–37.

161. Iida S, Rao PH, Nallasivam P, et al. The t(9;14)(p13;q32) chromosomal translocation associated with lymphoplasmacytoid lymphoma involves the PAX-5 gene. Blood 1996;88:4110–17.

162. Misiani R, Belllavita P, Fenili D, et al. Interferon alfa—a therapy in cryoglobulinemia associated with hepatitis C virus. N Engl J Med 1994;330:751.

163. Adams B, Dorfer P, Aguzzi A, et al. PAX-5 encodes the transcription factor BSAP and is expressed in B lymphocytes, the developing CNS, and adult testis. Genes Dev 1992;6:1589.

164. Warnke R, Levy R. Immunopathology of follicular lymphomas: a model of B-lymphocyte homing. N Engl J Med 1974;298:481–6.

165. Jaffe ES, Shevach EM, Frank MM, et al. Nodular lymphoma: evidence for origin from follicular B-lymphocytes. N Engl J Med 1974; 290:813–9.

166. Warnke RA, Kim H, Fuks Z, Dorfman RF. The coexistence of nodular and diffuse patterns in nodular non-Hodgkin's lymphomas: significance and clinicopathologic correlation. Cancer 1977;40:1229–33.

167. Mann RB, Jaffe ES, Braylan RC, et al. Non-endemic Burkitts's lymphoma. A B-cell tumor related to germinal centers. N Engl J Med 1976;295:685–91.

168. Nathwani BN, Winberg CD, Diamond LW, et al. Morphologic criteria for the differentiation of follicular lymphoma from florid reactive follicular hyperplasia: a study of 80 cases. Cancer 1981;48:1794–806.

169. Mann RB, Berard CW. Criteria for the cytologic su*bcl*assification of follicular lymphomas: a proposed alternative method. Hematol Oncol 1983;1:187–92.

170. Metter GE, Nathwani BN, Burke JS, et al. Morphological su*bcl*assification of follicular lymphoma: variability of diagnoses among hematopathologists: a collaborative study between the Repository Center and Pathology Panel for Lymphoma Clinical Studies. J Clin Oncol 1985;3:25–38.

171. Nathwani BN, Metter GE, Miller TP, et al. What should be the morphologic criteria for the subdivision of follicular lymphomas? Blood 1986;837–45.

172. Miller T, LeBlanc M, Grogan T, Fisher R. Follicular lymphomas: do histologic subtypes predict outcome? Hematol Oncol 1997;11:893–900.

173. Stein H, Berdes J, Mason DY. The normal and malignant germinal centre. Clin Haematol 1982;11:531.

174. Ngan BY, Chen-Levy Z, Weiss LM, et al. Expression in non-Hodgkin's lymphoma of the *bcl*-2 protein associated with the t(14;18) chromosomal translocation. N Engl J Med 1988;318:1638–44.

175. Tsujimoto Y, Cossman J, Jaffe E, Croce CM. Involvement of the *bcl*-2 gene in human follicular lymphoma. Science 1985;228:1440–3.

176. Hockenbery DM, Zutter M, Hickey W, et al. *Bcl*2 protein is topographically restricted in tissues characterized by apoptotic cell death. Proc Natl Acad Sci U S A 1991;88:6961–5.

177. Weiss LM, Strickler JG, Medeiros LJ, et al. Proliferative rates of non-Hodgkin's lymphomas as assessed by Ki-67 antibody. Hum Pathol 1987;18:1155–9.

178. Frizzera G, Murphy SB. Follicular (nodular) lymphoma in childhood: a rare clinical-pathological entity: report of eight cases from four cancer centers. Cancer 1979;44:2218–35.

179. Jones SE, Fuks Z, Bull M, et al. Non-Hodgkin's lymphomas. IV: Clinicopathologic correlation in 405 cases. Cancer 1973;31:806–23.

180. Ezdinli EZ, Costello WG, Kucuk O, Berard CW. Effect of the degree of nodularity on the survival of patients with nodular lymphomas. J Clin Oncol 1987;5:413–8.

181. Brittinger G, Bartels H, Common H, et al. Clinical and prognostic relevance of the Kiel classification of non-Hodgkin lymphomas: results of a prospective multicenter study by the Kiel Lymphoma Study Group. Hematol Oncol 1984;2:269–306.

182. Anderson T, Chabner BA, Young RC, et al. Malignant lymphoma 1: the history and staging of 473 patients at the National Cancer Institute. Cancer 1982;50:2699–707.

183. Chabner BA, Johnson RE, Young RC, et al. Sequential nonsurgical and surgical staging of non-Hodgkin's lymphoma. Ann Intern Med 1976;85:149–54.

184. Fisher RI, Hubbard SM, DeVita VT, et al. Factors predicting long-term survival in diffuse mixed, histiocytic, or undifferentiated lymphoma. Blood 1981;58:45–51.

185. Isaacson PG. Extranodal lymphomas: the MALT concept. Verh Dtsch Ges Pathol 1992;76:14–23.

186. Schmid C, Kirkham N, Diss T, Isaacson PG. Splenic marginal zone cell lymphoma. Am J Surg Pathol 1992;16:455–66.

187. Spencer J, Finn T, Pulford KA, et al. The human gut contains a novel population of B-lymphocytes, which resemble marginal zone cells. Clin Exp Immunol 1985;62:607–12.

188. van den Oord JJ, de Wolf-Peeters C, Desmet VJ. Marginal zone lymphocytes in the lymph node. Hum Pathol 1989;20:1225–7.

189. Cogliatti SB, Schmid U, Schumacher U, et al. Primary B-cell gastric lymphoma: a clinicopathological study of 145 patients. Gastroenterology 1991;101:1159–70.

190. Medeiros LJ, Harmon DC, Linggood RM, Harris NL. Immunohistologic features predict clinical behavior of orbital and conjunctival lymphoid infiltrates. Blood 1989;74:2121–9.

191. Li G, Hansmann ML, Zwingers T, Lennert K. Primary lymphomas of the lung: morphological, immunohistochemical and clinical features. Histopathology 1990;16:519–31.

192. Mattia AR, Ferry JA, Harris NL. Breast lymphoma: a B-cell spectrum including the low grade B-cell lymphoma of mucosa associated lymphoid tissue. Am J Surg Pathol 1993;17:574–87.

193. Hussell T, Isaacson PG, Crabtree JE, Spencer J. The response of cells from low-grade B-cell gastric lymphomas of mucosa-associated lymphoid tissue to *Helicobacter pylori*. Lancet 1993;342:571–4.

194. Wotherspoon AC, Doglioni C, Diss TC, et al. Regression of primary low-grade B-cell gastric lymphoma of mucosa-associated lymphoid tissue type after eradication of *Helicobacter pylori*. Lancet 1993;342:575–7.

195. Fisher RI, Dahlberg S, Nathwani BN, et al. A clinical analysis of two indolent lymphoma entities: mantle cell lymphoma and marginal zone lymphoma (including the mucosa-associated lymphoid tissue and monocytoid B-cell subcategories: a Southwest Oncology Group study. Blood 1995;85;1075–82.

196. So JCC, Ho FCS, Liang RHS. Lymphomas of mucosa-associated lymphoid tissue comprise only a proportion of primary gastric lymphomas and do not carry a better prognosis. Lab Invest 1994;70:121a.

197. Smith-Ravin J, Spencer J, Beverley PC, Isaacson PG. Characterization of two monoclonal antibodies (UCL4D12 and UCL3D3) that discriminate between human mantle zone and marginal zone B cells. Clin Exp Immunol 1990;82:181–7.

198. Fishleder A, Tubbs R, Hesse B, Levine H. Uniform detection of immunoglobulin-gene rearrangement in benign lymphoepithelial lesions. N Engl J Med 1987;316:1118–21.

199. Pan L, Diss TC, Cunningham D, Isaacson PG. The *bcl*-2 gene in primary B cell lymphoma of mucosa-associated lymphoid tissue (MALT). Am J Pathol 1989;135:7–11.

200. Finn T, Isaacson PG, Wotherspoon AC. Numerical abnormalities of

chromosomes 3, 7, 12 and 18 in low-grade lymphomas of MALT-type and splenic marginal zone cell lymphomas detected by interphase cytogenetics on paraffin embedded tissue. J Pathol 1993; 170:Suppl:335a.

201. Isaacson PG, Wotherspoon AC, Diss T, Pan LX. Follicular colonization in B-cell lymphoma of mucosa-associated lymphoid tissue. Am J Surg Pathol 1991;15:819–28.

202. Hyjek E, Smith WJ, Isaacson PG. Primary B-cell lymphoma of salivary glands and its relationship to myoepithelial sialadenitis. Hum Pathol 1988;19:766–76.

203. Zukerberg LR, Ferry JA, Southern JF, Harris NL. Lymphoid infiltrates of the stomach: evaluation of histologic criteria for the diagnosis of low-grade gastric lymphoma on endoscopic biopsy specimens. Am J Surg Pathol 1990;14:1087–99.

204. Harris NL. Extranodal lymphoid infiltrates and mucosa-associated lymphoid tissue (MALT): a unifying concept. Am J Surg Pathol 1991;15:879–84.

205. Sheibani K, Sohn CC, Burke JS, et al. Monocytoid B-cell lymphoma: a novel B-cell neoplasm. Am J Pathol 1986;124:310–8.

206. Sheibani K, Burke JS, Swartz WG, et al. Monocytoid B-cell lymphoma: clinicopathologic study of 21 cases of a unique type of low-grade lymphoma. Cancer 1988;62:1531–8.

207. Nathwani BN, Mohrmann RL, Brynes RK, et al. Monocytoid B-cell lymphomas: an assessment of diagnostic criteria and a perspective on histogenesis. Hum Pathol 1992;23:1061–71.

208. Ngan BY, Warnke RA, Wilson M, et al. Monocytoid B-cell lymphoma: a study of 36 cases. Hum Pathol 1991;22:409–21.

209. Nizze H, Cogliatti SB, von Schilling C, et al. Monocytoid B-cell lymphoma: morphological variants and relationship to low-grade B-cell lymphoma of the mucosa-associated lymphoid tissue. Histopathology 1991;18:403–14.

210. Shin SS, Sheibani K, Fishleder A, et al. Monocytoid B-cell lymphoma in patients with Sjogren's syndrome: a clinicopathologic study of 13 patients. Hum Pathol 1991;22:422–30.

211. Cogliatti SB, Lennert K, Hansmann ML, Zwingers TL. Monocytoid B cell lymphoma: clinical and prognostic features of 21 patients. J Clin Pathol 1990;43:619–25.

212. Carbone A, Gloghini A, Pinto A, et al. Monocytoid B-cell lymphoma with bone marrow and peripheral blood involvement at presentation. Am J Clin Pathol 1989;92:228–36.

213. Grogan T. Does nodal marginal zone lymphoma exist? In: Mason DY, Harris NL, eds. Human lymphoma: clinical implicaions of the REAL classification. London: Springer, 1999.

214. Tolksdorf G, Stein H, Lennert K. Morphological and immunological definition of a malignant lymphoma derived from germinal-centre cells with cleaved nuclei (centrocytes). Br J Cancer 1980;41:168–82.

215. Berard CW, Dorfman RF. Histopathology of malignant lymphomas. Clin Haematol 1974;3:39–76.

216. Weisenburger DD, Nathwani BN, Diamond LW, et al. Malignant lymphoma, intermediate lymphocytic type: a clinicopathologic study of 42 cases. Cancer 1981;48:1415–25.

217. Weisenburger DD, Kim H, Rappaport H. Mantle-zone lymphoma: a follicular variant of intermediate lymphocytic lymphoma. Cancer 1982;49:1429–38.

218. Banks PM, Chan J, Cleary ML, et al. Mantle cell lymphoma: a proposal for unification of morphologic, immunologic, and molecular data. Am J Surg Pathol 1992;16:637–40.

219. Lardelli P, Bookman MA, Sundeen J, et al. Lymphocytic lymphoma of intermediate differentiation: morphologic and immunophenotypic spectrum and clinical correlations. Am J Surg Pathol 1990;14:752–63.

220. Stein H, Lennert K, Feller AC, Mason DY. Immunohistological analysis of human lymphoma: correlation of histological and immunological categories. Adv Cancer Res 1984;42:67–147.

221. Rosenberg CL, Wong E, Petty EM, et al. PRAD1, a candidate *BCL1* oncogene: mapping and expression in centrocytic lymphoma. Proc Natl Acad Sci U S A 1991;88:9638–42.

222. O'Brian DS, Kennedy MJ, Daly PA, et al. Multiple lymphomatous polyposis of the gastrointestinal tract: a clinicopathologically distinctive form of non-Hodgkin's lymphoma of B-cell centrocytic type. Am J Surg Pathol 1989;13:691–9.

223. Warnke RA, Strauchen JA, Burke JS, et al. Morphologic types of diffuse large-cell lymphoma. Cancer 1982;50:690–5.

224. Spier CM, Lippman SM, Miller TP, Grogan TM. Lennert's lymphoma: a clinicopathologic study with emphasis on phenotype and its relationship to survival. Cancer 1988;61:517–24.

225. Jaffe ES, Strauchen JA, Berard CW. Predictability of immunologic phenotype by morphologic criteria in diffuse aggressive non-Hodgkin's lymphomas. Am J Clin Pathol 1982;77:46–9.

226. Cossman J, Jaffe ES, Fisher RI. Immunologic phenotypes of diffuse, aggressive, non-Hodgkin's lymphomas: correlation with clinical features. Cancer 1984;54:1310–17.

227. Doggett RS, Wood GS, Horning S, et al. The immunologic characterization of 95 nodal and extranodal diffuse large cell lymphomas in 89 patients. Am J Pathol 1984;115:245–52.

228. Spier CM, Grogan TM, Lippman SM, et al. The aberrancy of immunophenotype and immunoglobulin status as indicators of prognosis in B cell diffuse large cell lymphoma. Am J Pathol 1988;133:118–26.

229. Miller JB, Variakojis D, Bitran JDU, et al. Diffuse histiocytic lymphoma with sclerosis: a clinicopathologic entity frequently causing superior venacaval obstruction. Cancer 1981;47:748–56.

230. Gascoyne RD, Adomat SA, Krajewski S, et al. Prognostic significance of *bcl*-2 protein expression and *bcl*-2 gene rearrangement in diffuse aggressive non-Hodgkins lymphoma. Blood 1997;90:244.

231. Berard CW, O'Connor GI, Thomas LB. Histopathological definition of Burkitt's tumor. Bull WHO 1969;40:601.

232. Grogan TM, Warnke RA, Kaplan HS. A comparative study of Burkitt's and non-Burkitt's "undifferentiated" malignant lymphoma: immunologic, cytochemical, ultrastructural, cytologic, histopathologic, clinical and cell culture features. Cancer 1982;49:1817–28.

233. Miliauskas JR, Berard CW, Young RC, et al. Undifferentiated non-Hodgkin's lymphomas (Burkitt's and non-Burkitt's types): the relevance of making this histologic distinction. Cancer 1982;50:2115–21.

234. Ziegler JL, Beckstead JA, Volberding PA, et al. Non-Hodgkin's lymphoma in 90 homosexual men: relation to generalized lymphadenopathy and the acquired immunodeficiency syndrome. N Engl J Med 1984;311:565–70.

235. Krikorian JG, Burke JS, Rosenberg SA, Kaplan HS. Occurrence of non-Hodgkin's lymphoma after therapy for Hodgkin's disease. N Engl J Med 1979;300:452–8.

236. Swinin LJ, Costanzo-Nordin MR, Fisher R, et al. Increased incidence of lymphoproliferative disorder after immunosuppression with the monoclonal antibody OKT3 in cardiac transplant receipients. N Engl J Med 1990;323:1723.

237. Garcia CF, Weiss LM, Warnke RA. Small noncleaved cell lymphoma: an immunophenotypic study of 18 cases and comparison with large cell lymphoma. Hum Pathol 1986;17:454–61.

238. Payne CM, Grogan TM, Cromey DW, et al. An ultrastructural morphometric and immunophenotypic evaluation of Burkitt's and Burkitt's-like lymphomas. Lab Invest 1987;57:200–18.

239. Aiello A. Delia D. Fontanella E. et al. Expression of differentiation and adhesion molecules in sporadic Burkitt's lymphoma. Hematol Oncol 1990;8:229–38.

240. Verdi CJ, Grogan TM, Protell R, et al. Liver biopsy immunotyping to characterize lymphoid malignancies. Hepatology 1986;6:6–13.

241. Oliver JD, Grogan TM, Payne CM, et al. Burkitt's-like lymphoma of T-cell type. Mod Pathol 1988;1:15–22.

242. Yano T, van Krieken JH, Magrath IT, et al. Histogenetic correlations between subcategories of small noncleaved cell lymphomas. Blood 1992;79:1282–90.

243. Braziel R. A comparative study of Burkitt and Burkitt-like lymphoma. Blood (in press).

244. Lindahl T, Klein G, Reedman BM, et al. Relationship between Epstein-Barr virus (EBV) DNA and the EBV-determined nuclear antigen (EBNA) in Burkitt lymphoma biopsies and other lymphoproliferative malignancies. Int J Cancer 1974;13:764–72.

245. Ziegler JL, Andersson M, Klein G, Henle W. Detection of Epstein-Barr virus DNA in American Burkitt's lymphoma. Int J Cancer 1976;17:701–6.

246. Ballerini P, Gaidano G, Gong JZ, et al. Multiple genetic lesions in acquired immunodeficiency syndrome–related non-Hodgkin's lymphoma. Blood 1993;81:166–76.

247. Croce CM, Tsujimoto Y, Erikson J, Nowell P. Chromosome translocations and B cell neoplasia. Lab Invest 1984;51:258–67.

248. Magrath I. Biology and treatment of small non-cleaved cell lymphoma. Oncology 1989;3:41.

249. Burkitt D, O'Conner GT. Malignant lymphoma in African children. I: A clinical syndrome. Cancer 1961;14:258–69.

250. Flandrin G, Brouet JC, Daniel MT, Preud'homme JL. Acute leukemia with Burkitt's tumor cells: a study of six cases with special reference to lymphocyte surface markers. Blood 1975;45:183–8.

251. Ziegler JL, Drew WL, Miner RC, et al. Outbreak of Burkitt's-like lymphoma in homosexual men. Lancet 1982;2:631–3.

252. Hutchison RE, Murphy SB, Fairclough DL, et al. Diffuse small noncleaved cell lymphoma in children, Burkitt's versus non-Burkitt's types: results from the Pediatric Oncology Group and St. Jude Children's Research Hospital. Cancer 1989;64:23–8.

253. Bernstein JI, Coleman CN, Strickler JG, et al. Combined modality therapy for adults with small noncleaved cell lymphoma (Burkitt's and non-Burkitt's types). J Clin Oncol 1986;4:847–56.

254. Levine AM, Pavlova Z, Pockros AW, et al. Small noncleaved follicular center cell (FCC) lymphoma: Burkitt and non-Burkitt variants in the United States. I: Clinical features. Cancer 1983;52:1073–9.

255. Grogan T. A multi-institutional evaluation of lymphoma classification. In: Mason DY, Harris NL, eds. Human lymphoma: clinical implications of the REAL classification. London: Springer, 1999.

256. Nathwani BN, Kim H, Rappaport H. Malignant lymphoma, lymphoblastic. Cancer 1976;38:964–83.

257. Cossman J, Chused TM, Fisher RI, et al. Diversity of immunological phenotypes of lymphoblastic lymphoma. Cancer Res 1983;43:4486–90.

258. Weiss LM, Bindl JM, Picozzi VJ, et al. Lymphoblastic lymphoma: an immunophenotype study of 26 cases with comparison to T cell acute lymphoblastic leukemia. Blood 1986;67:474–8.

259. Sheibani K, Winberg CD, Burke JS, et al. Lymphoblastic lymphoma expressing natural killer cell-associated antigens: a clinicopathologic study of six cases. Leuk Res 1987;11:371–7.

260. Weiss LM, Crabtree GS, Rouse RV, Warnke RA. Morphologic and immunologic characterization of 50 peripheral T-cell lymphomas. Am J Pathol 1985;118:316–24.

261. Jaffe ES. Pathologic and clinical spectrum of post-thymic T-cell malignancies. Cancer Invest 1984;2:413–26.

262. Greer JP, York JC, Cousar JB, et al. Peripheral T-cell lymphoma: a clinicopathologic study of 42 cases. J Clin Oncol 1984;2:788–98.

263. Weis JW, Winter MW, Phyliky RL, Banks PM. Peripheral T-cell lymphomas: histologic immunohistologic, and clinical characterization. Mayo Clinic Proc. 1986;61:411–26.

264. Wright DH. T-cell lymphomas. Histopathology 1986;10:321–26.

265. Cossman J, Jaffe ES, Fisher RI. Diversity of immunologic phenotypes of T-cell lymphoma. Am J Surg Pathol 1982;6:72.

266. Horning SJ, Weiss LM, Crabtree GS, Warnke RA. Clinical and phenotypic diversity of T cell lymphomas. Blood 1986;67:1578–82.

267. Lippman SM, Miller TP, Spier CM, et al. The prognostic significance of the immunotype in diffuse large-cell lymphoma: a comparative study of the T-cell and B-cell phenotype. Blood 1988;72:436–41.

268. Coiffier B, Brousse N, Peuchmaur M, et al. Peripheral T-cell lymphomas have a worse prognosis than B-cell lymphomas: a prospective study of 361 immunophenotyped patients treated with the LNH-84 regimen: the GELA (Groupe d'Etude des Lymphomes Agressives). Ann Oncol 1990;1:45–50.

269. Lukes RJ, Collins RD. New approaches to the classification of the lymphomata. Br J Cancer 1975;31:Suppl 2:1–28.

270. Lennert K. Malignant lymphomas. Berlin: Springer-Verlag, 1978:196.

271. Shimoyama M, Mirato K, Saito H, et al. Immunoblastic lymphadenopathy (IBL)-like T-cell lymphoma. Jpn J Clin Oncol 1979; 9:Suppl:347–56.

272. Muller-Hermelink HK, Stein H, Steinmann G, Lennert K. Malignant lymphoma of plasmacytoid T-cells: morphologic and immunologic studies characterizing a special type of T-cell. Am J Surg Pathol 1983;7:849–62.

273. Stein H, Mason DY, Gerdes J, et al. The expression of the Hodgkin's disease associated antigen Ki-1 in reactive and neoplastic lymphoid tissue: evidence that Reed-Sternberg cells and histiocytic malignancies are derived from activated lymphoid cells. Blood 1985;66:848–58.

274. Kim H, Jacobs C, Warnke RA, Dorfman RF. Malignant lymphoma with a high content of epithelioid histiocytes: a distinct clinicopathologic entity and a form of so-called Lennert's lymphoma. Cancer 1978;41:620–35.

275. Patsouris E, Noel H, Lennert K. Lymphoplasmacytic/lymphoplasmacytoid immunocytoma with a high content of epithelioid cells: histologic and immunohistochemical findings. Am J Surg Pathol 1990;14:660–70.

276. Tamaki T, Katagiri S, Kanayama Y, et al. Helper T-cell lymphoma with marked plasmacytosis and polyclonal hypergammaglobulinemia: a case report. Cancer 1984;53:1590–5.

277. Whitcomb CC, Sternheim WL, Borowitz MJ, et al. T-cell lymphoma mimicking granulocytic sarcoma. Am J Clin Pathol 1985;84:760–3.

278. Kadin ME, Kamoun M, Lamberg J. Erythrophagocytic T gamma lymphoma: a clinicopathologic entity resembling malignant histiocytosis. N Engl J Med 1981;304:648–53.

279. Jaffe ES, Costa J, Fauci AS, et al. Malignant lymphoma and erythrophagocytosis simulating malignant histiocytosis. Am J Med. 1983;75:741–9.

280. Isaacson PG, O'Connor NT, Spencer J, et al. Malignant histiocytosis of the intestine: a T-cell lymphoma. Lancet 1985;2:688–91.

281. Greenberg BR, Grogan TM, Takasugi BJ, et al. A unique malignant T-cell lymphoproliferative disorder with neutropenia simulating hairy cell leukemia. Cancer 1985;56:2823–30.

282. Weiss LM, Strickler JG, Dorfman RF, et al. Clonal T-cell populations in angioimmunoblastic lymphadenopathy and angioimmunoblastic lymphadenopathy-like lymphoma. Am J Pathol 1986;122:392–7.

283. Lipford EH Jr, Margolick JB, Longo DL, et al. Angiocentric immunoproliferative lesions: a clinicopathologic spectrum of post-thymic T-cell proliferations. Blood 1988;5:1674–81.

284. Lippman SM, Grogan TM, Spier CM, et al. Lethal midline granuloma with a novel T-cell phenotype as found in peripheral T-cell lymphoma. Cancer 1987;59:936–9.

285. Uchiyama T, Yodoi J, Sagawa K, et al. Adult T-cell leukemia: clinical and hematologic features of 16 cases. Blood 1977;50:481–92.

286. Jaffe ES, Blattner WA, Blayney DW, et al. The pathologic spectrum of adult T-cell leukemia/lymphoma in the United States. Human T-cell leukemia/lymphoma virus–associated lymphoid malignancies. Am J Surg Pathol 1984;8:263–75.

287. Blattner WA, Kalyanaraman VS, Robert-Guroff M, et al. The human type-C retrovirus, HTLV, in blacks from the Caribbean region, and relationship to adult T-cell leukemia/lymphoma. Int J Cancer 1982;30:2457–64.

288. Mason DY, Bastard C, Rimokh R, et al. CD30-positive large cell lymphomas ("Ki-1 lymphoma") are associated with a chromosomal translocation involving 5q35. Br J Hematol 1990;74:161–8

289. Falini B, Pileri S, Stein H, et al. Variable expression of leucocyte-common (CD45) antigen in CD30 (Ki1)-positive anaplastic large-cell lymphoma: implications for the differential diagnosis between lymphoid and nonlymphoid malignancies. Hum Pathol 1990;21:624.

290. Herbst H, Tippelmann G, Anagnostopoulos I, et al. Immunoglobulin and T-cell receptor gene rearrangements in Hodgkin's disease and Ki-1-positive anaplastic large cell lymphoma: dissociation between phenotype and genotype. Leuk Res 1989;13:103.

291. Agnarsson B, Kadin ME. Ki-1 positive large cell lymphoma: a morphologic and immunologic study of 19 cases. Am J Surg Pathol 1988;12:264–274.

292. Delsol G, Blancher A, Al Saati T, et al. Antibody BNH9 detects red blood cell–related antigens on anaplastic large cell (CD30⁺) lymphomas. Br J Cancer 1991;64:321.

293. Delsol G, Al Saati T, Gatter K, et al. Coexpression of epithelial membrane antigen (EMA), Ki-1, and interleukin-2 receptor by anaplastic large cell lymphomas: diagnostic value in so-called malignant histiocytosis. Am J Pathol 1988;130:59.

294. Saati TA, Tkaczuk J, Krissansen G, et al. A novel antigen detected by the CBF.78 antibody further distinguishes anaplastic large cell lymphoma from Hodgkin's disease. Blood 1995;86:2741–46.

295. Mason D, Bastard C, Rimokh R, et al. CD30-positive large cell lymphomas ("Ki-1 lymphoma") are associated with a chromosomal translocation involving 5q35. Br J Haematol 1990;74:161.

296. Bitter MA, Franklin WA, Larson RA, et al. Morphology in Ki-1(CD30)–positive non-Hodgkin's lymphoma is correlated with clinical features and the presence of a unique chromosomal abnormality, t(2;5)(p23;q35). Am J Surg Pathol 1990;14:305–16.

297. Bullrich F, Morris SW, Hummel M, et al. Nucleophosmin (NPM) gene rearrangements in Ki-1-positive lymphomas. Cancer Res 199454:2873–7.

298. Downing JR, Shurtleff SA, Zielenska M, et al. Molecular detection of the (2;5) translocation of non-Hodgkin's lymphoma by reverse transcriptase-polymerase chain reaction. Blood 1995;85:3416–22.

299. de Bruin PC, Beljaards RC, Van Heerde P, et al. Differences in clinical behavior and immunophenotype between primary cutaneous and primary nodal anaplastic large cell lymphoma of T-cell or null cell phenotype. Histopathology 1993;23:127–35.

300. Kadin ME, Sako D, Berliner N, et al. Childhood Ki-1 lymphoma

presenting with skin lesions and peripheral lymphadenopathy. Blood 1986;68:1042–9.

301. Pileri S, Bocchia M, Baroni CD, et al. Anaplastic large cell lymphoma (CD30+/Ki-1+): results of a prospective clinico-pathological study of 69 cases. Br J Haematol 1994;86:513–23.

302. Uchiyama T, Yodoi J, Sagawa K, et al. Adult T-cell leukemia: clinical and hematologic features of 16 cases. Blood 1977;50:481.

303. Poiesz B, Ruscetti F, Gazdar A. Detection and isolation of type C retrovirus particles from fresh and cultured lymphocytes of a patient with cutaneous T-cell lymphoma. Proc Natl Acad Sci U S A 1980;77:7415.

304. Tokunaga M, Sato E. Non-Hodgkin's lymphomas in a southern prefecture in Japan: an analysis of 715 cases. Cancer 1980;46:1231.

305. Yamada Y. Phenotypic and functional analysis of leukemic cells from 16 patients with adult T cell leukemia/lymphoma. Blood 1983;61:192.

306. Jaffe E, Blattner W, Blayney D, et al. The pathologic spectrum of adult T-cell leukemia/lymphoma in the United States. Am J Surg Pathol 1984;8:263.

307. Swerdlow S, Habeshaw J, Rohatiner A, et al. Caribbean T-cell lymphoma/leukemia. Cancer 1984;54:687.

308. Duggan D, Elrlich G, Davey F, et al. HTLV-I induced lymphoma mimicking Hodgkin's disease: diagnosis by polymerase chain reaction amplification of specific HTLV-I sequences in tumor DNA. Blood 1988;71:1027.

309. Chadburn A, Athan E, Wieczorek R, Knowles D. Detection and characterization of HTLV-I associated T neoplasms in an HTLV-I non-endemic region by polymerase chain reaction. Blood 1991;70:1500.

310. Kikuchi M, Mitsui T, Takeshita M, et al. Virus associated adult T-cell leukemia (ATL) in Japan: clinical, histological and immunological studies. Hematol Oncol 1987;4:67.

311. Abrams M, Sidawy M, Novich M. Smoldering HTLV-associated T-cell leukemia. Arch Intern Med 1985;145:2257.

312. Kiyokawa T, Yamaguchi K, Takeya M, et al. Hypercalcemia and osteoclast proliferation in adult T-cell leukemia. Cancer 1987;59:1187–91.

313. Shibata D, Tokumaga M, Sasaki N, Nanba K. Detection of human T-cell leukemia virus type I proviral sequences from fixed tissues of seropositive patients. Am J Clin Pathol 1991;95:536–9.

314. Gonzales CL, Medeiros J, Braziel RM, Jaffe ES. T-cell lymphoma involving subcutaneous tissue: a clinicopathologic entity commonly associated with hemophagocytic syndrome. Am J Surg Pathol 1991;15:17–27.

315. Perniciaro C, Zalla MJ, White JW, Menke DM. Subcutaneous T-cell lymphoma: report of two additional cases and further observations. Arch Dermatol 1993;129:1171–6.

316. Aronson IK, West DP, Variakojis D, et al. Panniculitis associated with cutaneous T-cell lymphoma and cytophagocytic histiocytosis. Br J Dermatol 1985;112:87–96.

317. Burg G, Dummer R, Wilhelm M, et al. A subcutaneous delta-positive T-cell lymphoma that produces interferon gamma. N Engl J Med 1991;325:1078–81.

318. Chott A, Dragosics B, Radaszkiewicz T. Peripheral T-cell lymphomas of the intestine. Am J Pathol 1992;141:1361–71.

319. O'Farelly C, Feighery C, O'Brian DS, et al. Humoral response to wheat protein in patients with coeliac disease and enteropathy-associated T-cell lymphoma. Br Med J 1986;293:908–10.

320. Murray A, Cuevas EC, Jones DB, Wright DH. Study of the immunohistochemistry and T cell clonality of enteropathy-associated T cell lymphoma. Am J Pathol 1995;146:509–19.

321. Foucar K, Foucar E, Mitros F, et al. Epitheliotropic lymphoma of the small bowel: report of a fatal case with cytotoxic/suppressor T-cell immunotype Cancer 1984;54:54–60.

322. Spencer J, MacDonald TT, Diss TC, et al. Changes in intraepithelial lymphocyte subpopulations in coeliac disease and enteropathy associated T cell lymphoma (malignant histiocytosis of the intestine). Gut 1989;30:339–46.

323. Spencer J, Cerf-Bensussan N, Jarry A, et al. Enteropathy-associated T cell lymphoma (malignant histiocytosis of the intestine) is recognized by a monoclonal antibody (HML-1) that defines a membrane molecule on human mucosal lymphocytes. Am J Pathol 1988;132:1–5.

324. Wright DH, Jones DB, Clark H, et al. Is adult-onset coeliac disease due to a low-grade lymphoma of intraepithelial T lymphocytes? Lancet 1991;337:1373–74.

325. Möller P, Mielke B, Moldenhauer G. Monoclonal antibody HML-1: a marker for intraepithelial T cells and lymphomas derived thereof, also recognizes hairy cell leukemia and some B-cell lymphomas. Am J Pathol 1990;136:509–12.

326. Wong KF, Chan JKC, Matutes E, et al. Hepatosplenic? gamma delta T-cell lymphoma. A distinctive aggressive lymphoma type. Am J Surg Pathol 1995;19:718–26.

327. Mastovitch S, Ratech H, Ware RE, et al. Hepatosplenic T-cell lymphoma: an unusual case of a gamma delta T-cell lymphoma with a blast-like terminal transformation. Hum Pathol 1994;25:102–8.

328. Gaulard P, Bourqueltot P, Kanavaros P, et al. Expression of the alpha/beta and gamma/delta T-cell receptors in 57 cases of peripheral T-cell lymphomas: identification of a subset of gamma/delta T-cell lymphomas. Am J Surg Pathol 1990;137:617–28.

329. Carbone PP, Kaplan HS, Musshoff K, et al. Report of the Committee on Hodgkin's Disease Staging Classification. Cancer Res 1971;31:1860–1.

330. Bitran JD, Kinzie J, Sweet DL, et al. Survival of patients with localized histiocytic lymphoma. Cancer 1977;39:342–6.

331. Levitt SH, Bloomfield CD, Frizzera G, Lee CK. Curative radiotherapy for localized diffuse histiocytic lymphoma. Cancer Treat Rep 1980;64:175–7.

332. Miller TP, Jones SE. Is there a role for radiotherapy in localized diffuse lymphomas? Cancer Chemother Pharmacol 1980;4:67–70.

333. Goffinet DR, Warnke R, Dunnick NR, et al. Clinical and surgical (laparotomy) evaluation of patients with non-Hodgkin's lymphomas. Cancer Treat Rep 1977;61:981–92.

334. Lester JN, Fuller LM, Conrad FG, et al. The roles of staging laparotomy, chemotherapy, and radiotherapy in the management of localized diffuse large cell lymphoma: a study of 75 patients. Cancer 1982;49:1746–53.

335. Bonadonna G. Combined radiotherapy-chemotherapy in localized non-Hodgkin's lymphomas: 5-year results of a randomized study. In: Salmon SE, Jones SE, eds. Adjuvant therapy of cancer. II: New York: Grune & Stratton, 1979:145–53.

336. Kushlan P. Prognostic factors in stage II diffuse histiocytic lymphoma. Proc AACR and ASCO 1978;19:337.

337. Landberg TG, Hakansson LG, Moller TR, et al. CVP-remission-maintenance in stage I or II non-Hodgkin's lymphomas: preliminary results of a randomized study. Cancer 1979;44:831–8.

338. Miller TP, Jones SE. Chemotherapy of localised histiocytic lymphoma. Lancet 1979;1:358–60.

339. Miller TP. Lymphocytic lymphomas. In: DeVita VT Jr, Hellman S, Rosengerb SA, eds. Cancer: principles and practice of oncology updates. Vol. 3. No. 6. Philadelphia: JB Lippincott, 1989:1769.

340. Shipp MA, Harrington DP, Anderson JR. A predictive model of aggressive non-Hodgkin's lymphoma: the International Non-Hodgkin's Lymphoma Prognostic Factors Project. N Engl J Med 1993;329:987–94.

341. Dana BW, Dahlberg S, Nathwani BN, et al. Long-term follow-up of patients with low-grade malignant lymphomas treated with doxorubicin-based chemotherapy or chemoimmunotherapy. J Clin Oncol 1993;11:644–51.

342. Ciampi A, Bush RS, Gospodarowicz M, Till JE. An approach to classifying prognostic factors related to survival experience for non-Hodgkin's lymphoma patients: based on a series of 982 patients: 1967–1975. Cancer 1981;47:621–7.

343. Dixon DO, Neilan B, Jones SE, et al. Effect of age on therapeutic outcome in advanced diffuse histiocytic lymphoma: the Southwest Oncology Group experience. J Clin Oncol 1986;4:295–305.

344. Kwak LW, Halpern J, Olshen RA, Horning SJ. Prognostic significance of actual dose intensity in diffuse large-cell lymphoma: results of a tree-structured survival analysis. J Clin Oncol 1990;8:963–77.

345. Armitage JO, Dick FR, Corder MP, et al. Predicting therapeutic outcome in patients with diffuse histiocytic lymphoma treated with cyclophosphamide, Adriamycin, vincristine and prednisone (CHOP). Cancer 1982;50:1695–702.

346. Hoskins PJ, Ng V, Spinelli JJ, et al. Prognostic variables in patients with diffuse large-cell lymphoma treated with MACOP-B. J Clin Oncol 1991;9:220–6.

347. Stein RS, Greer JP, Flexner JM, et al. Large-cell lymphomas: clinical and prognostic features. J Clin Oncol 1990;8:1370–9.

348. Simon R, Durrleman S, Hoppe RT, et al. Prognostic factors for patients with diffuse large cell or immunoblastic non-Hodgkin's lymphomas: experience of the non-Hodgkin's Lymphoma Pathologic Classification Project. Med Pediatr Oncol 1990;18:89–96.

349. Fisher RI, Hubbard SM, DeVita VT, et al. Factors predicting long-term survival in diffuse mixed, histiocytic, or undifferentiated lymphoma. Blood 1981;58:45–51.

350. Jones SE, Miller TP, Connors JM. Long-term follow-up and analysis for prognostic factors for patients with limited-stage diffuse large-cell lymphoma treated with initial chemotherapy with or without adjuvant radiotherapy. J Clin Oncol 1989;7:1186–91.

351. Fisher RI, DeVita VT Jr, Johnson BL, et al. Prognostic factors for advanced diffuse histiocytic lymphoma following treatment with combination chemotherapy. Am J Med 1977;63:177–82.

352. Leopold KA, Canellos GP, Rosenthal D, et al. Stage IA–IIB Hodgkin's disease: staging and treatment of patients with large mediastinal adenopathy. J Clin Oncol 1989;7:1059–65.

353. Miller TP, Dahlberg S, Weick JK, et al. Unfavorable histologies of non-Hodgkin's lymphoma treated with ProMACE-CytaBOM: a groupwide Southwest Oncology Group study. J Clin Oncol 1990;8:1951–8.

354. Weick JK, Dahlberg S, Fisher RI, et al. Combination chemotherapy of intermediate-grade and high-grade non-Hodgkin's lymphoma with MACOP-B: a Southwest Oncology Group study. J Clin Oncol 1991;9:748–53.

355. Vose JM, Armitage JO, Weisenburger DD, et al. The importance of age in survival of patients treated with chemotherapy for aggressive non-Hodgkin's lymphoma. J Clin Oncol 1988;6:1838–44.

356. d'Amore F, Brincker H, Christensen BE, et al. Non-Hodgkin's lymphoma in the elderly: a study of 602 patients aged 70 or older from a Danish population-based registry. The Danish LYEO-Study Group. Ann Oncol 1992;3:379–86.

357. Coltman CA, Dahlberg S, Jones SE, et al. Southwest Oncology Group studies in diffuse large cell lymphoma: a subset analysis. In: Kimura K, ed. Cancer chemotherapy: challenges for the future. Vol 3. Tokyo: Excerpta Medica, 1988:194–210.

358. Jagannath S, Velasquez WS, Tucker SL, et al. Tumor burden assessment and its implication for a prognostic model in advanced diffuse large-cell lymphoma. J Clin Oncol 1986;4:859–65.

359. Coiffier B, Gisselbrecht C, Vose JM, et al. Prognostic factors in aggressive malignant lymphomas: description and validation of a prognostic index that could identify patients requiring a more intensive therapy: the Groupe d'Etudes des Lymphomes Agressifs. J Clin Oncol 1991;9:211–9.

360. Slymen DJ, Miller TP, Lippman SM, et al. Immunobiologic factors predictive of clinical outcome in diffuse large-cell lymphoma. J Clin Oncol 1990;8:986–93.

361. Danieu L, Wong G, Koziner B, Clarkson B. Predictive model for prognosis in advanced diffuse histiocytic lymphoma. Cancer Res 1986;46:5372–9.

362. Cowan RA, Jones M, Harris M, et al. Prognostic factors in high and intermediate grade non-Hodgkin's lymphoma. Br J Cancer 1989;59:276–82.

363. Bierman HR, Hill BR, Reinhardt L, Emory E. Correlation of serum lactic dehydrogenase activity with the clinical status of patients with cancer, lymphomas, and the leukemias. Cancer Res 1957;17:660–7.

364. Ferraris AM, Giuntini P, Gaetani GF. Serum lactic dehydrogenase as a prognostic tool for non-Hodgkin lymphomas. Blood 1979;54:928–32.

365. Schneider RJ, Seibert K, Passe S, et al. Prognostic significance of serum lactate dehydrogenase in malignant lymphoma. Cancer 1980;46:139–43.

366. Rooney MT. Molecular markers of malignant neoplasms. In: Henry JB, ed. Clinical diagnosis and management by laboratory methods. Philadelphia: WB Saunders, 1991:291

367. Cresswell P, Springer T, Strominger JL, et al. Immunological identity of the small subunit of HL-A antigens and beta2-microglobulin and its turnover on the cell membrane. Proc Natl Acad Sci U S A 1974;72:2123–27.

368. Shuster J, Gold P, Poulik MD. Beta 2-microglogulin levels in cancerous and other disease states. Clin Chem Acta 1976;67:307–13.

369. Hagberg H, Killander A, Simonsson B. Serum B2-microglobulin in malignant lymphoma. Cancer 1983;51:2220–5.

370. Amlot PL, Adinolfi M. B2-microglobulin: a tumour marker of lymphoproliferative disorders. Lancet 1978;2:476.

371. Litam P, Swan F, Cabanillas F, et al. Prognostic value of serum beta-2 microglobulin in low-grade lymphoma. Ann Intern Med 1991;114:855–60.

372. Swan F Jr, Velasquez WS, Tucker S, et al. A new serologic staging system for large-cell lymphomas based on initial beta 2-microglobulin and lactate dehydrogenase levels. J Clin Oncol 1989;7:1518–27.

373. Gerdes J, Schwab U, Lemke H, Stein H. Production of a mouse monoclonal antibody reactive with a human nuclear antigen associated with cell proliferation. Int J Cancer 1983;31:13–20.

374. Gerdes J, Lemke H, Baisch H, et al. Cell cycle analysis of a cell proliferation-associated human nuclear antigen defined by the monoclonal antibody Ki-67. J Immunol 1984;133:1710–5.

375. Klimecki WT, Futscher BW, Grogan TM, Dalton WS. P-glycoprotein expression and function in circulating blood cells from normal volunteers. Blood 1994;83: 2451–8.

376. Grogan TM, Spier CM, Salmon SE, et al. P-glycoprotein expression in human plasma cell myeloma: correlation with prior chemotherapy. Blood 1993;81:490–5.

377. Hoppe RT, Kushlan P, Kaplan HS, et al. The treatment of advanced stage favorable histology non-Hodgkin's lymphoma: a preliminary report of a randomized trial comparing single agent chemotherapy, combination chemotherapy, and whole body irradiation. Blood 1981;58:592–8.

378. Horning SJ. Durable remissions in stage III follicular lymphoma: interpret with caution. J Clin Oncol 1987;5:838–9.

379. Horning SJ, Rosenberg SA. The natural history of initially untreated low-grade non-Hodgkin's lymphomas. N Engl J Med 1984;311:1471–5.

380. Anderson T. Nodular mixed cell lymphoma: is there potential for a prolonged disease free survival and cure? In: Bennett JM, ed. Controversies in the management of lymphomas. Boston: Martinus Nijhoff, 1983:225–38.

381. Glick JH. Nodular mixed lymphoma: failure to demonstrate prolonged disease free survival and cure. In: Bennett JM, ed. Controversies in the management of lymphomas. Boston. Martinus Nijhoff, 1983:239–256.

382. Longo DL, Young RC, Hubbard SM, et al. Prolonged initial remission in patients with nodular mixed lymphoma. Ann Intern Med 1984;100:651–6.

383. Metter GE, Nathwani BN, Burke JS, et al. Morphological subclassification of follicular lymphoma: variability of diagnoses among hematopathologists: a collaborative study between the Repository Center and Pathology Panel for Lymphoma Clinical Studies. J Clin Oncol 1985;3:25–38.

384. Grogan T, Miller T, Fisher R. A Southwest Oncology Group perspective on the revised European-American Lymphoma Classification. Hematol Oncol 1997;11:819–46.

# CHAPTER 89

# LOW-GRADE LYMPHOMA

• NANCY L. BARTLETT • SANDRA J. HORNING

## Natural History

Chapter 88 presents the etiology, biology, pathology, and staging of all non-Hodgkin's lymphomas (NHLs). In this chapter, we briefly review these topics as they apply to low-grade lymphomas, but we focus primarily on prognosis and treatment. Recent advances in the therapy of low-grade lymphoma have included therapeutic monoclonal antibodies and radioimmunotherapy. Despite new therapies, low-grade lymphoma remains a challenging disease. Most patients are never cured with conventional treatment, and they eventually die of their disease.

## EPIDEMIOLOGY AND ETIOLOGY

Physicians diagnosed about 56,800 new cases of NHL in the United States in 1999, with approximately one quarter of these being low-grade lymphomas.[1, 2] The incidence of all subtypes of NHL has increased steadily since the 1940s.[3] The spread of the human immunodeficiency virus and an increase in organ transplantation account for only a small part of this increase.[3] These conditions are associated exclusively with intermediate- and high-grade lymphomas and do not explain the rise in the number of cases of low-grade lymphoma. Many studies have explored the association between occupational and environmental exposures and NHL. Most do not differentiate between the indolent and aggressive lymphomas. One occupational study found a sixfold increased risk of follicular lymphoma for construction workers—specifically painters, carpenters, masons, plumbers, and roofers—and an increased risk of all histologic subtypes of lymphoma for persons exposed to herbicides and pesticides.[4] Other epidemiologic studies suggest an association between follicular NHL and smoking, and between low-grade NHL and a previous history of blood transfusion.[5, 6] The Iowa Women's Health Study confirmed an association between NHL and a diet high in animal fat in older women.[7]

There are strong data to support a causative role for the infectious agent *Helicobacter pylori* in the development of low-grade gastric lymphomas of mucosa-associated lymphoid tissue (MALT).[8–12] These data include (1) the presence of *H. pylori* in the gastric mucosa of more than 90% of patients with gastric MALT lymphomas; (2) a high incidence of gastric lymphoma in areas with a high prevalence of *H. pylori* infection; (3) a case-control study suggesting an association between previous *H. pylori* infection and the development of primary gastric lymphoma; and (4) eradication of *H. pylori* with antibiotics, resulting in complete regression of most gastric MALT lymphomas.[8–12] Additional unidentified antigens may be responsible for the stimulation and growth of other low-grade lymphomas.

## BIOLOGY

Tremendous advances in our understanding of the biology of follicular low-grade lymphomas have occurred since the 1970s. Most low-grade lymphomas are B-cell neoplasms. As do non-neoplastic mature B cells, these lymphomas express immunoglobulin (Ig) on their cell surface. The surface Ig of each clone has a unique heavy and light chain variable region, referred to as the idiotype, which results from Ig gene rearrangements during normal development.[13] Demonstration of light chain–restricted surface Ig or clonal Ig gene rearrangements confirms the diagnosis of B-cell neoplasm in histologically equivocal cases. Most low-grade lymphomas are monoclonal. Rarely, as a result of secondarily acquired mutations in Ig rearrangements, biclonal or multiclonal populations that express different idiotypes can evolve from a common transformed progenitor cell.[14]

The t(14;18) chromosomal translocation is the cytogenetic hallmark of follicular lymphomas, and it occurs in more than 80% of cases.[15] This translocation juxtaposes the oncogene *bcl-2* on chromosome 18 with the Ig heavy chain locus on chromosome 14. Breakpoints occur in well-defined regions; the major breakpoint region (MBR) or minor cluster region (mcr) of the *bcl-2* gene is on chromosome 18, and one of the six joining segments of the heavy chain gene is on chromosome 14.[16] Each individual tumor has a unique junction sequence. The t(14;18) breakpoints have been cloned and sequenced, and they can now be detected by polymerase chain reaction techniques in as few as 1 in $10^5$ cells.[17]

Work by Korsmeyer and others has shown that translocation and deregulation of the *bcl-2* gene interfere with apoptosis or programmed cell death.[18, 19] Tumor cells enter $G_0/G_1$ but do not die. This proposed mechanism of neoplasia may explain both the slow growth rates of most low-grade lymphomas and the mechanism of transformation to more aggressive tumors. Extended cell survival may increase the opportunity of cells to acquire additional genetic defects in growth and proliferation genes or in tumor-suppressor genes.[19]

Additional translocations and genetic abnormalities identified in other low-grade lymphomas, such as the t(11;18) translocation and p53 mutations found in MALT lymphomas, may lead to the discovery of other genetic mechanisms involved in the pathogenesis of lymphoma.[20, 21] It must be hoped that an understanding of the molecular events associated with low-grade lymphoma will eventually lead to better treatments for this disease, just as it has already led to improvements in diagnosis.

## PATHOLOGY AND CLASSIFICATION

In 1994, the International Lymphoma Study Group proposed a new NHL classification system.[22] The Revised European-

American Classification of lymphoid neoplasms (REAL Classification) was developed to describe accurately all subtypes of non-Hodgkin's lymphoma confirmed by currently available morphologic, immunologic, and genetic techniques. The REAL classification expands on the International Working Formulation (IWF), which categorized lymphomas by morphology only.[23] The REAL classification does not use the terms *low-*, *intermediate-*, and *high-grade*. In this chapter, low-grade lymphoma will refer to those subtypes included in the IWF, as well as to the subtypes described in the REAL classification, which have a similar indolent but incurable natural history, primarily the marginal zone lymphomas.

The IWF describes three morphologic subtypes of low-grade lymphoma: (1) small lymphocytic (SL), which is composed of diffuse, small, round lymphocytes or plasmacytoid lymphocytes with uniform nuclear size and shape that efface the normal lymph node architecture; (2) follicular small cleaved cell (FSC), which consists of follicles of small- to medium-sized lymphocytes with irregular, indented nuclei with coarse chromatin; and (3) follicular mixed small cleaved and large cell (FM), which has a mixture of small cleaved cells and large cells with cleaved or noncleaved nuclei in a follicular pattern. Both the FSC and FM lymphomas may contain diffuse areas. The original pathologic criteria for differentiating between FSC and FM lymphoma were descriptive rather than quantitative. By definition, FSC lymphomas were composed "predominantly" of SC cells, and FM lymphomas had a mixture of neoplastic small lymphocytes and larger cells without a significant preponderance of either type. Others have suggested more objective criteria.[24, 25] Warnke and coworkers classified a tumor as FSC when less than 20% of the cells within the nodules were large, and as FM when 20 to 50% of the cells within the nodules were large.[24] Mann and Berard recommended a counting method.[25] Cases of FSC lymphoma should have fewer than five large cells per high-power field averaged over 20 fields, and FM lymphomas should have 5 to 15 large cells per high-power field. However, because of inherent difficulties in determination of both cell size and number, inconsistencies are common in the pathologic subclassification of the follicular lymphomas.[26]

REAL classification changes in the description of the IWF low-grade lymphomas include (1) use of the term *lymphoplasmacytoid lymphoma*, instead of the plasmacytoid variant of small lymphocytic lymphoma, to describe the distinct disorder of small lymphoid cells that show maturation to plasma cells, including most cases of Waldenström's macroglobulinemia and (2) use of the terms *follicle center cell lymphoma, follicular, grades I* (small cell), *II* (mixed small and large cell), and *III* (predominantly large cell) to replace FSC, FM, and follicular large cell, respectively.

Immunophenotypically, small lymphocytic and follicular lymphomas all express the pan–B-cell antigen CD20. The follicular lymphomas also uniformly express common acute lymphoblastic leukemia antigen (CALLA, CD10), and SL lymphomas express the pan–T-cell antigen CD5 but not CD10.[22] Lymphoplasmacytoid lymphomas are usually CD5 negative. CD23 expression is useful in distinguishing SL lymphoma (CD5$^+$, CD23$^+$) from mantle cell lymphoma (CD5$^+$, CD23$^-$).

Not included in the IWF, but described in the REAL classification, are the marginal zone B-cell lymphomas, a small subset of lymphomas with an indolent natural history. Clinically, marginal zone lymphomas have three distinct presentations: primarily extranodal (MALT), nodal, or splenic. All marginal zone lymphomas have similar pathologic features, including small- to medium-sized lymphocytes with abundant, pale-staining cytoplasm, which express CD20, but not CD5 or CD10, and often show plasmacytic differentiation.[22] In epithelial tissues, the lymphocytes infiltrate the epithelium, forming lymphoepithelial lesions. In lymph nodes, the abnormal lymphocytes may have a perisinusoidal, parafollicular, or marginal zone pattern. Splenic marginal zone lymphomas characteristically involve both the mantle and marginal zone of the splenic white pulp and the red pulp.

## CLINICAL FEATURES AND DIAGNOSIS

Low-grade lymphomas are generally a disease of middle-aged and older adults. The most common presentation is painless peripheral lymphadenopathy in an otherwise fit person.[27] A history of several months, or even years, of waxing and waning lymphadenopathy prior to diagnosis is not unusual. Most patients present with advanced-stage disease and bone marrow involvement. B symptoms, which include fevers, night sweats, and weight loss, occur in a minority of patients. Spontaneous regression, lasting for variable periods, occurs in up to 20% of patients, most commonly in the FSC subtype and usually during the first year following diagnosis.[28]

MALT lymphomas (also called MALTomas) typically present as localized stage I or II disease of the stomach or lung.[29] Less common primary sites include salivary glands, thyroid, breast, intestine, and skin. The bone marrow is rarely involved, and if the disease spreads, it is usually to other mucosal sites. Both extranodal and nodal marginal zone lymphomas occur more often in women, and many of these patients have a history of autoimmune disease, such as Sjögren's syndrome or Hashimoto's thyroiditis.[30] Most cases of gastric MALT lymphomas are associated with *H. pylori*. Transformation of low-grade MALT lymphomas may occur. Splenic marginal zone lymphomas present with splenomegaly and often have bone marrow and peripheral blood involvement, without adenopathy.

A precise diagnosis of low-grade lymphoma is made by excisional lymph node biopsy, which allows evaluation of both cell type and architecture. Pathologists are unable to differentiate follicular or nodular from diffuse patterns by fine-needle aspiration (FNA). Sampling errors associated with FNA may also limit determination of the predominant cell type. Repeat biopsies during the course of the disease may be necessary to rule out histologic transformation to an intermediate- or high-grade lymphoma. Clinical indications for repeat biopsy include rapidly progressive adenopathy or extranodal disease or lack of response to therapy. In a Stanford series of initially untreated patients with low-grade lymphoma, at a median follow-up of 50 months, 12% of patients had evidence of histologic transformation.[28] When only patients with repeat biopsies were considered, 44% of patients had transformed disease. Transformation can occur at any point following diagnosis, but the incidence appears to increase with time.

## STAGING

All patients with newly diagnosed low-grade lymphomas should undergo routine staging studies, including: (1) a thorough physical examination with special attention to all peripheral lymph node–bearing areas, liver, and spleen; (2) complete blood count with careful evaluation of the peripheral smear for circulating lymphoma cells; (3) serum chemistry panels, including lactate dehydrogenase (LDH); (4) computed tomography of the chest, abdomen, and pelvis; and (5) a bone marrow biopsy (bilateral for patients with clinical stage I or II disease). Although they are rarely performed outside a few select centers, lymphangiograms may improve the accuracy of staging for the small percentage of patients who appear to have stage I or stage II low-grade lymphoma. Serum $\beta_2$-microglobulin is part of the routine initial evaluation at some centers, and it may have prognostic significance when markedly elevated.

## PROGNOSIS

With the possible exception of a small subset of patients with localized disease, low-grade lymphomas are not curable with standard therapies. The disease responds well to both chemotherapy and radiotherapy, with 50 to 90% of patients achieving a good partial or complete remission with their first course of treatment.[31, 32] However, recurrence is the rule and most patients eventually die of their disease. Median survival with modern therapies is approximately 8 to 10 years.

Figure 89–1 shows the overall actuarial survival curve for 1021 patients with low-grade lymphomas seen at Stanford between 1960 and 1992.[32] Although current therapies are not curative, response to treatment is one of the most important determinants of survival time.[33–35] Gallagher and colleagues reported a 75% 5-year survival for patients with a complete or good partial response to initial therapy, compared with 38% for patients with a poor partial response, or none.[33] Longo and coworkers described a median survival of 13 years for complete responders with FM lymphoma versus 19 months for patients who had a partial response or none.[34]

Kalter and associates reported similar results for patients with FSC lymphoma: a median survival of 13 years for complete responders, and 2 years for patients achieving less than a complete response.[35] The median duration of first remission is 2 to 3 years in most studies, with shorter subsequent remission durations. Prognosis after first relapse depends on the duration of the first remission. More than half of patients with a first complete response lasting longer than 1 year are alive 5 years after relapse, compared with one third of those whose initial remission was less than 1 year.[36]

**Prognosis by Stage.** Extent of disease is an important prognostic factor in all low-grade lymphoma reports. Five- and ten-year relapse-free survivals of 55 to 82% and 44 to 73%, respectively, have been reported for patients with stage I or stage II disease treated with radiation therapy alone or with combined-modality therapy.[37, 38] Long-term failure-free survivals may be higher for young patients with localized disease.[37] Several series show a trend toward improved survival and remission duration in patients with stage III versus stage IV disease, but most do not reach statistical significance.[33, 39] One report demonstrates 5- and 10-year failure-free survival rates of 60% and 40%, respectively, for a selected subset of stage III patients with limited sites of disease.[40]

**Prognosis by Histology.** In the Southwest Oncology Group (SWOG) report of 415 low-grade lymphomas treated with CHOP (cyclophosphamide, doxorubicin, vincristine, and prednisone), FSC lymphoma had a significantly better 10-year survival than did FM or SL lymphoma (40% vs. 31% vs. 23%).[39] Other studies show no difference. For example, the long-term follow-up of 389 patients with low-grade lymphomas included in the IWF Classification Project shows no difference in the duration of complete remission or overall survival for FSC, FM, or SL lymphoma.[41] There was no definite survival plateau in any subgroup. Investigators at M.D. Anderson Cancer Center also found no difference in failure-free or overall survival for patients with stage IV FSC or FM lymphoma treated with CHOP-Bleo (bleomycin).[42]

Some studies have suggested that patients with FM lymphoma may enjoy a prolonged remission duration compared

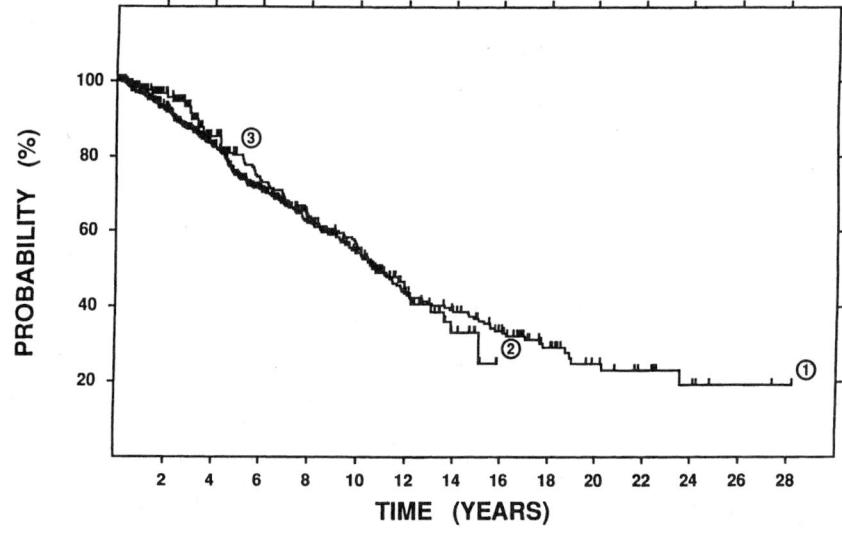

**Figure 89–1.** Actuarial survival of 1021 patients with low-grade lymphoma managed at Stanford University from 1960 to 1992. No difference in survival is seen over the three periods: 1960 to 1975 (1), 1976 to 1986 (2), and 1987 to 1992 (3). (From Horning SJ. Natural history of and therapy for the indolent non-Hodgkin's lymphomas. Semin Oncol 1993;20:suppl 5:77.)

with patients with FSC lymphoma.[33, 34] In these studies, survival curves appear to plateau, implying possible cure for a subset of patients. In the National Cancer Institute (NCI) trial, this was true of only the 24 patients receiving C-MOPP (cyclophosphamide, vincristine, procarbazine, and prednisone), not of those treated with CVP (cyclophosphamide, vincristine, and prednisone).[34] An Eastern Cooperative Oncology Group (ECOG) study failed to confirm durable complete remissions in patients with FM lymphoma treated with the COPP regimen (cyclophosphamide, vincristine, procarbazine, and prednisone).[43] Some of the differences among studies may be attributable to difficulty in making a precise diagnosis. As was mentioned previously, major disagreements exist about the subclassification of follicular lymphomas, regardless of the criteria used to differentiate FSC from FM lymphoma.

MALT and other marginal zone lymphomas have an indolent course, with long-term survival for most patients.[29, 44] Patients with stage III or stage IV MALT lymphoma have a prognosis similar to that of patients with other low-grade lymphomas.[44, 45] The majority of patients with gastric MALT present with stage I or stage II disease and are cured with either antibiotics or local radiotherapy.[12, 46]

**Prognosis After Transformation.** Histologic transformation to an aggressive lymphoma occurs in 10 to 60% of patients with low-grade lymphomas.[28, 47] The wide variation in reported incidence is likely due to differences in the length of follow-up, the number of serial biopsies performed, and whether the incidence is expressed as a percentage of patients having second biopsies or of all patients at risk. Median survivals in most series following transformation are less than 1 year.[33, 47] However, patients with nonbulky, limited-stage disease and no prior chemotherapy have a better prognosis.[48]

**Additional Prognostic Factors.** Several centers have attempted to identify prognostic factors other than stage and response to therapy that separate patients likely to have a more aggressive course from those who might be expected to have an extremely indolent course. Most of these analyses are limited to patients with follicular histology.

Gallagher and coworkers from St. Bartholomew's Hospital identified B symptoms—hepatosplenomegaly, anemia, and elevated liver function tests—as poor prognostic features in 148 patients with follicular lymphomas treated between 1972 and 1984.[33] Romaguera and associates from M.D. Anderson developed a tumor burden model to predict outcome for patients with stage IV follicular low-grade lymphoma.[42] Factors predicting a worse survival included more than one extranodal site, peripheral lymph nodes $\geq 5$ cm, more than 20% marrow involvement, and male sex. Patients with a low tumor burden (one extranodal site, peripheral lymph nodes $<5$ cm, and $<20\%$ marrow involvement) had a 72% 10-year cause-specific survival; patients with a high tumor burden (two or more extranodal sites and peripheral disease $\geq 5$ cm) had a 24% 10-year survival. Ten-year survivals were better for women than men in both the low (92% vs. 37%) and high (50% vs. 0%) tumor burden groups. Another report from this same institution demonstrated the importance of pretreatment $\beta_2$-microglobulin.[49] A level less than 3 mg/L predicted a high complete remission rate and prolonged failure-free survival. Bastion and colleagues identified bone marrow involvement, elevated LDH, $\beta_2$-micro-

globulin greater than 3.0 mg/L, and low serum albumin levels as poor prognostic features in 220 patients with previously untreated follicular lymphoma.[50]

Reports have shown that the International Prognostic Factors Index (IPI), developed for intermediate-grade lymphomas, is also applicable to patients with low-grade lymphomas.[51–53] Age greater than 59 years, performance status greater than 1, stage III or stage IV disease, elevated LDH levels, and more than one extranodal site are independent high-risk features that predict for both response and survival. In one series, no patient who had four or five high-risk features (11%) was alive at 10 years, and only 21% achieved a complete remission with therapy.[52] Use of the IPI and other prognostic factors helps in identifying subsets of patients who may benefit from innovative therapies.

## Treatment

### SURGERY

After the initial excisional biopsy, surgery is rarely indicated in the treatment of low-grade lymphoma. Effective management of NHL no longer requires staging laparotomy and splenectomy. The single exception to this may be the patient with severe hypersplenism, thus precluding safe administration of chemotherapy. Patients with splenic marginal zone NHL often require splenectomy for diagnosis. Surgical treatment of low-grade gastric lymphoma has been replaced by radiation therapy in most patients requiring treatment beyond antibiotics.[46]

### RADIATION THERAPY

Because low-grade lymphoma is almost always a systemic disease, radiation therapy is used less frequently than chemotherapy. The two most common indications for radiation therapy are (1) early-stage disease, for which potential cure is the intent and (2) palliation for local problems in patients with advanced-stage disease. These local problems may include bulky adenopathy, causing discomfort, hydronephrosis, or lymphedema; painful bone lesions; or extranodal disease in a critical location, such as the spinal cord or orbit. Local failure after radiation therapy is uncommon at total doses of 35 to 50 Gy. As was discussed earlier, radiation therapy alone or combined-modality therapy results in a high rate of prolonged remission for patients with localized low-grade lymphoma.[37, 38]

Randomized trials at Stanford University showed no difference in overall or relapse-free survival among advanced-stage patients treated with one of four different options: whole-body irradiation (1.5 Gy) with a 20-Gy boost to involved fields; split-course CVP with total lymphoid irradiation (TLI); single-alkylating-agent therapy; or CVP.[54] Patients tolerated the radical radiotherapy regimens well but continued to relapse. Extensive radiotherapy is rarely used for advanced-stage patients requiring systemic therapy because of concerns regarding prolonged bone marrow suppression and difficulties in administering future treatments. In another report from Stanford, Paryani and coworkers described a small group of patients with limited stage III disease who enjoyed an excellent overall survival (100%) and freedom from relapse (88%) 15 years after treatment with TLI.[40] Limited disease, as defined by fewer than five sites of involvement, adenopathy less than 10 cm, and no B symptoms, applied to only 12% of all stage III patients.

## CHEMOTHERAPY

**Alkylating Agents.** These agents, specifically chlorambucil and cyclophosphamide, have been the mainstay of therapy for low-grade lymphomas for more than three decades. A randomized trial at Stanford showed equivalent results for single-agent oral chlorambucil (0.1 to 0.2 mg/kg/day) or cyclophosphamide (1.5 to 2.5 mg/kg/day), and CVP (cyclophosphamide, 400 mg/m²/day orally days 1 to 5; vincristine, 2 mg intravenously day 1; prednisone, 100 mg/m² orally days 1 to 5; 21-day cycle).[54] The initial complete remission rate was higher for CVP than for single-agent therapy (90% vs. 78%), but the 8-year follow-up showed no difference in overall survival or freedom from relapse. The median time required to achieve a complete response was 12 months for daily single-agent chlorambucil or cyclophosphamide, and 5 months for CVP. Patients were treated for a median of 2 years. There is no benefit of maintenance therapy. It is now our policy to treat for two cycles beyond the best response and then observe.

The choice between single-agent therapy and CVP is somewhat arbitrary. Both are generally well tolerated. An alternative to daily low-dose chlorambucil is pulse chlorambucil (16 mg/m²/day orally days 1 to 5) with or without prednisone every 4 weeks.[55, 56] The advantages of chlorambucil include oral administration, no hair loss, little or no nausea, and minimal acute myelosuppression. This treatment is usually recommended for older patients who are minimally symptomatic or who have other medical problems. Concerns have been raised about the leukemogenic potential and residual marrow injury associated with continuous alkylator exposure.[57] One of 37 patients treated with daily alkylators on randomized trials at Stanford developed acute leukemia.[54] Because the time to complete response may be significantly shorter for CVP compared with daily oral alkylator therapy, we tend to choose CVP for patients who have systemic symptoms, very bulky disease, or disease in a critical location where a prompt response is essential.

**Alkylating Agents plus Doxorubicin.** The initial enthusiasm for adding doxorubicin to induction regimens for low-grade lymphoma has waned. The SWOG reported on 415 patients with low-grade lymphomas treated with CHOP in three different randomized trials.[39] With a median follow-up of 12.8 years, the median survival duration was 6.9 years, with no plateau in the survival curve. The results are comparable to those achieved with single-agent chlorambucil or CVP.[54] LePage and associates compared COPP to COPP plus doxorubicin and found no difference in the complete response rate or freedom from progression.[58] Both SWOG and the NCI tested ProMACE-MOPP (prednisone, methotrexate, doxorubicin, cyclophosphamide, etoposide, mechlorethamine, vincristine, procarbazine, prednisone) as induction therapy for low-grade lymphoma.[59, 60] The NCI trial includes

consolidative TLI following ProMACE-MOPP. Only preliminary results have been reported for these trials.

Outside the setting of a clinical trial, there appears to be no role for doxorubicin-based chemotherapy as initial treatment for low-grade lymphoma. However, doxorubicin is a reasonable alternative for patients refractory to alkylating agents.

**Purine Analogues.** Recent trials of two adenosine analogues, fludarabine phosphate and 2-chlorodeoxyadenosine (2-CdA, cladribine), have shown encouraging results in previously untreated and relapsed low-grade lymphomas.[61–65] The mechanism of action of these compounds is not fully understood. Both accumulate in lymphocytes and are resistant to adenosine deaminase. These agents kill both resting and dividing cells, which is ideal for neoplasms with low growth fractions.[66] Fludarabine and cladribine inhibit DNA synthesis in dividing cells and cause cleavage of DNA into oligonucleosomal fragments in resting cells, which leads to apoptosis.

Fludarabine and 2-CdA have overall response rates of approximately 50% in patients with relapsed or refractory low-grade lymphoma, with 25 to 45% of responses being complete.[61, 62] Single-agent response rates as high as 88% have been reported in previously untreated patients with low-grade NHL.[63, 64] FSC and FM lymphomas respond better than SL lymphomas. Median response duration is less than 6 months for relapsed disease, and 10 to 13 months for previously untreated patients. Time to nadir varies from 7 to 21 days. The standard dose of fludarabine is 25 mg/m² intravenously (IV) daily for 5 days every 4 to 5 weeks, and for 2-CdA, it is 0.1 mg/kg/day as a continuous IV infusion for 7 days every 4 to 5 weeks. To facilitate use of 2-CdA in the outpatient setting, doses of 0.14 mg/kg IV over 2 hours daily for 5 days have also been used.[65]

Results of combination regimens that include purine analogues have also been encouraging. Investigators from M.D. Anderson reported a 94% response rate (47% complete response, 47% partial response) to fludarabine (25 mg/m² IV days 1 to 3), mitoxantrone (10 mg/m² IV day 1), and dexamethasone (20 mg/day IV or PO days 1 to 5) in 51 patients with recurrent or refractory indolent lymphoma.[67] Investigators from ECOG reported results of a Phase II study of cyclophosphamide (600–1000 mg/m²) plus fludarabine (20 mg/m²/day IV days 1 to 5) every 4 weeks in patients with previously untreated follicular lymphoma.[68] The response rate was 100% (89% complete response) with 5-year freedom from progression and overall survival rates of 53% and 66%, respectively.

Myelosuppression and infection are the most significant toxicities associated with purine analogue therapy. Many of the infections are opportunistic, including fungal infections, *Pneumocystis carinii* pneumonia (PCP), cytomegalovirus, and herpes zoster. We recommend PCP prophylaxis for all patients treated with fludarabine or 2-CdA. Myelosuppression can be cumulative and prolonged, thus limiting the administration of further cycles and occasionally affecting the ability of patients to receive alternate therapies. The purine analogues do not cause hair loss, and less than 10% of patients experience nausea and vomiting.

## NO INITIAL THERAPY

Because of the indolent nature of most low-grade lymphomas, and our inability to cure advanced-stage disease with standard therapies, many physicians have adopted a "watch and wait" approach for asymptomatic patients. An initial report from Stanford showed no difference in overall survival for 44 patients who were relatively asymptomatic at presentation and had therapy withheld until required, compared with 112 patients who were treated on randomized clinical trials at the time of diagnosis.[69] Horning and Rosenberg expanded this report to include 83 initially untreated patients, and compared them with 73 protocol-treated patients who on retrospective review could have had therapy delayed.[28] Five-year survivals were identical in the two groups (84%). The median time until treatment was required was 3 years. Therapy was initiated for rapidly progressive or bulky adenopathy, systemic symptoms, anemia, thrombocytopenia, or disease in threatening locations such as the orbit or spinal cord.

NCI investigators randomized 89 patients either to a "watch and wait" approach, in which limited radiation therapy could be administered if necessary, or to aggressive combined-modality treatment with ProMACE-MOPP and TLI.[59] Patients who were initially being watched crossed over when systemic therapy was deemed necessary. Four-year survivals for the two randomized groups were nearly identical (83% vs. 84%). Comparison of disease-free survivals is not meaningful. Sixteen patients (39%) on the "watchful waiting" arm had limited radiation therapy. Median time to crossover was 34 months, with 35% of patients still not requiring chemotherapy at 5 years. The complete response rate was 78% in patients initially randomized to aggressive therapy and 43% in those who crossed over after initial assignment to the watch and wait arm. Four of 41 patients initially treated with ProMACE-MOPP-TLI developed myelodysplastic syndromes. Long-term follow-up of this study has never been published.

A more recent randomized trial comparing no initial treatment to single-agent prednimustine or single-agent interferon, in 193 patients with "low-tumor-burden" follicular lymphomas, showed no difference in 5-year overall survival among the three arms.[70] The median freedom-from-treatment interval was 2 years in the deferred treatment arm. The median time to second progression and the response rates at progression were the same for the three arms. Deferral of treatment did not seem to decrease response rates and survival after progression.

For selected, asymptomatic patients not participating in clinical studies, a watch and wait approach is appropriate. Watchful waiting requires close follow-up, at least bimonthly the first year and quarterly thereafter, to better understand the disease tempo in each patient and to intervene before serious problems arise. It has been our experience that, psychologically, most patients handle this approach well if they are informed of the supporting data.

## BONE MARROW TRANSPLANTATION

Because standard therapies have not been curative, bone marrow transplantation and peripheral blood stem cell transplantation (SCT) have both been tested for recurrent or refractory low-grade lymphoma. Realistically, this form of therapy is usually limited to patients younger than 65 years, which excludes more than half of patients with low-grade

lymphomas. There are no randomized trials of standard therapy versus high-dose therapy for relapsed low-grade lymphoma.

Several centers report extended disease-free survivals with high-dose therapy compared with historical controls treated with conventional therapy.[71–74] With median follow-up periods ranging from 5 to 8 years, the 5-year failure-free survivals range from 48% to 63% with autologous transplant.[71, 72] There is no definite evidence of a plateau in disease-free survival or of improvement in overall survival with high-dose therapy. Most patients in these trials represent a highly select group of young patients with an excellent performance status, who had achieved a complete response or minimal disease state with standard therapies. With improvements in supportive care, the mortality rate of autologous SCT is less than 5% in most series. A recent analysis from St. Bartholomew's Hospital suggests that treatment with high-dose therapy does not compromise outcome in patients who relapse after transplant.[75] Failure-free survivals with autologous transplant are significantly shorter in patients receiving more than two chemotherapy regimens before transplantation compared with those receiving one or two regimens.[73] Based on available data, it is reasonable to consider autologous transplantation for young patients in first or second relapse, with the understanding that it may not have an impact on overall survival.

A few small series on allogeneic transplantation for patients with relapsed low-grade lymphoma have been published.[76–78] Two single-institution studies each report on 10 extensively pretreated patients with recurrent low-grade lymphoma undergoing allogeneic transplantation.[76, 77] Two-year progression-free survivals were 68% and 80% percent, with two of 10, and three of 10 toxic deaths, respectively. Fifty centers participating in the International Bone Marrow Transplant Registry reported on 115 patients treated with allogeneic bone marrow transplantation for advanced low-grade lymphoma.[78] Three-year probabilities of recurrence and treatment-related mortality were 16% and 40%, respectively. Three-year probabilities of survival and disease-free survival were both 49%, with only one recurrence among 33 patients monitored for longer than 2 years. These low recurrence rates may be due to graft-versus-lymphoma effect or to lack of tumor contamination in the graft. Allogeneic transplantation may represent the first potentially curative therapy for low-grade lymphoma. However, given the high procedure-related mortality, currently this treatment should be recommended only to patients with symptomatic, refractory disease, or those with evidence of transformation or rapid progression following conventional therapy.

## BIOTHERAPY

**Interferon.** Phase II trials of single-agent human and recombinant interferon-α (INF) in both previously untreated and relapsed low-grade lymphomas have shown response rates of 30 to 70%.[70, 79, 80] Doses in these trials ranged from 1 million units (MU) daily to 50 MU/m² three times per week. The duration of therapy ranged from 4 weeks to 18 months. Responses were often slow, with at least one documented response occurring 3.5 months following completion of therapy.[80] No study documented a clear dose-response relationship, but most toxicities were dose dependent. Fever, chills, and myalgias occurred in the majority of patients but often subsided with continued treatment. Fatigue and anorexia were common with long-term therapy. Ninety percent of patients treated with 50 MU/m² three times weekly required dose reductions secondary to unacceptable side effects.[79] The highest reported response rates were seen in a trial of previously untreated patients with low tumor burden treated with 5 MU/day for 3 months, followed by 5 MU three times per week for 15 months.[70] The response rate was 70%, with 42% complete responses. Median time to progression was 35 months from the start of treatment.

The use of chemotherapy plus interferon as induction therapy, or maintenance interferon after chemotherapy, remains controversial. Several randomized trials testing chemotherapy with and without INF have reported conflicting results. Direct comparison of these studies is difficult because patient selection, chemotherapy regimens, and INF dose and schedule vary in each trial. Preliminary results of two large cooperative group trials showed no improvement in time to relapse or survival.[60, 81] Other studies have shown a prolonged time to progression with INF compared with chemotherapy alone, but no difference in overall survival.[82] Until recently, no study had shown a survival advantage. Because of the side effects and cost associated with INF, the possibility of a modest increase in remission duration without a survival advantage has not been enough for most physicians in the United States to incorporate this into the standard treatment of low-grade lymphoma. Results of selected trials are summarized in the following section.

**Trials with no Clinical Benefit.** The SWOG reported on 571 previously untreated low-grade lymphoma patients randomized to ProMACE-MOPP followed by INF or observation.[60] Complete and partial responders to ProMACE-MOPP were randomized to INF, 2 MU/m² three times per week for 24 months versus observation. With a median follow-up of 4.1 years, there was no difference in progression-free or overall survival. Preliminary results of an intergroup randomized trial of cyclophosphamide (100 mg/m² daily) with INF (2 MU three times per week) show no difference in response rate (89% vs. 84%) or time to relapse or death.[81] Treatment continued for 3 months past the best response. Toxicities were greater in the INF arm.

**Trials with Prolonged Time to Progression.** The European Organization for Research on the Treatment of Cancer (EORTC) randomized 331 patients to eight cycles of CVP and consolidative radiation therapy followed by 12 months of maintenance INF (3 MU three times per week) or observation.[82] Progression-free survival was prolonged in the interferon arm (median, 137 vs. 87 weeks), but there was no difference in overall survival. Price and colleagues reported on 160 previously untreated stage III to stage IV patients randomized to chlorambucil with INF (2 MU three times per week).[83] Responders were then randomized to maintenance INF or no maintenance. There was no difference in response rates or overall survival between treatment groups. Patients who received INF, both as induction and maintenance, had a significantly longer duration of response.

**Trials with Improved Survival.** ECOG randomized 291 patients with "clinically aggressive" low-grade lymphoma to eight cycles of COPA (cyclophosphamide, vincristine, prednisone, and doxorubicin) with or without INF (6 MU/m²

days 22 to 26 of a 28-day cycle).[84] Because of increased leukopenia, patients in the INF arm (I-COPA) received an average of 75% of the ideal cyclophosphamide and doxorubicin doses, compared with 95% in the COPA alone arm. The two regimens produced comparable objective response rates (86%), but the patients treated with INF had a prolonged time to treatment failure, duration of complete response, and overall survival. An update of this trial showed a median survival of 5.7 years for the COPA group and 7.8 years for the I-COPA group ($p = 0.04$). A Groupe D'Études des Lymphomes de l'Adulte (GELA) trial randomized 268 patients with advanced follicular lymphoma to CHVP alone (cyclophosphamide, doxorubicin, VM-26, and prednisone in 12 cycles over 18 months) or to CHVP with concomitant INF (5 MU three times per week).[85] There were higher response rates (85% vs. 69%) and a significantly longer disease-free and overall survival for the INF arm. The 5-year overall survival rate was 56.4% for the CHVP group versus 70.5% in the CHVP plus INF group.

Interestingly, the two trials that showed a survival benefit with the addition of INF were the only studies that used both an anthracycline-containing chemotherapy regimen and concomitant administration of INF. In addition, these two studies enrolled only patients who were believed to have clinically aggressive low-grade lymphoma. These factors raise the possibility that perhaps a synergy between doxorubicin and INF could explain the improved outcome in these two studies, compared with other randomized trials. Alternatively, the benefits of INF may be greater in patients with bulky, symptomatic disease than in those with a low tumor burden.

**Monoclonal Antibodies.** Initial monoclonal antibody (mAb) trials in lymphoma targeted the unique (idiotypic) variable region of the surface immunoglobulin on each B-cell lymphoma.[86] Despite initial enthusiasm engendered by anti-idiotypic antibodies, they are not a practical target for widespread use in lymphoma owing to prolonged production time, emergence of idiotype variants during treatment, high serum levels of idiotype protein, and development of human anti-mouse antibodies (HAMAs).[86, 87]

More recently, efforts have been directed at developing mAbs against pan-lymphocyte antigens such as CD20 and CDw52.[88–90] Although these mAbs also destroy normal lymphocytes, as long as the stem cell compartment is not damaged, normal lymphocytes will be replaced after treatment. In addition to new targets, genetic engineering techniques have resulted in the development of both chimeric and humanized mAbs. Chimeric mAbs contain a human constant region and a mouse variable region, and humanized mAbs have human constant and variable domains, with only mouse hypervariable regions.[91] These modified proteins interact more effectively with the human immune system, and HAMA responses are rare.

**Rituximab.** A chimeric monoclonal antibody directed against the pan–B-cell antigen CD20, rituximab is the first FDA-approved therapeutic monoclonal antibody. Phase II studies have shown response rates of 50% in patients with relapsed low-grade lymphoma.[92] Median remission duration is 10 to 12 months, and approximately half of previous responders will respond to a second course at the time of relapse. Follicular histologies respond better than do small lymphocytic lymphomas, and patients with tumors greater than 7 cm have lower response rates. Standard therapy is 375 mg/m² by slow IV infusion, once a week for 4 weeks. Toxicities are mild and are limited primarily to infusion-related reactions such as fevers, chills, myalgias, transient hypotension, and rarely bronchospasm. Trials are under way to better define the optimal dose and schedule of rituximab.

Based on in vitro studies demonstrating that the anti-CD20 monoclonal antibody potentiates the sensitivity of a lymphoma cell line to several cytotoxic agents,[93] Czuczman and colleagues tested the combination of rituximab and CHOP chemotherapy in patients with low-grade lymphoma.[94] Forty patients (31 previously untreated) received six infusions of rituximab and six cycles of CHOP, with an overall response rate of 95%. At a median follow-up of 29 months, 75% of patients remained in remission. While results are encouraging, this regimen should be tested against standard therapy in a randomized trial.

**Radiolabeled Monoclonal Antibodies.** mAbs conjugated with radioisotopes have potential advantages over mAbs alone. Radiolabeled antibodies introduce a second modality of therapy, which does not depend on the host immune system for activity. In addition, the radioisotope may kill cells up to 10 mm away from the target cell, potentially addressing the problems of antigen-negative cells and inhomogeneous deposition of antibody. Two approaches to the use of radiolabeled antibody in relapsed low-grade lymphoma have been reported. First, the use of myeloablative doses of iodine 131–anti-CD20 antibody with bone marrow or peripheral stem cell rescue resulted in an 86% response rate in 29 patients.[95] With a median follow-up of 42 months, the estimated overall and progression-free survivals were 68% and 42%, respectively. Encouraging results of nonmyeloablative radioimmunotherapy have also been reported. Response rates of approximately 80% have been achieved with ¹³¹I–anti-CD20 mAb and yttrium 90–anti-CD20 mAb.[96, 97] Side effects have been modest and self-limited. Although rituximab and nonmyeloablative radioimmunotherapy do not represent curative therapies for low-grade lymphoma, they are important advances in its treatment.

## COMBINED-MODALITY THERAPY

No studies have shown a clear benefit of combined-modality therapy in the treatment of low-grade lymphoma. Early trials of CVP plus TLI versus CVP alone showed no difference in response rates or survival.[54] Two nonrandomized trials suggested an improved disease-free survival with radiation therapy plus adjuvant chemotherapy for patients with early-stage low-grade lymphomas, compared with historical controls treated with radiation therapy alone.[38, 98] Currently, many autologous and allogeneic bone marrow transplantation trials for low-grade lymphoma use combined-modality therapy with total-body irradiation and high-dose chemotherapy.

## TREATMENT BY STAGE OF DISEASE

**Stages I and II.** Radiation is still the principal treatment modality for patients with limited-stage disease. Stanford investigators reported on 177 patients with stage I or stage II follicular lymphoma treated with TLI, or extended-field or involved-field radiation therapy. The 10- and 20-year relapse-free survivals were 44% and 37%, respectively.[37] Only 5 of 47 patients who reached 10 years without relapse subsequently developed recurrence. Freedom from relapse was significantly better for patients younger than 60 years than for those older than age 60 (Fig. 89–2). Figure 89–3 shows the overall survival of patients with stage I to stage II follicular lymphoma compared with age- and sex-matched controls.

Two nonrandomized trials from the M.D. Anderson Cancer Center and St. Bartholomew's Hospital showed improved relapse-free survival with involved-field radiation therapy and adjuvant chemotherapy, either CVP or CHOP-Bleo.[38, 98] Seymour and associates reported a 10-year freedom from relapse of 73% in 91 patients treated with COP/CHOP-Bleo and involved-field radiation therapy.[38]

Outside the setting of a clinical trial, we recommend 35 to 45 Gy regional radiotherapy for patients found to have

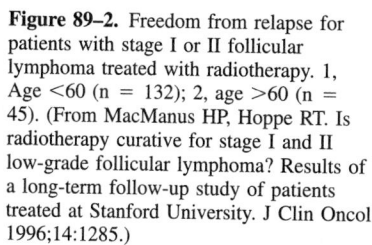

**Figure 89–2.** Freedom from relapse for patients with stage I or II follicular lymphoma treated with radiotherapy. 1, Age <60 (n = 132); 2, age >60 (n = 45). (From MacManus HP, Hoppe RT. Is radiotherapy curative for stage I and II low-grade follicular lymphoma? Results of a long-term follow-up study of patients treated at Stanford University. J Clin Oncol 1996;14:1285.)

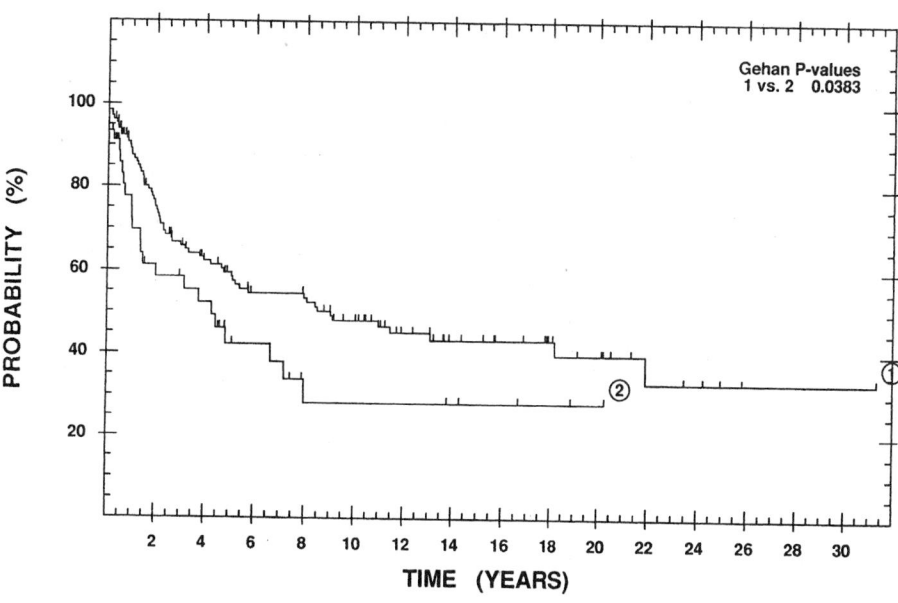

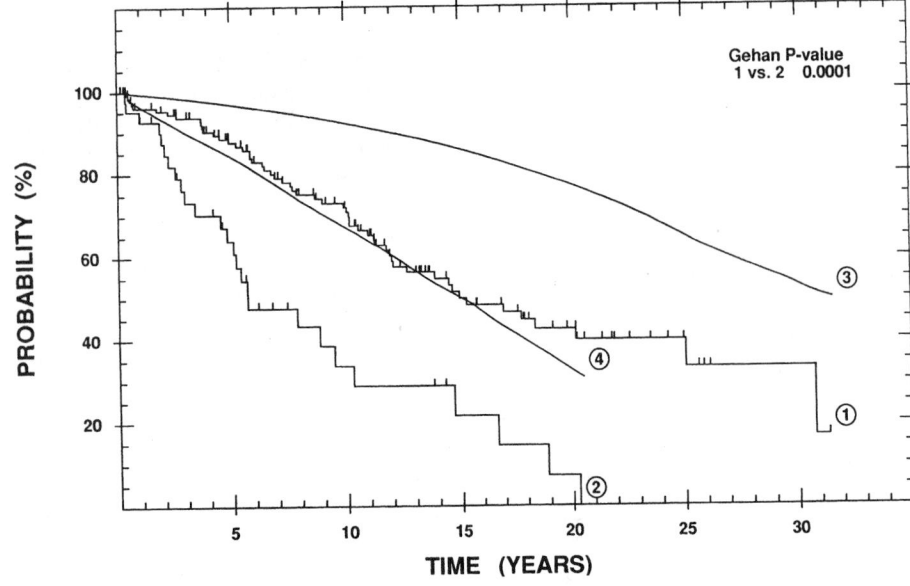

**Figure 89–3.** Survival for patients with stage I or II follicular lymphoma treated with radiotherapy compared with age- and sex-matched controls. 1, Age <60 (n = 132); 2, age ≥60 (n = 45); 3, controls <60 (n = 132); 4, controls ≥60 (n = 45). (From MacManus HP, Hoppe RT. Is radiotherapy curative for stage I and II low-grade follicular lymphoma? Results of a long-term follow-up study of patients treated at Stanford University. J Clin Oncol 1996;14:1284.)

stage I or stage II disease after careful clinical staging, including bilateral bone marrow biopsies and a lymphangiogram. The use of combined-modality therapy in this setting is also reasonable. For most patients with stage I gastric MALT, involved-field radiotherapy results in long-term remission.[46]

**Stages III and IV.** Previous sections outline in detail the treatment options for advanced-stage disease. Asymptomatic patients can be observed without treatment until symptoms develop or until problems related to disease progression appear imminent. Single-agent alkylators or CVP remains the first-line regimen when patients require therapy. Consideration should be given to entering patients into ongoing clinical trials of radioimmunotherapy or combination immunotherapy and chemotherapy.

## SUGGESTIONS FOR ADDITIONAL READING

Harris NL, Jaffe ES, Stein H, et al. A revised European-American classification of lymphoid neoplasms: a proposal from the International Lymphoma Study Group. Blood 1994;84:1361–92. *Concise summary of the new REAL lymphoma classification system with a brief description of both clinical and pathologic characteristics of each lymphoma subtype.*

Horning SJ. Natural history of and therapy for the indolent non-Hodgkin's lymphomas. Semin Oncol 1993;20:Suppl 5:75–88. *Comprehensive review of therapy for low-grade lymphoma.*

Brice P, Bastion Y, Lepage E, et al. Comparison in low-tumor-burden follicular lymphomas between an initial no-treatment policy, prednimustine, or interferon alfa: a randomized study from the Groupe D'Etude des Lymphomes Folliculaires. J Clin Oncol 1997;15:1110–17. *Recent randomized trial that supports continued use of the "watch and wait" approach in low-risk patients with low-grade lymphoma.*

Lopez-Guillermo A, Montserrat E, Bosch F, et al. Applicability of the International Index for aggressive lymphomas to patients with low-grade lymphoma. J Clin Oncol 1994;12:1343–8.

Maloney DG, Grillo-Lopez AJ, Bodkin DJ, et al. IDEC-C2B8: results of a phase I multiple-dose trial in patients with relapsed non-Hodgkin's lymphoma. J Clin Oncol 1997;15:3266–74.

## REFERENCES

1. Landis SH, Murray T, Bolden S, et al. Cancer statistics, 1999. CA Cancer J Clin 1999;49:8–31.
2. Greiner TC, Medeiros LJ, Jaffe ES. Non-Hodgkin's lymphoma. Cancer 1995;75:Suppl 1:370–80.
3. Hartge P, Devesa SS. Quantification of the impact of known risk factors on time trends in non-Hodgkin's lymphoma incidence. Cancer Res 1992;52:Suppl 19:5566s–9s.
4. Scherr PA, Hutchison GB, Neiman RS. Non-Hodgkin's lymphoma and occupational exposure. Cancer Res 1992;52:Suppl 19:5503s–9s.
5. Herrinton LJ, Friedman GD. Cigarette smoking and risk of non-Hodgkin's lymphoma subtypes. Cancer Epidemiol Biomarkers Prev 1998;7:25–8.
6. Brandt L, Brandt J, Olsson H, et al. Blood transfusion as a risk factor for non-Hodgkin's lymphoma. Br J Cancer 1996;73:1148–51.
7. Chiu BCH, Cerhan JR, Folsom AR, et al. Diet and risk of non-Hodgkin's lymphoma in older women. JAMA 1996;275:1315–21.
8. Wotherspoon AC, Ortiz-Hidalgo C, Falzon MR, et al. *Helicobacter pylori*–associated gastritis and primary B-cell gastric lymphoma. Lancet 1991;338:1175–6.
9. Parsonnet J, Hansen S, Rodriguez L, et al. *Helicobacter pylori* infection and gastric lymphoma. N Engl J Med 1994;330:1267–71.
10. Wotherspoon AC, Doglioni C, Diss TC, et al. Regression of primary low-grade B-cell gastric lymphoma of mucosa-associated lymphoid tissue type after eradication of *Helicobacter pylori*. Lancet 1993;342:575–7.
11. Roggero E, Zucca E, Pinotti G, et al. Eradication of *Helicobacter pylori* infection in primary low-grade gastric lymphoma of mucosa-associated lymphoid tissue. Ann Intern Med 1995;122:767–9.
12. Neubauer A, Thiede C, Morgner A, et al. Cure of *Helicobacter pylori* infection and duration of remission of low-grade gastric mucosa–associated lymphoid tissue lymphoma. J Natl Cancer Inst 1997;89:1350–5.
13. Cooper MD. Current concepts. B-lymphocytes. Normal development and function. N Engl J Med 1987;317:1452–6.
14. Cleary ML, Galili N, Trela M, et al. Single cell origin of bigenotypic and biphenotypic B-cell proliferations in human follicular lymphomas. J Exp Med 1988;167:582–97.
15. Yunis JJ, Frizzera G, Oken MM, et al. Multiple recurrent genomic defects in follicular lymphoma. A possible model for cancer. N Engl J Med 1987;316:79–84.
16. Cotter FE, Price C, Meerabux J, et al. Direct sequence analysis of 14q+ and 18q− chromosome junctions at the MBR and MCR revealing clustering within the MBR in follicular lymphoma. Ann Oncol 1991;2:Suppl 2:93–7.
17. Crescenzi M, Seto M, Herzig GP, et al. Thermostable DNA polymerase chain amplification of t(14;18) chromosome breakpoints and detection of minimal residual disease. Proc Natl Acad Sci USA 1988;85:4869–73.
18. Hockenbery D, Nunez G, Milliman C, et al. Bcl-2 is an inner mitochondrial membrane protein that blocks programmed cell death. Nature 1990;348:334–6.

19. Korsmeyer SJ. Bcl-2 initiates a new category of oncogenes: regulators of cell death. Blood 1992;80:879–86.
20. Auer IA, Gascoyne RD, Connors JM, et al. t(11;18) (q21;q21) is the most common translocation in MALT lymphomas. Ann Oncol 1997;8:979–85.
21. Du M, Peng H, Singh N, et al. The accumulation of p53 abnormalities is associated with progression of mucosa-associated lymphoid tissue lymphoma. Blood 1995;86:4587–93.
22. Harris NL, Jaffe ES, Stein H, et al. A revised European-American classification of lymphoid neoplasms: a proposal from the International Lymphoma Study Group. Blood 1994;84:1361–92.
23. The Non-Hodgkin's Lymphoma Pathologic Classification Project. National Cancer Institute sponsored study of classifications of non-Hodgkin's lymphomas. Cancer 1982;49:2112–35.
24. Warnke RA, Kim H, Fuks Z, et al. The coexistence of nodular and diffuse patterns in nodular non-Hodgkin's lymphomas: significance and clinicopathologic correlation. Cancer 1977;40:1229–33.
25. Mann RB, Berard CW. Criteria for the cytologic subclassification of follicular lymphomas: a proposed alternative method. Hematol Oncol 1983;1:187–92.
26. Metter GE, Nathwani BN, Burke JS, et al. Morphological subclassification of follicular lymphoma: variability of diagnoses among hematopathologists, a collaborative study between the Repository Center and Pathology Panel for Lymphoma Clinical Studies. J Clin Oncol 1985;3:25–38.
27. Rohatiner AZ, Lister TA. New approaches to the treatment of follicular lymphoma. Br J Haematol 1991;79:349–54.
28. Horning SJ, Rosenberg SA. The natural history of initially untreated low-grade non-Hodgkin's lymphomas. N Engl J Med 1984;311:1471–5.
29. Thieblemont C, Berger F, Coiffier B. Mucosa-associated lymphoid tissue lymphomas. Curr Opin Oncol 1995;7:415–20.
30. Royer B, Cazals-Hatem D, Sibilia J, et al. Lymphomas in patients with Sjogren's syndrome are marginal zone B-cell neoplasms, arise in diverse extranodal and nodal sites, and are not associated with viruses. Blood 1997;90:766–75.
31. Johnson PWM, Rohatiner AZS, Whelan JS, et al. Patterns of survival in patients with recurrent follicular lymphoma: a 20-year study from a single center. J Clin Oncol 1995;13:140–7.
32. Horning SJ. Natural history of and therapy for the indolent non-Hodgkin's lymphomas. Semin Oncol 1993;20:Suppl 5:75–88.
33. Gallagher CJ, Gregory WM, Jones AE, et al. Follicular lymphoma: prognostic factors for response and survival. J Clin Oncol 1986;4:1470–80.
34. Longo DL, Young RC, Hubbard SM, et al. Prolonged initial remission in patients with nodular mixed lymphoma. Ann Intern Med 1984;100:651–6.
35. Kalter S, Holmes L, Cabanillas F. Long-term results of treatment of patients with follicular lymphomas. Hematol Oncol 1987;5:127–38.
36. Weisdorf DJ, Andersen JW, Glick JH, et al. Survival after relapse of low-grade non-Hodgkin's lymphoma: implications for marrow transplantation. J Clin Oncol 1992;10:942–7.
37. MacManus MP, Hoppe RT. Is radiotherapy curative for stage I and II low-grade follicular lymphoma? Results of a long-term follow-up study of patients treated at Stanford University. J Clin Oncol 1996;14:1282–90.
38. Seymour JF, McLaughlin R, Fuller LM, et al. High rate of prolonged remissions following combined modality therapy for patients with localized low-grade lymphoma. Ann Oncol 1996;7:157–63.
39. Dana BW, Dahlberg S, Nathwani BN, et al. Long-term follow-up of patients with low-grade malignant lymphomas treated with doxorubicin-based chemotherapy or chemoimmunotherapy. J Clin Oncol 1993;11:644–51.
40. Paryani SB, Hoppe RT, Cox RS, et al. The role of radiation therapy in the management of stage III follicular lymphomas. J Clin Oncol 1984;2:841–8.
41. Simon R, Durrleman S, Hoppe RT, et al. The Non-Hodgkin Lymphoma Pathologic Classification Project. Long-term follow-up of 1153 patients with non-Hodgkin lymphomas. Ann Intern Med 1988;109:939–45.
42. Romaguera JE, McLaughlin P, North L, et al. Multivariate analysis of prognostic factors in stage IV follicular low-grade lymphoma: a risk model. J Clin Oncol 1991;9:762–9.
43. Glick JH, Barnes JM, Ezdinli EZ, et al. Nodular mixed lymphoma: results of a randomized trial failing to confirm prolonged disease-free survival with COPP chemotherapy. Blood 1981;58:920–5.
44. Fisher RI, Dahlberg S, Nathwani BN, et al. A clinical analysis of two indolent lymphoma entities: mantle cell lymphoma and marginal zone lymphoma (including the mucosa-associated lymphoid tissue and monocytoid B-cell subcategories): a Southwest Oncology Group study. Blood 1995;85:1075–82.
45. Montalban C, Castrillo JM, Abraira V, et al. Gastric B-cell mucosa-associated lymphoid tissue (MALT) lymphoma. Clinicopathological study and evaluation of the prognostic factors in 143 patients. Ann Oncol 1995;6:355–62.
46. Schechter NR, Portlock CS, Yahalom J. Treatment of mucosa-associated lymphoid tissue lymphoma of the stomach with radiation alone. J Clin Oncol 1998;16:1916–21.
47. Bastion Y, Sebban C, Berger F, et al. Incidence, predictive factors, and outcome of lymphoma transformation in follicular lymphoma patients. J Clin Oncol 1997;15:1587–94.
48. Yuen AR, Kamel OW, Halpern J, et al. Long-term survival after histologic transformation of low grade follicular lymphoma. J Clin Oncol 1995;13:1726–33.
49. Litam P, Swan F, Cabanillas F, et al. Prognostic value of serum beta-2 microglobulin in low-grade lymphoma. Ann Intern Med 1991;114:855–60.
50. Bastion Y, Berger F, Salles G, et al. Prognostic factors in follicular lymphomas: a retrospective analysis of 220 patients. Proc ASCO 1993;12:362. abstract.
51. The International Non-Hodgkin's Lymphoma Prognostic Factors Project. A predictive model for aggressive non-Hodgkin's lymphoma. N Engl J Med 1993;329:987–94.
52. Lopez-Guillermo A, Montserrat E, Bosch F, et al. Applicability of the International Index for aggressive lymphomas to patients with low-grade lymphoma. J Clin Oncol 1994;12:1343–8.
53. Hermans J, Krol ADG, van Groningen K, et al. International Prognostic Index for aggressive non-Hodgkin's lymphoma is valid for all malignancy grades. Blood 1995;86:1460–3.
54. Hoppe RT, Kushlan P, Kaplan HS, et al. The treatment of advanced stage favorable histology non-Hodgkin's lymphoma: a preliminary report of a randomized trial comparing single agent chemotherapy, combination chemotherapy, and whole body irradiation. Blood 1981;58:592–8.
55. Portlock CS, Fischer DS, Cadman E, et al. High-dose pulse chlorambucil in advanced, low-grade non-Hodgkin's lymphoma. Cancer Treat Rep 1987;71:1029–31.
56. Cadman E, Drislane F, Waldron JA Jr, et al. High-dose pulse chlorambucil: effective therapy for rapid remission induction in nodular lymphocytic poorly differentiated lymphoma. Cancer 1982;50:1037–41.
57. Greene MH, Young RC, Merrill JM, et al. Evidence of a treatment dose response in acute nonlymphocytic leukemias which occur after therapy of non-Hodgkin's lymphoma. Cancer Res 1983;43:1891–8.
58. LePage E, Sebban C, Gisselbrecht C, et al. Treatment of low-grade non-Hodgkin's lymphomas: assessment of doxorubicin in a controlled trial. Hematol Oncol 1990;8:31–9.
59. Young RC, Longo DL, Glatstein E, et al. The treatment of indolent lymphomas: watchful waiting v aggressive combined modality treatment. Semin Hematol 1988;25:Suppl 2:11–6.
60. Fisher RI, Dana BW, LeBlanc M, et al. Interferon alfa consolidation after intensive chemotherapy does not prolong progression-free survival of patients with low-grade non-Hodgkin's lymphoma: results of the Southwest Oncology Group randomized Phase III study 8809. J Clin Oncol 2000;18:2010–16.
61. Hochster HS, Kim KM, Green MD, et al. Activity of fludarabine in previously treated non-Hodgkin's low-grade lymphoma: results of an Eastern Cooperative Oncology Group study. J Clin Oncol 1992;10:28–32.
62. Kay AC, Saven A, Carrera CJ, et al. 2-Chlorodeoxyadenosine treatment of low-grade lymphomas. J Clin Oncol 1992;10:371–7.
63. Saven A, Emanuele S, Kosty M, et al. 2-Chlorodeoxyadenosine activity in patients with untreated, indolent non-Hodgkin's lymphoma. Blood 1995;86:1710–6.
64. Solal-Celigny P, Brice P, Brousse N, et al. Phase II trial of fludarabine monophosphate as first-line treatment in patients with advanced follicular lymphoma: a multicenter study by the Groupe D'Etude des Lymphomes de l'Adulte. J Clin Oncol 1996;14:514–9.
65. Tulpule A, Schiller G, Harvey-Buchanan LA, et al. Cladribine in the treatment of advanced relapsed or refractory low and intermediate grade non-Hodgkin's lymphoma. Cancer 1998;83:2370–6.
66. Saven A, Piro LD. 2-Chlorodeoxyadenosine: a newer purine analog active in the treatment of indolent lymphoid malignancies. Ann Intern Med 1994;120:784–91.

67. McLaughlin P, Hagemeister FB, Romaguera JE, et al. Fludarabine, mitoxantrone, and dexamethasone: an effective new regimen for indolent lymphoma. J Clin Oncol 1996;14:1262–8.
68. Hochster HS, Oken MM, Winter JN, et al. Phase I study of fludarabine plus cyclophosphamide in patients with previously untreated low grade lymphoma: results and the long-term follow-up—a report from the Eastern Cooperative Oncology Group. J Clin Oncol 1999;18:987–94.
69. Portlock CS, Rosenberg SA. No initial therapy for stage III and IV non-Hodgkin's lymphomas of favorable histologic types. Ann Intern Med 1979;90:10–3.
70. Brice P, Bastion Y, Lepage E, et al. Comparison in low-tumor-burden follicular lymphomas between an initial no-treatment policy, prednimustine, or interferon alfa: a randomized study from the Groupe D'Etude des Lymphomes Folliculaires. J Clin Oncol 1997;15:1110–7.
71. Freedman AS, Neuberg D, Mauch P, et al. Long-term follow-up of autologous bone marrow transplantation in patients with relapsed follicular lymphoma. Blood 1999;94:3325–33.
72. Apostolidis J, Gupta RR, Grenzelias D, et al. High-dose therapy with autologous bone marrow support as consolidation of remission in follicular lymphoma: long-term clinical and molecular follow-up. J Clin Oncol 2000;18:527–36.
73. Bierman PJ, Vose JM, Anderson JR, et al. High-dose therapy with autologous hematopoietic rescue for follicular low-grade non-Hodgkin's lymphoma. J Clin Oncol 1997;15:445–50.
74. Bastion Y, Brice P, Haioun C, et al. Intensive therapy with peripheral blood progenitor cell transplantation in 60 patients with poor-prognosis follicular lymphoma. Blood 1995;86:3257–62.
75. Apostolidis J, Foran JM, Johnson PWM, et al. Patterns of outcome following recurrence after myeloablative therapy with autologous bone marrow transplantation for follicular lymphoma. J Clin Oncol 1999;17:216–21.
76. van Besien KW, Khouri IF, Giralt SA, et al. Allogeneic bone marrow transplantation for refractory and recurrent low-grade lymphoma: the case for aggressive management. J Clin Oncol 1995;13:1096–1102.
77. Verdonck LF, Dekker AW, Lokhorst HM, et al. Allogeneic versus autologous bone marrow transplantation for refractory and recurrent low-grade non-Hodgkin's lymphoma. Blood 1997;90:4201–5.
78. van Besien K, Sobocinski KA, Rowlings PA, et al. Allogeneic bone marrow transplantation for low-grade lymphoma. Blood 1998;92:1832–6.
79. Foon KA, Sherwin SA, Abrams PG, et al. Treatment of advanced non-Hodgkin's lymphoma with recombinant leukocyte A interferon. N Engl J Med 1984;311:1148–52.
80. Horning SJ, Merigan TC, Krown SE, et al. Human interferon alpha in malignant lymphoma and Hodgkin's disease. Results of the American Cancer Society trial. Cancer 1985;56:1305–10.
81. Peterson BA, Petroni GR, Oken MM, et al. Cyclophosphamide versus cyclophosphamide plus interferon alfa-2b in follicular low-grade lymphomas: an intergroup phase III trial (CALGB 8691 and EST 7486). Proc Am Soc Clin Oncol 1997;16:14a. abstract.
82. Hagenbeek A, Carde P, Meerwaldt JH, et al. Maintenance of remission with human recombinant interferon alfa-2a in patients with stages III
and IV low-grade malignant non-Hodgkin's lymphoma. J Clin Oncol 1998;16:41–7.
83. Price CG, Rohatiner AZ, Steward W, et al. Interferon-alpha 2b in the treatment of follicular lymphoma: preliminary results of a trial in progress. Ann Oncol 1991;2:Suppl 2:141–5.
84. Smalley R, Weller E, Hawkins M, et al. α Interferon in non-Hodgkin's lymphoma—an update of the ECOG I-COPA trial (E6484). Blood 1998;92:486a. abstract.
85. Solal-Celigny P, Lepage E, Brousse N, et al. Doxorubicin-containing regimen with or without interferon alfa-2b for advanced follicular lymphomas: final analysis of survival and toxicity in the Groupe d'Etude des Lymphomes Folliculaires 86 trial. J Clin Oncol 1998;16:2332–8.
86. Meeker TC, Lowder J, Maloney DG, et al. A clinical trial of anti-idiotype therapy for B cell malignancy. Blood 1985;65:1349–63.
87. Meeker T, Lowder J, Cleary ML, et al. Emergence of idiotype variants during treatment of B-cell lymphoma with anti-idiotype antibodies. N Engl J Med 1985;312:1658–65.
88. Maloney DG, Grillo-Lopez AJ, Bodkin DJ, et al. IDEC-C2B8: results of a phase I multiple-dose trial in patients with relapsed non-Hodgkin's lymphoma. J Clin Oncol 1997;15:3266–74.
89. Maloney DG, Grillo-Lopez AJ, White CA, et al. IDEC-C2B8 (Rituximab) anti-CD20 monoclonal antibody therapy in patients with relapsed low-grade non-Hodgkin's lymphoma. Blood 1997;90:2188–95.
90. Lundin J, Osterborg A, Brittinger G, et al. CAMPATH-1H monoclonal antibody in therapy for previously treated low-grade non-Hodgkin's lymphomas: a phase II multicenter study. J Clin Oncol 1998;16:3257–63.
91. Riechmann L, Clark M, Waldmann H, et al. Reshaping human antibodies for therapy. Nature 1988;332:323–7.
92. McLaughlin P, Grillo-Lopez AJ, Link BK, et al. Rituximab chimeric anti-CD20 monoclonal antibody therapy for relapsed indolent lymphoma: half of patients respond to a four-dose treatment program. J Clin Oncol 1998;16:2825–33.
93. Demidem A, Lam T, Alas S, et al. Chimeric anti-CD20 (IDEC-C2B8) monoclonal antibody sensitizes a B cell lymphoma cell line to cell killing by cytotoxic drugs. Cancer Biother Radio 1997;12:177–86.
94. Czuczman MS, Grillo-Lopez AJ, White CA, et al. Treatment of patients with low-grade B-cell lymphoma with the combination of chimeric anti-CD20 monoclonal antibody and CHOP chemotherapy. J Clin Oncol 1999;17:268–76.
95. Liu SY, Eary JF, Petersdorf SH, et al. Follow-up of relapsed B-cell lymphoma patients treated with iodine-131–labeled anti-CD20 antibody and autologous stem-cell rescue. J Clin Oncol 1998;16:3270–8.
96. Witzig TE, White CA, Wiseman GA, et al. Phase I/II trial of IDEG Y2B8 radioimmunotherapy for treatment of relapsed or refractory CD20(+) B-cell non-Hodgkin's lymphoma. J Clin Oncol 1999;17:3793–803.
97. Kaminski MS, Zasadny KR, Francis IR, et al. Iodine-131–anti-B1 radioimmunotherapy for B-cell lymphoma. J Clin Oncol 1996;14:1974–81.
98. Richards MA, Gregory WM, Hall PA, et al. Management of localized non-Hodgkin's lymphoma: the experience at St. Bartholomew's Hospital 1972–1985. Hematol Oncol 1989;7:1–18.

# CHAPTER 90

# INTERMEDIATE- AND HIGH-GRADE LYMPHOMAS

• ELLEN R. GAYNOR • RICHARD I. FISHER

The non-Hodgkin's lymphomas (NHLs) are a diverse group of diseases, both in their natural history and in their response to therapy. Since 1982, the Working Formulation (WF) has been widely used to separate the various histologic types of NHL into low, intermediate, and high grade based on the natural histories of the various subtypes.[1] This grouping has

guided therapy and aided in predicting prognosis for the individual patient. There were, however, some inherent problems with the system; thus, it was never universally accepted by pathologists and clinicians. Furthermore, some important and distinct clinical entities were not identified at the time the WF was devised and therefore are not included in it.

*Table 90–1.* Major Non-Hodgkin's Lymphoma Types

| Category | Incidence (%) |
| --- | --- |
| Diffuse large B-cell | 31 |
| Follicular | 22 |
| Marginal zone B-cell, MALT | 8 |
| Peripheral T-cell | 7 |
| Small B-lymphocytic (CLL) | 7 |
| Mantle cell lymphoma | 6 |
| Primary mediastinal large B-cell | 2 |
| Anaplastic large T/null cell | 2 |
| High-grade B-cell, Burkitt-like | 2 |
| Marginal zone B-cell, nodal | 2 |
| Precursor T-lymphoblastic lymphoma | 2 |

MALT, mucosa-associated lymphoid tissue; CLL, chronic lymphocytic leukemia.
Adapted with permission from Armitage JO. The changing classification of non-Hodgkin's lymphomas. CA Cancer J Clin 1997;47:324.

The Revised European American Lymphoma classification (REAL) is a pathologically structured system that is more comprehensive than the WF; it also includes the newly identified entities (Table 90–1).[2]

Some of the newer entities that are recognized within the classification of intermediate-grade lymphoma include the following: anaplastic large cell lymphoma, primary mediastinal B-cell diffuse large cell lymphoma, and T-cell–rich B-cell lymphoma. Although each of these is a distinct clinicopathologic entity, each is managed in the same way as the more common B-cell diffuse large cell lymphoma. As treatment for lymphomas improves and as our knowledge of the biology of these diseases increases, treatments may be "tailored" to the distinct histologic type of intermediate-grade lymphoma.

A subtype of lymphoma that deserves special mention is mantle cell lymphoma (MCL). Despite being newly recognized, the disease itself is not new. In the 1970s, investigators recognized that some lymphomas of small cells did not fit well into previously used categories. In the United States, Berard and Dorfman proposed the term *lymphocytic lymphoma of intermediate differentiation*, and this entity constituted a large portion of what was previously diagnosed as diffuse small cleaved cell NHL.[3] MCL was not recognized as an independent entity when the WF was developed. However, it is included as an aggressive NHL in current classification systems because it shares the worst features of all lymphomas. Like the indolent lymphomas, MCL is not curable, and it may have a very aggressive clinical course.

MCL accounts for about 4 to 6% of all cases of NHL. Most patients present with enlarged lymph nodes, and biopsy leads to the diagnosis. There are, however, other presentations characteristic of this entity. For example, MCL may present with diffuse bowel involvement. In fact, MCL can present with isolated involvement of essentially any organ. Central nervous system (CNS) involvement, which is generally asymptomatic, has been noted in almost 20% of cases. Aggressive chemotherapy can induce a complete remission in more than 50% of patients. Responses tend to be transient, however, and the median survival of patients with MCL is 2.5 to 3 years. Factors that are associated with a particularly poor outcome have included (1) a blastic variant histology, (2) a high proliferative index (Ki-67), and (3) p53 gene mutations.

Diffuse large cell lymphoma is by far the most common histologic subtype encountered clinically. Treatment approaches for diffuse large cell lymphoma provide the basis for decisions regarding the management of patients with follicular large cell lymphoma, diffuse small cleaved cell lymphoma, and diffuse mixed cell lymphoma. High-grade lymphomas include immunoblastic lymphoma, which is a subtype of diffuse large cell lymphoma. Immunoblastic lymphomas are treated in the same way as diffuse large cell lymphomas of the intermediate category. The management of diffuse small noncleaved cell lymphoma is discussed elsewhere in this text. Lymphoblastic lymphoma is a rare type of aggressive lymphoma. Patients frequently present with bulky mediastinal masses and bone marrow and CNS involvement. The disease shares many features with, and treatment closely parallels that used for, acute lymphocytic leukemia. Details on the management of this type of lymphoma are beyond the scope of this chapter.

# Natural History and Pretreatment Planning

## STAGING AND PROGNOSTIC FACTORS

The purpose of any staging system for NHL is to identify patients who are more or less likely to respond to a proposed therapy. For many years, the most widely used staging system was the Ann Arbor System (Table 90–2), which is based on the anatomic extent of disease and the presence or absence of symptoms.[4] This system, which was devised for use in Hodgkin's lymphoma (HL), has proved inadequate for the staging of NHL because patterns of disease spread are different for HL and NHL. Unlike HL, the NHL do not commonly spread through contiguous groups of lymph nodes; frequently they are not localized at the time of diagnosis, and they often involve extranodal sites.

Because of the shortcomings associated with the Ann Arbor System, several other prognostic factors have been identified as useful in predicting outcome. These prognostic factors include patient age; the presence or absence of B symptoms; level of serum lactic dehydrogenase (LDH); performance status; tumor size, specifically the presence or

*Table 90–2.* The Ann Arbor Staging Classification*

**Stage I**
Involvement of a single lymph node region or of a single extranodal organ or site ($I_E$)
**Stage II**
Involvement of two or more lymph node regions on same side of diaphragm, or localized involvement of an extramodal site or organ ($II_E$) and of one or more lymph node regions on same side of diaphragm
**Stage III**
Involvement of lymph node regions on both sides of diaphragm, which may also be accompanied by localized involvement of an extranodal organ or site ($III_E$) or spleen ($III_S$), or both ($III_{SE}$)
**Stage IV**
Diffuse or disseminated involvement of one or more distant extranodal organs with or without associated lymph node involvement

*Fever >38°C, night sweats, and weight loss >10% of body weight during the 6 months preceding admission are defined as systemic symptoms and are denoted by the suffix "B." Asymptomatic patients are denoted by the suffix "A."

absence of bulky disease; the number of nodal and extra-nodal sites of disease; and the stage of disease, that is, localized (I and II) or extensive (III and IV).

Shipp and a large number of collaborators involved in the International Non-Hodgkin's Lymphoma Prognostic Factors Project (IPI) have proposed a predictive model for aggressive NHL based on the pretreatment characteristics of several thousand patients with aggressive NHL treated with doxorubicin (Adriamycin)-based combination chemotherapy.[5] Pretreatment characteristics that were independently statistically significant with respect to outcome included age ($\leq$60 years vs. >60 years), tumor stage I or II (localized) vs. stage III or IV (advanced), the number of extranodal sites of involvement ($\leq$1 vs. >1), patient performance status (0 or 1 vs. $\geq$2), and serum LDH (normal vs. abnormal).

According to these five pretreatment characteristics, patients could be assigned to one of four risk groups based on the number of presenting risk factors: low risk (0 or 1), low-intermediate risk (2), high-intermediate risk (3), and high risk (4 or 5). When patients were analyzed according to risk groups, they were found to have remarkably different rates of complete response (CR), relapse-free survival (RFS), and overall survival. For example, patients identified as low risk at the time of diagnosis had an 87% CR rate and a 5-year survival of 73%. In contrast, patients identified before therapy as being in the high-risk categories had a 44% CR rate and a 5-year survival of 26%.

The identified pretreatment prognostic factors are recognized to be surrogate markers of the biologic heterogeneity of the aggressive NHL. We are only beginning to understand this diversity as indices of cell proliferation (e.g., expression of the nuclear Ki-67 antigen, expression of cell surface adhesion molecules, and karyotypic abnormalities) are studied in large numbers of patients with these lymphomas.

As was noted earlier, the value of any staging system lies in its ability to predict the likelihood of response to a proposed treatment. Because the Ann Arbor System has proved inadequate in this regard, it is hoped that the use of a predictive model such as that proposed by Shipp and colleagues will allow clinicians to identify, before beginning therapy, the patient's chance of responding to conventional approaches to treatment. Patients whose predicted outcome is favorable could be spared the added toxicity frequently associated with more intensive experimental approaches. Those in whom an adequate response to standard therapy is unlikely would be identified as candidates for a more aggressive experimental approach.

## Treatment

Intermediate- and high-grade lymphomas are best viewed as systemic diseases; chemotherapy is therefore the mainstay of treatment. A summary of current therapy for these lymphomas is shown in Table 90–3.

### LOCALIZED DISEASE (STAGE I AND STAGE II NONBULKY)

By definition, localized disease includes patients with stage I or II disease that is nonbulky (no tumor mass $\geq$10 cm; no mediastinal mass >one third of the thoracic diameter). Cure rates in this subgroup of patients are high, and a variety of treatment approaches have been used successfully.

*Table 90–3.* Current Therapy for Intermediate-Grade and High-Grade NHL

| Patient | Regimen | 5-Yr Survival |
|---|---|---|
| **Untreated** | | |
| Stage I, I$_E$ | CHOP ($\times$3) plus RT[8] | 86% |
| Stage II, II$_E$ | CHOP[3] plus RT[8] | 74% |
| Stage Bulky II, II$_E$, III, IV | CHOP ($\times$8)[9] | 46% |
| **1st Relapse** | | |
| All Stages | Autotransplant[15] | 53% |
| All Stages | DHAP[15] | 32% |

CHOP (cyclophosphamide, 750 mg/m² IV day 1; doxorubicin, 50 mg/m² IV day 1; vincristine, 1.4 mg/m² IV day 1 [2 mg maximum]; prednisone, 100 mg/m² PO days 1–5 [cycle every 21 days $\times$8]).

DHAP (cisplatin, 100 mg/m² IV for 24 hr; cytarabine, 200 mg/m² on day 2 every 12 hr for two doses [1000 mg/m² $\times$ two doses for age >70 yr]; dexamethasone, 40 mg IV or PO days 1–4) (cycle every 3–4 wk). RT, radiation therapy.

One of the earliest reported studies of a doxorubicin-based chemotherapy regimen used either alone or in combination with radiation therapy (RT) was a nonrandomized trial conducted by Jones and colleagues.[6] All patients received CHOP (cyclophosphamide, doxorubicin, vincristine, prednisone) chemotherapy, usually for a total of eight cycles at 21-day intervals. Patients whose tumors responded poorly to chemotherapy or those in whom significant modification of chemotherapy doses was necessary received RT to an involved field (IFRT). When patients receiving chemotherapy alone were compared with those given combined-modality therapy, there was no significant difference in relapse rate or survival.

Connors and associates reported the use of a short course of chemotherapy (three cycles of CHOP) followed by IFRT in 78 patients with clinical stage I or II disease.[7] Among these patients, none of whom had poor prognostic characteristics such as bulky disease, 99% achieved CR and 85% were long-term survivors.

Miller and coworkers published the results of a randomized trial that compared eight cycles of CHOP chemotherapy alone with chemotherapy using three cycles of CHOP followed by IFRT.[8] All patients had localized intermediate- and high-grade NHL; lymphoblastic lymphoma patients were not included. The study demonstrated that three cycles of CHOP followed by IFRT was superior to eight cycles of CHOP alone for patients with I, I$_E$, and nonbulky II and II$_E$ disease. Patients treated with three cycles of CHOP plus RT had a significantly better progression-free survival (PFS) and overall survival than did patients treated with CHOP for eight cycles. The 5-year estimate of survival was 77% for patients receiving CHOP plus RT versus 64% for those receiving eight cycles of CHOP. The five-year estimate of PFS was 82% for CHOP plus RT versus 72% for CHOP given for eight cycles. In addition to superior results against disease, toxicity was less on the CHOP plus RT arm of the study. Life-threatening toxicity of any type was seen in 61 of 200 patients treated with CHOP plus RT, and in 80 of 200 patients treated with eight cycles of CHOP. A significant decrease in left ventricular function was seen in eight patients treated with CHOP alone; no cardiac events were observed in patients receiving only three cycles of chemotherapy plus RT. As a result of this study, three cycles of CHOP plus IFRT has been established as the standard therapy for patients with localized disease, and a new benchmark for future comparisons has been determined.

The authors also examined prognostic subgroups in their analysis of the data. Poor risk features included stage II disease, increased levels of LDH, performance status of 2 or more, and age older than 60. Five-year PFS was 94% for patients with no adverse risk factors versus 77%, 60%, and 34% for patients having one, two, or three poor prognostic factors, respectively. Thus, there is room for further study of new treatment approaches in patients with one or more risk factors. Outside of a clinical trial, three cycles of CHOP chemotherapy followed by IFRT is the standard of care.

## ADVANCED DISEASE (STAGE II BULKY, STAGE III, AND STAGE IV)

During the 1970s and 1980s, a series of phase II trials was begun, with regimens that were developed subsequent to the introduction of the CHOP chemotherapy regimen. These newer regimens seemed to demonstrate an improvement in CR rates and overall survival as compared with CHOP-type regimens, which had produced CR rates of 45 to 53% and long-term survival rates of 30 to 37%. Unfortunately, with longer follow-up, relapses continued to occur; therefore, the survival estimates decreased significantly. Furthermore, when these newer regimens that had been developed in single institutions were studied in cooperative group settings, the results were not as good as had been initially reported.

The Southwest Oncology Group (SWOG) conducted a randomized trial that compared standard therapy, CHOP, to three of the newer regimens—m-BACOD (methotrexate, bleomycin, doxorubicin, cyclophosphamide, vincristine, dexamethasone), ProMACE/CytaBOM (prednisone, doxorubicin, cyclophosphamide, etoposide, cytarabine, bleomycin, vincristine, methotrexate), and MACOP-B (methotrexate, doxorubicin, cyclophosphamide, vincristine, prednisone, bleomycin).[9] After 6 years of follow-up, there is still no difference in CR rate, time to treatment failure, or overall survival between CHOP and the newer regimens. However, the cost and toxicity of the new regimens have been higher. The Eastern Cooperative Oncology Group (ECOG) also conducted a randomized trial in which CHOP was compared with m-BACOD.[10] No difference in efficacy was found between the two regimens. Thus CHOP remains the best available standard of care. However, because of the fact that less than 50% of all patients are cured, it is absolutely essential that new and improved therapeutic approaches be developed for patients who at the time of diagnosis are predicted to do poorly with the CHOP regimen.

Investigators are currently using several different approaches to improve treatment outcome in high-risk subgroups of patients. These include (1) the identification of active new drugs for the treatment of lymphoma; (2) the use of colony-stimulating factors to allow dose escalation of myelotoxic drugs; (3) the use of strategies that may overcome the problem of resistance to chemotherapy, which is the ultimate cause of treatment failure in the majority of patients; and (4) the use of monoclonal antibodies such as rituximab along with the standard CHOP regimen.

Finding new drugs for the treatment of intermediate- and high-grade NHL remains a difficult task for several reasons. New drugs must be shown to have outstanding single-agent activity before they will be considered as front-line agents in the treatment of lymphoma. Drugs that might be considered active compared with available therapy for other solid tumors are rejected as minimally active in lymphomas. In addition, many patients who are not cured by initial therapy are now considered for high-dose salvage therapy at the time of initial relapse. Thus the pool of patients who might be candidates for phase II testing of new drugs is limited to those who are not eligible for high-dose therapy or who relapse following such therapy. Phase II testing of promising new drugs remains an important therapeutic strategy for improving prognosis in patients with diffuse aggressive NHLs.

The colony-stimulating factors have allowed the escalation of doses of marrow-toxic drugs such as doxorubicin and cyclophosphamide. The SWOG has completed a randomized phase II study of dose-intensified CHOP and dose-intensified ProMACE/CytaBOM, using granulocyte colony–stimulating factor (G-CSF) support. The ECOG has reported a successful phase I escalation study of ProMACE/CytaBOM and subsequently completed a phase II study of the augmented regimen.[11] Longer follow-up is needed before the results of these studies can be evaluated. Shipp and coworkers reported encouraging pilot data using G-CSF support to increase the doses of cyclophosphamide and doxorubicin in a CHOP-like regimen.[12] Subsequent testing of this regimen in a phase II study conducted by the Cancer and Acute Leukemia Group B (CALGB) did not seem to confirm the phase I promising results.

Because it has been demonstrated that pleiotropic drug resistance develops after treatment and relapse in a significant number of patients, the SWOG conducted phase II studies using infusional CHOP alone or in combination with verapamil and quinine. These regimens are given with the intent of overcoming this mechanism of drug resistance. To date, increased bone marrow toxicity has been seen with the use of verapamil and quinine, but there appears to be no benefit to infusional therapy alone or with chemosensitizers with regard to RFS when the results are compared with those of historical controls treated with CHOP alone.[13] Quinine and verapamil are first-generation multidrug resistance inhibitors; newer and more potent inhibitors of drug resistance are currently undergoing clinical trial. Whether the use of these newer agents will translate into better outcomes remains to be determined in these trials.

Rituximab is a monoclonal antibody directed against CD20, which is expressed on the majority of B cells, both malignant and benign. Rituximab has been shown to induce responses in up to 50% of patients with indolent lymphoma in a variety of studies. Information regarding its efficacy in treating diffuse aggressive B-cell lymphomas is more limited, but Coiffier and colleagues have reported an overall response rate of 31%, including 9% CR, in 54 patients with relapsing or refractory aggressive lymphoma.[14] This promising activity in the setting of relapsed or refractory disease has led to the design of several clinical trials incorporating the use of rituximab along with standard CHOP therapy as up-front treatment for intermediate- and high-grade B-cell lymphoma. Randomized phase III trials have been activated, which compare CHOP alone to CHOP plus rituximab. Results of these trials will be of interest to medical oncologists.

## HIGH-DOSE THERAPY WITH STEM CELL SUPPORT

The rationale for using high-dose therapy in previously untreated patients with aggressive NHL was initially provided by results of the PARMA trial.[15] In this study, patients younger than 60 years who had relapsed after an initial CR were treated with two cycles of the salvage regimen, DHAP (dexamethasone, high-dose cytarabine, cisplatin). Patients achieving CR or partial response to these two cycles were presumed to have chemosensitive disease and were subsequently randomized to high-dose carmustine, etoposide, cytarabine, cyclophosphamide, and IFRT with stem cell support versus DHAP for an additional 6 months followed by IFRT. The event-free survival of patients randomized to high-dose therapy was significantly better than for those patients randomized to continue DHAP (46% vs. 12%, respectively [$p$=0.001]). Overall survival was also superior on the high-dose arm ($p$=0.038). This study thus defined high-dose chemotherapy with stem cell support as the treatment of choice for patients with relapsed aggressive lymphoma who met the eligibility criteria of the study. The results of the study gave support to the hypothesis that earlier use of high-dose therapy in untreated patients might improve treatment outcome.

Gianni and colleagues conducted a trial of 75 patients with poor-risk aggressive NHL who were randomized to treatment with MACOP-B or with a novel high-dose regimen that required the use of stem cell support.[16] Patients who failed their initially assigned treatment were able to cross over to the other treatment arm. The toxic death rate on the high-dose arm was initially high (16%) but decreased with modification of the treatment regimen. After a median follow-up of 43 months, there was a statistically significant improvement in RFS (93% vs. 68%, $p$=0.05) and freedom from progression (88% vs. 41%, $p$=0.0001) in favor of high-dose therapy. Overall survival was not statistically different between the two arms. Following on this lead, the ECOG initially did a phase II trial of the high-dose Gianni regimen and then opened a phase III trial comparing the Gianni high-dose regimen with standard CHOP therapy. Despite encouraging results of the phase II trial, accrual to the phase III trial was extremely slow, and the study was closed before reaching its accrual goals.

Haioun and coworkers reported on a subset analysis of 727 patients treated on the LNH 87 protocol.[17] Three hundred seventy patients who had achieved a CR to induction therapy were randomized to sequential therapy or high-dose therapy with autotransplantation.[17] One patient died of transplant-related complications. Two-year overall survival and disease-free survial (DFS) did not differ between the consolidation arms ($p$=0.089). Because this trial was initiated before the publication of the IPI, patients were not stratified by IPI as an important prognostic factor. A subsequent retrospective analysis revealed both an RFS and overall survival benefit for patients with high-intermediate and high-risk IPI characteristics.[18]

A study conducted by Santini and associates lends support to the concept that high-dose therapy after standard induction therapy may be beneficial only for patients in the high-intermediate and high-risk IPI categories.[19] In their study, patients were randomized to receive either standard VACOP-B (vincristine, doxorubicin, cyclophosphamide, vincristine, prednisone, bleomycin) or VACOP-B followed by transplant. There was no difference in the DFS or PFS for the entire group of 124 patients participating in the study. There was, however, statistical improvement in DFS ($p$=0.008) and PFS ($p$=0.08) for patients with high-intermediate and high IPI scores who were randomized to the transplant arm when a subset analysis was performed. It is obvious that prospective randomized trials will be required to determine whether this subset of patients truly benefits from high-dose therapy as primary treatment.

A prospective randomized intergroup trial, including ECOG, CALGB, and SWOG, is ongoing and is comparing early versus delayed high-dose therapy in previously untreated patients with high-intermediate and high-risk IPI scores. Patients in these risk categories who are younger than 65 years are all treated with five cycles of CHOP chemotherapy. Following this, responding patients are randomized to receive one additional cycle of CHOP followed by high-dose autologous transplant, or to complete a total of eight cycles of CHOP. Patients randomized to the standard dose arm who subsequently relapse will receive the same high-dose therapy as is being given to those randomized to the experimental arm of the study. If this study confirms the benefit of early high-dose therapy in responsive patients with high-risk features, subsequent trials will attempt to increase the number of responding patients who become eligible for high-dose therapy.

## SALVAGE THERAPY

As was noted above, with the use of standard CHOP chemotherapy, approximately 55 to 65% of patients with advanced-stage intermediate- or high-grade NHL either will be refractory to, or will relapse after, initial chemotherapy. These patients should be considered for high-dose therapy with stem cell support, which offers an overall prolonged DFS of 20 to 25%. Although there has been considerable variability in selection criteria in transplant studies, there have been several consistent findings across studies. Patients who are likely to achieve CR and possible cure are those who had a good response to initial therapy and who enter high-dose therapy with no or minimal residual disease, having demonstrated a response to salvage chemotherapy. Such patients are said to have a "sensitive" relapse. Patients with disease progression on salvage therapy before stem cell transplant are unlikely to benefit. The same is true for patients who did not respond to initial therapy. A variety of preparative regimens have been used and have been shown effective.

Many patients are not candidates for high-dose salvage therapy owing to age, poor performance status, or poor medical condition. These individuals are usually given conventional-dose chemotherapy. Many of the reported salvage chemotherapy studies involve small numbers of patients with poor-risk factors (e.g., disease resistant to initial therapy, older age, bulky disease at relapse, high levels of LDH). To date, there are no randomized studies in the literature that compare different salvage regimens for aggressive NHL. Furthermore, it is not clear at present whether anyone with resistant or relapsed NHL can be cured with conventional-dose salvage chemotherapy, although a minority of patients may experience a prolonged DFS with such therapy.

## Conclusions

The intermediate- and high-grade lymphomas are among the most curable of all malignancies. Although progress has been made in their treatment, cure is achieved in only a minority of patients with advanced disease. Clearly, better treatment strategies are needed for those whom we can identify before therapy as being at risk of treatment failure. The ability to identify such patients and to develop appropriate therapies for them is dependent on the continuation of basic science research to further our understanding of these diseases.

## REFERENCES

1. National Cancer Institute sponsored study of classifications of non-Hodgkin's lymphomas: summary and description of a working formulation for clinical usage—The Non-Hodgkin's Lymphoma Pathologic Classification Project. Cancer 1982;49:2112–35.
2. Harris NL, Jaffe ES, Stein H, et al. A revised European-American classification of lymphoid neoplasms: a proposal from the International Lymphoma Study Group. Blood 1994;84(5):1361–92.
3. Berard CW, Dorfman RF. Histopathology of malignant lymphomas. Clin Hematol 1974;3:39.
4. Carbone PP, Kaplan HS, Musshoff K, et al. Report of the Committee on Hodgkin's Disease Staging Classification. Cancer Res 1971;31:1860–5.
5. Shipp MA, Harrington DP, Anderson JR, et al. A predictive model for aggressive NHL: The International NHL Prognostic Factors Project. N Engl J Med 1993;329:987–94.
6. Jones SE, Miller TP, Connors JMJ. Long term follow up and analysis for prognostic factors for patients with limited stage diffuse large cell lymphoma treated with initial chemotherapy with or without adjuvant radiotherapy. J Clin Oncol 1989;7:1186–91.
7. Connors JM, Klimo P, Fairey RN, et al. Brief chemotherapy and involved field radiation therapy for limited stage histologically aggressive lymphoma. Ann Intern Med 1987;107:25–30.
8. Miller TP, Dahlberg S, Cassady JR, et al. A randomized trial comparing chemotherapy alone to chemotherapy followed by radiotherapy for localized intermediate and high grade non-Hodgkin's lymphoma. N Engl J Med 1998;339:21–6.
9. Fisher RI, Gaynor ER, Dahlberg S, et al. Comparison of a standard regimen (CHOP) with three intensive chemotherapy regimens for advanced non-Hodgkin's lymphoma. N Engl J Med 1993;328:1002–6.
10. Gordon LI, Harrington D, Andersen J, et al. Comparison of a second generation combination chemotherapeutic regimen (m-BACOD) with a standard regimen (CHOP) for advanced diffuse non-Hodgkin's lymphoma. N Engl J Med 1992;327:1342–9.
11. Gordon LI, Andersen J, Habermann TM, et al. Phase I trial of dose escalation with growth factor support in patients with previously untreated diffuse aggressive lymphomas: determination of the maximum tolerated dose of ProMACE/CytaBOM. J Clin Oncol 1996;14:1275–81.
12. Shipp MA, Neuberg D, Janicek M, et al. High dose CHOP as initial therapy for patients with poor prognosis non-Hodgkin's lymphoma: a dose-finding pilot study. J Clin Oncol 1995;13:2916–23.
13. Gaynor ER, Miller TP, Dahlberg S, et al. Infusional therapy with first generation chemosensitizers results in increased toxicity without improved benefit in untreated lymphoma. Proc Am Soc Clin Oncol 1996;15:412.
14. Coiffier B, Haioun C, Ketterer N, et al. Rituximab (Anti-CD 20 monoclonal antibody) for the treatment of patients with relapsing or refractory aggressive lymphoma: a multicenter phase I study. Blood 1998;92(6):1927–32.
15. Philip T, Guglielmi C, Hagenbeek A, et al. Autologous bone marrow transplantation as compared with salvage chemotherapy in relapses of chemotherapy-sensitive non-Hodgkin's lymphoma. N Engl J Med 1995;333:1540–5.
16. Gianni AM, Bregni M, Siena S, et al. High dose chemotherapy and autologous bone marrow transplantation compared with MACOP-B in aggressive B-cell lymphoma. N Engl J Med 1997;336:1290–7.
17. Haioun C, Lepage E, Gisselbrecht C, et al. Comparison of autologous bone marrow transplantation with sequential chemotherapy for intermediate and high-grade non-Hodgkin's lymphoma in first complete remission: a study of 464 patients. J Clin Oncol 1994;12:2543–51.
18. Haioun C, Lepage E, Gisselbrecht C, et al. Benefit of autologous bone marrow transplantation over sequential chemotherapy in poor-risk aggressive non-Hodgkin's lymphoma: updated results of the prospective study LNH 87-2. J Clin Oncol 1997;15:1131–7.
19. Santini G, Salvagno L, Leoni, P, et al. VACOP-B versus VACOP-B plus autologous bone marrow transplantation for advanced diffuse non-Hodgkin's lymphoma: results of a prospective randomized trial by the non-Hodgkin's lymphoma studies group. J Clin Oncol 1998;16:2796–2802.

# CHAPTER 91

# BURKITT'S LYMPHOMA

• Gregory P. Sarna • A. Robert Kagan

## Natural History

Burkitt's lymphoma (BL) is a lymphoma that may arise in an endemic form (e.g., as a pediatric disease in Africa), in a sporadic form, in a form associated with acquired immunodeficiency syndrome (AIDS), and perhaps in a subendemic form (e.g., in Brazil[1, 2]). Although classic endemic BL is clearly defined histologically, there is fuzziness and variability in the histology of variants, and different classification schemes handle these variants differently. The *working formulation*[3] scheme for classifying lymphomas, derived in the early 1980s, classified BL as the major component of the small noncleaved cell lymphoma (SNCL) class, along with a variant *small noncleaved cell lymphoma, non-Burkitt's type*. The *REAL* classification scheme,[4] derived in the early 1990s, retains this variant *non-Burkitt's type* as a *provisional entity*, now called *high-grade B-cell lymphoma, Burkitt's-like*. With the provisional status came the expectation that the *Burkitt's-like* category was neither homogeneous nor reproducible. The World Health Organization (WHO) has developed a new classification scheme based on the REAL scheme and aiming for consensus and broad acceptance among hematopathologists.[5] This WHO scheme takes the position that entities formerly lumped in the Burkitt's-like category can usually be classified as either (true) BL or a large B-cell lymphoma. The WHO classification subclassifies BL into endemic, sporadic, AIDS associated, and *atypical or pleomorphic* variants. The last-mentioned variant encompasses some of the Burkitt's-like lymphomas. These lymphomas, previously classified as *undifferentiated lymphoma non-Burkitt's type* or *Burkitt's-like lymphoma*, were similar to sporadic BL as to growth rates, behavior, and response to therapy.[6–8]

The Burkitt's-like lymphoma may be genetically different from BL, lacking the characteristic c-*myc* oncogene abnormality, lacking the characteristic chromosomal translocations (t(8;14), t(8;22), or t (2;8), see subsequently), and—in a few cases—lacking a *bcl-2* oncogene rearrangement.[9] The *bcl-2* positive variants and variants with a low growth fraction can be classified as a diffuse large cell lymphoma, B-cell type[10] or *B-cell large cell lymphoma* by WHO systems. Lymphomas that resemble BL but are more heterogeneous as to nuclear size and shape are likely to be classified by the WHO system as atypical BL if the growth fraction (e.g., measured by Ki-67) is close to 100% and *bcl-2* expression is absent.[10]

Classic or endemic BL occurs largely as a pediatric disease and primarily in Africa (BL in Africa may also be nonendemic).[11] This form of BL is almost always associated with Epstein-Barr virus (EBV) exposure. The subendemic form of BL, also occurring in children and associated strongly with EBV, has been reported in Brazil. In that country, BL constitutes 12% of childhood lymphomas, versus 50% in Africa.[2] The sporadic form occurs in children and adults elsewhere and is less likely to be related to EBV. Sporadic BL is clinically similar to but not identical to the endemic form (e.g., more likely to have leukemic or bone marrow involvement, less likely to have jaw involvement). Sporadic BL may also occur in patients of any age, but the non-Burkitt's variant of SNCL (by working formulation or REAL classification) is more common in adults and may occur in children as well. The non-Burkitt's form of SNCL also occurs as one of the malignancies associated with AIDS.

BLs are rapidly growing tumors that may be essentially 100% in cell cycle. They are dramatically sensitive to chemotherapy—so sensitive, in fact, that a *tumor lysis syndrome* may be a severe or fatal consequence of effective therapy. BL is often curable by chemotherapy alone (at least in the non-AIDS group), but it may develop resistance to chemotherapeutic agents rapidly. Although BL is uncommon in the United States (outside the setting of AIDS), it is important that cases that do occur be diagnosed promptly and treated appropriately from the beginning. The rapid growth rate of this tumor makes undue delay in administering proper therapy a substantial hazard.

## ETIOLOGY AND EPIDEMIOLOGY

BL is endemic to tropical Africa, particularly the West Nile region of Uganda.[12] It is also endemic to Papua New Guinea. The incidence of endemic BL parallels that of malaria; BL is infrequent in the high-altitude regions of Uganda, where malaria is less common. BL appears most common in areas of dense rural populations of low socioeconomic status.[13] The peak incidence rate in Uganda has been estimated at 50 to 100 per 1 million per year.[14] BL is not endemic to South America but has an increased incidence in Brazil as compared with the United States and Europe.[1, 2]

BL also occurs in a sporadic fashion, with an estimated 200 to 300 cases diagnosed yearly in the 1970s in the United States.[15] BL has increased with the development of AIDS and AIDS-related lymphomas. Levine[16] has estimated that 4 to 10% of AIDS patients develop lymphomas. In AIDS patients with lymphoma, 20 to 40% of those tumors can be classified as BL.[17–20] BL is seen in sexually transmitted AIDS and AIDS attributed to intravenous drug abuse or to transfusion.

One of the factors that likely contributes to the causation of BL (at least the endemic African form) is infection with EBV. The relationship between EBV and BL has been reviewed by several authors.[21–25] Patients with endemic BL almost always have serologic evidence of past EBV infection. Titers of anti-EBV antibodies in such patients are usually substantially higher than positive titers in suitable control groups. The EBV genome can generally be expressed from the DNA of Burkitt's cells in such patients. EBV may exist in a replicative as well as an intact form in a few cases. It may be present either episomally or integrated, and, at least in one Burkitt's cell line, it may be integrated at the site of reciprocal chromosomal translocation.[26] Integration, however, may be less common in fresh tumors than in cell lines.[27] EBV is capable of *immortalizing* lymphoid cells in tissue culture, and EBV and related herpesviruses may cause clinically similar malignant lymphomas in primates.

In sporadic BL, however, serologic evidence of EBV infection may sometimes be lacking, and the EBV genome is found in the host DNA infrequently ($\leq$25%). Such data are consistent with a role for EBV in the causation of most cases of endemic BL and of some cases of nonendemic BL. It is possible that some of the cases analyzed previously for EBV as BL would now be found to be EBV-negative large cell lymphomas. This effect could artificially dilute the role of EBV in BL. Most individuals who are infected with EBV, however, do *not* develop this tumor, and the time course of serologic data suggests that BL tends to arise many years after an initial EBV infection. In AIDS-related non-Burkitt's SNCL, EBV has been found to be incorporated in the genome of some,[28, 29] but not all,[28, 30, 31] cases. An Italian study[19] found incorporation of EBV in 13 of 36 human immunodeficiency virus (HIV)–positive BLs versus in 4 of 20 sporadic cases. HIV and human T-cell lymphotropic virus type I genomic sequences have not been found in these studies.

Acutely, EBV infection may be asymptomatic or cause a mononucleosis type of illness. Although mononucleosis in general is a self-limited disease that does not evolve into BL, on at least one occasion a chronic recurrent mononuclear syndrome has been reported to transform into monoclonal BL, with EBV present in the BL genome.[32] In Asia, EBV infection is associated with nasopharyngeal carcinoma (and with BL[33]). Hodgkin's lymphoma, which may be EBV associated,[34, 35] has been reported to antedate BL in a least 19 patients,[36] and in one case BL was clonally related to the Hodgkin's lymphoma.[37]

Attempts to demonstrate different strains of EBV that vary as to malignant clinical manifestations have generally failed to show such differences, but this field is evolving.[38] Although it is possible that EBV is merely a passenger virus in patients with endemic BL, it seems more likely that it is one of several factors contributing to the causation of BL. It has been hypothesized that BL is most likely to develop from EBV infection if that infection occurs early (perinatally).[39]

Postulated cofactors, which may increase the likelihood of EBV resulting in BL, include malaria[13, 40] (perhaps related to chronic immunostimulation or immunosuppression) and viral infections other than EBV.[23]

Data suggest that a human B-cell lymphotropic virus may contribute to the cause of BL.[38] The role of coinfection with malaria is supported by the geographic pattern of endemic BL incidence as well as by immunologic differences in human T-cell immunity to EBV in groups of patients from malarial as opposed to nonmalarial regions.[41] Because patients with nonendemic BL may have no or scanty evidence of EBV infection, there may be factors or viruses other than EBV that can generate the transformation of normal lymphocytes into BL cells.

Genetic factors may be important in the genesis of BL. Familial clustering of BL has been observed.[42, 43] Because nonfamilial time-space clustering has also been noted, the genetic implication of this phenomenon is unclear. As a separate entity, however, kindreds have been reported with sex-linked recessive inability to handle EBV infection. This situation has led to a variety of sequelae, reportedly including nonendemic BL.[44] Because polyclonal B-cell lymphomas have also been noted with EBV infection,[45] however, this relationship may need clarification.

Characteristic chromosomal and oncogene abnormalities occur in BL. In overview, these tend to be predominantly t(8;14) and occasionally t(8;22) or t(2;8). The chromosomal abnormalities tend to juxtapose c-*myc* (normally on chromosome 8) with an immunoglobulin promoter, with subsequent overexpression of the translated c-*myc*. The normal c-*myc* locus tends to be inactivated,[46] and mutations in c-*myc* may occur.[47–49] This pattern of aberrant c-*myc* expression may allow virtually 100% of lymphoma cells to be in cycle, as detected by a high percent of cells staining positive for Ki-67, contributing to the aggressiveness of BL.[10] Patterns of chromosomal abnormalities and of c-*myc* expression and rearrangement in AIDS-related non-Burkitt's SNCL are similar to those in sporadic or endemic BL.[28, 31] Activation of the *Blym* oncogene has been reported in BL cell lines.[50] Mutations and accumulation of p53 may occur in 30 to 40% of BLs (and 70% of BL cell lines) but do not seem to indicate advanced disease or poor prognosis.[51]

Additionally, it has been shown that B-cell lymphoid lines derived from BL and other lymphoid lines transformed in vitro by EBV may produce a growth factor that is self-stimulating.[52] Characterization of this autogenous growth may lead to a better understanding of the biology and treatment of this tumor.

## HISTOLOGY

BL has been defined histologically by a panel of pathologists collaborating in a WHO project.[4, 53] The histologic features of BL have also been reviewed elsewhere.[4, 54] Fixed histologic sections of lymph nodes commonly form a starry-sky pattern, consisting of occasional macrophages in a background of lymphoid tumor cells that are relatively uniform, cohesive, and monotonous in size (generally medium sized) and shape. The cytoplasm is pyroninophilic; cytoplasmic lipid vacuoles are common. The nucleus, which is round to oval and at times indented, has abundant and clumped chromatin. Nucleoli are multiple and may be large. Cytologic preparations show more variation in size and shape. Deep basophilia is seen in Romanowsky-stained specimens. Vacuolization is common, and mitoses may be frequent.

The non-Burkitt's or Burkitt's-like variant of SNCL (if one uses the working formulation or REAL classification system) differs from BL in that the non-Burkitt's variant is pleomorphic as to cellular and nuclear shape and size, whereas BL is relatively uniform, and in that in BL multiple prominent basophilic nucleoli are common, whereas the non-Burkitt's variant commonly has a single eosinophilic nucleolus that is sometimes indistinct. The distinction between the non-Burkitt's variants and BL is not always clear, however, especially in pediatric patients.[55] The BL form of undifferentiated lymphoma was found by the Children's Cancer Study Group[55] to be more likely to be limited in stage than the non-Burkitt's variant. The opposite was noted, however, at the National Cancer Institute (NCI).[56, 57] The BL form is more likely than the non-Burkitt's variant to be extranodal or gastrointestinal and is less likely to have bone marrow involvement.[58, 59] Given age and prognostic factors, there is no clear difference in prognosis between the BL and non-BL variants.[6, 55, 56, 58] As discussed earlier, the non-Burkitt's variant has been reported to lack c-*myc* rearrangement and to have, in some cases with nodal presentation, a *bcl-2* rearrangement consistent with a follicular center cell origin.[20, 60]

BL cells are of B-cell origin, generally exhibiting surface immunoglobulin and occasionally showing complement and IgG Fc fragment receptors. The surface immunoglobulin has largely been monoclonal IgM,[61, 62] but IgG, IgA, IgD,[62] and surface membrane immunoglobulin negativity with cytoplasmic IgM (*pre–B cell* characteristics)[63] have also been reported. Light chains have been either kappa or lambda, and monoclonal serum immunoglobulins have been seen.[62] Tumor cells are often CD10 (common acute lymphocytic leukemia antigen) positive[64] and are CD5 and CD23 negative.[4] They lack *bcl-2* rearrangement[9] and by that criterion would not be classified as follicular center cells. Although architectural patterns of nodal involvement have suggested that BL might be of germinal center origin,[61] this has been questioned.[65]

## CYTOKINETICS

Endemic BL is presumably the fastest-growing human malignancy. Iversen and associates[66] have studied several cases of BL and found a mean potential doubling time of 25.6 hours and an actual doubling time of 66 hours. Cell cycle time was calculated at roughly 26 hours, and thymidine-labeling index was approximately 17%. The growth fraction was estimated at 90 to 100%, indicating a small to absent resting cell population. The cell loss factor was estimated at 69% (including 30% in G2). BL shows exuberant proliferative activity. This activity may relate both to sensitivity to therapy and to the tumor lysis syndrome that can result from effective treatment. The Burkitt's-like variant has not had extensive cytokinetic study, but data from Spina and colleagues[60] indicate that it grows comparably to the endemic form and that the sporadic form may be less cytokinetically active.

*Table 91–1.* **Clinical Features of Burkitt's Lymphoma at Presentation**

| Type | Age (yr) | Sex | Site (Most to Least Common) | Stage |
|------|----------|-----|------------------------------|-------|
| Endemic (African) | 8 (median) >15 (rare) | Predominantly male | Face, abdomen, CNS, lymph nodes, bone marrow | Advanced (30–50%) |
| Nonendemic (American) | 10 (median) >15 (25%) | Predominantly male (≤15 yrs) Equal (>15 yrs) | Abdomen (commonly ileocecal or ovarian), lymph nodes, CNS | Advanced (approximately 60%) |
| AIDS associated | Young adult | Predominantly male | Lymph nodes, bone marrow | Advanced (approximately 75%) |

AIDS, acquired immunodeficiency syndrome; CNS, central nervous system.

## CLINICAL FEATURES AND DIAGNOSIS

The clinical presentation of endemic BL is somewhat different from that of sporadic BL. Table 91–1 presents some salient features. Endemic BL is essentially a pediatric disease. The median and modal age of patients at diagnosis is approximately 8 years. Most patients are in the 6- to 9-year range, but the disease may appear in patients in early childhood and rarely (in <5% of cases) in the late teens or adulthood. Males predominate by a 2:1 to 3:1 ratio.[67, 68]

The most common site of disease presentation is the face (primarily the mandible and frequently multiple facial bones). The face may be involved in 55 to 75% of patients. The next most common area of involvement is the abdomen (30 to 50%), particularly involving the ovary, and involving the peritoneum (with ascites), ileocecum, mesentery, spleen, kidneys, liver, and pancreas. Orbital and meningeal involvement is not unusual (10 to 20%). Peripheral lymph node, testicular, and bone marrow involvement may occur but is not common at presentation. Disease is frequently bulky. Multiple sites of disease are often found at presentation, particularly when there is abdominal involvement. Of patients, 30 to 50% have advanced disease at diagnosis.[66, 69]

The profile of sporadic BL in the United States has been reviewed by Levine and coworkers.[70, 71] Sporadic BL is found in the United States in an older population than in Africa and may rarely be seen in patients in their 50s or 60s. The median age of patients at diagnosis is 10 years, with a mean age of 12 years. Approximately one third of patients are older than 15 years. Males predominate by a 3:1 ratio in the younger than 13 age group, but the sex ratio is equal in patients age 13 and older.

In sporadic BL, the most common site of presentation is the abdomen (digestive organs, particularly the ileocecum; genitourinary organs, particularly the ovaries in females aged 13 to 21; spleen; mesentery; peritoneum; and abdominal lymph nodes). Involvement of bone marrow, blood, pleura, or peripheral nodes (particularly cervical) is common. Presentation in the head and neck region occurs in 10 to 15% of patients, commonly including jaw, nasopharynx, and tonsils. Central nervous system (CNS) presentation is also seen in 10 to 15% of patients. Breast, nonfacial bones, and chest are sites of presentation as well. Approximately 60 to 70% of sporadic BL patients have advanced disease at diagnosis.[71, 72] AIDS-related BL is usually advanced and, as compared with sporadic BL, more likely to be nodal or to have liver or skin involvement.[19] Rarely, BL may present during pregnancy; the obstetric and gynecologic aspects of this problem have been reviewed.[73]

In Burkitt's-like SNCL, disease frequently presents extra-

nodally, particularly with gastrointestinal tract involvement.[74] Bone marrow and peripheral nodal disease are not rare, however.[56, 58, 63] Although non-Burkitt's SNCL may occur as a pediatric disease, it also occurs in adults (particularly when AIDS related).

The differential diagnosis of BL varies according to the mode of presentation of disease. Considerations based on sites of presentation alone include other lymphomas, Hodgkin's lymphoma, acute leukemia, Wilms' tumor, neuroblastoma, gastrointestinal and ovarian malignancies, embryonal rhabdomyosarcoma, retinoblastoma, osteosarcoma, plasmacytoma, and Ewing's sarcoma as well as benign tumors and reactive lymphadenopathy. Histologic differential diagnosis includes selected other lymphomas (particularly poorly differentiated lymphocytic lymphoma, lymphoblastic lymphoma, undifferentiated lymphoma, and large cell lymphoma), acute lymphoblastic and myeloid leukemias, extraosseous Ewing's sarcoma, and possibly embryonal rhabdomyosarcoma.

## STAGING AND DIAGNOSTIC STUDIES

Staging is currently more useful for assessing prognosis than for defining therapy because chemotherapy is the mainstay of treatment regardless of stage. One useful system from Ziegler[21] and Magrath and coworkers[75] is presented in Table 91–2. In nonendemic disease, patients may be grouped prognostically into good-risk (stages A, B, AR) or bad-risk (stages C and D) categories. Other staging systems have also been used.[15, 71]

In addition to history taking and physical examination, screening chemistries (including creatinine, uric acid, and lactate dehydrogenase), and chest radiography, staging studies should include bone marrow aspirate and biopsy and, in the absence of a leukemic phase, lumbar puncture. Staging studies should be performed rapidly so that therapy may be started promptly. Other useful studies include computed tomography scan of the abdomen[76] and abdominal ultra-

*Table 91–2.* **Staging System for Burkitt's Lymphoma**

| Stage | Description |
|-------|-------------|
| ABCD | Single extra-abdominal site, multiple abdominal sites, intra-abdominal tumor, intra-abdominal tumor with involvement of multiple extra-abdominal sites |
| AR | Stage C but with >90% of tumor surgically resected |

From Ziegler JL. Burkitt's lymphoma. N Engl J Med 1981;305:785.

sound. These techniques may assess whether or not renal obstruction, as well as disease, is present. Gallium scan has been found useful by some,[77, 78] but delaying therapy for 24- or 48-hour scan results seems unwise. Magnetic resonance imaging is of value for CNS evaluation particularly,[79] and positron emission tomography scanning has been reported to be positive for BL.[80]

Laboratory abnormalities are common with BL at presentation. Cohen and associates[81] studied 41 patients seen before 46 treatment episodes (29 studied before initial therapy). They found a 56% incidence of elevated levels of lactate dehydrogenase (>600 IU/L), a 33% incidence of hyperuricemia (>8.0 mg/dl), and a 15% incidence of azotemia (creatinine >1.6 mg/dl). Metabolic abnormalities correlated with increased creatinine. In this series, pretreatment derangements in phosphate and calcium were not substantial, but such abnormalities may occur. As previously discussed, positive antibody titers against EBV are common, particularly in the endemic form. Hematologic abnormalities are common when BL has a leukemic presentation.

## PROGNOSIS

In the 1970s, most patients with endemic or sporadic BL achieved a complete response with cyclophosphamide based chemotherapy, and many of these patients were cured. The overall relapse rate after a complete response was roughly 50% in endemic BL,[68, 82] with the rate of relapse increasing with increasing stage. Olweny and coworkers[82] reported in endemic BL roughly 80% disease-free survival in stage A, 50% in stage B, 45% in stage C, and 23% in stage D disease. In stage AR disease, they noted approximately an 85% relapse rate in 13 patients who survived 1 month past surgery. For stages A, B, C, and D, survival slightly exceeded disease-free survival (stage A, 86%; B and C, 50%; and D, 25%). This was likely due to an overall salvage rate of patients with relapse of approximately 32%. Salvage appeared to be better in patients with stage AR disease, who had a 56% long-term survival rate despite an 85% relapse rate. In those who experienced relapse, median time to relapse was roughly 3 months, and relapses were rare beyond 1 year. Three relapses were seen beyond 6 years in 201 patients who achieved a complete response.

In sporadic BL patients treated by combination-chemotherapy protocols at the NCI in the 1970s, stage-adjusted results of therapy were similar to those achieved in endemic BL,[15, 21, 72] although perhaps with some improvement in stage B disease. Levine and associates,[71] however, reporting results from more than 200 patients with American BL treated in a similar era at multiple institutions with a variety of approaches, presented less favorable results. Median overall survival was 7.4 months, with a 2-year survival rate of 33%. Two-year survival rates for stages A, B, C, and D were 47%, 27%, 33%, and 25%. Only two patients were stage AR in that series. In another series of BL in the United States, the median survival of 25 patients was 10.5 months.[58]

More modern data indicate overall complete response rates in the 70 to 90% range (see later). Long-term disease-free survival is roughly 50% overall and 80% or more in good-risk patients. Results are poorer in high-risk adults (e.g., lactate dehydrogenase >1000 IU/L, bone marrow

involvement, leukemic presentation, meningeal involvement), although children may fare better,[83, 84] and improved results in adults have been attributed to more recent and complex regimens.[85, 86] HIV-positive patients may fare similarly in terms of response rate and freedom from relapse but have poorer survival secondary to infectious complications and comorbid disease.

## Treatment

### SURGERY

Surgery may play a role in the management of bulky abdominal BL when at least 90% of the tumor can be removed so that the patient's disease can be reclassified to stage AR rather than stage C. Based on data from the 1970s and 1980s, patients whose abdominal tumors are initially debulked effectively fare better than those whose abdominal disease is not or cannot be resected.[72, 75, 87] The difference in survival was substantial, suggesting that it may have been a true therapeutic benefit. Such a benefit would be understandable because response to chemotherapy, chance of relapse, and risk of tumor lysis syndrome (see subsequent discussion) are related to tumor burden. It is also possible, however, that the presumed therapeutic benefit is an artifact of the selection of favorable patients as having resectable tumors and the exclusion of unfavorable patients as not having resectable disease or that improved chemotherapy mitigates against the role of surgery.

Retrospective data from the Mayo Clinic[88] show no clear benefit to surgical debulking in a small group of patients with abdominal BL. Data from Murphy and colleagues[89] suggest that intensive treatment with chemotherapy alone may be effective therapy for pediatric patients with bulky abdominal disease. More recent retrospective data from France support this premise.[90] Data from Shamberger and Weinstein[91] argue for debulking only of patients with limited ileocecal or mesenteric involvement, usually presenting with bowel obstruction or abdominal pain. Data from Libya argue for debulking only when disease is localized and mobile.[92]

Because studies of debulking surgery are retrospective and uncontrolled, the putative value of debulking must be weighed against the risks of surgery. In addition to the usual hazards of surgery, these risks include the growth of unresected tumor during the period in which the patient is recovering from surgery if chemotherapy is delayed and the risk of poor wound healing and secondary infection if chemotherapy is not delayed. An additional unusual surgical risk reported to be associated with BL is intraoperative malignant hyperthermia.[93] Surgical complications in BL have been described by Kemeny and coworkers.[87]

### RADIATION THERAPY

Radiation therapy given in daily fractions is not of great efficacy as a primary treatment for BL.[94, 95] This limited efficacy may be related to rapid tumor growth, which enables the tumor to "escape" from a daily radiation treatment, and to frequent dissemination of disease, which limits the feasibility of encompassing all disease effectively in radiation ports. In a small number of patients, *superfractionation* (three treatments a day) has been used,[91, 93] but this approach has largely been abandoned. Variations in radiation dose, tumor site and bulk, and previous therapy make firm conclusions difficult. Low-dose irradiation of the abdomen (21 Gy over 19 days), when added to chemotherapeutic treatment of patients with stage AR, C, or D disease, has not prevented substantial local relapse.[72] Radiation to the craniospinal axis has not by itself proved to be effective prophylaxis of meningeal spread of BL.[96, 97] Cranial irradiation may be given along with intrathecal chemotherapy in the treatment of meningeal BL. The relative contribution of the irradiation to therapeutic efficacy and toxicity in this setting is not clear. Possible indications for radiation therapy in SNCL include bulky CNS disease or bulky masses causing spinal cord compression, superior vena cava obstruction, tracheal obstruction, and pharyngeal obstruction.

## CHEMOTHERAPY

Chemotherapy is the major therapeutic modality for BL, regardless of stage. High-dose cyclophosphamide, administered either as a single agent or in combination with other drugs, is generally thought to be the cornerstone of effective chemotherapy.[21] High-dose cyclophosphamide has been reported to yield complete responses in approximately 80 to 95% of evaluable patients with African (endemic) BL.[21] These figures generally exclude approximately 10% of patients as unevaluable because of early death (within 28 days). A 75 to 85% complete response rate for all treated patients is likely to be a representative figure.

In sporadic BL, combination regimens appear to be superior. High response rates have been achieved with a variety of regimens. Table 91–3 outlines data from four regimens in adults. An early (1970s and early 1980s) NCI regimen (77-04)[98] and a Stanford regimen[74] are similar, basically a CHOP

(cyclophosphamide, hydroxydaunomycin, vincristine [Oncovin], and prednisone)–type regimen with an emphasis on cyclophosphamide and with CNS prophylaxis (plus radiation to bulky disease in the Stanford regimen). The Vanderbilt[99] regimen escalates the cyclophosphamide dose more substantially and uses high-dose etoposide. The second cycle of the Vanderbilt regimen adds doxorubicin (Adriamycin), which is not included in cycle 1. Results of these regimens in patients with favorable prognosis are in general comparable, but the high risk factor profile of patients in the Vanderbilt study suggests a benefit to the high cyclophosphamide dose approach (although with substantial toxicity). The putative importance of the alkylating agent dose is inferentially supported by the relative inactivity of a modest-dose cyclophosphamide regimen, MACOP-B (methotrexate, doxorubicin, cyclophosphamide, vincristine, prednisone, and bleomycin), in SNCL despite substantial activity in large cell lymphoma.[100] More recent results[86] (1989–1996) from a later NCI study[101] of a more complex and intensive regimen are of interest. That regimen (CODOX-M/IVAC), also shown in Table 91–3, alternates cyclophosphamide, doxorubicin, vincristine, and high-dose methotrexate and rescue with ifosfamide, etoposide, and high-dose cytosine arabinoside. This regimen achieved a 95% complete response rate in 41 evaluable patients (21 children, 20 adults). The adults achieved a 100% complete response rate, and all remain in remission at 2 years. The children did similarly well, with 90% complete response rate and 85% 2-year event-free survival. Other regimens not listed in Table 91–3 show promising results. A French study[85] of the LMB protocols (see subsequently) yielded 89% complete response and 74% 3-year survival in 65 adults (several of whom received high-dose therapy and bone marrow transplants in either remission or relapse).

In the pediatric group, regimens such as $LSA_2-L_2$, which are designed for childhood lymphomas, in general are less effective than regimens based on high-dose cyclophosphamide.[102] One such pediatric regimen is the St. Jude total therapy B regimen,[89] which yielded a 93% complete re-

*Table 91–3.* Selected Chemotherapy Regimens for Adult Burkitt's Lymphoma (Small Noncleaved Cell Lymphoma)

| Source | Regimen | Patient No. | Complete Response (%) | Overall Disease-Free Survival | Long-Term Survival in High-Risk Patients |
|---|---|---|---|---|---|
| NCI[98] (77-04) | CTX, VCR, Adr, Pred, MTX with rescue, IT MTX, ITAM-C | 72* | 89[72] | 56 | 30% LDH[72] >1000 IU/L BM positive<br>33% extensively intra-abdominal |
| Stanford[74] | CTX, VCR, MTX with rescue, Rad Tx BID to abdominal mass >10 cm | 18 | 71 | 67 | 38% stage D<br>20% LDH >500 IU/L |
| Vanderbilt[99] | (Cycle 1) CTX, etoposide, VCR, Bleo (CNS prophylaxis with MTX variable given) | 20 | 85 | 60 | Survival not analyzed by risk factors but 30% of group were BM positive, 35% had LDH >300 IU/L, 60% had ≥2 extranodal sites, 35% bulk >10 cm, and 80% stage IV |
| NCI[86, 101] (CODOX-M/IVAC) | (Cycle 2 adds Adr) CODOX-M (Ara-C IT, MTX IT, MTX with rescue, CTX, VCR, Adr) alternating with IVAC (high-dose Ara-C, ifosfamide, IT MTX, etoposide) | 41 | 95 | 92 | Includes 80% EFS in stage IV patients (BM and/or CNS) |

*33 children, 39 adults; results indistinguishable.

CTX, cyclophosphamide; VCR, vincristine; Adr, Adriamycin (doxorubicin); Pred, prednisone; MTX, methotrexate; Ara-C, cytarabine; Bleo, bleomycin; Rad Tx, radiation therapy; CNS, central nervous system; LDH, lactate dehydrogenase; BM, bone marrow; EFS, event-free survival; IT, intrathecal.

sponse rate and 81% 2-year disease-free survival in patients without CNS or marrow involvement (but only 2 of 10 long-term survivors with CNS or marrow involvement and only 36% 2-year disease-free survival with lactate dehydrogenase >1000 IU/L). Similar data with this regimen in good-risk patients have been reported elsewhere.[103] A variant of this regimen, using high-dose cytosine arabinoside, has also had good results.[83]

Another pediatric approach is the French LMB 89 protocol.[104] This complex approach used intensive six-drug or seven-drug regimens as treatment, with choice of therapy depending on extent of disease. With this strategy, 47 of 51 patients achieved a complete response, and 45 remained in first complete response with short (>9 month) follow-up. Of the 51 patients treated in this regimen, 30 had a peripheral blood leukemic phase, 20 had CNS involvement, and 42 had lactate dehydrogenase more than twice normal (nine >10 times normal). The results in this high-risk pediatric group are rather remarkable, and this may represent a superior approach. Earlier work with the six-drug regimen (LMB 84)[105] resulted in 78% event-free survival in 216 patients without CNS involvement (68% for stage IV and leukemic patients). Similar results have been seen with the seven-drug regimen (LMB 86)[106, 107] and with a Children's Cancer Group lymphoma regimen *(Orange)*.[107] This approach has been extended to adults with some promise but with significant toxicity.[108] Excellent results in children have been achieved with the CODOX-M/IVAC regimen discussed previously.[86]

Nonmyeloablative therapy, such as the regimens described previously, is effective in good-risk patients but may fail with a significant frequency in adult patients with high lactate dehydrogenase, bone marrow involvement, or CNS involvement. In refractory patients, high-dose therapy with autologous (or less likely allogeneic) bone marrow (or peripheral blood stem cell) transplantation as rescue may salvage a few patients, even with CNS disease.[109, 110] Better results are achieved with high-risk patients in responsive relapse or partial remission,[109–113] and data are available supporting transplantation of high-risk patients in first complete response.[113–115] Although such data are encouraging and high-dose therapy with autologous bone marrow or stem cell transplantation can be viewed as reasonable therapy for relapsed but chemotherapy-sensitive patients, the role of this approach is not yet clear. It may be relevant to note a large French randomized study of 370 patients, 16% of whom had BL or lymphoblastic lymphoma. This study found no advantage in survival or disease-free survival with autologous bone marrow transplantation consolidation of complete responders as compared with a more standard sequential consolidation schema.[116] Further studies using other conditioning regimens are necessary to clarify this issue.

Patients who fail to achieve a complete response frequently achieve a partial response. This situation has not commonly been associated with long-term survival, unless patients also received salvage high-dose therapy and transplantation. Early death, failure to achieve a complete response, and relapse from complete remission are more common in patients with advanced disease. Most patients who achieve a complete response do so after one to two courses of therapy, and multiple courses of chemotherapy are not clearly superior to treating one to two courses beyond a complete response[82] (although patients are commonly treated for ≥6 months).

BL in the setting of AIDS is responsive, but survival is poor. Typical complete response rates are 50%, and median survival is less than 1 year. Aggressive therapy is not more successful than modest dose therapy and may be less successful.[117] The experience from Italy is instructive.[19] In 46 HIV-positive patients with BL, treated variably, complete response rate was 40%, and median survival was 7 months. Freedom from relapse was 74% because 10 of 18 patients achieving complete response died of opportunistic infection. These results are in contrast to results in 29 HIV-negative patients with BL who achieved 65% complete response rate with roughly 52% long-term survival and 84% of patients achieving complete response alive and disease free. All of these data, however, may need re-evaluation in this era of improved antiretroviral therapy.

**Meningeal Disease.** Meningeal relapse in SNCL is a substantial problem if no CNS prophylaxis is given. In early data from endemic BL treated without prophylaxis, 31% of relapses were CNS only, and 21% were CNS plus systemic involvement.[82] Modern regimens using CNS prophylaxis have decreased the frequency of that problem. Haddy and colleagues[118] reviewed data on 120 patients treated on four NCI protocols. Seventeen patients (14%) presented with CNS disease. Five of these were long-term relapse-free survivors, and one additional patient was a long-term disease-free survivor after a subsequent relapse. Therapy included intrathecal methotrexate and cytarabine (but generally not radiation). Twelve patients (10%) relapsed with CNS disease as the first site. Three of these were long-term survivors after therapy that included CNS radiation. Risk factors for CNS involvement were bone marrow involvement and high lactate dehydrogenase. CNS prophylaxis decreased the risk of CNS relapses from 28 to 8%. Survival with CNS disease was not clearly different from survival without CNS disease, given other prognostic factors (lactate dehydrogenase, bone marrow).

**Tumor Lysis Syndrome.** Poor prognostic factors at the time of disease presentation include, in addition to advanced stage, high serum lactate dehydrogenase, high uric acid level, and high antibody titer to EBV early antigen.[119] In American BL, but not necessarily African BL, poor prognostic factors may include a low antibody titer to EBV viral capsid antigen[71] and possibly age greater than 13 years.[120] These variables seem generally to correlate with tumor mass.

Tumor mass contributes to a poor prognosis not only because of tumor resistance (failure to achieve a complete response and tendency toward early relapse), but also because of the substantial risk of tumor lysis syndrome. This risk also correlates with chemical tumor markers: High risk of tumor lysis syndrome is seen with a lactate dehydrogenase value greater than 1500 IU/L.[81, 121] Rapid tumor destruction, particularly in the setting of pretherapy azotemia (e.g., owing to dehydration, renal obstruction, or renal BL), may result in severe metabolic abnormalities, including hyperkalemia, hypocalcemia with hyperphosphatemia, lactic acidosis, hyperuricemia, and azotemia. Post-therapy azotemia may be secondary to intrarenal precipitation of calcium and phosphate, urate, xanthine, or hypoxanthine.

The metabolic sequelae of this event have been reported to cause renal failure in some patients and acute death in others, perhaps as a result of hypocalcemia or hyperkalemia, or both.[21, 121] Attempts to minimize this risk, in addition to debulking surgery for bulky abdominal disease,[74] include vigorous hydration (with diuretic use if necessary) and use of allopurinol. Alkalinization of the urine may increase the risk of renal tubular calcium phosphate precipitation and would seem contraindicated, unless uric acid levels cannot be controlled by hydration and allopurinol.[121] We recommend frequent monitoring of metabolic parameters (every 6 to 12 hours) in high-risk cases to make the diagnosis of the tumor lysis syndrome as early as possible. Dialysis may be necessary to control potassium levels in some patients, although hyperphosphate and hypocalcium may be less responsive to dialysis.

## SUMMARY OF TREATMENT

Once the diagnosis of SNCL is established, treatment should be started relatively promptly. Hydration and optimization of renal function should take place. If debulking surgery is to be considered, a decision should be made in a timely fashion. Surgery likely should be considered only for limited but bulky, mobile, and easily resectable disease. Computed tomography scanning may help to predict whether or not disease can be resected adequately. Disease confined to the ovary, omentum, or small bowel may be resected more easily than retroperitoneal disease. Guidelines as to when to start chemotherapy after cytoreductive surgery are not clear, but it seems reasonable to delay chemotherapy for approximately 10 to 14 days in patients without substantial residual disease, particularly if the lactate dehydrogenase value has returned to the normal range postoperatively and is not increasing. If substantial extra-abdominal or residual intra-abdominal disease is apparent or if the lactate dehydrogenase is rising rapidly postoperatively, the risks of more immediate postoperative chemotherapy may be accepted rather than allowing rapid tumor growth to occur.

In early endemic disease, high-dose cyclophosphamide alone may be adequate. Data suggest that in advanced disease or sporadic BL, an aggressive combination-chemotherapy regimen, such as the NCI CODOX-M regimen or, in a pediatric population, total therapy B[65] or LMB-89,[104] is superior. Further study of such regimens may help to clarify their role. Radiation therapy does not appear to play a primary role in the treatment of BL, unless CNS disease is present. Radiation may be useful in a palliative mode for local problems of treatment failure.

## SUGGESTIONS FOR ADDITIONAL READING

Griffin BE, Xue SA. Epstein-Barr virus infections and their association with human malignancies: some key questions. Ann Med 1998;30:249–59. *This article presents a cogent review.*

Barnes MN, Barrett JC, Kimberlin DF, Kilgore LC. Burkitt lymphoma in pregnancy. Obstet Gynecol 1998;92:4 Pt 2:675–8. *This article describes a case treated with immediate chemotherapy.*

## REFERENCES

1. Sandlund JT, Fonseca T, Leimig T, et al. Predominance and characteristics of Burkitt lymphoma among children with non-Hodgkin lymphoma in northeastern Brazil. Leukemia 1997;11:743–6.
2. Bacchi MM, Bacchi CE, Alvarenga M, et al. Burkitt's lymphoma in Brazil: strong association with Epstein-Barr virus. Mod Pathol 1996;9:63–7.
3. The Non-Hodgkin's Lymphoma Pathologic Classification Project. National Cancer Institute sponsored study of classifications of non-Hodgkin's lymphomas—summary and description of a Working Formulation for Clinical Usage. Cancer 1982;49:2112–35.
4. Harris NL, Jaffe ES, Stein H, et al. A revised European-American classification of lymphoid neoplasms: a proposal from the International Lymphoma Study Group. Blood 1994;84:1361–92.
5. Jaffe ES, Harris NL, Diebold J, Muller-Hermelink HK. World Health Organization classification of neoplastic diseases of the hematopoietic and lymphoid tissues: a progress report. Am J Clin Pathol 1999;111:Suppl 1:S8–12.
6. Pugh WC. Lymphoma: the next question, April 2–4, 1992. Orlando, FL, 1992.meeting abstract.
7. Hutchison RE, Murphy SB, Fairclough DL, et al. Diffuse small noncleaved cell lymphoma in children, Burkitt's versus non-Burkitt's types: results from the Pediatric Oncology Group and St. Jude Children's Research Hospital. Cancer 1989;64:23–8.
8. Jaffe ES, Diebold J, Harris NL, et al. Burkitt's lymphoma: a single disease with multiple variants: the World Health Organization classification of neoplastic diseases of the hematopoietic and lymphoid tissues. Blood 1999;93:1124.
9. Yano T, van Krieken JH, Magrath IT, et al. Histogenetic correlations between subcategories of small noncleaved cell lymphomas. Blood 1992;79:1282–90.
10. Harris NL, Jaffe ES, Armitage JO, Shipp M. Lymphoma classification: from REAL to WHO and beyond. Prin Pract Oncol 1999;13:1–14.
11. Wright DH. What is Burkitt's lymphoma and when is it endemic? Blood 1999;93:758.
12. Burkitt DP. The discovery of Burkitt's lymphoma. Cancer 1983;51:1777–86.
13. O'Connor GT. Persistent immunologic stimulation as a factor in oncogenesis, with special reference to Burkitt's tumor. Am J Med 1970;48:279–85.
14. Morrow RH, Kisuule A, Mafigiri J. Socioeconomic factors in Burkitt's lymphoma. Cancer Res 1974;34:1212.
15. Ziegler JL. Management of Burkitt's lymphoma: an update. Cancer Treat Rev 1979;6:95–105.
16. Levine AM. Non-Hodgkin's lymphomas and other malignancies in the acquired immune deficiency syndrome. Semin Oncol 1987;14:Suppl 3:34–9.
17. Ziegler JL, Beckstead JA, Volberding PA, et al. Non-Hodgkin's lymphoma in 90 homosexual men: relation to generalized lymphadenopathy and the acquired immunodeficiency syndrome. N Engl J Med 1984;311:565–70.
18. Knowles DM, Chamulak GA, Subar M, et al. Lymphoid neoplasia associated with the acquired immunodeficiency syndrome (AIDS): the New York University Medical Center experience with 105 patients (1981–1986). Ann Intern Med 1988;108:744–53.
19. Spina M, Tirelli U, Zagonel V, et al. Burkitt's lymphoma in adults with and without human immunodeficiency virus infection: a single-institution clinicopathologic study of 75 patients. Cancer 1998;82:766–74.
20. Davi F, Delecluse HJ, Guiet P, et al. Burkitt-like lymphomas in AIDS patients: characterization within a series of 103 human immunodeficiency virus-associated non-Hodgkin's lymphomas. Burkitt's Lymphoma Study Group. J Clin Oncol 1998;16:3788–95.
21. Ziegler JL. Burkitt's lymphoma. N Engl J Med 1981;305:735–45.
22. Klein G. The Epstein-Barr virus and neoplasia. N Engl J Med 1975;293:1353–7.
23. Ziegler JL, Magrath IT, Gerber P, Levine PH. Epstein-Barr virus and human malignancy. Ann Intern Med 1977;86:323–36.
24. Henle W, Henle G. Epidemiologic aspects of Epstein-Barr virus (EBV)–associated diseases. Ann N Y Acad Sci 1980;354:326–31.
25. Henderson A, Ripley S, Heller M, Kieff E. Chromosome site for Epstein-Barr virus DNA in a Burkitt tumor cell line and in lymphocytes growth-transformed in vitro. Proc Natl Acad Sci U S A 1983;80:1987–91.
26. Delecluse HJ, Bartnizke S, Hammerschmidt W, et al. Episomal and integrated copies of Epstein-Barr virus coexist in Burkitt lymphoma cell lines. J Virol 1993;67:1292–9.
27. Gulley ML, Raphael M, Lutz CT, et al. Epstein-Barr virus integration in human lymphomas and lymphoid cell lines. Cancer 1992;70:185–91.

28. Subar M, Neri A, Inghirami G, et al. Frequent c-myc oncogene activation and infrequent presence of Epstein-Barr virus genome in AIDS-associated lymphoma. Blood 1988;72:667–71.

29. Rechavi G, Ben-Bassat I, Berkowicz M, et al. Molecular analysis of Burkitt's leukemia in two hemophilic brothers with AIDS. Blood 1987;70:1713–7.

30. Ganser A, Carlo-Stella C, Bartram CR, et al. Establishment of two Epstein-Barr virus negative Burkitt cell lines from a patient with AIDS and B-cell lymphoma. Blood 1988;72:1255–60.

31. Bernheim A, Berger R. Cytogenetic studies of Burkitt lymphoma-leukemia in patients with acquired immunodeficiency syndrome. Cancer Genet Cytogenet 1988;32:67–74.

32. Abo W, Takada K, Kamada M, et al. Evolution of infectious mononucleosis into Epstein-Barr virus carrying monoclonal malignant lymphoma. Lancet 1982;1:1272–6.

33. Chao TY, Wang TY, Lee WH. Association between Epstein-Barr virus and Burkitt's lymphoma in Taiwan. Cancer 1997;80:121–8.

34. Andriko JA, Aguilera NS, Nandedkar MA, Abbondanzo SL. Childhood Hodgkin's disease in the United States: an analysis of histologic subtypes and association with Epstein-Barr virus. Mod Pathol 1997;10:366–71.

35. Glaser SL, Lin RJ, Stewart SL, et al. Epstein-Barr virus-associated Hodgkin's disease: epidemiologic characteristics in international data. Int J Cancer 1997;70:375–82.

36. Salloum E, Tallini G, Levy A, Cooper DL. Burkitt's lymphoma-leukemia in patients treated for Hodgkin's disease. Cancer Invest 1996;14:527–33.

37. Yoshinaga H, Ohashi K, Yamamoto K, et al. Clonal identification of Burkitt's lymphoma arising from lymphocyte-predominant Hodgkin's disease. Br J Haematol 1996;95:380–2.

38. Spring SB, Schluederberg A, Allen WP, Gruber J. Pathogenic diversity of Epstein-Barr virus. J Natl Cancer Inst 1989;81:13–20.

39. de-The G. Is Burkitt's lymphoma related to perinatal infection by Epstein-Barr virus? Lancet 1977;1:335–8.

40. Charmot G, Rodhain F, Roze JM. [Epidemiology of Burkitt's lymphoma in tropical areas—its relationship with malaria (author's transl)] Nouv Presse Med 1978;7:277–9.

41. Moss DJ, Burrows SR, Castelino DJ, et al. A comparison of Epstein-Barr virus-specific T-cell immunity in malaria-endemic and -nonendemic regions of Papua New Guinea. Int J Cancer 1983;31:727–32.

42. Judson SC, Henle W, Henle G. A cluster of Epstein-Barr-virus-associated American Burkitt's lymphoma. N Engl J Med 1977;297:464–8.

43. Winnett A, Thomas SJ, Brabin BJ, et al. Familial Burkitt's lymphoma in Papua New Guinea. Br J Cancer 1997;75:757–61.

44. Purtilo DT, DeFlorio D Jr, Hutt LM, et al. Variable phenotypic expression of an X-linked recessive lymphoproliferative syndrome. N Engl J Med 1977;297:1077–80.

45. Robinson JE, Brown N, Andiman W, et al. Diffuse polyclonal B-cell lymphoma during primary infection with Epstein-Barr virus. N Engl J Med 1980;302:1293–7.

46. Nishikura K, Murray JM. The mechanism of inactivation of the normal c-myc gene locus in human Burkitt lymphoma cells. Oncogene 1988;2:493–8.

47. Cesarman E, Dalla-Favera R, Bentley D, Groudine M. Mutations in the first exon are associated with altered transcription of c-myc in Burkitt lymphoma. Science 1987;238:1272–5.

48. Zajac-Kaye M, Gelmann EP, Levens D. A point mutation in the c-myc locus of a Burkitt lymphoma abolishes binding of a nuclear protein. Science 1988;240:1776–80.

49. Yano T, Sander CA, Clark HM, et al. Clustered mutations in the second exon of the MYC gene in sporadic Burkitt's lymphoma. Oncogene 1993;8:2741–8.

50. Diamond A, Cooper GM, Ritz J, Lane MA. Identification and molecular cloning of the human Blym transforming gene activated in Burkitt's lymphomas. Nature 1983;305:112–6.

51. Preudhomme C, Dervite I, Wattel E, et al. Clinical significance of p53 mutations in newly diagnosed Burkitt's lymphoma and acute lymphoblastic leukemia: a report of 48 cases. J Clin Oncol 1995;13:812–20.

52. Blazar BA, Sutton LM, Strome M. Self-stimulating growth factor production by B-cell lines derived from Burkitt's lymphomas and other lines transformed in vitro by Epstein-Barr virus. Cancer Res 1983;43:4562–8.

53. Berard CW, O'Connor GT, Thomas LB, Torloni H. Histopathological definition of Burkitt's tumor. Bull WHO 1969;40:601–7.

54. Wright DH. Burkitt's lymphoma: a review of the pathology, immunology, and possible etiologic factors. Pathol Annu 1971;6:337–63.

55. Wilson JF, Kjeldsberg CR, Sposto R, et al. The pathology of non-Hodgkin's lymphoma of childhood: II. reproducibility and relevance of the histologic classification of "undifferentiated" lymphomas (Burkitt's versus non-Burkitt's). Hum Pathol 1987;18:1008–14.

56. Miliauskas JR, Berard CW, Young RC, et al. Undifferentiated non-Hodgkin's lymphomas (Burkitt's and non-Burkitt's types): the relevance of making this histologic distinction. Cancer 1982;50:2115–21.

57. Grogan TM, Warnke RA, Kaplan HS. A comparative study of Burkitt's and non-Burkitt's "undifferentiated" malignant lymphoma: immunologic, cytochemical, ultrastructural, cytologic, histopathologic, clinical and cell culture features. Cancer 1982;49:1817–28.

58. Levine AM, Pavlova Z, Pockros AW, et al. Small noncleave follicular center cell (FCC) lymphoma: Burkitt and non-Burkitt variants in the United States: I. clinical features. Cancer 1983;52:1073–9.

59. Pavlova Z, Parker JW, Taylor CR, et al. Small noncleaved follicular center cell lymphoma: Burkitt's and non-Burkitt's variants in the US: II. pathologic and immunologic features. Cancer 1987;59:1892–902.

60. Spina D, Leoncini L, Megha T, et al. Cellular kinetic and phenotypic heterogeneity in and among Burkitt's and Burkitt-like lymphomas. J Pathol 1997;182:145–50.

61. Mann RB, Jaffe ES, Braylan RC, et al. Non-endemic Burkitt's lymphoma: a B-cell tumor related to germinal centers. N Engl J Med 1976;295:685–91.

62. Preud'homme JL, Brouet JC, Danon F, et al. Acute lymphoblastic leukemia with Burkitt's lymphoma cells: membrane markers and serum immunoglobulin. J Natl Cancer Inst 1981;66:261–4.

63. Ganick DJ, Finlay JL. Acute lymphoblastic leukemia with Burkitt cell morphology and cytoplasmic immunoglobulin. Blood 1980;56:311–4.

64. Foon KA, Todd RF 3d. Immunologic classification of leukemia and lymphoma. Blood 1986;68:1–31.

65. Wright DH, Isaacson P. Follicular center cell lymphoma of childhood: a report of three cases and a discussion of its relationship to Burkitt's lymphoma. Cancer 1981;47:915–25.

66. Iversen OH, Iversen U, Ziegler JL, Bluming AZ. Cell kinetics in Burkitt lymphoma. Eur J Cancer 1974;10:155–63.

67. Durodola JI. Burkitt's lymphoma in Ibadan: response to various doses of cyclophosphamide and long-term survivors. Eur J Cancer 1976;12:425–32.

68. Nkrumah FK, Perkins IV. Burkitt's lymphoma: a clinical study of 110 patients. Cancer 1976;37:671–6.

69. Ziegler JL, Magrath IT, Olweny CL. Cure of Burkitt's lymphoma: ten-year follow-up of 157 Ugandan patients. Lancet 1979;2:936–8.

70. Levine PH, Connelly RR, Berard CW, et al. The American Burkitt Lymphoma Registry: a progress report. Ann Intern Med 1975;83:31–6.

71. Levine PH, Kamaraju LS, Connelly RR, et al. The American Burkitt's Lymphoma Registry: eight years' experience. Cancer 1982;49:1016–22.

72. Ziegler JL. Treatment results of 54 American patients with Burkitt's lymphoma are similar to the African experience. N Engl J Med 1977;297:75–80.

73. Jones DE, d'Avignon MB, Lawrence R, Latshaw RF. Burkitt's lymphoma: obstetric and gynecologic aspects. Obstet Gynecol 1980;56:533–6.

74. Bernstein JI, Coleman CN, Strickler JG, et al. Combined modality therapy for adults with small noncleaved cell lymphoma (Burkitt's and non-Burkitt's types). J Clin Oncol 1986;4:847–58.

75. Magrath IT, Lwanga S, Carswell W, Harrison N. Surgical reduction of tumour bulk in management of abdominal Burkitt's lymphoma. Br Med J 1974;2:308–12.

76. Krudy AG, Dunnick NR, Magrath IT, et al. CT of American Burkitt lymphoma. AJR Am J Roentgenol 1981;136:747–54.

77. Richman SD, Appelbaum F, Levenson SM, et al. 67Ga radionuclide imaging in Burkitt's lymphoma. Radiology 1975;117:Pt 1:639–45.

78. Sandrock D, Lastoria S, Magrath IT, Neumann RD. The role of gallium-67 tumour scintigraphy in patients with small, non-cleaved cell lymphoma. Eur J Nucl Med 1993;20:119–22.

79. Johnson KA, Tung K, Mead G, Sweetenham J. The imaging of Burkitt's and Burkitt-like lymphoma. Clin Radiol 1998;53:835–41.

80. Barrington SF, Carr R. Staging of Burkitt's lymphoma and response to treatment monitored by PET scanning. Clin Oncol (R Coll Radiol) 1995;7:334–5.

81. Cohen LF, Balow JE, Magrath IT, et al. Acute tumor lysis syndrome: a review of 37 patients with Burkitt's lymphoma. Am J Med 1980;68:486–91.

82. Olweny CL, Katongole-Mbidde E, Otim D, et al. Long-term experience with Burkitt's lymphoma in Uganda. Int J Cancer 1980;26:261–6.

83. Bowman WP, Shuster JJ, Cook B, et al. Improved survival for children with B-cell acute lymphoblastic leukemia and stage IV small non-cleaved-cell lymphoma: a pediatric oncology group study. J Clin Oncol 1996;14:1252–61.

84. Gasparini M, Rottoli L, Massimino M, et al. Curability of advanced Burkitt's lymphoma in children by intensive short-term chemotherapy. Eur J Cancer 1993;29A:692–8.

85. Soussain C, Patte C, Ostronoff M, et al. Small noncleaved cell lymphoma and leukemia in adults: a retrospective study of 65 adults treated with the LMB pediatric protocols. Blood 1995;85:664–74.

86. Magrath I, Adde M, Shad A, et al. Adults and children with small non-cleaved-cell lymphoma have a similar excellent outcome when treated with the same chemotherapy regimen. J Clin Oncol 1996;14:925–34.

87. Kemeny MM, Magrath IT, Brennan MF. The role of surgery in the management of American Burkitt's lymphoma and its treatment. Ann Surg 1982;196:82–6.

88. Kaufman BH, Burgert EO, Jr, Banks PM. Abdominal Burkitt's lymphoma: role of early aggressive surgery. J Pediatr Surg 1987;22:671–4.

89. Murphy SB, Bowman WP, Abromowitch M, et al. Results of treatment of advanced-stage Burkitt's lymphoma and B cell (SIg +) acute lymphoblastic leukemia with high-dose fractionated cyclophosphamide and coordinated high-dose methotrexate and cytarabine. J Clin Oncol 1986;4:1732–9.

90. Miron I, Frappaz D, Brunat-Mentigny M, et al. Initial management of advanced Burkitt lymphoma in children: is there still a place for surgery? Pediatr Hematol Oncol 1997;14:555–61.

91. Shamberger RC, Weinstein HJ. The role of surgery in abdominal Burkitt's lymphoma. J Pediatr Surg 1992;27:236–40.

92. Gahukamble DB, Khamage AS. Limitations of surgery in intraabdominal Burkitt's lymphoma in children. J Pediatr Surg 1995;30:519–22.

93. Lees DE, Gadde PL, Macnamara TE. Malignant hyperthermia in association with Burkitt's lymphoma: report of a third case. Anesth Analg 1980;59:514–5.

94. Norin T, Clifford P, Einhorn J, et al. Conventional and superfractionated radiation therapy in Burkitt's lymphoma. Acta Radiol Ther Phys Biol 1971;10:545–57.

95. Norin T, Onyango J. Radiotherapy in Burkitt's lymphoma: conventional or superfractionated regime—early results. Int J Radiat Oncol Biol Phys 1977;2:399–406.

96. Norin T. Radiation therapy in Burkitt's lymphoma of the central nervous system. Acta Radiol Ther Phys Biol 1977;16:73–80.

97. Olweny CL, Atine I, Kaddu-Mukasa A, et al. Cerebrospinal irradiation of Burkitt's lymphoma: failure in preventing central nervous system relapse. Acta Radiol Ther Phys Biol 1977;16:225–31.

98. Magrath IT, Janus C, Edwards BK, et al. An effective therapy for both undifferentiated (including Burkitt's) lymphomas and lymphoblastic lymphomas in children and young adults. Blood 1984;63:1102–11.

99. McMaster ML, Greer JP, Greco FA, et al. Effective treatment of small-noncleaved-cell lymphoma with high-intensity, brief-duration chemotherapy. J Clin Oncol 1991;9:941–6.

100. Connors JM, Klimo P. MACOP-B 12 week chemotherapy for lymphoma: update and additional observations. Proc ASCO 1986;5:192.

101. Magrath IT, Adde M, Shad A, et al. Results in adults with small noncleaved cell (SNCL) lymphoma treated with a short duration intensive chemotherapy protocol also used in pediatric patients. Proc ASCO 1994;13:371.

102. Pichler E, Jürgenssen OA, Radaszkiewicz, et al. Results of LSA2-L2 therapy in 26 children with non-Hodgkin's lymphoma. Cancer 1982;50:2740–6.

103. Griffin TC, Bowman WP, Winick NJ, Buchanan GR. Treatment of advanced stage diffuse, small non-cleaved cell lymphoma in childhood: further experience with total therapy B. Med Pediatr Oncol 1994;23:393–9.

104. Patte C, Leverger G, Rubie H, et al. High cure rate in B-cell (Burkitt's) leukemia in the LMB 89 protocol of the SFOP (French Pediatric Oncology Society). Proc ASCO 1993;12:317.

105. Patte C, Philip T, Rodary C, et al. High survival rate in advanced-stage B-cell lymphomas and leukemias without CNS involvement with a short intensive polychemotherapy: results from the French Pediatric Oncology Society of a randomized trial of 216 children. J Clin Oncol 1991;9:123–32.

106. Patte C, Leverger G, Perel Y, et al. Updated results of the LMB 86 protocol of the French Pediatric Oncology Society (SFOP) for B-cell non-Hodgkin's lymphomas (B-NHL) with CNS involvement (CNS +) and B-ALL. Med Pediatr Oncol 1990;18:397.

107. Cairo MS, Krailo M, Hutchinson R, et al. Results of a phase II trial of "French" (F) (LMB-86) or "Orange" (O) (CCG-hybrid) in children with advanced non-lymphoblastic non-Hodgkin's lymphoma: an improvement in survival. Proc ASCO 1994;13:392.

108. Philip T, Meckenstock R, Deconnick E, et al. Treatment of poor prognosis Burkitt's lymphoma in adults with the Société Française d'Oncologie Pédiatrique LMB Protocol—a study of the Federation Nationale des Centres de Lutte Contre le Cancer (FNLCC). Eur J Cancer 1992;28A:1954–9.

109. Canellos GP, Nadler L, Takvorian T. Autologous bone marrow transplantation in the treatment of malignant lymphoma and Hodgkin's disease. Semin Hematol 1988;25:Suppl 2:58–65.

110. Philip T, Pinkerton R, Hartmann O, et al. The role of massive therapy with autologous bone marrow transplantation in Burkitt's lymphoma. Clin Haematol 1986;15:205–17.

111. Philip T, Hartmann O, Biron P, et al. High-dose therapy and autologous bone marrow transplantation in partial remission after first-line induction therapy for diffuse non-Hodgkin's lymphoma. J Clin Oncol 1988;6:1118–24.

112. Ladenstein R, Pearce R, Hartmann O, et al. High-dose chemotherapy with autologous bone marrow rescue in children with poor-risk Burkitt's lymphoma: a report from the European Lymphoma Bone Marrow Transplantation Registry. Blood 1997;90:2921–30.

113. Sweetenham JW, Pearce R, Taghipour G, et al. Adult Burkitt's and Burkitt-like non-Hodgkin's lymphoma—outcome for patients treated with high-dose therapy and autologous stem-cell transplantation in first remission or at relapse: results from the European Group for Blood and Marrow Transplantation. J Clin Oncol 1996;14:2465–72.

114. Troussard X, Leblond V, Kuentz M, et al. Allogeneic bone marrow transplantation in adults with Burkitt's lymphoma or acute lymphoblastic leukemia in first complete remission. J Clin Oncol 1990;8:809–12.

115. Nademanee A, Schmidt GM, O'Donnell MR, et al. High-dose chemoradiotherapy followed by autologous bone marrow transplantation as consolidation therapy during first complete remission in adult patients with poor-risk aggressive lymphoma: a pilot study. Blood 1992;80:1130–4.

116. Haioun C, Lepage E, Gisselbrecht C, et al. Autologous bone marrow transplantation (ABMT) versus sequential chemotherapy in first complete remission aggressive non-Hodgkin's lymphoma (NHL): 1st interim analysis on 370 patients (LNH87 protocol). Proc ASCO 1992;11:316.

117. Straus DJ. Treatment of Burkitt's lymphoma in HIV-positive patients. Biomed Pharmacother 1996;50:447–50.

118. Haddy TB, Adde MA, Magrath IT. CNS involvement in small non-cleaved-cell lymphoma: is CNS disease per se a poor prognostic sign? J Clin Oncol 1991;9:1973–82.

119. Magrath I, Lee YJ, Anderson T, et al. Prognostic factors in Burkitt's lymphoma: importance of total tumor burden. Cancer 1980;45:1507–15.

120. Ziegler JL, Magrath IT, Deisseroth AB, et al. Combined modality treatment of Burkitt's lymphoma. Cancer Treat Rep 1978;62:2031–4.

121. Tsokos GC, Balow JE, Spiegel RJ, Magrath IT. Renal and metabolic complications of undifferentiated and lymphoblastic lymphomas. Medicine 1981;60:218–29.

# CHAPTER 92

# NONCUTANEOUS T-CELL LYMPHOMAS AND NK NEOPLASMS

• PETER J. ROSEN • JONATHAN SAID

Previous classifications of the non-Hodgkin's lymphomas, such as the widely used Working Formulation, were devised without specific reference to the B-cell or T-cell origin of lymphomas.[1] Major advances in the ability to perform specialized studies on neoplastic tissue obtained from patients with non-Hodgkin's lymphoma now allow distinction between B-cell and T-cell lineage in most cases. These techniques include application of monoclonal antibodies to cell suspensions or frozen tissue as well as Southern blot analysis for immunoglobulin or T-cell receptor gene rearrangements. Cytogenetic analysis and polymerase chain reaction (PCR) amplification of specific chromosomal breakpoints are also of value in defining clinical pathologic entities, as is well known in subsets of B lineage non-Hodgkin's lymphoma, such as the follicular and Burkitt's types.

In addition to being relatively rare in comparison with B-cell lymphomas, the spectrum of T-cell and natural killer (NK)–cell neoplasms is highly diverse clinically and pathologically. In Western countries, greater than 85% of non-Hodgkin's lymphomas are of B lineage, whereas T-cell and NK lymphomas are more frequently found in Asian countries. The prevalence of T-cell lymphomas in Japan is only partially accounted for by the endemic adult T-cell leukemia and lymphoma (ATLL) syndrome. The heterogeneity of clinical and morphologic expressions of the T-cell (and NK) lymphomas has challenged pathologists and clinicians. Until the 1990s, no single pathologic classification had been adopted internationally, although the attempts by Lennert and Feller[2] (Kiel classification) were of seminal value and used throughout Europe. The approach in this chapter is syndrome based; the tumors are described as distinctive clinical and pathologic entities based on clinical, histologic, phenotypic, and genotypic features. This schema is in accordance with the more recent classifications included in the Revised European-American Lymphoma (REAL) proposal and the subsequent World Health Organization (WHO) modifications.[3, 4] Further refinements are sure to follow as these and other entities are characterized better in the future. The close interrelationships between T cells, NK cells, and NK-like T cells as well as the overlapping clinical presentations of the T-cell and NK lymphomas suggest that these entities are best considered together. Cutaneous T-cell lymphomas and ATLL are discussed elsewhere in this book.

## Classification

The current REAL and WHO proposed classifications for T-cell and NK-cell neoplasms are shown in Tables 92–1 and 92–2. T-cell and NK lymphomas can be divided between precursor T-cell malignancies and peripheral or mature T-cell and NK neoplasms. Precursor or thymic T-cell lymphomas are all high grade, and the term *lymphoblastic lymphoma* has been used conventionally to designate these cases. There is much overlap between lymphoblastic lymphoma and T-cell acute lymphoblastic leukemia (T-ALL). The peripheral T-cell lymphomas and NK tumors are a highly diverse group with varying clinical presentations and degrees of aggressiveness. Some peripheral T-cell lymphomas may evolve from relatively low grade to high grade analogous to the transformation of follicular lymphomas to high-grade B-cell neoplasms. In general, however, T-cell lymphomas behave in a clinically aggressive fashion relative to their B-cell histologic counterparts.

## Determination of T-Cell Origin of Lymphoma

Conclusive evidence for the T-cell derivation of lymphomas is hampered by the lack of simple markers of clonality. Although kappa or lambda light chain restriction permits strong inferential evidence for a clonal B-cell origin of lymphomas, no analogous marker susceptible to immunophenotypic characterization exists for the T-cell group. Demonstration of a preponderance of T cells in a pathologic specimen is inadequate evidence that one is dealing with a T-cell lymphoma. For example, it has been shown that some B-cell lymphomas are heavily infiltrated by reactive T cells that may outnumber the malignant B cells. The term

*Table 92–1.* REAL Classification of T/NK Neoplasms

*Precursor Cell Neoplasm*

Precursor T-cell lymphoblastic lymphoma/leukemia

*Peripheral (Mature) Cell Neoplasms*

T-cell chronic lymphocytic leukemia
Large granular lymphocytic leukemia (T or NK cell)
Mycosis fungoides
Peripheral T-cell lymphoma unspecified
Angioimmunoblastic T-cell lymphoma
Angiocentric lymphoma
Intestinal T-cell lymphoma (with or without enteropathy)
Adult T-cell lymphoma/leukemia HTLV-I[+]
Anaplastic large cell lymphoma, T-cell and null cell types

HTLV-I, human T-cell lymphotropic virus type I.

1401

*Table 92–2.* **WHO Classification of T-Cell Neoplasms**

*Precursor T-Cell Lymphoblastic Leukemia and Lymphoma*

*Peripheral T-cell and NK-Cell Neoplasms*

T-cell prolymphocytic leukemia
  Variants:  Small cell
        Cerebriform cell
T-cell large granular lymphocytic leukemia
Aggressive NK-cell leukemia
NK/T-cell lymphoma, nasal and nasal-type
Sézary's syndrome
Mycosis fungoides
  Variants:  Pagetoid reticulosis
        Mycosis fungoides–associated follicular mucinosis
        Granulomatous slack skin disease
Angioimmunoblastic T-cell lymphoma
Peripheral T-cell lymphoma (unspecified)
  Variants:  Lymphoepithelioid (Lennert's)
        T-zone
Adult T-cell leukemia/lymphoma (HTLV-I⁺)
  Variants:  Acute
        Lymphomatous
        Chronic
        Smoldering
        Hodgkin's-like
Anaplastic large cell lymphoma (T-cell and null-cell types)
  Variants:  Lymphohistiocytic
        Small cell
Primary cutaneous CD-30⁺ T-cell lymphoproliferative disorders
  Variants:  Lymphomatoid papulosis (type A and B)
        Primary cutaneous anaplastic large cell lymphoma
        Borderline lesions
Subcutaneous panniculitis-like T-cell lymphoma
Enteropathy-type intestinal T-cell lymphoma
Hepatosplenic gamma/delta T-cell lymphoma

HTLV-I, human T-cell lymphotropic virus type I.

*T cell–rich large B-cell lymphoma* has been introduced to describe this group.[5]

The categorization of a lymphoma as T cell in origin requires knowledge of the morphologic expression and certain immunophenotypic characteristics of T-cell lymphomas and, in some cases, application of T-cell receptor gene rearrangement techniques. Although the morphologic recognition of lymphoblastic lymphoma is relatively straightforward, the situation is more complex in the case of peripheral T-cell lymphomas. Certain morphologic features, although nonspecific, suggest that a lymphoma may be of a so-called peripheral or post-thymic T-cell origin and include (1) primary infiltration of T-cell regions (e.g., paracortical or T-zone); (2) increase in number and atypicality of high endothelial venules; (3) pleomorphic tumor cells (often exhibiting clear cytoplasm), frequently including giant cells and cells that may mimic Reed-Sternberg cells; and (4) coexisting mixtures of reactive epithelioid histiocytes, eosinophils, plasma cells, and interdigitating cells.[2]

In the context of these appropriate morphologic features, immunohistochemistry provides further evidence for T-cell origin (Fig. 92–1). Typical immunophenotypic findings include (1) T-cell predominance, (2) T-cell subset antigen restriction, (3) anomalous T-cell antigen expression, and (4) deletion of T-cell antigens. As noted, simple T-cell predominance is insufficient evidence for T-cell origin. Suspicion of a T-cell neoplasm is raised, however, when a single subset of T lymphocytes, often CD4 or CD8, predominates. Dele-

tion of one or more T-cell antigens (usually one or more of the pan-T antigens—CD2, CD3, CD5, CD7) or anomalous T-cell antigen expression (e.g., CD4⁺ and CD8⁺ or CD4⁻ and CD8⁻) is helpful in identifying cases of T-cell malignancy.

Combining morphology with immunohistochemistry allows identification of most T-cell lymphomas. In some cases, Southern blot or PCR analysis for T-cell receptor gene rearrangements using probes for the alpha/beta or gamma/delta receptors is required for final identification.

# Precursor T-Cell Lymphoblastic Leukemia and Lymphomas

## LYMPHOBLASTIC LYMPHOMA

Lymphoblastic lymphoma represents less than 2% of non-Hodgkin's lymphomas. Although a few examples of B-cell or NK-cell lymphoblastic lymphoma have been reported in the literature, greater than 85% of lymphomas with this histology are of T-cell origin.[6–8] This disorder is closely related to and often inseparable from T-ALL, which is covered in other sections of this book.

**Clinical Presentation.** Lymphoblastic lymphomas were first observed in the pediatric literature, where the term *Sternberg sarcoma* was used to describe cases of anterior mediastinal masses composed of primitive lymphoid cells in children and adolescents. The clinical and pathologic syn-

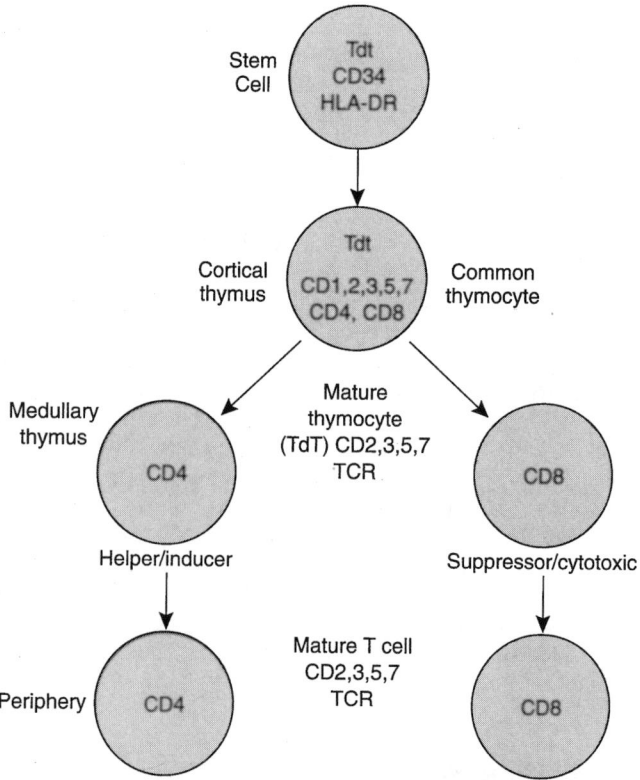

**Figure 92–1.** Schema of T-cell ontogeny. Lymphoblastic lymphomas are neoplasms corresponding to a stage of thymus development. Peripheral T-cell lymphomas are tumors of mature T cells.

drome was subsequently defined in detail by Barcos and Lukes,[9] and adult cases were recognized.[10] The disease is characteristically of explosive onset and usually occurs in teenagers and young adults, but examples of lymphoblastic lymphoma have been observed in all ages. There is a decided male predominance; in most series, the male/female ratio exceeds 3:1.

Patients often come to attention because of symptoms referable to a large anterior mediastinal (thymic) mass, which is observed in greater than 50% of cases. The most common presentations include symptoms secondary to tracheal compression, superior vena cava syndrome, or pleural and pericardial effusions. Lymphadenopathy, often supraclavicular, and splenomegaly are common findings.

Peripheral blood and bone marrow involvement are common, and some arbitrarily designate cases with major peripheral blood or bone marrow involvement (e.g., >25% bone marrow involvement) as T-ALL. During the course of the disease, meningeal involvement is seen in more than 50% of patients not undergoing central nervous system prophylaxis.

**Pathology.** Lymphoblastic lymphomas are derived from thymic T-cell precursor lymphoid cells. In 1975, Barcos and Lukes[9] described this entity as *convoluted lymphomas of the mediastinum*. The term *convoluted* referred to the morphologic appearance of the nuclei in most cases, but many examples without convolutions are seen. Lymphoblastic lymphomas usually present with involvement of the thymus, mediastinal soft tissues, and lymph nodes.

The pattern of infiltration is diffuse and consists of intermediate-size, blast-like lymphoid cells with frequent mitoses (Fig. 92–2). Nucleoli are not usually prominent. The nuclear chromatin is granular or finely stippled. Nuclear irregularity is variable, with some cases having round or oval nuclear outlines, whereas most have markedly convoluted or cerebriform nuclei. Convolutions may be subtle and best appreciated as branched lines when focusing on the nucleus. Characteristic cells have a *hand-in-glove* or *chicken's foot* nuclear outline. The cytoplasm is usually inconspicuous. Phagocytic macrophages are sometimes present but less prominent than in Burkitt's lymphoma.

In a small percentage (10%) of cases, variants consist of small and larger cells with more prominent nucleoli and no convolutions of the nucleoli. In these cases, the differential

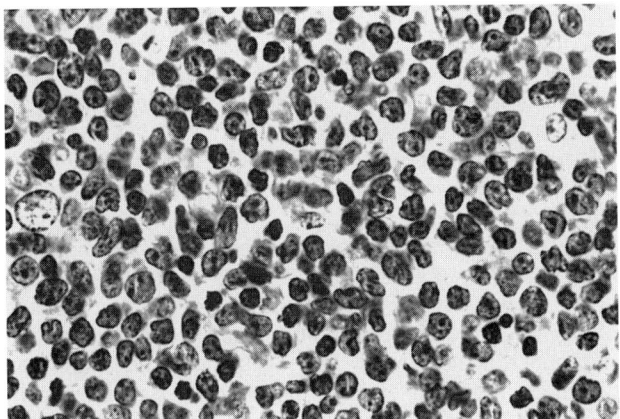

**Figure 92–2.** Lymphoblastic lymphoma. Note convoluted nuclei and inconspicuous nucleoli.

diagnosis includes Burkitt's lymphoma and the blastic variant of mantle cell lymphoma. Both of these entities are terminal deoxynucleotidyl transferase (TdT) negative, however, and of B lineage. Mantle cell lymphomas characteristically express *bcl-1*.

Immunologically the cells in precursor T-cell lymphomas are related to thymic T cells and are usually positive for TdT and one or more T-cell markers, including CD1, CD2, CD3, CD5, or CD7.[11] Common phenotypes include $CD4^+CD8^+$ as well as $CD4^-CD8^-$. There is punctate paranuclear staining for acid phosphastase. Of all the lymphoma subtypes, lymphoblastic lymphoma is the only one in which TdT positivity is seen, and this finding is of great diagnostic value.

Most cases have karyotypic abnormalities, including hyperdiploidy or near-tetraploidy. The specific translocations include chromosome 14 band q1 (site of the T-cell receptor alpha and delta genes), chromosome 7 at bands q34–36 (T-cell receptor beta gene), and chromosome 7 band p15 (T-cell receptor gamma gene).[12]

**Prognosis and Treatment.** Before the recognition of lymphoblastic lymphoma as a disorder closely related to ALL, patients were treated in a similar fashion to other aggressive non-Hodgkin's lymphomas with dismal results. The median survival was always less than 1 year, and leukemic and meningeal relapse were the rule.[10] On the basis of the similarity of the pathology and clinical course to T-ALL, a *leukemia strategy* was adopted for this disease in the late 1970s. Newer protocols used aggressive induction and consolidation therapy, central nervous system prophylaxis, and often a maintenance phase similar to that used in childhood ALL. Subsequently, long-term survival rates exceeding 40% have been observed in several series. Levine and colleagues[13] reported a small series of patients treated using a modified Memorial Sloan-Kettering childhood lymphoma protocol, LSA2–L2, which used induction therapy using cyclophosphamide, vincristine, doxorubicin, and prednisone combined with intrathecal methotrexate. Mediastinal radiation was also given. The consolidation phase included agents rarely used in adult lymphomas, such as cytarabine, L-asparaginase, and 6-thioguanine. Cranial radiation was delivered during consolidation. A maintenance program including complex cycles of alternating chemotherapy agents was given for 3 years. For a small group of 15 patients so treated, the median survival was 28.3 months, and the survival of complete responders exceeded 71 months. Median relapse-free survival was 41 months.

Coleman and coworkers[14] reported encouraging results employing cyclophosphamide, doxorubicin, vincristine, and prednisone induction; central nervous system prophylaxis; further consolidation therapy including L-asparaginase; and subsequent maintenance treatment with 6-mercaptopurine and methotrexate. Treatment was completed after 1 year. At 3 years, 56% of patients were projected to be alive and disease free. The addition of early central nervous system radiation to intrathecal chemotherapy dramatically reduced the rate of meningeal lymphoma from 31 to 3%. These authors subdivided their cases into low-risk and high-risk groups. High-risk patients manifested stage IV disease (Ann Arbor), often with bone marrow or central nervous system involvement or an elevated serum lactate dehydrogenase level (>300 IU). These patients had a poor outcome with only 19% freedom from relapse at 5 years. In contrast, patients without these adverse prognostic findings enjoyed 94% freedom from relapse. On the basis of these results, it was proposed that more aggressive treatment be given to the poor-prognosis group.

Other studies have not confirmed the sharp prognostic grouping noted by Coleman. A French study employing a variety of treatment protocols in 80 adults with lymphoblastic lymphoma found that age and lactate dehydrogenase level rather than bone marrow involvement were the important predictors of outcome,[15] whereas the Memorial Sloan-Kettering group observed that results for lymphoblastic lymphoma were essentially identical with those seen in adult ALL, with a 45% 5-year survival rate projected.[16] In the latter study, poor prognostic factors included age (>30 years), white blood cell count greater than 30,000/mm³, and failure to achieve or the slow development of complete remission. Multi-institutional trials of adult ALL note that T-ALL patients generally have a relatively favorable prognosis, suggesting that modern ALL management is the appropriate model for treatment of lymphoblastic lymphomas.

Although it is unclear whether a simple staging system can predict outcome for lymphoblastic lymphoma, the historically suboptimal results have led to trials of autologous and allogeneic bone marrow transplantation in first or subsequent remission. Nonrandomized trials suggest a superior outcome for poor-prognosis subgroups receiving autologous bone marrow transplantation in first complete remission.[17, 18] Retrospective studies indicate a possible superiority for allogeneic over autologous bone marrow transplantation.[19] A randomized trial conducted by the European Group for Blood and Bone Marrow Transplantation and the U.K. Lymphoma Group suggested a possible advantage for autologous stem cell transplantation in first remission for adult patients with lymphoblastic lymphoma.[20] In that study, 119 patients with lymphoblastic lymphoma from 33 European centers were studied. All patients received induction therapy, and responding patients were randomized to conventional therapy or high-dose chemotherapy with peripheral blood stem cell transplantation. Patients who relapsed after conventional therapy were eligible to receive peripheral blood stem cell transplants if they were responsive to salvage therapy. The results of the study are preliminary and hampered by the fact that only 65 of 119 patients were actually randomized. With a short median follow-up period of 12 months, a 45% reduction in the risk of relapse was observed following stem cell transplantation. At the time of reporting, there was no significant difference in overall survival between the groups, and this lack of difference may be due to the fact that relapsing patients could go on to autologous or allogeneic transplantation. The results of this trial, although randomized, appear insufficient to suggest the routine use of stem cell transplantation in first remission particularly when modern ALL-like treatment is applied. New agents undergoing development include compound 506U, a prodrug of 9-beta-D-arabinofuranosylguanine (ara-G). This agent induced remissions in 76% (complete response, 44%) of relapsed and refractory T-ALL cases.[21]

## Peripheral T-Cell and NK-Cell Leukemias

The peripheral T-cell and NK-cell leukemias are uncommon disorders, and classification has been confusing and inconsis-tently applied. Based on the WHO modifications of the REAL classification, major subsets of peripheral T-cell and NK-cell leukemias are recognized: (1) T-prolymphocytic leukemia (T-PLL), (2) T-cell large granular lymphocytic (LGL) leukemia, and (3) NK-cell leukemia.

### T-PROLYMPHOCYTIC LEUKEMIA

T-PLL is an extremely rare form of small cell lymphocytic leukemia and comprises less than 2% of all cases of chronic lymphocytic leukemia (CLL).[22] The disorder corresponding to B-CLL, in other words T-CLL, has not been easily recognized in the literature. Most cases previously described as T-CLL are subsumed under the designation T-PLL, and this disorder includes a spectrum of morphologic types.

**Clinical Presentation.** T-PLL probably accounts for 25% of all cases of prolymphocytic leukemia. Patients are generally older than age 30 and commonly present with splenomegaly, generalized lymphadenopathy, and cutaneous involvement. The more common B-PLL patients generally have only splenomegaly and do not manifest lymphadenopathy and cutaneous involvement. At presentation, the white blood count is generally markedly elevated, usually greater than 100,000/mm³, and the patients are often anemic and thrombocytopenic.

**Pathology.** There is a broad morphologic heterogeneity ranging from small lymphocytes to cases composed almost entirely of classic prolymphocytes (Fig. 92–3). The small lymphocytic form is often characterized by irregular or *knobby* nuclear outlines. The cytoplasm is basophilic and nongranular. Prolymphocytes have prominent nucleoli. In rare cases, the cells can be markedly irregular or cerebriform, resembling Sézary's syndrome.

The bone marrow is usually diffusely infiltrated, and the skin is involved by dermal infiltrates. In contrast to mycosis fungoides, there is no epidermotropism. Splenic involvement is common with infiltration of red and white pulp. Lymph nodes may show either diffuse infiltration or preferential involvement of the interfollicular or T-cell zones with sparing of the follicles.

Most cases have a mature T-helper phenotype, expressing CD4 and CD3, while showing negativity for CD8 and TdT.[22] The T lymphocytes stain strongly for acid phosphatase and α-naphthyl acetate esterase with a block-like paranuclear pattern. The most common cytogenetic abnormality is inversion of chromosome 14, with breakpoints in the long arms of q11 and q32. Other associated abnormalities are a reciprocal translocation t(9;14)(q11;q32), trisomy 8q, and deletion or translocations of chromosome 11.

**Prognosis and Treatment.** T-PLL in its various forms is a disease that is extremely resistant to treatment. Survivals have generally been less than 1 year. Only transient responses to a variety of cytotoxic agents have been noted. In addition to the alkylating agents and various anthracycline combinations, the purine nucleosides show some signs of activity. In particular, pentostatin (2-deoxycoformycin) may have preferential activity. This agent has been extensively studied by Mercieca and colleagues.[23] They reported a response rate of 45% in a series of 55 patients treated with pentostatin. Of the 25 responding patients, 5 achieved complete remissions. The duration of these remissions was rela-

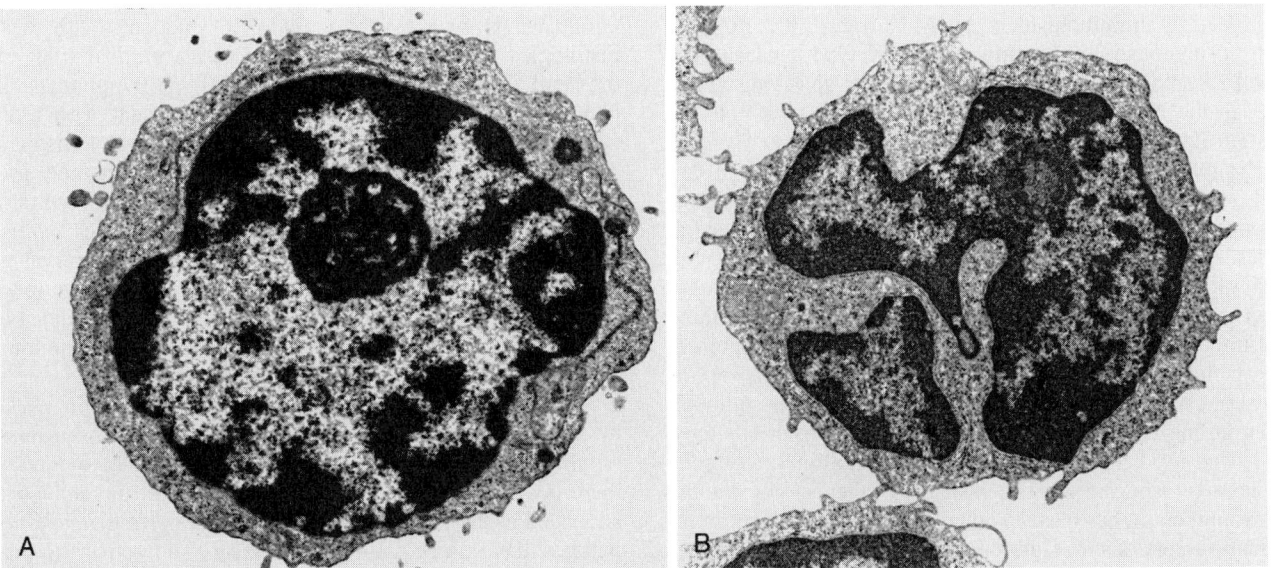

**Figure 92–3.** Morphologic spectrum of T-cell prolymphocytic leukemia. *A*, A typical prolymphocyte with large central nucleolus. *B*, A cell with a markedly irregular nucleus and less prominent nucleolus (electron micrograph, uranyl acetate and lead citrate, original ×11,000).

tively brief with a median of 6 months. Complete responders had longer remissions lasting a median of 10 months. Compound 506U (ara-G), mentioned in the discussion of lymphoblastic lymphoma, has also been studied in T-PLL with a 67% response rate observed in nine patients.[21]

CAMPATH-lH, a chimeric monoclonal antibody directed against CD52, a molecule expressed on T and B lymphocytes, deserves investigation in T-PLL.[24] Preliminary investigations show a high complete response rate in T-PLL.[24] Other treatments used with generally short-term palliation include splenic radiation and splenectomy.

## T-CELL LARGE GRANULAR LYMPHOCYTIC LEUKEMIA AND NK-CELL LEUKEMIAS

LGL leukemia is defined by a persistent increase in circulating LGLs—usually 2000 to 20,000/mm³—for more than 6 months without detectable cause.[25] Some series have described patients who have persistently elevated nonclonally expanded LGL, and patients with clonal expansion may manifest an indolent or nonprogressive condition over years.[26] The LGL leukemias can be divided into two major lineages: CD3⁻ (NK cells that mediate non–major histocompatibility complex [MHC] restricted cytotoxicity) and CD3⁺ T cells.

**Clinical Presentation.** LGL leukemias are uncommon and probably account for less than 3% of all cases of small lymphocytic leukemias. Within this group, the CD3⁺ T-cell type of LGL leukemia is more frequent. These patients generally present with neutropenia, which dominates their clinical course. They often have an associated autoimmune complex consisting of elevated rheumatoid factor, various autoantibodies, autoimmune hemolytic anemia or red cell aplasia, and, less commonly, thrombocytopenia.[27] Polyclonal hypergammaglobulinemia and monoclonal paraproteins have been described as well as hypogammaglobulinemia. The pathogenesis of the neutropenia has not been well defined.

It may be cyclic in some cases. The possibility of an inhibitory factor against colony forming unit–culture (CFU-C) has been postulated but not proved. Autoantibodies against neutrophils have also been proposed as the cause of the neutropenia.

The LGL leukemias that are CD3⁻ (NK cell) are less frequent and pursue a more fulminant course. The patients are usually young adults presenting with fever and hepatosplenomegaly. Their clinical course is generally downhill and is not affected by therapy, but occasional more indolent cases of NK-type LGL leukemias have also been reported in the literature.[28]

**Pathology.** The cells are characterized as circulating LGLs that have abundant clear cytoplasm and cytoplasmic granules that contain cytolytic proteins, such as TIAl, perforin, and granzyme. The bone marrow is usually diffusely infiltrated, but in some cases infiltration may be minimal. Splenomegaly is common, and the cells seem to infiltrate predominantly the red pulp. The skin and lymph nodes are not involved.[29]

In the CD3⁻ (NK-type) LGL leukemias, the cells resemble the more common T-cell variety, but nuclei are often more pleomorphic with prominent nucleoli, and cells are larger with more abundant cytoplasm. The white blood cell count is often higher than that seen in T-cell LGL leukemia.

The more common T-cell LGL leukemia is derived from mature suppressor-cytotoxic T lymphocytes (CD3⁺, T-cell receptor alpha/beta⁺, CD4⁻, CD8⁺). The cells characteristically express LGL antigens, CD16 and CD57. Most cases manifest rearrangements of the T-cell receptor alpha/beta genes; in rare cases, the gamma/delta genes are rearranged. In most cases, clonality is proved by T-cell receptor gene rearrangements using Southern blots or by cytogenetic studies.

The NK LGL leukemias exhibit a different phenotype. The cells are usually CD2⁺, CD3⁻, CD4⁻, and CD8⁻. In addition, most cases are CD16⁺ and CD56⁺ while CD57⁻. The cytolytic enzymes TIAl, perforin, and granzyme are expressed by immunohistochemistry. Currently, it is not possible to demonstrate clonality in the NK type because both T-cell receptor alpha/beta and gamma/delta genes are germline. In the NK-cell variant, the cells are often positive for Epstein-Barr virus (EBV), particularly in Asia.

**Prognosis and Treatment.** The more common T-cell LGL leukemia is often an indolent disorder frequently dominated by autoimmune phenomena and infection. In several series, survivals exceeding 10 years have been reported with 80% of patients surviving 10 years in one series. Management is often expectant and directed toward the autoimmune and infectious complications.[25, 27, 30] Single-agent chemotherapy, including alkylating agents and fludarabine, has reportedly controlled the leukemic aspects of the disorder, although often failing to correct the neutropenia. Corticosteroids have also been used for their antitumor and autoimmune effects, as has cyclosporine A. The benefit of splenectomy on the neutrophil count has been minimal in many cases. Neutrophil growth factors, such as granulocyte colony–stimulating factor and granulocyte-macrophage colony-stimulating factor, may correct the neutropenia.

The rarer NK LGL leukemia is generally a much more fulminant disorder as mentioned earlier. No consistent form of effective therapy has been described in the relatively few patients reported.

# Peripheral T-Cell and NK-Cell Lymphomas

## PERIPHERAL T-CELL LYMPHOMA (UNSPECIFIED)

Before considering the specific subcategories of the peripheral T-cell and NK-cell lymphomas, we emphasize that many cases cannot be subcategorized into specific clinical and pathologic syndromes, and the term *peripheral T-cell lymphoma (unspecified)* is used to encompass this group. This category includes a diverse population of peripheral T-cell lymphomas generally presenting with peripheral lymphadenopathy and represents the most common category of peripheral T-cell lymphomas seen in Western countries.[31–33] Because of the range of cell types, they have been subclassified in the REAL classification into small, large, and mixed subtypes. In the past, other terms have been used for variants in this category, including *lymphoepithelioid lymphoma (Lennert's lymphoma)*, *T-zone lymphoma*, and *pleomorphic T-cell lymphoma*. Subclassification of these latter entities has been problematic with poor interobserver reproducibility, however, and there appears to be relatively poor clinical correlation with these subtypes. Although the above-mentioned cell size spectrum suggests potential variation in clinical behavior, with the small cell variants exhibiting a less aggressive behavior, this generalization is only partially true. Most published studies of T-cell non-Hodgkin's lymphomas presented in the literature suggest a much poorer prognosis for all forms of peripheral T-cell lymphomas (except anaplastic large cell lymphoma) than their corresponding B-cell types. This poorer prognosis is particularly true in the more aggressive large cell variants of peripheral T-cell lymphoma. An example of a large series of prospectively studied patients with diffuse mixed and large cell non-Hodgkin's lymphoma (Working Formulation) was reported by the GELA

Group.[34] During a 6-year period, 1873 patients with these histologies were entered in a prospective clinical trial. Of the total, 278 (15%) had peripheral T-cell lymphomas. In that study, T-cell lymphomas tended to present with more advanced clinical stage, more frequent B symptoms, and a higher incidence of bone marrow involvement and skin involvement than their B-cell counterparts. T-cell lymphomas fared significantly worse than the B-cell types, with a 5-year overall survival of 42% and event-free survival of 33% in comparison with 52% and 45% for B-cell lymphomas. This difference was particularly evident in the 140 cases of pleomorphic large T-cell non-Hodgkin's lymphoma when compared with the diffuse large B-cell type.

**Clinical Presentation.** Peripheral T-cell lymphomas tend to occur in older adults, with a median age at diagnosis ranging from the late 50s to early 60s.[32, 33] In many series, there is a male preponderance. In most cases, the disease is advanced at the time of presentation, and more than 70% of patients have stage III to IV disease. The retroperitoneal lymph nodes appear to be preferentially involved. Constitutional symptoms (B symptoms) are noted in many patients.

In addition to lymphadenopathy, there is frequent hepatosplenomegaly and blood and bone marrow involvement. The skin is often involved. Eosinophilia and polyclonal hypergammaglobulinemia are common, and instances of the hemophagocytic syndrome have been noted. Occasionally, autoimmune or poorly defined pre-existing lymphoproliferative disorders may antedate the diagnosis of peripheral T-cell lymphoma.

**Pathology.** Lymph node architecture is usually diffusely effaced, but in the early stages, there may be involvement of the interfollicular areas with sparing of the follicles resulting in a T-zone pattern. The cells range in size from small lymphoid cells with irregular nuclei to intermediate or large cells (Fig. 92–4). The small cells often have characteristic irregular nuclear outlines termed *squiggly* or *corkscrew* appearing in the lymphoepithelioid variant as noted by Lukes. In addition to the neoplastic cell population, there is often infiltration by inflammatory cells, including epithelioid histiocytes and eosinophils, presumably the result of cytokine production by the T-cell population. The mixed background and presence of occasional large polyploid Reed-

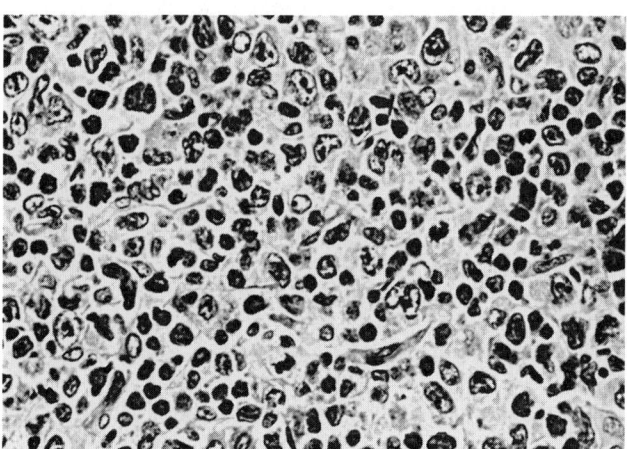

**Figure 92–4.** Peripheral T-cell lymphoma. Note pattern of mixed small cells with "irregular" nuclei and large cells with prominent nucleoli, a typical picture seen in peripheral T-cell lymphomas.

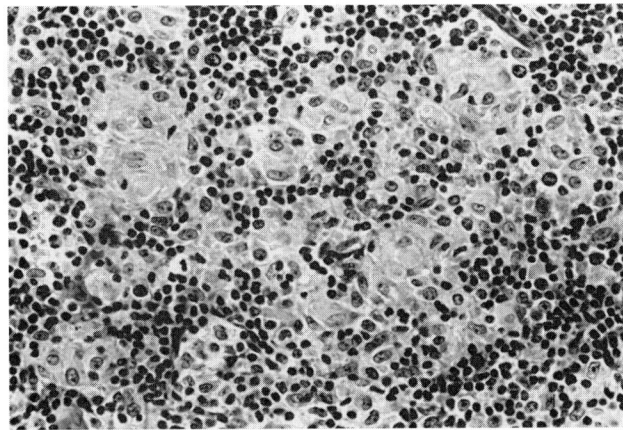

**Figure 92–5.** Lymphoepithelioid (Lennert's) lymphoma. Clusters of benign histiocytes are surrounded by small neoplastic T cells. On higher power, these T cells exhibit a "corkscrew" nucleus.

Sternberg–like cells may cause confusion with Hodgkin's lymphoma. The nuclear irregularity of the neoplastic cells in T-cell lymphomas usually exceeds that of Hodgkin's lymphoma, and immunophenotypic studies aid in the correct diagnosis (see later). In the lymphoepithelioid variant (Lennert's lymphoma), the histiocytes are numerous and cohesive, assuming a granulomatous appearance (Fig. 92–5).[35]

Cytologically the intermediate and larger cells have more open chromatin and prominent nucleoli in comparison with the small cell variants (Fig. 92–6). Both small and large cells tend to have a clear cytoplasm with well-defined cytoplasmic membranes, particularly in B5 fixed sections. Mitoses are increased and most numerous in the large cell varieties. Vascularity is generally increased, including the presence of atypical endothelial venules. In the peripheral T-cell lymphoma cases that resemble Hodgkin's lymphoma, the Hodgkin's-like or Reed-Sternberg–like cells are usually single and difficult to find, and the background cellular milieu differs from Hodgkin's lymphoma.[36]

The immunologic phenotype of the peripheral T-cell lymphomas often includes expression of CD2, CD3, CD4, and CD5, whereas preferential loss of CD7 is common.[37] The

cells are usually positive for the T-cell receptor antibody (βF1).[38] Large cells may be positive for CD30 (Ki-1). As opposed to Hodgkin's lymphoma, the Reed-Sternberg–like cells are positive for CD45 in most T-cell lymphomas, whereas CD15 is negative. Southern blot analysis characteristically exhibits alpha/beta T-cell receptor gene rearrangement. Complex karyotypes are seen in the mixed and large cell variants, whereas cases with the lymphoepithelioid morphology frequently exhibit trisomy 3.

The potential role of EBV infection in the pathogenesis of some variants of peripheral T-cell lymphoma is commented on in the specific sections. In the cases of peripheral T-cell lymphoma (unspecified), EBV expression as evidenced by EBV-encoded small nuclear RNA (EBER) was reported for a group of patients from Denmark, Nebraska, and British Columbia.[39] In that study, EBER positivity using in situ hybridization was seen in 40 of 130 (31%) cases of T-cell non-Hodgkin's lymphoma. Positive cases were restricted to some of the clinical pathologic syndromes to be described subsequently as well as Lennert's lymphoma and pleomorphic T-cell non-Hodgkin's lymphoma. EBER positivity conferred an adverse effect on overall prognosis.

The production of cytokines by the peripheral T-cell lymphomas may be responsible for some of the clinical manifestations of these disorders. For example, interleukin-4 and interleukin-6 may be implicated in the hypergammaglobulinemia and tissue plasmacytosis seen in some cases, whereas interferon-γ may be responsible for the epithelioid infiltration seen in Lennert's lymphoma.[40, 41]

**Prognosis and Treatment.** As mentioned, the lower-grade T-cell lymphomas in the Kiel classification and cases termed the *small cell variant* in the REAL classification exhibit a somewhat less aggressive behavior than their high-grade counterparts but still often pursue a progressive course. In general, the higher-grade B-cell lymphomas do considerably better than the peripheral T-cell lymphomas with respect to event-free and overall survival in most reported series.[34, 42–45] Some of the adverse prognosis associated with the T-lineage lymphoma may be secondary to advanced age, stage, and presence of clinical symptoms at the time of diagnosis. Direct comparisons between the B and the T lineage lymphomas are difficult because of the relative infrequency of the T-cell lymphomas, and, in most prospective series, T lineage was unreported for populations treated with standard therapies. More prospective data including immunophenotype are being accumulated now from the large cooperative groups, which should shed further light on the natural histories of the T lineage lymphomas and their specific clinical and pathologic subsets.

Current therapeutic strategies for the T lineage lymphoma have not been specified or differentiated from the programs commonly used for the B lineage lymphomas. Most patients with T-cell non-Hodgkin's lymphomas are treated with chemotherapeutic regimens designed predominantly for the B-cell lymphomas. Whether this policy is correct is unclear, but the poor treatment outcome observed in most T-cell lymphomas argues that much improvement is needed. Because T-cell lymphomas are often associated with other adverse prognostic factors as noted in the International Index,[46] it is possible that more aggressive treatment programs, such as the early implementation of high-dose chemotherapy with stem cell support, might be applicable in this group. At

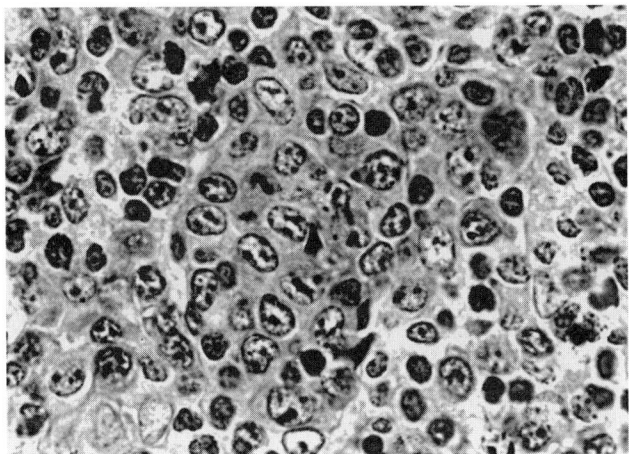

**Figure 92–6.** Peripheral T-cell lymphoma, large cell type. There are clusters of large transformed malignant cells with prominent nucleoli.

present, there are several anecdotal reports of favorable outcomes following stem cell transplantation for peripheral T-cell lymphomas. Nevertheless, it must be emphasized that most of the large prospectively randomized trials testing initial high-dose chemotherapy with stem cell support for newly diagnosed, predominantly B lineage lymphomas have failed to show a major benefit over standard therapy.[47, 48] It is anticipated that the further breakdown of the peripheral T-cell lymphomas into the specific clinical and pathologic entities described subsequently may facilitate the investigation of treatment programs unique to the individual disorder.

## Specific Post-Thymic T-Cell and NK Lymphoma Entities

### ANGIOIMMUNOBLASTIC T-CELL LYMPHOMA (ANGIOIMMUNOBLASTIC LYMPHADENOPATHY WITH DYSPROTEINEMIA–LIKE LYMPHOMA)

In the early 1970s, Lukes and Tindle[49] and Frizzera and coworkers[50] described a similar syndrome called *immunoblastic lymphadenopathy* and *angioimmunoblastic lymphadenopathy with dysproteinemia* (AILD). The term *lymphogranulomatosis X* was used by Knecht and associates.[51] Subsequently, this disorder has been characterized as a clinical and pathologic entity consisting of a systemic disease with characteristic symptoms associated with a distinct histologic pattern. In some cases, it may be difficult pathologically to differentiate an abnormal immune reaction from an instance of a true T-cell lymphoma, and the onset of disease may be preceded clinically by a viral-like syndrome or autoimmune disease. Often, successive lymph node biopsy specimens may evolve from an abnormal immune reaction into an obvious T-cell lymphoma. It is possible that some cases are non-neoplastic disorders, which share clinical and pathologic features currently inseparable from the lymphomatous counterpart.

**Clinical Presentation.** Patients generally present quite ill with constitutional symptoms of fever, night sweats, and weight loss. Examination frequently reveals generalized lymphadenopathy and hepatosplenomegaly associated with a diffuse erythematous skin rash. Patients frequently complain of generalized pruritus. Laboratory abnormalities include anemia, sometimes a Coombs'-positive hemolytic anemia, leukocytosis, eosinophilia, and hypergammaglobulinemia. Elevated levels of circulating immune complexes and rheumatoid factor have been noted as well as occasional monoclonal serum paraproteins. In some cases, the syndrome appears to be triggered by an allergen or drug, whereas most cases appear spontaneously. Spontaneous remissions have sometimes been observed, and significant responses to corticosteroid therapy have been noted (see later). A high fatality rate has been attributed to infectious complications and progression of high-grade disseminated lymphoma. Survival is typically less than 3 years.

**Pathology.** Nodal architecture is diffusely effaced by a vascular proliferation and polymorphous lymphoid cells ranging from small lymphocytes and plasma cells to immunoblasts. Immunoblasts often occur in sheets and clusters, which may help to differentiate true lymphomas from benign

or preneoplastic forms of AILD.[52] The immunoblasts are large with one or more prominent nucleoli and clear or basophilic cytoplasm. Germinal follicles are usually absent or regressive (so-called burnt-out germinal centers). The background often includes inflammatory cells, including plasma cells, eosinophils, histiocytes, and B immunoblasts. A characteristic histologic feature is the presence of prominent arborizing vessels with high endothelial venules (Fig. 92–7). Also present is a meshwork of dendritic cells usually surrounding the high endothelial venules in the background of the neoplastic cells. In some cases, there may be numerous epithelioid histiocytes resembling lymphoepithelioid lymphoma.[53]

The critical cells usually mark as CD3+, CD4+, and CD5+ T-helper lymphocytes, although rare cases may have a CD8+, CD4- phenotype.[54] CD7 is usually negative. Stains for dendritic cells, such as CD21 and fascin, characteristically reveal a prominent meshwork in the background, which may be helpful in diagnosis. The plasma cells are polyclonal.

Although most well-studied cases of AILD or angioimmunoblastic T-cell lymphoma exhibit evidence for T-cell clonality (usually T-cell receptor gene rearrangements of alpha-beta type),[55, 56] there remains a population of cases called AILD that fail to exhibit clear-cut characteristics sufficient to diagnose lymphoma. It is still conceivable that some cases exhibiting the clinical and pathologic features of AILD may be comprised of non-neoplastic conditions. In addition to the above-noted immunophenotypic features, EBV staining is frequently positive, and cytogenetic abnormalities, including trisomy 3, trisomy 5, and an additional X chromosome, have been reported.[57, 58]

**Prognosis and Treatment.** Currently, patients with angioimmunoblastic T-cell lymphoma have a poor prognosis, with survival less than 3 years in most cases. Treatment policies for angioimmunoblastic T-cell lymphoma are confounded by the concern that some cases may not be neoplastic. In a large German series, patients were treated with prednisone followed by chemotherapy using an intense multiagent regimen for relapse or with the same chemotherapy program given as first treatment.[59] In this nonrandomized trial, continuous complete response was infrequent (33%), and the median overall survival was short (15 months).

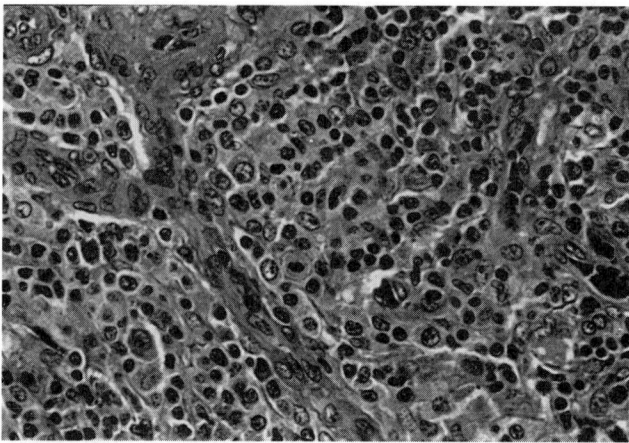

**Figure 92–7.** Angioimmunoblastic lymphadenopathy-like lymphoma. Note the prominent vessels. The larger cells with nucleoli are immunoblasts.

Other novel therapies have been inadequately studied but show potential promise. In one small series, 4 of 12 patients treated with low-dose interferon alfa obtained a complete response, whereas another four achieved a partial remission.[60] In another limited experience, two patients were treated successfully with cyclosporine A.[61] High-dose chemotherapy with autologous bone marrow or stem cell transplantation has produced prolonged disease-free survival in some patients with recurrent AILD-like lymphoma.[62]

## ANAPLASTIC LARGE CELL LYMPHOMA (Ki-1 LYMPHOMA)

In the course of examining the reaction of the monoclonal antibody Ki-1 (CD30) in a variety of tumor types, it became clear that a new lymphoma entity previously often misdiagnosed as carcinoma or melanoma could be recognized.[63] Anaplastic large cell lymphoma has been defined by expression of the CD30 epitope recognized with the antibodies Ki-1 or the more sensitive BerH2 in the setting of a characteristic morphologic appearance. The expression of CD30 is not specific for anaplastic large cell lymphoma, however, because this is an activation antigen present on other cell types, including some B cells and the Reed-Sternberg cells of Hodgkin's lymphoma. Not all cases of so-called anaplastic large cell lymphoma are actually anaplastic, with less common small cell and lymphohistiocytic variants described in the literature. Current discussion is primarily limited to Ki-1 anaplastic large cell lymphomas of T and null types. B-cell anaplastic large cell lymphomas have also been described as well as lymphomas of activated lymphoid cells, which secondarily express Ki-1, including those of T-cell and B-cell type. These lymphomas are excluded from this discussion. A primary cutaneous anaplastic large cell lymphoma syndrome has a distinctive clinical behavior and is discussed briefly.

**Clinical Presentation.** Anaplastic large cell lymphoma has a bimodal age distribution and is seen in children and relatively young adults, although all ages can be affected.[64, 65] Males predominate. Skin involvement is common in young patients and is apparently associated with an improved prognosis. Older patients generally present with lymphadenopathy and extranodal manifestations of disease. B symptoms and advanced stage are common, and involvement of the lung and skin is frequent.[66-68] A low frequency of bone marrow involvement despite frequent bone involvement has been described. The gastrointestinal tract appears to be rarely affected. In some of the adult series, patients with limited-stage disease (I or II) appear to be represented more frequently than in other types of peripheral T-cell lymphomas, in which stages III to IV predominate. The central nervous system is almost never involved. A primary cutaneous CD30 anaplastic large cell lymphoma characterized by spontaneous exacerbations and remissions, absence of the t(2;5) translocation, and a generally favorable prognosis has been described. This disorder resembles lymphomatoid papulosis and so-called regressing atypical histiocytosis.[69, 70]

**Pathology.** The characteristic neoplastic cell is a large anaplastic-appearing lymphoid cell with markedly irregular, lobated, or multiple nuclei (Fig. 92–8). Horseshoe-shaped nuclei with abundant cytoplasm, eccentric nuclei, and Golgi-

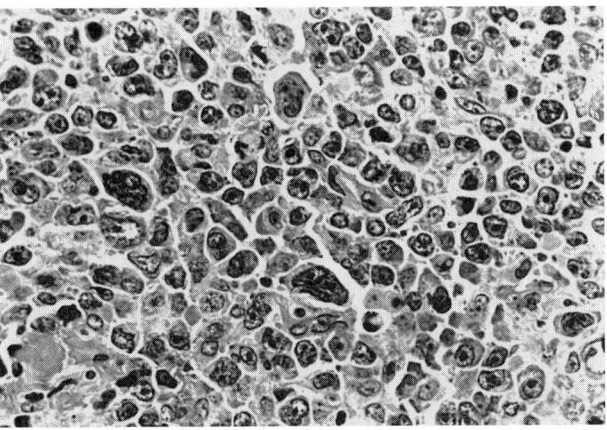

**Figure 92–8.** Ki-1 anaplastic large cell lymphoma. Note the presence of large, multinucleated giant cells and the highly pleomorphic cellular population.

like inclusions are commonly seen. Wreath-like forms and Reed-Sternberg–type cells are frequently noted. A characteristic feature of anaplastic large cell lymphoma is preferential involvement of lymph node sinuses. This distribution of involvement and the anaplastic characteristics of the cells may lead to diagnostic confusion with other malignancies, such as metastatic carcinoma or melanoma. The presence of Reed-Sternberg–like cells positive for CD30 has led to difficulty in the differential diagnosis of Hodgkin's lymphoma. Although many cases of lymphocyte-depletion Hodgkin's lymphoma have been shown retrospectively to be cases of anaplastic large cell lymphoma, there appear to remain a few cases of Hodgkin's-like anaplastic large cell lymphoma in which the differential diagnosis between Hodgkin's lymphoma may be subjective or resolved only by immunohistochemistry. The presence of Leu M-1 (CD15) staining argues for Hodgkin's lymphoma. The immunohistochemical detection of the ALK gene product (see later) may be a helpful differentiating factor, but not all cases of anaplastic large cell lymphoma express ALK, and anaplastic large cell lymphomas primary in the skin are always negative. Histologic variants of anaplastic large cell lymphoma include a lymphohistiocytic form, in which there is an intense reactive component of histiocytes and plasma cells, which can occasionally obscure the neoplastic component, and a small cell variant comprised of smaller, more uniform malignant cells. Transformation from the small to large cell type has been described, as has a sarcomatoid form with spindle or storiform cells.

Anaplastic large cell lymphoma may sometimes lack expression of CD45, while staining positively for activation antigens, such as CD25 and HLA-DR. Other markers variably expressed are CD45 RO (UCHL1), CD43, and CD3. In some cases, there is complete absence of T-cell and B-cell markers, leading to a null phenotype. The malignant cells by definition express CD30 at the cell membrane and within the cytoplasm in the region of the Golgi. The cells may also be positive for epithelial membrane antigen (EMA) but are negative for cytokeratins. T-cell anaplastic large cell lymphoma usually has alpha/beta or more rarely gamma/delta gene rearrangements of the T-cell receptor.

The discovery of an associated cytogenetic abnormality,

the t(2;5) translocation, and an available histochemical stain for the resultant ALK gene product of this translocation has led to increasing diagnostic specificity.[71] The t(2;5) translocation juxtaposes the ALK tyrosine kinase gene on chromosome 2p23 with the *NPM* (nucleophosmin) gene on chromosome 5q35. This translocation is seen in 20 to 65% of cases of T-cell and null anaplastic large cell lymphoma but is absent in B anaplastic large cell lymphoma, primary cutaneous anaplastic large cell lymphoma, or Hodgkin's lymphoma.[72] Cytogenetics, the PCR, and the above-mentioned antibody to the ALK gene product appear promising for characterizing these tumors. Not all cases of anaplastic large cell lymphoma manifest this translocation, however, and its absence cannot exclude the diagnosis.

CD30 expression, although characteristic of anaplastic large cell lymphoma, has been found in all major categories of non-Hodgkin's lymphoma except for lymphoblastic lymphoma. Among T-cell lymphomas, mycosis fungoides and peripheral T-cell lymphomas, including angioimmunoblastic T-cell lymphoma, human T-cell lymphotropic virus type I–positive ATLL, and pleomorphic peripheral T-cell lymphoma, have the highest incidence of CD30 expression. In most cases of mycosis fungoides, only a small proportion of cells corresponding to the large cerebriform cells are CD30$^+$.

**Treatment and Prognosis.** Several publications have pointed out the relatively favorable prognosis associated with the T and null anaplastic large cell lymphomas.[42] This improved prognosis is particularly evident when compared with the adverse outcome associated with other peripheral T-cell lymphomas and is particularly evident in cases with the t(2;5) translocation and ALK expression. Some series suggest that anaplastic large cell lymphoma may even have a superior prognosis to the B lineage large cell lymphomas. The treatment strategy for anaplastic large cell lymphoma has not been defined distinctly from treatment programs successful in other diffuse large cell lymphomas and rests predominantly on anthracycline combinations, such as CHOP (cyclophosphamide, hydroxydaunomycin, vinblastine sulfate [Oncovin], prednisone). The role of adjunctive radiation therapy also does not appear dissimilar to its role in other forms of large cell lymphoma. An anti-CD30 antibody has undergone therapeutic trials in another Ki-l-positive malignancy, Hodgkin's lymphoma, with some positive results.[73] Autologous stem cell transplantation has been mentioned in several series as an effective modality for relapsed patients with this disorder. The so-called B lineage anaplastic large cell lymphoma appears different in clinical presentation and prognosis from the T-cell and null types. A higher incidence of bone marrow involvement and a lower incidence of skin and pulmonary involvement have been observed in most series. Prognosis appears inferior to the T-cell and null types. A circulating form of CD30 (sCD30) can be detected in most cases of T-cell and null anaplastic large cell lymphoma.[74] This circulating protein may be useful diagnostically and in the follow-up of patients. Further correlative studies are indicated.

## NK/T-CELL LYMPHOMA, NASAL AND NASAL-TYPE

The category of unusual lymphomas underwent progressive redefinition in the 1990s from a basically inflammatory mid-line disease of the nasal cavity to an NK/T-cell lymphoma. This evolution underlines chronologic change in the terminology used to describe this disorder, including terms such as *lethal midline granuloma, malignant midline reticulosis, polymorphic reticulosis, angiocentric immunoproliferative lesion,* and *angiocentric T-cell lymphoma* in the REAL classification.[75–78] Lymphomatoid granulomatosis, a predominantly pulmonary disorder, was considered part of this spectrum of angiocentric destructive lesions, but studies suggest that it is usually a form of EBV-positive T cell–rich B-cell lymphoma.[79]

**Clinical Presentation.** There is a distinct geographic distribution of cases, with the most common presentations occurring in Asia, particularly China and Taiwan. Cases have also been seen in Central and South America and sporadically throughout the world.[80] There is a male predominance, and young to middle-aged individuals are affected. The most typical presentation appears to be a midline destructive lesion of the nasal cavity with associated involvement of the palate producing paranasal and periorbital swelling and erythema. In other cases, a mass effect (intranasal mass with obstruction) may predominate. Because of the predominantly nasal presentation of these cases, it is common for patients to be treated repetitively with antibiotics and other measures for a presumed inflammatory sinus disorder. This is particularly the case when biopsy specimens show an inflammatory-type infiltrate without distinctive neoplastic pathologic characteristics. Although most patients described present with localized disease, ultimate dissemination to other extranodal sites is common, particularly the skin, gastrointestinal tract, and testes. It has been speculated that the reason for this peculiar disease distribution may lie in the distinctive CD56$^+$ immunophenotype. CD56 represents neural cell adhesion molecule, which may confer this homing pattern. In contradistinction, lymph node involvement is uncommon. Less commonly, the disease may present in extranodal sites distinct from the nasal or upper aerodigestive tract. Such presentations often include the skin and mucous membranes as well as the gastrointestinal tract and testes similar to the patterns of distant dissemination of the nasal disorder.[81]

**Pathology.** Involved tissues are diffusely infiltrated and often destroyed by the neoplastic infiltrates, which are characteristically angiodestructive and angiocentric. Vascular damage often results in necrosis, which affects the tumor and normal tissues. Not all cases are marked by such angiocentricity, and yet necrosis is predominant. Speculation that expression of tumor necrosis factor-α and nuclear factor kappa/β by EBV-positive tumors may result in such necrosis has been presented.[82] There is a prominent inflammatory reaction that causes the above-mentioned confusion with inflammatory conditions, such as chronic sinusitis. Pleomorphism is variable in the neoplastic cells, which are characterized by irregular nuclei and clear cytoplasm. The size of the neoplastic lymphocytes is variable, ranging from a small irregular lymphocyte to a mixture of small and large cells as well as sheets of large malignant cells in occasional cases. At present, the prognostic significance of the different morphologic subtypes is uncertain. Cytoplasmic granules may be evident on Giemsa-stained imprints.

Although classified with the peripheral T-cell lymphomas, only approximately 20% of these nasal lymphomas react with antibodies to the T-cell receptor, βF1. These tumors usually lack CD3 and express NK antigens, such as CD56 and CD57. The characteristic phenotype is CD3⁻, CD2⁺, CD5⁻, CD56⁺. Some cases may be positive for CD7 and CD8. Although CD3 is usually negative in fresh tissues, polyclonal CD3 antibody used in paraffin sections may be positive because it reacts with the cytoplasmic epsilon epitope of the CD3 molecule that can be found in NK cells. The cells are usually positive for cytotoxic granules, such as perforin, TIAl, and granzyme.[83] Although most nasal angiocentric lymphomas have the CD3⁻, CD56⁺ phenotype, a few cases appear to be true T cells, expressing CD3 and usually CD57. The demonstration of T-cell gene rearrangements provides useful information regarding lineage because nasal NK lymphomas show a germline pattern for T-cell receptor and immunoglobulin gene rearrangements, whereas the T-cell variant generally shows T-cell receptor rearrangement. EBV expression is almost always seen in these cases (Fig. 92–9), particularly in Asian patients.[84] This observation is of differential diagnostic utility in instances in which the pathology may be inconclusive for malignancy. Most inflammatory conditions of the nasal cavity are negative for EBV.

**Prognosis and Treatment.** Although most patients with nasal NK lymphomas present with disease localized to the nasal cavity, the overall survival rate remains suboptimal. In a large study from Hong Kong of 113 patients presenting with primary lymphomas of the nose and nasopharynx, 45.5% were of the NK type.[85] The remainder expressed either T or B immunophenotype. Of the patients with NK nasal lymphomas, 62% were clinical stage IE, and only 17% were stage III or IV. Patients were treated in a variety of fashions, including radiation therapy alone and combined-modality chemoradiation therapy. In general, the chemotherapy consisted of CHOP or CHOP variations. The median dose of radiation therapy given was 50 Gy. In the NK-cell group, 56% of patients achieved complete remission. The 2-year disease-free survival, however, was only 31%, and overall survival was 43% at 2 years. It was not possible in the numbers of patients studied to ascertain the respective benefit of chemotherapy in addition to radiation. An additional study from Hong Kong showed that the median survival was only 12 months despite combined-modality management.[86] With such relatively poor statistics, there is much room for improvement, and newer approaches are needed. In some patients studied in Hong Kong, high-dose chemotherapy with peripheral stem cell support has proved useful in salvaging instances of relapsed nasal NK/T-cell lymphoma.[87]

A complication noted with significant frequency in these patients as well as patients with other EBV-associated NK/T-cell lymphomas and some EBV-negative T-cell lymphomas is the hemophagocytic syndrome.[88, 89] This syndrome is characterized by the constellation of fever, jaundice, hepatosplenomegaly, pancytopenia, altered coagulation parameters, and hypertriglyceridemia. The coagulation abnormalities include a low fibrinogen level presumably resulting from decreased hepatic synthesis. Although the pathogenesis of this syndrome is unclear, it has been associated with EBV and other viral infections. It has also been seen in a familial form. In general, the course is rapidly downhill over a period of several weeks. The bone marrow and other lymphatic tissues, such as liver, spleen, and lymph nodes, are involved by benign-appearing histiocytes exhibiting hemophagocytosis. Many therapeutic options have been examined, including trials of antiviral agents (acyclovir), interferon, and plasmapheresis. There is no consistent pattern to suggest the effectiveness of any of these modalities. In the familial form, bone marrow transplantation has proved life-saving in some cases. Occasional spectacular responses to cytotoxic chemotherapy, particularly etoposide, warrant further investigation.

## ENTEROPATHY-TYPE INTESTINAL T-CELL LYMPHOMA

In addition to the well-recognized immunoproliferative small intestinal disease occurring in the Middle East, North Africa, and the Southern Mediterranean, a second form of primary intestinal lymphoma appears with increased frequency in patients with a background of celiac disease and sometimes in patients with a background of nonspecific jejunoileal ulcerations. Although previously the disorder was believed to be a histiocytic malignancy, more recent evidence strongly identifies this as a T-cell lymphoma.

**Clinical Presentation.** Although these lymphomas characteristically occur in a patient with a prior diagnosis of celiac disease, the disorder has been identified in some cases concomitantly with the diagnosis of celiac disease and in rare instances may precede that diagnosis or may occur sporadically. As expected, this lymphoma is prevalent in areas with a high incidence of celiac disease, such as Great Britain and Ireland, and most cases have the associated HLA, DQA1* 0501 and DQB1* 0201 genotype. The clinical presentation is often elusive, and many cases come to diagnosis following intestinal catastrophes, such as hemorrhage and perforation, or in association with intractable abdominal pain and increasing malabsorption. Many cases remain undiagnosed for years with unavailable biopsy material, and some cases are diagnosed only at autopsy.[90, 91] The disorder should be suspected in any patient with known celiac disease who is exhibiting a progressive course despite gluten withdrawal.

**Pathology.** The lesions usually present in the jejunum or ileum and consist of ulcers or tumor masses. The histologic

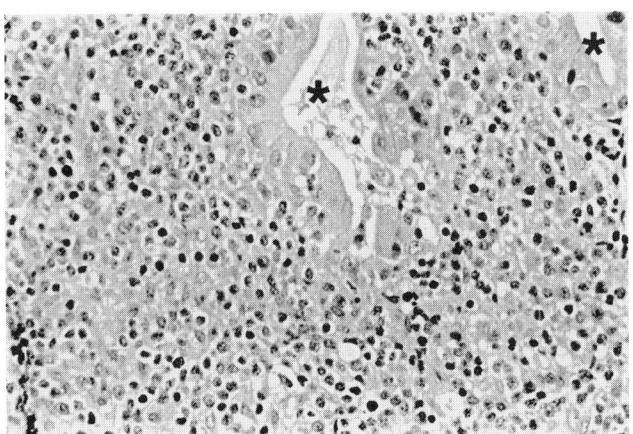

**Figure 92–9.** NK/T-cell lymphoma invading glands of the nasal sinus (*asterisk*). The neoplastic cells show nuclear hybridization (*black*) with probe to EBV encoded RNA (EBER).

spectrum ranges from small lymphocytes to large pleomorphic malignant cells. An inflammatory component is usually present. The adjacent mucosa usually, but not always, shows changes of celiac disease, including villous atrophy. The abnormal lymphoid cells often infiltrate the small intestinal epithelium forming lymphoepithelial lesions reminiscent of MALT-type lymphomas.

The tumor cells are CD3$^+$ and in many cases CD8$^+$ and CD4$^-$. Clonal rearrangements of T-cell receptor alpha/beta or gamma/delta genes are usually detected. These abnormalities may also be detected in the adjacent ulcerated or inflamed bowel wall, suggesting that these may be early lesions.

**Prognosis and Treatment.** Enteropathy-type intestinal T-cell lymphomas have a dire prognosis in most patients. Often the patients are already severely compromised because of perforation, malabsorption, and malnutrition and present as poor therapeutic candidates. As mentioned, the diagnosis is often reached after many months or years of a downhill course, and treatment is poorly tolerated. Surgical resection of affected areas is recommended, and no specific form of systemic therapy has been preferentially advised.

## HEPATOSPLENIC GAMMA/DELTA T-CELL LYMPHOMA

Hepatosplenic gamma/delta T-cell lymphoma is a rarely recognized form of lymphoma derived from T cells of gamma/delta type and is characterized morphologically by sinusoidal infiltration of the spleen, liver, and bone marrow.[92]

**Clinical Presentation.** The few reported cases identify a young male population presenting with hepatosplenomegaly without lymphadenopathy.[93] The patients frequently have dominant thrombocytopenia, often suggesting immune thrombocytopenia as well as evidence of hemolytic anemia. Fever and jaundice may also be present.

**Pathology.** The diagnosis is usually made on the basis of a liver biopsy specimen, bone marrow examination, or splenectomy. Tissues reveal an infiltration of the sinusoids of the liver or spleen by medium-size cells with irregular nuclei and pale cytoplasm. In the bone marrow, infiltration may be minimal and difficult to diagnose. Occasional cohesive aggregates of atypical cells may be seen. Circulating cells in the peripheral blood are often a late manifestation of disease and are rarely noted at diagnosis. In the spleen, the red pulp is preferentially involved.

The cells are CD2$^+$, CD3$^+$, CD5$^+$, CD7$^+$, CD56$^+$, and CD4$^-$ but may be positive or negative for CD8.[94] They characteristically stain with antibodies to the gamma/delta T-cell receptor and have rearrangements of the T-cell receptor gamma/delta genes. The cells may contain cytotoxic granules, such as TIA1 or granzyme. Cytoplasmic acid phosphatase staining has been noted. A characteristic isochromosome involving the long arm of chromosome 7 has been described.[93] EBV staining is usually absent.

**Prognosis and Treatment.** The clinical course of these patients has generally been downhill with death within 2 years for almost all patients described in the literature. Many patients are managed with corticosteroids initially and are believed to have an autoimmune disorder. Brief responses to such steroid therapy are typical. Splenectomy has also had a

brief ameliorating effect. Cytotoxic chemotherapy has generally produced brief remissions, although not enough patients have been studied. Autologous bone marrow transplantation has been attempted in at least one patient without permanent success.

## SUBCUTANEOUS PANNICULITIS-LIKE T-CELL LYMPHOMA

Subcutaneous panniculitis-like T-cell lymphoma is a rare lymphoma that distinctly involves the subcutaneous tissues of the skin and may be mistaken for benign panniculitis.[95] The disease is frequently complicated by a hemophagocytic syndrome, which is often lethal.

**Clinical Presentation.** Patients generally present with subcutaneous nodules preferentially affecting the extremities. The lesions are often diagnosed as benign inflammatory panniculitis in their early stages and remain undiagnosed until subsequent biopsy specimens reveal progression with morphologic evidence of lymphoma. These cases generally remain localized to the skin throughout the clinical course, although late dissemination has been occasionally described. Hemophagocytic syndrome may be a terminal event.[96]

**Pathology.** Malignant cells range from small to intermediate and large with variable nuclear pleomorphism. Neoplastic cells infiltrate the subcutaneous panniculus, characteristically surrounding adipocytes in a lace-like pattern (Fig. 92–10). The cells have irregular nuclei and clear cytoplasm, and there is commonly an inflammatory reaction, including frequent histiocytes. Fat necrosis and abundant karyorrhexis contribute to the diagnostic confusion with the inflammatory panniculitides, particularly in the low-grade lesions consisting of small lymphoid cells with minimal pleomorphism. Vascular invasion may occur. The cells are CD3$^+$ cytotoxic T cells and are usually positive for CD8. The cytoplasm usually contains cytotoxic granules that stain for TIA1, perforin, or granzyme. The cells are EBV negative, and usually alpha/beta and less commonly gamma/delta T-cell receptor gene rearrangements have been described.

**Treatment and Prognosis.** A defined recommendation regarding treatment is impossible. Responses to corticosteroids have been reported, although they are usually brief.

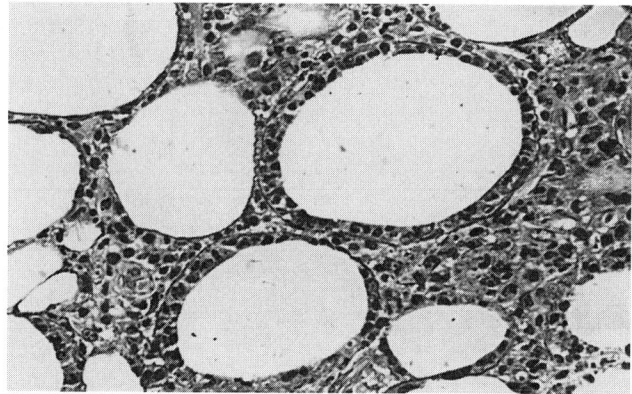

**Figure 92–10.** Subcutaneous panniculitis-like T-cell lymphoma involving the subcutaneous tissue of the skin. Neoplastic cells are infiltrating the subcutaneous panniculus, characteristically surrounding adipocytes in a lace-like pattern.

Combination chemotherapy regimens, such as CHOP, have been associated with durable remissions in occasional patients. The onset of hemophagocytic syndrome usually presages a downhill course.

## REFERENCES

1. The non-Hodgkin's lymphoma pathologic classification project: National Cancer Institute sponsored study of classifications of non-Hodgkin's lymphomas. Cancer 1982;49:2112–35.
2. Lennert K, Feller AC. Histopathology and diagnosis of non-Hodgkin's lymphomas. Berlin: Springer Verlag, 1992:165.
3. Harris NL, Jaffe ES, Stein H, et al. A revised European-American classification of lymphoid neoplasms: a proposal from the International Study Group. Blood 1994;84:1361–92.
4. Jaffe ES, Harris NL, Diebold J, et al. World Health Organization classification of neoplastic diseases of the hematopoietic and lymphoid tissues: a progress report. Am J Clin Pathol 1999;111:Suppl 1:S8–12.
5. Krishnan J, Wallberg K, Frizerra G. T-cell-rich large B-cell lymphoma: a study of 30 cases supporting its histologic heterogeneity and lack of clinical distinctness. Am J Surg Pathol 1994;18:455–65.
6. Sheibani K, Nathwani BN, Winberg CD, et al. Antigenically defined subgroups of lymphoblastic lymphoma: relationship to clinical presentation and biologic behavior. Cancer 1987;60:183–90.
7. Stroup R, Sheibani K, Misset JL, et al. Surface immunoglobulin-positive lymphoblastic lymphoma: a report of three cases. Cancer 1990;65:2559–63.
8. Sheibani K, Winberg CD, Burke JS, et al. Lymphoblastic lymphoma expressing natural killer cell-associated antigens: a clinicopathologic study of six cases. Leuk Res 1987;11:371–7.
9. Barcos MP, Lukes RJ. Malignant lymphoma of convoluted lymphocytes: a new entity of possible T-cell type. In: Sinks L, ed. Conflicts in childhood cancer. New York: Alan R Liss, 1975:175.
10. Rosen PJ, Feinstein DI, Pattengale PK, et al. Convoluted lymphocytic lymphoma in adults: a clincopathologic entity. Ann Intern Med 1978;89:319–24.
11. Weiss LM, Bindl JM, Picozzi VJ, et al. Lymphoblastic lymphoma: an immunophenotypic study of 26 cases with comparison to T-cell acute lymphoblastic leukemia. Blood 1986;67:474–8.
12. Carroll AJ, Crist WM, Link MP, et al. The t(1;14)(p34;q11) is nonrandom and restricted to T-cell acute lymphoblastic leukemia: a Pediatric Oncology Group study. Blood 1990;76:1220–4.
13. Levine AM, Forman SJ, Meyer PR, et al. Successful therapy of convoluted T-lymphoblastic lymphoma in the adult. Blood 1983;61:92–8.
14. Coleman CN, Picozzi VJ Jr, Cox RS, et al. Treatment of lymphoblastic lymphoma in adults. J Clin Oncol 1986;4:1628-37.
15. Morel P, Lepage E, Brice P, et al. Prognosis and treatment of lymphoblastic lymphoma in adults: a report on 80 patient. J Clin Oncol 1992;10:1078–85.
16. Slater DE, Mertelsmann R, Koziner B, et al. Lymphoblastic lymphoma in adults. J Clin Oncol 1986;4:57–67.
17. Verdonck LF, Dekker AW, de Gast GC, et al. Autologous bone marrow transplantation for adult poor-risk lymphoblastic lymphoma in first remission. J Clin Oncol 1992;10:644–6.
18. Milpied N, Ifrah N, Kuentz M, et al. Bone marrow transplantation for adult poor prognosis lymphoblastic lymphoma in first complete remission. Br J Haematol 1989;73:82–7.
19. Chopra R, Goldstone AH, Pearce R, et al. Autologous versus allogeneic bone marrow transplantation for non-Hodgkin's lymphoma: a case-controlled analysis of the European Bone Marrow Transplant Group Registry data. J Clin Oncol 1992;10:1690–5.
20. Sweetenham JW, Santini G, Simnet S, et al. Autologous stem cell transplantation in first remission improves relapse free survival in adult patients with lymphoblastic lymphoma: results from a randomized trial of the European Group for Blood and Bone Marrow Transplantation (EBMT) and the UK Lymphoma Group (UKLG). Proc ASCO 1998;17:17a.abstract.
21. Kurtzberg J, Keating M, Moore JO, et al. 2-amino-9-β-arabinosyl-6-methoxy-9H-guanine (GW 506U) is highly active in patients with T-cell malignancies: results of a Phase I trial in pediatric and adult patients with refractory hematological malignancies. Blood 1996; 88:699a.abstract.
22. Matutes E, Brito-Bapepulle V, Swansbury J, et al. Clinical and labora-
23. tory features of 78 cases of T-prolymphocytic leukemia. Blood 1991;78:3269–74.
24. Mercieca J, Matutes E, Dearden C, et al. The role of pentostatin in the treatment of T-cell malignancies: analysis of response rate in 145 patients according to disease subtype. J Clin Oncol 1994;12:2588–93.
25. Dearden CE, Matotes E, Dyer MJS, et al. CAMPATH-1H treatment of T-prolymphocytic leukemia. Blood 1999;94:Suppl 1:2929a. abstract.
26. Loughran Jr T. Clonal diseases of large granular lymphocytes. Blood 1993;82:1–14.
27. Dhodapkar MJ, Li C-Y, Lust JA, et al. Clinical spectrum of clonal proliferations of T-large granular lymphocytes: a T-cell clonopathy of undetermined significance. Blood 1994;84:1620–7.
28. Kingreen D, Siegert W. Chronic lymphatic leukemias of T and NK cell type. Leukemia 1997;11:Suppl 2:546–9.
29. Jaffe ES. Classification of natural killer (NK) cell and NK-like T-cell malignancies. Blood 1996;87:1207–10.
30. Agnarsson BA, Loughran TP, Starkebaum G, et al. The pathology of large granular lymphocyte leukemia. Hum Pathol 1989;20:643–51.
31. Berliner N. T gamma lymphocytosis and T cell chronic leukemias. Hematol Oncol Clin N Am 1990;4:473–86.
32. Suchi T, Lennert K, Tu L-Y, et al. Histopathology and immunohistochemistry of peripheral T cell lymphomas: a proposal for their classification. J Clin Pathol 1987;40:995–1015.
33. Armitage JO, Greer JP, Levine A, et al. Peripheral T cell lymphoma. Cancer 1989;63:158–63.
34. Pinkus GS, O'Hara CJ, Said JW. Peripheral/post thymic T cell lymphoma: a spectrum of disease: clinical, pathologic and immunotypic features of 78 cases. Cancer 1990;65:971–98.
35. Gisselbrecht C, Gaulard E, Lepage E, et al. Pleomorphic large T-cell lymphomas have a worse prognosis than diffuse large B cell lymphomas. Ann Oncol 1996;7:26.abstract.
36. Feller AC, Griesser GH, Mak TW, et al. Lymphoepithelioid lymphoma (Lennert's lymphoma) is a monoclonal proliferation of helper-inducer T cells. Blood 1986;68:663–7.
37. Patsouris E, Noel H, Lennert K. Cytohistologic and immunohistochemical findings in Hodgkin's disease, mixed cellularity type, with a high content of epithelioid cells. Am J Surg Pathol 1989;13:1014–22.
38. Weiss LM, Crabtree GS, Rouse RV, et al. Morphologic and immunologic characterization of 50 peripheral T cell lymphomas. Am J Pathol 1985;188:316–24.
39. Said JW, Shintaku IP, Parekh K, et al. Specific phenotyping of T-cell proliferations in formalin-fixed paraffin embedded tissues: use of antibodies to the T-cell receptor βFI. Am J Clin Pathol 1990;93:382–6.
40. d'Amore F, Johansen P, Mortensen LS, et al. Epstein-Barr virus in T-cell lymphomas: frequency, distribution pattern and prognostic significance. Ann Oncol 1996;7:10.abstract.
41. Ohnishi K, Ichikawa A, Kagami Y, et al. Interleukin 4 and gamma-interferon may play a role in the histopathogenesis of peripheral T-cell lymphoma. Cancer Res 1990;50:8028-33.
42. Hsu SM, Waldron JA Jr, Fink L, et al. Pathogenic significance of interleukin-6 in angioimmunoblastic lymphadenopathy-type T-cell lymphoma. Hum Pathol 1993;24:126–31.
43. Armitage JO, Weisenburger DD. New approach to classifying non-Hodgkin's lymphomas: clinical features of the major histologic subtypes. Non-Hodgkin's Lymphoma Classification Project. J Clin Oncol 1998;16:2780-95.
44. Lippman SM, Miller TP, Spier CM, et al. The prognostic significance of the immunophenotype in diffuse large cell lymphoma. Blood 1988;72:436–41.
45. Armitage JO, Vose JM, Linder J, et al. Clinical significance of immunophenotype in diffuse aggressive non-Hodgkin's lymphoma. J Clin Oncol 1989;7:1783–90.
46. Coiffier B, Brousse N, Peuchmaur M, et al. Peripheral T-cell lymphomas have a worse prognosis than B-cell lymphomas: a prospective study of 361 immunophenotyped patients treated with the LNH-84 regimen. Ann Oncol 1990;1:45–50.
47. A predictive model for aggressive non-Hodgkin's lymphoma. The International Non-Hodgkin's Lymphoma Prognostic Factors Project. N Engl J Med 1993;329:987–94.
48. Haroun C, Lepage E, Gisselbrecht C, et al. Comparison of autologous bone marrow transplantation with sequential chemotherapy for intermediate-grade and high-grade non-Hodgkin's lymphoma in first complete remission: a study of 464 patients. Groupe d'Etude des Lymphomes de l'Adulte. J Clin Oncol 1994;12:2543–51.
49. Reyes F, Lepage E, Morel P, et al. Failure of first-line induction high-

dose chemotherapy in poor risk patients with aggressive lymphoma: updated results of the randomized LNH 93–3 study. Blood 1997;90:Suppl 1:594a.abstract.

49. Lukes RJ, Tindle BH. Immunoblastic lymphadenopathy: a hyperimmune entity resembling Hodgkin's disease. N Engl J Med 1975;292:1–8.
50. Frizerra G, Moran EM, Rappaport H. Angio-immunoblastic lymphadenopathy with dysproteinaemia. Lancet 1974;l:1074–83.
51. Knecht H, Schwarze E, Lennert K. Histological, immunohistological and autopsy findings in lymphogranulomatosis X (including angioimmunoblastic lymphadenopathy). Virchow Arch (Pathol Anat) 1985;406:105–24.
52. Shimoyama M, Minato K, Saito H, et al. Immunoblastic lymphadenopathy (IBL)-like T cell lymphoma. Jpn J Clin Oncol 1979;9:437–56.
53. Patsouris E, Noel H, Lennert K. Angioimmunoblastic lymphadenopathy-type of T-cell lymphoma with a high content of epithelioid cells: histopathology and comparison with lymphoepithelioid cell lymphoma. Am J Surg Pathol 1989;13:262–75.
54. Namikawa R, Suchi T, Veda R, et al. Phenotyping of proliferating lymphocytes in angioimmunoblastic lymphadenopathy and related lesions by double immunoenzymatic staining technique. Am J Pathol 1987;127:279–87.
55. Weiss LM, Strikler J, Dorfman R, et al. Clonal T cell populations in angioimmunoblastic lymphadenopathy and angioimmunoblastic lymphadenopathy-like lymphoma. Am J Pathol 1986;122:392–7.
56. Feller AC, Griesser H, Schilling CV, et al. Clonal gene rearrangement patterns correlate with immunophenotype and clinical parameters in patients with angioimmunoblastic lymphadenopathy. Am J Pathol 1988;133:549–56.
57. Kaneko Y, Maseki N, Sakurai M, et al. Characteristic karyotypic pattern in T-cell lymphoproliferative disorders with reactive "angioimmunoblastic lymphadenopathy with dysproteinemia-type" features. Blood 1988;72:413–21.
58. Schlegelberger B, Zhang Y, Weber-Matthiessen K, et al. Detection of aberrant clones in nearly all cases of angioimmunoblastic lymphadenopathy with dysproteinemia-type T-cell lymphoma by combined interphase and metaphase cytogenetics. Blood 1994;84:2640–8.
59. Siegert W, Agthe A, Griesser H, et al. Treatment of angioimmunoblastic lymphadenopathy (AILD)-type lymphoma using prednisone with or without the COPBLAM/IMVP-16 regimen: a multicenter study. Kiel Lymphoma Study Group. Ann Intern Med 1992;117:364–70.
60. Siegert W, Nerl C, Meuthen I, et al. Recombinant human interferon-alpha in the treatment of angioimmunoblastic lymphadenopathy: results in 12 patients. Leukemia 1991;5:892–5.
61. Murayama T, Imoto A, Takahashi T, et al. Successful treatment of angioimmunoblastic lymphadenopathy with dysproteinemia with cyclosporin A. Cancer 1992;69:2567–70.
62. Schmitz N, Prange E, Haferlach T, et al. High-dose chemotherapy and autologous bone marrow transplantation in relapsing angioimmunoblastic lymphadenopathy with dysproteinemia (AILD). Bone Marrow Transplant 1991;8:503–6.
63. Stein H. Ki-1 anaplastic large cell lymphoma: is it a discrete entity. Leuk Lymphoma 1993;10:Suppl:81–4.
64. Stein H, Mason DY, Gerdes J, et al. The expression of the Hodgkin's disease associated antigen Ki-1 in reactive and neoplastic lymphoid tissue: evidence that Reed-Sternberg cells and histiocytic malignancies are derived from activated lymphoid cells. Blood 1985;66:848–58.
65. Kadin ME, Sako D, Berliner N, et al. Childhood Ki-1 lymphoma presenting with skin lesions and peripheral lymphadenopathy. Blood 1986;68:1042–9.
66. Fillipa DA, Ladanyi M, Wollner N, et al. CD30 (Ki-1)-positive malignant lymphomas: clinical, immunophenotypic, histologic, and genetic characteristics and differences with Hodgkin's disease. Blood 1996;87:2905–17.
67. Tilly H, Gaulard P, Lepage E, et al. Primary anaplastic large-cell lymphoma in adults: clinical presentation, immunophenotype and outcome. Blood 1997;90:3727–34.
68. Clavio M, Rossi E, Truini M, et al. Anaplastic large cell lymphoma: a clinicopathologic study of 53 patients. Leuk Lymphoma 1996;22:319–27.
69. DeCoteau JF, Butmarc JR, Kinney MC, et al. The t(2;5) chromosomal translocation is not a common feature of primary cutaneous CD30+ lymphoproliferative disorders: comparison with anaplastic large-cell lymphoma of nodal origin. Blood 1996;87:3437–41.
70. Beljaards RC, Meijer GJL, Van der Putte SCJ, et al. Primary cutaneous

T-cell lymphoma: clinicopathological features and prognostic parameters of 35 cases other than mycosis fungoides and CD30-positive large cell lymphoma. J Pathol 1994;172:53–60.
71. Pulford K, Lamant L, Morris SW, et al. Detection of anaplastic lymphoma kinase (ALK) and nucleolar protein nucleosphosmin in normal and neoplastic cells with the monoclonal antibody ALK1. Blood 1997;89:1394–1404.
72. Sarris AH, Luthra R, Papadimitropoulou V, et al. Long-range amplification of genomic DNA detects the (2;5) (p23;q35) in anaplastic large cell lymphoma but not in other non-Hodgkin's lymphomas, Hodgkin's disease or lymphomatoid papulosis. Ann Oncol 1997;8:Suppl 2:59–64.
73. Hartman F, Remner C, Jung W, et al. Treatment of refractory Hodgkin's disease with an anti-CD16/CD30 bispecfic antibody. Blood 1997;89:2042–7.
74. Nadali G, Vinante F, Stein H, et al. Serum levels of the soluble form of CD30 molecule as a tumor marker in CD30+ anaplastic large-cell lymphoma. J Clin Oncol 1995;13:1355–60.
75. Lipford EH, Margolick JB, Longo DL, et al. Angiocentric immunoproliferative lesions: a clinicopathologic spectrum of post-thymic T-cell proliferations. Blood 1988;72:1674–81.
76. Chan JKC, Ng CE, Lau WH, et al. Most nasal/nasopharyngeal lymphomas are peripheral T-cell neoplasms. Am J Surg Pathol 1987;11:418–29.
77. Ferry JA, Sklar J, Zukerberg LR, et al. Nasal lymphoma: a clinicopathologic study with immunophenotypic and genotypic analysis. Am J Surg Pathol 1991;15:268–79.
78. Strickler JG, Meneses MF, Habermann TM, et al. Polymorphic reticulosis: a reappraisal. Hum Pathol 1994;25:659–65.
79. Guinee P Jr, Jaffe E, Kingma D, et al. Pulmonary lymphomatoid granulomatosis: evidence for a proliferation of Epstein-Barr viral infected B-lymphocytes with a prominent T-cell component and vasculitis. Am J Surg Pathol 1994;18:753–64.
80. Kanavaros P, Leses MC, Briere J, et al. Nasal T-cell lymphoma: a clinicopathologic entity associated with peculiar phenotype and with Epstein-Barr virus. Blood 1993;81:2688–95.
81. Chan JKC, Sin VC, Wong KF, et al. Non-nasal lymphoma expressing natural killer marker CD56: a clinicopathologic study of 49 patients of an uncommon aggressive neoplasm. Blood 1997;89:4501–13.
82. Jaffe ES, Chen JKC, Su I-J, et al. Report of the workshop on nasal and related extranodal angiocentric T/natural killer cell lymphomas. An J Surg Pathol 1996;20:103–11.
83. Felgar RE, Macon WR, Kinney MC, et al. TIA-1 expression in lymphoid neoplasms: identification of subsets with cytotoxic T-lymphocyte or natural killer cell differentiation. Am J Pathol 1997;150:1893–1900.
84. Medeiros LJ, Jaffe ES, Chen Y-Y, et al. Localization of Epstein-Barr viral genomes in angiocentric immunoproliferative lesions. Am J Surg Pathol 1992;16:439–47.
85. Cheung MMC, Chan JKC, Lau WH, et al. Primary non-Hodgkin's lymphoma of the nose and nasopharynx: clinical features, tumor immunophenotype and treatment outcome in 113 patients. J Clin Oncol 1998;16:70–7.
86. Kwong YL, Chan ACL, Liang R, et al. CD56+ NK lymphomas: clinicopathologic features and prognosis. Br J Haematol 1997;97:821–9.
87. Liang R, Chen F, Lee CK, et al. Case report: autologous bone marrow transplantation for primary nasal T/NK cell lymphoma. Bone Marrow Transplant 1997;19:91–3.
88. Yao M, Cheng A-L, Su I-J, et al. Clinicopathologic spectrum of haemophagocytic syndrome in Epstein-Barr virus-associated peripheral T-cell lymphoma. Br J Haematol 1994;87:535–43.
89. Chang C-S, Wong C-H, Su I-J, et al. Hematophagic histiocytosis: a clinicopathologic analysis of 23 cases with special reference to the association with T-cell lymphoma. J Formos Med Assoc 1994;93:421–8.
90. Jaffe ES, Krenacs L, Raffeld M. Classification of the T-cell and NK-cell neoplasms based on the REAL classification. Ann Oncol 1997;8:Suppl 2:517–24.
91. Mathus-Vliegen EM, Van Halteren H, Tytgat GN. Malignant lymphoma in coeliac disease: various manifestations with distinct symptomatology and prognosis? J Intern Med 1994;236: 43–9.
92. Cooke CB, Krenecs L, Stetler-Stevenson M, et al. Hepatosplenic T-cell lymphoma: a distinct clinicopathologic entity of cytotoxic gamma delta T-cell origin. Blood 1996;88:4265–74.
93. Yao M, Tien HF, Lin MT, et al. Clinical and hematological characteristics of hepatosplenic T gamma/delta lymphoma with isochromosome for long arm of chromosome 7. Leuk Lymphoma 1996;22:495–500.

94. Wong KF, Chan JKC, Matutes E, et al. Hepatosplenic gamma/delta T-cell lymphoma: a distinctive aggressive lymphoma type. Am J Surg Pathol 1995;19:718–26.
95. Gonzalez CL, Medeiros LJ, Braziel RM, et al. T-cell lymphoma involv-ing subcutaneous tissue: a clinicopathologic entity commonly associ-ated with hemophagocytic syndrome. Am J Surg Pathol 1991;15:17–27.
96. Chan Y-F, Lee KC, Llewellyn H. Subcutaneous T-cell lymphoma pre-senting as panniculitis in children. Pediatr Pathol 1994;14:595–600.

# CHAPTER 93

# MYCOSIS FUNGOIDES AND OTHER CUTANEOUS LYMPHOMAS

• YOUN H. KIM • RICHARD T. HOPPE

The cutaneous lymphomas are a group of lymphomas that involve primarily the skin and affect other sites only second-arily. They include mycosis fungoides and Sézary's syn-drome as well as other T-cell or B-cell non-Hodgkin's lym-phomas. Most of this chapter discusses mycosis fungoides and Sézary's syndrome. The final section discusses the other cutaneous lymphomas.

## Mycosis Fungoides and Sézary's Syndrome

### NATURAL HISTORY

#### Etiology and Epidemiology

The cause of mycosis fungoides and Sézary's syndrome is unclear. Uncontrolled studies and case reports have sug-gested that the it may be related to chronic antigenic stimula-tion secondary to exposure to chemicals or pesticides[1]; how-ever, large case-controlled studies have failed to confirm this association, and the cause remains unknown.[2, 3]

A viral cause for mycosis fungoides has also been sug-gested. Although the human T-lymphotropic virus type I (HTLV-I) was first isolated from a patient thought to have mycosis fungoides, he actually suffered from a peripheral T-cell lymphoma involving the skin.[4] Nearly all patients with mycosis fungoides are HTLV-I seronegative. Nevertheless, using polymerase chain reaction (PCR) techniques, HTLV-I-related DNA sequences have been identified in the peripheral blood mononuclear cells and cutaneous lesions of some patients with mycosis fungoides, despite their seronegativ-ity.[5, 6] Other studies, however, have revealed further evidence against a role for HTLV-I.[7, 8] A similar virus, HTLV-V, was grown from a cell line derived from the peripheral blood lymphocytes of a patient with documented mycosis fun-goides.[9] Although the existence of this particular virus has not been confirmed, suspicion for a viral link remains.

Mycosis fungoides is an uncommon malignancy; about 500 to 600 new cases and 100 to 200 deaths are reported from the disease each year in the United States.[10] It accounts for less than 3% of new cases of non-Hodgkin's lymphomas. The diagnosis is most commonly made in older men. The average age at diagnosis is 60 years, and the male/female ratio is 2:1.

### Biology

The neoplastic cell of mycosis fungoides is well defined. Mycosis fungoides was among the first lymphomas to be well characterized immunologically.[11] Most cases of mycosis fungoides are of helper T-cell origin, based on functional assays and monoclonal antibody staining.[12] Mycosis fun-goides cells usually retain the CD4 cell surface antigen (helper T-cell phenotype) but may lose other mature T-cell antigens, such as CD7 or Leu-8.[13] These staining characteris-tics may be helpful in differentiating early mycosis fun-goides from benign infiltrates of the skin.

Southern blot and PCR analysis show monoclonal re-arrangements of the T-cell receptors in the skin, lymph nodes, and peripheral blood of patients with mycosis fun-goides.[14–17] These rearrangements are concordant about 80% of the time in multiple lesions from a single patient.[14, 18] Genotyping, the evaluation of skin biopsy specimens to detect T-cell receptor gene rearrangements, is sometimes helpful in the differential diagnosis of early mycosis fun-goides.

### Pathology

The classic histopathology of cutaneous mycosis fungoides includes an upper dermal mononuclear cell infiltrate, which is intimate with the epidermis and obscures the dermal-epidermal junction (Grenz zone). There is a variable admix-ture of histiocytes, eosinophils, and plasma cells.[19] The ab-normal mononuclear cells may infiltrate the epidermis as single cells or in characteristic clusters, called *Pautrier's microabscesses*. Abnormal cells must be present in the epi-dermis to make a firm diagnosis of mycosis fungoides. The density of the dermal infiltrate and extent of involvement of the epidermis may be much less in skin biopsy specimens from patients with Sézary's syndrome, making this diagnosis more difficult to establish. The recent use of topical cortico-steroids, especially in patch stage disease, may ablate the epidermal component of the infiltrate and obscure the diag-nosis.

Under oil emersion light microscopy, the nuclei of the mononuclear mycosis fungoides cells are hyperconvoluted. Ultrastructural studies show marked infolding of the nuclear membrane, which on three-dimensional reconstruction re-sembles the surface of the brain, so the cells are called *cerebriform.*[20] The nuclear contour index is a quantitative measure of the degree of nuclear irregularity as observed on electron photomicrographs and may be useful in the differential diagnosis between mycosis fungoides and benign skin diseases.[21]

The minimal criteria for establishing a diagnosis of mycosis fungoides vary among pathologists. Depending on the severity of the epidermal and dermal involvement, criteria considered *diagnostic of, consistent with,* and *suggestive of* mycosis fungoides have been proposed.[12, 19] Some pathologists have required monoclonal antibody–stained biopsy specimens to be consistent with the immunophenotype of mycosis fungoides before making a firm diagnosis. Treatment programs specific for the disease should not be used in patients who have a biopsy specimen merely suggestive of mycosis fungoides.

The pathology of extracutaneous disease is also important. Often, enlarged lymph nodes show only the changes of dermatopathic lymphadenitis, with sinus histiocytosis, an abundance of pigment-laden macrophages, and a small number of atypical lymphocytes. The National Cancer Institute (NCI) lymph node classification system reflects the degree of infiltration by these atypical cells.[22] Lymph nodes are classified as LN-0, LN-1, LN-2, LN-3, or LN-4 to correspond with lymph node involvement ranging from no atypical lymphocytes (LN-0) to partial or complete replacement of nodal architecture by atypical lymphocytes or frankly neoplastic cells (LN-4). This grading system has prognostic relevance.[22]

The detection of abnormal cells in skin, lymph node, or other biopsy specimens is facilitated by the use of special studies, such as T-cell cytology, electron microscopy, cytogenetic studies, and Southern blot and PCR analysis to detect rearrangements of the T-cell receptor.[15–17, 23, 24] Using these special techniques, neoplastic involvement may be shown even in lymph nodes that show only dermatopathic lymphadenitis on routine evaluation.[15] The clinical implication of lymph node involvement that is detectable only at the molecular level is unclear and is often not as severe as when involvement is detected by routine light microscopy.

## Clinical Features

Mycosis fungoides has a long natural history in many patients. The *premycotic* phase is characterized by nonspecific, slightly scaling skin lesions and nondiagnostic biopsy specimens. These lesions may wax and wane over a period of years, and a diagnosis of parapsoriasis en plaques is often made. During this phase of disease, patients may respond to treatment with topical corticosteroids. Some experience an evolution of their disease and develop more typical patches or infiltrated plaques with characteristic biopsy changes of mycosis fungoides. It is common for a history of skin lesions to precede a diagnosis of mycosis fungoides by 5 years or longer.[19] Repeated biopsy specimens must be obtained in patients suspected of having mycosis fungoides, even when an initial biopsy specimen is negative.

The typical patches of mycosis fungoides are erythematous and slightly scaling. Early involvement is often noted in the *bathing trunk* distribution, although any part of the body may be involved. Sites of disease may be curiously symmetric. The palms or soles may be heavily involved or spared. Scalp involvement may cause alopecia. Pruritus is the most common symptom and often prompts the initial visit to the dermatologist.

More infiltrated lesions present as palpable plaques, with variable shape and well-defined borders. Plaques may evolve into ulcerated or exophytic tumors. Ulcerated tumors may become infected; sepsis secondary to infection is the most common immediate cause of death in mycosis fungoides. Generalized dermal thickening from infiltrative disease may cause the appearance of the classic but rare leonine facies.

Another manifestation of skin involvement in mycosis fungoides is generalized erythroderma, with or without superimposed plaques or tumors. The skin may be atrophic or lichenified. The erythroderma is accompanied by cold intolerance and intense pruritus. These patients may also have lymphadenopathy and circulating abnormal cells in the peripheral blood. These cells have the same microscopic appearance, immunophenotyping, and genotyping characteristics as the cells that infiltrate the epidermis.[14] Patients with the complex of findings have Sézary's syndrome.[25]

Some patients may never show anything beyond the premycotic or patch phase of skin involvement. Many patients, however, have disease that progresses from patches to plaques and finally to tumorous involvement. The likelihood of developing extracutaneous disease correlates with the extent of skin involvement. It is exceedingly rare among patients with limited patch or plaque disease, relatively uncommon among those with generalized plaque (8%), and most likely among patients with tumorous involvement (30%).

Although mycosis fungoides may be a systemic disease from the outset, the clinical behavior seems to suggest that progressive skin involvement precedes extension to lymph nodes, then to viscera. The involved visceral sites of disease most commonly identified include the lungs, gastrointestinal tract, and liver, but virtually any organ may be involved at autopsy in patients who have died of the disease.[26]

## Staging

The standard staging classification system for mycosis fungoides is the TNMB system, first proposed at the Workshop on Mycosis Fungoides held at the NCI in 1978.[27] Tables 93–1 and 93–2 summarize the TNMB categories and staging classification.

The extent of skin involvement defines the *T* stage, which correlates closely with survival.[14] Lymph node involvement defines the *N* stage. Enlarged lymph nodes should always be biopsied because palpable enlargement is often associated only with changes of dermatopathic lymphadenitis, and these changes have only minor prognostic significance.[22, 28, 29] Only when frank lymph node involvement is detected is the prognosis substantially worse. The biopsy status of nodes should be designated by the appropriate subscripts.

Visceral disease defines the *M* category. Suspected sites of visceral involvement should always be confirmed histologically. Other neoplasms as well as benign diseases may be confused with mycosis fungoides if a diagnosis is based solely on imaging studies. This statement is important because the presence of visceral disease has severe prognostic

*Table 93–1.* **TNMB Classification for Mycosis Fungoides**

*T (Skin)*

T1  Limited patch/plaque (<10% of total skin surface)
T2  Generalized patch/plaque (≥10% of total skin surface)
T3  Tumors
T4  Generalized erythroderma

*N (Nodes)*

N0  Lymph nodes clinically uninvolved
N1  Lymph nodes enlarged, histologically uninvolved (includes reactive and dermatopathic nodes)
N2  Lymph nodes clinically uninvolved, histologically involved
N3  Lymph nodes enlarged and histologically involved

*M (Viscera)*

M0  No visceral involvement
M1  Visceral involvement

*B (Blood)*

B0  No circulating atypical (Sézary) cells (<5% of total lymphocytes)
B1  Circulating atypical (Sézary) cells (≥5% of total lymphocytes)

*Table 93–2.* **Clinical Staging System for Mycosis Fungoides**

| Clinical Stages | TNM Classification* | | |
|---|---|---|---|
| IA | T1 | N0 | M0 |
| IB | T2 | N0 | M0 |
| IIA | T1–2 | N1 | M0 |
| IIB | T3 | N0–1 | M0 |
| IIIA | T4 | N0 | M0 |
| IIIB | T4 | N1 | M0 |
| IVA | T1–4 | N2–3 | M0 |
| IVB | T1–4 | N0–3 | M1 |

*The *B* classification does not alter clinical stage.

implications. The *B* (blood) category signifies the absence or presence of abnormal cells in the peripheral blood. This does not appear to be an independent prognostic factor, other than in the erythrodermic (T4) subgroup,[28] but is closely linked with the extent of skin involvement and presence of extracutaneous disease.[22]

All patients with mycosis fungoides should undergo at least a limited staging evaluation, including a careful examination of the skin and lymph nodes, complete blood count, Sézary count, screening chemistries, and chest radiograph. Further staging studies are dictated by the results of those screening evaluations.[19] Any blood or radiographic abnormalities should be evaluated further as appropriate. If en-

larged lymph nodes are detected on physical examination, they should be biopsied. If nodes are involved by mycosis fungoides, additional staging studies, such as computed tomography (CT), should be performed to evaluate for the possibility of visceral disease.[19]

There is little value in completing radiographic imaging studies beyond a routine chest radiograph, unless indicated by the above-cited circumstances. Screening CT of the abdomen and pelvis, for example, is inevitably unrevealing unless there is known lymph node involvement.[30] Bone marrow biopsy specimens are rarely positive except in the presence of Sézary's syndrome; however, in this setting, marrow involvement is inconsequential.

## Prognosis

The median survival of patients with mycosis fungoides reported in large series is about 10 years.[19] Patient prognosis is linked closely to stage, more specifically to the extent of skin involvement and the presence of extracutaneous disease. Figure 93–1 shows the survival of a large group of patients from Stanford who had no known extracutaneous disease

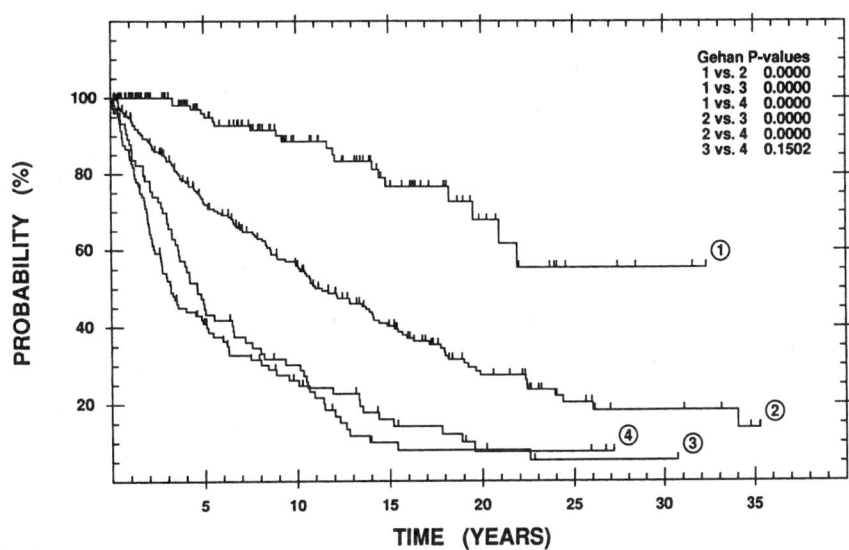

**Figure 93–1.** Actuarial survival of 543 patients with mycosis fungoides managed at Stanford University. All patients had disease apparently limited to the skin. Survival is calculated from the date of referral to Stanford (not from the date of diagnosis). 1 = 140 patients with limited patch/plaque disease; 2 = 219 patients with generalized patch/plaque disease; 3 = 108 patients with tumorous disease; and 4 = 76 patients with erythroderma.

and were treated with standard therapy. The outcome is displayed according to the extent of skin involvement. There is a clear difference in prognosis for T1 (limited patch or plaque) and T2 (generalized patch or plaque) disease, both of which have a substantially better prognosis than T3 (tumorous) or T4 (erythrodermic) disease. Although the prognosis for T3 and T4 is nearly identical, the different clinical appearance and natural history of these patients justify different T-stage designations.

The prognosis for patients with limited patch or plaque (T1) disease is excellent, with an overall long-term life expectancy that is similar to an age-matched, sex-matched, and race-matched control population.[31] Nearly all patients with T1 disease who die do so from causes other than mycosis fungoides. In the experience reported from Stanford, only 9% of patients treated at this stage progressed to a more advanced stage of disease. Patients who did progress had a lower complete response rate to initial therapy and an older mean age than did other patients with limited skin (T1) disease. Patients with generalized patch or plaque disease (T2) have a greater likelihood of disease progression (24%), and nearly 20% die from causes related to mycosis fungoides.[29] Most patients who present with tumorous disease (T3) ultimately die from mycosis fungoides.

The long-term outcome in patients with erythroderma (T4) is variable depending on patient age at presentation (<65 years vs. >65 years), overall stage (III vs. IV), and peripheral blood involvement (B0 vs. B1).[28] The median survival can vary widely depending on the combinations of these independent prognostic factors: Three distinct prognostic subgroups were identified, with median survivals of 10.2 years, 3.7 years, and 1.5 years. Mycosis fungoides patients with extracutaneous disease at presentation (stage IVA and stage IVB) regardless of extent of skin involvement have a median survival of only 1.4 years, and nearly all die of causes directly related to mycosis fungoides (Fig. 93–2).

## TREATMENT

Although the natural history of mycosis fungoides may be lengthy, even in the absence of specific therapy, prompt treatment is usually mandated by the presence of symptoms such as pruritus, the cosmetic disfigurement associated with the disease, or the threat of extracutaneous spread. Selection of a specific treatment plan is based on the clinical stage of the disease, the assessment of prognostic factors, the accessibility of different treatment approaches, the patient's age and other social and medical problems, and the cost/benefit ratio. In the absence of extracutaneous disease, control of the disease is most likely achieved by treatment directed at the skin, by means of phototherapy, topical chemotherapy, or irradiation.

For the treatment of the most limited extent of disease or cases in which the diagnosis may be in doubt, topical corticosteroids may achieve a good response and provide short-term palliation. Long-term complete responses are unlikely, however, and the long-term course of the disease is not altered.

## Phototherapy

Phototherapy was developed initially as a treatment for psoriasis. It involves using ultraviolet (UV) radiation in the form of UVA or UVB wavelengths, which can be used alone, together, or with psoralen, a photosensitizing agent, as psoralen plus UVA (PUVA). The long-wave UVA has the advantage over UVB in its greater depth of penetration into the dermal infiltrates of mycosis fungoides. For early limted diseases, UVB alone has been shown to be effective.[32]

PUVA, also referred to as *photochemotherapy*, is clearly the most commonly used form of phototherapy for patients with mycosis fungoides and Sezary's syndrome. Patients take the oral photosensitizing drug, usually 8-methoxypsoralen, then are exposed to long-wave UV light (UVA) in a specially designed box.[33] The psoralen intercalates with DNA in the presence of UVA, forming monofunctional and bifunctional adducts with DNA base pairs, and inhibits DNA synthesis. The UVA wavelength penetrates into the epidermis and upper dermis and so has its effect in the regions where the characteristic cellular infiltrate of mycosis fungoides is most likely to be located, especially in patients with patch or minimally infiltrated plaque disease.

Initially, patients are treated two to three times weekly for a period of 6 months to achieve skin clearance.[34] The dose (in joules) for each exposure is increased gradually and depends on the patient's skin type, severity of skin reaction, and degree of response. Once skin clearance has been achieved, patients continue on a maintenance program with a decreasing frequency of treatment, to as little as once per month. If disease progresses during the maintenance phase, the intensity of treatment is increased again to achieve better control.

Potential complications of PUVA therapy include erythema and blistering. These risks are greatest among patients with erythroderma, especially those with atrophic skin. Patients must shield their skin from sunlight for at least 24 hours following psoralen ingestion because sensitization of the skin by incorporation of the drug may continue that long. Cataract formation and secondary cutaneous malignancies are the most important potential long-term complications of PUVA.[35] Patients wear specially designed UV goggles while outdoors to reduce the risk of cataracts.

The results of PUVA therapy have been reported from several centers.[34, 36–38] The clearance rate is about 50% and varies with the initial extent of skin involvement. In a study of 82 patients with a mean follow-up period of 45 months, complete response was observed in 88% of patients with limited plaque (T1) disease and 52% with generalized plaque (T2) disease.[38] The response was less impressive in patients with tumor (T3) or erythrodermic (T4) disease. The response of patients with refractory plaques or tumors may be accelerated by the addition of localized irradiation. Patients with limited or generalized plaque disease may be good candidates for PUVA therapy. Patients with erythroderma are also suitable candidates for PUVA, provided that low daily exposures are used.[34] PUVA, combined with systemic therapy, such as interferon, may also be useful in patients with Sézary's syndrome.[38]

A variation of PUVA is photopheresis, known also as *extracorporeal PUVA*.[39] In photopheresis, the psoralen drug

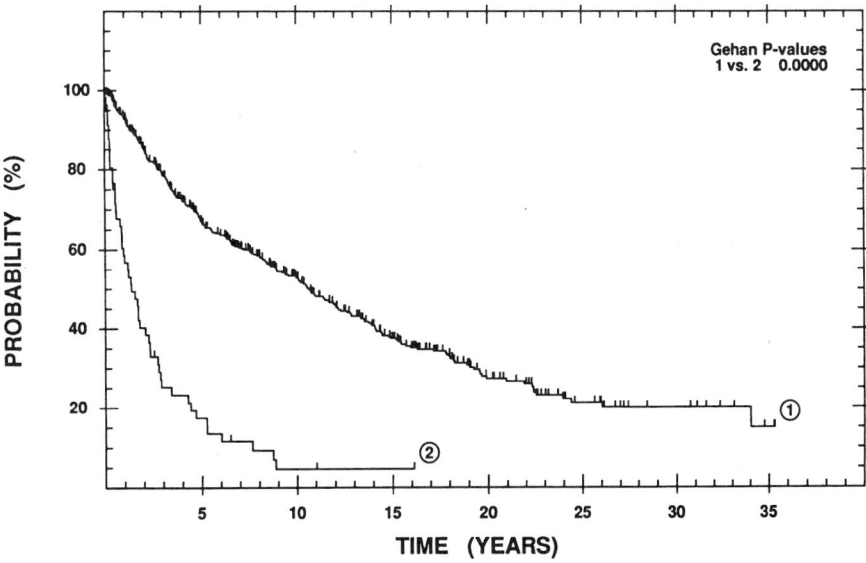

**Figure 93–2.** Actuarial survival of 600 patients with mycosis fungoides managed at Stanford University. Survival is calculated from the date of referral to Stanford (not from the date of diagnosis). 1 = 543 patients with disease apparently limited to the skin; 2 = 57 patients with extracutaneous disease at the time of presentation.

is administered orally, followed within 2 hours by pheresis of the white cells through an extracorporeal circuit. The lymphocyte-enriched fraction of the blood, combined with the psoralen-rich plasma, is exposed to UVA, then reinfused into the patient. The treatment schedule most commonly used is 2 consecutive days once a month. Usually, about 6 months of treatment is required before a response is seen. The mechanism of action of photopheresis is unclear. An immune-mediated effect has been proposed, although the efficacy may also be due to direct lymphotoxicity. Most patients are reported to respond to this therapy, with an overall response rate of 63%. Of patients, 41% showed at least a 50% improvement in their skin, and 20% of patients had a complete response.[40] The likelihood of response is greatest among patients with erythroderma, especially those with low CD4+/CD8+ ratios at the outset of therapy. Responses are less likely in patients who present with a large number of circulating Sézary cells.

### Topical Chemotherapy

Topical nitrogen mustard (mechlorethamine, HN2) is an effective and convenient form of treatment for mycosis fungoides. When used systemically, nitrogen mustard acts as an alkylating agent; however, when applied topically, nitrogen mustard probably acts by some method other than alkylation, perhaps an immune-mediated mechanism. There is no systemic absorption of topical nitrogen mustard so that hematologic monitoring is not necessary during therapy.

Nitrogen mustard is mixed in water or in an ointment base (Aquaphor), generally in a concentration of 10 to 20 mg/dl. It is applied at least once daily during the clearing phase, usually to the entire skin.[41, 42] If involvement is particularly limited, local treatment alone may be used. The concentration of the drug and frequency of application may be changed, depending on tolerance and response. The average time to skin clearance is about 6 months. Treatment is continued for at least 6 months after skin clearance.

The most common complication of topical nitrogen mustard therapy is a possible cutaneous hypersensitivity reaction, which occurs in 30% of patients treated with the aqueous solution and in about 5% of patients treated with the ointment base.[41] Hypersensitivity reactions may be overcome by a variety of topical or systemic desensitization programs.[41, 42] Secondary squamous and basal cell cancers have been associated with long-term nitrogen mustard use. This risk is greatest among patients who have had long-term sequential therapy with nitrogen mustard, PUVA, and irradiation.[35] Nearly all patients treated with topical nitrogen mustard achieve some response to therapy; complete response rates are 32 to 80%. The likelihood of a complete response depends on the initial extent of skin involvement.[29, 31, 41–43] Because of its efficacy and ease of application, topical nitrogen mustard is used widely in the management of patients with mycosis fungoides, especially those who have limited (T1) or generalized (T2) plaque phase of skin involvement.[29, 31] In long-term follow-up studies comparing efficacy of topical nitrogen mustard and total skin electron-beam therapy in patients with T1 and T2 disease, there was no survival benefit for patients treated with total skin radiation over those treated with nitrogen mustard despite superior complete response rates with radiation.[29, 31] As with PUVA, the response of patients with refractory plaques or tumors may be accelerated by the addition of localized irradiation. Although the overall response rate to topical nitrogen mustard is high, only a few patients (10 to 15%) maintain a long-term continuous complete response after the drug is discontinued.

Another drug that has been used as topical chemotherapy for mycosis fungoides is carmustine (BCNU).[44] Clearance rates are similar to those seen with nitrogen mustard; however, there is systemic absorption that requires hematologic monitoring, and patients treated with topical carmustine are especially prone to develop cutaneous telangiectasias, accentuated by exposure to irradiation.

## Radiation Therapy

Ionizing irradiation is the most effective single agent in the treatment of mycosis fungoides, as measured by its ability to achieve disease regression and total skin clearance.[45] Individual plaques or cutaneous tumors may be treated with small-field irradiation for palliation. Fractionated total doses of 15 to 25 Gy usually suffice. Occasionally, doses of 30 to 35 Gy are required. The exquisite radiosensitivity of mycosis fungoides permits the use of small daily doses (1.25 to 1.5 Gy) in areas such as the eyelids or face, to minimize normal tissue reactions. Larger size individual fractions may be used on other surfaces, but the use of fractions in excess of 2 Gy may result in the administration of a larger total dose than is really needed to achieve regression because the ability to titrate total dose to response is difficult when large daily fractions are used.

Because of the superficial nature of the disease, individual lesions can be treated most effectively with electrons (6 MeV), although orthovoltage x-rays (100 kV) may also be used. Electrons have the intrinsic advantage of a limited depth of penetration, dependent on their energy. Occasionally, patients present with disease that has extended into deeper tissue such as muscle, girdles an extremity, or involves large portions of a hand or foot. In these instances, megavoltage photons (4 to 10 MV) may be used most readily, to provide an adequate depth of penetration or delivery of a more homogeneous dose to the treatment volume than would be possible with electrons or orthovoltage x-rays. Tissue equivalent bolus on the surface may be necessary to avoid the *skin-sparing* effects of high-energy x-rays.

Megavoltage photon therapy may be effective palliative treatment for patients with extracutaneous mycosis fungoides, especially in lymph nodes. Nodal involvement may become extensive and symptomatic. Total doses similar to those used for cutaneous disease (30 Gy) are usually successful in controlling these sites. Other extracutaneous sites that may also be treated effectively in this fashion include the brain, oropharynx, and gastrointestinal tract.

Although the radiation responsiveness of mycosis fungoides has been appreciated since 1900, it was not until the late 1950s that techniques were developed to permit the treatment of large skin surfaces by means of electrons.[45, 46] Most widely used at this time are variations of the *Stanford technique*, using the electrons from a conventional linear accelerator. Patients are treated in the standing position about 3 m from the collimator of the linear accelerator, permitting the large field size. The patients stand in several (usually six) different positions, designed to expose virtually all of the skin surface to the electrons. At some centers, patients are treated on a rotating platform. Small daily fractions are used. At Stanford, the program is to deliver the equivalent of 1 Gy/day, 4 days per week, for a total of 36 Gy in 9 weeks.

In most patients, the only tissues that are shielded from the electrons are the lenses of the eyes. Lead external shields may be taped on the closed eyelids, or paraffin-coated, specially shaped lead shields may be placed under the lids (with the use of topical anesthesia). Other shielding may be used, as needed, in individual patients because of prior history of radiation exposure or to minimize normal tissue reactions that may develop during therapy.[45, 46] The scalp may be shielded after a dose of 24 Gy has been administered (provided that there is no involvement of the scalp) to reduce the likelihood of permanent alopecia.

Because of the position in which patients are treated, certain areas of the body are shadowed and do not receive an adequate dose of irradiation. Generally the soles of the feet and the perineum, which are completely protected, require supplemental treatment with electrons to a total dose of at least 20 Gy. The top of the scalp receives a reduced dose of irradiation, and if there is disease present on the scalp, this area must be boosted as well. Other areas that may require separate boost treatment include the inframammary regions, gluteal fold, and other skin fold areas.

Erythema, desquamation, and temporary epilation occur secondary to total skin electron-beam therapy. There is also temporary loss of fingernails and toenails (which occurs only after the completion of treatment) and an impaired ability to sweat for 6 to 12 months. Secondary squamous and basal cell cancers of the skin may develop in long-term follow-up, but this is most likely in patients who have received prolonged treatment with a variety of other topical therapies, including PUVA and topical nitrogen mustard.[35]

Many reports confirm the efficacy of total skin electron-beam therapy.[19, 29, 31, 47, 48] Nearly all patients respond to treatment, with complete response rates dependent on the extent of skin involvement. In our experience at Stanford, the complete response rates are 98%, 77%, 44%, and 36% for patients with T1, T2, T3, and T4 disease, respectively. Nearly 60% of patients with limited plaque disease (T1) and about 25% of patients with generalized plaque disease (T2) remain disease free more than 5 years after completion of a single course of electron-beam therapy.[29, 31] Although the curative potential of this treatment is debated, there is no doubt it provides an important palliative benefit, especially for patients with extensive disease. In addition, when disease recurs after electron-beam therapy, it is often in a more limited distribution and may be controlled more readily with limited topical therapy. Topical treatment with nitrogen mustard is often used as an adjuvant after completion of electron-beam therapy to prolong the response duration.[29, 49]

## Chemotherapy

Systemic chemotherapy, although effective in the management of nearly all lymphomas, has contributed little to the management of patients with mycosis fungoides.[19, 50] Virtually all drugs that are effective as single agents or in combination therapy in the treatment of patients with non-Hodgkin's lymphomas have been tested in mycosis fungoides. The largest experience is with combinations that include cyclophosphamide, vincristine, and prednisone, with or without doxorubicin (Adriamycin).[51–54] Complete response rates are only about 25% (range, 11 to 57%), and response durations are 3 to 20 months.[19, 50]

Some newer drugs show promise in early clinical trials. Fludarabine, a purine antimetabolite, which causes profound decreases in peripheral T-cell counts, has shown clinical activity against mycosis fungoides, chronic lymphocytic leukemia, and low-grade lymphomas.[55] Another drug that may be useful is pentostatin, which inhibits adenosine deaminase, an enzyme with a high level of activity in T cells. Adenosine deaminase inhibition leads to inhibition of DNA synthesis.

This drug has shown activity in mycosis fungoides and a variety of other non-Hodgkin's lymphomas as well as hairy cell leukemia. The response rate in mycosis fungoides may be 50%.[56, 57]

Although autologous bone marrow transplantation has been recognized as a potentially curative therapy for certain subsets of non-Hodgkin's lymphomas, its efficacy in mycosis fungoides and Sézary's syndrome has not been established. In one reported study, autologous bone marrow transplantation was used in six patients with advanced mycosis fungoides.[58] Five of the six patients had complete clinical responses, although three of these responses lasted less than 100 days.

## Biotherapy

The poor outcome of management of mycosis fungoides with traditional systemic therapy has led to trials of a variety of biologic agents. The interferons have antiproliferative, cytotoxic, and immunoregulatory functions. Interferon alfa was the first biologic agent tested in mycosis fungoides.[59–61] The overall response rates are reported to be 50 to 74%, with complete response rates of 21 to 35%. The likelihood of response correlates with stage of disease, intensity of prior therapy, and dose of interferon. The greatest likelihood of response is in patients with limited disease, little prior therapy, and interferon doses of $50 \times 10^6$ U/day for 5 days, every 3 weeks. With a high-dose regimen, patients often experience severe systemic adverse reactions, including severe fatigue, anorexia, decreased performance status, and leukopenia, necessitating dose reductions. Currently, interferon alfa is used at low doses of 3 to 5 million units given daily or three times a week. The dose is gradually increased depending on the clinical response and the severity of adverse reactions.

Another biologic therapy for mycosis fungoides is with anti–T cell monoclonal antibodies. Trials have been reported with a pan–T cell murine monoclonal antibody (anti-Leu-1)[62] as well as an iodine 131–radiolabeled version of a similar antibody (T101)[63] and a pan–T cell anti-CD5 antibody linked to ricin.[64] The responses reported are generally brief. Treatment is usually limited by the development of human antimouse antibodies. More recently, a chimeric anti–helper T cell (anti-CD4) antibody has been used to avoid the development of human antimouse antibodies and provide a more specific treatment against the mycosis fungoides subset of T cells.[65] The responses were generally modest and short-lived. Given even the minimal responses that have been observed so far, however, this modality deserves further study.

The retinoids are natural or synthetic analogues of vitamin A. Retinoids have multiple biologic effects that vary according to the biologic system and the drug concentration. They have been shown to promote differentiation and inhibit proliferation and to modulate immunologic function. Treatment with retinoids may achieve responses in patients with mycosis fungoides.[66–69] Overall response rates of approximately 45% with 20% complete response rates have been reported. The systemic retinoids are administered orally and are available as isotretinoin or acitretin. Newer retinoids (e.g., bexarotene) with potentially higher potency but without increased toxicity are currently undergoing clinical

trial.[70] Potential adverse effects of retinoids include photosensitivity, dryness of skin and mucous membranes, myalgia, arthralgia, fatigue, headaches, hepatotoxicity, and hyperlipidemic effects. The teratogenic effects of retinoids must be carefully addressed in female patients of childbearing age.

Cyclosporine, a potent anti–T cell drug used as an immunosuppressive agent in organ transplantation, has achieved some responses in mycosis fungoides. It inhibits the growth of mycosis fungoides cells by suppressing interleukin-2 production.[71]

Recombinant fusion toxins have been developed for use in mycosis fungoides and Sézary's syndrome.[72] This therapy involves the use of growth factor–cytotoxin fusion proteins designed specifically to kill defined neoplastic cell populations. The first example of this approach is the interleukin-2–diphtheria toxin fusion protein (Ontak, denileukin diftitox), which is currently approved for use in patients with refractory mycosis fungoides.[73]

## Combined-Modality Therapy

Combined-modality therapy has an important role in the management of patients with mycosis fungoides. Combined therapy may be in the form of sequential topical therapies, combined topical and systemic treatment, or combinations of systemic therapies.

As noted in the discussion of electron-beam therapy, the response rates to this treatment are high, but most patients relapse. For this reason, it is common to follow electron-beam therapy with a topical adjuvant, such as nitrogen mustard or PUVA. Adjuvant therapy prolongs the duration of the response; however, it is unclear whether it affects the ultimate relapse rate or overall survival.[49] In the Stanford study of patients with generalized plaque disease (T2), adjuvant topical nitrogen mustard improved the disease-free interval and freedom-from-relapse rates; however, there was no long-term survival benefit in the overall or disease-specific survivals.[29] Quiros and colleagues[74] reported that in their series of patients with T2 disease treated with total skin electron-beam therapy with or without adjuvant PUVA therapy, there were no significant differences in the overall survival between the two treatment groups, despite more favorable freedom-from-relapse survival results with adjuvant PUVA.

Combined topical therapies may be helpful in the palliative management of patients with persistent skin disease. For example, a program emphasizing topical nitrogen mustard therapy may be supplemented by the judicious use of irradiation to tumors or particularly refractory plaques. Occasionally, PUVA may be combined with topical nitrogen mustard. The main risk to consider in these cases is the potential for developing squamoproliferative lesions of the skin after prolonged therapy.[35]

Topical therapies may also be combined with biologic agents to enhance their response. Retinoids have been combined with PUVA in a program called *RePUVA*.[75] The clinical efficacy of combined PUVA and interferon alfa has been shown in mycosis fungoides and Sézary's syndrome.[38] In a series of patients primarily with stage I to II disease, a complete response rate of 80% was achieved; the responses were maintained for as long as maintenance PUVA and interferon were continued.[76]

Systemic therapies have been combined to maximize clinical response while maintaining tolerable toxicity risks. Oral retinoids have been combined with interferon alfa with an overall response rate of 42 to 77% in patients at stage I to IVB, with complete response rates of 15 to 54%.[77-79] Photopheresis can be combined with inteferon alfa.[80, 81] It is unclear whether this combined therapy is more effective than treatment with interferon alone.

Systemic chemotherapy has been combined with topical treatment in several reports.[19, 82-85] There is a wide range of responses reported, often reflective of differences in patient selection, and no single program has proved to be most effective. Responses may often be attributed to the topical component of therapy. The best test of a combined local-systemic approach was a trial reported from the NCI.[83] Patients were randomized to be treated aggressively with electron-beam therapy plus chemotherapy with cyclophosphamide, doxorubicin, VP-16, and vincristine or conservatively with sequential topical, then systemic therapies. After adjustment for stage of disease, both groups had a similar outcome. Specifically, there appeared to be no advantage to early systemic therapy for patients with limited disease.

## TREATMENT BY STAGE OF DISEASE

The most important factor in designing a treatment plan for patients with mycosis fungoides is their clinical stage. Patients with limited plaque disease (T1) can often be treated effectively with either topical nitrogen mustard or PUVA therapy. When nitrogen mustard is used, treatment with a 10 to 20 mg/dl ointment or solution is initiated to the entire skin because other areas of disease activity may become evident secondary to the inflammatory reaction that nitrogen mustard may provoke. After a period of several weeks, treatment may then be restricted to the affected region of the body. Treatment is continued on a daily basis until complete skin clearance and for 6 months thereafter. If response is particularly slow, the concentration of the nitrogen mustard may be increased to 30 to 40 mg/dl, especially to small areas, or the frequency of application may be increased to twice a day.

PUVA may also be used for limited plaque disease. Treatment is initiated on a three-times-weekly basis until skin clearance is achieved, after which the frequency of treatment is gradually decreased to as infrequently as once every 2 weeks. Maintenance therapy should be discontinued within 1 year.

Patients with generalized plaque disease (T2) may be treated with nitrogen mustard, PUVA, or total skin electron-beam therapy. Irradiation should be considered seriously for patients with thickened plaques because the depth of penetration of electron-beam therapy is more substantial than that of nitrogen mustard or PUVA. Irradiation should also be considered for patients with a recent history of rapid progression of disease. Patients treated with nitrogen mustard or PUVA should be followed closely, and treatment with electron-beam therapy should be initiated at the first evidence of disease progression. Generally, following completion of electron-beam therapy, adjuvant treatment with topical nitrogen mustard is appropriate and may be continued for 6 months or longer.

Patients with limited or generalized plaque disease who fail to respond to one therapy or who begin to progress after an initial response may be treated with an alternative topical therapy. There is no evidence that the development of resistance to one modality affects subsequent response to an alternative modality.

Most patients with tumorous involvement (T3) have generalized disease, and the greatest likelihood of a response is with electron-beam therapy, followed by adjuvant topical nitrogen mustard. Some patients, with a discrete number of tumors, may be treated with topical nitrogen mustard or PUVA, combined with localized irradiation to individual tumors.

Patients with erythroderma (T4) are challenging to manage. If there is no peripheral blood involvement, treatment may be initiated with low-dose PUVA (care must be taken to avoid phototoxic reactions). Photopheresis can be used as an effective initial monotherapy for patients with erythrodermic mycosis fungoides. In the presence of peripheral blood involvement (Sézary's syndrome), systemic management may play an important palliative role. One common treatment combines chlorambucil and prednisone.[86] Chlorambucil is administered at a dose of 2 mg/day and titrated according to response and toxicity (leukopenia and thrombocytopenia). Prednisone is given initially at a dose of 20 mg/day, decreasing as palliation is attained. Systemic retinoids or interferon alfa also can be used for erythrodermic mycosis fungoides and Sézary's syndrome, either alone or as part of a combined-modality regimen. If a systemic response is achieved, but cutaneous symptoms persist, topical therapy, such as corticosteroids, low-dose PUVA, or low concentrations of topical nitrogen mustard, may be added.

Patients with extracutaneous disease may be treated with megavoltage photon irradiation for palliation, especially for disease involving lymph nodes. Systemic chemotherapy and biologic response modifiers, alone or as a combined-modality regimen, are appropriate to consider in these patients as well. Because of the inadequacy of standard therapy, all patients with extracutaneous disease should be considered candidates for investigational therapies.

## Other Cutaneous Lymphomas

Patients with other primary cutaneous lymphomas represent only 5 to 7% of patients with extranodal non-Hodgkin's lymphoma.[87] There is a male predominance, and the median age is about 60 years. These lymphomas may be of B-cell or T-cell type and often are classified according to modified criteria of the Working Formulation[88] or newer classification systems.[89] These include low-grade B-cell lymphoma, diffuse large B-cell lymphoma, and intermediate-grade or high-grade B-cell and T-cell lymphomas. They may be categorized further according to the expression of cell surface antigens, such as CD-30 (Ki-1). The proportion of B-cell lymphomas in different series ranges from 50 to 75%.[90, 91] In contrast to mycosis fungoides, the T-cell types often lack some of the mature T-cell antigens and do not exhibit a T-helper or T-suppressor phenotype.

The pathology of the other cutaneous non-Hodgkin's lymphomas differs from that of mycosis fungoides in that they are nonepidermotropic. That is, neoplastic cells are not usually present in the epidermis but are limited to the dermis and subcutaneous tissues. The region between the dermis and epidermis is spared (the Grenz zone); however, relatively advanced lesions may ulcerate into the epidermis secondarily.

The most common histologic subtypes of primary cutaneous B-cell lymphoma are diffuse large cell and immunoblastic, which account for one half to two thirds of cases.[90, 92] It is important to differentiate the low-grade cutaneous lymphomas from benign lymphocytic proliferations, such as lymphocytoma cutis.[93] This is best done by immunophenotyping because lymphocytoma cutis is a polyclonal proliferation, in contrast to the monoclonal B-cell nature of the cutaneous lymphomas.

The clinical presentation of the primary cutaneous B-cell lymphomas is generally of nodules rather than the plaques or patches seen in mycosis fungoides. The predominant site is the head and neck area.[94] Regional lymph nodes are uncommonly affected.

The staging evaluation should include studies generally used for patients with non-Hodgkin's lymphomas in other sites. These should include a thorough physical examination, including detailed examination of the skin; complete blood counts; screening chemistries; a chest radiograph; computed tomographic scan of the chest, abdomen, and pelvis; and a bone marrow biopsy.

For patients who have localized involvement of the skin only (stage IE), treatment may be limited to local irradiation. A dose of 36 to 44 Gy generally suffices. At least half of these patients are cured with local treatment.[92, 94] Systemic treatment may be restricted to patients who have disease progression after localized radiation treatment. The most common site of failure is in skin sites distant from the primary site of involvement. The 10-year survival of patients who present with stage IE disease is 60 to 70%.[91, 92, 94]

Patients with stage IIE disease (regional lymph nodes involved) are best treated with combined-modality therapy, in a fashion analogous to that of other patients with stage II intermediate-grade or high-grade lymphoma.[95] In patients with stage III or IV disease, the cutaneous involvement should be considered incidental, unless it is particularly bulky and poses a problem for local control with chemotherapy, in which case adjuvant irradiation may be added to the primary chemotherapy program.

An entity called Ki-1 (CD30)-positive anaplastic large cell lymphoma of the skin has been described.[96] These lymphomas may arise de novo (primary) or develop in the setting of pre-existing lymphomatoid papulosis or cutaneous T-cell lymphoma of mycosis fungoides type (secondary). The behavior of primary anaplastic large cell lymphoma is relatively indolent, and the treatment approach may be similar to other nonaggressive cutaneous non-Hodgkin's lymphomas.[97] In the rare presentation in which there are multiple, generalized skin lesions, there is a higher risk of more extensive systemic involvement. The behavior of secondary cutaneous anaplastic large cell lymphoma, which arises in the setting of previous cutaneous T-cell lymphoma, such as mycosis fungoides, may be more aggressive and require more intensive local or systemic therapy.[96, 98]

Angiocentric T-cell or natural killer–cell and natural killer–like T-cell (CD56) lymphomas can also involve the skin. In these lymphomas, there is a high association of extracutaneous disease with an extremely aggressive clinical course and resistance to conventional chemotherapeutic agents.[99–101]

## SUGGESTIONS FOR ADDITIONAL READING

Hoppe RT, Wood GS, Abel EA. Mycosis fungoides and the Sezary syndrome: pathology, staging and treatment. Curr Prob Cancer 1990;14:295.

Wieselthier JS, Koh HK. Sezary syndrome: diagnosis, prognosis, and critical review of treatment options. J Am Acad Dermatol 1990;22:381.

Wood GS, Weiss LM, Warnke RA, et al. The immunopathology of cutaneous lymphomas: immunophenotypic and immunogenotypic characteristics. Semin Oncol 1986;5:334.

Sausville EA, Eddy JL, Makuch RW, et al. Histopathologic staging at initial diagnosis of mycosis fungoides and the Sezary syndrome: definition of three distinctive prognostic groups. Ann Intern Med 1988;109:372.

Rosenbaum MM, Roenigk HH, Caro WA, et al. Photochemotherapy in cutaneous T-cell lymphoma and parapsoriasis en plaques: long-term follow-up in forty-three patients. J Am Acad Dermatol 1985;13:613.

Heald P, Rook A, Perez M, et al. Treatment of erythrodermic cutaneous T-cell lymphoma with extracorporeal photochemotherapy. J Am Acad Dermatol 1992;27:427–33.

Vonderheid EC, Tan ET, Kantor AF, et al. Long-term efficacy, curative potential and carcinogenicity of topical mechlorethamine chemotherapy in cutaneous T cell lymphoma. J Am Acad Dermatol 1989;20:416.

Hoppe RT, Abel EA, Deneau DG, et al. Mycosis fungoides: management with topical nitrogen mustard. J Clin Oncol 1987;5:1796.

Olsen EA, Rosen ST, Vollmer RT, et al. Interferon alfa-2a in the treatment of cutaneous T cell lymphoma. J Am Acad Dermatol 1989;20:395.

Kaye FJ, Bunn PA, Steinberg SM, et al. A randomized trial comparing combination electron-beam radiation and chemotherapy with topical therapy in the initial treatment of mycosis fungoides. N Engl J Med 1989;321:1784.

Joly P, Charlotte F, Leibowitch M, et al. Cutaneous lymphomas other than mycosis fungoides: follow-up; study of 52 patients. J Clin Oncol 1991;9:1994.

Esche BA, Fitzpatrick PJ. Cutaneous malignant lymphoma. Int J Radiat Oncol Biol Phys 1986;12:2111.

Willemze R, Beljaards RC. Spectrum of primary cutaneous CD30 (Ki-1)-positive lymphoproliferative disorders: a proposal for classification and guidelines for management and treatment. J Am Acad Dermatol 1993;28:973.

Duvic M, Lemak NA, Redman JR, et al. Combined modality therapy for cutaneous T-cell lymphoma. J Am Acad Dermatol 1996;34:1022.

Kim YH, Bishop K, Varghese A, et al. Prognostic factors in erythrodermic mycosis fungoides and the Sezary syndrome. Arch Dermatol 1995;131:1003.

Kim YH, Jensen R, Watanabe G, et al. Clinical stage IA (limited patch and plaque) mycosis fungoides: a long-tern outcome analysis. Arch Dermatol 1996;132:1309.

Holloway K, Flowers F, Ramos-Caro F. Therpeutic alternatives in cutaneous T-cell lymphoma. J Am Acad Dermatol 1992;27:367.

## REFERENCES

1. Greene MH, Dalager NA, Lamberg SI, et al. Exposure to chemicals, physical agents and biologic agents in mycosis fungoides and the Sezary syndrome. Cancer Treat Rep 1979;63:596.
2. Whittemore AS, Holly EA, Lee IM, et al. Mycosis fungoides in relation to environmental exposures and immune response: a case control study. J Natl Cancer Inst 1989;81:1560.
3. Weinstock MA. A registry-based case-control study of mycosis fungoides. Ann Epidemiol 1991;1:533.
4. Poiesz BJ, Ruscetti FW, Gazdar AF, et al. Detection and isolation of type C retrovirus particles from fresh and cultured lymphocytes of a patient with cutaneous T-cell lymphoma. Proc Natl Acad Sci U S A 1980;77:7415.
5. Ranki A, Niemi KM, Nieminen P, et al. Antibodies against retroviral core proteins in relation to disease outcome in patients with mycosis fungoides. Arch Dermatol Res 1990;282:532.

6. Hall WW, Liu CR, Schneewind O, et al. Deleted HTLV-I provirus in blood and cutaneous lesions of patients with mycosis fungoides. Science 1991;253:317.

7. Wood GS, Salvekar A, Schaffer J, et al. Evidence against a role for HTLV-I in the pathogenesis of American cutaneous T-cell lymphoma. J Invest Dermatol 1996;107:301–7.

8. Li G, Vowels BR, Benoit BM, et al. Failure to detect human T-lymphotrphic virus type-I proviral DNA in cell lines and tissues from patients with cutaneous T-cell lymphoma. J Invest Dermatol 1996;107:308–13.

9. Manzari V, Gismondi A, Barillari G, et al. HTVL-V: a new human retrovirus isolated in a Tac-negative T-cell lymphoma/leukemia. Science 1987;238:1581.

10. Weinstock MA, Horm JW. Mycosis fungoides in the United States: increasing incidence and descriptive epidemiology. JAMA 1988;260:42.

11. Brouet JC, Flandrin G, Seligmann M. Indications of the thymus-derived nature of the proliferating cells in six patients with Sezary syndrome. N Engl J Med 1973;289:341.

12. Wood GS, Weiss LM, Warnke RA, et al. The immunopathology of cutaneous lymphomas: immunophenotypic and immunogenotypic characteristics. Semin Dermatol 1986;5:334.

13. Mitchie SA, Abel EA, Hoppe RT, et al. Expression of T-cell receptor antigens in mycosis fungoides and inflammatory skin lesions. J Invest Dermatol 1989;93:116.

14. Weiss LM, Wood GS, Hu E, et al. Detection of clonal T-cell receptor gene rearrangements in the peripheral blood of patients with mycosis fungoides/Sezary syndrome. J Invest Dermatol 1989;92:601.

15. Kern DE, Kidd PG, Moe R, et al. Analysis of T-cell receptor gene rearrangement in lymph nodes of patients with mycosis fungoides: prognostic implications. Arch Dermatol 1998;134:158.

16. Muche JM, Lukowsky A, Asadullah K, et al. Demonstration of frequent occurrence of clonal T-cells in the peripheral blood of patients with primary cutaneous T-cell lymphoma. Blood 1997;90:1636.

17. Ashton-Key M, Du MQ, Kirkham N, et al. The value of the polymerase chain reaction in the diagnosis of cutaneous T-cell infiltrates. Am J Surg Pathol 1997;21:743.

18. Bignon YJ, Souteyrand P, Roger H, et al. Clonotypic heterogeneity in cutaneous T-cell lymphomas. Cancer Res 1990;50:6620.

19. Hoppe RT, Wood GS, Abel EA. Mycosis fungoides and the Sezary syndrome: pathology, staging, and treatment. Curr Prob Cancer 1990;14:295.

20. Lutzner MA, Edelson RI, Schein P, et al. Cutaneous T-cell lymphomas: the Sezary syndrome, mycosis fungoides, and related disorders. Ann Intern Med 1975;83:534.

21. Meijer CJ, van der Loo EM, vanVloten WA, et al. Early diagnosis of mycosis fungoides and Sezary syndrome by morphometric analysis of lymphoid cells in the skin. Cancer 1980;45:2864.

22. Sausville EA, Eddy JL, Makuch RW, et al. Histopathologic staging at initial diagnosis of mycosis fungoides and the Sezary syndrome: definition of three distinctive prognostic groups. Ann Intern Med 1988;109:372.

23. Bunn PA, Huberman MS, Whang-Peng J, et al. Prospective staging evaluation of patients with cutaneous T-cell lymphomas: demonstration of a high frequency of extracutaneous dissemination. Ann Intern Med 1980;93:223.

24. Weiss, LM, Hu E, Wood GS, et al. Clonal rearrangements of the T-cell receptor gene in mycosis fungoides and dermatopathic lymphadenopathy. N Engl J Med 1985;315:539.

25. Wieselthier JS, Koh HK. Sezary syndrome: diagnosis, prognosis, and critical review of treatment options. J Am Acad Dermatol 1990;22:381.

26. Epstein EH, Devin DL, Croft JD, et al. Mycosis fungoides: survival, prognostic features, response to therapy, and autopsy findings. Medicine 1972;15:61.

27. Bunn PA, Lamberg SI. Report of the committee on staging and classification of cutaneous T-cell lymphomas. Cancer Treat Rep 1979;63:725.

28. Kim YH, Bishop K, Varghese, et al. Prognostic factors in erythrodermic mycosis fungoides and the Sezary syndrome. Arch Dermatol 1995;131:1003.

29. Kim YH, Chow S, Varghese A, et al. Clinical characteristics and long-term outcome of patients with generalized patch and plaque (T2) mycosis fungoides. Arch Dermatol 1999;135:26.

30. Kulin PA, Marglin SI, Shuman WP, et al. Diagnostic imaging in the initial staging of mycosis fungoides and Sezary syndrome. Arch Dermatol 1990;126:914.

31. Kim YH, Jensen RA, Watanabe GL, et al. Clinical stage IA (limited patch and plaque) mycosis fungoides. Arch Dermatol 1996;132:1309.

32. Ramsay D, Lish K, Yalowitz C, et al. Ultraviolet-B phototherapy for early-stage cutaneous T-cell lymphoma. Arch Dermatol 1992;128:931.

33. Gilchrest BA, Parrish JA, Tanenbaum L, et al. Oral methoxsalen photochemotherapy of mycosis fungoides. Cancer 1976;38:683.

34. Abel EA, Sendagorta E, Hoppe RT, et al. PUVA treatment of erythrodermic and plaque-type mycosis fungoides: ten-year follow-up study. Arch Dermatol 1987;123:897.

35. Abel EA, Sendagorta E, Hoppe RT. Cutaneous malignancies and metastatic squamous cell carcinoma following topical therapies for mycosis fungoides. J Am Acad Dermatol 1986;14:1029.

36. Honigsmann H, Brenner W, Rauschmeier W, et al. Photochemotherapy for cutaneous T-cell lymphoma. J Am Acad Dermatol 1984;10:238.

37. Rosenbaum MM, Roenigk HJ, Caro WA, et al. Photochemotherapy in cutaneous T-cell lymphoma and parapsoriasis en plaques: long term follow-up in forty-three patients. J Am Acad Dermatol 1985;13:613.

38. Roenigk H, Kuzel T, Skoutelis A, et al. Photochemotherapy alone or combined with interferon alpha-2a in the treatment of cutaneous T-cell lymphoma. J Invest Dermatol 1990;95:98S–205S.

39. Edelson R, Berger C, Gasparro F, et al. Treatment of cutaneous T-cell lymphoma by extracorporeal photochemotherapy: preliminary results. N Engl J Med 1987;316:297.

40. Heald P, Rook A, Perez M, et al. Treatment of erythrodermic cutaneous T-cell lymphoma with extracorporeal photochemotherapy. J Am Acad Dermatol 1992;27:427.

41. Hoppe RT, Abel EA, Deneau DG, et al. Mycosis fungoides: management with topical nitrogen mustard. J Clin Oncol 1987;5:1796.

42. Vonderheid EC, Tan ET, Kantor AF, et al. Long term efficacy, curative potential, and carcinogenicity of topical mechlorethamine chemotherapy in cutaneous T-cell lymphoma. J Am Acad Dermatol 1989;20:416.

43. Ramsay DL, Halperin PS, Zeleniuch JA. Topical mechlorethamine therapy for early stage mycosis fungoides. J Am Acad Dermatol 1988;9:684.

44. Zackheim HS, Epstein EH, Crain WR. Topical carmustine (BCNU) for cutaneous T-cell lymphoma: a 15-year experience in 143 patients. J Am Acad Dermatol 1990;22:802.

45. Hoppe RT, Fuks Z, Bagshaw MA. Radiation therapy in the management of cutaneous T-cell lymphomas. Cancer Treat Rep 1979;63:625.

46. Hoppe RT. Total skin electron beam therapy in the management of mycosis fungoides. Front Radiat Ther Oncol 1990;25:140.

47. Lo TCM, Salzman FA, Moschella SJ, et al. Whole body surface electron irradiation in the treatment of mycosis fungoides: an evaluation of 200 patients. Radiology 1979;130:453.

48. Tadros AAM, Tepperman BS, Hryniuk WM, et al. Total skin electron irradiation for mycosis fungoides: failure analysis and prognostic factors. Int J Radiat Oncol Biol Phys 1983;9:1279.

49. Price NM, Hoppe RT, Constantine VS, et al. The treatment of mycosis fungoides: adjuvant topical mechlorethamine after electron beam therapy. Cancer 1977;40:2851.

50. Broder S, Bunn PA. Cutaneous T-cell lymphomas. Semin Oncol 1980;7:310.

51. Case DC Jr. Combination chemotherapy for mycosis fungoides with cyclophosphamide, vincristine, methotrexate, and prednisone. Am J Clin Oncol 1984;7:453.

52. Molin L, Thomsen K, Volden G, et al. Combination chemotherapy in the tumor stage of mycosis fungoides with cyclophosphamide, vincristine, VP-16, adriamycin and prednisolone (COP, CHOP, CA-VOP): a report from the Scandinavian Mycosis Fungoides Study Group. Acta Derm Venerol 1980;60:542.

53. Raafat J, Oster MW, LoGerfo P, et al. Combination chemotherapy for advanced cutaneous T-cell lymphomas. Cancer Treat Rep 1980;64:1371.

54. Tirelli U, Carbone A, Veronesi, et al. Combination chemotherapy with cyclophosphamide, vincristine, and prednisone (CVP) in TNM-classified stage IV mycosis fungoides. Cancer Treat Rep 1982;66:167.

55. Von Hoff DD, Dahlberg S, Hartstock RJ, et al. Activity of fludarabine monophosphate in patients with advanced mycosis fungoides: a Southwest Oncology Group study. J Natl Cancer Inst 1990;82:1353.

56. Cummings FJ, Kim K, Neiman RC, et al. Phase II trial of pentostatin in refractory lymphomas and cutaneous T-cell disease. J Clin Oncol 1991;9:565.

57. Merciecaq J, Matutes E, Dearden C, et al. The role of pentostatin in

the treatment of T-cell malignancies: analysis of response rate in 145 patients according to disease subtype. J Clin Oncol 1994;12:2588.

58. Bigler R, Crilley P, Micaily B, et al. Autologous bone marrow transplantation for advanced stage mycosis fungoides. Bone Marrow Transplant 1991;7:133.

59. Kohn EC, Steis RG, Sausville EA, et al. Phase II trial of intermittent high-dose recombinant interferon alfa-2a in mycosis fungoides and the Sezary syndrome. J Clin Oncol 1990;8:155.

60. Olsen EA, Rosen ST, Vollmer RT, et al. Interferon alfa-2a in the treatment of cutaneous T-cell lymphoma. J Am Acad Dermatol 1989;20:395.

61. Vegna ML, Papa G, Defazio D, et al. Interferon alpha-2a in cutaneous T-cell lymphoma. Eur J Haematol 1990;45:32.

62. Miller RA, Oseroff AR, Stratte PT, et al. Monoclonal antibody therapeutic trials in seven patients with T-cell lymphoma. Blood 1983;62:988.

63. Dillman RO, Beauregard J, Shawler DL, et al. Continuous infusion of T101 monoclonal antibody in chronic lymphocyte leukemia and cutaneous T-cell lymphoma. J Biol Response Mod 1986;5:394.

64. LeMaistre CF, Rosen S, Frankel A, et al. Phase I trial of H65-RTA immunoconjugate in patients with cutaneous T-cell lymphoma. Blood 1991;78:1173.

65. Knox SJ, Levy R, Hodgkinson S, et al. Observations on the effect of chimeric anti-CD4 monoclonal antibody in patients with mycosis fungoides. Blood 1991;77:20.

66. Molin L, Thomsen K, Volden G, et al. Oral retinoids in mycosis fungoides and Sezary syndrome: a comparison of isotretinoin and etretinate: a study from the Scandinavian Mycosis Fungoides Group. Acta Derm Venereol (Stockh) 1987;67:232.

67. Claudy A, Rouchouse B, Boucheron S, et al. Treatment of cutaneous lymphoma etretinate. Br J Dermatol 1983;109:49.

68. Tousignant J, Raymond G, Light M. Treatment of cutaneous T-cell lymphoma with the arotinoid Ro 13-6298. J Am Acad Dermatol 1987;16:167.

69. Hoting E, Meissner K. Arotinoid-ethylester effectiveness in refractory cutaneous T-cell lymphoma. Cancer 1988;62:1044.

70. Miller VA, Benedetti FM, Rigas JR, et al. Initial clinical trial of a selective retinoid X receptor (RXR) ligand, 3-methyl TTNEB (LGD1069). Proc ASCO 1995;14:172.

71. Jensen JR, Thestrup-Pedersen K, Zachariae H, et al. Cyclosporin A therapy for mycosis fungoides. Arch Dermatol 1987;123:161.

72. Hesketh P, Caguioa P, Koh H, et al. Clinical activity of a cytotoxic fusion protein in the treatment of cutaneous T-cell lymphoma. J Clin Oncol 1993;11:1682.

73. LeMaistre CF, Saleh MN, Kuzel TM, et al. Phase I trial of a ligand fusion-protein (DAB389IL-2) in lymphomas expressing the receptor for interleukin-2. Blood 1998;91:399.

74. Quiros P, Jones G, Kacinski B, et al. Total skin electron beam therapy followed by adjuvant psoralen/ultraviolet-A light in the management of patients with T1 and T2 cutaneous T-cell lymphoma (mycosis fungoides). Int J Radiat Oncol Biol Phys 1997;38:1027.

75. Thomsen K, Hammar H, Molin L, et al. Retinoid plus PUVA (Re-PUVA) and PUVA in mycosis fungoides, plaque stage. Acta Derm Venereol (Stockh) 1989;69:536.

76. Kuzel TM, Gilyon K, Springer E, et al. Interferon alfa-2a combined with phototherapy in the treatment of cutaneous T-cell lymphoma. J Natl Cancer Inst 1990;82:203.

77. Dreno B. Roferon-A (interferon alpha 2a) combined with Tegason (etretinate) for treatment of cutaneous T-cell lymphomas. Stem Cells 1993;11:269.

78. Dreno B, Claudy A, Meynadier J, et al. The treatment of 45 patients with cutaneous T-cell lymphoma with low doses of interferon alpha 2a and etretinate. Br J Dermatol 1991;125:456.

79. Altomare G, Capella G, Pigatto P, et al. Intramuscular low dose alpha-2b interferon and etretinate for treatment of mycosis fungoides. Int J Dermatol 1993;32:138.

80. Rook A, Prystowsky M, Cassin M, et al. Combined therapy for Sezary syndrome with extracorporeal photochemotherapy and low-dose interferon alfa therapy. Arch Dermatol 1991;127:1535.

81. Gottlieb SL, Wolfe JT, Fox FE, et al. Treatment of cutaneous T-cell lymphoma with extracorporeal photopheresis monotherapy and in combination with recombinant interferon alfa: a 10-year experience at a single institution. J Am Acad Dermatol 1996;35:946.

82. Braveman IM, Klein S, Grant A. Electron microscopic and immunolabeling studies of the lesional and normal skin of patients with mycosis fungoides treated by total body electron beam irradiation. J Am Acad Dermatol 1987;16:45.

83. Kaye FJ, Bunn PA, Steinberg SM, et al. A randomized trial comparing combination electron-beam radiation and chemotherapy with topical therapy in the initial treatment of mycosis fungoides. N Engl J Med 1989;321:1784.

84. Zakem MH, Davis BR, Adelstein DJ, et al. Treatment of advanced stage mycosis fungoides with bleomycin, doxorubicin, and methotrexate with topical nitrogen mustard (BAM-M). Cancer 1986;58:2611.

85. Duvic M, Lemak NA, Redman JR, et al. Combined modality therapy for cutaneous T-cell lymphoma. J Am Acad Dermatol 1996;34:1022.

86. Winklelmann RK, Diaz-Perez JL, Buechner SA. The treatment of Sezary syndrome. J Am Acad Dermatol 1984;10:1000.

87. Paryani S, Hoppe RT, Burke JS, et al. Extralymphatic involvement in diffuse non-Hodgkin's lymphoma. J Clin Oncol 1983;1:682.

88. Non-Hodgkin's Lymphoma Pathology Classification Project. National Cancer Institute–sponsored study of classifications of non-Hodgkin's lymphomas: summary and description of a working formulation for clinical usage. Cancer 1982;49:2112.

89. Armitage JO, Weisenburger DD, for the Non-Hodgkin's Lymphoma Classification Project. New approach to classifying non-Hodgkin's lymphomas: clinical features of the major histologic subtypes. J Clin Oncol 1998;16:2780.

90. Wood GS, Burke JS, Horning S, et al. The immunologic and clinicopathologic heterogeneity of cutaneous lymphomas other than mycosis fungoides. Blood 1983;62:464.

91. Joly P, Charlotte F, Leibowitch M, et al. Cutaneous lymphomas other than mycosis fungoides: follow-up study of 52 patients. J Clin Oncol 1991;9:1994.

92. Esche BA, Fitzpatrick PJ. Cutaneous malignant lymphoma. Int J Radiat Oncol Biol 1986;12:2111.

93. Garcia CF, Weiss LM, Warnke RA, et al. Cutaneous follicular lymphoma. Am J Surg Pathol 1986;10:454.

94. Burke JS, Hoppe RT, Cibull ML, et al. Cutaneous malignant lymphoma: a pathologic study of 50 cases with clinical analysis of 37. Cancer 1981;47:300.

95. Prestidge BR, Horning SJ, Hoppe RT. Combined modality therapy for stage I–II large cell lymphoma. Int J Radiat Oncol Biol Phys 1988;15:633.

96. Kaudewitz P, Stein H, Dallenbach F, et al. Primary and secondary Ki-1 (CD30+) anaplastic large cell lymphomas: morphologic, immunohistologic and clinical characteristics. Am J Pathol 1989;135:359.

97. Beljaards RC, Kaudewitz P, Berti E, et al. Primary cutaneous large cell lymphomas: definition of a new type of cutaneous lymphoma with a favorable prognosis: an European multicenter study on 47 patients. Cancer 1993;71:2097.

98. Wood G, Bahler D, Hoppe R, et al. Transformation of mycosis fungoides: T-cell receptor beta-gene analysis demonstrates a common clonal origin for plaque-type mycosis fungoides and CD30+ large cell lymphoma. J Invest Dermatol 1993;101:296.

99. Chan JKC, Ng CS, Ngan KC, et al. An aggressive lymphoma distinct from mycosis fungoides. Am J Surg Pathol 1988;12:861.

100. Chan JKC, Sin VC, Wong KF, et al. Nonnasal lymphoma expressing the natural killer cell marker CD45: a clinicopathologic study of 49 cases of an uncommon aggressive neoplasm. Blood 1997;89:4501.

101. Nakamura S, Suchi T, Koshikawa T, et al. Clinicopathologic study of CD56 (NCAM)-positive angiocentric lymphoma occurring in sites other than the upper and lower respiratory tract. Am J Surg Pathol 1996;19:284.

# CHAPTER 94

# EXTRANODAL LYMPHOMAS

• GREGORY P. SARNA • A. ROBERT KAGAN

Lymphomas commonly present as extranodal primary tumors. Roughly 25% of lymphomas in the United States[1, 2] and about 40% of lymphomas elsewhere[3–5] have been reported to be of extranodal origin. These figures are imprecise because there is often inconsistency in the classification of a patient with a solitary extranodal site and diffuse lymphadenopathy (IIE or IIIE vs. IV) and of a patient with multiple extranodal sites in one or more organs (multiple IE or IIE vs. IV). The most common sites of extranodal primary tumors are in the head and neck region (commonly Waldeyer's ring, orbit, brain), skin, and gastrointestinal tract (commonly stomach, small bowel). Myriads of other sites exist, and several are discussed subsequently.

The above-mentioned 25 to 40% incidence refers to lymphomas arising in the immunocompetent host. In the setting of acquired immunodeficiency syndrome (AIDS) (and probably organ transplantation), extranodal lymphomas are the rule rather than the exception. Of AIDS-related lymphomas, 56 to 85% appear extranodal at diagnosis, frequently with multiple extranodal sites of involvement.[6, 7] In the AIDS setting, the most common sites of involvement are the brain and gastrointestinal tract. Other sites, often bizarre in non-AIDS patients (e.g., heart, anus, effusions[8]), frequently are noted.[6, 7] This chapter focuses on the noncutaneous extranodal lymphomas. The reader is also referred to *Seminars of Oncology*, Volume 26, Number 3 (June 1999), which is devoted to extranodal lymphomas.

## Natural History

### HISTOLOGY

Most extranodal lymphomas are diffuse rather than nodular[9, 10] in architecture with, by Rappaport criteria, diffuse histiocytic the most common histologic appearance followed by diffuse mixed or poorly differentiated lymphocytic. By Working Formulation criteria, a Danish study of 463 cases of extranodal lymphoma[11] has reported 44% to be high grade; 17%, intermediate grade; 27%, low grade; and 12%, unclassified.

Many extranodal lymphomas are now recognized histologically and clinically as mucosa-associated lymphoid tissue (MALT) lymphomas (MALTomas, marginal zone B-cell lymphomas of MALT type). These are B-cell lymphomas originating in the mucosa of gastrointestinal tract organs and probably other organs, including lung, thyroid, salivary gland, and larynx.[12] Other sites also exist. The occurrence of MALTomas may be related to chronic inflammation (e.g., gastric lymphoma related to *Helicobacter pylori* gastritis,[13] salivary gland lymphoma related to Sjögren's syndrome, or

thyroid lymphoma related to Hashimoto's thyroiditis),[14] and the growth of these tumors, particularly gastric MALTomas, may be antigen driven.[15] Histologically, these tend to be low-grade tumors showing lymphoplasmacytic infiltration and lymphoepithelial cells. The malignant lymphocytes have features of *centrocyte-like* cells similar to marginal zone B cells.[14] Follicles may be present but are generally reactive or composed of centrocyte-like cells that have colonized a reactive follicle, rather than follicular center cells.[16] In lymph nodes, these cells may appear monocytoid.[14] Consistent with the concept that the malignant cells are not follicular center B cells is the absence of the *bcl-2* gene rearrangement[17] and of the t(14;18) translocation.[18, 19] These lymphomas tend to be indolent and stay localized, and early-stage disease may be curable. In some cases, though, late relapse may occur, as may transformation to a higher grade; some lymphomas may be aggressive and multifocal. Genetic studies suggest that these are more likely to be *homing* to other mucosa-associated tissue than to be multiple concurrent primary lymphomas.[20]

Mantle cell lymphomas are commonly extranodal. These lymphomas may, in *typical* variants, consist histologically of small to intermediate size cells that resemble low-grade lymphomas. The *blastic* variant consists of more variable intermediate to large size cells and appears higher grade.[21] Both variants are characterized by t(11;14)(q13;q32) translocation, overexpression of cyclin D1, and *bcl-1* rearrangement.[21] Similar to small lymphocytic lymphoma or chronic lymphocytic leukemia, these variants may coexpress CD5 and B cell antigens, but in contrast to those diseases, they tend to be negative for CD23.[22]

In the AIDS setting, lymphomas are generally high grade. Levine,[23] reporting the University of Southern California (USC) experience with AIDS lymphoma, found 61% to be small noncleaved (including 10% Burkitt's) and 35% to be B-cell immunoblastic. Levine[23] also cited data from the AIDS Clinical Trial Unit, in which 41 patients from eight institutions had 83% high-grade B-cell tumors and 10% had intermediate-grade tumors. Although these data refer to nodal and extranodal presentations, most of these patients had extranodal disease. In the New York University (NYU) Medical Center series of 89 patients with AIDS lymphoma,[7] 69% had high-grade lymphomas (small noncleaved, 40%; large cell immunoblastic/plasmacytoid, 28%), and 31% showed intermediate-grade lymphoma (large noncleaved). Of these 89 patients, 87% had extranodal lymphoma at presentation. Gastrointestinal tract involvement was seen in 25% of patients and was commonly (52%) large cell immunoblastic/plasmacytic. Additionally, 36% of this group had a large noncleaved histologic appearance. Only 12% had small noncleaved tumors. With central nervous system involvement, these three histologic types were similarly represented.

Davi and colleagues[24] have reported on 103 patients with AIDS lymphoma. Nineteen of these (18.4%) had Burkitt's-like lymphoma, whereas 25 (24.3%) were believed to have (true) Burkitt's lymphoma. Of 32 patients with these two histologies in whom site of disease was noted, 3 had extranodal disease only, and 20 had disease in nodal and extranodal (other than liver, spleen, and bone marrow) sites.

Although extranodal lymphomas, in the non-AIDS and AIDS settings, are generally B cell, T-cell extranodal lymphomas also occur. Nasal, and to a lesser degree nasopharyngeal, lymphomas are frequently of T or natural killer (NK) cell origin and part of the spectrum of angiocentric lymphoproliferative disorders of the upper and lower respiratory tracts. These lymphomas generally appear to be large cell or immunoblastic.[25, 26] Human T-cell leukemia/lymphoma virus type 1 (HTLV-1)–associated extranodal T-cell lymphomas have also been reported.[27] Mycosis fungoides and other cutaneous lymphomas may be T cell in origin, as may small bowel lymphomas related to inflammatory enteropathy.

## CLINICAL FEATURES

Although extranodal lymphomas are heterogeneous, their nature and behavior varying with site, histology, stage, and other factors, certain generalizations are useful, as follows:

1. Extranodal lymphomas in the AIDS setting may be stage IE but are commonly disseminated. In the NYU Medical Center series,[7] only 25% of patients with extranodal involvement had stage IE disease, and the USC group reported stage I or II disease (nodal and extranodal) in only 5 to 10% of patients. Patients with AIDS and stage IE non–central nervous system lymphomas may benefit from radiation.[28, 29] Long-term lymphoma-free survival is possible but not common, and chemotherapy designed for AIDS-related lymphomas (see Chapter 101) should be considered as appropriate.

2. MALT extranodal lymphomas are generally localized and indolent. They may also spread to other mucosa-associated sites and may transform to a more aggressive grade.

3. Low-grade, localized, extranodal stage IE disease or *geographic* stage IIE (spread of disease limited to adjacent nodes only) may be cured with local therapy alone (radiation therapy or, occasionally, surgery). Benefits of the combined-modality approach are uncertain.

4. Combined-modality therapy (chemotherapy plus local therapy, e.g., CHOP [cyclophosphamide, doxorubicin (hydroxydaunomycin), vincristine (Oncovin), prednisone] followed by involved-field radiation[30, 31]) appears superior to local therapy for patients with early-stage extranodal disease characterized by unfavorable histology, site, or stage. Bulky disease or disease extending through the capsule or serosa of the primary organ site has a high local and distant recurrence rate with local therapy alone.

5. Mantle cell lymphoma, particularly the blastic variant, is more aggressive than low-grade lymphoma. The optimal regimen for early extranodal mantle cell disease is not defined, but a combined-modality approach is preferable to radiation therapy alone.

With these generalizations in mind, extranodal lymphomas are considered by site.

## Head and Neck Lymphomas

### WALDEYER'S RING LYMPHOMAS

Waldeyer's ring lymphomas account for roughly 50% of head and neck lymphomas and about 80% of aerodigestive lymphomas. The palatine tonsils account for about 50 to 70% of Waldeyer's ring primary tumors.[32–34] Waldeyer's ring disease tends to be of unfavorable histology (primarily large cell lymphoma) about 70 to 90% of the time but may be low-grade disease (e.g., follicular small cleaved or small lymphocytic) 10 to 30% of the time. T-lymphoblastic lymphomas may occur in the tonsil and carry a poor prognosis.[35] Approximately 50% of unfavorable-histology disease in the aerodigestive tract is stage III or IV at presentation; favorable-histology disease is usually stage III or IV at presentation.[32, 36] Waldeyer's ring involvement may be diagnosed in staging a patient who presents nodally. High cervical node presentation is a clue to potential Waldeyer's ring involvement.

Overall 5-year survival in stage I and II patients treated by irradiation approximates 40 to 50%, with survival in stage II disease similar to that in stage I in some series but inferior in others. Survival may be 75% in favorable-histology disease.[32–34, 37]

Results in patients with stage I and II intermediate-grade or high-grade lymphomas of Waldeyer's ring treated with the combined-modality approach (e.g., CHOP plus radiation) appear superior to results from radiation alone. Forty-one of 44 patients were reported to be disease free after such therapy in one series from Japan,[38] and 77% of stage II patients were reported as survivors (vs. 32% treated with radiation alone) in another series.[39] Similar data have been reported from Hong Kong.[40] A study from Mexico[41] randomized more than 300 patients with stage I Waldeyer's ring lymphomas to extended-field radiation alone, chemotherapy alone (CHOP or CHOP-like therapy), or radiation followed by chemotherapy. Best results were seen with combined-modality therapy. Survival at 5 years with combined-modality therapy was 90% (83% failure free) versus 58% (45% failure free) with chemotherapy and 56% (48% failure free) with radiation therapy. Roughly one third of relapses were in the gastrointestinal tract. Upper gastrointestinal series with small bowel follow-through may be a reasonable staging procedure, but yield is uncertain.

### SINUS LYMPHOMAS

Sinus lymphomas may have a particularly poor prognosis, perhaps related to bulk of disease and local extension. In the Stanford experience,[42] paranasal sinus lymphoma is usually of unfavorable histology, is often locally extensive, and has a propensity to spread to the meninges. Five-year survival in the Stanford series for paranasal sinus primary tumors (treated before 1985, primarily with irradiation) is approximately 20%. Poor prognosis for sinus lymphomas has been confirmed in some series[43] but not in others.[35, 44, 45] Failure after radiation treatment for aerodigestive lymphomas is usually in nonirradiated sites, including other extranodal sites (such as the gastrointestinal tract) and marginal sites.[32, 33] Lumbar puncture for sinus primary tumors may be a reasonable staging procedure. The yield in asymptomatic patients at presentation is unclear, however.[46]

Stanford[47] reported data in 16 patients with stage I or II paranasal sinus lymphomas treated more recently with combined-modality therapy (including central nervous system prophylaxis in 12). Five-year survival was only 29% with median survival 18 months. Canadian data[48] in 29 patients with a combined-modality therapy and central nervous system prophylaxis approach are a bit better, however, with 53% survival (68% disease-specific survival) at 5 and 10 years. Retrospective data from M.D. Anderson Cancer Center[49] also support a benefit for the combined-modality approach. In 70 patients with nasal cavity (14) or sinus (56) lymphoma, combined-modality therapy (with central nervous system prophylaxis) resulted in 5-year freedom from progression of 71% (87% stage $I_E$) versus 38% with radiation alone (59% $I_E$). A trend, not statistically significant, was seen for improved survival with combined-modality treatment (58% vs. 43% at 5 years).

## SALIVARY GLAND LYMPHOMAS

Lymphomas of the salivary glands are usually low-grade MALTomas,[50] although true nodular lymphomas with t(14;18) and *bcl-2* gene rearrangements have been reported.[51] Because some salivary gland lymphomas may be nodal lymphomas arising in a lymph node within the gland, this heterogeneity may be expected. High-grade and T-cell lymphomas have been reported but are uncommon.[52, 53] Salivary gland lymphomas may arise in the setting of sialadenitis or Sjögren's disease.[54] With limited disease, prognosis after radiation therapy for salivary gland lymphoma is good, with a 5-year survival of 50 to 90%.[32, 42, 55–57] These figures probably would not apply to high-grade salivary gland lymphomas, however.

## THYROID LYMPHOMAS

Thyroid lymphomas often occur in the setting of previous thyroiditis.[58–62] They may be low grade, either MALT[63, 64] or follicular center cell in origin,[65] or intermediate or high grade,[66] usually diffuse large cell. Thyroidectomy has been performed for this entity, but there may be no clear advantage over biopsy followed by nonsurgical therapy.[66, 67] Prognosis is a function of histology, stage, presence or absence of extracapsular disease, and age. In the most favorable groups, 5-year survival is 70% after radiation therapy alone. In the unfavorable-histology groups, 5-year survival may be 10 to 35%, although better results may be obtained with a combined-modality approach for intermediate-grade or high-grade tumors.[66, 68] Combined-modality treatment may be indicated in patients presenting with stridor, dysphagia, or vocal cord paralysis in addition to other poor prognostic factors mentioned earlier and has been advocated by some for most thyroid lymphomas.[69, 70] Thyroid lymphoma has been reviewed by Ansell and colleagues.[71]

## NASAL AND NASOPHARYNGEAL LYMPHOMAS

Lymphomas may present involving both sinus and nasal cavity, and the site of origin may be difficult to ascertain. It is apparent that nasal cavity lymphomas, most common in Asians, are likely to be of T-cell or NK-cell origin (CD2+, CD56+), are angiocentric, and are Epstein-Barr virus related.[72] Nasopharyngeal lymphomas may be a form of Waldeyer's ring presentation and are more likely to be B-cell than nasal lymphomas.[73] Nasal lymphomas in Westerners are more commonly B cell in origin. The T/NK variant is an aggressive disease, causing local necrosis of the nasal septum, nose, and palate. It may spread locally or distantly to skin and subcutaneous tissue and may metastasize to the gastrointestinal tract. It may spread in a leukemic fashion. The T/NK variant also frequently is associated with a hemophagocytic leukemia (similar to that which may be seen in large granular lymphocyte leukemia). Prognosis for patients with stage $I_E$ disease limited to the nasal cavity has been reported to be good (roughly 90% survival at 5 years with radiation therapy with or without chemotherapy). Prognosis is poorer with more extensive stage $I_E$ disease (57% survival at 5 years with combined-modality therapy) or stage $II_E$ disease (35% 5-year survival).[74] Similar results (66% 5-year survival stage I, 33% for II) have been reported from Hong Kong.[75] Comparable results have been reported from Japan.[76, 77]

## OCULAR ADNEXAL LYMPHOMAS

Ocular adnexal lymphomas occur most commonly in the orbit and less commonly in conjunctivae and eyelids. The lacrimal gland may also be a primary site. These tumors tend to be low grade, often MALToma,[78, 79] and indolent. They may be bilateral and may relapse in extraocular sites. With local therapy (excision plus radiation), long-term disease-free survival is common, even with bilateral disease. Low-dose radiation ($\leq$35 Gy) is effective and not associated strongly with the dry eye, retinitis, and neuritis seen at higher doses. In patients who relapse, the course is frequently indolent, although lymphoma-induced death may occur. Patients with polyclonal or reactive ocular adnexal lymphoid infiltrates often later develop lymphoma or act similarly to those with clear histologic evidence of lymphoma. These issues were studied in 1990 by Knowles and colleagues[80] and earlier by Kim and Fayos.[81] Comparable data have been reported elsewhere.[78, 79, 82, 83]

## OCULAR LYMPHOMAS

Ocular lymphomas (including those in the vitreous, retina, or choroid) are frequently manifestations of central nervous system (brain, spinal cord) lymphoma but may occur independently. Peterson and associates[84] have presented data and reviewed literature indicating that 20% of central nervous system lymphomas have ocular involvement and that 60 to 80% of patients with ocular lymphoma develop central nervous system involvement. With radiation therapy or chemotherapy, responses are common but temporary. The optimal treatment is not clear. Peterson and associates[84] recommended that therapy include radiation to both eyes. Whole-brain radiation and chemotherapy, fashioned after the treatment of brain lymphoma,[85] would seem reasonable treatment, but optimal therapy is uncertain.

# CENTRAL NERVOUS SYSTEM LYMPHOMAS

Primary lymphoma of the central nervous system (brain or spinal cord) occurs, as mentioned earlier, with increased frequency in patients with AIDS[86, 87] and in renal transplant patients.[88] Although brain parenchymal lymphoma may occur secondarily, this is unusual if the lymphoma initially presented nodally. A mass in the brain of such a patient may commonly be of different origin (e.g., infection). The histologic aspects of primary central nervous system lymphomas are protean, but these tumors are most often diffuse histiocytic lymphomas or diffuse, poorly differentiated lymphocytic lymphomas by Rappaport criteria[89–92] (large cell or diffuse small cleaved by Working Formulation criteria). Central nervous system lymphomas most commonly present in the cerebrum but may be in the brain stem, cerebellum, or spinal cord.[91] They are frequently multicentric and commonly associated with meningeal spread.[91, 92] Survival with surgery alone or with no therapy approximates 2 to 3 months.[90, 93] Radiation may prolong survival to a median of roughly 12 to 18 months in the noncompromised host,[89, 91–95] with local recurrence a substantial problem. The local recurrence rate may be higher than in irradiated lymphomas of other sites, raising the issue of possible biologic differences between central nervous system and other lymphomas. Spinal cord compression syndromes are more likely to be due to extradural lymphoma, extending from or independent of bone. This complication implies a poor prognosis and is an indication for combined-modality therapy to maximize and accelerate decompression.

Results in patients with AIDS may be poorer, with median survival less than 1 year.[96, 97] Lymphomas in the brain may respond to chemotherapy, including high-dose methotrexate with leucovorin rescue,[97–101] high-dose cytarabine,[101] or multiagent chemotherapy with[102] or without[103] osmotic disruption of the blood-brain barrier. The osmotic disruption approach is unwieldy but has been reported to achieve, without radiation therapy, a median survival of about 45 months with decreased late central nervous system toxicity from that seen in survivors who received high-dose radiation. That risk is substantial in patients 50 years of age and older.[103] A simpler approach has been reported,[104] using combined-modality therapy but limiting radiation to 40 Gy whole-brain radiation plus a 1440-cGy boost and delaying radiation therapy until after methotrexate (high-dose systemic with rescue plus intrathecal) administration. High-dose cytarabine is also used. This regimen has resulted in a 43-month median survival with a modest (10%) risk of late neurologic toxicity, although that figure may be higher in older patients and patients at risk for longer periods. In one small series (four patients) of AIDS-related central nervous system lymphomas, combined chemotherapy and radiation resulted in 11- to 16-month survival.[105] More recent series of combined-modality therapy have not been clearly superior to prior studies.[106–109] Maher and Fine[110] have reviewed central nervous system lymphoma.

## Abdominal Lymphomas

### GASTRIC LYMPHOMAS

Gastric lymphomas are commonly high grade, but low-grade and mixed-histology tumors are also seen.[111–113] Although earlier literature classifies these lymphomas as diffuse histiocytic or poorly differentiated lymphocytic lymphomas and identifies the cells of origin as B cells of follicular center cell origin,[114] these are currently thought to be predominantly MALTomas, with the high-grade lymphomas evolving from transformation of a low-grade component.[115] Isaacson and associates[116] have suggested a specialized classification scheme for gastrointestinal lymphomas, stressing the MALT origin of most such lymphomas. Follicular lymphomas of the stomach and other gastrointestinal sites are seen but are rare.[117] Gastric lymphomas of mantle cell origin are also seen, particularly in the setting of multiple lymphoproliferative polyposis of the gastrointestinal tract, in which case the lymphoma is usually multifocal through the gastrointestinal tract and often disseminated.[118, 119] Follicular lymphoma of the gastrointestinal tract may also present as multiple lymphomatous polyps.

Prognosis is largely a function of the size of the primary tumor and the local extent of disease as well as histology and patient age. In a mixed series of histologic types reported by Lim and associates,[111] the TNM system was a useful predictor of survival in patients treated with surgery, with or without radiation. Patients with stage IA or IB disease (focal gastric wall involvement and no serosal penetration, nodal spread, or metastases) had 75 to 90% long-term survival. Patients with diffuse involvement of the stomach wall, regional nodal involvement, or serosal involvement had roughly 35% long-term survival. Postoperative radiation decreased the recurrence rate in patients resected for cure in this series.

A large review of gastrointestinal lymphomas[120] (76 stomach, 15 small bowel, 13 large bowel) from Memorial Sloan-Kettering showed long-term survival to vary substantially with the size of the primary (80% at 5 to 10 years for <5 cm vs. 30% for >5 cm), stage (60 to 70% survival for stage I vs. 40% for stage II), involvement of adjacent tissue (70% survival without invasion vs. 30% with invasion), and histology (90% well-differentiated lymphocytic lymphoma vs. 20% diffuse histiocytic vs. 50% other). Separating stage II disease into stage IIIe (contiguous lymph nodes) or stage II2e (distant regional lymph nodes) is also predictive of long-term survival (60% vs. 18%). Gastric lymphoma is frequently advanced at presentation. The likelihood of this advanced presentation has varied among series.[120–122] Radiation therapy has the capacity of providing long-term disease-free survival in unresected cases of gastric lymphoma, with reported 5-year survival exceeding 50% for stages I and II disease.[43, 123–125] Data support the role of adjuvant radiation therapy in the treatment of resected gastric lymphoma,[111, 126] although not all studies show a benefit from such adjuvant treatment.[125, 127, 128] Results with adjuvant chemotherapy (CVP [cyclophosphamide, vincristine, prednisone], COPP [cyclophosphamide, Oncovin, procarbazine, prednisone], or CHOP) have yielded high disease-free survival rates for resected gastric and gastrointestinal lymphoma[114, 129–133] and suggest a role for such therapy, at least in poor-risk patients. In retrospective studies, patients with stage II or worse disease who were treated by resection and subsequent chemotherapy fared better than those given chemotherapy alone.[114] This difference may be largely due to complications of successful therapy (perforation, hemorrhage) when bulky transmural disease is present and rapidly lyses. In series in which such complications are uncommon, the role of surgery has been questioned. Surgery may be indicated for obstruction, perforation, hemorrhage, or an uncertain diagnosis, however.[134, 135] Gastrectomy results in a substantial obligatory morbidity (and some risk of mortality), and chemotherapy and radiation in this setting may be tolerated poorly. A patient regarded as at low risk of perforation reasonably may be treated with chemotherapy, with or without radiation.[134–136]

The previous data reflect experience in heterogeneous series, with many patients with adverse stage or histology. The low-stage, low-grade MALT lymphoma, however, is a distinct entity.[137] It is usually *H. pylori* positive, is indolent, and may be managed in a variety of manners. Treatment of the *H. pylori*–positive patient for the *H. pylori* infection may engender a durable complete response in 60 to 80% of T1 N0 tumors[138, 139] but is less effective in bulky tumors, diffusely infiltrative tumors, or regional lymph node–positive tumors. Endoscopic ultrasonography is useful to determine initial stage, and blind biopsies and ultrasonography are useful for following response to therapy. Relapse from complete response can occur. Low-dose radiation therapy (e.g., 30 Gy) has been found useful in patients with stage I or II low-grade gastric MALT lymphomas who are *H. pylori* negative or who fail to enter a complete remission with therapy to eradicate *H. pylori*.[140]

## SMALL BOWEL LYMPHOMAS

Small bowel lymphomas of the Western type are of B-cell origin approximately two thirds of the time, and the remainder are of T-cell origin.[141] T-cell small bowel lymphomas are associated with celiac disease and histologically resemble a histiocytic malignancy.[141, 142] B-cell lymphomas tend to be found in the distal small bowel and are roughly 60% high grade, 30% low grade, and 10% mixed; T-cell lymphomas tend to be proximal and about 80% high grade.[141] Small bowel lymphomas also may present as multiple lymphomatous polyposis, often of mantle cell origin.

Similar to gastric lymphoma, small bowel lymphoma may occur in the setting of advanced-stage disease.[43, 121, 122] In general, prognosis as a function of histology, stage, and treatment is not well defined (although T-cell lymphomas may have a poorer prognosis).[141] Small bowel lymphomas are generally treated in the same way as gastric lymphomas with similar results, stage for stage. Small bowel lymphomas, however, may be more advanced at presentation, with a subsequently poorer prognosis overall. Two- to 5-year survival for limited disease appears to be about 40 to 50%.[43, 127] In patients with advanced disease, the value of surgical debulking is an uncertain but relevant issue, the goal of that procedure being to prevent local complications, including perforation or bleeding as a consequence of therapy-induced tumor lysis.[121, 122]

Mediterranean small bowel lymphomas may evolve from an immunoproliferative small intestinal disease (IPSID). IPSID is manifested by diarrhea, malabsorption, clubbing, and plasma cell infiltration of the small bowel. It has been seen frequently in the Middle East, the Mediterranean region, and Africa. IPSID commonly is associated with the presence of monoclonal alpha chains in the serum. The cause may be related to parasitic or other infections as well as racial and genetic factors.[143] The resultant lymphomas are varied in histologic type and include immunoblastic sarcomas, presumably of B-cell origin; diffuse undifferentiated lymphomas; small lymphocytic plasmacytoid lymphomas; and others.[144] In some[145] but not all cases,[146] the lymphomatous cells have been shown to have the immunologic characteristics of the plasma cells producing alpha chains. Presumably, Mediterranean lymphoma generally occurs as a clonal lymphomatous evolution of lymphoplasmacytic intestinal infiltration. Not all cases of Mediterranean lymphoma are characterized by alpha-chain production, however, and this phenomenon is absent in the Western type of intestinal lymphoma.[147]

In Mediterranean small bowel lymphomas, the involvement of mesenteric nodes is common. Peripheral node involvement occurs occasionally, and liver and spleen involvement occur rarely.[147, 148] Total abdominal irradiation appears to be capable of inducing frequent complete responses and disease-free survival beyond 1 year in this disease, and combination chemotherapy may also be effective.[149–151] These data are preliminary, however, and less favorable results have been noted, with typical survival of less than 1 year.[149] In Mediterranean or enteropathy-associated small bowel lymphomas, diarrhea or malabsorption may mask symptoms of lymphoma, with resultant advanced local disease at diagnosis, often with perforation and abscess formation.

Optimal therapy for small bowel lymphoma is not well defined. It is probably reasonable to treat low-grade, early-stage lymphomas locally (resection with or without radiation) and to use chemotherapy alone or the combined-modality approach for high-grade, mantle cell, or extensive lesions.

## LARGE BOWEL AND ANORECTAL LYMPHOMAS

Lymphomas of the colon and rectum constitute 10% of gastrointestinal lymphomas, and approximately half of these are rectal.[152–154] Overall long-term survival tends to be around 50% for early-stage disease treated surgically, with or without radiation therapy.[153, 155–157] Disease that mimics polyposis on presentation tends to be low grade, with a better prognosis than a large ulcerating or obstructing lesion, which tends to be high grade. Treatment as for small bowel lymphomas seems reasonable.

Anorectal lymphomas tend to be of varied histology but are primarily B cell in origin.[154] This entity now apparently is increasing in frequency as a complication of AIDS.[158] Treatment with radiation therapy (plus chemotherapy if high grade) seems reasonable.

## HEPATIC LYMPHOMAS

Hepatic primary lymphomas are rare. They may be associated with immunosuppression,[159] hepatitis C,[160, 161] and primary biliary cirrhosis.[162, 163] They generally present as a solitary hepatic mass, but there may be multiple masses. Histologically, they are typically large cell or diffuse histiocytic. They may be of B-cell or T-cell origin.[158, 164, 165] The T-cell type may include the *hepatosplenic T gamma/delta lymphoma,*[166] a disorder perhaps related to large granular lymphocyte leukemia or nasal T-cell or NK-cell lymphoma. It is an aggressive disease, with survival often less than 1 year. It may present with cytopenias and *B symptoms* as well as hepatosplenomegaly and has been characterized by chromosomal abnormalities, including isochrome 7q and trisomy 8.[167–170] For intermediate-grade or high-grade hepatic lymphomas, combination chemotherapy, with or without surgical resection, may result in prolonged disease-free survival in most patients.[171, 172] Low-grade hepatic lymphomas have been reported as well. They may be MALTomas,[173, 174] which may be more indolent and treated more conservatively.

## SPLENIC LYMPHOMAS

It is debatable whether primary splenic lymphomas should be considered extranodal or nodal and whether lymphoma limited to the spleen and regional nodes should be considered primary to the spleen or not. Lymphomas limited to the spleen have been infrequently reported, and the marginal zone variant is likely truly extranodal. The pattern of regional spread may be geographic (e.g., limited to splenic hilar nodes), and long-term disease-free survival after splenectomy alone has been reported.[175] The histologic appearance of splenic lymphomas is variable. In 46 patients identified at M.D. Anderson Cancer Center,[176] the most common types were diffuse small lymphocytic (20 cases) and diffuse large cell (11 cases), with other types also seen. It is likely that many cases of splenic diffuse small lymphocytic lymphoma are early presentations of chronic lymphocytic leukemia. Many of the cases reported with that histology were bone marrow positive, and CD5$^+$ B-cell lymphomas may so present.[177] Other lymphoid malignancies presenting with dominant spleen and bone marrow and blood involvement include hairy cell leukemia and a similar but distinct disease, splenic lymphoma with circulating villous lymphocytes.[178–180] The splenic lymphoma with circulating villous lymphocytes is likely on a continuum with splenic marginal zone lymphoma (which lacks an overt leukemic phase). This disease resembles chronic lymphocytic leukemia and hairy cell leukemia. It is often controlled by splenectomy. If more treatment is needed, fludarabine appears useful.[180, 181] When no leukemic phase is present, this disease at times resembles a splenic mantle cell lymphoma.[180] Large cell lymphoma of the spleen also occurs and is frequently stage II by virtue of involvement of splenic hilar or retroperitoneal nodes.[176–179, 182] Older data suggest that patients who have undergone splenectomy fare better than those who have not undergone splenectomy and that 5-year survival for splenic lymphomas (all histologic types) approximates 30% with splenectomy plus radiation or alkylating agent chemotherapy, or both.[183]

## RENAL LYMPHOMAS

Renal involvement with disseminated lymphoma is common and may occasionally lead to renal failure[184]; primary renal lymphoma has also been reported[185, 186] and in one study composed 3% of renal masses.[187] In the Mayo Clinic experience with roughly 6400 patients with lymphoma, 176 had renal involvement, and 5 had primary renal lymphoma.[188]

This disease rapidly disseminates, often to other extranodal sites, and has a poor prognosis, although long-term disease-free survival can occur. Renal lymphoma is commonly of high-grade or diffuse histiocytic histology and should probably be treated with nephrectomy (when unilateral) followed by combination chemotherapy or with combination chemotherapy followed by radiation (again when unilateral). Renal dysfunction in this setting may require adjustments in choice of chemotherapy and dosages. If renal failure is present, nitrogen mustard can be substituted for cyclophosphamide to avoid problems with renal clearance of the alkylating agent.

## Chest Lymphomas

### PULMONARY LYMPHOMAS

Primary lymphomas of the lung may vary in histologic type, but 70 to 90% are low grade, generally with pathologic features and behavior consistent with MALTomas.[189–191] They may at times be categorized erroneously as pseudolymphomas or lymphoid interstitial pneumonia.[192–195] Pulmonary lymphomas may also be part of the angiocentric T-cell lymphoproliferative disorder spectrum, classified as lymphomatoid granulomatosis. Epstein-Barr virus has been related to these lymphomas.[196] In general, pulmonary lymphomas carry a good prognosis. Anatomically, they may be lymphangitic, parenchymal, or endobronchial in location.[197, 198] A few MALTomas of the lung may arise in the setting of autoimmune interstitial lung disease.[199] In cases of lymphocytic histology without nodal involvement, surgery alone may be sufficient therapy. Radiation may play some role for stage IIE disease or intermediate-grade or high-grade tumors. Overall 5-year survival ranges from 40 to 80%.[186] Early stage and lymphocytic histology are favorable prognostic factors, with greater than 90% 5-year survival in low-grade tumors in one series.[190]

In a large series (161 cases) of patients reported from the Armed Forces Institute of Pathology,[200] overall recurrence rate (varied histologies) was roughly 50% at 5 years, with 10-year survival of 75%. Of 65 patients with localized disease treated with surgical excision alone, 15 had relapsed (6 of these died), 38 were reported alive and well, and 12 died of unrelated causes. Thirty-one patients with more extensive disease (generally multicentric or with pleural effusion) received radiation or chemotherapy, or both. Eight of these patients were reported alive and well (7 of 17 who had complete excision of tumor vs. 1 of 14 who had biopsy only). Systemic symptoms and pleural effusion were predictive of poor prognosis. Primary pulmonary lymphoma has been reviewed by Habermann and coworkers.[201]

### MEDIASTINAL AND THYMIC LYMPHOMAS

Although lymphoma in the anterior mediastinum may be nodal in some circumstances, when localized, it tends to be diffuse large cell lymphoma of thymic B-cell origin.[202–205] This disease entity differs from the usual B-cell large cell lymphoma in that it is seen predominantly in young women, commonly characterized by sclerosis histologically, and, although CD20+, tends to be CD21– and surface immunoglobulin negative. It is CD5– and often is CD30+.[205–207] The disease acts similarly to other B-cell large cell lymphomas, with increasing bulk a poor prognostic factor. Mediastinal lymphoma appears to be best treated with a combined-modality approach.[207-211] Anterior mediastinal lymphoma may also be lymphoblastic histologically, but this tends to be disseminated at presentation. MALTomas are sometimes seen.[204, 212]

## CARDIAC LYMPHOMAS

Although cardiac involvement is not a rare consequence of advanced disseminated lymphoma,[213] primary cardiac lymphoma has been a rare disease.[214] Cardiac involvement with lymphomas appears to be increasing in the setting of AIDS as well as in immunocompetent patients. Cardiac lymphoma frequently presents with heart failure[215] and may present with heart block.[216, 217] Pericardial effusion is common.[213] Transesophageal echocardiography, magnetic resonance imaging, and pericardiocentesis (if effusion is present) are useful diagnostic tools.[215] Gill and associates[218] reported nine patients who presented with cardiac lymphoma from 1977 to 1985. Four of these cases were AIDS related. Histologic features were all of high or intermediate grade: small noncleaved (four), immunoblastic sarcoma (one), and diffuse large cell (four). Seven of these patients had disseminated disease, and in these cases the cardiac involvement may or may not have been primary. Despite aggressive combination chemotherapy, median survival was 1.5 months, and maximal reported survival was 6 months. Diagnosis is often late because disease may not be recognized until heart failure ensues. It is possible to have longer survival (e.g., ≥8 months) in patients diagnosed early and given combination chemotherapy, however.[219]

## BREAST LYMPHOMAS

Primary lymphomas of the breast are generally intermediate-grade or high-grade B-cell lymphomas,[220–223] but there may be other types, including low-grade MALTomas.[223,224] In a review of breast lymphomas, Brogi and Harris[225] tabulated 209 cases from 12 reported series and found 71% of the reported cases to be high grade and 29% to be low grade. Mastectomy is not generally necessary for local control; excision or irradiation, or both, may suffice. Chemotherapy may be appropriate for high-grade or intermediate-grade lymphomas. With varied therapies for varied histologies and stages, median survival of 4 to 6 years has been reported.[220, 226] Giardini and colleagues,[227] in a series of 35 Italian women with breast lymphoma, reported overall survival at 5 years to be 43%, with 61% survival and 50% disease-free survival for stage I disease.

## Other Extranodal Lymphomas

### LYMPHOMA OF BONE

As in other extranodal lymphomas, diverse histologic types are seen.[228, 229] Ostrowski and associates[229] reported the 75-

year experience with bone lymphoma at the Mayo Clinic. Over that period, 422 patients were seen, of whom 42% presented with disease limited to unifocal bone involvement and 19% with disease limited to multifocal involvement. The other 39% had or proximately developed soft tissue or nodal involvement; this broke down to 13% with such involvement 6 months or more after presentation and 26% after an interval of less than 6 months. Histologies were diverse, with diffuse mixed (28%) and diffuse large cell (30%) the most common. With variable treatment (>75 years), survival was best in the unifocal bone group (58% at 5 years, 53% at 10 years) and intermediate in the multiple bone group (42% at 5 years, 35% at 10 years). The nodal and soft tissue group fared the poorest (22% at 5 years, 12.5% at 10 years). Bacci and coworkers[230, 231] reported a series of 30 patients; 4 received radiation alone, and 26 received radiation plus chemotherapy. With a 3-year median follow-up, only 1 of 4 patients treated with radiation and 3 of 26 patients given combined-modality therapy had experienced relapse. Baar and coworkers,[232] in their review of lymphoma of bone, updated their earlier data.[233] They report on 28 patients (64% stage IE) treated primarily (75%) with combined-modality therapy. Overall response rate was 86% (29% complete response), and overall survival was 79%. Eighteen of 21 patients treated with combined-modality therapy remain relapse free. These data and data reported elsewhere[234–236] suggest a role for chemotherapy in this disease, compared with the Mayo Clinic data[229] (most patients not treated primarily with chemotherapy) and other data reporting 40 to 60% survival at 5 years after radiation therapy for stage IE disease.[237, 238] The combined-modality approach was reported by Barbieri[239] to be less successful, and data from M.D. Anderson Cancer Center show no clear difference in results between radiation alone and combined-modality therapy, however.[240] Osteoradionecrosis and pathologic fracture may occur when doses of 5000 cGy are added to chemotherapy.

### TESTICULAR LYMPHOMA

Testicular lymphoma has been reviewed by Shahab and Doll[241] (and previously by Doll and Weiss[242]). Shahab and Doll[241] tabulated stage at presentation in 317 patients from 13 series and found roughly 50% to be stage I and 24% to be stage IV. Histology is usually intermediate grade or high grade (B cell) and diffuse in pattern. For localized disease treated with radiation, they found in 14 series relapse rates of 50 to 100%, with a median figure of close to 70%. Surgery alone has also been shown to have a high failure rate.[242] With chemotherapy (with or without radiation) for early-stage disease, results were also poor, with (in 11 series reviewed) a pooled relapse rate of 40 to 50% and typical median survival of 1 to 3 years. Median survival for advanced disease generally has been a few months with rare long-term survival. Spread to central nervous system, contralateral testis, skin, Waldeyer's ring, and lung is common. Aggressive treatment seems warranted.

### OTHER SITES

Primary extranodal lymphomas may occur in many other sites. Literature regarding extranodal lymphomas of these sites largely consists of case reports and small series. References are available for ovarian (non-Burkitt's) lymphoma,[243–246] uterine and cervical lymphoma,[247, 248] vulvar lymphoma,[249] vaginal lymphoma,[250, 251] prostatic lymphoma,[252, 253] urethral lymphoma,[254–256] bladder lymphoma,[257, 258] adrenal lymphoma,[259] pancreatic lymphoma,[260–264] and lymphoma primary to muscle.[265–266]

## Summary

Patients younger than 60 years old with stage $I_E$ or geographic $II_E$ extranodal lymphoma of low grade, small bulk, and favorable site may fare well ($\geq 75\%$ long-term survival) with radiation therapy alone, particularly those with lymphoma of MALT origin. Extranodal lymphomas of orbit, lung, salivary gland, and breast commonly present in this fashion. Bulky or high-grade disease or disease in a high-risk site may be an indication for the combined-modality approach. Extranodal lymphomas of gonad, sinus, small bowel, and nasal tract commonly present in this fashion. Mantle cell extranodal lymphoma may require aggressive therapy. Lymphomas of the central nervous system and ocular lymphomas require specialized, usually combined-modality, therapy.

### SUGGESTIONS FOR ADDITIONAL READING

Newton R, Ferlay J, Beral V, Devesa SS. The epidemiology of non-Hodgkin's lymphoma: comparison of nodal and extra-nodal sites. Int J Cancer 1997;72:923–30.

Economopoulos T, Asprou N, Stathakis N, et al. Primary extranodal non-Hodgkin's lymphoma in adults: clinicopathological and survival characteristics. Leuk Lymphoma 1996;21:131–6.

### REFERENCES

1. Rosenberg SA, Diamond HD, Jaslowitz B, Craver LF. Lymphosarcoma: a review of 1269 cases. Medicine 1961;40:31–84.
2. Freeman C, Berg JW, Cutler SJ. Occurrence and prognosis of extranodal lymphomas. Cancer 1972;29:252–60.
3. Rosen PJ, Feinstein DI, Pattengale PK, et al. Convoluted lymphocytic lymphoma in adults: a clinicopathologic entity. Ann Intern Med 1978;89:319–24.
4. d'Amore F, Christensen BE, Brincker H, et al. Clinicopathological features and prognostic factors in extranodal non-Hodgkin lymphomas. Danish LYFO Study Group. Eur J Cancer 1991;27:1201–8.
5. Otter R, Gerrits WB, v d Sandt MM, et al. Primary extranodal and nodal non-Hodgkin's lymphoma: a survey of a population-based registry. Eur J Cancer 1989;25:1203–10.
6. Levine AM. Epidemiology, clinical characteristics, and management of AIDS-related lymphoma. Hematol Oncol Clin North Am 1991;5:331–42.
7. Knowles DM, Chamulak GA, Subar M, et al. Lymphoid neoplasia associated with the acquired immunodeficiency syndrome (AIDS). Ann Intern Med 1988;108:744–53.
8. Kaplan LD. Clinical management of human immunodeficiency virus–associated non-Hodgkin's lymphoma. J Natl Cancer Inst Monograph 1998;23:101–105.
9. Paryani S, Hoppe RT, Burke JS, et al. Extralymphatic involvement in diffuse non-Hodgkin's lymphoma. J Clin Oncol 1983;1:682–8.
10. Gospodarowicz MK, Sutcliffe SB, Brown TC, et al. Patterns of disease in localized extranodal lymphomas. J Clin Oncol 1987;5:875–80.
11. d'Amore F, Christensen BE, Brincker H, et al. Clinicopathological features and prognostic factors in extranodal non-Hodgkin lymphomas. Danish LYFO Study Group. Eur J Cancer 1991;27:1201–8.
12. Isaacson PG, Spencer J. Malignant lymphoma of mucosa-associated lymphoid tissue. Histopathology 1987;11:445–62.
13. Wotherspoon AC, Ortiz-Hidalgo C, Falzon MR, Isaacson PG. Helicobacter pylori-associated gastritis and primary B-cell gastric lymphoma. Lancet 1991;338:1175–6.
14. Isaacson PG. Extranodal lymphomas: the MALT concept. Verh Dtsch Ges Pathol 1992;76:14–23.
15. Isaacson PG. Mucosa-associated lymphoid tissue lymphoma. Semin Hematol 1999;36:139–47.
16. Isaacson PG, Wotherspoon AC, Diss T, Pan LX. Follicular colonization in B-cell lymphoma of mucosa-associated lymphoid tissue. Am J Surg Pathol 1991;15:819–28.
17. Pan L, Diss TC, Cunningham D, Isaacson PG. The bcl-2 gene in primary B lymphoma of mucosa-associated lymphoid tissue (MALT). Am J Pathol 1989;135:7–11.
18. Clark HM, Jones DB, Wright DH. Cytogenetic and molecular studies of t(14;18) and t(14;19) in nodal and extranodal B-cell lymphoma. J Pathol 1992;166:129–37.
19. Isaacson PG, Androulakis-Papachristou A, Diss TC, et al. Follicular colonization in thyroid lymphoma. Am J Pathol 1992;141:43–52.
20. Diss TC, Peng H, Wotherspoon AC, et al. Brief report: a single neoplastic clone in sequential biopsy specimens from a patient with primary gastric-mucosa-associated lymphoid-tissue lymphoma and Sjögren's syndrome. N Engl J Med 1993;329:172–5.
21. Campo E, Raffeld M, Jaffe ES. Mantle-cell lymphoma. Semin Hematol 1999;36:115–27.
22. Frizzera G, Wu CD, Inghirami G. The usefulness of immunophenotypic and genotypic studies in the diagnosis and classification of hematopoietic and lymphoid neoplasms: an update. Am J Clin Pathol 1999;111:Suppl 1:S13–39.
23. Levine AM. Epidemiology, clinical characteristics, and management of AIDS-related lymphoma. Hematol Oncol Clin North Am 1991;5:331–42.
24. Davi F, Delecluse HJ, Guiet P, et al. Burkitt-like lymphomas in AIDS patients: characterization within a series of 103 human immunodeficiency virus-associated non-Hodgkin's lymphomas. Burkitt's Lymphoma Study Group. J Clin Oncol 1998;16:3788–95.
25. Ye YL, Zhou MH, Lu XY, et al. Nasopharyngeal and nasal malignant lymphoma: a clinicopathological study of 54 cases. Histopathology 1992;20:511–6.
26. Ferry JA, Sklar J, Zukerberg LR, Harris NL. Nasal lymphoma: a clinicopathologic study with immunophenotypic and genotypic analysis. Am J Surg Pathol 1991;15:268–79.
27. Shimamoto Y, Yamaguchi M. HTLV-I induced extranodal lymphomas. Leuk Lymphoma 1992;7:37–45.
28. DeWeese TL, Hazuka MB, Hommel DJ, et al. AIDS-related non-Hodgkin's lymphoma: the outcome and efficacy of radiation therapy. Int J Radiat Oncol Biol Phys 1991;20:803–8.
29. Goldstein J, Woods W, Valentine E, Davis E. Radiation therapy (RT) in acquired immunodeficiency syndrome (AIDS) related systemic non-Hodgkins lymphoma (NHL): a retrospective analysis. Proc ASCO 1990;9:A13.
30. Connors JM, Klimo P, Fairey RN, Voss N. Brief chemotherapy and involved field radiation therapy for limited-stage, histologically aggressive lymphoma. Ann Intern Med 1987;107:25–30.
31. Tondini C, Zanini M, Lombardi F, et al. Combined modality treatment with primary CHOP chemotherapy followed by locoregional irradiation in stage I or II histologically aggressive non-Hodgkin's lymphoma. J Clin Oncol 1993;11:720–5.
32. Jacobs C, Hoppe RT. Non-Hodgkin's lymphomas (NHL) of the head and neck. Proc ASCO 1983;2:221.
33. Brugére J, Dumont J, Jaulerry C, Schwaab G. Invasion of the upper respiratory and digestive tract in adult lymphoid neoplasias. Recent Results Cancer Res 1978;65:58–62.
34. Brugére J, Schlienger M, Gérard-Marchant R, et al. Non-Hodgkin's malignant lymphomata of upper digestive and respiratory tract: natural history and results of radiotherapy. Br J Cancer 1975;31:Suppl II:435–40.
35. Shima N, Kobashi Y, Tsutsui K, et al. Extranodal non-Hodgkin's lymphoma of the head and neck: a clinicopathologic study in the Kyoto-Nara area of Japan. Cancer 1990;66:1190–7.
36. Bonadonna G, Castellani R, Narduzzi C, et al. Pathological staging in adult previously untreated non-Hodgkin's lymphomas. Recent Results Cancer Res 1978;65:41–50.

37. Kim YH, Fayos JV, Schnitzer B. Extranodal head and neck lymphomas: result of radiation therapy. Int J Radiat Oncol Biol Phys 1978;4:789–94.
38. Uematsu M. [Limited chemotherapy and radiotherapy for stage I–II intermediate or high grade lymphoma of nodal sites or Waldeyer's ring.] Nippon Igaku Hoshasen Gakkai Zasshi 1991;51:962–9.
39. Hiramatsu H, Kondo M, Shigematsu N, et al. Improved survival of non-Hodgkin's lymphoma of the Waldeyer's ring. Proc ASCO 1989;8:268.
40. Liang R, Ng RP, Todd D, et al. Management of stage I–II diffuse aggressive non-Hodgkin's lymphoma of the Waldeyer's ring: combined modality therapy versus radiotherapy alone. Hematol Oncol 1987;5:223–30.
41. Aviles A, Delgado S, Ruiz H, et al. Treatment of non-Hodgkin's lymphoma of Waldeyer's ring: radiotherapy versus chemotherapy versus combined therapy. Eur J Cancer B Oral Oncol 1996;32B:19–23.
42. Jacobs C, Hoppe RT. Non-Hodgkin's lymphomas of head and neck extranodal sites. Int J Radiat Oncol Biol Phys 1985;11:357–64.
43. Van der Werf-Messing B. Radiotherapy of extranodal non-Hodgkin's lymphoma. Recent Results Cancer Res 1978;65:111–28.
44. Sofferman RA, Cummings CW. Malignant lymphoma of the paranasal sinuses. Arch Otolaryngol 1975;101:287–92.
45. Shibuya H, Kamiyama R, Watanabe I, et al. Stage I and II Waldeyer's ring and oral-sinonasal non-Hodgkin's lymphoma. Cancer 1987;59:940–4.
46. Cooper DL, Ginsberg SS. Brief chemotherapy, involved field radiation therapy, and central nervous system prophylaxis for paranasal sinus lymphoma. Cancer 1992;69:2888–93.
47. Hausdorff J, Davis E, Long G, et al. Non-Hodgkin's lymphoma of the paranasal sinuses: clinical and pathological features, and response to combined-modality therapy. Cancer J Sci Am 1997;3:303–11.
48. Connors JM. Problems in lymphoma management: special sites of presentation. Oncology 1998;12:185–91.
49. Logsdon M, Ha CS, Kavadi VS. Lymphoma of the nasal cavity and paranasal sinuses: improved outcome and altered prognostic factors with combined modality therapy. Cancer 1997;80:477–88.
50. Takahashi H, Cheng J, Fujita S, et al. Primary malignant lymphoma of the salivary gland: a tumor of mucosa-associated lymphoid tissue. J Oral Pathol Med 1992;21:318–25.
51. Kerrigan DP, Irons J, Chen IM. bcl-2 gene rearrangement in salivary gland lymphoma. Am J Surg Pathol 1990;14:1133–8.
52. James M, Norton AJ. Primary T-cell lymphoma of salivary gland. J Pathol 1992;167:Suppl:122A.
53. Takahashi H, Tsuda N, Tezuka F, et al. Non-Hodgkin's lymphoma of the major salivary gland: a morphologic and immunohistochemical study of 15 cases. J Oral Pathol Med 1990;19:306–12.
54. Harris NL. Lymphoid proliferations of the salivary glands. Am J Clin Pathol 1999;111:Suppl 1:S94–S103.
55. Nime FA, Cooper HS, Eggleston JC. Primary malignant lymphomas of the salivary glands. Cancer 1976;37:906–12.
56. Gleeson MJ, Bennett MH, Cawson RA. Lymphomas of salivary glands. Cancer 1986;58:699–704.
57. Avilés A, Delgado S, Huerta-Guzmán J. Marginal zone B cell lymphoma of the parotid glands: results of a randomised trial comparing radiotherapy to combined therapy. Eur J Cancer B Oral Oncol 1996;32B:420–2.
58. Aozasa K, Inoue A, Tajima K, et al. Malignant lymphomas of the thyroid gland: analysis of 79 patients with emphasis on histologic prognostic factors. Cancer 1986;58:100–4.
59. Aozasa K, Ueda T, Katagiri S, et al. Immunologic and immunohistologic analysis of 27 cases with thyroid lymphomas. Cancer 1987;60:969–73.
60. Aozasa K, Tajima K, Tominaga N, et al. Immunologic and immunohistochemical studies on chronic lymphocytic thyroiditis with or without thyroid lymphoma. Oncology 1991;48:65–71.
61. Scholefield JH, Quayle AR, Harris SC, Talbot CH. Primary lymphoma of the thyroid, the association with Hashimoto's thyroiditis. Eur J Surg Oncol 1992;18:89–92.
62. Pedersen RK, Pedersen NT. Primary non-Hodgkin's lymphoma of the thyroid gland: a population based study. Histopathology 1996;28:25–32.
63. Fellbaum C, Sträter J, Hansmann ML, Fischer R. [Follicular dendritic cells in extranodal non-Hodgkin's lymphomas.] Verh Dtsch Ges Pathol 1992;76:213–8.
64. Laing RW, Hoskin P, Hudson BV, et al. The significance of MALT histology in thyroid lymphoma: a review of patients from the BNLI and Royal Marsden Hospital. Clin Oncol (R Coll Radiol) 1994;6:300–4.
65. Logue JP, Hale RJ, Stewart AL, et al. Primary malignant lymphoma of the thyroid: a clinicopathological analysis. Int J Radiat Oncol Biol Phys 1992;22:929–33.
66. Skarsgard ED, Connors JM, Robins RE. A current analysis of primary lymphoma of the thyroid. Arch Surg 1991;126:1199–203.
67. Pyke CM, Grant CS, Habermann TM, et al. Non-Hodgkin's lymphoma of the thyroid: is more than biopsy necessary? World J Surg 1992;16:604–9.
68. Pledge S, Bessell EM, Leach IH, et al. Non-Hodgkin's lymphoma of the thyroid: a retrospective review of all patients diagnosed in Nottinghamshire from 1973 to 1992. Clin Oncol (R Coll Radiol) 1996;8:371–5.
69. Doria R, Jekel JF, Cooper DL. Thyroid lymphoma: the case for combined modality therapy. Cancer 1994;73:200–6.
70. Tsang RW, Gospodarowicz MK, Sutcliffe SB, et al. Non-Hodgkin's lymphoma of the thyroid gland: prognostic factors and treatment outcome. The Princess Margaret Hospital Lymphoma Group. Int J Radiat Oncol Biol Phys 1993;27:599–604.
71. Ansell SM, Grant CS, Habermann TM. Primary thyroid lymphoma. Semin Oncol 1999;26:316–23.
72. Jaffe ES, Chan JK, Su IJ, et al. Report of the workshop on nasal and related extranodal angiocentric T/natural killer cell lymphomas: definitions, differential diagnosis, and epidemiology. Am J Surg Pathol 1996;20:103–11.
73. Ye YL, Zhou MH, Lu XY, et al. Nasopharyngeal and nasal malignant lymphoma: a clinicopathological study of 54 cases. Histopathology 1992;20:511–6.
74. Li YX, Coucke PA, Li JY, et al. Primary non-Hodgkin's lymphoma of the nasal cavity: prognostic significance of paranasal extension and the role of radiotherapy and chemotherapy. Cancer 1998;83:449–56.
75. Liang R, Todd D, Chan TK, et al. Treatment outcome and prognostic factors for primary nasal lymphoma. J Clin Oncol 1995;13:666–70.
76. Shikama N, Izuno I, Oguchi M, et al. Clinical stage IE primary lymphoma of the nasal cavity: radiation therapy and chemotherapy. Radiology 1997;204:467–70.
77. Nakamura S, Katoh E, Koshikawa T, et al. Clinicopathologic study of nasal T/NK-cell lymphoma among the Japanese. Pathol Int 1997;47:38–53.
78. White WL, Ferry JA, Harris NL, Grove AS Jr. Ocular adnexal lymphoma: a clinicopathologic study with identification of lymphomas of mucosa-associated lymphoid tissue type. Ophthalmology 1995;102:1994–2006.
79. Baldini L, Blini M, Guffanti A, et al. Treatment and prognosis in a series of primary extranodal lymphomas of the ocular adnexa. Ann Oncol 1998;9:779–81.
80. Knowles DM, Jakobiec FA, McNally L, Burke JS. Lymphoid hyperplasia and malignant lymphoma occurring in the ocular adnexa (orbit, conjunctiva, and eyelids): a prospective multiparametric analysis of 108 cases during 1977 to 1987. Hum Pathol 1990;21:959–73.
81. Kim YH, Fayos JV. Primary orbital lymphoma: a radiotherapeutic experience. Int J Radiat Oncol Biol Phys 1976;1:1099–105.
82. Galieni P, Polito E, Leccisotti A, et al. Localized orbital lymphoma. Haematologica 1997;82:436–9.
83. Chao CK, Lin HS, Deviveni VR, Smith M. Radiation therapy for primary orbital lymphoma. Int J Radiat Oncol Biol Phys 1995;31:929–34.
84. Peterson K, Gordon KB, Heinemann MH, DeAngelis LM. The clinical spectrum of ocular lymphoma. Cancer 1993;72:843–9.
85. Valluri S, Moorthy RS, Khan A, Rao NA. Combination treatment of intraocular lymphoma. Retina 1995;15:125–9.
86. Payan MJ, Gambarelli D, Routy JP, et al. Primary lymphoma of the brain associated with AIDS: a study of one case. Acta Neuropathol 1984;64:78–80.
87. Loureiro C, Gill PS, Meyer PR, et al. Autopsy findings in AIDS-related lymphoma. Cancer 1988;62:735–9.
88. Schneck SA, Penn I. De-novo brain tumours in renal-transplant recipients. Lancet 1971;1:983–6.
89. Henry JM, Heffner RR Jr, Dillard SH, et al. Primary malignant lymphomas of the central nervous system. Cancer 1974;34:1293–302.
90. Taylor CR, Russell R, Lukes RJ, Davis RL. An immunohistological study of immunoglobulin content of primary central nervous system lymphomas. Cancer 1978;41:2197–205.

91. Bonnín JM, Garcia JH. Primary malignant non-Hodgkin's lymphoma of the central nervous system. Pathol Annu 1987;22:353–75.

92. Gonzalez DG, Schuster-Uitterhoeve AL. Primary non-Hodgkin's lymphoma of the central nervous system: results of radiotherapy in 15 cases. Cancer 1983;51:2048–52.

93. Freeman CR, Shustik C, Brisson ML, et al. Primary malignant lymphoma of the central nervous system. Cancer 1986;58:1106–11.

94. Nelson DF, Martz KL, Bonner H, et al. Non-Hodgkin's lymphoma of the brain: can high dose, large volume radiation therapy improve survival? Report on a prospective trial by the Radiation Therapy Oncology Group (RTOG): RTOG 8315. Int J Radiat Oncol Biol Phys 1992;23:9–17.

95. Laperriere NJ, Cerezo L, Milosevic MF, et al. Primary lymphoma of brain: results of management of a modern cohort with radiation therapy. Radiother Oncol 1997;43:247–52.

96. Formenti SC, Gill PS, Lean E, et al. Primary central nervous system lymphoma in AIDS: results of radiation therapy. Cancer 1989;63:1101–7.

97. Jacomet C, Girard PM, Lebrette MG, et al. Intravenous methotrexate for primary central nervous system non-Hodgkin's lymphoma in AIDS. AIDS 1997;11:1725–30.

98. Ervin T, Canellos GP. Successful treatment of recurrent primary central nervous system lymphoma with high-dose methotrexate. Cancer 1980;45:1556–7.

99. Skarin AT, Zuckerman KS, Pitman SW, et al. High-dose methotrexate with folinic acid in the treatment of advanced non-Hodgkin lymphoma including CNS involvement. Blood 1977;50:1039–47.

100. Gabbai AA, Hochberg FH, Linggood RM, et al. High-dose methotrexate for non-AIDS primary central nervous system lymphoma: report of 13 cases. J Neurosurg 1989;70:190–4.

101. Hochberg FH, Loeffler JS, Prados M. The therapy of primary brain lymphoma. J Neurooncol 1991;10:191–201.

102. Neuwelt EA, Goldman DL, Dahlborg SA, et al. Primary CNS lymphoma treated with osmotic blood-brain barrier disruption: prolonged survival and preservation of cognitive function. J Clin Oncol 1991;9:1580–90.

103. Freilich RJ, Delattre JY, Monjour A, DeAngelis LM. Chemotherapy without radiation therapy as initial treatment for primary CNS lymphoma in older patients. Neurology 1996;46:435–9.

104. DeAngelis LM, Yahalom J, Thaler HT, Kher U. Combined modality therapy for primary CNS lymphoma. J Clin Oncol 1992;10:635–43.

105. Chamberlain MC. Long survival in patients with acquired immune deficiency syndrome-related primary central nervous system lymphoma. Cancer 1994;73:1728–30.

106. Bessell EM, Graus F, Punt JA, et al. Primary non-Hodgkin's lymphoma of the CNS treated with BVAM or CHOD/BVAM chemotherapy before radiotherapy. J Clin Oncol 1996;14:945–54.

107. Glass J, Shustik C, Hochberg FH, et al. Therapy of primary central nervous system lymphoma with pre-irradiation methotrexate, cyclophosphamide, doxorubicin, vincristine, and dexamethasone (MCHOD). J Neurooncol 1996;30:257–65.

108. Brada M, Hjiyiannakis D, Hines F, et al. Short intensive primary chemotherapy and radiotherapy in sporadic primary CNS lymphoma (PCL). Int J Radiat Oncol Biol Phys 1998;40:1157–62.

109. O'Neill BP, O'Fallon JR, Earle JD, et al. Primary central nervous system non-Hodgkin's lymphoma: survival advantages with combined initial therapy? Int J Radiat Oncol Biol Phys 1995;33:663–73.

110. Maher E, Fine HA. Primary CNS lymphoma. Semin Oncol 1999;26:346–56.

111. Lim FE, Hartman AS, Tan EG, et al. Factors in the prognosis of gastric lymphoma. Cancer 1977;39:1715–20.

112. Isaacson P, Wright DH, Judd MA, Mepham BL. Primary gastrointestinal lymphomas: a classification of 66 cases. Cancer 1979;43:1805–9.

113. d'Amore F, Brincker H, Grønbaek K, et al. Non-Hodgkin's lymphoma of the gastrointestinal tract: a population-based analysis of incidence, geographic distribution, clinicopathologic presentation features, and prognosis. Danish Lymphoma Study Group. J Clin Oncol 1994;12:1673–84.

114. List AF, Greer JP, Cousar JC, et al. Non-Hodgkin's lymphoma of the gastrointestinal tract: an analysis of clinical and pathologic features affecting outcome. J Clin Oncol 1988;6:1125–33.

115. Chan JKC, Ng CS, Isaacson PG. Relationship between high-grade lymphoma and low-grade B-cell mucosa-associated lymphoid tissue lymphoma (MALToma) of the stomach. Am J Pathol 1990;136:1153–64.

116. Isaacson PG, Spencer J, Wright DH. Classifying primary gut lymphomas. Lancet 1988;2:1148–9.

117. LeBrun DP, Kamel OW, Cleary ML, et al. Follicular lymphomas of the gastrointestinal tract: pathologic features in 31 cases and bcl-2 oncogenic protein expression. Am J Pathol 1992;140:1327–35.

118. Ruskoné-Fourmestraux A, Delmer A, Lavergne A, et al. Multiple lymphomatous polyposis of the gastrointestinal tract: prospective clinicopathologic study of 31 cases. Groupe D'étude des Lymphomes Digestifs. Gastroenterology 1997;112:7–16.

119. Crump M, Gospodarowicz M, Shepherd FA. Lymphoma of the gastrointestinal tract. Semin Oncol 1999;26:324–37.

120. Weingrad DN, Decosse JJ, Sherlock P, et al. Primary gastrointestinal lymphoma: a 30-year review. Cancer 1982;49:258–65.

121. Rosenfelt F, Rosenberg SA. Diffuse histiocytic lymphoma presenting with gastrointestinal tract lesions: the Stanford experience. Cancer 1980;45:2188–93.

122. Hande KR, Fisher RI, DeVita VT, et al. Diffuse histiocytic lymphoma involving the gastrointestinal tract. Cancer 1978;41:1984–9.

123. Burnett HW, Herbert EA. The role of irradiation in the treatment of primary malignant lymphoma of the stomach. Radiology 1956;67:723–8.

124. Rao AR, Kagan AR, Potyk D, et al. Management of gastrointestinal lymphoma. Am J Clin Oncol 1984;7:213–9.

125. Brooks JJ, Enterline HT. Primary gastric lymphomas: a clinicopathologic study of 58 cases with long-term follow-up and literature review. Cancer 1983;51:701–11.

126. Bush RS, Ash CL. Primary lymphoma of the gastrointestinal tract. Radiology 1969;92:1349–54.

127. Blackledge G, Bush H, Dodge OG, Crowther D. A study of gastrointestinal lymphoma. Clin Oncol 1979;5:209–19.

128. Shimm DS, Dosoretz DE, Anderson T, et al. Primary gastric lymphoma: an analysis with emphasis on prognostic factors and radiation therapy. Cancer 1983;52:2044–8.

129. Sheridan WP, Medley G, Brodie GN. Non-Hodgkin's lymphoma of the stomach: a prospective pilot study of surgery plus chemotherapy in early and advanced disease. J Clin Oncol 1985;3:495–500.

130. Connors JM, Klimo P, Fairey RN, Voss N. Brief chemotherapy and involved field radiation therapy for limited-stage, histologically aggressive lymphoma. Ann Intern Med 1987;107:25–30.

131. Shepherd FA, Evans WK, Kutas G, et al. Chemotherapy following surgery for stages IE and IIE non-Hodgkin's lymphoma of the gastrointestinal tract. J Clin Oncol 1988;6:253–60.

132. Shiu MJ, Nisce LZ, Pinna A, et al. Recent results of multimodal therapy of gastric lymphoma. Cancer 1986;58:1389–99.

133. Maor MH, Maddux B, Osborne BM, et al. Stages IE and IIE non-Hodgkin's lymphomas of the stomach: comparison of treatment modalities. Cancer 1984;54:2330–7.

134. Maor MH, Velasquez WS, Fuller LM, Silvermintz KB. Stomach conservation in stages IE and IIE gastric non-Hodgkin's lymphoma. J Clin Oncol 1990;8:266–71.

135. Gobbi PG, Dionigi P, Barbieri F, et al. The role of surgery in the multimodal treatment of primary gastric non-Hodgkin's lymphomas: a report of 76 cases and review of the literature. Cancer 1990;65:2528–36.

136. Blazquez M, Haioun C, Chaumette MT, et al. Low grade B cell mucosa associated lymphoid tissue lymphoma of the stomach: clinical and endoscopic features, treatment, and outcome. Gut 1992;33:1621–5.

137. Roggero E, Zucca E, Cavalli F. Gastric mucosa-associated lymphoid tissue lymphomas: more than a fascinating model. J Natl Cancer Inst 1997;89:1328–30.

138. Steinbach G, Ford R, Glober G, et al. Antibiotic treatment of gastric lymphoma of mucosa-associated lymphoid tissue: an uncontrolled trial. Ann Intern Med 1999;131:88–95.

139. Neubauer A, Thiede C, Morgner A, et al. Cure of Helicobacter pylori infection and duration of remission of low-grade gastric mucosa-associated lymphoid tissue lymphoma. J Natl Cancer Inst 1997;89:1350–5.

140. Schechter NR, Portlock CS, Yahalom J. Treatment of mucosa-associated lymphoid tissue lymphoma of the stomach with radiation alone. J Clin Oncol 1998;16:1916–21.

141. Domizio P, Owen RA, Shepherd NA, et al. Primary lymphoma of the small intestine: a clinicopathological study of 119 cases. Am J Surg Pathol 1993;17:429–42.

142. Isaacson PG, O'Connor NT, Spencer J, et al. Malignant histiocytosis of the intestine: a T-cell lymphoma. Lancet 1985;2:688–91.

143. Khojasteh A, Haghshenass M, Haghighi P. Current concepts immuno-proliferative small intestinal disease: a "Third-World lesion." N Engl J Med 1983;308:1401–5.

144. Salem P, el-Hashimi L, Anaissie E, et al. Primary small intestinal lymphoma in adults: a comparative study of IPSID versus non-IPSID in the Middle East. Cancer 1987;59:1670–6.

145. Brouet JC, Mason DY, Danon F, et al. Alpha-chain disease: evidence for common clonal origin of intestinal immunoblastic lymphoma and plasmacytic proliferation. Lancet 1977;1:861.

146. Cohen HJ, Gonzalvo A, Krook J, et al. New presentation of alpha heavy chain disease: North American polypoid gastrointestinal lymphoma: clinical and cellular studies. Cancer 1978;41:1161–9.

147. Lewin KJ, Kahn LB, Novis BH. Primary intestinal lymphoma of "Western" and "Mediterranean" type, alpha chain disease and massive plasma cell infiltration: a comparative study of 37 cases. Cancer 1976;38:2511–28.

148. Salem PA, Nassar VH, Shahid MJ, et al. "Mediterranean abdominal lymphoma," or immunoproliferative small intestinal disease: part I. clinical aspects. Cancer 1977;40:2941–7.

149. Galian A, Lecestre MJ, Scotto J, et al. Pathological study of alpha-chain disease, with special emphasis on evolution. Cancer 1977;39:2081–101.

150. Khojasteh A, Saalabian MJ, Haghshenass M. Randomized comparison of abdominal irradiation (AI) vs CHOP vs C-MOPP for the treatment of immunoproliferative small intestinal disease (IPSID) associated lymphoma (AL). Proc ASCO 1983;2:207.

151. El Saghir N, Mass R, Fawzy E, et al. Chemotherapy (CT) for primary small intestinal lymphoma: excellent response and minimal complications. Proc ASCO 1987;6:191.

152. Naqvi MS, Burrows L, Kark AE. Lymphoma of the gastrointestinal tract: prognostic guides based on 162 cases. Ann Surg 1969;170:221–31.

153. Loehr WJ, Mujahed Z, Zahn FD, et al. Primary lymphoma of the gastrointestinal tract: a review of 100 cases. Ann Surg 1969;170:232–8.

154. Vanden Heule B, Taylor CR, Terry R, Lukes RJ. Presentation of malignant lymphoma in the rectum. Cancer 1982;49:2602–7.

155. Wychulis AR, Beahrs OH, Woolner LB. Malignant lymphoma of the colon: a study of 69 cases. Arch Surg 1966;93:215–25.

156. Renard TH, Morton RL, Mathews R, Poulos E. Primary lymphoma of the rectum. Am Surg 1992;58:634–7.

157. Devine RM, Beart RW Jr, Wolff BG. Malignant lymphoma of the rectum. Dis Colon Rectum 1986;29:821–4.

158. Ioachim HL, Weinstein MA, Robbins RD, et al. Primary anorectal lymphoma: a new manifestation of the acquired immune deficiency syndrome (AIDS). Cancer 1987;60:1449–53.

159. Avlonitis VS, Linos D. Primary hepatic lymphoma: a review. Eur J Surg 1999;165:725–9.

160. Chowla A, Malhi-Chowla N, Chidambaram A, Surick B. Primary hepatic lymphoma in hepatitis C: case report and review of the literature. Am Surg 1999;65:881–3.

161. Rubbia-Brandt L, Bründler MA, Kerl K, et al. Primary hepatic diffuse large B-cell lymphoma in a patient with chronic hepatitis C. Am J Surg Pathol 1999;23:1124–30.

162. Sato S, Masuda T, Oikawa H, et al. Primary hepatic lymphoma associated with primary biliary cirrhosis. Am J Gastroenterol 1999;94:1669–73.

163. Prabhu RM, Medeiros LJ, Kumar D, et al. Primary hepatic low-grade B-cell lymphoma of mucosa-associated lymphoid tissue (MALT) associated with primary biliary cirrhosis. Mod Pathol 1998;11:404–10.

164. Scoazec JY, Degott C, Brousse N, et al. Non-Hodgkin's lymphoma presenting as a primary tumor of the liver: presentation, diagnosis and outcome in eight patients. Hepatology 1991;13:870–5.

165. Anthony PP, Sarsfield P, Clarke T. Primary lymphoma of the liver: clinical and pathological features of 10 patients. J Clin Pathol 1990;43:1007–13.

166. Sallah S, Smith SV, Lony LC, et al. Gamma/delta T-cell hepatosplenic lymphoma: review of the literature, diagnosis by flow cytometry and concomitant autoimmune hemolytic anemia. Ann Hematol 1997;74:139–42.

167. Cooke CB, Krenacs L, Stetler-Stevenson M, et al. Hepatosplenic T-cell lymphoma: a distinct clinicopathologic entity of cytotoxic gamma delta T-cell origin. Blood 1996;88:4265–74.

168. Francois A, Lesesve JF, Stamatoullas A, et al. Hepatosplenic gamma/delta T-cell lymphoma: a report of two cases in immunocompromised

169. Jonveaux P, Daniel MT, Martel V, et al. Isochromosome 7q and trisomy 8 are consistent primary, non-random chromosomal abnormalities associated with hepatosplenic T gamma/delta lymphoma. Leukemia 1996;10:1453–5.

170. Yao M, Tien HF, Lin MT, et al. Clinical and hematological characteristics of hepatosplenic T gamma/delta lymphoma with isochromosome for long arm of chromosome 7. Leuk Lymphoma 1996;22:495–500.

171. Ryan J, Straus DJ, Lange C, et al. Primary lymphoma of the liver. Cancer 1988;61:370–5.

172. Osborne BM, Butler JJ, Guarda LA. Primary lymphoma of the liver: ten cases and a review of the literature. Cancer 1985;56:2902–10.

173. Isaacson PG, Banks PM, Best PV, et al. Primary low-grade hepatic B-cell lymphoma of mucosa-associated lymphoid tissue (MALT)-type. Am J Surg Pathol 1995;19:571–5.

174. Kirk CM, Lewin D, Lazarchick J. Primary hepatic B-cell lymphoma of mucosa-associated lymphoid tissue. Arch Pathol Lab Med 1999;123:716–9.

175. Montanaro A, Patton R. Primary splenic malignant lymphoma, histiocytic type, with sclerosis: report of a case with long-term survival. Cancer 1976;38:1625–8.

176. Kraemer BB, Osborne BM, Butler JJ. Primary splenic presentation of malignant lymphoma and related disorders: a study of 49 cases. Cancer 1984;54:1606–19.

177. Baldini L. In 5th International Symposium on Therapy of Acute Leukemias. Roma, November 1–6, 1991. Book of abstracts. Haematologica 1991;76:Suppl 4:22.

178. Melo JV, Robinson DS, Gregory C, Catovsky D. Splenic B cell lymphoma with "villous" lymphocytes in the peripheral blood: a disorder distinct from hairy cell leukemia. Leukemia 1987;1:294–8.

179. Mulligan SP, Matutes E, Dearden C, Catovsky D. Splenic lymphoma with villous lymphocytes: natural history and response to therapy in 50 cases. Br J Haematol 1991;78:206–9.

180. Catovsky D, Matutes E. Splenic lymphoma with circulating villous lymphocytes/splenic marginal-zone lymphoma. Semin Hematol 1999;36:148–54.

181. Bolam S, Orchard J, Oscier D. Fludarabine is effective in the treatment of splenic lymphoma with villous lymphocytes. Br J Haematol 1997;99:158–61.

182. Harris NL, Aisenberg AC, Meyer JE, et al. Diffuse large cell (histiocytic) lymphoma of the spleen: clinical and pathologic characteristics of ten cases. Cancer 1984;54:2460–7.

183. Ahmann DL, Kiely JM, Harrison EG Jr, Payne WS. Malignant lymphoma of the spleen: a review of 49 cases in which the diagnosis was made at splenectomy. Cancer 1966;19:461–9.

184. Glicklich D, Sung MW, Frey M. Renal failure due to lymphomatous infiltration of the kidneys: report of three new cases and review of the literature. Cancer 1986;58:748–53.

185. Kandel LB, McCullough DL, Harrison LH, et al. Primary renal lymphoma: does it exist? Cancer 1987;60:386–91.

186. Richards MA, Mootoosamy I, Reznek RH, et al. Renal involvement in patients with non-Hodgkin's lymphoma: clinical and pathological features in 23 cases. Hematol Oncol 1990;8:105–10.

187. Dimopoulos MA, Moulopoulos LA, Costantinides C, et al. Primary renal lymphoma: a clinical and radiological study. J Urol 1996;155:1865–7.

188. Okuno SH, Hoyer JD, Ristow K, Witzig TE. Primary renal non-Hodgkin's lymphoma: an unusual extranodal site. Cancer 1995;75:2258–61.

189. Fiche M, Caprons F, Berger F, et al. Primary pulmonary non-Hodgkin's lymphomas. Histopathology 1995;26:529–37.

190. Cordier JF, Chailleux E, Lauque D, et al. Primary pulmonary lymphomas: a clinical study of 70 cases in nonimmunocompromised patients. Chest 1993;103:201–8.

191. Tamura A, Komatsu H, Yanai N, et al. Primary pulmonary lymphoma: relationship between clinical features and pathologic findings in 24 cases. The Japan National Chest Hospital Study Group for Lung Cancer. Jpn J Clin Oncol 1995;25:140–52.

192. Addis BJ, Hyjek E, Isaacson PG. Primary pulmonary lymphoma: a re-appraisal of its histogenesis and its relationship to pseudolymphoma and lymphoid interstitial pneumonia. Histopathology 1988;13:1–17.

193. Marchevsky A, Padilla M, Kaneko M, Kleinerman J. Localized lymphoid nodules of lung: a reappraisal of the lymphoma versus pseudolymphoma dilemma. Cancer 1983;51:2070–7.

patients, associated with isochromosome 7q. Am J Surg Pathol 1997;21:781–90.

194. Turner RR, Colby TV, Doggett RS. Well-differentiated lymphocytic lymphoma: a study of 47 patients with primary manifestation in the lung. Cancer 1984;54:2088–96.
195. Kennedy JL, Nathwani BN, Burke JS, et al. Pulmonary lymphomas and other pulmonary lymphoid lesions: a clinicopathologic and immunologic study of 64 patients. Cancer 1985;56:539–52.
196. Katzenstein AL, Peiper SC. Detection of Epstein-Barr virus genomes in lymphomatoid granulomatosis: analysis of 29 cases by the polymerase chain reaction technique. Mod Pathol 1990;3:435–41.
197. Colby TV, Carrington CB. Pulmonary lymphomas: current concepts. Hum Pathol 1983;14:884–7.
198. Rose RM, Grigas D, Strattemeir E, et al. Endobronchial involvement with non-Hodgkin's lymphoma: a clinical-radiologic analysis. Cancer 1986;57:1750–5.
199. Nicholson AG, Wotherspoon AC, Jones AL, et al. Pulmonary B-cell non-Hodgkin's lymphoma associated with autoimmune disorders: a clinicopathological review of six cases. Eur Respir J 1996;9:2022–5.
200. Koss MH, Hochholzer L, Nichols PW, et al. Primary non-Hodgkin's lymphoma and pseudolymphoma of lung: a study of 161 patients. Hum Pathol 1983;14:1024–38.
201. Habermann TM, Ryu JH, Inwards DJ, Kurtin PJ. Primary pulmonary lymphoma. Semin Oncol 1999;26:307–15.
202. Levitt LJ, Aisenberg AC, Harris NL, et al. Primary non-Hodgkin's lymphoma of the mediastinum. Cancer 1982;50:2486–92.
203. Möller P, Moldenhauer G, Momburg F, et al. Mediastinal lymphoma of clear cell type is a tumor corresponding to terminal steps of B cell differentiation. Blood 1987;69:1087–95.
204. Addis BJ, Isaacson PG. Large cell lymphoma of the mediastinum: a B-cell tumour of probable thymic origin. Histopathology 1986;10:379–90.
205. Aisenberg AC. Primary large cell lymphoma of the mediastinum. Semin Oncol 1999;26:251–8.
206. Higgins JP, Warnke RA. CD30 expression is common in mediastinal large B-cell lymphoma. Am J Clin Pathol 1999;112:241–7.
207. Lazzarino M, Orlandi E, Paulli M, et al. Treatment outcome and prognostic factors for primary mediastinal (thymic) B-cell lymphoma: a multicenter study of 106 patients. J Clin Oncol 1997;15:1646–53.
208. Martelli MP, Martelli M, Pescarmona E, et al. MACOP-B and involved field radiation therapy is an effective therapy for primary mediastinal large B-cell lymphoma with sclerosis. Ann Oncol 1998;9:1027–9.
209. Cazals-Hatem D, Lepage E, Brice P, et al. Primary mediastinal large B-cell lymphoma: a clinicopathologic study of 141 cases compared with 916 nonmediastinal large B-cell lymphomas, a GELA ("Groupe d'Etude des Lymphomes de l'Adulte") study. Am J Surg Pathol 1996;20:877–88.
210. Zinzani PL, Bendandi M, Frezza G, et al. Primary mediastinal B-cell lymphoma with sclerosis: clinical and therapeutic evaluation of 22 patients. Leuk Lymphoma 1996;21:311–6.
211. Rodriguez J, Pugh WC, Romaguera JE, Cabanillas F. Primary mediastinal large cell lymphoma. Hematol Oncol 1994;12:175–84.
212. Isaacson PG, Chan JK, Tang C, Addis BJ. Low-grade B-cell lymphoma of mucosa-associated lymphoid tissue arising in the thymus: a thymic lymphoma mimicking myoepithelial sialadenitis. Am J Surg Pathol 1990;14:342–51.
213. McDonnell PJ, Mann, RB, Bulkley BH. Involvement of the heart by malignant lymphoma: a clinicopathologic study. Cancer 1982;49:944–51.
214. Chou ST, Arkles LB, Gill GD, et al. Primary lymphoma of the heart: a case report. Cancer 1983;52:744–7.
215. Ceresoli GL, Ferreri AJ, Bucci E, et al. Primary cardiac lymphoma in immunocompetent patients: diagnostic and therapeutic management. Cancer 1997;80:1497–506.
216. Nagano M, Uike N, Suzumiya J, et al. Successful treatment of a patient with cardiac lymphoma who presented with a complete atrioventricular block. Am J Hematol 1998;59:171–4.
217. Nakayama Y, Uchimoto S, Tsumura K, Morii H. Primary cardiac lymphoma with infiltration of the atrioventricular node: remission with reversal of the atrioventricular block induced by chemotherapy. Cardiology 1997;88:613–6.
218. Gill PS, Chandraratna PA, Meyer PR, Levine AM. Malignant lymphoma: cardiac involvement at initial presentation. J Clin Oncol 1987;5:216–24.
219. Nand S, Mullen GM, Lonchyna VA, Moncada R. Primary lymphoma of the heart: prolonged survival with early systemic therapy in a patient. Cancer 1991;68:2289–92.
220. Smith MR, Brustei S, Straus DJ. Localized non-Hodgkin's lymphoma of the breast. Cancer 1987;59:351–4.
221. Bobrow LG, Richards MA, Happerfield LC, et al. Primary breast lymphoma: a clinicopathological review. J Pathol 1992; 167:Suppl: 139A.
222. Jeon HJ, Akagi T, Hoshida Y, et al. Primary non-Hodgkin malignant lymphoma of the breast: an immunohistochemical study of seven patients and literature review of 152 patients with breast lymphoma in Japan. Cancer 1991;70:2451–9.
223. Aozasa K, Ohsawa M, Saeki K, et al. Malignant lymphoma of the breast: immunologic type and association with lymphocytic mastopathy. Am J Clin Pathol 1992;97:699–704.
224. Hennessy C, Henry JA, Patterson DA, et al. Primary lymphoma of the breast: the Scottish and Newcastle experience. Proc ASCO 1991;10:276.
225. Brogi E, Harris NL. Lymphomas of the breast: pathology and clinical behavior. Semin Oncol 1999;26:357–64.
226. Talbot D, Rayter Z, Beck N, et al. Primary lymphoma of the breast—the Royal Marsden experience since 1959. Br J Cancer 1991;63:Suppl 13:10.
227. Giardini R, Piccolo C, Rilke F. Primary non-Hodgkin's lymphomas of the female breast. Cancer 1992;69:725–35.
228. Reimer RR, Chabner BA, Young RC, et al. Lymphoma presenting in bone: results of histopathology, staging, and therapy. Ann Intern Med 1977;87:50–5.
229. Ostrowski ML, Unni KK, Banks PM, et al. Malignant lymphoma of bone. Cancer 1986;58:2646–55.
230. Bacci G, Jaffe N, Emiliani E, et al. Therapy for primary non-Hodgkin's lymphoma of bone and a comparison of results with Ewing's sarcoma: ten years' experience at the Istituto Ortopedico Rizzoli. Cancer 1986;57:1468–72.
231. Bacci G, Ferraro A, Casadei R, et al. Primary lymphoma of bone: long term results in patients treated with vincristine-Adriamycin-cyclophosphamide and local radiation. J Chemother 1991;3:189–93.
232. Baar J, Burkes R, Gospodarowicz M. Primary non-Hodgkin's lymphoma of bone. Semin Oncol 1999;26:270–5.
233. Baar J, Burkes RL, Bell R, et al. Primary non-Hodgkin's lymphoma of bone: a clinicopathologic study. Cancer 1994;73:1194–9.
234. Christie DR, Barton MB, Bryant G, et al. Osteolymphoma (primary bone lymphoma): an Australian review of 70 cases. Australasian Radiation Oncology Lymphoma Group (AROLG). Aust N Z J Med 1999;29:214–9.
235. Fairbanks RK, Bonner JA, Inwards CY, et al. Treatment of stage IE primary lymphoma of bone. Int J Radiat Oncol Biol Phys 1994;28:363–72.
236. Mendenhall NP, Jones JJ, Kramer BS, et al. The management of primary lymphoma of bone. Radiother Oncol 1987;9:137–45.
237. Dosoretz DE, Murphy GF, Raymond AK, et al. Radiation therapy for primary lymphoma of bone. Cancer 1983;51:44–6.
238. Boston HC Jr, Dahlin DC, Ivins JC, Cupps RE. Malignant lymphoma (so-called reticulum cell sarcoma) of bone. Cancer 1974;34:1131–7.
239. Barbieri E. Ninth Ann Mtg Eur Soc Therapeutic Radiol Oncol, Montecatini Terme, Italy. September 12–15, 1990.
240. Dubey P, Ha CS, Besa PC, et al. Localized primary malignant lymphoma of bone. Int J Radiat Oncol Biol Phys 1997;37:1087–93.
241. Shahab N, Doll DC. Testicular lymphoma. Semin Oncol 1999;26:259–69.
242. Doll DC, Weiss RB. Malignant lymphoma of the testis. Am J Med 1986;81:515–24.
243. Paladugu RR, Bearman RM, Rappaport H. Malignant lymphoma with primary manifestation in the gonad: a clinicopathologic study of 38 patients. Cancer 1980;45:561–71.
244. Imaizumi E, Seki K, Kikuchi Y, et al. Primary ovarian lymphoma: a case report. Arch Gynecol Obstet 1993;252:209–13.
245. Rotmensch J, Woodruff JD. Lymphoma of the ovary: report of twenty new cases and update of previous series. Am J Obstet Gynecol 1982;143:870–5.
246. Dimopoulos MA, Daliani D, Pugh W, et al. Primary ovarian non-Hodgkin's lymphoma: outcome after treatment with combination chemotherapy. Gynecol Oncol 1997;64:446–50.
247. Aozasa K, Saeki K, Ohsawa M, et al. Malignant lymphoma of the uterus: report of seven cases with immunohistochemical study. Cancer 1993;72:1959–64.
248. Makarewicz R, Kuzminska A. Non-Hodgkin's lymphoma of the uterine cervix: a report of three patients. Clin Oncol (R Coll Radiol) 1995;7:198–9.

249. Bagella MP, Fadda G, Cherchi PL. Non-Hodgkin lymphoma: a rare primary vulvar localization. Eur J Gynaecol Oncol 1990;11:153–6.

250. Prevot S, Hugol D, Audouin J, et al. Primary non Hodgkin's malignant lymphoma of the vagina: report of 3 cases with review of the literature. Pathol Res Pract 1992;188:78–85.

251. Höffkes HG, Schumann A, Uppenkamp M, et al. Primary non-Hodgkin's lymphoma of the vagina: case report and review of the literature. Ann Hematol 1995;70:273–6.

252. Kerbl K, Pauer W. Primary non-Hodgkin lymphoma of prostate. Urology 1988;32:347–9.

253. Bostwick DG, Iczkowski KA, Amin MB, et al. Malignant lymphoma involving the prostate: report of 62 cases. Cancer 1998;83:732–8.

254. Nabholtz JM, Friedman S, Tremeaux JC, et al. Non-Hodgkin's lymphoma of the urethra: a rare extranodal entity. Gynecol Oncol 1989;35:110–1.

255. Vapnek JM, Turzan CW. Primary malignant lymphoma of the female urethra: report of a case and review of the literature. J Urol 1992;147:701–3.

256. Hofmockel G, Dämmrich J, Manzanilla Garcia H. Primary non-Hodgkin's lymphoma of the male urethra: a case report and review of the literature. Urol Int 1995;55:177–80.

257. Patel A. Primary lymphoma of the bladder (PLB): a case report and review of literature. Proc ASCO 1992;11:322.

258. Kempton CL, Kurtin PJ, Inwards DJ, et al. Malignant lymphoma of the bladder: evidence from 36 cases that low-grade lymphoma of the MALT-type is the most common primary bladder lymphoma. Am J Surg Pathol 1997;21:1324–33.

259. Harris GJ, Tio FO, Von Hoff DD. Primary adrenal lymphoma. Cancer 1989;63:799–803.

260. Joly I, David A, Payan MJ, et al. A case of primary non-Hodgkin lymphoma of the pancreas. Pancreas 1992;7:118–20.

261. Cappell MS, Yao F, Cho KC, Axiotis CA. Lymphoma predominantly involving the pancreas. Dig Dis Sci 1989;34:942–7.

262. Fischer MG, Kabakow B. Lymphoma of the pancreas. Mt Sinai J Med 1987;54:423–6.

263. Salvatore JR, Ross RS. Primary bilateral adrenal lymphoma. Leuk Lymphoma 1999;34:111–7.

264. Bouvet M, Staerkel GA, Spitz FR, et al. Primary pancreatic lymphoma. Surgery 1998;123:382–90.

265. Jeffery GM, Golding PF, Mead GM. Non-Hodgkin's lymphoma arising in skeletal muscle. Ann Oncol 1991;2:501–4.

266. Samuel LM, White J, Lessells AM, et al. Primary non-Hodgkins lymphoma of muscle. Clin Oncol (R Coll Radiol) 1999;11:49–51.

---

## CHAPTER 95

# ACUTE LYMPHOBLASTIC LEUKEMIA

• STANLEY R. FRANKEL • WENDY STOCK • JOHN BYRD • CLARA D. BLOOMFIELD

---

## Natural History

Acute lymphoblastic leukemia (ALL) is biologically and clinically a heterogeneous group of diseases characterized by a malignant proliferation of immature lymphoid cells in the bone marrow. Advances in our understanding of the biology of ALL have enabled the application of laboratory technology to improve diagnosis and treatment. Indeed, appropriate treatment of ALL is now dependent on the availability of laboratories to determine the karyotype, immunophenotype, and molecular genetic abnormalities of the patient's leukemia cells.

Progress in understanding and treating ALL has come primarily from studies of the disease in children. Many of the lessons learned from pediatric trials are applicable to adults; however, age-related biologic differences result in a striking difference in outcome. Although the cure rate is better than 60% in children, only one third of adults survive this disease.

### EPIDEMIOLOGY

The worldwide incidence of ALL ranges between 10 and 65 cases per million individuals, and is rising slowly.[1] The incidence of ALL in the United States is 17 cases per million individuals. Of the 30,800 new cases of leukemia forecast to occur in the United States in 2000, approximately 3200

were ALL.[2] At least 1300 deaths occur each year in the United States from ALL. The incidence of ALL follows a bimodal pattern as a function of age. The incidence of ALL is 5.7 cases per 100,000 in children younger than 5 years and falls to 3 cases per 100,000 between ages 5 and 9.[3] The median age at diagnosis of ALL is 11 years. Incidence of ALL remains relatively high through the teens but falls during the next two decades and increases steadily beyond 45 years. Up to one third of adult patients with ALL may be diagnosed at age 60 or older.[4]

Seventy percent of ALL cases occur in children younger than age 20. ALL accounts for 25% of malignancies in children younger than 15 years. ALL accounts for only 15 to 20% of adult acute leukemia but 80% of childhood leukemias.[5] Approximately 1000 new cases of ALL are diagnosed annually in individuals age 20 years or older.[2, 5] Both incidence and mortality are slightly higher in males.[2, 6]

### ETIOLOGY

Heredity, viruses, and environmental factors have been implicated in the etiology of ALL.[7–20] However, for most ALL patients, no causal conditions or exposures are found. When associated conditions have been identified, the mechanisms by which these factors influence the development of leukemia are unknown. However, advances in the understanding of malignant transformation at the molecular level suggest that the activation of oncogenes represents a mechanism common to many causative factors.[21] Retrospective molecular studies provide evidence that leukemogenesis in young

Supported in part by the Coleman Leukemia Research Fund

patients may occur in utero; however, the causative agents remain to be identified.[22, 23]

**Congenital Disorders and Heredity.** A number of congenital or inherited syndromes, particularly in children, are associated with an increased incidence of ALL.[7, 11–13, 16, 24] These include syndromes associated with somatic cell chromosome aneuploidy such as Down syndrome (trisomy 21) and Klinefelter's syndrome (XXY and variants). The risk of developing acute leukemia in Down syndrome is nearly 20 times greater than expected and is increased for all ages, but particularly during the neonatal period.[24] Although neonates and older patients usually have acute myeloid leukemia (AML), younger patients with Down syndrome usually have ALL.

Inherited diseases characterized by excessive chromosomal fragility and rearrangement such as Bloom syndrome[25] and ataxia telangiectasia[26] are also associated with a higher incidence of acute leukemia. Other inherited diseases that appear associated with an increased incidence of ALL include Li-Fraumeni syndrome,[27] Shwachman syndrome,[28] and neurofibromatosis.[29, 30]

Other genetic factors probably also influence the occurrence of acute leukemia.[7, 11, 12, 16] When one monozygotic twin develops leukemia, the chance that the second twin will also is estimated at 20 to 25%. In utero transmission of a leukemic progenitor cell between twins has been suggested.[31, 32] Acute leukemia is also more likely to occur in dizygotic twins and other family members of patients with acute leukemia; thus it is not possible to distinguish genetic and environmental contributions.[12, 13, 16] However, a role for genetic factors is supported by the observation that the incidence of leukemia differs in relation to human leukocyte antigen (HLA) type and ethnic group.[7, 33–35] Inherited mutations in p53 also may be associated with a predisposition to the development of ALL.[36] Increasing birth weight increased the relative risk of developing ALL.

**Viruses.** Retroviruses account for most of the known leukemia viruses in animals. In human carcinogenesis, retroviruses have been identified as causative agents of certain types of adult T-cell leukemia/lymphoma (see Chapter 96). The possibility that viruses play a role in common ALL of childhood is suggested by epidemiologic data linking increased risk with higher socioeconomic status and other community characteristics that lead to delayed exposure to the usual infections of infancy.[11, 15, 19] In utero infection has also been proposed as an initiating factor.[37] JC polyomavirus may fit the model for a potential etiologic agent.[38]

Epstein-Barr virus (EBV) has been associated with the development of Burkitt's lymphoma and may also be associated with B-cell ALL, the leukemic form of this disease.[12, 39, 40] How EBV infection leads to lymphoid malignancy remains unknown.[10, 12, 41] EBV-associated membrane proteins play a pathogenetic role in at least some of the lymphoproliferative disorders.[42] Measles infection at a young age was associated with an increased likelihood of ALL developing.[43] Psoriasis, but not other immune-related disorders, has been associated with a higher incidence of ALL in adults.[43]

**Environmental Factors.** Little is known about associations between environmental exposures and ALL. The risk of the disease may be increased by the interaction of immunologic and genetic characteristics, and possibly retroviruses, with environmental factors.[7]

Radiation is a definite causative factor for AML.[9, 12] Fewer cases of ALL secondary to radiation have been identified. However, the incidence of ALL has been reported to be increased in young survivors of the atomic bomb and in young children exposed to radioactive fallout from nuclear weapons testing.[44] A marked increase in the incidence of leukemia in children of fathers who worked at a nuclear processing plant has been reported.[45]

Data suggest that environmental exposure is more important than previously recognized in adult ALL. An increased risk of ALL has been associated with residence within 5 miles of an industrial site.[46] Particularly important industrial exposures were paper and allied products and primary metal industries including iron, steel, and aluminum. Although exposure to extremely low frequency electromagnetic fields from electricity transmission lines has been hypothesized to increase the incidence of leukemia, this association has not been substantiated.[47–49]

Living on a farm as an adult has been associated with a significantly increased risk of ALL.[46] Although there is extensive literature linking farming with leukemia risk,[50] the explanation for the association with living on a farm is unknown. Possible reasons include exposure to pesticides and animal viruses.

Smoking appears to increase the risk of ALL, especially in older patients.[51, 52] Persons older than age 60 who smoked had three times the risk of developing ALL compared with those who never smoked. A significant association with permanent and semipermanent hair dye use has been identified by some[53] but not all investigators.[54, 55]

Trichloroethylene contamination of drinking water has been associated with an increased incidence of ALL.[56]

Although there is a higher incidence of childhood ALL among whites than is seen in African Americans, age differences in childhood ALL incidence may not be solely accounted for by socioeconomic status differences.[57]

**Secondary Acute Lymphoblastic Leukemia.** ALL has been reported in patients with an antecedent myelodysplastic syndrome, as a blastic transformation of chronic myelogenous leukemia (CML),[58] and following chemotherapy for other malignancies including childhood cancers.[59–61] ALL that develops after administration of topoisomerase II inhibitors has been associated with a specific cytogenetic abnormality, t(4;11)(q21;q23).[62, 63] ALL has on occasion been reported following bone marrow transplantation for other diseases.[64, 65]

## PATHOLOGY AND CLASSIFICATION

Although historically, the diagnosis of acute leukemia was based solely on bone marrow morphology, cytochemical, immunologic, cytogenetic, and molecular genetic studies are now also used to subclassify ALL and distinguish it from AML. Examination of the marrow aspirate smear using routine Romanowsky stains (May-Grünwald-Giemsa, Wright, or Wright-Giemsa) remains the first step. The marrow is usually hypercellular, with replacement of fat and normal marrow cells by the leukemic population. Remaining myeloid and erythroid elements and megakaryocytes usually have normal morphologic characteristics. When the marrow cannot be aspirated, examination of circulating blasts may allow the diagnosis of ALL.

The nuclear and cytoplasmic features of the leukemic cell should be assessed on marrow or blood smears. The nuclear chromatin in lymphoblasts is clumped and irregularly distributed and often condensed along the nuclear and nucleolar membranes, making the nucleoli apparent. Unlike AML, granules are usually absent, the cytoplasm is scant, and Auer rods are not seen.

Three categories of lymphoblasts (L1, L2, L3) have been defined by the French-American-British (FAB) group (Table 95–1).[66–68] Two thirds of adult disease has L2 morphology.[69, 70] L1 cells predominate in childhood ALL.[71] Often a combination of L1 and L2 lymphoblasts is present.

**Cytochemistry and Immunohistochemistry.** Classification of the acute leukemias is facilitated by evaluating various cytoplasmic constituents with cytochemical techniques.[72–74] Myeloperoxidase is the most useful stain for separating ALL from AML. A positive myeloperoxidase reaction (i.e., presence of myeloperoxidase in >3% of the blast cells) distinguishes M1 AML from L2 ALL. Sudan black B activity parallels that of peroxidase, but occasionally is positive in ALL.[75] The periodic acid–Schiff (PAS) reaction can also be helpful because lymphoblasts may contain coarse granules or large blocks of PAS reactivity, whereas myeloblasts are usually PAS negative.[76] However, only 11% of ALL cases are strongly PAS positive.[77] A strong acid phosphatase reaction localized in the Golgi region of the cytoplasm may help to identify T-cell ALL (T-ALL).[69, 72]

Terminal deoxynucleotidyl transferase (TdT), a nuclear DNA polymerase, inserts nucleotide sequences at splice sites required for recombination of the immunoglobulin and T-cell receptor (TCR) genes. High concentrations of TdT are found in normal cortical thymocytes and in a small percentage of normal marrow progenitor cells, but not in circulating lymphocytes.[78–82] Most cases of ALL other than L3 are TdT positive, but so are 20% of AML.[74, 83–88]

**Immunophenotype.** The characterization of cell-surface molecules expressed on lymphoid and myeloid cells has increased our understanding of the biologic and clinical heterogeneity of ALL.[89, 90] Based on expression of T, B, and myeloid lineage-restricted antigens, it is now possible to assign stages of T, B, and myeloid differentiation of leukemic cells. Patterns of marker expression may identify subsets of ALL patients with characteristic clinical presentations and disease courses. Moreover, preliminary data suggest that aberrant patterns of antigen expression demonstrated by multiparameter flow cytometry may be used to detect minimal residual disease (MRD).[91–103] With the exception of surface immunoglobulin expression in FAB-L3, there is no concordance between FAB subtype and immunophenotype.

Prior to the availability of antibodies directed against lineage-restricted surface antigens, the subclassification of ALL relied on the expression of sheep erythrocyte receptors (E rosette receptor) to define T-ALL and demonstration of surface immunoglobulin (SIg) to define B-cell ALL. The remaining cases were classified as "null-ALL" or "non-B, non-T ALL." A fourth category, common ALL (cALL), was defined by reactivity of lymphoblasts from a subgroup of "null-ALL" with antisera raised against the common acute lymphocytic leukemia antigen (CALLA).

Studies using monoclonal antibodies allowed further subclassification. To facilitate classification, antibodies were segregated into cluster designation (CD) groups based on binding to similar cell-surface antigens.[104–106] For example, CALLA, previously defined by polyclonal sera, is designated CD10.

Using monoclonal antibodies, the vast majority of "null-ALL" were shown to be of B-cell origin.[90, 107] Because the term *B-cell ALL* historically referred to cells expressing SIg, these cases are designated B-lineage or B-precursor ALL. ALL immunophenotype has been refined further by the application of antibodies to detect co-expression of myeloid antigens.

Non–lineage-associated antigens useful in defining leukemia immunophenotype include HLA-DR, CD34, and CD45. HLA-DR (Ia) antigens are part of the major histocompatibility complex class II antigen system.[108] Although absent from the most primitive hematopoietic stem cells identified, HLA-DR is expressed on early hematopoietic progenitor cells. It is lost with T-cell and granulocytic maturation and terminal B-cell differentiation.[82, 109, 110] HLA-DR expression in ALL favors a diagnosis of B-lineage disease, but activated or immature T-lineage cells and myeloid cells also may express this antigen.[111]

The CD34$^+$ normal marrow compartment contains early stem cells and progenitor cells of all lymphohematopoietic lineages, including all TdT-positive cells.[81, 112, 113] The co-expression of CD34, TdT, and CD10 defines a lymphoid stem cell capable of differentiation into either B- or T-lineage cells.[81] CD34 is found on the majority of early B- or T-lineage ALL but is not present on mature B- or T-cell ALL.[114]

CD45, the leukocyte common antigen, is expressed on all

*Table 95–1.* **The French-American-British (FAB) Classification of Acute Lymphoblastic Leukemia**[66–68]

L1: A relatively homogeneous cell population with 75% or more small cells having scanty cytoplasm, finely dispersed chromatin, and regular nuclear shape. Nucleoli are inconspicuous in more than 75% of the cells.*

L2: A heterogeneous cell population with regard to size, chromatin pattern, and nuclear shape. The cells are usually large, with the cytoplasm occupying 20% or more of the surface area of the cell. Nucleoli are large in 25% or more of the cells.

L3: A large and relatively homogeneous cell population with regular nuclei and a fine chromatin pattern. Nucleoli are prominent. Cytoplasm is moderately abundant with vacuolization and deep basophilia. Lymphoblasts resemble those seen in Burkitt's lymphoma.

| Criterion | Score |
|---|---|
| 1. High N/C ratio in ≥75% of cells | +1 |
| 2. Low N/C ratio in ≥25% of cells | −1 |
| 3. Nucleoli: 0 to 1 (small) | +1 |
| 4. Nucleoli: 1 or more (prominent) | −1 |
| 5. Irregular nuclear membrane | −1 |
| 6. Large cells compose ≥50% of total | −1 |

| Subtype | Sum of Scores |
|---|---|
| L1 | 0 to 2+ |
| L2 | −1 to −4 |

*See scoring system, which assists in separating L1 from L2.[68]
N/C, Nuclear-cytoplasmic.
From Frankel SR. In: Abeloff M, et al (eds). Clinical oncology. New York: Churchill Livingstone, 1995.

normal hematopoietic cells except platelets and erythrocytes.[115] In children, CD45 expression is nearly universal in T-ALL but is detected in only 84% of B-lineage ALL.[116, 117]

Immunophenotypic classification of ALL is based on expression of combinations of antigens associated with B-, T-, and myeloid lineages. Delineation of the ontogeny of normal lymphoid markers has allowed subclassification of normal B- and T-lineage cells based on the stage of maturation. Classification of B-lineage ALL and T-ALL is based on the degree of maturation.[89, 90, 111, 118-129] A new complex classification system based on a weighted scoring system for individual markers has been proposed.[128] The frequencies of the various immunophenotypes in large series of adult and pediatric patients are shown in Table 95–2. T-ALL is uncommon in elderly patients, whereas the frequency of B-cell ALL may be twice that seen in the younger adult age group.[4] The criteria for each classification are described in the discussion that follows.

*T*-Acute Lymphoblastic Leukemia. The hierarchy of normal T-cell differentiation defined by surface marker expression serves as the template for assigning T-lineage and classifying T-cell maturation stages in ALL.[90, 118, 130-133] Most T-ALL cases express CD7, CD2, and CD5. Although these cells express CD45, they usually lack HLA-DR.

The most immature normal marrow T-cell precursor expresses CD34 in combination with CD7, TdT, and cytoplasmic CD3 (cCD3).[134] This population of "pre-T" cells does not express CD2, the sheep erythrocyte receptor.[135] CD7 expression precedes TdT expression and TCR gene rearrangements.[136-140] Maturing cells sequentially gain expression of CD2, CD1, and CD5, followed by CD4, CD8, and membrane CD3.[130, 133]

CD7, the most sensitive surface marker for T-ALL, is present in most cases.[141, 142] However, it is not specific for T-ALL, occurring in AML and natural killer cell leukemia.[143-147] Cytoplasmic CD3 expression is the most lineage-specific marker for T-cell differentiation,[148-151] but cytoplasmic antigens are not analyzed by routine flow cytometry.

Patients with T-ALL frequently present with a high white blood cell (WBC) count, a mediastinal mass, lymphadenopathy, and splenomegaly. They tend to have aggressive disease characterized by central nervous system (CNS) and testicular

relapses and a relatively brief survival with conventional therapy. Adults with T-ALL tend to be younger and more commonly male than are adults with B-lineage (non–SIg-positive) ALL, whereas children with T-ALL tend to be older than other childhood ALL patients.[111] Adults with a "pre-T" immunophenotype (cCD3+, CD7+, E-rosette, CD1−, CD4−, CD8− with variable CD2 expression) are less likely to present with a mediastinal mass, lymphadenopathy, or thrombocytopenia than are patients with more mature T-ALL.[152, 153] Although no apparent relationship between particular translocations and level of thymocyte maturation has been identified, a higher frequency of normal karyotypes in cases with more immature thymocytes and of pseudodiploidy in more mature cases has been reported.[154]

***B-Cell Acute Lymphoblastic Leukemia.*** Approximately 5% of adults and 3% of children with ALL are classified as B-cell ALL based on expression of SIg, usually IgM (see Table 95–2). Morphologically, these cases are typically L3 leukemias.[69, 155, 156] The cells are low in TdT and are usually acid phosphatase negative. Children with B-cell ALL tend to be older.[122, 128] The proportion of patients older than age 60 who present with B-cell ALL may be increased. Adults and children with B-ALL are predominantly male. At presentation, hepatosplenomegaly and CNS leukemia are common, as are low WBC counts with few circulating lymphoblasts.[69, 122, 128]

***B-Lineage (B-Precursor) Acute Lymphoblastic Leukemia.*** B-lineage ALL usually expresses CD19 and HLA-DR. Cytoplasmic CD22 (cCD22) is a sensitive and specific marker of B-precursor ALL.[148] Between 50% and 72% of adult and 80% and 85% of childhood ALL is B-lineage (see Table 95–2).

B-lineage ALL can be subdivided into early pre-B (also called *pre-pre B* or *null-ALL*), common ALL, pre-B ALL, and transitional B-ALL based on normal B-cell ontogeny.[90, 107, 118, 121-123, 126, 127, 148, 157-160] In normal ontogeny, the early pre-B cells have Ig heavy chain (IgH) gene rearrangements and express HLA-DR, CD34, TdT, CD19, cCD22, and CD24 without cytoplasmic Ig expression.[122] With further maturation, CD34 and TdT expression are lost. The appearance of CD10 may either precede or follow CD19 expression.[107, 126, 157]

Early pre-B ALL, the earliest lineage-specific subgroup, is defined by the addition of CD19, CD24, and cCD22 expression to the progenitor phenotype consisting of CD34, HLA-DR, and TdT expression. The IgH gene is rearranged, but the Ig light chain genes remain germline. Common ALL is distinguished by the expression of CD10 with or without CD19. Pre-B ALL is identified by the expression of cIg heavy chain (cμ); light chain genes may be either rearranged or germline. Transitional pre-B ALL co-expresses cytoplasmic and surface IgH chains but lacks surface light chain expression.[161] CD20 is another B-lineage–associated antigen that may be used to assign lineage. Although usually found on more mature normal B-lineage cells, CD20 status does not define a specific stage of maturation in ALL.

***Acute Lymphoblastic Leukemia with Myeloid Antigens (Mixed Lineage or Biphenotypic Acute Leukemia).*** The co-expression of lymphoid and myeloid surface markers on blast cells that are morphologically lymphoblasts and are myeloperoxidase negative defines myeloid antigen–positive ALL. When characteristics of two different cell lineages are

*Table 95–2.* **Frequency of Immunophenotypic Groups in ALL***

| Category | Defining Antigens | Approximate Frequency (%) | |
| --- | --- | --- | --- |
| | | ADULTS | CHILDREN |
| B cell | CD19, CD20, or cCD22 and SIg | 5 | 3 |
| B lineage | CD19, CD20, or cCD22 | 70 | 80 |
| Common | CD10 | 50 | 60 |
| Pre-B | cμ | 10 | 20 |
| T cell | CD5, CD7, or cCD3 with CD1, 2, 3, 4, or 8 | 25 | 17 |
| Myeloid co-expression | CD13 or CD33 (CD14, CD15)† | 20 | 15 |

*See references 71, 111, 123, 124, 127, 128, 158, 170, 174, 374, 404, 405, 409, 485.

†CD14 and CD15 alone do not define myeloid lineage.

CD, cluster designation; cCD, cytoplasmic cluster designation; SIg, surface immunoglobulin.

identified on a single cell, the case is designated mixed-lineage or biphenotypic acute leukemia. Biclonal (bilineage) leukemia demonstrates two separate cell populations with distinct phenotypes.[162] Multiparameter flow cytometry techniques that directly measure antigen co-expression and distinguish contaminating normal lymphocytes from leukemic cells should establish the true frequency and the clinical characteristics of mixed-lineage and biclonal ALL.

CD13 and CD33 are the most useful markers of myeloid lineage. Although in adult ALL, as many as 35% of cases express myeloid antigens,[163–166] the incidence of childhood ALL expressing myeloid antigens is less than 24%.[122, 163, 167–169] The co-expression of myeloid antigens in ALL is frequently found in infants.[170] Mixed-lineage ALL can be subclassified as B-myeloid or T-myeloid based on the lymphoid antigen expressed. B-myeloid ALL has presenting clinical and hematologic characteristics similar to those of B-lineage ALL, except that adult patients with B-lineage ALL may be somewhat younger. Rare cases of AML that stain positively for myeloperoxidase and Sudan black B lack typical myeloid antigen expression but express CD19.[171, 172] When cases of adult T-ALL were studied using uniparameter flow cytometry to infer co-expression of myeloid (CD13, CD33) and B antigens (CD19, CD20), 28% of cases expressed T and myeloid antigens (T+, My+, B-), 22% T and B antigens (T+, B+, My-), and 6% all three antigens.[173] The expression of myeloid markers in T-lineage ALL may be more common in the earlier stage of T-cell differentiation.[124, 174, 175]

**Immunoglobulin and T-Cell Receptor Gene Rearrangements.** The formation of functional Ig and TCR genes require rearrangement and juxtaposition of discrete segments of DNA. Individual germline segments recombine to form unique DNA sequences. For Ig genes, as part of each splicing step, nucleotides are removed from the junctions of these regions and new nucleotides (termed *N nucleotides*) are inserted.[176] These gene rearrangements are the initial steps lymphoid precursor cells follow during differentiation ultimately to produce proteins capable of recognizing the diversity of antigens they may encounter.[177] The genetic sequence produced by the recombined VDJ alleles with the intervening N nucleotides is known as the third complementarity-determining region (CDR III).[177–179] The light chain genes, kappa and lambda, rearrange after heavy chain genes.[180] Kappa chain genes usually rearrange prior to lambda genes.[181–183]

The T-cell receptor is somewhat homologous in its structure to the immunoglobulin gene.[184] Two heterodimers of subunits of the TCR genes are present on the surface of the T cell in association with the CD3 protein: TCR-$\alpha$/$\beta$ or TCR-$\delta$/$\gamma$.[180, 185–188] Rearrangements of the TCR loci lead to variable cytoplasmic and surface expression of their respective proteins.[189]

Clonal rearrangements of either IgH or TCR genes are present in virtually all ALL patients. IgH gene rearrangements characterize most B-precursor ALLs.[190, 191] TCR-$\beta$ and TCR-$\delta$ rearrangements are found in virtually all T-ALL.[192–196] However, IgH and TCR gene rearrangements are not lineage specific.[190] IgH rearrangements can be seen in AML and T-ALL, and TCR rearrangements can be seen in B-lineage ALL.[91, 194, 196–199] The rearrangement patterns in adult patients may be more immature than those seen in

children.[200] The small number of patients who have germline IgH and TCR genes appear to have an unfavorable outcome.[190] Different recombination patterns in TCR-$\delta$ may have prognostic importance.[201]

There is enormous diversity of genomic sequences created by immune receptor gene rearrangements. As a result, the individual DNA sequences can be viewed as specific for a given patient's leukemic clone. These rearrangements are detectable by Southern blot analysis when a clone expands to more than 1% of the population of cells tested.[202] Because many leukemia clones have a relatively limited repertoire of rearrangements, a small number of oligonucleotide primers can be used to amplify DNA from a leukemic patient using the polymerase chain reaction (PCR). The resulting DNA can then be used to prepare a clonospecific probe. The application of these techniques to study MRD is discussed later.

**Cytogenetics and Molecular Genetics.** The careful analysis of clonal chromosomal abnormalities, including translocations, has provided great insight into the pathobiology of ALL, and into the molecular changes involved in leukemogenesis of this diverse group of diseases.[203–205] Recurring cytogenetic abnormalities and molecular genetic changes define distinct subsets of ALL with distinctive morphologic and clinical features, response to treatment, and survival.[57, 206–212]

*Incidence of Cytogenetic Abnormalities.* The cytogenetics at diagnosis in childhood ALL have been studied in series of more than 1000 cases,[57, 213, 214] whereas few series of more than 150 adult patients have been reported.[207, 210, 212, 215–220] Both structural and numerical chromosome abnormalities are found. The frequency at diagnosis of the more common cytogenetic abnormalities in adult and childhood ALL is shown in Table 95–3. The relative frequencies of specific abnormalities differ between children and adults. The t(9;22)(q34;q11) is the most common abnormality in adults, occurring in 25 to 30%; it occurs in less than 5% of childhood cases.[214, 221, 222] Trisomy 21 occurs in 10 to 15% of adult patients, but about 30% of children. The t(1;19)(q23;p13), which occurs in approximately 5% of children with ALL, is rare in adults in the United States. Abnormalities of the short arm of chromosome 9 have been reported in some pediatric series to occur in about 10% of cases,[159] and in up to 15% of adults.[208] Abnormalities of

*Table 95–3.* **Frequency of Most Common Clonal Cytogenetic Abnormalities in ALL**[206, 213, 217, 223–225, 235]

| Cytogenetic Abnormality | Adults (%) | Children (%) |
|---|---|---|
| t(9;22)(q34;q11) or variant | 27 | 3–5 |
| Trisomy 21 | 10 | 30 |
| t(4;11)(q21;q23) or variant | 7 | 3 |
| Trisomy 8 | 7 | NA |
| Monosomy 7 | 6 | NA |
| t(8;14)(q24;q32) or variant | 6 | 2–5 |
| t(1;19)(q23;p13) | NA | 3–6 |
| Abnormalities of 12p11-p13 | 5 | 10–12 |
| Abnormalities of 14q11-q13 | 3 | 4 |
| del(9)(p13-p24) | 3 | 7–12 |
| Abnormalities of 14q32 other than t(8;14) | 3 | NA |
| del(6)(q13-q22) | 2 | 4–13 |

NA, not available.

11q23, 14q11, 6q, 12p, trisomy 8, monosomy 7, and t(8;14)(q24;q32) each occur in 3 to 10%.[207, 208, 212]

Ploidy is a distinctive cytogenetic feature in childhood ALL that may predict clinical outcome.[206, 216, 223, 224] Up to 40% of childhood ALL cases have pseudodiploid karyotypes (i.e., structural abnormalities but 46 chromosomes). Hyperdiploid cases with more than 50 chromosomes account for up to 30% of childhood ALL. Coexistent structural chromosomal abnormalities are seen in 62% of this group. Hyperdiploid cases with 47 to 50 chromosomes account for 15% of cases. Hypodiploidy is found in 8% of cases of childhood ALL.[206, 224, 225] The frequency of cytogenetically normal cases varies by series from 10 to 40%. Hyperdiploidy (>50 chromosomes) without structural abnormalities, which occurs in 30% of children, is much less frequent in adults and occurs in 2 to 5% of cases. The good prognosis found in children with hyperdiploid ALL has not been demonstrated convincingly in adult ALL with hyperdiploidy.[212, 220]

*Clinical, Hematologic, and Immunologic Associations with Cytogenetic Abnormalities.* Several of the primary chromosome abnormalities seen in ALL have been associated with distinctive clinical or hematologic features including presenting age, WBC count, FAB type, and immunophenotype (Table 95–4).[217, 226] Associations with response to therapy and survival are particularly striking, and will be discussed subsequently, along with other prognostic features. In general, specific cytogenetic syndromes are similar whether found in children or adults.

Philadelphia chromosome–positive ALL (Ph+ ALL) is defined by the presence of an abnormal chromosome 22 with a deletion of the terminal end of the long arm; the most common cytogenetic rearrangement is t(9;22)(q34;q11). Features associated with Ph+ ALL include older age, male preponderance, high WBC count, FAB L2 morphology, and a B-lineage phenotype.[221] More than one third of patients express myeloid antigens in addition to B-lineage antigens.[217] Expression of CD25 has been reported to occur more frequently in Ph+ cases than in other subtypes of ALL.[227]

The t(4;11)(q21;q23) in adults is associated with younger age. In childhood ALL, 30 to 60% of cases are found in infants.[228, 229] The majority of infants younger than 1 year of age with ALL possess this cytogenetic abnormality or its molecular correlate.[230, 231] Clinically cases are commonly female patients with high WBC counts and L1 predominance.[217, 228, 229] Patients with this chromosomal aberration

may have myeloid or stem cell features.[232] Most of these patients possess a CD19+, HLA-DR+, CD10- early B-lineage immunophenotype and many also express CD15.[128, 228, 233, 234] The t(11;19)(q23;p13) also is associated with a presentation in infants younger than 1 year old and is characterized by a high WBC count, organomegaly, CNS disease, a CD19+, HLA-DR+, CD10- early B-lineage immunophenotype and poor prognosis.[235]

The t(8;14)(q24;q32) or one of its variants [t(8;22)(q24;q11), t(2;8)(p12;q24)] is associated with older age, male predominance, frequent CNS involvement, a modestly elevated WBC count, expression of SIg, and L3 morphology.[217, 226]

The t(1;19)(q23;p13) is associated with a pre-B cell immunophenotype. It is found in 5 to 6% of pediatric ALL cases and makes up 25% of the pre-B cell cases in children.[122, 234] Different molecular breakpoint sites may have distinct prognostic importance.[236]

Associations between karyotype and immunophenotype have been recognized for many of the less common chromosome abnormalities (Table 95–5). Most of the data come from childhood series.[165, 206, 210, 225, 237, 238] Associations include t(1;19)(q23;p13) with a pre-B phenotype, rearrangements of 11q23 and 12p12 with B lineage, and rearrangements involving 14q11 and 7q32-36 with T lineage. Many of the chromosomal aberrations associated with T-ALL involve the loci of genes encoding the TCR. The TCR-α and -δ genes have been mapped to 14q11. Translocations involving 14q11 include t(1;14)(p32;q11),[239] t(10;14)(q24;q11),[240, 241] t(11;14)(p13;q11),[242] and t(11;14)(p15;q11).[243–245] Only the t(10;14)(q24;q11) is commonly seen in adults.[207, 217, 218] Approximately 25% of T-ALL cases have a normal karyotype.[218] Deletions of 6q, 9p, or 12p have not been found to correlate with a molecular or immunophenotypic subgroup of ALL.[223]

*Molecular Abnormalities Associated with Cytogenetic Findings.* Recurrent cytogenetic abnormalities found in ALL patients identify locations in the genome of potential target genes whose alteration may contribute to pathogenesis.[203, 206, 246]

With the development of positional cloning techniques, the identification of the genes involved in these chromosomal breakpoints has occurred rapidly. In addition, the application of sophisticated techniques such as PCR and fluorescence in situ hybridization (FISH) has revealed an

**Table 95–4.** Comparison of Clinical and Laboratory Features Associated with the More Common Primary Cytogenetic Abnormalities in Adult and Childhood ALL[206, 217, 425]

| Presenting Features | t(9;22) | t(4;11) | t(8;14) | t(1;19) |
|---|---|---|---|---|
| Relative age | Older | Younger* | Older | Children |
| Predominant sex | Male | Female | Male | Neither |
| WBC | High | Very high | Moderately elevated | Elevated |
| Percent blood blasts | High | High | Low | Intermediate |
| Predominant FAB type | L2 | L1, L2 | L3 | L1, L2 |
| Immunophenotype | B lineage | B lineage | B cell (SIg+) | B lineage |
| CD33 or CD13 expression | One third | 15 percent | No | No |
| DNA ploidy | | | | Normal |
| CNS involvement | 5% | 20% | 22% | 12% |

*Common in younger adults and infants. WBC, white blood cell count; FAB, French-American-British; CD, cluster designation; CNS, central nervous system; SIg, surface immunoglobulin.

| Chromosomal Aberration | Immunophenotype |
|---|---|
| t(2;8)(p12;q24) | B cell |
| t(8;14)(q24;q32) | B cell |
| t(8;22)(q24;q11) | B cell |
| t(1;11)(p32;q23) | B lineage |
| t(1;19)(q23;p13) | Pre-B, early pre-B |
| t(4;11)(q21;q23) | B lineage, My |
| t(5;14)(q31;q32) | B lineage |
| dic(7;9)(p13;p11) | B lineage |
| dic(7;12)(p11;12) | B lineage |
| t(8;14)(q11;q32) | B lineage |
| dic(9;12)(p11–12;p12) | B lineage |
| t(9;22)(q34;q11) | B lineage, rare T |
| t(10;11)(p14–p15;q22) | B lineage |
| t(11;19)(q23;p13) | B lineage, My |
| t(12;17)(p12–p13;q12) | B lineage |
| t(14;22)(q32;q11) | B lineage |
| t(17;19)(q21–22;p13) | Early pre-B lineage |
| t(1;7)(p34;q34) | T |
| t(1;14)(p32;q11) | T |
| t(7;9)(q34;q32) | T, ?B lineage |
| t(7;9)(q35;q34) | T |
| t(7;10)(q35;q34) | T |
| t(7;11)(q35;q13) | T |
| t(7;14)(q34–36;q11) | T |
| t(7;19)(q35;p13) | T |
| t(8;14)(q24;q11) | T |
| t(10;14)(q24;q11) | T |
| t(11;14)(p13;q11) | T |
| t(11;14)(p15;q11) | T |

expanding number of molecular rearrangements in leukemia. For example, the t(12;21)(p12;q22) was considered to be a relatively rare translocation. However, with the use of FISH and PCR techniques, the TEL-AML1 fusion gene has now been identified in approximately 30% of children with B-precursor ALL, although its incidence in adult ALL is low.[209, 247, 248]

Many of the target genes altered by the chromosomal translocations in ALL have now been identified. The function of some of these genes has been elucidated and their role in the pathogenesis of ALL is the focus of active study. Studies using mouse models have demonstrated that the genes involved in these translocations interfere with the normal regulation of hematopoiesis and may provide the stimulus for leukemic transformation.[138, 145]

Chromosome translocations in the acute leukemias most frequently affect genes that encode transcription factors, the critical regulatory proteins that control blood cell development.[249, 250] Translocation can juxtapose an intact transcription unit from one chromosome to an enhancer element from a gene on another chromosome, or form chimeric fusion proteins.[204] In ALL, the transcription unit is frequently translocated into the vicinity of genes encoding discrete chains of the immunoglobulin molecule or T-cell receptor, resulting in inappropriate expression of the translocated gene. For example, in the t(8;14) in B-ALL, the *myc* proto-oncogene translocates into the IgH locus, leading to the inappropriate expression of *myc*. However, the *myc* gene product is identical to the "wild type" protein. In general, the translocations involved in T-ALL are characterized by dysregulated expression of a gene.

Alternatively, chromosome translocations can disrupt two genes within their coding sequences, leading to the creation of a chimeric fusion protein. For example, the t(9;22) in ALL and CML results in the formation of a chimeric BCR-ABL fusion protein, which encodes a cytoplasmic protein containing the activated ABL tyrosine kinase domain. In general, translocations in B-lineage ALL result in chimeric fusion proteins.

### Chimeric Fusion Genes

***BCR/ABL and t(9;22).*** In a prospective study, pulsed-field gel electrophoresis and Southern blotting detected the BCR/ABL fusion gene in 30% of adult ALL compared with cytogenetic detection of the Ph chromosome in 23%.[251] Most cases (76%) were the p190 subtype.[251, 252] Using a more sensitive PCR assay, BCR/ABL chimeric products were detected in 43% of 179 newly diagnosed adult ALL patients.[253] The rearrangements were restricted to patients with B-lineage ALL and occurred in 55% of adults with cALL. The reciprocal gene product (ABL/BCR) also may be detected and may contribute to the biologic heterogeneity of Ph+ ALL.[254]

Experiments in mice using either retroviral transmission of the p210 and p190 BCR/ABL fusion genes or transgenic mice have clearly shown that the presence of the fusion gene leads to both myeloproliferative disease (CML) and ALL.[255, 256] It is not yet known whether structural differences in the p190 and p210 proteins correspond to functional differences in the leukemia cells. Both the p190 and p210 proteins, which are located on the cytoplasmic surface of the cell membrane, function in the transmission of growth regulatory signals from the cell surface to the nucleus via the RAS signal transduction pathway.[257, 258] Studies suggest that the BCR/ABL fusion protein also has an inhibitory role in mediation of apoptotic cell death.[259, 260]

It has been suggested that in CML, the BCR/ABL fusion gene affects a pluripotent hematopoietic stem cell, whereas in ALL it affects a more committed progenitor; however, definitive studies of the target cell for BCR/ABL transformation remain to be done. Patients with ALL and restriction of the BCR/ABL fusion gene to the lymphoblasts appear to have a shorter survival when compared with patients with BCR/ABL expression in both lymphoid and myeloid cells.[261] Interestingly, mice transplanted with cells transfected with the p190 BCR/ABL protein develop tumors more rapidly than those transplanted with p210 BCR/ABL.[262]

***The MLL Gene in Translocations Involving Chromosome Band 11q23.*** Translocations involving chromosome band 11q23 occur frequently in both ALL and AML. There are at least 30 different partner chromosomal sites involved in recurring reciprocal 11q23 translocations.[263] This exceeds the number of known translocations affecting the Ig loci and suggests that the 11q23 breakpoint region may contain genomically unstable sequences that lead to chromosomal recombination events. In ALL, the t(4;11) and the t(11;19)(q23;p13.3) occur predominantly. MLL gene translocations are the most frequent abnormality reported in ALL in infants and also occur commonly in therapy-related leukemias following exposure to chemotherapeutic agents that inhibit topoisomerase II.[264] As mentioned earlier, in ALL, these leukemias often express myeloid or monocytoid markers in addition to B-cell markers. The MLL gene was isolated from the 11q23 breakpoint by several groups and is referred to by other names including *HRX*, *ALL-1*, and *Htrx*.[265–268] MLL (myeloid-lymphoid or mixed-lineage leukemia) was so named because the rearrangements of MLL may affect a pluripotential stem cell or, alternatively, that disruption of MLL may affect a common differentiation pathway shared by lymphoid and myeloid progenitor cells.

In 11q23 translocations, the chromosomal breakpoints in both ALL and AML cluster within an 8.3-kb genomic region within MLL; therefore, all MLL gene rearrangements can be identified on Southern blot analysis using a single 0.74-kb *Bam*H1 cDNA fragment that contains the exons that span the breakpoint cluster region.[263] For this reason, Southern blot analysis has become a useful and sensitive tool for the identification of MLL gene abnormalities in clinical samples.[231, 269, 270]

Abnormalities of MLL have been associated with early treatment failure and poor survival.[269] Among patients with MLL rearrangements, the t(4;11) may confer a particularly poor prognosis,[231] and current recommendations include aggressive therapy, including allogeneic stem cell transplantation for this group of patients, as discussed in the treatment section of this chapter.

MLL encodes a large protein, with a predicted molecular weight of 430 kd, that contains two regions of extensive homology to the *Drosophila* trithorax gene.[271] The MLL protein contains transcriptional activation and repression domains.[272] A knockout mouse model shows that disruption of the MLL gene causes lethality at embryonic day 10.5.[273] MLL heterozygous mice exhibit growth retardation and skeletal malformations. These MLL knockout mice also have been demonstrated to have disrupted HOX gene expression, suggesting that MLL is a positive regulator of HOX gene expression. HOX genes, or homeobox-containing genes, play important roles in axial morphogenesis and patterning, and their expression in blood cell progenitors is tightly regulated and presumed critical to normal hematopoietic differentiation.[205] The disruption of the normal sequence of hematopoiesis mediated by HOX genes and other critical regulators of hematopoiesis may be one of the mechanisms by which MLL gene abnormalities contribute to leukemogenesis.

In ALL, two fusion genes, MLL/AF4 (FEL) and MLL/ENL, have been described as a result of the t(4;11) and t(11;19), respectively.[267, 274] Interestingly, the two partner genes that contribute their C-terminal sequences to the fusion, AF4 and ENL, share sequence homology; both encode serine- and proline-rich proteins containing nuclear localization sequences. Based on their structure, it has been suggested that the resultant fusion genes function as chimeric transcription factors.[275, 276] In a mouse model, retroviral bone marrow infection of the MLL/ENL fusion gene resulted in immortalization of the transduced cells, whereas transduction with either MLL or ENL alone was not sufficient to maintain proliferative capacity.[277] This mouse model provides persuasive evidence that the expression of MLL fusion genes contributes to leukemogenesis and that the partner genes are a critical component of this process.

***E2A/PBX1 and t(1;19).*** The t(1;19) results in fusion of the basic helix-loop-helix (bHLH) transcription factor E2A on chromosome 19 to the homeobox protein PBX1 on chromosome 1.[278–282] The fusion transcript occurs in 5 to 6% of all childhood ALL, and in up to 30% of pre-B ALL of childhood, although as noted earlier, it is less common in adult ALL.[206, 212] The E2A/PBX1 fusion protein causes transcriptional dysregulation of a number of candidate genes, and its ability to produce a lymphoid malignancy has been demonstrated in transgenic mouse models.[283] However, the specific target genes that are dysregulated by E2A/PBX1 and responsible for leukemic transformation have not yet been identified. A similar, but rare, translocation associated with precursor-B cell ALL, the t(17;19)(q21–22;p13), results in fusion of E2A to another transcription factor, HLF, that may have a role in regulation of apoptosis.[284]

***TEL/AML1 and t(12;21).*** The t(12;21)(p12;q22) is one of the most recently described translocations associated with ALL and fuses the Ets-related transcription factor TEL (ETV6) to the transcription factor AML1 (CBFA2).[247, 285] The TEL gene, like MLL, is rearranged in both lymphoid and myeloid malignancies through chromosomal translocation.[205] As mentioned earlier, the t(12;21) is not typically visible by routine cytogenetic analysis; however, using FISH, Southern blotting, or reverse transcriptase-PCR (RT-PCR), the molecular rearrangement is detected and is the single most common fusion gene identified in pediatric ALL, accounting for almost 25% of cases.[209] The TEL/AML1 fusion gene is rare in adult ALL, representing only about 3% of cases in retrospective analyses.[248, 286]

The TEL/AML1 fusion gene appears restricted to B-lineage ALL. The chimeric protein contains the first 336 amino acids of TEL and virtually the entire coding sequence of AML1, an oncogene that encodes one of the DNA-binding subunits of the transcription factor complex core-binding factor.[247] Disruption of one of the members of the core-binding factor complex by translocation occurs in both AML and ALL.[287] Transcriptional activation assays in cell culture systems suggest that TEL/AML1 may act as a dominant inhibitory protein, thereby blocking normal AML1 function[288, 289] Fusion proteins generated by these translocations are dominant repressors of genes regulated by the Runt-domain factors.[290, 291]

Another interesting observation about the TEL gene in patients with the t(12;21) has been made. In addition to one TEL allele being disrupted through fusion to AML1, the other TEL allele on the apparently normal (nontranslocated) copy of chromosome 12 is almost always deleted and thus results in complete loss of wild-type TEL function in the leukemic cells.[292] This double allele loss suggests a tumor-suppressor function for TEL.

***Breakpoints Within Immunoglobulin or T-Cell Receptor Genes.*** Several of the recurring chromosomal aberrations seen in ALL are associated with breakpoints that correspond to Ig or TCR gene loci. In the t(8;14)(q24;q32) and its variant translocations, t(2;8)(p12;q24) and t(8;22)(q24;q11), the IgH locus at 14q32, or the light chain loci, kappa at 2p12 or lambda at 22q11, are translocated to the proto-oncogene *myc* locus at 8q24.[39, 293–297] These three translocations result in constitutive activity of the *myc* gene, which encodes a bHLH protein that acts in the nucleus and appears to be involved in the regulation of the transition cells from a resting to a proliferative state, and may alter cellular proliferation.[298, 299] The pathogenetic role of deregulated *myc* expression in human Burkitt's lymphoma and B-cell ALL is supported by the induction of B-cell neoplasms in transgenic mice that carry the *myc* oncogene driven by an Ig gene enhancer.[298, 300]

Similarly, translocations or deletions at 14q11 at the TCR-α[301] and TCR-δ chain loci,[244] 7q35 at the TCR-β chain locus,[302] and 7p15 at the TCR-γ chain locus[303] have been identified[154] (see Table 95–5). The proto-oncogenes activated by chromosomal translocations involving the TCR loci can be assigned to 1 of 4 families of proteins: homeodomain (HOX11); bHLH, (TAL1/SCL, TAL2, LYL1, CMYC); LIM domain (RBTN1, RBTN2); or kinase (LCK).[242, 304] In the t(10;14)(q24;q11), the putative proto-oncogene HOX11 (TCL3) at 10q24 is rearranged with TCR-δ.[241] The HOX11 proto-oncogene is not transcribed in normal T cells, but its expression may be dysregulated by translocation of the TCR-δ constant region and its enhancer to the derivative chromosome 10.[305–309] This gene encodes a homeodomain protein that can bind DNA and transactivate transcription.[310] Similar to the other genes noted earlier, the gene is not expressed in normal T cells; therefore, the HOX11 protein may well activate target genes in T cells with a 10q24 translocation, contributing to leukemogenesis in T-ALL. The TCL-3 gene product may function as a nuclear transcription factor for G1 progression in the cell cycle.[311] Study of t(1;14)(p32;q11) led to the identification of a gene on chromosome 1 known as TAL1, SCL, or TCL5 that encodes a transcription factor with DNA-binding capacity. TAL1 rearrangements may also occur with the TCR-β locus on chromosome 7.[312] TAL1 rearrangements have been reported in up to 25% of childhood T-ALL cases but in fewer adult patients.[239, 304, 313–320] These rearrangements may involve a site-specific chromosomal deletion of a locus called *SIL* (for SCL interrupting locus).[314] TAL1/SCL expression may activate a specific set of target genes that are normally silent in T cells and contribute to leukemogenesis. In transgenic mouse models, inappropriately expressed TAL1/SCL can cause aggressive T-cell malignancies in collaboration with another transcription factor found in translocations involving the TCR in T-ALL, RBTN2.[321, 322] RBTN2 is a cysteine-rich zinc finger protein with a LIM motif, as is RBTN1, another member of this gene family involved in TCR translocations in T-ALL.[323] Both TAL1/SCL and RBTN2 are required for normal erythroid differentiation in mouse models. The TAL2 oncogene located at 9q34 encodes another bHLH phosphoprotein that is unable to directly bind to DNA but forms bHLH heterodimers with DNA-binding activity.[324] Two proteins with similar structure, RBTN1 located at 11p15 and RBTN2 located at 11p13, contain two cysteine-rich motifs that have been dubbed LIM domains.[242, 325] The alteration of these genes by translocation is hypothesized to alter transcriptional regulation of differentiation.[242]

**Tumor-Suppressor Genes.** A number of tumor-suppressor genes whose protein products suppress tumor formation in differentiating cells of a particular lineage have been identified within commonly deleted genomic regions. In ALL, a number of different tumor-suppressor genes have been implicated in the pathogenesis and progression of the disease. Many of these genes encode proteins involved in regulation of the cell cycle.

***p16 (CDKN2, MTS1, p16^INK4A).*** A candidate tumor-suppressor gene, p16, has been localized to chromosome 9p21, a frequent site of allelic loss in many human malignancies including ALL.[326–329] The p16 gene encodes a 156–amino acid protein that blocks progression through the cell cycle by binding to either cyclin-dependent kinase (CDK) 4 or 6

and inhibiting the action of cyclin D.[326, 327] The major function of D cyclins is to drive the cell cycle forward by binding to CDKs and forming a catalytically active complex that phosphorylates the retinoblastoma protein, which results in release of E2F and new transcription of important cell regulatory genes. Thus, the major biochemical effect of p16 is to halt cell cycle progression at the G1/S stage of the cell cycle. The loss of p16 function may lead to cancer progression by allowing unregulated cell proliferation. In vitro biologic studies of p16 suggest a regulatory role in cell senescence.[328, 330] p16 knockout mice develop normally into adulthood; however, these mice develop spontaneous tumors at an early age and are highly susceptible to tumorigenesis after treatment with chemical carcinogens and ultraviolet radiation.[331]

Homozygous deletions of p16 appear to be the most common mechanism of gene inactivation in both pediatric and adult patients with ALL, although transcriptional inactivation of p16 in adult ALL has also been reported as an alternative means of gene inactivation.[332–335] Deletions of p16 have been reported in as many as 25 to 40% of newly diagnosed ALL cases in adults and children and occur most frequently in T-ALL, in which the incidence may be as high as 90%.[336] Two other putative tumor-suppressor genes, p15 (MTS2, p15^ink4B) and p16β (which is the alternative transcript to p16), are also frequently inactivated by deletions occurring at the 9p21 locus in ALL.[337–339] The high incidence of p16 abnormalities implicates p16 inactivation in pathogenesis of ALL; however, no clear prognostic nificance has been noted when clinical outcomes of adult patients with and without a p16 abnormality are compared.[334, 340] The methylation pattern of p15 may be a useful diagnostic and prognostic tool in ALL.[341]

***Rb and p53.*** The Rb (retinoblastoma) gene located on chromosome 13q14 is a prototypic tumor-suppressor gene whose protein product, pRB, has a critical role in control of cell proliferation.[342] Deletions of Rb have been linked to the development of both hereditary and a wide variety of sporadic tumors, either through germline or acquired mutations. The main function of pRB is to act as a signal transducer connecting elements of the cell cycle with the transcriptional machinery of the cell. In ALL, pRB is inactivated in up to 64% of newly diagnosed adult cases and in a similar percentage of relapsed-refractory patients.[343] In most adult ALL patients, the mechanism by which the failed pRB expression is generated is unknown. In cytogenetic studies of a limited number of evaluable cases, no abnormalities of chromosome 13q were noted and Rb gene rearrangements were detected in only some of these cases.[343] Alternative explanations for pRB inactivation include the possibility that point mutations generate an unstable protein that is rapidly degraded, or that hypermethylation of the Rb gene promoter may reduce its expression.[344, 345]

Mutations of the p53 gene, located on chromosome band 17p13, have also been reported in ALL, although at a lower frequency than abnormalities of either p16 or Rb. In the largest series of p53 mutations in adults with ALL, 21% of newly diagnosed, and 42% of relapsed-refractory patients had a p53 mutation that was not accompanied by any identifiable cytogenetic abnormality of 17p.[343] Others have reported a correlation between p53 mutations and acute leukemias with rearrangements of the MLL gene.[346] In childhood

ALL, the frequency of p53 mutations has been reported less frequently than in the adult series[347]; p53 mutation or overexpression of the mdm-2 protein, which also results in p53 inactivation, has been linked to early treatment failure in ALL of children.[348] One proposed mechanism for the poor clinical outcome of this group of children is the finding that a p53 mutation, perhaps as a consequence of deregulated cell cycle control, correlates with amplification of the dihydrofolate reductase gene in patients with ALL and results in the acquisition of resistance to methotrexate.[349] The presence of p53 mutations correlates with drug resistance and poor outcome in a wide variety of malignancies.[350] In series of adults with ALL, however, no clear prognostic significance has been established regarding the presence of either p53 or Rb mutations.[343, 351] Some pediatric studies suggest a negative prognostic import of low levels of Rb expression.[352] Nevertheless, it is possible that inactivation or overexpression of a combination of these, or other tumor-suppressor genes, including BCL-2, with critical cell cycle regulatory and survival roles, may have an impact on response to treatment and survival in ALL.[353–356]

## CLINICAL FEATURES

Most patients with ALL present with signs and symptoms attributable to expansion of the leukemic clone in the marrow or extramedullary sites. Anemia may manifest as malaise, fatigue, weakness, pallor, tachycardia, or chest pain. Thrombocytopenia may result in ecchymoses, epistaxis, or petechiae. Neutropenia may lead to fever, chills, or other signs of infection. Up to 15% of patients may present with symptoms attributed to leukocytosis. The proliferation of leukemic cells may lead to hyperuricemia and an elevated lactate dehydrogenase level. Hepatosplenomegaly or adenopathy may be present at initial examination, but they are rarely symptomatic. Chest radiography reveals a mediastinal mass in up to 10% of cases, usually associated with a T-ALL.

The CNS is involved at diagnosis in 2 to 10% of patients, often without symptoms.[357–365] The diagnosis of CNS leukemia is made when the spinal fluid mononuclear cell count is greater than 5/μL with blasts identifiable on cytocentrifuge preparations.[366] An abnormal cytospin as an isolated finding, in the absence of cerebrospinal fluid pleiocytosis or elevated cerebrospinal fluid protein, is of uncertain significance but may define a group of patients with an increased risk of CNS relapse.[363, 364, 367]

## DIAGNOSIS

When the diagnosis of acute leukemia is suspected, rapid evaluation and initiation of appropriate therapy should follow. In addition to establishing the type of leukemia, initial studies should evaluate the overall functional integrity of the cardiovascular, pulmonary, hepatic, and renal systems. Suggestions for the appropriate evaluation at diagnosis are outlined in Table 95–6.

The major issues in making the correct diagnosis of ALL are to distinguish non-neoplastic proliferations of lymphoid cells and to exclude myeloid leukemias. If significant adenopathy is present, the diagnosis of high-grade lymphoma

**Table 95–6.** Diagnostic Evaluation of Patients with ALL

**History**
Family history of ALL
Occupational exposures
Tobacco or hair dye use
Symptoms of anemia or thrombocytopenia
Symptoms of infection
Headache, vision, and neurologic status

**Physical Examination**
Fundoscopy
Pallor
Tachycardia
Gingival and pharyngeal petechiae or infiltration
Adenopathy
Hepatosplenomegaly
Testicular masses
Thorough neurologic assessment

**Laboratory Studies**
CBC with differential
Chemistry profile
    Electrolytes, uric acid, calcium, phosphorus
    LDH, creatinine, hepatic enzymes
Coagulation studies
    PT, PTT, fibrinogen, fibrin split products
Chest radiograph
ECG
Cardiac ejection fraction by nuclear scan or echocardiogram
Lumbar puncture: cell count, glucose, protein cytology on cytospin
    preparation
Bone marrow aspirate and biopsy for
    Morphology
    Cytochemistry
    Cytogenetics
    Immunophenotype
    Molecular studies: BCR/ABL, IgH, TCR, ALL-1
HLA type if age <60
Blood type
Cytomegalovirus serology

ALL, acute lymphoblastic leukemia; CBC, complete blood count; LDH, lactate dehydrogenase; PT, prothrombin time; PTT, partial thromboplastin time; ECG, electrocardiogram; TCR, T-cell receptor; HLA, human leukocyte antigen.
From Frankel SR. In: Abeloff M, et al (eds). Clinical Oncology. New York: Churchill Livingstone, 1995.

must be considered; however, the distinction between ALL and lymphoblastic or Burkitt's lymphoma is largely semantic. By convention, if more than 25% of the marrow is involved with malignant lymphoid cells, the diagnosis of ALL is favored.

On occasion, the morphologic, cytochemical, and immunologic evaluation will suggest that both lymphoid and myeloid lineages are involved. Cases with strong myeloperoxidase or Sudan black B reactivity, or Auer rods, should be classified as AML despite morphologic features suggestive of ALL or the presence of lymphoid surface markers. Cases that fail to react with myeloperoxidase or Sudan black B, but express only myeloid surface markers, should be classified as AML-FAB M0.[368, 369]

## PROGNOSTIC FACTORS

Identification of groups of ALL patients with differing prognoses based on the biology of the malignant cell and clinical patterns of disease has altered therapeutic strategy. More than two decades ago, large clinical trials in childhood ALL adjusted therapy based on prognostic factors at diagno-

*Table 95-7.* Poor Prognostic Factors in Adult ALL

| Achievement of CR | CR Duration | Survival |
|---|---|---|
| Increasing age | Increasing age[387, 388, 432, 485, 500, 528, 529] | Increasing age[217, 485, 499, 527] |
| Elevated WBC[358, 378–380, 387, 388, 432, 446, 499, 527, 528] | Elevated WBC[378, 388, 446, 485, 499, 500, 528, 529] | Elevated WBC[217, 485] |
| B-cell phenotype[380] | Blast count[217, 380, 528] | Percent BM blasts[217] |
| | Marrow or blood | |
| Low albumin[378, 432] | Karyotypic abnormalities[216, 217, 378, 447, 485] | Karyotypic abnormalities[217, 485] |
| | Philadelphia chromosome | Philadelphia chromosome |
| | t(4;11) | t(4;11) |
| | Prolonged time to CR[358, 378, 388, 447] beyond 4–5 weeks of | |
| Hepatomegaly or splenomegaly[388, 528] | initiation of induction | Beta 2-microglobulin (β2M)>4 mg/l[530] |
| Undifferentiated morphology[432] | L2 subtype[378, 379, 499] | |
| | B-cell phenotype[378, 379] | |
| | Platelet count[485]<100×10⁹/L | Platelet count[485]<100×10⁹/L |

ALL, acute lymphoblastic leukemia; CR, complete remission; WBC, white blood cell count; BM, bone marrow.

sis.[370, 371] Treatment tailored to individual risk groups has dramatically improved the outcome in childhood ALL,[372, 373] and risk-adapted therapy is now being applied to adults.

Initial multivariate analyses of prognostic factors included only clinical features. As more sophisticated laboratory techniques became available, additional variables were examined, including immunophenotype, ploidy, and cytogenetic group. Clinical and biologic variables that have been reported in studies to correlate with achievement of complete remission (CR), CR duration, or survival in adult ALL are shown in Table 95–7 and event-free survival in childhood ALL in Table 95–8. These risk factors differ slightly between adults and children and may reflect the biologic differences in the subtypes of disease that present in the different age groups and the ability of older patients to tolerate intensive therapy.

Although the relative power of individual prognostic factors varies as a function of the therapy administered, several have been consistently identified as important in ALL. Two universal predictive factors are age and WBC count.[365, 370, 374–377] In pediatric ALL, children age 2 to 10 have a better outcome than do older children or infants.[374, 375] Remission duration is shorter for children with a higher WBC count, although the level varies by study (10,000, 50,000, 100,000).[374] DNA index, the presence of CNS disease, and either t(1;19) or t(9;22) have been added to stratify children into appropriate risk groups.[234] Risk factors that are consistently identified by multivariate analysis of outcome of large adult ALL trials are WBC count, age, and specific cytogenetic translocations, including t(9;22), t(4;11), and t(8;14). Time to achieve CR may be important as a variable for predicting the length of remission.

*Table 95-8.* Poor Prognostic Factors in Childhood ALL

Age <1 or >10 years[127, 373, 452, 454, 472, 476, 531]
Elevated WBC[127, 361, 373, 472, 476, 478, 531, 532]
Pseudodiploidy/hypodiploidy[127, 225, 361, 429, 436, 454, 478]
Karyotypic abnormalities[225, 423, 454]
    Philadelphia chromosome
    t(4;11)
CNS involvement[476]
T-cell immunophenotype[127, 476]
Male sex[373, 454, 478, 531]

ALL, acute lymphoblastic leukemia; WBC, white blood cell count; CNS, central nervous system.

**Immunophenotype.** Immunophenotype identifies subsets of ALL (i.e., T cell and mature B cell) that respond favorably when specific therapeutic agents or regimens are used. Because this technique can be applied successfully to virtually all patients presenting with ALL, widespread clinical use of flow cytometry at diagnosis of ALL is required.

The prognostic value of specific immunophenotypes has changed over time. Early studies demonstrated a lower CR rate and CR duration for patients with B-ALL (SIg⁺).[374, 378–380] When treated with new therapeutic approaches, outcome of this group of patients has markedly improved.[381–386] Similarly, adults with T-ALL formerly had inferior CR and disease-free survival (DFS) rates,[387] but with newer regimens the CR rate has improved so that it is better than that achieved in adult B-lineage ALL.[164, 388–392] Similar improvements in CR rate for T-lineage ALL in children have been reported.[170, 361, 393–395] The poor prognosis of T lineage may vanish when multivariate analysis is performed and more aggressive treatment regimens are used.[374, 396] Subgroups of B-lineage ALL have been defined in children, which may have prognostic importance. With less aggressive treatment regimens, as in the Pediatric Oncology Group (POG) ALinC 13 trial, children with pre-B ALL fared worse than those with early pre-B disease.[397] However, the outcome for patients with pre-B ALL who lacked the t(1;19) was not significantly different from that of children with early pre-B ALL.[234, 398] Patients whose blasts express CD20 fared more poorly in another large trial.[170]

Prognostic subgroups within adult T-ALL have been identified. The maturational stage of T-ALL may be prognostically important. The more mature T-lineage ALL cases have a better prognosis whether separated into ontogenic stage or based on number of T-lineage markers expressed.[164, 399] Thiel and coworkers classified adult patients with T-ALL into three immunophenotypic groups: pre-T (E-rosette⁻), thymocytic (CD1⁺), and mature T (CD1⁻).[153] Median CR duration was 17.2 months and median survival 24.6 months for the pre-T group compared with 34.2 months and 50.7 months, respectively, in the other two groups combined (p=0.02).[152, 153] Other studies confirm that adults with more immature T-lineage patterns (e.g., HLA-DR⁺ pre-T ALL, or T–stem cell phenotypes) do poorly.[124, 143, 175, 400] Expression of more than six T-lineage markers may have a favorable prognosis compared with T-lineage disease with fewer than three markers expressed.[164] The prognostic value of these subgroups is debatable in pediatric T-ALL.[395, 401–403] The prognostic role of CD10 (CALLA) expression is controversial.[374, 380, 391, 404–407] Particularly in children, the poor prognostic value of absent CD10 expression may lie in the association of this immunophenotype with adverse cytogenetic or other clinical characteristics.[164, 374, 401, 407] For example, in one study, half of the CD10⁻ B-lineage cases possessed an 11q23 breakpoint that appeared to account for their poor prognosis.[407] Although myeloid antigen expression was an adverse prognostic feature in earlier studies in adults and children,[163, 173, 408–410] this does not appear to be true with contemporary multiagent chemotherapy in adults or in children.[164, 167, 168, 170, 234, 411–414] In pediatric ALL, it has been suggested that the presence of CD34 is associated with improved event-free survival (EFS).[234, 415] Although most ALL cases are CD45⁺, those pediatric patients with CD45⁻ blasts appear to have a more favorable outcome.[116]

Immunophenotyping may identify distinct biologic subgroups of ALL and may be important even in the setting of multivariate analysis of prognostic factors.[374] However, the true importance of immunophenotypic analysis will require additional follow-up of patients studied using more sophisticated techniques that can identify prognostic subgroups within broad lineages.[234] Broad immunophenotypic subgroups are heterogeneous. In an analysis of the interaction of other prognostic factors in T-cell ALL, age 15 years or older, L2 lymphoblast morphology, abnormal karyotype, and membrane CD3 expression were found to confer an increased risk of treatment failure.[416]

**Karyotype and Molecular Genetics.** Cytogenetic abnormalities are among the most important factors for predicting the outcome of adult ALL.[207, 208, 210, 212, 215, 216, 406, 417, 418] The t(9;22) and t(4;11) are indicators of poor overall prognosis, reflected by short CR duration and survival even for patients treated with current intensive chemotherapy regimens.[208, 229, 418–420] In contrast, patients with the t(10;14) have durable remissions. Using multivariate analysis, karyotype adds prognostic significance to age when adults with the t(9;22) and t(4;11) are combined.[217, 252] In children, the Ph chromosome and t(1;19) have been reported as independent prognostic factors for poor outcome.[234, 421, 422] The presence of specific translocations, t(4;11) or t(9;22), have been reported to be associated with a relatively poor EFS.[423] The presence or absence of nonspecific translocations was not an independent predictor of EFS when effective intensive therapy was used.[423] Cases where the Ph chromosome is found only in lymphoid cells appear to have a shorter EFS than those where the pluripotent stem cell is involved.[424] Although t(1;19) was an adverse prognostic factor in patients treated with antimetabolite-based or nonintensive older treatment programs protocols,[398] EFS is 80% in more intensively treated patients.[425] Although children with t(4;11) may also fare poorly, most of these children would be considered at high risk of treatment failure based on the associations with hyperleukocytosis and infancy. In one study, 88% of children age 1 to 9 who had t(4;11) had durable remissions.[228] In one report, a dicentric translocation involving the short arms of chromosomes 9 and 12 in pediatric ALL was associated with an excellent prognosis.[426]

Adult patients with BCR/ABL recombination detected by PCR have been reported to have significantly shorter CR duration and survival. However, because these patients were also older and presented with high WBC count, PCR analysis did not add significantly to the prediction of treatment outcome.[253] Among patients with BCR/ABL recombination, the location of the breakpoint in BCR has not been associated with a difference in prognosis.[252, 253] Although children with variant translocations that are associated with BCR/ABL involvement may have clinical outcomes similar to those with the classic Ph chromosome, those children with variant translocations without BCR/ABL involvement may not have a poor outcome.[427]

Those structural aberrations commonly found as sole abnormalities in pediatric ALL have been reported to be associated with decreased EFS.[223] Probability of remaining in continuous CR (CCR) was more than 70% in patients without such structural karyotypic abnormalities but fell to less than 30% in patients with such structural aberrations.[223]

Ploidy as determined by flow cytometry DNA index may be complementary to standard karyotype analysis. DNA aneuploidy has been found to be associated with a low WBC count, pre-B immunophenotype, CD10 expression, female sex, age 2 to 10 and a low risk classification.[428] Although DNA aneuploidy studies cannot define the specific chromosomal aberrations, more samples are evaluable by this technique than by standard karyotyping.[428] Hyperdiploidy has been reported to be a favorable prognostic finding in childhood ALL.[423, 428, 429] Intensive treatment may abrogate the prognostic significance of cytogenetic ploidy in pediatric patients.[421] Furthermore, there is no significant difference in EFS among abnormal ploidy groups in childhood T-cell ALL.[430] Hyperdiploidy is not a favorable prognostic factor for adults because hyperdiploidy without structural rearrangements is rare in adults.[431] Hyperdiploid adults also frequently possess the t(9;22) translocation.[217]

**Prognostic Factors to Define Risk Groups.** Combinations of prognostic factors have been used to stratify patients into risk groups.[432] To predict CR duration and DFS, the German Multimodality ALL Group (GMALL) separated adult patients based on the number of the following adverse prognostic factors present: time to CR greater than 4 weeks, age older than 35 years, WBC count greater than 30,000/μL, and null ALL phenotype. Among patients with no adverse factors, the median CR duration has not yet been reached, and long-term DFS may reach a plateau as high as 60%, compared with a median CR duration of only 9.6 months and less than 10% long-term DFS in the poor prognosis group with two or three adverse factors.[388]

Combinations of risk factors have been applied to assign therapy for children with ALL.[234, 433–436] Most large pediatric cooperative groups and institutions have used age and WBC count as the initial basis for risk classification (Table 95–9). A uniform risk classification proposed at a 1993 National Cancer Institute–sponsored workshop separates children based on three age groups (<1, 1 to 9, >9 years) and WBC count (<50,000/mm³ or >50,000/mm³).[371] Using these criteria, standard-risk patients are defined as age 1 to 9 with a WBC count at diagnosis less than 50,000/mm³. These patients represent two thirds of B-lineage ALL patients and have an expected 4-year EFS of approximately 80%.[433] The Berlin-Frankfurt-Münster (BFM) group has used a risk factor index that includes blast count and extent of organomegaly.[437] In addition to these clinical factors, DNA index, early response to therapy, cytogenetics, immunophenotype,

*Table 95–9.* **Low-Risk Group Definitions for Childhood ALL**

| Group/Institution | Age and WBC | Other Requirements |
|---|---|---|
| Pediatric Oncology Group[127, 402, 429, 435] | 1–9 yrs with WBC <10,000/mm³; or 3–5 yrs with WBC <100,000 Any WBC if DNA index >1.16 | No CNS disease No t(9;22) or t(1;19) No T-cell ALL |
| Children's Cancer Group[439, 474] | 2–9 yrs with WBC <10,000 (if girl) 2–9 yrs with WBC <10,000 and platelets >100,000 (if boy) | No "lymphoma" syndrome |
| St. Jude Study XIII | Age 1–10 yrs with WBC <25,000 | No CNS leukemia No t(9;22) or t(1;19) DNA index ≥1.16; <1.60 |
| Dana-Farber[452, 475, 476] | Age 2–8 yrs with WBC <20,000 | Remission by day 31 No CNS leukemia No mediastinal mass No T-cell ALL No t(9;22) |

ALL, acute lymphoblastic leukemia; WBC, white blood cell count; CNS, central nervous system.

From Smith M. Towards a more uniform approach to risk-classification and treatment assignment for children with acute lymphoblastic leukemia. Am Soc Clin Oncol Educational Booklet 1994;124–30.

and CNS involvement may further modify risk. Children with hyperdiploid blast cells (DNA index >1.16) have a favorable prognosis.[428, 429] The rapidity of blast cytoreduction may also correlate with DFS.[438] Children with increased numbers of residual blasts in the bone marrow on days 7, 14, or 30 of therapy fare poorly.[434, 438, 439] The response of the blood blast count to prednisone by day 8 may also predict outcome.[440]

## Treatment

### CHEMOTHERAPY

Treatment of the newly diagnosed patient with ALL comprises four phases: remission induction, CNS prophylaxis, postremission consolidation or intensification, and maintenance. The initial goal is the induction of a complete remission. CR is defined as recovery of normal hematopoiesis (platelet count greater than 100,000/μL and neutrophil count greater than 1500/μL without circulating lymphoblasts) accompanied by bone marrow with a cellularity of greater than 20% and less than 5% blasts.[368] At the time of CR, it is assumed that residual leukemia cells persist because relapses occur in virtually all patients in the absence of further treatment. Postremission therapy usually includes a consolidation phase that is similar in intensity to induction therapy, or an intensification phase of greater dose intensity. The goal of these two phases is to include the most effective agents early to eliminate the leukemic population rapidly and possibly reduce the emergence of drug resistance. Specific CNS therapy is usually given shortly after achievement of CR to prevent recurrence in this sanctuary site. Finally, a prolonged maintenance phase using drugs at low-dose intensity is often

administered to eliminate residual leukemic cells that have survived induction and consolidation therapy.

Many different regimens are currently used to treat adult and childhood ALL. One trial schema representative of the current approach to the treatment of childhood ALL is outlined in Table 95–10. One adult regimen is shown in Table 95–11. A summary of the results of adult ALL trials appears in Table 95–12, and childhood ALL trials are summarized in Table 95–13. It can be seen that current therapy results in CR for most patients, with rates ranging from 58 to 88% in adults and more than 90% in children.[441] The efficacy of a given ALL treatment program is measured not only by its ability to induce CR but also by CR duration and overall survival. At best, only 40% of adult patients have long-term DFS, compared with 70% of children.

Comparisons between regimens reported in different studies must be interpreted with caution. Regimens using the same drugs may differ in the number of injections, dose, and mode of administration of chemotherapeutic agents. Studies also vary greatly in the composition of the patient population, so outcome must be evaluated for specific risk groups.

*Table 95–10.* **St. Jude Total Therapy XI Regimen for Childhood ALL[361, 363, 373, 473]**

| | Dose | Days |
|---|---|---|
| **Induction (8 weeks)** | | |
| Prednisone | 40 mg/m² PO | 1–29 |
| Vincristine | 1.5 mg/m² IV | 1, 8, 15, 22 |
| Daunorubicin | 25 mg/m² IV | 2, 8, ±15 |
| L-Asparaginase | 10,000 U/m² IM | 3, 4, 6, 8, 10, 12, ±15, ±17, ±19 |
| Teniposide | 200 mg/m² IV | 22, 25, 29 |
| Cytarabine | 300 mg/m² IV | 22, 25, 29 |
| Methotrexate | 12 mg* IT | 2, 22, 43 |
| Hydrocortisone | 24 mg* IT | 2, 22, 43 |
| Cytarabine | 36 mg* IT | 2, 22, 43 |
| Methotrexate† | 2 g/m² IV | 44, 51 |
| **Postremission for high-risk patients: (120 weeks) 4-week cycles** | | |
| Each pair of drugs rotated weekly | | |
| Week 1 | | |
| Etoposide | 300 mg/m² IV | Day 1 |
| Cyclophosphamide | 300 mg/m² IV | Day 1 |
| Week 2 | | |
| 6-Mercaptopurine | 75 mg/m² PO | Days 8–14 |
| Methotrexate | 40 mg/m² IV/IM | Day 8 |
| Week 3 | | |
| Teniposide | 150 mg/m² IV | Day 15 |
| Cytarabine | 300 mg/m² IV | Day 15 |
| Week 4 | | |
| Prednisone | 40 mg/m² PO | Days 22–28 |
| Vincristine | 1.5 mg/m² IV | Day 22 |
| **Postremission for standard-risk patients: (120 weeks) 4-week cycles** | | |
| Mercaptopurine | 75 mg/m² PO | Days 1–21 |
| Methotrexate | 40 mg/m² IV/IM | Days 1, 8, 15 |
| Prednisone | 40 mg/m² PO | Days 22–28 |
| Vincristine | 1.5 mg/m² IV | Day 22 |

*All doses were adjusted for children less than 3 years old.
†Given the leucovorin rescue as consolidation of remission treatment.
± Additional doses administered if blasts persisted.
IV, intravenously; IM, intramuscularly; IT, intrathecally.

*Table 95–11.* Cancer and Leukemia Group B Adult ALL Treatment Regimen 9111[411, 508]

**Induction**

| | | |
|---|---|---|
| Prednisone | 60 mg/m² PO | Days 1–21 |
| age >60 | | Days 1–7 |
| L-Asparaginase | 6000 U/m² | Days 4, 8, 11, 15, 18, 22 |
| Vincristine | 2 mg IV | Days 1, 8, 15, 22 |
| Daunorubicin | 45 mg/m² IV | Days 1–3 |
| age >60 | 30 mg/m² | |
| Cyclophosphamide | 1200 mg/m² IV | Day 1 |
| age >60 | 800 mg/m² | |

**Consolidation: Two Courses**

| | | |
|---|---|---|
| Cytarabine | 75 mg/m² SC | Days 1–4, 8–11 |
| Methotrexate | 15 mg IT | Day 1 |
| 6-Mercaptopurine | 60 mg/m² PO | Days 1–14 |
| L-Asparaginase | 6000 U/m² | Days 15, 18, 22, 25 |
| Vincristine | 2 mg IV | Days 15, 22 |

**CNS Therapy**

| | | |
|---|---|---|
| CNS irradiation | 2400 cGy | 12 fractions in 3 wks |
| Methotrexate | 15 mg IT | Day 1, 8, 15, 22, 29 |
| 6-Mercaptopurine | 60 mg/m² PO | Days 1–71 |
| Methotrexate | 20 mg/m² PO | Days 36, 43, 50, 57, 64 |
| TMP/SMZ* | 160 mg/800 mg PO BID | 3 Days per week |

**2 Weeks Off Therapy**
**Late "Intensification"**
Phase I

| | | |
|---|---|---|
| Dexamethasone | 10 mg/m² PO | Days 1–14 |
| Vincristine | 2 mg IV | Days 1, 8, 15 |
| Adriamycin | 30 mg/m² IV | Days 1, 8, 15 |

Phase II

| | | |
|---|---|---|
| Cyclophosphamide | 1000 mg/m² IV | Day 1 |
| Cytarabine | 75 mg/m² SC | Days 1–4, 8–11 |
| 6-Thioguanine | 60 mg/m² PO | Days 1–14 |

**2 Weeks Off Therapy**
**Maintenance†** *4-Week Cycles* *For 102 weeks*

| | | |
|---|---|---|
| 6-Mercaptopurine | 60 mg/m² PO | Daily |
| Methotrexate | 20 mg/m² PO | Weekly |
| Prednisone | 60 mg/m² PO | Days 1–5 |
| Vincristine | 2 mg IV | Day 1 |

*TMP/SMZ (trimethoprim/sulfamethoxazole) continues until end of maintenance.
†Maintenance continues for a total of 2 years of therapy.
ALL, acute lymphoblastic leukemia; IV, intravenously, SC, subcutaneously; IT, intrathecally.

**Remission Induction Therapy.** Vincristine and prednisone have served as the backbone of induction therapy for ALL. This combination induces CR in 85 to 95% of children and up to two thirds of adults.[442, 443] In adults, the addition of an anthracycline, daunorubicin, or doxorubicin increases the CR rate to between 72% and 92%.[357, 378, 442, 444–450] Pediatric trials have added asparaginase or an anthracycline as a third agent without changes in CR rate but with prolongation of remission duration.[451–453] Other active agents that are often added to induction regimens for adult ALL and high-risk childhood ALL include cyclophosphamide, cytarabine, methotrexate (MTX), thioguanine, and mercaptopurine (6-MP). Given the high remission rate for the combination of vincristine, prednisone, and asparaginase or an anthracycline, it has been difficult to demonstrate improvement with additional drugs.[454, 455] However, the actual dosage of daunorubicin delivered during induction may play a role in long-term DFS of adult ALL.[456] Most current trials continue to use four or more drugs for induction therapy in high-risk children and adults with the hope of improving DFS even if the CR rate is not improved.[452, 457]

Current studies in Cancer and Leukemia Group B

(CALGB) use the five-drug induction regimen shown in Table 95–11.[392, 411, 458, 459] This combination induces CR in more than 90% of adults.[460] GMALL has divided induction therapy into two phases to include more drugs at high dose. In the GMALL 01/81 trial, the first phase of induction included prednisone, vincristine, daunorubicin, and L-asparaginase, followed by a second phase with cyclophosphamide, cytarabine, MTX, and 6-MP.[457] This treatment plan induced CR in 74% of adults. Minor modification of this induction plan occurred in the subsequent trial GMALL 02/84 with similar results.[457, 461] Although the two-phase induction has not been directly compared with other four- or five-drug induction regimens, it sets a baseline for induction therapy in a large group of adults to which other approaches can be compared. These eight drugs are administered early in other adult trials.[462, 463]

It may be possible to improve the outcome of induction therapy, especially in adults, by administration of hematopoietic growth factors to ameliorate the myelosuppression of intensive multiagent chemotherapy. The routine addition of granulocyte colony–stimulating factor (G-CSF) during induction reduces the intensity and duration of neutropenia and allows increased delivery of chemotherapy on schedule.[458, 464–466] Administration of G-CSF during induction has also been shown to decrease the death rate and reduce the number of hospital days.[458] However, in this study, growth factors did not shorten the time to complete induction and early consolidation, thus negating its ability to allow further intensification of currently used induction therapies in ALL. This study did demonstrate a reduced rate of death during induction for elderly (age >60 years) ALL patients (5% vs. 31%), an area highly exploitable to intervention.

Although a single dose of L-asparaginase given during induction of adults with ALL failed to demonstrate improvement in either CR rate or overall survival, different dose schedules and types of asparaginase remain under study.[455] No difference in outcome was seen in a retrospective analysis of number of doses of asparaginase received in adult ALL.[467] Optimization of *Escherichia coli*–derived L-asparaginase pharmacokinetics with prolonged asparagine depletion combined with improvements in the toxicity profile has been made possible using the polyethylene glycol conjugate form of this agent. Phase II studies with the polyethylene glycol form of *E. coli* L-asparaginase have been completed by the CALGB[459] and others. However, before substitution of this agent occurs in standard treatment regimens, extended follow-up will be needed to ensure similar long-term outcomes with historical control series.

Another approach has been to intensify the dose or type of anthracycline administered during induction therapy. Use of idarubicin has yielded high CR rates (85%) in a large phase II study.[468] Phase II studies of intensified daunorubicin induction in adult ALL patients have noted promising results.[469] Another approach has been to intensify anthracycline dose with high-dose cytarabine and delay the use of vincristine and prednisone.[470, 471] At present, data strongly support the inclusion of an anthracycline such as daunorubicin into the initial induction schema of adult ALL patients. Current CALGB phase II trials have used a starting dose of 60 mg/m² of daunorubicin given for 3 days and escalated to 80 mg/m²/day.

In pediatric ALL, the goal of current therapy is not

*Table 95–12.* **Recent Results of Chemotherapy in Adult ALL**

| Group[ref.] | No. | Median Age | CR% | Median CR (mo.) | Median Survival (mo.) | Relapse-Free Survival @60 mo. | Overall Survival @60 mo. |
|---|---|---|---|---|---|---|---|
| Bay Area LSG[447] | 109 | 25 | 88 | 37 | | 35% | 40% |
| EORTC ALL-2[445, 533] | 106 | 27 | 74 | 32 | 28 | 40% @ 84 | 30% @ 84 |
| HDAC arm | 50 | | 74 | 58 | | 55% | 40% |
| SAKK 33/86[500] | 63 | 27 | 81 | 32 | | 40% @ 36 | |
| Verona[456] | 88 | 33 | 79 | 32 | 11 | 24% | 26% |
| MSKCC[432, 497] | 199 | | 81 | 28 | 30.7 | 35% | 31% |
| CALGB 8811[411]* | 199 | 32 | 85 | 28 | 32 | 43% @ 36 | 50% @ 36 |
| GATLA-GLATHEM ALL-82[527] | 145 | 29 | 78 | 28 | 34.0 | 34% | 35 |
| GMALL 02/84[457, 461] | 569 | 28 | 75 | 27 | 26 | 39% @ 84 | 36% |
| GMALL 01/81[457, 461] | 368 | 25 | 74 | 24 | 26 | 35% @ 120 | 33% @ 132 |
| SWOG 8001[446] | 168 | 28 | 68 | 23 | 18 | | 26% |
| MDAC[378] | 105 | 30 | 84 | 22 | 19 | 40% @ 36 | 32% @ 36 |
| CALGB 8011[358] | 277 | 33 | 64 | 21 | 16 | 29% | 25% |
| GIMEMA 0288[496] | 343 | 30 | 84 | 20 | NA | 45% @ 26 | NA |
| GIMEMA 0183[499] | 358 | 31 | 79 | 19 | 21.7 | 21.9% @ 50.6 | 29.4% @ 55 |
| CALGB 8513[498] | 164 | 31 | 64 | 19 | 11.2 | 32% @ 36 | 20% @ 36 |
| FGTALL[485] LALA87 | 467† | 33 | 76 | 17 | 18 | 37% @ 36 | 37% @ 36 |
| Age 15–50 | 96† | | | | 20 | 28 | 32% @ 36 | 42% @ 36 |
| Age >50 | 58‡ | | | | 14 | 22 | 24% @ 36 | 28% @ 36 |
| ECOG 3486[482]§ | 125 | 32 | 58 | 11 | | 35% @ 24 | |
| GATLA-GLATHEM ALL-79[527] | 137 | 30 | 80 | 10 | 14.0 | 20% | 22% |
| ECOG 2483[482] | 89 | | | | | | |
| EORTC ALL-3[533] | 120 | 31 | 78 | | | | |
| High risk | 91 | 40 | 75 | | | 45% @ 36 | 32% @ 36 |
| Sweden[463] | 113 | 38 | 77 | | | 37–60% @ 14¶ | |
| MRC UKALL XA[534] | 621 | 26 | 84 | | | 29% | |
| JALSG ALL-87[535] | 117 | 38 | 81 | | | % @ 27 | 21% @ 27 |
| SWOG 8417[536] | 354 | | 64 | | | 25% | 29% |

*Larson RA, personal communication.
†Results for all patients including bone marrow transplantation (BMT).
‡Patients who received only chemotherapy without BMT.
§Best arm only.
¶Range for standard- and high-risk patients.

ALL, acute lymphoblastic leukemia; CR, complete remission; CALGB, Cancer and Leukemia Group B; ECOG, Eastern Cooperative Oncology Group; EORTC, European Organization for Research and Treatment of Cancer; FGTALL, French Group on Therapy for Adult Acute Lymphoblastic Leukemia; GATLA-GLATHEM, Argentine Group for Treatment of Acute Leukemias, Latin American Group for Treatment of Malignant Hemopathies; GIMEMA, Gruppo Italiano Malattie Ematologiche Maligne dell'Adulto; GMALL, German Multicenter ALL Group; JALSG, Japanese Acute Leukemia Study Group; MDAC, M.D. Anderson Cancer Center; MRC, Medical Research Council; MSKCC, Memorial Sloan-Kettering Cancer Center; SAKK, Swiss Group for Epidemiologic and Clinical Cancer Research; SWOG, Southwest Oncology Group.

solely to maintain the high cure rates achieved by intensive regimens but also to diminish serious acute and long-term toxicity. To that end, the POG treated children with standard-risk ALL with induction therapy composed of vincristine, prednisone, and asparaginase and with triple intrathecal chemotherapy (MTX, hydrocortisone, cytarabine). Four different intensification regimens were used composed of varying doses of MTX, L-asparaginase, and cytarabine. Continuation therapy comprised 6-MP and MTX with vincristine plus prednisone pulses. Patients with T-cell or B-cell ALL or infants younger than than 1 year were treated on separate, very intensive, multiagent therapy protocols. With this approach, which spares the majority of children exposure to alkylating agents, anthracyclines, epipodophylotoxins, and irradiation, the 4-year EFS for all patients was 66%.[127]

**Postremission Therapy.** The addition of either increased doses of drugs used in induction or the addition of non–cross-resistant new agents termed *intensification* or *consolidation* is required to prolong the EFS in most patients. Other approaches to initial postremission therapy include continuing low-dose therapy over several weeks, periodic pulses of MTX with or without other agents, concentrating a group of drugs into a 5-day block, or use of complex rotating schedules.

The choice and dose of drugs for initial postremission therapy may vary by risk group. However, a 20% decrease in EFS that occurred when an intensification phase was omitted for low-risk children suggests that even this group requires this type of therapy.[437] Repeated intensifications may prolong EFS beyond that achieved by a single course of therapy. The strategy of early and late intensification at 5 and 20 weeks using daunorubicin, cytarabine, etoposide, vincristine, prednisolone, and thioguanine administered over 5 days was superior to either no intensification or only early or late intensification.[472]

The St. Jude Study XI delivered the seven-drug induction regimen shown in Table 95–10 to all risk groups. Low-risk children were treated with prednisone, vincristine, MTX, and 6-MP maintenance, whereas high-risk children were stratified to delivery of drug combinations rotated either weekly or every 6 weeks. This approach yielded a 5-year EFS of 72% but only a 51% EFS in children with T-cell disease.[473] The Children's Cancer Group Study 106 demonstrated that high-risk patients benefit from intensive therapy, which includes improved consolidation and intensification.[474] A two-phase induction, which included an initial administration of vincristine, prednisone, daunorubicin, and L-asparaginase followed by cyclophosphamide, cytarabine,

*Table 95–13.* **Results of Selected Childhood ALL Trials**

| Group(ref) (dates of study) | No. of Children | CR | Event-Free Survival Rate |
|---|---|---|---|
| Dana-Farber 85-01 (1985–1987)[476] | 220 | 99% | 78% @ 7 yrs |
| Dutch (1984–1988)[71] | 291 | | 73% @ 5 yrs |
| BFM 86[393, 440] | 998 | 99% | 72% @ 5 yrs |
| Dana-Farber 81-01 (1981–1985)[452, 479] | 289 | | 72% @ 7 yrs |
| St. Jude Study XI (1984–1988)[373, 473] | 358 | 97% | 71% @ 5 yrs |
| CCG 100 series (1983–1989)[71] | 3712 | | 66% @ 5 yrs |
| MRC UKALL X (1985–1990)[472] | 1614 | NA | 66% @ 4 yrs |
|   Double intensification arm | | | 75% |
| POG protocols (1986–1990) risk-stratified trials[127] | 2404 | NA | 66% @ 4 yrs |
|   B precursor | | | 72% |
|   T-ALL | | | 50% |
|   B-ALL | | | 60% |
| Infants | | | 16.5% |
| TCCSG L84-11 (1984–1989)[71, 593] | 490 | 97% | 64% @ 7 yrs |
| BFM 83 (1983–1986)[537] | 677 | 96% | 64% @ 7 yrs |
| AIEOP ALL82, ALL87, ALL88 (1982–1990)[71, 538] | 2010 | | 62% @ 5 yrs |
| CCG-106 (1983–1987)[474] | 477 | 95% | 61% @ 7 yrs |
| FRALLE 83 (1983–1987)[493] | 559 | 93% | 57% @ 7 yrs |
|   Low risk | 120 | 99% | 64% |
|   Intermediate risk | 265 | 94% | 56% |
|   High risk | 174 | 89% | 49% |
| GATLA/GLATHEM[539] (1984–1987) | 703 | 89% | 49% @ 5 yrs |
|   Good risk | 240 | 90% | 52% |
|   Intermediate risk | 324 | 87% | 48% |
|   Poor risk | 139 | 91% | 44% |

ALL, acute lymphoblastic leukemia; NA, not available; CR, complete remission; BFM, Berlin-Fraukfurt-Münster; CCG, Children's Cancer Group; MRC, Medical Research Council; POG, Pediatric Oncology Group; TCCSG, Tokyo Children Cancer Study Group; AIEOP, Associazione Italiana Ematologia Oncologia Pediatrica; FRALLE, ; GATLA/GLATHEM, Argentine Group for Treatment of Acute Leukemias, Latin American Group for Treatment of Malignant Hemopathies.

and mercaptopurine similar to that shown in the CALGB regimen in Table 95–11, resulted in a 7-year EFS of 63% compared with only 47% for children treated with vincristine, prednisone, L-asparaginase induction without intensification.[474] A 71% EFS for higher risk children was achieved by the Dana-Farber group using MTX, doxorubicin, vincristine, and prednisone induction followed by intensive asparaginase therapy.[452] Subsequent BFM trials and trials from Boston have resulted in similar EFS for high-risk children.[475, 476] The POG found that a four-drug induction followed by 30 weeks of intensification using alternating drug pairs including MTX, intravenous 6-MP, leucovorin, daunorubicin, cytarabine, and teniposide for patients with high-risk childhood ALL resulted in a 55% EFS at 4 years.[435] Infants appear to benefit particularly from intensified remission induction therapy and intensification with high-dose MTX and cytarabine.[476]

Multiagent intensification may not be required for standard-risk childhood ALL. A less aggressive, relatively innocuous approach using pulses of intravenous 6-MP and MTX produced an EFS of 94% at 4 years and 82% at 7 years.[436, 477] When a similar drug regimen was used for higher risk patients, the 4-year EFS was 57%.[436] The use of high-dose methotrexate (HDMTX) without cranial irradiation for patients with standard-risk childhood ALL resulted in a 64% 9-year EFS compared with 52% of those who received cranial irradiation and alternating regimens of doxorubicin-cyclophosphamide and teniposide-cytarabine ($p = 0.03$).[478] The role of HDMTX (6 to 8 g/m²) as systemic consolidation and CNS prophylaxis is undergoing evaluation in the UKALL XI trial.[472] HDMTX may be an effective induction agent when given at the beginning of therapy.[479]

Although pediatric ALL trials have established superior

long-term EFS compared with trials conducted in the 1980s, the majority of patients relapse, even when consolidation therapy is given. One approach in adult ALL and high-risk childhood ALL has been to intensify postremission treatment. Dose intensification may overcome inherent or acquired drug resistance, and increased drug delivery may allow penetration into sanctuary sites such as the CNS and the testes. The potential therapeutic gains from intensive therapy must be weighed against the increased toxicity. The presence of adverse prognostic factors can be used to identify patients for whom aggressive postremission therapy is justified. The optimal balance between efficacy and toxicity has yet to be established. Thus, children with ALL should continue to be enrolled in clinical trials.

Postremission intensification may consist of chemotherapy either alone or with marrow transplantation. For adults, the consolidation program used in the GMALL 1/81 trial serves as a good standard for comparison of newer approaches attempting to improve postremission therapy. The GMALL consolidation phase included two regimens: the first consisted of dexamethasone, vincristine, and doxorubicin and the second consisted of cyclophosphamide, cytarabine, and thioguanine. Mediastinal irradiation was delivered to patients with mediastinal tumors. Median CR duration was 24 months, and probability of CCR at 10 years was 35%. Overall survival was 33% at 11 years.[388, 457, 461, 480]

GMALL Protocol 02/84 added four nonintensive consolidation cycles of VM26 and cytarabine twice weekly for 4 weeks for high-risk patients (CR >4 weeks, age >35 years, WBC count >30,000, non-T or cALL immunophenotype).[457] The addition of the VM26/cytarabine consolidation tended to improve outcome in the high-risk subgroup.[481] For patients age 36 to 50, the CCR rate at 7 years rose from 22% to

38%, and similar improvement in CCR was seen in the 51- to 65-year group.

GMALL 03/87 administered VM26 and cytarabine to all patients and added high-dose cytarabine (HDAC)/mitoxantrone intensification for high-risk patients as defined in GMALL 02/84. Preliminary results suggest a slight improvement in outcome compared with GMALL 02/84.[481] The CCR rate was 43% at 4 years for the high-risk patients who received the HDAC/mitoxantrone, with DFS at 3 years of nearly 50%.[461] Unfortunately, even with an attenuated cytarabine dose of 1 g/m², only 49% of patients older than age 50 could receive the planned intensification therapy.[481] HDAC intensification may benefit some poor prognosis groups but increases toxicity and early mortality without long-term benefit in good-risk patients and high-risk patients with advanced age.[482, 483]

GMALL 04/89 assigned treatment based on a different grouping of prognostic factors than used in previous GMALL trials. Immunophenotype, presence of the Ph chromosome, WBC count greater than 30,000, and time to CR more than 4 weeks were used to define a high-risk group among patients 50 years or younger. Patients with null or myeloid antigen–positive ALL were considered high risk, as were patients age 36 to 50 with cALL phenotype. High-risk patients were randomly assigned to receive intensification therapy with either HDAC/mitoxantrone or HDMTX/L-asparaginase. To avoid excessive toxicity, all patients older than age 50 were treated with VM26/cytarabine rather than the preceding intensification, as were patients who had a T-ALL phenotype or a cALL phenotype and age younger than 36 years.[461] The CCR rate at 3 years for patients older than age 50 improved to 31% with the VM26/cytarabine regimen. There was no significant difference between the HDAC/mitoxantrone and the HDMTX/L-asparaginase regimens for high-risk patients.

Despite dose intensification as delivered by even the best of the published regimens, the relapse rate for adult ALL remains high. Patients should continue to be enrolled in clinical trials testing new agents or drug combinations as postremission therapy.

The role of allogeneic bone marrow transplantation (BMT) as intensification therapy is under investigation by several large cooperative groups including CALGB, the Eastern Cooperative Oncology Group, the Medical Research Council,[484] the French Group on Therapy for Adult Acute Lymphoblastic Leukemia,[485] and the European Organization for Research and Treatment of Cancer. Patients without donors are randomized to receive either autologous BMT or postremission chemotherapy.

**Central Nervous System Therapy.** The approach to CNS-directed treatment has been derived largely from the extensive experience reported in children. The interaction between systemic and CNS-directed therapy combined with lack of randomized trials for which CNS-directed therapy is the only variable clouds the assignment of a best treatment approach.[486] Cranial irradiation combined with intrathecal MTX has been the most widely used regimen and remains the standard with which newer approaches should be compared. Therapy is modified by the patient's risk group and body habitus. The cumulative incidence of CNS relapse in 518 children (excluding SIg⁺ ALL) treated with cranial irradiation and intrathecal MTX was 6%—2.5% in the stan-

dard risk group and 8.2% in the high-risk group.[487] The incidence of CNS relapse in adults has been as high as 50%.[488] CNS prophylaxis using intrathecal MTX and 24 Gy of cranial irradiation decreases the risk of CNS relapse in adults to less than 20%.[358, 489] The type and intensity of systemic chemotherapy administered alters the incidence of CNS relapse irrespective of the specific CNS therapy delivered.[490] More aggressive systemic therapy, when combined with this intrathecal MTX and cranial irradiation, has reduced the incidence of CNS leukemia to 10%.[358] The use of more intensive induction and postremission therapy also appears to reduce the frequency of CNS relapses, even without administration of CNS prophylactic therapy.[360] Prophylactic treatment with 18 Gy of cranial irradiation is equally efficacious as higher doses.[476]

Cranial irradiation combined with intrathecal chemotherapy may result in late neurologic sequelae in children[491]; the effect on adults is uncertain.[492] Pediatric cooperative groups have evaluated the replacement of cranial irradiation with systemic or intrathecal chemotherapy in an attempt to reduce neurotoxicity. Alternative strategies for CNS prophylaxis have included intrathecal MTX alone, triple intrathecal chemotherapy (MTX, cytarabine, and hydrocortisone), intrathecal MTX with intermediate- to high-dose systemic MTX or cytarabine, or systemic chemotherapy using high doses of MTX or cytarabine.[366, 490]

Intermediate doses of parenteral MTX appear ineffective in substituting for cranial irradiation or intrathecal therapy in the absence of other intensive systemic therapy in two pediatric trials.[437, 493] Triple intrathecal therapy without cranial irradiation appears to be effective CNS prophylaxis for children who are not in high-risk groups.[366, 494] Cranial radiation also may be unnecessary for low-risk pediatric patients when aggressive systemic and intrathecal therapies are administered.[495]

The best regimen for CNS prophylaxis in adults is uncertain. Intrathecal and intraventricular MTX without cranial irradiation may allow for as low as a 5% CNS relapse rate.[357] Italian trials indicate a 4% CNS relapse rate after prophylactic treatment with intrathecal MTX and intermediate doses of systemic MTX without CNS irradiation.[496] HDAC without other CNS therapy also resulted in only a 4% incidence of CNS relapse.[482] In the absence of CNS prophylaxis, even "low-risk" patients had greater than a 10% incidence of CNS relapse.[360]

**Maintenance Therapy.** The optimal drugs, dose, and duration of maintenance therapy remain to be established. The maintenance phase typically consists of daily 6-MP and weekly MTX for 18 to 36 months, often with the addition of periodic vincristine and prednisone pulses. A more intensive maintenance scheme adds cycles of doxorubicin, carmustine, and cyclophosphamide for at least 2 years.[497] Evaluation of different approaches is difficult because few randomized trials have examined alternative maintenance regimens without changes in other aspects of therapy. Results favor the use of maintenance therapy combined with consolidation over consolidation alone.[482, 498] Maintenance therapy of 3 years' duration was no better than only 2 years' duration in children.[454] If intensive induction and postinduction therapies are used, maintenance may not be necessary[499, 500]; however, maintenance therapy probably should continue to be given until prospective trials show otherwise.

**Treatment of B-Cell Acute Lymphoblastic Leukemia.**
When adults and children with B-cell ALL were treated with standard ALL protocols, long-term survival was virtually nonexistent.[501, 502] The poor outcome motivated the investigation of alternative approaches based on Burkitt's lymphoma remission induction regimens. Studies in childhood B-cell ALL incorporating high doses of cyclophosphamide, MTX, and cytarabine in addition to vincristine, dexamethasone or prednisone, ifosfamide, doxorubicin, and vincristine-prednisone (VP)-16 or vinblastine-mitomycin (VM)-26 led to CR rates of better than 80%.[381, 382, 503] Although CNS irradiation was included in the early studies, the use of triple intrathecal chemotherapy in combination with HDAC and high-dose cyclophosphamide appears to offer adequate CNS prophylaxis. DFS has been better than 40% and approaches 80% in more recent pediatric trials.[381, 382, 503, 504] The presence of residual disease after the first two courses has correlated with an increased risk of therapy failure. Most relapses occur while patients are still receiving therapy or shortly thereafter. Thus, repeated courses of intensive therapy delivered within a 4-month period are highly effective in the treatment of childhood B-cell ALL.

The treatment approaches pioneered in childhood B-cell ALL have been successfully applied to adults.[389, 505] Using the BFM B-NHL 86 protocol (shown in Table 95–14), 71% of adults achieved a CR with a 44% 5-year survival.[461] It is now recommended that all adult and childhood ALL patients with L3 morphology, expression of SIg, or t(8;14)(q24;q32) or its variants be treated according to protocols designed specifically for this subtype.

Dose-intensive therapy using allogeneic BMT has also been successful in the treatment of L3 ALL.[506] However, given the marked improvement in EFS with newer chemo-therapy regimens, deferring allogeneic BMT until first relapse or second remission (CR2) may be preferable.

**Treatment of T-Cell Acute Lymphoblastic Leukemia.**
Pediatric patients with T-cell ALL should be treated with intensive regimens.[476] Cranial irradiation should be included in the treatment plan because of a 15% frequency of CNS relapse when this modality is omitted.[361, 507] Adults with T-ALL require multiagent intensive induction and postremission regimens that include cyclophosphamide, cytarabine, MTX, and L-asparaginase. Only 39% of adults with T-ALL treated on trials that did not include the use of cyclophosphamide and L-asparaginase during induction therapy entered remission. With the addition of these two agents, the CR rate increased to 82%, and DFS improved to 45 to 60% in the German trials summarized in Table 95–13.[390] Similarly, the CALGB five-drug induction regimen (see Table 95–11) raised the CR rate for T-cell ALL from 67 to 93%.[411, 508]

**Treatment of Ph⁺ Acute Lymphoblastic Leukemia.**
The patient with Ph⁺ ALL currently poses the greatest problem in the treatment of ALL, especially in adults. Although CR can be achieved in up to 80% of patients with contemporary regimens, the median CR duration is generally less than 1 year, with less than 10% surviving leukemia-free at 5 years.[216, 217, 509–512] To date, allogeneic BMT is the only postinduction therapy that has consistently improved long-term DFS, at least in adults.[509] For patients with an HLA-matched donor, allogeneic BMT offers prolonged DFS for as many as 40 to 50%.[513–516] Although there is general agreement that allogeneic BMT should be performed in first CR if an HLA-compatible donor is available, transplantation in relapse or subsequent remission also may be curative. Second remissions are often difficult to achieve, however, because these patients may be refractory to salvage chemo-

*Table 95–14.* **BFM B-NHL 86 for Adult B-ALL**[382, 389]

| **Cytoreductive prephase** | | |
|---|---|---|
| Prednisone | 60 mg/m² PO | Days 1–5 |
| Cyclophosphamide | 200 mg/m² IV | Days 1–5 |
| **Course A** | | |
| Vincristine | 2 mg IV | Day 1 |
| Ifosfamide | 800 mg/m² IV | Days 1–5 |
| Mesna | 200 mg/m² IV | q4h×3, days 1–5 |
| Methotrexate | 1.5 g/m² IV | Day 1 by infusion over 24 hours; 150 mg/m² given as a loading dose over 30 minutes |
| Leucovorin | 50 mg/m² | 12h post MTX |
| | 12 mg/m² | Continue q6h until [MTX]<5×10⁸ M |
| Dexamethasone | 10 mg/m² PO | Days 1–5 |
| VM-26 | 100 mg/m² IV | Days 4–5 |
| Cytarabine | 150 mg/m² IV | Days 4–5 q12h |
| **Course B** | | |
| Vincristine | 1.5 mg/m² IV | Day 1 |
| Cyclophosphamide | 200 mg/m² IV | Days 1–5 |
| Methotrexate | 1.5 g/m² IV | Given as in Course A |
| Leucovorin | 50 mg/m² | As in Course A |
| | 12 mg/m² | As in Course A |
| Dexamethasone | 10 mg/m² PO | Days 1–5 |
| Doxorubicin | 25 mg/m² IV | Days 4 5 |
| **Courses A and B alternate for six cycles** | | |
| **Intrathecal therapy: Administered in each of six cycles** | | |
| Methotrexate | 15 mg | Days 1, 5 |
| Cytarabine | 40 mg | |
| Dexamethasone | 4 mg | |

WBC >1.0, absolute neutrophil count >.2, platelets >50 to start courses 2–4.
WBC >2.0, absolute neutrophil count >.5 for courses 5–6.
BFM, Berlin-Frankfurt-Münster; B-NHL, No. 86; B-ALL, B-cell acute lymphoblastic leukemia; MTX, Methotrexate; VM, Vinblastine, Mitomycin; WBC, white blood cell count.

therapy.[517] The International Bone Marrow Transplant Registry (IBMTR) reported DFS at 2 years for 41% of patients in relapse or subsequent remission and 25% of patients with primary refractory disease.[513]

If an HLA-compatible sibling donor is unavailable, a search for a matched unrelated donor (MUD) should be initiated as soon after diagnosis as possible. The availability of HLA typing using DNA allows accurate typing, including that of the D-region, even before remission is achieved. Marrow transplantation from an MUD is best planned for first remission because the time required to identify a compatible donor and obtain marrow for transplantation (several months) precludes transplant at the time of relapse for most patients. If an allogeneic transplant is not possible, autologous marrow obtained during remission may allow dose intensification or treatment at relapse. The use of monoclonal antibody–treated autologous marrow for BMT appears promising.[516, 518]

Intensive postremission therapy for Ph$^+$ or BCR/ABL$^+$ ALL patients who are not transplant candidates with HDAC and possibly HDMTX may improve outcome. The use of HDAC and mitoxantrone or HDMTX and L-asparaginase for adults with Ph$^+$ ALL led to a 19% survival at 4 years according to a preliminary report from Germany.[481] Pediatric ALL patients with t(9;22) who received an aggressive seven-drug induction-consolidation including early intensification with MTX and cytarabine followed by rotational combination chemotherapy had a 40% CCR beyond 6 years.[361, 519] Future studies are needed to determine whether intensified cytotoxic therapy with these agents can improve the prognosis of Ph$^+$ adult ALL.

**Chemotherapy of Refractory or Relapsed Acute Lymphoblastic Leukemia.** The pattern of failure following first remission has been similar in most adult ALL trials. Most patients relapse within 3 years, and few relapses occur after 6 years.[358, 447, 457, 497] Relapses in children tend to develop within 2 years after completing therapy, but may occur up to a decade later.[520–522] The prognostic significance and the management of relapse are influenced by the duration of the first remission, the intensity of the initial regimen used, and the site of relapse. Postrelapse survival increases with longer duration of first remission, less intensive initial therapy, and relapse limited to one site.[432, 497, 522, 523] Because most data on retreatment were derived from patients who relapsed after low- to moderate-intensity therapy, as more intensive initial regimens are used, it is likely that retreatment with chemotherapy alone will be less successful.

The approach to the patient who relapses in the bone marrow depends on the duration of the initial remission. For late relapses (>18 months off therapy), two thirds of adult patients may enter CR with the use of vincristine, prednisone, asparaginase, and an anthracycline.[523–525] Second CR may be obtained in 75 to 95% of children with intensive retreatment.[520, 521, 526] For patients who relapse while on therapy or shortly after its completion, drugs not previously received are required. Common regimens include moderate-to high-dose MTX with L-asparaginase or folinic acid rescue, cytarabine and teniposide, or HDAC combined with an anthracycline, amsacrine, or other agents.[520, 521] Because CNS relapses as second events after bone marrow relapse occur, these patients require institution of CNS-directed therapy. CNS irradiation, intrathecal therapy, and HDMTX may have

additive effects in this setting.[520, 527] Consolidation and intensive maintenance therapy have been reported to be successful in prolonging the duration of second remissions.[525] Unfortunately, most patients who achieve a second remission subsequently relapse. In the era of intensive initial therapy, few adults, less than 20% of children who relapse early, and only one third of children who relapse late can be cured by chemotherapy after relapse.[520, 527, 528] For these patients, allogeneic BMT remains the best hope for long-term DFS. During second remission, it may be possible to find a compatible donor for an allogeneic BMT or harvest marrow for an autologous transplant.

Children with isolated extramedullary relapses following intensive initial therapy have at best a 72% EFS at 5 years with reinstitution of chemotherapy.[520] Patients with isolated CNS relapse require additional systemic therapy.[529, 530] Patients with testicular relapses can achieve a prolonged second remission with reinduction and maintenance chemotherapy, including CNS prophylaxis and testicular irradiation.[531]

Cytarabine has been used extensively in the retreatment of ALL as a single agent in high dosage or in combination with asparaginase, etoposide, amsacrine, mitoxantrone, or anthracyclines. The CR rate for single-agent cytarabine in relapsed or refractory ALL has been reported to be 38%, with a median CR duration of 6 months.[532, 533] Variation between studies precludes critical analysis, but in toto it appears that combinations of HDAC (1 to 3 g/m$^2$ × 4 to 12 doses) with mitoxantrone, m-AMSA VP-16, or daunorubicin-idarubicin appear to be more effective than HDAC alone in refractory and relapsed patients, with CR rates of approximately 60% in adults and up to 80% in children.[445, 523, 532, 534–539] Continuous-infusion cyclophosphamide may be a useful agent in this setting.[540] In general, CR durations following these salvage regimens are between 3 and 6 months, and further therapy, usually involving BMT, is typically required for long-term survival.

Another promising regimen is high-dose VP-16 (2.4 to 4.2 g/m$^2$) by continuous infusion followed by 4 days of cyclophosphamide (50 mg/kg/day). This "transplant" level dose-intensive regimen may induce remissions in patients who are refractory to or relapse from HDAC-containing regimens.[541] Lower doses of VP-16 combined with ifosfamide and mitoxantrone can also induce brief remissions in refractory patients.[542] Early inclusion of etoposide improved the rapidity of achieving remission but had no survival benefit.[543]

Topotecan has been studied in a window of opportunity in previously untreated patients with only modest results.[544]

## BONE MARROW TRANSPLANTATION

The infusion of autologous or allogeneic marrow following high-dose conditioning regimens using chemotherapy, sometimes with total body irradiation (TBI), is the most dose-intensive approach to ALL. The antileukemic activity of BMT results from the increased efficacy of intensive cytotoxic therapy and probably from an additional immunologically mediated graft-versus-leukemia effect associated with allogeneic marrow engraftment. Advances in supportive care make analysis of BMT trials conducted before 1988 of limited value.[545] The availability of growth factors, new antibiotic agents, and ganciclovir has reduced treatment-related mortality without increasing the relapse rate.

The optimal timing of BMT depends on the balance between the increased risk of resistant disease when transplant is applied late and the risk of treatment-related mortality for patients who undergo transplantation in first remission (CR1) who may already have been cured with chemotherapy. An appropriate balance can best be achieved by using prognostic factors to identify patients in CR1 who are at high risk of relapse and thus should undergo transplantation. Children and adults with standard- or low-risk ALL should have transplantation deferred until CR2 or possibly first relapse. After the first relapse, the low probability of long-term DFS with chemotherapy alone justifies the risk of BMT in adults.[523] In children, the decision to proceed with BMT in CR2 is less clear. Although children with bone marrow relapses of T-cell ALL or non–T-lineage ALL with initial remission durations of less than 18 months have survival rates less than 5% when treated with chemotherapy alone, children with longer initial remissions have an EFS of 30% when retreated with chemotherapy.[520] However, children who have a relapse in bone marrow earlier than 6 months after completing maintenance therapy have a 56% EFS and a 69% relapse-free interval at 7 years that is superior to results seen with chemotherapy.[546]

The results of BMT depend on patient status at the time of transplantation. In adults, transplantation in CR1 produces a higher proportion of durable CRs, but some of these patients would have remained in remission without BMT. For adults without adverse prognostic factors, the superiority of BMT in CR1 is uncertain. There are no mature randomized trials comparing chemotherapy with BMT for adults with ALL.[547] An ongoing French multicenter trial compares the relative efficacy of allogeneic BMT, autologous BMT, or consolidation plus maintenance chemotherapy in adult ALL.[485, 548] When analyzed by intention to treat, early results suggest superior outcome for patients who undergo allogeneic BMT. At 3 years, the actuarial median survival was 43% for the allogeneic BMT group, 39% for the autologous BMT arm, and 32% for the chemotherapy arm. Preliminary results of an Italian study confirm these findings.[549]

There is no consensus as to the best transplant regimen for ALL. The two most widely used regimens are cyclophosphamide plus TBI (Cy/TBI),[550] and busulfan plus cyclophosphamide (Bu/Cy).[551] Other regimens include HDAC/TBI,[552] VP-16/TBI,[553] busulfan/VP-16 (Bu/VP),[554] HDAC/Cy/TBI,[555] TBI/HDAC/melphalan,[556] and melphalan/TBI.[557] In a randomized comparison of VP-16/TBI with Bu/Cy, no significant difference was detected.[558]

Comparisons among reported trials are difficult because of variations in transplant regimens, patient selection, and definition of risk groups. Salient BMT series are classified by timing of BMT, patient age group, high-risk factors, and type of graft in Table 95–15.

A representative overview of the efficacy of allogeneic BMT in ALL is provided by the reports of the IBMTR.[559-563] Data for the combined experience with adult and pediatric cases of ALL from 1985 to 1991 indicate that up to 50% of patients who undergo transplantation in CR1 may become long-term disease-free survivors.[562, 563] Similar results have been reported by others.[545, 550] If the analysis is restricted to patients in CR1 who are at "high risk" of relapse, IBMTR

data indicate a 4-year actuarial DFS of 45%, compared with 22% for patients in CR2[560]; the probability of relapse at 4 years is 26% and 56%, respectively. Considering only adults in CR1, the IBMTR results indicate a 5-year DFS rate of 39%.[561] Transplant in second or subsequent remission results in a 33% 4-year DFS, and, for patients transplanted in relapse, long-term survival falls to 18% or less.[562, 564] More recent studies appear to have better transplant outcomes than the IBMTR data.[565-567] The EFS at 7 years for children who undergo allogeneic BMT in CR2 is a function of time to initial relapse: 56% for early relapses compared with 47% for late relapses.[546] Children with either extramedullary or late marrow relapses may do as well with chemotherapy as with BMT.[546]

BMT remains the best treatment for primary refractory patients. In a IBMTR report, DFS was seen in 23% of primary refractory patients who underwent transplantation using a matched sibling donor.[568] The results, however, were highly dependent on age and performance status at the time of BMT.

The improved outcome following allogeneic BMT for high-risk patients in first CR indicates that adverse prognostic factors do not affect this treatment strategy to the same degree that they affect chemotherapy. BMT, however, does not entirely nullify these factors. Patients with slow responses to induction chemotherapy fare more poorly when undergoing transplantation than do those who show a faster response.[569] In addition, older age and high WBC count at diagnosis remain unfavorable prognostic factors despite BMT.[561]

The role of MUD transplants for ALL is uncertain. Based on the overall experience with MUD transplants, it is reasonable to consider this option for any patient (<age 55) for whom an allogeneic transplant is indicated, when a fully matched donor is identified.

For patients who lack an allogeneic donor, autologous transplantation provides another means by which potentially curative dose-intensive therapy can be administered. The major reason for treatment failure in autologous transplants is relapse. A retrospective analysis of 233 patients who underwent autologous BMT in CR1 before 1989 reported a 5-year DFS of 40%.[570] The range of long-term DFS in other reports of autologous BMT for ALL patients in CR1 is from 30 to 65%.[571-576] Time-to-treatment bias, exclusion of older patients and those with comorbid conditions, and physician selection of patients for BMT who are at high risk cloud the results of uncontrolled trials. Several trials have failed to show a benefit of autologous BMT over chemotherapy in CR1.[378, 484, 485, 572, 577]

Long-term DFS falls to approximately 25% in patients undergoing autologous BMT in CR2, although selected trials report DFS as high as 40%.[556, 572, 575, 576, 578-580] For patients who do not have the option of an allogeneic BMT in CR2, autologous BMT may be preferable to chemotherapy alone.

Three approaches have been taken to improve the outcome in autologous transplants. First, preparative regimens have been modified and post-BMT maintenance chemotherapy has been given to improve leukemic cytoreduction.[557] Second, methods to purge the infused autologous product of residual leukemic cells have been pursued.[580-582] Finally, techniques to produce an autologous graft-versus-leukemia effect have been investigated.[583]

*Table 95–15.*  **Bone Marrow Transplantation Trials in ALL**

| Report[ref] Year | Age Median Range | Risk Group | No. | Rx | Disease-Free Survival (% @ yrs) | | | | | | |
|---|---|---|---|---|---|---|---|---|---|---|---|
| | | | | | CR1 | CR2 | CR1+2 | CR≥2 | Rel 1 | CR≥2+ Rel/Ref | Rel≥1+ Refr |
| IBMTR[563] 1993 | A+C | All | 623 | Allo | 50 @ 5 | | | | | | |
| | | | 694 | | | | | 32 @ 5 | | | |
| | | | 323 | | | | | | | | 18 @ 5 |
| IBMTR[561] 1989 | 15 1–49 | All | 391 | Allo | | | | 26 @ 5 | | | |
| IBMTR[563, 568] 1993 | 32 1–50 | High | 38 | Allo | | | | | | | 21* @ 5 |
| IBMTR[513] 1992 | 28 5–49 | High | 67 | Allo | 38 @ 2 | | | | | 41 @ 2 | 25 @ 2 |
| IBMTR[560] 1987 | 22 1–48 | High | 236 | Allo | 45 @ 4 | | | | | | |
| | | | 208 | | | 22 @ 4 | | | | | |
| IBMTR[547] 1991 | A 15–45 | All | 251 | Allo | 44 @ 5 | | | | | | |
| IBMTR[561] 1989 | 24 16–48 | All | 243 | Allo | 39 @ 5 | | | | | | |
| IBMTR[561] 1989 | 13 1–15 | All | 56 | Allo | 56 @ 5 | | | | | | |
| Germany[546] 1991 | 8 1–18 | All | 51 | Allo | | 52 @ 7 | | | | | |
| FGTALL[485, 548] 1993 | 26 15–40 | All | 92 | Allo | 47 @ 3 | | | | | | |
| Spain[566] 1992 | 17 5–36 | High | 30 | Allo | | | 69 @ 4 | | | 15 @ 4 | |
| City of Hope/ Stanford[565] 1991 | 24 0–45 | High | 53 | Allo | 64 @ 5 | | | | | | |
| Seattle[564] 1991 | 22 18–53 | All | 41 | Allo | 21 @ 5 | | | | | | |
| | | | 48 | | | | | 15 @ 5 | | | |
| | | | 103 | | | | | | | | 12 @ 5 |
| Hopkins[567] 1990 | 15 3–41 | All | 18 | Allo | 42 @ 5 | | | | | | |
| | | | 36 | | | 43 @ 5 | | | | | |
| | | | 20 | | | | | | | 25 @ 5 | |
| GEGMO[550] 1988 | 24 15–36 | All | 27 | Allo | 59 @ 3 | | | | | | |
| MRC[484] 1991 | A | All | 44 | Allo | 42 @ 3 | | | | | | |
| | | | | Auto | 44 @ 3 | | | | | | |
| Italy[578] 1991 | A+C | High | 168 | Allo | | | | 52 @ 5 | | | |
| | | | | Auto | | | | 29 @ 5 | | | |
| Japan[518] 1993 | 19 4–51 | High | 17 | Auto+P | 75 @ 3 | | | | 14 @ 3 | | |
| EBMT[540] 1992 | A+C 65% <20 | Std | 280 | Auto | 42 @ 8 | | | | | | |
| | | High | 174 | | 40 @ 8 | | | | | | |
| | | All | 357 | | | 37 @ 8 | | | | | |
| Italy[577] 1992 | 22 16–45 | All | 61 | Auto | 40 @ 8 | | | | | | |
| | | | 39 | +P | 31–45 | | | | | | |
| | | | 22 | −P | 50 | | | | | | |
| London[571] 1991 | 18 11–45 | High | 27 | Auto+P | 32 @ 7 | | | | | | |
| GEGMO[550] 1988 | 25 15–50 | All | 63 | Auto+P | 51 @ 3 | | | | | | |

*All with primary refractory disease.

A, Adults; C, children; High, high risk by prognostic factors; All, all risk groups; Std, standard risk group; r, refractory only, Allo, allogeneic; Auto, autologous; +P, purged; −P, unpurged; IBMTR, International Bone Marrow Transplant Registry; FGTALL, French Group on Therapy for Adult Acute Lymphoblastic Leukemia; GEGMO, Groupe d'Études de la Greffe de Moelle Osseuse; MRC, Medical Research Council; EMBT, retrospective results of bone marrow transplantation in Europe; Rel, relapse; Refr, refractory.

Autologous BMT with ex vivo purging may be a viable alternative for patients who require transplantation but do not have a marrow donor identified. For patients who underwent BMT in CR1 using autologous marrow purged ex vivo with a trio of antibodies and a cyclophosphamide, cytarabine, TBI conditioning regimen, DFS at 5 years was 75%.[518] To date, no randomized trial has demonstrated a benefit to purging.

A novel approach to purging is to use peripheral blood stem cells rather than autologous marrow. High-risk patients receive cytotoxic chemotherapy during remission, and peripheral blood stem cells are collected by apheresis beginning with the early phase of marrow recovery, often with the additional stimulation of cytokines (e.g., G-CSF). Under these conditions, normal pluripotent stem cells enter the circulating blood in large numbers, and it may be possible to collect them without significant contamination by leukemic progenitors, even if residual leukemia is present in the marrow.[584] After collection of an adequate supply of stem cells, patients can be treated with ablative chemoradiotherapy and then infused with peripheral blood stem cells for hematopoietic reconstitution. Initial results from such approaches are promising.[585]

## COMPLICATIONS OF THERAPY FOR ALL

The administration of combination chemotherapy and radiation therapy engenders myriad potential problems. Early deaths may result from bleeding or infection. In one large adult study, 11% of patients developed major bleeding and another 6% had thrombosis.[586] Thrombosis may be due to toxic effects of L-asparaginase or the release of procoagulants.[587] Laboratory evidence of disseminated intravascular coagulation can be detected in more than 75% of patients during remission induction therapy but is rarely clinically significant.[588] Acute parotitis and pancreatitis attributable to asparaginase may develop.[589] Patients are at risk for the development of *Pneumocystis carinii* pneumonia and require prophylactic antibiotic therapy.[590]

Delayed sequelae observed in survivors of ALL include second neoplasms, neuropsychological changes, endocrine dysfunction,[591, 592] and cardiomyopathy.[593] Survivors of childhood ALL have a 7-fold excess of all cancers and a 22-fold excess of CNS neoplasms that may be attributable in large part to radiation therapy.[594] Up to 5% of patients may develop secondary AML that may be linked to the use of epipodophyllotoxins.[595, 596] Alterations in the white matter have been detected by magnetic resonance imaging in children after CNS therapy.[597] Long-term neurologic and neuropsychological functioning may be impaired following CNS therapy even when irradiation is avoided.[598, 599] Children who received anthracycline therapy may have a 10% incidence of clinical congestive heart failure.[600]

## The Future

The major issue in the therapy of ALL is how to improve the outcome of high-risk children and adults. Current investigations have focused on the use of newer therapeutic agents and interventions based on the persistence of MRD. Additional insights into drug resistance and the pathogenesis of ALL may provide further clues that will lead us to the cure of this disease. Of increasing importance is the development of effective and safe therapy for the elderly patient with ALL.[601–603]

## NEWER THERAPEUTIC OPTIONS

Newer chemotherapeutic agents undergoing trials in ALL include carboplatin[604] and the combination of ifosfamide and etoposide.[605] Teniposide has been used extensively in childhood ALL but to a limited degree in adult ALL. Infusional delivery of anthracyclines may improve killing of

leukemic cells.[606] Immunologic therapy continues to be studied. Interferon[607, 608] or interleukin-2 may be useful.[609–613]

New insight into the cause of ALL and regulation of leukemic cell growth may lead to further therapeutic breakthroughs. The association between the BCL2 gene and apoptosis led to the investigation of this protein's expression in ALL. Bcl-2 protein levels were 10-fold higher in B-lineage ALL than in normal human B-cell progenitors. The cells with increased bcl-2 expression had prolonged survival in vitro.[614] This may convey a growth advantage to leukemic lymphoblasts. Thus, methods that regulate bcl-2 expression may be therapeutically useful in the therapy of ALL. The role of multidrug resistance in ALL remains to be determined.[615–622]

The use of monoclonal antibodies to deliver toxins directly to the leukemic cell is undergoing active exploration.[623] These antibodies can be targeted against the surface antigens that are associated with the appropriate lineage. Early targets have included CD19, CD20, CD2, and CD7.[624, 625] The combination of cytotoxic chemotherapy and immunotoxins attached to monoclonal antibodies directed at leukemic cells has been highly effective in an immunodeficient mouse model and will be entering clinical trials.[626, 627] Monoclonal antibodies may also be useful in improving the results of purging of autologous marrow.[581, 628]

## DETECTION AND PROGNOSTIC ROLE OF MINIMAL RESIDUAL DISEASE

A subclinical level of leukemia beyond the detection of conventional methods is termed *MRD*. Four general approaches to detect residual leukemic cells at a frequency of less than 1 in 100 are being investigated: in situ cytogenetics,[629, 630] immunologic methods to detect aberrant antigen expression,[631, 632] in vitro colony assays,[633] and molecular diagnostics.[91]

In situ cytogenetics uses fluorochrome conjugated DNA probes to hybridize to the cytogenetic abnormality of interest. These include probes for individual chromosomes that can delineate either monosomies or trisomies or probes whose sequences are targeted for individual translocation breakpoints. The immunologic detection of MRD is accomplished by flow cytometry or fluorescence microscopy. This technique depends on identifying an immunophenotypic pattern that is distinct for the leukemic cells that can then be used as a template to screen remission samples for cells occurring at low frequency. Molecular studies to screen for genetic rearrangements specific for the leukemic clone may be performed on DNA by the Southern blotting technique or in some cases on RNA by a RT-PCR. DNA fingerprinting using minisatellite probes may be useful in some leukemic patients to detect impending relapse, but it has the same sensitivity as other Southern blot techniques.[634] Although a Southern blot can at best reliably detect 1 abnormal cell in 100, PCR methods may improve the sensitivity to 1 in $10^5$.

For patients with known chromosomal translocations, the advent of molecular identification of the cytogenetic abnormalities has made it possible to screen patients at diagnosis and after therapy. To date, the most sensitive method to detect aberrant transcripts uses RT-PCR. It is theoretically possible to apply this method to screen for cells that express chimeric nucleotide sequences associated with any cytogenetic rearrangement. The BCR/ABL fusion gene associated with t(9;22)[635, 636] and the ALL-1/AF4 fusion gene associated with t(4;11)[637] have been used for diagnosis and to follow patients' responses to therapy.

Although PCR-based methods to detect leukemia-specific sequences due to translocations are highly specific and sensitive, the majority of patients with ALL do not have such translocations that can be followed. The use of the genomic diversity of the immune receptor supergene family allows almost universal application of PCR techniques to follow ALL patients for MRD. Specific rearrangement of IgH or TCR serves as a clonal marker for individual leukemia cases.

Clonospecific probes prepared by PCR amplification of the DNA fragment containing the N-junctional sequences that specifically characterize a VD or VDJ recombination of the TCR-δ or TCR-γ loci can detect rearrangements that differentiate clonal cells from polyclonal T cells, distinguish between different T-cell clones, and detect residual clonal populations at $10^{-4}$ to $10^{-5}$ dilution.[638] Because the junctional regions of TCR-δ genes are more diverse than the junctional regions of TCR-γ genes, PCR-mediated amplification of TCR genes will be more sensitive if TCR-δ junction specific probes are used instead of TCR-γ probes.[639] V-J junction sequences are clone specific in both B- and T-lineage ALL. V-(D)-J nucleotide sequences of rearrangements are usually identical at presentation and relapse.[640]

With the methodology described earlier, the clinical significance of persistence of a leukemia-specific or leukemia-associated marker has been investigated. Preliminary studies of molecular residual disease status at the end of chemotherapy suggest that correlations with clinical outcome may be confusing. Most patients in hematologic remission who had yet to complete their planned course of therapy had evidence of residual leukemic cells, whereas the majority of patients analyzed 6 months after completing all planned therapy had no evidence of residual leukemia.[195] In another study of children with ALL, the amount of residual disease quantitated in first remission marrows at the end of induction chemotherapy predicted clinical outcome.[641] Serial analyses of remission samples show two patterns: loss of detectable leukemia or persistence of disease. These patterns have been reported using different PCR clonal markers: IgH CDR III[642, 643] or TCR-δ sequences.[195, 644–646] The absence of detectable residual leukemia by PCR at the end of chemotherapy may not be sufficient to ensure that the patient is cured.[647] Furthermore, the presence of detectable residual disease may not always predict relapse.[91, 195, 648, 649] Molecular evidence of a residual leukemic clone can be detected in marrow for as long as 9 years following therapy without a clinical relapse.[649] However, an increase in the level of MRD detected while patients remain on therapy may precede clinical relapse.[646, 649, 650] Similarly, a gradual loss of signal may correlate with persistent remission.[642, 643, 646, 650] False-negative results, although rare, may result from clonal change in IGH or TCR and therefore limit the predictive power of a negative result.[643, 646, 649, 651] Serial monitoring of residual disease at regular intervals is likely necessary to predict relapse off therapy.[643, 646, 647] Regrowth of the leukemic clone and changes in the PCR signal can occur within as short a period as 3 months.[650]

These techniques have been applied to bone marrow samples but will need to be applied to blood samples to monitor residual disease more easily in the future. Prospective randomized trials that include serial testing throughout remission are required to define the utility of this technique.[647] Ultimately, it will be necessary to show that intervention based on the detection of MRD increases DFS.

## SUGGESTIONS FOR ADDITIONAL READING

Greaves M. Molecular genetics, natural history and the demise of childhood leukaemia. Eur J Cancer 1999;35(2):173–85.

Finiewicz KJ, Larson, RA. Dose-intensive therapy for adult acute lymphoblastic leukemia. Semin Oncol 1999;26(1):6–20

O'Connor OA, Weiss M. Recent advances in the biology and management of acute lymphoblastic leukemia in adults. Cancer Treat Res 1999;99:307–33.

Ohno R. Granulocyte colony-stimulating factor, granulocyte-macrophage colony-stimulating factor and macrophage colony-stimulating factor in the treatment of acute myeloid leukemia and acute lymphoblastic leukemia. Leuk Res 1998;22(12):1143–54.

## REFERENCES

1. Whelan SL, Parkin DM, Masuyer E. Patterns of cancer in five continents. Lyon: International Association for Research on Cancer, 1990.
2. Greenlee RT, Murray T, Bolden S, Wingo PA. Cancer statistics, 2000. CA Cancer J Clin 2000;50:7–33. abstract.
3. Borings CC, Squires TS, Tong T, Montgomery S. Cancer statistics, 1994. CA Cancer J Clin 1994;44:7–26.
4. Taylor PRA, Reid MM, Bown N, et al. Acute lymphoblastic leukemia in patients aged 60 years and over: a population-based study of incidence and outcome. Blood 1992;80:1813–7.
5. Miller BA, Ries LAG, Hankey BF, et al. Cancer statistics review 1973–1985. Bethesda: NIH Pub. No. 92-2789, 1992.
6. Pendergrass TW. Epidemiology of acute lymphoblastic leukemia. Semin Oncol 1985;12:80–91.
7. Linet M. The leukemias: epidemiologic agents. New York: Oxford University Press, 1985.
8. Sandler DP. Epidemiology and etiology of leukemia. Curr Opin Oncol 1990;2:3–9.
9. Cartwright RA, Staines A. Acute leukaemias. In: Fleming AF, ed. Bailliere's clinical haematology international practice and research. London: Bailliere Tindall, 1992:1–26.
10. Alexander FE. Viruses, clusters and clustering of childhood leukaemia: a new perspective? Eur J Cancer Clin Oncol 1993;29A:1424–43.
11. Greaves M. A natural history for pediatric acute leukemia. Blood 1993;82:1043–51.
12. Sullivan AK. Classification, pathogenesis, and etiology of neoplastic diseases of the hematopoietic system. In: Lee GR, Bithell TC, Foerster J, et al., eds. Wintrobe's clinical hematology. 9th ed. Philadelphia: Lea & Febiger, 1993:1725–91.
13. Mulvihill JJ. Childhood cancer, the environment, and heredity. In: Pizzo PA, Poplack DG, eds. Principles and practice of pediatric oncology. 2nd ed. Philadelphia: JB Lippincott, 1993:11–27.
14. Gartenhaus RB, Gallo RC. Etiology of acute leukemia: molecular genetics and viral oncology. In: Wiernik PH, Canellos GP, Kyle RA, Schiffer CA, eds. Neoplastic diseases of the blood. 2nd ed. New York: Churchill Livingstone, 1991:145–55.
15. Greaves MF, Alexander FE. An infectious etiology for common acute lymphoblastic leukemia in childhood? Leukemia 1993;7:349–60.
16. Li FP. Epidemiology of cancer in childhood. In: Nathan DG, Oski FA, eds. Hematology of infancy and childhood. 4th ed. Philadelphia: WB Saunders, 1993:1102–19.
17. Sandler DP, Ross JA. Epidemiology of acute leukemia in children and adults. Semin Oncol 1997;24:3–16.
18. Greaves MF. Aetiology of acute leukaemia. Lancet 1997;349:344–9.
19. Westergaard T, Andersen PK, Pedersen JB, et al. Birth characteristics, sibling patterns, and acute leukemia risk in childhood: a population-based cohort study. J Natl Cancer Inst 1997;89:939–47.

20. Severson RK, Ross JA. The causes of acute leukemia. Curr Opin Oncol 1999;11:20–4.
21. Rabbitts TH. Translocations, master genes, and differences between the origins of acute and chronic leukemias. Cell 1991;67:641–4.
22. Gale KB, Ford AM, Repp R, et al. Backtracking leukemia to birth: identification of clonotypic gene fusion sequences in neonatal blood spots. Proc Natl Acad Sci U S A 1997;94:13950–4.
23. Rowley JD. Backtracking leukemia to birth [news]. Nat Med 1998;4:150–1.
24. Fong C, Brodeur GM. Down's syndrome and leukemia: epidemiology, genetics, cytogenetics and mechanisms of leukemogenesis. Cancer Genet Cytogenet 1987;28:55–76.
25. German J, Gardin C. Bloom's syndrome. XV. The instances of acute myelogenous leukemia in the Bloom's syndrome registry. In: Gale RP, ed. Acute myelogenous leukemia: progress and controversies. New York: Wiley-Liss, 1990:35–49.
26. Sugimoto T, Kodiwaki T, Sawada T, et al. Ataxia-telangiectasia associated with non-T, non-B cell acute lymphocytic leukemia. Acta Paediatr Scand 1982;71:509–10.
27. Horwitz M. The genetics of familial leukemia. Leukemia 1997;11:1347–59.
28. Woods WG, Roloff JS, Lukens JN, Krivit W. The occurrence of leukemia in patients with the Shwachman syndrome. J Pediatr 1981;99:425–8.
29. Bader JL, Miller RW. Neurofibromatosis and childhood leukemia. J Pediatr 1978;92:925–9.
30. Klopfenstein KJ, Sommer A, Ruymann FB. Neurofibromatosis-Noonan syndrome and acute lymphoblastic leukemia: a report of two cases. J Pediatr Hematol Oncol 1999;21:158–60.
31. Ford AM, Pombo-de-Oliveira MS, McCarthy KP, et al. Monoclonal origin of concordant T-cell malignancy in identical twins. Blood 1997;89:281–5.
32. Gill Super HJ, Rothberg PG, Kobayashi H, et al. Clonal, nonconstitutional rearrangements of the MLL gene in infant twins with acute lymphoblastic leukemia: in utero chromosome rearrangement of 11q23. Blood 1994;83:641–4.
33. Greaves MF, Colman SM, Beard ME, et al. Geographical distribution of acute lymphoblastic leukaemia subtypes: second report of the collaborative group study. Leukemia 1993;7:27–34.
34. Bortin MM, D'Amaro J, Bach FH, et al. HLA associations with leukemia. Blood 1987;70:227–32.
35. Taylor GM. The genetics of human leukemia. In: Whittaker JA, Delamore IW, eds. Leukemia. Oxford: Blackwell, 1987:39–63.
36. Felix CA, Nau MM, Takahashi T, et al. Hereditary and acquired p53 gene mutations in childhood acute lymphoblastic leukemia. J Clin Invest 1992;89:640–7.
37. Smith MA, Chen T, Simon R. Age-specific incidence of acute lymphoblastic leukemia in U.S. children: in utero initiation model. J Natl Cancer Inst 1997;89:1542–4.
38. Smith M. Considerations on a possible viral etiology for B-precursor acute lymphoblastic leukemia of childhood. J Immunother 1997;20:89–100.
39. Magrath I. The pathogenesis of Burkitt's lymphoma. Advances in Cancer Research 1990;55:133–270.
40. Ambinder RF. Human lymphotropic viruses associated with lymphoid malignancy: Epstein-Barr and HTLV-1. Hematol Oncol Clin North Am 1990;4:821–33.
41. zur Hausen H. Viruses in human cancers. Science 1991;254:1167–73.
42. Liebowitz D. Epstein-Barr virus and a cellular signaling pathway in lymphomas from immunosuppressed patients [see comments]. N Engl J Med 1998;338:1413–21.
43. Cooper GS, Kamel F, Sandler DP, et al. Risk of adult acute leukemia in relation to prior immune-related conditions. Cancer Epidemiol Biomarkers Prev 1996;5:867–72.
44. Stevens W, Thomas DC, Lyon JL, et al. Leukemia in Utah and radioactive fallout from the Nevada test site. JAMA 1990;264:585–91.
45. Gardner MJ, Snee MP, Hall AJ, et al. Results of case-control study of leukaemia and lymphoma among young people near Sellafield nuclear plant in West Cumbria. Br Med J 1990;300:425–9.
46. Shore DL, Sandler DP, Davey FR, et al. Acute leukemia and residential proximity to potential sources of environmental pollutants. Arch Env Health 1993;48:414–30.
47. Coleman MP, Bell CMJ, Taylor H-L, Primic-Zakelj M. Leukaemia and residence near electricity transmission equipment: a case-control study. Br J Cancer 1989;60:793–8.
48. Green LM, Miller AB, Villeneuve PJ, et al. A case-control study of childhood leukemia in southern Ontario, Canada, and exposure to magnetic fields in residences. Int J Cancer 1999;82:161–70.
49. Linet MS, Hatch EE, Kleinerman RA, et al. Residential exposure to magnetic fields and acute lymphoblastic leukemia in children [see comments]. N Engl J Med 1997;337:1–7.
50. Blair A, Mulker H, Cantor K, et al. Cancer among farmers: a review. Scand J Work Environ Health 1985;11:397–407.
51. Sandler DP, Shore DL, Anderson JR, et al. Cigarette smoking and risk of acute leukemia: associations with morphology and cytogenetic abnormalities in bone marrow. J Natl Cancer Inst 1993;85:1994–2003.
52. Brownson RC, Novotny TE, Perry MC. Cigarette smoking and adult leukemia: a meta-analysis. Arch Intern Med 1993;153:469–75.
53. Sandler DP, Shore DL, Bloomfield CD. Hair dye use and leukemia. Am J Epidemiol 1993;138:636–7. abstract.
54. Grodstein F, Hennekens CH, Colditz GA, et al. A prospective study of permanent hair dye use and hematopoietic cancer. J Natl Cancer Inst 1994;86:1466–70.
55. Thun MJ, Altekruse SF, Namboodiri MM. Hair dye use and risk of fatal cancers in U.S. women [see comments]. J Natl Cancer Inst 1994;86:210–5.
56. Cohn P, Klotz J, Bove F, et al. Drinking water contamination and the incidence of leukemia and non-Hodgkin's lymphoma. Environ Health Perspect 1994;102:556–61.
57. Chessels JM, Swansbury GJ, Reeves B, et al. Cytogenetics and prognosis in childhood lymphoblastic leukaemia: results of MRC UKALL X. Medical Research Council Working Party in Childhood Leukaemia. Br J Haematol 1997;99:93–100.
58. Hernandez JM, Sanchez I, Gonzalez M, et al. Acute lymphoid leukemias following either a previous chronic myelongenous leukemia or myelodysplastic syndrome: phenotypic and genomic differences. Am J Hematol 1993;43:256–8.
59. Hunger SP, Sklar J, Link MP. Acute lymphoblastic leukemia occurring as a second malignant neoplasm in childhood: report of three cases and review of the literature. J Clin Oncol 1992;10:156–63.
60. Geetha N, SreedeviAmma N, Kusumakumary P, et al. Acute lymphoblastic leukemia occurring as a second malignancy: report of a case and review of literature. Pediat Hematol Oncol 1999;16:267–70.
61. Travis LB, Curtis RE, Storm H, et al. Risk of second malignant neoplasms among long-term survivors of testicular cancer [see comments]. J Natl Cancer Inst 1997;89:1429–39.
62. Pedersen-Bjergaard J. Acute lymphoid leukemia with t(4;11) (q21;q23) following chemotherapy with cytostatic agents targeting at DNA-topoisomerase II. editorial. Leuk Res 1992;16:733–5.
63. Kobayashi Y, Yang J, Shindo E, et al. HRX gene rearrangement in acute lymphoblastic leukemia after adjuvant chemotherapy of breast cancer. letter. Blood 1993;82:3220–1.
64. Witherspoon RP, Fisher LD, Schock G, et al. Secondary cancers after bone marrow transplantation for leukemia or aplastic anemia. N Engl J Med 1989;321:784–9.
65. Deeg HJ, Witherspoon RP. Risk factors for the development of secondary malignancies after marrow transplantation. Hematol Oncol Clin North Am 1993;7:417–29.
66. Bennett JM, Catovsky D, Daniel MT, et al. Proposals for the classification of the acute leukaemias. Br J Haematol 1976;33:451–8.
67. First MIC Cooperative Study Group. Morphologic, immunologic, and cytogenetic (MIC) working classification of acute lymphoblastic leukemia. Cancer Genet Cytogenet 1986;23:189–197.
68. Bennett JM, Catovsky D, Daniel MT, et al. The morphological classification of acute lymphoblastic leukaemia: concordance among observers and clinical correlations. Br J Haematol 1981;47:553–60.
69. Bloomfield CD. The clinical relevance of lymphocyte surface markers in adult acute lymphoblastic leukemia. In: Bloomfield CD, ed. Adult leukemias 1. The Hague: Marinus Nijhoff, 1982:265.
70. Loffler H, Kayser W, Schmitz N. Morphological and cytochemical classification of adult acute leukemias in two multicenter studies in the Federal Republic of Germany. Haematol Blood Transfus 1987;30:21–7.
71. Pui CH, Crist WM. Biology and treatment of acute lymphoblastic leukemia. J Pediatr 1994;124:491–503.
72. Huhn D, Thiel E, Rodt H, Andreewa P. Cytochemistry and membrane markers in acute lymphatic leukaemia. Scand J Haematol 1981;26:311–20.
73. Behm FG. Morphologic and cytochemical characteristics of childhood lymphoblastic leukemia. Hematol Oncol Clin North Am 1990;4:715–41.

74. Hirsch-Ginsberg C, Hug YO, Kagan J, et al. Advances in the diagnosis of acute leukemia. Hematol Oncol Clin North Am 1993;7:1–46.

75. Tricot G, Broeckaert-Van Orshoven A, Van Hoof A, Verwilghen RL. Sudan black B positivity in acute lymphoblastic leukaemia. Br J Haematol 1982;51:615–21.

76. Humphrey GB, Nesbit ME, Brunning RD. Prognostic value of the periodic acid-Schiff (PAS) reaction in acute lymphoblastic leukemia. Am J Clin Pathol 1974;61:393.

77. Boros L, Bennett JM. Morphology and cytochemistry. In: Henderson ES, Lister TA, eds. Leukemia. 5th ed. Philadelphia: WB Saunders, 1990:361–84.

78. McCaffrey R, Harrison TA, Parkman P, Baltimore D. Terminal deoxynucleotidyl transferase activity in human leukemic cells and in normal thymocytes. N Engl J Med 1975;292:775–80.

79. Kung PC, Long JC, McCaffrey RP, et al. Terminal deoxynucleotidyl transferase in the diagnosis of leukemia and malignant lymphoma. Am J Med 1978;64:788–94.

80. Smith RG, Kitchens RL. Phenotypic heterogeneity of TDT+ cells in the blood and bone marrow: implications for surveillance of residual leukemia. Blood 1989;74:312–9.

81. Gore SD, Kastan MB, Civin CI. Normal human bone marrow precursors that express terminal deoxynucleotidyl transferase include T-cell precursors and possible lymphoid stem cells. Blood 1991;77:1681–90.

82. van Dongen JJM, Hooijkaas H, Comans-Bitter M. Human bone marrow cells positive for terminal deoxynucleotidyl transferase. HLA-DR, and a T cell marker may represent prothymocytes. J Immunol 1985;135:3144–50.

83. Hofbrand AV, Drexler HG, Ganeshaguru K, et al. Biochemical aspects of acute leukaemia. Clin Haematol 1986;15:669.

84. Drexler HG, Menon M, Minowada J. Incidence of TdT positivity in cases of leukemia and lymphoma. Acta Haematol 1986;75:12–7.

85. Drexler HG, Sperling C, Ludwig WD. Terminal deoxynucleotidyl tranferase expression in acute myeloid leukaemia. Leukemia 1993;7:1142–50.

86. Stark AN, MacKarill ID, Limbert HJ, et al. TdT expression in acute myeloid leukaemia. Blut 1988;56:33–8.

87. Adriaansen HJ, van Dongen JJM, Kappers-Klunne MC, et al. Terminal deoxynucleotidyl transferase positive subpopulations occur in the majority of ANLL: Implications for the detection of minimal disease. Leukemia 1990;4:404–10.

88. Paietta E, Racevskis J, Bennett JM, Wiernik PH. Differential expression of terminal transferase in acute lymphocytic leukaemia expressing myeloid antigens and TdT positive acute myeloid leukaemia as compared to myeloid antigen negative acute lymphocytic leukaemia. Br J Haematol 1993;84:416–22.

89. Mirro J Jr. Pathology and immunology of leukemia. Curr Opin Oncol 1990;2:18–25.

90. Vaickus L, Foon KA. Immunobiology of acute leukemia. In: Wiernik PH, Canellos GP, Kyle RA, Schiffer CA, eds. Neoplastic diseases of the blood. 2nd ed. New York: Churchill Livingstone, 1991.

91. Potter MN. The detection of minimal residual disease in acute lymphoblastic leukaemia. Blood Rev 1992;6:68–82.

92. Drach J, Drach D, Glassl H, et al. Flow cytometric determination of atypical antigen expression in acute leukemia for the study of minimal residual disease. Cytometry 1992;13:893–901.

93. Drach J, Gattringer C, Huber H. Combined flow cytometric assessment of cell surface antigens and nuclear TdT for the detection of minimal residual disease in acute leukaemia. Br J Haematol 1991;77:37–42.

94. Neale GA, Coustan-Smith E, Pan Q, et al. Tandem application of flow cytometry and polymerase chain reaction for comprehensive detection of minimal residual disease in childhood acute lymphoblastic leukemia. Leukemia 1999;13:1221–6.

95. Campana D, Coustan-Smith E. Detection of minimal residual disease in acute leukemia by flow cytometry. Cytometry 1999;38:139–52.

96. Kallakury BV, Hartmann DP, Cossman J, et al. Posttherapy surveillance of B-cell precursor acute lymphoblastic leukemia. Value of polymerase chain reaction and limitations of flow cytometry. Am J Clin Pathol 1999;111:759–66.

97. Dworzak MN, Stolz F, Froschl G, et al. Detection of residual disease in pediatric B-cell precursor acute lymphoblastic leukemia by comparative phenotype mapping: a study of five cases controlled by genetic methods. Exp Hematol 1999;27:673–81.

98. Lucio P, Parreira A, van den Beemd MW, et al. Flow cytometric analysis of normal B cell differentiation: a frame of reference for the detection of minimal residual disease in precursor-B-ALL. Leukemia 1999;13:419–27.

99. Ciudad J, San Miguel JF, Lopez-Berges MC, et al. Prognostic value of immunophenotypic detection of minimal residual disease in acute lymphoblastic leukemia. J Clin Oncol 1998;16:3774–81.

100. Farahat N, Morilla A, Owusu-Ankomah K, et al. Detection of minimal residual disease in B-lineage acute lymphoblastic leukaemia by quantitative flow cytometry. Br J Haematol 1998;101:158–64.

101. Coustan-Smith E, Behm FG, Sanchez J, et al. Immunological detection of minimal residual disease in children with acute lymphoblastic leukaemia [see comments]. Lancet 1998;351:550–4.

102. Nagler A, Condiotti R, Rabinowitz R, et al. Detection of minimal residual disease (MRD) after bone marrow transplantation (BMT) by multi-parameter flow cytometry (MPFC). Med Oncol 1999;16:177–87.

103. Griesinger F, Piro-Noack M, Kaib N, et al. Leukaemia-associated immunophenotypes (LAIP) are observed in 90% of adult and childhood acute lymphoblastic leukaemia: detection in remission marrow predicts outcome. Br J Haematol 1999;105:241–55.

104. Anonymous. Leukocyte typing IV: white cell differentiation antigens. 1st ed. Oxford: Oxford University Press, 1989.

105. Anonymous. Leukocyte typing V: white cell differentiation antigens. London: Oxford Press, 1994.

106. Schlossman SF, Boumsell L, Gilks W, et al. CD antigens 1993. Blood 1994;83:879–80.

107. Nadler LM, Korsmeyer SJ, Anderson KC, et al. B cell origin of non-T acute lymphoblastic leukemia. A model for discrete stages of neoplastic and normal pre-B cell differentiation. J Clin Invest 1984;74:332–49.

108. Nadler LM, Stashenko P, Hardy R. Monoclonal antibody identifies a new Ia-like polymorphic system linked to the HLA-D/DR region. Nature 1981;290:591–3.

109. Moore MAS, Broxmeyer HE, Sheridan APC, et al. Continuous human bone marrow culture: Ia antigen characterization of probable pluripotential stem cells. Blood 1980;55:682–90.

110. Fitchen JH, LeFevre C, Ferrone S, Cline M. Expression Ia-like and HLA-A,B antigens on human multipotential hematopoietic progenitor cells. Blood 1982;59:188–90.

111. Borowitz MJ. Immunologic markers in childhood acute lymphoblastic leukemia. Hematol Oncol Clin North Am 1990;4:743–65.

112. Huang S, Terstappen LWMM. Formation of haematopoietic microenvironment and haematopoietic stem cells from single human bone marrow stem cells. Nature 1992;360:745–9.

113. Civin CI, Trischmann TM, Fackler MJ, et al. Report on the CD34 cluster workshop. In: Knapp W, Dorken B, Rieber EP, et al, eds. Leukocyte typing IV: white cell differentiation antigens. 1st ed. Oxford: Oxford University Press, 1989:818–25.

114. Batinic D, Tindle R, Boban D, et al. Expression of haematopoietic progenitor cell-associated antigen BI-3C5/CD34 in leukaemia. Leukemia Res 1989;13:83–5.

115. Shah VO, Civin CI, Loken MR. Flow cytometric analysis of human bone marrow. IV. Differential quantitative expression of T-200 common leukocyte antigen during normal hemopoiesis. J Immunol 1988;140:1861–7.

116. Behm FG, Raimondi SC, Schell MJ, et al. Lack of CD45 antigen on blast cells in childhood acute lymphoblastic leukemia is associated with chromosomal hyperdiploidy and other favorable prognostic features. Blood 1992;79:1011–6.

117. Behm FG, Raimondi SC, Schell MJ, et al. Response to "CD45 expression and prognosis in acute lymphoblastic leukemia." Blood 1993;81:563.

118. Knowles DM, Chadburn A, Inghirami G. Immunophenotypic markers useful in the diagnosis and classification of hematopoietic neoplasms. In: Knowles DM, ed. Neoplastic hematopathology. 1st ed. Baltimore: Williams & Wilkins, 1992:73–167.

119. Traweek ST. Immunophenotypic analysis of acute leukemia. Am J Clin Pathol 1993;99:504–12.

120. Sobol RE, Bloomfield CD, Royston I. Immunophenotyping in the diagnosis and classification of acute lymphoblastic leukemia. Clin Lab Med 1988;1:151–62.

121. Garand R, Vannier JP, Bene MC, et al. Correlations between acute lymphoid leukemia immunophenotype and clinical and laboratory data at presentation. Cancer 1989;64:1437–46.

122. Pui CH, Behm FG, Crist WM. Clinical and biologic relevance of immunologic marker studies in childhood acute lymphoblastic leukemia. Blood 1993;82:343–62.

123. van't Veer MB, van Putten WLJ, Verdonck LF, et al. Acute lymphoblastic leukaemia in adults: immunological subtypes and clinical features at presentation. Ann Hematol 1993;66:277–82.

124. Garand R, Bene MC. Incidence, clinical and laboratory features, and prognostic significance of immunophenotypic subgroups in acute lymphoblastic leukemia: the GEIL experience. Recent Results Cancer Res 1993;131:283–95.

125. Deegan MJ. Membrane antigen analysis in the diagnosis of lymphoid leukemias and lymphomas. Arch Pathol Lab Med 1989;113:606–18.

126. Uckun FM. Regulation of human B-cell ontogeny. Blood 1990;76:1908–23.

127. Crist W, Shuster J, Look T, et al. Current results of studies of immunophenotype-, age- and leukocyte-based therapy for children with acute lymphoblastic leukemia. The Pediatric Oncology Group. Leukemia 1992;6:Suppl 2:162–6.

128. Garand R, Bene MC, the GEIL. A new approach of acute lymphoblastic leukemia immunophenotypic classification: 1984–1994 the GEIL experience. Leuk Lymphoma 1994;13:Suppl 1:1–5.

129. De Rossi G, Grossi C, Foa R, et al. Immunophenotype of acute lymphoblastic leukemia cells: the experience of the Italian Cooperative Group (Gimema). Leuk Lymphoma 1993;9:221–8.

130. Haynes BF, Denning SM, Singer KH, Kurtzberg J. Ontogeny of T-cell precursors: a model for the initial stages of human T-cell development. Immunol Today 1989;10:87–91.

131. Reinherz EL, Kung PC, Goldstein G, et al. Discrete stages of human intrathymic differentiation: analysis of normal thymocytes and leukemic lymphoblasts of T-cell lineage. Proc Natl Acad Sci U S A 1980;77:1588–92.

132. LeBien TW, Villablancea JG. Ontogeny of normal human B-cell and T-cell precursors and its relation to leukemogenesis. Hematol Oncol Clin North Am 1990;4:835–47.

133. Terstappen LWMM, Huang S, Picker LJ. Flow cytometric assessment of human T-cell differentiation in thymus and bone marrow. Blood 1992;79:666–77.

134. Galy A, Verma S, Barcena A, Spits H. Precursors of CD3$^+$, CD4$^+$, CD8$^+$ cells in the human thymus are defined by expression of CD34. Delineation of early events in human thymic development. J Exp Med 1993;178:391–401.

135. Borowitz MJ, Dowell BL, Boyett JM, et al. Clinicopathologic aspects of E rosette negative T cell acute lymphocytic leukemia: a pediatric oncology group study. J Clin Oncol 1986;4:170–7.

136. Furley AJ, Mizutani K, Weilbaecher K, et al. Developmentally regulated rearrangement and expression of genes encoding the T-cell receptor T3 complex. Cell 1986;46:75.

137. Lafaille JJ, DeCloux A, Boneville M, et al. Junctional sequences of T cell receptor XgXδ genes: implications for XgXδ T cell lineages and for a novel intermediate of V-(D)-J joining. Cell 1989;59:859.

138. Haynes BE, Martin ME, Kay HH, Kurtzberg J. Early events in human T cell ontogeny. Phenotypic characterization and immunohistologic localization of T cell precursors in early human fetal tissues. J Exp Med 1988;168:1061.

139. Tasaka T, Nagai M, Murao S, et al. CD7, CD34-positive stem cell leukemia arising in agnogenic myeloid metaplasia. Am J Hematol 1993;44:53–7.

140. Jacobs JC, Rearden A. CD7-postive acute leukemia lacking T cell receptor gene rearrangements and terminal dexoynucleotidyl transferase expression suggesting pre-T cell origin. Am J Hematol 1989;32:212.

141. Borowitz MJ, Dowell BL, Boyett JM, et al. Monoclonal antibody definition of T cell acute leukemia: a Pediatric Oncology Group study. Blood 1985;65:785–8.

142. Pittaluga S, Raffield M, Lipford EH, Cossmann J. 3A1 (CD7) Expression precedes Tβ gene rearrangements in precursor T (lymphoblastic) neoplasms. Blood 1986;68:134–9.

143. Kurtzberg J, Waldmann TA, Davey MP, et al. CD7$^+$, CD4$^-$, CD8$^-$ acute leukemia: a syndrome of malignant pluripotent lymphohematopoietic cells. Blood 1989;73:381–90.

144. Kita K, Miwa H, Nakase K, et al. Clinical importance of CD7 expression in acute myelocytic leukemia. Blood 1993;81:2399–405.

145. Barcena A, Muench MO, Galy AHM, et al. Phenotypic and functional analysis of T-cell precursors in the human fetal liver and thymus: CD7 expression in the early stages of T- and myeloid-cell development. Blood 1993;82:3401.

146. Bradstock KF, Kirk J, Grimsley PG, et al. Unusual immunophenotypes in acute leukaemias: incidence and clinical correlations. Br J Haematol 1989;72:512–8.

147. Zutter MM, Martin PJ, Hanke D, Kidd PG. CD7 + acute non-lymphocytic leukemia: evidence for an early multipotential progenitor. Leukemia Res 1990;14:23.

148. Janossy G, Coustan-Smith E, Campana D. The reliability of cytoplasmic CD3 and CD22 antigen expression in the immunodiagnosis of acute leukemia: a study of 500 cases. Leukemia 1989;3:170–81.

149. Del Vecchio LD, Schiavone EM, Ferrara F, et al. Immunodiagnosis of acute leukemia displaying ectopic antigens: proposal for classification of promiscuous phenotypes. Am J Hematol 1989;31:173–80.

150. van Dongen JJM, Krissansen GW, Wolvers-Tettero IL, et al. Cytoplasmic expression of the CD3 antigen as a diagnostic marker for immature T-cell malignancies. Blood 1988;71:603–12.

151. Campana D, Thompson JS, Amlot P, et al. The cytoplasmic expression of CD3 antigens in normal and malignant cells of the T lymphoid lineage. J Immunol 1987;138:648–55.

152. Ludwig WD, Thiel E, Bartram CR, et al. Clinical importance of T-ALL subclassification according to thymic or prethymic maturation stage. In: Buchner T, Schellong G, Hiddemann W, Ritter J, eds. Acute leukemias II. Berlin: Springer-Verlag, 1990:419–27.

153. Thiel E, Franz BR, Raghavachar A. Prethymic phenotype and genotype of pre-T (CD7 + /ER-) -cell leukemia and its clinical significance within adult lymphoblastic leukemia. Blood 1989;73:1247–58.

154. Raimondi SC, Behm FG, Roberson PK, et al. Cytogenetics of childhood T-cell leukemia. Blood 1988;72:1560–6.

155. Gill PS, Meyer PR, Pavolva Z, Levine AM. B cell acute lymphoblastic leukemia in adults. Clinical, morphologic, and immunologic findings. J Clin Oncol 1986;4:737–43.

156. Davey FR, Lawrence D, MacCallum J, et al. Morphologic characteristics of acute lymphoblastic leukemia (ALL) with abnormalities of chromosome 8, band q24. Am J Hematol 1992;40:183–91.

157. Hurwitz CA, Gore SD, Stone KD, Civin CI. Flow cytometric detection of rare normal human marrow cells with immunophenotypes characteristic of acute lymphoblastic leukemia cells. Leukemia 1992;6:233–9.

158. McKinney PA, Alexander FE, Cartwright RA, et al. Acute lymphoblastic leukaemia incidence in the UK by immunophenotype. Leukemia 1993;7:1630–4.

159. Rieder H, Ludwig WD, Gassmann W, et al. Chromosomal abnormalities in adult acute lymphoblastic leukemia: results of the German ALL/AUL Study Group. Recent Results in Cancer Research 1993;131:133–8.

160. Krause JR, Penchansky L, Contis L, Kaplan SS. Flow cytometry in the diagnosis of acute leukemia. Am J Clin Pathol 1988;89:341–6.

161. Koehler MQ, Behm FG, Shuster J, et al. Transitional pre-B-cell acute lymphoblastic leukemia of childhood is associated with favorable prognostic clinical features and an excellent outcome: a Pediatric Oncology Group study. Leukemia 1993;7:2064–8.

162. Greaves MF, Chan LC, Furley AJ, et al. Lineage promiscuity in hemopoietic differentiation and leukemia. Blood 1986;67:1–11.

163. Drexler HG, Thiel E, Ludwig W-D. Review of the incidence and clinical relevance of myeloid antigen-positive acute lymphoblastic leukemia. Leukemia 1991;5:637–45.

164. Czuczman MS, Dodge RK, Stewart CC, et al. Value of immunophenotype in intensively treated adult acute lymphoblastic leukemia: cancer and leukemia Group B study 8364. Blood 1999;93:3931–9.

165. Khalidi HS, Chang KL, Medeiros LJ, et al. Acute lymphoblastic leukemia. Survey of immunophenotype, French-American-British classification, frequency of myeloid antigen expression, and karyotypic abnormalities in 210 pediatric and adult cases. Am J Clin Pathol 1999;111:467–76.

166. Boucheix C, David B, Sebban C, et al. Immunophenotype of adult acute lymphoblastic leukemia, clinical parameters, and outcome: an analysis of a prospective trial including 562 tested patients (LALA87). French Group on Therapy for Adult Acute Lymphoblastic Leukemia. Blood 1994;84:1603–12.

167. Pui C-H, Raimondi SC, Head DR, et al. Characterization of childhood acute leukemia with multiple myeloid and lymphoid markers at diagnosis and relapse. Blood 1991;78:1327–37.

168. Borowitz MJ, Schuster JJ, Land VJ, et al. Myeloid-antigen expression in childhood acute lymphoblastic leukemia. letter to the editor. N Engl J Med 1991;325:1379–80.

169. Uckun FM, Sather HN, Gaynon PS, et al. Clinical features and treatment outcome of children with myeloid antigen positive acute lymphoblastic leukemia: a report from the Children's Cancer Group. Blood 1997;90:28–35.

170. Basso G, Rondelli R, Putti MC, et al. Incidence and prognostic significance of immunophenotypic subgroups in childhood acute lymphoblastic leukemia: the experience of the AIEOP Cooperative

Study. Associazione Italiana Ematologia Oncologia Pediatrica. Recent Results Cancer Res 1993;131:297–307.

171. Khalil SH, Jackson JM, Qari MH, Pyle H. Acute myeloblastic leukemia (AML-M2) expressing CD19 B-cell lymphoid antigen without myeloid surface antigens. Leukemia Res 1994;18:145.

172. Tsuchiya H, ElSonbaty SS, Nagano K, et al. Acute myeloblastic leukemia (ANLL-M2) with t(8;21)(q22;;q22) variant expressing lymphoid but not myeloid surface antigens with a high number of G-CSF receptors. Leukemia Res 1993;17:375–7.

173. Sobol RE, Mick R, Royston I, et al. Clinical importance of myeloid antigen expression in adult acute lymphoblastic leukemia. N Engl J Med 1987;316:1111–7.

174. Ludwig W-D, Reiter A, Loffler H, et al. Immunophenotypic features of childhood and adult acute lymphoblastic leukemia (ALL): experience of the German multicentre trials ALL-BFM and GMALL. Leuk Lymphoma 1994;13:Suppl 1:71–76.

175. Huh YO, Kantarjian H, Childs CC, et al. Classification of adult ALL by immunophenotype. Blood 1990;76:Suppl 1:282a.

176. Steward CG, Goulden NJ, Potter MN, Oakhill A. The use of the polymerase chain reaction to detect minimal residual disease in childhood acute lymphoblastic leukaemia. Eur J Cancer 1993;29A:1192–8.

177. Yamada M, Hudson S, Tournay O, et al. Detection of minimal disease in hematopoietic malignancies of the B-cell lineage by using third-complementarity-determining region-specific probes. Proc Natl Acad Sci U S A 1989;86:5123–7.

178. Steward CG, Potter MN, Oakhill A. Third complementarity determining region (CDR III) sequence analysis in childhood B-lineage acute lymphoblastic leukaemia: implications for the design of oligonucleotide probes for use in monitoring minimal residual disease. Leukemia 1992;6:1213–9.

179. Steenbergen EJ, Verhagen OJ, van Leeuwen EF, et al. B precursor acute lymphoblastic leukemia third complementarity-determining regions predominantly represent an unbiased recombination repertoire: leukemic transformation frequently occurs in fetal life. Eur J Immunol 1994;24:900–8.

180. Griesser H, Tkachuk D, Reis MD, Mak TW. Gene rearrangements and translocations in lymphoproliferative diseases. Blood 1989;73:1402–15.

181. Tang JQ, Bëne MC, Faure GC. Alternative rearrangements of immunoglobulin light chain genes in human leukemia. Leukemia 1991;5:651–6.

182. Beishuizen A, Hahlen K, Hagemeijer A, et al. Multiple rearranged immunoglobulin genes in childhood acute lymphoblastic leukemia of precursor B-cell origin. Leukemia 1991;5:657–67.

183. Kawakami K, Kita K, Miwa H, et al. Rearrangement patterns of immunoglobulin heavy chain (IgH) and light chain genes in acute lymphoblastic leukemia and chronic myelocytic leukemia lymphoid crisis cells showing oligoclonal IgH gene rearrangements. Int J Hematol 1992;55:61–9.

184. Marchalonis JJ, Schluter SF, Edmundson AB. The T-cell receptor as immunoglobulin: paradigm regained. Proc Soc Exp Biol Med 1997;216:303–18.

185. Marrack P, Kappler J. The T cell receptor. Science 1987;238:1073–79.

186. Winoto A, Baltimore D. Separate lineages of T cells expressing the αβ and XgXδ receptors. Nature 1989;338:430.

187. Foroni L, Laffan M, Boehm T, et al. Rearrangements of the T-cell receptor δ genes in human T-cell leukemias. Blood 1989;73:559–65.

188. Davis MM, Bjorkman PJ. T-cell antigen genes and T-cell recognition. Nature 1988;334:395–402. review.

189. Secker-Walker LM, Campana D, Hawkins JM, et al. Karyotype and T-cell receptor expression in T-lineage acute lymphoblastic leukemia. Genes Chromosomes Cancer 1992;4:41–5.

190. Felix CA, Poplack DG, Reaman GH, et al. Characterization of immunoglobulin and T-cell receptor gene patterns in B-cell precursor acute lymphoblastic leukemia of childhood. J Clin Oncol 1990;8:431–42.

191. Schardt C, Hoelzer D, Ganser A. Presence of more than two rearranged immunoglobulin heavy-chain genes in adult precursor B-cell acute lymphoblastic leukemia. Ann Hematol 1992;64:72–77.

192. Knowles DM. Immunophenotypic and antigen receptor gene rearrangement analysis in T cell neoplasia. Am J Pathol 1989;134:761.

193. Mirro J Jr, Kitchingman G, Behm FG, et al. T cell differentiation stages identified by molecular and immunologic analysis of the T cell receptor complex in childhood lymphoblastic leukemia. Blood 1987;69:908–12.

194. Griesinger F, Greenberg JM, Kersey JH. T cell receptor gamma and delta rearrangements in hematologic malignancies. relationship to lymphoid differentiation. J Clin Invest 1989;84:506–16.

195. Yokota S, Hansen-Hagge TE, Ludwig WD, et al. Use of polymerase chain reactions to monitor minimal residual disease in acute lymphoblastic leukemia patients. Blood 1991;77:331–9.

196. Breit TM, Wolvers-Tettero IL, Beishuizen A, et al. Southern blot patterns, frequencies, and junctional diversity of T-cell receptor-cδ gene rearrangements in acute lymphoblastic leukemia. Blood 1993;82:3063–74.

197. Taylor JJ, Rowe D, Williamson IK, et al. Detection of T-cell receptor gamma chain V gene rearrangements using the polymerase chain reaction: application to the study of clonal disease cells in acute lymphoblastic leukemia. Blood 1991;77:1989–95.

198. Goasguen JE, Kitchingman GR, Mirro J Jr, Stass SA. Lineage heterogeneity in acute leukemia. In: Knowles DM, editor. Neoplastic hematopathology. 1st ed. Baltimore: Williams & Wilkins, 1992:1351–65.

199. Szczepanski T, Beishuizen A, Pongers-Willemse MJ, et al. Cross-lineage T cell receptor gene rearrangements occur in more than ninety percent of childhood precursor-B acute lymphoblastic leukemias: alternative PCR targets for detection of minimal residual disease. Leukemia 1999;13:196–205.

200. Szczepanski T, Langerak AW, Wolvers-Tettero IL, et al. Immunoglobulin and T cell receptor gene rearrangement patterns in acute lymphoblastic leukemia are less mature in adults than in children: implications for selection of PCR targets for detection of minimal residual disease. Leukemia 1998;12:1081–8.

201. Diaz MA, Garcia-Sanchez F, Vicario JL, et al. Clinical relevance of T-cell receptor delta gene rearrangements in childhood B-precursor cell acute lymphoblastic leukaemia [see comments]. Br J Haematol 1997;99:308–13.

202. Wright JJ, Poplack DG, Bakhshi A, et al. Gene rearrangements as markers of clonal variation and minimal residual disease in acute lymphoblastic leukemia. J Clin Oncol 1987;5:735–41.

203. Mitelman F, Kaneko Y, Berger R. Report of the committee on chromosome changes in neoplasia. Genome Priority Reports 1993;1:700–26.

204. Rabbitts TH. Chromosomal translocations in human cancer. Nature 1994;372:143–9.

205. Look AT. Oncogenic transcription factors in the human acute leukemias. Science 1997;278:1059–64.

206. Raimondi SC. Current status of cytogenetic research in childhood acute lymphoblastic leukemia. Blood 1993;81:2237–51.

207. Anonymous. Cytogenetic abnormalities in adult acute lymphoblastic leukemia: correlations with hematologic findings outcome. A Collaborative Study of the Group Francais de Cytogenetique Hematologique [published erratum appears in Blood 1996 Oct 1;88(7):2818]. Blood 1996;87:3135–42.

208. Wetzler M, Dodge RK, Mrozek K, et al. Prospective karyotype analysis in adult acute lymphoblastic leukemia: the cancer and leukemia Group B experience. Blood 1999;93:3983–93.

209. Rubnitz JE, Downing JR, Pui CH, et al. TEL gene rearrangement in acute lymphoblastic leukemia: a new genetic marker with prognostic significance. J Clin Oncol 1997;15:1150–7.

210. Secker-Walker LM, Prentice HG, Durrant J, et al. Cytogenetics adds independent prognostic information in adults with acute lymphoblastic leukaemia on MRC trial UKALL XA. MRC Adult Leukaemia Working Party [see comments]. Br J Haematol 1997;96:601–10.

211. Anonymous. Cytogenetic abnormalities in adult acute lymphoblastic leukemia: correlations with hematologic findings outcome. A Collaborative Study of the Group Francais de Cytogenetique Hematologique [published erratum appears in Blood 1996;88(7):2818]. Blood 1996;87:3135–42.

212. Faderl S, Kantarjian HM, Talpaz M, Estrov Z. Clinical significance of cytogenetic abnormalities in adult acute lymphoblastic leukemia. Blood 1998;91:3995–4019.

213. Watson MS, Carroll AJ, Shuster JJ, et al. Trisomy 21 in childhood adult lymphoblastic leukemia: a Pediatric Oncology Group Study (8602). Blood 1993;82:3098–102.

214. Harbott J, Ritterbach J, Ludwig W-D, et al. Clinical significance of cytogenetic studies in childhood acute lymphoblastic leukemia: experience of the BFM trials. In: Ludwig W-D, Thiel E, eds. Recent results in cancer research. 131st ed. Heidelberg: Springer-Verlag Berlin, 1993:123–32.

215. Bloomfield CD, Secker-Walker LM, Goldman AI, et al. Six-year follow-up of the clinical significance of karyotype in acute lymphoblastic leukemia. Cancer Genet Cytogenet 1989;40:171–85.

216. Bloomfield CD, Goldman AI, Alimena G, et al. Chromosomal abnormalities identify high risk and low-risk patients with acute lymphoblastic leukemia. Blood 1986;67:415–20.

217. Frankel SR, Wurster-Hill DH, Lawrence D, et al. Cytogenetics is the most important prognostic factor in adult acute lymphoblastic leukemia. Blood 1992;80:Suppl 1:257a.

218. Charrin C, Groupe Francais de Cytogenetique Hematologique (GFCH). Karyotypes of 433 adults with acute lymphoblastic leukemia: a prospective collaborative study. Blood 1993;82:Suppl 1:57a. abstract.

219. Wetzler M, Dodge RK, Mrozek K, et al. Prospective karyotype analysis in adult acute lymphoblastic leukemia: the cancer and leukemia Group B experience. Blood 1999;93:3983–93.

220. Fenaux P, Lai JL, Morel P, et al. Cytogenetics and their prognostic value in childhood and adult acute lymphoblastic leukemia (ALL) excluding L3. Hematol Oncol 1989;7:307–17.

221. Crist W, Carroll A, Shuster J, et al. Philadelphia chromosome positive childhood acute lymphoblastic leukemia: clinical and cytogenetic characteristics and treatment outcome. A Pediatric Oncology Group study. Blood 1990;76:489–94.

222. Schlieben S, Borkhardt A, Reinisch I, et al. Incidence and clinical outcome of children with BCR/ABL-positive acute lymphoblastic leukemia (ALL). A prospective RT-PCR study based on 673 patients enrolled in the German pediatric multicenter therapy trials ALL-BFM-90 and CoALL-05-92. Leukemia 1996;10:957–63.

223. Harbott J, Ritterbach J, Janka-Schaub G, et al. Cytogenetics of childhood acute lymphoblastic leukemia in multicenter trials. In: Buchner T, Schellong G, Hiddemann W, Ritter J, eds. Acute leukemias II. Berlin: Springer-Verlag, 1994:451–8.

224. Secker-Walker LM. Prognostic and biological importance of chromosome findings in acute lymphoblastic leukemia. Cancer Genet Cytogenet 1990;49:1–13.

225. Harbott J, Ritterbach J, Ludwig WD, et al. Clinical significance of cytogenetic studies in childhood acute lymphoblastic leukemia: experience of the BFM trials. Recent Results Cancer Res 1993;131:123–32.

226. Anonymous. Third international workshop on chromosomes in leukemia, 1980: clinical significance of chromosomal abnormalities in acute lymphoblastic leukemia. Cancer Genet Cytogenet 1981;4:111–37.

227. Paietta E, Racevskis J, Neuberg D, et al. Expression of CD25 (interleukin-2 receptor alpha chain) in adult acute lymphoblastic leukemia predicts for the presence of BCR/ABL fusion transcripts: results of a preliminary laboratory analysis of ECOG/MRC Intergroup Study E2993. Eastern Cooperative Oncology Group/Medical Research Council. Leukemia 1997;11:1887–90.

228. Pui C, Frankel LS, Carroll AJ, et al. Clinical characteristics and treatment outcome of childhood acute lymphoblastic leukemia with the t(4;11)(q21;q23): a collaborative study of 40 cases. Blood 1991;77:440–7.

229. Johansson B, Moorman AV, Haas OA, et al. Hematologic malignancies with t(4;11)(q21;q23)—a cytogenetic, morphologic, immunophenotypic and clinical study of 183 cases. European 11q23 Workshop participants. Leukemia 1998;12:779–87.

230. Heerema NA. Cytogenetic abnormalities and molecular markers of acute lymphoblastic leukemia. Hematol Oncol Clin North Am 1990;4:795–820.

231. Rubnitz JE, Link MP, Shuster JJ, et al. Frequency and prognostic significance of *HRX* rearrangements in infant acute lymphoblastic leukemia: a Pediatric Oncology Group Study. Blood 1994;84:570–73.

232. Childs CC, Hirsch-Ginsberg C, Culbert SJ, et al. Lineage heterogeneity in acute leukemia with the t(4;11) abnormality. Implications of acute mixed lineage leukemia. Hematol Pathol 1993;2:145–51.

233. Mirro J, Kitchingman G, Williams D, et al. Clinical and laboratory characteristics of acute leukemia with the (4;11) translocation. Blood 1986;67:689–97.

234. Borowitz MJ, Carroll AJ, Shuster JJ, et al. Use of clinical and laboratory features to define prognostic subgroups in B-precursor acute lymphoblastic leukemia: experience of the Pediatric Oncology Group. Recent Results Cancer Res 1993;131:257–67.

235. Gibbons B, Katz FE, Ganly P, Chessells JM. Infant acute lymphoblastic leukaemia with t(11;19). Br J Haematol 1990;74:264–9.

236. Privitera E, Kamps MP, Hayashi Y, et al. Different molecular consequences of the 1;19 chromosomal translocation in childhood B-cell precursor acute lymphoblastic leukemia. Blood 1992;79:1781–8.

237. Sandberg AA. The chromosomes in human cancer and leukemia. 2nd ed. New York: Elsevier, 1991.

238. Uckun FM, Gajl-Peczalska KJ, Provisor AJ, Heerema NA. Immunophenotype-karyotype associations in human acute lymphoblastic leukemia. Blood 1989;73:271–80.

239. Carroll AJ, Crist WM, Link MP, et al. The t(1;14)(p34;q11) is nonrandom and restricted to T-cell acute lymphoblastic leukemia: a Pediatric Oncology Group study. Blood 1990;76:1220–4.

240. Dube ID, Raimondi SC, Pi D, Kalousek DK. A new translocation, t(10;14)(q24;q11), in T cell neoplasia. Blood 1986;67:1181–4.

241. Zutter M, Hockett RD, Roberts CW, et al. The t(10;14)(q24;q11) of T-cell acute lymphoblastic leukemia juxtaposes the delta T-cell receptor with TCL3, a conserved and activated locus at 10q24. Proc Natl Acad Sci U S A 1990;87:3161–5.

242. Sanchez-Garcia I, Rabbitts TH. LIM domain proteins in leukaemia and development. Semin Cancer Biol 1993;4:349–58.

243. McGuire EA, Rintoul CE, Sclar GM, Korsmeyer SJ. Thymic overexpression of Ttg-1 in transgenic mice results in T-cell acute lymphoblastic leukemia/lymphoma. Mol Cell Biol 1992;12:4186–96.

244. Boehm T, Baer R, Lavenir I, et al. The mechanism of chromosomal translocation t(11;14) involving the T-cell receptor Cδ locus on human chromosome 14q11 and a transcribed region of chromosome 11p15. EMBO J 1988;7:385–94.

245. McGuire EA, Hockett RD, Pollock KM, et al. The t(11;14)(p15;q11) in a T-cell acute lymphoblastic leukemia cell line activates multiple transcripts, including TTG-1, a gene including a potential zinc finger. Mol Cell Biol 1989;9:2124–32.

246. Berger R. Molecular cytogenetics of acute lymphoblastic leukemia. Nouv Rev Fr Hematol 1991;33:86–91.

247. Golub TR, Barker GF, Bohlander SK, et al. Fusion of the TEL gene on 12p13 to the AML1 gene on 21q22 in acute lymphoblastic leukemia. Proc Natl Acad Sci U S A 1995;92:4917–21.

248. Aguiar RC, Sohal J, van Rhee F, et al. TEL-AML1 fusion in acute lymphoblastic leukaemia of adults. M.R.C. Adult Leukaemia Working Party. Br J Haematol 1996;95:673–7.

249. Orkin SH. Transcription factors and hematopoietic development. J Biol Chem 1995;270:4955–8.

250. Shivdasani RA, Orkin SH. The transcriptional control of hematopoiesis [see comments]. Blood 1996;87:4025–39.

251. Westbrook CA, Hooberman AL, Spino C, et al. Clinical significance of the BCR-ABL fusion gene in adult acute lymphoblastic leukemia: a Cancer and Leukemia Group B Study (8762). Blood 1992;80:2983–90.

252. Secker-Walker LM, Craig JM, Hawkins JM, Hoffbrand AV. Philadelphia positive acute lymphoblastic leukemia in adults: age distribution, BCR breakpoint and prognostic significance. Leukemia 1991;5:196–9.

253. Maurer J, Janssen JWG, Thiel E, et al. Detection of chimeric BCR-ABL genes in acute lymphoblastic leukaemia by the polymerase chain reaction. Lancet 1991;337:1055–8.

254. Melo JV, Gordon DE, Tuszynski A, et al. Expression of the ABL-BCR fusion gene in Philadelphia-positive acute lymphoblastic leukemia. Blood 1993;81:2488–91.

255. Daley GQ, Van Etten RA, Baltimore D. Induction of chronic myelogenous leukemia in mice by the P210bcr/abl gene of the Philadelphia chromosome. Science 1990;247:824–30.

256. Heisterkamp N, Jenster G, ten Hoeve J, et al. Acute leukaemia in bcr/abl transgenic mice. Nature 1990;344:251–3.

257. Goga A, McLaughlin J, Afar DE, et al. Alternative signals to RAS for hematopoietic transformation by the BCR-ABL oncogene. Cell 1995;82:981–8.

258. Sawyers CL, McLaughlin J, Witte ON. Genetic requirement for Ras in the transformation of fibroblasts and hematopoietic cells by the Bcr-Abl oncogene. J Exp Med 1995;181:307–13.

259. Sanchez-Garcia I, Martin-Zanca D. Regulation of Bcl-2 gene expression by BCR-ABL is mediated by Ras. J Mol Biol 1997;267:225–8.

260. Dubrez L, Eymin B, Sordet O, et al. BCR-ABL delays apoptosis upstream of procaspase-3 activation. Blood 1998;91:2415–22.

261. Anastasi J, Feng J, Dickstein JI, et al. Lineage involvement by BCR/ABL in Ph+ lymphoblastic leukemias: chronic myelogenous leukemia presenting in lymphoid blast vs Ph+ acute lymphoblastic leukemia. Leukemia 1996;10:795–802.

262. Voncken JW, Kaartinen V, Pattengale PK, et al. BCR/ABL P210 and P190 cause distinct leukemia in transgenic mice. Blood 1995;86:4603–11.

263. Thirman MJ, Gill HJ, Burnett RC, et al. Rearrangement of the MLL gene in acute lymphoblastic and acute myeloid leukemias with 11q23 chromosomal translocations [see comments]. N Engl J Med 1993;329:909–14.

264. Chen CS, Sorensen PH, Domer PH, et al. Molecular rearrangements on chromosome 11q23 predominate in infant acute lymphoblastic leukemia and are associated with specific biologic variables and poor outcome. Blood 1993;81:2386–93.

265. Zieman-van der Poel S, McCabe NR, Gill HJ, et al. Identification of a gene, MLL, that spans the breakpoint in 11q23 translocations associated with human leukemias. Proc Natl Acad Sci U S A 1991; 88:10735–9.

266. Gu Y, Cimino G, Alder H, et al. The (4;11)(q21;q23) chromosome translocations in acute leukemias involve the VDJ recombinase. Proc Natl Acad Sci U S A 1992;89:10464–8.

267. Tkachuk DC, Kohler S, Cleary ML. Involvement of a homolog of Drosophila trithorax by 11q23 chromosomal translocations in acute leukemias. Cell 1992;71:691–700.

268. Djabali M, Selleri L, Parry P, et al. A trithorax-like gene is interrupted by chromosome 11q23 translocations in acute leukaemias. Nat Genet 1992;2:113–8.

269. Stock W, Thirman MJ, Dodge RK, et al. Detection of MLL gene rearrangements in adult acute lymphoblastic leukemia (CALGB 8762). Blood 1993;82:Suppl 1:58a. abstract.

270. Hilden JM, Frestedt JL, Moore RO, et al. Molecular analysis of infant acute lymphoblastic leukemia: MLL gene rearrangement and reverse transcriptase-polymerase chain reaction for t(4;11)(q21;q23). Blood 1995;86:3876–82.

271. Mazo AM, Huang DH, Mozer BA, Dawid IB. The trithorax gene, a trans-acting regulator of the bithorax complex in Drosophila, encodes a protein with zinc-binding domains. Proc Natl Acad Sci U S A 1990;87:2112–6.

272. Zeleznik-Le NJ, Harden AM, Rowley JD. 11q23 translocations split the "AT-hook" cruciform DNA-binding region and the transcriptional repression domain from the activation domain of the mixed-lineage leukemia (MLL) gene. Proc Natl Acad Sci U S A 1994;91:10610–4.

273. Yu BD, Hess JL, Horning SE, et al. Altered Hox expression and segmental identity in Mll-mutant mice. Nature 1995;378:505–8.

274. Gu Y, Nakamura T, Alder H, et al. The t(4;11) chromosome translocation of human acute leukemias fuses the ALL-1 gene, related to Drosophila trithorax, to the AF-4 gene. Cell 1992;71:701–8.

275. Nakamura T, Alder H, Gu Y, et al. Genes on chromosomes 4, 9, and 19 involved in 11q23 abnormalities in acute leukemia share sequence homology and/or common motifs. Proc Natl Acad Sci U S A 1993;90:4631–5.

276. Corral J, Forster A, Thompson S, et al. Acute leukemias of different lineages have similar MLL gene fusions encoding related chimeric proteins resulting from chromosomal translocation. Proc Natl Acad Sci U S A 1993;90:8538–42.

277. Lavau C, Szilvassy SJ, Slany R, Cleary ML. Immortalization and leukemic transformation of a myelomonocytic precursor by retrovirally transduced HRX-ENL. EMBO J 1997;16:4226–37.

278. Kamps MP, Murre C, Sun X-H, Baltimore D. A new homeobox gene contributes the DNA binding domain of the t(1;19) translocation protein in pre-B ALL. Cell 1990;60:547–55.

279. Hunger SP, Galili N, Carroll AJ, et al. The t(1;19)(q23;p13) results in consistent fusion of E2A and PBX1 coding sequences in acute lymphoblastic leukemias. Blood 1991;77:687–93.

280. Nourse J, Melletin JD, Galili N, et al. Chromosomal translocation t(1;19) results in synthesis of a homeobox fusion mRNA that codes for a potential chimeric transcription factor. Cell 1990;60:535–45.

281. Kamps MP, Look AT, Baltimore D. The human t(1;19) translocation in pre-B ALL produces multiple nuclear E2A-Pbx1 fusion proteins with differing transforming potential. Genes Dev 1991;5:358–68.

282. Izraeli S, Henn T, Strobl H, et al. Expression of identical E2A/PBX1 fusion transcripts occurs in both pre-B and early pre-B immunological subtypes of childhood acute lymphoblastic leukemia. Leukemia 1993;7:2054–6.

283. Dedera DA, Waller EK, LeBrun DP, et al. Chimeric homeobox gene E2A-PBX1 induces proliferation, apoptosis, and malignant lymphomas in transgenic mice [published erratum appears in Cell 1993;75(4):826]. Cell 1993;74:833–43.

284. Inaba T, Inukai T, Yoshihara T, et al. Reversal of apoptosis by the leukaemia-associated E2A-HLF chimaeric transcription factor. Nature 1996;382:541–4.

285. Romana SP, Mauchauffe M, Le Coniat M, et al. The t(12;21) of acute lymphoblastic leukemia results in a tel-AML1 gene fusion. Blood 1995;85:3662–70.

286. Shih LY, Chou TB, Liang DC, et al. Lack of TEL-AML1 fusion transcript resulting from a cryptic t(12;21) in adult B lineage acute lymphoblastic leukemia in Taiwan. Leukemia 1996;10:1456–8.

287. Okuda T, van Deursen J, Hiebert SW, et al. AML1, the target of multiple chromosomal translocations in human leukemia, is essential for normal fetal liver hematopoiesis. Cell 1996;84:321–30.

288. Friedman AD. Leukemogenesis by CBF oncoproteins. Leukemia 1999;13:1932–42.

289. Hiebert SW, Sun W, Davis JN, et al. The t(12;21) translocation converts AML-1B from an activator to a repressor of transcription. Mol Cell Biol 1996;16:1349–55.

290. Lutterbach B, Westendorf JJ, Linggi B, et al. A mechanism of repression by acute myeloid leukemia-1, the target of multiple chromosomal translocations in acute leukemia. J Biol Chem 2000;275:651–6.

291. Westendorf JJ, Hiebert SW. Mammalian runt-domain proteins and their roles in hematopoiesis, osteogenesis, and leukemia. J Cell Biochem 1999;Suppl 32–33:51–58.

292. Raynaud S, Cave H, Baens M, et al. The 12;21 translocation involving TEL and deletion of the other TEL allele: two frequently associated alterations found in childhood acute lymphoblastic leukemia. Blood 1996;87:2891–9.

293. Berger R, Bernheim A. Cytogenetic studies in Burkitt's lymphoma-leukemia. Cancer Genet Cytogenet 1982;7:231–44.

294. Berger R, Bernheim A, Brouet JC, et al. t(8;14) translocation in a Burkitt's type of lymphoblastic leukaemia (L3). Br J Haematol 1979;43:87–90.

295. Mitelman F, Andersson-Anvret M, Brandt L. Reciprocal 8;14 translocation in an EBV negative B cell acute lymphocytic leukemia with Burkitt's type cells. Int J Cancer 1979;24:27–33.

296. Taub R, Kirsch I, Morton C, et al. Translocation of the c-myc gene into the immunoglobulin heavy chain locus in human Burkitt's lymphoma and murine plasmacytoma cells. Proc Natl Acad Sci U S A 1982;79:7837–41.

297. Dalla-Favera R, Bregni M, Erikson J, et al. Human c-myc onc gene is located in the region of chromosome 8 that is translocated in Burkitt's lymphoma cells. Proc Natl Acad Sci U S A 1982;79:7824–7.

298. Adams JM, Harris AW, Pinkert CA, et al. The c-myc oncogene driven by immunoglobulin enhancers induces lymphoid malignancy in transgenic mice. Nature 1985;318:533–8.

299. Davis TA, Maloney DG, Czerwinski DK, et al. Anti-idiotype antibodies can induce long-term complete remissions in non-Hodgkin's lymphoma without eradicating the malignant clone. Blood 1998;92:1184–90.

300. Langdon WY, Harris AW, Cory S, Adams JM. The c-myc oncogene perturbs B lymphocyte development in E-mu-myc transgenic mice. Cell 1986;47:11–18.

301. Croce CM, Isobe M, Palumbo A, et al. Gene for alpha-chain of human T-cell receptor: location of chromosome 14 region involved in T-cell neoplasms. Science 1985;227:1044–7.

302. Raimondi SC, Pui C-H, Behm FG, Williams DL. 7q32–36 translocations in childhood T cell leukemia: cytogenetic evidence for involvement of the T cell receptor β-chain gene. Blood 1987;67:131–4.

303. Kaneko Y, Maseki N, Homma C, et al. Chromosomal translocations involving band 7q35 or 7p15 in childhood T-cell leukemia/lymphoma. Blood 1988;72:534–8.

304. Baer R. TAL1, TAL2 and LYL1: a family of basic helix-loop-helix proteins implicated in T cell acute leukaemia. Semin Cancer Biol 1993;4:341–7.

305. Park JK, Le Beau MM, Shows TB, et al. A complex genetic rearrangement in a t(10;14)(q24;q11) associated with T-cell acute lymphoblastic leukemia. Genes Chromosomes Cancer 1992;4:32–40.

306. Dube ID, Kamel-Reid S, Yuan CC, et al. A novel human homeobox gene lies at the chromosome 10 breakpoint in lymphoid neoplasias with chromosomal translocation t(10;14). Blood 1991;78:2996–3003.

307. Hatano M, Roberts CW, Minden M, et al. Deregulation of a homeobox gene, HOX11, by the t(10;14) in T cell leukemia. Science 1991;253:79–82.

308. Kagan J, Finan J, Letofsky J, et al. Alpha-chain locus of the T-cell antigen receptor is involved in the t(10;14) chromosome translocation of T-cell acute lymphocytic leukemia. Proc Natl Acad Sci U S A 1987;84:4543–6.

309. Lu M, Dube I, Raimondi S, et al. Molecular characterization of the t(10;14) translocation breakpoints in T-cell acute lymphoblastic leukemia: further evidence for illegitimate physiological recombination. Genes Chromosomes Cancer 1990;2:217–22.

310. Dear TN, Sanchez-Garcia I, Rabbitts TH. The HOX11 gene encodes

a DNA-binding nuclear transcription factor belonging to a distinct family of homeobox genes. Proc Natl Acad Sci U S A 1993;90:4431–5.

311. Zhang N, Gong ZZ, Minden M, Lu M. The HOX-11 (TCL-3) homeobox proto-oncogene encodes a nuclear protein that undergoes cell cycle-dependent regulation [published erratum appears in Oncogene 1994 Apr;9(4):1305]. Oncogene 1993;8:3265–70.

312. Fitzgerald TJ, Neale GA, Raimondi SC, Goorha RM. c-tal, a helix-loop-helix protein, is juxtaposed to the T-cell receptor-beta chain gene by a reciprocal chromosomal translocation: t(1;7)(p32;q35). Blood 1991;78:2686–95.

313. Borkhardt A, Repp R, Harbott J, et al. Frequency and DNA sequence of tal-1 rearrangement in children with T-cell acute lymphoblastic leukemia. Ann Hematol 1992;64:305–8.

314. Aplan PD, Lombardi DP, Reaman GH, et al. Involvement of the putative hematopoietic transcription factor SCL in T-cell acute lymphoblastic leukemia. Blood 1992;79:1327–33.

315. Stock W, Sher D, Sobol RE, et al. Absence of TAL1 rearrangements in adult T-cell acute lymphoblastic leukemia. Blood 1992;80:Suppl 1:194a.

316. Kikuchi A, Hayashi Y, Kobayashi S, et al. Clinical significance of TAL1 gene alteration in childhood T-cell acute lymphoblastic leukemia and lymphoma. Leukemia 1993;7:933–8.

317. Bash RO, Crist WM, Shuster JJ, et al. Clinical features and outcome of T-cell acute lymphoblastic leukemia in childhood with respect to alterations at the TAL1 locus: a Pediatric Oncology Group study. Blood 1993;81:2110–7.

318. Janssen HWG, Ludwig W, Sterry W, Bartram CR. SIL-TAL1 deletion in T-cell acute lymphoblastic leukemia. Leukemia 1993;7:1204–10.

319. Goldfarb AN, Goueli S, Michelson D, Greenberg JM. T-cell acute lymphoblastic leukemia—the associated gene SCL/tal codes for a 42-Kd nuclear phosphoprotein. Blood 1992;80:2858–66.

320. Stock W, Westbrook CA, Sher DA, et al. Low incidence of TAL1 gene rearrangements in adult acute lymphoblastic leukemia: a cancer and leukemia group B study (8762). Clin Cancer Res 1995;1:459–63.

321. Larson RC, Lavenir I, Larson TA, et al. Protein dimerization between Lmo2 (Rbtn2) and Tal1 alters thymocyte development and potentiates T cell tumorigenesis in transgenic mice. EMBO J 1996;15:1021–7.

322. Aplan PD, Jones CA, Chervinsky DS, et al. An scl gene product lacking the transactivation domain induces bony abnormalities and cooperates with LMO1 to generate T-cell malignancies in transgenic mice. EMBO J 1997;16:2408–19.

323. Foroni L, Boehm T, White L, et al. The rhombotin gene family encode related LIM-domain proteins whose differing expression suggests multiple roles in mouse development. J Mol Biol 1992;226:747–61.

324. Xia Y, Hwang LY, Cobb MH, Baer R. Products of the TAL2 oncogene in leukemic T cells: bHLH phosphoproteins with DNA-binding activity. Oncogene 1994;9:1437–46.

325. Rabbitts TH, Boehm T. LIM domains. Nature 1990;346:418.

326. Serrano M, Hannon GJ, Beach D. A new regulatory motif in cell-cycle control causing specific inhibition of cyclin D/CDK4 [see comments]. Nature 1993;366:704–7.

327. Kamb A, Gruis NA, Weaver-Feldhaus J, et al. A cell cycle regulator potentially involved in genesis of many tumor types [see comments]. Science 1994;264:436–40.

328. Alcorta DA, Xiong Y, Phelps D, et al. Involvement of the cyclin-dependent kinase inhibitor p16 (INK4a) in replicative senescence of normal human fibroblasts. Proc Natl Acad Sci U S A 1996;93:13742–7.

329. Nobori T, Miura K, Wu DJ, et al. Deletions of the cyclin-dependent kinase-4 inhibitor gene in multiple human cancers. Nature 1994;368:753–6.

330. Hara E, Smith R, Parry D, et al. Regulation of p16CDKN2 expression and its implications for cell immortalization and senescence. Mol Cell Biol 1996;16:859–67.

331. Serrano M, Lee H, Chin L, et al. Role of the INK4a locus in tumor suppression and cell mortality. Cell 1996;85:27–37.

332. Okuda T, Shurtleff SA, Valentine MB, et al. Frequent deletion of p16INK4a/MTS1 and p15INK4b/MTS2 in pediatric acute lymphoblastic leukemia. Blood 1995;85:2321–30.

333. Rasool O, Heyman M, Brandter LB, et al. p15ink4B and p16ink4 gene inactivation in acute lymphocytic leukemia. Blood 1995;85:3431–6.

334. Quesnel B, Preudhomme C, Philippe N, et al. p16 gene homozygous deletions in acute lymphoblastic leukemia. Blood 1995;85:657–63.

335. Stock W, Sher D, Dodge R, et al. Transcriptional silencing is an alternative means of p16 inactivation: further evidence for p16 role in pathogenesis of adult acute lymphoblastic leukemia, a Cancer and Leukemia Group B study (8762). Proc Am Soc Clin Oncol 1997;16:1992. abstract.

336. Batova A, Diccianni MB, Yu JC, et al. Frequent and selective methylation of p15 and deletion of both p15 and p16 in T-cell acute lymphoblastic leukemia. Cancer Res 1997;57:832–6.

337. Quelle DE, Zindy F, Ashmun RA, Sherr CJ. Alternative reading frames of the INK4a tumor suppressor gene encode two unrelated proteins capable of inducing cell cycle arrest. Cell 1995;83:993–1000.

338. Liggett WHJ, Sidransky D. Role of the p16 tumor suppressor gene in cancer. J Clin Oncol 1998;16:1197–1206.

339. Faderl S, Estrov Z, Kantarjian HM, et al. The incidence of chromosome 9p21 abnormalities and deletions of tumor suppressor genes p15(INK4b)/p16(INK4a)/p14(ARF) in patients with acute lymphoblastic leukemia. Cytokines Cell Mol Ther 1999;5:159–63.

340. Faderl S, Kantarjian HM, Manshouri T, Chan CY, Pierce S, Hays KJ, et al. The prognostic significance of p16INK4a/p14ARF and p15INK4b deletions in adult acute lymphoblastic leukemia. Clin Cancer Res 1999;5:1855–61.

341. Wong IH, Ng MH, Huang DP, Lee JC. Aberrant p15 promoter methylation in adult and childhood acute leukemias of nearly all morphologic subtypes: potential prognostic implications. Blood 2000;95:1942–9.

342. Weinberg RA. The retinoblastoma protein and cell cycle control. Cell 1995;81:323–30.

343. Tsai T, Davalath S, Rankin C, et al. Tumor suppressor gene alteration in adult acute lymphoblastic leukemia (ALL). Analysis of retinoblastoma (Rb) and p53 gene expression in lymphoblasts of patients with de novo, relapsed, or refractory ALL treated in Southwest Oncology Group studies. Leukemia 1996;10:1901–10.

344. Sakai T, Toguchida J, Ohtani N, et al. Allele-specific hypermethylation of the retinoblastoma tumor-suppressor gene. Am J Hum Genet 1991;48:880–8.

345. Ohtani-Fujita N, Fujita T, Aoike A, et al. CpG methylation inactivates the promoter activity of the human retinoblastoma tumor-suppressor gene. Oncogene 1993;8:1063–7.

346. Lanza C, Gaidano G, Cimino G, et al. p53 gene inactivation in acute lymphoblastic leukemia of B cell lineage associates with chromosomal breakpoints at 11q23 and 8q24. Leukemia 1995;9:955–9.

347. Wada M, Bartram CR, Nakamura H, et al. Analysis of p53 mutations in a large series of lymphoid hematologic malignancies of childhood. Blood 1993;82:3163–9.

348. Marks DI, Kurz BW, Link MP, et al. Altered expression of p53 and mdm-2 proteins at diagnosis is associated with early treatment failure in childhood acute lymphoblastic leukemia. J Clin Oncol 1997;15:1158–62.

349. Goker E, Waltham M, Kheradpour A, et al. Amplification of the dihydrofolate reductase gene is a mechanism of acquired resistance to methotrexate in patients with acute lymphoblastic leukemia and is correlated with p53 gene mutations. Blood 1995;86:677–84.

350. Wattel E, Preudhomme C, Hecquet B, et al. p53 mutations are associated with resistance to chemotherapy and short survival in hematologic malignancies. Blood 1994;84:3148–57.

351. Preudhomme C, Dervite I, Wattel E, et al. Clinical significance of p53 mutations in newly diagnosed Burkitt's lymphoma and acute lymphoblastic leukemia: a report of 48 cases. J Clin Oncol 1995;13:812–20.

352. Sauerbrey A, Stammler G, Zintl F, Volm M. Expression and prognostic value of the retinoblastoma tumour suppressor gene (RB-1) in childhood acute lymphoblastic leukaemia. Br J Haematol 1996;94:99–104.

353. Findley HW, Gu L, Yeager AM, Zhou M. Expression and regulation of Bcl-2, Bcl-xl, and Bax correlate with p53 status and sensitivity to apoptosis in childhood acute lymphoblastic leukemia. Blood 1997;89:2986–93.

354. Coustan-Smith E, Kitanaka A, Pui CH, et al. Clinical relevance of BCL-2 overexpression in childhood acute lymphoblastic leukemia. Blood 1996;87:1140–6.

355. Maung ZT, MacLean FR, Reid MM, et al. The relationship between bcl-2 expression and response to chemotherapy in acute leukaemia. Br J Haematol 1994;88:105–9.

356. Marks DI, Kurz BW, Link MP, et al. Altered expression of p53 and mdm-2 proteins at diagnosis is associated with early treatment failure in childhood acute lymphoblastic leukemia. J Clin Oncol 1997;15:1158–62.

357. Clarkson B, Ellis S, Little C, et al. Acute lymphoblastic leukemia in adults. Semin Oncol 1985;12:160–79.

358. Ellison RR, Mick R, Cuttner J, et al. The effects of postinduction intensification treatment with cytarabine and daunorubicin in adult acute lymphocytic leukemia: a prospective randomized clinical trial by Cancer and Leukemia Group B. J Clin Oncol 1991;9:2002–15.

359. Linker CA, Levitt LJ, O'Donnell M, et al. Improved results of treatment of adult acute lymphoblastic leukemia. Blood 1987;69:1242–8.

360. Kantarjian HM, Walters RS, Smith TL, et al. Identification of risk groups for development of central nervous system leukemia in adults with adult lymphocytic leukemia. Blood 1988;72:1784–9.

361. Rivera GK, Raimondi SC, Hancock ML, et al. Improved outcome in childhood acute lymphoblastic leukaemia with reinforced early treatment and rotational combination chemotherapy. Lancet 1991;337:61–6.

362. Gaynon PS, Bleyer WA, Àlbo VC, et al. Intensive therapy for children with acute lymphoblastic leukaemia and unfavourable presenting features. Lancet 1988;2:8617.

363. Mahmoud HH, Rivera GK, Hancock ML, et al. Low leukocyte counts with blast cells in cerebrospinal fluid of children with newly diagnosed acute lymphoblastic leukemia. N Engl J Med 1993;329:314–9.

364. Bleyer WA. Central nervous system leukemia. In: Henderson ES, Lister TA, eds. Leukemia. 5th ed. Philadelphia: WB Saunders, 1990:733–68.

365. Larson RA, Dodge RK, Burns CP, et al. A five-drug remission induction regimen with intensive consolidation for adults with acute lymphoblastic leukemia: cancer and leukemia group B study 8811. Blood 1995;85:2025–37.

366. Pullen J, Boyett J, Shuster J, et al. Extended triple intrathecal chemotherapy trial for prevention of CNS relapse in good-risk and poor-risk patients with B-progenitor acute lymphoblastic leukemia: a Pediatric Oncology Group study. J Clin Oncol 1993;11:839–49.

367. Tubergen DG, Cullen JW, Boyett JM, et al. Blasts in CSF with a normal cell count do not justify alteration of therapy for acute lymphoblastic leukemia in remission: a Children's Cancer Group study. J Clin Oncol 1994;12:273–8.

368. Cheson BD, Cassileth PA, Head DR, et al. Report of the National Cancer Institute-sponsored workshop in definitions of diagnosis and response in acute myeloid leukemia. J Clin Oncol 1990;8:813–9.

369. Bennett JM, Catovsky D, Daniel MT, et al. Proposal for the recognition of minimally differentiated acute myeloid leukaemia (AML-M0). Br J Haematol 1991;78:325–9.

370. Bleyer WA. Acute lymphoblastic leukemia in children. Cancer 1990;65:689–95.

371. Smith M, Arthur D, Camitta B, et al. Uniform approach to risk classification and treatment assignment for children with acute lymphoblastic leukemia [see comments]. J Clin Oncol 1996;14:18–24.

372. Pui CH, Evans WE. Acute lymphoblastic leukemia. N Engl J Med 1998;339:605–15.

373. Rivera GK, Pinkel D, Simone JV, et al. Treatment of acute lymphoblastic leukemia. N Engl J Med 1993;329:1289–95.

374. Holowiecki J, Koehler M, Zintl Z, et al. Childhood acute lymphoblastic leukemia immunophenotypes and their prognostic significance: experience of the IGCI-study in 389 children. Leuk Lymphoma 1992;7:225–34.

375. Sather HN. Age at diagnosis in childhood acute lymphoblastic leukemia. Med Pediatr Oncol 1986;14:166–72.

376. Chessells JM, Hall E, Prentice HG, et al. The impact of age on outcome in lymphoblastic leukaemia; MRC UKALL X and XA compared: a report from the MRC Paediatric and Adult Working Parties. Leukemia 1998;12:463–73.

377. Mandelli F, Annino L, Rotoli B. The GIMEMA ALL 0183 trial: analysis of 10-year follow-up. GIMEMA Cooperative Group, Italy. Br J Haematol 1996;92:665–72.

378. Kantarjian HM, Walters RS, Keating MJ, et al. Results of the vincristine, doxorubicin, and dexamethasone regimen in adults with standard- and high-risk acute lymphocytic leukemia. J Clin Oncol 1990;8:994–1004.

379. Lazzarino M, Morra E, Alessandrino EP, et al. Adult acute lymphoblastic leukemia. Response to therapy according to presenting features in 62 patients. Eur J Cancer 1982;18:813–9.

380. Barnett MJ, Greaves MF, Amess JAL, et al. Treatment of acute lymphoblastic leukaemia in adults. Br J Haematol 1986;64:455–68.

381. Patte C, Philip T, Rodary C, et al. High survival rate in advanced-stage B-cell lymphomas and leukemias without CNS involvement with a short intensive polychemotherapy: results from the French Pediatric Oncology Society of a randomized trial of 216 children. J Clin Oncol 1991;9:123–32.

382. Reiter A, Schrappe M, Ludwig W-D, et al. Favorable outcome of B-cell acute lymphoblastic leukemia in childhood: a report of three consecutive studies of the BFM group. Blood 1992;80:2471–8.

383. Hoelzer D, Ludwig WD, Thiel E, et al. Improved outcome in adult B-cell acute lymphoblastic leukemia. Blood 1996;87:495–508.

384. Soussain C, Patte C, Ostronoff M, et al. Small noncleaved cell lymphoma and leukemia in adults. A retrospective study of 65 adults treated with the LMB pediatric protocols. Blood 1995;85:664–74.

385. Magrath I, Adde M, Shad A, et al. Adults and children with small non-cleaved-cell lymphoma have a similar excellent outcome when treated with the same chemotherapy regimen. J Clin Oncol 1996;14:925–34.

386. Guo SX, Taki T, Ohnishi H, et al. Hypermethylation of p16 and p15 genes and RB protein expression in acute leukemia. Leuk Res 2000;24:39–46.

387. Marcus RE, Catowsky D, Johnson SA, et al. Adult acute lymphoblastic leukemia: a study of prognostic features and response to treatment over a ten year period. Br J Cancer 1986;53:175–80.

388. Hoelzer D, Thiel E, Loffler H, et al. Prognostic factors in a multicenter study for treatment of acute lymphoblastic leukemia in adults. Blood 1988;71:123–31.

389. Hoelzer DF. Therapy of the newly diagnosed adult with acute lymphoblastic leukemia. Hematol Oncol Clin North Am 1993;7:139–60.

390. Hoelzer D. Prognostic factors in acute lymphoblastic leukemia. Leukemia 1992;6:Suppl 4:49–51.

391. Boucheix C, Racadot E, Sigaux F, et al. Immunophenotype of adult acute lymphoblastic leukemia characteristics and outcome of 562 patients included in a prospective trial (LALA 87). Br J Haematol 1994;84:Suppl 1:4. abstract.

392. Larson RA, Dodge RK, Burns CP, et al. A five drug remission induction regimen with intensive consolidation for adults with acute lymphoblastic leukemia: Cancer and Leukemia Group B Study 8811. Blood 1995;85:2025–37.

393. Feickert HJ, Bettoni C, Schrappe M, et al. Event-free survival of children with T-cell acute lymphoblastic leukemia after introduction of high dose methotrexate in multicenter trial ALL-BFM 86. Proc Am Soc Clin Oncol 1993;12:317. abstract.

394. Lauer SJ, Pinkel D, Buchanan GR, et al. Cytosine arabinoside/cyclophosphamide pulses during continuation therapy for childhood acute lymphoblastic leukemia. Cancer 1987;60:2366–71.

395. Uckun FM, Gaynon PS, Sensel MG, et al. Clinical features and treatment outcome of childhood T-lineage acute lymphoblastic leukemia according to the apparent maturational stage of T-lineage leukemic blasts: a Children's Cancer Group study. J Clin Oncol 1997;15:2214–21.

396. Uckun FM, Reaman G, Steinherez PG, et al. Improved clinical outcome for children with T-lineage acute lymphoblastic leukemia after contemporary chemotherapy: a Children's Cancer Group Study. Leuk Lymphoma 1996;24:57–70.

397. Crist W, Boyett J, Jackson J, et al. Prognostic importance of the pre-B-cell immunophenotype and other presenting features in B-lineage childhood acute lymphoblastic leukemia: a Pediatric Oncology Group Study. Blood 1989;74:1252–9.

398. Crist WM, Carroll AJ, Shuster JJ, et al. Poor prognosis of children with pre-B acute lymphoblastic leukemia is associated with the t(1;19)(q23;p13): a Pediatric Oncolcogy Group study. Blood 1990;76:117–22.

399. Uckun FM, Steinherz PG, Sather H, et al. CD2 antigen expression on leukemic cells as a predictor of event-free survival after chemotherapy for T-lineage acute lymphoblastic leukemia: a Children's Cancer Group study. Blood 1996;88:4288–95.

400. Ferrara F, Cimino R, Antinolfi I, et al. Clinical relevance of immunological dissection in T-ALL: a report on 20 cases with stem cell (CD7+, CD4-, CD8-, CD1-) phenotype. Am J Hematol 1992;40:98–102.

401. Ludwig WD, Harbott J, Bartram CR, et al. Incidence and prognostic significance of immunophenotypic subgroups in childhood acute lymphoblastic leukemia: experience of the BFM study 86. Recent Results Cancer Res 1993;131:269–82.

402. Shuster JJ, Falletta JM, Pullen J, et al. Prognostic factors in childhood T-cell acute lymphoblastic leukemia: a Pediatric Oncology Group Study. Blood 1990;75:166–73.

403. Crist WM, Shuster JJ, Falletta J, et al. Clinical features and outcome in childhood T-cell leukemia-lymphoma according to stage of thymocyte differentiation: a Pediatric Oncology Group study. Blood 1988;72:1891–7.

404. Pagnucco G, Santagostino A, Livraghi A, et al. Clinical importance of the immunophenotype in adult acute lymphoblastic leukemia. Haematologica 1991;76:Suppl 4:13. abstract.

405. Gomez E, San Miguel JF, Gonzalez M, et al. The value of the immunological subtypes and individual markers compared to classical parameters in the prognosis of acute lymphoblastic leukemia. Hematol Oncol 1991;9:33–42.

406. Bassan R, Battista R, Montaldi A, et al. Reinforced HEAV'D therapy for adult acute lymphoblastic leukemia: improved results and revised prognostic criteria. Hematol Oncol 1993;11:169–77.

407. Pui CH, Rivera GK, Hancock ML, et al. Clinical significance of CD10 expression in childhood acute lymphoblastic leukemia. Leukemia 1993;7:35–40.

408. Kurec AS, Belair PB, Stefanu C, et al. Significance of aberrant immunophenotypes in childhood acute lymphoid leukemia. Cancer 1991;67:3081–6.

409. Wiersma SR, Ortega J, Sobel E, Weinberg KI. Clinical importance of myeloid-antigen expression in acute lymphoblastic leukemia of childhood. N Engl J Med 1991;324:800–8.

410. Guyotat D, Campos L, Shi Z-H, et al. Myeloid surface antigen expression in adult acute lymphoblastic leukemia. Leukemia 1990;9:664–6.

411. Larson RA, Burns CP, Dodge RK, et al. A 5-drug induction regimen with intensive consolidation for adult acute lymphoblastic leukemia (ALL): Cancer and Leukemia Group B. Proc Am Soc Clin Oncol 1992;11:263. abstract.

412. Pui C-H, Behm FG, Singh B, et al. Myeloid-associated antigen expression lacks prognostic value in childhood acute lymphoblastic leukemia treqated with intensive multiagent chemotherapy. Blood 1990;75:198–202.

413. Cantu-Rajnoldi A, Putti C, Saitta M, et al. Co-expression of myeloid antigens in childhood acute lymphoblastic leukaemia: relationship with the stage of differentiation and clinical significance. Br J Haematol 1991;79:40–3.

414. Pui C-H, Schell MJ, Raimondi SC, et al. Myeloid-antigen expression in childhood acute lymphoblastic leukemia. N Engl J Med 1991;325:1378–81.

415. Borowitz MJ, Shuster JJ, Civin CI, et al. Prognostic significance of CD34 expression in childhood B-precursor acute lymphoblastic leukemia: a Pediatric Oncology Group study. J Clin Oncol 1990;8:1389–98.

416. Pui CH, Behm FG, Singh B, et al. Heterogeneity of presenting features and their relation to treatment outcome in 120 children with T-cell acute lymphoblastic leukemia. Blood 1990;75:174–9.

417. Hoelzer D. Acute lymphoblastic leukemia in adults. In: Hoffman R, Benz EJ Jr, Shattil SJ, et al, eds. Hematology: basic principles and practice. 1st ed. New York: Churchill Livingstone, 1991:793–804.

418. Walters R, Kantarjian HM, Keating MJ, et al. The importance of cytogenetic studies in adult acute lymphocytic leukemia. Am J Med 1990;89:579–87.

419. Faderl S, Kantarjian HM, Thomas DA, et al. Outcome of Philadelphia chromosome-positive adult acute lymphoblastic leukemia. Leuk Lymphoma 2000;36:263–73.

420. Rambaldi A, Attuati V, Bassan R, et al. Molecular diagnosis and clinical relevance of t(9;22), t(4;11) and t(1;19) chromosome abnormalities in a consecutive group of 141 adult patients with acute lymphoblastic leukemia. Leuk Lymphoma 1996;21:457–66.

421. Fletcher JA, Lynch EA, Kimball VA, et al. Translocation (9;22) is associated with extremely poor prognosis in intensively treated children with acute lymphoblastic leukemia. Blood 1991;77:435–9.

422. Fletcher JA, Kimball VM, Lynch E, et al. Prognostic implications of cytogenetic studies in an intensively treated group of children with acute lymphoblastic leukemia. Blood 1989;74:2130–5.

423. Rubin CM, Le Beau MM, Mick R, et al. Impact of chromosomal translocations on prognosis in childhood acute lymphoblastic leukemia. J Clin Oncol 1991;9:2183–92.

424. Secker-Walker LM, Craig JM. Prognostic implications of breakpoint and lineage heterogeneity in Philadelphia-positive acute lymphoblastic leukemia: a review. Leukemia 1993;7:147–51.

425. Raimondi SC, Behm FG, Roberson PK, et al. Cytogenetics of pre-B-cell acute lymphoblastic leukemia with emphasis on prognostic implications of the t(1;19). J Clin Oncol 1990;8:1380–8.

426. Mahmoud H, Carroll AJ, Behm F, et al. The non-random dic(9;12) translocation in acute lymphoblastic leukemia is associated with B-progenitor phenotype and an excellent prognosis. Leukemia 1992;6:703–7.

427. Latham JA, Bown N, Cain G, et al. Molecular heterogeneity of variant Philadelphia translocations in childhood acute lymphoblastic leukaemia. Leukemia 1994;8:292–4.

428. Hiddemann W, Harbott J, Ludwig WD, et al. DNA aneuploidy in childhood acute lymphoblastic leukemia: relation to clinical determinants and prognosis within four consecutive BFM trials. Recent Results Cancer Res 1993;131:113–21.

429. Trueworthy R, Shuster J, Look T, et al. Ploidy of lymphoblasts is the strongest predictor of treatment outcome in B-progenitor cell acute lymphoblastic leukemia of childhood: a Pediatric Oncology Group study. J Clin Oncol 1992;10:606–13.

430. Katz J, Shuster J, Schneider N, et al. The significance of ploidy in childhood T-cell acute lymphoblastic leukemia (T-ALL): a Pediatric Oncology Group (POG) study. Proc Am Soc Clin Oncol 1993;12:316. abstract.

431. Machnicki JL, Bloomfield CD. Clinical significance of the cytogenetics of acute leukemias. Oncology 1990;10:23–30.

432. Gaynor J, Chapman D, Little C, et al. A Cause-specific hazard rate analysis of prognostic factors among 199 adults with acute lymphoblastic leukemia: the Memorial Hospital experience since 1969. J Clin Oncol 1988;6:1014–30.

433. Smith M. Towards a more uniform approach to risk-classification and treatment assignment for children with acute lymphoblastic leukemia. Am Soc Clin Oncol Educational Booklet 1994;124–30.

434. Miller DR, Coccia PF, Bleyer WA, et al. Early response to induction therapy as a predictor of disease-free survival and late recurrence of childhood acute lymphoblastic leukemia: a report from the Children's Cancer Study Group. J Clin Oncol 1989;7:1807–15.

435. Lauer SJ, Camitta BM, Leventhal BG, et al. Intensive alternating drug pairs for treatment of high risk childhood acute lymphoblastic leukemia. Cancer 1993;71:2854–61.

436. Camitta B, Mahoney D, Leventhalt B, et al. Intensive intravenous methotrexate and mercaptopurine treatment of higher-risk non-T, non-B acute lymphocytic leukemia: a Pediatric Oncology Group study. J Clin Oncol 1994;12:1383–9.

437. Riehm H, Gadner H, Henze G, et al. Results and significance of six randomized trials in four consecutive ALL-BFM studies. In: Buchner T, Schellong G, Hiddemann W, Ritter J, eds. Acute leukemias II. Berlin: Springer-Verlag, 1990:439–50.

438. Janka-Schaub GE, Stuehrk H, Kortuem B, et al. Bone marrow blast count at day 28 as the single most important prognostic factor in childhood acute lymphoblastic leukemia. Hamatol Bluttransfus 1992;34:233–7.

439. Gaynon PS, Bleyer WA, Steinherz PG, et al. Day 7 marrow response and outcome for children with acute lymphoblastic leukemia and unfavorable presenting features. Med Pediatr Oncol 1990;18:273–9.

440. Reiter A, Kuhl JS, Schrappe M, et al. The multicenter trials of ALL/NHL-BFM 86: treatment strategy and results of pediatric non-B acute lymphoblastic leukemia. Proc Am Soc Clin Oncol 1993;12:317. abstract.

441. Ribeiro RC, Pui C. Prognostic factors in childhood acute lymphoblastic leukemia. Hematol Pathol 1993;7:121–42.

442. Hoelzer DF. Therapy of the newly diagnosed adult with acute lymphoblastic leukemia. Hematol Oncol Clin North Am 1993;7:139–60.

443. Komp DM, George SL, Falletta J, et al. Cyclophosphamide-asparaginase-vincristine-prednisone induction therapy in childhood acute lymphocytic and nonlymphocytic leukemia. Cancer 1976;37:1243–7.

444. Gottlieb AJ, Weinberg V, Ellison RR, et al. Daunorubicin in the therapy of adult acute lymphoblastic leukemia—a prospective randomized trial by Cancer and Leukemia Group B. Blood 1984;64:267–74.

445. Stryckmans P, Debusscher L. Chemotherapy of adult acute lymphoblastic leukaemia. Baillieres Clin Haematol 1991;4:115–30.

446. Hussein KK, Dahlberg S, Head D, et al. Treatment of acute lymphoblastic leukemia in adults with intensive induction, consolidation, and maintenance chemotherapy. Blood 1989;73:57–63.

447. Linker CA, Levitt LJ, O'Donnell M, et al. Treatment of adult acute lymphoblastic leukemia with intensive cyclical chemotherapy: a follow-up report. Blood 1991;78:2814–22.

448. Radford JE Jr, Burns CP, Jones MP, et al. Adult acute lymphoblastic leukemia: results of the Iowa HOP-L protocol. J Clin Oncol 1989;7:58–66.

449. Schauer P, Arlin ZA, Mertelsmann R, et al. Treatment of acute lymphoblastic leukemia in adults: results of the L-10 and L-10M protocols. J Clin Oncol 1983;1:462–70.

450. Champlin R, Gale RP. Acute lymphoblastic leukemia: recent advances in biology and therapy. Blood 1989;73:2051–66.

451. Sallan SE, Hitchcock-Bryan S, Gelber R, et al. Influence of intensive asparaginase in the treatment of childhood non-T-cell acute lymphoblastic leukemia. Cancer Res 1983;43:5601–7.

452. Clavell LA, Gelber R, Cohen HJ, et al. Four-agent induction and intensive asparaginase therapy for treatment of childhood acute lymphoblastic leukemia. N Engl J Med 1986;315:657–63.

453. Hitchcock-Bryan S, Gelber R, Cassady JR, Sallan SE. The impact of induction anthracycline on long-term failure-free survival in childhood acute lymphoblastic leukemia. Med Pediatr Oncol 1986;14:211–5.

454. Eden OB, Lilleyman JS, Richards S, et al. Results of Medical Research Council childhood leukaemia trial UKALL VIII (report to the Medical Research Council on behalf of the Working Party on Leukaemia in Childhood). Br J Haematol 1991;78:187–96.

455. Nagura E, Kimura K, Yamada K, et al. Nation-wide randomized comparative study of doxorubicin, vincristine and prednisolone combination therapy with and without L-asparaginase for adult acute lymphoblastic leukemia. Cancer Chemother Pharmacol 1994;33:359–65.

456. Todeschini G, Meneghini V, Pizzolo G, et al. Relationship between daunorubicin dosage delivered during induction therapy and outcome in adult acute lymphoblastic leukemia. Leukemia 1994;8:376–81.

457. Hoelzer D, Thiel E, Ludwig WD, et al. Follow-up of the first two successive German multicentre trials for adult ALL (01/81 and 02/84). Leukemia 1993;7:Suppl 2:S130–4.

458. Larson RA, Dodge RK, Linker CA, et al. A randomized controlled trial of filgrastim during remission induction and consolidation chemotherapy for adults with acute lymphoblastic leukemia: CALGB study 9111. Blood 1998;92:1556–64.

459. Frankel SR, Kurtzberg J, DeOleivera D, et al. Toxicity and pharmacokinetics of PEG-asparaginase in newly diagnosed adult acute lymphoblastic leukemia: CALGB 9511. Blood 1996;88:669a. abstract.

460. Larson RA, Linker CA, Dodge RK, et al. Granulocyte-colony stimulating factor (filgrastim; G-CSF) reduces the time to neutrophil recovery in adults with acute lymphoblastic leukemia receiving intensive remission induction chemotherapy: Cancer and Leukemia Group B Study 9111. Proc Am Soc Clin Oncol 1994;13:305.

461. Hoelzer D, Thiel E, Ludwig WD, et al. The German multicentre trials for treatment of acute lymphoblastic leukemia in adults. The German Adult ALL Study Group. Leukemia. 1992;6:Suppl 2:175–7.

462. Crist W, Pullen J, Boyett J, et al. Acute lymphoid leukemia in adolescents: clinical and biologic features predict a poor prognosis—a Pediatric Oncology Group Study. J Clin Oncol 1988;6:34–43.

463. Smedmyr B, Simonsson B, Fjorkholm M, et al. Treatment of adult acute lymphoblastic and undifferentiated leukemia, according to a national protocol, in Sweden. Haematologica 1991;76:Suppl 4:107. abstract.

464. Scherrer R, Geissler K, Kyrle PA, Gisslinger H, et al. Granulocyte colony-stimulating factor (G-CSF) as an adjunct to induction chemotherapy of adult acute lymphoblastic leukemia (ALL). Ann Hematol 1993;66:283–9.

465. Ottmann OG, Hoelzer D, Gracien E, et al. Concomitant r-methu G-CSF (filgrastim) and intensive chemoradiotherapy as induction treatment in adult ALL: a randomized multicenter phase III trial. Blood 1993;82:193a.

466. Bassan R, Lerede T, Di Bona E, et al. Granulocyte colony-stimulating factor (G-CSF, filgrastim) after or during an intensive remission induction therapy for adult acute lymphoblastic leukaemia: effects, role of patient pretreatment characteristics, and costs. Leuk Lymphoma 1997;26:153–61.

467. Larson RA, Fretzin MH, Dodge RK, Schiffer CA. Hypersensitivity reactions to L-asparaginase do not impact on the remission duration of adults with acute lymphoblastic leukemia. Leukemia 1998;12:660–5.

468. Bassan R, Battista R, Corneo G, et al. Idarubicin in the inital treatment of adults with acute lymphoblastic leukemia: the effect of drug schedule on outcome. Leuk Lymphoma 1993;11:105–10.

469. Todeschini G, Tecchio C, Meneghini V, et al. Estimated 6-year event-free survival of 55% in 60 consecutive adult acute lymphoblastic leukemia patients treated with an intensive phase II protocol based on high induction dose of daunorubicin. Leukemia 1998;12:144–9.

470. Weiss MA, Drullinsky P, Maslak P, et al. A phase I trial of a single high dose of idarubicin combined with high-dose cytarabine as induction therapy in relapsed or refractory adult patients with acute lymphoblastic leukemia. Leukemia 1998;12:865–8.

471. Weiss M, Maslak P, Feldman E, et al. Cytarabine with high-dose mitoxantrone induces rapid complete remissions in adult acute lymphoblastic leukemia without the use of vincristine or prednisone. J Clin Oncol 1996;14:2480–5.

472. Chessells JM, Bailey CC, Richards S. MRC UKALL X. The UK protocol for childhood ALL: 1985–1990. The Medical Research Council Working Party on Childhood Leukaemia. Leukemia 1992;6:Suppl 2:157–61.

473. Rivera GK, Pui CH, Hancock ML, et al. Update of St Jude Study XI for childhood acute lymphoblastic leukemia. Leukemia 1992;6:Suppl 2:153–6.

474. Gaynon PS, Steinherz PG, Bleyer WA, et al. Improved therapy for children with acute lymphoblastic leukemia and unfavorable presenting features: a follow-up report of the Children's Cancer Group study CCG-106. J Clin Oncol 1993;11:2234–42.

475. Niemeyer CM, Reiter A, Riehm H, et al. Comparative results of two intensive treatment programs for childhood acute lymphoblastic leukemia: The Berlin-Frankfurt-Münster and Dana-Farber Cancer Institute protocols. Ann Oncol 1991;2:745–9.

476. Schorin MA, Blattner S, Gelber RD, et al. Treatment of childhood acute lymphoblastic leukemia: results of Dana-Farber Cancer Institute/Children's Hospital Acute Lymphoblastic Leukemia Consortium Protocol 85-01. J Clin Oncol 1994;12:740–7.

477. Camitta B, Leventhal B, Lauer S, et al. Intermediate dose intravenous methotrexate and mercaptopurine therapy for non-T, non-B acute lymphocytic leukemia of childhood: a Pediatric Oncology Group Study. J Clin Oncol 1989;7:1539–44.

478. Pui CH, Simone JV, Hancock ML, et al. Impact of three methods of treatment intensification on acute lymphoblastic leukemia in children: long-term results of St Jude total therapy study X. Leukemia 1992;6:150–7.

479. Niemeyer CM, Gelber RD, Tarbell NJ, et al. Low-dose versus high-dose methotrexate during remission induction in childhood acute lymphoblastic leukemia (Protocol 81-01 update). Blood 1991;78:2514–9.

480. Hoelzer D, Thiel E, Loffler H, et al. Intensified therapy in acute lymphoblastic and acute undifferentiated leukemia in adults. Blood 1984;64:38–47.

481. Hoelzer D, Arnold R, Aydemir U, et al. Results of intensified consolidation therapy in four consecutive German multicentre studies for adult ALL. Blood 1993;82:193a.

482. Cassileth PA, Andersen JW, Bennett JM, et al. Adult acute lymphocytic leukemia: the Eastern Cooperative Oncology Group experience. Leukemia 1992;6:Suppl 2:178–81.

483. Rohatiner AZS, Bassan R, Battista R, et al. High dose cytosine arabinoside in the initial treatment of adults with acute lymphoblastic leukaemia. Br J Cancer 1990;62:454–8.

484. Durrant J, Richards S, Bell P, Prentice HG. Bone marrow transplantation in first remission in adults with acute lymphoblastic leukaemia. Haematologica 1991;76:Suppl 4:109. abstract.

485. Fière D, Lepage E, Sebban C, et al. Adult acute lymphoblastic leukemia: a multicentric randomized trial testing bone marrow transplantation as postremission therapy. The French Group on Therapy for Adult Acute Lymphoblastic Leukemia. J Clin Oncol 1993;11:1990–2001.

486. Hann IM. CNS-directed therapy in childhood acute lymphoblastic leukemia. Br J Haematol 1992;82:2–5.

487. Gelber RD, Sallan SE, Cohen HJ, et al. Central nervous system treatment in childhood acute lymphoblastic leukemia. Cancer 1993;72:261–70.

488. Law IP, Blom J. Adult acute leukemia—frequency of CNS involvement in long-term survivors. Cancer 1977;40:1306–6.

489. Omura GA, Moffitt S, Vogler WR, Salter MM. Combination chemotherapy of adult acute lymphoblastic leukemia with randomized central nervous system prophylaxis. Blood 1980;55:199–204.

490. Tubergen DG, Gilchrist GS, O'Brien RT, et al. Prevention of CNS disease intermediate-risk acute lymphoblastic leukemia: comparison of cranial radiation and intrathecal methotrexate and the importance of systemic therapy: a childrens cancer group report. J Clin Oncol 1993;11:520–6.

491. Chessells JM. Childhood acute lymphoblastic leukaemia: the late effects of treatment. Br J Haematol 1983;53:369–78.

492. Tucker J, Prior PF, Green CR, et al. Minimal neuropsychological sequelae following prophylactic treatment of the central nervous system in adult leukaemia and lymphoma. Br J Cancer 1989;60:775–80.

493. Schaison G, Sommelet D, Bancillon A, et al. Treatment of acute lymphoblastic leukemia French protocol Fralle 83–87. Leukemia. 1992;6:Suppl 2:148–52.

494. Komp DM, Fernandez CH, Falletta JM, et al. CNS prophylaxis in acute lymphoblastic leukemia. Comparison of two methods. A Southwest Oncology Group Study. Cancer 1982;50:1031–6.

495. Buhrer C, Henze G, Hoffman J, et al. Central nervous system relapse prevention in 1165 standard-risk children with acute lymphoblastic leukemia in five BFM trials. Haem Blood Transf 1990;33:500–3.

496. Mandelli F, Annino L, Vegna ML, et al. GIMEMA ALL 0288: a multicentric study on adult acute lymphoblastic leukemia. Preliminary results. Leukemia 1992;6:Suppl 2:182–5.

497. Clarkson B, Gaynor J, Little C, et al. Clinical trials in adults with acute lymphoblastic leukemia at Memorial Sloan-Kettering Cancer Center. In: Gale RP, Hoelzer D, eds. Acute lymphoblastic leukemia. New York: Alan R. Liss, 1990:231–52.

498. Cuttner J, Mick R, Budman DR, et al. Phase III trial of brief intensive treatment of adult acute lymphocytic leukemia comparing daunorubicin and mitoxantrone: a CALGB study. Leukemia 1991;5:425–31.

499. GIMEMA Cooperative Group. GIMEMA ALL 0183: a multicentric study on adult acute lymphoblastic leukaemia in Italy. Br J Haematol 1989;71:377–86.

500. Wernli M, Tichelli A, von Fliedner V, et al. Intensive induction/consolidation therapy without maintenance in adult acute lymphoblastic leukaemia: a pilot assessment. Br J Haematol 1994;87:39–43.

501. Henderson ES, Hoelzer D, Freeman AI. The treatment of acute lymphoblastic leukemia. In: Henderson ES, Lister TA, eds. Leukemia. 5th ed. Philadelphia: WB Saunders, 1990:443–84.

502. Preti A, Kantarjian HM. Management of adult acute lymphocytic leukemia: present issues and key challenges. J Clin Oncol 1994;12:1312–22.

503. Schwenn MR, Blattner SR, Lynch E, Weinstein HJ. HiC-COM: a 2-month intensive chemotherapy regimen for children with stage III and IV Burkitt's lymphoma and B-cell acute lymphoblastic leukemia. J Clin Oncol 1991;9:133–8.

504. Patte C, Leverger G, Rubie H, et al. High cure rate in B-cell (Burkitt's) leukemia in the LMB 89 protocol of the French Pediatric Oncology Society. Proc Am Soc Clin Oncol 1993;12:317. abstract.

505. Fenaux P, Lai JL, Miaux O, et al. Burkitt cell acute leukaemia (L3 ALL) in adults: a report of 18 cases. Br J Haematol 1989;71:371–6.

506. Troussard X, LeBlond V, Kuentz M, et al. Allogeneic bone marrow transplantation in adults with Burkitt's lymphoma or acute lymphoblastic leukemia in first complete remission. J Clin Oncol 1990;8:809–12.

507. Baruchel A, Leverger G, Schaison G, for the FRALLE group. Use of immunophenotype as part of the prognostic stratification for childhood ALL in the FRALLE 93 protocol. Leuk Lymphoma 1994;13:Suppl 1:91–3.

508. Schiffer CA, Larson RA, Bloomfield CD, for the CALGB. Cancer and Leukemia Group B (CALGB) studies in adult acute lymphocytic leukemia. Leukemia 1992;6:Suppl 2:171–4.

509. Götz G, Weh HJ, Walter TA, et al. Clinical and prognostic significance of the Philadelphia chromosome in adult patients with acute lymphoblastic leukemia. Ann Hematol 1992;64:97–100.

510. Grigg AP. Approaches to the treatment of Philadelphia-positive acute lymphoblastic leukemia. Bone Marrow Transplant 1993;12:431–5.

511. Fiere D, Castaigne S, Huguet F, et al. Characteristics and therapeutic results of 48 adult Philadelphia positive (Ph 1) acute lymphoblastic leukemias (ALL). Blood 1990;76:270a. abstract.

512. Annino L, Ferrari A, Cedrone M, et al. Adult Philadelphia-chromosome-positive acute lymphoblastic leukemia: experience of treatments during a ten-year period. Leukemia 1994;8:664–7.

513. Barrett AJ, Horowitz MM, Ash RC, et al. Bone marrow transplantation for Philadelphia chromosome-positive acute lymphoblastic leukemia. Blood 1992;79:3067–70.

514. Brennan C, Weisdorf D, Kersey J, et al. Bone marrow transplantation (BMT) for Philadelphia chromosome-positive acute lymphoblastic leukemia (Ph + ALL). Proceedings of American Society of Clinical Oncology 1991;10:222.

515. Forman SJ, O'Donnell MR, Nademanee AP, et al. Bone marrow transplantation for patients with Philadelphia chromosome-positive acute lymphoblastic leukemia. Blood 1987;70:587–8.

516. Miyamura K, Tanimoto M, Morishima Y, et al. Detection of Philadelphia chromosome-positive acute lymphoblastic leukemia by polymerase chain reaction: possible eradication of minimal residual disease by marrow transplantation. Blood 1992;79:1366–70.

517. Arlin Z, Feldman EJ, Ahmed T, et al. Philadelphia chromosome-positive acute lymphoblastic leukemia is resistant to effective therapy for Ph¹-negative ALL. Acta Haematol 1989;81:217–8.

518. Morishima Y, Miyamura K, Kojima S, et al. Autologous BMT in high risk patients with CALLA-positive ALL: possible efficacy of ex vivo

519. Roberts WM, Rivera GK, Raimondi SC, et al. Intensive chemotherapy for Philadelphia-chromosome-positive acute lymphoblastic leukaemia. Lancet 1994;343:331–2.

520. Henze G, Fengler R, Hartmann R, et al. Six-year experience with a comprehensive approach to the treatment of recurrent childhood acute lymphoblastic leukemia (ALL-REZ BFM 85). A relapse study of the BFM group. Blood 1991;78:1166–72.

521. Sadowitz PD, Smith SD, Shuster J, et al. Treatment of late bone marrow relapse in children with acute lymphoblastic leukemia: a Pediatric Oncology Group study. Blood 1993;81:602–9.

522. Buchanan GR, Rivera GK, Boyett JM, et al. Reinduction therapy in 297 children with acute lymphoblastic leukemia in first bone marrow relapse: a Pediatric Oncology Group study. Blood 1988;72:1286–92.

523. Freund M, Diedrich H, Ganser A, et al. Treatment of relapsed or refractory adult acute lymphocytic leukemia. Cancer 1992;69:709–16.

524. Woodruff RK. Combination chemotherapy for haematological relapse in adult acute lymphoblastic leukemia. Am J Hematol 1978;4:173–7.

525. Bassan R, Cornelli PE, Battista R, et al. Intensive retreatment of adults and children with acute lymphoblastic leukemia. Hematol Oncol 1992;10:105–10.

526. von der Weid N, Wagner B, Angst R, et al. Treatment of relapsing acute lymphoblastic leukemia in childhood. III. Experiences with 54 first bone marrow, nine isolated testicular, and eight isolated central nervous system relapses observed 1985–1989. Med Pediatr Oncol 1994;22:361–9.

527. Chessells JM. Treatment of childhood acute lymphoblastic leukaemia: present issues and future prospects. Blood Rev 1992;6:193–203.

528. Behrendt H, van Leeuwen EF, Schuwirth C, et al. Bone marrow relapse occurring as first relapse in children with acute lymphoblastic leukemia. Med Pediatr Oncol 1990;18:190–6.

529. Behrendt H, van Leeuwen EF, Schuwirth C, et al. The significance of an isolated central nervous system relapse occurring as first relapse in children with acute lymphoblastic leukemia. Cancer 1989;63:2066.

530. Winick NJ, Smith SD, Shuster J, et al. Treatment of CNS relapse in children with acute lymphoblastic leukemia: a Pediatric Oncology Group study. J Clin Oncol 1993;11:271–8.

531. Wofford MM, Smith SD, Shuster JJ, et al. Treatment of occult or late overt testicular relapse in children with acute lymphoblastic leukemia: a Pediatric Oncology Group Study. J Clin Oncol 1992;10:624–30.

532. Hoelzer D. High-dose chemotherapy in adult acute lymphoblastic leukemia. Semin Hematol 1991;28:84–9.

533. Kantarjian HM, Walters RL, Keating MJ, et al. Mitoxantrone and high-dose cytosine arabinoside for treatment of refractory acute lymphocytic leukemia. Cancer 1990;65:5–8.

534. Arlin ZA, Feldman E, Kempin S, et al. Amsacrine with high-dose cytarabine is highly effective therapy for refractory and relapsed acute lymphoblastic leukemia in adults. Blood 1988;72:433–5.

535. Whelan JS, Davis CL, Rohatiner AZ, et al. Etoposide in combination with intermediate dose cytosine arabinoside (ID ARA C) given with the intention of further myeloablative therapy for the treatment of refractory or recurrent hematological malignancy. Hematol Oncol 1992;10:87–94.

536. Arlin ZA, Feldman EJ, Finger LR, et al. Short course high dose mitoxantrone with high dose cytarabine is effective therapy for adult lymphoblastic leukemia. Leukemia 1991;5:712–4.

537. Milpied N, Gisselbrecht C, Harousseau JL, et al. Successful treatment of acute lymphoblastic leukemia after relapse with prednisone, intermediate dose cytarabine, mitoxantrone, and etoposide (PAME) chemotherapy. Cancer 1990;66:627–31.

538. Martino R, Brunet S, Sureda A, et al. Treatment of refractory and relapsed adult acute leukemia using a uniform chemotherapy protocol. Leuk Lymphoma 1993;11:393–8.

539. Testi AM, Moleti ML, Giona F, et al. Treatment of primary refractory or relapsed acute lymphoblastic leukemia (ALL) in children. Ann Oncol 1992;3:765–7.

540. Ciolli S, Leoni F, Caporale R, et al. Continuous-infusion cyclophosphamide plus vincristine, cytosine-arabinoside and prednisone for refractory acute lymphoblastic leukemia in adults. Haematologica 1991;76:293–7.

541. Brown RA, Herzig RH, Wolff SN, et al. High-dose etoposide and cyclophosphamide without bone marrow transplantation for resistant hematologic malignancy. Blood 1990;76:473–9.

542. Schiller G, Lee M, Territo M, et al. Phase II study of etoposide,

ifosfamide, and mitoxantrone for the treatment of resistant adult acute lymphoblastic leukemia. Am J Hematol 1993;43:195–9.

543. Kaufmann SH, Karp JE, Burke PJ, Gore SD. Addition of etoposide to initial therapy of adult acute lymphoblastic leukemia: a combined clinical and laboratory study [published erratum appears in Leuk Lymphoma 1997;24(5–6):553]. Leuk Lymphoma 1996;23:71–83.

544. Gore SD, Rowinsky EK, Miller CB, et al. A phase II "window" study of topotecan in untreated patients with high risk adult acute lymphoblastic leukemia [see comments]. Clin Cancer Res 1998;4:2677–89.

545. Frassoni F, Labopin M, Palut-Mzali P, et al. Evolution of allogeneic bone marrow transplantation in Europe: improved results for patients with acute leukemia in first remission. Blood 1993;82:291a. abstract.

546. Dopfer R, Henze G, Bender-Götze C, et al. Allogeneic bone marrow transplantation for childhood acute lymphoblastic leukemia in second remission after intensive primary and relapse therapy according to the BFM- and CoALL-protocols: results of the German Cooperative Study. Blood 1991;78:2780–4.

547. Horowitz MH, Messerer D, Hoelzer D, et al. Chemotherapy compared with bone marrow transplantation for adults with acute lymphoblastic leukemia in first remission. Ann Intern Med 1991;115:113–8.

548. Fiere D, Gisselbrecht C, Chauvin P, et al. Adult acute lymphoblastic leukemia. First interim analysis of the evolution of 467 patients (French Multicentric Trial LALA 87). Haematologica 1991;76:Suppl 4:108. abstract.

549. Bernasconi C, Lazzarino M, Morra E, et al. Early intensification followed by allo-BMT or auto-BMT or a second intensification in adult ALL: a randomized multicenter study. Leukemia. 1992;6:Suppl 2:204–8.

550. Vernant JP, Marit G, Maraninchi D, et al. Allogeneic bone marrow transplantation in adults with acute lymphoblastic leukemia in first complete remission. J Clin Oncol 1988;6:227–31.

551. Copelan EA, Biggs JC, Avalos BR, et al. Radiation-free preparation for allogeneic bone marrow transplantation in adults with acute lymphoblastic leukemia. J Clin Oncol 1992;10:237–42.

552. Weyman C, Graham-pole J, Emerson S, et al. Use of cytosine arabinoside and total body irradiation as conditioning for allogeneic marrow transplantation in patients with acute lymphoblastic leukemia: a multicenter survey. Bone Marrow Transplant 1993;11:43–50.

553. Blume KG, Forman SJ, O'Donnell MR, et al. Total body irradiation and high-dose etoposide: a new preparatory regimen for bone marrow transplantation in patients with advanced hematologic malignancies. Blood 1987;69:1015–20.

554. Chao NJ, Stein AS, Long GD, et al. Busulfan/etoposide—initial experience with a new preparatory regimen for autologous bone marrow transplantation in patients with acute nonlymphocytic leukemia. Blood 1993;81:319–23.

555. Lambertenghi Deliliers G, Mozzana R, Annaloro C, et al. Long-term results of autologous bone marrow transplantation in adult acute lymphoblastic leukemia. Leuk Lymphoma 1993;11:419–25.

556. Cahn JY, Bordigoni P, Souillet G, et al. The TAM regimen prior to allogeneic and autologous bone marrow transplantation for high-risk acute lymphoblastic leukemias: a cooperative study of 62 patients. Bone Marrow Transplant 1991;7:1–4.

557. Tiley C, Powles R, Treleaven J, et al. Feasibility and efficacy of maintenance chemotherapy following autologous bone marrow transplantation for first remission acute lymphoblastic leukaemia. Bone Marrow Transplant 1993;12:449–55.

558. Blume KG, Kopecky KJ, Henslee-Downey JP, et al. A prospective randomized comparison of total body irradiation-etoposide versus busulfan-cyclophosphamide as preparatory regiens for bone marrow transplantation in patients with leukemia who were not in first remission: a Southwest Oncology Group study. Blood 1993;81:2187–93.

559. Bortin MM, Horowitz MM, Gale RP, et al. Changing trends in allogeneic bone marrow transplantation for leukemia in the 1980s. JAMA 1992;268:607–12.

560. Herzig R, Barrett AJ, Gluckman E, et al. Bone marrow transplantation in high-risk acute lymphoblastic leukaemia in first and second remission. Lancet 1987;1:786–9.

561. Barrett AJ, Horowitz MM, Gale RP, et al. Marrow transplantation for acute lymphoblastic leukemia: factors affecting relapse and survival. Blood 1989;74:862–71.

562. Bortin MM, Horowitz MM, Rimm AA, for the Advisory Committee of the International Bone Marrow Transplant Registry. Progress report from the International Bone Marrow Transplant Registry. Bone Marrow Transplant 1992;10:113–22.

563. Bortin MM, Horowitz MM, Rowlings PA, et al. 1993 Progress report from the International Bone Marrow Transplant Registry. Bone Marrow Transplant 1994;12:97–104.

564. Doney K, Fisher LD, Appelbaum FR, et al. Treatment of adult acute lymphoblastic leukemia with allogeneic bone marrow transplantation. Multivariate analysis of factors affecting acute graft-versus-host disease, relapse, and relapse-free survival. Bone Marrow Transplant 1991;7:453–9.

565. Chao NJ, Forman SJ, Schmidt GM, et al. Allogeneic bone marrow transplantation for high risk acute lymphoblastic leukemia during first complete remission. Blood 1991;78:1923–7.

566. De la Camara R, Figuera A, Steegmann JL, et al. Allogeneic bone marrow transplantation for high risk acute lymphoblastic leukemia. Results from a single institution. Bone Marrow Transplant 1992;9:433–8.

567. Wingard JR, Piantadosi S, Santos GW, et al. Allogeneic bone marrow transplantation for patients with high-risk acute lymphoblastic leukemia. J Clin Oncol 1990;8:820–30.

568. Biggs JC, Horowitz MM, Gale RP, et al. Bone marrow transplants may cure patients with acute leukemia never achieving remission with chemotherapy. Blood 1992;80:1090–3.

569. Niederwieser D, Granena A, Hermans J, et al. Slow response to induction chemotherapy is an indicator of poor survival after bone marrow transplantation for acute lymphoblastic leukemia. The Leukemia Working Party of the European Group of Bone Marrow Transplantation (EBMT). Bone Marrow Transplant 1992;9:439–43.

570. Gorin NC, Aegerter P, Auvert B. Autologous bone marrow transplantation for acute leukemia in remission: an analysis of 1322 cases. In: Buchner T, Schellong G, Hiddemann W, Ritter J, eds. Haematology and blood transfusion. Vol. 33. Acute leukemias II. Berlin: Springer-Verlag, 1990:660–74.

571. Gilmore MJML, Hamon MD, Prentice HG, et al. Failure of purged autologous bone marrow transplantation in high risk acute lymphoblastic leukaemia in first complete remission. Bone Marrow Transplant 1991;8:19–26.

572. Dicke KA. Role of bone marrow transplant in acute lymphocytic leukemia. Leukemia 1992;6:Suppl 4:56–8.

573. Cahn JY, Flesch M, Vernant JP, Fiere D. Autologous bone marrow transplantation for intensification of first remission in adult patients with acute lymphoblastic leukemia. Leukemia 1992;6:Suppl 4:100–2.

574. Gorin NC, Herve P, Aegerter P, et al. Autologous bone marrow transplantation for acute leukaemia in remission. Br J Haematol 1986;64:385–95.

575. Dicke KA, Hoelzer DF, Gorin NC, et al. The role of bone marrow transplantation in adult acute lymphocytic leukemia. Ann Oncol 1993;4:Suppl 1:81–90.

576. Simonsson B, Burnett AK, Prentice HG, et al. Autologous bone marrow transplantation with monoclonal antibody purged marrow for high risk acute lymphoblastic leukemia. Leukemia 1989;3:631–6.

577. Rizzoli V, Carlo-Stella C, Almici C, et al. Autologous bone marrow transplantation for acute myeloid and lymphoid leukemia. Leukemia 1992;6:Suppl 4:103–5.

578. Arcese W, Amadori S, Meloni G, et al. Allogeneic or autologous bone marrow transplantation for intensification of salvage therapy in patients with high-risk advanced acute lymphoblastic leukemia. The AIEOP/GIMEMA Groups. Semin Hematol 1991;28:116–21.

579. Blaise D, Gaspard MH, Stoppa AM, et al. Allogeneic or autologous bone marrow transplantation for acute lymphoblastic leukemia in first complete remission. Bone Marrow Transplant 1990;5:7–12.

580. Soiffer RJ, Roy DC, Gonin R, et al. Monoclonal antibody-purged autologous bone marrow transplantation in adults with acute lymphoblastic leukemia at high risk of relapse. Bone Marrow Transplantation 1993;12:243–51.

581. Gulati SC, Lemoli RM, Acaba L, et al. Purging in autologous and allogeneic bone marrow transplantation. Curr Opin Oncol 1992;4:264–71.

582. Uckun FM, Myers DE. Allograft and autograft purging using immunotoxins in clinical bone marrow transplantation for hematologic malignancies. J Hematother 1993;2:155–63.

583. Hess AD, Jones RJ, Morris LE, et al. Autologous graft-versus-host disease: a new frontier in immunotherapy. Bone Marrow Transplant 1992;10:Suppl 1:16–21.

584. Martin H, Atta J, Bruecher J, et al. In patients with BCR-ABL-positive ALL in CR peripheral blood contains less residual disease than bone marrow: implications for autologous BMT. Ann Hematol 1994;68:85–7.

585. Carella AM. High-risk acute lymphoblastic leukemia (ALL): is there an alternative approach for increasing the number of cures? Haematologica 1992;77:348–51.

586. Barbui T, Finazzi G, Falanga A, et al. Bleeding and thrombosis in acute lymphoblastic leukemia. Leuk Lymphoma 1993;11:Suppl 2:43–7.

587. Leroy P, Krust A, Zelent A, et al. Multiple isoforms of the mouse retinoic acid receptor *alpha* are generated by alternative splicing and differential induction by retinoic acid. EMBO J 1991;10:59–69.

588. Katz JA, Taylor LD, Carroll A, et al. Cytogenetic features of childhood acute lymphoblastic leukemia. A Concordance Study and a Pediatric Oncology Group study. Cancer Genet Cytogenet 1991;55:249–56.

589. Sica S, Pagano L, Salutari P, et al. Acute parotitis during induction therapy including L-asparaginase in acute lymphoblastic leukemia. Ann Hematol 1994;68:91–2.

590. Bleyer WA, Sather HN, Nickerson HJ, et al. Monthly pulses of vincristine and prednisone prevent bone marrow and testicular relapse in low-risk childhood acute lymphoblastic leukemia: a report of the CCG-161 study by the Children's Cancer Study Group. J Clin Oncol 1991;9:1012–21.

591. Hokken-Koelega ACS, van Doorn JWD, Hahlen K, et al. Long-term effects of treatment for acute lymphoblastic leukemia with and without cranial irradiation on growth and puberty: a comparative study. Pediatr Res 1993;33:577–82.

592. Kreuser ED, Hetzel WD, Heit W, et al. Reproductive and endocrine gonadal functions in adults follwing multidrug chemotherapy for acute lymphoblastic or undifferentiated leukemia. J Clin Oncol 1988;6:588–95.

593. Yamamoto M, Fukunaga Y, Tsukimoto I, et al. Late effects of childhood acute leukemia and its treatment. Acta Paediatr Jpn 1991;33:573–88.

594. Neglia JP, Meadows AT, Robison LL, et al. Second neoplasms after acute lymphoblastic leukemia in childhood. N Engl J Med 1991;325:1330–6.

595. Pui C-H, Ribeiro RC, Hancock ML. Secondary acute myeloid leukemia in children treated with epipodophyllotoxins for acute lymphoblastic leukemia. N Engl J Med 1991;325:1682–7.

596. Winick NJ, McKenna RW, Shuster JJ, et al. Secondary acute myeloid leukemia in children with acute lymphoblastic leukemia treated with etoposide [see comments]. J Clin Oncol 1993;11:209–17.

597. Pääkkö E, Vainionpää L, Lanning M, et al. White matter changes in children treated for acute lymphoblastic leukemia. Cancer. 1992; 70:2728–33.

598. Giralt J, Ortega JJ, Olive T, et al. Long-term neuropsychologic sequelae of childhood leukemia: comparison of two CNS prophylactic regimens. Int J Radiat Oncol Biol Phys 1992;24:49–53.

599. Ochs J, Mulhern R, Fairclough F, et al. Comparison of neuropsychologic functioning and clinical indicators of neurotoxicity in long-term survivors of childhood leukemia given cranial radiation or parenteral methotrexate: a prospective study. J Clin Oncol 1991;9:145–51.

600. Lipshultz SE, Colan SD, Gelber RD, et al. Late cardiac effects of doxorubicin therapy for acute lymphoblastic leukemia in childhood. N Engl J Med 1991;324:808–14.

601. Virgilio JF, Moscinski LC, Ballester OF, et al. Acute lymphocytic leukemia in elderly patients. Hematol Oncol 1993;11:121–6.

602. Durand JM, Lefevre P. Mitomycin-induced thrombotic thrombocytopenic purpura: possible successful tretment with vincristine and cyclophosphamide. Haematologica 1991;76:421–3.

603. Preti A, O'Brien S, Robertson L, et al. Acute lymphocytic leukemia in the elderly: characteristics and outcome with the vincristine-adriamycin-dexamethasone regimen. Blood 1993;82:57a.

604. Ettinger LJ, Krailo MD, Gaynon PS, Hammond GD. A phase I study of carboplatin in children with acute leukemia in bone marrow relapse. Cancer 1993;72:917–22.

605. Bernstein ML, Whitehead VM, Devine S, et al. Ifosfamide with mesna uroprotection and etoposide in recurrent, refractory acute leukemia in childhood. Cancer 1993;72:1790–4.

606. Steinherz P, Redner A, Steinherz L, et al. Intensive therapy for acute lymphoblastic leukemia (ALL) in children at increased risk of early relape—the MSK-NY-II protocol. Proc Am Soc Clin Oncol 1993;12:317.

607. Ohyashiki K, Ohyashiki JH, Tauchi T, et al. Treatment of Philadelphia chromosome-positive acute lymphoblastic leukemia: a pilot study which raises important questions. Leukemia 1991;5:611–4.

608. Ochs J, Brecher ML, Mahoney D, et al. Recombinant interferon alfa

609. Arienti F, Gambacorti-Passerini C, Borin L, et al. Increased susceptibility to lymphokine activated killer (LAK) lysis of relapsing vs. newly diagnosed acute leukemic cells without changes in drug resistance or in the expression of adhesion molecules. Ann Oncol 1992;3:155–62.

610. Charak BS, Choudhary GD, Tefft M, Mazumder A. Interleukin-2 in bone marrow transplantation: preclinical studies. Bone Marrow Transplant 1992;10:103–11.

611. Parrado A, Rodriguez-Fernandez JM, Casares S, et al. Generation of LAK cells in vitro in patients with acute leukemia. Leukemia 1993;7:1344–8.

612. Dickinson AM, Lennard AL, Cartner R, Proctor SJ. Interleukin-2 induction of lymphokine-activated killer activity in the peripheral blood of an acute lymphoblastic leukaemia patient—case study. Leukemia 1992;6:957–60.

613. Weisdorf DJ, Anderson PM, Blazar BR, et al. Interleukin 2 immediately after autologous bone marrow transplantation for acute lymphoblastic leukemia—a phase I study. Transplantation 1993;55:61–6.

614. Campana D, Coustan-Smith E, Manabe A, et al. Prolonged survival of B-lineage acute lymphoblastic leukemia cells is accompanied by overexpression of bcl-2 protein. Blood 1993;81:1025–31.

615. Goasguen JE, Dossot J-M, Fardel O, et al. Expression of the multidrug resistance-associated P-glycoprotein (P-170) in 59 cases of de novo acute lymphoblastic leukemia: prognostic implications. Blood 1993;81:2394–8.

616. Kuwazuru Y, Yoshimura A, Hanada S, et al. Expression of the multidrug transporter, P-glycoprotein, in acute leukemia cells and correlation to clinical drug resistance. Cancer 1990;66:868–73.

617. Pieters R, Hongo T, Loonen AH, et al. Different types of non-P-glycoprotein mediated multiple drug resistance in children with relapsed acute lymphoblastic leukaemia. Br J Cancer 1992;65:691–7.

618. Musto P, Melillo L, Lombardi G, et al. High risk of early resistant relapse for leukaemic patients with presence of multidrug resistance associated P-glycoprotein positive cells in complete remission. Br J Haematol 1991;77:50–3.

619. Savignano C, Geromin A, Michieli M, et al. The expression of the multidrug resistance related glycoprotein in adult acute lymphoblastic leukemia. Haematologica 1993;78:261–3.

620. Ludescher C, Hilbe W, Eisterer W, et al. Low incidence of activity of P-glycoprotein (P-170) in de novo acute lymphoblastic leukemia determined by a flow cytometric assay [letter; comment]. Blood 1993;82:3505–7.

621. Fenneteau O, Marie JP, Lescoeur B, et al. Expression of the multidrug resistance-associated P-glycoprotein (P-170) in acute lymphoblastic leukemia [letter]. Blood 1993;82:3787–9.

622. List AF. Multidrug resistance: clinical relevance in acute leukemia. Oncology (Huntingt) 1993;7:23–8, 32; disc.

623. Grossbard ML, Press OW, Appelbaum RR, et al. Monoclonal antibody-based therapies of leukemia and lymphoma. Blood 1992;80:863–78.

624. Tazzari PL, Bolognesi A, de Totero D, et al. Immunotoxins containing saporin linked to different CD2 monoclonal antibodies: in vitro evaluation. Br J Haematol 1994;86:97–105.

625. Uckun FM, Chelstrom LM, Irvin JD, et al. In vivo efficacy of B43 (anti-CD19)-pokeweed antiviral protein immunotoxin against BCL-1 murine B-cell leukemia. Blood 1992;79:2649–61.

626. Jansen B, Kersey JH, Jaszcz WB, et al. Effective immunochemnotherapy of human t(4;11) leukemia in mice with severe combined immunodeficiency using B43 (anti-CD19)-pokeweed antiviral protein immunotoxin plus cyclophosphamide. Leukemia 1993;7:290–7.

627. Morland BJ, Barley J, Boehm D, et al. Effectiveness of HB2 (anti-CD7)-saporin immunotoxin in an in vivo model of human T-cell leukaemia developed in severe combined immunodeficient mice. Br J Cancer 1994;69:279–85.

628. Uckun FM, Kersey JH, Haake R, et al. Autologous bone marrow transplantation in high-risk remission B-lineage acute lymphoblastic leukemia using a cocktail of three monoclonal antibodies (BA-1/CD24, BA-2/CD9, and BA-3/CD10) plus complement and 4-hydroperoxycyclophosphamide for ex vivo bone marrow purging. Blood 1992;79:1094–1104.

629. Heerema NA, Argyropoulos G, Weetman R, et al. Interphase in situ hybridization reveals minimal residual disease in early remission and

return of the diagnostic clone in karyotypically normal relapse of acute lymphoblastic leukemia. Leukemia 1993;7:537–43.

630. Dewald GW, Schad CR, Christensen ER, et al. The application of fluorescent in situ hybridization to detect Mbcr/abl fusion in variant Ph chromosomes in CML and ALL. Cancer Genet Cytogenet 1993;71:7–14.

631. Imamura N, Kuramoto A. Detection of minimal residual disease in acute lymphoblastic leukemia by flow cytometry with monoclonal antibodies. Am J Hematol 1991;38:332–4.

632. Orfao A, Ciudad J, Lopez-Berges MC, et al. Acute lymphoblastic leukemia: detection of minimal residual disease at flow cytometry. Leuk Lymphoma 1994;13:Suppl 1:87–90.

633. Uckun FM, Kersey JH, Haake R, et al. Pretransplantation burden of leukemic progenitor cells as a predictor of relapse after bone marrow transplantation for acute lymphoblastic leukemia. N Engl J Med 1993;329:1296–1301.

634. Pakkala S. DNA fingerprinting in the detection of residual disease in acute leukemia. Leukemia 1991;5:437–40.

635. Gehly GB, Bryant EM, Lee AM, et al. Chimeric BCR-abl messenger RNA as a marker for minimal residual disease in patients transplanted for Philadelphia chromosome-positive acute lymphoblastic leukemia. Blood 1991;78:458–65.

636. Miyamura K, Takeo T, Kataoka T, et al. Detection of minimal residual disease in Philadelphia chromosome positive acute lymphoblastic leukemia: rationale for bone marrow transplantation from the polymerase chain reaction point of view. Leuk Lymphoma 1993;11:181–9.

637. Biondi A, Rambaldi A, Rossi V, et al. Detection of ALL-1/AF4 fusion transcript by reverse transcription-polymerase chain reaction for diagnosis and monitoring of acute leukemias with the t(4;11) translocation. Blood 1993;82:2943–7.

638. Macintyre EA, d'Auriol L, Duparc N, et al. Use of oligonucleotide probes directed against T cell antigen receptor gamma delta variable-(diversity)-joining junctional sequences as a general method for detecting minimal residual disease in acute lymphoblastic leukemias. J Clin Invest 1990;86:2125–35.

639. Breit TM, Wolvers-Tettero IL, Hahlen K, et al. Extensive junctional diversity of XgXδ T-cell receptors expressed by T-cell acute lymphoblastic leukemias: implications for the detection of minimal residual disease [published erratum appears in Leukemia 1992;6(2):169–70]. Leukemia 1991;5:1076–86.

640. Burnett RC, David J, Harden AM, et al. The LCK gene is involved in the t(1;7)(p34;q34) in the T-cell acute lymphoblastic leukemia derived cell line, HSB-2. Genes Chromosomes Cancer 1991;3:461–7.

641. Brisco MJ, Condon J, Hughes E, et al. Outcome prediction in childhood acute lymphoblastic leukaemia by molecular quantification of residual disease at the end of induction. Lancet 1994;343:196–200.

642. Yamada M, Wasserman R, Lange B, et al. Minimal residual disease in childhood B-lineage lymphoblastic leukemia. Persistence of leukemic cells during the first 18 months of treatment [see comments]. N Engl J Med 1990;323:448–55.

643. Nizet Y, Van Daele S, Lewalle P, et al. Long-term follow-up of residual disease in acute lymphoblastic leukemia patients in complete remission using clonogeneic IgH probes and the polymerase chain reaction. Blood 1993;82:1618–25.

644. Neale GA, Menarguez J, Kitchingman GR, et al. Detection of minimal residual disease in T-cell acute lymphoblastic leukemia using polymerase chain reaction predicts impending relapse. Blood 1991;78:739–47.

645. Langlands K, Eden OB, Micallef-Eynaud P, et al. Direct sequence analysis of TCR V delta 2-D delta 3 rearrangements in common acute lymphoblastic leukaemia and application to detection of minimal residual disease. Br J Haematol 1993;84:648–55.

646. Biondi A, Yokota S, Hansen-Hagge TE, et al. Minimal residual disease in childhood acute lymphoblastic leukemia: analysis of patients in continuous complete remission or with consecutive relapse. Leukemia 1992;6:282–88.

647. Ito Y, Wasserman R, Galili N, et al. Molecular residual disease status at the end of chemotherapy fails to predict subsequent relapse in children with B-lineage acute lymphoblastic leukemia. J Clin Oncol 1993;11:546–53.

648. Wasserman R, Galili N, Ito Y, et al. Residual disease at the end of induction therapy as a predictor of relapse during therapy in childhood B-lineage acute lymphoblastic leukemia. J Clin Oncol 1992;10:1879–88.

649. Potter MN, Steward CG, Oakhill A. The significance of detection of minimal residual disease in childhood acute lymphoblastic leukaemia. Br J Haematol 1993;83:412–8.

650. Kitchingman GR. Residual disease detection in multiple follow-up samples in children with acute lymphoblastic leukemia. Leukemia 1994;8:395–401.

651. Taylor JJ, Rowe D, Kylefjord H, et al. Characterisation of nonconcordance in the T-cell receptor gamma chain genes at presentation and clinical relapse in acute lymphoblastic leukemia. Leukemia 1994;8:60–66.

# CHAPTER 96

# ADULT T-CELL LEUKEMIA/LYMPHOMA

• CHARLES L. MAURER • WILLIAM J. HARRINGTON JR.
• PARKASH GILL • CARSTEN E. KAMPE • JOSEPH D. ROSENBLATT

Adult T-cell leukemia/lymphoma (ATL) is a rare lymphoproliferative disorder of CD4+ T cells characterized by an aggressive course and a poor response to standard chemotherapy. ATL is frequently associated with hypercalcemia, skin manifestations, visceral involvement, and occasionally lytic bone lesions.[1–3] It was first recognized as a discrete clinical syndrome by Takatsuki and coworkers.[4] The causative agent of this disease is a retrovirus, human T-cell lymphotropic virus type I (HTLV-I),[5–7] a member of a unique family of oncogenic lymphotropic type C retroviruses that includes the closely related HTLV-II as well as bovine leukemia virus. The discovery of ATL provided the first proven link between retroviruses and disease in humans.[5, 6]

## Role of Human T-Cell Lymphotropic Virus I in the Pathogenesis of Adult T-Cell Leukemia/Lymphoma

The discovery of the serologic and molecular link between HTLV-I and ATL has led to intense investigation of potential pathogenic mechanisms. The initial link was established by identification of the retrovirus in a T-cell line derived from a patient thought to have Sézary's syndrome[5] and by demonstration of patient antibodies directed against viral antigens in a virally infected cell line.[6] A hallmark of ATL is an oligoclonally integrated provirus in leukemic cells as detected by Southern blotting.[8] As opposed to other leukemogenic animal retroviruses, however, HTLV-I appears to integrate randomly, and no evidence for activation of adjacent cellular proto-oncogenes has been shown.[9] HTLV-I and HTLV-II sequences bear little or no homology to cellular sequences, and the virus does not transduce a cellular oncogene. Leukemogenesis by HTLV is likely to involve novel mechanisms. In comparison with other animal retroviruses, the human HTLV-I and HTLV-II as well as the bovine leukemia virus (a cause of leukemia and lymphoma in cattle) have a more complex genome, which encodes additional mRNA species. In addition to the unspliced *gag/pol* and singly spliced *env* mRNA, splicing events may generate eight new mRNA species for HTLV-I, and at least four additional proteins are known to be encoded by these multiply spliced RNAs.[10, 11] The molecular organization of HTLV-I is illustrated in Figure 96–1. Some of these proteins act as transcriptional and post-transcriptional regulators of viral gene expression. The pX region, located at the 3′ end of the genome, contains at least four open reading frames.[9] Proteins encoded by mRNA from the HTLV pX region include Tax, Rex, p21rex, p12, p13, and p30.[10–13]

The *tax* gene in HTLV-I and HTLV-II is a regulator of transcription; in HTLV-I, it encodes a 40-kd nuclear phosphoprotein, and in HTLV-II, it encodes a 37-kd nuclear phosphoprotein.[10, 14, 15] The Tax protein acts as a transcriptional regulator but does not bind to DNA directly. Tax promotes enhanced HTLV transcription through indirect interactions with DNA transcription factors that bind to Tax-responsive elements (TRE-1 and TRE-2) within the HTLV long terminal repeat (LTR).[16] These transcription factors include the cyclic adenosine monophosphate (cAMP)–responsive element (CRE)–binding protein (CREB) and CRE modulator (CREM) and are members of the CRE/activated transcription factor (ATF) family (leucine zipper protein). Tax interacts directly with CREB and the KIX domain of the coactivator CREB binding protein (CBP) to form a stable nucleoprotein complex on viral CREs.[17, 18]

Once bound to the HTLV promoter, CBP can activate transcription.[18] A second protein known as Rex is a post-transcriptional regulator of RNA transport and splicing; it migrates with an apparent molecular weight of 27 kd in HTLV-I and 26 kd in HTLV-II.[11, 19, 20] Use of an alternative methionine initiation codon has been shown to account for a truncated Rex protein of 21-kd size in HTLV-I; in HTLV-II, Rex has been shown to be phosphorylated on serine residues, and a hypophosphorylated 24-kd protein has been noted.[21]

Other proteins encoded in the pX region include p21[rexIII], p12[I], p13[II], and p30[II]/tof. Expression of p21[rexIII] has been found in uncultured ATL cells.[22] p12[I] is a 12-kd, 99–amino acid protein encoded by double-spliced and single-spliced mRNA in open reading frame 1.[23] The p12[I] protein structurally resembles the bovine papillomavirus E5 protein and is considered to be a weak oncogene.[24] The p12[I] protein also reportedly interacts with and downregulates the expression of beta and gamma chains of interleukin-2 (IL-2) receptors.[25] This downregulation may alter cellular responses to IL-2 and have a role in T-cell transformation.[25]

The interactions of Tax with cellular transcription factors have been suggested as a mechanism for T-cell transformation by HTLV-I and HTLV-II. In addition to transcriptional enhancement from the viral promoters, Tax appears to affect transcriptional activity from a wide variety of cellular promoters. There are now numerous examples of cellular gene promoters directly or indirectly transactivated by Tax. Some of the interactions with cellular transcription factors observed for Tax appear to account for many of the phenotypic characteristics of HTLV-transformed T cells. Some of these genes affected by *tax* are linked to regulation of T-cell growth. The cellular genes transactivated by Tax can be separated into several categories: proto-oncogenes, cytokines and growth factors, transcriptional factors, and miscellaneous cellular factors. These include the promoter for the IL-2 gene; the promoter for the alpha chain of the IL-2 receptor[26];

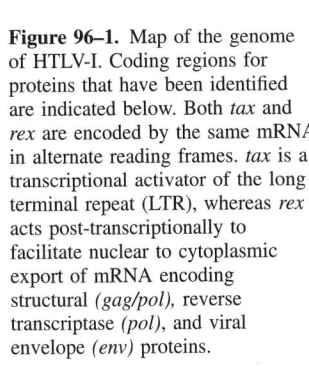

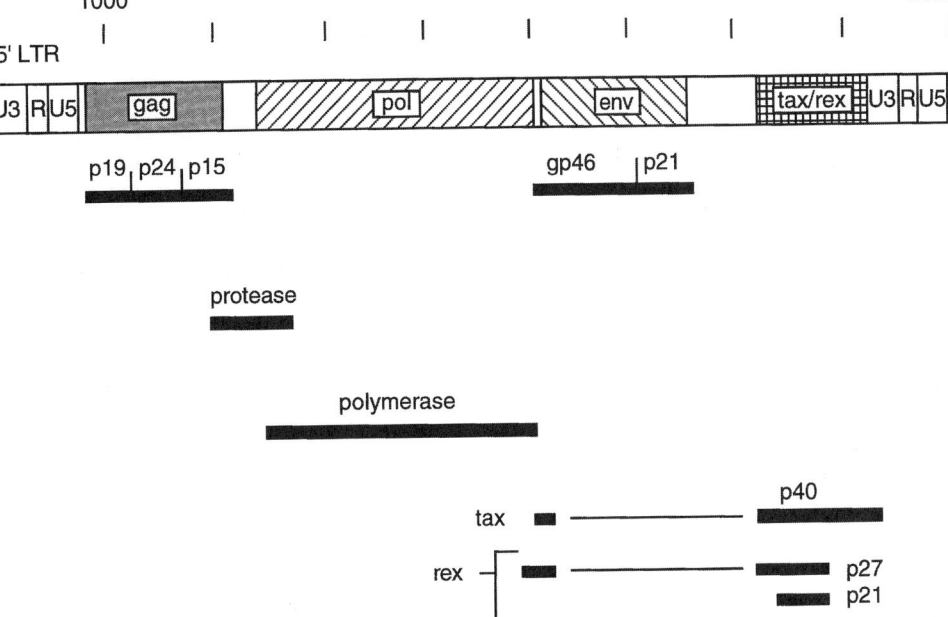

**Figure 96–1.** Map of the genome of HTLV-I. Coding regions for proteins that have been identified are indicated below. Both *tax* and *rex* are encoded by the same mRNA in alternate reading frames. *tax* is a transcriptional activator of the long terminal repeat (LTR), whereas *rex* acts post-transcriptionally to facilitate nuclear to cytoplasmic export of mRNA encoding structural (*gag/pol*), reverse transcriptase (*pol*), and viral envelope (*env*) proteins.

and the promoters for the cellular c-*fos* oncogene,[27] c-*myc*, and cytokines such as granulocyte-macrophage colony-stimulating factor (GM-CSF)[28] and gamma interferon.[29] Enhanced expression of the CD25 antigen encoding the p55 alpha chain of the high-affinity IL receptor may be due to the effects of *tax* on the IL-2 receptor promoter.[26] Several cellular genes that can be induced by Tax by the *nuclear factor kappa B (NF-kB)* pathways, such as the IL-2 receptor gene, could conceivably lead to T-cell stimulation.[26] *Tax* expression has also been postulated to account for constitutive expression of a variety of cytokines or hormones, or both, in HTLV-transformed cells, such as GM-CSF and parathyroid hormone–related protein (PTHrP).[28, 30–32] PTHrP has been implicated in humoral hypercalcemia and in a variety of solid tumors as well as in ATL. Watanabe and coworkers[30] demonstrated PTHrP expression in peripheral blood mononuclear cells of patients with ATL. Pleural and ascites fluid from patients with ATL has been noted to contain elevated levels of PTHrP.[31] The *tax* gene of HTLV-I and HTLV-II strongly activates the PTHrP promoter.[32] Transactivation of PTHrP appears to be cell type specific and has been observed in transfections of T cells but not B cells or fibroblasts. This transactivation appears to depend on the transcription factor AP-2 and is another example of promiscuous transactivation by *tax* (Prager D, unpublished results). Investigators have linked *tax* to genesis of the T-cell transformed phenotype and to a possible direct role in the hypercalcemia of ATL. *Promiscuous* transactivating activity by Tax is considered to play a significant role in the proliferation and transformation of HTLV-I–infected T cells.

Several lines of evidence suggest a role for *tax* in the transformation of HTLV-I–infected CD4[+] T cells. NIH 3T3 and Rat-1 cells transfected with HTLV-I *tax* show increased growth in vitro, and the *tax*-transduced Rat-1 cells form tumors in nude mice.[33] HTLV-I *tax*, under the control of the LTR, appears to induce nonlymphoid tumors (neurofibromas) in transgenic mice.[34] The LTR-*tax* transgenics also developed thymic atrophy, suggesting a possible toxic effect of *tax* expression on lymphocyte differentiation and development. Infection of fresh peripheral blood lymphocytes (PBLs) with a replication-competent, nontransforming herpesvirus saimiri vector expressing *tax* produced immortalized but IL-2–dependent T cells in tissue culture. Transgenic mice have also been developed that target expression of Tax to the mature T-cell compartment by using the human granzyme B promoter.[35] These transgenic mice developed a large granular cell–like leukemia or lymphoma of T-cell or natural killer–cell origin.[36] These and other studies suggest that *tax* is involved in, but is not sufficient for, transformation by HTLV-I. Although investigators have described a potential role for *tax* in T-cell transformation and mitogenesis, this role is not clear.

As opposed to *tax*, the *rex* gene has not been directly implicated in transformation. Evidence has shown that *rex* may act in concert with *tax* to increase the stability or export of IL-2 receptor mRNA in HTLV-I–infected cells.[37] These studies suggest that *rex* may alter the expression of cellular genes and may play a role in potentiating T-cell transformation. Rex is an RNA-binding protein that has been localized to the nucleus and principally the nucleolus of infected cells, and it recognizes a cognate RNA recognition sequence in the HTLV LTR.[20, 38] Whether *rex* can affect transport and

expression of other cellular RNAs, affecting gene expression and T cells, is not known. Additional investigation suggests that HTLV virions may well be directly mitogenic to T cells.[39] Whether mitogenic effects are mediated by soluble *tax* directly, by the env protein of HTLV, or by other HTLV products is not known.

The molecular understanding of HTLV biology does not explain the long latent period between initial infection and subsequent leukemogenesis. Cytogenetic evidence suggests that in advanced ATL, multiple cytogenetic abnormalities are often present.[40] These cytogenetic abnormalities often include translocations involving the T-cell receptor alpha chain locus and other translocations that may lead to aberrant expression of cellular proto-oncogenes or oncogene fusion proteins in HTLV-infected cells. The prolonged latency period suggests that an accumulation of cytogenetic abnormalities may lead to full-blown malignancy. Hatta and colleagues[41] found homozygous and hemizygous deletions in at least one exon of the p15 and p16 tumor-suppressor genes in 10 of 37 patients with ATL. The p15 and p16 genes located on chromosome 9p are considered tumor-suppressor genes. They inhibit the activity of CDK4 and CDK6, which inactivate the retinoblastoma protein. Patients with ATL and deletions of p15 or p16, or both, have significantly shorter survival times than those without the deletions.[42]

In some cases, abnormalities may also include mutations in the p53 tumor-suppressor gene.[43] Mutations in p53 genes have been found in only one fourth of cases of ATL, however.[43] More recent data reveal the wild-type p53 to be stabilized and functionally inactive in most HTLV-transformed cells.[44] Tax is thought to inactivate p53 through phosphorylation, preventing p53 interaction with transcription factors.[45, 46] DNA repair may also be affected adversely through Tax-mediated downregulation of the DNA β-polymerase gene. ATL cells have also been shown to have a higher incidence of microsatellite instability.[47] Microsatellite instability has been associated with tumor formation and represents defects in the DNA mismatch repair system.

The frequent demonstration of defective HTLV genomes in ATL suggests that active viral replication is not required for maintenance of established ATL. HTLV-I probably acts at an early stage, leading to T-cell expansion, and may predispose the individual to leukemia. Further understanding of the role played by HTLV-I and HTLV-II in T-cell transformation in the laboratory may clarify the role of these viruses in leukemogenesis.

## Epidemiology of Human T-Cell Lymphotropic Virus I and Adult T-Cell Leukemia/Lymphoma

ATL has a unique geographic distribution that coincides with the distribution of HTLV-I and probably reflects the origin and transmission of the virus. The prevalence as well as the geographic distribution of HTLV-I is widely variable throughout the world. Based on patterns of genetic drift, the origin of HTLV-I has been postulated to have occurred in the Indo-Malay region or Asia with subsequent spread to Africa. It is hypothesized that slave traders and European travelers disseminated HTLV-I from Africa and the Indo-

Malay region to the New World.[48–50] HTLV-I infection is highly prevalent in Southern Japan,[2, 51] where approximately 20% of the adult population is seropositive. HTLV-I occurs in endemic populations in Central and West Africa, the Caribbean basin,[52] Central and South America,[53, 54] and Melanesia.[55] HTLV-I is not indigenous to Europe or North America, but immigration has carried HTLV-I throughout the world. The infection has been shown in West Indians living in England, Japanese living in Hawaii, and African Americans from the southeastern United States living in New York City.[56–58] In the United States, most cases of HTLV-I infection are seen in southeastern Florida and among Caribbean immigrants to the Eastern seaboard.[1, 3, 59] The seroprevalence of HTLV-I, HTLV-II, and human immunodeficiency virus type 1 (HIV-1) in more than 480,000 random blood donations from five U.S. centers tested is shown in Table 96–1. The frequency of seropositivity with HTLV-I and HTLV-II was approximately three times higher than that of HIV-1 (0.043% vs. 0.013%) from December 1988 to May 1989.[60] The seroprevalence of HIV-1 during the first 6 months of antibody screening in 1985 from the same centers was 0.54%, indicating that seroprevalence rates of HTLV-I and HTLV-II and of HIV-1 in previously unscreened blood donor populations were similar. More than 50% of the seronegative blood donors harbored HTLV-II rather than HTLV-I and were detected as a result of serologic cross-reactivity of the HTLV-I–based enzyme-linked immunosorbent assay.[60]

HTLV-I infection appears to require prolonged, close contact between infected and uninfected individuals. Cell-free HTLV-I seems to be considerably less infectious than HIV-1. For example, although cell-free HIV can transmit viral infection, transmission by free HTLV-I rarely occurs.[61–68] Transmission of HTLV-I occurs primarily through mother-to-child transfer, blood products, and sexual intercourse. Mother-to-child transmission occurs through maternal HTLV-I–infected T cells in breast milk with an efficiency of approximately 20%.[69, 70] Less commonly, transmission can occur vertically from mothers to non–breast-fed infants.[69–71] Factors associated with a higher risk of HTLV-I transmission include the duration of breast-feeding, level of maternal viral load, and maternal antibody titer.[59, 71–73] Infants breast-fed for fewer than 6 months have a rate of infection similar to that of bottle-fed infants.[69–71, 74]

Sexual transmission of HTLV-I is bidirectional, although more commonly transmitted from male to female rather than female to male.[62, 74–76] The length of the sexual relationship, viral load, titers of anti-HTLV, and presence of genital ulcers are important risk factors for HTLV transmission.[74, 77] Semen is thought to be the primary vehicle for transmission in sexual contacts because of the presence of virus-positive mononuclear cells within seminal fluid.[78]

HTLV transmission can occur through blood transfusions containing infected T cells[68, 79, 80] and through shared needles among intravenous drug abusers. This virus is transmitted through cellular blood products, including whole blood, packed red blood cells, and platelet concentrates. It is not transmitted through plasma derivatives. If red cells are stored for more than 14 days, the rate of transmission falls to negligible levels.[81] In the United States, the prevalence of HTLV seropositivity is approximately 0.05% among asymptomatic blood donors.[60, 61] Owing to serologic cross-reactivity between HTLV-I and HTLV-II, this does not reflect true HTLV-I infection, and more than half of seropositive U.S. blood donors are infected with HTLV-II rather than HTLV-I.[60] African Americans and Hispanics have the highest seroprevalence. Increased seroprevalence is also found in intravenous drug abusers and patients in clinics for sexually transmitted diseases. Most seropositive intravenous drug abusers in the United States appear to be infected with HTLV-II rather than HTLV-I. Certain Native American populations in New Mexico as well as in Central and South America have been found to harbor HTLV-II.[82] There is no evidence to suggest that transmission of HTLV-I occurs by other means, such as by insect vectors.

## Natural History

### CLINICAL FEATURES AND CLASSIFICATION

ATL generally has its onset in adulthood, 20 to 40 years after the initial infection with HTLV-I. An analysis of Japanese ATL patients found an age distribution of 17 to 78 years with a mean age of 53 years for both sexes.[83] Most patients were 50 to 59 years old (men) or 60 to 69 years old (women). The male/female ratio in patients with ATL was 1.3:1. Although HTLV-I infection is necessary for the devel-

*Table 96–1.* **Prevalence of HTLV-I and HTLV-II Antibodies in U.S. Blood Donors***

| Site | December 1988–May 1989 Confirmed Seropositive | | April 1985–September 1985 Confirmed Seropositive | |
|---|---|---|---|---|
| | DONORS | HTLV-I/II (%) | HIV (%) | DONORS | HIV (%) |
| Los Angeles, Orange County | 188,237 | 110 (0.058) | 31 (0.016) | 183,686 | 156 (0.085) |
| New Orleans | 42,377 | 11 (0.026) | 8 (0.019) | 39,472 | 21 (0.053) |
| Pennsylvania, New Jersey | 158,410 | 51 (0.032) | 23 (0.015) | 166,639 | 64 (0.038) |
| Kansas City | 46,181 | 8 (0.017) | 2 (0.004) | 49,482 | 7 (0.014) |
| Sacramento | 49,414 | 27 (0.055) | 0 | 41,858 | 11 (0.026) |
| *Total* | 484,619 | 207 (0.043) | 64 (0.013) | 481,137 | 259 (0.054) |

*Although serologic evidence for HTLV-I infection was obtained by enzyme-linked immunosorbent assay or Western blot, greater than 50% of seropositive individuals were actually infected by HTLV-II (details in text).

HTLV-I, HTLV-II; human T-cell lymphotropic virus types I and II; HIV, human immunodeficiency virus.

From Lee HH, Swanson P, Rosenblatt JD, et al. Relative prevalence and risk factors of HTLV-I and HTLV-II infection in US blood donors. Lancet 1991;337:1436. With permission from The Lancet Ltd.

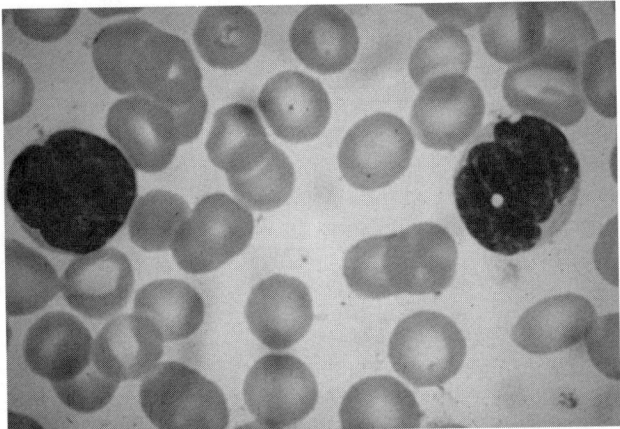

**Figure 96–2.** Abnormal lymphocytes in a patient with acute adult T-cell leukemia/lymphoma (ATL). Some cells show characteristic multilobulation of the nucleus. (From Rosenblatt JD, Chen IS, Wachsman W. Infection with HTLV-I and HTLV-II: evolving concepts. Semin Hematol 1988;25:232.)

opment of ATL, the disease develops in only a few infected individuals. Approximately 95% of persons infected with HTLV-I are likely to remain asymptomatic carriers.[53, 84, 85] In the Japanese population, in which about 1% are carriers of HTLV-I,[86] the lifetime risk for ATL is estimated to be 2 to 4% among carriers.[86, 87]

Most HTLV-I–infected individuals are carriers of the virus and do not manifest any overt signs or symptoms.[84–87] Fresh PBLs from HTLV-I carriers produce little or no detectable virus by Southern blotting. Oligoclonal integration of the HTLV genome into cellular DNA is generally not observed.[84] These individuals are still able to transmit the virus, however, because proviral genome is integrated into host-cell DNA sequences as detected by polymerase chain reaction.

The Lymphoma Study Group of Japan has proposed a classification system based on four defined clinical subtypes[88–91]: smoldering, chronic, lymphoma, and acute types.[88–91] A preleukemic phase of ATL (pre-ATL) has also been well described.[92–95] These patients with pre-ATL are asymptomatic and identified by the finding of modest leukocytosis or of abnormal PBLs with characteristic lobulated *flower* nuclei as seen in ATL (Fig. 96–2).[88, 92] DNA extracted from the PBLs of pre-ATL patients contains oligoclonally integrated HTLV-I.[92] In addition to abnormal PBLs, Hisada and colleagues[95] found a positive correlation between the level of anti-HTLV antibody titer and risk of developing ATL. There is a 1.6-fold increase in risk of ATL per 2-fold increase in anti–HTLV-I titer. In approximately half of these cases, the abnormal T cells regress spontaneously. In the remaining cases, especially those with elevated white blood cell counts, the pre-ATL progresses to one of four defined clinical subtypes of ATL.

The smoldering type of ATL is characterized by low levels of circulating leukemic cells, presence of skin lesions, absence of hypercalcemia, and absence of visceral and lymph node involvement. Pulmonary lesions may be present. Chronic ATL is defined by an absolute lymphocytosis ($\geq$4 $\times$ 10$^9$/L) with a T lymphocytosis of 3.5 $\times$ 10$^9$ or greater and elevated lactate dehydrogenase levels. There may be lymphadenopathy and involvement of liver, spleen, skin, and

lungs, and 5% or more abnormal T lymphocytes are often seen in the peripheral blood. The calcium level is not elevated; there is no involvement of central nervous system, bone, and gastrointestinal tract; and there is neither ascites nor pleural effusion. The smoldering and chronic forms of ATL are generally less aggressive than the acute form of the disease.[90, 91, 96] These disease subtypes may represent a transitional state in evolution of the malignant clone before the development of the acute syndrome.[90, 96]

Most patients presenting with ATL fall into the category of acute ATL.[90, 91, 97–99] These patients have an elevated white blood cell count, with many morphologically atypical circulating mature T-helper lymphocytes that express the CD4 antigen and the p55 chain of the IL-2 receptor. They have clonally rearranged T-cell receptor V genes and monoclonal integration of HTLV-I into the genome, indicating that the malignant T cells originate from a single HTLV-I–infected clone.[8, 100, 101] There may be eosinophilia and neutrophilia.[102–104] In contrast to lymphoblastic lymphoma, patients with acute ATL often present with lymphadenopathy that characteristically spares the mediastinum and with hepatosplenomegaly and skin lesions resulting from an infiltration of leukemia cells (Fig. 96–3). Interstitial pneumonitis, also caused by leukemic cell infiltration, is sometimes present.[105] Serum chemistry studies often show elevated lactate dehydrogenase and bilirubin levels.

Approximately 50% of patients with acute ATL have hypercalcemia, with or without lytic bone lesions. The com-

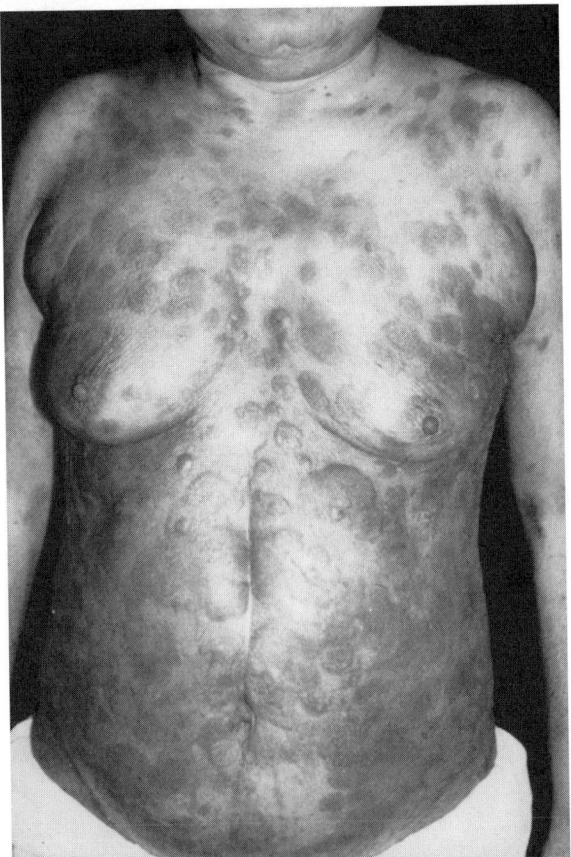

**Figure 96–3.** Lytic lesions in a Japanese patient with ATL. (From Rosenblatt JD, Chen IS, Wachsman W. Infection with HTLV-I and HTLV-II: evolving concepts. Semin Hematol 1988;25:232.)

plex mechanisms underlying this humoral hypercalcemia syndrome are not completely understood; however, PTHrP is most strongly implicated as a potential mediator, as with other malignancies.[30–32] Studies have shown that the PTHrP promoter is transactivated by the HTLV-I Tax protein.[30, 32] The presence of hypercalcemia indicates a poor prognosis, and this is difficult to control unless there is a good antitumor response to chemotherapy. Patients may or may not have osteolytic bone lesions, abnormal bone scans, and elevated alkaline phosphatase levels. The characteristically intense uptake evident in the joints and skull as seen on radionuclide bone scans in ATL is in contrast to other lymphomas and leukemias, in which these findings are rare.[91, 106]

Some ATL patients present with clinical features suggestive of a T-cell lymphoma rather than a leukemia.[91, 99, 107] Lymphomatous ATL is characterized by lymphadenopathy with or without extranodal lesions in the absence of lymphocytosis. In these patients, 1% or less of abnormal T lymphocytes may be present in the blood. Hepatosplenomegaly and cutaneous lesions can also be present.[91] In a U.S. study of ATL in patients with Japanese and Caribbean ancestry, those of Caribbean descent were generally younger and more frequently presented with lymphoma-type ATL.[108] The histopathology of lymph nodes from ATL patients is heterogeneous, but most fall into the large cell, immunoblastic classification.[88, 109] Lymph node biopsy specimens contain oligoclonally integrated HTLV-I, as determined by Southern blot hybridization.[8, 110] The various histopathologic grades of lymphomatous ATL do not appear to affect prognosis.[111] It is important, however, to distinguish patients with lymphoma-type ATL from those with non–HTLV-I-related T-cell lymphoma because the prognosis and therapeutic response in ATL are different from that in other T-cell lymphomas. A study of 572 cases of nodal T-cell lymphoma from Japan reported that 77% of patients with clonal integration of HTLV-I proviral DNA by Southern blotting had pleomorphic-type histopathology.[112]

The immune system in patients with ATL appears to be compromised, as evidenced by the high incidence of opportunistic infections, including *Pneumocystis carinii* pneumonia; cytomegalovirus pneumonia; cryptococcal meningitis; disseminated fungal infections; parasitic infections, including strongyloidiasis; bacterial lung abscesses; and bacterial sepsis.[113–116] T-cell–mediated immunity is impaired in HTLV-I carriers and in those with ATL.[91] Of the opportunistic organisms, *Strongyloides stercoralis* has often been found concurrently with HTLV-I infection.[114, 117] Nakada and colleagues[115] found that 58% of patients with *Strongyloides* infection were HTLV-I positive, and 66% of those had monoclonal integration of HTLV-I proviral DNA in their blood lymphocytes. This finding has initiated speculation regarding *Strongyloides* infection as a cofactor in the development of ATL. Leukemic cell production and secretion of large quantities of transforming growth factor-$\beta_1$ may also contribute to the immunosuppression seen in this disease.[118, 119]

## DIAGNOSIS

The differential diagnosis of ATL includes other T-cell malignancies, such as the non-Hodgkin's lymphomas, mycosis fungoides (cutaneous T-cell lymphoma), Sézary's syndrome,

and T-cell chronic lymphocytic leukemia. A variety of laboratory studies can assist in the diagnosis of ATL, including a positive HTLV-I serologic panel, elevated serum calcium levels, negative staining for terminal deoxynucleotidyl transferase (TdT), and immunologic phenotyping of ATL cells, which characteristically express both the CD4 and the Tac (IL-2 receptor) antigens. Serologic assay for HTLV-I is performed using commercially available enzyme-linked immunosorbent assay and Western blot assays. HTLV-I–infected and some HTLV-II–infected individuals are identified by standard serologic testing. Discrimination between HTLV-I and HTLV-II can be difficult given the high degree of amino acid homology between the two viruses.[120] Polymerase chain reaction or peptide-based serologic tests can be used to distinguish between HTLV-I and HTLV-II.[121] Definitive evidence for the disease is shown by the presence of monoclonally or oligoclonally integrated HTLV-I in the malignant T-cell clone.[8, 9, 122–124] There is continued controversy over whether HTLV-I may also be implicated in cases of seronegative mycosis fungoides from nonendemic regions. Defective HTLV-I genomes have been detected in some cases by polymerase chain reaction, and *virion*-like particles have been noted in T-cell lines by electron microscopy.[117, 125] Because this finding is not yet confirmed, HTLV-I–seronegative cases of cutaneous T-cell lymphoma are best operationally classified as cutaneous T-cell lymphoma, whereas seropositive cases should be regarded as ATL.

## PROGNOSIS

The median survival for the acute and lymphoma types of ATL is less than 1 year despite aggressive chemotherapy.[88, 90, 91] Nevertheless, about 18% of patients with aggressive types of ATL survive for more than 2 years. The eventual cause of death in most patients is related to hypercalcemia, infection, or tumor progression.[3, 4, 126, 127]

Several reports have described cases of spontaneous regression of ATL, but this is considered to be a rare event.[128–132] Infection and biopsy were believed to have triggered spontaneous regression in most of these patients, a phenomenon previously described in non-Hodgkin's lymphoma[133, 134] and in African Burkitt's lymphoma.[135, 136] Whether such spontaneous regressions are immunologically mediated is unknown.

Tsukasaki and colleagues[137] reported the outcome of 114 ATL patients with various forms of ATL. Survival data are shown in Figure 96–4. Median survival time was 5.5 months for acute ATL, 8.7 months for lymphoma-type ATL, and 37.9 months for chronic ATL and was not reached for the smoldering type. Eight of 11 patients with smoldering ATL were alive greater than 10 years. Differences in survival between these groups of patients were statistically significant, arguing favorably for the usefulness of this classification scheme. A multivariate analysis performed in 90 patients with aggressive ATL revealed that poor performance status and renal insufficiency were significant prognostic factors for shortened survival. Unexpectedly the presence of ascites was found to correlate with a good prognosis,[137] in contrast to other lymphomas.[138] An earlier, smaller study showed a strong predictive relationship between serum lactate dehydrogenase, calcium, and total protein levels and

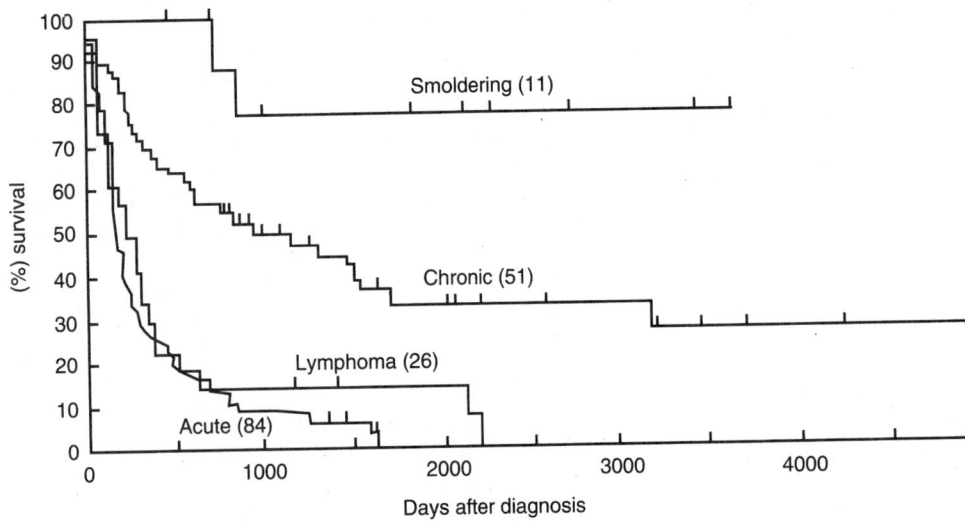

**Figure 96–4.** Survival of patients with ATL according to clinical subtype. The numbers of patients are in parentheses. (From Tsukasaki K, Ikeda S, Murata K, et al. Characteristics of chemotherapy-induced clinical remission in long survivors with aggressive adult T-cell leukemia/lymphoma. Leuk Res 1993;17:159.)

survival in patients with the lymphoma type of ATL.[139] A third study performed by the Lymphoma Study Group from Japan also reported the major prognostic factors of patients with ATL. In their study of 854 patients, they found five factors to have a statistically significant association with decreased survival: (1) poor performance status, (2) high lactate dehydrogenase value, (3) age of 40 years or more, (4) increased number of total involved areas, and (5) hypercalcemia.[140] Environmental factors may also affect survival. Concurrent *Strongyloides* infection and hypereosinophilia in ATL has been associated with longer survival.[116] Genetic alterations are heterogeneous in ATL, and their impact on survival are not yet well understood. Deletions of the p15 and p16 gene may confer shorter survival.[42]

## Treatment

ATL is a highly malignant disease with a median survival measured in months in the subacute and acute forms.[90, 91] Because the smoldering and chronic ATL forms can persist for years with few symptoms, no chemotherapy is recommended for these. For acute ATL, there is no known specific treatment, and a variety of regimens have been used.

For patients with acute and lymphoma subtypes of ATL, treatment with standard chemotherapy regimens can produce varying initial response rates. Single-agent chemotherapy gives overall complete response rates of less than 10%.[104] Deoxycoformycin was used as a single agent in five Caribbean patients with ATL refractory to chemotherapy and produced one partial and two mixed responses lasting 2 to 4 weeks.[141] In one case, a partial response was obtained with the use of 2-chloro-2'-deoxyadenosine monthly for three cycles.[142] Other reports indicate variable degrees of efficacy.[143–146] Kojima and colleagues[147] published a case report of a 74-year-old woman with ATL in acute phase in whom a 16-month complete remission was achieved by daily oral low-dose etoposide.

Standard chemotherapy regimens designed for treatment of aggressive non-Hodgkin's lymphoma or acute lymphoblastic leukemia have been used with some success in a few

patients.[143–146, 148] In the largest study to date, a complete remission rate of 35.8% was reported from a multi-institutional study of CHOP (cyclophosphamide, hydroxydaunomycin, vincristine [Oncovin], prednisone) plus etoposide, ranimustine, and mitoxantrone with granulocyte colony–stimulating factor support in 81 patients with acute and lymphoma subtypes of ATL.[149] Complete, but transient, remissions have been observed in about 50% of patients given intensive combination chemotherapy regimens, such as ProMACE/CytaBOM (prednisone, methotrexate, doxorubicin [Adriamycin], cyclophosphamide, etoposide/cytarabine, bleomycin, vincristine, methotrexate) or M-BACOD (methotrexate, bleomycin, doxorubicin, cyclophosphamide, vincristine, dexamethasone).[3]

The role of bone marrow or stem cell transplantation in ATL is yet to be determined. Because bone marrow involvement is common in the acute and lymphoma subtypes of ATL, autologous transplantation is not a curative procedure. Autologous peripheral blood stem cell rescue may prove to be an effective option because CD34+ progenitor cells are reportedly not infected with HTLV-I.[150] Pawson and colleagues[151] reported two patients treated with BEAC (bleomycin, etoposide, doxorubicin, cyclophosphamide) conditioning followed by peripheral blood stem cell rescue. One patient was alive with smoldering disease at 18 months.

Many novel agents have been used to treat ATL. The unusual combination of zidovudine (AZT), an antiretroviral agent, and interferon alfa has been described in previously untreated and treated patients.[152–154] In a multi-institutional study by Gill and colleagues,[153] the overall and complete response rates were 58% and 26%. The median survival of patients achieving either a complete or partial response was 13 months. Of patients who responded to this combination, approximately 50% achieved a response within 30 days. Patients were treated with AZT 200 mg five times per day and interferon gamma 5 million units per day. If tolerated, the interferon gamma was increased to 10 million units daily. The superiority of interferon gamma and AZT to standard cytotoxic chemotherapy as well as the optimal dosing regimen remains to be determined. Other antiviral agents may also be effective in ATL. One case of a coincidental response to administration of foscarnet was noted in a patient treated for cytomegalovirus retinitis.[155]

Anti-Tac antibody is another novel therapeutic agent in development.[156–160] In contrast to normal resting cells, HTLV-I–infected T cells express large numbers of high-affinity IL-2 receptors in ATL.[156–163] Anti-Tac is a monoclonal antibody that binds to the IL-2 receptor, preventing its interaction with IL-2.[159, 160] In a preliminary study, Waldmann and colleagues[164] reported a measurable response in 7 of 19 patients. Durable remissions were not achieved in most of these patients, however. The addition of a radiolabeled conjugate to the anti-Tac antibody is under investigation. There has also been work in the development of anti–IL-2 receptor monoclonal antibody conjugated to liposomes containing cytotoxic drugs aimed at the malignant cells.[165] Other novel agents being tested include interferon beta, interferon gamma, a new topoisomerase II inhibitor, and MST-16.[166–170] Okamura and associates[171] reported successful treatment of the chronic form of ATL with the biologic response modifier ubenimex.

The difficulty in achieving clinical success in the treatment of ATL is severalfold. One explanation for the early relapse after standard chemotherapy is the expression of the multidrug resistance by the malignant cells. Overexpression of a membrane glycoprotein, P-glycoprotein, occurs in various multidrug-resistant cell lines. Kuwazuru and colleagues[172] showed P-glycoprotein expression in all samples of relapsed ATL. Additionally, there is evidence that HTLV-I Tax protein increases the expression of the *MDR-1* gene.[173]

Laboratory studies are hampered by the lack of an ATL animal model. Some ATL cells, but not in vitro HTLV-I–transformed T-cell lines, have been found to grow in severe combined immunodeficient mice, providing a potential model.[174] Achieving adequate enrollment into controlled clinical studies remains a challenge. With the exception of smoldering ATL and pre-ATL, this disease is uniformly fatal, and new therapeutic approaches are needed.

## Other Diseases Associated with Human T-Cell Lymphotropic Virus I

Several reports suggest that HTLV-I infection may be associated with other hematologic malignancies in addition to ATL.[175–181] These reports have described cases of T-cell non-Hodgkin's lymphoma, T-cell angiocentric lymphoma, prolymphocytic leukemia, Sézary's syndrome, large granular lymphocytic leukemia (T-gamma lymphoproliferative disease),[182] and B-cell chronic lymphocytic leukemia in some Caribbean patients that were associated, either serologically or molecularly, with HTLV-I. A causal role for HTLV-I in these diseases, however, remains speculative.

HTLV-I–associated myelopathy (HAM) is a chronic progressive demyelinating disease strongly associated with HTLV-I infection.[183–189] Tropical spastic paraparesis (TSP), first recognized as a clinical disorder by Montgomery and colleagues,[190] and HAM are now considered identical diseases. Patients characteristically present with symmetric, slowly progressive weakness of the lower extremities. They may also complain of dysesthesias and paresthesias. They may have spasticity of the extremities, hyperreflexia, exten-

sor plantar reflexes, urinary and fecal incontinence, and mild peripheral sensory loss.[191, 192] Antibodies to HTLV-I are found in the serum and cerebrospinal fluid.[193, 194] Cerebrospinal fluid protein is often elevated. Atypical T cells resembling ATL cells may also be seen in the blood and cerebrospinal fluid,[71, 193, 195, 196] but most patients do not have lymphocytosis or significant pleocytosis. In Japan, women are affected more often than men.[190] Magnetic resonance imaging of the brain may be normal or may show areas of increased intensity in the periventricular white matter, reminiscent of multiple sclerosis.[197] HAM/TSP can be distinguished clinically from multiple sclerosis on the basis of a paucity of extraocular movement abnormalities, the absence of a history of exacerbations and remissions, and the frequent accompaniment of peripheral nervous system involvement.[198] In contrast to ATL, HAM/TSP is seen after acquisition of HTLV-I infection by transfusion.[199] The incubation period appears to be considerably shorter, on the order of several months. Treatment of HAM/TSP with corticosteroids is reported to produce modest neurologic improvement in more than 50% of patients.[200–202] HAM/TSP is reported to respond favorably to danazol, an anabolic steroid with immunomodulatory qualities. Increased strength and improvement in bowel and bladder control have been reported.[203] In our experience, although incontinence and motor strength may improve, problems with severe spasticity persist with use of danazol. Patients who acquired HTLV-I infection through blood transfusions appear to respond better to corticosteroids than other patients.[201] Sheremata and colleagues[204] showed that high doses of AZT (2 g daily for 4 weeks followed by 1 g/day for 20 weeks) can be given safely to patients with HTLV-I–associated myelopathy. Seven of 10 ambulatory patients showed objective neurologic improvement while on therapy, and 4 of these regressed after treatment was withdrawn. Further investigations into the efficacy of antiretroviral therapy in HTLV-I–associated diseases are under way. The role of interferon beta, reported to be efficacious in multiple sclerosis, has not been investigated adequately in HAM/TSP. No specific treatment is known to be uniformly effective in this disease.

An arthritic disease known as HTLV-I–associated arthropathy has also been described, often in association with myelopathy.[205–207] The arthritis is characteristically inflammatory in nature, and atypical ATL-like cells can be found in the peripheral blood as well as in synovial fluid. HTLV-I provirus can be identified in peripheral blood cells and synovial cells.

HTLV-I has been associated with uveitis,[208, 209] polymyositis,[210–212] and a pediatric syndrome called *infectious dermatitis*.[213] As for HTLV-I–associated arthropathy, uveitis appears to be more prevalent in patients with HAM/TSP. A causal role for HTLV-I in each of these diseases remains to be shown.

## Prevention

The connection between HTLV-I and leukemia, myelopathy, and arthropathy has led to vigorous efforts in preventing transmission of the virus. Because both ATL and HAM are at best poorly treatable, the best strategy for dealing with

HTLV-I is to prevent infection. As described previously, the established routes of HTLV-I transmission include breast milk, blood, and sexual contacts. Large-scale screening of the blood supply is now standard practice in the United States and other developed countries and can largely prevent transfusion-related infection. Such screening identifies HTLV-I–infected carriers as well as some HTLV-II–infected carriers. Organized efforts to decrease HTLV-I transmission in Japan began in 1987 with the commencement of the ATL Prevention Program in Nagasaki.[214] Of 90% of gravid mothers enrolled and screened, the seroprevalence of HTLV-I was 4%. This group found that formula-fed children of supportive mothers had an HTLV-I seroprevalence of 3.6%, whereas children breast-fed for at least 12 months had a seroprevalence of 15.7%. Identification of female carriers and the recommendation to formula feed these infants would lead to a significant decline in HTLV-associated illnesses. Such a recommendation poses challenges for less developed countries, however, where breast milk remains the primary source of nutrition.[215] Passive immunization as prophylaxis against HTLV-I conversion is another area of investigation. Preliminary animal studies have found evidence for the use of hyperimmune globulin derived from healthy blood donors with high antibody titers to HTLV-I.[216] The prevention of HTLV transmission is feasible and the most effective approach in reducing the morbidity and mortality associated with HTLV infection.

## SUGGESTIONS FOR ADDITIONAL READING

Franchini G. Molecular mechanisms of human T-cell leukemia/lymphotropic virus type 1 infection. Blood 1995;86:3619–39.

Pawson R, Mufti GJ, Pagliuca A. Management of adult T-cell leukemia/lymphoma. Br J Haematol 1998;100:453–8.

Newman C, Rosenblatt D. Human T-cell lymphotropic viruses. In: McCance DJ, ed. Human tumor viruses. Washington, D.C.: ASM Press, 1998:331–57.

Gessain A, Gout O. Chronic myelopathy associated with human T-lymphotropic virus type I (HTLV-I). Ann Intern Med 1992;117:933–46. *This article provides a comprehensive review of the clinical, epidemiologic, immunologic, and virologic aspects of the chronic myelopathy associated with HTLV-I.*

Höllsberg P, Hafler DA. Pathogenesis of diseases induced by human lymphotropic virus type I infection. N Engl J Med 1993;328:1173–82.

Rosenblatt JD, Danon Y, Black AC. A decade with HTLV-I/HTLV-II: lessons in viral leukemogenesis. Leukemia 1992;6:18–23.

Rosenblatt JD. Human T-lymphotropic virus types I and II. West J Med 1993;158:379–84. *This article summarizes epidemiologic and clinical findings related to the presence of HTLV-I and HTLV-II in the Americas and explores how these viruses might be implicated in leukemogenesis and in the development of neurologic disease in humans.*

## REFERENCES

1. Blayney DW, Jaffe ES, Blattner WA, et al. The human T-cell leukemia/lymphoma virus associated with American T-cell leukemia/lymphoma. Blood 1983;62:401–15.
2. Blattner WA, Blayney DW, Robert-Guroff M, et al. Epidemiology of human T-cell leukemia/lymphoma virus. J Infect Dis 1983;147:406–16.
3. Bunn PA, Schechter GP, Jaffe E, et al. Clinical course of retrovirus-associated adult T-cell lymphoma in the United States. N Engl J Med 1983;309:257–64.
4. Takatsuki K, Uchiyama T, Sagawa K, Yodoi J. Adult T-cell leukemia: clinical and hematologic features of 16 cases. Blood 1977;50:481–92.
5. Poiesz BJ, Ruscetti FW, Gazdar AF, et al. Detection and isolation of type C retrovirus particles from fresh and cultured lymphocytes of a patient with cutaneous T-cell lymphoma. Proc Natl Acad Sci U S A 1980;77:7415–9.
6. Hinuma Y, Nagata K, Hanaoka M, et al. Adult T-cell leukemia: antigen in an ATL cell line and detection of antibodies to the antigen in human sera. Proc Natl Acad Sci U S A 1981;78:6476–80.
7. Broder S. Cutaneous T-cell lymphomas. Semin Oncol 1980;7:310–31.
8. Yoshida M, Seiki M, Yamaguchi K, Takatsuki K. Monoclonal integration of human T-cell leukemia provirus in all primary tumors of adult T-cell leukemia suggests causative role of human T-cell leukemia virus in the disease. Proc Natl Acad Sci U S A 1984;81:2534–7.
9. Seiki M, Eddy R, Shows TB, Yoshida M. Nonspecific integration of the HTLV provirus genome into adult T-cell leukemia cells. Nature 1984;309:640.
10. Cann AJ, Rosenblatt JD, Wachsman W, et al. Identification of the gene responsible for human T-cell leukemia virus transcriptional regulation. Nature 1985;318:571–4.
11. Kiyokawa T, Seiki M, Iwashita S, et al. P27×-III and p21×-III proteins encoded by the pX sequence of human T-cell leukemia virus type I. Proc Natl Acad Sci U S A 1985;82:8359–63.
12. Koralnik IJ, Fullen J, Franchini G. The p12I, p13II, and p30II proteins encoded by human T-cell leukemia/lymphotropic virus type I open reading frames I and II are localized in three different cellular compartments. Lancet 1993;2:240. letter.
13. Koralnik IJ, Gessain A, Klotman ME, et al. Protein isoforms encoded by the pX region of human T-cell leukemia/lymphotropic virus type I. Proc Natl Acad Sci U S A 1992;89:8813–7.
14. Slamon DJ, Press MF, Souza LM, et al. Studies of the putative transforming protein of the type I human T-cell leukemia virus. Science 1985;228:1427–30.
15. Seiki M, Inoue J, Takeda T, Yoshida M. Direct evidence that p40× of human T-cell leukemia virus type I is a trans-acting transcriptional activator. EMBO J 1986;5:561–5.
16. Wagner S, Green MR. HTLV-I tax protein stimulation of DNA binding of bZIP proteins by enhancing dimerization. Science 1993;262:395–9.
17. Giebler HA, Loring JE, van Orden K, et al. Anchoring of CREB binding protein to the human T-cell leukemia virus type I promoter: a molecular mechanism of Tax transactivation. Mol Cell Biol 1997;17:5156–64.
18. Lenzmeier BA, Giebler HA, Nyborg JK. Human T-cell virus type 1 Tax requires direct access to DNA for recruitment of CREB binding protein to the viral promoter. Mol Cell Biol 1998;18:721–31.
19. Sagata N, Yasunaga T, Ikawa Y. Two distinct polypeptides may be translated from a single spliced mRNA of the X genes of human T-cell leukemia and bovine leukemia viruses. FEBS Lett 1985;192:37–42.
20. Inoue J, Yoshida M, Seiki M. Transcriptional (p40×) and post-transcriptional (p27×-III) regulators are required for the expression and replication of human T-cell leukemia virus type genes. Proc Natl Acad Sci U S A 1987;84:3653–7.
21. Green PL, Xie YM, Chen IS. The rex proteins of human T-cell leukemia virus type II differ by serine phosphorylation. J Virol 1991;65:546–50.
22. Berneman ZN, Gartenhaus RB, Reitz MS Jr, et al. Expression of alternatively spliced human T-lymphotropic virus type I (HTLV-I) pX mRNA in infected T-cell lines and in primary uncultured cells from patients with adult T-cell leukemia/lymphoma and healthy carriers. Proc Natl Acad Sci U S A 1992;89:3005–9.
23. Koralnik IJ, Fullen J, Franchini G. The p12I p13II, and p30II proteins encoded by human T-cell leukemia/lymphotropic virus type I open reading frames I and II are localized in three different cellular compartments. J Virol 1993;67:2360–6.
24. Franchini G, Mulloy JC, Koralnik IJ. The human T-cell leukemia/lymphotropic virus type I p12I protein cooperates with the E5 oncoprotein and binds the 16-kilodalton subunit of the vacuolar H$^+$ATPase. J Virol 1993;67:7701–4.
25. Mulloy JC, Crownley RW, Fullen J, et al. The human T-cell leukemia/lymphotropic virus type I p12I protein binds the interleukin-2 receptor β and γ chains and affects their expression on the cell surface. J Virol 1996;70:599–605.
26. Greene WC, Leonard WJ, Depper JM, et al. The human interleukin-2 receptor: normal and abnormal expression in T cells and in leukemias induced by the human T-lymphotropic retroviruses. Ann Intern Med 1986;105:560–72.
27. Wisdon R, Verma IM. Transformation by Fos proteins requires a C-terminal transactivation domain. Mol Cell Biol 1993;13:7429–38.

28. Nimer S. Tax responsiveness of the GM-CSF promoter is mediated by the mitogen-inducible sequences other than kappa B. New Biol 1991;3:997–1004.

29. Brown DA, Nelson FB, Reinherz EL, Diamond DJ. The human interferon gamma gene contains an inducible promoter that can be transactivated by tax I and II. Eur J Immunol 1991;21:1879–85.

30. Watanabe T, Yamaguchi K, Takatsuki K, et al. Constitutive expression of parathyroid hormone-related protein gene in human T-cell leukemia virus type I (HTLV-I) carriers and adult T cell leukemia patients that can be trans-activated by HTLV-I tax gene. J Exp Med 1990;172:759–65.

31. Motokura T, Fukumoto S, Matsumoto T, et al. Parathyroid hormone-related protein in adult T-cell leukemia-lymphoma. Ann Intern Med 1989;111:484–8.

32. Ejima E, Rosenblatt JD, Massari M, et al. Cell-type-specific transactivation of the parathyroid hormone-related protein gene promoter by the human T-cell leukemia virus type I (HTLV-I) tax and HTLV-II tax proteins. Blood 1993;81:1017–24.

33. Yamaoka S, Tobe T, Hatanaka M. Tax protein of human T-cell leukemia virus type I is required for maintenance of the transformed phenotype. Oncogene 1992;7:433–7.

34. Nerenberg M, Heinrichs SH, Reynolds RK, et al. The tat gene of human T-lymphotropic virus type I induces mesenchymal tumors in mice. Science 1987;237:1324–9.

35. Grossman WJ, Kimata JT, Wong FH, et al. Development of leukemia in mice transgenic for the tax gene of human lymphotropic virus type I. Proc Natl Acad Sci U S A 1995;92:2057–61.

36. Grossman WJ, Ratner L. Cytokine expression and tumorigenicity of large granular lymphocytic leukemia cells from mice transgenic for the Tax gene of human T-cell leukemia virus type I. Blood 1997;90:783–94.

37. McGuire KL, Curtis VE, Larson EL, Haseltine WA. Influence of human T-cell leukemia virus type I tax and rex on interleukin-2 gene expression. J Virol 1993;67:1590–9.

38. Black AC, Ruland CT, Yip MT, et al. Human T-cell leukemia virus type II Rex binding and activity require an intact splice donor site and a specific RNA secondary structure. J Virol 1991;65:6645–53.

39. Duc Dodon M, Gazzolo L. Loss of interleukin-2 requirement for the generation of T colonies defines an early event of human T-lymphotropic virus type I infection. Blood 1987;69:12–7.

40. Sadamori N. Cytogenetic implication in adult T-cell leukemia: a hypothesis of leukemogenesis. Cancer Genet Cytogenet 1991;51:131–6.

41. Hatta Y, Hirama T, Miller CW, et al. Homozygous deletions of the p15 (MTS2) and p16 (CDKN2/MTS1) genes in adult T-cell leukemia. Blood 1995;85:2699–704.

42. Yamada Y, Hatta Y, Murata K, et al. Deletions of p15 and/or p16 genes as a poor-prognosis factor in adult T-cell leukemia. J Clin Oncol 1997;15:1778–85.

43. Sakashita A, Hattori T, Miller CW, et al. Mutations in the p53 gene in adult T-cell leukemia. Blood 1992;79:477–80.

44. Reid RL, Lindholm PF, Mireskandari A, et al. Stabilization of wild-type p53 in human T-lymphocytes transformed by HTLV-1. Oncogene 1993;8:2029–36.

45. Pise-Masison CA, Choi KS, Radonovich M, et al. Inhibition of the p53 transactivation function by the human T-cell lymphotropic virus type I tax protein. J Virol 1998;72:1165–70.

46. Pise-Masison CA, Radonovich M, Sakaguchi K, et al. Phosphorylation of p53: a novel pathway for p53 inactivation in human T-cell lymphotropic virus type transformed cells. J Virol 1998;72:6348–55.

47. Hatta Y, Yamada Y, Tomonaga M, et al. Microsatellite instability in adult T-cell leukemia. Br J Haematol 1998;101:341–4.

48. Gessain AF, Boeri E, Yanagihara R, et al. Complete nucleotide sequence of a highly divergent human T-cell leukemia (lymphotropic) virus type I (HTLV) variant from Melanesia: genetic and phylogenetic relationship to HTLV strains from other geographical regions. J Virol 1993;67:1015–23.

49. Gessain AF, Gallo RC, Franchini G. Low degree of human T-cell leukemia/lymphoma virus type I genetic drift in vivo as means of monitoring viral transmission and movement of ancient populations. J Virol 1992;66:2288–95.

50. Saksena NK, Sherman MP, Yanagihara R, et al. LTR sequence and phylogenetic analyses of a newly discovered variant of HTLV-1 isolated from the Hagahai of Papua New Guinea. Virology 1992;189:1–9.

51. Hinuma Y, Komoda H, Chosa T, et al. Antibodies to adult T-cell leukemia-virus associated antigen (ATLA) in sera from patients with ATL and controls in Japan: a nationwide sero-epidemiologic study. Int J Cancer 1982;29:631–5.

52. Blattner WA, Kalyanaraman VS, Robert-Guroff M, et al. The human type-c retrovirus, HTLV, in blacks, from the Caribbean region, and relationship to adult T-cell leukemia/lymphoma. Int J Cancer 1982;30:257–64.

53. Reeves WC, Saxinger C, Brenes MM, et al. Human T-cell lymphotropic virus type 1 (HTLV-1) seroepidemiology and risk factors in metropolitan Panama. Am J Epidemiol 1988;127:532–9.

54. Maloney EM, Ramirez H, Levin A, Blattner WA. A survey of human T-cell lymphotropic virus type 1 (HTLV-1) in Southwestern Colombia. Int J Cancer 1989;44:419–23.

55. Yanagihara R, Jenkins CL, Alexander SS, et al. Human T lymphotropic virus type I infection in Papua New Guinea: high prevalence among the Hagahai confirmed by Western analysis. J Infect Dis 1990;162:649–54.

56. Blattner WA, Nomura A, Clark JW, et al. Modes of transmission and evidence for viral latency from studies of human T-cell lymphotropic virus type 1 in Japanese migrant populations in Hawaii. Proc Natl Acad Sci U S A 1986;83:4895–8.

57. Dosik H, Denic S, Patel N, et al. Adult T-cell leukemia/lymphoma in Brooklyn. JAMA 1988;259:2255–7.

58. Catovsky D, Greaves MF, Rose M, et al. Adult T-cell lymphoma-leukemia in blacks from the West Indies in Southeastern Florida and among Caribbean immigrants to the Eastern seaboard. Lancet 1982;1:639–43.

59. Hino S, Katamine S, Miyamoto T, et al. Association between maternal antibodies to the external envelope glycoprotein, and vertical transmission of human T-lymphotropic virus type 1. J Clin Invest 1995;95:2920–5.

60. Lee HH, Swanson P, Rosenblatt JD, et al. Relative prevalence and risk factors of HTLV-I and HTLV-II infection in US blood donors. Lancet 1991;337:1435–9.

61. Williams AE, Fang CT, Slamon DJ, et al. Seroprevalence and epidemiological correlates of HTLV-1 infection in US blood donors. Science 1988;240:643–6.

62. Bartholomew C, Saxinger WC, Clark JW. Transmission of HTLV-1 and HIV among homosexual men in Trinidad. JAMA 1987;257:2604–8.

63. Yamamoto N, Matsumoto T, Koyanagi Y, et al. Unique cell lines harbouring both Epstein-Barr virus and adult T-cell leukaemia virus, established from leukaemia patients. Nature 1982;299:367–9.

64. Clapham P, Nagy K, Cheinsong-Popov R, et al. Productive infection and cell free transmission of human T-cell leukemia virus in a non-lymphoid cell line. Science 1983;222:1125–7.

65. Seto A, Isono T, Ogawa K. Infection of inbred rabbits with cell-free HTLV-1. Leuk Res 1991;15:105–10.

66. Yamamoto N, Chosa T, Koyanagi Y, et al. Binding of adult T-cell leukemia virus to various hematopoietic cells. Cancer Lett 1984;21:261–8.

67. Yamade I, Isono T, Ishiguro T, Yoshida Y. Comparative study of human and rabbit cell infection with cell-free HTLV-1. J Med Virol 1993;39:75–9.

68. Okochi K, Sato H, Hinuma Y. A retrospective study on transmission of adult T-cell leukemia virus by blood transfusion: seroconversion in recipients. Vox Sang 1984;46:245–53.

69. Hino S: Mother-to-child transmission of human T-cell leukemia virus type-1. Jpn J Cancer Res 1985;76:474–80.

70. Kinoshita K, Hino S, Amagaski T, et al. Demonstration of adult T-cell leukemia virus antigen in milk from three sero-positive mothers. Gann 1984;75:103–5.

71. Takahashi K, Takazeki T, Oki T, et al. Inhibitory effect of maternal antibody on mother-to-child transmission of human T-lymphotropic virus type I: the Mother-to-Child Study Group. Int J Cancer 1991;49:673–7.

72. Hino S, Sugiyama H, Doi H, et al. Breaking the cycle of HTLV-I transmission via carrier mothers' milk. Lancet 1987;2:158–9.

73. Wiktor SZ, Pate EJ, Murphy EL, et al. Mother to child transmission of human T-cell lymphotropic virus type I (HTLV-I) in Jamaica: association with antibodies to glycoprotein (gp46) epitopes. J Acquir Immune Defic Syndr 1993;6:1162–7.

74. Murphy EL, Figueroa JP, Gibbs WN, et al. Sexual transmission of human T-lymphotropic virus type-1. Ann Intern Med 1989;111:555–60.

75. Hirai K, Takemori K, Onodera R, et al. Possibility of transmission from wife with ATL to husband. Int J Hematol 1992;55:305–6.

76. Tajima K, Tominaga S, Suchi T, et al. Epidemiological analysis of the distribution of antibody to adult T-cell leukemia-virus-associated antigen: possible horizontal transmission of adult T-cell leukemia virus. Gann 1982;73:893–901.

77. Kaplan JE, Murphy EL, Khabbaz RF, et al. Male to female transmission of human T-cell lymphotropic virus types I and II: association with viral load. The Retrovirus Epidemiology Donor Study Group. J Acquir Immune Defic Syndr Hum Retrovirol 1996;12:193–201.

78. Nakano S, Ando Y, Ichijo M, et al. Search for possible routes of vertical and horizontal transmission of adult T-cell leukemia virus. Jpn J Cancer Res 1984;75:1044–5.

79. Osame M, Izumo S, Igata A, et al. Blood transfusion and HTLV-1 associated myelopathy. Lancet 1986;2:104–5.

80. Gout O, Baulac M, Gessain A, et al. Rapid development of myelopathy after HTLV-1 infection acquired by transfusion during cardiac transplantation. N Engl J Med 1990;322:383–8.

81. Kleinman S, Swanson P, Allain JP, Lee H. Transfusion transmission of human T-lymphotropic virus types I and II: serologic and polymerase chain reaction results in recipients identified through look-back investigations. Transfusion 1993;33:14–8.

82. Hjelle G, Scalf R, Swenson S. High frequency of human T-cell leukemia-lymphoma virus type II infection in New Mexico blood donors: determination by sequence specific oligonucleotide hybridization. Blood 1990;76:450–4.

83. Tajima K, Tominaga S. Epidemiology of adult T-cell leukemia/lymphoma in Japan. Curr Top Microbiol Immunol 1985;115:53–66.

84. Gotoh YI, Sugamura K, Hinuma Y. Healthy carriers of a human retrovirus, adult T-cell leukemia virus (ATLV): demonstration by clonal culture of ATLV-carrying T cells from peripheral blood. Proc Natl Acad Sci U S A 1982;79:4780–2.

85. Hinuma Y, Nagata K, Hanaoka M, et al. Adult T-cell leukemia: antigen in an ATL cell line and detection of antibodies to the antigen in human sera. Proc Natl Acad Sci U S A 1981;78:6476–80.

86. Tajima K. In: Blattner WA, ed. Human Retrovirology: HTLV. New York: Raven Press, 1990:267.

87. Tokudome S, Tokunaga O, Shimamoto Y, et al. Incidence of adult T-cell leukemia/lymphoma among human T-lymphotropic virus type I carriers in Saga, Japan. Cancer Res 1989;49:226–8.

88. Jaffe ES, Blatner WA, Blayney DW, et al. The pathologic spectrum of adult T-cell leukemia/lymphoma in the United States: human T-cell leukemia/lymphoma virus–associated lymphoid malignancies. Am J Surg Pathol 1984;8:263–75.

89. Yamaguchi K, Nishimura H, Kohrogi H, et al. A proposal for smoldering adult T-cell leukemia: a clinicopathologic study of five cases. Blood 1983;62:758–66.

90. Kawano F, Yamaguchi K, Nishimura H. Variation in the clinical courses of adult T-cell leukemia. Cancer 1985;55:851–6.

91. Shimoyama M. Diagnostic criteria and classification of clinical subtypes of adult T-cell leukemia-lymphoma: a report from the Lymphoma Study Group. Br J Haematol 1991;79:428–37.

92. Kinoshita K, Amagasaki T, Ikeda S, et al. Preleukemic state of adult T-cell leukemia: abnormal T lymphocytosis induced by human adult T-cell leukemia-lymphoma virus. Blood 1985;66:120–7.

93. Taguchi H, Miyoshi I. Three cases of pre-adult T-cell leukemia. Jpn J Clin Oncol 1983;13:209–14.

94. Ikeda S, Momita S, Amagasaki T, et al. Detection of preleukemic state of adult T-cell leukemia (pre-ATL) in HTLV-1 carriers. Cancer Detect Prev 1990;14:431–5.

95. Hisada M, Okayama A, Shioiri S, et al. Risk factors for adult T-cell leukemia among carriers of human T-lymphotropic virus type I. Blood 1998;92:3557–61.

96. Ikeda S, Momita S, Kinoshita K, et al. Clinical course of human T-cell lymphotropic virus type I carriers with molecularly detectable monoclonal proliferation of T-lymphocytes: defining a low- and high-risk population. Blood 1993;82:2017–24.

97. Blayney DW, Jaffe ES, Fisher RI, et al. The human T-cell leukemia/lymphoma virus, lymphoma, lytic bone lesions, and hypercalcemia. Ann Intern Med 1983;98:144–51.

98. Shimoyama M, Minato K, Tobinai K, et al. Atypical adult T-cell leukemia-lymphoma: diverse clinical manifestations of adult T-cell leukemia-lymphoma. Jpn J Clin Oncol 1983;13:165–87.

99. Yamaguchi K, Yoshioka R, Kiyokawa T, et al. Lymphoma type adult T-cell leukemia—a clinicopathologic study of HTLV-related T cell type malignant lymphoma. Hematol Oncol 1986;4:59–65.

100. Jarrett RF, Mitsuya H, Mann DL, et al. Configuration and expression of the T cell receptor beta chain gene in human T-lymphotropic virus I–infected cells. J Exp Med 1986;163:383–99.

101. Matsuoka M, Hagiya M, Hattori T, et al. Gene rearrangements of T cell receptor beta and gamma chains in HTLV-I infected primary neoplastic T cells. Leukaemia 1988;2:84.

102. Murata K, Yamada Y, Kamihira S, et al. Frequency of eosinophilia in adult T-cell leukemia/lymphoma. Cancer 1992;69:966.

103. Yamamoto S, Hattori T, Asou N, et al. Absolute neutrophilia in adult T cell leukemia. Jpn J Cancer Res 1986;77:858–61.

104. Yano A, Yasukawa M, Yanaisawa K. Adult T cell leukemia associated with eosinophilia: analysis of eosinophil-stimulating factors produced by leukemic cells. Acta Haematol 1992;88:207.

105. Tamura K, Yokota T, Mashita R, Tamura S. Pulmonary manifestations in adult T-cell leukemia at the time of diagnosis. Respiration 1993;60:115.

106. Broder S, Bunn PA Jr, Jaffe ES, et al. NIH conference: T-cell lymphoproliferative syndrome associated with human T-cell leukemia/lymphoma virus. Ann Intern Med 1984;100:543.

107. Cappell MS, Chow J. HTLV-I associated lymphoma involving the entire alimentary tract and presenting with an acquired immune deficiency. Am J Med 1987;82:649.

108. Levine PH, Cleghorn F, Manns A, et al. Adult T-cell leukemia/lymphoma: a working point score classification for epidemiological studies. Int J Cancer 1994;59:491–3.

109. O'Brien C, Lampert IA, Catovsky D. The histopathology of adult T-cell lymphoma in blacks from the Caribbean. Histopathology 1983;7:349.

110. Yamaguchi K, Seiki M, Yoshida M, et al. The detection of human T cell leukemia virus proviral DNA and its application for classification and diagnosis of T cell malignancy. Blood 1984;63:1235.

111. Davey FR, Hutchison RE. Pathology and immunology of adult T-cell leukemia/lymphoma. Curr Opin Oncol 1991;3:13–20.

112. Ohshima K, Suzumiaya J, Sato K, et al. Nodal T-cell lymphoma in an HTLV-1 DNA, histological classification and clinical evaluation. Br J Haematol 1998;101:703–11.

113. Plumelle Y, Pascaline N, Nguyen D, et al. Adult T-cell leukemia-lymphoma: a clinico-pathologic study of twenty-six patients from Martinique. Hematol Pathol 1993;7:251–62.

114. Newton RC, Limpuangthip P, Greenberg S, et al. *Strongyloides stercoralis* hyperinfection in a carrier of HTLV-I virus with evidence of selective immunosuppression. Am J Med 1992;92:202–8.

115. Nakada K, Yamaguchi K, Furugen S, et al. Monoclonal integration of HTLV-I proviral DNA in patients with *Strongyloides*. Int J Cancer 1987;40:145–8.

116. Plumelle Y, Gonin C, Edouard A, et al. Effect of *Strongyloides stercoralis* infection with eosinophilia on age at onset and prognosis of adult T-cell leukemia. Am J Clin Pathol 1997;107:81–7.

117. Patey O, Gessain A, Breuil J, et al. Seven years of recurrent severe strongyloidiasis in an HTLV-I-infected man who developed adult T-cell leukemia. AIDS 1992;6:575.

118. Kim SJ, Kehrl JH, Burton J, et al. Transactivation of the transforming growth factor beta 1 (TGF-beta 1) gene by human T lymphotropic virus type 1 tax: a potential mechanism for the increased production of TGF-beta 1 in adult T cell leukemia. J Exp Med 1990;172:121.

119. Tendler CL, Greenberg SJ, Burton JD, et al. Cytokine induction in HTLV-I associated myelopathy and adult T-cell leukemia: alternate molecular mechanisms underlying retroviral pathogenesis. J Cell Biochem 1991;46:302.

120. Shimotohno K, Takahashi Y, Shimizu N, et al. Complete nucleotide sequence of an infectious clone of human T-cell leukemia virus type II: an open reading frame for the protease gene. Proc Natl Acad Sci U S A 1985;82:3101–5.

121. Rosenblatt JD, Zack JA, Chen ISY, Lee H. Recent advances in the detection of human T-cell leukemia viruses type I and II infection. Nat Immun 1990;9:143–9.

122. Ueda N, Iwata K, Tokuoka H, et al. Adult T-cell leukemia with generalized cytomegalic inclusion disease and *Pneumocystis carinii* pneumonia. Acta Pathol Jpn 1979;29:221.

123. Yoshioka R, Yamaguchi K, Yoshinaga T, Takatsuki K. Pulmonary complications in patients with adult T-cell leukemia. Cancer 1985;55:2491.

124. Wong-Staal F, Hahn B, Manzari V, et al. A survey of human leukaemias for sequences of a human retrovirus. Nature 1983;302:626–8.

125. Hall WW, Liu CR, Schneewind O, et al. Deleted HTLV-I provirus in blood and cutaneous lesions of patients with mycosis fungoides. Science 1991;253:317.

126. Neely S. Adult T-cell leukemia-lymphoma. West J Med 1989;100:557.
127. Uchiyama T. Adult T-cell leukemia. Blood Rev 1988;2:232.
128. Shimamoto Y, Kikuchi M, Funai N, et al. Spontaneous regression in adult T-cell leukemia/lymphoma. Cancer 1993;72:735.
129. Schnitzer B, Lovett EJ 3d, Kahn LE. Adult T-cell leukaemia with spontaneous remission. Lancet 1983;2:1030. letter.
130. Kimura I, Tsubota T, Hayashi K, Ohnoshi T. Spontaneous complete remission in adult T-cell leukemia: a case report. Jpn J Clin Oncol 1983;13:231.
131. Kawano F, Tsuda H, Yamaguchi K, et al. Unusual clinical courses of adult T-cell leukemia in siblings. Cancer 1984;54:131.
132. Murakawa M, Shibuya T, Teshima T, et al. Spontaneous remission from acute exacerbation of chronic adult T-cell leukemia. Blut 1990;61:346.
133. Poppema S, Postma L, Briner M, de Jong B. Spontaneous regression of a small non-cleaved cell malignant lymphoma (non-Burkitt's lymphoblastic lymphoma): morphologic, immunohistological, and immunoglobulin gene analysis. Cancer 1988;62:791.
134. Drobyski WR, Qazi R. Spontaneous regression in non-Hodgkin's lymphoma: clinical and pathogenetic considerations. Am J Hematol 1989;31:138.
135. McClain KM, Warkentin P, Kay N. Spontaneous remission of Burkitt's lymphoma associated with herpes zoster infection. Am J Pediatr Hematol Oncol 1985;7:9.
136. Zeigler JL. Spontaneous remission in Burkitt's lymphoma. Natl Cancer Inst Monogr 1976;44:61–5.
137. Tsukasaki K, Ikeda S, Murata K, et al. Characteristics of chemotherapy-induced clinical remission in long survivors with aggressive adult T-cell leukemia/lymphoma. Leuk Res 1993;17:157.
138. Carbone PP, Kaplan HS, Musshoff K, et al. Report of the Committee on Hodgkin's Disease Staging Classification. Cancer Res 1971;31:1860.
139. Shimamoto Y, Suga K, Nishimura J, et al. Major prognostic factors of Japanese patients with lymphoma-type adult T-cell leukemia. Am J Hematol 1990;35:232.
140. Major prognostic factors of patients with adult T-cell leukemia-lymphoma: a cooperative study. Lymphoma Study Group (1984–1987). Leuk Res 1991;15:81.
141. Lofters WS, Campbell M, Gibbs WN, Cheson BD. 2′-Deoxycoformycin therapy in adult T-cell leukemia/lymphoma. Cancer 1987;60:2605.
142. Uike N, Choi I, Tokoro A, et al. Adult T-cell leukemia-lymphoma successfully treated with 2-chlorodeoxyadenosine. Intern Med 1998;37:411–3.
143. Shimoyama M, Daenen S, Rojer RA, et al. Successful chemotherapy with deoxycoformycin in adult T-cell lymphoma-leukaemia. J Clin Oncol 1988;6:1088.
144. Shimoyama M, Oyama A, Tajima K, et al. Differences in clinicopathological characteristics and major prognostic factors between B-lymphoma and peripheral T-lymphoma excluding adult T-cell leukemia/lymphoma. Leuk Lymphoma 1990;3:335.
145. Yamaguchi K, Kiyokawa T, Futami G, et al. Pathogenesis of adult T-cell leukemia from clinical pathologic features. In: Blattner WA, ed. Human retrovirology: HTLV. New York: Raven Press, 1990:163–70.
146. Daenen S, Rojer RA, Smit JW, et al. Successful chemotherapy with deoxycoformycin in adult T-cell lymphoma-leukaemia. Br J Haematol 1984;58:723.
147. Kojima H, Hori M, Shibuya A, et al. Successful treatment of a patient with adult T-cell leukemia by daily oral administration of low-dose etoposide: decrease in the amount of HTLV-I proviral DNA revealed by the polymerase chain reaction method. Cancer 1993;72:614.
148. Shimoyama M, Ota K, Kikuchi M, et al. Chemotherapeutic results and prognostic factors in patients with advanced non-Hodgkin's lymphoma treated with VEPA or VEPA-M. J Clin Oncol 1988;6:128.
149. Taguchi H, Kinoshita KI, Takatsuki K, et al. An intensive chemotherapy of adult T-cell leukemia/lymphoma: CHOP followed by etoposide, vindesine, ranimustine, and mitoxantrone with granulocyte colony-stimulating factor support. J Acquir Immune Defic Syndr Hum Retrovirol 1996;12:182–6.
150. Nagafuji K, Harada M, Teshima T, et al. Hematopoietic progenitor cells from patients with adult T-cell leukemia-lymphoma are not infected with human T-cell leukemia virus type 1. Blood 1993;82:2823–8.
151. Pawson R, Mufti GJ, Pagliuca A. Management of adult T-cell leukemia/lymphoma. Br J Haematol 1998;100:453–8.
152. Broniscer A, Ribeiro RC, Srinivas RV, et al. An adolescent with HTLV-I-associated adult T-cell leukemia treated with interferon-alfa and zidovudine. Leukemia 1996;10:1244–8.
153. Gill PS, Harrington W Jr, Kaplan MH, et al. Treatment of adult T-cell leukemia-lymphoma with a combination of interferon alfa and zidovudine. N Engl J Med 1995;332:1744–8.
154. Hermne O, Bouscary D, Gessain A, et al. Brief report: treatment of adult T-cell leukemia-lymphoma with zidovudine and interferon alfa. N Engl J Med 1995;332:1749–51.
155. Takimoto Y. Improvement of adult T-cell lymphoma/leukaemia by antiviral drugs incuding foscarnet. Br J Haematol 1998;102:872–7.
156. Waldmann TA. IL-2 receptor expression in the haematologic malignancies: a target for immunotherapy. Cancer Surv 1989;8:891.
157. Waldmann TA, Greene WC, Sarin PS, et al. Functional and phenotypic comparison of human T cell leukemia/lymphoma virus positive adult T cell leukemia with human T cell leukemia/lymphoma virus negative Sezary leukemia, and their distinction using anti-Tac monoclonal antibody identifying the human receptor for T cell growth factor. J Clin Invest 1982;73:1711.
158. Waldmann TA, Goldman CK, Bongiovanni KF, et al. Therapy of patients with human T-cell lymphotrophic virus I-induced adult T-cell leukemia with anti-Tac, a monoclonal antibody to the receptor for interleukin-2. Blood 1988;72:1805.
159. Waldmann TA, White JD, Goldman CK, et al. The interleukin-2 receptor: a target for monoclonal antibody treatment of human T-cell lymphotrophic virus I-induced adult T-cell leukemia. Blood 1993;82:1701.
160. Waldmann TA. The multichain interleukin 2 receptor: a target for immunotherapy in lymphoma, autoimmune disorders, and organ allografts (clinical reference). JAMA 1990;263:272.
161. Greene WC, Leonard WJ, Depper JM, et al. The human interleukin-2 receptor: normal and abnormal expression in T cells and in leukemias induced by the human T-lymphotropic retroviruses (clinical conference). Ann Intern Med 1986;105:560.
162. Uchiyama T, Hori T, Tsudo M. Interleukin-2 receptor (Tac antigen) expressed on adult T cell leukemia cells. J Clin Invest 1985;76:446.
163. Depper JM, Leonard WJ, Kronke M, et al. Augmented T cell growth factor receptor expression in HTLV-1-infected human leukemic T cells. J Immunol 1984;133:1691.
164. Waldmann T, White J, Carrasquillo JA, et al. Radioimmunotherapy of interleukin-2Ra-expressing adult T-cell leukemia with Yttrium-90-labeled anti-Tac. Blood 1995;86:4063–75.
165. Hege KM, Daleke DL, Waldmann TA, Matthay KK. Comparison of anti-Tac and anti-transferrin receptor conjugated liposomes for specific drug delivery to adult T-cell leukemia. Blood 1989;74:2043.
166. Matsushima M, Yoneyama A, Nakamura T, et al. A first case of complete remission of beta interferon sensitive adult T-cell leukemia. Eur J Haematol 1987;39:282.
167. Tamura K, Makino S, Araki Y, et al. Recombinant interferon beta and gamma in the treatment of adult T-cell leukemia. Cancer 1987;59:1059.
168. Tamura K, Makino S, Araki Y, et al. A case of CD4 + /CD8 − adult T-cell leukemia with good response to interferon-beta terminating as a CD4 + /CD8 + adult T-cell lymphoma. Leuk Res 1987;11:665.
169. Ichihashi T, Kiyoi H, Fukutani H, et al. Effective treatment of adult T cell leukemia/lymphoma with a novel oral antitumor agent, MST-16. Oncology 1992;49:333.
170. Ohno R, Masaoka T, Shirakawa S, et al. Treatment of adult T-cell leukemia/lymphoma with MST-16, a new oral antitumor drug and a derivative of bis(2,6-dioxopiperazine): the MST-16 Study Group. Cancer 1993;71:2217.
171. Okamura T, Shibuya T, Harada M, Niho Y. Successful treatment of chronic adult T-cell leukemia with ubenimex. Acta Haematol 1992;87:94.
172. Kuwazuru Y, Hanada S, Furukawa T, et al. Expression of P-glycoprotein in adult T-cell leukemia cells. Blood 1990;76:2065–71.
173. Chuang SE, Doong SI, Lin MT, Cheng AL. Tax of the human T-lymphotropic virus type transactivates promoter of the MDR-1 gene. Biochem Biophys Res Commun 1997;238:482–6.
174. Feuer G, Zack JA, Harrington WJ Jr, et al. Establishment of human T-cell leukemia virus type I T-cell lymphomas in severe combined immunodeficient mice. Blood 1993;82:722.
175. Gessain A, Jouannelle A, Escarmant P, et al. HTLV antibodies in patients with non-Hodgkin lymphomas in Martinique. Lancet 1984;1:1183. letter.

176. Gibbs WN, Lofters WS, Campbell M, et al. Non-Hodgkin lymphoma in Jamaica and its relation to adult T-cell leukemia-lymphoma [published erratum appears in Ann Intern Med 1987;106(6):917]. Ann Intern Med 1987;106:361.

177. Matsuzaki H, Asou N, Kawaguchi Y, et al. Human T-cell leukemia virus type 1 associated with small cell lung cancer. Cancer 1990;66:1763.

178. Saxinger WC, Wantzin GL, Thomsen K, et al. Occurrence of HTLV-I antibodies in Danish patients with cutaneous T-cell lymphoma. Scand J Haematol 1985;31:455.

179. Sohn CC, Blayney DW, Misset JL, et al. Leukopenic chronic T cell leukemia mimicking hairy cell leukemia: association with human retroviruses. Blood 1986;67:949.

180. Starkebaum G, Loughran TP Jr, Kalyanaraman VS, et al. Serum reactivity to human T-cell leukaemia/lymphoma virus type I proteins in patients with large granular lymphocytic leukaemia. Lancet 1984;1:596.

181. Yamada Y, Kamihira S, Amagasaki T, et al. Adult T cell leukemia with atypical surface phenotypes: clinical correlation. J Clin Oncol 1985;3:782.

182. Warzynski MJ, Rosen MH, Golightly MG, et al. An acute form of T gamma lymphoproliferative disease presenting with massive splenomegaly: importance of immunophenotyping for diagnosis. Clin Immunol Immunopathol 1993;67:100.

183. Cruickshank JK. A aeropathic syndrome of uncertain origin: a review of 100 cases. West Indian Med J 1956;5:147–58.

184. Gessain A, Barin F, Vernant JC, et al. Antibodies to human T-lymphotropic virus type-I in patients with tropical spastic paraparesis. Lancet 1985;2:407.

185. Rodgers-Johnson P, Gajdusek DC, Morgan OS, et al. HTLV-I and HTLV-III antibodies and tropical spastic paraparesis. Lancet 1985;2:1247. letter.

186. Bartholomew C, Cleghorn F, Charles W, et al. HTLV-I and tropical spastic paraparesis. Lancet 1986;2:99. letter.

187. Román G, Spencer PS, Schoenberg BS, et al. Tropical spastic paraparesis: HTLV-I antibodies in patients from the Seychelles. N Engl J Med 1987;316:51. letter.

188. Gessain A, Francis H, Sonan T, et al. HTLV-I and tropical spastic paraparesis in Africa. Lancet 1986;2:698. letter.

189. Newton M, Cruickshank JK, Miller D, et al. Antibody to human T-lymphotropic virus type 1 in West-Indian-born UK residents with spastic paraparesis. Lancet 1987;1:415.

190. Montgomery RD, Cruickshank JK, Robertson WB, McMenemey WH. Clinical and pathological observations on Jamaican neuropathy. Brain 1964;87:425.

191. Bhigjee AI, Wiley CA, Wachsman W, et al. HTLV-I-associated myelopathy: clinicopathologic correlation with localization of provirus to spinal cord. Neurology 1991;41:1990.

192. Shibasaki H, Endo C, Kuroda Y, et al. Clinical picture of HTLV-I associated myelopathy. J Neurol Sci 1988;87:15.

193. Cruickshank JK, Rudge P, Dalgleish AG, et al. Tropical spastic paraparesis and human T cell lymphotropic virus type 1 in the United Kingdom. Brain 1989;112:1057.

194. Bhagavati S, Ehrlich G, Kula RW, et al. Detection of human T-cell lymphoma/leukemia virus type I DNA and antigen in spinal fluid and blood of patients with chronic progressive myelopathy. N Engl J Med 1988;318:1141.

195. Dalgleish A, Richardson J, Matutes E, et al. HTLV-1 infection in tropical spastic paraparesis: lymphocyte culture and serologic response. AIDS Res Hum Retroviruses 1988;4:475.

196. Sarin PS, Rodgers-Johnson P, Sun DK, et al. Comparison of a human T-cell lymphotropic virus type I strain from cerebrospinal fluid of a Jamaican patient with tropical spastic paraparesis with a prototype human T-cell lymphotropic virus type I. Proc Natl Acad Sci U S A 1989;86:2021.

197. Rudge P, Ali A, Cruickshank JK. Multiple sclerosis, tropical spastic paraparesis and HTLV-1 infection in Afro-Caribbean patients in the United Kingdom. J Neurol Neurosurg Psychiatry 1991;54:689.

198. Ehrlich GD, Glaser JB, Bryz-Gornia V, et al. Multiple sclerosis, retroviruses, and PCR. The HTLVMS Working Group. Neurology 1991;41:335.

199. Saxton EH, Lee H, Swanson P, et al. Detection of human T-cell leukemia/lymphoma virus type I in a transfusion recipient with chronic myelopathy. Neurology 1989;39:841.

200. Osame M, Usuku K, Izumo S, et al. HTLV-I associated myelopathy, a new clinical entity. Lancet 1986;1:1031. letter.

201. Osame M, Matsumoto M, Usuku K, et al. Chronic progressive myelopathy associated with elevated antibodies to human T-lymphotropic virus type I and adult T-cell leukemia–like cells. Ann Neurol 1987;22:116.

202. Duncan J, Rudge P. Methylprednisolone therapy in tropical spastic paraparesis. J Neurol Neurosurg Psychiatry 1990;53:173. letter.

203. Harrington WJ, Sheremata WA, Snodgrass SR, et al. Tropical spastic paraparesis/HTLV-1-associated myelopathy (TSP/HAM): treatment with an anabolic steroid danazol. AIDS Res Hum Retroviruses 1991;7:1031.

204. Sheremata WA, Benedict D, Squilacote DC, et al. High-dose zidovudine induction in HTLV-I-associated myelopathy: safety and possible efficacy. Neurology 1993;43:2125.

205. Nishioka K, Maruyama I, Sato K, et al. Chronic inflammatory arthropathy associated with HTLV-I. Lancet 1989;1:441. letter.

206. Kitajima I, Yamamoto K, Sato K, et al. Detection of human T cell lymphotropic virus type I proviral DNA and its gene expression in synovial cells in chronic inflammatory arthropathy. J Clin Invest 1991;88:1315.

207. Ijichi S, Matsuda T, Maruyama I, et al. Arthritis in a human T lymphotropic virus type I (HTLV-I) carrier. Ann Rheum Dis 1990;49:718.

208. Merle H, Smadja D, Bera O, et al. [Uveo-papillitis associated with paraparesis caused by HTLV-1 virus]. Presse Med 1993;22:1179.

209. Mochizuki M, Watanabe T, Yamaguchi K, et al. HTLV-I uveitis: a distinct clinical entity caused by HTLV-I. Jpn J Cancer Res 1992;83:236.

210. Morgan OS, Rodgers-Johnson P, Mora C, Char G. HTLV-1 and polymyositis in Jamaica. Lancet 1989;2:1184.

211. Wiley CA, Nerenberg M, Cros D, Soto-Aguilar MC. HTLV-I polymyositis in a patient also infected with the human immunodeficiency virus. N Engl J Med 1989;320:992.

212. Mattos K, Queiroz C, Pecanha-Martins AC. Lymphocyte alveolitis in HAM/TSP patients: preliminary report. Arq Neuropsiquiatr 1993;51:134.

213. LaGrenade L, Hanchard B, Fletcher V, et al. Infective dermatitis of Jamaican children: a marker for HTLV-I infection. Lancet 1990;336:1345.

214. Hino S, Katamine S, Miyata H, et al. Primary prevention of HTLV-1 in Japan. Leukemia 1997;11:Suppl 3:57–65.

215. Tazeki T, Tajima K, Ito M, et al. Short-term breast-feeding may reduce the risk of vertical transmission of HTLV-1. Leukemia 1997;11:Suppl 3:60–2.

216. Murata N, Hakoda Emachida H, Ikezoe T, et al. Prevention of human T-cell lymphotropic virus type 1 infection in Japanese macaques by passive immunization. Leukemia 1996;10:1971–4.

# CHAPTER 97

# CHRONIC LYMPHOCYTIC LEUKEMIA

• DOROTHY J. PARK • H. PHILLIP KOEFFLER

Chronic lymphocytic leukemia (CLL) is a clonal lympho-proliferative disorder characterized by increased numbers of morphologically mature-appearing lymphocytes in the peripheral blood, bone marrow, spleen, and lymph nodes. The malignant cells in CLL are most often B cells, and despite their mature appearance, they are immunologically incompetent. CLL is the most commonly occurring leukemia in adults in Western countries but is rarely found in Asians. It occurs in persons older than 50 years of age (median age, 55 to 60 years) and is rare in persons younger than 30 years of age. Men outnumber women 2:1 to 3:1.

The cause of CLL is unknown. In contrast to many of the other leukemias, radiation exposure and chemicals do not appear to play a significant role in the development of this disease. A familial tendency has been suggested, but no consistent pattern of inheritance is observed to suggest a genetic predisposition.[1, 2] Evidence shows that leukemic cells from patients with adult T-cell leukemia have a unique human retrovirus, human T-cell lymphotropic virus type I (HTLV-I).[3] Epstein-Barr virus (EBV) infection may also be related to a rare form of natural killer (NK)–cell leukemia. Clonal integration of EBV DNA has been found in cells from NK large granular lymphocytic (LGL) leukemia patients but not in cells from patients with polyclonal expansion of LGL cells.[4, 5] No direct evidence exists, however, that a virus plays a role in classic CLL.

## Natural History, Diagnosis, and Staging

### CLINICAL FEATURES

In more than one fourth of patients with CLL, the disease is discovered as an incidental finding on peripheral blood examination. Because blood counts are done with increasing frequency as part of routine medical examinations, asymptomatic patients are identified at a younger age and earlier stage of the disease process. Some patients seek attention because of symptoms of anemia or enlarged lymph nodes. At diagnosis, the spleen is only moderately enlarged, and the liver is minimally enlarged in about 50% of individuals.

In normal adults, the absolute lymphocyte count does not exceed 4 × 10⁹/L. Persistent lymphocytosis greater than 10 × 10⁹/L is usually considered sufficient for diagnosis, but the definition of lymphocytosis in CLL varies from 5 × 10⁹/L to 15 × 10⁹/L.[6, 7] Most cells are small, mature-appearing lymphocytes, although occasional prolymphocytes can be seen. Cell surface marker analysis is clearly helpful in making a specific diagnosis of CLL and in differentiating CLL from other related disorders, such as prolymphocytic leukemia, hairy cell leukemia, and LGL leukemia.

The total peripheral blood white blood cell (WBC) count at diagnosis usually ranges from 15 × 10⁹/L to 200 × 10⁹/L, with 70 to 95% of these cells being lymphocytes. In contrast to chronic myelogenous leukemia, the WBC count does not correlate well with symptomatic disease. Lymphocyte counts greater than 100 × 10⁹/L are frequently tolerated without symptoms. The bone marrow shows infiltration with small, well-differentiated lymphocytes. The red blood cell (RBC) and platelet counts are generally slightly reduced at diagnosis.

Autoimmune complications of the hematopoietic system occur frequently in patients with CLL. Approximately 10 to 20% of patients with CLL develop Coombs' test–positive autoimmune hemolytic anemia.[8] The autoantibody is usually of the warm-reacting immunoglobulin G (IgG) class against RBCs. These patients have numerous spherocytes and polychromatophilic macrocytes on their blood smear, elevated reticulocyte counts, and erythroid hyperplasia in their bone marrow. Less frequently, CLL patients may develop immune thrombocytopenia,[9] pure RBC aplasia,[10] or neutropenia.[11]

Hypogammaglobulinemia is a common feature in patients with CLL. It becomes more severe as the disease advances and is present in 50 to 75% of patients with CLL. This condition appears to be due to an intrinsic defect in the malignant B lymphocyte.[12] These individuals may also have a decreased ability to activate the complement system.[13] Impaired immunity predisposes to frequent infections, especially to encapsulated organisms and gram-negative bacteria, which accounts for nearly 50% of the deaths of patients with CLL.[14, 15] Patients with CLL have impaired antibody and cell-mediated immunity to recall antigens.

As the disease advances, patients with CLL frequently develop constitutional symptoms, such as weakness, easy fatigue, night sweats, fever, and weight loss. A small proportion of patients may have a sudden change in clinical course and develop Richter's syndrome.[16] This clinicopathologic entity is characterized by sudden progression of systemic symptoms and rapid increase in the size of lymph nodes. A biopsy specimen of the lymph nodes shows diffuse large cell or immunoblastic lymphoma; it represents a clonal evolution of the original leukemia.[17, 18] Prolymphocytic transformation may occur in the terminal stages of CLL. Therapy for these transformations is frequently unsuccessful, and overall survival is extremely poor.

### MOLECULAR, CYTOGENETIC, AND IMMUNOPHENOTYPIC FEATURES

CLL is considered to be the result of an expanded clone of neoplastic lymphoid cells that is produced mainly by cell accumulation rather than cell proliferation.[19, 20] The expanded clone usually is blocked at a relatively uniform stage of differentiation, but the clone often contains some cells with different degrees of differentiation.[21]

In 95% of cases, the CLL cells express monoclonal immunoglobulins at low intensity on their cell surface, most commonly IgM, either with or without IgD.[21-23] Approximately 5% of CLL patients have an associated prominent monoclonal immunoglobulin (usually IgM) in the serum. The CLL cells possess a receptor for the Fc portion of IgG, and complement receptors are variably present.[24, 25] The B-CLL cells typically stain positively for a pan T-cell marker, CD5 and B-cell markers, CD19, CD20, or CD24. These cells may also express CD25, CD23, and CD11c, but their expression levels are heterogeneous.

Malignant transformation occurs as a result of cumulative genetic alterations. To date, no specific molecular alterations have been shown to cause CLL; however, specific, nonrandom chromosomal abnormalities (Table 97–1), such as trisomy 12, 13q−, and t(11;14), occur in CLL and are associated with a poor prognosis.[26] Trisomy 12 is the most frequent karyotypic abnormality in these patients and is associated with increased number of prolymphocytes, but the relevant genes on this chromosome are unknown.[27] t(11;14) (q13:q32) juxtaposes *bcl-1*, a putative oncogene, to the region of the immunoglobulin heavy chain enhancer sequences, leading to overexpression of the *bcl-1* gene.[28, 29] In contrast to classic CLL, lymphocytes in B-CLL with t(11;14) are CD5⁻, a combination that may indicate that this subgroup of CLL has a distinct pathogenetic background.[30] Studies of the clinical relevance of the translocation of *bcl-1* are under way. Inactivation of tumor-suppressor genes is associated with tumorigenicity.

The high frequency (30%) of deletions of chromosome 13 at 13q14 suggests that a tumor-suppressor gene at this locus may be involved in the multistep pathogenesis of CLL. The retinoblastoma (Rb) tumor-suppressor gene is located at 13q14. No abnormalities of its expression have been noted in CLL, but fluorescent in situ hybridization (FISH) suggests that one Rb allele is frequently deleted in CLL.[31, 32] Often a transformed cell with an abnormal tumor-suppressor gene has mutation of one allele and loss of the remaining normal allele. Data suggest that 13q14 may contain a new tumor-suppressor gene whose inactivation contributes to the pathogenesis of CLL.[33-35] The 13q12 locus encompassing *BRCA2* has also been found to be frequently lost.[36] Studies suggested that the *BRCA2* may not be the key gene involved because its expression appears to be intact.[37] An intense search for a new tumor-suppressor gene is under way. p53 mutations have been reported in a small percentage of B-CLL, usually

associated with transformation to a more aggressive disease, such as Richter's syndrome.[38, 39]

## DIFFERENTIAL DIAGNOSIS

The adult with CLL usually has prominent lymphocytosis on repeated blood cell counts over several monthly examinations. The morphology and cytochemistry of the leukemic lymphocytes are similar to those of normal cells. Occasionally, CLL is difficult to diagnose early in the course of the disease. Determination of the percentage of B and T lymphocytes in blood can be useful, and the expression of CD5 antigen on circulating lymphocytes is essential. The best confirmation of a monoclonal B-lymphoproliferative disorder is the demonstration of a single class of light chain immunoglobulin on circulating lymphocytes. Also, Southern blot analysis shows monoclonal rearrangement of the immunoglobulin heavy and light chain genes. This molecular analysis is often not readily available, however. These tests are important in patients with modest but persistent lymphocytosis. Other diseases can readily be excluded by clinical findings and morphologic cytochemical and immunologic studies (Table 97–2). The following sections include examples of some of these diseases.

**Reactive Lymphocytosis.** Infectious mononucleosis and other viral illnesses that occur in children and young adults can transiently elevate the lymphocyte count in the peripheral blood. The lymphocyte morphology is distinguished easily from that seen in CLL. Most of the lymphocytes are T cells; the B lymphocytes do not have monoclonal antibodies on their surfaces. Also, normal mature B lymphocytes do not express CD5 antigens on their surface. Hyposplenism has been occasionally associated with lymphocytosis in patients.[40] This is clearly a benign condition that should be distinguished from the early phases of CLL.

**Prolymphocytic Leukemia.** Prolymphocytic leukemia (PLL) is a variant of CLL that can be T-cell or B-cell type.[41] The natural course of PLL is usually more aggressive than that of CLL, and response to chemotherapy is poor. The absolute lymphocyte count tends to be high at diagnosis, usually greater than 100 to 200 × 10⁹/L. The spleen is often massive, and bone marrow infiltration is extensive; the lymph nodes are usually not greatly enlarged. The cells are larger than regular lymphocytes with prominent nucleoli and coarsely condensed chromatin and may resemble activated lymphocytes. Rarely, CLL may undergo transformation to PLL.[42, 43]

B-PLL cells are CD5⁻ and CD19⁺, CD20⁺, CD22⁺, and FMC7⁺, and surface immunoglobulin is strongly positive. The surface marker analysis of T-PLL is consistent with post-thymic T-cell phenotype; they are CD2⁺, CD3⁺, and CD4⁺, but CD8 expression may be negative.[44, 45] Aberrations of chromosomes are common; inversions and translocations of chromosome 14 with breakpoints at q11 and q32 are found in 76% of cases of T-PLL and rarely in other forms of T-cell malignancies.[46, 47] Trisomy 8 is also common in T-PLL.

**Leukemic Phase of Non-Hodgkin's Lymphoma.** Poorly differentiated lymphocytic lymphomas can have peripheral blood involvement.[48] These patients often have prominent lymphadenopathy. The cells are large, and the nuclei are

*Table 97–1.* **Common Chromosomal Abnormalities Associated with Chronic Lymphocytic Leukemia**

| Chromosome Change | Comments |
| --- | --- |
| Trisomy 12 | Most common abnormality in CLL |
| 13q deletions | Site of unknown tumor-suppressor genes |
| 11q23 translocations | *bcl-1* inactivation |
| 17p | p53 inactivation |

CLL, chronic lymphocytic leukemia.

*Table 97–2.* **Features of Selected Lymphoproliferative Conditions**

| Disease | Clinical Features | Lymphocyte Morphology | Immunologic Marker |
|---|---|---|---|
| CLL | Usually lymphadenopathy and splenomegaly | Small, mature with scanty cytoplasm (occasionally polymorphic in size with more abundant cytoplasm) | B cell<br>Weak surface immunoglobulin staining; single light chain types; weak complement receptors; CD5[+], CD19[+], CD20[+], CD23[+] |
| Leukemic phase/NHL | Prominent lymphadenopathy and splenomegaly | Large cells with notched nucleus | B cell<br>Strong surface immunoglobulin staining; strong complement receptors; CD10[+], CD19[+], CD20[+], CD21[+], FMC7[+], CD22[+] |
| Prolymphocytic leukemia | Massive splenomegaly, usually no lymphadenopathy | Large cells with large nuclei, prominent nucleoli | B cell<br>CD5[-], CD19[+], CD20[+], CD22[+], FMC7[+]; strong surface immunoglobulin staining<br>T cell<br>CD2[+], CD3[+], CD4[+], ± CD8 |
| Hairy cell leukemia | Prominent splenomegaly, usually no lymphadenopathy | Lymphocytoid cells with occasional hairy projections, tartrate-resistant acid phosphatase stain positive, pancytopenia | B cell<br>CD19[+], CD20[+], CD25[+], CD11c[+], B-ly7[+] |

CLL, chronic lymphocytic leukemia; NHL, non-Hodgkin's lymphoma.

typically notched. Monoclonal immunoglobulin is usually present on the cell surface; in contrast to CLL, the immunoglobulin staining is intense, frequently with spontaneous capping.[49]

**T-Lymphocytic Leukemias.** Patients with T-cell CLL have been described as having lymphocytes of CLL morphology but possessing T-lymphocyte cell markers.[50] A diverse group of diseases probably exists under the classification of T-CLL, and these cases may be classified into two main groups: (1) de novo leukemias, such as T-PLL and LGL leukemia, and (2) lymphomas with a leukemic blood picture representing various types of T-cell non-Hodgkin's lymphoma, including Sézary's syndrome and adult T-cell leukemia.

**Large Granular Lymphocyte Leukemias.** Rarely, T-cell leukemia may involve LGL cells with properties of either NK or suppressor T cells: NK-LGL leukemia is characterized by clonal proliferation of CD3[-] cells, and T-LGL is composed of CD3[+] leukemia cells (see review by Loughran[51]). NK-LGL leukemia has an acute clinical presentation with splenomegaly, in contrast to polyclonal CD3[-] lymphocytosis, which is a chronic disease. T-LGL is associated with chronic neutropenia and autoimmune features. The distinction between T-PLL and different forms of LGL leukemia is clinically important because T-PLL is an aggressive disease requiring active therapy, whereas T-LGL leukemia usually has a benign course.

**Adult T-Cell Leukemia.** Adult T-cell leukemia is most prevalent in Asia, especially the southwestern part of Japan, Okinawa, and Taiwan, and in the Caribbean basin and Central Africa.[52] In the acute form of the disease, the patient typically presents with leukemia, lymphadenopathy, hepatosplenomegaly, and skin lesions containing leukemic infiltration. The WBC count is elevated, with many malignant lymphocytes and eosinophils. Often the patient has hypercalcemia associated with bone lesions. The morphology of the abnormal lymphocytes is characterized by highly lobulated or cloverleaf nucleoli. The cells usually express the CD4

antigen, but functionally they often behave as suppressor cells. These cells carry integrated HTLV, and in vitro HTLV can transform normal T cells. Treatment of adult T-cell leukemia is generally ineffective. Patients with acute disease have a short survival.

Other forms of adult T-cell leukemia exist: a preleukemic state, smoldering adult T-cell leukemia, and chronic adult T-cell leukemia.[53] The preleukemic state is marked by a lymphocytosis, and the patients are seropositive for HTLV. Half of these patients lose their lymphocytosis and have no further problems; the remaining patients develop a smoldering, chronic, or acute phase of the disease. Patients with the smoldering phase have skin lesions and modest marrow involvement; patients with the chronic phase have a lymphocytosis. After months, these patients often develop the acute phase of disease.

**Hairy Cell Leukemia.** Hairy cell leukemia (leukemic reticuloendotheliosis) usually presents as splenomegaly and pancytopenia with atypical lymphocytoid cells in the peripheral blood and other organs.[54–56] These *hairy* cells frequently have wispy edges, moderately abundant cytoplasm, and homogeneous chromatin. These cells stain strongly for the tartrate-resistant isoenzyme-5 of acid phosphatase.[57, 58] The cells have B-lymphocyte cell markers, and studies have shown that they can produce immunoglobulin.[55, 56, 59] Experimentally the cellular features of hairy cell leukemia can be induced in CLL cells in vitro.[60] This feature suggests a close relationship between these entities.

## STAGING

In 1975, based on easily obtainable clinical and hematologic data, Rai and colleagues[61] proposed a staging system for CLL consisting of five stages (Rai 0 to IV) (Table 97–3). Rai stage 0 included patients with lymphocytosis in blood and bone marrow only, and Rai stage I included patients with lymphadenopathy. If splenomegaly or hepatomegaly

**Table 97–3.**  Clinical Staging of Chronic Lymphocytic Leukemia

| Staging System | Stage | Risk Groups | Criteria | Median Survival (yr) |
|---|---|---|---|---|
| Rai[61] | 0 | Low | Lymphocytosis in blood and bone marrow | >10 |
| | I | Intermediate | + Lymphadenopathy | 7 |
| | II | | + Hepatomegaly, splenomegaly, or both | |
| | III | High | + Anemia (hemoglobin <11 g/dL) | 1.5 |
| | IV | | + Thrombocytopenia (platelets <100 × $10^9$/L) | |
| Binet[62] | A | N/A | <3 lymph node groups* | >10 |
| | B | | ≥3 lymph node groups* | 6 |
| | C | | Anemia (hemoglobin <10 g/dL), thrombocytopenia (platelets <100 × $10^9$/L), or both | 2 |

*Lymph node groups include spleen, liver, and lymph nodes in the cervical, axillary, and inguinal area.

were present, these patients were staged to II. Non–immune-mediated anemia or thrombocytopenia were staged as III or IV. This system was later modified into three risk groups, low (Rai 0), intermediate (Rai I to II) and high (III to IV), because no real difference in survival was observed between stages I and II as well as between stages III and IV. Although other investigators have confirmed the value of this method of staging in predicting survival time, a limitation exists because the intermediate group is heterogeneous with respect to prognosis.

The other staging system that is widely used in clinical practice was developed by Binet and coworkers.[62] Data from more than 900 CLL patients were analyzed by the International Workshop, and a three-stage system (Binet A, B, and C) was recommended (see Table 97–3). Patients with anemia (hemoglobin, 10 g/dl) or thrombocytopenia (platelets, 100 × $10^9$/L), or both, have the poorest prognosis and compose group C. The prognosis of the remaining patients is correlated with the number of lymph node groups that are involved with leukemia. Clinical enlargement of the spleen, liver, and lymph nodes in the cervical, axillary, and inguinal regions represents five separate areas of possible involvement. Patients with involvement of fewer than three areas are placed in group A and have the best prognosis; patients with three or more involved areas constitute group B and have an intermediate prognosis.

Few other staging systems for CLL have been proposed, but their merits relative to the Rai and Binet staging systems are as yet undefined. The National Cancer Institute–sponsored Working Group (NCI-WG) recommended using the modified Rai staging system for future clinical trials,[63] and the International Workshop on Chronic Lymphocytic Leukemia (IWCLL) suggested that the Binet and Rai staging systems be integrated[7]; generally, this has proved difficult, and most investigators and physicians use one or the other system.[64]

## PROGNOSTIC FACTORS

The best predictor of survival in patients with CLL remains the clinical stage at the time of diagnosis. Numerous clinical and laboratory factors have been reported to correlate with prognosis (Table 97–4); however, few have been shown to be independent of clinical stage. Although series differ, in general, older age[14, 65] and male sex probably correlate with

a shorter survival. Once the patient with CLL develops a hemoglobin concentration of less than 10 g/dl or a platelet count of less than 100 × $10^9$/L, his or her survival is about 20 to 25 months. This poor prognosis does not hold, however, for patients with anemia as a result of autoimmune hemolysis[66] or thrombocytopenia as a result of hypersplenism.[67]

Lymphocyte size in CLL probably does not affect survival,[68] although earlier reports suggested a worse prognosis for patients with *large-cell CLL*.[69] One study suggested that CLL patients in whom more than 35% of the lymphocytes resemble benign atypical lymphocytes had longer survivals than those in whom most of the lymphocytes had the typical narrow rims of cytoplasm and coarsely clumped chromatin.[70] The patients with increased number of prolymphocytes in the peripheral blood tend to have a clinical course similar to the CLL variant, PLL. PLL may be refractory to conventional chemotherapy and is associated with poorer prognosis, with a median survival of 4 months.[71]

Other factors that predict clinical outcome more consistently include the pattern of bone marrow involvement, lymphocyte doubling time, and abnormal cytogenetics. Individuals with a diffuse pattern of bone marrow involvement compared with a nondiffuse (nodular, interstitial, or mixed) pattern have a worse prognosis. Although peripheral blood lymphocyte counts have not been shown consistently to reflect disease activity, a blood lymphocyte doubling time of less than 12 months has been shown to predict shorter survival.[72–74] Chromosomal abnormalities involving chromosomes 12, 13q, 11q, and 17p as well as complex and multiple chromosomal abnormalities have also been associated with poor prognosis. Other prognostic factors reported in the

**Table 97–4.**  Factors Associated with Poor Prognosis in Chronic Lymphocytic Leukemia

Older age
Male sex
Anemia (hemoglobin <10–11 g/dL)
Thrombocytopenia (platelets <100 × $10^9$/L)
Increased prolymphocytes
Lymphocyte doubling time ≤12 mo
Diffuse bone marrow involvement
Chromosomal abnormality
p53 mutation
High lactate dehydrogenase
Increased soluble CD23

literature include high lactate dehydrogenase, low CD23 expression, high surface immunoglobulin staining, and increased serum-soluble CD23 receptors.[75]

## Treatment

In contrast to acute leukemias, CLL is an indolent disease and does not require an immediate institution of chemotherapy in all individuals. It is not a curable illness with currently available therapy, and the decision to start therapy should be individualized. A subgroup of Binet stage A patients have *smoldering CLL*, which can be defined as a hemoglobin greater than 12 g/dl and a lymphocyte count less than 30 × 10⁹/L. Studies have shown that these patients have life expectancies similar to that of a sex-matched and age-matched control population and have a much lower risk of disease progression.[76, 77] Approximately 50% of these patients did not require any therapy. The French Cooperative Group on Chronic Lymphocytic Leukemia reported on long-term follow-up of two large clinical trials in which good-prognosis (Binet stage A) patients were randomized to receive either no therapy or chlorambucil with or without prednisone.[78] As suggested in the earlier report, no difference in overall survival was detected in this long-term follow-up. Treatment was effective, however, in controlling troublesome symptoms. Results of these studies indicate that outside of a clinical trial, patients with early disease can be observed without therapy until disease progression. The usual indications for therapy are as follows: (1) systemic constitutional symptoms (e.g., weight loss, night sweats, fever without the evidence of infection, severe fatigue, anorexia); (2) bulky lymphadenopathy or massive hepatosplenomegaly producing obstruction, discomfort, disfigurement, or organ dysfunction; (3) presence of either acquired autoimmune hemolytic anemia or thrombocytopenia; (4) evidence of progressive bone marrow failure with granulocytopenia, thrombocytopenia, or anemia; (5) rapid disease progression as measured by lymphocyte doubling time less than 12 months; and (6) recurrent infections. Rate of progression needs to be determined in each patient because of the highly heterogeneous nature of the disease.

The three standard forms of therapy are chemotherapy (usually an alkylating agent or purine analogues) (Table 97–5), adrenocorticosteroids, and radiation therapy. Splenectomy and leukapheresis are other less frequently used modalities. Because of wide variability in survival (1 to ≥20 years), assessment of the effects of the different forms of therapy is difficult. Chemotherapy with an alkylating agent, with or without an adrenocorticosteroid, constitutes the usual initial treatment for CLL patients. These patients should often be treated with allopurinol orally 300 mg/day and should be well hydrated before the initiation of therapy. Most patients should receive pneumococcal vaccine because of their depressed immune status. A randomized trial of intravenous immunoglobulin in patients with CLL and hypogammaglobulinemia showed that intravenous immunoglobulin can prevent infections in this patient group.[79] The long-term benefit of intravenous immunoglobulin is unclear, and administration of intravenous immunoglobulin for a long

**Table 97–5. Chemotherapeutic Regimens for Chronic Lymphocytic Leukemia**

Chlorambucil continuous dosing 0.1 mg/kg/day PO daily

Chlorambucil intermittent pulse dosing 0.4 mg/kg PO every 2 wk or 0.7 mg/kg PO every 3–4 wk

Fludarabine 25–30 mg/m² IV daily for 5 days repeated every 4 wk

Pentostatin 4 mg/m² IV every 2 wk

Cladribine 0.1 mg/kg/day by continuous IV infusion for 1 wk or 0.14 mg/kg/day IV over 2 hr for 5 days repeated every 4 wk

CHOP (modified): Cyclophosphamide 300 mg/m²/day PO at days 1–5; doxorubicin 25 mg/m² IV at day 1; vincristine 1.4 mg/m² (maximal dose, 2 mg) IV at day 1; prednisone 40 mg/m²/day PO at days 1–5 repeated every 3–4 wk

IV, intravenous.

duration is expensive and is not recommended as routine therapy.[80]

## CHEMOTHERAPY

**Alkylating Agents.** Chlorambucil is the alkylating agent most frequently used in CLL. Chlorambucil is administered orally and is rarely emetogenic. Commonly used dosing schedules include continuous daily dosing of 0.1 mg/kg/day or intermittent pulse dosing of 0.4 mg/kg every 2 weeks or 0.7 mg/kg every 3 to 4 weeks.[81, 82] Although no survival advantage has been shown with the different dosing schedules, pulse therapy is preferred; the advantages of this approach are ease in monitoring the WBC count and convenience to the patient.[81] Reversible myelosuppression is the dose-limiting toxicity; the neutrophil, platelet, and RBC counts are monitored closely to ensure that dangerous cytopenia does not result from the therapy. In general, therapy should be continued until maximal response or severe toxicity occurs. When the desired response is reached, institution of a low daily maintenance dose of chlorambucil does not appear to be better than discontinuation of therapy until early progression occurs. Even though the peripheral WBC count may be decreased readily with therapy, lymphocytosis in the blood and bone marrow, hypogammaglobulinemia, lymphadenopathy, and splenomegaly often persist.[14]

Few clinical trials have been performed comparing the efficacy of different alkylating agents in CLL. Chlorambucil has been shown to be better than busulfan,[65] and cyclophosphamide is probably as effective as chlorambucil. Cyclophosphamide may be effective when resistance develops to chlorambucil. Alkylating agents are powerful mutagens, and CLL patients receiving these agents have developed secondary acute myelogenous leukemia or myelodysplastic syndrome.[83]

**Adrenocorticosteroids.** Glucocorticosteroids should not be used routinely in CLL. They are not highly lympholytic in humans and have minimal activity as a single agent. Many serious side effects are associated with their use, including severe immune suppression causing marked increase in opportunistic infections. Glucocorticosteroid therapy has been frequently combined in the past with chlorambucil as an initial therapy. This combination regimen gave improved response rates, but subsequent studies have reported no significant difference in survival.[78]

Coombs' test–positive hemolytic anemia or immune thrombocytopenia constitutes a clear indication for glucocorticosteroid therapy. Patients usually respond favorably to this treatment, but they generally require continued therapy to maintain the response. Chemotherapy frequently is started with the corticosteroids. Patients who require high doses of steroid or do not respond to the drug should be considered for splenectomy.

A major cause of morbidity and mortality in CLL patients is infection. If steroids are administered for a long time, more frequent and severe infections tend to develop.[83] To lessen the infectious complications, the drug should be used only when necessary and should be given in intermittent schedules if possible.

**Combination Chemotherapies.** CVP (cyclophosphamide, vincristine, and prednisone) administered at 3- to 4-week intervals may be effective in patients who are refractory to daily alkylating agents.[84, 85] This combined chemotherapy is not more effective than conventional therapy as an initial treatment, however. Neither response rate nor survival of patients receiving CVP was superior to those receiving chlorambucil plus a steroid.[86] When used as a single agent, vincristine does not appear to be effective in CLL.[87] Early studies suggested using CVP with the addition of doxorubicin (25 mg/m²) every 3 weeks (modified CHOP [cyclophosphamide, hydroxydaunomycin, vincristine (Oncovin), prednisone]) was beneficial in stages III and IV of CLL.[88] Subsequent studies have not supported this approach, however.[89] Overall, no evidence exists that modified CHOP therapy prolongs survival.

**Purine Analogues.** Fludarabine is a fluorinated purine analogue and is phosphorylated by deoxycytidine kinase in vivo to 2-fluoro-ara-ATP, which inhibits DNA polymerase and ribonucleotide reductase. The recommended dose of fludarabine is 25 to 30 mg/m²/day intravenously for 5 days, repeated every 4 weeks until maximal response or toxicity. Usual number of cycles given is six. The dose-limiting toxicity is myelosuppression, and prolonged treatment with fludarabine may produce profound, irreversible cytopenias. Careful monitoring of blood counts is necessary. Rare occurrences of autoimmune hemolytic anemia have been reported after fludarabine therapy.[90] These patients should not be rechallenged with fludarabine because it can be fatal. Another common toxicity is severe immune suppression with prolonged CD4 lymphopenia and frequent opportunistic infections, such as *Pneumocystis* pneumonia, listeriosis, and herpes zoster. This complication can be exacerbated by concurrent use of steroids and should be avoided if possible. Tumor lysis syndrome is an uncommon complication occurring in less than 1% of CLL patients treated with fludarabine.[91] Prophylaxis against tumor lysis syndrome should be administered, however, because of significant morbidity and mortality.

Overall response rates with fludarabine treatment may be comparable to those with chlorambucil, but clinical studies have shown that fludarabine treatment can result in a complete response in significant number of untreated and previously treated CLL patients.[92, 93] In a series of 113 patients treated with fludarabine alone, the disease-free survival of those who were previously untreated was markedly improved by achieving a complete response compared with a partial response.[93] In this study, the prior responsiveness to alkylating agents in previously treated patients had a marked impact on the results. The response rate of those who were responsive to conventional alkylating therapy was 93%; the response rate of those who had become refractory to alkylating agents was 38%. After relapse, only patients who had been previously responsive to alkylating agents benefited from a second course of fludarabine; salvage therapy in the refractory group was unsuccessful. Despite its impressive response rate and prolonged progression-free survival with fludarabine therapy, when compared with chlorambucil (40 mg/m² every 4 weeks), patients who were treated with fludarabine had similar overall survival.

When fludarabine was used as a single agent or in combination with prednisone as an initial therapy in patients with CLL, the overall response rate was 78% (29% complete response, 32% partial response—nodular, and 17% partial response), and the median survival was 63 months.[94] The addition of prednisone did not affect the overall response rate. The complete response rate for fludarabine and prednisone was significantly less than for fludarabine alone (23% vs. 38%). Patients who received fludarabine and prednisone had a shorter survival compared with patients who received fludarabine as a single agent (54 months vs. 74 months; $p = 0.06$). At the time of relapse after receiving fludarabine, 67% of patients responded to a fludarabine-containing regimen again, whereas only 25% responded to another regimen.

2′-Deoxycoformycin (DCF, pentostatin) is a potent inhibitor of adenosine deaminase (ADA). ADA is an enzyme essential for purine nucleoside metabolism; when it is inhibited, cells die through apoptosis. Normal and malignant B lymphocytes have low levels of ADA activity, and low concentrations of DCF inhibit this enzyme markedly in the peripheral blood of patients with CLL.[95] Treatment of CLL patients with a relatively nontoxic, low-dose regimen (4 mg/m² intravenously every 1 to 2 weeks) resulted in complete or partial remission in 15 to 25% of patients, and an additional 20 to 30% experienced some clinical improvement. Patients who do not respond to fludarabine may respond to DCF, but the two agents should not be combined because of the increased risk of pulmonary toxicity.[96]

2-Chloro-2′-deoxyadenosine (CdA, cladribine) is a purine nucleoside analogue resistant to inactivation by ADA. Accumulation of CdA nucleotides in leukemic cells inhibits DNA polymerase and DNA repair, causing single-strand breaks, DNA fragmentation, and apoptosis. CdA is equally cytotoxic against resting and proliferating cells and has an effect on low-grade lymphoid malignancies.[97] CdA is administered 0.1 mg/kg/day by continuous intravenous infusion for a week or 0.14 mg/kg/day over 2 hours for 5 days. Median number of CdA administered is two courses. In a small series of 18 patients who had been treated previously with other chemotherapeutic agents, the total response rate to CdA was 67%. Thrombocytopenia was the dose-limiting toxicity and seemed to be cumulative and long lasting.[98]

## BONE MARROW TRANSPLANTATION

Allogeneic or autologous hematopoietic stem cell transplantation is used in an attempt to cure patients with CLL.

Allogeneic bone marrow transplant after conditioning with high-dose chemotherapy or total-body irradiation (TBI), or both, in a small number of relatively young patients has produced encouraging results.[99–103] Given the long natural history of this disease, follow-up times of these studies are extremely short, and durability of remissions remains to be determined. Also, few patients are young enough to receive an allogeneic bone marrow transplant. Allogeneic and autologous hematopoietic stem cell transplantation remain an investigational therapy and should be used only in the setting of clinical trials.

## RADIATION THERAPY

**Total-Body Irradiation.** TBI had been used in the treatment of CLL in the past.[104] Therapy with TBI generally consists of daily fractions of 0.05 to 0.1 Gy, three to five times weekly, with a total dose usually between 1 and 4 Gy. The course of therapy is interrupted by a rest period of a few weeks to several months to avoid serious cytopenias. Toxicity is modest, with anemia and thrombocytopenia developing in about 15% of patients.

Johnson[104, 105] reported on the efficacy of TBI. One third of his patients had complete resolution of symptoms and palpable disease, correction of anemia, near-normalization of the bone marrow, and some restitution of immunologic competence. The median survival of the group was 57 months from diagnosis to death, almost twice that of a much smaller control group of patients treated with daily chlorambucil or cyclophosphamide and local irradiation. The assignment of Johnson's patients to either treatment modality was not random, and the extent to which corticosteroids were used in the TBI group is unclear, so analysis of the data is difficult. TBI was inferior to treatment with intermittent chlorambucil and prednisone for remission induction in a small series of CLL patients reported by the Eastern Cooperative Oncology Group.[106] No data are available comparing TBI with new purine analogues. Although this form of therapy appears to be effective in selected patients, TBI is not recommended for general use because of toxicity.

**Local Irradiation.** Local radiotherapy should be considered when splenic or lymph node enlargement causes pain, symptoms of obstruction, or intolerable cosmetic disfigurement. Splenic irradiation usually relieves painful splenomegaly within 7 days and frequently has the added effect of transiently lowering the peripheral blood lymphocyte counts and increasing the platelet and RBC counts.[107] The enlarged lymph nodes and spleen are usually treated with 1 to 2.5 Gy, and diminution of tumor size lasts from several weeks to months. Splenic irradiation is usually given in 0.25- to 0.5-Gy fractions to prevent serious cytopenia with the risk of infection.

## SPLENECTOMY

Splenectomy may be of some value for patients with CLL if either the spleen is massively enlarged and symptomatic[108, 109] or hypersplenism has caused thrombocytopenia.[67, 110] Although peripheral blood lymphocyte counts do not change, the hemoglobin and platelet counts often increase after the spleen is removed. The operative mortality rate may be 4 to 10%, however, if the procedure is done late in the course of the disease.[108, 111] Splenectomy does not appear to change the natural history of the disease. CLL patients with autoimmune hemolytic anemia who are refractory to steroids or require high doses of the drug may respond to splenectomy. Splenectomy may be useful in treating pure RBC aplasia associated with CLL.[112]

## LEUKAPHERESIS

Continuous-flow blood cell separators provide a method of reducing the total lymphocyte mass because the circulating lymphocytes are in communication with all the other lymphocyte compartments.[113] When CLL becomes resistant to conventional therapy, repeated leukapheresis may allow some clearing of lymphocytes from the bone marrow and improve the platelet and RBC counts. This form of therapy offers only temporary improvement, however, so it is not generally recommended.

## BIOLOGIC THERAPY

Immunotherapy for this disease is only moderately successful. Treatment with interferon alfa has resulted in 15 to 67% partial responses in CLL patients. Hematologic responses have been documented in untreated early-stage patients and in patients pretreated with chlorambucil.[114, 115] Whether interferon alfa has beneficial effects on the survival of these patients is unknown. Chimeric antibody directed against CD20 (rituximab, IDEC-C2B8), which is expressed in most B-cell lymphoproliferative disorders, was used to treat low-grade non-Hodgkin's lymphoma. Overall response rate was 50% in relapsed low-grade non-Hodgkin's lymphoma.[116, 117] Rituximab is a promising new class of therapy for CLL, and further studies using this agent alone or in combination with other agents, such as fludarabine, is necessary.

Campath 1H is an antibody against CD52 that is expressed in most B and T lymphocytes as well as CLL cells. A trial in previously treated CLL patients reported a 42% response rate.[118] This study reported a high frequency of opportunistic infections, however, as a result of profound cellular immune suppression. Further studies are necessary to find ways to decrease toxicity. Monoclonal anti-idiotypic antibody therapy is a tumor-specific approach to treatment, but responses have been minimal.[113] Antibody therapy was also attempted with a monoclonal antibody (T101) that recognizes an antigen expressed on normal mature T lymphocytes as well as on malignant T and B lymphocytes, including CLL cells. No clinical responses were noted when this antibody was given alone or conjugated to a toxin, ricin.[119] The variable domain of immunoglobulin molecule directed against the interleukin-2 receptor has been fused to diphtheria toxin to produce recombinant immunotoxins that kill interleukin-2 receptor–bearing cells. In vitro, these immunotoxins are effective against CLL cells, but in vivo data are unavailable.[120] Also, levamisole, an immunomodulatory agent, did not improve the outcome of CLL patients.[121]

## SUMMARY OF TREATMENT

For early-stage CLL patients, treatment may not be necessary. The patient is instructed regarding possible adverse symptoms and is followed every 3 or 4 months. For regional symptomatic problems, local radiotherapy is the treatment of choice. For advanced-stage, symptomatic disease, intermittent or daily chlorambucil or fludarabine could be used as an initial therapy. Fludarabine is preferred if the goal of the therapy is to achieve a complete response, especially in a young patient in preparation for bone marrow transplant. Once maximal response is achieved, therapy should be discontinued, and the patient is followed clinically for any progression.

Fludarabine is the treatment of choice for second-line therapy in patients who have failed therapy with an alkylating agent. Fludarabine can be reused in patients who failed fludarabine as an initial therapy because more than two thirds of patients respond again. Drug combinations (e.g., CHOP) may be effective in the patient in whom resistance to therapy with a single alkylating agent develops. Alternatively, DCF and CdA may be used, but they should be used with caution because of the possibility of developing long-lasting cytopenias, especially after fludarabine therapy. Infections and autoimmune complications should be dealt with promptly and vigorously. The patient should receive pneumococcal vaccination. Above all, the physician should be guided by the fact that CLL is an incurable disease of relatively long duration in an older age group, and the therapeutic morbidity and mortality must be carefully balanced against the therapeutic benefit, and all patients should be encouraged to enter clinical trials.

## REFERENCES

1. Blattner WA, Strober W, Muchmore AV, et al. Familial chronic lymphocytic leukemia: immunologic and cellular characterization. Ann Intern Med 1976;84:554–7.
2. Schwartz RS, Andre-Schwartz J. Malignant lymphoproliferative diseases: interactions between immunological abnormalities and oncogenic viruses. Annu Rev Med 1968;19:269–82.
3. Poiesz BJ, Ruscetti FW, Mier JW, et al. T-cell lines established from human T-lymphocytic neoplasias by direct response to T-cell growth factor. Proc Natl Acad Sci U S A 1980;77:6815–9.
4. Kawa-Ha K, Ishihara S, Ninomiya T, et al. CD3-negative lymphoproliferative disease of granular lymphocytes containing Epstein-Barr viral DNA. J Clin Invest 1989;84:51–5.
5. Loughran TPJ, Zambello R, Ashley R, et al. Failure to detect Epstein-Barr virus DNA in peripheral blood mononuclear cells of most patients with large granular lymphocyte leukemia. Blood 1993;81:2723–7.
6. Bennett JM, Catovsky D, Daniel MT, et al. Proposals for the classification of chronic (mature) B and T lymphoid leukaemias. French-American-British (FAB) Cooperative Group. J Clin Pathol 1989;42:567–84.
7. Chronic lymphocytic leukemia: recommendations for diagnosis, staging, and response criteria. International Workshop on Chronic Lymphocytic Leukemia. Ann Intern Med 1989;110:236–8.
8. Pirofsky B. Immune haemolytic disease: the autoimmune haemolytic anaemias. Clin Haematol 1975;4:167–80.
9. Duhrsen U, Augener W, Zwingers T, Brittinger G. Spectrum and frequency of autoimmune derangements in lymphoproliferative disorders: analysis of 637 cases and comparison with myeloproliferative diseases. Br J Haematol 1987;67:235–9.
10. Abeloff MD, Waterbury L. Pure red blood cell aplasia and chronic lymphocytic leukemia. Arch Intern Med 1974;134:721–4.
11. Hamblin TJ, Oscier DG, Young BJ. Autoimmunity in chronic lymphocytic leukaemia. J Clin Pathol 1986;39:713–6.
12. Fernandez LA, MacSween JM, Langley GR. Immunoglobulin secretory function of B cells from untreated patients with chronic lymphocytic leukemia and hypogammaglobulinemia: role of T cells. Blood 1983;62:767–74.
13. Heath ME, Cheson BD. Defective complement activity in chronic lymphocytic leukemia. Am J Hematol 1985;19:63–73.
14. Boggs DR, Sofferman SA, Wintrobe MM, Cartwright GE. Factors influencing the duration of survival of patients with chronic lymphocytic leukemia. Am J Med 1966;40:243–54.
15. Hansen MM. Chronic lymphocytic leukaemia: clinical studies based on 189 cases followed for a long time. Scand J Haematol 1973;18:Suppl:3–286.
16. Richter MN. Generalized reticular cell sarcoma of lymph nodes associated with lymphatic leukemia. Am J Pathol 1928;4:285.
17. Nowell P, Finan J, Glover D, Guerry D. Cytogenetic evidence for the clonal nature of Richter's syndrome. Blood 1981;58:183–6.
18. Delsol G, Laurent G, Kuhlein E, et al. Richter's syndrome: evidence for the clonal origin of the two proliferations. Am J Clin Pathol 1981;76:308–15.
19. Dormer P, Theml H, Lau B. Chronic lymphocytic leukemia: a proliferative or accumulative disorder? Leuk Res 1983;7:1–10.
20. Reed JC. Molecular biology of chronic lymphocytic leukemia. Semin Oncol 1998;25:11–8.
21. Rubartelli A, Sitia R, Zicca A, et al. Differentiation of chronic lymphocytic leukemia cells: correlation between the synthesis and secretion of immunoglobulins and the ultrastructure of the malignant cells. Blood 1983;62:495–504.
22. Preud'homme JL, Seligmann M. Surface bound immunoglobulins as a cell marker in human lymphoproliferative diseases. Blood 1972;40:777–94.
23. Gordon J, Mellstedt H, Aman P, et al. Phenotypes in chronic B-lymphocytic leukemia probed by monoclonal antibodies and immunoglobulin secretion studies: identification of stages of maturation arrest and the relation to clinical findings. Blood 1983;62:910–7.
24. Pincus S, Bianco C, Nussenzweig V. Increased proportion of complement-receptor lymphocytes in the peripheral blood of patients with chronic lymphocytic leukemia. Blood 1972;40:303–10.
25. Ross GD, Polley MJ, Rabellino EM, Grey HM. Two different complement receptors on human lymphocytes: one specific for C3b and one specific for C3b inactivator-cleaved C3b. J Exp Med 1973;138:798–811.
26. Juliusson G. Immunologic and cytogenetic studies improve prognosis prediction in chronic B-lymphocytic leukemia: a multivariate analysis of 24 variables. Cancer 1986;58:688–93.
27. Escudier SM, Pereira-Leahy JM, Drach JW, et al. Fluorescent in situ hybridization and cytogenetic studies of trisomy 12 in chronic lymphocytic leukemia. Blood 1993;81:2702–7.
28. Withers DA, Harvey RC, Faust JB, et al. Characterization of a candidate bcl-1 gene. Mol Cell Biol 1991;11:4846–53.
29. Rimokh R, Berger F, Delsol G, et al. Rearrangement and overexpression of the BCL-1/PRAD-1 gene in intermediate lymphocytic lymphomas and in t(11q13)-bearing leukemias. Blood 1993;81:3063–7.
30. Raghoebier S, van Krieken JH, Kluin-Nelemans JC, et al. Oncogene rearrangements in chronic B-cell leukemia. Blood 1991;77:1560–4.
31. Stilgenbauer S, Dohner H, Bulgay-Morschel M, et al. High frequency of monoallelic retinoblastoma gene deletion in B-cell chronic lymphoid leukemia shown by interphase cytogenetics. Blood 1993;81:2118–24.
32. Ginsberg AM, Raffeld M, Cossman J. Inactivation of the retinoblastoma gene in human lymphoid neoplasms. Blood 1991;77:833–40.
33. Brown AG, Ross FM, Dunne EM, et al. Evidence for a new tumour suppressor locus (DBM) in human B-cell neoplasia telomeric to the retinoblastoma gene. Nat Genet 1993;3:67–72.
34. Kalachikov S, Migliazza A, Cayanis E, et al. Cloning and gene mapping of the chromosome 13q14 region deleted in chronic lymphocytic leukemia. Genomics 1997;42:369–77.
35. Bullrich F, Veronese ML, Kitada S, et al. Minimal region of loss at 13q14 in B-cell chronic lymphocytic leukemia. Blood 1996;88:3109–15.
36. Garcia-Marco JA, Caldas C, Price CM, et al. Frequent somatic deletion of the 13q12.3 locus encompassing BRCA2 in chronic lymphocytic leukemia. Blood 1996;88:1568–75.
37. Catovsky D. The search for genetic clues in chronic lymphocytic leukemia. Hematol Cell Ther 1997;39:Suppl 1:S5–11.
38. Fenaux P, Preudhomme C, Lai JL, et al. Mutations of the p53 gene

in B-cell chronic lymphocytic leukemia: a report on 39 cases with cytogenetic analysis. Leukemia 1992;6:246–50.

39. Newcomb EW, el Rouby S, Thomas A. A unique spectrum of p53 mutations in B-cell chronic lymphocytic leukemia distinct from that of other lymphoid malignancies. Mol Carcinog 1995;14:227–32.

40. Wilkinson LS, Tang A, Gjedsted A. Marked lymphocytosis suggesting chronic lymphocytic leukemia in three patients with hyposplenism. Am J Med 1983;75:1053–6.

41. Galton DA, Goldman JM, Wiltshaw E, et al. Prolymphocytic leukaemia. Br J Haematol 1974;27:7–23.

42. Ghani AM, Krause JR, Brody JP. Prolymphocytic transformation of chronic lymphocytic leukemia: a report of three cases and review of the literature. Cancer 1986;57:75–80.

43. Galton DA. Terminal transformation in B-cell chronic lymphocytic leukaemia. Bone Marrow Transplant 1989;4:Suppl 1:156–7.

44. Volk JR, Kjeldsberg CR, Eyre HJ, Marty J. T-cell prolymphocytic leukemia: clinical and immunologic characterization. Cancer 1983;52:2049–54.

45. Coiffier B, Haioun C, Ketterer N, et al. Rituximab (Anti-CD20 monoclonal antibody) for the treatment of patients with relapsing or refractory aggressive lymphoma: a multicenter phase II study. Blood 1998;92:1927–32.

46. Fujita K, Fukuhara S, Nasu K, et al. Recurrent chromosome abnormalities in adult T-cell lymphomas of peripheral T-cell origin. Int J Cancer 1986;37:517–24.

47. Sanger WG, Weisenburger DD, Armitage JO, Purtilo DT. Cytogenetic abnormalities in noncutaneous peripheral T-cell lymphoma. Cancer Genet Cytogenet 1986;23:53–9.

48. Jaffe ES, Shevach EM, Frank MM, et al. Nodular lymphoma—evidence for origin from follicular B lymphocytes. N Engl J Med 1974;290:813–9.

49. Aisenberg AC, Wilkes B. Lymphosarcoma cell leukemia: the contribution of cell surface study to diagnosis. Blood 1976;48:707–15.

50. Lille I, Desplaces A, Meeus L, et al. Thymus-derived proliferating lymphocytes in chronic lymphocytic leukaemia. Lancet 1973;2:263–4.

51. Loughran TPJ. Clonal diseases of large granular lymphocytes. Blood 1993;82:1–14.

52. Wachsman W, Golde DW, Chen IS. HTLV and human leukemia: perspectives 1986. Semin Hematol 1986;23:245–56.

53. Ratner L, Griffith RC, Marselle L, et al. A lymphoproliferative disorder caused by human T-lymphotropic virus type I: demonstration of a continuum between acute and chronic adult T-cell leukemia/lymphoma. Am J Med 1987;83:953–8.

54. Katayama I, Finkel HE. Leukemic reticuloendotheliosis: a clinicopathologic study with review of the literature. Am J Med 1974;57:115–26.

55. Catovsky D, Pettit JE, Galton DA, et al. Leukaemic reticuloendotheliosis ('Hairy' cell leukaemia): a distinct clinico-pathological entity. Br J Haematol 1974;26:9–27.

56. Golde DW, Stevens RH, Quan SG, Saxon A. Immunoglobulin synthesis in hairy cell leukaemia. Br J Haematol 1977;35:359–65.

57. Yam LT, Li CY, Lam KW. Tartrate-resistant acid phosphatase isoenzyme in the reticulum cells of leukemic reticuloendotheliosis. N Engl J Med 1971;284:357–60.

58. Katayama I, Li CY, Yam LT. Histochemical study of acid phosphatase isoenzyme in leukemic reticuloendotheliosis. Cancer 1972;29:157–64.

59. Golde DW, Saxon A, Stevens RH. Macroglobulinemia and hairy-cell leukemia. N Engl J Med 1977;296:92–3.

60. Ziegler-Heitbrock HW, Munker R, Dorken B, et al. Induction of features characteristic of hairy cell leukemia in chronic lymphocytic leukemia and prolymphocytic leukemia cells. Cancer Res 1986;46:2172–8.

61. Rai KR, Sawitsky A, Cronkite EP, et al. Clinical staging of chronic lymphocytic leukemia. Blood 1975;46:219–34.

62. Binet JL, Auquier A, Dighiero G, et al. A new prognostic classification of chronic lymphocytic leukemia derived from a multivariate survival analysis. Cancer 1981;48:198–206.

63. Cheson BD, Bennett JM, Rai KR, et al. Guidelines for clinical protocols for chronic lymphocytic leukemia: recommendations of the National Cancer Institute-sponsored working group. Am J Hematol 1988;29:152–63.

64. Foon KA, Gale RP. Staging and therapy of chronic lymphocytic leukemia. Semin Hematol 1987;24:264–74.

65. Phillips EA, Kempin S, Passe S, et al. Prognostic factors in chronic lymphocytic leukaemia and their implications for therapy. Clin Haematol 1977;6:203–22.

66. Geisler C, Hansen MM. Chronic lymphocytic leukaemia: a test of a proposed new clinical staging system. Scand J Haematol 1981;27:279–86.

67. Rubinstein DB, Longo DL. Peripheral destruction of platelets in chronic lymphocytic leukemia: recognition, prognosis and therapeutic implications. Am J Med 1981;71:729–32.

68. Knospe WH, Gregory SA, Trobaugh FEJ, et al. Chronic lymphocytic leukemia: correlation of clinical course and therapeutic response with in vitro testing and morphology of lymphocytes. Am J Hematol 1977;2:73–101.

69. Peterson LC, Bloomfield CD, Sundberg RD, et al. Morphology of chronic lymphocytic leukemia and its relationship to survival. Am J Med 1975;59:316–24.

70. Peterson LC, Bloomfield CD, Brunning RD. Relationship of clinical staging and lymphocyte morphology to survival in chronic lymphocytic leukemia. Br J Haematol 1980;44:563–7.

71. Brouet JC, Flandrin G, Seligmann M. Indications of the thymus-derived nature of the proliferating cells in six patients with Sezary's syndrome. N Engl J Med 1973;289:341–4.

72. Molica S. Prognostic value of biological variables in B-cell chronic lymphocytic leukemia: can we improve upon clinical parameters? Haematologica 1997;82:705–9.

73. Vallespi T, Montserrat E, Sanz MA. Chronic lymphocytic leukaemia: prognostic value of lymphocyte morphological subtypes: a multivariate survival analysis in 146 patients. Br J Haematol 1991;77:478–85.

74. Dhodapkar M, Tefferi A, Su J, Phyliky RL. Prognostic features and survival in young adults with early/intermediate chronic lymphocytic leukemia (B-CLL): a single institution study. Leukemia 1993; 7:1232–5.

75. Geisler CH, Larsen JK, Hansen NE, et al. Prognostic importance of flow cytometric immunophenotyping of 540 consecutive patients with B-cell chronic lymphocytic leukemia. Blood 1991;78:1795–1802.

76. Montserrat E, Vinolas N, Reverter JC, Rozman C. Natural history of chronic lymphocytic leukemia: on the progression and prognosis of early clinical stages. Nouv Rev Fr Hematol 1988;30:359–61.

77. Natural history of stage A chronic lymphocytic leukaemia untreated patients. French Cooperative Group on Chronic Lymphocytic Leukaemia. Br J Haematol 1990;76:45–57.

78. Dighiero G, Maloum K, Desablens B, et al. Chlorambucil in indolent chronic lymphocytic leukemia. French Cooperative Group on Chronic Lymphocytic Leukemia. N Engl J Med 1998;338:1506–14.

79. Intravenous immunoglobulin for the prevention of infection in chronic lymphocytic leukemia: a randomized, controlled clinical trial. Cooperative Group for the Study of Immunoglobulin in Chronic Lymphocytic Leukemia. N Engl J Med 1988;319:902–7.

80. Weeks JC, Tierney MR, Weinstein MC. Cost effectiveness of prophylactic intravenous immune globulin in chronic lymphocytic leukemia. N Engl J Med 1991;325:81–6.

81. Knospe WH, Loeb VJ, Huguley CMJ. Proceedings: bi-weekly chlorambucil treatment of chronic lymphocytic leukemia. Cancer 1974;33:555–62.

82. Sawitsky A, Rai KR, Glidewell O, Silver RT. Comparison of daily versus intermittent chlorambucil and prednisone therapy in the treatment of patients with chronic lymphocytic leukemia. Blood 1977;50:1049–59.

83. Stern N, Shemesh J, Ramot B. Chronic lymphatic leukemia terminating in acute myeloid leukemia: review of the literature. Cancer 1981;47:1849–51.

84. Desal DV, Ezdinli EZ, Stutzman L. Vincristine therapy of lymphomas and chronic lymphocytic leukemia. Cancer 1970;26:352–9.

85. Liepman M, Votaw ML. The treatment of chronic lymphocytic leukemia with COP chemotherapy. Cancer 1978;41:1664–9.

86. Montserrat E, Alcala A, Parody R, et al. Treatment of chronic lymphocytic leukemia in advanced stages: a randomized trial comparing chlorambucil plus prednisone versus cyclophosphamide, vincristine, and prednisone. Cancer 1985;56:2369–75.

87. Oken MM, Kaplan ME. Combination chemotherapy with cyclophosphamide, vincristine, and prednisone in the treatment of refractory chronic lymphocytic leukemia: effectiveness of "CHOP" regimen in advanced untreated chronic lymphocytic leukaemia. French Cooperative Group on Chronic Lymphocytic Leukaemia. Lancet 1986; 1:1346–9.

88. Therapy of chronic lymphocytic leukemia patients: results from the French cooperative trials. French Cooperative Group on Chronic Lymphocytic Leukemia. Nouv Rev Fr Hematol 1988;30:443–8.

89. Dighiero G. Chronic lymphocytic leukemia treatment. Hematol Cell Ther 1997;39:Suppl 1:S31–S40.

90. Weiss RB, Freiman J, Kweder SL, et al. Hemolytic anemia after fludarabine therapy for chronic lymphocytic leukemia. J Clin Oncol 1998;16:1885–9.

91. Cheson BD, Frame JN, Vena D, et al. Tumor lysis syndrome: an uncommon complication of fludarabine therapy of chronic lymphocytic leukemia. J Clin Oncol 1998;16:2313–20.

92. Robertson LE, Huh YO, Butler JJ, et al. Response assessment in chronic lymphocytic leukemia after fludarabine plus prednisone: clinical, pathologic, immunophenotypic, and molecular analysis. Blood 1992;80:29–36.

93. Keating MJ, O'Brien S, Kantarjian H, et al. Long-term follow-up of patients with chronic lymphocytic leukemia treated with fludarabine as a single agent. Blood 1993;81:2878–84.

94. Keating MJ, O'Brien S, Lerner S, et al. Long-term follow-up of patients with chronic lymphocytic leukemia (CLL) receiving fludarabine regimens as initial therapy. Blood 1998;92:1165–71.

95. Grever MR, Siaw MF, Jacob WF, et al. The biochemical and clinical consequences of 2'-deoxycoformycin in refractory lymphoproliferative malignancy. Blood 1981;57:406–17.

96. Juliusson G, Elmhorn-Rosenborg A, Liliemark J. Response to 2-chlorodeoxyadenosine in patients with B-cell chronic lymphocytic leukemia resistant to fludarabine. N Engl J Med 1992;327:1056–61.

97. Piro LD, Carrera CJ, Carson DA, Beutler E. Lasting remissions in hairy-cell leukemia induced by a single infusion of 2-chlorodeoxyadenosine. N Engl J Med 1990;322:1117–21.

98. Juliusson G, Liliemark J. High complete remission rate from 2-chloro-2'-deoxyadenosine in previously treated patients with B-cell chronic lymphocytic leukemia: response predicted by rapid decrease of blood lymphocyte count. J Clin Oncol 1993;11:679–89.

99. Rabinowe SN, Soiffer RJ, Gribben JG, et al. Autologous and allogeneic bone marrow transplantation for poor prognosis patients with B-cell chronic lymphocytic leukemia. Blood 1993;82:1366–76.

100. Khouri IF, Przepiorka D, van Besien K, et al. Allogeneic blood or marrow transplantation for chronic lymphocytic leukaemia: timing of transplantation and potential effect of fludarabine on acute graft-versus-host disease. Br J Haematol 1997;97:466–73.

101. Khouri IF, Keating MJ, Vriesendorp HM, et al. Autologous and allogeneic bone marrow transplantation for chronic lymphocytic leukemia: preliminary results. J Clin Oncol 1994;12:748–58.

102. Dreger P, von Neuhoff N, Kuse R, et al. Early stem cell transplantation for chronic lymphocytic leukaemia: a chance for cure? Br J Cancer 1998;77:2291–7.

103. Michallet M, Archimbaud E, Bandini G, et al. HLA-identical sibling bone marrow transplantation in younger patients with chronic lymphocytic leukemia. European Group for Blood and Marrow Transplantation and the International Bone Marrow Transplant Registry. Ann Intern Med 1996;124:311–5.

104. Johnson RE. Total body irradiation of chronic lymphocytic leukemia: incidence and duration of remission. Cancer 1970;25:523–30.

105. Johnson RE. Total body irradiation of chronic lymphocytic leukemia: relationship between therapeutic response and prognosis. Cancer 1976;37:2691–6.

106. Rubin P, Bennett JM, Begg C, et al. The comparison of total body irradiation vs chlorambucil and prednisone for remission induction of active chronic lymphocytic leukemia: an ECOG study: Part I. total body irradiation-response and toxicity. Int J Radiat Oncol Biol Phys 1981;7:1623–32.

107. Guiney MJ, Liew KH, Quong GG, Cooper IA. A study of splenic irradiation in chronic lymphocytic leukemia. Int J Radiat Oncol Biol Phys 1989;16:225–9.

108. Adler S, Stutzman L, Sokal J, Mittelman A. Splenectomy for hematologic depression in lymphocytic lymphoma and leukemia. Cancer 1975;35:521–8.

109. Christensen BE, Hansen MM, Videbaek A. Splenectomy in chronic lymphocytic leukaemia. Scand J Haematol 1977;18:279–87.

110. Merl SA, Theodorakis ME, Goldberg J, Gottlieb AJ. Splenectomy for thrombocytopenia in chronic lymphocytic leukemia. Am J Hematol 1983;15:253–9.

111. Neal TFJ, Tefferi A, Witzig TE, et al. Splenectomy in advanced chronic lymphocytic leukemia: a single institution experience with 50 patients. Am J Med 1992;93:435–40.

112. Radosevich CA, Gordon LI, Weil SC, et al. Complete resolution of pure red cell aplasia in a patient with chronic lymphocytic leukemia following antithymocyte globulin therapy. JAMA 1988;259:723–5.

113. Miller RA, Maloney DG, Warnke R, Levy R. Treatment of B-cell lymphoma with monoclonal anti-idiotype antibody. N Engl J Med 1982;306:517–22.

114. Ziegler-Heitbrock HW, Schlag R, Flieger D, Thiel E. Favorable response of early stage B CLL patients to treatment with IFN-alpha 2. Blood 1989;73:1426–30.

115. Montserrat E, Villamor N, Urbano-Ispizua A, et al. Treatment of early stage-B chronic lymphocytic leukemia with alpha-2b interferon after chlorambucil reduction of the tumoral mass. Ann Hematol 1991;63:15–9.

116. McLaughlin P, Grillo-Lopez AJ, Link BK, et al. Rituximab chimeric anti-CD20 monoclonal antibody therapy for relapsed indolent lymphoma: half of patients respond to a four-dose treatment program. J Clin Oncol 1998;16:2825–33.

117. Maloney DG, Liles TM, Czerwinski DK, et al. Phase I clinical trial using escalating single-dose infusion of chimeric anti-CD20 monoclonal antibody (IDEC-C2B8) in patients with recurrent B-cell lymphoma. Blood 1994;84:2457–66.

118. Osterborg A, Dyer MJ, Bunjes D, et al. Phase II multicenter study of human CD52 antibody in previously treated chronic lymphocytic leukemia. European Study Group of CAMPATH-1H Treatment in Chronic Lymphocytic Leukemia. J Clin Oncol 1997;15:1567–74.

119. Foon KA, Schroff RW, Bunn PA, et al. Effects of monoclonal antibody therapy in patients with chronic lymphocytic leukemia. Blood 1984;64:1085–93.

120. Kreitman RJ, Chaudhary VK, Kozak RW, et al. Recombinant toxins containing the variable domains of the anti-Tac monoclonal antibody to the interleukin-2 receptor kill malignant cells from patients with chronic lymphocytic leukemia. Blood 1992;80:2344–52.

121. Aymard JP, Janot C, Thibaut G, et al. Levamisole in chronic lymphocytic leukaemia: a prospective study of 15 patients. Acta Haematol 1984;71:316–21.

# CHAPTER 98

# HAIRY CELL LEUKEMIA

• LAWRENCE D. PIRO • DAVID W. GOLDE

Hairy cell leukemia (HCL) is now a well-defined and well-recognized lymphoid malignancy with a usual clinical picture of pancytopenia, splenomegaly, and characteristic abnormal mononuclear lymphoid cells. These hairy cells have a typical morphologic appearance with cytoplasmic projections, and they circulate in the blood and infiltrate the bone marrow. Approximately 600 new patients with HCL are diagnosed each year in the United States. The disease affects four times as many males as females, with Ashkenazi Jewish men being more frequently afflicted. The disease is predominantly found in middle-aged men, with a median age at presentation of 52 years.

Historically, HCL has been an interesting clinical disorder because of difficulties identifying the cell of origin, unique cellular morphologic features, and the uncertainty of its site of origin in the spleen or the marrow. It is now a well-characterized entity, known to be principally of B-cell lineage and bearing B-cell markers demonstrating the capability of immunoglobulin synthesis.[1-4] Although T-cell variants of HCL have been reported, it has been difficult to establish whether a T-cell form of disease really exists.[5, 6] Investigators described an association with human T-cell leukemia virus type II in two cases, but later showed that this virus was not directly related to the disease process.[5, 7] Patients with HCL, however, can suffer from severe T-cell dysfunction.[8] No distinctive cytogenetic abnormalities are seen in patients with HCL. Familial cases[9] and geographic clustering[10] have been described, but are rare. The cause of HCL remains unknown.

The history of treatments developed for HCL is perhaps the most fascinating aspect of this disease. The first consistently useful treatment was splenectomy, which had the curious property of having a salutary effect remotely on the bone marrow, often resulting in clinical stabilization. Traditional chemotherapy and radiation had little positive effect on the clinical course and were generally associated with considerable toxicity. Interferon (the first Food and Drug Administration (FDA)–approved biologic therapy) was approved for use in HCL, giving this disease another important place in medical history. Although a higher percentage of patients went into remission with interferon therapy than with splenectomy, complete remissions were unusual. Further studies led to dramatic clinical results with the newer purine analogues 2-chlorodeoxyadenosine (2-CdA, cladribine, Leustatin; Ortho Biotech) and deoxycoformycin (DCF, pentostatin, Nipent; Parke-Davis), which produce high rates of complete remission. In light of these newer therapies, HCL has emerged as a highly treatable disease, underscoring the importance of distinguishing it from other low-grade lymphoproliferative disorders.

## Natural History

### CLINICAL FEATURES

HCL is a lymphoaccumulative disorder, and patients with the disease may go for long periods without symptoms. Symptoms most commonly occur as a result of developing splenomegaly, anemia, neutropenia, or immune dysregulation resulting in infections and may dictate a need for therapy. Because of the routine use of standard blood counts in clinical screening, many patients are identified while still asymptomatic, with mild leukopenia, anemia, or thrombocytopenia detected on such routine examinations. Once an asymptomatic patient is identified, physical examination yields evidence of splenomegaly in more than 80%, usually without lymphadenopathy or hepatomegaly.[11]

In addition to presentations with leukopenia, anemia, and splenomegaly, more unusual presentations such as bulky lymphadenopathy, cutaneous vasculitis, and lytic bone lesions are occasionally seen. Patients with HCL are particularly vulnerable to opportunistic infections, especially atypical mycobacteria. Rarely, patients present with dual hematologic malignancies such as myeloma, and patients with HCL have a higher incidence of second malignancies.[11-16]

Laboratory evaluations typically reveal pancytopenia. Morphologically typical hairy cells are present in the blood in most cases but usually represent less than half of the white cells present.[11] Although most patients have some circulating hairy cells, some may present with splenomegaly and marrow infiltration and no detectable hairy cells in the peripheral blood. Bone marrow is typically difficult to aspirate, and biopsy generally shows infiltration with lymphocytes that have oval nuclei and abundant foamy cytoplasm with indistinct borders. The morphologic appearance of cells in the bone marrow is similar to a series of "fried eggs" adjacent to one another, resulting in the use of this descriptive term in characterizing bone marrow from patients with HCL.[17-20] Lymphocytes in the peripheral blood usually have the tartrate-resistant isoenzyme-5 of acid phosphatase, demonstrable by "TRAP" staining.[21, 22] The classic morphologic appearance of hairy cells in the peripheral blood, the fried egg appearance of hairy cells in the bone marrow, and TRAP positivity on peripheral blood lymphocytes all confirm the diagnosis of HCL.

A computed tomographic scan of the abdomen helps establish the presence or absence of splenomegaly. In some cases, splenectomy may be required for diagnostic purposes. A diffuse, red pulp pattern of splenic infiltration is seen with HCL.[23] In problematic cases, quantitation of soluble interleukin-2 (IL-2) receptor levels may be useful. The detection of high serum levels of soluble IL-2 receptors supports the diagnosis and may also be used to monitor therapy. Increased soluble IL-2 receptor levels have also been observed in patients with autoimmune diseases and certain B- and T-cell malignancies, limiting its diagnostic specificity.

Immunophenotypic analysis has been helpful in characterizing HCL. Hairy cells have a mature B-cell phenotype and typically express single or multiple immunoglobulin heavy chains with monotypic light chains.[24–29] They also express receptors for the Fc portion of IgG and IgM but do not express the complement receptor.[1, 30–33] Hairy cells form rosettes with mouse erythrocytes and express the pan B-cell antigens CD19, CD20, and CD22.[34] Hairy cells do not express CD21, an antigen lost in the later stages of B-cell ontogeny. Hairy cells also commonly express PCA-1, an early plasma cell antigen, perhaps reflective of its malignant origin arising late in lymphocyte ontogeny, similar to multiple myeloma. HCL has a characteristic pattern of staining, with a panel of multiple monoclonal antibodies by two-color flow cytometric analysis as applied to peripheral blood or bone marrow samples. This pattern is best visualized by a combination of the pan B-cell markers (CD19 and CD20) with CD11c, CD25, CD103, HC2 and B-ly7.[35, 36]

Immunohistochemical staining of bone marrow biopsy sections may also be supportive of the diagnosis of HCL. Hairy cells stain with L26, which accentuates the ruffled abundant cytoplasm of the hairy cells, and DBA.44, an undefined antigen that stains hairy cells in cytoplasmic, granular, and membranous patterns.

## DIFFERENTIAL DIAGNOSIS

The differential diagnosis of HCL includes an HCL variant as well as numerous other low-grade B-cell lymphoproliferative disorders such as chronic lymphocytic leukemia, splenic lymphoma with circulating villous lymphocytes, marginal zone lymphoma of the spleen, and monocytoid B-cell lymphoma. Hypoplastic HCL may be confused with aplastic anemia. Although all these entities can present with clinical pictures that may be confused with HCL, the mentioned diagnostic studies can be helpful in trying to differentiate these disorders. Such differentiation has become extremely important, given the high therapeutic success in treating HCL.

# Treatment

## INDICATIONS FOR TREATMENT

About 10% of patients may never require therapy, but most will. Standard hematologic indications have been developed for initiation of therapy for HCL. In general, treatment is initiated for significant anemia manifested as a hemoglobin level less than 8 to 10 g/dl; thrombocytopenia, seen as a platelet count less than 50 to 100 $\times$ 10$^9$/L; or severe neutropenia, seen as an absolute neutrophil count less than 0.05 to 1.0 $\times$ 10$^9$/L. Less common indications for the initiation of therapy have included leukocytosis with a high proportion of hairy cells, repeated infections, symptomatic splenomegaly, bulky or painful lymphadenopathy, vasculitis, and bony

involvement. In the proper clinical setting, an evaluation to exclude infection should be performed before initiating systemic therapy.

Given the progress in the treatment of HCL with interferon and purine analogues, much attention has been paid to the issue of early treatment. In view of the attendant risks of blood product administration, weighed against the capability of achieving durable complete remissions, it may be prudent to initiate therapy earlier than outlined by these criteria, especially in patients who have never been previously transfused with blood products. Since the results of long-term follow-up of patients after many of these therapies remain to be determined, one must still be cautious in deciding how aggressively to treat asymptomatic patients.

## SPLENECTOMY

Splenectomy was the first standard modality used to treat HCL, and it rapidly corrects peripheral cytopenias in most patients.[37, 38] Patients with clinical splenomegaly are more likely to respond to splenectomy than are those not found to have an enlarged spleen. Spleen size, however, is not always a good predictor of response to splenectomy.[38, 39] Patients with only patchy involvement of the marrow by HCL appear to respond more favorably to removal of the spleen, irrespective of splenic size. The lack of a consistent correlation between spleen weight and response to splenectomy may be explained by the prominent splenic red blood cell pooling that occurs in HCL, in excess of that in other lymphoproliferative disorders with comparable splenomegaly.[40] Given the current availability of effective systemic agents in the treatment of HCL and the fact that 50% of splenectomized patients require systemic therapy an average of 8.3 months after splenectomy,[41] this procedure is not commonly used as primary treatment today. In general, this treatment is reserved for patients with active infection or those in whom systemic therapies have failed.

## TREATMENTS OF HISTORICAL INTEREST

A number of chemotherapeutic treatments are of no or limited significant benefit, and their interest is largely historical.[42] The alkylating agents *triethylenemelamine, nitrogen mustard,* and *cyclophosphamide,* as well as *6-mercaptopurine, vincristine,* and *steroids* were all largely unsuccessful. Chronic, low-dose *chlorambucil* (4 mg/day orally for 6 months) induces a significant number of peripheral hematologic responses. The absolute neutrophil count, however, does not often increase to greater than 1000 cells/μL with chlorambucil, making this treatment of limited value. Radiation has been used on occasion for focal HCL infiltration in bone.

## INTERFERON

Alfa interferon administration was the first systemic therapy to show consistent efficacy in HCL, including the eradication of hairy cells from bone marrow. The first successful use of partially purified human alfa interferon was in 1984.[43]

Subsequently, recombinant alfa-2a (Roferon; Hoffmann-La Roche) and alfa-2b interferon (Intron A; Schering Corporation) have proved highly effective in inducing remission in patients with HCL. These results led the FDA to approve the use of alfa interferon for the treatment of HCL, representing the first approval of the use of a biologic agent to treat cancer. Recombinant alfa-2a interferon is similar to alfa-2b interferon with the exception of a cysteine residue for arginine in position 23. Studies with both recombinant forms of interferon in as many as 195 patients have shown a 70% partial and complete response achieved with 12 months of therapy at a dosage of 2 MU/m² three times weekly.[44] These results were confirmed in two large cooperative group studies in both previously untreated[45] and splenectomized[46] patients. Studies have indicated that 12 months of therapy is optimal and that more protracted treatment does not substantially improve response rates or diminish relapse rates; it does, however, increase toxicity.[47, 48] The median time to treatment failure after discontinuation of interferon therapy is 18 to 25 months, and reinstitution of interferon at relapse achieves a 77% overall response rate.[49] The presence of splenomegaly does not adversely affect response rates to interferon therapy.

The mechanism by which interferon induces remissions in HCL is poorly understood. Interferon stimulates natural killer cell activity, which is known to be suppressed in HCL; has a growth-inhibitory effect on lymphoma cell lines; and stimulates differentiation of leukemic cell lines.[50–52] How any of these effects relate to the therapeutic efficacy of interferon against HCL is not known. Specifically, it is not certain whether its therapeutic action is due to a direct antiproliferative effect or to an immunomodulatory mechanism.

The standard recommended dose for interferon is 2 MU/m² administered subcutaneously three times a week for 12 months. Although this is the recommended treatment plan, clearing of hairy cells from the bone marrow has been reported more often in patients using daily induction treatment than in those receiving a three-times-a-week schedule. Toxic effects of interferon therapy include a flu-like syndrome of fever, myalgia, and malaise, which occurs in most patients. Tachyphylaxis often develops, and acetaminophen can ameliorate symptoms in a majority of patients. Maculopapular rashes and gastrointestinal complaints occur in about 50% of patients. Central and peripheral nervous system complaints, hepatitis, alopecia, small joint arthritis, and decreased libido have been reported.

## GRANULOCYTE COLONY–STIMULATING FACTOR

Granulocyte colony–stimulating factor (G-CSF) abolishes the early myelosuppressive effects of interferon and reverses neutropenia in some HCL patients. The role of G-CSF in the management of HCL is to ameliorate neutropenia in infected neutropenic patients with HCL and to be adjunctive to effective systemic treatments during remission induction therapy. One patient with HCL was reported to develop acute neutrophilic dermatosis after G-CSF administration.[53] The adjunctive role of G-CSF to 2-CdA has been studied by evaluating the effect of G-CSF on 2-CdA–induced neutropenia when administered as priming for 2-CdA administration and following therapy with this agent.[54] When compared

with historical controls, there was no reduction in the percentage of febrile patients, number of febrile days, or frequency of admissions, although it did raise the absolute neutrophil count and shorten the duration of severe neutropenia after 2-CdA administration. Therefore the routine use of G-CSF with 2-CdA cannot be recommended, but its use may have application in certain patients with concomitant infection or prolonged neutropenia following treatment.

## PURINE ANALOGUES

After the observation that 30% of children with severe combined immunodeficiency syndrome were deficient in the purine catabolic enzyme adenosine deaminase,[55] pentostatin (DCF) and cladribine (2-CdA) were identified as useful agents for the treatment of a variety of lymphoid malignancies. In phase II testing, both drugs were shown to induce dramatic responses in patients with HCL.[56, 57] DCF is an irreversible inhibitor of adenosine deaminase, whereas 2-CdA is a purine substrate analogue resistant to the action of adenosine deaminase.

**Pentostatin.** Pentostatin (DCF) is a natural product isolated from the culture broth of *Streptomyces antibioticus.* In 1983, it was first shown to have activity in a single patient with HCL.[57] Successful administration of low-dose DCF at 5 mg/m² for 2 to 3 days, and then weekly for 15 to 16 doses, was reported in 1984.[58] Although DCF was introduced into clinical trials about the same time as was interferon, published trials and accrued numbers of patients are fewer. The Eastern Cooperative Oncology Group treated HCL patients with DCF administered at 5 mg/m² for 2 days every other week until complete remission was achieved.[59] Of 27 evaluable patients with HCL, 16 (59%) achieved complete remission and 10 (37%) achieved a partial response. Updates of these results with higher numbers of accrued patients demonstrate similar response rates.[60] Two large cooperative group studies in previously untreated[45] and splenectomized[46] patients also yielded similar results. Long-term follow-up studies estimate a relapse-free survival at 8 years of 76% ± 4%.[61]

The European Organization for Research and Treatment of Cancer conducted a study of DCF as salvage therapy for HCL patients resistant to or failing alfa interferon treatment.[62] Of 33 evaluable patients, 33% achieved complete remission and 45% attained partial remission, with a median duration of response of 12 months. Preliminary results have been published from the United States Cooperative Group study comparing interferon with DCF in previously untreated HCL patients.[63] Of 154 patients randomized to DCF, 76% entered complete remission and 3% had partial remission. Ten of the 117 patients who experienced complete remission relapsed at 13 to 44 months. Three patients died in complete remission. Of the 159 patients randomized to alfa interferon, 11% experienced complete remission and 26% partial remission. Twelve of the 17 patients who had complete responses relapsed between 9 and 27 months. Accordingly, this study showed a higher overall activity of DCF than of alfa interferon in inducing complete responses in HCL patients.

DCF therapy may be complicated by fever, nausea, vomiting, photosensitivity, and keratoconjunctivitis.[58, 64] Severe myelosuppression occurs soon after the initiation of DCF

*Table 98–1.* **Responses to Treatment with 2'-Deoxycoformycin (Pentostatin) in Patients with Hairy Cell Leukemia**

| Study | No. of Patients | Dose | Responses (%) | | |
|---|---|---|---|---|---|
| | | | COMPLETE | PARTIAL | NONE |
| Cassileth et al[60] | 50 | 5 mg/m² for 2 days every other week | 32 (64) | 10 (20) | 8 (16) |
| Kraut et al[85] | 23 | 4 mg/m² every other week | 20 (87) | 1 (4) | 2 (9) |
| Ho et al[86] | 33 | 4 mg/m²/wk × 3 wk, then every other week for 6 wk, then variable | 11 (33) | 15 (46) | 7 (21) |
| Johnston et al[87] | 28 | 4 mg/m²/wk × 3 wk, then variable | 25 (89) | 3 (11) | 0 (0) |
| Grever et al[63] | 150 | 4 mg/m² every other week | 103 (69) | 9 (6) | 38 (25) |
| Total | 284 | | 191 (67) | 38 (13) | 55 (19) |

therapy, especially in patients with pre-existing marrow compromise. Patients with better pretreatment hematologic parameters have less myelosuppression after DCF administration.[60, 64, 65] Serious infections, including disseminated herpes zoster and *Escherichia coli, Haemophilus influenzae,* and pneumococcal infections, have been documented after administration of DCF.[64] Therefore, it is generally recommended that DCF is best avoided in patients with active infection, poor performance status, or impaired renal function.[59]

DCF is potently immunosuppressive. During DCF therapy and for at least 14 months afterward, CD4 and CD8 lymphocytes may decrease to levels less than 200 cells/μL.[66, 67] Despite the severity of the immunosuppression, its significance in terms of late infections or secondary malignancies is not clear thus far. The recommended dose of DCF for patients with HCL is 4 mg/m² body surface area every other week for 3 to 6 months until maximal response is obtained (Table 98–1).

**Cladribine.** In 1990, data on the first 12 HCL patients with a single 7-day course of 2-CdA at 0.1 mg/kg/day by continuous infusion were reported by Piro and colleagues.[68] An overall response rate of 94% was achieved, with an 82% complete response rate and a 12% partial response rate. These data were confirmed by studies worldwide[70–74] (Table 98–2) and in the publication of the long-term follow-up of 349 patients treated at Scripps Clinic, which showed complete remission was achieved in 91% of patients.[69] Responses are independent of prior therapy. Twenty-four percent of complete responders relapsed at a median of 30 months. Patients who relapse can be retreated successfully with 2-CdA. Eighty-eight percent of 53 evaluable patients who

relapsed after complete remission responded to treatment with a 62% complete response rate and a 26% partial response rate.[69]

Fever has been the principal toxicity, occurring in 43% of patients treated. Its occurrence appears to be related to the disappearance of hairy cells and seems to be most marked in patients with the greatest pretreatment disease burden, manifested principally as splenomegaly. Documented infections, with the exception of catheter infections, are uncommon. Given the rarity of infection and the frequency of fever, it has been postulated that these febrile episodes are probably cytokine mediated in most cases rather than infectious in nature. Like DCF, 2-CdA is also immunosuppressive. Treatment with 2-CdA causes lymphopenia, and T-cell levels often fall to less than 200 cells/μL. Recovery appears to occur over the subsequent 12 to 24 months, although the suppression may be prolonged.[75–78] Relapse rates with 2-CdA have been low at approximately 4%. When the results of all studies that involve a single infusion of 2-CdA are combined, the overall response rate is 98% after a single infusion, with 81% complete remissions and 16% partial remissions. In these studies, 2-CdA was administered at 0.1 mg/kg/day by continuous intravenous infusion for a single 7-day cycle.

## MINIMAL RESIDUAL DISEASE

Following either DCF or 2-CdA treatment, immunohistochemical (IHC) techniques have been used to detect minimal residual disease (MRD) in both the bone marrow and peripheral blood of patients with complete response as defined by

*Table 98–2.* **Responses to Treatment with 2'-Chlorodeoxyadenosine (Cladribine) in Patients with Hairy Cell Leukemia**

| Study | No. of Patients | Dose | Responses (%)* | | |
|---|---|---|---|---|---|
| | | | COMPLETE | PARTIAL | NONE |
| Piro et al[68] | 144 | 0.1 mg/kg/day by CI × 7 days | 123 | 17 | 3 |
| Estey et al[71] | 46 | 4 mg/m²/day by CI × 7 days | 36 | 5 | 5 |
| Juliusson et al[74] | 73 | 0.1 mg/kg/day by CI × 7 days | 59 | 10 | 4 |
| Hoffman et al[73] | 49 | 0.1 mg/kg/day by CI × 7 days | 37 | 12 | 0 |
| Tallman et al[70] | 50 | 0.1 mg/kg/day by CI × 7 days | 40 | 9 | 1 |
| Lauria et al[72] | 40 | 0.1 mg/kg/day by CI × 7 days | 30 | 10 | 0 |
| Total | 402 | | 325 (81) | 63 (16) | 13 (3) |

*Responses according to peripheral blood and bone marrow criteria.
CI, continuous infusion.

routine morphologic (hematoxylin and eosin) examination.[79-81] Various combinations of antibodies against CD11c, CD25, CD103, HC2, CD45RO, CD20, and DBA.44 have been used in IHC techniques. Twenty-five to 50% of patients in complete remission may show evidence of MRD by IHC technique. IHC positivity in morphologic complete response may be associated with a higher incidence of morphologic relapse in long-term follow-up.[79] As such, the detection of MRD may be helpful in the early identification of patients at risk for relapse in whom additional therapy may be beneficial.

## SECOND MALIGNANCIES AFTER TREATMENT OF HAIRY CELL LEUKEMIA

The immunosuppressive nature of interferon and the purine analogues have raised concern about the potential for second malignancies developing in patients with HCL who receive such therapies. Patients with HCL are said to have an increased risk of such malignancies independent of therapy.[84] Treatment of HCL with purine analogues and interferon has been associated in some studies with an increased risk of second malignancy.[61, 69, 82, 83] Further follow-up and longer term observation will be required to confirm whether these treatments are truly associated with development of second neoplasms. As yet there is no clear consensus, and therefore achieving complete responses with the minimal drug exposure is still advised.

## TREATMENT CONSIDERATIONS

Specific treatment considerations for patients with HCL are currently in evolution. Splenectomy, the first standard treatment, is not commonly used because of the availability of systemic agents capable of inducing pathologic complete remissions. The three systemic agents, alfa interferon, DCF, and 2-CdA, all have substantial activity in the treatment of HCL. Although alfa interferon is associated with high overall response rates, complete remissions are uncommon, and therefore this agent when used alone is unlikely to have curative potential. Interferon still has a specific role in the treatment of HCL, but the exact order of therapy as it relates to the purine analogues remains to be determined. The relapse rate after 2CdA treatment at the Scripps Clinic was 26% after a median of 29 months.[69] After DCF treatment, 22% of 23 patients relapsed after a median of 59 months.[81] Complete remissions are inducible again in the majority of patients who relapse after purine analogue therapy. The response rate to interferon or splenectomy following relapse after either 2-CdA or DCF treatment is not well studied.[85-87] Although both DCF and 2-CdA commonly induce durable, complete responses, 2-CdA has largely been the treatment of choice because of its high complete response rate after only brief exposure to therapy and because of its favorable toxicity spectrum. Cross-resistance between 2-CdA and DCF is also not well studied, but responses to 2-CdA following DCF administration have been reported.[85] The optimal treatment after failure of primary therapy with a purine nucleoside is not well understood. In one study, three of nine patients receiving interferon after 2-CdA responded

and six of seven patients receiving dCF after 2-CdA responded.

In general, once a patient meets the indications for treatment, purine analogues are recommended as first-line therapy. Patients who fail therapy with purine analogues can undergo splenectomy or receive interferon therapy. Studies with a number of anti CD-20 B-cell monoclonal antibodies are under way, especially for patients who have failed after therapy with purine analogues.

Because HCL is an indolent disease, protracted follow-up is necessary to determine both relapse and true cure rates. Before the introduction of systemic therapy for this disease, the median survival for patients was only 53 months.[11] Interferon has had a favorable impact on the survival of patients with HCL, and the dramatic effects of the newer purine analogues seem likely to have substantially altered survival rates in this disease.

## SUGGESTIONS FOR ADDITIONAL READING

Saven A, Burian C, Koziol JA, Piro LD. Long-term follow-up of patients with hairy cell leukemia after cladribine treatment. Blood 1998;92:1918–26.
Saven A, Piro LD. Drug therapy: newer purine analogues for the treatment of hairy cell leukemia. N Engl J Med 1994;330:691–7.
Saven A, Piro LD: The treatment of hairy cell leukemia. Blood 1992;79:1111–20.

## REFERENCES

1. Jansen J, Schuit HR, Meijer CJ, et al. Cell markers in hairy cell leukemia studied in cells from 51 patients. Blood 1982;59:52–60.
2. Debusscher L, Bernheim JL, Collard-Ronge E, et al. Hairy cell leukemia: functional, immunologic, kinetic, and ultrastructural characterization. Blood 1975;46:495–507.
3. Golde DW, Stevens RH, Quan SG, et al. Immunoglobulin synthesis in hairy cell leukaemia. Br J Haematol 1977;35:359–65.
4. Cawley JC, Burns GF, Bevan A, et al. Typical hairy-cell leukaemia with IgGk paraproteinemia. Br J Haematol 1979;43:215–21.
5. Rosenblatt JD, Golde DW, Wachsman W, et al. A second isolate of HTLV-II associated with atypical hairy-cell leukemia. N Engl J Med 1986;315:372–7.
6. Saxon A, Stevens RH, Golde DW. T-lymphocyte variant of hairy-cell leukemia. Ann Intern Med 1978;88:323–6.
7. Chen IS, McLaughlin J, Gasson JC, et al. Molecular characterization of genome of a novel human T-cell leukaemia virus. Nature 1983;305:502–5.
8. Van De Corput L, Falkenburg JHF, Kluin-Nelemans JC. T-cell dysfunction in hairy cell leukemia: an updated review. Leuk Lymphoma 1998;30:31–9.
9. Makower D, Marino P, Frank M, Wiernik PH. Familial hairy cell leukemia. Leuk Lymphoma 1998;29:193–7.
10. Ruiz-Arguelles GJ, Cantu-Rodriguez OG, Gomez-Almaguer D, et al. Hairy cell leukemia is infrequent in Mexico and has a geographic distribution. Am J Hematol 1996;52:316–8.
11. Golomb HM, Catovsky D, Golde DW. Hairy cell leukemia: a clinical review based on 71 cases. Ann Intern Med 1978;89:677–83.
12. Quesada JR, Keating MJ, Libshitz HI, et al. Bone involvement in hairy cell leukemia. Am J Med 1983;74:228–31.
13. Elkon KB, Hughes GR, Catovsky D, et al. Hairy-cell leukaemia with polyarteritis nodosa. Lancet 1979;2:280–2.
14. Rudolph RI. Vasculitis associated with hairy cell leukemia. Arch Dermatol 1980;116:1077–8.
15. Pope A, Lazarchick J, Hoyer L, et al. Hairy cell leukemia and vasculitis. J Rheumatol 1980;7:895–9.
16. Westbrook CA, Golde DW. Autoimmune disease in hairy-cell leukaemia: clinical syndromes and treatment. Br J Haematol 1985;61:349–56.

17. Bartl R, Frisch B, Hill W, et al. Bone marrow histology in hairy cell leukemia: identification of subtypes and their prognostic significance. Am J Clin Pathol 1983;79:531–45.

18. Katayama I. Bone marrow in hairy cell leukemia. Hematol Oncol Clin North Am 1988;2:585–602.

19. Burke JS. The value of the bone-marrow biopsy in the diagnosis of hairy cell leukemia. Am J Clin Pathol 1978;70:876–84.

20. Naeim F, Jacobs AD. Bone marrow changes in patients with hairy cell leukemia treated by recombinant alpha 2-interferon. Hum Pathol 1985;16:1200–5.

21. Yam LT, Janckila AJ, Li CY, et al. Cytochemistry of tartrate-resistant acid phosphatase: 15 years' experience. Leukemia 1987;1:285–8.

22. Li CY, Yam LT, Lam KW. Studies of acid phosphatase isoenzymes in human leukocytes demonstration of isoenzyme cell specificity. J Histochem Cytochem 1970;18:901–10.

23. Arber DA, Rappaport H, Weiss LM. Non-Hodgkin's lymphoprolifera-tive disorders involving the spleen. Mod Pathol 1997;10:18–32.

24. Korsmeyer SJ, Greene WC, Cossman J, et al. Rearrangement and expression of immunoglobulin genes and expression of Tac antigen in hairy cell leukemia. Proc Natl Acad Sci USA 1983;80:4522–6.

25. Hsu SM, Yang K, Jaffe ES. Hairy cell leukemia: a B cell neoplasm with a unique antigenic phenotype. Am J Clin Pathol 1983;80:421–8.

26. Melo JV, San Miguel JF, Moss VE, et al. The membrane phenotype of hairy cell leukemia: a study with monoclonal antibodies. Semin Oncol 1984;11:381–5.

27. Anderson KC, Boyd AW, Fisher DC, et al. Hairy cell leukemia: a tumor of pre-plasma cells. Blood 1985;65:620–9.

28. Falini B, Pulford K, Erber WN, et al. Use of a panel of monoclonal antibodies for the diagnosis of hairy cell leukaemia. Histopathology 1986;10:671–87.

29. Falini B, Schwarting R, Erber W, et al. The differential diagnosis of hairy cell leukemia with a panel of monoclonal antibodies. Am J Clin Pathol 1985;83:289–300.

30. Fu SM, Winchester RJ, Rai KR, et al. Hairy cell leukemia: proliferation of a cell with phagocytic and B-lymphocyte properties. Scand J Immunol 1974;3:847–51.

31. Jaffe ES, Shevach EM, Frank MM, et al. Leukemic reticuloendothel-iosis: presence of a receptor for cytophilic antibody. Am J Med 1974;57:108–14.

32. Burns GF, Cawley JC, Worman CP, et al. The distribution of a receptor for IgM (muFcR) on haemic cells. Am J Hematol 1979;6:243–51.

33. Burns GF, Cawley JC, Barker CR, et al. Absence of a receptor for fixed C3 on the hairy cells of leukaemic reticuloendotheliosis. Clin Exp Immunol 1977;29:442–6.

34. Catovsky D, Cherchi M, Okos A, et al. Mouse red-cell rosettes in B-lymphoproliferative disorders. Br J Haematol 1976;33:173–7.

35. Robbins BA, Ellison DJ, Spinosa JC, et al. Diagnostic application of two-color flow cytometry in 161 cases of hairy cell leukemia. Blood 1993;82:1277–87.

36. Visser L, Shaw A, Slupsky J, et al. Monoclonal antibodies reactive with hairy cell leukemia. Blood 1989;74:320–5.

37. Mintz U, Golomb HM. Splenectomy as initial therapy in twenty-six patients with leukemic reticuloendotheliosis (hairy cell leukemia). Cancer Res 1979;39:2366–70.

38. Jansen J, Hermans J. Splenectomy in hairy cell leukemia: a retrospec-tive multicenter analysis. Cancer 1981;47:2066–76.

39. Golomb HM, Vardiman JW. Response to splenectomy in 65 patients with hairy cell leukemia: an evaluation of spleen weight and bone marrow involvement. Blood 1983;61:349–52.

40. Lewis SM, Catovsky D, Hows JM, et al. Splenic red cell pooling in hairy cell leukaemia. Br J Haematol 1977;35:351–7.

41. Golde DW. Therapy of hairy-cell leukemia. N Engl J Med 1982;307:495–6.

42. Huang AT. Hairy cell and chronic lymphocytic leukemia. New York: Elsevier Science, 1987:55–61.

43. Quesada JR, Reuben J, Manning JT, et al. Alpha interferon for induction of remission in hairy-cell leukemia. N Engl J Med 1984;310:15–18.

44. Golomb HM, Fefer A, Golde DW, et al. Report of a multi-institutional study of 193 patients with hairy cell leukemia treated with interferon-alfa2b. Semin Oncol 1988;15:Suppl 5:7–9.

45. Grever M, Kopecky K, Foucar MK, et al. Randomized comparison of pentostatin versus interferon alfa-2a in previously untreated patients with hairy cell leukemia: an intergroup study. J Clin Oncol 1995;13:974–82.

46. Rai KR. Comparison of pentostatin and alpha interferon in splenecto-

mized patients with active hairy cell leukemia: an intergroup study. Leuk Lymphoma 1994;14:Suppl 1:107–8.

47. Golomb HM, Ratain MJ, Fefer A, et al. Randomized study of the duration of treatment with interferon alfa-2B in patients with hairy cell leukemia. J Natl Cancer Inst 1988;80:369–73.

48. Berman E, Heller G, Kempin S, et al. Incidence of response and long-term follow-up in patients with hairy cell leukemia treated with recombinant interferon alfa-2a. Blood 1990;75:839–45.

49. Ratain MJ, Golomb HM, Vardiman JW, et al. Relapse after interferon alfa-2b therapy for hairy-cell leukemia: analysis of prognostic variables. J Clin Oncol 1988;6:1714–21.

50. Ruco LP, Procopio A, Maccallini V, et al. Severe deficiency of natural killer activity in the peripheral blood of patients with hairy cell leuke-mia. Blood 1983;61:1132–37.

51. Lee SH, Kelley S, Chiu H, et al. Stimulation of natural killer cell activity and inhibition of proliferation of various leukemic cells by purified human leukocyte interferon subtypes. Cancer Res 1982;42:1312–6.

52. Lieberman D, Voloch Z, Aviv H, et al. Effects of interferon on hemo-globin synthesis and leukemia virus production in Friend cells. Mol Biol Rep 1974;1:447–51.

53. Glaspy JA, Baldwin GC, Robertson PA, et al. Therapy for neutropenia in hairy cell leukemia with recombinant human granulocyte colony–stimulating factor. Ann Intern Med 1988;109:789–9.

54. Saven A, Burian C, Adusumalli J, et al. Filgrastim for cladribine-induced neutropenic fever in patients with hairy cell leukemia. Blood 1999;93:2471–7.

55. Giblett ER, Anderson JE, Cohen F, et al. Adenosine-deaminase defi-ciency in two patients with severely impaired cellular immunity. Lancet 1972;2:1067–9.

56. Piro LD, Carrera CJ, Carson DA, et al. Complete remission in hairy cell leukemia after treatment with 2-chlorodeoxyadenosene. Blood 1988;72:Suppl 1:220A.

57. Spiers ASD, Parekh SJ. Pentostatin (2'-deoxycoformycin, DCF) is active in hairy cell leukemia (HCL). Blood 1983;62:Suppl:208.

58. Spiers AS, Parekh SJ, Bishop MB. Hairy-cell leukemia: induction of complete remission with pentostatin (2'-deoxycoformycin). J Clin On-col 1984;2:1336–42.

59. Spiers AS, Moore D, Cassileth PA, et al. Remissions in hairy-cell leukemia with pentostatin (2'deoxycoformycin). N Engl J Med 1987;316:825–30.

60. Cassileth PA, Cheuvart B, Spiers AS, et al. Pentostatin induces durable remissions in hairy cell leukemia. J Clin Oncol 1991;9:243–6.

61. Flinn IW, Kopecky KJ, Foucar MK, et al. Long-term results in hairy cell leukemia (HCL) treated with pentostatin. Blood 1997;90:Suppl 1:578a.

62. Ho AD, Thaler J, Stryckmans P, et al. Pentostatin in resistant chronic lymphocytic leukemia—a phase II trial of the European Organization for Research and Treatment of Cancer. Proc ASCO 1990;9:206.

63. Grever M, Kopecky K, Foucar MK, et al. Randomized comparison of pentostatin versus interferon alfa-2a in previously untreated patients with hairy cell leukemia: an intergroup study. J Clin Oncol 1995;13:974–82.

64. Johnston JB, Glazer RI, Pugh L, Israels LG. The treatment of hairy-cell leukaemia with 2'-deoxycoformycin. Br J Haematol 1986;63:525–34.

65. Ho AD, Thaler J, Stryckmans P, et al. Pentostatin in refractory chronic lymphocytic leukemia: a phase II trial of the European Organization for Research and Treatment of Cancer. J Natl Cancer Inst 1990;82:1416–20.

66. Kraut EH, Neff JC, Bouroncle BA, et al. Immunosuppressive effects of pentostatin. J Clin Oncol 1990;8:848–55.

67. Urba WJ, Baseler MW, Kopp WC, et al. Deoxycoformycin-induced immunosuppression in patients with hairy cell leukemia. Blood 1989;73:38–46.

68. Piro LD, Carrera CJ, Carson DA, Beutler E. Lasting remissions in hairy-cell leukemia induced by a single infusion of 2-chlorodeoxyade-nosine. N Engl J Med 1990;322:1117–21.

69. Saven A, Burian C, Koziol JA, Piro LD. Long-term follow-up of patients with hairy cell leukemia after cladribine treatment. Blood 1998;92:1918–26.

70. Tallman MS, Hakimian D, Rademaker AW, et al. Relapse of hairy cell leukemia after 2-chlorodeoxyadenosine: long-term follow-up of the Northwestern University experience. Blood 1996;88:1954–59.

71. Estey EH, Kurzrock R, Kantarjian HM, et al. Treatment of hairy cell leukemia with 2-chlorodeoxyadenosine (2-CdA). Blood 1992;79:882–7.

72. Lauria F, Rondelli D, Zinzani PL, et al. Long-lasting complete remission in patients with hairy cell leukemia treated with 2-CdA: a 5-year survey. Leukemia 1997;11:629–32.

73. Hoffman MA, Janson D, Rose E, Rai KR. Treatment of hairy-cell leukemia with cladribine: response, toxicity, and long-term follow-up. J Clin Oncol 1997;15:1138–42.

74. Juliusson G, Heldal D, Hippe E, et al. Subcutaneous injections of 2-chlorodeoxyadenosine for symptomatic hairy cell leukemia. J Clin Oncol 1995;13:989–95.

75. Carrera CJ, Piro LD, Saven A, et al. Restoration of lymphocyte subsets following 2-chlorodeoxyadenosine remission induction in hairy cell leukemia. Blood 1990;76:Suppl 1:260a.

76. Juliusson G, Lilemark J. Rapid recovery from cytopenia in hairy cell leukemia after treatment with 2-chloro-2-deoxyadenosine (CDA): relationship to opportunistic infections. Blood 1992;79:888.

77. Seymour JF, Kurzrock R, Freireich EJ, et al. 2-Chlorodeoxyadenosine induces durable remissions and prolonged suppression of CD4$^+$ lymphocyte counts in patients with hairy cell leukemia. Blood 1994;83:2906–11.

78. Ellison DJ, Sharpe RW, Robbins BA, et al. Immunomorphologic analysis of bone marrow biopsies after treatment with 2-chlorodeoxyadenosine for hairy cell leukemia. Blood 1994;84:4310–5.

79. Wheaton S, Tallman MS, Hakimian D, et al. Minimal residual disease may predict bone marrow relapse in patients with hairy cell leukemia treated with 2-chlorodeoxyadenosine. Blood 1996;87:1556–60.

80. Matutes E, Meeus P, McLennan K, et al. The significance of minimal residual disease in hairy cell leukaemia treated with deoxycoformycin: a long-term follow-up study. Br J Haematol 1997;98:375–83.

81. Au WY, Klasa RJ, Gallagher R, et al. Second malignancies in patients with hairy cell leukemia in British Columbia: a 20-year experience. Blood 1998;92:1160–64.

82. Kampmeier P, Spielberger R, Dichstein J, et al. Increased incidence of second neoplasms in patients treated with interferon alpha 2b for hairy cell leukemia: a clinicopathologic assessment. Blood 1994;83:2931–8.

83. Kuzrock R, Strom SS, Estey E, et al. Second cancer risk in hairy cell leukemia: analysis of 350 patients. J Clin Oncol 1997;15:1803.

84. Saven A, Piro LD. Complete remissions in hairy cell leukemia with 2-chlorodeoxyadenosine after failure with 2′-deoxycoformycin. Ann Intern Med 1993;119:278–83.

85. Kraut EH, Bouroncle BA, Grever MR. Pentostatin in the treatment of advanced hairy cell leukemia. J Clin Oncol 1989;7:168–72.

86. Ho AD, Thaler J, Mandelli F, et al. Response to pentostatin in hairy-cell leukemia refractory to interferon-alpha. J Clin Oncol 1989;7:1533–8.

87. Johnston JB, Eisenhauer E, Corbett WE, et al. Efficacy of 2′-deoxycoformycin in hairy-cell leukemia: a study of the National Cancer Institute of Canada Clinical Trials Group. J Natl Cancer Inst 1988;80:765–9.

# CHAPTER 99

# MYELOMA, MACROGLOBULINEMIA, AND AMYLOIDOSIS

• ROBERT A. VESCIO • JAMES R. BERENSON

The primary function for the most differentiated B lymphocyte, the plasma cell, is the secretion of large quantities of immunoglobulin (Ig) to aid in host defense. For this to be effective, a large variety of Ig proteins must be produced to combat the multitude of infectious pathogens that an individual encounters during life. In a normal individual, this heterogeneity is noted within the electrophoretic pattern of serum protein, in which a bell-shaped curve of migration occurs within the agarose gel resulting from the different mobilities of these thousands of Ig molecules. When a clonal population of plasma cells accumulates, a monoclonal Ig or Ig protein fragment can be found. These monoclonal proteins (M proteins or paraproteins) either accumulate within the serum, or if incomplete, collect within the urine of a patient with a malignant plasma cell dyscrasia. Nevertheless, the mere presence of a paraprotein is not diagnostic of neoplasia. In fact, the majority of patients with a detectable M protein have a pre-malignant condition termed *monoclonal gammopathy of undetermined significance* (MGUS). Finally, patients with autoimmune disease, those with infections, and those recovering from bone marrow transplantation may develop mild paraproteinemia due to an aberrant proliferation of plasma cells. The majority of patients with a malignancy and a detectable M protein within the urine or blood have multiple myeloma or Waldenström's macroglobulinemia (WM). However, patients with other malignancies involving less differentiated B cells, such as chronic lymphocytic leukemia and non-Hodgkin's lymphoma, may also have a detectable M spike resulting from its production by the malignant clone.

The clinical characteristics of a particular plasma cell dyscrasia depend on the level of B-lymphocyte maturation predominating in the neoplastic clone and on the nature of its secretory products (Table 99–1). The predominant tumor cell in myeloma is a bone marrow–based plasma cell. The secretion of nephrotoxic light chains and osteoclast-activating factors (OAFs) and the suppression of polyclonal plasma cell numbers and function are responsible for the classic symptom complex of renal insufficiency, bone disease, and susceptibility to infection. Tumor infiltration of soft tissues gives rise to isolated or multiple plasmacytomas.

In contrast, the tumor cell of WM is morphologically described as a plasmacytoid lymphocyte that secretes whole IgM molecules whose size and tendency to aggregate lead to the hyperviscosity syndrome. Lymphadenopathy and hepatosplenomegaly are due to infiltration of lymphoid tissues with tumor cells.

Heavy chain disease (HCD) is a plasmacytic-lymphocytic neoplasm in which symptoms primarily relate to infiltration of tissues by malignant cells. In alpha HCD, the small intestine is diffusely infiltrated; in mu and gamma HCD, peripheral lymphoid tissues are predominantly affected.

Amyloidosis develops in patients when a clone of B lymphocytes or plasma cells proliferates and produces a monoclonal Ig protein that then deposits in interstitial tissue, resulting in organ destruction.

## Multiple Myeloma

### EPIDEMIOLOGY

Multiple myeloma is the second most common hematologic malignancy, accounting for 1% of all nonskin cancers diag-

*Table 99–1.* Spectrum of Malignant Plasma Cell Dyscrasias

| Type | M Components | Tumor Location | Symptom Complex |
|---|---|---|---|
| Multiple myeloma | Igg<br>IgA<br>IgD<br>IgM<br>IgE<br>Free light chains | Bone marrow<br>Plasmacytomas | Renal insufficiency<br>Bone disease<br>Susceptibility to infection |
| Waldenström's macroglobulinemia | IgM | Marrow<br>Spleen<br>Nodes<br>Liver | Hyperviscosity syndrome<br>Hepatosplenomegaly<br>Lymphadenopathy |
| Heavy chain disease | Alpha heavy chain<br>Mu heavy chain<br>Gamma heavy chain | Small intestine<br>Peripheral lymphoid tissue<br>Peripheral lymphoid tissue | Malabsorption<br>Hepatosplenomegaly<br>Lymphadenopathy |

From Durie BG: Staging and kinetics of multiple myeloma. In: Wiernik PH, Canellos GP, Kyle RA, Schiffer CA, eds. Neoplastic Diseases of the Blood. 2nd ed. New York: Churchill Livingstone, 1991:440.

nosed in the United States.[1] Since the 1970s, the number of patients diagnosed with this cancer has increased substantially, but much of this change may be attributed to improved detection and the aging of the population. The lack of a real change is supported by a report from Olmsted County, Minnesota, where a population-based study failed to reveal an increase in incidence rate within a given age group.[2] In a second study of mortality rates from multiple myeloma, the incidence of the disease increased steadily from 1960 to 1989, but the rate of increase slowed in the 1980s.[3] Much of this increased incidence was attributed to improved recognition and, thus, documentation of this disease in elderly patients. Nevertheless, small increased incidence rates have occurred in most countries in recent times, particularly in locales where baseline rates of disease are low, such as Japan.[4]

Myeloma is more common in males (approximately 60% of all cases), and its incidence increases strikingly with advancing age.[4] Peak rates are found in the 70- to 80-year-old age group, with a mean age at diagnosis of 62 years. The disease is uncommon in young adults, with only 6 of 12,000 cases occurring in adults younger than age 25 in a 15-year U.S. registry study.[4, 5]

The disease also has a distinct racial distribution. It is the most common hematologic malignancy in the black population, occurring twice as frequently as it does in whites.[6] It is unclear whether the high incidence in blacks is due to genetic, cultural, or environmental factors. A pseudogene with sequences highly homologous to poly(ADP-ribose)polymerase, a nuclear enzyme thought to play a role in DNA repair,[7] shows increased frequency of an allelic polymorphism containing deleted DNA (the B allele) in several B-cell malignancies. There is a higher incidence of the B-allele polymorphism in the black population, and an even higher incidence of the B allele was noted in germline DNA from blacks who developed myeloma and MGUS.[8] In contrast, Asians generally have a low incidence of myeloma, similar to the infrequent occurrence of chronic lymphocytic leukemia in these populations, and the prevalence of the poly(ADP-ribose)polymerase B allele in this population is lowest of all.[9] Plasmacytoma-susceptible BALB/c mice also have an abnormality of this gene; consequently, the presence

or absence of the B allele may explain the racial differences in incidence. Conversely, the allele may simply be a genetic marker for the disease with no relevance to pathophysiology. Similar associations with the human leukocyte antigen (HLA-Cw2) allele have also been described.[10]

Race per se has no bearing on stage at diagnosis or survival.[11] One retrospective study, using 1970 census block information to access socioeconomic status, indicated that impoverished patients presented with greater tumor burden and had a lower response rate to therapy and shorter survival compared with patients from higher socioeconomic status groups.[11] In a second study[12] in which socioeconomic status was directly assessed by interviews, these conclusions could not be confirmed.

## ETIOLOGY

**Hereditary Factors.** The occurrence of familial immunopathies is now well documented, with more than 75 families described in the literature.[13] Most affected individuals in the reported families are siblings, which suggests that genetic factors are more important than environmental ones. Genetic marker studies tend to support this view.[14, 15] When both parent and child have been diagnosed with this disease, the onset of myeloma tends to occur earlier in the child.[13]

Familial occurrence is not confined to myeloma and has been reported in patients with WM and MGUS. In a prospective study of 76 relatives of subjects with plasma cell dyscrasia,[16] three cases of asymptomatic paraproteinemias were discovered, suggesting a higher frequency of these disorders among family members than that observed in the general population. Another study described a fourfold increase in multiple myeloma incidence when a first-degree relative also had the disease.[6] Additional support for genetic influences comes from the murine myeloma model in which certain specific inbred strains, such as BALB/c, have a more marked incidence.

**Radiation Exposure.** An excess of myeloma has also been found in several cohorts of patients exposed to irradiation, such as atomic bomb survivors, radiologists, and radium dial painters.[1, 17–19] In contrast to the experience with radiation-induced acute leukemia, in which an increased incidence occurs 2 to 15 years after exposure, the increase in the incidence of myeloma occurs 10 to 30 years after exposure.

**Environmental Factors.** Prior occupational exposure to petroleum (relative risk of 3.7)[20] and agricultural and chemical products (relative risk of 1.8)[21] has been associated with a higher rate of myeloma, as has the use of black hair dye.[22] However, conflicting negative studies almost always exist. Benzene exposure, which has been widely found to contribute to leukemia development, does not appear to lead to multiple myeloma.[23] In fact, at present, there is no proven association between environmental exposures and increased multiple myeloma development. However, the most consistently identified association has been noted in farmers and those exposed to pesticides. Numerous studies have noted an increased relative risk of multiple myeloma in these population cohorts,[24–27] and a meta-analysis has confirmed this association.[28]

**Antigenic Stimulation.** Early studies[29–31] suggested that excessive antigenic stimulation played a role in the pathogenesis of myeloma. The "two-hit" hypothesis of Salmon and Seligmann[31a] theorizes that B-cell neoplasia evolves from a premalignant stimulation of a lymphocyte clone by a specific antigen. During the period of antigenic stimulation, the clone remains under some regulatory control but is susceptible to a second oncogenic event. Once this occurs, the clone could become malignant, and overt myeloma would develop. In support of this theory, some myeloma paraproteins have antibody activity to well-defined antigens,[32, 33] suggesting a prior specific antigenic stimulation. Although results from case-control studies[20, 34] have been somewhat contradictory, a prospective study[35] noted increased disease incidence in patients with chronic antigenic exposure due to infectious, allergic, autoimmune, or inflammatory disorders. Chronicity of exposure was important, as the increased relative risk was primarily evident in patients with conditions that were present for at least 5 years.[35] The most convincing relationship exists between rheumatoid arthritis and multiple myeloma. Relative risk ratios of 3 to 9 have been described for the development of multiple myeloma in these patients.[36, 37]

We[38] and others[39] have examined the Ig heavy chain sequence expressed by the myeloma cells to search for differences in comparison with the germline gene. A high degree of somatic mutation had occurred in most patients, and the majority of nucleotide mutations leading to amino acid replacements occurred in the regions of the sequence conferring antigenic specificity ($p<0.001$).[38] Thus, the myeloma precursor cell must have passed through a stage of antigenic selection pressure whereby increased antigenic specificity improved the likelihood of cell survival. The importance of antigenic stimulation is also suggested by studies in the murine model.[40] Induction of murine myeloma is impossible when mice are raised under germ-free conditions. This observation, coupled with the fact that murine myeloma usually originates from the gastrointestinal tract, suggests that antigenic stimulation by enteric bacteria plays a role in the genesis of the neoplasm.

## BIOLOGY

**Myeloma Cell of Origin.** The terminally differentiated cell of the B-lymphocyte lineage, the plasma cell, is the predominant morphologically identified tumor cell in myeloma. Because these bone marrow plasma cells have a low proliferative rate, the existence of a more rapidly dividing and less differentiated B-lymphocyte precursor cell has been thought to account for this rapidly progressive disease. Evidence in support of such a precursor cell includes the expression of shared idiotypes by the myeloma cell and IgM-producing lymphocytes,[41–43] the expression of myeloid and megakaryocytic markers on the aneuploid cell population in myeloma patients,[44] and the identification of an IgM-producing cell with terminal complementarity determining region 3 (CDR3) sequence homology with the myeloma clone.[45, 46] These results remain inconclusive, however. First, anti-idiotypic antibodies are probably not specific enough to prove clonality because of cross-reactivity. Second, the presence of myeloid and megakaryocytic markers has been noted on normal plasma cells, reflecting the frequent aberrant expression of these cell surface antigens.[47] Finally, the terminal CDR3 region (which is composed of the D/JH junction) may not be unique, as there is a lack of N-region nucleotide insertion in myeloma.[48]

To further address myeloma pathophysiology, the Ig heavy chain variable region (VH) was sequenced in 40 patients with multiple myeloma and compared with germline VH sequences.[38] We[38] and others[39, 49] found a lack of VH gene intraclonal diversity among tumor clones, the presence of a high degree of VH gene somatic mutation, and the existence of prior antigenic selection pressure. These processes could occur only if the malignancy developed from a postgerminal center cell such as a memory B cell, plasmablast, or plasma cell. Because this sequence does not vary among tumor cells in an individual patient, oligonucleotide primers can be designed that will be specific for the myeloma clone when used in the polymerase chain reaction (PCR). When IgM-producing B lymphocytes that used the same VH germline gene sequence as the myeloma clone were analyzed in these same patients, there was never evidence of VH sequence identity to the myeloma clones,[38] nor was there ever evidence of clonal cells in an extremely pure population of bone marrow cells expressing the CD34 hematopoietic stem cell antigen.[50] These results make it unlikely that a malignant clonal stem cell or pre-Ig class switch cell exists in multiple myeloma.

### Myeloma Growth Factors

*Interleukin-6.* Interleukin-6 (IL-6) appears to function as the primary growth factor for multiple myeloma. This cytokine is produced in large amounts in the bone marrow microenvironment and has been reported to function as both an autocrine and paracrine growth factor, although the latter is likely more predominant clinically.[51–53] The bone marrow stromal cells that compose the microenvironment for the malignant plasma cells secrete large quantities of IL-6, and this production is enhanced by the adhesion of myeloma cells to stromal cell cultures.[54] This synergism is evident in vitro, as the initiation of myeloma cell lines often requires the exogenous administration of IL-6 or adherence to bone marrow stroma co-cultures.[55, 56] The importance of this cytokine is also evident in vivo, as transgenic mice carrying an activated IL-6 gene develop polyclonal plasmacytosis.[57] Furthermore, elevated levels of IL-6 are often noted in patients with multiple myeloma and are associated with poor prognosis.[58, 59] This cytokine appears to protect plasma cells from undergoing chemotherapy-induced apoptosis.[60–62] Finally, patients treated with anti–IL-6 monoclonal antibodies have responded to treatment, although at present this approach has been limited by the development of neutralizing human anti-mouse antibodies.[63, 64] Clearly, given these findings, IL-6 has an important role in multiple myeloma pathogenesis.

***Interleukin-1β.*** Interleukin-1β (IL-1β) is a potent bone resorption factor and can be produced by the myeloma cells directly.[65, 66] By using in situ hybridization, IL-1β secretion was found to be increased in bone marrow aspirates from patients with MGUS and multiple myeloma when compared with normal controls.[67, 68] Patients with lytic bone lesions were more likely to have elevated IL-1β transcripts. This factor can also induce IL-6 stromal cell production and thus can serve as a mediator of paracrine-induced myeloma cell growth.[66]

***Tumor Necrosis Factor Alpha.*** Tumor necrosis factor alpha (TNF-α) has been found to protect myeloma cells deprived of IL-6 from apoptosis and can induce the growth of some myeloma cell lines.[66, 69, 70] TNF-α serum levels are often increased in patients with monoclonal gammopathies, and these levels may be predictive of transformation from MGUS to multiple myeloma.[71, 72] The drug thalidomide may exert some of its beneficial effect by its inhibition of this cytokine.

***Other Factors.*** Insulin-like growth factor also appears to have a stimulatory role in myeloma cell growth.[73, 74] This factor may increase the sensitivity of tumor cells to IL-6[75] and inhibit dexamethasone-induced apoptosis.[76] IL-10,[77] hepatocyte growth factor (HGF),[78] granulocyte-macrophage colony-stimulating factor (GM-CSF),[55, 79] and, paradoxically, interferon-α (interferon alfa) have all been found in some in vitro and in vivo studies to stimulate myeloma cell growth. INF-α can be both inhibitory[80] and stimulatory[81] in some myeloma cell line models, which may explain our experience with occasional patients who developed profound tumor cell growth following its administration after autologous transplantation.

***Human Herpesvirus 8.*** Kaposi's sarcoma–associated herpesvirus is a new member of the gamma herpesvirus family most homologous to the human pathogen Epstein-Barr virus. This virus (now more correctly termed *human herpesvirus 8 [HHV-8]*) was discovered by using a technique called *representational difference analysis* on Kaposi's sarcoma tumor tissue to identify genes unique to the tissue of interest.[82] The viral genome has been sequenced and found to contain numerous homologues to human cytokines, including a viral form of IL-6 (v-IL-6).[83, 84] Because of the importance of this cytokine on multiple myeloma cell growth, we looked for viral contamination of myeloma bone marrow and peripheral blood specimens. HHV-8 was detected in the majority of bone marrow stromal cell cultures from multiple myeloma patients and in a subset of cultures derived from patients with MGUS, yet only rarely in normal individuals.[85] In situ hybridization demonstrated that the virus was not within the plasma cell but instead was within the supporting dendritic cells in the bone marrow microenvironment.[86] Although some groups have failed to corroborate our findings,[87–90] other groups have found similar evidence of HHV-8 in myeloma patient material.[91–93] Whether this viral infection is an epiphenomenon or important in myeloma pathogenesis

remains to be determined. Certainly, our finding that the strain of HHV-8 present in myeloma patients may be restricted and differ from that found in patients with Kaposi's sarcoma suggests the importance of HHV-8 in these patients' malignancies.[94]

***Cytogenetic Abnormalities.*** There is growing evidence that rearrangement, alteration, or amplification of cellular oncogenes leads to human malignancy. Moreover, these changes are often correlated with specific chromosomal abnormalities at the oncogenic sites. In contrast with other B-cell malignancies, no specific cytogenetic abnormalities have been identified in multiple myeloma. Numerous structural and numeric abnormalities are typically found in the myeloma cell. Detectable karyotypic abnormalities occur in approximately 40% of patients[95, 96] but are more commonly noted in patients with advanced disease. The study of cytogenetic abnormalities in multiple myeloma has been hampered by the low proliferative rate of these malignant cells. Consequently, conventional cytogenetics, which requires cells in metaphase, is often unrewarding and definitely underestimates the true prevalence of the genetic abnormalities that exist. Numeric abnormalities of chromosomes 3, 7, 9, 11, and 15 and deletions of chromosome 13 are most frequently noted. The loss of the long arm of 13 (13q) has been strongly associated with shortened survival. In a retrospective analysis by Barlogie's group in Arkansas, the presence of a 13q abnormality was found to be the single most important prognostic indicator for patients undergoing autologous transplantation. Similar adverse survival was noted for patients with 17p deletions, presumably from the loss of the p53 tumor-suppressor gene.

The most common translocations in multiple myeloma involve the Ig heavy chain locus on chromosome 14 and have been found in 60 to 73% of patients.[97, 98] The chromosomal breakpoints often occur within the Ig heavy chain switch region located at 14q32 and use the nonexpressed allele. Numerous partner chromosomes have been noted, with the most common being chromosomes 11, 4, 8, and 16. Potential oncogenes include cyclin D,[99] FGFR,[100] c-*myc*,[101] and c-*maf*[102] for these translocations, respectively. N-*ras*,[103] p53,[104] and Rb1[105] gene mutations have also been noted in patients and in myeloma cell lines and play a role in disease pathogenesis and aggressiveness.

We do not routinely perform cytogenetic analysis on myeloma bone marrow aspirates because the knowledge of adverse prognosis does lead to a change in the treatment approach for a given patient. However, recent improvements in the identification of karyotypic abnormalities using fluorescence in situ hybridization and spectral karyotypic imaging may change this approach.[106] These techniques are capable of more discretely identifying the abnormalities that exist within the malignant cell in the hope that subclassification of myeloma patients will be possible. Ultimately, targeted therapeutics based on the genetic abnormalities within a patient's tumor clone may be possible as was demonstrated for patients with chronic myelogenous leukemia.

## NATURAL HISTORY

### Clinical Findings and Diagnosis

The diagnosis of myeloma is based on the presence of a plasmacytoma or atypical plasma cells in the bone marrow, coupled with a detectable serum or urine monoclonal protein on electrophoresis. Occasionally plasmacytosis may not be found in patients with patchy marrow involvement. Suggested criteria for the diagnosis of myeloma are outlined in Table 99–2. When serum protein electrophoresis is performed, 80% of myeloma patients have evidence of a detectable monoclonal protein. Although there are occasional pa-

*Table 99–2.* **Diagnostic Criteria for Multiple Myeloma, Indolent Myeloma, Smoldering Multiple Myeloma, and Monoclonal Gammopathy of Undetermined Significance (MGUS)**

*Major Criteria*

I. Plasmacytoma on tissue biopsy
II. Bone marrow plasmacytosis >30% with plasma cells
III. Monoclonal globulin spike on serum electrophoresis exceeding 3.5 g% for G peaks or 2.0 g% for A peaks, ≥1.0 g/24 hr of κ- or λ-light chain excretion on urine electrophoresis in the absence of amyloidosis

*Minor Criteria*

a. Bone marrow plasmacytosis 10–30% plasma cells
b. Monoclonal globulin spike present, but less than the levels defined above
c. Lytic bone lesions
d. Normal IgM <50 mg%, IgA <100 mg%, or IgG <600 mg%
   Diagnosis will be confirmed when any of the following features are documented in symptomatic patients with clearly progressive disease. The diagnosis of myeloma requires a *minimum* of one major + one minor criterion *or* three minor criteria, which must include a + b:
   1. I + b, I + c, I + d (I + a not sufficient)
   2. II + b, II + c, II + d
   3. III + a, III + c, III + d
   4. a + b + c, a + b + d

*Criteria for MGUS, Indolent Myeloma, and Smoldering Myeloma (Stage I or IIA)*

*MGUS*

I. Monoclonal gammopathy
II. M-component level
    IgG <3.5 g/dl
    IgA <2.0 g/dl
    BJ protein ≤1.0 g/24 hr
III. Bone marrow plasma cells <10%
IV. No bone lesions
V. No symptoms

*Indolent Myeloma: Criteria as for Myeloma (I Above) Except (all the Following)*

I. No bone lesions or only limited bone lesions (≥3 lytic lesions); no compression fractures
II. M-component levels: (a) IgG <7 g/dl; (b) IgA <5 g/dl
III. No symptoms or associated disease features
    a. Performance status >70%
    b. Hemoglobin >10 g/dl
    c. Serum calcium normal
    d. Serum creatinine <2.0 mg/dl
    e. No infections

*Smoldering Myeloma: Criteria as for Indolent Myeloma Except*

I. *No* bone lesions
II. Bone marrow plasma cells ≤30%

BJ, Bence Jones; IgA, immunoglobulin A; IgG, immunoglobulin G; IgM, immunoglobulin M.
From Durie BG: Staging and kinetics of multiple myeloma. In: Neoplastic Diseases of the Blood, 2nd ed. Wiernik PH, Canellos GP, Kyle RA, Schiffer CA, eds. New York: Churchill Livingstone, 1991:440.

tients with nonsecretory disease (<1%), the majority of the remaining patients have light chain–only disease (Bence Jones proteinuria), necessitating urine protein electrophoresis for diagnosis. Conditions that strongly suggest the diagnosis include azotemia, bone pain, and hypercalcemia. Other abnormalities that frequently occur but are of a nonspecific nature include hypoalbuminemia, a low anion gap, hyperuricemia, anemia, and osteoporosis.

Patients usually present with weakness, bone pain, or symptoms of renal failure. Occasionally, asymptomatic patients are diagnosed by a fortuitous electrophoresis and, under observation, develop the classic symptoms of myeloma. These patients must be distinguished from the asymptomatic patients with MGUS or smoldering myeloma, who do not require immediate treatment. Careful observation is warranted for patients with disease overlapping the diagnoses of MGUS and multiple myeloma, as there is no evidence that early treatment of myeloma improves survival, and the morbidity from chemotherapy may be delayed in these patients.

Occasionally, symptoms can develop because of the biologic properties of the secreted M protein.[107] Cryoprecipitability of the paraprotein can lead to Raynaud's phenomenon, and interactions between paraproteins and lipids can result in hyperlipidemia and xanthoma formation.[108] Acquired factor VIII deficiency has also been described in a few patients and can be treated with porcine factor VIII replacement.[109] The incidence of the hyperviscosity syndrome in multiple myeloma is approximately 5 to 10%, although symptoms rarely occur unless the viscosity level rises to greater than 4 CP.[110, 111] Most cases are associated with myeloma of the IgA and IgG3 subclasses resulting from the tendencies of these paraproteins to aggregate and form high-molecular-weight complexes.[110, 111] Although IgA and IgG are distributed between intravascular and extravascular spaces, plasma exchange[110, 112, 113] is usually successful in decreasing symptoms, and repeated plasmapheresis is rarely needed.

**Bone Disease.** At diagnosis, 60% of patients have lytic bone lesions, and another 20% have osteoporosis or pathologic fractures, or both.[114] Indeed, the major clinical manifestation of this malignancy is related to osteolytic bone destruction.[114, 115] Even patients who respond to chemotherapy may have progression of skeletal disease,[116, 117] and once the lytic bone lesion develops, recalcification and radiologic improvement are rare. Mundy and coworkers originally found that myeloma plasma cells produce factors called *OAFs* that stimulate osteoclast bone resorption.[118] Although early work suggested that IL-1β and lymphotoxin (TNF-β) were these factors,[119, 120] other factors have been implicated from more recent studies, including TNF-α, IL-6,[121] transforming growth factor-β,[122] HGF,[123] metalloproteinases,[124] and other molecules yet to be characterized. Corticosteroids strongly inhibit IL-1β production, which may explain some of their effectiveness in patients.[125]

Obviously, enhanced osteoclast activity would not be associated with enhanced bone loss if there was not an accompanying loss in bone formation.[126] This uncoupling bone process (i.e., increased bone resorption in the presence of a reduction in bone formation) is the hallmark of multiple myeloma with osteolytic disease. Osteocalcin, a marker of bone formation activity, has been shown to be decreased in patients with lytic bone disease in comparison with myeloma patients without bony lesions.[127] In support of the important relationship of bone disease to overall outcome in these patients, serum osteocalcin levels have been shown to be inversely related to survival.[128]

Because the major clinical manifestations of myeloma are related to bone disease, the importance of assessing its status cannot be overestimated. Early detection of lesions at risk to fracture or lead to cord compression allows prompt use of prophylactic surgery or radiotherapy. The roentgenographic bone survey is far more specific and sensitive than scintigraphy for detecting bone involvement, and the gold standard for detection of myeloma bone disease has been plain radiographs of the skull, spine, and pelvis and long bones of the upper and lower extremities.[129] Because myelomatous lesions are usually purely lytic with little blastic component, the reactive bone formation detected by bone scan may not be present, leading to a falsely negative result. Nevertheless, studies suggest that bone scans may be useful in lesions that are difficult to interpret with plain radiographs, for example, lesions of the sternum, ribs, and vertebral bodies.[130] Occasional patients with features of the POEMS syndrome (*p*olyneuropathy, *o*rganomegaly, *e*ndocrinopathy, *m*onoclonal gammopathy, and *s*kin changes), in which bone lesions are usually sclerotic, may also best be followed by bone scans.

Bone densitometry using dual-energy x-ray absorptiometry (DEXA) clearly has been helpful in the management of osteoporosis. DEXA scans are almost always abnormal in patients with multiple myeloma and often correlate with the risk of future fractures.[131] We have used this procedure to help determine the need for bisphosphonate administration and to guide therapeutic decisions for patients with osteoporosis and MGUS or smoldering myeloma.

Magnetic resonance imaging (MRI) can also detect myelomatous bony involvement and is much more sensitive than plain radiographs. An abnormal MRI scan generally demonstrates three patterns, including diffuse involvement without the appearance of normal marrow signal, nodular or focal areas of replacement of normal marrow, or multiple tiny areas of replacement.[132] Studies demonstrate that patients with diffuse involvement have the worst prognosis and have associated increased plasma cell loads.[133] MRI may be most useful, however, in determining which patients with solitary plasmacytomas will progress and develop disease dissemination.[134] Radiotherapy to the solitary tumor bed can be curative in some patients, but patients with other bone lesions seen on screening MRI scans of the spine are much more likely to develop progressive multiple myeloma.[135]

Radiologic surveys should be repeated periodically to assess response to therapy or progression of disease. Bone healing occurs infrequently, however, with only 30% of patients with responsive disease showing radiologic improvement.[136] Clearly, patients with progressive disease and new bone pain should have radiologic assessments performed to identify any new impending fractures that can be prevented by measures such as radiation or surgical therapy.

**Infection.** Patients with myeloma are particularly susceptible to infection. The incidence ranges from 1.4 to 2 per patient per year,[137, 138] and infectious complications are still the major cause of death.[139] Patients are most susceptible to encapsulated organisms and often develop sinusitis and pneumonias from agents such as *Streptococcus pneumoniae.*

The greatest period of risk for infection is during the first 2 months after chemotherapy is begun, and the infection rate is lowest when the patient is in remission.

There are many abnormalities of host defenses in patients with myeloma. Nonparaprotein levels of serum Ig are depressed in most patients, and there is an impaired antibody response to many antigens. Conceivable reasons for this deficiency include circulating immunologic suppressor cells,[140–142] possibly activated by tumor cell products, and an RNA-rich extract that prevents immunocompetent lymphocytes from expressing surface Ig, their putative antigen receptor.[143] The granulocytopenic effects of chemotherapy and the immunosuppressive effects of steroids also contribute to the increased susceptibility to serious infections. In addition, the adherence properties of polymorphonuclear leukocytes are decreased,[144] intracellular lysozyme levels are deficient,[145] serum complement levels are depressed,[146] and heat-labile and heat-stable opsonic activity in myeloma serum is deficient.[147] The clinical significance of these latter abnormalities is less clear. Finally, many patients have indwelling catheters for chemotherapy administration, which are associated with increased rates of infections from staphylococci. Herpes zoster infections are particularly frequent in these patients and can predate disease diagnosis in some patients.[148]

**Renal Disease.** Renal involvement complicates the course of myeloma in approximately 50% of patients,[149] is present in 20% of patients at diagnosis, and is the second most frequent cause of death.[139] The pathologic findings that correlate best with renal insufficiency are tubular atrophy and degeneration.[150, 151] Intratubular casts can also be found in a significant number of patients. Although many complications of myeloma (hypercalcemia, hyperuricemia, hyperviscosity syndrome, infection, and amyloidosis) may contribute to renal injury, the most important factor is the presence of Bence Jones (free light chain) proteinuria. Patients with Bence Jones proteinuria are much more likely to have decreased creatinine clearances,[151, 152] and there is a general inverse correlation between the level of Bence Jones proteinuria and the creatinine clearance. However, there are occasional patients who, despite high levels of light chain proteinuria, maintain normal renal function.[153] Thus, the level of Bence Jones proteinuria is not the sole determinant of renal injury, and individual light chains differ in their nephrotoxic potential.[154] These Bence Jones proteins can damage the kidneys by forming tubular casts (myeloma cast nephropathy), fibrils (seen in amyloidosis), or crystals (adult Fanconi's syndrome) or by their precipitation within the basement membrane (light chain deposition disease). Certain light chain subtypes are particularly associated with nephropathy in multiple myeloma patients. In one animal model, only light chains obtained from patients with renal disease were pathogenic to mouse kidneys after intraperitoneal injection.[155] Further molecular analysis of Ig gene sequences from patients has revealed that the use of Vk1 and Vk4 gene families by the myeloma clone is more frequent in patients with light chain deposition disease and adult Fanconi's syndrome.[156]

Acute renal failure occurs in patients with myeloma, usually in the setting of Bence Jones proteinuria and hypercalcemia.[149] Dehydration, significant gastrointestinal bleeding with hypovolemia, use of nephrotoxic antibiotics, or recent intravenous pyelography are frequent inciting causes. Intravenous pyelography, even in the absence of clinical dehydration, can precipitate acute renal failure, and extreme caution must be used before performing this procedure. Although older reports emphasized the extremely poor prognosis of myeloma patients with acute renal failure, more recent reviews suggest that recovery of renal function and prolonged survival are possible with effective chemotherapy and aggressive supportive care.[157, 158] In one series, 6 of 10 patients recovered renal function and 5 survived beyond 1 year.[157]

The adult Fanconi's syndrome (proximal tubular dysfunction) can be associated with myeloma, and these patients can have the classic findings of glycosuria, aminoaciduria, phosphaturia, acidosis, and osteomalacia. Many patients with myeloma and Bence Jones proteinuria have concentrating and acidification defects in the absence of reduced glomerular filtration, suggesting a distal tubular dysfunction.[151] A report has also documented a case of distal renal tubular acidosis in a patient with multiple myeloma.[159] Renal biopsy is the only definitive method of diagnosis. Often, as the patient's urinary M protein improves, renal function improves as well. Thus, renal biopsy is not typically required for patient management but is occasionally needed to differentiate between myeloma-associated kidney disease and other potential causes (diabetic, hypertensive, or drug-induced nephropathy) when a specific biopsy finding will alter patient treatment.

## Pretreatment Prognostic Factors and Staging

A clinical staging system developed by Durie and Salmon was designed to estimate total body myeloma cell mass by the severity of various disease features such as M component level, hypercalcemia, anemia, and lytic bone lesions (Table 99–3).[160] Patients are classified according to myeloma cell mass—low (stage I), intermediate (stage II), or high (stage III)—and several studies have confirmed the prognostic importance of this staging system.[161] One retrospective analysis showed a median survival of 64, 32, and 6 months for low, intermediate, and high tumor cell mass groups, respectively.[162]

Since renal function correlated poorly with myeloma cell mass[161] but was felt to be an important prognostic variable, it was included as a subclassification of each stage into A (normal) or B (abnormal) renal function. One prospective study of 150 patients demonstrated a median survival of 61 months for stage IA, 54.5 months for stages IIA and IIB, 30 months for stage IIIA, and 15 months for stage IIIB. A summary of other studies assessing the prognostic value of this staging system is outlined in Table 99–4.

The Durie-Salmon staging system does not include two important prognostic variables: (1) the inherent biology and proliferative rate of the tumor and (2) its sensitivity to chemotherapy. Thus, several other variables have been examined in attempts to provide more accurate prognostic information.

One variable that appears particularly promising is the serum level of β2-microglobulin.[163] β2-microglobulin represents the "light chain" of HLA on the membranes of all nucleated cells. As a consequence of membrane turnover or cell death (especially of lymphoid cells), it is released into the serum and subsequently excreted by the kidneys. Thus, the serum β2-microglobulin level is dependent on production, that is, cell turnover or death, and excretion, that is, renal function. An increased serum β2-microglobulin concentration has been found in 80 to 90% of patients with myeloma,[164, 165] and myeloma cells secrete serum β2-microglobulin in vitro. Thus, the serum β2-microglobulin level has been investigated as a prognostic variable.

As would be expected, serum β2-microglobulin levels correlate with tumor mass and serum creatinine in myeloma

*Table 99–3.* **Staging of Myeloma**

| Stage | Clinical Staging System Criteria | Myeloma Cell Mass (Cells × 10¹²/m²) |
|---|---|---|
| I | All of the following:<br>1. Hemoglobin >10 g/dl<br>2. Serum calcium value normal (≤12 mg/dl)<br>3. On radiograph, normal bone structure or solitary bone plasmacytoma only<br>4. Low M-component production rates<br>  a. IgG value <5 g/dl<br>  b. IgA value <3 g/dl<br>  c. Urine light chain M component on electrophoresis <4 g/24 hr | $<0.6 \times 10^{12}$ (low) |
| II | Fitting neither stage I nor stage III | $0.6–1.2 \times 10^{12}$ (intermediate) |
| III | One or more of the following:<br>1. Hemoglobin <8.5 g/dl<br>2. Serum calcium >12 g/dl<br>3. Advanced lytic bone lesions<br>4. High M-component production rates<br>  a. IgG value >7 g/dl<br>  b. IgA value >5 g/dl<br>  c. Urine light chain M component on electrophoresis >12 g/24 hours | $>1.2 \times 10^{12}$ (high) |
| A or B | A = creatinine ≤2 mg/dl<br>B = creatinine >2 mg/dl | |

From Durie BG, Salmon SE: A clinical staging system for multiple myeloma: correlation of measured myeloma cell mass with presenting clinical features, response to treatment, and survival. Cancer 1975;36:842–54.

*Table 99–4.* Median Survival in Relation to Stage at Diagnosis

| Investigations | No. of Patients | Median Survival (mo) STAGE | | | | |
| --- | --- | --- | --- | --- | --- | --- |
| | | I | II | III | A | B |
| Durie and Salmon[160] | 71 | >60 | 50 | 26 | | |
| Alexanian et al[197] | 343 | 39 | 27 | 17 | | |
| Woodruff et al[167] | 237 | 64 | 32 | 6 | 21 | 2 |
| Merlini et al[500] | 123 | 76 | 41 | 12 | | |
| Belpomme et al[501] | 118 | >60 | 28 | 7 | >60 | 12 |
| Gobbi et al[502] | 91 | >79 | 51 | 33 | | |
| Santoro et al[503] | 81 | 48 | 41 | 23 | 35 | 7 |
| Bergsagel et al[504] | 364 | 46 | 32 | 23 | 32 | 11 |
| Summary | 1428 | >60 | 41 | 23 | | |

From Salmon SE, Cassady JR: Plasma cell neoplasms. In: DeVita VT, Jr., Hellman S, Rosenberg SA, eds. Cancer: Principles and practice of oncology. 4th ed. Philadelphia: JB Lippincott, 1993:1995.

patients.[164–167] Because stage and survival depend on both these variables, it is not surprising that serum β2-microglobulin levels also correlate with initial stage and prognosis. In fact, several studies identified serum β2-microglobulin levels at diagnosis as the most powerful single determinant of prognosis.[165, 167, 168] Further support for its strength as a clinically useful tool comes from inspection of Durie-Salmon stage IIIA patients. The largest number of patients are diagnosed with this stage of disease, and it is somewhat heterogeneous with regard to prognosis. Several investigators[166, 169] have shown that serum β2-microglobulin levels can differentiate stage IIIA patients into good- and poor-risk groups. Even in one dissenting study[170] in which the results of serum β2-microglobulin levels did not add predictive value to the Durie-Salmon system for all patients, those within stage IIIA were more accurately assessed. Nineteen patients with a serum β2-microglobulin level less than 2 mg/ml had a median survival of 41 months, whereas 19 patients with a level greater than 2 mg/ml had a median survival of 14 months. Unfortunately, the overlap between serum β2-microglobulin levels in stage I or smoldering myeloma patients and MGUS precludes its value as a useful discriminant between these disorders. β2-microglobulin levels are also one of the best predictors of outcome following autologous transplantation.[171, 172] Although most studies demonstrate a good correlation between serum β2-microglobulin levels and clinical response to therapy,[164, 165, 168, 173, 174] there is no indication that the assay can add to following the serum protein electrophoresis and other clinical parameters during treatment. Therefore, the test is best used as an initial indicator of prognosis and not as a prognosticator while in the midst of treatment.

The plasma cell labeling index (PCLI)[175, 176] is another useful prognostic factor in multiple myeloma, but it is not available at most centers. This test measures the percentage of plasma cells in S phase based on incorporation of bromodeoxyuridine. Numerous retrospective studies have verified the usefulness of this marker, with levels greater than 1% predictive of an adverse outcome. Flow cytometry can also be used to determine the percentage of cells in S phase. Patients with more than 3% of their plasma cells in S phase had a poor prognosis based on multivariant analysis.[177] Combining a marker for tumor mass and renal function (serum β2-microglobulin) with the PCLI, which measures

tumor proliferation rate, can provide better prognostic information than can clinical staging alone (Fig. 99–1).[178] Patients with both a PLCI less than 1% and a serum β2-microglobulin level less than 2.7 mg/L had a median survival of 71 months versus 17 months for patients with elevations of both markers in one study.[179]

Because the PCLI is not widely available, other biologic markers have been evaluated for prognostic value. Serum C-reactive protein (CRP) levels accurately reflect the activity of the myeloma growth factor IL-6 and show independent prognostic value when compared with serum β2-microglobulin.[174] Patients who are fortunate to have low CRP and serum β2-microglobulin levels (50% of patients) had a median survival of 54 months versus 6 months for the 15% of patients with elevations in both markers ($p<0.0001$). Since these measurements are quick and simple to obtain, this prognostic system can be useful (Fig. 99–2). In our experience, however, only rare patients have CRP elevations, thus adding little to the value of the serum β2-microglobulin level.

Plasmablastic morphology is another useful prognostic factor,[180] occurring when greater than 2% of bone marrow plasma cells have this phenotype on microscopic analysis. Although less than 10% of patients have this characteristic, such patients have a markedly reduced overall median survival following standard chemotherapy (<2 years vs. 3.7 years).[181] Patients with plasmablastic morphology were also found to have a markedly shortened survival following autologous transplantation in a study performed by the Mayo group.[182]

Cytogenetic abnormalities are also useful indicators of prognosis in multiple myeloma. Unfortunately, because of the slow proliferative rate in multiple myeloma, standard cytogenetic techniques identify abnormal karyotypic features in only 20 to 50% of patients.[95, 183] The use of fluorescence in situ hybridization can identify these abnormalities in up to 90% of cases. In one study of multiple myeloma patients undergoing tandem autologous transplantation, patients found to have an abnormality of chromosome 11q or a deletion of chromosome 13 had a median overall survival of only 21 months versus 55 months in the remaining cohort. These adverse karyotypes were found to be the most important prognostic factor on multivariate analysis in this large

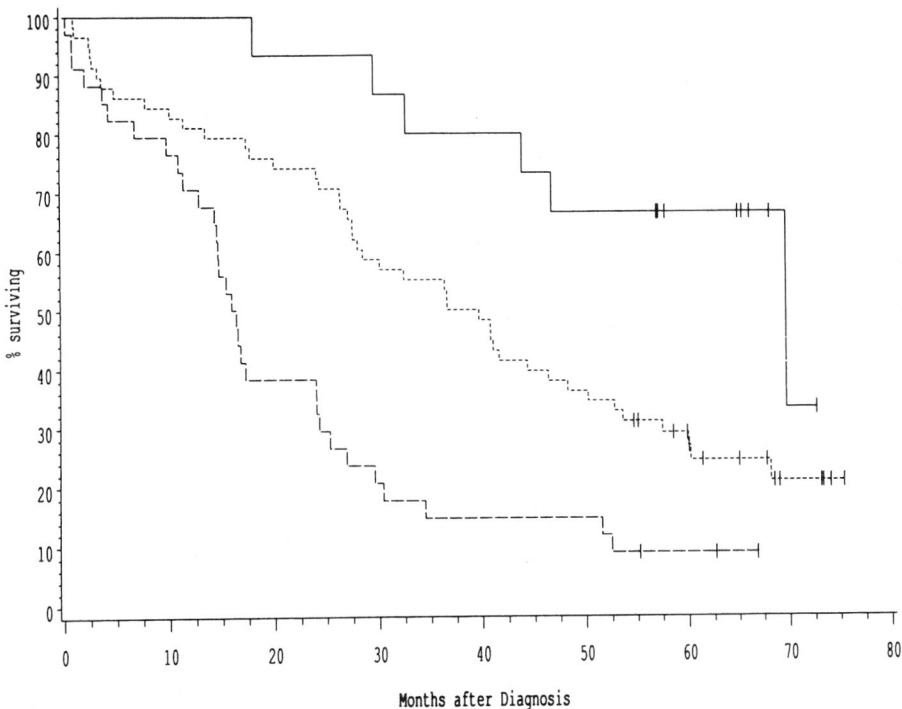

**Figure 99–1.** Kaplan-Meier survival curves for patients grouped by PCLI and β₂M (mg/L). *Upper curve,* PCLI <1 and β₂M <2.7, n = 15. Median survival was 71 months; nine patients were alive at the latest follow-up. Symbols indicate censored events. *Middle curve,* PCLI ≥1 or β₂M ≥2.7, n = 58. Median survival was 40 months, with 14 patients alive at the latest follow-up. *Lower curve,* PCLI ≥1 and β₂M ≥2.7, n = 34. Median survival was 17 months, with 3 patients alive at the latest follow-up. (From Greipp PR, Lust JA, D'Fallon WM, et al: Value of beta 2-microglobulin level and plasma cell labeling indices as prognostic factors in patients with newly diagnosed myeloma. Blood 1993;81:3385.)

427-patient trial.[184] Other investigators have confirmed the adverse outcome for patients with chromosome 13 deletions.[185] This adverse outcome is believed to be related to the deletion of the Rb gene, which is located on chromosome 13. Patients with Rb gene deletions had a median survival of 14 months versus 60 months (p=0.0012) in a study of 63 patients with multiple myeloma treated with standard chemo-

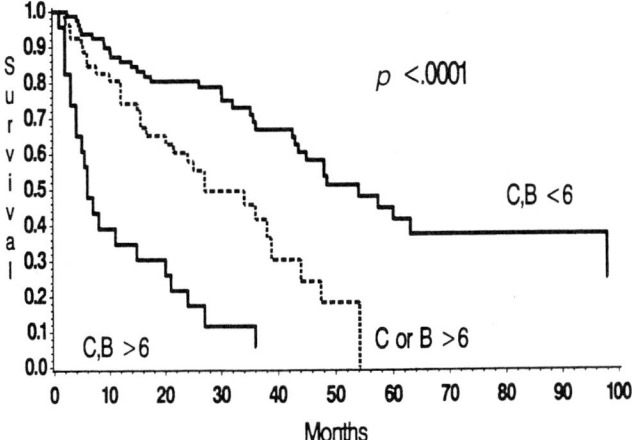

**Figure 99–2.** Actuarial survival of 162 multiple myeloma patients according to serum C-reactive protein (CRP) and β₂M levels at diagnosis. C,B <6 = CRP and β₂M <6 mg/L; C or B >6 = CRP or β₂M ≥6 mg/L; C,B >6 = CRP and β₂M ≥6 mg/L. (From Bataille R, Boccadoro M, Klein B, et al: C-reactive protein and beta-2 microglobulin produce a simple and powerful myeloma staging system. Blood 1992;80:733–7.)

therapy.[186] Patients with trisomies 6, 9, and 17 had improved survival times in this same Spanish study.

Other factors associated with poor survival include poor performance status,[187] anemia,[188] thrombocytopenia,[189] hypoalbuminemia, hypercalcemia,[190] p53 deletions,[191] and increased serum levels of lactate dehydrogenase (LDH),[192] thymidine kinase,[193] circulating plasma cells,[194] or soluble IL-6 receptor.[195] Younger patients (<40 years) appear to have improved median survival times of greater than 50 months.[196] Prognosis may also depend on the heavy and light chain isotype class of the paraprotein. Some studies have shown that patients with the IgA type of myeloma have a worse prognosis than do those with the IgG type.[197] However, azotemia and hypercalcemia occur more frequently in patients with IgA myeloma,[197] and when this is taken into consideration, heavy chain isotype carries less significance as an independent variable. Several reports indicate that patients with light chain myeloma (without serum M protein) carry a significantly worse prognosis than do those with serum paraproteins,[198] although others have challenged this finding.[197]

The degree of response to initial chemotherapy does not appear to influence outcome for patients treated with standard chemotherapy.[199, 200] Patients achieving a complete response (CR) do not substantially outlive those attaining only a partial or minimal response to chemotherapy. In contrast, patients with progressive disease during initial chemotherapy do poorly. Thus, the lack of progressive disease is the most important characteristic identifying patients with a good outcome. A rapid response to initial chemotherapy has been identified by some studies as a poor prognostic sign.[152, 201] Presumably, this is related to a more aggressive phenotype in these patients. One study supporting this notion revealed that patients with rapid responses had high PCLIs, indicative of tumors with rapid proliferative rates, and consequently they experienced short remissions.[161] These individuals were also more likely to have lambda light chain class, hyperuricemia, advanced disease (stage III), and a significant incidence of central nervous system relapse.

In summary, numerous factors can be used to determine prognosis in patients with multiple myeloma. Although the Durie-Salmon staging system is most widely used in the community, combinations of serum β2-microglobulin and CRP levels, PCLI, and cytogenetics may be more definitive. Nevertheless, the importance of these variables in clinical practice is less clear because it has never been shown that treatment decision-making based on these factors is of value. In general, we typically use the finding of early Durie-Salmon stage coupled with low serum β2-microglobulin levels to identify patients in whom high-dose chemotherapy can be delayed.

## TREATMENT

### Decision to Treat

Patients with *symptomatic* multiple myeloma should be treated as soon as the diagnosis is established. Because myeloma is an incurable disease with standard chemotherapy, except in rare cases,[202] such therapy is generally given for palliative purposes only. Despite the rarity of cure, however, responses to chemotherapy are high (50 to 75%), and treated patients have median survival times of 24 to 40 months compared with less than 12 months for untreated patients. It is less clear whether patients with asymptomatic and indolent disease require immediate therapy. Patients with smoldering myeloma have slowly progressive disease, and many have advocated a "watch and wait" policy for such patients to prevent treatment-related morbidity. A Swedish prospective study was performed in which 50 patients with asymptomatic stage IA disease were randomized between melphalan plus prednisone (MP) therapy initiated at diagnosis and deferred treatment until the time of disease progression. No differences in survival were noted, and there was a 12-month median chemotherapy deferral time in the watch-and-wait group. Two patients died of leukemia, both of whom were in the initial treatment arm.[203] Clearly, patients with MGUS should not be treated and should simply be observed periodically for signs of malignancy.

Appropriate management of myeloma patients has two major components: management of disease complications and the specific use of antineoplastic therapy. During therapy, the patient must be followed for both subjective and objective signs of response. In the disease complication category, the relief of pain and an increase in patient activity are important goals. Objective criteria of response to treatment include a decrease in serum myeloma protein concentration and daily excretion of light chain (Bence Jones) protein, improvement in anemia, and control of renal insufficiency and hypercalcemia. Since the serum and urine concentrations of the monoclonal protein reflect the size of the

malignant plasma cell mass, it is usually unnecessary to repeat bone marrow biopsies to determine if there is a reduction in marrow plasmacytosis. Although additional lytic bone lesions should not develop during effective chemotherapy, recalcification and bone healing of old lesions occur relatively infrequently.

### Management of Disease Complications

**Bone Disease.** Severe bone pain is a disabling symptom in many patients with myeloma. Adequate analgesia is mandatory to allow resumption of function and prevent immobilization. Supporting braces can be of great benefit in the management of bone pain. Pathologic fractures of long bones can be treated by fixation with intramedullary rods. These rods should also be placed preventatively into bones with such extensive destruction that a pathologic fracture is imminent. Modest doses of local palliative radiotherapy are successful in alleviating pain from bony lesions in 90% of cases.[204] However, this modality should be used only sparingly because the irradiation of large areas of hematopoietically active bone marrow can make future chemotherapy intolerable or high-dose chemotherapy impossible. Instead, treatment of the underlying disease process with chemotherapy and the use of other useful adjuncts discussed further on may be a better tactic because the entire disease process can be treated at once in this way. When radiotherapy is required, doses of 10 to 20 Gy in 2- to 2.5-Gy fractions appears adequate for this radiosensitive tumor.[205] In a study by Leigh and colleagues, even doses lower than 10 Gy were effective at relieving symptoms in 12 of 13 patients, and no dose response curve was noted.[206] These authors suggested that a total dose of 10 Gy should adequately provide durable symptom relief in the majority of patients.

Early attempts to slow bony destruction in multiple myeloma patients looked at fluoride and calcium supplementation. Unfortunately, randomized studies showed no clear benefit for these treatments.[207, 208] Intranasal calcitonin shows promise and demonstrated reductions in bone resorption markers compared with calcium supplementation in a small study of multiple myeloma patients.[209]

The bisphosphonates make up a new class of drugs that inhibit osteoclast function. Several pilot studies showed effective blocking of bone resorption in patients with myeloma, as evidenced by decreased bone pain, decreased serum calcium, and decreased calcium and hydroxyproline excretion.[210, 211] The initial studies completed in multiple myeloma used relatively weak agents such as etidronate and clodronate. In the Canadian study involving etidronate, 166 patients were randomized to etidronate (5 mg/kg) or placebo in addition to primary chemotherapy with melphalan and prednisone.[116] No significant difference in clinically meaningful events such as new fractures, hypercalcemic episodes, and bone pain were noted between the two arms.

Three large randomized trials have been published using oral clodronate in myeloma patients. In the Finnish trial, 336 newly diagnosed and previously untreated patients were randomized to receive either clodronate (2.4 g) or placebo daily for 2 years.[212] All patients were also treated with intermittent oral melphalan and prednisolone. Patients treated with clodronate were less likely to have progression of lytic bone lesions (12%) compared with the placebo group

(24%) ($p = 0.026$). However, pathologic fractures, hypercalcemia, analgesic use, and pain index scores were not significantly different between the two arms.

Clodronate has also been evaluated in an open-label randomized German trial.[213] In this study, 170 previously untreated patients were randomized to receive oral clodronate (1.6 g) daily for 1 year in addition to chemotherapy. There was a trend toward a reduction in the number of new progressive sites in the clodronate-treated group after 6 ($p = 0.06$) and 12 ($p = 0.09$) months. Furthermore, the percentage of patients without pain and not using analgesics was higher in the treatment arm. However, there was no difference in bone disease progression, nor was there an improvement in performance status for the treated patients.

The Medical Research Council published the results of a large randomized trial involving 549 patients with recently diagnosed myeloma.[214] Patients received either 1.6 g/day of oral clodronate or placebo in addition to alkylator-based chemotherapy. Treated patients developed less hypercalcemia and nonvertebral fractures ($p = 0.021$). Back pain and poor performance status were not significantly different between the two groups except at one time point (24 months), and the proportion of patients requiring radiotherapy was similar between the two arms. Overall, these three studies suggest that oral clodronate has a mild to modest beneficial effect on bone pain and fracture development in multiple myeloma. Although there are advantages to oral administration, the poor and variable absorption (approximately 1%), high cost, and gastrointestinal side effects make the clinical benefit marginal for these patients.

Pamidronate is 100-fold and 10-fold more potent in preventing bone resorption in vitro when compared with etidronate and clodronate, respectively. In multiple myeloma patients, results of open-label trials lasting up to 24 months suggested that pamidronate disodium might be effective in reducing skeletal complications. Thus, a randomized, double-blind study was conducted to determine whether monthly 90-mg infusions of pamidronate compared with placebo reduced skeletal events in patients with multiple myeloma who were receiving chemotherapy.[215] Patients were eligible for enrollment if they had Durie-Salmon stage III multiple myeloma and at least one osteolytic lesion. The 392 patients were stratified into two groups: stratum 1 = first-line chemotherapy; and stratum 2 = patients with relapsed disease, who were then randomized to receive placebo or 90 mg of pamidronate. A total of 377 patients were evaluated for efficacy and after the preplanned initial time point of 9 months, the proportions of myeloma patients having a skeletal event was 41% in patients receiving placebo but only 24% in pamidronate-treated patients ($p < 0.001$). In addition, the number of skeletal events per year was reduced by approximately half in the patients treated with pamidronate ($p < 0.001$). The patients randomized to receive pamidronate also had significant decreases in bone pain and, in contrast with patients receiving the placebo, showed no deterioration in performance status and quality of life at the end of 9 months. These benefits continued for the remaining 12 months of the study. Although overall survival was not significantly different between the two treatment groups, the median survival time for the patients with more advanced disease (stratum 2 patients) was 21 months if they received

pamidronate versus 14 months for those on the placebo arm ($p = 0.04$).[216]

All the bisphosphonates are poorly absorbed orally (usually <1%). Similar to results with other oral bisphosphonates (see earlier discussion), oral pamidronate (300 mg/day) does not have a beneficial effect on skeletal complications in myeloma patients.[217] These drugs bind strongly to hydroxyapatite in bones and concentrate in areas where active bone remodeling occurs.[218] Once the drug becomes part of the bone that is not remodeling, it is biologically inactive. As a result, continued administration of bisphosphonates is required to achieve the desired lasting inhibition of bone resorption; we generally continue to administer these drugs to patients with multiple myeloma for the duration of their lives. Bisphosphonates are actively excreted by the kidneys and can cause renal insufficiency. This process appears to be related to dose and rate of infusion, with the newer, more potent generation of agents less likely to cause this toxicity because of the lower dosages required to achieve desirable clinical effects. Despite the possibility of toxicity, published results show the safety of infusing this agent monthly to patients with severe renal impairment.[219]

Evaluation of two other potent bisphosphonates has been completed as part of larger randomized clinical trials, and the results have been published in abstract form. In a randomized phase III trial, 198 patients with multiple myeloma who received monthly bolus injections of 2 mg of ibandronate did not have fewer skeletal events in comparison with patients who received a placebo. This poor result may have been due to an inadequate drug dose. Zoledronate appears to be the most potent bisphosphonate developed to date. It is at least 100 times as potent as pamidronate in mouse models and in one study was more effective at controlling hypercalcemia when compared with pamidronate. Trials comparing zoledronate at doses up to 8 mg to pamidronate as adjunctive treatment for multiple myeloma bone disease are currently under way.

In summary, these studies imply that bisphosphonates, and in particular intravenous (IV) pamidronate, can reduce the skeletal complications that occur in these patients and improve the quality of life. Whether patients with earlier stages of disease or patients without bone disease should be treated remains unclear. For these patients, we often use bone densitometry as a guide for treatment necessity. Nevertheless, there may be reasons to use these drugs in myeloma patients even when control of bone resorption is not essential. In vitro studies demonstrate that the bisphosphonates may possess direct antitumor properties. These drugs can induce apoptosis of myeloma cells[220] and suppress the production of IL-6 (an important myeloma growth factor) by bone marrow stromal cells from myeloma patients.[221] This may explain the prolonged survival that was seen in patients treated with pamidronate in the randomized IV study. Studies are currently under way to evaluate high-dose pamidronate (90 to 180 mg every 2 weeks) and zoledronate as monotherapy for patients with multiple myeloma to see if a direct antitumor effect can be demonstrated.

**Hypercalcemia.** Hypercalcemia occurs in approximately one third of all patients with myeloma and should be suspected in patients with symptoms of fatigue, constipation, polyuria, dehydration, nausea, or confusion. Myeloma patients with hypercalcemia should be treated aggressively because they are particularly prone to renal failure under these conditions. Rehydration with saline should begin to correct the dehydration induced by calciuresis and will also lower serum calcium levels in many patients. IV fluids should not be the sole means of therapy, however, as the condition will rapidly recur in most patients if the underlying causative factors are not alleviated. Corticosteroids (e.g., prednisone, 60 to 100 mg/day) are frequently beneficial because of a tumoricidal effect on the myeloma cells and their inhibitory effects on OAFs such as IL-1β.[125, 222] Calcitonin is frequently effective and has the advantage of a more rapid onset of action (2 to 4 hours) when compared with other available therapies. The salmon form of the drug is given subcutaneously at a dose of 4 IU/kg every 12 hours but can be associated with allergic reactions, and tachyphylaxis limits its long-term benefit. Since it is only of modest benefit, calcitonin should never be relied on as the sole mode of treatment. Bisphosphonates provide the mainstay of treatment, and a single infusion of 90 mg of pamidronate leads to normocalcemia in most patients after 4 to 5 days.[223] Repeated doses can be given every other week if necessary to maintain normocalcemia. Zoledronate is currently under Food and Drug Administration review for approval in patients with tumor-induced hypercalcemia based on data showing its superiority to pamidronate in a randomized phase III study. Inorganic phosphates are too toxic for routine parenteral use but can be administered orally in patients with hypophosphatemia. Mithramycin and gallium nitrate are other drugs that could be used in resistant patients. It is important that chemotherapy not be delayed because of hypercalcemia since a good response to antitumor therapy is the most important factor in maintaining normal calcium levels.

**Infection.** The best means of preventing infectious complications is by achieving a good remission. Patients experiencing objective responses to chemotherapy have a decreased risk of infection for the duration of their response.[137] In addition, the depressed levels of polyclonal Ig may resolve with successful therapy.[224] Infection should be treated aggressively, but nephrotoxic antibiotics should be avoided if other effective alternatives are available. Three studies have shown that patients with myeloma have a poor overall response to polyvalent pneumococcal vaccination.[225–227] However, up to 30% of patients demonstrate potentially protective antibody titers to some pneumococcal serotypes.[225] Because there are few serious side effects from the immunization, it is recommended that pneumococcal vaccination be administered to patients with myeloma.

For patients with recurrent bacterial infections, replacement therapy with monthly IV immunoglobulin can be extremely beneficial. One randomized study demonstrated a significant reduction in serious infections for patients receiving IV IgG. Monthly doses of 500 mg/kg are recommended.

**Renal Insufficiency.** Prevention of dehydration and hypotension, rapid correction of hypercalcemia and hyperuricemia, treatment of infections, and caution in the use of nephrotoxic antibiotics and IV pyelography are all important measures for preserving renal function in patients with myeloma. Patients with high tumor mass should be given allopurinol for the first few cycles of therapy, and all patients should maintain high fluid intake. In many cases (39 of 49 in a previous study), renal failure can be at least partially

corrected if the tumor is responsive to therapy and adequate hydration is maintained. We favor the use of VAD (vincristine, Adriamycin [doxorubicin], dactinomycin) in a newly diagnosed patient with renal failure. Since these agents do not need adjustment for renal disease and the regimen is one of the most rapidly effective, most patients can avoid permanent dialysis if treated quickly. Plasmapheresis has also proved useful in some studies of patients with acute renal failure.[228–230] The prompt removal of the pathogenic light chains may be particularly helpful in patients with an acute onset of renal failure. Peritoneal dialysis is also capable of removing light chains and has been used successfully in several patients with acute renal failure and myeloma,[231] although it is much less efficient.[232]

Long-term hemodialysis in some patients with myeloma and chronic renal failure has been used advantageously.[233] In the rare patient who has an excellent response to chemotherapy, with reversal of all symptoms except renal failure, renal transplantation can be considered.[234] One must be confident that light chain production has been sufficiently reduced so that the transplanted kidney will not become affected with light chain nephropathy.

### Chemotherapy

**General Principles.** With the technology available for determining the in vitro synthetic rate of paraprotein per myeloma cell, the total body tumor cell mass can be estimated.[235] Studies using these techniques demonstrate that patients presenting with myeloma usually have a tumor cell burden of $10^{11}$ to $10^{12}$ cells. They also suggest that myeloma tumor cell growth follows gompertzian kinetics.[236] The initial doubling time may be short (2 to 3 days), but as the clone grows to a mass of approximately $10^{11}$ to $10^{12}$ cells, the doubling time becomes longer and the growth slows down.

During successful induction therapy, there is a rapid decrease in tumor cell mass. After reaching a certain level, usually 1 or 2 logs lower than the original tumor mass, the disease enters a plateau phase in which continuing chemotherapy has no effect on tumor mass. Although the growth fraction of the tumor increases after induction chemotherapy,[237] it has been shown that for the majority of patients, this increase may not persist into the plateau phase[238] and, in fact, the tumor does not grow during this phase. It is not known what factors control tumor cell proliferation during the plateau phase.

The pattern of frequent initial responses but virtually no cures that is seen in myeloma patients treated with chemotherapy suggests the emergence of drug resistance as a major obstacle to successful treatment. In vitro studies suggest resistance to chemotherapy may be due to decreased cellular uptake,[239] protection by intracellular glutathione,[240] increased efflux from target cells,[241, 242] resistance to Fas-mediated apoptosis,[243] mutations of the glucocorticoid receptor,[244] or an enhanced DNA repair mechanism.[245] Most of the current therapeutic attempts to disrupt tumor resistance have focused on P-glycoprotein inhibition. This protein pump is responsible for drug efflux of numerous chemotherapeutic agents (most notably doxorubicin) from plasma cells. Unfortunately, this protein may be inherently active on plasma cells even prior to malignant transformation. In one study, P-glycoprotein expression was noted on plasma cells derived from 42 of 43 patients with MGUS, myeloma, and amyloidosis.[246] Nevertheless, the recurrent administration of pulse doses of chemotherapeutic drugs often selects for the most resistant clones.[247] Patients with progressive disease are often found to have plasma cells with high P-glycoprotein expression.[248, 249] Verapamil and quinine can block P-glycoprotein function and have been tested for activity in clinical trials. Unfortunately, neither of these drugs was found to improve outcome compared with standard chemotherapy regimens when used alone or in combination.[250–252] Third-generation agents, most notably PSC-833,[253] are currently undergoing clinical trials.[254, 255]

### Individual Chemotherapy Agents

*Corticosteroids.* The corticosteroids are the most important drug class in the treatment of multiple myeloma. Steroids can induce the apoptotic death of myeloma cells in culture[62] and also have secondary beneficial effects on hematopoiesis, hypercalcemia, bone disease (secondary to inhibitory effects on OAFs), and renal function. Dexamethasone also inhibits the autocrine production of IL-6, the predominant growth factor for multiple myeloma.[256, 257]

The beneficial effects of this class of drug have been demonstrated in numerous randomized trials. Prednisone, when added to melphalan as primary therapy, reproducibly prolongs patient survival (Table 99–5).[258] In fact, monotherapy with high-dose steroids (dexamethasone 20 mg/m² daily for 4 days every 2 weeks) provided response rates only 15% less than seen with VAD combination chemotherapy and was associated with similar overall survival in a randomized trial.[259] In fact, high-dose dexamethasone is currently the most active single agent in the treatment of myeloma. Since there is no long-term hematologic toxicity from steroid ther-

apy, the use of steroids may be the treatment of choice for many patients with multiple myeloma.[260] Steroids also have a key role in the maintenance of plateau phase, as is discussed further on.

*Alkylating Agents.* The alkylating agents are also effective as chemotherapeutic agents.[261]

MELPHALAN. Of these drugs, melphalan is the most widely used and the most intensively studied. Response rates (defined as a 50 to 75% reduction in M spike) with melphalan therapy range from 20 to 50% in various studies, whereas median survival approximates 2 years.[258] For responders, median survival is 30 months, and in one series 2.2% of patients survived 10 years or longer.[262] Melphalan is usually administered orally, 0.25 mg/kg/day for 4 days, and repeated every 4 to 6 weeks.[263] Patients can also be treated with continuous daily administration of melphalan, and although the response rate is lower compared with pulse intermittent schedules, survival is comparable (see Table 99–5).[258]

There is variability in the absorption of orally administered melphalan,[264, 265] and the results of one study suggested that IV administration produces a greater antitumor effect.[182] However, follow-up studies have disputed this notion.[183] Because the absorption of melphalan is variable, the hemogram should be followed to ensure that at least a moderate degree of myelotoxicity occurs during chemotherapy. To ensure adequate dosing, the daily oral dosage should be increased by 20% increments every cycle until the absolute neutrophil count reaches a nadir of 1000 to 2000 cells/$\mu$L or thrombocytopenia ($<100,000/\mu$L) develops. High-dose melphalan (140 to 200 mg/kg) is the cornerstone of most autologous transplantation regimens and is discussed later in this chapter.

*Table 99–5.* **Randomized Studies of Induction Chemotherapy: Melphalan, Cyclophosphamide, and Prednisone**

| Author | Study | Doses | % Response | | Median Survival (Months) | |
|--------|-------|-------|------------|--|--------------------------|--|
| Alexanian[258] | (1) M, continuous | Melph, 0.025 mg/kg/day | 17 | | 18 | |
| | vs. | | | | | |
| | (2) M, intermittent | Melph, 0.25 mg/kg/day × 4, q 4 wk | 32* | | 18 | |
| | vs. | | | | | |
| | (3) M + P | Melph as in (2); pred, 2 mg/kg/day × 4, q 4 wk | 60* | | 24* | |
| MRC[266] | (1) M, continuous | Melph, 4 mg/day | — | | 23 | |
| | vs. | | | | | |
| | (2) C, continuous | Ctx, 150 mg/day | — | | 27 | |
| MRC[505] | (1) C, continuous | Ctx, 150 mg/day | — | | | |
| | vs. | | | | approx. 20 mo | |
| | (2) M, intermittent | Melph, 10 mg/day × 4–7 days, q 6 wk | — | | | |
| | vs. | | | | | |
| | (3) M + P | Melph as in (2); pred, 40 mg/day × 4–7 days, q 6 wk | — | | | |
| Ahre[315] | (1) M | Melph, 0.07 mg/kg/day × 3 wk; rest 1–2 wk; continue at 1–2 mg/day | 31* | | 29† | |
| | vs. | | | | | |
| | (2) M + P | Melph, 0.25 mg/kg/day × 4 days; pred, 2 mg/kg/day × 4 days } repeat q 6 wk | 45* | | 36† | |

| | | | GR | PR | GR | PR |
|--|--|--|----|----|----|----|
| Costa[314] | (1) M | Melph, 0.15 mg/kg/day × 7 days; rest; then, 0.05 mg/kg/day | 23* | 28 | 30* | 21* |
| | vs. | | | | | |
| | (2) M + P | Melph, as in (1); pred, 1.25 mg/kg/day × 2 wk, then gradual taper over 8 wk | 55* | 31 | 53* | 9* |

*Groups significantly different from each other, $p<0.05$.
†$p<0.05$ only for stage I and II patients.
M, Melph, melphalan; P, pred, prednisone; C, Ctx, cyclophosphamide; MRC, Medical Research Council Working Party on Leukemia (United Kingdom); GR, good risk; PR, poor risk.

CYCLOPHOSPHAMIDE. The antitumor effect of cyclophosphamide (Cytoxan) has been confirmed in a number of studies. Randomized trials of continuous cyclophosphamide versus continuous melphalan therapy have shown no significant difference in response rate or survival (see Table 99–5).[266] One potential advantage for cyclophosphamide over melphalan is that the latter drug is more toxic to resting cells. Thus, the prolonged use of melphalan may be more damaging to the resting stem cell compartment, making future therapy more difficult. Initial reports suggested that cyclophosphamide had efficacy in patients who were resistant to melphalan,[267] but later studies have not confirmed these findings.[268, 269] Most investigators feel that there is significant cross-resistance between melphalan and cyclophosphamide, and the latter drug is usually ineffective in truly melphalan-resistant patients. One regimen using weekly pulse doses of cyclophosphamide (200 to 300 mg/m²—500 mg maximum) coupled with prednisone 50 mg every other day can be effective and is well tolerated, even in elderly patients.[270] High-dose cyclophosphamide can also be effective for refractory patients,[271] and this agent is also used in many preparative regimens for autologous transplantation.[272]

CHLORAMBUCIL. This drug appears to have antitumor effects in patients with myeloma.[273] Compared with melphalan, however, response rates are lower, even though survival rates are similar.

*Nitrosoureas.* IV bis-chloroethyl-nitrosourea (BCNU, carmustine) in a dose of 150 mg/m² every 6 weeks with prednisone produced a response rate and duration of survival similar to those of melphalan and prednisone in previously untreated patients.[274] However, in a more recent study,[275] the combination of melphalan and prednisone was superior to either BCNU and prednisone or chloroethyl cyclohexylnitrosourea (CCNU, lomustine) and prednisone in producing objective responses and in prolonging survival in good-risk patients.

*Procarbazine.* Procarbazine has demonstrated good antitumor activity[276] but has not been used extensively as a single agent in this disease.

*Anthracyclines.* Doxorubicin has been used as a single agent in melphalan-resistant myeloma and has shown antitumor activity.[277] This drug is most commonly used in combination with other agents, such as vincristine in the VAD regimen. Idarubicin has demonstrated modest activity either alone or in combination with dexamethasone and has the advantage of an available oral formulation.[278, 279]

*Vinca Alkaloids.* Although response rates are increased by approximately 15% when vincristine is included in multiagent combinations (compared with melphalan and prednisone-treated historical controls; see SWOG studies under the section Multiagent Combination Chemotherapy), the specific contribution of vincristine is unclear. In a randomized trial by the British Medical Research Council's Working Party,[280] the addition of vincristine to melphalan and prednisone induction therapy offered no survival benefit. Furthermore, vincristine as a single agent given by continuous infusion to alkylator-refractory patients is ineffective.[281] Vinblastine appears to be inactive in myeloma. Although an initial report[282] indicated significant responses in melphalan-resistant patients treated with vindesine and prednisone, a follow-up study by Alexanian and colleagues[283] demonstrated that efficacy was due to the high-dose prednisone, as

vindesine alone was ineffective. A second study detected a 17% response rate when resistant patients were treated with vindesine, melphalan, cyclophosphamide, and prednisone.[284] Single-agent vinorelbine (Navelbine) yields occasional but brief responses in our experience.

*Interferons.* Interferon alfa is probably the most widely studied drug in multiple myeloma. Studies have demonstrated up to a 50% response rate in untreated patients with myeloma.[285] However, in more recent randomized studies comparing interferon alfa to chemotherapy in untreated patients, response rates of only 14 to 36% were reported.[286, 287] In these two reports, interferon seemed to be more effective in IgA than IgG myeloma. Studies on previously treated refractory patients are even less promising. Response rates range between 11 and 21%,[288, 289] and remission duration tends to be short, although approximately 30% of responders (only 5% of treated patients) may achieve relatively long remission.[290] The mechanism of action remains unclear, but in vitro it can induce apoptosis in cell lines[291] and decrease the tumor labeling index, self-renewal capacity, and M protein secretion in other studies.[292] This latter point is important because the M protein is often the sole marker used to assess tumor response. Since interferon alfa can suppress M protein excretion directly, an apparent response may, in fact, not correspond to an actual reduction in tumor cell burden. This feature clouds the interpretation of some studies. Paradoxically, a growth-promoting effect is occasionally noted in vitro.[291, 293] We have witnessed this phenomenon in occasional patients, particularly after transplantation. Induction of stimulatory cytokines may lead to this paradoxical effect.[294] There is probably a dose-response curve, because in a retrospective analysis of one trial the median dose given to partially responding patients was 12 MU/day compared with only 6.5 MU/day given to the minimally responsive and nonresponding patients.[295] Overall, the toxicity and expense of this agent make it of little value in the initial management of multiple myeloma patients.

*Thalidomide.* Barlogie and colleagues in Arkansas used thalidomide to treat a multiple myeloma patient who was refractory to numerous salvage chemotherapy regimens; they achieved a dramatic response. The drug was given based on publicity surrounding the beneficial effects of antiangiogenesis medications in oncology. A phase II trial was subsequently performed, and 32% of the patients treated with thalidomide achieved a response.[296] The drug was started at 200 mg/day and escalated every 2 weeks to a maximum of 800 mg/day. Side effects were common and consisted of sedation, constipation, and neuropathy. Since this seminal publication, thalidomide has become a widely used agent in the treatment of multiple myeloma. In addition to antiangiogenic effects, the drug also suppresses TNF[297] and IL-12[298] and alters the expression of other cytokines as well. It remains unclear which of these actions is most important in multiple myeloma. Even smaller doses of thalidomide have been useful, and we and others have found doses as low as 50 mg per day to be effective.[299] In our own experience, the combination of steroids and thalidomide seems particularly active. This has also been noticed by Alexanian's group.[300] Newer agents have been developed that will, hopefully, improve the activity and lessen some of the side effects associated with this medication. These drugs are currently in phase I and II trials.

***Other Agents.*** The plant alkaloid acronine,[301] high-dose cytosine arabinoside,[302] etoposide,[303] fludarabine,[304] and paclitaxel[305, 306] have little efficacy in multiple myeloma. Peptichemio, an agent popular in Europe, can produce a significant antitumor effect,[307] even in pretreated resistant patients.[308] The CD20 antigen is only rarely expressed by myeloma cells but rituximab (Rituxan) can be useful for patients with tumors that express this antigen.[309]

**Combination Chemotherapy.** Multiple studies have used combination chemotherapy in an attempt to improve response rates and survival. Many of these studies have used historical controls. This may be particularly misleading in myeloma because most patients succumb to medical complications, and the management of these complications has improved substantially over the past 15 years. Improvements in salvage therapy of patients refractory to initial agents also complicates the use of historical controls. Good examples of this phenomenon are (1) the increased survival of patients treated similarly with melphalan and prednisone as control

arms of Cancer and Leukemia Group B (CALGB) protocols from 1972 to 1977[310, 311] and (2) the increased median survival (from 28 to 36 months) of patients treated identically with BCNU, cyclophosphamide, and prednisone by the Southeastern Cancer Study Group between 1972 and 1976.[208] For these reasons, we have emphasized randomized, prospective studies of induction therapy (Tables 99–6 and 99–7; see also Table 99–5).

***Melphalan and Prednisone.*** The combination of melphalan and prednisone is considered optimal therapy by many oncologists, especially for the elderly and patients with minimal disease.[312, 313] The addition of prednisone to melphalan increases response rates and appears to prolong survival by 6 to 9 months, although this difference has not always reached statistical significance (18 months vs. 24 months in one study[258] and 26 months vs. 35 months in another[314]). Similar conclusions were drawn from a randomized trial from the Myeloma Group of Central Sweden.[315] The median survival was again increased in the combination therapy

*Table 99–6.* **Randomized Studies of Induction: Combination Chemotherapy Versus Melphalan and Prednisone**

| Author | Study | Dose | % Response | Median Survival |
|---|---|---|---|---|
| Pavlovsky[323] | MPCCV | (M 8 mg/m²/day × 4 days; P 40 mg/m²/day × 7 days; C 600 mg/m² × 1; V 0.6 mg/m² × 1) q 4 wk + methyl-CCNU 100 mg/m² × 1 q 8 wk | 69 | 43 |
| | M + P | M 8 mg/m²/day × 4 days; P 40 mg/m²/day × 7 days | 58 | 43 |
| Pavlovsky[506] | MeCP | (C 600 mg/m²; P 40 mg/m²/day × 7 days) q 4 wk + methyl-CCNU 100 mg/m² q 8 wk | 67 | 32 |
| | M + P | M 8 mg/m²/day × 4 days; P 40 mg/m²/day × 7 days | 62 | 32 |
| Palva[317] | MOCCA | V 0.03 mg/kg × 1 day; CCNU, 40 mg × 1 day; M 0.25 mg/kg/day × 4 days; Mp 0.8 mg/kg/day × 7 days; C 10 mg/kg × 1 day | 75 | 41 |
| | M + P | M 9–12 mg/m²/day × 4 days; P 1 mg/kg/day × 4 days | 54 | 45 |
| Salmon[274] | VMCP/VBAP | VMCP = [V 1 mg/m² + (M 6 mg/m²; C 125 mg/m²; P 60 mg/m²) × 4 days] q 3 wk VBAP = [V 1 mg/m²; B 30 mg/m²; A 30 mg/m²; P 60 mg/m²/day × 4 days] q 3 wk | 53 | 43 |
| | M + P | M 8 mg/m²/day × 4 days; P 60 mg/m²/day × 4 days | 32 | 23 |
| Abramson[507] | BCP | B 75 mg/m²; C 400 mg/m²; P 75 mg/m²/day × 7 days | 50 | 25 |
| | M + P | M 8 mg/m²/day × 4 days; P 75 mg/day × 7 days | 43 | 19 |
| Harley[508] | BCMP | [M 8 mg/m²; C 300 mg/m²; B 100 mg/m²] q 6 wk + P 1–2 mg/kg/day × 7 days; tapered over 10 wk | 68 | 25 |
| | M + P | M 0.15 mg/kg/day × 7 days then L-PAM 0.05 mg/kg/day; P 1–2 mg/kg/day × 7 days; tapered over 10 wk | 56 | 25 |
| Cohen[208] | BCP | B 75 mg/m²; C 400 mg/m²; P 75 mg/day × 7 days | 49 | 36 |
| | M + P | M 8 mg/m²/day × 4 days; P 75 mg/day × 7 days | 52 | 36 |
| Cooper[328] | MCBP | M 8 mg/m²; C 300 mg/m²; B 100 mg/m²; P 0.8 mg/kg/day × 14 days and taper over 4 wk | 43 | 29 |
| | MCBPA | M 8 mg/m²; C 300 mg/m²; B 100 mg/m²; A 45 mg/m² q 100 days beginning day 85; P 0.8 mg/kg/day × 14 days and taper over 4 wk | 38 | 26 |
| | M + P | M 16 mg/m² on days 1, 15, 29, 43, and q 28 days thereafter; P 0.8 mg/kg/day × 14 days and taper over 4 wk | 40 | 34 |
| Boccadoro[509] | VMCP/VBAP | VMCP = [V 1 mg + (M 6 mg/m²; P 60 mg/m²; C 120 mg/m²) × 7 days] q 4 wk VBAP = (V 1 mg; A 30 mg/m²; B 30 mg/m²; P 60 mg/m²/day × 7 days) q 4 wk | 59 | 32 |
| | M + P | M 6 mg/m²/day × 7 days; P 60 mg/m²/day × 7 days | 47 | 37 |
| Tribalto[327] | VMCP | (V 1 mg; M 6 mg/m²/day × 7; C 125 mg/m²/day × 7; P 60 mg/m²/day × 7 days) q mo | 46 | 45 |
| | M + P | (M 0.1 mg/kg/day × 7 days; P 40 mg/m²/day × 7 days) q mo | 35 | 30 |
| Peest[510] | VCMP | [(M 5 mg/m²; C 100 mg/m²; P 60 mg/m²) × 4 days + V 1 mg] q 4 wk | 33 | 42 |
| | M + P | M 8 mg/m²/day × 4 days; P 60 mg/m²/day × 4 days | 33 | 50 |
| Hjorth[511] | VCMP or VCMP/VBAP | VCMP = [(M 5 mg/m²; C 100 mg/m²; P 60 mg/m²) × 4 days + V 1 mg] q 4 wk VBAP = (V 1 mg; B 30 mg/m²; A 30 mg/m², P 60 mg/m² day × 4 days) q 4 wk | 56 | 27 |
| | M + P | (M 0.25 mg/kg/day × 4 days + P 2 mg/kg/day × 4 days) q 6 wk | 62 | 33 |
| Blade[330] | VCMP/VBAP | VBAP as above; VCMP = (V 1 mg; C 500 mg/m²; M 6 mg/m²/day × 4 days; P 60 mg/m²/day × 4 days) q 4 wk | 63 | 32 |
| | M + P | (M 9 mg/m²/day × 4 days; P 60 mg/m²/day × 4 days) q 4 wk | 52 | 27 |
| Keldsen[512] | NOP | (Mitoxantrone 16 mg/m²; V 2 mg/m²; Mp 250 mg/day days 1–4 and 17–20) q 4 wk | 60 | 14 |
| | M + P | (M 0.25 mg/kg/day × 4 days; Mp ~150 mg/day × 4 days) q 4 wk | 64 | 31 |

Only randomized trials with a minimum of 100 enrolled patients are included. Survival is in months. Response rates between different studies are not directly comparable because of patient selection and different criteria for response.

M, melphalan; P, prednisone; B, BCNU (carmustine); C, cyclophosphamide; V, vincristine; Mp, methylprednisolone; A, Adriamycin (doxorubicin).

*Table 99–7.* **Randomized Studies of Induction Chemotherapy: Combination Chemotherapy Versus Non-Melphalan/Prednisone Regimens**

| Author | Study | Dose | % Response | Median Survival |
|--------|-------|------|------------|-----------------|
| Durie[329] | VMCP/VBAP + Lev | VMCP × 3 cycles then VBAP × 3 cycles per Table 99–8 + Lev 50 mg QID days 8, 9, 15, 16 | 44 | 33 |
| | VMCP/VBAP − Lev | VMCP × 3 cycles then VBAP × 3 cycles per Table 99–8 | 54 | 48 |
| | VCP + Lev | V 1 mg day 1; C 180 mg/m²/day × 4 days; P 60 mg/m²/day × 4 + Lev 50 mg QID days 8, 9, 15, 16 | 28 | 26 |
| | VCP − Lev | V 1 mg day 1; C 180 mg/m²/day × 4 days; P 60 mg/m²/d × 4 | 28 | 29 |
| MRC V[513] | ABCM | [A 30 mg/m² day 1; B 30 mg/m² day 1; C 100 mg/m²/day; M 6 mg/m²/day days 22–25] q 6 wk | 61 | 32 |
| | M7 | M 7 mg/m² PO × 4 days q 3 wk | 59 | 24 |

Survival is reported in months.
PO, by mouth; A, Adriamycin; B, BCNU (carmustine); C, cyclophosphamide; M, melphalan; Lev, levamisole; P, prednisone.

group (36 months vs. 29 months), but this difference did not achieve statistical significance. In the study by Costa,[314] the addition of prednisone improved survival in good-risk patients but reduced survival in poor-risk patients. A trial evaluating substitution of prednisone with high-dose dexamethasone is warranted to determine if the improved response rates with increased steroid doses will translate into further survival improvement.

**Multiagent Combination Chemotherapy.** In an attempt to improve the 50% response rates with melphalan and prednisone, and hopefully affect overall survival, more intensive chemotherapy regimens have been devised that incorporate multiple active agents. Phase II studies using various regimens have frequently demonstrated improvement in the rapidity and duration of response and have suggested overall improvements in survival.

The M-2 protocol of the Sloan-Kettering Cancer Center uses melphalan, cyclophosphamide, prednisone, BCNU, and vincristine in 5-week cycles.[316] The reported response rate obtained with this regimen was 87% in 46 previously untreated patients, with a median survival time of more than 50 months. These results are better than those achieved with any other protocol. However, the study has been criticized for the following reasons: It was a uni-institutional, uncontrolled study; the patients may have been selected for good performance status because the mean age was low and few patients experienced early death; and survival was computed from diagnosis rather than treatment. Nevertheless, nonrandomized studies from other institutions have presented similar results with the M-2 protocol.[317–320] In general, most studies have computed survival from onset of treatment and patients appeared less selected, as determined by performance status and mortality during the first 12 to 15 months. However, when the M-2 regimen has been compared in randomized studies, response rates are occasionally better but survival has not been prolonged compared with that achieved with melphalan and prednisone.[321–323]

Only a few studies have demonstrated a survival benefit based on the choice of induction chemotherapy. The Southwest Oncology Group (SWOG) conducted a series of studies with multiagent combination chemotherapy.[324, 325] In general, response rates were increased by approximately 15% when vincristine was included in the regimen and the drugs were administered every 3 weeks instead of every 6 weeks. These protocols were associated with a survival advantage of approximately 5 to 7 months, but they suffered from the use of historical controls. Later, the SWOG compared melphalan and prednisone with alternating combinations of multiagent chemotherapy in a randomized trial.[326] The combination therapy using vincristine, doxorubicin, prednisone, and alkylating agents induced a response more frequently than did melphalan and prednisone (53% vs. 32%) and resulted in a survival advantage (median survival 43 months vs. 23 months for all patients). When analyzed by pretreatment prognostic factors, however, a significant survival advantage was detected only in patients with stage III disease who did not have severe hypercalcemia or impaired renal function. A major criticism of this study is that melphalan and prednisone were administered every third week instead of every sixth week, and treatment cycles may have been delayed or omitted because of cytopenias that peaked at 3 weeks. An additional problem is that the median survival of the control melphalan and prednisone group (23 months) is somewhat lower (30 to 36 months) than that obtained by other investigators.[208, 315, 321, 327, 328]

This SWOG study remains the only study showing a statistically significant advantage in survival between combination chemotherapy and MP. The fifth Medical Research Council trial also showed an improvement in overall survival using ABCM (Adriamycin [doxorubicin], carmustine, cyclophosphamide, melphalan), but this was compared with melphalan alone (median survival 32 months vs. 24 months). Because the addition of prednisone to melphalan has also shown a 6- to 9-month improvement in survival,[315, 324] it is unlikely that the ABCM regimen is significantly better than MP. A randomized SWOG study comparing VCP (vincristine, cyclophosphamide, prednisone) versus alternating cycles of VMCP (vincristine, melphalan, cyclophosphamide, prednisone) and VBAP (vincristine, BCNU, Adriamycin [doxorubicin], prednisone) demonstrated improved response rates and overall median survival (29 months vs. 48 months) for the alternating schedule.[329] However, this latter regimen has been compared by a number of groups with standard melphalan and prednisone chemotherapy in randomized trials and has not improved survival. The most recent study comparing VCMP/VBAP to MP analyzed 449 randomized patients and found higher response rates in the alternating regimen (63% vs. 52%) but no significant difference in survival (32 months vs. 27 months).[330] Finally, in 1992 a meta-analysis was performed on the 18 trials comparing MP with combination chemotherapy and included outcomes from 3814 patients.[331] Equivalent 2-year survival rates were noted (57.5% for MP regimens vs. 55.5% for combination regimens). Subgroup analysis implied improved results with MP when given to good-prognosis patients, and there is a suggestion from the meta-analysis and the Spanish study[330] that combination chemotherapy is better for patients with IgA myeloma. Explanations for these findings are not obvious,[332] and therefore these results will need prospective confirmation by a future trial. A more recent analysis looked at 27 trials that randomized more than 6500 patients with multiple myeloma between combination chemotherapy and MP.[333] No significant survival advantage was noted between the groups. Subgroup analysis also failed to detect survival advantages based on dose intensity or patient performance status. Nevertheless, some investigators argue that the more aggressive combination chemotherapy regimens lead to greater early toxicity but better long-term survival. In an Eastern Cooperative Oncology Group study (E2479), patients were randomized to VBMCP (vincristine, BCNU, melphalan, cyclophosphamide, prednisone) versus MP.[321] Median survival was no different between groups (29 months for VBMCP vs. 27 months for MP), but the percentage of patients alive at 5 years was slightly higher for the more aggressively treated group (26% vs. 19%). These authors argue that for patients who can tolerate the chemotherapy initially, there could be a modest long-term benefit from this more aggressive regimen. Similar arguments have been made by other respected investigators.[334]

Other randomized trials have been performed without MP as the control arm. In a SWOG study published in 1994, 522 previously untreated multiple myeloma patients were randomized to three chemotherapy regimens with differing glucocorticoid intensities.[335] Patients randomized to receive VAD or VMCP/VBAP plus alternate-day prednisone at 50 mg every other day had improved survival compared with patients receiving the standard VMCP/VBAP regimen. Median survival times were 35 and 40 months for the steroid-intensive arms, respectively, compared with 31 months for the standard VMCP/VBAP regimen ($p = 0.02$). This beneficial effect of glucocorticoids was comparable to that noted in trials comparing melphalan alone with melphalan plus prednisone discussed earlier. In addition, trials with maintenance prednisone have also shown beneficial effects on survival, as is discussed later.

Because of its efficacy as a single agent and different mechanism of action, natural interferon was combined with MP[336] in a randomized study of stage II and stage III patients to assess response rate and overall survival. Although response rates were higher (68% vs. 42%), especially in patients with IgA myeloma (85%), the addition of $7 \times 10^6$ IU/m²/day of natural alfa-interferon (given days 1 to 5 and 22 to 26 of a 42-day cycle) did not increase overall survival. Two other randomized studies showed no benefit of adding alfa interferon to MP with respect to response rates or survival.[249, 337] One more recent study demonstrated improved progression-free (23 months vs. 16 months) and overall survival times (39 months vs. 30 months) for patients randomized to receive alfa interferon in addition to VMCP, but these differences were not statistically significant.[338] In summary, alfa interferon may improve response rates for patients with multiple myeloma but at considerable expense

and morbidity that does not translate into a meaningful prolongation in survival. Therefore, its use cannot be recommended in the initial management of most multiple myeloma patients.

**High-Dose Chemotherapy with Bone Marrow Transplantation.** Because myeloma is sensitive to cytotoxic agents in most patients, dose-intensive chemotherapy with marrow transplantation has been used in an attempt to induce complete remission and improve disease-free survival.[339–341]

*Allogeneic Transplantation.* Initial trials focused on the use of allogeneic bone marrow transplantation, and more than 200 have been performed worldwide to date.[342] An early review of the European Group for Bone Marrow Transplantation experience[343] demonstrated a high rate of CRs, 39 of 67 cases after transplantation. The likelihood of achieving a CR correlated inversely with the number of prior chemotherapy regimens given (61% if only one previous regimen was given, 31% if three or more regimens had been administered). In addition, advanced stage at diagnosis predicted for lower CR rates (79% stage I, 37% stage II or stage III). As would be expected, patients achieving a CR had improved survival rates, and survival was not dependent on age. Long-term survival was 36% (60% in patients attaining CR after transplant) in an updated analysis of these results.[344] The Seattle experience using allogeneic transplantation was similar.[345] Eighty patients underwent transplantation in this study, most using sibling HLA-matched donors. Thirty-five patients (44%) died of transplant-related causes within 100 days, and the overall survival rate was 24% at 4.5 years. In a multivariate analysis, some adverse risk factors for outcome end points included transplantation more than 1 year from diagnosis; serum $\beta_2$-microglobulin levels greater than 2.5 mg/L at transplantation; female transplant recipients receiving transplants from male donors; patients who had received more than eight cycles of chemotherapy before transplantation, and Durie stage III disease at the time of transplantation. In both studies, there appeared to be a few patients who achieved long disease-free survival, suggesting possible curative treatment. In fact, two patients treated with syngeneic transplants remained free of disease 12 and 14 years after transplantation, although detectable monoclonal proteins remained. However, because of treatment-related mortality, allogeneic transplantation is typically limited to patients younger than age 55 who also have an HLA-identical sibling. Because myeloma is a disease of the elderly, less than 5% of all patients would be eligible for this procedure. Given the 40 to 50% transplant-related mortality[346, 347] we are reluctant to perform this procedure even though there may be a small percentage of patients with long-term disease-free survival. If treatment-related mortality can be improved by the use of nonmyeloablative regimens now undergoing clinical trials,[348] this procedure may become more acceptable.

*Syngeneic Transplantation.* In contrast, the beneficial outcome for patients treated with syngeneic transplantation has been corroborated.[349] The median overall survival time of 73 months was significantly better for patients who received a syngeneic transplant when compared with matching patients receiving autologous or allogeneic transplants (each < 44 months). Progression-free survival time was prolonged as well in these patients (median = 72 months) and was comparable to that obtained for patients following allogeneic transplantation who survive the initial treatment. Therefore, for those few patients with an available identical twin, syngeneic transplantation in multiple myeloma appears to be the treatment of choice.

*Autologous Transplantation.* Myeloablative chemotherapy with autologous transplantation is now widely performed for patients with multiple myeloma and has become part of the standard of care for patients with advanced disease who are younger than 65 years. Nonetheless, the potential problems of autologous transplantation include the following: First, even with high doses of chemotherapy and radiation, the myeloma cell clone may be difficult to eliminate. Second, both the bone marrow and the peripheral blood are involved by the disease, so tumor cells will be reinfused after conditioning chemotherapy. Third, there is no potentially beneficial graft-versus-myeloma effect. Initial trials were developed in patients with advanced and refractory disease. Although cytoreduction was achieved, progression-free survival was short. Factors predictive for poor outcome included chemotherapy-resistant disease[350] and prolonged exposure to alkylator-containing regimens.[351] To avoid these risks, patients were treated earlier in the disease course, and apparently beneficial outcomes were noted in phase II studies.[352–356]

To prove benefit, randomized trials are required; thus, a large phase III study was initiated in France comparing standard doses of chemotherapy with autologous transplantation.[357, 358] Two hundred patients with stage II or stage III multiple myeloma received an initial 4 months of VMCP alternating with VBAP. Patients were then randomized to receive an additional 8 months of chemotherapy or 140 mg/m$^2$ of melphalan plus total-body irradiation followed by autologous bone marrow transplantation. The study was analyzed on an intent-to-treat analysis even though only 74 of the 100 patients assigned to high-dose therapy actually received the autologous bone marrow transplant. As might be expected, response rates were higher for the more aggressive approach (CR = 22% vs. 5%, partial response (PR) + CR = 81% vs. 57% respectively). Event-free survival (EFS) was also prolonged in the patients randomized to transplantation (median EFS = 27 months vs. 18 months). Overall survival was improved for these patients as well. Five-year survival was only 12% for the patients who received standard chemotherapy yet was 57% for the patients who were randomized to autologous transplantation. This difference was statistically significant and was most pronounced in the subgroup of patients younger than age 60. A more recent update of this study continues to demonstrate a doubling of overall survival after 5 years.

This study has been criticized because the outcome for patients receiving standard chemotherapy is poor. Two other trials have looked at outcome for standard chemotherapy when compared with autologous transplantation.[359] In the Nordic Myeloma Study Group trial, a group of 274 patients treated with high-dose chemotherapy were compared with a historical population of 313 patients. Survival was prolonged in the intensive-therapy group compared with the control group (4-year survival of 61% vs. 46%, respectively). Finally, a second French group compared early versus late autologous transplantation. One hundred eight-five patients were randomized to receive autologous transplantation at presentation (following some initial chemotherapy) or at the

time of disease relapse.[360] Overall survival was similar between both groups. However, because of the additional chemotherapy needed to reattain a remission state following progressive disease, the quality of life was judged better for the patients who received early high-dose chemotherapy. A similar trial is accruing patients in the United States and should again address whether early versus late autologous transplantation is preferable.

Bone marrow was used as the hematologic support in the early transplant studies but is rarely used today. The use of peripheral blood progenitor cells (PBPCs) is advantageous because patients have a shortened duration of neutropenia and hospitalization, avoid the operating room for bone marrow harvesting, and receive a reduced load of reinfused tumor cells following cytoreductive chemotherapy.[352–356] Our group compared multiple myeloma tumor burden in PBPC and back-up bone marrow harvests from patients undergoing autologous transplantation. In almost every case, tumor burden was less in the PBPC product, translating into a median 14-fold reduction in contaminating tumor cells.[361] Unfortunately, this reduction in tumor burden does not seem to have made a significant impact on progression-free or overall survival.[362] The majority of patients continue to relapse within 4 years, with median survival times varying between 36 and 65 months.[171, 363–367]

In an attempt to improve these results, efforts have been made to eliminate contaminating tumor cells from the reinfused autograft products. We have previously demonstrated that the stem cell antigen CD34 is not expressed by the malignant cells in patients with multiple myeloma.[50] Consequently, a phase III study was initiated comparing CD34-selected autografts to unmanipulated PBPC autografts for patients with multiple myeloma.[368] The CD34 selection procedure was safe, with equivalent neutrophil nadirs (median 12 days) and only a 2-day delay in platelet engraftment (median 11 days vs. 9 days). Infections were also comparable between groups. Using PCR analysis of myeloma-specific Ig gene sequences, the purging procedure resulted in a median 3.1 log reduction in autograft tumor burden. Nevertheless, no improvement in progression-free or overall survival has been noted to date. Consequently, the study demonstrates that the reinfusion of malignant cells is not the main contributor to disease relapse in patients following autologous transplantation.[369]

**Choosing Chemotherapy for the Newly Diagnosed Patient.** How does the clinician choose among this bewildering array of combinations? This is clearly a controversial subject, but the initial decision should be based on the age of the patient and the stage of disease at diagnosis.

Patients with stage I disease and patients who are asymptomatic should generally be observed. Since no treatment appears capable of curing the disease, there does not appear to be a benefit for early treatment in these patients, which may lead to early morbidity and mortality or late complications such as myelodysplasia or leukemia. This latter point is particularly important because some of these patients can survive for 10 years or more. Treatment with bisphosphonates should also be considered to prevent the bony complications that eventually develop in all patients with multiple myeloma.

Young patients (<65 years) with Durie-Salmon stage II or stage III disease or with other adverse prognostic factors (elevated $\beta_2$-microglobulin levels) should generally receive an autologous peripheral blood stem cell transplant following several courses of conventional chemotherapy without alkylating agents. Although this treatment is not curative, it offers the best hope of long-term survival and also allows most patients a chance at a prolonged plateau state at which quality of life is high. The procedure should be performed at large experienced referral centers, where transplant-related mortality should be less than 2%.[368] Patients between the ages of 65 and 70 and even older patients can be considered for high-dose chemotherapy depending on their performance status. These elderly patients may benefit from this more aggressive approach as well,[370] but they tend to have slightly higher treatment-related mortality and more prolonged recovery times that can adversely affect the quality of life. If an autologous transplant is planned, the initial chemotherapy used to achieve disease response should avoid alkylating drugs. Melphalan in particular can damage the primordial stem cell compartment, making adequate stem cell collection impossible. We generally treat these patients with VAD because this regimen does not include stem cell–damaging drugs and is one of the most active regimens. Three to six cycles of chemotherapy are typically given, and even patients with stable or minimal responses to treatment can benefit from high-dose chemotherapy. High-dose dexamethasone therapy is another potential initial treatment regimen to use prior to autologous transplantation.

For the remaining patients, the choice of the initial chemotherapy regimen is more extensive. MP remains the gold standard and is certainly useful because of its ease, reasonable cost, and comparable efficacy. We tend to use high-dose dexamethasone or VAD in these patients as well because the initial use of melphalan may make future chemotherapy at the time of disease relapse less tolerable because of limited bone marrow reserve. However, elderly patients tend to tolerate these high glucocorticoid doses poorly, so MP or one of the other combination chemotherapy regimens may be a better choice. Because drug regimens such as VAD or VMCP have higher and more rapid response rates than MP, these regimens may also be useful for symptomatic patients in whom a rapid clinical improvement is desirable. The VAD regimen, in particular, should be strongly considered for patients presenting with renal failure. The details of selected regimens of chemotherapy are given in Table 99–8.

## Maintenance Therapy

Since few patients with myeloma will have a CR to chemotherapy (normal bone marrow plasmacytosis and absent urine and serum immunofixation analysis), most responding patients will reach a time point in their disease at which the M protein level remains constant (plateau phase). Because of initial reports of an increase in the growth fraction of myeloma cells during successful induction chemotherapy, the plateau phase was thought to represent a balance between the continuing cytoreductive effects of chemotherapy and the increased proliferative rate of the tumor clone. However, most studies have shown that continued chemotherapy in patients who have achieved a stable remission offers no advantage in terms of duration of remission or survival. Although relapses occur more quickly in the untreated population, these patients frequently respond to reinstitution of chemotherapy.[371] A re-evaluation of the cytokinetics of the plateau phase offers an explanation for these results.[238] Although expansion of the tumor growth fraction may occur during remission induction, it does not extend into the plateau phase, and the tumor clone of most patients during this time is in a relatively inactive state.

The continuation of chemotherapy in patients who have responded to MP offers no survival benefit.[324, 325] Terminating chemotherapy during the plateau phase in patients successfully induced with the M-2 protocol was followed by rapid relapse in a few patients,[311] but the need for maintenance therapy was not studied prospectively.

Alexanian and colleagues[371] have identified characteristics of patients likely to exhibit long unmaintained remissions after successful induction therapy. Patients with a low pretreatment tumor cell mass or with disappearance of the M protein irrespective of pretherapy tumor mass were likely to have long unmaintained remissions. Limiting exposure to chemotherapy in these patients is important in view of the increased risk of acute leukemia in myeloma patients treated for a long duration.

Because tumor burden has an impact on the efficacy of

*Table 99–8.* **Common Drug Regimens Used in Multiple Myeloma**

| Drug Regimen | Dosage | Cycle Time |
|---|---|---|
| M + P | M 0.25 mg/kg/day × 4 days; P 2 mg/kg/day × 4 days* | q 4–6 wk |
| VMCP[326] | V 1 mg/m² IV day 1 (1.5 mg max); (M 6 mg/m²; C 125 mg/m²; P 60 mg/m²) PO days 1–4 | q 3 wk |
| VBAP[335] | V 1 mg/m² IV day 1 (1.5 mg max); B 30 mg/m² IV day 1; A 30 mg/m² IV day 1; P 60 mg/m² PO days 1–4 | q 3 wk |
| M-2[316] | V 0.03 mg/kg IV day 1; M 0.25 mg/kg PO days 1–4; C 10 mg/kg IV day 1; B 0.5 mg/kg IV day 1; P 1 mg/kg PO days 1–7 | q 4–5 wk |
| VAD[514] | V 0.4 mg/day IV by CI × days 1–4; A 9 mg/m²/day IV by CI days 1–4; Dex 40 mg/day PO days 1–4, days 9–12†, days 17–20† | q 4 wk |
| Dex only | Dex 40 mg/day PO × 4 days | q 2 wk |
| Interferon | 3–5 million U/m² SC daily or 3 times/wk | |

\*The dosage of melphalan should be increased by 20% increments every cycle until the absolute neutrophil count reaches a nadir of 1000–2000 cells/μL or thrombocytopenia (<100,000/μL) develops.

†Days 9–12 and 17–21 of dexamethasone are given on odd cycles only.

M, melphalan; P, prednisone; B, BCNU (carmustine); C, cyclophosphamide; V, vincristine; Dex, dexamethasone; A, Adriamycin; CI, continuous infusion; SC, subcutaneously; IV, intravenously; PO, by mouth.

α-INF, numerous trials have searched for a potential role in myeloma treatment after induction as maintenance therapy. In an Italian multicenter trial, 101 patients who had attained a response to induction therapy were randomized to receive interferon or no therapy.[372] Interferon alfa-2b was given at a dose of 3 MU/m$^2$ three times a week, and improved response duration (26 months vs. 14 months; $p = 0.0002$) and overall survival (52 months vs. 39 months, $p = 0.05$) were detected. Similar results were found in a Swedish trial of 120 patients, with improved remission durations in the treated group using 5 MU of interferon alfa-2b three times a week (59 weeks vs. 26 weeks) and fewer deaths in the treatment arm (10 vs. 21).[373] Canadian[374] and Austrian[375] trials using lower doses of interferon (Canadian study = 2 MU/m$^2$ three times per week; Austrian study = 2 MU/m$^2$ three times per week) showed only slight survival improvements. A recent study randomized 193 patients who had a 75% or greater response to chemotherapy to a fixed dose of 3 MU of interferon alfa-2b three times a week or placebo. No survival benefit was shown.[335] A recent meta-analysis of all trials in which patients in remission were randomized to placebo versus α-INF was completed. Although interferon alfa can prolong the duration of the plateau phase, the improvement in survival is minimal (<3 months). Given the cost and significant morbidity that this drug causes, these modest benefits are probably insufficient to recommend the use of this drug in most patients.[376] A review of these studies suggests there may be a slight dose-related effect. Consequently, if interferon alfa is used, doses of at least 3 MU/m$^2$/day 3 times per week should be given.

Since glucocorticoids are important components of induction therapy, they have also been studied as therapeutic agents during the plateau phase. One SWOG study randomized patients attaining remission following VAD chemotherapy to either interferon alfa plus prednisone (50 mg every other day) or interferon alfa alone.[251] The patients receiving the combination had improved progression-free survival (median, 19 months vs. 9 months; $p = 0.008$) and overall survival (57 months for interferon alfa + prednisone vs. 46 months for interferon alfa). European studies suggested similar beneficial effects from the combination of interferon alfa and steroids.[377] Two hundred sixty-two patients with multiple myeloma were enrolled in a SWOG group study assessing the addition of quinine to VAD chemotherapy and moderate-dose prednisone as disease maintenance.[377a] Although the quinine added no significant benefit to patient outcome, 127 patients who achieved at least a PR were randomized to maintenance therapy with either 10 or 50 mg of prednisone every other day in the second phase of the study. Progression-free survival was increased from 6 to 16 months for the patients taking the higher steroid dose. Median overall survival time was extended from 26 to 42 months ($p = 0.02$) by this well-tolerated and inexpensive treatment. This landmark study suggests that all patients should be treated with prednisone maintenance therapy as a means of prolonging the duration of remission.

## Therapy for Refractory Myeloma

Thirty to 50% of patients do not respond to initial alkylator-based chemotherapy. In addition, all responders, if they live long enough, relapse because there is no plateau apparent in survival curves. Management decisions concerning these "alkylator-refractory" patients are complicated by the heterogeneity of this group. In all studies, previously unresponsive patients have much lower response rates and survival with second-line therapy when compared with those who relapse after an initial remission. The former group can be further subdivided into those who clearly progress during induction therapy and those who remain stable but without attaining a definite response. As described by Bergsagel,[378] the "progressors" have a poor prognosis (median survival of 15 months in a National Cancer Institute of Canada study[379]), whereas the "stable" patients have a good prognosis (median of 49 months).[380] It is also clear that patients who relapse while receiving alkylator-based therapy are less likely to respond to second-line therapy when compared with those who relapse during an unmaintained remission. A second issue is the lack of information on the natural history of relapsing patients. Their current survival without treatment is unknown, and this makes it difficult to evaluate any survival data from studies of second-line therapy. There are clearly relapsing patients who still may have relatively indolent disease that is compatible with prolonged survival. Current staging procedures do not allow identification of these individuals, although serum β2-microglobulin or PCLI, or both, may prove to be of some value in this regard.

Patients who relapse after unmaintained remissions of greater than 6 months' duration are often still responsive to the agents used initially. Response rates (>50% reduction in M component serum or urine concentration) of 50 to 80% have been achieved by re-treatment of such patients with melphalan and prednisone[371]; vincristine, melphalan, cyclophosphamide, and prednisone[325]; or the M-2 protocol.[319] Responses are, in general, less impressive and of shorter duration than those seen with initial therapy but are still significant. A second remission induced by re-treatment with the M-2 regimen[319] or melphalan and prednisone[371] lasted 11 and 8 months, respectively (median).

Patients who relapse during therapy or within 6 months of stopping maintenance therapy should not be re-treated with the same agents because they are unlikely to respond. These and the primary resistant patients ("previously unresponsive") are difficult to treat. Those without progressive disease (stable M protein, no increase in bone disease, or renal insufficiency) should be watched closely without therapy.

For patients whose disease is progressing, high-dose glucocorticoids with or without continuous-infusion vincristine and doxorubicin (VAD) offer the best chance for a meaningful response. The VAD protocol[380] was based on the original observation of Alexanian[283] that significant responses in refractory patients could be achieved with frequent pulses of high-dose prednisone. VAD uses doses of dexamethasone (40 mg/day for 4 days beginning on days 1, 9, and 17 of each 28- to 35-day cycle), which are the equivalent of a sixfold increase in prednisone, as initially used by Alexanian. In addition, continuous infusions of vincristine (0.4 mg/day for 4 days) and doxorubicin (9 mg/m$^2$/day for 4 days) are administered through an indwelling venous catheter, with the rationale that the slowly cycling tumor cells of myeloma are more likely to be injured by constant exposure to these agents. In the initial report,[380] 73% of relapsing and 43% of previously unresponsive patients responded to VAD.

Responses were seen rapidly, usually within the first two cycles of therapy. Some of the patients may have been preselected for good prognosis, as evidenced by low tumor burden (28% were stage I) and the fact that half the previously unresponsive patients who subsequently responded to VAD had demonstrated a stable tumor mass while receiving initial chemotherapy. Nevertheless, the magnitude and frequency of the responses are impressive. With documented responses, the patients demonstrated clinical benefit with increased hemoglobin levels and performance status, and decreased bone pain and hypercalcemia. The major side effect was infection, documented in 8 of 29 patients and causing unexplained fever in 3 others.

Several studies from other institutions confirm the promising results of the VAD protocol.[381, 382] Response rates were similar to the initial report and toxicity was just as severe, with a 20 to 30% incidence of serious infection and occasional cases of steroid-induced psychosis or gastrointestinal toxicity. Most investigators administered prophylactic cimetidine and trimethoprim–sulfa drugs during VAD therapy. Patients receiving VAD who develop steroid-induced psychosis may improve if the dexamethasone is changed to prednisone 100 mg every other day.[290]

A follow-up study by Alexanian and coworkers[383] used dexamethasone alone (in doses identical to the VAD protocol) and compared it with the experience with VAD. In previously unresponsive patients, VAD and dexamethasone alone were comparable (32% and 27% response rates, respectively). However, in relapsing patients, VAD induced a response in 65% and dexamethasone in only 21% of patients. These data suggest an advantage for VAD in relapsing patients. However, the difference between treatments becomes less certain in view of the fact that (1) 9 of 49 patients treated with dexamethasone alone experienced a 50 to 74% reduction in tumor mass (not scored as a response), whereas only 2 of 39 VAD patients were in this category; (2) the median duration of response was 9 months for both groups; (3) the median survival was 14 months for both groups; and (4) the two groups of patients were not randomized.

Treatment options for patients resistant to VAD are limited but include high-dose cyclophosphamide (3 g/m²) and etoposide (900 mg/m²) followed by GM-CSF,[384] EDAP (etoposide, dexamethasone, ara-C [cytarabine], Platinol [cisplatin])[385] or high-dose melphalan.[339] Elevated serum β2-microglobulin and LDH are factors associated with a poor response to salvage chemotherapy.[385]

Although there are still some questions concerning the toxicity, expense, and efficacy of VAD and high-dose pulse administration of glucocorticoids, we believe they are the best available therapies for truly refractory patients. In previously unresponsive patients, dexamethasone alone appears as good as VAD. In patients who relapse during maintenance therapy or within 6 months of stopping initial therapy, we recommend the VAD regimen. In both categories, only patients with clearly progressive disease should be treated. Finally, thalidomide with or without steroids is another useful treatment regimen. Although experience with thalidomide is limited, occasional patients treated with this regimen can have dramatic responses even if they have been otherwise refractory to chemotherapy. This latter treatment is also beneficial for patients who relapse following high-dose chemotherapy because bone marrow reserve may be limited in these patients. Since thalidomide causes only mild cytopenias, this drug can be particularly useful in this setting.

**Systemic Radiotherapy.** Sequential hemibody irradiation (8 Gy midplane dose in a single dose to each half with a 4- to 6-week interval) and total bone irradiation (10 Gy or 15 Gy to the bones of each body segment sequentially) has been successful in producing relief of bone pain and some objective remissions.[386–390] Myelotoxicity was a significant complication in many treated patients and also limited tolerance to future chemotherapy. A prospective randomized phase III trial compared the efficacy of hemibody irradiation versus further chemotherapy after complete remissions were obtained in patients treated with standard chemotherapy.[391] Disease-free intervals and overall survival times were shorter for patients treated with irradiation. In general, hemibody or systemic irradiation is seldom the treatment of choice, although occasional patients are identified with multiple localized plasmacytomas that may benefit. Holmium 166 has been given to patients with refractory and advanced disease because of its skeletal homing and short radiation half-life (27 hours) properties. This may permit increased bone marrow radiation doses with limited systemic radiation toxicity when combined with stem cell reinfusion.[392]

## Myeloma Variants

Several variants of myeloma have been described that may require a different therapeutic approach.

### MONOCLONAL GAMMOPATHY OF UNDETERMINED SIGNIFICANCE

MGUS, also known as *benign monoclonal gammopathy (BMG)*, is a condition characterized by the presence of a monoclonal immunoglobulin in asymptomatic individuals who have no evidence of myeloma, WM, or other related diseases. It is relatively common in elderly individuals; by age 80, routine serum protein electrophoresis reveals that approximately 3% of individuals have asymptomatic M spikes.[393] Using more sensitive techniques of high-resolution agarose gel electrophoresis,[394] immunofixation, or immunoisoelectric focusing,[395] M proteins can be detected in 10 to 14% of individuals older than age 70. Asymptomatic M components also occur with increased frequency in renal allograft recipients undergoing immunosuppression (30% of patients[396]). In 74% of those individuals, the M component was transient, and in the others it remained stable. These data suggest that aging and suppressive treatment allow the development of MGUS through immunosuppression. A detailed case report[397] further supports this hypothesis. During the immediate period following transplantation of a severe combined immunodeficiency patient with haploidentical bone marrow that had been depleted of T lymphocytes, three separate M components appeared. The levels of these paraproteins significantly decreased as T-lymphocyte numbers and function returned to the patient.

Because of their advanced age, patients with MGUS may have radiologically detectable osteoporosis. In addition, anemia or azotemia may be present because of other conditions.

Thus, on occasion the differential diagnosis between early myeloma and MGUS may be difficult. The height of the M component may allow some distinction because most patients with MGUS have a monoclonal protein less than 3 g/dl.[398] Significant levels of Bence Jones proteinuria[399, 400] suggest the diagnosis of myeloma over MGUS, but there is significant overlap between the two entities. The plasma cell labeling index has also been proposed as a tool for differential diagnosis.[175] A labeling index of 0 is probably confirmatory of a diagnosis of MGUS or smoldering myeloma (see next section).[401] A labeling index of 0 to 1 is highly suggestive of these two diagnoses, as only 3 of 13 patients with overt early stage I myeloma had indices less than 1. When there is still doubt whether an M spike reflects true myeloma or MGUS, the most practical and accurate test is that of time. In patients with MGUS, the M component remains stable, whereas it rises in untreated patients with myeloma.

There are well-documented cases of patients whose disease evolved into multiple myeloma up to 24 years after an initial diagnosis of MGUS was made.[402] However, other studies demonstrate that most patients do not develop malignant disease. Kyle prospectively followed 241 patients with MGUS for a median of 22 years (range 20 to 35 years) to determine the incidence of a malignant event developing.[403] Because the median age at presentation was 64 years, 47% of patients died during this extended follow-up without evidence of a B-cell malignancy or related disorder. Of the remaining patients, 19% had stable benign monoclonal gammopathy, 10% had M protein levels greater than 3 g/dl but never required treatment, and 24% developed a related malignancy of myeloma (16.1%), amyloidosis (3.3%), macroglobulinemia (2.9%), or lymphoma (2.0%). The rate of conversion to a malignant disorder remained constant throughout the follow-up period, and there were no factors (Ig type, M-protein level) that distinguished between patients with an ultimate benign or malignant course. Thus, although most patients remain asymptomatic with lengthy follow-up, one fourth develop malignant disease. These factors make serial M-protein measurements and examinations necessary for the detection of early malignant disease.

One clinical problem that can occur in MGUS without evidence of overt malignant disease is the development of a severe sensorimotor peripheral neuropathy.[404] This syndrome is similar to that present with malignant plasma cell dyscrasia and is discussed later.

## SMOLDERING (INDOLENT) MYELOMA

An entity somewhere between MGUS and overt myeloma has been termed *indolent*[405] or *smoldering myeloma*.[406] Patients with this syndrome (2% of all patients with myeloma) fulfill the diagnostic criteria for myeloma but have a tumor clone and M component that remain stable for long periods. They are asymptomatic at diagnosis and lack significant bone disease, anemia, hypercalcemia, or renal insufficiency. They can be followed without therapy, although some eventually need treatment. Additional survival after starting therapy is no different from patients who are treated at diagnosis. The syndrome must be distinguished from aggressive myeloma fortuitously diagnosed at an early stage. Close observation and repeated electrophoretic studies enable an accu-

rate differentiation. Although not yet clinically available, the labeling index can aid in differential diagnosis.[401] In Alexanian's series,[405] the median time from diagnosis to the initiation of chemotherapy was 3 years.

## SOLITARY PLASMACYTOMA OF BONE

Five percent of patients with myeloma present with a single plasmacytoma of bone.[405] By definition, none of these patients has anemia, more than one bone lesion, or marrow plasmacytosis. Only 50% have serum or urine M components and, if present, the M component is usually less than 1.5 g/dl in serum and less than 500 mg/day in urine. Given enough time, most patients' disease will disseminate either to multiple myeloma or a syndrome of recurrent isolated plasmacytomas at different sites of the bony skeleton. Twenty to 30% of patients will have dissemination in the first few years[405, 407, 408] and up to 85% by 10 years of follow-up. After progression to myeloma, further survival is comparable to patients with stage I myeloma (median of 47 months)[409]; therefore, overall survival from the initial diagnosis of plasmacytoma is long (median >10 years).[410] The treatment of choice is radiation therapy, which usually eradicates the bone lesion and often markedly reduces any M component, although small peaks persist in some patients. Because of intramedullary spread, the entire medullary cavity of the involved bone should be encompassed by the radiation field.[334] In one review of 45 consecutive patients, there was no correlation between the dosage of radiation therapy and prolonged survival,[410] although doses of at least 45 Gy are recommended by most authorities.[204] In this series, all nine patients with an initial M protein that disappeared after radiation therapy remained disease free at 10 years, compared with 15% disease-free survival for those patients with a persistent M protein after radiation therapy. Presumably, the patients with a stable M protein after radiation therapy had an isolated conversion of a myeloma subclone to a more aggressive state, which was then eradicated by the local irradiation. In other studies, the existence of an M protein after irradiation had less prognostic significance.[411] Tumor size greater than 5 cm, age older than 40 years,[412] and evidence of spinal involvement on MRI[134] are other adverse predictors of disease relapse. We tend to perform the latter screening test to identify patients who, in fact, have disseminated disease. Patients with abnormal MRI studies required therapy within a median of 16 months compared with a median delay of 43 months for patients with a normal imaging study in the aforementioned study.

Localized extramedullary plasmacytomas differ considerably from solitary plasmacytoma of bone. The former usually presents as a submucosal mass in the tissues of the upper airway passages.[413] Metastatic spread is frequently to soft tissues,[413] whereas spread of solitary plasmacytoma of bone is typically to other bony sites. In addition, conversion to myeloma occurs much less commonly in patients with extramedullary plasmacytomas,[414, 415] and these patients have a better prognosis than do patients with solitary bone plasmacytomas. Treatment with radiotherapy using doses greater than 40 Gy appears to be curative in many patients.[415] In one series, 71% of patients with this problem were progression free at 10 years, and the median overall survival was

101 months.[416] For patients with presentations within the head and neck, irradiation of adjacent lymph nodes has been advocated.[417]

## PLASMA CELL DYSCRASIA WITH POLYNEUROPATHY, ORGANOMEGALY, ENDOCRINOPATHY, MONOCLONAL GAMMOPATHY, AND SKIN CHANGES (POEMS)

A rare variant of plasma cell neoplasia is associated with severe sensorimotor peripheral polyneuropathy. Although most earlier cases were reported from Japan, this syndrome is becoming recognized more frequently in the United States. Patients are relatively young, predominantly male, and usually have neurologic symptoms.[418] If present, bone lesions are sclerotic instead of lytic.[419] Organomegaly (hepatosplenomegaly, lymphadenopathy), endocrinopathies (diabetes mellitus, gonadal failure, or hypothyroidism, or a combination),[420] and skin changes (hypertrichosis, hyperpigmentation, and thickened skin)[421] have been present in many of these patients. Although initial reports described brief survival times (Driedger and Pruzanski reported a median survival of 20 months in their series[418]), other studies have suggested better long-term survival for patients with multiple myeloma associated with POEMS features. Treatment of isolated sclerotic bone lesions with radiation or systemic chemotherapy for patients with more diffuse disease can often lead to improvements in endocrine, cutaneous, and neurologic manifestations presumably due to the paracrine effects these tumors inflict.[422] Finally, patients with POEMS symptoms often have markedly elevated serum levels of proinflammatory cytokines such as TNF, IL-1β and IL-6.[423, 424] IL-6 in particular plays a prominent role in disease pathogenesis for these patients, and clinical responses have been noted for patients treated with IL-6–blocking antibodies.

## PARAPROTEIN-ASSOCIATED NEUROPATHIES

All patients presenting with an unexplained neuropathy should have serum and urine electrophoresis performed to look for monoclonal proteins. Up to 10% of patients have a detectable M protein.[425] Although the pathogenesis of paraprotein-associated neuropathies is poorly understood, these symptoms can occur not only in patients with multiple myeloma and Waldenström's disease but also in patients with MGUS. In 20 of 430 patients with IgM paraproteins who had an unexplained neuropathy, 12 carried the diagnosis of MGUS.[404] In Sherman and colleagues' series of 10 patients,[426] 7 had normal bone marrow examinations and no evidence of malignant disease. Osby and colleagues[427] detected clinical or electrophysiologic evidence of neuropathy in 15 of 21 patients with MGUS. Latov and colleagues[428] showed that in some patients, the monoclonal protein demonstrates antibody activity to peripheral nerve components such as the myelin-associated glycoprotein[429] or chondroitin sulfate[430] and binds to nerves in vitro. This provides a rationale for therapeutic plasmapheresis, which induced marked improvement in 6 patients and stabilization in 3 of 10 patients.[426] Citrate should be used as the anticoagulant because in some patients with polyneuropathy, the paraprotein interacts with heparin. Other beneficial therapies include cortico-

steroids, intravenous Ig, and other immunosuppressive therapies.[431–434] Associated malignant plasma cell dyscrasias should be treated with appropriate chemotherapy,[422] whereas patients with MGUS who respond to plasmapheresis may be followed without chemotherapy. Some of these latter patients may have a decreased requirement for plasmapheresis with time.

## AMYLOIDOSIS

Amyloidosis is a multisystem illness in which insoluble fibrillar protein with a beta-pleated configuration is deposited extracellularly into many organs. In primary amyloidosis, the protein consists of the Ig light chain and is designated *AL*. In amyloidosis secondary to chronic infection, autoimmune disease, or familial Mediterranean fever, the protein represents an alpha globulin derived from a normal serum component and is termed *AA* or *amyloid A protein*. Only primary amyloidosis is considered here.

Primary amyloidosis is caused by an underlying plasma cell dyscrasia with secretion of monoclonal light chains that are "amyloidogenic." In other words, some characteristic or characteristics of the light chains produced allows them to be processed in a particular way by macrophages[435] or to be attracted to and deposited in certain tissue sites after their production, or both. There are no consistent differences in organ distribution or dysfunction between primary (AL) and secondary (AA) amyloidosis. Although all patients with primary amyloidosis have overproduction of monoclonal light chains, clinically and histologically proven myeloma is present in only 20% of patients.[436] Conversely, of all patients with myeloma, approximately 10% have associated amyloidosis.[329] An M component is present in up to 90% of patients with primary amyloidosis, but because this is a light chain disease, many patients have only excessive light chain production. Thus, the serum protein electrophoresis shows an M spike in only 25% of cases,[437] immunoelectrophoresis of serum is positive (for atypical arcs with light chain antisera) in approximately 65% of cases,[437] and urine immunoelectrophoresis is positive in 75% of cases. Lambda light chains are more likely to be amyloidogenic (λ:κ ratio = 2:1).[438] Furthermore, 41% of cases of lambda light chain amyloidosis used the Vλ$_{VI}$ gene family subgroup compared with only 3% use of this subgroup by normal B cells.[155] This suggests that certain lambda chains may be more pathogenic than others. In support of this, repeated injections of Bence Jones light chains derived from patients with amyloidosis can produce amyloid deposits in mice. Similar injections of light chains derived from multiple myeloma patients without amyloidosis do not cause this phenomenon.[439] Further analysis of 39 patients with amyloidosis found patterns of association between light chain variable gene use and the organ of primary amyloid deposition. Patients whose clones were derived from lambda VI IGLV6S1 more commonly had renal involvement, whereas other lambda light chain gene families were used in patients with primary cardiac involvement.[440]

### Incidence

Amyloidosis AL is uncommon, occurring at an incidence of 6 to 10 per million person-years. Like multiple myeloma, the disease is more common in men (65%), but the median age at diagnosis is somewhat older (73 years).[441] Patients with the disease often complain of generalized fatigue and light-headedness and present with one or more of the following symptom complexes: nephrotic syndrome, congestive heart failure, hepatomegaly, peripheral neuropathy, macroglossia, and skin purpura. A serum and urine immunoelectrophoresis should be performed for patients with these features. More than 90% of patients have a detectable monoclonal protein. To confirm the diagnosis, fat aspiration and bone marrow biopsies should be performed and stained using Congo red. Although rectal,[436] skin,[442] and small bowel biopsies are often positive, abdominal fat pad aspirations are least invasive and are positive nearly 80% of the time.[443] The bone marrow biopsy can also be stained for amyloid. Combined with the fat aspiration, the two tests have a sensitivity of nearly 90%.[444] Biopsies of the involved organ will be positive in the remaining cases.

## Prognosis

The median survival of all patients is short, ranging from 12 to 22 months.[436, 445, 446] The presence of congestive heart failure, urinary free light chains, hepatomegaly, or related myeloma are associated with poor prognosis.[436] Heart failure, in particular, is a grave finding at diagnosis, associated with a median survival of less than 6 months,[436] although patients with isolated cardiac amyloidosis (so-called senile amyloidosis) have a better prognosis. A useful measure of cardiac involvement is the Doppler-derived index, which can be obtained during routine echocardiography. Patients with a restrictive ventricular physiology (deceleration times <150 msec) have 1-year survival rates of 49% compared with 92% for those with longer deceleration times.[447, 448] Patients presenting with only peripheral neuropathy do better and have a median survival of more than 3 years.

## Treatment

The treatments available for amyloidosis often parallel the options available for multiple myeloma. This makes sense, of course, since the pathogenic cell type is comparable. Unfortunately, responses are much less frequent and are also more difficult to document because many months are typically required before the involved organ improves. Definitions of response include a 50% reduction in urinary protein, reduction in serum alkaline phosphatase, or a 2-mm reduction in cardiac wall thickness for patients with renal, hepatic, and cardiac amyloidosis, respectively.[447] In addition, a reduction in urinary amyloid protein also is predictive of response because this correlates with improved outcome.

Patients treated with colchicine between 1976 and 1983 had longer survival times (median = 17 months) compared with untreated patients followed from 1961 through 1973 (median = 6 months) in one retrospective study.[445] Colchicine blocks amyloid production in mice,[449] has efficacy in familial Mediterranean fever[450] and, theoretically, may prevent macrophage processing of amyloidogenic protein. However, a substantial portion of the survival gain may have been due to improvements in supportive care between these periods and the higher percentage of patients with congestive heart failure in the untreated group.

Kyle and Greipp[437] randomized patients to receive either melphalan and prednisone or placebo. Patients treated with chemotherapy appeared to have a delay or slowing in progression of disease and a significant improvement in nephrotic syndrome. However, survival was identical. A second study by these investigators compared melphalan and prednisone to colchicine in 101 randomly assigned patients.[446] Although there were only a few instances of clear responses, when patients treated with only one or the other regimen were considered (i.e., excluding patients crossed over to the alternative modality), a significant survival advantage was shown with chemotherapy. In addition, "progression-free" median survival was significantly greater in patients treated with chemotherapy (16 vs. 6 months). Unfortunately, 8% of patients developed acute nonlymphocytic leukemia after 23 to 39 months of melphalan therapy.

High-dose dexamethasone can also be beneficial and is not leukemogenic. We tend to use this agent for patients for this reason, switching to maintenance doses of prednisone (50 mg every other day), which can be tolerated better long term. Finally, high-dose therapy with autologous transplantation shows promise. Treatment-related complications tend to be higher in patients with amyloidosis when compared with multiple myeloma patients.[451] Nevertheless, the initial results with this form of therapy (melphalan 200 mg/m$^2$) seem favorable, with a 68% 2-year survival rate and a 62% CR rate. Eleven of 17 patients had disease-related organ improvement following the procedure.[452] Given the rarity of the disease, a randomized study is not possible. However, we tend to perform autologous transplantation for patients who are younger than age 60 with good performance status and no evidence of cardiac involvement. For such patients, prolonged courses of melphalan should be avoided so that sufficient stem cells can be collected for the procedure. High-dose dexamethasone or VAD chemotherapy can be used before transplantation instead.

In summary, melphalan and prednisone remain the mainstay of treatment for most patients with amyloidosis. However, to prevent the development of acute leukemia, we advise discontinuation of melphalan after 1 year of therapy if there has been no indication of any response. Chemotherapy can help decrease light chain production and, if successful, the balance of protein deposition versus resorption can be reversed and organ damage can improve. Given the slowly progressive nature of the untreated disease, responses tend to be slow as well. Regrettably, most patients are not so fortunate. Younger patients should be considered for autologous transplantation. Studies looking at agents useful in multiple myeloma, such as thalidomide, are being initiated and appear promising anecdotally. Enbrel (etanercept), which can inhibit TNF, also showed promise in a small phase II study. Finally, organ transplantation can be of benefit for patients with isolated organ (kidney or cardiac) involvement and can lead to improved survival and quality of life.[453]

# Waldenström's Macroglobulinemia

## NATURAL HISTORY

WM was first described in 1944[454] and is characterized by a proliferation of B cells, which are morphologically intermediate between plasma cells and lymphocytes, which secrete a monoclonal IgM. Presenting symptoms are related either to tumor infiltration of lymphoid tissues (adenopathy, splenomegaly) or to the effects of the circulating (hyperviscosity syndrome, cryoglobulinemia) or tissue monoclonal gammopathy (neuropathy, amyloidosis). In many patients, the disease runs an indolent course. However, not all cases of plasma cell dyscrasia and IgM paraprotein are associated with the clinical picture of WM. Although rare, there are well-documented cases of IgM myeloma with multiple osteolytic bone lesions and a more aggressive course.[152, 455]

The average age of patients with WM at diagnosis is 60 years, but there may be an asymptomatic period of several years prior to diagnosis. Because the early stages of the disease are often asymptomatic and the natural history is prolonged, it may be particularly difficult to distinguish the disease from benign monoclonal IgM gammopathy.[404] In the series of 241 Mayo Clinic patients, 2.9% of patients with MGUS developed WM during 20 years of follow-up.[403] Consequently, benign IgM gammopathy may be a harbinger of symptomatic disease, and these patients should be followed closely. Familial patterns of development have been described,[456, 457] most recently in a Lebanese family in which two sisters had WM and four other family members had elevated serum IgM levels.[458]

## CLINICAL FEATURES

**Anemia.** Many patients present with symptoms secondary to severe anemia. The cause is commonly multifactorial and related to decreased erythropoiesis from marrow tumor involvement, renal insufficiency, and increased plasma volume.[459] Some patients have coexisting cold agglutinin hemolytic anemia, which is typically due to an IgM κ antibody to the Ia antigen.[460, 461]

**Hyperviscosity.** The hyperviscosity syndrome results in a constellation of signs and symptoms that includes visual disturbances, tinnitus, hearing loss, ataxia, decreased level of consciousness, and high-output cardiac failure. A clue to the diagnosis can be found in examination of the optic fundi. The retinal veins are dilated in an irregular pattern ("sausage effect") with associated hemorrhages and exudates. The level of serum viscosity at which symptoms occur varies among patients and probably depends on the integrity of the vascular supply to target organs as well as the speed at which the viscosity rises. However, a serum viscosity greater than four times normal, which usually requires an IgM concentration greater than 3 g/dl, should be considered dangerous.[462]

**Tumor Infiltration.** Lymphadenopathy, splenomegaly, and hepatomegaly develop in a variable percentage of patients. Examination of the bone marrow reveals an increase in lymphocytic-plasmacytic forms. Malignant cells can be found in the peripheral blood,[463] and in some patients the peripheral smear resembles chronic lymphocytic leukemia (CLL). Tumor cells are typically CD19, CD20, and CD22 positive but like CLL can be CD5 positive.[462]

**Peripheral Neuropathy.** Up to 46% of patients with WM develop peripheral neuropathy.[464] Patients typically complain of foot numbness, paresthesia, or ataxia. Muscle weakness occurs late in the course. The patients with this problem are

somewhat heterogeneous, and in many cases the neuropathy antedates a diagnosis of macroglobulinemia. In such patients, studies have shown that the monoclonal IgM antibody frequently reacts with myelin of the peripheral nerves.[465] Injections of the monoclonal IgM antibody from patients with neuropathy has induced a demyelinating condition in felines, implicating a direct causative effect.[466, 467]

**Cryoglobulinemia.** Cryoglobulins are formed by the precipitation of monoclonal IgM (type I) or mixed monoclonal IgM and polyclonal IgG complexes (type II). Type I cryoglobulins are associated with WM, and although they are frequently detected, only 5% of patients develop associated symptoms (Raynaud's syndrome, arthralgias). For diagnostic purposes, blood should be maintained at 37°C prior to laboratory separation.[462] Patients with mixed cryoglobulinemias should be evaluated for a coexistent hepatitis C infection, as they may respond to interferon alfa therapy.[468]

**Skin Involvement.** Infiltration of the dermis with malignant cells can cause maculopapular lesions,[469] whereas flesh-colored papules and nodules can be related to intraepidermal deposits of IgM.[470]

## PROGNOSIS

Although slow growing for much of its course, WM eventually becomes progressive and refractory to chemotherapy. Median survival times have been estimated at 5 years but more than 20% of patients can survive longer than 10 years.[471] Death usually results from exacerbation of the disease. In some patients, there is an apparent transformation to an aggressive lymphoma resembling immunoblastic sarcoma.[472–474] The development of acute myelogenous leukemia in patients with WM has also been documented but may be related to prior leukemogenic chemotherapy.[475] A retrospective analysis of 167 French patients with WM found that age older than 60, male sex, and neutropenia correlated with poor prognosis on multivariate regression analysis.[476] A scoring system has been devised for prognostic purposes. One point is given for the following: age older than 65, albumin less than 40 g/dl, and isolated cytopenia. A second point is given if two cytopenias are present, for a maximum score of 4. Patients with low risk (0 or 1 point) had 5-year survival times of 86%. Those with intermediate (2 points) or high risk (3 to 4 points) fared more poorly (5-year survival times of 61% and 26%, respectively).[477]

## TREATMENT

Because there is no curative treatment, asymptomatic patients should be followed without therapy. Symptoms secondary to the hyperviscosity syndrome are indications for plasmapheresis as a temporary measure, and plasmapheresis can also be used as the sole therapy for some patients.[478] Plasmapheresis should be continued until the symptoms resolve and the serum viscosity has decreased to acceptable levels. Repeated plasmapheresis may be required until the antitumor effects of chemotherapy become evident. Plasmapheresis should also be considered for patients with cryoglobulinemia or peripheral neuropathy, but 3 months of treatment may be necessary before a beneficial effect is achieved.[479, 480]

Because WM is so rare, there have been few adequate studies comparing different chemotherapeutic regimens. Furthermore, because the natural history is prolonged and patients often succumb to other conditions of advanced age, it is difficult to assess the impact of therapeutic intervention.

In general, the chemotherapeutic agents effective for CLL are also effective for WM. The alkylating agents, chlorambucil (Leukeran) in particular, have significant activity.[481] Up to 55% of patients have a substantial decrease in M component while receiving alkylator or alkylator plus prednisone treatment.[482] More aggressive chemotherapeutic regimens can improve response rates: (65%) for CHOP (cyclophosphamide, hydroxydaunorubicin, Oncovin [vincristine], plus prednisone) and 82% for the M-2 protocol,[483] but the impact on overall survival is uncertain without randomized studies.

The nucleoside analogues, fludarabine and cladribine (2-CdA), have shown promising activity and are probably the drugs of choice for alkylator-resistant disease. Fludarabine at a dose of 20 to 30 mg/m$^2$ for 5 consecutive days every 4 weeks leads to a 31% response rate in alkylator-resistant patients with median 38-month remission rates.[484] Treatment with 2-CdA for two courses of 0.1 mg/kg of continuous intravenous infusion for 7 days led to a 40% response rate in patients whose disease was progressing with initial therapy.[485] Treatment with nucleoside analogues should be limited to prevent prolonged hematologic suppression and T-cell–mediated immunity. Determining whether the incorporation of these drugs into early treatment of WM will affect survival will require a randomized study. Rituximab (an anti-CD20 monoclonal antibody) can be helpful even in refractory patients because most tumors express the CD20 antigen.[486] PRs were noted in three of the seven heavily pretreated patients and the treatment was well tolerated. High-dose therapy with autologous transplantation has also shown promise in anecdotal cases.

Our recommendations are for the prompt use of plasmapheresis for symptoms of hyperviscosity and the institution of chlorambucil with or without prednisone for long-term control in symptomatic patients. When the disease has clearly become resistant to chlorambucil, a nucleoside analogue should be given. We have found the use of low intermittent doses of fludarabine to be beneficial.

## Heavy Chain Disease

The HCDs are neoplastic proliferations of plasma cells that secrete heavy chains unattached to light chains. Although the clinical syndrome associated with alpha HCD is distinct, the presentation of gamma HCD can be heterogeneous, and it has been argued that mu HCD is not a distinct entity at all. These diseases are rare, and little is known about their prognoses or responses to therapy.

The molecular biology of HCD has been investigated.[487] The heavy chains produced by malignant cells are truncated and lack most of the VH.[488] The initially synthesized heavy chain proteins are abnormally small, indicating that postsynthetic degradation is not a likely cause of the truncated polypeptides. In some cases, portions of the VH of the heavy chain genes have been deleted,[489] with the resulting production of the abnormal heavy chain. In contrast, other studies[490] have demonstrated abnormal RNA splicing sites in DNA, which lead to elimination of the VH of the heavy chain. Thus, the pathology at the molecular level is heterogeneous.

### ALPHA HEAVY CHAIN DISEASE

The most frequently occurring HCD is alpha HCD. It primarily affects individuals of low socioeconomic status in their second or third decade of life, and there is a slight male predominance.[491] Although early reports involved individuals living in the Mediterranean region, patients from the Middle East, South America, and Asia have now been described.[492] Seligmann has suggested that intestinal infestation with parasites plays a role in pathogenesis.[491]

The entity primary Mediterranean lymphoma, described earlier by Israeli authors, is probably identical to alpha HCD. Presenting symptoms include severe malabsorption with chronic diarrhea, weight loss, generalized abdominal pain, edema, and clubbing. Although palpable abdominal masses are present in late stages, hepatosplenomegaly, peripheral adenopathy, and marrow involvement are rare. At laparotomy, the entire small bowel and mesenteric nodes are involved, with a diffuse infiltration of plasma cells, lymphocytes, and transitional forms. In a few cases, patients have presented with pulmonary symptoms from infiltration of the lungs by tumor.[493] Three stages of disease have been described. Patients with stage A disease typically have a plasmacytic or lymphoplasmacytic infiltrate invading the intestinal mucosal lamina propria. Patients with more advanced stage C disease have discrete ulcerating tumors corresponding to an immunoblastic lymphoma. Stage B patients have intermediate disease.[487, 494]

The abnormal alpha chain can be difficult to detect. Serum protein electrophoresis usually demonstrates hypoimmunoglobulinemia or an abnormal broad band in the alpha$_2$ and beta regions.[491] The immunochemical diagnosis depends on detection of an abnormal component on immunoelectrophoresis reactive with anti–IgA antiserum but not with anti–light chain antiserum. High concentrations of the abnormal heavy chain are present in jejunal fluid,[491] and small amounts can be found in concentrated urine. Bence Jones proteinuria is never found; in fact, the tumor cells are usually incapable of secreting light chains.[491]

Alpha HCD may represent a continuum of plasmacytic-lymphocytic proliferation. In a few patients, treatment with antibiotics resulted in complete remission,[495] suggesting a premalignant early stage related to microbial infestation. Patients with stage A disease should be treated for 6 months with antibiotics chosen on the basis of intestinal bacterial cultures.[487] Parasitic infections should be sought and treated as well. In late stages of the disease, combinations of an alkylating agent, prednisone, and broad-spectrum antibiotics may be successful in inducing remissions.[492] Doxorubicin-based regimens may also be useful.[487]

### GAMMA HEAVY CHAIN DISEASE (FRANKLIN'S DISEASE)

Although the earliest cases of gamma HCD appeared to represent a distinct clinical entity resembling WM or non-

Hodgkin's lymphoma, this disease has now been detected in patients with rheumatoid arthritis[496] as well as in those with myeloma.[497] Kyle and Greipp[437] have reviewed the characteristics of 48 patients. The disease has a median age of onset of 62 years,[378] and patients present with weakness, fever, adenopathy, hepatosplenomegaly, autoimmune hemolytic anemia, idiopathic thrombocytopenic purpura, or edema and erythema of the tongue, palate, and uvula. Biopsy of the lymph nodes or bone marrow, or both, reveals infiltration with plasma cells, lymphocytes, and intermediate forms. Light chains usually are not produced by the tumor.[498] Immunochemical diagnosis depends on accurate immunoelectrophoresis. The median survival in Kyle's series was 12 months. Treatment with cyclophosphamide, vincristine, and prednisone has been recommended.

## MU HEAVY CHAIN DISEASE

The rarest of the HCDs, this syndrome is not associated with a specific clinical picture and has been found in patients with chronic lymphocytic leukemia, large cell non-Hodgkin's lymphoma, and myeloma.[499] In contrast with alpha and gamma HCDs, monoclonal light chains (usually the kappa type) are produced and secreted in many cases. The malignant plasma cell is incapable of joining heavy and light chains intracellularly, and both are secreted independently. Immunoelectrophoresis is crucial in making the diagnosis because serum protein electrophoresis usually does not demonstrate the abnormal heavy chain.

The natural history and response to therapy are unknown. It appears that mu HCD can appear in several different plasmacytic-lymphocytic neoplasms, and treatment should be tailored to the underlying disorder.

## SUGGESTIONS FOR ADDITIONAL READING

Riedel DA, Pottern LM. The epidemiology of multiple myeloma. Hematol Oncol Clin North Am 1992;6:225–47.

Singhal S, Mehta J, Desikan R, et al. Antitumor activity of thalidomide in refractory multiple myeloma. N Engl J Med 1999;341:1565–71. *This is the original article describing the beneficial effect of thalidomide in multiple myeloma treatment.*

Hu K, Yahalom J. Radiotherapy in the management of plasma cell tumors. Oncology 2000;14:101–9. *This is an excellent overview on the rationale behind dosages and methodology of the primary and palliative treatment of myeloma bone disease.*

Dalton WS, Salmon SE. Drug resistance in myeloma mechanisms and approaches to circumvention. Hematol Oncol Clin North Am 1992;6:383–93.

Attal M, Harousseau JL, Stoppa AM, et al. A prospective, randomized trial of autologous bone marrow transplantation and chemotherapy in multiple myeloma. Intergroupe Français du Myelome. N Engl J Med 1993;335:91–7. *This article describes a randomized study demonstrating improved outcome for multiple myeloma patients who receive autologous bone marrow transplantation.*

Dimopoulos MA, Panayiotidis P, Moulopoulos LA, et al. Waldenström's macroglobulinemia: clinical features, complications, and management. J Clin Oncol 2000;18:214–26. *This is an outstanding and up-to-date review of the disease.*

Kyle RA. "Benign" monoclonal gammopathy—after 20 to 35 years of follow-up. Mayo Clin Proc 1993;68:26–36. *This article presents a summary of disease development in 241 patients with MGUS.*

Gertz MA, Lacy MQ, Dispenzieri A. Amyloidosis. Hematol Oncol 1999;1211–33. *This article presents an overview of amyloidosis by the leading experts in the field.*

Fermand J-P, Brouet J-C. Heavy-chain diseases. Hematol Oncol 1999;1281–94.

## REFERENCES

1. Riedel DA, Pottern LM. The epidemiology of multiple myeloma. Hematol Oncol Clin North Am 1992;6:225–47.
2. Kyle RA, Beard CM, O'Fallon WM, Kurland LT. Incidence of multiple myeloma in Olmsted County, Minnesota: 1978 through 1990, with a review of the trend since 1945. J Clin Oncol 1994;12:1577–83.
3. Cuzick J. Multiple myeloma. Cancer Surv 1994;20:455–74.
4. Hernandez JA, Land KJ, McKenna RW. Leukemias, myeloma, and other lymphoreticular neoplasms. Cancer 1995;75:381–94.
5. Hewell GM, Alexanian R. Multiple myeloma in young persons. Ann Intern Med 1976;84:441–3.
6. Brown LM, Linet MS, Greenberg RS, et al. Multiple myeloma and family history of cancer among blacks and whites in the U.S. Cancer 1999;85:2385–90.
7. Thraves PJ, Kasid U, Smulson ME. Selective isolation of domains of chromatin proximal to both carcinogen-induced DNA damage and poly-adenosine diphosphate-ribosylation. Cancer Res 1985;45:386–91.
8. Cao J, Hong CH, Rosen L, et al. Deletion of genetic material from a poly(ADP-ribose) polymerase-like gene on chromosome 13 occurs frequently in patients with monoclonal gammopathies. Cancer Epidemiol Biomarkers Prev 1995;4:759–63.
9. Bhatia KG, Cherney BW, Huppi K, et al. A deletion linked to a poly(ADP-ribose) polymerase gene on chromosome 13q33-qter occurs frequently in the normal black population as well as in multiple tumor DNA. Cancer Res 1990;50:5406–13.
10. Pottern LM, Gart JJ, Nam JM, et al. HLA and multiple myeloma among black and white men: evidence of a genetic association. Cancer Epidemiol Biomarkers Prev 1992;1:177–82.
11. Savage D, Lindenbaum J, Van Ryzin J, et al. Race, poverty, and survival in multiple myeloma. Cancer 1984;54:3085–94.
12. Weston B, Grufferman S, MacMillan JP, Cohen HJ. Effects of socio-economic and clinical factors on survival in multiple myeloma. J Clin Oncol 1987;5:1977–84.
13. Deshpande HA, Hu XP, Marino P, et al. Anticipation in familial plasma cell dyscrasias. Br J Haematol 1998;103:696–703. see comments.
14. Leech SH, Bryan CF, Elston RC, et al. Genetic studies in multiple myeloma. 1: Association with HLA-Cw5. Cancer 1983;51:1408–11.
15. Ludwig H, Mayr W. Genetic aspects of susceptibility to multiple myeloma. Blood 1982;59:1286–91.
16. Zawadzki ZA, Aizawa Y, Kraj MA, et al. Familial immunopathies: report of nine families and survey of literature. Cancer 1977;40:2094–101.
17. Boice JD Jr, Morin MM, Glass AG, et al. Diagnostic x-ray procedures and risk of leukemia, lymphoma, and multiple myeloma. JAMA 1991;265:1290–4 [published erratum appears in JAMA 1991;5:265:2810].
18. Cuzick J. Radiation-induced myelomatosis. N Engl J Med 1981;304:204–10.
19. Ichimaru M, Ishimaru T, Mikami M, Matsunaga M. Multiple myeloma among atomic bomb survivors in Hiroshima and Nagasaki, 1950–76: relationship to radiation dose absorbed by marrow. J Natl Cancer Inst 1982;69:323–8.
20. Linet MS, Harlow SD, McLaughlin JK. A case-control study of multiple myeloma in whites: chronic antigenic stimulation, occupation, and drug use. Cancer Res 1987;47:2978–81.
21. Cuzick J, De Stavola B. Multiple myeloma—a case-control study. Br J Cancer 1988;57:516–20.
22. Brown LM, Everett GD, Burmeister LF, Blair A. Hair dye use and multiple myeloma in white men. Am J Public Health 1992;82:1673–4.
23. Bergsagel DE, Wong O, Bergsagel PL, et al. Benzene and multiple myeloma: appraisal of the scientific evidence. Blood 1999;94:1174–82.
24. Demers PA, Vaughan TL, Koepsell TD, et al. A case-control study of multiple myeloma and occupation. Am J Ind Med 1993;23:629–39.
25. Fritschi L, Siemiatycki J. Lymphoma, myeloma and occupation: results of a case-control study. Int J Cancer 1996; 67:498–503.
26. Nanni O, Falcini F, Buiatti E, et al. Multiple myeloma and work in agriculture: results of a case-control study in Forli, Italy. Cancer Causes Control 1998;9:277–83.
27. Swaen GM, van Vliet C, Slangen JJ, Sturmans F. Cancer mortality

among licensed herbicide applicators. Scand J Work Environ Health 1992;18:201–4.

28. Khuder SA, Mutgi AB. Meta-analyses of multiple myeloma and farming. Am J Ind Med 1997;32:510–6.

29. Isobe T, Osserman EF. Pathologic conditions associated with plasma cell dyscrasias: a study of 806 cases. Ann NY Acad Sci 1971;190:507–18.

30. Rosenblatt J, Hall CA. Plasma-cell dyscrasia following prolonged stimulation of reticuloendothelial system. Lancet 1970;1:301–2.

31. Goldenberg GJ, Paraskevas F, Israels LG. The association of rheumatoid arthritis with plasma cell and lymphocytic neoplasms. Arthritis Rheum 1969;12:569–79.

31a. Salmon SE, Seligmann M. B-cell neoplasia in man. Lancet 1974;2:1230–4.

32. Potter M. Myeloma proteins (M-components) with antibody-like activity. N Engl J Med 1971;284:831–8.

33. Seligmann M, Danon F, Basch A, Bernard J. IgG myeloma cryoglobulin with antistreptolysin activity. Nature 1968;220:711–2.

34. Cohen HJ, Bernstein RJ, Grufferman S. Role of immune stimulation in the etiology of multiple myeloma: a case control study. Am J Hematol 1987;24:119–26.

35. Bourguet CC, Logue EE. Antigenic stimulation and multiple myeloma. A prospective study. Cancer 1993;72:2148–54.

36. Eriksson M. Rheumatoid arthritis as a risk factor for multiple myeloma: a case-control study. Eur J Cancer 1993;2:259–63.

37. Katusic S, Beard CM, Kurland LT, et al. Occurrence of malignant neoplasms in the Rochester, Minnesota, rheumatoid arthritis cohort. Am J Med 1985;78:50–5.

38. Vescio RA, Cao J, Hong CH, et al. Myeloma Ig heavy chain V region sequences reveal prior antigenic selection and marked somatic mutation but no intraclonal diversity. J Immunol 1995;155:2487–97.

39. Bakkus MH, Van Riet I, Van Camp B, Thielemans K. Evidence that the clonogenic cell in multiple myeloma originates from a pre-switched but somatically mutated B cell. Br J Haematol 1994;87:68–74.

40. Potter M. The developmental history of the neoplastic plasma cell in mice: a brief review of recent developments. Semin Hematol 1973;10:19–32.

41. Kubagawa H, Vogler LB, Capra JD, et al. Studies on the clonal origin of multiple myeloma: use of individually specific (idiotype) antibodies to trace the oncogenic event to its earliest point of expression in B-cell differentiation. J Exp Med 1979;150:792–807.

42. Boccadoro M, Van Acker A, Pileri A, Urbain J. Idiotypic lymphocytes in human monoclonal gammopathies. Ann Immunol (Paris) 1981;132C:9–19.

43. Osterborg A, Steinitz M, Lewin N, et al. Establishment of idiotype bearing B-lymphocyte clones from a patient with monoclonal gammopathy. Blood 1991;78:2642–9.

44. Epstein J, Xiao HQ, He XY. Markers of multiple hematopoietic-cell lineages in multiple myeloma. N Engl J Med 1990;322:664–8. see comments.

45. Billadeau D, Ahmann G, Greipp P, Van Ness B. The bone marrow of multiple myeloma patients contains B cell populations at different stages of differentiation that are clonally related to the malignant plasma cell. J Exp Med 1993;178:1023–31.

46. Corradini P, Boccadoro M, Voena C, Pileri A. Evidence for a bone marrow B cell transcribing malignant plasma cell VDJ joined to C mu sequence in immunoglobulin (IgG)- and IgA-secreting multiple myelomas. J Exp Med 1993;178:1091–6.

47. Terstappen LW, Johnsen S, Segers-Nolten IM, Loken MR. Identification and characterization of plasma cells in normal human bone marrow by high-resolution flow cytometry. Blood 1990;76:1739–47.

48. Kunkel LA, Vescio R, Cao J, et al. Analysis of multiple myeloma third complementarity–determining regions reveals characteristics of prenatal B cells. Ann NY Acad Sci 1995;764:519–22.

49. Ralph QM, Brisco MJ, Joshua DE, et al. Advancement of multiple myeloma from diagnosis through plateau phase to progression does not involve a new B-cell clone: evidence from the Ig heavy chain gene. Blood 1993;82:202–6.

50. Vescio RA, Hong CH, Cao J, et al. The hematopoietic stem cell antigen, CD34, is not expressed on the malignant cells in multiple myeloma. Blood 1994;84:3283–90.

51. Kawano M, Hirano T, Matsuda T, et al. Autocrine generation and requirement of BSF-2/IL-6 for human multiple myelomas. Nature 1988;332:83–5.

52. Klein B, Zhang XG, Jourdan M, et al. Paracrine rather than autocrine regulation of myeloma-cell growth and differentiation by interleukin-6. Blood 1989;73:517–26.

53. Klein B, Zhang XG, Lu ZY, Bataille R. Interleukin-6 in human multiple myeloma. Blood 1995;85:863–72.

54. Uchiyama H, Barut BA, Mohrbacher AF, et al. Adhesion of human myeloma–derived cell lines to bone marrow stromal cells stimulates interleukin-6 secretion. Blood 1993;82:3712–20.

55. Zhang XG, Bataille R, Jourdan M, et al. Granulocyte-macrophage colony-stimulating factor synergizes with interleukin-6 in supporting the proliferation of human myeloma cells. Blood 1990;76:2599–605. see comments.

56. Jernberg H, Pettersson M, Kishimoto T, Nilsson K. Heterogeneity in response to interleukin 6 (IL-6), expression of IL-6 and IL-6 receptor mRNA in a panel of established human multiple myeloma cell lines. Leukemia 1991;5:255–65 [published erratum appears in Leukemia 1991;5:following 530].

57. Suematsu S, Matsuda T, Aozasa K, et al. IgG1 plasmacytosis in interleukin 6 transgenic mice. Proc Natl Acad Sci U S A 1989;86:7547–51.

58. Bataille R, Jourdan M, Zhang XG, Klein B. Serum levels of interleukin 6, a potent myeloma cell growth factor, as a reflection of disease severity in plasma cell dyscrasias. J Clin Invest 1989;84:2008–11.

59. Ludwig H, Nachbaur DM, Fritz E, et al. Interleukin-6 is a prognostic factor in multiple myeloma. Blood 1991; 77:2794–5. letter; see comments.

60. Lichtenstein A, Tu Y, Fady C, et al. Interleukin-6 inhibits apoptosis of malignant plasma cells. Cell Immunol 1995;162:248–55.

61. Xu FH, Sharma S, Gardner A, et al. Interleukin-6-induced inhibition of multiple myeloma cell apoptosis: support for the hypothesis that protection is mediated via inhibition of the JNK/SAPK pathway. Blood 1998;92:241–51.

62. Chauhan D, Pandey P, Ogata A, et al. Dexamethasone induces apoptosis of multiple myeloma cells in a JNK/SAP kinase independent mechanism. Oncogene 1997;15:837–43.

63. Klein B, Wijdenes J, Zhang XG, et al. Murine anti-interleukin-6 monoclonal antibody therapy for a patient with plasma cell leukemia. Blood 1991;78:1198–204.

64. Bataille R, Barlogie B, Lu ZY, et al. Biologic effects of anti-interleukin-6 murine monoclonal antibody in advanced multiple myeloma. Blood 1995;86:685–91.

65. Cozzolino F, Torcia M, Aldinucci D, et al. Production of interleukin-1 by bone marrow myeloma cells. Blood 1989;74:380–7.

66. Carter A, Merchav S, Silvian-Draxler I, Tatarsky I. The role of interleukin-1 and tumour necrosis factor-alpha in human multiple myeloma. Br J Haematol 1990;74:424–31.

67. Donovan KA, Lacy MQ, Kline MP, et al. Contrast in cytokine expression between patients with monoclonal gammopathy of undetermined significance or multiple myeloma. Leukemia 1998;12:593–600.

68. Lacy MQ, Donovan KA, Heimbach JK, et al. Comparison of interleukin-1 beta expression by in situ hybridization in monoclonal gammopathy of undetermined significance and multiple myeloma. Blood 1999;93:300–5.

69. Jourdan M, Tarte K, Legouffe E, et al. Tumor necrosis factor is a survival and proliferation factor for human myeloma cells. Eur Cytokine Netw 1999;10:65–70.

70. Borset M, Waage A, Brekke OL, Helseth E. TNF and IL-6 are potent growth factors for OH-2, a novel human myeloma cell line. Eur J Haematol 1994;53:31–7.

71. Filella X, Blade J, Montoto S, et al. Impaired production of interleukin 6 and tumour necrosis factor alpha in whole blood cell cultures of patients with multiple myeloma. Cytokine 1998;10:993–6.

72. Filella X, Blade J, Guillermo AL, et al. Cytokines (IL-6, TNF-alpha, IL-1 alpha) and soluble interleukin-2 receptor as serum tumor markers in multiple myeloma. Cancer Detect Prev 1996;20:52–6.

73. Jelinek DF, Witzig TE, Arendt BK. A role for insulin-like growth factor in the regulation of IL-6–responsive human myeloma cell line growth. J Immunol 1997;159:487–96.

74. Georgii-Hemming P, Wiklund HJ, Ljunggren O, Nilsson K. Insulin-like growth factor I is a growth and survival factor in human multiple myeloma cell lines. Blood 1996;88:2250–8.

75. Jelinek DF. Mechanisms of myeloma cell growth control. Hematol Oncol Clin North Am 1999;13:1145–57.

76. Xu F, Gardner A, Tu Y, et al. Multiple myeloma cells are protected against dexamethasone-induced apoptosis by insulin-like growth factors. Br J Haematol 1997;97:429–40.

77. Lu ZY, Zhang XG, Rodriguez C, et al. Interleukin-10 is a proliferation factor but not a differentiation factor for human myeloma cells. Blood 1995;85:2521–7.
78. Seidel C, Borset M, Turesson I, et al. Elevated serum concentrations of hepatocyte growth factor in patients with multiple myeloma. The Nordic Myeloma Study Group. Blood 1998;91:806–12.
79. Celsing F, Hast R, Stenke L, et al. Extramedullary progression of multiple myeloma following GM-CSF treatment—grounds for caution? Eur J Haematol 1992;49:108. letter.
80. Schwabe M, Brini AT, Bosco MC, et al. Disruption by interferon-alpha of an autocrine interleukin-6 growth loop in IL-6–dependent U266 myeloma cells by homologous and heterologous down-regulation of the IL-6 receptor alpha- and beta-chains. J Clin Invest 1994;94:2317–25.
81. Jourdan M, Zhang XG, Portier M, et al. IFN-alpha induces autocrine production of IL-6 in myeloma cell lines. J Immunol 1991;147:4402–7.
82. Chang Y, Cesarman E, Pessin MS, et al. Identification of herpesvirus-like DNA sequences in AIDS-associated Kaposi's sarcoma. Science 1994;266:1865–9. see comments.
83. Moore PS, Boshoff C, Weiss RA, Chang Y. Molecular mimicry of human cytokine and cytokine response pathway genes by KSHV. Science 1996;274:1739–44.
84. Neipel F, Albrecht JC, Ensser A, et al. Human herpesvirus 8 encodes a homolog of interleukin-6. J Virol 1997;71:839–42.
85. Rettig MB, Ma HJ, Vescio RA, et al. Kaposi's sarcoma–associated herpesvirus infection of bone marrow dendritic cells from multiple myeloma patients. Science 1997;276:1851–4. see comments.
86. Said JW, Rettig MR, Heppner K, et al. Localization of Kaposi's sarcoma–associated herpesvirus in bone marrow biopsy samples from patients with multiple myeloma. Blood 1997;90:4278–82. see comments.
87. Bellos F, Cremer FW, Ehrbrecht E, et al. Leukapheresis cells of patients with multiple myeloma collected after mobilization with chemotherapy and G-CSF do not bear Kaposi's sarcoma associated herpesvirus DNA. Br J Haematol 1998;103:1192–7.
88. Tarte K, Olsen SJ, Yang Lu Z, et al. Clinical-grade functional dendritic cells from patients with multiple myeloma are not infected with Kaposi's sarcoma–associated herpesvirus. Blood 1998;91:1852–7. see comments.
89. Yi Q, Ekman M, Anton D, et al. Blood dendritic cells from myeloma patients are not infected with Kaposi's sarcoma–associated herpesvirus (KSHV/HHV-8). Blood 1998;92:402–4.
90. Rask C, Kelsen J, Olesen G, et al. Danish patients with untreated multiple myeloma do not harbour human herpesvirus 8. Br J Haematol 2000;108:96–8.
91. Chauhan D, Bharti A, Raje N, et al. Detection of Kaposi's sarcoma herpesvirus DNA sequences in multiple myeloma bone marrow stromal cells. Blood 1999;93:1482–6.
92. Raje N, Gong J, Chauhan D, et al. Bone marrow and peripheral blood dendritic cells from patients with multiple myeloma are phenotypically and functionally normal despite the detection of Kaposi's sarcoma herpesvirus gene sequences. Blood 1999;93:1487–95.
93. Belec L, Mohamed AS, Authier FJ, et al. Human herpesvirus 8 infection in patients with POEMS syndrome–associated multicentric Castleman's disease. Blood 1999;93:3643–53.
94. Vescio RA, Wu CH, Zheng L, et al. Human herpesvirus 8 (KSHV) contamination of peripheral blood and autograft products from multiple myeloma patients. Bone Marrow Transplant 2000;25:153–60.
95. Dewald GW, Kyle RA, Hicks GA, Greipp PR. The clinical significance of cytogenetic studies in 100 patients with multiple myeloma, plasma cell leukemia, or amyloidosis. Blood 1985;66:380–90.
96. Gould J, Alexanian R, Goodacre A, et al. Plasma cell karyotype in multiple myeloma. Blood 1988;71:453–6.
97. Nishida K, Tamura A, Nakazawa N, et al. The Ig heavy chain gene is frequently involved in chromosomal translocations in multiple myeloma and plasma cell leukemia as detected by in situ hybridization. Blood 1997;90:526–34.
98. Avet-Loiseau H, Li JY, Facon T, et al. High incidence of translocations t(11;14)(q13;q32) and t(4;14)(p16;q32) in patients with plasma cell malignancies. Cancer Res 1998;58:5640–5.
99. Chesi M, Bergsagel PL, Brents LA, et al. Dysregulation of cyclin D1 by translocation into an IgH gamma switch region in two multiple myeloma cell lines. Blood 1996;88:674–81. see comments.
100. Chesi M, Nardini E, Lim RS, Smith KD, et al. The t(4;14) transloca-

tion in myeloma dysregulates both FGFR3 and a novel gene, MMSET, resulting in IgH/MMSET hybrid transcripts. Blood 1998;92:3025–34.
101. Selvanayagam P, Blick M, Narni F, et al. Alteration and abnormal expression of the c-myc oncogene in human multiple myeloma. Blood 1988;71:30–5.
102. Chesi M, Bergsagel PL, Shonukan OO, et al. Frequent dysregulation of the c-maf proto-oncogene at 16q23 by translocation to an Ig locus in multiple myeloma. Blood 1998;91:4457–63.
103. Neri A, Murphy JP, Cro L, et al. Ras oncogene mutation in multiple myeloma. J Exp Med 1989;170:1715–25.
104. Mazars GR, Portier M, Zhang XG, et al. Mutations of the p53 gene in human myeloma cell lines. Oncogene 1992;7:1015–8 [published erratum appears in Oncogene 1993;8:1107].
105. Dao DD, Sawyer JR, Epstein J, et al. Deletion of the retinoblastoma gene in multiple myeloma. Leukemia 1994;8:1280–4.
106. Rao PH, Cigudosa JC, Ning Y, et al. Multicolor spectral karyotyping identifies new recurring breakpoints and translocations in multiple myeloma. Blood 1998;92:1743–8.
107. Osterland CK, Espinoza LR. Biological properties of myeloma proteins. Arch Intern Med 1975;135:32–6.
108. Kilgore LL, Patterson BW, Parenti DM, Fisher WR. Immune complex hyperlipidemia induced by an apolipoprotein-reactive immunoglobulin A paraprotein from a patient with multiple myeloma: characterization of this immunoglobulin. J Clin Invest 1985;76:225–32.
109. Bovill EG, Ershler WB, Golden EA, et al. A human myeloma–produced monoclonal protein directed against the active subpopulation of von Willebrand factor. Am J Clin Pathol 1986;85:115–23.
110. Preston FE, Cooke KB, Foster ME, et al. Myelomatosis and the hyperviscosity syndrome. Br J Haematol 1978;38:517–30.
111. Pruzanski W, Watt JG. Serum viscosity and hyperviscosity syndrome in IgG multiple myeloma: report on 10 patients and a review of the literature. Ann Intern Med 1972;77:853–60.
112. Reinhart WH, Lutolf O, Nydegger UR, et al. Plasmapheresis for hyperviscosity syndrome in macroglobulinemia Waldenström and multiple myeloma: influence on blood rheology and the microcirculation. J Lab Clin Med 1992;119:69–76.
113. Kes P, Pecanic Z, Getaldic B, Ratkovic-Gusic I. Treatment of hyperviscosity syndrome in the patients with plasma cell dyscrasias. Acta Med Croatica 1996;50:173–7.
114. Kyle RA. Multiple myeloma: review of 869 cases. Mayo Clin Proc 1975;50:29–40.
115. Mundy GR, Bertolini DR. Bone destruction and hypercalcemia in plasma cell myeloma. Semin Oncol 1986;13:291–9 [published erratum appears in Semin Oncol 1986;13:lxiii].
116. Belch AR, Bergsagel DE, Wilson K, et al. Effect of daily etidronate on the osteolysis of multiple myeloma. J Clin Oncol 1991;9:1397–402.
117. Kyle RA, Jowsey J, Kelly PJ, Taves DR. Multiple myeloma bone disease: the comparative effect of sodium fluoride and calcium carbonate or placebo. N Engl J Med 1975;293:1334–8.
118. Mundy GR, Raisz LG, Cooper RA, et al: evidence for the secretion of an osteoclast stimulating factor in myeloma. N Engl J Med 1974;291:1041–6.
119. Kawano M, Yamamoto I, Iwato K, et al. Interleukin-1 beta rather than lymphotoxin as the major bone resorbing activity in human multiple myeloma. Blood 1989;73:1646–9.
120. Mandelli F, Avvisati G, Tribalto M. Biology and treatment of multiple myeloma. Curr Opin Oncol 1992;4:73–86.
121. Hughes FJ, Howells GL. Interleukin-6 inhibits bone formation in vitro. Bone Miner 1993;21:21–8.
122. Urashima M, Ogata A, Chauhan D, et al. Transforming growth factor-beta 1: differential effects on multiple myeloma versus normal B cells. Blood 1996;87:1928–38.
123. Hjertner O, Torgersen ML, Seidel C, et al. Hepatocyte growth factor (HGF) induces interleukin-11 secretion from osteoblasts: a possible role for HGF in myeloma-associated osteolytic bone disease. Blood 1999;94:3883–8.
124. Barille S, Akhoundi C, Collette M, et al. Metalloproteinases in multiple myeloma: production of matrix metalloproteinase-9 (MMP-9), activation of proMMP-2, and induction of MMP-1 by myeloma cells. Blood 1997;90:1649–55.
125. Ishikawa H, Tanaka H, Iwato K, et al. Effect of glucocorticoids on the biologic activities of myeloma cells: inhibition of interleukin-1 beta osteoclast activating factor–induced bone resorption. Blood 1990;75:715–20.
126. Taube T, Beneton MN, McCloskey EV, et al. Abnormal bone remod-

elling in patients with myelomatosis and normal biochemical indices of bone resorption. Eur J Haematol 1992;49:192–8.

127. Bataille R, Delmas PD, Chappard D, Sany J. Abnormal serum bone Gla protein levels in multiple myeloma: crucial role of bone formation and prognostic implications. Cancer 1990;66:167–72.

128. Carlson K, Ljunghall S, Simonsson B, Smedmyr B. Serum osteocalcin concentrations in patients with multiple myeloma—correlation with disease stage and survival. J Intern Med 1992;231:133–7.

129. Woolfenden JM, Pitt MJ, Durie BG, Moon TE. Comparison of bone scintigraphy and radiography in multiple myeloma. Radiology 1980;134:723–8.

130. Agren B, Lonnqvist B, Bjorkstrand B, et al. Radiography and bone scintigraphy in bone marrow transplant multiple myeloma patients. Acta Radiol 1997;38:144–50.

131. Abildgaard N, Brixen K, Kristensen JE, et al. Assessment of bone involvement in patients with multiple myeloma using bone densitometry. Eur J Haematol 1996;57:370–6.

132. Moulopoulos LA, Dimopoulos MA. Magnetic resonance imaging of the bone marrow in hematologic malignancies. Blood 1997;90:2127–47. see comments.

133. Kusumoto S, Jinnai I, Itoh K, et al. Magnetic resonance imaging patterns in patients with multiple myeloma. Br J Haematol 1997;99:649–55.

134. Moulopoulos LA, Dimopoulos MA, Smith TL, et al. Prognostic significance of magnetic resonance imaging in patients with asymptomatic multiple myeloma. J Clin Oncol 1995;13:251–6.

135. Moulopoulos LA, Dimopoulos MA, Weber D, et al. Magnetic resonance imaging in the staging of solitary plasmacytoma of bone. J Clin Oncol 1993;11:1311–5.

136. Rodriguez LH, Finkelstein JB, Shullenberger CC, Alexanian R. Bone healing in multiple myeloma with melphalan chemotherapy. Ann Intern Med 1972;76:551–6.

137. Perri RT, Hebbel RP, Oken MM. Influence of treatment and response status on infection risk in multiple myeloma. Am J Med 1981;71:935–40.

138. Shaikh BS, Lombard RM, Appelbaum PC, Bentz MS. Changing patterns of infections in patients with multiple myeloma. Oncology 1982;39:78–82.

139. Kapadia SB. Multiple myeloma: a clinicopathologic study of 62 consecutively autopsied cases. Medicine (Baltimore) 1980;59:380–92.

140. Broder S, Humphrey R, Durm M, et al. Impaired synthesis of polyclonal (non-paraprotein) immunoglobulins by circulating lymphocytes from patients with multiple myeloma: role of suppressor cells. N Engl J Med 1975;293:887–92.

141. Paglieroni T, Mackenzie MR. Multiple myeloma: an immunologic profile. Cytotoxic and suppressive effects of the EA rosette-forming cell. J Immunol 1980;124:2563–70.

142. Mills KH, Cawley JC. Abnormal monoclonal antibody–defined helper/suppressor T-cell subpopulations in multiple myeloma: relationship to treatment and clinical stage. Br J Haematol 1983;53:271–5.

143. Chen Y, Bhoopalam N, Yakulis V, Heller P. Changes in lymphocyte surface immunoglobulins in myeloma and the effect of an RNA-containing plasma factor. Ann Intern Med 1975;83:625–31.

144. MacGregor RR, Negendank WG, Schreiber AD. Impaired granulocyte adherence in multiple myeloma: relationship to complement system, granulocyte delivery, and infection. Blood 1978;51:591–9.

145. Karle H, Hansen NE, Plesner T. Neutrophil defect in multiple myeloma: studies on intraneutrophilic lysozyme in multiple myeloma and malignant lymphoma. Scand J Haematol 1976;17:62–70.

146. Spitler LE, Spath P, Petz L, et al. Phagocytes and C4 in paraproteinaemia. Br J Haematol 1975;29:279–92.

147. Cheson BD, Plass RR, Rothstein G. Defective opsonization in multiple myeloma. Blood 1980;55:602–6.

148. Gramenzi A, Buttino I, D'Avanzo B, et al. Medical history and the risk of multiple myeloma. Br J Cancer 1991;63:769–72.

149. DeFronzo RA, Humphrey RL, Wright JR, Cooke CR. Acute renal failure in multiple myeloma. Medicine (Baltimore) 1975;54:209–13.

150. Levi DF, Williams RC Jr, Lindstrom FD. Immunofluorescent studies of the myeloma kidney with special reference to light chain disease. Am J Med 1968;44:922–33.

151. DeFronzo RA, Cooke CR, Wright JR, Humphrey RL. Renal function in patients with multiple myeloma. Medicine (Baltimore) 1978;57:151–66.

152. Hobbs JR. Immunochemical classes of myelomatosis: including data from a therapeutic trial conducted by a Medical Research Council working party. Br J Haematol 1969;16:599–606.

153. Woodruff R, Sweet B. Multiple myeloma with massive Bence Jones proteinuria and preservation of renal function. Aust N Z J Med 1977;7:60–2.

154. Khamlichi AA, Aucouturier P, Silvain C, et al. Primary structure of a monoclonal kappa chain in myeloma with light chain deposition disease. Clin Exp Immunol 1992;87:122–6.

155. Solomon A, Weiss DT, Kattine AA. Nephrotoxic potential of Bence Jones proteins. N Engl J Med 1991;324:1845–51. see comments.

156. Rocca A, Khamlichi AA, Touchard G, et al. Sequences of V kappa L subgroup light chains in Fanconi's syndrome: light chain V region gene usage restriction and peculiarities in myeloma-associated Fanconi's syndrome. J Immunol 1995;155:3245–52.

157. Cohen DJ, Sherman WH, Osserman EF, Appel GB. Acute renal failure in patients with multiple myeloma. Am J Med 1984;76:247–56.

158. Bernstein SP, Humes HD. Reversible renal insufficiency in multiple myeloma. Arch Intern Med 1982;142:2083–6.

159. Lazar GS, Feinstein DI. Distal renal tubular acidosis in multiple myeloma. Arch Intern Med 1981;141:655–6.

160. Durie BG, Salmon SE. A clinical staging system for multiple myeloma. Correlation of measured myeloma cell mass with presenting clinical features, response to treatment, and survival. Cancer 1975;36:842–54.

161. Durie BG, Salmon SE, Moon TE. Pretreatment tumor mass, cell kinetics, and prognosis in multiple myeloma. Blood 1980;55:364–72.

162. Woodruff RK, Wadsworth J, Malpas JS, Tobias JS. Clinical staging in multiple myeloma. Br J Haematol 1979;42:199–205.

163. Bataille R, Durie BG, Grenier J, Sany J. Prognostic factors and staging in multiple myeloma: a reappraisal. J Clin Oncol 1986;4:80–7.

164. Garewal H, Durie BG, Kyle RA, et al. Serum beta 2-microglobulin in the initial staging and subsequent monitoring of monoclonal plasma cell disorders. J Clin Oncol 1984;2:51–7.

165. Alexanian R, Barlogie B, Fritsche H. Beta 2 microglobulin in multiple myeloma. Am J Hematol 1985;20:345–51.

166. Scarffe JH, Anderson H, Palmer MK, Crowther D. Prognostic significance of pretreatment serum beta 2-microglobulin levels in multiple myeloma. Eur J Cancer Clin Oncol 1983;19:1361–4.

167. Bataille R, Durie BG, Grenier J. Serum beta 2 microglobulin and survival duration in multiple myeloma: a simple reliable marker for staging. Br J Haematol 1983;55:439–47.

168. Cuzick J, Cooper EH, MacLennan IC. The prognostic value of serum beta 2 microglobulin compared with other presentation features in myelomatosis. Br J Cancer 1985;52:1–6.

169. Bataille R, Grenier J, Sany J. Beta-2-microglobulin in myeloma: optimal use for staging, prognosis, and treatment—a prospective study of 160 patients. Blood 1984;63:468–76.

170. van Dobbenburgh OA, Rodenhuis S, Ockhuizen T, et al. Serum beta 2-microglobulin: a real improvement in the management of multiple myeloma? Br J Haematol 1985;61:611–20.

171. Majolino I, Vignetti M, Meloni G, et al. Autologous transplantation in multiple myeloma: a GITMO retrospective analysis on 290 patients: Gruppo Italiano Trapianti di Midollo Osseo. Haematologica 1999;84:844–52.

172. Bjorkstrand B, Goldstone AH, Ljungman P, et al. Prognostic factors in autologous stem cell transplantation for multiple myeloma: an EBMT Registry Study: European Group for Bone Marrow Transplantation. Leuk Lymphoma 1994;15:265–72.

173. Child JA, Crawford SM, Norfolk DR, et al. Evaluation of serum beta 2-microglobulin as a prognostic indicator in myelomatosis. Br J Cancer 1983;47:111–4.

174. Bataille R, Boccadoro M, Klein B, et al. C-reactive protein and beta-2 microglobulin produce a simple and powerful myeloma staging system. Blood 1992;80:733–7.

175. Greipp PR, Kyle RA. Clinical, morphological, and cell kinetic differences among multiple myeloma, monoclonal gammopathy of undetermined significance, and smoldering multiple myeloma. Blood 1983;62:166–71.

176. Durie BG, Young LA, Salmon SE. Human myeloma in vitro colony growth: interrelationships between drug sensitivity, cell kinetics, and patient survival duration. Blood 1983;61:929–34.

177. San Miguel JF, Garcia-Sanz R, Gonzalez M, et al. A new staging system for multiple myeloma based on the number of S-phase plasma cells. Blood 1995;85:448–55.

178. Greipp PR, Katzmann JA, O'Fallon WM, Kyle RA. Value of beta 2-microglobulin level and plasma cell labeling indices as prognostic factors in patients with newly diagnosed myeloma. Blood 1988;72:219–23.

179. Greipp PR, Lust JA, O'Fallon WM, et al. Plasma cell labeling index and beta 2-microglobulin predict survival independent of thymidine kinase and C-reactive protein in multiple myeloma. Blood 1993;81:3382–7. see comments.
180. Bartl R, Frisch B, Burkhardt R, et al. Bone marrow histology in myeloma: its importance in diagnosis, prognosis, classification and staging. Br J Haematol 1982;51:361–75.
181. Greipp PR, Leong T, Bennett JM, et al. Plasmablastic morphology—an independent prognostic factor with clinical and laboratory correlates: Eastern Cooperative Oncology Group (ECOG) myeloma trial E9486 report by the ECOG Myeloma Laboratory Group. Blood 1998;91:2501–7.
182. Rajkumar SV, Fonseca R, Lacy MQ, et al. Plasmablastic morphology is an independent predictor of poor survival after autologous stem-cell transplantation for multiple myeloma. J Clin Oncol 1999;17:1551–7.
183. Sawyer JR, Waldron JA, Jagannath S, Barlogie B. Cytogenetic findings in 200 patients with multiple myeloma. Cancer Genet Cytogenet 1995;82:41–9.
184. Tricot G, Sawyer JR, Jagannath S, et al. Unique role of cytogenetics in the prognosis of patients with myeloma receiving high-dose therapy and autotransplants. J Clin Oncol 1997;15:2659–66.
185. Seong C, Delasalle K, Hayes K, et al. Prognostic value of cytogenetics in multiple myeloma. Br J Haematol 1998;101:189–94.
186. Perez-Simon JA, Garcia-Sanz R, Tabernero MD, et al. Prognostic value of numerical chromosome aberrations in multiple myeloma: a FISH analysis of 15 different chromosomes. Blood 1998;91:3366–71.
187. Bergsagel DE. Treatment of plasma cell myeloma. Annu Rev Med 1979;30:431–43.
188. Party MRCW. Report on the first myelomatosis trial. I: Analysis of presenting features of prognostic importance. Br J Haematol 1973;24:123–39.
189. Cavo M, Galieni P, Zuffa E, et al. Prognostic variables and clinical staging in multiple myeloma. Blood 1989;74:1774–80.
190. Peest D, Coldewey R, Deicher H, et al. Prognostic value of clinical, laboratory, and histological characteristics in multiple myeloma: improved definition of risk groups. Eur J Cancer 1993;7:978–83.
191. Drach J, Ackermann J, Fritz E, et al. Presence of a p53 gene deletion in patients with multiple myeloma predicts for short survival after conventional-dose chemotherapy. Blood 1998;92:802–9.
192. Dimopoulos MA, Barlogie B, Smith TL, Alexanian R. High serum lactate dehydrogenase level as a marker for drug resistance and short survival in multiple myeloma. Ann Intern Med 1991;115:931–5.
193. Brown RD, Joshua DE, Nelson M, et al. Serum thymidine kinase as a prognostic indicator for patients with multiple myeloma: results from the MRC (UK) V trial. Br J Haematol 1993;84:238–41.
194. Witzig TE, Gertz MA, Lust JA, et al. Peripheral blood monoclonal plasma cells as a predictor of survival in patients with multiple myeloma. Blood 1996;88:1780–7. see comments.
195. Greipp PR. Prognosis in myeloma. Mayo Clin Proc 1994;69:895–902.
196. Blade J, Kyle RA, Greipp PR. Presenting features and prognosis in 72 patients with multiple myeloma who were younger than 40 years. Br J Haematol 1996;93:345–51.
197. Alexanian R, Balcerzak S, Bonnet JD, et al. Prognostic factors in multiple myeloma. Cancer 1975;36:1192–201.
198. A cooperative study by Acute Leukemia Group B. Correlation of abnormal immunoglobulin with clinical features of myeloma. Arch Intern Med 1975;135:46–52.
199. Blade J, Lopez-Guillermo A, Bosch F, et al. Impact of response to treatment on survival in multiple myeloma: results in a series of 243 patients. Br J Haematol 1994;88:117–21.
200. Oivanen TM, Kellokumpu-Lehtinen P, Koivisto AM, et al. Response level and survival after conventional chemotherapy for multiple myeloma: a Finnish Leukaemia Group study. Eur J Haematol 1999;62:109–16.
201. Hansen OP, Jessen B, Videbaek A. Prognosis of myelomatosis on treatment with prednisone and cytostatics. Scand J Haematol 1973;10:282–90.
202. van Hoeven KH, Reed LJ, Factor SM. Autopsy-documented cure of multiple myeloma 14 years after M2 chemotherapy. Cancer 1990; 66:1472–4.
203. Hjorth M, Hellquist L, Holmberg E, et al. Initial versus deferred melphalan-prednisone therapy for asymptomatic multiple myeloma stage I—a randomized study. Myeloma Group of Western Sweden. Eur J Haematol 1993; 50:95–102.
204. Mill WB, Griffith R. The role of radiation therapy in the management of plasma cell tumors. Cancer 1980; 45:647–52.
205. Hu K, Yahalom J. Radiotherapy in the management of plasma cell tumors [In Process Citation]. Oncology (Huntingt) 2000; 14:101–8, 111; discussion 111–2, 115.
206. Leigh BR, Kurtts TA, Mack CF, et al. Radiation therapy for the palliation of multiple myeloma. Int J Radiat Oncol Biol Phys 1993; 25:801–4. see comments.
207. Harley JB, Schilling A, Glidewell O. Ineffectiveness of fluoride therapy in multiple myeloma. N Engl J Med 1972;286:1283–8.
208. Cohen HJ, Silberman HR, Tornyos K, Bartolucci AA. Comparison of two long-term chemotherapy regimens, with or without agents to modify skeletal repair, in multiple myeloma. Blood 1984;63:639–48.
209. Rico H, Hernandez ER, Diaz-Mediavilla J, et al. Treatment of multiple myeloma with nasal spray calcitonin: a histomorphometric and biochemical study. Bone Miner 1990;8:231–7.
210. van Breukelen FJ, Bijvoet OL, van Oosterom AT. Inhibition of osteolytic bone lesions by (3-amino-1-hydroxypropylidene)-1,1-bisphosphonate (A.P.D.). Lancet 1979;1:803–5.
211. Siris ES, Sherman WH, Baquiran DC, et al. Effects of dichloromethylene diphosphonate on skeletal mobilization of calcium in multiple myeloma. N Engl J Med 1980;302:310–5.
212. Lahtinen R, Laakso M, Palva I, et al. Randomised, placebo-controlled multicentre trial of clodronate in multiple myeloma: Finnish Leukaemia Group. Lancet 1992; 340:1049–52 [published erratum appears in Lancet 1992;340:1420]. see comments.
213. Heim ME, Clemens MR, Queisser W, et al. Prospective randomized trial of dichloromethylene bisphosphonate (clodronate) in patients with multiple myeloma requiring treatment: a multicenter study. Onkologie 1995;18:439–48.
214. McCloskey EV, MacLennan IC, Drayson MT, et al. A randomized trial of the effect of clodronate on skeletal morbidity in multiple myeloma: MRC Working Party on Leukaemia in Adults. Br J Haematol 1998;100:317–25.
215. Berenson JR, Lichtenstein A, Porter L, et al. Efficacy of pamidronate in reducing skeletal events in patients with advanced multiple myeloma: Myeloma Aredia Study Group. N Engl J Med 1996;334:488–93. see comments.
216. Berenson JR, Lichtenstein A, Porter L, et al. Long-term pamidronate treatment of advanced multiple myeloma patients reduces skeletal events: Myeloma Aredia Study Group. J Clin Oncol 1998;16:593–602. see comments.
217. Brincker H, Westin J, Abildgaard N, et al. Failure of oral pamidronate to reduce skeletal morbidity in multiple myeloma: a double-blind placebo-controlled trial: Danish-Swedish co-operative study group. Br J Haematol 1998;101:280–6.
218. Troehler U, Bonjour JP, Fleisch H. Renal secretion of diphosphonates in rats. Kidney Int 1975;8:6–13.
219. Berenson JR, Rosen L, Vescio R, et al. Pharmacokinetics of pamidronate disodium in patients with cancer with normal or impaired renal function. J Clin Pharmacol 1997;37:285–90.
220. Aparicio A, Gardner A, Tu Y, et al. In vitro cytoreductive effects on multiple myeloma cells induced by bisphosphonates. Leukemia 1998;12:220–9.
221. Savage AD, Belson DJ, Vescio RA, et al. Pamidronate reduces IL-6 production by bone marrow stroma from multiple myeloma patients. Blood 1996;88:105a.
222. Raisz LG, Luben RA, Mundy GR, et al. Effect of osteoclast activating factor from human leukocytes on bone metabolism. J Clin Invest 1975;56:408–13.
223. Body JJ, Magritte A, Seraj F, et al. Aminohydroxypropylidene bisphosphonate (APD) treatment for tumor-associated hypercalcemia: a randomized comparison between a 3-day treatment and single 24-hour infusions. J Bone Miner Res 1989;4:923–8.
224. Alexanian R, Bonnet J, Gehan E, et al. Combination chemotherapy for multiple myeloma. Cancer 1972;30:382–9.
225. Lazarus HM, Lederman M, Lubin A, et al. Pneumococcal vaccination: the response of patients with multiple myeloma. Am J Med 1980;69:419–23.
226. Shildt RA, Rubin RR, Schiffman G, Giolma P. Polyvalent pneumococcal immunization of patients with plasma cell dyscrasias. Cancer 1981;48:1377–80.
227. Birgens HS, Espersen F, Hertz JB, et al. Antibody response to pneumococcal vaccination in patients with myelomatosis. Scand J Haematol 1983;30:324–30.
228. Misiani R, Remuzzi G, Bertani T, et al. Plasmapheresis in the treatment of acute renal failure in multiple myeloma. Am J Med 1979;66:684–8.

229. Johnson WJ, Kyle RA, Pineda AA, et al. Treatment of renal failure associated with multiple myeloma: plasmapheresis, hemodialysis, and chemotherapy. Arch Intern Med 1990;150:863–9.

230. Kes P, Pecanic Z, Getaldic B. Plasmapheresis and hemodialysis in the treatment of acute renal failure in multiple myeloma. Acta Med Croatica 1995;49:39–42.

231. Bear RA, Cole EH, Lang A, Johnson M. Treatment of acute renal failure due to myeloma kidney. Can Med Assoc J 1980;123:750–3.

232. Rosansky SJ, Richards FW. Use of peritoneal dialysis in the treatment of patients with renal failure and paraproteinemia. Am J Nephrol 1985;5:361–5.

233. Johnson WJ, Kyle RA, Dahlberg PJ. Dialysis in the treatment of multiple myeloma. Mayo Clin Proc 1980;55:65–72.

234. Humphrey RL, Wright JR, Zachary JB, et al. Renal transplantation in multiple myeloma: a case report. Ann Intern Med 1975;83:651–3.

235. Salmon SE, Smith BA. Immunoglobulin synthesis and total body tumor cell number in IgG multiple myeloma. J Clin Invest 1970;49:1114–21.

236. Salmon SE. Immunoglobulin synthesis and tumor kinetics of multiple myeloma. Semin Hematol 1973;10:135–44.

237. Salmon SE. Expansion of the growth fraction in multiple myeloma with alkylating agents. Blood 1975;45:119–29.

238. Durie BG, Russell DH, Salmon SE. Reappraisal of plateau phase in myeloma. Lancet 1980;2:65–8.

239. Redwood WR, Colvin M. Transport of melphalan by sensitive and resistant L1210 cells. Cancer Res 1980;40:1144–9.

240. Hamilton TC, Winker MA, Louie KG, et al. Augmentation of Adriamycin, melphalan, and cisplatin cytotoxicity in drug-resistant and -sensitive human ovarian carcinoma cell lines by buthionine sulfoximine mediated glutathione depletion. Biochem Pharmacol 1985;34:2583–6.

241. Dalton WS, Durie BG, Alberts DS, et al. Characterization of a new drug-resistant human myeloma cell line that expresses P-glycoprotein. Cancer Res 1986;46:5125–30.

242. Hazlehurst LA, Foley NE, Gleason-Guzman MC, et al. Multiple mechanisms confer drug resistance to mitoxantrone in the human 8226 myeloma cell line. Cancer Res 1999;59:1021–8.

243. Landowski TH, Gleason-Guzman MC, Dalton WS. Selection for drug resistance results in resistance to Fas-mediated apoptosis. Blood 1997;89:1854–61.

244. Moalli PA, Rosen ST. Glucocorticoid receptors and resistance to glucocorticoids in hematologic malignancies. Leuk Lymphoma 1994;15:363–74.

245. Hofmann V, Salmon SE, Durie BG. Drug resistance in multiple myeloma associated with high in vitro incorporation of 3H-thymidine. Blood 1981;58:471–6.

246. Mongkonsritragoon W, Kimlinger T, Ahmann G, Greipp PR. Is multi-drug resistance (P-glycoprotein) an intrinsic characteristic of plasma cells in patients with monoclonal gammopathy of undetermined significance, plasmacytoma, multiple myeloma and amyloidosis? Leuk Lymphoma 1998;29:577–84.

247. Wyler B, Shao Y, Schneider E, et al. Intermittent exposure to doxorubicin in vitro selects for multifactorial non–P-glycoprotein–associated multidrug resistance in RPMI 8226 human myeloma cells. Br J Haematol 1997;97:65–75.

248. Grogan TM, Spier CM, Salmon SE, et al. P-glycoprotein expression in human plasma cell myeloma: correlation with prior chemotherapy. Blood 1993;81:490–5.

249. Musto P, Lombardi G, Matera R, Carotenuto M. The expression of the multidrug transporter P-170 glycoprotein in remission phase is associated with early and resistant relapse in multiple myeloma. Haematologica 1991;76:513–6.

250. Dalton WS, Crowley JJ, Salmon SS, et al. A phase III randomized study of oral verapamil as a chemosensitizer to reverse drug resistance in patients with refractory myeloma: a Southwest Oncology Group study. Cancer 1995;75:815–20.

251. Salmon SE, Crowley JJ, Balcerzak SP, et al. Interferon versus interferon plus prednisone remission maintenance therapy for multiple myeloma: a Southwest Oncology Group Study. J Clin Oncol 1998;16:890–6.

252. Raje N, Powles R, Kulkarni S, et al. A comparison of vincristine and doxorubicin infusional chemotherapy with methylprednisolone (VAMP) with the addition of weekly cyclophosphamide (C-VAMP) as induction treatment followed by autografting in previously untreated myeloma. Br J Haematol 1997;97:153–60.

253. Jonsson B, Nilsson K, Nygren P, Larsson R. SDZ PSC-833—a novel potent in vitro chemosensitizer in multiple myeloma. Anticancer Drugs 1992;3:641–6.

254. Sonneveld P, Marie JP, Huisman C, et al. Reversal of multidrug resistance by SDZ PSC 833, combined with VAD (vincristine, doxorubicin, dexamethasone) in refractory multiple myeloma: a phase I study. Leukemia 1996;10:1741–50.

255. Dalton WS, Jove R. Drug resistance in multiple myeloma: approaches to circumvention. Semin Oncol 1999;26:23–7.

256. Shiao RT, Miglietta L, Khera SY, et al. Dexamethasone and suramin inhibit cell proliferation and interleukin-6–mediated immunoglobulin secretion in human lymphoid and multiple myeloma cell lines. Leuk Lymphoma 1995;17:485–94.

257. Smith MR, Xie T, Joshi I, Schilder RJ. Dexamethasone plus retinoids decrease IL-6/IL-6 receptor and induce apoptosis in myeloma cells. Br J Haematol 1998;102:1090–7.

258. Alexanian R, Haut A, Khan AU, et al. Treatment for multiple myeloma: combination chemotherapy with different melphalan dose regimens. JAMA 1969;208:1680–5.

259. Alexanian R, Dimopoulos MA, Delasalle K, Barlogie B. Primary dexamethasone treatment of multiple myeloma. Blood 1992;80:887–90.

260. Alexanian R, Dimopoulos M. The treatment of multiple myeloma. N Engl J Med 1994;330:484–9.

261. Woodruff R. Treatment of multiple myeloma. Cancer Treat Rev 1981;8:225–70.

262. Kyle RA. Long-term survival in multiple myeloma. N Engl J Med 1983;308:314–6.

263. Alexanian R, Bergsagel DE, Migliore PJ, et al. Melphalan therapy for plasma cell myeloma. Blood 1968;31:1–10.

264. Alberts DS, Chang SY, Chen HS, et al. Oral melphalan kinetics. Clin Pharmacol Ther 1979;26:737–45.

265. Bosanquet AG, Gilby ED. Pharmacokinetics of oral and intravenous melphalan during routine treatment of multiple myeloma. Eur J Cancer Clin Oncol 1982;18:355–62.

266. Medical Research Council. Myelomatosis: comparison of melphalan and cyclophosphamide therapy. Br Med J 1971;1:640–1.

267. Bergsagel DE, Cowan DH, Hasselback R. Plasma cell myeloma: response of melphalan-resistant patients to high-dose intermittent cyclophosphamide. Can Med Assoc J 1972;107:851–5.

268. Kyle RA, Gailani S, Seligman BR, et al. Multiple myeloma resistant to melphalan: treatment with cyclophosphamide, prednisone, and BCNU. Cancer Treat Rep 1979;63:1265–9.

269. Blade J, Feliu E, Rozman C, et al. Cross-resistance to alkylating agents in multiple myeloma. Cancer 1983;52:786–9.

270. Brandes LJ, Israels LG. Weekly low-dose cyclophosphamide and alternate-day prednisone: an effective low toxicity regimen for advanced myeloma. Eur J Haematol 1987;39:362–8.

271. Palumbo A, Boccadoro M, Bruno B, et al. Cyclophosphamide (3.6 g/m$^2$) therapy with G-CSF support for resistant myeloma. Haematologica 1994;79:513–8.

272. Schiller G, Vescio R, Freytes C, et al. Transplantation of CD34$^+$ peripheral blood progenitor cells after high-dose chemotherapy for patients with advanced multiple myeloma. Blood 1995;86:390–7.

273. Southeastern Cancer Study Group. Treatment of myeloma: comparison of melphalan, chlorambucil, and azathioprine. Arch Intern Med 1975;135:157–62.

274. Salmon SE. Nitrosoureas in multiple myeloma. Cancer Treat Rep 1976;60:789–94.

275. Cornwell GGD, Pajak TF, Kochwa S, et al. Comparison of oral melphalan, CCNU, and BCNU with and without vincristine and prednisone in the treatment of multiple myeloma: Cancer and Leukemia Group B experience. Cancer 1982;50:1669–75.

276. Moon JH, Edmonson JH. Procarbazine (NSC-77213) and multiple myeloma. Cancer Chemother Rep 1970;54:245–8.

277. Alberts DS, Salmon SE. Adriamycin (NSC-123127) in the treatment of alkylator-resistant multiple myeloma: a pilot study. Cancer Chemother Rep 1975;59:345–50.

278. Cook G, Sharp RA, Tansey P, Franklin IM. A phase I/II trial of Z-Dex (oral idarubicin and dexamethasone), an oral equivalent of VAD, as initial therapy at diagnosis or progression in multiple myeloma. Br J Haematol 1996;93:931–4.

279. Sumpter K, Powles RL, Raje N, et al. Oral idarubicin as a single agent therapy in patients with relapsed or resistant multiple myeloma. Leuk Lymphoma 1999;35:593–7.

280. MacLennan IC, Cusick J. Objective evaluation of the role of vincristine in induction and maintenance therapy for myelomatosis: Medical Research Council Working Party on Leukaemia in Adults. Br J Cancer 1985;52:153–8.

281. Jackson DV, Case LD, Pope EK, et al. Single agent vincristine by infusion in refractory multiple myeloma. J Clin Oncol 1985;3:1508–12.

282. Houwen B, Ockhuizen T, Marrink J, Nieweg HO. Vindesine therapy in melphalan-resistant multiple myeloma. Eur J Cancer 1981;17:227–32.

283. Alexanian R, Yap BS, Bodey GP. Prednisone pulse therapy for refractory myeloma. Blood 1983;62:572–7.

284. van der Lelie H, Monasch E, Pegels HG, von dem Borne AE. Vindesine in refractory multiple myeloma. Cancer 1986;7:226–9.

285. Quesada JR, Alexanian R, Hawkins M, et al. Treatment of multiple myeloma with recombinant alpha-interferon. Blood 1986;67:275–8.

286. Ahre A, Bjorkholm M, Osterborg A, et al. High doses of natural alpha-interferon (alpha-IFN) in the treatment of multiple myeloma—a pilot study from the Myeloma Group of Central Sweden (MGCS). Eur J Haematol 1988;41:123–30.

287. Ludwig H, Cortelezzi A, Scheithauer W, et al. Recombinant interferon alfa-2C versus polychemotherapy (VMCP) for treatment of multiple myeloma: a prospective randomized trial. Eur J Cancer Clin Oncol 1986;22:1111–6.

288. Costanzi JJ, Cooper MR, Scarffe JH, et al. Phase II study of recombinant alpha-2 interferon in resistant multiple myeloma. J Clin Oncol 1985;3:654–9.

289. Wagstaff J, Loynds P, Scarffe JH. Phase II study of rDNA human alpha-2 interferon in multiple myeloma. Cancer Treat Rep 1985;69:495–8.

290. Buzaid AC, Durie BG. Management of refractory myeloma: a review. J Clin Oncol 1988;6:889–905.

291. Otsuki T, Yamada O, Sakaguchi H, et al. Human myeloma cell apoptosis induced by interferon-alpha. Br J Haematol 1998;103:518–29.

292. Bergsagel DE, Haas RH, Messner HA. Interferon alfa-2b in the treatment of chronic granulocytic leukemia. Semin Oncol 1986;13:29–34.

293. Ferlin-Bezombes M, Jourdan M, Liautard J, et al. IFN-alpha is a survival factor for human myeloma cells and reduces dexamethasone-induced apoptosis. J Immunol 1998;161:2692–9.

294. Brass U, Tretter T, Schneller F, et al. IFN-alpha stimulates proliferation and cytokine secretion of CD40-stimulated B cell chronic lymphocytic leukemia cells in vitro. J Interferon Cytokine Res 1999;19:335–43.

295. Ohno R, Kimura K. Treatment of multiple myeloma with recombinant interferon alfa-2a. Cancer 1986;57:1685–8.

296. Singhal S, Mehta J, Desikan R, et al. Antitumor activity of thalidomide in refractory multiple myeloma. N Engl J Med 1999;341:1565–71. see comments.

297. Sastry PS. Inhibition of TNF-alpha synthesis with thalidomide for prevention of acute exacerbations and altering the natural history of multiple sclerosis. Med Hypotheses 1999;53:76–7.

298. Moller DR, Wysocka M, Greenlee BM, et al. Inhibition of IL-12 production by thalidomide. J Immunol 1997;159:5157–61.

299. Larkin M. Low-dose thalidomide seems to be effective in multiple myeloma. Lancet 1999;354:925.

300. Weber DM, Gavino M, Delsalle K, et al. Thalidomide alone or with dexamethasone for multiple myeloma. Blood 1999;94:Suppl 1:604a.

301. Scarffe JH, Beaumont AR, Crowther D. Phase I–II evaluation of acronine in patients with multiple myeloma. Cancer Treat Rep 1983;67:93–4.

302. Kantarjian H, Dreicer R, Barlogie B, et al. High-dose cytosine arabinoside in multiple myeloma. Eur J Cancer Clin Oncol 1984;20:227–31.

303. Gockerman JP, Bartolucci AA, Nelson MO, et al. Phase II evaluation of etoposide in refractory multiple myeloma: a Southeastern Cancer Study Group Trial. Cancer Treat Rep 1986;70:801–2.

304. Kraut EH, Crowley JJ, Grever MR, et al. Phase II study of fludarabine phosphate in multiple myeloma: a Southwest Oncology Group study. Invest New Drugs 1990;8:199–200.

305. Dimopoulos MA, Arbuck S, Huber M, et al. Primary therapy of multiple myeloma with paclitaxel (Taxol). Ann Oncol 1994;5:757–9.

306. Miller HJ, Leong T, Khandekar JD, et al. Paclitaxel as the initial treatment of multiple myeloma: an Eastern Cooperative Oncology Group study (E1A93). Am J Clin Oncol 1998;21:553–6.

307. Merlini G, Gobbi PG, Riccardi A, et al. Peptichemio induction therapy in myelomatosis. Cancer Chemother Pharmacol 1982;8:9–16.

308. Paccagnella A, Salvagno L, Chiarion-Sileni V, et al. Peptichemio in pretreated patients with plasma cell neoplasms. Eur J Cancer Clin Oncol 1986;22:1053–8.

309. Hussein MA, Karan MA, McLain DA, et al. Biologic and clinical evaluation of Rituxan (RT) in the management of newly diagnosed multiple myeloma (MM) patients (Pts). Blood 1999;94:Suppl 1:313a.

310. Sporn JR, McIntyre OR. Chemotherapy of previously untreated multiple myeloma patients: an analysis of recent treatment results. Semin Oncol 1986;13:318–25.

311. Cohen HJ, Silberman HR, Larsen WE, et al. Combination chemotherapy with intermittent 1-3-bis(2-chloroethyl)1-nitrosourea (BCNU), cyclophosphamide, and prednisone for multiple myeloma. Blood 1979;54:824–36.

312. Bergsagel DE. Is aggressive chemotherapy more effective in the treatment of plasma cell myeloma? Eur J Cancer Clin Oncol 1989;25:159–61.

313. Boccadoro M, Pileri A. Standard chemotherapy for myelomatosis: an area of great controversy. Hematol Oncol Clin North Am 1992;6:371–82.

314. Costa G. Unknown. Am J Med 1973;54:589.

315. Ahre A, Bjorkholm M, Mellstedt H, et al. Intermittent high-dose melphalan/prednisone vs continuous low-dose melphalan treatment in multiple myeloma. Eur J Cancer Clin Oncol 1983;19:499–506.

316. Case DC Jr, Lee DJD, Clarkson BD. Improved survival times in multiple myeloma treated with melphalan, prednisone, cyclophosphamide, vincristine and BCNU: M-2 protocol. Am J Med 1977;63:897–903.

317. Palva IP, Ahrenberg P, Ala-Harja K, et al. Treatment of multiple myeloma with an intensive 5-drug combination or intermittent melphalan and prednisone; a randomised multicentre trial: Finnish Leukaemia Group. Eur J Haematol 1987;38:50–4.

318. Casey DE. Tardive dyskinesia: nondopaminergic treatment approaches. Psychopharmacology 1985;2:Suppl:137–44.

319. Paccagnella A, Cartei G, Fosser V, et al. Treatment of multiple myeloma with M-2 protocol and without maintenance therapy. Eur J Cancer Clin Oncol 1983;19:1345–51.

320. Tirelli U, Crivellari D, Carbone A, et al. Combination chemotherapy for multiple myeloma with melphalan, prednisone, cyclophosphamide, vincristine, and carmustine (BCNU) (M-2 protocol). Cancer Treat Rep 1982;66:1971–3.

321. Oken MM, Harrington DP, Abramson N, et al. Comparison of melphalan and prednisone with vincristine, carmustine, melphalan, cyclophosphamide, and prednisone in the treatment of multiple myeloma: results of Eastern Cooperative Oncology Group Study E2479. Cancer 1997;79:1561–7.

322. Hansen OP, Clausen NA, Drivsholm A, Laursen B. Phase III study of intermittent 5-drug regimen (VBCMP) versus intermittent 3-drug regimen (VMP) versus intermittent melphalan and prednisone (MP) in myelomatosis. Scand J Haematol 1985;35:518–24.

323. Pavlovsky S, Saslavsky J, Tezanos Pinto M, et al. A randomized trial of melphalan and prednisone versus melphalan, prednisone, cyclophosphamide, MeCCNU, and vincristine in untreated multiple myeloma. J Clin Oncol 1984;2:836–40.

324. Alexanian R, Salmon S, Bonnet J, et al. Combination therapy for multiple myeloma. Cancer 1977;40:2765–71.

325. Alexanian R, Salmon S, Gutterman J, et al. Chemoimmunotherapy for multiple myeloma. Cancer 1981;47:1923–9.

326. Salmon SE, Haut A, Bonnet JD, et al. Alternating combination chemotherapy and levamisole improves survival in multiple myeloma: a Southwest Oncology Group Study. J Clin Oncol 1983;1:453–61.

327. Tribalto M, Amadori S, Cantonetti M, et al. Treatment of multiple myeloma: a randomized study of three different regimens. Leuk Res 1985;9:1043–9.

328. Cooper MR, McIntyre OR, Propert KJ, et al. Single, sequential, and multiple alkylating agent therapy for multiple myeloma: a CALGB Study. J Clin Oncol 1986;4:1331–9.

329. Durie BG, Dixon DO, Carter S, et al. Improved survival duration with combination chemotherapy induction for multiple myeloma: a Southwest Oncology Group Study. J Clin Oncol 1986;4:1227–37.

330. Blade J, San Miguel JF, Alcala A, et al. Alternating combination VCMP/VBAP chemotherapy versus melphalan/prednisone in the treatment of multiple myeloma: a randomized multicentric study of 487 patients. J Clin Oncol 1993;11:1165–71.

331. Gregory WM, Richards MA, Malpas JS. Combination chemotherapy versus melphalan and prednisolone in the treatment of multiple myeloma: an overview of published trials. J Clin Oncol 1992;10:334–42. see comments.

332. Bergsagel DE. Myeloma, melphalan, and meta-analysis J Clin Oncol 1992;10:178–9. editorial; comment.

333. Group MTC. Combination chemotherapy versus melphalan plus prednisone as treatment for multiple myeloma: an overview of 6,633 patients from 27 randomized trials: Myeloma Trialists' Collaborative Group. J Clin Oncol 1998;16:3832–42.

334. Salmon SE, Cassidy JR. Plasma cell neoplasms. In: DeVita VT, et al. Cancer: principles and practice of oncology. Philadelphia: JB Lippincott, 1993:1995.

335. Salmon SE, Crowley JJ, Grogan TM, et al. Combination chemotherapy, glucocorticoids, and interferon alfa in the treatment of multiple myeloma: a Southwest Oncology Group study. J Clin Oncol 1994;12:2405–14. see comments.

336. Osterborg A, Bjorkholm M, Bjoreman M, et al. Natural interferon-alpha in combination with melphalan/prednisone versus melphalan/prednisone in the treatment of multiple myeloma stages II and III: a randomized study from the Myeloma Group of Central Sweden. Blood 1993;81:1428–34.

337. Cooper MR, Dear K, McIntyre OR, et al. A randomized clinical trial comparing melphalan/prednisone with or without interferon alfa-2b in newly diagnosed patients with multiple myeloma: a Cancer and Leukemia Group B study. J Clin Oncol 1993;11:155–60.

338. Ludwig H, Cohen AM, Polliack A, et al. Interferon-alpha for induction and maintenance in multiple myeloma: results of two multicenter randomized trials and summary of other studies. Ann Oncol 1995;6:467–76.

339. Barlogie B, Jagannath S, Dixon DO, et al. High-dose melphalan and granulocyte-macrophage colony-stimulating factor for refractory multiple myeloma. Blood 1990;76:677–80.

340. Buckner CD, Fefer A, Bensinger WI, et al. Marrow transplantation for malignant plasma cell disorders: summary of the Seattle experience. Eur J Haematol 1989;51:Suppl:186–90.

341. Copelan EA, Tutschka PJ. Marrow transplantation following busulfan and cyclophosphamide in multiple myeloma. Bone Marrow Transplant 1988;3:363–5.

342. Barlogie B, Gahrton G. Bone marrow transplantation in multiple myeloma. Bone Marrow Transplant 1991;7:71–9.

343. Gahrton G, Tura S, Flesch M, et al. Bone marrow transplantation in multiple myeloma: report from the European Cooperative Group for Bone Marrow Transplantation. Blood 1987;69:1262–4.

344. Gahrton G. Allogeneic bone marrow transplantation in multiple myeloma. Br J Haematol 1996;92:251–4.

345. Bensinger WI, Buckner CD, Anasetti C, et al. Allogeneic marrow transplantation for multiple myeloma: an analysis of risk factors on outcome. Blood 1996;88:2787–93.

346. Tura S, Cavo M. Allogeneic bone marrow transplantation in multiple myeloma. Hematol Oncol Clin North Am 1992;6:425–35.

347. Gahrton G. Allogeneic bone marrow transplantation in multiple myeloma. Pathol Biol (Paris) 1999;47:188–91.

348. Slavin S, Nagler A, Naparstek E, et al. Nonmyeloablative stem cell transplantation and cell therapy as an alternative to conventional bone marrow transplantation with lethal cytoreduction for the treatment of malignant and nonmalignant hematologic diseases. Blood 1998;91:756–63.

349. Gahrton G, Svensson H, Bjorkstrand B, et al. Syngeneic transplantation in multiple myeloma—a case-matched comparison with autologous and allogeneic transplantation: European Group for Blood and Marrow Transplantation. Bone Marrow Transplant 1999;24:741–5.

350. Jagannath S, Barlogie B. Autologous bone marrow transplantation for multiple myeloma. Hematol Oncol Clin North Am 1992;6:437–49.

351. Schiller G, Nimer S, Vescio R, et al. Phase I–II study of busulfan and cyclophosphamide conditioning for transplantation in advanced multiple myeloma. Bone Marrow Transplant 1994;14:131–6.

352. Reiffers J, Marit G, Boiron JM. Autologous blood stem cell transplantation in high-risk multiple myeloma. Br J Haematol 1989; 72:296–7. letter.

353. Fermand JP, Chevret S, Ravaud P, et al. High-dose chemoradiotherapy and autologous blood stem cell transplantation in multiple myeloma: results of a phase II trial involving 63 patients. Blood 1993;82:2005–9.

354. Vesole DH, Jagannath S, Glenn L, Barlogie B. Autotransplantation in multiple myeloma. Hematol Oncol Clin North Am 1993;7:613–30.

355. Cunningham D, Paz-Ares L, Gore ME, et al. High-dose melphalan for multiple myeloma: long-term follow-up data. J Clin Oncol 1994;12:764–8.

356. Schiller G, Vescio R, Freytes C, et al. Autologous CD34-selected blood progenitor cell transplants for patients with advanced multiple myeloma. Bone Marrow Transplant 1998;21:141–5. see comments.

357. Attal M, Harousseau JL, Stoppa AM, et al. A prospective, randomized trial of autologous bone marrow transplantation and chemotherapy in multiple myeloma: Intergroupe Français du Myelome. N Engl J Med 1996;335:91–7. see comments.

358. Harousseau JL, Attal M. The role of autologous hematopoietic stem cell transplantation in multiple myeloma. Semin Hematol 1997; 34:61–6.

359. Lenhoff S, Hjorth M, Holmberg E, et al. Impact on survival of high-dose therapy with autologous stem cell support in patients younger than 60 years with newly diagnosed multiple myeloma: a population-based study: Nordic Myeloma Study Group. Blood 2000;95:7–11.

360. Fermand JP, Ravaud P, Chevret S, et al. High-dose therapy and autologous peripheral blood stem cell transplantation in multiple myeloma: up-front or rescue treatment? Results of a multicenter sequential randomized clinical trial. Blood 1998;92:3131–6.

361. Vescio RA, Han EJ, Schiller GJ, et al. Quantitative comparison of multiple myeloma tumor contamination in bone marrow harvest and leukapheresis autografts. Bone Marrow Transplant 1996;18:103–10.

362. Raje N, Powles R, Horton C, et al. Comparison of marrow vs blood-derived stem cells for autografting in previously untreated multiple myeloma. Br J Cancer 1997;75:1684–9.

363. Jagannath S, Tricot G, Barlogie B. Autotransplants in multiple myeloma: pushing the envelope. Hematol Oncol Clin North Am 1997;11:363–81.

364. Goldschmidt H, Hegenbart U, Wallmeier M, et al. High-dose chemotherapy in multiple myeloma. Leukemia 1997;11:Suppl 5:S27–31.

365. Vesole DH. Bone marrow and stem cell transplantation for multiple myeloma. Cancer Treat Res 1999;99:171–94.

366. Fermand JP, Brechignac S. The role of autologous stem cell transplantation in the management of multiple myeloma. Pathol Biol (Paris) 1999;47:199–202.

367. Tribalto M, Amadori S, Cudillo L, et al. Autologous peripheral blood stem cell transplantation as first line treatment of multiple myeloma: an Italian multicenter study. Haematologica 2000;85:52–8.

368. Vescio R, Schiller G, Stewart AK, et al. Multicenter phase III trial to evaluate CD34(+) selected versus unselected autologous peripheral blood progenitor cell transplantation in multiple myeloma. Blood 1999;93:1858–68.

369. Vescio R, Berenson J. Autologous transplantation: purging and the impact of minimal residual disease. Hematol Oncol Clin North Am 1999;13:969–86.

370. Siegel DS, Desikan KR, Mehta J, et al. Age is not a prognostic variable with autotransplants for multiple myeloma. Blood 1999;93:51–4.

371. Alexanian R, Gehan E, Haut A, et al. Unmaintained remissions in multiple myeloma. Blood 1978;51:1005–11.

372. Mandelli F, Avvisati G, Amadori S, et al. Maintenance treatment with recombinant interferon alfa-2b in patients with multiple myeloma responding to conventional induction chemotherapy. N Engl J Med 1990;322:1430–4.

373. Westin J. Interferon therapy during the plateau phase of multiple myeloma: an update of a Swedish multicenter study. Semin Oncol 1991;18:37–40.

374. Browman GP, Bergsagel D, Sicheri D, et al. Randomized trial of interferon maintenance in multiple myeloma: a study of the National Cancer Institute of Canada Clinical Trials Group. J Clin Oncol 1995;13:2354–60.

375. Ludwig H, Cohen AM, Huber H, et al. Interferon alfa-2b with VMCP compared to VMCP alone for induction and interferon alfa-2b compared to controls for remission maintenance in multiple myeloma: interim results. Eur J Cancer 1991; 27:S40–5.

376. Zee B, Cole B, Li T, et al. Quality-adjusted time without symptoms or toxicity analysis of interferon maintenance in multiple myeloma. J Clin Oncol 1998;16:2834–9. see comments.

377. Palumbo A, Boccadoro M, Garino LA, et al. Interferon plus glucocorticoids as intensified maintenance therapy prolongs tumor control in relapsed myeloma. Acta Haematol 1993;90:71–6.

377a. Berenson J, Crowley J, Barlogie B, et al. Alternate day prednisone maintenance therapy improves progression-free and overall survival in multiple myeloma patients. Blood 1998;92:Suppl 1:318a.

378. Bergsagel DE. Use a gentle approach for refractory myeloma patients. J Clin Oncol 1988;6:757–8. editorial.

379. Belch A, Shelley W, Bergsagel D, et al. A randomized trial of maintenance versus no maintenance melphalan and prednisone in responding multiple myeloma patients. Br J Cancer 1988;57:94–9.

380. Barlogie B, Smith L, Alexanian R. Effective treatment of advanced multiple myeloma refractory to alkylating agents. N Engl J Med 1984;310:1353–6.

381. Monconduit M, Le Loet X, Bernard JF, Michaux JL. Combination chemotherapy with vincristine, doxorubicin, dexamethasone for refractory or relapsing multiple myeloma. Br J Haematol 1986;63:599–601. letter.

382. Sheehan T, Judge M, Parker AC. The efficacy and toxicity of VAD in the treatment of myeloma and related disorders. Scand J Haematol 1986;37:425–8.

383. Alexanian R, Barlogie B, Dixon D. High-dose glucocorticoid treatment of resistant myeloma. Ann Intern Med 1986;105:8–11.

384. Dimopoulos MA, Delasalle KB, Champlin R, Alexanian R. Cyclophosphamide and etoposide therapy with GM-CSF for VAD-resistant multiple myeloma. Br J Haematol 1993;83:240–4.

385. Barlogie B, Vesole DH, Jagannath S. Salvage therapy for multiple myeloma: the University of Arkansas experience. Mayo Clin Proc 1994;69:787–95.

386. Tobias JS, Richards JD, Blackman GM, et al. Hemibody irradiation in multiple myeloma. Radiother Oncol 1985;3:11–6.

387. Singer CR, Tobias JS, Giles F, et al. Hemibody irradiation: an effective second-line therapy in drug-resistant multiple myeloma. Cancer 1989;63:2446–51.

388. Thomas PJ, Daban A, Bontoux D. Double hemibody irradiation in chemotherapy-resistant multiple myeloma. Cancer Treat Rep 1984;68:1173–5.

389. McSweeney EN, Tobias JS, Blackman G, et al. Double hemibody irradiation (DHBI) in the management of relapsed and primary chemoresistant multiple myeloma. Clin Oncol 1993;5:378–83.

390. Plesnicar A, Jereb B, Zaletel-Kragelj L. Half-body irradiation in the treatment of multiple myeloma: a report of nine cases. Tumori 1996;82:588–91.

391. Salmon SE, Tesh D, Crowley J, et al. Chemotherapy is superior to sequential hemibody irradiation for remission consolidation in multiple myeloma: a Southwest Oncology Group study. J Clin Oncol 1990;8:1575–84. see comments.

392. Bayouth JE, Macey DJ, Kasi LP, et al. Pharmacokinetics, dosimetry and toxicity of holmium-166-DOTMP for bone marrow ablation in multiple myeloma. J Nucl Med 1995;36:730–7.

393. Axelsson U, Bachmann R, Hallen J. Frequency of pathological proteins (M-components) in 6,995 sera from an adult population. Acta Med Scand 1966;179:235–47.

394. Crawford J, Eye MK, Cohen HJ. Evaluation of monoclonal gammopathies in the "well" elderly. Am J Med 1987;82:39–45.

395. Sinclair D, Sheehan T, Parrott DM, Stott DI. The incidence of monoclonal gammopathy in a population over 45 years old determined by isoelectric focusing. Br J Haematol 1986;64:745–50.

396. Radl J, Valentijn RM, Haaijman JJ, Paul LC. Monoclonal gammopathies in patients undergoing immunosuppressive treatment after renal transplantation. Clin Immunol Immunopathol 1985;37:98–102.

397. Ghory H, Schiff S, Buckley R. Appearance of multiple benign paraproteins during early engraftment of soy lectin T cell–depleted haploidentical bone marrow cells in severe combined immunodeficiency. J Clin Immunol 1986;6:161–9.

398. Kyle RA. Monoclonal gammopathy of undetermined significance. Blood Rev 1994;8:135–41.

399. Hobbs JR. Paraproteins, benign or malignant? Br Med J 1967;3:699–704.

400. Dammacco F, Waldenstrom J. Bence Jones proteinuria in benign monoclonal gammopathies: incidence and characteristics. Acta Med Scand 1968;184:403–9.

401. Boccadoro M, Gavarotti P, Fossati G, et al. Low plasma cell 3(H) thymidine incorporation in monoclonal gammopathy of undetermined significance (MGUS), smouldering myeloma and remission phase myeloma: a reliable indicator of patients not requiring therapy. Br J Haematol 1984;58:689–96.

402. Norgaard O. Three cases of multiple myeloma in which the preclinical asymptomatic phases persisted throughout 15 to 24 years. Br J Cancer 1971;25:417–22.

403. Kyle RA. "Benign" monoclonal gammopathy—after 20 to 35 years of follow-up. Mayo Clin Proc 1993;68:26–36.

404. Kyle RA, Garton JP. The spectrum of IgM monoclonal gammopathy in 430 cases. Mayo Clin Proc 1987;62:719–31.

405. Alexanian R. Localized and indolent myeloma. Blood 1980;56:521–5.

406. Kyle RA, Greipp PR. Smoldering multiple myeloma. N Engl J Med 1980;302:1347–9.

407. Meis JM, Butler JJ, Osborne BM, Ordonez NG. Solitary plasmacytomas of bone and extramedullary plasmacytomas: a clinicopathologic and immunohistochemical study. Cancer 1987;59:1475–85.

408. Bataille R, Sany J. Solitary myeloma: clinical and prognostic features of a review of 114 cases. Cancer 1981;48:845–51.

409. Chak LY, Cox RS, Bostwick DG, Hoppe RT. Solitary plasmacytoma of bone: treatment, progression, and survival. J Clin Oncol 1987;5:1811–5.

410. Wollersheim HC, Holdrinet RS, Haanen C. Clinical course and survival in 16 patients with localized plasmacytoma. Scand J Haematol 1984;32:423–8.

411. Frassica DA, Frassica FJ, Schray MF, et al. Solitary plasmacytoma of bone: Mayo Clinic experience. Int J Radiat Oncol Biol Phys 1989;16:43–8.

412. Holland J, Trenkner DA, Wasserman TH, Fineberg B. Plasmacytoma: treatment results and conversion to myeloma. Cancer 1992;69:1513–7.

413. Wiltshaw E. The natural history of extramedullary plasmacytoma and its relation to solitary myeloma of bone and myelomatosis. Medicine (Baltimore) 1976;55:217–38.

414. Tong D, Griffin TW, Laramore GE, et al. Solitary plasmacytoma of bone and soft tissues. Radiology 1980;135:195–8.

415. Corwin J, Lindberg RD. Solitary plasmacytoma of bone vs. extramedullary plasmacytoma and their relationship to multiple myeloma. Cancer 1979;43:1007–13.

416. Knowling MA, Harwood AR, Bergsagel DE. Comparison of extramedullary plasmacytomas with solitary and multiple plasma cell tumors of bone. J Clin Oncol 1983;1:255–62.

417. Dimopoulos MA, Kiamouris C, Moulopoulos LA. Solitary plasmacytoma of bone and extramedullary plasmacytoma. Hematol Oncol Clin North Am 1999;13:1249–57.

418. Driedger H, Pruzanski W. Plasma cell neoplasia with peripheral polyneuropathy: a study of five cases and a review of the literature. Medicine (Baltimore) 1980;59:301–10.

419. Kelly JJ Jr, Kyle RA, Miles JM, Dyck PJ. Osteosclerotic myeloma and peripheral neuropathy. Neurology 1983;33:202–10.

420. Bardwick PA, Zvaifler NJ, Gill GN, et al. Plasma cell dyscrasia with polyneuropathy, organomegaly, endocrinopathy, M protein, and skin changes: the POEMS syndrome: report on two cases and a review of the literature. Medicine (Baltimore) 1980;59:311–22.

421. Waldenstrom JG, Adner A, Gydell K, Zettervall O. Osteosclerotic "plasmacytoma" with polyneuropathy, hypertrichosis and diabetes. Acta Med Scand 1978;203:297–303.

422. Parra R, Fernandez JM, Garcia-Bragado F, et al. Successful treatment of peripheral neuropathy with chemotherapy in osteosclerotic myeloma. J Neurol 1987;234:261–3.

423. Rose C, Mahieu M, Hachulla E, et al. POEMS syndrome. Rev Med Interne 1997;18:553–62.

424. Feinberg L, Temple D, de Marchena E, et al. Soluble immune mediators in POEMS syndrome with pulmonary hypertension: case report and review of the literature. Crit Rev Oncog 1999;10:293–302.

425. Nemni R, Gerosa E, Piccolo G, Merlini G. Neuropathies associated with monoclonal gammopathies. Haematologica 1994;79:557–66. see comments.

426. Sherman WH, Olarte MR, McKiernan G, et al. Plasma exchange treatment of peripheral neuropathy associated with plasma cell dyscrasia. J Neurol Neurosurg Psychiatry 1984;47:813–9.

427. Osby E, Noring L, Hast R, et al. Benign monoclonal gammopathy and peripheral neuropathy. Br J Haematol 1982;51:531–9.

428. Latov N, Sherman WH, Nemni R, et al. Plasma-cell dyscrasia and peripheral neuropathy with a monoclonal antibody to peripheral-nerve myelin. N Engl J Med 1980;303:618–21.

429. Saito T, Sherman WH, Latov N. Specificity and idiotype of M-proteins that react with MAG in patients with neuropathy. J Immunol 1983;130:2496–8.

430. Sherman WH, Latov N, Hays AP, et al. Monoclonal IgM kappa antibody precipitating with chondroitin sulfate C from patients with axonal polyneuropathy and epidermolysis. Neurology 1983;33:192–201.

431. Niemierko E, Weinstein R. Response of patients with IgM- and IgA-associated peripheral polyneuropathies to "off-line" immunoadsorp-

tion treatment using the Prosorba protein A column. J Clin Apheresis 1999;14:159–62.

432. Notermans NC, Lokhorst HM, Franssen H, et al. Intermittent cyclophosphamide and prednisone treatment of polyneuropathy associated with monoclonal gammopathy of undetermined significance. Neurology 1996;47:1227–33.

433. Simmons Z. Paraproteinemia and neuropathy. Curr Opin Neurol 1999;12:589–95.

434. Kelly JJ. Neuropathies of monoclonal gammopathies of undetermined significance. Hematol Oncol Clin North Am 1999;13:1203–10.

435. Durie BG, Persky B, Soehnlen BJ, et al. Amyloid production in human myeloma stem-cell culture, with morphologic evidence of amyloid secretion by associated macrophages. N Engl J Med 1982;307:1689–92.

436. Kyle RA, Greipp PR, O'Fallon WM. Primary systemic amyloidosis: multivariate analysis for prognostic factors in 168 cases. Blood 1986;68:220–4.

437. Kyle RA, Greipp PR. Primary systemic amyloidosis: comparison of melphalan and prednisone versus placebo. Blood 1978;52:818–27.

438. Fielder K, Durie BG. Primary amyloidosis associated with multiple myeloma: predictors of successful therapy. Am J Med 1986;80:413–8.

439. Solomon A, Weiss DT, Pepys MB. Induction in mice of human light-chain-associated amyloidosis. Am J Pathol 1992;140:629–37.

440. Comenzo RL, Wally J, Kica G, et al. Clonal immunoglobulin light chain variable region germline gene use in AL amyloidosis: association with dominant amyloid-related organ involvement and survival after stem cell transplantation. Br J Haematol 1999;106:744–51.

441. Kyle RA, Linos A, Beard CM, et al. Incidence and natural history of primary systemic amyloidosis in Olmsted County, Minnesota, 1950 through 1989. Blood 1992;79:1817–22. see comments.

442. Scott PP, Scott WW Jr, Siegelman SS. Amyloidosis: an overview. Semin Roentgenol 1986;21:103–12.

443. Duston MA, Skinner M, Shirahama T, Cohen AS. Diagnosis of amyloidosis by abdominal fat aspiration: analysis of four years' experience. Am J Med 1987;82:412–4.

444. Gertz MA, Lacy MQ, Lust JA, et al. Prospective randomized trial of melphalan and prednisone versus vincristine, carmustine, melphalan, cyclophosphamide, and prednisone in the treatment of primary systemic amyloidosis. J Clin Oncol 1999;17:262–7.

445. Cohen AS, Rubinow A, Anderson JJ, et al. Survival of patients with primary (AL) amyloidosis: colchicine-treated cases from 1976 to 1983 compared with cases seen in previous years (1961 to 1973). Am J Med 1987;82:1182–90.

446. Kyle RA, Greipp PR, Garton JP, Gertz MA. Primary systemic amyloidosis: comparison of melphalan/prednisone versus colchicine. Am J Med 1985;79:708–16.

447. Gertz MA, Lacy MQ, Dispenzieri A. Amyloidosis. Hematol Oncol Clin North Am 1999;13:1211–33, ix. review.

448. Klein AL, Hatle LK, Taliercio CP, et al. Prognostic significance of Doppler measures of diastolic function in cardiac amyloidosis: a Doppler echocardiography study. Circulation 1991;83:808–16.

449. Shirahama T, Cohen AS. Blockage of amyloid induction by colchicine in an animal model. J Exp Med 1974;140:1102–7.

450. Zemer D, Pras M, Sohar E, Gafni J. Colchicine in familial Mediterranean fever. N Engl J Med 1976;294:170–1. letter.

451. Moreau P, Leblond V, Bourquelot P, et al. Prognostic factors for survival and response after high-dose therapy and autologous stem cell transplantation in systemic AL amyloidosis: a report on 21 patients. Br J Haematol 1998;101:766–9.

452. Comenzo RL, Vosburgh E, Falk RH, et al. Dose-intensive melphalan with blood stem-cell support for the treatment of AL (amyloid light-chain) amyloidosis: survival and responses in 25 patients. Blood 1998;91:3662–70.

453. Turkmen A, Yildiz A, Erkoc R, et al. Transplantation in renal amyloidosis. Clin Transplant 1998;12:375–8.

454. Waldenstrom J. Incipient myelomatosis or "essential" hyperglobulinemia with fibrinogenopenia—a new syndrome? Acta Med Scand 1944;117:216.

455. Zarrabi MH, Stark RS, Kane P, et al. IgM myeloma, a distinct entity in the spectrum of B-cell neoplasia. Am J Clin Pathol 1981;75:1–10.

456. Fine JM, Muller JY, Rochu D, et al. Waldenstrom's macroglobulinemia in monozygotic twins. Acta Med Scand 1986;220:369–73.

457. Renier G, Ifrah N, Chevailler A, et al. Four brothers with Waldenstrom's macroglobulinemia. Cancer 1989;64:1554–9.

458. Taleb N, Tohme A, Abi Jirgiss D, et al. Familial macroglobulinemia in a Lebanese family with two sisters presenting Waldenstrom's disease. Acta Oncol 1991;30:703–5.

459. Kopp WL, MacKinney AA Jr, Wasson G. Blood volume and hematocrit value in macroglobulinemia and myeloma. Arch Intern Med 1969;123:394–6.

460. Crisp D, Pruzanski W. B-cell neoplasms with homogeneous cold-reacting antibodies (cold agglutinins). Am J Med 1982;72:915–22.

461. Pruzanski W, Shumak KH. Biologic activity of cold-reacting autoantibodies (first of two parts). N Engl J Med 1977;297:538–42.

462. Dimopoulos MA, Alexanian R. Waldenstrom's macroglobulinemia. Blood 1994;83:1452–9.

463. Smith BR, Robert NJ, Ault KA. Waldenstrom's macroglobulinemia: the quantity of detectable circulating monoclonal B lymphocytes correlates with clinical course. Blood 1983;61:911–4.

464. Nobile-Orazio E, Marmiroli P, Baldini L, et al. Peripheral neuropathy in macroglobulinemia: incidence and antigen-specificity of M proteins. Neurology 1987;37:1506–14.

465. Dellagi K, Dupouey P, Brouet JC, et al. Waldenstrom's macroglobulinemia and peripheral neuropathy: a clinical and immunologic study of 25 patients. Blood 1983;62:280–5.

466. Hays AP, Latov N, Takatsu M, Sherman WH. Experimental demyelination of nerve induced by serum of patients with neuropathy and an anti-MAG IgM M-protein. Neurology 1987;37:242–56.

467. Willison HJ, Trapp BD, Bacher JD, et al. Demyelination induced by intraneural injection of human antimyelin-associated glycoprotein antibodies. Muscle Nerve 1988;11:1169–76.

468. Ferri C, Marzo E, Longombardo G, et al. Interferon-alpha in mixed cryoglobulinemia patients: a randomized, crossover-controlled trial. Blood 1993;81:1132–6.

469. Bergroth V, Reitamo S, Konttinen YT, Wegelius O. Skin lesions in Waldenstrom's macroglobulinaemia: characterization of the cellular infiltrate. Acta Med Scand 1981;209:129–31.

470. Hanke CW, Steck WD, Bergfeld WF, et al. Cutaneous macroglobulinosis. Arch Dermatol 1980;116:575–7.

471. Dimopoulos MA, Galani E, Matsouka C. Waldenstrom's macroglobulinemia. Hematol Oncol Clin North Am 1999;13:1351–66.

472. Lichtenstein A, Levine AM, Lukes RJ, et al. Immunoblastic sarcoma: a clinical description. Cancer 1979;43:343–52.

473. Leonhard SA, Muhleman AF, Hurtubise PE, Martelo OJ. Emergence of immunoblastic sarcoma in Waldenstrom's macroglobulinemia. Cancer 1980;45:3102–7.

474. Abe M, Takahashi K, Mori N, Kojima M. "Waldenstrom's macroglobulinemia" terminating in immunoblastic sarcoma: a case report. Cancer 1982;49:2580–6.

475. Rosner F, Grunwald HW. Multiple myeloma and Waldenstrom's macroglobulinemia terminating in acute leukemia: review with emphasis on karyotypic and ultrastructural abnormalities. N Y State J Med 1980;80:558–70.

476. Facon T, Brouillard M, Duhamel A, et al. Prognostic factors in Waldenstrom's macroglobulinemia: a report of 167 cases. J Clin Oncol 1993;11:1553–8.

477. Morel P, Monconduit M, Jacomy D, et al. A new scoring system in Waldenstrom's macroglobulinemia: description of 232 patients with validation on 167 other patients. Blood 1997;90:Suppl 1:243a.

478. Buskard NA, Galton DA, Goldman JM, et al. Plasma exchange in the long-term management of Waldenstrom's macroglobulinemia. Can Med Assoc J 1977;117:135–7.

479. Gorevic PD, Kassab HJ, Levo Y, et al. Mixed cryoglobulinemia: clinical aspects and long-term follow-up of 40 patients. Am J Med 1980;69:287–308.

480. Kelly JJ, Adelman LS, Berkman E, Bhan I. Polyneuropathies associated with IgM monoclonal gammopathies. Arch Neurol 1988;45:1355–9.

481. McCallister BD, Bayrd ED, Harrison EG, et al. Primary macroglobulinemia. Am J Med 1967;43:394.

482. MacKenzie MR, Fudenberg HH. Macroglobulinemia: an analysis for forty patients. Blood 1972;39:874–89.

483. Case DC Jr, Ervin TJ, Boyd MA, Redfield DL. Waldenstrom's macroglobulinemia: long-term results with the M-2 protocol. Cancer Invest 1991;9:1–7.

484. Dimopoulos MA, O'Brien S, Kantarjian H, et al. Fludarabine therapy in Waldenstrom's macroglobulinemia. Am J Med 1993;95:49–52.

485. Dimopoulos MA, Kantarjian H, Estey E, et al. Treatment of Waldenstrom macroglobulinemia with 2-chlorodeoxyadenosine. Ann Intern Med 1993;118:195–8.

486. Byrd JC, White CA, Link B, et al. Rituximab therapy in Waldenstrom's macroglobulinemia: preliminary evidence of clinical activity. Ann Oncol 1999;10:1525–7.

487. Fermand JP, Brouet JC. Heavy-chain diseases. Hematol Oncol Clin North Am 1999;13:1281–94.

488. Frangione B, Franklin EC. Heavy chain diseases: clinical features and molecular significance of the disordered immunoglobulin structure. Semin Hematol 1973;10:53–64.

489. Alexander A, Steinmetz M, Barritault D, et al. Gamma heavy chain disease in man: cDNA sequence supports partial gene deletion model. Proc Natl Acad Sci U S A 1982;79:3260–4.

490. Bakhshi A, Guglielmi P, Siebenlist U, et al. A DNA insertion/deletion necessitates an aberrant RNA splice accounting for a mu heavy chain disease protein. Proc Natl Acad Sci U S A 1986;83:2689–93.

491. Seligmann M. Immunochemical, clinical, and pathological features of alpha-chain disease. Arch Intern Med 1975;135:78–82.

492. Doe WF. Alpha chain disease clinicopathological features and relationship to so-called Mediterranean lymphoma. Br J Cancer 1975;31:Suppl 2:350–5.

493. Stoop JW, Ballieux RE, Hijmans W, Zegers BJ. Alpha-chain disease with involvement of the respiratory tract in a Dutch child. Clin Exp Immunol 1971;9:625–35.

494. Galian A, Lecestre MJ, Scotto J, et al. Pathological study of alpha-chain disease, with special emphasis on evolution. Cancer 1977;39:2081–101.

495. Roge J, Druet P, Marche C. [Mediterranean lymphoma with alpha chain disease: triple chemical anatomic and immunological remission]. Pathol Biol 1970;18:851–8.

496. Zawadzki ZA, Benedek TG, Ein D, Easton JM. Rheumatoid arthritis terminating in heavy-chain disease. Ann Intern Med 1969;70:335–47.

497. Solling K, Askjaer SA. Multiple myeloma with urinary excretion of heavy chain components of IgG and nodular glomerulosclerosis. Acta Med Scand 1973;1–2:23–30.

498. Kyle RA, Greipp PR, Banks PM. The diverse picture of gamma heavy-chain disease: report of seven cases and review of literature. Mayo Clin Proc 1981;56:439–51.

499. Pruzanski W, Hasselback R, Katz A, Parr DM. Multiple myeloma (light chain disease) with rheumatoid-like amyloid arthropathy and mu-heavy chain fragment in the serum. Am J Med 1978;65:334–41.

500. Merlini G, Waldenstrom JG, Jayakar SD. A new improved clinical staging system for multiple myeloma based on analysis of 123 treated patients. Blood 1980;55:1101–9.

501. Belpomme D, Simon F, Pouillart P, et al. Prognostic factors and treatment of multiple myeloma: interest of a cyclic sequential chemohormonotherapy combining cyclophosphamide, melphalan, and prednisone. Recent Results Cancer Res 1978;65:28–40.

502. Gobbi M, Cavo M, Savelli G, et al. Prognostic factors and survival in multiple myeloma: analysis of 91 cases treated by melphalan and prednisone. Haematologica 1980;65:437–45.

503. Santoro A, Schieppati G, Franchi F, et al. Clinical staging and therapeutic results in multiple myeloma. Eur J Cancer Clin Oncol 1983;19:1353–9.

504. Bergsagel DE, Bailey AJ, Langley GR, et al. The chemotherapy on plasma-cell myeloma and the incidence of acute leukemia. N Engl J Med 1979;301:743–8.

505. MacLennan IC, Cusick J. Objective evaluation of the role of vincristine in induction and maintenance therapy for myelomatosis. Medical Research Council Working Party on Leukaemia in Adults. Br J Cancer 1985;52:153–8.

506. Pavlovsky S, Corrado C, Santarelli MT, et al. An update of two randomized trials in previously untreated multiple myeloma comparing melphalan and prednisone versus three- and five-drug combinations: an Argentine Group for the Treatment of Acute Leukemia study. J Clin Oncol 1988;6:769–75.

507. Abramson N, Lurie P, Mietlowski WL, et al. Phase III study of intermittent carmustine (BCNU), cyclophosphamide, and prednisone versus intermittent melphalan and prednisone in myeloma. Cancer Treat Rep 1982;66:1273–7.

508. Harley JB, Pajak TF, McIntyre OR, et al. Improved survival of increased-risk myeloma patients on combined triple-alkylating-agent therapy: a study of the CALGB. Blood 1979;54:13–22.

509. Boccadoro M, Marmont F, Tribalto M, et al. Multiple myeloma: VMCP/VBAP alternating combination chemotherapy is not superior to melphalan and prednisone even in high-risk patients. J Clin Oncol 1991;9:444–8.

510. Peest D, Deicher H, Coldewey R, et al. Induction and maintenance therapy in multiple myeloma: a multicenter trial of MP versus VCMP. Eur J Cancer Clin Oncol 1988;24:1061–7.

511. Hjorth M, Hellquist L, Holmberg E, et al. Initial treatment in multiple myeloma: no advantage of multidrug chemotherapy over melphalan-prednisone. The Myeloma Group of Western Sweden. Br J Haematol 1990;74:185–91.

512. Keldsen N, Bjerrum OW, Dahl IM, et al. Multiple myeloma treated with mitoxantrone in combination with vincristine and prednisolone (NOP regimen) versus melphalan and prednisolone: a phase III Study. Nordic Myeloma Study Group (NMSG). Eur J Haematol 1993;51:80–5.

513. MacLennan IC, Chapman C, Dunn J, Kelly K. Combined chemotherapy with ABCM versus melphalan for treatment of myelomatosis: The Medical Research Council Working Party for Leukaemia in Adults. see comments. Lancet 1992;339:200–5.

514. Samson D, Gaminara E, Newland A, et al. Infusion of vincristine and doxorubicin with oral dexamethasone as first-line therapy for multiple myeloma. see comments. Lancet 1989;2:882–5.

# XXI

# NEOPLASMS RELATED TO THE ACQUIRED IMMUNODEFICIENCY SYNDROME (AIDS)

# AIDS AND SOLID TUMORS

..............................................

## AIDS AND CANCER

• Alice Reier • Ronald T. Mitsuyasu

Acquired immunodeficiency syndrome (AIDS) was first described in 1981. The causative virus, the human immunodeficiency virus (HIV), was identified by Barre-Sinoussi and colleagues in 1982.[1] HIV, transmitted by sexual intercourse and through exposure to infected blood products, preferentially infects $CD4^+$ lymphocytes and monocytes and macrophages, causing profound immunodeficiency with increased risk not only for opportunistic infections but also for some cancers. According to United Nations AIDS data, at the end of 1998, there were an estimated 33.4 million individuals worldwide and approximately 890,000 individuals in North America infected with the AIDS virus.[2] An estimated 10 to 30% of these infected persons will ultimately develop Kaposi's sarcoma (KS) and an estimated 2 to 10% will be diagnosed with non-Hodgkin's lymphoma (NHL) at some time during the course of their disease. Of the estimated 178,000 HIV-infected women in North America in December 1998, approximately 2300 (1.3%) will be diagnosed with invasive cervical cancer during their lifetime, although most of the estimated 14.4 million HIV-infected women worldwide live in developing countries, and their risk of being diagnosed with invasive cervical cancer is much greater.

Although KS, NHL and invasive cervical cancer are the only "official" AIDS-defining malignancies, U.S. reference data reveal that HIV-infected individuals have an increased risk for other cancers as well. These cancers include anal cancer (relative risk [RR] = 31.7), leukemias other than lymphoid and myeloid (RR = 11), Hodgkin's lymphoma (RR = 7.6), soft tissue sarcomas (RR = 7.2), multiple myeloma (RR = 4.5), primary brain cancers other than primary central nervous system (CNS) lymphoma (RR = 3.5), testicular cancer (RR = 2.9), and lung adenocarcinomas (RR = 2.5).[3]

Research in the field of AIDS has led to a greater understanding of the pathogenesis of HIV-related immune dysregulation and viral-mediated cancers. Effective protease inhibitors have been developed to treat HIV and are now routinely used in treatment regimens combined with reverse transcriptase inhibitors. When taken with prophylactic antibiotics, these multidrug "cocktails," also known as highly active antiretroviral therapy (HAART), have resulted in improved control of HIV replication, increased $CD4^+$ lymphocyte counts, and a decline in the incidence of opportunistic infections. Moreover, as HIV-infected patients are living longer, healthier lives, there is growing evidence that suppression of HIV replication may result in partial immune reconstitution and a reduced incidence of some HIV-related malignancies. Based on Centers for Disease Control (CDC) data of nearly 18,000 cases of HIV-infected individuals in the United States comparing January to June, 1994 with July to December,

1996, the incidence of KS decreased from 53.4 to 10.3/1000 patient-years ($p<0.001$), and the incidence of primary CNS lymphoma has decreased from 8.5 to 0.9/1000 patient-years ($p<0.04$).[4] During the same period, the incidence of NHL in HIV-infected individuals decreased by one-third, although this was not a significant decline, and the incidence of invasive cervical cancer showed no change.[4] Patients in the Multicenter AIDS Cohort Study (MACS) showed a similar decline in the incidence of KS during 1996 to 1997 and no change in the incidence of NHL.[5]

Several of the malignancies seen more frequently in the HIV-infected population are strongly associated with viruses other than the AIDS virus. The Epstein-Barr virus is found in the tumor tissue of 100% of patients with HIV-related primary central nervous system lymphoma as well as in the tissue of some of the other HIV-related non-Hodgkin's lymphomas. Human papillomavirus (HPV) serotypes 16, 18, 31, 33, and 35, which are known to have a causal relationship with intraepithelial neoplasia and invasive cervical cancer, are now known to be commonly associated with and may well have a causal relationship with anal epithelial neoplasia and anal cancer.[6–12]

Because of the epidemiology of KS, a viral cause for this malignancy has long been suspected. In 1994, Chang and colleagues identified the genome of the herpesvirus that is now known to be associated with KS.[13] Viral genomes of this newly identified virus, human herpesvirus 8, also known as *Kaposi's sarcoma herpesvirus* (KSHV), has been found in the spindle cells and endothelial cells of nearly all KS tumor samples from both HIV-infected and non–HIV-infected patients.[14] KSHV has also been found in the lymph nodes of patients with multicentric Castleman's disease and in the lymphoma cell lines of patients with primary effusion lymphoma (PEL), also called *body cavity–based lymphoma,* a rare type of non-Hodgkin's lymphoma.[15–19] KSHV has been found in the dendritic cells of HIV-infected and non–HIV-infected patients with multiple myeloma, although it has not been found in myeloma cells.[20]

The increased risk for developing cancer in the HIV-infected population is likely related to the underlying immunodeficiency and prior exposure to oncogenic pathogens. When cancer is diagnosed in HIV-infected patients, the cancer usually presents at a more advanced stage and follows a more aggressive course than in their HIV-negative counterparts. Despite the more advanced and aggressive presentation of cancer in these patients, until recently, HIV-infected cancer patients were routinely treated with lower doses of chemotherapy because of their greater susceptibility to opportunistic infections and overall poor prognosis for survival. At present, however, with the use of antibiotic prophylaxis against opportunistic infections, effective antiretroviral treatment, and growth factors, most HIV-infected patients with cancer can now tolerate, and are routinely given, standard-dose chemotherapy. In some cases, HIV-infected patients have tumor remission rates and tumor-free survival intervals that approach those of non–HIV-infected cancer patients.

In addition to using standard chemotherapy regimens to treat HIV-infected cancer patients, new treatment strategies, such as the use of antitumor antibodies, angiogenesis inhibitors, and antiviral drugs as well as cytokine and gene therapies, are being evaluated and may prove useful in the prevention or treatment of HIV-related tumors.

## REFERENCES

1. Barré-Sinoussi F, Chermann JC, Rey F, et al. Isolation of a T-lymphotropic retrovirus from a patient at risk for acquired immune deficiency syndrome (AIDS). Science 1983;220:868–71.
2. UNAIDS/WHO Report on the Global HIV/AIDS epidemic. June 1998.
3. Goedert JJ, Coté TR, Virgo P, et al. Spectrum of AIDS-associated malignant disorders. Lancet 1998;351:1833–9.
4. Johnson CC, Wilcosky T, Kvale P, et al. Cancer incidence among an HIV-infected cohort: Pulmonary Complications of HIV Infection Study Group. Am J Epidemiol 1997;146:470–5.
5. Jacobson LP, Yamashita TE, Detels R, et al. Impact of potent antiretroviral therapy on the incidence of Kaposi's sarcoma and non-Hodgkin's lymphomas among HIV-1-infected individuals: Multicenter AIDS Cohort Study. J Acquir Immune Defic Syndr 1999;21:Suppl 1:S34–41.
6. Palefsky JM, Gonzales J, Greenblatt RM, et al. Anal intraepithelial neoplasia and anal papillomavirus infection among homosexual males with group IV HIV disease. JAMA 1990;263:2911–6.
7. Frisch M, Glimelius B, van den Brule AJ, et al. Sexually transmitted infection as a cause of anal cancer. N Engl J Med 1997;337:1350–8.
8. Palefsky JM, Holly EA, Ralston ML, Jay N. Prevalence and risk factors for human papillomavirus infection of the anal canal in human immunodeficiency virus (HIV)-positive and HIV-negative homosexual men. J Infect Dis 1998;177:361–7.
9. Melbye M, Coté TR, Kessler L, et al. High incidence of anal cancer among AIDS patients: The AIDS/Cancer Working Group. Lancet 1994;343:636–9.
10. Melbye M, Rabkin C, Frisch M, Biggar RJ. Changing patterns of anal cancer incidence in the United States, 1940–1989. Am J Epidemiol 1994;139:772–80.
11. Shah KV. Human papillomaviruses and anogenital cancers. N Engl J Med 1997;337:1386–8.
12. Sun XW, Kuhn L, Ellerbrock TV, et al. Human papillomavirus infection in women infected with the human immunodeficiency virus. N Engl J Med 1997;337:1343–9.
13. Chang Y, Cesarman E, Pessin MS, et al. Identification of herpesvirus-like DNA sequences in AIDS-associated Kaposi's sarcoma. Science 1994;266:1865–9.
14. Gao SJ, Kingsley L, Li M, et al. KSHV antibodies among Americans, Italians and Ugandans with and without Kaposi's sarcoma. Nature Med 1996;2:925–8.
15. Said JW, Tasaka T, Takeuchi S, et al. Primary effusion lymphoma in women: report of two cases of Kaposi's sarcoma herpes virus–associated effusion-based lymphoma in human immunodeficiency virus–negative women. Blood 1996;88:3124–8.
16. Said J. Kaposi's sarcoma-associated herpesvirus (KSHV): a new viral pathogen associated with Kaposi's sarcoma, primary effusion lymphoma, and multicentric Castleman's disease. West J Med 1997;167:37–8.
17. O'Leary JJ, Kennedy MM, McGee JO. Kaposi's sarcoma associated herpes virus (KSHV/HHV 8): epidemiology, molecular biology and tissue distribution. Mol Pathol 1997;50:4–8.
18. Chang Y. Kaposi's sarcoma and Kaposi's sarcoma associated herpesvirus (human herpesvirus 8): where are we now? J Natl Cancer Inst 1997;89:1829–31.
19. Brooks LA, Wilson AJ, Crook T. Kaposi's sarcoma–associated herpesvirus (KSHV)/human herpesvirus 8 (HHV8)–a new human tumor virus. J Pathol 1997;182:262–5.
20. Rettig MB, Ma HJ, Vescio RA, et al. Kaposi's sarcoma–associated herpesvirus infection of bone marrow dendritic cells from multiple myeloma patients. Science 1997;276:1851–4.

# KAPOSI'S SARCOMA

• Alice Reier • Steven A. Miles

When Kaposi's sarcoma (KS) was initially described, it was a rare tumor mainly affecting elderly males of Mediterranean or Eastern European Jewish descent. In this population, "classic" KS presented as vascular plaques and nodules limited to the lower extremities and adjacent lymph nodes. Rarely, mucous membranes and visceral organs were involved. Later, it was discovered that KS is also an endemic malignancy of equatorial Africa, more common in males and sometimes affecting prepubescent boys. The "endemic" form can be seen in four distinct variations: a nodular form, similar to classic KS; a more aggressive fungating and invasive form; a widely disseminated invasive type that may affect visceral organs; and a virulent lymphadenopathic type. KS has also been identified in patients with renal allografts and in other immunocompromised patients.[1, 2]

## Natural History

### EPIDEMIOLOGY

As early as 1977, an excess of KS cases was reported in New York and California. In 1981, KS was recognized as a major manifestation of acquired immunodeficiency syndrome (AIDS), heralding the start of the AIDS epidemic. KS is the most common malignancy in the human immunodeficiency virus (HIV)-infected patient, affecting 10 to 30% of all HIV-infected males and 1% of all HIV-infected females at some time during the course of their disease.[2–8] Using reference data from the pre-AIDS epidemic (1975–79) AIDS-Cancer Match Registry, there is an increased relative risk (RR) of patients with AIDS being diagnosed with KS of approximately 100,000 fold. Using U.S. reference data from 1985 to 1989, the RR is lower (310).[9] Other studies have estimated the RR of KS in HIV-infected patients to be approximately 1000 to 73,000.[10–12] Now referred to as "epidemic" KS, this malignancy more commonly develops in men who have had sex with other men than in men who have contracted HIV through blood products. It is also more common in women who have bisexual partners than in women who have contracted HIV through injection drug use.

### ETIOLOGY

In 1994, Moore and Chang identified a previously undescribed gamma II herpes virus in Kaposi's sarcoma tissue.[13]

Genomes of this virus, now referred to as human herpes virus (HHV)-8 or Kaposi's sarcoma herpes virus (KSHV), are found in virtually all KS lesion spindle and endothelial cells. They are also found in cells isolated from the tissue of all subtypes of the disease (classic, endemic, and epidemic) and from the KS tumor tissue of HIV-uninfected immunocompromised patients.[13–16] KSHV has also been identified in primary effusion lymphomas, in lymph nodes of patients with multicentric Castleman's disease, and in the dendritic cells of patients with multiple myeloma.[13, 15, 17, 18] Current data strongly support a causative role for HHV-8 in the development of KS, although the mechanism of oncogenesis is incompletely understood. It has been proposed that an HHV-8–encoded G protein–coupled receptor or other HHV-8 gene products such as viral interleukin (IL)-6 may act as oncogenes by stimulating the production of angiogenic growth factors.[1, 19–21]

## PATHOGENESIS

KS is a spindle cell cancer. Inflammatory lymphocytes, ectatic endothelial cells, and the histologic hallmark of chaotic vascular slits with extravasated red blood cells characterize the mesenchymal tumor pathologically. The endothelial cells lining the lumens of these microvessels may be the origin of the tumor spindle cells.[22–24] HIV, although not necessary for the development of KS, facilitates the growth of the KS tumor. By infecting CD4 lymphocytes, HIV leads to suppression of immune function and decreased tumor surveillance. In addition, advanced HIV disease leads to the release of multiple cytokines, which have been closely associated with the development of KS. These include IL-10, transforming growth factor-β, tumor necrosis factor α (TNF-α), and IL-6.[1, 5, 22, 23, 25] Other cytokines that are thought to regulate KS growth are angiogenic growth factors, such as platelet-derived growth factor, IL-8, vascular endothelial growth factor (VEGF), basic fibroblast growth factor (BFGF), and oncostatin M.[23–29] VEGF is also thought to cause the vascular permeability that leads to the debilitating edema seen in advanced KS disease and is the target of several angiogenesis inhibitors currently in clinical trials for the treatment of KS. In addition to increased cytokine release resulting from HIV infection, the AIDS virus produces a protein, tat, that is essential for HIV replication. Ensoli and colleagues have reported that HIV-infected CD4 lymphocytes and monocytes may release biologically active tat that can stimulate the proliferation of spindle cells and may also be involved in endothelial migration, thus playing an integral role in the pathogenesis of AIDS-related KS.[30, 31] Corticosteroid treatment has been associated with the development of KS in immunocompromised patients, with or without HIV infection, and with the exacerbation of KS in patients with established KS tumors. This association may be the result of a synergistic effect between glucocorticoids and various growth factors.[6, 27]

## CLINICAL FEATURES AND DIAGNOSIS

In the HIV-infected patient, KS can present with single or multiple cutaneous lesions on the face, extremities, or trunk, with or without clinically obvious lymph node involvement. Mucocutaneous lesions of the oral cavity are seen in 30% of patients.[6] Lesions of the eyelid and conjunctiva, which may be mistaken for conjunctival hemorrhages, can lead to ocular irritation, infection, trichiasis, and visual obstruction.[32, 33] Cutaneous lesions may be plaque-like, nodular, or pedunculated. They can appear as violaceous nodules, clear fluid-filled papules, or fungating lesions. Facial lesions can be cosmetically disturbing, and lesions on the extremities can be accompanied by mild or severe and often debilitating edema.

Especially in the early stages of KS, mucocutaneous KS tumors can be confused with lesions of other diseases. Bacillary angiomatosis, caused by *Bartonella* spp. bacteria can result in raised red papules or nodules with an appearance that is similar to KS tumors both clinically and histologically. Angiomas, nevi, and dermatofibromas can also be mistaken for KS lesions. Although a clinical diagnosis can often be made by physical examination, a small punch biopsy of the lesion should always be performed to confirm the diagnosis prior to treatment.

Visceral disease affecting the gastrointestinal tract and lungs and, less commonly, the kidneys, adrenal glands, spleen, testes, bones, bone marrow, and heart can be present in the absence of cutaneous lesions.[2, 6, 32, 34] Asymptomatic gastrointestinal tract lesions may be found in more than 50% of patients. Gastric outlet obstruction, small bowel enteropathy, and rarely gastrointestinal bleeding have been reported. Patients who present with extensive clinical disease should have a chest radiograph, and a bronchoscopy or endoscopy with biopsies should be performed on patients who have radiologic or clinical evidence of pulmonary or gastrointestinal disease.

Although extensive KS is seen more frequently in patients who are severely immunocompromised, it can be present at any stage of HIV infection, including in HIV-infected patients with normal CD4 lymphocyte counts. Commonly, KS develops soon after the onset of an opportunistic infection. Also, when there is a rapid increase in HIV viral replication, patients with established KS may experience more rapid tumor progression. Complete resolution of opportunistic infections and aggressive antiretroviral treatment that successfully decreases HIV replication results in tumor regression in most patients and sometimes the clinical disappearance of the KS.[35] When patients present with progressive, unresponsive KS, clinicians should rule out concurrent opportunistic infections and uncontrolled HIV replication.

Prior to the widespread use of multiagent chemotherapy for HIV infection and prophylactic antibiotics, survival of patients with AIDS-related KS generally paralleled the survival of patients after any AIDS-defining illness. This ranged from 3 months to 3 years, with a better survival in patients with CD4 lymphocyte counts greater than 300 cells/μL, no prior opportunistic infections, and no systemic symptoms.[36] In a retrospective study of 688 patients with AIDS-related KS seen at a single institution from 1981 to 1990, four variables predicted survival: CD4 lymphocyte count, hematocrit, number of KS lesions, and body mass index. In that study, the overall median survival was 13 months, with a 65% reduction in mortality across all prognostic categories in patients presenting after 1987.[37] This decrease in mortality is thought to be attributable to the commercial availability of zidovudine and the use of *Pneumocystis carinii* pneumonia prophylaxis, the mainstays of HIV therapy at the time. Today, even more effective and less toxic KS therapy, combined with more potent antiretroviral therapy, routine *Pneumocystis carinii* pneumonia prophylaxis, and improved treatments for cytomegalovirus and other opportunistic infections, is believed to have greatly improved the survival of HIV-infected patients with KS.

## Treatment

There is currently no cure for KS, although death directly related to this malignancy is unusual. The goals of KS management, therefore, are to improve the appearance of cosmetically unappealing lesions, decrease lymphatic obstruction and extremity edema, and relieve the symptoms of visceral disease. A greater understanding of the viral and immune pathogenesis of KS has led to advances in the development of effective and minimally toxic KS therapy. Control of HIV viral replication and treatment of opportunistic infections are fundamental to the successful treatment of KS. Moreover, acute progression of KS should signal an aggressive search for a new or inadequately treated opportunistic infection or increased HIV viral replication. KS is a systemic disease and should be treated with systemic therapy except in cases in which the KS clinical presentation is limited to a few small cutaneous lesions. Proven effective systemic therapies include interferon alfa, liposomal anthracyclines, and paclitaxel. Other promising agents include angiogenesis inhibitors, systemic retinoids, and other biomodulators (Table 100–1).

### LOCAL THERAPIES

Local therapy is usually performed for cosmetic reasons, and the benefits are always confined to the locally treated area. Tumor regrowth usually occurs at the perimeter or within the treated area. The risks of local treatment include infection at the tumor site, pain, pigmentation changes, scarring, and tissue fibrosis. If performed incorrectly, local therapy can cause a worse cosmetic result than the original KS lesion. Local therapies include topical retinoid creams, cryotherapy with liquid nitrogen, intralesional chemotherapy with vinblastine injections, laser therapy, and radiation therapy.

Topical 9-*cis*-retinoic acid is approved for the treatment of cutaneous KS. Two placebo-controlled trials show that approximately 40% of HIV-infected patients will respond within 12 weeks. Response rates of greater than 70% are seen with long-term use (>6 months). The drug is applied as a thick gel twice a day as tolerated and allowed to dry before applying clothes. Pain, redness, scaling, and occasional ulceration that resolves with decreased dosing are the most frequent side effects. Cryotherapy with liquid nitrogen is the treatment of choice for small mucocutaneous lesions anywhere on the body, including the eyelid, conjunctiva, sclera, oral mucous membranes, glans penis, and perirectal area. The freeze time is approximately 20 to 60 seconds. It can be divided and given at weekly intervals until the lesion

is adequately treated.[38] Hypopigmentation can result when using this treatment modality on dark-skinned patients.

Intralesional injections of vinblastine, 0.1 mg in 0.1 ml of sterile water have also been used successfully to treat small mucocutaneous lesions.[39] Local vinblastine injections can be painful, and repeated injections are often required. Hyperpigmentation and depressed scars at the injection site can result. Lasers have been used to treat small KS lesions as well.[40–42] In addition to scarring and hyperpigmentation, post-treatment infections may result with prolonged tissue healing time. Pulsed dye laser treatment may have more minimal treatment-associated side effects, although large population studies have not been done.[42]

KS tumor tissue is exquisitely sensitive to radiation, and palliative radiotherapy has been used successfully to treat isolated mucocutaneous lesions presenting in all areas of the body. Doses of 7 to 22 Gy in divided doses can be given to treat oral and periorbital lesions.[43–45] Radiation can also be used for large involved lymph nodes to relieve lymphatic drainage obstruction. As with other local therapies, radiation can result in severe and long-lasting side effects. Overlap of radiation ports can be difficult to avoid and can result in tissue necrosis. Radiation of lymph nodes can cause sclerosis of the lymphatics and result in further drainage obstruction or fibrosis of muscle and connective tissue and lead to joint immobility, muscle contractures, and disuse atrophy. KS tumors can regrow in previously irradiated areas or around the perimeter of an irradiated area. In addition, a phenomenon termed *radiation recall* has been documented in patients treated with systemic anthracyclines and taxanes after having been treated with radiation. Although the mechanism is unknown, severe damage can occur in previously irradiated sites and can result in full-thickness ulcers.

### CHEMOTHERAPY

Systemic therapy is the treatment of choice for KS patients who present with more than a few small cutaneous lesions and for patients with visceral KS involvement. Until 1996, combination cytotoxic chemotherapy with bleomycin and vincristine or doxorubicin (Adriamycin), bleomycin, and vincristine was considered to be the most effective chemotherapy for KS, with reported response rates of 23 to 80%.[46, 47] Etoposide was used as salvage chemotherapy, administered intravenously or orally, with a reported response rate of 32%.[48] All these regimens had a high incidence of severe adverse reactions. In addition to dose-limiting bone marrow suppression, there were often cardiac, pulmonary, and neurologic toxicities that made it difficult to deliver effective doses for extended periods.

In 1996, two liposomal anthracyclines were approved by the U.S. Food and Drug Administration for the treatment of AIDS-related KS. Both liposomal doxorubicin and liposomal daunorubicin are anthracyclines encapsulated in microscopic vesicles composed of one or more lipid bilayers enclosing an aqueous phase that contains the drug. Liposome encapsulation prolongs the plasma half-life of the drug, increases drug concentrations in KS tissue, and causes less organ toxicity.[49, 50] Phase II studies using liposomal doxorubicin at a dose of 20 mg/m², administered every 2 to 3 weeks in patients with AIDS-related KS, showed response rates of 66

*Table 100–1.* **Management of Human Immunodeficiency Virus–Associated Kaposi's Sarcoma**

| Treatment | Indications and Comments | Side Effects |
|---|---|---|
| *Local Therapy* | Patients who have a few cutaneous lesions, including on the eyelid, conjunctiva, sclera, oral mucous membranes, glans penis, or perirectal area | KS lesions may regrow in field of treatment or in perimeter except with retinoids |
| Topical retinoids | Treatment of choice<br>Apply BID to lesions only | Hypersensitivity to sunlight, erythema, scaling, ulceration |
| Cryotherapy | May replace retinoids as treatment of choice; 20–60 sec freeze time<br>May be divided and given every week | Hypopigmentation |
| Vinblastine intralesional | Small, cosmetically disfiguring lesions<br>Repeated injections of 0.1 mg in 0.1 ml of sterile water often needed | Painful injection<br>Hyperpigmentation |
| Lasers | | Infections<br>Scarring<br>Hyperpigmentation |
| Radiotherapy | Cosmetically disfiguring lesions that are too large for effective cryotherapy for periorbital and oral lesions, KS-involved lymph nodes to relieve obstruction of lymphatic drainage 7–22 Gy in divided doses | Tissue necrosis in overlapping fields<br>"Radiation recall"<br>Sclerosis of the lymphatics<br>Fibrosis of muscle, connective tissue |
| *Systemic Therapy* | Treatment of choice for patients with more than a few small cutaneous lesions | |
| Liposomal doxorubicin | 20 mg/m² IV every 2–4 wk | Mild hair thinning<br>Occasional nausea<br>Mild myelosuppression<br>Hand-foot syndrome |
| Liposomal daunorubicin | 40 mg/m² IV every 24 wk | Same as liposomal doxorubicin except no reported hand-foot syndrome |
| Paclitaxel | Liposomal anthracycline-resistant KS 135–175 mg/m² IV over 3–96 hr every 24 wk | Severe alopecia<br>Myelosuppression<br>Neuropathy |
| Interferon-alfa | As an adjunct to liposomal anthracyclines<br>Will also decrease Kaposi's sarcoma pigmentation<br>3–9 MIU SC every day | Hair thinning<br>Mild myelosuppression<br>Headache<br>Flu-like symptoms<br>Mucositis |

KS, Kaposi's sarcoma; BID, twice daily; IV, intravenously; MIU, million international units; SC, subcutaneously.

to 90%. In a multicenter phase III trial, 241 patients with AIDS-related KS were randomized to receive liposomal doxorubicin, 20 mg/m² given intravenously over 30 minutes, or bleomycin and vincristine, at standard doses of bleomycin, 15 units/m² given intravenously over 30 minutes, and vincristine, 1.4 mg/m² (maximum 2 mg) as an intravenous bolus every 3 weeks for six cycles. Of the 218 evaluable patients, 58.7% responded to the liposomal doxorubicin, compared with 23.3% responding to bleomycin and vincristine.[49]

Since the widespread use of protease inhibitors over the past several years, some investigators are reporting greater than 90% response rates and increased survival in patients with pulmonary KS.[51] Because of the excellent efficacy and modest side effect profile, liposomal anthracyclines are now considered to be first-line therapy for AIDS-related KS. At a dose of 20 mg/m² of liposomal doxorubicin or 40 mg/m² of liposomal daunorubicin given every 2 to 3 weeks, patients may experience mild myelosuppression, hand-foot syndrome and, rarely, hair thinning and mild nausea. Some patients have had hypersensitivity reactions during the infusions, resulting in dyspnea, hypotension, flushing, and a mild choking sensation. Slowing the infusion from 60 minutes to 90 minutes usually prevents this infusion reaction. Patients who

have had infusion reactions can be given hydrocortisone, 25 mg, and diphenhydramine, 25 mg, prior to subsequent infusions. Prochlorperazine, 10 mg orally, given as a premedication usually prevents nausea. Hand-foot syndrome, which is a painful erythema of the hands or plantar surfaces of the feet, occurs more commonly when patients are treated in 2-week dosing cycles. Increasing the dosing interval to 3 or 4 weeks and decreasing the dose to 15 mg/m² normally allows hand-foot syndrome to resolve without a break in treatment. After the resolution of hand-foot syndrome, chemotherapy can often be resumed at 20 mg/m² and at an increased dosing interval. Pyridoxine, 50 mg orally twice daily on the day of chemotherapy and for the next 2 to 3 days, may be of some benefit in preventing or decreasing the severity of hand-foot syndrome.

Liposomal daunorubicin given at a dose of 40 mg/m² every 2 weeks, although not reported to cause hand-foot syndrome, does result in slightly lower KS tumor response rates as compared with liposomal doxorubicin. In a phase II study, liposomal daunorubicin, 60 mg/m² given every 2 weeks, was administered to 53 patients who had a median CD4 lymphocyte count of less than 20 cells/μL and symptomatic pulmonary KS. Median survival for the treated patients was 7.1 months as compared with 1 to 4 months for historical controls. Of the treated patients, reversible grade 3 or 4 neutropenia, severe anemia, and thrombocytopenia were reported in 85%, 32%, and 17% of patients, respectively. Nonhematologic toxicities, such as alopecia and mucositis, occurred in 11% and 6% of patients, respectively. [52] Anthracycline-related cardiotoxicity has not been reported in patients receiving liposomal anthracyclines, and there is as yet no established cumulative dose limit.

Paclitaxel, also used as a single agent, was approved for treatment of AIDS-related KS in 1997. A phase II study demonstrated that when given in the recommended dose of 135 mg/m$^2$ infused over 3 hours in 3-week cycles, there was a major response in more than 70% of patients, including those in whom other agents had been ineffective. Response rates greater than 80% were reported when the infusion was given over 96 hours.[53] Side effects of paclitaxel include significant myelosuppression and severe alopecia. Prolonged paclitaxel therapy can also cause peripheral neuropathy. In addition, because paclitaxel is delivered in the excipient cremophor, some patients experience characteristic hypersensitivity reactions, including dyspnea, chest pain, hypotension, flushing, angioedema, and urticaria, which may be severe. Hypersensitivity reactions can be eliminated or diminished by pretreatment with prednisone 10 to 20 mg orally 12 hours and 6 hours prior to each paclitaxel dose in addition to dexamethasone (Decadron), 10 mg intravenously with an H$_2$ blocker, such as famotidine or ranitidine, and diphenhydramine, 25 to 50 mg intravenously within an hour prior to the paclitaxel infusion. Because of its more severe side effect profile, paclitaxel is considered to be second-line systemic therapy for AIDS-related KS. Although there are currently no large population studies documenting response rates in KS patients treated with liposomal anthracyclines or paclitaxel who are also receiving highly active antiretroviral therapy regimens and prophylactic antibiotics, there have been anecdotal reports of nearly 100% response rates in this population.

## IMMUNOMODULATORS

Interferon alfa has been used for the treatment of AIDS-related KS since the beginning of the epidemic and has long been recognized for its antiproliferative and antiretroviral effects.[32, 54] Early studies involved doses as high as 50 million IU/m$^2$/day. Although response rates of 32 to 40% were reported, side effects such as flu-like symptoms, including chills, fever, headaches, myalgias, anorexia, and diarrhea as well as thrombocytopenia, neutropenia, and hepatic enzyme abnormalities often precluded long-term therapy. Investigators have reported that for patients with AIDS-related KS taking effective antiretroviral chemotherapy, lower doses of interferon alfa alone or after chemotherapy with anthracyclines or paclitaxel appear to extend the benefit of the chemotherapy. This benefit has been seen with doses of interferon alfa-2a or -2b at 2 to 6 million IU/m$^2$/day. Subjective toxicities may be experienced even with the lower doses of interferon and can be mitigated by taking anti-inflammatory agents, such as naproxen, 250 mg orally, 1 hour before and 4 hours after each interferon dose.

The mechanism of action of IFN-$\alpha$ in KS therapy is unclear. When given in lower doses, it may act by indirectly inhibiting the activity of TNF-$\alpha$ and IL-1 and by inhibition of angiogenesis by downregulation of BFGF.[55] In higher doses, it may have additional antiretroviral or tumor properties, or both. Interferon beta and interferon gamma have been studied and have not been shown to be effective against KS.[56, 57] Other immunomodulators, such as IL-4, which is known to inhibit IL-6 production, and specific inhibitors of TNF-$\alpha$, have not proved to be effective therapeutic agents for patients with KS.[58, 59] An IL-1 antagonist has been observed to inhibit KS cell proliferation competitively in a dose-dependent manner in vitro but was not shown to be effective clinically when given to KS patients in a phase I/II trial as soluble human IL-1 receptor.[60]

## HORMONES

Despite the fact that AIDS-related KS is seen primarily in men, it is unclear whether sex hormones play a significant role in this disease. Investigators have found that impure preparations of human chorionic gonadotropin (hCG) can induce apoptosis of KS cell lines in vitro by a mechanism that is not yet understood. Small clinical trials using hCG administered by local intralesional injections and parenteral injection have yielded conflicting results.[61-63] There have also been a few anecdotal reports of worsening KS with androgen therapy, but there have been no large controlled studies of androgen deprivation or of purified hCG therapy for AIDS-related KS.

## NEW TREATMENT APPROACHES

Because KS is a vascular tumor and angiogenic factors are believed to be at least partially responsible for the growth and proliferation of KS cells, angiogenesis inhibition is currently an area of great interest in the treatment of KS. VEGF and BFGF are present in great abundance in KS tissue. VEGF is thought to be associated with the vascular permeability found in KS tumor tissue as well as being an angiogenic growth factor. When VEGF binds to growth factor receptors on endothelial and spindle cells, the receptors dimerize, causing tyrosine kinase activation, which, in turn, causes autophosphorylation of the receptors. This leads to a cascade of signaling events within the cells, resulting in proliferation and differentiation of the endothelial and spindle cells and formation of new blood vessels.[28] SU5416, a twice-weekly, intravenously administered VEGF inhibitor is a promising new treatment for KS. It works by inhibiting autophosphorylation of the VEGF-mediated receptor. Preliminary data from an ongoing phase I/II study show SU5416 to be well tolerated and effective in treating AIDS-related KS at doses of 17 to 145 mg/m$^2$, decreasing tumor growth as well as the extremity edema associated with KS. The major side effect at the higher doses is a migraine headache that can be relieved with sumatriptan.

IM862 is an angiogenesis inhibitor that is administered intranasally. It is currently being studied in a phase I/II clinical trial for AIDS-related KS. Preliminary results reveal that it is well tolerated and 8 of 15 evaluable patients have had a partial response lasting a median of 7.4 months when given 5 mg intranasally in regimens of 5 days on and 5 days off or on alternate days. The mechanism of action is not fully understood. Thalidomide, known for its teratogenic effects, has been shown to inhibit production of TNF-α as well as adhesion molecules, and it has been shown to interfere with basement membrane formation. It has also been shown to inhibit blood vessel formation and is currently being studied for possible use in the treatment of KS.

Retinoids are known to regulate proliferation and differentiation in many types of normal cells and tumor cells. Cultured KS cells express abundant retinoic acid receptors, and both all-*trans*-retinoic acid and 13-*cis*-retinoic acid inhibit growth of KS cells both in vitro and in vivo in a dose-dependent manner. In small clinical trials, retinoids given orally have been shown to produce some tumor response. In a phase II trial treating 24 patients with oral all-*trans*-retinoic acid at a target dose of 150 mg/m²/day, there was a 17% partial response, 13% minor response, and 29% stable disease for 4 months or more. Headache was the most frequent adverse side effect, followed by nausea and vomiting, skin dryness, hypertriglyceridemia, anemia, and neutropenia.[64] The mechanism of action of the retinoids is thought to be through downregulation of IL-6 by way of ligand-dependent receptor transcription interactions and by downregulation of BFGF and inhibition of growth-promoting effects of oncostatin-M and TNF-α.[65–67] Oral 9-*cis*-retinoic acid may be a superior agent to study based on the higher response rate when used topically and the better pharmacodynamics.

Since the identification of HHV-8 (KSHV) in KS tumor tissue, there has been interest in treating or preventing KS by inhibiting KSHV replication. KSHV found in KS tumor tissue is primarily in the latent (episomal) stage, with only small numbers of cells infected with replicating virus.[68] Because the episomal-phase virus is not generally sensitive to antiviral drugs, it has been suggested that HHV-8 could be controlled by inducing replication of the virus in latently infected cells followed by antiviral therapy. It may be possible to prevent HHV-8 induction of KS by prophylaxis with antiretroviral agents. HHV-8 has been shown in vitro to be susceptible to foscarnet, ganciclovir, cidofovir, adefovir and lobucavir.[69, 70]

## Summary of Treatment

The treatment of KS has changed enormously since 1997, and the future appears to hold many more changes in our approach to this devastating disease. Minimal disease is still best treated with local therapies such as the retinoid creams or liquid nitrogen. Radiation therapy is no longer the treatment of choice for these patients. For patients with more advanced disease or rapid progression, the liposomal anthracyclines followed by paclitaxel are the drugs of choice. Regimens using bleomycin, vinca alkaloids, and free anthracyclines are no longer recommended. Interferons at low doses with aggressive antiretroviral therapy remain an attractive treatment option for patients with HIV infection or in patients with classic KS after inducing a response with liposomal anthracyclines. In the future, with improved serologic tests for KSHV infection and a better understanding of the factors that lead to tumor formation, it may be possible to initiate pre-emptive prophylaxis against the development of KS in high-risk individuals.

## SUGGESTIONS FOR ADDITIONAL READING

Blauvelt A. The role of human herpesvirus 8 in the pathogenesis of Kaposi's sarcoma. Adv Dermatol 1999;14:167–206.

Murakami-Mori K, Mori S, Bonavida B. Molecular pathogenesis of AIDS-associated Kaposi's sarcoma: growth and apoptosis. Adv Cancer Res 2000;78:159–97.

Yarchoan R. Therapy for Kaposi's sarcoma: recent advances and experimental approaches. J Acquir Immune Defic Syndr 1999;21:Suppl 1:S66–73.

Nasti G, Errante D, Santarossa S, et al. A risk and benefit assessment of treatment for AIDS-related Kaposi's sarcoma. Drug Safety 1999; 20:403–25.

## REFERENCES

1. Boshoff C, Moore PS. Kaposi's sarcoma-associated herpesvirus: a newly recognized pathogen. AIDS Clin Rev 1997–98;323–47.
2. Friedman-Kien AE, Saltzman BR. Clinical manifestations of classical, endemic African, and epidemic AIDS-associated Kaposi's sarcoma. J Am Acad Dermatol 1990;22(Pt 2):1237–50.
3. Mitsuyasu RT. Clinical variants and staging of Kaposi's sarcoma. Semin Oncol 1987;14(Suppl 3):13–8.
4. Biggar RJ, Rabkin CS. The epidemiology of AIDS-related neoplasms. Hematol Oncol Clin North Am 1996;10:997–1010.
5. Miles SA. Pathogenesis of HIV-related Kaposi's sarcoma. Curr Opin Oncol 1994;6:497–502.
6. Dezube BJ. Clinical presentation and natural history of AIDS-related Kaposi's sarcoma. Hematol Oncol Clin North Am 1996;10:1023–9.
7. Haverkos HW, Friedman-Kien AE, Drotman DP, Morgan WM. The changing incidence of Kaposi's sarcoma among patients with AIDS. J Am Acad Dermatol 1990;22(Pt 2):1250–3.
8. Cooley TP, Hirschhorn LR, O'Keane JC. Kaposi's sarcoma in women with AIDS. AIDS 1996;10:1221–5.
9. Goedert JJ, Coté TR, Virgo P, et al. Spectrum of AIDS-associated malignant disorders. Lancet 1998;351:1833–9.
10. Johnson CC, Wilcosky T, Kvale P, et al. Cancer incidence among an HIV-infected cohort. Pulmonary Complications of HIV Infection Study Group. Am J Epidemiol 1997;146:470–5.
11. Schulz TF, Boshoff CH, Weiss RA. HIV infection and neoplasia. Lancet 1996;348:587–91.
12. Speck CE. 2nd Natl AIDS Malignancy Conference (Abstract 12), 1998.
13. Moore PS, Chang Y. Detection of herpesvirus-like DNA sequences in Kaposi's sarcoma in patients with and without HIV infection. N Engl J Med 1995;332:1181–5.
14. Boshoff C, Whitby D, Hatziioannou T, et al. Kaposi's-sarcoma-associated herpesvirus in HIV-negative Kaposi's sarcoma. Lancet 1995; 345:1043–4.
15. O'Leary JJ, Kennedy MM, McGee JO. Kaposi's sarcoma associated herpes virus (KSHV/HHV 8): epidemiology, molecular biology and tissue distribution. Mol Pathol 1997;50:4–8.
16. Gillison ML, Ambinder RF. Human herpesvirus-8. Curr Opin Oncol 1997;9:440–9.
17. Said J. Kaposi's sarcoma-associated herpesvirus (KSHV): a new viral pathogen associated with Kaposi's sarcoma, primary effusion lymphoma, and multicentric Castleman's disease. West J Med 1997; 167:37–8.
18. Rettig MB, Ma HJ, Vescio RA, et al. Kaposi's sarcoma-associated herpesvirus infection of bone marrow dendritic cells from multiple myeloma patients. Science 1997;276:1851–4.
19. Guo HG, Browning P, Nicholas J, et al. Characterization of a chemokine receptor-related gene in human herpesvirus 8 and its expression in Kaposi's sarcoma. Virology 1997;228:371–8.
20. Bais C, Santomasso B, Coso O, et al. G-protein-coupled receptor of Kaposi's sarcoma-associated herpesvirus is a viral oncogene and angiogenesis activator. Nature 1998;391(6662):86–9; 392:210.
21. Boshoff C. Kaposi's sarcoma. Coupling herpesvirus to angiogenesis. Nature 1998;391:24–5.

22. Ganem D. KSHV and Kaposi's sarcoma: the end of the beginning? Cell 1997;91:157–60.
23. Cornali E, Zietz C, Benelli R, et al. Vascular endothelial growth factor regulates angiogenesis and vascular permeability in Kaposi's sarcoma. Am J Pathol 1996;149:1851–69.
24. Rabkin CS, Janz S, Lash A, et al. Monoclonal origin of multicentric Kaposi's sarcoma lesions. N Engl J Med 1997;336:988–93.
25. Neipel F, Albrecht JC, Ensser A, et al. Human herpesvirus 8 encodes a homology of interleukin-6. J Virol 1997;71:839–42.
26. Miles SA. Pathogenesis of AIDS-related Kaposi's sarcoma. Evidence of a viral etiology. Hematol Oncol Clin North Am 1996;10:1011–21.
27. Cai J, Zheng T, Lotz M, et al. Glucocorticoids induce Kaposi's sarcoma cell proliferation through the regulation of transforming growth factor-beta. Blood 1997;89:1491–500.
28. Nakamura S, Murakami-Mori K, Rao N, et al. Vascular endothelial growth factor is a potent angiogenic factor in AIDS-associated Kaposi's sarcoma-derived spindle cells. J Immunol 1997;158:4992–5001.
29. Karp JE, Pluda JM, Yarchoan R. AIDS-related Kaposi's sarcoma. A template for the translation of molecular pathogenesis into targeted therapeutic approaches. Hematol Oncol Clin North Am 1996;10:1031–49.
30. Ensoli B, Buonaguro L, Barillari G, et al. Release, uptake, and effects of extracellular human immunodeficiency virus type 1 Tat protein on cell growth and viral transactivation. J Virol 1993;67:277–87.
31. Ensoli B, Gendelman R, Markham P, et al. Synergy between basic fibroblast growth factor and HIV-1 Tat protein in induction of Kaposi's sarcoma. Nature 1994;371:674–80.
32. Mitsuyasu RT, Miles SA. Biotherapy with interferon in AIDS-related Kaposi's sarcoma. Oncol Nurs Forum 1987;14:Suppl:27–31.
33. Shuler JD, Holland GN, Miles SA, et al. Kaposi sarcoma of the conjunctiva and eyelids associated with the acquired immunodeficiency syndrome. Arch Ophthalmol 1989;107:858–62.
34. Chyu KY, Birnbaum Y, Naqvi T, et al. Echocardiographic detection of Kaposi's sarcoma causing cardiac tamponade in a patient with acquired immunodeficiency syndrome. Clin Cardiol 1998;21:131–3.
35. Murphy M, Armstrong D, Sepkowitz KA, et al. Regression of AIDS-related Kaposi's sarcoma following treatment with an HIV-1 protease inhibitor. AIDS 1997;11:261–2.
36. Chachoua A, Krigel R, Lafleur F, et al. Prognostic factors and staging classification of patients with epidemic Kaposi's sarcoma. J Clin Oncol 1989;7:774–80.
37. Miles SA, Wang H, Elashoff R, Mitsuyasu RT. Improved survival for patients with AIDS-related Kaposi's sarcoma. J Clin Oncol 1994;12:1910–6.
38. Tappero JW, Berger TG, Kaplan LD, et al. Cryotherapy for cutaneous Kaposi's sarcoma (KS) associated with acquired immune deficiency syndrome (AIDS): a phase II trial. J Acquir Immune Defic Syndr 1991;4:839–46.
39. Newman SB. Treatment of epidemic Kaposi's sarcoma (KS) with intralesional vinblastine injection (IL-VLB). ASCO 1988;7:5.
40. Wheeland RG, Bailin PL, Norris MJ. Argon laser photocoagulative therapy of Kaposi's sarcoma: a clinical and histologic evaluation. J Dermatol Surg Oncol 1985;11:1180–5.
41. Webster GF. Local therapy for mucocutaneous Kaposi's sarcoma in patients with acquired immunodeficiency syndrome. Dermatol Surg 1995;21:205–8.
42. Marchell N, Alster TS. Successful treatment of cutaneous Kaposi's sarcoma by the 585-nm pulsed dye laser. Dermatol Surg 1997;23:973–5.
43. Nisce LZ, Safai B. Radiation therapy of Kaposi's sarcoma in AIDS. Memorial Sloan-Kettering experience. Front Radiat Ther Oncol 1985;19:133–7.
44. Nobler MP, Leddy ME, Huh SH. The impact of palliative irradiation on the management of patients with acquired immune deficiency syndrome. J Clin Oncol 1987;5:107–12.
45. Kirova YM, Belembaogo E, Frikha H, et al. Radiotherapy in the management of epidemic Kaposi's sarcoma: a retrospective study of 643 cases. Radiother Oncol 1998;46:19–22.
46. Gompels MM, Hill A, Jenkins P, et al. Kaposi's sarcoma in HIV infection treated with vincristine and bleomycin. AIDS 1992;6:1175–80; 6:1410.
47. Gill PS, Miles SA, Mitsuyasu RT, et al. Phase I AIDS Clinical Trials Group (075) study of Adriamycin, bleomycin and vincristine chemo-

48. Schwartsmann G, Sprinz E, Kromfield M, et al. Clinical and pharmaco-kinetic study of oral etoposide in patients with AIDS-related Kaposi's sarcoma with no prior exposure to cytotoxic therapy. J Clin Oncol 1997;15:2118–24.
49. Stewart S, Jablonowski H, Goebel FD, et al. Randomized comparative trial of pegylated liposomal doxorubicin versus bleomycin and vincris-tine in the treatment of AIDS-related Kaposi's sarcoma. International Pegylated Liposomal Doxorubicin Study Group. J Clin Oncol 1998;16:683–91.
50. Amantea MA, Forrest A, Northfelt DW, Mamelok R. Population phar-macokinetics and pharmacodynamics of pegylated-liposomal doxorubi-cin in patients with AIDS-related Kaposi's sarcoma. Clin Pharmacol Ther 1997;61:301–11.
51. Grünaug M, Bogner JR, Loch O, Goebel FD. Liposomal doxorubicin in pulmonary Kaposi's sarcoma: improved survival as compared to patients without liposomal doxorubicin. Eur J Med Res 1998;3:13–9.
52. Tulpule A, Yung RC, Wernz J, et al. Phase II trial of liposomal daunorubicin in the treatment of AIDS-related pulmonary Kaposi's sarcoma. J Clin Oncol 1998;16:3369–74.
53. Welles L, Saville MW, Lietzau J, et al. Phase II trial with dose titration of paclitaxel for the therapy of human immunodeficiency virus-associated Kaposi's sarcoma. J Clin Oncol 1998;16:1112–21.
54. Volberding PA, Mitsuyasu R. Recombinant interferon alpha in the treatment of acquired immune deficiency syndrome-related Kaposi's sarcoma. Semin Oncol 1985;12:Suppl 5:2–6.
55. Fidler IJ, Singh RK, Gutman M, et al. Interferons alpha and beta downregulate the expression of basic fibroblast growth factor (bFGF) in human carcinomas. Proc Am Assoc Cancer Res 1994;35:57.
56. Miles SA, Wang HJ, Cortes E, et al. Beta-interferon therapy in patients with poor-prognosis Kaposi sarcoma related to the acquired immunode-ficiency syndrome (AIDS). A phase II trial with preliminary evidence of antiviral activity and low incidence of opportunistic infections. Ann Intern Med 1990;112:582–9.
57. Mitsuyasu RT. Hematopoietic growth factors in the treatment of patients with HIV infection. Biotherapy 1988;2:173–82.
58. Aboulafia D, Miles SA, Saks SR, Mitsuyasu RT. Intravenous recombi-nant tumor necrosis factor in the treatment of AIDS-related Kaposi's sarcoma. J Acquir Immune Defic Syndr 1989;2:54–8.
59. Tulpule A, Joshi B, DeGuzman N, et al. Interleukin-4 in the treatment of AIDS-related Kaposi's sarcoma. Ann Oncol 1997;8:79–83.
60. Krown SE, Paredes J, Polsky B, et al. Phase I/II trial of soluble recombinant human interleukin-1 receptor (rhu IL-1R) in patients with human immunodeficiency virus-1 (HIV-1) infection. Proc Am Soc Clin Oncol 1995;14:292.
61. Lang ME, Lottersberger C, Roth B, et al. Induction of apoptosis in Kaposi's sarcoma spindle cell cultures by the subunits of human chori-onic gonadotropin. AIDS 1997;11:1333–40.
62. Gill PS, Lunardi-Ishkandar Y, Louie S, et al. The effects of preparations of human chorionic gonadotropin on AIDS-related Kaposi's sarcoma. N Engl J Med 1996;335:1261–9; 1997;336:670.
63. Krown SE. Kaposi's sarcoma—what's human chorionic gonadotropin got to do with it? N Engl J Med 1996;335:1309–10.
64. Gill PS, Espina BM, Moudgil T, et al. All-*trans* retinoic acid for the treatment of AIDS-related Kaposi's sarcoma: results of a pilot phase II study. Leukemia 1994;8:Suppl 3:S26–32.
65. Guo WX, Gill PS, Antakly T. Inhibition of AIDS-Kaposi's sarcoma cell proliferation following retinoic acid receptor activation. Cancer Res 1995;55:823–9.
66. Corbeil J, Rapaport E, Richman DD, Looney DJ. Antiproliferative effect of retinoid compounds on Kaposi's sarcoma cells. J Clin Invest 1994;93:1981–6.
67. Nagpal S, Cai J, Zheng T, et al. Retinoid antagonism of NF-IL6: insight into the mechanism of antiproliferative effects of retinoids in Kaposi's sarcoma. Mol Cell Biol 1997;17:4159–68.
68. Zhong W, Wang H, Herndier B, Ganem D. Restricted expression of Kaposi sarcoma-associated herpesvirus (human herpesvirus 8) genes in Kaposi sarcoma. Proc Natl Acad Sci U S A 1996;93:6641–6.
69. Medveczky MM, Horvath E, Lund T, Medveczky PG. In vitro antiviral drug sensitivity of the Kaposi's sarcoma-associated herpesvirus. AIDS 1997;11:1327–32.
70. Panyutich EA, Said JW, Miles SA. Infection of primary dermal micro-vascular endothelial cells by Kaposi's sarcoma-associated herpesvirus. AIDS 1998;12:467–72.

# CHAPTER 101

# ACQUIRED IMMUNODEFICIENCY SYNDROME–RELATED LYMPHOMA

• ANIL TULPULE • ALEXANDRA M. LEVINE

## Natural History, Diagnosis, and Staging

### ETIOLOGY AND BIOLOGY

More than 40% of all patients with human immunodeficiency virus (HIV) infection develop malignant disease at some time during the course of their illness. Further, as survival in HIV disease has increased, greater numbers of patients with neoplastic disease are being diagnosed. This increase is well documented with regard to lymphoma. The incidence of AIDS-related lymphoma has been shown by Pluda and colleagues, who followed a group of 116 such patients, to be 19% at 3 years after development of symptomatic HIV disease.[1]

The cancers that occur in acquired immunodeficiency syndrome (AIDS) are highly reminiscent of those that are known to develop in organ transplant patients, who receive immunosuppressive drugs to prevent graft rejection. The first cancer seen in this setting is Kaposi's sarcoma, which occurs at a relative risk of 500 times over that expected in the general population, with an average latent period of 20 months from transplantation. The second malignancy that may develop is lymphoma, at a relative risk of 28- to 49-fold, occurring at an average latent period of 32 months. Various cancers of the anogenital tract, such as vulvar and cervical carcinomas, are seen at a relative risk of 100-fold and 14-fold, respectively, with a latent period of approximately 107 months.

Other disorders of immune dysregulation are also associated with an increased risk of lymphoma, as documented for various autoimmune diseases and for certain congenital immunodeficiency diseases such as Wiskott-Aldrich syndrome, ataxia telangiectasia, and the X-linked lymphoproliferative syndrome.

With these facts in mind, it does not seem surprising that the incidence of lymphoma would also be significantly increased in patients with the underlying immune dysregulation induced by chronic HIV infection.

### EPIDEMIOLOGY

The incidence of lymphoma doubled in the United States between 1940 and 1970. The AIDS epidemic has resulted in an additional risk of lymphoma of approximately 100 times that expected.[2] Unfortunately, the Centers for Disease Control and Prevention (CDC) collect data only on initial AIDS-defining illnesses. The precise U.S. prevalence and incidence rates of AIDS-related lymphoma are thus likely to be significantly underestimated by the CDC; in France, 33% of lymphoma cases have occurred after an earlier AIDS-defining illness. In an attempt to obtain a more precise estimate of the impact of HIV on the incidence of lymphoma, Cote and associates[3] reported results from an epidemiologic linkage study, in which cases from population-based cancer registries in the United States were linked to AIDS registries in the same areas. The risk of immunoblastic lymphoma after an earlier AIDS diagnosis was found to be increased by 652-fold, whereas that of small noncleaved lymphoma was increased 261-fold, and intermediate grade large cell lymphoma was increased 113-fold. Even low-grade lymphoma was found to be increased in this linkage study—by 14-fold among persons with earlier AIDS diagnoses. It is apparent from these data that lymphoma is frequently a later manifestation of HIV disease, occurring after earlier AIDS-defining conditions.

The use of highly active combination antiretroviral therapy (HAART) has resulted in significant declines in the incidence of essentially all opportunistic infections, as well as Kaposi's sarcoma. Although the incidence of lymphoma has declined to a lesser extent in some studies, other studies report a continued increase.

In the United States, lymphoma accounts for approximately 3% of all new cases of AIDS. All population groups appear equally likely to develop the disease. Further, AIDS-related lymphoma is seen in all age groups, among all risk groups for acquisition of HIV infection, and in all geographic regions. The incidence in women is somewhat lower than in men, being similar to the usual distribution of lymphoma in patients without HIV infection.

A prospective study of 1295 HIV-infected patients with hemophilia has demonstrated a 5.5% incidence of lymphoma, at a median interval of 59 months from initial HIV infection. The relative risk of lymphoma was 36.5 times higher than that seen in HIV-negative hemophiliacs and 29 times higher than expected in the general population. The mean CD4 cell count at diagnosis of lymphoma was 64/mm$^3$. All clinical and pathologic characteristics were similar to those described in other AIDS risk groups.

### PATHOLOGY

Most AIDS-related lymphomas are B-cell tumors of high-grade pathologic type, consisting primarily of immunoblastic lymphoma and small noncleaved lymphoma. The latter may be of either the Burkitt's or non-Burkitt's subtype. Approximately 80 to 90% of patients are diagnosed with one of these pathologic types of disease. It is interesting that only 10 to 15% of patients with de novo lymphoma, unassociated with HIV, are diagnosed with one of these rather unusual forms of lymphoma. Aside from these high-grade lymphomas, intermediate-grade, diffuse large cell lymphoma has also been reported with some regularity in the setting of underlying HIV infection. There is no strong evidence to suggest that patients with intermediate-grade large cell lymphoma fare any differently from those with high-grade disease. A new type of AIDS-related lymphoma has been recognized, termed *primary effusion lymphoma* (PEL) or *body cavity–based lymphoma*. This entity is uniformly associated with human herpes virus-8-infection within tumor cells. Histologically, the lymphoma consists of large anaplastic cells that also harbor Epstein-Barr virus sequences. Clinically, patients with PEL present with effusions, in the absence of mass lesions. Prognosis is poor, with a median survival of 2 months despite treatment.

Although the designation of AIDS-related lymphoma is confined to the pathologic types discussed, cancer-AIDS linkage studies have found a 14-fold increase in low-grade lymphoma among patients with AIDS. Further, the incidence of multiple myeloma has been shown to be significantly increased among HIV-infected homosexual men when compared with HIV-negative controls. HIV-infected patients with low-grade lymphoma or multiple myeloma seem to fare similarly to individuals without underlying HIV infection, and standard modalities and concepts of treatment are used.

Various T-cell lymphomas have been described in HIV-infected patients, although there has been no epidemiologic increase in these cases, and they are not considered AIDS defining.[3]

## CLINICAL FEATURES

Patients with newly diagnosed AIDS-related lymphoma may first present with systemic B symptoms consisting of fever, drenching night sweats, weight loss, or a combination. These symptoms occur in approximately 80% of patients with systemic AIDS-related lymphoma and in 90% of those with lymphoma primary to the central nervous system (CNS).[3, 4] The presence of such symptoms in an HIV-infected patient should alert the clinician to the possibility of lymphoma.

Most patients (60 to 90%) present with far-advanced disease in extranodal sites. This is in sharp distinction to patients with de novo lymphoma, of whom approximately 40% present with extranodal disease.

Virtually any anatomic site may be involved, with lymphoma reported in the myocardium, ear lobe, gallbladder, rectum, gingival area, popliteal fossa, and elsewhere. The more common reported sites of initial extranodal disease include the CNS (approximately 30%), gastrointestinal tract (about 25%), bone marrow (21 to 33%), and liver (about 10%).

## STAGING EVALUATION

Staging evaluation should begin with a computed tomographic scan of the chest, abdomen, and pelvis. In a series of 112 patients with AIDS-related lymphoma, 64% were found to show evidence of intra-abdominal lymphomatous disease, which most commonly involved lymph nodes, gastrointestinal tract, liver, kidney, and adrenal glands. In patients with predominant signs and symptoms related to the

abdomen, 58 of 59 (98%) were found to have abnormalities on computed tomographic scan of this region. Neither hepatic nor splenic enlargement was seen as an isolated finding in the absence of other intra-abdominal abnormalities.

Gallium-67 scanning is also an important staging tool and may be particularly useful in evaluating residual stable masses after the completion of systemic chemotherapy. Thus, an initial gallium-avid lymphomatous mass may be seen to decrease significantly in size on postchemotherapy computed tomographic scanning, with residual enlargement still present. A repeat gallium scan may help differentiate residual fibrosis from remaining active disease; in the former situation the gallium scan should be negative, whereas it will remain positive in the presence of residual lymphoma.

Bone marrow aspiration and biopsy should be performed, as the likelihood of marrow involvement ranges from 21 to 33% in various series.

Although not required in most patients with de novo lymphoma, lumbar puncture (LP) should be performed routinely as part of the staging evaluation of a patient with AIDS-related lymphoma. Approximately 20% of HIV-infected patients are found to have leptomeningeal involvement even when completely asymptomatic with regard to the CNS. Since prophylactic intrathecal chemotherapy has become an integral part of initial therapy, it is now common practice to inject the first dose of methotrexate or cytosine arabinoside (ara-C) at the time of this initial staging LP in an attempt to prevent isolated CNS relapse.[5]

## DIAGNOSIS

The initial diagnosis of AIDS-related lymphoma requires tissue biopsy, with definitive pathologic review. No study other than biopsy can yield specific diagnostic information, which is mandatory before the institution of multiagent chemotherapy, especially in these immunosuppressed individuals.

Aside from simple histologic review, immunophenotypic or genotypic studies are often helpful to confirm the monoclonality (and thus malignant nature) of the process and to exclude the possibility of a reactive lymphoid lesion.

## PROGNOSIS

In patients with lymphoma unrelated to HIV, certain factors have been associated with decreased survival, including higher tumor burden and decreased patient vigor. In HIV-infected patients with lymphoma, additional factors related to the degree of immunodeficiency appear to have significance. Thus, both lymphoma- and HIV-related factors appear important in predicting patient survival.

In a group of 49 HIV-positive patients with systemic lymphoma treated with curative intent, decreased survival was associated with a history of AIDS prior to the lymphoma, Karnofsky performance status less than 70%, involvement of bone marrow, and low CD4 cells as a continuous variable. In another retrospective study, stage IV disease was also independently associated with shorter survival, as was treatment with a more dose-intensive regimen. In a prospective therapeutic trial using the intensive LNH-84 regimen in 141 good-risk patients (Eastern Cooperative Oncology Group performance status less than 2 and absence of an active opportunistic infection at the time of therapy), four factors were associated with shorter survival on multivariate analysis: CD4 count less than $100/mm^3$, performance status greater than 1, immunoblastic lymphoma, and a history of AIDS before the lymphoma.[6] A prospective study of 192 patients identified age older than 35 years and injection drug use as factors associated with shortened survival, in addition to CD4 count less than $100/mm^3$ and stage III/IV disease.

In comparing patients with AIDS-related systemic lymphoma with those who have lymphoma primary to the CNS (P-CNS), it is apparent that patients with P-CNS disease fare significantly worse, with a median survival of only 2 to 3 months despite therapy. The shorter survival in these patients appears to be related to the far-advanced degree of HIV disease, with median CD4 cell count of $30/mm^3$, and a history of AIDS before the diagnosis of P-CNS lymphoma in approximately 75%.

Leptomeningeal involvement in patients with AIDS-related systemic lymphoma is not a poor prognostic indicator; long-term survival is possible in these individuals provided that specific therapy is given.

## Treatment

### SYSTEMIC AND LEPTOMENINGEAL LYMPHOMA

**Chemotherapy.** In the 1980s, multiple dose-intensive chemotherapeutic regimens were designed and tested in patients with de novo large cell lymphoma. Although initially promising, such regimens have been shown to have no real advantage over the earlier, less intensive CHOP (cyclophosphamide, doxorubicin, vincristine, prednisone) regimen. Nonetheless, at the outset of the AIDS epidemic in 1981, when physicians were faced with patients who had far-advanced, high-grade disease, it seemed reasonable to use dose-intensive regimens. Many such regimens were tested, including COMP (cyclophosphamide, vincristine, methotrexate, prednisone), which resulted in a complete remission (CR) rate of 28% and a median survival of only 3 months, and ProMACE-MOPP (prednisone, methotrexate, doxorubicin, cyclophosphamide, etoposide, mechlorethamine, vincristine, procarbazine, prednisone), which resulted in a CR rate of 20%, with complicating opportunistic infections in 27% and a median survival of 5 months. Novel regimens were also used with agents such as high-dose ara-c, high-dose methotrexate, and high-dose cyclophosphamide. Unfortunately, these regimens were also found to be ineffective (CR rate of 33%) and associated with high rates of complicating opportunistic infections (78%), often leading to early patient demise. The results of one such regimen, COMET-A (cyclophosphamide, vincristine, methotrexate, etoposide, doxorubicin), were compared with those obtained from various standard, less intensive regimens. On multivariate analysis, patients who received the more dose-intensive COMET-A regimen were found to have a statistically shorter survival.

With these facts in mind, the AIDS Clinical Trials Group (ACTG), sponsored by the National Institutes of Allergy and

Infectious Disease, embarked on a study of a low-dose modification of the M-BACOD (methotrexate, bleomycin, doxorubicin, cyclophosphamide, vincristine, dexamethasone) regimen in an attempt to evaluate the hypothesis that "less might be better" in patients with AIDS-related lymphoma (Table 101–1). In this national, multi-institutional prospective trial, intrathecal ara-C was administered once weekly for 4 weeks during the first cycle of therapy in an attempt to prevent isolated CNS relapse, and prophylactic therapy for *Pneumocystis carinii* pneumonia (PCP) was mandated. After two cycles, a restaging evaluation was performed; with CR, the patient received two additional cycles, at which time all chemotherapy was discontinued and zidovudine administration was begun. With 35 evaluable patients, a CR rate of approximately 50% was achieved, with long-term, lymphoma-free survival in 75% of complete responders. No patient experienced isolated CNS relapse. CRs were seen equally in all pathologic types. Despite the low-dose chemotherapy and the use of prophylaxis for PCP, this infection occurred in 20% of patients, representing the only complicating opportunistic infection. Further, again despite the low doses of chemotherapy, approximately 60% of patients experienced nadir granulocyte counts less than $1000 \times 10^6/L$, whereas 21% had nadirs of $500 \times 10^6/L$ or less. The median survival of complete responders was 15 months, whereas that of all evaluable patients was 6.5 months.

**Hematopoietic Growth Factors.** In an attempt to improve the toxicity profile, granulocyte-macrophage colony-stimulating factor (GM-CSF) was added to the M-BACOD regimen, with subsequent escalation of M-BACOD to full doses. This regimen was found tolerable, with no documented upregulation of HIV despite the use of GM-CSF. The efficacy of this approach was compared with the low-dose M-BACOD regimen. A subsequent prospective trial conducted by the ACTG randomized patients between this low-dose modification of M-BACOD and standard-dose M-BACOD with GM-CSF after stratification for prognostic

*Table 101–1.* **Low-Dose M-BACOD**

| Treatment | Regimen |
|---|---|
| Bleomycin | 4 mg/m² day 1 IV |
| Doxorubicin | 25 mg/m² day 1 IV |
| Cyclophosphamide | 300 mg/m² day 1 IV |
| Vincristine sulfate | 1.4 mg/m² day 1 IV (not to exceed 2 mg) |
| Dexamethasone | 3 mg/m² days 1–5 PO |
| Methotrexate (MTX) | 500 mg/m² day 15 IV, with folinic acid rescue, 25 mg PO q 6 hr × 4, beginning 6 hr after completion of MTX |
| Cytosine arabinoside | 50 mg days 1, 8, 21, 28 intrathecally |
| Helmet-field radiotherapy | 24 Gy with marrow involvement; 40 Gy with known CNS involvement |
| Zidovudine | 200 mg q 4 hr for 1 yr, starting after chemotherapy |
| *Total treatment* | 4–6 cycles at 28-day intervals |

IV, intravenously; PO, orally; CNS, central nervous system.

From Levine AM, Wernz JC, Kaplan L, et al. Low-dose chemotherapy with central nervous system prophylaxis and zidovudine maintenance in AIDS-related lymphoma: a prospective multi-institutional trial. JAMA 1991;266:84–8. Copyright 1991, American Medical Association.

factors. A total of 192 patients were evaluated. Although efficacy was similar, the standard-dose regimen was significantly more toxic, despite the use of GM-CSF. Standard-dose therapy was not found advantageous in patients with good- or those with poor-risk prognostic features.

**Addition of Antiretroviral Agents.** Antiretroviral agents have been used in an attempt to ameliorate the immune dysfunction of HIV while chemotherapy is administered. Unfortunately, zidovudine is associated with significant bone marrow suppression, and regimens consisting of zidovudine with concomitant chemotherapy (even low doses) have been associated with significant bone marrow suppression and short survival. However, a significant partial remission of mixed small and large cell lymphoma of the lung lasting approximately 9 months has been reported after the use of zidovudine alone in one patient.

The simultaneous use of chemotherapy and other antiretroviral agents such as dideoxycytidine (zalcitabine, ddC) has also been reported by Levine and colleagues, who noted a CR rate of 56% in a group of 25 patients treated with low-dose M-BACOD and ddC. Opportunistic infections occurred in 12%. Significant bone marrow suppression was less than that reported in earlier studies using chemotherapy alone, and response rates were similar in patients with poor prognostic indicators.[7] Combination infusion chemotherapy (CDE [cyclophosphamide, doxurubicin {Adriamycin}, etoposide]) with didanosine (ddI; Videx) has been used by Sparano and colleagues, who noted lesser degrees of hematologic suppression than seen with CDE alone, with a CR rate of 58%.[8] Use of HAART with CHOP chemotherapy has been studied by the ACTG. Although results concerning pharmacokinetic interactions are currently pending, anecdotal reports have not shown increased toxicity with the use of CHOP and HAART therapy.

**Dose-Intensive Regimens.** Occasional reports of efficacy with dose-intensive regimens have been published. For example, the MACOP-B (methotrexate, doxorubicin, cyclophosphamide, vincristine, prednisone, bleomycin, cotrimoxazole) regimen was found effective and tolerable in a small group of HIV-infected patients. This series was characterized by the chance inclusion of patients who had presented with good prognostic indicators, such as excellent performance status and no history of AIDS before the lymphoma. It is possible, then, that patients with disease of good prognosis may be able to tolerate the dose-intensive regimens, whereas these same regimens are too toxic in patients with poor prognostic features.

Gisselbrecht and associates[6] reported the use of a dose-intensive LNH-84 regimen given to 141 patients as part of a French-Italian consortium. HIV-seropositive patients with no active opportunistic infection and with a performance status less than 3 were eligible. The regimen consisted of three cycles of doxorubicin (75 mg/m$^2$), cyclophosphamide (1200 mg/m$^2$), vindesine (2 mg/m$^2$ × 2 days), bleomycin (10 mg × 2 days), and prednisone (60 mg/m$^2$ × 5 days). This was followed by a consolidation phase of high-dose methotrexate plus leucovorin, ifosfamide, etoposide, asparaginase, and ara-C. CNS prophylaxis with intrathecal methotrexate was also used, and zidovudine was added as maintenance therapy after completion of chemotherapy. There were 10 treatment-related deaths during the initial induction period, and only 30% of patients received the induction regi-

men at the correct interval, owing to hematologic toxicity and slow recovery. CR was achieved in 63%, with median disease-free survival of 16.7 months. Median survival for all patients was 9.3 months. The CR rate was significantly less in patients with B symptoms, poor performance status, disseminated stage, bone marrow involvement, more than two extranodal sites of disease, elevated lactate dehydrogenase levels, or CD4 count less than 100/mm$^3$.[6]

Another report has documented the efficacy of infusional chemotherapy (cyclophosphamide, hydroxydaunorubicin, and etoposide), administered over 4 days to a group of 14 patients with poor prognostic indicators.[9] Complete remissions were achieved in 71%, whereas opportunistic infections occurred in 36%.

**Summary of Systemic Treatment Options.** It is apparent that further progress is needed to define the optimal therapy for patients with AIDS-related lymphoma. However, it is clear that low-dose regimens (such as the one described in Table 101–1) are at least as effective as standard- or high-dose intensity combinations, and toxicity may be less. Patients with disease of good prognosis may be able to tolerate the various dose-intensive regimens, but there is no clear information to prove that such regimens are more effective. Intrathecal chemotherapy appears important in an attempt to prevent CNS relapse. Use of hematopoietic growth factors may ameliorate the bone marrow toxicity of systemic chemotherapy, without significant upregulation of HIV. Use of marrow-sparing antiretroviral agents, including HAART, may be associated with improved marrow tolerance and a decrease in opportunistic infections.

## PRIMARY CENTRAL NERVOUS SYSTEM LYMPHOMA

Patients with P-CNS lymphoma present with far-advanced HIV disease, median CD4 cells less than 50/mm$^3$, and a history of AIDS prior to the lymphoma in approximately 75%. Initial symptoms and signs may be variable, with seizures, headache, or focal neurologic dysfunction, or a combination. Subtle changes in personality or behavior may also be seen as the only presenting complaint.

Radiographic scanning reveals mass lesions in the brain, occurring at any site. These are likely to be relatively large (2 to 4 cm) and relatively few in number (one to three lesions); ring enhancement may be seen. There is no specific radiographic picture of P-CNS lymphoma, and definitive diagnosis requires tissue biopsy.

A review of the literature by Fine and Mayer indicates that optimal therapy of primary CNS lymphoma in patients with AIDS has yet to be defined.[10] Although radiation is associated with CR in 20 to 50%, median survival has been only 2 to 3 months, with death often due to opportunistic infection. Although radiation may not improve the duration of survival, the quality of life does improve in approximately 75% of patients, often dramatically. The combined use of chemotherapy and radiation improves survival in P-CNS lymphoma unrelated to AIDS, but this has not yet been studied in AIDS-related disease. Protocols to test this hypothesis are in progress. A case of spontaneous remission has been reported in a patient with P-CNS lymphoma who received HAART alone. This case serves to illustrate the importance of immune deficiency in the development of AIDS- related P-CNS lymphoma.

## SUGGESTIONS FOR ADDITIONAL READING

Nasir S, DeAngelis LM. Update on the management of primary CNS lymphoma. Oncology 2000;14:228–34; discussion 237–42, 244.

O'Brien P, Roos D, Pratt G, et al. Phase II multicenter study of brief single-agent methotrexate followed by irradiation in primary CNS lymphoma. J Clin Oncol 2000;18:519–526.

## REFERENCES

1. Pluda JM, Venzon DJ, Tosato G, et al. Parameters affecting the development of non-Hodgkin's lymphoma in patients with severe human immunodeficiency virus infection receiving antiretroviral therapy. J Clin Oncol 11:1099–107, 1993.
2. Beral V, Peterman T, Berkelman R, Jaffe H. AIDS-associated non-Hodgkin's lymphoma. Lancet 337:805–9, 1991.
3. Levine AM. Acquired immunodeficiency syndrome–related lymphoma. Blood 1992;80:8–20.
4. Levine AM, Sullivan-Halley J, Pike MC, et al. Human immunodeficiency virus–related lymphoma; prognostic factors predictive of survival. Cancer 1991;68:2466–24.
5. Levine AM, Wernz JC, Kaplan L, et al. Low dose chemotherapy with central nervous system prophylaxis and zidovudine maintenance in AIDS-related lymphoma. A prospective multi-institutional trial. JAMA 1991;266:84–8.
6. Gisselbrecht C, Oksenhendler E, Tirelli U, et al. Human immunodeficiency virus-related lymphoma treatment with intensive combination chemotherapy: French-Italian Cooperative group. Am J Med 1993;95:188–96,.
7. Levine AM, Tulpule A, Espina B, et al. Low dose methotrexate, bleomycin, doxorubicin, cyclophosphamide, vincristine, and dexamethasone with zalcitabine in patients with acquired immunodeficiency syndrome–related lymphoma. Cancer 1996;78:517–26,.
8. Sparano JA, Wiernik PH, Hu X, et al. Pilot trial of infusional cyclophosphamide, doxorubicin, and etoposide plus didanosine and filgrastin in patients with human immunodeficiency virus–associated non-Hodgkin's lymphoma. J Clin Oncol 1996;14:3026–35.
9. Sparano JA, Wiernik PH, Strack M, et al. Infusional cyclophosphamide, doxorubicin, and etoposide in human immunodeficiency virus– and human T-cell leukemia virus type I–related non-Hodgkin's lymphoma: a highly active regimen. Blood 1993;81:2810–5.
10. Fine HA, Mayer RJ. Primary central nervous system lymphoma. Ann Intern Med 1993;119:1093–1103.

# CHAPTER 102

# METASTASIS OF UNKNOWN ORIGIN

• DENNIS A. CASCIATO

## Natural History

### DEFINITION

*Metastasis of unknown origin (MUO)* is defined as a metastatic solid tumor (hematopoietic and lymphoproliferative malignancies are excluded) for which the site of origin is not suggested by a thorough history and physical examination, chest radiographs, routine blood and urine studies, or detailed evaluation of biopsy specimens. Pathologists should be provided with all relevant clinical information before the term *MUO* is applied.

### DILEMMA

Despite its common occurrence, the MUO syndrome creates a dilemma for the clinician in nearly every case and for many reasons. First, malignant tumors presenting as MUO often behave atypically compared with similar tumors with an evident primary site. This aberrant natural history prevents a prediction of the primary site based on metastatic patterns. Second, with certain notable exceptions, the detection of MUO represents the discovery of a far-advanced malignancy that is rarely curable and is usually resistant even to palliative chemotherapy. Tumors that may present as MUO and are potentially responsive to systemic treatment are found in only about 20% of all patients. Third, the medical literature abundantly documents that the diagnostic work-ups of these patients are models of excessiveness and futility. The futility, rather than the utility, of radiographic studies in elucidating the primary site in patients with MUO is stressed. The time required to complete the studies represents a significant portion of the patient's life expectancy; that fact, the monetary cost, and the discomfort of diagnostic studies should be considered seriously when formulating plans to manage these patients.

### EPIDEMIOLOGY

Before 1970,[1] little was published about the MUO syndrome. Since the early 1980s, the literature on this syndrome has expanded significantly. Several published series have resulted in the recognition of MUO as a distinct and frequently occurring oncologic phenomenon, have helped define its natural history, and have permitted the development of guidelines for diagnostic and therapeutic interventions in affected patients.[2–16]

Approximately 3 to 7% of patients with noncutaneous cancers present with the MUO syndrome. Its incidence ranks only below that of cancers of the lung, prostate, breast, cervix, stomach, and large intestine. Tumor registry figures and epidemiologic data, however, grossly understate the actual frequency of primary tumors originating from an unknown site because primary sites are often assigned to patients on a "best guess" basis, without proof of a tumor's origin.

The median age of patients with the MUO syndrome is 56 to 60 years. Men and women are affected about equally, with men predominating in certain series. About 10% of patients have a history of another antecedent cancer.[4, 17]

### HISTOPATHOLOGY

The frequency of histologic subtypes in the MUO syndrome varies somewhat among the large reported series.[1, 2, 10, 14, 15] Adenocarcinoma accounts for 35 to 55% of MUO syndrome cases; undifferentiated carcinoma, for 30 to 45%; squamous cell carcinoma, for 5 to 15%; malignant melanoma, for 2 to 5%; neuroendocrine carcinoma, for 1 to 3%; and all others for less than 5%. If patients presenting with cervical lymphadenopathy alone were excluded, the incidence of squamous cell carcinoma would be reduced to less than 5%.

### PROGNOSIS

The prognosis for most patients with the MUO syndrome is dismal. The median survival is 1 to 4 months in most series (excluding the treatable subsets), and more than 80% of patients die within 1 year.[1–14, 18, 19] Nearly all long-term survivors are found in two groups: (1) patients who presented with peripheral lymphadenopathy alone and (2) patients who had cancers that were extremely sensitive to chemotherapy. The latter group includes poorly differentiated or neuroendocrine carcinomas, women with peritoneal carcinomatosis, and men with poorly differentiated carcinoma in a midline lymphadenopathic distribution. Unfavorable prognostic groups are those with multiple metastatic sites, supraclavicular lymphadenopathy, and histology of well-differentiated or moderately differentiated adenocarcinoma.[15, 20]

Age and performance status clearly affect prognosis. The median survival in one series was 2 months for patients older than age 57 years and 5 months for patients younger than age 57.[3] Men younger than 40 years old, particularly those with poorly differentiated malignancies, have a relatively favorable prognosis (see later). In another series, the median survival was 6 to 10 months for patients with a good performance status and 2 months for patients with a poor performance status.[21] Van der Gaast and colleagues[22] observed a simple prognostic model for patients with undifferentiated or poorly differentiated adenocarcinomas based on the most important prognostic factors: performance status and serum alkaline phosphatase levels, the latter reflecting metastases to liver or bone, or both. Patients with a World Health Organization performance status of 0 and alkaline phosphatase value less than 1.25 times the upper limits of normal had a median survival of more than 4 years. Patients with a World Health Organization performance status of more than 1 and elevated alkaline phosphatase had a median survival of 4 months. Importantly, a nearly universal observation in the medical literature is that the prognosis in patients with MUO is not improved by discovering the primary lesion.

## MANIFESTATIONS

Of patients with the MUO syndrome, 97% present with symptoms of metastasis; the remainder are detected by means of routine evaluations or serendipity.[1] Symptoms are commonly multiple and present for 1 to 4 months before the diagnosis of metastatic carcinoma. In one series, symptoms were present for less than 1 month in more than half of the patients.[23]

The frequencies of predominant manifestations are shown in Table 102–1 and vary with the referral bias of the reporting institutions. The major problem is lymphadenopathic in approximately 30% of patients, abdominal in 20%, pulmonary in 20%, bony in 15%, and neurologic in 5%. Other less frequent manifestations include cutaneous and soft tissue nodules, cryptogenic cachexia, fever of unknown origin, and migratory thrombophlebitis. Thromboembolic episodes occur frequently in patients with adenocarcinomatous MUO.

The frequencies of reported manifestations vary with the distribution of histologic features. In series that report all histopathologic subtypes of MUO, the predominant feature is lymphadenopathic in 30% and abdominal in 15% of cases. In series that report only adenocarcinomatous MUO, the predominant feature is abdominal in 30% and lymphadenopathic in 15%. The frequencies of other predominant manifestations were not affected by histologic type.

**Supraclavicular Lymph Nodes.** In MUO cases involving supraclavicular lymph nodes at presentation and in which the primary tumor was eventually identified, the ultimate primary sites proved to be the lung, stomach, pancreas, and kidney.[14, 24] The median survival of patients with metastasis to this nodal chain is less than 6 months. Patients with MUO to supraclavicular (and lower cervical) lymph nodes should

*Table 102–1.* **Predominant Presenting Manifestations in the Metastasis of Unknown Origin Syndrome***

| Manifestations | Patients (%) | Range (%) |
|---|---|---|
| Lymphadenopathy | 28 | 14–37 |
| Thoracic abnormalities | 21 | 18–27 |
| Abdominal abnormalities | 20 | 9–37 |
| Bone pain or fracture | 16 | 6–26 |
| Neurologic symptoms | 6 | 6–17 |
| Skin nodules | 2 | 0–9 |
| Other manifestations | 2 | 1–10 |

*Data were collected from reports from four centers involving a total of 714 patients.[7–10]

be evaluated and managed as patients with MUO to nonlymphatic tissues.

**Intrathoracic Metastasis.** MUO presenting as a solitary pulmonary nodule is rare but is most frequently associated with colorectal carcinoma or sarcoma when it does occur. Pleural effusions in adults are caused by malignant disease in 50% of cases and occur in 20% of MUO cases.[10, 25] Thoracic computed tomographic scanning appeared to detect a primary tumor in the lung in one third of MUO patients in one series,[26] but the clinical value of that information was limited. Pericardial metastasis is rarely the predominant manifestation of MUO.

**Intra-abdominal Metastasis.** Hepatomegaly, abdominal carcinomatosis, malignant ascites, and any combination of these are frequent manifestations of the MUO syndrome. Prostate and ovarian carcinoma metastasize to the liver more frequently when they present as unknown primary tumors than when they occur as known primaries.[27] In a survey of malignant ascites, 6 to 11% of patients had the MUO syndrome, and the median survival of those patients was 2 weeks.[28] Owing to the poor prognosis of male patients with malignant ascites resulting from MUO, aggressive management is not recommended. For women with malignant ascites, however, a variant of ovarian cancer should be suspected; the prognosis for these patients is substantially improved with appropriate therapy.

**Brain Metastasis.** MUO is second in frequency only to bronchogenic carcinoma as the cause of brain metastasis.[10] Conversely, neurologic symptoms are the most frequent manifestation of lung cancer when presenting as an MUO syndrome. In cases that presented as MUO to the brain, the primary site eventually became evident while the patient was alive in approximately 40% of cases and was lung carcinoma about 90% of the time.[5, 29–32] The remainder of cases of MUO to the brain comprise malignant melanoma and carcinomas of the breast, colon, and kidney.

Metastatic brain lesions may be single or multiple. Most series of patients who had single brain lesions that were excised, however, usually had the same poor survival (3 to 7 months) as other patients with the MUO syndrome.[32–35]

**Epidural Metastasis.** Occasionally, MUO may present with spinal cord compression. The diagnostic and therapeutic considerations follow the same general principles as cord compression resulting from known causes except that laminectomy has been traditionally recommended as the first step to establish the histopathologic diagnosis. Two series of patients presenting with metastatic adenocarcinoma to the spine (with nearly half of patients with neurologic dysfunction) reported median survivals of only 2 months, however.[36, 37] Nonsurgical therapy should be the guideline for patients with MUO causing spinal cord compression, and laminectomy should be offered only to carefully selected patients.

**Cutaneous Metastasis.** When cutaneous metastasis represents the initial manifestation of cancer, carcinoma of the lung or kidney is the most likely possibility. Patients with MUO who present with cutaneous metastasis represent 10% of all cases of the MUO syndrome. They have a median survival of about 7 months if the primary lesion ultimately does not prove to be in the lung.

**Bone Metastasis.** Bone metastasis is second only to intra-abdominal metastasis as the most frequent extralymphatic site of presentation for patients with the MUO syndrome.

When a primary tumor is found, carcinoma of the lung is the most frequent cause of MUO presenting with bony manifestations.[14, 38] When presenting as an unknown primary tumor, pancreatic carcinoma frequently involves the skeleton.[27] Carcinomas of the lung, prostate, and ovary are found in 85% of patients with MUO presenting with pathologic fractures.[5]

Surveys of patients with MUO to bone confirm that the primary sites were determined in only 14% of patients, even with computed tomographic scanning of the abdomen.[39] The median survival of these patients in one series was 3 months.[39] Certain investigators have claimed that the primary site of origin can be detected in 30 to 50% of cases presenting as MUO to bone by using thorough radiographic evaluation[40, 41] (more than double the rate of the general experience); most of these patients, however, did *not* have MUO according to the definition given at the beginning of this chapter.

**Bone Marrow Metastasis.** The bone marrow is involved in 10 to 15% of cases of MUO as evaluated by aspiration or biopsy techniques.[38, 42] Autopsy techniques involving the thoracolumbar spine or bilateral hip biopsy specimens increase the yield of positive results by twofold or threefold in patients with carcinoma.[43] The highest rates of positive results are found in patients with carcinomas of the lung, breast, or prostate.[1]

In about half of the patients with solid tumors, a positive bone marrow biopsy specimen is associated with an abnormal peripheral blood smear or an abnormal bone scan.[44] Only 50% of patients with a positive bone scan had a positive marrow biopsy. Although patients with metastasis to the bone marrow frequently had leukocytosis, monocytosis, or thrombocytosis, leukoerythroblastosis was the most accurate barometer of bone marrow involvement (all cases had positive biopsy results).[44, 45] At the University of Missouri, 11% of bone marrow biopsy specimens containing metastatic carcinomas proved the diagnosis to be MUO[45]; the median survival of those patients was only 18 days after diagnosis.

## BIOLOGY

Several hypothetical mechanisms could explain the existence of occult primary neoplasms. First, unrecognized primary lesions may have been removed years before the appearance of metastatic lesions (e.g., in the case of a malignant skin lesion removed by electrocautery or freezing or an incompletely examined uterus removed for a leiomyoma). Second, the primary cancer may have shed metastases, then undergone spontaneous regression (as is known to happen with melanoma). Third, the primary tumor may grow too slowly and be too small to be detected, even at postmortem examination. Finally, the site of origin may be obscured by the extensiveness of metastases or by the atypical pattern of dissemination. The inference to be drawn from these possible mechanisms is that the primary tumor has changed its phenotype and presumably its genotype subsequent to malignant transformation.

Metastasis is a complex, multistep process involving numerous interactions between tumor cells and the host's extracellular matrix and immune system. Metastatic foci are derived from only a small subpopulation of the primary tumor. Proposals to explain how tumor cells leave a primary site and subsequently invade tissues at a secondary site include the ability of tumor cells to produce proteases, to express certain surface adhesion molecules, to express histocompatibility antigens, to induce clotting, to develop resistance to natural killer cell lysis, and to have enhanced growth response to cytokines as well as other factors.[46]

The specific organ microenvironment can influence profoundly whether the metastatic colony grows in the first place, its pattern of growth, and the phenotypic expression of the metastasis, such as its morphology. For example, brain, liver, and lung metastases from the same primary tumor frequently do not resemble one another histologically or biochemically. Conversely, certain metastatic sites seem to induce a common histologic pattern that obfuscates the differing primary neoplasms (e.g., an intense desmoplastic reaction).

Although the distribution of metastases from tumors of known origin often follows a remarkably reproducible pattern, metastasis to one organ without metastasis to another organ implies a selective process. Frost[47] described two patterns of tumor progression. Type 1 progression develops through a histologically defined malignant cascade. The best example of type 1 progression is colon carcinoma with sequential changes from a benign polyp to liver metastases, with parallel changes in histology, karyotype, oncogene expression, and DNA methylation. Type 2 progression is accelerated: a malignant phenotype is acquired directly or soon after the transformation event. The most dramatic examples of type 2 progression are MUO tumors.[47]

The tumors of many patients with MUO have been shown to have abnormalities in chromosome 1p that could explain the accelerated type 2 progression.[48, 49] Theoretically the 1p chromosome could contain an important tumor suppressor gene needed for the expression of the metastatic phenotype and could lead to cells that dominate the primary tumor and all subsequent metastases. The clonally dominant cells with altered 1p metastasize, grow, and then diversify. Mutation of the p53 gene does not appear to play a major role in the development and progression of MUO, however.[50]

Although MUO shows a high degree of vascularization and is presumably highly angiogenic, angiogenesis itself does not appear to have a biologic role in the metastatic phenotype of the MUO.[51] Patients with MUO do highly overexpress certain oncogenes (e.g., c-*myc*, *ras*, c-*erb*B2), but the biologic role of overexpression is also unknown.[52]

The discussed dissimilarities between the metastatic focus and the primary tumor make the determination of site of origin difficult and often impossible. From a clinical perspective, an understanding of how metastasis occurs is unlikely to provide a basis for prevention in terms of current knowledge.[46]

## Histopathologic Clues to Tumor Origin

The histopathologic diagnosis of cancer should be made expeditiously at the site of least possible morbidity to eliminate undirected diagnostic tests. Defining the histology is the most important factor in suggesting the site of origin, in determining treatability and prognosis, and in directing diagnostic tests. In two studies of patients with the MUO syndrome that sought this information, the median time from the initiation of a metastatic work-up to the performance of a biopsy was 8 to 10 days.[5, 53]

Tissue of good quality in adequate amounts is necessary to maximize the efforts at histopathologic diagnosis. Needle biopsies may be inadequate in establishing the type of malignancy. Open biopsy of accessible tumors is the procedure of choice when there is a diagnostic problem because this method rarely results in the retrieval of inadequate tissue. The only exception to obtaining a direct biopsy is in patients who have potentially malignant lymph nodes in the cervical chain alone (see later discussion). The diagnosis may also be established by cytologic studies in 5 to 15% of cases if ascites or pleural effusion is present.[3, 14]

In cases of suspected MUO syndrome, biopsy specimens should be reviewed carefully with a pathologist. Ideally the pathologist should receive biopsy specimens before the material is placed in a fixative. This practice permits the performance of histochemistry, immunohistochemistry, hormone receptor studies, or electron microscopy, if warranted. Histopathologic clues of tumor origin are shown in Table 102–2.

Microscopic diagnosis is not an exact science. The interpretations of histologic specimens are subjective opinions, not facts. In one study of 100 lymph nodes involved with carcinomatous metastases, the opinions of a panel of reviewing pathologists were unanimous regarding histopathologic classification in only 57% of cases.[54] Disagreements were common with undifferentiated neoplasms and nonkeratinizing squamous cell carcinomas. In this study, the most likely primary site (usually the lungs) was correctly identified in 59% of cases with a blind review of slides and no clinical information. Interpreter bias was also shown in a study of MUO in which 27% of the primary sites were identified correctly on morphologic criteria alone and 46% with knowledge of the metastatic site.[55] In another report of 100 cases of adenocarcinomatous MUO, two separate pathologists agreed on the primary site less than half the time; this series had the highest agreement for cancers of the breast, prostate, and ovary, which are neoplasms that often have idiotypic histologic features.[56]

The limitations of light microscopy in identifying primary sites were emphasized in a study by Le Chevalier and colleagues[2] of 257 cases of MUO that were initially biopsied and later autopsied. The primary site was *suggested* in 123 cases, but the suggestion was incorrect in 73 (59%) of these cases. They also noted that the histologic appearance was misleading in 134 cases (52%) and concluded that the initial biopsy specimen was not contributory as to the origin of the malignant neoplasm in 207 of the 257 MUO cases (80%).

## HISTOLOGY

**Squamous Cell Carcinoma.** No further information can be obtained by special studies of the biopsy specimen be-

*Table 102–2.* **Microscopic Clues to Tumor Origin**

| Potentially Helpful Findings | Probable Primary Site or Tumor Type |
|---|---|
| *Histopathology* | |
| Signet-ring cells | Gastrointestinal tract, ovary, breast (lobular carcinoma) |
| Psammoma bodies | Ovary, thyroid, breast |
| Papillary | Thyroid, ovary, mesothelioma |
| Nonacinar cell nests | Carcinoid, melanoma, paraganglioma |
| Rosettes and areas of ganglion cell–like differentiation | Neuroblastoma |
| *Histochemistry* | |
| Mucin stains (e.g., mucicarmine) | Adenocarcinoma |
| Glycogen stains (PAS-positive removed by diastase) | Abundant in renal cell carcinoma, germ cell tumors, and some adrenocortical carcinomas (small quantities not helpful) |
| Silver impregnation (e.g., Fontana-Masson, Grimelius, Sevier-Munger) | Tumors of polypeptide-forming endocrine cells, enterochromaffin cells, melanoma |
| *Electron Microscopy* | |
| Lamellar surfactant bodies | Alveolar carcinoma (lung) |
| Cells united by well-developed cell junctions (desmosomes), intercellular bridges, tonofilaments | Squamous cell carcinoma |
| Premelanosomes, melanosomes, tubular arrays | Melanoma |
| Abundant polyribosomes, absence of intercellular junctions | Lymphoma, leukemia |
| Myofibrils, extracellular osteoid, dilated rough endoplasmic reticulum | Sarcoma |
| Long surface microvilli | Mesotheliomas (some) |
| Cytoplasmic neuroendocrine secretory granules | Neuroendocrine tumors, including carcinoid |
| Apical terminal webs | Gut epithelial cells |
| Acinar spaces, junctional complex, tight junctions, microvilli, desmosomes | Adenocarcinomas |
|    Microvilli, glycocaliceal bodies, terminal webs, apical mucus granules |    Colon |
|    Intracellular neolumina, prominent tonofilaments |    Breast |
|    Staghorn microvilli |    Ovary |
|    Tubulofilamentous structures of cytoplasm |    Kidney |

PAS, periodic acid–Schiff.

cause squamous cell carcinomas appear similar histologically, regardless of their site of origin. They originate most commonly from the head and neck, lung, or uterine cervix but may also arise from the esophagus, rectum, anus, penis, or skin. The most likely site of the primary lesion depends on the location of the metastasis.

**Adenocarcinoma.** The histologic features of well-differentiated hepatocellular, renal clear cell, and thyroid follicular carcinomas are pathognomonic. Infiltrating duct carcinoma of the breast and carcinoma of the colon have fairly characteristic patterns that may suggest their origin.

Mucin production is characteristic of many types of adenocarcinoma, but the presence or absence of gland formation is not a specific indicator of tumor origin. A positive mucin stain excludes renal cell carcinoma, for example, but a negative mucin stain does not rule out adenocarcinoma from any site. Signet-ring cells are found in adenocarcinoma of the gastrointestinal tract, ovary, and (rarely) breast. Psammoma bodies may be present in adenocarcinoma of the thyroid, ovary, or breast.

**Undifferentiated and Poorly Differentiated Large Cell Neoplasms.** Undifferentiated neoplasms and poorly differentiated adenocarcinomas frequently present challenging clinical problems. They may represent carcinoma, lymphoma, malignant melanoma, or extragonadal germ cell tumors. Many patients with these histopathologic diagnoses have achieved excellent responses to cisplatin-based combination chemotherapy.[57]

Lymphoma or melanoma is a common diagnosis when the initial histologic diagnosis is undifferentiated or poorly differentiated neoplasm. Gastric lymphoma, for example, is frequently misdiagnosed as carcinoma. Another example, Ki-1 lymphoma, is a T-cell malignancy that is commonly confused with carcinomas but is characterized by long survival times and spontaneous remissions. The tissue should be examined with special techniques to clarify the diagnosis of poorly differentiated neoplasms and evaluate fully the tumor for treatable possibilities.

**Undifferentiated Small Cell Neoplasms.** Small cell carcinomas may originate from a variety of sites and may be difficult to distinguish even with studies of ultrastructure. The following are included in the differential diagnosis of undifferentiated small cell neoplasms: neuroendocrine carcinomas, hematologic neoplasms (lymphoma and plasmacytoma), pediatric neoplasms (rhabdomyoblastoma and Ewing's sarcoma), anaplastic seminoma, and amelanotic melanoma.

Primary oat cell carcinomas have been described in the thymus, thyroid, esophagus, stomach, small and large bowel, pancreas, nasal cavity, paranasal sinuses, larynx, hypopharynx, salivary glands, uterine cervix, endometrium, breast, prostate, urinary bladder, and skin. These tumors are indistinguishable from bronchogenic oat cell carcinoma. The multiplicity of sites in which extrapulmonary small cell neoplasms are found suggests that a common ancestral cell derived from neural crest tissue migrates to various epithelial sites within the body. An alternative suggestion is that the cell of origin is an endodermally derived stem cell that can result in neuroendocrine and epithelial differentiation.

**Clear Cell Tumors.** Polygonal cells with clear cytoplasm can represent artifactual changes, benign neoplasms, or malignancies. Clear cytoplasm can occur with ex vivo hydropic degeneration or by an abundance of glycogen, mucin, mucopolysaccharides, lipid, or phagocytosed foreign material in the cytoplasm of tumor cells. Neoplastic proliferation of epithelial, mesenchymal, melanocytic, and hematopoietic lineage may manifest a virtually identical clear cell appearance, regardless of whether they are benign or malignant in nature.

This pathologic dilemma of clear cell tumors[58] is exceptionally important for patients with MUO because seminomas, nonseminomatous germ cell carcinomas, and lymphomas can be clear cell tumors. Differentiation of the various types of malignancies in these circumstances requires detailed analysis of clinical, histologic, immunohistochemical, and occasionally electron microscopic features. Renal cell clear cell carcinoma, for example, may not be distinguished by any of these approaches, but may be defined by magnetic resonance imaging (MRI) findings. Direct communication between the clinician and pathologist is essential in these cases.

**Malignant Melanoma.** Approximately 12% of patients with melanoma MUO have amelanotic tumors.[59] The problem in detecting amelanotic melanoma is compounded by its misclassification on light microscopy as undifferentiated carcinoma. Because cures are still possible if metastatic disease is limited to the peripheral lymph nodes, it is imperative that undifferentiated carcinomas be evaluated by histochemical studies for melanoma markers and by electron microscopy, if possible, to search for premelanosomes.[60] S-100 cytoplasmic protein is specific for tissues of the nervous system and is present on human malignant melanoma cell lines. HMB-45 and Epl-3 are antigens that are also highly specific for the melanocyte lineage.[61]

## IMMUNOHISTOLOGY

Antigen-antibody reactions can be elicited by enzyme-labeled antibodies in sections that are fixed, processed, and embedded by conventional histologic methods, particularly those using the horseradish peroxidase-antiperoxidase method. Potentially useful markers that are detectable by immunoperoxidase staining (IPS) techniques are shown in Table 102–3. Few antibodies, however, identify a specific primary tumor site.

Endocrine tumors may be established by identification of their hormonal products, such as calcitonin, thyroglobulin, gastrin, insulin, and somatostatin. Neuroendocrine tumors can be defined by the appropriate light microscopic findings in combination with pan-neuroendocrine markers (neuron-specific enolase, synaptophysin, and chromogranin).[62] Tumors derived from certain tissues may also be classified by this technique (e.g., with antibodies to myoglobulin for sarcoma, to factor VIII–related antigen for endothelium-derived tumors, or to keratin for squamous cell carcinomas). Epithelial membrane antigens (cytokeratins) are normally expressed by exocrine gland cells and a wide range of adenocarcinomas. Results from IPS using carcinoembryonic antigen (CEA) antibody have been nonspecific, while giving variable results.[62] CA-125 antibody for IPS stains better for serous than for mucinous ovarian adenocarcinomas.[62] IPS is rarely helpful in evaluating malignant effusions.

IPS appears to have three useful purposes in poorly differentiated neoplasms: (1) to confirm the diagnosis of carcinoma, (2) to identify patients with other neoplasms (e.g.,

*Table 102–3.* Selected Immunohistologic Tumor Markers

| Detectable Antigen | Tumor Type |
|---|---|
| Alpha-fetoprotein (AFP) | Germ cell (particularly yolk sac) and trophoblastic tumors; hepatocellular carcinoma, hepatoblastoma |
| $\beta_1$-antitrypsin | Hepatocellular carcinoma |
| BCA-225 | Breast, lung, ovary |
| CA-125 | Ovary, lung, upper gastrointestinal tract |
| CA-19-9 | Pancreas, colon, breast |
| Carcinoembryonic antigen (CEA) | Bowel, stomach, pancreas, liver, cervix uteri, lung, ovary, breast, urinary tract, thyroid (medullary) |
| Chromogranin | NET, thyroid (medullary) |
| Cytokeratin (e.g., CK7, CK20, CK34) | Broad range of carcinomas and sarcomas |
| Desmin | Sarcomas (smooth or skeletal muscle, glomus tumors); corpus uteri (connective tissue part) |
| Factor VIII; CD31, CD34 | Sarcomas (vascular) |
| Gross cystic disease fluid protein (GCDFP-15, BRST-2) | Breast, salivary gland |
| Hormones (specific to gland) | Endocrine gland, gastrointestinal or pancreatic tumors |
| Human chorionic gonadotropin (hCG) | Trophoblastic, nonseminomatous testicular, breast, and other tumors |
| Human placental lactogen | Trophoblastic tumors |
| Immunoglobulin molecules | Lymphomas/leukemias |
| Involucrin | Squamous epithelia |
| Laminin; type IV collagen | Sarcomas (neurogenic, smooth muscle) |
| Leukocyte common antigen (LCA) | Lymphomas/leukemias, histiocytic tumors |
| Lymphoid cell epitopes and activation markers | Lymphomas/leukemias |
| Milk fat globules | Breast, lung |
| Muramidase (lysozyme); CD68 | Histiocytic tumors, myelogenous leukemia |
| Myelin base protein | Sarcomas (neurogenic), neurilemoma |
| Myoglobin | Sarcomas (neurogenic, skeletal muscle), corpus uteri |
| Muscle-specific actin | Sarcomas (leiomyosarcoma, MFH) |
| Neurofilaments | NET; lung (small cell carcinoma), brain, olfactory neuroblastoma |
| Neuron-specific enolase | NET; lung (small cell carcinoma); melanoma; breast (some); lymphoma (some); neuroblastoma, medulloblastoma, retinoblastoma, other brain tumors, meningioma, neurilemoma, chordoma, pituitary adenoma |
| NKI/C3 or MB-5 | Melanoma |
| Pancreatic carcinoma antigen | Pancreas, gut |
| Prostate-specific acid phosphatase, prostate antigen (PAP, PSA) | Prostate, salivary gland |
| S100 protein | Brain tumors: astrocytoma, oligodendroglioma, ependymoma, choroid plexus papilloma, ganglioneuroblastoma, meningioma, medulloepithelioma, hemangioblastoma, craniopharyngioma, chordoma |
| | Peripheral neuroblastoma; Schwann cell tumors (neurilemoma, neurofibroma, granular cell tumor) |
| | Melanoma; sarcomas (neurogenic, cartilage); histiocytic tumors; breast; mixed sweat gland tumor, pleomorphic salivary gland adenoma, eosinophilic granulomas |
| Thyroglobulin | Thyroid |
| Villin | Adenocarcinoma of gastrointestinal tract and lung |
| Vimentin | Sarcomas (muscle, cartilage, vessels, bone, synovial, epithelioid, MFH); renal cell carcinoma; melanoma; lymphomas/leukemias |

NETs, neuroendocrine tumors (including neuroblastic, Merkel cell, and carcinoid tumors; paraganglioma; pheochromocytoma); MFH, malignant fibrous histiocytoma.

lymphoma), and (3) to identify a site of recognized cancer (e.g., prostate). The most useful IPS markers in the MUO syndrome appear to be leukocyte common antigen, cytokeratins, S-100 protein, vimentin, and prostate-specific antigen (PSA).[62–65] In one series of referred biopsy specimens, malignant lymphoma was identified by IPS in 8 of 24 specimens (33%) that were initially diagnosed as unclassifiable and in 29 of 43 specimens (66%) that were initially thought to be undifferentiated carcinoma.[65] Hainsworth and colleagues[63] studied 89 patients with poorly differentiated carcinoma; IPS confirmed the pathologic diagnosis in 56%, established an alternative diagnosis (melanoma, lymphoma, prostate cancer, or yolk sac tumor) in 16%, and was inconclusive in 28% of specimens.

Formerly the IPS method was projected to be helpful in identifying germ cell tumors with β-human chorionic gonadotropin (β-hCG) and alpha-fetoprotein (AFP). IPS using AFP, β-hCG, and neuron-specific enolase did not yield substantial information in a large series of patients with poorly differentiated carcinomas of unknown origin.[63] Even PSA determinations may give false-positive results[66] and may be found in men with salivary gland adenocarcinomas.[67]

Immunocytochemical techniques are helpful when staining results are positive but less useful when results are negative. With the rapid proliferation of commercially available antisera, caution in the interpretation of results is advisable. Considerable technical expertise is required to perform these tests accurately and reproducibly. The reliability of results depends on rigorous quality control, review of the slides by experienced pathologists, and awareness of the limitations and pitfalls of the findings. Regardless of the relatively high specificity of several immunoperoxidase markers, false-positive as well as false-negative staining may be expected. Differences in fixation techniques and in the kind of antigen used are responsible for the observed differences in sensitivity and specificity.

In the setting of undifferentiated cancers and poorly differentiated adenocarcinomas, IPS could be useful to verify the histologic diagnosis of treatable entities (e.g., lymphoma, prostate carcinoma, and neuroendocrine carcinoma). Panels of antigens have been used to try to identify the primary sites in patients with MUO[68, 69]; however, the discriminatory ability of such panels (e.g., using CEA, vimentin, CA-125, and several cytokeratins) has not been established.

## ELECTRON MICROSCOPY

Electron microscopy may improve identification of specimens with undifferentiated histologic features but is not widely available, is expensive, and is limited by the need for specially fixed tissues when generally only formalin-fixed tissues are available. Although formalin-fixed tissue can be used or transferred into glutaraldehyde, the loss in quality of the sample precludes identification of subtle features.

Potentially discriminating findings of electron microscopy are shown in Table 102–2. The presence of lamellar surfactant bodies (for alveolar carcinoma of the lung) or apical terminal webs (for gut epithelial cells) may be useful in evaluating cases of MUO.[70] Electron microscopy can be extremely helpful in the evaluation of small round cell tumors and lymphomas or to provide evidence of neuroendocrine differentiation. When cell differentiation is sufficient, the presence of cytoplasmic organelles, membrane specialization, intercellular relationships, and a variety of secretory granules may be helpful in the differential diagnosis of several tumors. With dedifferentiation, however, poorly differentiated tumors lose specific morphologic and ultrastructural features. For example, malignant melanoma that does not contain premelanosomes may be indistinguishable from undifferentiated carcinoma, even when the ultrastructure is studied.

## ESTROGEN RECEPTOR DETERMINATION

The determination of estrogen receptors (ERs) may be useful for the identification of possible breast cancer in patients with adenocarcinoma of unknown origin, and assay of the initial biopsy specimen may be the sole opportunity to determine the tumor's hormonal receptor status. The human malignancies found to exhibit specific estrogen-binding protein with any frequency are malignant melanoma, germ cell tumors, and carcinomas of the breast, endometrium, ovary, colon, pancreas, and kidney. Routine determination of ER by IPS has not been helpful, however, in identifying the primary site or in prescribing therapy of patients with MUO.[16, 71]

## Searching for the Primary Site

The primary site of malignancy is determined before the death of the patient in only 13% of carcinomas presenting as MUO, no matter what diagnostic efforts are expended. Table 102–4 shows the results of searching for the primary site in patients with the MUO syndrome before and after death.[2–19] About half are detected at the initial diagnostic evaluation and half on following the patient's clinical course. Postmortem examination fails to detect the primary tumor in 22% of patients.

When the primary site is eventually determined (Table 102–5), either during the clinical course or at autopsy, carcinomas of the pancreas and lung predominate.[2–12] Solid tumors that are currently considered treatable in advanced stages (germ cell neoplasms and carcinomas of the ovary, breast, prostate, and thyroid) are found in about 15% of patients presenting with the MUO syndrome.

The expected frequencies of malignancies are skewed in cases of MUO. Although breast carcinoma accounts for 25% of all cancer-related deaths, it causes less than 3% of deaths resulting from carcinoma presenting with unknown primary

*Table 102–4.* **Results of Searching for the Primary Site in the Metastasis of Unknown Origin Syndrome**

| Institution | Before Death | | After Death | |
|---|---|---|---|---|
| | NO. PATIENTS | NO. PS FOUND | NO. AUTOPSIES | NO. PS NOT FOUND |
| M.D. Anderson Hospital[16] | 840 | 122 (14%) | — | — |
| Tulane U.[10] | 453 | 14 (3%) | — | — |
| France[2] | 302 | 82 (27%)* | 302 | 48 (16%) |
| U. Southern California[6] | 266 | 22 (8%)* | 130 | 23 (18%) |
| Roswell Park Memorial Inst.[14] | 254 | 6 (2%) | 97 | 26 (27%) |
| Boston U.[4] | 106 | 33 (31%)* | — | — |
| Ludwig Inst., Australia[3] | 87 | 23 (26%) | 16 | 2 (12%) |
| Harvard U.[5] | 67 | 17 (25%)* | 9 | 2 (22%) |
| Southwest Oncology Group[8] | 51 | 6 (12%) | 13 | 2 (15%) |
| Mayo Clinic[12] | — | — | 162 | 42 (26%) |
| UCLA[13] | — | — | 34 | 20 (55%) |
| Italy[19] | — | — | 31 | 8 (26%) |
| Brooke Army Hospital[11] | — | — | 18 | 5 (28%) |
| U. South Florida[7] | — | — | 11 | 2 (20%) |
| *Totals (Mean)* | 2426 | 325 (13%) | 823 | 180 (22%) |

*Approximately half were diagnosed on following the clinical course.
PS, primary site.

*Table 102–5.* Ultimately Determined Primary Sites in Patients Presenting with the Metastasis of Unknown Origin Syndrome*

| Origin of Tumor | Diagnosed Patients (%) |
|---|---|
| Pancreas | 25.5 |
| Lung | 23.0 |
| Lower bowel | 8.1 |
| Hepatobiliary tract | 7.8 |
| Kidney, urinary tract | 7.0 |
| Upper bowel | 6.5 |
| Ovary | 5.4 |
| Prostate | 4.0 |
| Breast | 2.4 |
| Thyroid | 2.4 |
| Adrenal | 2.4 |
| Germ cells | 1.0 |
| Other sites | 4.5 |
| *Total* | 100.0 |

*Data are collated from reports from 10 centers[2–12] at which the primary site of origin for the malignancy was determined during life or at autopsy in 627 of 1675 patients. Patients with primary neoplasms of the head and neck are excluded. All histopathologic subtypes of carcinoma are included.

sites. Carcinomas of the prostate and large bowel are common cancers that become manifest infrequently as an occult primary tumor. Carcinomas of the pancreas account for 1.5% of cancer deaths in a general population but for more than 25% of deaths in patients presenting with MUO.

The probable sites of origin for various metastatic presentations can usually be predicted according to their usual natural histories. Cancers that present as MUO often do not behave accordingly. The pattern of dissemination in tumors presenting as MUO is variable and does not follow typical pathways.[19, 25, 27] For example, bony metastases develop in 30 to 50% of cases when lung carcinoma presents with an evident primary site but in only 5% of cases that present with MUO. Carcinomas of the pancreas and liver involve bone in only 5 to 10% of cases, but when they present as MUO, they involve the skeleton in 30% of cases. The lung and liver are uncommonly involved by metastatic prostate carcinoma, unless the tumor presents as MUO, in which case these organs are involved in more than half of the patients. These aberrant metastatic behavioral patterns seriously compromise the prediction of primary site of disease in patients presenting with metastases and an occult site of origin.

Whatever the explanation for occult primary sites of carcinoma, insufficient vigor in diagnostic pursuit is not a factor. In the classic epidemiologic study of the MUO syndrome undertaken in 1970, the authors quizzically noted as an aside that "the scope, expense, and hazard of the searches for primary tumors were impressive; often staggering."[1] In a 1992 study of the diagnostic behavior of internists, patients with adenocarcinomatous MUO had a substantially higher and *striking* mean number of investigations than patients with eventually identified primary sites.[53] These same internists delayed biopsy of clinically evident lesions in adenocarcinomatous MUO by a median 8 days while in pursuit of the "prebiopsy prolonged investigative pathway."

Table 102–6 shows the frequency of diagnostic studies performed in patients with MUO at 11 teaching hospitals reporting this information.[2–8, 14, 72–74] Of patients, 60 to 80%

underwent radiologic evaluation of the upper and lower gastrointestinal tracts and the urinary tracts, often repeatedly. In addition to the radiologic studies listed, patients were frequently subjected to gallium scans or radionuclide imaging of the pancreas, kidney, brain, and lung; random endoscopies; arteriography; and exploratory laparotomy. This attention to diagnosis resulted in prolongation of the median stay by 10 to 35 days compared with that for patients admitted for the evaluation of cancer emanating from a clinically known site.[4, 14]

## RADIOGRAPHS

Chest radiographs, which are taken in virtually all patients with MUO, are frequently abnormal. They can be misleading in identifying the primary site, however. In Le Chevalier's series,[2] the chest radiographs identified the lung as the primary site in 96 cases, but that designation was ultimately wrong in 31 of the cases.

No chest x-ray pattern can differentiate a metastasis from a primary lung cancer. Although multiple nodules and infiltrates suggest metastasis, patterns suggestive of a primary lung carcinoma (coin lesions, malignant effusions, or hilar masses) represent metastasis in 45% of cases.[6] Pulmonary metastasis may be solitary, and primary lesions may be multifocal. In a report of lung carcinoma presenting as the MUO syndrome, most chest radiographs did not detect the lesion, even in retrospect, despite a mean tumor size of nearly 3 cm.[75]

Of patients with epigastric symptoms, 70 to 85% had abnormal findings in upper gastrointestinal studies, but most of these results added no new information beyond the clinical evaluation[4, 5]; in the absence of symptoms, 8% of patients had abnormal results. Likewise, 55% of the patients with abdominal symptoms or occult blood in the stools had abnormal findings in barium enema examinations, whereas 5% of those without these symptoms had abnormal results[4, 5]; in only about 6% of cases were malignant lesions of the bowel identified.[5, 6] Similarly, intravenous pyelograms frequently gave abnormal results without useful information (organ

*Table 102–6.* Frequency of Diagnostic Studies in Patients with the Metastasis of Unknown Origin Syndrome*

| Diagnostic Study (No. Reporting Series) | No. Patients at Risk | % Patients Undergoing Test |
|---|---|---|
| Upper GI series (10) | 1187 | 67 |
| Barium enema (10) | 1187 | 58 |
| Intravenous pyelogram (9) | 1173 | 58 |
| Mammogram in women (7) | 295 | 35 |
| Cholecystogram (4) | 666 | 11 |
| CT scan and/or ultrasound, abdomen-pelvis (5) | 281 | 58 |
| Bone scan (4) | 303 | 43 |
| Thyroid scan (4) | 686 | 18 |
| Bronchoscopy (6) | 494 | 31 |
| Sigmoidoscopy or colonoscopy (5) | 471 | 14 |
| Upper GI endoscopy (3) | 432 | 12 |

*Data collected from 11 reported series.[2–8, 14, 72–74]
GI, gastrointestinal; CT, computed tomography.

displacement by exogenous tumor) and frequently missed the few true cases of primary renal carcinoma.[3, 5, 6]

Four separate reports on patients with MUO have indicated that the results of upper gastrointestinal series, barium enema, and intravenous pyelography each suggest a malignant primary lesion in 5 to 10% of cases, but that only about half are true-positive results.[2, 3, 5, 6] In addition to providing results that are frequently misleading, these studies missed at least an equal number of primary lesions confirmed at autopsy (this represents a minimal number because all patients did not undergo postmortem examination except in the series of Le Chevalier and colleagues[2]). The contrast-enhanced radiographic techniques for the gastrointestinal and upper urinary tracts provide about equal numbers of true-positive, false-positive, and false-negative results for diagnosing primary malignancies.

## SCANS

The use of computed tomography (CT) has not improved the diagnostic yield.[8, 16, 72, 76, 77] When CT does detect primary sites of malignancy (such as lung or pancreas), the condition usually responds poorly to therapy, and the information becomes moot. One series of 31 MUO patients claimed that CT found the primary site in 58% of their patients but was unhelpful or wrong in 23%.[78] CT of the chest, abdomen, and pelvis costs about $4700.[16] An abdominal computed tomographic scan alone, however, may be the most cost-effective single test in evaluating patients with the MUO syndrome because patients and their families rarely accept the recommendation that no diagnostic testing at all is necessary.

Bone scans are commonly abnormal in patients with MUO in the absence of bone pain. The incidence of positivity varies with the patient population in the different reported series. Bone scans have been abnormal in 48% of patients with MUO but without symptoms and in 91% of patients with bone pain.[3–5] Patients with MUO by definition have disseminated disease that is usually refractory to treatment; the complete staging of asymptomatic sites in this population is a dubious practice.

Thyroid scans were performed in 113 of 643 cases of MUO in three reports.[2, 3, 14] Although thyroid carcinoma is frequently suggested by histologic appearance, it accounts for less than 1% of adenocarcinomatous MUO. These scans resulted in identifying only three cases of thyroid carcinoma correctly, identifying it wrongly in three cases, and missing four true cases that were found at autopsy. Gallium scans as well as thyroid scans are useless in the evaluation of patients with the MUO syndrome.[4]

## SERUM TUMOR MARKERS

Pavlidis and colleagues[79] showed that more than 40% of 85 patients with MUO had elevation of *all five* serum tumor markers that were assayed (CEA, CA-15-3, CA-125, CA-19-9, and β-hCG). Measurements of CEA, CA-125, and CA-19-9 are generally of little use in determining the primary site in patients with the MUO syndrome because of their lack of specificity (as opposed to their established

values in monitoring patients with known primary sites). CA-125 specifically also has been shown not to be helpful as a guide to treatment in female patients with MUO, even when the presentation suggests variants of ovarian carcinoma.[80] Routine use of these tests offers neither diagnostic nor prognostic assistance for patients with MUO because the syndrome is associated with a nonspecific overexpression of several serum tumor markers. A wide variety of other tumor markers have been described, but none has achieved clinical usefulness for patients with the MUO syndrome.

Acid phosphatase levels, particularly when measured by radioimmunoassay, may be helpful in identifying patients with prostatic carcinoma who have an atypical clinical presentation. In one series, only 14% of 444 patients with elevations of prostatic acid phosphatase were subsequently found to have prostate cancer.[81] Transient elevations in the level of serum acid phosphatase may be noted after prostatic surgery, prostatic infarction, urinary retention, and catheterization (but probably not after rectal examination). Other causes of an elevated serum acid phosphatase level include bone diseases with osteoclastic activity (including metastatic carcinoma) and diseases of the kidney, hepatobiliary system, and reticuloendothelial system. A patient with small cell carcinoma MUO who had high serum values of prostatic acid phosphatase and PSA in the absence of prostate cancer has been reported.[66] In the autopsy series of MUO cases by Le Chevalier and colleagues,[2] measurement of prostatic acid phosphatase in 45 men resulted in four true-positive, three false-positive, and six false-negative results. An elevated serum acid phosphatase or PSA level is insufficient by itself to establish the diagnosis of prostate cancer.

The measurement of AFP and β-hCG is essential in patients with germ cell neoplasms. Each test must be interpreted, however, in light of the knowledge of other conditions that are associated with elevated values and in the clinical context of patients with MUO. AFP is elevated in patients with testicular carcinomas that contain yolk sac elements (teratocarcinoma and embryonal cell carcinoma); hepatocellular carcinomas; liver metastasis; cancers of the stomach, pancreas, lung, or colon; or benign liver disease. β-hCG is produced by nonseminomatous testicular cancers; cancers of the lung, ovary, breast, or gastrointestinal tract; certain lymphoproliferative disorders; melanomas; and rarely seminomas. Elevations of β-hCG may also occur in benign diseases, including pregnancy, inflammatory bowel or duodenal ulcer disease, and cirrhosis of the liver. At least three large series[2, 57, 82] of patients with MUO have shown that measurement of AFP and β-hCG was not helpful in identifying either the primary site or patients who would benefit from chemotherapy. Both AFP and β-hCG are associated with malignant and nonmalignant conditions; neither AFP nor β-hCG is de facto evidence for germ cell neoplasms.

## OTHER STUDIES

Screening bronchoscopy, sigmoidoscopy, colonoscopy, gastroscopy, and arteriography are too invasive and rarely helpful in the MUO syndrome. No report has shown that these or other invasive procedures enhance the diagnostic yield. Even mammography in women with the MUO syndrome appears to be useless.[2, 4, 71, 83]

The autopsy series of Le Chevalier and colleagues[2] emphasized the high frequency of misleading results from endoscopic searching for the primary site in patients with the MUO syndrome. Upper gastrointestinal endoscopy was performed in 35 patients and resulted in three true-positive, five false-positive, and two false-negative results. Sigmoidoscopy in 28 patients resulted in two true-positive, one false-positive, and no false-negative results. Combining the findings of chest radiography and bronchoscopy performed in 105 patients, 32 bronchogenic carcinomas were diagnosed, but 13 were proved wrong at autopsy.

## AUTOPSIES

The penultimate diagnostic test to identify a primary site is postmortem examination. Recapitulating what was shown in Table 102–4, however, autopsy still fails to detect the primary site in approximately one quarter of patients with the MUO syndrome.

## SUMMARY

Despite the extensive assault with the diagnostic armamentarium, the primary neoplasm is diagnosed before death in less than 15% of cases, often while the patient is being followed clinically (see Table 102–4). The irony of this recurrent theme is that many of the diagnostic tests are misleading as often as they are helpful.[2–6, 19] Prospectively, given this poor degree of accuracy, clinicians cannot place much confidence in the results of any study that attempts to identify the origin of the metastasis in patients with the MUO syndrome. Yet, physicians continue to expose patients with MUO to persistent searches for the primary site. The quest is exhaustive emotionally for the patient and the physician, physically for the patient, and financially for the patient or third-party payer. Schapira and Jarrett[18] estimated that the cost of work-up for patients with MUO is about $18,000 per patient and extrapolated the national annual expenditure for this effort to be $1.5 billion. Many investigators have recanted in many ways: finding the primary site has no bearing on the patient's treatment or survival.

## Management

The MUO syndrome clearly contains two major subdivisions: conditions that are treatable and those that are not. Approximately 80% of patients with MUO have expected median survivals of less than 1 year (usually <5 months) and rare long-term survivals. The patients with MUO who may respond to treatment and hope for long-term survival have metastases that involve lymph nodes alone or are sensitive to chemotherapy. These treatable groups are organized in this chapter as follows:

1. Lymph node metastases alone, including
   a. Melanoma to peripheral lymph nodes alone.
   b. Squamous or undifferentiated carcinoma to lymph nodes in the upper two thirds of the neck.
   c. Adenocarcinoma to unilateral axillary lymph nodes, particularly in women.
   d. Carcinoma to unilateral groin nodes alone.
2. Metastases that are exquisitely responsive to chemotherapy, including
   a. Neuroendocrine (small cell) carcinoma.
   b. Peritoneal carcinomatosis in women.
   c. Poorly differentiated carcinoma to the peripheral lymph nodes, mediastinum, or retroperitoneum, particularly in men.

## MELANOMA METASTASIS OF UNKNOWN ORIGIN TO PERIPHERAL LYMPH NODES

**Background.** Malignant melanoma presents without a detectable primary lesion in 4 to 6% of cases[59, 84–87] and accounts for 2 to 5% of cases of the MUO syndrome.[1, 10] Most series show male preponderance. The prevalence of dysplastic nevi was 22.5% in one series,[88] intermediate between that reported among patients with primary melanoma (39%) and among the general population (7%).

Melanoma arises in lymph nodes as MUO because the primary lesion was eradicated, underwent spontaneous regression (a well-supported hypothesis), or arose de novo in a lymph node region. Axillary involvement appears to predominate, although cervical and inguinal lymph node involvement occurs with about the same relative frequency as in instances in which the primary lesion is known.[85, 86]

**Prognosis.** The clinical disease course of melanoma MUO is similar to that of patients with known primaries when the same clinical stages of the disease are compared. The 5-year survival rate of patients with melanoma presenting as MUO and superficial lymph node involvement only (stage II disease) is 30 to 50% and no worse than the rate of patients with known primary lesions.[59, 84–89] Most series report 5-year survival rates of about 50%. The 5-year and 10-year disease-free survival rates are nearly identical. Some series observe that patients with unknown primary lesions survive longer than patients diagnosed with lymph node metastasis concurrent with a known cutaneous primary melanoma.[88, 90]

Survival is not affected by whether or not there is a history of a pre-existing lesion, by sex or age of the patient, or by whether the lesion is melanotic or amelanotic.[84, 85, 89–92] It is affected by the number of lymph nodes involved[84, 90] and by the promptness and aggressiveness of surgery.[85] Some reports[89, 90, 92] suggested a worse prognosis for patients with cervical node metastases compared with other sites of metastases, but others have observed similar survival rates as patients with MUO to axillary or groin lymph nodes.

**Treatment.** Authorities recommend radical lymphadenectomy as the treatment of choice for stage II malignant melanoma presenting as MUO. The 5-year and 10-year survival rates were 65% and 57% for patients treated promptly and 18% for patients treated after a delay of 3 or more months.[85]

**Recommendations.** When patients present with apparently stage II malignant melanoma as MUO, the skin should be carefully searched for a possible primary lesion, and any suspicious mole or nevus should be biopsied. Visceral metastases should be excluded by history, physical examination, ophthalmoscopy, chest radiographs, liver function tests (CT if there are abnormalities on physical examination or laboratory studies), and brain computed tomographic scan. If no other metastases are evident, the patient should undergo radical lymphadenectomy of the affected nodes, which should be repeated on occasions when disease recurs locally. Adjuvant therapy with interferon appears to improve survival in patients with stage II melanoma and known primary site; similar systemic treatment could be a logical choice for melanoma and unknown primary site.

## METASTASIS OF UNKNOWN ORIGIN TO NECK LYMPH NODES

**Background.** The occurrence of MUO in cervical lymph nodes is five to seven times higher in men than in women. Patients are usually heavy smokers and heavy drinkers who have noted the mass for several months. MUOs are found in 3 to 9% of patients with head and neck cancers in large reported series. Despite the absence of a detected primary site, long-term survival and cures are observed in a significant percentage of patients in nearly all reported series.

Metastases are located in the upper jugular chain in most patients and bilaterally in about 20% of cases. Approximately 50% of metastases contain squamous cell carcinoma, and 25% contain undifferentiated carcinoma. Most of the remainder contain adenocarcinoma from various sites or melanoma. Multiple adenopathies in the posterior cervical areas are usually lymphoma or metastases from infraclavicular sites or the nasopharynx.

**Diagnosis.** The contemporary approach to diagnosis of MUO involving cervical lymph nodes alone is to obtain a computed tomographic or MRI scan of the neck followed by cytologic evaluation by fine-needle aspiration (FNA). If cytologic results show malignant melanoma, the scalp, conjunctiva, and ear should be examined carefully for a primary lesion, and the patient should be managed as previously discussed. If they show an adenocarcinoma, the patient should be evaluated for MUO to any other site. Regardless of the primary tumor, the outlook for adenocarcinomatous metastasis to cervical lymph nodes is essentially hopeless (see Prognosis, later). If the cytologic findings reveal a squamous cell or undifferentiated carcinoma, management for a primary head and neck cancer should proceed.

Before *unknown primary* is designated, a thorough search for a primary lesion should be made, including examination of the head and neck, indirect laryngoscopy, and radiography of the chest and sinuses. If no primary is found, the patient should be examined while under general anesthesia with nasopharyngoscopy, laryngoscopy, bronchoscopy, and esophagoscopy. If no primary is found at panendoscopy, traditionally random biopsy specimens of the nasopharynx, tonsillar fossae, base of the tongue, and piriform sinuses have been obtained. Although the yield for random biopsy specimens is low, these sites are statistically most likely to harbor a primary source. Some surgeons recommend tonsillectomy rather than blind biopsies of the tonsillar region, particularly in patients with involvement of the high neck nodes.[93, 94] If the tonsillectomy specimen contained no malignancy, radiation ports would not include all potential sites of primary cancer.

Ultrasonographically guided FNA cytology is associated with an accuracy of 90%, sensitivity of 76 to 93%, and specificity of nearly 100%.[95, 96] The major concern with FNA cytology is an insufficient amount of specimen for the diagnosis of lymphoma or undifferentiated carcinoma. When FNA cytology fails to yield a diagnosis, biopsy should be performed and should be excisional rather than incisional, unless the tumor is unresectable. Several traditional concerns with open biopsy have been raised, including increased risk of inducing tumor spread and impairment of results of subsequent surgical therapy by scarring or vascular impairment. Data regarding the true risk of an open biopsy procedure are lacking, however. Some authorities no longer believe that pretreatment excisional biopsy affects the prognosis for survival or local disease control in patients with head and neck MUO.

Positron emission tomography (PET) using fludeoxyglucose (FDG) has been evaluated in patients with head and neck primary cancers,[97, 98] including patients with MUO to this region.[99] PET may detect more metastatic sites and provide a higher rate of positive biopsy results during panendoscopy, but the clinical relevance of this information is limited. Clinical examination and high-resolution computed tomographic and MRI studies provide good accuracy for information that is required for treatment and is unavailable with FDG PET images. For patients with MUO to cervical nodes or with primary head and neck cancers with metastasis to cervical nodes, FDG PET scans appear to provide high accuracy at high cost with only a small marginal gain of little relevance.[98, 99]

**Prognosis.** Because the usual head and neck squamous cell carcinoma tends to remain regional for long periods, MUO to cervical lymph nodes does not carry a hopeless prognosis. Five-year survivals for all patients with squamous cell carcinoma MUO to cervical lymph nodes range from 35 to 50% in reported series.[94, 100–119] Five-year and 10-year survival rates are nearly identical. Prognosis is predominantly affected by the N stage of neck disease, by the histopathology, and by whether the primary site is ever found.

All large series show a clear deterioration in prognosis from NX (excised node with no residual cancer) to N3 (nodes that are bilateral or > 6 cm in diameter). The 5-year survival appears to be about 70 to 80% for N1 and N2 disease and 15 to 25% for N3 disease.[105, 118] The involvement of supraclavicular lymph nodes nearly always indicates a far-advanced malignant disease from a distant primary site rather than local disease from the head and neck region.

Histopathologic prognostic factors include cell type and, probably more important for squamous cell carcinoma, the presence or absence of nodal capsular invasion into connective tissue. Many large series have confirmed the important poor-prognosis finding of extracapsular invasion into connective tissue[102, 103, 112, 118, 119] and have emphasized the importance of adding radiotherapy for this condition. Although many patients with squamous cell carcinomas enjoy long survival, the median survival of patients with adenocarcinomas (except those of thyroid origin) is 8 months, and only 20% survive for 2 years.[24, 108] The supraclavicular fossa is the site of metastasis in 76% of patients with adenocarcinomatous MUO to the neck, and 86% of these patients have metastases to other body sites.[24]

Although some reports disagree, most series show that survival is significantly improved if the primary tumor never becomes manifested.[94, 100–104, 107, 113, 116] The 5-year survival rate was about 60% if the primary went undetected and about 30% if it was detected. Generally, the administration of radiation therapy appears to reduce the rate of ultimately found primary sites. At 10 years after treatment, however, the risk of finding a primary site is about 30%, which is the same as the odds of developing a second cancer after successful treatment.[113]

**Treatment.** All reports of treatment results in patients with neck lymph node MUO have been retrospective analyses of relatively small numbers of patients treated in a nonuniform manner. Many studies included patients with supraclavicular lymphadenopathy, which often represented a primary lung cancer. Most studies comprise an admixture of histopathologic subtypes, often including adenocarcinoma or melanoma. Some studies do not adhere to the definition of unknown primary sites as defined previously; many of the patients reported really had identifiable primary sites. Few studies have specified survival rates separately for each of the important prognostic factors, especially nodal substages and extracapsular invasion. No study compared different treatment modalities directly in randomized trials. Definitive conclusions regarding optimal therapy are difficult to make.

The forms of treatment available are high-dose radiation therapy, electron-beam irradiation, excisional lymph node biopsy alone, radical neck dissection, and combinations of these. If radiation therapy is given, fields traditionally included everything from the base of the skull to the clavicles to encompass a small primary that may be present somewhere within the head and neck, especially in the oropharynx or hypopharynx. Critical reviews of the literature, however, concluded that there was no convincing evidence that irradiating the entire mucosa of the upper aerodigestive tract improves local control or overall survival.[94, 103, 106, 113] Radiotherapy to such extensive fields can cause significant acute toxicity and chronic morbidity, mainly xerostomia and its associated complications. Modern imaging substantially eliminates the indication for comprehensive elective mucosal irradiation. Radiation to ipsilateral nodes alone is indicated, unless nasopharyngeal carcinoma is suspected on histologic or clinical grounds.[100, 106]

For patients with N1 disease, most investigators agree that good results can be achieved with a single treatment modality (neck dissection or radiotherapy). Several series involving a total of 226 patients have reported their experience in treating N1 and N2a disease with surgery alone.[101–104] The primary tumor eventually developed in less than 15% of patients, and the disease recurred in the treated neck in less than 20% of cases. The 5-year and 10-year survival rates of these patients are both approximately 80%. Similar results for low-stage squamous cell carcinoma MUO have been achieved by treating N1 and N2a disease with radiotherapy to the ipsilateral neck only, with or without surgery,[100, 103, 106] as well as with radiotherapy to the bilateral neck and mucosa, with and without surgery.[100–105, 120] Patients with N1 disease and unfavorable prognostic factors, such as extracapsular invasion, are usually given combined-modality therapy.[100, 112]

For patients with substages N2b and higher, effective therapy remains problematic. Patients with N3 disease constitute 20 to 60% in various series[104–107, 109–112]; the 5-year survival rate in these reports is 14 to 36% (average 19%). Most investigators have recommended combined-modality therapy for these patients.

Two studies have reported encouraging results from combining cisplatin-based chemotherapy with radiotherapy, with or without neck dissection.[121, 122] In both small series, the complete remission rate for the chemotherapy combination was more than 70% with median survivals of approximately 32 months. These results are encouraging, but too few patients have been studied to justify incorporating chemotherapy into the standard treatment of squamous cell carcinoma MUO to cervical lymph nodes.

**Recommendations.** The appropriate extent of surgery, the optimal radiation field, and the optimal sequence of treatment modalities are unknown for patients with cervical node MUO containing squamous cell or undifferentiated carcinoma. The following general recommendations seem most appropriate.

The approach to cervical lymph node MUO involves MRI of the neck, FNA, and panendoscopy with random biopsy specimens for most patients. Tonsillectomy can be considered for patients with unilateral high cervical nodes. Therapy is focused on the best chance to achieve local disease control and long-term survival despite the metastatic presentation. Treatment must be comprehensive at the outset because salvage treatment has a low yield.

A single nodal metastasis, particularly if less than 3.0 cm in diameter, can be treated with neck dissection alone; if pathologic evaluation reveals extracapsular invasion or multiple node metastases, radiotherapy must be added. More advanced disease (N2b, N2c, or N3) can be treated with radiotherapy to the involved neck, while avoiding full doses to the oropharynx or hypopharynx. Total mucosal irradiation can be administered if there is strong suspicion of a primary nasopharyngeal carcinoma (i.e., involvement of posterior cervical nodes, especially if bilateral; the histologic picture of lymphoepithelioma; or the clinical associations of a nasopharyngeal primary tumor). After radiotherapy, neck dissection can be performed in selected patients. Cisplatin-based chemotherapy can be considered in patients with massive or bilateral disease in the neck.

## METASTASIS OF UNKNOWN ORIGIN TO AXILLARY LYMPH NODES

**Background.** Surgically removed, isolated axillary lymphadenopathy demonstrated benign disease in 75% of cases.[123] The most likely sites of origin of a malignancy metastasizing to the axilla are the breast, lung, gastrointestinal tract, thyroid, arm, and regional trunk. The primary site of carcinoma, however, remains occult in more than half of the cases of isolated malignant axillary lymphadenopathy.[124, 125]

**Prognosis.** In one excellent analysis of 60 patients presenting with carcinomatous axillary lymphadenopathy,[124] 30% of the patients were ultimately diagnosed as having breast cancer, and 15% died with the primary site determined to be elsewhere (usually by postmortem examination). All 33 patients (55%) with undetectable primary sites had poorly differentiated histopathology; on review, half of these were possibly either amelanotic melanoma or squamous cell carcinoma. Excluding the patients in whom breast cancer was ultimately diagnosed, 21% of the 42 patients with MUO were alive without evidence of disease 2 to 10 years (median, 5 years) after either excisional biopsy alone (7 patients) or axillary dissection (2 patients); only 3 of these patients received adjuvant radiotherapy. Other reports indicate high percentages of long-term survivals (median survivals of 42 to 92 months) in patients treated with excisional biopsy alone or node dissection with or without axillary radiation therapy.[126–128] Long-term survival in patients with axillary MUO is possible with or without the possibility of breast cancer. This relatively favorable prognosis appears to be restricted to women; men with MUO to axillary lymph nodes have the same prognosis as those with metastases to other lymph node sites.

**Occult Breast Cancer.** The most controversial situation involves the woman with adenocarcinoma in axillary lymph nodes alone. Of women with malignant axillary lymph nodes and a negative breast examination, 30 to 50% have been shown to have occult breast carcinoma.[10, 124] Occult breast cancer presenting with axillary metastasis accounts for 0.3 to 0.5% of all breast cancer patients.[71, 129, 130] Approximately 25% of these patients have a history of breast cancer in maternal first-degree relatives.[83] Mammography is abnormal in less than half of these patients, but there is no consistent correlation between the location of the radiologic abnormality and the site at which a carcinoma is ultimately located. MRI of the breast can detect breast cancers in cases in which the mammogram was negative,[131] but the clinical relevance of this information is moot.

The treatment for this condition traditionally has been radical or modified radical mastectomy,[132] usually with adjuvant postoperative radiation therapy to the axilla, because it was assumed that this represented breast cancer with an occult primary tumor.[124, 126, 130] Alternatively, upper outer quadrant sector mastectomy was proposed as the treatment most likely to detect and eradicate an occult primary lesion presenting with regional nodal metastasis.[125] These recommendations, however, contradict the current state of knowledge of the natural history of breast cancer. Diagnostic modified radical mastectomy for possible breast carcinoma is no longer tenable.[129]

Five series involving 52 patients treated with mastectomy and 93 patients without mastectomy have been published.[133–137] Primary tumors have been found in 5 to 85% of mastectomy specimens, depending on the series. The 5-year and 10-year survival rates are approximately the same with and without mastectomy[133–137]; the 10-year survival rates are 50 to 71%. Primary tumors developed eventually in less than 20% of patients given radiation therapy to the retained breast.[134, 135] These survival rates were not altered significantly in patients whose primary tumor was found compared with those in whom it was not found.[71, 137] Because ER activity was negative in 44% of patients tested in one series,[137] the absence of that activity does not rule out occult breast cancer.

Virtually all authors of these series recommend systemic therapy for these patients, as is customarily given for stage II breast cancer. The anomaly is that only some of these authors state directly that mastectomy is unnecessary in this rare presentation of breast cancer.[134–136] What argument can be presented for mastectomy to treat a lesion that is not palpable when a lumpectomy is sufficient for a palpable lesion?

**Recommendations.** The major treatable malignancies presenting in axillary lymph nodes are breast carcinoma, malignant melanoma, amelanotic melanoma masquerading as undifferentiated carcinoma, and malignant lymphoma masquerading as undifferentiated carcinoma. All histopathologies should be reviewed carefully and special studies performed as indicated.

For women with adenocarcinoma or poorly differentiated carcinoma in the axilla, ER analysis of tumor specimens and mammography should be performed with the realization that the results may not be helpful. If breast carcinoma is detected or highly suspected, the patient should be treated for stage II disease, the expectations of survival being the same as for known breast cancer.

Patients with melanoma (proved or suspected) should undergo radical axillary dissection for improved prognosis and possible cure, as discussed earlier. All other patients probably should undergo superficial axillary dissection, particularly if the biopsy was not excisional. This approach attempts to provide local control of disease and has been reported to achieve a 20 to 25% long-term survival rate. This high rate of success is probably due to a high proportion of patients who have occult amelanotic melanoma and to the rare cases of squamous cell carcinoma apparently arising de novo in lymph node sites.

## METASTASIS OF UNKNOWN ORIGIN TO GROIN LYMPH NODES

**Background.** Lymph nodes in the femoral triangle and inguinal regions are less frequently involved in the MUO syndrome than are the cervical or axillary lymph nodes because the primary tumor is found in 99% of patients having malignant groin lymphadenopathy.[138] Although pelvic viscera do not drain primarily to the inguinal lymph nodes, they may do so with advanced malignant disease. When the primary site is detectable, the tumors that metastasize to groin nodes most frequently originated in genital and reproductive organs (40% of cases), skin (32%, especially from the lower extremity and lower half of the trunk), rectum or anus (6%), or urinary bladder (3%); all remote parts of the body are represented in the remaining 20% of cases.[138, 139] When no primary lesion is found, malignant lymphoma or Hodgkin's lymphoma is present most commonly.

In patients with a detected primary site, malignant melanoma (one third of all cases), squamous cell carcinoma, and adenocarcinoma constitute more than 75% of the histopathologic diagnoses.[138] Conversely, more than 50% of the patients who present with MUO in groin lymph nodes have unclassifiable carcinomas[138, 140] (the remainder are squamous cell carcinoma or adenocarcinoma). A major question relative to these patients is the determination of how many of the unclassifiable carcinomas are truly stage II amelanotic melanomas.

Metastatic malignancies may be incidentally and rarely detected in the hernia sac at the time of herniorrhaphy. Of 22,816 patients undergoing inguinal herniorrhaphy at the Mayo Clinic over four decades, 15 (0.07%) had metastatic tumors within their hernias, including two patients with

MUO.[141] Because of the rarity of this location, however, routine histologic examination of hernia sacs and their contents is not warranted.

**Treatment.** Eleven of 22 patients (50%) with MUO to groin nodes alone were treated with excisional biopsy or superficial groin dissection alone and survived more than 2 years.[138] In another report[140] of 17 patients given radical radiation therapy, 47% were alive at 3 years and 35% at 5 years; of 12 patients treated with local excision or lymph node dissection, the median survival was more than 20 months, whereas 3 patients were alive more than 9 years after treatment. The overall 5-year survival rate in this study was 40%. These results indicate that the groin lesions may have been solitary and may have originated in the lymph node.

**Recommendations.** Authorities recommend the following sequence in the management of patients presenting with isolated malignant lymphadenopathy in the groin. First, the physician should clinically search for a primary site on the skin, anus, rectum, pelvis, and lower genitourinary tract. Second, if no primary lesion is found, a diagnostic excisional biopsy should be performed. Third, if the node reveals carcinoma of any histologic type, a superficial groin node dissection should be performed or radiation therapy should be given. Superficial groin dissection is preferred to radical dissection if no primary lesion is found because it may afford local control with less morbidity and mortality from the procedure. Adjuvant radiotherapy does not appear to be necessary in these patients.

## SMALL CELL (NEUROENDOCRINE) CARCINOMA METASTASIS OF UNKNOWN ORIGIN

**Background.** Neuroendocrine carcinomas accounted for 3% of all patients with MUO at M.D. Anderson Hospital.[15] Approximately 0.2% of all cancers and 2.5% of all small cell cancers occur in extrapulmonary sites.[142] The association with cigarette smoking, the histologic picture, many of the tumor's biologic features, and the apparent chemosensitivity are similar among small cell tumors that arise in the lung and extrapulmonary sites. In contrast to its pulmonary counterpart, however, extrapulmonary small cell carcinoma is not characterized by the 3p chromosomal deletion and may be complicated by hypercalcemia.[143]

**Treatment.** Small cell carcinomas are another potentially chemotherapy-responsive subcategory of MUO. Although the biologic features of extrapulmonary and pulmonary small cell carcinomas are similar, there are some important differences. For example, in contrast to pulmonary small cell carcinoma, local therapy alone with surgery or radiotherapy, or both, results in prolonged survival for extrapulmonary small cell carcinomas that present as primary tumors in minor salivary glands and paranasal sinuses and as MUO to cervical lymph nodes.[142]

Treatment of 18 patients with anaplastic neuroendocrine carcinomas with a 3-day infusion of cisplatin and etoposide at the Mayo Clinic[143] was associated with a response of 67%, a median duration of regression of 8 months, and a median survival of 19 months. This high response rate was confirmed in another study of 11 patients with extrapulmonary undifferentiated small cell carcinomas given combination chemotherapy in whom an objective response rate of 82% was observed[144]; long-term survival was seen in patients with limited disease who achieved a complete response after chemotherapy followed by radiotherapy. Treatment of neuroendocrine MUO at M.D. Anderson Hospital resulted in a median survival of 27 months.[15]

**Recommendations.** Patients with undifferentiated small cell carcinomas of unknown origin who have consistent histologic findings by light microscopy should be evaluated with appropriate immune staining or electron microscopy. Synaptophysin, chromogranin, and neuron-specific enolase are useful pan-neuroendocrine markers for immunohistochemical investigation in these patients. If the diagnosis is confirmed, patients should be treated with combination chemotherapy. An exception to this approach could be small metastases to cervical lymph nodes alone, which may be treated with neck dissection, radiotherapy, or both.

## PERITONEAL CARCINOMATOSIS IN WOMEN

**Background.** Malignant ascites caused by MUO has a grave prognosis, with a reported median survival of 8 days.[28] Peritoneal carcinomatosis of unknown origin (PCUO) in women may reflect variants of ovarian carcinoma because the prognosis is improved substantially. The clinical picture of abdominal pain, distention, and ascites is typical of advanced ovarian carcinoma and PCUO; many of these neoplasms also had histopathologic features suggesting ovarian cancer, such as psammoma bodies and papillary configuration. Synonyms of PCUO include papillary serous carcinoma of the peritoneum, papillary carcinoma arising from extraovarian tissue, extraovarian papillary serous carcinoma, and malignant müllerian degeneration of the peritoneum. Differential diagnosis includes abdominal carcinomatosis from a gastrointestinal primary site and malignant mesothelioma. IPS is helpful in differentiation of PCUO from mesothelioma.[145] CA-125 values have not been helpful for diagnosis or prognosis in women with PCUO.[80]

Seven series involving 195 women with PCUO have been reported.[145-151] These patients underwent exploratory laparotomy, total abdominal hysterectomy with bilateral salpingo-oophorectomy, and cytoreductive surgery without intrinsic ovarian malignancy being found. One half to two thirds of patients were left with small residual disease (nodules < 2 or 3 cm in diameter) after surgery. Nearly all patients were then given cisplatin-based combination chemotherapy, and most achieved clinical responses. The median survival of patients in these series was 17 to 27 months. The completeness of cytoreductive surgery appears to affect survival. In the Vanderbilt series,[148] the median survival of patients was 31 months with limited residual disease after debulking surgery and 11 months with extensive residual disease. Of patients with PCUO, 10 to 26% survived at least 3 years after diagnosis.[147-149]

**Recommendations.** PCUO in women represents another treatable subset of patients with MUO. The overall median survival and the percentage of long-term disease-free survivors are similar to those reported in patients with ovarian cancer. Although no firm conclusions can be made about the superiority of one treatment over another from these retrospective studies, we agree with other authors that these patients should be treated as if they have ovarian cancer. If other sources of malignancy are reasonably excluded, exploratory laparotomy is indicated even if the pelvic examination, pelvic computed tomographic scan, and pelvic ultrasonographic examination are otherwise normal. If PCUO is confirmed, total abdominal hysterectomy with bilateral salpingo-oophorectomy and aggressive cytoreductive surgery should be carried out, followed by cisplatin-based combination chemotherapy. Second-look laparotomy has no proven therapeutic benefit, and salvage therapy in this group of patients remains undefined.

## POORLY DIFFERENTIATED CARCINOMA WITH LYMPHADENOPATHY

**Background.** Most patients with proven extragonadal germ cell tumors have anterior mediastinal or retroperitoneal masses as the predominant feature and have often been misdiagnosed as having undifferentiated carcinoma, poorly differentiated carcinoma, or poorly differentiated adenocarcinoma.[152] Vanderbilt researchers[57] have described many patients who on presentation had a histopathologic diagnosis of undifferentiated carcinoma, poorly differentiated carcinoma, or poorly differentiated adenocarcinoma and who achieved excellent responses to cisplatin-based combination chemotherapy. This group of patients consisted predominantly of young men with rapidly growing tumor masses and symptoms or signs that began less than 2 months before diagnosis. The male/female ratio was 3:1, and the median age was 39 years. The predominant sites of metastases were the mediastinum, retroperitoneum, and peripheral lymph nodes in 84% of the initial 32 patients who achieved complete remission.

The Vanderbilt investigators' criteria for histopathologic classification were defined as follows:[57] *Poorly differentiated carcinomas* consisted of a pleomorphic population of large, cohesive, malignant cells growing with no definable histologic pattern. *Poorly differentiated adenocarcinomas* had the same characteristics with any adenomatous differentiation (e.g., rudimentary gland formation or strongly positive histochemical stains for mucin). *Well-differentiated adenocarcinomas*, which were excluded from these treatment studies, contained well-formed glandular structures, ducts with lumina, and mucin evident by hematoxylin and eosin staining.

With retrospective use of IPS, some of these initially reported complete responders were reclassified as having lymphoma or melanoma.[63] The question as to whether the remainder of these responsive neoplasms were unrecognized germinal tumors remains unresolved.

**Treatment.** In the Vanderbilt experience,[57] 220 patients with poorly differentiated malignancies had confirmation by IPS, electron microscopy, or both, in 80% of cases. Measurement of serum levels of β-hCG or AFP was not helpful in identifying patients who would respond to therapy. All patients were treated with cisplatin in combination with etoposide or vinblastine (with or without bleomycin or doxorubicin [Adriamycin]). The response rate of patients in whom the dominant sites of metastases were the mediastinum, retroperitoneum, and peripheral lymph nodes (48% of this series' patients) was 74%. The complete response rate of patients in the latter group was 52%, with two thirds of

these patients enjoying long-term disease-free survival. The 5-year disease-free survival (and 10-year actuarial survival) was 37% for patients with disease confined to the retroperitoneum and peripheral lymph nodes and 16% for those with disease affecting predominantly the mediastinum. In contrast, the response rate of patients with metastasis to liver, bone, pleura, peritoneum, or other visceral sites was only 22%, with a 7% 5-year disease-free survival. In a 1997 update for long-term follow-up of these patients, the median survival for patients who achieved a complete remission was 4.5 years.[153] Of the original 220 patients, 12% remained alive with a minimum follow-up of 6.5 years. Despite exhaustive review, the tumor origin, cell lineage, and biology of these malignancies remain an enigma. Motzer and colleagues[154] have proposed that abnormalities in the 12p chromosome supports the diagnosis of germ cell tumors in patients with poorly differentiated carcinoma or undifferentiated carcinoma and predicts a good response to cisplatinbased treatment.

Other institutions have confirmed these excellent response rates to cisplatin-based combinations for metastatic undifferentiated carcinoma, poorly differentiated carcinoma, and poorly differentiated adenocarcinoma to lymph node regions and relatively poor response rates of short duration for poorly differentiated carcinoma metastatic to other sites.[22, 79, 80, 155] Other drug combinations that did not include cisplatin also were associated with relatively high response rates for poorly differentiated carcinoma and poorly differentiated adenocarcinoma with lymph node metastases.[156, 157] These data are included in Table 102–7.

The prolongation of survival to the degree reported by Hainsworth, Greco, and colleagues[57, 153] has not been recapitulated in other series. Median duration of responses is usually 4 to 5 months. Several researchers have emphasized that the impact of chemotherapy on survival has been minimal despite excellent response rates[20, 80, 155] and have warned about selection bias in analysis of subgroups of patients. Van der Gaast and colleagues[22] showed that for patients with poorly differentiated adenocarcinoma and undifferentiated carcinoma treated with cisplatin and etoposide, the median survival was more than 4 years in patients who were asymptomatic and had no evidence of liver or bone metastases and was 4 months for patients with a lower performance status and increased serum alkaline phosphatase levels.

**Recommendations.** Patients with unknown primary poorly differentiated carcinoma or poorly differentiated adenocarcinoma metastatic predominantly to lymph nodes, particularly young men with a midline distribution of metastases, should be given a cisplatin-based combination chemotherapy regimen. Evidence suggests that these patients gain important clinical benefit and perhaps may even have prolonged survival.

## METASTASIS OF UNKNOWN ORIGIN TO ALL OTHER SITES

**Background.** Metastases of unknown origin to sites other than lymph nodes account for more than 75% of cases of the MUO syndrome. The median survival of these patients is 3 to 6 months. These patients are the least likely to benefit

*Table 102–7.* Chemotherapy Regimens Used in Adenocarcinoma Metastases of Unknown Origin

| Author, Year | FU | DOX | CYC | MI | PLAT | ETO | OTHER | NO. PATIENTS | RESPONSES % | COMPLETE RESPONSES % | NOTES† |
|---|---|---|---|---|---|---|---|---|---|---|---|
| Kelsen,[163] 1988 | X | | | | | | Leuc, HD Mtx | 21 | 5 | 0 | |
| Nole,[164] 1993 | X | | | | | | Leuc | 17 | 0 | 0 | NLN |
| Rigg,[165] 1997 | X | | | | | | Leuc, Carb | 30 | 30 | | 1 |
| Woods,[21] 1980‡ | X | | X | | | | Mtx | 22 | 5 | 0 | |
| Walach,[157] 1987 | X | | X | | | | Mtx, Vcr | 10 | 90 | 60 | LNO |
| Walach,[157] 1987 | X | | X | | | | Mtx, Vcr | 11 | 9 | 0 | NLN |
| Valentine,[76] 1979 | X | X | X | | | | | 14 | 14 | 7 | |
| Schildt,[8] 1983‡ | X | X | X | | | | | 16 | 0 | 0 | NLN |
| Jordan,[9] 1985 | X | X | X | | | | | 19 | 10 | 0 | |
| Pasterz,[23] 1986 | X | X | X | | X | | | 47 | 28 | 13 | 1 |
| Bedikian,[166] 1983 | | X | X | | X | | ± Ftor | 13 | 15 | 0 | |
| Anderson,[156] 1983 | | X | X | | | | Vcr | 8 | 62 | 50 | 1A, 2, LNO |
| Anderson,[156] 1983 | | X | X | | | | Vcr | 12 | 42 | 0 | 1A, 2 |
| Pasterz,[23] 1986 | | X | X | | | | Vcr, Dcz | 14 | 36 | | 1A |
| Goldberg,[72] 1986 | X | X | | X | | | | 43 | 30 | 9 | |
| Pasterz,[23] 1986 | X | X | | X | | | | 9 | 22 | | |
| Van der Gaast,[159] 1988 | X | X | | X | | | | 22 | 14 | 0 | |
| al Idrissi,[168] 1990 | X | X | | X | | | | 29 | 10 | 0 | NLN |
| Sulkes,[160] 1988‡ | X | X | | X | | | | 15 | 13 | 0 | |
| Sulkes,[160] 1988‡ | | X | | X | | | Vbl | 14 | 28 | 7 | 1A |
| Eagan,[161] 1987‡ | | X | | X | | | | 28 | 14 | 0 | |
| Woods,[21] 1980‡ | | X | | X | | | | 25 | 36 | 4 | 1 |
| Milliken,[162] 1987‡ | | X | | X | | | | 51 | 39 | 0 | 1 |
| Kambhu,[169] 1990 | | X | | X | | | Vnd | 57 | 30 | 5 | |
| Fiore,[158] 1985 | | X | | | | | Vnd | 38 | 16 | 3 | |
| Eagan,[161] 1987‡ | | X | | X | X | | | 27 | 26 | 0 | |
| Falkson,[155] 1998‡ | | | | X | | | | 39 | 18 | 8 | |
| Falkson,[155] 1998‡ | | | | X | X | | Epi | 41 | 49 | 20 | 1A |
| Wegener,[171] 1991 | | | | X | | | | 21 | 19 | | |
| Milliken,[162] 1987‡ | | | | X | | | Vbl, Bleo | 50 | 30 | 2 | 1 |
| Van der Gaast,[22] 1995 | | | | X | | X | ± Bleo | 77 | 43 | 12 | 1A, LNO |
| Raber,[170] 1991 | X | | | | X | X | | 36 | 22 | 11 | 1 |
| de Campos,[167] 1994 | | X | X | | X | X | Vcr | 50 | 10 | | |
| Gill,[172] 1991 | | | | | X | X | | 16 | 19 | 6 | NLN |
| Farrugia,[80] 1996 | | | | | X | | + Various | 22 | 59 | 4 | 1A |
| Farrugia,[80] 1996 | | | | | X | | + Various | 64 | 30 | 3 | |
| Pavlidis,[146] 1992 | | | | | X | | + Various | 44 | 29 | 16 | 1, LNO |
| Hainsworth,[57] 1992 | | | | | X | | + 2 others | 105 | 74 | 43 | 1A, 2, LNO |
| Hainsworth,[57] 1992 | | | | | X | | + 2 others | 115 | 22 | 17 | 1A, 2, NNL |
| Hainsworth,[173] 1997 | | | | | | X | Pacl, Carb | 13 | 69 | 31 | LNO |
| Hainsworth,[173] 1997 | | | | | | X | Pacl, Carb | 40 | 40 | 7 | NLN |

*Abbreviations for drugs: Bleo, bleomycin; Carb, carboplatin; Cyc, cyclophosphamide; Dcz, dacarbazine; Dox, doxorubicin; Epi, epirubicin; Eto, etoposide; Ftor, ftorafur; FU, 5-fluorouracil; HD, high dose; Leuc, leucovorin; Mi, mitomycin C; Mtx, methotrexate; Pacl, paclitaxel; Plat, cisplatin; Vbl, vinblastine; Vcr, vincristine; Vnd, vindesine.

†Abbreviations for notes: 1, authors identify a significant proportion of patients with undifferentiated carcinoma or poorly differentiated adenocarcinoma; 1A, all patients have undifferentiated carcinoma or poorly differentiated adenocarcinoma; 2, median age of patients less than 40 years, with a preponderance of men; LNO, metastases to lymph nodes only, often in a midline distribution; NLN, metastases were not restricted to lymph nodes.

‡Randomized trial.

from chemotherapy of any kind and are unlikely to survive for 1 year.

**Surgery.** Surgical resection of metastases is considered under certain circumstances. Resection of upper cervical lymph nodes, resection of other peripheral lymph nodes alone, and cytoreduction surgery for PCUO have already been discussed. With the exception of solitary metastases to the brain without evidence of a primary site, surgical excision of other metastases has no role in treatment of MUO. Most series report survivals of 3 to 7 months for patients with a single MUO to the brain treated with surgical excision, usually followed by whole-brain radiotherapy.[32–35] Occasional reports claim much better survivals, showing that patient selection has had a great influence on reported results.

**Chemotherapy.** The results of chemotherapy for adenocarcinoma of unknown primary site have been generally disappointing. Except for specific subgroups of patients discussed earlier, chemotherapy has resulted in low response rates and unimproved survival. The median survival for all patients treated with chemotherapy is 3 to 7 months. Many authors have reported that responders with the MUO syndrome survive longer than nonresponders.[9, 12, 14, 21, 23, 76, 158, 159] This method of reporting survival data, however, has been regularly discredited.

Response rates and survival for patients with the MUO syndrome treated with chemotherapy have correlated with the presence or absence of symptoms (i.e., performance status [PS]). Most reports on the responses to chemotherapy regimens fail to analyze the PS of treated subjects. Woods and coworkers[21] showed that the median survival in patients with the MUO syndrome was 7 weeks for those with a poor PS, 26 weeks for those with a good PS and no response to chemotherapy, and more than 40 weeks for those with a good PS and an objective response to chemotherapy. Pasterz and colleagues[23] observed that the response rates to chemotherapy were 75% for patients who were asymptomatic, 19% for those who were symptomatic, 42% for those who had a good PS, and 11% for those who had a poor PS. The relationship of PS and survival was also discussed earlier (under Prognosis) for patients with undifferentiated and poorly differentiated carcinomas; survival was clearly related to PS for those histologic subtypes.[22]

Single-agent therapy with 5-fluorouracil, cyclophosphamide, methotrexate, doxorubicin, mitomycin C, vincristine, etoposide, semustine, and other drugs is associated with objective response rates of 6 to 18%.[7, 12, 14, 76, 154] Published reports on combination chemotherapy regimens used to treat patients with MUO and adenocarcinomas are summarized in Table 102–7.[8, 9, 21–23, 57, 72, 76, 80, 146, 155–173]

The most frequently used combinations were FDC (5-fluorouracil, doxorubicin, cyclophosphamide), FDMI (5-fluorouracil, doxorubicin, mitomycin C), DMI (doxorubicin, mitomycin C), and cisplatin combination regimens. Collating the results from reports using the same combinations of drugs, 9% of 49 patients responded to FDC, 20% of 118 patients responded to FDMI, and 32% of 104 patients responded to DMI. The DMI combination appears to be the most effective of these regimens; however, two of the three reports of the use of DMI included significant numbers of patients with undifferentiated carcinomas, which have been clearly associated with higher response rates than the other varieties of carcinoma in MUO.

Six studies to date have prospectively randomized patients between two treatment alternatives. Woods and colleagues[21] randomized 47 patients with adenocarcinomatous MUO syndrome to receive either DMI or CMF (cyclophosphamide, methotrexate, 5-fluorouracil). The response rate was 36% with DMI and 5% with CMF, but the DMI group contained several patients with poorly differentiated malignancies; survival was clearly related to performance status. Sulkes and colleagues[160] randomized 29 patients to treatment with either DMI or FDMI. The response rates were 28% and 13%, respectively, and the DMI group had more patients with poorly differentiated malignancies. Eagan and colleagues[161] randomized 55 patients to receive DMI alone or DMI with cisplatin; the response rates were 16% and 26%; the DMI group with cisplatin contained more patients with poorly differentiated malignancies. Similarly, Milliken and coworkers[162] randomized 101 patients to receive DMI or cisplatin, vinblastine, and bleomycin. Response rates were comparable (39% and 30%), but hematologic toxicity was predominant in patients treated with DMI, and gastrointestinal toxicity was predominant in patients given the cisplatin regimen; both groups contained patients with poorly differentiated malignancies. In contrast, the Southwest Oncology Group (SWOG)[8] randomized 36 patients with adenocarcinomatous MUO syndrome to receive 5-fluorouracil alone or FDC; no patient responded to either regimen, but the toxicity of the FDC regimen was substantially greater than that of 5-fluorouracil alone. Falkson and Cohen[155] randomized 80 patients to receive mitomycin C alone or combined with cisplatin and epirubicin. Response rates were 18% and 49%; the patients with poorly differentiated neoplasms were disproportionately included in the combination chemotherapy group.

Response rates and survival for patients with the MUO syndrome treated with combination chemotherapy should be reported with caution because data have depended greatly on (1) the sites involved with metastases and (2) the histopathology. Reports showing the higher response rates almost invariably included significant numbers of patients with predominantly nodal metastases or undifferentiated or poorly differentiated histology. With consultative review of the biopsy specimen or performance of immunohistochemical staining, a significant number of responding patients turned out to have lymphoma. Many series reporting encouraging results of chemotherapy contained MUO presentations that we now consider to be treatable, such as lymphoma or peritoneal carcinomatosis in women.

Patients with metastases involving lymph nodes only do much better than those with metastases involving viscera or bone.[6, 17, 20–23, 57, 76, 146, 156–158] In one series,[23] the response rate to combination chemotherapy regimens was 70% in patients with metastases involving only lymph node or soft tissue sites and 22% in patients with metastases involving other sites. Walach and Horn[157] found that 90% of patients who responded to chemotherapy had metastases that involved lymph nodes only. Complete remissions after chemotherapy appear to occur only in patients with metastases involving lymph nodes, soft tissue, or bone marrow.[57, 146, 156, 157]

Attention to histopathology is also exceptionally important in interpreting the published results of treatment with cytotoxic agents. More recent series have excluded patients with germ cell malignancies or possible neuroendocrine tumors. Several older series included many patients with *anaplastic* or *undifferentiated* neoplasms, which may explain why certain series[6, 21, 23, 160, 162, 170] report response rates that are inordinately high compared with the general experience (see "Notes" column in Table 102–7). Complete responses accounted for 31 to 60% of the observed responses. In two of these series,[57, 157] the median age of the patients was less than 40 years (two decades younger than the median age of all patients with the MUO syndrome), all patients had poorly differentiated or anaplastic neoplasms, and all complete remissions were seen in patients who did not have visceral or bony metastases. If investigators were careful to exclude anaplastic or undifferentiated carcinomas that ultimately were diagnosed as being lymphoma by use of immunohistochemistry, the response rates to chemotherapy and the survival times for all other patients were poor.

Hainsworth and colleagues[173] published an intriguing report showing a high response rate in all histopathologic subtypes and a wide variety of nonlymphatic sites, in contrast to most of the previous reports. Paclitaxel was combined in a regimen with carboplatin and oral etoposide. The response rates were 45% for 29 patients with adenocarcinoma and 48% for 21 patients with poorly differentiated adenocarcinoma or undifferentiated carcinoma. The complete response rate was about 12% for both histologic groups, 31% for patients with metastases to lymph nodes only, and 7% for patients with metastases to other sites. With a median duration of follow-up of 12 months, the actuarial median survival for the whole group was 13 months.

**Chemotherapy Overview.** Responsive subtypes of MUO are now identified. Response rates for the whole group of MUO patients no longer have meaning. Response rates must be defined relative to the anatomic distribution of metastasis (particularly separating patients with metastases to lymph nodes alone) and to the histologies involved (particularly separating undifferentiated or poorly differentiated subtypes), as determined by the appropriate use of immunohistochemical and ultrastructural techniques.

Few studies have analyzed critical patient factors, such as PS, and no studies have compared one form of treatment with no treatment. Consequently the significance of partial responses, stable disease, and survival time of responding patients is impossible to evaluate. Most studies report short durations of response and minimal impact on survival from the most enthusiastic proponents of combination therapy. The superiority of platinum-based treatments reported in selected subgroups cannot be applied to the whole spectrum of MUO.

Given the toxicity of cytotoxic agents and the notoriously poor response and survival rates of patients with the MUO syndrome (with the exception of those with the treatable forms of MUO, as discussed earlier), the real question is whether any antitumor therapy is better than none at all.

**Recommended Evaluation.** Because of the low frequency of detection of the primary site in patients with the MUO syndrome and because of the frequently misleading results of radiologic studies, x-ray or radionuclide studies are justified only in the presence of either specific abnormalities in the screening evaluation or possibilities suggested by review of the histopathology. The screening evaluation includes a complete history and physical examination, routine serum chemistry panel, urinalysis, stool for occult blood, and chest radiograph. Women with adenocarcinoma or undifferentiated carcinoma should undergo careful pelvic examination and probably mammography, although the latter has not proved helpful. Men with adenocarcinoma or undifferentiated carcinoma should be evaluated for prostate carcinoma and germ cell neoplasms. All patients with poorly differentiated neoplasms should be evaluated thoroughly for the possibility of lymphoma.

If this approach does not suggest a primary organ site, further evaluation is usually fruitless and not indicated. Even when the primary site can be determined, therapy is not likely to be effective. With the exception of the recognized treatable malignancies, documenting a primary site is probably more important to the patient (or physician) psychologically than therapeutically. Intellectual curiosity on the part of the physician is no justification for launching an aggressive search to locate a primary tumor when finding the primary site serves no useful purpose.

**Recommended Treatment.** Patients with metastases to sites other than peripheral lymph nodes, by definition, rarely have curable disease. Removal of primary tumors that have already disseminated is of no curative value; regression of metastases after removal of the primary tumor has been well publicized in anecdotal reports but has never been documented histologically. Surgery may be helpful in these patients for palliation of rapidly progressive symptoms of urinary or gastrointestinal tract obstructions or of other se-

lected problems of disseminated malignancy (such as solitary brain metastases). Radiation therapy may be important for the palliation of pain from bone lesions, osteolytic metastasis in weight-bearing regions, brain metastasis, superior vena caval obstruction, and perhaps spinal cord compression. The salient questions, however, relate to the role of chemotherapy in the management of these patients.

Treatment for patients with the MUO syndrome should be cautious, benevolent, and palliative. For patients who have clinicopathologic findings consistent with a responsive malignancy, appropriate treatment should be instituted accordingly. Combination chemotherapy should be strongly considered for women with peritoneal carcinomatosis, for patients with neuroendocrine carcinomas, and for patients with metastases that are distributed to peripheral lymph nodes, mediastinum, and retroperitoneum, but not to bone or viscera (other than lung, perhaps). For these patients, a cisplatin-based regimen is reasonable. If the Hainsworth report[173] is confirmed, the carboplatin-paclitaxel regimen can be used.

For other patients, chemotherapy is generally not recommended. Cytotoxic agents are usually ineffective for disseminated malignant melanomas and squamous cell carcinomas. For patients with adenocarcinomas or undifferentiated carcinomas who request therapy and who have a good performance status, 5-fluorouracil with leucovorin or doxorubicin with mitomycin C may be tried. For patients who request therapy and have a poor performance status, 5-fluorouracil alone or nontoxic drug dosages may be administered; although poor response rates should be expected, drug toxicities and costs are minimal, and treatment may provide psychological support for the patient, in that at least "something is being done."

## Summary and Conclusions

Figure 102–1 is a flow chart depicting the management of patients with the MUO syndrome based on the data and principles discussed in this chapter. The following points summarize these principles:

1. The MUO syndrome is common, accounting for 7% of all cancer patients.

2. The natural histories of these malignancies are aberrant in that metastatic patterns often differ from those expected when the primary site is evident at the time of presentation.

3. The histopathologic diagnosis should be established quickly with a biopsy specimen of a clinically evident metastasis by the least dangerous technique. For poorly differentiated neoplasms, definitive diagnosis requires adequate amounts of good tissue and integration of the clinical findings with light microscopy, immunohistochemical findings, and possibly ultrastructural features or molecular studies.

4. Searching for the primary site usually requires uncomfortable, expensive, unrewarding, and meddlesome procedures. The primary site is found in less than 15% of patients before death and frequently goes undiscovered at postmortem examination. Contrast radiographs are just as frequently misleading as they are helpful. Computed tomographic scanning of the abdomen as the only radiographic test appears to be cost-effective even though the diagnostic yield is small.

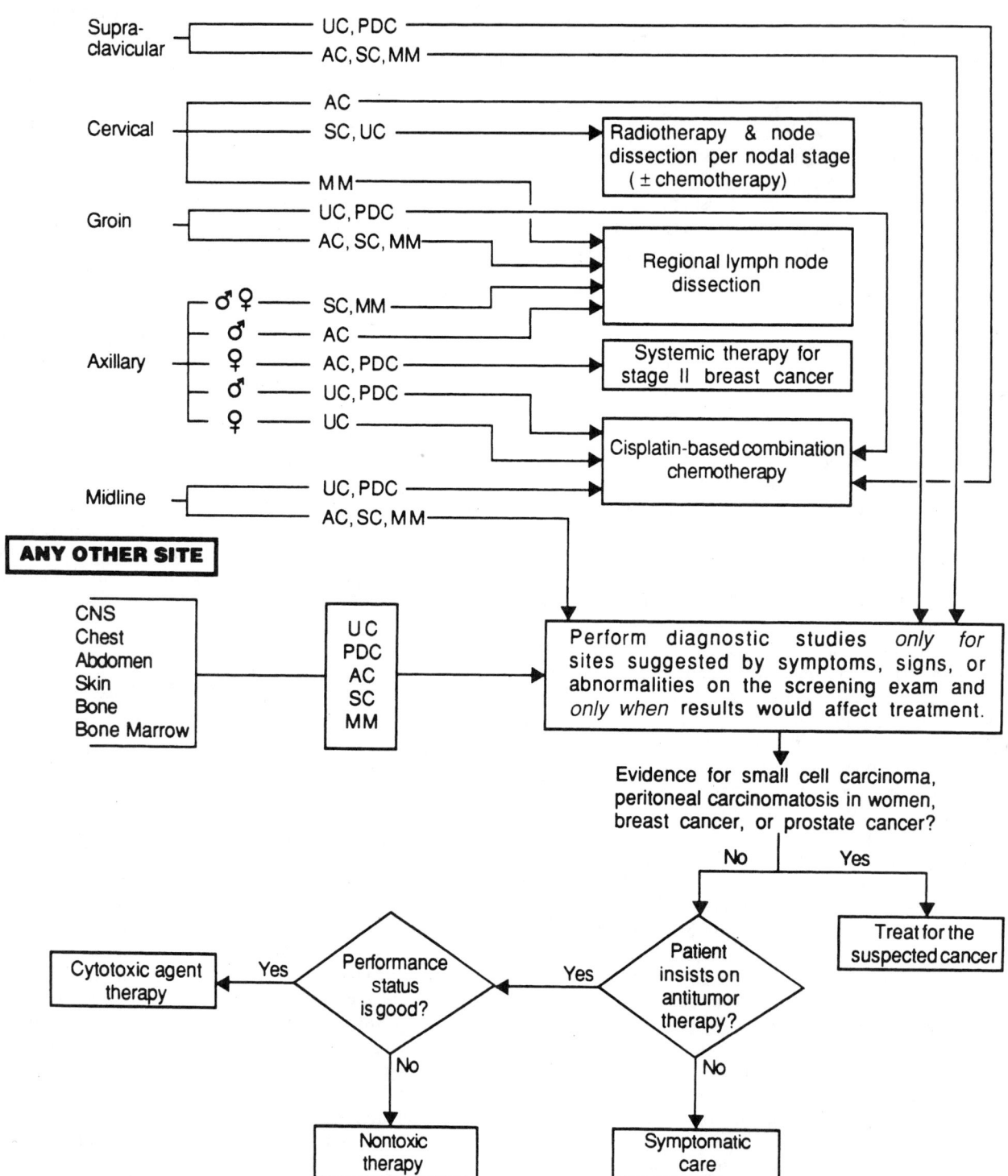

**Figure 102–1.** An approach to the treatment of patients with metastases of unknown origin. AC, adenocarcinoma; MM, malignant melanoma; PDC, poorly differentiated carcinoma; SC, squamous cell carcinoma; UC, undifferentiated carcinoma. (From Casciato DA. In: Casciato DA, Lowitz BB, eds. Manual of clinical oncology. 3rd ed. Boston: Little, Brown, 1995.)

5. Staging of asymptomatic sites with scans and radiographs in patients who have unresponsive malignancies is a dubious practice at best.

6. Prognosis depends on the involved site and is unaffected by whether or not the primary site is ever found.

7. For patients presenting with metastasis to peripheral lymph nodes, node dissection may be curative. The extent of the dissection depends on the nodal region involved and the histologic type of tumor.

8. For patients presenting with small cell malignancies, peritoneal carcinomatosis (in women), or poorly differentiated carcinomas involving external lymph nodes, mediastinum, or retroperitoneum, but without metastases to viscera or bone, objective long-term responses are possible with combination chemotherapy.

9. For all other patients, toxic therapies are recommended only for patients with good functional status, for palliation of symptoms when they develop, and for continuous support of the quality of life.

## SUGGESTIONS FOR ADDITIONAL READING

Abbruzzese JL, Abbruzzese MC, Lenzi R, et al. Analysis of a diagnostic strategy for patients with suspected tumors of unknown origin. J Clin Oncol 1995;13:2094–103. *Pathologic review is the most important test to identify tumors in patients with MUO that potentially have improved survival. Detailed and critical review of the biopsy specimen is more important than extensive and expensive radiologic investigations and the use of large panels of immunohistochemistry.*

Kemeny MM. Mastectomy: is it necessary for occult breast cancer? N Y State J Med 1992;92:516–7. *This article provides an eloquent discussion of the controversies in treating women with occult breast cancer (axillary nodal metastases with adenocarcinoma of unknown origin).*

Le Chevalier T, Cvitkovic E, Caille P, et al. Early metastatic cancer of unknown primary presentation: a clinical study of 302 consecutive autopsied patients. Arch Intern Med 1988;148:2035–9. *This landmark study of MUO patients shows the severe limitations of pathology and radiology in identifying correctly primary sites in patients with MUO. The original biopsy specimens and diagnostic study results were compared with the findings at postmortem examination.*

Pavlidis N, Kalef-Ezra J, Briassoulis E, et al. Evaluation of six tumor markers in patients with carcinoma of unknown primary. Med Pediatr Oncol 1994;22:162–7. *Patients with MUO have a nonspecific overexpression of several commonly used tumor markers. Routine use of these markers provides neither diagnostic nor prognostic assistance in patients with MUO.*

Van der Gaast A, Verwij J, Planting AS, et al. The value of immunohistochemistry in patients with poorly differentiated adenocarcinomas and undifferentiated carcinomas of unknown primary. Cancer Res Clin Oncol 1996;122:181–5. *This article offers a fine discussion of the contribution of immunohistochemical techniques to the identification of treatable, otherwise occult malignancies in patients with MUO and poorly characterized malignancies.*

## REFERENCES

1. Holmes FF, Fouts TL. Metastatic cancer of unknown primary site. Cancer 1970;26:816–20.
2. Le Chevalier T, Cvitkovic E, Caille P, et al. Early metastatic cancer of unknown primary origin at presentation: a clinical study of 302 consecutive autopsied patients. Arch Intern Med 1988;148:2035–9.
3. Stewart JF, Tattersall MH, Woods RL, Fox RM. Unknown primary adenocarcinoma: incidence of overinvestigation and natural history. Br Med J 1979;1:1530–3.
4. Gaber AO, Rice P, Eaton C, et al. Metastatic malignant disease of unknown origin. Am J Surg 1983;145:493–7.
5. Osteen RT, Kopf G, Wilson RE. In pursuit of the unknown primary. Am J Surg 1978;135:494–7.
6. Nystrom JS, Weiner JM, Wolf RM, et al. Identifying the primary site in metastatic cancer of unknown origin: inadequacy of roentgenographic procedures. JAMA 1979;241:381–3.
7. Lyman GH, Preisler HD. Carcinoma of unknown primary: natural history and response to therapy. J Med 1978;9:445–59.
8. Schildt RA, Kennedy PS, Chen TT, et al. Management of patients with metastatic adenocarcinoma of unknown origin. A Southwest Oncology Group study. Cancer Treat Rep 1983;67:77–9.
9. Jordan WE 3rd, Shildt RA. Adenocarcinoma of unknown primary site. The Brooke Army Medical Center experience. Cancer 1985;55:857–60.
10. Krementz ET, Cerise EJ, Foster DS, Morgan LR Jr. Metastases of undetermined source. Curr Probl Cancer 1979;4:4–37.
11. Maiche AG. Cancer of unknown primary: a retrospective study based on 109 patients. Am J Clin Oncol 1993;16:26–9.
12. Moertel CG, Reitemeier RJ, Schutt AJ, Hahn RG. Treatment of the patient with adenocarcinoma of unknown origin. Cancer 1972;30:1469–72.
13. Steckel RJ, Kagan AR. Diagnostic persistence in working up metastatic cancer with an unknown primary site. Radiology 1980;134:367–9.
14. Didolkar MS, Fanous N, Elias EG, Moore RH. Metastatic carcinomas from occult primary tumors: a study of 254 patients. Ann Surg 1977;186:625–30.
15. Abbruzzese JL, Abbruzzese MC, Hess KR, et al. Unknown primary carcinoma: natural history and prognostic factors in 657 consecutive patients. J Clin Oncol 1994;12:1272–80.
16. Abbruzzese JL, Abbruzzese MC, Lenzi R, et al. Analysis of a diagnostic strategy for patients with suspected tumors of unknown origin. J Clin Oncol 1995;13:2094–103.
17. Altman E, Cadman E. An analysis of 1539 patients with cancer of unknown primary site. Cancer 1986;57:120–4.
18. Schapira DV, Jarrett AR. The need to consider survival, outcome, and expense when evaluating and treating patients with unknown primary carcinoma. Arch Intern Med 1995;155:2050–4.
19. Mayordomo JI, Guerra JM, Guijarro C, et al. Neoplasms of unknown primary site: a clinicopathological study of autopsied patients. Tumori 1993;79:321–4.
20. Lenzi R, Hess KR, Abbruzzese MC, et al. Poorly differentiated carcinoma and poorly differentiated adenocarcinoma of unknown origin: favorable subsets of patients with unknown primary carcinoma? J Clin Oncol 1997;12:2056–66.
21. Woods RL, Fox RM, Tattersall MHN. Metastatic adenocarcinomas of unknown primary site: a randomized study of two combination chemotherapy regimens. N Engl J Med 1980;303:87.
22. van der Gaast A, Verweij J, Planting AS, et al. Simple prognostic model to predict survival in patients with undifferentiated carcinoma of unknown primary site. J Clin Oncol 1995;13:720–5.
23. Pasterz R, Savaraj N, Burgess M. Prognostic factors in metastatic carcinoma of unknown primary. J Clin Oncol 1986;4:1652–7.
24. Lee NK, Byers RM, Abbruzzese JL, Wolf P. Metastatic adenocarcinoma to the neck from an unknown primary source. Am J Surg 1991;162:306–9.
25. Nissenblatt MJ. The CUP syndrome (carcinoma unknown primary). Cancer Treat Rev 1981;8:211–24.
26. Bonnefoi H, Smith IE. How should cancer presenting as a malignant pleural effusion be managed? Br J Cancer 1996;74:832–5.
27. Nystrom JS, Weiner JM, Heffelfinger-Juttner J, et al. Metastatic and histologic presentations in unknown primary cancer. Semin Oncol 1977;4:53–8.
28. Ringenberg QS, Doll DC, Loy TS, Yarbro JW. Malignant ascites of unknown origin. Cancer 1989;64:753–5.
29. van de Pol M, van Aalst VC, Wilmink JT, Twijnstra A. Brain metastases from an unknown primary tumour: which diagnostic procedures are indicated? J Neurol Neurosurg Psychiatry 1996;61:321–3.
30. Zimm S, Wampler GL, Stablein D, et al. Intracerebral metastases in solid-tumor patients: natural history and results of treatment. Cancer 1981;48:384–94.
31. Debevec M. Management of patients with brain metastases of unknown origin. Neoplasma 1990;37:601–6.
32. Ebels EJ, van der Meulen JD. Cerebral metastasis without known primary tumour: a retrospective study. Clin Neurol Neurosurg 1978;80:195–7.
33. Chee CP. Brain metastasis of unknown origin. Singapore Med J 1990;31:48–50.

34. Eapen L, Vachet M, Catton G, et al. Brain metastases with an unknown primary: a clinical perspective. J Neurooncol 1988;6:31–5.

35. Khansur T, Routh A, Hickman B. Brain metastases from unknown primary site. J Miss State Med Assoc 1997;38:238–42.

36. Doll DC, Ringenberg QS, Bickel JT, Yarbro JW. Epidural spinal cord compression as the presenting manifestation of tumor of unknown origin. Med Pediatr Oncol 1990;18:280–2.

37. Saengnipanthkul S, Jirarattanaphochai K, Rojviroj S, et al. Metastatic adenocarcinoma of the spine. Spine 1992;17:427–30.

38. Anner RM, Drewinko B. Frequency and significance of bone marrow involvement by metastatic solid tumors. Cancer 1977;39:1337–44.

39. Barón MG, de la Gándara I, Espinosa E, et al. Bone metastases as the first manifestation of a tumour. Int Orthop 1991;15:373–6.

40. Simon MA, Bartucci EJ. The search for the primary tumor in patients with skeletal metastases of unknown origin. Cancer 1986;58:1088–95.

41. Rougraff BT, Kneisl JS, Simon MA. Skeletal metastases of unknown origin: a prospective diagnostic strategy. J Bone Joint Surg Am 1993;75:1276–81.

42. Cohen Y, Gershoni-Baruch R, Lichtic C. Bone marrow biopsy in patients with malignant neoplasms other than lymphomas or leukemia. Acta Haematol 1979;62:181–4.

43. Suprun H, Rywlin AM. Metastatic carcinoma in histologic sections of aspirated bone marrow: a comparative autopsy study. South Med J 1976;69:438–9.

44. Brochamer WL Jr, Keeling MM. The bone marrow biopsy, osteoscan, and peripheral blood in non-hematopoietic cancer. Cancer 1977;40:836–40.

45. Ringenberg QS, Doll DC, Yarbro JW, Perry MC. Tumors of unknown origin in the bone marrow. Arch Intern Med 1986;146:2027–8.

46. Frost P, Levin B. Clinical implications of metastatic process. Lancet 1992;339:1458–61.

47. Frost P. Unknown primary tumors: an example of accelerated (type 2) tumor progression. Basic Life Sci 1991;57:233–7.

48. Bell CW, Pathak S, Frost P. Unknown primary tumors: establishment of cell lines, identification of chromosomal abnormalities, and implications for a second type of tumor progression. Cancer Res 1989;49:4311–5.

49. Abbruzzese JL, Lenzi R, Raber MN, et al. The biology of unknown primary tumors. Semin Oncol 1993;20:238–43.

50. Bar-Eli M, Abbruzzese JL, Lee-Jackson D, Frost P. p53 gene mutation spectrum in human unknown primary tumors. Anticancer Res 1993;1619–23.

51. Hillen HF, Hak LE, Joosten-Achjanie SR, Arends JW. Microvessel density in unknown primary tumors. Int J Cancer 1997;74:81–5.

52. Pavlidis N, Briassoulis E, Bai M, et al. Overexpression of C-myc, Ras and C-erbB2 oncoproteins in carcinoma of unknown primary origin. Anticancer Res 1995;15:2563–7.

53. Farag SS, Green MD, Morstyn G, et al. Delay by internists in obtaining diagnostic biopsies in patients with suspected cancer. Ann Intern Med 1992;116:473–8.

54. Kern WH, Abbott M. The determination of unknown primary sites based upon the histologic appearance of metastases. Surg Gynecol Obstet 1980;151:73–6.

55. Sheahan K, Abramowitz A, Carlson JA, et al. Accuracy of pathologic evaluation of metastatic adenocarcinomas of unknown primary sites: an analysis using a computerized image storing system. Lab Invest 1990;62:112A.

56. Sheahan K, O'Keane JC, Abramowitz A, et al. Metastatic adenocarcinoma of an unknown primary site: a comparison of the relative contributions of morphology, minimal essential clinical data and CEA immunostaining status. Am J Clin Pathol 1993;99:729–35.

57. Hainsworth JD, Johnson DH, Greco FA. Cisplatin-based combination chemotherapy in the treatment of poorly differentiated carcinoma and poorly differentiated adenocarcinoma of unknown primary site: results of a 12-year experience. J Clin Oncol 1992;10:912–22.

58. Nappi O, Mills SE, Swanson PE, Wick MR. Clear cell tumors of unknown nature and origin: a systematic approach to diagnosis. Semin Diagn Pathol 1997;14:164–74.

59. Velez A, Walsh D, Karakousis CP. Treatment of unknown primary melanoma. Cancer 1991;68:2579–81.

60. Gaynor R, Herschman HR, Irie R, et al. S100 protein: a marker for human malignant melanomas? Lancet 1981;1:869–71.

61. Mottolese M, Venturo I, Benevolo M, et al. Immunocytochemical diagnosis of amelanotic metastatic melanoma using monoclonal antibodies HMB-45 and Epl-3. Melanoma Res 1994;4:53–8.

62. Gamble AR, Bell JA, Ronan JE, et al. Use of tumour marker immunoreactivity to identify primary site of metastatic cancer. Br Med J 1993;306:295–8.

63. Hainsworth JD, Wright EP, Johnson DH, et al. Poorly differentiated carcinoma of unknown primary site: clinical usefulness of immunoperoxidase staining. J Clin Oncol 1991;9:1931–8.

64. van der Gaast A, Verwij J, Planting AS, et al. The value of immunohistochemistry in patients with poorly differentiated adenocarcinomas and undifferentiated carcinomas of unknown primary. J Cancer Res Clin Oncol 1996;122:181–5.

65. Gatter KC, Alcock C, Heryet A, Mason DY. Clinical importance of analysing malignant tumours of uncertain origin with immunohistological techniques. Lancet 1985;1:1302–5.

66. Freeman NJ, Doolittle C. Elevated prostate markers in metastatic small cell carcinoma of unknown primary. Cancer 1991;68:1118–20.

67. van Krieken JH. Prostate marker immunoreactivity in salivary gland neoplasms: a rare pitfall in immunohistochemistry. Am J Surg Pathol 1993;17:410–4.

68. Lagendijk JH, Mullink H, Van Diest PJ, et al. Tracing the origin of adenocarcinomas with unknown primary using immunohistochemistry: differential diagnosis between colonic and ovarian carcinomas as primary sites. Hum Pathol 1998;29:491–7.

69. Brown RW, Campagna LB, Dunn JK, Cagle PT. Immunohistochemical identification of tumor markers in metastatic adenocarcinoma: a diagnostic adjunct in the determination of primary site. Am J Clin Pathol 1997;107:12–9.

70. Dvorak AM, Monahan RA. Metastatic adenocarcinoma of unknown primary site: diagnostic electron microscopy to determine the site of tumor origin. Arch Pathol Lab Med 1982;106:21–4.

71. Baron PL, Moore MP, Kinne DW, et al. Occult breast cancer presenting with axillary metastases: updated management. Arch Surg 1990;125:210–4.

72. Goldberg RM, Smith FP, Ueno W, et al. 5-Fluorouracil, Adriamycin, and mitomycin in the treatment of adenocarcinoma of unknown primary. J Clin Oncol 1986;4:395–9.

73. Lleander VC, Goldstein G, Horsley JS 2d. Chemotherapy in the management of metastatic cancer of unknown primary site. Oncology 1972;26:265–70.

74. Steck WD, Helwig EB. Tumors of the umbilicus. Cancer 1965;18:907–15.

75. Clary CF, Michel RP, Wang NS, Hanson RE. Metastatic carcinoma: the lung as the site for the clinically undiagnosed primary. Cancer 1983;51:362–6.

76. Valentine I, Rosenthal S, Arseneau JC. Combination chemotherapy for adenocarcinoma of unknown primary origin. Cancer Clin Trials 1979;2:265.

77. Hamilton CS, Langlands AO. ACUPS (adenocarcinoma of unknown primary site): a clinical and cost benefit analysis. Int J Radiat Oncol Biol Phys 1987;13:1497–503.

78. Görich J, Beyer-Enke SA, Müller M, et al. [The value of computed tomography in the search for an unknown primary tumor.] Rofo Fortschr Geb Rontgenstr Nuklearmed 1988;149:277–9.

79. Pavlidis N, Kalef-Ezra J, Briassoulis E, et al. Evaluation of six tumor markers in patients with carcinoma of unknown primary. Med Pediatr Oncol 1994;22:162–7.

80. Farrugia DC, Norman AR, Nicolson MC, et al. Unknown primary carcinoma: randomised studies are needed to identify optimal treatments and their benefits. Eur J Cancer 1996;32A:2256–61.

81. Cooper JF. The radioimmunochemical measurement of prostatic acid phosphatase: current state of the art. Urol Clin North Am 1980;7:653–65.

82. Currow DC, Findlay M, Cox K, Harnett PR. Elevated germ cell markers in carcinoma of uncertain primary site do not predict response to platinum based chemotherapy. Eur J Cancer 1996;32A:2357–9.

83. Rosen PP. Occult carcinoma presenting with axillary lymph node metastases. 12th Annual International Breast Cancer Conference, Miami, Fla., March 16–18, 1995. abstract.

84. Milton GW, Shaw HM, McCarthy WH. Occult primary malignant melanoma: factors influencing survival. Br J Surg 1977;64:805–8.

85. Chang P, Knapper WH. Metastatic melanoma of unknown primary. Cancer 1982;49:1106–11.

86. Giuliano AE, Moseley HS, Morton DL. Clinical aspects of unknown primary melanoma. Ann Surg 1980;191:98–104.

87. Schlagenhauff B, Stroebel W, Ellwanger U, et al. Metastatic melanoma of unknown primary origin shows prognostic similarities to regional

metastatic melanoma: recommendations for initial staging examinations. Cancer 1997;80:60–5.

88. Anbari KK, Schuchter LM, Bucky LP, et al. Melanoma of unknown primary site: presentation, treatment, and prognosis—a single institution study. University of Pennsylvania Pigmented Lesion Study Group. Cancer 1997;79:1816–21.

89. Jonk A, Kroon BB, Rümke P, et al. Lymph node metastasis from melanoma with an unknown primary site. Br J Surg 1990;77:665–8.

90. Nasri S, Namazie A, Dulguerov P, Mickel R. Malignant melanoma of cervical and parotid lymph nodes with an unknown primary site. Laryngoscope 1994;104:1194–8.

91. Akslen LA, Hartveit F. Metastatic melanoma of unknown origin at autopsy. Eur J Surg Oncol 1988;14:379–82.

92. Balm AJ, Kroon BB, Hilgers FJ, et al. Lymph node metastases in the neck and parotid gland from an unknown primary melanoma. Clin Otolaryngol 1994;19:161–5.

93. Lapeyre M, Malissard L, Peiffert D, et al. Cervical lymph node metastasis from an unknown primary: is tonsillectomy necessary? Int J Radiat Oncol Biol Phys 1997;39:291–6.

94. Weir L, Keane T, Cummings B, et al. Radiation treatment of cervical lymph node metastases from an unknown primary: an analysis of outcome by treatment volume and other prognostic factors. Radiother Oncol 1995;35:206–11.

95. van den Brekel MW, Castelijns JA, Stel HV, et al. Occult metastatic neck disease: detection with US and US-guided fine-needle aspiration cytology [published erratum appears in Radiology 1992;182:288]. Radiology 1991;180:457–61.

96. Birchall MA, Stafford ND, Walsh-Waring GP. Malignant neck lumps: a measured approach. Ann R Coll Surg Engl 1991;73:91–5.

97. Mukherji SK, Drane WE, Mancuso AA, et al. Occult primary tumors of the head and neck: detection with 2-[F-18]-fluoro-2-deoxy-D-glucose SPECT. Radiology 1996;199:761–6.

98. Keyes JW Jr, Watson NE Jr, Williams DW 3rd, et al. PDG PET in head and neck cancer. AJR Am J Roentgenol 1997;169:1663–9.

99. Kole AC, Nieweg OE, Pruim J, et al. Detection of unknown occult primary tumors using positron emission tomography. Cancer 1998;82:1160–6.

100. Marcial-Vega VA, Cardenes H, Perez CA, et al. Cervical metastases from unknown primaries: radiotherapeutic management and appearance of subsequent primaries. Int J Radiat Oncol Biol Phys 1990;19:919–28.

101. Coker DD, Casterline PF, Chambers RG, Jaques DA. Metastases to lymph nodes of the head and neck from an unknown primary site. Am J Surg 1977;134:517–22.

102. Wang RC, Goepfert H, Barber AE, Wolf P. Unknown primary squamous cell carcinoma metastatic to the neck. Arch Otolaryngol Head Neck Surg 1990;116:1388–93.

103. Coster JR, Foote RL, Olsen KD, et al. Cervical nodal metastasis of squamous cell carcinoma of unknown origin: indications for withholding radiation therapy. Int J Radiat Oncol Biol Phys 1992;23:743–9.

104. Jesse RH, Perez CA, Fletcher GH. Cervical lymph node metastasis: unknown primary cancer. Cancer 1973;31:854–9.

105. Nguyen C, Shenouda G, Black MJ, et al. Metastatic squamous cell carcinoma to cervical lymph nodes from unknown primary mucosal sites. Head Neck 1994;16:58–63.

106. Glynne-Jones RG, Anand AK, Young TE, Berry RJ. Metastatic carcinoma in the cervical lymph nodes from an occult primary: a conservative approach to the role of radiotherapy. Int J Radiat Oncol Biol Phys 1990;18:289–94.

107. Bataini JP, Rodriguez J, Jaulerry C, et al. Treatment of metastatic neck nodes secondary to an occult epidermoid carcinoma of the head and neck. Laryngoscope 1987;97:1080–4.

108. Glynne-Jones RG, Anand AK, Young TE, Berry RJ. Metastatic adenocarcinoma in the cervical lymph nodes from an occult primary. Clin Oncol (R Coll Radiol) 1989;1:19–21.

109. Lefebvre JL, Coche-Dequeant B, Van JT, et al. Cervical lymph nodes from an unknown primary tumor in 190 patients. Am J Surg 1990;160:443–6.

110. Nordstrom DG, Tewfik HH, Latourette HB. Cervical lymph node metastases from an unknown primary. Int J Radiat Oncol Biol Phys 1979;5:73–6.

111. Yang ZY, Hu YH, Yan JH. Lymph node metastases in the neck from an unknown primary: report on 113 patients. Acta Radiol Oncol 1983;22:17–22.

112. Davidson BJ, Spiro RH, Patel S, et al. Cervical metastases of occult origin: the impact of combined modality therapy. Am J Surg 1994;168:395–9.

113. Sinnathamby K, Peters LJ, Laidlaw C, Hughes PG. The occult head and neck primary: to treat or not to treat? Clin Oncol (R Coll Radiol) 1997;9:322–9.

114. Reddy SP, Marks JE. Metastatic carcinoma in the cervical lymph nodes from an unknown primary site: results of bilateral neck plus mucosal irradiation vs ipsilateral neck irradiation. Int J Radiat Oncol Biol Phys 1997;37:797–802.

115. Talmi YP, Wolf GT, Hazuka M, Krause CJ. Unknown primary of the head and neck. J Laryngol Otol 1996;110:353–6.

116. Jakobsen J, Aschenfeldt P, Johansen J, Jørgensen K. Lymph node metastases in the neck from unknown primary tumour. Acta Oncol 1992;31:653–5.

117. Oen AL, de Boer MF, Hop WC, Knegt P. Cervical metastasis from unknown primary tumor. Eur Arch Otorhinolaryngol 1995;252:222–8.

118. Medini E, Medini AM, Lee CK, et al. The management of metastatic squamous cell carcinoma in cervical lymph nodes from an unknown primary. Am J Clin Oncol 1998;21:121–5.

119. Maulard C, Housset M, Brunel P, et al. Postoperative radiation therapy for cervical lymph node metastases from an occult squamous cell carcinoma. Laryngoscope 1992;102:884–90.

120. McCunniff AJ, Raben M. Metastatic carcinoma of the neck from an unknown primary. Int J Radiat Oncol Biol Phys 1986;12:1849–52.

121. de Braud F, Heilbrun LK, Ahmed K, et al. Metastatic squamous cell carcinoma of an unknown primary localized to the neck: advantages of an aggressive treatment. Cancer 1989;64:510–5.

122. Jeremic B, Zivic DJ, Matovic M, Marinkovic J. Cisplatin and 5-fluorouracil as induction chemotherapy followed by radiation therapy in metastatic squamous cell carcinoma of an unknown primary tumor localized to the neck: a phase II study. J Chemother 1993;5:262–5.

123. Pierce EH, Gray HK, Dockerty MB. Surgical significance of isolated axillary adenopathy. Ann Surg 1957;145:104–7.

124. Copeland EM, McBride CM. Axillary metastases from unknown primary sites. Ann Surg 1973;178:25–7.

125. Feigenberg Z, Zer M, Dintsman M. Axillary metastases from an unknown primary source. Isr J Med Sci 1976;12:1153–8.

126. Westbrook KC, Gallager HS. Breast carcinoma presenting as an axillary mass. Am J Surg 1971;122:607–11.

127. Jackson B, Scott-Conner C, Moulder J. Axillary metastasis from occult breast carcinoma: diagnosis and management. Am Surg 1995;61:431–4.

128. van Ooijen B, Bontenbal M, Henzen-Logmans SC, Koper PC. Axillary nodal metastases from an occult primary consistent with breast carcinoma. Br J Surg 1993;80:1299–300.

129. Kemeny MM. Mastectomy: is it necessary for occult breast cancer? N Y State J Med 1992;92:516–7.

130. Feuerman L, Attie JN, Rosenberg B. Carcinoma in axillary lymph nodes as an indicator of breast cancer. Surg Gynecol Obstet 1962;114:5–8.

131. Tilanus-Linthorst MM, Obdeijn AI, Bontenbal M, Oudkerk M. MRI in patients with axillary metastases of occult breast cancer. Breast Cancer Res Treat 1997;44:179–82.

132. Halstead WS. The results of radical operations for the cure of cancer of the breast. Ann Surg 1907;46:1–19.

133. Campana F, Fourquet A, Ashby MA, et al. Presentation of axillary lymphadenopathy without detectable breast primary (T0 N1b breast cancer): experience at Institut Curie. Radiother Oncol 1989;15:321–5.

134. Ellerbroek N, Holmes F, Singletary E, et al. Treatment of patients with isolated axillary nodal metastases from an occult primary carcinoma consistent with breast origin. Cancer 1990;66:1461–7.

135. Whillis D, Brown PW, Rodger A. Adenocarcinoma from an unknown primary presenting in women with an axillary mass. Clin Oncol (R Coll Radiol) 1990;2:189–92.

136. Kemeny MM, Rivera DE, Terz JJ, Benfield JR. Occult primary adenocarcinoma with axillary metastases. Am J Surg 1986;152:43–7.

137. Fortunato L, Sorrento JJ, Golub RA, Cantu R. Occult breast cancer: a case report and review of the literature. N Y State J Med 1992;92:555–7.

138. Zaren HA, Copeland EM III. Inguinal node metastases. Cancer 1978;41:919–23.

139. Albers CA, Johnson RH Jr, Mansberger AR Jr. The management of patients with metastatic cancer from an unknown primary site. Am Surg 1981;47:162–6.

140. Guarischi A, Keane TJ, Elhakim T. Metastatic inguinal nodes from

an unknown primary neoplasm: a review of 56 cases. Cancer 1987;59:572–7.

141. Nicholson CP, Donohue JH, Thompson GB, Lewis JE. A study of metastatic cancer found during inguinal hernia repair. Cancer 1992;69:3008–11.

142. Remick SC, Ruckdeschel JC. Extrapulmonary and pulmonary small-cell carcinoma: tumor biology, therapy, and outcome. Med Pediatr Oncol 1992;20:89–99.

143. Moertel CG, Kvols LK, O'Connell MJ, Rubin J. Treatment of neuro-endocrine carcinomas with combined etoposide and cisplatin: evidence of major therapeutic activity in the anaplastic variants of these neoplasms. Cancer 1991;68:227–32.

144. Van Der Gaast A, Verwey J, Prins E, Splinter TA. Chemotherapy as treatment of choice in extrapulmonary undifferentiated small cell carcinomas. Cancer 1990;65:422–4.

145. Zhou J, Iwasa Y, Konishi I, et al. Papillary serous carcinoma of the peritoneum in women: a clinicopathologic and immunohistochemical study. Cancer 1995;76:429–36.

146. Pavlidis N, Kosmidis P, Skarlos D, et al. Subsets of tumors responsive to cisplatin or carboplatin combinations in patients with carcinoma of unknown primary site. Ann Oncol 1992;3:631.

147. Ransom DT, Patel SR, Keeney GL, et al. Papillary serous carcinoma of the peritoneum: a review of 33 cases treated with platin-based chemotherapy. Cancer 1990;66:1091–4.

148. Strnad CM, Grosh WW, Baxter J, et al. Peritoneal carcinomatosis of unknown primary site in women: a distinctive subset of adenocarcinoma. Ann Intern Med 1989;111:213–7.

149. Lele SB, Piver MS, Matharu J, Tsukada Y. Peritoneal papillary carcinoma. Gynecol Oncol 1988;31:315–20.

150. Fromm GL, Gershenson DM, Silva EG. Papillary serous carcinoma of the peritoneum. Obstet Gynecol 1990;75:89–95.

151. Dalrymple JC, Bannatyne P, Russell P, et al. Extraovarian peritoneal serous papillary carcinoma: a clinicopathologic study of 31 cases. Cancer 1989;64:110–5.

152. Richardson RL, Schoumacher RA, Fer MF, et al. The unrecognized extragonadal germ cell cancer syndrome. Ann Intern Med 1981; 94:181–6.

153. Greco FA, Thomas M, Hainsworth JD. Poorly differentiated carcinoma (PDC) or adenocarcinoma (PDA) of unknown primary site: Long-term follow-up after cisplatin-based chemotherapy. Proc ASCO 1997;16:A974. abstract.

154. Motzer RJ, Rodriguez E, Reuter VE, et al. Molecular and cytogenetic studies in the diagnosis of patients with poorly differentiated carcinomas of unknown primary site. J Clin Oncol 1995;13:274–82.

155. Falkson CI, Cohen GL. Mitomycin C, epirubicin and cisplatin versus mitomycin C alone as therapy for carcinoma of unknown primary origin. Oncology 1998;55:116–21.

156. Anderson H, Thatcher N, Rankin E, et al. VAC (vincristine, Adriamycin, cyclophosphamide) chemotherapy for metastatic carcinoma from an unknown primary site. Eur J Cancer Clin Oncol 1983;19:49.

157. Walach N, Horn Y. Combination chemotherapy in the treatment of adenocarcinoma of unknown primary origin. Cancer Treat Rep 1987;71:605.

158. Fiore JJ, Kelsen DP, Gralla RJ, et al. Adenocarcinoma of unknown primary origin: treatment with vindesine and doxorubicin. Cancer Treat Rep 1985;69:591.

159. van der Gaast A, Verweij J, Planting AS, Stoter G. 5-Fluorouracil, doxorubicin and mitomycin C (FAM) combination chemotherapy for metastatic adenocarcinoma of unknown primary. Eur J Cancer Clin Oncol 1988;24:765.

160. Sulkes A, Uziely B, Isacson R, et al. Combination chemotherapy in metastatic tumors of unknown origin. Isr J Med Sci 1988;24:604.

161. Eagan RT, Therneau TM, Rubin J, et al. Lack of value for cisplatin added to mitomycin-doxorubicin combination chemotherapy for carcinoma of unknown primary site. Am J Clin Oncol 1987;10:82.

162. Milliken ST, Tattersall MHN, Woods RL, et al. Metastatic adenocarcinoma of unknown primary site: a randomized study of two combination regimens. Eur J Cancer Clin Oncol 1987;23:1645.

163. Kelsen D, Martin DS, Colofiore J, et al. A phase II trial of biochemical modulation using N-phosphonacetyl-L-aspartate, high-dose methotrexate, high-dose 5-fluorouracil, and leucovorin in patients with adenocarcinoma of unknown primary site. Cancer 1992;70:1988.

164. Nole F, Colleoni M, Buzzoni R, Bajetta E. Fluorouracil plus folinic acid in metastatic adenocarcinoma of unknown primary site suggestive of a gastrointestinal primary. Tumori 1993;79:116–8.

165. Rigg A, Cunningham D, Gore M, et al. A phase I/II study of leucovorin, carboplatin and 5-fluorouracil (LCF) in patients with carcinoma of unknown primary site or advanced esophagogastric/pancreatic adenocarcinomas. Br J Cancer 1997;75:101–5.

166. Bedikian AY, Bodey GP, Valdivieso M, Burgess MA. Sequential chemotherapy for adenocarcinoma of unknown primary. Am J Clin Oncol 1983;6:219.

167. de Campos ES, Menasce LP, Radford J, et al. Metastatic carcinoma of uncertain primary site: a retrospective review of 57 patients treated with vincristine, doxorubicin, cyclophosphamide (VAC) or VAC alternating with cisplatin and etoposide. Cancer 1994;73:470–5.

168. al-Idrissi HY. Combined 5-fluorouracil, Adriamycin and mitomycin C in the management of adenocarcinoma metastasizing to the liver from an unknown primary site. J Intern Med Res 1990;18:425.

169. Kambhu SA, Kelsen DP, Fiore J, et al. Metastatic adenocarcinomas of unknown primary site: prognostic variables and treatment results. Am J Clin Oncol 1990;13:55.

170. Raber MN, Faintuch J, Abbruzzese JL. Continuous infusion 5-fluorouracil, etoposide and cis-diamminedichloroplatinum in patients with metastatic carcinoma of unknown primary origin. Ann Oncol 1991;2:519.

171. Wagener DJ, de Mulder PH, Burghouts JT, Croles JJ. Phase II trial of cisplatin for adenocarcinoma of unknown primary site. IKZ/IKO Clinical Research Group. Eur J Cancer 1991;27:755–7.

172. Gill I, Guaglianone P, Grunberg SM, et al. High dose intensity of cisplatin and etoposide in adenocarcinoma of unknown primary. Anticancer Res 1991;11:1231.

173. Hainsworth JD, Erland JB, Kalman LA, et al. Carcinoma of unknown primary site: treatment with 1-hour paclitaxel, carboplatin, and extended schedule etoposide. J Clin Oncol 1997;15:2385–93.

# CHAPTER 103

# MALIGNANT EFFUSIONS

• DONNA L. WALKER • DENNIS A. CASCIATO

## Malignant Pleural Effusions

Malignancy accounts for 25 to 50% of pleural effusions in adults and is the most common cause of exudative pleural effusions in patients older than 60 years. Virtually all malignancies, except primary brain tumors, can result in the accumulation of fluid in the pleural cavity. Pleural effusions are most commonly caused by the following malignancies: lung cancer (approximately 35% of cases), breast cancer (25%), lymphoma (10%), and adenocarcinoma of unknown primary site (10%); all other cancers compose the remaining 20% of cases.[1–3] Lymphoma is the most common cause of chylothorax.[3] Approximately 100,000 new cases of malignant pleural effusion are diagnosed annually in the United States.

## PATHOGENESIS

The pleural space is a potential compartment defined by the visceral pleura, which covers the lungs, and the parietal pleura, which lines the chest wall, the diaphragm, and the mediastinum. The pleural membranes are composed of a single layer of mesothelial cells, blood vessels, lymphatics, and connective tissue. In normal individuals, it is estimated that up to 10 L of fluid is produced each day, with the majority being reabsorbed so that this space contains 5 to 40 ml of fluid at any one time.[2]

The secretion and reabsorption of pleural fluid are governed in part by the same Starling's forces that influence the movement of fluid from intravascular to interstitial compartments.[4] Imbalances in the rates of secretion and reabsorption lead to the formation of pleural effusions. Increases in secretion may be caused by increased capillary hydrostatic pressure (e.g., congestive heart failure) or by decreases in capillary oncotic pressure (e.g., hypoalbuminemia). Increases in negative pleural pressure from atelectasis and increased pleural fluid oncotic pressures from necrotic material shed by the pleura also result in excess fluid in the pleural space.

The most important factors in the formation of malignant pleural effusions appear to be increased capillary permeability from tumor-induced pleural inflammation and obstruction of lymphatic channels.[5] Lymphatic openings (stomas) located between the mesothelial cells in the parietal pleura drain approximately 90% of the pleural fluid, primarily to mediastinal lymph nodes.[3] The development of pleural effusion is directly related to carcinomatous infiltration of these lymph nodes and is not related to the extent of pleural involvement by metastases.[6]

## DIAGNOSIS

**Signs and Symptoms.** Patients with pleural effusions commonly present with dyspnea, cough, or chest pain. Less than 25% of patients are asymptomatic at the time of diagnosis.[6] Dullness to percussion, decreased breath sounds, and reduced tactile fremitus are the typical signs. It is thought that the physical examination can detect effusions of about 500 ml.[1]

**Radiology.** Posteroanterior and lateral chest films may detect effusions as small as 200 ml,[7] whereas lateral decubitus films may detect effusions greater than 100 ml.[8, 9] Ultrasonography can identify effusion pockets containing as little as 3 to 5 ml and has a sensitivity of 89.2% and a specificity of 100% in detecting pleural effusions.[10] Computed tomography (CT) performed to delineate abnormalities seen on chest films often reveals clinically unsuspected pleural effusions. Magnetic resonance imaging (MRI) has a limited role in the evaluation of the pleura but does provide the ability to image the thorax in the axial, sagittal, and coronal planes. Studies are currently ongoing to determine if the use of triple-echocardiographic pulse sequencing MRI can differentiate transudates from exudates.[11]

**Thoracentesis.** Pleural fluid should be sampled in patients with suspected malignant or infectious pleural effusions. If the effusion is small or loculated, thoracentesis should be performed with ultrasonographic or CT guidance. The fluid should be routinely evaluated with cytologic studies, and staining and cultures for pyogenic bacteria, mycobacteria, and fungi. The pH, specific gravity, leukocyte and erythrocyte counts, and glucose, protein, and lactate dehydrogenase (LDH) concentrations should be determined. The characteristics of pleural fluid in common disorders are listed in Table 103–1.

The separation of effusions into transudates and exudates may suggest the cause. A malignant effusion is more likely, but not necessarily, an exudate. Approximately 5% of malignant pleural effusions are transudates.[6] Light's criteria and their modifications are often used to determine if a pleural effusion is exudative. Pleural effusions are considered to be exudates rather than transudates if the pleural LDH level is greater than two thirds of the upper limit of normal for the serum value, if the ratio of pleural LDH to serum LDH is greater than 0.6, or if the ratio of pleural fluid protein to serum protein is greater than 0.5. Other criteria commonly used to define exudates include a pleural protein concentration greater than 3 g/dl, a pleural fluid to serum albumin gradient of at least 1.2 g/dl, a pleural to serum bilirubin ratio of greater than 0.6, and a pleural to serum cholesterol ratio of greater than 0.3.[12]

The total leukocyte count in malignant pleural effusions varies widely and is usually composed predominantly of lymphocytes. A low pleural pH (<7.3) may be associated with empyema or malignant effusions. When associated with empyema, a pleural fluid pH of less than 7.2 may indicate the need for prompt, aggressive drainage procedures. A low glucose concentration (<60 mg/dl or a pleural to serum glucose ratio <0.5) may have prognostic and therapeutic significance in malignant effusions but may also be found in tuberculous and collagen vascular effusions.[1, 13] Amylase may be elevated in 10% of malignant pleural effusions but can be misleading and may not warrant routine determination.[12, 13] High pleural fluid amylase concentrations are also associated with pancreatitis, pancreatic carcinoma, and esophageal rupture.[13]

True chylous effusions have high levels of chylomicrons and triglycerides. Chemical analysis of the lipid content in milky pleural fluids is necessary to prove that the effusion is chylous because it may be pseudochylous (high cholesterol concentration) or chyliform (rich in degenerated cells and debris). Milky fluid should also be stained with Sudan III to demonstrate the presence of fat microscopically.[7]

The concentration of tumor markers has been evaluated for their ability to signify that a pleural effusion is malignant. To date no ideal marker or combination of markers has proved useful. Elevated pleural fluid carcinoembryonic antigen (CEA) levels may be seen with both malignant and benign effusions. The latter has been associated with CEA levels as high as 20 to 30 ng/ml.[14, 15] CA-125 may be produced by benign mesothelial cells and has no value in differentiating benign from malignant effusions.[16] CA 27.29 (also known as CA 15.3) assay in effusions neither enhances the sensitivity of cytologic diagnosis nor predicts a breast cancer primary lesion.[18]

Concentrations of acid mucopolysaccharide, hyaluronic acid, haptoglobin, complement factors C3 and C4, $\alpha_1$-antitrypsin, ferritin, the GLUT1 glucose transporter, and many other substances have been tested for their ability to predict a malignant cause of effusion. Although some small studies look promising for the predictive value of very high ferritin

*Table 103–1.* **Pleural Effusion Characteristics**

| Etiology | Appearance | Cytology | Cell Count* | Glucose Ratio (Effusion/Serum) | Lactate Dehydrogenase Ratio (Effusion/Serum) | pH | Protein (g/dl) | Specific Gravity | Other |
|---|---|---|---|---|---|---|---|---|---|
| Cancer | Serosanguineous or bloody | Positive in 50% | Variable | 0.5–0.75 | >0.6 | < or ≥ 7.32 | >3.0 | >1.018 | |
| Chylous effusion | Cloudy, yellow | Negative | Variable | >0.5 | >0.6 | >7.32 | >3.0 | >1.018 | High triglycerides, low cholesterol |
| Postirradiation effusion | Serosanguineous or serous | Dysplastic MCs (class 3–4) | Variable with atypical MCs | >0.5 | >0.6 | >7.32 | >3.0 | >1.018 | |
| Pulmonary embolus with infarction | Serosanguineous or bloody | Negative | Erythrocytes, some neutrophils | >0.5 | >0.6 | >7.32 | >3.0 | >1.018 | |
| Congestive heart failure | Serous | Negative | Few MCs | >0.5 | <0.6 | >7.32 | <2.5 | <1.015 | |
| Bacterial infection (empyema) | Purulent or cloudy | Negative | Neutrophils | ≤0.5 | >0.6 | <7.32 | >3.0 | >1.018 | Cultures usually positive |
| Tuberculosis | Serofibrinous or serous to cloudy | Negative | >1000 mononuclear cells is suggestive | ≤0.5 | >0.6 | >7.32 | >3.0 | >1.018 | Cultures usually positive |
| Rheumatoid arthritis | Serous to cloudy | Negative | Variable | <0.5 | >0.6 | < or ≥ 7.32 | >3.0 | >1.018 | |

*Eosinophilia is nonspecific in pleural effusions and can be associated with cancer, infection, trauma, pulmonary embolism, and even prior thoracentesis. MC, mesothelial cells.

Adapted from Tabbarah HJ, Casciato DA. In: Casciato DA, Lowitz BB, eds. Manual of clinical oncology. 3rd ed. Boston: Little, Brown, 1995:487.

levels and elevated GLUT1, none can be thought of as a standard diagnostic tool.[1, 18–20] Chromosome analysis may be helpful in identifying hyperploid cells or cells containing abnormal chromosomes, but these techniques are expensive and are not universally available.

The diagnosis of malignancy can be established only by demonstrating the presence of malignant cells in the fluid or pleural tissue. Cytologic studies are more sensitive than percutaneous pleural needle biopsy because the latter is a blind sampling procedure. Cytologic tests have the ability to diagnose malignant pleural effusions in about two thirds of cases.[2] Pleural biopsy is positive in only 50 to 60% of proven malignant effusions; however, the likelihood of obtaining the diagnosis is increased to 80 to 90% when biopsy is combined with cytologic studies.[2, 21, 22] Thoracoscopy can provide the diagnosis in 93 to 96% of patients with malignant pleural effusion but should be reserved for cases that cannot be diagnosed by less invasive means because of the increased risk of morbidity.[1, 2]

## PROGNOSIS

A malignant pleural effusion usually signifies advanced disease and a poor prognosis. The median survival after the onset of malignant effusion varies significantly with the type of cancer. For example, the mean survival time for patients with breast cancer–associated effusions is 7 to 15 months; 20% of patients survive 3 years after the diagnosis of pleural effusion.[6] The mean survival time for patients with non–small cell lung cancer–associated effusion is only 2 months; two thirds of these patients die within 3 months.[6] The results of treatment for malignant pleural effusions must be measured not only in terms of survival but also with regard to the patient's discomfort from the effusion, the time the patient is confined to the hospital, and the morbidity caused by therapy.

## MANAGEMENT

A critical analysis of the many reports describing the efficacy of therapeutic modalities is difficult for several reasons. The criteria for response, the contribution of concurrent systemic therapies, the prevalence of previous treatments, and the rigor with which the cause of the effusions is proved vary among reports. Prognostic factors that are patient related (e.g., performance status, age, sex) and those that are tumor related (e.g., histologic characteristics, tumor load, response to previous therapy) are certainly important in assessment of the response rate but are infrequently analyzed.

**Thoracentesis.** Therapeutic thoracentesis is the initial procedure in the treatment of malignant pleural effusions. Initial evacuation should not remove more than 1500 ml of pleural fluid at one time to minimize the risk of re-expansion pulmonary edema. The results of thoracentesis alone are usually short-lived, with reaccumulation of fluid in almost all patients. Frequent repeated thoracenteses should be used only for patients with a life expectancy of less than 1 month because there are associated risks of pneumothorax, empyema, fluid loculation, and an increasing rate of fluid accumulation from hypoproteinemia.

**Tube Thoracostomy.** A small number of patients treated with tube thoracostomy alone may remain fluid free. In most cases, however, pleural effusion recurs, and more definitive methods of therapy should be attempted.

**Systemic Chemotherapy.** Effusions that develop early in the course of lymphoma, breast cancer, small cell lung cancer, or germ cell tumors are usually sensitive to chemotherapy and may respond dramatically. The response to chemotherapy of malignant pleural effusions caused by other malignancies, however, has been disappointing.

**Radiation Therapy.** Radiation to the hemithorax is generally contraindicated in the treatment of malignant pleural effusions because the side effects usually outweigh the benefits. Conversely, pleural effusions caused by lymphoma or mediastinal lymphadenopathy may best be treated with radiation therapy, particularly if the underlying disease is relatively radiosensitive.

**Radioactive Isotopes.** Radioactive gold ($^{198}$Au) and colloidal radioactive phosphorus ($^{32}$P) are the two radioactive isotopes most frequently instilled into the pleural space for the treatment of malignant pleural effusion. Technical difficulties of radioactive fluid collection and disposal make the instillation of these substances cumbersome. Response rates range from 55 to 65% in patients receiving such treatment. Mild myelosuppression and nausea are the most common side effects observed following the administration of these agents.

**Pleurodesis.** Pleurodesis or sclerotherapy is the most frequently used method of treating malignant pleural effusions. The goal of pleurodesis is the obliteration of the pleural space to prevent reaccumulation of fluid. Pleurodesis is accomplished by putting the chemically irritated visceral and parietal pleurae in close contact, thereby promoting viscero-parietal symphysis with firm adhesions. Patients subjected to pleurodesis should meet the following criteria: (1) dyspnea has been documented to be relieved by thoracentesis, (2) the pleural effusion has recurred after two or three aspirations or has recurred rapidly (within a few days), and (3) the patient's life expectancy is estimated to be more than 1 month.

Dozens of agents have been used as sclerosing agents for pleurodesis. Considerations in choosing a sclerosing agent must include not only efficacy but also cost, difficulty of administration, and frequency of adverse effects. See Table 103–2 for recommended doses of frequently employed substances.

*Procedure.* After the chest tube is inserted in the most dependent location, preferably in the anterior axillary line, the pleural fluid is first allowed to drain slowly by means of gravity and a water seal. Suction ($-20$ cm $H_2O$) may be applied later if necessary. When less than 100 ml of fluid drains in 24 hours, a chest film is obtained to document complete evacuation of the fluid and re-expansion of the underlying lung. After the patient is premedicated for pain, the sclerosing drug is injected into the cross-clamped chest tube and flushed into the pleural space with 50 ml of normal saline; the chest tube should remain cross-clamped from 1 to several hours after the drug instillation, depending on the agent used. When nitrogen mustard is used, the patient's position should be changed every 30 seconds for a few minutes; when other agents are used, such changing of position is probably not necessary. The chest tube is then

*Table 103–2.* Intracavitary Agents for Malignant Effusions

| Drug | Dosage |
|---|---|
| Talc, dry powder or 50-ml suspensions | 1–2 g (intrapericardial) 2–6 g (intrapleural) |
| Doxycycline | 500 mg (may be repeated) |
| Bleomycin | 1 unit/kg (not to exceed 40 units in the elderly) |
| Nitrogen mustard | 10–40 mg |
| Thiotepa | 30–45 mg (15 mg intrapericardial) |
| Cisplatin | 100 mg/m² (intrapleural) |
| Cytarabine | 1200 mg (intrapleural) |
| Fluorouracil | 750–1000 mg |
| Doxorubicin | 30 mg |
| Mitoxantrone | 6–10 mg/m² (intraperitoneal) |
| ³²P | 15–25 mCi (intraperitoneal) 5 mCi (intrapericardial) |

unclamped and the pleural fluid allowed to drain, preferably with suction ($-20$ cm $H_2O$). When less than 100 ml drains in 24 hours, the chest tube is removed.

*Complications.* General complications that may occur with any sclerosing agent include pain, fever, cough, fluid loculation, and infection. Pain may result from the chest tube insertion or from the drug instillation. It is generally recommended that analgesics be used prophylactically. Fever usually lasts 2 to 3 days and may be caused by pleural inflammation or infection. If there is no suggestion of infection, antipyretics may be used. Cough due to lung re-expansion is self-limited and may be helpful in clearing atelectasis. Fluid loculation is not uncommon, and lysis of adhesions may be performed via video-assisted thoracosopy if necessary. Small studies of fibrinolytic agents show promise. Infection is uncommon, but empyema should be considered in any patient having persistent fever.

### Antibiotic Sclerosing Agents

TETRACYCLINE. Tetracycline has been widely used and is often the substance to which new agents are compared. However, the parenteral form of this agent is no longer produced. A critical review of the literature reveals response rates that vary between 25% and 100%, with an average of 72%.[23] Fever and pain are the most commonly reported side effects.[24]

DOXYCYCLINE. This agent has been considered as a replacement for tetracycline but often requires multiple instillations (mean of three), with response rates of 60 to 88%, with an average of 73%.[25, 26] The need for repeated instillations increases costs and makes it less desirable for patients.

MINOCYCLINE. This agent was associated with a response rate of 86% in one small series. Experimental models, however, have demonstrated vestibular symptoms and a high incidence of hemothorax with this drug.[27]

*Immune Modulator Sclerosing Agents.* There are limited data on the use of interferons and cytokines as sclerosing agents. Interferons alfa, beta, and gamma have all been tried, but response rates are low and side effects vary from flu-like symptoms and hematologic reactions with interferon alfa to pain and fever with interferon beta.[23, 28] Recombinant interleukin-2 is commercially available and one small study that used daily instillation for 24 days resulted in a 100% response rate, with relapse occurring after an average of 16

months.[29] Fever and a transient increase in the size of the effusion were the most commonly reported side effects in that study. Using recombinant tumor necrosis factor (TNF), Rauthe and Sistermanns[30] reported no reaccumulation of pleural effusion over the remainder of the patients' lives in 14 (78%) of 18 patients treated with one to three instillations. The most commonly reported side effects were flu-like symptoms and fever.

### Biologic Sclerosing Agents

CORYNEBACTERIUM PARVUM. Extracts of this anaerobic gram-positive bacterium have been used with an average response rate of 76%.[31] The lipopolysaccharide cell wall is thought to prompt inflammation and pleural adhesion.

PICIBANIL (OK-432, OK-142, OKY-142). Experimental studies with these dried streptococcal preparations have yielded response rates in the range of 70%. The proposed mechanism of action involves causing an immune reaction to the increased expression of ICAM-1 molecules on tumor cells.[32]

### Miscellaneous Sclerosing Agents

QUINACRINE (ATABRINE). This antiparasitic agent has been used in Scandinavia but has been associated with serious central nervous system toxicity as well as severe chest pain, fever, hypotension, oliguria, and skin discoloration.[24] Response rates range from 64 to 100%, with a mean of 86%.[23]

FIBRIN GLUE. Although this substance has efficacy as a sclerosant in treating pneumothorax, it has a high failure rate in treating malignant pleural effusions because of the increase of fibrinolysis in malignant effusions.[33]

IODOPOVIDONE. This readily available and inexpensive substance was noted to promote dense pleural adhesions when used to "wash out" the chest cavity at thoracotomy. In one small trial, 20 ml diluted in normal saline instilled via chest tube up to three times had a response rate of approximately 64%.[34]

TALC. This trilayered magnesium sheet silicate was first reported as a pleural sclerosant in 1935 by Bethune.[35] USP asbestos-free talc must be sterilized with dry heat, gamma irradiation, or ethylene oxide gas prior to use. Traditionally, this agent has been administered as a powder (poudrage) or by insufflation during open thoracotomy or via rigid thoracoscope using general anesthesia. The expense of operating room time and the morbidity and mortality of open procedures (reaching 9% in some studies) made talc a less desirable agent than other agents, despite its consistently high success rate. The successful control of malignant pleural effusions with talc has been reported to be 100% with open thoracotomy, 97% with thoracoscopic insufflation, and 93% with closed-tube thoracostomy. More recent studies have shown that talc can be administered as a slurry via chest tube with efficacies of 91 to 100%.[24, 36] Complications of talc pleurodesis include fatal cases of adult respiratory distress syndrome. A review of the literature suggests that most cases of respiratory distress have occurred with doses of 10 g or more, when bilateral pleurodesis has been performed, or when pleural or lung biopsy has been performed in conjunction with pleurodesis.[9]

### Chemotherapeutic Sclerosing Agents

NITROGEN MUSTARD, THIOTEPA, AND FLUOROURACIL. When nitrogen mustard is instilled, the patient's position should be changed every 30 seconds for a few minutes. In most studies, fluid accumulation was reduced or stopped in 25 to 95% of patients treated, with a mean response rate of only 44%.[23]

Nitrogen mustard, fluorouracil, and thiotepa may cause tumor lysis, but the sclerosing action is mostly the result of pleural irritation. These chemotherapeutic drugs are well absorbed from the pleural cavity and may cause systemic side effects such as nausea, vomiting, and leukopenia.

DOXORUBICIN AND MITOXANTRONE. These agents have achieved objective responses in 39 to 80% of patients, with the most common adverse effects being pain, nausea and vomiting, and fever.[5] Early trials with mitoxantrone show results similar to that of tetracycline or bleomycin with only mild toxicity.[5]

CISPLATIN AND CYTARABINE. The combination of these two drugs has been used based on studies suggesting synergism. Rusch and colleagues[37] reported success with this combination in 49% of lung cancer patients, with minimal toxicity and an encouraging duration of response.

PACLITAXEL. A small phase II trial[38] in patients with non–small cell lung cancer found a response rate of 93% at 1 month. Pain, fever, flushing, and nausea were the most common side effects; one occurrence of grade IV neutropenia was reported.

BLEOMYCIN. This antineoplastic antibiotic from *Streptomyces verticillus* has been used extensively in the treatment of malignant pleural effusions. Most studies report a 30-day success rate in controlling effusions between 63% and 85%.[36, 39–42] Nearly 50% of intrapleural bleomycin is systemically absorbed, but only rare cases of toxicity have been reported. Bleomycin is not myelosuppressive, but cases of severe toxicity were seen in patients with renal impairment.[23, 36] The two most common adverse effects are pain and fever. Bleomycin appears to be as efficacious when instilled in soft, small-bore chest tubes as it is via standard chest tubes. The major drawback of this agent is its expense.

**Pleurectomy.** Partial pleurectomy and decortication have been attempted in patients with malignant pleural effusions, but 6 to 10% of patients die of the procedure, and 23% develop postoperative complications.[43] Thus, pleurectomy should not be considered except for a small subset of patients who are exceptionally healthy, whose primary tumor is under good control, and in whom more conservative measures have failed to control the pleural effusion. Video-assisted thoracoscopic techniques may decrease risks, but the learning curve for the procedure is steep.

**Pleural-Peritoneal Shunts.** Internal drainage of malignant pleural effusions into the abdomen was first described in 1984.[44] Such shunts have been reported to control refractory pleural effusions in patients with trapped lung but require manual pumping of a subcutaneously placed chamber hundreds of times per day. Shunt failure from clogging is common, and only patients with good performance status who have failed other methods should be considered for this procedure.

## SUMMARY OF TREATMENT

The purpose of treatment of malignant pleural effusions in the majority of patients is to relieve dyspnea. The patient's discomfort, the complication rate, and the success rate for each possibility must be considered in the selection of treatment methods. For most patients, we recommend chest tube drainage with pleurodesis using talc, bleomycin, or doxycy-

cline as the treatment of choice for recurrent malignant effusions.

## Malignant Pericardial Effusion

Pericardial tamponade from malignant pericardial effusion accounts for more than half the pericardial effusions requiring intervention.[2] Malignant pericardial effusion is usually, but not always, associated with poor life expectancy. In autopsy series, pericardial disease is present in 8 to 21% of patients dying of malignancy.[45–47] Malignancy is the most common cause of cardiac tamponade, even in patients without previously diagnosed cancer.[48] The most common malignancies associated with pericardial effusion are lung cancer, breast cancer, and lymphoma, and there are case reports of nearly all tumor types causing malignant pericardial effusions.

### PATHOGENESIS

Pericardial metastasis can enter the pericardium in a variety of ways. Direct extension of the tumor can involve the pericardium, with or without involvement of the heart. Hematogenous or lymphatic dissemination, or both, can result in the pericardium's being studded with tumor nodules or diffusely infiltrated. Constrictive pericarditis can develop, particularly if thickening and fibrosis of the pericardium are associated with tumor infiltration.

Normally the pericardial sac contains less than 10 ml of fluid. Fluid accumulation in the pericardial cavity can be caused by mediastinal lymphatic obstruction and by secretion from tumor nodules studding the pericardial surfaces. Cardiac tamponade is caused by the accumulation of fluid in the pericardium in an amount sufficient to seriously obstruct the inflow of blood to the ventricle. The amount of fluid necessary to produce this critical state may be small (250 ml) when fluid accumulates rapidly or may be more than 1000 ml when the effusion accumulates slowly.

### DIAGNOSIS

**Signs and Symptoms.** Approximately 15% of patients with pericardial metastasis develop cardiac tamponade, but about 70% have no cardiac symptoms during life. Symptoms that do develop most frequently result from the fall in cardiac output and systemic venous congestion. The frequencies of manifestations are shown in Table 103–3.

The most common symptoms of pericardial effusion are dyspnea, fatigue and malaise, cough, chest pain, orthopnea, palpitations, and dizziness. The symptoms of slowly developing tamponade resemble those of congestive heart failure. Patients may find maximal relief from symptoms in the upright forward-leaning position. Signs include bilateral neck vein distention, which may increase on inspiration (Kussmaul's sign). Palpation of the precordium may reveal weakness or absence of the cardiac impulse. Percussion delineate an increase in cardiac dullness. Heart sound be distant or weak except when there is excessiv

*Table 103–3.* **Manifestations of Malignant Pericardial Effusion**

| Proportion of Patients | Manifestations |
| --- | --- |
| 80–90 | Dyspnea |
| 45–65 | Cough |
| 40–50 | Pleural effusion, hepatomegaly, chest pain, orthopnea |
| 25–35 | Cyanosis, cardiomegaly, venous distention, leg edema |
| 15–20 | Pulmonary rales, dysphagia, splenomegaly |
| 5–10 | Systolic murmur, hemoptysis, paradoxical pulse, ascites |
| <5 | Syncope, hiccough, palpitation, paroxysmal nocturnal dyspnea, friction rub, diastolic gallop, distant heart sounds, paroxysmal ventricular tachycardia, pulsus alternans |

involvement or constrictive pericarditis. Atrial arrhythmias, early diastolic sounds, and a pericardial friction rub may also be heard.

An important sign of cardiac tamponade is the presence of a paradoxical pulse, which is a weakening of the pulse with a fall in systolic blood pressure of more than 10 mm Hg during and at the end of inspiration (paradoxical pulse may also occasionally occur from severe myocardial failure, hemorrhagic shock, chronic obstructive airway disease, and severe asthma). With severe tamponade, facial plethora, profuse perspiration, confusion or impaired consciousness, rapid and shallow breathing, peripheral cyanosis, and cardiovascular collapse may develop.

**Radiology.** Chest films may be completely normal or may show simple cardiomegaly, a globular heart shadow with water-bottle configuration, or an irregular nodular cardiac contour. Mediastinal or hilar abnormalities may be noted. CT is sensitive and may suggest malignant pericardial disease when the pericardial effusion is of high density, the pericardium is locally or diffusely thickened, masses are seen within or contiguous with the pericardium, or normal tissue planes are obliterated between a paracardiac mass and the heart or pericardium.

**Echocardiography.** This is the least invasive and most sensitive method for the diagnosis of pericardial effusion and can be performed at the bedside. Echocardiography can detect pericardial effusions as small as 15 ml,[49] masses, loculations, and pericardial thickening. The diagnosis of cardiac tamponade may be established by invagination of the ventricular walls and by motion abnormalities of the anterior leaflet of the mitral valve.[50]

**Electrocardiography.** The electrocardiogram may demonstrate low-voltage and other nonspecific changes. Total (or simultaneous) electrical alternans, involving both atrial and ventricular complexes arising from the same pacemaker independent of periodic extracardiac phenomena, is considered virtually pathognomonic of cardiac tamponade.[51] Ventricular alternans (involving QRS complexes only) is more common and less specific and occurs in patients with myocardial failure of various causes.

**Right Heart Catheterization.** This is the gold standard for the diagnosis and monitoring of cardiac function in pericardial effusion. Equalization of diastolic pressures across the cardiac chambers defines tamponade.

**Fluid Studies.** When pericardiocentesis is performed, the fluid should be examined for cell count and differential, total

protein, glucose, LDH levels, and cytologic characteristics. Malignant pericardial effusions are typically exudates and are often hemorrhagic. Bloody effusions may also be associated with tuberculosis, uremia, anticoagulant therapy, and mediastinal radiation therapy. Cytologic examination for malignant cells is essential, with 50 to 60% sensitivity and 100% specificity.[52]

Differentiation between radiation-induced pericarditis and pericardial metastasis is difficult in patients who have received prior mediastinal radiation therapy; both may produce bloody effusions with negative cytologic findings. Radiation pericarditis may occur after 35 to 40 Gy of fractionated radiation therapy to the heart. The injury to the pericardium may present as acute pericarditis during the course of radiation therapy or weeks, months, or years after the completion of therapy. Acute radiation pericarditis is frequently self-limited and often subsides without residual constriction. Chronic radiation pericarditis may lead to constriction or tamponade.

## PROGNOSIS

The presence of malignant pericardial effusion is usually associated with a poor prognosis. A number of small studies have looked at survival in patients with malignant pericardial effusion. Most studies report a median overall survival of 3 to 4 months.[24, 53–58] A survival difference has been noted between patients with cytologically positive (median 1.4 months) and cytologically negative (5.8 months) pericardial effusions.[24, 57] A longer survival has been observed in patients with breast cancer.[53–55] Some patients (up to 28% in one study[54]) will be alive 2 years after the diagnosis of malignant pericardial effusion.

## MANAGEMENT

The presence of pericardial effusion is not in itself an indication for treatment. The indications for malignant pericardial fluid aspiration include[51] signs and symptoms of tamponade, rising peripheral venous pressure of about 13 cm $H_2O$, measured pulsus paradoxus exceeding 50% of the pulse pressure, or falling pulse pressure to less than 20 mm Hg.

**Pericardiocentesis.** Pericardiocentesis was first introduced by Schuh in 1841.[49] The needle is inserted to the left of the xiphoid process under the costal margin at a 45-degree angle in the direction of the top of the left shoulder. An electrocardiographic chest lead may be attached to the needle to monitor for any signs of cardiac injury. Echocardiography or fluoroscopic guidance can lower complication rates and increase diagnostic yields.[59] Patients with loculated posterior effusions cannot undergo drainage via the usual approaches. The complications of pericardiocentesis, although unusual, include laceration of the heart or coronary artery, laceration of the internal mammary artery, penetration of the pleural cavity, tension pneumothorax, and ventricular tachycardia. Pericardiocentesis alone is not sufficient to prevent recurrence of malignant pericardial effusions. Cardiac tamponade may recur within 24 to 48 hours unless catheter drainage is instituted. Therefore, additional therapeutic approaches should be initiated.

**Pericardial Catheter Drainage.** A pigtail angiographic catheter may be inserted at the time of pericardiocentesis. Drainage usually requires 24 to 72 hours when the catheter is put to gravity. A few patients have achieved control of their effusions at 1 month using catheter drainage alone.[60]

**Sclerotherapy.** Several substances have been used to produce adhesion between the visceral and parietal pericardial membranes in an attempt to obliterate the pericardial space. Most agents significantly decrease intrapericardial fluid reaccumulation in 50 to 75% of patients.[58, 61–66] The development of constrictive pericarditis and refractory cardiac failure over the long term has been reported.

Chemotherapeutic agents that are used include bleomycin, nitrogen mustard, thiotepa, cisplatin, vinblastine, and fluorouracil. Bleomycin and thiotepa are used most frequently. In small studies, bleomycin was noted to be more costly than thiotepa; neither resulted in significant pain or fever after intrapericardial instillation.[49]

[198]Au, [32]P, and radioactive yttrium ([90]Y) have yielded encouraging results. In one report, 20 of 28 patients had no subsequent effusions.[62] Meaningful conclusions cannot be drawn because of the small numbers of patients with a variety of tumors that were so treated. Managing radioactive leakage and waste is problematic with these agents.

Other agents that have been used include quinacrine, OK-432, talc, interferon, tetracycline (no longer commercially available), and doxycycline. Doxycycline has been reported to cause fevers in 50% of patients as well as intense pain after instillation.[58, 66] Dosages are given in Table 103–2.

**Systemic Chemotherapy.** Chemotherapy may be effective in slowly developing pericardial effusions caused by responsive tumors. This response has been observed in patients with lymphoma and breast carcinoma early in the disease, when the tumor is still sensitive to the chemotherapeutic agents.

**Radiation Therapy.** External-beam irradiation appears to control malignant pericardial effusion in radio-responsive tumor types. Dosages of 25 to 40 Gy are usually used. The highest success rates are seen in patients with leukemia or lymphoma.

**Surgery.** Surgical treatments for pericardial effusions include balloon pericardiotomy, subxiphoid pericardial window, anterolateral thoracotomy with partial pericardiectomy, and video-assisted thoracoscopic surgery (VATS)-created pericardial windows.

The development of percutaneous balloon pericardiotomy has provided a safe and effective means of relieving pericardial effusions in many small series. Success rates range from 91 to 100%, with few complications.[67, 68]

The creation of a subxiphoid window (inferior pericardiotomy) using local anesthesia was originally described by Larrey in 1829.[69] The procedure carries a low morbidity rate (10 to 15%) in patients with malignant pericardial effusions and has an 86% success rate at 3 months.[55, 57, 70] Tumor encasement can preclude the conversion of the pericardial incision to a window. These windows may close within a short period because of adhesions and obliteration by the overlying lung.

Pericardial windows created via thoracotomy or VATS have success rates of 90 to 95%.[52, 71, 72] However, these procedures are associated with increased rates of morbidity and mortality that may not be justified in patients with limited survival.

## SUMMARY OF TREATMENT

As with pleural effusions, studies of the treatment of pericardial effusions are difficult to compare. Press and Livingstone[49] reviewed 10 reported series (308 patients) with malignant pericardial effusion, treated with radiation therapy (66 patients), subxiphoid pericardiotomy (100 patients), pleuropericardial window (55 patients), or tetracycline sclerosis (87 patients). They suggested that subxiphoid pericardiotomy may be the initial procedure of choice. With the increased experience and availability of percutaneous pericardiotomy, we feel that the experiences of the individual physician and institution along with the condition of the patient should dictate the choice of treatment for malignant pericardial effusions.

## Malignant Ascites

Malignancy accounts for approximately 10% of all cases of ascites. Ascites is the presenting symptom of malignancy in approximately half of all patients with malignant ascites. Most cases of malignant ascites are due to intra-abdominal tumors. Ovarian cancer is the most frequent cause and makes up 28 to 54% of cases in most series.[73–75] Carcinoma of unknown primary site is the second largest group and makes up 13 to 22% of cases in most series.[73–76] Other common intra-abdominal primary tumor sites include endometrium, colon, stomach, liver, and pancreas. The most common extra-abdominal malignancies to cause malignant ascites are breast cancer, lung cancer, and lymphoma. Rare cases of ascites have been reported to occur in patients with prostate carcinoma, multiple myeloma, and malignant melanoma.[77–79]

## PATHOGENESIS

The healthy peritoneal cavity contains approximately 50 ml of fluid. The influx and efflux rates of pleural fluid are normally 4 to 5 ml/hr.[80] Absorption of fluid from the peritoneal cavity is directly proportional to increasing intra-abdominal pressures, and the rate of absorption can increase more than 10-fold in the presence of malignant ascites.

Lymphatic obstruction plays a major role in the formation of malignant ascites as demonstrated by radiolabeled technetium colloid and other studies.[81] Abdominal neoplasms, usually lymphoma, cause more than 80% of cases of chylous ascites in adults through lymphatic obstruction.

Malignant ascites is usually associated with peritoneal metastases, which increase peritoneal fluid formation through a variety of mechanisms. Locally mediated vasoactive substances promote increased permeability of microvessels, including new vessels from tumor angiogenesis. Similar to findings in ascites caused by cirrhosis, plasma renin activity may be elevated in patients with malignant ascites, causing sodium conservation and water retention via the renin-angiotensin-aldosterone pathway.[82, 83]

# DIAGNOSIS

**Signs and Symptoms.** Ascites is usually first noticed because of abdominal distention. The appearance of abdominal or inguinal hernia may also be noted. Abdominal discomfort or pain, often with nausea and anorexia, is common. Associated symptoms may include weight gain with manifestations of muscle wasting, symptoms of gastroesophageal reflux, general discomfort, a sensation of pulling at the flanks or groin, or vague low back pain. Localized pain in patients with malignant ascites usually results from involvement of abdominal organs. Dyspnea, orthopnea, or tachypnea may result from elevation of the diaphragm. A coexistent pleural effusion, usually on the right side, may contribute to the respiratory compromise.

The physical examination has limited sensitivity (60 to 80%) and specificity (65 to 90%) in ascites.[84] Ascites is usually demonstrable clinically when 500 ml of fluid or more has accumulated in the peritoneal cavity. Bulging flanks and an everted umbilicus may be present. Flank dullness that shifts with changing position and fluid wave may be noted. Palpation is often difficult with massive ascites, and ballottement may be the only method of palpating enlarged organs or masses.

Careful auscultation of the liver may reveal a souffle (bruit) of a vascular tumor such as hepatoma, or metastases from renal cell carcinoma, leiomyosarcoma, or carcinoid or islet cell tumors. A venous hum at the umbilicus may signify portal hypertension.

**Radiologic Studies.** Supine and upright radiographs of the abdomen may demonstrate abdominal haziness, the loss of psoas margins, increased density that shifts to the pelvis on the upright film, and poor definition of the major abdominal organs, but plain films are generally unreliable in detecting ascites.

Ultrasonography can be performed at the bedside and is able to detect as little as 100 ml of ascitic fluid.[85] Ultrasonography can also detect liver metastases and peritoneal carcinomatosis.[137]

CT is the most reliable method of evaluating the liver, spleen, and retroperitoneum. MRI is also useful. Early studies of contrast-enhanced fast multiplanar spoiled gradient recalled MRI imaging show promise for detecting peritoneal disease.[86] No radiologic studies can accurately determine if ascitic fluid is benign or malignant.

**Paracentesis.** Diagnostic paracentesis is important in the routine evaluation of ascites. Careful aspiration of 50 to 100 ml from a flank or low midline site should be attempted, and the ascitic fluid should be examined for its appearance, color, cell count, protein content, and the presence of microorganisms or malignant cells. Turbid or purulent ascites favors pyogenic peritonitis but may also be the result of large numbers of malignant cells or leukocytes emanating from noninfectious causes. Turbid ascitic fluid should not be confused with chylous fluid. Mucinous ascitic fluid may suggest pseudomyxoma peritonei or, rarely, a colloid carcinoma of the stomach or colon with peritoneal implants.

Some features of ascitic fluid may suggest certain diagnostic possibilities. Protein values are rarely greater than 2.5 g/dl in ascites caused by cirrhosis and are usually greater than 2.5 g/dl in ascites caused by tuberculosis or malignancy. Bloody fluid with more than 2.5 g/dl of protein is consistent with malignancy or tuberculous peritonitis. If the fluid is a typical transudate but contains more than 250 white blood cells/mm³, a search for a tumor or infection is warranted.

A malignant cause for ascites is usually determined by cytologic examination of fluid or peritoneal biopsy. Cytologic examination alone detects malignant cells in 40 to 70% of effusions caused by tumors.[73, 74, 87, 88] The specificity of cytologic examination approaches 100%. Biopsy of the peritoneum with a side-biting hook-type needle (Abrams' or Cope's needle) in patients with exudative ascites results in the correct diagnosis in more than 50% of patients with malignant ascites. The ideal combination of fluid tests to detect malignant ascites has not been determined. Ascitic fluid CEA values elevated to greater than 12 ng/ml occur in approximately 50% of patients with malignant ascites and rarely with ascites caused by benign disease.[89] The sensitivities for the β subunit of human chorionic gonadotropin greater than 10 mIU/ml and cholesterol greater than 45 mg/dl have been reported to be 61% and 83%, with specificities of 94% and 81%, respectively.[90]

**Laparoscopy.** When simple investigation fails to make the diagnosis, 86 to 94% of cases can be diagnosed with laparoscopy and biopsy.[91, 92] This procedure may be performed using local anesthesia and sedation and allows direct inspection of the liver and peritoneal cavity. Morbidity from the procedure has been reported to be about 6%, with leakage at the trocar site and infection reported most commonly.

# PROGNOSIS

Overall survival from the time of diagnosis of malignant ascites averages about 20 weeks[73, 74] but varies greatly with the tumor of origin. Patients with malignant ascites caused by lymphoma tend to have the longest survival (58 to 78 weeks). Patients with primary tumors originating in the gastrointestinal tract have a mean survival of 12 to 20 weeks, with most studies reporting mean survivals of approximately 3 months. Malignant ascites associated with cancers of unknown primary site carries the worst prognosis, with an average survival of less than 3 months.[76] However, women with papillary serous carcinoma of the peritoneum have survival times of about 2 years when they are treated like patients with stage III ovarian carcinoma (see Chapter 102).

# MANAGEMENT

Ovarian carcinoma with ascites is generally managed with cytoreductive surgical resection and adjuvant chemotherapy. In abdominal malignant lymphoma, long-term survival may also be achieved following treatment with chemotherapy or radiation, or a combination of these. For the remainder of patients, malignant ascites usually signifies far-advanced disease with a poor prognosis.

**Paracentesis.** Repeated large-volume paracenteses are generally the mainstay of treatment in symptomatic malignant ascites. Five to 7 L may be removed safely without colloidal support.[93–95] In ovarian carcinoma studies, removal of 2400 to 11,000 ml during a short time (30 minutes) did not lead to significant changes in hemodynamics, hematocrit values, or serum electrolyte concentrations during the procedure and the ensuing 24 to 48 hours; however, serum protein concentrations fell to approximately two thirds of the baseline level in each patient. Complete drainage may become difficult over time because adhesions and loculations may develop. Rare complications of paracentesis include peritonitis, pulmonary embolism, and hypotension.

**Diuretic Therapy.** Because secondary hyperaldosteronism often plays a role in perpetuating edema and ascites, an aldosterone antagonist (spironolactone), used alone or with proximal-segment diuretics (thiazides or furosemide), can be effective in controlling malignant ascites.[83, 96] Diuretics may mobilize ascites caused by hepatic metastasis. Diuretics are rarely helpful, however, for ascites caused by peritoneal carcinomatosis or chylous malignant ascites.

**Systemic Chemotherapy.** Chemotherapy may be effective early in the course of disease for patients with lymphoma or breast carcinoma. Systemic chemotherapy is used almost universally in ovarian cancer patients without contraindications.

**Intraperitoneal Chemotherapy.** Chemotherapeutic drugs have been used intraperitoneally, with the major toxicities being nausea, local pain, fever, and leukopenia. The rate of drug absorption across the peritoneal membrane varies with the lipid solubility and molecular weight of the drug. Much higher concentrations of the drug can be achieved because the clearance of drugs from the peritoneal cavity is slow (<20 ml/min). The drug concentration achieved can be up to 25 times the concentration in the serum.[97] Drugs administered intraperitoneally are generally absorbed via the portal circulation with large first-pass effects leading to low systemic concentrations. The tissue penetration of most chemotherapeutic agents given intraperitoneally is generally 1 to 3 mm, so bulky carcinomatous masses are not likely to be affected.[98]

Many different chemotherapeutic agents have been used intraperitoneally. No study has proved the superiority of any particular agent. Thiotepa, fluorouracil, bleomycin, nitrogen mustard, doxorubicin, cisplatin, mitoxantrone, and mitomycin C have been used most extensively; dosages are given in Table 103–2. The response rates to each drug vary from series to series. Reduction or complete cessation of peritoneal fluid production has been reported in approximately 35% of patients treated with fluorouracil, 35 to 60% of those treated with bleomycin, 30% of those treated with thiotepa, and 50% of patients treated with nitrogen mustard or cisplatin.[99–102] Doxorubicin has also been shown efficacious in small studies but appears to be associated with more abdominal pain.[76, 101] Intraperitoneal mitoxantrone 10 mg/m² total dose, was well tolerated and provided palliation for malignant ascites in 30 to 79% of patients with gynecologic malignancy.[103–105] Mitomycin C conferred a survival advantage in patients with gastric cancer and serosal involvement in one study.[106]

Heat and mitomycin C appear to act synergistically against tumor cells in vitro. Intraperitoneal hyperthermic chemotherapy (IPHC) is administered through intraperitoneal catheters placed surgically. The chemotherapeutic agents are infused into the peritoneum with inflow temperatures between 42° C and 49° C with or without cooling measures to maintain the patients core body temperature at less than 39.5° C. When intraperitoneal shunts and IPHC were used in several small studies, there was no increase in

perioperative mortality. Response rates vary between 75% and 90% over the remainder of the patients' lives.[107, 108]

**Intraperitoneal Radiocolloids.** The first reported use of radioactive colloids for malignant ascites was in 1945. Since that time $^{32}P$ has been studied extensively. $^{32}P$ emits beta radiation that penetrates peritoneal tissues to a depth of 4 to 8 mm and has a long half-life of 14 days. Response rates for colloidal $^{32}P$ range from 40% to 58%.[109, 110] Complications are usually mild and include nausea, pain, vomiting, diarrhea, and low-grade fever. More serious complications include bowel obstruction and bowel perforation, which have been reported to occur in up to 1.5% of patients.[110] Colloidal $^{198}Au$ may result in depression of the hematopoietic system. Colloidal radioactive zinc ($^{63}Zn$) has been associated with a higher rate of bowel necrosis. No trial has proved one agent to be superior to another. Loculation is a relative contraindication to the instillation of radioactive isotopes.

**Intraperitoneal Immune Modifiers.** Experiments using intraperitoneal interferons and cytokines abound, but studies are small and response rates equivocal. Interferon alfa may result in an objective response in 36% of patients with advanced ovarian cancer. Its side effects include malaise, fever, and flu-like symptoms. In one study, interferon plus cisplatin proved more effective than cisplatin alone (response rate of 77% vs. 22%).[111] A small number of cases showed responses to interferon beta. In one small study, the combination of TNF and interferon gamma was shown to have a response rate of 54%.[112]

Interleukins 2, 4, 6, and 7 have been used for a variety of tumor types and can induce tumor-specific immunity,[113] but no study has shown a clinically significant response in malignant ascites. Combinations of immune modifiers with chemotherapy are being evaluated.

Intraperitoneal injection of OK-432, the heat- and penicillin-treated lyophilized powder of the Su strain of *Streptococcus pyogenes* A3, has been shown to cause the influx of immune cells and the destruction of tumor cells with a decrease in ascites production. This agent has been studied most extensively in Japan for gastric cancer and reduces symptoms of ascites in up to 63% of patients at 6 weeks.[114] *C. parvum* has also been used in the treatment of malignant ascites with some success in several small studies.

**Radiation Therapy.** External-beam irradiation may be used to control a primary tumor producing ascites in lymphoma or ovarian carcinoma. The moving-strip technique allows the delivery of a higher dose of radiation but apparently does not result in improved tumor control when compared with traditional methods. In one study, the moving-strip technique was associated with major complications in 13% of patients (small-bowel perforation, acute colitis, abdominocutaneous fistula, rectal ulcer) and minor complications in 60% (usually leukopenia).[115]

**Peritoneovenous Shunts.** LaVeen introduced peritoneovenous (PV) shunts in 1974 and Denver soon followed. One end of a special collecting catheter is inserted into the peritoneal cavity, and the other end is inserted into the superior vena cava via the internal jugular vein; a pressure-sensitive one-way valve permits fluid flow when the intraperitoneal pressure exceeds the central venous pressure by 3 to 5 cm $H_2O$. The Denver shunt has a subcutaneous compressible valve chamber that allows daily manual flushing for nonoperative clearing of obstruction by the physician,

*Table 103–4.* Contraindications for Peritoneovenous Shunts

*Ascitic Fluid Characteristics*

Hemorrhagic *or*
Protein concentration >4.5 g/dl *or*
Large number of malignant cells *or*
Thick or tenacious (e.g., pseudomyxoma peritonei) *or*
Loculated

*Patient Factors*

Recent or concurrent infection
Preoperative overt or subclinical coagulopathy
Liver failure (bilirubin concentration >10 mg/dl)
Present or prior cardiac or renal disease
Simultaneous bowel surgery

nurse, or patient; it also allows a rapid determination of patency on physical examination (a stiff chamber indicates occlusion). PV shunts have been reported to provide palliation in 64 to 88% of cases of malignant ascites.[116–121]

Shunts fail mostly because of occlusion. They function for a median of 20 weeks in patients with negative findings on cytologic examination of ascitic fluid for malignant cells compared with 3 to 4 weeks in patients with positive cytologic studies. The complication rate for PV shunts in one analysis was 25%[117] and resulted from shunt occlusion and transient congestive heart failure due to increased intravascular volume. Other well-described complications include coagulopathy, which appears to be less common with malignant ascites than with cirrhotic ascites.[120] Elevated fibrin degradation products are considered an index of shunt function. Other complications that have been reported rarely include tumor dissemination, pulmonary embolism, and superior vena cava thrombosis.

The contraindications to insertion of PV shunts are summarized in Table 103–4. In the absence of these contraindications, the technique may be used in patients with intractable symptomatic malignant ascites when other means for control have failed.

**Surgery.** Surgery has often been considered contraindicated for massive ascites associated with nongynecologic malignancies. Some institutions have reported good success in major cytoreductive surgery for nonovarian primary tumors in the face of malignant ascites,[107] and we would recommend that the individual surgeon and institution determine the need for surgical intervention. Less extensive surgical procedures to relieve ascites have been used in small numbers of patients. One approach involves the formation of a pedicle flap of intestinal mucosa to create an absorptive surface for the ascitic fluid. Another approach is to devise peritoneovesicular drainage so that ascitic fluid can be voided.

## SUMMARY OF TREATMENT

The purpose of treatment for malignant ascites is to relieve patient discomfort. Following paracentesis, systemic chemotherapy is given if the tumor is recognized to be responsive (lymphoma, breast carcinoma, or ovarian carcinoma). If the malignancy is unresponsive to systemic chemotherapy, intraperitoneal administration of chemotherapeutic agents or $^{32}$P

may be tried. PV shunts may be considered in patients who are symptomatic and in whom there are no contraindications to the procedure.

## REFERENCES

1. Sahn SA. Pleural diseases related to metastatic malignancies. Eur Respir J 1997;10:1907–13.
2. De Camp MM, Mentzer SJ, Sugarbaker DJ. Malignant effusive disease of the pleura and pericardium. Chest 1997;112:291s–5s.
3. Sahn SA. Malignancy metastatic to the pleura. Clin Chest Med 1998;19:351–61.
4. Black LF. The pleural space and pleural fluid. Mayo Clin Proc 1972;47:493–506.
5. Grossi F, Pennucci MC, Tixi L, et al. Management of malignant pleural effusions. Drugs 1998;55:47–58.
6. Chernow B, Sahn SA. Carcinomatous involvement of the pleura: an analysis of 96 patients. Am J Med 1977;63:695–702.
7. Woodring JH. Recognition of pleural effusion on supine radiographs: how much fluid is required? AJR Am J Roentgenol 1984;142:642–6.
8. Tattersal M. Pleural effusions. Curr Opin Oncol 1992;4:642–6.
9. Ruckdeschel JC. Management of malignant pleural effusions: an overview. Semin Oncol 1993;15:Suppl 3:24–8.
10. Mathis G. Thorax sonography. Part I: Chest wall and pleura. Ultrasound Med Biol 1997;23:1131–9.
11. McLoud TC. CT and MR in pleural disease. Clin Chest Med 1998;19:261–76.
12. Heffner JE. Evaluating diagnostic tests in the pleural space. Clin Chest Med 1998;19:277–93.
13. Light RW, Ball WC. Glucose and amylase in pleural effusions. JAMA 1973;225:257–9.
14. Martinez-Vea A, Gatell JM, Segura F, et al. Diagnostic value of tumoral markers in serous effusions: CEA, alpha-1 acidglycoprotein, alpha-feto-protein, phosphohexose isomerase, and beta-2 microglobulin. Cancer 1982;50:1783–8.
15. Milano G, Krebs BP, Duplay H, et al. Use of tumor markers as a supplement to cytology in diagnosis of malignant effusions. Clin Chem 1980;26:1632.
16. Miles DW, Knight RK. Diagnosis and management of malignant pleural effusion. Cancer Treat Rev 1993;19:151–68.
17. Pinto MM. CA-15.3 assay in effusions. comparison of CEA and CA-125 assay and cytologic diagnosis. Acta Cytol 1996;40:437–42.
18. Alexandrakis M, Coulocheri S, Kyriakou D, et al. Diagnostic value of ferritin, haptoglobin, alpha-antitrypsin, LDH, and complement factors C3 and C4 in pleural effusion differentiation. Respir Med 1997;91:517–23.
19. Burstein DE, Reder I, Weiser K, et al. GLUT1 glucose transporter: a highly sensitive marker of malignancy in body cavity effusions. Mod Pathol 1998;11:392–6.
20. Cascinu S, Del Ferro E, Barbanti I, et al. Tumor markers in the diagnosis of malignant serous effusions. Am J Clin Oncol 1997;20:247–50.
21. Hsu C. Cytologic detection of malignancy in pleural effusion: a review of 5,255 samples from 3,811 patients. Diagn Cytopathol 1987;3:8–12.
22. Prakash UBS, Reinman HM. Comparison of needle biopsy with cytologic analysis for the evaluation of pleural effusion: analysis of 414 cases. Mayo Clin Proc 1985;60:158–64.
23. Belani CP, Pajeau TS, Bennett CL. Treating malignant pleural effusions cost consciously. Chest 1998;113:78s–85s.
24. Rodriguez-Panadero F, Antony VB. Pleurodesis: state of the art. Eur Respir J 1997;10:1648–54.
25. Heffner JE, Standerfer RJ, Torstveit J, Unruh L. Clinical efficacy of doxycycline for pleurodesis. Chest 1994;105:1743–7.
26. Seaton KG, Patz EF, Goodman PC. Palliative treatment of malignant pleural effusions: value of small-bore catheter thoracostomy and doxycycline sclerotherapy. AJR Am J Roentgenol 1995;164:589–91.
27. Light RW, Wang NS, Sassoon CS, et al. Comparison of the effectiveness of tetracycline and minocycline as pleural sclerosing agent in rabbits. Chest 1994;106:577–82.
28. Yanagawa H, Haku T, Hiramatsu K, et al. Intrapleural instillation of interferon-gamma in patients with malignant pleurisy due to lung cancer. Cancer Immunol Immunother 1997;45:93–9.
29. Suzuki H, Abo S, Kitamura M, et al. The intrapleural administration

of recombinant interleukin-2 (rIL-2) to patients with malignant pleural effusion: clinical trials. Surg Today 1993;23:1053–9.

30. Rauthe G, Sistermanns J. Pleurodesis with recombinant tumor necrosis factor in gynaecological neoplasms. Eur J Gynaecol Oncol 1998;19:108–12.

31. Ostrowsky MJ, Priestman TJ, et al. A randomized trial of intracavitary bleomycin and *Corynebacterium parvum* in the control of malignant pleural effusions. Radiother Oncol 1989;14:19–26.

32. Luh KT, Yang PC, Kuo SH, et al. Comparison of OK-432 and mitomycin C pleurodesis for malignant pleural effusions caused by lung cancer: a randomized trial. Cancer 1992;69:674–9.

33. Rodriguez-Panadero F, Segado A, Martin Juan J, et al. Failure of talc pleurodesis is associated with increased pleural fibrinolysis. Am J Respir Crit Care Med 1995;151:3 Pt 1:785–90.

34. Kelly-Garcia J, Roman-Berumen JF, Ibarra-Perez C. Iodopovidone and bleomycin pleurodesis for effusions due to malignant epithelial neoplasms. Arch Med Res 1997;28:583–5.

35. Bethune N. Pleural poudrage: a new technique for the deliberate production of pleural adhesions as a preliminary to lobectomy. J Thorac Surg 1935;4:251–61.

36. Zimmer PW, Hill M, Casey K, et al. Prospective randomized trial of talc slurry vs. bleomycin in pleurodesis for symptomatic malignant pleural effusions. Chest 1997;112:430–4.

37. Rusch VW, Figlin R, Godwin D, et al. Intrapleural cisplatin and cytarabine in the management of malignant pleural effusions: a lung cancer study group trial. J Clin Oncol 1991;9:313–9.

38. Perng RP, Chen YM, Wu MF, et al. Phase II trial of intrapleural paclitaxel injection for non–small cell lung cancer patients with malignant pleural effusions. Respir Med 1998;92:473–9.

39. Martinez-Moragon E, Aparicio J, Rogado MC, et al. Pleurodesis in malignant pleural effusions: a randomized study of tetracycline vs. bleomycin. Eur Respir Med 1997;10:2380–83.

40. Ruckdeschel JC, Moores D, et al. Intrapleural therapy for malignant pleural effusions: a randomized comparison of bleomycin and tetracycline. Chest 1991;100:1528–35.

41. Emad A, Rezaian GR. Treatment of malignant pleural effusions with a combination of bleomycin and tetracycline. Cancer 1996;78:2498–501.

42. Hartman DL, Gaither JM, Kesler KA, et al. Comparison of insufflated talc under thoracoscopic guidance with standard tetracycline and bleomycin pleurodesis for control of malignant pleural effusions. J Thorac Cardiovasc Surg 1993;105:743–7.

43. Martini N, Bains MS, Beattie EJ. Indications for pleurectomy in malignant effusion. Cancer 1975;35:734–8.

44. Dorsey JS, Cogordan JA. Pleuroperitoneal shunt for intractable effusion. Can J Surg 1984;27:598–9.

45. Hawkins JW, Vacek JL. What constitutes definitive therapy of malignant pericardial effusion? "Medical" vs. surgical treatment. Am Heart J 1989;118:428–32.

46. Olufunmilayo IO, Ultmann JE. Malignant effusions. Cancer J Clin 1991;41:167–79.

47. Bisel HF, Wroblewski F, La Due JS. Incidence and clinical manifestations of cardiac metastases. JAMA 1953;153:712–5.

48. Groeger JS, Keefe D. Cardiac tamponade. In: Groeger JS, ed. Critical care of the cancer patient. 2nd ed. St. Louis: CV Mosby, 1991:250–60.

49. Press OW, Livingstone R. Management of malignant pericardial effusion and tamponade. JAMA 1987;257:1088–92.

50. D'Cruz IA, Cohen HE, Prabhu R, et al. Diagnosis of cardiac tamponade by echocardiography: changes in mitral valve motion and ventricular dimensions with special reference to paradoxical pulse. Circulation 1975;52:460–5.

51. Spodick DH. Acute cardiac tamponade: pathologic pathophysiology, diagnosis and management. Prog Cardiovasc Dis 1967;10:64–96.

52. Wiener HG, Kristensen IB, Haubek A, et al. The diagnostic value of pericardial cytology: an analysis of 95 cases. Acta Cytol 1991;35:149–53.

53. Okamoto H, Shinkai T, Yamakido M. Cardiac tamponade caused by primary lung cancer and the management of pericardial effusion. Cancer 1993;71:93–8.

54. Celermajer DS, Boyer MJ, Bailey BP, Tattersall MH. Pericardiocentesis for symptomatic malignant pericardial effusion: a study of 36 patients. Med J Austr 1991;154:19–22.

55. Mills SA, Julian S, Holliday RH, et al. Subxiphoid pericardial window for pericardial effusive disease. J Cardiovasc Surg 1989;768–73.

56. Park JS, Rentschler R, Wilbur D. Surgical management of pericardial effusion in patients with malignancies. Cancer 1991;67:76–80.

57. Moores DWO, Allen KB, Faber LP, et al. Subxiphoid pericardial drainage for pericardial tamponade. J Thorac Cardiovasc Surg 1995;109:546–52.

58. Maher EA, Shephard FA, Todd TJR. Pericardial sclerosis as the primary management of malignant pericardial effusion and cardiac tamponade. J Thorac Cardiovasc Surg 1996;112:637–43.

59. Callahan JA, Seward JB, Nishimura RA, et al. Two-dimensional echocardiography-guided pericardiocentesis: experience in 117 consecutive patients. Am J Cardiol 1985;55:476–9.

60. Kopecky SL, Callahan JA, Tajik SA, Seward JB. Percutaneous pericardial catheter drainage: report of 42 consecutive cases. Am J Cardiol 1986;58:633–5.

61. Girardi LN, Ginsberg RJ, Burt ME. Pericardiocentesis and intrapericardial sclerosis: effective therapy for malignant pericardial effusions. Ann Thorac Surg 1997;64:1422–8.

62. Martini N, Freiman AH, Watson RC, Hilaris BS. Intrapericardial instillation of radioactive chromic phosphate in malignant effusion. AJR Am J Roentgenol 1977;128:639–41.

63. Shepherd FA, Ginsberg JS, Evans WK, et al. Tetracycline sclerosis in the management of pericardial effusion. J Clin Oncol 1985;3:1678–82.

64. Vaitkus PT, Hemann HC, Le Winter MM. Treatment of malignant pericardial effusions. JAMA 1994;272:59–64.

65. Yano T, Yokoyamama H, Inoue T, et al. A simple technique to manage pericardial effusion with local instillation of bleomycin in non–small cell carcinoma of the lung. Oncology 1994;51:507–9.

66. Liu G, Crump M, Goss PE, et al. Prospective comparison of the sclerosing agents doxycycline and bleomycin for the primary management of malignant pericardial effusion and cardiac tamponade. J Clin Oncol 1996;14:3141–7.

67. Chow WH, Chow TC, Yip AS, Cheung KL. Inoue balloon pericardiotomy for patients with recurrent pericardial effusion. Angiology 1996;47:57–60.

68. Ziskind AA, Pearce AC, Lemmon CC, et al. Percutaneous balloon pericardiotomy for the treatment of cardiac tamponade and large pericardial effusions: description of technique and report of the first 50 cases. J Am Coll Cardiol 1993;21:1–5.

69. Larrey D. Clin Chir 1829;36:393.

70. Van Trigt P, Douglas J, Smith PK, et al. A prospective trial of subxiphoid pericardiotomy in the diagnosis and treatment of large pericardial effusion: a follow-up report. Ann Surg 1993;218:777–82.

71. Hazelrigg SR, Mack MJ, Landreneau RJ, et al. Thoracoscopic pericardectomy for effusive pericardial disease. Am Thorac Surg 1993;56:792–5.

72. Piehler J, Pluth J, Schaff HV, et al. Surgical management of effusive pericardial disease: influence of extent of pericardial resection on clinical course. J Thorac Cardiovasc Surg 1985;90:506–16.

73. Runyon BA. Care of patients with ascites. N Engl J Med 1994;330:337–42.

74. Parsons SL, Lang MW, Steel RJC. Malignant ascites: a two-year review from a teaching hospital. Eur J Surg Oncol 1996;22:237–9.

75. Malik I, Abubakar S, Rizwana I, et al. Clinical features and management of malignant ascites. J Pakist Med Assoc 1991;41:38–40.

76. Ringenberg QS, Doll DC, Loy TS, Yarbro NJW. Malignant ascites of unknown origin. Cancer 1989;64:753–5.

77. Megalli MR, Gursel EO, Veenema RJ. Ascites as an unusual presentation of carcinoma of the prostate. J Urol 1973;110:232–4.

78. Koeffler HP, Cline MJ. Multiple myeloma presenting as ascites. West J Med 1977;127:248–50.

79. Einhorn LH, Burgess MA, Vallejos C, et al. Prognostic correlations and response to treatment in metastatic malignant melanoma. Cancer Res 1974;34:1995–2004.

80. Hirabayshi K, Graham J. Genesis of ascites in ovarian carcinoma. Am J Obstet Gynecol 1970;106:492–7.

81. Coates G, Bush RS, Aspin N. A study of ascites using lymphoscintigraphy with 99m Tc-sulfur colloid. Radiology 1973;107:577–83.

82. Bosch J, Arroyo V, Betriu A, et al. Hepatic hemodynamics and the renin-angiotensin-aldosterone system in cirrhosis. Gastroenterology 1980;78:92–9.

83. Greenway B, Johnson PJ, Williams R. Control of malignant ascites with spironolactone. Br J Surg 1982;69:441–2.

84. Williams JW, Simel DL. Does this patient have ascites? How to divine fluid in the abdomen. JAMA 1992;267:2645–8.

85. Michaud MR. Sonographic detection of peritoneal carcinomatosis: a prospective study of 37 cases. Abdom Imaging 1995;20:47–51.

86. Low RN, Sigeti JS. MR imaging of peritoneal disease: comparison of

contrast-enhanced fast multiplanar spoiled gradient-recalled and spin echo imaging. AJR Am J Roentgenol 1994;163:1131–40.

87. Runyon BA, Hoefs JC, Morgan TR. Ascitic fluid analysis in malignancy-related ascites. Hepatology 1988;8:1104–9.

88. Sears D, Hajdu SI. The cytologic diagnosis of malignant neoplasms in pleural and peritoneal effusions. Acta Cytol 1987;31:85–97.

89. Loewenstein MS, Rittgers RA, Feinerman AE, et al. Carcinoembryonic antigen assay of ascites and detection of malignancy. Ann Intern Med 1978;88:635–8.

90. Gerbes AL, Hoermann R, Mann K, et al. Human chorionic gonadotropin-beta in the differentiation of malignancy-related and non-malignant ascites. Digestion 1996;57:113–7.

91. Chu CM, Lin SM, Peng SM, et al. The role of laparoscopy in the evaluation of ascites of unknown origin. Gastrointest Endosc 1994;40:285–9.

92. Menzies RI, Fitzgerald JM, Mulpeter K. Laparoscopic diagnosis of ascites in Lesotho. Br Med J 1985;291:473–5.

93. Pinto PC, Amerian J, Reynolds TB. Large-volume paracentesis in nonedematous patients with tense ascites: its effect on intravascular volume. Hepatology 1988;8:207–10.

94. Kao HW, Rakov NE, Savage E, et al. The effect of large-volume paracentesis on plasma volume: a cause of hypovolemia? Hepatology 1985;5:403–7.

95. Halpin TF, McCann TO. Dynamics of body fluids following the rapid removal of large volumes of ascites. Am J Obstet Gynecol 1971;110:103–6.

96. Pockros PJ, Esrason KT, Nguyen C, et al. Mobilization of malignant ascites with diuretics is dependent on ascitic fluid characteristics. Gastroenterology 1992;103:1302–6.

97. Markman M. Intracavitary chemotherapy for malignant disease confined to body cavities. West J Med 1985;142:364–8.

98. Fujimoto S, Takahashi M, Kobayashi K, et al. Cytohistologic assessment of antitumor effects of intraperitoneal hyperthermic perfusion with mitomycin-C for patients with gastric cancer and peritoneal metastases. Cancer 1992;70:2754–60.

99. Bitran JD, Brown C, Desser RK, et al. Intracavitary bleomycin for the control of malignant effusions. J Surg Oncol 1981;16:273–7.

100. Bitran J. Intraperitoneal bleomycin: pharmacokinetics and results of a phase II trial. Cancer 1985;56:2420–3.

101. Kefford RF, Woods RL, Fox RM, et al. Intracavitary Adriamycin, nitrogen mustard, and tetracycline in the control of malignant effusions: a randomized study. Med J Aust 1980;2:447–8.

102. Schilsky RL, Choi KE, Grayhack J, et al. Phase I clinical and pharmacologic study of intraperitoneal cisplatin and fluorouracil in patients with advanced intraabdominal cancer. J Clin Oncol 1990;8:2054–61.

103. Markman M, Hakes T, Reichman B, et al. Phase II trial of weekly or biweekly intraperitoneal mitoxantrone in epithelial ovarian cancer. J Clin Oncol 1991;9:978–82.

104. Lorusso V, Catino A, Gargano A, et al. Mitoxantrone in the treatment of recurrent ascites of pre-treated ovarian cancer. Eur J Gynaecol Oncol 1994;15:75–80.

105. Link KH, Hepp G, Staib L, et al. Intraperitoneal regional chemotherapy with mitoxantrone. Cancer Treat Res 1996;81:31–40.

106. Hagiwara A, Takahashi T, Kojima O, et al. Prophylaxis with carbon-absorbed mitomycin against peritoneal recurrence of gastric cancer. Lancet 1992;339:629–31.

107. Loggie BW, Perini M, et al. Treatment and prevention of malignant ascites associated with disseminated intraperitoneal malignancies by aggressive combined-modality therapy. Am Surg 1997;63:137–43.

108. Gilly FN, Carry PY, Sayag AC, et al. Regional chemotherapy (with mitomycin C) and intraoperative hyperthermia for digestive cancers with peritoneal carcinomatosis. Hepatogastroenterology 1994;41:124–9.

109. Jackson GL, Blosser NM. Intracavitary chromic phosphate ($^{32}$P) colloidal suspension therapy. Cancer 1981;48:2596–8.

110. Van Nostrand D, Siberstein EB. Therapeutic uses of $^{32}$P. In: Freeman LM, Weissmann HS, eds. Nuclear medicine annual. New York: Raven Press, 1985:285–344.

111. Bezwoda WR, Golombick T, Dansey R, Keeping J. Treatment of malignant ascites due to recurrent/refractory ovarian cancer: the use of interferon-alpha or interferon-alpha and chemotherapy in vivo and in vitro. Eur J Cancer 1991;27:1423–9.

112. Ott MG, Mannel DN, Gallati H, et al. Peripheral natural killer cell activity and intraperitoneal soluable p55 tumor necrosis factor receptor in patients with malignant ascites: two possible indicators for response to intraperitoneal combined tumor necrosis factor-alpha and interferon-gamma treatment. Cancer Immunol Immunother 1996;42:31–7.

113. Heike Y, Takahashi M, Ohira T, et al. Genetic immunotherapy by intrapleural, intraperitoneal, and subcutaneous injection of IL-2 gene modified Lewis lung carcinoma cells. Int J Cancer 1997;73:844–9.

114. Katano M, Torisu M. New approach to management of malignant ascites with a streptococcal preparation of OK-432 I, II: intraperitoneal inflammatory cell-mediated tumor cell destruction. Surgery 1983;93:357–73.

115. Perez CA, Korba A, Zivnuska F, et al. $^{60}$Co moving strip technique in the management of carcinoma of the ovary: analysis of tumor control and morbidity. Int J Radiat Oncol Biol Phys 1978;4:379–88.

116. Gough IR, Balderson GA. Malignant ascites: a comparison of peritoneovenous shunting and non-operative management. Cancer 1993;71:2377–82.

117. Helzberg JH, Greenberger NJ. Peritoneovenous shunt in malignant ascites. Dig Dis Sci 1985;30:1104–7.

118. Edney JA, Hill A, Armstrong D. Peritoneovenous shunts palliate malignant ascites. Am J Surg 1989;158:598–601.

119. Faught W, Kirkpatrick JR, Krepart GV, et al. Peritoneovenous shunt for palliation of gynecologic malignant ascites. J Am Coll Surg 1995;180:472–4.

120. Scott-Coombes DM, Whawell SA, Vipond MN, et al. Fibrinolytic activity of ascites caused by alcoholic cirrhosis and peritoneal malignancy. Gut 1993;34:1120–2.

121. Fildes J, Narvaez GP, Baig KA, et al. Pulmonary tumor embolization after peritoneovenous shunting for malignant ascites. Cancer 1988;61:1973–6.

---

# CHAPTER 104

# MANAGEMENT OF LIVER METASTASES

• NANCY KEMENY

## Natural History and Diagnosis

The liver is the primary site of metastasis for many malignant neoplasms. Gastrointestinal malignancies are especially prone to spread to the liver because of its portal venous drainage. Fifteen percent of patients with colorectal cancer already have liver metastases at the time of diagnosis[1] and 60% have liver metastases sometime during the course of their illness. Extra-abdominal tumors such as bronchogenic carcinoma, breast cancer, and malignant melanoma often spread hematogenously to the liver.

For gastrointestinal tumors, differences occur in the natural history of the hepatic metastases. In some circumstances, hepatic metastases are a sign of disseminated disease. When gastric and pancreatic cancers metastasize to the liver, the mean survival is short, and widespread metastases often exist so that radical measures such as hepatic resection or hepatic artery infusion (HAI) usually are not appropriate. In contrast, when a patient has colorectal cancer, the liver may be the sole site of metastatic disease, and a significant fraction of these patients may have isolated liver metastasis. In this setting, progress has been made in the areas of hepatic resection, regional chemotherapy, and radiation therapy, as discussed in this chapter.

The diagnosis of symptomatic liver metastases generally is not difficult. In a patient who has previously undergone treatment for colorectal malignancy, the presence of pain, weight loss, anorexia, fatigue, malaise, unexplained fever, jaundice, or virtually any unexplained symptom demands further evaluation.

The diagnosis of asymptomatic liver metastases can be more difficult. Liver function tests and determination of alkaline phosphatase (AP), prothrombin time, lactic dehydrogenase (LDH), and serum transaminases are not very sensitive.[2–4] Measurement of carcinoembryonic antigen (CEA) remains the most sensitive test for metastatic colorectal cancer, but even these results can be normal in the presence of liver metastases, especially with minimal hepatic disease or poorly differentiated tumors. In a prospective study at the City of Hope Hospital in patients with metastatic liver disease (deemed resectable by computed tomography [CT]), the average AP and LDH levels were within normal limits, whereas CEA levels were elevated in 73% of the patients.[5]

### IMAGING TECHNIQUES

The imaging modalities currently available are CT, magnetic resonance imaging (MRI), ultrasonography, computed tomographic angiography, and positron emission tomography (PET).

**Computed Tomography.** These images should be routinely evaluated by two different window settings. A soft tissue window allows evaluation of adjacent abdominal architecture, but a narrow window and a lower width (100 to 150 HU) must be used to evaluate the liver because this setting increases contrast differences between the normal liver parenchyma and abnormalities.

Contrast scanning is better than noncontrast CT for detecting tumors that are hypovascular, such as colorectal carcinomas. One problem with this modality is that lesions may not be distinguishable from liver parenchyma during the equilibrium phase of the contrast injection (when the intravascular and interstitial concentrations equilibrate).[6] Even with contrast, some benign lesions may appear malignant, such as cysts, fatty infiltration, hamartomas, adenomas, hemangiomas, and focal nodular hyperplasia.

Computed tomographic angiography uses a bolus of contrast medium that is injected into the hepatic artery (computed tomographic angiography) or via the superior mesenteric artery (computed tomographic portography). Liver imaging during the arterial phase is critical for detection of hepatocellular carcinoma. Computed tomographic portography dramatically enhances the liver parenchyma because dye returned via the portal vein gives excellent contrast to the normal liver so that metastases appear as filling defects.[6]

**Magnetic Resonance Imaging.** MRI uses T1- or T2-weighted spin echo. The T1 images generally show metastases as low-intensity lesions; in T2-weighted images, metastases are areas of high-signal intensity, which is generally superior for detection and characterization of liver masses. Benign cysts and hemangiomas are generally homogeneous and have a bright appearance (termed *a light bulb sign*), whereas metastatic lesions are more heterogeneous and not as bright.[6, 7]

**Positron Emission Tomography.** PET is an imaging modality that allows direct evaluation of cellular glucose metabolism. Studies are being performed to evaluate its usefulness for detecting early disease, finding disease missed by other diagnostic tests, and evaluating treatment. In 27 patients undergoing liver resection, PET detected disease in 11 patients whose disease was missed by conventional radiology.[8]

## Liver Resection

The experience of resecting metastatic lesions from the liver is mostly confined to colorectal cancer.[9–18] In a registry of hepatic resections for colorectal metastases compiled from multiple institutions by Hughes and colleagues,[10] the 5-year survival for those undergoing complete resection of solitary metastases was 33% (Table 104–1). No randomized study comparing resection to any other treatment modality has been performed. However, in two studies of 120 patients with solitary hepatic lesions without resection, none was alive after 3 years.[19, 20] In patients with multiple metastases, the median survival is 3 to 8 months without resection (Table 104–2).[21–23]

Many studies have demonstrated that resecting two or three hepatic lesions gives the same survival as resecting a solitary metastasis.[11, 12, 14, 16] However, in the large tumor registry,[10] the 5-year survival for patients with more than three tumors was 18% (Table 104–3).

The value of resecting four or more lesions remains debatable. In the Mayo Clinic study, only 9% of patients with three or more lesions survived 5 years,[12] whereas in the Rotterdam report, no patients with three or more lesions were alive at 5 years. In the study from Milan, the median survival for patients with solitary lesions was 36 months versus 28 months for patients with four or more lesions. In a French study[16] of 1500 patients, the 5-year survival for those with four lesions was 14% versus 30% for three or less

*Table 104–1.* **Results of Hepatic Resection for Metastatic Colorectal Cancer**

| Study | n | 5-Year Survival |
|---|---|---|
| Adson et al[132] | 141 | 25 |
| Hughes et al[10] | 607 | 33 |
| Schlag et al[133] | 122 | 30 |
| Doci et al[18] | 100 | 30 |
| Scheele et al[134] | 219 | 39 |
| Rosen et al[135] | 280 | 25 |
| Foster[136] | 78 | 22 |
| Fortner et al[137] | 75 | 35 |
| Butler et al[138] | 62 | 34 |
| Iwatsuki et al[30] | 60 | 45 |
| Nordlinger et al[16] | 80 | 25 |

*Table 104–2.* **Natural History of Untreated Colorectal Cancer**

| Reference | Stage | Survival (mo) Median* or Mean |
|---|---|---|
| Wood et al[141] | Solitary | 17 |
| | Several, one lobe | 11 |
| | Widespread, both lobes | 3 |
| Bengtsson et al[23] | <25%, one lobe | 6* |
| | 25–75% | 6 |
| | >75%, both lobes | 3 |
| Wagner et al[142] | Solitary | 21* |
| | Several, one lobe | 15 |
| | Multiple, both lobes | 10 |
| Adson[143] | Few metastases | 18 |
| | Several | 9 |
| | Multiple | 5 |
| | Solitary | 22 |
| | Widespread | 12 |
| Lahr et al[39] | Unilobar | 12 |
| | Bilobar | 4 |

nodules ($p = 0.001$). Thus the number of lesions amenable to resection remains controversial.

Prognostic variables that may affect survival include stage of primary cancer (Dukes C being worse), a high preoperative CEA level, a disease-free interval of less than 1 year, a positive margin of resection, and the size of the tumor (see Table 104–3). Extrahepatic disease and the presence of positive hepatic nodes are generally considered contraindications to hepatic resection. In one series, of patients who exhibited positive hilar lymph nodes, none was alive at 3 years.[24] Although extrahepatic disease is generally considered a contraindication for surgery, there is a report of resection of both hepatic and pulmonary metastases with a 44% 5-year survival in 30 patients.[25] The prognostic value

of the disease-free interval from the time of resection of the colorectal primary to the appearance of the hepatic metastases remains controversial. More recent studies using a 12-month or 24-month cutoff period have also found that there is a difference in survival[14, 16]; in one study, an interval of greater than 1 year produced a 5-year survival of 42% versus 24% for those with a shorter interval ($p = 0.01$).[26]

The importance of a clear margin of resection between the tumor and normal liver parenchyma has been documented.[19] Survival is definitely worse in patients with no margin,[11, 27] but there are conflicting reports on how narrow the margin can be, with some studies suggesting no difference in survival with 1 mm, 10 mm, or greater (see Table 104–3).[12]

One of the major advances in the last 15 years is that more hepatic resections are now being performed along nonanatomic lines, that is, by removal of tumor plus a rim of hepatic tissue, rather than by a formal lobectomy. With greater familiarity of the anatomic hepatic segments (Fig. 104–1),[28] resections are more frequently performed with a reduction in the amount of normal liver removed, and disease is being resected from both lobes. Operative techniques using total vascular exclusion and ultrasonic dissection (i.e., Cavitron, laser dissector, or autotransfuser) have improved results in some studies.[29]

Complications of liver resections include the following: liver insufficiency, 3 to 8%; bile leaks, 4%; perihepatic abscesses, 2 to 10%; hemorrhage, 1 to 3%; pleural effusions, 5 to 10%; and overall complications in the 20% range.[27] Mortality for experienced surgeons is less than 5% but increases greatly with less experience. Approximately 40 to 50% of patients who have hepatic resections have recurrent disease in the liver as the first sign of relapse. In the Milan study, 41% had relapse in the liver only, 28% had only extra-abdominal relapse, 13% had intra-abdominal extrahepatic relapse, and 19% had relapse in both the liver and an extrahepatic site.[30]

*Table 104–3.* **Prognostic Factors After Liver Resection**

| | Five-Year Survival (%) | | | | |
|---|---|---|---|---|---|
| | Nordlinger et al[139] | Hughes et al[10] | Scheele et al[134] | Doci et al[18] | Ooijen et al[140] |
| Dukes' B | 35* | 47* | 52* | 47* | 26 |
| Dukes' C | 26 | 23 | 31 | 24 | 11 |
| Size | | | | | |
| <5 cm | 30* | 38 | 43* | — | — |
| >5 cm | 26 | 27 | 34 | — | — |
| Disease-free interval | | | | | |
| <2 yr | 26* | — | 35 | — | — |
| >2 yr | 32 | — | 27 | — | — |
| Synchronous | — | 27* | 32* | 31 | 15* |
| Metachronous | | (>12 months) 42 | 45 | 28 | 22 |
| No. of metastases | | | | | |
| Solitary | (<3) 30 | 37* | 40 | 38 | 26* |
| Multiple | 14 | 18 | 39 | 40 | 0 |
| Margin | | | | | |
| <1 | 32* | 20 | (1–4 cm) 28* | | 13* |
| >1 | 16 | 30 | (>10 cm) 39 | | 20 |
| Margin positive | — | — | | | 11 |
| CEA | | | | | |
| <5 | 70* (2 yr) | 47* | | | |
| >30 | 56 (2 yr) | 28 | | | |

*Significant factors.
CEA, carcinoembryonic antigen.

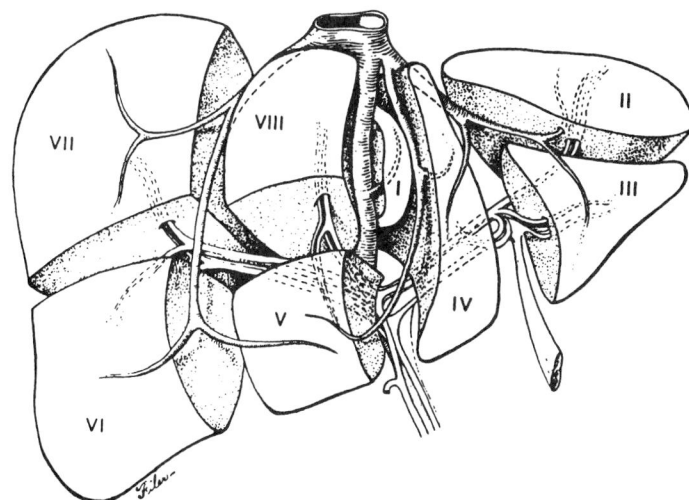

**Figure 104–1.** Couinaud's eight hepatic segments. (From Iwatsuki S, Sheahan DG, Starzl TE. The changing face of hepatic resection. Curr Probl Surg 1989;26:281–379.)

Approximately 10% of patients who have had hepatic resection can have a repeat resection, with reported survivals of 33% (50% at 3 years).[27] Some report improved survival if the interval between resections is greater than 1 year.[31]

## ADJUVANT THERAPY AFTER LIVER RESECTION

Because the recurrence of metastases is high, with 50% recurring in the liver, the use of HAI or chemotherapy after liver resection has been studied in two large randomized studies, one at Memorial Sloan-Kettering Cancer Center and one conducted by the Eastern Cooperative Oncology Group. Both studies have been completed. The first study compared HAI coupled with systemic chemotherapy to systemic therapy alone after liver resection; the second compared therapy with HAI plus systemic treatment to no further treatment after resection. Both these studies used floxuridine (FUDR) HAI versus systemic therapy or control, and in both studies there was a definite increase in survival free of hepatic metastases with the use of HAI. In the first study, the objective was an increase in 2-year survival (which was obtained—86% for HAI plus systemic vs. 72% for systemic alone, *p* = 0.03).[32] Survival free of hepatic progression was markedly improved with HAI as opposed to systemic chemotherapy (*p* < 0.001, Fig. 104–2). The results of the second

study are available only in abstract form and are still being analyzed.[32a] In two retrospective studies, there was an increase in survival and a decrease in recurrence with chemotherapy.[33, 34] In a randomized study from Germany using fluorouracil (FU) instead of FUDR for HAI chemotherapy,[35] there was no increase in survival in the HAI group.

Factors that inhibit hepatic carcinogenesis may also be useful as adjuvant therapies.[36] A study of an acyclic retinoid after resection decreased the development of new tumors in patients with hepatocellular cancer.

## FACTORS THAT HELP PREDICT SURVIVAL

The volume of disease will predict survival. In one study of patients with less than 20% involvement, the median survival was greater than 25 months, whereas for those with more than 60% involvement, the median survival was only 4 months.[37] Baseline laboratory parameters that influence survival include LDH and CEA.[22] In one study, patients whose initial LDH and CEA levels were normal had a median survival of 32 months versus only 8 months for those with abnormal values. Other studies have also shown that patients with an elevated AP level, elevated white blood cell count, or extensive liver involvement, or a combination, have worse survival rates.[22, 38, 39]

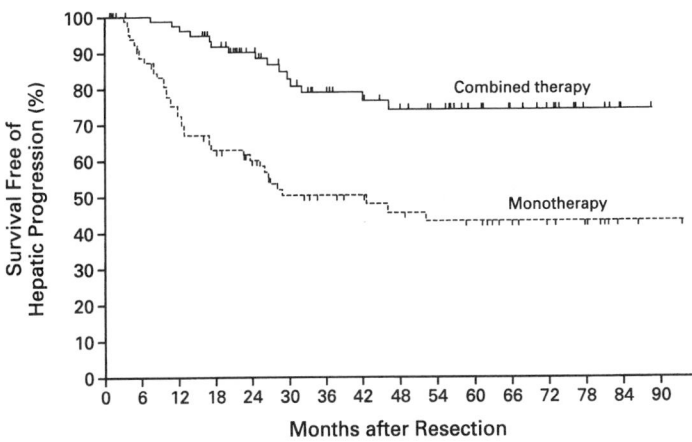

**Figure 104–2.** Kaplan-Meier estimates of survival free of hepatic progression in the group assigned to hepatic arterial infusion plus systemic chemotherapy (combined therapy) and the group assigned to systemic chemotherapy alone (monotherapy). (From Kemeny N, Huang Y, Cohen AM, et al. Hepatic arterial infusion of chemotherapy after resection of hepatic metastases from colorectal cancer. N Engl J Med 1999;341:2039–48.)

*Table 104–4.* Treatment of Metastatic Colorectal Carcinoma

| Drugs and Reference | No. of Patients | Total Response (%) | No. with Liver Metastases | Response for Liver Metastases (%) |
|---|---|---|---|---|
| 5-FU[144] | 42 | 10 | 11 | 0 |
| 5-FU[145] | 31 | 23 | 31 | 23 |
| MeCCNU + 5-FU[144] | 152 | 32 | 41 | 31 |
| MeCCNU + 5-FU[146] | 133 | 16 | 93 | 18 |
| MeCCNU + 15-FU[147] | 69 | 11 | 41 | 11 |
| MOF-Strep[147] | 75 | 32 | 60 | 37 |
| 5-FU + interferon[148] | 35 | 26 | 24 | 29 |
| 5-FU + interferon[149] | 17 | 76 | 13 | 76 |
| 5-FU + leucovorin[150] | 63 | 33 | 46 | — |
| 5-FU + low-dose leucovorin[151] | 115 | 19 | 39 | — |
| 5-FU + leucovorin[152] | 36 | 44 | 24 | — |
| CPT-11[153] | 41 | 33 | 35 | 28 |
| CPT-11[154] | 48 | 10 | 32 | 25 |
| CPT-11[155] | 121 | 13.3 | 41 | 34 |

5-FU, 5-fluorouracil; MeCCNU, methyl chloroethyl hexylnitrosourea; CPT-11, camptothecin-11 (irinotecan); MOF, methyl CCNU, vincristine, and 5-FU.

## Systemic Chemotherapy

Responses of liver metastases to systemic chemotherapy are variable, usually reflecting the response of the primary tumor. Most studies using systemic therapy for metastatic disease do not differentiate patients who have only liver metastases from those with generalized metastatic disease, making it difficult to draw conclusions about the usefulness of systemic chemotherapy to treat liver metastases; however, from the data available, the response to systemic chemotherapy is low.

In breast cancer, one[40] review demonstrated a 20% response in liver metastases versus 32% and 27% in soft tissue and osseous metastases, respectively. Although combination chemotherapy has substantially improved the response rates obtained in treating breast cancer, liver metastases from the breast still have a lower response rate than does soft tissue or pulmonary disease.

In patients with colorectal cancer, the liver is the most common site of dissemination, and up to 70% of patients with any metastatic disease develop liver metastases.[41] Table 104–4 lists chemotherapy trials in patients with colorectal cancer; the response of liver metastases is listed separately. The overall response rate shown in Table 104–4 is usually low, as is the response of liver metastases to systemic therapy. In other gastrointestinal tumors that metastasize to the liver, such as gastric and pancreatic cancer, the response rates for liver metastases are similar to the overall response rate.

## Hepatic Arterial Chemotherapy

The rationale for hepatic arterial chemotherapy has an anatomic and pharmacologic basis:

1. Liver metastases are perfused almost exclusively by the hepatic artery, whereas normal hepatocytes derive their blood supply mainly from the portal vein.[42]

2. Certain drugs are extracted by the liver during the first pass, resulting in high local concentrations with minimal systemic toxicity. There is a 400-fold extraction advantage for FUDR when it is infused into the hepatic artery rather than intravenously. The pharmacologic advantages of various chemotherapeutic agents (Table 104–5) have been reported.[43–45]

3. Drugs with a high total body clearance are more useful for hepatic infusion[46] because drugs that are not cleared rapidly recirculate through the systemic circulation.

4. The liver is often the first site of metastatic disease through hematogenous spread via the portal vein; thus, aggressive treatment of metastases confined to the liver may increase survival.[47]

Regional hepatic arterial therapy can be performed by using either a hepatic arterial port or a percutaneously placed catheter connected to an external pump or to a totally implantable pump. Early studies with percutaneously placed hepatic artery catheters produced high response rates, but complications such as clotting of the catheters and bleeding led physicians to abandon this method. New and old studies using this technique are listed in Tables 104–6 and 104–7.

When percutaneous placement of the hepatic artery catheter is compared with surgical placement of a catheter or a reservoir, the number of days chemotherapy can be administered will be 25, 34, or 115 days, respectively.[48] The develop-

*Table 104–5.* Drugs for Hepatic Arterial Infusion

| Drug | Half-life (min) | Estimated Increased Exposure by Hepatic Arterial Infusion |
|---|---|---|
| 5-FU | <10 | 5- to 10-fold |
| 5-FUDR | <10 | 100- to 400-fold |
| BCNU | <5 | 6- to 7-fold |
| Mitomycin C | <10 | 6- to 8-fold |
| Cisplatin | 20–30 | 4- to 7-fold |
| Doxorubicin (Adriamycin) | 60 | 2-fold |
| Dichloromethotrexate (DCMTX) | — | 6- to 8-fold |

5-FU, 5-fluorouracil; 5-FUDR, floxuridine; BCNU, bis-chloroethyl-nitrosourea (carmustine).

*Table 104–6.* Hepatic Artery Infusion with External Pump and Fluorouracil Infusion

| Reference | No. of Patients | Dose of Fluorouracil | Response (%) | Catheter Complications or Bleed (%) |
|---|---|---|---|---|
| Tandon et al[156] | 122 | 25 mg/kg × 9 days | 65 | 42 |
| Ansfield et al[157] | 419 | 25 mg/kg × 4 days | 55 | 21 |
| Watkins et al[158] | 184 | 2 mg/kg × 10 days | 71 | 28 |
| Smiley et al[159] | 166 | 25 mg/kg × 4 days | 25 | 30 |
| Metzger et al[160] | 30 | 2 g/m² × 5 days | 57 | 33 |
| Denck et al[161] | 50 | 6 g/m² × 3 days | 58 | 5 |
| Schlag et al[133] | 33 | 1 g/m² × 5 days | 27 | 20 |
| Rougier et al[162] | 43 | 1 g/m² weekly | 56 | 65 |
| Borner et al[163] | 28 | 750 mg/m² × 5 days | 50 | 61 |

ment of a totally implantable pump has allowed long-term HAI with good patency of the catheter and a low incidence of infection.[49] Table 104–8 lists some of the phase II studies using an implantable pump with FUDR infusion for the treatment of colorectal carcinoma.

**Randomized Studies.** To assess the impact of HAI on tumor response and survival, randomized studies have been conducted (Table 104–9). At Memorial Sloan-Kettering Cancer Center,[50] HAI using FUDR was compared with systemic FUDR infusion. In patients randomized to systemic therapy, crossover from systemic therapy to HAI was permitted. Of the 99 evaluable patients, partial responses were seen in 53% and 21% of the HAI and systemic groups, respectively ($p = 0.001$). Of the patients who crossed over from systemic to HAI therapy, 25% had a partial response after the crossover and 60% had a decrease in CEA levels. The median survivals for the HAI and systemic groups were 17 and 12 months, respectively ($p = 0.424$). The interpretation of survival is difficult because 60% of the patients receiving systemic therapy crossed over. Those who did not cross over had a median survival of 8 months compared with 18 months for those who crossed over to HAI ($p = 0.04$) (Fig. 104–3).

In a similar randomized study conducted by the Northern California Oncology Group,[51] of the 117 eligible patients, 42% responded to HAI and 10% responded to the systemic therapy ($p < 0.001$). The median time to progression was 401 and 201 days for HAI and systemic groups, respectively ($p = 0.009$), whereas median survivals were 503 days and

484 days, respectively. Although a crossover design was not built into the study, 43% of the patients receiving systemic therapy eventually received HAI, which may have obscured survival differences because the crossover patients had a doubling of survival in comparison to the noncrossover group.

Of the 64 patients in a National Cancer Institute study,[52] the response rates were 62% and 17% for the HAI and systemic groups, respectively ($p < 0.003$). Interpretation of survival data is difficult, because 34% of the HAI group never received chemotherapy, and 38% of the HAI group had positive portal lymph nodes. Despite these limitations, in the subset of patients without extrahepatic disease, the 2-year survival was 47% in the HAI group versus 13% in the systemic group ($p = 0.03$).

In another small study conducted by the Mayo Clinic (69 patients),[53] objective tumor response was observed in 48% and 21% of patients in the HAI and systemic groups, respectively ($p = 0.02$), and the time to hepatic progression was 15.7 and 6 months, respectively ($p = 0.001$). Despite the increase in response rate and time to hepatic progression, survival was similar in the two groups (12.6 and 10.5 months, respectively). However, this survival information is difficult to interpret because 48% of the HAI groups either were not adequately treated or had extrahepatic disease.

A French trial of 163 patients reported response rates of 49% in the HAI group and 14% in the systemic groups.[54] Median time to hepatic progression was 15 and 6 months,

*Table 104–7.* Hepatic Arterial Therapy with Combination Therapy

| Investigator | No. of Patients | Dose (mg/m²) | % Response | Median Survival (mo) |
|---|---|---|---|---|
| Cortesi et al[164] | 109 | FU 500 × 5 days Cisplatin 24 × 5 days | 46 | 16 |
| Warren et al[165] | 31 | FU 1500 × 24 hr LV 400 weekly × 6 days | 48 | 17 |
| Sugihara[166] | 58 | FU 360 × 7 days then 100 × 7 days | 50 | 11 |
| Kerr et al[167] | 43 | LV 200 FU 400 then FU 1800-22 hr | 36 | — |
| Howell et al[168] | 40 | LV 200 FU 400 then FU 1600-22 hr q 2 wk | 46 | 19 |
| Patt et al[62] | 48 | Interferon 5 mU FU 1000 × 5 hr q wk | 33 | 15 |
| Arai et al[169] | 32 | FU 1000 × 5 hr q wk | 78 | 25 |
| Hidalgo et al[170] | 31 | Carbo 55 FU 900 × 5 days | 51 | 26 |

*Table 104–8.* Hepatic Arterial FUDR Infusion with Internal Pump: Response and Toxicity

| Reference | No. of Patients | Partial Response | Ulcer (%) | ↑ Bilirubin (%) | Median Survival (mo) |
|---|---|---|---|---|---|
| Niederhuber et al[49] | 70 | 83 | 8 | 24 | 25 |
| Balch et al[171] | 50 | 83 | 6 | 23 | 20 |
| Kemeny et al[172] | 41 | 73 | 29 | 22 | 12 |
| Shepard et al[173] | 53 | 42 | 20 | 24 | 17 |
| Cohen et al[174] | 50 | 32 | 40 | 25 | — |
| Weiss et al[175] | 17 | 51 | 11 | 23 | 13 |
| Schwartz et al[176] | 23 | 29 | — | 20 | 18 |
| Johnson et al[177] | 40 | 15 | 8 | 13 | 12 |
| Kemeny et al[55] | 31 | 47 | 6 | — | 22 |

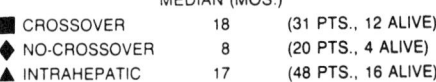

| | MEDIAN (MOS.) | |
|---|---|---|
| ■ CROSSOVER | 18 | (31 PTS., 12 ALIVE) |
| ◆ NO-CROSSOVER | 8 | (20 PTS., 4 ALIVE) |
| ▲ INTRAHEPATIC | 17 | (48 PTS., 16 ALIVE) |

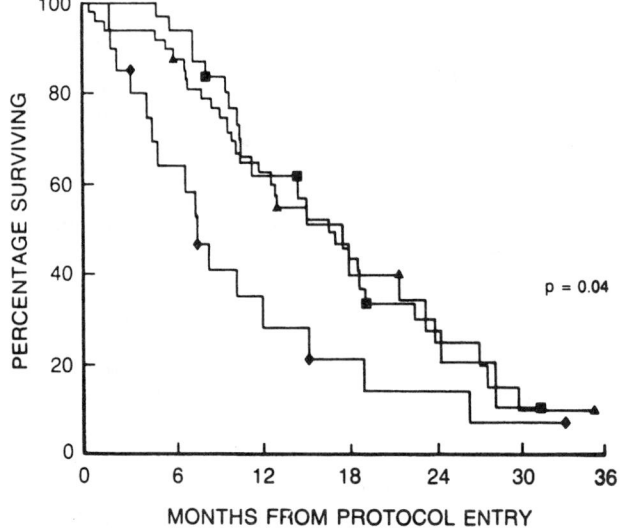

**Figure 104–3.** Kaplan-Meier survival curves from a Memorial Sloan–Kettering Study of hepatic artery infusion versus systemic infusion chemotherapy for liver metastases from colorectal cancer. (From Kemeny N, Daly J, Reichman B, et al. Intrahepatic or systemic infusion of fluorodeoxyuridine in patients with liver metastases from colorectal carcinoma. Ann Intern Med 1987;107:459.)

*Table 104–9.* Randomized Studies of Intrahepatic Versus Systemic Chemotherapy for Hepatic Metastases from Colorectal Cancer: Response

| Study | No. of Patients | Response | | Survival | |
|---|---|---|---|---|---|
| | | HAI | SYSTEMIC | HAI | SYSTEMIC |
| Memorial Sloan-Kettering[50] | 162 | 52 | 20 | 18 | 12 |
| NCOG[51] | 143 | 42* | 10 | 16.6 | 16 |
| NCI[52] | 64 | 62* | 17 | 20 | 11 |
| Consortium[179] | 43 | 58* | 38 | — | — |
| City of Hope[180] | 41 | 56 | 0 | — | — |
| Mayo Clinic[53] | 69 | 48* | 21 | 12.6 | 10.5 |
| French[54] | 163 | 49* | 14 | 15* | 11 |
| English[181] | 100 | 50* | 0 | 13* | 6.3 |

*Significant difference.
HAI, hepatic arterial infusion; NCOG, Northern California Oncology Group; NCI, National Cancer Institute.

and median survival was 14 and 10 months for the HAI and systemic groups, respectively. The 2-year survival was 22% for HAI and 10% for the systemic group ($p<0.02$). One of the criticisms of this trial is that some patients in the systemic group received chemotherapy only when they became symptomatic.

In a similar study carried out in England, quality of life and survival were significantly improved for the HAI group. Median survival was 405 and 198 days in the HAI and systemic groups, respectively ($p = 0.03$). The number of days with good quality of life was doubled in the HAI group. However, this study was also flawed because patients in the systemic arm were given chemotherapy only when they became symptomatic.

**Toxicity of Hepatic Arterial Floxuridine Infusion.** The most serious problem with the use of FUDR via HAI is hepatic toxicity (Table 104–10; see also Table 104–8).[55, 56] The bile ducts derive their blood supply almost exclusively from the hepatic artery and thus are undoubtedly perfused with high doses of chemotherapeutic agents.[57, 178]

In patients who develop jaundice, endoscopic retrograde cholangiopancreatography may demonstrate lesions resembling idiopathic sclerosing cholangitis in 5 to 29% of these patients.[55] Since the ducts are sclerotic, sonograms usually do not show dilatation. In some patients, the strictures may be focal, at the hepatic duct bifurcation, and drainage procedures may be helpful.[56] Duct obstruction from metastases should first be excluded by CT of the liver. To avoid biliary complications, it is necessary to closely monitor liver function. If the serum bilirubin increases to 3 mg/dl or higher, no further treatment should be given.

Severe ulcer disease results from inadvertent perfusion of the stomach and duodenum with drugs via small collateral branches from the hepatic artery; this outcome can be prevented via careful dissection of these collaterals at the time of pump placement. Myelosuppression, nausea, vomiting, and diarrhea normally do not occur; thus, if there is diarrhea, shunting to the bowel should be suspected.[58]

Three approaches have been used to decrease hepatic toxicity: (1) hepatic infusion of dexamethasone, (2) the use of FU instead of FUDR, and (3) the use of circadian rhythm. In a randomized study of FUDR with dexamethasone (Dex) versus FUDR alone, there was a trend toward decreased bilirubin elevation and an increase in the response rate. With FUDR and Dex versus FUDR alone, the response rate was 71% and 45%, respectively.[59] A weekly hepatic arterial bolus of FU does not cause hepatobiliary toxicity; however, it frequently produces treatment-limiting systemic toxicity or arteritis. Two studies that alternated FUDR HAI and FU HAI reported a low rate of biliary sclerosis.[60, 61] Patt and colleagues, using HAI of FU and interferon in FU- and leucovorin-refractory patients, produced a 33% response rate with a median survival of 15 months and no hepatobiliary toxicity.[62]

In a nonrandomized study at the University of Minnesota, a comparison was conducted of constant (flat) infusion versus circadian-modified hepatic arterial FUDR infusion. The group with circadian modification received 68% of each daily dose between 3:00 PM and 9:00 PM. The patients with circadian-modified infusion tolerated almost twice the daily dose of FUDR, with decreased hepatic toxicity, as did patients receiving flat infusions, but it was not a prospective randomized study.[63]

**Technical Aspects.** It is necessary to mobilize the entire gastroduodenal (GDA) artery from its takeoff from the common hepatic artery to the first portion of the duodenum; all branches distal to the catheter that supply the stomach, duodenum, bile duct, or pancreas must be identified and ligated. Frequently, branches to the pancreas and duodenum arise from the posterior aspect of the GDA.

The GDA is ligated with a nonabsorbable tie at the level of the first portion of the duodenum, the catheter inserted up to but not beyond the junction of the hepatic artery. If the catheter protrudes into the common hepatic artery, turbulence of the blood flow can lead to thrombosis of the vessel. Perfusion of both lobes of the liver is confirmed at the end of the procedure by infusing 5 ml half-strength fluorescein through the side port and then flushing the side port with heparinized saline. Following surgery and prior to beginning chemotherapy, a macroaggregated albumin scan should be performed to identify extrahepatic or incomplete perfusion. Patients with portal vein occlusion are excluded because of the risk of liver infarction if the hepatic artery should occlude during surgery or while the patient is receiving chemotherapy. A common technical error during pump insertion is placing the pump catheter tip too far from the junction of the GDA and hepatic artery. The segment of GDA is then continuously exposed to full-dose chemotherapy and may eventually thrombose.

**New Studies.** The use of other agents with FUDR has increased response rates. The addition of leucovorin to HAI FUDR produced an overall response rate of 62%, but 15% of patients developed biliary sclerosis. The toxicity of the combination was higher than FUDR alone, but the survival was improved: 86% of the patients were alive at 1 year, 62% at 2 years, 33% at 3 years, and 10% at 5 years (see Table 104–11).[64, 65]

*Table 104–10.* **Randomized Studies of Hepatic Arterial Infusion Versus Systemic Toxicity**

| Study | Hepatic Arterial Infusion (%) | Systemic (%) |
|---|---|---|
| Memorial Sloan-Kettering Cancer Center | | |
| Ulcer | 16 | 6 |
| Bil >3 | 18 | 4 |
| Diarrhea | 2 | 70 |
| Northern California Oncology Group | | |
| Bil grade 3 | 16 | 0 |
| Diarrhea | 0 | 18 |
| National Cancer Institute | | |
| Bil >3 | 33 | 0 |
| Ulcer | 16 | 0 |
| Diarrhea | 0 | 59 |
| Mayo Clinic | | |
| Hepatitis | 26 | 0 |
| Gastritis | 13 | 0 |
| Diarrhea | 0 | 18 |
| French Trial | | |
| Sclerosing cholangitis | 35 | 0 |

Bil, bilirubin (mg/dL).

*Table 104–11.* **Previously Untreated Patients with Colorectal Cancer: Comparison of Systemic and Hepatic Arterial Infusion Trials**

| Treatment | No. of Patients | % Response | Survival 1 YEAR | Survival 2 YEARS |
|---|---|---|---|---|
| Systemic | | | | |
| FU + LV[182] | 803 | 11 | 45 | 20 |
| FU + LV[183] | 422 | 18 | 45 | 25 |
| CPT-11[153] | 41 | 30 | 40 | 25 |
| HAI | | | | |
| FUDR + LV[65] | 64 | 66 | 82 | 71 |
| FUDR + Dex + LV[69] | 32 | 78 | 91 | 76 |
| FUDR + Dex[59] | 25 | 71 | 85 | 45 |
| Mit + FUDR + Dex[68] | 37 | 73 | 80 | 38 |
| FUDR Alone[50] | 50 | 50 | 76 | 42 |

FU, fluorouracil; LV, leucovorin; CPT-11, camptothecin-11; FUDR, floxuridine; Dex, dexamethasone; Mit, mitomycin C.

New agents such as irinotecan have shown no advantage when given by HAI. Some alkylating agents such as fotemustine may have a regional advantage because of a high total-body clearance and a short plasma half-life.[66] A randomized trial of mitomycin-C, bischloroethylnitrosourea (BCNU), and FUDR versus FUDR alone in previously treated patients[67] produced a 48% and 24% response rate, respectively, in those who were previously treated for metastatic disease.

The use of high-dose mitomycin C via the side port, with FUDR and dexamethasone in the body of the pump, increased response rate, especially in previously treated patients (i.e., 65% of previously treated patients responded). The toxicity, however, was increased, with 16% developing biliary sclerosis[68] and some patients also developing biliary abscesses or bilomas.

To further increase response rate without an increase in toxicity, Dex was added to the combination of FUDR and leucovorin.[69] The response rate was 78% in previously untreated patients, with only 3% developing sclerosing cholangitis. In patients who had received previous chemotherapy, the response rate was 52%. The median survival was 24.8 months and the 1- and 2-year survivals were 91% and 57%, respectively (Tables 104–11 and 104–12). Although hepatic arterial therapy is applicable to a minority of patients with metastatic colorectal carcinoma (those with hepatic metastases only), it may be the best available therapy for these patients. Therefore, the Cancer and Leukemia Group B is conducting a study comparing HAI to systemic therapy without a crossover. The trial will also include a detailed analysis of both cost and quality of life; it must also obtain molecular markers—such as thymidylate synthetase and mutated p53—to address whether these markers affect survival or response. Patients with other tumors may also benefit from HAI. Patients with breast cancer can have reasonable responses to HAI after disease progresses on systemic therapy. Responses range from 19 to 73%, with six of nine studies reporting responses greater than 50% (Table 104–13). HAI therapy for liver metastases from gastric cancer is not used frequently because gastric cancer usually metastasizes to other areas. However, responses of 62% have been reported, with a median survival of 12 months.[70]

## Hepatic Arterial Embolization

Hepatic arterial ligation (HAL) and embolization have been used to reduce the tumor's blood supply because hepatic metastases as well as primary liver tumors derive their blood supply from the hepatic artery.[71] HAL may produce a benefit of only short duration because of the rapid development of collateral vessels. By using transient or particle occlusion of the hepatic artery (hepatic artery embolization [HAE]), the development of a collateral blood supply may be minimized;

*Table 104–12.* **Previously Treated Patients with Colorectal Cancer**

| Treatment | No. of Patients | % Response | Survival 1 YEAR | Survival 2 YEARS |
|---|---|---|---|---|
| Systemic | | | | |
| CPT-11[184] | 127 | 4 | 45 | |
| CPT-11[185] | 189 | 13 | 36 | |
| HAI | | | | |
| FUDR + Dex + LV | 29 | 50 | 66 | 28 |
| Mit + FUDR + Dex[68] | 37 | 64 | 74 | 32 |
| Mit + BCNU + FUDR[67] | 37 | 47 | 60 | 21 |
| FUDR alone[67] | | 33 | 60 | 10 |

CPT-11, camptothecin-11; HAI, hepatic arterial infusion; FUDR, floxuridine; Dex, dexamethasone; Mit, mitomycin C; BCNU, bis-chloroethyl-nitrosourea.

*Table 104–13.* Hepatic Arterial Infusion for Breast Cancer*

| Investigators | No. of Patients | Partial Response (%) | Median Survival (mo) |
|---|---|---|---|
| Fraschini et al[186] | 34 | 33 | 11 |
| Estape et al[187] | 16 | 50 | 16 |
| Lange and Minton[188] | 9 | 89 | |
| Fraschini et al[189] | 25 | 52 | 11† |
| Fraschini et al[190] | 26 | 19 | 11 |
| Fraschini et al[191] | 15 | 73 | |
| Maral et al[192] | 17 | 53 | 18‡ |
| Maral et al[192] | 45 | 37 | 7.5 |
| Arai et al[193] | 56 | 81 | 12.5 |

*Most studies consist of patients whose tumor progressed after previous systemic chemotherapy.
†Median survival for responders.
‡Includes colon cancer.

this also provides the opportunity for retreatment because only the microvasculature is occluded.[72]

HAE has a definite role in highly vascular tumors such as neuroendocrine tumors of the liver.[73] These tumors usually grow slowly, and a reduction in tumor bulk can result in significant palliation. Some of the studies using HAE are listed in Table 104–14; all demonstrate an improvement in symptoms and a decrease in hormone levels. Gelfoam (absorbable gelatin sponge; size 1 to 2 mm), one of the agents used for embolization, does not lead to peripheral vascular occlusion and has an inconsistent duration of occlusion (owing to absorption), whereas polyvinyl sponge (Ivalon) (size 150 to 500 μm), a smaller particle, allows more peripheral occlusion and is not absorbable, producing a more persistent arterial occlusion.[74–76] A collagen particle (Angiostat, size 20 to 250 μm) and a biodegradable albumin microsphere (size 15 to 40 μm) are currently being tested, especially in combination with chemotherapy.

The complications of embolization are nausea, vomiting, fever, pain, and changes in liver function test results. Problems less commonly encountered include (1) injury of the gallbladder by retrograde flow through the cystic artery, (2) ischemic necrosis of the bowel by embolization of one of the vessels to the intestinal tract, (3) pancreatic infarction and pancreatitis by embolization of one of the pancreatic vessels, and (4) dyspnea by embolization of the lungs.[74–79] Interference with hepatic blood flow can exacerbate the underlying liver disease and can be dangerous in patients

with portal venous thrombosis, which is present more often in patients with primary liver tumors than in those with metastatic disease. Rarely, embolization will cause a reversal of tumor-induced portal vein thrombus. In neuroendocrine tumors responding to HAE, rapid cell death may result in tumor lysis syndrome, with symptomatic hyperuricemia leading to uric acid nephropathy and oliguria. Vigorous hydration and prophylactic allopurinol may prevent this problem. In carcinoid tumors, HAE may cause a life-threatening carcinoid crisis from the rapid release of hormones from tumor cells. Somatostatin analogues may be given prior to the procedure or if a carcinoid crisis occurs.[80] To avoid some of the serious complications of HAE, patients with cirrhosis, portal vein occlusion, and biliary tract obstruction are usually excluded from such treatment.

## Chemoembolization

A local entrapment of drug in the embolization agent (chemoembolization) provides a prolonged exposure of the tumor to the drug with less systemic drug circulation. Nonrandomized studies have suggested that the addition of chemotherapy to the embolic agent (Angiostat) produced an increase in response rate over the embolic agent alone.[81] In a study by Venook and colleagues,[82] patients with unresectable hepatocellular carcinoma were treated with Gelfoam and

*Table 104–14.* Neuroendocrine Tumors

| References | Agent | No. of Patients | Biochemical or Symptomatic Response (%) | Tumor Response (%) |
|---|---|---|---|---|
| *Hepatic Artery Ligation* | | | | |
| Martin et al[77] | | 8 | 76 | |
| Moertel[78] | | 10 | 70 | |
| Melia et al[79] | | 6 | 50 | 17 |
| *Hepatic Artery Embolization* | | | | |
| Carrasco et al[75] | Gelfoam | 23 | 87 | — |
| Ajani et al[74] | Ivalon + Gelfoam | 22 | | 60 |
| Marlink et al[76] | Gelfoam | 10 | 100 | 90 |
| Maton et al[194] | Lyodura | 13 | 76 | — |

*Table 104–15.* Chemoembolization for Colon Cancer

| Reference | No. of Patients | Agent | Partial Response (%) | Median Survival (mo) |
|---|---|---|---|---|
| Daniels et al[195] | 55 | Mit C Collagen Cisplatin Doxorubicin | 34 | |
| Stuart et al[196] | 20 | Mit C FU | 59 | 7 |
| Tellez et al[197] | 30 | Mit C Ethiodized oil Gelatin Angiostat | 62 | 8 |
| Link et al[198] | 17 | Cisplatin Doxorubicin (Adriamycin) Mit C Lipiodol | 0 | 7 |
| Lang and Brown[199] | 46 | Doxorubicin (Adriamycin) Lipiodol | 17 | |
| Stagg et al[200] | 12 | Doxorubicin Gelfoam | 0 | |
| Martinelli et al[201] | 13 | Doxorubicin Mit C Cisplatin Polyvinyl Alcohol | 24 | 9.3 |
| Hidalgo et al[170] | 31 | FU Interferon Carboplatin FU | 51 | 26 |

Mit C, mitomycin C; FU, fluorouracil.

a mixture of three drugs—doxorubicin, mitomycin C, and cisplatin—given via a percutaneous hepatic artery catheter. Twelve (24%) had a partial response, and a 50% reduction in alpha-fetoprotein was seen in 68% of patients. Using this technique for neuroendocrine tumors, there was a 33% partial response, with a reduction in hormone levels,[83] and a median survival of 7 months (range, 3 months to 3 years). The response rates and survival in trials of chemoembolization for colorectal metastases are listed in Table 104–15.

Lipiodol (iodized oil contrast) has been found to remain selectively in the primary and secondary liver cancers when injected into the hepatic artery, allowing visualization of tumors as small as 4 mm. Thus, Lipiodol can be used to deliver either chemotherapy or local radiation such as irradiation with iodine 131 ($^{131}$I).[84] In a study of three groups of patients treated with (1) gelatin sponge, Lipiodol, and doxorubicin, (2) doxorubicin and Lipiodol, or (3) doxorubicin alone,[85] the lowest systemic doxorubicin plasma area under the curve:plasma decay curve concentration versus time (AUC) was seen in the first group. The mean AUC of doxorubicin was 740, 1400, and 1430 ng/ml for the three groups, respectively. The group receiving all three substances also had the highest tumor necrosis rate. Other investigators using Lipiodol also saw reasonable response rates and survival (Table 104–16). In a retrospective analysis of 343 patients with hepatocellular cancer who underwent

*Table 104–16.* Chemoembolization with Lipiodol for Hepatocellular Carcinoma

| Reference | No. of Patients | Agents | Partial Response (%) | % Survival (Yr) 1 | 2 | 3 |
|---|---|---|---|---|---|---|
| Konno[202] | 323 | Neocarzinostatin | 58 | 84 | 47 | 37 |
| Ichida et al[203] | 50 | Epi Cisplatin TAE | | 80 | 67 | |
| Civalleri et al[204] | 37 | Mitoxantrone Lipiodol Gelfoam | 33 | 79 | | |
| Inoue et al[205] | 76 | Lipiodol Adr Mito Cisplatin | 51 | 68 | 41 | |
| Yodono[206] | 45 | VP16, Cisplatin, FU | 46 | 68 | 44 | 35 |
| Ngan et al[207] | 80 | Cisplatin | 80 | 55 | 38 | |
| Stuart et al[208] | 52 | Dox gelatin | 43 | 60 | 45 | |
| Rougier et al[209] | 232 | Dox Gelfoam Lipiodol | 41 | | | |

Epi, epirubicin; TAE, transcatheter embolization; Adr, Adriamycin; Mito, mitomycin C; FU, fluorouracil; dox, doxorubicin.

chemoembolization, those who received Lipiodol had a significantly longer survival.[86] Whether chemotherapy adds to Lipiodol embolization is not clear. A large retrospective analysis found no benefit when chemotherapy was added to embolization.[87] A similar study using cisplatin and embolization versus embolization alone showed no differences in survival.[88] Raoul and colleagues randomized 142 patients with hepatocellular cancer to receive [131]I and Lipiodol or chemoembolization with cisplatin. The 1- and 2-year survivals were 42% and 22%, and 38% and 22%, respectively. Tolerance was reported to be better with [131]I.[84]

There are reports that embolization does not increase survival.[89, 90] Pelletier and colleagues randomized patients to chemoembolization versus symptomatic treatment and found no difference in 1- and 2-year survivals.[89] Another, larger French study also concluded that embolization does not improve survival.[90]

Another form of chemoembolization is to enclose the chemotherapeutic agents in a microsphere. Degradable starch microspheres injected intra-arterially are trapped in an extra-capillary network formed in liver metastases and can be used for chemoembolization.[91, 92] Drugs or monoclonal antibodies[93] dissolved in the microsphere suspension will be retained in the blood vessels of the target organ as long as the blood flow is blocked, and they will then gradually release the chemotherapeutic agents, resulting in a longer duration of tumor exposure to the drug. The most appropriate agents for microspheres include agents such as mitomycin C, which are preferentially toxic to cells under hypoxic conditions. In a rabbit study, the mean tumor drug level was significantly higher when the drug was used with the microsphere when compared with the drug alone.[94] Radioembolization attempts have been made using glass microspheres containing yttrium 90,[95–97] or [131]I-labeled Lipiodol.[98]

## Cryosurgery

Cryosurgery is a selective safe freezing of tumors by in situ destruction of tissue using subzero temperatures. The rapid freeze-thaw of tissues results in cellular damage and death, and cancer cells cannot exist through the stages of cooling, freezing, and thawing.[99] One advantage of cryosurgery is the ability to use local treatment without sacrificing normal tissue. Two technical developments improved the use of cryosurgery: (1) cryoprobes cooled by liquid nitrogen allowed more precise freezing even within the liver and (2) intraoperative ultrasonography allowed precise placement of the cryoprobe and more accurate monitoring of the freezing process. In a series of 32 patients with liver tumors (24 with colorectal carcinoma),[100] 28% remained free of disease from 5 to 60 months. Onik and associates[101] reported that 4 of 18 patients had complete remission, with a median survival of 28 months, whereas 14 patients were considered inadequately treated and had a 21-month median survival.

Morris and Ross[102] reported 67 patients undergoing cryosurgery; 75% had an increase in CEA by 6 months. Occasionally the surgeon believes that all disease has been destroyed, but PET after cryosurgery can demonstrate that tumor is left behind. The 2-year survival after cryosurgery has been reported to be as high as 72%. The series with the

highest survival may reflect the type of patients selected, that is, those with smaller tumors and fewer metastases.[103]

Adam and colleagues[104] reported a 2-year survival of 50% for patients with colorectal metastases versus 67% for patients with hepatocellular carcinoma, with a local recurrence rate of 44%. Since local recurrence is high, the use of HAI after cryosurgery may be useful. One small, nonrandomized study doubled survival by using HAI after cryosurgery.[105] Other trials are now evaluating the use of HAI with or without systemic therapy.

Cryoablation can also be used following hepatic resection with close margins or to remove central lesions. Cryoprobes can be used as a handle to assist in segmental resections. An ice ball is produced with 1 cm margins around the tumor, and the probe is then used for traction so that a segmental resection can be performed.[106]

Technical issues involving cryosurgery include (1) adequate hydration before surgery because myoglobinuria and tumor lysis may occur, (2) attention to bile ducts because biliary fistula may occur, (3) two freeze-thaw cycles are preferred, and (4) the probe should not be pulled or twisted vigorously because that may cause cracking.[100]

Complications include hepatic cracking secondary to the thermal stresses that occur during rapid freezing; these are usually associated with hemorrhage, which may require packing. Other complications include biliary fistula, requiring percutaneous drainage and myoglobinuria, resulting in acute tubular necrosis.

Except in clinical trials,[107] cryosurgery should not replace surgical resection if resection is feasible.

## Percutaneous Ethanol Injection

In percutaneous ethanol injection therapy (PEIT), up to 30 ml of absolute ethanol is injected into the lesion under ultrasonographic guidance.[108] In patients with primary hepatocellular carcinoma, this treatment can produce 5-year survivals of 43%. Susuki and colleagues[109] assigned 42 patients with hepatocellular carcinoma smaller than 3 cm to three groups: (1) chemotherapy and Lipiodol (C-LIP), (2) C-LIP followed by gelatin sponge transcatheter embolization (TAE), or (3) PEIT. They demonstrated a decrease in local recurrence with PEIT. Local recurrences at 1 year were 61%, 29%, and 20% for groups 1, 2 and 3, respectively. In pooled data on 11,000 patients with hepatocellular carcinoma from Japan, the 3-year survival for surgical resection, PEIT, or embolization was 58%, 53%, and 20%, respectively. However, others report a higher recurrence rate after PEIT versus surgical resection.[110]

The size of the lesion also affects outcome. In an Italian study on 26 patients with metastatic disease, 5 patients with lesions smaller than 2 cm had responses, whereas no response was seen in the 6 patients with lesions greater than 4 cm.[111] In a randomized study of TAE versus TAE and PEIT, the 3-year survival was 20% and 50%, respectively ($p = 0.05$)[112]

## New Therapies

Some new therapies that are being developed include isolation perfusion, microwave coagulation, and gene therapy.

The liver can be isolated by clamping the hepatic arteries, vena cava, and portal vein and then placing a catheter in the hepatic artery to perfuse the liver. Trials using the technique have been performed with L-phenylalanine mustard (melphalan, L-PAM), FU, and mitomycin C.[113] Hyperthermic isolation perfusion of tumor necrosis factor and melphalan produced a 75% response rate.[114]

Because cancer cells may be more sensitive to heat owing to decreased vasodilation capacity of the neurovascular bed,[115] microwave coagulation can also be used. In one study, 28 of 31 nodules from hepatocellular carcinoma underwent complete tumor ablation, and 10 of the 19 patients are still free of disease (follow-up 14 to 64 months).[116]

Gene therapies have been hampered by the ability to get the therapy to the tumor. Tumors largely restricted to the liver (primary or metastatic) can potentially be treated by gene therapy because gene transfer agents can be injected locally into tumor or via the hepatic artery. One trial involves the use of an adenovirus vector carrying the wild-type p53 gene. Alteration in p53 function is present in more than half of all malignancies and re-expression of wild-type p53 can result in apoptosis and tumor shrinkage in rodents. A phase I study of recombinant adenovirus encoding wild-type p53 administered via the hepatic artery produced no responses in 19 patients.[117] Other gene therapies involve (1) the use of prodrug genes to convert innocuous drugs[118] into active chemotherapeutic agents; (2) directed immunotherapy, such as HLA-B7 gene on a liposomal vector;[119] or (3) injecting genes that express thymidine kinase and then using ganciclovir.[120]

## Radiation

The traditional approach of using whole-liver irradiation has been limited by the low tolerance of the liver to irradiation. Doses greater than 30 to 35 Gy given to the entire liver produces radiation hepatitis.[121] Patients will present with this complication 1 to 3 months after the completion of radiation therapy with ascites and painful hepatomegaly. Laboratory evaluation demonstrates a marked elevation of AP levels, and liver biopsy reveals veno-occlusive disease. Although the majority of patients recover in 1 to 2 months, a small fraction develop overt liver failure.[122, 123]

In an attempt to improve the modest results of whole-liver irradiation, radiation treatment has been combined with either systemic or regional chemotherapy. The fluoropyrimidines have been the most widely used because they are radiation sensitizers.[124] The objective response rates and reported survival after combined modality therapy appears to be superior to that obtained by radiation alone, and the tolerance of the liver does not appear to be markedly affected by the addition of chemotherapy.[125] One method of delivering high-dose localized radiation is through the use of yttrium 90 ($^{90}$Y) microspheres. $^{90}$Y is a pure beta emitter and has a half-life of 64.5 hours and an average electron range of approximately 2.5 cm.[95] $^{90}$Y microspheres can be infused into the hepatic artery as a form of regional therapy for well-vascularized tumors.[96, 97] Technical problems include pulmonary shunting, which can lead to radiation pneumonitis.[126]

Other methods of delivering high doses of radiation to parts of the liver include interstitial brachytherapy (placement of radioactive sources inside the tumor), a high-dose-rate iridium 192 afterloader placed at the time of laparotomy,[127] and $^{125}$I seed implants, which deliver low-dose–rate irradiation (< about 0.15 Gy/hr) over several months.[128]

Although interstitial brachytherapy is a promising technique, a relative disadvantage of this approach is that sources can be placed only at laparotomy. Furthermore, a homogenous dose distribution is difficult to obtain with interstitial brachytherapy techniques when the tumor exceeds 3 to 5 cm. If sufficient normal liver is spared, parts of the liver may be treated with high doses of radiation without causing toxicity. Conformal three-dimensional treatment planning, in which beams can enter the patient from almost any angle, can substantially reduce irradiation of normal liver.[129, 130] Treatment with HAI FUDR combined with up to 72.6 Gy $^{131}$I (given by conformal three-dimensional technique) produced an objective response rate of 50%, with an overall median survival of 20 months.

## Summary

Liver metastases, especially from colorectal primaries, are treatable and potentially curable. Imaging techniques such as CT, MRI, and ultrasonography have advanced, leading to increased sensitivity and specificity in the diagnosis of liver metastases. When properly applied, the techniques are nearly as sensitive as surgical exploration in detecting hepatic lesions and in differentiating benign processes from malignant ones.

Liver surgery has been revolutionized since 1980. Dissections along nonanatomic lines have permitted the resection of multiple lesions that may previously have been considered unresectable. The new technique of vascular exclusion may improve the safety of major hepatic resections. Resection of solitary hepatic metastases (or two to four metastases from colorectal carcinoma) should be regarded as the best treatment for this condition. In older patients (> 70 years) or in patients with medical conditions preventing surgery, expectant follow-up can be endorsed. Withholding treatment is acceptable as long as the tumor remains stable, but if the tumor starts growing rapidly and local techniques cannot be used, systemic chemotherapy should be considered. In patients with progressive metastatic disease in the liver, systemic therapy or HAI may be initiated. In young patients with metastatic disease, even when disease is indolent or symptomatic, it may be difficult not to treat. These patients may be considered for either local regional therapy (resection or regional infusion) or systemic chemotherapy followed by regional therapy.

For patients who fail first-line treatment, external localized radiation or interstitial radiation can be used, perhaps in concert with chemotherapy. In patients with neuroendocrine tumors metastatic to the liver, the first approach is not to treat, since there may be a long period of stable disease. Symptoms may be treated with octreotide (Sandostatin). If the tumor progresses and the symptoms are not controlled, these vascular tumors can be treated by embolization or chemoembolization, with high expectations of response. Newer approaches to liver metastases such as cryosurgery, chemoembolization, interstitial radiation, or alcohol injections are available. The benefit of these techniques compared with surgery or regional therapy is being investigated as are other newer approaches, such as gene therapy and isolation perfusion.

## SUGGESTIONS FOR ADDITIONAL READING

Cromheecke M, de Jong KP, Hoekstra HJ. Current treatment for colorectal cancer metastatic to the liver. Eur J Surg Oncol 1999;25:451–63.

Kemeny N, Fata F. Arterial, portal, or systemic chemotherapy for patients with hepatic metastasis of colorectal carcinoma. J Hepatobiliary Pancreatic Surg 1999;6:39–49.

Kemeny N, Huang Y, Cohen AM, et al. Hepatic arterial infusion of chemotherapy after resection of hepatic metastases from colorectal cancer. N Engl J Med 1999;341:2039–48.

Nakamura S, Suzuki S, Baba S. Resection of liver metastases of colorectal carcinoma. World J Surg 1997;21:741–7.

Scheele J, Altendorf-Hofmann A. Resection of colorectal liver metastases. Langenbecks Arch Surg 1999;384:313–27.

Tellez C, Benson AB 3rd, Lyster MT, et al. Phase II trial of chemoembolization for the treatment of metastatic colorectal carcinoma to the liver and review of the literature. Cancer 1998;82:1250–9.

## REFERENCES

1. Boring C, Squires T, Tong T. Cancer Statistics 1992. CA Cancer J Clin 1992;42:30–1.
2. Kemeny M, Subarbaker PH, Smith TJ, et al. A prospective analysis of laboratory tests and imaging studies to detect hepatic lesions. Ann Surg 1982;195:163–7.
3. Tartter P, Slater G, Gelernt I, Aufses AH Jr. Screening for liver metastases from colorectal cancer with carcinoembryonic antigen and alkaline phosphatase. Ann Surg 1981;193:357–60.
4. Ranson J, Adams P, Localio S. Preoperative assessment for hepatic metastases in carcinoma of the colon and rectum. Surg Gynecol Obstet 1973;137:435–8.
5. Kemeny M, Hogan J, Ganteaume B, et al. Preoperative staging with computerized axial tomography and biochemical laboratory tests in patients with hepatic metastases. Ann Surg 1986;203:69–172.
6. Baron RL, Freeny PC, Moss AA. The liver. In: Moss AA, Gamsu G, Genant HK, eds. Computed tomography of the body with magnetic resonance imaging. Philadelphia: WB Saunders, 1991:735–821.
7. Phillips V, Bernardino M. The liver and spleen. In: Putman D, Ravin C, eds. Diagnostic imaging. Vol. 1. Philadelphia: WB Saunders, 1988:937.
8. Lai D, Fulham M, Stephen M, et al. The role of whole-body positron emission tomography with [18F] fluorodeoxyglucose in identifying operable colorectal cancer metastasis to the liver. Arch Surg 1996;131:703–7.
9. Fegiz G, Ramacciato G, Gennari L, et al. Hepatic resection for colorectal metastases: the Italian multicenter experience. J Surg Oncol 1991;2:144–54.
10. Hughes KS, Simon R, Songhorabodi S, et al. Resection of the liver for colorectal carcinoma metastases: a multi-institutional study of patterns of recurrence. Surgery 1986;100:278–84.
11. Gayowski T, Iwatsuki S, Madariaga J, et al. Experience in hepatic resection for metastatic colorectal cancer: analysis of clinical and pathologic risk factors. Surg 1994;116:703–11.
12. Jamison R, Donohur J, Nagorney D, et al. Hepatic resection for metastatic colorectal cancer results in cure for some patients. Arch Surg 1997;132:505–11.
13. Rees M, Plant G, Bygrave S. Late results justify resection for multiple hepatic metastases from colorectal cancer. Br J Surg 1997;84:1136–40.
14. Fong Y, Cohen AM, Fortner JG, et al. Liver resection for colorectal metastases. J Clin Oncol 1987;15:938–46.
15. D'Angelica M, Brennan M, Fortner J, et al. Ninety-six five-year survivors after liver resection for metastatic colorectal cancer. J Am Coll Surg 1997;185:554–9.
16. Nordlinger B, Guigiet M, Vaillant J, et al. Surgical resection of colorectal carcinoma metastases to the liver. Cancer 1996;77:1254–62.
17. Scheele J, Stangl R, Altendorf-Hofmann A, et al. Indicators of prognosis after hepatic resection for colorectal secondaries. Surgery 1991;110:13–29.
18. Doci R, Gennari L, Bignami P, et al. One hundred patients with hepatic metastases from colorectal cancer treated by resection: analysis of prognostic determinants. Br J Surg 1991;78:797–801.
19. Scheele J, Stang R, Altendorf-Hofmann A. Hepatic metastases from colorectal carcinoma: impact of surgical resection on the natural history. Br J Surg 1990;77:1241–46.
20. Wilson S, Adson M. Surgical treatment of hepatic metastases from colorectal cancers. Arch Surg 1976;111:330–334.
21. Rougier P, Ducreux M, Pignon J, et al. Prognostic factors in patients with liver metastases from colorectal carcinoma treated with discontinous intra-arterial hepatic chemotherapy. Eur J Cancer 1991;27:1226–30.
22. Kemeny N, Braun D. Prognostic factors in advanced colorectal carcinoma: the importance of lactic dehydrogenase, performance status, and white blood cell count. Am J Med 1983;74:786–94.
23. Bengtsson G, Carlsson G, Hafstrom L. Natural history of patients with untreated liver metastases from colorectal cancer. Am J Surg 1981;141:586–9.
24. Beckurts K, Holscher A, Thorban S, et al. Significance of lymph node involvement at the hepatic hilum in the resection of colorectal liver metastases. Br J Surg 1997;84:1081–4.
25. Murata S, Moriya Y, Akasu T, et al. Resection of both hepatic and pulmonary metastases in patients with colorectal cancer. Cancer 1998;83:1096–93.
26. Registry of Hepatic Metastases. Resection of the liver for colorectal carcinoma metastases: a multi-institutional study of indications for resection. Surgery 1988;103:278–88.
27. Fong Y, Kemeny N, Paty P, et al. Treatment of colorectal cancer: hepatic metastasis. Semin Surg Oncol 1996;12:219–52.
28. Couinaud C. Le foie; études anatomiques et chirugicales. Paris: Mason, 1957:400–9.
29. Bismuth H, Castaing D, Garden J. Major hepatic resection under total vascular exclusion. Ann Surg 1989;210:13–9.
30. Iwatsuki S, Shaw B, Starzl T. Experience with 150 liver resections. Ann Surg 1983;197:247–253.
31. Adam R, Bismuth H, Castaing D, et al. Repeat hepatectomy for colorectal liver metastases. Ann Surg 1997;225:51–60.
32. Kemeny N, Huang Y, Cohen AM, et al. Hepatic arterial infusion of chemotherapy after resection of hepatic metastases from colorectal cancer. N Engl J Med 1999;341:2039–48.
32a. Kemeny MM, Adak S, Lipsitz S, et al. Results of the Intergroup (Eastern Cooperative Oncology Group [ECOG] and Southwest Oncology Group [SWOG]) prospective randomized study of surgery alone versus continuous hepatic artery infusion of FUDR and continuous systemic infusion of 5FU after hepatic resection for colorectal liver metastases. Proc ASCO 1999;18:264a. abstract 1012.
33. Lorenz M, Staib-Sebler E, Koch B, et al. The value of postoperative hepatic arterial infusion following curative liver resection. Anticancer Res 1997;17:3825–34.
34. Nonami T, Takeuchi Y, Yasui M, et al. Regional adjuvant chemotherapy after partial hepatectomy for metastatic colorecal carcinoma. Semin Oncol 1997;24:56–130.
35. Lorenz M, Muller H-H, Schramm H, et al. Randomized trial of surgery versus surgery followed by adjuvant hepatic arterial infusion with 5-fluorouracil and folinic acid for liver metastases of colorectal cancer. Surgery 1998;228:756–62.
36. Muto Y, Moriwaki H, Ninomiya M, et al. Prevention of second primary tumors by an acyclic retinoid, polyprenoid acid, in patients with hepatocellular carcinoma. N Engl J Med 1996;334:1561–7.
37. Kemeny N, Daly J, Oderman P, et al. Prognostic variables in patients with hepatic metastases from colorectal cancer: importance of medical assessment of liver involvement. Cancer 1989;63:742–7.
38. Finan P, Marshall R, Cooper E, Giles G. Factors affecting survival in patients presenting with synchronous hepatic metastases from colorectal cancer: a clinical and computer analysis. Br J Surg 1985;72:373.
39. Lahr C, Soong S-J, Cloud G, et al. A multifactorial analysis of prognostic factors in patients with liver metastases from colorectal carcinoma. J Clin Oncol 1983;1:720–6.
40. Carter S. Single and combination nonhormonal chemotherapy in breast cancer. Cancer 1972;30:1543–55.
41. Kemeny N, Yagoda A, Braun D, et al. Therapy for metastatic colorectal carcinoma with combination of methyl-CCNU, 5-fluorouracil, vincristine and streptozotocin (MOF-Strep). Cancer 1980;45:876–81.

42. Breedis C, Young C. The blood supply of neoplasms in the liver. Am J Pathol 1954;30:969.
43. Ensminger WD, Rosowsky A, Raso V. A clinical pharmacological evaluation of hepatic arterial infusions of 5-fluoro-2-deoxyuridine and 5-fluorouracil. Cancer Res 1978;38:3789–92.
44. Van Groeningen C, Van derVijgh W, Giaccone G, et al. Phase I clinical and pharmacokinetic study of 5 day CPT-11 hepatic arterial infusion (HAI) chemotherapy. Proc ASCO 1997;16:A768. meeting abstract.
45. Van Tellingen O, Kuck M, Vlasveld L, et al. Unchanged pharmacokinetics of etoposide given by intra-arterial hepatic infusion as compared with IV infusion. Cancer Chemother Pharmacol 1996;38:387–90.
46. Collins J. Pharmacologic rationale for regional drug delivery. J Clin Oncol 1984;2:498–504.
47. Weiss L. Metastatic inefficiency and regional therapy for liver metastases from colorectal carcinoma. Regional Cancer Treat 1989;2:77–81.
48. Yasuda S, Noto T, Ikeda M, et al. Hepatic arterial infusion chemotherapy using implantable reservoir in colorectal liver metastasis. Gan To Kagaku Ryoho 1990;8:1815–19.
49. Niederhuber J, Ensminger W, Gyves J, et al. Regional chemotherapy of colorectal cancer metastatic to the liver. Cancer 1984;53:1336.
50. Kemeny N, Daly J, Reichman B, et al. Intrahepatic or systemic infusion of fluorodeoxyuridine in patients with liver metastases from colorectal carcinoma—a randomized trial. Ann Intern Med 1987;107:459–67.
51. Hohn D, Stagg R, Friedman M, et al. A randomized trial of continuous versus hepatic intra-arterial floxuridine in patients with colorectal cancer metastatic to the liver: the Northern California Oncology Group trial. J Clin Oncol 1989;7:1646–54.
52. Chang AE, Schneider PD, Sugarbaker PH. A prospective randomized trial of regional versus systemic continuous 5-fluoroxyuridine chemotherapy in the treatment of colorectal liver metastases. Ann Surg 1987;206:685–93.
53. Martin JKJ, O'Connell MG, Wieland HS, et al. Intra-arterial floxuridine vs systemic fluorouracil for hepatic metastases from colorectal cancer: a randomized trial. Arch Surg 1990;125:1022.
54. Rougier P, Laplanche A, Huguier M, et al. Hepatic arterial infusion of floxuridine in patients with liver metastases from colorectal carcinoma: long-term results of a prospective randomized trial. J Clin Oncol 1992;10:1112–8.
55. Kemeny M, Battifora H, Flayney D, et al. Sclerosing cholangitis after continuous hepatic artery infusion of FUDR. Ann Surg 1985;202:176.
56. Brown K, Kemeny N, Berger M, et al. Obstructive jaundice in patients receiving hepatic artery infusional chemotherapy: etiology, treatment implications, and complications after transhepatic biliary drainage. J Vasc Interv Radiol 1997;8:229–34.
57. Northover J, Terblance J. A new look at the arterial supply of the bile duct in man and its surgical implications. Br J Surg 1979;66:379–84.
58. Gluck W, Akwari O, Kelvin F, et al. A reversible enteropathy complicating continuous hepatic artery infusion chemotherapy with 5-fluoro 2-deoxyuridine. Cancer 1985;56:2424.
59. Kemeny N, Steiter K, Diedzweiecki D, et al. A randomized trial of intrahepatic infusion of fluorouridine (FUDR) with dexamethasone versus FUDR alone in the treatment of metastatic colorectal cancer. Cancer 1992;69:327–34.
60. Stagg R, Venook A, Chase J, et al. Alternating hepatic intra-arterial floxuridine and fluorouracil: a less toxic regimen for treatment of liver metastases from colorectal cancer. J Natl Cancer Inst 1991;83:423–8.
61. Davidson B, Izzo F, Chase J, et al. Alternating floxuridine and 5-fluorouracil hepatic arterial chemotherapy for colorectal liver metastases minimizes biliary toxicity. Am J Surg 1996;172:244–7.
62. Patt Y, Charnsangavej C, Yoffe B, et al. Hepatic arterial infusion of floxuridine, leucovorin, doxorubicin, and cisplatin for hepatocellular carcinoma: effects of hepatitis B and C viral infection on drug toxicity and patient survival. J Clin Oncol 1994;12:1204–11.
63. Hrushesky W, Von Roemelling R, Lanning R, Rabtini J. Circadian-shaped infusions of fluoxuridine for progressive metastatic renal cell carcinoma. J Clin Oncol 1990;8:1504–13.
64. Kemeny N, Cohen A, Bertino J, et al. Continuous intrahepatic infusion of floxuridine and leucovorin through an implantable pump for the treatment of hepatic metastases from colorectal carcinoma. Cancer 1990;65:2446–50.
65. Kemeny N, Seiter K, Conti J, et al. Hepatic arterial floxuridine and leucovorin for unresectable liver metastases from colorectal carcinoma. Cancer 1994;73:1134–42.
66. Hartmann J, Schmoll E, Bokemeyer C, et al. Phase I pharmacological study of intra-arterially infused fotemustine for colorectal liver metastases. Eur J Cancer 1998;34:87–91.
67. Kemeny N, Cohen A, Steiner K, et al. Randomized trial of hepatic arterial FUDR, mitomycin and BCNU versus FUDR alone: effective salvage therapy for liver metastases of colorectal cancer. J Clin Oncol 1993;11:330–5.
68. Kemeny N, Conti J, Blumgart L, et al. Hepatic arterial infusion of floxuridine (FUdR), dexamethasone (Dex) and high dose mitomycin-C: comparable response to FUdR/leucovorin/Dex but with greater toxicity. Proc ASCO 1995;14:201.
69. Kemeny N, Conti JA, Cohen A, et al. Phase II study of hepatic arterial floxuridine, leucovorin, and dexamethasone for unresected liver metastases from colorectal carcinoma. J Clin Oncol 1994;12:2288–95.
70. Uemura T, Kawasaki S, Kawai H, et al. Evaluation of hepatic arterial infusion chemotherapy for gastric cancer (Japanese). Gan To Kagaku Ryoho 1996;23:1787–91.
71. Markowitz J. The hepatic artery. Surg Gynecol Obstet 1952;95:644–6.
72. Allison D, Modlin I, Jenkins W, et al. Treatment of carcinoid liver metastases by hepatic artery embolization. Lancet 1977;2:1323–25.
73. Martenson H, Nobin A, Bengmark S, et al. Embolization of the liver in the management of metastatic carcinoid tumors. J Surg Oncol 1984;27:152–8.
74. Ajani J, Carrasco CH, Charnsanpavej C, et al. Islet cell tumors metastatic to the liver: effective palliation by sequential hepatic artery embolization. Ann Intern Med 1988;108:340–4.
75. Carrasco C, Charnsanpavej C, Ajani J, et al. The carcinoid syndrome: palliation by hepatic artery embolization. AJR 1986;147:149–54.
76. Marlink R, Lokich J, Robins J, Clouse M. Hepatic arterial embolization for metastatic hormone-secreting tumors. Cancer 1990;65:2227–32.
77. Martin J, Moertel C, Adson M, et al. Surgical treatment of functioning metastatic carcinoid tumors. Arch Surg 1983;118:537–41.
78. Moertel C. Treatment of the carcinoid tumor and the malignant carcinoid syndrome. J Clin Oncol 1983;1:727–40.
79. Melia W, Nunnerley H, Johnson P, Williams R. Use of arterial devascularization and cytotoxic drugs in 30 patients with the carcinoid syndrome. Br J Cancer 1982;46:331–39.
80. Kvols L, Buck M, Moertel C, et al. Treatment of metastatic islet cell carcinoma with a somatostatin analogue (SMS 201–995). Ann Intern Med 1987;107:162–68.
81. Daniels J, Daniels A, Quinn M, et al. Phase I trial with cisplatin or mitomycin hepatic chemoembolization (CE) with Angiostat collagen for embolization (CFE) in patients with colorectal cancer. Proc ASCO 1988;7:101.
82. Venook A, Stagg R, Lewis B, et al. Chemoembolization for hepatocellular carcinoma. J Clin Oncol 1990;8:1108–14.
83. Venook A, Stagg R, Frye J, et al. Embolization of patients with liver metastases from carcinoid and islet cell tumors. Proc ASCO 1991;10:A386.
84. Raoul J, Bourquet P, Bretagne J, et al. Hepatic artery injection of I-131 labeled lipiodol. Part 1: Biodistribution study in patients with hepatocellular carcinoma and liver metastases. Radiology 1988;168:541–45.
85. Raoul J, Heresbach D, Bretagne J, et al. Chemoembolization of hepatocellular carcinomas. Cancer 1992;70:585–90.
86. Nakao N, Uchida H, Kamino K, et al. Effectiveness of lipiodol in transcatheter arterial embolization of hepatocellular carcinoma. Cancer Chemother Pharmacol 1992;31:Suppl:S72–6.
87. Nakao N, Kamino K, Miura K, et al. Transcatheter arterial embolization in hepatocellular carcinoma: a long-term follow-up. Radiat Med 1992;10:13–18.
88. Chang J-M, Tzeng W-S, Pan H-B, et al. Transcatheter arterial embolization with or without cisplatin treatment of hepatocellular carcinoma: a randomized controlled study. Cancer 1994;74:2449–59.
89. Pelletier G, Roche A, Ink O, et al. A randomized trial of hepatic arterial chemoembolization in patients with unresectable hepatocellular carcinoma. J Hepatol 1990;11:181–4.
90. Anonymous. A comparison of lipidol chemoembolization and conservative treatment for unresectable hepatocellular carcinoma. N Engl J Med 1995;332:1256–61.
91. Aronsen K, Hellekant C, Holmberg J, et al. Controlled blocking of hepatic artery flow with enzymatically degradable microspheres combined with oncolytic drugs. Eur J Surg Res 1979;11:99–106.
92. McVie J, Hoefnagel C, Burger J. Tumor targeting of cytostatic com-

pounds using intra-arterial biodegradable microspheres. Ann Rep Netherlands Cancer Inst 1985;83.

93. Ball A. Regional chemotherapy for colorectal hepatic meatastases using degradable starch microspheres. Acta Oncol 1991;30:309.

94. Sigurdson E, Ridge J, Daly J. Intra-arterial infusion of doxorubicin with degradable starch microspheres. Arch Surg 1986;121:1277–81.

95. Gray B, Anderson J, Burton MA, et al. Regression of liver metastases following treatment with yttrium-90 microspheres. Aust N Z J Surg 1992;62:105–110.

96. Tian J, BX X, Zhang J, et al. Ultrasound-guided internal radiotherapy using yttrium-90 glass microspheres for liver malignancies. J Nucl Med 1996;37:958–63.

97. Ho S, Lau W, Leung T, et al. Clinical evaluation of the partition model for estimating radiation doses from yttrium-90 microspheres in the treatment of hepatic cancer. Eur J Nucl Med 1997;24:293–8.

98. Bretagne J, Raoul J, Bourguet P, et al. Hepatic artery injection of I-131–labeled lipiodol. Part II: Preliminary results of therapeutic use in patients with hepatocellular carcinoma and liver metastases. Radiology 1988;168:547–50.

99. Ravikumar T, Kane R, Cady B, et al. A 5-year study of cryosurgery in the treatment of liver tumors. Arch Surg 1991;126:1520–24.

100. Ravikumar TS, Steele GJ, Kane R, et al. Experimental and clinical observations on hepatic cryosurgery for colorectal metastases. Cancer Res 1991;51:6233–7.

101. Onik G, Rubinsky B, Zemel R, et al. Ultrasound-guided hepatic cryosurgery in the treatment of metastatic colon carcinoma. Cancer 1991;67:901–7.

102. Morris D, Ross W. Australian experience of cryoablation of liver tumors: metastases. Surg Oncol Clin North Am 1996;5:391–7.

103. Steele G Jr, Ravikumar T, Benotti P. New surgical treatments for recurrent colorectal cancer. Cancer 1990;65:723–30.

104. Adam R, Akpinar E, Johann M, et al. Place of cryosurgery in the treatment of malignant liver tumors. Ann Surg 1997;225:39–47.

105. Preketes A, Caplehorn J, King J, et al. Effect of hepatic artery chemotherapy on survival of patients with hepatic metastases from colorectal carcinoma treated with cryotherapy. World J Surg 1995;19:768–71.

106. Welling R, Lamping K. Cryoprobe as a "handle" for resection of metastatic liver tumors. J Surg Oncol 1990;45:227–28.

107. Tandan V, Harmantas A, Gallinger S. Long-term survival after hepatic cryosurgery versus surgical resection for metastatic colorectal carcinoma: a critical review of the literature. Can J Surg 1997;40:175–81.

108. Livraghi T, Baietta E, Matricardi L, et al. Fine needle percutaneous intratumoral chemotherapy under ultrasound guidance: a feasibility study. Tumori 1986;72:81–7.

109. Suzuki M, Suzuki H, Yamamoto T, et al. Indication of chemoembolization therapy without gelatin sponge for hepatocellular carcinoma. Semin Oncol 1997;24:Suppl 6:56–110.

110. Shiina S, Imamura M, Obi S, et al. Percutaneous ethanol injection therapy for small hepatocellular carcinoma. Gan To Kagaku Ryoho 1996;23:835–9.

111. Livraghi T, Vettori C, Lazaroni S. Liver metastases: results of percutaneous ethanol injection in 14 patients. Radiology 1991;179:709–12.

112. Yamamoto K, Masuzawa M, Kato M, et al. Evaluation of combined therapy with chemoembolization and ethanol injection for advanced hepatocellular carcinoma. Semin Oncol 1997;24:Suppl 6:50–5.

113. Van Zuidewign D, de Brauw L, Marinelli A, et al. Isolated liver perfusion with mitomycin C or melphalan in patients with hepatic metastases. Soc Surg Oncol 1993;46:198.

114. Alexander H, Bartlett D, Libutti S, et al. Isolated hepatic perfusion with tumor necrosis factor and melphalan for unresectable cancers confined to the liver. J Clin Oncol 1998;16:1479–89.

115. Sugiyama A, Katayama M, Matsuda T, et al. Hepatic arterial infusion chemotherapy combined with hyperthermia for metastatic liver tumors of colorectal cancer. Semin Oncol 1997;24:Suppl 6:135–38.

116. Sato M, Watanabe Y, Ueda S, et al. Microwave coagulation therapy for hepatocellular carcinoma. Gastroenterology 1996;110:1507–14.

117. Venook A, Bergsland E, Ring E, et al. Gene therapy of colorectal liver metastases using a recombinant adenovirus encoding wt p53 (SCH 58500) via hepatic artery infusion: a phase I study. Proc ASCO 1998;17:431a.

118. Crystal R, Hirschowitz E, Lieberman M, et al. Phase I study of direct administration of a replication of deficient adenovirus vector containing the E. coli cytosine deaminase gene to metastatic colon carcinoma of the liver in association with the oral administration of the prodrug 5-fluorocytosine. Hum Gene Ther 1997;8:985–1001.

119. Rubin J, Galanis E, Pitot H, et al. Phase I study of immunotherapy of hepatic metastases of colorectal carcinoma by direct gene transfer of an allogeneic histocompatibility antigen, HLA-B7. Gene Ther 1997;4:419–25.

120. Trinh Q, Austin E, Murray D, et al. Enzyme/prodrug gene therapy: comparison of cytosine deaminase/5-fluorocytosine versus thymidine kinase/ganciclovir enzyme/prodrug systems in a human colorectal carcinoma cell line. Cancer Res 1995;55:4808–12.

121. Reed G, Cox A. The human liver after radiation injury. Am J Pathol 1966;48:597–612.

122. Lawrence T, Robertson J, Ensminger W, et al. Hepatic toxicity resulting from cancer treatment. Int J Radiat Oncol Biol Phys 1995;31:1237–48.

123. Jirtle R, Anscher M, Alati T. Radiation sensitivity of the liver. Adv Radiat Biol 1990;14:269–311.

124. Byfield J, Calabro-Jones P, Klisak I, Kulhanian F. Pharmacologic requirements for obtaining sensitization of human tumor cells in vitro to combined 5-fluorouracil or ftorafur and x-rays. Int J Radiat Oncol Biol Phys 1982;8:1923–33.

125. McCracken J, Weatherall T, Oishi N, et al. Adjuvant intrahepatic chemotherapy with mitomycin and 5-FU combined with hepatic irradiation in high risk patients with carcinoma of the colon: a Southwest Oncology Group Phase II pilot study. Cancer Treat Rep 1985;69:129–31.

126. Leung T, Lau W, Ho S, et al. Radiation pneumonitis after selective internal radiation treatment with intraarterial 90-yttrium microspheres for inoperable hepatic tumors. Int J Radiat Oncol Biol Phys 1995;33:919–24.

127. Thomas D, Nauta R, Rodgers J, et al. Intraoperative high dose rate interstitial irradiation of hepatic metastases from colorectal carcinoma: results of a phase I–II trial. Cancer 1993;71:1977–81.

128. Donath D, Nori D, Turnbull A, et al. Brachytherapy in the treatment of solitary colorectal metastases to the liver. J Surg Oncol 1990;44:55–61.

129. Ten Haken R, Lawrence T, McShan D, et al. Technical considerations in the use of 3-D beam rearrangements in the abdomen. Radiother Oncol 1991;22:19–28.

130. Lawrence T, Tesser R, Ten Haken R. An application of dose volume histograms to the treatment of intrahepatic malignancies with radiation therapy. Int J Radiat Oncol Biol Phys 1990;19:1041–47.

131. Robertson J, Lawrence T, Walker S, et al. The treatment of colorectal liver metastases with conformal radiation therapy and regional chemotherapy. Int J Radiat Oncol Biol Phys 1995;32:445–50.

132. Adson M, Van Heerden J, Adson M, et al. Resection of hepatic metastases from colorectal cancer. Arch Surg 1984;119:647–51.

133. Schlag P, Hohenberger P, Herfath C. Resection of liver metastases in colorectal cancer—competitive analysis of treatment results in synchronous versus metachronous metastases. Eur J Surg Oncol 1990;16:360–5.

134. Scheele J, Stang R, Altendorf-Hofmann A, et al. Resection of colorectal liver metastases. World J Surg 1995;19:59–71.

135. Rosen D, Nagorney D, Taswell H, et al. Perioperative blood transfusion and determinants of survival after liver resection for metastatic colorectal carcinoma. Ann Surg 1992;216:493–505.

136. Foster J. Survival after liver resection for secondary tumors. Am J Surg 1978;135:389–94.

137. Fortner J, Silva J, Cox E, et al. Multivariate analysis of a personal series of 247 patients with liver metastases from colorectal cancer. Ann Surg 1984;199:317–23.

138. Butler J, Attiyeh F, Daly J. Hepatic resection for metastases of the colon and rectum. Surg Gynecol Obstet 1986;162:109–13.

139. Nordlinger B, Vaillant J, Guiguet M, et al. A scoring system to select candidates for resection of colorectal liver metastases based on 1568 cases. Soc Surg Oncol Abstract Book 1996;17:11.

140. Van Ooijen B, Wiggers T, Meijer S, et al. Hepatic resections for colorectal metastases in the Netherlands—a multi-institutional 10-year study. Cancer 1992;70:28–34.

141. Wood C, Gillis C, Blumgart L. A retrospective study of the natural history of patients with liver metastases from colorectal cancer. Clin Oncol 1976;2:285–8.

142. Wagner J, Adson M, Heerden J, et al. The natural history of hepatic metastases from colorectal cancer. Ann Surg 1984;199:502.

143. Adson M. Diagnosis and surgical treatment of primary and secondary solid tumors in the adult. Surg Clin North Am 1981;61:181–96.

144. Baker L, Talley R, Maiter R, et al. Phase III comparison of the

treatment of advanced gastrointestinal cancer with bolus weekly 5-FU vs methyl CCNU plus bolus weekly 5-FU. Cancer 1976;38:1–7.

145. Grage T, Vassilopoulos P, Shingleton W, et al. Results of a prospective randomized study of hepatic artery infusion with 5-fluorouracil vs intravenous 5-fluorouracil in patients with hepatic metastases from colorectal cancer: a Central Oncology Group study. Surgery 1979;86:550–5.

146. Buroker T, Kim PN, Groppe C, et al. 5-FU infusion with methyl-CCNU in the treatment of advanced colon cancer. Cancer 1978;42:1228–33.

147. Kemeny N, Yagoda A, Braun DJ, Golbey R. A randomized study of two different schedules of methyl CCNU, 5-FU and vincristine for metastatic colorectal carcinoma. Cancer 1979;43:78–82.

148. Kemeny N, Younes A, Seiter K, et al. Combination fluorouracil (FU) and recombinant alpha interferon (IFN) in advanced colorectal carcinoma: activity but significant toxicity. Cancer 1990;66:2470–5.

149. Wadler S, Schwartz E, Goldman M, et al. Fluorouracil and recombinant alpha-2a interferon: an active regimen against advanced colorectal carcinoma. J Clin Oncol 1989;7:1769–75.

150. Ehrlichman C, Fine S, Wong A, Elhakim T. Randomized trial of fluorouracil and folinic acid in patients with metastatic colorectal carcinoma. J Clin Oncol 1988;6:469–75.

151. Petrelli N, Douglas H, Herrera L, et al. The modulation of fluorouracil with leucovorin in metastatic colorectal carcinoma: a prospective randomized phase III trial. J Clin Oncol 1989;7:1419–26.

152. Doroshow J, Multhauf P, Leong L, et al. Prospective randomized comparison of fluorouracil versus fluorouracil and high-dose continuous infusion leucovorin calcium for the treatment of advanced measurable colorectal cancer in patients previously unexposed to chemotherapy. J Clin Oncol 1990;8:491–501.

153. Conti J, Kemeny N, Saltz L, et al. Irinotecan is an active agent in untreated patients with metastatic colorectal cancer. J Clin Oncol 1996;14:709–15.

154. Rothenberg ML, Eckardt JR, Kuhn JG, et al. Phase II trial of irinotecan in patients with progress of rapidly recurrent colorectal cancer. J Clin Oncol 1996;14:1128–35.

155. Pitot H, Wonder D, O'Connell M, et al. Phase II trial of irinotecan in patients with metastatic colorectal carcinoma. J Clin Oncol 1997;15:2910–19.

156. Tandon RN, Bunnell IL, Cooper RG. The treatment of metastatic carcinoma of the liver by percutaneous selective hepatic artery infusion of 5-fluorouracil. Surgery 1973;73:118–21.

157. Ansfield FJ, Ramirez G, Davis HLJ, et al. Further clinical studies with intrahepatic arterial infusion with 5-fluorouracil. Cancer 1975;36:2413–7.

158. Watkins E Jr, Khazei AM, Nahra KS. Surgical basis for arterial infusion chemotherapy of disseminated carcinoma of the liver. Surg Gynecol Obstet 1970;130:581–605.

159. Smiley S, Schouten J, Chang A, et al. Intrahepatic arterial infusion with 5-FU for liver metastases of colorectal carcinoma. Proc ASCO 1981;22:391.

160. Metzger U, Weder W, Rothlin M, Largiader F. Phase II study of intraarterial fluorouracil and mitomycin-C for liver metastases of colorectal cancer. Recent Results Cancer Res 1991;121:198–204.

161. Denck H. Results of intermittent intra-arterial chemotherapy with 5-FU in liver metastases and inoperable tumors of the gastrointestinal and urogenital tracts. Onkologie 1984;7:167–76.

162. Rougier P, Laser P, Elias D, et al. Intraarterial hepatic chemotherapy (IAHC) for liver metastases (LM) from colorectal (CR) origin. Proc ASCO 1987;6:369.

163. Borner M, Laffer U, Ludwig C, et al. Effectiveness and low toxicity of hepatic artery infusion with fluorouracil and mitomycin for metastatic colorectal cancer confined to the liver: from the Swiss Group for Clinical and Epidemiological Cancer Research (SAKK). Ann Oncol 1990;1:227–8.

164. Cortesi E, Capussotti L, DiTora P, et al. Bolus vs continuous hepatic arterial infusion of cisplatin plus intravenous 5-fluorouracil chemotherapy for unresectable colorectal metastases. Dis Colon Rectum 1994;37:S138–43.

165. Warren H, Anderson J, O'Gorman P, et al. A phase II study of regional 5-fluorouracil infusion with intravenous folinic acid for colorectal liver metastases. Br J Cancer 1994;70:677–80.

166. Sugihara K. Continuous hepatic arterial infusion of 5-fluorouracil for unresectable colorectal liver metastases: phase II study. Surgery 1995;117:624–8.

167. Kerr D, Ledermann J, McArdle C, et al. Phase I clinical and pharmacokinetic study of leucovorin and infusional hepatic arterial fluorouracil. J Clin Oncol 1995;13:2968–72.

168. Howell J, McArdle C, Kerr D, et al. A phase I study of regional 2-weekly 5-fluorouracil infusion with intravenous folinic acid in the treatment of colorectal liver metastases. Br J Cancer 1997;76:1390–3.

169. Arai Y, Inaba Y, Takeuchi Y, Ariyoshi Y. Intermittent hepatic arterial infusion of high dose 5-FU on a weekly schedule for liver metastases from colorectal cancer. Cancer Chemother Pharmacol 1997;40:526–30.

170. Hidalgo O, Rebollo J, Vieitez J, et al. Intra-arterial hepatic treatment with carboplatin (CBDCA) and 5-fluorouracil (5-FU) in metastases from colorectal carcinoma. Am J Cliin Oncol 1993;16:30–3.

171. Balch C, Urist M. Intra-arterial chemotherapy for colorectal liver metastases and hepatomas using a totally implantable drug infusion pump. Recent Results Cancer Res 1986;100:123–47.

172. Kemeny N, Daly J, Oderman P, et al. Hepatic artery pump infusion toxicity and results in patients with metastatic colorectal carcinoma. J Clin Oncol 1984;2:595–600.

173. Shepard KV, Levin B, Karl RC, et al. Therapy for metastatic colorectal cancer with hepatic artery infusion chemotherapy using a subcutaneous implanted pump. J Clin Oncol 1985;3:161–9.

174. Cohen A, Kaufman S, Wood W, et al. Regional hepatic chemotherapy using an implantable drug infusion pump. Am J Surg 1983;145:529–33.

175. Weiss G, Garnick M, Osteen R, et al. Long-term arterial infusion of 5-fluorouracil for liver metastases using an implantable infusion pump. J Clin Oncol 1983;1:337–44.

176. Schwartz S, Jones L, McCune C. Assessment of treatment of intrahepatic malignancies using chemotherapy via an implantable pump. Ann Surg 1985;201:560–7.

177. Johnson L, Wasserman P, Rivkin S. FUDR hepatic arterial infusion via an implantable pump for treatment of hepatic tumors. Proc ASCO 1983;2:119.

178. Hohn D, Stagg R, Price D, et al. Avoidance of gastroduodenal toxicity in patients receiving hepatic arterial 5-fluoro-2-deoxyuridine. J Clin Oncol 1985;3:1257–60.

179. Niederhuber J. Arterial chemotherapy for metastatic colorectal cancer in the liver. Conference on the advances in regional cancer therapy. Giessen, West Germany, 1985.

180. Wagman L, Kemeny M, Leong L, et al. A prospective randomized evaluation of the treatment of colorectal cancer metastatic to the liver. J Clin Oncol 1990;8:1885–93.

181. Allen-Mersh T, Earlam S, Fordy C, et al. Quality of life and survival with continuous hepatic artery floxuridine infusion for colorectal liver metastases. Lancet 1994;344:1255–60.

182. Project ACCM-A. Modulation of fluorouracil by leucovorin in patients with advanced colorectal cancer: evidence in terms of response rate. J Clin Oncol 1992;10:896–903.

183. Labianca R, Cascinu S, Frontini L, et al. High versus low-dose levo-leucovorin as a modulator of 5-fluorouracil in advanced colorectal cancer: a "GISCAD" phase II study. Ann Oncol 1997;8:169–74.

184. Rougier P, Van Cutbem E, Bujetta E, et al. Randomized trial of irinotecan versus fluorouracil by continuous infusion after fluorouracil failure in patients with metastatic colorectal cancer. Lancet 1998;352:1407–12.

185. Cunningham D, Pyrhonen S, James R, et al. Randomised trial of irinotecan plus supportive care versus supportive care alone after fluorouracil failure for patients with metastatic colorectal cancer. Lancet 1998;352:1413–8.

186. Fraschini G, Charngangavej C, Carrasco C, et al. Percutaneous hepatic arterial infusion of cisplatin-vinblastine for refractory cancer metastatic to the liver. Am J Clin Oncol 1988;11:34–8.

187. Estape J, Daniels M, Vinolas N, et al. Combination chemotherapy with oral etoposide plus intravenous cyclophosphamide in liver metastases of breast cancer. Am J Clin Oncol 1990;13:98–100.

188. Lange M, Minton J. Intrahepatic chemotherapy salvage following systemic chemotherapy failure for metastatic breast cancer to the liver. Proc ASCO 1990;9:A116.

189. Fraschini G, Fleishman G, Charnsangavej C, et al. Continuous 5-day infusion of vinblastine for percutaneous hepatic arterial chemotherapy for metastatic breast cancer. Cancer Treat Rep 1987;71:1001–5.

190. Fraschini G, Fleishman G, Yap H-Y, et al. Percutaneous hepatic arterial infusion of cisplatin for metastatic breast cancer. Cancer Treat Rep 1987;71:313–5.

191. Fraschini G, Holmes F, Wallace S, Hortobagyi G. Hepatic arterial

infusion (HAI) of mitomycin-C (M) and floxuride (F) + adriamycin (A) for breast cancer metastatic to the liver. Breast Cancer Res Treat 1986;8. abstract 53.

192. Maral J, Baumer R, Curet P, et al. Intra-arterial chemotherapy for liver metastases of colon and breast cancer. Third European Conference on Clinical Oncology and Cancer Nursing, Stockholm, 1985. abstract.

193. Arai Y, Sone Y, Inaba Y, et al. Hepatic arterial infusion chemotherapy for liver metastases from breast cancer. Cancer Chemother Pharmacol 1994;33(S):142–4.

194. Maton P, Camilleri M, Griffin G, et al. Role of hepatic arterial embolization in the carcinoid syndrome. Br Med J 1983;287:932–5.

195. Daniels J, Pentecost M, Teitelbaum G, et al. Hepatic artery chemoembolization (HAE) for carcinoma of colon using Angiostat collagen and cisplatin, mitomycin, and doxorubicin: response, survival, and serum drug levels. Proc ASCO 1992;11:171.

196. Stuart K, Huberman M, Posner M, et al. Chemoembolization for colorectal liver metastases. Proc ASCO 1995;14:190.

197. Tellez C, Benson AL, Lyster M, et al. Chemoembolization for colorectal metastases to the liver. Proc ASCO 1995;14:198.

198. Link M, Ross W, Clingan P, et al. Treatment of liver metastases with intra-arterial lipiodol-Adriamycin. Reg Cancer Treat 1993;3:121–4.

199. Lang E, Brown CJ. Colorectal metastases to the liver: selective chemoembolization. Radiology 1993;189:417–22.

200. Stagg R, Venook A, Chase J, et al. Chemoembolization of primary and metastatic liver tumors. Reg Cancer Treat 1992;1:53–7.

201. Martinelli D, Wadler S, Bakal C, et al. Utility of embolization or chemoembolization as second-line treatment in patients with advanced or recurrent colorectal carcinoma. Cancer 1994;74:1706–12.

202. Konno T. Targeting chemotherapy for hepatoma: arterial administration of anticancer drugs dissolved in lipiodol. Eur J Cancer 1992;28:403–9.

203. Ichida T, Kato M, Hayakawaw A, et al. Therapeutic effect of a CDDP-epirubicin-lipiodol emulsion on advanced hepatocellular carcinoma. Cancer Chemother Pharmacol 1994;33:S74–8.

204. Civalleri D, Pellicci R, Decaro G, et al. Palliative chemoembolization of hepatocellular carcinoma with mitoxantrone, lipiodol, and Gelfoam: a phase II study. Anticancer Res 1996;16:937–41.

205. Inoue H, Miyazono N, Hori A, et al. Treatment of hepatocellular carcinoma by intraarterial injection of Adriamycin/mitomycin C oil suspension (ADMOS) alone or combined with cis-diaminodichloroplatinum (CDDP). Acta Radiol 1993;34:388–91.

206. Yodono H, Takekawa SD, Tarasawa K, et al. Combination therapy consisting of arterial infusion chemotherapy (EPF, EAP) and transcatheter arterial embolization (TAE). Cancer Chemother Pharmacol 1994;33:Suppl:79–83.

207. Ngan H, Lai C, Fan S, et al. Treatment of inoperable hepatocellular carcinoma by transcatheter arterial chemoembolization using an emulsion of cisplatin in iodized oil and Gelfoam. Clin Radiol 1993;47:315–20.

208. Stuart K, Stokes K, Jenkins R, et al. Treatment of hepatocellular carcinoma using doxorubicin/ethiodized oil/gelatin powder chemoembolization. Cancer 1993;72:3202–9.

209. Rougier P, Roche A, Pelletier G, et al. Efficacy of chemoembolization for hepatocellular carcinomas: experience from the Gustave Roussy Institute and the Bicentre Hospital. J Surg Oncol 1993;3:Suppl:94–6.

# CHAPTER 105

# MANAGEMENT OF PULMONARY METASTASES

• CAROL NISHIKUBO

Pulmonary metastases are a common site of spread for a variety of solid tumors. Approaches to treatment include chemotherapy or immunotherapy for the systemic disease, radiation therapy to symptomatic lesions, and surgery for selected subsets of patients. The responses to these therapies vary depending on the underlying tumor type and extent of disease. Chemotherapy, immunotherapy, and radiation therapy are discussed in greater detail in the sections on the specific tumor types. The remainder of this discussion reviews surgical approaches to pulmonary metastases.

The first reported cases of resection of solitary pulmonary metastases date back to the 19th century[1]; however, more widespread use has occurred only since the 1970s. The logic behind metastasectomy comes from the observation that in autopsy series of patients who die of pulmonary metastases, the lungs are often the only site of distant disease.[2] Therefore, if one can achieve control of the primary site of disease, theoretically a patient can be cured if the pulmonary metastases are eliminated. The likelihood of cure in this setting obviously depends on the site of origin of the primary tumor. The most common type of tumors treated in this fashion, and with the most success, are soft tissue sarcomas and colorectal tumors. In other tumor types, including melanoma,[1, 3, 4] renal cell carcinoma,[5, 6] head and neck tumors,[7–11] breast cancer,[12] meningioma,[13, 14] endocrine tumors,[15, 16] gastric tumors, and other tumors of gastrointestinal origin,[17–19] resection has met with variable success. Resection of resid-

ual tumors, including pulmonary disease in germ cell tumors, is a well-established practice.

Soft tissue and bone sarcomas spread to the lung as the only site of metastatic disease in up to 40 to 70% of patients with metastases in some series.[20, 21] Surgical resection of pulmonary disease has resulted in 5-year survival rates of 14 to 38%.[20, 22] Factors that may favorably affect the prognosis for these patients include a prolonged disease-free interval before the development of pulmonary metastases, fewer metastatic lesions, low tumor histologic grade, absence of microscopic margins of resection, and patient age younger than 40 years, although not all studies have shown all these factors to be of importance.[3, 4, 20, 23]

For patients with colorectal cancer undergoing resection of pulmonary metastases, the 5-year survival rates have been in the 20 to 60% range.[24–28] As is the case for sarcomas, there is debate about which factors, if any, predict for a better outcome for surgical treatment. Possible predictive factors include the preoperative carcinoembyonic antigen level, the number of metastases, and the ability to achieve a complete resection.[25–29] However, unlike the sarcomas, the disease-free interval from diagnosis of the primary lesion to development of metastases is less commonly associated with overall prognosis.[25–29] Also dissimilar from the treatment of sarcomas, attempts have been made to resect disease in patients with a greater number of both hepatic and pulmonary metastases. Long-term survival has been observed in several smaller series reported in the literature of patients who have undergone resection of both hepatic and pulmonary metastases.[30, 31]

Another area of some controversy is the surgical approach to resection in these patients. Some authors have used a thoracoscopic approach or video-assisted thoracic surgery (VATS) for patients with one or two pulmonary lesions, with survival outcomes similar to those achieved historically with thoracotomy.[32] Most authors, however, feel that thoracotomy is required because up to 56% of patients are understaged by computed tomographic scan alone.[33, 34]

In summary, resection of pulmonary metastases is being used more commonly for selected patients with solid tumors having the lung as the sole site of metastatic disease and with few lesions. Large prospective, randomized studies comparing surgery to systemic therapy alone are not available, although outcomes using surgery are improved compared with historical controls, and long-term survival is observed with surgery alone. In selected patients with colorectal cancer with both pulmonary and hepatic metastases, again with few lesions at each site, resection at both sites may result in long-term survival. The accepted surgical approach at this time is thoracotomy with direct palpation of the lungs to assess for occult disease not detected by radiographic techniques.

## SUGGESTIONS FOR ADDITIONAL READING

Lin JC, Wiechmann RJ, Szwerc MF, et al. Diagnostic and therapeutic video-assisted thoracic surgery resection of pulmonary metastases. Surgery 1999;126:636–41. *The authors compared their results with VATS of pulmonary metastases and standard open thoracotomy. They concluded that the results were comparable provided that preoperative high-resolution helical computed tomographic scanning was performed to rule out the presence of disease that could not be resected by the VATS technique.*

Murata S, Moriya Y, Akasu T, et al. Resection of both hepatic and pulmonary metastases in patients with colorectal carcinoma. Cancer 1998;83:1086–93. *The articles by Robinson and Murata and their colleagues support the resection of both hepatic and pulmonary metastases in highly selected patients. Factors favoring a beneficial outcome included younger age, limited extent of metastases, and a long disease-free interval between the time of initial diagnosis and the subsequent development of metachronous metastases.*

Robinson BJ, Rice TW, Strong SA, et al. Is resection of pulmonary and hepatic metastases warranted in patients with colorectal cancer? J Thorac Cardiovasc Surg 1999;117:66–75.

## REFERENCES

1. Pastorino U. Lung metastasectomy: why, when, how. Crit Rev Oncol Hematol 1997;26:137–45.
2. Farrell JT. Pulmonary metastases: pathological, clinical roentgenological study based on 78 cases at necropsy. Radiology 1935;24:444–50.
3. Robert JH, Ambrogi V, Mermillod B, et al. Factors influencing long-term survival after lung metastasectomy. Ann Thorac Surg 1997;63:777–84.
4. Pastorino U, Buyse M, Friedel G, et al. International Registry of Lung Metastases. Long-term results of lung metastasectomy: prognostic analyses based on 5206 cases. J Thorac Cardiovasc Surg 1997;113:37–49.
5. Fourquier P, Regnard JF, Rea S, et al. Lung metastases of renal cell carcinoma: results of surgical resection. Eur J Cardiothorac Surg 1997;11:17–21.
6. Thomita Y, Imai T, Tanikawa T, et al. Treatment of bilateral renal cell cancer and multiple lung metastasis: nephron-sparing surgery and resection of lung tumors after interleukin-2 therapy. Eur Urol 1998;33:238–40.
7. Wedman J, Balm AJ, Hart AA, et al. Value of resection of pulmonary metastases in head and neck cancer patients. Head Neck 1996;18:311–16.
8. Chou CW, Liu JM, Wu MF, et al. Prolonged survival in a nasopharyngeal carcinoma patient with multiple metastases: a case report and review of the literature. Jpn J Clin Oncol 1997;27:336–9.
9. Younes RN, Gross JL, Silva JF, et al. Surgical treatment of lung metastases of head and neck tumors. Am J Surg 1997;174:499–502.
10. Nibu K, Nakagawa K, Kamata S, et al. Surgical treatment for pulmonary metastases of squamous cell carcinoma of the head and neck. Am J Otolaryngol 1997;18:391–5.
11. Cheng LC, Chiu CSW, Lee JWT. Surgical resection of pulmonary metastases. J Cardiovasc Surg 1998;39:503–7.
12. Simpson R, Kennedy C, Carmalt H, et al. Pulmonary resection for metastatic breast cancer. Aust N Z J Surg 1997;67:717–9.
13. Shin MS, Holman WL, Herrera GA, Ho KJ. Extensive pulmonary metastasis of an intracranial meningioma with repeated recurrence: radiographic and pathologic features. South Med J 1996;89:313–8.
14. Murrah CP, Ferguson ER, Jennelle RL, et al. Resection of multiple pulmonary metastases from a recurrent intracranial meningioma. Ann Thorac Surg 1996;61:1823–4.
15. Van Haaren ER, Kievit J, Huysmans HA, van de Velde CJ. Successful resection of hepatic and pulmonary metastases in a patient with parathyroid carcinoma. Jpn J Clin Oncol 1996;26:99–102.
16. Khan JH, McElhinney DB, Rahman SB, et al. Pulmonary metastases of endocrine origin: the role of surgery. Chest 1998;114:526–34.
17. Urabe M, Sakakibara T, Daibo M, et al. Two cases of recurrent pulmonary metastasis resected after operation for gastric cancer. Nippon Geka Hokan 1996;65:22–9.
18. Lam CM, Lo CM, Yuen WK, et al. Prolonged survival in selected patients following surgical resection for pulmonary metastasis from hepatocellular carcinoma. Br J Surg 1998;85:1198–200.
19. Kanemitsu Y, Kondo H, Katai H, et al. Surgical resection of pulmonary metastases from gastric cancer. J Surg Oncol 1998;69:147–50.
20. Van Geel AN, Pastorino U, Jauch KW, et al. Surgical treatment of lung metastases: the European Organization for Research and Treatment of Cancer—soft tissue and bone sarcoma group study of 255 patients. Cancer 1996;77:675–82.
21. Paulussen M, Ahrens S, Craft AW, et al. Ewing's tumors with primary lung metastases: survival analysis of 114 (European Intergroup) cooperative Ewing's sarcoma studies patients. J Clin Oncol 1998;16:3044–52.
22. Ellis PM, Tattersall MHN, McCaughan B, Stalley P. Osteosarcoma and pulmonary metastases: 15-year experience from a single institution. Aust N Z J Surg 1997;67:625–9.
23. Alvegard TA, Saeter G. The role of pulmonary metastasectomy for soft tissue sarcoma. Acta Orthop Scand 1997;68:Suppl 273:145–7.
24. Zanella A, Marchet A, Mainente P, et al. Resection of pulmonary metastases from colorectal carcinoma. Eur J Surg Oncol 1997;23:424–7.
25. Girard P, Ducreux M, Baldeyrou P, et al. Surgery for lung metastases from colorectal cancer: analysis of prognostic factors. J Clin Oncol 1996;14:2047–53.
26. Van Halteren HK, van Geel AN, Hart AAM, Zoetmulder FAN. Pulmonary resection for metastases of colorectal origin. Chest 1995;107:1526–31.
27. Okumura S, Kondo H, Tsuboi M, et al. Pulmonary resection for metastatic colorectal cancer: experiences with 159 patients. J Thorac Cardiovasc Surg 1996;112:867–74.
28. Baron O, Amini M, Duveau D, et al. Surgical resection of pulmonary metastases from colorectal carcinoma: five-year survival and main prognostic factors. Eur J Cardiothorac Surg 1996;10:347–51.
29. Yano T, Fukuyama Y, Yokoyama H, et al. Failure in resection of multiple pulmonary metastases from colorectal cancer. J Am Coll Surg 1997;185:120–2.
30. Ambiru S, Miyazaki M, Ito H, et al. Resection of hepatic and pulmonary metastases in patients with colorectal carcinoma. Cancer 1998;82:274–8.
31. Regnard JF, Grunenwald D, Spaggiari L, et al. Surgical treatment of hepatic and pulmonary metastases from colorectal cancers. Ann Thorac Surg 1998;66:214–9.
32. Watanabe M, Deguchi H, Sato M, et al. Midterm results of thoracoscopic surgery for pulmonary metastases especially from colorectal cancers. J Laparoend Adv Surg Tech. Part A 1998;8:195–200.

33. Van der Veen AH, van Geel AN, Hop WC, Wiggers T. Median sternotomy: the preferred incision for resection of lung metastases. Eur J Surg 1998;164:507–12.

34. McCormack PM, Bains MS, Begg CB, et al. Role of video-assisted thoracic surgery in the treatment of pulmonary metastases: results of a prospective trial. Ann Thorac Surg 1996;62:213–7.

# APPENDIX A

# NOMOGRAPH FOR CALCULATING THE BODY SURFACE AREA OF ADULTS

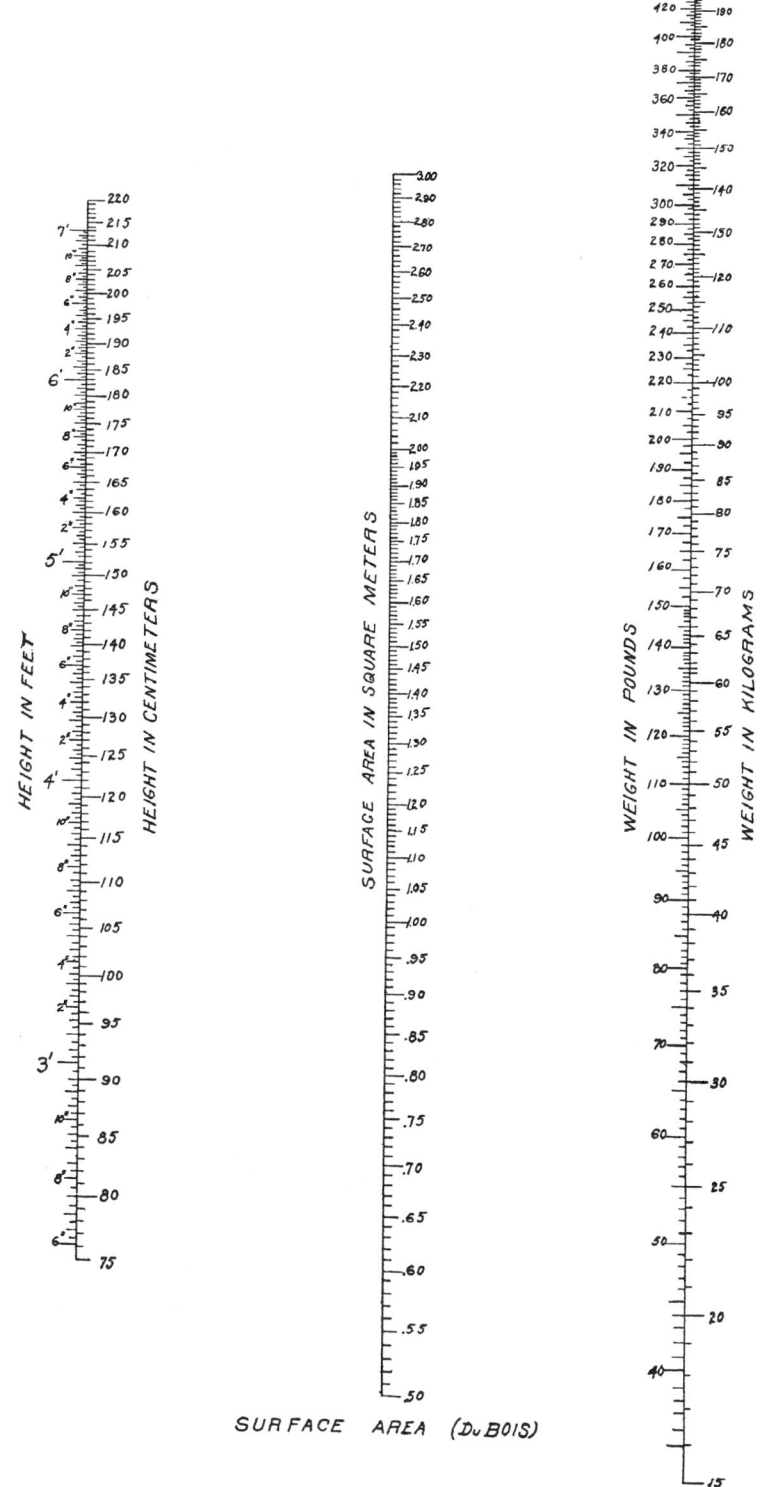

SURFACE AREA (DuBOIS)

From Boothby WM, Sandiford RB: Nomographic charts for the calculation of the metabolic rate by the gasometer method. Boston Med Surg J Sept 22, 1921; 185(12):337. Based on the formula of DuBois and DuBois: BSA in $m^2$ = [71.84] [$kg^{0.425}$] [$cm^{0.725}$] [$10^{-4}$].

# NATIONAL CANCER INSTITUTE/SOUTHWEST ONCOLOGY GROUP GUIDELINES FOR GRADING TOXICITY

| | Grade | | | | |
|---|---|---|---|---|---|
| **Adverse Event** | 0 | 1 | 2 | 3 | 4 |

## ALLERGY/IMMUNOLOGY

| | | | | | |
|---|---|---|---|---|---|
| Allergic reaction/ hypersensitivity (including drug fever) | None | Transient rash, drug fever <38° C (<100.4° F) | Urticaria, drug fever ≥38° C (≥100.4° F), and/or asymptomatic bronchospasm | Symptomatic bronchospasm, requiring parenteral medication(s), with or without urticaria; allergy-related edema/angioedema | Anaphylaxis |

Note: Isolated urticaria, in the absence of other manifestations of an allergic or hypersensitivity reaction, is graded in the DERMATOLOGY/SKIN category.

| | | | | | |
|---|---|---|---|---|---|
| Allergic rhinitis (including sneezing, nasal stuffiness, postnasal drip) | None | Mild, not requiring treatment | Moderate, requiring treatment | — | — |
| Autoimmune reaction | None | Serologic or other evidence of autoimmune reaction but patient is asymptomatic (e.g., vitiligo), all organ function is normal, and no treatment is required | Evidence of autoimmune reaction involving a nonessential organ or function (e.g., hypothyroidism), requiring treatment other than immunosuppressive drugs | Reversible autoimmune reaction involving function of a major organ or other adverse event (e.g., transient colitis or anemia), requiring short-term immunosuppressive treatment | Autoimmune reaction causing major grade 4 organ dysfunction; progressive and irreversible reaction; long-term administration of high-dose immunosuppressive therapy required |

Also consider Hypothyroidism, Colitis, Hemoglobin, Hemolysis.

| | | | | | |
|---|---|---|---|---|---|
| Serum sickness | None | — | — | Present | |

Urticaria is graded in the DERMATOLOGY/SKIN category if it occurs as an isolated symptom. If it occurs with other manifestations of allergic or hypersensitivity reaction, grade as "allergic reaction/hypersensitivity" above.

| | | | | | |
|---|---|---|---|---|---|
| Vasculitis | None | Mild, not requiring treatment | Symptomatic, requiring medication | Requiring steroids | Ischemic changes or requiring amputation |
| Allergy/ immunology—other (specify, _____) | None | Mild | Moderate | Severe | Life-threatening or disabling |

## AUDITORY/HEARING

Conductive hearing loss is graded as "middle ear/hearing" in the AUDITORY/HEARING category.

Earache is graded in the PAIN category.

| | | | | | |
|---|---|---|---|---|---|
| External auditory canal | Normal | External otitis with erythema or dry desquamation | External otitis with moist desquamation | External otitis with discharge, mastoiditis | Necrosis of the canal soft tissue or bone |

Note: Changes associated with radiation to external ear (pinnae) are graded under "radiation dermatitis" in the DERMATOLOGY/SKIN category.

| | | | | | |
|---|---|---|---|---|---|
| Inner ear/hearing | Normal | Hearing loss on audiometry only | Tinnitus or hearing loss, not requiring hearing aid or treatment | Tinnitus or hearing loss, correctable with hearing aid or treatment | Severe unilateral or bilateral hearing loss (deafness), not correctable |

| Adverse Event | Grade | | | | |
|---|---|---|---|---|---|
| | 0 | 1 | 2 | 3 | 4 |
| Middle ear/hearing | Normal | Serous otitis without subjective decrease in hearing | Serous otitis or infection requiring medical intervention; subjective decrease in hearing; rupture of tympanic membrane with discharge | Otitis with discharge, mastoiditis, or conductive hearing loss | Necrosis of the canal soft tissue or bone |
| (Auditory/ hearing—other (specify, _____) | Normal | Mild | Moderate | Severe | Life-threatening or disabling |

## BLOOD/BONE MARROW

| Adverse Event | Grade | | | | |
|---|---|---|---|---|---|
| | 0 | 1 | 2 | 3 | 4 |
| Bone marrow cellularity | Normal for age | Mildly hypocellular or ≤25% reduction from normal cellularity for age | Moderately hypocellular or >25–≤50% reduction from normal cellularity for age or >2 but <4 weeks to recovery of normal bone marrow cellularity | Severely hypocellular or >50–≤75% reduction in cellularity for age or 4–6 weeks to recovery of normal bone marrow cellularity | Aplasia or >6 weeks to recovery of normal bone marrow cellularity |

Normal ranges:

| | |
|---|---|
| Children (≤18 years) | 90% cellularity average |
| Younger adults (19–59 years) | 60–70% cellularity average |
| Older adults (≥60 years) | 50% cellularity average |

Note: Grade "bone marrow cellularity" only for changes related to treatment not disease.

| Adverse Event | 0 | 1 | 2 | 3 | 4 |
|---|---|---|---|---|---|
| CD4 count | WNL | <LLN–500/mm³ | 200–<500/mm³ | 50–<200/mm³ | <50/mm³ |
| Haptoglobin | Normal | Decreased | — | Absent | — |
| Hemoglobin (Hgb) | WNL | <LLN–10.0 g/dl<br><LLN–100 g/L<br><LLN–6.2 mmol/L | 8.0—<10.0 g/dl<br>80—<100 g/L<br>4.9—<6.2 mmol/L | 6.5–<8.0 g/dl<br>65—<80 g/L<br>4.0—<4.9 mmol/L | <6.5 g/dl<br><65 g/L<br><4.0 mmol/L |
| For leukemia studies or bone marrow infiltrative/ myelophthisic processes, if specified in the protocol. | WNL | 10–<25% decrease from pretreatment | 25–<50% decrease from pretreatment | 50–<75% decrease from pretreatment | ≥75% decrease from pretreatment |
| Hemolysis (e.g., immune hemolytic anemia, drug-related hemolysis, other) | None | Only laboratory evidence of hemolysis (e.g., direct antiglobulin test [DAT, Coombs'] schistocytes) | Evidence of red blood cell destruction and ≥2 g decrease in hemoglobin, no transfusion | Requiring transfusion and/or medical intervention (e.g., steroids) | Catastrophic consequences of hemolysis (e.g., renal failure, hypotension, bronchospasm, emergency splenectomy) |

Also consider Haptoglobin, Hemoglobin.

| Adverse Event | 0 | 1 | 2 | 3 | 4 |
|---|---|---|---|---|---|
| Leukocytes (total WBC) | WNL | <LLN–3 × 10⁹/L<br><LLN–3000/mm³ | ≥2.0–<3.0 × 10⁹/L<br>≥2000–<3000/mm³ | ≥1.0–<2 × 10⁹/L<br>≥1000–<2000/mm³ | <1.0 × 10⁹/L<br><1000/mm³ |

| Adverse Event | Grade | | | | |
|---|---|---|---|---|---|
| | 0 | 1 | 2 | 3 | 4 |
| For BMT studies, if specified in the protocol. | WNL | ≥2–<3 × 10⁹/L ≥2000–<3000/mm³ | ≥1.0–<2.0 × 10⁹/L ≥1000–<2000/mm³ | ≥0.5–<1.0 × 10⁹/L ≥500–<1000/mm³ | <0.5 × 10⁹/L <500/mm³ |
| For pediatric BMT studies (using age, race, and sex normal values), if specified in the protocol. | | ≥75–<100% LLN | ≥50–<75% LLN | ≥25–50% LLN | <25% LLN |
| Lymphopenia | WNL | <LLN–1.0 × 10⁹/L <LLN—1000/mm³ | ≥05.–<1.0 × 10⁹/L ≥500–<1000/mm³ | <0.5 × 10⁹/L <500/mm³ | |
| For pediatric BMT studies (using age, race and sex normal values), if specified in the protocol. | | ≥75%–<100% LLN | ≥50–<75% LLN | ≥25–<50% LLN | <25% LLN |
| Neutrophils/ granulocytes (ANC/ AGC) | WNL | ≥1.5–<2.0 × 10⁹/L ≥1500–<2000/mm³ | ≥1.0–<1.5 × 10⁹/L ≥1000–<1500/mm³ | ≥0.5–<1.0 × 10⁹/L ≥500–<1000/mm³ | <0.5 × 10⁹/L <500/mm³ |
| For BMT studies, if specified in the protocol. | WNL | ≥1.0–<1.5 × 10⁹/L ≥1000–<1500/mm³ | ≥0.5–<1.0 × 10⁹/L ≥500–<1000/mm³ | ≥0.1–<0.5 × 10⁹/L ≥100–<500/mm³ | <0.1 × 10⁹/L <100/mm³ |
| For leukemia studies or bone marrow infiltrative/ myelophthisic process, if specified in the protocol. | WNL | 10–<25% decrease from baseline | 25–<50% decrease from baseline | 50–<75% decrease from baseline | ≥75% decrease from baseline |
| Platelets | WNL | <LLN–75.0 × 10⁹/L <LLN–75,000/mm³ | ≥50.0–<75.0 × 10⁹/L ≥50,000–<75,000/mm³ | ≥10.0–<50.0 × 10⁹/L ≥10,000–<50,000/mm³ | <10.0 × 10⁹/L <10,000/mm³ |
| For BMT studies, if specified in the protocol. | WNL | ≥50.0–<75.0 × 10⁹/L ≥50,000–<75,000/mm³ | ≥20.0–<50.0 × 10⁹/L ≥20,000–<50,000/mm³ | ≥10.0–<20.0 × 10⁹/L ≥10,000–<20,000/mm³ | <10.0 × 10⁹/L <10,000/mm³ |
| For leukemia studies or bone marrow infiltrative/ myelophthisic process, if specified in the protocol. | WNL | 10–<25% decrease from baseline | 25–<50% decrease from baseline | 50–<75% decrease from baseline | ≥75% decrease from baseline |
| Transfusion: platelets | None | — | — | Yes | Platelet transfusions and other measures required to improve platelet increment; platelet transfusion refractoriness associated with life-threatening bleeding (e.g., HLA or cross-matched platelet transfusions) |
| For BMT studies, if specified in the protocol. | None | 1 platelet transfusion in 24 hours | 2 platelet transfusions in 24 hours | ≥3 platelet transfusions in 24 hours | Platelet transfusions and other measures required to improve platelet increment; platelet transfusion refractoriness associated with life-threatening bleeding (e.g., HLA or cross-matched platelet transfusions) |

| Adverse Event | Grade | | | | |
|---|---|---|---|---|---|
| | 0 | 1 | 2 | 3 | 4 |
| Also consider Platelets. | | | | | |
| Transfusion: PRBCs | None | — | — | Yes | — |
| For BMT studies, if specified in the protocol. | None | ≥2 units—PRBCs in 24 hours, elective or planned | 3 units—PRBCs in 24 hours, elective or planned | ≥4 units PRBCs in 24 hours | Hemorrhage or hemolysis associated with life-threatening anemia; medical intervention required to improve hemoglobin |
| For pediatric BMT studies, if specified in the protocol. | None | ≥15 mL/kg in 24 hours, elective or planned | >15–≤30 mL/kg in 24 hours, elective or planned | >30 mL/kg in 24 hours | Hemorrhage or hemolysis associated with life-threatening anemia; medical intervention required to improve hemoglobin |
| Also consider Hemoglobin. | | | | | |
| Blood/bone marrow—other (specify, _____) | None | Mild | Moderate | Severe | Life-threatening or disabling |

## CARDIOVASCULAR (ARRHYTHMIA)

| Adverse Event | Grade | | | | |
|---|---|---|---|---|---|
| | 0 | 1 | 2 | 3 | 4 |
| Conduction abnormality/ atrioventricular heart block | None | Asymptomatic, not requiring treatment (e.g., Mobitz type I second-degree AV block, Wenckebach) | Symptomatic, but not requiring treatment | Symptomatic and requiring treatment (e.g., Mobitz type II second-degree AV block, third-degree AV block) | Life-threatening (e.g., arrhythmia associated with CHF, hypotension, syncope, shock) |
| Nodal/junctional arrhythmia/ dysrhythmia | None | Asymptomatic, not requiring treatment | Symptomatic, but not requiring treatment | Symptomatic, but not requiring treatment | Life-threatening (e.g., arrhythmia associated with CHF, hypotension, syncope, shock) |
| Palpitations | None | Present | — | — | — |

Note: Grade palpitations *only* in the absence of a documented arrhythmia.

| Adverse Event | Grade | | | | |
|---|---|---|---|---|---|
| | 0 | 1 | 2 | 3 | 4 |
| Prolonged QTc interval (QTc >0.48 second) | None | Asymptomatic, not requiring treatment | Symptomatic, but not requiring treatment | Symptomatic and requiring treatment | Life-threatening (e.g., arrhythmia associated with CHF, hypotension, syncope, shock) |
| Sinus bradycardia | None | Asymptomatic, not requiring treatment | Symptomatic, but not requiring treatment | Symptomatic and requiring treatment | Life-threatening (e.g., arrhythmia associated with CHF, hypotension, syncope, shock) |
| Sinus tachycardia | None | Asymptomatic, not requiring treatment | Symptomatic, but not requiring treatment | Symptomatic and requiring treatment of underlying cause | — |
| Supraventricular arrhythmias (SVT/ atrial fibrillation/ flutter) | None | Asymptomatic, not requiring treatment | Symptomatic, but not requiring treatment | Symptomatic and requiring treatment | Life-threatening (e.g., arrhythmia associated with CHF, hypotension, syncope, shock) |

| Adverse Event | Grade 0 | 1 | 2 | 3 | 4 |
|---|---|---|---|---|---|

Syncope (fainting) is graded in the NEUROLOGY category.

| Adverse Event | 0 | 1 | 2 | 3 | 4 |
|---|---|---|---|---|---|
| Vasovagal episode | None | — | Present without loss of consciousness | Present with loss of consciousness | — |
| Ventricular arrhythmia (PVCs/bigeminy/ trigeminy/ ventricular tachycardia) | None | Asymptomatic, not requiring treatment | Symptomatic, but not requiring treatment | Symptomatic and requiring treatment | Life-threatening (e.g., arrhythmia associated with CHF, hypotension, syncope, shock) |
| Cardiovascular arrhythmia—other (specify, _____) | None | Asymptomatic, not requiring treatment | Symptomatic, but not requiring treatment | Symptomatic and requiring treatment of underlying cause | Life-threatening (e.g., arrhythmia associated with CHF, hypotension, syncope, shock) |

## CARDIOVASCULAR (GENERAL)

| Adverse Event | 0 | 1 | 2 | 3 | 4 |
|---|---|---|---|---|---|
| Acute vascular leak syndrome | Absent | — | Symptomatic, but not requiring fluid support | Respiratory compromise or requiring fluids | Life-threatening; requiring pressor support and/or ventilatory support |
| Cardiac—ischemia/ infarction | None | Nonspecific T-wave flattening or changes | Asymptomatic, ST- and T-wave changes suggesting ischemia | Angina without evidence of infarction | Acute myocardial infarction |
| Cardiac left ventricular function | Normal | Asymptomatic decline of resting ejection fraction of ≥10% but <20% of baseline value; shortening fraction ≥24% but <30% | Asymptomatic but resting ejection fraction below LLN for laboratory or decline of resting ejection fraction ≥20% of baseline value; <24% shortening fraction | CHF responsive to treatment | Severe or refractory CHF or requiring intubation |

CNS cerebrovascular ischemia is graded in the NEUROLOGY category.

| Adverse Event | 0 | 1 | 2 | 3 | 4 |
|---|---|---|---|---|---|
| Cardiac troponin I (cTnI) | Normal | — | — | Levels consistent with unstable angina as defined by the manufacturer | Levels consistent with myocardial infarction as defined by the manufacturer |
| Cardiac troponin T (cTnT) | Normal | ≥0.03–<0.05 ng/ml | ≥0.05–<0.1 ng/ml | ≥0.1–<0.2 ng/ml | ≥0.2 ng/ml |
| Edema | None | Asymptomatic, not requiring therapy | Symptomatic, requiring therapy | Symptomatic edema limiting function and unresponsive to therapy or requiring drug discontinuation | Anasarca (severe generalized edema) |
| Hypertension | None | Asymptomatic, transient increase by >20 mm Hg (diastolic) or to >150/100* if previously WNL; not requiring treatment | Recurrent or persistent or symptomatic increase by >20 mm Hg (diastolic) or to >150/100* if previously WNL; not requiring treatment | Requiring therapy or more intensive therapy than previously | Hypertensive crisis |

*Note: For pediatric patients, use age- and sex-appropriate normal values >95th percentile ULN.

| Adverse Event | 0 | 1 | 2 | 3 | 4 |
|---|---|---|---|---|---|
| Hypotension | None | Changes, but not requiring therapy (including transient orthostatic hypotension) | Requiring brief fluid replacement or other therapy but not hospitalization; no physiologic consequences | Requiring therapy and sustained medical attention, but resolves without persisting physiologic consequences | Shock (associated with acidemia and impairing vital organ function due to tissue hypoperfusion) |

| Adverse Event | Grade | | | | |
|---|---|---|---|---|---|
| | 0 | 1 | 2 | 3 | 4 |

Also consider Syncope (fainting).

Notes: Angina or MI is graded as Cardiac-ischemia/infarction in the CARDIOVASCULAR (GENERAL) category.
For pediatric patients, systolic BP 65 mm Hg or less in infants up to 1 year old and 70 mm Hg or less in children older than 1 year, use two successive or three measurements in 24 hours.

| Adverse Event | 0 | 1 | 2 | 3 | 4 |
|---|---|---|---|---|---|
| Myocarditis | None | — | — | CHF responsive to treatment | Severe or refractory CHF |
| Operative injury of vein/artery | None | Primary suture repair for injury, but not requiring transfusion | Primary suture repair for injury, requiring transfusion | Vascular occlusion requiring surgery or bypass for injury | Myocardial infarction; resection or organ (e.g., bowel, limb) |
| Pericardial effusion/ pericarditis | None | Asymptomatic effusion, not requiring treatment | Pericarditis (rub, ECG changes, and/or chest pain) | With physiologic consequences | Tamponade (drainage or pericardial window required) |
| Peripheral arterial ischemia | None | — | Brief episode of ischemia managed nonsurgically and without permanent deficit | Requiring surgical intervention | Life-threatening or with permanent functional deficit (e.g., amputation) |
| Phlebitis (superficial) | None | — | Present | | |

Notes: Injection site reaction is graded in the DERMATOLOGY/SKIN category.
Thrombosis/embolism is graded in the CARDIOVASCULAR (GENERAL) category.

Syncope (fainting) is graded in the NEUROLOGY category.

| Adverse Event | 0 | 1 | 2 | 3 | 4 |
|---|---|---|---|---|---|
| Thrombosis/embolism | None | — | Deep vein thrombosis, not requiring anticoagulant therapy | Deep vein thrombosis, requiring anticoagulant therapy | Embolic event including pulmonary embolism |

Vein/artery operative injury is graded as "operative injury of vein/artery" in the CARDIOVASCULAR (GENERAL) category.

| Adverse Event | 0 | 1 | 2 | 3 | 4 |
|---|---|---|---|---|---|
| Visceral arterial ischemia (nonmyocardial) | None | — | Brief episode of ischemia managed nonsurgically and without permanent deficit | Requiring surgical intervention | Life-threatening or with permanent functional deficit (e.g., resection of ileum) |
| Cardiovascular/ genera—other (specify, _____) | None | Mild | Moderate | Severe | Life-threatening or disabling |

## COAGULATION

Note: See the HEMORRHAGE category for grading the severity of bleeding events.

| Adverse Event | 0 | 1 | 2 | 3 | 4 |
|---|---|---|---|---|---|
| DIC (disseminated intravascular coagulation) | Absent | — | — | Laboratory findings present with *no* bleeding | Laboratory findings *and* bleeding |

Also consider Platelets.

Note: Must have increased fibrin split products or D-dimer in order to grade as DIC.

| Adverse Event | 0 | 1 | 2 | 3 | 4 |
|---|---|---|---|---|---|
| Fibrinogen | WNL | ≥0.75–<1.0 × LLN | ≥0.5–<0.75 × LLN | ≥0.25–<0.5 × LLN | <0.25 × LLN |
| For leukemia studies or bone marrow infiltrative/ myelophthisic process, if specified in the protocol. | WNL | <20% decrease from pretreatment value or LLN | ≥20–<40% decrease from pretreatment value or LLN | ≥40–<70% decrease from pretreatment value or LLN | <50 mg |
| Partial thromboplastin time (PTT) | WNL | >ULN–≤1.5 × ULN | >1.5–≤2 × ULN | >2 × ULN | |

| Adverse Event | Grade | | | | |
|---|---|---|---|---|---|
| | 0 | 1 | 2 | 3 | 4 |
| Phlebitis is graded in the CARDIOVASCULAR (GENERAL) category. | | | | | |
| Prothrombin time (PT) | WNL | >ULN–≤1.5 × ULN | >1.5–≤2 × ULN | >2 × ULN | |
| Thrombosis/embolism is graded in the CARDIOVASCULAR (GENERAL) category. | | | | | |
| Thrombotic microangiopathy (e.g., thrombotic thrombocytopenic purpura [TTP] or hemolytic uremic syndrome [HUS]) | Absent | — | — | Laboratory findings present without clinical consequences | Laboratory findings and clinical consequences, (e.g., CNS hemorrhage/ bleeding or thrombosis/ embolism or renal failure) requiring therapeutic intervention |
| For BMT studies, if specified in the protocol. | — | Evidence of RBC destruction (schistocytosis) without clinical consequences | Evidence of RBC destruction with elevated creatinine (≤3 × ULN) | Evidence of RBC destruction with creatinine (>3 × ULN) not requiring dialysis | Evidence of RBC destruction with renal failure requiring dialysis and/or encephalopathy |

Also consider Hemoglobin, Platelets, Creatinine.

Note: Must have microangiopathic changes on blood smear (e.g., schistocytes, helmet cells, red cell fragments).

| Coagulation—other (specify, _____) | None | Mild | Moderate | Severe | Life-threatening or disabling |
|---|---|---|---|---|---|

## CONSTITUTIONAL SYMPTOMS

| Adverse Event | 0 | 1 | 2 | 3 | 4 |
|---|---|---|---|---|---|
| Fatigue (lethargy, malaise, asthenia) | None | Increased fatigue over baseline, but not altering normal activities | Moderate (e.g., decrease in performance status by 1 ECOG level or 20% Karnofsky or Lansky) or causing difficulty performing some activities | Severe (e.g., decrease in performance status by ≥2 ECOG levels or 40% Karnofsky or Lansky) or loss of ability to perform some activities | Bedridden or disabling |
| Fever (in the absence of neutropenia, where neutropenia is defined as AGC <1.0 × 10⁹/L) | None | 38–39° C (100.4–102.2° F) | 39.1–40° C (102.3–104° F) | >40° C (>104° F) for <24 hours | >40° C (>104° F) for >24 hours |

Also consider Allergic reaction/hypersensitivity.

Note: The temperature measurements listed above are oral or tympanic. Hot flashes/flushes are graded in the ENDOCRINE category.

| Rigors, chills | None | Mild, requiring symptomatic treatment (e.g., blanket) or non-narcotic medication | Severe and/or prolonged, requiring narcotic medication | Not responsive to narcotic medication | — |
| Sweating (diaphoresis) | Normal | Mild and occasional | Frequent or drenching | — | — |
| Weight gain | <5% | 5–<10% | 10–<20% | ≥20% | — |

Also consider Ascites, Edema, Pleural effusion (nonmalignant).

| Weight gain associated with veno-occlusive disease (VOD) for BMT studies, if specified in the protocol. | <2% | ≥2–<5% | ≥5–<10% | ≥10% or as ascites | ≥10% or fluid retention resulting in pulmonary failure |
|---|---|---|---|---|---|

Also consider Ascites, Edema, Pleural effusion (nonmalignant).

| Adverse Event | Grade | | | | |
|---|---|---|---|---|---|
| | 0 | 1 | 2 | 3 | 4 |
| Weight loss | <5% | 5–<10% | 10–<20% | ≥20% | — |

Also consider Vomiting, Dehydration, Diarrhea.

| | | | | | |
|---|---|---|---|---|---|
| Constitutional symptoms—other (specify, _____) | None | Mild | Moderate | Severe | Life-threatening or disabling |

## DERMATOLOGY/SKIN

| Adverse Event | 0 | 1 | 2 | 3 | 4 |
|---|---|---|---|---|---|
| Alopecia | Normal | Mild hair loss | Pronounced hair loss | — | — |
| Bruising (in absence of grade 3 or 4 thrombocytopenia) | None | Localized or in dependent area | Generalized | — | — |

Note: Bruising *resulting from grade 3 or 4 thrombocytopenia* is graded as Petechiae/purpura *and* Hemorrhage/bleeding with grade 3 or 4 thrombocytopenia in the HEMORRHAGE category, *not* in the DERMATOLOGY/SKIN category.

| Adverse Event | 0 | 1 | 2 | 3 | 4 |
|---|---|---|---|---|---|
| Dry skin | Normal | Controlled with emollients | Not controlled with emollients | — | — |
| Erythema multiforme (e.g., Stevens-Johnson syndrome, toxic epidermal necrolysis) | Absent | — | Scattered, but not generalized eruption | Severe or requiring IV fluids (e.g., generalized rash or painful stomatitis) | Life-threatening (e.g., exfoliative or ulcerating dermatitis or requiring enteral or parenteral nutritional support) |
| Flushing | Absent | Present | — | — | — |
| Hand-foot skin reaction | None | Skin changes or dermatitis without pain (e.g., erythema, peeling) | Skin changes with pain, not interfering with function | Skin changes with pain, interfering with function | — |
| Injection site reaction | None | Pain or itching or erythema | Pain or swelling, with inflammation or phlebitis | Ulceration or necrosis that is severe or prolonged, or requiring surgery | — |
| Nail changes | Normal | Discoloration or ridging (koilonychia) or pitting | Partial or complete loss of nail(s) or pain in nailbeds | — | — |

Petechiae is graded in the HEMORRHAGE category.

| Adverse Event | 0 | 1 | 2 | 3 | 4 |
|---|---|---|---|---|---|
| Photosensitivity | None | Painless erythema | Painful erythema | Erythema with desquamation | — |
| Pigmentation changes (e.g., vitiligo) None | Localized pigmentation changes | Generalized pigmentation changes | — | — | |
| Pruritus | None | Mild or localized, relieved spontaneously or by local measures | Intense or widespread, relieved spontaneously or by systemic measures | Intense or widespread and poorly controlled despite treatment | — |

Purpura is graded in the HEMORRHAGE category.

| Adverse Event | 0 | 1 | 2 | 3 | 4 |
|---|---|---|---|---|---|
| Radiation dermatitis | None | Faint erythema or dry desquamation | Moderate to brisk erythema or a patchy, moist desquamation, mostly confined to skin folds and creases; moderate edema | Confluent moist desquamation ≥1.5 cm diameter and not confined to skin folds; pitting edema | Skin necrosis or ulceration of full-thickness dermis; may include bleeding not induced by minor trauma or abrasion |

| Adverse Event | Grade | | | | |
|---|---|---|---|---|---|
| | 0 | 1 | 2 | 3 | 4 |
| Note: Pain associated with radiation dermatitis is graded separately in the PAIN category as Pain due to radiation. | | | | | |
| Radiation recall reaction (reaction following chemotherapy in the absence of additional radiation therapy that occurs in a previous radiation port) | None | Faint erythema or dry desquamation | Moderate to brisk erythema or a patchy, moist desquamation, mostly confined to skin folds and creases; moderate edema | Confluent moist desquamation ≥1.5 cm diameter and not confined to skin folds; pitting edema | Skin necrosis or ulceration of full-thickness dermis; may include bleeding not induced by minor trauma or abrasion |
| Rash/desquamation | None | Macular or papular eruption or erythema without associated symptoms | Macular or papular eruption or erythema with pruritus or other associated symptoms covering <50% of body surface or localized desquamation or other lesions covering <50% of body surface area | Symptomatic generalized erythroderma or macular, papular, or vesicular eruption or desquamation covering ≥50% of body surface area | Generalized exfoliative dermatitis or ulcerative dermatitis |

Also consider Allergic reaction/hypersensitivity.

Note: Stevens-Johnson syndrome is graded separately as Erythema multiforme in the DERMATOLOGY/SKIN category.

| Adverse Event | Grade | | | | |
|---|---|---|---|---|---|
| Rash/dermatitis associated with high-dose chemotherapy or BMT studies. | None | Faint erythema or dry desquamation | Moderate to brisk erythema or a patchy, moist desquamation, mostly confined to skin folds and creases; moderate edema | Confluent moist desquamation ≥1.5 cm diameter and not confined to skin folds; pitting edema | Skin necrosis or ulceration of full-thickness dermis, may include spontaneous bleeding not induced by minor trauma or abrasion |
| Rash/desquamation associated with graft versus host disease (GVHD) for BMT studies, if specified in the protocol. | None | Macular or papular eruption or erythema covering <25% of body surface area without associated symptoms | Macular or papular eruption or erythema with pruritus or other associated symptoms covering ≥25–<50% of body surface or localized desquamation or other lesions covering ≥25–<50% of body surface area | Symptomatic generalized erythroderma or symptomatic macular, papular, or vesicular eruption, with bullous formation, or desquamation covering ≥50% of body surface area | Generalized exfoliative dermatitis or ulcerative dermatitis or bullous formation |

Also consider Allergic reaction/hypersensitivity.
Note: Stevens-Johnson syndrome is graded separately as Erythema multiforme in the DERMATOLOGY/SKIN category.

| Adverse Event | Grade | | | | |
|---|---|---|---|---|---|
| Urticaria (hives, welts, wheals) | None | Requiring no medication | Requiring PO or topical treatment or IV medication or steroids for <24 hours | Requiring IV medication or steroids for ≥24 hours | — |
| Wound—infectious | None | Cellulitis | Superficial infection | Infection requiring IV antibiotics | Necrotizing fasciitis |
| Wound—noninfectious | None | Incisional separation | Incisional hernia | Fascial disruption without evisceration | Fascial disruption with evisceration |
| Dermatology/skin—other (specify, _____) | None | Mild | Moderate | Severe | Life-threatening or disabling |

## ENDOCRINE

| Adverse Event | Grade | | | | |
|---|---|---|---|---|---|
| Cushingoid appearance (e.g., moon face, buffalo hump, centripetal obesity, cutaneous striae) | Absent | — | Present | — | — |

| Adverse Event | Grade | | | | |
|---|---|---|---|---|---|
| | 0 | 1 | 2 | 3 | 4 |
| Also consider Hyperglycemia, Hypokalemia. | | | | | |
| Feminization of male | Absent | — | — | Present | — |
| Gynecomastia | None | Mild | Pronounced or painful | Pronounced or painful and requiring surgery | — |
| Hot flashes/flushes | None | Mild or no more than 1 per day | Moderate and greater than 1 per day | — | — |
| Hypothyroidism | Absent | Asymptomatic, TSH elevated, no therapy given | Symptomatic or thyroid replacement treatment given | Patient hospitalized for manifestations of hypothyroidism | Myxedema coma |
| Masculinization of female | Absent | — | — | Present | — |
| SIADH (syndrome of inappropriate antidiuretic hormone) | Absent | — | — | Present | — |
| Endocrine—other (specify, _____) | None | Mild | Moderate | Severe | Life-threatening or disabling |

## GASTROINTESTINAL

Amylase is graded in the METABOLIC/LABORATORY category.

| | 0 | 1 | 2 | 3 | 4 |
|---|---|---|---|---|---|
| Anorexia | None | Loss of appetite | Oral intake significantly decreased | Requiring IV fluids | Requiring feeding tube or parenteral nutrition |
| Ascites (nonmalignant) | None | Asymptomatic | Symptomatic, requiring diuretics | Symptomatic, requiring therapeutic paracentesis | Life-threatening physiologic consequences |
| Colitis | None | — | Abdominal pain with mucus and/or blood in stool | Abdominal pain, fever, change in bowel habits with ileus or peritoneal signs, and radiographic or biopsy documentation | Perforation or requiring surgery or toxic megacolon |

Also consider Hemorrhage/bleeding with grade 3 or 4 thrombocytopenia, Hemorrhage/bleeding without grade 3 or 4 thrombocytopenia, Melena/GI bleeding, Rectal bleeding/hematochezia, Hypotension.

| | 0 | 1 | 2 | 3 | 4 |
|---|---|---|---|---|---|
| Constipation | None | Requiring stool softener or dietary modification | Requiring laxatives | Obstipation requiring manual evacuation or enema | Obstruction or toxic megacolon |
| Dehydration | None | Dry mucous membranes and/or diminished skin turgor | Requiring IV fluid replacement (brief) | Requiring IV fluid replacement (sustained) | Physiologic consequences requiring intensive care; or hemodynamic collapse |

Also consider Diarrhea, Vomiting, Stomatitis/pharyngitis (oral/pharyngeal mucositis), Hypotension.

| | 0 | 1 | 2 | 3 | 4 |
|---|---|---|---|---|---|
| Diarrhea patients without colostomy | None | Increase of <4 stools/ day over pretreatment | Increase of 4–6 stools/ day, or nocturnal stools | Increase of ≥7 stools/ day or incontinence; or need for parenteral support for dehydration | Physiologic consequences requiring intensive care; or hemodynamic collapse |

| Adverse Event | Grade | | | | |
|---|---|---|---|---|---|
| | 0 | 1 | 2 | 3 | 4 |
| Patients with a colostomy | None | Mild increase in loose, watery colostomy output compared with pretreatment | Moderate increase in loose, watery colostomy output compared with pretreatment, but not interfering with normal activity | Severe increase in loose, watery colostomy output compared with pretreatment, interfering with normal activity | Physiologic consequences, requiring intensive care; or hemodynamic collapse |
| Diarrhea associated with graft versus host disease (GVHD) for BMT studies, if specified in the protocol. | None | >500–≤1000 ml of diarrhea/day | >1000–≤1500 ml of diarrhea/day | >1500 ml of diarrhea/day | Severe abdominal pain with or without ileus |
| For pediatric BMT studies, if specified in the protocol. | >5–≤10 ml/kg of diarrhea/day | >10–≤15 ml/kg of diarrhea/day | >15 ml/kg of diarrhea/day | — | |

Also consider Hemorrhage/bleeding with grade 3 or 4 thrombocytopenia. Hemorrhage/bleeding without grade 3 or 4 thrombocytopenia, Pain, Dehydration, Hypotension.

| Adverse Event | 0 | 1 | 2 | 3 | 4 |
|---|---|---|---|---|---|
| Duodenal ulcer (requires radiographic or endoscopic documentation) | None | — | Requiring medical management or nonsurgical treatment | Uncontrolled by outpatient medical management; requiring hospitalization | Perforation or bleeding, requiring emergency surgery |
| Dyspepsia/heartburn | None | Mild | Moderate | Severe | — |
| Dysphagia, esophagitis, odynophagia (painful swallowing) | None | Mild dysphagia, but can eat regular diet | Dysphagia, requiring predominantly pureed, soft, or liquid diet | Dysphagia, requiring IV hydration | Complete obstruction (cannot swallow saliva requiring enteral or parenteral nutritional support, or perforation |

Note: If the adverse event is radiation-related, grade *either* under Dysphagia—esophageal related to radiation *or* Dysphagia—pharyngeal related to radiation.

| Adverse Event | 0 | 1 | 2 | 3 | 4 |
|---|---|---|---|---|---|
| Dysphagia—*esophageal* related to radiation | None | Mild dysphagia, but can eat regular diet | Dysphagia, requiring predominantly pureed, soft, or liquid diet | Dysphagia, requiring feeding tube, IV hydration, or hyperalimentation | Complete obstruction (cannot swallow saliva); ulceration with bleeding not induced by minor trauma or abrasion or perforation |

Also consider Pain due to radiation, Mucositis due to radiation.
Note: fistula is graded separately as Fistula—esophageal.

| Adverse Event | 0 | 1 | 2 | 3 | 4 |
|---|---|---|---|---|---|
| Dysphagia—*pharyngeal* related to radiation | None | Mild dysphagia, but can eat regular diet | Dysphagia, requiring predominantly pureed, soft, or liquid diet | Dysphagia, requiring feeding tube, IV hydration, or hyperalimentation | Complete obstruction (cannot swallow saliva); ulceration with bleeding not induced by minor trauma or abrasion or perforation |

Also consider Pain due to radiation, Mucositis due to radiation.
Note: Fistula is graded separately as Fistula—pharyngeal.

| Adverse Event | 0 | 1 | 2 | 3 | 4 |
|---|---|---|---|---|---|
| Fistula—esophageal | None | — | — | Present | Requiring surgery |
| Fistula—intestinal | None | — | — | Present | Requiring surgery |
| Fistula—pharyngeal | None | — | — | Present | Requiring surgery |
| Fistula—rectal/anal | None | — | — | Present | Requiring surgery |
| Flatulence | None | Mild | Moderate | — | — |

| Adverse Event | Grade | | | | |
|---|---|---|---|---|---|
| | 0 | 1 | 2 | 3 | 4 |
| Gastric ulcer (requires radiographic or endoscopic documentation) | None | | Requiring medical management or nonsurgical treatment | Bleeding without perforation, uncontrolled by outpatient medical management; requiring hospitalization or surgery | Perforation or bleeding, requiring emergency surgery |

Also consider Hemorrhage/bleeding with grade 3 or 4 thrombocytopenia, Hemorrhage/bleeding without grade 3 or 4 thrombocytopenia.

| | | | | | |
|---|---|---|---|---|---|
| Gastritis | None | — | Requiring medical management or nonsurgical treatment | Uncontrolled by outpatient medical management; requiring hospitalization or surgery | Life-threatening bleeding, requiring emergency surgery |

Also consider Hemorrhage/bleeding with grade 3 or 4 thrombocytopenia, Hemorrhage/bleeding without grade 3 or 4 thrombocytopenia.
Hematemesis is graded in the HEMORRHAGE category.
Hematochezia is graded in the HEMORRHAGE category as Rectal bleeding/hematochezia.

| | | | | | |
|---|---|---|---|---|---|
| Ileus (or neuroconstipation) | None | — | Intermittent, not requiring intervention | Requiring nonsurgical intervention | Requiring surgery |
| Mouth dryness | Normal | Mild | Moderate | — | — |

Mucositis

Notes: Mucositis *not due to radiation* is graded in the GASTROINTESTINAL category for specific sites: Colitis, Esophagitis, Gastritis, Stomatitis/pharyngitis (oral/pharyngeal mucositis), and Typhlitis; or the RENAL/GENITOURINARY category for Vaginitis.
Radiation-related mucositis is graded as Mucositis due to radiation.

| | | | | | |
|---|---|---|---|---|---|
| Mucositis due to radiation | None | Erythema of the mucosa | Patchy pseudomembranous reaction (patches generally ≤1.5 cm in diameter and noncontiguous) | Confluent pseudomembranous reaction (contiguous patches generally >1.5 cm in diameter) | Necrosis or deep ulceration; may include bleeding not induced by minor trauma or abrasion |

Also consider Pain due to radiation.
Notes: Grade radiation Mucositis of the larynx here.
Dysphagia related to radiation is also graded as *either* Dysphagia—esophageal related to radiation *or* Dysphagia—pharyngeal related to radiation, depending on the site of treatment.

| | | | | | |
|---|---|---|---|---|---|
| Nausea | None | Able to eat | Oral intake significantly decreased | No significant intake, requiring IV fluids | — |
| Pancreatitis | None | — | — | Abdominal pain with pancreatic enzyme elevation | Complicated by shock (acute circulatory failure) |

Also consider Hypotension.

Note: Amylase is graded in the METABOLIC/LABORATORY category.

Pharyngitis is graded in the GASTROINTESTINAL category as Stomatitis/pharyngitis (oral/pharyngeal mucositis).

| | | | | | |
|---|---|---|---|---|---|
| Proctitis | None | Increased stool frequency, occasional blood-streaked stools, or rectal discomfort (including hemorrhoids) not requiring medication | Increased stool frequency, bleeding, mucous discharge, or rectal discomfort requiring medication; anal fissure | Increased stool frequency/diarrhea requiring parenteral support; rectal bleeding requiring transfusion; or persistent mucous discharge, necessitating pads | Perforation, bleeding or necrosis, or other life-threatening complication requiring surgical intervention (e.g., colostomy) |

Also consider Hemorrhage/bleeding with grade 3 or 4 thrombocytopenia, Hemorrhage/bleeding without grade 3 or 4 thrombocytopenia. Pain due to radiation.

Notes: Fistula is graded separately as Fistula—rectal/anal.
Proctitis occurring more than 90 days after the start of radiation therapy is graded in the RTOG/EORTC Late Radiation Morbidity Scoring Scheme.

| Adverse Event | Grade | | | | |
|---|---|---|---|---|---|
| | 0 | 1 | 2 | 3 | 4 |
| Salivary gland changes | None | Slightly thickened saliva; may have slightly altered taste (e.g., metallic); additional fluids may be required | Thick, ropy, sticky saliva; markedly altered taste; alteration in diet required | — | Acute salivary gland necrosis |
| Sense of smell | Normal | Slightly altered | Markedly altered | — | — |
| Stomatitis/pharyngitis (oral/pharyngeal mucositis) | None | Painless ulcers, erythema, or mild soreness in the absence of lesions | Painful erythema, edema, or ulcers, but can eat or swallow | Painful erythema, edema, or ulcers requiring IV hydration | Severe ulceration or requires parenteral or enteral nutritional support or prophylactic intubation |
| For BMT studies, if specified in the protocol. | None | Painless ulcers, erythema, or mild soreness in the absence of lesions | Painful erythema, edema, or ulcers but can swallow | Painful erythema, edema, or ulcers preventing swallowing or requiring hydration or parenteral (or enteral) nutritional support | Severe ulceration requiring prophylactic intubation or resulting in documented aspiration pneumonia |

Note: Radiation-related mucositis is graded as Mucositis due to radiation.

| Adverse Event | Grade | | | | |
|---|---|---|---|---|---|
| Taste disturbance (dysgeusia) | Normal | Slightly altered | Markedly altered | — | — |
| Typhlitis (inflammation of the cecum) | None | — | — | Abdominal pain, diarrhea, fever, and radiographic or biopsy documentation | Perforation, bleeding or necrosis, or other life-threatening complication requiring surgical intervention (e.g., colostomy) |

Also consider Hemorrhage/bleeding with grade 3 or 4 thrombocytopenia, Hemorrhage/bleeding without grade 3 or 4 thrombocytopenia, Hypotension, Febrile neutropenia.

| Adverse Event | Grade | | | | |
|---|---|---|---|---|---|
| Vomiting | None | 1 episode in 24 hours over pretreatment | 2–5 episodes in 24 hours over pretreatment | ≥6 episodes in 24 hours over pretreatment; or need for IV fluids | Requiring parenteral nutrition; or physiologic consequences requiring intensive care; hemodynamic collapse |

Also consider Dehydration.

Weight gain is graded in the CONSTITUTIONAL SYMPTOMS category.

Weight loss is graded in the CONSTITUTIONAL SYMPTOMS category.

| Adverse Event | Grade | | | | |
|---|---|---|---|---|---|
| Gastrointestinal—other (specify, _____) | None | Mild | Moderate | Severe | Life-threatening or disabling |

## HEMORRHAGE

Notes: Transfusion in this section refers to PRBC infusion.

For *any* bleeding with grade 3 or 4 platelets (<50,000), *always* grade Hemorrhage/bleeding with grade 3 or 4 thrombocytopenia. Also consider Platelets, Transfusion: PRBCs, and Transfusion: platelets in addition to grading severity by grading the site or type of bleeding.

If the site or type of hemorrhage/bleeding is listed, also use the grading that incorporates the site of bleeding: CNS Hemorrhage/bleeding, Hematuria, Hematemesis, Hemoptysis, Hemorrhage/bleeding with surgery, Melena/lower GI bleeding, Petechiae/purpura (Hemorrhage/bleeding into skin), rectal bleeding/hematochezia, Vaginal bleeding.

If the platelet count is ≥50,000 and the site or type of bleeding is listed, grade the specific site. If the site or type is *not* listed and the platelet count is ≥50,000, grade Hemorrhage/bleeding without grade 3 or 4 thrombocytopenia and specify the site or type in the "other" category.

| Adverse Event | Grade | | | | |
|---|---|---|---|---|---|
| | 0 | 1 | 2 | 3 | 4 |
| Hemorrhage/bleeding with grade 3 or 4 thrombocytopenia | None | Mild without transfusion | | Requiring transfusion | Catastrophic bleeding, requiring major nonelective intervention |

Also consider Platelets, Hemoglobin, Transfusion: platelets, Transfusion: PRBCs, site or type of bleeding. If the site is not listed, grade as Hemorrhage—other (specify site, _____).

Note: This adverse event must be graded for any bleeding with grade 3 or 4 thrombocytopenia.

| | | | | | |
|---|---|---|---|---|---|
| Hemorrhage/bleeding without grade 3 or 4 thrombocytopenia | None | Mild without transfusion | | Requiring transfusion | Catastrophic bleeding requiring major nonelective intervention |

Also consider Platelets, Hemoglobin, Transfusion: platelets, Transfusion: PRBCs, Hemorrhage—other (specify site, _____).

Note: Bleeding in the absence of grade 3 or 4 thrombocytopenia is graded here only if the specific site or type of bleeding is not listed elsewhere in the HEMORRHAGE category. Also grade as "other" in the HEMORRHAGE category.

| | | | | | |
|---|---|---|---|---|---|
| CNS hemorrhage/ bleeding | None | — | — | Bleeding noted on CT or other scan with no clinical consequences | Hemorrhagic stroke or hemorrhagic vascular event (CVA) with neurologic signs and symptoms |
| Epistaxis | None | Mild without transfusion | — | Requiring transfusion | Catastrophic bleeding requiring major nonelective intervention |
| Hematemesis | None | Mild without transfusion | — | Requiring transfusion | Catastrophic bleeding, requiring major nonelective intervention |
| Hematuria (in the absence of vaginal bleeding) | None | Microscopic only | Intermittent gross bleeding, no clots | Persistent gross bleeding or clots; may require catheterization or instrumentation, or transfusion | Open surgery or necrosis or deep bladder ulceration |
| Hemoptysis | None | Mild without transfusion | — | Requiring transfusion | Catastrophic bleeding, requiring major nonelective intervention |
| Hemorrhage/bleeding associated with surgery | None | Mild without transfusion | — | Requiring transfusion | Catastrophic bleeding, requiring major nonelective intervention |

Note: Expected blood loss at the time of surgery is not graded as an adverse event.

| | | | | | |
|---|---|---|---|---|---|
| Melena/GI bleeding | None | Mild without transfusion | — | Requiring transfusion | Catastrophic bleeding, requiring major nonelective intervention |
| Petechiae/purpura (hemorrhage/ bleeding into skin or mucosa) | None | Rare petechiae of skin | Petechiae or purpura in dependent areas of skin | Generalized petechiae or purpura of skin or petechiae of any mucosal site | — |
| Rectal bleeding/ hematochezia | None | Mild without transfusion or medication | Persistent, requiring medication (e.g., steroid suppositories) and/or break from radiation treatment | Requiring transfusion | Catastrophic bleeding, requiring major nonelective intervention |
| Vaginal bleeding | None | Spotting, requiring <2 pads per day | Requiring ≥2 pads per day, but not requiring transfusion | Requiring transfusion | Catastrophic bleeding, requiring major nonelective intervention |
| Hemorrhage—other (specify site, _____) | None | Mild without transfusion | — | Requiring transfusion | Catastrophic bleeding, requiring major nonelective intervention |

| Adverse Event | Grade | | | | |
|---|---|---|---|---|---|
| | 0 | 1 | 2 | 3 | 4 |

## HEPATIC

| Adverse Event | 0 | 1 | 2 | 3 | 4 |
|---|---|---|---|---|---|
| Alkaline phosphatase | WNL | >ULN–2.5 × ULN | >2.5–5 × ULN | >5–20 × ULN | >20 × ULN |
| Bilirubin | WNL | >ULN–1.5 × ULN | >1.5–3 × ULN | >3–10 × ULN | >10 × ULN |
| Bilirubin associated with graft versus host disease (GVHD) for BMT studies, if specified in the protocol. | Normal | ≥2–<3 mg/100 ml | ≥3–<6 mg/100 ml | ≥6–<15 mg/100 ml | ≥15 mg/100 ml |
| GGT (γ-Glutamyl transpeptidase) | WNL | >ULN–2.5 × ULN | >2.5–5 × ULN | >5–20 × ULN | >20 × ULN |
| Hepatic enlargement | Absent | — | — | Present | — |

Note: Grade Hepatic enlargement only for treatment-related adverse event including veno-occlusive disease.

| Adverse Event | 0 | 1 | 2 | 3 | 4 |
|---|---|---|---|---|---|
| Hypoalbuminemia | WNL | <LLN–3 g/dl | ≥2–<3 g/dl | <2 g/dl | — |
| Liver dysfunction/ failure (clinical) | Normal | — | — | Asterixis | Encephalopathy or coma |
| Portal vein flow | Normal | — | Decreased portal vein flow | Reversal/retrograde portal vein flow | — |
| SGOT (AST) (serum glutamic oxaloacetic transaminase) | WNL >ULN–2.5 × ULN | >2.5–5 × ULN | >5–20 × ULN | >20 × ULN | |
| SGPT (ALT) | WNL | >ULN–2.5 × ULN | >2.5–5 × ULN | >5–20 × ULN | >20 × ULN |
| Hepatic—other (specify, _____) | None | Mild | Moderate | Severe | Life-threatening or disabling |

## INFECTION/FEBRILE NEUTROPENIA

| Adverse Event | 0 | 1 | 2 | 3 | 4 |
|---|---|---|---|---|---|
| Catheter-related infection | None | Mild, no active treatment | Moderate, localized infection, requiring local or oral treatment | Severe, systemic infection, requiring IV antibiotic or antifungal treatment or hospitalization | Life-threatening sepsis (e.g., septic shock) |
| Febrile neutropenia (fever of unknown origin without clinically or microbiologically documented infection) (ANC <1.0 × 10⁹/L, fever ≥38.5° C) | None | — | — | Present | Life-threatening sepsis (e.g., septic shock) |

Also consider Neutrophils.
Note: Hypothermia instead of fever may be associated with neutropenia and is graded here.

| Adverse Event | 0 | 1 | 2 | 3 | 4 |
|---|---|---|---|---|---|
| Infection (documented clinically or microbiologically) with grade 3 or 4 neutropenia (ANC <1 × 10⁹/L) | None | — | — | Present | Life-threatening sepsis (e.g., septic shock) |

Also consider Neutrophils.
Notes: Hypothermia instead of fever may be associated with neutropenia and is graded here.
    In the absence of documented infection grade 3 or 4, neutropenia with fever is graded as Febrile neutropenia.

| Adverse Event | 0 | 1 | 2 | 3 | 4 |
|---|---|---|---|---|---|
| Infection with unknown ANC | None | — | — | Present | Life-threatening sepsis (e.g., septic shock) |

Note: This adverse event criterion is used in the rare case when ANC is unknown.

| Adverse Event | 0 | 1 | 2 | 3 | 4 |
|---|---|---|---|---|---|
| Infection without neutropenia | None | Mild, no active treatment | Moderate, localized infection, requiring local or oral treatment | Severe, systemic infection, requiring IV antibiotic or antifungal treatment, or hospitalization | Life-threatening sepsis (e.g., septic shock) |

Also consider Neutrophils.
Wound—infectious is graded in the DERMATOLOGY/SKIN category.

| Adverse Event | 0 | 1 | 2 | 3 | 4 |
|---|---|---|---|---|---|
| Infection/febrile neutropenia—other (specify, _____) | None | Mild | Moderate | Severe | Life-threatening or disabling |

| Adverse Event | Grade | | | | |
|---|---|---|---|---|---|
| | 0 | 1 | 2 | 3 | 4 |

## LYMPHATICS

| Adverse Event | 0 | 1 | 2 | 3 | 4 |
|---|---|---|---|---|---|
| Lymphatics | Normal | Mild lymphedema | Moderate lymphedema requiring compression; lymphocyst | Severe lymphedema limiting function; lymphocyst requiring surgery | Severe lymphedema limiting function with ulceration |
| Lymphatics—other (specify, _____) | None | Mild | Moderate | Severe | Life-threatening or disabling |

## METABOLIC/LABORATORY

| Adverse Event | 0 | 1 | 2 | 3 | 4 |
|---|---|---|---|---|---|
| Acidosis (metabolic or respiratory) | Normal | pH <normal, but ≥7.3 | — | pH <7.3 | pH <7.3 with life-threatening physiologic consequences |
| Alkalosis (metabolic or respiratory) | Normal | pH >normal, but ≤7.5 | — | pH >7.5 | pH >7.5 with life-threatening physiologic consequences |
| Amylase | WNL | >ULN–1.5 × ULN | >1.5–2 × ULN | >2–5 × ULN | >5 × ULN |
| Bicarbonate | WNL | <LLN–16 mEq/dl | 11–15 mEq/dl | 8–10 mEq/dl | <8 mEq/dl |
| CPK (creatine phosphokinase) | WNL | >ULN–2.5 × ULN | >2.5–5 × ULN | >5–10 × ULN | >10 × ULN |
| Hypercalcemia | WNL | >ULN–11.5 mg/dl >ULN–2.9 mmol/L | >11.5–12.5 mg/dl >2.9–3.1 mmol/L | >12.5–13.5 mg/dl >3.1–3.4 mmol/L | >13.5 mg/dl >3.4 mmol/L |
| Hypercholesterolemia | WNL | >ULN–300 mg/dl >ULN–7.75 mmol/L | >300–400 mg/dl >7.75–10.34 mmol/L | >400–500 mg/dl >10.34–12.92 mmol/L | >500 mg/dl >12.92 mmol/L |
| Hyperglycemia | WNL | >ULN–160 mg/dl >ULN–8.9 mmol/L | >160–250 mg/dl >8.9–13.9 mmol/L | >250–500 mg/dl >13.9–27.8 mmol/L | >500 mg/dl >27.8 mmol/L or acidosis |
| Hyperkalemia | NWL | >ULN–5.5 mmol/L | >5.5–6 mmol/L | >6–7 mmol/L | >7 mmol/L |
| Hypermagnesemia | WNL | >ULN–3 mg/dl >ULN–1.23 mmol/L | — | >3–8 mg/dl >1.23–3.3 mmol/L | >8 mg/dl >3.3 mmol/L |
| Hypernatremia | WNL | >ULN–150 mmol/L | >150–155 mmol/L | >155–160 mmol/L | >160 mmol/L |
| Hypertriglyceridemia | WNL | >ULN–2.5 × ULN | >2.5–5 × ULN | >5–10 × ULN | >10 × ULN |
| Hyperuricemia | WNL | >ULN–≤10 mg/dl ≤0.59 mmol/L without physiologic consequences | | >ULN–≤10 mg/dl ≤0.59 mmol/L with physiologic consequences | >10 mg/dl >0.59 mmol/L |

Also consider Tumor lysis syndrome, Renal failure, Creatinine, Hyperkalemia.

| Adverse Event | 0 | 1 | 2 | 3 | 4 |
|---|---|---|---|---|---|
| Hypocalcemia | WNL | <LLN–8 mg/dl <LLN–2 mmol/L | 7–<8 mg/dl 1.75–<2 mmol/L | 6–<7 mg/dl 1.5–<1.75 mmol/L | <6 mg/dl <1.5 mmol/L |
| Hypoglycemia | WNL | <LLN–55 mg/dl <LLN–3 mmol/L | 40–<55 mg/dl 2.2–<3 mmol/L | 30–<40 mg/dl 1.7–<2.2 mmol/L | <30 mg/dl <1.7 mmol/L |
| Hypokalemia | WNL | <LLN–3 mmol/L | — | 2.5–<3 mmol/L | <2.5 mmol/L |
| Hypomagnesemia | WNL | <LLN–1.2 mg/dl <LLN–0.5 mmol/L | 0.9–<1.2 mg/dl 0.4–<0.5 mmol/L | 0.7–<0.9 mg/dl 0.3–<0.4 mmol/L | <0.7 mg/dl <0.3 mmol/L |
| Hyponatremia | WNL | <LLN–130 mmol/L | — | 120–<130 mmol/L | <120 mmol/L |
| Hypophosphatemia | WNL | <LLN–2.5 mg/dl <LLN–0.8 mmol/L | ≥2–<2.5 mg/dl ≥0.6–<0.8 mmol/L | ≥1–<2 mg/dl ≥0.3–<0.6 mmol/L | <1.0 mg/dl <0.3 mmol/L |

Hypothyroidism is graded in the ENDOCRINE category.

| Adverse Event | 0 | 1 | 2 | 3 | 4 |
|---|---|---|---|---|---|
| Lipase | WNL | >ULN–1.5 × ULN | >1.5–2 × ULN | >2–5 × ULN | >5 × ULN |
| Metabolic/laboratory—other (specify, _____) | None | Mild | Moderate | Severe | Life-threatening or disabling |

## MUSCULOSKELETAL

Arthralgia is graded in the PAIN category.

| Adverse Event | 0 | 1 | 2 | 3 | 4 |
|---|---|---|---|---|---|
| Arthritis | None | Mild pain with inflammation, erythema, or joint swelling but not interfering with function | Moderate pain with inflammation, erythema, or joint swelling interfering with function but not interfering with activities of daily living | Severe pain with inflammation, erythema, or joint swelling and interfering with activities of daily living | Disabling |

| Adverse Event | Grade | | | | |
|---|---|---|---|---|---|
| | 0 | 1 | 2 | 3 | 4 |
| Muscle weakness (not due to neuropathy) | Normal | Asymptomatic with weakness on physical examination | Symptomatic and interfering with function but not interfering with activities of daily living | Symptomatic and interfering with activities of daily living | Bedridden or disabling |

Myalgia (tenderness or pain in muscles) is graded in the PAIN category.

| Adverse Event | 0 | 1 | 2 | 3 | 4 |
|---|---|---|---|---|---|
| Myositis (inflammation/ damage of muscle) | None | Mild pain not interfering with function | Pain interfering with function, but not interfering with activities of daily living | Pain interfering with function and interfering with activities of daily living | Bedridden or disabling |

Also consider CPK.
Note: Myositis implies muscle damage (i.e., elevated CPK).

| Adverse Event | 0 | 1 | 2 | 3 | 4 |
|---|---|---|---|---|---|
| Osteonecrosis (avascular necrosis) | None | Asymptomatic and detected by imaging only | Symptomatic and interfering with function, but not interfering with activities of daily living | Symptomatic and interfering with activities of daily living | Symptomatic; or disabling |
| Musculoskeletal—other (specify, _____) | None | Mild | Moderate | Severe | Life-threatening or disabling |

## NEUROLOGY

Aphasia, receptive and/or expressive, is graded under Speech impairment in the NEUROLOGY category.

| Adverse Event | 0 | 1 | 2 | 3 | 4 |
|---|---|---|---|---|---|
| Arachnoiditis/ meningismus/ radiculitis | Absent | Mild pain not interfering with function | Moderate pain interfering with function, but not interfering with activities of daily living | Severe pain interfering with activities of daily living | Unable to function or perform activities of daily living; bedridden; paraplegia |

Also consider Headache, Vomiting, Fever.

| Adverse Event | 0 | 1 | 2 | 3 | 4 |
|---|---|---|---|---|---|
| Ataxia (incoordination) | Normal | Asymptomatic but abnormal on physical examination and not interfering with function | Mild symptoms interfering with function, but not interfering with activities of daily living | Moderate symptoms interfering with activities of daily living | Bedridden or disabling |
| CNS cerebrovascular ischemia | None | — | — | Transient ischemic attack (TIA) or event | Permanent event (e.g., cerebral-vascular accident) |

CNS hemorrhage/bleeding is graded in the HEMORRHAGE category.

| Adverse Event | 0 | 1 | 2 | 3 | 4 |
|---|---|---|---|---|---|
| Cognitive disturbance/ learning problems | None | Cognitive disability; not interfering with work/school performance; preservation of intelligence | Cognitive disability; interfering with work/ school performance; decline of 1 SD (standard deviation) or loss of developmental milestones | Cognitive disability; resulting in significant impairment of work/ school performance; cognitive decline >2 SD | Inability to work/frank mental retardation |
| Confusion | Normal | Confusion or disorientation or attention deficit or brief duration; resolves spontaneously with no sequelae | Confusion or disorientation or attention deficit interfering with function, but not interfering with activities of daily living | Confusion or delirium interfering with activities of daily living | Harmful to others or self; requiring hospitalization |

Cranial neuropathy is graded in the NEUROLOGY category as Neuropathy—cranial.

| Adverse Event | 0 | 1 | 2 | 3 | 4 |
|---|---|---|---|---|---|
| Delusions | Normal | — | — | Present | Toxic psychosis |
| Depressed level of consciousness | Normal | Somnolence or sedation not interfering with function | Somnolence or sedation interfering with function, but not interfering with activities of daily living | Obtundation or stupor; difficult to arouse; interfering with activities of daily living | Coma |

Note: Syncope (fainting) is graded in the NEUROLOGY category.

| Adverse Event | 0 | 1 | 2 | 3 | 4 |
|---|---|---|---|---|---|
| Dizziness/ lightheadedness | None | Not interfering with function | Interfering with function, but not interfering with activities of daily living | Interfering with activities of daily living | Bedridden or disabling |

| Adverse Event | Grade | | | | |
|---|---|---|---|---|---|
| | 0 | 1 | 2 | 3 | 4 |

Dysphasia, receptive and/or expressive, is graded under Speech impairment in the NEUROLOGY category.

| Adverse Event | 0 | 1 | 2 | 3 | 4 |
|---|---|---|---|---|---|
| Extrapyramidal/ involuntary movement/ restlessness | None | Mild involuntary movements not interfering with function | Moderate involuntary movements interfering with function, but not interfering with activities of daily living | Severe involuntary movements or torticollis interfering with activities of daily living | Bedridden or disabling |
| Hallucinations | Normal | — | — | Present | Toxic psychosis |

Headache is graded in the PAIN category.

| Adverse Event | 0 | 1 | 2 | 3 | 4 |
|---|---|---|---|---|---|
| Insomnia | Normal | Occasional difficulty sleeping not interfering with function | Difficulty sleeping interfering with function, but not interfering with activities of daily living | Frequent difficulty sleeping, interfering with activities of daily living | — |

Note: This adverse event is graded when insomnia is related to treatment. If pain or other symptoms interfere with sleep do *not* grade as insomnia.
>ULN–2.5 × ULN

| Adverse Event | 0 | 1 | 2 | 3 | 4 |
|---|---|---|---|---|---|
| Irritability (children <3 years of age) | Normal | Mild; easily consolable | Moderate; requiring increased attention | Severe; inconsolable | |
| Leukoencephalopathy-associated radiologic findings | None | Mild increase in SAS (subarachnoid space) and/or mild ventriculomegaly; and/or small (± multiple) focal T2 hyperintensities, involving periventricular white matter or <⅓ of susceptible areas of cerebrum | Moderate increase in SAS; and/or moderate ventriculomegaly; and/or focal T2 hyperintensities extending into centrum ovale; or involving ⅓ to ⅔ of susceptible areas of cerebrum | Severe increase in SAS; severe ventriculomegaly; near total white matter T2 hyperintensities or diffuse low attenuation (CT); focal white matter necrosis (cystic) | Severe increase in SAS; severe ventriculomegaly; diffuse low attenuation with calcification (CT); diffuse white matter necrosis (MRI) |
| Memory loss | Normal | Memory loss not interfering with function | Memory loss interfering with function, but not interfering with activities of daily living | Memory loss interfering with activities of daily living | Amnesia |
| Mood alteration— anxiety, agitation | Normal | Mild mood alteration not interfering with function | Moderate mood alteration interfering with function, but not interfering with activities of daily living | Severe mood alteration interfering with activities of daily living | Suicidal ideation or danger to self |
| Mood alteration— depression | Normal | Mild mood alteration not interfering with function | Moderate mood alteration interfering with function, but not interfering with activities of daily living | Severe mood alteration interfering with activities of daily living | Suicidal ideation or danger to self |
| Mood alteration— euphoria | Normal | Mild mood alteration not interfering with function | Moderate mood alteration interfering with function, but not interfering with activities of daily living | Severe mood alteration interfering with activities of daily living | Danger to self |

Neuropathic pain is graded in the PAIN category.

| Adverse Event | 0 | 1 | 2 | 3 | 4 |
|---|---|---|---|---|---|
| Neuropathy—cranial | Absent | — | Present, not interfering with activities of daily living | Present, interfering with activities of daily living | Life-threatening, disabling |
| Neuropathy—motor | Normal | Subjective weakness but no objective findings | Mild objective weakness interfering with function, but not interfering with activities of daily living | Objective weakness interfering with activities of daily living | Paralysis |
| Neuropathy—sensory | Normal | Loss of deep tendon reflexes or paresthesia (including tingling) but not interfering with function | Objective sensory loss or paresthesia (including tingling), interfering with function, but not interfering with activities of daily living | Sensory loss or paresthesia interfering with activities of daily living | Permanent sensory loss that interferes with function |

| Adverse Event | Grade | | | | |
|---|---|---|---|---|---|
| | 0 | 1 | 2 | 3 | 4 |
| Nystagmus Also consider Vision—double vision. | Absent | Present | — | — | — |
| Personality/behavioral | Normal | Change, but not disruptive to patient or family | Disruptive to patient or family | Disruptive to patient and family; requiring mental health intervention | Harmful to others or self; requiring hospitalization |
| Pyramidal tract dysfunction (e.g., ↑ tone, hyperreflexia, positive Babinski, ↓ fine motor coordination) | Normal | Asymptomatic with abnormality on physical examination | Symptomatic or interfering with function but not interfering with activities of daily living | Interfering with activities of daily living | Bedridden or disabling; paralysis |
| Seizure(s) | None | — | Seizure(s) self-limited and consciousness is preserved | Seizure(s) in which consciousness is altered | Seizures of any type that are prolonged, repetitive, or difficult to control (e.g., status epilepticus, intractable epilepsy) |
| Speech impairment (e.g., dysphasia or aphasia) | Normal | — | Awareness of receptive or expressive dysphasia, not impairing ability to communicate | Receptive or expressive dysphasia, impairing ability to communicate | Inability to communicate |
| Syncope (fainting) Also consider CARDIOVASCULAR (ARRHYTHMIA), Vasovagal episode, CNS cerebrovascular ischemia. | Absent | — | — | Present | — |
| Tremor | None | Mild and brief or intermittent but not interfering with function | Moderate tremor interfering with function, but not interfering with activities of daily living | Severe tremor interfering with activities of daily living | — |
| Vertigo | None | Not interfering with function | Interfering with function, but not interfering with activities of daily living | Interfering with activities of daily living | Bedridden or disabling |
| Neurology—other (specify, _____) | None | Mild | Moderate | Severe | Life-threatening or disabling |

## OCULAR/VISUAL

| Cataract | None | Asymptomatic | Symptomatic, partial visual loss | Symptomatic, visual loss requiring treatment or interfering with function | — |
|---|---|---|---|---|---|
| Conjunctivitis | None | Abnormal ophthalmologic changes, but asymptomatic or symptomatic without visual impairment (i.e., pain and irritation) | Symptomatic and interfering with function, but not interfering with activities of daily living | Symptomatic and interfering with activities of daily living | — |
| Dry eye | Normal | Mild, not requiring treatment | Moderate or requiring artificial tears | — | — |
| Glaucoma | None | Increase in intraocular pressure but no visual loss | Increase in intraocular pressure with retinal changes | Visual impairment | Unilateral or bilateral loss of vision (blindness) |
| Keratitis (corneal inflammation/ corneal ulceration) | None | Abnormal ophthalmologic changes but asymptomatic or symptomatic without visual impairment (i.e., pain and irritation) | Symptomatic and interfering with function, but not interfering with activities of daily living | Symptomatic and interfering with activities of daily living | Unilateral or bilateral loss of vision (blindness) |
| Tearing (watery eyes) | None | Mild: not interfering with function | Moderate: interfering with function, but not interfering with activities of daily living | Interfering with activities of daily living | — |

| Adverse Event | Grade | | | | |
|---|---|---|---|---|---|
| | 0 | 1 | 2 | 3 | 4 |
| Vision—blurred vision | Normal | — | Symptomatic and interfering with function, but not interfering with activities of daily living | Symptomatic and interfering with activities of daily living | — |
| Vision—double vision (diplopia) | Normal | — | Symptomatic and interfering with function, but not interfering with activities of daily living | Symptomatic and interfering with activities of daily living | — |
| Vision—flashing lights/ floaters | Normal | Mild: not interfering with function | Symptomatic and interfering with function, but not interfering with activities of daily living | Symptomatic and interfering with activities of daily living | — |
| Vision—night blindness (nyctalopia) | Normal | Abnormal electroretinography but asymptomatic | Symptomatic and interfering with function, but not interfering with activities of daily living | Symptomatic and interfering with activities of daily living | — |
| Vision—photophobia | Normal | — | Symptomatic and interfering with function, but not interfering with activities of daily living | Symptomatic and interfering with activities of daily living | — |
| Ocular/visual—other (specify, _____) | Normal | Mild | Moderate | Severe | Unilateral or bilateral loss of vision (blindness) |

## PAIN

| Adverse Event | Grade | | | | |
|---|---|---|---|---|---|
| | 0 | 1 | 2 | 3 | 4 |
| Abdominal pain or cramping | None | Mild pain not interfering with function | Moderate pain: pain or analgesics interfering with function, but not interfering with activities of daily living | Severe pain: pain or analgesics severely interfering with activities of daily living | Disabling |
| Arthralgia (joint pain) | None | Mild pain not interfering with function | Moderate pain: pain or analgesics interfering with function, but not interfering with activities of daily living | Severe pain: pain or analgesics severely interfering with activities of daily living | Disabling |

Arthritis (joint pain with clinical signs of inflammation) is graded in the MUSCULOSKELETAL category.

| Adverse Event | Grade | | | | |
|---|---|---|---|---|---|
| Bone pain | None | Mild pain not interfering with function | Moderate pain: pain or analgesics interfering with function, but not interfering with activities of daily living | Severe pain: pain or analgesics severely interfering with activities of daily living | Disabling |
| Chest pain (noncardiac and nonpleuritic) | None | Mild pain not interfering with function | Moderate pain: pain or analgesics interfering with function, but not interfering with activities of daily living | Severe pain: pain or analgesics severely interfering with activities of daily living | Disabling |
| Dysmenorrhea | None | Mild pain not interfering with function | Moderate pain: pain or analgesics interfering with function, but not interfering with activities of daily living | Severe pain: pain or analgesics severely interfering with activities of daily living | Disabling |
| Dyspareunia | None | Mild pain not interfering with function | Moderate pain interfering with sexual activity | Severe pain preventing sexual activity | — |

| Adverse Event | Grade | | | | |
|---|---|---|---|---|---|
| | 0 | 1 | 2 | 3 | 4 |
| Dysuria is graded in the RENAL/GENITOURINARY category. | | | | | |
| Earache (otalgia) | None | Mild pain not interfering with function | Moderate pain: pain or analgesics interfering with function, but not interfering with activities of daily living | Severe pain: pain or analgesics severely interfering with activities of daily living | Disabling |
| Headache | None | Mild pain not interfering with function | Moderate pain: pain or analgesics interfering with function, but not interfering with activities of daily living | Severe pain: pain or analgesics severely interfering with activities of daily living | Disabling |
| Hepatic pain | None | Mild pain not interfering with function | Moderate pain: pain or analgesics interfering with function, but not interfering with activities of daily living | Severe pain: pain or analgesics severely interfering with activities of daily living | Disabling |
| Myalgia (muscle pain) | None | Mild pain not interfering with function | Moderate pain: pain or analgesics interfering with function, but not interfering with activities of daily living | Severe pain: pain or analgesics severely interfering with activities of daily living | Disabling |
| Neuropathic pain (e.g., jaw pain, neurologic pain, phantom limb pain, postinfectious neuralgia, or painful neuropathies) | None | Mild pain not interfering with function | Moderate pain: pain or analgesics interfering with function, but not interfering with activities of daily living | Severe pain: pain or analgesics severely interfering with activities of daily living | Disabling |
| Pain due to radiation | None | Mild pain not interfering with function | Moderate pain: pain or analgesics interfering with function, but not interfering with activities of daily living | Severe pain: pain or analgesics severely interfering with activities of daily living | Disabling |
| Pelvic pain | None | Mild pain not interfering with function | Moderate pain: pain or analgesics interfering with function, but not interfering with activities of daily living | Severe pain: pain or analgesics severely interfering with activities of daily living | Disabling |
| Pleuritic pain | None | Mild pain not interfering with function | Moderate pain: pain or analgesics interfering with function, but not interfering with activities of daily living | Severe pain: pain or analgesics severely interfering with activities of daily living | Disabling |
| Rectal or perirectal pain (proctalgia) | None | Mild pain not interfering with function | Moderate pain: pain or analgesics interfering with function, but not interfering with activities of daily living | Severe pain: pain or analgesics severely interfering with activities of daily living | Disabling |
| Tumor pain (onset or exacerbation of tumor pain due to treatment) | None | Mild pain not interfering with function | Moderate pain: pain or analgesics interfering with function, but not interfering with activities of daily living | Severe pain: pain or analgesics severely interfering with activities of daily living | Disabling |
| Tumor flare is graded in the SYNDROME category. | | | | | |
| Pain—other (specify, _____) | None | Mild | Moderate | Severe | Disabling |

## PULMONARY

| Adverse Event | Grade | | | | |
|---|---|---|---|---|---|
| Adult respiratory distress syndrome (ARDS) | Absent | — | — | — | Present |

| Adverse Event | Grade 0 | Grade 1 | Grade 2 | Grade 3 | Grade 4 |
|---|---|---|---|---|---|
| Apnea | None | — | — | Present | Requiring intubation |
| Carbon monoxide diffusion capacity (DLCO) | ≥90% of pretreatment or normal value | ≥75–<90% of pretreatment or normal value | ≥50–<75% of pretreatment or normal value | ≥25–<50% of pretreatment or normal value | <25% of pretreatment or normal value |
| Cough | Absent | Mild, relieved by nonprescription medication | Requiring narcotic antitussive | Severe cough or coughing spasms, poorly controlled or unresponsive to treatment | — |
| Dyspnea (shortness of breath) | Normal | — | Dyspnea on exertion | Dyspnea at normal level of activity | Dyspnea at rest or requiring ventilator support |
| FEV$_1$ | ≥90% of pretreatment or normal value | ≥75–<90% of pretreatment or normal value | ≥50–<75% of pretreatment or normal value | ≥25–<50% of pretreatment or normal value | <25% of pretreatment or normal value |
| Hiccoughs (hiccups, singultus) | None | Mild, not requiring treatment | Moderate, requiring treatment | Severe, prolonged, and refractory to treatment | — |
| Hypoxia | Normal | — | Decreased O$_2$ saturation with exercise | Decreased O$_2$ saturation at rest, requiring supplemental oxygen | Decreased O$_2$ saturation, requiring pressure support (CPAP) or assisted ventilation |
| Pleural effusion (nonmalignant) | None | Asymptomatic and not requiring treatment | Symptomatic, requiring diuretics | Symptomatic, requiring O$_2$ or therapeutic thoracentesis | Life-threatening (e.g., requiring intubation) |

Pleuritic pain is graded in the PAIN category.

| Adverse Event | Grade 0 | Grade 1 | Grade 2 | Grade 3 | Grade 4 |
|---|---|---|---|---|---|
| Pneumonitis/ pulmonary infiltrates | None | Radiographic changes but asymptomatic or symptoms not requiring steroids | Radiographic changes and requiring steroids or diuretics | Radiographic changes and requiring oxygen | Radiographic changes and requiring assisted ventilation |
| Pneumothorax | None | No intervention required | Chest tube required | Sclerosis or surgery required | Life-threatening |

Pulmonary embolism is graded as Thrombosis/embolism in the CARDIOVASCULAR (GENERAL) category.

| Adverse Event | Grade 0 | Grade 1 | Grade 2 | Grade 3 | Grade 4 |
|---|---|---|---|---|---|
| Pulmonary fibrosis | None | Radiographic changes, but asymptomatic or symptoms not requiring steroids | Requiring steroids or diuretics | Requiring oxygen | Requiring assisted ventilation |

Note: Radiation-related pulmonary fibrosis is graded in the RTOG/EORTC Late Radiation Morbidity Scoring Scheme—Lung.

| Adverse Event | Grade 0 | Grade 1 | Grade 2 | Grade 3 | Grade 4 |
|---|---|---|---|---|---|
| Voice changes/stridor/ larynx (e.g., hoarseness, loss of voice, laryngitis) | Normal | Mild or intermittent hoarseness | Persistent hoarseness, but able to vocalize; may have mild to moderate edema | Whispered speech, not able to vocalize; may have marked edema | Marked dyspnea/stridor requiring tracheostomy or intubation |

Notes: Cough from radiation is graded as cough in the PULMONARY category.
Radiation-related hemoptysis from larynx/pharynx is graded as Grade 4 Mucositis due to radiation in the GASTROINTESTINAL category.
Radiation-related hemoptysis from the thoracic cavity is graded as Grade 4 Hemoptysis in the HEMORRHAGE category.

| Adverse Event | Grade 0 | Grade 1 | Grade 2 | Grade 3 | Grade 4 |
|---|---|---|---|---|---|
| Pulmonary—other (specify, _____) | None | Mild | Moderate | Severe | Life-threatening or disabling |

## RENAL/GENITOURINARY

| Adverse Event | Grade 0 | Grade 1 | Grade 2 | Grade 3 | Grade 4 |
|---|---|---|---|---|---|
| Bladder spasms | Absent | Mild symptoms, not requiring intervention | Symptoms requiring antispasmodic | Severe symptoms requiring narcotic | |
| Creatinine | WNL | >ULN–1.5 × ULN | >1.5–3 × ULN | >3–6 × ULN | >6 × ULN |

Note: Adjust to age-appropriate levels for pediatric patients.

| Adverse Event | Grade 0 | Grade 1 | Grade 2 | Grade 3 | Grade 4 |
|---|---|---|---|---|---|
| Dysuria (painful urination) | None | Mild symptoms requiring no intervention | Symptoms relieved with therapy | Symptoms not relieved despite therapy | — |
| Fistula or GU fistula (e.g., vaginal, vesicovaginal) | None | — | — | Requiring intervention | Requiring surgery |
| Hemoglobinuria | — | Present | — | — | — |

Hematuria (in the absence of vaginal bleeding) is graded in the HEMORRHAGE category.

| Adverse Event | Grade 0 | Grade 1 | Grade 2 | Grade 3 | Grade 4 |
|---|---|---|---|---|---|
| Incontinence | None | With coughing, sneezing, and so on | Spontaneous, some control | No control (in the absence of fistula) | — |

| Adverse Event | Grade | | | | |
|---|---|---|---|---|---|
| | 0 | 1 | 2 | 3 | 4 |
| Operative injury to bladder and/or ureter | None | — | Injury of bladder with primary repair | Sepsis, fistula, or obstruction requiring secondary surgery; loss of one kidney; injury requiring anastomosis or reimplantation | Septic obstruction of both kidneys or vesicovaginal fistula requiring diversion |
| Proteinuria | Normal or <0.15 g/24 hours | 1 + or 0.15–1 g/24 hours | 2+ to 3+ or 1–3.5 g/24 hours | 4+ or >3.5 g/24 hours | Nephrotic syndrome |
| Note: If there is an inconsistency between absolute value and dipstick reading, use the absolute value for grading. | | | | | |
| Renal failure | None | — | — | Requiring dialysis, but reversible | Requiring dialysis and irreversible |
| Ureteral obstruction | None | Unilateral, not requiring surgery | — | Bilateral, not requiring surgery | Stent, nephrostomy tube, or surgery |
| Urinary electrolyte wasting (e.g., Fanconi's syndrome, renal tubular acidosis) | None | Asymptomatic, not requiring treatment | Mild, reversible, and manageable with oral replacement | Reversible but requiring IV replacement | Irreversible, requiring continued replacement |
| Also consider Acidosis, Bicarbonate, Hypocalcemia, Hypophosphatemia. | | | | | |
| Urinary frequency/ urgency | Normal | Increase in frequency or nocturia up to 2× normal | Increase >2× normal but <hourly | Hourly or more with urgency, or requiring catheter | — |
| Urinary retention | Normal | Hesitancy or dribbling, but no significant residual urine; retention occurring during the immediate postoperative period | Hesitancy requiring medication or occasional in/out catheterization (<4× per week), or operative bladder atony requiring indwelling catheter beyond immediate postoperative period but for <6 weeks | Requiring frequent in/ out catheterization (≥4× per week) or urological intervention (e.g., TURP, suprapubic tube, urethrotomy) | Bladder rupture |
| Urine color change (not related to other dietary or physiologic cause e.g., bilirubin, concentrated urine, hematuria) | Normal | Asymptomatic, change in urine color | — | — | — |
| Vaginal bleeding is graded in the HEMORRHAGE category. | | | | | |
| Vaginitis (not due to infection) | None | Mild, not requiring treatment | Moderate, relieved with treatment | Severe, not relieved with treatment, or ulceration not requiring surgery | Ulceration requiring surgery |
| Renal/ genitourinary—other (specify, _____) | None | Mild | Moderate | Severe | Life-threatening or disabling |

## SECONDARY MALIGNANCY

| | | | | | |
|---|---|---|---|---|---|
| Secondary malignancy—other (specify type, _____) excludes metastasis from initial primary | None | — | — | — | Present |

## SEXUAL/REPRODUCTIVE FUNCTION

Dyspareunia is graded in the PAIN category.
Dysmenorrhea is graded in the PAIN category.

| | | | | | |
|---|---|---|---|---|---|
| Erectile impotence | Normal | Mild (erections impaired but satisfactory) | Moderate (erections impaired, unsatisfactory for intercourse) | No erections | — |
| Female sterility | Normal | — | — | Sterile | — |

| Adverse Event | Grade | | | | |
|---|---|---|---|---|---|
| | 0 | 1 | 2 | 3 | 4 |
| Feminization of male is graded in the ENDOCRINE category. | | | | | |
| Irregular menses (change from baseline) | Normal | Occasionally irregular or lengthened interval, but continuing menstrual cycles | Very irregular, but continuing menstrual cycles | Persistent amenorrhea | — |
| Libido | Normal | Decrease in interest | Severe loss of interest | — | — |
| Male infertility | — | — | Oligospermia (low sperm count) | Azoospermia (no sperm) | — |
| Masculinization of female is graded in the ENDOCRINE category. | | | | | |
| Vaginal dryness | Normal | Mild | Requiring treatment and/ or interfering with sexual function, dyspareunia | — | — |
| Sexual/reproductive function—other (specify, _____) | None | Mild | Moderate | Severe | Disabling |

## SYNDROMES (not included in previous categories)

Acute vascular leak syndrome is graded in the CARDIOVASCULAR (GENERAL) category.
ARDS (adult respiratory distress syndrome) is graded in the PULMONARY category.
Autoimmune reactions are graded in the ALLERGY/IMMUNOLOGY category.
DIC (disseminated intravascular coagulation) is graded in the COAGULATION category.
Fanconi's syndrome is graded as Urinary electrolyte wasting in the RENAL/GENITOURINARY category.
Renal tubular acidosis is graded as Urinary electrolyte wasting in the RENAL/GENITOURINARY category.
Stevens-Johnson syndrome (erythema multiforme) is graded in the DERMATOLOGY/SKIN category.
SIADH (syndrome of inappropriate antidiuretic hormone) is graded in the ENDOCRINE category.
Thrombotic microangiopathy (e.g., thrombotic thrombocytopenic purpura [TTP] or hemolytic uremic syndrome [HUS] is graded in the COAGULATION category.

| | | | | | |
|---|---|---|---|---|---|
| Tumor flare | None | Mild pain not interfering with function | Moderate pain; pain or analgesics interfering with function, but not interfering with activities of daily living | Severe pain; pain or analgesics interfering with function and interfering with activities of daily living | Disabling |

Also consider Hypercalcemia.
Note: Tumor flare is characterized by a constellation of symptoms and signs in direct relation to initiation of therapy (e.g., antiestrogens/androgens or additional hormones). The symptoms/signs include tumor pain, inflammation of visible tumor, hypercalcemia, diffuse bone pain, and other electrolyte disturbances.

| | | | | | |
|---|---|---|---|---|---|
| Tumor lysis syndrome | Absent | — | — | Present | — |

Also consider Hyperkalemia, Creatine.
Urinary electrolyte wasting (e.g., Fanconi's syndrome, renal tubular acidosis) is graded in the RENAL/GENITOURINARY category.

| | | | | | |
|---|---|---|---|---|---|
| Syndromes—other (specify, _____) | None | Mild | Moderate | Severe | Life-threatening or disabling |

Adapted from Cancer Therapy Evaluation Program, Common Toxicity Criteria, Version 2.0, Division of Cancer Treatment and Diagnosis (DCTD), National Cancer Institute, National Institutes of Health, Department of Health and Human Services, March 1998. Additional information can be found on the Internet at ⟨http://ctep.info.nih.gov/CTC3/ctc.htm⟩.

WNL, within normal limits; LLN, lower limit of normal; WBC, white blood cell; BMT, bone marrow transplantation; ANC, absolute neutrophil count; AGC, absolute granulocyte count; PRBCs, packed red blood cells; AV, atrioventricular; CHF, congestive heart failure; SVT, supraventricular tachycardia; PVCs, premature ventricular contractions; CNS, central nervous system; ULN, upper limits of normal; MI, myocardial infarction; BP, blood pressure; ECG, electrocardiographic; ECOG, Eastern Cooperative Oncology Group; IV, intravenous; PO, orally; TSH, thyroid-stimulating hormone; CT, computed tomography; CVA, cerebrovascular accident; CPK, creatine phosphokinase; MRI, magnetic resonance imaging; CPAP, continuous positive airway pressure; GU, genitourinary; TURP, transurethral prostatectomy.

# APPENDIX C

# SELECTED ABBREVIATIONS

## ORGANIZATIONS, SOCIETIES, JOURNALS, AND PROCEEDINGS*

| | |
|---|---|
| AACR | American Association for Cancer Research |
| ACCC | Association of Community Cancer Center |
| AJCC | American Joint Committee on Cancer |
| ARS | American Radium Society |
| ASCO | American Society of Clinical Oncology |
| ASH | American Society of Hematology |
| ASTRO | American Society for Therapeutic Radiology and Oncology |
| BCRC | Baltimore Cancer Research Center |
| BCTF | Breast Cancer Task Force |
| BTSG | Brain Tumor Study Group |
| CALGB | Cancer and Leukemia Cooperative Group B |
| CCG | Children's Cancer Group |
| COG | Central Oncology Group |
| ECOG | Eastern Cooperative Oncology Group |
| EORTC | European Organization for Research on Treatment of Cancer |
| GITSG | Gastrointestinal Tumor Study Group |
| GOG | Gynecologic Oncology Group |
| IBMTR | International Bone Marrow Transplant Registry |
| LALA | French Group on the Therapy of Adult ALL |
| LCSG | Lung Cancer Study Group |
| MDA | M.D. Anderson Hospital and Tumor Institute |
| MRC | Medical Research Council of Great Britain |
| MSKCC | Memorial Sloan-Kettering Cancer Center |
| NBCCGA | National Bladder Cancer Collaborative Group A |
| NCCTG | North Central Cancer Treatment Group |
| NCI | National Cancer Institute—USA |
| NPCP | National Prostatic Cancer Project |
| NSABP | National Surgical Adjuvant Breast and Bowel Project |
| NWTSG | National Wilms' Tumor Study Group |
| ONS | Oncology Nursing Society |
| PDQ | Physician's Data Query program of the NCI |
| POG | Pediatric Oncology Group |
| Proc AACR | Proceedings of AACR |
| Proc ASCO | Proceedings of ASCO |
| RPMI | Roswell Park Memorial Institute |
| RTOG | Radiation Therapy Oncology Group |
| SAKK | Swiss Group for Clinical Cancer Research |
| SEG, SEOG | Southeastern Cancer Study Group |
| SSO | Society of Surgical Oncology |
| SWOG | Southwest Oncology Group |
| UICC | International Union Against Cancer |
| VALG | Veterans Administration Lung Cancer Study Group |
| VASAG | Veterans Administration Surgical Adjuvant Group |
| WCSG | Western Cancer Study Group |

## DRUG ABBREVIATIONS†

| | |
|---|---|
| ADR, ADRIA, D, H, DOXO | doxorubicin (Adriamycin), hydroxy-daunomycin |
| AMSA | amsacrine |
| ARA-C | cytarabine (Cytosar) |
| ASP OR L-ASP | L-asparaginase, Elspar |
| ATRA | tretinoin, all-*trans* retinoic acid |
| BCNU | carmustine, BiCNU |
| BLEO | bleomycin sulfate, Blenoxane |
| BSF | busulfan, Myleran |
| CBDCA, JM-8 | carboplatin, Paraplatin |
| CCNU | lomustine, CeeNU |
| CSA, 2-CDA | 2-chloro-2-deoxyadenosine, Leustatin |
| CHL | chlorambucil, Leukeran |
| CPT-11 | irinotecan |
| CYC, CTX, CPM | cyclophosphamide, Cytoxan, Neosar, Endoxan |
| D, DNR | daunomycin, daunorubicin, Cerubidine |
| DACT, ACT-D | dactinomycin, Cosmegen |
| DDP | *cis*-dichlorodiammineplatinum (II), cisplatin (Platinol) |
| DES | diethylstilbestrol |
| DEF | pentostatin, 2′-deoxycoformycin, Nipent |
| DEX, DXM | dexamethasone, Decadron |
| DHAD, DHAQ | mitoxantrone, Novantrone |
| DTIC | dimethyltriazenoimidazole carboxamide, dacarbazine, DTIC-Dome |
| ETOP, VP-16 | etoposide, VePesid |
| FAMP | fludarabine phosphate, Fludara |
| FUDR | floxuridine |
| Fu, 5-FU | fluorouracil, 5-fluorouracil |
| HIDAC | high-dose ara-C (Cytarabine) |
| HMM, HXM | hexamethylmelamine, altretamine, Hexalen |

| | |
|---|---|
| **HN2, M, MUST** | mechlorethamine, Mustargen, nitrogen mustard |
| **ICRF-187** | desrazoxane |
| **INF, IFN** | interferon |
| **IFOS** | ifosfamide, Ifex |
| **LEV** | levamisole, Ergamisol |
| **LV** | leucovorin |
| **MECCNU** | semustine |
| **MEG** | megestrol acetate, Megace |
| **MGBG** | mitoguazone |
| **MMC** | mitomycin-C, Mutamycin |
| **MP, 6-MP** | 6-mercaptopurine, Purinethol |
| **MTX** | methotrexate |
| **OH-UREA** | hydroxyurea, Hydrea |
| **o,p′-DDD** | mitotane, Lysodren |
| **PALA** | *N*-phosphonacetyl-L-aspartic acid |
| **PAM, L-PAM** | melphalan, Alkeran |
| **PRED** | prednisone |
| **PROC** | procarbazine, Matulane |
| **STZ** | streptozocin, Zanosar |
| **TAM** | tamoxifen, Nolvadex |
| **TAXOL** | paclitaxel |
| **TG, 6-TG** | 6-thioguanine, Thioguanine Tabloid brand |
| **TSPA** | thiotepa |
| **UFT** | uracil-ftorafur |
| **VBL** | vinblastine, Velban |
| **VCR, O** | vincristine, Oncovin |
| **VM-26** | teniposide, Vumon |
| **VP-16 (ETOP)** | etoposide, Vepeside |

## SELECTED DRUG COMBINATIONS (ACRONYMS)

| Acronym | Drugs |
|---|---|
| **ABVD** | ADR, BLEO, VBL, DTIC |
| **BACON** | BELO, ADR, CCNU, VER, M |
| **BACOP** | BLEO, ADR, CYC, VER, PRED |
| **B-CAVe** | BLEO, CCNU, ADR, VBL |
| **BCVPP** | BCNU, CYC, VBL, PROC, PRED |
| **B-DOPA** | BLEO, DTIC, VCR, PRED, ADR |
| **CAF** | CYC, ADR, 5-FU |
| **CAMP** | CYC, ADR, MTX, PROC |
| **CHOP** | CYC, ADR, VER, PRED |
| **ChlVPP** | CHLOR, VBL, PROC, PRED |
| **CHOP-BLEO** | BELO, ADR, CYC, VER, PRED |
| **CMF** | CYC, MTX, 5-FU |
| **CMFVP** | CYC, MTX, 5-FU, VCR, PRED |
| **COAP** | CYC, VCR, ARA-C, PRED |
| **COB-MAM** | CYC, VCR, BLEO, MTX, ADR, MECCNU |
| **COMB** | CYC, VCR, MECCNU, BLEO |
| **COP** | CYC, VCR, PRED |
| **COPP, C-MOPP** | CYC, VCR, PROC, PRED |
| **CVP** | CYC, VCR, PRED |
| **CyVADIC** | CYC, VCR, ADR, DTIC |
| **EVA** | ETOP, VCR, ADRI |
| **EVAP** | ETOP, VBL, ARA-C, DDP |
| **FAM** | FU, ADRI, MMC |

| | |
|---|---|
| **MIME** | MGBG, IFOS, MTX, ETOP |
| **MOCA** | MTX, VCR, CYC, ADR |
| **MOPP** | M, VCR, PROC, PRED |
| **MVPP** | M, VBL, PROC, PRED |
| **POMP** | PRED, VCR, MTX, 6-MP |
| **TAD** | 6-TG, ARA-C, DUR |
| **VAC** | VCR, DACT, CYC |
| **VAMP** | VCR, MTX, 6-MP, PRED |

## MISCELLANEOUS ABBREVIATIONS

| | |
|---|---|
| **ACTH** | Adrenocorticotropic hormone |
| **AFP** | Alpha-fetoprotein |
| **APUD** | Cells of the amine precursor uptake and decarboxylation system |
| **BCG** | Bacillus Calmette-Guérin |
| **β-hCG** | Beta-human chorionic gonadotropin |
| **CCR** | Continuous complete response |
| **CD** | Cluster designation for monoclonal antibodies |
| **CI** | Continuous infusion |
| **CEA** | Carcinoembryonic antigen |
| **CLL** | Chronic lymphocytic leukemia |
| **CML** | Chronic myelogenous leukemia |
| **CR** | Complete response or remission |
| **CR1, CR2** | Complete response 1, 2 |
| **CS** | Clinical stage |
| **DFS** | Disease-free survival |
| **DH or DHL** | Diffuse histiocytic lymphoma |
| **DM or DML** | Diffuse mixed histiocytic-lymphocytic lymphoma |
| **DPDL** | Diffuse poorly differentiated lymphocytic lymphoma |
| **DU** | Diffuse undifferentiated lymphoma |
| **DWDL** | Diffuse well-differentiated lymphocytic lymphoma |
| **EFS** | Event-free survival |
| **EGB** | Eosinophilic granuloma of bone |
| **ER** | Estrogen receptor |
| **FCC** | Follicular center cell |
| **GFCL** | Giant follicular cell lymphoma |
| **GVL** | Graft-versus-leukemia (or lymphoma) disease |
| **HAI** | Hepatic chorionic gonadotropin |
| **HD** | Hodgkin's disease |
| **5HIAA** | 5-Hydroxyindoleacetic acid |
| **HMR** | Histiocytic medullary reticulosis |
| **HSC** | Hand-Schüller-Christian disease |
| **5HT** | 5-Hydroxytryptamine (serotonin) |
| **IA** | Intra-arterial |
| **IV** | Intravenous |
| **kVp** | Peak kilovoltage on the x-ray tube |
| **LAF** | Laminar airflow room |
| **LAG** | Lymphangiogram |
| **LCL** | Large cell lymphoma |
| **LD** | Lymphocyte-depleted HD |
| **LET** | Linear energy transfer |
| **LLN** | Lower limit of normal |
| **LMM** | Lentigo maligna melanoma |
| **LP** | Lymphocyte-predominant HD |

| | | | |
|---|---|---|---|
| **LS** | Lymphosarcoma | **PO** | By mouth (oral medication) |
| **LSD** | Letterer-Siwe disease | **PR** | Partial response ($\geq$50% reduction in |
| **MC** | Mixed-cellularity HD | | sum of the products of greater and |
| **MDR** | Multiple drug resistance | | lesser diameter of tumor and without |
| **MEN** | Multiple endocrine neoplasia | | new lesions) |
| **MeV** | Million electron volts potential on x-ray tube | **PS** | Pathologic stage |
| | | **PTH** | Parathyroid hormone |
| **MRD** | Minimal residual disease | **RCS** | Reticulum cell sarcoma |
| **MTD** | Maximally tolerated dose of an agent | **RFS** | Relapse-free survival |
| **MUD** | Matched unrelated donor (for transplantation) | **SIADH** | Syndrome of inappropriate adrenocorticotropic hormone secretion |
| **NED** | No evidence of disease | | |
| **NGF** | Nerve growth factor | **SSM** | Superficial spreading melanoma |
| **NH or NHL** | Nodular histiocytic lymphoma | **SVC** | Superior vena cava |
| **NK cell** | Natural killer cell | **TdT** | Terminal deoxynucleotidyl transferase |
| **NM or NML** | Nodular mixed histiocytic-lymphocytic lymphoma | **T1 N0 M0** | TNM format for versions of the TNM system since 1988 |
| **NM** | Nodular melanoma | **$T_1 N_0 M_0$** | TNM format for versions before 1988 |
| **NPDL** | Nodular poorly differentiated lymphocytic lymphoma | **TSH** | Thyroid-stimulating hormone |
| | | **TTF** | Time to treatment failure |
| **NSD** | Nominal single dose (of radiation) | **ULN** | Upper limit of normal |
| **NWDL** | Nodular well-differentiated lymphocytic lymphoma | **VIP** | Vasoactive intestinal polypeptide |
| | | **WDHA** | Syndrome of watery diarrhea with hypokalemic alkalosis |
| **PCR** | Polymerase chain reaction | | |
| **PgR** | Progesterone receptor | **WNL** | Within normal limits |

*Unless otherwise listed here, journal citations are abbreviated according to the style used in Index Medicus.

†Please note that the abbreviation for individual drugs may also start with a capital letter followed by lowercase letters. This facilitates the recognition of abbreviation for individual drugs from acronyms used for various drug combinations.

# APPENDIX D

# CANCER AND THE INTERNET

Physicians have traditionally used medical textbooks, journals, meetings, and consultations with colleagues to maintain their medical knowledge. In the past, patients have largely relied on their physicians for counseling and education about medical concerns. Today, the educational needs of both groups are being transformed by the Internet, which provides ready access to an enormous amount of information regarding all facets of cancer. This includes the ability to locate information about patients with exceedingly rare diseases.[1] Many medical journals are available online and new electronic journals are proliferating.[2] Most major medical organizations and federal agencies maintain websites for health care professionals and the general public. Commercial organizations have embraced the Internet because its users are a large potential market. Cancer patients can use the Internet to obtain information about a particular malignancy and to find support groups of various types, including formal support groups in their communities or "chat rooms" on the Internet.

Internet access to medical information has created new opportunities and challenges. Foremost among concerns about this innovation is the fact that some Internet sites are of uncertain quality and credibility.[3] In general, sites that are sponsored by the United States federal government (e.g., the PDQ Search Service for Health Professionals maintained by the National Cancer Institute,[4] the Medline database maintained by the National Library of Medicine,[5, 6] and information provided by the Food and Drug Administration[7]) and major oncologic organizations (e.g., the American Society for Clinical Oncology[8] and the American Cancer Society[9]) are more credible than sites that are sponsored by for-profit organizations.

Guidelines for assessing the quality and credibility of health care–related websites have been established by the Health On the Net Foundation in Geneva, Switzerland.[10] This nonprofit organization has evaluated a large number of websites using eight principles. These principles are as follows:

1. *Authority.* Any medical or health advice provided and hosted on this site will be given only by medically trained and qualified professionals unless a clear statement is made that a piece of advice offered is from a nonmedically qualified individual or organization.

2. *Complementarity.* The information provided on this site is designed to support, not replace, the relationship that exists between a patient–site visitor and his or her existing physician.

3. *Confidentiality.* Confidentiality of data relating to individual patients and visitors to a medical-health website, including their identity, is respected by this website. The website owners undertake to honor or exceed the legal requirements of medical-health information privacy that apply in the country and state where the website and mirror sites are located.

4. *Attribution.* When appropriate, information contained on this site will be supported by clear references to source data and, when possible, have specific HTML links to those data. The date when a clinical page was last modified will be clearly displayed (e.g., at the bottom of the page).

5. *Justifiability.* Any claims relating to the benefits-performance of a specific treatment, commercial product, or service will be supported by appropriate, balanced evidence in the manner outlined above in principle 4.

6. *Transparency of Authorship.* The designers of this website will seek to provide information in the clearest possible manner and provide contact addresses for visitors who seek further information or support. The webmaster will display his or her e-mail address clearly throughout the website.

7. *Transparency of Sponsorship.* Support for this website will be clearly identified, including the identities of commercial and noncommercial organizations that have contributed funding, services, or material for the site.

8. *Honesty in Advertising and Editorial Policy.* If advertising is a source of funding, it will be clearly stated. A brief description of the advertising policy adopted by the website owners will be displayed on the site. Advertising and other promotional material will be presented to viewers in a manner and context that facilitates differentiation between it and the original material created by the institution operating the site.

*Charles M. Haskell*

## REFERENCES

1. DeGroen PC, Barry JA, Schaller WJ. Applying world wide web technology to the study of patients with rare diseases. Ann Intern Med 1998;129:107–113.
2. McKie M. Oncology journals and the internet: a shared resource. Cancer Control: Moffitt Cancer Center 1999;6:627–635. *http://www.moffitt.usf.edu/ccjournal/index.html*
3. Biermann JS, Golladay GJ, Greenfield MLVH, Baker LH. Evaluation of cancer information on the Internet. Cancer 1999;86:381–90.
4. PDQ Search Service by telephone: 1-800-345-3300; PDQ Search Service by Fax: 1-800-380-1575 (313-831-8292 if outside the United States); PDQ Search Service on the Internet: *pdqsearch@icicc.nci.nih.gov.*
5. *http://www.nlm.nih.gov.*
6. Hutchinson DB. Medline for health professionals: how to search PubMed on the Internet. Sacramento, Calif: New Wind, 1998, 170 pp.
7. *http://www.fda.gov/cder/drug.htm.*
8. *http://www.asco.org.*
9. *http://www.cancer.org.*
10. *http://www.hon.ch/HONcode/HONcode_check.html*

# INDEX

Note: Page numbers in *italics* refer to illustrations;
page numbers followed by (t) refer to tables.

Exocrine pancreas, cancer of, 752–766
  chemotherapy for, 763(t), 763–765,
      764(t)
    radiation therapy plus surgery com-
        bined with, 758–762, 759(t),
        760(t)
  diagnosis of, 754
  epidemiology of, 752–753
  etiology of, 752–753
  molecular pathogenesis of, 753
  natural history of, 752–755
  palliative therapy for, 757–758
  pathology of, 753, 753(t)
  radiation therapy for, surgery com-
      bined with, 759(t), 761
    surgery plus chemotherapy com-
        bined with, 758–762, 759(t),
        760(t)
  risk factors for, 752–753
  staging of, 755(t)
    treatment in relation to, 766
  surgery for, 756–758, *757*
    radiation therapy combined with,
        759(t), 761
    radiation therapy plus chemother-
        apy combined with, 758–762,
        759(t), 760(t)
  tumor markers for, 754
External beam radiation therapy, 54. See
    also *Radiation therapy.*
  for pancreatic cancer, 758, 759, 759(t),
      760(t), 761
  for prostate cancer, 817–818
External-beam radiation therapy, for
    retinoblastoma, 1200–1201
  late effects of, 1202
Extranodal lymphomas, 1426–1433
Extrapleural pneumonectomy, for
    mesothelioma, 642
Extravasation, of chemotherapeutic agents,
    74, 74(t)
Extremities, bones of, sarcomas of. See
    *Ewing's sarcoma; Osteogenic
    sarcoma.*
Eye(s), chemotherapeutic agents harmful
    to, 76, 219
  malignant tumors of, 1178–1186, 1198–
      1203, 1428. See also *Melanoma,
      uveal* and *Retinoblastoma.*
Eyelid(s), melanoma of, 1179–1180
  treatment of, 1181


FAB (French-American-British)
    classification, of acute lymphoblastic
      leukemia, 1440(t)
  of acute myeloid leukemia, 1281(t),
      1281–1282
  of myeloproliferative disorders, progno-
      ses in relation to, 1298–1299,
      1299(t)
FAC chemotherapy regimen, for breast
    cancer, 568
Fallopian tube(s), cancer of, 925–926,
    926(t)
  resection of, with oophorectomy. See
    *Oophorectomy.*
FAM chemotherapy regimen, for stomach
    cancer, 693

Familial adenomatous polyposis (FAP),
    704
Familial melanoma, of skin, 1158–1159
  of uvea, 1179
Familial pancreatic cancer, 752
Family problems, of cancer patients, 385
Family therapy, in psychosocial support of
    cancer patient, 397
FAP (familial adenomatous polyposis), 704
FDMI chemotherapy regimen, for MUO
    syndrome, 1572
Female patient(s). See also sex organ-
    specific cancer entries, e.g., *Vaginal
    cancer.*
  age of, and incidence of cancer, by tu-
      mor site, *437*
  breast cancer in. See *Breast cancer.*
  genital cancer in. See site-specific en-
      tries, e.g., *Vaginal cancer.*
  hereditary nonpolyposis colorectal can-
      cer in, as risk factor for other neo-
      plasms, 901
  pregnant. See *Pregnancy.*
  race of, and incidence of cancer, by tu-
      mor site, 415(t)
    and lethality of cancer, by tumor site,
        415(t)
  urethra in, 854, *854*
    cancer of, 854–856, 855(t)
    resection of, for cancer, 856
Femur, osteogenic sarcoma of, *1245*
  surgery for, 1250, *1251*
Fenretinide, for neuroblastoma, 1229
Ferritin, in diagnosis of neuroblastoma,
    1220
Fetus. See also *Pregnancy.*
  exposure of, to DES, and breast cancer,
      510
    and cervical cancer, 944, 992
    and vaginal cancer, 944, 992
  metastasis to, 428
Fever, in cancer patients, 342. See also
    *Infection, in cancer patients.*
Fibroadenoma, of breast, ultrasonography
    of, 519, *520*
Fibrocystic disease, of breast, 511
Fibrosarcomatous osteogenic sarcoma,
    1245
Fibrosis, pulmonary, due to bleomycin, 75,
    113, 894
Fibrous tumor, benign, of pleura, 639
FIGO staging, of Bartholin's gland cancer,
    prognostic significance of, 981(t)
  of endometrial cancer, 955(t)
  of fallopian tube cancer, 926(t)
  of ovarian cancer, 904(t)
  of uterine cancer, 955(t)
  of vaginal cancer, 990(t)
  of vulvar cancer, 973(t)
Floor of mouth, cancer of, 1007–1008
Flow cytometry, in assessment of breast
    cancer, 512
Floxuridine, 148–149
  for metastatic liver cancer, 1595
  for renal cell carcinoma, 870
  toxicity of, 1597
Fludarabine, 149–151
  emetogenic potential of, 328(t)
  for chronic lymphocytic leukemia, 1492

Fludarabine *(Continued)*
  for low-grade lymphoma, 1380
  for non-Hodgkin's lymphoma, 1380
Fluoropyrimidines, 477–478
  in chemotherapy for colorectal cancer,
      732–733, 733(t)
5-Fluorouracil, 151–154
  continuous infusion of, 229–230
  dosage of, 153–154
    for patients with renal insufficiency,
        70(t)
  emetogenic potential of, 328(t)
  for anal canal cancer, 747, 747(t), 748,
      748(t), 749, 750
  for colorectal cancer, 728–732
    use of leucovorin with, 728–732,
        729(t), 732(t), 733(t)
  for cutaneous carcinoma, 1193
  for esophageal cancer, 674, 674(t), 675,
      677, 677(t)
    preoperative use of, 672, 673(t),
        678(t)
  for gastric cancer, 691(t)–695(t), 692,
      693, 694, 696, 700(t)
  for head and neck cancer, 1031,
      1031(t)–1035(t), 1032, 1033, 1034,
      1035
  for hepatocellular carcinoma, 779(t),
      780, 780(t), 782(t), 783(t)
  for liver cancer, arising as primary tu-
      mor, 779(t), 780, 780(t), 782(t),
      783(t)
  for MUO syndrome, 1572
  for nasopharyngeal cancer, 1037, 1038
  for neck and head cancer, 1031,
      1031(t)–1035(t), 1032, 1033, 1034,
      1035
  for skin cancer, 1193
  for stomach cancer, 691(t)–695(t), 692,
      693, 694, 696, 700(t)
  for vulvar intraepithelial neoplasia, 969
  oral mucositis induced by, 331, 332
  use of leucovorin with, for colorectal
      cancer, 728–732, 729(t), 732(t),
      733(t)
    for head and neck cancer, 1033,
        1034(t)
    for stomach cancer, 691, 695(t),
        700(t)
  use of levamisole with, for colorectal
      cancer, 728–730, 729(t)
Flutamide, 155–156
Follicular lymphoma, 1353, *1353*
  cell proliferation in, *1349*
  radiation therapy for, results of, *1383,
      1384*
  vs. reactive lymph node, *1345*
Follicular thyroid carcinoma, 1056
Foreskin, penile cancer risk associated
    with, 859
Franklin's disease, 1528–1529
French-American-British (FAB)
    classification, of acute lymphoblastic
      leukemia, 1440(t)
  of acute myeloid leukemia, 1281(t),
      1281–1282
  of myeloproliferative disorders, progno-
      ses in relation to, 1298–1299,
      1299(t)